MW01153031

BARASH, CULLEN, AND STOELTING'S

Clinical Anesthesia

NINTH EDITION

BARASH, CULLEN, AND STOELTING'S

Clinical Anesthesia

NINTH EDITION

Bruce F. Cullen, MD
Professor Emeritus
Department of Anesthesiology and Pain Medicine
University of Washington School of Medicine
Seattle, Washington

M. Christine Stock, MD
Professor Emerita
Department of Anesthesiology
Northwestern University Feinberg School of Medicine
Chicago, Illinois

Rafael Ortega, MD
Professor and Chair
Department of Anesthesiology
Boston University Chobanian & Avedisian School of Medicine
Boston, Massachusetts

Sam R. Sharar, MD
Professor
Vice Chair for Faculty Affairs and Development
Department of Anesthesiology and Pain Medicine
University of Washington School of Medicine
Seattle, Washington

Natalie F. Holt, MD, MPH
Adjunct Professor
Department of Anesthesiology
Yale School of Medicine
Medical Director
Ambulatory Procedures Unit
VA Connecticut Healthcare System
West Haven, Connecticut

Christopher W. Connor, MD, PhD
Associate Professor
Department of Anaesthesia
Harvard Medical School
Brigham and Women's Hospital
Boston, Massachusetts

Naveen Nathan, MD
Department of Anesthesiology, Critical Care and Pain Medicine
University of Chicago Pritzker School of Medicine
NorthShore University Health System
Chicago, Illinois

Wolters Kluwer

Philadelphia • Baltimore • New York • London
Buenos Aires • Hong Kong • Sydney • Tokyo

Senior Acquisitions Editor: Keith Donnellan
Senior Developmental Editor: Ashley Fischer
Editorial Coordinator: Marisa Solorzano-Taylor
Production Project Manager: Bridgett Dougherty
Design Coordinator: Stephen Druding
Senior Manufacturing Coordinator: Lisa Bowling
Marketing Manager: Kristen Watrud
Prepress Vendor: Aptara, Inc.

Ninth Edition

9 8 7 6 5 4 3 2 1

Printed in Mexico

Library of Congress Cataloging-in-Publication Data

Names: Cullen, Bruce F., editor.
Title: Barash, Cullen, and Stoelting's clinical anesthesia / edited by Bruce F. Cullen, M. Christine Stock, Rafael Ortega, Sam R. Sharar, Natalie F. Holt, Christopher W. Connor, Naveen Nathan.
Other titles: Clinical anesthesia (Barash)
Description: Ninth edition. | Philadelphia, PA : Wolters Kluwer, [2024] | Preceded by Clinical anesthesia / edited by Paul G. Barash, Bruce F. Cullen, Robert K. Stoelting, Michael K. Cahalan, M. Christine Stock, Rafael Ortega, Sam R. Sharar, Natalie F. Holt. Eighth edition. [2017] | Includes bibliographical references and index.
Identifiers: LCCN 2023020337 (print) | LCCN 2023020338 (ebook) | ISBN 9781975199074 (hardback) | ISBN 9781975199081 (epub)
Subjects: MESH: Anesthesia | Anesthesiology | Anesthetics | BISAC: MEDICAL / Anesthesiology
Classification: LCC RD81 (print) | LCC RD81 (ebook) | NLM WO 200 | DDC 617.9/6–dc23/eng/20230531
LC record available at https://lccn.loc.gov/2023020337
LC ebook record available at https://lccn.loc.gov/2023020338

shop.lww.com

QUADM0823

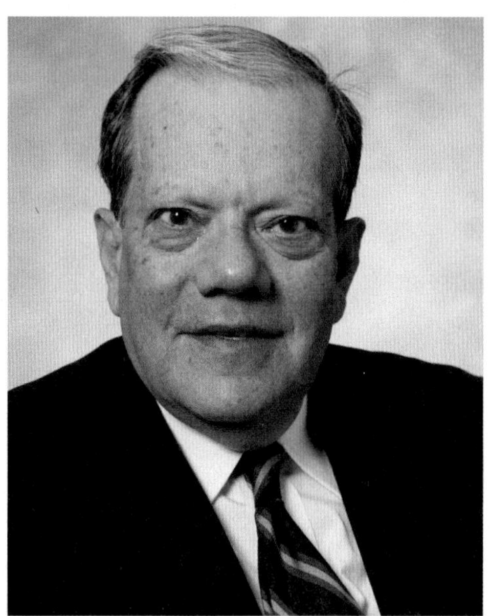

Paul G. Barash, MD

1942–2020

Editor Emeritus and Co-Founder, Clinical Anesthesia and Clinical Anesthesia Fundamentals
Former Chair of Anesthesiology and Associate Dean of Clinical Affairs,
Yale University School of Medicine,
Gifted Clinician and Academic Physician,
Award-Wining Educator, Tireless Editor, Generous Mentor, Yankees Fan,
Charismatic and Kind Family Man and Friend

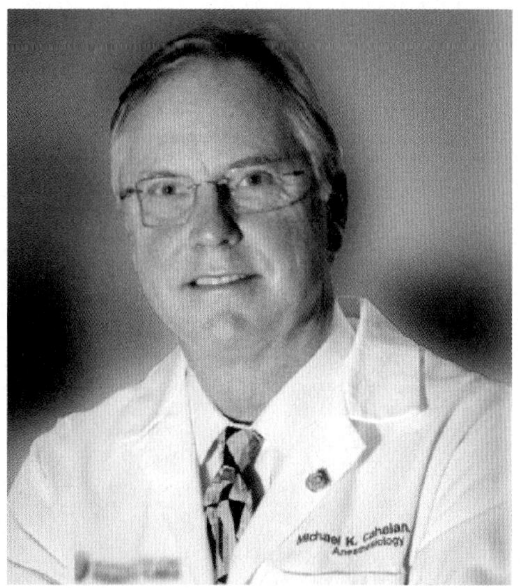

Michael K. Cahalan, MD

1949–2019

Editor Emeritus, Clinical Anesthesia and Clinical Anesthesia Fundamentals
Former Chair of Anesthesiology, University of Utah,
Pioneer and Recognized Global Expert in Clinical Echocardiography,
Gifted Author, Editor and Mentor
Congenial and Fair-minded Leader Guided by Compassion and a Strong Moral Compass

Preface

We welcome you to the ninth edition of *Clinical Anesthesia.* Since its first edition was published in 1990, the editorial team—led by founding editors Paul G. Barash, Bruce F. Cullen, and Robert K. Stoelting—has published new editions approximately every 4 years, responding to the rapid pace of evolving knowledge and clinical practice in our specialty. Each new edition included not only updated conventional print content in the form of written text, tables, and figures but also several novel learning tools, including a clinical handbook, multiple choice questions/answer collections, podcasts, and a growing spectrum of innovative, multimedia content in a fully interactive and portable eBook format (e.g., tutorial videos, narrated clinical vignettes, and comprehensive atlas of ultrasound and echocardiography).

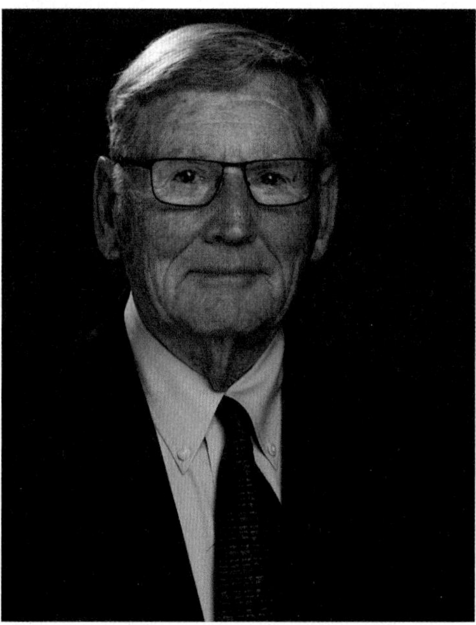

Bruce F. Cullen, MD

When the eighth edition of *Clinical Anesthesia* was published in 2017, none of us could have predicted two unanticipated events on the horizon that would greatly impact our personal, professional, and publishing lives, thereby delaying production of this ninth edition. First and without question, the COVID-19 pandemic extracted a devastating toll on several fronts, but particularly those of us who work in health care systems. These disruptions—from which we are only now starting to emerge—resulted in significant mortality, health-threatening impediments to routine health care delivery for patients, and both physically and emotionally demanding increases in workload, occupational risk, and burnout among those of us who are health care workers. Under these circumstances, updating *Clinical Anesthesia* obviously took a backseat to these much higher priorities.

The second challenge faced was the unexpected death of two indelible forces behind the *Clinical Anesthesia* and companion *Clinical Anesthesia Fundamentals* series—cofounding editor Paul Barash and long-time editor Michael Cahalan. Paul passed away peacefully in June 2020 leaving a legacy of excellence in his professional life as Professor Emeritus of Anesthesiology, former department Chair and Associate Dean of Clinical Affairs at Yale University, among many national leadership roles. He was a gifted and award-winning teacher who selflessly mentored numerous chairs, section chiefs, and a wide spectrum of trainees, as well as each of us, his coeditors. Paul was the driving force behind each of the first eight editions of *Clinical Anesthesia,* all editions of *The Handbook of Clinical Anesthesia,* and the inaugural edition of *Clinical Anesthesia Fundamentals.* Recruited by a publisher to author a comprehensive textbook on anesthesiology, he took it upon himself to recruit Bob Stoelting and Bruce Cullen to assist him as founding editors of *Clinical Anesthesia.* He was also the *de facto* Managing Editor of all editions, and he was instrumental in instituting publication of the *Handbook of Clinical Anesthesia* and most of the multimedia components of digital versions of the original textbook. Mike passed away after a short illness in 2019, having served as a coeditor for three editions of *Clinical Anesthesia* and the inaugural edition of *Clinical Anesthesia Fundamentals.* A widely acclaimed expert in cardiac anesthesia and pioneer in echocardiography, he served as Chief of Anesthesia for the Pediatric and Adult Cardiac service for most of his 22 years at the University of California San Francisco, then as Professor and Chair of Anesthesiology at the University of Utah for 15 years. Mike was instrumental in overseeing all aspects of cardiac-related material in the *Clinical Anesthesia* series and personally oversaw inclusion of the video atlas of ultrasound and echocardiography appendices. Paul and Mike will be sorely missed, yet fondly remembered.

This ninth edition marks one additional major transition in the *Clinical Anesthesia* series, as cofounding editor Bruce Cullen marks his final page proofs. Bruce's name has been synonymous with the series for almost four decades, beginning with its conception in the mid-1980s. Since then, Bruce has pulled far more than his share of editorial weight for all nine editions of *Clinical Anesthesia,* all editions of *The Handbook of Clinical Anesthesia,* and both editions of *Clinical Anesthesia Fundamentals.* Long regarded as a broadly skilled practitioner and learner-centered clinical educator, his exceptional scientific writing, contributor networking, and editorial skills have defined the creation and continuous evolution of this series, always targeting the students and clinical practitioners of anesthesiology. For us as coeditors, Bruce has been our role model, our confidant, and our friend—and we are forever indebted to his grace and generosity.

With that, what are the key changes and improvements readers should expect from this ninth edition? First, in recognition of the mammoth commitment and dedication of the series' founding editors, the title of the textbook has been revised to *Barash, Cullen, and Stoelting's Clinical Anesthesia.* In addition, two new editors—Christopher W. Connor and Naveen Nathan—have joined our team, specifically selected for their internationally recognized expertise in novel educational formats, multimedia teaching platforms, and as exceptional clinical educators. Because one hallmark of *Clinical Anesthesia* is the presentation of both long-standing and newly emerging concepts in an easily accessible, understandable, clinically useful, and "fresh" manner, we have also updated our team of contributors—seven of the text's 59 chapters were written *de novo* by new author teams of emerging experts in their fields. At the same time, returning authors have significantly revised their chapters with newly recognized concepts and evidence, particularly those topics experiencing swift and paradigm-shifting expansions in knowledge and understanding, such as perioperative genomics (Chapter 6: Genomic Basis of Perioperative Precision Medicine) and both pathophysiology and clinical care related to COVID-19 conditions (Chapter 57: Critical Care Medicine).

Last, the interactive multimedia content of this edition, which can be conveniently accessed via the eBook bundled with the print version of this text on desktops, laptops, and portable devices, has been significantly expanded with new topics and is presented in a refreshed color scheme. A series of icons are present throughout chapters to alert readers to associated multimedia content (and "key" features):

Video
Narrative Interactive Clinical Vignette (NICV)
Key Point 1

The ninth edition contains over 300 Videos and 192 NICVs—accessed via the eBook—across the entire content spectrum. Each NICV consists of a short case presentation followed by a series of questions prompting the learner to generate their own responses. The types of questions include multiple choice, true/false, and other interactive formats, such as identifying elements in a figure and matching lists of items. Both correct and incorrect answers result in immediate feedback and provide the learner with the opportunity to compare their responses with an appropriate explanation.

Of utmost importance, we wish to express our extreme gratitude to the individual contributors whose hard work and dedication—particularly when superimposed upon the COVID-19 pandemic—made production of this edition possible. Despite what has been one of the most physically and emotionally demanding epochs for anesthesiologists and related specialists, our contributors' concurrent commitment to our trainees and colleagues is truly exceptional. Finally, thank you to our colleagues at Wolters Kluwer who continually demonstrate their commitment to excellence in medical publishing, who provide valuable editorial support, and who make the final stages of production a joy.

Bruce F. Cullen, MD

M. Christine Stock, MD

Rafael Ortega, MD

Sam R. Sharar, MD

Natalie F. Holt, MD, MPH

Christopher W. Connor, MD, PhD

Naveen Nathan, MD

Contributing Authors

Ramon E. Abola, MD
Clinical Associate Professor of Anesthesiology
Department of Anesthesiology
Renaissance School of Medicine at Stony Brook University
Stony Brook, New York

Abey Abraham, MD
Chief Fellow
Department of Cardiothoracic Anesthesiology
Cleveland Clinic Foundation
Cleveland, Ohio

Pudkrong K. Aicholz, MD
Assistant Professor
Department of Anesthesiology and Pain Medicine
University of Washington School of Medicine
Harborview Medical Center
Seattle, Washington

Shamsuddin Akhtar, MBBS
Professor
Department of Anesthesiology and Pharmacology
Yale School of Medicine
New Haven, Connecticut

Trefan Archibald, MD
Acting Assistant Professor of Anesthesiology and Critical Care Medicine
Department of Anesthesiology
University of Washington School of Medicine
Seattle, Washington

Ruben J. Azocar, MD, MHCM, FASA, FCCM
VP Perioperative Services
Beth Israel Deaconess Medical Center
Boston, Massachusetts

Douglas R. Bacon, MD, MA
Professor and Chair (Retired)
Department of Anesthesiology
University of Mississippi Medical Center
Jackson, Mississippi

Gina Cleopatra Badescu, MD
Anesthesiologist, Cardiothoracic Anesthesiology
Everett, Washington

Christopher R. Barnes, MD, FCCM
Assistant Professor
Department of Anesthesiology and Critical Care Medicine
Harborview Medical Center
Seattle, Washington

John Patrick F. Bebawy, MD
Professor of Anesthesiology & Neurological Surgery
Chief of Neurosurgical Anesthesiology
Program Director, Neurosurgical Anesthesiology Fellowship Program
Northwestern University Feinberg School of Medicine
Chicago, Illinois

Itay Bentov, MD, PhD
Associate Professor Anesthesiology and Pain Medicine
Adjunct Associate Professor Department of Medicine
Department of Anesthesiology and Pain Medicine
University of Washington School of Medicine
Harborview Medical Center
Seattle, Washington

Honorio T. Benzon, MD
Professor Emeritus of Anesthesiology
Northwestern University Feinberg School of Medicine
Chicago, Illinois

Robert Bishop, MD
Assistant Clinical Professor of Anesthesiology
Department of Anesthesiology and Pain Medicine
UC Davis School of Medicine
UC Davis Medical Center
Sacramento, California

Jessica R. Black, MD
Associate Professor of Anesthesiology
Department of Anesthesiology and Critical Care
UC San Diego School of Medicine
San Diego, California

Brent T. Boettcher, DO
Associate Professor of Anesthesiology
Medical College of Wisconsin
Milwaukee, Wisconsin

Michelle Y. Braunfeld, MD
Clinical Professor of Anesthesiology (Retired)
Division of Anesthesiology and Perioperative Medicine
David Geffen School of Medicine at UCLA
Los Angeles, California

Karolina Brook, MD
Assistant Professor of Anesthesiology
Department of Anesthesiology
Boston University Chobanian & Avedisian School of Medicine
Boston Medical Center
Boston, Massachusetts

Brenda A. Bucklin, MD, MEHP, FASA
Professor of Anesthesiology
Associate Dean for Continuing Medical Education
Department of Anesthesiology
University of Colorado School of Medicine
Aurora, Colorado

Nelson Burbano-Vera, MD
Chief, Division of Pediatric Cardiothoracic Anesthesiology
Department of Pediatric Anesthesiology
Cleveland Clinic Foundation
Cleveland, Ohio

Louanne M. Carabini, MD, MA
Associate Professor of Anesthesiology
Section of Anesthesiology and Critical Care Medicine
Northwestern University Feinberg School of Medicine
Chicago, Illinois

Maurizio Cereda, MD
Member of the Faculty of Anesthesia
Department of Anesthesia, Critical Care and Pain Medicine
Harvard Medical School
Massachusetts General Hospital
Boston, Massachusetts

Amy Chen, MD
Assistant Clinical Professor of Anesthesiology
Department of Anesthesiology and Pain Medicine
UC Davis School of Medicine
UC Davis Medical Center
Sacramento, California

Surendrasingh Chhabada, MD
Assistant Professor
Departments of Pediatric Anesthesiology and Outcomes Research
Cleveland Clinic Foundation
Cleveland, Ohio

Christine Choi, MD
Assistant Clinical Professor
Department of Anesthesiology
UC San Diego School of Medicine
La Jolla, California

Sung-Wook Choi, MD
Assistant Professor
Department of Anesthesia and Perioperative Medicine
Division of Pediatric Anesthesia
Medical University of South Carolina
Shawn Jenkins Children's Hospital
Charleston, South Carolina

Adam J. Claessens, DO
Acting Assistant Professor of Anesthesiology
Department of Anesthesiology and Pain Medicine
University of Washington School of Medicine
Seattle, Washington

Amalia Cochran, MD
Professor and Vice Chair of Professional Development
Department of Surgery
University of Florida College of Medicine
Gainesville, Florida

Steven P. Cohen, MD
Professor of Anesthesiology and Critical Care Medicine; Neurology; Physical Medicine and Rehabilitation; Psychiatry and Behavioral Sciences
Department Anesthesiology and Critical Care Medicine
Johns Hopkins School of Medicine
Professor of Physical Medicine and Rehabilitation; Anesthesiology
Uniformed Services University of the Health Sciences
Walter Reed National Military Medical Center
Baltimore, Maryland

Edmond Cohen, MD, FASA
Professor of Anesthesiology and Thoracic Surgery
Director of Thoracic Anesthesia
Department of Anesthesiology, Perioperative and Pain Medicine
Icahn School of Medicine at Mount Sinai
New York, New York

Melissa L. Coleman, MD
Associate Professor of Anesthesiology
Division of Anesthesiology and Perioperative Medicine
Penn State University College of Medicine
Milton S. Hershey Medical Center
Hershey, Pennsylvania

Christopher M. Conley, MD
Clinical Associate Professor of Anesthesiology and Pediatrics
Department of Anesthesiology
Boston University Chobanian & Avedisian School of Medicine
Boston Medical Center
Boston, Massachusetts

Christopher W. Connor, MD, PhD
Associate Professor
Department of Anaesthesia
Harvard Medical School
Brigham and Women's Hospital
Boston, Massachusetts

C. Michael Crowder, MD, PhD
Professor of Anesthesiology and Pain Medicine
Department of Anesthesiology and Pain Medicine
Adjunct Professor of Genome Sciences
Mitochondrial and Metabolism Center
University of Washington School of Medicine
Seattle, Washington

Albert Dahan, MD, PhD
Professor
Head of Research
Head and Founder, Anesthesia and Pain Research Unit
Department of Anesthesiology
Leiden University Medical Center
Leiden, The Netherlands

Karen B. Domino, MD, MPH
Professor
Department of Anesthesiology and Pain Medicine
University of Washington School of Medicine
University of Washington Medical Center
Seattle, Washington

Thomas J. Ebert, MD, PhD
Professor of Anesthesiology
Department of Anesthesiology
Medical College of Wisconsin
Milwaukee, Wisconsin

Jan Ehrenwerth, MD
Professor Emeritus of Anesthesiology
Department of Anesthesiology
Yale School of Medicine
Yale New Haven Hospital
New Haven, Connecticut

James B. Eisenkraft, MD
Professor
Department of Anesthesiology, Perioperative and Pain Medicine
Icahn School of Medicine at Mount Sinai
Mount Sinai Medical Center
New York, New York

Holly B. Ende, MD
Associate Professor of Anesthesiology
Department of Anesthesiology
Vanderbilt University School of Medicine
Vanderbilt University Medical Center
Nashville, Tennessee

Alex S. Evers, MD
Henry E. Mallinckrodt Professor of Anesthesiology
Department of Anesthesiology
Washington University School of Medicine
St. Louis, Missouri

Rachel M. Feldman, MD
Assistant Professor of Anesthesiology
Department of Anesthesiology and Pain Medicine
University of Washington School of Medicine
Seattle Children's Hospital
Seattle, Washington

Ana Fernandez-Bustamante, MD, PhD
Associate Professor of Anesthesiology
Department of Anesthesiology
University of Colorado School of Medicine
Aurora, Colorado

Gabrielle Fisher, MD
Assistant Professor
Department of Anesthesia and Perioperative Medicine
Medical University of South Carolina
Charleston, South Carolina

Michael A. Fowler, MD, MBA
Associate Professor of Anesthesiology
Division of Transplant Anesthesia
University of Florida College of Medicine
UF Health Shands Hospital
Gainesville, Florida

Julie K. Freed, MD, PhD
Associate Professor of Anesthesiology and Physiology
Medical College of Wisconsin
Milwaukee, Wisconsin

Tong Joo (TJ) Gan, MD, MBA, MHS
Professor and Division Head
Division of Anesthesiology, Critical Care and Pain Medicine
The University of Texas, MD Anderson Cancer Center
Houston, Texas

Timothy G. Gaulton, MD, MSc
Faculty of Anesthesia
Harvard Medical School
Department of Anesthesia, Critical Care and Pain Medicine
Massachusetts General Hospital
Boston, Massachusetts

Steven Gayer, MD, MBA, FASA
Professor of Anesthesiology and Ophthalmology
Department of Anesthesiology
Bascom Palmer Eye Institute
University of Miami Miller School of Medicine
Miami, Florida

Katherine R. Gentry, MD, MA
Associate Professor of Anesthesiology
Department of Anesthesiology and Pain Medicine
Seattle Children's Hospital
University of Washington School of Medicine
Seattle, Washington

Sofia Geralemou, MD
Clinical Assistant Professor of Anesthesiology
Department of Anesthesiology
Renaissance School of Medicine at Stony Brook University
Stony Brook, New York

Rafael Mauricio Gonzalez, MD
Clinical Associate Professor
Department of Anesthesiology
Boston University Chobanian & Avedisian School of Medicine
Boston, Massachusetts

Stuart Alan Grant, MD
Professor and Chief of Regional Anesthesia
Department of Anesthesiology
University of North Carolina School of Medicine
Chapel Hill, North Carolina

Nikolaus Gravenstein, MD
Jerome H. Modell, MD, Professor of Anesthesiology
Professor of Neurosurgery and Periodontology
Department of Anesthesiology
University of Florida College of Medicine
UF Health Shands Hospital
Gainesville, Florida

Dennis Grech, MD
Vice Chairman Clinical Affairs
Associate Professor of Anesthesiology
Department of Anesthesiology and Perioperative Medicine
Rutgers Robert Wood Johnson Medical School
New Brunswick, New Jersey
University Hospital, Rutgers
Newark, New Jersey

Loreta Grecu, MD
Associate Professor of Anesthesiology
Cardiothoracic Anesthesiology and Critical Care Division
Duke University School of Medicine
Duke University Medical Center
Durham, North Carolina

Benjamin F. Gruenbaum, MD, PhD
Assistant Professor of Anesthesiology
Department of Anesthesiology and Perioperative Medicine
Mayo Clinic College of Medicine and Science
Jacksonville, Florida

Stella Haddadin, BS, PharmD
Clinical Pharmacist
Department of Pharmacy
Advent Health
Orlando, Florida

Carin A. Hagberg, MD, FASA
Chief Academic Officer
Bud Johnson Clinical Distinguished Chair
Division of Anesthesiology, Critical Care and Pain Medicine
The University of Texas MD Anderson Cancer Center
Houston, Texas

Michael L. Hall, MD
Associate Professor of Anesthesiology and Pain Medicine
Department of Anesthesiology and Pain Medicine
University of Washington School of Medicine
Seattle, Washington

Matthew R. Hallman, MD, MS
Associate Professor
Department of Anesthesiology and Pain Medicine
University of Washington School of Medicine
Seattle, Washington

Dustin Hang, MD
Assistant Professor of Anesthesiology
Medical College of Wisconsin
Milwaukee, Wisconsin

Elizabeth E. Hansen, MD, PhD
Assistant Professor
Department of Anesthesiology and Pain Medicine
University of Washington School of Medicine
Pediatric Anesthesiologist
Seattle Children's Hospital
Seattle, Washington

Jennifer M. Hargrave, DO, FAOCA, FASA
CTA Fellowship Program Director
Vice-Chair of Education
Department of Cardiothoracic Anesthesiology
Cleveland Clinic Foundation
Cleveland, Ohio

Stephen C. Haskins, MD
Clinical Associate Professor of Anesthesiology
Weill Cornell Medical College
Department of Anesthesiology, Critical Care & Pain Management
Hospital for Special Surgery
New York, New York

Tara M. Hata, MD
Vice Chair, Department of Pediatric Anesthesia
Anesthesiology Institute
Cleveland Clinic Foundation
Cleveland, Ohio

Laurence M. Hausman, MD
Vice Chairman Academic Affiliations
Medical Director Ambulatory Anesthesia
Professor of Anesthesiology and Perioperative and Pain Medicine
Department of Anesthesiology, Perioperative and Pain Medicine
Icahn School of Medicine at Mount Sinai
New York, New York

Christopher L. Heine, MD
Assistant Professor
Department of Anesthesia and Perioperative Medicine
Medical University of South Carolina
Charleston, South Carolina

Laura B. Hemmer, MD, FASA
Associate Professor of Anesthesiology and Neurological Surgery
Department of Anesthesiology
Northwestern University Feinberg School of Medicine
Northwestern Memorial Hospital
Chicago, Illinois

Thomas K. Henthorn, MD
Professor of Anesthesiology
Department of Anesthesiology
University of Colorado School of Medicine
Adjoint Professor of Pharmaceutical Sciences
University of Colorado Skaggs School of Pharmacy and Pharmaceutical Sciences
University of Colorado Hospital
Aurora, Colorado

Erica L. Holland, MD
Assistant Professor of Pediatric Anesthesiology and Pain Medicine
Department of Anesthesiology and Pain Medicine
University of Washington School of Medicine
Seattle Children's Hospital
Seattle, Washington

Robert S. Holzman, MD, MA (Hon), FAAP
Professor of Anaesthesia
Harvard Medical School
Senior Associate in Anesthesiology
Department of Anesthesiology, Critical Care and Pain Medicine
Boston Children's Hospital
Boston, Massachusetts

Harriet W. Hopf, MD
Professor
Departments of Anesthesiology and Biomedical Engineering
Spencer Fox Eccles School of Medicine at the University of Utah
Salt Lake City, Utah

Keith A. Howell, MD
Associate Professor of Anesthesiology
Department of Anesthesiology
University of Florida College of Medicine
UF Health
Gainesville, Florida

Michelle L. Humeidan MD, PhD
Associate Professor of Clinical Anesthesiology
Department of Anesthesiology
The Ohio State University College of Medicine
The Ohio State University Wexner Medical Center
Columbus, Ohio

Robert W. Hurley, MD, PhD, FASA
Associate Dean, Faculty Development
Professor, Department of Anesthesiology
Professor, Department of Neurobiology and Anatomy
Wake Forest University School of Medicine
Executive Director, Pain Service Line
Atrium Health
Winston-Salem, North Carolina

Jaime B. Hyman, MD
Associate Professor of Anesthesiology
Department of Anesthesiology
Yale School of Medicine
New Haven, Connecticut

Jerry Ingrande, MD, MS
Clinical Professor
Department of Anesthesiology
UC San Diego School of Medicine
Staff Anesthesiologist
Department of Anesthesiology
San Diego VA Medical Center
San Diego, California

Adam K. Jacob, MD
Associate Professor of Anesthesiology and Perioperative Medicine
Department of Anesthesiology and Perioperative Medicine
Mayo Clinic College of Medicine and Science
Rochester, Minnesota

Rebecca L. Johnson, MD, FASA
Associate Professor of Anesthesiology
Department of Anesthesiology and Perioperative Medicine
Mayo Clinic College of Medicine and Science
Rochester, Minnesota

Sarah S. Joo, MD
Clinical Professor of Anesthesiology
Department of Anesthesiology, Perioperative and Pain Medicine
Icahn School of Medicine at Mount Sinai
Mount Sinai Morningside and West Hospitals
New York, New York

Sharma E. Joseph, MD, MPH
Assistant Professor of Anesthesiology
Department of Anesthesiology and Perioperative Medicine
Tufts University School of Medicine
Tufts Medical Center
Boston, Massachusetts

Jonathan D. Katz, MD
Clinical Professor of Anesthesiology
Department of Anesthesiology
Yale School of Medicine
New Haven, Connecticut

Christopher D. Kent, MD
Professor
Department of Anesthesiology & Pain Medicine
University of Washington School of Medicine
University of Washington Medical Center
Seattle, Washington

Sandeep Khanna, MD, FASA
Associate Program Director, Anesthesiology Residency
Department of Cardiothoracic Anesthesiology, General Anesthesiology & Outcomes Research
Cleveland Clinic Foundation
Cleveland, Ohio

Meghan A. Kirksey, MD, PhD
Clinical Assistant Professor of Anesthesiology
Weill Cornell Medical College
Department of Anesthesiology, Critical Care & Pain Management
Hospital for Special Surgery
New York, New York

Sandra L. Kopp, MD
Professor of Anesthesiology
Department of Anesthesiology and Perioperative Medicine
Mayo Clinic College of Medicine and Science
Rochester, Minnesota

Sundar Krishnan, MBBS
Associate Professor of Anesthesiology
Divisions of Cardiac Anesthesia and Critical Care Medicine
Duke University School of Medicine
Durham, North Carolina

Catherine M. Kuhn, MD
Professor of Anesthesiology, Associate Dean for Graduate Medical Education
Department of Anesthesiology
Duke University School of Medicine
Duke University Health System
Durham, North Carolina

Jerrold H. Levy, MD, FAHA, FCCM
Professor of Anesthesiology, Critical Care, and Surgery (Cardiothoracic)
Duke University School of Medicine
Durham, North Carolina

Michael Hua-Gen Li, MD, MPHTM, GCCT, FANZCA
Adult Cardiac Anesthesia Fellow
Division of Cardiac Anesthesiology
Duke University Hospital
Durham, North Carolina

Lauren Kemp Licina, MD
Staff Anesthesiologist
Department of Pediatric and Congenital Cardiac Anesthesiology
Cleveland Clinic Foundation
Cleveland, Ohio

Yi Lin, MD, PhD
Clinical Assistant Professor of Anesthesiology
Department of Anesthesiology, Critical Care & Pain Management
Hospital for Special Surgery
New York, New York

Scott Lindberg, MD, FASA
Clinical Assistant Professor
Department of Anesthesiology and Critical Care
Houston Methodist Hospital
Houston, Texas

Justin B. Long, MD, MHI
Associate Professor of Anesthesiology and Pediatrics
Emory University School of Medicine
Director, Pediatric Cardiac Anesthesiology
Children's Healthcare of Atlanta
Atlanta, Georgia

Isaac Luria, MS, MD
Assistant Professor of Anesthesiology
Departments of Anesthesiology and Acute Pain Service
University of Florida College of Medicine
UF Health Shands Hospital
Gainesville, Florida

Stephen M. Macres, Pharm D, MD
Clinical Professor of Anesthesiology
Director of Perioperative Pain Services
Department of Anesthesiology and Pain Medicine
UC Davis School of Medicine
UC Davis Medical Center
Sacramento, California

Yasdet Maldonado, MD, MMM, FASE
Associate Professor
Department of Cardiothoracic Anesthesiology
Cleveland Clinic Foundation
Cleveland, Ohio

Peter Mancini, MD
Assistant Professor of Clinical Anesthesiology
Yale School of Medicine
New Haven, Connecticut

Gerard R. Manecke, MD
Professor Emeritus
Department of Anesthesiology
UC San Diego School of Medicine
La Jolla, California

Joseph H. McIsaac III, MD, MS, MBA, CPE, FASA
Clinical Professor Anesthesiology
Department of Anesthesiology
University of Connecticut School of Medicine
Chief of Trauma Anesthesia
Department of Anesthesiology
Hartford Hospital
Hartford, Connecticut

Sara E. Meitzen, MD
Associate Professor of Anesthesiology
Department of Anesthesiology and Critical Care
UC San Diego School of Medicine
La Jolla, California

Shawn L. Mincer, MSW
Research Coordinator
Department of Anesthesiology and Pain Medicine
University of Washington School of Medicine
University of Washington Medical Center
Seattle, Washington

Candice K. Morrissey, MD, MSPH
Associate Professor
Department of Anesthesiology
Spencer Fox Eccles School of Medicine at the University of Utah
Salt Lake City, Utah

Shivani G. Mukkamala, MD
Assistant Professor of Anesthesiology and Pediatrics
Emory University School of Medicine
Department of Pediatric Anesthesiology
Children's Healthcare of Atlanta
Atlanta, Georgia

Michael J. Murray, MD, PhD, MCCM, FASA
Professor of Anesthesiology and Internal Medicine (Cardiology)
University of Arizona College of Medicine
Director of ICU Integration
Medical Director CV ICU
Banner University Medical Center Phoenix
Phoenix, Arizona

Ariana M. Nelson, MD
Clinical Associate Professor of Anesthesiology
Division of Pain Medicine
UCI School of Medicine
Irvine, California

Marieke Niesters, MD, PhD
Anesthesiologist—Pain specialist
Department of Anesthesiology
Leiden University Medical Center
Leiden, The Netherlands

Mark C. Norris, MD
Clinical Professor of Anesthesiology
Department of Anesthesiology
Boston University Chobanian & Avedisian School of Medicine
Boston Medical Center
Boston, Massachusetts

Benjamin O'Brien, MD, FRCA, FFICM, FFMLM, MHBA
Professor of Cardiac Anesthesiology and Intensive Care Medicine
Department of Cardiac Anesthesiology and Intensive Care Medicine
Deutsches Herzzentrum der Charité
Berlin/Germany

E. Andrew Ochroch, MD, MSCE
Professor of Anesthesiology
Department of Anesthesiology and Critical Care
Perelman School of Medicine at the University of Pennsylvania
University of Pennsylvania Health System
Philadelphia, Pennsylvania

Bukola Ojo, MD
Assistant Professor of Anesthesiology
Department of Anesthesiology and Pain Medicine
University of Washington School of Medicine
Seattle Children's Hospital
Seattle, Washington

Charles W. Otto, MD, FCCM
Professor Emeritus of Anesthesiology
Department of Anesthesiology
University of Arizona College of Medicine
Tucson, Arizona

Frank J. Overdyk, MSEE, MD
Adjunct Professor of Anesthesiology
Donald and Barbara Zucker School of Medicine at Hofstra/Northwell
Hempstead, New York

Nathan Leon Pace, MD, MStat
Professor of Anesthesiology
Department of Anesthesiology, Perioperative and Pain Medicine
Spencer Fox Eccles School of Medicine at the University of Utah
Salt Lake City, Utah

Paul S. Pagel, MD, PhD
Staff Physician, Anesthesiology Service
Clement J. Zablocki Veterans Affairs Medical Center
Professor of Anesthesiology
Medical College of Wisconsin
Milwaukee, Wisconsin

Ben J. A. Palanca, MD, PhD, MSCI
Associate Professor
Department of Anesthesiology
Washington University School of Medicine in St. Louis
St. Louis, Missouri

Raymond S. Park, MD
Assistant Professor of Anaesthesia
Harvard Medical School
Department of Anesthesiology, Critical Care and Pain Medicine
Boston Children's Hospital
Boston, Massachusetts

Jeffrey J. Pasternak, MS, MD
Professor of Anesthesiology
Department of Anesthesiology and Perioperative Medicine
Mayo Clinic College of Medicine and Science
Rochester, Minnesota

Feyce M. Peralta, MD, MS
Associate Professor and Vice Chair for Faculty Development & Diversity, Equity, and Inclusion
Department of Anesthesiology
Northwestern University Feinberg School of Medicine
Chicago, Illinois

Dasun S. Peramunage, MD
Acting Assistant Professor
Department of Anesthesiology and Pain Medicine
University of Washington School of Medicine
Harborview Medical Center
Seattle, Washington

James M. Peyton, MBChB, MRCP, FRCA
Assistant Professor of Anaesthesia
Harvard Medical School
Department of Anesthesiology, Critical Care and Pain Medicine
Boston Children's Hospital
Boston, Massachusetts

Mihai V. Podgoreanu, MD
Associate Professor and Chief, Cardiothoracic Anesthesiology
Department of Anesthesiology
Duke University School of Medicine
Durham, North Carolina

Angela L. Pollak, MD
Assistant Professor of Anesthesiology
Division of Cardiothoracic Anesthesiology
Duke University School of Medicine
Duke University Medical Center
Durham, North Carolina

Jamie R. Privratsky, MD, PhD
Assistant Professor
Department of Anesthesiology
Duke University School of Medicine
Durham, North Carolina

Bridget P. Pulos, MD, FASA
Assistant Professor of Anesthesiology
Department of Anesthesiology and Perioperative Medicine
Mayo Clinic College of Medicine and Science
Rochester, Minnesota

William P. Qiao, MD
Assistant Attending Anesthesiologist
Department of Anesthesiology, Critical Care & Pain Management
Hospital for Special Surgery
New York, New York

Sally E. Rampersad, BM, DCH, FRCA
Attending Anesthesiologist and Professor
Department of Anesthesiology and Pain Medicine
University of Washington School of Medicine
Seattle Children's Hospital
Seattle, Washington

Glenn Ramsey, MD
Professor of Pathology
Northwestern University Feinberg School of Medicine
Medical Director, Patient Blood Management Program
Northwestern Memorial Hospital
Chicago, Illinois

Kevin T. Riutort, MD, MS
Assistant Professor of Anesthesiology
Department of Anesthesiology and Perioperative Medicine
Mayo Clinic College of Medicine and Science
Jacksonville, Florida

Gerardo Rodriguez, MD
Associate Professor of Anesthesiology
Department of Anesthesiology and Perioperative Medicine
Division of Critical Care Medicine
Rutgers Robert Wood Johnson Medical School
Robert Wood Johnson University Hospital
New Brunswick, New Jersey

William H. Rosenblatt, MD
Professor
Department of Anesthesiology
Yale School of Medicine
New Haven, Connecticut

Richard W. Rosenquist, MD
Chairman
Department of Pain Management
Cleveland Clinic Foundation
Cleveland, Ohio

Usha Saldanha, MD
Assistant Professor of Anesthesiology and Pain Medicine
Department of Anesthesiology and Pain Medicine
UC Davis School of Medicine
UC Davis Medical Center
Sacramento, California

Jeffrey J. Schwartz, MD
Associate Professor
Department of Anesthesiology
Yale School of Medicine
Yale New Haven Hospital
New Haven, Connecticut

Sam R. Sharar, MD
Professor
Vice Chair for Faculty Affairs and Development
Department of Anesthesiology and Pain Medicine
University of Washington School of Medicine
Seattle, Washington

Elizabeth H. Sinz, MD, MEd, FCCM, FSSH
Professor of Anesthesiology and Perioperative Medicine
Associative Dean for Clinical Simulation
Department of Anesthesiology and Perioperative Medicine
Penn State College of Medicine
Penn State Health Milton S. Hershey Medical Center
Hershey, Pennsylvania

Nikolaos J. Skubas, MD, DSc
Professor and Chair
Department of Cardiothoracic Anesthesiology
Cleveland Clinic Foundation
Cleveland, Ohio

Ian R. Slade, MD
Assistant Professor
Department of Anesthesiology and Pain Medicine
University of Washington School of Medicine
Harborview Medical Center
Seattle, Washington

Hugh M. Smith, MD, PhD
Anesthesiologist
Department of Anesthesiology and Perioperative Medicine
Mayo Clinic College of Medicine and Science
Rochester, Minnesota

Terry Smith, PhD
Associate Professor
Department of Anesthesiology
Leiden University Medical Center
Leiden, The Netherlands

Jennifer Smith, MD
Assistant Professor
Department of Anesthesia and Perioperative Medicine
Medical University of South Carolina
Charleston, South Carolina

Ellen M. Soffin, MD, PhD
Clinical Associate Professor of Anesthesiology
Weill Cornell Medical College
Department of Anesthesiology, Critical Care & Pain Management
Hospital for Special Surgery
New York, New York

Nicole Z. Spence, MD
Assistant Professor of Anesthesiology, Director of Acute Pain Service
Department of Anesthesiology
Boston University Chobanian & Avedisian School of Medicine
Boston Medical Center
Boston, Massachusetts

Mark Stafford-Smith, MD, CM FRCP(C), MBA, FASE
Professor of Anesthesiology
Duke University School of Medicine
Duke University Medical Center
Durham, North Carolina

Andrew F. Stasic, MD
Associate Professor Emeritus
Department of Anesthesia—Pediatric Anesthesia
Indiana University School of Medicine
Indianapolis, Indiana

Randolph H. Steadman, MD, MS
Professor and Carole Walter Looke Centennial Chair
Department of Anesthesiology and Critical Care
Houston Methodist Hospital
Houston, Texas

Alecia L. S. Stein, MD
Associate Professor of Clinical Anesthesia
Division of Anesthesiology, Perioperative Medicine and Pain Management
University of Miami Miller School of Medicine
Bascom Palmer Eye Institute
Miami, Florida

David F. Stowe, MD, PhD
Professor of Anesthesiology and Physiology
Medical College of Wisconsin
Milwaukee, Wisconsin

Madhav Swaminathan, MD, MMCi, FASE
Professor and Vice-Chair
Department of Anesthesiology
Duke University School of Medicine
Durham, North Carolina

Martin Szafran, MD
Partner Anesthesiologist, Board Member
Department of Dupage Valley Anesthesiologists
Edward-Elmhurst Health
Naperville, Illinois

Anthony Tanella, MD
Assistant Professor of Anesthesiology
Department of Anesthesiology
Yale School of Medicine
New Haven, Connecticut

Stephan R. Thilen, MD, MS
Associate Professor
Department of Anesthesiology and Pain Medicine
University of Washington School of Medicine
Seattle, Washington

Joshua M. Tobin, MD, MSc
Professor of Anesthesiology
Division of Trauma Anesthesiology
University of Texas Health—San Antonio
San Antonio, Texas

Klaus D. Torp, MD
Assistant Professor of Anesthesiology
Department of Anesthesiology and Perioperative Medicine
Mayo Clinic College of Medicine and Science
Jacksonville, Florida

Chi-Ho Ban Tsui, MD, MSc
Professor of Anesthesiology
Department of Anesthesiology, Perioperative and Pain Medicine
Stanford University School of Medicine
Stanford, California

Cristiane M. Ueno, MD, FACS
Associate Professor
Department of Plastic Surgery
The Ohio State University College of Medicine
Columbus, Ohio

Elizabeth A. Valentine, MD
Associate Professor of Clinical Anesthesiology
Department of Anesthesiology and Critical Care
Perelman School of Medicine at the University of Pennsylvania
University of Pennsylvania Health System
Philadelphia, Pennsylvania

Amy E. Vinson, MD
Assistant Professor of Anaesthesia
Harvard Medical School
Department of Anesthesiology, Critical Care and Pain Medicine
Boston Children's Hospital
Boston, Massachusetts

Daniel L. Wang, MD
Resident Physician of Anesthesiology
Department of Anesthesiology and Critical Care
UC San Diego School of Medicine
La Jolla, California

Wade A. Weigel, MD
Staff Anesthesiologist
Department of Anesthesiology
Virginia Mason Franciscan Health
Seattle, Washington

Cynthia A. Wong, MD
Professor and Chair of Anesthesia
Department of Anesthesia
University of Iowa Carver College of Medicine
Iowa City, Iowa

Susan Wright, MB, BS, FRCA, FFICM
Consultant Anaesthetist
Department of Perioperative Medicine
St. Bartholomew's Hospital
London, United Kingdom

Daniel J. Wyler, MS, MD
Assistant Professor of Anesthesiology
Department of Anesthesiology and Perioperative Medicine
Case Western Reserve University School of Medicine
University Hospitals Cleveland Medical Center
Cleveland, Ohio

Victor W. Xia, MD
Clinical Professor
Division of Anesthesiology and Perioperative Medicine
David Geffen School of Medicine at UCLA
Ronald Reagan UCLA Medical Center
Los Angeles, California

Jon Y. Zhou, MD
Anesthesiologist
Department of Anesthesia
Kaiser Roseville Medical Center
The Permanente Medical Group
Roseville, California

Contents

Section 5

PREOPERATIVE ASSESSMENT AND PERIOPERATIVE MONITORING

Section 6

BASIC ANESTHETIC MANAGEMENT

Section 7

ANESTHESIA SUBSPECIALITY CARE

Section 8

ANESTHESIA FOR SELECTED SURGICAL SERVICES

Multimedia Contents

Chapter-Based Narrated Interactive Clinical Vignettes (NICVs)

Supplementary Narrated Interactive Clinical Vignettes (NICVs)

Chapter-Based Tutorial Videos

Supplemental Tutorial Videos

Hemodynamic Simulations

Appendix 2 Videos

Section 1

INTRODUCTION AND OVERVIEW

1 The History of Anesthesia

MELISSA L. COLEMAN • ADAM K. JACOB • SANDRA L. KOPP • HUGH M. SMITH • DOUGLAS R. BACON

KEY POINTS

1. Anesthesiology is a young specialty historically, especially when compared with surgery or internal medicine.
2. Discoveries in anesthesiology have taken decades to build upon the observations and experiments of many people, and in some instances, we are still searching. For example, the ideal volatile anesthetic has yet to be discovered.
3. Much of our current anesthesia equipment is the direct result of anesthesiologists being unhappy with existing tools and needing better ones to properly anesthetize patients.
4. Many safety standards have been established through the work of anesthesiologists who were frustrated by the status quo.
5. Regional anesthesia is the direct outgrowth of a chance observation by an intern who would go on to become a successful ophthalmologist.
6. Pain medicine began as an outgrowth of regional anesthesia.
7. Organizations of anesthesia professionals have been critical in establishing high standards in education and proficiency, which in turn has defined the specialty.
8. Respiratory critical care medicine started as the need by anesthesiologists to use positive-pressure ventilation to help polio victims.
9. Surgical anesthesia and physician specialization in its administration have allowed for increasingly complex operations to be performed on increasingly ill patients.

Surgery without adequate pain control may seem cruel to the modern reader, and in contemporary practice, we are prone to forget the realities of surgery without anesthesia. Fanny Burney, a well-known literary artist from the early 19th century, described a mastectomy she endured after receiving a "wine cordial" as her sole anesthetic. As seven male assistants held her down, the surgery commenced: "When the dreadful steel was plunged into the breast-cutting through veins-arteries-flesh–nerves, I needed no injunction not to restrain my cries. I began a scream that lasted unintermittently during the whole time of the incision–and I almost marvel that it rings not in my Ears still! So excruciating was the agony. Oh Heaven!–I then felt the knife racking against the breast bone–scraping it! This performed while I yet remained in utterly speechless torture."[1] Burney's description illustrates the difficulty of overstating the impact of anesthesia on the human condition. An epitaph on a monument to William Thomas Green Morton, one of the founders of anesthesia, summarizes the contribution of anesthesia: "BEFORE WHOM in all time Surgery was Agony."[2] Although most human civilizations evolved some method for diminishing patient discomfort, *anesthesia*, in its modern and 1 effective meaning, is a comparatively recent discovery with traceable origins in the mid-19th century. How we have changed perspectives, from one in which surgical pain was terrible and expected to one in which patients reasonably assume they will be safe, pain free, and unaware during extensive operations, is a fascinating story and the subject of this chapter.

Anesthesiologists are like no other physicians: We are experts at controlling the airway and at emergency resuscitation; we are real-time cardiopulmonologists achieving hemodynamic and respiratory stability for the anesthetized patient; we are pharmacologists and physiologists, calculating appropriate doses and desired responses; we are gurus of postoperative care and patient safety; we are internists performing perianesthetic medical evaluations and therapy; we are the pain experts across all medical disciplines and apply specialized techniques in pain clinics and labor wards; we manage the severely sick and injured in critical care units; we are neurologists, selectively blocking sympathetic, sensory, or motor functions with our regional techniques; and we are trained researchers exploring scientific mystery and clinical phenomena.

Anesthesiology is an amalgam of specialized techniques, equipment, drugs, and knowledge that like the growth rings of a tree have built up over time. Current anesthesia practice is the summation of the individual efforts and fortuitous discoveries of centuries. Every component of modern anesthesia was at some point a new discovery and reflects the experience, knowledge, and inventiveness of our predecessors. Historical examination enables understanding of how these individual components of anesthesia evolved. Knowledge of the history of anesthesia enhances our appreciation of current practice and foretells where our specialty might be headed.

Anesthesia Before Ether

Physical and Psychological Anesthesia

The Edwin Smith Surgical Papyrus, the oldest known written surgical document, describes 48 cases performed by an Egyptian surgeon from 3000 to 2500 BC. Although this remarkable surgical treatise contains no direct mention of measures to lessen patient pain or suffering, Egyptian pictographs from the same era show a surgeon compressing a nerve in a patient's antecubital fossa while operating on the patient's hand. Another image displays a patient compressing his own brachial plexus while a procedure is performed on his palm.[3] In the 16th century, military surgeon Ambroise Paré became adept at nerve compression as a means of creating anesthesia.

Medical science has benefited from the natural refrigerating properties of ice and snow as well. For centuries, anatomic dissections were performed only in winter because colder temperatures delayed deterioration of the cadaver. In the 17th century, Marco Aurelio Severino described the technique of "refrigeration anesthesia" in which snow was placed in parallel lines across the incisional plane such that the surgical site became insensate within minutes. The technique never became widely used, likely because of the challenge of maintaining stores of snow year-round.[4] Severino is also known to have saved numerous lives during an epidemic of diphtheria by performing tracheostomies and inserting trocars to maintain patency of the airway.[5]

Formal manipulation of the psyche to relieve surgical pain was undertaken by French physicians Charles Dupotet and Jules Cloquet in the late 1820s with hypnosis, then called *mesmerism*. Although the work of Anton Mesmer was discredited by the French Academy of Science after formal inquiry several decades earlier, proponents like Dupotet and Cloquet continued with mesmeric experiments and pleaded to the Academie de Medicine to reconsider its utility.[6] In a well-attended demonstration in 1828, Cloquet removed the breast of a 64-year-old patient while she reportedly remained in a calm, mesmeric sleep. This demonstration made a lasting impression on British physician John Elliotson, who became a leading figure of the mesmeric movement in England in the 1830s and 1840s. Innovative and quick to adopt new advances, Elliotson performed mesmeric demonstrations and in 1843, published *Numerous Cases of Surgical Operations Without Pain in the Mesmeric State.* Support for mesmerism faded when in 1846 renowned surgeon Robert Liston performed the first operation using ether anesthesia in England and remarked, "This Yankee dodge beats mesmerism all hollow."[7]

Early Analgesics and Soporifics

Dioscorides, a Greek physician from the first century AD, commented on the analgesia of mandragora, a drug prepared from the bark and leaves of the mandrake plant. He observed that the plant substance could be boiled in wine, strained, and used "in the case of persons... about to be cut or cauterized, when they wish to produce anesthesia."[8] Mandragora was still being used to benefit patients as late as the 17th century. From the 9th to the 13th centuries, the *soporific sponge* was a dominant mode of providing pain relief during surgery. Mandrake leaves, along with black nightshade, poppies, and other herbs, were boiled together and cooked onto a sponge. The sponge was then reconstituted in hot water and placed under the patient's nose before surgery. Prior to the hypodermic syringe and routine venous access, ingestion and inhalation were the only known routes for administering medicines to gain systemic effects. Prepared as indicated by published reports of the time, the sponge generally contained morphine and scopolamine—drugs used in modern anesthesia—in varying amounts.[9]

Alcohol was another element of the pre-ether armamentarium because it was thought to induce stupor and blunt the impact of pain. Although alcohol is a central nervous system depressant, in the amounts administered, it produced little analgesia in the setting of true surgical pain. Fanny Burney's account underscores the ineffectiveness of alcohol as an anesthetic. Not only did alcohol provide minimal pain control, but it also did nothing to dull her recollection of events. Laudanum was an alcohol-based solution of opium first compounded by Paracelsus in the 16th century. It was wildly popular in the Victorian and Romantic periods and prescribed for a wide variety of ailments, from the common cold to tuberculosis. Although appropriately used as an analgesic in some instances, it was frequently misused and abused. Laudanum was given by nursemaids to quiet wailing infants and abused by many upper-class women, poets, and artists who fell victim to its addictive potential.

In the first three decades of the 19th century, in Japan, Seisyu Hanaoka performed operations under what has been described as general anesthesia.[10] In the late 1900s, the manuscript "On the Use of Mafutsuto," the name given to the anesthetic method by Hanaoka, was translated into English. Written by Hajime Matsuoka, the manuscript details preanesthetic evaluation, the timing of anesthesia, and the proposed duration of surgery. The manuscript stated that care should be taken to ensure that lighting is appropriate; therefore, it recommended that operations be performed at noon. Similarly, it stated that operations should not last more than 2 hours, because there was no way to replace intraoperative fluid or blood losses. The manuscript also contains a section on postoperative care.[11]

Inhaled Anesthetics

For many years, nitrous oxide was known for its ability to induce lightheadedness, and it was often inhaled by those seeking a thrill. It was made by heating ammonium nitrate in the presence of iron filings. The evolved gas was passed through water to eliminate toxic oxides of nitrogen before being stored. Nitrous oxide was first prepared in 1773 by Joseph Priestley, an English clergyman and scientist, who ranks among the great pioneers of chemistry. Without formal scientific training, Priestley prepared and examined several gases, including nitrous oxide, ammonia, sulfur dioxide, oxygen, carbon monoxide, and carbon dioxide.

At the end of the 18th century in England, there was a strong interest in the supposed wholesome effects of mineral water and gases, particularly with regard to treatment of scurvy, tuberculosis, and other diseases. Thomas Beddoes opened his Pneumatic Institute close to the small spa of Hotwells, in the city of Bristol, to study the beneficial effects of inhaled gases. He hired Humphry Davy in 1798 to conduct research projects for the institute. Davy performed brilliant investigations of several gases but focused much of his attention on nitrous oxide. His human experimental results, combined with research on the physical properties of the gas, were published in *Nitrous Oxide,* a 580-page book published in 1800. This impressive treatise is now best remembered for a few incidental observations. Davy commented that nitrous oxide transiently relieved a severe headache, obliterated a minor headache, and briefly quenched an aggravating toothache. The most frequently quoted passage was a casual entry: "As nitrous oxide in its extensive operation appears capable of destroying physical pain, it may probably be used with advantage during surgical operations in which no great effusion of blood takes place."[12] This is perhaps the most famous of the "missed opportunities" to discover surgical anesthesia. Davy's lasting nitrous oxide legacy was coining the phrase "laughing gas" to describe its unique property.

Almost Discovery: Hickman, Clarke, Long, and Wells

2 As the 19th century progressed, societal attitudes toward pain changed, perhaps best exemplified in the writings of the Romantic poets.[13] Thus, efforts to relieve pain were undertaken, and several more near-breakthroughs that occurred deserve mention. An English surgeon named Henry Hill Hickman searched intentionally for an inhaled anesthetic to relieve pain in his patients.[14] Hickman used high concentrations of carbon dioxide in his studies on mice and dogs. Carbon dioxide has some anesthetic properties, as shown by the absence of response to an incision in the animals of Hickman's study, but it was never determined whether the animals were insensate because of hypoxia rather than anesthesia. Hickman's concept was magnificent; his choice of agent was regrettable.

The discovery of surgical anesthetics in the modern era remains linked to inhaled anesthetics. The compound now known as *diethyl ether* had been known for centuries; it may have been synthesized first by 8th-century Arabian philosopher Jabir ibn Hayyan or possibly by Raymond Lully, a 13th-century European alchemist. But diethyl ether was certainly known in the 16th century, to both Valerius Cordus and Paracelsus, who prepared it by distilling sulfuric acid (oil of vitriol) with fortified wine to produce an *oleum vitrioli dulce* (sweet oil of vitriol). In one of the first "missed" observations on the effects of inhaled agents, Paracelsus observed that ether caused chickens to fall asleep and awaken unharmed. He must have been aware of its analgesic qualities because he reported that it could be recommended for use in painful illnesses.

For three centuries thereafter, this simple compound remained a therapeutic agent with only occasional use. Some of its properties were examined but without sustained interest by distinguished British scientists Robert Boyle, Isaac Newton, and Michael Faraday, none of whom made the conceptual link to surgical anesthesia. Its only routine application came as an inexpensive recreational drug among the poor of Britain and Ireland, who sometimes drank an ounce or two of ether when taxes made gin prohibitively expensive.[15] An American variation of this practice was conducted by groups of students who held ether-soaked towels to their faces at nocturnal "ether frolics."

William E. Clarke, a medical student from Rochester, New York, may have given the first ether anesthetic in January 1842. From techniques learned as a chemistry student in 1839, Clarke entertained his companions with nitrous oxide and ether. Emboldened by these experiences, he administered ether, from a towel, to a young woman named Hobbie. One of her teeth was then extracted without pain by a dentist named Elijah Pope.[16] However, it was suggested that the woman's unconsciousness was due to hysteria, and Clarke was advised to conduct no further anesthetic experiments.[17]

Two months later, on March 30, 1842, Crawford Williamson Long administered ether with a towel for surgical anesthesia in Jefferson, Georgia. His patient, James M. Venable, was a young man who was already familiar with ether's exhilarating effects, for he reported in a certificate that he had previously inhaled it and was fond of its use. Venable had two small tumors on his neck but refused to have them excised because he feared the pain that accompanied surgery. Knowing that Venable was familiar with ether's action, Dr Long proposed that ether might alleviate pain and gained his patient's consent to proceed. After inhaling ether from the towel and having the procedure successfully completed, Venable reported that he was unaware of the removal of the tumors.[18] In determining the first fee for anesthesia and surgery, Long settled on a charge of $2.00.[19]

A common mid-19th century problem facing dentists was that patients refused beneficial treatment of their teeth for fear of the pain of the procedure. From a dentist's perspective, pain was not so much life-threatening as it was livelihood-threatening. One of the first dentists to engender a solution was Horace Wells of Hartford, Connecticut, whose great moment of discovery came on December 10, 1844. He observed a lecture–exhibition on nitrous oxide by an itinerant "scientist," Gardner Quincy Colton, who encouraged members of the audience to inhale a sample of the gas. Wells observed a young man injure his leg without pain while under the influence of nitrous oxide. Sensing that it might provide pain relief during dental procedures, Wells contacted Colton and boldly proposed an experiment in which Wells was to be the subject. The following day, Colton gave Wells nitrous oxide before a fellow dentist, William Riggs, extracted a tooth.[20] Afterward, Wells declared that he had not felt any pain and deemed the experiment a success. Colton taught Wells to prepare nitrous oxide, which the dentist administered with success to patients in his practice. His apparatus probably resembled that used by Colton: a wooden tube placed in the mouth through which nitrous oxide was breathed from a small bag filled with the gas.

Public Demonstration of Ether Anesthesia

Another New Englander, William Thomas Green Morton, briefly shared a dental practice with Wells in Hartford. Wells' daybook shows that he gave Morton a course of instruction in anesthesia, but Morton apparently moved to Boston without paying for the lessons.[21] In Boston, Morton continued his interest in anesthesia

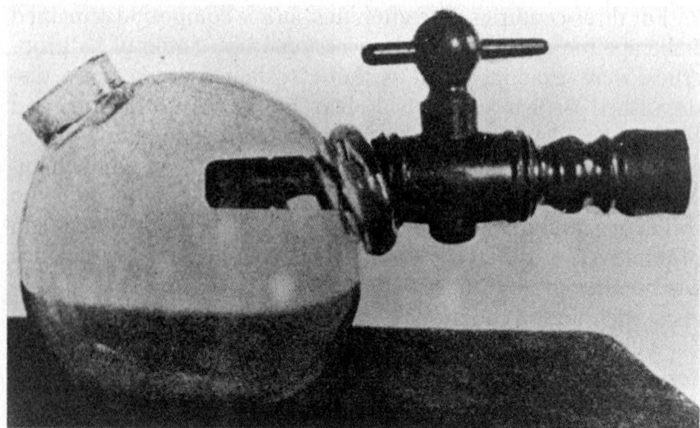

Figure 1-1 Morton's ether inhaler (1846).

and sought instruction from chemist and physician Charles T. Jackson. After learning that ether dropped on the skin provided analgesia, he began experiments with inhaled ether, an agent that proved to be much more versatile than nitrous oxide. Bottles of liquid ether were easily transported, and the volatility of the drug permitted effective inhalation. The concentrations required for surgical anesthesia were so low that patients did not become hypoxic when breathing ether vaporized in air. It also possessed what would later be recognized as a unique property among all inhaled anesthetics: the quality of providing surgical anesthesia without causing respiratory depression. These properties, combined with a slow rate of induction, gave the patient a significant safety margin even in the hands of relatively unskilled anesthetists.[22]

After anesthetizing a pet dog, Morton became confident of his skills and anesthetized patients with ether in his dental office (NICV 1-1). Encouraged by his success, Morton sought an invitation to give a public demonstration in the Bullfinch amphitheater of the Massachusetts General Hospital (the site where Wells' failed demonstration of the efficacy of nitrous oxide as a complete surgical anesthetic was incorrectly also thought to have occurred).[23] Many details of the October 16, 1846, demonstration are well known. Morton secured permission to provide an anesthetic to Edward Gilbert Abbott, a patient of surgeon John Collins Warren. Warren planned to excise a vascular lesion from the left side of Abbott's neck and was about to proceed when Morton arrived late. He had been delayed because he was obliged to wait for an instrument maker to complete a new inhaler (Fig. 1-1, 1 Video 1-1). It consisted of a large glass bulb containing a sponge soaked with oil of orange mixed with ether and a spout that was placed in the patient's mouth. An opening on the opposite side of the bulb allowed air to enter and be drawn over the ether-soaked sponge with each breath.[23,24]

The conversations of that morning were not accurately recorded; however, popular accounts state that the surgeon responded testily to Morton's apology for his tardy arrival by remarking, "Sir, your patient is ready." Morton directed his attention to his patient and first conducted a much-abbreviated preoperative evaluation. He inquired, "Are you afraid?" Abbott responded that he was not and took the inhaler in his mouth. After a few minutes, Morton turned to the surgeon and said, "Sir, your patient is ready." Gilbert Abbott later reported that he was aware of the surgery but experienced no pain. It has been alleged that when the procedure ended, Warren immediately turned to his audience and uttered the statement, "Gentlemen, this is no humbug," but this has since been disputed.[23,25]

What would be recognized as America's greatest contribution to 19th century medicine had occurred. However, Morton, wishing to capitalize on his "discovery," refused to divulge what agent was in his inhaler. Some weeks passed before Morton admitted that the active component of the colored fluid, which he had called "Letheon," was simple diethyl ether. Morton, Wells, Jackson, and their supporters soon became drawn into a contentious, protracted, and fruitless debate over priority for the discovery (2 Video 1-2).[26] This debate has subsequently been termed *the ether controversy*. In short, Morton had applied for a patent for Letheon and, when it was granted, tried to receive royalties for the use of ether as an anesthetic.[27]

When the details of Morton's anesthetic technique became public knowledge, the information was transmitted by train, stagecoach, and coastal vessels to other North American cities and by ship to the world. As ether was easy to prepare and administer, anesthetics were performed in Britain, France, Russia, South Africa, Australia, and other countries almost as soon as surgeons heard the welcome news of the extraordinary discovery. Even though surgery could now be performed with "pain put to sleep," the frequency of operations did not rise rapidly, and several years would pass before anesthesia was universally recommended.

Chloroform and Obstetrics

James Young Simpson was a successful obstetrician in Edinburgh, Scotland, and among the first to use ether for the relief of labor pain. Dissatisfied with ether, Simpson soon sought a more pleasant, rapid-acting anesthetic. He and his junior associates conducted a bold search by inhaling samples of several volatile chemicals collected for Simpson by British apothecaries. David Waldie suggested chloroform, which had first been prepared in 1831. Simpson and his friends inhaled it after dinner at a party in Simpson's home on the evening of November 4, 1847. They promptly fell unconscious and, when they awoke, were delighted with their success. Simpson quickly set about encouraging the use of chloroform. Within 2 weeks, he submitted his first account of its use for publication in *The Lancet*.

In the 19th century, the relief of obstetric pain had significant social ramifications and made anesthesia during childbirth a controversial subject. Simpson argued against the prevailing view, which held that relieving labor pain opposed God's will. The pain of the parturient was viewed as both a component of punishment and a means of atonement for Original Sin. Less than a year after administering the first anesthesia during childbirth, Simpson addressed these concerns in a pamphlet entitled *Answers to the Religious Objections Advanced Against the Employment of Anaesthetic Agents in Midwifery and Surgery and Obstetrics*. In it, Simpson recognized the Book of Genesis as being the root of this sentiment and noted that God promised to relieve the descendants of Adam and Eve of the curse. In addition, Simpson asserted that labor pain was a result of scientific and anatomic causes and not the result of religious condemnation. He stated that the upright position of humans necessitated strong pelvic muscles to support the abdominal contents. As a result, he argued that the uterus necessarily developed strong musculature to overcome the resistance of the pelvic floor and that great contractile power caused great pain. Simpson's pamphlet probably did not have a significant impact on the prevailing attitudes, but he did articulate many concepts that his contemporaries were debating at the time.[28]

Chloroform gained considerable notoriety after John Snow used it to deliver the last two children of Queen Victoria. The Queen's consort, Prince Albert, interviewed John Snow before he was called to Buckingham Palace to administer chloroform at the request of the Queen's obstetrician. During the monarch's labor, Snow gave analgesic doses of chloroform on a folded handkerchief. This technique was soon termed *chloroform à la reine*.

Victoria abhorred the pain of childbirth and enjoyed the relief that chloroform provided. She wrote in her journal, "Dr. Snow gave that blessed chloroform and the effect was soothing, quieting, and delightful beyond measure."[29] When the Queen, as head of the Church of England, endorsed obstetric anesthesia, religious debate over the management of labor pain terminated abruptly.

John Snow, already a respected physician, took an interest in anesthetic practice and was soon invited to work with many leading surgeons of the day. In 1848, Snow introduced a chloroform inhaler. He had recognized the versatility of the new agent and came to prefer it in his practice. At the same time, he initiated what was to become an extraordinary series of experiments that were remarkable in their scope and for anticipating sophisticated research performed a century later. Snow realized that successful anesthetics should abolish pain and unwanted movements. He anesthetized several species of animals with varying strengths of ether and chloroform to determine the concentration required to prevent reflex movement from sharp stimuli. This work approximated the modern concept of minimum alveolar concentration.[30] Snow assessed the anesthetic action of several potential anesthetics but did not find any to rival chloroform or ether. His studies led him to recognize the relationship between solubility, vapor pressure, and anesthetic potency, which was not fully appreciated until after World War II. Snow published two remarkable books, *On the Inhalation of the Vapour of Ether* (1847) and *On Chloroform and Other Anaesthetics* (1858). The latter was almost completed when he died of a stroke at the age of 45, and it was published posthumously.

3 Anesthesia Principles, Equipment, and Standards

Control of the Airway

Definitive control of the airway is a skill anesthesiologists now consider paramount. However, it was not until many patients died or nearly escaped death because of partial or complete airway obstruction that safe and reliable airway management techniques were developed. Toward the end of the 19th century, prior to the introduction of tracheal intubation, several important techniques were proposed that remain integral to anesthesiology education and practice. Joseph Clover was the first Englishman to urge the now-universal practice of thrusting the patient's jaw forward to overcome obstruction of the upper airway by the tongue. Clover also published a landmark case report in 1877 in which he created a surgical airway. Once his patient was asleep, Clover discovered that his patient had a tumor of the mouth that obstructed the airway completely, despite his trusted jaw-thrust maneuver. He averted disaster by inserting a small curved cannula of his design through the cricothyroid membrane. He continued anesthesia via the cannula until the tumor was excised. Clover, the model of the prepared anesthesiologist, remarked, "I have never used the cannula before although it has been my companion at some thousands of anaesthetic cases."[31]

Tracheal Intubation

The development of techniques and instruments for tracheal intubation ranks among the major advances in the history of anesthesiology. The first tracheal tubes were developed for the resuscitation of drowning victims but were not used in anesthesia until 1878. The first use of elective oral intubation for an anesthetic was undertaken by Scottish surgeon William Macewan. He had practiced passing flexible metal tubes through the larynx of a cadaver before attempting the maneuver on an awake patient with an oral tumor at the Glasgow Royal Infirmary on July 5, 1878.[32] Because topical anesthesia was not yet known, the experience must have demanded fortitude on the part of Macewan's patient. Once the tube was correctly positioned, an assistant began a chloroform-air anesthetic via the tube. Once anesthetized, the patient soon stopped coughing. Unfortunately, Macewan abandoned the practice following a fatality in which a patient had been successfully intubated while awake but the tube became dislodged once the patient was asleep. After the tube was removed, an attempt to provide chloroform by mask anesthesia was unsuccessful and the patient died.

An American surgeon named Joseph O'Dwyer is remembered for his extraordinary dedication to the advancement of tracheal intubation. In 1885, O'Dwyer designed a series of metal laryngeal tubes, which he inserted blindly between the vocal cords of children suffering a diphtheritic crisis. Three years later, O'Dwyer designed a second rigid tube with a conical tip that occluded the larynx so effectively that it could be used for artificial ventilation when applied with the bellows and T-piece tube designed by George Fell. The Fell–O'Dwyer apparatus, as it came to be known, was used during thoracic surgery by Rudolph Matas of New Orleans. Matas was so pleased with it that he predicted, "The procedure that promises the most benefit in preventing pulmonary collapse in operations on the chest is… the rhythmical maintenance of artificial respiration by a tube in the glottis directly connected with a bellows."[33]

After O'Dwyer's death, the outstanding pioneer of tracheal intubation was Franz Kuhn, a surgeon of Kassel, Germany. From 1900 until 1912, Kuhn[34] published several articles and a classic monograph, "*Die perorale Intubation*," which were not well known in his lifetime but have since become widely appreciated. His work might have had a more profound impact if it had been translated into English. Kuhn described techniques of oral and nasal intubation that he performed with flexible metal tubes composed of coiled tubing similar to those now used for the spout of metal gasoline cans. After applying cocaine to the airway, Kuhn introduced his tube over a curved metal stylet that he directed toward the larynx with his left index finger. Although he was aware of the subglottic cuffs that had been used briefly by Victor Eisenmenger, Kuhn preferred to seal the larynx by positioning a supralaryngeal flange near the tube's tip before packing the pharynx with gauze. Kuhn even monitored the patient's breath sounds continuously through a monaural earpiece connected to an extension of the tracheal tube by a narrow tube.

Intubation of the trachea by palpation was an uncertain and sometimes traumatic act; surgeons even believed that it would be anatomically impossible to visualize the vocal cords directly. This misapprehension was overcome in 1895 by Alfred Kirstein in Berlin, who devised the first direct-vision laryngoscope.[35] Kirstein was motivated by a friend's report that a patient's trachea had been accidentally intubated during esophagoscopy. Kirstein promptly fabricated a handheld instrument that at first resembled a shortened cylindrical esophagoscope. He soon substituted a semicircular blade that opened inferiorly. Kirstein could now examine the larynx while standing behind his seated patient, whose head had been placed in an attitude approximating the currently termed "sniffing position." Although Alfred Kirstein's "autoscope" was not used by anesthesiologists, it was the forerunner of all modern laryngoscopes. Endoscopy was refined by Chevalier Jackson in Philadelphia, who designed a U-shaped laryngoscope by adding a handgrip that was parallel to the blade. The Jackson blade has remained a standard instrument for endoscopists but was not favored by anesthesiologists. Two laryngoscopes that closely resembled modern L-shaped instruments were designed in 1910 and 1913 by two American surgeons, Henry Janeway and George Dorrance, but neither instrument achieved lasting use despite their excellent designs.[36]

Before the introduction of muscle relaxants in the 1940s, intubation of the trachea could be challenging. This challenge was made somewhat easier, however, with the advent of laryngoscope blades specifically designed to increase visualization of the vocal cords. Robert Miller of San Antonio, Texas, and Robert Macintosh of Oxford University created their respectively named blades within an interval of 2 years. In 1941, Miller brought forward the slender, straight blade with a slight curve near the tip to ease the passage of the tube through the larynx. Although Miller's blade was a refinement, the technique of its use was identical to that of earlier models as the epiglottis was lifted to expose the larynx.[37]

The Macintosh blade, which is placed in the vallecula rather than under the epiglottis, was invented as an incidental result of a tonsillectomy. Sir Robert Macintosh later described the circumstances of its discovery in an appreciation writing regarding the career of his technician, Mr. Richard Salt, who constructed the blade. As Sir Robert recalled, "A Boyle-Davis gag, a size larger than intended, was inserted for tonsillectomy, and when the mouth was fully opened, the cords came into view. This was a surprise since conventional laryngoscopy, at that depth of anaesthesia, would have been impossible in those pre-relaxant days. Within a matter of hours, Salt had modified the blade of the Davis gag and attached a laryngoscope handle to it; and streamlined (after testing several models), the end result came into widespread use."[38] Macintosh underestimated the popularity of the blade, as it is likely that nearly a million of the original, or many special-purpose versions, have been produced and marketed.

The most distinguished innovator in tracheal intubation was the self-trained British anaesthetist Ivan (later, Sir Ivan) Magill.[39] In 1919, while serving in the Royal Army as a general medical officer, Magill was assigned to a military hospital near London. Although he had only rudimentary training in anesthesia, Magill was obliged to accept an assignment to the anesthesia service, where he worked with another neophyte, Stanley Rowbotham.[40] Together, Magill and Rowbotham attended casualties disfigured by severe facial injuries who underwent repeated restorative operations. These procedures required that the surgeon, Harold Gillies, have unrestricted access to the face and airway. These patients presented formidable challenges, but both Magill and Rowbotham became adept at tracheal intubation and quickly understood its current limitations. Because they learned from fortuitous observations, they soon extended the scope of tracheal anesthesia.

They gained expertise with blind nasal intubation after they learned to soften semirigid insufflation tubes for passage through the nostril. Even though their original intent was to position the tips of the nasal tubes in the posterior pharynx, the slender tubes frequently ended up in the trachea. Stimulated by this chance experience, they developed techniques of deliberate nasotracheal intubation. In 1920, Magill devised an aid to manipulating the catheter tip, the "Magill angulated forceps," which continues to be manufactured according to his original design over 90 years ago.

With the war over, Magill entered civilian practice and set out to develop a wide-bore tube that would resist kinking but be conformable to the contours of the upper airway. While in a hardware store, he found mineralized red rubber tubing that he cut, beveled, and smoothed to produce tubes that clinicians around the world would come to call "Magill tubes." His tubes remained the universal standard for more than 40 years until rubber products were supplanted by inert plastics. Magill also rediscovered the advantage of applying cocaine to the nasal mucosa, a technique that greatly facilitated awake blind nasal intubation.

In 1926, Arthur Guedel began a series of experiments that led to the introduction of the cuffed tracheal tube. Guedel transformed the basement of his Indianapolis home into a laboratory, where he subjected each step of the preparation and application of his cuffs to a vigorous review.[41] He fashioned cuffs from the rubber of dental dams, condoms, and surgical gloves that were glued onto the outer wall of tubes. Using animal tracheas donated by the family butcher as his model, he considered whether the cuff should be positioned above, below, or at the level of the vocal cords. He recommended that the cuff be positioned just below the vocal cords to seal the airway. Ralph Waters later recommended that cuffs be constructed of two layers of soft rubber cemented together. These detachable cuffs were first manufactured by Waters' children, who sold them to the Foregger Company.

Guedel sought ways to show the safety and utility of the cuffed tube. He first filled the mouth of an anesthetized and intubated patient with water and showed that the cuff sealed the airway. Even though this exhibition was successful, he searched for a more dramatic technique to capture the attention of those unfamiliar with the advantages of intubation. He reasoned that if the cuff prevented water from entering the trachea of an intubated patient, it should also prevent an animal from drowning, even if it were submerged under water. To encourage physicians attending a medical convention to use his tracheal techniques, Guedel prepared the first of several "dunked dog" demonstrations (Fig. 1-2). An anesthetized and intubated dog, Guedel's own pet, "Airway," was immersed in an aquarium. After the demonstration was completed, the anesthetic was discontinued before the animal was removed from the water. According to legend, Airway awoke promptly, shook water over the onlookers, saluted a post, then trotted from the hall to the applause of the audience.

After a patient experienced an accidental endobronchial intubation, Ralph Waters reasoned that a very long cuffed tube could be used to isolate the lungs. The dependent lung could be ventilated while the upper lung was being resected.[42] On learning of his friend's success with intentional one-lung anesthesia, Arthur Guedel proposed an important modification for chest surgery, the double-cuffed single-lumen tube, which was introduced by Emery Rovenstine. These tubes were easily positioned, an advantage over bronchial blockers that had to be inserted by a skilled bronchoscopist. In 1953, single-lumen tubes were supplanted by double-lumen endobronchial tubes. The double-lumen tube currently most popular was designed by Frank Robertshaw of Manchester, England, and is prepared in both right- and left-sided versions. Robertshaw tubes were first manufactured from mineralized red rubber but are now made of extruded plastic, a technique refined by David Sheridan. Sheridan was also the first person to embed centimeter markings along the side of tracheal

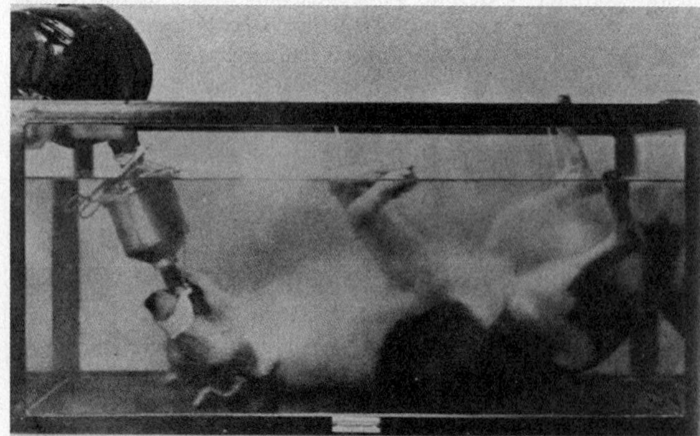

Figure 1-2 The "dunked dog."

tubes, a safety feature that reduced the risk of the tubes being incorrectly positioned.

Advanced Airway Devices

Conventional laryngoscopes proved inadequate for patients with "difficult airways." A few clinicians credit harrowing intubating experiences as the incentive for invention. In 1928, a rigid bronchoscope was specifically designed for examination of the large airways. Rigid bronchoscopes were refined and used by pulmonologists. Although it was known in 1870 that a thread of glass could transmit light along its length, technologic limitations were not overcome until 1964, when Shigeto Ikeda developed the first flexible fiberoptic bronchoscope. Fiberoptic-assisted tracheal intubation has become a common approach in the management of patients with difficult airways having surgery. The image of the airway can be viewed by looking directly through the scope or by being displayed on a screen.

Roger Bullard desired a device to simultaneously examine the larynx and intubate the vocal cords. He had been frustrated by failed attempts to visualize the larynx of a patient with Pierre Robin syndrome. In response, he developed the Bullard laryngoscope, whose fiberoptic bundles lie beside a curved blade. Similarly, the Wu-scope was designed by Tzu-Lang Wu in 1994 to combine and facilitate visualization and intubation of the trachea in patients with difficult airways.[43]

Dr A. I. J. "Archie" Brain first recognized the principle of the *laryngeal mask airway* (LMA) in 1981 when, like many British clinicians, he provided dental anesthesia via a Goldman nasal mask. However, unlike any before him, he realized that just as the dental mask could be fitted closely about the nose, a comparable mask attached to a wide-bore tube might be positioned around the larynx. He not only conceived of this radical departure in airway management, which he first described in 1983,[44] but also spent years in single-handedly fabricating and testing several incremental modifications. Scores of Brain's prototypes are displayed in the Royal Berkshire Hospital, Reading, England, where they provide a detailed record of the evolution of the LMA. He fabricated his first models from Magill tubes and Goldman masks, then refined their shape by performing postmortem studies of the hypopharynx to determine the form of cuff that would be most functional. Before silicone rubber was selected, Brain had even mastered the technique of forming masks from liquid latex. Every detail of the LMA, the number and position of the aperture bars and the shape and the size of the masks, required repeated modification.[45]

Early Anesthesia Delivery Systems

The transition from ether inhalers and chloroform-soaked handkerchiefs to more sophisticated anesthesia delivery equipment occurred gradually, with incremental advances supplanting older methods. One of the earliest anesthesia apparatus designs was that of John Snow, who had realized the inadequacies of ether inhalers through which patients rebreathed via a mouthpiece. After practicing anesthesia for only 2 weeks, Snow created the first of his series of ingenious ether inhalers.[46] His best-known apparatus featured unidirectional valves within a malleable, well-fitting mask of his own design, which closely resembles the form of a modern face mask. The face piece was connected to the vaporizer by a breathing tube, which Snow deliberately designed to be wider than the human trachea so that even rapid respirations would not be impeded. A metal coil within the vaporizer ensured that the patient's inspired breath was drawn over a large surface area to promote the uptake of ether. The device also incorporated a warm water bath to maintain the volatility of the agent (Fig. 1-3). Snow did not attempt to capitalize on his creativity, in contrast to William Morton; he closed his account of its preparation with the generous observation, "There is no restriction respecting the making of it."[47]

Joseph Clover, another British physician, was the first anaesthetist to administer chloroform in known concentrations through the "Clover bag." He obtained a 4.5% concentration of chloroform in air by pumping a measured volume of air with a bellows through a warmed evaporating vessel containing a known volume of liquid chloroform.[48] Although it was realized that nitrous oxide diluted in air often gave a hypoxic mixture and that the oxygen–nitrous oxide mixture was safer, Chicago surgeon Edmund Andrews complained about the physical limitations of delivering anesthesia to patients in their homes. The large bag was conspicuous and awkward to carry along busy streets. He observed that "In city practice, among the higher classes, however, this is no obstacle as the bag can always be taken in a carriage, without attracting attention."[49] In 1872, Andrews was delighted to report the availability of liquefied nitrous oxide compressed under 750 pounds of pressure, which allowed a supply sufficient for three patients to be carried in a single cylinder.

Critical to increasing patient safety was the development of a machine capable of delivering a calibrated amount of gas and volatile anesthetic. In the late 19th century, demands in dentistry instigated development of the first freestanding anesthesia machines. Three American dentist–entrepreneurs, Samuel S. White,

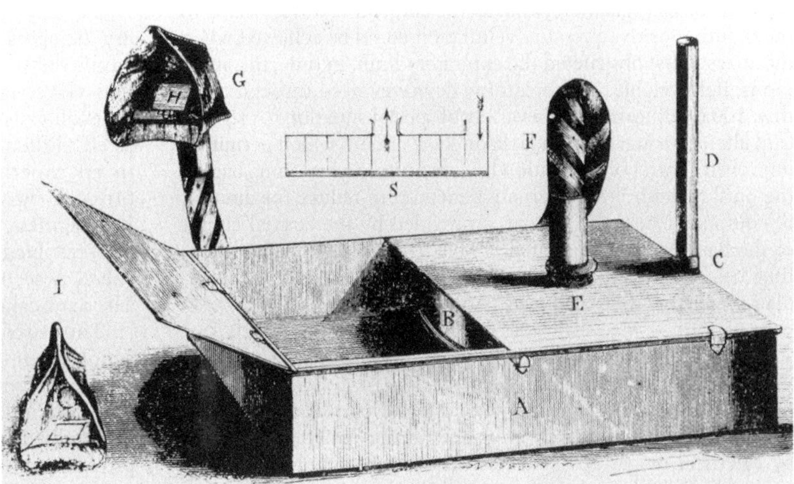

Figure 1-3 John Snow's inhaler (1847). The ether chamber (*B*) contained a spiral coil so that the air entering through the brass tube (*D*) was saturated by ether before ascending the flexible tube (*F*) to the face mask (*G*). The ether chamber rested in a bath of warm water (*A*).

Charles Teter, and Jay Heidbrink, developed the original series of U.S. instruments that used compressed cylinders of nitrous oxide and oxygen. Before 1900, the S. S. White Company modified Frederick Hewitt's apparatus and marketed its continuous-flow machine, which was refined by Teter in 1903. Heidbrink added reducing valves in 1912. In the same year, physicians initiated other important developments. Water-bubble flowmeters, introduced by Frederick Cotton and Walter Boothby of Harvard University, allowed the proportion of gases and their flow rate to be approximated. The Cotton and Boothby apparatus was transformed into a practical portable machine by James Tayloe Gwathmey of New York. The Gwathmey machine caught the attention of London anaesthetist Henry E. G. "Cockie" Boyle, who acknowledged his debt to the American when he incorporated Gwathmey's concepts in the first of the series of "Boyle" machines that were marketed by Coxeter and British Oxygen Corporation. During the same period in Lubeck, Germany, Heinrich Draeger and his son, Bernhaard, adapted compressed gas technology, which they had originally developed for mine rescue equipment, to manufacture ether and chloroform–oxygen machines.

In the years after World War I, several U.S. manufacturers continued to bring forward widely admired anesthesia machines. Richard von Foregger was an engineer who was exceptionally receptive to clinicians' suggestions for additional features for his machines. Elmer McKesson became one of the country's first specialists in anesthesiology in 1910 and developed a series of gas machines. In an era of flammable anesthetics, McKesson carried nitrous oxide anesthesia to its therapeutic limit by performing inductions with 100% nitrous oxide and thereafter adding small volumes of oxygen. If the resultant cyanosis became too profound, McKesson depressed a valve on his machine that flushed a small volume of oxygen into the circuit. Even though his techniques of primary and secondary saturation with nitrous oxide are no longer used, the oxygen flush valve is part of McKesson's legacy.

Alternative Circuits

A valveless device, the Ayre's T-piece, has found wide application in the management of intubated patients. Phillip Ayre practiced anesthesia in England when the limitations of equipment for pediatric patients produced what he described as "a protracted and sanguine battle between surgeon and anaesthetist, with the poor unfortunate baby as the battlefield."[50] In 1937, Ayre introduced his valveless T-piece to reduce the effort of breathing in neurosurgical patients. The T-piece soon became particularly popular for cleft palate repairs, as the surgeon had free access to the mouth. Positive-pressure ventilation could be achieved when the anaesthetist obstructed the expiratory limb. In time, this ingenious, lightweight, nonrebreathing device evolved through more than 100 modifications for a variety of special situations. A significant alteration was Gordon Jackson Rees' circuit, which permitted improved control of ventilation by substituting a breathing bag on the outflow limb.[51] An alternative method to reduce the amount of equipment near the patient is provided by the coaxial circuit of the Bain–Spoerel apparatus.[52] This lightweight tube-within-a-tube has served very well in many circumstances since its Canadian innovators described it in 1972.

Ventilators

Mechanical ventilators are now an integral part of the anesthesia machine. Patients are ventilated during general anesthesia by electrical or gas-powered devices that are simple to control yet sophisticated in their function. The history of mechanical positive-pressure ventilation began with attempts to resuscitate victims of drowning by a bellows attached to a mask or tracheal tube. These experiments found little role in anesthetic care for many years. At the beginning of the 20th century, however, several modalities were explored before intermittent positive-pressure machines evolved.

A series of artificial environments were created in response to the frustration experienced by thoracic surgeons who found that the lung collapsed when they incised the pleura. Between 1900 and 1910, continuous positive- or negative-pressure devices were created to maintain inflation of the lungs of a spontaneously breathing patient once the chest was opened. Brauer (1904) and Murphy (1905) placed the patient's head and neck in a box in which positive pressure was continually maintained. Sauerbruch (1904) created a negative-pressure operating chamber encompassing both the surgical team and the patient's body and from which only the patient's head projected.[53]

In 1907, the first intermittent positive-pressure device, the Draeger "Pulmotor," was developed to rhythmically inflate the lungs. This instrument and later American models such as the E & J Resuscitator were used almost exclusively by firefighters and mine rescue workers. In 1934, a Swedish team developed the "Spiropulsator," which C. Crafoord later modified for use during cyclopropane anesthesia.[54] Its action was controlled by a magnetic control valve called *the flasher,* a type first used to provide intermittent gas flow for the lights of navigational buoys. When Trier Morch, a Danish anesthesiologist, could not obtain a Spiropulsator during World War II, he fabricated the Morch "Respirator," which used a piston pump to rhythmically deliver a fixed volume of gas to the patient.[53]

A major stimulus to the development of ventilators came as a consequence of a devastating epidemic of poliomyelitis that struck Copenhagen in 1952. As scores of patients were admitted, the only effective ventilatory support that could be provided to patients with bulbar paralysis was continuous manual ventilation via tracheostomy employing devices such as Waters' "to-and-fro" circuit. This succeeded only through the dedicated efforts of hundreds of volunteers. The Copenhagen crisis stimulated a broad European interest in the development of portable ventilators in anticipation of another epidemic of poliomyelitis. At this time, the common practice in North American hospitals was to place polio patients with respiratory involvement in "iron lungs," metal cylinders that encased the body below the neck. Inspiration was caused by intermittent negative pressure in the chamber created by an electric motor acting on a piston-like device.

Some early American ventilators were adaptations of respiratory-assist machines originally designed for the delivery of aerosolized drugs for respiratory therapy. Two types employed the Bennett or Bird "flow-sensitive" valves. The Bennett valve was designed during World War II when a team of physiologists at the University of Southern California encountered difficulties in separating inspiration from expiration in an experimental apparatus designed to provide positive-pressure breathing for aviators at high altitudes. An engineer, Ray Bennett, visited their laboratory, observed their problem, and resolved it with a mechanical flow-sensitive automatic valve. A second valving mechanism was later designed by an aeronautical engineer, Forrest Bird.

The use of the Bird and Bennett valves gained anesthetic application when the gas flow from the valve was directed into a rigid plastic jar containing a breathing bag or bellows as part of an anesthesia circuit. These "bag-in-bottle" devices mimicked the action of the clinician's hand as the gas flow compressed the bag, thereby providing positive-pressure inspiration. Passive exhalation was promoted by the descent of a weight on the bag or bellows.

Carbon Dioxide Absorption

Carbon dioxide (CO_2) absorption is a basic element of modern anesthetic machines. It was initially developed to allow rebreathing of gas and minimize loss of flammable gases into the room, thereby reducing the risk of explosion. In current practice, it permits decreased utilization of oxygen and anesthetic, thus reducing cost. The first CO_2 absorber in anesthesia came in 1906 from the work of Franz Kuhn, a German surgeon. Unfortunately, his circuit had significant limitations: exceptionally narrow breathing tubes and a large dead space. Kuhn's device was soon ignored.

A few years later, the first American machine with a CO_2 absorber was independently fabricated by a pharmacologist named Dennis Jackson. In 1915, he developed an early technique of CO_2 absorption that permitted the use of a closed anesthesia circuit. He used solutions of sodium and calcium hydroxide to absorb CO_2. As his laboratory was located in an area of St. Louis, heavily laden with coal smoke, Jackson reported that the apparatus allowed him the first breaths of absolutely fresh air he had ever enjoyed in that city. The complexity of Jackson's apparatus limited its use in hospital practice, but his pioneering work in this field encouraged Ralph Waters to introduce a simpler device using soda lime granules 9 years later. Waters positioned a soda lime canister (Fig. 1-4) between a face mask and an adjacent breathing bag to which was attached the fresh gas flow. As long as the mask was held against the face, only small volumes of fresh gas flow were required and no valves were needed.[55]

Waters' device featured awkward positioning of the canister close to the patient's face. Brian Sword[56] overcame this limitation in 1930 with a freestanding machine with unidirectional valves to create a circle system and an inline CO_2 absorber. James Elam and his coworkers at the Roswell Park Cancer Institute in Buffalo, further refined the CO_2 absorber, increasing the efficiency of CO_2 removal with a minimum of resistance for breathing.[57] Consequently, the circle system introduced by Sword in the 1930s, with a few refinements, became the standard anesthesia circuit in North America.

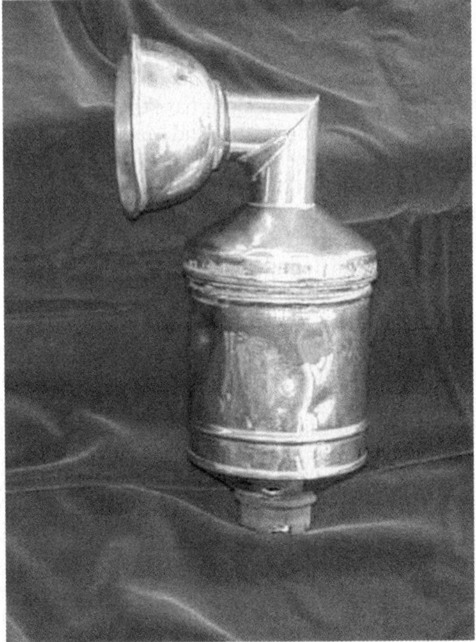

Figure 1-4 Waters' carbon dioxide absorbance.

Flowmeters

As closed and semiclosed circuits became practical, gas flow could be measured with greater accuracy. Bubble flowmeters were replaced with dry bobbins or ball-bearing flowmeters, which, although they did not leak fluids, could cause inaccurate measurements if they adhered to the glass column. In 1910, M. Neu had been the first to apply rotameters in anesthesia for the administration of nitrous oxide and oxygen, but his machine was not a commercial success, perhaps because of the great cost of nitrous oxide in Germany at that time. Rotameters designed for use in German industry were first employed in Britain in 1937 by Richard Salt; but as World War II approached, the English were denied access to these sophisticated flowmeters. After World War II, rotameters became regularly employed in British anesthesia machines, although most American equipment still featured nonrotating floats. The now-universal practice of displaying gas flow in liters per minute was not a customary part of American machines until more than a decade after World War II.

Vaporizers

The art of a smooth induction with a potent anesthetic was a great challenge, particularly if the inspired concentration could not be determined with accuracy. Even the clinical introduction of halothane after 1956 might have been thwarted except for a fortunate coincidence: the prior development of calibrated vaporizers. Two types of calibrated vaporizers designed for other anesthetics had become available in the half-decade before halothane was marketed. The prompt acceptance of halothane was in part because of an ability to provide it in carefully titrated concentrations.

The *Copper Kettle* was the first temperature-compensated, accurate vaporizer. It had been developed by Lucien Morris at the University of Wisconsin in response to Ralph Waters' plan to test chloroform by giving it in controlled concentrations.[58] Morris achieved this goal by passing a metered flow of oxygen through a vaporizer chamber that contained a sintered bronze disk to separate the oxygen into minute bubbles. The gas became fully saturated with anesthetic vapor as it percolated through the liquid. The concentration of the anesthetic inspired by the patient could be calculated by knowing the vapor pressure of the liquid anesthetic, the volume of oxygen flowing through the liquid, and the total volume of gases from all sources entering the anesthesia circuit. Although experimental models of Morris' vaporizer used a water bath to maintain vaporizer temperature stability, the excellent thermal conductivity of copper, especially when the device was attached to a metal anesthetic machine, was substituted in later models.[59] The Copper Kettle (Foregger Company) and the Vernitrol (Ohio Medical Products) were universal vaporizers that could be charged with any anesthetic liquid, and, provided that its vapor pressure and temperature were known, the inspired concentration could be calculated quickly.

When halothane was first marketed in Britain, an effective temperature-compensated, agent-specific vaporizer had recently been placed in clinical use. The TECOTA (TEmperature COmpensated Trichloroethylene Air) vaporizer featured a bimetallic strip composed of brass and a nickel–steel alloy, two metals with different coefficients of expansion. As the anesthetic vapor cooled, the strip bent to move away from the orifice, thereby permitting more fresh gas to enter the vaporizing chamber. This maintained a constant inspired concentration despite changes in temperature and vapor pressure. After their TECOTA vaporizer was accepted into anesthetic practice, the technology was used to create the "Fluotec," (Fluothane was the trade name for halothane) the first of a series of agent-specific "tec" vaporizers for use in the operating room (OR).

Patient Monitors

In many ways, the history of late-19th and early-20th century anesthesiology is the quest for the safest anesthetic. The discovery and widespread use of electrocardiography, pulse oximetry, blood gas analysis, capnography, and neuromuscular blockade monitoring have reduced patient morbidity and mortality and revolutionized anesthesia practice. Although safer machines assured clinicians that appropriate gas mixtures were delivered to the patient, monitors provided an early warning of acute physiologic deterioration before patients suffered irrevocable damage.

Joseph Clover was one of the first clinicians to routinely perform basic hemodynamic monitoring. Clover developed the habit of monitoring his patients' pulses, but, surprisingly, this was a contentious issue at the time. Prominent Scottish surgeons scorned Clover's emphasis on the action of chloroform on the heart. Baron Lister and others preferred that senior medical students give anesthetics and urged them to "strictly carry out certain simple instructions, among which is that of never touching the pulse, in order that their attention may not be distracted from the respiration."[60] In contrast, although attention to respiration was justified, Clover had observed the effect of chloroform on animals and urged other anesthetists to monitor the pulse at all times and to discontinue the anesthetic temporarily if any irregularity or weakness was observed in the strength of the pulse.

Two American surgeons, George W. Crile and Harvey Cushing, developed a strong interest in measuring blood pressure during anesthesia. Both men wrote thorough and detailed examinations of blood pressure monitoring; however, Cushing's contribution is better remembered because he was the first American to apply the Riva Rocci blood pressure cuff, which he saw while visiting Italy. Cushing introduced the concept in 1902 and had blood pressure measurements recorded on anesthesia records.[61] In 1894, Cushing and a fellow student at Harvard Medical School, Charles Codman, initiated a system of recording patients' pulses to assess the course of the anesthetics they administered. In 1902, Cushing continued the practice of monitoring and recording patient blood pressures and pulses. The transition from manual to automated blood pressure devices, which first appeared in 1936 and operate on an oscillometric principle, was gradual but there use now is almost universal.

The first precordial stethoscope, placed on the patient's chest, was believed to have been used by S. Griffith Davis at Johns Hopkins University. He adapted the technique to enable medical students to listen to bruits from cardiac valve lesions created in dogs. Davis' technique was forgotten until rehabilitated by Dr Robert Smith, an energetic pioneer of pediatric anesthesiology in Boston in the 1940s. A Canadian contemporary, Albert Codesmith, of the Hospital for Sick Children, Toronto, became frustrated by the repeated dislodging of the chest piece under the surgical drapes and fabricated his first esophageal stethoscope from urethral catheters and Penrose drains.[62]

Electrocardiography, Pulse Oximetry, and Capnography

Clinical electrocardiography began with Willem Einthoven's application of the string galvanometer in 1903. Within two decades, Thomas Lewis had described its role in the diagnosis of disturbances of cardiac rhythm, whereas James Herrick and Harold Pardee first drew attention to the changes produced by myocardial ischemia. After 1928, cathode ray oscilloscopes were available, but the risk of explosion owing to the presence of flammable anesthetics forestalled the introduction of the electrocardiogram into routine anesthetic practice until after World War II. At that time, the small screen of the heavily shielded "bullet" oscilloscope displayed only 3 seconds of data, but that information was highly prized.

Pulse oximetry, the optical measurement of oxygen saturation in tissues, is one of the more recent additions to the anesthesiologist's array of routine monitors. Although research in this area began in 1932, its first practical application came during World War II. An American physiologist, Glen Millikan, responding to a request from British colleagues in aviation, prepared a series of devices to improve the safety of pilots flying at high altitudes in unpressurized aircraft. To monitor oxygen delivery and to prevent the pilot from succumbing to an unrecognized failure of his oxygen supply, Millikan created an oxygen-sensing monitor worn on the pilot's earlobe and coined the name *oximeter* to describe its action. Refinements of oximetry by a Japanese engineer, Takuo Aoyagi, led to the development of *pulse oximetry*. As John Severinghaus recounted the episode, Aoyagi had attempted to eliminate the changes in a signal caused by pulsatile variations when he realized that this fluctuation could be used to measure both the pulse and oxygen saturation.[63]

Anesthesiologists have recognized a need for breath-by-breath measurement of respiratory and anesthetic gases. The ability to confirm endotracheal intubation and monitor ventilation, as reflected by concentrations of CO_2 in respired gas, began in 1943. At that time, Luft[64] described the principle of infrared absorption by CO_2 and developed an apparatus for measurement. Routine application of capnography in anesthesia practice was pioneered by Smalhout and Kalenda in the Netherlands. Breath-to-breath continuous monitoring and a waveform display of CO_2 levels help anesthesiologists recognize abnormalities in metabolism, ventilation, and circulation. More recently, infrared analysis has been perfected to enable breath-by-breath measurement of anesthetic gases as well. This technology has replaced mass spectrometry, which initially had only industrial applications before Albert Faulconer of the Mayo Clinic first used it to monitor the concentration of an exhaled anesthetic in 1954.

Safety Standards

The introduction of safety features was coordinated by the American National Standards Institute (ANSI) Committee Z79, which was sponsored from 1956 until 1983 by the American Society of Anesthesiologists. Since 1983, representatives from industry, government, and health care professions have met on Committee Z79 of the American Society for Testing and Materials. They establish voluntary goals that may become accepted national standards for the safety of anesthesia equipment. 5

Ralph Tovell voiced the first call for standards during World War II while he was the U.S. Army Consultant in Anesthesiology for Europe. Tovell found that because there were four different dimensions for connectors, tubes, masks, and breathing bags, supplies dispatched to field hospitals might not match their anesthesia machines. As Tovell[65] observed, "When a sudden need for accessory equipment arose, nurses and corpsmen were likely to respond to it by bringing parts that would not fit." Although Tovell's reports did not gain an immediate response, after the war, Vincent Collins and Hamilton Davis took up his concern and formed ANSI Committee Z79. One of the committee's most active members, Leslie Rendell-Baker,[66] wrote an account of the committee's domestic and international achievements. He reported that Tovell encouraged all manufacturers to select the now-uniform orifice of 22 mm for all adult and pediatric face masks and to make every tracheal tube connector 15 mm in diameter. For the first time, a Z79-designed mask-tube elbow adapter would fit every mask and tracheal tube connector.

The Z79 Committee introduced other advances. Tracheal tubes of nontoxic plastic bear a Z79 or IT (implantation tested) mark. The committee also mandated touch identification of the oxygen flow control knob on the anesthesia machine at the suggestion of Roderick Calverley,[67] which reduced the risk that the wrong gas would be selected before internal mechanical controls prevented the selection of a hypoxic mixture. Pin indexing reduced the hazard of attaching a wrong cylinder in the place of oxygen. Diameter indexing of connectors prevented similar errors in high-pressure tubing. For many years, however, errors committed in reassembling hospital oxygen supply lines led to a series of tragedies before polarographic oxygen analyzers were added to the inspiratory limb of the anesthesia circuit.

The History of Anesthetic Agents and Adjuvants

Inhaled Anesthetics

Throughout the second half of the 19th century, other compounds were examined for their anesthetic potential. The pattern of fortuitous discovery that brought nitrous oxide, diethyl ether, and chloroform forward between 1844 and 1847 continued. The next inhaled anesthetics to be used routinely, ethyl chloride and ethylene, were also discovered as a result of unexpected observations. Ethyl chloride and ethylene were first formulated in the 18th century. Ethyl chloride was used as a topical anesthetic and counterirritant; it was so volatile that the skin transiently "froze" after ethyl chloride was sprayed on it. Its rediscovery as an anesthetic came in 1894, when a Swedish dentist named Carlson sprayed ethyl chloride into a patient's mouth to "freeze" a dental abscess. Carlson was surprised to discover that his patient suddenly lost consciousness.

As the mechanisms to deliver drugs were refined, entirely new classes of inhaled medications were also developed. Ethylene gas was the first alternative to ether and chloroform. Its rediscovery also came from a serendipitous observation. After it was learned that ethylene gas had been used to inhibit the opening of carnation buds in Chicago greenhouses, it was speculated that a gas that put flowers to sleep might also have an anesthetic action on humans. Arno Luckhardt was the first to publish a clinical study in February 1923 and within a month, Isabella Herb in Chicago and W. Easson Brown in Toronto presented two other independent studies. Ethylene was not a successful anesthetic because high concentrations were required and it was explosive. An additional significant shortcoming was a particularly unpleasant smell, which could only be partially disguised by the use of oil of orange or a cheap perfume. When cyclopropane was introduced, ethylene was abandoned.

The anesthetic action of cyclopropane was inadvertently discovered in 1929.[68] Brown and Henderson had previously shown that propylene had desirable properties as an anesthetic when freshly prepared, but after storage in a steel cylinder, it deteriorated to create a toxic material that produced nausea and cardiac irregularities in humans. Velyien Henderson, a professor of pharmacology at the University of Toronto, suggested that the toxic product be identified. After a chemist, George Lucas, identified cyclopropane among the chemicals in the tank, he prepared a sample in low concentration with oxygen and administered it to two kittens. The animals fell asleep quietly but quickly recovered unharmed. Rather than being a toxic contaminant, Lucas saw that cyclopropane was a potent anesthetic. After its effects in other animals were studied and cyclopropane proved to be stable after storage, human experimentation began.

Henderson was the first volunteer; Lucas followed. They then arranged a public demonstration in which Frederick Banting, a Nobel laureate for the discovery of insulin, was anesthetized before a group of physicians. Despite this promising beginning, further research was abruptly halted. Several anesthetic deaths in Toronto had been attributed to ethyl chloride, and concern about Canadian clinical trials of cyclopropane prevented human studies from proceeding. Rather than abandoning the study, Henderson encouraged an American friend, Ralph Waters, to use cyclopropane at the University of Wisconsin. The Wisconsin group investigated the drug thoroughly and reported its clinical success in 1934.[69]

In 1930, Chauncey Leake and MeiYu Chen performed successful laboratory trials of Vinethene (divinyl ether) but were thwarted in its further development by a professor of surgery in San Francisco. Ironically, Canadians, who had lost cyclopropane to Wisconsin, learned of Vinethene from Leake and Chen in California and conducted the first human study in 1932 at the University of Alberta. International research collaboration enabled early anesthetic use of both cyclopropane and divinyl ether, advances that may not have occurred independently in either the United States or Canada.

All potent anesthetics of this period were explosive save for chloroform, whose hepatic and cardiac toxicity limited use in America. Anesthetic explosions remained a rare but devastating risk to both anesthesiologist and patient. To reduce the danger of explosion during the incendiary days of World War II, British anaesthetists turned to trichloroethylene. This nonflammable anesthetic found limited application in America, as it decomposed to release phosgene when warmed in the presence of soda lime. Shortly after the end of World War II, however, another class of nonflammable anesthetics, fluorinated hydrocarbons, was prepared for laboratory trials and soon was tested clinically and revolutionized inhalation anesthesia.

Fluorine, the lightest and most reactive halogen, forms exceptionally stable bonds. These bonds, although sometimes created with explosive force, resist separation by chemical or thermal means. For that reason, many early attempts to fluorinate hydrocarbons in a controlled manner were frustrated by the marked chemical activity of fluorine. In 1930, the first commercial application of fluorine chemistry came in the form of the refrigerant, Freon. This was followed by the first attempt to prepare a fluorinated anesthetic by Harold Booth and E. May Bixby in 1932. Although their drug, monochlorodifluoromethane, was devoid of anesthetic action, as were other drugs studied in that decade, their report predicted future developments. "A survey of the properties of 166 known gases suggested that the best possibility of finding a new noncombustible anesthetic gas lay in the field of organic fluoride compounds. Fluorine substitution for other halogens lowers the boiling point, increases stability, and generally decreases toxicity."[70]

A team at the University of Maryland under professor of pharmacology John C. Krantz, Jr, investigated the anesthetic properties of dozens of hydrocarbons over a period of several years, but only one, ethyl vinyl ether, entered clinical use in 1947. Because it was flammable, Krantz requested that it be fluorinated. In response, Julius Shukys prepared several fluorinated analogs. One of these, trifluoroethyl vinyl ether (fluroxene), became the first fluorinated anesthetic. Fluroxene, which was nonflammable in concentrations needed for anesthesia, was marketed from 1954 until 1974. Despite its flammability at high concentrations, it was popular because, unlike halothane, it had favorable respiratory and circulatory depressant properties similar to its "cousin" diethyl ether.

In 1951, Charles Suckling, a British chemist at Imperial Chemical Industries, was asked to create a new anesthetic. Suckling, who already had an expert understanding of fluorination, began by asking clinicians to describe the properties of an ideal anesthetic. He learned from this inquiry that his search must consider several limiting factors, including the volatility, flammability, stability, and potency of the compounds. After 2 years of research and testing, Suckling created halothane. He first determined that halothane possessed anesthetic action by anesthetizing mealworms and houseflies before he forwarded it to pharmacologist James Raventos. Suckling also made accurate predictions as to the concentrations required for anesthesia in higher animals. After Raventos completed a favorable review, halothane was offered to Michael Johnstone, a respected anaesthetist of Manchester, England, who recognized its great advantages over other anesthetics available in 1956. After Johnstone's endorsement, halothane (Fluothane) use spread quickly and widely within the practice of anesthesia.[71]

Halothane was followed in 1960 by methoxyflurane (Penthrane), an anesthetic that remained popular for a decade. By 1970, however, it was learned that dose-related nephrotoxicity following protracted methoxyflurane anesthesia was caused by inorganic fluoride. Similarly, because of persisting concern that rare cases of hepatitis following anesthesia might be a result of a metabolite of halothane, the search for newer inhaled anesthetics focused on the resistance to metabolic degradation.

Two fluorinated liquid anesthetics, enflurane (Ethrane) and its isomer isoflurane (Forane), were results of the search for increased stability. They were synthesized by Ross Terrell in 1963 and 1965, respectively. Because enflurane was easier to create, it preceded isoflurane. Its application was restricted after it was shown to be a marked cardiovascular depressant and to have some convulsant properties. Isoflurane was nearly abandoned because of difficulties in its purification, but after Louise Speers overcame this problem, several successful trials were published in 1971. The release of isoflurane for clinical use was delayed again for more than half a decade by calls for repeated testing in lower animals, owing to an unfounded concern that the drug might be carcinogenic. As a consequence, isoflurane received more thorough testing than any other drug heretofore used in anesthesia. The era when an anesthetic could be introduced following a single fortuitous observation had given way to a cautious program of assessment and reassessment. Remarkably, no anesthetics were introduced into clinical use for another 20 years. Finally, desflurane was released in 1992 and sevoflurane was released in 1994. Xenon, a gas having many properties of the ideal anesthetic, was administered to a few patients in the early 1950s but it never gained popularity because of the extreme costs associated with its removal from air. However, interest in xenon has been renewed now that gas concentrations can be accurately measured when administered at low flows, and devices are available to scavenge and reuse the gas.

Intravenous Anesthetics

Prior to William Harvey's description of a complete and continuous intravascular circuit in *De Motu Cordis* (1628), it was widely held that blood emanated from the heart and was propelled to the periphery where it was consumed. The idea that substances could be injected intravascularly and travel systemically probably originated with Christopher Wren who in 1657, injected aqueous opium into a dog through a goose quill attached to a pig's bladder, rendering the animal "stupefied."[72] Wren similarly injected intravenous *crocus metallorum*, an impure preparation of antimony, and observed the animals to vomit and then die. Knowledge of a circulatory system and intravascular access spurred investigations in other areas, and Wren's contemporary, Richard Lower, performed the first blood transfusions of lamb's blood into dogs and other animals.

In the mid-19th century, equipment necessary for effective intravascular injections was conceived. Vaccination lancets were used in the 1830s to puncture the skin and force morphine paste subcutaneously for analgesia.[73] The hollow needle and hypodermic syringe were developed in the following decades but were not initially designed for intravenous use. In 1845, Dublin surgeon Francis Rynd created the hollow needle for injection of morphine into nerves in the treatment of "neuralgias." Similarly, Charles Gabriel Pravaz designed the first functional syringe in 1853 for perineural injections. Alexander Wood, however, is generally credited with perfecting the hypodermic glass syringe. In 1855, Wood published an article on the injection of opiates into painful spots by the use of hollow needle and his glass syringe.[74]

In 1872, Pierre Oré of France performed what is perhaps the first successful intravenous surgical anesthesia by injecting chloral hydrate immediately prior to incision. His 1875 publication describes its use in 36 patients, but several postoperative deaths lent little to recommend this method to other practitioners.[75] In 1909, Ludwig Burkhardt produced surgical anesthesia by intravenous injections of chloroform and ether in Germany. Seven years later, Elisabeth Bredenfeld of Switzerland reported the use of intravenous morphine and scopolamine. The trials failed to show an improvement over inhaled anesthetics. Intravenous anesthesia found little application or popularity, primarily because of a lack of suitable drugs. But, in the following decades, this would change.

The first barbiturate, barbital, was synthesized in 1903 by Fischer and von Mering. Phenobarbital and all other successors of barbital had very protracted action and found little use in anesthesia. After 1929, oral pentobarbital was used as a sedative before surgery, but when it was given in anesthetic concentrations, long periods of unconsciousness followed. The first short-acting oxybarbiturate was hexobarbital (Evipal), available clinically in 1932. Hexobarbital was enthusiastically received by the anesthesia communities in Europe and North America because its abbreviated induction time was unrivaled by any other technique. A London anaesthetist, Ronald Jarman, found that it had a dramatic advantage over inhalation inductions for minor procedures. Jarman instructed his patients to raise one arm while he injected hexobarbital into a vein of the opposite forearm. When the upraised arm fell, indicating the onset of hypnosis, the surgeon could begin. Patients were also amazed in that many awoke unable to believe they had been anesthetized.[76]

Even though the prompt action of hexobarbital had a dramatic effect on the conduct of anesthesia, it was soon replaced by two thiobarbiturates. In 1932, Donalee Tabern and Ernest H. Volwiler of the Abbott Company synthesized thiopental (Pentothal) and thiamylal (Surital). The sulfated barbiturates proved to be more satisfactory, potent, and rapid acting than were their oxybarbiturate analogs. Thiopental was first administered to a patient at the University of Wisconsin in March 1934, but the successful introduction of thiopental into clinical practice followed a thorough investigation conducted by John Lundy and his colleagues at the Mayo Clinic in June 1934.

When first introduced, thiopental was often given in repeated increments as the primary anesthetic for protracted procedures. Its hazards were soon appreciated. At first, depression of respiration was monitored by the simple method of observing the motion of a wisp of cotton placed over the nose. Only a few skilled practitioners were prepared to pass a tracheal tube if the patient stopped breathing. Such practitioners realized that thiopental without supplementation did not suppress airway reflexes, and they, therefore, encouraged the prophylactic provision of topical anesthesia of the airway beforehand. The vasodilatory effects of thiobarbiturates were widely appreciated only when thiopental caused cardiovascular collapse in hypovolemic burned civilian and military patients in World War II. In response, fluid replacement was used more aggressively and thiopental administered with greater caution.

In 1962, ketamine (Ketalar) was synthesized by Dr Calvin Stevens at the Parke Davis Laboratories in Ann Arbor, Michigan. One of the cyclohexylamine compounds that includes phencyclidine, ketamine was the only drug of this group that gained clinical utility. The other compounds produced undesirable postanesthetic delirium and psychotomimetic reactions. In 1966, the neologism "dissociative anesthesia" was created by Guenter Corrsen and Edward Domino to describe the trancelike state of profound analgesia produced by ketamine.[77] It was released for use in 1970, and although it remains primarily an agent for anesthetic induction, its analgesic and psychedelic properties are increasingly studied and used for treatment of pain and other purposes.

Etomidate was first described by Paul Janssen and his colleagues in 1964 and originally given the name hypnomidate. Its key advantages, minimal hemodynamic depression and lack of histamine release, account for its ongoing utility in clinical practice. It was released for use in 1974 and despite its drawbacks (pain on injection, myoclonus, postoperative nausea and vomiting (PONV), and inhibition of adrenal steroidogenesis), etomidate is often the drug of choice for anesthetizing hemodynamically unstable patients.

Propofol, or 2,6-diisopropylphenol, was first synthesized by Imperial Chemical Industries and tested clinically in 1977. Investigators found that it produced hypnosis quickly with minimal excitation and that patients awoke promptly once the drug was discontinued. In addition to its excellent induction characteristics, the antiemetic action of propofol made it an agent of choice in patient populations prone to nausea and emesis. Regrettably, Cremophor EL, the solvent with which it was formulated, produced several severe anaphylactic reactions, and it was withdrawn from use. Once propofol was reformulated with egg lecithin, glycerol, and soybean oil, the drug re-entered clinical practice and gained great success. Its popularity in Britain coincided with the introduction of the LMA, and it was soon noted that propofol suppressed pharyngeal reflexes to a degree that permitted the insertion of an LMA without a need for either muscle relaxants or potent inhaled anesthetics.

Local Anesthetics

Centuries after the conquest of Peru, Europeans became aware of the stimulating properties of a local, indigenous plant that the Peruvians called *khoka. Khoka,* which meant *the plant,* quickly became known as *coca* in Europe. In 1860, shortly after the Austrian Carl von Scherzer imported enough coca leaves to allow for analysis, German chemists Albert Niemann and Wilhelm Lossen isolated the main alkaloid and named it *cocaine.* Twenty-five years later, at the recommendation of his friend Sigmund Freud, Carl Koller undertook several animal experiments and then successfully demonstrated the analgesic properties of cocaine applied to the eye in a patient with glaucoma.[78] Unfortunately, nearly simultaneous with the first reports of cocaine use, there were reports of central nervous system and cardiovascular toxicity.[79,80] As the popularity of cocaine grew, so did the frequency of toxic reactions and cocaine addictions.[81] Skepticism about the use of cocaine quickly grew within the medical community, forcing the pharmacologic industry to develop alternative local anesthetics.

In 1898, Alfred Eihorn synthesized nivaquine, the first amino amide local anesthetic.[82] Nirvaquine proved to be an irritant to tissues, and its use was immediately stopped. Returning his attention to the development of amino ester local anesthetics, Eihorn synthesized benzocaine in 1900 and procaine (Novocaine) shortly after in 1905. Amino esters were commonly used for local infiltration and spinal anesthesia despite their low potency and high likelihood to cause allergic reactions. Tetracaine, the last (and probably safest) amino ester local anesthetic developed, proved to be quite useful for many years.

In 1944, Nils Löfgren and Bengt Lundquist developed lidocaine (Xylocaine), an amino amide local anesthetic.[81] Lidocaine gained immediate popularity because of its potency, rapid onset, decreased incidence of allergic reactions, and overall effectiveness for all types of regional anesthetic blocks. Since the introduction of lidocaine, all local anesthetics developed and marketed have been of the amino amide variety.

Because of the increase in lengthy and sophisticated surgical procedures, the development of a long-acting local anesthetic took precedence. From that demand, bupivacaine was introduced in 1965. Synthesized by B. Ekenstam[83] in 1957, bupivacaine was initially discarded after it was found to be highly toxic. By 1980, several years after being introduced to the United States, there were several reports of almost simultaneous seizures *and* cardiovascular collapse following unintended intravascular injection.[84] Shortly after this, as a result of the cardiovascular toxicity associated with bupivacaine and the profound motor block associated with etidocaine, the pharmaceutical industry began searching for a new long-acting alternative. Introduced in 1996, ropivacaine is structurally similar to mepivacaine and bupivacaine.[85] The potential safety of ropivacaine is controversial because ropivacaine is approximately 25% less potent than bupivacaine. Therefore, at equal-potent doses, the margin of safety between ropivacaine and bupivacaine becomes less apparent, although systemic toxicity with ropivacaine may respond more quickly to conventional resuscitation.[86]

Each local anesthetic developed has had its own positive and negative attributes, which is why some are still used today and others have fallen out of favor. The pharmaceutical industry is in the process of developing extended-release local anesthetics using liposomes and microspheres.[86–88]

Opioids

Opioids (historically referred to as *narcotics,* although semantically incorrect—see Chapter 20) remain the analgesic workhorse in anesthesia practice. They are used routinely in the perioperative period, in the management of acute and chronic pain. The availability of short-, medium-, and long-acting opioids, as well as the many routes of administration, gives physicians considerable flexibility in the use of these agents. The analgesic and sedating properties of opium have been known for more than two millennia. Greek and Chinese civilizations harnessed these properties in medical and cultural practices. Opium is derived from the seeds of the poppy (*Papaver somniferum*) and is an amalgam of more than 25 pharmacologic alkaloids. The first alkaloid isolated, morphine, was extracted by Prussian chemist Freidrich A. W. Sertürner in 1803. He named this alkaloid after the Greek god of dreams, Morpheus. Morphine became commonly used as a supplement to inhaled anesthesia and for postoperative pain control during the latter half of the 19th century. Codeine, another alkaloid of opium, was isolated in 1832 by Robiquet, but its relatively weaker analgesic potency and nausea at higher doses limit its role in managing moderate-to-severe perioperative surgical pain.

Meperidine (Demerol) was the first synthetic opioid and was developed in 1939 by two German researchers, Otto Eisleb and O.

Schaumann. Although many pharmacologists are remembered for the introduction of a single drug, one prolific Belgian researcher, Paul Janssen, has since 1953 brought forward more than 70 agents from among 70,000 chemicals created in his laboratory. His products have had profound effects on disciplines as disparate as parasitology and psychiatry. The pace of productive innovation in Janssen's research laboratory is astonishing. Chemical R4263 (fentanyl), synthesized in 1960, was followed only a year later by R4749 (droperidol), and then etomidate in 1964. Innovar, the fixed combination of fentanyl and droperidol, is less popular now but Janssen's phenylpiperidine derivatives, fentanyl, sufentanil, and alfentanil, are staples in the anesthesia pharmacopeia. Remifentanil, an ultrashort-acting opioid introduced by Glaxo Wellcome in 1996, is a departure from other opioids in that it has very rapid onset and equally rapid offset owing to metabolism by nonspecific tissue esterases. Ketorolac (Toradol), a nonsteroidal anti-inflammatory drug (NSAID) approved for use in 1990, was the first parenteral NSAID indicated for postoperative pain. With analgesic potency equivalent to 6 to 8 mg of morphine, Ketorolac provides significant postoperative pain control and has particular use when an opioid-sparing approach is essential. However, its use is limited by side effects.

Muscle Relaxants

Muscle relaxants entered anesthesia practice nearly a century after inhalational anesthetics. Curare, the first known neuromuscular blocking agent, was discovered in South America where natives were using it in hunting and tribal warfare. The curares are alkaloids prepared from plants native to equatorial rain forests. The harmless sap of several species of vines was made lethal (through total muscular paralysis and apnea) but only when injected through the skin by a warrior's arrow blown through a blowpipe. This was an extraordinary triumph introduced by paleopharmacologists in loincloths. Their discovery was more remarkable because it was independently repeated on three separate continents—South America, Africa, and Asia. Moreover, the American Indians knew of the juice of an herb that would counteract the effects of the poison if administered in time.[89]

The earliest clinical use of curare in humans was to ameliorate the tortuous muscle spasms of infectious tetanus. In 1858, New York physician Louis Albert Sayres reported two cases in which he attempted to treat severe tetanus with curare at the Bellevue Hospital. Both his patients died. Similar efforts were undertaken to use muscle relaxants to treat epilepsy, rabies, and choreiform disorders. Treatment of Parkinson-like rigidity and the prevention of trauma from seizure therapy also preceded the use of curare in anesthesia.[90]

Interestingly, curare antagonists were developed well before muscle relaxants were ever used in surgery. In 1900, Jacob Pal, a Viennese physician, recognized that curare could be antagonized by physostigmine. This substance had been isolated from the Calabar bean some 36 years earlier by Scottish pharmacologist Sir T. R. Fraser. Neostigmine methylsulfate was synthesized in 1931 and was significantly more potent in antagonizing the effects of curare.[91]

In 1938, Richard and Ruth Gill returned to New York from South America, bringing with them 11.9 kg of crude curare collected near their Ecuadorian ranch. Their motivation was a mixture of personal and altruistic goals. Some months before, while on an earlier visit to the United States, Richard Gill learned that he had multiple sclerosis. His physician, Dr Walter Freeman, mentioned the possibility that curare might have a therapeutic role in the management of spastic disorders. When the Gills returned to the United States with their supply of crude curare, they encouraged scientists at E. R. Squibb & Co. to take an interest in its unique properties. Squibb soon offered semirefined curare to two groups of American anesthesiologists, who assessed its action but quickly abandoned their studies when it caused total respiratory paralysis in two patients and the death of laboratory animals.

The earliest effective clinical application of curare in medicine occurred in physiatry. After A. R. McIntyre refined a portion of the raw curare in 1939, Abram E. Bennett of Omaha, Nebraska, injected it into children with spastic disorders. Although no persistent benefit could be observed in these patients, he next administered it to patients about to receive metrazol, a precursor to electroconvulsive therapy. Because it eliminated seizure-induced fractures, they termed it a "shock absorber." By 1941, other psychiatrists followed this practice and, when they found that the action of curare was protracted, occasionally used neostigmine as an antidote.

Curare was used initially in surgery by Arthur Lawen in 1912, but the published report was written in German and was ignored for decades. Lawen, a physiologist and physician from Leipzig, used curare in his laboratory before boldly producing abdominal relaxation at a light level of anesthesia in a surgical patient. Lawen's efforts were not appreciated for decades, and although his pioneering work anticipated later clinical application, safe use would have to await the introduction of regular intubation of the trachea and controlled ventilation of the lungs.[92]

Thirty years after Lawen, Harold Griffith, the chief anesthetist of the Montreal Homeopathic Hospital, learned of A. E. Bennett's successful use of curare and resolved to apply it in anesthesia. Because Griffith was already a master of tracheal intubation, he was much better prepared than were most of his contemporaries to attend to potential complications. On January 23, 1942, Griffith and his resident, Enid Johnson, anesthetized and intubated the trachea of a young man before injecting curare early in the course of his appendectomy. Satisfactory abdominal relaxation was obtained, and the surgery proceeded without incident. Griffith and Johnson's report of the successful use of curare in the 25 patients of their series launched a revolution in anesthetic care.[93]

Anesthesiologists who practiced before muscle relaxants recall the anxiety they felt when a premature attempt to intubate the trachea under cyclopropane caused persisting laryngospasm. Before 1942, abdominal relaxation was possible only if the patient tolerated high concentrations of an inhaled anesthetic, which might bring profound respiratory depression and protracted recovery. Curare and the drugs that followed transformed anesthesia profoundly. Because intubation of the trachea could now be taught in a deliberate manner, a neophyte could fail on a first attempt without compromising the safety of the patient. For the first time, abdominal relaxation could be attained when curare was supplemented by light planes of inhaled anesthetics or by a combination of intravenous agents providing "balanced anesthesia." New frontiers opened. Sedated and paralyzed patients could now successfully undergo the major physiologic trespasses of cardiopulmonary bypass, deliberate hypothermia, or long-term respiratory support after surgery.

Credit for successful and safe introduction of curare and d-tubocurarine into anesthesia must in part be given to a Squibb researcher named H. A. Holladay. Crude, unstandardized preparations of curare produced uncertain clinical effects and undesirable side effects related to various impurities. Isolation of d-tubocurarine in 1935 renewed clinical interest, but a method for standardizing "Intocostrin" and its purer derivative, d-tubocurarine, had yet to be devised. In the early 1940s, in part as a result of Griffith and Johnson's successful trials, Squibb embarked on wide-scale production. Holaday developed a reliable, easily reproducible

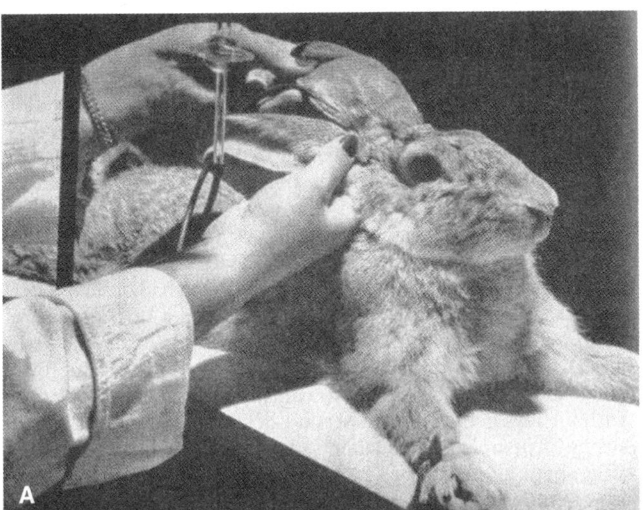

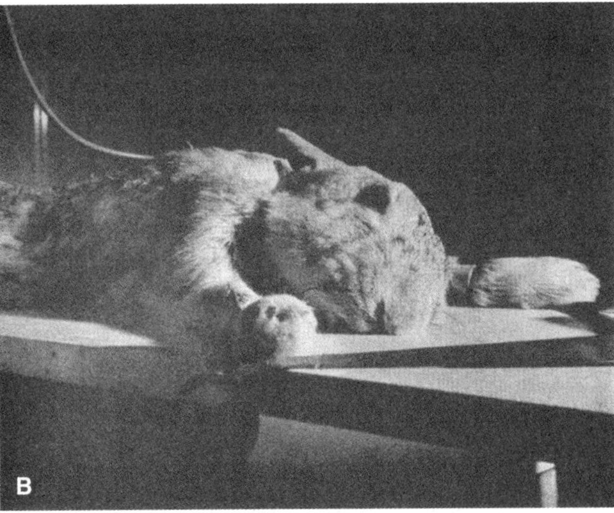

Figure 1-5 The rabbit head-drop assay. H. A. Halladay of Squibb pharmaceutical company developed a method of standardizing doses of curare and d-tubocurarine. A normal rabbit (**A**) had 0.1 mL of aqueous cecurane solution injected every 15 seconds until it could no longer raise its head (**B**).

method for standardizing curare doses that became known as the rabbit head-drop assay (Fig. 1-5). The assay consisted of aqueous curare solution injected intravenously in 0.1-mL doses every 15 seconds until the end point, when the rabbit became unable to raise its head, was reached.[94]

Successful clinical use of curare led to the introduction of other muscle relaxants. By 1948, gallamine and decamethonium had been synthesized. Succinylcholine was prepared by the Nobel laureate Daniel Bovet in 1949 and was in wide international use before historians noted that the drug had been synthesized and tested long beforehand. In 1906, Reid Hunt and R. Taveaux prepared succinylcholine among a series of choline esters, which they had injected into rabbits to observe their cardiac effects. If their rabbits had not been previously paralyzed with curare, the depolarizing action of succinylcholine might have been recognized decades earlier.

The ability to monitor intraoperative neuromuscular blockade with nerve stimulators began in 1958. Working at St. Thomas' Hospital in London, T. H. Christie and H. Churchill-Davidson developed a method for monitoring peripheral neuromuscular blockade during anesthesia. It was not until 1970, however, that H. H. Ali et al.[95] devised the technique of delivering four supramaximal impulses delivered at 2 Hz (0.5 seconds apart), or a "train of four," as a method of quantifying the degree of residual neuromuscular blockade.

Research in relaxants was rekindled in 1960 when researchers became aware of the action of maloetine, a relaxant from the Congo basin. It was remarkable in that it had a steroidal nucleus. Investigations of maloetine led to pancuronium in 1968. In the 1970s and 1980s, research shifted toward identification of specific receptor biochemistry and development of receptor-specific drugs. From these isoquinolines, four related products emerged: vecuronium, pipecuronium, rocuronium, and rapacuronium. Rapacuronium, released in the early 1990s, was withdrawn from clinical use after several cases of intractable bronchospasm led to brain damage or death. Four clinical products based on the steroid parent drug d-tubocurarine (atracurium, mivacurium, doxacurium, and *cis*-atracurium) also made it to clinical use. Recognition that atracurium and *cis*-atracurium undergo spontaneous degradation by Hoffmann elimination has defined a role for these muscle relaxants in patients with liver and renal insufficiency.

Antiemetics

Effective treatment for PONV evolved relatively recently and has been driven by incentives to limit hospitalization expenses and improve patient satisfaction. But PONV is an old problem for which late-19th century practitioners recognized many causes including anxiety, severe pain, sudden changes in blood pressure, ileus, ingestion of blood, and the residual effects of opioids and inhalational anesthetics. Risk of pulmonary aspiration of gastric contents and subsequent death from asphyxia or aspiration pneumonia was a feared consequence of anesthesia, especially preceding use of cuffed endotracheal tubes. Vomiting and aspiration during anesthesia led to the practice of maintaining an empty stomach preoperatively, a policy that continues today despite evidence that clear fluids up to 3 hours before surgery do not increase gastric volumes, change gastric pH, or increase the risk of aspiration.

A variety of treatments for nausea and vomiting were proposed by early anesthetists. James Gwathemy's 1914 publication, *Anesthesia*, commented that British surgeons customarily gave tincture of iodine in a teaspoonful of water every half hour for three or four doses. Inhalation of vinegar fumes and rectal injection of 30 to 40 drops of tincture of opium with 60 grains of sodium bromide were also thought to quiet the vomiting center.[96] Other practitioners attempted olfactory control by placing a piece of gauze moistened with essence of orange or an aromatic oil on the upper lip of the patient.[97] A 1937 anesthesia textbook encouraged treatment of PONV with lateral positioning, "iced soda water, strong black coffee, and chloretone (a mixture of chloroform and acetone)." Counterirritation, such as mustard leaf on the epigastrium, was also believed useful in limiting emesis.[98] As late as 1951, anesthesia texts recommended oxygen administration, whiffs of ammonia spirits, and control of blood pressure and positioning.[99] The complex central mechanisms of nausea and vomiting were largely unaffected by most of these treatments. Newer drugs capable of intervening at specific pathways were needed. As more short-acting anesthetics were developed, the problem received sharper focus in awake postoperative patients in the recovery room. The nausea accompanying use of newer chemotherapy agents provided additional impetus to the development of antiemetic medications.

In 1955, a nonrandomized study of patients demonstrated that the antihistamine cyclizine significantly reduced PONV. The following year, a more rigorous study by Knapp and Beecher reported a significant benefit from prophylaxis with the neuroleptic chlorpromazine. In 1957, promethazine (Phenergan) and chlorpromazine were both found to reduce PONV when used prophylactically. Thirteen years later, a double-blind study evaluating metoclopramide was published, and that drug became a first-line drug in the management of PONV. Droperidol, released in the early 1960s, became widely used until 2001, when concerns regarding prolongation of QT intervals prompted a warning from the Food and Drug Administration about its continued use.

The antiemetic effects of corticosteroids were first recognized by oncologists treating intracranial edema from tumors.[100] Subsequent studies have borne out the antiemetic properties of this class of drugs in treating PONV. Recognition of the serotonin 5-HT3 pathway in PONV has led to a unique class of drugs devoted only to addressing this particular problem. Ondansetron, the first representative of this drug class, was approved by the Food and Drug Administration in 1991. Additional serotonin 5-HT3 antagonists have been approved and are available today.

Anesthesia Subspecialties

Regional Anesthesia

As described above, cocaine, was the first effective local anesthetic. It was noted that cocaine provided topical anesthesia and even produced local insensibility when injected, but Carl Koller, a Viennese surgical intern, first recognized the utility of cocaine in clinical practice. In 1884, Koller was completing his medical training at a time when many operations on the eye were performed without general anesthesia. Almost four decades after the discovery of ether, general anesthesia by mask still had limitations for ophthalmic surgery: lack of patient cooperation, interference of the anesthesia apparatus with surgical access, and a high incidence of PONV. At that time, because fine sutures were not available and surgical incisions of the eye were not closed, postoperative vomiting threatened the extrusion of the globe's contents, putting the patient at risk for irrevocable blindness.[101]

While a medical student, Koller had worked in a Viennese laboratory in a search of a topical ophthalmic anesthetic to overcome the limitations of general anesthesia. Unfortunately, the suspensions of morphine, chloral hydrate, and other drugs that he had used had been ineffectual. In 1884, Koller's friend, Sigmund Freud, became interested in the cerebral-stimulating effects of cocaine and gave him a small sample in an envelope, which he placed in his pocket. When the envelope leaked, a few grains of cocaine stuck to Koller's finger and he absentmindedly licked it
6 with his tongue. When his tongue became numb, Koller instantly realized that he had found the object of his search. In his laboratory, he made a suspension of cocaine crystals that he and a laboratory associate tested in the eyes of a frog, a rabbit, and a dog. Satisfied with the anesthetic effects seen in the animal models, Koller dropped the solution onto his own cornea. To his amazement, his eyes were insensitive to the touch of a pin.[102] As an intern, Carl Koller could not afford to attend the Congress of German Ophthalmologists in Heidelberg. So on September 15, 1884, a friend presented his findings at the meeting, and a revolution in ophthalmic surgery and other surgical disciplines began. Within the next year, more than 100 articles supporting the use of cocaine appeared in European and American medical journals. In 1888, Koller immigrated to New York, where he practiced ophthalmology for the remainder of his career.

The first reports of the subcutaneous injection of cocaine were published in December 1884 by two young surgeons, William Halsted and Richard Hall, who described blocks of the sensory nerves of the face and arm. Halsted[103] even performed a brachial plexus block but did so under direct vision while the patient received an inhaled anesthetic. Unfortunately, self-experimentation with cocaine was hazardous, as both surgeons became addicted.[104] Addiction was an ill-understood but frequent problem in the late 19th century, especially when cocaine and morphine were present in many patent medicines and folk remedies.

Other regional anesthetic techniques were attempted before the end of the 19th century. The term *spinal anesthesia* was coined in 1885 by Leonard Corning, a neurologist who had observed Hall and Halsted. After first assessing its action in a dog, producing a blockade of rapid onset that was confined to the animal's rear legs, Corning performed a neuraxial block using cocaine on a man "addicted to masturbation." Corning administered one dose without effect, then after a second dose, the patient's legs "felt sleepy." The man had impaired sensibility in his lower extremity after about 20 minutes and left Corning's office "none the worse for the experience."[105] Although Corning did not describe escape of cerebrospinal fluid (CSF) in either case, it is likely that the dog had a spinal anesthetic and that the man had an epidural anesthetic. No therapeutic benefit was described, but Corning closed his account and his attention to the subject by suggesting that cocainization might in time be "a substitute for etherization in genitourinary or other branches of surgery."[106]

Two other authors, August Bier and Theodor Tuffier, described authentic spinal anesthesia, with mention of CSF, injection of cocaine, and an appropriately short onset of action. In a comparative review of the original articles by Bier, Tuffier, and Corning, it was concluded that Corning's injection was extradural, and Bier merited the credit for introducing spinal anesthesia.[107]

Fourteen years passed before spinal anesthesia was performed for surgery. In the interval, Heinrich Quincke of Kiel, Germany, had described his technique of lumbar puncture. He offered the valuable observation that it was most safely performed at the level of the third or fourth lumbar interspace because entry at that level was below the termination of the spinal cord. Quincke's technique was used in Kiel for the first deliberate cocainization of the spinal cord in 1899 by his surgical colleague, August Bier. Six patients received small doses of cocaine intrathecally, but because some cried out during surgery and others vomited and experienced headaches, Bier considered it necessary to conduct further experiments before continuing this technique for surgery.

Professor Bier permitted his assistant, Dr Hildebrandt, to perform a lumbar puncture, but after the needle penetrated the dura, Hildebrandt could not fit the syringe to the needle, and a large volume of the professor's spinal fluid escaped. They were at the point of abandoning the study when Hildebrandt volunteered to be the subject of a second attempt. Their persistence was rewarded with an astonishing success. Twenty-three minutes after the spinal injection, Bier noted: "A strong blow with an iron hammer against the tibia was not felt as pain. After 25 minutes: Strong pressure and pulling on a testicle were not painful."[97] They celebrated their success with wine and cigars. That night, both developed violent headaches, which they attributed at first to their celebration. Bier's headache was relieved after 9 days of bed rest. Hildebrandt, as a house officer, did not have the luxury of continued rest. Bier postulated that their headaches were a result of the loss of large volumes of CSF and urged that this be avoided if possible. The high incidence of complications following lumbar puncture with wide-bore needles and the toxic reactions attributed to cocaine explain his later loss of interest in spinal anesthesia.[108]

Surgeons in several other countries soon practiced spinal anesthesia, and progress occurred by many small contributions to the technique. Theodor Tuffier published the first series of 125 spinal anesthetics from France and later counseled that the solution should not be injected before CSF was seen. The first American report was by Rudolph Matas of New Orleans, whose first patient developed postanesthetic meningismus, a frequent complication that was overcome in part by the use of hermetically sealed sterile solutions recommended by E. W. Lee of Philadelphia and sterile gloves as advocated by Halsted. During 1899, Dudley Tait and Guidlo Caglieri of San Francisco performed experimental studies in animals and therapeutic spinals for orthopedic patients. They encouraged the use of fine needles to lessen the escape of CSF and urged that the skin and deeper tissues be infiltrated beforehand with local anesthesia.[109] This had been suggested earlier by William Halsted and the foremost advocate of infiltration anesthesia, Carl Ludwig Schleich of Berlin. An early American specialist in anesthesia, Ormond Goldan, published an anesthesia record appropriate for recording the course of "intraspinal cocainization" in 1900. In the same year, Heinrich Braun learned of a newly described extract of the adrenal gland, epinephrine, which he used to prolong the action of local anesthetics with great success. Braun developed several new nerve blocks, coined the term *conduction anesthesia,* and is remembered by European writers as the "father of conduction anesthesia." Braun was the first person to use procaine, which, along with stovaine, was one of the first synthetic local anesthetics produced to reduce the toxicity of cocaine.

Before 1907, anesthesiologists were sometimes disappointed to observe that their spinal anesthetics were incomplete. Most believed that the drug spread solely by local diffusion before the property of baricity was investigated by Arthur Barker, a London surgeon.[110] Barker constructed a glass tube shaped to follow the curves of the human spine and used it to demonstrate the limited spread of colored solutions that he had injected through a T-piece in the lumbar region. Barker applied this observation to use solutions of stovaine made hyperbaric by the addition of 5% glucose, which worked in a more predictable fashion. After the injection was complete, Barker placed his patient's head on pillows to contain the anesthetic below the nipple line. Lincoln Sise acknowledged Barker's work in 1935 when he introduced the use of hyperbaric solutions of tetracaine (Pontocaine). John Adriani advanced the concept further in 1946 when he used a hyperbaric solution to produce "saddle block," or perineal anesthesia. Adriani's patients remained seated after injection as the drug descended to the sacral nerves.

Tait, Jonnesco, and other early masters of spinal anesthesia used a cervical approach for thyroidectomy and thoracic procedures, but this radical approach was supplanted in 1928 by the lumbar injection of hypobaric solutions of "light" nupercaine by G. P. Pitkin. Although the use of hypobaric solutions is now limited primarily to patients positioned in the jackknife position, their former use for thoracic procedures demanded skill and precise timing. The enthusiasts of hypobaric anesthesia devised formulas to attempt to predict the time in seconds needed for a warmed solution of hypobaric nupercaine to spread in patients of varying size from its site of injection in the lumbar area to the level of the fourth thoracic dermatome.

The recurring problem of inadequate duration of single-injection spinal anesthesia led a Philadelphia surgeon, William Lemmon, to devise an apparatus for continuous spinal anesthesia in 1940.[111] Lemmon began with the patient in the lateral position. The spinal tap was performed with a malleable silver needle, which was left in position. As the patient was turned supine, the needle was positioned through a hole in the mattress and table. Additional injections of local anesthetic could be performed as required. Malleable silver needles also found a less cumbersome and more common application in 1942 when Waldo Edwards and Robert Hingson encouraged the use of Lemmon's needles for continuous caudal anesthesia in obstetrics. In 1944, Edward Tuohy of the Mayo Clinic introduced two important modifications of the continuous spinal techniques. He developed the now familiar Tuohy needle[112] as a means of improving the ease of passage of lacquered silk ureteral catheters through which he injected incremental doses of local anesthetic.[113]

In 1949, Martinez Curbelo of Havana, Cuba, used Tuohy's needle and a ureteral catheter to perform the first continuous epidural anesthetic. Silk and gum elastic catheters were difficult to sterilize and sometimes caused dural infections before being superseded by disposable plastics. Yet deliberate single-injection peridural anesthesia had been practiced occasionally for decades before continuous techniques brought it greater popularity. At the beginning of the 20th century, two French clinicians experimented independently with caudal anesthesia. Neurologist Jean Athanase Sicard applied the technique for a nonsurgical purpose, the relief of back pain. Fernand Cathelin used caudal anesthesia as a less dangerous alternative to spinal anesthesia for hernia repairs. He also demonstrated that the epidural space terminated in the neck by injecting a solution of India ink into the caudal canal of a dog. The lumbar approach was first used solely for multiple paravertebral nerve blocks before the Pagés–Dogliotti single-injection technique became accepted. Because they worked separately, the technique carries the names of both men. Captain Fidel Pagés prepared an elegant demonstration of segmental single-injection peridural anesthesia in 1921, but died soon after his article appeared in a Spanish military journal.[114] Ten years later, Achille M. Dogliotti of Turin, Italy, wrote a classic study that made the epidural technique well known.[77] Whereas Pagés used a tactile approach to identify the epidural space, Dogliotti identified it by the loss-of-resistance technique.

Surgery on the extremities lent itself to other regional anesthesia techniques. In 1902, Harvey Cushing coined the phrase *regional anesthesia* for his technique of blocking either the brachial or sciatic plexus under direct vision during general anesthesia to reduce anesthesia requirements and provide postoperative pain relief.[64] Fifteen years before his publication, George Crile advanced a similar approach to reduce the stress and shock of surgery. Crile, a dedicated advocate of regional and infiltration techniques during general anesthesia, coined the term *anociassociation.*[115]

An intravenous regional technique with procaine was reported in 1908 by August Bier, the surgeon who had pioneered spinal anesthesia. Bier injected procaine into a vein of the upper limb between two tourniquets. Even though the technique is termed the *Bier block,* it was not used for many decades until it was reintroduced 55 years later by Mackinnon Holmes, who modified the technique by introducing exsanguination before applying a single proximal cuff. Holmes used lidocaine, the very successful amide local anesthetic synthesized in 1943 by Lofgren and Lundquist of Sweden.

Several investigators achieved upper extremity anesthesia by percutaneous injections of the brachial plexus. In 1911, based on his intimate knowledge of the anatomy of the axillary area, Hirschel promoted a "blind" axillary injection. In the same year, Kulenkampff described a supraclavicular approach in which the operator sought out paresthesias of the plexus while keeping the needle at a point superficial to the first rib and the pleura. The risk of pneumothorax with Kulenkampff's approach led Mulley to attempt blocks more proximally by a lateral paravertebral approach, the precursor of what is now popularly known as the *Winnie block* (after Alon Winnie from Chicago).

Heinrich Braun wrote the earliest textbook of local anesthesia, which appeared in its first English translation in 1914. After 1922, Gaston Labat's *Regional Anesthesia* dominated the American market. Labat migrated from France to the Mayo Clinic in Minnesota, where he served briefly before taking a permanent position at the Bellevue Hospital in New York. He formed the first American Society for Regional Anesthesia.[116] After Labat's death, Emery A. Rovenstine was recruited to Bellevue to continue Labat's work, among other responsibilities. Rovenstine created the first American clinic for the treatment of chronic pain, where he and his associates refined techniques of lytic and therapeutic injections and used the American Society of Regional Anesthesia to further the knowledge of pain management across the United States.[117]

7 The development of the multidisciplinary pain clinic was one of the many contributions to anesthesiology made by John J. Bonica, a renowned teacher of regional techniques. During his periods of military, civilian, and university service at the University of Washington, Bonica formulated a series of improvements in the management of patients with chronic pain. His classic text *The Management of Pain* is regarded as a standard of the literature of anesthesia.

Cardiovascular Anesthesia

The earliest attempts to operate on the heart were limited to repairing cardiac wounds. These attempts generally failed until German surgeon Ludwig Rehn repaired a right ventricular stab wound in September 1896.[118] Despite this success, the field was not ready to advance. The taboo of cardiac surgery was summarized by Theodore Billroth when he supposedly said "any surgeon who would attempt an operation on the heart should lose the respect of his colleagues."[119] The resistance to such operations was partly because of fledgling anesthetic medications, lack of adequate monitors, and even a clear understanding of cardiovascular physiology that pervades modern anesthesia practice.

Fortunately, the turn of the 20th century saw many advances in anesthesia practice, blood typing, and transfusion, anticoagulation, and antibiosis as well as surgical instrumentation and technique. Some continued to attempt procedures like closed mitral valvotomy in the midst of these technologic advancements, but outcomes were still very poor with mortality rates exceeding 80%. Many believe that the successful ligation of a 7-year-old girl's patent ductus arteriosus by Robert Gross in 1938 served as the landmark case for modern cardiac surgery. Soon after Gross' achievement, a host of new procedures were developed for repairing congenital cardiac lesions, including the first Blalock-Taussig shunt performed on a 15-month-old "blue baby" in 1944.[73] Although the shunt had been successfully demonstrated in animal models, Austin Lamont, Chief of Anesthesia at Johns Hopkins, was not supportive of the procedure. He emphatically stated "I will not put that child to death" and left the open drop ether-oxygen anesthetic to resident anesthesiologist Merel Harmel.[120] Lamont attended on the second Blalock–Taussig shunt 2 months later. Together, Harmel and Lamont[121] would publish the first article on anesthesia for cardiac surgery in 1946 based on 100 cases with Alfred Blalock and repair of congenital pulmonic stenosis.

Closed cardiac surgery ensued, and anesthesia pioneers like William McQuiston and Kenneth Keown worked side by side with surgeons during procedures like the first aortic-pulmonary anastomosis and the first transmyocardial mitral commissurotomy. Never before had anesthesia providers worked as intimately with surgeons for the patient's welfare. Anesthesiologist and World War II physician Max Samuel Sadove remarked, "the small-arms fire of the anesthesiologist joins the spy system of the lab to back up the surgeon's big artillery in a coordinated attack to conquer disease."[122]

Through the 1930s and 1940s, John Gibbon had been experimenting with several extracorporeal circuit designs and by 1947 was able to successfully place dogs on heart–lung bypass. The first successful use of Gibbon's cardiopulmonary bypass machine in humans in May 1953 was a monumental advance in the surgical treatment of complex cardiac pathology that stimulated international interest in open heart surgery and the specialty of cardiac anesthesia.

Over the next decade, rapid growth and expanded applications of cardiac surgery, including artificial valves and coronary artery bypass grafting, required many more anesthesiologists acquainted with these specialized techniques. In 1967, J. Earl Wynands published one of the first articles on anesthetic management of patients undergoing surgery for coronary artery disease.

As cardiac surgery evolved, so did the perioperative monitoring and care of patients undergoing cardiac surgery. Postoperative mechanical ventilation and surgical intensive care units appeared by the late 1960s. Devices like the left atrial pressure monitor and the intra-aortic balloon pump offered new methods of understanding cardiopulmonary physiology and treating postoperative ventricular failure. Cardiac anesthesiologists were quick to bring the pulmonary artery catheter (PAC) into the OR, permitting more precise hemodynamic monitoring and intervention. Joel Kaplan, already known for using the V_5 lead to monitor for myocardial ischemia and nitroglycerin infusions to treat ischemia, popularized the use of the PAC to detect myocardial ischemia. At Texas Heart Institute, Stephen Slogoff and Arthur Keats demonstrated the negative impact of myocardial ischemia on clinical outcome. By the end of the 1980s, the same duo would reveal that the choice of anesthetic agent had little impact on outcome, challenging the earlier paradigm of "isoflurane steal" proposed by Sebastian Reiz.

Developments like cold potassium cardioplegia, monitoring and reversal of heparin, and reduction of blood loss with aprotinin would change the practice of cardiac anesthesia. Transesophageal echocardiography, introduced into cardiac surgery by Roizen, Cahalan, and Kremer in the 1980s, helped to further define the subspecialty of cardiac anesthesia.

Pediatric Anesthesia

Wells and Snow documented pediatric cases where they administered ether or chloroform for surgical anesthesia in the United States and Europe.[18,123] Though some pediatric patients underwent anesthesia, 19th century practice was a far cry from the specialized care of modern pediatric anesthesiologists.

In the years surrounding the World Wars, a handful of physicians pursued anesthetic considerations for pediatric patients. In 1923, C. Langton Hewer wrote the first textbook dedicated to pediatric practice.[124] The content included the use of inhalational agents employing equipment designed for adults, reflecting that Hewer's practice was not limited to pediatrics. Charles H. Robson became the earliest anesthesiologist to dedicate his clinical practice to pediatrics as the Chief Anesthetist at Toronto's Hospital for Sick Children in 1919. Robson recognized children as more than small adults and advocated for properly sized equipment, pain control for neonates, preoperative anxiolysis, and preoperative fasting.[125] His clinical observations on administering anesthesia to children were accurate despite the limited knowledge of pediatric physiology at the time.

In 1937, Philip Ayre, an honorary anesthetist at Babies Hospital in Newcastle upon Tyne, noted that expiratory valves on the usual "closed circuit" techniques created extra work of breathing in infants which led to respiratory failure. He made a landmark modification to pediatric inhalational technique by creating a connecting piece to supply oxygen between the endotracheal tube and the circuit by "opening the anesthetic circuit to the outside air and discarding both rebreathing bag and exhaling valve."[126] Ayre's T-piece decreased the work of breathing and was perhaps the first documented specialized equipment for pediatric anesthesia.

By the 1940s and 50s, physiologists uncovered substantial differences between infants and adults, providing a foundation for advances in surgery and anesthesia.[127–129] Pediatric anesthesia and surgical specialists emerged who capitalized on this information to push the limits of pediatric surgical care. Their efforts resulted in publications to better guide general anesthesiologists in standard cases and improved anesthetic techniques for treating complex congenital conditions in specialized pediatric hospitals.[130,131]

While leading the pediatric anesthesia division at Children's Memorial Hospital in Montreal, Canada, in the 1940s, M. Digby Leigh and M. Kathleen Belton wrote an influential textbook on pediatric anesthesia published in 1948.[132] Two decades after Hewer's instructional book, Leigh and Belton's work demonstrated significant clinical progress due to an increased variety of anesthetics, the use of neuromuscular blockade, fluid therapy, and intravenous techniques.[133] In addition to significant contributions to the literature, they trained skilled pediatric anesthesiologists like Margery van Deming, who founded the pediatric anesthesia department at the Children's Hospital of Philadelphia (CHOP) and worked alongside pediatric surgeon C. Everett Koop. Deming and Koop would push anesthesia practice forward, pioneering anesthetics for complex surgeries like repair of tracheal esophageal fistula.[134]

Further strides in pediatric anesthesia were made by leaders such as Robert M. Smith at Boston Children's, who described the implications of congenital heart diseases on anesthetics, outlined the physiology, and discussed the anesthetic requirements in these patients.[135–137] Ultimately, he trained over 800 residents and fellows in pediatric anesthesia, beginning in 1953 with his first fellow and future intensive care pioneer, Leonard Bachman.[138]

The first anaesthetist to dedicate his practice solely to pediatrics in the United Kingdom, Gordon Jackson Reese, published the influential paper: "Anaesthesia in the Newborn" in 1950, connecting principles of anesthetic practice directly to neonatal physiology.[51] He also modified Ayre's T-piece setup to monitor spontaneous respiration and adapted the "Liverpool technique" for pediatric patients which consisted of nitrous oxide, muscle relaxants, and positive pressure ventilation.[51]

Collaboration between anesthesiologists and pediatric specialists across children's hospitals sparked significant progress toward specialized units to care for critically ill children outside the OR. Virginia Apgar, director of the division of anesthesia at Babies Hospital in New York City, joined with other pediatric physicians to create a unit designated strictly for neonatal care. She also developed the eponymous APGAR score in 1953 to assess newborn infants' appearance, pulse, grimace, activity, and respiration. This was perhaps one of the broadest contributions of anesthesiology to medicine.[131,139]

The first documented pediatric intensive care unit (PICU) was in the Children's Hospital of Goteburg, Sweden, founded by Goran Haglund.[140] Leonard Bachman and Jack Downes at CHOP pioneered the first PICU In the United States in 1967.[141] While caring for critically ill pediatric patients at the University of California, San Francisco, George Gregory impacted the survival of premature infants suffering from respiratory distress syndrome (RDS) by applying continuous positive airway pressure (CPAP)—a common technique utilized to maintain the upper airway during mask anesthesia in adults.[142]

Neuroanesthesia

Brain surgery is considered by some to be the oldest of the practiced medical arts. Evidence of trephination, a form of neurosurgery in which a hole is drilled or scraped into the skull to access the dura, was discovered in skulls dating back to 6500 BC at a French burial site. Prehistoric brain surgery was also practiced by civilizations in South America, Africa, and Asia.[143]

With the introduction of inhalational anesthesia in the mid-1800s, Scottish surgeon and neurosurgery pioneer Sir William Macewen used this novel practice while performing the first successful craniotomy for tumor removal in 1879. Macewen, well known for introducing the technique of orotracheal intubation, promoted the idea of teaching medical students at Glasgow Royal Infirmary the art of chloroform anesthesia.

Like Macewen, Sir Victor Horsely was a neurosurgeon with an interest in anesthesia. His experiments of how ether, chloroform, and morphine affected intracranial contents led him to conclude that "the agent of choice was chloroform and that morphine had some value because of its cerebral constriction effects."[144] He first published his anesthetic technique for brain surgery in the *British Medical Journal* in 1886.[145] Later, he omitted morphine from his regimen after discovering its tendency to produce respiratory depression.

Meanwhile, Harvard medical student and aspiring neurosurgeon Harvey Cushing developed the first charts to record heart rate, temperature, and respiration during anesthesia. Soon after, he would add blood pressure readings to the record. Cushing was one of the first surgeons to recognize the importance of dedicated, specially trained anesthesia personnel versed in neurosurgery. Charles Frazier,[146] a neurosurgical contemporary of Cushing, also recognized this need, stating that "no [cranial] operation be undertaken unless the services of a skilled anesthetizer are available."

Because ether and chloroform anesthesia had significant drawbacks, beginning in 1918, Cushing and his contemporaries explored the advantages of regional or local anesthesia for intracranial surgery. Part of the motivation driving this change was the increased duration in surgical time. Cushing and colleagues used a "slow" surgical technique for most surgical procedures, where the average duration for cranial operations was 5 hours.[147] In contrast, early neurosurgeons like Horseley and Sir Percy Sargeant could perform similar procedures in less than 90 minutes. Therefore, prolonged patient exposure to chloroform or ether anesthesia was likely to result in increased bleeding, postoperative headache, confusion, and/or vomiting. Cushing and his contemporaries thought the use of local or regional anesthesia lessened the risk of these complications.

After a decade, it was realized that the remote positioning of the anesthetist was troublesome when managing the airway of an awake or lightly sedated patient undergoing cranial surgery with regional anesthesia. Also, endotracheal tubes, although introduced at the beginning of the century, had become popular instruments for securing a patient's airway and providing inhalation anesthesia. Combined, these circumstances led to the rapid resurgence of popularity in general anesthesia for cranial surgery, a trend that would continue to the present day.

Although the introduction of agents like thiopental, curare, and halothane advanced the practice of anesthesiology in general, the development of methods to measure brain electrical activity, cerebral blood flow, and metabolic rate by Kety and Schmidt and intracranial pressure by Lundburg "put neuroanesthesia practice on a scientific foundation and opened doors to neuroanesthesia research."[148] Clinician–scientists like John D. (Jack) Michenfelder, later known as the father of neuroanesthesia, conducted basic science and clinical research on cerebral blood flow and brain function and protection in response to various anesthetic agents and techniques. Many lessons learned during this period of ground-breaking research are still commonly used in modern neuroanesthesia practice.

Obstetric Anesthesia

Social attitudes about pain associated with childbirth began to change in the 1860s, and women started demanding anesthesia for childbirth. Societal pressures were so great that physicians, although unconvinced of the benefits of analgesia, felt obligated to offer this service to their obstetric patients.[149] In 1907, an Austrian physician, Richard von Steinbüchel, used a combination of morphine and scopolamine to produce *dämmerschlaff* or "twilight sleep."[150] Although these two drugs were well known, physicians remained skeptical that twilight sleep was essential to labor and delivery, which unfortunately contrasted with the opinion of most women. This method gained popularity after German obstetricians Carl Gauss and Bernhardt Krönig widely publicized the technique. Numerous advertisements touted the benefits of twilight sleep (analgesia, partial pain relief, and amnesia) as compared to ether and chloroform, which resulted in total unconsciousness.[151] Gauss recognized the narrow therapeutic margin of these medications and gave precise instructions on its use: The first injection (morphine 10 mg and scopolamine) was to be given shortly after active labor began—this was intended to blunt the pain of labor—and subsequent injections consisted of only scopolamine, which was dosed to obliterate the memory of labor. Because of the effects of scopolamine, many patients became disoriented and would scream and thrash about during labor and delivery. Gauss believed that he could minimize this reaction by decreasing the sensory input; therefore, he would put patients in a dark room, cover their eyes with gauze, and insert oil-soaked cotton into their ears. The patients were often confined to a padded bed and restrained with leather straps during the delivery.[152] Over time, the doses of morphine administered seemed to increase, although there were few, if any, reports of adverse neonatal effects. Virginia Apgar's landmark 1953 publication of a system for evaluating newborns (the Apgar Score) helped to demonstrate that there actually was a difference in the neonates of mothers who had general versus regional anesthesia.[153]

The bulk of the interest in twilight sleep appears to have been popular rather than medical and, for a brief period, was intensely followed in the United States.[154] Public enthusiasm for twilight sleep quickly subsided after a prominent advocate of the method died during childbirth. Her physicians claimed her death was not related to complications from the method of twilight sleep that was used.[155]

The first articles describing the obstetric application of spinal, epidural, caudal, paravertebral, parasacral, and pudendal nerve blocks appeared between 1900 and 1930. However, their benefits were underappreciated for many years because the obstetricians seldom used these techniques.[155] Continuous caudal anesthesia was introduced in 1944 by Hingson and Edwards,[156] and spinal anesthesia became popular shortly thereafter. Initially, spinal anesthesia could be administered by inexperienced personnel without monitoring. The combination of inexperienced providers and lack of patient monitoring led to higher rates of morbidity and mortality than those observed for general anesthesia.[157] Therefore, the use of spinal anesthesia was highly discouraged in the 1950s, leading to the "dark ages of obstetric anesthesia" when pain relief in obstetrics was essentially abandoned and women were forced to endure "natural childbirth" to avoid serious anesthesia-related complications.

With an increased understanding of neuraxial anesthesia, involvement by well-trained anesthesiologists, and an appreciation for the physiologic changes during pregnancy, maternal and fetal safety greatly improved. At the onset of the 21st century, anesthesia-related deaths during cesarean sections performed under general anesthesia were reported as being more likely than those performed during neuraxial anesthesia. Thus regional anesthesia became the method of choice.[158] With the availability of safe and effective options for pain relief during labor and delivery, today's focus is on improving the quality of the birth experience for expectant parents.

Transfusion Medicine

Blood transfusion was first attempted in 1667 by the physician to Louis XIV, Jean Baptiste Denis. Denis had learned of Richard Lower's transfusion of lamb's blood into a dog the previous year. Lamb's blood was most frequently used because the donating animal's essential qualities were thought to be transferred to the recipient. Despite this dangerous transspecies transfusion, Denis' first patient got better. His next two patients were not as fortunate, however, and Denis avoided further attempts. Given the poor outcomes of these early blood transfusions, and heated religious controversy regarding the implications of transferring animal-specific qualities across species, blood transfusion in humans was banned for more than 100 years in both France and England beginning in 1670.[73]

In 1900, Karl Landsteiner and Samuel Shattock independently helped lay the scientific basis of all subsequent transfusions by recognizing that blood compatibility was based on different blood groups. Landsteiner, an Austrian physician, originally organized human blood into three groups based on substances present in the red blood cells. The fourth type, AB group, was identified in 1902 by two students, Decastrello and Sturli. On the basis of these findings, Reuben Ottenberg performed the first type-specific blood transfusion in 1907. Transfusion of physiologic solutions occurred in 1831, independently performed by O'Shaughnessy and Lewins in Great Britain. In his letter to *The Lancet,* Lewins described transfusing large volumes of saline solutions into patients with cholera. He reported that he would inject into adults 5 to 10 pounds of saline solution and repeat as needed.[159] Despite its publication in a prominent journal, Lewins' technique was apparently overlooked for decades, and balanced physiologic solution availability would have to await the coming of analytical chemistry.

Professionalism and Anesthesia Practice

Organized Anesthesiology

Physician anesthetists sought to obtain respect among their surgi- 8
cal colleagues by organizing professional societies and improving the quality of training. The first American organization was founded by nine members on October 6, 1905, and called the Long Island Society of Anesthetists with annual dues of $1.00. In 1911, the Long Island Society became the New York Society of Anesthetists. Although the new organization still carried a local title, it drew members from several states and had a membership of 70 physicians in 1915.[160]

One of the most noteworthy figures in the struggle to professionalize anesthesiology was Francis Hoffer McMechan. McMechan had been a practicing anesthesiologist in Cincinnati until 1911, when he suffered a severe first attack of rheumatoid arthritis, which eventually left him confined to a wheelchair and forced his retirement from the OR in 1915. McMechan had been in practice for only 15 years, but he had written 18 clinical articles in this short time. A prolific researcher and writer, McMechan did not permit his crippling disease to sideline his career. Instead of pursuing goals in clinical medicine, he applied his talents to establishing anesthesiology societies.[161]

McMechan supported himself and his devoted wife, Laurette, through editing the *Quarterly Anesthesia Supplement* from 1914 until August 1926. He became editor of the first journal devoted to anesthesia, *Current Researches in Anesthesia and Analgesia,* the precursor of *Anesthesia and Analgesia,* the oldest journal of the specialty. As well as fostering the organization of the International Anesthesia Research Society (IARS) in 1925, McMechan and his wife became overseas ambassadors of American anesthesia. Because Laurette was French, it was understandable that McMechan combined his own ideas about anesthesiology with concepts from abroad.[148]

In 1926, McMechan held the Congress of Anesthetists in a joint conference with the Section on Anaesthetics of the British Medical Association. Subsequently, he traveled throughout Europe, giving lectures and networking with physicians in the field. On his final return to America, he was gravely ill and was confined to bed for 2 years. His hard work and constant travel paid dividends, however: In 1929, the IARS, which McMechan founded in 1922, and which celebrated its 100th anniversary in 2022, had members not only from North America but also from Europe, Japan, India, Argentina, and Brazil.[144] In 1929, McMechan also met a young Australian anesthesiologist, Geoffry Kaye. Kaye became a devoted follower of McMechan, and in the following decades helped establish the Australian Society of Anesthesiologists, and to support the society he created a meeting space, workshop, library, and museum in the first floor of his home.[162]

In the 1930s, McMechan expanded his mission from organizing anesthesiologists to promoting the academic aspects of the specialty. In 1931, work began on what would become the International College of Anesthetists; a body which began to award fellowships in 1935. For the first time, physicians were recognized as specialists in anesthesiology. The College's certification qualifications were universal, and fellows were recognized as specialists in several countries. Although the criteria for certification were not strict, the college was a success in raising the standards of anesthesia practice in many nations.[163]

Academic Anesthesiology

Among the many Americans who promoted the growth of organized anesthesiology, Ralph Waters was unique. His greatest contribution to the specialty was raising its academic standards. After completing his internship in 1913, he entered medical practice in Sioux City, Iowa, where he gradually limited his practice to anesthesia. His personal experience and extensive reading were supplemented by the only postgraduate training available, a 1-month course conducted in Ohio by E. I. McKesson. At that time, the custom of becoming a self-proclaimed specialist in medicine and surgery was common. Waters, who was frustrated by low standards and who would eventually have a great influence on establishing both anesthesia residency training and the formal examination process, recalled that before 1920, "The requirements for specialization in many Midwestern hospitals consisted of the possession of sufficient audacity to attempt a procedure and persuasive power adequate to gain the consent of the patient or his family."[164]

In 1925, Waters relocated to Kansas City with a goal of gaining an academic post at the University of Kansas, but the professor of surgery failed to support his proposal. The larger city did allow him to initiate his freestanding outpatient surgical facility, "The Downtown Surgical Clinic," which featured one of the first post-anesthetic recovery rooms.[155] In 1927, Erwin Schmidt, professor of surgery at the University of Wisconsin's medical school, encouraged Dean Charles Bardeen to recruit Waters to join the faculty in Madison.

In accepting the first American academic position in anesthesia, Waters described four objectives that have been since adopted by many other academic departments. His goals were as follows: "(1) to provide the best possible service to patients of the institution, (2) to teach what is known of the principles of Anesthesiology to all candidates for their medical degree, (3) to help long-term graduate students not only to gain a fundamental knowledge of the subject and to master the art of administration, but also to learn as much as possible of the effective methods of teaching, (4) to accompany these efforts with the encouragement of as much cooperative investigation as is consistent with achieving the first objectives."[154]

Waters' personal and professional qualities impressed talented young men and women who sought residency posts in his department. He encouraged residents to initiate research interests in which they collaborated with two pharmacologists whom Waters had known before arriving in Wisconsin, Arthur Loevenhart and Chauncey Leake, as well as others with whom he became associated in Madison. Clinical concerns were also investigated. As an example, anesthesia records were coded onto punch cards to form a database that was used to analyze departmental activities. Morbidity and mortality meetings, now a requirement of all training programs, also originated in Madison. Members of the department and distinguished visitors from other centers attended these meetings. As a consequence of their critical reviews of the conduct of anesthesia, responsibility for an operative tragedy gradually passed from the patient to the physician. Prior to this, in more casual times, a practitioner could complain, "The patient died because he did not take a good anesthetic." Alternatively, the death might be attributed to a mysterious force such as "status lymphaticus," of which Arthur Guedel, a master of sardonic humor, observed, "Certainly status lymphaticus is at times a great help to the anesthetist. When he has a fatality under anesthesia with no other cleansing explanation he is glad to recognize the condition as an entity."[154]

Another prominent physician in early organized anesthesiology was John Lundy who in 1929, while at the Mayo Clinic organized the Anesthetists' Travel Club whose members were leading American or Canadian teachers of anesthesia. Each year, one member was the host for a group of 20 to 40 anesthesiologists who gathered for a program of informal discussions. There were demonstrations of promising innovations for the OR and laboratory, which were all subjected to what is remembered as a "high-spirited, energetic, critical review."[152] The Travel Club would later be critical in the upcoming battle to form the American Board of Anesthesiology (ABA).

Even during the lean years of the Depression, international guests also visited Waters' department. For Geoffrey Kaye of Australia, Torsten Gordh of Sweden, Robert Macintosh and Michael Nosworthy of England, and scores of others, Waters' department was their "mecca of anesthesia." Ralph Waters trained 60 residents during the 22 years he was the "Chief." From 1937 onward, the alumni, who declared themselves the "Aqualumni" in his honor, returned annually for a professional and social reunion. Thirty-four Aqualumni took academic positions and, of these, 14 became chairpersons of departments of anesthesia. They maintained Waters' professional principles and encouraged teaching careers for many of their own graduates.[165] His enduring legacy was once recognized by the dean who had recruited him in 1927, Charles Bardeen, who observed, "Ralph Waters was the first person the University hired to put people to sleep, but, instead, he awakened a world-wide interest in anesthesia."[166]

Establishing a Society

Waters and Lundy, along with Paul Wood of New York City, had an important role in establishing organized anesthesia and the definition of the specialty (3 Video 1-3). In the heart of the Great Depression, these three physicians realized that anesthesiology needed to have a process to determine who was an anesthetic specialist with American Medical Association (AMA) backing. Using the New York Society of Anesthetists, of which Paul Wood was secretary–treasurer, a new class of members, "Fellows," was created. The Fellows criteria followed established AMA guidelines for specialty certification. However, the AMA wanted a national organization to sponsor a specialty board. The New York Society of Anesthetists changed its name to the American Society of Anesthetists (ASA) in 1936. Combined with the American Society of Regional Anesthesia, whose president was Emery Rovenstine, the ABA was organized as a subordinate board to the American Board of Surgery in 1938. With McMechan's death in 1939, the AMA
9 favored independence for the ABA, and in 1940, independence was granted.[163]

A few years later, the officers of the ASA were challenged by Dr M. J. Seifert, who wrote, "An Anesthetist is a technician and an Anesthesiologist is the specific authority on anesthesia and anesthetics. I cannot understand why you do not term yourselves the American Society of Anesthesiologists." Ralph Waters was declared the first president of the newly named American Society of Anesthesiologists in 1945. In that year, when World War II ended, 739 (37%) of 1977 ASA members were in the armed forces. In the same year, the ASA's first Distinguished Service Award was presented to Paul M. Wood for his tireless service to the specialty, one element of which can be examined today in the extensive archives preserved in the Society's Wood Library-Museum at ASA headquarters, Park Ridge, Illinois.[166]

Conclusions

This overview of the development of anesthesiology is but a brief outline of the innovative, important, interesting, and exciting roles in which anesthesiologists have served in hospitals, clinics, and laboratories. It also outlines the many contributions made by anesthesiologists to advance medicine and the care of patients. Today, the OR and obstetric delivery suite remain the central interest of most anesthesiologists, where the complexities of patient illness, surgical procedures, patient monitoring, and computer technology have increased significantly. Yet, anesthesiologists have also ventured into an expanding list of arenas such as pain clinics, radiology suites, the ICU, outpatient surgery centers, and administrative positions such as heads of perioperative services. Anesthesiologists have played a fundamental role in advancing the specialty of anesthesiology, and the future for the specialty is bright.

For additional information please see 4 Video 1-4 in the eBook bundled with this text.

For further review and interactivities, please see the videos and narrative interactive clinical vignettes (NICVs) accessible in the complimentary eBook bundled with this text. Access instructions are located on the inside front cover.

REFERENCES

1. Joyce H. The journals and letters of Fanny Burney. Clarendon; 1975. As quoted in: Papper EM. Romance, Poetry, and Surgical Sleep. Westport, CT: Greenwood Press; 1995:12.
2. Epitaph to W.T.G. Morton on a Memorial from the Mt. Auburn Cemetery. Cambridge.
3. These Egyptian pictographs are dated approximately 2500 BC. *See Ellis ES: Ancient Anodynes: Primitive Anaesthesia and Allied Conditions*. WM Heinemann Medical Books; 1946:80.
4. Bacon DR. Regional anesthesia and chronic pain therapy: a history. In: Brown DL, ed. *Regional Anesthesia and Analgesia*. WB Saunders; 1996:11.
5. Rutkow I. *Surgery, an Illustrated History*. Mosby; 1993:215.
6. Winter A. *Mesmerized: Powers of Mind in Victorian Britain*. University of Chicago Press; 1998:42.
7. Marmer MJ. Hypnosis in Anesthesiology. Charles C Thomas; 1959:10.
8. Dioscorides. On mandragora. In: *Dioscorides Opera Libra*. Quoted in: Bergman N. The Genesis of Surgical Anesthesia. Wood Library-Museum of Anesthesiology; 1998:11.
9. Dote K. General anesthesia in Japan around 1830. *J Anesth Hist*. 2015;1:88.
10. Dote K. Mafutsutoron. Ehime University School of Medicine; 2016.
11. Dote K, Ikemune K, Desaki Y, Yorozuya T, Makino H. Mafutsuto-Ron: the first anesthesia textbook in the world. bibliographic review and English translation. *J Anesth Hist*. 2015;1(4):102–110.
12. Davy H. *Researches Chemical and Philosophical Chiefly Concerning Nitrous Oxide or Dephlogisticated Nitrous Air, and Its Respiration*. J Johnson; 1800:533.
13. Papper EM. *Romance, Poetry, and Surgical Sleep*. Greenwood Press; 1995.
14. Hickman HH. A letter on suspended animation, containing experiments showing that it may be safely employed during operations on animals, with the view of ascertaining its probable utility in surgical operations on the human subject, addressed to T.A. Knight, Esq. Imprint Ironbridge, W. Smith, 1824.
15. Strickland RA. Ether drinking in Ireland. *Mayo Clin Proc*. 1996;71:1015.
16. Lyman HM. *Artificial Anaesthesia and Anaesthetics*. William Hood; 1881:6.
17. Desai SP, Desai MS, Pandav CS. The discovery of modern anaesthesia-contributions of Davy, Clarke, Long, Wells and Morton. *Indian J Anaesth*. 2007;51(6):472–476.
18. Long CW. An account of the first use of sulphuric ether by inhalation as an anaesthetic in surgical operations. *South Med Surg J*. 1849;5:705.
19. Robinson V. *Victory Over Pain*. Henry Schuman; 1946:91.
20. Smith GB, Hirsch NP. Gardner Quincy Colton: pioneer of nitrous oxide anesthesia. *Anesth Analg*. 1991;72:382.
21. Menczer LF. Horace Wells's "day book A": a transcription and analysis. In: Wolfe RJ, Menczer LF, eds. *IAwaken to Glory*. Boston Medical Library; 1994:112.
22. Greene NM. A consideration of factors in the discovery of anesthesia and their effects on its development. *Anesthesiology*. 1971;35:515–522.
23. Fenster J. *Ether Day*. Harper Collins; 2001:76.
24. Haridas RP, Mifflin JA. Researches regarding the Morton ether inhaler at Massachusetts General Hospital, Boston. *Anesth Analg*. 2013;117(5):1230–1235.
25. Haridas RP. "Gentlemen! This Is no humbug!": did John Collins Warren, M.D., proclaim these words on October 16, 1846, at Massachusetts General Hospital, Boston? *Anesthesiology*. 2016;124:553–560.
26. Haridas RP, Gionfriddo M, Bause GS. Etymology of Letheon: nineteenth-century linguistic effervescence. *Anesthesiology*. 2019;131(6):1210–1222.
27. Haridas RP, Mather LE, Bause GS. William TG. Morton's English patent for etherization: patently pointless? *Anesth Analg*. 2022;134(6):1326–1336.
28. Caton D. *What a Blessing She Had Chloroform*. Yale University Press; 1999:103.
29. Journal of Queen Victoria. In: Strauss MB, ed. *Familiar Medical Quotations*. Little Brown; 1968:17.
30. Eger EI 2nd, Saidman LJ, Brandstater B. Minimum alveolar anesthetic concentration: a standard of anesthetic potency. *Anesthesiology*. 1965;26:756–763.
31. Clover JT. Laryngotomy in chloroform anesthesia. *Br Med J*. 1877;1:132–133.
32. Macewan W. Clinical observations on the introduction of tracheal tubes by the mouth instead of performing tracheotomy or laryngotomy. *Br Med J*. 1880;2(1022):163–165.
33. Matas RI. On the management of acute traumatic pneumothorax. *Ann Surg*. 1899;29:409–434.
34. Thierbach A. Franz Kuhn, his contribution to anaesthesia and emergency medicine. *Resuscitation*. 2001;48(3):193–197.
35. Hirsch NP, Smith GB, Hirsch PO. Alfred Kirstein: pioneer of direct laryngoscopy. *Anaesthesia*. 1986;41:42–45.
36. Burkle CM, Zepeda FA, Bacon DR, Rose SH. A historical perspective on use of the laryngoscope as a tool in anesthesiology. *Anesthesiology*. 2004;100:1003–1006.
37. Miller RA. A new laryngoscope. *Anesthesiology*. 1941;2:317.
38. Macintosh RR. Richard Salt of Oxford, anaesthetic technician extraordinary. *Anaesthesia*. 1976;31:855.
39. McLachlan G. Sir Ivan Magill KCVO, DSc, MB, BCh, BAO, FRCS, FFARCS (Hon), FFARCSI (Hon), DA, (1888-1986). *Ulster Med J*. 2008;77(3):146–152.
40. Condon HA, Gilchrist E. Stanley Rowbotham: twentieth century pioneer anaesthetist. *Anaesthesia*. 1986;41:46–52.
41. Calverley RK. Classical file. *Surv Anesth*. 1984;28:70.
42. Gale JW, Waters RM. Closed endobronchial anesthesia in thoracic surgery: preliminary report. *Curr Res Anesth Analg*. 1932;11:283.
43. Wu TL, Chou HC. A new laryngoscope: the combination intubating device. *Anesthesiology*. 1994;81:1085–1087.

44. Brain AIJ. The laryngeal mask: a new concept in airway management. *Br J Anaesth*. 1983;55: 801–805.
45. Van Zundert TCRV, Briacombe JR, Ferson DZ, Bacon DR, Wilkinson DJ. Archie brain: celebrating 30 years of development in laryngeal mask airways. *Anaesthesia*. 2012;67(12): 1375–1385.
46. Mather LE. Dr Snow killed a bird: the genesis of pharmacokinetics and pharmacodynamics in anaesthesia. *Anaesth Intensive Care*. 2017;45(7):37–44.
47. Snow J. *On the Inhalation of the Vapour of Ether*. J Churchill; 1847:23. Reprinted by the Wood Library-Museum of Anesthesiology.
48. Ball CM. *The Chloroformist*. Melbourne University Press, 2021:113–116,119–120.
49. Andrews E. The oxygen mixture, a new anaesthetic combination. *Chicago Med Exam*. 1868;9:656.
50. Obituary of T. Philip Ayre. *Br Med J*. 1980;280:125.
51. Rees GJ. Anaesthesia in the newborn. *Br Med J*. 1950;2:1419–1422.
52. Bain JA, Spoerel WE. A streamlined anaesthetic system. *Can Anaesth Soc J*. 1972;19:426–435.
53. Mushin WW, Rendell-Baker L. *Thoracic Anaesthesia Past and Present*. Charles C Thomas; 1953:44. Reprinted by the Wood Library-Museum of Anesthesiology, 1991.
54. Shephard DAE. Harvey Cushing and anaesthesia. *Can Anaesth Soc J*. 1965;12:431–442.
55. Waters RM. Clinical scope and utility of carbon dioxide filtration in inhalation anesthesia. *Curr Res Anesth Analg*. 1923;3:20.
56. Sword BC. The closed circle method of administration of gas anesthesia. *Curr Res Anesth Analg*. 1930;9:198.
57. Sands RP Jr, Bacon DR. An inventive mind: The career of James O. Elam, M.D. (1918–1995). *Anesthesiology*. 1998;88:1107–1112.
58. Morris LE. A new vaporizer for liquid anesthetic agents. *Anesthesiology*. 1952;13:587–593.
59. Sands RP Jr, Bacon DR. The copper kettle: a historical perspective. *J Clin Anesth*. 1996;8:528–532.
60. Duncum BM. *The Development of Inhalation Anaesthesia*. Oxford University Press; 1947:540.
61. Cushing H. On the avoidance of shock in major amputations by cocainization of large nerve trunks preliminary to their division: with observations on blood-pressure changes in surgical cases. *Ann Surg*. 1902;36:321–345.
62. Codesmith A. An endo-esophageal stethoscope. *Anesthesiology*. 1954;15:566.
63. Severinghaus JW, Honda Y. Pulse oximetry. *Int Anesthesiol Clin*. 1987;25:205–214.
64. Luft K. Methode der registrieren gas analyse mit hilfe der absorption ultraroten Strahlen ohne spectrale Zerlegung. *Z Tech Phys*. 1943;24:97.
65. Tovell RM. Problems in supply of anesthetic gases in the European Theater of Operations, U.S. Army. *Anesthesiology*. 1947;8:303–311.
66. Rendell-Baker L. History of standards for anesthesia equipment. In: Rupreht J, van Lieburg MJ, Lee JA, Erdmann W, eds. *Anaesthesia: Essays on Its History*. Springer-Verlag; 1985:161.
67. Calverley RK. A safety feature for anaesthesia machines: touch identification of oxygen flow control. *Can Anaesth Soc J*. 1971;18:225–229.
68. Lucas GH. The discovery of cyclopropane. *Anesth Analg*. 1961;40:15–27.
69. Seevers MH, Meek WJ, Rovenstine EA, et al. Cyclopropane study with special reference to gas concentration, respiratory and electrocardiographic changes. *J Pharmacol Exp Ther*. 1934;51:1.
70. Calverley RK. Fluorinated anesthetics. I. The early years. *Surv Anesth*. 1986;29:170.
71. Suckling CW. Some chemical and physical factors in the development of fluothane. *Br J Anaesth*. 1957;29:466–472.
72. Wren PC. *Philosophical Transactions. Vol 1*. Anno; 1665 and 1666.
73. Keys TE. *The History of Surgical Anesthesia*. Dover Publications; 1945:38.
74. Dundee J, Wyant G. *Intravenous Anesthesia*. Churchill Livingstone; 1974:1.
75. Oré PC. *Etudes, cliniques sur l'anesthésie chirurgicale par la methode des injection de choral dans les veines*. JB Balliere et Fils; 1875. As quoted in: Hemelrijck JV, Kissin I. History of intravenous anesthesia. In: White PF, ed. Textbook of Intravenous Anesthesia. Baltimore: Williams & Wilkins; 1997:3.
76. Macintosh RR. Modern anaesthesia, with special reference to the chair of anaesthetics in Oxford. In: Rupreht J, van Lieburg MJ, Lee JA, Erdmann W, eds. *Anaesthesia: Essays on Its History*. Springer-Verlag; 1985:352.
77. Hemelrijck JV, Kissin I. History of intravenous anesthesia. In: White PF, ed. *Textbook of Intravenous Anesthesia*. Williams & Wilkins; 1997:3.
78. Fink BR. Leaves and needles: the introduction of surgical local anesthesia. *Anesthesiology*. 1985;63:77–83.
79. Koller C. Über die Verwendung des Cocain zur Anästhesirung am Auge. *Wien Med Wochenschr*. 1884;34:1276.
80. Calatayud J, González A. History of the development and evolution of local anesthesia since the coca leaf. *Anesthesiology*. 2003;98:1503–1508.
81. Fink BR. History of local anesthesia. In: Cousins MJ, Bridenbaugh PO, eds. *Neural Blockade*. JB Lippincott; 1980:12.
82. Ruetsch YA, Boni T, Borgeat A. From cocaine to ropivacaine: the history of local anesthetic drugs. *Curr Top Med Chem*. 2001;1:175.
83. Ekenstam B, Egnev B, Pettersson G. Local anaesthetics: I. N-alkyl pyrrolidine and N-alkyl piperidine carboxylic acid amides. *Acta Chem Scand*. 1957;11:1183.
84. Albright GA. Cardiac arrest following regional anesthesia with etidocaine or bupivacaine. *Anesthesiology*. 1979;51:285.
85. Aberg G. Toxicological and local anaesthetic effects of optically active isomers of two local anaesthetic compounds. *Acta Pharmacol Toxicol (Copenh)*. 1972;31:273–286.
86. Polley LS, Santos AC. Cardiac arrest following regional anesthesia with ropivacaine: here we go again! *Anesthesiology*. 2003;99:1253–1254.
87. Castillo J, Curley J, Hotz J, et al. Glucocorticoids prolong rat sciatic nerve blockade in vivo from bupivacaine microspheres. *Anesthesiology*. 1996;85:1157–1166.
88. Mowat JJ, Mok MJ, MacLeod BA, Madden TD. Liposomal bupivacaine: extended duration nerve blockade using large unilamellar vesicles that exhibit a proton gradient. *Anesthesiology*. 1996;85:635–643.
89. McIntyre AR. *Curare, Its History, Nature, and Clinical Use*. University of Chicago Press; 1947;6:131.
90. Thomas BK. *Curare: Its History and Usage*. JB Lippincott Company; 1963:90.
91. Rushman GB, Davies NJH, Atkinson RS. *A Short History of Anaesthesia*. Butterworth-Heinemann; 1996:78.
92. Knoefel PK. *Felice Fontana: Life and Works*. Societa de Studi Trentini; 1985:284.
93. Griffith HR, Johnson GE. The use of curare in general anesthesia. *Anesthesiology*. 1942;3:418.
94. McIntyre AR. Historical background, early use and development of muscle relaxants. *Anesthesiology*. 1959;20:409–415.
95. Ali HH, Utting JE, Gray TC. Quantitative assessment of residual antidepolarizing block. II. *Br J Anaesth*. 1971;43:478–485.
96. Gwathmey JT. *Anesthesia*. Appleton and Company; 1914:379.
97. Flagg PJ. *The Art of Anaesthesia*. JB Lippincott Company; 1918:80.
98. Hewer CL. *Recent Advances in Anaesthesia and Analgesia*. P Blakiston's Son & Co. Inc; 1937:237.
99. Collins VJ. *Principles and Practice of Anesthesiology*. Lea & Febiger; 1952:327.
100. Raeder J. History of postoperative nausea and vomiting. *Int Anesthesiol Clin*. 2003;41:1–12.
101. Koller C. Personal reminiscences of the first use of cocaine as local anesthetic in eye surgery. *Curr Res Anesth Analg*. 1928;7:9.
102. Becker HK. Carl Koller and cocaine. *Psychoanal Q*. 1963;32:309–373.
103. Halsted WS. Practical comments on the use and abuse of cocaine; suggested by its invariably successful employment in more than a thousand minor surgical operations. *N Y Med J*. 1885;42:294.
104. Olch PD, William S. Halstead and local anesthesia: contributions and complications. *Anesthesiology*. 1975;42:479–486.
105. Marx GF. The first spinal anesthesia: who deserves the laurels? *Reg Anesth*. 1994;19:429–430.
106. Corning JL. Spinal anaesthesia and local medication of the cord. *N Y Med J*. 1885;42:483.
107. Bier AKG. Experiments in cocainization of the spinal cord, 1899. In: Faulconer A, Keys TE (trans), eds. *Foundations of Anesthesiology*. Charles C Thomas; 1965:854.
108. Goerig M, Agarwal K, Schulte am Esch J. The versatile August Bier (1861-1949), father of spinal anesthesia. *J Clin Anesth*. 2000;12:561–569.
109. Larson MD. Tait and Caglieri. The first spinal anesthetic in America. *Anesthesiology*. 1996; 85:913–919.
110. Lee JA. Arthur Edward James Barker, 1850-1916: British pioneer of regional anaesthesia. *Anaesthesia*. 1979;34:885–891.
111. Lemmon WT. A method for continuous spinal anesthesia: a preliminary report. *Ann Surg*. 1940;111:141–144.
112. Martini JA, Bacon DR, Vasdev GM. Edward Tuohy: the man, his needle, and its place in obstetric anesthesia. *Reg Anesth Pain Med*. 2002;27:520–523.
113. Tuohy EB. Continuous spinal anesthesia: its usefulness and technique involved. *Anesthesiology*. 1944;5:142.
114. Pagés F. Metameric anesthesia, 1921. In: Faulconer A, Keys TE (trans), eds. *Foundations of Anesthesiology*. Charles C Thomas; 1965:927.
115. Crile GW, Lower WE. *Anoci-Association*. WB Saunders Company; 1915.
116. Brown DL, Winnie AP. Biography of Louis Gaston Labat, M.D. *Reg Anesth*. 1992;17:249–262.
117. Bacon DR, Darwish H. Emery A. Rovenstine and regional anesthesia. *Reg Anesth*. 1997; 22:273–279.
118. Rehn L. On penetrating cardiac injuries and cardiac suturing. *Arch Klin Chir*. 1897;55:315.
119. Naef AP. The mid-century revolution in thoracic and cardiovascular surgery: part 1. *Interact Cardiovasc Thorac Surg*. 2003;2:219–226.
120. Baum VC. Pediatric cardiac surgery: an historical appreciation. *Pediatr Anesth*. 2006;16: 1213–1225.
121. Harmel M, Lamont A. Anesthesia in the treatment of congenital pulmonary stenosis. *Anesthesiology*. 1948;7:477–498.
122. With gas & needle. Time. Monday, October 19, 1953.
123. Warde D. Dr. John Snow (1813–1858)- his work with infants and children. *Proceedings of the History of Anesthesia Society*. 2016;49:131–140.
124. Hewer CL. *Anaesthesia in Children*. H.K. Lewis & Co; 1923.
125. Robson CH. Anesthesia in children. *Curr Res Anesth Analg*. 1925;4:235–240.
126. Ayre P. Endotracheal Anesthesia for Babies with Special Reference to Hare-lip and Cleft Palate Operations. *Curr Res Anesth Analg*. 1937;16(6):330–333.
127. Smith CA. *Physiology of the Newborn Infant*. Charles Thomas; 1946.
128. Cross KW. The respiratory rate and ventilation in the newborn baby. *J Physiol*. 1949;109:459.

129. Cook CD, Cherry RB, O'Brien D, Karlberg P, Smith CA. Studies of respiratory physiology in the newborn infant: I. observations on normal premature and full term infants. *J Clin Invest.* 1955;34:975–982.
130. Leigh MD, Belton MK, Lewis GB. Pediatric Anesthesia. *Curr Res Anes Analg.* 1956;35(1):1–17.
131. Smith RM. Some reasons for the high mortality in pediatric anesthesia. *Anesth Analg.* 1957; 36(3):105–112.
132. Leigh MD, Belton MK. *Pediatric Anesthesia.* The Macmillan Company; 1948.
133. Warde, D. Pediatric anaesthesia. *The History of Anesthesia Society Proceedings.* Vol 51:29–47.
134. Zindler M, Van Deming MN. The anesthetic management of infants for the surgical repair of congenital atresia of the esophagus with tracheo-esophageal fistula. *Curr Res Anesth Analg.* 1953;32(3):180–190.
135. Smith RM. Circulatory Factors affecting anesthesia in surgery for congenital heart disease. *Anesthesiology.* 1952;13:38–61.
136. Smith RM, Engineer EH. Problems Related to Open-hearth operations in children: Part 1. *Anesth Analg.* 1960;39(2):104–109.
137. Smith RM, Engineer EH. Problems Related to Open-hearth operations in children: Part 2. *Anesth Analg.* 1960;39(3):262–272.
138. Holzman RS. An appreciation of Robert Moors Smith MD, an icon of pediatric anesthesiology. *Pediatric Anesthesia.* 2010;20:767–770.
139. Calmes SH. Dr. Virginia Apgar and the Apgar score: how the Apgar score came to be. *Anesth Analg.* 2015;120(5):1060–1064.
140. Mai CL, Coté CJ. A history of pediatric anesthesia: a tale of pioneers and equipment. *Paediatr Anaesth.* 2012;22:511–520.
141. Bachman L, Downes JJ, Richards CC, Coyle D, May E. Organization of an intensive care unit in a children's hospital. *Anesth Analg.* 1967;46:570–574.
142. Gregory GA, Kitterman JA, Phibbs RH, Tooley WH, Hamilton WK. Treatment of the idiopathic respiratory-distress syndrome with continuous positive airway pressure. *N Engl J Med.* 1971;284:1333–1340.
143. Tracy PT, Hanigan WC. The history of neuroanesthesia. In: Greenblatt SH, ed. *The History of Neurosurgery.* Thieme; 1997:213.
144. Samuels SI. The history of neuroanesthesia: a contemporary review. *Int Anesthesiol Clin.* 1996;34:1–20.
145. Horsley V. Brain surgery. *Br Med J.* 1886;2:670.
146. Frazier C. Problems and procedures in cranial surgery. *JAMA.* 1909;52:1805.
147. Bacon DR. The World Federation of Societies of Anesthesiologists: McMechan's final legacy? *Anesth Analg.* 1997;84:1130–1135.
148. Seldon TH. Francis Hoeffer McMechan. In: Volpitto PP, Vandam LD, eds. *Genesis of American Anesthesiology.* Charles C Thomas; 1982:5.
149. Canton D. The history of obstetric anesthesia. In: Chestnut DH, ed. *Obstetric Anesthesia: Principles and Practice.* Elsevier Mosby; 2004.
150. Barnett R. A horse named 'Twilight Sleep': the language of obstetric anaesthesia in 20th century Britain. *Int J Obstet Anesth.* 2005;14:310–315.
151. Canton D. *What a Blessing She Had Chloroform.* Yale University Press; 1999.
152. MacKenzie RA, Bacon DR, Martin DP. The Anaesthetists' Travel Club: a transformation of the Society of Clinical Surgery? *Bull Anesth Hist.* 2004;22:7–10.
153. Apgar V. A proposal for a new method of evaluation of the newborn infant. *Curr Res Anesth Analg.* 1953;32:260–267.
154. Guedel AE. *Inhalation Anesthesia: A Fundamental Guide.* Macmillan; 1937:129.
155. Waters RM. The down-town anesthesia clinic. *Am J Surg.* 1919;33:71.
156. Hingson RA. Continuous caudal analgesia in obstetrics, surgery, and therapeutics. *Br Med J.* 1949;2:777–781.
157. Gogarten W, Van Aken H. A century of regional analgesia in obstetrics. *Anesth Analg.* 2000;91:773–775.
158. Hawkins JL. Anesthesia-related maternal mortality. *Clin Obstet Gynecol.* 2003;46: 679–687.
159. Jenkins MT. *Epochs in Intravenous Fluid Therapy: From the Goose Quill and Pig Bladder to Balanced Salt Solutions.* The Lewis H. Wright Memorial Lecture, Wood Library-Museum Collection; 1993:4.
160. Betcher AM, Ciliberti BJ, Wood PM, Wright LH. The jubilee year of organized anesthesia. *Anesthesiology.* 1956;17:226–264.
161. Bacon DR. The promise of one great anesthesia society. The 1939-1940 proposed merger of the American Society of Anesthetists and the International Anesthesia Research Society. *Anesthesiology.* 1994;80:929–935.
162. Edwards ML, Waisel DB. 49 Mathoura Road: Geoffrey Kaye's letters to Paul M. Wood, 1939-1955. *Anesthesiology.* 2014;121:1150–1157.
163. Bacon DR, Lema MJ. To define a specialty: a brief history of the American Board of Anesthesiology's first written examination. *J Clin Anesth.* 1992;4:489–497.
164. Waters RM. Pioneering in anesthesiology. *Postgrad Med.* 1948;4:265–270.
165. Bacon DR, Ament R. Ralph Waters and the beginnings of academic anesthesiology in the United States: the Wisconsin template. *J Clin Anesth.* 1995;7:534–543.
166. Bamforth BJ, Siebecker KL, Ralph M. Waters. In: Volpitto PP, Vandam LD, eds. *Genesis of American Anesthesiology.* Charles C Thomas; 1982.

2 The Practice of Anesthesiology

RAFAEL MAURICIO GONZALEZ • MARK C. NORRIS • KAROLINA BROOK • RUBEN J. AZOCAR

KEY POINTS

1. Organization, self-regulation, and setting standards mark the transition from artisanal to professional practice in any trade. Anesthesiology's journey to full recognition as a medical specialty ended in 1941 when the American Board of Medical Specialties approved the American Board of Anesthesiology as an independent body.
2. The increasing number and variety of subspecialty training programs reflect the growing scope of practice of anesthesiology.
3. The American Society of Anesthesiologists introduced the perioperative surgical home (PSH) concept as a means to achieve the triple aim and value care goals.
4. Well implemented enhanced recovery after surgery (ERAS) protocols are associated with shortened hospital stays, decreased costs and fewer complications. ERAS incorporated into PSH models may yield the best results.
5. Anesthesiologists are well positioned to serve in senior leadership roles even beyond the operating room.
6. Certification by the American Board of Anesthesiology (ABA) demonstrates expertise in our specialty. Graduates are eligible for initial certification upon completion of an accredited residency program and for recertification every 5 years through the ABA MOCA program. The ABA also offers certifications in several subspecialties of anesthesiology.
7. Reimbursement for any patient encounter requires a diagnosis code, a procedure code, with matching anesthesia code, and, for operating room anesthesia, an anesthesia start time, and anesthesia end time.
8. Because of longstanding insufficient reimbursement for anesthesia services by government payers (Medicare and Medicaid) in addition to recent restrictions on balance billing of privately insured patients, many anesthesia groups now rely on hospital subsidies to balance their budgets.
9. Anesthesiology was the first medical specialty to develop a systematic approach to patient safety resulting in a dramatic decrease in anesthesia-related mortality. Consequently, anesthesiologists increasingly focus on decreasing patient morbidity, such as decreasing postoperative wound infection, postoperative cognitive decline, and opioid-related harm.
10. While it is necessary that hospital and department leaders promote psychological safety in their departments, individual clinicians remain key stakeholders in establishing and maintaining a culture of safety.
11. Regulatory agency surveyors closely scrutinize anesthesia departments. Indepth knowledge of, and careful compliance with, federal and state rules and regulations are essential to avoid citations and penalties.
12. A well-organized anesthesia department needs the support of a variety of staff and services to allow clinicians to deliver patient care safely and efficiently.
13. Although difficult to predict with certainty, current trends suggest continued growth in both the supply of and demand for anesthesiologists.
14. Clinicians continue to report high levels of burnout. A multipronged approach is necessary to mitigate burnout and promote physician wellness.
15. A basic understanding of personal finances is essential for all physicians, including debt management, saving for retirement and protecting assets. While a financial advisor may be helpful, it is important to understand their compensation structure as it could influence the advice they provide.

Introduction

A full account of the evolution of anesthesiology as a specialty is beyond the reach of this chapter. However, a review of some of the milestones on this journey will help us understand the many aspects that comprise the specialty today.

Mankind has long strived to relieve surgical pain. Centuries of records document different cultures' attempts to achieve this goal. William T. G. Morton, a dentist, performed the first public demonstration of ether anesthesia at the Massachusetts General Hospital on October 16, 1846.[1] This act would change the course of medicine and surgery. At first, anesthetists were little more than technicians and most advances in the field came from chemists and other scientists.[2] However, the increasing in length and complexity of surgical operations created a need for true anesthesia professionals.

1 Organization, self-regulation, and the setting of standards mark the transition from artisanal to professional practice in any trade. The Long Island Society of Anesthetists was formed in 1905 under the leadership of A. F. Erdmann. As membership grew, the name changed to the New York Society of Anesthetists in 1912. In 1936, the name changed again to the American Society of Anesthetists. The Advisory Board for Medical Specialties approved the American Board of Anesthesiology (ABA) as an affiliate of the American Board of Surgery in 1938. Subsequently, the House of Delegates of the American Medical Association recognized the Section on Anesthesiology in 1940. The Society changed its name one last time to the American Society of Anesthesiologists (ASA) to indicate those formally trained in the administration of anesthesia. In 1941, the American Board of Medical Specialties (ABMS) approved the ABA as an independent body, and Anesthesiology became fully recognized as a medical specialty in the United States.[3]

Dr. Ralph Waters established the first anesthesiology residency at the University of Wisconsin in 1927. Dr. Waters' illustrious alumni went on to found and lead many other U.S. anesthesiology training programs. At first, the number programs grew slowly.[4] World War II dramatically changed this trend and by 1948, there were 214 accredited anesthesia residencies in the United States. The number of U.S. anesthesia residency programs peaked in 1964 at 296 and declined thereafter.[4] However, from 2017 to 2022, the number of programs increased by 22%. As of 2022, there were 159 U.S. anesthesiology residency programs training over 6,000 physicians.[5]

The evolution of anesthesiology into a recognized medical specialty included a struggle for equitable the compensation. In the mid-1950s, Dr. Joseph Falling of California introduced a method for calculating anesthetic fees based on complexity of the procedure, skills required of the anesthesiologist, and the length of the procedure. He called his system the "Anesthetic Value Unit." His method was adopted in 1962 by the ASA and is known today as the "Relative Value Guide." This fee schedule is currently accepted by many component societies, third party payers, and regulatory agencies.[3]

As is the case with other medical specialties, the unfortunate events of war have contributed to the advancement of anesthesiology. Anesthesia made its first appearance in battlefield medicine in the Mexican-American war, shortly after Morton's public demonstration. Although used sparingly at first, providing anesthesia for injured soldiers became steadily more common. Some of the lessons learned in each conflict were forgotten during the interwar periods, only to be relearned and built upon in the next war. World War II saw the first systematic studies of trauma care in the Mediterranean theater. Specialized anesthetists became a necessity as the complexity of surgical care increased, progressing from mainly amputations to wound control, the precursor of what is known now as damage control surgery. Anesthesia providers played a significant role in improving the care of the severely wounded. They observed the effects of anesthetics on the physiology of these patients and began developing a body of knowledge pertaining to the management of hypovolemic shock. Many of the techniques and practices we employ today either appeared or advanced in times of conflict. Some examples include airway management, controlled ventilation, transfusion medicine, the use of intravenous anesthetics, regional anesthesia, triage and transport of trauma victims, and the refinement of anesthesia delivery equipment.[6]

Anesthesiology was the first medical specialty to develop a systematic approach to patient safety. Rapidly changing technology and the perception of high anesthesia-related morbidity and mortality galvanized the specialty. In 1984, Ellison C. Pearce, then President of the ASA, established a standing committee on Patient Safety and Risk Management. One year later, the Anesthesia Patient Safety Foundation (APSF) was born as an independent, multidisciplinary, non-for-profit organization with the vision that "no one shall be harmed by anesthetic care." APSF contributions include a newsletter (the mostly widely read anesthesia publication in the world), research grants, and education on topics like operating room (OR) fire safety and medication safety. Later, the American Medical Association and others launched the National Patient Safety Foundation following the APSF model.[7]

Creating and maintaining a diverse and inclusive workforce is vital to the future of our specialty, but much work remains to be done before we achieve our goals. In 2021, more than half of U.S. medical students were women, but only one-third of U.S. anesthesia residents were female.[8] The gender gap is even greater in academic anesthesia. In 2015, women accounted for about 14% of academic anesthesia chairs and 6.9% of full professors.[9] Physicians who are of Black, Hispanic, or Native American origin also continue to be underrepresented in medicine in general and anesthesiology in particular.[10] The benefits of a diverse workforce have been reported extensively in the business literature and increasingly in medical literature. Diverse teams are not only more productive and innovative, but they also promote wellness and help recruit and retain the best talent. Significant advantages exist when the medical team composition mirrors that of their patient population (concordance). Individual and population health outcomes improve as does access to care. A diverse physician workforce also fosters research focused on conditions that disproportionately affect minorities. A diverse anesthesiology workforce will make us better physicians, educators, and researchers and will help us serve our communities.[11,12]

The Practice of Anesthesiology

The 21st century has seen anesthesia practice expand far beyond 2
its traditional reaches, in both location and the type of patients we serve. This expansion in geography, complexity, and scope has created both opportunities and challenges. The increasing number and variety of subspecialty training programs reflect this growing scope of practice (Table 2-1).[13]

Cardiothoracic and vascular anesthesiologists care for patients undergoing myocardial revascularization, heart valve replacement or repair, the repair of congenital cardiac abnormalities, heart and lung transplantation, implantation of cardiac assist devices, and those requiring extracorporeal membrane oxygenation (ECMO). Their expertise includes anesthetic management for advanced lung surgeries, tracheal procedures, and surgery on the thoracic aorta. These specialists care for patients throughout

Table 2-1 Subspecialty Fellowships in Anesthesiology and Available American Board of Anesthesiology Certification Examinations

Fellowship	ABA Subspecialty Certification
Adult cardiothoracic anesthesiology	Yes
Pediatric cardiac anesthesiology	
Pediatric anesthesiology	Yes
Obstetric anesthesiology	
Anesthesiology critical care medicine	Yes
Pain medicine	Yes
Neuro anesthesia	
Neuro critical care	Yes
Regional anesthesiology and acute pain medicine	
Sleep medicine	Yes
Perioperative medicine	
Hospice and palliative medicine	Yes
Addiction medicine	
Clinical informatics	
Ambulatory anesthesiology	
Trauma anesthesiology	
Liver transplantation anesthesiology	
Global anesthesiology	

their perioperative course. They may offer neuraxial or other advanced regional anesthesia techniques for postoperative pain management and often provide postoperative critical care. They have a thorough understanding of cardiovascular physiology and pathology. They plan and conduct anesthetics that are adapted for both the patient and the surgery. The subspecialty continues to evolve in response to changing surgical techniques, including robotically assisted surgery and endovascular repair of structural cardiac lesions.[14]

Today, cardiothoracic anesthesiologists receive extensive training in the use and interpretation of transesophageal echocardiography (TEE), which has become an essential part of modern cardiac surgery. Cardiac anesthesiologists can become certified in basic or advanced TEE. Basic certification recognizes proficiency in TEE monitoring during the conduct of any anesthetic. Advanced TEE certification requires proficiency in the full diagnostic capabilities of TEE, especially during invasive and interventional cardiac procedures.[15]

Pediatric cardiac anesthesiologists care for children with a wide variety of congenital cardiac anomalies. Pediatric cardiac anesthesiologists have also completed a fellowship in pediatric anesthesiology or adult cardiothoracic anesthesiology. Fellows in pediatric cardiac anesthesiology receive training in postoperative critical care medicine and perioperative echocardiography. They are frequently called upon to care for patients with congenital cardiac diseases undergoing noncardiac procedures.[16]

Children, particularly neonates and infants, are not simply small adults. Even healthy children, have distinct anatomic and physiologic features. Their immature organ systems and metabolic pathways can alter their response to anesthetic and adjuvant medications. Most anesthetic drugs have narrow therapeutic windows and require precise dosing to avoid harming these tiny patients. Differences in airway anatomy and cardiopulmonary physiology make neonates and infants challenging to intubate their tracheas and more likely to develop oxygen desaturation. Some children have unusual congenital malformations or metabolic syndromes. Young children especially may have difficulty comprehending and coping with the surgical experience. Separation from parents, induction, and emergence can trigger crying, struggling, and other disruptive behaviors. The skilled pediatric anesthesiologist adapts and responds to these challenges with a combination of medical knowledge, empathy, and play as they ease little ones safely in and out the anesthetic state.

Obstetric anesthesiology is one of the newest fields in our specialty. The original obstetric anesthetics and analgesics were inhaled vapors, like ether and chloroform and opioids such as meperidine and morphine. Modern neuraxial techniques have proven safer and more effective at both relieving labor pain and providing anesthesia for cesarean delivery. While most anesthesiologists should be able to care for a healthy mother and baby, those with extra training and expertise in obstetric anesthesia are often called upon to care for our increasingly older and sicker pregnant patients.[17] Obstetric anesthesiologists have an important role in addressing the high levels of maternal morbidity and mortality seen in the United States. The American College of Obstetrics and Gynecology has issued a consensus statement advocating for the establishment of risk-based maternal levels of care within health systems (ACOG maternal levels of care).[18] This document recommends that hospitals providing subspecialty obstetric care have a fellowship-trained obstetric anesthesiologist serving as the director of obstetric anesthesia. Hospitals serving as regional perinatal health care centers should always have obstetric anesthesia fellowship–trained anesthesiologists on site.[18]

There are many paths to training and certification in critical care medicine. Completion of a residency in anesthesiology followed by an anesthesiology critical care medicine fellowship is one. A critical care anesthesiologist combines the knowledge and skills learned during residency, like airway management and regional anesthesia, with those acquired during critical care training, to provide a broader array of services than other critical care specialists can offer. Anesthesiologist-intensivists are specialists in the perioperative management of critically ill surgical patients. They typically work in an intensive care unit (ICU) as part of a multidisciplinary team of medical and allied health professionals. Anesthesiologist-intensivists possess expertise in all aspects of life support including advanced cardiac support with assist devices and ECMO, airway management, ventilator management, point-of-care ultrasound (POCUS), invasive monitoring, central venous access, nutritional support, antimicrobial therapies, renal replacement therapies, pain management, and sedation. Additionally, they have a deep understanding of the rehabilitation needs of critically ill patients, and are trained to manage end-of-life issues, compassionately, ethically, and with dignity.[19]

The quest to alleviate surgical pain gave birth to anesthesiology. As the specialty matured, anesthesiologists began using their skills to manage pain beyond the OR. The first pain medicine programs were accredited by the ACGME in 1992 and the first subspecialty certification examination was administered by the ABA 1 year later. As with critical care medicine, there are multiple paths to a career in pain medicine. Physicians trained in neurology, physical medicine and rehabilitation, and psychiatry may pursue training in pain medicine. All currently accredited pain medicine fellowship programs are affiliated with anesthesiology.[20]

Although pain medicine began with a focus on regional anesthesia techniques, today's practitioners are also experts in pharmacotherapy, physical therapy, and psychological approaches to chronic pain. Some pain medicine specialists have begun performing more invasive procedures like implanting spinal cord stimulators and intrathecal infusion pumps. Others may offer percutaneous spinal stabilization techniques.

Anesthesiologists trained in pain medicine typically work in outpatient settings and manage chronic pain syndromes and cancer-related pain. These physicians usually have a long-term relationship with patients similar to that of other medical specialties. Today, only a few pain medicine anesthesiologists also provide surgical anesthesia care. Instead, new subspecialties of regional anesthesiology and acute pain medicine have developed. These experts practice in hospital settings and care for patients suffering from postsurgical pain, trauma, or other pathologies (e.g., sickle cell crises). Acute pain specialists also may help manage inpatients with complex chronic pain syndromes. The current U.S. opioid epidemic has amplified the value of these anesthesiologists who can offer ways to effectively manage pain while minimizing the use of potentially addicting medications.[20]

The central nervous system is the most complex and least understood part of the human body. The growing complexity of neurologic surgery, including stereotactic surgery, awake craniotomies, and advanced neuromonitoring techniques, has led some anesthesiologists to specialize in neuro anesthesia and neuro critical care.[21] These specialists care for patients suffering cerebrovascular accidents, traumatic brain injury, status epilepticus, inflammatory and infectious diseases, spinal cord pathology, central nervous system neoplasia, and more with the goal of improving survival and functional recovery.[22]

Trauma is the leading cause of death for individuals under the age of 45, and the third overall leading cause of death in the United States. The care of trauma victims requires integration of local and regional emergency services with multidisciplinary teams working in the trauma centers. The anesthesiologist is a fundamental member of any trauma service. Trauma anesthesiologists are often cross trained in critical care and are experts in the management of hemorrhagic shock and the treatment of patients suffering devastating injuries. Additionally, they are skilled in advanced airway management, vascular access, acute pain management, and invasive monitoring.[23] Trauma anesthesiologists care for a variety of critically ill patients and also can provide leadership in emergency management and transfusion medicine.

Liver transplants are among today's most complicated surgeries. Transplant anesthesiologists manage coagulopathy, acid–base derangements, multiorgan system failure,[24] and massive transfusion. They are skilled in vascular access and invasive monitoring. These anesthesiologists also care for patients undergoing multiorgan transplants and complex hepatobiliary surgeries. Transplant anesthesiologists often participate in transplant selection committees and can provide preoperative and postoperative care.

Economics and the development of minimally invasive techniques are driving more and more procedures and anesthetics to outpatient and office-based settings. Today, more than half of the anesthetics administered in the United States are for either ambulatory or 23-hour stay procedures. Even patients who traditionally spent several days in the hospital, such as those receiving cardiac interventions or total joint replacements are now going home on the day of surgery. All anesthesiologists care for ambulatory patients and need to adjust their techniques accordingly.[25]

Many of today's invasive procedures take place outside of the traditional operating suite. Patients undergo many increasingly complex catheter-based, endoscopic, and image-guided diagnostic and therapeutic techniques. These interventions are often offered to older and sicker patients, who cannot tolerate more invasive procedures. Successful interventional procedures are associated with faster recovery, fewer ICU admissions, and shorter hospital stays.[26] Today, anesthesia personnel are routinely deployed to interventional or diagnostic radiology suites, magnetic resonance imaging (MRI) scanners, cardiac catheterization and electrophysiology laboratories, and endoscopy centers.[27] This trend will only increase as nonoperating room anesthesia (NORA) is currently growing faster than OR anesthesia.

Anesthesiologists are venturing into areas of medicine beyond the traditional reach of the specialty. In 2011, The ABA began offering a certification sleep medicine. Candidates must have completed a 1-year accredited fellowship in sleep medicine.[28] Anesthesiologists are particularly well suited to manage patients in terminal stages of disease given their expertise in pain management and life support. The palliative and hospice medicine specialist endeavors to provide comfort, dignity, and appropriate care to dying patients. These physicians also support families as they make difficult decisions about their loved one's end-of-life care. Interested anesthesiologists can obtain subspecialty certification after completing a 1-year fellowship program in palliative and hospice medicine.[29] Anesthesiologists specializing in addiction medicine care for patients struggling with substance use disorders and their associated comorbidities.[30] Combined residency programs provide joint training in anesthesiology and either emergency medicine, pediatrics, or internal medicine.[31]

Anesthesiologists also may pursue other opportunities that combine clinical and administrative skills. Perioperative medicine is a developing specialty that aims to improve the health outcomes of surgical patients, beginning in the preparatory stages and extending throughout recovery. Perioperative medicine specialists develop and apply evidence-based clinical pathways aimed at mitigating risk and enhancing functional recovery of surgical patients.[32] Perioperative medicine fellowships should provide experience in perioperative medicine, clinical leadership, quality improvement, and clinical research.[33]

Clinical Informatics is a subspecialty approved by the ABMS under the sponsorship of the American Board of Preventive Medicine. This certification is available to diplomates of any of the ABMS-approved boards including anesthesiology. The first certification examination was offered in 2012. The clinical informaticians analyze and manage data, study and refine workflows, design clinical support aids, and lead in the acquisition, implementation, and maintenance of information and communication systems, including electronic health records (EHRs) necessary to support the mission of a health care organization.[34,35]

In the United States, anesthesia-related morbidity and mortality has been steadily improving. This degree of safety is often not achieved in low- and middle-income countries. Fellowships in Global Anesthesia train candidates to develop systems that facilitate the sustainable delivery of safe, high quality anesthesia care within an individual country's unique economic and cultural confines. Some global anesthesia programs allow fellows to earn a Master's in Public Health (MPH) degree.[36]

The specialty of anesthesiology rests on the three pillars of teaching, clinical care, and research. For decades, multiple barriers have limited research in anesthesiology. There has been a lack of money to support new researchers and a shortage of research mentors. External funding to provide space, resources, and nonclinical time is vanishingly hard to find.[37] Fewer than 60 of the 159 U.S. anesthesiology residency programs currently receive research funding from the National Institutes of Health (NIH).[38] Despite these barriers, some anesthesiology departments have built robust research training programs.[39–41] Anesthesiologists interested in pursuing a research career also can obtain early career funding through the Foundation for Anesthesia Education and Research, the ASA, and other affiliated organizations.[42,43] With perseverance, mentoring, and hard work, the interested anesthesiologist can build a successful and rewarding career advancing the medicine and science of our specialty.

The Value of Anesthesiologists

Perioperative Surgical Home

The United States ranks last among developed countries in access to medical care, administrative efficiency, health care equity, and outcomes despite spending a much larger proportion of its gross domestic product on medical services.[44] The "Triple Aim" of health care has become a useful framework to address this problem.[45] The premise of the triple aim is that by improving the health of populations, enhancing the patient experience of care, and reducing the per capita cost of health care, providers and institutions will enhance and optimize health care delivery. While some have advocated for the quadruple aim (assuring wellness of the providers)[46] and the quintuple aim (addressing disparities in health care),[47] we will limit the scope of this discussion to the original triple aim. The concepts of the triple aim resemble the idea of value, which aims to improve care while decreasing costs by moving reimbursements from volume to value.[48]

3 Anesthesiologists are uniquely positioned to achieve triple aim and value-care goals. The current state of fragmented perioperative care increases cost, risk, and adverse outcomes. To address this problem, ASA introduced the concept of the perioperative surgical home (PSH), in which "the patient's experience of care is coordinated by a physician-led, interdisciplinary team" with the goal of "improved operational efficiencies, decreased resource utilization, a reduction in length of stay and readmission, and a decrease in complications and mortality-resulting in a better patient experience of care."[49]

In 2014, the University of California Irvine established the feasibility of the PSH and published their experience with patients undergoing total joint arthroplasty.[50] Subsequent publications have shown that the PSH can decrease hospital length of stay and admission to skilled nurse facilities.[51] A financial analysis revealed that the PSH was associated with lower direct hospital costs.[52] Since 2014, hundreds of publications have touted both clinical and financial benefits of the PSH.[53] The ASA offers resources and tools for those interested in learning more about PSH and its implementation.[49]

Enhanced Recovery after Surgery

In the 1990's, Professor Henrik Kehlet, a surgeon working at the University of Copenhagen in Denmark, and others began advocating for the use of multimodal clinical pathways in the care of surgical patients. The ideas became the foundation of multiple enhanced recovery after surgery (ERAS) protocols.[54] These protocols are evidence-informed clinical pathways that aim to stan-
4 dardize perioperative care. Well-implemented ERAS protocols are associated with shortened hospital stays, decreased costs, and fewer complications.[55] ERAS protocols can be incorporated into PSH models to address the triple aim goals of population health, patient experience, and cost. Currently, published ERAS protocols address bariatric, breast, plastic, cardiac, colorectal, esophageal, head and neck, hepatic, gynecologic, neurologic, obstetric, orthopedic, pancreatic, thoracic, and urologic surgeries.[56]

Practice Parameters: Standards, Guidelines, and Advisories

A key contribution of the ASA has been the development, approval, and dissemination of practice standards, guidelines, and advisories. The ASA Committee on Standards and Practice Parameters supervises the creation and revision of practice parameters, which are then reviewed and approved by the ASA House of Delegates.[57]

These parameters are defined as follows[57]:

> "A. Practice **standards** provide rules or minimum requirements for clinical practice. They are regarded as generally accepted principles of patient management. Standards may be modified only under unusual circumstances; for example, extreme emergencies or unavailability of equipment.
>
> B. Practice **guidelines** provide recommendations for patient care that describe a basic management strategy or a range of basic management strategies. Practice guidelines include recommendations that are developed based on a systematic review that assesses the quality, quantity, and consistency of evidence. Evidence-based practice guidelines are not offered or intended as standards or minimum requirements.
>
> C. Practice **advisories** provide guidance to assist decision making in areas of patient care where there is insufficient published research. Practice advisories are based on a systematic review but supported by evidence of limited quality, quantity, or consistency. Practice advisories are not offered or intended as standards, minimum requirements, or guidelines."*

The practice parameters are reviewed periodically as medical knowledge evolves. While these parameters provide a framework for practice, they are not designed to serve as unique indicators of appropriate care. Hence, the judgment of the anesthesiologist in each circumstance might warrant deviation from the parameters. A departure from practice parameter guidance may be appropriate if the facts and circumstances of the case demonstrate that the rendered care met the physician's duty to the patient.[57]

Operating Room Management

Anesthesiologists are well positioned and trained to become leaders in managing the complexity of surgical services. Our specialty has a strong commitment to patient safety and quality improvement. As natural inhabitants of ORs, anesthesiologists are exposed to the importance of efficiently and effectively managing these limited and expensive resources. These skills allow us to improve OR efficiency, productivity, and evaluate operational and financial performance. In addition, anesthesiologists can bring light to OR design and construction, which influence efficiency and productivity.

Physician Executive Roles and Additional Training

While good OR management can stem from a mix of personal leadership skills (i.e., emotional intelligence) and experience, additional training can complement these assets. Developing an understanding of finance (budgeting, balance statements), legal considerations, enhanced negotiation skills, and other aspects from the business world add to the armamentarium of

*Excerpted from Policy Statement on Practice Parameters (Updated October 13, 2021) © 2023 of the American Society of Anesthesiologists. A copy of the full text can be obtained from ASA, 1061 American Lane Schaumburg, IL 60173-4973 or online at www.asahq.org.

the anesthesiologist in a leadership position. Furthermore, these
5 positions are no longer limited to the OR. Anesthesiologists serve in many senior leadership roles including hospital chief executive officer, chief medical officer, chief operating officer, and vice chair for perioperative services.[58]

Advocacy/Participation

With more than 55,000 members, the ASA is the largest anesthesiology association in the world. The ASA provides educational content, sets practice parameters, and supports research. In addition, the ASA actively engages in political advocacy, educating members, legislators, and the public on issues related to reimbursement, scope of practice, challenges in health care delivery (i.e., drug shortages) and, most recently, physician wellness.[59] At the state level, component societies, under the umbrella of the ASA, play a similar role.

Accreditation, Training, and Certification

Founded in 1981, the Accreditation Council for Graduate Medical Education (ACGME) is a U.S.-based organization that provides accreditation to graduate medical education (residency and fellowship) programs and the institutions that sponsor them. This voluntary accreditation is achieved by demonstrating compliance with published standards called the common program requirements.[60] Recently, the ACGME has expanded their scope into other countries with an international arm.[61] In addition to core anesthesiology residency programs, the ACGME provides accreditation to 10 anesthesiology subspecialties (Table 2-1).[62] Currently, there are 159 anesthesiology residency programs in the United States[5] with approximately 1,774 first year,[63] and over 6,000 active, anesthesiology residents.[8]

Initial Certification

Physicians who successfully complete training on an accredited anesthesiology residency program are eligible for certification by
6 the ABA.[64] Board certification is a way to demonstrate expertise. While voluntary, state licensing boards, health care facilities, and the public view board certification as a quality standard. Most health care facilities and states require board eligibility or certification for credentialing and licensing.

For those who completed training before June 30, 2016, the certification process entailed a written (part 1) and a subsequent oral examination (part 2).[65] Those graduating after 2016 must pass the BASIC, ADVANCED, and APPLIED staged examinations. The BASIC examination, usually taken at the end of the first year of anesthesia training, focuses on the scientific basis of anesthesiology practice. The ADVANCED examination focuses on clinical aspects of anesthetic practice and emphasizes subspecialty-based practice and advanced clinical issues. Anesthesiologists take this examination after completing their residency training. Last, candidates must pass the APPLIED examination, which includes two components—the traditional standardized oral examination (SOE) and the objective structured clinical examination (OSCE).[66]

The ABA also offers written examinations leading to certification in critical care medicine, pain medicine, hospice and palliative care medicine, sleep medicine, pediatric anesthesiology, and neurocritical care medicine.[67] Most recently, the ABA added the Anesthesiology Special Purpose Examination (ASPEX) for diplomates who need to establish that they passed a secure, medical-knowledge examination within the last 10 years to gain a state medical license.[68]

Maintenance of Certification

At the behest of the ABMS, the ABA established the Maintenance of Certification in Anesthesiology (MOCA) program as a mechanism to ensure that the standard achieved at initial certification is maintained. The MOCA program focuses on lifelong learning and quality patient care. There are four requirements that need to be met every 10 years to maintain certification:

- Maintain an unrestricted medical license in the United States or Canada.
- Earn 250 Continuing Medical Education credits (125 every 5 years).
- Earn 50 quality improvement points (25 every 5 years).
- Complete 125 MOCA-minute questions every calendar year.

The MOCA minute is an innovation that replaces the earlier requirement of passing a written recertification examination. With the MOCA minute, the ABA diplomate has access to an interactive lifelong learning platform that allows self-assessment and acquisition of new knowledge while fulfilling MOCA requirements.[69] New ABMS standards taking effect in 2024 require that the ABA renew certification every 5 years instead of every 10 years.[70]

Financial Aspects of Anesthesia Practice

Introduction

Medicine is a service industry. Physicians provide services to patients and expect payment in return. Who pays, how they pay, and how much they pay are in constant flux. This section reviews the basics of anesthesia billing and reimbursement. It discusses the relationships among anesthesiologists and other qualified anesthesia providers including anesthesia residents, certified registered nurse anesthetists (CRNAs) and certified anesthesiologist assistants (CAAs). Then, we will discuss some of the financial pressures faced by anesthesiologists. Among them, the low rates paid by government programs (Medicare and Medicaid) and the more recent practice by private insurers of using newly enacted limitations on balance billing to unilaterally decrease reimbursement. Last, we will discuss how some anesthesia groups are responding to these pressures.

Basics of Anesthesia Billing and Reimbursement

Coding

Every medical encounter has a reason (the diagnosis) and a procedure (the nature of the encounter). Diagnoses can range from "well-child visit" or "preconception counseling" to "myocardial infarction" and beyond. Diagnoses are standardized in the international classification of diseases (ICD). The ICD derives from efforts beginning in the mid-19th century to create a common language to allow the systematic collection and comparison of health, disease, and hospitalization information. Today, the ICD has become a global tool for epidemiology, health management, and clinical purposes. The ICD is maintained by the World Health Organization (WHO).[71] U.S. health care providers currently use ICD-10, which contains 14,400 diagnosis codes. ICD-10 was released in 1992 but not adopted for United States use until 2015. The latest ICD version, ICD-11, contains 55,000 diagnosis codes. It was released in January 2022 and U.S. implementation is scheduled for 2025.[72]

Medical services (procedures) are categorized by current procedural technology (CPT) codes. The CPT code set was developed by and is owned and maintained by the American Medical

Table 2-2 Common Coding Acronyms and Their Uses

Code	Owner	Use
International disease classification (ICD)	World Health Organization	Global diagnostic tool for epidemiology, health management and clinical purposes. The 10th iteration (ICD-10) contains approximately 14,400 diagnostic codes. The 11th edition, ICD-11, was released in January 2022 and contains 55,000 diagnosis codes.
Current procedural terminology (CPT)	American Medical Association	Nomenclature used to report medical services and procedures to Medicare and commercial insurers. Also called the Healthcare Common Procedures Coding System (HCPCS) when used by the Center for Medicare and Medicaid Services (CMS).
Relative value guide (RVG)	American Society of Anesthesiologists	Index of anesthesia base units plus guidance on proper anesthesia billing including start/stop time, field avoidance, and labor analgesia services. The RVG is usually used in conjunction with CROSSWALK, which cross links anesthesia RVG codes to corresponding CPT codes.

Association. It provides a common nomenclature that is used to report medical, surgical, radiology, laboratory, and anesthesiology services to public and private health insurance programs.[73] Currently there are CPT codes for more than 10,000 medical services. The CPT is regularly evaluated and updated. There were 329 code changes in 2021, including 206 additions, 54 deletions, and 69 revisions.[73] The CPT coding system is used by the Center for Medicare and Medicaid Services (CMS), where it is called the Healthcare Common Procedures Coding System (HCPCS). Table 2-2 reviews common billing-related acronyms.

Billing

Medicare and Medicaid

Understanding anesthesia billing and reimbursement starts with understanding Medicare and Medicaid, the predominant payers for health care in the United States. The legislation creating Medicare and Medicaid, officially, Title XVIII and Title XIX of the Social Security Act, was signed into law by President Lyndon B. Johnson on July 30, 1965. Medicare was originally intended to provide health insurance to Americans aged 65 and older who were receiving social security or other federal retirement benefits. It has since been expanded to include almost all U.S. residents aged 65 and older, younger residents with certain disabilities, and all patients with end-stage renal disease. Medicaid funds are allocated to individual states to provide health insurance for low-income families, pregnant persons, people with disabilities, and those needing long-term care. The Children's Health Insurance Program (CHIP) was signed into law in 1997 and provides federal matching funds to states that provide health coverage to children in families with incomes too high to qualify for Medicaid, but who cannot afford

Table 2-3 Customary, Reasonable, and Prevailing Definitions

Customary	Median of a physician's charges for a specific service for a specific time period
Reasonable	The 90th percentile of all customary charges of physicians in the same peer group (specialty) in a specific locale
Prevailing	The lower of the actual payment or the customary charge for a particular service in a defined locale

From Morewood G, Cohen NH, Merrick SK. Anesthesia Practice Finances, 2030. *ASA Monit.* 2021;85(S10):24–26.

private coverage. Approximately 41% of the U.S. population, over 144 million people, are covered by Medicare or Medicaid.[44]

Originally, Medicare payments to providers were based on customary, reasonable, and prevailing (CRP) charges (Table 2-3).[74] Limitations of the CRP system included lack of standardization, variations in payments to different specialties for the same service, and inability to control the growth of Medicare spending. The resource-based relative value system (RBRVS) was developed to standardize payments for medical services.[75] The RVRBS assigns relative value units (RVUs) to each service or procedure. RVUs are based on the resources or "work" required to provide any service. Each service is divided into three components:

- Physician work: the time, skill, mental and physical effort needed to provide the service.
- Practice expense, which varies with the site of the service. For instance, inpatient surgery is reimbursed at a higher rate than outpatient or office-based surgery.
- Professional liability insurance.

RVUs are assigned to each CPT code. RVUs are reviewed and often adjusted by CMS based on input from the American Medical Association's Specialty Society Relative Value Scale Update Committee (RUC). Payment for medical services is based on the RVU value assigned to that service times a conversion factor (CF), which determines the dollar value of a single RVU. The value of the CF is determined by the United States Congress for government-paid services or by contract between providers and health care insurance companies.

Anesthesia Billing Basics

NORA services are billed and reimbursed using the RVU methodology. These activities include the evaluation and management of a critically ill patient or providing pain management services. Most peripheral nerve blocks, spinal injections, or additional services (i.e., intra-arterial catheters, central venous catheters, and echocardiography) are also valued and billed by RVU.

However, OR anesthesia is different. Because anesthesiologists do not control the length of any given surgery, the ASA has consistently and successfully advocated for time-based payment. A bill for anesthesia services consists of "base units," which vary with the complexity of the surgery, "time units," usually 10- to 15-minute increments, and qualifying circumstances, additional units that reflect more complex anesthetics. Table 2-4 shows accepted ASA physical status modifiers. Table 2-5 shows commonly reimbursed qualifying circumstances.[76] Base units and modifiers are determined by the ASA and published in their Relative Value

Table 2-4 ASA Physical Status Modifiers and Base Unit Assignments

Descriptor	ASA Physical Status Classification	ASA Provided Examples	Base Units
A normal healthy patient	ASA I	Healthy, nonsmoking, no or minimal alcohol use	0
A patient with mild systemic disease	ASA II	Mild diseases only without substantive functional limitations. Examples include (but not limited to): current smoker, social alcohol drinker, pregnancy, obesity (30 < BMI < 40), well-controlled DM/HTN, mild lung disease	0
A patient with severe systemic disease	ASA III	Substantive functional limitations; one or more moderate to severe diseases. Examples include (but not limited to): poorly controlled DM or HTN, COPD, morbid obesity (BMI ≥ 40), active hepatitis, alcohol dependence or abuse, implanted pacemaker, moderate reduction of ejection fraction, ESRD, undergoing regularly scheduled dialysis, premature infant PCA < 60 wk, history (>3 mo) of MI, CVA, TIA or CAD/stents	1
A patient with severe systemic disease that is a constant threat to life	ASA IV	Examples include (but not limited to): recent (<3 mo) MI, CVA, TIA, or CAD/stents, ongoing cardiac ischemia or severe valve dysfunction, severe reduction of ejection fraction, sepsis, DIC, ARD or ESRD not undergoing regularly scheduled dialysis	2
A moribund patient who is not expected to survive without the operation	ASA V	Examples include (but not limited to): ruptured abdominal/thoracic aneurysm, massive trauma, intracranial bleed with mass effect, ischemic bowel in the face of significant cardiac pathology, or multiple organ/system dysfunction	3
A declared brain-dead patient whose organs are being removed for donor purposes	ASA VI		0

Modified from American Society of Anesthesiologists. *Anesthesia Payment Basics Series: #4 Physical Status.* Document created in 2019. Accessed 2/3/2023. https://www.asahq.org/quality-and-practice-management/managing-your-practice/timely-topics-in-payment-and-practice-management/anesthesia-payment-basics-series-4-physical-status

Guide book (RVG). The ASA also publishes and sells CROSSWALK to link anesthesia RVG codes with the appropriate CPT code.[77] Every bill for OR anesthesia services needs a diagnosis (ICD-10), a compatible procedure (CPT code), and a matching ASA code from the RVG. Table 2-6 shows some representative invoices for anesthesia care.

Table 2-5 Qualifying Circumstances CPT Code and Base Unit Assignments

CPT/HCPCS Code	Descriptor	Base Units
+99100	Anesthesia for a patient of extreme age (<1 y or >70 y)	1
+99116	Anesthesia complicated by the utilization of total body hypothermia	5
+99135	Anesthesia complicated by the utilization of controlled hypotension	5
+99140	Anesthesia complicated by emergency conditions (specify)	2

Modified with permission from Merrick SK. Physical status and qualifying circumstances. *ASA Monitor.* 2021;85:38. doi: https://doi.org/10.1097/01.ASM.0000803364.48940.0e

There are several exceptions and variations to this methodology. One of the most common is billing for epidural labor analgesia. There is no universally accepted method of charging for time for labor analgesia. The RVG advises: "Professional charges...should reasonably reflect the costs of providing labor analgesia services as well as the intensity and time involved...."[78] Common approaches include base units plus time to delivery, subject to a cap; base units plus one unit per hour (plus direct patient contact time); incremental time-based fees (i.e., 0 to 2 hours, 2 to 6 hours, etc.); or a single fee.[78]

Billing for spinal or epidural injections and peripheral nerve blocks depends on the primary purpose of the procedure. If the epidural or nerve block will serve as the primary anesthetic (i.e., wrist fracture repair under supraclavicular block with sedation), the time needed to perform the block is added to the total anesthesia time. However, if the block or injection is primarily for postoperative pain (i.e., an adductor canal block for analgesia after a total knee arthroplasty or a thoracic epidural catheter for postoperative analgesia), then the procedure is billed using the RVU system. Table 2-7 shows some common procedure CPT codes and their work RVU values.

Although the RVU and RVG methodology remain robust ways to quantify the work or productivity of individual providers, the actual reimbursement for anesthesia services, especially by Medicare and Medicaid is subject to constant revision. The Medicare Access and CHIP Reauthorization Act of 2015 (MACRA) is the

Table 2-6 Representative Anesthesia Invoices

Procedure	Diagnosis (ICD-10)	Procedure (CPT Code)	ASA CPT Code (RVG)	Base Units	Time (min)	Time Units	Total ASA Units
Cataract extraction	H26.9 unspecified cataract	66984: cataract surgery w/IOL	00142: anesthesia for Lens surgery	4	53	4	8
Breast reduction	N62: hypertrophy of breast	19318: breast reduction	00402: anesthesia, surgery of breast	5	162	11	16
Neovaginoplasty	F64.0: Transexualism	57291: Construction of vagina	00904: anesthesia, perineal surgery	7	431	29	36
Labor Analgesia	O80-O82: encounter for delivery	59409: obstetrical care	01967: neuraxial anesthesia/analgesia for planned vaginal delivery	5	860	57[a]	63[a]

[a]Time billed according to "local standards." See text.

latest attempt to ensure quality care while controlling or decreasing the growth of U.S. health care spending. MACRA attempts to reward clinicians for quality, outcomes, and value, not volume. MACRA requires providers to participate in one of two payment alternatives: The merit-based incentive payments program (MIPS) or eligible Alternative Payment Models (APMs).[79]

MIPS allows providers or groups to earn up to 100 points based on performance in four quality-related categories (Table 2-8). Those exceeding a predefined performance threshold receive a payment adjustment of up to 9%. Providers not meeting the goal see a payment decrease of up to 9%. In 2022, the threshold to receive a positive adjustment was 75 points. Those scoring below 75 points will receive a negative adjustment in 2024. Practices scoring exactly 75 points will receive a neutral adjustment. Providers and practices scoring 89 points or above will earn an "exceptional bonus."[80]

APMs attempt to incentivize quality, cost-efficiency, and effectiveness by providing bundled payments for a specific clinical condition, care episode, or patient population. In 2016, the comprehensive care for joint replacement (CJR) model was the first episode-based bundled payment model. The CJR model has been implemented in 67 geographic regions. Advanced APMs are a subset of APMs that allow clinicians to earn greater rewards for taking on some risk related to their patient outcomes. Practices that enroll in advanced APMs are eligible for lump-sum bonuses in the initial years and enhanced annual Medicare payment increases compared to those enrolled in MIPS programs.[51]

Table 2-7 Representative Anesthesia Procedures and Their Corresponding Relative Value Units

CPT Code	CPT Descriptor	Work RVU[a]
64415	Injection anesthetic agents; brachial plexus	1.35
36620	Arterial catheterization or cannulation for sampling, monitoring or transfusion; percutaneous	1.00
31500	Intubation, endotracheal, emergency procedure	3.00
99291	Critical care, evaluation and management of the critically ill or critically injured patient; first 30–74 min	
62323	Injection(s)—interlaminar, epidural or subarachnoid, lumbar of sacral; with imaging guidance (i.e., fluoroscopy or CT)	1.80

From *2020 Relative Value Guide® A Guide for Anesthesia Values*. American Society of Anesthesiologists®.
[a]The Centers for Medicare and Medicaid Services 2022 physician fee schedule conversion factor was $34.6062 per RVU.

The ASA's PSH model (Fig. 2-1) is one approach to achieving value-based goals. "In the PSH model, the patient's experience of care is coordinated by a physician-led, interdisciplinary team. The expected metrics include improved operational efficiencies, decreased resource utilization, a reduction in length of stay and readmission, and a decrease in complications and mortality resulting in a better patient experience of care."[49] The PSH provides a systematic approach that expands the opportunities for anesthesiologists to demonstrate quality and participate in advanced APMs.[81]

Although ever more U.S. health care dollars are paid through APMs, evidence that this approach to value-based purchasing improves quality or decreases cost is sparce.[82] Value-based payment systems also may fail to account for uncaptured clinical status and social determinants of health. As a result, scoring systems may be biased against physicians caring for large numbers of underserved patients.[83,84] In 2021, most health care providers were still paid for volume not value.[85]

Coding and Billing Summary

Although the details will continue to evolve, the basics of anesthesia coding and billing will likely remain unchanged. Reimbursement for any patient encounter will require a diagnosis code, a procedure code with matching anesthesia code, and, for OR anesthesia, an anesthesia start time and anesthesia end time. These codes must exactly match the codes submitted by the proceduralist. Close attention to these details will both ensure that you get paid promptly for your work and protect you in the case of an audit. 7

Medical Direction and the Anesthesia Care Team Model

What are Medical Direction and Medical Supervision?

In the United States, most anesthetics are administered personally by a physician anesthesiologist, or by another, nonphysician, anesthesia provider (i.e., a CRNA or a CAA in an anesthesia care

Table 2-8 Merit Based Incentive Payments Program Performance Categories

Category	Points	Examples	Data Source(s)
Cost performance	30	Population-based measures: Medicare spending per beneficiary; procedure-based cost measures: knee arthroplasty, hip arthroplasty, cataract removal, etc.	Medicare claims data
Improvement activities	15	Select among 100 clinical practice improvement activities	Qualified clinical data registry (QCDR); that is, the ASA's National Anesthesia Clinical Outcomes Registry (NACOR)
Promoting interoperability	25	Patient engagement and electronic exchange of health information using certified electronic health record technology. (Note: Most anesthesiologists and their groups will *not* have to submit the promoting interoperability category. Anesthesia practices are designated as nonpatient facing, hospital-based, or ambulatory surgery center-based and are automatically exempt. Instead, the 25% weighting of this category will be reallocated to the quality performance category	N/A
Quality performance	30	Anesthesiology measure set for performance year 2022: Prevention of CVC-related bloodstream infections Anesthesiology smoking abstinence Perioperative temperature management Prevention of PONV—combination therapy Prevention of postoperative vomiting (POV)—combination therapy (pediatrics) Multimodal pain management	Electronic medical record, QCDR, Medicare claims

From American Society of Anesthesiologists. The Merit-based Incentive Payment System (MIPS). Accessed February 14, 2022. https://www.asahq.org/macra/qualitypaymentprogram/mips

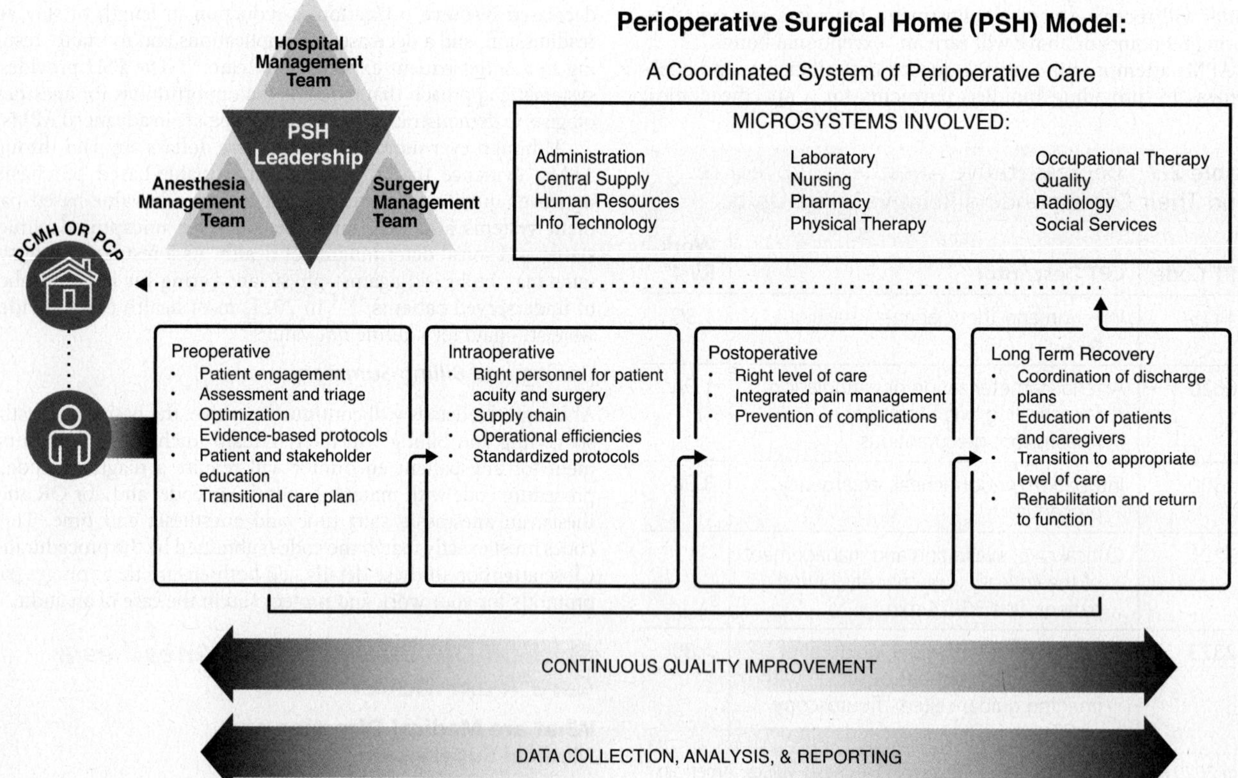

Figure 2-1 Overview of the perioperative surgical home model. (© 2020 is reprinted with permission of the American Society of Anesthesiologists,1061 American Lane, Schaumburg, Illinois 60173–4973.)

Table 2-9 The Seven Elements of Medical Direction

1.	Perform a preanesthetic examination and evaluation.
2.	Prescribe the anesthesia plan.
3.	Personally, participate in the most demanding procedures in the anesthesia plan, including (if applicable) induction and emergence.
4.	Ensure a qualified individual performs any procedures in the anesthesia plan that the anesthesiologist does not personally perform.
5.	Monitor the course of anesthesia administration at frequent intervals.
6.	Remain physically present for all key and critical portions of the procedure, and be available for immediate diagnosis and treatment of emergencies.[a]
7.	Provide postanesthesia care as indicated.

[a]Medicare considers an anesthesiologist "immediately available" when they are: physically within the same area as the CRNA or AA and not otherwise occupied in a way that prevents an immediate hands-on intervention.[1]

Reprinted from Robinson DH, Toledo AH. Historical development of modern anesthesia. *J Invest Surg*. 2012;25(3):141–149. With permission.

team model. Terms like "medical direction," "medical supervision," or "without medical direction of a physician" have specific meanings when used to describe the interactions among members of the anesthesia care team. These meanings have implications for the coding, billing, and reimbursement of anesthesia services.

Medical direction describes anesthesia care delivered by one to four "qualified anesthesia providers" under the direction of an anesthesiologist. To bill for medical direction, CMS mandates that the anesthesiologist fulfill seven criteria (Table 2-9). The CMS requirements are very specific. From the Medicare Claims Processing Manual: "The physician must *document* (emphasis added) in the medical record that he or she performed the preanesthetic examination and evaluation. Physicians must also document that they provided indicated post anesthesia care, were present during some portion of the anesthesia monitoring, and were present during the most demanding procedures in the anesthesia plan, including induction and emergence, where indicated."[86] Failure to *document* your compliance with each of the seven elements of medical direction may make you subject to penalties under the False Claims Act.[87] When medically directing other anesthesia providers, the anesthesiologist can only personally provide a limited number of anesthesia-related services (Table 2-10). Anesthesiologists may medically direct a maximum of four certified anesthesia providers or two trainees at any one time.

Table 2-10 Services That an Anesthesiologist Can Perform Without Breaking the Medical Direction Rules:

- Addressing an emergency of short duration
- Administering labor epidural
- Periodically (rather than continuously) monitoring an obstetrical patient
- Receiving patients entering the operating suite for surgery
- Checking on or discharging patients in the recovery room
- Handling scheduling matters

Modified from Medicare Claims Processing Manual Chapter 12–Physicians/Nonphysician Practitioners. (Rev. 11181, 01-14-22)

Medical supervision describes situations where a single anesthesiologist is responsible for more than four concurrent procedures. The distinction between medical direction and medical supervision has billing implications that will be discussed below.

Who are "Qualified Individuals"?

In the United States, there are three main types of anesthesia providers. Physician anesthesiologists hold an MD or DO degree and undergo at least 4 years of postgraduate training. Anesthesiologists may personally provide anesthesia care or may medically direct or supervise other providers or trainees. For more information, visit the ASA (www.asahq.org).

CRNAs earn a bachelor's degree in nursing (BSN), have at least 1 year of critical care nursing experience, and train for 2 to 3 years in a nurse anesthesia program. CMS requires that CRNAs be supervised by the operating practitioner performing the procedure or an immediately available anesthesiologist. However, CMS allows individual states to opt out of these supervision requirements. In 2022, 30 states had opted out of these supervision requirements. For more information, visit the American Association of Nurse Anesthetists (www.aana.com).

CAAs hold a bachelor's degree and have 2 to 3 years of training in a Master's of Medical Science program. CAAs only work under the medical direction of an anesthesiologist as a member of the anesthesia care team. Seventeen states currently license CAAs to administer anesthesia. For more information, visit the American Academy of Anesthesiologist Assistants (www.anesthetist.org).

Payment for Anesthesia Care

How Does Medical Direction or Supervision Affect Reimbursement?

Differing combinations of qualified providers influence coding, billing, and reimbursement for anesthesia care. Medicare requires that each claim include specific payment modifiers that denote the number and types of anesthesia providers (Table 2-11). A physician personally providing anesthesia care would include the AA modifier in their bill. When using the AA modifier, the anesthesiologist is paid 100% of the allowable charge. Under medical direction, both the anesthesiologist and the qualified anesthesia provider

Table 2-11 Medical Direction: Ratios and Modifiers

Modifier	Ratio	Definition
AA		An anesthesiologist personally performed the service
AD		Medical supervision by an anesthesiologist of more than four concurrent procedures
QY	1:1	Medical direction of a qualified provider by an anesthesiologist
QK or	1:2, 1:3, or 1:4	Medical direction of anesthesia trainees or qualified providers by an anesthesiologist[a]
QX		CRNA medically directed by an anesthesiologist
QZ		CRNA service without medical direction

[a]An anesthesiologist may medically direct a maximum of two trainees or four qualified providers.[2]

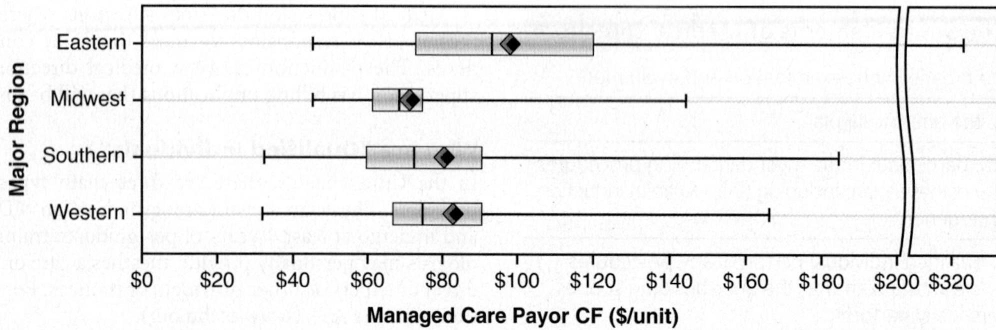

Figure 2-2 2020 Anesthesia conversion factors by U.S. geographical area. (Reprinted with permission from Stead SW, Merrick SK. ASA Survey Results: Commercial Fees Paid for Anesthesia Services, 2020. *ASA Monit*. 2020;84(10):1–29. doi: 10.1097/01.ASM.0000718828.55472.1a)

(CRNA/CAA) submit a bill for their services using a QK, QX, or QY modifier. Medicare reimburses the physician 50% of the total allowed amount and the CRNA/CAA is paid the other 50% of the total. If the anesthesiologist's bill includes the AD modifier (medical supervision of more than four qualified providers), Medicare only pays three base units (four if the anesthesiologist was present for induction) plus time. The CRNA is still paid 50% of the total allowable amount.[88] The QZ modifier denotes that the CRNA was not supervised or medically directed by a physician (CAAs cannot bill under the QZ modifier, nor can a supervising anesthesiologist use the AD modifier when working with a CAA). When billing under the QZ modifier, the CRNA receives 100% of the allowable payment. Some groups use the QZ modifier when the anesthesiologist fails to document compliance with the seven elements of medical direction. Although a CRNA can bill Medicare using the QZ (unsupervised) modifier, the anesthesiologist would likely still be held medically responsible, should a complication occur.

Government versus Commercial Insurance Payments

The charge for anesthesia care is determined by the number of ASA units (base units + time + modifiers) times a CF. Each CF is adjusted depending on whether the payer is an individual patient, a commercial insurance company, or a government insurer (i.e., Medicare or Medicaid). In 2016–2017, commercial insurance *charged* CFs were between $104 to $231 per ASA unit with a median charge of $149 per ASA unit.[89] In 2020, the U.S. commercial *paid* CF varied widely among insurers and geographic location (Fig. 2-2) with a median value of $73 per ASA unit.[90] In contrast, 2022 national Medicare CF was $21.5623 per ASA unit, or less than 33% of the median commercial CF.[86] This large difference in CF stems from the challenges encountered when trying to incorporate anesthesia time into the RVRBS billing methodology.[91] The value of an anesthesia unit was set at $13.68 for 1992, the first year of RBRVS. This value was a 29% reduction from the 1991 Medicare CF and approximately 40% of the prevailing commercial CF at that time.[92] Despite vigorous lobbying efforts by the ASA, the Medicare CF for anesthesia care continues to lag the commercial CF (Fig. 2-3).

The undervaluing of anesthesia services by government payers has significant implications for anesthesiologists. The most obvious is that practices with significant Medicare and Medicaid patient populations are unable to meet their expenses based solely on their insurance collections. In response, many anesthesia practices now rely on hospital subsidies to balance their budgets. From 2002 to 2014, the percentage of California hospitals

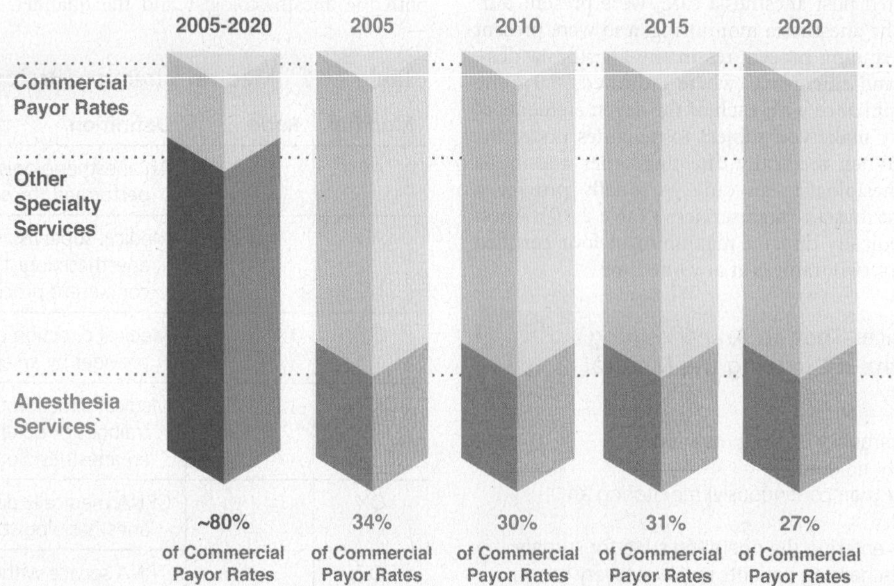

Figure 2-3 Trends in Medicare. Payment for anesthesia services versus Medicare payments for other specialties and commercial payor rates. (Medicare Payment Reform: 33% Problem Infographic © 2023 is reprinted with permission of the American Society of Anesthesiologists, 1061 American Lane, Schaumburg, Illinois 60173–4973.)

that made direct payments to anesthesia providers increased from 52% to 69%, with a median subsidy of $1,295,369 in 2018 U.S. dollars.[93] Hospitals receiving a larger fraction of their anesthesia revenues from government payers were more likely to make direct payments to anesthesia groups.[93] Other estimates suggest that 85% to 95% of hospitals provide direct or indirect anesthesia subsidies.[94]

Balance Billing and the No Surprises Act

An important consequence of the low government payment for anesthesia services is its effect on negotiated commercial insurance payment rates. Commercial insurance companies often base their reimbursement on a percentage of Medicare allowable charges. For most physicians, a payment of 110% of Medicare is fair and reasonable. However, because of the low Medicare CF for anesthesia services, rates pegged to that CF fail to adequately compensate for anesthesia care. Still, commercial insurers have been aggressively demanding lower rates from anesthesia providers. In some cases, anesthesia providers and insurance companies have been unable to come to agreement. As a result, anesthesia providers may be "out-of-network" even though surgeons and facilities remain "in-network." Patients may then receive a "surprise" bill for the, often significant, difference between the insurance payment and the provider charge. Many states have regulated this practice of balance billing for out-of-network services. In December 2020, the U.S. Congress passed the "No Surprises Act" as a part of the Consolidated Appropriations Act of 2021.[95] The No Surprises Act bans balance billing by out-of-network anesthesiologists. If an anesthesiologist feels that a commercial insurer's out-of-network payment is inadequate, they may appeal through a newly created independent dispute resolution (IDR) process. The IDR process allows an independent arbiter to select either the payment rate offered by the insurer, or the payment rate sought by the physician. One proposed factor that the arbiter can consider is the insurer's self-calculated median in-network rate, or qualifying payment amount (QPA). Many medical societies, including the ASA, fear that this mechanism will allow insurers to drive down their reimbursement by offering progressively lower in-network rates.[96] A November 2021 correspondence from Blue Cross Blue Shield of North Carolina demanding that participating providers accept an immediate 15% reduction in contracted rates suggests that these fears are not unfounded.[97] An informal survey of anesthesia practices in 2021 found that 50% to 70% had experienced a unilateral decrease in contracted rates or contract termination.[98] Significant decreases in commercial reimbursement for both in network and out of network anesthesia services has followed the enactment of similar balance billing laws in California, Florida, and New York.[99]

Summary and Future Directions

Anesthesiologists have long been well-compensated by direct payments from patients and insurers. However, over the past 20 years, trends in payment for health care services have con-
8 verged to challenge this model. Underpayment for anesthesia care by government payers (Medicare and Medicaid) has threatened the financial stability of many anesthesia groups. They are forced to rely more heavily on subsidies from hospitals and other health care facilities. The recently enacted "No Surprises Act" is likely to further reduce reimbursement for anesthesia care. These trends will likely change the relationships among anesthesia practices, insurers, and health care systems. Morewood et al. predict that many anesthesia practices will shift from contracting with commercial and government insurers to contracting directly with hospitals and health care systems to provide a comprehensive package of anesthesia services.[74] In this model, anesthesiologists will collaborate with other health care providers to provide service lines, procedural teams, and patient-centered homes. While collaborating and cooperating with other specialties to optimize clinical care, anesthesia practices will still need to document the value of each provider's services across the continuum of care to ensure fair compensation.[74] Unfortunately, not all hospitals and health care systems will be willing or able to meet these financial demands. Recent news items describe a variety of approaches to lower the cost of anesthesia care:

- Contract with an anesthesia group that will provide services for a lower or no hospital subsidy.
- Add CRNAs to a current physician-only practice.
- Use only CRNAs (in a state that has opted out of the Medicare supervision rule).
- Opt for a "Zone" model of anesthesia coverage relying on medical supervision or the unsupervised QZ modifier.[94]

These trends make it clear that all anesthesiologists and their professional organizations must remain actively engaged by staying informed, supporting their colleagues, lobbying their representatives, and more. Only through concerted advocacy, emphasizing the value that anesthesiologists bring to U.S. health care, will we ensure equitable payments for our services and influence policy to sustain the economic viability our specialty.[100]

Quality and Safety

The successful public demonstration of ether anesthesia on October 16, 1846, revolutionized surgical care. A short time later came the first death attributed to anesthesia.[101] In the subsequent century, death due to anesthesia remained distressingly common. Beecher and Todd estimated that between 1948 and 1952, anesthetics killed more people in the United States than poliomyelitis.[102] The subsequent three decades saw rapid advances in surgical care and, with the arrival of Medicare and Medicaid, a vast increase in the number of patients who could access medical care. The continued risk of patient harm was accompanied by a steady increase in the number of malpractice actions against anesthesiologists and rapidly increasing insurance costs.[103] In 1982, the television show "The Deep Sleep: 6,000 Will Die or Suffer Brain Damage" added public pressure to the malpractice crisis and accelerated the efforts of the ASA to address patient safety (Fig. 2-4).[104] These actions, spearheaded by then ASA president, Ellison C. Pierce, Jr, M.D., included the founding of the Closed Claims Project and the APSF and the approval of the ASA's Basic Standards for Intraoperative Monitoring.[105]

The ASA and the University of Washington at Seattle started the Closed Claims Project in 1984 to analyze closed malpractice claims and examine trends in anesthesia-related patient safety.[106] The project reviewed 4,000 claims by 1999[107] and almost 9,000 by 2011.[108] These reviews have led to more than 60 peer review publications covering topics from airway management to obstetric anesthesia to chronic pain management and monitored anesthesia care.[109] Information obtained from the Closed Claims Project was instrumental in promoting standards for pulse oximetry and end-tidal carbon dioxide monitoring as well as guiding the development of the ASA's difficult airway algorithm.[107] Closed Claims reviews have led to a better understanding of rare, but serious, events like postoperative visual loss[110] and burns.[111] Over time, the nature of malpractice claims against anesthesiologists has evolved. In the 1970s, 64% of claims involved permanent or disabling injuries or death. This number decreased to 41% by the

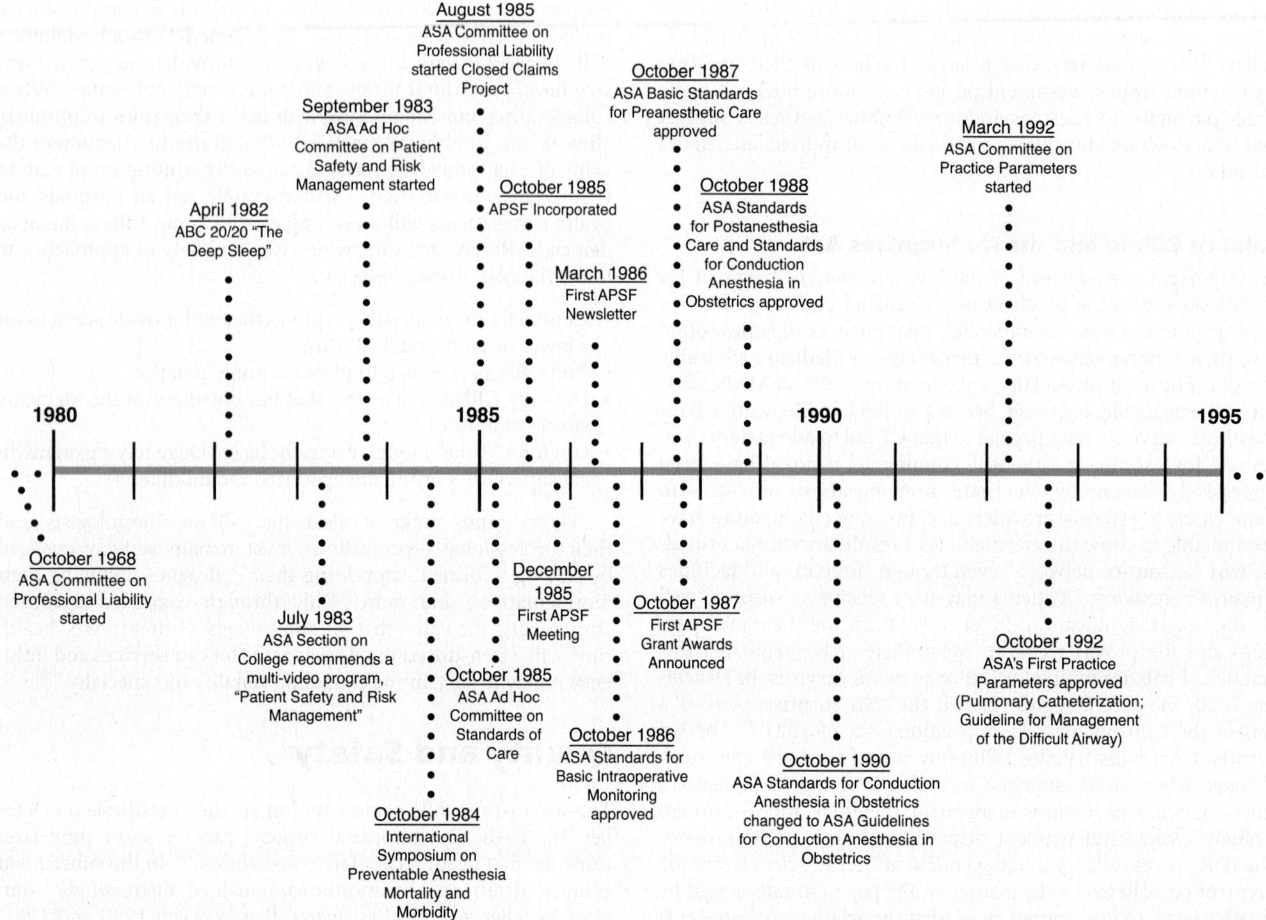

Figure 2-4 This timeline depicts major events that contributed to anesthesiology's lead role in improving patient safety during the years 1968 to 1992. ABC, American Broadcasting Corporation; APSF, Anesthesia Patient Safety Foundation; ASA, American Society of Anesthesiologists. (Reprinted with permission from Warner MA, Warner ME. The evolution of the anesthesia patient safety movement in America: lessons learned and considerations to promote further improvement in patient safety. *Anesthesiology*. 2021;135:963–974.)

1990's.[112] But death and permanent brain damage still accounted for 35% of claims between 1990 and 2007.[108] Meanwhile, claims for nerve injuries and those related to acute and chronic pain management have increased.[108] Recent publications have focused on the importance of communication during adverse events[113] and the increasing number of claims arising from events in non-OR locations.[114]

The ASPF was founded in 1985 with the goal "that no patient shall be harmed by anesthesia."[7] This organization has been a leader of the patient safety movement. In 1996, the American Medical Association and corporate partners founded the National Patient Safety Foundation, based on the APSF model.[115] Its efforts were also acknowledged in the landmark 1999 report from the Institute of Medicine, "Too err is Human,"[116] and in a 2005 front page article in the Wall Street Journal.[117] Today, the ASPF remains a leader of the anesthesia patient safety movement. It sets priorities, funds research, and disseminates information. Its newsletter is one of the most widely read anesthesia-related publications in the world.[118]

The anesthesia patient safety movement, through technology, like pulse oximetry and capnography, research, education, and advocacy is credited with reducing the anesthesia-related mortality rate from 64 per 100,000 to an estimated 0.5 per 100,000 patients.[119]

9 Because of these substantial gains, the quality lens has shifted from individual anesthetics to the entire perioperative period. Anesthesia providers effect surgical morbidity and mortality in many ways. Timely administration of perioperative prophylactic antibiotics significantly decreases the risk of postoperative wound infection.[120] Careful hand hygiene and disinfection of the anesthesia work station, both during and between cases, may decrease the risk of postoperative infection.[121] Interventions to address postoperative cognitive decline and opioid-related harm are current top ASPF safety priorities.[122] National registries such as National Anesthesia Clinical Outcomes Registry (NACOR)[123] and Multicenter Perioperative Outcomes Group (MPOG)[124] are collecting data to help understand postoperative kidney and myocardial injury.

While many patient safety goals have quantifiable metrics, others focus on the quality of human interactions. Two current APSF priorities are encouraging anesthesiology departments to establish and maintain a "culture of safety" (Table 2-12), and to improve teamwork by collegial communication and multidisciplinary collaboration.[122] While these goals are fundamental, they can be incredibly hard to establish and are even more difficult to measure. National organizations can only define "culture of safety" and encourage individual anesthesiology departments to create such an environment. It is hospital systems, departments,

Table 2-12 Definitions

Culture of safety	The sum of what an organization is and does in the pursuit of safety.[3] A culture of safety is the "product of individual and group beliefs, values, attitudes, perceptions, competencies, and patterns of behavior that determine the organization's commitment to quality and patient safety."[4]
Psychological safety[5]	Individuals working in a psychologically safe environment feel comfortable admitting a mistake or asking for help and expect not to be punished. Speaking up, asking questions or presenting new ideas are welcomed, not undermined.[6]
Just culture	Imperfect humans function in imperfect systems. A core principle of just culture is shared accountability. Just cultures hold individual accountable, but avoid blaming them for system errors.[7,8]

and department leaders who must do the work of implementing and maintaining an environment that allows all providers to feel safe and secure when reporting and analyzing medical errors.

Focusing on the triple aim of health care, improving patient experience and population health while decreasing the per capita cost can place excessive emphasis on efficiency and productivity at the expense of patient safety. Production-focused organizations emphasize optimization and standardization but they can be resistant to change and error prone. They treat adverse events as anomalies and often respond by blaming the providers involved.[125] In contrast, high-reliability organizations (HROs) prioritize safety. They build redundant systems that are adaptable and flexible. They treat adverse events as information about potential system dysfunctions and reward the messenger. HROs recognize that humans are imperfect and work in imperfect settings.[126] They use principles of human factors engineering to optimize systems and processes to improve quality and safety and thereby prevent future adverse events.[127] Central to these efforts is an emphasis on psychological safety[128] and just culture.[129]

While committed leadership and well-designed systems are 10
crucial to creating and maintaining a robust safety culture, individual clinicians are key stakeholders and must be engaged in this process. For example, while it is up to department leaders to create easy-to-use reporting systems, establish the importance of reporting all nonroutine events, praise (and not punish) individuals for reporting, and then provide feedback on system changes based on reported events,[130,131] it is up to individual clinicians to recognize the importance of reporting these nonroutine events—and to actually do so.[125,132,133]

Regulatory

Anesthesia practices and health care facilities must comply with a multitude of standards and regulations set forth by various governmental and private organizations. In this section, we will review the implications of the rules proscribed by the Centers for Medicare and Medicaid Services (CMS), The Joint Commission (TJC), the Health Insurance Portability and Accountability Act of 1996 (HIPAA), and state agencies.

Center for Medicare and Medicaid Services

CMS conditions of participation defines and regulates all anesthesia services provided in a health care facility. CMS requires that anesthetic services must be appropriately organized under the guidance of a qualified doctor in medicine or osteopathy. The anesthesia director oversees the provision of all types of anesthesia and moderate sedation by qualified anesthesia care providers and nonanesthesia care providers alike (Fig. 2-5). The anesthesia

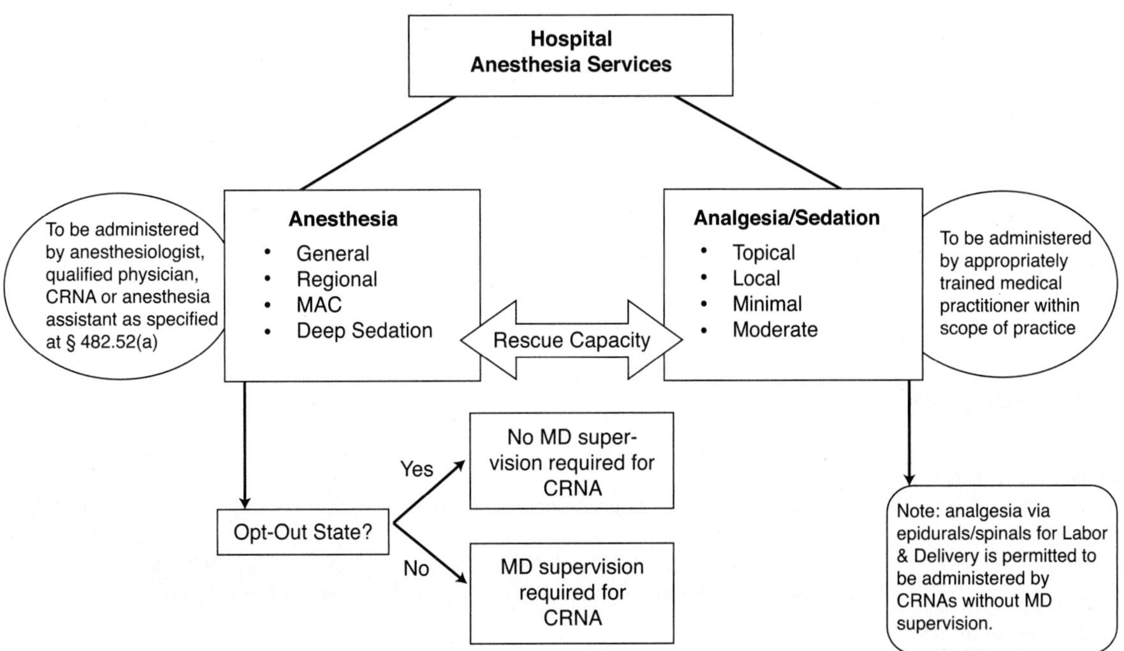

Figure 2-5 Organization of Hospital Anesthesia Services. (From CMA Manual System. Accessed from CMS.gov on June 1, 2022.)

director is responsible for all policies and procedures related to anesthesia services. This charge includes ensuring adequate staffing and aligning quality and improvement activities with those of the facility. The anesthesia director is also required to set minimal qualifications for nonanesthesia providers administering moderate sedation and approve their rescue plans.[134] Health care facilities must meet the conditions of participation to receive reimbursement from Medicare and Medicaid for services provided.

The conditions of participation also provide specific definitions of the elements of anesthesia care:

- Preanesthesia evaluation to be completed by an individual qualified to administer anesthesia within 48 prior to the induction of anesthesia. The preanesthesia evaluation is comprised of a review of the medical and anesthetic history, and the patient's medications and allergies. Interview and a focused physical examination of the patient that includes at least the airway and the cardiac and pulmonary systems. Documentation of the ASA physical status. Identification of potential anesthesia problems and contraindications. Ordering and review of any applicable tests. Last, documentation of the anesthesia plan detailing technique and medications to be used, additional procedures that may be necessary and discussion of risks and benefits with the patient or their surrogate.[134]
- Intraoperative anesthesia record for all general, regional, or monitored anesthesia care (MAC) cases. This anesthesia record must include the patient's name and medical record number, name(s) of all members of the anesthesia care team, an accurate report of all medications administered (name, dose, route, and time), anesthetic technique, patient's position, vascular access, airways, administration of intravenous fluids and blood products when applicable, and documentation of the vital signs on a time grid according to the ASA Standards of Monitoring. All complications and unexpected reactions must be clearly described in the anesthesia record including their management.[134]
- A postanesthesia evaluation to be completed by a qualified anesthesia provider once the patient has recovered sufficiently from the anesthetic to participate in the evaluation or is back at baseline. This evaluation must include assessment of airway patency, respiratory and cardiac functions, mental status, temperature, pain, nausea and vomiting, and hydration status. It must be completed within 48 hours after transfer to the recovery area or ICU, and once the above criteria are met.[134]

The Joint Commission

The Joint Commission (TJC) is an independent, not-for-profit organization founded in 1951. TJC sets standards for and accredits hospitals and a variety of health care facilities. Each accredited hospital is surveyed every 3 years. The surveyors evaluate a facility's compliance with the CMS and TJC standards to ensure that the care provided is safe, efficient, and effective. Recent surveys have focused compliance with National Patient Safety Goals (Table 2-13).[135] TJC also certifies hospitals as "Centers of Excellence" in areas like cardiovascular medicine, stroke care, and total joint arthroplasties. When reviewing anesthesia services, the TJC focuses on medication safety, infection control, and safe

Table 2-13 National Patient Safety Goals

Identify patients correctly NPSG.01.01.01	Use at least two ways to identify patients. For example, use the patient's name and date of birth. This is done to make sure that each patient gets the correct medicine and treatment.
Improve staff communication NPSG.02.03.01	Get important test results to the right staff person on time.
Use medicines safely	
NPSG.03.04.01	Before a procedure, label medicines that are not labeled. For example, medicines in syringes, cups and basins. Do this in the area where medicines and supplies are set up.
NPSG.03.05.01	Take extra care with patients who take medicines to thin their blood.
NPSG.03.06.01	Record and pass along correct information about a patient's medicines. Find out what medicines the patient is taking. Compare those medicines to new medicines given to the patient. Give the patient written information about the medicines they need to take. Tell the patient it is important to bring their up-to-date list of medicines every time they visit a doctor.
Use alarms safely NPSG.06.01.01	Make improvements to ensure that alarms on medical equipment are heard and responded to on time.
Prevent infection NPSG.07.01.01	Use the hand cleaning guidelines from the Centers for Disease Control and Prevention or the World Health Organization. Set goals for improving hand cleaning. Use the goals to improve hand cleaning.
Identify patient safety risks NPSG.15.01.01	Reduce the risk for suicide.
Prevent mistakes in surgery	
UP.01.01.01	Make sure that the correct surgery is done on the correct patient and at the correct place on the patient's body.
UP.01.02.01	Mark the correct place on the patient's body where the surgery is to be done.
UP.01.03.01	Pause before the surgery to make sure that a mistake is not being made.

2022 Hospital National Patient Safety Goals
The purpose of the National Patient Safety Goals is to improve patient safety. The goals focus on problems in health care safety and how to solve them.
From The Joint commission. *Who We Are.* Accessed June 2, 2022. www.jointcommission.org.

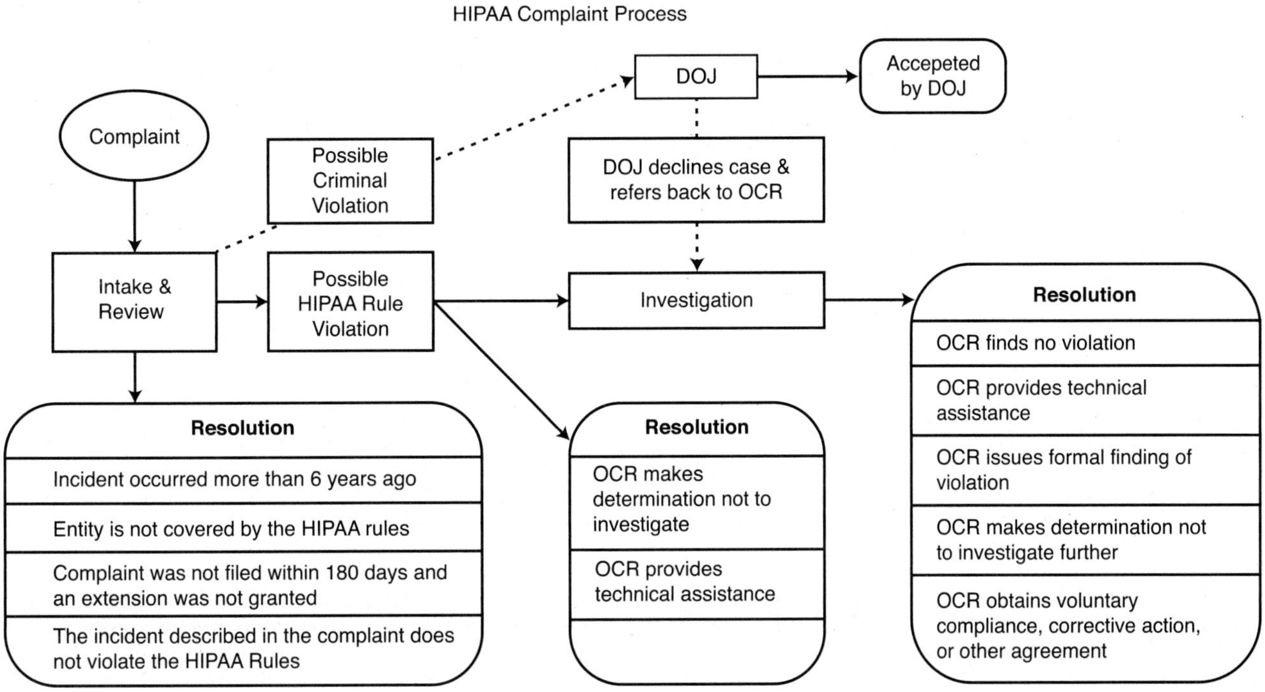

HIPAA Complaint Process

Complaint
Intake & Review
Possible Criminal Violation
Possible HIPAA Rule Violation
DOJ
Accepeted by DOJ
DOJ declines case & refers back to OCR
Investigation

Resolution
Incident occurred more than 6 years ago
Entity is not covered by the HIPAA rules
Complaint was not filed within 180 days and an extension was not granted
The incident described in the complaint does not violate the HIPAA Rules

Resolution
OCR makes determination not to investigate
OCR provides technical assistance

Resolution
OCR finds no violation
OCR provides technical assistance
OCR issues formal finding of violation
OCR makes determination not to investigate further
OCR obtains voluntary compliance, corrective action, or other agreement

Figure 2-6 HIPAA Complaint Process. Created by the Office for Civil Rights (OCR). (Last reviewed September 17, 2021. Viewed on HHS.gov on June 2, 2022.)

periprocedural care (i.e., right procedure for the right patient—Universal Protocol).

Health Insurance Portability and Accountability Act

Health matters are deeply personal. Physicians and other health care providers have a duty to protect a patient's privacy. The Health Insurance Portability and Accountability Act (HIPAA) of 1996 mandates the creation of standards to prevent personal health information (PHI) from being disseminated without a patient's consent. The law defines PHI and codifies the situations in which it can be shared.[136] HIPAA rules apply to health insurers, health care facilities, allied organizations (i.e., pharmacies), individual providers, and more. HIPAA is a living regulation that is constantly adapting to the changes in biomedical innovation, public health, and medical informatics.[137] Possible HIPAA violations may be investigated by the Federal Office of Civil Rights or the Department of Justice (Fig. 2-6).[138] Violators can face severe professional consequences, financial penalties, or criminal charges.

State Regulations

Health care organizations are also subject to individual state rules and regulations. These requirements are usually overseen by a Department of Public Health or equivalent. At times, state authorities can act on behalf of CMS.

Conclusion

11 Anesthesiology is unique among medical specialties. We work with complex machines, perform invasive procedures, and deliver potent medications. Only anesthesia providers prescribe, prepare, and administer potentially lethal medications without direct involvement of a pharmacist or other health care provider. For these reasons, and more, anesthesia departments are closely scrutinized by CMS, TJC, and state surveyors. Indepth knowledge of, and careful compliance with, federal and state rules and regulations are essential to avoid citations, penalties, and worse.

Support

The modern practice of anesthesia spans the continuum of health care. Anesthesia services are provided in ORs, obstetric units, interventional suites and radiology suites, ICUs, endoscopy units, pain clinics, free-standing ambulatory centers, and doctor's offices. Highly sophisticated equipment, including anesthesia machines, airway management tools, ultrasound machines, monitoring devices, rapid infusers, warming devices, smart infusion pumps, and computers (hardware and specialized software) are fundamental to the delivery of anesthetic care. In addition, delivering anesthetic care requires an extensive inventory of soft goods. Some reusable equipment requires high-level disinfection
or sterilization. A well-organized anesthesia department needs 12
the support of a variety of staff and services to allow clinicians to deliver patient care safely and efficiently.

Anesthesia technicians and technologists provide vital support. These personnel ensure that anesthetizing locations and equipment are cleaned, well-stocked, and ready for use.[139] They manage the inventory of the anesthesia supplies in coordination with a facility's materials and management staff. Depending on local, regional, and hospital regulations, training, and certification, they may have more critical duties including performing quality control and point-of-care testing, setting up and operating cell-saver devices, and disinfection or sterilization of reusable equipment. Until recently, these skills were learned on the job, often passed down from technician to technician. Anesthesia technicians often only completed high school, and few had specialized training. The American Society of Anesthesia Technologists and Technicians (ASATT) is working to raise the professional standards and education of these critical personnel.[140,141] As of December of 2021, there were 14 anesthesia technician schools offering degrees or certificates. However, only five are accredited by the Commission on Accreditation of Allied Health Education Programs (CAAHEP). Graduates from accredited programs can become certified by the ASATT.[141,142]

Modern anesthesia equipment is highly sophisticated and complex. It includes a wide range of machines and devices. Although anesthesia technicians often perform routine maintenance and troubleshooting, the complete care of the anesthesia equipment, both preventative and repairs, should be conducted by trained biomedical engineers.

Environmental Services staff, handle specialized disposal of all types of medical waste including needles, syringes, and other types of potentially dangerous or contaminated items. Central processing or sterilization departments perform high-level disinfection or sterilization of reusable anesthesia equipment that comes in contact with patient mucosae and body cavities including laryngoscopes, bronchoscopes, and transesophageal echocardiogram probes.

Every anesthesia department should have a close working relationship with their institution's informational technology (IT) and EHRs departments. Anesthesia information management systems (AIMS) better known as electronic anesthesia records should interface with all anesthesia delivery systems and monitoring equipment. Ideally a facility's AIMS will be fully integrated into its system-wide EHR. This arrangement can provide decision support and streamline workflows, freeing clinicians to concentrate on patient care instead of charting. AIMS are critical to the delivery of anesthetic care but must be appropriately supported by readily available and knowledgeable staff.

Pharmacy support is instrumental to safe anesthesia practice. Pharmacists are an excellent source of knowledge and advice. They can collaborate in the design and implementation of clinical pathways and protocols (i.e., ERAS), help with development of order sets, analyze new medications, and develop mitigation strategies for medication shortages. Pharmacists can also work with IT to integrate warnings and contraindications into the EHR/AIMS, collaborate on research projects, and more.

Finally, a full complement of professional office staff allows a well-structured anesthesia department to thrive clinically and financially. Their responsibilities include budgeting, billing, staffing, recruitment, and payroll. Other staff may be needed to support residency training or a research program.

In summary, a 21st century anesthesia department requires a variety of support to provide safe, timely, efficient, effective, equitable, and patient-centered care. Having a strong support system allows the anesthesia department to be a sustainable enterprise that adds value to the health system in which it operates.

Employment Markets

The future supply of and demand for anesthesiologists will likely be affected by changes in health care coverage, an aging population, the increasing number of women in the physician workforce, increasing cost pressures, and shifting modes of health care delivery. However, predicting the future employment prospects for anesthesiologists is a fraught exercise. A 1983 report predicted a shortfall of 2,700 anesthesiologists by 1990.[143] A few years later, the ASA commissioned a report by Abt Associates, Inc. entitled "Estimation of Physician Work Force Requirements in Anesthesiology."[144] Released in 1994, the so-called Abt Report predicted a gross oversupply of anesthesiologists. As a result, the number of U.S. medical school graduates choosing anesthesiology plummeted from 1609 in 1992 to a nadir of 493 in 1997. The number of anesthesia trainees subsequently rebounded, but the United States was still experiencing a significant shortage of anesthesiologists in 2004.[144] Subsequent reports suggested an ongoing shortage of anesthesiologists in 2007 but a small surplus in 2013.[145,146] Since then, the U.S. supply of anesthesiologists has steadily increased. Between 2016 and 2020, the number of U.S. anesthesiologists grew by 9%, outpacing the growth of other specialties (Fig. 2-7).[147] Although regional differences exist,[148] current reports suggest continued growth in both the supply of and demand for anesthesiologists (Figs. 2-8 and 2-9).[149]

13

Anesthesiologists with subspecialty training will likely also remain in high demand. However, employment prospects may vary by subspecialty. An analysis from 2018 predicted that the supply of pediatric anesthesiologists will increase from 5.4 anesthesiologists per 100,000 children to 7.4 pediatric anesthesiologists per 100,000 children by 2035. As a result, the average number of inpatient pediatric cases per pediatric anesthesiologist was predicted to decrease from 262 per year to 191 per year.[150] This trend may make it more difficult for new graduates to find employment in settings where they can care exclusively for pediatric patients. In contrast, the proposed stratification of maternal levels of care currently recommended by the American College

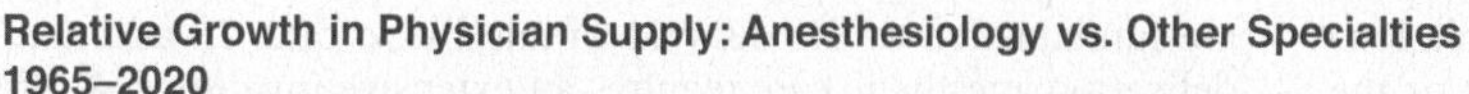

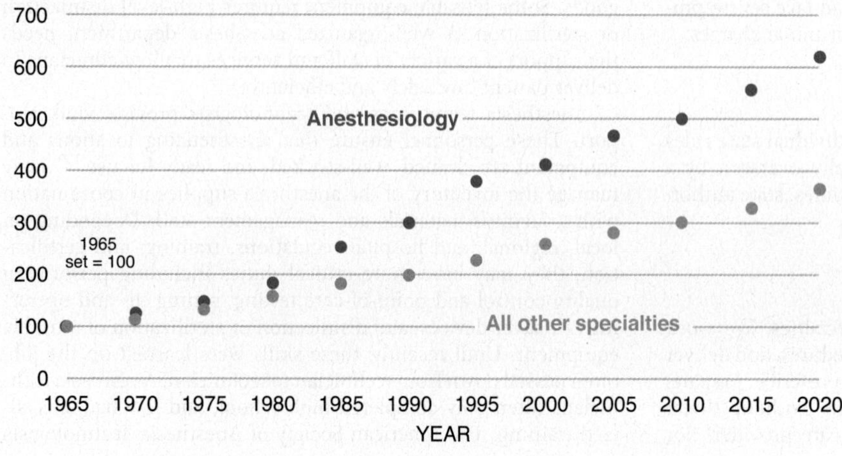

Figure 2-7 Relative growth in physician supply: Anesthesiology vs. other specialties. (Reprinted from Robinson DH, Toledo AH. Historical Development of Modern Anesthesia. *J Invest Surg*. 2012;25(3):141–149. With permission.)

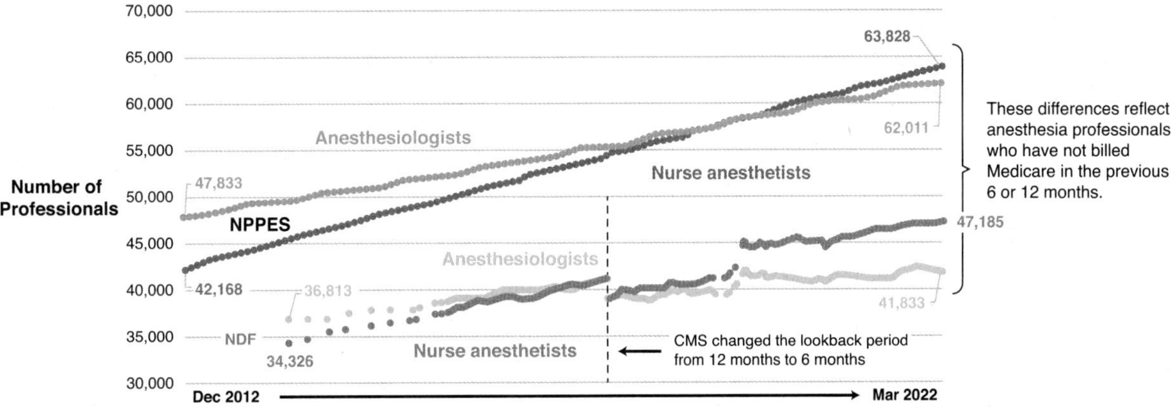

Figure 2-8 Growth in the number of anesthesiologists and nurse anesthetists from December 2012 to March 2022. (From ASA Open Forum—ASA Community. Accessed July 27, 2022. https://community.asahq.org/viewdocument/caws-anesthesia-workforce-trends.[2])

of Obstetrics and Gynecology is expected to markedly increase the demand for anesthesiologists with obstetric anesthesia fellowship training.[151]

Choosing a Practice

While the choice of your first practice is important, your first practice is unlikely to be your last. Up to 70% of physicians leave their first position within 5 years.[152] There are many resources that can help guide and inform your job search. Your personal network, be it friends, colleagues, family, or alumni, can introduce you to possible employers. Websites like Gaswork.com and the Anesthesiology Career Center[153] post active job listings. Journal advertisements and recruitment agencies provide other opportunities.

Carefully consider your personal and family priorities as you conduct your search. Where do you want to practice? East Coast? West Coast? City? Suburb? Rural? Are you interested in an academic or private practice? Do you want to work full-time or part-time? Will you be an independent contractor, partner, or employee? Will you be doing your own cases or supervising CRNAs or CAAs? Will you be teaching residents? What kind of cases will you be doing? Will you have nonclinical duties? If you want to do research, what kind of support is available?

Be sure you understand the financial terms of any job offer. What are the base salary and retirement benefits? Does your employer contribute to your retirement account? When do you qualify for those contributions? When are you vested? Will your employer provide health insurance? How much vacation time and sick time? Is there a sign-on bonus? What are the terms of the sign on bonus? Is there a moving stipend? How much "Continuing Medical Education" (CME) money is provided per year? If you are considering a practice that offers partnership, understand

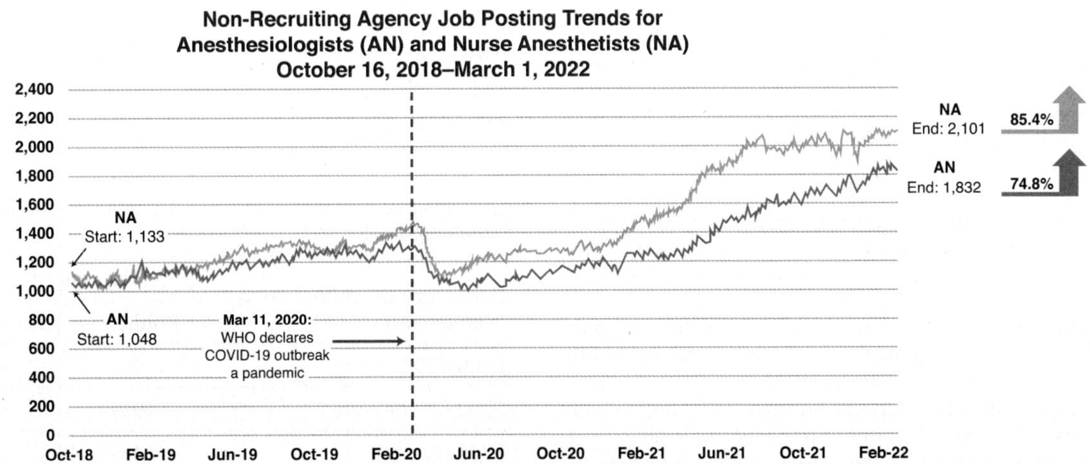

Figure 2-9 Monthly trends in Internet job postings for anesthesiologists and nurse anesthetists from October 2018 to February 2022. (Derived from ASA Open Forum—ASA Community. Accessed July 27, 2022. https://community.asahq.org/viewdocument/caws-anesthesia-workforce-trends.)

the terms. How long before partnership is offered? Is there a buy-in? How is the buy-in determined? Are there different classes of partner?

Those not ready to commit to a permanent position may work as a *locum tenens* (Latin meaning "to hold a place"). Here, the physician is a temporary worker. Locums positions may last from a week or two to several years. They may be full-time or part-time. Their major advantage is flexibility. Most locum tenens physicians are considered independent contractors, not employees. Unlike employees, independent contractors typically do not have taxes and benefits deducted from their pay. They are responsible for arranging and paying their own health insurance, retirement, and taxes.[154]

Regardless of the type of job or the location you choose, carefully read and understand your contract. A local health care attorney or a national service can help. One particular item to understand is a possible noncompete clause, which could limit your options for future employment should you choose to leave.[155]

Job offers are negotiable. Some items in the contract may be fixed (such as base salary), but other items might be negotiable. If using a recruitment agency, the agent can negotiate on your behalf; otherwise, it is acceptable to negotiate for yourself.[156] There are many resources available to help you refine your negotiation skills.[157]

Life Outside of Clinical Practice

Wellness and Burnout

Wellness and the prevention of burnout have become much-discussed topics. The Covid-19 pandemic only heightened the attention paid to these concerns.[158–160] The diagnosis of burnout, defined as "problems related to life management difficulty" first appeared in the 10th Revision of the World Health Organization's ICD-10.[161] The updated ICD-11 defines burnout as an occupational phenomenon resulting from chronic workplace stress. Burnout is characterized by three dimensions: (1) feelings of energy depletion; (2) increased mental distance from one's job; and (3) reduced professional efficacy.[162]

Risk factors for burnout include being a young physician, being female, and having children. Residents suffer higher rates of burnout compared to medical students and those who have completed their training. Some studies have reported that midcareer physicians have the highest rates of burnout, related to longer work hours, higher call burden and higher rates of emotional exhaustion. Late career physicians consistently report less burnout, felt to be a "survivor effect." Factors that can increase burnout include long work hours, number of nights on call per week, unclear job expectations, and a workplace culture that promotes bullying. Finally, personality traits such as neuroticism, anxiety, and use of negative coping strategies are associated with higher rates of burnout.[163]

14 Preventing or mitigating burnout requires a multitiered approach, and truly effective prevention and treatment strategies are yet to be identified.[164] Interventions are generally divided into individual or systems-based strategies. Examples of systems-based or institutional strategies include debriefing or peer support programs, ensuring anesthesiologists have access to mental health resources and substance use treatment resources. Institutions should promote culture of equity and wellness. Providing backup childcare has become an important response to pandemic-related school closures. Work-hour flexibility may also increase job satisfaction and prevent burnout.[165,166] Individual approaches to burnout include exercising regularly, eating a healthy diet, practicing meditation or mindfulness, resilience training, or using specific coping mechanisms. These individual strategies can help with burnout, but they are unlikely to be successful in isolation.[164]

Financial Wellness

Financial stress can be a major contributor to burnout. Many medical students are graduating with staggering amounts of debt, and some anesthesiologists delay saving for retirement for decades. In this environment, all physicians need a basic understanding 15 of personal finance. Although a detailed discussion is beyond the scope of this chapter, we will provide a brief overview and some helpful resources.

Important topics include:

1. Debt: student debt, mortgages, and high-interest credit card loans
2. Savings: retirement accounts, and taxable accounts
3. Protecting assets: personal and professional insurance

Useful resources include books, websites, and blogs.[167–170] In addition, professional financial advisors will be eager to help you manage your money. If you opt for professional assistance, understand how your advisor is paid. Some earn commission on the products they sell; others charge an annual percentage of the assets you have them manage, and others charge an hourly or annual retainer. These different financial arrangements can affect your advisor's incentives and may influence the advice you receive.[171]

Debt Burden and Debt Repayment

Attending college and medical school is expensive.[172] In 2021, approximately 73% of medical students graduated owing money. Their mean debt was $203,062. Almost 20% owed $300,000 or more (Table 2-14).[173] Managing this debt requires

Table 2-14 Medical Student Education: Costs, Debt, and Loan Repayment

Cost (in-state)	Public	Private
Tuition and fees, first-year (median)	$40,562	$65,650
Cost of attendance (COA), first-year (median)	$65,025	$90,138
4-y COA, class of 2022 (median)	$263,488	$357,868
Education debt	**Public**	**Private**
Percentage with education Debt	74%	70%
Median educational debt of indebted only	$195,000	$220,000
Education Debt (Including Premedical)	**Percentage of Graduates**	
	Public	**Private**
$100,000 or more	84%	82%
$200,000 or more	49%	59%
$300,000 or more	14%	27%

Source: American Association of Medical Colleges, Tuition and Student Fees Reports, 2021.[1]

careful planning and a thorough understanding of the available options.[174,175] Both the federal government and private organizations offer student loans. Federal loans often have lower interest rates than private loans and offer a variety of flexible repayment and loan-forgiveness options.[176] Federal loans may qualify for certain income-driven repayment (IDR) plans, which base monthly payments on income.[177] Physicians employed by a U.S. federal, state, local, or tribal government or not-for-profit organization, might quality for the Public Service Loan Forgiveness Program.[178] Private loans may offer fixed or variable interest rates and usually offer fewer options for deferred repayment. But, in some circumstances, private loans may be less expensive than federal ones.[179]

Savings, Budgeting, and Retirement Planning

Every anesthesiologist should have a basic understanding of saving, budgeting, and retirement planning. Albert Einstein allegedly called compound interest the eighth wonder of the world. Whether or not he was the source of this quote,[180] compound interest is a mechanism by which an individual can amass wealth. But compound interest requires time. Saving for retirement should start on your first day of work. Unfortunately, medical school graduates often start saving for retirement years after their fellow college graduates. The additional years of residency may further delay the time when most anesthesiologists start saving money. As a result, anesthesiologists must be even *more* financially savvy and save even more money to ensure a comfortable and timely retirement.

Learning to budget requires diligence. Newly graduated practitioners frequently spend too much of their increased income. When making a budget, consider your debt burden, total yearly expenses (both currently and anticipated in retirement), and the number of years you plan to work before retiring. Decide how much money to allocate to debt repayment and retirement savings. A simple rule suggests saving least 20% of your gross salary to ensure having enough money to retire comfortably.

Common retirement savings vehicles include individual retirement accounts (IRA), 401(k), 403(b), and 457(b) accounts. These accounts are funded by "pretax" dollars, money that is deducted from your salary **before** you pay income taxes. Instead, you will pay income taxes as you withdraw money from these accounts in retirement. In contrast, Roth accounts are funded with "post tax" dollars and subsequent withdrawals are tax free. Consider contributing to a Roth account when your current tax rate is lower than the expected tax rate in retirement (i.e., during training). Employers will often match your contributions to certain retirement accounts. Take full advantage of this "free-money." Health savings accounts, available to those with high-deductible health insurance plans, are another tax advantaged savings vehicle that can provide money for current and future medical expenses. Remember, money placed in retirement accounts is not available for other expenses. Early withdrawal will incur income taxes and penalties.[181]

Not all savings is for retirement. Consider setting aside enough money to cover 3 to 6 months of expenses in case of emergency (e.g., loss of job, unanticipated medical expenses). Owning a home can be an excellent way to build wealth but may require saving for a down payment. If you have children, consider contributing to a tax advantaged 529 savings plan.[182]

Most money set aside for savings should be invested in something other than a money market or savings account. Target funds, which adjust the ratio money invested in stocks or bonds over time are available for college and retirement savings accounts. These funds allocate more money to riskier, but potentially more profitable, stocks in the early years and then increase holdings in more stable, but lower yielding, bonds as the target date nears.[183] Target funds, while simple, are more expensive to own (i.e., they charge higher management fees, usually a percentage of the assets in the account), and do not provide the owner with any control over specific assets.

Mutual funds are a popular alternative to target funds. A mutual fund is a company that pools money from many investors to buy stocks, bonds, and short-term debt. The holdings of the mutual fund are known as its portfolio. Investors buy shares in mutual fund portfolios. Each share represents an investor's part ownership in the fund and the income it generates.[184] Mutual funds may be actively managed (active funds) or track a specific stock or bond index (index funds). Active funds use various investment strategies to try to maximize investment returns. Active funds charge higher management fees than index funds and have not proven to outperform the market over the long term.[185] In contrast, index funds match the investments in specific financial market (i.e., Standard & Poor's 500 Index (S&P 500) or the National Association of Securities Dealers Automated Quotations (NASDAQ) 100). Because they require less oversight, index funds usually charge lower management fees. Funds may invest in the broad stock market or in specific sectors (i.e., technology, health care, energy, etc.). When choosing a mutual fund, consider your risk tolerance and your timeline. Stocks outperform bonds over time but are more volatile. When choosing individual funds, consider their management fees.[186] Some investment firms currently offer index funds with no management fees.[187] Regardless of the funds you choose, remember, the best investment strategy is to "set it and forget it."[188,189]

Protecting Assets: Insurance

Most physicians do not think twice about obtaining automobile, homeowner's, or renter's insurance, yet they fail to insure their most valuable asset, themselves. To that end, there are a few types of insurance that all anesthesiologists should have.

Disability Insurance

Disability insurance pays you a percentage of your income if you are unable to work for an extended period because of an illness or injury. As many as one in seven physicians has to use disability insurance.[190] Disability policies usually exclude preexisting medical conditions. As a result, you should purchase your policy when you are young and, hopefully, healthy. Many disability insurance carriers offer discounts to trainees, allowing them to purchase the minimum monthly coverage with the option to add coverage as salary increases.

Both group and individual policies are available. Employers and professional organizations offer group disability insurance.[191] Group disability insurance is generally cheaper and can be a good option for those with a preexisting medical condition. Individual disability insurance has the advantage of being "portable" (it belongs to you, regardless of where you work). Many companies sell individual disability insurance. An independent insurance agent can help you choose among the many options. Understand the terms of your individual policy. Is it noncancelable? Is the premium guaranteed? Does it cover your occupation (i.e., a physician) or your specialty (anesthesiologist)? How long must you be unable to work before benefits begin? How long do the benefits last? Is the benefit taxable income? Does it cover disability due to mental health or substance use disorders? Does it offer a future increase option? Partial disability coverage? Inflation protection? Catastrophic disability coverage? Disability policies can be more expensive for women, a 'unisex' policy may be less expensive.[190]

Life Insurance

A life insurance policy pays money if you die. That money can be used to support those (partner, children, etc.) who rely on your income. There are different types of life insurance policies. Whole life, variable life, or universal life insurance policies blend insurance and investing and are more expensive than term-life insurance. A term policy insures your life for a set number of years (usually 30), for a fixed premium. The premium is based on your age at the time of purchase. There are different views as to what type of life insurance policy is best for physicians. While an independent insurance agent can help you choose among the many options,[192,193] you need to be well informed and understand your particular situation to make the best decision.

Malpractice Insurance

Medical malpractice insurance, also known as professional liability insurance, protects physicians against lawsuits related to acts and omissions that occur while caring for patients. Policies are often in the millions of dollars, described as (for example) $2 million/$4 million—where the first number applies to the coverage per case and the second number is the total amount the insurance company could pay out per year.[194]

For most physicians, the malpractice insurance provider is selected by and paid for by their employer. There are two main types of malpractice insurance: claims-made and occurrence. Claims-made policies are more common and cover events that occur while the policy is active (starting with the date the policy went into effect) and are also reported while the policy is still active. Occurrence policies cover events that take place while the policy is active but may be reported after the policy is no longer in force. Since claims-made policies cover only events that both occur and are reported while the policy is in effect, you will also need prior acts ("nose") and extended reporting ("tail") coverage. The "nose" covers events that occurred before the period of coverage while the "tail" insures events occurring during the period of coverage but reported after the coverage ends. If your employer has a claims-made policy, understand who is responsible for "nose" and "tail" coverage. Confirm that the employer will cover the tail policy if you leave.[195]

Umbrella Insurance

Umbrella insurance is extra liability insurance that provides protection beyond existing limits and coverages of your other policies. Umbrella insurance also can provide coverage for claims that are to be excluded by your other liability policies. Umbrella insurance policies are relatively inexpensive. Discounts are often available if you purchase auto, home, and umbrella policies from the same company.[196]

The Future

Global and Public Health

The Lancet Commission on Global Surgery from 2015 highlighted the disparities that limit access to surgical and anesthetic care in low-to-middle-income countries (LMICs). A major deficiency is a lack of trained anesthesia providers.[197] Consequently, global health organizations have shifted their focus from short-term "mission" trips to building education and training programs for clinicians living and working in LMICs with the goal building sustainable capacity in the local health care system.[198–200] U.S. trained anesthesiologists participate in these global health efforts for many reasons. First is simple altruism, believing that every patient deserves safe anesthesia care. Engaging in global health educational projects also provides professional benefit. One not only teaches others, but also learns the perspective of those practicing in a vastly different setting. Finally, participating in cross-cultural activities enriches one's own life.[201] Local, national, and international organizations provide avenues for engaging in global health projects.[202–204]

In the aftermath of the COVID-19 pandemic, it should be clear that global health is public health. Addressing worldwide health care disparities requires confronting U.S. health care inequities as well.[205,206] Including a health equity curriculum in residency training is an important step in solving these problems.[207–209]

Green or "Clean" Anesthesia

Climate change is a global reality. Health care produces 5% to 8% of global greenhouse gas emissions.[210,211] National and international anesthesia societies have begun to address this problem.[212] Inhaled anesthetics, including nitrous oxide, are potent greenhouse gases and account for about 3% of the total health care-related climate footprint and up to 50% of the climate impact of surgical care.[213,214] Atmospheric lifetimes of inhaled agents range from 1 to 5 years for sevoflurane to 114 years for nitrous oxide (Table 2-15).[213,212] Strategies to reduce the environmental impact of inhaled anesthetics include using efficient ventilation and scavenging systems, ensuring anesthesia equipment is well-maintained, avoiding the use of desflurane and nitrous oxide, minimizing fresh gas flow rates, and using total intravenous anesthesia.[214]

US hospitals produce over 5 million tons of waste each year. An estimated 20% to 30% of that waste is produced in the OR.[212,210,215] Single-use plastics used to provide anesthesia care, including face masks, breathing circuits, and intravenous tubing, comprise about one quarter of this environmentally damaging waste.[216] Up to 60% of this waste is recyclable.[210,217,218] The mantra "reduce, reuse, recycle" can provide a useful framework for addressing the problem of medical waste (Fig. 2-10).[216,210,219,220]

Artificial Intelligence and the Future of Anesthesia Care

Artificial intelligence (AI) and machine learning are emerging technologies that will likely have significant future impacts on the provision of anesthesia care. AI is study of algorithms that give machines the ability to problem-solve and make decisions.[221] Machine learning is a tool that is helping drive the development of AI.[222] Current anesthesia-related AI research is focusing on:[223]

- depth of anesthesia monitoring,
- control of anesthesia,
- event and risk prediction (for example, prediction of postoperative mortality or prediction of hypotension)[224]
- ultrasound guidance,[225]
- pain management, and
- OR logistics.

While AI can provide a staggering amount of information, precisely what to do with this data and when and how to act on it are still largely unknown. The accuracy of an algorithm is only as good as its inputs.[226] Obtaining reliable information can be challenging when caring for complex patients in dynamic surgical situations.[227] In a specialty where mistakes can be deadly, any machine-learning approach must be perfect.[222] A potential downside to the widespread adoption of AI is the "deskilling" of clinicians as practice shifts to rely on automated processes.[226] Nonetheless, AI and machine learning will be a part of our future as practicing anesthesiologists.

Table 2-15 Greenhouse Gas Emissions of Common Inhaled Anesthetics

1 MAC Agent at Various Fresh Gas Flows (FGF)	Atmospheric Life (y)	100-y Global Warming Potential (GWP)[a]	CO_2 Equivalents	Equivalent Auto Miles per Hour of Anesthetic Use
Sevoflurane @ 2L FGF	1.1	130	1.0	8
Sevoflurane @ 1L FGF			0.5	4
Isoflurane @ 2L FGF	3.2	510	2.2	18
Isoflurane @ 1L FGF			1.1	9
Desflurane @ 2L FGF	14	2,540	49.2	400
Desflurane @ 1L FGF			24.6	200
60% N2O @ 1L FGF	114	298		61

[a]BWP per kg compared with CO_2, where CO_2 = 1.
MAC, minimum alveolar concentration.
Modified from Axelrod D, et al. Greening the Operating Room. https://www.asahq.org/about-asa/governance-and-committees/asa-committees/environmental-sustainability/greening-the-operating-room

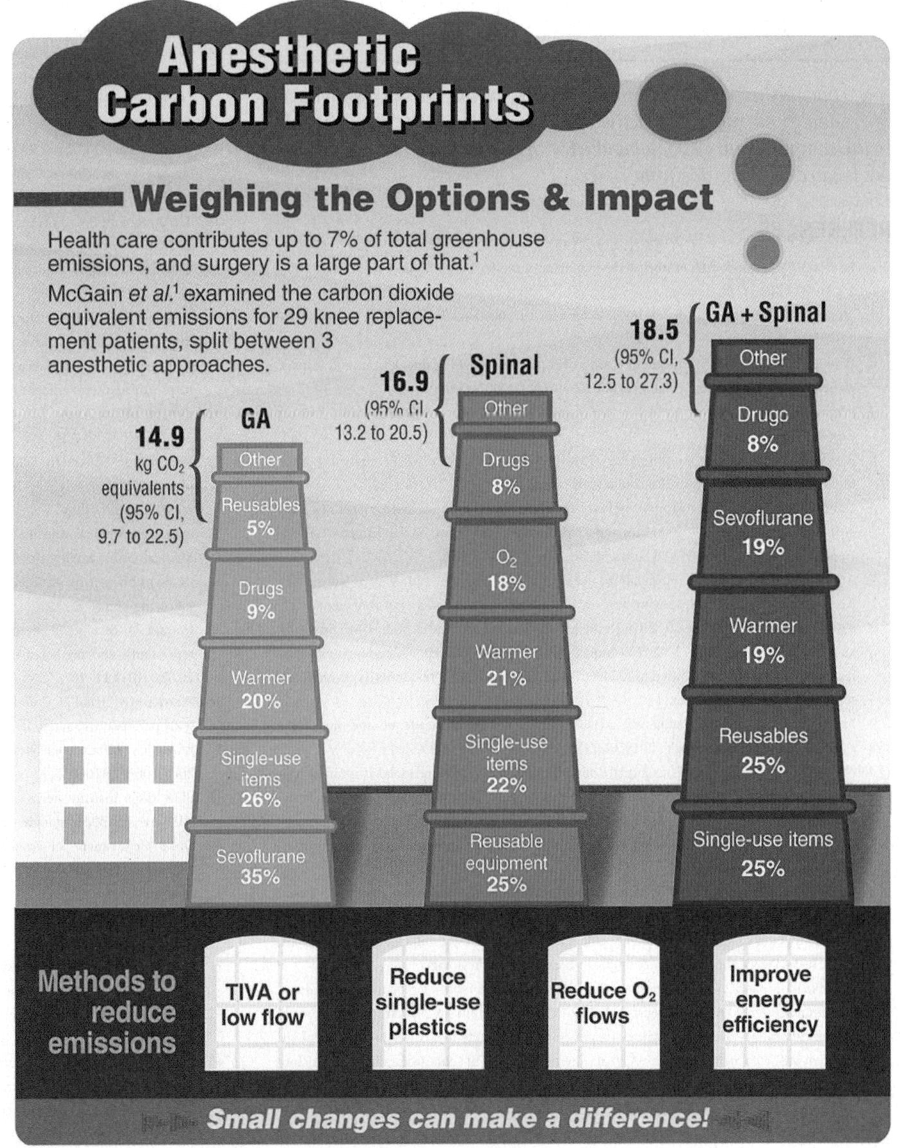

Figure 2-10 Anesthetic carbon footprints: weighing the options and impact. (Reprinted with permission from Wanderer JP, Rathmell JP. Anesthetic carbon footprints: Weighing the options and impact. *Anesthesiology*. 2021;135:A15. doi: https://doi.org/10.1097/ALN.0000000000004070)

Conclusion

It has been a fruitful journey in the years since Morton's demonstration at the Ether Dome in Massachusetts. Much has been accomplished yet more remains to be done. Anesthesiology today is stronger than ever, with multiple accredited and nonaccredited subspecialties that span the continuum of medical care. We no longer confine ourselves to the operating theater. In the coming years, we must continue to expand our sphere of influence beyond the surgical act. We must focus on relieving all types of pain, while decreasing the role of opiates. Just as advancements in anesthesia helped advance of surgical care, we will now do the same for other interventional fields. We should collaborate with surgeons in developing and instituting ERAS protocols and use our broad understanding of patient care to become leaders of PSHs. While we continue to advance and evolve as a specialty that prioritizes the safety and functional recovery of our patients, we must not forget to care for our most precious resource, ourselves. We need to promote wellness in the workplace. The future presents challenges, yet it is bright, so long as we as a specialty rise to the task and adapt to the ever-changing environment of health care.

For additional information please see NICV 2-1 in the eBook bundled with this text.

For further review and interactivities, please see the videos and narrative interactive clinical vignettes (NICVs) accessible in the complimentary eBook bundled with this text. Access instructions are located on the inside front cover.

REFERENCES

1. Robinson DH, Toledo AH. Historical development of modern anesthesia. *J Invest Surg*. 2012; 25(3):141–149.
2. McGoldrick KE. The history of professionalism in anesthesiology. *AMA J Ethics*. 2015; 17(3):258–264.
3. Wanderer JP, Rathmell JP. Anesthetic Carbon Footprints: Weighing the Options and Impact. *Anesthesiology*. 2021;135:A15. doi.org/10.1097/ALN.0000000000004070
4. Ahmad M, Tariq R. History and Evolution of Anesthesia Education in United States. *J Anesth Clin Res*. 2017;8:734.
5. Residency Programs List. Anesthesiology Residency Programs. Accessed February 17, 2022. https://www.residencyprogramslist.com/anesthesiology2022
6. Condon-Rall ME. A brief history of military anesthesia. In: *Anesthesia and Perioperative Care of the Combat Casualty*. R. Zaitchuk and C.M Grande, eds. Office of the Surgeon General Department of the Army, United States of America; 1995:855–896.
7. Anesthesia Patient Safety Foundation. APSF History, Mission and Vision Statements. Accessed June 2, 2022. https://www.apsf.org/about-apsf/mission-and-vision-statements/
8. AAMC. Table B3. Number of Active Residents, by Type of Medical School, GME Specialty, and Sex. Accessed June 2, 2022. https://www.aamc.org/data-reports/students-residents/interactive-data/report-residents/2021/table-b3-number-active-residents-type-medical-school-gme-specialty-and-sex
9. Bissing MA, Lange EM, Davila WF, et al. Status of women in academic anesthesiology: a 10-year update. *Anesth Analg*. 2019;128(1):137–143.
10. Nwokolo OO, Coombs AAT, Eltzschig HK, Butterworth JFI. Diversity and inclusion in anesthesiology. *Anesth Analg*. 2022;134(6):1166–1174. https://journals.lww.com/anesthesia-analgesia/Fulltext/2022/06000/Diversity_and_Inclusion_in_Anesthesiology.9.aspx
11. Malinzak EB, Thompson A, Straker T. Examining diversity in anesthesiology grand rounds. *ASA Monit*. 2020;84(5):38–40.
12. Stanford FC. The importance of diversity and inclusion in the healthcare workforce. *J Natl Med Assoc*. 2020;112(3):247–249.
13. American Board of Medical Specialties. American Board of Anesthesiology. Accessed May 16, 2022. https://www.abms.org/board/american-board-of-anesthesiology/
14. Kukafka JD, Milas BL. Cardiac Anesthesiology. In: *A Guide to Anesthesiology for Medical Students*. American Society of Anesthesiologists; 2018:32–33. Accessed June 23, 2022. https://www.asahq.org/education-and-career/asa-medical-student-component/guide-to-a-career-in-anesthesiology
15. Cahalan MK, Stewart W, Pearlman A, et al. American society of echocardiography and society of cardiovascular anesthesiologists task force guidelines for training in perioperative echocardiography. *J Am Soc Echocardiogr*. 2002;15(6):647–652.
16. Boston Children's Hospital. Cardiac Anesthesia Services. Accessed July 7, 2022. https://dme.childrenshospital.org/cardiac-anesthesia-services-fellowship/
17. American Society of Anesthesiologists. Guide to a Career in Anesthesiology. Accessed July 11, 2022. https://www.asahq.org/education-and-career/asa-medical-student-component/guide-to-a-career-in-anesthesiology
18. American College of Obstetricians and Gynecologists. Levels of Maternal Care. Accessed July 10, 2022. https://www.acog.org/en/clinical/clinical-guidance/obstetric-care-consensus/articles/2019/08/levels-of-maternal-care
19. Hernandez A, Behringer EC. Critical care anesthesiolgists. In: *A Guide to Anesthesiology for Medical Students*. American Society of Anesthesiologists; 2018:43–44. Accessed June 23, 2022. https://www.asahq.org/education-and-career/asa-medical-student-component/guide-to-a-career-in-anesthesiology
20. Rathmell JP. Pain medicine. In: *A Guide to Anesthesiology for Medical Students*. American Society of Anesthesiologists; 2018:36–37. Accessed June 24, 2022. https://www.asahq.org/education-and-career/asa-medical-student-component/guide-to-a-career-in-anesthesiology
21. Jaffe RA. Neuroanesthesia. In: *A Guide to Anesthsiology for Medical Students*. American Society of Anesthesiologists; 2018:34. Accessed June 24, 2022. https://www.asahq.org/education-and-career/asa-medical-student-component/guide-to-a-career-in-anesthesiology
22. Neurocritical Care Society. About the NCS. Accessed June 23, 2022. https://www.neurocriticalcare.org/about/about-ncs
23. American Society of Anesthesiologists. What is trauma anesthesiology. Accessed June 28, 2022. https://www.asahq.org/about-asa/governance-and-committees/asa-committees/committee-on-trauma-and-emergency-preparedness-cotep/trauma-anesthesiology/what-is-trauma-anesthesiology
24. Adelmann D, Kronish K, Ramsay MA. Anesthesia for liver transplantation. *Anesthesiol Clin*. 2017;35(3):491–508.
25. Walsh MT. Ambulatory anesthesia. *Anesthesiol Clin*. 2019;37(2):xv–xvi.
26. Anesthesia Patient Safety Foundation. Safety in Non-Operating Room Anesthesia (NORA). Accessed May 12, 2022. https://www.apsf.org/article/safety-in-non-operating-room-anesthesia-nora/
27. Nagrebetsky A, Gabriel RA, Dutton RP, Urman RD. Growth of nonoperating room anesthesia care in the United States: A contemporary trends analysis. *Anesth Analg*. 2017;124(4): 1261–1267.
28. The American Board of Anesthesiology. Subspecialty Certification Exams. Accessed June 23, 2022. https://theaba.org/subspecialty%20certification%20exams.html
29. Gebauer S. Hospice and palliative medicine as a specialty option for anesthesiologists. *ASA Monit*. 2016;80(10):8–9.
30. Brigham and Women's Hospital. Addiction Medicine Fellowship. Accessed June 23, 2022. https://www.brighamandwomens.org/psychiatry/fellowships/addiction-medicine-fellowship
31. The American Board of Anesthesiology. Combined Training Programs. Accessed July 7, 2022. https://theaba.org/combined%20training%20programs.html
32. Grocott MPW, Pearse RM. Perioperative medicine: the future of anaesthesia? *Br J Anaesth*. 2012;108(5):723–726.
33. Washington University School of Medicine in St. Louis. Fellowship Overview. Anesthesiology. Accessed July 13, 2022. https://anesthesiology.wustl.edu/patient-care/perioperative-medicine/fellowship/
34. American Medical Informatics Association. Clinical Informatics Becomes a Board-certified Medical Subspecialty Following ABMS Vote. Accessed July 5, 2022. https://amia.org/news-publications/clinical-informatics-becomes-board-certified-medical-subspecialty-following-abms
35. Detmer D, Munger B, Lehmann C. Clinical informatics board certification: history, current status, and predicted impact on the clinical informatics workforce. *Appl Clin Inform*. 2010;01(01):11–18.
36. Warner MA, Arnal D, Cole DJ, et al. Anesthesia patient safety: next steps to improve worldwide perioperative safety by 2030. *Anesth Analg*. 2022;135(1):6–19.
37. Reves JG. We are what we make: transforming research in anesthesiology. *Anesthesiology*. 2007;106(4):826–835.
38. Blue Ridge Institute for Medical Research. Accessed July 19, 2022. https://www.brimr.org/NIH_Awards/2021/#google_vignette
39. Duke Department of Anesthesiology. Integrated Training in Anesthesiology Research (NIH T32 GM08600). Accessed July 19, 2022. https://anesthesiology.duke.edu/research/integrated-training
40. Washington University in St. Louis. Research. Accessed July 19, 2022. https://anesthesiology.wustl.edu/research/
41. American Society of Anesthesiologists. Training Grants. Accessed July 19, 2022. https://www.asahq.org/research-and-publications/research-and-grant-funding/training-grants
42. American Society of Anesthesiologists (ASA). Grants. Accessed July 19, 2022. https://www.asahq.org/faer/grants
43. IARS. Grants and Awards. Accessed July 19, 2022. https://iars.org/research-awards/
44. Schneider EC, Shah A, Doty MM, Tikkanen R, Fields K, Williams II RD. *Mirror, Mirror 2021: Reflecting Poorly*. Commonwealth Fund; 2021.

45. Berwick DM, Nolan TW, Whittington J. The triple aim: care, health, and cost. *Health Aff (Millwood)*. 2008;27(3):759–769.
46. Bodenheimer T, Sinsky C. From triple to quadruple aim: care of the patient requires care of the provider. *Ann Fam Med*. 2014;12(6):573–576.
47. Nundy S, Cooper LA, Mate KS. The quintuple aim for health care improvement: a new imperative to advance health equity. *JAMA*. 2022;327(6):521–522.
48. Porter ME. What Is Value in Health Care? *N Engl J Med*. 2010;363(26):2477–2481.
49. American Society of Anesthesiologists. Perioperative Surgical Home (PSH) Overview. Accessed June 2, 2022. https://www.asahq.org/psh/aboutpsh
50. Garson L, Schwarzkopf R, Vakharia S, et al. Implementation of a total joint replacement- focused perioperative surgical home: a management case report. *Anesth Analg*. 2014;118(5):1081–1089.
51. Qiu C, Rinehart J, Nguyen VT, et al. An Ambulatory surgery perioperative surgical home in Kaiser permanente settings: practice and outcomes. *Anesth Analg*. 2017;124(3):768–774.
52. Raphael DR, Cannesson M, Schwarzkopf R, et al. Total joint perioperative surgical home: an observational financial review. *Perioper Med Lond*. 2014;3(1):6–6.
53. Elhassan A, Elhassan I, Elhassan A, et al. Perioperative surgical home models and enhanced recovery after surgery. *J Anaesthesiol Clin Pharmacol*. 2019;35(Suppl 1):S46–S50.
54. ERAS Society. History. Accessed June 2, 2022. https://erassociety.org/about/history/
55. Smith TW, Wang X, Singer MA, Godellas CV, Vaince FT. Enhanced recovery after surgery: a clinical review of implementation across multiple surgical subspecialties. *Am J Surg*. 2020;219(3):530–534.
56. ERAS Society. Specialties. Accessed June 2, 2022. https://erassociety.org/specialties/
57. American Society of Anesthesiologists. Policy Statement on Practice Parameters. Accessed June 2, 2022. https://www.asahq.org/standards-and-guidelines/policy-statement-on-practice-parameters
58. Conroy JM, Lubarsky D, Newman MF. Anesthesiologists as Health System Leaders: Why It Works. *Anesth Analg*. 2022;134(2):235–240. https://journals.lww.com/anesthesia-analgesia/Fulltext/2022/02000/Anesthesiologists_as_Health_System_Leaders__Why_It.3.aspx
59. American Society of Anesthesiologists. ASA Home. Accessed June 2, 2022. https://www.asahq.org/
60. Accreditation Council for Graduate Medical Education. Overview. Accessed June 2, 2022. https://www.acgme.org/what-we-do/overview/
61. ACGME. ACGME International Home. Accessed June 2, 2022. https://www.acgme-i.org/
62. ACGME. Overview. Accessed June 2, 2022. https://www.acgme.org/specialties/anesthesiology/overview/
63. American Medical Association. Anesthesiology programs with the most residency positions. Accessed June 2, 2022. https://www.ama-assn.org/residents-students/residency/anesthesiology-programs-most-residency-positions
64. The American Board of Anesthesiology. ABA Home. Accessed June 4, 2022. https://theaba.org/index.html
65. The American Board of Anesthesiology. Traditional Certification Exams. Accessed June 4, 2022. https://theaba.org/traditional%20certification%20exams.html
66. The American Board of Anesthesiology. Staged Exams. Accessed June 4, 2022. https://theaba.org/staged%20exams.html
67. The American Board of Anesthesiology. Certification Exams. Accessed June 4, 2022. https://theaba.org/certifications%20and%20exms.html
68. The American Board of Anesthesiology. Certification Exams. Accessed June 4, 2022. https://theaba.org/certifications%20and%20exms.html#ASPEX
69. The American Board of Anesthesiology. MOCA. Accessed June 4, 2022. https://theaba.org/moca.html
70. The American Board of Anesthesiology. The ABA's Statement on ABMS Standards for Continuing Certification. Published November 10, 2021. Accessed June 4, 2022. https://abathelatest.org/2021/11/the-abas-statement-on-abms-standards-for-continuing-certification/
71. World Health Organization. International Classification of Diseases (ICD). Accessed February 14, 2022. https://www.who.int/standards/classifications/classification-of-diseases
72. AAPC. US gets the ball rolling on ICD-11. AAPC Knowledge Center. 2019. Accessed February 14, 2022. https://www.aapc.com/blog/48275-us-gets-the-ball-rolling-on-icd-11/
73. Journal Of AHIMA. Highlights of the 2021 CPT Code Updates. Published January 11, 2021. Accessed February 14, 2022. https://journal.ahima.org/highlights-of-the-2021-cpt-code-updates/
74. Morewood G, Cohen NH, Merrick SK. Anesthesia Practice Finances, 2030. *ASA Monit*. 2021;85(S10):24–26.
75. Becker ER, Dunn D, Braun P, Hsiao WC. Refinement and expansion of the Harvard Resource-Based Relative Value Scale: the second phase. *Am J Public Health*. 1990;80(7):799–803.
76. Merrick SK. Physical status and qualifying circumstances. *ASA Monit*. 2021;85(12):38.
77. American Society of Anesthesiologists. Anesthesia Payment Basics Series: #2 Anesthesia Coding Resources. Published July 2019. Accessed February 14, 2022. https://www.asahq.org/quality-and-practice-management/managing-your-practice/timely-topics-in-payment-and-practice-management/anesthesia-payment-basics-series-2-anesthesia-coding-resources
78. *2020 Relative Value Guide® A Guide for Anesthesia Values*. American Society of Anesthesiologists®; 2019.
79. American Society of Anesthesiologists. MACRA and You. Accessed February 14, 2022. https://www.asahq.org/macra/macraandyou
80. American Society of Anesthesiologists. MIPS. Accessed February 14, 2022. https://www.asahq.org/macra/qualitypaymentprogram/mips
81. Martin DP, Salcedo V, Merrick SK. Rescanning the alternative payment model horizon for physician anesthesiologists. *ASA Monit*. 2021;85(6):38–39.
82. Werner RM, Emanuel E, Pham HH, Navathe AS. The Future of Value Based Payment: A Road Map to 2030. White Paper. Feb 2021. Published online February 2021.
83. Byrd JN, Chung KC. Evaluation of the merit-based incentive payment system and surgeons caring for patients at high social risk. *JAMA Surg*. 2021;156(11):1018–1024.
84. Khullar D, Schpero WL, Bond AM, Qian Y, Casalino LP. Association between patient social risk and physician performance scores in the first year of the merit-based incentive payment system. *JAMA*. 2020;324(10):975–983.
85. Advisory Board. How do physicians get paid? (Hint: It's mostly not value-based.). Published February 1, 2022. Accessed February 3, 2023. https://www.advisory.com/Daily-Briefing/2022/02/01/physician-compensation
86. CMS. Anesthesiologists Center. Accessed February 14, 2022. https://www.cms.gov/Center/Provider-Type/Anesthesiologists-Center
87. Deaprtment of Justice. The False Claims Act. Published June 17, 2019. Accessed February 17, 2022. https://www.justice.gov/civil/false-claims-act
88. Anesthesia Billing. Anesthesia modifier Modifier QK, Modifier QS, Modifier QX, Modifier QY & Modifier QZ. Accessed February 14, 2022. http://www.anesthesiabilling.org/2010/05/anethesia-billing-modifier-qk-qx-and.html
89. Erin L, Duffy P, Bich Ly BA, Loren Adler MS, Erin Trish P. Commercial and Medicare Advantage Payment for Anesthesiology Services. Published June 16, 2021. Accessed February 14, 2022. https://www.ajmc.com/view/commercial-and-medicare-advantage-payment-for-anesthesiology-services
90. Stead SW, Merrick SK. ASA survey results: commercial fees paid for anesthesia services, 2020. *ASA Monit*. 2020;84(10):1–29.
91. Pauker KY. A History of RBRVS as a Perspective on P4P. Published 2006. Accessed February 14, 2022. https://www.csahq.org/docs/default-source/history-of-anesthesia-articles/history-articles/pauker-a-history-of-rbrvs-part2-2006.pdf?sfvrsn=d864c146_2
92. Pregler J, Saluja V, Vaidyanathan M, et al. The 33% problem: Origins and Actions Committee on Economics 33% Workgroup Report ASA Economic Strategic Plan Initiative—October 2020. *ASA Monit*. 2020;84(12):28–33.
93. O'Connell C, Dexter F, Mauler DJ, Sun EC. Trends in direct hospital payments to anesthesia groups: a retrospective cohort study of nonacademic hospitals in California. *Anesthesiology*. 2019;131(3):534–542. doi:10.1097/ALN.0000000000002819
94. A Penned Point. Anesthesia practices in peril when hospitals lose money. Accessed February 14, 2022. https://apennedpoint.com/anesthesia-practices-in-peril-when-hospitals-lose-money/
95. Cuellar H. H.R.133 - Consolidated Appropriations Act, 2021. Published December 27, 2020. Accessed February 14, 2022. https://www.congress.gov/bill/116th-congress/house-bill/133/text
96. American Society of Anesthesiologists. American Society of Anesthesiologists, American College of Emergency Physicians, and American College of Radiology File Lawsuit Against the Federal Government's Implementation Rules for 'No Surprises Act.' Accessed February 14, 2022. https://www.asahq.org/about-asa/newsroom/news-releases/2021/12/lawsuit-against-no-surprises-act
97. Blue Cross Blue Shield of North Carolina Rate Reduction Notice. Published online November 5, 2021.
98. Nalley C. Payment Progress Series, Part 3: ASA initiatives to secure your economic future: abusive insurer negotiation techniques. *ASA Monit*. 2021;85(7):18–18.
99. La Forgia A, Bond AM, Braun RT, Kjaer K, Zhang M, Casalino LP. Association of surprise-billing legislation with prices paid to in-network and out-of-network anesthesiologists in California, Florida, and New York: an economic analysis. *JAMA Intern Med*. 2021;181(10):1324–1331.
100. American Society of Anesthesiologists. Payment Progress. Accessed February 25, 2022. https://www.asahq.org/advocating-for-you/payment-progress
101. Knight PR, Bacon DR. An unexplained death: Hannah Greener and Chloroform. *Anesthesiology*. 2002;96(5):1250–1253.
102. Beecher HK, Todd DP. A study of the deaths associated with anesthesia and surgery: based on a study of 599, 548 anesthesias in ten institutions 1948–1952, inclusive. *Ann Surg*. 1954;140(1):2–35.
103. Warner MA, Warner ME. The evolution of the anesthesia patient safety movement in america: lessons learned and considerations to promote further improvement in patient safety. *Anesthesiology*. 2021;135(6):963–974.
104. Pierce EC Jr. The 34th Rovenstine Lecture: 40 Years behind the mask: safety revisited. *Anesthesiology*. 1996;84(4):965–975.
105. American Society of Anesthesiologists. Standards for Basic Anesthetic Monitoring. Accessed June 9, 2022. https://www.asahq.org/standards-and-guidelines/standards-for-basic-anesthetic-monitoring

106. Anesthesia Quality Institute. About closed claims program. Accessed June 13, 2022. https://www.aqihq.org/ACCMain.aspx
107. Cheney FW. The American Society of Anesthesiologists Closed Claims Project: What have we learned, how has it affected practice, and how will it affect practice in the future? *Anesthesiology*. 1999;91(2):552–556.
108. Metzner J, Posner KL, Lam MS, Domino KB. Closed claims' analysis. *Saf Anaesth.* 2011;25(2):263–276.
109. Anesthesia Quality Institute. Publications. Accessed June 13, 2022. https://www.aqihq.org/ACCPublications.aspx
110. The Postoperative Visual Loss Study Group. Risk factors associated with ischemic optic neuropathy after spinal fusion surgery. *Anesthesiology*. 2012;116(1):15–24.
111. Mehta SP, Bhananker SM, Posner KL, Domino KB. Operating room fires: a closed claims analysis. *Anesthesiology*. 2013;118(5):1133–1139.
112. Anesthesia Patient Safety Foundation. Closed Claims Project Shows Safety Evolution. Accessed June 13, 2022. https://www.apsf.org/article/closed-claims-project-shows-safety-evolution/
113. Douglas RN, Stephens LS, Posner KL, et al. Communication failures contributing to patient injury in anaesthesia malpractice claims☆. *Br J Anaesth.* 2021;127(3):470–478.
114. Woodward ZG, Urman RD, Domino KB. Safety of non-operating room anesthesia: a closed claims update. *Anesth Clin.* 2017;35(4):569–581.
115. National Patient Safety Foundation. About the National Patient Safety Foundation. Accessed June 13, 2022. https://npsf.digitellinc.com/npsf/
116. Kohn LT, Corrigan J, Donaldson MS. *To Err Is Human: Building a Safer Health System*. National Academy Press;2000.
117. The Wall Street Journal. Once Seen as Risky, One Group Of Doctors Changes Its Ways. Published June 21, 2005. Accessed June 13, 2022. https://www.wsj.com/articles/SB111931728319164845.
118. APSF Newsletter. Anesthesia Patient Safety Foundation. Accessed June 13, 2022. https://www.apsf.org/apsf-newsletter/
119. Pollard RJ, Hopkins T, Smith CT, et al. Perianesthetic and anesthesia-related mortality in a Southeastern United States Population: a longitudinal review of a prospectively collected quality assurance data base. *Anesth Analg.* 2018;127(3):730–735. https://journals.lww.com/anesthesia-analgesia/Fulltext/2018/09000/Perianesthetic_and_Anesthesia_Related_Mortality_in.24.aspx
120. Liu Z, Dumville JC, Norman G, et al. Intraoperative interventions for preventing surgical site infection: an overview of Cochrane Reviews. *Cochrane Database Syst Rev.* 2018;2(2):CD012653.
121. Loftus RW, Koff MD, Birnbach DJ. The Dynamics and implications of bacterial transmission events arising from the anesthesia work area. *Anesth Analg.* 2015;120(4):853–860. https://journals.lww.com/anesthesia-analgesia/Fulltext/2015/04000/The_Dynamics_and_Implications_of_Bacterial.24.aspx
122. Anesthesia Patient Safety Foundation. Perioperative Patient Safety Priorities. Accessed June 9, 2022. https://www.apsf.org/patient-safety-priorities/
123. Anesthesia Quality Institute. National Anesthesia Clinical Outcomes Registry (NACOR). Accessed June 9, 2022. https://www.aqihq.org/introduction-to-nacor.aspx
124. MPOG. MPOG. Accessed June 9, 2022. https://mpog.org/
125. Anesthesia Patient Safety Foundation. Safety vs. Quality—The 2020 APSF/ASA Ellison C. Pierce, Jr., MD, Memorial Safety Lecture. Anesthesia Patient Safety Foundation. Published 2020. Accessed February 3, 2023. https://www.apsf.org/article/safety-vs-quality-the-2020-apsf-asa-ellison-c-pierce-jr-md-memorial-safety-lecture/
126. Landau M, Chisholm D. The arrogance of optimism: notes on failure-avoidance management. *J Contingencies Crisis Manag.* 1995;3(2):67–80.
127. Weinger MB, Gardner-Bonneau D, Wiklund ME, Kelly LM. *Handbook of Human Factors in Medical Device Design*. CRC Press/Taylor & Francis Group; 2011.
128. Edmondson A. Psychological Safety and Learning Behavior in Work Teams. *Adm Sci Q.* 1999;44(2):350–383.
129. Reason J. *Managing the Risks of Organizational Accidents*. 1st ed. Routledge; 1997. https://doi.org/10.4324/9781315543543
130. Peterfreund RA, Driscoll WD, Walsh JL, et al. Evaluation of a Mandatory Quality Assurance Data Capture in Anesthesia: a secure electronic system to capture quality assurance information linked to an automated anesthesia record. *Anesth Analg.* 2011;112(5):1218–1225. https://journals.lww.com/anesthesia-analgesia/Fulltext/2011/05000/Evaluation_of_a_Mandatory_Quality_Assurance_Data.50.aspx
131. Cooper JB. Is Voluntary Reporting of Critical Events Effective for Quality Assurance? *Anesthesiology*. 1996;85(5):961–964.
132. Liberman JS, Slagle JM, Whitney G, et al. Incidence and classification of nonroutine events during anesthesia care. *Anesthesiology*. 2020;133(1):41–52.
133. Clarke JR. How a system for reporting medical errors can and cannot improve patient safety. *Am Surg.* 2006;72(11):1088–1091.
134. CMS Manual System. Anesthesia Services. Published May 21, 2010. Accessed June 1, 2022. https://www.cms.gov/regulations-and-guidance/guidance/transmittals/downloads/r59soma.pdf.
135. The Joint Commission. Hospital: 2022 National Patient Safety Goals. Accessed June 4, 2022. https://www.jointcommission.org/standards/national-patient-safety-goals/hospital-national-patient-safety-goals/
136. CDC. Health Insurance Portability and Accountability Act of 1996 (HIPAA). Published February 21, 2019. Accessed June 3, 2022. https://www.cdc.gov/phlp/publications/topic/hipaa.html
137. Allen AL. HIPAA at 25—a work in progress. *N Engl J Med.* 2021;384(23):2169–2171.
138. HHS.gov. Enforcement Process. Published May 7, 2008. Accessed June 3, 2022. https://www.hhs.gov/hipaa/for-professionals/compliance-enforcement/enforcement-process/index.html
139. Shallik NA, Ismail A, Al Hariri O, eds. *Improving Anesthesia Technical Staff's Skills*. Springer International Publishing; 2022.
140. ASATT. About ASATT. Accessed June 9, 2022. https://www.asatt.org/index.php/about-us/about-asatt
141. MTS. Anesthesia Technician Schools. Accessed June 9, 2022. https://www.medicaltechnologyschools.com/anesthesia-technician
142. Axelrod D, et al. Greening the Operating Room. Accessed February 3, 2023. https://www.asahq.org/about-asa/governance-and-committees/asa-committees/environmental-sustainability/greening-the-operating-room
143. Bowman MA, Katzoff JM, Garrison LP Jr, Wills J. Estimates of Physician Requirements for 1990 for the Specialties of Neurology, Anesthesiology, Nuclear Medicine, Pathology, Physical Medicine and Rehabilitation, and Radiology: a further application of the GMENAC methodology. *JAMA.* 1983;250(19):2623–2627.
144. Grogono AW. The Abt Report: what was it, and what happened? *ASA Newsl.* 2004;68(9):20–21.
145. Daugherty L, Fonseca R, Kumar KB, Michaud PC. An analysis of the labor markets for anesthesiology. *Rand Health Q.* 2011;1(3):18.
146. Baird MD, Daugherty L, Kumar KB, Arifkhanova A. *The Anesthesiologist Workforce in 2013: A Final Briefing to the American Society of Anesthesiologists*. RAND Corporation; 2014. https://www.rand.org/pubs/research_reports/RR650.html
147. American Society of Anesthesiologists. 2021 Anesthesia Almanac. Published September 8, 2021. Accessed June 29, 2022. www.asahq.org › analytics-research-services › 2021-anesthesia-almanac
148. Baird M, Daugherty L, Kumar KB, Arifkhanova A. Regional and Gender Differences and Trends in the Anesthesiologist Workforce. *Anesthesiology*. 2015;123(5):997–1012.
149. American Society of Anesthesiologists. ASA Open Forum–ASA Community. Accessed July 27, 2022. https://community.asahq.org/viewdocument/caws-anesthesia-workforce-trends
150. Muffly MK, Singleton M, Agarwal R, et al. The pediatric anesthesiology workforce: projecting supply and trends 2015–2035. *Anesth Analg.* 2018;126(2):568–578. https://journals.lww.com/anesthesia-analgesia/Fulltext/2018/02000/The_Pediatric_Anesthesiology_Workforce__Projecting.33.aspx
151. Gelber K, Kahwajian H, Geller AW, Zakowski MI. Obstetric Anesthesiology in the United States: current and future demand for fellowship-trained subspecialists. *Anesth Analg.* 2018;127(6):1445–1447. https://journals.lww.com/anesthesia-analgesia/Fulltext/2018/12000/Obstetric_Anesthesiology_in_the_United_States_.25.aspx
152. InvestingDoc. Higher Job Turnover In Medicine Than Expected. Published August 9, 2017. Accessed June 8, 2022. https://investingdoc.com/higher-job-turnover-in-medicine-than-expected/
153. American Society of Anesthesiologists. Recent Jobs. Accessed June 8, 2022. https://careers.asahq.org/jobs/
154. The White Coat Investor. Investing & Personal Finance for Doctors. Locum Tenens: What You Need to Know. Published November 27, 2020. Accessed June 8, 2022. https://www.whitecoatinvestor.com/locum-tenens/
155. Thomson Reuters. The basics of non-compete agreements. Accessed June 8, 2022. https://legal.thomsonreuters.com/en/insights/articles/the-basics-of-non-compete-agreements
156. The White Coat Investor. Things to Ask for in a Physician Contract. Published August 9, 2021. Accessed June 8, 2022. https://www.whitecoatinvestor.com/things-to-ask-for-in-a-physician-contract/
157. Malhotra D, Bazerman M. *Negtiation Genius*. Bantam Books; 2007.
158. Siddiqui S, Tung A, Kelly L, et al. Anxiety, worry, and job satisfaction: effects of COVID-19 care on critical care anesthesiologists. *Can J Anesth Can Anesth.* 2022;69(4):552–554.
159. Aron R, Pawlowski J, Shukry M, Shillcutt S. The Impact of COVID-19 on the Status of the Anesthesiologists' Well-Being. *Adv Anesth.* 2021;39:149–167.
160. O'Brien JM, Goncin U, Ngo R, Hedlin P, Chakravarti A. Professional fulfillment, burnout, and wellness of anesthesiologists during the COVID-19 pandemic. *Can J Anaesth J Can Anesth.* 2021;68(5):734–736.
161. ICD10Data.com. 2022 ICD-10-CM Diagnosis Code Z73.0: Burn-out. Accessed June 12, 2022. https://www.icd10data.com/ICD10CM/Codes/Z00-Z99/Z69-Z76/Z73-/Z73.0
162. ICD-11 for Mortality and Morbidity Statistics. QD85 Burnout. Accessed June 12, 2022. https://icd.who.int/browse11/l-m/en#/http://id.who.int/icd/entity/129180281
163. Romito BT, Okoro EN, Ringqvist JRB, Goff KL. Burnout and Wellness: The Anesthesiologist's Perspective. *Am J Lifestyle Med.* 2020;15(2):118–125.
164. Wiederhold BK, Cipresso P, Pizzioli D, Wiederhold M, Riva G. Intervention for physician burnout: a systematic review. *Open Med Wars Pol.* 2018;13:253–263.
165. Almeida M. Burnout and the mental health impact of COVID-19 in anesthesiologists: a call to action. *J Clin Anesth.* 2021;68:110084–110084.
166. Khan A, Vinson AE. Physician well-being in practice. *Anesth Analg.* 2020;131(5):1359–1369. https://journals.lww.com/anesthesia-analgesia/Fulltext/2020/11000/Physician_Well_Being_in_Practice.8.aspx

167. Dahle JM. *The White Coat Investor: A Doctor's Guide to Personal Finance and Investing (The White Coat Investor Series)*. The White Coat Investor, LLC; 2014.
168. Stanley TJ, Danko WD. *The Millionaire Next Door*. Gallery Books; 1998.
169. Physician on FIRE. Home. Published April 30, 2016. Accessed June 12, 2022. https://www.physicianonfire.com/
170. The White Coat Investor. Home. Accessed June 12, 2022. https://www.whitecoatinvestor.com/
171. The White Coat Investor. How to Choose a Financial AdvisorPublished March 16, 2021. Accessed June 12, 2022. https://www.whitecoatinvestor.com/12-things-you-should-know-about-choosing-a-financial-adviser/
172. AAMC. Tuition and Student Fees Reports. Accessed June 20, 2022. https://www.aamc.org/data-reports/reporting-tools/report/tuition-and-student-fees-reports
173. AAMC Store. Medical Student Education: Debt, Costs, and Loan Repayment Fact Card for the Class of 2021. Accessed June 20, 2022. https://store.aamc.org/medical-student-education-debt-costs-and-loan-repayment-fact-card-for-the-class-of-2021.html
174. FIRST (Financial Information, Resources, Services, and Tools). AAMC. Accessed June 20, 2022. https://students-residents.aamc.org/financial-aid
175. Physician on FIRE. The Student Loan Resource Page. Published September 23, 2019. Accessed June 20, 2022. https://www.physicianonfire.com/loans/
176. Federal Student Aid. Federal Versus Private Loans. Accessed June 20, 2022. https://studentaid.gov/understand-aid/types/loans/federal-vs-private
177. Federal Student Aid. Income-Driven Repayment Plans. Accessed June 20, 2022. https://studentaid.gov/manage-loans/repayment/plans/income-driven
178. Federal Student Aid. Public Service Loan Forgiveness. Accessed June 20, 2022. https://studentaid.gov/manage-loans/forgiveness-cancellation/public-service
179. AAMC. Should I Refinance My Student Loans? Accessed June 20, 2022. https://students-residents.aamc.org/financial-aid-resources/should-i-refinance-my-student-loans
180. Soschner C. Did Einstein Ever Say Compound Interest Is the 8th Wonder of The World? Medium. Published August 19, 2021. Accessed June 20, 2022. https://medium.datadriveninvestor.com/did-einstein-ever-say-compound-interest-is-the-8th-wonder-of-the-world-75ca2f200dd7
181. Internal Revenue Service. Here's what people should know about taking early withdrawals from retirement plans. Accessed June 22, 2022. https://www.irs.gov/newsroom/heres-what-people-should-know-about-taking-early-withdrawals-from-retirement-plans
182. SEC.gov. An Introduction to 529 Plans. Accessed June 22, 2022. https://www.sec.gov/reportspubs/investor-publications/investorpubsintro529htm.html
183. MarketWatch. What are target-date funds and how do they work? Accessed June 22, 2022. https://www.marketwatch.com/story/what-are-target-date-funds-and-how-do-they-work-11654798024
184. Investor.gov. Mutual Funds. Accessed June 22, 2022. https://www.investor.gov/introduction-investing/investing-basics/investment-products/mutual-funds-and-exchange-traded-1
185. Vanguard. Index funds vs. actively managed funds. Accessed June 22, 2022. https://investor.vanguard.com/investor-resources-education/understanding-investment-types/index-funds-vs-actively-managed-funds
186. Vanguard. Vanguard mutual fund fees and minimums. Accessed June 22, 2022. https://investor.vanguard.com/investment-products/mutual-funds/fees
187. Fidelity. Fidelity Mutual Funds. Accessed June 22, 2022. https://www.fidelity.com/mutual-funds/fidelity-funds/overview
188. Lindauer M, Larimore T, LeBeouf M. *The Bogleheads' Guide to Investing*. 2nd ed. Wiley; 2021.
189. NASDAQ. Here's Your Set It and Forget It Investing Strategy. Accessed June 22, 2022. https://www.nasdaq.com/articles/heres-your-set-it-and-forget-it-investing-strategy-2018-10-24
190. The White Coat Investor. Understanding Disability Insurance for Doctors. Published December 1, 2021. Accessed June 22, 2022. https://www.whitecoatinvestor.com/what-you-need-to-know-about-disability-insurance/
191. AMA Insurance. AMA-Sponsored Disability Income Insurance. Accessed June 22, 2022. https://amainsure.com/insurance-products/physician-disability-insurance/disabilitypro/
192. The White Coat Investor. Whole Life Insurance For Doctors – Your Questions Answered. Published June 22, 2021. Accessed June 22, 2022. https://www.whitecoatinvestor.com/what-you-need-to-know-about-whole-life-insurance/
193. The White Coat Investor. How to Buy Life Insurance. Published March 15, 2022. Accessed June 22, 2022. https://www.whitecoatinvestor.com/how-to-buy-life-insurance/
194. The White Coat Investor. 10 Things You Want to Know About Medical Malpractice. Published April 26, 2021. Accessed June 22, 2022. https://www.whitecoatinvestor.com/medical-malpractice/
195. The White Coat Investor. How to Buy Medical Malpractice Insurance. Published July 12, 2016. Accessed June 22, 2022. https://www.whitecoatinvestor.com/how-to-buy-medical-malpractice-insurance/
196. The White Coat Investor. Umbrella Insurance for Doctors. Published December 3, 2021. Accessed June 22, 2022. https://www.whitecoatinvestor.com/umbrella-insurance/
197. Meara JG, Leather AJM, Hagander L, et al. Global Surgery 2030: evidence and solutions for achieving health, welfare, and economic development. *The Lancet*. 2015;386(9993):569–624.
198. Tuyishime E, Powell WF Jr, Evans FM. Anesthesiology training in LMICs: defining the problem, challenges, and solutions. *ASA Monit*. 2021;85(10):35–36.
199. Duperrault MR, McGoldrick RR, Crawford AM. Considerations in developing thoughtful anesthesia global health programs. *ASA Monit*. 2018;82(4):50–51.
200. Bridenbaugh PO. Role of anesthesiologists in global health: can one volunteer make a difference? *Int Anesthesiol Clin*. 2010;48(2):165–175. https://journals.lww.com/anesthesiaclinics/Fulltext/2010/04820/Role_of_Anesthesiologists_in_Global_Health__Can.15.aspx
201. Ardon AE. Why participate in global health educational projects? One anesthesiologist's viewpoint. *ASA Monit*. 2018;82(12):28–30.
202. Drum ET, Gelb AW, Peel F. ASA and WFSA: partners for uniting anesthesiologists around the world. *ASA Monit*. 2021;85(7):14–15.
203. SOAP. SOAP/Kybele International Outreach Grant. Accessed June 22, 2022. https://www.soap.org/soap-kybele-international-outreach-grants
204. Kybele. For Safe Childbirth Worldwide. Accessed June 22, 2022. https://kybeleworldwide.org/
205. Crawford AM, Jensen A. Global includes local. *ASA Monit*. 2021;85(2):21–22.
206. Couillard BK, Foote CL, Gandhi K, Meara E, Skinner J. Rising geographic disparities in US mortality. *J Econ Perspect*. 2021;35(4):123–146.
207. Wollner E, Law T, Sullivan K, Lipnick MS. Why every anesthesia trainee should receive global health equity education. *Can J Anesth Can Anesth*. 2020;67(8):924–935.
208. Missett RM, Kynes JM. Emphasis on Equity: moving global health education forward. *ASA Monit*. 2021;85(10):33–34. doi:10.1097/01.ASM.0000795112.39055.1b
209. Johnson C, Rastetter M, Olayiwola JN. Pathways to equity: a pilot study implementing a health equity leadership curriculum in residency education as an antidote to systemic racism. *J Natl Med Assoc*. 2022;114(2):141–146.
210. Chung JW, Meltzer DO. Estimate of the carbon footprint of the US Health Care Sector. *JAMA*. 2009;302(18):1970–1972.
211. Lenzen M, Malik A, Li M, et al. The environmental footprint of health care: a global assessment. *Lancet Planet Health*. 2020;4(7):e271–e279.
212. American Society of Anesthesiologists. Greening the Operating Room. Accessed June 27, 2022. https://www.asahq.org/about-asa/governance-and-committees/asa-committees/environmental-sustainability/greening-the-operating-room
213. Sherman JD, Sulbaek Andersen MP, Renwick J, McGain F. Environmental sustainability in anaesthesia and critical care. *Response to Br J Anaesth*. 2021;126:e195–e197. *Br J Anaesth*. 2021;126(6):e193–e195.
214. Gaya da Costa M, Kalmar AF, Struys MMRF. Inhaled anesthetics: environmental role, occupational risk, and clinical use. *J Clin Med*. 2021;10(6):1306.
215. Babu MA, Dalenberg AK, Goodsell G, Holloway AB, Belau MM, Link MJ. Greening the operating room: results of a scalable initiative to reduce waste and recover supply costs. *Neurosurgery*. 2019;85(3):432–437.
216. Xiao MZX, Abbass SAA, Bahrey L, Rubinstein E, Chan VWS. A roadmap for environmental sustainability of plastic use in anesthesia and the perioperative arena. *Anesthesiology*. 2021;135(4):729–737.
217. Hutchins DCJ, White SM. Coming round to recycling. *BMJ*. 2009;338:b609.
218. McGain F, Hendel SA, Story DA. An audit of potentially recyclable waste from anaesthetic practice. *Anaesth Intensive Care*. 2009;37(5):820–823.
219. Struys MMRF, Eckelman MJ. Environmental footprint of anesthesia: more than inhaled anesthetics! *Anesthesiology*. 2021;135(6):937–939.
220. Wanderer JP, Rathmell JP. Anesthetic carbon footprints: weighing the options and impact. *Anesthesiology*. 2021;135(6):A15–A15.
221. Bellman R. *Artificial Intelligence: Can Computers Think?* Boyd & Fraser Publishing Company; 1978. https://books.google.com/books?id=g9AO65QphqIC
222. Mathis MR, Kheterpal S, Najarian K. Artificial intelligence for anesthesia: what the practicing clinician needs to know: more than black magic for the art of the dark. *Anesthesiology*. 2018;129(4):619–622.
223. Hashimoto DA, Witkowski E, Gao L, Meireles O, Rosman G. Artificial intelligence in anesthesiology: current techniques, clinical applications, and limitations. *Anesthesiology*. 2020;132(2):379–394.
224. Etemadi M, Hogue CW. Preventing intraoperative hypotension: artificial intelligence versus augmented intelligence? *Anesthesiology*. 2020;133(6):1170–1172.
225. Bowness JS, El-Boghdadly K, Woodworth G, Noble JA, Higham H, Burckett-St Laurent D. Exploring the utility of assistive artificial intelligence for ultrasound scanning in regional anesthesia. *Reg Anesth Amp Pain Med*. 2022;47(6):375.
226. London MJ. Back to the OR of the future: how do we make it a good one? *Anesthesiology*. 2021;135(2):206–208.
227. Aldwinckle RJ. Can we trust the black box? *Reg Anesth Amp Pain Med*. 2022;47(5):338.

3 Occupational Health and Well-Being

AMY E. VINSON • ROBERT S. HOLZMAN • JONATHAN D. KATZ

KEY POINTS

1. The strain imposed by the COVID-19 pandemic on health care workers and the health care system has highlighted the critical role of both occupational health and well-being in medicine and the specialty of anesthesiology.
2. Vigilance is one of the most critical tasks performed by anesthesiologists and may be adversely affected by several occupationally related issues including poor equipment engineering and design, excessive noise, interpersonal conflict, production pressures, and fatigue.
3. Exposure to waste anesthetic gases can be reduced to levels below those recommended by the National Institute for Occupational Safety and Health by using waste gas scavenging equipment, routinely maintaining anesthesia machines, and following appropriate work practices.
4. Sleep deprivation and fatigue are common among anesthesiologists and can adversely affect patient safety due to deleterious effects on the physician's cognition, mood, and health.
5. Substance use disorder, or chemical dependency, is a significant, often lethal, occupational hazard among anesthesiologists. An incidence of controlled substance abuse of 1% to 2% has been repeatedly reported within anesthesia training programs. Rates have not changed despite educational and systematic interventions.
6. The risk of exposure to infectious pathogens can be reduced by the routine use of standard precautions, transmission-based precautions for infected patients, and safety devices designed to prevent needlestick injuries.
7. Hepatitis B vaccine is recommended for all anesthesia personnel because of the increased risk for occupational transmission of this blood-borne pathogen.
8. Anesthesiologists have a disproportionately high rate of suicide. Factors include pre-existing personality traits, substance use disorder, and stress.
9. Physician well-being is integral to occupational health and patient safety. There is an evolving professional commitment to optimizing physician work style and lifestyle, as well as physical health (e.g., through better nutrition, fitness, and rest).
10. Creating a culture of well-being and support for physicians and other medical personnel through organizational, systemic, and policy-level interventions has become an imperative of many governmental bodies and professional organizations.

Introduction

Prior to the COVID-19 pandemic, most anesthesiologists viewed occupational health as something of infrequent concern. It was seen as the entity ensuring tuberculosis (TB) testing, mask fitting and vaccination compliance, and the one to call in situations of pathogen exposure, such as accidental needle stick injuries and
1 splash events. However, with the dawning of a global pandemic, the safety of the anesthesiologist's work environment and the availability of personal protective equipment (PPE) took on an immediate and salient focus within their collective consciousness. Most clinicians are now well versed in forms and levels of PPE, as well as the risks and hazards encompassed by the COVID-19 virus.

However, occupational health reaches much further than threats posed by pathogen exposure. The health care industry has the dubious distinction of being one of the most hazardous places to work in the United States. According to the U.S. Bureau of Labor, workers in the health care and social assistance industry in 2020 had the highest rate and greatest number of nonfatal occupational injuries among all workers in the private industry sector.[1] Unfortunately, in contrast to other well-known hazardous workplaces, such as agriculture and construction, the frequency of occupational injuries in the health care sector continues to rise.

In addition to the occupational risks incurred by other members of the health care team, commonly recognized workplace hazards specifically affecting anesthesia personnel include exposure to waste anesthetic gases (WAGs), ionizing radiation, fires, and infectious agents, to name a few. In addition, anesthesia personnel are susceptible to emotional and psychological conditions such as burnout and substance use disorder (SUD), all within a culture where clinicians seeking mental health care are still met with stigma.

Despite heightened awareness and concerted efforts to minimize these occupational maladies, many continue to occur at disproportionate rates among our colleagues. This chapter will explore the ways in which the anesthesiologist's workplace affects anesthesia personnel physically and psychologically, and the work that is being done to mitigate occupational risks and to promote well-being and a supportive work culture.

Physical Hazards

Ergonomics

The International Ergonomics Association defines ergonomics as the scientific discipline concerned with the promotion of efficient and safe use of interactions among humans and other elements of a system. While ergonomic analysis has gained its widest acceptance in industries such as aviation and nuclear power, where many well-publicized catastrophes have been linked to human error, the work performed by anesthesiologists shares many of the characteristics found in these industries, including the intricacy of the tasks, the narrow safety margin, and the vulnerability to human error. The serious nature of surgical procedures and critical care may account for up to 79% of adverse events in health care.[2]

Several human factor shortcomings exist in the anesthesiologist's workplace. Anesthesia equipment is often poorly designed or positioned. Anesthesia monitors and computers for electronic medical records are frequently placed so that the anesthesiologist's attention is diverted away from the patient and the surgical field. Poor engineering of monitor displays can increase the difficulty in extracting and interpreting pertinent information and adversely influence the operator's conclusions, and therefore, performance.

Even alarms that were developed with the specific goal of augmenting safety can produce unintended and conflicting reports. In general, alarms are nonspecific and are susceptible to artifacts and false positives that can cause alarm fatigue and distract the observer from more clinically significant information. It is not unusual for distractive alarms to be ignored or inactivated.[3] A positive trend that is emerging in alarm technology is the development of "knowledge-based alarms" that can integrate information from more than one monitor and suggest a list of diagnostic and therapeutic possibilities.[2]

The thermal environment of the operating room affects workers and patients in significant ways. Thermal vulnerability of patients is well recognized, however, thermal effects on operating room staff are often acknowledged but not well studied. Beyond room temperature, additional thermal effects consist of the quality and velocity of air exchanges, humidity, the activity of the occupants, and clothing worn. Performance of vigilance tasks can be lowest in warm environments, such as the pediatric operating room, due to soporific effects. Tasks that some caregivers perform comfortably in street clothes or hospital uniforms become "warmth discomfort" tasks when carried out in isolation garb (as experienced during the COVID-19 pandemic) or lead aprons over scrubs and under sterile gowns. Likewise, the effects of cold on health care providers' performance are often ignored, and while there are few effects on mental performance, cold can act as a "secondary task," that is, shivering, or physical movement to keep warm. Moreover, the effects of cold may slow movement due to stiffening of joints and slowing of muscle reaction. Degradation of dexterity and performance at manual tasks may result. Draft has been identified as one of the most annoying environmental factors in workplaces[4] and is of special concern in the operating room and critical care areas (ICU, PACU) with heating, ventilation, and air conditioning (HVAC) systems requiring rapid air exchange or utilizing high-efficiency particulate air (HEPA) filtration for patient isolation techniques.

The operating room surrounds its personnel with illumination of many wavelengths, intensities, and brightness. The measurement of brightness is complex. The *source* of light may be characterized by its *luminous intensity*, while the actual amount of this energy that strikes the surface of an object to be seen is described as the *illuminance*. How much *illuminance* an object receives depends on the distance of the object from the light source. *Glare* is produced by brightness within the field of vision that is sufficiently greater than the luminance to which the eyes are adapted. Although everyone has had the experience of having a light source shine in their eyes (operating room light, laparoscope, optical telescope), reflected glare (a high-intensity light source reflecting off a polished steel instrument container) can also cause annoyance, discomfort, or degradation of visual performance. *Ambient light* recommendations for the operating room are as great as double that of other examination areas, with *task lighting* recommendations 10- to 20-fold higher. The human factors approach prompts further consideration of the interaction of differently visually equipped human perception, which has not only a genetic basis (i.e., color blindness) but also effects of aging and comorbidities (i.e., glaucoma, cataracts, diabetes, macular degeneration).

Collisions with the ever-proliferating and enlarging pieces of equipment in the operating room have increased as screen technology has improved with high- and ultra–high-definition screens. In addition, there are now multiple boom and wall-mounted screens to provide optimal viewing angles for endoscopic techniques for every specialty and every body cavity. Often, these devices are wired so that they can communicate with recording and communication lines. Commonly, these cables are simply laying on the operating room floor, which is frequently wet and slippery. In this hazardous situation, rushed personnel, paying attention to something else rather than their hazardous environment, may suffer a variety of injuries such as crushing, cutting, fracturing, shearing, abrading, and puncturing. Collisions with suspended, ceiling-mounted, or dangling objects, sometimes known as "boom strikes," can result in head injuries, even concussions, which can be both acutely incapacitating as well as disabling in the long term.

Inhalation Anesthetics

Levels of Waste Anesthetic Gases

In the absence of adequate air exchange and scavenging of WAGs, high levels of anesthetic vapors can be detected in the ambient air surrounding anesthetizing locations. In 1969, prior to the routine use of scavenging devices, Linde and Bruce[5] observed an average concentration of halothane of 10 ppm and nitrous oxide of 130 ppm in the air surrounding an active anesthesia machine, with end-expired air samples from anesthesiologists as high as 12 ppm of halothane. Subsequent studies have reported even

Table 3-1 NIH-Set Occupational Exposure Limits (OELs)

NIH-Set Occupational Exposure Limits (OELs)		
Anesthetic Gas	**NIH-Set OEL as a TWA in Parts per million (ppm)**	**Additional Notes**
Isoflurane/Forane	**2.0** ppm (based on CalOSHA, NIOSH, and ALARA)	Effects on pregnancy under study
Enflurane	**75.0** ppm (based on ACGIH)	FDA Pregnancy Risk Group C
Desflurane	**2.0** ppm (Set similar to Iso and Sevo; similar health impacts)	Effects on pregnancy under study
Halothane	Replace with safer anesthetic gas where possible. **2.0** ppm TWA otherwise (NIOSH REL)	Liver damage
Nitrous oxide	**25.0** ppm (NIOSH REL)	Prolonged exposure may inhibit DNA synthesis; avoid in the first trimester
Sevoflurane	**2.0** ppm (NIOSH REL)	Effects on pregnancy under study
ACGIH	American Conference of Governmental Industrial Hygienists	
NIOSH	National Institute for Occupational Safety and Health	
FDA	Food and Drug Administration	
CalOSHA	California Division of Occupational Safety and Health	
Pregnancy risk groups (based upon FDA research and information):		
Category A	Adequate and well-controlled studies have failed to demonstrate a risk to the fetus in the first trimester of pregnancy (and there is no evidence of risk in later trimesters).	
Category B	Animal reproduction studies have failed to demonstrate a risk to the fetus and there are no adequate and well-controlled studies in pregnant women.	
Category C	Animal reproduction studies have shown an adverse effect on the fetus and there are no adequate and well-controlled studies in humans, but potential benefits may warrant use of the chemical in pregnant women despite potential risks.	
Category D	There is positive evidence of human fetal risk based on adverse reaction data from investigational or marketing experience or studies in humans, but potential benefits may warrant use of the chemical in pregnant women despite potential risks.	

TWA, time-weighted average.

higher concentrations in poorly ventilated and/or unscavenged locations.

Citing health concerns, the National Institute for Occupational Safety and Health (NIOSH) in 1977 recommended exposure limits (RELs) of 2 ppm for halogenated anesthetic agents when used alone or 0.5 ppm for a halogenated agent and 25 ppm of nitrous oxide when used together (time-weighted average [TWA] during the period of anesthetic administration). The latest available recommendations continue to support these guidelines.[6]

In 1994, NIOSH issued an alert to health care personnel that exposure to inhalation anesthetic agents, especially nitrous oxide, may produce “harmful effects” and included recommendations to monitor the air in operating rooms, implement appropriate engineering controls, enact certain work practices and equipment maintenance procedures, and institute a worker education program (Table 3-1).

Concentrations of WAGs can usually be reduced to acceptable levels through strict compliance with the NIOSH recommendations.[7] However, there remain unavoidable situations, such as a mask induction (most common in pediatric anesthesia), where levels of WAGs will briefly, but frequently, exceed these limits. Elevated levels of WAGs have also been identified in the PACU, typically occurring due to exhaled gases from recovering patients.[8] Levels of WAGs in the PACU can be reduced by ensuring adequate room ventilation and by discontinuing anesthetic gases in sufficient time before leaving the operating room.

Health Consequences of WAG Exposure

The first published report of specific toxic effects from chronic occupational exposure to WAGs appeared in a 1967 article that described a high incidence of fatigue, nausea, headaches, and miscarriage among female Russian anesthesiologists.[9] Although the study methodology has subsequently been questioned, it opened an ongoing dialogue about whether chronic exposure to WAGs renders anesthesia providers more vulnerable to cellular injury, organ toxicity, adverse reproductive outcomes, impairment of psychomotor skills, SUD, and premature death.

It is not surprising that chemicals with such profound physiologic effects as anesthetic agents would exhibit toxic properties if applied in adequate concentrations to tissues. For example, there is ample evidence that cellular damage can be caused by chronic exposure of cultured cells and experimental animals to high concentrations of anesthetic gases.[10] However, the clinical literature remains inconclusive regarding causality between adverse health effects and the level of occupational exposure to WAGs experienced by most anesthesia personnel. Limitations to many of the clinical studies include occupational exposure in the study population to other risk factors such as radiation, long work hours, stress, and unhealthy personal habits, as well as potential reporter bias that can occur in retrospective studies.

Most of the studies of possible health consequences to humans with occupational exposure to WAGs have focused on cytotoxic changes, cancer, and reproductive outcomes. The reports on possible genotoxic effects of trace anesthetic exposure are conflicting. For example, in one study, occupational exposure to sevoflurane (8.9 +/– 5.6 ppm) and nitrous oxide (119 +/– 39 ppm) was associated with increased levels of sister chromatid exchange (a marker of genotoxicity) with abnormal cytology returning to normal after 2 months of leave from the operating room.[11] However, other studies have reported no findings of cellular damage among clinicians exposed to the levels of anesthetic gases that are encountered in an adequately ventilated and scavenged operating room.[12] A conclusion that can be drawn from these conflicting reports is that the risk of genotoxicity is minimal under the low exposure to WAGs usually experienced in a well-scavenged operating room in compliance with current recommendations.

The possibility of adverse reproductive outcomes has been the most intensively researched aspect of occupational WAG exposure. Early reports suggested an association between long-term occupational exposure to WAGs and infertility, spontaneous abortions, and congenital abnormalities. The American Society of Anesthesiologists (ASA) and NIOSH published a retrospective analysis in 1974 in which 49,585 operating room personnel with occupational WAG exposure were compared with a nonexposed group of 23,911 health care professionals.[13] Among the findings in this study was an increased risk of spontaneous abortion and congenital abnormalities in children of women who worked in the operating room and an increased risk of congenital abnormalities in offspring of unexposed wives of male operating room personnel.

In 1985, in response to criticism of the methodology and data analysis in this and other earlier reports, and in recognition of the fact that many of the studies were conducted prior to routine WAG scavenging, the ASA commissioned a meta-analysis of the existing data.[14] This study reported that the relative risks of spontaneous abortion for female physicians and female nurses working in the operating room were 1.4 and 1.3, respectively. The increased relative risk for congenital abnormalities was of borderline statistical significance for exposed physicians only. The overall risk created by WAG exposure was small compared with other, better-documented maternal risk factors, such as cigarette smoking and long working hours. The review also pointed out that duration and levels of anesthetic exposure were not measured in any of the studies and that other confounding factors were not adequately controlled.

The importance of adequate scavenging was highlighted in a subsequent meta-analysis of the risk of spontaneous abortion among hospital workers, dental assistants, veterinarians, and veterinary assistants.[15] The study identified a significant risk of spontaneous abortion in those studies conducted prior to the era of scavenging but no increased risk among personnel who worked in environments where WAGs were scavenged.

Reports of elevated risks for adverse reproductive outcomes have continued to appear. Most of these reports concern health care personnel in locations where adequate scavenging of WAGs is not universally practiced. Female dental assistants[15] and female veterinarians who work in large animal hospitals have been specifically identified as at risk for adverse reproductive outcomes.

It is likely that other job-associated conditions besides exposure to trace anesthetic gases, such as stress, infections, long work hours, shift work, and radiation exposure, may account for many of the adverse reproductive outcomes. A survey of 3,985 Swedish midwives demonstrated that night work was significantly associated with spontaneous abortions after the 12th week of pregnancy (odds ratio 3.33), while exposure to nitrous oxide appeared to have no effect.[16] Preterm birth in obstetric and neonatal nurses was associated with increased work hours, hours worked while standing, and occupational fatigue.[17] In addition, in a study of female veterinarians, the risks of birth defects were highest among those exposed to radiation and to long working hours (>45 h/wk) but not to those exposed to WAG.[12]

Table 3-2 Proper Work Practices for the Management of Waste Anesthetic Gases

Ensure tight fit of anesthetic mask
Ensure tight fit of endotracheal tube cuff or laryngeal mask airway
Ensure absence of leaks in anesthetic machine and tubing
Use low-flow techniques when appropriate (e.g., during maintenance phase of anesthetic)
Do not administer inhaled anesthetic until scavenging system is active
Ensure that anesthetic vaporizer(s) are turned off when anesthetic machine not in use

The literature on this subject remains inconclusive. However, the concern it generates persists. Many of the epidemiologic studies continue to suffer from important design flaws. For example, the level of exposure to WAGs is frequently unknown or not reported and the retrospective nature of the questionnaire lends itself to reporter bias. Still, the evidence suggests that there is a slight increase in the relative risk of spontaneous abortion and congenital abnormalities in offspring of female health care workers (HCWs) exposed to WAGs. This risk is minimized when appropriate waste gas scavenging technology and other commonsense work practices are applied (Table 3-2).[18]

One of the principal reasons identified by NIOSH in their original publication on WAGs was concern about decrements in performance, cognition, audiovisual ability, and dexterity. One study found transient psychomotor and cognitive abnormalities after exposure to subanesthetic concentrations (30% N_2O, 0.2% to 0.4% isoflurane) of anesthetic gases.[19] but the effect of these gases at concentrations found in operating rooms with scavenged WAGs was not tested.

Although the contribution of volatile anesthetics to total greenhouse gas (GHG) emissions is small (0.1%) compared with CO_2 (82.2%), it is still important to consider the long-term, cumulative impact of inhaled anesthetics on climate change and pursue strategies to minimize the introduction of these agents into the environment. Nitrous oxide is the greatest contributor to this effect because of the relatively large volumes that are used, the longer time period that it has been in use compared to other inhalation anesthetics, and the fact that nitrous oxide from a number of nonmedical sources is currently the dominant ozone-depleting gas. Nitrous oxide from anesthetic use represents only a small fraction of that found in the stratosphere but nevertheless does contribute to the greenhouse effect. Atmospheric lifetimes vary among volatile anesthetics. Sevoflurane has the shortest lifetime (1 to 5 years) and a lower estimated global warming potential (GWP) compared with isoflurane (3 to 6 years) or desflurane (9 to 21 years). Overall, life-cycle GHG emissions with desflurane are 15 times larger than those with sevoflurane and 20 times higher than those with isoflurane.[20]

Notwithstanding inconclusive evidence over decades at this point, it is prudent to mitigate the readily identifiable contributions to WAGs in anesthetizing locations.

Surgical Smoke

Tissue evaporation by electrical, laser, and ultrasonic techniques causes smoke, which contains tissue debris, malignant cells, and microorganisms. Electrocautery smoke can contain mutagenic, carcinogenic, and toxic compounds.[21] Laser smoke contains benzene, formaldehyde, hydrogen cyanide, and bioaerosols consisting of solid and liquid particles. An N95 mask can remove up to 95% of 0.3 μm size particles, including most of the bacteria, however, many particles in smoke are smaller. Smoke-evacuating equipment with an ultra–low particulate air (ULPA) filter should be used. Although these can remove up to 99.999% of 0.12-micron size particles, smoke includes many smaller particles.

Greater than one-half million HCWs including surgeons, anesthesia care providers, nurses, surgical technologists, and others are exposed to surgical smoke each year. While little is known about the chronic health effects of exposure to surgical smoke, acute health effects include eye, nose, and throat irritation, headache, cough, nasal congestion, and asthma. Furthermore, surgical smoke has been shown to contain toxic gases, vapors and particulates, viable and nonviable cellular material, viruses, and bacteria. A 2016 survey found that local exhaust ventilation (LEV), a widely recommended engineering control, is only used 47% of the time, that 49% of laser surgery respondents and 44% of electrosurgery respondents said that they never had training that addressed the hazards of surgical smoke, and that 90% of laser respondents and 98% of electrosurgery respondents used laser masks or surgical masks, which do not provide respiratory protection.[22]

Smoke-vacuuming systems as well as PPE are recommended when personnel are in proximity to surgical smoke.[23,24] The smoke-vacuuming systems should be held as close as 1 cm. to the target. HEPA or ultra–low penetration air filters and charcoal filters should be used for odor and gas absorption. Venting should be to the outdoors, if possible, and venting systems should have the ability to detect filter overloading (i.e., pressure drop). These filtration guidelines do not address fluid aspiration, which must be carried out independently. In addition, operating room personnel working in the vicinity of the laser plume should wear gloves, goggles, and high-efficiency filter masks (N95 respirators).

Radiation

Ionizing radiation consists of high-energy photons that have sufficient energy to eject electrons from exposed atoms. When the exposed matter is living tissue, molecular damage and cellular injury is the direct result.

The Occupational Safety and Health Administration (OSHA) and the Environmental Protection Agency (EPA) have published occupational limits for workers exposed to ionizing radiation.[25] The recommended annual limit is 50 mSv with an allowable lifetime limit of 10 mSv multiplied by the individual's age in years. The maximum permissible occupational exposure to a pregnant or lactating worker should not exceed a monthly limit of 5 mSv (excluding medical and natural background radiation).

Anesthesia personnel frequently work in locations where they are at risk of excessive radiation exposure. Occupational exposure can occur from being in the direct line of fire of the emitting beam or indirectly from scattered radiation reflected off surfaces such as tables, other equipment, and the patient.

Early studies reported that the exposure to radiation among anesthesia personnel is safely below OSHA limits. However, studies conducted subsequent to the increased utilization of ionizing radiation in operating rooms and in cardiac catheterization and interventional radiology suites, have revealed a worrisome trend toward increased exposure among anesthesia personnel.[26] In one study, there was a doubling of the aggregate radiation exposure to members of a department of anesthesiology in a community hospital in the year following the introduction of an electrophysiology laboratory.[27] Another report observed that anesthesiologists working in a neurointerventional suite received three times the facial exposure to radiation as did the radiologist.[28]

The biologic consequences of radiation exposure vary depending on age, gender, and the specific organ that is exposed. Different tissues have different susceptibilities to radiation injury, based on their rate of cellular proliferation, their degree of cellular metabolism, and cellular differentiation. Thus, stem cells, bone marrow, intestinal epithelium, and reproductive tissues, which all have rapid cell turnover, are the most sensitive. Bone and muscle, with little cell turnover, are the least sensitive.

The adverse consequences of radiation exposure can be deterministic or stochastic, or both. Deterministic effects refer to direct cell injury and death that occurs when the dose of radiation exceeds a threshold. Examples of these kinds of injuries include skin erythema ("sun burn"), gonadal injury, and cataract formation. Stochastic effects refer to radiation-induced DNA injury that results in genetic damage. Stochastic effects have a long latency period and the probability of this type of injury increases with cumulative dose. The development of cancer is an example of a stochastic injury.

Cumulative data suggests an increased incidence of various cancers among health care personnel. For example, reports have appeared identifying an increased incidence of brain cancer among interventional cardiologists with the tumor first appearing on the side of the brain closest to their procedural field.[29] However, due to the elevated background incidence of cancer in the general population (almost 50% lifetime risk of developing cancer and close to 25% risk of a fatal malignancy) and the long latency period before clinical presentation of cancer, a direct correlation to occupational exposure among HCWs has not been definitively established.

Awareness of radiation risks is critical to mitigate the risks of injury due to occupational radiation exposure. Unfortunately, this potential hazard has not received adequate attention.[30] Preventative strategies are critical to minimize the risk of radiation-induced injury. The basic principle is to keep exposure as low as reasonably practical (ALARP). In practice, this means to limit the intensity and exposure time to the x-ray beam, to distance oneself as much as possible from the source of the radiation, and to use maximal shielding from all sources of radiation.

A second form of radiation with potential health consequences comes in the form of chronic exposure to low-frequency electromagnetic fields such as those emitted by magnetic resonance imaging (MRI) equipment. Transient symptoms such as vertigo, nausea, dizziness, and visual phosphenes have all been reported. The severity of these symptoms is a function of the field strength of the scanner, the proximity to the scanner, and the rate of movement of the individual within the magnetic field.

There are currently no published regulations in the United States that limit occupational exposure to electromagnetic fields. Guidelines from the International Commission on Non-Ionizing Radiation Protection offer some suggestions regarding technique and worker practices to limit neurobehavioral effects.[31] Studies to date have not identified any chronic adverse health effects from long-term exposure to high-intensity magnetic fields. However, until more information is available, and especially in light of the increasing use of magnets with stronger electromagnetic fields, it would seem prudent to conform to the general admonition regarding all forms of radiation exposure: keep it as low as reasonably achievable.

Noise

A definition of "noise" that is particularly germane to the operating room setting is "the wrong sound at the wrong place." This

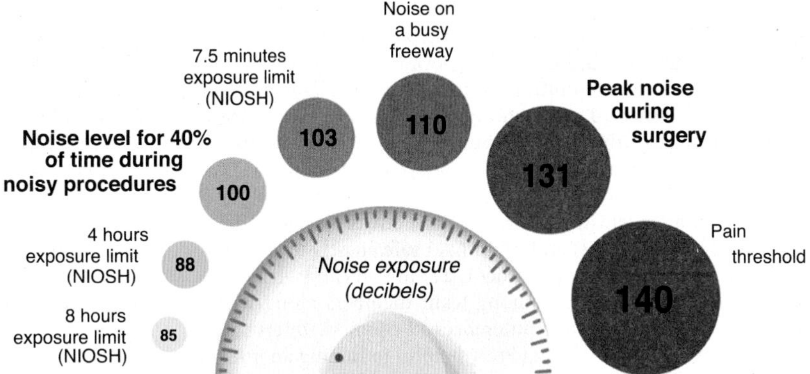

Figure 3-1 Noise. This schematic illustrates the relative intensities of different noises and the acceptable time limits of exposure. The noise levels commonly experienced in a modern operating room frequently exceed limits established by the National Institute for Occupational Safety and Health (NIOSH). (Reproduced with permission from Katz JD. Noise in the operating room. *Anesthesiology*. 2014;121(4): 894–898.)

emphasizes the important point that sounds that might be tolerable in one environment (such as a construction site) can be disruptive and even harmful in another (such as an operating room).

Noise is measured by the intensity and frequency of the sound waves and the duration during which these waves hit the ear. The unit commonly used to measure the volume of sound is the decibel (Db) which is reported on a logarithmic scale so that an increase of 10 Db corresponds roughly to a doubling of the intensity. A frequently accepted standard for the maximum level of safe noise exposure is 90 Db for 8 hours (Fig. 3-1). This level of background noise makes it necessary for a speaker to raise their voice in order to be heard at a distance of 3 feet. Each increase in ambient noise of 5 Db above 90 Db halves the permissible exposure time, so that 100 Db is acceptable for just 2 hours per day. The maximum peak allowable exposure in an industrial setting is 115 Db.

A considerably quieter environment is recommended for hospital settings. The EPA recommends that background noise levels in hospitals remain below 45 Db.[32] Recommendations for operating room noise levels by the World Health Organization are even more strict, requiring that it be maintained below 35 Db, which is approximately equivalent to the noise in a quiet library.[33]

These desirable limits for noise are routinely exceeded in an anesthesiologist's workplace. A modern operating room is often the noisiest place in a hospital. Noise routinely exceeds the TWA limit at which hearing protection is required by the OSHA. Machinery such as high-capacity heating and air conditioning systems, ventilators, suction equipment, forced air patient-warming devices, music, and conversations can produce ambient noise levels greater than 90 Db. Sporadic clatter from dropped instruments, surgical saws and drills, and anesthetic alerts and alarms add to this background noise so that in some operating rooms, noise levels of 100 Db or greater occur for 40% of the time, with peak levels exceeding 120 Db. The beginning and the end of surgery, when surgical equipment is being prepared or dismantled and casual conversations between staff members occur, and which coincides with anesthetic induction and emergence, are especially noisy periods.[34]

Excessive noise can adversely impact the operating room experience in many ways.[35] At the very least, it is a nuisance and distracting, especially to trainees and inexperienced clinicians. Noise also interferes with clinicians' critical ability to maintain meaningful communication, hear and interpret vital tones and alarms, perform complex psychomotor tasks, and accurately communicate with surgical team members.[36] One study suggested that excessive noise can contribute to increased surgical site infections.[37]

Exposure to excessive noise imposes several health hazards. Hearing loss is the most frequently reported medical consequence.[38] The hearing loss can be the result of a single exposure to an extremely loud sound (such as an explosion) or by repeated exposures to chronic loud noises (such as blaring music). The hearing loss occurs gradually and is frequently not recognized until significant damage has already occurred and is irreversible. There is growing evidence that HCWs who consistently work in noisy operating rooms are susceptible to noise-induced hearing loss. Substantial hearing loss has been demonstrated among anesthesiologists, especially those younger than age 55 years.[39] In 7% of anesthesiologists studied, the hearing impairment could potentially interfere with their ability to hear standard operating room alerts and alarms. Surgeons who consistently work in particularly noisy operating rooms are also reported to suffer an elevated risk of hearing loss.[40] Other health hazards commonly associated with exposure to excess noise include cardiovascular disease, impairment of cognitive function, and various psychological disorders.

The role of music in the operating room deserves special consideration. An individual's response to music can vary from calmed to agitated, depending upon other environmental factors and coexisting circumstances. When properly selected, background music can be soothing and contribute toward work efficiency. However, music also adds substantially to the already considerable ambient noise levels in the operating room. To many members of the surgical team, music that is not self-selected is distracting and serves as a hindrance to optimal performance.[41] Anesthesiologists frequently report that music can interfere with performance of several of their tasks. In one study, 26% of anesthesiologists felt that music reduced their vigilance and impaired their communication with other staff members and 51% felt that music was distracting when a problem was encountered.[42] The majority felt that music that they disliked was the most distracting. On the other hand, a subsequent study by the same group found that self-selected or classical music did not adversely affect the performance of anesthesiology residents on various psychomotor tests.[43] The bottom line is that, if music is to be played in the operating room, the selection, volume, and timing should all be determined by mutual consent.

Interpersonal Issues

Organizational issues, such as failed communication with other team members, can adversely impact an anesthesiologist's performance. The potential for disaster because of poor communication has been well illustrated in several airline catastrophes. The possibility for miscommunication and resultant error is heightened in the operating room because of the overlapping realms of professional responsibility, which may be at odds with established hierarchy, for example, when a problem noted by a nurse—or anesthesiologist—may have a consequence that only the surgeon can control. Poor communication can lead to conflict and compromised patient safety and has been identified as a root cause of many anesthesia-related sentinel events. Crisis resource management training, well established in the aerospace industry, has emerged to address this issue.

Effective conflict resolution is an important element of the teamwork necessary for successful surgical outcomes. Some degree of conflict occurs during the management of as many as 78% of patients in high-intensity areas such as operating rooms or critical care units.[44] Conflict and unpleasant interpersonal interactions among team members are among the most stressful aspects of the job of an anesthesiologist and can hinder safe anesthetic care.

Successful resolution of conflict is a skill that can be learned.[45] Mutual respect is required among team members along with a willingness to acknowledge differences of opinion. Intervention by a neutral third party is frequently helpful in finding an innovative solution. The airline industry has successfully implemented crew resource management programs to improve the performance of cockpit teams.[46]

"Production pressure" has the potential to create an environment in which issues of productivity supersede those of safety resulting in errors due directly to haste and/or deliberate deviations from safe practices.[47] The routine use of a preoperative checklist can help prevent those potential sources of error directly related to production pressure.[48]

Night Call, Sleepiness, and Fatigue

A circadian pattern of alertness and sleep is a basic component of human physiology. A common requirement for continued health is for 7 to 9 hours of sleep per 24-hour period, although this varies considerably among individuals and across one individual's life span.

Inadequate sleep, causing sleepiness (or drowsiness) results from a decreased quantity or a compromised quality of sleep. This can be caused by a multitude of factors including circadian rhythm disturbances following an extended period of wakefulness, obstructive sleep apnea, or disruptive work schedules. A related circumstance, physical or mental fatigue, can be caused by a number of factors in the workplace, especially time-on-task and the severity of the workload.

Many adverse health consequences have been associated with chronic sleep deprivation and fatigue including psychological illness, cardiovascular disease, immunodeficiency, reduced well-
4 being, and increased risk of premature death.[49] Cognitive impairment and specifically behavioral alertness and vigilant attention, which are critical tasks necessary to administer a safe anesthetic, are among the most prominent of the adverse consequences of sleep deprivation. And sleep deprivation and chronic fatigue have been identified among the major contributors to the growing epidemic of burnout among physicians in all specialties.

Sleep deprivation and fatigue are also closely associated with impaired worker performance. The psychomotor changes that are observed in the workplace are similar in many ways to those seen with alcohol or drug intoxication.[50] Sleep-deprived workers are at increased risk of committing workplace errors and suffer more work-related accidents. For example, fatigue has been recognized as a probable cause in approximately one-quarter of all major commercial aviation accidents.[51] It has also been identified as a major factor in many of the well-publicized industrial catastrophes, including those at Chernobyl, Three Mile Island, Exxon Valdez, and the Challenger space shuttle tragedy. Accident susceptibility extends beyond work hours to other activities of daily living, such as driving.[52]

There are significant individual variations in the impairment resulting from fatigue. Older individuals are particularly susceptible to the adverse effects of sleep deprivation and many older physicians find it difficult to manage the challenges of night call.[53]

Reports have identified sleep deprivation and fatigue as contributing factors in errors occurring within the health care setting.[54] An early report by Friedman[55] observed that interns reading electrocardiograms committed twice as many errors after an extended work shift than after a night of sleep. Several subsequent studies have reported that sleep-deprived physicians demonstrated increased vulnerability to such impairments as diminished intubation skills, increased error rates during laparoscopy, and poorer communication with patients and family members.[56] In one study that examined the management by medical interns during admissions to a medical service, 35.9% more medical errors occurred while on a "traditional" schedule (>24-hour work shifts) than when working a schedule that eliminated extended work shifts and reduced the number of hours worked per week.[57] Reports have also demonstrated an elevated risk for preventable adverse surgical events attributable to surgeon fatigue.[58]

However, other studies have reported little or no evidence of suboptimal clinical management or poorer outcomes from sleep-deprived clinicians. Koda et al.[59] conducted a meta-analysis covering the years 2010 to 2020 to determine the effects of surgeon fatigue on postoperative complications. They reported no significant differences between rested and fatigued surgeons in their rates of postoperative morbidity or mortality for both elective and nonelective surgeries. Other studies of surgeons and critical care specialists agree with these findings.[60,61]

Anesthesiologists who take night calls commonly suffer from each of the three well-defined classes of sleep deprivation: total, partial, and selective sleep deprivation. Interruption of sleep during call frequently occurs between the hours of 2 AM and 4 AM when humans are most vulnerable to fatigue-induced errors.

The role of fatigue specifically on anesthetic outcomes remains unclear. Several studies have identified consequences of sleep deprivation and fatigue that could adversely impact the conduct of a safe anesthetic, including impairments to cognition, short-term memory, and clinical decision making, prolonged reaction time, and reduced attention, vigilance, and performance. In an early study of American anesthesiologists, more than 50% admitted to having committed an error in medical judgment that they attributed to fatigue.[62] Howard et al.[63] examined how sleep-deprived anesthesiology residents managed a 4-hour simulated anesthetic and demonstrated progressive impairment of alertness, mood, and performance and a longer response latency to vigilance probes. A single-site study reporting on various adverse anesthetic events found that clinical outcomes are better for patients anesthetized at the beginning of the workday when compared to those later in the afternoon.[64] Several factors, including anesthesiologists' fatigue, were hypothesized to be contributory. Further, 58% of New Zealand anesthesiologists reported that they had exceeded their self-defined limit for safe continuous administration of anesthesia, with 86% admitting that they had committed a fatigue-related error.[65]

However, these are largely surrogate markers and/or subjective reporting that do not conclusively link fatigue with actual medical errors or adverse clinical outcomes. Several factors help to explain the difficulty in definitively establishing this relationship. Sleep deprivation is often arbitrarily defined, with varying criteria for both the control and the fatigued state. Similarly, the tasks being studied vary widely, so that reports measuring cognitive function (more sensitive to fatigue) are likely to demonstrate more impairment than those examining technical skills (less sensitive). Also, it is difficult to eliminate confounding variables such as the impact of loss of continuity of care, errors occurring during "hand-offs" of patients, and the reallocation of many medical tasks from physicians to colleagues and to nonphysician providers. An illustrative example was seen in a study that found that an increased number of medical errors were committed by ICU residents when working in a schedule that eliminated extended shifts (>24 hours).[66] As an unintended consequence of reducing consecutive duty hours, each resident had to care for a greater number of patients during their shift, with an increased number of handoffs, which may have contributed to medical errors. Finally, it can be difficult to extrapolate findings from simulation studies using volunteers in a laboratory to clinicians in real-life work conditions.

The health care industry is slowly catching up with other business enterprises that impact public health in identifying and regulating work practices that require excessively long shifts. It was not until the well-publicized Libby Zion case in 1984 (which alleged that fatal, avoidable mistakes were made by exhausted, unsupervised residents) that medical organizations and state legislatures acted to limit excessive work hours among residents. In 2003, the Accreditation Council for Graduate Medical Education (ACGME) established the first set of standards to limit resident duty hours. These standards have been revised several times, most recently in 2020. Among other guidance, these standards impose several work hours restrictions, including the well-known limit of 80 weekly work hours with the longest consecutive period being 30 hours. The imposition and effectiveness of these standards have been controversial, and several authors have commented on a perceived failure of these changes to improve resident education or clinical outcomes.[67] A contradiction that is inherent in the ACGME work hours restrictions is that they apply only to trainees and work hours remain unregulated for their attending physicians and for the same trainees when they enter medical practice.

Prolonged work hours and sleep deprivation are a ubiquitous component of many anesthesiologists' professional lives. Many academic faculty members now work longer hours than they did prior to house staff work hour limitations because of a shift of work from residents to faculty. In addition, the commonly recognized demands contributing to clinicians' fatigue were exacerbated by the challenges imposed by the COVID viral pandemic.

The only way to completely avoid sleep deprivation and related fatigue is to allow time and opportunity for adequate sleep. It is important to recognize that a single night of recovery sleep may not be adequate to counteract all the adverse neurobiologic effects caused by an extended period of sleep deprivation. When long work periods are unavoidable, several strategies have been devised to mitigate the adverse effects. Recommendations include minimizing sleep debt by maximizing sleep before on-call shifts and utilizing maneuvers to overcome sleep inertia such as increasing ambient light levels, stretching, taking frequent breaks, and napping when possible.[68] A number of pharmaceutical aids, such as caffeine and modafinil (a schedule intravenous [IV] drug), have been approved for military use and, if used under supervision and carefully monitored, could play some role for clinicians with shift-work sleep disorder.[51]

Substance Use Disorders

Although drug proclivities have changed over time, society continues to struggle with SUDs.[69] SUDs include abuse (in which the use of a substance continues despite negative consequences) and addiction (involving compulsive use, psychological dependence, or physiologic dependence). Many physicians will, at some point in their careers, develop a form of SUD, with anesthesiologists in the particularly vulnerable position of having access and expertise for use of potent anesthetic and opiate medications. The most common substance abused by the general physician population remains alcohol. A 2015 study reported 12.9% of male and 21.4% of female physicians espoused alcohol abuse or dependence.[70] However, among anesthesiologists, Warner found that the most commonly abused substances were opiates, followed by alcohol, followed by anesthetics/hyponotics.[71]

The medical community has held a long-standing concern for SUD among physicians that, intriguingly, has not spared the luminaries of medicine.[72] Improved data collection began in the 1980s when the Medical Association of Georgia's Impaired Physician Program found that, among their first 1,000 participants, anesthesiologists were disproportionately represented (12.1% of participants while only 3.9% of U.S. physicians; 33.7% of resident participants while 4.6% of US residents).[73] Further, anesthesiologists were much more likely to abuse narcotics, multiple substances and utilize the intravenous route than other physicians, who were more likely to abuse ethanol. Propofol has since emerged as a drug of abuse, highlighting the more treacherous nature of the substances abused by anesthesiologists.[74] Unlike alcohol abuse, intravenous narcotic and hypnotic abuse has a short initiation to discovery phase, a high mortality, and involves drug diversion. Unfortunately, the initial discovery of abuse is too often an overdose event.

Early recognition of addiction is critical to implementing lifesaving interventions. Anesthesiologists must be able to recognize the constellation of physiologic, behavioral, and relational characteristics exhibited in SUDs (Table 3-3). Professional and personal

Table 3-3 Signs of Substance Abuse and Dependence Within the Practice of Anesthesia

Within the practice of anesthesia:

- Signing out increasing quantities of narcotics/hypnotics (often inappropriately high for the case)
- Volunteering for cases requiring high-dose narcotics
- Arriving early, staying late, taking extra call, and offering extra breaks to gain access to drugs (or calling in sick in the case of alcoholics)
- Refusing lunch or breaks, personally administering medications in the recovery room, and preferring to work alone to mask drug diversion behavior
- Asking for additional bathroom breaks, or staying in bathroom for long periods to use drugs
- Being difficult to locate after breaks, as naps often follow drug use
- Wearing long sleeves to hide needle marks
- Illegible or sloppy charting
- Frequent changes in job to maintain the secret

Behavioral changes:

- Mood swings and emotional lability
- Social withdrawal (from people and previously enjoyed activities)
- Increased impulsivity
- Leaving drug paraphernalia (bloody swabs, needles, etc.) in common areas
- Decreased sexual drive
- Increased domestic strife

Physical signs:

- Pinpoint pupils
- Long sleeves worn due to cold sensitivity (associated with narcotics)
- Alcohol odor on the breath or witnessing IV drug use
- Weight loss and pallor
- Narcotic withdrawal (sweating, tremors)
- Coma and death—unfortunately a not uncommon presenting symptom

withdrawal, while maintaining a façade of normality at work to preserve the access to drugs, is a typical early sign. By the time impairment is evident to most colleagues, the disease is often in its fatal end stages.

Compared to internists, anesthesiologists also have an increased relative rate (RR) of mortality from suicide (RR 1.45), drug-related suicide (RR 2), and drug-related death (RR 2.79).[75] Strikingly, in a study of 601 physicians who were found to have SUD during anesthesiology residency between 1977 and 2013, 114 (19%) 5 died from a SUD-related cause during the follow-up period. As such, if one is to consider SUD-related death an occupational hazard of anesthesia, the profession is more dangerous than being a firefighter.[71]

There exist many state-specific legal ramifications to physician chemical impairment. In many cases, the legal jeopardy can be mitigated if the involved physician voluntarily seeks treatment, many of which are closely affiliated with State Medical Boards. By federal law, the National Practitioner Data Bank must be notified of disciplinary action taken against an impaired physician. A physician who fails to report an impaired colleague may be subject themselves to disciplinary and criminal penalties in certain states. The reluctance to seek help is deeply rooted in physician culture, reinforced by years of self-denial required to complete training and practice medicine. A well-developed defense mechanism enables many physician addicts to minimize evolving impairment and delay treatment, with often devastating consequences.

Recently, the Federation of State Medical Boards (FSMB) has issued guidance for how states should approach mental health and SUD in their licensure processes to include the following:

1. Analyze whether probing questions related to physician mental health, addiction, and substance use are necessary
2. Carefully differentiate between presenting illness and the resulting impairments
3. Limit questions of impairment to the past 2 years
4. Consider offering the option of "safe haven nonreporting" for physicians actively engaged in appropriate treatment for mental health or addiction[76]

Further, the National Academy of Medicine (NAM)'s Action Collaborative on Clinician Well-Being and Resilience recently released a consensus report, "Taking Action Against Clinician Burnout: A Systems Approach to Professional Well-being," which outlines multiple policy and systemic level interventions, including the destigmatization of mental health and SUDs.[77] This collaborative continues, with support from the U.S. Department of Health and Human Services, to advocate for and provide tools to further destigmatize clinician mental health.

One strategy aimed at prevention and early detection of SUDs is compulsory pre-employment and random drug screening (RDS) of anesthesiologists, a practice standard in other high-profile industries (aviation, military, nuclear). While RDS is an element of reentry contracts, few anesthesia departments randomly screen anesthesiologists. Data at one institution employing a system of RDS indicates a reduction in SUDs in residents.[78] Experience has shown that the spouse of an abusing anesthesiologist, who is educated and alert to the signs of the illness, can often recognize and confront the affected anesthesiologist well before that person's health care colleagues or an institution's RDS.

Controversy persists over the appropriate disposition of an anesthesiologist who has successfully completed SUD treatment. While the prognosis for sustained recovery is higher for physicians than the general public, relapse is often fatal among those returning to practice in anesthesia, fueling the argument that it is a risk too great to take. Countering that argument is that a risk stratification approach may be used, taking into account the three greatest factors linked to relapse: family history of substance abuse, a major opioid as the abused drug, and a coexisting psychiatric disorder.[79]

Reentry into practice for a recovering physician must be collaborative, involving the recovering physician, the treating addiction counselor, occupational health, department leadership, organizational credentialing board, and others. Federal laws, such as the Americans with Disabilities Act, impose additional considerations. A carefully worded contract is essential and should include the following:

- Continued monitoring of sobriety
- Continued maintenance treatment
- A period of supervised or modified practice

Despite precautions, relapse must be anticipated, and the advice of a physician treatment center can be helpful. Those with the highest chance of successful reentry into practice accept and understand their disease, have no concomitant psychiatric illness, have strong social support, are sponsored, are committed to their recovery. and have bonded with Alcoholics Anonymous (AA; http://www.aa.org/) or Narcotics Anonymous (NA; http:/www.na.org/). In addition, their department and hospital must support their return. Those with active disease, severe psychiatric comorbidities, prolonged intravenous substance use, or with prior relapses or treatment failures should be redirected to another specialty.[79]

SUD prevention requires strict control of substances of abuse. Meticulous controlled substance regulation and accounting is essential, especially with the advent of conveniences like satellite pharmacies and automated drug-dispensing machines.

While there is no clear link between SUD and poor patient care, there are cases of patient harm involving an impaired anesthesiologist. A 1994 inquiry of the ASA's Closed Claims Database revealed seven cases citing "substance abuse" or "chemical dependence" in the anesthesiologist reviewer claim summary. Five of these involved an anesthesiologist shown to be abusing substances.[80]

The burden of SUD is great in anesthesiology and does not appear to be abating. Efforts must be made on multiple fronts to decrease this tragic occupational hazard, including education, controlled substance accounting, and systems of prevention, discovery, treatment, and recovery.

Infectious Hazards

Anesthesia personnel are at risk for acquiring infections from patients, their families, and from numerous other personnel in the health care workforce (Video 3-1). This risk is clearly increasing because evolutionary biology encourages new survival strategies for these pathogens. Increasingly, immune-compromised patients become vectors for these resistant, opportunistic organisms. Furthermore, globalization brings increasing spread of organisms from less-developed areas in the world, such as the 1999 outbreak in New York of West Nile Virus encephalitis, the 2003 epidemic of severe acute respiratory syndrome (SARS) in Hong Kong, and the more recent SARS COVID-19 pandemic, the initial infections for which were reported in Wuhan, China. Finally, diseases that were once thought to be noninfectious such as peptic ulcer disease (*Helicobacter pylori*), invasive cervical cancer (human papillomavirus), Kaposi sarcoma (human herpesvirus type 8), and certain lymphomas such as Burkitt and non-Hodgkin (Epstein–Barr virus [EBV]) are now better understood as a long-term consequence of infection, making occupational health precautions even more important.

Viral infections are the most significant threat to HCWs. Most commonly, these are spread through the respiratory route. Other infections are spread by hand-to-hand transmission and hand washing is the single most important protection strategy.[81] Immunity against some viral pathogens, such as hepatitis B, can be provided through vaccination. Transmission of blood-borne pathogens such as hepatitis (HBV, HCV) and human immunodeficiency virus (HIV) can be prevented
6 with mechanical barriers. Current recommendations from the Centers for Disease Control and Prevention (CDC) for pre-employment screening, infection control practices, vaccination, postexposure treatment, and work restrictions for infected personnel should be consulted for specific information related to each pathogen.[82,83]

Standard and Transmission-Based Precautions

In the late 1980s, the CDC formulated recommendations ("universal precautions") for preventing transmission of blood-borne infections to HCWs. The guidelines were based on the epidemiology of HBV as a worst-case model for transmission of blood-borne infections and available knowledge of the epidemiology of HIV and HCV. Since asymptomatic carriers of many blood-borne viruses cannot be identified, universal precautions were recommended for use during all patient contact. This strategy was broadened to include saliva, semen, vaginal secretions, human tissues, and cerebrospinal, synovial, pleural, peritoneal, pericardial, and amniotic fluids. Subsequently, the CDC aggregated the major features of universal precautions into standard infection control guidelines that should be applied to all patients (Tables 3-4 to 3-6). *Transmission-based precautions* are the second tier of infection control and are

Table 3-4 CDC Infection Control Guidelines

Infection Control Guidelines	Link
Perform hand hygiene	
Website for hand hygiene	https://www.cdc.gov/handhygiene/index.html
Guideline for hand hygiene	https://www.cdc.gov/handhygiene/providers/guideline.html
Training course for hand hygiene	https://www.cdc.gov/handhygiene/training/interactiveEducation/
Posters and brochures for hand hygiene	https://www.cdc.gov/handhygiene/campaign/index.html?CDC_AA_refVa https%3A%2F%2Fwww.cdc.gov%2Fhandhygiene%2Fresources.html
Use personal protective equipment (PPE) whenever there is an expectation of possible exposure to infectious material	https://www.cdc.gov/infectioncontrol/guidelines/isolation/index.html
Protecting health care personnel	https://www.cdc.gov/HAI/prevent/ppe.html
Training slides and posters for protecting health care personnel	https://www.cdc.gov/HAI/prevent/ppe.html
Follow respiratory hygiene/cough etiquette principles	
Guideline for isolation precautions	https://www.cdc.gov/infectioncontrol/guidelines/isolation/index.html
Respiratory hygiene/cough etiquette in health care settings	https://www.cdc.gov/flu/professionals/infectioncontrol/resphygiene.htm
Cover your cough	https://www.cdc.gov/flu/business/prevent-flu-workplace.html
Ensure appropriate patient placement	
Guideline for isolation precautions	https://www.cdc.gov/infectioncontrol/guidelines/isolation/index.html
Properly handle and properly clean and disinfect patient care equipment and instruments/devices	
Clean and disinfect the environment appropriately	
Guidelines for environmental infection control	https://www.cdc.gov/infectioncontrol/guidelines/environmental/index.html
Guidelines for disinfection and sterilization	https://www.cdc.gov/infectioncontrol/guidelines/disinfection/index.html
Toolkit evaluating environmental cleaning	https://www.cdc.gov/hai/toolkits/Evaluating-Environmental-Cleaning.html
Handle textiles and laundry carefully	
Environmental infection control guidelines	https://www.cdc.gov/infectioncontrol/guidelines/environmental/index.html
Follow safe injection practices	
Wear a surgical mask when performing lumbar punctures	
Injection safety	https://www.cdc.gov/injectionsafety/index.html
Guideline for isolation precautions	https://www.cdc.gov/infectioncontrol/guidelines/isolation/index.html
One & only campaign	https://www.cdc.gov/injectionsafety/one-and-only.html

Table 3-5 Updated CDC Transmission-Based Precautions

Ensure appropriate patient placement
Use personal protective equipment (PPE) appropriately
Limit transport and movement of patients
***Airborne Precautions*: use airborne precautions for patients known or suspected to be infected with pathogens transmitted by the airborne route (e.g., tuberculosis, measles, chickenpox, disseminated herpes zoster)**
Source control: put a mask on the patient
Ensure appropriate patient placement in an airborne infection isolation room (AIIR)
Restrict susceptible health care personnel from entering the room
Use personal protective equipment (PPE) appropriately
Limit transport and movement of patients
Immunize susceptible persons as soon as possible following unprotected contact

https://www.cdc.gov/infectioncontrol/basics/transmission-based-precautions.html

used in addition to standard precautions for infected or colonized patients. They consist of three tiers—contact precautions, droplet precautions, and airborne precautions.

OSHA's Bloodborne Pathogens Standard (29 CFR 1910.1030) prescribes safeguards to protect workers against the health hazards caused by blood-borne pathogens.[84] These standards require an exposure control plan specifically detailing the methods that the employer is providing to reduce employees' risk of exposure to blood-borne pathogens. The employer must encourage strategies to reduce blood exposures, furnish appropriate PPE, offer the HBV vaccine at no charge to personnel, and provide an annual education program to inform employees of their risk for blood-borne infections. Congressional testimony by OSHA reported an order-of-magnitude decrease in HBV infection in a span of 8 years (1987 to 1995).[85]

The institution's employee health service is required to obtain and record a contagious disease history from new employees. Annual TB testing of health care personnel is not recommended unless there is a known exposure or ongoing transmission.[86] In addition, the employee health service must have protocols for dealing with workers exposed to contagious diseases and those exposed to the blood of patients infected with HIV or hepatitis B or C virus. Free consultation regarding HIV is available from the CDC Post-Exposure Prophylaxis Hotline (PEPline) at 1-888-448-4911.

Respiratory Viruses

Even in nonpandemic times, respiratory viruses accounted for half or more of all acute illnesses. Every year across the globe, there are an estimated 1 billion cases of influenza, of which 3 to 5 million are severe cases, resulting in 290,000 to 650,000 influenza-related respiratory deaths. This problem was significantly exacerbated by the COVID-19 pandemic, with over 472 million cases and more than 6 million deaths worldwide from 2019 to 2022. Small-particle aerosols from viruses such as influenza, corona viruses, and measles are produced by coughing, sneezing, or talking and can be propelled over large distances. Large droplets that have been produced by coughing or sneezing can contaminate the donor's hands or an inanimate surface. The virus is then transferred to the oral, nasal, or conjunctival mucous membranes of a susceptible person by self-inoculation. Rhinovirus and human respiratory syncytial virus (HRSV) are also spread by this process.

Influenza Viruses

There are four types of influenza viruses: A, B, C, and D. They are distinguished based on characteristics of the nucleoprotein (NP) and matrix (M) protein antigens. Influenza A viruses are subtyped based on the surface hemagglutinin (H) and neuraminidase (N) antigens. Individual strains are designated according to the site of origin, isolate number, year of isolation, and subtype, for example, influenza A/California/07/2009 (the infamous H1N1 of 2009). Influenza A has 18 H subtypes and 11 N subtypes, of which H1-3, H5-7, H9-10, N1-2, and N5-9 have caused disease in humans. Influenza B viruses are not divided into subtypes but rather lineages and strains. Influenza C virus infections generally cause mild illness and are not thought to cause human epidemics. Influenza D viruses primarily affect cattle and are not known to infect or cause illness in people. Acutely ill patients shed virus for as long as 5 days after the onset of symptoms via small-particle aerosols. Because of their contact with patient's nasopharyngeal secretions, anesthesiologists can easily become victims as well as vectors in the spread of influenza.

Influenza A (H1N1), A (H3N2), and one or two influenza B viruses (depending on the vaccine) are included in each year's influenza vaccine. The CDC recommends that all U.S. HCWs be immunized annually with the inactivated (killed virus) influenza vaccine. Through the efforts of the Society for Healthcare Epidemiology of America (SHEA), there is established precedent to make this a condition of employment and medical staff credentialing.[87] Since the vaccine used in the United States and many other countries is produced in eggs, individuals with true hypersensitivity to egg products either should be desensitized or not be vaccinated. A live attenuated influenza vaccine, approved for use in healthy nonpregnant persons 2 to 49 years of age and administered by intranasal spray, is now available. It is quadrivalent as well in order to provide protection against the two influenza A (H1N1 and H3N2) and influenza B viruses.

Influenza outbreaks occur almost every year, although their extent and severity vary widely. In the past century, there have been three influenza pandemics (1918, 1957, and 1968) with the "Great Influenza" in 1918 killing between 40 and 50 million people worldwide. The most recent pandemic emerged in March 2009 and was caused by an influenza A/H1N1 virus that rapidly spread worldwide over several months. Containment requires early identification and isolation of infected individuals. NIOSH-certified respirators (N95 or higher) should be used by personnel during activities or procedures likely to generate infectious respiratory aerosols.

Avian Influenza A

In 1997, human cases of influenza caused by avian influenza viruses (A/H5N1) were detected in Hong Kong during an extensive outbreak of influenza in poultry. Domestic poultry may be infected with highly pathogenic avian influenza (HPAI) A viruses or low-pathogenic avian influenza (LPAI) A viruses. This classification refers to the ability of the virus to cause disease in chickens in the laboratory, not in humans. Human infection with low-pathogenic and highly pathogenic avian influenza A viruses have resulted in a range of symptoms from mild to severe, although rarely. A vaccine for prophylaxis against avian influenza H5N1 was approved for use in the United States in 2007.

Table 3-6 COVID-19—American Society of Anesthesiologists Recommendations for Infection Control

Topic	Link
COVID-19 and clinical care (home page)	https://www.asahq.org/in-the-spotlight/coronavirus-covid-19-information/clinical-care
Videolaryngoscopy	
Intubating COVID-19 or suspected COVID-19 patients	https://www.asahq.org/about-asa/governance-and-committees/asa-committees/committee-on-occupational-health/coronavirus
Care for COVID-19 patients in the intensive care unit	https://www.asahq.org/in-the-spotlight/coronavirus-covid-19-information/caesar
Critical care drug recommendations for COVID-19 during times of drug shortages	https://www.asahq.org/about-asa/newsroom/news-releases/2020/06/critical-care-drug-recommendations-for-covid-19-during-times-of-drug-shortages
Purposing anesthesia machines as ICU ventilators	https://www.asahq.org/in-the-spotlight/coronavirus-covid-19-information/purposing-anesthesia-machines-for-ventilators
Tracheotomies and COVID-19 patients	https://journals.lww.com/anesthesia-analgesia/fulltext/2020/08000/perioperative_considerations_for_tracheostomies_in.10.aspx
Blood management and COVID-19 patients	https://www.asahq.org/in-the-spotlight/coronavirus-covid-19-information/pandemics-andpatient-blood-management
EGD procedures and COVID-19 patients	https://www.giejournal.org/article/S0016-5107(20)34306-6/fulltext
LMA usage and MAC anesthesia	https://gi.org/2020/03/15/joint-gi-society-message-on-covid-19/
MAC cases with an open airway	https://www.asahq.org/in-the-spotlight/coronavirus-covid-19-information/clinical-care
Using an LMA with positive pressure ventilation vs. an endotracheal tube in a standard operating room (positive pressure room)	https://www.asahq.org/in-the-spotlight/coronavirus-covid-19-information/clinical-care
Delivering supplemental oxygen to a COVID+ or PUI patient wearing a mask	https://www.asahq.org/in-the-spotlight/coronavirus-covid-19-information/clinical-care
Steroid injections in the elderly with COVID	https://www.asahq.org/in-the-spotlight/coronavirus-covid-19-information/clinical-care
ECT and COVID-19 patients	https://www.asahq.org/in-the-spotlight/coronavirus-covid-19-information/clinical-care
Treatment of stroke patients during the COVID-19 pandemic? (SNACC Consensus)	https://journals.lww.com/jnsa/Fulltext/2020/07000/Anesthetic_Management_of_Endovascular_Treatment_of.4.aspx
Safety of regional anesthesia vs. general anesthesia for COVID-19 and PUIs	https://www.asahq.org/about-asa/governance-and-committees/asa-committees/committee-on-occupational-health/coronavirus
Recommendations for pediatric airway management in COVID-19 Patients	https://journals.lww.com/anesthesia-analgesia/fulltext/2020/07000/pediatric_airway_management_in_covid_19_patients_.11.aspx
Recommendations on anesthetizing a patient who previously had COVID-19	https://www.asahq.org/about-asa/newsroom/news-releases/2022/02/asa-and-apsf-joint-statement-on-elective-surgery-procedures-and-anesthesia-for-patients-after-covid-19-infection
COVID-19 and occupational safety and wellness	https://www.asahq.org/in-the-spotlight/coronavirus-covid-19-information/occupational-safety-and-wellness

Human Respiratory Syncytial Virus

HRSV is the most common cause of serious bronchiolitis and lower respiratory tract disease in infants and young children worldwide. In the United States, HRSV is responsible for 57,000 hospitalizations annually and 500,000 emergency department visits among children <5 years old. Ironically, reports from around the world have revealed up to a 98% reduction in HRSV cases during the COVID-19 pandemic. Large amounts of virus are present in respiratory secretions of infected children. Viable virus can be recovered for up to 6 hours on contaminated environmental surfaces. The virus is readily inactivated with soap and water and disinfectants. Infection of susceptible people occurs by self-inoculation when HRSV in secretions is transferred to the hands, which then contact the mucous membranes of the eyes or nose. Although most children have been exposed to HRSV early in life, immunity is not permanent, and reinfection is common. HRSV may also be a significant cause of illness in healthy elderly patients and those with chronic cardiac or pulmonary disease. HRSV is shed for approximately 7 days after infection. Careful hand washing and the use of standard precautions have been shown to reduce HRSV infection in hospital personnel.

Severe Acute Respiratory Syndrome

SARS is a respiratory tract infection produced by SARS-associated coronavirus (SARS-CoV). The coronavirus SARS-CoV-2, the infective agent of COVID-19, shares more than 70% genetic similarity with SARS-CoV-1, the origin of 2003 SARS outbreak. Infection-associated symptoms are very similar between SARS and COVID-19 diseases. SARS typically presents with a fever greater than 38.0 °C followed by symptoms of headache, generalized aches, and cough. Severe pneumonia may lead to acute respiratory distress syndrome and death. The mechanisms of transmission of SARS are incompletely understood. Spread may occur by both large and small aerosols and perhaps by the fecal–oral route, as well as close person-to-person contact. The virus can also be spread when an individual touches a contaminated object and then inoculates their own mouth, nose, or eyes. Aerosolization of respiratory secretions during airway procedures has been a recognized risk to HCWs including anesthesiologists and critical care nurses since the first SARS infections.[88] The cytokine storm, identified in both SARS and COVID-19 severe cases, is generated through inflammasome activation.

After the first cases of SARS-CoV-1 were reported from Asia in late 2002, the disease quickly spread globally in 2003 before being controlled. In most cases, the infection was transmitted from human to human. The overall case fatality rate was 9.5%. Cases appeared to be somewhat milder in the United States with less severity among children. Since 2004, global surveillance for SARS-CoV-1 has detected no confirmed cases.

That has not been the case for SARS-CoV-2, or COVID-19. One of the key differences from the prior SARS and Middle Eastern respiratory syndrome (MERS) outbreaks has been a requirement to consider on a global scale the provision of infection control and HCW protective equipment. Within the context of an almost daily change in the landscape of evolving knowledge, numerous clinical, personal, and occupational health concerns for HCWs have emerged. Multiple U.S. and international organizations have published recommendations for infection control and the use of PPE during anesthesia for patients with COVID-19 (Table 3-6). Most precautions are based on guidance from the CDC and prior experience with other infectious agents such as SARS-CoV or MERS-CoV viruses. At this time, airborne precautions (N95 or higher respirator, or powered air purifying respirator [PAPR]) are recommended for all patients who require airway management, since patients may be asymptomatic or minimally symptomatic, and COVID-19 may not be suspected.

During the early years of the COVID-19 pandemic, a relative consensus developed around the efficacy of measures for personal and patient care precautions, as well as overall agreement about the efficacy of vaccination and boosters. However, at the time this chapter was written (2022), diagnostic testing was undergoing an evolving process of understanding, discovery, advances in technology, and utilization. In particular, rapid diagnostic (antigen) self-testing was being deployed at the patient/citizen level to address public health concerns and thereby "democratize" the process of population protection and supplementing the intense efforts of clinicians, allowing symptomatic people to quarantine while awaiting test results, retest while maintaining their quarantine if symptomatic, and self-performed follow-up testing 5 to 7 days later if negative.[89] Antigen self-testing correlates with the level of antigenemia and enables more rapid diagnosis while conferring as much protection as possible to further contacts (Fig. 3-2).

Enteric Infections

Diarrheal disease is second only to lower respiratory tract infections as the most common infectious cause of death worldwide. Infectious agents include viruses, bacteria, and parasites, acting via noninflammatory (enterotoxin), inflammatory (cytotoxin), or penetrating mechanisms. Traveler's diarrhea is the most common travel-related infectious illness (20% to 50%), with *Escherichia coli* the most common organism. Rotavirus is most common among children less than 2 years of age, especially children in day

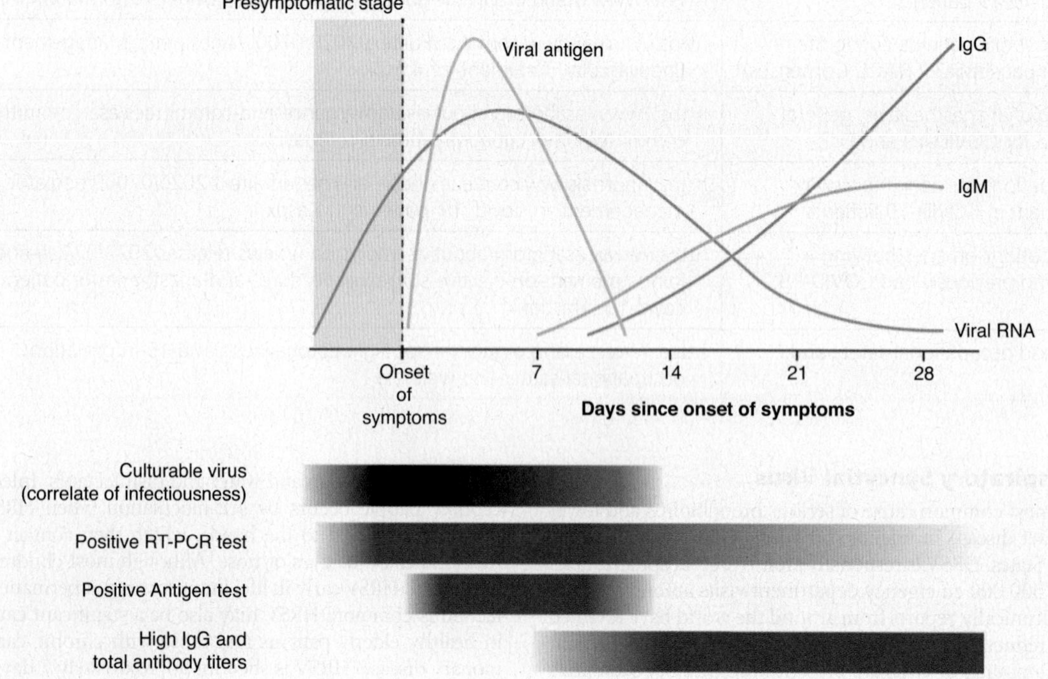

Figure 3-2 Timeline of viremia, antigenemia, and immune response during acute SARS-CoV-2 infection. (Derived from Drain PK. Rapid diagnostic testing for SARS-CoV-2. *N Engl J Med.* 2022;386(3):264–272.)

care. Rotavirus can spread rapidly in day care centers and pediatric wards. *Giardia lamblia* is more common in older children, as is norovirus, and there is a high rate of secondary cases among family members. *Clostridium difficile* is the main cause of nosocomial diarrhea among adult inpatients in the United States. One-third of elderly patients in nursing homes develop a significant diarrheal illness each year, and more than half of these are caused by *C. difficile*, especially following antibiotic therapy. Personal hygiene on the part of clinicians is directed to limiting secondary fecal–oral spread (Table 3-7).

Table 3-7 Prevention of Occupational-Acquired Infections

Infection/Condition	Precautions	Comments
Abscess		
Draining/major	Contact	
Draining/minor	Standard	
Acquired immune deficiency virus (HIV)	Standard	Postexposure prophylaxis (PEP) for some exposures
Avian influenza	Standard+Contact+ Airborne	Enhanced precautions
Bronchiolitis	Contact	
Clostridium		
Botulinum	Standard	Not transmitted person to person
Difficile	Contact	
Perfringens	Standard	Not transmitted person to person
Conjunctivitis		
Bacterial	Standard	
Viral	Contact	Most commonly: adenovirus, enterovirus, coxsackie virus A24.
Creutzfeldt–Jakob disease	Standard	Single-use equipment preferred, special cleaning (NaOH, heat, and time requirements) for contaminated instruments and environment
Diptheria pharyngeal	Droplet	Until 2 cultures >24 h apart are negative
E. coli	Standard	Contact precautions if patient incontinent
Haemophilus influenza		
Seasonal	Droplet	Single-patient room or cohort, gown and glove
Pandemic	Droplet	Enhanced precautions (airborne may be recommended)
Hepatitis, viral		
A	Standard	Contact precautions for incontinent patients
B	Standard	
C	Standard	
E	Standard	Contact precautions for incontinent patients
Herpes, zoster (varicella-zoster)		
Disseminated	Airborne, contact	Health care workers (HCWs) without immunity should not care for patient if immune HCW available. For susceptible exposed persons for whom vaccine is contraindicated, provide varicella zoster immune globulin as soon as possible after exposure and within 10 d
Localized	Standard	
Impetigo	Contact	
Legionnaires disease	Standard	Not transmitted person to person
Lice		
Head	Contact	
Body	Standard	
Pubic	Standard	
Lyme disease	Standard	
Malaria	Standard	

Table 3-7 Prevention of Occupational-Acquired Infections (CONTINUED)

Infection/Condition	Precautions	Comments
Measles	Airborne	Management of exposed health care personnel with presumptive evidence of immunity: postexposure prophylaxis is not necessary; work restrictions are not necessary; daily monitoring for signs and symptoms of measles infection for 21 d after the last exposure; have awareness that previously vaccinated individuals may have a modified disease presentation. • For HCW without presumptive evidence of immunity to measles: administer postexposure prophylaxis in accordance with CDC and ACIP recommendations; exclude from work from the 5th day after the first exposure until the 21st day after the last exposure; HCW who received the first dose of MMR vaccine prior to exposure may remain at work and should receive the second dose of MMR vaccine, at least 28 d after the first dose; implement daily monitoring for signs and symptoms of measles infection for 21 d after the last exposure.
Meningitis		
Bacterial	Standard	
Fungal	Standard	
Neisseria	Droplet	
Streptococcus	Standard	PEP available
Multidrug-resistant organisms (MDROs: MRSA, VRE, VISA/VRSA, ESBL-resistant *S. pneumoniae*)	Standard/Contact	In acute care facilities: Implement contact precautions routinely for all patients infected with target MDROs and for patients that have been previously identified as being colonized with target MDROs.
Mumps	Droplet	Susceptible HCWs should not care for patient if immune HCW available.
Mycoplasma	Droplet	
Mycobacterium tuberculosis	Airborne	
Norovirus gastroenteritis	Contact+Standard	
Parainfluenza	Contact	
Pertussis	Droplet	Single-patient room or cohort. PEP available. Tdap recommended.
Poliomyelitis	Contact	
Rabies	Standard	
Respiratory syncytial virus	Contact	Standard mask should be worn.
Rhinovirus	Droplet	
Rubella	Droplet	Susceptible HCW should not care for patient if immune HCW available. Vaccine available. Non–immune-exposed individuals may be contagious from day 5–21 after exposure.
Salmonella	Standard	Contact precautions for incontinent patients.
SARS-CoV-1	Airborne+Droplet+ Contact+Standard	Maintain precautions until 10 d after resolution of fever.
SARS-CoV-2 (COVID-19)	Airborne+Droplet+ Contact+Standard	
Shigella	Standard	Contact precautions for incontinent patients.
Smallpox	Contact/Airborne	Maintain precautions until all scabs have crusted and separated (3–4 wk). Nonvaccinated HCW should not care for patient if immune HCW available.
Staphylococcal		
Major, wound	Contact	
Streptococcal		
Major, wound	Contact, droplet	

ESBL, extended-spectrum beta-lactamase–producing organisms; MRSA, methicillin-resistant Staphylococcus aureus; VISA/VRSA, vancomycin-intermediate/resistant Staphylococcus aureus; VRE, vancomycin-resistant Enterococci.
Adapted from CDC Guideline for Isolation Precautions: Preventing Transmission of Infectious Agents in Healthcare Settings 2007 (last updated July 2019). For a complete list of organisms, see Appendix A. Type and duration of precautions recommended for selected infections and conditions. https://www.cdc.gov/infectioncontrol/guidelines/isolation/index.html

DNA Viruses

Herpes simplex viruses (HSV-1, HSV-2; *Herpesvirus hominis*) produce a variety of infections involving mucocutaneous surfaces, central nervous system (CNS), and visceral organs. Exposure to HSV at mucosal surfaces or abraded skin allows entry of the virus and initiation of viral replication. The primary infection with HSV type 1 is usually clinically inapparent but may involve severe oral lesions, fever, and adenopathy. After the primary infection subsides, the latent virus persists within the sensory nerve ganglion. Gingivostomatitis and pharyngitis are the most common clinical manifestations of first-episode HSV-1 infection, while recurrent herpes labialis is the most common clinical manifestation of reactivation HSV-2. Herpetic whitlow—HSV infection of the finger—may occur as a complication of primary oral or genital herpes by inoculation of virus through a break in the epidermal surface or by direct introduction of virus into the hand, a particularly important point for HCWs. HSV infection of the eye is the most common cause of corneal blindness in the United States. Of all HSV-infected populations, infants younger than 6 weeks have the highest frequency of visceral and/or CNS infection. Of note for obstetrical anesthesia practice, antibody to HSV-2 has been detected in 32% of pregnant women with no history of genital herpes. Asymptomatic HSV shedding was detected in 0.43% of women in late pregnancy and during delivery, and a first episode of clinical genital herpes was recognized by 16% of women during their pregnancy.[90] HCWs can be inoculated by direct contact with body fluids laden with either HSV type 1 or 2.

Varicella–zoster virus (VZV) causes two distinct clinical diseases: varicella (chickenpox) and zoster (shingles). Chickenpox, ubiquitous and highly contagious, is usually a benign illness of childhood with transmission by the respiratory route. Reactivation of latent VZV (herpes zoster), most common after the sixth decade of life, presents as a markedly painful dermatomal vesicular rash. Infection during pregnancy may result in fetal death or (rarely) congenital defects. Patients and medical personnel with active VZV infection can transmit the virus to others. Anesthesiologists working in pain clinics can be exposed to VZV when caring for patients who have discomfort from herpes zoster. Communicability begins 1 to 2 days before the onset of the rash and ends when all the lesions are crusted, usually 4 to 6 days after the rash appears. Following initial recommendations, postexposure prophylaxis (PEP) has been extended, particularly for neonates and immunocompromised patients.[83,91] Respiratory isolation should be used for patients with chickenpox or disseminated herpes zoster. Use of gloves to avoid contact with vesicular fluid is adequate to prevent VZV spread from patients with localized herpes zoster.

Most adults in the United States have protective antibodies to VZV. Since there have been many reports of nosocomial transmission of VZV, it is recommended that all HCWs have immunity to the virus. Anesthesia personnel should be questioned about prior VZV infection, and those with a negative or unknown history of infection should consider being serologically tested.[91] All employees with negative titers should be restricted from caring for patients with active VZV infection and should be offered immunization with two doses of the live, attenuated varicella vaccine.

Susceptible personnel with a significant exposure to an individual with VZV infection are potentially infective from 10 to 21 days after exposure and should not contact patients during this period. The postexposure period during which a patient may receive varicella zoster immune globulin (VariZIG) recently increased from 4 to 10 days, although VariZIG should be administered as soon as possible after exposure.[83]

EBV, also a member of the family *Herpesviridae*, is the cause of heterophile-positive infectious mononucleosis, characterized by fever, sore throat, lymphadenopathy, and atypical lymphocytosis. About 15% of cases of Burkitt lymphoma in the United States and 90% of those in Africa are associated with EBV. Anaplastic nasopharyngeal carcinoma is common in southern China and is uniformly associated with EBV. EBV has also been associated with Hodgkin disease, especially the mixed-cellularity type.

EBV is spread by contact with oral secretions. The virus is frequently transmitted from asymptomatic adults to infants and among young adults by transfer of saliva during kissing. Transmission by less intimate contact is rare. EBV has been transmitted by blood transfusion and bone marrow transplantation. More than 90% of asymptomatic seropositive individuals shed the virus in oropharyngeal secretions.

Cytomegalovirus (CMV) infects between 50% and 85% of individuals in the United States before age 40, with most infections producing minimal symptoms.[92] After the primary infection, the virus remains dormant, and recurrent disease only occurs with compromise of the individual's immune system. CMV is not readily spread by casual contact but rather by repeated or prolonged intimate exposure. It is unlikely that aerosols or small droplets play a role in CMV transmission.

Primary or recurrent CMV infection during pregnancy results in a fetal infection rate of up to 35%.[93] Congenital CMV syndrome may be found in up to 10% of infected infants. Thus, although CMV infection usually does not result in morbidity in healthy adults, it may have significant sequelae in pregnant women, and therefore becomes an occupational health concern.

The two major populations with CMV infection in the hospital include affected infants and immunocompromised patients. Routine infection control procedures (standard precautions) are sufficient to prevent CMV infection in health care personnel. Pregnant personnel should be made aware of the risks associated with CMV infection during pregnancy and of appropriate infection control precautions to be used when caring for high-risk patients.

Rubella

Although most adults in the United States are immune to rubella, up to 20% of women of childbearing age are still susceptible, allowing the potential for viral replication in the placenta and infection of fetal organs (congenital rubella syndrome-CRS). The infection is persistent throughout fetal development and for up to 1 year after birth. Therefore, only individuals immune to rubella should have contact with infants who have CRS or who are congenitally infected with rubella virus but are not showing signs of CRS.[94]

Rubella is transmitted by contact with nasopharyngeal droplets spread by infected individuals through coughing or sneezing. Patients are most contagious while the rash is erupting but can transmit the virus from 1 week before to 5 to 7 days after the onset of the rash. Droplet precautions should be used to prevent transmission (Table 3-7).[95]

History is a poor indicator of immunity. Therefore, ensuring immunity at the time of employment (evidence of prior vaccination with live rubella vaccine or serologic confirmation) should prevent nosocomial transmission of rubella to personnel. A live, attenuated rubella virus vaccine (measles, mumps, rubella [MMR]) is available to produce immunity in susceptible personnel.[96] Many state or local health departments mandate rubella immunity for all HCWs, and local regulations should be consulted.

Measles (Rubeola)

Measles virus is highly transmissible by large droplets and by the airborne route. The virus is found in the mucus of the nose and pharynx of the infected individual and is spread by coughing and sneezing. The disease can be transmitted from 4 days prior to the onset of the rash to 4 days after its onset. Airborne precautions should be used for infected patients (Table 3-7).[95] Secondary attack rates in susceptible household and institutional contacts generally exceed 90%. The United States experienced a record number of measles cases during 2014, with 668 cases from 27 states reported to CDC's National Center for Immunization and Respiratory Diseases (NCIRD).[97] This is the greatest number of cases since measles elimination was prematurely reported in the United States in 2000.

Medical settings are well-recognized sites of measles virus transmission. Highly infectious children may present to health care facilities during the prodrome when the diagnosis is not yet obvious. HCWs are at increased risk for acquiring measles and transmitting the virus to susceptible coworkers and patients. The CDC recommends that medical personnel have adequate immunity to measles, as documented by one of the following: evidence of two doses of live measles vaccine, a record of physician-diagnosed measles, or serologic evidence of measles immunity (Table 3-7).[96] Susceptible personnel born in or after 1957 should receive two doses of the live measles vaccine at the time of employment.[96]

Viral Hepatitis

Many viruses produce hepatitis. The most common are type A (infectious hepatitis), type B (HBV, serum hepatitis), and type C (HCV and non-A, non-B hepatitis [NANBH]), which are responsible for most cases of parenterally transmitted hepatitis in the United States. Delta hepatitis (HDV), caused by an incomplete virus, occurs only in people infected with HBV. HEV, previously labeled epidemic or enterically transmitted NANBH, is an enterically transmitted virus that occurs primarily in India, Asia, Africa, and Central America. In these locations, HEV is the most common cause of acute hepatitis. All types of viral hepatitis produce clinically similar illnesses. These range from asymptomatic and unapparent to fulminant and fatal infections, as well as subclinical to chronic persistent liver disease with cirrhosis and hepatocellular carcinoma, common to the blood-borne types (HBV, HCV, and HDV). The greatest risks of occupational transmission to anesthesia personnel are associated with HBV and HCV.

Hepatitis A virus is the cause of about 20% to 40% of viral hepatitis in adults in the United States and has increased dramatically since 2017 (Fig. 3-3). Hepatitis A is usually a self-limited illness, and no chronic carrier state exists. Spread is predominantly by the fecal–oral route, either by person-to-person contact or by ingestion of contaminated food or water. Outbreaks are usually found in institutions or other closed groups where there has been a breakdown in normal sanitary conditions. Hospital personnel do not appear to be at increased risk for hepatitis A and nosocomial transmission is rare. Personnel exposed to patients with hepatitis A should receive immune globulin intramuscularly as soon as possible but not more than 2 weeks after the exposure to reduce the likelihood of infection.[98] Immune globulin provides protection against hepatitis A through passive transfer of antibodies and is used for PEP. Hepatitis A vaccine is not routinely recommended for health care personnel except for those who may be working in countries where hepatitis A is endemic.

Hepatitis B virus is a significant occupational hazard for nonimmune anesthesiologists and other medical personnel who have frequent contact with blood and blood products. The prevalence of hepatitis B in the United States during 1999 to 2006 (anti-HBc = 4.7% and hepatitis B surface antigen [HBsAg] = 0.27%) was not statistically different from what it was during 1988 to 1994 (5.4% and 0.38%, respectively).

Acute HBV infection may be asymptomatic and usually resolves without significant hepatic damage. Less than 1% of acutely infected patients develop fulminant hepatitis.[99] Approximately 10% become chronic carriers of HBV (serologic evidence for >6 months). Within 2 years, half of the chronic carriers resolve their infection without significant hepatic impairment. Chronic active hepatitis, which may progress to cirrhosis and is linked to hepatocellular carcinoma, is most common in individuals with chronic viral infection for >2 years.

The diagnosis and staging of HBV infection is made based on serologic testing. The first marker is detectable in serum within 1 to 12 weeks (HBsAg). HBsAg becomes undetectable 1 to 2 months after the onset of jaundice and rarely persists beyond 6 months. After HBsAg disappears, antibody to HBsAg (anti-HBs) becomes detectable in serum and remains detectable indefinitely. Antibody to the surface antigen (anti-HBs) appears with resolution of the acute infection and confers lasting immunity against subsequent HBV infections. Chronic HBV carriers are likely to have HBsAg and antibody to the core antigen (anti-HBc) present in serum samples. The presence of hepatitis Be antigen (HBeAg) in serum is indicative of active viral replication in hepatocytes.

Anesthesia personnel are at risk for occupationally acquired HBV infection because of accidental percutaneous or mucosal contact with blood or body fluids from infected patients. Patient groups with a high prevalence of HBV include immigrants from endemic areas, users of illicit parenteral drugs, homosexual men, and patients on hemodialysis.[99] Carriers are frequently not identified during hospitalization because the clinical history and routine preoperative laboratory tests may be insufficient for diagnosis. The risk for infection after an HBV-contaminated percutaneous exposure, such as an accidental needlestick, is 37% to 62% if the source patient is HBeAg positive and 23% to 37% if HBeAg negative.[99] HBV can be found in saliva, but the rate of transmission is significantly less after mucosal contact with infected oral secretions than after percutaneous exposures to blood. HBV is a hardy virus that may be infectious for at least 1 week in dried blood on environmental surfaces.

Hepatitis B vaccine is the primary strategy to prevent occupational transmission of HBV to anesthesia personnel and other health personnel at increased risk. Administration of three doses of vaccine results in the production of protective antibodies (anti-HBs) in >90% of healthy personnel. Hospitals and anesthesia departments should have policies for educating, screening, and counseling personnel about their risk of acquiring HBV infection and should make vaccination available for susceptible personnel.[99] If adequate postvaccination immunity is not confirmed, a second three-dose vaccine series should be administered. Nonresponders to vaccination remain at risk for HBV infection and should be counseled on strategies to prevent infections and the need for PEP. Vaccine-induced antibodies decline over time. The CDC states that for vaccinated adults with normal immune status, routine booster doses are not necessary and periodic monitoring of antibody concentration is not recommended.[99]

Hepatitis C virus causes most cases of parenterally transmitted NANBH and is a leading cause of chronic liver disease in the United States. Although antibody to HCV (anti-HCV) can be detected in most patients with hepatitis C, its presence does not correlate with resolution of the acute infection or progression of hepatitis, and it does not confer immunity against HCV infection. Seropositivity for HCV RNA is a marker of chronic infection and continued viral presence. Around 30% (15% to 45%) of infected persons spontaneously clear the virus within 6 months of infection without any treatment. The remaining 70% (55% to 85%) of persons will develop chronic HCV infection. Of those with chronic HCV infection, the risk of cirrhosis ranges from 15% to 30% within 20 years.[100]

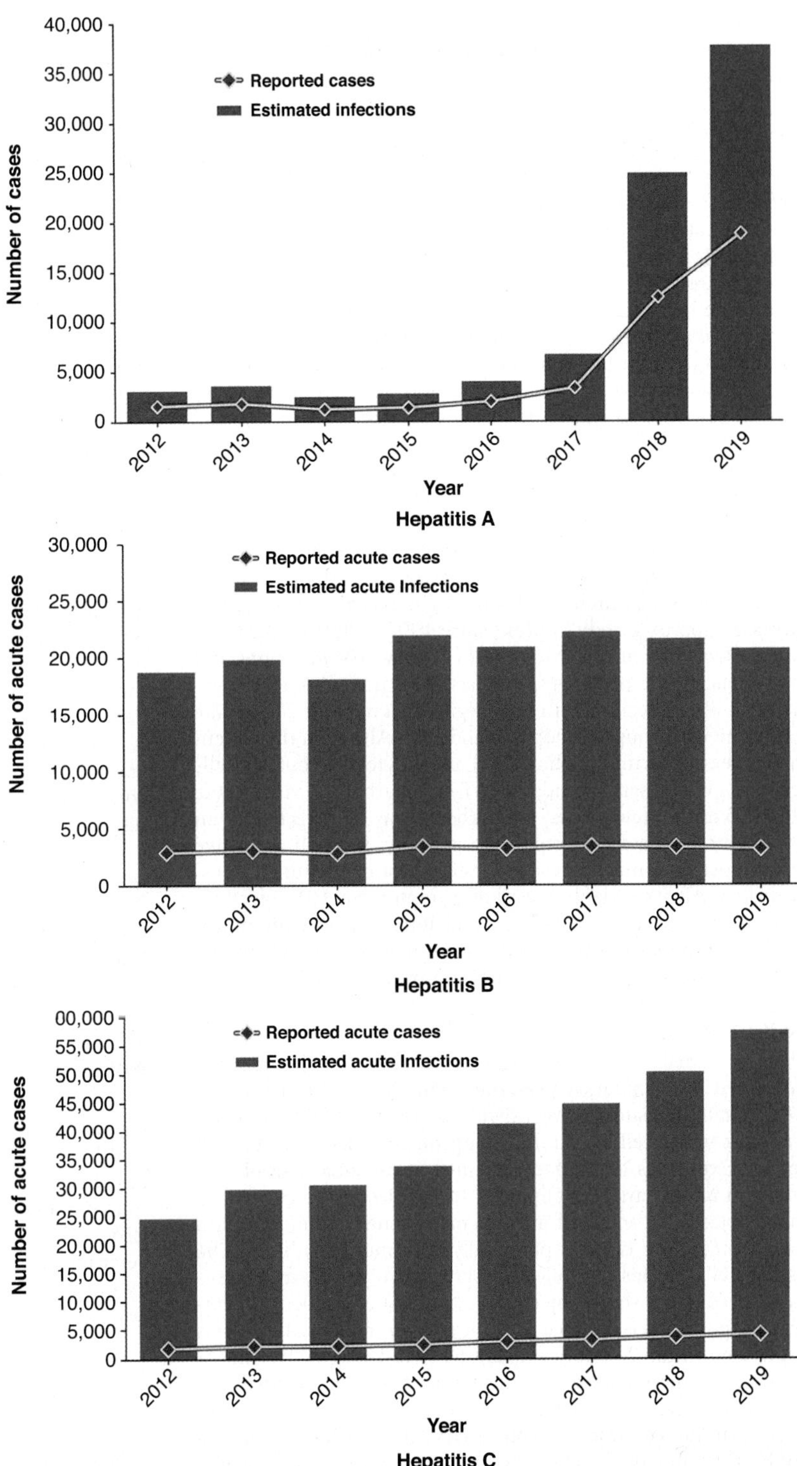

Figure 3-3 Number of reported acute hepatitis virus infection cases and estimated infections in the United States, 2012–2019. (From Centers for Disease Control and Prevention. 2019 Viral Hepatitis Surveillance Report. Published July 2021. Accessed May10,2022.https://www.cdc.gov/hepatitis/statistics/SurveillanceRpts.htm)

Like HBV, HCV is transmitted through blood, but the rate of occupational HCV infection is less than for HBV. Although HCV transmission has been documented in health care settings, the prevalence of anti-HCV in HCWs in the United States is not greater than that found in the general population (1.6%). The greatest risk of occupational HCV transmission is associated with exposure to blood from an HCV-positive source. HCV has been transmitted through blood splashes to the eye and with exposure via nonintact skin. HCV in dried blood on environmental surfaces may remain infectious for up to 16 hours, but environmental contamination does not appear to be a common route of transmission. HCV can be found in the saliva of infected individuals, but it is not believed to represent a great risk for occupational transmission.

Prevention of exposure remains the primary strategy for protection against HCV infection. Personnel who have had a percutaneous or mucosal exposure to HCV-positive blood should have counseling and serologic testing in accordance with available guidelines.[101]

Pathogenic Human Retroviruses

The family *Retroviridae*, positive-stranded enveloped RNA viruses that reverse transcribe their RNA into a DNA intermediate during viral replication (hence the name "retroviruses") includes seven subfamilies, two of which produce disease in humans, human T lymphotropic viruses (HTLV)-I and HTLV-II, which are transforming retroviruses, and HIV-1 and HIV-2, which cause cytopathic effects either directly or indirectly. Tissue destruction may result directly from the viral infection or indirectly from malignant transformation of infected cells and an immune-deficient state in response to the virus, leading to neoplastic and infectious disease. HTLV-I infection is transmitted in at least three ways: from mother to child (especially via breast milk), through sexual activity, and parenterally via contaminated transfusions or contaminated needles. Between 2010 and 2015, worldwide new HIV infections decreased from around 2.2 million to fewer than 2 million, in parallel with a decrease in deaths from about 1.15 million to just under 900,000.[102] The global prevalence has increased approximately fourfold since 1990, reflecting the combined effects of continued high rates of new HIV infections and the beneficial (life-prolonging) impact of antiretroviral therapy.

The initial infection with HIV begins as a mononucleosis-like syndrome with lymphadenopathy and rash. Although the patient then enters an asymptomatic period, monocyte–macrophage cells serve as a viral reservoir and CD4+ T cells harbor the virus in the blood. Within a few weeks, an antibody may be detected by an enzyme immunoassay or rapid HIV antibody test, but a positive result must be confirmed using Western blot or immunofluorescent assay. After a variable period of asymptomatic HIV infection, there is an increase in viral titer and impaired host immunity, resulting in opportunistic infections and malignancies characteristic of Acquired immune deficiency syndrome (AIDS).

Risk of Occupational HIV Infection

There is a small but definite occupational risk of HIV transmission to HCWs, laboratory personnel, and others who work with HIV-containing materials. Worldwide, more than 2 million HCWs are stuck with needles or other sharp medical instruments each year.[103] Exposures that place personnel at potential risk of HIV infection are percutaneous injuries (a needlestick or cut with a sharp object) or contact of mucous membrane or nonintact skin with blood, tissue, or other potentially infectious body fluids. The risk of HIV transmission following skin puncture from a contaminated needle or a sharp object is 0.3% and after a mucous membrane exposure, it is 0.09% if the injured and/or exposed person is not treated within 24 hours with antiretroviral drugs.[82] HIV transmission after nonintact skin exposure has been documented, but the average risk for transmission by this route has not been precisely determined. Transmission of HIV through intact skin has not been documented. While the principles of exposure management remain unchanged, recommended HIV PEP regimens and the duration of HIV follow-up testing for exposed personnel have been updated to include PEP medication regimens that contain three (or more) antiretroviral drugs for all occupational exposures to HIV and if a newer fourth-generation combination HIV p24 antigen–HIV antibody test is utilized for follow-up HIV testing of exposed HCWs, HIV testing may be concluded at 4 months after exposure. If a newer testing platform is not available, follow-up HIV testing is typically concluded at 6 months after an HIV exposure.[82]

In the United States between 1985 and 2013, 58 HCWs, for whom case investigations were completed, had confirmed seroconversions to HIV following occupational exposures; an additional 150 possible cases of occupationally acquired HIV infection were reported to CDC.[104] Since 1999, only one case has been reported. The routes of exposure were 49 percutaneous (puncture/cut injury); 5 mucocutaneous (mucous membrane and/or skin); 2 both percutaneous and mucocutaneous; and 2 of unknown route. The individuals with documented seroconversions included 20 laboratory workers, 24 nurses, 6 physicians (nonsurgical), 2 surgical technicians, and 6 others.[104]

Anesthesia personnel are frequently exposed to blood and body fluids during invasive procedures such as insertion of vascular catheters, arterial punctures, and endotracheal intubation. Although many exposures are mucocutaneous and can be prevented using PPE, these barriers do not prevent percutaneous exposures. Because of the tasks they perform, anesthesia personnel are likely to use and be injured by large-bore, hollow needles such as intravenous catheter stylets and needles on syringes. Needleless or protected needle safety devices can be used to replace standard devices to reduce the risk of needlestick injuries.

The occupational risk of HIV infection is a function of the annual number of blood exposures, the rate of HIV transmission with each exposure to infected blood, and the prevalence of HIV infection in the specific patient population. Specifically, regarding anesthesia personnel, Greene et al.[105] prospectively collected data on 138 contaminated percutaneous injuries. The rate of contaminated percutaneous injuries per year per full-time equivalent anesthesia worker was 0.42, and the average annual risk of HIV and HCV infection was estimated to be 0.0016% and 0.015%, respectively.

Although HIV can be recovered in low titers from saliva in a small number of infected subjects, there is no convincing evidence that saliva can transmit HIV infection, either through kissing or through other exposures, such as those that occur occupationally. Moreover, there is no evidence that HIV transmission can occur as a result of exposure to tears, sweat, or urine.

Postexposure Treatment and Prophylactic Antiretroviral Therapy

When personnel have been exposed to patients' blood or body fluids, the incident should immediately be reported to the employee health service or the designated individual within the institution. Based on the nature of the injury, the exposed worker and the source individual should be tested for serologic evidence of HIV, HBV, and HCV infection. Current local laws must be consulted to determine policies for testing the source patient, and confidentiality must be maintained. U.S. Public Health Service recommendations include the following[82]:

1. PEP is recommended when occupational exposures to HIV occur.
2. Determine the HIV status of the exposure source patient to guide need for HIV PEP, if possible.
3. Start PEP medication regimens as soon as possible after occupational exposure to HIV and continue them for a 4-week duration.
4. PEP medication regimens should contain three (or more) antiretroviral drugs for all occupational exposures to HIV.
5. Expert consultation is recommended for any occupational exposures to HIV. Provide close follow-up for exposed personnel that includes counseling, baseline and follow-up HIV testing, and monitoring for drug toxicity. Follow-up appointments should begin within 72 hours of an HIV exposure.

6. If a newer fourth-generation combination HIV p24 antigen–HIV antibody test is utilized for follow-up HIV testing of exposed HCP, HIV testing may be concluded at 4 months after exposure. If a newer testing platform is not available, follow-up HIV testing is typically concluded at 6 months after an HIV exposure.

Failure of PEP has been attributed to a large viral inoculum, use of a single antiviral agent, drug resistance in the virus from the source patient, and delayed initiation or short duration of PEP therapy. For consultation on the treatment of occupational exposures to HIV and other blood-borne pathogens, the clinician managing the exposed patient can call the National Clinicians' Post-Exposure Prophylaxis Hotline (PEPline) at 1-888-448-4911.

Prion Diseases

Prions (from *pro*tein + infect*ion*) are composed of misfolded protein without nucleic acid. They are responsible for the transmissible spongiform encephalopathies: Bovine spongiform encephalopathy or "mad cow disease" in cattle and Creutzfeldt–Jakob disease (CJD) in humans. All are untreatable and fatal. When a prion enters a healthy organism, it provides a template to guide the misfolding of normal protein into the extremely stable prion form, highly resistant to denaturation by chemical and physical agents. This makes disinfection and sterilization of reusable medical instruments a unique challenge because effective prion decontamination relies upon protein hydrolysis or destruction of protein tertiary structure.

Prions cause neurodegenerative disease by aggregating extracellularly within the CNS to form amyloid plaques resulting in the histologically characteristic spongy architecture. CJD, caused by an infectious protein or prion, may be unsuspected in patients presenting with dementia. There are specific guidelines for the disinfection and sterilization of prion-contaminated medical instruments.[106]

Tuberculosis

TB is a major cause of death worldwide and, if properly treated, almost always curable. When untreated, TB can be fatal within 5 years in 50% to 65% of cases.[107] More than 1.6 million die annually. A fourth of the world's population—nearly 2 billion people—are infected with TB; 95% of cases are reported from developing countries.[108]

Mycobacterium tuberculosis is most commonly transmitted from a person with infectious pulmonary TB to others by aerosolized droplet nuclei via coughing, sneezing, or speaking. As many as 3,000 infectious nuclei per cough can remain suspended in the air for several hours and can reach the terminal air passages when inhaled. The most infectious patients have cavitary pulmonary disease or, much less commonly, laryngeal TB, and produce sputum containing as many as 10^5 to 10^7 acid-fast bacilli (AFB)/mL. Other routes of transmission are uncommon. Clinical illness directly following infection is classified as *primary TB* and is common among children in the first few years of life and among immune-compromised persons.

The best way to prevent TB is to diagnose and isolate infectious cases rapidly and to administer appropriate treatment until patients are noninfectious, usually 2 to 4 weeks after the start of proper treatment. In low-prevalence countries with adequate resources, screening of high-risk groups such as immigrants from high-prevalence countries, migratory workers, prisoners, homeless individuals, substance abusers, and HIV-seropositive persons is recommended.

Outbreaks of TB in health care facilities have been attributed to delayed diagnosis of TB in the source patient, delayed initiation or inadequate deployment of airborne precautions, lapses in precautions during aerosol-generating procedures, and lack of adequate respiratory protection in health care personnel.

Effective prevention of spread to medical personnel requires early identification of infected patients and immediate initiation of airborne infection isolation (Table 3-7). Patients must remain in isolation until adequate treatment is documented. Personnel should wear fit-tested respiratory protective devices when they enter an isolation room or when performing procedures that may induce coughing, such as endotracheal intubation or tracheal suctioning.[109] HEPA respirators (classified as N95) are NIOSH-approved devices that meet the CDC criteria for respiratory protective devices against TB.[110] It is reasonable to postpone elective surgery until infected patients have had an adequate course of chemotherapy. If surgery prior to the completion of treatment is required, bacterial filters (HEPA filters) should be used on the anesthetic breathing circuit for patients with TB. Patients must be recovered in a room that meets all the requirements for airborne precautions.

A systematic review found a low percentage of HCWs have a positive TB test at baseline and upon serial testing. Updated recommendations for screening and testing HCWs include an individual baseline (preplacement) risk assessment, symptom evaluation and testing of persons without prior TB or latent TB infection (LTBI), no routine serial testing in the absence of exposure or ongoing transmission, treatment for HCWs diagnosed with LTBI, annual symptom screening for persons with untreated LTBI, and annual TB education of all HCWs.[86]

Impairment and Disability

The safe administration of anesthesia demands that the anesthesiologist possess a large store of current medical knowledge and have the judgment and skill to competently apply that knowledge in performing a myriad of intricate cognitive and technical tasks. Any degree of impairment* carries the potential to disrupt these processes and can threaten the successful conduct of the anesthetic.

Etiologies of impairment include mental, emotional, sensory, physical, or developmental sources. The onset can be sudden, as occurs with injury or acute illness, or gradual, as is the case with chronic disease. It can be of a temporary nature, with spontaneous recovery, or more protracted or permanent. Some impairments are associated with a high mortality rate whereas others do not affect life expectancy. Many impairments are capable of evoking feelings of compassion among colleagues and acquaintances, while others can elicit blame and stigma.

Not all impairments result in disability.† A condition that is disabling to one individual might be an inconvenience to another individual or to the same person at another time or under different circumstances. Work disability is a complex interaction between the individual and the work environment in which an impairment hampers a worker's ability to perform the required tasks in a safe or acceptable manner. An impaired physician‡ might be fully competent in accomplishing the activities of daily

*Impairment is any loss of use of any body part, organ system, or organ function.

†Disability is an impairment that substantially limits one or more major life activities.

‡An impaired physician is one whose performance as a professional person and as a practitioner of the healing arts is impaired because of alcoholism, drug abuse, mental illness, senility, or disabling disease.

living but disabled regarding work because of an inability to perform the intricate tasks required for safe medical practice. The work of an anesthesiologist is so demanding that the inability or failure to remain current in the medical literature can be considered a disabling impairment.

Data regarding the number of impaired physicians are difficult to obtain. Physicians are frequently unaware when their own skills are failing and are reluctant to report disability among themselves or their colleagues.[111]

Many cases of physician impairment are the result of SUDs (see Substance Use Disorder above). At some point in their career, as many as 15% of practicing anesthesiologists are thought to suffer from SUD.[70] SUD-impaired anesthesiologists are at increased risk of inflicting patient injury if they administer anesthetics while under the influence. A 1994 report from the ASA's Closed Claims Database identified seven cases involving "substance abuse" or "chemical dependence."[80] Moreover, the authors commented that the role of SUD in other medical liability claims might be concealed and therefore underreported.

Other factors that can result in physician impairment include various forms of mental illness. Psychiatric illness, including anxiety, depression, personality disorders, and disruptive behavior are common findings among impaired physicians.[112] Risk factors for these mental illnesses include many of the personality traits that ensure success as a physician, such as self-sacrifice, competitiveness, achievement orientation, denial of feelings, and intellectualization of emotions.

Cognitive aging and age-related neurodegenerative disorders account for a large incidence of impairment observed among physicians (see The Aging Anesthesiologist below). As many as 64% of physicians who have been referred "for cause" to licensing or credentialing organizations are found to have significant, previously undiagnosed, cognitive impairment.[113,114]

It can be very challenging for colleagues to appropriately respond to many of the problems imposed by the impaired or unsafe anesthesiologist. Helpful suggestions for dealing with impaired physicians can be found in the literature.[113]

The Aging Anesthesiologist

Aging is a natural process that occurs in all living organisms, including anesthesiologists. Among the consequences of normal aging are important physical, functional, psychological, spiritual, and social changes. In the aggregate, aging can transform a healthy and resilient person into one who is increasingly vulnerable to injury and illness. Among the ultimate results of aging are senescence and death.

Cognitive and sensory decline are among the most extensively studied of the physiologic changes associated with aging. Commonly observed are reduced short-term memory, decreased processing speed, limited ability to complete complex tasks, increased difficulty in filtering out irrelevant information, reduced hearing and visual acuity, and decreased manual dexterity and visuospatial ability. One striking observation is a wide variability concerning cognitive decline among older physicians. Many demonstrate fully intact cognition while an equal number show signs of significant cognitive decline.[115]

Each of these changes and others can impact the practice of anesthesiology.[116] Some important qualities and skills, such as expertise, experience, and wisdom, are frequently enhanced. Others, such as creative thinking, reaction time, and on-the-spot reasoning, may be compromised. These changes may be accompanied by other physiologic changes that can exacerbate any coexisting sensory or cognitive impairment. The older anesthesiologist who is experiencing these neurologic changes is potentially more prone to difficulties in performing some of the critical processes necessary for safe anesthetic management, including rapid processing of information, assimilation and application of new knowledge, complex decision making, and proper response initiation.

There are also important changes in the cardiovascular and musculoskeletal systems that commonly occur and can influence the practice of an aging anesthesiologist. Older anesthesiologists may lack adequate strength to perform some of the more physically demanding aspects of practice. Night call can be especially challenging for older physicians who tend to be more vulnerable to the adverse effects of sleep deprivation and may be more susceptible to late-night errors.[53]

The relationship between age-related physiologic changes and professional competence is unclear. Older physicians have been reported to experience an increased incidence of complications and disciplinary actions by state licensing boards.[117] And a meta-analysis that examined the relationship between years in practice and markers of quality of care reported that 73% of the studies demonstrated decreasing performance with some or all the outcomes assessed among physicians of advanced age.[118] On the other hand, 22% of the studies reported no association, or an improvement in performance with age.

The correlation between physicians' age and actual clinical outcomes is even less clear because of wide variability in research design including differences in procedure, procedure volume, and practice site. The question of age-related competency has been studied extensively in the surgical specialties with various findings of improved, unchanged, or worse outcomes when older surgeons are compared with younger colleagues.[119]

Neither has the relationship between advanced age and clinical outcomes among anesthesiologists been definitively established. Suggestions of poorer outcomes come from studies that track surrogates such as the frequency of complaints against senior anesthesiologists and the risk of being found responsible in professional litigation.[120] One study that employed high-frequency simulation to create a mock "cannot intubate/cannot ventilate" scenario found an association between decreased proficiency in establishing an emergency cricothyroidotomy and increased operator age and years from residency.[121]

Aging among anesthesiologists raises complex legal and ethical issues. Several federal laws are relevant to the aging anesthesiologist's rights and responsibilities regarding continuation of work. These include the Age Discrimination Act, Title VII of the Civil Rights Act, the Medical and Family Leave Act, the Fair Labor Standards Act, and the Employee Retirement Income Security Act. Both the American Medical Association and the American College of Surgeons have issued statements that call for proactive steps to be taken toward monitoring their aging members' competency.[115] However, both proposals rely on voluntary action by physicians, unlike many other industries which impact public health, where advanced chronologic age automatically triggers limitations on the range of professional activities. In many cases, the decision to limit or retire from practice remains at the sole discretion of the individual anesthesiologist.

Age is one of the most important factors in decisions about retirement.[122] The median age of retirement for anesthesiologists as of 2012 was approximately 64 years.[123] Commonly cited reasons for retirement among older anesthesiologists include on-call responsibilities, financial considerations, lack of professional satisfaction, health concerns, and changes in governmental policies and the health care operating environment. The decision to retire from anesthesiology is frequently precipitated by concerns about deteriorating clinical skills. In many cases, the retiring anesthesiologist just "felt it was time." Older anesthesiologists who postpone retirement cite career satisfaction, unmet financial obligations, and the need to maintain health insurance for family members as the primary reason to remain in the workforce.

Mortality Among Anesthesiologists

There have been conflicting reports regarding the common causes of death among anesthesiologists. As discussed below (see section on Suicide), many studies have reported an increased rate of suicide.[75,124] Some earlier studies also reported an increased incidence of cancer, specifically leukemia and lymphoma, attributed at the time to chronic exposure to WAG, radiation, and stress.[14] Subsequent reports have failed to confirm an increased risk for cancer-related mortality but continue to cite a disproportionate number of drug-related deaths and suicide.[75]

There are also contradictory reports about the average longevity of anesthesiologists. Using different databases, control populations, and methodologies, these studies have variously reported a shortened,[75] average,[125] or prolonged life expectancy.[124] A 2006 study reported a significant increase in longevity among anesthesiologists who had died throughout the 10-year study period 1992 to 2001, such that the average age at death in the last year of the study was 78 years, the same as the national average for all Americans at that time.[126]

Suicide

There is a disproportionately high incidence of suicide among
8 physicians, especially female physicians.[127] Anesthesiologists have been singled out in the medical literature as well as the lay press as being particularly vulnerable.[128] A meta-analysis in 2020 reported that anesthesiologists were among the top two specialties at risk for suicide.[127] A partial explanation for this alarming observation lies with the high degree of stress that is an integral part of the job, including risk of malpractice litigation.

SUD among anesthesia personnel is another potential contributor to the increased suicide rate, though intentionality of overdose is often difficult to demonstrate. (See Substance Use Disorder above.) Death from an inadvertent drug overdose can be difficult to distinguish from suicide. Drug abuse is among the highest causes of death and the most frequent method of suicide among anesthesiologists.[75,129] Physicians whose privileges to practice medicine have been suspended or revoked due to substance abuse are also at heightened risk for attempting suicide.[130]

As with SUD, the societal stigma associated with mental health conditions is real, and a significant cause of nontreatment in the medical community. Not only do physicians avoid seeking help secondary to societal stigma, but there are substantial licensure and credentialing implications to carrying out a mental health diagnosis. The practice of state licensure boards inquiring about mental health conditions in a disproportionate manner compared to physical health conditions likely violates the Americans with Disabilities Act and is the target of interventions proposed by organizations like the FSMB and the NAM.[76,131]

Psychological Considerations

Stress

Occupational stress is unavoidable and often motivating, but when it exceeds the capabilities of the worker, it can lead to poor mental and physical health, accidents, and burnout. Stress has been linked to cardiovascular, musculoskeletal, and gastrointestinal disease, sleep and mood disturbances, and disruption of personal relationships, as well as higher absenteeism, injuries, disability, and decreased productivity.

Anesthesia practice can be mentally, emotionally, and physically stressful. The perioperative environment provides constant low-level stress, unpredictably punctuated by episodes of extreme stress, which are largely not controllable by anesthesiologists. Anesthesiologists frequently cite the following as particularly stressful: unpredictability of work, fear of litigation, need for sustained vigilance, production pressure, economic uncertainty, and strained relationships. Several aspects of practice are predictably stressful: a perioperative catastrophe, medical malpractice, and interpersonal conflict. Anesthesiologists have demonstrated objective evidence of stress at certain critical stages during anesthetic management.[132] To a great extent, the stress of anesthetic practice is continuous and changes dynamically across life and career stages. For example, the COVID-19 pandemic, with its attendant significant personal and psychological ramifications, added stress to an already stressful profession.[133]

Impact of Adverse Events

An adverse event with a bad outcome is among the most significant stressors for an anesthesiologist. The description of a "second victim" being the involved medical provider and the "third victim" being subsequently cared-for patients, was proposed by Wu in a 2000 editorial.[134]

In a 2012 study of ASA members, 84% had encountered a "perioperative catastrophe," with 88% requiring time to recover, 19% never fully recovering, 12% considering changing careers, 67% feeling care in the subsequent 4 hours was compromised and only 7% being given any time off.[135] Following a medical error, an intense emotional response is the norm and conversations with peers are often cited as the most helpful coping mechanism. A study of anesthesiology residents reported that peer support and individual meetings with department leadership were the most efficacious support modalities following an adverse event.[136]

The support available after an adverse event is tightly linked to organizational culture. In the 2018 Hospital Survey on Patient Safety Culture, encompassing more than 600 hospitals, most respondents felt that their events and mistakes were kept in an employee file and held against them.[137] Countering this are programs enhancing psychological safety, like the Resilience in Stressful Events (RISE) program at Johns Hopkins Hospital[138] and the Schwartz Center Rounds,[139] which seek to further debrief medical experiences and normalize the appropriate humanistic responses experienced.

Well-Being, Burnout, and Workplace Culture

Burnout

Stress and burnout, while causally related, are distinct entities. The concept of burnout as an occupational phenomenon in service industries was originally studied in the 1970s[140] with quantitative investigation beginning in the 1980s with the Maslach Burnout Inventory (MBI),[141] which classified burnout into three domains: emotional exhaustion, depersonalization/cynicism, and a low sense of personal accomplishment. Freudenberger describes a cascade of events culminating in the "burnout syndrome."[140] Ironically, the initial steps are essentially requisite for successful medical school matriculation, underscoring the cultural vulnerability to burnout clinicians face.

The effects of burnout on medicine and anesthesia are signifi- 9
cant. Shanafelt[142] published the first large study (7,288 respondents) of U.S. physicians' burnout levels, finding that 45.8% of

physicians expressed one or more major symptoms of burnout, a level much higher than the background rate of U.S. nonphysicians. Among all physicians, anesthesiologists scored above the mean for burnout and near the mean for work–life balance. Recently, large, targeted studies of burnout in anesthesiologists have shown high rates of burnout, disproportionate rates of burnout in chronic pain physicians, and a tight link between burnout and sense of support in the workplace.[143,144] In fact, expressing little to no support in one's work–life carried an odd's ratio of 6.7 for being at high risk for burnout in attending anesthesiologists.[144] The health consequences of burnout, including cardiovascular, musculoskeletal, and psychological maladies, SUD, and altered cortisol expression, have been well documented. A correlation has been shown among physicians between burnout and medical malpractice, quality of patient care, medical errors, and career satisfaction.[145]

10 Reducing occupational burnout has become an imperative for the medical community, demonstrated by high-level engagement by professional societies, credentialing bodies, and governmental health entities. One example is the continued work of the NAM's Action Collaborative on Clinician Well-Being and Resilience, currently co-chaired by the U.S. Surgeon General. This organization is working to engage stakeholders at all levels of health care infrastructure and has created organizational tools and roadmaps for medical entities to implement.[131]

Well-Being

Sir William Osler said that "in no relationship is the physician more often derelict than in his duty to himself."[146] An emphasis on well-being has emerged as a codified component of anesthesia training; for instance, in the United States, the adoption of the ACGME Milestones Project,[147] mandates that a trainee should demonstrate a "responsibility to maintain personal emotional, physical, and mental health." This begins with the acknowledgment that external stressors, such as disease, disability, divorce, death, malpractice, and financial distress, may provoke maladaptive coping mechanisms with profound short- and long-term consequences.[148]

Nutrition, Diet, and Fitness

Half of the deaths in the United States are estimated to be premature and potentially "deferrable" with the modification of 10 behaviors: tobacco use, dietary pattern, physical activity level, alcohol consumption, exposure to microbial agents, exposure to toxic agents, use of firearms, sexual behavior, motor vehicle crashes, and illicit use of drugs.[148] More than a quarter (27.7%) of U.S. workers fulfill body mass index (BMI) criteria for obesity, with working greater than 40 hours per week and in the health care setting being independent risk factors for obesity.[149]

In contrast to the documented negative impacts of a lack of exercise, physical activity has been shown to improve perceptions of daily life, self-esteem, and mental health.[150] If the thought of becoming an elite athlete is daunting, there exists encouraging data that longer periods of moderate physical activity (e.g., walking) carry a similar overall survival benefit to shorter extremes of activity (e.g., running), with fewer injuries.[151] The U.S. Department of Health and Human Services recommends at least 150 minutes of moderate-intensity or 75 minutes of vigorous-intensity activity weekly.[152]

Regarding nutrition, an unhealthy diet is associated with cognitive deficits, poorer attention, memory impairment, and reduced work performance.[153] As such, one may argue that proper nutrition and attention to physical well-being is a professional duty owed to patients.

Mindfulness

Mindfulness, with its roots in Buddhist meditation practice, is an intentional, nonjudgmental practice of attention meant to cultivate awareness of the present moment.[154] The introduction of mindfulness-based stress reduction (MBSR) techniques to improve quality of life, decrease burnout, and supplement integrative approaches to medical therapy began appearing in the medical literature in the 1980s due largely to the work of Jon Kabat-Zinn.[155] Meditation techniques have been shown to change transcription profiles and the biochemical milieu, particularly in buffering oxidative stress and repairing cellular damage, as well as affecting cortical structure and function (particularly relating to learning, memory, emotional stability, and positivity).[156] The use of MBSR with health care providers has shown promise in decreasing burnout and improving physical and mental health and the argument has even been made that, in the name of patient safety and high reliability, mindful practice is our ethical responsibility as anesthesiologists.[156]

Creating a Culture of Support

Many physicians spend more waking hours at work than at home, emphasizing the personal impact of work culture on well-being. Afonso et al.[144] demonstrated a tight link between perceived sense of support in the workplace and burnout, further accentuating the systemic nature of physician burnout and well-being. In 2018, Schwenk[157] likened the physician to a canary in a coal mine, highlighting that the burnout crisis was being fueled not by poorly resilient physicians, but by a toxic work environment. This editorial punctuated the moment when multiple state and national organizations began to approach well-being from a systems and policy standpoint. Pointedly, the NAM created an Action Collaborative on Clinician Well-Being and Resilience that, after publishing a major report on burnout in HCWs, has continued to work toward positive systems and policy change.[77]

Several models have been developed to approach organizational well-being. One such model, the Stanford Model of Professional Fulfillment (Fig. 3-4) centers professional fulfillment in the center of three major factors: culture of wellness, efficiency of

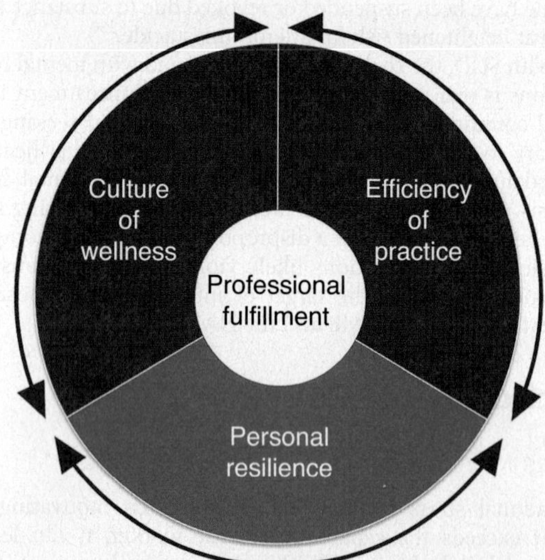

Figure 3-4 Professional Fulfillment Index from the Stanford WellMD center outlining three main areas of foci for improving well-being and engagement. (© 2016 Board of Trustees of the Leland Stanford Junior University. All rights reserved.)

practice, and personal resilience. Notably, two out of three factors are systems based, not individual, placing the onus more on organizations than clinicians.[158]

The ASA has similarly developed organizational approaches to well-being. For instance, The ASA Statement on Creating a Culture of Well-Being for Health Care Workers, which was approved by the House of Delegates at the 2021 ASA Annual Meeting, outlines an approach taking into consideration factors of scheduling flexibility, care provider support, destigmatization of clinician mental illness, systemic life imbalances, the impact of COVID-19 on careers, and general well-being initiatives.[159]

Conclusion

The lessons learned from the COVID-19 pandemic have dramatized how the state of the anesthesiologist's workplaces, both in terms of physical and psychological safety, is paramount to the anesthesiologist's own well-being and ultimately the quality of care provided to their patients. As such, HCW well-being ought to be a key quality metric for any health care organization desiring long-term success. An understanding and regard for these considerations across a wide range of sources and remedies is a good start for those endeavoring to create cultures of support and well-being.

For additional information please see NICV 3-1 in the eBook bundled with this text.

For further review and interactivities, please see the videos and narrative interactive clinical vignettes (NICVs) accessible in the complimentary eBook bundled with this text. Access instructions are located on the inside front cover.

REFERENCES

1. Bureau of Labor Statistics. U.S. Department of Labor. Employer-reported workplace injuries and illnesses–2020. 2020. Accessed May 10, 2022. https://www.bls.gov/news.release/pdf/osh.pdf
2. Torralba-Rodriguez FJ, Bixquert-Montagud V, Fernández-Breis JT, Martínez-BéjarR. An incremental knowledge acquisition-based system for supporting decisions in biomedical domains. *Comput Methods Programs Biomed.* 2010;98(2):161–171.
3. Edworthy J, Hellier E. Alarms and human behaviour: implications for medical alarms. *Br J Anaesth.* 2006;97(1):12–17.
4. Sanders MS, McCormick EJ. *Human Factors in Engineering and Design.* 7th ed. McGraw-Hill; 1993:80–82.
5. Linde HW, Bruce DL. Occupational exposure of anesthetists to halothane, nitrous oxide and radiation. *Anesthesiology.* 1969;30(4):363–368.
6. National Institutes of Health. Office of Research Services. Waste Anesthetic Gas. Bethesda, MD, 2019. Accessed January 17, 2022. https://ors.od.nih.gov/sr/dohs/Documents/WAG%20Fact%20Sheet%20FV.pdf
7. Panni MK, Corn SB. Scavenging in the operating room. *Curr Opin Anaesthesiol.* 2003;16(6):611–617.
8. Sessler DI, Badgwell JM. Exposure of postoperative nurses to exhaled anesthetic gases. *Anesth Analg.* 1998;87(5):1083–1088.
9. Vaisman AI. Working conditions in the operating room and their effect on the health of anesthetists. *Eksp Khir Anesteziol.* 1967;12(3):44–49.
10. Sanders RD, Weimann J, Maze M. Biologic effects of nitrous oxide: a mechanistic and toxicologic review. *Anesthesiology.* 2008;109(4):707–722.
11. Eroglu A, Celep F, Erciyes N. A comparison of sister chromatid exchanges in lymphocytes of anesthesiologists to nonanesthesiologists in the same hospital. *Anesth Analg.* 2006;102(5):1573–1577.
12. Wiesner G, Hoerauf K, Schroegendorfer K, Sobczynski P, Harth M, Ruediger HW. High-level, but not low-level, occupational exposure to inhaled anesthetics is associated with genotoxicity in the micronucleus assay. *Anesth Analg.* 2001;92(1):118–122.
13. Occupational disease among operating room personnel: a national study. Report of an Ad Hoc Committee on the Effect of Trace Anesthetics on the Health of Operating Room Personnel, American Society of Anesthesiologists. *Anesthesiology.* 1974;41(4):321–340.
14. Buring JE, Hennekens CH, Mayrent SL, Rosner B, Greenberg ER, Colton T. Health experiences of operating room personnel. *Anesthesiology.* 1985;62(3):325–330.
15. Boivin JF. Risk of spontaneous abortion in women occupationally exposed to anaesthetic gases: a meta-analysis. *Occup Environ Med.* 1997;54(8):541–548.
16. Axelsson G, Ahlborg G Jr, Bodin L. Shift work, nitrous oxide exposure, and spontaneous abortion among Swedish midwives. *Occup Environ Med.* 1996;53(6):374–378.
17. Luke B, Mamelle N, Keith L, et al. The association between occupational factors and preterm birth: a United States nurses' study. Research Committee of the Association of Women's Health, Obstetric, and Neonatal Nurses. *Am J Obstet Gynecol.* 1995;173(3 Pt 1):849–862.
18. Lawson CC, Rocheleau CM, Whelan EA, et al. Occupational exposures among nurses and risk of spontaneous abortion. *Am J Obstet Gynecol.* 2012;206(4):327.e1–8.
19. Zacny JP, Yajnik S, Lichtor JL, et al. The acute and residual effects of subanesthetic concentrations of isoflurane/nitrous oxide combinations on cognitive and psychomotor performance in healthy volunteers. *Anesth Analg.* 1996;82(1):153–157.
20. Varughese S, Ahmed R. Environmental and occupational considerations of anesthesia: a narrative review and update. *Anesth Analg.* 2021;133(4):826–835.
21. Tramontini CC, Galvão CM, Claudio CV, Ribeiro RP, Martins JT. Composição da fumaça produzida pelo bisturi elétrico: revisão integrativa da literature [Composition of the electrocautery smoke: integrative literature review]. *Rev Esc Enferm USP.* 2016 Feb;50(1):148–157. Portuguese. doi: 10.1590/S0080-623420160000100019. PMID: 27007432.
22. Steege AL, Boiano JM, Sweeney MH. Secondhand smoke in the operating room? Precautionary practices lacking for surgical smoke. *Am J Ind Med.* 2016;59(11):1020–1031.
23. National Institute for Occupational Safety and Health. Control of Smoke from Laser/Electric Surgical Procedures. Publication No. 96-128. 1996. Accessed January 17, 2022. https://www.cdc.gov/niosh/docs/hazardcontrol/hc11.html
24. Sehulster L, Chinn RYW; CDC, HICPAC. Guidelines for environmental infection control in health-care facilities. Recommendations of CDC and the Healthcare Infection Control Practices Advisory Committee (HICPAC). *MMWR Recomm Rep.* 2003;52(RR-10):1–42.
25. Hussey P, Wu I, Johnston T. 2018 ACC/HRS/NASCI/SCAI/SCCT Expert Consensus document on optimal use of ionizing radiation in cardiovascular imaging: best practices for safety and effectiveness-a review for the cardiac anesthesiologist. *J Cardiothorac Vasc Anesth.* 2019;33(11):2902–2908.
26. Ismail S, Khan F, Sultan N, Naqvi M. Radiation exposure to anaesthetists during interventional radiology. *Anaesthesia.* 2010;65(1):54–60.
27. Katz JD. Radiation exposure to anesthesia personnel: the impact of an electrophysiology laboratory. *Anesth Analg.* 2005;101(6):1725–1726.
28. Anastasian ZH, Strozyk D, Meyers PM, Wang S, Berman MF. Radiation exposure of the anesthesiologist in the neurointerventional suite. *Anesthesiology.* 2011;114(3):512–520.
29. Roguin A, Goldstein J, Bar O, Goldstein JA. Brain and neck tumors among physicians performing interventional procedures. *Am J Cardiol.* 2013;111(9):1368–1372.
30. Whitney GM, Thomas JJ, Austin TM, Fanfan J, Yaster M. Radiation safety perceptions and practices among pediatric anesthesiologists: a survey of the physician membership of the Society for Pediatric Anesthesia. *Anesth Analg.* 2019;128(6):1242–1248.
31. International Commission on Non-Ionizing Radiation Protection (ICNIRP). Guidelines on limits of exposure to static magnetic fields. *Health Phys.* 2009;96(4):504–514.
32. de Lima Andrade E, da Cunha E Silva DC, de Lima EA, de Oliveira RA, Zannin PHT, Martins ACG. Environmental noise in hospitals: a systematic review. *Environ Sci Pollut Res Int.* 2021;28(16):19629–19642.
33. Clark C, Paunovic K. WHO environmental noise guidelines for the European region: a systematic review on environmental noise and quality of life, wellbeing and mental health. *Int J Environ Res Public Health.* 2018;15(11):2400.
34. Ginsberg SH, Pantin E, Kraidin J, Solina A, Panjwani S, Yang G. Noise levels in modern operating rooms during surgery. *J Cardiothorac Vasc Anesth.* 2013;27(3):528–530.
35. Katz JD. Noise in the operating room. *Anesthesiology.* 2014;121(4):894–898.
36. McLeod R, Myint-Wilks L, Davies SE, Elhassan HA. The impact of noise in the operating theatre: a review of the evidence. *Ann R Coll Surg Engl.* 2021;103(2):83–87.
37. Kurmann A, Peter M, Tschan F, Mühlemann K, Candinas D, Beldi G. Adverse effect of noise in the operating theatre on surgical-site infection. *Br J Surg.* 2011;98(7):1021–1025.
38. Fritsch MH, Chacko CE, Patterson EB. Operating room sound level hazards for patients and physicians. *Otol Neurotol.* 2010;31(5):715–721.
39. Wallace MS, Ashman MN, Matjasko MJ. Hearing acuity of anesthesiologists and alarm detection. *Anesthesiology.* 1994;81(1):13–28.
40. Palmer JS, Wilson C, Fraig H, Wilson D, Garrett S. Hearing Evaluation of ARthroplasty Surgeons: results from the HEARS study. *Ann R Coll Surg Engl.* 2021;103(9):673–677.
41. Miskovic D, Rosenthal R, Zingg U, Oertli D, Metzger U, Jancke L. Randomized controlled trial investigating the effect of music on the virtual reality laparoscopic learning performance of novice surgeons. *Surg Endosc.* 2008;22(11):2416–2420.
42. Hawksworth C, Asbury AJ, Millar K. Music in theatre: not so harmonious. A survey of attitudes to music played in the operating theatre. *Anaesthesia.* 1997;52(1):79–83.
43. Hawksworth CR, Sivalingam P, Asbury AJ. The effect of music on anaesthetists' psychomotor performance. *Anaesthesia.* 1998;53(2):195–197.
44. Breen CM, Abernethy AP, Abbott KH, Tulsky JA. Conflict associated with decisions to limit life-sustaining treatment in intensive care units. *J Gen Intern Med.* 2001;16(5):283–289.
45. Katz JD. Conflict and its resolution in the operating room. *J Clin Anesth.* 2007;19(2):152–158.

46. Helmreich RL, Merritt AC, Wilhelm JA. The evolution of Crew Resource Management training in commercial aviation. *Int J Aviat Psychol*. 1999;9(1):19–32.
47. Gaba DM, Howard SK, Jump B. Production pressure in the work environment. California anesthesiologists' attitudes and experiences. *Anesthesiology*. 1994;81(2):488–500.
48. Russ S, Rout S, Sevdalis N, Moorthy K, Darzi A, Vincent C. Do safety checklists improve teamwork and communication in the operating room? A systematic review. *Ann Surg*. 2013;258(6): 856–871.
49. Shi H, Huang T, Schernhammer ES, Sun Q, Wang M. Rotating night shift work and healthy aging after 24 years of follow-up in the nurses' health study. *JAMA Network Open*. 2022;5(5): e2210450.
50. Huizinga CRH, de Kam ML, Stockmann H, van Gerven JMA, Cohen AF, van der Bogt KEA. Evaluating fitness to perform in surgical residents after night shifts and alcohol intoxication: the development of a "fit-to-perform" test. *J Surg Educ*. 2018;75(4):968–977.
51. Wingelaar-Jagt YQ, Wingelaar TT, Riedel WJ, Ramaekers JG. Fatigue in aviation: safety risks, preventive strategies and pharmacological interventions. *Front Physiol*. 2021;12:712628.
52. Barger LK, Cade BE, Ayas NT, et al; Harvard Work Hours, Health, and Safety Group. Extended work shifts and the risk of motor vehicle crashes among interns. *N Engl J Med*. 2005;352(2):125–134.
53. Reid K, Dawson D. Comparing performance on a simulated 12 hour shift rotation in young and older subjects. *Occup Environ Med*. 2001;58(1):58–62.
54. Gates M, Wingert A, Featherstone R, Samuels C, Simon C, Dyson MP. Impact of fatigue and insufficient sleep on physician and patient outcomes: a systematic review. *BMJ Open*. 2018; 8(9):e021967.
55. Friedman RC, Bigger JT, Kornfeld DS. The intern and sleep loss. *N Engl J Med*. 1971;285(4): 201–203.
56. Abrams RM. Sleep Deprivation. *Obstet Gynecol Clin North Am*. 2015;42(3):493–506.
57. Landrigan CP, Rothschild JM, Cronin JW, et al. Effect of reducing interns' work hours on serious medical errors in intensive care units. *N Engl J Med*. 2004;351(18):1838–1848.
58. Rothschild JM, Keohane CA, Rogers S, et al. Risks of complications by attending physicians after performing nighttime procedures. *JAMA*. 2009;302(14):1565–1572.
59. Koda N, Oshima Y, Koda K, Shimada H. Surgeon fatigue does not affect surgical outcomes: a systematic review and meta-analysis. *Surg Today*. 2021;51(5):659–668.
60. Ellman PI, Law MG, Tache-Leon C, et al. Sleep deprivation does not affect operative results in cardiac surgery. *Ann Thorac Surg*. 2004;78(3):906–911; discussion 906–911.
61. Yaghoubian A, Kaji AH, Putnam B, de Virgilio C. Trauma surgery performed by "sleep deprived" residents: are outcomes affected? *J Surg Educ*. 2010;67(6):449–451.
62. Gravenstein JS, Cooper JB, Orkin FK. Work and rest cycles in anesthesia practice. *Anesthesiology*. 1990;72(4):737–742.
63. Howard SK, Gaba DM, Smith BE, et al. Simulation study of rested versus sleep-deprived anesthesiologists. *Anesthesiology*. 2003;98(6):1345–1355; discussion 5A.
64. Wright MC, Phillips-Bute B, Mark JB, et al. Time of day effects on the incidence of anesthetic adverse events. *Qual Saf Health Care*. 2006;15(4):258–263.
65. Gander PH, Merry A, Millar MM, Weller J. Hours of work and fatigue-related error: a survey of New Zealand anaesthetists. *Anaesth Intensive Care*. 2000;28(2):178–183.
66. Landrigan CP, Rahman SA, Sullivan JP, et al; ROSTERS Study Group. Effect on patient safety of a resident physician schedule without 24-hour shifts. *N Engl J Med*. 2020;382(26):2514–2523.
67. Awan M, Zagales I, McKenney M, Kinslow K, Elkbuli A. ACGME 2011 duty hours restrictions and their effects on surgical residency training and patients outcomes: a systematic review. *J Surg Educ*. 2021;78(6):e35–e46.
68. Janhofer DE, Lakhiani C, Song DH. Addressing surgeon fatigue: current understanding and strategies for mitigation. *Plast Reconstr Surg*. 2019;144(4):693e–699e.
69. Centers for Disease Control and Prevention. National Center for Health Statistics. WONDER. 2020. Accessed May 1, 2022. http://wonder.cdc.gov
70. Oreskovich MR, Shanafelt T, Dyrbye LN, et al. The prevalence of substance use disorders in American physicians. *Am J Addict*. 2015;24(1):30–38.
71. Warner DO, Berge K, Sun H, Harman A, Wang T. Substance use disorder in physicians after completion of training in anesthesiology in the United States from 1977 to 2013. *Anesthesiology*. 2020;133(2):342–349.
72. Morris SD, Morris AJ, Rockoff MA. Freeman Allen: Boston's pioneering physician anesthetist. *Anesth Analg*. 2014;119(5):1186–1193.
73. Talbott GD, Gallegos KV, Wilson PO, Porter TL. The Medical Association of Georgia's Impaired Physicians Program. Review of the first 1000 physicians: analysis of specialty. *JAMA*. 1987; 257(21):2927–2930.
74. Earley PH, Finver T. Addiction to propofol: a study of 22 treatment cases. *J Addict Med*. 2013; 7(3):169–176.
75. Alexander BH, Checkoway H, Nagahama SI, Domino KB. Cause-specific mortality risks of anesthesiologists. *Anesthesiology*. 2000;93(4):922–930.
76. Supplemental Resource: Report and Recommendations of the FSMB Workgroup on Physician Wellness and Burnout. *Journal of Medical Regulation*. 2018;104(2):37–48.
77. National Academy of Medicine. *Taking Action Against Clinician Burnout: A Systems Approach to Professional Well-being*. The National Academies Press; 2019.
78. Fitzsimons MG, Baker K, Malhotra R, Gottlieb A, Lowenstein E, Zapol WM. Reducing the incidence of substance use disorders in anesthesiology residents: 13 years of comprehensive urine drug screening. *Anesthesiology*. 2018;129(4):821–828.
79. Fitzsimons MG, Baker KH. Not all strikes are easy to call. *Anesth Analg*. 2009;109(3):693–694.
80. Sivarajan M, Posner KL, Caplan RA, Gild WM, Cheney FW. Substance abuse among anesthesiologists. *Anesthesiology*. 1994;80(3):704.
81. Katz JD. Hand washing and hand disinfection: more than your mother taught you. *Anesthesiol Clin North America*. 2004;22(3):457–471, vi.
82. Kuhar DHD, Struble K, Heneine W, et. al. Updated U.S. Public Health Service Guidelines for the Management of Occupational Exposures to HIV and Recommendations for Postexposure Prophylaxis. 2018. Accessed January 17, 2022. https://stacks.cdc.gov/view/cdc/20711
83. Centers for Disease Control and Prevention (CDC). FDA approval of an extended period for administering VariZIG for postexposure prophylaxis of varicella. *MMWR Morb Mortal Wkly Rep*. 2012;61(12):212.
84. U.S. Government Printing Office. Occupational Exposure to Bloodborne Pathogens; Needlestick and Other Sharps Injuries. Final Rule. 2001. 29 CFR Part 1910. Accessed January 17, 2022. https://www.osha.gov/laws-regs/federalregister/2001-01-18
85. Statement of Charles N. Jeffress, Assistant Secretary, Occupational Safety and Health Administration. June 22, 2000. Accessed May 10, 2022. https://www.osha.gov/news/testimonies/06222000
86. Sosa LE, Njie GJ, Lobato MN, et al. Tuberculosis screening, testing, and treatment of U.S. health care personnel: recommendations from the National Tuberculosis Controllers Association and CDC, 2019. *MMWR Morb Mortal Wkly Rep*. 2019;68(19):439–443.
87. Quach S, Pereira JA, Kwong JC, et al; Public Health Agency of Canada/Canadian Institutes of Health Research Influenza Research Network (PCIRN) Program Delivery and Evaluation Theme Group. Immunizing health care workers against influenza: a glimpse into the challenges with voluntary programs and considerations for mandatory policies. *Am J Infect Control*. 2013; 41(11):1017–1023.
88. Kamming D, Gardam M, Chung F. Anaesthesia and SARS. *Br J Anaesth*. 2003;90(6):715–718.
89. Drain PK. Rapid diagnostic testing for SARS-CoV-2. *N Engl J Med*. 2022;386(3):264–272.
90. Frenkel LM, Garratty EM, Shen JP, Wheeler N, Clark O, Bryson YJ. Clinical reactivation of herpes simplex virus type 2 infection in seropositive pregnant women with no history of genital herpes. *Ann Intern Med*. 1993;118(6):414–418.
91. Marin M, Guris D, Chaves SS, Schmid S, Seward JF; Centers for Disease Control and Prevention (CDC). Prevention of varicella: recommendations of the Advisory Committee on Immunization Practices (ACIP). *MMWR Recomm Rep*. 2007;56(RR-4):1–40.
92. National Center for Immunization and Respiratory Diseases. Cytomegalovirus (CMV) and Congenital CMV Infection. 2020. Accessed January 24, 2022. http://www.cdc.gov/cmv/index.html
93. Pass RF, Arav-Boger R. Maternal and fetal cytomegalovirus infection: diagnosis, management, and prevention. *F1000Res*. 2018;7:255.
94. Watson JC, Hadler SC, Dykewicz CA, Reef S, Phillips L. Measles, mumps, and rubella–vaccine use and strategies for elimination of measles, rubella, and congenital rubella syndrome and control of mumps: recommendations of the Advisory Committee on Immunization Practices (ACIP). *MMWR Recomm Rep*. 1998;47(RR-8):1–57.
95. Siegel JD, Rhinehart E, Jackson M, Chiarello L; Health Care Infection Control Practices Advisory Committee. 2007 guideline for isolation precautions: preventing transmission of infectious agents in health care settings. *Am J Infect Control*. 2007;35(10 Suppl 2):S65–S164.
96. Advisory Committee on Immunization Practices, Centers for Disease Control and Prevention. Immunization of health-care personnel: recommendations of the Advisory Committee on Immunization Practices (ACIP). *MMWR Recomm Rep*. 2011;60(RR-7):1–45.
97. Clemmons NS, Gastanaduy PA, Fiebelkorn AP, Redd SB, Wallace GS; Centers for Disease Control and Prevention (CDC). Measles - United States, January 4-April 2, 2015. *MMWR Morb Mortal Wkly Rep*. 2015;64(14):373–376.
98. Advisory Committee on Immunization Practices; Fiore AE, Wasley A, Bell BP. Prevention of hepatitis A through active or passive immunization: recommendations of the Advisory Committee on Immunization Practices (ACIP). *MMWR Recomm Rep*. 2006;55(RR-7):1–23.
99. U. S. Public Health Service. Updated U.S. Public Health Service guidelines for the management of occupational exposures to HBV, HCV, and HIV and recommendations for postexposure prophylaxis. *MMWR Recomm Rep*. 2001;50(RR-11):1–52.
100. World Health Organization. Hepatitis C. July 27, 2021. Accessed January 23, 2022. https://www.who.int/news-room/fact-sheets/detail/hepatitis-c
101. Moorman AC, de Perio MA, Goldschmidt R, et al. Testing and clinical management of health care personnel potentially exposed to hepatitis C virus - CDC Guidance, United States, 2020. *MMWR Recomm Rep*. 2020;69(6):1–8.
102. Joint United Nations Programme on HIV/AIDS. Global AIDS Update 2020. 2020. Accessed February 1, 2022. https://www.unaids.org/en/resources/documents/2020/global-aids-report
103. Bouya S, Balouchi A, Rafiemanesh H, et al. Global prevalence and device related causes of needle stick injuries among health care workers: a systematic review and meta-analysis. *Ann Glob Health*. 2020;86(1):35.
104. Joyce MP, Kuhar D, Brooks JT. Notes from the field: occupationally acquired HIV infection among health care workers - United States, 1985-2013. *MMWR Morb Mortal Wkly Rep*. 2015;63(53):1245–1246.

105. Greene ES, Berry AJ, Jagger J, et al. Multicenter study of contaminated percutaneous injuries in anesthesia personnel. *Anesthesiology*. 1998;89(6):1362–1372.
106. Rutala WA, Weber DJ; Society for Healthcare Epidemiology of America. Guideline for disinfection and sterilization of prion-contaminated medical instruments. *Infect Control Hosp Epidemiol*. 2010;31(2):107–117.
107. Blumberg HM, Burman WJ, Chaisson RE, et al; American Thoracic Society, Centers for Disease Control and Prevention and the Infectious Diseases Society. American Thoracic Society/Centers for Disease Control and Prevention/Infectious Diseases Society of America: treatment of tuberculosis. *Am J Respir Crit Care Med*. 2003;167(4):603–662.
108. Centers for Diseae Control and Prevention. Tuberculosis Data and Statistics. 2020. Accessed January 23, 2022. https://www.cdc.gov/tb/statistics/default.htm
109. Jensen PA, Lambert LA, Iademarco MF, Ridzon R; CDC. Guidelines for preventing the transmission of Mycobacterium tuberculosis in health-care settings, 2005. *MMWR Recomm Rep*. 2005;54(RR-17):1–141.
110. Centers for Disease Control and Prevention. NIOSH Respiratory Protective Device Information. June 2021. Accessed January 23, 2022. https://www.cdc.gov/niosh/npptl/resources/pressrel/letters/respprotect/CA-2021-1033-R1.html
111. DesRoches CM, Rao SR, Fromson JA, et al. Physicians' perceptions, preparedness for reporting, and experiences related to impaired and incompetent colleagues. *JAMA*. 2010;304(2):187–193.
112. Rose GL, Brown RE Jr. The impaired anesthesiologist: not just about drugs and alcohol anymore. *J Clin Anesth*. 2010;22(5):379–384.
113. Soonsawat A, Tanaka G, Lammando MA, Ahmed I, Ellison JM. Cognitively impaired physicians: how do we detect them? How do we assist them? *Am J Geriatr Psychiatry*. 2018;26(6):631–640.
114. Del Bene VA, Brandt J. Identifying neuropsychologically impaired physicians. *Clin Neuropsychol*. 2020;34(2):318–331.
115. Dellinger EP, Pellegrini CA, Gallagher TH. The aging physician and the medical profession: a review. *JAMA Surg*. 2017;152(10):967–971.
116. Katz JD. The aging anesthesiologist. *Curr Opin Anaesthesiol*. 2016;29(2):206–211.
117. Kohatsu ND, Gould D, Ross LK, Fox PJ. Characteristics associated with physician discipline: a case-control study. *Arch Intern Med*. 2004;164(6):653–658.
118. Choudhry NK, Fletcher RH, Soumerai SB. Systematic review: the relationship between clinical experience and quality of health care. *Ann Intern Med*. 2005;142(4):260–273.
119. Weininger G, Mori M, Brooks C 2nd, et al. Association between cardiac surgeons' number of years in practice and surgical outcomes in New York cardiac centers. *JAMA Netw Open*. 2020;3(11):e2023671.
120. Tessler MJ, Shrier I, Steele RJ. Association between anesthesiologist age and litigation. *Anesthesiology*. 2012;116(3):574–579.
121. Siu LW, Boet S, Borges BCR, et al. High-fidelity simulation demonstrates the influence of anesthesiologists' age and years from residency on emergency cricothyroidotomy skills. *Anesth Analg*. 2010;111(4):955–960.
122. Garfield JM, Garfield FB. The ageing anaesthetist: lessons from the North American experience. *BJA Educ*. 2021;21(1):20–25.
123. Orkin FK, McGinnis SL, Forte GJ, et al. United States anesthesiologists over 50: retirement decision making and workforce implications. *Anesthesiology*. 2012;117(5):953–963.
124. Carpenter LM, Swerdlow AJ, Fear NT. Mortality of doctors in different specialties: findings from a cohort of 20000 NHS hospital consultants. *Occup Environ Med*. 1997;54(6):388–395.
125. Katz JD. Do anesthesiologists die at a younger age than other physicians? Age-adjusted death rates. *Anesth Analg*. 2004;98(4):1111–1113.
126. Katz JD, Slade MD. Anesthesiologists are living longer: mortality experience 1992 to 2001. *J Clin Anesth*. 2006;18(6):405–408.
127. Duarte D, El-Hagrassy MM, Couto TCE, Gurgel W, Fregni F, Correa H. Male and female physician suicidality: a systematic review and meta-analysis. *JAMA Psychiatry*. 2020;77(6):587–597.
128. Dutheil F, Aubert C, Pereira B, et al. Suicide among physicians and health-care workers: a systematic review and meta-analysis. *PLoS One*. 2019;14(12):e0226361.
129. Mayall R. Substance abuse in anaesthetists. *BJA Educ*. 2016;16(7):236–241.
130. Iannelli RJ, Finlayson AJR, Brown KP, et al. Suicidal behavior among physicians referred for fitness-for-duty evaluation. *Gen Hosp Psychiatry*. 2014;36(6):732–736.
131. National Academy of Medicine. Resource Compendium for Health Care Worker Well-being. Accessed May 1, 2022. https://nam.edu/compendium-of-key-resources-for-improving-clinician-well-being/
132. Eisenach JH, Sprung J, Clark MM, et al. The psychological and physiological effects of acute occupational stress in new anesthesiology residents: a pilot trial. *Anesthesiology*. 2014;121(4):878–893.
133. Shanafelt T, Ripp J, Trockel M. Understanding and addressing sources of anxiety among health care professionals during the COVID-19 pandemic. *JAMA*. 2020;323(21):2133–2134.
134. Wu AW. Medical error: the second victim. The doctor who makes the mistake needs help too. *BMJ*. 2000;320(7237):726–727.
135. Gazoni FM, Amato PE, Malik ZM, Durieux ME. The impact of perioperative catastrophes on anesthesiologists: results of a national survey. *Anesth Analg*. 2012;114(3):596–603.
136. Vinson AE, Mitchell JD. Assessing levels of support for residents following adverse outcomes: a national survey of anesthesia residency programs in the United States. *Med Teach*. 2014;36(10):858–866.
137. Agency for Healthcare Research and Quality. Patient Safety Network. Hospital Survey on Patient Safety Culture: 2018 User Database Report. 2018. Accessed May 10, 2022. https://psnet.ahrq.gov/issue/hospital-survey-patient-safety-culture-2018-user-database-report
138. Edrees H, Connors C, Paine L, Norvell M, Taylor H, Wu AW. Implementing the RISE second victim support programme at the Johns Hopkins Hospital: a case study. *BMJ Open*. 2016;6(9):e011708.
139. Lown BA, Manning CF. The Schwartz Center Rounds: evaluation of an interdisciplinary approach to enhancing patient-centered communication, teamwork, and provider support. *Acad Med*. 2010;85(6):1073–1081.
140. Freudenberger HJ. Staff Burn-Out. *J Soc Issues*. 1974;30:159–165.
141. Maslach C, Jackson SE, Leiter MP. *Maslach Burnout Inventory Manual*. 3rd ed. Consulting Psychologists Press; 1996.
142. Shanafelt TD, Boone S, Tan L, et al. Burnout and satisfaction with work-life balance among US physicians relative to the general US population. *Arch Intern Med*. 2012;172(18):1377–1385.
143. Hyman SA, Card EB, De Leon-Casasola O, Shotwell MS, Shi Y, Weinger MB. Prevalence of burnout and its relationship to health status and social support in more than 1000 subspecialty anesthesiologists. *Reg Anesth Pain Med*. 2021;46(5):381–387.
144. Afonso AM, Cadwell JB, Staffa SJ, Zurakowski D, Vinson AE. Burnout rate and risk factors among anesthesiologists in the United States. *Anesthesiology*. 2021;134(5):683–696.
145. Khan A, Vinson AE. Physician well-being in practice. *Anesth Analg*. 2020;131(5):1359–1369.
146. Osler WS1-1 SM, Murray TJ, Bryan CS. *The quotable Osler*. American College of Physicians; 2008.
147. The anesthesiology milestone project. *J Grad Med Educ*. 2014;6(1 Suppl 1):15–28.
148. McGinnis JM, Foege WH. Actual causes of death in the United States. *JAMA*. 1993;270(18):2207–2212.
149. Luckhaupt SE, Cohen MA, Li J, Calvert GM. Prevalence of obesity among U.S. workers and associations with occupational factors. *Am J Prev Med*. 2014;46(3):237–248.
150. Gupta S. *Keep Sharp: Build a Better Brain at Any Age*. Simon & Schuster; 2021.
151. Wen CP, Wai JPM, Tsai MK, Chen CH. Minimal amount of exercise to prolong life: to walk, to run, or just mix it up? *J Am Coll Cardiol*. 2014;64(5):482–484.
152. Physical Activity Guidelines for Americans. 2nd edition. 2018. Accessed May 10, 2022. https://health.gov/sites/default/files/2019-09/Physical_Activity_Guidelines_2nd_edition.pdf
153. Hamidi MS, Boggild MK, Cheung AM. Running on empty: a review of nutrition and physicians' well-being. *Postgrad Med J*. 2016;92(1090):478–481.
154. Rapgay L, Bystrisky A. Classical mindfulness: an introduction to its theory and practice for clinical application. *Ann N Y Acad Sci*. 2009;1172:148–162.
155. Kabat-Zinn J, Massion AO, Kristeller J, et al. Effectiveness of a meditation-based stress reduction program in the treatment of anxiety disorders. *Am J Psychiatry*. 1992;149(7):936–943.
156. Vinson AE, Wang J. Is mindful practice our ethical responsibility as anesthesiologists? *Int Anesthesiol Clin*. 2015;53(3):1–11.
157. Schwenk TL. Physician well-being and the regenerative power of caring. *JAMA*. 2018;319(15):1543–1544.
158. The Stanford Model of Professional FulfillmentTM. Accessed March 18, 2022. https://wellmd.stanford.edu/about/model-external.html
159. American Society of Anesthesiologists. Statement on Creating a Culture of Well-being for Health Care Workers. Accessed March 18, 2022. https://www.asahq.org/standards-and-guidelines/asa-statement-on-creating-a-culture-of-well-being-for-health-care-workers

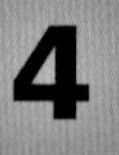

4 Anesthetic Risk, Quality Improvement, and Liability

IAN R. SLADE • CHRISTOPHER D. KENT • SHAWN L. MINCER • KAREN B. DOMINO

KEY POINTS

1. Anesthetic mortality has decreased, but potentially preventable deaths and disabling complications still occur.
2. Risk management programs are broadly oriented toward reducing the liability exposure of the organization. Risk management programs complement quality improvement programs in minimizing liability exposure while maximizing quality of patient care.
3. Continuous quality improvement is a systems approach to identifying and improving quality of care. Quality improvement programs focus on improving the structure, process, and outcome of care.
4. Quality improvement programs are generally guided by the requirements of the Joint Commission that accredits health care organizations and the reporting and performance requirements of the Centers for Medicare and Medicaid Services.
5. Medical malpractice refers to the legal concept of professional negligence. The patient-plaintiff must prove that the anesthesiologist owed the patient a duty and failed to fulfill this duty, that the anesthesiologist's actions caused an injury, and that the injury resulted from a breach in the standard of anesthesia care.
6. The most common lawsuits against anesthesiologists (excluding dental injuries) are for death, brain damage, nerve damage, and airway injury. Chronic pain management is the source of an increasing number of malpractice claims against anesthesiologists.

In anesthesia, as in other areas of life, everything does not always go as planned. Undesirable outcomes can occur regardless of the quality of care provided. Continuous quality improvement (CQI) programs are intended to maximize the collective learning from past near misses and undesirable outcomes to prevent their future occurrence. An anesthesia risk management program can work in conjunction with a program for quality improvement to minimize the liability risk of practice. Payers such as the Centers for Medicare and Medicaid Services (CMS) are increasingly depending on accreditation through bodies such as the Joint Commission to ensure that mechanisms are in place to deliver quality and safe care to all patients. In addition, there has been a move toward linking reimbursement to performance measurement and reporting. The legal aspects of American medical practice are important to the anesthesia community as the public turns to the courts for economic redress when their expectations of medical treatment are not met.

This chapter discusses anesthetic mortality and morbidity, risk management, CQI, performance measurement, and medical liability. The chapter provides background for the practitioner concerning the role of risk management activity in minimizing and managing liability exposure. Also described are the medical-legal system, the most frequent causes of lawsuits for anesthesiologists, and appropriate actions for physicians to take in the event of a malpractice suit.

Anesthesia Risk

Mortality and Major Morbidity Related to Anesthesia

Estimates of anesthesia-related morbidity and mortality are difficult to quantify (1 Video 4-1). Not only are there difficulties obtaining data on complications, but also different methods yield different estimates of anesthesia risk. Studies differ in their definitions of complications, in length of follow-up, and especially in approaches to evaluation of the contribution of anesthesia care to patient outcomes. A comprehensive review of anesthesia complications is beyond the scope of this chapter. A sampling of studies of anesthesia mortality and morbidity will be presented to provide historical perspective plus a limited overview of relatively recent findings.

Early studies estimated the anesthesia-related mortality rate as 1 per 1,560 anesthetics.[1] More recent studies use data from the 1990s and later estimate the anesthesia-related death rate in the United States to be lower than 1 per 10,000 anesthetics (Table 4-1).[2–9] Differences in estimates may be influenced by different reporting methods, definitions, anesthesia practices, and patient populations, as well as actual differences in underlying complication rates. A systematic review and meta-analysis of mortality attributable to general anesthesia (GA) from before the 1970s through 1

Table 4-1 Estimates of Anesthesia-Related Death

Reference	Country	Time	Data Sources/Methods	Rate of Death
Bainbridge et al.[2]	Global	1940s–2011 a. pre-1970s b. 1970s–1980s c. 1990s–2000s	Systematic review and meta-analysis of published studies in any language with a sample size over 3,000 of rates of anesthesia-related mortality of surgical patients who had undergone general anesthesia. (n = 87 studies including 21.4 million general anesthetics for patients undergoing surgery)	Anesthetic solely attributable mortality: a. 3.57/10,000 b. 0.52/10,000 c. 0.34/10,000 Anesthetic contributory mortality: a. 6.5/10,000 b. 3.23/10,000 c. 1.43/10,000
			Anesthetic mortality by national development status using the United Nations Human Development Index (HDI) over time to assess impact of country development on anesthetic mortality	Anesthetic solely attributable mortality: a. High HDI 3.57/10,000, Low HDI not reported b. High HDI 0.32/10,000, Low HDI 1.01/10,000 c. High HDI 0.25/10,000, Low HDI 1.41/10,000 Anesthetic contributory mortality: a. High HDI 6.84/10,000, Low HDI 3.26/10,000 b. High HDI 2.34/10,000, Low HDI 4.32/10,000 c. High HDI 0.85/10,000, Low HDI 4.67/10,000
Li et al.[3]	USA	1999–2005	Deaths with anesthesia-related complication codes from death certificate data a. Population data from census records b. National hospital discharge survey data (inpatients)	Anesthesia-related deaths a. 1.1/million population/y b. 8.2/million hospital surgical discharges
Ellis et al.[4]	USA	1999–2009	Cardiac arrests within 24 h of surgery (n = 217,365 anesthetics) in a single hospital	Death due to anesthesia-attributable cardiac arrest—0.2/10,000 anesthetics Death due to anesthesia-contributable cardiac arrest—0.7/10,000 anesthetics
Gibbs[5]	Australia	2003–2005	Deaths reported to Anesthesia Mortality Committees (n = 5,983,704 anesthetics)	Anesthesia-related deaths 0.19/10,000
Pollard et al.[6] Stefani et al.[7] van der Griend et al.[8]	USA Brazil Australia	2011–2016 2012–2013 2003–2008	Quality database from 20 facilities Deaths in University Hospital Anesthesia-related deaths in children ≤18 y from a single pediatric hospital (n = 101,885)	Anesthetic-related death 0.051/10,000 Anesthetic contributory 0.23/10,000 Anesthesia contributory 1.72/10,000 Anesthetic-related death 0.98/10,000
de Bruin et al.[9]	Netherlands	2006–2012	Reported 30-d postoperative in-hospital mortality children <18 y from a single pediatric hospital (n = 45,182 anesthetics)	Partially anesthesia-related mortality within 24 h 0.7/10,000 Partially anesthesia-related mortality within 30 d 1.1/10,000

2011 suggested a decrease worldwide, especially in developed countries.[2] This lends support to the generally accepted belief that anesthesia safety has improved over the past 50+ years.

Other complications related to anesthesia include postoperative nerve injury, awareness during GA, eye injuries, and dental injury (Table 4-2).[10–26] Most peripheral nerve injuries have multifocal etiologies where underlying neuronal reserve plays an important role in the injury (see also Chapter 29).[27] The incidence of ulnar neuropathy has been estimated to be 47 per 10,000 patients.[10] Lower-extremity neuropathy following surgery in the lithotomy position was observed in 151 per 10,000 patients, with 30 per 10,000 for the sciatic and common peroneal nerves, 40 per 10,000 for the lateral cutaneous nerve of the thigh, and 50 per 10,000 for the obturator nerve.[11] Permanent neurologic injury following neuraxial anesthesia was estimated at 0.15 per 10,000 spinal anesthetics and 0.015 to 0.09 per 10,000 epidural anesthetics.[13] Peripheral nerve injury following peripheral nerve blocks (PNBs) was estimated to occur at a rate up to 4.2 per 10,000 anesthetics.[15] Postoperative neurologic symptoms related to ultrasound-guided PNBs were estimated to occur at a rate of 18/10,000 and 9/10,000 for symptoms lasting shorter than 5 days and greater than 6 months, respectively.[14] Awareness during GA has been estimated to occur in 15 to 100 per 10,000 patients.[16–19]

Eye injuries are a risk of anesthesia, including corneal abrasions as well as more rare complications such as blindness from ischemic optic neuropathy (ION) or central retinal artery occlusion.[20–23] Corneal abrasion has occurred at a rate of 15.1 per 10,000 procedures, with a marked decrease in rate with a performance initiative to 4.7 per 10,000 procedures.[23] ION has been observed at 0.57 to 2.8 per 10,000 spine surgeries.[21,22] Risk factors for ION after spinal fusion have been identified and include a variety of patient, surgical, and anesthetic factors.[28] Among these include use of a Wilson surgical bed frame, obesity, and long anesthetic durations. All can contribute to increased venous congestion in the optic canal and potentially reduce optic nerve perfusion pressure. There was insufficient evidence to conclude that intraoperative anemia or transient periods of hypotension were causative factors. Fortunately, the incidence of postoperative visual loss has been decreasing in the United States.[22]

Damage to teeth or dentures is the most common injury leading to anesthesia malpractice claims. Dental injury complaints are usually resolved by a hospital risk management department. Dental injuries after general endotracheal anesthesia were observed in approximately 1 per 2,000 to 3,000 patients in the United States.[24,25] A prospective study of dental damage diagnosed by a dentist after classic direct laryngoscopy in Portugal reported a high rate of 2,500/10,000.[26]

Risk Management

Conceptual Introduction

Risk management and quality improvement programs work hand in hand to minimize liability exposure while maximizing quality of patient care (2 Video 4-2). Although the functions of these programs vary from one institution to another, they overlap in their focus on patient safety. A hospital risk management program is broadly oriented toward reducing the liability exposure of the organization. This includes not only professional malpractice liability (and therefore patient safety) but also contracts, employee safety, public safety, and any other liability exposure of the institution. Quality improvement programs have as their main goal the continuous maintenance and improvement of the quality of patient care. These programs may be broader in their patient safety focus than strictly risk management. Quality improvement (sometimes called *patient safety*) departments are responsible for providing the resources to provide safe, patient-centered, timely, efficient, effective, and equitable patient care.[29]

Risk Management in Anesthesia

Those aspects of risk management that are most directly relevant 2
to the liability exposure of the anesthesiologist include prevention of patient injury, adherence to standards of care, documentation, and patient relations.

Key factors in the prevention of patient injury include provider vigilance, adequate monitoring, up-to-date knowledge, and systems that facilitate optimal individual and team performance and communication between care providers.[30]

The American Society of Anesthesiologists (ASA) published *Standards for Basic Anesthetic Monitoring* in 1986. The introduction of these standards was temporally enmeshed with other improvements in anesthesia care, so their precise impact is difficult to quantify, but there was a substantial reduction in patient injury and anesthesiology malpractice premiums in the years following their introduction.[31] Detailed information on anesthesia monitoring techniques can be found in Chapter 26.

The ASA website is an accessible resource that can be reviewed periodically for any changes in the published *Guidelines and Statements*.[32] It should be noted that although membership in the ASA is not required for the practice of anesthesiology, expert witnesses will, with virtual certainty, hold any practitioner to the ASA standards. It is also possible that as a risk management strategy, a professional liability insurer or hospital may hold an individual anesthesiologist to standards higher than those promulgated by the ASA.

Another process tool that has had great utility in risk management and patient safety is the use of checklists. The first formal practice of using checklists was developed for pilots in the military. Since then, checklists have been adopted by many industries wherein processes are too numerous and/or complex to rely solely on human memory. A checklist is a simple, yet powerful, tool that ensures no important detail is forgotten, reducing variability, enhancing consistency, and decreasing the likelihood of error. Checklists help to remind providers of key steps and thus work to facilitate safe and effective health care delivery.[33]

Historically, checklists have been first used in anesthesia for anesthesia machine checkout procedures. Information pertaining to anesthesia workstation preuse procedures as well as safety considerations for workstations can be found in Chapter 25. The use of checklists in clinical care has been expanded beyond workstation preparation and has been promoted in clinical settings such as central venous catheterization, intraoperative emergencies, and perioperative care. Catheter-related bloodstream infections were reduced significantly with the implementation of a standardized process that included a checklist for catheter placement and management.[34] During simulated emergency scenarios, checklists have improved performance in the management of local anesthetic systemic toxicity[35] and improved the management of intraoperative crises such as malignant hyperthermia, massive hemorrhage, air embolism, and cardiac arrest.[36,37]

Perioperative use of surgical safety checklists in a variety of global hospital settings has reduced surgical complications and mortality.[38] These communication tools have been implemented in a staged fashion at critical points of care (prior to induction, prior to skin incision, prior to wound closure, and prior to patient leaving the operating room), to confirm patient information, presence of personnel, and address potential case-specific concerns. Checklists incorporate significant processes ranging from a

Table 4-2 Rates of Selected Anesthesia Complications

Complication	Reference	Country	Time	Specific Complication	Results
Nerve injury	Warner et al.[10]	USA	1995	Ulnar neuropathy in adults following noncardiac surgery (*n* = 1,502)	47/10,000
	Warner et al.[11]	USA	1997–1998	Lower extremity neuropathy in adult patients ≥18 y under general anesthesia (GA) while in lithotomy position (*n* = 991)	151/10,000
	Welch et al.[12]	USA	1997–2007	Peripheral nerve injury within 48 h of sedation or anesthesia (*n* = 380,680)	2.9/10,000
	de Sèze et al.[13]	France	2000	Incapacitating neurologic complications lasting ≥3 mo after central neuraxial blockade	Nonobstetric SBs (*n* = 67,884): 0.15/10,000; Nonobstetric epidural blocks (EBs) (*n* = 65,464): 0.015/10,000 Obstetric EBs (*n* = 116,639): 0.09/10,000
	Sites et al.[14]	USA	2003–2011	Postoperative sensory or motor dysfunction after ultrasound-guided PNB with anatomic basis to support possible block contribution (*n* = 12,668)	Symptoms lasting >5 d 18/10,000 Symptoms lasting >6 mo 9/10,000
	Barrington et al.[15]	USA	2006–2008	Late neurologic complications after PNB or plexus block (*n* = 7,156 blocks)	4.2/10,000 PNBs
Awareness	Sandin et al.[16]	Sweden	1997–1998	Awareness associated with GA (*n* = 11,785)	15.3/10,000 procedures
	Sebel et al.[17]	USA	2001–2002	Awareness in patients ≥18 y old in seven academic medical centers (*n* = 19,575)	12.8/10,000
	Avidan et al.[18]	USA	2005–2006	Single-center prospective study in patients ≥18 y old (*n* = 1,941)	20.0/10,000
	Xu et al.[19]	China	NA	Multicenter cohort study of awareness after GA with muscle relaxants (*n* = 11,101)	41.4/10,000
Vision loss and eye injuries	Shen et al.[20]	USA	1996–2005	Vision loss in surgery	Overall: 2.35/10,000 Cardiac surgery: 8.64/10,000 Spinal fusion: 3.09/10,000 Cholecystectomy 0.66/10,000 Appendectomy: 0.12/10,000
	Nandyala et al.[21]	USA	2002–2009	Postoperative visual loss after spinal fusion surgery from a national inpatient sample (*n* = 541,485)	1.9/10,000
	Rubin et al.[22]	USA	1998–2012	Postoperative visual loss after spinal fusion surgery using Nationwide Inpatient Sample	1.02/10,000
	Martin et al.[23]	USA	2005	Postoperative corneal injury (*n* = 84,796) Baseline	15.1/10,000
			2006–2007	Performance initiative postoperative corneal injury	7.9/10,000
			2007–2008	Follow-up postoperative corneal injury	4.7/10,000

Table 4-2 Rates of Selected Anesthesia Complications (CONTINUED)

Complication	Reference	Country	Time	Specific Complication	Results
Dental injury	Martin et al.[24]	USA	2001–2009	Dental injuries in adult nonoperating room emergent intubations at a tertiary care hospital (n = 3,423)	17.5/10,000
	Vallejo et al.[25]	USA	2001–2008	Dental injuries in patients receiving anesthesia care at multiple locations of a large university hospital system (n = 816,690)	Overall incidence 4.4/10,000 GA 5.7/10,000 Monitored anesthesia care 0.8/10,000
	Mourao et al.[26]	Portugal	2011	Prospective study of dental damage diagnosed by a dentist after classic direct laryngoscopy at a university hospital (n = 536)	2,500/10,000

surgical time-out to a postprocedural briefing (Table 4-3). Specific anesthesia preinduction checklists have also been developed and tested to improve information exchange and patient safety.[39]

Informed Consent

Informed consent regarding anesthesia should be documented with a general surgical consent and should include a statement to the effect that the patient affirms an understanding that anesthetics involve risks of complications, serious injury, or, rarely, death from both known and unknown causes. In addition, there should be a note in the patient's record that the risks of anesthesia and alternatives were discussed and that the patient accepted the proposed anesthetic plan. Including a brief documentation in the record that the common complications and material risks of the proposed technique were discussed is helpful. In some institutions and states, a separate written anesthesia consent form must be used, which may include more detail about risks. If it is necessary to change the agreed-on anesthesia plan significantly after the patient is premedicated or anesthetized, the reasons for the change should be documented in the record. Aspects of informed consent obtained after the patient has received analgesic or anxiolytic medication are not automatically invalid, rather a patient's capacity for consent must be assessed by the provider at the time they are engaging with the patient in the informed consent process. Withholding medication with the explicit message to the patient that they can receive it only after consent is signed or verbally agreed to can be perceived as coercive and therefore potentially more suspect than consent obtained after the administration of any medication.[40]

Informed consent can be problematic in that standard forms are often difficult for patients to understand, and patients often differ from physicians in their expectations and understanding of the risks and benefits associated with their treatments.[41–43] Patient complaints are commonly grounded in elements of the informed consent process that are perceived by patients as incomplete or have been misremembered or were misunderstood. Complaints arising from problems with informed consent absorb valuable health care system resources even if they do not lead to a malpractice complaint.[44] Patient complaints can be leveraged to identify high-risk providers to target for interventions to improve communication skills.[45,46]

Shared decision making is an enhanced form of informed consent applicable in elective situations when different options for treatment are available to the patient. Shared decision making is a strategy to empower the patient to actively make an evidence-based choice in their treatment.[47] In shared decision making, evidence-based information is shared with the patient using educational materials ("decision aids"), and patient preferences and values are elicited during the decision-making process. When all parties are satisfied that they understand the options and expectations, an informed decision can be made regarding treatment.[48,49]

Table 4-3 World Health Organization Surgical Safety Checklist Elements

Preinduction
Patient confirms identity, site, procedure, and consent
Site marked
Anesthesia machine and medication check
Pulse oximeter on and functioning
Does the patient have:
Known allergy?
Risk for difficult airway or aspiration?
Before Incision
Team members introduce themselves by name and role
Confirm patient identity, procedure, and incision site
Antibiotics within last 60 min
Anticipated critical events:
Critical or nonroutine steps in procedure
Anticipated duration of surgery
Anticipated blood loss
Anesthesia concerns
Sterility confirmed
Equipment issues or concerns
Essential imaging displayed
Before Patient Leaves Operating Room
Confirm procedure
Complete instrument, sponge, and needle counts
Specimens labeled
Address equipment problems
What are the key concerns for recovery?

Adapted with permission from the WHO Surgical Safety Checklist, http://whqlibdoc.who.int/publications/2009/9789241598590_eng_Checklist.pdf.

Record Keeping

Good records can form a strong defense if they are adequate; however, records can be disastrous if inadequate. The anesthesia record itself should be as accurate, complete, and in the increasingly uncommon case of handwritten records, as neat as possible. In addition to documenting vital signs at least every 5 minutes, special attention should be paid to ensure that the patient's ASA classification, monitors used, fluids administered, and doses and times of all administered drugs are accurately charted. Because the principal causes of hypoxic brain damage and death during anesthesia are related to ventilation and/or oxygenation, all respiratory variables that are monitored should be documented accurately. Captured data that includes monitoring artifacts should be labeled and identified in the record when feasible. It is important to note when there is a change of anesthesia personnel during the conduct of a case. Sloppy, inaccurate anesthesia records, with gaps during critical events, can be extremely damaging to the defense when enlarged and placed before a jury. Litigation is a lengthy process, and a court appearance to explain the incident and the record to a jury may be years away, when memories have faded. Although the adage "if it wasn't documented it didn't happen" is an oversimplification of the complex process of review of records in malpractice cases, it can be problematic in deposition or at trial to rely repeatedly, or entirely, on the statement "As I recall my usual and customary practice at that time was . . ." to fill in important information missing from an incomplete record.

The use of electronic health records (EHRs) has been mandated in health care, and currently in the U.S. anesthesia information management systems (AIMS) have almost entirely supplanted the traditional anesthesia paper record in most anesthetizing sites. Basic AIMS are connected to the patient monitors and the anesthesia machine and capture perioperative data specific to anesthesia (e.g., vital signs, times of induction, intubation and emergence, medications and fluids). There is improved patient care and cost savings at institutions where EHR are fully incorporated.[50] When properly configured, AIMS can increase provider efficiency,[51] improve quality of care,[52] improve coding and billing accuracy,[53,54] decrease paperwork, and be a legible, chronologic documentation of clinical care. Use of AIMS has substantial potential as a clinical decision support mechanism.[55] AIMS can process information from multiple devices and the EHR, incorporate algorithms to remind physicians to perform critical clinical processes on time,[56,57] and alert physicians to changes in patient status.[58]

Some physicians, whose entry into practice predated the use of EHRs, are wary of the possible increased risk of exposure to litigation the EHR might present. Concerns have been raised about the profuse amounts of data and the risk of electronic discovery being used in litigation.[59,60] Further concerns have also been raised about the EHR since the passing of a law in 2016 in the United States that requires immediate release of records to patients potentially bypassing an opportunity for providers to help interpret the record and place data from the record in context.[61] Inaccurate medical records, which are common with EHRs, are also a source of patient complaints to state medical boards. Although there is a growing body of data and opinion, no definitive conclusions can yet be made regarding the impact of EHRs and the risk of malpractice.[62] EHRs were associated with fewer paid malpractice claims in one study.[63] The digital data reviewed in court may be detrimental to the physician-defendant case when shortcuts are taken and anomalies in time-stamped entries cast doubt on the integrity of the record; for example, engaging in the practice of documenting events before they actually occur.[64] In the documentation of preoperative assessments, consents, pain management, and critical care consultation notes, the EHR presents an additional medico-legal and billing compliance risk if the practitioner engages in the use of copying and pasting, cloning, or carrying forward information from other notes without very careful review of those notes for accuracy and relevance to the care encounter they purport to document.

What to Do After an Adverse Outcome

If a critical incident occurs during the conduct of an anesthetic, the anesthesiologist should document, in narrative form, what happened, which drugs and procedures were used, the time sequence, and who was present. If there is no format appropriate to adequately summarize a complex catastrophic intra-anesthetic event in the usual anesthesia record, it should be documented in the patient's progress notes. The critical incident note should be written as soon as possible after the event. For events where the etiology is unclear, speculation in the health record regarding causation should be limited only to the generation of a differential diagnosis that might contribute to the immediate ongoing care of the patient. The report should be as consistent as possible with concurrent records, such as the anesthesia, operating room, recovery room, and cardiac arrest records. If significant inconsistencies exist, they should be explained. If an error is made in a handwritten record, a line should be drawn through the error, leaving it legible, and the correction should be initialed and timed. AIMS typically track edits to the record made by the provider who is logged into the EHR so any post-hoc edits have the potential to be scrutinized for accuracy and legitimacy. If the institution or anesthesia department has a database set up for tracking and documentation of events for peer-review quality improvement activities, distinct entries into that database should be made without any linking reference in the EHR. Institutional peer-review quality improvement processes are generally, but not absolutely, protected from legal discovery by federal common law and state statutes and that variable degree of protection could be undermined by a provider's statement in the EHR referencing any information entered into a quality improvement database.[29]

Whenever an anesthetic complication becomes apparent, appropriate consultation should be obtained quickly, and the departmental or institutional risk management group should be notified. If the complication is apt to lead to prolonged hospitalization or permanent injury, the liability insurance carrier should be notified. The patient should be followed closely while in the hospital, with telephone follow-up, if indicated, after discharge. The anesthesiologist(s), surgeon(s), consulting physicians, and the institution should coordinate and be consistent in their explanations to the patient or the patient's family as to the cause of any complication.

If anesthetic complications occur, the anesthesiologist should be honest with both the patient and the family about the cause, recognizing that there are limits to the accuracy of any individual's perceptions and memories. The providers should provide the facts about the event, but limit speculation about ultimate causes in events where these are unclear.

There is an increasing body of evidence to suggest that sharing of information with patients, particularly when there may have been an adverse outcome, perhaps involving a medical error, can be beneficial. Effective disclosure can improve doctor–patient relations, facilitate better understanding of systems, and potentially decrease medical malpractice costs.[49,65] Some states have laws mandating disclosure of serious adverse events to patients, and disclosure has been incorporated into quality reporting. The statutes addressing the legal status of expressions of condolences or sympathy after an adverse event have been called apology laws.[66] These laws vary state by state across the United States and have been further classified as full and partial apology laws. A full apology law is a statute that prohibits the use of a provider's expression of condolences or sympathy as grounds for a malpractice suit and explicitly prohibits any statement of fault that was made in the context of that apology from being admitted as evidence. A partial apology law may protect a statement such as "I'm sorry this happened to you" or "your loved one," from constituting an admission of guilt in a court of law, but the partial nature of that law might permit the apology to be used in a malpractice suit if it was also accompanied by an admission of wrongdoing or fault. Disclosure is considered the ethically right thing to do, and secondarily may reduce malpractice risk,[67] although malpractice risk reduction through disclosure is still subject to debate.[68] Some institutions, health systems, and insurers have adopted formal "communication and resolution" approaches to adverse events.[69,70] These approaches vary in their details but share the underlying premise that early disclosure and an offer of compensation may provide satisfactory resolution to the patient and avoid formal litigation proceedings.[71]

Special Circumstances: "Do Not Resuscitate"

It is important to recognize that patients have well-established rights, and that among these is the right to refuse specific treatments. Two situations most relevant to anesthesia care are "do-not-resuscitate" (DNR) orders and the special circumstance of blood transfusion for Jehovah's Witnesses. The care of Jehovah's Witnesses as it relates to the use of blood products is covered in detail in Chapter 17 so the focus in this section will be on the impact of DNR orders in perioperative and critical care settings.

Patients with severe medical conditions may elect to forgo resuscitation attempts in the event of cardiac arrest. Such DNR orders may be specified at hospital admission or may be in place in the form of an advance directive prior to admission. DNR orders or advance directives may be general or specific, such as refusal of tracheal intubation or mechanical ventilation. When a patient with DNR status presents for procedural or operative anesthesia care, it is important to discuss this with the patient or patient's surrogate to clarify the patient's intentions. In many hospitals, the institutional policy historically has been to automatically suspend the DNR order during the immediate perioperative period since the cause for a cardiac arrest may be easily identified and treated, but DNR suspension should not be considered to be automatic and each patient's thoughts about and goals for a procedure should be explored and explicit consent for suspension of a DNR order should be sought if it is thought to be in a patient's best interests. The patient may choose to suspend the DNR order during the entire perioperative period, but best practice is to clarify with the patient when the DNR order should be reinstated (e.g., discharge from recovery or possibly later, when the patient has recovered from the procedure) and documented in the patient's record. The perioperative status of DNR orders should also be clarified with the surgeon and other providers who will be involved in the patient's perioperative care. The ASA has published *Ethical Guidelines of the Anesthesia Care of Patients with Do-Not-Resuscitate Orders or Other Directives That Limit Treatment*.[72]

As a general rule, physicians are not obligated to treat all patients who apply for treatment in elective situations. It is well within the rights of a physician to decline to care for any patient who wishes to place burdensome constraints on the physician or to unacceptably limit the physician's ability to provide optimal care.

National Practitioner Data Bank

It is usually the obligation of the hospital risk management department to make reports and inquiries to the National Practitioner Data Bank (NPDB),[73] a nationwide information system that provides licensing boards and hospitals a means of detecting adverse information about physicians.[74] Theoretically, the databank prevents physicians with especially problematic ethical and/or legal histories from hiding their past simply by moving from state to state.

The NPDB requires notification of various adverse actions including medical malpractice payments, license actions by medical boards or states, negative actions or findings by a peer review organization or private accreditation entity, adverse clinical privilege actions, and adverse professional membership society actions.[75] There has been a great deal of effort to establish a minimum malpractice payment below which no report is necessary, but to date, any payment made on behalf of a physician in response to a written complaint or claim must be reported. Settlements made by cancellation of bills or settlements made on verbal complaints are not considered reportable payments.

Once a report has been submitted, the physician is notified and may dispute the accuracy of the report. At this time, the reporting entity may correct the form or void it. Failing that, the physician has the option of putting a brief statement in the file or appealing to the U.S. Secretary of Health and Human Services, who may also either correct or void the form. A practitioner may make a query about their file at any time. A physician may also add a statement to a report at any time. Such statements will be included in any reports that are sent in response to inquiries. The existence of the NPDB reporting requirements has made physicians reluctant to allow settlement of nuisance suits because it will cause their names to be added to the data bank.

Quality Improvement and Patient Safety in Anesthesia

Quality is a concept defined by the Institute of Medicine (IOM) as "the degree to which health care services for individuals and populations increase the likelihood of desired health outcomes and are consistent with current professional knowledge."[76] The IOM characterizes six domains for assessing quality of a process or system: effectiveness, efficiency, equity, patient centeredness, safety, and timeliness.[76] Quality improvement (QI) focuses on studying and measuring factors that influence each of these domains and designing targeted interventions to improve performance over time. Patient safety, while targeting adverse event prevention and harm reduction, has a foundation in scientific principles for system design that consider the intersections of interprofessional culture, communication, and human factors. A number of professional and regulatory groups, discussed later in this chapter, seek to impact the safety, quality, and outcomes of anesthesia care through data analysis, defined performance targets, dissemination of safety science, and educational initiatives.

Structure, Process, and Outcome: The Building Blocks of Quality

Quality of care is often framed in a three-component model: structure, process, and outcome.[77] *Structure* refers to the setting in which care was provided, for example, personnel and facilities used to provide health care services and the way they are organized. This includes the qualifications and licensing of personnel, ratio of practitioners to patients, standards for the facilities and equipment used to provide care, and organizational structure. The *process* of care includes the sequence and coordination of patient care activities, that is, what is actually done. Was a preanesthetic evaluation performed and documented? Were established safety processes followed? *Outcome* of care refers to changes in health status of the patient following the delivery of medical care. This three-part model is sometimes presented as unidirectionally related: structural elements form the foundation for processes, which in turn are expected to produce a desired outcome. While these domains can be convenient for measurability, the roles of patient and practitioner variability are vital inputs to processes and outcomes. Improving quality focuses on relationships between all these components to develop more reliable systems of care.

Continuous Quality Improvement

3 Individual practitioners are just one part of a complex system, and in the absence of recklessness or deliberate disregard for safety practices, it is misguided to assert that individuals are solely responsible for errors or undesired outcomes. CQI involves monitoring current practices to inform systems-based strategies to improve quality of care.[78,79] An important premise is that system failures should be controllable and strategies to minimize them should be within reach.

A CQI process has a variety of inputs, typically starting with evidence of an error, process deviation, or undesirable outcome. Sources of this information include reports from directly involved practitioners, patient feedback, chart review, and systematic data analysis. CQI programs acknowledge that not all undesired outcomes result from error, just as not all errors result in a poor outcome. This view forms the context for untangling the system factors that contribute to non–patient-related variability, rather than assigning individual blame. For example, instead of asking which practitioners have the highest patient mortality rates, a CQI program may focus on the relationship between the process of care and patient mortality. What proportion of deaths were related to the patient's disease process or debilitated condition? Are these patients being appropriately evaluated for anesthesia and surgery? Were there any controllable causes, such as lack of extra help during resuscitation? The latter may lead to a modification of personnel resources (structure) or assignments (process) to be sure that adequate personnel are always available.

While the description above implies that CQI activities are largely *reactive* to something undesired, attention to *proactively* redesigning processes that are vulnerable to failure is essential, even though luck may have averted any recent instances of breakdown. This work is driven from the bottom up, by those who are most involved in the process to be improved, rather than from the top down by administrators. Structured sessions for process mapping, brainstorming, and failure mode analysis can highlight areas of vulnerability that may not have been previously recognized. Framing problems in relation to the IOM domains of quality can help clarify specific improvement goals. As in any QI work, understanding the measurable aspects of the current state is vital to assessing whether an implemented change has been successful, and supports iterative improvement cycles.

Tracking Adverse Events for Anesthesia CQI Programs

One approach in measuring quality of care is tracking the rate of adverse outcomes. However, major adverse outcomes are relatively rare in anesthesia. For example, if an institution lowers its mortality rate of surgery patients from 1 in 1,000 to 0.5 in 1,000, this difference may not be statistically significant. This can make it impossible to know if the difference resulted from changes in care or simply random fluctuation. Many adverse outcomes in anesthesia are sufficiently rare to render them problematic as quality improvement measures. Even desired outcomes, such as effective postoperative pain management, are very difficult to define and reliably measure. Like many important outcome measures in the perioperative setting, there are so many inputs, patient factors, and temporal characteristics that it is difficult or impossible to quantify the contributions of anesthetic care.[80]

To complement outcome measurement, anesthesia CQI programs can focus on structural and process measures as intermediate outcomes more immediate to anesthetic care. This involves examining critical incidents, sentinel events, and human errors. *Critical incidents* are events that cause, or have the potential to cause (near misses), patient injury if not noticed and corrected in a timely manner. For example, a partial disconnect of the breathing circuit may be corrected before patient injury occurs yet has the potential for causing hypoxic brain injury or death. Critical incidents are more common than adverse outcomes. Measurement of the occurrence rate of critical incidents may serve as a proxy for rare outcomes in anesthesia.

Sentinel events are a subset of high-severity critical incidents that are unexpected occurrences involving death or serious physical or psychological injury (or risk thereof) and that may indicate a systemic problem. The Joint Commission has requirements for analyzing sentinel events that will be discussed later. Examples include a syringe swap with administration of a potentially lethal dose of medication that was noted and treated promptly, avoiding catastrophe, or an unexpected significant patient injury such as intraoperative death. In either case, a CQI program investigates sentinel events to uncover correctable systemic problems in the care delivery. A syringe swap may be analyzed for confusing or unclear labeling of medications or unnecessary medications routinely stocked on the anesthesia cart, setting the scene for unintended mix-up. In the case of death, all aspects of the patient's hospital course from selection for surgery to anesthetic management may be analyzed to determine if similar deaths can be prevented by a change in the care delivery system.

Human error has garnered much attention since a 1999 government report that 98,000 Americans may die annually from medical errors in hospitals.[81] Human errors are inevitable yet potentially preventable by appropriate system safeguards. Errors of planning involve use of a wrong plan to achieve an aim. Errors of execution are the failure of a planned action to be completed as intended. Modern anesthesia equipment is designed with safeguards such as alarm systems to detect errors that could lead to harm. Other anesthesia care processes are also amenable to human factors design principles such as standardized drug labeling and bar coding. A CQI program looks for human errors to institute safety systems that aid in error prevention.

Many institutions have implemented "Communication and Resolution Programs" as a way to improve transparency, communication, and patient satisfaction after medical errors. Instead of a "shame and blame" treatment of involved personnel, it is centered around a nonpunitive "just culture" approach.[82] When an error has occurred, the involved parties (including medical personnel, risk management, medical liability insurers, and the patient) immediately communicate, the cause of the error is thoroughly investigated, the patient is rapidly remunerated financially (if necessary), and mechanisms are instituted to prevent recurrence of a similar error. These programs are patient and family centered, improve patient satisfaction, and reduce liability claims. They potentially reduce the incidence of error, likely through improved safety culture, which could lead to a greater chance of system correction.[82]

Joint Commission Requirements for Quality Improvement

The Joint Commission is a nonprofit organization providing accreditation of hospitals and surgery centers. While participation is officially voluntary, Joint Commission accreditation is a requirement to participate in Medicaid billing in many states. Joint Commission accreditation visits are unannounced or conducted on short notice and involve the inspection team watching patient care to see that safe and acceptable practices are routinely followed. Surveyors may talk to any staff member about organizational policies and procedures.

Joint Commission requirements for quality improvement activities are updated on an annual basis and are available online. In general, a hospital must adopt a method for systematically assessing and improving important functions and processes of care and their outcomes in a cyclical fashion. The general outline of this CQI process is to design a process or function, measure performance, assess performance measures through statistical analysis or comparison with other data sources, and iteratively improve the process or function. The Joint Commission provides specific standards and examples of appropriate measures of performance, with the goal of improving patient safety and quality of care.

The Joint Commission outlines National Patient Safety Goals annually.[83] These include performance elements for all aspects of hospital care including the perioperative phase, such as medication labeling, the prevention of infections via hand hygiene, surgical site marking, and the preprocedure time-out.[83] The time-out is meant to ensure that the entire team (anesthesiologist, surgeon, nursing staff) agrees that the procedure, patient, and procedural details, including surgical site, are correct. The surgical checklist, described earlier in this chapter, is often used for this purpose.

The Joint Commission also requires all sentinel events, as defined earlier in this chapter, to undergo a timely systematic analysis and plan for corrective action.[84] A root cause analysis is typically facilitated by the hospital and includes everyone involved in the care of the affected patient in reconstructing the events to identify system process failures and human factors that facilitated medical error. Sentinel events in the perioperative area include any invasive procedure on the wrong patient or wrong body part, unintentionally retained foreign objects, fire during direct patient care caused by equipment, and transfusion errors resulting in harm. The Joint Commission publishes sentinel event alerts so that health care organizations can learn from the experiences of others and prevent future medical errors.

Alternative Payment Models and Pay for Performance

Among many factors influencing health care groups to develop QI infrastructure have been initiatives by payers to create positive and negative incentives based on measures of quality, value, and efficiency. Such systems are referred to as Alternative Payment Models (APMs) and Pay for Performance (P4P). These programs indicate a desire to shift away from traditional volume-driven fee-for-service systems to other payment formulas that aim to share risk between payers and providers. The models expect reporting of health care progress in attaining specific goals and standards for processes and outcomes. The risk of excess costs due to complications and inefficient care is partially shifted to providers through capitation and/or bundled payments. Some models also reward the benefits of cost savings gained through improved efficiency. A full exploration of this trend in reimbursement and its potential impact on the future practice of anesthesiologists is beyond the scope of this chapter and is mentioned here due to its importance as part of the forces shaping QI programs.

There are many initiatives in the private sector but historically the best-known P4P programs have been those of the CMS; the Value-Based Purchasing program for hospitals and institutions and the Physician Quality Reporting System (PQRS) for individual health professionals and group practices. Within these programs, performance parameters were divided into the domains of clinical process of care, structure, outcome, efficiency, and patient experience. The initial phase introduced a formula that paid a percentage bonus to institutions and providers for having reported and met applicable performance goals. Over time, negative payment adjustments or penalties were introduced for participants that failed to report data or did not meet performance goals. Performance parameters directly applicable to the delivery of perioperative care are only a small subset of all the parameters in these programs and continue to change over time.[85]

The concept of P4P has been around long enough that there is literature accumulating on how well the idea has performed in meeting the intended goals. The evidence is mixed as to whether processes and practitioner behavior are changed by P4P initiatives. A large assessment[86] of CMS Merit-Based Incentive Payment System (MIPS) physician quality scores showed an association of better surgical outcomes of certain cardiac and vascular surgery patients under the care of surgeons with higher MIPS quality scores.[87] For anesthesiologists participating in the first 2 years of the MIPS program (2017 to 2018), there was a higher likelihood of meeting bonus payment criteria for physicians who reported performance through a practice group or APMs, compared to reports by individuals.[88] A Cochrane review did not find clear evidence that P4P impacted quality or outcomes at the hospital level in a sustainable long-term fashion but concluded that nonpayments might be more effective than bonus payments. Regardless of any present equivocal evidence for the effectiveness of APMs and P4P, they will remain part of the health care landscape and anesthesiologists should adopt a proactive approach to shaping and improving any future P4P programs.

Clinical Outcomes Registries in Anesthesiology

Two major resources to collect anesthesiology quality and outcome data in the United States are spearheaded by the Anesthesia Quality Institute (AQI) and the Multicenter Perioperative Outcome Group (MPOG). AQI was chartered by ASA in 2009 and has developed a National Anesthesia Clinical Outcomes Registry (NACOR) to which participating members electronically transfer digital data from billing and health records, HER, AIMS, etc. MPOG also receives electronic data from participating organizations, aimed at assembling a large dataset to permit multicenter retrospective analyses of focused clinical topics. NACOR focuses on helping participants meet payer reporting requirements, including P4P programs. MPOG promulgates anesthesia-specific process and outcome measures in over a dozen clinical domains that are available for members to use for performance comparison within and between participating organizations.[89] Both NACOR and MPOG data can be used for benchmarking and have a role in outcomes analysis to drive ongoing quality improvement at a national and local level.

Professional Liability

This section addresses the basic concepts of medical liability.

The Tort System

5 Although physicians may become involved in the criminal law system in a professional capacity, they more commonly become involved in the legal system of civil laws. Civil law is broadly divided into *contract law* and *tort law*. A tort may be loosely defined as a civil wrongdoing; negligence is one type of tort. *Malpractice* refers to any professional misconduct, but its use in legal terms typically refers to professional negligence.

To be successful in a malpractice suit, the patient-plaintiff must prove four things:

1. Duty: that the anesthesiologist owed the patient a duty
2. Breach of duty: that the anesthesiologist failed to fulfill their duty
3. Causation: that a reasonably close causal relation exists between the anesthesiologist's acts and the resultant injury
4. Damages: that actual damage resulted because of a breach of the standard of care

Failure to prove any one of these four elements will result in a decision for the defendant-anesthesiologist.

Duty

As a physician, the anesthesiologist establishes a duty to the patient when a doctor–patient relationship exists. When the patient is seen preoperatively and the anesthesiologist agrees to provide anesthesia care for the patient, a duty to the patient has been established. In the most general terms, the duty the anesthesiologist owes to the patient is to adhere to the *standard of care* for the treatment of the patient. Because it is virtually impossible to delineate specific standards for all aspects of medical practice and all eventualities, the courts have created the concept of the *reasonable and prudent* physician. For all specialties, there is a national standard that has displaced the local standard.

Breach of Duty

In a malpractice action, expert witnesses will review the medical records of the case and determine whether the anesthesiologist acted in a reasonable and prudent manner in the specific situation and fulfilled their duty to the patient. If they find that the anesthesiologist either did something that should not have been done or failed to do something that should have been done, then the duty to adhere to the standard of care has been breached. Therefore, the second requirement for a successful suit will have been met.

Causation

Judges and juries are interested in determining whether the breach of duty was the *proximate cause* of the injury. If the odds are better than even that the breach of duty led, however circuitously, to the injury, this requirement is met. The standard of proof for causation in malpractice cases is not, as it is in criminal cases of proof "beyond a reasonable doubt", rather it is "is it more likely than not."

There are two common tests employed to establish causation. The first is the *but for* test and the second is the *substantial factor* test. If the injury would not have occurred but for the action of the defendant-anesthesiologist, or if the act of the anesthesiologist was a substantial factor in the injury despite other causes, then proximate cause is established.

Although the burden of proof of causation ordinarily falls on the patient-plaintiff, it may, under special circumstances, be shifted to the physician-defendant under the doctrine of *res ipsa loquitur* (literally, "the thing speaks for itself"). Applying this doctrine requires proving the following:

1. The injury is of a kind that typically would not occur in the absence of negligence.
2. The injury must be caused by something under the exclusive control of the anesthesiologist.
3. The injury must not be attributable to any contribution on the part of the patient.
4. The evidence for the explanation of events must be more accessible to the anesthesiologist than to the patient.

Because anesthesiologists render patients insensible to their surroundings and unable to protect themselves from injury, the doctrine of *res ipsa loquitur* may be invoked in anesthesia malpractice cases. If the plaintiff can successfully argue that the injury would not have occurred in the absence of negligence, then the defendant-anesthesiologist must prove that they were not negligent in the case under consideration.

Damages

The law allows for three different types of damages. *General damages* are those such as pain and suffering that directly result from the injury. *Special damages* are those actual damages that are a consequence of the injury, such as medical expenses, lost income, and funeral expenses. *Punitive damages* are intended to punish the physician for negligence that was reckless, wanton, fraudulent, or willful. Punitive damages are exceedingly rare in medical malpractice cases. More likely in the case of gross negligence is a loss of the license to practice anesthesia. In extreme cases, criminal charges may be brought against the physician, although this is rare. Determination of the dollar amount is usually based on some assessment of the plaintiff's condition versus the condition they would have been in had there been no negligence. Plaintiffs' attorneys generally charge a percentage of the damages and will, therefore, seek to maximize the award given. Some states have legislated caps on damages. Such caps are more common for general damages, although some states cap total compensation for malpractice awards.

Standard of Care

Because medical malpractice usually involves issues beyond the comprehension of lay jurors and judges, the court establishes the standard of care in a particular case by the testimony of *expert witnesses*. These witnesses differ from factual witnesses mainly in that they may give opinions. The trial court judge has sole discretion in determining whether a witness may be qualified as an expert. Although any licensed physician may be an expert, information will be sought regarding the witness's education and training, the nature and scope of the person's practice, memberships and affiliations, and publications. The purpose in gathering this information is not only to establish the qualifications of the witness to provide expert testimony but also to determine the weight to be given to that testimony by the jury. In many cases, the success of a lawsuit depends primarily on the stature and believability of the expert witnesses.

Unfortunately, there is a tendency for experts to link severe injury with inappropriate care (i.e., a bias that "bad outcomes mean bad care"). To investigate the influence of the severity of the injury on the assessment of standard of care, a group of 112 practicing anesthesiologists judged appropriateness of care in 21 cases involving adverse anesthetic outcomes.[90] The original outcome in each case was either temporary or permanent. For each original case, a matching alternate case was created that was identical to the original in every respect, except that a plausible outcome of the opposite severity was substituted. Reviewers judged the standard of care in each case. Knowledge of the severity of injury produced a significant inverse effect on the judgment of appropriateness of care.[90] The proportion of ratings for appropriate care decreased when the outcome was changed from temporary to permanent and increased when the outcome was changed from permanent to temporary. These results suggest that outcome

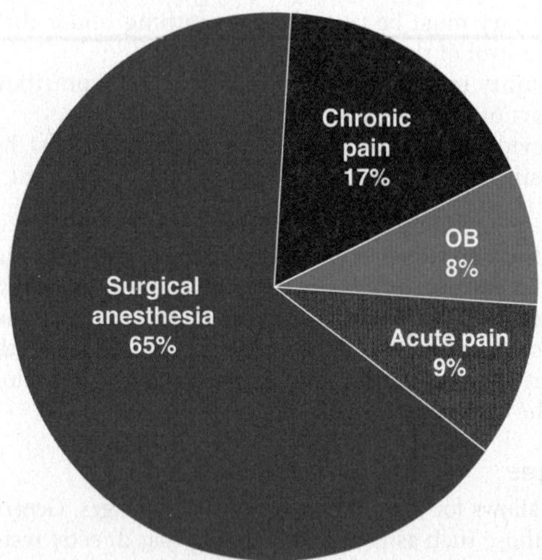

Figure 4-1 Types of anesthesia care in malpractice claims in the year 2005–2014. Most claims are associated with surgical anesthesia care. Anesthesia Closed Claims Project (n = 11,306). OB, obstetric.

bias in the assessment of standard of care may contribute to the frequency and size of payments.

The ASA has developed basic standards of preoperative, intraoperative, and postoperative anesthesia care.[32] In certain circumstances, the standard of care may also be determined from written policies of a hospital or department, or from textbooks and monographs. In contrast, practice guidelines developed by the ASA are not intended as standards or absolute requirements. These recommendations may be adopted, modified, or rejected by a practicing anesthesiologist according to clinical needs and constraints. In addition, guidelines are not intended to replace local institutional policies.

Causes of Anesthesia-Related Lawsuits

Relatively few adverse outcomes end up in a malpractice suit. It has been estimated that less than 1 of 25 patient injuries result in malpractice litigation.[91] The Anesthesia Closed Claims Program, funded by the ASA since 1985 and transferred to the AQI in 2019, has conducted a nationwide analysis of malpractice claims against anesthesiologists, excluding dental damage.[92] While most malpractice claims continue to be associated with surgical anesthesia care, obstetric anesthesia, acute pain management, and chronic pain management together represent one-third of anesthesia malpractice claims (Fig. 4-1).

The leading injuries in anesthesia-related malpractice claims for adverse events from 2005 to 2014 were death (30%), nerve damage (21%), permanent brain damage (9%), and airway injury (7%) (Fig. 4-2). Burns from on-patient fires during monitored anesthesia care were also important patient injuries.[93] The causes of death and permanent brain damage were predominantly problems in airway management (e.g., inadequate ventilation, difficult intubation, premature extubation, aspiration of gastric contents) and other complications such as pulmonary embolism, inadequate fluid therapy, stroke, hemorrhage, and myocardial infarction.[94] Nerve damage often occurs despite apparently adequate positioning.[27] Nerve injury was also the most common complication leading to claims after PNBs.[95] Aspiration of gastric contents occurred in 5% of closed claims, mostly in patients at high risk for delayed gastric emptying, especially acute gastrointestinal processes.[96] Chronic pain management is an important source of malpractice claims against anesthesiologists, relating to neuraxial blocks, implanted devices, and opioid medication management.[97–99] Recent closed claims studies have highlighted the importance of situational awareness errors and communication failures in causing medical errors and subsequent malpractice claims.[100,101] Future improvements in anesthesia patient safety will need to improve the human factors skills of anesthesiologists, including communication, leadership, teamwork, situational awareness, and decision making. 6

What to Do When Sued

A lawsuit begins when the patient-plaintiff's attorney files a *complaint* and demands for jury trial with the court. The anesthesiologist is then served with the complaint and a summons requiring an answer to the complaint. Until this happens, no lawsuit has been filed. Insurance carriers must be notified immediately after the receipt of the complaint. The anesthesiologist will need assistance in answering the complaint, and there is a time limit placed on the response.

Specific actions at this point include the following:

1. Do not discuss the case with anyone, including colleagues who may have been involved, operating room personnel, or friends. (Although in many jurisdictions the courts will look favorably upon a physician who speaks to the patient soon after an adverse outcome occurs and offers sympathy and an apology without necessarily admitting guilt.)[81]
2. Never alter any records.
3. Gather together all pertinent records, including a copy of the anesthetic record, billing statements, and correspondence concerning the case.
4. Make notes recording all events recalled about the case.
5. Cooperate fully with the attorney provided by the insurer.

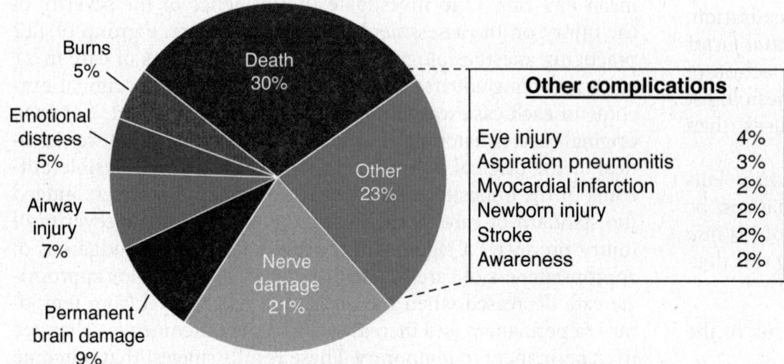

Figure 4-2 The most common injuries leading to anesthesia malpractice claims in the year 2005–2014. Damage to teeth and dentures excluded. Anesthesia Closed Claims Project (n = 11,306).

The first task the anesthesiologist must perform with an attorney is to prepare an answer to the complaint. The complaint contains certain facts and allegations with which the defense may either agree or disagree. Defense attorneys rely on the frank and totally candid observations of the physician in preparing an answer to the complaint. Physicians should be willing to educate their attorneys about the medical facts of the case, although most medical malpractice attorneys will be knowledgeable and medically sophisticated.

The next phase of the malpractice suit is called *discovery*. The purpose of discovery is the gathering of facts and clarification of issues in advance of the trial. In all likelihood, the anesthesiologist will initially receive a written interrogatory, which will request factual information. In consultation with the defense attorney, the interrogatory should be answered in writing because carelessly or inadvertently misstated facts can become troublesome later.

Depositions are a second mechanism of discovery. The defendant-anesthesiologist will be deposed as a fact witness, and depositions will be obtained from other anesthesiologists who will act as expert witnesses. A nationally recognized expert in the area in question, recommended by the defendant but who is not a personal friend, and who agrees with the defense position, may be very valuable.

The plaintiff's attorney, not the defense attorney, will depose the anesthesiologist. Despite the apparent informality of the deposition, the anesthesiologist must be constantly aware that what is said during the deposition carries as much weight as what would be said in court. It is important to be factually prepared for the deposition by review of personal notes, the anesthetic record, and the medical record. Regardless of a physician's usual style and approach to fashion, it is advisable to dress conservatively and professionally. Image and appearance have been shown to be important in this context. The opposition is assessing the physician to see how they will appear to a jury. Answer only the question asked, and do not volunteer information. Rely on one's attorney for assistance when preparing for a deposition.

There will be depositions from expert witnesses, both for the plaintiff and for the defense. The anesthesiologist should work with their attorney to suggest questions and rebuttals. The better educated the attorney is about the medical facts, the reasons the anesthesiologist did what was done, and the alternative approaches, the better able the attorney will be to conduct these expert depositions.

If there is some merit in the case but the damages are minimal, or if proof of innocence will be difficult, there will probably be a settlement offer. There is a high cost incurred by both plaintiffs and defendants in pursuing a malpractice claim up through a jury trial. Unless there is a strong probability of a large dollar award, reputable plaintiffs' attorneys are not likely to pursue the claim. Thus, even if physicians believe that they are totally innocent of any wrongdoing, they should not be offended or angered about settling of the case: This is primarily a matter of money, not medicine.

If a settlement is not reached during the discovery phase, a trial will occur. Only about 1 in 20 malpractice cases ever reach the point of a jury trial. Only those cases in which both sides think they can win, and which are likely to have significant financial impact, will proceed to trial.

The discussion of deposition testimony also applies to testimony in court, but there are a few additional points to consider during the trial. The members of the jury will not be as sophisticated medically as the attorneys who deposed the anesthesiologist during discovery. However, do not underestimate the intelligence of the jury. Talking down to them will create an unfavorable impression. If the answer to a question is not known, avoid guessing. If specific facts cannot be remembered, say so. Nobody expects total recall of events that may have occurred years before.

The defendant-physician should be present during the entire trial, even when not testifying, and should dress professionally. Displays of anger, remorse, relief, or hostility will hurt the physician in court. The physician should be able to give their testimony without using notes or documents. When it is necessary to refer to the medical record, it will be admitted into evidence. The anesthesiologist's goal is to convince the jury that they behaved in this case as any other competent and prudent anesthesiologist would have behaved.

It is important to keep in mind that *proof* in a malpractice case means only "more likely than not." The patient-plaintiff must "prove" the four elements of negligence, not to absolute certainty, but only to a probability greater than 50%. On the positive side, this means that the defendant-anesthesiologist must only show that their actions were, more likely than not, within an acceptable standard of care.

Malpractice litigation commonly follows a patient experiencing an adverse event. For anesthesiologists, having a patient harmed as a result of their direct care is extremely stressful. To subsequently be sued for that event further accentuates that stress. Such extreme stress has been identified as a potential cause for anesthesiologists to experience a mental breakdown, to stop practice or change specialties, or even to commit suicide. This topic is discussed in more detail in Chapter 3.[102]

Acknowledgments

We greatly acknowledge the contributions of Drs F. W. Cheney, D. A. Kroll, and K. L. Posner whose material from previous editions of this chapter has been retained in the current edition.

For further review and interactivities, please see the videos and narrative interactive clinical vignettes (NICVs) accessible in the complimentary eBook bundled with this text. Access instructions are located on the inside front cover.

REFERENCES

1. Beecher HK, Todd DP. A study of the deaths associated with anesthesia and surgery: based on a study of 599,548 anesthesias in ten institutions 1948–1952, inclusive. *Ann Surg*. 1954; 140:2–35.
2. Bainbridge D, Martin J, Arango M, Cheng D; Evidence-based Peri-operative Clinical Outcomes Research (EPiCOR) Group. Perioperative and anesthesia-related mortality in developed and developing countries: a systematic review and meta-analysis. *Lancet*. 2012;380: 1075–1081.
3. Li G, Warner M, Lang BH, Huang L, Sun LS. Epidemiology of anesthesia-related mortality in the United States, 1999–2005. *Anesthesiology*. 2009;110(4):759–765.
4. Ellis SJ, Newland MC, Simonsen JA, et al. Anesthesia-related cardiac arrest. *Anesthesiology*. 2014;120;829–838.
5. Gibbs N, ed. *Safety of Anaesthesia: A Review of Anaesthesia-Related Mortality Reporting in Australia and New Zealand 2003–2005. Report of the mortality working group convened under the auspices of the Australian and New Zealand College of Anaesthetists*. Melbourne: Australian and New Zealand College of Anaesthetists; 2009.
6. Pollard RJ, Hopkins T, Smith CT, et al. Perianesthetic and anesthesia-related mortality in a Southeastern United States population: a longitudinal review of a prospectively collected quality assurance data base. *Anesth Analg*. 2018;127:730–735.
7. Stefani LC, Gamermann PW, Backof A, et al. Perioperative mortality related to anesthesia within 48 h and up to 30 days following surgery: a retrospective cohort study of 11,562 anesthetic procedures. *J Clin Anesth*. 2018;49:79–86.
8. van der Griend BF, Lister NA, McKenzie IM, et al. Postoperative mortality in children after 101,885 anesthetics at a tertiary pediatric hospital. *Anesth Analg*. 2011;112:1440–1447.
9. de Bruin L, Pasma W, van der Werff DBM, et al. Perioperative hospital mortality at a tertiary paediatric institution. *Br J Anaesth*. 2015;115:608–615.

10. Warner MA, Warner DO, Matsumoto JY, Harper CM, Schroeder DR, Maxson PM. Ulnar neuropathy in surgical patients. *Anesthesiology*. 1999;90:54–59.
11. Warner MA, Warner DO, Harper CM, Schroeder DR, Maxson PM. Lower extremity neuropathies associated with lithotomy positions. *Anesthesiology*. 2000;93:938–942.
12. Welch MB, Brummett CM, Welch TD, et al. Perioperative peripheral nerve injuries: a retrospective study of 380,680 cases during a 10-year period at a single institution. *Anesthesiology*. 2009;111:490–497.
13. de Sèze MP, Sztark F, Janvier G, Joseph PA. Severe and long-lasting complications of the nerve root and spinal cord after central neuraxial blockade. *Anesth Analg*. 2007;104:975–979.
14. Sites BD, Taenzer AH, Herrick MD, et al. Incidence of local anesthetic systemic toxicity and postoperative neurologic symptoms associated with 12,668 ultrasound-guided nerve blocks: an analysis from a prospective clinical registry. *Reg Anesth Pain Med*. 2012;37:478–482.
15. Barrington MJ, Watts SA, Gledhill SR, et al. Preliminary results of the Australasian Regional Anaesthesia Collaboration: a prospective audit of more than 7000 peripheral nerve and plexus blocks for neurologic and other complications. *Reg Anesth Pain Med*. 2009;34:534–541.
16. Sandin RH, Enlund G, Samuelsson P, Lennmarken C. Awareness during anaesthesia: a prospective case study. *Lancet*. 2000;355:707–711.
17. Sebel PS, Bowdle TA, Ghoneim MM, et al. The incidence of awareness during anesthesia: a multicenter United States study. *Anesth Analg*. 2004;99:833–839.
18. Avidan MS, Zhang L, Burnside BA, et al. Anesthesia awareness and the bispectral index. *N Engl J Med*. 2008;358:1097–1108.
19. Xu L, Wu AS, Yue Y. The incidence of intra-operative awareness during general anesthesia in China: a multi-center observational study. *Acta Anaesthesiol Scand*. 2009;53:873–882.
20. Shen Y, Drum M, Roth S. The prevalence of perioperative visual loss in the United States: a 10-year study from 1996 to 2005 of spinal, orthopedic, cardiac, and general surgery. *Anesth Analg*. 2009;109:1534–1545.
21. Nandyala SV, Marquez-Lara A, Fineberg SJ, Singh R, Singh K. Incidence and risk factors for perioperative visual loss after spine fusion. *Spine J*. 2014;14:1866–1872.
22. Rubin DS, Parakati I, Lee LA, Moss HE, Joslin CE, Roth S. Perioperative visual loss in spine fusion surgery: ischemic optic neuropathy in the United States from 1998 to 2012 in the nationwide inpatient sample. *Anesthesiology*. 2016;125:457–464.
23. Martin DP, Weingarten TN, Gunn PW, et al. Performance improvement system and postoperative corneal injuries: incidence and risk factors. *Anesthesiology*. 2009;111:320–326.
24. Martin LD, Mhyre JM, Shanks AM, Tremper KK, Kheterpal S. 3,423 emergency tracheal intubations at a university hospital: airway outcomes and complications. *Anesthesiology*. 2011;114:42–48.
25. Vallejo MC, Best MW, Phelps AL, et al. Perioperative dental injury at a tertiary care health system: an eight-year audit of 816,690 anesthetics. *J Healthc Risk Manag*. 2012;31:25–32.
26. Mourão J, Neto J, LuísC, et al. Dental injury after conventional direct laryngoscopy: a prospective observational study. *Anaesthesia*. 2013;68:1059–1065.
27. Chui J, Murkin JM, Posner KL, Domino KB. Perioperative peripheral nerve injury after general anesthesia: a qualitative systematic review. *Anesth Analg*. 2018;127:134–143.
28. The Postoperative Visual Loss Study Group. Risk factors associated with ischemic optic neuropathy after spinal fusion surgery. *Anesthesiology*. 2012;116:15–24.
29. Institute of Medicine (US) Committee on Quality of Health Care in America, Chapter 6, Protecting Voluntary Reporting Systems from Legal Discovery. In To Err is Human: Building a Safer Health System. Kohn LT, Corrigan JM, Donaldson MS, eds. Washington (DC): National Academies Press (US); 2000.
30. Gaba DM, Maxwell M, DeAnda A. Anesthetic mishaps: breaking the chain of accident evolution. *Anesthesiology*. 1987;66:670–676.
31. Eichhorn JH. Monitoring standards: role of monitoring in reducing risk of anesthesia. *Problems in Anesthesia*. 2001;13:430–443.
32. American Society of Anesthesiologists website. Standards & Guidelines. Accessed June 3, 2022. https://www.asahq.org/standards-and-guidelines/resources-from-asa-committees#Quality
33. Krombach JW, Marks JD, Dubowitz G, Radke OC. Development and implementation of checklists for routine anesthesia care: a proposal for improving patient safety. *Anesth Analg*. 2015;121:1097–1103.
34. Provonost P, Needham D, Berenholtz S, et al. An intervention to decrease catheter-related bloodstream infections in the ICU. *N Engl J Med*. 2006;355:2725–2732.
35. Neal JM, Hsiung RL, Mulroy MF, Halpern BB, Dragnich AD, Slee AE. ASRA checklist improves trainee performance during a simulated episode of local anesthetic systemic toxicity. *Reg Anesth Pain Med*. 2012;37:8–15.
36. Ziewacz JE, Arriaga AF, Bader AM, et al. Crisis checklists for the operating room: development and pilot testing. *J Am Coll Surg*. 2011;213:212–217.
37. Arriga AF, Bader AM, Wong JM, et al. Simulation-based trial of surgical trial checklists. *N Engl J Med*. 2013;368:246–253.
38. Haynes AB, Weiser TG, Berry WR, et al; Safe Surgery Saves Lives Study Group. A surgical safety checklist to reduce morbidity and mortality in a global population. *N Engl J Med*. 2009;360:491–499.
39. Tscholl DW, Weiss M, Kolbe M, et al. An anesthesia preinduction checklist to improve information exchange, knowledge of critical information, perception of safety, and possibly perception of teamwork in anesthesia teams. *Anesth Analg*. 2015;121:948–956.
40. Tait AR, Teig MK, Voepel-Lewis T. Informed consent for anesthesia: a review of practice and strategies for optimizing the consent process. *Can J Anaesth*. 2014;61(9):832–842.
41. Etchells E, Ferrari M, Kiss A, Martyn N, Zinman D, Levinson W. Informed decision-making in elective major vascular surgery: analysis of 145 surgeon-patient consultations. *Can J Surg*. 2011;54:173–178.
42. Ankuda CK, Block SD, Copper Z, et al. Measuring critical deficits in shared decision making before elective surgery. *Patient Educ Couns*. 2014;94:328–333.
43. Whittle J, Conigliaro J, Good CB, Kelley ME, Skanderson M. Understanding of the benefits of coronary revascularization procedures among patients who are offered such procedures. *Am Heart J*. 2007;154:662–668.
44. Posner KL, Seversson JR, Domino KB. The role of informed consent in patient complaints: reducing hidden health system costs and improving patient engagement through shared decision-making. *J Healthc Risk Manag*. 2015;35:38–45.
45. Hickson GB, Jenkins AD. Identifying and addressing communication failures as a means of reducing unnecessary malpractice claims. *N C Med J*. 2007;68:362–364.
46. Pichert JW, Moore IN, Karrass J, et al. An intervention model that promotes accountability: peer messengers and patient/family complaints. *Jt Comm J Qual Patient Saf*. 2013;39:435–446.
47. Charles C, Gafni A, Whelan T. Shared decision-making in the medical encounter: what does it mean? (Or it takes at least two to tango). *Soc Sci Med*. 1997;44:681–692.
48. Cooper Z, Sayal P, Abbett SK, Neuman MD, Rickerson EM, Bader AM. A conceptual framework for appropriateness in surgical care: reviewing past approaches and looking ahead to patient-centered shared decision making. *Anesthesiology*. 2015;123:1450–1454.
49. Souter KJ, Gallagher TH. The disclosure of unanticipated outcomes of care and medical errors: what does this mean for anesthesiologists? *Anesth Analg*. 2012;114:615–621.
50. Hillestad R, Bigelow J, Bower A, et al. Can electronic medical record systems transform health care? Potential health benefits, savings and costs. *Health Aff (Millwood)*. 2005;24:1103–1117.
51. McLellan S, Galvin M, McMaugh D. Benefits measurement from the use of an automated anaesthetic record keeping system (AARK). *Electron J Health Inform*. 2011;6(1):e6.
52. Chaudhry B, Wang J, Wu S, et al. Systematic review: impact of health information technology on quality, efficiency, and costs of medical care. *Ann Intern Med*. 2006;144:742–752.
53. Reich DL, Kahn RA, Wax D, Palvia T, Galati M, Krol M. Development of a module for point-of-care charge capture and submission using an anesthesia information management system. *Anesthesiology*. 2006;105:179–186.
54. Spring SF, Sandberg WS, Anupama S, Walsh JL, Driscoll WD, Raines DE. Automated documentation error detection and notification improves anesthesia billing performance. *Anesthesiology*. 2007;106:157–163.
55. Wanderer JP, Sandberg WS, Ehrenfeld JM. Real-time alerts and reminders using information systems. *Anesthesiol Clin*. 2011;29:389–396.
56. Nair BG, Grunzweig K, Peterson GN, et al. Intraoperative blood glucose management: impact of a real-time decision support system on adherence to institutional protocol. *J Clin Monit Comput*. 2016;30:301–312.
57. Nair BG, Newman SF, Peterson GN, Wu WY, Schwid HA. Feedback mechanisms including real-time electronic alerts to achieve near 100% timely prophylactic antibiotic administration in surgical cases. *Anesth Analg*. 2010;111:1293–1300.
58. Nair BG, Horibe M, Newman SF, Wu WY, Peterson GN, Schwid HA. Anesthesia information management system-based near real-time decision support to manage intraoperative hypotension and hypertension. *Anesth Analg*. 2014;118:206–214.
59. Vigoda MM, Lubarsky DA. Failure to recognize loss of incoming data in an anesthesia record-keeping system may have increased medical liability. *Anesth Analg*. 2006;102:1798–1802.
60. Miller AR, Tucker CE. Electronic discovery and the adoption of information technology. *J Law Econ Organ*. 2014;30:217–243.
61. Salmi L, Blease C, Hägglund M, Walker J, DesRoches CM. US policy requires immediate release of records to patients. *BMJ*. 2021;372:n426.
62. Mangalmurti SS, Murtagh L, Mello MM. Medical malpractice liability in the age of electronic health records. *N Engl J Med*. 2010;363:2060–2067.
63. Virapongse A, Bates DW, Shi P, et al. Electronic health records and malpractice claims in office practice. *Arch Intern Med*. 2008;168:2362–2367.
64. Vigoda MM, Lubarsky DA. The medicolegal importance of enhancing timeliness of documentation when using an anesthesia information system and the response to automated feedback in an academic practice. *Anesth Analg*. 2006;103:131–136.
65. Gallagher TH, Studdert D, Levinson W. Disclosing harmful medical errors to patients. *N Engl J Med*. 2007;356:2713–2719.
66. Ross NE, Newman WJ. The role of apology laws in medical malpractice. *J Am Acad Psychiatry Law*. 2021;49:406–414.
67. Kachalia A, Bates DW. Disclosing medical errors: the view from the USA. *Surgeon*. 2014;12:64–67.
68. Studdert DM, Mello M, Gawande AA, Brennan TA, Wang YC. Disclosure of medical injury to patients: an improbable risk management strategy. *Health Aff*. 2007;26:215–226.
69. Mello MM, Gallagher TH. Malpractice reform: opportunities for leadership by health care institutions and liability insurers. *N Engl J Med*. 2010;362:1353–1356.
70. Boothman RC, Blackwell AC, Campbell DA Jr, Commiskey E, Anderson S. A better approach to medical malpractice claims? The University of Michigan experience. *J Health Life Sci Law*. 2009;2:125–159.

71. Quinn RE, Iechler MC. The 3Rs program: the Colorado experience. *Clin Obstet Gynecol.* 2008;51:709–718.
72. American Society of Anesthesiologists website. Ethical Guidelines of the Anesthesia Care of Patients with Do-Not-Resuscitate Orders or Other Directives That Limit Treatment. Reaffirmed October 17, 2018. Accessed May 22, 2022. https://www.asahq.org/standards-and-guidelines/ethical-guidelines-for-the-anesthesia-care-of-patients-with-do-not-resuscitate-orders-or-other-directives-that-limit-treatment
73. Code of Federal Regulations. Title 45, Subtitle A, Subchapter A, Part 60 (2013). National Practitioner Data Bank for Adverse Information on Physicians and Other Health Care Practitioners. Accessed May 22, 2022. https://www.ecfr.gov/current/title-45/subtitle-A/subchapter-A/part-60
74. Baldwin LM, Hart LG, Oshel RE, Fordyce MA, Cohen R, Rosenblatt RA. Hospital peer review and the National Practitioner Data Bank: clinical privileges action reports. *JAMA.* 1999;282:349–355.
75. Health Resources and Services Administration (HRSA), HHS. National Practitioner Data Bank for adverse information on physicians and other health care practitioners: reporting on adverse and negative actions. Final rule. *Fed Regist.* 2010;75(18):4655–4682.
76. Agency for Healthcare Research and Quality website. Six Domains of Health Care Quality. Accessed May 25, 2022. https://www.ahrq.gov/talkingquality/measures/six-domains.html
77. Donabedian A. The quality of care: how can it be assessed? *JAMA.* 1988;260:1743–1748.
78. Deming WE. *Out of the Crisis.* Massachusetts Institute of Technology; 1986.
79. Juran JM. *Juran on Planning for Quality.* Free Press; 1988.
80. Tung A. Challenges in outcome reporting. *Anesthesiol Clin.* 2018;36:191–199.
81. Kohn LT, Corrigan JM, Donaldson MS, eds. Committee on Quality of Health Care in America, Institute of Medicine. To Err is Human: Building a Safer Health System. Washington (DC): National Academies Press; 2000.
82. Gallagher TH, Mello MM, Sage WM, Bell SK, McDonald TB, Thomas EJ. Can communication-and-resolution programs achieve their potential? Five key questions. *Health Aff (Millwood).* 2018;37:1845–1852.
83. The Joint Commission website. National patient safety goals. Accessed May 25, 2022. https://www.jointcommission.org/standards/national-patient-safety-goals/
84. The Joint Commission website. Sentinel event policy and procedures. Accessed May 25, 2022. https://www.jointcommission.org/resources/patient-safety-topics/sentinel-event/sentinel-event-policy-and-procedures/
85. The Centers for Medicare & Medicaid Services website. Hospital value-based purchasing. Accessed May 25, 2022. https://www.cms.gov/Medicare/Quality-Initiatives-Patient-Assessment-Instruments/Value-Based-Programs/HVBP/Hospital-Value-Based-Purchasing
86. Uri O, Folman Y, Laufer G, Behrbalk E. A reimbursement system based on a 48-hour target time for surgery shortens the waiting time for hip fracture fixation in elderly patients. *J Orthop Trauma.* 2020;34:248–251.
87. Glance LG, Thirukumaran CP, Feng C, Lustik SJ, Dick AW. Association between the physician quality score in the merit-based incentive payment system and hospital performance in hospital compare in the first year of the program. *JAMA Netw Open.* 2021;4:e2118449.
88. Gal JS, Morewood GH, Mueller JT, Popovich MT, Caridi JM, Neifert SN. Anesthesia provider performance in the first two years of merit-based incentive payment system: Shifts in reporting and predictors of receiving bonus payments. *J Clin Anesth.* 2022;76:110582.
89. Multicenter Perioperative Outcomes Group website. QI Measures. Accessed May 25, 2022. https://spec.mpog.org/Measures/Public
90. Caplan RA, Posner KL, Cheney FW. Effect of outcome on physician judgments of appropriateness of care. *JAMA.* 1991;265:1957–1960.
91. Localio AR, Lawthers AG, Brennan TA, et al. Relation between malpractice claims and adverse events due to negligence: results of the Harvard Medical Practice Study III. *N Engl J Med.* 1991;325:245–251.
92. Cheney FW. The American Society of Anesthesiologists Closed Claims Project: what have we learned, how has it affected practice, and how will it affect practice in the future? *Anesthesiology.* 1999;91:552–556.
93. Mehta SP, Bhananker SM, Posner KL, Domino KB. Operating room fires: a closed claims analysis. *Anesthesiology.* 2013;118:1133–1139.
94. Cheney FW, Posner KL, Lee LA, Caplan RA, Domino KB. Trends in anesthesia-related death and brain damage: a closed claims analysis. *Anesthesiology.* 2006;105:1081–1086.
95. Lee LA, Posner KL, Kent CD, Domino KB. Complications associated with peripheral nerve blocks: lessons from the ASA Closed Claims Project. *Int Anesthesiol Clin.* 2011;49:56–67.
96. Warner MA, Meyerhoff KL, Warner ME, Posner KL, Stephens L, Domino KB. Pulmonary aspiration of gastric contents: a closed claims analysis. *Anesthesiology.* 2021;135(2): 284–291.
97. Pollak KA, Stephens LS, Posner KL, et al. Trends in pain medicine liability. *Anesthesiology.* 2015;123:1133–1141.
98. Rathmell JP, Michna E, Fitzgibbon DR, Stephens LS, Posner KL, Domino KB. Injury and liability associated with cervical procedures for chronic pain. *Anesthesiology.* 2011;114: 918–926.
99. Fitzgibbon DR, Rathmell JP, Michna E, Stephens LS, Posner KL, Domino KB. Malpractice claims associated with medication management for chronic pain. *Anesthesiology.* 2010;112:948–956.
100. Schulz CM, Burden A, Posner KL, et al. The frequency and type of situational awareness errors contributing to death and brain damage: a closed claims analysis. *Anesthesiology.* 2017;127(2):326–337.
101. Douglas RN, Stephens LS, Posner KL, et al. Communication failures contributing to patient injury in anesthesia malpractice claims. *Brit J Anaesth.* 2021;127(3):470–478.
102. Gazoni FM, Amato PE, Malik ZM, Durieux ME. The impace of perioperative catastrophies on anesthesiologists: results of a national survey. *Anesth Analg.* 2012;114:596–603.

5 Electrical Safety and Fires in the Operating Room

ISAAC LURIA • JAN EHRENWERTH • NIKOLAUS GRAVENSTEIN

KEY POINTS

1. To receive a shock, the electrical circuit must contact the person at two points and there must be a voltage source to cause the current to flow.
2. A microshock hazard is conductive wiring or an electrolyte solution–filled catheter that starts outside the patient's body and terminates near the patient's heart.
3. Cardiac fibrillation can be induced by a current as low as 100 μA directly across the heart.
4. The sensory perception threshold for an electrical current at 60 Hz is 1 mA.
5. A typical operating room circuit has a capacity for only 15 or 20 A and is therefore easily overwhelmed by multiple high-current draw devices (e.g., fluid warmer, forced air warmer, rapid infusion system) on a single circuit.
6. Line isolation monitors notify operating room personnel about potentially unsafe equipment so that it can be serviced at a time that is safe for patient care.
7. Some degree of fire hazard is present in virtually every operating room. The fire triad is necessary for a fire to ignite and consists of an oxidizing agent, a fuel, and an ignition source.
8. A nasal cannula delivering 2 L/min O_2 is delivering 100% oxygen out of the nasal cannula.
9. An air:oxygen ratio of at least 7:1 is required to keep the ambient oxygen concentration around the open oxygen source outlet no higher than 30%.
10. The most common type of fire is an on-patient fire and happens during upper-body monitored anesthesia care (MAC) cases with nasal cannula or face mask oxygen supplementation.

Modern operating rooms (ORs) are full of electrical and electronic devices with uses ranging from convenience to mission-critical, life-sustaining equipment for patient care. The electrical system and individual devices in ORs need to be designed to reduce the risk of electrical hazards to providers and patients. The mix of electricity, vulnerable patients, and a "wet" environment (i.e., bodily fluids and electrolyte solutions) creates a potentially dangerous combination. Understanding these safety features and how electricity can interact with the human body and other devices is of great importance to the anesthesia provider.

Fundamental Principles of Electricity

It is useful to review some basic physics terms from mechanics before describing their electrical analogs. A **force** imparted on an object tends to induce motion. As a mental model, consider pushing a car across a parking lot. This requires the application of a force in the direction of the desired motion. Pushing with greater force imparts a higher acceleration to the car. The energy imparted to the object is called **work**; if pushing the car uphill, one expects it to roll down again on its own if it is released halfway up. The car releases the gravitational potential energy imparted to it by the work pushing it uphill. The rate at which work is done on the car is called **power**; one expects that pushing a car across a parking lot more quickly requires more power, meaning the same amount of work needs to be done in less time.

These same principles apply when considering the motion of charged objects under the influence of electromotive forces. Within a conductive electrical circuit, these principles simplify to the well-known Ohm's law and its derivatives.

$$V = I \times R$$

In this equation, V is electromotive **force** (or circuit voltage) measured in volts, I is current measured in amperes (A), and R is resistance measured in ohms. The equation can be rearranged to make it more intuitive to understand:

$$I = V/R$$

In this arrangement, it is easier to see that current (the rate at which the electrical charge flows through a circuit) is proportional to voltage (how hard energy is pushed through the circuit) and inversely proportional to resistance (how strongly the circuit resists the movement of electrical charge). To return to the example of the car, pushing with more force is expected to increase the speed of the car, while someone in the driver's seat pressing the brakes (adding resistance to rolling) is expected to slow the car or require more force to maintain the same speed.

$$P = V \times I = (I \times R) \times I = I^2 \times R$$

Power is the rate at which the circuit transfers electrical energy in watts. A 100-W light bulb is brighter than a 60-W bulb and also consumes more electrical energy per unit time to produce that brighter light. Electrical **work** is the power multiplied by time and is measured in watt-seconds (also known as joules). A more familiar unit of work may be the kilowatt-hour which is used to measure electrical work done by the power grid in supplying energy to a home. Watt-hours or kilowatt-hours are also used to describe the electrical energy storage capacity of batteries, for example, in a mobile phone or electric vehicle.

Electrical Circuits with Oscillating Voltages

The properties of an electrical circuit can vary dramatically based on how electrical energy is delivered to the circuit. Direct current (DC) involves a constant unidirectional flow of charge through the circuit wherein the electromotive force is always in the same direction. It is an oversimplification, but one can think of electrons or other charge carriers moving in the same continuous direction through the circuit. Alternating current (AC) involves a circuit voltage that oscillates between a positive and negative voltage with some frequency (for mains power in the United States, this frequency is 60 Hz). This circuit can be oversimplified as one where electrons or other charge carriers move "forward" and then "backward" in the circuit with the frequency of the AC current delivery (Fig. 5-1).

The concept of impedance becomes important now because all real-world electrical circuits also have some degree of capacitance and inductance, terms that are defined below. The common formulation of Ohm's law described above is a simplified version of the more general formulation, which includes a variable for impedance (Z) rather than resistance (R). Whereas resistance is a static term that describes a tendency of a circuit component to resist any flow of current in any direction, impedance is a dynamic term. It describes a component's tendency to resist the flow of current on the basis of time and current frequency (cycles per second). The impedance of a component can change rapidly based on circuit conditions and the frequency of applied voltage. Although mathematical descriptions involving impedance exceed the scope of this text, a conceptual understanding is relevant to much of electrical safety in the OR.

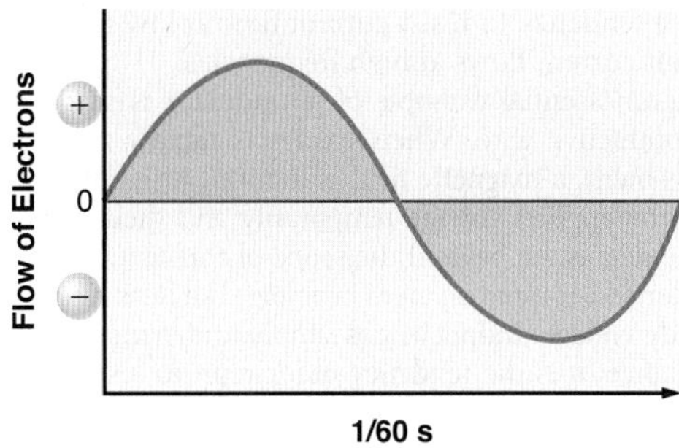

Figure 5-1 Sine wave flow of electrons in a 60-Hz AC.

$$V = I \times Z$$

The relevance of impedance as a concept will become clearer with a discussion of capacitance and inductance. The quintessential example of a capacitor is shown in Figure 5-2 in which two conductive plates oppose each other and have an insulating material in between them. When DC voltage is applied to the capacitor, opposite charges accumulate on each plate as the driving force of the voltage pushes charges in one direction. As this charge accumulates, the driving forces equilibrate and the current eventually stops flowing. Imagine a battery in a circuit with a capacitor. The voltage of the battery will drive a charge difference between the two plates until enough of a charge difference has accumulated that the capacitor and the battery have equal and opposite voltages across their respective poles. Essentially, the charged capacitor has a voltage that "pushes back" against the battery's voltage. When they are equal, there is no longer a net driving force to move charges in the circuit. This situation is analogous to applying a mechanical force to a spring. Compressing the spring causes it to push back on the compressing force until they are balanced. The spring stops compressing and remains in equilibrium until the compressing force changes and a new equilibrium forms. The spring also stores mechanical energy, which can be released later by allowing the force of the spring to move something and thus do work as described above. Similarly, a capacitor stores electrical energy and can produce a current-driving voltage when it is charged.

It may now be clear that a capacitor represents a large impedance to current flow when that current is DC. AC will, however, pass more easily through a capacitor. Current flows in the circuit as the capacitor charges; if the direction changes, then current flows in the opposite direction again until the capacitor is charged. Thus, the higher the frequency of a current, the more easily it will pass through a capacitor, that is, capacitance in a

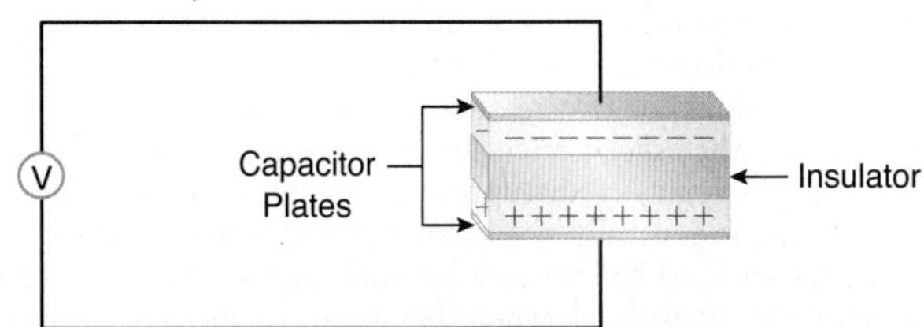

Figure 5-2 A capacitor consists of two parallel conductors separated by an insulator. The capacitor is capable of storing charge supplied by a voltage source.

circuit is a tendency to resist current flow at low frequencies and to transmit current flows at high frequencies.

The quintessential example of an inductor is that of a helical coil of conductive wire. When voltage is rapidly applied to such an arrangement, a magnetic field is induced inside the coil, which counters the applied voltage temporarily and then gradually subsides. The details are beyond the scope of this text, but put simply, an inductor resists rapid changes in voltage but does little to interfere with steady voltage. Inductance is simply understood as the inverse of capacitance; it is the tendency of a circuit to resist current flow at high frequencies and transmit current flows at low frequencies.

All electrical systems exhibit some amount of capacitance and inductance; therefore, some degree of frequency-dependent behavior is inevitable. This may appear in the form of a frequency-dependent current leakage through parts of a circuit that may have been thought of as impermeable. However, the relevance of these concepts might be best understood when considering the behavior of current in the context of an electrolyte fluid such as normal saline. DC applied across a body of saline causes the oppositely charged sodium and chlorine ions to pull away from each other and toward opposite sides of the fluid volume. The charge separation within the saline ions eventually creates its own countervailing voltage and current no longer flows. Alternatively, a high-frequency current such as that provided by an electrosurgical unit (ESU; commonly referred to by the eponymous inventor, William T. Bovie) will flow easily through saline as the ions are pulled back and forth rapidly and never allowed to separate enough to produce the countervailing voltage. If this sounds a lot like capacitance, it is because it is exactly capacitance.

One final point to consider before discussing more specific topics of electrical safety is the universality of the physics of electricity and magnetism. Although it is often convenient to imagine the rules of electricity as governing behavior only within a conductive electrical circuit, the movement of electrical charge, electric fields, and magnetic fields is not bound by wires. Rather, electrical charges can interact with environments around a flow of electricity. Given the immense difference in conductivity between copper wire in a circuit and the air, rubber, and plastic that lies between, it is convenient to think of these rules of electricity as applying only within the circuit. However, many safety considerations involve the unexpected ways that a constructed and intended pathway for current flow can be disrupted or diverted and expose workers and patients to potential harm. The environment around a flow of electricity remains a contributing component of the system even though, under normal circumstances, its contribution would be negligible.

Electrical Shock

1 Hazardous electrical shock is a potentially dangerous flow of electricity through a human body. Such flows can be caused by unintended contact between a person and a voltage source, normal contact with equipment in the setting of an equipment fault, or a fault that causes otherwise harmless current flows (e.g., electrosurgery) to become harmful. These current flows can be considered hazardous for two reasons, often called microshock and
2 macroshock. *Microshock* refers to small current flows that can become physiologically disruptive, inducing ventricular fibrillation. Tissue is generally not injured in microshock; rather, the current causes it to behave in a harmful way. Patients are more susceptible to microshock when they have conductive pathways toward electrically sensitive tissues, such as pacing wires or electrolyte solution–filled catheters in the heart. *Macroshock* refers to the more common understanding of hazardous electrical shock in which larger current flows dissipate energy in the form of heat, causing thermal injury to tissues. Macroshock occurs when the current exceeds skin resistance.[1]

The severity of an electrical shock depends on the current density within affected tissues and the frequency and duration of the current. Current density is often simplified to just current within a conductive circuit of wires because the precise spatial distribution of current flow within the wire core is often not relevant to the behavior of the circuit. However, within the ion-rich fluids of the human body, current needs to be thought of as having a three-dimensional flow from source to sink with a broad distribution of current densities. For example, a Bovie electrosurgery device has a narrow blade-like heating tool and a broad flat return pad. All the current that leaves the blade must be traveling through the patient and exiting through the return pad. Normally only the tissue next to the blade is heated to burning because the small blade produces a much higher current density than the broad return pad. If a similarly narrow conductor is used for the current return, tissues are heated at both contact points, showing the importance of proper and complete application of the electrocautery return pad.

Given the above example, it should be clear that bringing a source of electrical voltage closer to electrically susceptible tissues
such as the heart greatly increases the risk of shock. A current 3
of 100 mA or greater (60 Hz) at the skin is generally required to induce ventricular fibrillation in a patient. However, if it is applied directly to the myocardium (via a pacing wire or saline-filled catheter), only 0.1 mA is required to produce the same outcome. The current density within the heart is unchanged between these two scenarios, but the same density can be achieved with substantially less current when the electrodes are brought closer to the relevant
tissue. This is particularly important because the threshold of 4
sensation at the skin is 1 mA.[2] A provider can cause a dangerous microshock with an electrical current close to a patient's heart, a current that they cannot feel. Table 5-1 shows relevant current

Table 5-1 Effects of 60-Hz Current on an Average Human for a 1-Second Contact

Current	Effect
Macroshock	
1 mA (0.001 A)	Threshold of perception
5 mA (0.005 A)	Accepted as maximum harmless current intensity
10–20 mA (0.01–0.02 A)	"Let-go" current before sustained muscle contraction
50 mA (0.05 A)	Pain, possible fainting, mechanical injury; heart and respiratory functions continue
100–300 mA (0.1–0.3 A)	Ventricular fibrillation will start, but respiratory center remains intact
6,000 mA (6 A)	Sustained myocardial contraction, followed by normal heart rhythm; temporary respiratory paralysis; burns if current density is high
Microshock	
100 μA (0.1 mA)	Ventricular fibrillation
10 μA (0.01 mA)	Recommended maximum 60-Hz leakage current

A, amperes; mA, milliamperes; μA, microamperes.

thresholds at 60 Hz. Of note, the "let-go" current refers to a macroshock threshold beyond which sustained muscle contraction is induced. Thus, if a person grabs an energized wire and their body conducts electricity beyond the "let-go" current, they will be unable to release their grip on the wire. For this reason, such a threshold is of particular importance for designing safe electrical systems.[3–5]

The effect of frequency on the severity of shock can also be appreciated with common OR equipment. A peripheral nerve stimulator for assessing train of four will easily stimulate a sustained skeletal muscle contraction with a 50-Hz or 100-Hz frequency when used to assess sustained tetany. However, the >500,000-Hz frequency of Bovie electrosurgery generally does not stimulate muscle contraction.[6] Very high–frequency currents do not stimulate cellular depolarization or action potentials because the voltage changes so rapidly that charges are not separated enough to actuate voltage gates on cell membranes. Therefore, very high–frequency currents are unlikely to cause macroshock or microshock, but they can still interfere with implanted electrical devices, a topic discussed in more detail later.

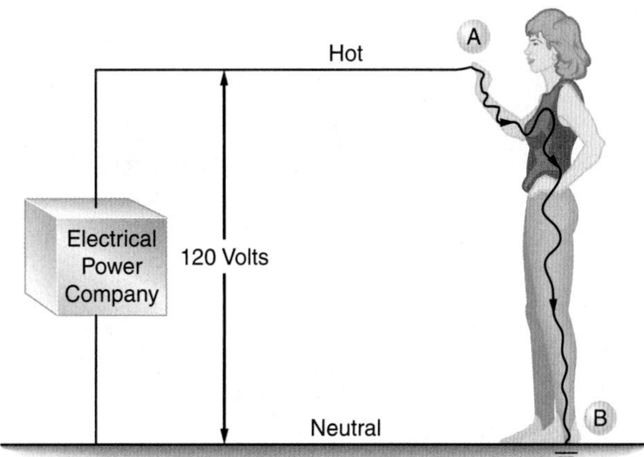

Figure 5-4 An individual can complete an electric circuit and receive a shock by coming in contact with the hot side of the circuit (point *A*). This is because they are standing on the ground (point *B*) and the contact point *A* and the ground point *B* provide the two contact points necessary for a completed circuit. The severity of the shock that the individual receives depends on their skin resistance.

Causes of Electric Shock

The driving force of charges through a circuit is often called the voltage differential. This concept is a circuit-based simplification of electric potential, a field in space that describes the direction and force with which a charged particle is pushed by the electromotive force at any given point in the field. In the context of electrical circuits, the complexity of the forces involved can be simplified and it is assumed that charges travel only through the conductor. Thus, the three-dimensional electric potential field becomes a simple comparison between voltages at different points in the circuit. As seen in Figure 5-3, a power source applies different voltages to each end of the circuit, which pushes current through the impedance. The two lines driving current through the circuit are often referred to as the "hot" line and the "neutral" line. Completing a circuit across the hot and neutral lines allows the voltage differential to drive a current through an electrical device (Fig. 5-3). Should a person complete such a circuit it will conduct potentially harmful current through their body.

Many electrical hazards are caused by a *short circuit*, which is a (often unintended) low-resistance connection between the hot and neutral lines of a circuit. This is called a short circuit because it can be thought of as a current shortcut. The low-resistance shunt pathway allows current to flow easily from the hot line directly to the neutral line with minimal resistance. Although not necessarily a source of shock to providers or patients, electrical shorts can cause a variety of additional hazards. Short circuits can cause overheated or melted wires, sparks and fires, inadequate current flow through vital devices, or, most commonly, a triggering of safety measures that will disconnect power from the circuit, potentially leaving vital equipment unpowered.

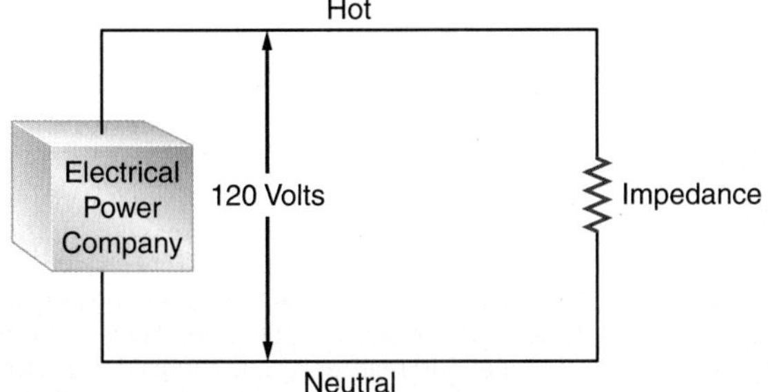

Figure 5-3 A typical AC circuit where there is a potential difference of 120 V between the hot and neutral sides of the circuit. The current flows through a resistance, which in AC circuits is more accurately referred to as impedance, and then returns to the electrical power company.

Unintended pathways to electrical ground are a significant contributor to electric shock. Much of the remainder of this chapter is devoted to describing how electrical ground interacts with electrical systems and can lead to shock hazards. The use of the term ground or grounded is itself a significant source of confusion when discussing electrical safety. The term has slightly different meanings in different contexts. It can be used to describe a type of electrical system; types of electrical equipment that might be connected to an electrical system; any conductor that is at a neutral voltage compared to the driving voltage of the circuit (most accurately called circuit ground, although "circuit" is often omitted); and the literal ground wherein a conductive spike driven into the earth acts as a neutral line in an electrical system (most accurately called earth ground). At its most basic, the term refers to the fact that the earth can be considered a universal neutral electric potential against which other electric potentials can be compared and as a practically unlimited sink for excess electrical charge. Many electrical system arrangements take advantage of this behavior intentionally; however, unintentional connections between earth ground and a live electrical line can also be a source of a shock hazard (Fig. 5-4) or a *ground fault*, which will be discussed in more detail later in this chapter.

Grounded Electrical Power

An electrical system can be either grounded or ungrounded (also called a floating ground). The OR environment gains many safety benefits from being ungrounded or ground isolated. To understand the implications of this, it is useful to review how a grounded electrical system works. Along with a discussion of grounded electrical systems, this section also discusses the difference between grounded and ungrounded electrical devices. As already mentioned, the context-sensitive use of the word "ground" can be a source of confusion. The following discussion will both make it clear what these terms specifically refer to and why the word "ground" is featured so prominently.

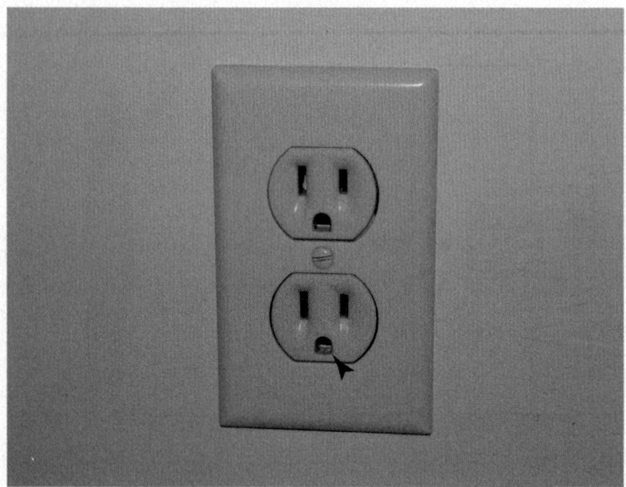

Figure 5-5 Modern electrical outlet in which the ground wire is present. The *arrowhead* points to the part of the receptacle where the ground wire connects.

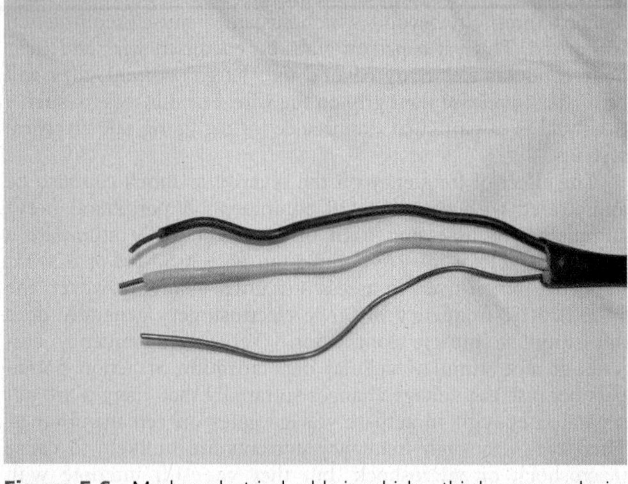

Figure 5-6 Modern electrical cable in which a third, or ground wire has been added.

A typical home power outlet features three ports to match the two or three prongs of an electrical device's power cord (Fig. 5-5, Video 5-1). The two slotted ports connect to the hot and neutral lines at the breaker box, where utility power connects to the building. Within the walls, these wires are most often black and white. The black wire is the "hot" line, which carries the driving voltage from the power utility, and the white wire is the "neutral" line where current returns to the source in the circuit. The third port of the outlet (green or bare metal wire inside the walls) is the ground port. Figure 5-6 shows these three wires as they are commonly found in a residential power system. What defines the system as grounded is that the neutral (white) line is connected to earth ground at the point of entry to the house. This connection most often happens at the circuit breaker box. The ground connection is a metal pipe that runs through the ground or sometimes a metal spike driven into the earth specifically to function as an electrical ground. Figure 5-7 demonstrates this wiring. The power utility maintains earth ground connections on the neutral line at many points during the transmission of power to prevent charge buildup in the neutral line. Without these connections, a thunderstorm could, for example, induce an excessive charge buildup in the lines from the power company, causing a voltage differential between the neutral line and earth ground. This could allow potentially dangerous current to flow between the neutral line and ground. To prevent these voltage differences between the neutral line and the earth ground, the neutral line is connected to the earth ground at multiple points.

This description and Figure 5-7 might suggest that current is flowing to a house via the hot line from the power utility and then flowing into the earth via the grounding line in the circuit breaker box. In practice, this is not what happens. The connection between the neutral line and the earth is relatively high resistance; although some current will leave the circuit into the ground, the majority will follow the low-resistance neutral line back to the source at the power utility. Thus the "ground" line in the outlet and the "ground" line in the circuit breaker box are connected to each other. Both are called ground but are fundamentally performing two different jobs. The earth grounding of the neutral line in the circuit breaker box prevents excessive charge buildup and keeps the neutral line at approximately the same electric potential as the earth to prevent instability and discharges between neutral and the earth. These connections are analogous to an overflow drain in a reservoir. Water may enter and leave

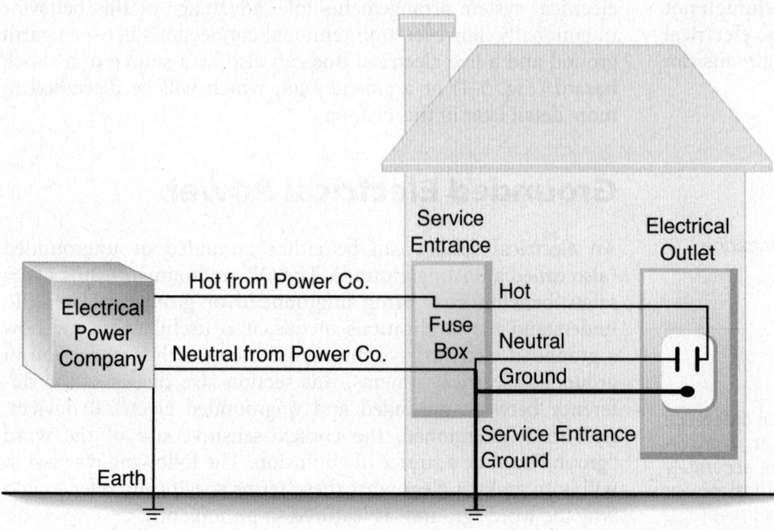

Figure 5-7 In a neutral grounded power system, the electric company supplies two lines to the typical home. The neutral wire is connected to ground by the power company and again connected to a service entrance ground when it enters the fuse box. Both the neutral and ground wires are connected together in the fuse box at the neutral bus bar, which is also attached to the service entrance ground.

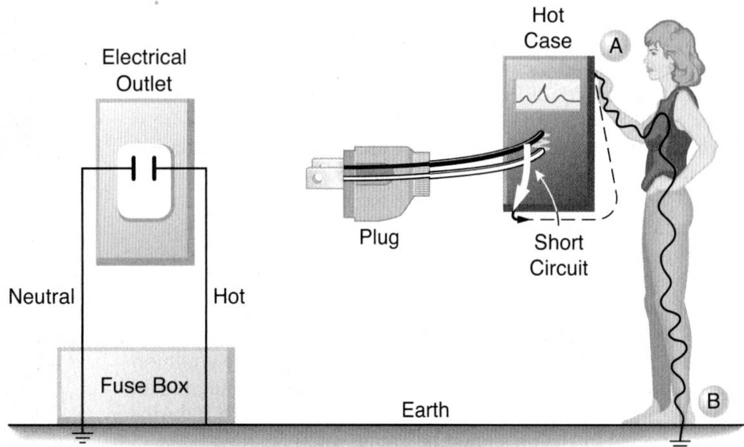

Figure 5-8 When a faulty piece of equipment without an equipment ground wire is plugged into an electrical outlet not containing a ground wire, the case of the instrument will become hot. An individual touching the hot case (point *A*) will receive a shock because they are standing on the earth (point *B*) and completes the circuit. The current (*dashed line*) will flow from the instrument through the individual touching the hot case.

a reservoir simultaneously under normal use, but if an unusual event (such as a hurricane) adds more water to the reservoir than would normally flow in, an overflow channel will allow the reservoir to dump the extra water via an emergency flow path rather than exceed the safe filling volume. The ground connections along the neutral line of a power grid function similarly.

The function of the ground port on a power outlet is better understood less as a path to the earth and more as a backup neutral connection. The ground wire is connected to the casing of an electrical device, and under normal circumstances, no current flows through it. If a fault occurs and the hot line within a device gains contact with the casing, the ground line connected to the casing will provide a safe, low-resistance pathway back to the neutral (and incidentally grounded) portion of the circuit breaker (2 Video 5-2). This serves two purposes. First, it gives the current a safer pathway to flow than through a person. Second, it drives a high current through the breaker or fuse, causing it to disconnect from the circuit with the faulty equipment on it. Without the ground line connection on the device, a faulty connection between the case and the hot line energizes the case, causing a grounded person who touches it to conduct current through their body (Fig. 5-8). Figure 5-9 depicts the same scenario when a grounded device has the same fault and the person is unlikely to be harmed. In addition, an ungrounded case can become energized without tripping a circuit breaker. The grounded case will provide a low-resistance (and thus high-current) circuit back to the breaker, which will cause it to trip and disconnect. Such a disconnection is the safest outcome when a device has failed in this way. This behavior may not be desirable for a piece of life support equipment in an OR environment, and this distinction will be further discussed later in the chapter.

If the neutral line and the ground line are connected at the breaker box, then why bother having two lines in the first place? Why not simply connect the neutral line to a device casing? The answer is that the neutral line is intended to carry current. If it is connected to the case, then the case would be in circuit with the mains power and a grounded person could still conduct current from it to ground. It is true that most of the current would still flow through the normal pathway back through the neutral prong of the power plug. While current is often described as taking "the path of least resistance," it must always be remembered that electric potential and current flows are three-dimensional. Current does not simply take a single linear path from an area of high potential to one of low potential. Some of the current will still flow through higher-resistance pathways in proportion to the difference in resistance of the pathways. This means that even if "backtracking" through the case rather than driving straight through the neutral line is not an optimal current path, some of the current will still take this path. This can cause anything from harmful shocks to noticeable and annoying tingling or zapping sensations (i.e., >1 mA) if someone touches a metal casing that is connected to the neutral line rather than a separate ground line. The ground line ensures that the case carries no current during normal operation but still maintains a backup pathway to the neutral side of the breaker box in the event of a fault.

This discussion naturally leads to the following question: what about devices with only two-pronged plugs? These are ungrounded devices, also called double-insulated devices. As

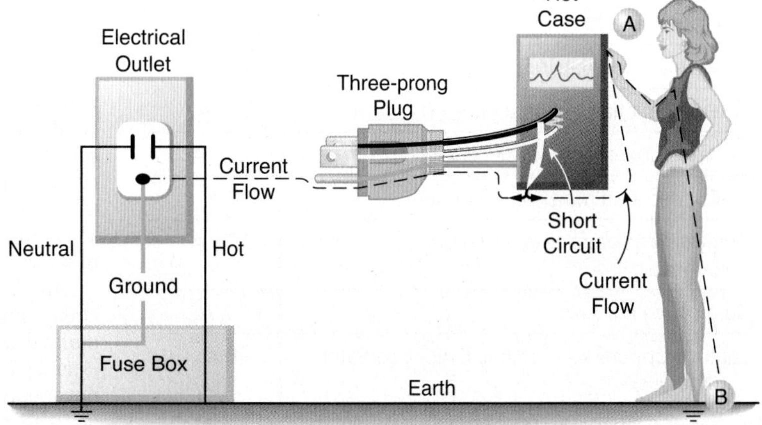

Figure 5-9 When a faulty piece of equipment containing an equipment ground wire is properly connected to an electrical outlet with a grounding connection, the current (*dashed line*) will preferentially flow down the low-resistance ground wire. An individual touching the case (point *A*) while standing on the ground (point *B*) will still complete the circuit; however, only a small part of the current will go through the individual.

described above, the primary purpose of the ground wire is to protect the user when a device develops a faulty connection between a conductive case and the hot wire. If a device is "double insulated" and has two sources of insulation that must separately fail before a user could be exposed to mains voltage, then the ground wire is deemed unnecessary in normal home use. This double insulation most frequently takes the form of insulated internal wires, which almost every electrical device has. The "second" layer of insulation is a plastic or other nonconductive casing. A common cellphone charger needs only two prongs because it is fully encased in plastic with no external metal on its case. These different appliance types are also called Class I (single insulated with a ground wire) and Class II (double insulated with no ground wire) appliances. It should be noted that electrolyte solution intrusion is a common way in which insulation is bypassed in an OR setting, rendering an appliance more susceptible to shocking the user. As such, a device with suspected intrusion should be unplugged if possible.[7]

Common Safety Features of a Grounded Electrical Power System

Circuit breakers or fuses are an important piece of any electrical power delivery system. The electrical wiring system in a building always has some intrinsic resistance; thus, it will generate some amount of heat as current flows through it. Thicker wires can conduct more current without heating up because they have less resistance than thinner wires. Thus, every electrical circuit in a building (multiple outlets often reside on a single circuit) has a maximum electrical load that it can safely tolerate. Most outlets in a home will be 120 V and 15 or 20 A of maximum current (clothes dryers, HVAC systems, water heaters, and other large appliances may have outlets up to 240 V/50 A). If a device (or more often multiple devices) attempts to draw more than 15 A of current on a 15-A circuit, the fuse will melt and need to be replaced or the breaker will trip and need to be manually reset. Roommates who often need to use hair dryers at the same time probably have figured out the hard way which outlets are on the same circuit as two hair dryers used simultaneously will generally draw more than 15 A and trip a circuit breaker. A typical OR circuit is 120 V/15 or 20 A (National Electrical Manufacturers Association [NEMA] 5-15 or 5-20; see below for further discussion). Table 5-2 shows common current draws

Table 5-2 Common Operating Room Current Draw

Device	Maximum Current Draw
Forced air warmer (Bair Hugger)	11.7 A
Anesthesia machine	10 A
Infusion pump (Alaris)	1.25 A
Tourniquet inflation pump (Stryker)	1.5 A
OR table underbody warmer (Gaymar)	11.5 A
POC ultrasound machine (Sonosite)	8 A
Surgical headlamp—external mount, fiberoptic (Sunoptic)	3.75 A
Surgical ice maker	12 A
Laparoscopy stack—(camera, lamp, insufflator (Olympus)	8 A

OR, operating room; POC, point-of-care ultrasound.

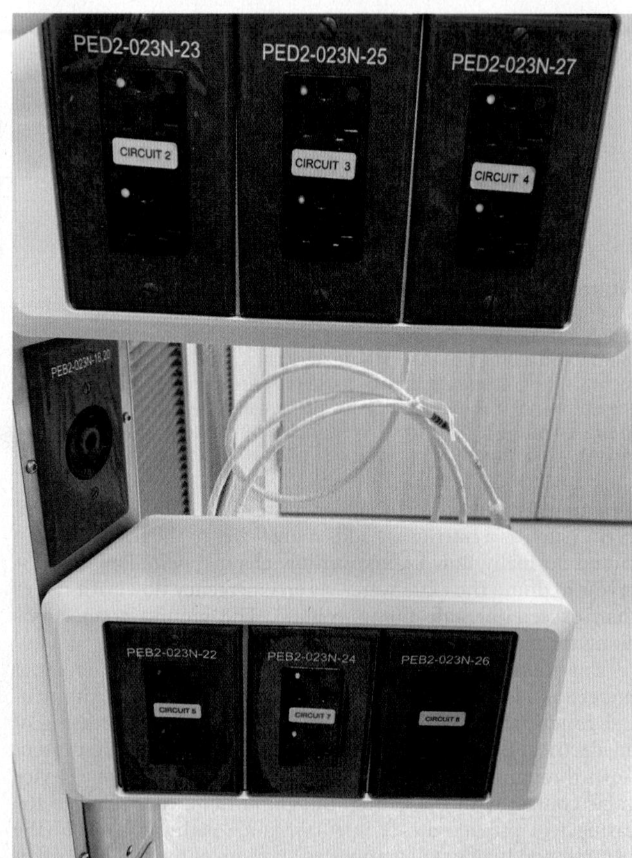

Figure 5-10 Operating room receptacles with circuit labeling.

of a variety of OR devices. It is easy to envision how plugging an upper body and lower body forced-air warmer (combined current of greater than 20 A) into a multiple port electrical adapter plugged into one OR circuit can be made to fail. This is also why it is useful to label the circuit that a plug is connected to in the OR (Fig. 5-10). An additional consideration regarding overloaded circuits is that Table 5-2 specifies the *maximum* current draw of the listed devices. This current draw is often variable based on the device's settings and environmental factors. A circuit can become overloaded even if all connected devices have been in use if conditions change or multiple devices enter an "active" state simultaneously. Safe circuit load should be determined based on the maximum possible load of each device to avoid sudden midsurgery overload.

In addition, many OR and home devices will have their own internal fuses or breakers to protect their internal wiring from overheating in a fault state. It is worth noting that 120 V/15 A is enough electrical power to cause serious harm to a person. Recall that 100 mA of current can cause ventricular fibrillation. The circuit breaker is intended to protect wiring from melting and/or catching fire or shut off appliances with dangerous short circuits. Such systems are not intended to protect a person who contacts both the hot and neutral lines simultaneously; power should always be shut off before interacting with a home electrical system in a way that makes such contact more likely.

Another common electrical safety device is the ground fault circuit interrupter (GFCI). The word "circuit" is occasionally omitted with such devices being erroneously called ground fault interrupters (GFIs), which is a different device altogether and one not found within indoor electrical circuitry. Many will be familiar with these devices in their home bathrooms and kitchens

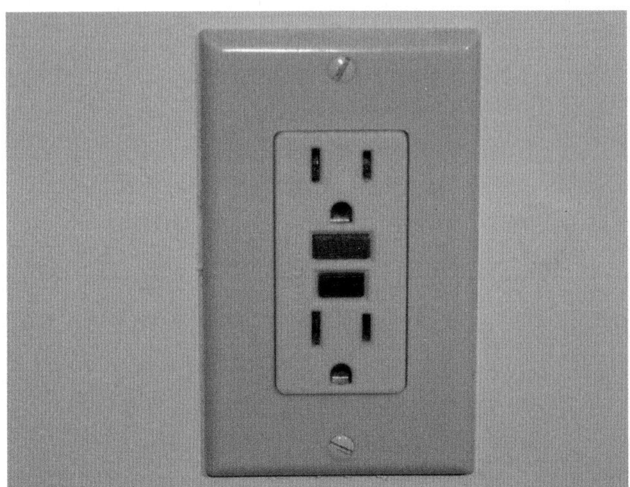

Figure 5-11 A GFCI electrical outlet with integrated test (*black*) and reset (*red*) buttons.

(Fig. 5-11). These devices are particularly important in parts of a building that are both wet and have good electrical conduction to earth ground (often a drainpipe with flowing water as in a sink or bathtub). A wet person has lower skin resistance and thus conducts electricity more easily with hot line contact. If that person is in contact with earth ground via a water drain, they will readily conduct electricity between the hot line and earth ground. Any unintended connection between the hot line and earth ground is generally called a ground fault. A GFCI continuously measures the current flow on the hot and neutral lines of the outlet, and if they are not closely in balance, the GFCI will disconnect the circuit. It should be noted that although the voltage decreases from 120v to 0v from the hot to the neutral side, the current remains the same in both limbs of the circuit. A GFCI has no way of calculating the amount of current flowing to ground. It is assuming that current leaving the hot line but not returning via the neutral line must be exiting the circuit somewhere else and will trigger the disconnect.

In general, GFCIs can be expected to disconnect a circuit with between 5 and 6 mA of current leakage within 25 to 40 milliseconds. These devices are used in some ORs but not all, and their use poses special considerations discussed later in this chapter. As a side note, some devices can trigger a GFCI when they are first turned on. Certain types of appliances (compact fluorescent bulbs were well known for this) need to charge their internal electrical system before steady-state electricity flow. As a result, under normal operation, they will draw more current than they return immediately upon activation. This may be a wide enough gap that lasts long enough to trip a GFCI device even without a ground fault present. As stated above, the GFCI does not know where the current is going; it only knows that less comes back than leaves and assumes the worst-case scenario.

Power Receptacles

Power receptacles (outlets) come in many different shapes and sizes. Different parts of the world have different and often incompatible electrical systems and receptacles. Within North America, receptacle standards are specified by the NEMA. There are many categories of NEMA standard outlets, the vast majority of which are either deprecated, reserved for possible future uses, or used only in specialized industrial applications. The three most common categories in North America are NEMA 5, 6, and 14. NEMA standard receptacles are designed to prevent accidental connections between a device and a power source with incompatible supply voltage or current requirements. This is achieved with many variations of pin spacing, size, and orientation to ensure incompatible plugs do not fit into the wrong receptacle type.[8]

The receptacle likely to be most familiar is the NEMA 5-15 receptacle (Fig. 5-5). This receptacle is so called because it is part of the NEMA 5 standard, which includes three pins (one earth ground, one neutral, and one hot 120-V AC) and is also limited to 15 A of current. While they can be found in residential environments, the NEMA 5-20 is more commonly found in commercial settings and are likely to be seen in health care and OR environments (Fig. 5-10). The NEMA 5-20 plug is similar to the 5-15, but the hot pin is rotated 90° to prevent plugging into a 15-A–limited receptacle. The T-shaped hot port on the NEMA 5-20 receptacle is so shaped such that it can accommodate a NEMA 5-15 or 5-20 plug.

There are some further useful concepts demonstrated in Figure 5-10. The NEMA 5-20 receptacles are installed "upside down" relative to what most people may be used to. NEMA does not specify a "correct" orientation for receptacles, so there is no such thing as "right side up" or "upside down." Ground pin down is standard in residential environments by convention only. In working environments (like the OR from which the picture was taken), receptacles are often installed ground pin up because of the potential safety benefit. Should a conductive object fall onto a receptacle with a plug inside and slightly exposed pins, it would contact the ground pin first. As a result, it may be less likely to contact hot and neutral pins simultaneously than the usual ground pin down orientation. Such contact between hot and neutral pins would create a short circuit, possibly spark or ignite, and likely trip an overcurrent breaker or fuse. It is also common in residential environments for receptacles to be installed ground pin up to visually distinguish them from others in the house, as in receptacles that are controlled by a wall switch.

In addition, as mentioned above, the individual outlets are labeled with the electrical circuit they are on. A NEMA 5-15 outlet simply designates that it is part of a 15-A–limited circuit. If multiple outlets are on the same circuit, one can still easily overload the circuit by plugging in multiple devices that each draw less than 15 A but exceed that amount in combination. It should be kept in mind that overload is possible even in the example figure in which each individual outlet is on a separate circuit. Since each outlet offers two plugs, it can still be overloaded by plugging in two high-current devices to the same outlet (e.g., forced air and fluid warmers).

Considering the vital importance of intact ground wire connections and the abuse that plugs often receive in a hospital environment, it may be no surprise that the durability of plugs and receptacles is of special consideration to hospitals. While NEMA specifies standards for plug and receptacle shape and size, an organization formally known as Underwriters Laboratories (UL) maintains a testing specification specifically for "hospital-grade" plugs and outlets. UL is one of the few companies approved by the U.S. Occupational Safety and Health Administration (OSHA) to perform safety testing and certification on electrical appliances. The circular "UL" logo can be seen on many electrical devices. Figure 5-12 shows both a hospital-grade plug and receptacle that are easily denoted by a green dot.[9] The figure shows that the ground pin on a grounded plug is actually a bit longer than the other two pins to ensure that it contacts the ground line before the other two pins are connected when plugged in. Hospital-grade plugs are required to have solid pins and thicker plug bodies to reduce the risk of breaking and bending pins or plug bodies coming loose from the wire when pulled or bent, among many other specifications. These specifications make such plugs and receptacles more durable and thus almost certainly safer in a hospital

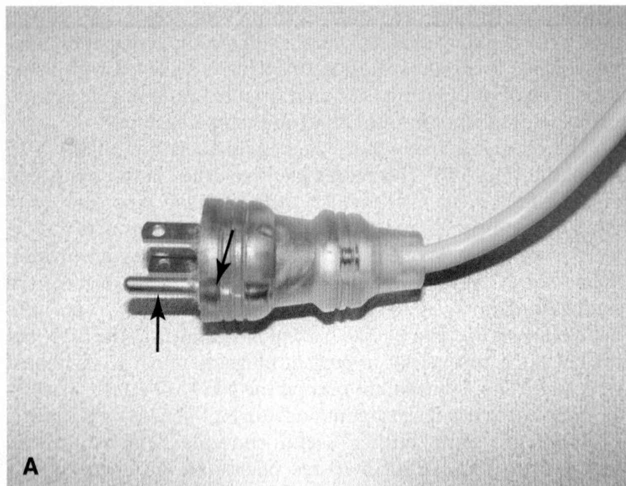

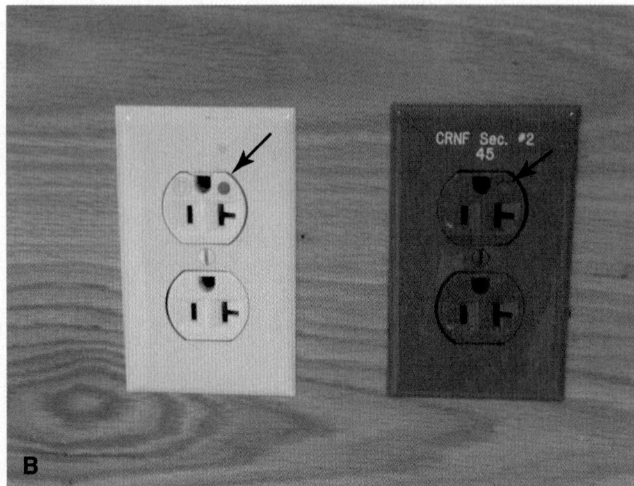

Figure 5-12 **A:** A hospital-grade plug that can be visually inspected. The arrow points to the equipment ground wire whose integrity can be readily verified. Note that the prong for the ground wire (*arrow*) is longer than the hot or neutral prong, so that it is the first to enter the receptacle. **B:** The *arrows* point to the *green dot* denoting a hospital-grade power outlet. The *red* outlet on the **right** is connected to the emergency power (generator) system.

environment.[10] In addition, many modern ORs prioritize keeping electrical wires and power strips off the floor with ceiling-mounted arms for outlets and power strips mounted on surfaces or poles off the floor.[11] In at least one case, a power strip on an OR floor became doused in saline and tripped a breaker, which cut power to the entire OR.[12] Power strips with splash-resistant receptacle covers and water intrusion-resistant external casings are commonly used in modern ORs for just this reason (Fig. 5-13).

Ground-Isolated Electrical Power

ORs are unusually hazardous places when it comes to electrical safety. These environments are prone to electrical accidents because of the frequent use of mission-critical electrical equipment (much of which draws significant current; Table 5-2), a high chance for spilling or pooling of electrolyte solutions such as intravenous fluids or surgical irrigation, and staff who have patient care tasks that may divert their attention from seemingly mundane details such as electrical power delivery. Thus, it is hardly surprising that despite accounting for a relatively small portion of an average hospital, ORs account for 40% of all electrical accidents reported in hospitals.[13] To mitigate the electrical risks, most ORs are built with an *isolated power system* (IPS). This is an ungrounded power delivery system, also called a floating ground. As the name floating ground might imply, the neutral line of an IPS is not tied to earth ground. The same 120-V differential exists between the hot line and the neutral line as in a grounded system, but since the neutral line is not grounded, there is no potential circuit path between the hot line and earth ground (3 Video 5-3).

This feat is accomplished with the use of a *line isolation transformer* (pictured for educational purposes only in Fig. 5-14 as anesthesia providers should not be directly interacting with an OR power system at this level). Electrical transformers are devices that can modify the voltage and current of an electrical power source within the same power envelope. For example, a 1,800-W standard power outlet (120 V/15 A) can drive a transformer to deliver 240 V, but that transformer would then be able to output only 7.5 A because the transformer can deliver only as much power as it receives. The 1,800-W limitation would still apply despite the increased output voltage.

A line isolation transformer is simply a transformer with equal coil windings on each side so that the output voltage and current is the same as the input. Since electrical power is transferred across the transformer via a magnetic field, there is no direct electrical flow between the source circuit and the output circuit. The line isolation transformer is so named because it is used only for isolation and not voltage transformation. As described above, the

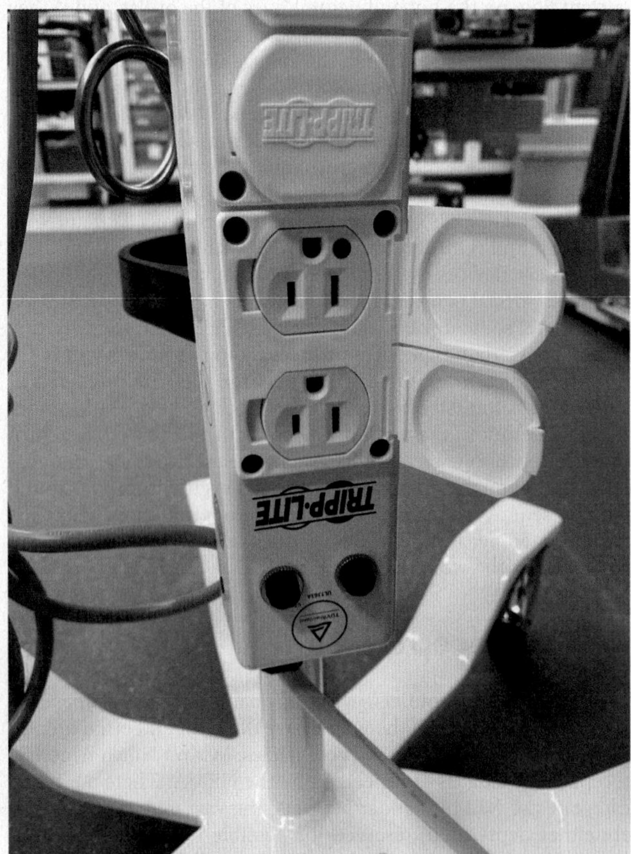

Figure 5-13 Power strip on an IV pole with splash-resistant covers.

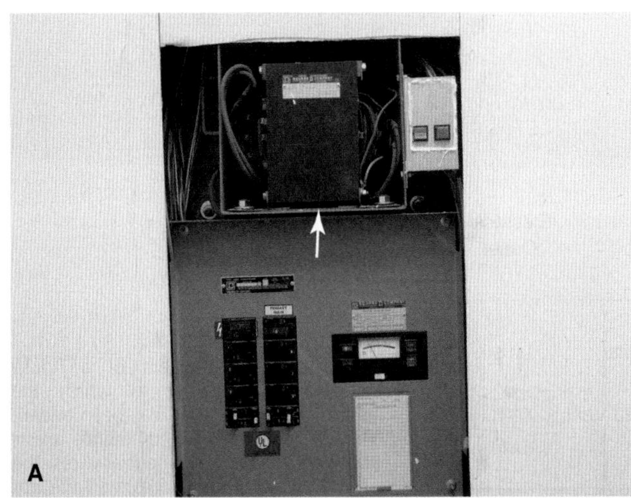

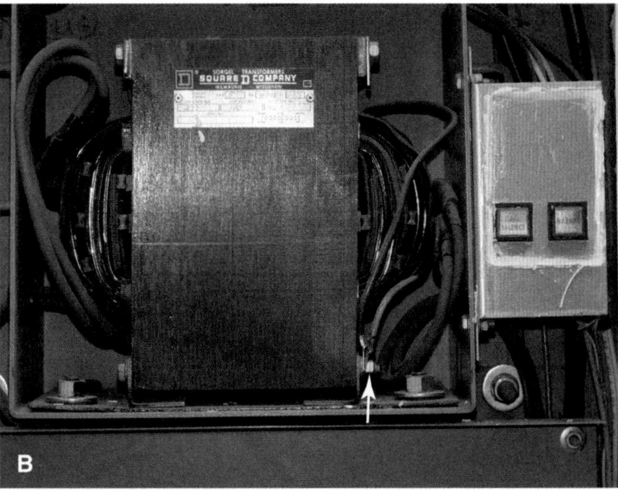

Figure 5-14 **A:** Isolated power panel showing circuit breakers, LIM, and isolation transformer (*arrow*). **B:** Detail of an isolation transformer with the attached warning lights. The *arrow* points to ground wire connection on the primary side of the transformer. Note that no similar connection exists on the secondary side of the transformer.

neutral line of a power grid is connected to earth ground at many points, so the isolating aspect of the many transformers used in a power grid is removed. Because the OR is behind a line isolation transformer and also ungrounded, its power system remains isolated from the mains power system. Figure 5-15 shows how an IPS is arranged. Within the secondary circuit, the terms hot line and neutral line become instead line 1 and line 2. The 120-V potential exists between the two lines, but without a ground reference, neither is considered neutral. Compare this arrangement to Figure 5-16 where the 120-V potential exists between the hot line and the neutral line, ground line, and earth ground.

It may not be immediately obvious why this arrangement is meaningful in an OR. As an example, if a light bulb is connected to only the hot line of a home power outlet and the other pole of the bulb to a wire in the ground, the bulb would light up. The grounded power system is driving an electric potential between the hot line and a grounded neutral line. Thus, a potential current path exists between the hot line and earth ground. As shown in Figure 5-17, no such path exists between the IPS and earth ground, so a similar connection of a light bulb in an IPS would not light up the bulb. Only a connection across lines 1 and 2 will drive current because the system is not directly connected to earth ground at any point. In a grounded power system, a person who has a low-impedance connection to ground is at a higher risk of shock because they only need to contact the hot line to create a viable circuit path for electricity flow, as discussed in an earlier section regarding GFCIs. The IPS protects even a well-grounded person from such a shock risk. However, this will not protect a person who simultaneously contacts both lines of the IPS. In that case, the 120-V potential will still drive hazardous current through a person.

There is a second benefit of an IPS in this context in addition to protecting a grounded person from macroshock with only a single point of contact to the electrical circuit. This second benefit manifests in how a faulty piece of equipment interacts with the system. In a home power system, a piece of equipment with an errant connection between the hot line and the grounded casing will cause a short circuit between hot and neutral, which trips the breaker. This is an important safety feature in the context of a power system wherein a grounded person can receive a macroshock from a single point contact with the hot line. In the IPS, faulty equipment with the same errant connection to the grounded casing will not cause a short circuit and trip a breaker. Because this faulty equipment is the only connection to ground for the isolated circuit, there is no low-impedance loop in which current will flow unimpeded. There are two ramifications of this connection (Fig. 5-18). First, because the unintended ground connection does not cause a breaker to trip, a single piece of faulty equipment will not take down a whole power circuit, potentially shutting down critical and life-sustaining equipment. Such a faulty piece of equipment can even be used uneventfully during surgery if it is critical to patient safety, with

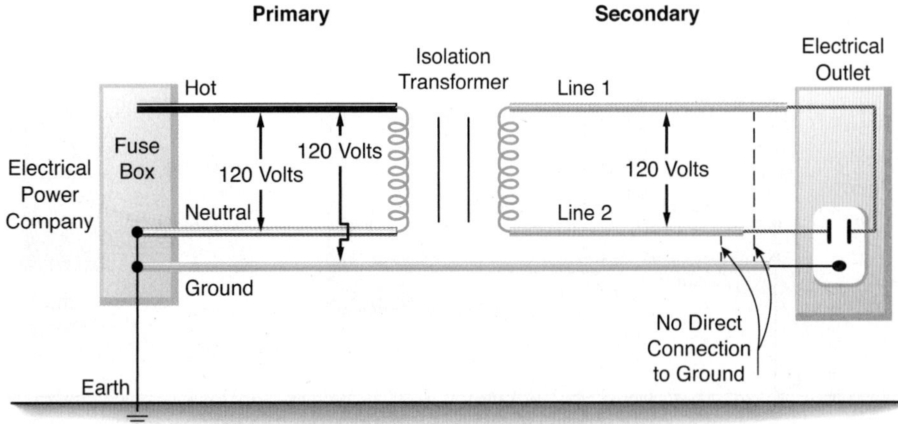

Figure 5-15 In the OR, the isolation transformer converts the grounded power on the primary side to an ungrounded power system on the secondary side of the transformer. A 120-V potential difference exists between line 1 and line 2. There is no direct connection from the power on the secondary side to ground. The equipment ground wire, however, is still present.

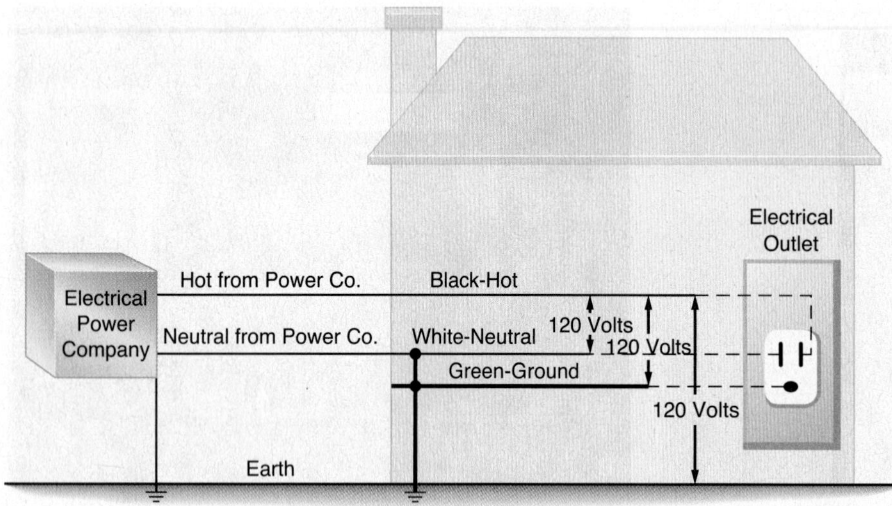

Figure 5-16 Diagram of a house with modern wiring in which the third, or ground, wire has been added. The 120-V potential difference exists between the hot and neutral wires, the hot and the ground wires, and the hot wire and the earth.

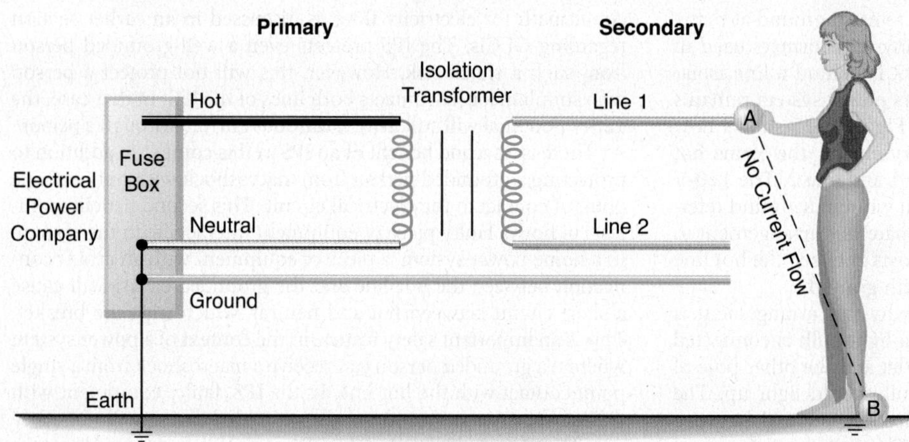

Figure 5-17 A safety feature of the isolated power system is illustrated. An individual contacting one side of the isolated power system (point *A*) and standing on the ground (point *B*) will not receive a shock. In this instance, the individual is not contacting the circuit at two points and thus is not completing the circuit. Point *A* is part of the isolated power system, and point *B* is part of the primary or grounded side of the circuit.

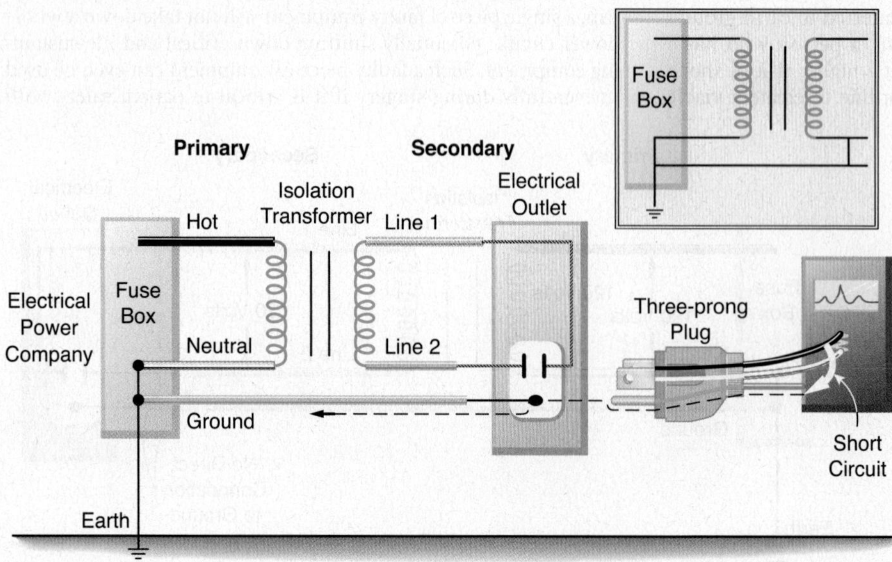

Figure 5-18 A faulty piece of equipment plugged into the isolated power system does not present a shock hazard. It merely converts the isolated power system into a grounded power system. The figure inset illustrates that the isolated power system is now identical to the grounded power system. The *dashed line* indicates current flow in the ground wire.

an important caveat that constitutes the second ramification of the errant connection to ground: the IPS is now no longer isolated and will behave just as a grounded home power system would. If a second piece of faulty equipment were to be plugged into the now grounded power system, a grounded person in contact with it would receive a macroshock and/or a breaker could be tripped, cutting power to important devices.

This phenomenon is often referred to as the "second fault." It is important for anesthesia providers to understand this concept to make vital decisions about the safety of patients who may depend on the equipment, as well as the safety of everyone else in the OR who may be interacting with electrical equipment. As described above, losing the isolation of the OR power system with a faulty piece of equipment is not in itself hazardous, but it does remove an important layer of protection and creates a situation where a second fault could cause problems that the IPS would otherwise prevent. Making decisions about how to manage these situations requires an understanding of the line isolation monitor (LIM) and the information it conveys about the status of an IPS.

The Line Isolation Monitor

The LIM is fundamentally an ohmmeter (resistance meter) between earth ground and each line of the IPS. It measures the impedance between these two lines and earth ground to assess the extent to which the IPS is isolated. The discussion of the topic thus far may have suggested that a power system is either fully isolated or fully grounded, but this is not truly the case. As discussed earlier, electric fields do not simply follow wires in a linear path; rather, the whole three-dimensional environment contributes to the flow of electrical current. As such, there is *always* some connection between an electrical system and earth ground. Even the air between two wires is technically a possible electrical connection, just one with extremely high impedance. Wires in proximity will develop a small amount of capacitance between them, which can allow a flow of ACs in a frequency-dependent manner just as any capacitor would. Coils generating magnetic fields in transformers can induce small voltage changes in nearby conductors. Put more simply, any real-world electrical system will demonstrate what is called *leakage current*, or very small amounts of current through very high–impedance pathways to earth ground (Fig. 5-19). This is all to explain that a LIM is not a simple measurement of a line being "isolated" or "not isolated"; there is a variable amount of impedance between the IPS and ground that can be considered normal and an amount that is considered potentially problematic. Understanding how various factors affect this measurement of line isolation is important to appropriately manage OR electrical systems.

Another potential point of confusion about the LIM is that despite measuring impedance between the IPS and earth ground, the monitor will generally report this impedance not in ohms but in milliamperes of *potential* current (in this context also called hazard current) (4 Video 5-4). The "potential" is important here; the LIM is not reporting an actual flow of current. Rather, it is reporting (based on impedance to earth ground) how much current *would* flow through a direct connection between the IPS and earth ground. Therefore, it represents a maximum possible current that a person could be exposed to during a ground fault. For example, a reading of 1 mA of hazard current means that if a single piece of faulty equipment were connected to the IPS with an errant connection between either of the IPS lines and ground, a well-grounded person touching the device might be exposed to up to 1 mA of current. This is a small amount of current, likely to be barely perceptible and not dangerous. If the same monitor reports 50 mA of hazard current, a person could be exposed to current exceeding the "let-go" threshold of 20 mA. The threshold of safety beyond which an alarm will sound is generally set at 5 mA for modern LIMs and possibly lower (2 mA) for older LIM devices (Fig. 5-20).

There are two primary contributions to the hazard current reading on the LIM, which increases as impedance between the IPS and ground decreases. The first contributor is the connection of faulty equipment. A piece of equipment with a grounded conductive casing and an unintended connection between either line 1 or line 2 of the IPS and its casing will thus introduce a direct connection between the IPS and the ground line. The impedance of that connection will be largely driven by the impedance of the physical connection within the device, such as a loose wire or melted solder joint. In this circumstance, the LIM alarm will likely be triggered with a new low-impedance ground fault, leading to a sudden increase in hazard current on the LIM. This represents the classic scenario of the "first fault" and is the scenario that most will think of when contemplating the purpose and function of a LIM.

The second scenario is less often considered when anesthesia providers manage line isolation but no less important to understand. As described above, all electrical circuits and devices have some amount of intrinsic capacitance to ground and thus leakage current. This leakage current is extremely small but non-zero in properly functioning devices. If too many properly functioning devices are plugged in simultaneously, the hazard current on the LIM will gradually creep up to the limit and the alarm can be triggered even without a faulty device on the IPS. The increasing abundance of electrical devices used in modern ORs often leads

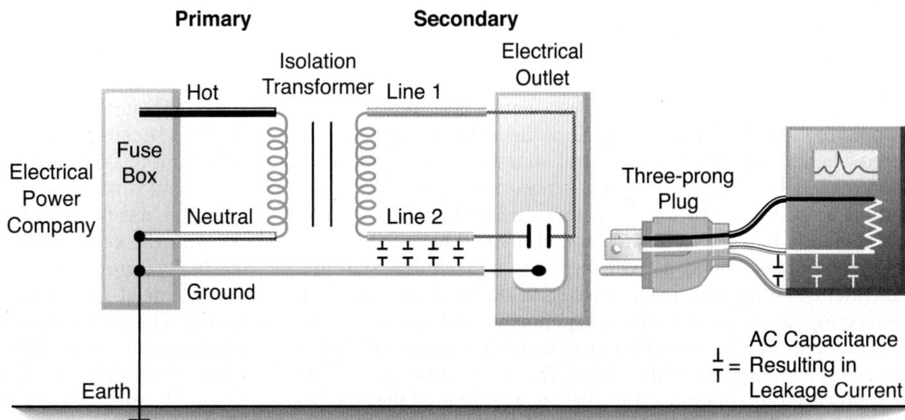

Figure 5-19 The capacitance that exists in alternating current (AC) power lines and AC-operated equipment results in small "leakage currents" that partially degrade the isolated power system.

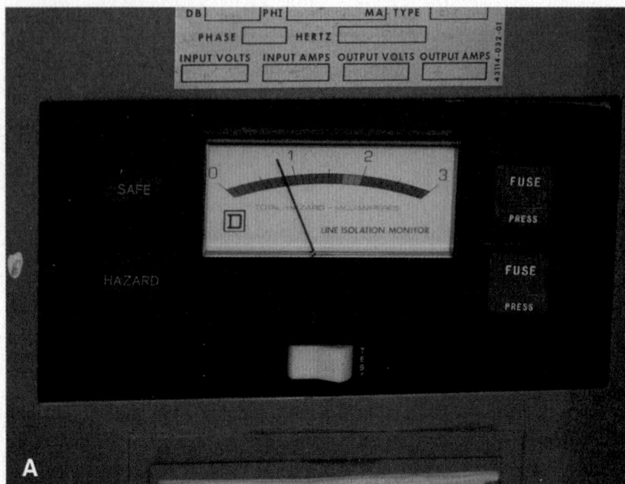

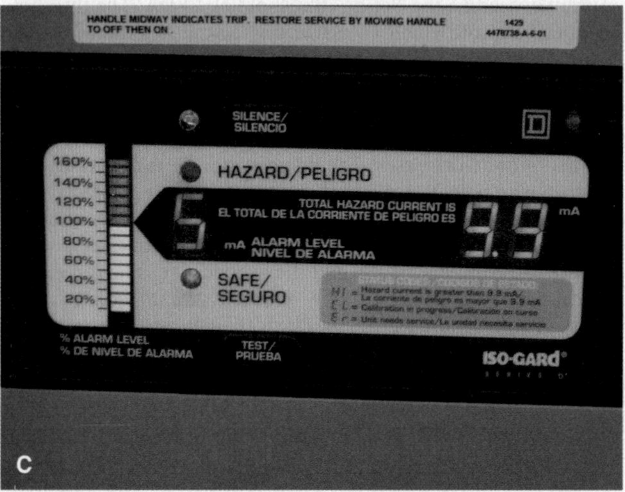

Figure 5-20 The meter of the LIM is calibrated in milliamperes. If the isolation of the power system is degraded such that more than 2 mA (5 mA in newer systems) of current could flow, the hazard light will illuminate and a warning buzzer will sound. Note the button for testing the hazard warning system. **A:** Older LIM that will trigger an alarm at 2 mA. **B:** Newer LIM that will trigger an alarm at 5 mA. **C:** The LIM alarm is triggered, and the red hazard stripe is illuminated, and the number on the right shows 9.9 mA of potential current flow.

to false alarms and is the reason that newer LIM devices generally trigger an alarm state at a 5-mA hazard current rather than the 2 mA that was typical with older devices.[14] Another important implication of this leakage current is that if the LIM alarm is triggered when a new device is plugged in, there is no way to know without directly observing the LIM hazard current before and after whether the device is faulty or whether the OR is overburdened with devices on a circuit. For this reason, when calling a service technician or clinical engineer about a device that triggered a LIM alarm, it is important to inform the servicer about the device and the OR in which the alarm occurred. The device may be functioning normally and simply be in an OR overburdened with electrical equipment (Table 5-2).

Putting this all together leads to some best practices for responding to LIM alarms in the OR. If the isolation alarm is triggered when plugging in a new piece of nonessential equipment (or even essential equipment if a case is not in progress), the alarm should be addressed by disconnecting the offending equipment. Then, ensure that the isolation alarm clears and have the offending device serviced and the OR inspected by technical staff at a time that is safe for patients. If an isolation alarm is triggered when connecting an essential piece of equipment, that device can be safely used for the duration of surgery with the understanding that the IPS is no longer ground isolated. This is the "first fault" in an IPS, which should not cause any direct danger beyond the fact that a "second fault" can lead to shock hazard. The offending device should be serviced as soon as patient safety allows, and the risk of a second fault should be reduced as much as possible by avoiding connecting any more devices to the alarm state IPS circuit unless necessary. This point is worth repeating: A single ground fault 6
introduced to an IPS is not inherently dangerous; it simply reverts the IPS to a grounded system just like the ones encountered virtually everywhere power outlets are in use. The danger lies in the fact that the wet environment of the OR justifies an extra layer of security, a layer which should be restored as soon as possible should the system lose isolation and become grounded.

An intact grounding wire in an OR device is essential for maintaining safety. If the ground wire in a piece of equipment is broken, the device can have a faulty connection to the casing, which will not disrupt its normal functioning or be detected by the LIM because there is no longer a connection to ground. Put more simply, such a device will act as a silent first fault. A second fault would have the same shock risk ramifications, but in this case, the first fault would not trigger an alarm state on the LIM. Without the errant connection to ground, the LIM cannot "see" the faulty connection in the device. Many medical devices have a small metal peg on their casing near where the power is connected. This peg is intended to serve as an easy connection point to confirm the continuity of the ground wire and the device casing when a technician is testing it.

GFCIs are also used as electrical safety devices in certain OR settings, but they are used less often than LIMs and IPSs. GFCI

Figure 5-21 Special GFCI circuit breaker. The *arrowhead* points to the distinguishing *red* test button.

function was discussed earlier in the chapter, but there are some special considerations that limit their applicability for OR use. GFCIs can be applied to individual outlets (Fig. 5-11) or entire circuits at the breaker level (Fig. 5-21). Just as in the home environment, GFCIs are intended to cut power to devices that may have a ground fault; however, in an OR environment, the sudden loss of power to a device without warning can be a significant hazard to patient care. A LIM will give the anesthesia provider a warning about a ground fault and allow the provider to decide about the use of a device while considering patient safety. A GFCI will simply cut power to an appliance that may be essential for patient care. An additional consideration is that GFCIs can be applied to a whole circuit rather than a single outlet. A case report by Courtney et al.[15] demonstrates why this should not be done in an OR. When a warming blanket with a ground fault present was plugged in, power was cut without warning to multiple devices, including the anesthesia machine and patient monitors. The confusion and distraction of trying to solve a problem like this in the middle of surgery can be just as harmful as the power loss itself. For these reasons, GFCIs are not a popular choice for electrical safety in modern ORs. Current NFPA 99 code requires that if they are to be used at all, they can only protect a single outlet at a time and never a whole circuit unless that circuit has only one outlet. Similarly, they must not be "daisy chained" such that a single GFCI outlet cuts power to multiple outlets.

Microshock

While still relevant to microshock, much of the chapter thus far has focused on preventing macroshock. Some electrical safety considerations unique to preventing microshock merit a discussion separate from macroshock. As discussed earlier, voltage applied across a person's skin will generate a current that disperses and spreads out within the body between the two points of circuit contact. Current density is highest at the skin where contact is made (and even higher if the contact point is very small as in the tip of an electrosurgery blade) and lower within the body where current flows can disperse within ion-rich tissues.[16] This explains why, in Table 5-1, the current threshold for inducing ventricular fibrillation is much higher at the skin than if that same current is applied directly across the myocardium (100 to 300 mA vs. 0.1 mA, respectively). This difference is not just of degree, but also of kind; the skin current required to induce microshock is well above what is perceptible to a person, whereas the current directly at the heart that is needed to induce microshock is much lower than the threshold of perception at the skin. Thus, microshock in an electrically susceptible patient remains a risk even when a provider is exposed to current flows that they cannot feel themselves. Wires (e.g., pacing or catheter guide wires) and saline-filled catheters in contact with or near the heart create a DC path to the heart and produce a state of electrical susceptibility in a patient.[17]

The exact amount of current needed to induce ventricular fibrillation in an electrically susceptible patient is not predictable or static. It varies with factors such as minute environmental conditions, precise timing of shock, or precise placement of a catheter. As such, studies seeking a current threshold tend to report a wide range in numbers. Whalen et al.[18] reported a threshold of 20 µA in a dog study. Raftery et al.[19] reported 80 µA in human patients. Hull reported that on average, 50% of patients fibrillated with a threshold of 200 µA. Despite this uncertainty in current threshold data, the constant is that all reported thresholds are well below the approximately 1,000-µA (i.e., 1 mA) threshold of sensory perception for a person with a 60-Hz AC current. Electrical devices can generate these amounts of current as leakage current, stray capacitance, or electrostatic charge buildup when they have moving parts such as cooling fans. There are many documented cases of microshock phenomena inducing ventricular fibrillation.[20–22] A functioning ground wire remains the best safety precaution against these sources of excess charge buildup.

Figure 5-22 demonstrates how a ground wire can protect an electrically susceptible patient by having a very low–resistance

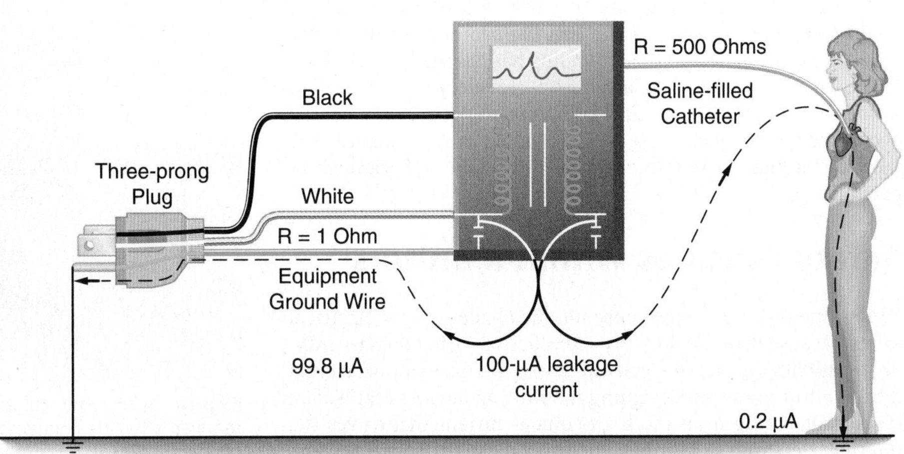

Figure 5-22 The electrically susceptible patient is protected from microshock by the presence of an intact equipment ground wire. The equipment ground wire provides a low-impedance path in which the majority of the leakage current (*dashed lines*) can flow. R, resistance.

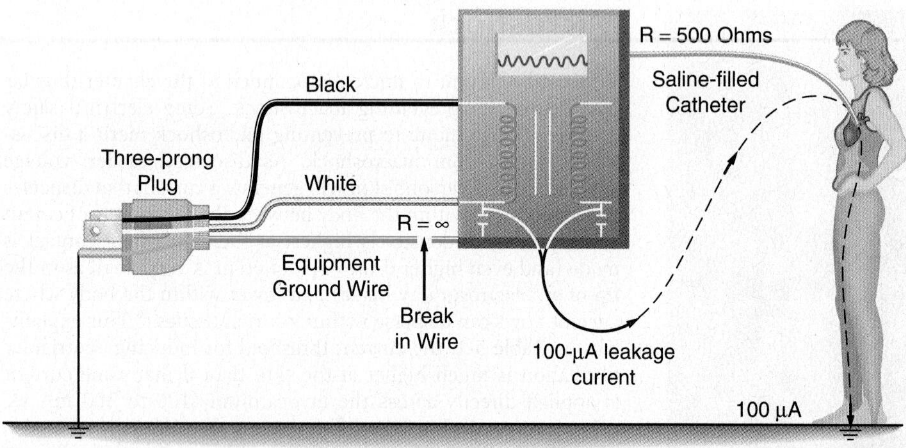

Figure 5-23 A broken equipment ground wire results in a significant hazard to the electrically susceptible patient. In this case, the entire leakage current can be conducted to the heart and may result in ventricular fibrillation. R, resistance.

pathway to ground. In the diagram, a potentially hazardous amount of leakage current is available to flow to ground and possibly through a grounded patient with a catheter near their heart. However, given two pathways to ground, each will divert a proportion of the available current based on their relative resistances. A saline catheter and a patient with skin contact to a source of earth ground is unlikely to come close to presenting as low a resistance pathway as a copper wire leading directly to a reliable source of earth ground. Thus, only a tiny fraction of the hazard current travels through the patient despite their state of electrical susceptibility. Figure 5-23 demonstrates the same scenario but with an interrupted ground wire. In this case, all the hazard current flows through the patient despite their poor conductance to earth ground.

Beyond proper grounding of equipment, there are some risk mitigation behaviors that anesthesia providers can practice such as wearing of protective gloves to reduce the risk to electrically susceptible patients. It is good practice to avoid handling a patient's central or pulmonary artery catheter while simultaneously touching a piece of plugged-in electrical equipment. Also, because a high resistance to ground is, as demonstrated above, a risk-mitigating factor, OR staff should be cognizant of the degree to which they may have an abnormally low resistance to earth ground, such as if their shoes are drenched in saline and they are standing in a puddle or near a drain or grounded power strip.

Microshock has an insidious nature; it is imperceptible to skin contact by providers, it can be caused by even properly functioning equipment, the LIM provides no protective alarms, and it is highly responsive to the extent to which a provider or patient might be grounded, such that it can happen even during commonly repeated actions if the grounding has changed. Given these factors, it is important that anesthesia providers remain vigilant to the risks of microshock and take steps to reduce its potential occurrence, even when those actions are likely to be unnecessary most of the time. The rare occurrence can still be hazardous to patients.

Safety Features within Monitors

Patient monitoring devices pose unique challenges for electrical safety because they often involve conductive wiring directly linking a patient's skin to an electrical device. Because of this, a great deal of effort goes into designing monitoring devices that isolate the sensor wiring from the high-voltage current that drives the internal electronics. Multiple methods exist to isolate sensors from high voltage including very high resistance between sensors and power supply voltage, which ensures that a power surge will direct only a small fraction of surge current to the sensor wires.[23] Another such option is the use of optical isolators (also called optocouplers or optoisolators), which involve converting an electrical signal into an optical signal with an LED and then back to electronic again with a phototransistor. These signal transmission couplings allow a signal to pass to a high-voltage system within a device without establishing a conductive pathway for high-voltage current. The optical portion of the transmission acts as a break in what would otherwise be a continuous electrical pathway.

Even with well-isolated electronics, human factors can still lead to unforeseen problems. Between 1985 and 1994, the U.S. Food and Drug Administration (FDA) was notified of 24 incidents of children and infants being electrocuted by electrocardiography (ECG) or apnea monitoring wires (5 cases were fatal).[24,25] In these cases, electrodes were accidentally plugged into mains power instead of the correct connecting cable for the monitor. To address this, in 1997, the FDA began requiring that exposed male connectors for such devices be deprecated and replaced with cabling that features female connectors only on the patient side. On the monitor side, male connectors must be housed within a protective casing (Fig. 5-24). This significantly reduces the risk of

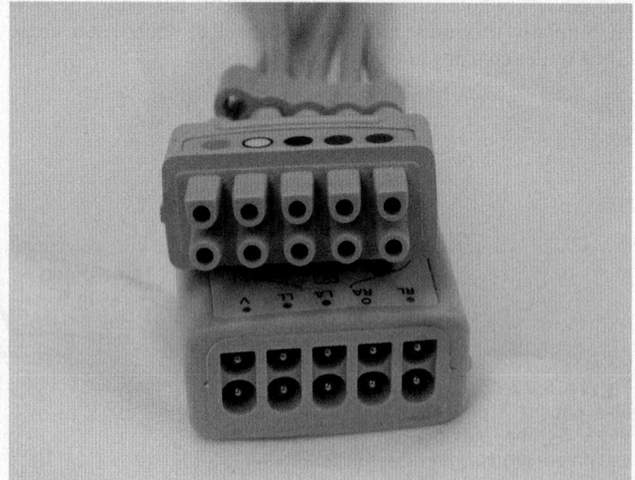

Figure 5-24 The current standard for patient lead wires (**top**) requires a female connector. The patient cable (**bottom**) has shielded connector pins that the lead wires plug into.

exposed conductors on either side of the connector and reduces the risk of connections to high voltage either by human error or equipment fault.

Electrosurgery

Electrosurgery is ubiquitous in the modern OR, often referred to by the eponymous inventor, William Bovie, or (erroneously) as electrocautery.[26] An ESU provides many surgical benefits to patients and surgeons, but it presents some hazards that OR staff must understand. It should not be surprising that a device intended to heat and cauterize tissues can serve as an ignition source if oxygen and combustion fuel are in proximity. The fire risks that electrosurgery presents are discussed in more detail later in this chapter. Interference with OR monitors and electrical-sensing implanted devices (e.g., pacemakers) is extremely common. Faulty or improperly used ESU instruments can also lead to patient burns at the return pad electrode or other metal in contact with the patient. Finally, while specifically designed to avoid inducing or interfering with cellular action potentials, electrosurgery can in some circumstances cause harmful microshock and ventricular fibrillation.

Electrosurgery functions on relatively simple principles. High-frequency AC voltage is applied across two electrodes that are in contact with the patient. Current flows through the patient from one electrode to the other. The only factor that distinguishes the cutting blade electrode from the harmless return electrode is relative size (Fig. 5-25). Heat generated within tissue is a factor of current density. Although the same amount of current flows through both the small cutting blade and the large return pad, the current density at the blade is much higher than at the return pad. This difference is more than enough to result in tissue burning and coagulating at the blade (small electrode) and passing harmlessly into the return pad (large electrode) (5 Video 5-5).[27] Radio frequency AC (500,000 to 1,000,000 Hz) is important for this use. As discussed earlier in the chapter, a lower-frequency current such as 60 Hz will excite cellular action potentials, cause muscle contraction, and potentially induce harmful arrythmias in the myocardium. However, radio frequency voltage means that voltage across voltage-gated ion channels in cell membranes is not sustained long enough to trigger their opening and radio frequency current will pass through tissues without stimulating muscle contraction or nerve conduction. This effect can be overcome with very high current density, which is why small areas of muscle contraction can be seen immediately adjacent to the ESU active electrode (blade) when in use.[28]

Although it should theoretically not be possible, there have been cases of ventricular fibrillation apparently induced by an ESU.[29–31] Although such case reports leave many unanswered questions, faulty or inadequate mains isolation may have allowed a 50-Hz or 60-Hz frequency to overlie the radiofrequency output of the ESU, rendering the current capable of inducing cellular action potentials. The use of coagulation mode near the heart in an electrically susceptible patient (e.g., one with an indwelling central catheter) seems to increase this risk.

The safety of electrosurgery is contingent on the presence of a predictable current flow pathway through the patient, which ends in a large contact area with an electrode to produce a low current density (NICV 5-1). As shown in Figure 5-26, an improperly placed, partially nonadherent, or faulty return pad with only a small contact area can create a high current density, which leads to burns at that site, and many case studies can be found to this effect.[32–36] Modern ESUs mitigate this risk with contact quality-monitoring return pads that are actually two separate conductive pads. The current from the ESU active electrode will flow to both adjacent return contacts as if they were one circuit. However, the separate conductors allow the ESU to monitor the impedance between the two conductive portions of the pad and alarm if the impedance is too high as it would indicate an improperly placed/skin-contacted pad. Patient contact to earth ground is also a risk factor for ESU-related injuries. This may seem confusing given that the return pad of an ESU is often colloquially referred to as a "ground pad" or "grounding pad." It is not connected to earth ground and the safety of the patient as well as the providers in contact with the patient would be substantially harmed if it were. Prior to 1968, ESUs did connect their return lines to the earth ground pin of the power outlet and alternate site burns were much more common until the introduction of isolated ESUs. This failure mode may serve as a reprisal of all the issues already discussed relating to the grounding versus isolation of OR power systems. An ESU that drives its output voltage against earth ground renders any earth ground contact almost as good a return pathway as the intended return pad. This dramatically increases the risk to the patient that current will return to the ESU via an unexpected pathway. A low-impedance ground contact to the patient will always increase their risk of injury somewhat when electrosurgery is used, but if that ESU power system is also grounded, then the risk is substantially greater. To make matters worse, the ESU would appear to function normally in this circumstance and the problem may not be noticed until surgery is completed. To address this, modern ESUs (just as modern ORs) isolate their internal power systems from earth ground. This ensures that the

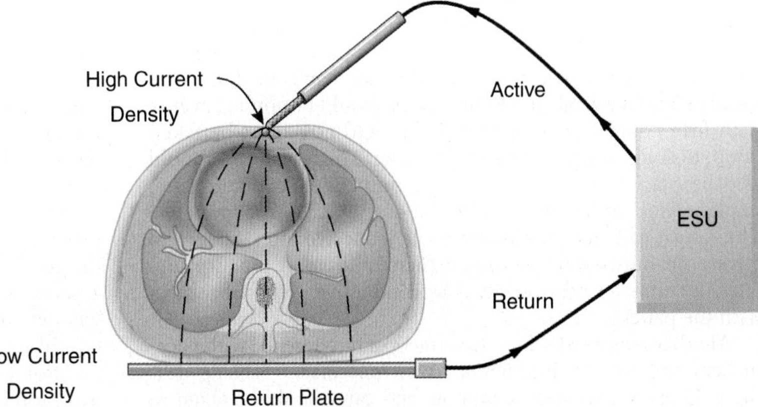

Figure 5-25 A properly applied electrosurgical unit (ESU) return plate. The current density at the return plate is low, resulting in no danger to the patient.

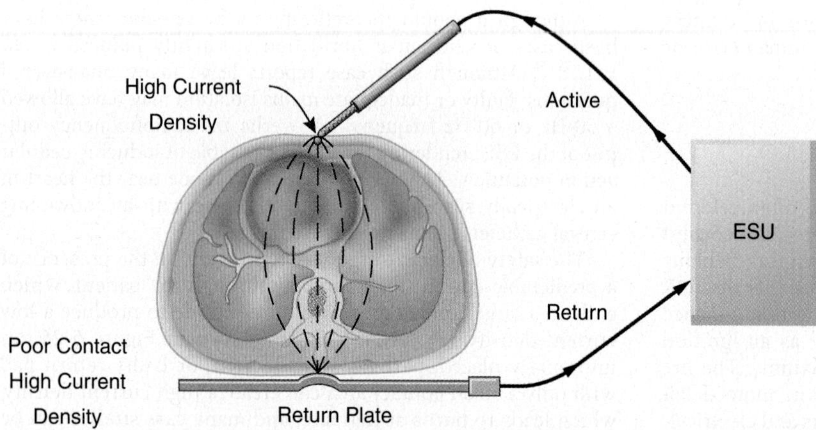

Figure 5-26 An improperly applied electrosurgical unit (ESU) return plate. Poor contact with the return plate results in a high current density and a possible burn to the patient.

lowest impedance route for current to return to the ESU will always be via the intended return pad.[37] Despite being isolated, there are still some circumstances where the ESU current can possibly return via alternate pathways. If the return pad is left in contact with the conductive casing of the ESUs (which should be connected to earth ground like all equipment conductive casing) and if the return pad is in electrical contact with a conductive OR table, then the risk of alternative return pathways is dramatically increased.

With the two safety features discussed above (contact quality-monitoring return pads and ground-isolated ESU power), alternate site burns have become relatively rare, including when metal jewelry is involved. Although removal of metal jewelry is often mandated in perioperative settings to reduce risks of ESU burns, there are actually no published case reports of alternate site burns caused by metal piercings.[38] Laboratory testing with ex vivo animal tissue demonstrates no significant heating of metal piercings between the ESU active electrode and the return pad, or even when the return pad is in direct contact with the piercing. Only direct contact or proximity with the active electrode (5 to 10 mm) demonstrated significant heating of the piercings.[39] While it is hard to argue with the safety benefit of extracting easily removed metal jewelry, when jewelry is not easily removed, anesthesia providers should weigh the risks of canceled surgeries or traumatized skin against the extremely low risk of ESU burns when such jewelry is to be distant from the active electrode.

A properly functioning ESU with an isolated power supply does not render the patient immune to ESU-related burns. Providers in the room need to remain vigilant about the proper placement of return pads, the placement of equipment with earth ground casing, and other hazards that are present even without errant ESU current pathways, such as flammable alcohol vapor near the ESU surgical site. Return pads should be applied evenly with firm contact to the patient's skin and care must be taken not to dislodge them when repositioning. The return pad should also be placed far from ECG leads and pacemaker/automatic implantable cardioverter defibrillators (AICDs) if possible. The return pad site should always be inspected after surgery to ensure no burns were sustained there, and good practice dictates the same for other electrically conductive points of contact with the patient.

Another major risk of electrosurgery is interference with pacemakers and AICDs. Interference with pacemaker sensing during ESU use is extremely common, and care should be taken in patients using pacers to mitigate the risk of interference. Avoidance of ESU entirely is a good way to prevent pacer problems in susceptible patients if surgical considerations allow. In addition, bipolar ESU produces little interference compared to unipolar. With bipolar ESU, the two electrodes are next to each other in the surgical field without a return pad. Interference can also be minimized if ESU use is below the umbilicus and the return pad can also be placed below the umbilicus.[40] However, patients should still be monitored closely for signs of hemodynamic instability caused by pacer interference even under these circumstances. If pacer interference cannot be reduced, it must usually be managed by placing a pacer into a nonsensing pacer mode such that it will continue to pace even with sensing interference from the ESU. Placing a magnet over a pacemaker generator will usually put it into a nonsensing paced rhythm, although this is not guaranteed, and pacers can be programmed to exhibit other behaviors with a magnet.

AICDs create specific considerations because interference in their sensing capability can "trick" them into defibrillating erroneously. The high-frequency electrical noise of the ESU can be misinterpreted as a tachydysrhythmia and lead to AICD shocks, which can be harmful to the patient, as well as to providers who may be in contact with the patient at the time. Although intended to fix a tachydysrhythmia, an erroneous defibrillation can put a patient into such a rhythm. The electrical interference from electroconvulsive therapy can also induce an erroneous shock from an AICD.[41] In any case where ESU or ECT interference is expected, an anesthesia provider should consider disabling the defibrillation functionality of an AICD temporarily either with a magnet or temporarily reprogramming it before the procedure.[40] When disabling defibrillator functionality in a patient's implanted device (which they were presumably given because of their intrinsic risk of tachydysrhythmia), an external defibrillator should be available. If defibrillation is needed, a provider should first attempt to remove the magnet from an AICD and observe for a therapeutic response from the AICD and only defibrillate from the external source if the AICD does not respond.[42]

Safe use of electrosurgery is everyone's concern in an OR. All providers should feel empowered to speak frankly about risks to the patient such as the extent to which ESU may interfere with a pacer, whether a return pad appears to be placed correctly, or whether increasing amplitude of ESU settings beyond what is typical might be a sign that something is wrong with the equipment or setup. ESU-related burns and microshock can be insidious problems that are not always obvious until real damage has been done to a patient. Patients benefit when everyone in the OR is vigilant to these potential problems.

Electromagnetic Interference

Electrical interference of implanted and external medical devices takes two common forms. The first is current flows directly across a device's sensing electrodes, as was discussed in the previous section on electrosurgery. The second form will be discussed here and is caused by electromagnetic radiation. Such radiation can be produced intentionally, as with a radio transmitter, or incidentally as with high-voltage transmission of ACs or high-frequency current switching in modern computers. Electromagnetic radiation is a general term that encompasses all wavelengths of photon transmission. Thus, the light emitting from a nearby light source and producing an image on the retina is electromagnetic radiation, as are the harmless radio signals conveying data to a phone. Some wavelengths of this radiation are of high enough energy to knock electrons away from their stable state and ionize a molecule or atom. This process can be harmful if it happens within the body of a living organism, which has led to cultural distrust of anything using the word "radiation." However, the word simply means any form of energy transmission through empty space or propagation through a medium.

Wireless communication devices that emit electromagnetic radiation have proliferated rapidly through society, and hospitals are no exception. Rather than just being common but incidentally held devices, they are often considered essential components of communication within health care teams in modern practice. Providers frequently communicate via SMS messaging, electronic medical records often have a smartphone app, and the massive increase in the use of videoconferencing since the COVID-19 pandemic began has made joining a meeting from a mobile device a common occurrence in any workplace. All of these factors have pushed powerful mobile communication devices into the pockets of almost everyone in the hospital and OR. Electromagnetic interactions between these devices and medical devices will become increasingly common.

Electromagnetic interference (EMI) is a difficult topic to study for a variety of reasons. When connecting devices to sensitive electrical probing instruments in a laboratory setting, an EMI impact is generally easy to find on almost any electrical system. Determining whether a slight blip or deviation on a voltage tracing actually matters in the real-world use of a device is often much harder to assess. Incidents of EMI disrupting medical equipment or implanted devices are rare, and like any rare incident, strong data are expensive and time consuming to collect. In addition, rarity often leads research dollars to be spent on more common problems. Finally, the EMI landscape is rapidly changing; in the time it would take a researcher to collect good data on clinically significant interference of 3G mobile communications devices with pacemakers, 4G networks may be appearing. As a result, clear and specific guidelines about EMI risk are unlikely to exist, and to the extent that they do, they are unlikely to remain relevant for long.

Although a variety of individual case studies exist, they do not shed much light on a risk assessment for such rare adverse events. Few large-scale studies assess these risks. One such study by Hayes et al.[43] ran 5,533 tests on 980 patients with implanted pacemakers using mobile phones as a source of EMI. In worst-case scenarios (phones set to maximum transmission power and placed close to the pacer), 20% of tests demonstrated detectable interference, and 6.6% of patients had clinically significant interference. With the phones used at the ear under normal operating conditions, no clinically significant interference was detected. Another study by von Olshausen et al.[44] studied 2,940 patients with implantable cardioverter defibrillators over a span of years, finding a detectable EMI event rate of 1.87% per patient per year and a clinically significant or potentially significant event rate of just 0.27% per patient per year. Keep in mind the discussion above about how rapidly these technologies change: the study by Hayes was published in 1997 and von Olshausen collected data from 2005 to 2013. Even with these large studies, these risk assessments may no longer be relevant in today's electrical device environment.

Devices tend to be more sensitive to low-frequency EMI, such as that given off by local two-way radio (walkie-talkie) and high-voltage power switching in industrial settings. Higher-frequency EMI tends to be less problematic for medical devices. Local two-way radio operates in the MHz radio frequencies, whereas wireless networking (WiFi) and mobile broadband operate within the GHz range. Newer wireless standards also trend toward using higher frequencies to increase bandwidth for faster data transfer, such as WiFi transitioning from 2.4 to 5 GHz and mobile broadband transitioning through multiple generations (e.g., 2G/GSM, 3G, 4G/LTE, 5G), increasing from 900 MHz up to approximately 40 GHz in modern standards. Bluetooth wireless communications can extend down to 2 MHz but are also extremely low transmission power. Given all this, the EMI risk to implanted devices is much lower from modern wireless communication devices than in decades past.[45] Although not related to EMI specifically, it is notable that many modern mobile devices and accessories use neodymium magnets for both structural attachment between devices and cases or accessories, as well as aligning charging connections. Such magnets can trigger magnet placement functionality in implantable devices. Just as with EMI, users should avoid keeping such devices too close to an implantable device.[46]

Putting this all together leads to some reasonable takeaways and conclusions. The FDA recommends keeping mobile electronic devices at least 6 inches away from cardiac implantable electronic devices.[47] Studies suggest that the normal use of such devices is extremely unlikely to result in clinically significant EMI. As wireless transmissions transition to higher-frequency radios and electronics become better shielded and maintain more of their internal signal chain as a digital signal (which is much less susceptible to EMI than an analog signal), it can be expected that interactions between modern devices will be less prone to significant EMI than the already small risks demonstrated in past decades. As such, clinically significant EMI is likely something an anesthesia provider does not need to worry about under normal circumstances. However, such EMI is possible under abnormal conditions, so providers should remain mindful of potential impacts and additional non-EMI interactions such as devices with magnetic connections.

Emergency Backup Power

Given that modern health care requires electricity to function, it should be no surprise that hospitals and many other health care facilities are required to maintain a source of emergency backup power. Backup power should be available within 10 seconds of main utility power loss, according to National Fire Protection Association (NFPA) 99 and 110 building codes.[48,49] Such backup systems often take the form of fuel-powered generators that turn on when loss of utility power is detected. In some cases, batteries or flywheel systems may be in place to provide instantaneous coverage of an outage during the time it takes generators to start. The NFPA maintains practice standards for hospitals that include regular testing of backup power systems.[48,49] Such systems should also be able to run for at least 2 days without utility power. Because emergency backup power is unlikely to cover the full normal power load of the hospital, outlets serviced by backup power are red to denote that they should remain active in a power loss. Mission-critical equipment should always be plugged into red outlets, and equipment that is not essential should be plugged in elsewhere if there is another option. This will ensure that critical equipment is powered in an emergency and precious emergency electrical load capacity is not wasted on noncritical equipment such as coffee makers and entertainment devices.

Although natural disasters are a common cause of power loss to hospitals, it is important to remember that construction is another major cause of power loss. In fact, construction mishaps can be more problematic than natural disasters because they often result in broken connections within the hospital power system and emergency backup power designed to turn on when utility power is lost will not activate. Hospitals should have a contingency plan for loss of power in every location that anesthesia is provided. The plan should include the possibility that backup power may not be readily available. Battery-powered light sources, anesthesia machines with internal battery backup power, and provider education about how to manage a power loss are vital components to navigating a power loss emergency.[50] Even an anesthesia machine that is electronically controlled should fail over into a manual ventilation state in the event of power and battery failure. This allows the anesthesia provider to manually ventilate a patient with oxygen and deliver anesthetic vapor, although desflurane, which requires a powered vaporizer, will not be available. It is important not only that resources are available, but also that staff are trained in how to use them and where to find them in an emergency. Anesthesia providers should remain aware that they can still manually ventilate and anesthetize a patient even with an anesthesia machine that normally requires electronic input to switch to a manual ventilation mode.

Regulations and Building Codes

What happens within hospitals presents significant health and safety implications on a societal level: not just for patients with dangerous health conditions, but also for health care providers who are potentially exposed to radiation, infectious diseases, collisions with heavy and mobile equipment, and other hazards. As such, it should be no surprise that there is a substantial regulatory framework in place to set minimum standards for hazard prevention and response. The NFPA maintains a national collection of building codes, including those that cover health care facilities, life safety, and emergency power systems (NFPA 99, 101, and 110, respectively). The history of building codes for electrical systems within ORs can largely be understood as a discussion of three separate questions: (1) Are flammable gases used routinely in ORs? (2) Is an OR a wet procedure location? and (3) Is it safe to interrupt power in an OR?

The first of these three questions is the most straightforward. Before the introduction of halothane, almost all inhalational anesthetics used in ORs were flammable; since then, none are. Nitrous oxide is worth mentioning because it is often erroneously considered flammable. Nitrous oxide is not flammable, but it can support combustion just as oxygen does and should be avoided in the same situations where a high oxygen concentration is a combustion risk. Due to the previously common use of flammable anesthetic gases, electrical safety code for ORs required the use of an IPS and LIM. The relevant NFPA 99 code was revised in 1984 to remove this requirement because of the dearth of flammable anesthetics in use since then.[51,52]

The next two questions become relevant with subsequent revisions of NFPA 99, which specify that the following "wet procedure locations shall be provided with special protection against electrical shock." A subsection defines special protection as a "(1) power distribution system that inherently limits the possible ground-fault current due to a first fault to a low value, without interrupting the power supply, (2) power distribution system in which the power supply is interrupted if the ground-fault current does, in fact, exceed the trip value of a Class A GFCI."[48] At this point in the chapter, it should be easy to identify system (1) as an Isolated Power System and system (2) as a GFCI. Additional language in this code describes this choice more plainly: "the use of an isolated power system shall be permitted as a protective means capable of limiting ground-fault current without power interruption." Thus, the fundamental electrical regulatory questions about the modern OR come into focus. Is special protection needed at all? If so, is an IPS required or is a GFCI sufficient? The language of the code reduces these two questions to those mentioned at the start of this section: is an OR a wet procedure space, meaning special protection is required? If so, can power be interrupted? If not, an IPS is required.

The consequences of reliance on GFCIs were discussed in detail earlier. Reviewing briefly, GFCIs are components that protect users only from a "hazard in progress," which need to actuate beyond their resting state to achieve that protection, and achieve that protection only by cutting power to potentially mission-critical equipment. An IPS, on the other hand, prevents a hazard state for a first fault, does so without needing to actuate anything, and offers this protection without a surprise power loss to vital equipment. As for an IPS not needing to actuate, recall that the LIM (which is an active component that can fail) is not needed to protect users from a first fault. It is only needed to alert users to the presence of the first fault so that they can take appropriate action before a second fault.

This issue attracts the attention of stakeholders who are concerned about the cost of installing and maintaining equipment whose safety features are needed only infrequently, as well as stakeholders who are concerned about the safety of their patients and themselves. Such stakeholders often find themselves on opposite sides of the debate about the necessity or lack thereof of an IPS in an OR. While such debates are ongoing, the current state of NFPA 99 standards was revised in 2012 and 2015 to state the following: "ORs shall be considered to be a wet procedure location, unless a risk assessment conducted by the health care governing body determines otherwise." However, the standards go on to state that "operating rooms defined as wet procedure locations shall be protected by either isolated power or ground fault circuit interrupters."[48] In addition, the 2015 standards added a stipulation that if a GFCI is used to protect ORs, then each outlet should have its own separate GFCI. These standards remain in the latest 2021 edition of NFPA 99.[48]

This leaves the current status of this regulatory framework requiring that ORs are designated wet procedure areas necessitating special protection unless separate approval is granted to declare an OR dry. When an OR is designated as a wet area, either an IPS or GFCI is required. The purpose of this section is not to advocate one way or the other. Certainly, it is possible to imagine a theoretical safety measure that incurs the same costs as the installation of an IPS but has a larger safety impact. Similarly, some may suggest that it is obvious that ORs are a wet procedural area and that IPSs are doubtless the best way to protect them. The purpose of this section is to bring attention to this ongoing debate about the regulations that many physicians consider "someone else's problem to sort out." As stakeholders in this regulatory framework (in the most literal sense as we are individually affected by electrocution risk), anesthesia providers should understand the importance of these safety regulations and insist that other stakeholders take seriously the tradeoffs inherent to these questions. It is important to understand the implications of a hospital attempting to classify ORs as dry locations and the risks of such a change.[53]

Operating Room Fires

The original concern for fires in the OR derived from the presence of highly flammable or explosive (ether, cyclopropane, ethylene, ethyl chloride) volatile anesthetics. In the past, static electricity was the most common ignition source.[54] The concern for fire was once so high that conductive flooring was required for ORs and everyone in an OR was advised to wear grounded shoes to reduce the risk of a static electricity spark. This was because the flammable anesthetics were typically delivered by mask and were therefore not contained within a closed system. With these anesthetics no longer in clinical use, conductive flooring to prevent static electricity sparks is no longer an OR construction requirement.[48] However, static electricity can still spark a fire in the presence of an alcohol-based skin preparation in 21% oxygen without electrocautery, as has been reported.[55,56]

In modern ORs, significant fire risks persist because other risks have replaced those eliminated by removing flammable anesthetics. These include the transition from nonflammable skin preparation solutions such as povidone–iodine to flammable isopropyl alcohol-based ones and the substitution of cloth drapes with more flammable paper drapes. In addition, the advent of laser procedures in the OR has created its own fire risks.

To put the modern OR fire risk in perspective, in 2013, the Emergency Care Research Institute included OR fires as one of the top 10 technology hazards. For context, to become an identified technology hazard, the hazard must have resulted in death, occurred frequently, or have a high profile.[57] The institute estimated that there were at least 600 OR fires annually.[57] That averages to approximately 12 fires per week, that is, more than 2 per weekday, occurring somewhere in the United States. Despite much attention to the topic of fire awareness and prevention led by the American Society of Anesthesiologists (ASA) and the Anesthesia Patient Safety Foundation (APSF), the most recent estimates still describe a current annual incidence of at least 100 fires.[56,58,59] However, these remain rough estimates that likely represent a significant underestimation because many states do not have mandatory reporting. The lower, more recent OR fire incidence estimate represents substantial progress but certainly not an elimination of this serious adverse event. OR fires are sentinel events, yet they still occur at least twice weekly despite being considered overwhelmingly avoidable with well-disseminated knowledge regarding prevention.[60,61]

American Society of Anesthesiologists Fire Prevention Practice Advisory

The most recent ASA practice advisory on the "Prevention and Management of Operating Room Fires" was published in 2013.[61] The recommendations are detailed in Figure 5-27. The APSF has also made an excellent instructive video, titled "Prevention and Management of Operating Room Fires."[62]

Several points bear particular emphasis when there is a fire risk and an open oxygen source: (1) Does the patient really need supplemental oxygen? Room air is preferred if oxygen saturation remains acceptable without supplemental oxygen; (2) If a high fire risk is present and >0.3 FIO_2 is needed for adequate oxygenation, secure the airway; and (3) If there is a high fire risk, do not give nasal cannula or face mask supplemental oxygen via the barbed oxygen flowmeter because it can only deliver 100% oxygen. Instead, use the air and oxygen flowmeters or a blender to deliver a reduced oxygen concentration.

Fire Triangle/Tetrahedron

To better appreciate the risk of fire, it is useful to consider what is required to start a fire (6 Video 5-6). The triad of com- 7
ponents necessary for fire initiation is termed the fire triangle (Fig. 5-28). More recently a fourth component, required for a fire to continue to burn and make the triangle a tetrahedron, has been added. This fourth component becomes the floor of the fire triangle (Fig. 5-29) and is an uninhibited chemical chain reaction between fuel(s) and oxidizer(s). This is required for the fire to continuously oxidize more fuel to sustain itself, thereby making it a fire instead of a flash or explosion.[63] The sides of the triangle are oxidizer, fuel, and ignition (heat/spark) source, while the tetrahedron adds a sustaining chemical reaction enabled by the continued availability of the oxidizer and fuel. As abundantly evident from Table 5-3, the modern OR is replete with elements from all three triangle components. One should think of each component as both an element of fire risk and an opportunity to be aware of and mitigate that risk. Within the OR team, the anesthesia provider, surgeon, and circulating nurse/scrub technician typically each control a component. The anesthesia provider determines how much and what oxidizer is/are present (FIO_2/N_2O), the surgeon operates the ignition source(s) and settings (electrosurgery/laser), and the nurse/scrub technician manages many of the fuels (alcohol-based skin preparation, preparation drying time, draping, and whether the electrosurgical unit is turned on and gauze and sponges are moistened). The anesthesia provider additionally determines whether the airway is open (nasal cannula/mask) or sealed (cuffed endotracheal tube/laryngeal mask).

Flammability, Oxygen Concentration, Gas Density, and Nitrous Oxide

The flammability of a combustible object is a measurement of how easily it burns. Flammability increases with any oxygen enrichment. A flammable drape that will burn in 21% oxygen will ignite slightly quicker in 25% oxygen, even quicker in 30%, and so on. Culp et al., using a variety of common flammable OR materials, demonstrated a nonlinear increase in flammability with an increase in ambient oxygen concentration.[64] Using a bench model with a match as the ignition source and 21%, 50%, and 100% oxygen, the study found that the median [minimum, maximum] ignition time in 21% oxygen was 0.9 seconds [0.3, 1.9], 0.4 seconds [0.1, 1.2] in 50% oxygen, and 0.2 seconds [0.0, 0.4] in 100% oxygen.[64] Some items such as the utility drape or surgical gown that did not burn in room air ignited in less than 0.5 s in 50% oxygen. With each doubling of the oxygen concentration, there

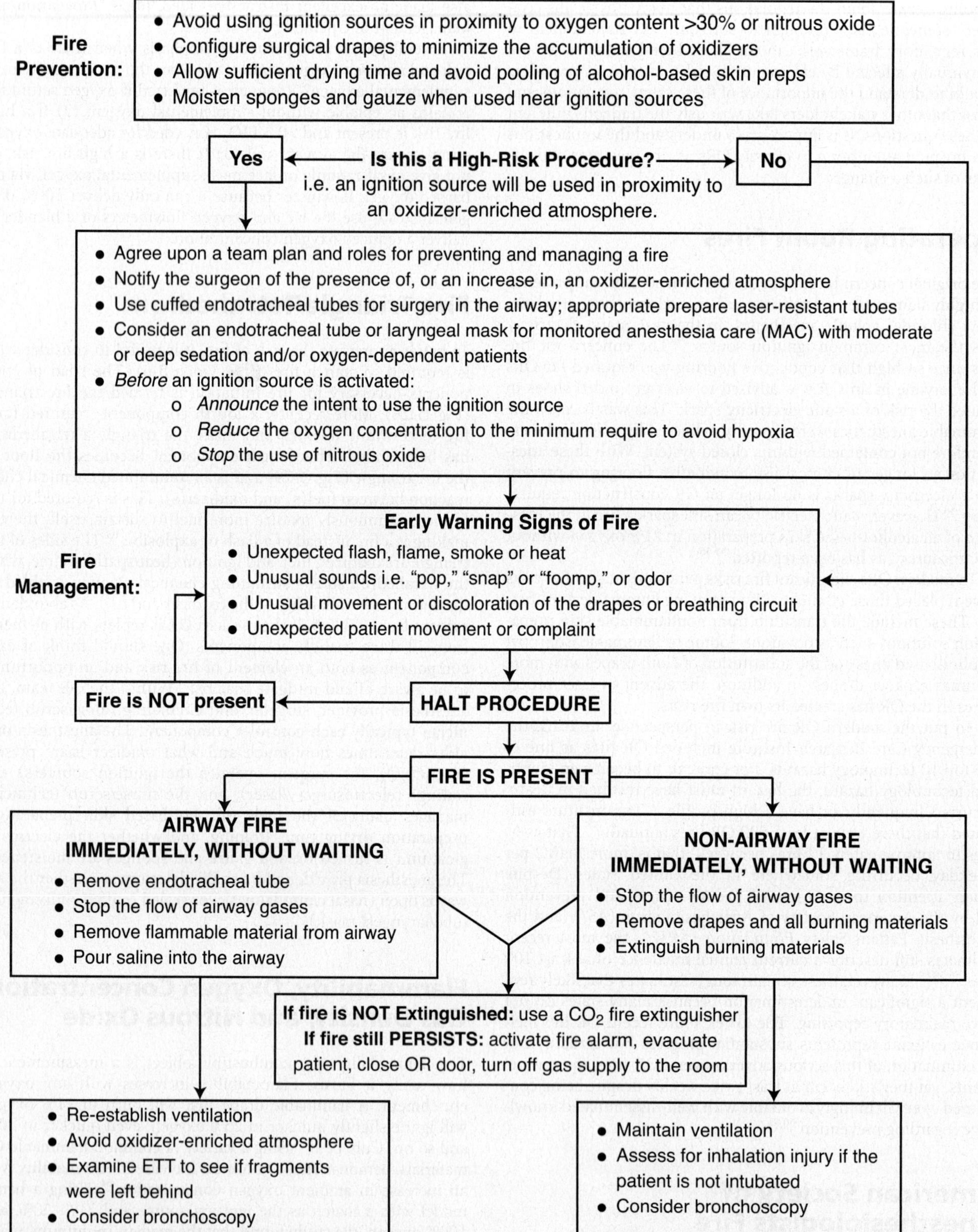

Figure 5-27 American Society of Anesthesiologists fire safety algorithm. (Reprinted with permission from An Updated Report by the American Society of Anesthesiologists Task Force on Operating Room Fires. *Anesthesiology* 2013;118:271–290. doi: https://doi.org/10.1097/ALN.0b013e31827773d2.)

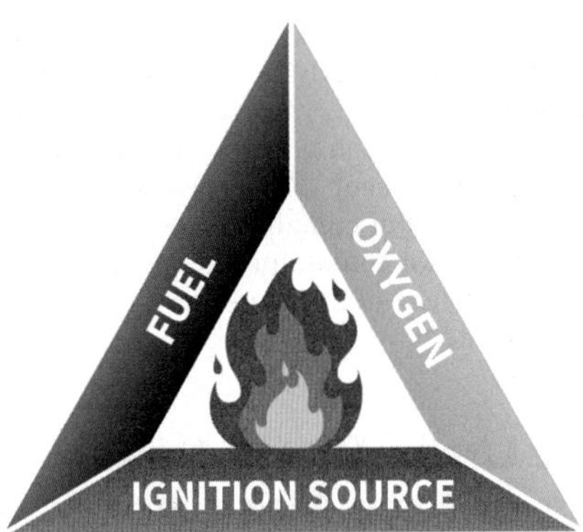

Figure 5-28 The fire triangle. (Reprinted with permission, Copyright, Emergency Care Research Institute d/b/a ECRI. www.ecri.org. 5200 Butler Pike, Plymouth Meeting, PA 19462. This Material is protected by copyright laws and may not in whole, in part, or by reference be used in any advertising or promotional material, or to compete with ECRI.)

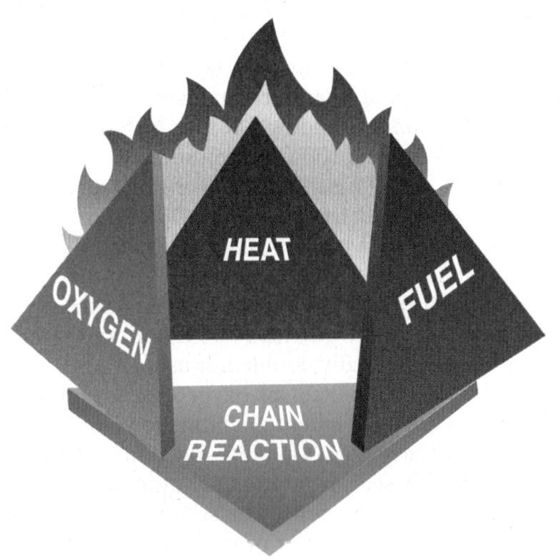

Figure 5-29 The fire tetrahedron.

Table 5-3 Examples of Operating Room Fire Triangle Components

Oxidizers
- Air
- Oxygen
- Nitrous oxide

Fuels
- Alcohol
- Drape (paper > cloth)
- Gauze
- Hair
- Nasal cannula
- Face mask
- Endotracheal tube
- Laryngeal mask airway
- Breathing circuit hoses
- Intestinal gases

Ignition Sources
- Electrosurgery
- Laser
- Bipolar ESU

Table 5-4 Flammability of Surgical Materials

Materials	Ignition Time in 21% O_2 (s)	Ignition Time in 50% O_2 (s)	Ignition Time in 100% O_2 (s)
Laparotomy sponge	0.9 [0.8, 1.4]	0.3 [0.1, 1.0]	0.1 [0.0, 0.1]
Utility drape	Did not ignite	0.2 [0.1, 0.4]	0.2 [0.1, 0.4]
Surgical gown	Did not ignite	0.4 [0.3, 0.4]	0.3 [0.2, 0.4]
Blue operating room towel	1.6 [1.3, 1.9]	0.5 [0.4, 0.5]	0.1 [0.1, 0.2]

Ignition times for each sample type in room air, 50% oxygen, and 100% oxygen environments, expressed as mean [minimum, maximum].
Modified with permission from Culp WC Jr, Kimbrough BA, Luna S. Flammability of surgical drapes and materials in varying concentrations of oxygen. *Anesthesiology*. 2013;119:770–776.

was an approximate halving of the time to ignition (Table 5-4). A general recommendation is to not allow the ambient oxygen concentration to exceed 30% where a fire risk exists.[61,62] It is an interesting fact that fire will generally not propagate if the oxygen concentration is less than 16%, but it is obviously not clinically practical to do that.[65] One of the benefits of using carbon dioxide as the insufflation gas in thoracoscopic and laparoscopic procedures is that the carbon dioxide replaces or dilutes any oxidizing gases in the operative site and carbon dioxide is in and of itself fire quenching. Because oxygen with a molar mass of 15.9994 g/mol has a higher density than nitrogen at 14.0067 g/mol, it will sink and risks accumulating in a patient's pillow or hair and under a drape. This is a relevant consideration during open delivery of supplemental oxygen via a nasal cannula or mask and another reason to avoid configuring drapes around the head and neck in a way that promotes oxygen accumulation under the drapes. A suction under the drapes near the face significantly speeds dissipation of accumulated oxygen when supplemental oxygen administration is stopped.[66]

Like oxygen, nitrous oxide is an oxidizer; as such, it is an additive oxidizer to oxygen. The flammability index of a material is the minimum fraction of oxidant (oxygen or nitrous oxide) in which it will burn.[67] The polyvinyl chloride (PVC) laser ignition flammability index of nitrous oxide is approximately twice that of oxygen, that is, the oxygen flammability index for a PVC endotracheal tube is 0.25 and for nitrous oxide it is 0.45. For a Salem sump nasogastric tube, the oxygen flammability index is 0.229 and for nitrous oxide it is 0.43.[67,68] Despite nitrous oxide being a less potent oxidizer than oxygen, a conservative heuristic when assessing fire risk is to treat the concentrations of oxygen and nitrous oxide as additive. Even better, simply avoid nitrous oxide when there is a fire risk.

Assessing Fire Risk during the Presurgical Timeout

Prior to any procedure, a fire-risk assessment should be performed. An example of basic questions to be asked and considered during a presurgical timeout is shown in Table 5-5. A score of three or higher is considered high risk and special attention should be paid to fire prevention. A fundamental step includes mandating that an alcohol-containing skin preparation is allowed to dry for at least 3 minutes. The skin preparation should be allowed to completely dry and the evaporated alcohol vapors

Table 5-5 Fire-Risk Assessment

	Score
1: Procedure above xiphoid	1 (yes) 0 (no)
2: Alcohol-based skin preparation used prior to incision	1 (yes) 0 (no)
3: Open oxidizer (O_2/N_2O) source nasal cannula, face mask, uncuffed ETT	1 (yes) 0 (no)
4: Ignition source (cautery, laser, fiberoptic light)	1 (yes) 0 (no)

Modified from Fire prevention: avoid oxygen to face. *OR Manager*. 2010; 26(1):19–21.

dissipated before draping. In addition, ensure that no puddle of alcohol-containing preparation solution has formed, which could subsequently evaporate under the drape and create a fuel vapor bomb that can be ignited. Some areas of the body, such as hair, can take considerably longer to completely dry.[69]

If an open (e.g., nasal cannula, face mask) oxidizer source will be used during a procedure above the xiphoid, there should also be confirmation that there is no tunneling space under the drapes between the oxygen source and the surgical field. Then, and consistent with patient needs, the oxygen concentration should be limited to 30% or less; otherwise, it is advised to seal the airway.[62]

In addition, for high–fire-risk procedures, moistened sponges should be used because they are less flammable, a basin or bottle of sterile irrigating fluid should be readily available, and ignition sources should be kept away from the drapes. When a high fire risk is identified during the timeout, all parties, who each control a limb of the fire triangle, should acknowledge their awareness and preemptive plan. This communication is essential. The fire risk for a procedure may increase or decrease as the procedure evolves.

OR Fires and Lessons from Closed Claims and Review Findings

The most recent closed claims analysis of OR fires was published in 2013 and includes cases dating to 1985.[70] The findings remain instructive because most of the underlying hazards still exist. In that analysis of 103 fires, electrosurgery was the heat/ignition source in 90% of cases. Most fires (81%) occurred during monitored anesthesia care or regional anesthesia care. A recurring theme was that supplemental oxygen was administered via an open system (nasal cannula or face mask). Of the fires in the closed claims analysis, 85% occurred during head, neck, or upper chest procedures. Significantly, the authors observed that oxygen was often administered at flow rates and/or concentrations higher than what were likely needed to maintain an acceptable oxygen saturation. For fires occurring under general anesthesia, tracheostomy and tonsillectomy were the two most common operations.[70] The recurring etiology appears to be electrosurgery in the presence of an elevated oxidizer concentration at the operative site, that is, an oxygen ± nitrous oxide concentration >30% from a leak into the operative site, for example, an uncuffed tube. In a separate review of fires associated with tonsillectomy, an uncuffed tube and oxygen concentration >30% were noted in 35 of 36 reported cases.[71,72] A series of images from a manikin simulation set up to duplicate a case where a fire occurred during a burr hole placement with supplemental oxygen by face mask and monopolar electrosurgery provide a vivid demonstration of the speed and intensity of the fire (Fig. 5-30). In this case simulation, Barker and Polson observed through a series of trials in their manikin model that fire did not occur if: (1) there was no supplemental oxygen, or (2) no alcohol-containing preparation solution was used, or (3) the alcohol-containing preparation was allowed to dry for 5 minutes instead of 2 minutes, or (4) the drapes did not create a closed space.[73]

Why Is 2 L/min O_2 via Nasal Cannula or Face Mask Not Safe for High–Fire-Risk Cases?

Historical teaching is the heuristic that for each liter per minute of nasal cannula O_2 flow, the patient's inspired oxygen concentration increases 3% to 4%.

Using this formula, 2 L/min of supplemental O_2 administered via nasal cannula should typically yield an inspired oxygen concentration of 27% to 29%. It does in fact do that, but that is the oxygen concentration **at the alveolar level**. The fundamentally 8 important point to understanding OR fires is that at 2 L/min, the nasal cannula is delivering 100% oxygen at 2,000 mL/min into the space around the face of a patient who is resting at one MET and therefore only consuming less than 4 mL O_2/kg/min.[74] This leaves an excess of over 1,500 mL/min O_2 that is denser than nitrogen and can accumulate around a patient's head, hair, and neck, thereby making this area substantially oxygen enriched. If giving 4 L/min of supplemental O_2 instead of 2 L/min, the ambient oxygen enrichment is essentially doubled. If using a nasal mask–type device or supplying supplemental oxygen via a high-flow nasal cannula, this oxygen enrichment phenomenon is magnified even further.[75,76] It is an easy trap to fall into, but add in a drape, beard, or residual alcohol-based preparation solution and a cautery and the risk of fire becomes obvious. The seemingly routine practice of always giving at least 2 L/min of supplemental O_2 during any sedation case should be seriously reconsidered, particularly for high–fire-risk cases such as those where cautery is used near the upper chest or head. As the ASA and APSF advise: "*reduce* the delivered oxygen concentration to the minimum required to avoid hypoxia."[61,77] Effective workarounds to achieve a lower delivered oxygen concentration are to instead connect the nasal cannula using a 15-mm adapter (e.g., the adapter from a 4.5 endotracheal tube) to the breathing circuit elbow (with the APL valve closed) or to the auxiliary common gas outlet of the anesthesia machine. Then the air and oxygen flowmeters or FIO_2 selection on the anesthesia machine can be used to provide 30% oxygen or less (Fig. 5-31).[78] It is important to be aware of how surprisingly little oxygen it takes in an air-oxygen mixture to increase the delivered oxygen concentration to 30% (Table 5-6). A 2 L/min fresh gas flow, using 200 mL/min O_2 and 1.8 L/min air (i.e., a 1:9 O_2:air ratio) creates a delivered oxygen concentration of 29%.[62] Any air:oxygen ratio less than 7:1 yields a greater than 30% deliv- 9 ered oxygen. A comfortable nasal cannula flow rate is 4 L/min: using 3.5 L/min air with 0.5 L/min O_2 (a 7:1 ratio) results in delivery of 30% oxygen. Reducing oxygen further, such as 0.25 L/min O_2 with 3.5 L/min air, yields a lower delivered O_2 of 26% and a further reduction in flammability.

Even though it is clinically affirming to give supplemental oxygen routinely to sedated patients, there is no medical care requirement to give supplemental oxygen to a sedated patient who has an otherwise clinically acceptable oxygen saturation.[77] Supplemental oxygen is often unnecessary, and can be avoided if there

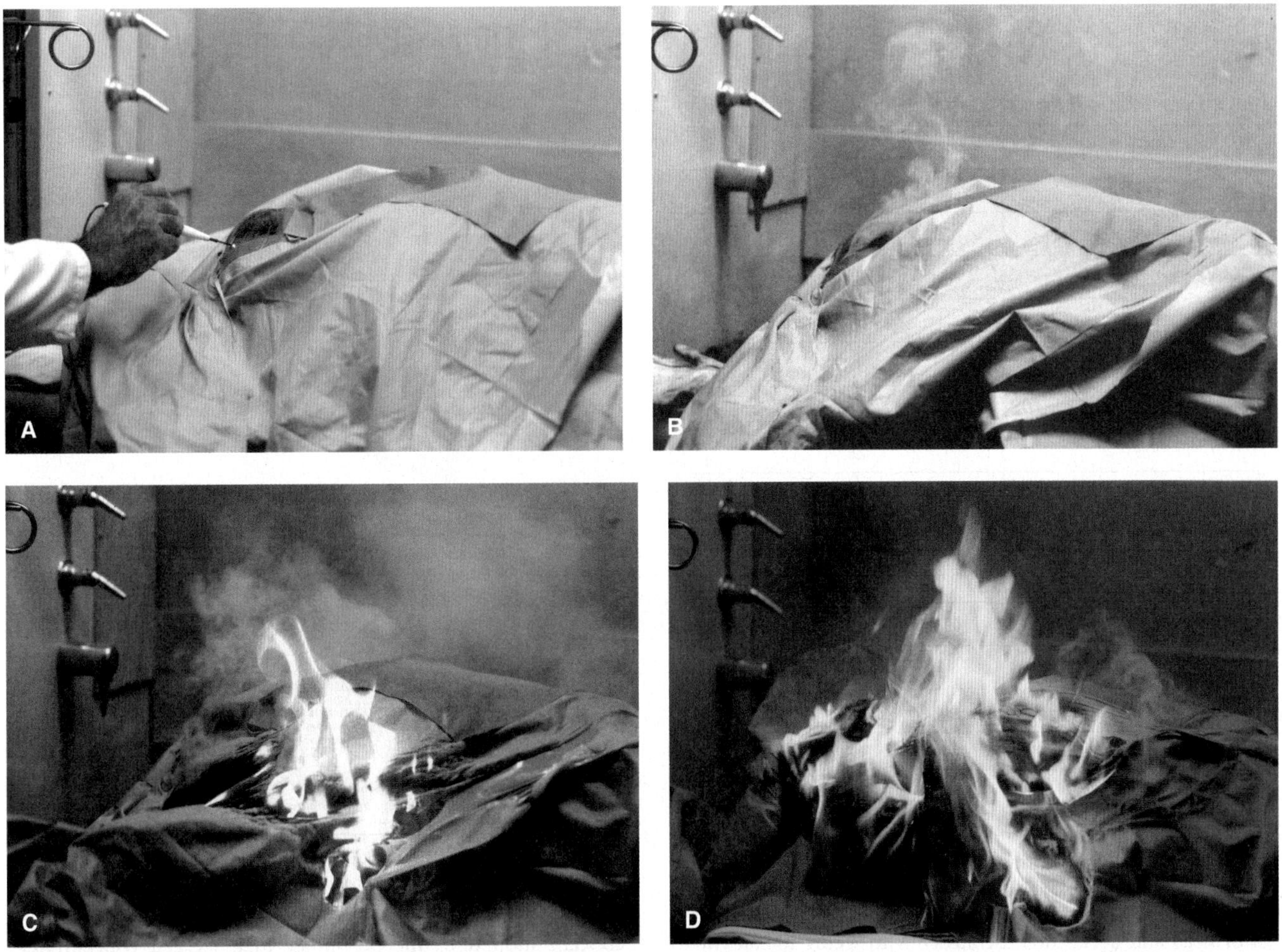

Figure 5-30 Simulation of fire caused by ESU electrode during surgery. **A:** Mannequin prepared and draped for surgery. Electrosurgical unit monopolar pencil electrode applied to operative site at the start of surgery. **B:** Six seconds after electrosurgical unit application. Smoke appears from under the drapes. **C:** Fourteen seconds after electrosurgical unit application. Flames burst through the drapes. **D:** Twenty-four seconds after electrosurgical unit application. Entire patient head and drapes in flames. (Reprinted with permission from Barker SJ, Polson JS. Fire in the operating room: A case report and laboratory study. *Anesth Analg*. 2001;93:960. Copyright © 2001, International Anesthesia Research Society.)

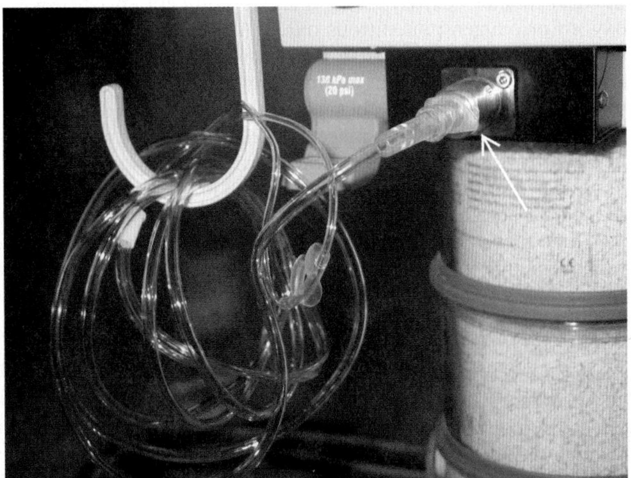

Figure 5-31 A nasal cannula connected to the alternate fresh gas outlet (*arrow*) on a GE-Datex-Ohmeda Aestiva anesthesia machine.

is a fire risk. Beginning from a 7:1 supplemental air:oxygen ratio via a nasal cannula or face mask, it is advisable to titrate down to room air or to the lowest amount of supplemental oxygen that maintains an adequate oxygen saturation. It is helpful to maintain some fresh gas flow over the face of a draped patient, even if only of room air, as otherwise the oxygen concentration under the drape can decrease and carbon dioxide can accumulate.[79] Placing a source of suction near the patient's face is another method for producing a flow of fresh room air.

It is a truism that when giving supplemental oxygen via a face mask or nasal cannula under a drape, oxygen can and will accumulate around the patient's head. The choice of surgical field drapes and draping in an upper body procedure also impacts oxygen accumulation. Surgical towels are porous and allow the supplemental oxygen to diffuse into the operative field. This decreases the oxygen accumulation around the face but increases it in the field. With a plastic drape, the opposite happens: There is less of an oxygen increase on the surgical side of the drape but more underneath the drape.[80] Thus, with an open oxygen source and a high–fire-risk procedure, the fire risk persists regardless of the draping material choice. Oxygen under the drape can

Table 5-6 Impact of Air:Oxygen Flow Ratios on Delivered Oxygen Concentration

Air : Oxygen Ratio (L/min)	Resulting Oxygen Concentration
1:1	60%
1:2	47%
1:3	40%
1:4	36%
1:5	34%
1:6	32%
1:7	30%
1:8	29%
1:9	28%
1:10	28%
1:11	27%
1:12	27%
1:13	26%
1:14	26%
1:15	26%

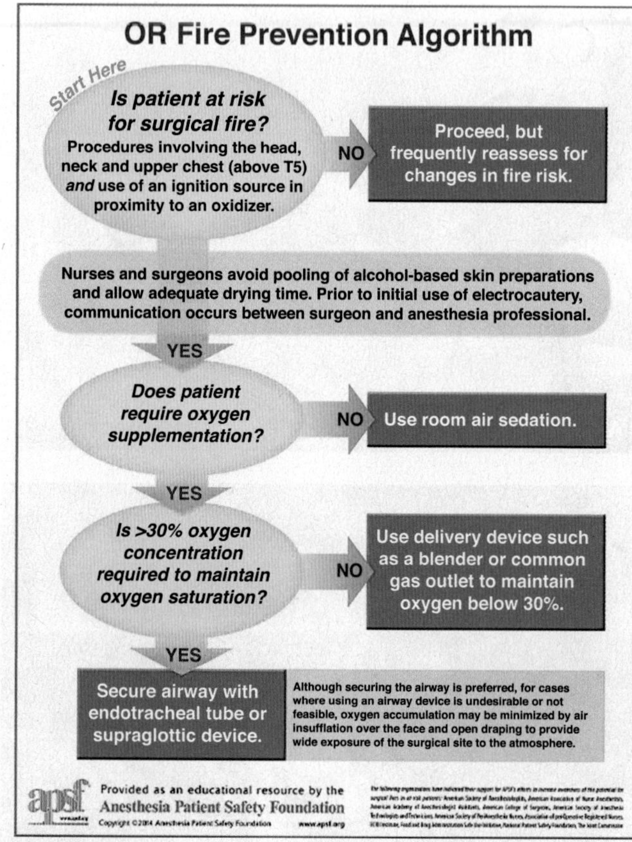

Figure 5-32 Anesthesia Patient Safety Foundation fire prevention algorithm.

contaminate the operative field either through permeability of the drape or imperfect sealing of the operative site with a plastic drape. If a patient is expected to require or requires a delivered oxygen concentration >30% during a procedure on the upper thorax or head and neck, then the advice is to secure the airway to isolate the higher FIO_2 from the ignition source (Fig. 5-32).

On-Patient versus In-Patient Fires

10 Most fires occur on the patient and are most commonly associated with an open airway and delivery of supplemental oxygen by nasal cannula or face mask (NICV 5-2).[70] A supraglottic airway, for the purposes of fire prevention considerations, qualifies as a closed airway. On-patient fires are overwhelmingly associated with procedures where cautery is used around the upper thorax, head, and neck.[70]

Common examples of such procedures are port placement, temporal artery biopsy, and blepharoplasty. These fires typically involve surgical drapes and/or hair. It is a mistake to assume that because the patient is draped that the cautery is isolated from the presence of open administration of oxygen. Furthermore, when open administration of supplemental oxygen flow to the patient under the drapes is stopped, it can take many minutes for the ambient oxygen concentration to reduce to 30% or less.[66]

A significant time delay to achieve a reduced circuit oxygen concentration is also evident with intubated patients. As an example, it is important to reduce the breathing circuit oxygen concentration from a higher FIO_2 to no higher than 30% for fire-risk reduction during an oropharyngeal or airway case. Depending on the starting FIO_2, fresh gas flow rate, breathing circuit configuration, and minute ventilation, it will usually take several minutes for the circuit concentration to reach <30% oxygen. The decline in expired oxygen concentration significantly lags the inspired concentration until the previously high oxygen concentration in the functional residual capacity of the patient is progressively washed out.[81]

Airway Fires

An airway fire can occur when a source of ignition such as an electrosurgery unit or a laser interacts with a fuel such as an endotracheal tube or charred tissue in an environment enriched with oxygen or oxygen plus nitrous oxide. A PVC endotracheal tube will burn in 25% O_2.[68] These fires occur because fuel, ignition, and an oxidizer are present in proximity and in a sufficient quantity to initiate a fire and then sustain the chemical chain reaction: the fire tetrahedron is present. These fires can be particularly devastating not only because of the thermal injury and associated tissue destruction, but also because of the inhalation injury from the toxic materials released by combustion.[82]

Three prevalent airway fire case scenarios to consider are airway laser surgery, tracheostomy, and tonsillectomy procedures. An airway fire is a fire that is within the airway or breathing circuit. Breathing circuit fires are extremely rare and may come from an electrical short in a breathing circuit warmer or from an exothermic chemical reaction between a desiccated strong alkali carbon dioxide absorbent like soda lime and sevoflurane.[83,84] The risk of desiccated absorbent is markedly reduced by stopping the fresh gas flow through the anesthesia machine to prevent drying of the absorbent when it is not in use. The interaction between sevoflurane and absorbent is also eliminated by using an absorbent such as Amsorb (Armstrong Medical Limited, Coleraine, Northern Ireland) that

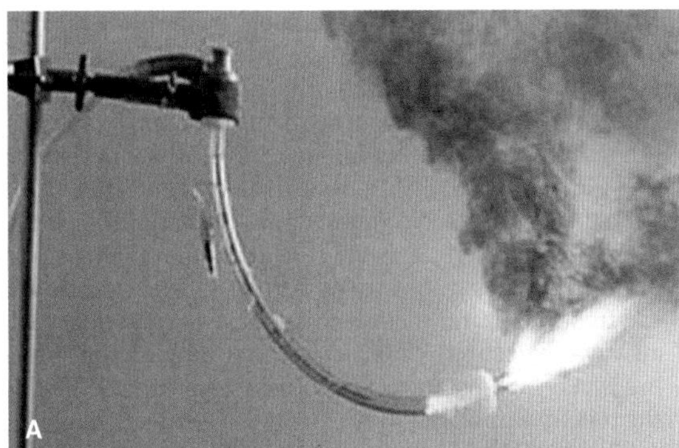

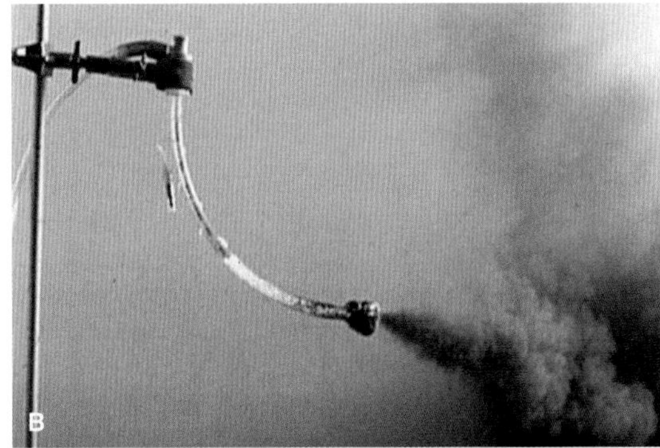

Figure 5-33 **A:** A burning ET tube with a high concentration of O_2 or O_2/N_2O will exhibit a "blowtorch" effect. (**A.** Reprinted with permission, Copyright, Emergency Care Research Institute d/b/a ECRI. www.ecri.org. 5200 Butler Pike, Plymouth Meeting, PA 19462. This Material is protected by copyright laws and may not in whole, in part, or by reference be used in any advertising or promotional material, or to compete with ECRI.) **B:** A burning ET tube will produce a large amount of debris. (**B.** Reprinted with permission, Copyright, Emergency Care Research Institute d/b/a ECRI. www.ecri.org. 5200 Butler Pike, Plymouth Meeting, PA 19462. This Material is protected by copyright laws and may not in whole, in part, or by reference be used in any advertising or promotional material, or to compete with ECRI.)

does not contain a strong alkali like potassium hydroxide. Other weak base absorbents include Medisorb EF (Vyaire Medical, Chicago, IL, USA), Dragersorb Free (Drager, Lübeck, Germany), LoFloSorb and Spherasorb (Intersurgical, Wokingham, United Kingdom), LithoLyme (Allied Healthcare, St. Louis, MO, USA), and SpiraLithCa (Micropore, Middlesbrough, England).

Laser-Related Airway Fires

The most common etiology of an airway fire is secondary to laser use. Laser is the acronym for light amplification of stimulated emission of radiation. A laser emits a collimated beam of light that therefore does not disperse and can be focused to deliver a high-power density of heat to tissue. The lasers used around the airway are usually carbon dioxide lasers (also known as CO_2 lasers), potassium titanyl phosphate (also known as KTP lasers), blue light, or neodymium: yttrium aluminum garnet (also known as Nd:YAG lasers), among others.[85] They differ in wavelength and tissue penetration as a function of their lasing medium. CO_2 lasers are used primarily during airway procedures. It is important for an anesthesia provider to know that a CO_2 laser interacts with water and any surface and therefore everyone in the room, including the patient, requires eye protection with goggles or glasses. Clear lens safety glasses are adequate for CO_2 lasers. KTP, blue light, and Nd:YAG lasers interact with tissue pigment and therefore special tinted safety glasses are required for eye protection. These lasers do not interact with glass and can, therefore, be delivered via clear flexible glass fibers through a bronchoscope into the trachea or distal airways.

A laser can serve as the ignition source in the fire triad. An airway laser-related fire can occur when a laser beam contacts a fuel such as a flammable PVC endotracheal tube or cuff, a dry sponge, or even charred tissue in the presence of an oxidizer (i.e., oxygen ± nitrous oxide).[68] An endotracheal tube fire is the most feared and a well-described complication of airway laser surgery.[86–88] The mechanism for a laser-induced endotracheal tube fire is that the heat-generating laser beam contacts the endotracheal tube or the endotracheal tube is ignited by adjacent flaming tissue.[89,90] The fire looks like a blowtorch (Fig. 5-33). The entire fire tetrahedron is present because there is abundant fuel and oxidizer to sustain the fire. In the event of an endotracheal tube fire, immediately remove the endotracheal tube from the patient, stop the flow of gases, remove any other flammable materials from the airway, and pour saline into the airway (Fig. 5-27).[61] Unintended laser strikes happen frequently: in a series of 50 laryngeal laser cases where the endotracheal tube was examined for CO_2 laser contact after extubation, half of the tubes showed evidence of a laser strike having occurred during the procedure.[91] Damage to the endotracheal tube cuff increases the risk for a leak of gas around the now deflated cuff, causing a more oxygen-enriched environment to form around the endotracheal tube. If an endotracheal tube is required, such as during microlaryngoscopy lasering procedures, then it is advisable to use a double-cuffed tube that is specifically resistant to the laser being used.

One option to guard against a laser-induced airway fire is to avoid using an endotracheal tube altogether during lasering, for example, intermittent apnea and mask ventilation or intermittent manual or low-frequency jet ventilation with a Sanders injector via a rigid bronchoscope. With these approaches, a high FIO_2 can be used because there is no flammable material in the airway.[92–94] High-frequency jet ventilation is another option.[95,96] Regarding the risk of fire and FIO_2, Huang et al. used a KTP laser (which does not generate as much heat as a CO_2 laser) and found that the fire risk increased by a factor of 2.3 for every 10% increase in oxygen concentration above 60%.[97] Continuous lasing for longer than 5 seconds increased the risk by a factor of 72, whereas lasing charred tissue increased the risk of flame by a factor of 98. The authors recommended using the pulsed lasing mode at a low power, in a reduced oxygen concentration environment, and avoiding lasering adipose and charred tissue.[89] When lasering via a flexible bronchoscope, the actual lasering is distal to the endotracheal tube, so a laser-resistant endotracheal tube is not required. However, a fire risk from charred tissue may still arise when lasering via a bronchoscope where, as has been reported, the flexible bronchoscope itself caught fire.

There are a variety of manufacturer approaches to make endotracheal tubes laser resistant including copper foil coating, aluminum foil coating, and a corrugated flexible stainless-steel wrapper (Fig. 5-34).[98] Such tubes are not resistant to all laser types, so attention must still be paid to the manufacturer's instructions for use. These specialized endotracheal tubes are referred to as laser resistant instead of laser immune because they still have flammable cuffs and PVC at the tip and inside the endotracheal tube.

During laser surgery, the FIO_2 should be limited to no greater than 0.3, only moistened gauze sponges should be used, and the exterior of the endotracheal tube should be moistened if it has a hydratable coating, for example, Merocel (Medtronic Inc., Minneapolis, MN, USA). The endotracheal cuffs should be inflated with colored saline (e.g., methylene blue tinted) rather than air: this will make a cuff strike and leak more immediately apparent, prolong

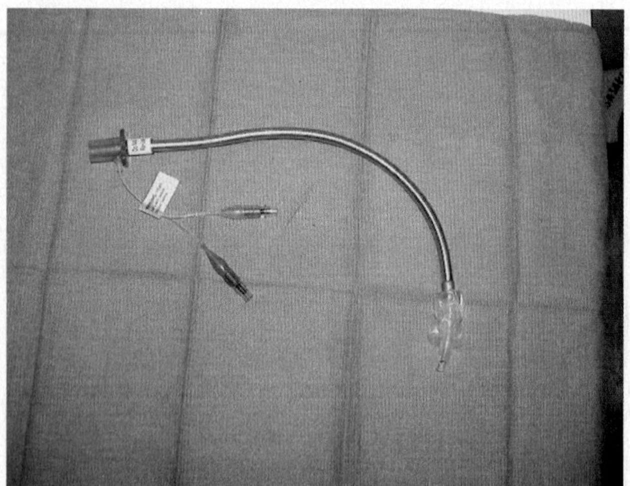

Figure 5-34 Laser-Flex® laser resistant ET tube Mallinckrodt (Pleasanton CA).

the time to cuff deflation, and delay the subsequent potential leak of oxygen into the lasing field.[99] Finally, the laser should be set on intermittent mode at the lowest clinically useful energy level.

The management of young children presents a unique challenge as laser-resistant tubes do not come in the smallest sizes and the smallest laser-resistant tubes are not cuffed. This allows oxygen-enriched air to leak into the operative field, especially if the leak pressure is less than 12 cmH_2O.[100,101] The significant likelihood of a leak around an uncuffed endotracheal tube is unavoidable, and so there is a premium on maintaining as low a circuit oxygen concentration and peak inspiratory pressure as possible while preserving an adequate oxygen saturation and avoiding the use of nitrous oxide.[102] Consequently, the alternative approaches of intermittent apneic technique or low-frequency jet ventilation via a rigid laryngoscope and manually controlled Sanders injector are commonly used in these patients.

Tracheostomy Fires

The concern for fire during tracheostomy is obvious as again there is colocation of ignition (electrosurgery), fuel (endotracheal tube, drapes, tissue), and oxidizer (oxygen-enriched environment). A patient requiring a tracheostomy will virtually always require supplemental oxygen and may present either with an endotracheal tube in place, or with a natural airway that is managed with a face mask or nasal cannula supplementation during the tracheostomy. In the case of the patient with a natural airway proceeding directly to tracheostomy, the recommendations are to supply the minimum clinically tolerable supplemental oxygen via a breathing circuit or common gas outlet connection to the anesthesia machine, drape widely, avoid drape tunneling, place suction under the drape to inhibit oxygen accumulation, and to encourage bipolar over monopolar cautery because there is less sparking with the latter. During surgery, the trachea should be entered with a knife without any cautery to eliminate the ignition source.[103] If using the high-flow nasal cannula THRIVE technique (transnasal humidified rapid-insufflation ventilatory exchange), the entire area around the patient's face will have approximately the same oxygen concentration that the high-flow device is delivering, although the humidification of the gases may serve as a fire retardant.[104,105] The gases released by electrosurgery from adipose tissue can also burn; thus, the fire triangle/tetrahedron remains ever present.[106]

Similar considerations apply for intubated patients undergoing tracheostomy. Not only are elevated fire risks present, but there is also an endotracheal tube (fuel) in the airway. The tracheostomy procedure begins with closed administration of supplemental oxygen, which becomes open administration as the trachea is entered surgically, and subsequently becomes closed again once the tracheostomy cuff is inflated. An additional risk factor is that the FIO_2 is normally increased before entering the trachea to enable tolerance of the interruption in ventilation that accompanies entering the trachea and securing the tracheostomy. The key point again is that the airway is entered with a knife and not with electrosurgery, and that electrosurgery is not used again until the airway is resecured. This places a premium on the surgeon obtaining a very hemostatic field prior to entering the trachea to avoid the reflexive application of cautery for hemostasis during the critically vulnerable time while the trachea is open.[107,108]

Tonsillectomy Fires

Fire during tonsillectomy procedures is fortunately rare but also well described. Again, the fire tetrahedron is present and all elements are in close proximity. If an ignition occurs, the fuel source can be either the endotracheal tube or the tonsil tissue bed.[107] The risk is elevated with the use of an uncuffed endotracheal tube, especially if the peak inspiratory pressure is 12 cmH_2O or greater.[100] If there is a leak around the endotracheal tube, the pharyngeal oxygen concentration will be similar to the oxygen concentration in the breathing circuit.[100,109,110] Hence, the recurring recommendation is to use a cuffed endotracheal tube, with FIO_2 no greater than 30%, avoiding nitrous oxide, and to wait patiently for the expired oxygen concentration to decrease to the target level before electrosurgery begins.[81] During an elevated fire-risk procedure like tonsil and/or adenoid resection, ventilation with room-air is clinically reasonable in an otherwise healthy patient while cautery is in use.

Eye Surgery Fires

The fire triad/tetrahedron is often present during periocular surgery. A closed claims review and survey of 168 eye surgeons revealed familiar findings: 88% of fires occurred in the presence of supplemental oxygen, 59% under monitored anesthesia care, and 41% with monopolar cautery. In another 41%, high-temperature thermal cautery was the ignition source.[111] Hair was the most common fuel (40%) and ignition of cotton gauze was second (19%). Twelve percent of the fires occurred in room air, which is a reminder that there can be a fire risk even without supplemental oxygen because of the flammability of fuels such as paper drapes and hair in room air. However, injury was not as severe in the room air fires. This can be interpreted to mean that the oxidizer limb of the fire triangle was not as potent, making the fire slower to burn and more easily extinguished. This finding discourages the use of supplemental oxygen as a routine practice in these cases.[112] Bipolar cautery appeared less likely to cause a fire than monopolar cautery, which is in keeping with the ECRI recommendations.[113]

It was noteworthy that 44% of these surgeons and presumably their accompanying anesthesia provider had already experienced at least one OR fire, with on average only 17.7 years in practice, and 12.5% of the surgeons had already experienced more than one fire.[111] Another survey of 258 oculoplastic surgeons found that 32% of surgeons had experienced at least one fire in the OR and 10 as many as three fires. Eyelid surgeries were the most common (90%) eye surgery associated with fire. Based on these numbers, this study estimated there would be 14 fires each year related to oculoplastic surgery alone.[112]

Abdominal Surgery/ Colonoscopy Fires

During open abdominal procedures and colonoscopy, even room air provides adequate oxidizer for flammable intestinal gases (e.g., hydrogen, methane) to burn.[114–116] Similar conditions exist in open abdominal surgery with either a bowel perforation and release of gas into the peritoneal cavity or during entry into a viscus with a cautery.[117] In modern practice, carbon dioxide is increasingly used as the insufflating gas during gastrointestinal endoscopy because it is more comfortable for patients and recognized as safer than air in the event of a gas embolus. It has the incidental benefit of reducing fire risk.[118]

Intrabdominal surgical procedures are increasingly performed laparoscopically. Because the insufflation gas is 100% carbon dioxide, which is fire quenching, the fire risk from the abdominal gases is low. However, if oxygen is accidentally used for insufflation, fire can and has occured.[119]

Thoracic Surgery Fires

An operation using cautery in the chest may also result in an in-the-patient fire.[120,121] These fires generally follow some violation of the lung parenchyma, resulting in an enriched oxygen environment within the thorax or mediastinum accompanied by cautery and dry lap sponges.

The typically higher FiO_2 used in thoracic and cardiac surgery patients increases the risk when there is an opening in the lung. This is also true during pulmonary surgery with lung isolation where the operative side may have a deflated lung with apneic oxygenation to that lung. In thoracoscopic surgery, the insufflated carbon dioxide provides some protection against fire.

Electrical Equipment Fire

The OR is a nest of electrical wires, cables, and equipment. Wires are vulnerable to wear and tear, contain flammable materials, are in a room air-oxidizing environment, and contain or are adjacent to fuel sources, for example, the wire insulation. The ignition heat in such fires typically comes from a short circuit.[122] In another case, a forced air warmer caught on fire, presumably from an internal device failure: the device was unplugged and doused with water to extinguish it.[123]

Fire Prevention

Fire prevention comes down to communication at the beginning of each case as to the assessed degree of fire risk and the OR team's plans to mitigate it. If an alcohol-based skin preparation is being used, the fire risk is never zero.[48] The degree of fire risk is established by assigning a point for each risk element: open source of oxygen administration (nasal cannula, face mask), an ignition/heat source (cautery, laser), surgery location above the xiphoid, and alcohol-based skin preparation (Table 5-5). After establishing the risk, the team should have a discussion to articulate the plan for the anesthesia provider, surgeon, and nurse/technician to manage the risk and plan a response should a fire occur. As individual team member examples, the anesthesia provider may then decide to secure the airway with a supraglottic device or endotracheal tube. The surgeon may choose to use a knife. If it is necessary to use an ESU, then a lower energy setting may be employed. The nurse and surgical technician can ensure that the preparation has adequate time to dry and that no preparation solution has pooled before draping, as well as that moistened sponges and extinguishing solution are immediately available on the field. As noted earlier, the fire risk may change during a case and become greater (e.g., a patient's open oxygen requirement increases, or the skin is reprepped with an alcohol-based solution during a case), or it may diminish (e.g., after a tracheostomy is secured).

Fire Response

The best plan is to maintain a heightened awareness during high–fire-risk procedures, as established during the preincision time-out, and avoid a fire in the first place. However, if a fire occurs, it is imperative to have a well-trained OR team response. The team should know where the fire extinguisher is and what their individual roles are in the event of a fire (Fig. 5-27).[61,124]

The mnemonic ERASE captures the essential elements of any fire response: Extinguish, Rescue, Activate, Shut, and Evaluate. The extinguish step includes a combination of rapid removal of the burning fuel from the patient, using water or saline or smothering to extinguish any flame. This action is normally successful and does not require a fire extinguisher. If an extinguisher is used, a carbon dioxide extinguisher is the preferred type; it can also be used on energized electrical equipment. The rescue step of the mnemonic comes into play only if the extinguish step is not successful and includes evacuating the patient and personnel from the OR, activating the fire alarm, closing the OR door(s), and shutting off the medical gas supply to the OR. Evaluating and treating the patient is the last step, or follows successful extinguishing (Fig. 5-27).

For additional information please see NICVs 5-3 and 5-4 in the eBook bundled with this text.

For further review and interactivities, please see the videos and narrative interactive clinical vignettes (NICVs) accessible in the complimentary eBook bundled with this text. Access instructions are located on the inside front cover.

REFERENCES

1. Mana S. Electrical safety. In: Pal K, Kraatz HB, Khasnobish A, Bag S, Banerjee I, Kuruganti U, eds. *Bioelectronics and Medical Devices*. Elsevier; 2019:313–330.
2. Effect of current on human beings and livestock–Part 1: General aspects. IEC 60479-1. 2005. 4th ed.
3. Harpell TR. Electrical shock hazards in the hospital environment. Their causes and cures. *Can Hosp*. 1970;47(11):48–53.
4. Wald A. Electrical safety in medicine. In: Shalak R, Chien S, ed. *Handbook of Bioengineering*. McGraw-Hill; 1987.
5. Dalziel revisited 75 years later; analysis of mixed bipolar and monopolar waveforms. 2019 IEEE International Symposium on Product Compliance Engineering (ISPCE). IEEE, 2019.
6. Munro MG. Fundamentals of electrosurgery part I: principles of radiofrequency energy for surgery. In: Feldman L, Fuchshuber P, Jones DB, eds. *The SAGES Manual on the Fundamental Use of Surgical Energy (FUSE)*. Springer; 2012:15–59.
7. Gibby GL. Shock and electrocution. https://aneskey.com/shock-and-electrocution/
8. NSI/NEMA WD 6-2016: *Wiring Devices–Dimensional Specifications*. National Electrical Manufacturer's Association. 2016. p. 17. Accessed August 20, 2022.
9. Cromwell L, Weibell FJ, Pfeiffer EA. *Biomedical Instrumentation and Measurements*. Prentice-Hall; 1973.
10. Edwards NK. Specialized electrical grounding needs. *Clin Perinatol*. 1976;3:367–374.
11. McLaughlin AJ, Campkin NT. Electrical safety-a reminder. *Anaesthesia*. 1998;53(6):608–609.
12. Nixon MC, Ghurye M. Electrical failure in theatre—a consequence of complacency? *Anaesthesia*. 1997;52(1):88–89.
13. Bruner JM, Aronow S, Cavicchi RV. Electrical incidents in a large hospital: a 42 month register. *J Assoc Adv Med Instrum*. 1972;6(3):222–230.
14. Bernstein MS. Isolated power and line isolation monitors. *Biomed Instrum Technol*. 1990; 24(3):221–223.

15. Courtney NM, McCoy EP, Scolaro RJ, Watt PA. A serious and repeatable electrical hazard–compressed electrical cord and an operating table. *Anaesth Intensive Care*. 2006;34(3):392–396.
16. Weinberg DI, Artley JL, Whalen RE, McIntosh HD. Electric shock hazards in cardiac catheterization. *Circ Res*. 1962;11:1004–1009.
17. Starmer CF, Whalen RE. Current density and electrically induced ventricular fibrillation. *Med Instrum*. 1973;7(2):158–161.
18. Whalen RE, Starmer CF, McIntosh HD. Electrical hazards associated with cardiac pacemaking. *Ann N Y Acad Sci*. 1964;111:922–931.
19. Raftery EB, Green HL, Yacoub MH. Disturbances of heart rhythm produced by 50 Hz leakage currents in human subjects. *Cardiovasc Res*. 1975;9(2):263–265.
20. Noordijk JA, Oey FT, Tebra W. Myocardial electrodes and the danger of ventricular fibrillation. *Lancet*. 1961;1(7184):975–977.
21. Pengelly LD, Klassen GA. Myocardial electrodes and the danger of ventricular fibrillation. *Lancet*. 1961;277:1234.
22. Rowe GG, Zarnstorff WC. Ventricular fibrillation during selective angiocardiography. *JAMA*. 1965;192:947–950.
23. Leeming MN. Protection of the "electrically susceptible patient": a discussion of systems and methods. *Anesthesiology*. 1973;38(4):370–383.
24. ECRI Institute. Medical devices; establishment of a performance standard for electrode lead wires and patient cables. *Federal Register*. 1997;62:25477.
25. ECRI Institute. FDA establishes performance standards for electrode lead wires. *Health Devices*. 1998;27:34.
26. Goldwyn RM. Bovie: the man and the machine. *Ann Plast Surg*. 1979;2(2):135–153.
27. Dornette WHL. An electrically safe surgical environment. *Arch Surg*. 1973;107(4):567–573.
28. Lacourse JR, Miller WT 3rd, Vogt M, Selikowitz SM. Effect of high-frequency current on nerve and muscle tissue. *IEEE Trans Biomed Eng*. 1985;32(1):82–86.
29. Klop WMC, Lohuis PJFM, Strating RP, Mulder W. Ventricular fibrillation caused by electrocoagulation during laparoscopic surgery. *Surg Endosc*. 2002;16(2):362.
30. Fu Q, Cao P, Mi WD, Zhang H. Ventricular fibrillation caused by electrocoagulation during thoracic surgery. *Acta Anaesthesiol Scand*. 2010;54(2):256.
31. Dalibon N, Pelle-Lancien E, Puyo P, Leclerc JF, Fischler M. Recurrent asystole during electrocauterization: an uncommon hazard in common situations. *Eur J Anaesthesiol*. 2005;22(6):476–478.
32. Meathe EA. Electrical safety for patients and anesthetists. In: Saidman LJ, Smith NT, eds. *Monitoring in Anesthesia*. 2nd ed. Butterworth-Heinemann; 1984.
33. Parker EO 3rd. Electrosurgical burn at the site of an esophageal temperature probe. *Anesthesiology*. 1984;61(1):93–95.
34. Schneider AJ, Apple HP, Braun RT. Electrosurgical burns at skin temperature probes. *Anesthesiology*. 1977;47(1):72–74.
35. Becker CM, Malhotra IV, Hedley-Whyte J. The distribution of radiofrequency current and burns. *Anesthesiology*. 1973;38(2):106–122.
36. Russell MJ, Gaetz M. Intraoperative electrode burns. *J Clin Monit Compute*. 2004;18(1):25–32.
37. Jones CM, Pierre KB, Nicoud IB, Stain SC, Melvin WV 3rd. Electrosurgery. *Curr Surg*. 2006;63(6):458–463.
38. Blumenstein N, Wickemeyer J, Rubenfeld A. Bringing to light the risk of burns from retained metal jewelry piercings during electrosurgery—torching the myth. *JAMA Surg*. 2022;157(5):455–456.
39. Deml MC, Goost H, Schyma C, Kabir K, Hoppe S, Deborre C. Thermic effect on metal body piercing by electrosurgery: an ex vivo study on pig skin and bovine liver. *Technol Health Care*. 2018;26(2):239–247.
40. Rosero EB, Rajan N, Joshi GP. Pro-con debate: are patients with a cardiovascular implantable electronic device suitable to receive care in a free-standing ambulatory surgery center? *Anesth Analg*. 2022;134(5):919–925.
41. Carr CM, Whiteley SM. The automatic implantable cardioverter-defibrillator. Implications for anaesthetists. *Anaesthesia*. 1991;46(9):737–740.
42. Practice advisory for the perioperative management of patients with cardiac implantable electronic devices: pacemakers and implantable cardioverter–defibrillators 2020: an updated report by the American Society of Anesthesiologists Task Force on perioperative management of patients with cardiac implantable electronic devices. *Anesthesiology*. 2020;132:225–252.
43. Hayes DL, Wang PJ, Reynolds DW, et al. Interference with cardiac pacemakers by cellular telephones. *N Engl J Med*. 1997;336(21):1473–1479.
44. von Olshausen G, Rondak IC, Lennerz C, et al. Electromagnetic interference in implantable cardioverter defibrillators: present but rare. *Clin Res Cardiol*. 2016;105(8):657–665.
45. Burri H, Mondouagne Engkolo LP, Dayal N, et al. Low risk of electromagnetic interference between smartphones and contemporary implantable cardioverter defibrillators. *Europace*. 2016;18(5):726–731.
46. Nadeem F, Tran CT, Torbey E, Philbin D, Morales C, Wu M. Interference by modern smartphones and accessories with cardiac pacemakers and defibrillators. *Curr Cardiol Rep*. 2022;24(4):347–353.
47. Magnets in cell phones and smart watches may affect pacemakers and other implanted medical devices. FDA [Internet]. 2021 May 13. Accessed 26 June 2022. https://www.fda.gov/radiation-emitting-products/cell-phones/magnets-cell-phones-and-smart-watches-may-afect-pacemakers-and-other-implanted-medical-devices
48. National Fire Protection Association. *NFPA-99, Health Care Facilities Code, Electrical Systems, Chapter 6*. 2021 Edition. Quincy, MA.
49. National Fire Protection Association. *NFPA-110, Standard for Emergency and Standby Power Systems*. Chapter 8. 2022 Edition. Quincy, MA.
50. Holland EL, Hoaglan CD, Carlstead MA, Beecher RP, Porteous GH. How do I prepare for OR power failure? *Anesthesia Patient Safety Foundation Newsletter*. 2016;30(3):58–62. https://www.apsf.org/article/how-do-i-prepare-for-or-power-failure/
51. Kermit E, Staewen WS. Isolated power systems: historical perspective and update on regulations. *Biomed Tech Today*. 1986;1:86.
52. NFPA-99 Healthcare Facilities Code. 2021 edition: Article 6.7.4.1.1. *Maintenance and Testing of Alternate Power Source and Transfer Switches. Quincy, MA.*
53. Wills JH, Ehrenwerth J, Rogers D: Electrical Injury to a Nurse Due to Conductive Fluid in an Operating Room Designated as a Dry Location. *Anesth Analg*. 2010;110:1647–1649.
54. Ciliberti BJ, Wood PM. Survey of fires and explosions in hospitals of the United States. *Am J Surg*. 1952;83(4):527–530.
55. Kim JB, Jung HJ, Im KS. Operating room fire using an alcohol-based skin preparation but without electrocautery. *Can J Anaesth*. 2013;60:413–414.
56. Rinder CS. Fire safety in the operating room. *Curr Opin Anesthesiol*. 2008;21:790–795.
57. Emergency Care Research Institute. Top 10 Health Technology Hazards for 2013. *Health Devices*. 2012;41(11);342–365. https://www.ecri.org/Resources/Whitepapers_and_reports/2013_Health_Devices_Top_10_Hazards.pdf
58. Kaye AD, Kolinsky D, Urman RD. Management of a fire in the operating room. *J Anesth*. 2014;28(2):279–287.
59. Ehrenwerth J. Operating room fires: comment. *Anesthesiology*. 2019;131(4):946–947.
60. American College of Surgeons. Monitoring OR fires to improve patient safety. Accessed June 20, 2022. https://bulletin.facs.org/2015/05/monitoring-or-fires-to-improve-patient-safety/
61. Apfelbaum JL, Caplan RA, Barker SJ, et al; American Society of Anesthesiologists Task Force on Operating Room Fires. Practice advisory for the prevention and management of operating room fires: an updated report by the American Society of Anesthesiologists Task Force on Operating Room Fires. *Anesthesiology*. 2013;118(2):271–290.
62. Anesthesia Patient Safety Foundation. Operating Room Fire Safety Video. 2010. Accessed June 17, 2022. https://www.apsf.org/videos/or-fire-safety-video/
63. Gann RG, Friedman R. Combustion, fire, and flammability. In: Gann R, Friedman R, eds. *Principles of Fire Behavior and Combustion*. 4th ed. Jones & Bartlett Learning; 2015:77–94.
64. Culp WC Jr, Kimbrough BA, Luna S. Flammability of surgical drapes and materials in varying concentrations of oxygen. *Anesthesiology*. 2013;119(4):770–776.
65. Elements of Fire. Accessed June 20, 2022. https://smokeybear.com/en/about-wildland-fire/fire-science/elements-of-fire
66. Kung TA, Kong SW, Aliu O, Azizi J, Kai S, Cederna PS. Effects of vacuum suctioning and strategic drape tenting on oxygen concentration in a simulated surgical field. *J Clin Anesth*. 2016;28:56–61.
67. Simpson JI, Wolf GL. Flammability of esophageal stethoscopes, nasogastric tubes, feeding tubes, and nasopharyngeal airways in oxygen-and nitrous oxide-enriched atmospheres. *Anesth Analg*. 1988;67(11):1093–1095.
68. Simpson JI, Wolf GL, Rosen A, Krespi Y, Schiff GA. The oxygen and nitrous oxide indices of flammability of endotracheal tubes determined by laser ignition. *Laryngoscope*. 1991;101(9):981–984.
69. Chloraprep One-Step. Accessed June 20, 2022. https://www.drugs.com/pro/chloraprep-one-step.html
70. Mehta SP, Bhananker SM, Posner KL, Domino KB. Operating room fires: a closed claims analysis. *Anesthesiology*. 2013;118(5):1133–1139.
71. Day AT, Rivera E, Farlow JL, Gourin CG, Nussenbaum B. Surgical fires in otolaryngology: a systematic and narrative review. *Otolaryngol Head Neck Surg*. 2018;158(4):598–616.
72. Yamasaki A, Bhattacharyya N. Rare electrosurgical complications in tonsillectomy: analysis of national adverse event reporting. *Laryngoscope*. 2020;130(5):1138–1143.
73. Barker SJ, Polson JS. Fire in the operating room: a case report and laboratory study. *Anesth Analg*. 2001;93(4):960–965.
74. Leal-Martín J, Muñoz-Muñoz M, Keadle SK, et al. Resting oxygen uptake value of 1 metabolic equivalent of task in older adults: a systematic review and descriptive analysis. *Sports Med*. 2022;52(2):331–348.
75. Vyaire Medical. Products: Anesthesiology. Accessed 8 October 2022. https://www.vyaire.com/products?specialties%5B83%5D=83
76. Cooper J, Griffiths B, Ehrenwerth J. Safe use of high-flow nasal oxygen (HFNO) with special reference to difficult airway management and fire risk. *Anesthesia Patient Safety Foundation Newsletter*. 2018;33(2):51–53. https://www.apsf.org/article/safe-use-of-high-flow-nasal-oxygen-hfno-with-special-reference-to-difficult-airway-management-and-fire-risk/

77. Cowles C, Lake C, Ehrenwerth J. Surgical fire prevention: a review. *Anesthesia Patient Safety Foundation Newsletter*. 2020;35(3):82–84. https://www.apsf.org/article/surgical-fire-prevention-a-review/
78. Lampotang S, Gravenstein N, Paulus DA, Gravenstein D. Reducing the incidence of surgical fires: supplying nasal cannulae with sub-100% O2 gas mixtures from anesthesia machines. *Anesth Analg*. 2005;101(5):1407–1412.
79. Schlager A, Luger TJ. Oxygen application by a nasal probe prevents hypoxia but not rebreathing of carbon dioxide in patients undergoing eye surgery under local anaesthesia. *Br J Ophthalmol*. 2000;84(4):399–402.
80. Culp WC Jr, Muse KW. Preventing operating room fires: impact of surgical drapes on oxygen contamination of the operative field. *J Patient Saf*. 2021;17(8):e1846–e1850.
81. Remz M, Luria I, Gravenstein M, et al. Prevention of airway fires: do not overlook the expired oxygen concentration. *Anesth Analg*. 2013;117(5):1172–1176.
82. Ward P, Airway fire. Poon C, Lilaonitkul M, eds. World Federation of Societies of Anaesthesiologists Anesthesia Tutorial of the Week. 2017. https://resources.wfsahq.org/wp-content/uploads/353_english.pdf
83. Do W, Kang D, Hong P, Kim HJ, Baik J, Lee D. Incidental operating room fire from a breathing circuit warmer system: a case report. *BMC Anesthesiol*. 2021;21(1):271.
84. Bailey CR. Fires from the interaction of anesthetics with desiccated absorbent. *Survey of Anesthesiology*. 2005;49(3):131. doi:10.1097/01.sa.0000165226.67470.3d
85. Tong JY, Pasick LJ, Benito DA, Sataloff RT. Adverse events associated with laser use in the upper airway. *Otolaryngol Head Neck Surg*. 2021;164(5):911–917.
86. Burgess GE, Lejeune FE, Thompson DS. Endotracheal tube ignition during laser surgery of the larynx. *Survey of Anesthesiology*. 1981;25(3):157.
87. Marinov Ts, Belitova M, Popov T, et al. Anesthetic challenges during laser surgery of the larynx part 2. operating room fire. *International Bulletin of Otorhinolaryngology*. 2019;15(3):14–19.
88. Krawtz S, Mehta AC, Wiedemann HP, DeBoer G, Schoepf KD, Tomaszewski MZ. Nd-YAG laser-induced endobronchial burn: management and long-term follow-up. *Chest*. 1989;95(4):916–918.
89. Simonini A, Brogi E, Mazzei O, et al. Airway fire during laser surgery of the vocal cords in children: a case report. *Turk J Anaesthesiol Reanim*. 2021;49(3):257–260.
90. Hirshman CA, Smith J. Indirect ignition of the endotracheal tube during carbon dioxide laser surgery. *Arch Otolaryngol*. 1980;106(10):639–641.
91. Pashayan AG, Gravenstein N. High incidence of CO2 laser beam contact with the tracheal tube during operations on the upper airway. *J Clin Anesth*. 1989;1(5):354–357.
92. Weisberger EC, Miner JD. Apneic anesthesia for improved endoscopic removal of laryngeal papillomata. *Laryngoscope*. 1988;98(7):693–697.
93. Syamal MN, Hanisak J, Macfarlan J, Ortega B, Sataloff RT, Benninger MS. To tube, or not to tube: comparing ventilation techniques in microlaryngeal surgery. *Laryngoscope*. 2021;131(12):2773–2781.
94. Ebeling CG, Riccio CA. Apneic oxygenation with high-flow nasal cannula and transcutaneous carbon dioxide monitoring during airway surgery: a case series. *A A Prac*. 2019;12(10):366–368.
95. Naik SP. High-frequency jet ventilation: an invaluable tool for anesthesia in microlaryngoscopy with carbon dioxide laser. *J Laryngol Voice*. 2018;8(2):46–469.
96. Philips R, deSilva B, Matrka L. Jet ventilation in obese patients undergoing airway surgery for subglottic and tracheal stenosis. *Laryngoscope*. 2018;128(8):1887–1892.
97. Huang L, Badenoch A, Vermeulen M, et al. Risk of airway fire with the use of KTP laser and high flow humidified oxygen delivery in a laryngeal surgery model. *Sci Rep*. 2022;12(1):543.
98. Doroshenko M, Guerra A, Vu L. Airway for Laser Surgery. [Updated 2022 May 15]. In: *StatPearls [Internet]*. StatPearls Publishing; 2022. https://www.ncbi.nlm.nih.gov/books/NBK564406/
99. Sosis MB, Dillon FX. Saline-filled cuffs help prevent laser-induced polyvinylchloride endotracheal tube fires. *Anesth Analg*. 1991;72(2)187–189.
100. Raman V, Tobias JD, Bryant J, et al. Effect of cuffed and uncuffed endotracheal tubes on the oropharyngeal oxygen and volatile anesthetic agent concentration in children. *Int J Pediatr Otorhinolaryngol*. 2012;76(6):842–844.
101. Mattucci KF, Militana CJ. The prevention of fire during oropharyngeal electrosurgery. *Ear Nose Throat J*. 2003;82(2):107–109.
102. Akhtar N, Ansar F, Baig MS, Abbas A. Airway fires during surgery: management and prevention. *J Anaesthesiol Clin Pharmacol*. 2016;32(1):109–111.
103. Radmilović-Radjenović M, Radjenović D, Radjenović B. The effect of the design of surgical electrodes on the formation of sparking enhanced burns. *Journal of Engineering and Science in Medical Diagnostics and Therapy*. 2021;4(3):031001.
104. Chang MY, Chen JH, Lin SP, et al. Fire safety study on high-flow nasal oxygen in shared-airway surgeries with diathermy and laser: simulation based on a physical model. *J Clin Monit Comput*. 2022;36(3):649–655.
105. Adams TRP, Ricciardelli A. Airway fire during awake tracheostomy using high-flow nasal oxygen. *Anaesth Rep*. 2020;8(1):25–27.
106. ECRI. Preventing, preparing for, and managing surgical fires. *Health Devices*. 1992;21: 24–30.
107. Rogers ML, Nickalls RW, Brackenbury ET, Salama FD, Beattie MG, Perks AG. Airway fire during tracheostomy: prevention strategies for surgeons and anaesthetists. *Ann R Coll Surg Engl*. 2001;83(6):376–380.
108. Niskanen M, Purhonen S, Koljonen V, Ronkainen A, Hirvonen E. Fatal inhalation injury caused by airway fire during tracheostomy. *Acta Anaesthesiol Scand*. 2007;51(4):509–513.
109. Kaddoum RN, Chidiac EJ, Zestos MM, Ahmed Z. Electrocautery-induced fire during adenotonsillectomy: report of two cases. *J Clin Anesth*. 2006;18(2):129–131.
110. Keller C, Elliott W, Hubbell RN. Endotracheal tube safety during electrodissection tonsillectomy. *Arch Otolaryngol Head Neck Surg*. 1992;118(6):643–645.
111. Connor MA, Menke AM, Vrcek I, Shore JW. Operating room fires in periocular surgery. *Int Ophthalmol*. 2018;38(3):1085–1093.
112. Maamari RN, Custer PL. Operating room fires in oculoplastic surgery. *Ophthalmic Plast Reconstr Surg*. 2018;34(2):114–122.
113. Emergency Care Research Institute. New clinical guide to surgical fire prevention. *Health Devices*. 2009;38:314-332.
114. Avgerinos A, Kalantzis N, Rekoumis G, Pallikaris G, Arapakis G, Kanaghinis T. Preparation and the risk of explosion during colonoscopic polypectomy. *Gut*. 1984;25(4):361–364.
115. Ladas SD, Karamanolis G, Ben-Soussan E. Colonic gas explosion during therapeutic colonoscopy with electrocautery. *World J Gastroenterol*. 2007;13(40):5295–5298.
116. Kusada R, Ida Y, Matsumura H. Iatrogenic burns caused by gastrointestinal gas explosion during use of a holmium YAG laser. *Burns Open*. 2018;4(2):181–184.
117. Raghavan K, Lagisetty KH, Butler KL, Cahalane MJ, Gupta A, Odom SR. Intraoperative fires during emergent colon surgery. *Am Surg*. 2015;81(2):E82–E83.
118. Dellon ES, Hawk JS, Grimm IS, Shaheen NJ. The use of carbon dioxide for insufflation during GI endoscopy: a systematic review. *Gastrointest Endosc*. 2009;69(4):843–849.
119. Shadangi BK, Khanna S, Mehta Y. Wrong gas: risk of intra-abdominal fire during laparoscopic surgery. *Indian J Anaesth*. 2012;56(6):599–600.
120. Katz JA, Campbell L. Fire during thoracotomy: a need to control the inspired oxygen concentration. *Anesth Analg*. 2005;101(2):612.
121. Kim TJ, Mascetti C, Ramsingh D. Airway fire during left internal mammary dissection in cardiac surgery: a case report. *A A Pract*. 2018;11(12):348–350.
122. Lepiane SE. Fire in the OR: this can't be happening to me. *ORL Head Neck Nurs*. 2001;19(2):18–19.
123. Stucky CH, Wolf JM. Fire in the operating room: surgical case report from a forced-air warming device equipment fire. *J Perianesthes Nurs*. 2022;37(6):766–769.
124. Flowers J. Code red in the OR—implementing an OR fire drill. *AORN J*. 2004;79:797–805.

Section 2

BASIC SCIENCE AND FUNDAMENTALS

6 Genomic Basis of Perioperative Precision Medicine

MIHAI V. PODGOREANU

KEY POINTS

1. Phenotype-driven classification fails to accurately predict perioperative outcomes or treatment response. An increasing number of genetic association studies suggest that susceptibility to a range of common adverse perioperative events and ensuing critical illness is genetically and epigenetically determined. Ongoing emphasis is placed on prioritizing genetic variants that warrant clinical action, assessing their combined predictive ability through polygenic risk scores, and integration with the electronic health record data for clinical decision support.
2. Emerging approaches utilizing "omics," physiomarkers, and imaging allow precise perioperative diagnosis and therapy. Potential applications of biomarkers in perioperative medicine and critical illness include prognosis, diagnosis, and monitoring of adverse events, as well as informing therapeutic decisions along the surgical patient journey. Very few have been rigorously evaluated to demonstrate incremental discriminatory accuracy when added to existing risk stratification models (clinical validity), or change therapy (clinical utility). Among the most promising remain natriuretic peptides and C-reactive protein (CRP) for cardiovascular risk prediction, postoperative troponin surveillance to diagnose myocardial injury, and procalcitonin to assess infection in the critically ill.
3. Interindividual variability in response to anesthetic agents is as high as 24% and has underlying genetic mechanisms.
4. Individual variability in analgesic responsiveness is attributed to genetic control of peripheral nociceptive pathways and descending central pain modulatory pathways.
5. Pharmacogenomic variation in genes modulating drug actions explains part of the variability in drug response and has shown promising clinical utility for several classes of drugs used perioperatively.
6. To facilitate translation to medical practice, systematic evaluation of existing genomic evidence for clinical decisions in the perioperative continuum, updating the practice guidelines, as well as identifying the revenue sources to reimburse the generation and use of genomic information are still required. Deliverables of this approach include classification of patients to enhance clinical trial design both in the acute perioperative period and during long-term recovery; biomarkers to select candidates for therapeutic intervention and track the efficacy of the intervention; and predictive models to increase discrimination of recovery probabilities in surgical patients.

Scientific Rationale for Perioperative Precision Medicine

Intrinsic variability exists across the human population in morphology, behavior, physiology, development, and disease susceptibility. Of particular relevance to our specialty, responses to stressful stimuli and drug therapy are also variable. As we appreciate in our daily practices in the operating rooms and intensive care units, one hallmark of perioperative physiology is the wide range of patient responses to the acute and sometimes repeated exposures to a collection of robust perturbations to homeostasis induced by surgical injury, hemodynamic challenges, vascular cannulations, mechanical circulatory support, intra-aortic balloon

Table 6-1 Categories of Perioperative Phenotypes

Immediate perioperative outcomes	• Inhospital mortality • Perioperative myocardial infarction/myocardial injury after noncardiac surgery (MINS) • Perioperative low cardiac output syndrome/acute decompensated heart failure/ventricular dysfunction • Perioperative vasoplegic syndrome • Perioperative arrhythmias (atrial fibrillation, QTc prolongation) • Postoperative bleeding • Perioperative venous thromboembolism • Acute postoperative stroke • Postoperative delirium • Perioperative acute kidney injury • Acute perioperative lung injury/acute respiratory distress syndrome/prolonged postoperative mechanical ventilation • Primary graft dysfunction/acute rejection • Postoperative infection and sepsis • Multiple organ dysfunction syndrome • Organ support-free days • Postoperative nausea and vomiting • Acute postoperative pain • Variability in response to anesthetics, analgesics, and other perioperative drugs/adverse drug reactions • Variability in degree of perioperative thromboinflammation • Intermediate phenotypes (plasma biomarker levels); metabolic phenotypes, metabolic trajectory
Long-term postoperative outcomes	• Event-free survival/major adverse cardiac events • Progression of vein graft disease • Chronic allograft dysfunction/rejection • Postoperative cognitive dysfunction/postoperative Alzheimer disease and related dementias • Postoperative depression • Chronic postsurgical pain • Cancer progression • Quality of life

Complex perioperative and critical illness phenotypes listed above are highly heterogeneous in nature, with multiple *subphenotypes*, and therefore will require a new translational classification system focused on causal biologic pathways that characterize an individual patient's response to injury in order to enable precision medicine.

counterpulsation, mechanical ventilation, partial/total organ resection, transient limb/organ ischemia-reperfusion, transfusions, anesthetic agents, and the pharmacopoeia used in the perioperative period (the *perioperative exposome*). This translates into substantial interindividual variability in immediate adverse perioperative events (mortality or incidence/severity of organ dysfunction), recovery trajectories during a surgical patient journey, as well as long-term outcomes (i.e., phenotypes; Table 6-1). For decades, we have attributed this variability only to a combination of inherent patient factors that increase an individual's biologic susceptibility or reduce resilience to surgical trauma (such as age, gender, frailty, cardiopulmonary fitness, nutritional state, comorbidities)—what we colloquially call "protoplasm"—or to heterogeneity in the intensity of exposure to perioperative stressors. In recent years, we are increasingly appreciating that genomic and epigenomic variation is also partially responsible for this observed variability in patient vulnerability and outcomes.[1] An individual's susceptibility to adverse perioperative events and critical illness stems not only from genomic contributions to the development of comorbid risk factors (such as coronary artery disease [CAD] or reduced preoperative cardiopulmonary reserve) during their lifetime, but also from genomic variability in specific biologic pathways participating in the host response to surgical injury, heterogeneity of treatment effect,[2] or in resilient responses to trauma and stress (Fig. 6-1). With increasing evidence suggesting that genomic and epigenomic regulation can significantly modulate risk of adverse perioperative events by influencing the host responses to surgery and trauma, host–device interactions, host-allograft interactions, and host-tumor interactions,[1,3,4] the emerging field of *perioperative genomics* aims to apply functional genomic approaches to uncover biologic mechanisms that explain why similar patients have such dramatically different outcomes after surgery, and is justified by a unique combination of exposures to environmental insults and postoperative phenotypes that characterize surgical trauma and critically ill patient populations. Indeed, underlying perioperative genomics is the *perioptome* concept,[5] which highlights the intersection of an individual's genome with exposure to surgical stressors and anesthetics leading to a set of phenotypic entities in that individual patient collectively referred to as the *perioperative phenome*.

Traditional epidemiologic approaches have been limiting our ability to examine factors contributing to such differential individual susceptibility to adverse perioperative events, often having to generalize from otherwise limited homogenous cohorts to the effects on the overall population. However, it has become apparent that heterogeneity in response to stressors at the individual level tends to "stretch out" the population-level response distribution curve, such that average treatment effects may not be representative of the heterogeneity of individual treatment effects (Fig. 6-1).[2,6] *Precision medicine* (or in this case, precision surgery, precision perioperative care, and precision critical care)[7] is an emerging approach for disease prevention and treatment that takes into account individual variability in genes, environment, preference, and lifestyle for each patient.[8,9] Although not new, this concept has been recently brought within our reach by three converging opportunities: a rapid and significant expansion of large-scale biologic databases (such as the reference human genome, catalogs of human genetic variation, increased characterization of genetic variant pathogenicity, RNA and protein databases, curated biologic pathway databases, and expansion of biobanks); powerful methods to characterize and monitor patients (including the ability to conduct molecular profiles at the genome, proteome, metabolome and microbiome levels, cellular assays, multiparameter physiologic data streaming, mobile health technologies, patient-activated social networks); and refinement of computational tools for managing and analyzing large datasets ("Big Data" analytics, machine learning, and augmented intelligence).[10] Spearheaded by a presidential Precision Medicine Initiative, the National Institutes of Health launched in 2016 the All of Us Research Program, which seeks to extend precision medicine to all diseases by building a national research cohort of more than 1 million participants reflecting the diversity of the U.S. population, with commitment to protecting participant privacy, regulatory modernization, and public–private partnerships.[11]

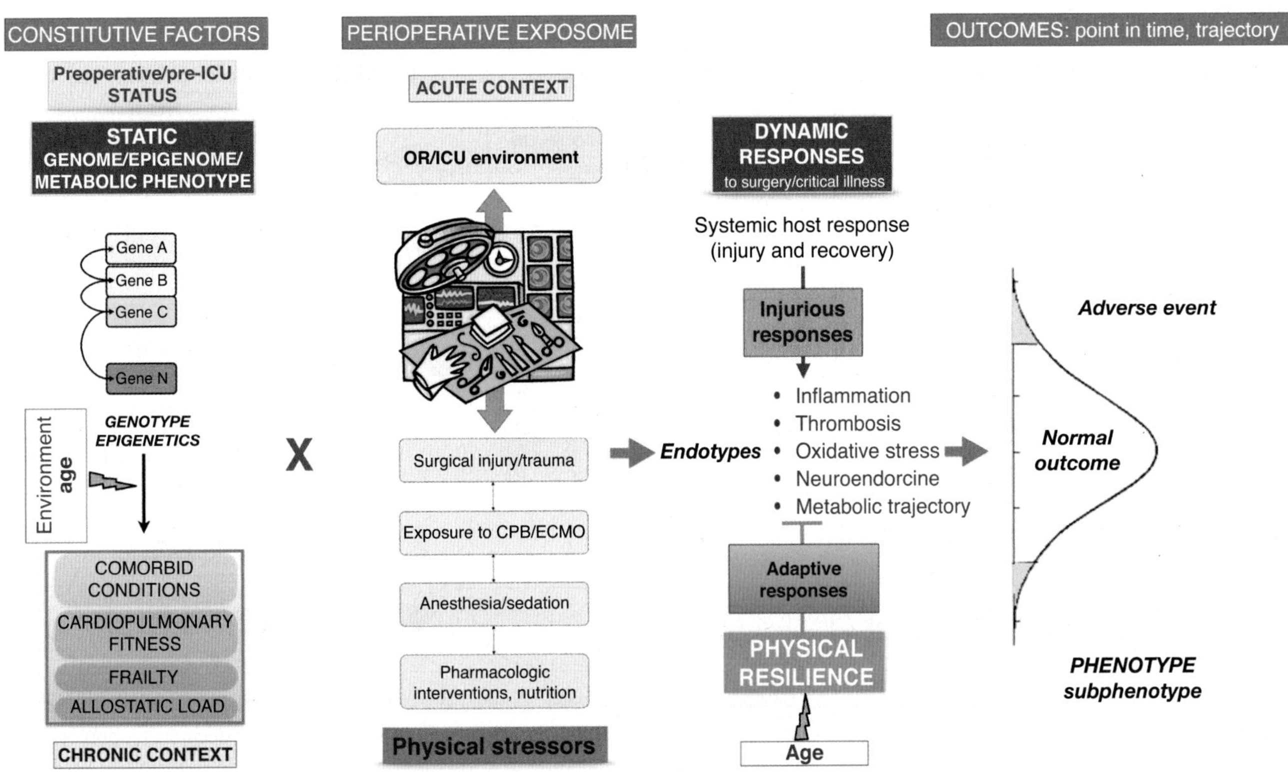

Figure 6-1 The perioperative period represents a unique and extreme example of gene–environment interactions. Perioperative adverse events are complex traits, characteristically involving an interaction between acute exposures to robust operative environmental perturbations (surgical trauma, hemodynamic challenges, exposure to extracorporeal circulation, drug administration, nutritional challenges—the *perioperative exposome*) occurring on a landscape of susceptibility determined by an individual's clinical and genetic characteristics (constitutive factors). The observed variability in perioperative outcomes can be in part attributed to genetic and epigenetic variability modulating the dynamic host responses to surgical injury. Adverse outcomes will develop only in patients whose combined burden of genetic and environmental risk factors exceeds a certain threshold, which may vary with age. In fact, physiologic stress associated with life-threatening injury exposes genetic anomalies that might otherwise go unnoticed. Identification of such genetic contributions not only to disease causation and susceptibility but also to the individual patient's *responses* to disease and drug therapy, and incorporation of genetic risk information in clinical decision making, may lead to improved health outcomes and reduced costs. However, some individuals are more sensitive than others to any given exposure to perioperative stressors, making them more susceptible to develop adverse events. Heterogeneity in response at the individual level tends to "stretch out" the population-level dose–response curve for any perioperative stress exposure. Under an emerging concept of *physical resilience*, the occurrence of perioperative adverse events is further determined by the effectiveness of adaptive (hormetic) responses to perioperative stressors, which can mitigate injurious systemic host responses. OR, operating room; CPB, cardiopulmonary bypass.

Several unique characteristics of the perioperative continuum suggest that it may represent an ideal acute care paradigm to implement precision medicine strategies. First, as a planned event (for the most part), surgery allows for preemptive molecular or genomic profiling that can inform preoperative optimization strategies. Second, the perioperative environment involves intense perturbations and stressors that can unmask underlying genetic susceptibilities. A third unique feature of the perioperative setting is the dynamic decision-making process, which involves multiple decision points over a relatively short period of time, several medications amenable to pharmacogenomics-driven decision support in order to improve their efficacy and safety, and a clinical need for such guidance regarding patient-specific drug choices and dosing (Fig. 6-2). Fourth, the acuity of the initial surgical episode is similarly followed by a rapid convalescence period or a short time to developing adverse events, thus allowing for rapid assessment of clinical outcomes and interventions.[1] Perioperative physicians are generally familiar with risk prediction tools, their implementation in clinical practice including incorporating interindividual variability into risk decisions, communicating risks, and the intricacies of managing longitudinal care transitions throughout the perioperative continuum. Finally, perioperative health care delivery systems have been early adopters of electronic health records (EHRs), with several large multi-institutional data integration efforts like the Multicenter Perioperative Group (www.mpogresearch.org) and the Anesthesiology Performance Improvement and Reporting Exchange (www.aspirecqi.org) well underway to enable perioperative medicine research, improve adherence to evidence-based standards of care, and reduce variability in both clinical practice and in common adverse postoperative outcomes, hospital length of stay, and cost.

Precision perioperative medicine aims to provide tailored management and/or prevention of perioperative complications according to the specific characteristics of a stratified individual, subpopulation, or population to enhance care of surgical, critically ill, and injured patients. These characteristics are derived from the integrated evaluation of phenotype, genotype, and treatment bioresponses realized through a systems biomedicine "omics" approach.[7] Decisions regarding preventive or therapeutic interventions, informed by precision medicine molecular and analytical approaches, would then be concentrated on patients likely to benefit, sparing expense and side effects for those who

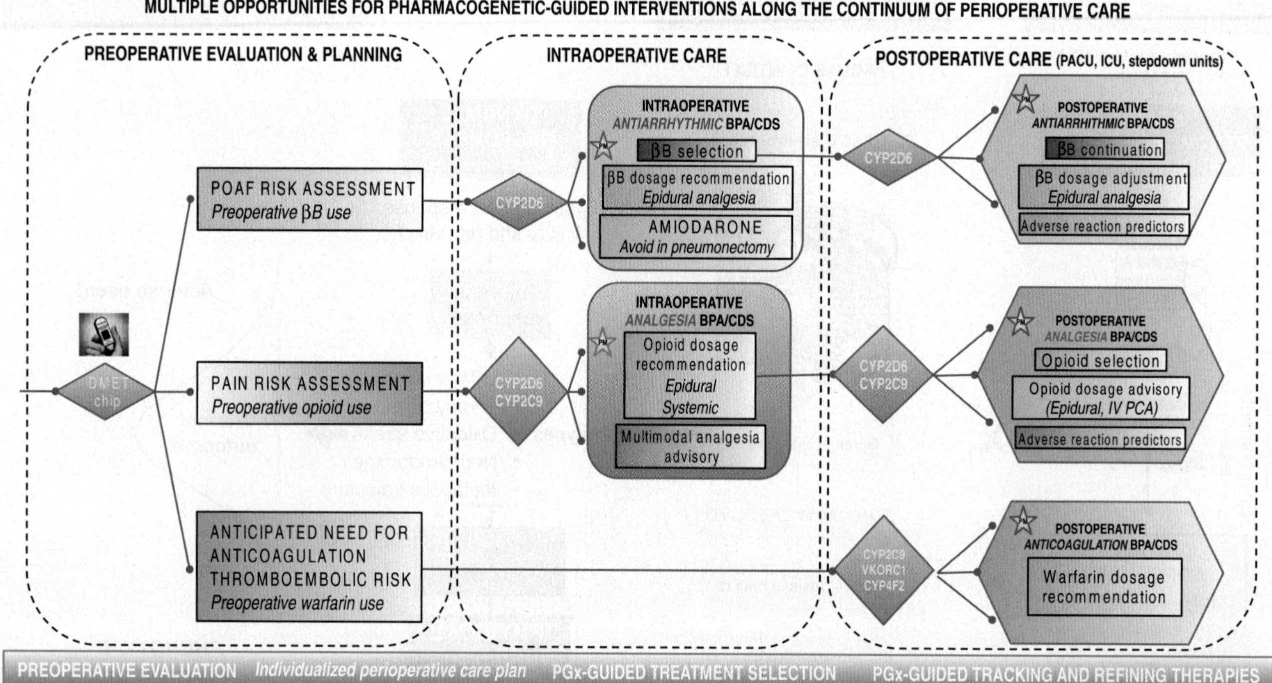

Figure 6-2 Multiple opportunities exist for implementation of a set of actionable, accessible, and sustainable clinical decision support tools to provide pharmacogenomics (PGx)-guided drug prescription along the continuum of perioperative care, under a new clinical paradigm to reduce hospital length of stay and cost. POAF, postoperative atrial fibrillation; βB, beta-blocker; PACU, postanesthesia care unit; ICU, intensive care unit; PCA, patient-controlled analgesia.

will not. Future implementation of perioperative precision medicine is conceptually viewed as an automated feedback loop, relying on several interdependent cogs (precision *science*-precision *integration*-precision *delivery*) to enable rapid acquisition, analysis, and end-user delivery of stratified or personalized therapeutic interventions.[8] Adoption of this new generation of molecular tests into clinical practice is predicated, however, on perioperative physicians becoming increasingly familiar with several key concepts, including patterns of human genome variation, gene regulation, basic population genetic methodology, gene and protein expression analysis, and most importantly the general principles for evaluating biomarker performance, in addition to digital literacy. This chapter serves as a primer in genomic and precision perioperative medicine by highlighting the evolving applications of genomic technologies to refine perioperative risk stratification, outcome prediction, understanding the complex biologic mechanisms underlying responses to surgical stress and critical illness, as well as identification and validation of novel targets for perioperative organ protection.

Human Genomic Variation

In elucidating the genetic basis of disease, much of what has been investigated in the pre–Human Genome Project era focused on identifying rare genetic variants (*mutations*) responsible for more than 1,500 monogenic disorders such as hypertrophic cardiomyopathy, long QT syndrome, sickle cell anemia, cystic fibrosis, or familial hypercholesterolemia. However, most of the genetic diversity in the population is attributable to more widespread DNA sequence variations (*polymorphisms*), typically single nucleotide base substitutions (*single nucleotide polymorphisms*, SNPs), or to a broader category of *structural genetic variants* which include short sequence repeats (*microsatellites*), insertion/deletion (I/D) of one or more nucleotides (*indels*), inversions, and copy number variants (*CNVs*, large segments of DNA that vary in number of copies), all of which may or may not be associated with a specific phenotype (Fig. 6-3). In addition to the nuclear genome, the mitochondrial genome encodes for 37 genes essential to mitochondrial function. Variability in the mitochondrial DNA is implicated in a growing number of diseases including neurodegenerative, myopathic, cardiovascular, and metabolic conditions, with important implications for perioperative and critical care management.[12] Twenty-two years since the release of the first draft of the human genome, the publication of a truly complete gap-free sequence of the human genome in 2022 by the Telomere-to-Telomere Consortium revealed what has been missing.[13] This complete assembly corrected structural errors in the prior references, introducing nearly 200 million base pairs of sequence containing biologically important regions such as the centromeres (the constricted region of a chromosome), including more than 1,900 new genes, 99 of which are predicted to be protein coding, leading to improved characterization of human genetic variation, which will better support precision medicine, population genome analysis, evolutionary biology, and genome editing. This effort will further be complemented by the ongoing Human Pangenome Project, aiming to catalog all-inclusive human genomic diversity by sequencing genomes of distinct populations from around the world.[14] It is also noteworthy that the 2022 Nobel Prize in Physiology and Medicine was awarded for work on sequencing the genomes of Neanderthals and Denisovans. About 1% to 4% of the genomes of modern humans come from Neanderthals, information that is not only relevant to understanding human evolution, but also disease susceptibility such as risk of serious complications from contracting COVID-19.[15]

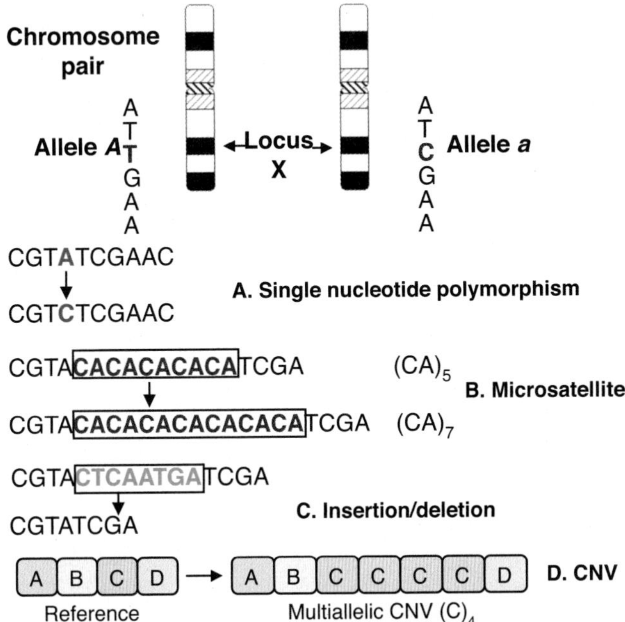

Figure 6-3 Categories of common human genetic variation. **A:** *Single nucleotide polymorphisms (SNP)* can be silent or have functional consequences: changes in amino acid sequence or premature termination of protein synthesis (if they occur in the coding regions of the gene) or alterations in the expression of the gene, resulting in more or less protein (if they occur in regulatory regions of the gene such as the promoter region or the intron/exon boundaries). Structural genetic variants include the following: **B:** *Microsatellites* with varying number of dinucleotide $(CA)_n$ repeats; **C:** *Insertions–deletions;* **D:** Copy number variation (CNV), A-D are long DNA segments, segment D shows variation in copy number. Glossary: *locus,* the location of a gene/genetic marker in the genome; *alleles,* alternative forms of a gene/genetic marker; *genotype,* the observed alleles for an individual at a genetic locus; *heterozygous,* two different alleles are present at a locus; *homozygous,* two identical alleles are present at a locus. An SNP at position 1691 of a gene, with alleles G and A would be written as 1691G>A.

To be classified as a polymorphism, the DNA sequence alternatives (i.e., *alleles*) must exist with a frequency greater than 1% in the population. About 15 million SNPs are estimated to exist in the human genome, approximately once every 300 base pairs, located in genes as well as in the surrounding regions of the genome. Polymorphisms may directly alter the amino acid sequence and therefore potentially alter protein function or alter regulatory DNA sequences that modulate protein expression. Sets of nearby SNPs on a chromosome are inherited in blocks, referred to as *haplotypes.* As it will be shown later, haplotype analysis is a useful way of applying genotype information in disease gene discovery. With increased identification of novel sequence variants in the course of testing patient specimens for a rapidly increasing number of genes associated with medical conditions, the American College of Human Genetics and Genomics (ACMG) has issued guidelines for evidence-based classification of genetic variants for clinical interpretation into pathogenic, benign, or variants of unknown significance.[16] Furthermore, ACMG has also assembled a list of 73 genes for which specific variants are known to be causative of disorders with defined phenotypes that are clinically actionable by an accepted intervention, including several with direct implications for perioperative medicine (malignant hyperthermia, long QT syndrome, and other cardiovascular phenotypes), along with guidance for reporting secondary findings in the context of clinical exome and genome sequencing.[17]

Profiling the Regulatory Genome to Understand Perioperative Biology and Discover Biomarkers of Organ Injury and Adverse Outcomes

Genomic approaches are anchored in the "central dogma" of molecular biology, the concept of transcription of messenger RNA (mRNA) from a DNA template, followed by translation of RNA into protein (Fig. 6-4). Since transcription is a key regulatory step that may eventually signal many other cascades of events, the study of RNA abundance in a cell or organ (i.e., quantifying gene expression) can improve the understanding of a wide variety of biologic systems. Furthermore, although the human genome contains only about 26,000 genes, functional variability at the protein level is far more diverse, resulting from extensive post-transcriptional and posttranslational modifications. It is believed that there are approximately 200,000 distinct proteins in humans, further subjected to a wide array of dynamic posttranslational modifications (such as phosphorylation, glycosylation, acetylation, S-nitrosylation, carbonylation, SUMOylation, and disulfide structures, among others), which are implicated in protein stability, coordinate protein–protein interactions, and serve key regulatory functions. Increasing evidence suggests that variability in gene expression levels underlies complex disease and is determined by regulatory DNA polymorphisms affecting transcription, splicing, and translation efficiency in a tissue- and stimulus-specific manner.[18] Thus, in addition to the assessment of genetic variability at the DNA sequence level (*static genomics*), analysis of large-scale variability in the pattern of RNA and protein expression both at baseline and in response to exposure to the multidimensional perioperative stimuli (*dynamic genomics*) using microarray, next-generation sequencing (NGS), and proteomic approaches provides a much needed understanding of the overall regulatory networks involved in the pathophysiology of adverse postoperative outcomes (Table 6-2). Such dynamic genomic markers can be incorporated in genomic classifiers and used clinically to improve perioperative risk stratification or monitor postoperative recovery, including transplant rejection surveillance.[7,19–21] An example of

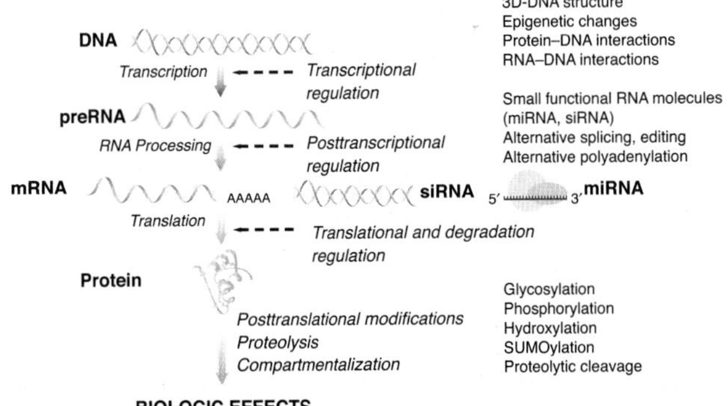

Figure 6-4 Increasing complexity of the central dogma of molecular biology. Protein expression involves two main processes: RNA synthesis (*transcription*) and protein synthesis (*translation*), with many intermediate regulatory steps. A single gene can give rise to multiple protein products (isoforms) via processing of preRNA molecules yielding multiple RNA products, including microRNA (miRNA) and small interfering RNA (siRNA) molecules, as well as alternative splicing and RNA editing. Thus, functional variability at the protein level, ultimately responsible for biologic effects, is the cumulative result of genetic variability as well as extensive transcriptional, posttranscriptional, translational, and posttranslational modifications.

Table 6-2 Summary of Gene and Protein Expression Studies with Implications for Perioperative and Critical Illness Outcomes

Tissue	Stimulus/Method	Genomic Signature: Number/Types of Genes	Reference
Myocardium	CPB/circulatory arrest/μA	58 (inflammation, transcription activators, apoptosis, stress response)-adults 50 (cardioprotective, antiproliferative, antihypertrophic)-neonates	37 38
Myocardium	CPB/cold cardioplegia-induced ischemia/ RNA-seq	Downregulation of 3,724 transcripts (90%), including humoral immune response and complement pathway genes; upregulation of 374 transcripts (9.1%), including hemoglobin genes	39
Myocardium	APC, OPCAB, postoperative LV function/μA	319 upregulated and 281 downregulated gene sets in response to OPCAB; deregulation of fatty acid oxidation, DNA-damage signaling, and G-CSF survival (perioperative) and PGC-1α (constitutive) pathways predict improved LV function in sevoflurane-treated patients	42
PBMC	APC, sevoflurane/μA	Deregulation of late preconditioning, PGC-1α, fatty acid oxidation, and L-selectin pathways	41
Atrial myocardium	AF/μA	1,434 (ventricular-like genomic signature)	216
PBMC	Cardiac surgery, PoAF/μA	1,302 genes uniquely deregulated in PoAF/401 upregulated (oxidative stress), 902 downregulated	34
PBMC	Cardiac surgery, POCD/μA	1,201 genes uniquely deregulated in POCD/531 upregulated, 670 downregulated (inflammation, antigen presentation, cell adhesion, and apoptosis)	33
Serum	Cardiac surgery, POD/P	23 proteins upregulated and 11 proteins downregulated in POD group after CPB (cytokine-receptor interaction and metabolism)	47
Myocardium	LVAD, myocardial recovery/ RNA-seq, P	Unique signature of 29 transcripts and 93 phosphopeptides that distinguished responders to LVAD unloading from nonresponders (cell cycle regulation and extracellular matrix/focal adhesions)	49
PBMC	Heart transplant rejection/ RT-PCR	11 (AlloMap, AlloMap score)	283, 284
PBMC	Racial differences after heart transplant/RT-PCR	11 (AlloMap)	21
Myocardium	Heart transplant rejection/P	2 (increased αB-crystallin and tropomyosin serum levels)	285
PBMC, plasma	TAAA/μA+P	138 genes and 7 plasma proteins predicted MODS	23
PBMC	Obstructive CAD in nondiabetic patients/ RT-PCR	23-gene expression signature	286, 287
PBMC	COVID-19 pneumonia/ digital fluorescent detection	33-messenger RNA classifier accurately assigned disease endotypes into inflammopathic, adaptive, or coagulopathic	26
Plasma	ARDS	8 plasma biomarkers (PC, PAI-1, IL6, IL6, sTNFR1, sIACM1, SPD, vWFa) in latent class analysis identified hyperinflammatory and hypoinflammatory ARDS subphenotypes	30
PBMC/Plasma	Bowel resection, SSCs/ single-cell mass cytometry+P	Multiomic immune signature (coregulated proinflammatory and immunosuppressive signaling responses) accurately predicted SSCs	71

AF, atrial fibrillation; APC, anesthetic preconditioning, APostC, anesthetic postconditioning; ARDS, acute respiratory distress syndrome; CPB, cardiopulmonary bypass; CAD, coronary artery disease; G-CSF, granulocyte colony stimulating factor; IL6, interleukin-6; IL8, interleukin-8; IPC, ischemic preconditioning; LV, left ventricle; LVAD, left ventricular assist device; μA, microarray; MCL-2, myosin light chain 2; MODS, multiple organ dysfunction syndrome; OPCAB, off-pump coronary artery bypass; P, proteomics; PBMC, peripheral blood mononuclear cells; PC, protein C; PGC-1α, peroxisome proliferators-activated receptor γ cofactor-1α; PoAF, postoperative atrial fibrillation; POCD, postoperative cognitive decline; POD, postoperative delirium; RT-PCR, real time polymerase chain reaction; sICAM1, soluble intercellular adhesion molecule-1; SPD, surfactant protein D; SSC, surgical site complication; sTNFR1, soluble tumor necrosis factor receptor-1; TAAA, thoracoabdominal aortic aneurysm repair; vWFa, von Willebrand factor antigen.

using the interplay between static genomic and dynamic genomic information for perioperative risk prediction in the case of thoracic aortic disease follows. Although surgical repair of thoracic aortic aneurysms is typically recommended when the aortic diameter reaches 5.0 to 5.5 cm, studies indicate that 60% of aortic dissections occur at aortic diameters smaller than 5.5 cm. However, DNA variants in specific genes (static genomics) can not only distinguish patients at risk for thoracic aortic disease but also predict the risk of early dissection at diameters smaller than 5.0 cm, thus potentially personalizing the timing of aortic surgery.[22] Moreover, combined genomic and proteomic analysis (dynamic genomics) using expression patterns of 138 genes from peripheral blood leukocytes and levels of seven circulating plasma proteins accurately discriminated patients who developed multiple organ dysfunction syndrome (MODS) after thoracoabdominal aortic aneurysm repair from those who did not. Importantly, these genome-wide gene expression and plasma protein concentration patterns were observed *before* surgical trauma and visceral ischemia-reperfusion injury, suggesting that patients who developed MODS differed preoperatively in either their genetic predisposition or pre-existing inflammatory state.[23]

In addition to their applications for risk prediction, dynamic genomic markers can improve mechanistic understanding of perioperative stress, by evaluating and cataloging organ-specific responses to surgical injury and severe systemic stimuli such as cardiopulmonary bypass (CPB), ischemia-reperfusion, and endotoxemia, which can be subsequently used to *subphenotype* patients into specific subgroups (*endotypes*) and identify and validate novel targets for organ protective or enhanced recovery strategies. This adds to ongoing efforts to standardize surgical outcome assessments,[24] including organ- and procedure-specific (e.g., transplantation)[25] severity of complications. Individual endotypes of critical illness syndromes or postoperative complications were identified using classifiers developed using combinations of clinical and molecular markers,[7] including COVID-19 viral sepsis endotypes (inflammopathic, coagulopathic, or adaptive),[26] immunologic endotypes after sepsis[27] and trauma,[28] as well as subphenotypes of delirium,[29] acute respiratory distress syndrome (ARDS),[30] and acute kidney injury (AKI).[31] We further illustrate such applications with several examples from the perioperative period. Using an integrated approach of transcriptomic and proteomic analyses of peripheral blood, the molecular response signatures to cardiac surgery with and without CPB have been characterized,[32] offering novel insights into the concepts of contact activation and compartmentalization of inflammatory responses to major surgery. Although CPB has been traditionally thought to be a robust trigger of systemic inflammation, similar systemic levels of key inflammatory mediators were in fact seen following off-pump cardiac surgery, but with a delayed onset. Rather than being the primary source of serum cytokines as previously believed, peripheral blood leukocytes only assume a primed phenotype upon contact with the extracorporeal circuit which facilitates their trapping and subsequent tissue-associated inflammatory response. Yet, other studies have identified genomic differences in circulating blood leukocytes between patients developing postoperative neurocognitive decline[33] or new-onset postoperative atrial fibrillation (AF).[34] Using circulating blood cells as a sentinel or reporter tissue is complemented by a large number of reports describing gene expression changes directly in myocardial tissue in response to acute ischemia, such as alterations in immediate early genes (c-*fos*, *jun*B), genes coding for calcium-handling proteins (calsequestrin, phospholamban), extracellular matrix, and cytoskeletal proteins in ischemic myocardium,[35] as well as upregulation of transcripts involved in cytoprotection (heat shock proteins), resistance to apoptosis, and cell growth in areas of stunned myocardium.[36] Moreover, cardiac gene expression profiling after CPB and cardioplegic arrest has identified age-related upregulation of inflammatory and transcription activators, apoptosis, and stress genes.[37,38] Conversely, next-generation RNA sequencing of human ventricular myocardium during cold cardioplegia-induced ischemia identified significant downregulation of immune inflammatory and complement genes, and interesting targets in transcription factors regulating reactive oxygen species production, apoptosis, and inflammatory response.[39] Whole-genome expression analysis has also been utilized to study molecular changes associated with myocardial preconditioning. The main functional categories of genes identified as potentially involved in cardioprotective pathways include a host of transcription factors, heat shock proteins, antioxidant genes (heme-oxygenase, glutathione peroxidase), and growth factors, but different gene programs were found to be activated in ischemic versus anesthetic preconditioning, resulting in two distinct molecular cardioprotective phenotypes.[40] Notably, transcriptional response pattern consistent with late preconditioning has been reported in peripheral blood leukocytes following sevoflurane administration in healthy volunteers, characterized by reduced expression of L-selectin as well as downregulation of genes involved in fatty acid oxidation and the PCG1α (peroxisome activated receptor gamma coactivator 1α) pathway,[41] which mirrors changes observed in the myocardium from patients undergoing off-pump coronary artery bypass grafting (CABG) (Table 6-2).[42] Deregulation of these conserved survival pathways thus appears to generalize across tissues, making them important targets for cardioprotection, but further studies are needed to correlate perioperative gene expression response patterns in end organs such as the myocardium to those in readily available surrogate tissues such as peripheral blood leukocytes.

A limitation of gene expression studies evaluating RNA abundance like those described earlier is that changes in the *transcriptome* (the complete collection of transcribed elements of the genome) is not fully representative of the *proteome* (the complement of proteins encoded by the genome), since many transcripts are not targeted for translation, as evidenced by the concept of gene silencing by RNA interference. Alternative splicing, a wide variety of posttranslational modifications, and protein–protein interactions responsible for biologic function, would therefore remain undetected by gene expression profiling (Fig. 6-4). This has led to the emergence of *proteomics*, a field seeking to study the sequence, abundance, modification, localization, and function of proteins in a biologic system at a given time and in response to a disease state, trauma, stress, or therapeutic intervention.[43] Thus, proteomics offers a more global and integrated view of biology, complementing other functional genomic approaches. Several proteomic studies relevant to perioperative medicine have characterized the temporal changes in brain protein expression in response to various inhaled anesthetics,[44,45] following experimental cardiac surgery with hypothermic circulatory arrest,[46] or in serum proteins associated with postoperative delirium.[47] This may focus further studies aimed to identify new anesthetic binding sites, and the development of neuroprotective strategies. The natural cardioprotective adaptations invoked by mammalian hibernators to cope with ischemia-reperfusion injury have been characterized using comparative proteomic approaches, and involve extensive metabolic remodeling with increased expression of fatty acid metabolic proteins and reduced levels of toxic lipid metabolites, offering insights into novel strategies for metabolic optimization as a transformative approach for perioperative organ protection.[48] Recently, combined transcriptomic and proteomic profiling was used to understand host–device interactions, identifying a signature of transcripts and phosphopeptides in left ventricular tissue from patients with advanced heart failure receiving left ventricular assist device (LVAD) that was unique to the patients with complete and sustained ventricular recovery following mechanical circulatory support (i.e., responders) compared to nonresponders.[49] By providing insight into the underlying biologic mechanisms for recovery in responders, these findings could guide patient selection for LVAD support and help identify new pharmacologic therapies for heart failure. Finally, detailed knowledge of the plasma proteome has profound implications in perioperative transfusion medicine, in particular related to peptide and protein changes that occur during blood product storage.[50]

Unique *metabolic phenotypes* characterize individual patients, reflecting a composite readout of host genetic-controlled metabolic processes, diet and lifestyle responses, and microbial activity. Nowhere is this more important than in surgery, where the metabolic phenotype is modified by anesthetic drugs, neoadjuvant therapies, microbial contamination and decontamination, perioperative nutritional strategies, heterogeneous pathologies, and varying surgical techniques, approaches, and hospital environments.[51,52] Because metabolic phenotypes can be measured from the composition of accessible biofluids, gases, and tissues sampled longitudinally in the perioperative course, applications spanning from population-based disease risk studies for surgical conditions to precision health care and surgical stratification have been proposed.[52,53] Nicholson et al. have proposed the concept of "phenotypically augmented patient journey," in which longitudinal or dynamic metabolic phenotyping (the metabolic trajectory) enables improved diagnosis, stratification, optimization (including enhanced recovery protocols), and outcome prediction by mapping and monitoring a patient's response to a therapeutic intervention.[52] Deviations from the recovery trajectory can occur at any point in the patient journey, at which point biologic samples can be obtained again to refine assessment of differential diagnosis, therapeutic responses, and long-term outcome prediction. Emerging *metabolomic* tools have created the opportunity to establish metabolic signatures of tissue injury. Biofluids such as plasma or urine represent snapshots of a patient's metabolic state and reflect biochemical processes occurring in multiple organs and tissues. In a population of patients undergoing alcohol septal ablation for hypertrophic obstructive cardiomyopathy, a human model of planned myocardial infarction (MI), targeted mass spectrometry-based metabolite profiling identified changes in circulating levels of metabolites participating in pyrimidine metabolism, the TCA cycle, and the pentose phosphate pathway as early as 10 minutes after MI in an initial derivation group and were validated in a second, independent group. Coronary sinus sampling distinguished cardiac derived from peripheral metabolic changes. To assess generalizability, the planned MI-derived metabolic signature (consisting of aconitic acid, hypoxanthine, trimethylamine N-oxide, and threonine) differentiated with high-accuracy patients with spontaneous MI.[54] We applied a similar approach to cardiac surgical patients undergoing planned global myocardial ischemia/reperfusion, and identified clear differences in metabolic fuel uptake based on the pre-existing ventricular state (left ventricular dysfunction, CAD, or neither) as well as altered metabolic signatures predictive of postoperative hemodynamic course and perioperative MI.[55] Although simultaneous assessment of coronary sinus effluent in addition to the peripheral blood improves cardiac specificity of the observed signatures, complementary measurements of metabolites directly in myocardial tissue allow marked enrichment and easier detection of potential biomarkers compared to plasma, as well as mechanistic insight by assessing how metabolic substrates are utilized in the tissue of interest. Such studies are possible in cardiac surgical patients where atrial tissues are routinely removed; for example, one study using high-resolution ^{1}H-NMR spectroscopy identified alterations in myocardial ketone metabolism associated with persistent AF, and the ratio of glycolytic to lipid metabolism end products correlated positively with time of onset of postoperative AF.[56] Applications of metabolic phenotyping for surgical outcome prediction have been reported for cardiac surgery,[57] abdominal organ transplantation,[58] and major trauma,[59] with specific prognostic signatures for critical illness outcomes[60] including prediction of intensive care unit (ICU) length of stay.[61] Bariatric surgery represents the model for studying surgical metabolism, however, where metabolic profiling has been reported to predict long-term response to different procedures both in terms of weight loss and remission of type 2 diabetes.[62] Potentially complementing metabolic phenotyping, prediction of weight loss after bariatric surgery is also improved using body mass index–associated polygenic risk scores (PRS) in a cost-effective manner, suggesting that genetic testing could be used in the preoperative assessment of patients with severe obesity.[63] However, clinical implementation is still limited by lack of standardization of both study design and analytic approaches.[64] Furthermore, a new paradigm for using *pharmacometabonomics* has been proposed, which involves longitudinal and dynamic measurement of an individual's metabolic profiles prior to, during, and after a therapeutic intervention (e.g., surgery, perioperative drug administration, nutritional support) in order to stratify patients and predict response to future treatments or likelihood of adverse events.[52,65] This will be discussed further in the Pharmacogenomics and Anesthesia section.

Integration of multiple static and dynamic "omic" profiles through *multiomics analysis* approaches can connect functional layers to improve prediction, understanding of complex mechanisms, and biomarker identification. Here, we briefly summarize this approach to study innate and adaptive immune host responses to surgery, which play key roles in the pathogenesis of perioperative organ injury and dysfunction. This was facilitated by recent advances in single-cell transcriptomic and proteomic technologies, enabling a comprehensive characterization of human immune response to surgery for both predictive and mechanistic understanding.[66] Previously, comprehensive immune monitoring via *flow cytometry* (exact quantification of surface marker expression on blood immune cells) was used in combination with cytokine determination for outcome prediction. Monocytic HLA-DR surface expression and plasma IL-10 were the best predictors of infection risk after cardiac surgery,[67] whereas surface expression of CD99 and CD47 (markers of neutrophil migratory responses) predict AKI and, when combined with the EuroSCORE, improve prediction of postoperative ICU length of stay after cardiac surgery.[68] More recently, high-dimensional *single-cell mass cytometry* applied to longitudinally collected blood samples identified a uniform surgical immune signature and also correlated with surgical recovery trajectories in patients undergoing hip replacement.[69] Importantly, a patient-specific "immune phenotype" assessed in samples obtained preoperatively and stimulated exogenously *in vitro* with lipopolysaccharide and other inflammatory ligands predicted postoperative individual recovery across patient-centered domains like pain, dysfunction, and disability.[70] This presurgical immune signature, involving toll-like receptor 4 signaling responses in CD14 monocytes, offers a new paradigm and potentially actionable insight for manipulating the speed of postoperative recovery. Integrated single-cell mass cytometry and proteomic analyses conducted on samples collected perioperatively identified specific systemic immune signatures preceding the development of surgical site complications in patients undergoing noncancer bowel resection.[71] Moreover, a similar mass cytometry systems immunology approach was used to identify a specific immune signature in immature neutrophils differentiating sepsis severity from aseptic inflammatory responses associated with cardiac surgery, an old clinical dilemma in sepsis diagnosis timing and accuracy.[72] Given the complexity of the host responses to surgery and critical illness, such multiomic approaches can provide insight into whether a derangement in biomarker level may be epiphenomenal rather than integral to a causative pathway, or may even be part of an adaptive pathway.[73]

Epigenetics: The Link between Environment and Genes

In response to outside stimuli, the genome can undergo potentially heritable alterations that can substantially affect gene expression and regulation without altering the DNA sequence—hence termed epigenetic. Whereas DNA is the blueprint, epigenetic information provides the instruction for using that blueprint. The epigenetic code—consisting of DNA-based modifications (e.g., DNA methylation), post-translational modifications of histone proteins (e.g., acetylation), and a growing array of noncoding RNAs (e.g., micro-RNA)—is responsive to the environment, differs between cell types, and is susceptible to change, thus representing an excellent target to impact health outcomes. Evidence from animal and human studies suggests that epigenetic mechanisms can explain susceptibility to acute and chronic pain, making them potential therapeutic targets. Specific epigenetic mechanisms relevant to perioperative analgesia involve the developmental expression of opioid receptors and opioid-induced hyperalgesia. In general, opiates tend to increase global DNA methylation levels, whereas local anesthetics conversely have a demethylating effect. This local anesthetic effect may have potential in the development of chronic pain and perioperative cancer medicine.[74] Furthermore, important pathophysiologic processes relevant to the perioperative period like stress-induced proinflammatory responses are regulated by epigenetic factors such as histone acetylation. Again, lidocaine has been shown to both demethylate DNA and have strong anti-inflammatory properties, but a direct epigenetic link has not yet been investigated. Finally, the ability of noncoding RNAs to mediate important organ protective phenomena like anesthetic preconditioning has recently been reported.[75]

Recently, *circulating cell-free nucleic acids* have been increasingly recognized as epigenetic plasma cell-free DNA (cfDNA) has been increasingly recognized as epigenetic biomarkers in precision medicine. They are a mixture of single- or double-standed nucleic acids, released into the blood plasma by different tissues via necrosis, apoptosis, and secretions. These include DNA, RNA, microRNA (miRNA), long noncoding RNA (lncRNA), fetal DNA/RNA, and mitochondrial DNA/RNA, which act as potential biomarkers in various clinical conditions. [76] In particular, several studies have characterized total *cfDNA* levels as a sensitive acute-phase biomarker for surgical damage or severity of injury, including following penetrating trauma and surgery.[77,78] Of note, while changes in cfDNA levels differed with magnitude of surgery, no correlations were found with conventional markers of surgical damage, including surgical time, estimated blood loss, postoperative white blood count, or postoperative C-reactive protein (CRP) level. In surgical oncology, perioperative changes in cfDNA concentrations were associated with surgical complications and tumor recurrence following curative resection for colon and other gastrointestinal cancers,[79] and nonmetastatic breast cancer.[80] In cardiac surgery, cfDNA predicted development of late AKI in adults[81] and mortality in infants.[82] But the most robust application of cfDNA is in transplant surgery, for surveillance of allograft injury, dysfunction, and rejection. In this case, *donor-derived cell-free DNA (ddcfDNA)* can be assayed in a transplant recipient's blood without the need for donor or recipient genotyping. The key incremental value of ddcfDNA over peripheral gene expression testing in cardiac transplantation is its ability to detect and distinguish both acute cellular rejection and antibody-mediated rejection, in addition to identifying graft dysfunction, a true "liquid biopsy."[20,83] Similar performance reports exist for lung,[84] liver, and kidney allograft surveillance.[85] Remaining challenges include validating the threshold values for clinical use and their roles in differentiating alternative (nonrejection) forms of allograft injury.

Next, we review the common genomic strategies used to study disease and drug responses.

Overview of Genetic Epidemiology and Functional Genomic Methodology

Most ongoing research on complex disorders focuses on identifying genetic variants that modify susceptibility to given conditions or drug responses. Often the design of such studies is complicated by the presence of multiple risk factors, gene–environment interactions, and a lack of even rough estimates of the number of genes underlying such complex traits. Genetic association studies examine the frequency of specific genetic or epigenetic variants in a population-based sample of unrelated diseased individuals and appropriately matched unaffected controls. The nature of most complex diseases in general, and perioperative adverse outcomes in particular (surgical patients are typically elderly), makes the study of extended multigenerational family pedigrees impractical (with few exceptions, e.g., malignant hyperthermia), due to the lack of availability of pedigree information and/or DNA samples. Even a detailed family history, the first tool in the genomic toolbox, is seldom available for most categories of adverse perioperative events. Feasibility without requiring family-based sample collections, and the increased statistical power to uncover small clinical effects of multiple genes constitute the main advantages of the genetic association approach over traditional linkage analysis methodology.

Two broad strategies have been employed to identify complex trait loci through association analysis. The *candidate gene* approach is motivated by what is known about the trait biologically, with genes selected because of *a priori* hypotheses about their potential etiologic role in disease based on current understanding of the disease pathophysiology,[86] and can be characterized as a hypothesis-testing approach but is intrinsically biased. In the early stages of perioperative genomics, most significant results were gathered from candidate gene association studies. As it will be presented in more detail later, this includes most published reports on specific genotypes associated with a variety of organ-specific perioperative adverse outcomes, including MI,[87,88] neurocognitive dysfunction,[89–91] renal compromise,[92–94] vein graft restenosis,[95,96] postoperative thrombosis,[97] vascular reactivity and vasoplegia,[98,99] severe sepsis,[100] transplant rejection,[101] and death (for reviews, see references 1 and 102).

The second strategy is the *genome-wide scan,* in which thousands of markers uniformly distributed throughout the genome or epigenome are used to locate regions that may harbor genes or regulatory regions influencing phenotypic variability. Examples include genome-wide association studies (GWAS) or epigenome-wide association studies (EWAS), as well as NGS technologies involving whole-exome sequencing (all the protein-coding genes in a genome) or whole-genome sequencing. These are unbiased approaches, in the sense that no prior assumptions are being made about the biologic processes involved and no weight is given to known genes, thus allowing the detection of previously unknown trait loci. Within the past decades, an explosion of adequately powered and successfully replicated GWAS has identified very significant genetic contributors to risk for common polygenic diseases like CAD,[103] MI,[104] heart failure,[105] diabetes (type I and II),[106,107] AF,[108] obesity, blood pressure,[109] asthma, common cancers, rheumatoid arthritis, Crohn disease, and others. In the last decade, the GWAS methodology has also been extended to study key perioperative adverse outcomes like MI,[110] AF,[111] ventricular dysfunction,[112] and AKI.[113] Although the ability to predict disease remains limited, the newly discovered genetic associations have provided insight into unsuspected mechanisms for disease, many of them located in known drug targets. These studies were facilitated by the completion of several key extensions of the Human Genome Project—the International HapMap Project (a high-resolution map of human genetic variation and haplotypes),[114] the 1,000 Genomes Project (an initial catalog of human genetic variation across ethnically diverse populations),[115] the 100,000 Genomes Project,[116] and the Encyclopedia of DNA Elements (ENCODE, a map of functional elements in the human genome, their tissue distribution, and their roles in affecting gene function and regulation)[117]—coupled with advances in high-throughput genotyping technologies. At the time of this publication, the NHGRI-EBI GWAS Catalog (www.ebi.ac.uk/gwas) included approximately 6,000 publications and 400,000 polymorphisms-trait associations, with the list growing every day.[118] Several important themes have emerged from GWAS. First, most SNPs associated with common diseases collectively explain only a small proportion of the observed contribution of heredity to the risk of disease (e.g., 6% for type 2 diabetes), or other complex traits (e.g., 2% for body mass index and 5% for height). This "*missing heritability*" problem is in part explained by the underlying rationale for GWAS—the "Common Disease-Common Variant" hypothesis—postulating that common diseases may arise secondary to cumulative effects of common variants. Most genes, however, lack a common functional coding variant with a detectable functional effect, yet they typically contain several rare variants. A counterhypothesis has emerged stating that there are additional novel genes harboring such low-frequency variants (possibly with larger effects) that may be the primary drivers of common disease. Currently, these variants are poorly detected by genotyping microarrays, but with the advent of next-generation sequencing technologies, the potential exists to revolutionize complex traits genetics by identifying and typing rare variants and thus rendering virtually every gene susceptible for genetic analysis. Nevertheless, GWAS results also underscored that small genetic effect sizes do not necessarily translate into limited therapeutic effectiveness of intervening in the respective biologic pathways. Case in point, although the risk variant in HMG CoA reductase was associated in GWAS with only 2.3 mg/dL variability in low density lipoproten (LDL) cholesterol,[119] up to 60% reductions in LDL levels can be achieved by intervening in the LDL metabolic pathway. Second, more than two-thirds of the variants identified so far are located either in intergenic regions or in genes of unknown function. This, among other findings, has challenged the very concept of "gene" as the traditional unit of heredity. Instead of directly driving disease and complex phenotypes, many genetic variants regulate the activity of genes, influencing how much RNA is being transcribed and ultimately how much protein is being produced. Pinpointing these regulatory regions, known as expression quantitative trait loci (eQTL), enables better understanding of genetic drivers of disease risk. A recent seminal study has systematically cataloged regulatory gene locations adjacent to a gene of interest (known as *cis*-eQTL), as well as regions more distant to the gene or on another chromosome (known as *trans*-eQTL), which exerted strong influence on gene expression primarily through regulation of transcription factors.[120] This is the mechanistic underpinning the use of PRS to summarize genome-wide combined risk for a complex disease into a single metric that can be used to stratify individuals,[121,122] which will be further discussed in subsequent sections. Discovery of the diverse and ubiquitous roles of new classes of RNA (including *microRNAs* and *short interfering RNAs*) led to an emerging picture of gene regulation as interdependent layers of control consisting of interactions of DNA with regulatory proteins and RNA (Fig. 6-4).[123] Moreover, as discussed earlier, on top of the DNA sequence lays another (*epigenetic*) code, that influences when and what genes should be transcribed or silenced. The epigenome is laid down during pre- and postnatal development and is heritable through cell divisions.

One of the main weaknesses of the genetic association approach is that, unless the marker of interest "travels" (i.e., is in *linkage disequilibrium*) with a functional variant, or the marker allele is the actual functional (causal) variant, the power to detect and map complex trait loci will be reduced. Newer ("next-generation") approaches based on direct *whole-genome sequencing* depart from the concept of linkage by attempting to directly identify causal alleles.[124] One particular application of genome-scale sequencing is *whole-exome sequencing*. The *exome*, defined as the protein-coding portion of the genome, is comprised in humans of approximately 30 megabases (1%) split among approximately 200,000 exons. Aside from the ability to identify rare variants and the obvious substantial cost reduction (~ 20-fold), this approach has the advantage of focusing on nonsynonymous variants in coding genes for which there are well-established methods of functional validation and interpretation of biologic effects, thus enabling their implication as causal variants. However, it completely misses noncoding and structural variation in the genome. Early results suggest that whole-exome sequencing is an effective approach to identify causal mutations for monogenic disorders but also to distinguish signal (causal rare variants) from noise (background rate of rare mutations) for complex traits. Successful studies so far (e.g., early-onset MI) sequenced individuals informed by the following key observations: the younger the age when developing MI, the greater the heritability; selecting extremes of the phenotype distribution (e.g., young with MI vs. old without MI as a "hypernormal" control group) is likely to improve power, under the scientific rationale that phenotypic extremes are enriched for either deleterious or protective variants[125]; and that genetic discovery may be enhanced by studying multiple ethnicities. These studies have demanded the development of novel statistical methods to associate rare variants with the phenotype. One such promising solution for overcoming the statistical challenges revolving around sequencing low-frequency variants is to combine all nonsynonymous SNPs (by gene or biologic pathway) into a single statistical test. The first integrated analysis of a complete human genome in a clinical context, in a patient with a family history of vascular disease and early sudden death has been reported in 2010.[126] The analysis revealed increased genetic risk for CAD, MI, type 2 diabetes, and some cancers, as well as rare variants in three genes clinically associated with sudden cardiac death. Furthermore, the patient had variants associated with clopidogrel resistance, a positive response to lipid-lowering therapies, and a low initial dosing requirement for warfarin, suggesting that routine whole-genome sequencing can yield clinically relevant information for individual patients. Several additional advantages of next-generation technologies involve sequencing of multiple genomes per person, such as matched tumor and blood DNA samples from 20 common types of cancer in the Cancer Genome Atlas, which enable development of targeted therapeutics based on a detailed molecular understanding of pathogenesis and host–tumor interactions. Equally important for medical progress is the sequencing of genomes of the billions of microorganisms that dwell within us as part of the Human Microbiome Project.

Other known limitations of genetic association studies include potential false positive findings resulting from population stratification (i.e., admixture of different ethnic or genetic backgrounds in the case and control groups), and multiple comparison issues when large numbers of genes or variants are being assessed.[127] Replication of findings across different populations or related phenotypes remains the most reliable method of validating a true relationship between genetic polymorphisms and disease, but poor reproducibility in subsequent studies has been one of the main criticisms of the candidate gene association approach.[128] Therefore, it is particularly important to follow initial association analysis results with functional analyses using in silico, in vitro, and in vivo experiments aimed at identifying the causal genetic variants, causal epigenetics, and affected biologic pathways.

Translation of genomic findings to the clinic ultimately revolves around either new disease mechanisms (better disease definition or disease stratification) or new therapeutic strategies (new targets, drug repurposing, or drug response stratification). A particular focus of recent efforts to translate genome sequence information into clinical decision making revolves around the "actionability" of specific genetic variants, and the level of evidence required to establish whether a variant is actionable. In the context of incidental findings or in an asymptomatic individual, *clinical actionability* represents the degree to which an intervention exists that can mitigate harm before a clinical diagnosis is made. Related terms are *clinical validity,* the accuracy and reliability of a variant in identifying or predicting an event with biologic or medical significance in an asymptomatic individual, and *clinical utility,* the usefulness of information in clinical decision making and improving health outcomes.[129] The National Institutes of Health has created the Clinical Genome Resource (ClinGen) to serve as an authoritative public portal defining the clinical relevance of genomic variants for use in precision medicine (www.clinicalgenome.org).[130] Several applications to perioperative medicine are presented in the following sections.

Genomics and Perioperative Risk Profiling

1 More than 40 million patients undergo surgery annually in the United States at a cost of $450 billion. This global burden of surgery[131] continues to challenge society with a large corpus of unmet medical needs. Each year, approximately 1 million patients sustain medical complications after surgery, resulting in costs of $25 billion annually. The proportion of the U.S. population above 65 years of age is estimated to double in the next two decades, adding multimorbidity to the world of surgery and critical care[132] and leading to a 25% increase in the number of surgeries, a 50% increase in surgery-related costs, and a 100% increase in complications from surgery. Although many preoperative predictors have been identified and are constantly being refined, risk stratification based on clinical, procedural, and biologic markers explains only a small part of the variability in the incidence of perioperative complications. As mentioned earlier, it is becoming increasingly recognized that perioperative morbidity arises as a direct result of the environmental stress of surgery occurring on a landscape of susceptibility that is determined by an individual's clinical and genetic characteristics, and may even occur in otherwise healthy individuals. Such adverse outcomes will develop only in patients whose combined burden of genetic and environmental risk factors exceeds a certain threshold, which may vary with age. Identification of such genetic contributions not only to disease causation and susceptibility but also to the *response* to disease and drug therapy, and incorporation of genetic risk information in clinical decision making, may lead to improved health outcomes and reduced costs. For instance, understanding the role of genetic variation in proinflammatory and prothrombotic pathways (thromboinflammation), the main pathophysiologic mechanisms responsible for perioperative complications, may contribute to the development of target-specific therapies, thereby limiting the incidence of adverse events in high-risk patients. Genomic variability has not only been identified in the host responses to surgery and trauma, but also in host–device interactions, host–allograft interactions, and host–tumor interactions, all with a potential to impact the surgical patient journey. To increase clinical relevance for the practicing perioperative physician, we summarize next existing evidence by specific outcome while highlighting candidate genes in relevant mechanistic pathways (Tables 6-3 through 6-5).

Predictive Biomarkers for Perioperative Adverse Cardiac Events

Perioperative Myocardial Infarction and Ventricular Dysfunction

Patients with underlying cardiovascular disease can be at increased risk for perioperative cardiac complications. Over the last few decades, several multifactorial risk indices have been developed and validated for both noncardiac (e.g., Lee's revised cardiac risk index [RCRI]) and cardiac surgical patients (e.g., Hannan scores), with the specific aim of stratifying risk for perioperative adverse events. However, these multifactorial risk indices have only limited predictive value for identifying patients at the highest risk of postoperative MI (PMI).[133] In this context, it has been proposed that genomic approaches could aid in refining an individual's risk profile. The incidence of PMI following cardiovascular surgery remains between 7% and 19%,[134] despite advances in surgical, cardioprotective, and anesthetic techniques, and is consistently associated with reduced short- and long-term survival in these patients. The pathophysiology of PMI after cardiac surgery involves systemic and local inflammation, "vulnerable" blood, and neuroendocrine stress.[1] In noncardiac surgery, PMI occurs as a result of two distinct mechanisms: (1) coronary plaque rupture and subsequent thrombosis triggered by a number of perioperative stressors including catecholamine surges, proinflammatory, and prothrombotic states; and (2) myocardial oxygen supply–demand imbalance.[135] Interindividual genetic variability in these mechanistic pathways is extensive, which may combine in any given patient to modulate overall susceptibility to perioperative stress and ultimately the magnitude of myocardial injury. Nevertheless, until recently, only a few studies have explored the role of genetic factors in the development of PMI,[95,136,137] mainly conducted in patients undergoing CABG surgery (Table 6-3).

Inflammation biomarkers and perioperative adverse cardiac events. Although the role of inflammation in cardiovascular disease biology has long been established, we are just beginning to understand the relationship between genetically controlled variability in inflammatory responses to surgery and PMI pathogenesis. Several studies reported independent predictive value for incident PMI after cardiac surgery with CPB of polymorphisms in proinflammatory genes interleukin-6 (*IL6*), intercellular adhesion molecule-1 (*ICAM1*), and E-selectin (*SELE*),[87] or a combined haplotype in the mannose-binding lectin gene (*MBL2* LYQA secretor haplotype), an important recognition molecule in the complement pathway.[88] Similarly, genetic variants in *IL6* and *TNFA* have also been described in association with increased incidence of postoperative cardiovascular complications including PMI after lung surgery for cancer.[138] Several polymorphisms in key proinflammatory genes have been associated with robust increases in

Table 6-3 Representative Genetic Polymorphisms and Polygenic Risk Scores Associated with Altered Susceptibility to Adverse Perioperative Cardiovascular Events

Gene	Polymorphism	Type of Surgery	Effect Size	Reference
Perioperative Myocardial Infarction, Ventricular Dysfunction, Early Vein Graft Failure				
IL6	−572G>C −174G>C	Cardiac/CPB Thoracic	2.47 1.8	87 138
ICAM1	E469 L	Cardiac/CPB	1.88	87
SELE	98G>T		0.16	87
MBL2	LYQA secretor haplotype	CABG/CPB	3.97	88
ITGB3	L33P (Pl^{A1}/Pl^{A2})	CABG/CPB Major vascular	2.5[a] 2.4	173 176
GP1 BA	T145M	Major vascular	3.4	176
TNFA	−308G>A	Thoracic	2.5	138
TNFB (LTA)	TNFB2	Cardiac/CPB	3.84	144
IL10	−1082G>A		n.r.	148
F5	R506Q(FVL)	CABG/CPB	3.29	178
CMA1	−1905 A>G		n.r.	95
ANRIL	rs10116277 G>T (9p21)		1.7	198
NPR3	rs700923 A>G rs16890196 A>G rs765199 C>T		4.28 4.09 4.27	184
NPPA_NPPB	rs700926 A>C rs632793 T>C rs6668352 G>A rs549596 T>C rs198388 C>T rs198389 A>G		3.89 0.52 0.44 0.48 0.51 0.54	184
PAI1	4G/5G		n.r.	171
PAR4	rs773857		2.4	175
PAPPA2[f]	rs10454444 rs10913237		0.46[b] 0.46[b]	110
HDAC4[f]	rs10200850		2.23[b]	
SEC24D[f]	rs4834703 rs6822035		1.98[b] 1.65[b]	
3p22.3[f]	rs17691914		2.01[b]	112
PRS_{CAD}			1.17[b]	200
Perioperative Vasoplegia, Vascular Reactivity, Coronary Tone				
DDAH II	−449G>C	Cardiac/CPB	0.4	188
NOS3	E298D		n.r.	187, 288
ACE	In/del		n.r.	98, 289
AGTRAP	rs11121816	CABG/CPB, septic shock	1.42[d]	189
ADRB2	Q27E	Tracheal intubation	11.7[c]	194
GNB3	825 C>T	Response to α-AR agonists	n.r.	288
PON1	Q192R	Resting coronary tone	n.r.	288
TNFB	rs909253 A>G	Hyperdynamic state		290
Postoperative Arrhythmias: Atrial Fibrillation, Qtc Prolongation				
IL6	−174G>C	CABG/CPB β-Blocker failure Thoracic	3.25 n.r. 1.8	203, 204 291 138
RANTES	−403G>A	β-Blocker failure	n.r.	291
TNFA	−308G>A	Thoracic	2.5	138
ATFB5 (4q25)	rs2200733 C>T rs2220427 T>G rs10033464	Cardiac/CPB	1.97[b] 1.76[b] 1.28[d]	200, 292

Table 6-3 Representative Genetic Polymorphisms and Polygenic Risk Scores Associated with Altered Susceptibility to Adverse Perioperative Cardiovascular Events (*Continued*)

Gene	Polymorphism	Type of Surgery	Effect Size	Reference
IL1B	−511 T>C 5810G>A		1.44 0.66	293
ADRB1	rs1801253 (Arg389Gly)		2.63[b]	208
GRK5	rs3740563	CABG/CPB	2.6[b]	209
LY96[f]	rs10504554	CABG/CPB	0.48[b]	111
PRS_{AF}		CABG+valve/CPB	1.63[b]	212
PRS_{AF}		CABG, PCI	1.15, 1.22[c]	213
Postoperative MACE, Late Vein Graft Failure				
ADRB1	R389G	Noncardiac with spinal block	1.87[d]	186
ACE	In/del	CABG/CPB	3.1[e]	136
ITGB3	L33P	4.7	117	
MTHFR	A222 V	PTCA and CABG/CBP	2.8	294
ADRB2	R16G Q27E	Cardiac surgery/CPB	1.96 2.82	218
HP	Hp1/Hp2	CABG	n.r.	137
CR1, KDR		CABG/CPB	n.r.	96
MICA				
HLA-DPB1				
VTN				
LPL	HindIII		n.r.	295
THBD	A455 V		2.78	219
ATFB5 (4q25)	rs2200733		1.57[d]	292
IL6	−174G>C nt565 G>A	Noncardiac vascular surgery	2.14 1.84	149 149
IL10	−1082 G>A −819 C>T −592 C>A ATA haplotype		2.16	
Cardiac Allograft Rejection				
TNFA	−308G>A	Cardiac transplant	n.r.	296
IL10	−1082G>A		n.r.	296
ICAM1	K469E		n.r.	297
IL1RN	86-bp VNTR	Thoracic transplant	2.02	298
IL1B	3953 C>T		20.5[f]	298
TGFB	915G>C	Cardiac transplant	n.r.	299

ACE, angiotensin converting enzyme; ADRB1, β_1 adrenergic receptor; ADRB2, β_2 adrenergic receptor; AF, atrial fibrillation; AGTRAP, angiotensin II type 1 receptor-associated protein; ANRIL, antisense noncoding RNA in the INK4 locus; ATFB5, Atrial fibrillation, familial 5; CABG, coronary artery bypass grafting; CAD, coronary artery disease; CMA1, heart chymase; CPB, cardiopulmonary bypass; CR1, complement component 3b/4b receptor 1; DDAH II, dimethylarginine dimethylaminohydrolase II; F5, factor V; GNB3, G-protein β_3 subunit; GP1 BA, glycoprotein Ibα; HLA-DPB1, β chain of class II major histocompatibility complex; HP, haptoglobin; ICAM1, intercellular adhesion molecule 1; IL1B, interleukin 1β; IL1RN, interleukin 1 receptor antagonist; IL6, interleukin 6; IL10, interleukin 10; ITGB3, glycoprotein IIIa; KDR, kinase inert domain receptor; LPL, lipoprotein lipase; MACE, major adverse cardiac event; MBL2, mannose binding lectin 2; MICA, MHC I polypeptide; MTHFR, methylenetetrahydrofolate reductase; NOS3, endothelial nitric oxide synthase; NPPA/NPPB, natriuretic peptide precursor A/B; NPR3, natriuretic peptide receptor 3 precursor; n.r., not reported; OR, odds ratio; PAI-1, plasminogen activator inhibitor 1; PCI, percutaneous coronary intervention; PON1, paraoxonase 1; PRS, polygenic risk scores; RANTES, regulated upon activation normally T-expressed and secreted; SELE, E-selectin; SELP, P-selectin; TGFB, transforming growth factor-beta; TNFA, tumor necrosis factor α; TNFB, tumor necrosis factor β; VNTR, variable number tandem repeat; VTN, vitronectin.

[a]relative risk;
[b]odds ratio;
[c]F-value;
[d]hazard ratio;
[e]β-coefficient;
[f]in haplotype with IL1RN VNTR;
[g]locus identified in perioperative GWAS.

Table 6-4 Representative Genetic Polymorphisms Associated with Altered Susceptibility to Adverse Perioperative Neurologic Events

Gene	Polymorphism	Type of Surgery	OR	Reference
Perioperative Stroke				
IL6	−174G>C	Cardiac/CPB	3.3	220
CRP	1846 C>T			
Perioperative Cognitive Dysfunction, Neurodevelopmental Dysfunction				
SELP	E298D	Cardiac/CPB	0.51	89
CRP	1059G>C	Cardiac/CPB	0.37	89
ITGB3	L33P (PI^{A1}/PI^{A2})	Cardiac/CPB	n.r.	90
APOE	ε4 ε2	CABG/CPB (adults) Cardiac/CPB (children)	n.r. 7; 11	221 231, 300
APOE	ε4	CABG/CPB	1.26	301
Postoperative Delirium				
APOE	ε4	Major noncardiac Critically ill	3.64 7.32	228 229
SLC6A3	rs393795	Cardiac and noncardiac, elderly	0.4	302

APOE, apolipoprotein E; CPB, cardiopulmonary bypass; CRP, C-reactive protein; IL6, interleukin 6; ITGB3, platelet glycoprotein IIIa; n.r., not reported; OR, odds ratio; SELP, P-selectin; SLC6A3, solute carrier family 6, member 3.

perioperative inflammatory responses in patients undergoing cardiac surgery with CPB. These include the promoter SNPs in *IL6* (-572G>C and -174G>C),[139] also shown to prolong the hospital length of stay[140]; the apolipoprotein E genotype (the *ε4* allele)[141]; SNPs in the tumor necrosis factor genes (*TNFA*-308G>A and -863 C>A, *LTA*+250G>A),[142,143] further associated with postoperative left ventricular dysfunction[144]; and a functional genetic variant in macrophage migration inhibitory factor (MIF)[145] and toll-like receptor 4.[146] Conversely, a genetic variant is modulating the release of the anti-inflammatory cytokine interleukin-10 (*IL10*–1082G>A) in response to CPB, with high levels of IL10 surprisingly being associated with postoperative cardiovascular dysfunction.[147,148] In patients undergoing elective surgical revascularization for peripheral vascular disease, several SNPs in *IL6* (-174 G>C, nt565 G>A) and *IL10* (-1082 G>A, -819 C>T, -592 C>A, and the ATA haplotype) were associated with endothelial dysfunction and an increased risk of a composite endpoint of acute postoperative cardiovascular events.[149]

CRP is the prototypical acute-phase reactant and the most extensively studied inflammatory marker in clinical studies, and high-sensitivity CRP (hs-CRP) has emerged as a robust predictor of cardiovascular risk at all stages, from healthy subjects to patients with acute coronary syndromes and acute decompensated heart failure.[150] Whether CRP is merely a marker or also a mediator of inflammatory processes is yet unclear, but several lines of evidence support the latter theory. In perioperative medicine, elevated preoperative CRP levels have been associated with increased short- and long-term morbidity and mortality in patients undergoing primary elective CABG (cutoff >3 mg/L)[151] as well as in higher-acuity CABG patients (cutoff >10 mg/L).[152] Interestingly, in a retrospective analysis of patients with elevated baseline hs-CRP levels undergoing off-pump CABG surgery, preoperative statin therapy was associated with reduced postoperative myocardial injury and need for dialysis.[153] In elective major noncardiac surgery patients, preoperative CRP levels (cutoff >3.4 mg/L) independently predicted perioperative major cardiovascular events (composite of MI, pulmonary edema, cardiovascular death) and significantly improved the predictive power of RCRI in receiver operating characteristic analysis.[154] While baseline plasma CRP levels have an estimated heritability around 50%,[155] intriguingly the acute-phase rise in postoperative plasma CRP levels is also genetically determined. The *CRP*1059G>C polymorphism was associated with lower peak postoperative serum CRP following both elective CABG with CPB,[156] as well as esophagectomy for thoracic esophageal cancer.[157] Furthermore, *CRP*-717 C>T polymorphism was associated with stress hyperglycemia in patients undergoing esophagectomy for cancer, leading to increased postoperative infectious complications and ICU length of stay.[158] Using PRS methodology, it is possible to index an individual's genetic susceptibility to systemic inflammation. A calculated PRS for CRP level based on genome-wide meta-analysis results from the CHARGE Consortium[159] was differentially associated with response to antidepressant drugs.[160] Bolstered by breakthroughs in the scale of GWAS and accessibility to large biobank datasets, additional studies have focused on the clinical utility and remaining challenges for PRS in predicting inflammatory diseases and evaluating putative causal relationships with magnitude of inflammatory responses.[161] A clinical-PRS model including 11 clinical risk factors and 7 SNPs was trained and validated to predict severe COVID-19,[162] whereas another 6 SNP PRS were independently associated with severe COVID-19 and improved predictions of both risk of hospitalization and risk of severe disease.[163]

The COVID-19 pandemic brought *cytokine storm* syndrome back to the forefront, with increased understanding of its immunopathology, genetic determinism, and importantly therapeutic targeting.[164–166] The central role played by IL6 in this immune hyperactivation condition has prompted targeted immunomodulatory treatment with anti-IL6 receptor monoclonal antibody (tocilizumab) in patients with severe COVID-19,[167,168] which

Table 6-5 Representative Genetic Polymorphisms Associated with Other Adverse Perioperative Outcomes

Gene	Polymorphism	Type of Surgery	Effect Size	Reference
Perioperative Thrombotic Events				
F5	FVL	Noncardiac, cardiac	n.r.	97
Perioperative Bleeding				
F5	R506Q(FVL)	Cardiac/CPB	−1.25[a]	177
PAI1	4G/5G		10^{b}	303
ITGA2	−52 C>T, 807 C>T		−0.15[a]	304, 305
GP1 BA	T145M		−0.22[a]	304
TF	−603 A>G		−0.03[a]	304
TFPI	−399 C>T		−0.05[a]	304
F2	20210G>A		0.38[a]	304
ACE	In/del		0.15[a]	304
ITGB3	L33P (PI^{A1}/PI^{A2})		n.r.	306
PAI1	4G/5G		10^{b}	303
ELAM1	98 G>T, 561 A>C	CABG/CPB	n.r.	307
PROC	rs1799809	Cardiac/CPB	1.97[b]	305
ABO	rs630014		1.83[b]	305
F9	rs6048		1.72[b]	305
TNFA	−238G>A	Brain AVM treatment	3.5[c]	308
APOE	ε2		10.9[c]	308
Perioperative Acute Kidney Injury				
IL6	−572G>C	CABG/CPB	20.04[d]	92
AGT	M235 T		32.19[d]	92
NOS3	E298D		4.29[d]	92
APOE	ε4		−0.13[a]	92, 94
3p21.6[f]	rs13317787	Cardiac/CPB	21.7[a]	113
BBS9[f]	rs10262995		12.8[a]	
PHLPP2[f]	rs78064607	Cardiac/CPB		
Perioperative Severe Sepsis				
APOE	ε3		0.28[e]	100

ABO, ABO blood group; ACE, angiotensin converting enzyme; AGT, angiotensinogen; APOE, apolipoprotein E; AVM, arteriovenous malformation; BBS9, Bardet–Biedl Syndrome 9; CPB, cardiopulmonary bypass; CRP, C-reactive protein; ELAM-1, endothelial-leukocyte adhesion molecule-1; F2, prothrombin; F5, factor V; FVL, factor V Leiden; F9, factor IX; GP1 BA, glycoprotein Ibα; IL6, interleukin 6; ITGA2, glycoprotein Ialla; ITGB3, glycoprotein IIIa; NOS3, endothelial nitric oxide synthase; n.r., not reported; OR, odds ratio; PHLPP2, PH domain and leucine rich repeat protein phosphatase 2; PROC, protein C; TF, tissue factor; TFPI, tissue factor pathway inhibitor.

[a]β-coefficient;
[b]odds ratio;
[c]hazard ratio;
[d]F-value;
[e]relative risk;
[f]locus identified in perioperative GWAS.

demonstrated increased efficacy in patients' high baseline IL6 levels and highlighted the challenges of refining a window of therapeutic opportunity. Given that significant cytokine release can complicate cardiac surgery, and absent proven benefits of routine administration of corticosteroids, the clinical utility of targeted anticytokine therapies (pharmacologic, hemoadsorbtion) in at-risk cardiac surgical patients (infective endocarditis, genetic susceptibility for exaggerated inflammatory response) should be reappraised as a perioperative precision medicine strategy.[169]

Hemostatic biomarkers and perioperative adverse cardiac events. The host response to surgery is also characterized by alterations in the coagulation system, manifested as increased fibrinogen concentration, platelet adhesiveness, and plasminogen activator inhibitor-1 (PAI-1) production. These changes can be more pronounced after cardiac surgery, where the complex and multifactorial effects of hypothermia, hemodilution, and CPB-induced activation of coagulation, fibrinolytic, and inflammatory pathways are combined. Dysfunction of the coagulation system following cardiac surgery may manifest on a continuum ranging from increased thrombotic complications such as coronary graft thrombosis, PMI, stroke, and pulmonary embolism at one end of the spectrum, to excessive bleeding as the other extreme. The balance between normal hemostasis, bleeding, and thrombosis is markedly influenced by the rate of thrombin formation and platelet activation, with genetic variability known to modulate each of these mechanistic pathways,[170] suggesting significant heritability of the prothrombotic state (see Table 6-5 for an overview of genetic variants associated with postoperative bleeding). Several genotypes in hemostatic genes have been associated with increased risk of coronary graft thrombosis and myocardial injury following CABG. A genetic variant in the promoter of the *PAI1* gene, consisting of an insertion (5G)/deletion (4G) polymorphism, has been associated with changes in the plasma levels of PAI-1. Since PAI-1 is an important negative regulator of fibrinolytic activity, its polymorphism has been associated with increased risk of early graft thrombosis after CABG,[171] and in a meta-analysis, with increased incidence of MI.[172] Functional genetic variants regulating platelet activation have also been associated with adverse postoperative outcomes. These include a polymorphism in the platelet glycoprotein IIIa gene (*ITGB3*), resulting in increased platelet aggregation (Pl^{A2} polymorphism), associated with increased perioperative myocardial injury,[173] risk of thrombotic coronary graft occlusion, MI, and 1-year mortality,[174] as well as a variant in the protease-activated receptor-4 (*PAR4*) gene associated with PMI after CABG.[175] Advanced heart failure patients requiring ventricular mechanical support represent a unique population that might benefit from a thorough preoperative risk profiling, given that implantation of ventricular assist devices can unmask previously undiagnosed thrombophilia. In the setting of noncardiac surgery, two polymorphisms in platelet glycoprotein receptors (*ITGB3* and *GP1 BA*) have been shown to be independent risk predictors of PMI in patients undergoing major vascular surgery, and resulted in improved discrimination of an ischemia risk assessment tool when added to historic and procedural risk factors.[176] Finally, a point mutation in coagulation factor V (1691G>A) resulting in resistance to activated protein C (factor V Leiden) was also associated with various postoperative thrombotic complications following noncardiac surgery.[97] Conversely, in patients undergoing cardiac surgery, factor V Leiden was associated with significant reductions in postoperative blood loss and overall risk of transfusion.[177] Nevertheless, in a prospective study of CABG patients with routine 3-month postoperative angiographic follow-up, carriers of factor V Leiden had a higher incidence of graft occlusion.[178]

Natriuretic peptides and perioperative adverse cardiac events. Circulating B-type natriuretic peptide (BNP) is a powerful biomarker of cardiovascular outcomes in many circumstances. Produced mainly in the ventricular myocardium, BNP is formed by cleavage of its prohormone by the enzyme corin into the biologically active C-terminal fragment (BNP), and an inactive N-terminal fragment (NT-proBNP). Known stimuli of BNP activation are myocardial mechanical stretch (from volume or pressure overload), acute ischemic injury, and a variety of other proinflammatory and neurohormonal stimuli inducing myocardial stress. Although secreted in 1:1 ratio, circulating levels of BNP and NT-proBNP differ considerably due to different clearance characteristics. A large number of studies have reported consistent associations of baseline plasma BNP or NT-proBNP levels with a variety of postoperative short- and long-term morbidity and mortality end points, independent of the traditional risk factors. For noncardiac surgery, these have been summarized in two meta-analyses that overall indicate an approximately 20-fold increase in risk of adverse perioperative cardiovascular outcomes.[179] Similarly, for cardiac surgery patients, preoperative BNP was a strong independent predictor of inhospital postoperative ventricular dysfunction, hospital length of stay, and 5-year mortality following primary CABG,[180] performing better than peak postoperative BNP.[181] Perioperative plasma corin concentrations decrease in patients undergoing CABG surgery, and larger relative decreases are associated with risk of long-term heart failure hospitalization and death.[181] The current guidelines for preoperative cardiac risk assessment in noncardiac surgery list BNP and NT-proBNP measurements as class IIb/level B indications.[182] However, despite the large number of studies conducted in both cardiac and noncardiac surgery, precise cut-off levels for BNP still need to be determined and adjusted for age, gender, and renal function. Similarly, no BNP-based goal-directed therapies have been reported in the perioperative period, although a role for BNP assays in monitoring aortic valve disease for optimal timing of surgery has been proposed.[183] Furthermore, Fox et al.[184] found genetic variation in natriuretic peptide precursor genes (*NPPA/NPPB*) to be independently associated with decreased risk of postoperative ventricular dysfunction following primary CABG, whereas variants in natriuretic peptide receptor *NPR3* were associated with an increased risk (Table 6-3), offering additional clues into the molecular mechanisms underlying postoperative ventricular dysfunction.

Genetic variation in vascular reactivity and perioperative adverse cardiac events. The perioperative period is characterized by robust activation of the sympathetic nervous system, which plays an important role in the pathophysiology of PMI. Thus, patients with CAD who carry specific polymorphisms in adrenergic receptor (AR) genes can be at high risk for catecholamine toxicity and cardiovascular complications. Several functionally important SNPs modulating the AR pathways have been described.[185] One of them is the Arg389Gly polymorphism in β_1-AR gene (*ADRB1*), an SNP associated with increased risk of composite cardiovascular morbidity at 1 year after noncardiac surgery under spinal anesthesia.[186] Of note, perioperative β-blockade had no effect. These findings prompted the investigators to suggest that stratification on AR genotype in future trials may help identify patients likely to benefit from perioperative β-blocker (BB) therapy. Significantly increased vascular responsiveness to α-adrenergic stimulation (phenylephrine) has been observed in carriers of the endothelial nitric oxide synthase (*NOS3*) 894>T polymorphism,[187] and angiotensin-converting enzyme (*ACE*) I/D polymorphism[98] undergoing cardiac surgery with CPB. Conversely, certain patients, especially those undergoing CPB for cardiac surgery, exhibit a form of vasodilatory shock known as vasoplegic syndrome, with a reported incidence of

8% to 20%. Although the precise mechanisms remain unclear, vasoplegic syndrome and vasopressor requirements have been associated with a common polymorphism in the dimethylarginine dimethyl-aminohydrolase II (*DDAH II*) gene, an important regulator of nitric oxide synthase activity,[188] whereas a functional SNP in angiotensin II type 1 receptor-associated protein (*AGTRAP*), the negative regulator of angiotensin II receptor type 1, is associated with decreased postoperative blood pressure following CABG as well as increased mortality in septic shock.[189] Regulation of pulmonary vascular tone is also subject to genetic regulation, and pediatric patients carrying the Glu298Asp polymorphism in *NOS3* are more likely to develop acute postoperative pulmonary hypertension following intracardiac repair of congenital cardiac disease with CPB.[190] Significant alterations in postoperative endothelial function are observed following on-pump cardiac surgery, and are associated with pronounced changes in biomarkers of endothelial origin like soluble P-selectin and SELE, tetranectin, von Willebrand factor, and ACE activity.[191] Moreover, plasma concentrations of IL1β, soluble TREM-1, endocan, and cfDNA are early predictive biomarkers of sterile-SIRS after cardiovascular surgery.[192] In addition to variability in perioperative vascular tone, a genetic susceptibility to disturbed fluid handling following cardiac surgery has also been identified, with a common polymorphism in uromodulin (*UMOD*) gene as well as a genetic risk score comprising 14 SNPs related to inflammatory and hemodynamic pathways associated with risk of postoperative fluid overload.[193] Differences in perioperative vascular reactivity in relation to genetic variants of the β_2-AR (*ADRB2*) have similarly been noted in patients undergoing noncardiac surgery. A common functional *ADRB2* SNP (Glu27) was associated with increased blood pressure responses to endotracheal intubation,[194] whereas the incidence and severity of maternal hypotension and response to treatment in obstetric patients following spinal anesthesia for cesarean delivery was affected by *ADRB2* genotype (Gly16 and/or Glu27 led to lower vasopressor use for the treatment of hypotension).[195,196]

GWAS and PRS for perioperative myocardial adverse events. A common SNP at the 9p21 locus has been identified in several replicated GWAS analyses to be associated with a wide array of vascular phenotypes in ambulatory populations, including CAD, MI, carotid atherosclerosis, abdominal aortic aneurysms, and intracranial aneurysms. Two studies have validated the association of polymorphisms at the 9p21 locus with both perioperative myocardial injury[197] and all-cause mortality after primary CABG.[198] The mechanism of action of this SNP in the development of PMI and mortality is not completely understood, but involves altered regulation of cell proliferation, senescence, and apoptosis. It seems that cardiac surgery with CPB may trigger the effects of the 9p21 gene variant leading to accumulation of senescent cells or cells that show evidence of necrotic death with cellular edema and lysis.

More recently, polymorphisms in the pregnancy-associated plasma protein A2 (*PAPPA2*), histone deacetylase-4 (*HDAC4*), and SEC24 family, member D (*SEC24D*, a member of the cytoplasmatic coat protein complex II), and two intergenic regions were identified as part of a GWAS in patients undergoing CABG to be associated with postoperative MI.[110] These novel findings implicate regulation of insulin-like growth factor bioavailability and repair processes (*PAPPA2*), myocardial cell cycle progression, differentiation, and apoptosis, with potential use in predicting individual patient responsiveness to HDAC inhibition (*HDAC4*), and endoplasmic reticulum trapping of misfolded proteins under conditions of endoplasmic reticulum stress such as ischemia and oxidative injury (*SEC24D*). Although these observations are intriguing, future follow-up studies will be needed to translate these initial findings into biologic insights that could lead to predictive and therapeutic advances in perioperative care.

As discussed above, PRS allow us to test the aggregate effects of multiple variants across the genome, weighted by their effect sizes, on a given phenotype.[199] The Michigan Genomics Initiative investigative team tested the performance of a previously developed PRS for CAD (PRS_{CAD}) in predicting myocardial injury after noncardiac surgery (MINS), defined as new troponin elevation within 30 days postoperatively.[200,201] While independently associated with MINS and contributing to reclassification of up to 3.6% of patients into a new outcome category, addition of PRS_{CAD} did not significantly improve discrimination in models including the benchmark RCRI, preoperative variables alone, or a combination of preoperative and intraoperative variables, However, the results point out the value of integrating genetic and EHR data in assessing risk of postoperative adverse events.

Perioperative Atrial Fibrillation

Perioperative atrial fibrillation (PoAF) remains a significant clinical problem after cardiac and noncardiac thoracic procedures. With an incidence of 27% to 40%, PoAF is associated with increased morbidity, hospital length of stay, rehospitalization, health care costs, and reduced survival. This has prompted several investigators to develop comprehensive indices for PoAF risk prediction based on demographic, clinical, electrocardiographic, and procedural risk factors. Nevertheless, the predictive accuracy of these risk indices remains limited, suggesting that genetic variation may play a significant role in the occurrence of PoAF. Heritable forms of AF have been described in the ambulatory nonsurgical population, and it appears both monogenic forms like "lone" AF as well as polygenic predisposition to more common acquired forms like PoAF do exist. A GWAS found two polymorphisms on chromosome 4q25 to be significantly associated with AF,[108] findings replicated in other patient groups from Sweden, the United States, and Hong Kong. Subsequently, this locus was also associated with new-onset PoAF after cardiac surgery with CPB (CABG with or without concurrent valve surgery).[202] The mechanism of action of this genetic locus is not fully elucidated, but it lies close to several genes involved in the development of pulmonary myocardium (in particular, the transcription factor PITX2c), or the sleeve of cardiomyocytes extending from the left atrium into the initial portion of the pulmonary veins.

Other candidate susceptibility genes for PoAF include those determining the duration of action potential (voltage-gated ion channels, ion transporters), responses to extracellular factors (adrenergic and other hormone receptors, heat shock proteins), remodeling processes, and magnitude of inflammatory and oxidative stress. It has been described that inflammation, reflected by elevated baseline CRP or IL6 levels and exaggerated postoperative leukocytosis, predicts the occurrence of PoAF. A link between inflammation and the development of PoAF is also supported by evidence that postoperative administration of nonsteroidal anti-inflammatory drugs may reduce the incidence of PoAF. Several studies implicated a functional SNP in the *IL6* promoter (-174G>C) to be associated with higher perioperative plasma IL-6 levels and adverse outcomes after CABG, including PoAF.[203–205] Activation of innate immune responses has also recently been suggested by results from the first GWAS of PoAF following CABG, which identified a variant in lymphocyte antigen 96 (*LY96*) to be associated with decreased incidence of new-onset PoAF after adjustment for clinical and procedural risk factors.[111] In noncardiac surgery, candidate polymorphisms in *IL6* and *TNFA* genes have been shown to be associated with an increased risk of postoperative morbidity, including new-onset arrhythmias.[138] There is, however, a contradictory lack of association between

CRP levels (strongly regulated by IL-6) and PoAF in women undergoing cardiac surgery,[206] which may reflect gender-related differences. On the other hand, both pre- and postoperative PAI-1 levels were independently associated with development of PoAF following cardiac surgery.[207]

Polymorphisms in adrenergic pathway genes have also been implicated in susceptibility to develop new-onset PoAF after CABG. A functional variant in the β_1-AR gene (*ADRB1* Arg389Gly) was associated with PoAF, with effects modulated by BB therapy, being stronger among patients without BB prophylaxis compared to those receiving BBs.[208] Furthermore, in patients undergoing CABG, polymorphisms in G-protein–coupled kinase 5 (*GRK5*) were associated with PoAF despite perioperative BB therapy.[209,210] GRK5 is expressed in the normal human heart, and regulates cardiac inotropic and chronotropic actions of catecholamines by physiologically modulating β-AR activity through receptor phosphorylation, β-arrestin recruitment, uncoupling from G proteins, and β-AR desensitization. Although the mechanism of action is incompletely understood, functional variants in *GRK5* modify the β_1-adrenergic receptor signaling pathway similar to partial receptor antagonism by BBs, thus altering their effectiveness. In summary, these polymorphisms may provide new insights into new-onset PoAF pathogenesis and differential responses to BB therapy, which can inform development of personalized perioperative treatment strategies for this common complication.

Most recently, the performance of a previously published polygenic risk score of AF (PRS_{AF})[211] was tested for prediction of PoAF after cardiac surgery.[212] In a cohort of 1,047 patients of White European ancestry undergoing CABG or valve surgery, addition of PRS_{AF} to conventional clinical predictors improved discrimination, calibration, and risk reclassification of PoAF. Another recent report investigated the association of 5 PRSs (AF, MI, stroke, intracranial bleeding, and gastrointestinal bleeding) with corresponding adverse events after coronary revascularization in a large cohort of patients with CAD participating in the Finnish FinnGen study. Only the PRS_{AF} was independently associated with PoAF across the three cohorts of patients undergoing percutaneous coronary intervention, CABG, or any revascularization, improving model discrimination when added to clinical risk factors.[213] Furthermore, PRSs associated with higher incidence of AF recurrence following direct current cardioversion,[214] or after catheter ablation[215] have been reported, suggesting potentially distinct genetic susceptibilities for AF onset and AF recurrence.

Investigations in the transcriptional responses to AF in human atrial appendage myocardium collected at the time of cardiac surgery or in preclinical models (Table 6-2) have identified a ventricular-like genomic signature in fibrillating atria, with increased ratios of ventricular to atrial isoforms, suggesting dedifferentiation.[216] It remains unclear whether this "ventricularization" of atrial gene expression reflects cause or effect of AF, but likely represents an adaptive energy-saving process to the high metabolic demand of fibrillating atrial myocardium, akin to chronic hibernation. Because atrial tissue gene expression profiling may help to determine how differentially expressed genes in the human atrium before CPB are related to subsequent biologic pathway activation patterns, and whether specific expression profiles are associated with an increased risk for PoAF or altered response to BB therapy after CABG surgery, we recently reported an eQTL analysis of PoAF.[217] We found significant upregulation of *VOPP1* gene (vesicular overexpressed in cancer-prosurvival protein 1) in patients with PoAF, which was associated with transactivating variants in *GRK5*, suggesting potential pathophysiologic roles of VOPP1 in PoAF despite perioperative BB therapy. Patients who exhibit PoAF after cardiac surgery also display a differential genomic response to CPB in their peripheral blood leukocytes, characterized by upregulation of oxidative stress genes correlated with a significant increase in oxidant stress both systemically (as measured by total peroxide levels) as well as at the myocardial level (as measured in the right atrium).[34] Finally, one study used high-resolution ^{1}H-NMR spectroscopy to conduct combined metabolomic and proteomic analyses of atrial tissue samples obtained at the time of cardiac surgery identified alterations in myocardial ketone metabolism associated with persistent AF, and the ratio of glycolytic end products to end products of lipid metabolism correlated positively with time of onset of PoAF.[56]

Genetic Variants and Postoperative Event-Free Survival

Large randomized clinical trials examining the benefits of CABG surgery and percutaneous coronary interventions relative to medical therapy and/or to one another have refined our knowledge of early and long-term survival after CABG. Although these studies have helped define subgroups of patients who benefit from surgical revascularization, they also revealed substantial variability in long-term survival after CABG, altered by important demographic and environmental risk factors. Increasing evidence suggests that the *ACE* gene indel polymorphism may influence post-CABG complications, with carriers of the *D* allele having higher mortality and restenosis rates after CABG surgery compared with the *I* allele.[136] As discussed earlier, a prothrombotic amino acid alteration in the β_3-integrin chain of the glycoprotein IIb/IIIa platelet receptor (the Pl^{A2} polymorphism) is associated with an increased risk for major adverse cardiac events (composite of MI, coronary bypass graft occlusion, or death) following CABG surgery (Table 6-3).[174] And variation at the chromosome 9p21 locus described earlier was associated with 5-year all-cause mortality following CABG, and improved the predictive ability of the EuroSCORE.[198] We found preliminary evidence for association of two functional SNPs modulating β_2-AR activity (Arg16Gly and Gln27Glu) with incidence of death or major adverse cardiac events following cardiac surgery,[218] and further identified a functional polymorphism in thrombomodulin gene (*THBD* Ala455Val) associated with increased 5-year mortality after CABG independent of EuroSCORE.[219]

Genetic Susceptibility to Adverse Perioperative Neurologic Outcomes

Despite advances in surgical and anesthetic techniques, significant neurologic morbidity continues to occur following cardiac surgery, ranging in severity from coma and focal stroke (incidence 1% to 3%) to more subtle cognitive deficits (incidence up to 69%), with a substantial impact on the risk of perioperative death, quality of life, and resource utilization. Variability in the reported incidence of both early and late neurologic deficits remains poorly explained by procedural risk factors, suggesting that environmental (operative) and genetic factors may interact to determine disease onset, progression, and recovery. The pathophysiology of perioperative neurologic injury is thought to involve complex interactions between primary pathways associated with atherosclerosis and thrombosis, and secondary response pathways like inflammation, vascular reactivity, and direct cellular injury. Many functional genetic variants have been reported in each of these mechanistic pathways involved in modulating the magnitude and the response to neurologic injury, which may have implications in chronic as well as acute perioperative neurocognitive outcomes.

For example, the interaction of minor alleles of the CRP (1846 C>T) and IL-6 promoter SNP -174G>C significantly increases the risk of acute stroke after cardiac surgery.[220] Similarly, P-selectin and CRP genes, both modulate the susceptibility to postoperative cognitive decline (POCD) following cardiac surgery.[89] Specifically, the loss-of-function minor alleles of *CRP* 1059G>C and *SELP* 1087G>A are independently associated with a *reduction* in the observed incidence of POCD after adjustment for known clinical and demographic covariates (Table 6-4).

Our group has initially reported an association between the apolipoprotein E (*APOE*) E4 genotype and adverse cerebral outcomes in cardiac surgery patients.[221,222] This is consistent with the role of the *APOE* genotype in recovery from acute brain injury, such as intracranial hemorrhage,[223] closed head injury,[224] and stroke,[225] as well as experimental models of cerebral ischemia and ischemia-reperfusion injury[226,227]; two subsequent studies in CABG patients, however, have not replicated these initial findings. Furthermore, the incidence of postoperative delirium following major noncardiac surgery in the elderly[228] and in critically ill patients[229] is increased in carriers of the *APOE* ε4 allele. Unlike adult cardiac surgery patients, infants possessing the *APOE* ε2 allele are at increased risk for developing adverse neurodevelopmental sequelae following cardiac surgery.[230,231] The mechanisms by which the *APOE* genotypes might influence neurologic outcomes have yet to be determined, but do not seem to be related to alterations in global cerebral blood flow or oxygen metabolism during CPB[232]; however, genotypic effects in modulating the inflammatory response,[141] extent of aortic atheroma burden,[233] and risk for premature coronary atherosclerosis[234] may play a role.

Consistent with the observed role of platelet activation in the pathophysiology of adverse neurologic sequelae, genetic variants in surface platelet membrane glycoproteins, important mediators of platelet adhesion and platelet–platelet interactions, increase the susceptibility to prothrombotic events. Among these, the Pl^{A2} polymorphism in glycoprotein IIb/IIIa has been related to various adverse thrombotic outcomes, including acute coronary thrombosis[235] and atherothrombotic stroke.[236] Notably, the Pl^{A2} allele is to be associated with more severe neurocognitive decline after CPB,[90] which could represent exacerbation of platelet-dependent thrombotic processes associated with plaque embolism.

Cardiac surgical patients who develop POCD demonstrate inherently different genetic responses to CPB from those without POCD, as evidenced by acute deregulation of gene expression pathways involving inflammation, antigen presentation, and cellular adhesion in peripheral blood leukocytes.[33] These findings corroborate with proteomic changes, in which patients with POCD similarly have significantly higher serologic inflammatory indices compared with those patients without POCD,[237,238] and adds to the increasing level of evidence that CPB does not cause an indiscriminate variation in gene expression, but rather distinct patterns in specific pathways that are highly associated with the development of postoperative complications such as POCD. The implications for perioperative medicine include identifying populations at risk who might benefit not only from an improved informed consent, stratification, and resource allocation, but also from targeted anti-inflammatory strategies.

In noncardiac surgery, a study conducted in patients undergoing carotid endarterectomy concluded that preoperative plasma levels of fibrinogen and hs-CRP were independently associated with new periprocedural cerebral ischemic lesions caused by microembolic events, as determined by MRI diffusion-weighted imaging.[239]

Genetic Susceptibility to Adverse Perioperative Kidney Outcomes

AKI is a common, serious complication of cardiac surgery; about 8% to 15% of patients develop moderate renal injury (>1.0 mg/dL peak creatinine rise), and up to 5% of them develop renal failure requiring dialysis.[240] AKI is independently associated with inhospital mortality rates, exceeding 60% in patients requiring dialysis.[241] Several studies have demonstrated that inheritance of genetic polymorphisms in the APOE gene (ε4 allele)[94] and in the promoter region of the *IL6* gene (-174 C allele)[205] are associated with AKI following CABG surgery (Table 6-5). We have reported that major differences in peak postoperative serum creatinine rise after CABG are predicted by carrying combinations of polymorphisms that interestingly differ by race: the angiotensinogen (*AGT*) 842 T>C and *IL6* -572G>C variants in Caucasians, and the endothelial nitric oxide synthase (*NOS3*) 894G>T and *ACE* I/D in African Americans are associated with more than 50% reduction in postoperative glomerular filtration rate.[92] A recent GWAS of cardiac surgery–associated AKI identified two novel susceptibility loci, one located in the Bardet–Biedl syndrome 9 (*BBS9*) gene, potentially implicating abnormalities in the primary renal cilia function in the pathogenesis of AKI.[113] An additional susceptibility locus for AKI after cardiac surgery was reported in PH Domain and Leucine Repeat Protein Phosphatase 2 (*PHLPP2*) gene, involved in regulation of the prosurvival kinase pathway.[242] Conversely, a two-institution GWAS analysis found no significant association with postoperative AKI following noncardiac surgery.[243] Moreover, a previously published PRS of estimated glomerular filtration rate[244] was not significantly associated with postoperative AKI in this cohort, with an overall low estimated heritability around 4.5%.[243] Nevertheless, further identification of genotypes predictive of adverse perioperative renal outcomes may facilitate individually tailored therapy, risk stratify the patients for interventional trials targeting the gene product itself, and aid in medical decision making (e.g., selecting medical over surgical management).

Genetic Variants and Risk for Postoperative Acute Lung Injury

Prolonged mechanical ventilation (inability to extubate patient by 24 hours postoperatively) is a significant complication following cardiac surgery, occurring in 5.6% and 10.5% of patients undergoing first and repeat CABG surgery, respectively.[245] Several pulmonary and nonpulmonary causes have been identified, and scoring systems based on preoperative and procedural risk factors have been proposed and validated. Recently, genetic variants in the renin–angiotensin pathway and in proinflammatory cytokine genes have been associated with respiratory complications post-CPB. The *D* allele of a common functional I/D polymorphism in the *ACE* gene, accounting for 47% of variance in circulating ACE levels,[246] is associated with prolonged mechanical ventilation following CABG,[247] and with susceptibility to and prognosis of ARDS.[248] Furthermore, a hyposecretor haplotype in the neighboring genes tumor necrosis factor alpha (*TNFA*) and lymphotoxin alpha (*LTA*) on chromosome 6 (*TNFA-308G/LTA+250G* haplotype)[249] and a functional polymorphism modulating postoperative interleukin-6 levels (*IL6*–174G>C)[205] are independently associated with higher risk of prolonged mechanical ventilation post-CABG. The association is more dramatic in patients undergoing conventional CABG than in those undergoing off-pump CABG (OPCAB), suggesting that in high-risk patients identified by preoperative genetic screening OPCAB may be the optimal surgical procedure. In children, plasma gelsolin and sRAGE have been reported to improve prediction of CPB-induced acute lung injury.[250,251]

Pharmacogenomics and Anesthesia

Interindividual variability in response to drug therapy, both in terms of efficacy and safety, is a rule by which anesthesiologists live. In fact, much of the art of anesthesiology is the astute clinician being prepared to deal with outliers. The term *pharmacogenomics* is used to describe how inherited variations in genes modulating drug actions are related to interindividual variability in drug response. Such variability in drug action may be *pharmacokinetic* or *pharmacodynamic* (Fig. 6-5). Pharmacokinetic variability refers to variability in a drug's absorption, distribution, metabolism, and excretion that mediates its efficacy and/or toxicity. The molecules involved in these processes include drug-metabolizing enzymes (such as members of the cytochrome P450, or CYP, superfamily), and drug transport molecules that mediate drug uptake into, and efflux from, intracellular sites. Pharmacodynamic variability refers to variable drug effects despite equivalent drug delivery to molecular sites of action. This may reflect variability in the function of the molecular target of the drug, or in the pathophysiologic context in which the drug interacts with its receptor target (e.g., affinity, coupling, expression).[252] Thus, pharmacogenomics investigates complex, polygenically determined phenotypes of drug efficacy or toxicity, with the goal of identifying novel therapeutic targets and customizing drug therapy.

Historically, characterization of the genetic basis for plasma pseudocholinesterase deficiency in 1956 was of fundamental importance to anesthesia and the further development and understanding of genetically determined differences in drug response. Moreover, research to refine the genetic underpinnings of malignant hyperthermia, a rare autosomal-dominant genetic disease of skeletal muscle calcium metabolism triggered by administration of general anesthesia with volatile anesthetic agents or succinylcholine in susceptible individuals, revealed that MH susceptibility results from a complex interaction between multiple genes and environment.[253] Although direct DNA testing in the general population for susceptibility to MH is currently not recommended, testing individuals with a positive family history has the potential to greatly reduce mortality and morbidity.[254]

Genetic Variability in Response to Anesthetic Agents

3

Anesthetic potency, defined by the minimum alveolar concentration (MAC) of an inhaled anesthetic that abolishes purposeful movement in response to a noxious stimulus, varies among individuals, with a coefficient of variation (the ratio of standard deviation to the mean) of approximately 10% (NICV 6-1). This observed variability may be explained by interindividual differences in multiple genes that underlie responsiveness to anesthetics, by environmental or physiologic factors (brain temperature, age), or by measurement errors. With growing public concern over intraoperative awareness, understanding the mechanisms responsible for this variability may facilitate implementation of patient-specific preventative strategies. Evidence of a genetic basis for increased anesthetic requirements is beginning to emerge, suggested for instance by variability in the immobilizing dose of sevoflurane (as much as 24%) in populations with different ethnic (and thus genetic) backgrounds.[255]

Based on combined pharmacologic and genetic in vivo studies to date, several receptors are unlikely to be direct mediators of MAC, including the gamma aminobutyric acid ($GABA_A$) (despite their compelling role in IV anesthetic-induced immobility), 5-HT_3, AMPA, kainate, acetylcholine and α_2-ARs, and potassium channels.[256] Glycine, NMDA receptors, and sodium channels remain likely candidates.[257] These conclusions, however, do not apply to other anesthetic end points, such as hypnosis, amnesia, and analgesia. Several preclinical proteomic analyses have identified in a more unbiased way a group of potential anesthetic targets for halothane,[43] desflurane,[44] and sevoflurane,[45] which should provide the basis for more focused studies of anesthetic binding sites. Such "omic" approaches have the potential to evolve into preoperative screening profiles useful in guiding individualized therapeutic decisions, such as prevention of anesthetic awareness in patients with a genetic predisposition to increased anesthetic requirements.

Genetic Variability in Pain Response

Similar to the observed variability in anesthetic potency, the response to painful stimuli and analgesic manipulations varies among individuals. Increasing evidence suggests that pain

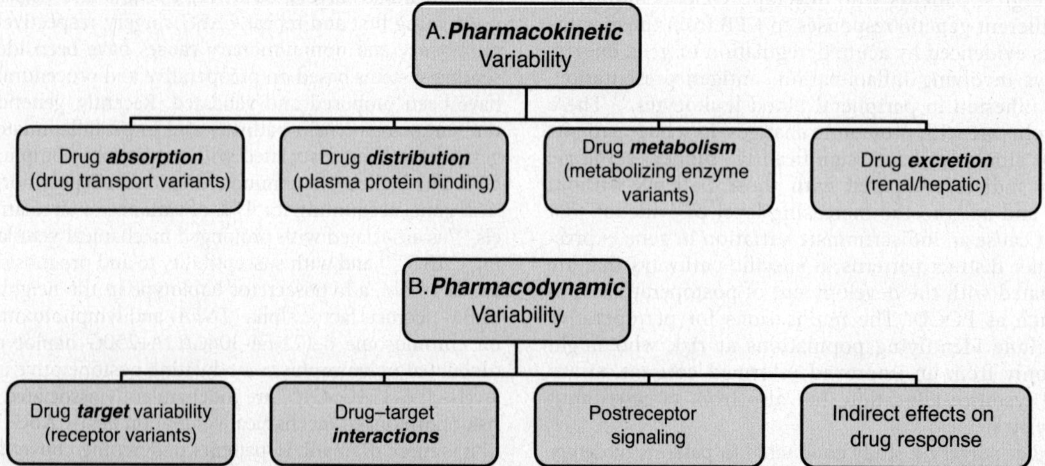

Figure 6-5 Pharmacogenomic determinants of individual drug response operate by pharmacokinetic and pharmacodynamic mechanisms. A: Genetic variants in *drug transporters* (e.g., ATP-binding cassette subfamily B member 1 or *ABCB1* gene) and *drug-metabolizing enzymes* (e.g., cytochrome P450 2D6 or *CYP2D6* gene, *CYP2C9* gene, N-acetyltransferase or *NAT2* gene, plasma cholinesterase or *BCHE* gene) are responsible for *pharmacokinetic* variability in drug response. **B:** Polymorphisms in *drug targets* (e.g., β_1 and β_2-adrenergic receptor *ADRB1, ADRB2* genes; angiotensin-I converting enzyme *ACE* gene), *postreceptor signaling molecules* (e.g., guanine nucleotide binding protein β_3 or *GNB3* gene), or *molecules indirectly affecting drug response* (e.g., various ion channel genes involved in drug-induced arrhythmias) are sources of *pharmacodynamic* variability.

behavior in response to noxious stimuli and its modulation by the central nervous system in response to drug administration or environmental stress, as well as the development of persistent pain conditions through pain amplification, are strongly influenced by genetic factors.[258–260] Results from studies in twins[261] and inbred mouse strains[262] indicate a moderate heritability for chronic pain syndromes and nociceptive sensitivity, which appears to be mediated by multiple genes. Various strains of knockout mice lacking target genes like neurotrophins and their receptors (e.g., nerve growth factor), peripheral mediators of nociception and hyperalgesia (e.g., substance P), opioid and nonopioid transmitters and their receptors, and intracellular signaling molecules have significantly contributed to the understanding of pain processing mechanisms.[263] A locus responsible for 28% of phenotypic variance in magnitude of systemic morphine analgesia in mouse has been mapped to chromosome 10, in or near the *OPRM* (μ-opioid receptor) gene. The μ-opioid receptor is also subject to pharmacodynamic variability; polymorphisms in the promoter region of the *OPRM* gene modulating interleukin-4–mediated gene expression have been correlated with morphine antinociception. The much quoted *OPRM* 188 A>G polymorphism is associated with decreased responses to morphine-6-glucuronide, resulting in altered analgesic requirements, but also reduced incidence of postoperative nausea and vomiting, and reduced risks of toxicity in renal failure patients. Conversely, variants of the melanocortin 1 receptor (*MC1R*) gene, which produce a red hair–fair skin phenotype, are associated with increased analgesic responses to κ-opioid agonists in women but not men, providing evidence for a gene-by-gender interaction in regulating analgesic response (for a review, see Somogyi et al.[264]). Previous reports suggest that peripherally located β_2-ARs (*ADRB2*) also contribute to basal pain sensitivity and the development of chronic pain states, as well as opioid-induced hyperalgesia.[260] Functionally important haplotypes in the *ADRB2*[259] and catechol-O-methyltransferase (*COMT*)[265] genes are associated with enhanced pain sensitivity in humans. Pain sensitivity has been established as a predictor of acute postoperative pain, and for risk for developing chronic pain conditions. A recent large GWAS of pain sensitivity assessed by questionnaire and a cold pressor test identified a new susceptibility locus in the *EIPR1* (endosome-associated recycling protein) gene and confirmed previous findings that females with red hair were more sensitive to pain, with genetic variation in *MC1R* associated with an increase in self-perceived pain sensitivity.[266]

4

In addition to the genetic control of peripheral nociceptive pathways, considerable evidence exists for genetic variability in the descending central pain modulatory pathways, further explaining the interindividual variability in analgesic responsiveness. One good example relevant to analgesic efficacy is cytochrome P450D6 (*CYP2D6*), a member of the superfamily of microsomal enzymes that catalyze phase I drug metabolism, and responsible for the metabolism of a large number of therapeutic compounds. The relationship between the *CYP2D6* genotype and the enzyme metabolic rate has been extensively characterized, with at least 12 known mutations leading to a tetramodal distribution of CYP2D6 activity: ultrarapid metabolizers (5% to 7% of the population), extensive metabolizers (60%), intermediate metabolizers (25%), and poor metabolizers (10%). Currently, pharmacogenomic screening tests predict CYP2D6 phenotype with more than 95% reliability. The consequences of inheriting an allele that compromises CYP2D6 function include the inability to metabolize codeine (a prodrug) to morphine by O-demethylation, leading to lack of analgesia but increased side effects from the parent drug (e.g., fatigue) in poor metabolizers.[253,258] Based on the known large effects of allelic variation at the *CYP2D6* locus on metabolism of at least codeine and tramadol, and possibly oxycodone and hydrocodone, and more limited data for *OPRM1* and *COMT* loci, guidelines for dosing are now provided by the Clinical Pharmacogenetic Implementation Consortium (CPIC).[267]

In an insightful analysis of the potential role of PRS for prediction of therapeutic responses in patients with opioid use disorder, Gibson[268] reviewed three potential targets for prediction of opioid response: identification of individuals at high risk of addiction, identification of poor metabolizers, and identification of ultrarapid metabolizers.

Genetic Variability in Response to Other Drugs Used Perioperatively

A wide variety of drugs used in the perioperative period display significant pharmacokinetic or pharmacodynamic variability that is genetically modulated (Table 6-6). Although such genetic variation in drug-metabolizing enzymes or drug targets usually results in unusually variable drug response, genetic markers associated with rare but life-threatening side effects have also been described. Of note, the most commonly cited categories of drugs involved in adverse drug reactions include cardiovascular, antibiotic, psychiatric, and analgesic medications, and interestingly, each category has a known genetic basis for increased risk of adverse reactions.

There are more than 30 families of drug-metabolizing enzymes in humans, most with genetic polymorphisms shown to influence enzymatic activity. Of special importance to the anesthesiologist is the *CYP2D6*, one of the most intensively studied and best understood examples of pharmacogenetic variation, involved in the metabolism of several drugs including analgesics (codeine, dextromethorphan), BBs, antiarrhythmics (flecainide, propafenone, quinidine), and diltiazem. *CYP2D6* is also involved in the biotransformation of ondansetron, and its genetic variation resulting in the so-called ultrarapid metabolizing phenotype has been associated with increased incidence of ondansetron failure for the prevention of postoperative vomiting but not nausea,[269] which was even more pronounced if tropisetron was used as an antiemetic treatment.[270] Joint assessment of genotype-dependent CYP2D6 and CYP3A4 activities revealed that ondansetron metabolism is enantioselective, and doubling the ondansetron dose is ineffective in patients with high CYP2D6/3A4 activity.[271]

Another important pharmacogenetic variation has been described in cytochrome P450C9 (*CYP2C9*), involved in metabolizing anticoagulants (warfarin), anticonvulsants (phenytoin), antidiabetic agents (glipizide, tolbutamide), and nonsteroidal anti-inflammatory drugs (celecoxib, ibuprofen), among others. Three known *CYP2C9* variant alleles result in different enzyme activities (extensive, intermediate, and slow metabolizer phenotypes), and have clinical implications in the increased risk of life-threatening bleeding complications in slow metabolizers during standard warfarin therapy. This illustrates the concept of "high-risk pharmacokinetics," which applies to drugs with low therapeutic ratios eliminated by a single pathway (in this case, CYP2C9-mediated oxidation); genetic variation in that pathway may lead to large changes in drug clearance, concentrations, and effects.[252] Dose adjustments based on the pharmacogenetic phenotype have been proposed for drugs metabolized via both CYP2D6 and CYP2C9 pathways,[253] and a commercially available, FDA-approved test (CYP450 AmpliChip, Roche Molecular Diagnostics) allows clinicians for the first time to test patients for a wide spectrum of genetic variation in drug-metabolizing enzymes. The strongest evidence to date for use of pharmacogenomic testing is to aid in the determination of warfarin dosage by using genotypes in the *CYP2C9* and vitamin K epoxide reductase complex 1 (*VKORC1*) genes, with four FDA-approved tests now commercially available. Furthermore, *CYP2C9* genotypes and age could be used in patients on chronic warfarin therapy awaiting elective surgery to inform the time required to discontinue the

Table 6-6 Examples of Genetic Polymorphisms Involved in Variable Responses to Drugs Used in the Perioperative Period

Drug Class	Gene Name (Gene Symbol)	Effect of Polymorphism
Pharmacokinetic Variability		
β-blockers	Cytochrome P450 2D6 (*CYP2D6*)	Enhanced drug effect
Codeine, dextromethorphan	*CYP2D6*	Decreased drug effect
Ca-channel blockers	Cytochrome P450 3A4 (*CYP3A4*)	Uncertain
Alfentanil	*CYP3A4*	Enhanced drug response
Angiotensin-II receptor type 1 blockers	Cytochrome P450 2C9 (*CYP2C9*)	Enhanced blood pressure response
Warfarin	*CYP2C9*	Enhanced anticoagulant effect, risk of bleeding
Phenytoin	*CYP2C9*	Enhanced drug effect
ACE-inhibitors	Angiotensin-I converting enzyme (*ACE*)	Blood pressure response
Procainamide	N-acetyltransferase 2 (*NAT2*)	Enhanced drug effect
Succinylcholine	Butyrylcholinesterase (*BCHE*)	Enhanced drug effect
Digoxin	P-glycoprotein (*ABCB1, MDR1*)	Increased bioavailability
Pharmacodynamic Variability		
β-Blockers	β_1 and β_2 adrenergic receptors (*ADRB1, ADRB2*)	Blood pressure and heart rate response, airway responsiveness to β_2-agonists
QT-prolonging drugs (antiarrhythmics, cisapride, erythromycin, etc.)	Sodium and potassium ion channels (*SCN5 A, KCNH2, KCNE2, KCNQ1*)	Long QT syndrome, risk of torsade de pointes
Aspirin, glycoprotein IIb/IIIa inhibitors	Glycoprotein IIIa subunit of platelet glycoprotein IIb/IIIa (*ITGB3*)	Variability in antiplatelet effects
Phenylephrine	Endothelial nitric oxide synthase (*NOS3*)	Blood pressure response

drug preoperatively (rather than uniformly applying the 5-day recommended guidelines) and thus potentially avoiding the costs associated with surgical delays.[272]

Genetic variation in drug targets (receptors) can have profound effect on drug efficacy, and over 25 examples have already been identified. For example, functional polymorphisms in the β_2-AR (Arg16Gly, Gln27Glu) influence the bronchodilator and vascular responses to β-agonists, and β_1-AR variants (Arg389Gly) modulate responses to BBs and may impact postoperative cardiovascular adverse events.[185,186] An excellent review by Nagele[273] provides a strong rationale for using pharmacogenomic variation in BB metabolism (*CYP2D6*) and receptor signaling pathways (both *ADRB1, ADRB2*, and downstream genes) to determine the effectiveness and safety of perioperative β-blockade for prevention of perioperative MI, particularly given the conflicting results raised by the POISE trial.[274] Finally, clinically important genetic polymorphisms with indirect effects on drug response have been described. These include variants in candidate genes like sodium (*SCN5 A*) and potassium ion channels (*KCNH2, KCNE2, KCNQ1*), which alter susceptibility to drug-induced long QT syndrome and ventricular arrhythmias (torsade de pointes) associated with the use of drugs like erythromycin, terfenadine, disopyramide, sotalol, cisapride, or quinidine. Carriers of such susceptibility alleles have no manifest QT-interval prolongation or family history of sudden death until QT-prolonging drug challenge is superimposed.[252] Predisposition to QT-interval prolongation (considered a surrogate for risk of life-threatening ventricular arrhythmias) has been responsible for more drug withdrawals from the market than any other category of adverse event in recent times, so understanding genetic predisposing factors constitutes one of the highest priorities of current pharmacogenomic efforts.

Leveraging genetic information to improve prediction of perioperative complications through implementation of pharmacogenomic-guided interventions requires integration of genotypes into the EHR for clinicians to contextualize the information as part of clinical decision support tools. In a proof of principle study, Douville et al. analyzed pharmacogenes associated with three anesthetic complications with well-characterized genetic inheritance—butyrylcholinesterase deficiency, factor V Leiden, and malignant hyperthermia—using an open-source script designed for clinican use. Although they found strong associations between genotypes and EHR-derived phenotypes, many genetic susceptibilities were not documented in the EHR either as part of the family history or clinical features of the conditions.[275]

Complementary to pharmacogenomics, *pharmacometabonomics* describes the use of metabolic profiling of biofluids, tissues, and tissue extracts to predict, prior to dosing, the beneficial and adverse effects of an intervention such as drug administration.[276] This has been proposed as a potential significant development for precision medicine because of its ability to longitudinally sample both genetic and environmental factors (surgical stress, rapid fluid shifts, alterations in gut microbiome) that influence drug transport, metabolism, efficacy, and toxicity in a patient.

Pharmacogenomics is emerging as an additional modifying 5
component to anesthesia along with age, gender, comorbidities, and medication usage. Specific testing and treatment guidelines

allowing clinicians to appropriately modify drug utilization (e.g., adjust dose or change drug) already exist for a few compounds,[253] and will likely be expanded to all relevant therapeutic compounds (Fig. 6-2), together with identification of novel therapeutic targets.

Conclusions and Future Directions

The Human Genome Project has revolutionized all aspects of medicine, allowing us to assess the impact of genetic variability on disease taxonomy, characterization, and outcome, and individual responses to various drugs and injuries. Mechanistically, information gleaned through genomic approaches is already unraveling long-standing mysteries behind general anesthetic action and adverse responses to drugs used perioperatively. To take full advantage of the unique opportunities offered by the genomic revolution and begin implementing precision medicine concepts, the cycle of innovation in perioperative medicine must shift to a new framework which includes comprehensive and standardized definitions of the phenotypes of interest (including short- and long-term adverse outcomes such as organ injury/dysfunction, organ support-free days, adverse drug responses, transition to chronic pain, as well as novel intermediate outcomes that may not be considered patient centric by current standards)[7,277] by developing and refining EHR-driven phenotyping algorithms,[278] followed by identification of the underlying genes and dynamic genomic markers, characterization of the mechanism from DNA to phenotype, robust data integration and data science tools, and rigorous development and validation of actionable companion diagnostics implemented at the point of care using EHR-integrated clinical decision support tools (Fig. 6-2).[279] For the anesthesiologist, this may soon translate into prospective risk assessment incorporating genetic profiling of markers important in thrombotic, inflammatory, vascular, and neurologic responses to perioperative stress, with implications ranging from individualized additional preoperative testing and physiologic optimization to choice of perioperative monitoring strategies and critical care resource utilization. Furthermore, genetic profiling of drug-metabolizing enzymes, carrier proteins, and receptors, using currently available high-throughput molecular technologies, will enable personalized choice of drugs and dosage regimens tailored to suit a patient's pharmacogenetic profile. At that point, perioperative physicians will have far more robust information to use in designing the most appropriate and safest anesthetic plan for a given patient. At the same time, considerable progress should be made in understanding risks and benefits of personalization versus protocolization. Theoretically, homogenizing the treatment given to a highly heterogeneous patient population falling under a wide syndromic umbrella (e.g., sepsis)[73] or subject to various surgical procedures through the use of bundles and protocols may result in compromised outcomes in an individual patient. Benefit from an intervention in one subset may be negated by harm in another, or diluted out by noneffect in a majority subset.[280]

Although one of the aims of the Human Genome Project is to improve therapy through genome-based prediction, the birth of personal genomics opens up a Pandora's box of ethical issues, including privacy and the risk for discrimination against individuals who are genetically predisposed for a medical disorder. Such discrimination may include barriers to obtaining health, life, or long-term care insurance, or obtaining employment. Thus, extensive efforts are made to protect patients participating in genetic research from prejudice, discrimination, or uses of genetic information that will adversely affect them. To address the concerns of both biomedical research and health communities, the U.S. Senate has approved in 2003 the Genetic Information and Nondiscrimination Act, which provides the strong safeguards required to protect the public participating in human genome research. Another ethical concern is the transferability of genetic tests across ethnic groups, particularly in the prediction of adverse drug responses. It is known that most polymorphisms associated with variability in drug response show significant differences in allele frequencies among populations and racial groups. Furthermore, the patterns of linkage disequilibrium are markedly different between ethnic groups, which may lead to spurious findings when markers, instead of causal variants, are used in diagnostic tests extrapolated across populations. In exploring racial disparities in health and disease outcomes, considerable debate has focused on whether race and ethnic identity are primarily social or biologic constructs, and the contribution of genetic variability in explaining observed differences in the rates of disease between racial groups. With the goal of personalized medicine being the prediction of risk and treatment of disease on the basis of an individual's genetic profile, some have argued that biologic consideration of race will become obsolete. However, in this discovery phase of the postgenome era, continuing to incorporate racial information in genetic studies should improve our understanding of the architecture of the human genome, and its implications for novel strategies aiming at identifying variants protecting against, or conferring susceptibility to, common diseases and modulating drug effects.[281,282]

For further review and interactivities, please see the videos and narrative interactive clinical vignettes (NICVs) accessible in the complimentary eBook bundled with this text. Access instructions are located on the inside front cover.

REFERENCES

1. Podgoreanu MV, Schwinn DA. New paradigms in cardiovascular medicine: emerging technologies and practices: perioperative genomics. *J Am Coll Cardiol*. 2005;46:1965–1977.
2. Iwashyna TJ, Burke JF, Sussman JB, Prescott HC, Hayward RA, Angus DC. Implications of heterogeneity of treatment effect for reporting and analysis of randomized trials in critical care. *Am J Respir Crit Care Med*. 2015;192:1045–1051.
3. Neudecker V, Brodsky KS, Kreth S, Ginde AA, Eltzschig HK. Emerging roles for micrornas in perioperative medicine. *Anesthesiology*. 2016;124:489–506.
4. Eckhoff AM, Connor AA, Thacker JKM, et al. A multidimensional bioinformatic platform for the study of human response to surgery. *Ann Surg*. 2022;275:1094–1102.
5. Shaw A, Vandeven T. Secrets of the perioptome: new tools for a new concept. *Curr Opin Crit Care*. 2010;16(4):365–370
6. National academies of sciences engineering, and medicine; division on earth and life studies; Board on life sciences: Interindividual variability. *New Ways to Study and Implications for Decision Making: Workshop in Brief*. National Academies Press (US); 2016.
7. Maslove DM, Tang B, Shankar-Hari M, et al. Redefining critical illness. *Nat Med*. 2022;28: 1141–1148.
8. Pal N, Kertai MD. Future of perioperative precision medicine: integration of molecular science, dynamic health care informatics, and implementation of predictive pathways in real time. *Anesth Analg*. 2022;134:900–908.
9. Wagner M, Brandenburg JM, Bodenstedt S, et al. Surgomics: personalized prediction of morbidity, mortality and long-term outcome in surgery using machine learning on multimodal data. *Surg Endosc*. 2022;36:8568–8591.
10. Collins FS, Doudna JA, Lander ES, Rotimi CN. Human molecular genetics and genomics – important advances and exciting possibilities. *N Engl J Med*. 2021;384:1–4.
11. The All of Us Research Program Investigators; Denny JC, Rutter JL, Goldstein DB, et al. The "All of Us" research program. *N Engl J Med*. 2019;381:668–676.
12. Niezgoda J, Morgan PG. Anesthetic considerations in patients with mitochondrial defects. *Paediatr Anaesth*. 2013;23:785–793.
13. Nurk S, Koren S, Rhie A, et al. The complete sequence of a human genome. *Science*. 2022; 376:44–53.
14. Khamsi R. A more-inclusive genome project aims to capture all of human diversity. *Nature*. 2022;603:378–381.
15. Zeberg H, Pääbo S. The major genetic risk factor for severe COVID-19 is inherited from Neanderthals. *Nature*. 2020;587:610–612.
16. Richards S, Aziz N, Bale S, et al; ACMG Laboratory Quality Assurance Committee. Standards and guidelines for the interpretation of sequence variants: a joint consensus recommendation of the American College of Medical Genetics and Genomics and the Association for Molecular Pathology. *Genet Med*. 2015;17:405–424.

17. Miller DT, Lee K, Abul-Husn NS, et al; ACMG Secondary Findings Working Group. ACMG SF v3.1 list for reporting of secondary findings in clinical exome and genome sequencing: a policy statement of the American College of Medical Genetics and Genomics (ACMG). *Genet Med.* 2022;24:1407–1414.
18. Stranger BE, Nica AC, Forrest MS, et al. Population genomics of human gene expression. *Nat Genet.* 2007;39:1217–1224.
19. Hopf HW. Molecular diagnostics of injury and repair responses in critical illness: what is the future of "monitoring" in the intensive care unit. *Crit Care Med.* 2003;31:S518–S523.
20. Holzhauser L, DeFilippis EM, Nikolova A, et al. The end of endomyocardial biopsy? A practical guide for noninvasive heart transplant rejection surveillance. *JACC Heart Fail.* 2023; 11(3):263–276.
21. Khush KK, Pham MX, Teuteberg JJ, et al. Gene expression profiling to study racial differences after heart transplantation. *J Heart Lung Transplant.* 2015;34:970–977.
22. Milewicz DM, Regalado ES. Use of genetics for personalized management of heritable thoracic aortic disease: how do we get there? *J Thorac Cardiovasc Surg.* 2015;149:S3–S5.
23. Feezor RJ, Baker HV, Xiao W, et al. Genomic and proteomic determinants of outcome in patients undergoing thoracoabdominal aortic aneurysm repair. *J Immunol.* 2004;172: 7103–7109.
24. Balvardi S, St-Louis E, Yousef Y, et al. Systematic review of grading systems for adverse surgical outcomes. *Can J Surg.* 2021;64:E196–E204.
25. Daoud D, Chacon Alberty L, Wei Q, et al. Incidence of primary graft dysfunction is higher according to the new ISHLT 2016 guidelines and correlates with clinical and molecular risk factors. *J Thorac Dis.* 2021;13:3426–3442.
26. Sweeney TE, Liesenfeld O, Wacker J, et al. Validation of inflammopathic, adaptive, and coagulopathic sepsis endotypes in coronavirus disease 2019. *Crit Care Med.* 2021;49:e170–e178.
27. Fenner BP, Darden DB, Kelly LS, et al. Immunological endotyping of chronic critical illness after severe sepsis. *Front Med (Lausanne).* 2021;7:616694.
28. Brakenridge SC, Wang Z, Cox M, et al. Distinct immunologic endotypes are associated with clinical trajectory after severe blunt trauma and hemorrhagic shock. *J Trauma Acute Care Surg.* 2021;90:257–267.
29. Bowman EML, Cunningham EL, Page VJ, McAuley DF. Phenotypes and subphenotypes of delirium: a review of current categorisations and suggestions for progression. *Crit Care.* 2021; 25:334.
30. Calfee CS, Delucchi K, Parsons PE, Thompson BT, Ware LB, Matthay MA; NHLBI ARDS Network. Subphenotypes in acute respiratory distress syndrome: latent class analysis of data from two randomised controlled trials. *Lancet Respir Med.* 2014;2:611–620.
31. Reddy K, Sinha P, O'Kane CM, Gordon AC, Calfee CS, McAuley DF. Subphenotypes in critical care: translation into clinical practice. *Lancet Respir Med.* 2020;8:631–643.
32. Tomic V, Russwurm S, Möller E, et al. Transcriptomic and proteomic patterns of systemic inflammation in on-pump and off-pump coronary artery bypass grafting. *Circulation.* 2005; 112:2912–2920.
33. Ramlawi B, Otu H, Rudolph JL, et al. Genomic expression pathways associated with brain injury after cardiopulmonary bypass. *J Thorac Cardiovasc Surg*, 2007;134:996–1005.
34. Ramlawi B, Otu H, Mieno S, et al. Oxidative stress and atrial fibrillation after cardiac surgery: a case-control study. *Ann Thorac Surg.* 2007;84:1166–1172; discussion 1172.
35. Sehl PD, Tai JT, Hillan KJ, et al. Application of cDNA microarrays in determining molecular phenotype in cardiac growth, development, and response to injury. *Circulation.* 2000; 101:1990–1999.
36. Depre C, Tomlinson JE, Kudej RK, et al. Gene program for cardiac cell survival induced by transient ischemia in conscious pigs. *Proc Natl Acad Sci U S A.* 2001;98:9336–9341.
37. Ruel M, Bianchi C, Khan TA, et al. Gene expression profile after cardiopulmonary bypass and cardioplegic arrest. *J Thorac Cardiovasc Surg.* 2003;126:1521–1530.
38. Konstantinov IE, Coles JG, Boscarino C, et al. Gene expression profiles in children undergoing cardiac surgery for right heart obstructive lesions. *J Thorac Cardiovasc Surg.* 2004;127:746–754.
39. Muehlschlegel JD, Christodoulou DC, McKean D, et al. Using next-generation RNA sequencing to examine ischemic changes induced by cold blood cardioplegia on the human left ventricular myocardium transcriptome. *Anesthesiology.* 2015;122:537–550.
40. Sergeev P, da Silva R, Lucchinetti E, et al. Trigger-dependent gene expression profiles in cardiac preconditioning: evidence for distinct genetic programs in ischemic and anesthetic preconditioning. *Anesthesiology.* 2004;100:474–488.
41. Lucchinetti E, Aguirre J, Feng J, et al. Molecular evidence of late preconditioning after sevoflurane inhalation in healthy volunteers. *Anesth Analg.* 2007;105:629–640.
42. Lucchinetti E, Hofer C, Bestmann L, et al. Gene regulatory control of myocardial energy metabolism predicts postoperative cardiac function in patients undergoing off-pump coronary artery bypass graft surgery: inhalational versus intravenous anesthetics. *Anesthesiology.* 2007;106:444–457.
43. Atkins JH, Johansson JS. Technologies to shape the future: proteomics applications in anesthesiology and critical care medicine. *Anesth Analg.* 2006;102:1207–1216.
44. Fütterer CD, Maurer MH, Schmitt A, Feldmann RE Jr, Kuschinsky W, Waschke KF. Alterations in rat brain proteins after desflurane anesthesia. *Anesthesiology.* 2004;100:302–308.
45. Kalenka A, Hinkelbein J, Feldmann RE Jr, Kuschinsky W, Waschke KF, Maurer MH. The effects of sevoflurane anesthesia on rat brain proteins: a proteomic time-course analysis. *Anesth Analg.* 2007;104:1129–1135, tables of contents.
46. Sheikh AM, Barrett C, Villamizar N, et al. Proteomics of cerebral injury in a neonatal model of cardiopulmonary bypass with deep hypothermic circulatory arrest. *J Thorac Cardiovasc Surg.* 2006;132:820–828.
47. Rhee J, Kuznetsov A, McKay T, et al. Serum proteomics of older patients undergoing major cardiac surgery: identification of biomarkers associated with postoperative delirium. *Front Aging Neurosci.* 2021;13:699763.
48. Quinones QJ, Zhang Z, Ma Q, et al. Proteomic profiling reveals adaptive responses to surgical myocardial Ischemia-Reperfusion in hibernating arctic ground squirrels compared to rats. *Anesthesiology.* 2016;124:1296–1310.
49. Drakos SG, Badolia R, Makaju A, et al. Distinct transcriptomic and proteomic profile specifies patients who have heart failure with potential of myocardial recovery on mechanical unloading and circulatory support. *Circulation.* 2023;147(5):409–424.
50. Queloz PA, Thadikkaran L, Crettaz D, Rossier JS, Barelli S, Tissot JD. Proteomics and transfusion medicine: future perspectives. *Proteomics.* 2006;6:5605–5614.
51. Kinross J, Muirhead L, Takats Z. Precision surgery and surgical spectroscopy. Holmes E, Nicholson JK, Darzi AW, Lindon JC (eds): *Metabolic Phenotyping in Personalized and Public Healthcare.* Elsevier; 2016;75–109.
52. Nicholson JK, Holmes E, Kinross JM, Darzi AW, Takats Z, Lindon JC. Metabolic phenotyping in clinical and surgical environments. *Nature.* 2012;491:384–392.
53. Mirnezami R, Kinross JM, Vorkas PA, et al. Implementation of molecular phenotyping approaches in the personalized surgical patient journey. *Ann Surg.* 2012;255:881–889.
54. Lewis GD, Wei R, Liu E, et al. Metabolite profiling of blood from individuals undergoing planned myocardial infarction reveals early markers of myocardial injury. *J Clin Invest.* 2008;118: 3503–3512.
55. Turer AT, Stevens RD, Bain JR, et al. Metabolomic profiling reveals distinct patterns of myocardial substrate use in humans with coronary artery disease or left ventricular dysfunction during surgical ischemia/reperfusion. *Circulation.* 2009;119:1736–1746.
56. Mayr M, Yusuf S, Weir G, et al. Combined metabolomic and proteomic analysis of human atrial fibrillation. *J Am Coll Cardiol.* 2008;51:585–594.
57. Shah AA, Craig DM, Sebek JK, et al. Metabolic profiles predict adverse events after coronary artery bypass grafting. *J Thorac Cardiovasc Surg.* 2012;143:873–878.
58. Kim CD, Kim EY, Yoo H, et al. Metabonomic analysis of serum metabolites in kidney transplant recipients with cyclosporine A- or tacrolimus-based immunosuppression. *Transplantation.* 2010;90:748–756.
59. Mao H, Wang H, Wang B, et al. Systemic metabolic changes of traumatic critically ill patients revealed by an NMR-based metabonomic approach. *J Proteome Res.* 2009;8:5423–5430.
60. Wu J, Cyr A, Gruen DS, et al; PAMPer study group. Lipidomic signatures align with inflammatory patterns and outcomes in critical illness. *Nat Commun.* 2022;13:6789.
61. Acharjee A, Hazeldine J, Bazarova A, et al. Integration of metabolomic and clinical data improves the prediction of intensive care unit length of stay following major traumatic injury. *Metabolites.* 2021;12:29.
62. Vaz M, Pereira SS, Monteiro MP. Metabolomic signatures after bariatric surgery – a systematic review. *Rev Endocr Metab Disord.* 2022;23:503–519.
63. de Toro-Martín J, Guénard F, Tchernof A, Pérusse L, Marceau S, Vohl MC. Polygenic risk score for predicting weight loss after bariatric surgery. *JCI Insight.* 2018;3:122011.
64. Khan TA, Loftus TJ, Filiberto AC, et al. Metabolomic profiling for diagnosis and prognostication in surgery: a scoping review. *Ann Surg.* 2021;273:258–268.
65. Everett JR. Pharmacometabonomics: the prediction of drug effects using metabolic profiling. *Handb Exp Pharmacol.* 2019;260:263–299.
66. Verdonk F, Einhaus J, Tsai AS, et al. Measuring the human immune response to surgery: multiomics for the prediction of postoperative outcomes. *Curr Opin Crit Care.* 2021;27:717–725.
67. Strohmeyer JC, Blume C, Meisel C, et al. Standardized immune monitoring for the prediction of infections after cardiopulmonary bypass surgery in risk patients. *Cytometry B Clin Cytom.* 2003;53:54–62.
68. Kennedy SA, McEllistrem B, Kinsella A, et al. EuroSCORE and neutrophil adhesion molecules predict outcome post-cardiac surgery. *Eur J Clin Invest.* 2012;42:881–890.
69. Gaudillière B, Fragiadakis GK, Bruggner RV, et al. Clinical recovery from surgery correlates with single-cell immune signatures. *Sci Transl Med.* 2014;6:255ra131.
70. Fragiadakis GK, Gaudillière B, Ganio EA, et al. Patient-specific immune states before surgery are strong correlates of surgical recovery. *Anesthesiology.* 2015;123:1241–1255.
71. Rumer KK, Hedou J, Tsai A, et al. Integrated single-cell and plasma proteomic modeling to predict surgical site complications: a prospective cohort study. *Ann Surg.* 2022;275:582–590.
72. Meghraoui-Kheddar A, Chousterman BG, Guillou N, et al. Two new neutrophil subsets define a discriminating sepsis signature. *Am J Respir Crit Care Med.* 2022;205:46–59.
73. Singer M. Sepsis: personalization v protocolization. *Crit Care.* 2019;23:127.
74. Lirk P, Fiegl H, Weber NC, Hollmann MW. Epigenetics in the perioperative period. *Br J Pharmacol.* 2015;172:2748–2755.
75. Stary CM, Patel HH, Roth DM. Epigenetics: the epicenter for future anesthesia research. *Anesthesiology.* 2015;123:743–744.
76. Rahat B, Ali T, Sapehia D, Mahajan A, Kaur J. Circulating cell-free nucleic acids as epigenetic biomarkers in precision medicine. *Front Genet.* 2020;11:844.
77. Gögenur M, Burcharth J, Gögenur I. The role of total cell-free DNA in predicting outcomes among trauma patients in the intensive care unit: a systematic review. *Crit Care.* 2017;21:14.

78. Henriksen TV, Reinert T, Christensen E, et al; IMPROVE Study Group. The effect of surgical trauma on circulating free DNA levels in cancer patients-implications for studies of circulating tumor DNA. *Mol Oncol*. 2020;14:1670–1679.
79. Hsu PJ, Singh K, Dhiman A, et al. Utility of perioperative measurement of Cell-Free DNA and circulating tumor DNA in informing the prognosis of GI cancers: a systematic review. *JCO Precis Oncol*. 2022;6:e2100337.
80. Hassan F, Wang JH, Cullinane C, et al. Assessment of cell-free DNA (cfDNA) concentrations in the perioperative period can predict risk of recurrence in patients with non-metastatic breast cancer. *Surg Oncol*. 2022;42:101753.
81. Merkle J, Daka A, Deppe AC, et al. High levels of cell-free DNA accurately predict late acute kidney injury in patients after cardiac surgery. *PLoS One*. 2019;14:e0218548.
82. Scott JP, Tanem JM, Tomita-Mitchell A, et al. Elevated nuclear and mitochondrial cell-free deoxyribonucleic acid measurements are associated with death after infant cardiac surgery. *J Thorac Cardiovasc Surg*. 2022;164:367–375.
83. Agbor-Enoh S, Shah P, Tunc I, et al; GRAfT Investigators. Cell-free DNA to detect heart allograft acute rejection. *Circulation*. 2021;143(12):1184–1197.
84. Jang MK, Tunc I, Berry GJ, et al. Donor-derived cell-free DNA accurately detects acute rejection in lung transplant patients, a multicenter cohort study. *J Heart Lung Transplant*. 2021; 40:822–830.
85. Kohut TJ, Barandiaran JF, Keating BJ. Genomics and liver transplantation: genomic biomarkers for the diagnosis of acute cellular rejection. *Liver Transpl*. 2020;26:1337–1350.
86. Tabor HK, Risch NJ, Myers RM. Candidate-gene approaches for studying complex genetic traits: practical considerations. *Nat Rev Genet*. 2002;3:391–397.
87. Podgoreanu MV, White WD, Morris RW, et al; Perioperative Genetics and Safety Outcomes Study (PEGASUS) Investigative Team. Inflammatory gene polymorphisms and risk of postoperative myocardial infarction after cardiac surgery. *Circulation*. 2006;114:I275–I281.
88. Collard CD, Shernan SK, Fox AA, et al. The MBL2 'LYQA secretor' haplotype is an independent predictor of postoperative myocardial infarction in whites undergoing coronary artery bypass graft surgery. *Circulation*. 2007;116:I106–I112.
89. Mathew JP, Podgoreanu MV, Grocott HP, et al; PEGASUS Investigative Team. Genetic variants in P-selectin and C-reactive protein influence susceptibility to cognitive decline after cardiac surgery. *J Am Coll Cardiol*. 2007;49:1934–1942.
90. Mathew JP, Rinder CS, Howe JG, et al. Platelet PlA2 polymorphism enhances risk of neurocognitive decline after cardiopulmonary bypass. Multicenter Study of Perioperative Ischemia (McSPI) Research Group. *Ann Thorac Surg*. 2001;71:663–666.
91. Bartels K, Li YJ, Li YW, et al. Apolipoprotein epsilon 4 genotype is associated with less improvement in cognitive function five years after cardiac surgery: a retrospective cohort study. *Can J Anaesth*. 2015;62:618–626.
92. Stafford-Smith M, Podgoreanu M, Swaminathan M, et al; Perioperative Genetics and Safety Outcomes Study (PEGASUS) Investigative Team. Association of genetic polymorphisms with risk of renal injury after coronary bypass graft surgery. *Am J Kidney Dis*. 2005;45: 519–530.
93. Chew ST, Newman MF, White WD, et al. Preliminary report on the association of apolipoprotein E polymorphisms, with postoperative peak serum creatinine concentrations in cardiac surgical patients. *Anesthesiology*. 2000;93:325–331.
94. Mackensen GB, Swaminathan M, Ti LK, et al; Perioperative Outcomes Research Group, Cardiothoracic Anesthesiology Research Endeavors (C.A.R.E.) Investigators of the Duke Heart Center. Preliminary report on the interaction of apolipoprotein E polymorphism with aortic atherosclerosis and acute nephropathy after CABG. *Ann Thorac Surg*. 2004;78:520–526.
95. Ortlepp JR, Janssens U, Bleckmann F, et al. A chymase gene variant is associated with atherosclerosis in venous coronary artery bypass grafts. *Coron Artery Dis*. 2001;12:493–497.
96. Ellis SG, Chen MS, Jia G, Luke M, Cassano J, Lytle B. Relation of polymorphisms in five genes to long-term aortocoronary saphenous vein graft patency. *Am J Cardiol*. 2007;99:1087–1089.
97. Donahue BS. Factor V Leiden and perioperative risk. *Anesth Analg*. 2004;98:1623–1634.
98. Lasocki S, Iglarz M, Seince PF, et al. Involvement of renin-angiotensin system in pressure-flow relationship: role of angiotensin-converting enzyme gene polymorphism. *Anesthesiology*. 2002;96:271–275.
99. Nielsen M, Staalsoe JM, Ullum H, Secher NH, Nielsen HB, Olsen NV. The Gly16 allele of the Gly16Arg single-nucleotide polymorphism in the β_2-adrenergic receptor gene augments perioperative use of vasopressors: a retrospective cohort study. *Anesth Analg*. 2016;122:1385–1393.
100. Moretti EW, Morris RW, Podgoreanu M, et al; Perioperative Genetics and Safety Outcomes Study (PEGASUS) Investigative Team. APOE polymorphism is associated with risk of severe sepsis in surgical patients. *Crit Care Med*. 2005;33:2521–2526.
101. Slavcheva E, Albanis E, Jiao Q, et al. Cytotoxic T-lymphocyte antigen 4 gene polymorphisms and susceptibility to acute allograft rejection. *Transplantation*. 2001;72:935–940.
102. Ziegeler S, Tsusaki BE, Collard CD. Influence of genotype on perioperative risk and outcome. *Anesthesiology*. 2003;99:212–219.
103. Samani NJ, Erdmann J, Hall AS, et al; WTCCC and the Cardiogenics Consortium. Genomewide association analysis of coronary artery disease. *N Engl J Med*. 2007;357:443–453.
104. Helgadottir A, Thorleifsson G, Manolescu A, et al. A common variant on chromosome 9p21 affects the risk of myocardial infarction. *Science*. 2007;316:1491–1493.
105. Shah S, Henry A, Roselli C, et al; Regeneron Genetics Center. Genome-wide association and Mendelian randomisation analysis provide insights into the pathogenesis of heart failure. *Nat Commun*. 2020;11:163.
106. Todd JA, Walker NM, Cooper JD, et al; Genetics of Type 1 Diabetes in Finland, Wellcome Trust Case Control Consortium. Robust associations of four new chromosome regions from genome-wide analyses of type 1 diabetes. *Nat Genet*. 2007;39:857–864.
107. Diabetes Genetics Initiative of Broad Institute of Harvard and MIT, Lund University, and Novartis Institutes of BioMedical Research; Saxena R, Voight BF, Lyssenko V, et al. Genomewide association analysis identifies loci for type 2 diabetes and triglyceride levels. *Science*. 2007;316:1331–1336.
108. Gudbjartsson DF, Arnar DO, Helgadottir A, et al. Variants conferring risk of atrial fibrillation on chromosome 4q25. *Nature*. 2007;448:353–357.
109. The International Consortium for Blood Pressure Genome-Wide Association Studies, CARDIoGRAM consortium, CKDGen Consortium, KidneyGen Consortium, EchoGen consortium, CHARGE-HF consortium; Ehret GB, Munroe PB, Rice KM, et al. Genetic variants in novel pathways influence blood pressure and cardiovascular disease risk. *Nature*. 2011;478: 103–109.
110. Kertai MD, Li YJ, Li YW, et al; Duke Perioperative Genetics and Safety Outcomes (PEGASUS) Investigative Team. Genome-wide association study of perioperative myocardial infarction after coronary artery bypass surgery. *BMJ Open*. 2015;5:e006920.
111. Kertai MD, Li YJ, Ji Y, et al; Duke Perioperative Genetics and Safety Outcomes (PEGASUS) Investigative Team. Genome-wide association study of new-onset atrial fibrillation after coronary artery bypass grafting surgery. *Am Heart J*. 2015;170:580–590.e28.
112. Fox AA, Pretorius M, Liu KY, et al. Genome-wide assessment for genetic variants associated with ventricular dysfunction after primary coronary artery bypass graft surgery. *PLoS One*. 2011;6:e24593.
113. Stafford-Smith M, Li YJ, Mathew JP, et al; Duke Perioperative Genetics and Safety Outcomes (PEGASUS) Investigative Team. Genome-wide association study of acute kidney injury after coronary bypass graft surgery identifies susceptibility loci. *Kidney Int*. 2015;88:823–832.
114. International HapMap Consortium; Frazer KA, Ballinger DG, Cox DR, et al. A second generation human haplotype map of over 3.1 million SNPs. *Nature*. 2007;449:851–861.
115. 1000 Genomes Project Consortium; Abecasis GR, Auton A, Brooks LD, et al. An integrated map of genetic variation from 1,092 human genomes. *Nature*. 2012;491:56–65.
116. 100,000 Genomes Project Pilot Investigators; Smedley D, Smith KR, Martin A, et al. 100,000 Genomes pilot on rare-disease diagnosis in health care – preliminary report. *N Engl J Med*. 2021;385:1868–1880.
117. ENCODE Project Consortium; Moore JE, Purcaro MJ, Pratt HE, et al. Expanded encyclopaedias of DNA elements in the human and mouse genomes. *Nature*. 2020;583:699–710.
118. Sollis E, Mosaku A, Abid A, et al. The NHGRI-EBI GWAS Catalog: knowledgebase and deposition resource. *Nucleic Acids Res*. 2023;51:D977–D985.
119. Kathiresan S, Willer CJ, Peloso GM, et al. Common variants at 30 loci contribute to polygenic dyslipidemia. *Nat Genet*. 2009;41:56–65.
120. Võsa U, Claringbould A, Westra HJ, et al. Large-scale cis- and trans-eQTL analyses identify thousands of genetic loci and polygenic scores that regulate blood gene expression. *Nat Genet*. 2021;53:1300–1310.
121. Kullo IJ, Lewis CM, Inouye M, Martin AR, Ripatti S, Chatterjee N. Polygenic scores in biomedical research. *Nat Rev Genet*. 2022;23:524–532.
122. Boyle EA, Li YI, Pritchard JK. An expanded view of complex traits: from polygenic to omnigenic. *Cell*. 2017;169:1177–1186.
123. Feero WG, Guttmacher AE, Collins FS. Genomic medicine–an updated primer. *N Engl J Med*. 2010;362:2001–2011.
124. Wheeler DA, Srinivasan M, Egholm M, et al. The complete genome of an individual by massively parallel DNA sequencing. *Nature*. 2008;452:872–876.
125. Amanat S, Requena T, Lopez-Escamez JA. A systematic review of extreme phenotype strategies to search for rare variants in genetic studies of complex disorders. *Genes (Basel)*. 2020;11:987.
126. Ashley EA, Butte AJ, Wheeler MT, et al. Clinical assessment incorporating a personal genome. *Lancet*. 2010;375:1525–1535.
127. Cardon LR, Bell JI. Association study designs for complex diseases. *Nat Rev Genet*. 2001; 2:91–99.
128. Hirschhorn JN, Lohmueller K, Byrne E, Hirschhorn K. A comprehensive review of genetic association studies. *Genet Med*. 2002;4:45–61.
129. Roundtable on Translating Genomic-Based Research for Health, Board on Health Sciences Policy, Institute of Medicine: Assessing Genomic Sequencing Information for Health Care Decision Making: Workshop Summary. 2014.
130. Rehm HL, Berg JS, Brooks LD, et al; ClinGen. ClinGen–the clinical genome resource. *N Engl J Med*. 2015;372:2235–2242.
131. Dobson GP. Addressing the global burden of trauma in major surgery. *Front Surg*. 2015;2:43.
132. Miller PE, Thomas A, Breen TJ, et al. Prevalence of noncardiac multimorbidity in patients admitted to two cardiac intensive care units and their association with mortality. *Am J Med*. 2021;134:653–661.e5.
133. Howell SJ, Sear JW. Perioperative myocardial injury: individual and population implications. *Br J Anaesth*. 2004;93:3–8.
134. Mahaffey KW, Roe MT, Kilaru R, et al. Creatine kinase-MB elevation after coronary artery bypass grafting surgery in patients with non-ST-segment elevation acute coronary syndromes predict worse outcomes: results from four large clinical trials. *Eur Heart J*. 2007;28:425–432.
135. Landesberg G, Beattie WS, Mosseri M, Jaffe AS, Alpert JS. Perioperative myocardial infarction. *Circulation*. 2009;119:2936–2944.

136. Völzke H, Engel J, Kleine V, et al. Angiotensin I-converting enzyme insertion/deletion polymorphism and cardiac mortality and morbidity after coronary artery bypass graft surgery. *Chest*. 2002;122:31–36.
137. Delanghe J, Cambier B, Langlois M, et al. Haptoglobin polymorphism, a genetic risk factor in coronary artery bypass surgery. *Atherosclerosis*. 1997;132:215–219.
138. Shaw AD, Vaporciyan AA, Wu X, et al. Inflammatory gene polymorphisms influence risk of postoperative morbidity after lung resection. *Ann Thorac Surg*. 2005;79:1704–1710.
139. Brull DJ, Montgomery HE, Sanders J, et al. Interleukin-6 gene -174g>c and -572g>c promoter polymorphisms are strong predictors of plasma interleukin-6 levels after coronary artery bypass surgery. *Arterioscler Thromb Vasc Biol*. 2001;21:1458–1463.
140. Burzotta F, Iacoviello L, Di Castelnuovo A, et al. Relation of the -174 G/C polymorphism of interleukin-6 to interleukin-6 plasma levels and to length of hospitalization after surgical coronary revascularization. *Am J Cardiol*. 2001;88:1125–1128.
141. Grocott HP, Newman MF, El-Moalem H, Bainbridge D, Butler A, Laskowitz DT. Apolipoprotein E genotype differentially influences the proinflammatory and anti-inflammatory response to cardiopulmonary bypass. *J Thorac Cardiovasc Surg*. 2001;122:622–623.
142. Roth-Isigkeit A, Hasselbach L, Ocklitz E, et al. Inter-individual differences in cytokine release in patients undergoing cardiac surgery with cardiopulmonary bypass. *Clin Exp Immunol*. 2001; 125:80–88.
143. Boehm J, Hauner K, Grammer J, et al. Tumor necrosis factor-α-863 C/A promoter polymorphism affects the inflammatory response after cardiac surgery. *Eur J Cardiothorac Surg*. 2011; 40(1):e50–e54.
144. Tomasdottir H, Hjartarson H, Ricksten A, Wasslavik C, Bengtsson A, Ricksten SE. Tumor necrosis factor gene polymorphism is associated with enhanced systemic inflammatory response and increased cardiopulmonary morbidity after cardiac surgery. *Anesth Analg*. 2003;97:944–949.
145. Lehmann LE, Schroeder S, Hartmann W, et al. A single nucleotide polymorphism of macrophage migration inhibitory factor is related to inflammatory response in coronary bypass surgery using cardiopulmonary bypass. *Eur J Cardiothorac Surg*. 2006;30:59–63.
146. Koch A, Hamann L, Schott M, et al. Genetic variation of TLR4 influences immunoendocrine stress response: an observational study in cardiac surgical patients. *Crit Care*. 2011;15:R109.
147. Allen ML, Hoschtitzky JA, Peters MJ, et al. Interleukin-10 and its role in clinical immunoparalysis following pediatric cardiac surgery. *Crit Care Med*. 2006;34:2658–2665.
148. Galley HF, Lowe PR, Carmichael RL, Webster NR. Genotype and interleukin-10 responses after cardiopulmonary bypass. *Br J Anaesth*. 2003;91:424–426.
149. Stoica AL, Stoica E, Constantinescu I, Uscatescu V, Ginghina C. Interleukin-6 and interleukin-10 gene polymorphism, endothelial dysfunction, and postoperative prognosis in patients with peripheral arterial disease. *J Vasc Surg*. 2010;52:103–109.
150. Willerson JT, Ridker PM. Inflammation as a cardiovascular risk factor. *Circulation*. 2004;109: II2–II10.
151. Perry TE, Muehlschlegel JD, Liu KY, et al; CABG Genomics Investigators. Preoperative C-reactive protein predicts long-term mortality and hospital length of stay after primary, nonemergent coronary artery bypass grafting. *Anesthesiology*. 2010;112:607–613.
152. Kangasniemi OP, Biancari F, Luukkonen J, et al. Preoperative C-reactive protein is predictive of long-term outcome after coronary artery bypass surgery. *Eur J Cardiothorac Surg*. 2006;29:983–985.
153. Song Y, Kwak YL, Choi YS, Kim JC, Heo SB, Shim JK. Effect of preoperative statin therapy on myocardial protection and morbidity endpoints following off-pump coronary bypass surgery in patients with elevated C-reactive protein level. *Korean J Anesthesiol*. 2010;58:136–141.
154. Choi JH, Cho DK, Song YB, et al. Preoperative NT-proBNP and CRP predict perioperative major cardiovascular events in non-cardiac surgery. *Heart*. 2010;96:56–62.
155. Sas AA, Vaez A, Jamshidi Y, et al. Genetic and environmental influences on stability and change in baseline levels of C-reactive protein: a longitudinal twin study. *Atherosclerosis*. 2017; 265:172–178.
156. Perry TE, Muehlschlegel JD, Liu KY, et al; CABG Genomics Investigators. C-Reactive protein gene variants are associated with postoperative C-reactive protein levels after coronary artery bypass surgery. *BMC Med Genet*. 2009;10:38.
157. Motoyama S, Miura M, Hinai Y, et al. C-reactive protein 1059G>C genetic polymorphism influences serum C-reactive protein levels after esophagectomy in patients with thoracic esophageal cancer. *J Am Coll Surg*. 2009;209:477–483.
158. Motoyama S, Miura M, Hinai Y, Maruyama K, Murata K, Ogawa JI. C-reactive protein -717C>T genetic polymorphism associates with esophagectomy-induced stress hyperglycemia. *World J Surg*. 2010;34:1001–1007.
159. Dehghan A, Dupuis J, Barbalic M, et al. Meta-analysis of genome-wide association studies in >80 000 subjects identifies multiple loci for C-reactive protein levels. *Circulation*. 2011;123:731–738.
160. Zwicker A, Fabbri C, Rietschel M, et al. Genetic disposition to inflammation and response to antidepressants in major depressive disorder. *J Psychiatr Res*. 2018;105:17–22.
161. Hübenthal M, Löscher BS, Erdmann J, et al. Current developments of clinical sequencing and the clinical utility of polygenic risk scores in inflammatory diseases. *Front Immunol*. 2020;11:577677.
162. Dite GS, Murphy NM, Allman R. Development and validation of a clinical and genetic model for predicting risk of severe COVID-19. *Epidemiol Infect*. 2021;149:e162.
163. Horowitz JE, Kosmicki JA, Damask A, et al; Regeneron Genetics Center. Genome-wide analysis provides genetic evidence that ACE2 influences COVID-19 risk and yields risk scores associated with severe disease. *Nat Genet*. 2022;54:382–392.
164. Fricke-Galindo I, Falfán-Valencia R. Genetics insight for COVID-19 susceptibility and severity: a review. *Front Immunol*. 2021;12:622176.
165. Fajgenbaum DC, June CH. Cytokine Storm. *N Engl J Med*. 2020;383:2255–2273.
166. Sagris M, Theofilis P, Antonopoulos AS, Oikonomou E, Tsioufis K, Tousoulis D. Genetic predisposition and inflammatory inhibitors in COVID-19: where do we stand. *Biomedicines*. 2022;10:242.
167. REMAP-CAP Investigators; Gordon AC, Mouncey PR, Al-Beidh F, et al. Interleukin-6 receptor antagonists in critically Ill patients with Covid-19. *N Engl J Med*. 2021;384:1491–1502.
168. Writing Committee of the REMAP-CAP Investigators; Higgins AM, Berry LR, Lorenzi E, et al. Long-term (180-Day) outcomes in critically Ill patients with COVID-19 in the REMAP-CAP randomized clinical trial. *JAMA*. 2023;329:39–51.
169. Margraf A, Ludwig N, Zarbock A, Rossaint J. Systemic inflammatory response syndrome after surgery: mechanisms and protection. *Anesth Analg*. 2020;131:1693–1707.
170. Voetsch B, Loscalzo J. Genetic determinants of arterial thrombosis. *Arterioscler Thromb Vasc Biol*. 2004;24:216–229.
171. Rifón J, Páramo JA, Panizo C, Montes R, Rocha E. The increase of plasminogen activator inhibitor activity is associated with graft occlusion in patients undergoing aorto-coronary bypass surgery. *Br J Haematol*. 1997;99:262–267.
172. Iacoviello L, Burzotta F, Di Castelnuovo A, Zito F, Marchioli R, Donati MB. The 4G/5G polymorphism of PAI-1 promoter gene and the risk of myocardial infarction: a meta-analysis. *Thromb Haemost*. 1998;80:1029–1030.
173. Rinder CS, Mathew JP, Rinder HM, et al; Multicenter Study of Perioperative Ischemia Research Group. Platelet PlA2 polymorphism and platelet activation are associated with increased troponin I release after cardiopulmonary bypass. *Anesthesiology*. 2002;97:1118–1122.
174. Zotz RB, Klein M, Dauben HP, Moser C, Gams E, Scharf RE. Prospective analysis after coronary-artery bypass grafting: platelet GP IIIa polymorphism (HPA-1b/PIA2) is a risk factor for bypass occlusion, myocardial infarction, and death. *Thromb Haemost*. 2000;83:404–407.
175. Muehlschlegel JD, Perry TE, Liu KY, et al. Polymorphism in the protease-activated receptor-4 gene region associates with platelet activation and perioperative myocardial injury. *Am J Hematol*. 2011;87(2):161–166.
176. Faraday N, Martinez EA, Scharpf RB, et al. Platelet gene polymorphisms and cardiac risk assessment in vascular surgical patients. *Anesthesiology*. 2004;101:1291–1297.
177. Donahue BS, Gailani D, Higgins MS, Drinkwater DC, George AL Jr. Factor V Leiden protects against blood loss and transfusion after cardiac surgery. *Circulation*. 2003;107:1003–1008.
178. Moor E, Silveira A, van't Hooft F, et al. Coagulation factor V (Arg506–>Gln) mutation and early saphenous vein graft occlusion after coronary artery bypass grafting. *Thromb Haemost*. 1998;80:220–224.
179. Rodseth RN, Biccard BM, Le Manach Y, et al. The prognostic value of pre-operative and post-operative B-type natriuretic peptides in patients undergoing noncardiac surgery: B-type natriuretic peptide and N-terminal fragment of pro-B-type natriuretic peptide: a systematic review and individual patient data meta-analysis. *J Am Coll Cardiol*. 2014;63:170–180.
180. Fox AA, Shernan SK, Collard CD, et al. Preoperative B-type natriuretic peptide is as independent predictor of ventricular dysfunction and mortality after primary coronary artery bypass grafting. *J Thorac Cardiovasc Surg*. 2008;136:452–461.
181. Fox AA, Muehlschlegel JD, Body SC, et al. Comparison of the utility of preoperative versus postoperative B-type natriuretic peptide for predicting hospital length of stay and mortality after primary coronary artery bypass grafting. *Anesthesiology*. 2010;112:842–851.
182. Kristensen SD, Knuuti J, Saraste A, et al. 2014 ESC/ESA Guidelines on non-cardiac surgery: cardiovascular assessment and management: The Joint Task Force on non-cardiac surgery: cardiovascular assessment and management of the European Society of Cardiology (ESC) and the European Society of Anaesthesiology (ESA). *Eur Heart J*. 2014;35:2383–2431.
183. Shaw SM, Lewis NT, Williams SG, Tan LB. A role for BNP assays in monitoring aortic valve disease for optimal timing of surgery. *Int J Cardiol*. 2008;127:328–330.
184. Fox AA, Collard CD, Shernan SK, et al. Natriuretic peptide system gene variants are associated with ventricular dysfunction after coronary artery bypass grafting. *Anesthesiology*. 2009; 110:738–747.
185. Zaugg M, Schaub MC. Genetic modulation of adrenergic activity in the heart and vasculature: implications for perioperative medicine. *Anesthesiology*. 2005;102:429–446.
186. Zaugg M, Bestmann L, Wacker J, et al. Adrenergic receptor genotype but not perioperative bisoprolol therapy may determine cardiovascular outcome in at-risk patients undergoing surgery with spinal block: the Swiss Beta Blocker in Spinal Anesthesia (BBSA) study: a double-blinded, placebo-controlled, multicenter trial with 1-year follow-up. *Anesthesiology*. 2007;107:33–44.
187. Philip I, Plantefeve G, Vuillaumier-Barrot S, et al. G894T polymorphism in the endothelial nitric oxide synthase gene is associated with an enhanced vascular responsiveness to phenylephrine. *Circulation*. 1999;99:3096–3098.
188. Ryan R, Thornton J, Duggan E, et al. Gene polymorphism and requirement for vasopressor infusion after cardiac surgery. *Ann Thorac Surg*. 2006;82:895–901.
189. Nakada TA, Russell JA, Boyd JH, et al. Association of angiotensin II type 1 receptor-associated protein gene polymorphism with increased mortality in septic shock. *Crit Care Med*. 2011; 39:1641–1648.
190. Loukanov T, Hoss K, Tonchev P, et al. Endothelial nitric oxide synthase gene polymorphism (Glu298Asp) and acute pulmonary hypertension post cardiopulmonary bypass in children with congenital cardiac diseases. *Cardiol Young*. 2011;21:161–169.
191. Panagiotopoulos I, Palatianos G, Michalopoulos A, Chatzigeorgiou A, Prapas S, Kamper EF. Alterations in biomarkers of endothelial function following on-pump coronary artery revascularization. *J Clin Lab Anal*. 2010;24:389–398.
192. Stoppelkamp S, Veseli K, Stang K, Schlensak C, Wendel HP, Walker T. Identification of predictive early biomarkers for sterile-SIRS after cardiovascular surgery. *PLoS One*. 2015;10:e0135527.

193. Enger TB, Pleym H, Stenseth R, Wahba A, Videm V. Genetic and clinical risk factors for fluid overload following open-heart surgery. *Acta Anaesthesiol Scand*. 2014;58:539–548.
194. Kim NS, Lee IO, Lee MK, Lim SH, Choi YS, Kong MH. The effects of beta2 adrenoceptor gene polymorphisms on pressor response during laryngoscopy and tracheal intubation. *Anaesthesia*. 2002;57:227–232.
195. Odekon L, Landau R, Blouin JL, Brodow D, Wang S, Smiley RM. The Effect of β2-adrenoceptor genotype on phenylephrine dose administered during spinal anesthesia for cesarean delivery. *Anesth Analg*. 2015;120:1309–1316.
196. Smiley RM, Blouin JL, Negron M, Landau R. beta2-adrenoceptor genotype affects vasopressor requirements during spinal anesthesia for cesarean delivery. *Anesthesiology*. 2006;104:644–650.
197. Liu KY, Muehlschlegel JD, Perry TE, et al. Common genetic variants on chromosome 9p21 predict perioperative myocardial injury after coronary artery bypass graft surgery. *J Thorac Cardiovasc Surg*. 2010;139:483–488, 488.e1.
198. Muehlschlegel JD, Liu KY, Perry TE, et al; CABG Genomics Investigators. Chromosome 9p21 variant predicts mortality after coronary artery bypass graft surgery. *Circulation*. 2010; 122:S60–S65.
199. Torkamani A, Wineinger NE, Topol EJ. The personal and clinical utility of polygenic risk scores. *Nat Rev Genet*. 2018;19:581–590.
200. Douville NJ, Surakka I, Leis A, et al. Use of a polygenic risk score improves prediction of myocardial injury after non-cardiac surgery. *Circ Genom Precis Med*. 2020;13:e002817.
201. Mathew JP, Fontes ML, Tudor IC, et al. A multicenter risk index for atrial fibrillation after cardiac surgery. *JAMA*. 2004;291:1720–1729.
202. Body SC, Collard CD, Shernan SK, et al. Variation in the 4q25 chromosomal locus predicts atrial fibrillation after coronary artery bypass graft surgery. *Circ Cardiovasc Genet*. 2009;2:499–506.
203. Gaudino M, Andreotti F, Zamparelli R, et al. The -174G/C interleukin-6 polymorphism influences postoperative interleukin-6 levels and postoperative atrial fibrillation. Is atrial fibrillation an inflammatory complication. *Circulation*. 2003;108(Suppl 1):II195–199.
204. Motsinger AA, Donahue BS, Brown NJ, Roden DM, Ritchie MD. Risk factor interactions and genetic effects associated with post-operative atrial fibrillation. *Pac Symp Biocomput*. 2006;584–595.
205. Gaudino M, Di Castelnuovo A, Zamparelli R, et al. Genetic control of postoperative systemic inflammatory reaction and pulmonary and renal complications after coronary artery surgery. *J Thorac Cardiovasc Surg*. 2003;126:1107–1112.
206. Hogue CW, Palin CA, Kailasam R, et al. C-reactive protein levels and atrial fibrillation after cardiac surgery in women. *Ann Thorac Surg*. 2006;82:97–102.
207. Pretorius M, Donahue BS, Yu C, Greelish JP, Roden DM, Brown NJ. Plasminogen activator inhibitor-1 as a predictor of postoperative atrial fibrillation after cardiopulmonary bypass. *Circulation*. 2007;116:I1–17.
208. Jeff JM, Donahue BS, Brown-Gentry K, et al. Genetic variation in the β1-adrenergic receptor is associated with the risk of atrial fibrillation after cardiac surgery. *Am Heart J*. 2014;167:101–108.e1.
209. Kertai MD, Li YW, Li YJ, et al; Duke Perioperative Genetics and Safety Outcomes (PEGASUS) Investigative Team. G protein-coupled receptor kinase 5 gene polymorphisms are associated with postoperative atrial fibrillation after coronary artery bypass grafting in patients receiving β-blockers. *Circ Cardiovasc Genet*. 2014;7:625–633.
210. El Gindy DMK, Solayman MH, Khorshid R, Schaalan MF, El Wakeel LM. Effect of clinical and genetic factors on the development of postoperative atrial fibrillation after coronary artery bypass grafting (CABG) in Egyptian patients receiving beta-blockers. *Cardiovasc Drugs Ther*. 2022.
211. Choi SH, Jurgens SJ, Weng LC, et al. Monogenic and polygenic contributions to atrial fibrillation risk: results from a National Biobank. *Circ Res*. 2020;126:200–209.
212. Kertai MD, Mosley JD, He J, et al. Predictive accuracy of a polygenic risk score for postoperative atrial fibrillation after cardiac surgery. *Circ Genom Precis Med*. 2021;14(2):e003269.
213. Aittokallio J, Kauko A, Vaura F, et al. Polygenic risk scores for predicting adverse outcomes after coronary revascularization. *Am J Cardiol*. 2022;167:9–14.
214. Vogel S, Rudaka I, Rots D, et al. A higher polygenic risk score is associated with a higher recurrence rate of atrial fibrillation in direct current cardioversion-treated patients. *Medicina (Kaunas)*. 2021;57:1263.
215. Choe WS, Kang JH, Choi EK, et al. A genetic risk score for atrial fibrillation predicts the response to catheter ablation. *Korean Circ J*. 2019;49:338–349.
216. Barth AS, Merk S, Arnoldi E, et al. Reprogramming of the human atrial transcriptome in permanent atrial fibrillation: expression of a ventricular-like genomic signature. *Circ Res*. 2005;96:1022–1029.
217. Kertai MD, Qi W, Li YJ, et al; Duke Perioperative Genetics and Safety Outcomes (PEGASUS) Investigative Team. Gene signatures of postoperative atrial fibrillation in atrial tissue after coronary artery bypass grafting surgery in patients receiving β-blockers. *J Mol Cell Cardiol*. 2016;92:109–115.
218. Podgoreanu MV, Booth JV, White WD, et al. Beta adrenergic receptor polymorphisms and risk of adverse events following cardiac surgery. *Circulation*. 2003;108:434.
219. Lobato RL, White WD, Mathew JP, et al; Duke Perioperative Genetics and Safety Outcomes (PEGASUS) Investigative Team. Thrombomodulin gene variants are associated with increased mortality after coronary artery bypass surgery in replicated analyses. *Circulation*. 2011;124:S143–S148.
220. Grocott HP, White WD, Morris RW, et al; Perioperative Genetics and Safety Outcomes Study (PEGASUS) Investigative Team. Genetic polymorphisms and the risk of stroke after cardiac surgery. *Stroke*. 2005;36:1854–1858.
221. Tardiff BE, Newman MF, Saunders AM, et al. Preliminary report of a genetic basis for cognitive decline after cardiac operations. The Neurologic Outcome Research Group of the Duke Heart Center. *Ann Thorac Surg*. 1997;64:715–720.
222. Newman MF, Booth JV, Laskowitz DT, et al. Genetic predictors of perioperative neurological and cognitive injury and recovery. *Best Practice & Research Clinical Anaesthesiology*. 2001;15:247–276.
223. Biffi A, Anderson CD, Jagiella JM, et al; International Stroke Genetics Consortium. APOE genotype and extent of bleeding and outcome in lobar intracerebral haemorrhage: a genetic association study. *Lancet Neurol*. 2011;10:702–709.
224. Teasdale GM, Nicoll JA, Murray G, Fiddes M. Association of apolipoprotein E polymorphism with outcome after head injury. *Lancet*. 1997;350:1069–1071.
225. Slooter AJ, Tang MX, van Duijn CM, et al. Apolipoprotein E epsilon4 and the risk of dementia with stroke. A population-based investigation. *JAMA*. 1997;277:818–821.
226. Mori T, Kobayashi M, Town T, Fujita SC, Asano T. Increased vulnerability to focal ischemic brain injury in human apolipoprotein E4 knock-in mice. *J Neuropathol Exp Neurol* 2003 62:280–291.
227. Sheng H, Laskowitz DT, Bennett E, et al. Apolipoprotein E isoform-specific differences in outcome from focal ischemia in transgenic mice. *J Cereb Blood Flow Metab*. 1998;18:361–366.
228. Leung JM, Sands LP, Wang Y, et al. Apolipoprotein E e4 allele increases the risk of early postoperative delirium in older patients undergoing noncardiac surgery. *Anesthesiology*. 2007; 107:406–411.
229. Ely EW, Girard TD, Shintani AK, et al. Apolipoprotein E4 polymorphism as a genetic predisposition to delirium in critically ill patients. *Crit Care Med*. 2007;35:112–117.
230. Fuller S, Nord AS, Gerdes M, et al. Predictors of impaired neurodevelopmental outcomes at one year of age after infant cardiac surgery. *Eur J Cardiothorac Surg*. 2009;36:40–47.
231. Gaynor JW, Gerdes M, Zackai EH, et al. Apolipoprotein E genotype and neurodevelopmental sequelae of infant cardiac surgery. *J Thorac Cardiovasc Surg*. 2003;126:1736–1745.
232. Ti LK, Mathew JP, Mackensen GB, et al. Effect of apolipoprotein E genotype on cerebral autoregulation during cardiopulmonary bypass. *Stroke*. 2001;32:1514–1519.
233. Ti LK, Mackensen GB, Grocott HP, et al; Neurologic Outcome Research Group. Apolipoprotein E4 increases aortic atheroma burden in cardiac surgical patients. *J Thorac Cardiovasc Surg*. 2003;125:211–213.
234. Newman MF, Laskowitz DT, White WD, et al. Apolipoprotein E polymorphisms and age at first coronary artery bypass graft. *Anesth Analg*. 2001;92:824–829.
235. Weiss EJ, Bray PF, Tayback M, et al. A polymorphism of a platelet glycoprotein receptor as an inherited risk factor for coronary thrombosis. *N Engl J Med*. 1996;334:1090–1094.
236. Carter AM, Catto AJ, Bamford JM, Grant PJ. Platelet GP IIIa PlA and GP Ib variable number tandem repeat polymorphisms and markers of platelet activation in acute stroke. *Arterioscler Thromb Vasc Biol*. 1998;18:1124–1131.
237. Ramlawi B, Rudolph JL, Mieno S, et al. C-reactive protein and inflammatory response associated to neurocognitive decline following cardiac surgery. *Surgery*. 2006;140:221–226.
238. Ramlawi B, Rudolph JL, Mieno S, et al. Serologic markers of brain injury and cognitive function after cardiopulmonary bypass. *Ann Surg*. 2006;244:593–601.
239. Heider P, Poppert H, Wolf O, et al. Fibrinogen and high-sensitive C-reactive protein as serologic predictors for perioperative cerebral microembolic lesions after carotid endarterectomy. *J Vasc Surg*. 2007;46:449–454.
240. Brown JR, Baker RA, Shore-Lesserson L, et al. The Society of Thoracic Surgeons/Society of Cardiovascular Anesthesiologists/American Society for Extracorporeal Technology Clinical Practice guidelines for the prevention of adult cardiac surgery-associated acute kidney injury. *Anesth Analg*. 2023;136:176–184.
241. Thakar CV, Worley S, Arrigain S, Yared JP, Paganini EP. Influence of renal dysfunction on mortality after cardiac surgery: modifying effect of preoperative renal function. *Kidney Int*. 2005;67:1112–1119.
242. Westphal S, Stoppe C, Gruenewald M, et al; RIPHeart-Study Collaborators. Genome-wide association study of myocardial infarction, atrial fibrillation, acute stroke, acute kidney injury and delirium after cardiac surgery – a sub-analysis of the RIPHeart-Study. *BMC Cardiovasc Disord*. 2019;19:26.
243. Larach DB, Lewis A, Bastarache L, et al. Limited clinical utility for GWAS or polygenic risk score for postoperative acute kidney injury in non-cardiac surgery in European-ancestry patients. *BMC Nephrol*. 2022;23:339.
244. Wuttke M, Li Y, Li M, et al; Lifelines Cohort Study, V. A. Million Veteran Program. A catalog of genetic loci associated with kidney function from analyses of a million individuals. *Nat Genet*. 2019;51:957–972.
245. Yende S, Wunderink R. Causes of prolonged mechanical ventilation after coronary artery bypass surgery. *Chest*. 2002;122:245–252.
246. Rigat B, Hubert C, Alhenc-Gelas F, Cambien F, Corvol P, Soubrier F. An insertion/deletion polymorphism in the angiotensin I-converting enzyme gene accounting for half the variance of serum enzyme levels. *J Clin Invest*. 1990;86:1343–1346.
247. Yende S, Quasney MW, Tolley EA, Wunderink RG. Clinical relevance of angiotensin-converting enzyme gene polymorphisms to predict risk of mechanical ventilation after coronary artery bypass graft surgery. *Crit Care Med*. 2004;32:922–927.
248. Marshall RP, Webb S, Bellingan GJ, et al. Angiotensin converting enzyme insertion/deletion polymorphism is associated with susceptibility and outcome in acute respiratory distress syndrome. *Am J Respir Crit Care Med*. 2002;166:646–650.
249. Yende S, Quasney MW, Tolley E, Zhang Q, Wunderink RG. Association of tumor necrosis factor gene polymorphisms and prolonged mechanical ventilation after coronary artery bypass surgery. *Crit Care Med*. 2003;31:133–140.
250. Shi S, Chen C, Zhao D, et al. The role of plasma gelsolin in cardiopulmonary bypass induced acute lung injury in infants and young children: a pilot study. *BMC Anesthesiol*. 2014;14:67.

251. Liu X, Chen Q, Shi S, et al. Plasma sRAGE enables prediction of acute lung injury after cardiac surgery in children. *Crit Care*. 2012;16:R91.
252. Roden DM, Van Driest SL, Wells QS, Mosley JD, Denny JC, Peterson JF. Opportunities and challenges in cardiovascular pharmacogenomics: from discovery to implementation. *Circ Res*. 2018;122:1176–1190.
253. Rosenberg H, Pollock N, Schiemann A, Bulger T, Stowell K. Malignant hyperthermia: a review. *Orphanet J Rare Dis*. 2015;10:93.
254. Bukaveckas BL, Valdes R Jr, Linder MW. Pharmacogenetics as related to the practice of cardiothoracic and vascular anesthesia. *J Cardiothorac Vasc Anesth*. 2004;18:353–365.
255. Ezri T, Sessler D, Weisenberg M, et al. Association of ethnicity with the minimum alveolar concentration of sevoflurane. *Anesthesiology*. 2007;107:9–14.
256. Gerstin KM, Gong DH, Abdallah M, Winegar BD, Eger EI 2nd, Gray AT. Mutation of KCNK5 or Kir3.2 potassium channels in mice does not change minimum alveolar anesthetic concentration. *Anesth Analg*. 2003;96:1345–1349.
257. Sonner JM, Antognini JF, Dutton RC, et al. Inhaled anesthetics and immobility: mechanisms, mysteries, and minimum alveolar anesthetic concentration. *Anesth Analg*. 2003;97:718–740.
258. Sternberg WF, Mogil JF. Genetic and hormonal basis of pain states. Best *Practice & Research Clinical Anaesthesiology*. 2001;15:229–245.
259. Diatchenko L, Anderson AD, Slade GD, et al. Three major haplotypes of the beta2 adrenergic receptor define psychological profile, blood pressure, and the risk for development of a common musculoskeletal pain disorder. *Am J Med Genet B Neuropsychiatr Genet*. 2006;141B:449–462.
260. Diatchenko L, Nackley AG, Tchivileva IE, Shabalina SA, Maixner W. Genetic architecture of human pain perception. *Trends Genet*. 2007;23:605–613.
261. Bengtsson B, Thorson J. Back pain: a study of twins. *Acta Genet Med Gemellol (Roma)*. 1991; 40:83–90.
262. Mogil JS, Wilson SG, Bon K, et al. Heritability of nociception I: responses of 11 inbred mouse strains on 12 measures of nociception. *Pain*. 1999;80:67–82.
263. Lacroix-Fralish ML, Ledoux JB, Mogil JS. The Pain Genes Database: an interactive web browser of pain-related transgenic knockout studies. *Pain*. 2007;131:3.e1–e4.
264. Somogyi AA, Barratt DT, Coller JK. Pharmacogenetics of opioids. *Clin Pharmacol Ther*. 2007; 81:429–444.
265. Diatchenko L, Nackley AG, Slade GD, et al. Catechol-O-methyltransferase gene polymorphisms are associated with multiple pain-evoking stimuli. *Pain*. 2006;125:216–224.
266. Fontanillas P, Kless A, Bothmer J, Tung JY; 23andMe Research Team. Genome-wide association study of pain sensitivity assessed by questionnaire and the cold pressor test. *Pain*. 2022;163:1763–1776.
267. Crews KR, Monte AA, Huddart R, et al. Clinical Pharmacogenetics implementation consortium guideline for CYP2D6, OPRM1, and comt genotypes and select opioid therapy. *Clin Pharmacol Ther*. 2021;110:888–896.
268. Gibson G. On the utilization of polygenic risk scores for therapeutic targeting. *PLoS Genet*. 2019;15:e1008060.
269. Candiotti KA, Birnbach DJ, Lubarsky DA, et al. The impact of pharmacogenomics on postoperative nausea and vomiting: do CYP2D6 allele copy number and polymorphisms affect the success or failure of ondansetron prophylaxis? *Anesthesiology*. 2005;102:543–549.
270. Kaiser R, Sezer O, Papies A, et al. Patient-tailored antiemetic treatment with 5-hydroxytryptamine type 3 receptor antagonists according to cytochrome P-450 2D6 genotypes. *J Clin Oncol*. 2002;20:2805–2811.
271. Stamer UM, Lee EH, Rauers NI, et al. CYP2D6- and CYP3A-dependent enantioselective plasma concentrations of ondansetron in postanesthesia care. *Anesth Analg*. 2011;113: 48–54.
272. Abohelaika S, Wynne H, Cope L, Kamali F. The impact of genetics on the management of patients on warfarin awaiting surgery. *Age Ageing*. 2015;44:721–722.
273. Nagele P, Liggett SB. Genetic variation, β-blockers, and perioperative myocardial infarction. *Anesthesiology*. 2011;115:1316–1327.
274. POISE Study Group; Devereaux PJ, Yang H, Yusuf S, et al. Effects of extended-release metoprolol succinate in patients undergoing non-cardiac surgery (POISE trial): a randomised controlled trial. *Lancet*. 2008;371:1839–1847.
275. Douville NJ, Kheterpal S, Engoren M, et al. Genetic mutations associated with susceptibility to perioperative complications in a longitudinal biorepository with integrated genomic and electronic health records. *Br J Anaesth*. 2020;125:986–994.
276. Nicholson JK, Everett JR, Lindon JC. Longitudinal pharmacometabonomics for predicting patient responses to therapy: drug metabolism, toxicity and efficacy. *Expert Opin Drug Metab Toxicol*. 2012;8:135–139.
277. Gajic O, Ahmad SR, Wilson ME, Kaufman DA. Outcomes of critical illness: what is meaningful? *Curr Opin Crit Care*. 2018;24:394–400.
278. Liao KP, Cai T, Savova GK, et al. Development of phenotype algorithms using electronic medical records and incorporating natural language processing. *BMJ*. 2015;350:h1885.
279. Castaneda C, Nalley K, Mannion C, et al. Clinical decision support systems for improving diagnostic accuracy and achieving precision medicine. *J Clin Bioinforma*. 2015;5:4.
280. Andreis DT, Singer M. Catecholamines for inflammatory shock: a Jekyll-and-Hyde conundrum. *Intensive Care Med*. 2016;42:1387–1397.
281. Phimister EG. Medicine and the racial divide. *N Engl J Med*. 2003;348:1081–1082.
282. Lucchinetti E, da Silva R, Pasch T, et al. Anaesthetic preconditioning but not postconditioning prevents early activation of the deleterious cardiac remodelling programme: evidence of opposing genomic responses in cardioprotection by pre- and postconditioning. *Br J Anaesth*. 2005;95:140–152.
283. Lai LP, Lin JL, Lin CS, et al. Functional genomic study on atrial fibrillation using cDNA microarray and two-dimensional protein electrophoresis techniques and identification of the myosin regulatory light chain isoform reprogramming in atrial fibrillation. *J Cardiovasc Electrophysiol*. 2004;15:214–223.
284. Pham MX, Teuteberg JJ, Kfoury AG, et al. Gene-expression profiling for rejection surveillance after cardiac transplantation. *N Engl J Med*. 2010;362:1890–1900.
285. Borozdenkova S, Westbrook JA, Patel V, et al. Use of proteomics to discover novel markers of cardiac allograft rejection. *J Proteome Res*. 2004;3:282–288.
286. Rosenberg S, Elashoff MR, Beineke P, et al. Multicenter validation of the diagnostic accuracy of a blood-based gene expression test for assessing obstructive coronary artery disease in nondiabetic patients. *Ann Intern Med*. 2010;153:425–434.
287. Matkovich SJ, Van Booven DJ, Youker KA, et al. Reciprocal regulation of myocardial micro RNAs and messenger RNA in human cardiomyopathy and reversal of the microRNA signature by biomechanical support. *Circulation*. 2009;119:1263–1271.
288. Heusch G, Erbel R, Siffert W. Genetic determinants of coronary vasomotor tone in humans. *Am J Physiol Heart Circ Physiol*. 2001;281:H1465–8.
289. Henrion D, Benessiano J, Philip I, et al. The deletion genotype of the angiotensin I-converting enzyme is associated with an increased vascular reactivity in vivo and in vitro. *J Am Coll Cardiol*. 1999;34:830–836.
290. Iribarren JL, Sagasti FM, Jimenez JJ, et al. TNFbeta+250 polymorphism and hyperdynamic state in cardiac surgery with extracorporeal circulation. *Interact Cardiovasc Thorac Surg*. 2008;7:1071–1074.
291. Donahue BS, Roden D. Inflammatory cytokine polymorphisms are associated with beta-blocker failure in preventing postoperative atrial fibrillation (abstr). *Anesth Analg*. 2005;100:SCA30.
292. Virani SS, Brautbar A, Lee VV, et al. Usefulness of single nucleotide polymorphism in chromosome 4q25 to predict in-hospital and long-term development of atrial fibrillation and survival in patients undergoing coronary artery bypass grafting. *Am J Cardiol*. 2011;107:1504–1509.
293. Kertai MD, Ji Y, Li YJ, et al. Interleukin-1β gene variants are associated with QTc interval prolongation following cardiac surgery: a prospective observational study. *Can J Anaesth*. 2016;63:397–410.
294. Botto N, Andreassi MG, Rizza A, et al. C677T polymorphism of the methylenetetrahydrofolate reductase gene is a risk factor of adverse events after coronary revascularization. *Int J Cardiol*. 2004;96:341–345.
295. Taylor KD, Scheuner MT, Yang H, et al. Lipoprotein lipase locus and progression of atherosclerosis in coronary-artery bypass grafts. *Genet Med*. 2004;6:481–486.
296. Holweg CT, Weimar W, Uitterlinden AG, et al. Clinical impact of cytokine gene polymorphisms in heart and lung transplantation. *J Heart Lung Transplant*. 2004;23:1017–1026.
297. Borozdenkova S, Smith J, Marshall S, et al. Identification of ICAM-1 polymorphism that is associated with protection from transplant associated vasculopathy after cardiac transplantation. *Hum Immunol*. 2001;62:247–255.
298. Vamvakopoulos JE, Taylor CJ, Green C, et al. Interleukin 1 and chronic rejection: possible genetic links in human heart allografts. *Am J Transplant*. 2002;2:76–83.
299. Benza RL, Coffey CS, Pekarek DM, et al. Transforming growth factor-beta polymorphisms and cardiac allograft rejection. *J Heart Lung Transplant*. 2009;28:1057–1062.
300. Zeltser I, Jarvik GP, Bernbaum J, et al. Genetic factors are important determinants of neurodevelopmental outcome after repair of tetralogy of Fallot. *J Thorac Cardiovasc Surg*. 2008;135:91–97.
301. McDonagh DL, Mathew JP, White WD, et al. Cognitive function after major noncardiac surgery, apolipoprotein E4 genotype, and biomarkers of brain injury. *Anesthesiology*. 2010;112:852–859.
302. van Munster BC, de Rooij SEJA, Yazdanpanah M, et al. The association of the dopamine transporter gene and the dopamine receptor 2 gene with delirium, a meta-analysis. *Am J Med Genet B Neuropsychiatr Genet*. 2010;153B:648–655.
303. Duggan E, O'Dwyer MJ, Caraher E, et al. Coagulopathy after cardiac surgery may be influenced by a functional plasminogen activator inhibitor polymorphism. *Anesth Analg*. 2007;104:1343–1347.
304. Welsby IJ, Podgoreanu MV, Phillips-Bute B, et al. Genetic factors contribute to bleeding after cardiac surgery. *J Thromb Haemost*. 2005;3:1206–1212.
305. Greiff G, Pleym H, Stenseth R, et al. Genetic variation influences the risk of bleeding after cardiac surgery: novel associations and validation of previous findings. *Acta Anaesthesiol Scand*. 2015 59:796–806.
306. Morawski W, Sanak M, Cisowski M, et al. Prediction of the excessive perioperative bleeding in patients undergoing coronary artery bypass grafting: role of aspirin and platelet glycoprotein IIIa polymorphism. *J Thorac Cardiovasc Surg*. 2005;130:791–796.
307. Welsby IJ, Podgoreanu MV, Phillips-Bute B, et al. Association of the 98T ELAM-1 polymorphism with increased bleeding after cardiac surgery. *J Cardiothorac Vasc Anesth*. 2010; 24:427–433.
308. Achrol AS, Kim H, Pawlikowska L, et al. Association of tumor necrosis factor-alpha-238G>A and apolipoprotein E2 polymorphisms with intracranial hemorrhage after brain arteriovenous malformation treatment. *Neurosurgery*. 2007;61:731–739; discussion 740.

7 Experimental Design and Statistics

NATHAN LEON PACE

KEY POINTS

1 Statistics and mathematics are the language of scientific medicine.

2 Good research planning includes a clear biologic hypothesis, the specification of outcome variables, the choice of anticipated statistical methods, and sample size planning.

3 The crucial elements of good research design include concurrent control groups; random allocation of subjects to treatment groups; concealment of random allocation; blinding of treatment assignment to patients, caregivers, and outcome assessors; and full reporting of outcomes for all study patients. These techniques minimize the risk of bias in clinical research.

4 The use of graphs, descriptive statistics (e.g., mean, standard deviation), and inferential statistics (e.g., *t*-test, confidence interval) are important methods for the presentation of research results.

5 Bayesian statistical methods report research results as a function of both observed data and historical (prior) knowledge; the more common frequentist statistical methods report research results only as a function of observed data.

6 Multivariable logistic regression and propensity score matching are statistical techniques for identifying associations between risk factors and outcomes in nonrandomized studies.

7 Systematic review and meta-analysis summarize the results of individual studies and permit more powerful inferences for the comparison of interventions.

8 Anesthesia data does not yet have the Volume, Velocity, and Variety characteristics of Big Data.

9 Resources and guidance for experimental design and statistical methods include policy statements, textbooks, journal articles, and public domain software.

Introduction

1 If physicians are to be practitioners of scientific medicine, they must read the language of science to be able to independently assess and interpret the scientific report. Without exception, the language of medicine is increasingly statistical. This chapter provides a brief review of some of the most important elements of experimental design and statistical analysis for the clinical anesthesiologist.

Foundations

Statistics is a method for working with *sets* of numbers. A typical scientific hypothesis asks which of two interventions is better, *X* or *Y*. Statistical methods are necessary because there are sources of variation in any data set, including random biologic variation and measurement error. These errors in the data cause difficulties in avoiding bias and in being precise. Bias keeps the true value from being known and fosters incorrect decisions; precision deals with the problem of data scatter and with quantifying the uncertainty about the value in the population from which a sample is drawn. These statistical methods are relatively independent of the particular field of study.

Data Structure

Data collected in an experiment include the defining characteristics of the experiment and the values of events or attributes that vary over time or conditions. The former are called *explanatory variables* and the latter are called *response variables*. Variables such as gender, age, and doses of accompanying drugs reflect the variability of the experimental subjects. Explanatory variables, it is 2
hoped, describe the systematic variations in the response variables.

Table 7-1 Data Types

Data Type	Definition	Examples
Interval		
Discrete	Data measured with an integer-only scale	Parity, number of teeth
Continuous	Data measured with a constant scale interval	Blood pressure, temperature
Categorical		
Dichotomous	Binary data	Mortality, gender
Nominal	Qualitative data that cannot be ordered or ranked	Eye color, drug category
Ordinal	Data ordered, ranked, or measured without a constant scale interval	American Society of Anesthesiologists (ASA) physical status score, pain score

Response variables are also called *dependent variables.* Response variables reflect the primary properties of experimental interest in the subjects. Research in anesthesiology is particularly likely to have repeated measurement variables; that is, a particular measurement recorded more than once for each individual. Some variables can be both explanatory and response; these are called *intermediate response variables.* Suppose an experiment is conducted comparing electrocardiography and myocardial responses between five doses of an opioid. One might analyze how ST segments depended on the dose of opioids; here, maximum ST-segment depression is a response variable. Maximum ST-segment depression might also be used as an explanatory variable to address the subtler question of the extent to which the effect of an opioid dose on postoperative myocardial infarction can be accounted for by ST-segment changes.

The mathematical characteristics of the possible values of a variable fit into five classifications (Table 7-1). Properly assigning a variable to the correct data type is essential for choosing the correct statistical technique. For *interval variables,* there is equal distance between successive intervals; the difference between 15 and 10 is the same as the difference between 25 and 20. *Discrete interval data* can have only integer values; for example, number of living children. *Continuous interval data* are measured on a continuum and can be a decimal fraction; for example, blood pressure can be described as accurately as desired (e.g., 136, 136.1, or 136.14 mm Hg). The same statistical techniques are used for discrete and continuous data.

Putting observations into two or more discrete subsets describes the concept of categorical *variables*; for statistical analysis, numeric values are assigned as labels to the categories. *Dichotomous data* allow only two possible values; for example, male versus female. *Ordinal data* have three or more categories that can logically be ranked or ordered; however, the ranking or ordering of the variable indicates only relative and not absolute differences between values; for example, there is not necessarily the same difference between American Society of Anesthesiologists Physical Status score I and II as there is between III and IV. Although ordinal data are often treated as interval data in choosing a statistical technique, alternative techniques for ordinal data are available and may in fact be preferable. *Nominal variables* are placed into categories that have no logical ordering. The eye colors blue, hazel, and brown might be assigned the numbers 1, 2, and 3, but these values have no meaning.

Descriptive Statistics

There are concise ways of summarizing the data from any experiment called descriptive statistics. These numbers are called *sample* or *summary statistics.*[1,2] By convention, the symbols of summary statistics are Roman letters. The two summary statistics most frequently used for interval variables are the *central location* and the *variability,* but there are others. Different data types have analogous summary statistics. Although the first purpose of descriptive statistics is to describe the numbers obtained in a sample, there is also the desire to use the summary statistics from the sample to characterize the population from which the sample was derived. The population also has measures of central location and variability called the *parameters* of the population; Greek letters denote population parameters. Usually, the population parameters cannot be directly calculated because data from all population members cannot be obtained. The beauty of properly chosen summary statistics is that they are the best possible estimators of the population parameters.

These sampling statistics can be used in conjunction with a probability density function to provide additional descriptions of the sample and its population. Also commonly described as a probability distribution, a probability density function is an algebraic equation, $f(x)$, which gives a theoretical percentage distribution of x. Each value of x has a probability of occurrence given by $f(x)$. The most important probability distribution is the *normal* or *Gaussian function* $f(x) = \frac{1}{\sqrt{2\pi\sigma^2}} \exp\left[-\frac{1}{2}\left(\frac{x-\mu}{\sigma}\right)^2\right]$. There are two parameters (population mean and population variance) in the equation of the normal function that are denoted μ and σ^2. Often called the *normal equation,* it can be plotted and produces the familiar bell-shaped curve. Why are the mathematical properties of this curve so important to biostatistics? First, it has been empirically noted that when a biologic variable is sampled repeatedly, the pattern of the numbers plotted as a histogram resembles the normal curve; thus, most biologic data are said to follow or to obey a normal distribution. Second, if it is reasonable to assume that a sample is from a normal population, the mathematical properties of the normal equation can be used with the sampling statistic estimators of the population parameters to describe the sample and the population. Third, a mathematical theorem (the central limit theorem) allows the use of the assumption of normality for certain purposes, even if the population is not normally distributed.

Central Location

The three most common summary statistics of central location for interval variables are the arithmetic *mean, median,* and *mode.* The mean is merely the average of the numbers in the data set. Being a summary statistic of the sample, the arithmetic mean is denoted by the Roman letter x under a bar or $\bar{x} = \frac{1}{n}\sum_{i=1}^{n} x_i$ where i is the index of summation and n is the count of objects in the sample. If all values in the population could be obtained, then the population mean μ could be calculated similarly. Because all values of the population cannot be obtained, the sample mean is used. (Statisticians describe the sample mean as the unbiased, consistent, minimum variance, sufficient estimator of the population mean. Thus, the sample mean $\overline{x}$ is the estimator of the population mean μ.)

The median is the middlemost number or the number that divides the sample into two equal parts after first ranking the sample values from lowest to highest and then counting halfway to obtain the median. The concept of ranking is used in nonparametric statistics. A virtue of the median is that it is hardly affected by a few extremely high or low values.

The mode is the most popular number in a sample; that is, the number that occurs most frequently. A sample may have more than one value that is most common, that is, it may be bi- or polymodal; these modes may be widely separated or adjacent. The raw data should be inspected for this unusual appearance. The mode is often mentioned in discussions of descriptive statistics, but it is rarely used in statistical practice.

Spread or Variability

Any set of interval data has variability unless all the numbers are identical. Variability is specified by calculating the *deviation* or *deviate* of each individual x_i from the center (mean) for all the x_is. The *sum of the squared deviates* is always positive unless all set values are identical. This sum is then divided by the number of individual measurements. The result is the *averaged squared deviation;* the average squared deviation is ubiquitous in statistics.

The concept of describing the spread of a set of numbers by calculating the average distance from each number to the center of the numbers applies to both a sample and a population; this average squared distance is called the *variance.* The population variance is a parameter and is represented by σ^2. As with the population mean, the population variance is not usually known and cannot be calculated. Just as the sample mean is used in place of the population mean, the sample variance is used in place of the population variance. The sample variance is $VAR = SD^2 = \frac{\sum_{i=1}^{n}(x_i - \overline{x})^2}{(n-1)}$. Statistical theory demonstrates that if the divisor in the formula for SD^2 is $(n - 1)$ rather than n, the sample variance is an unbiased estimator of the population variance. While the variance is used extensively in statistical calculations, the units of variance are squared units of the original observations. The square root of the variance has the same units as the original observations; the square roots of the sample and population variances are called the *sample* (*SD*) and *population* (σ) *standard deviations.*

It was previously mentioned that most biologic observations appear to come from populations with normal distributions. By accepting this assumption of a normal distribution, further meaning can be given to the sample summary statistics (mean and SD) that have been calculated. This involves the use of the expression $\overline{x} \pm k \times SD$ where $k = 1, 2, 3$, and so forth. If the population from which the sample is taken is unimodal and roughly symmetric, then the bounds for $k = 1, 2$, and 3 encompass roughly 68%, 95%, and 99%, respectively, of the sample and population members.

Types of Research Design

Ultimately, research design consists of choosing what subjects to study, what experimental conditions and constraints to enforce, and which observations to collect at what intervals.[3,4] A few key features in this research design largely determine the strength of scientific inference that can be made based on the collected data. These key features allow the classification of research reports

Table 7-2 Classification of Clinical Research Reports

I. Longitudinal studies
  A. Prospective (cohort) studies
    1. Studies of deliberate intervention
      a. Concurrent controls
      b. Historical controls
    2. Observational studies
  B. Retrospective (case-control) studies
II. Cross-sectional studies

(Table 7-2). This classification reveals the variety of experimental approaches and indicates strengths and weaknesses of the same design applied to many research problems.

The first distinction is between *longitudinal* and *cross-sectional* studies. The former is the study of changes over time, whereas the latter describes a phenomenon at a certain point in time. For example, reporting the frequency with which certain drugs are used during anesthesia is a cross-sectional study, whereas investigating the hemodynamic effects of different drugs during anesthesia is a longitudinal analysis.

Longitudinal studies are next classified by the method with which the research subjects are selected. The methods for choosing research subjects can be either *prospective* or *retrospective;* these two approaches are also known as *cohort* (prospective) or *case-control* (retrospective). A prospective study assembles groups of subjects by some input characteristic that is thought to change an output characteristic; a typical input characteristic would be the opioid drug administered during anesthesia; for example, remifentanil or fentanyl. A retrospective study gathers subjects by an output characteristic; an output characteristic is the status of the subject after an event; for example, the occurrence of a myocardial infarction. A prospective (cohort) study would be one in which a group of patients undergoing neurologic surgery was divided into two groups, given two different opioids (remifentanil or fentanyl), and followed for the development of a perioperative myocardial infarction. In a retrospective (case-control) study, patients who suffered a perioperative myocardial infarction would be identified from hospital records; a group of subjects of similar age, gender, and disease who did not suffer a perioperative myocardial infarction also would be chosen, and the two groups would then be compared for the relative use of the two opioids (remifentanil or fentanyl). Retrospective studies are a primary tool of epidemiology. A case-control study can often identify an association between an input and output characteristic, but the causal link or relationship between the two is more difficult to specify.

Prospective studies are further divided into those in which the investigator performs a deliberate intervention and those in which the investigator merely observes. In a study of *deliberate intervention,* the investigator would choose several anesthetic maintenance techniques and compare the incidence of postoperative nausea and vomiting (NICV 7-1). If it was performed as an *observational study,* the investigator would observe a group of patients receiving anesthetics chosen at the discretion of each patient's anesthesiologist and compare the risk of postoperative nausea and vomiting among the anesthetics used. Obviously, in this example of an observational study, there has been an intervention; an anesthetic has been given. The crucial distinction is whether the investigator controlled the intervention. An observational study may reveal differences among treatment groups, but whether such differences are the consequence of the treatments or of other differences among the patients receiving the treatments will remain obscure. The comparison of cohorts with interventions not assigned under experimental control is a prominent technique of epidemiology.

Studies of deliberate intervention are further subdivided into those with concurrent controls and those with historical controls. Concurrent controls are either a simultaneous parallel control group or a self-control study; historical controls include previous studies and literature reports. A *randomized controlled trial* (RCT) is thus a longitudinal, prospective study of deliberate intervention with concurrent controls.

Innovative clinical trialists and statisticians have added several novel variations of clinical trial design including adaptive design,[5] platform trials,[6] stepped-wedge trials,[7] noninferiority[8] and equivalence trials,[9] pragmatic trials,[10] and others[11]; these new trial designs are increasingly used. Although most of this discussion about experimental design has focused on human experimentation, the same principles apply and should be followed in animal experimentation. The randomized, controlled clinical trial is the most potent scientific tool for evaluating medical treatment; randomization into treatment groups is relied on to equally weight the subjects of the treatment groups for baseline attributes that might predispose or protect the subjects from the outcome of interest.

Experimental Medicine: Management of Bias

Case reports engender interest, suspicion, doubt, wonder, and perhaps the desire to experiment; however, the case report is not sufficient evidence to advance scientific medicine. The experimenter attempts to constrain and control, as much as possible, the environment in which they collect numbers to find associations and relationships. The elements of experimental design are intended to prevent and minimize the possibility of bias, that is, a deviation of results or inferences from the true state of nature.

Sampling

In statistical language, *population* and *sample* have specialized meanings. Instead of referring only to the count of individuals in a geographic or political region, population refers to any target group of things (animate or inanimate) in which there is interest. A typical target population might be mothers in the first stage of labor or head-trauma victims undergoing craniotomy. A target population could also be cell cultures or hospital bills. A sample is a subset of the target population. Samples are taken because of the impossibility of observing the entire population; it is generally not affordable, convenient, or practical to examine more than a relatively small fraction of the population. Nevertheless, the researcher wishes to generalize from the results of the small sample group to the entire population.

Alike in at least one way, population members are generally quite diverse in other ways. The researcher desires that the sample of subjects in the experiment is representative of the population's diversity. Head-injury patients can have open or closed wounds, a variety of coexisting diseases, and normal or increased intracranial pressure. These subgroups within a population are called *strata*. Often the researcher wishes to increase the sameness or homogeneity of the target population by further restricting the sample and the population to just a few strata. However, restricting the target population to eliminate too much diversity must be balanced against the desire to have the results be applicable to the broadest possible population of patients.

The best hope for a representative sample of the population would be realized if every subject in the population had the same chance of being observed; this is called *simple random sampling*. If there were several strata of importance, *stratified random sampling* from each stratum would be appropriate. Other types of sampling including cluster and systematic methods are also used. In most clinical anesthesia studies, researchers are limited to using those patients who happen to show up at their hospitals; this is called *convenience sampling*. Convenience sampling is subject to the nuances of the surgical schedule, the goodwill of the referring physician and attending surgeon, and the willingness of the patient to cooperate. At best, the convenience sample is representative of patients at that institution, with no assurance that these patients are similar to those elsewhere. Convenience sampling is also the rule in studying new anesthetic drugs; such studies are typically performed on healthy, young volunteers.

Experimental Constraints

The researcher must define the conditions to which the sample members will be exposed. Particularly in clinical research, one must decide whether these conditions should be rigidly standardized or whether the experimental circumstances should be adjusted or individualized to the patient. In anesthetic drug research, should a fixed dose be given to all members of the sample or should the dose be adjusted to produce an effect or to achieve a specific end point? Standardizing the treatment groups by fixed doses simplifies the research work. There are risks to this standardization. They include the following: (1) a fixed dose may produce excessive numbers of side effects in some patients; (2) a fixed dose may be therapeutically insufficient in others; and (3) a treatment standardized for an experimental protocol may be so artificial that it has no broad clinical relevance, even if demonstrated to be superior. The researcher should carefully choose and report the adjustment/individualization of experimental treatments.

Control Groups

Even if a researcher is studying just one experimental group, the results of the experiment are usually not interpreted solely in terms of that one group but are also contrasted and compared with other experimental groups. Examining the effects of a new drug on blood pressure during anesthetic induction is important, but what is more important is comparing those results with the effects of one or more standard drugs commonly used in the same situation. Where can the researcher obtain these comparative data? There are several possibilities: (1) each patient could receive the standard drug under identical experimental circumstances at another time; (2) another group of patients receiving the standard drug could be studied simultaneously; (3) a group of patients could have been studied previously with the standard drug under similar circumstances; and (4) literature reports of the effects of the drug under related but not necessarily identical circumstances could be used. Under the first two possibilities, the control group is contemporaneous—either a *self-control* (crossover) or *parallel control* group. The second two possibilities are examples of the use of *historical controls*.

Because historical controls already exist, they are convenient and seemingly cheap to use. Unfortunately, the history of medicine is littered with the "debris" of therapies enthusiastically accepted on the basis of comparison with past experience. A classic example is operative ligation of the internal mammary artery for the treatment of angina pectoris—a procedure now known to be of no value. Proposed as a method to improve coronary artery blood flow, the lack of benefit was demonstrated in a trial where some patients had the procedure and some had a sham procedure; both groups showed benefit.[12] There is now firm empirical evidence that studies using historical controls usually show a favorable outcome for a new therapy, whereas studies with concurrent controls, that is, parallel control group or self-control, less often reveal a benefit.[13] Nothing seems to increase the enthusiasm for a new treatment as much as the omission of a concurrent control group. If the outcome with an old treatment is not studied simultaneously with the outcome of a new treatment, one cannot know if any differences in results are a consequence of the two treatments, or of unsuspected and unknowable differences between the patients, or of other changes over time in the general medical environment. One possible exception would be in studying a disease that is uniformly fatal (100% mortality) over a very short time.

Random Allocation of Treatment Groups

3 How should each subject be assigned to a specified experimental group? Should it depend on the whim of the investigator, the day of the week, the preference of a referring physician, the wish of the patient, the assignment of the previous subject, the availability of a study drug, a hospital chart number, or some other arbitrary criterion? All such methods have been used, but all can ruin the usefulness of the experiment. It is important to remember the purpose of sampling: by exposing a small number of subjects from the target population to the various experimental conditions, one hopes to make inferences about the entire population. Thus, the experimental groups should be as similar as possible to each other in reflecting the target population; if the groups are systematically different, selection bias is introduced into the experiment. Although randomly allocating subjects of a sample to one or another of the experimental groups requires additional work, this principle prevents selection bias by the researcher, minimizes (but cannot always prevent) the possibility that systematic differences exist among the experimental groups, and disarms critics' complaints about research methods. Random allocation is most commonly accomplished by the use of computer-generated random numbers. Even with a random allocation process, selection bias can occur if research personnel are allowed knowledge of the group assignment of the next patient to be recruited for a study. Failure to conceal random allocation leads to biases in the results of clinical studies.[14] Well-described techniques (centralized random allocation, opaque sealed envelopes, etc.) are successful in preventing this form of selection bias.[15] RCTs are the appropriate standard for establishing efficacy. Nevertheless, observational studies often will report the same magnitude of effect.[16,17]

Blinding

Blinding refers to the masking from the view of patient and experimenters the experimental group to which the subject has been or will be assigned. In clinical trials, the necessity for blinding starts even before a patient is enrolled in the research study; this is called the *concealment of random allocation*. There is good evidence that, if the process of random allocation is accessible to view, the referring physicians, the research team members, or both are tempted to manipulate the entrance of specific patients into the study to influence their assignment to a specific treatment group.[18]

They do so having formed a personal opinion about the relative merits of the treatment groups and desiring to get the "best" for someone they favor. This creates selection bias in the experimental groups.

Each subject should remain, if possible, ignorant of the assigned treatment group after entrance into the research protocol. The patient's expectation of improvement, a placebo effect, is a real and useful part of clinical care. But when studying a new treatment, one must ensure that the fame or infamy of the treatments does not induce a bias in outcome by changing patient expectations. A researcher's knowledge of the treatment assignment can bias their ability to administer the research protocol and to observe and record data faithfully; this is true for clinical, animal, and in vitro research. If the treatment group is known, those who observe data cannot trust themselves to record the data impartially and dispassionately. The appellations *single-blind* and *double-blind* to describe blinding are commonly used in research reports, but often applied inconsistently; the researcher should carefully plan and report exactly who is blinded.

Experimental Medicine: Data Analysis

The researcher starts work with some intuition about the phenomenon to be studied. Whether stated explicitly or not, this is the *biologic hypothesis;* it is a statement of observational or experimental expectations to be accomplished by using observations, tools, instruments, or methods accessible to the research team. An example would be the hope that isoflurane would produce less myocardial ischemia than fentanyl; the experimental method might be the electrocardiography determination of ST-segment changes. The researcher measures quantities that can vary—variables such as heart rate or temperature or ST-segment change—in samples from populations of interest. The workflow of data analysis consists of descriptive statistics (see above) to describe the properties of the observed sample data and inferential statistics to infer properties of the population. The most common method of inferential statistics is the use of P values in null significance hypothesis testing (NSHT).[19] The biologic hypothesis of the researcher becomes a *statistical hypothesis* during research planning.

Null Significance Hypothesis Test Formulation

In a statistical hypothesis, statements are made about the relationship among parameters of one or more populations. (To restate, a *parameter* is a number estimated from variables in a sample that describes a population; Roman letters label variables and Greek letters are used to denote parameters.) The typical statistical hypothesis can be established in a somewhat rote fashion for every research project, regardless of the methods, materials, or goals. The most frequently used method of setting up the algebraic formulation of the statistical hypothesis is to create two mutually exclusive statements about some parameters of the study population (Table 7-3); estimates for the values for these parameters are acquired by sampling data. In the hypothetical example comparing isoflurane and fentanyl, f_1 and f_2 would represent the ST-segment changes with isoflurane and with fentanyl. The

Table 7-3 Algebraic Statement of Statistical Hypotheses

H_0: $f_1 = f_2$ (null hypothesis)
H_a: $f_1 \neq f_2$ (alternative hypothesis)
f_1 = Parameter estimated from sample of first population
f_2 = Parameter estimated from sample of second population

null hypothesis is the hypothesis of no difference of ST-segment changes between isoflurane and fentanyl. The *alternative hypothesis* is usually nondirectional, that is, either $f_1 < f_2$ or $f_1 > f_2$; this is known as a *two-tail alternative hypothesis*. This is a more conservative alternative hypothesis than assuming that the inequality can only be either less than or greater than.

Logic of Proof

One particular decision strategy is used most commonly to choose between the null and alternative hypothesis. The approach is to assume that the null hypothesis is true even though the goal of the experiment is to show that there is a difference. One examines the consequences of this assumption by examining the actual sample values obtained for the variable(s) of interest. This is done by calculating what is called a *sample test statistic*; sample test statistics are calculated from the sample numbers. Associated with a sample test statistic is a *probability*, usually designated the *P value*. One also chooses the *level of significance;* the level of significance is the probability level considered too low to warrant support of the null hypothesis being tested. If sample values are sufficiently unlikely to have occurred by chance (i.e., the probability of the sample test statistic is less than the chosen level of significance), the null hypothesis is rejected; otherwise, the null hypothesis is not rejected.

It is often assumed that only the observed sample values are relevant for making inferences from the value of the test statistic and the associated P value. In fact, all statistical inferences depend on a complex web of assumptions. This is commonly labeled a *statistical model*. Typical assumptions of a statistical model include (1) measurements are independent of each other; (2) variability is constant across measurements; and (3) sample values actually represent the population of interest. Assumptions are usually difficult to verify. The P value becomes a logical test of all the assumptions, not just is $\phi_1 = \phi_2$. The P value may be large or small because the assumptions are incorrect.[20]

Because the statistics deal with probabilities, not certainties, there is a chance that the decision concerning the null hypothesis is erroneous. These errors are best displayed in table form (Table 7-4); condition 1 and condition 2 could be different drugs, two doses of the same drug, or different patient groups. Of the four possible outcomes, two decisions are clearly undesirable. The error of wrongly rejecting the null hypothesis (false-positive) is called the *type I* or *alpha error.* The experimenter should choose a probability value for alpha before collecting data; the experimenter decides how cautious to be against falsely claiming a difference. The most common choice for the value of alpha is 0.05. What are the consequences of choosing an alpha of 0.05? Assuming that there is, in fact, no difference between the two conditions and that the experiment is to be repeated 20 times, then during one of these experimental replications (5% of 20), a mistaken conclusion that there is a difference would be made. The probability of a type I error depends on the chosen level of significance and the existence or nonexistence of a difference between the two experimental conditions. The smaller the chosen alpha, the smaller will be the risk of a type I error.

The error of failing to reject a false null hypothesis (false-negative) is called a *type II* or *beta error.* (The power of a test is 1 minus beta.) The probability of a type II error depends on four factors. Unfortunately, the smaller the alpha, the greater the chance of a false-negative conclusion; this fact keeps the experimenter from automatically choosing a very small alpha. Also, the more variability there is in the populations being compared, the greater the chance of a type II error. This is analogous to listening to a noisy radio broadcast; the more static there is, the harder it will be to discriminate between words. In addition, increasing the number of subjects will lower the probability of a type II error. The fourth and most important factor affecting the probability of a type II error is the magnitude of the difference between the two experimental conditions. The probability of a type II error varies from very high, when there is only a small difference, to extremely low, when the two conditions produce large differences in population parameters.

Sample Size Calculations

Formerly, researchers typically ignored type II errors in experimental design. The practical importance of worrying about type II errors reached the consciousness of the medical research community several decades ago. Some controlled clinical trials that claimed to find no advantage of new therapies compared with standard therapies lacked sufficient statistical power to discriminate between the experimental groups and would have missed an important therapeutic improvement. As an example, the formula for calculating the size of each sample in a study comparing the means of two populations is: $n = 2\left[\frac{(z_\alpha - z_\beta)\sigma}{\mu_1 - \mu_2}\right]^2$. The z values are taken from the normal probability distribution and represent assumptions about the prespecified alpha and beta; the sigma (σ) is the assumed common SD; the mu's (μ) are the assumed population values. There are four options for decreasing type II error (increasing statistical power): (1) raise alpha; (2) reduce population variability; (3) make the sample bigger; and (4) make the difference between the conditions greater. Under most circumstances, only the sample size can be varied. Sample size planning has become an important part of research design for controlled clinical trials.[21] Some published research still fails the test of adequate sample size planning.

Table 7-4 Errors in Hypothesis Testing: The Two-Way Truth Table

		Reality (Population Parameters)	
		Conditions 1 and 2 Equivalent	**Conditions 1 and 2 Not Equivalent**
Conclusion from sample (sample statistics)	**Conditions 1 and 2 equivalent**[a]	Correct conclusion	False-negative type II error (beta error)
	Conditions 1 and 2 not equivalent[b]	False-positive type I error (alpha error)	Correct conclusion

[a]Do not reject the null hypothesis: condition 1 = condition 2.
[b]Reject the null hypothesis: condition 1 ≠ condition 2.

Sample Test Statistics

4 NSHT has been the main focus of inferential statistics. Hypothesis testing allows the experimenter to use data from the sample to make inferences about the population. Statisticians have created formulas that use the values of the samples to calculate test statistics. Statisticians have also explored the properties of various theoretical probability distributions. Depending on the assumptions about how data are collected, the appropriate probability distribution is chosen as the source of critical values to accept or reject the null hypothesis. If the value of the test statistic calculated from the sample(s) is greater than the critical value, the null hypothesis is rejected. The critical value is chosen from the appropriate probability distribution after the magnitude of the type I error is specified.

There are parameters within the equation that generate any particular probability distribution; for the normal probability distribution, the parameters are μ and σ^2. For the normal distribution, each set of values for μ and σ^2 will generate a different shape for the bell-like normal curve. All probability distributions contain one or more parameters and can be plotted as curves; these parameters may be discrete (integer only) or continuous. Each value or combination of values for these parameters will create a different curve for the probability distribution being used. Thus, each probability distribution is actually a family of probability curves. Some additional parameters of theoretical probability distributions have been given the special name *degrees of freedom* and are represented by Roman letters such as *m, n,* and *s*.

Associated with the formula for computing a test statistic is a rule for assigning integer values to the degrees of freedom. The number of degrees of freedom and the value for each degree of freedom depend on (1) the number of subjects; (2) the number of experimental groups; (3) the specifics of the statistical hypothesis; and (4) the type of statistical test. The correct curve of the probability distribution from which to obtain a critical value for comparison with the value of the test statistic is obtained with the values of one or more degrees of freedom.

To accept or reject the null hypothesis, the following steps are performed: (1) confirm that experimental data conform to the assumptions of the intended statistical test; (2) choose a significance level (alpha); (3) calculate the test statistic; (4) determine the degree(s) of freedom; and (5) find the critical value for the chosen alpha and the degree(s) of freedom from the appropriate probability distribution. If the test statistic exceeds the critical value, reject the null hypothesis; if the test statistic does not exceed the critical value, do not reject the null hypothesis.

The Fickle P Value

There is an extremely common misapprehension about the meaning of the P value in the typical null hypothesis/alternative hypothesis testing format.[22,23] If a statistical test is declared to be significant at $P < 0.05$, most physicians will state that there is 95% or greater certainty that the null hypothesis is incorrect. As Steven Goodman has stated: "This is an understandable but categorically wrong interpretation because the P value is calculated on the assumption that the null hypothesis is true. It cannot, therefore, be a direct measure of the probability that the null hypothesis is false."[22] The odds that the desired outcome—the alternative hypothesis—is true will depend not just on the data of the experiment, but also on how plausible was the hypothesis. This interaction of hypothesis plausibility and statistical results can be displayed graphically. (See Fig. 7-1.)[24] An implausible hypothesis (19-to-1 odds against) stills remains implausible (11% chance of a real effect) even if the P value of the experiment is 0.05.

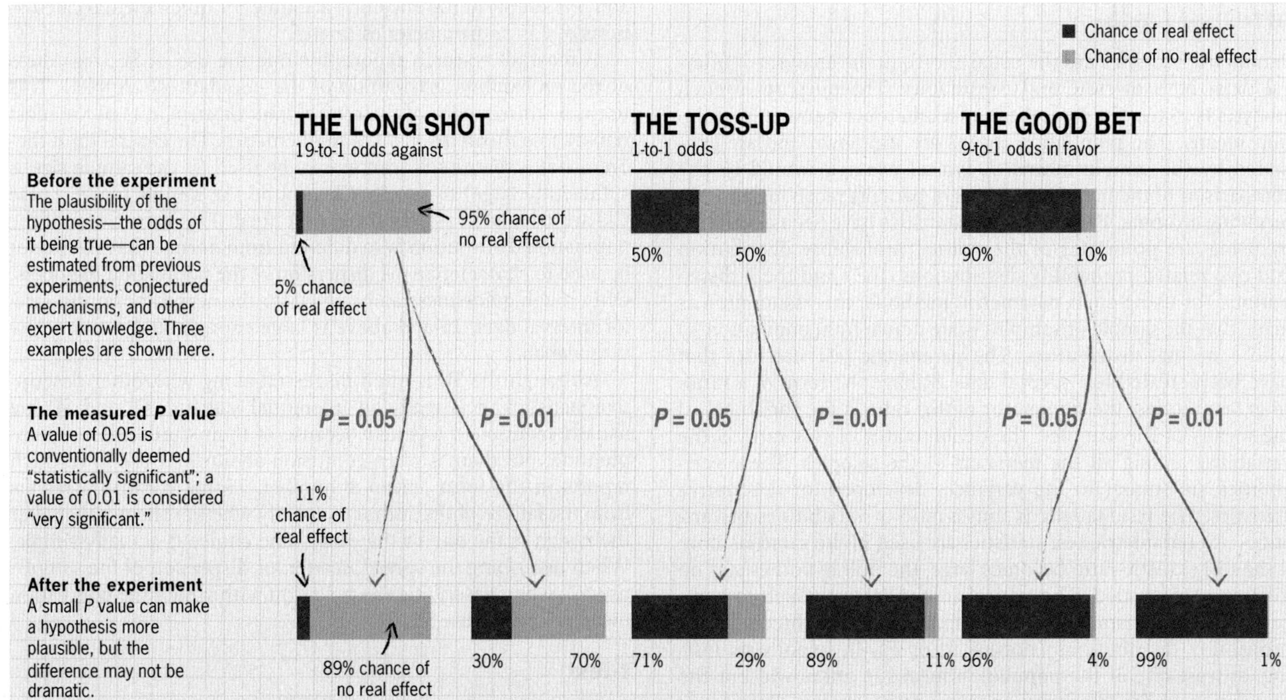

Figure 7-1 A *P* value measures whether an observed result can be attributed to chance. It cannot answer a researcher's real question—what are the odds that a hypothesis is correct? Those odds depend on the strength of the result and, most importantly, on how plausible the hypothesis was in the first place. (Reprinted with permission from Nuzzo R. Statistical errors. P values, the 'gold standard' of statistical validity, are not as reliable as many scientists assume. *Nature.* 2014;506:150–152. Copyright © 2014 Nature, with permission from Macmillan Publishers Ltd.)[25]

The Bayesian Alternative

Be it an RTC or an observational study report, the results and claims of medical research are not and should not be considered in isolation from prior knowledge. Yet, the most commonly used methods of statistical inference applied to medical research explicitly use only the newly obtained data. This is the frequentist approach or inference, so called because the precise definition of probability values depends on assumptions about hypothetical repeated replication of data collection. The new information of a study is a function only of the data.

5 A competing approach is called Bayesian inference that explicitly reports the new information of a study as a function of both observed data and historical (prior) knowledge. Both frequentist and Bayesian inferences make statements about parameters. But Bayesian methods involve the multiplication of the prior knowledge represented as a probability distribution of the parameter(s) times the likelihood of the observed data; the product is the new (posterior) probability distribution of the parameter.[26–30] Bayesian methods have been proposed to resolve the conundrum that some highly cited clinical research whose evidence is interpreted by a frequentist P value is later contradicted or found to be excessively optimistic in the magnitude of effect.[31–34] Among reasons for the slower adoption of Bayesian methods are concerns about the subjectivity in defining the prior probability distribution and the considerably greater computational difficulty in performing an analysis. Many public domain software packages have become available for Bayesian analyses, resolving some of the computational challenges.[35]

Experimental Medicine: Statistical Tests

Interval Data

Parametric statistics are the usual choice in the analysis of interval data, both discrete and continuous. The purpose of such analysis is to test the hypothesis of a difference between population means. The population means are unknown and are estimated by the sample means. A typical example would be the comparison of the mean heart rates of patients receiving and not receiving atropine. Parametric test statistics have been developed by using the properties of the normal probability distribution and two related probability distributions, the *t* and the *F* distributions. In using such parametric methods, the assumption is made that the sample or samples is/are drawn from population(s) with a normal distribution. The parametric test statistics that have been created for interval data all have the form of a ratio. In general terms, the numerator of this ratio is the variability of the means of the samples; the denominator of this ratio is the variability among all the members of the samples. These variabilities are similar to the variances developed for descriptive statistics. The test statistic is thus a ratio of variabilities or variances. All parametric test statistics are used in the same fashion; if the test statistic ratio becomes large, the null hypothesis of no difference is rejected. The critical values against which to compare the test statistic are taken from tables of the three relevant probability distributions (normal, *t*, or *F*). In hypothesis testing, at least one of the population means is unknown, but the population variance(s) may or may not be known. Parametric statistics can be divided into two groups according to whether or not the population variances are known. If the population variance is known, the test statistic used is called the *z* score; critical values are obtained from the normal distribution. In most biomedical applications, the population variance is unknown, and the *z* score is little used.

Confidence Intervals

The other major areas of statistical inference are the estimation of parameters with associated *confidence intervals* (CIs). In statistics, a CI is an interval estimate of a population parameter. A CI describes how likely it is that the population parameter is estimated by any particular sample statistic such as the mean. (The technical definition of the CI of the mean is more rigorous. A 95% CI implies that if the experiment were done over and over again, 95 of each 100 CIs would be expected to contain the true value of the mean.) CIs are a range of the following form: summary statistic ± (confidence factor) × (precision factor).

The *precision factor* is derived from the sample itself, whereas the *confidence factor* is taken from a probability distribution and also depends on the specified confidence level chosen. For a sample of interval data taken from a normally distributed population for which CIs are to be chosen for $\bar{x}$, the precision factor is called the *standard error of the mean* and is obtained by dividing SD by the square root of the sample size or

$$SE = \frac{SD}{\sqrt{n}} = \sqrt{\sum_{i=1}^{n}(x_i - \bar{x})^2/n(n-1)}.$$

The confidence factors are the same as those used for the dispersion or spread of the sample and are obtained from the normal distribution. The CIs for confidence factors 1, 2, and 3 have roughly a 68%, 95%, and 99% chance of containing the population mean. Strictly speaking, when the SD must be estimated from sample values, the confidence factors should be taken from the *t distribution*, another probability distribution. These coefficients will be larger than those used previously. This is usually ignored if the sample size is reasonable; for example, $n > 25$. Even when the sample size is only five or greater, the use of the coefficients 1, 2, and 3 is simple and sufficiently accurate for quick mental calculations of CIs on parameter estimates.

Almost all research reports include the use of SE, regardless of the probability distribution of the populations sampled. This use is a consequence of the *central limit theorem*, one of the most remarkable theorems in all of mathematics. The central limit theorem states that the SE can always be used (if the sample size is sufficiently large) to specify CIs around the sample mean. These CIs are calculated as previously described. This is true even if the population distribution is so different from normal that SD cannot be used to characterize the dispersion of the population members. Only rough guidelines can be given for the necessary sample size; for interval data, 25 and above is large enough, and 4 and below is too small.

Although the SE is often discussed along with other descriptive statistics, it is really an inferential statistic. SE and SD are usually mentioned together because of their similarities of computation, but there is often confusion about their use in research reports in the form "mean ± number." Some confusion results from the failure of the author to specify whether the number after the ± sign is the one or the other. The choice is actually simple. When describing the spread, scatter, or dispersion of the sample, use SD; when describing the precision with which the population mean is known, use SE.

t-Test

An important advance in statistical inference came early in the 20th century with the creation of the *Student's t-test statistic* and the *t distribution,* which allowed the testing of hypotheses when the population variance is not known. The most common use of the Student's *t*-test is to compare the mean values of two populations. There are two types of *t*-tests. If each subject has two measurements taken, for example, one before (x_i) and one after (y_i) a drug, then a one-sample or *paired t-test* procedure is used; each control measurement taken before drug administration is paired with a measurement in the same patient after drug administration. Of course, this is a self-control experiment. This pairing of measurements in the same patient reduces variability and increases statistical power. The difference $d_i = x_i - y_i$ of each pair of values is calculated and the average $\bar{d}$ is calculated. In the formula for the Student's *t* statistic, the numerator is $\bar{d}$, whereas the denominator is the SE of $\bar{d}$ denoted $(SE_{\bar{d}})$ so the test statistic is $t = \dfrac{\bar{d}}{SE_{\bar{d}}}$.

All *t* statistics are created in this way; the numerator is the difference of two means, whereas the denominator is the SE of the two means. If the difference between the two means is large compared with their variability, then the null hypothesis of no difference is rejected. The critical values for the *t* statistic are taken from the *t* probability distribution. The *t* distribution is symmetric and bell shaped but more spread out than the normal distribution. The *t* distribution has a single integer parameter; for a paired *t*-test, the value of this single degree of freedom is the sample size minus one. There can be some confusion about the use of the letter *t*. It refers both to the value of the test statistic calculated by the formula and to the critical value from the theoretical probability distribution. The critical *t* value is determined by looking in a *t* table after a significance level is chosen and the degree of freedom is computed.

More commonly, measurements are taken on two separate groups of subjects. For example, one group receives blood pressure treatment with sample values x_i, whereas no treatment is given to a control group with sample values y_i. The number of subjects in each group might or might not be identical; regardless of this, in no sense is an individual measurement in the first group matched or paired with a specific measurement in the second group. In this scenario, an *unpaired* or *two-sample t-test* is used to compare the means of the two groups. The numerator of the *t* statistic is $\bar{x} - \bar{y}$. The denominator is a weighted average of the SDs of each sample so that the test statistic *t* is

$$t = \frac{\bar{x} - \bar{y}}{\sqrt{\left(\frac{1}{n_x} + \frac{1}{n_y}\right)\left(\frac{(n_x - 1)s_x^2 + (n_y - 1)s_y^2}{n_x + n_y - 2}\right)}}.$$

The degree of freedom for an unpaired *t*-test is calculated as the sum of the subjects of the two groups minus two. As with the paired *t*-test, if the *t* ratio becomes large, the null hypothesis is rejected.

The results of a comparison of samples from two populations should be complete. In addition to displaying the individual mean values of $\bar{x}$ and $\bar{y}$ with their CIs and the results of the *t*-test, the mean difference, $\bar{x} - \bar{y}$ is also included with its associated CI. This difference of means is the effect size, a quantitative measure of the magnitude of effect.[36] The reporting of the effect size facilitates the interpretation of the clinical importance, as opposed to the statistical significance, of a research result.[37,38]

Analysis of Variance

Experiments in anesthesia, whether they are with humans or with animals, may not be limited to one or two groups of data for each variable. It is very common to follow a variable longitudinally; heart rate, for example, might be measured five times before and during anesthetic induction. These are also called *repeated measurement experiments*; the experimenter will wish to compare changes between the initial heart rate measurement and those obtained during induction. The experimental design might also include several groups receiving different induction drugs; for example, comparing heart rate across groups immediately after laryngoscopy. Researchers have mistakenly handled these analysis problems with just the *t*-test. If heart rate is collected five times, these collection times could be labeled *A, B, C, D,* and *E*. Then *A* could be compared with *B, C, D,* and *E*; *B* could be compared with *C, D,* and *E*; and so forth. The total of possible pairings is 10; thus, 10 paired *t*-tests could be calculated for all the possible pairings of *A, B, C, D,* and *E*. A similar approach can be used for comparing more than two groups for unpaired data.

The use of *t*-tests in this fashion is inappropriate. In testing a statistical hypothesis, the experimenter sets the level of type I error; this is usually chosen to be 0.05. When using many *t*-tests, as in the example given earlier, the chosen error rate for performing all these *t*-tests is much higher than 0.05, even though the type I error is set at 0.05 for each individual comparison. In fact, the type I error rate for all *t*-tests simultaneously; that is, the chance of finding at least one of the multiple *t*-test statistics significant merely by chance is given by the formula $\alpha = 1 - 0.95^{\kappa}$. If 13 *t*-tests are performed ($\kappa = 13$), the real error rate is 49%. Applying *t*-tests over and over again to all the possible pairings of a variable will misleadingly identify statistical significance when in fact there is none.

The most versatile approach for handling comparisons of means between more than two groups or between several measurements in the same group is called *analysis of variance* and is frequently cited by the acronym ANOVA. Analysis of variance consists of rules for creating test statistics on means when there are more than two groups. These test statistics are called *F ratios*, after statistician Ronald Fisher; the critical values for the *F* test statistic are taken from the *F* probability distribution that Fisher derived.

Suppose that data from three groups are obtained. What can be said about the mean values of the three target populations? The *F* test is actually asking several questions simultaneously: is group 1 different from group 2?; is group 2 different from group 3?; and is group 1 different from group 3? As with the *t*-test, the *F*-test statistic is a ratio; in general terms, the numerator expresses the variability of the mean values of the three groups, whereas the denominator expresses the average variability or difference of each sample value from the mean of all sample values. The formulas to create the test statistic are computationally elegant but are rather hard to appreciate intuitively. The *F* statistic has two degrees of freedom, denoted *m* and *n;* the value of *m* is a function of the number of experimental groups; the value for *n* is a function of the number of subjects in all experimental groups. The analysis of multigroup data is not necessarily finished after the ANOVAs are calculated. If the null hypothesis is rejected and it is accepted that there are differences among the groups tested, how can it be decided where the differences are? A variety of techniques are available to make what are called *multiple comparisons* after the ANOVA test is performed.

Robustness and Nonparametric Tests

All statistical tests depend on certain assumptions; these include the distribution of values in the underlying populations from which experimental samples are taken and the distribution of the test statistic. For the parametric statistics, that is, *t*-tests and analysis of variance, it is assumed that the populations follow the normal distribution. However, for some data, experience or historical reasons suggests that these assumptions of a normal distribution do not hold; some examples include proportions, percentages, and response times. What should the experimenter do if they fear that the data are not normally distributed?

Table 7-5 Choice of Statistical Test

Variable Type	One-sample Tests	Two-sample Tests	Multiple-sample Tests
Dichotomous or nominal	Binomial distribution	Chi-square test, Fisher's exact test	Chi-square test
Ordinal	Chi-square test	Chi-square test, nonparametric tests	Chi-square test, nonparametric tests
Continuous or discrete	*z* distribution or *t* distribution	Unpaired *t*-test, paired *t*-test, nonparametric tests	Analysis of variance, nonparametric analysis of variance

The experimenter might choose to ignore the problem of nonnormal data and inhomogeneity of variance, hoping that everything will work out. Such insouciance is actually a very practical and reasonable approach to the problem. Parametric statistics are called *robust* statistics; they stand up to much adversity. To a statistician, robustness implies that the magnitude of type I errors is not seriously affected by ill-conditioned data. Parametric statistics are sufficiently robust that the accuracy of decisions reached by means of *t*-tests and analysis of variance remains very credible, even for moderately severe departures from the assumptions.

Another possibility would be to use statistics that do not require any assumptions about probability distributions of the populations. Such statistics are known as *nonparametric tests;* they can be used whenever there is very serious concern about the shape of the data. Nonparametric statistics are also the tests of choice for ordinal data. The basic concept behind nonparametric statistics is the ability to rank or order the observations; nonparametric tests are also called *order statistics.*

Most nonparametric statistics still require the use of theoretical probability distributions; the critical values that must be exceeded by the test statistic are taken from the binomial, normal, and chi-square distributions, depending on the nonparametric test being used. The *nonparametric sign test, Mann–Whitney rank sum test,* and *Kruskal–Wallis one-way analysis of variance* are analogous to the paired *t*-test, unpaired *t*-test, and one-way analysis of variance, respectively. The currently available nonparametric tests are not used more commonly because they do not adapt well to complex statistical models and because they are less able than parametric tests to distinguish between the null and alternative hypotheses if the data are, in fact, normally distributed. There are general guidelines that relate the variable type and the experimental design to the choice of statistical test (Table 7-5).

Binary Variables

Confidence Intervals on Proportions

Categorical binary data, also called *enumeration data,* provide counts of subject responses. Given a sample of subjects of whom some have a certain characteristic (e.g., death, female sex), a ratio of responders to the number of subjects can be easily calculated as $p = x/n$; this ratio or rate can be expressed as a decimal fraction or as a percentage. It should be clear that this is a measure of central location of binary data. In the population from which the sample is taken, the ratio of responders to total subjects is a population parameter, denoted π. (This is not related to the geometry constant $\pi = 3.14159\ldots$). The sample proportion p is the estimator ($\hat{\pi}$) of the population proportion π. As with other data types, π is usually not known but must be estimated from the sample. The sample ratio *p* is the best estimate of π.

Because the population parameter is not generally known, the experimenter usually wishes to estimate π by the sample ratio *p* and to specify with what precision π is known. If the sample is sufficiently large ($n \times p \geq 5$; $n \times (1 - p) \geq 5$), advantage is taken of the central limit theorem to derive an SE analogous to that derived for interval data—$SE = \sqrt{\frac{p \times (1-p)}{n}}$. This sample SE is exactly analogous to the sample SE of the mean for interval data, except that it is an SE of the proportion. Just as a 95% CI of the mean was calculated, so may a CI on the proportion may be obtained. Larger samples will make the CI more precise.

If nothing goes wrong, is everything all right? This question was proposed by Henley and Lippman-Hand to discuss the interpretations of zero numerators using the 3 over n rule.[39] Consider an observational study that reports no morbidity in a 167 patients receiving a new intravenous anesthetic. Is there really no risk? While the best estimate of the population parameter π is 0/167 or 0%, an upper bound on the 95% CI is relevant to consider how high the rate of adverse events might be. As the probability of binary data is provided by the *binomial probability distribution function,* this upper bound may be derived from $1 - (0.05)^{1/n}$ where n is the denominator; for n > 30, this is well approximated by 3/n = 3/167 ≈ 1.8%.

The zero numerator example can be used to illustrate a difference between a Bayesian and frequentist approach. If there is no prior information (Bayes–Laplace *beta probability distribution function*), the upper bound is 3/(n + 1) = 3/168 ≈ 1.8%; the Bayesian equivalent of a CI is called a credible interval (CrI).[40] As the sample size increases, 3/n and 3/(n + 1) becomes closer and closer. By contrast, when there is prior information, Bayesian inference will provide a smaller CrI than a frequentist approach CI. Suppose a prior study with the same new anesthetic had found 15 morbid events in 10,000 (0.15%) patients. Then, with the new data, the estimate of the population rate of morbidity is 0.12% (upper bound 95% CrI = 0.36%).[40] Using prior information and the new data of zero events in 167 patients, the population rate estimate has been reduced from 0.15% to 0.12%, and the upper bound of the 95% CrI is much lower (0.36% vs. 1.8%) than by frequentist estimation.

Hypothesis Testing

In an RCT comparing hyperbaric bupivacaine versus hyperbaric lidocaine for spinal anesthesia, 9 of the 35 patients (26%) in the lidocaine group had transient neurologic symptoms (TNS) while only 1 of the 35 (3%) patients in the bupivacaine had this result, as shown in a two-by-two table (Table 7-6).[41] Is this difference real? The null hypothesis is that there is no association between the rows and the columns; the alternative hypothesis is that there is an association. A variety of statistical techniques allow a comparison of the TNS rate. These include *Fisher's exact test* and *(Pearson's) chi-square test,* and the null hypothesis is rejected for this data. The chi-square test offers the advantage of being computationally simpler; it can also analyze contingency tables with more than two rows and two columns; however, certain assumptions of sample size and response rate are not achieved here, and the Fisher's exact test is preferred.

Table 7-6 Metrics of Binary Treatment Effect

	Transient Neurologic Symptoms	
Treatment	Yes	No
Lidocaine	A = 9	B = 26
Bupivacaine	C = 1	D = 34

Keld et al.[41]
Pearson's chi-square test = 5.72, degrees of freedom = 1, P value = .0168
Fisher's exact test = 11.4, P value = .0134
Risk difference (RD) = A/(A + B) – C/(C + D) = 9/35 – 1/35 = 0.23 (0.07–0.38)
Risk ratio (OR) = (A/(A + B))/(C/(C + D)) = (9/(35)/(1/(35)) = 9 (1.20–67)
Odds ratio (OR) = (A/B)/(C/D) = (9/35)/(1/35) = 11.8 (1.40–98.9)
Number needed to treat (NNT) = 1/RD = 4.4 (2.6–13.6)
Statistic point estimates are presented with 95% confidence intervals.
For ratio statistics when a cell has a zero value, 0.5 is added to all cells.

The results of such experiments are often presented as an effect size: the risk ratio (RR), the odds ratio (OR), the risk difference (RD), and the number needed to treat or harm (NNT, NNH).[42–44] In this trial, patients were much more likely to have developed TNS when receiving lidocaine (RR = 9, OR = 11.8). With the NNH equal to 4.6, for every four to five patients receiving lidocaine, one additional patient would suffer TNS. RCTs concerning lidocaine versus other local anesthetics for spinal anesthesia have not necessarily found similar effect sizes. Statistical methods of meta-analysis (MA) can synthesize effect sizes from multiple trials to achieve greater precision and resolve inconsistencies in reported literature (see below).

Linear Regression

Often, a goal of an experiment is to find relationships between two variables so that in new patients the prediction of the value of one characteristic may be made by knowledge of another characteristic. The most commonly used technique for this purpose is linear regression analysis. Experiments for this purpose collect data pairs (x_i, y_i); these data pairs may be captured in either clinical trials or observational studies. The y variable is called the dependent or response variable while the x variable is denoted the independent or explanatory variable. These data should be displayed in a scatter plot; in the simplest type, a straight line (linear relationship) is assumed between two variables; the *y* variable is considered a function of the *x* variable. This is expressed as the linear regression equation $y = a + bx$; the parameters of the regression equation are *a* and *b*. The parameter *b* is the slope of the straight line relating *x* and *y*; for each 1 unit change in *x*, there are *b* unit changes in *y*. The parameter *a* is the intercept (value of *y* when *x* equals 0). Estimates of the parameters are obtained from a least squares method that sets the slope *b* value to minimize the sum of the vertical distances from the data pairs to the regression line: $b = \frac{\sum_{i=1}^{n}(x_i - \bar{x})(y_i - \bar{y})}{\sum_{i=1}^{n}(x_i - \bar{x})^2}$; $a = \bar{y} + b\bar{x}$. The parameter of greatest interest in regression is usually the slope, especially whether the slope is nonzero; a zero-value slope implies that *x* and *y* are not linearly related. With the additional assumption of bivariate normality (both *x* and *y* normally distributed), a *t*-test statistic is used to check the statistical significance of the slope.

The same (x_i, y_i) data pairs are usually subjected to correlation analysis. The correlation coefficient *r* is a measure of the linear covariation of *x* and *y*; *r* ranges from −1 to 1. There is no linear correlation between *x* and *y* if r is zero valued. It is estimated by $r = \frac{\sum_{i=1}^{n}(x_i - \bar{x})(y_i - \bar{y})}{\sqrt{\sum_{i=1}^{n}(x_i - \bar{x})^2 \sum_{i=1}^{n}(y_i - \bar{y})^2}}$. The test of the statistical significance of *r* is equivalent to the test for the significance of the regression slope *b*. The squared value of *r* known as the coefficient of determination (r^2) varies between 0 or 1 and is sometimes expressed as a percentage. The coefficient of determination has a very useful interpretation: the fraction of the variation of *y* explained by the variation of *x*.

As a hypothetical example, suppose that age and a plasma biomarker of physical maturity are collected in 11 children. The (x_i, y_i) values recorded are (10, 8.04), (8, 6.95), (13, 7.58), (9, 8.81), (11, 8.33), (14, 9.96), (6, 7.24), (4, 4.26), (12, 10.84), (7, 4.82), and (5, 5.68). Neither an inspection of these values nor of the summary statistics $\bar{x} = 9.00$, $\bar{y} = 7.50$, permits the reader to detect any relationship. The calculation of the coefficient of determination ($r^2 = 0.67$) does allow the inference that 67% of the variation in the biomarker is explained by the variation in age.[45]

A researcher or reader should not be satisfied to see only the statistical results of regression and correlation. The statistician Anscombe created four hypothetical data sets to illustrate the importance of visual inspection of data.[46] Each data set has 11 paired (x_i, y_i) observations (Fig. 7-2). The hypothetical example (listed above) is displayed in the upper left quadrant; a linear relationship is illustrated. For the data in the upper right quadrant, the relationship between *x* and *y* is curvilinear (quadratic). For the lower right quadrant, there is no relationship between *x* and *y*; with one exception all data pairs have the same x value. For the lower left quadrant, there is a near-perfect correlation between x and y except for one data pair with a much higher y value. Nevertheless, all summary statistics, regression and correlation values of the four data sets including means, SDs, slopes, intercepts, standard errors of regression parameters, statistical significance of regression parameters, and correlation coefficients are equal. There are clearly four different patterns that can only be detected by visual inspection. Even this simplest form of regression and correlation analysis is based on the strong assumption of an underlying linear relationship between *x* and *y*; failure of that assumption leads to erroneous statistical inference. Using just the summary, regression and correlation statistics, the four data sets would have been thought to have very similar/identical underlying relationships. Reports of linear regression should always include scatter plots of raw data.

Epidemiology

Epidemiology is the study of the patterns, causes, and effects of health and disease conditions. Epidemiology is based on observations collected systematically but without the interventions (anesthetic drugs and techniques) being allocated to patients under experimental control. Major areas of epidemiologic study relevant to anesthesia care are nonrandomized studies (NRSs) of the effectiveness of anesthetic drugs and techniques on outcomes following anesthesia and surgery, the properties of diagnostic tests for the identification of perioperative complications, the determination of risk factors for outcomes, and the estimation of risk prognosis models for individual predication. Systematic reviews (SRs) and MA also come under the banner of epidemiology as does the advent of "Big Data."

A fundamental axiom of epidemiology is that an "association does not necessarily imply causation." In 1965, the epidemiologist Bradford Hill suggested guidelines for assessing evidence of

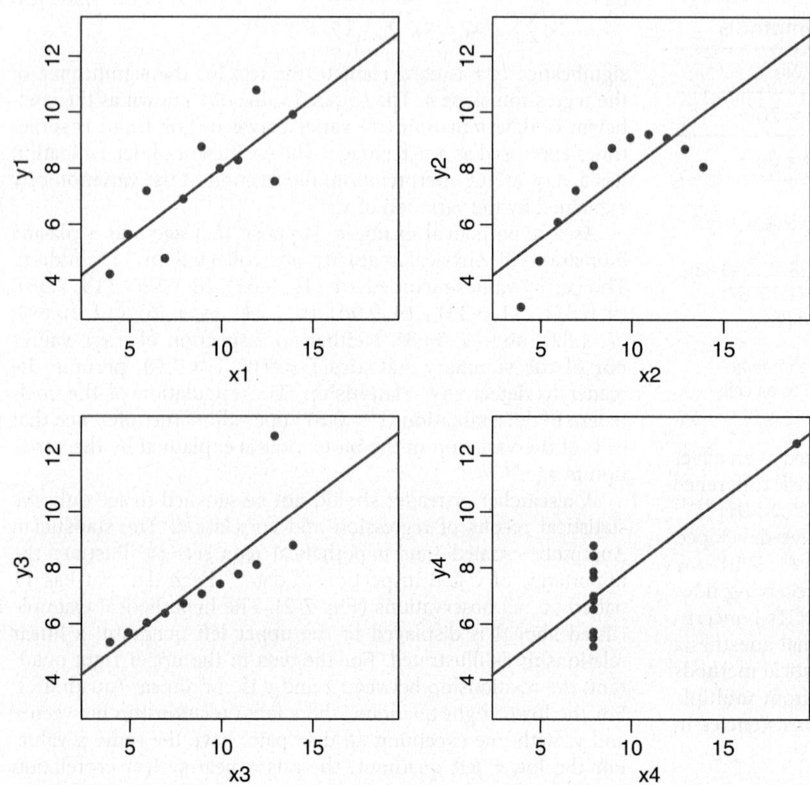

Figure 7-2 Four scatter plots from the Anscombe data sets. For each data set, $n = 11$, $\bar{x} = 9.00$, $SD_x = 3.31$, $\bar{y} = 7.50$, $SD_y = 2.03$, $y = 3.00 + 0.50x$, $SE_a = 1.12$, $SE_b = 0.12$, $r^2 = 0.67$, and so forth. All statistics are equal up to the fourth decimal place.

causation when presented with an observed association between the environment and disease.[47] Fifty years later, Ioannidis revisited these criteria, assessed which of these had worked, and identified two: consistency and experiment.[48] Of the former, Hill offered this question "Has it (an association) been repeatedly observed by different persons, in different places, circumstances and times?"[47] However, nothing can replace experiment. Ioannidis reported: "Among the most highly cited papers in the biomedical literature, five out of six observational studies have been 'refuted' by subsequent randomized trials . . . ."[31] Be it an RCT or an observational study report, the results and claims of medical research are not and should not be considered in isolation from prior knowledge. The precision with which the P value is calculated by statistical software by itself should not replace a consideration of all evidence.

Multivariable Linear Regression

Regression methods can be extended to data sets in which one response variable is linearly related to many explanatory variables. This regression includes methods for choosing which of the explanatory variables have a statistically significant (i.e., nonzero) regression slope. Multivariable linear regression is the creation of a model relating some continuous response such as heart rate to any number of k explanatory variables; these are also called covariates. This regression starts with data from n patients of the form $(y_i, x_{i,1}, x_{i,2}, \ldots, x_{i,k})$ where the subscript i denotes the *ith* patient, y_i is the response in the *ith* patient, x_i is the value of a covariate in the *ith* patient, and the second subscript of x_i denotes the 1 to k covariates. The linear model equation for the *ith* individual is: $\mu_i = \beta_0 + \beta_1 x_{i,1} + \beta_2 x_{i,2} + \cdots + \beta_k x_{i,k} = \sum_{j=1}^{k} \beta_j x_{i,j}$.

The β_js are the unknown coefficients (parameters) of the model that will be estimated from the observed data. For the *ith* individual, the expected value of the model, μ_i, is the linear sum of each covariate value multiplied by its coefficient. The difference between the observed (y_i) and expected value (μ_i) reflects biologic variability, measurement error, and other such factors.

Univariable and Multivariable Logistic Regression

If the response variable is binary (alive/dead, complication/no complication), linear regression has been extended. Thus, there is the typical sigmoidally shaped regression of a binary outcome (e.g., movement) versus anesthetic dose. There are multiple methods for regression of binary outcomes, the most common being logistic regression. The most commonly used format of the logistic method is the multivariable logistic regression model. The response variable y_i denotes the value of the binary outcome in the *ith* individual and is generally coded as 0 or 1 representing the absence or presence of an event (e.g., day-of-surgery mortality). Letting π represent the probability that the response variable has value 1, then the logit transformation, log of the odds ratio $= \ln\left(\frac{\pi}{1-\pi}\right)$, allows π to be expressed as the linear combination of the covariates:

$$\ln\left(\frac{\pi_i}{1-\pi_i}\right) = \beta_0 + \beta_1 x_{i,1} + \beta_2 x_{i,2} + \cdots + \beta_k x_{i,k} = \sum_{j=1}^{k} \beta_j x_{i,j}.$$

The logit transformation is the link function relating the sum of the covariates to the probability of the binary outcome.

Multivariable regression is used to control for confounding. Confounding occurs when the apparent association between a covariate and an outcome is affected by the relationship of a third variable to the covariate and to the outcome; the third variable is a confounder. As contrasted to sequentially regressing each covariate against the response variable, multivariable regression is performed by simultaneously fitting all explanatory variables.[49] For example, in exploring the relationship between tobacco and myocardial infarction, male sex, poverty, and sedentary lifestyle could be confounders because they are associated with both smoking and coronary heart disease.

Each year, thousands of reports are published in the medical literature using stepwise, multivariable logistic regression on observational data to identify "independent" predictors for various clinical outcomes.[50] Stepwise, multivariable logistic regression is an automatic procedure where there are a large number of potential explanatory variables and no underlying theory on which to base the selection of prediction model risk factors.[51,52] In the anesthesia literature, postoperative nausea and vomiting has been a very common topic for such statistical modeling.[53–55] Once these predictive models have been created, there is a framework for assessing their performance.[56–58] This mandates the acquisition of new patients at a different time and place. There is a widely used predictive model of sepsis in hospitalized patients implemented in hundreds of hospitals; it was developed from a proprietary database of over 400,000 patient encounters; it had poor discrimination and calibration in predicting sepsis onset.[59] Great skepticism should be shown for most of these prognostic models, especially those concerning mortality and critical illness, as they usually have not been validated, have modest accuracy, and do not have documented clinical utility.[60,61]

Propensity Score Matching and Analysis

6 Another approach for providing estimation of treatment effect in NRSs is the methodology of propensity score matching.[62,63] This use of NRS data is intended to investigate the effect of treatment X on a specified dichotomous outcome Y; the good outcome can be denoted Y^+, for example, survival, with Y^- being the opposite. It is usually the case that one or more baseline prognostic covariates (confounders $C_1, C_2, \ldots, C_k$) may be imbalanced between the patients that did (X^+) and did not (X^-) receive the treatment of interest. The favorable outcome, conditional on receiving treatment X^+, is denoted $Y^+|X^+$ with $Y^+|X^-$ being a favorable outcome in those not receiving the treatment. Any difference between interventions on the outcome Y may be a consequence of the confounders influencing both the treatment and the outcome; a failure to observe a difference in outcome may also be a consequence of confounding. As an example, pulmonary artery catheterization (PAC) in the care of the critically ill was adopted about 40 years ago and widely disseminated without rigorous evaluation. The enthusiasm of intensivists for such monitoring even forced the cessation of an RCT comparing care with and without PACs because of the unwillingness of physicians to allow patient participation in the study.[64] Using data of 5,735 critically ill patients, Connors et al. reported lower 6-month survival in the 2,184 patients with PACs ($Y^+|X^+ = 46.3\%$ vs. $Y^+|X^- = 53.7\%$), but far more X^+ patients had multiorgan system failure (MOSF: 57% vs. 35%) at the time of PAC placement; there were other imbalances of initial covariates.[65] Was the higher mortality attributable to the use of PACs or to a greater severity of illness? Using propensity matching, Connors created a pair of subsets (1,008 patients vs. 1,008 patients) with similar proportions of prognostic factors in both groups (e.g., MOSF: 34%); 6-month survival was still lower ($Y^+|X^+ = 46.0\%$ vs. $Y^+|X^- = 51.2\%$).

Propensity score matching is a statistical technique within the general concept of matching. If only one prognostic factor was important, for example, sex, then a pair of matched subsets could be created easily by repeatedly and randomly placing one man and one woman into each subset—matching the groups just by sex. However, there is usually a great deal of baseline information about patients observed in an NRS; Connors had details for about 40+ baseline covariates.[36] In addition, it is often not evident which baseline characteristics are predictive of outcome. Creating groups by simple matching is not generally possible using more than a very few covariates.

The propensity score is defined as a subject's probability of receiving a specific treatment, conditional on the many baseline covariates. The propensity score is usually estimated by multivariable logistic regression. In contrast to the attempt to create of parsimonious model with a few independent predictors of outcome by logistic regression modeling of NRS data, all available covariates are left in the model for a propensity score, regardless of whether they are statistically significant. These covariates must be restricted to those that are known prior to the intervention. In the study by Connors, the presence/absence of MOSF on hospital admission should be included in the propensity score; MOSF developing a week later should not.

For each patient in the data set, the z score obtained from the sum of each covariate times its regression coefficient is calculated: $z = \beta_0 + \beta_1 C_{i,1} + \beta_2 C_{i,2} + \cdots + \beta_k C_{i,k} = \sum_{j=1}^{k} \beta_j C_{i,j}$. Taking the antilogit of the z score $\left(p = \dfrac{1}{1+e^{-z}}\right)$ yields the probability that a patient with those covariate values received the intervention. Of course, it is in fact known whether or not a patient received the intervention. Propensity-matched subsets of patients are created by randomly choosing and matching one patient receiving the intervention to one patient not receiving the intervention with the same probability from the z score; usually, the propensity probabilities (scores) are matched to the third or greater decimal place. The success of propensity score matching in balancing many covariates was well displayed in an observational comparison of epidural anesthesia for intermediate- to high-risk noncardiac surgery by Wijeysundera et al.[66] As graphed by Gayat et al. (Fig. 7-3), 45 baseline characteristics of two matched subsets of about 44,000 patients each became extremely well balanced.[67] In the original data set, an arterial line was used in 59% versus 33%; after balancing, an arterial line was used in 48% for both. The total of patients in the two matched subsets will always be less than the total count of patients in the NRS data set; some patients can't be matched. Simple paired statistics are used to compare the outcomes of the two subsets.

Propensity score methods are being used in NRSs to reduce the effect of selection bias in estimating causal treatment effects. Besides propensity score matching, the effect of selection bias can also be reduced by using propensity scores for stratification, regression adjustment, and weighting. It is now routine to see NRS using propensity analysis in the intensive care and anesthesia literature—most commonly using matching. A propensity score matching analysis should include (1) details of propensity score building; (2) matching method; and (3) demonstration of covariate balancing by tabular or graphical display.[38] The propensity score can reduce bias due to observed covariates.

As useful as they are, propensity score methods cannot replace the RCT, since randomization minimizes covariate imbalance between treatment groups for observed, unobserved, and unobservable covariates. In 2007, Murphy et al. reported outcomes following cardiac surgery using a database of operations on about 8,700 patients; propensity scores estimated from preoperative risk factors and intraoperative events were used to adjust all statistical comparisons for this potential confounding.[68] Mortality, morbidity,

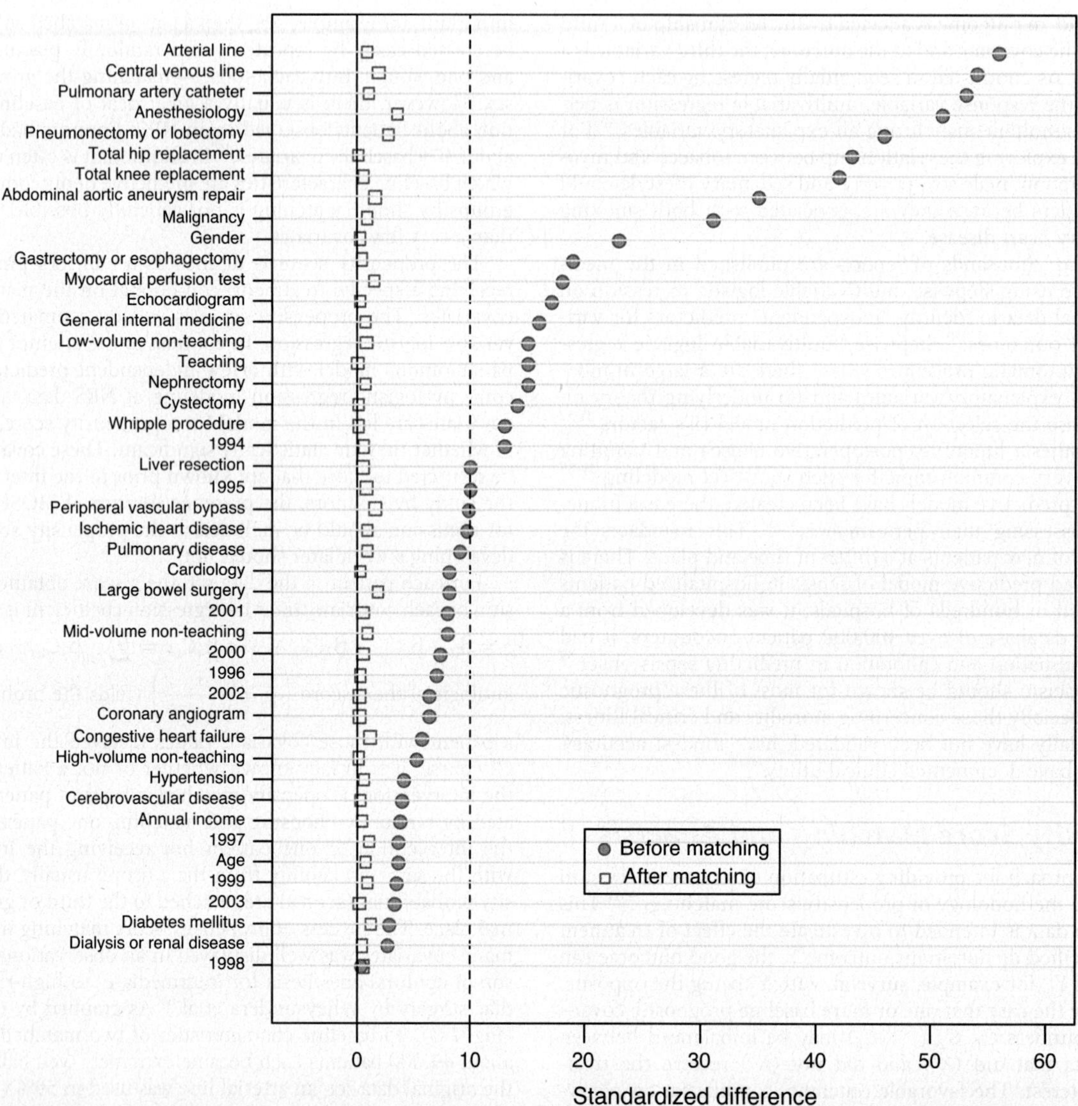

Figure 7-3 Graphical representation of 45 baseline covariates before and after propensity score matching using data from Wijeysundera et al.[66] The standardized difference for each covariate is the average difference between groups divided by the average standard deviation of the two groups. The standardized difference increases directly with increasing imbalance between groups. With propensity score matching, the standardized difference is close to zero for all covariates. (Reprinted from Gayat E, Pirracchio R, Resche-Rigon M, et al. Propensity scores in intensive care and anaesthesiology literature: a systematic review. *Intensive Care Medicine*. 2010;36;1997.[67] With kind permission from Springer Science+Business Media.)

and cost of care was increased in patients receiving blood. In 2015, Murphy et al. reported the 2,000-patient TITRe2 trial with the hypothesis that a restrictive threshold for red-cell transfusion would reduce postoperative morbidity.[69] There was no difference by transfusion strategy in the primary, composite outcome (serious infections or ischemic events); indeed, mortality was higher (4.2% vs. 2.6%) at 3 months in the restrictive-threshold group. The authors concluded: "The difference is probably due to the fact that observational analyses are confounded by prognostic factors that influence the decision to transfuse red cells." Even a well-conducted, propensity-adjusted analysis cannot remove confounding for unobserved or unobservable covariates.

Systematic Reviews and Meta-Analyses

7 It is over 30 years since the first systematic review (SR) with an accompanying meta-analysis (MA) was published in an anesthesia journal[70] and reports using these research methods are now commonplace in anesthesia journals.[71–73] The focused question of an SR of interventions can subsumed by the acronym PICO: P = Population, I = Intervention, C = Comparison, and O = Outcome. The structured title of an SR usually contains most of the PICO elements.

Data are obtained from controlled trials (usually randomized) already in the medical literature rather than from newly conducted clinical trials; the basic unit of analysis of this observational research is the published study. A structured protocol is followed that includes in part (1) choice of study inclusion/exclusion criteria; (2) explicitly defined literature searching; (3) abstraction of data from included studies; (4) appraisal of risk bias within each study; (5) systematic pooling of data; and (6) discussion of inferences. This structured protocol is intended to minimize bias. Even RCTs may have sources of bias such as (1) selection bias: systematic differences between the patients receiving each intervention;

(2) performance bias: systematic differences in care being given to study patients other than the preplanned interventions being evaluated; (3) attrition bias: systematic differences in the withdrawal of patients from each of the two intervention groups; and (4) detection bias: systematic differences in the ascertainment and recording of outcomes. The main focus of bias detection in the trials incorporated into an SR is the (1) randomization process; (2) concealment of random allocation; (3) use of blinding; and (4) the reporting/analysis of dropouts.

Binary outcomes (yes/no, alive/dead, presence/absence) within a study are usually compared by the risk ratio (RR) or odds ratio (OR) effect size; for continuous variables, the effect size is the mean difference. If there is sufficient clinical similarity among the included studies, a summary value of the overall effect size of the intervention versus comparison treatments is estimated by MA. MA is a set of statistical techniques for combining results from different studies. The results of an MA are usually present in a figure called a *Forest plot* (Fig. 7-4). The far left column identifies the included studies; the center-left columns display the observed data. The center-right columns list the RRs with 95% CIs for the individual studies and the summary statistics. The horizontal lines and diamond shapes in the figures of the far right column are graphical representations of individual study RR and summary RR, respectively. There are also descriptive and inferential statistics concerning the statistical heterogeneity of the MA and the significance of the summary statistics. Interestingly, it has been noted that the initial estimates of benefit in an SR are generally inflated when compared to the effect size estimated when the SR is later updated.[74]

An examination of Figure 7-4 shows that 11 of 15 individual comparisons had wide, nonsignificant CIs that touched or crossed the RR of identity (RR = 1). However, the overall consistency of effect is easily seen with lidocaine being "favored" in only one study. The RR calculated from all studies was 7.31 with a 95% CI [4.16, 12.86]. In this example, the power of summary statistics to combine evidence is clear. About every seventh patient (92/637) who had a lidocaine spinal block had TNS; the risk of TNS was about seven times higher compared to other local anesthetics.[75]

The production of SRs comes from several sources. Many come from the individual initiative of researchers who publish their results as stand-alone reports in the journals of medicine and anesthesia. The American Society of Anesthesiologists has developed a process for the creation of practice parameters that includes, among other things, a variant form of SRs. A prominent proponent of SRs is the Cochrane Collaboration: an international network of more than 30,000 volunteers from over 100 countries that have published about 9,000 SRs online in The Cochrane Library.[a] An SR should be considered provisional, an update with new evidence always being possible. One distinction between Cochrane and non-Cochrane SRs is the updating of Cochrane SRs periodically as new research reports become available; for example, the SR concerning TNS has been recently updated.[76] Methods for MA continue to be refined to include multiple treatment comparisons,[77] diagnostic tests,[78,79] the use of random effects models,[80] trial sequential analysis to maintain the Type I error rate with MA updating,[81] and many approaches to statistical heterogeneity. The R statistical platform offers over 50 packages to estimate and display MAs.[b] The Cochrane Collaboration has extensive documentation, tutorials, and software available that electronically explains the techniques of SRs and MA.[c]

[a]See https://www.cochranelibrary.com

[b]https://cran.r-project.org/web/views/MetaAnalysis.html

[c]https://training.cochrane.org/handbook

Big Data

Big Data has the attributes of the three "V"s (Volume, Velocity, and Variety). How big is Big Data? The volume usually cited is billions of records produced at a velocity of millions each day encompassing many variable types. The computer storage of Big Data requires a new nomenclature beyond gigabyte (GB) and terabyte: petabyte = 10^6 GBs; exabyte = 10^9 GBs; and even higher. Big Data can be also defined to include studies that required new approaches to the collection, management, and analysis of data beyond those commonly used or available; historically, two epidemiology reports in anesthesia published 50 or more years ago can claim inclusion within Big Data. The first was a 5-year (1948 to 1952) study of all postoperative deaths following about 600,000 anesthetics at 10 academic medical centers distributed across the United States.[82] The other was the National Halothane Study that reported the rate of deaths and fatal hepatic necrosis during 4 years (1959 to 1962) following about 850,000 anesthetics at 34 hospitals.[83] Both studies required a scaling up of resources for data collection and management and both included new statistical methods.

What does Big Data promise? Messages posted to social media and inquiries on web search engines tally in the millions each day. The logs of this activity have been called the digital exhaust of our age. Is there usable health content therein? Authors from the search engine company Google reported that by tallying search topics, for example, "cold/flu remedy" or "Influenza complication," this social media data predicted accurately influenza flu trends across several years of flu epidemics; these predictions mirrored official health statistics of the rise and fall of infections.[84] It was proposed that by harnessing the collective intelligence of millions of users, even faster surveillance of disease activity was possible. A more skeptical reexamination of these social media models found them not sufficient to replace timely local and national surveillance of health trends.[85]

Whither goes Big Data in anesthesia and pain care?[86–89] There is much use of institutional and governmental administrative and billing databases in epidemiology reports of anesthesia. And there are now several national repositories of perioperative data including the National Clinical Outcomes Registry (NACOR), the Multicenter Perioperative Outcomes Group (MPOG), the National Surgery Quality Program (NSQIP), and the Society of Thoracic Surgeons National Database.[88] While all have millions of patient records, only MPOG routinely captures all physiologic monitoring data at 5-minute or more frequent intervals. Even with this perioperative data, no repository or administrative database meets the definition of Big Data. The routine digitation of waveforms (e.g., electrocardiogram) at high resolution with storage in a national repository would quickly create Big Data.[90,91] The use of prospective genotyping of patients prior to anesthesia and surgery would also create Big Data.[88,92] Until then, Big Data does not yet apply to anesthesia research.

Conclusions

Interpretation of Results

Scientific studies do not end with the statistical test.[93] Whether the primary outcome of a new treatment succeeds or fails, the experimenter must submit an opinion as to the generalizability of their work to the rest of the world.[94,95] Even if there is a statistically significant difference, the experimenter must decide if this difference is medically or physiologically important. Statistical significance does not always equate with biologic or clinical relevance. The questions an experimenter should ask about the interpretation of results are highly dependent on the specifics of the experiment. First, even small, clinically unimportant differences

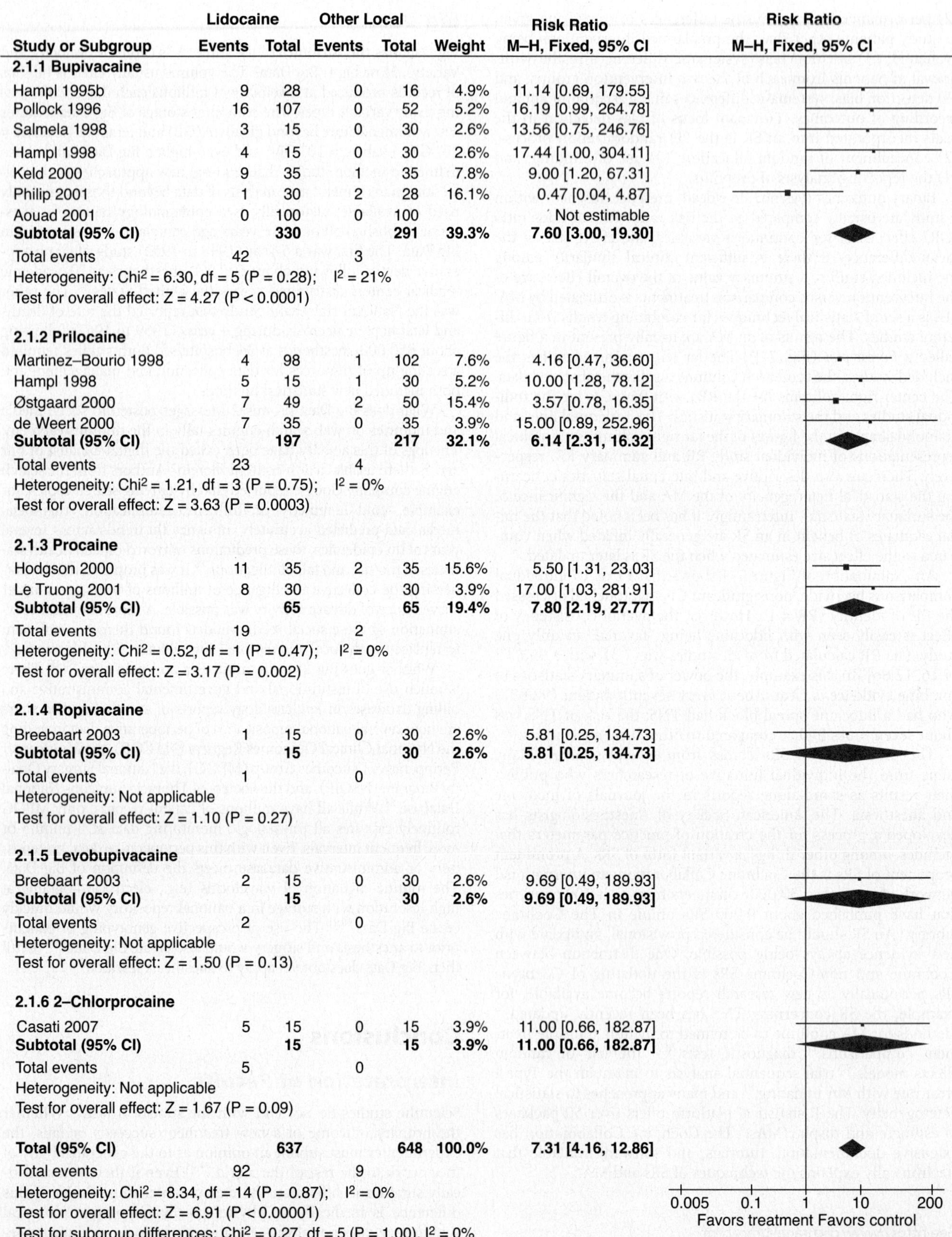

Study or Subgroup	Lidocaine Events	Lidocaine Total	Other Local Events	Other Local Total	Weight	Risk Ratio M–H, Fixed, 95% CI
2.1.1 Bupivacaine						
Hampl 1995b	9	28	0	16	4.9%	11.14 [0.69, 179.55]
Pollock 1996	16	107	0	52	5.2%	16.19 [0.99, 264.78]
Salmela 1998	3	15	0	30	2.6%	13.56 [0.75, 246.76]
Hampl 1998	4	15	0	30	2.6%	17.44 [1.00, 304.11]
Keld 2000	9	35	1	35	7.8%	9.00 [1.20, 67.31]
Philip 2001	1	30	2	28	16.1%	0.47 [0.04, 4.87]
Aouad 2001	0	100	0	100		Not estimable
Subtotal (95% CI)		**330**		**291**	**39.3%**	**7.60 [3.00, 19.30]**
Total events	42		3			
Heterogeneity: Chi² = 6.30, df = 5 (P = 0.28); I² = 21%						
Test for overall effect: Z = 4.27 (P < 0.0001)						
2.1.2 Prilocaine						
Martinez–Bourio 1998	4	98	1	102	7.6%	4.16 [0.47, 36.60]
Hampl 1998	5	15	1	30	5.2%	10.00 [1.28, 78.12]
Østgaard 2000	7	49	2	50	15.4%	3.57 [0.78, 16.35]
de Weert 2000	7	35	0	35	3.9%	15.00 [0.89, 252.96]
Subtotal (95% CI)		**197**		**217**	**32.1%**	**6.14 [2.31, 16.32]**
Total events	23		4			
Heterogeneity: Chi² = 1.21, df = 3 (P = 0.75); I² = 0%						
Test for overall effect: Z = 3.63 (P = 0.0003)						
2.1.3 Procaine						
Hodgson 2000	11	35	2	35	15.6%	5.50 [1.31, 23.03]
Le Truong 2001	8	30	0	30	3.9%	17.00 [1.03, 281.91]
Subtotal (95% CI)		**65**		**65**	**19.4%**	**7.80 [2.19, 27.77]**
Total events	19		2			
Heterogeneity: Chi² = 0.52, df = 1 (P = 0.47); I² = 0%						
Test for overall effect: Z = 3.17 (P = 0.002)						
2.1.4 Ropivacaine						
Breebaart 2003	1	15	0	30	2.6%	5.81 [0.25, 134.73]
Subtotal (95% CI)		**15**		**30**	**2.6%**	**5.81 [0.25, 134.73]**
Total events	1		0			
Heterogeneity: Not applicable						
Test for overall effect: Z = 1.10 (P = 0.27)						
2.1.5 Levobupivacaine						
Breebaart 2003	2	15	0	30	2.6%	9.69 [0.49, 189.93]
Subtotal (95% CI)		**15**		**30**	**2.6%**	**9.69 [0.49, 189.93]**
Total events	2		0			
Heterogeneity: Not applicable						
Test for overall effect: Z = 1.50 (P = 0.13)						
2.1.6 2–Chlorprocaine						
Casati 2007	5	15	0	15	3.9%	11.00 [0.66, 182.87]
Subtotal (95% CI)		**15**		**15**	**3.9%**	**11.00 [0.66, 182.87]**
Total events	5		0			
Heterogeneity: Not applicable						
Test for overall effect: Z = 1.67 (P = 0.09)						
Total (95% CI)		**637**		**648**	**100.0%**	**7.31 [4.16, 12.86]**
Total events	92		9			
Heterogeneity: Chi² = 8.34, df = 14 (P = 0.87); I² = 0%						
Test for overall effect: Z = 6.91 (P < 0.00001)						
Test for subgroup differences: Chi² = 0.27, df = 5 (P = 1.00), I² = 0%						

Figure 7-4 A Forest plot illustrates the relative strength of treatment effect across multiple studies. The point estimate for each study is represented by a square with 95% CIs represented by horizontal lines. In a Forest plot of RRs or ORs, the x-axis of the graph is on a logarithmic scale so that CIs are symmetrical about the point estimate. The vertical line of no effect is at 1. The area of each square is proportional to the weight of that study in the summary RR. The summary RRs are diamonds whose lateral points indicate the 95% CI of the summary value. (Reprinted by permission from Zaric D, Pace NL. Transient neurologic symptoms (TNS) following spinal anaesthesia with lidocaine versus other local anaesthetics. *Cochrane Database Syst Rev.* 2009;CD003006(2). Copyright © John Wiley & Sons.[75])

between groups can be detected if the sample size is sufficiently large. On the other hand, if the sample size is small, one must always worry that identified or unidentified confounding variables may explain any difference; as the sample size decreases, randomization is less successful in assuring homogenous groups. Second, if the experimental groups are given three or more doses of a drug, do the results suggest a steadily increasing or decreasing dose-response relationship? Suppose the observed effect for an intermediate dose is either much higher or much lower than that for both the highest and lowest dose; a dose-response relationship may exist, but some skepticism about the experimental methods is warranted. Third, for clinical studies comparing different drugs, devices, and operations on patient outcome, are the patients, clinical care, and studied therapies sufficiently similar to those provided at other locations to be of interest to a wide group of practitioners? This is the distinction between *efficacy*—does it work under the best (research) circumstances—and *effectiveness*—does it work under the typical circumstances of routine clinical care?

Finally, in comparing alternative therapies, the confidence that a claim for a superior therapy is true depends on the study design. The strength of the evidence concerning efficacy will be least for an anecdotal case report; next in importance will be a retrospective study, then a prospective series of patients compared with historical controls, and finally a randomized, controlled clinical trial. The greatest strength for a therapeutic claim is a series of randomized, controlled clinical trials confirming the same hypothesis.

Statistical Resources

Accompanying the exponential growth of medical information has been the creation of a wealth of biostatistical knowledge. The increased emphasis on evidence-based medicine creates a great need for educating future and current physicians in quantitative reasoning, probability, and statistics. Textbooks oriented toward medical statistics and with expositions of basic, intermediate, and advanced statistics abound. There are journals of biomedical statistics, including *Epidemiology*, *Research Synthesis Methods*, *Systematic Reviews*, *Statistics in Medicine*, and *Statistical Methods in Medical Research*, whose audiences are both statisticians and biomedical researchers. Some medical journals, for example, the *British Medical Journal*, *JAMA*, *New England Journal of Medicine*, regularly publish expositions of both basic and newer advanced statistical methods. Journals of anesthesia including *Anesthesiology* and *Anesthesia & Analgesia* now frequently publish details of research design and statistical methods. Extensive internet resources including free online courses on data analysis methods, electronic textbooks of basic statistical methods, online statistical calculators, standard data sets, and reviews of statistical software can be easily found. High-performance statistical software is freely available from the R Foundation for Statistical Computing, Vienna, Austria.[d] There is continuing expansion in the resources giving guidance in methodology. Much of the improvement has been driven by epidemiologists and statisticians associated with the Cochrane Collaboration[e] and the Equator (Enhancing the QUAlity and Transparency Of health Research) network. There is a centralized resource for obtaining these and other reporting guidelines at the Equator network that includes over 500 entries.[f] Another resource is the GRADE (Grading of Recommendations Assessment, Development and Evaluation) working group that develops methods to rate the certainty of evidence and strength of recommendations in SRs.[g]

[d]See http://www.R-project.org
[e]See http://www.cochrane.org
[f]See http://www.equator-network.org/
[g]See http://www.gradeworkinggroup.org

Statistics and Anesthesia

Academic anesthesia needs more individuals well trained in statistical fundamentals. Statistically knowledgeable academic anesthesiologists will be positioned not only to improve their own research projects, but also to assist their colleagues, to strengthen the editorial review of journal manuscripts, and to know when to seek guidance from a professional statistician. Readers of the clinical literature should also expand their effort to acquire basic statistical skills, as journals are increasingly difficult to understand without basic statistical knowledge. Finally, understanding principles of experimental design and statistical inference can prevent premature acceptances of new therapies from faulty studies.

For further review and interactivities, please see the videos and narrative interactive clinical vignettes (NICVs) accessible in the complimentary eBook bundled with this text. Access instructions are located on the inside front cover.

REFERENCES

1. Vetter TR. Descriptive statistics: reporting the answers to the 5 basic questions of who, what, why, when, where, and a sixth, so what? *Anesth Analg.* 2017;125(5):1797–1802.
2. Vetter TR. Fundamentals of research data and variables: the devil is in the details. *Anesth Analg.* 2017;125(4):1375–1380.
3. Vetter TR. Magic mirror, on the wall-which is the right study design of them all?-Part I. *Anesth Analg.* 2017;124(6):2068–2073.
4. Vetter TR. Magic mirror, on the wall-which is the right study design of them all?-Part II. *Anesth Analg.* 2017;125(1):328–332.
5. Bhatt DL, Mehta C. Adaptive designs for clinical trials. *N Engl J Med.* 2016;375(1):65–74.
6. Park JJH, Detry MA, Murthy S, Guyatt G, Mills EJ. How to use and interpret the results of a platform trial: users' guide to the medical literature. *JAMA.* 2022;327(1):67–74.
7. Ellenberg SS. The stepped-wedge clinical trial: evaluation by rolliong deployment. *JAMA.* 2018;319(6):607–608.
8. Mauri L, D'Agostino RB Sr. Challenges in the design and interpretation of noninferiority trials. *N Engl J Med.* 2017;377(14):1357–1367.
9. Schober P, Vetter TR. Noninferiority and equivalence trials in medical. *Anesth Analg.* 2020;131(1):208–209.
10. Ford I, Norrie J. Pragmatic trials. *N Engl J Med.* 2016;375(5):454–463.
11. Sessler DI, Myles PS. Novel clinical trial designs to improve the efficiency of research. *Anesthesiology.* 2020;132(1):69–81.
12. Cobb LA, Thomas GI, Dillard DH, Merendino KA, Bruce RA. An evaluation of internal-mammary-artery ligation by a double-blind technic. *N Engl J Med.* 1959;260(22):1115–1118.
13. Sacks H, Chalmers TC, Smith H Jr. Randomized versus historical controls for clinical trials. *Am J Med.* 1982;72(2):233–240.
14. Kunz R, Oxman AD. The unpredictability paradox: review of empirical comparisons of randomised and non-randomised clinical trials. *BMJ.* 1998;317(7167):1185–1190.
15. Herbison P, Hay-Smith J, Gillespie WJ. Different methods of allocation to groups in randomized trials are associated with different levels of bias. A meta-epidemiological study. *J Clin Epidemiol.* 2011;64(10):1070–1075.
16. Concato J, Shah N, Horwitz RI. Randomized, controlled trials, observational studies, and the hierarchy of research designs. *N Engl J Med.* 2000;342(25):1887–1892.
17. Benson K, Hartz AJ. A comparison of observational studis and randomized, controlled trials. *N Engl J Med.* 2000;342(25):1878–1886.
18. Schulz KF, Chalmers I, Hayes RJ, Altman DG. Empirical evidence of bias. Dimensions of methodological quality associated with estimates of treatment effects in controlled trials. *JAMA.* 1995;273(5):408–412.
19. Wasserstein RL, Lazar NA. The ASA statement on p-values: context, process, and purpose. *Am Stat.* 2016;70(2):129–133.
20. Greenland S, Senn SJ, Rothman KJ, et al. Statistical test, P-values, confidence intervals, and power: a guide to misinterpretations. *Eur J Epidemiol.* 2016;31(4):337–350.
21. Mascha EJ, Vetter TR. Significance, errors, power, and sample size: The blocking and tackling of statistics. *Anesth Analg.* 2018;126(2):691–698.
22. Goodman SN. Toward evidence-based medical statistics. 1: the P value fallacy. *Ann Intern Med.* 1999;130(12):995–1004.
23. Goodman SN. Toward evidence-based medical statistics. 2: the bayes factor. *Ann Intern Med.* 1999;130(12):1005–1013.
24. Goodman SN. Of P-values and Bayes: a modest proposal. *Epidemiology.* 2001;12(3):295–297.
25. Nuzzo R. Scientific method: statistical errors. *Nature.* 2014;506(7487):150–152.
26. Little RJ. Calibrated Bayes: a Bayes/Frequentist roadmap. *Am Stat.* 2006;60:213–223.

27. Sterne JA, Davey SG. Sifting the evidence-what's wrong with significance tests? *BMJ*. 2001; 322(7280):226–231.
28. Wei Z, Yang A, Rocha L, Miranda MF, Nathoo FS. A review of Bayesian hypothesis testing and its practical implementations. *Entropy (Basel)*. 2022;24(2):161.
29. van de Schoot R, Depaoli S, King R, et al. Bayesian statistics and modelling. *Nat Rev Methods Primers*. 2021;1(1).
30. McGlothlin AE, Viele K. Bayesian hierarchical models. *JAMA*. 2018:320(22):2365–2366.
31. Ioannidis JPA. Contradicted and initially stronger effects in highly cited clinical research. *JAMA*. 2005;294(2):218–228.
32. Ioannidis JPA. Effect of formal statistical significance on the credibility of observational associations. *Am J Epidemiol*. 2008;168(4):374–383; discussion 384–390.
33. Ioannidis JPA. Why most published research findings are false. *PLoS Med*. 2005;2(8):e124.
34. Katki HA. Invited commentary: evidence-based evaluation of p values and Bayes factors. *Am J Epidemiol*. 2008;168:384–388.
35. Cameletti M, Gómez-Rubio V. Software for bayesian statistics. *J Stat Softw*. 2021;100(1):1–7.
36. Goodman SN, Berlin JA. The use of predicted confidence intervals when planning experiments and the misuse of power when interpreting results. *Ann Intern Med*. 1994;121(3):200–206.
37. Schober P, Bossers SM, Schwarte LA. Statistical significance versus clinical importance of observed effect sizes: what do P values and confidence intervals really represent? *Anesth Analg*. 2018;126(3):1068–1072.
38. Hawkins AT, Samuels LR. Use of confidence intervals in intnerpreting nonstatistically significant results. *JAMA*. 2021;236(20):2068–2069.
39. Hanley JA, Lippman-Hand A. If nothing goes wrong, is everything all right? Interpreting zero numerators. *JAMA*. 1983;249(13):1743–1745.
40. Tuyl F, Gerlach R, Mengersen K. A comparison of Bayes–Laplace, Jeffreys, and other priors: the case of zero events. *Am Stat*. 2008;62:40–44.
41. Keld DB, Hein L, Dalgaard M, Krogh L, Rodt SA. The incidence of transient neurologic symptoms (TNS) afterspinal anaesthesia in patients undergoing surgery in thesupine position. Hyperbaric lidocaine 5% versus hyperbaricbupivacaine 0.5%. *Acta Anaesthesiol Scand*. 2000;44(3):285–290.
42. Norton EC, Dowd BE, Maciejewski ML. Odds ratios – current best practice and use. *JAMA*. 2018;320(1):84–85.
43. Holmberg MJ, Andersen LW. Estimating risk ratios and risk differences: alternatives to odds ratios. *JAMA*. 2020;324(11):1098–1099.
44. Vetter TR, Jesser CA. Fundamental epidemiology terminology and measures: it really is all in the name. *Anesth Analg*. 2017;125(6):2146–2151.
45. Schober P, Mascha EJ, Vetter TR. Statistics from a (agreement) to z (z score): a guide to interpreting common measures of association, agreement, diagnostic accuracy, effect size, heterogeneity, and reliability in medical research. *Anesth Analg*. 2021;133(6):1633–1641.
46. Anscombe FJ. Graphs in statistical analysis. *Am Stat*. 1973;27:17–21.
47. Hill AB. The Environment and Disease: Association or Causation? *Proc R Soc Med*. 1965;58:295–300.
48. Ioannidis JPA. Exposure-wide epidemiology: revisiting Bradford Hill. *Stat Med*. 2015;35:1749–1762.
49. Katz MH. Multivariable analysis: a primer for readers of medical research. *Ann Intern Med*. 2003; 138(8):644–650.
50. Brotman DJ, Walker E, Lauer MS, O'Brien RG. In search of fewer independent risk factors. *Arch Intern Med*. 2005;165(2):138–145.
51. Pace NL. Independent predictors from stepwise logistic regression may be nothing more than publishable P values. *Anesth Analg*. 2008;107:1775–1778.
52. Smith G. Step away from stepwise. *J Big Data*. 2018;5:32.
53. Kranke P. Effective management of postoperative nausea and vomiting: let us practise what we preach! *Eur J Anaesthesiol*. 2011;28(3):152–154.
54. Eberhart LHJ, Morin AM. Risk scores for predicting postoperative nausea and vomiting are clinically useful tools and should be used in every patient: con – 'life is really simple, but we insist on making it complicated.' *Eur J Anaesthesiol*. 2011;28:155–159.
55. Pierre S. Risk scores for predicting post-operative nausea and vomiting are clinically useful tools and should be used in every patient: 'don't throw the baby out with the bathwater.' *Eur J Anaesthesiol*. 2011;28:160–163.
56. Cook NR. Statistical evaluation of prognostic versus diagnostic models: beyond the ROC curve. *Clin Chem*. 2008;54:17–23.
57. Cook NR, Ridker PM. Advances in measuring the effect of individual predictors of cardiovascular risk: the role of reclassification measures. *Ann Intern Med*. 2009;150(11):795–802.
58. Steyerberg EW, Vickers AJ, Cook NR, et al. Assessing the performance of prediction models: a framework for traditional and novel measures. *Epidemiology*. 2010;21(1):128–138.
59. Wong A, Otles E, Donnelly JP, et al. external validation of a widely implemented proprietary sepsis prediction model in hospitalized patients. *JAMA Intern Med*. 2021;181(8):1065–1070.
60. Siontis GCM, Tzoulaki I, Ioannidis JPA. Predicting death: an empirical evaluation of predictive tools for mortality. *Arch Intern Med*. 2011;171(19):1721–1726.
61. Wyatt JC, Altman DG. Prognostic models: clinically useful or quickly forgotten? *BMJ*. 1995;311:1539–1541.
62. Staffa SJ, Zurakowski D. Five steps to successfully implement and evaluate propensity score matching in clinical research studies. *Anesth Analg*. 2018;127(4):1066–1073.
63. Schulte PJ, Mascha EJ. Propensity score methods: theory and practice for anesthesia research. *Anesth Analg*. 2018;127(4):1074–1084.
64. Guyatt G. A randomized control trial of right-heart catheterization in critically ill patients. Ontario Intensive Care Study Group. *J Intensive Care Med*. 1991;6:91–95.
65. Connors AF Jr., Speroff T, Dawson NV, et al. The effectiveness of right heart catheterization in the initial care of critically ill patients. SUPPORT Investigators. *JAMA*. 1996;276(11):889–897.
66. Wijeysundera DN, Beattie WS, Austin PC, Hux JE, Laupacis A. Epidural anaesthesia and survival after intermediate-to-high risk non-cardiac surgery: a population-based cohort study. *Lancet*. 2008;372(9638):562–569.
67. Gayat E, Pirracchio R, Resche-Rigon M, Mebazaa A, Mary JY, Porcher R. Propensity scores in intensive care and anaesthesiology literature: a systematic review. *Intensive Care Med*. 2010;36(12):1993–2003.
68. Murphy GJ, Reeves BC, Rogers CA, Rizvi SIA, Culliford L, Angelini GD. Increased mortality, postoperative morbidity, and cost after red blood cell transfusion in patients having cardiac surgery. *Circulation*. 2007;116(22):2544–2552.
69. Murphy GJ, Pike K, Rogers CA, et al; TITRe2 Investigators. Liberal or restrictive transfusion after cardiac surgery. *N Engl J Med*. 2015;372(11):997–1008.
70. Pace NL. Prevention of succinylcholine myalgias: a meta-analysis. *Anesth Analg*. 1990;70: 477–483.
71. Pace NL. Research methods for meta-analyses. *Best Pract Res Clin Anaesthesiol*. 2011;25(4): 523–533.
72. Møller AM, Myles PS. What makes a good systematic review and meta-analysis? *Br J Anaesth*. 2016;117(4):428–430.
73. Schober P, Vetter TR. Meta-analysis in clinical research. *Anesth Analg*. 2020;131(4):1090–1091.
74. Pereira TV, Ioannidis JPA. Statistically significant meta-analyses of clinical trials have modest credibility and inflated effects. *J Clin Epidemiol*. 2011;64(10):1060–1069.
75. Zaric D, Pace NL. Transient neurologic symptoms (TNS) following spinal anaesthesia with lidocaine versus other local anaesthetics. *Cochrane Database Syst Rev*. 2009;(2): CD003006.
76. Forget P, Borovac JA, Thackeray EM, Pace NL. Transient neurological symptoms (TNS) following spinal anaesthesia with lidocaine versus other local anaesthetics in adult surgical patients: a network meta-analysis. *Cochrane Database Syst Rev*. 2019;12:CD003006.
77. Mills EJ, Ioannidis JPA, Thorlund K, Schunemann HJ, Puhan MA, Guyatt GH. How to use an article reporting a multiple treatment comparison meta-analysis. *JAMA*. 2012;308(12): 1246–1253.
78. Leeflang MMG. Systematic reviews and meta-analyses of diagnostic test accuracy. *Clin Microbiol Infect*. 2014;20(2):105–113.
79. McInnes MDF, Moher D, Thombs BD, et al. Preferred reporting items for a systematic review and meta-analysis of diagnostic test accuracy studies: The PRISMA-DTA Statement. *JAMA*. 2018;319(4):388–396.
80. Serghiou S, Goodman SN. Random-effects meta-analysis: summarizing evidence with caveats. *JAMA*. 2019;321(3):301–302.
81. Imberger G, Gluud C, Boylan J, Wetterslev J. Systematic reviews of anesthesiologic interventions reported as statistically significant: problems with power, precision, and type 1 error protection. *Anesth Analg*. 2015;121(6):1611–1622.
82. Beecher HK, Todd DP. A study of the deaths associated with anesthesia and surgery: based on a study of 599, 548 anesthesias in ten institutions 1948–1952, inclusive. *Ann Surg*. 1954; 140(1):2–35.
83. Summary of the national Halothane Study. Possible association between halothane anesthesia and postoperative hepatic necrosis. *JAMA*. 1966;197(10):775–788.
84. Ginsberg J, Mohebbi MH, Patel RS, Brammer L, Smolinski MS, Brilliant L. Detecting influenza epidemics using search engine query data. *Nature*. 2009;457(7232):1012–1014.
85. Olson DR, Konty KJ, Paladini M, Viboud C, Simonsen L. Reassessing Google Flu Trends data for detection of seasonal and pandemic influenza: a comparative epidemiological study at three geographic scales. *PLoS Comput Biol*. 2013;9(10):e1003256.
86. Liem VGB, Hoeks SE, van Lier F, de Graaff JC. What we can learn from Big Data about factors influencing perioperative outcome. *Curr Opin Anaesthesiol*. 2018;31(6):723–731.
87. Simpao AF, Ahumada LM, Rehman MA. Big data and visual analytics in anaesthesia and health care. *Br J Anaesth*. 2015;115(3):350–356.
88. Levin MA, Wanderer JP, Ehrenfeld JM. Data, big data, and metadata in anesthesiology. *Anesth Analg*. 2015;121(6):1661–1667.
89. Müller-Wirtz LM, Volk T. Big Data in studying acute pain and regional anesthesia. *J Clin Med*. 2021;10(7):1425.
90. Liu D, Görges M, Jenkins SA. University of Queensland vital signs dataset: development of an accessible repository of anesthesia patient monitoring data for research. *Anesth Analg*. 2012;114(3):584–589.
91. Lee HC, Jung CW. Vital Recorder-a free research tool for automatic recording of high-resolution time-synchronised physiological data from multiple anaesthesia devices. *Sci Rep*. 2018;8(1):1527.
92. Pulley JM, Denny JC, Peterson JF, et al. Operational implementation of prospective genotyping for personalized medicine: the design of the Vanderbilt PREDICT project. *Clin Pharmacol Ther*. 2012;92(1):87–95.
93. Sutherland WJ, Spiegelhalter D, Burgman MA. Policy: Twenty tips for interpreting scientific claims. *Nature*. 2013;503(7476):335–337.
94. Pocock SJ, Stone GW. The primary outcome fails – what next? *N Engl J Med*. 2016;375(9): 861–870.
95. Pocock SJ, Stone GW. The primary outcome is positive – is that good enough? *N Engl J Med*. 2016;375(10):971–979.

8 Inflammation, Wound Healing, and Infection

HARRIET W. HOPF • AMALIA COCHRAN • CRISTIANE M. UENO • CANDICE K. MORRISSEY

KEY POINTS

1. The most crucial component of infection prevention is frequent and effective hand hygiene. Wearing gloves does not reduce the need for hand hygiene.
2. The ideal hand hygiene agent kills a broad spectrum of microbes, has antimicrobial activity that persists for at least 6 hours after application, is simple to use, and has few side effects.
3. There is no compelling evidence that single-use disposables reduce infections, except where adequate disinfection is not (currently) possible (e.g., vascular catheters, duodenoscopes). While the cost of acquisition is lower for disposables, the per-use cost is almost always orders of magnitude greater. In addition, life-cycle analyses have shown that disposables cause demonstrable public health harm (in the range of that caused by medical errors) by increasing waste, pollution, and greenhouse gas emissions, offsetting any theoretical protection from infection.
4. Antibiotic prophylaxis has become standard for surgeries in which there is more than a minimum risk of infection. The most commonly used antibiotic for surgical prophylaxis is cefazolin, a first-generation cephalosporin, as the potential pathogens for most surgeries are gram-positive cocci from the skin.
5. The exact timing for the administration of preoperative antibiotic prophylaxis depends on the pharmacology and half-life of the drug, but should generally be 0 to 60 minutes before incision. Anesthesiologists should work in consultation with surgeons to take initiative for administering prophylactic antibiotics because they have access to the patient during the 60 minutes prior to incision and can optimize timing of administration.
6. The standard teaching that oxygen delivery depends more on hemoglobin-bound oxygen (oxygen content) than on arterial PO_2 may be true for working muscle, but it is not true for wound healing. Although oxygen consumption is relatively low in wounds, it is consumed by processes that require oxygen at a high concentration. Delivery of oxygen to wounds depends on arterial PO_2 rather than hemoglobin-bound oxygen (oxygen content).
7. Peripheral vasoconstriction, which results from central sympathetic control of subcutaneous vascular tone, is probably the most frequent and clinically the most important impediment to wound oxygenation and wound healing. All vasoconstrictive stimuli must be corrected simultaneously to allow optimal healing. Modifiable risks for wound infections include smoking, malnutrition, obesity, hyperglycemia, hypercholesterolemia, and hypertension. These should be assessed and corrected (when possible) prior to surgery.
8. Prevention or correction of hypothermia has been shown to decrease wound infections and increase collagen deposition in patients undergoing major abdominal surgery. Maintenance of a high room temperature or active warming before, during, and after the operation is significantly more effective than other methods of warming, such as application of warmed blankets, circulating water blankets placed on the surface of the operating table, and humidification of the breathing circuit.
9. Optimizing the volume of perioperative fluid administration to minimize morbidity and mortality remains a significant and controversial challenge. Current best recommendations for volume management include replacing fluid losses based on standard recommendations for the type of surgery, replacement of blood loss, and replacement of other ongoing fluid losses (e.g., high urine output due to diuretic or dye administration, hyperglycemia, or thermoregulatory vasoconstriction).
10. Administration of supplemental oxygen via face mask or nasal cannula increases safety in patients receiving systemic opioids. As a side benefit, it may also improve wound healing. Pain control also appears important since it favorably influences both pulmonary function and vascular tone.
11. In patients with moderate to high risk of surgical site infection, anesthesiologists have the opportunity to enhance wound healing and reduce the incidence of wound infections by simple, inexpensive, and readily available means.

Introduction

Despite major advances in the management of patients undergoing surgery—including aseptic technique, prophylactic antibiotics, and advances in surgical approaches such as laparoscopic surgery—surgical site infection (SSI) and wound failure remain common complications of surgery (Table 8-1).[1] SSIs account for about 20% of health care–associated infections are associated with prolonged hospitalization (~10 days) and mortality, and an annual cost of about $3 billion.[1] In recent years, focused efforts have had some measure of success. The Centers for Disease Control and Prevention (CDC) estimates that the rate of health care–associated infections in surgical patients decreased from 4% in 2011 to 3.2% in 2015.[1] A primary driver is the reduction in SSIs and urinary tract infections.[2] While reducing bacterial contamination has been the primary focus of SSI prevention efforts, a growing body of literature supports the concept that patient factors are also a major determinant of wound outcome following surgery.

Table 8-1 Criteria for Defining a Surgical Site Infection (SSI)

Superficial Incisional SSI

- Infection occurs within 30 d after the operation

And

- Infection involves only skin or subcutaneous tissue of the incision

And

- At least *one* of the following:
  1. Purulent drainage, with or without laboratory confirmation, from the superficial incision
  2. Organisms isolated from an aseptically obtained culture of fluid or tissue from the superficial incision
  3. At least one of the following signs or symptoms of infection: pain or tenderness, localized swelling, redness, or heat *and* superficial incision is deliberately opened by the surgeon, *unless* the incision is culture negative
  4. Diagnosis of superficial incisional SSI by the surgeon or attending physician
- Do *not* report the following conditions as superficial incisional SSI:
  1. Stitch abscess (minimal inflammation and discharge confined to the points of suture penetration)
  2. Infection of an episiotomy or newborn circumcision site
  3. Infected burn wound
  4. Incisional SSI that extends into the facial and muscle layers (see "Deep Incisional SSI")

Note: Specific criteria are used for identifying infected episiotomy and circumcision sites and burn wounds

Deep Incisional SSI

- Infection occurs within 30 d after the operation if no implant is left in place or within 1 y if implant is in place and the infection appears to be related to the operation

And

- Infection involves deep soft tissues (e.g., fascial and muscle layers) of the incision

And

- At least *one* of the following:
  1. Purulent drainage from the deep incision but not from the organ/space component of the surgical site
  2. A deep incision spontaneously dehisces or is deliberately opened by a surgeon when the patient has at least one of the following signs or symptoms: fever (> 38°C), localized pain, or tenderness, unless site is culture negative
  3. An abscess or other evidence of infection involving the deep incision is found on direct examination, during reoperation, or by histopathologic or radiologic examination
  4. Diagnosis of a deep incisional SSI by a surgeon or attending physician

Notes:

1. Report infection that involves both superficial and deep incision sites as deep incisional SSI
2. Report an organ/space SSI that drains through the incision as a deep incisional SSI

Organ/Space SSI

- Infection occurs within 30 d after the operation if no implant is left in place or within 1 y if implant is in place and the infection appears to be related to the operation

And

- Infection involves any part of the anatomy (e.g., organs or spaces), other than the incision, which was opened or manipulated during an operation

And

- At least *one* of the following:
  1. Purulent drainage from a drain that is placed through a stab wound into the organ/space
  2. Organisms isolated from an aseptically obtained culture of fluid or tissue in the organ/space
  3. An abscess or other evidence of infection involving the organ/space that is found on direct examination, during reoperation, or by histopathologic or radiologic examination
  4. Diagnosis of an organ/space SSI by a surgeon or attending physician

From Centers for Disease Control National Healthcare Safety Network Surgical Site Infection Event (SSI) Procedure-Associated Module, January 2023. Accessed online February 7, 2023. chrome-extension://efaidnbmnnnibpcajpcglclefindmkaj/https://www.cdc.gov/nhsn/pdfs/pscmanual/9pscssicurrent.pdf

Comorbidities such as diabetes and cardiac disease clearly contribute; a patient's genetic make-up may also have a role.[3] In addition, environmental stressors and the individual response to stress are important. In particular, wounds are exquisitely sensitive to hypoxia, which is both common and preventable. Perioperative management can be adapted to promote postoperative wound healing and resistance to infection. Along with aseptic technique and prophylactic antibiotics, maintaining perfusion and oxygenation of the wound is paramount. This chapter discusses how knowledge of the principles of infection control and the physiology of wound repair and resistance to infection can improve outcomes.

Infection Control

Hand Hygiene

1 The most crucial component of infection prevention is frequent and effective hand hygiene. In 1847, Ignaz Semmelweis made the observation that women who delivered their babies in the First Clinic at the General Hospital of Vienna, staffed by medical students and physicians, had a mortality rate of 5% to 15%, largely the result of puerperal infections; this was substantially higher than the 2% rate of women who delivered at Clinic 2, which was staffed by midwife students and midwives.[4] Students and physicians at Clinic 1 usually started the day performing autopsies (including on patients who died of puerperal fever) and then moved on to the clinic, where they performed examinations on women in labor. Semmelweis made the connection, and although germ theory was some years off, he insisted that physicians and medical students wash their hands in a chlorinated solution when leaving the pathology laboratory. This reduced the rate of puerperal fever to the same rate as at Clinic 2. Soon, Semmelweis identified cases of transmission from an infected to an uninfected patient and instituted the use of chlorinated solution hand washing between cases as well. He also demonstrated that the chlorinated solution was more effective than soap and water. Unfortunately, his innovation was not widely adopted, resulting from a combination of factors, including delay in publishing his results, reluctance of his colleagues to accept that they might be responsible for transmitting disease, and his lower social standing as a Hungarian living in the Austrian Empire. Despite our current knowledge of germ theory, hand hygiene remains an inexplicably neglected component of infection control. Studies consistently demonstrate about a 40% rate of adherence (range, 5% to 81%) to hand hygiene guidelines,[4] and compliance by anesthesiologists in the operating room (OR) is notably lower.[5]

Bacteria are resident in the skin and can never be completely eliminated.[6] Resident flora are embedded in the deeper folds of the skin and are more resistant to removal, but are also infrequently pathogenic. Coagulase-negative staphylococci and diphtheroids are the most common. Transient flora colonizes the superficial layers of the skin and thus are easier to remove with hand hygiene. Transient flora is also the source of most health care–associated infections, as health care worker's skin can become contaminated from patient contact or contact with contaminated surfaces. Contamination from surfaces is most common with organisms such as staphylococci and enterococci, both of which are resistant to drying. Even "clean" activities such as taking a patient's pulse or applying monitors can lead to hand contamination. In one study, 100 to 1,000 colony-forming units of *Klebsiella* species were measured on nurses' hands following such activities.[6] No studies have related hand contamination to actual transmission of infection to patients; however, numerous studies, starting with those of Semmelweis, have demonstrated a reduction in health care–associated infections following institution of hand hygiene or improved adherence to hand hygiene.[6]

A number of products are available for hand hygiene. The ideal 2
agent kills a broad spectrum of microbes, has antimicrobial activity that persists for at least 6 hours after application, is simple to use, and has few side effects.

Plain (not antiseptic) soap and water are generally the least effective at reducing hand contamination.[6] Although obvious dirt is removed by the detergent effect of soap and the mechanical action of washing, bacterial load is not greatly reduced. Further, soap and water hand hygiene is associated with high rates of skin irritation and drying, both of which are risk factors for an increased bacterial load. Soap and water are, however, the most effective at removing spores, and, therefore, should be used when contamination with *Clostridium difficile* or *Bacillus anthracis* is a concern.[6]

The antimicrobial activity of alcohol-based rinses, gels, and foams comes from their ability to denature proteins.[6] Ethanol is most commonly used because it has more antiviral activity than isopropanol. Antiseptics containing 60% to 95% ethanol with a water base are germicidal and effective against gram-positive and gram-negative bacteria, lipophilic viruses such as herpes simplex, human immunodeficiency, influenza, respiratory syncytial, and vaccinia viruses, and hepatitis B and C viruses. They have little persistent activity, although regrowth of bacteria does occur slowly after use of alcohol-based products. Combination with low doses of other agents such as chlorhexidine, quaternary ammonium compounds, or triclosan can confer persistent activity. Efficacy depends on volume applied (3 mL is superior to 1 mL) and duration of contact (ideally, 30 seconds).

Chlorhexidine is a cationic bisbiguanide that disrupts cytoplasmic membranes, resulting in precipitation of cellular contents.[6] It is germicidal against gram-positive bacteria and lipophilic viruses, with somewhat less activity against gram-negative bacteria and fungi and minimal activity against tubercle bacilli. It has substantial persistence on the skin. The CDC has identified chlorhexidine as the topical agent of choice. It may cause severe corneal damage after direct contact with the eye, ototoxicity after direct contact with the inner or middle ear, and neurotoxicity after direct contact with the brain or meninges. There are reports of bacteria that have acquired reduced susceptibility to chlorhexidine, but these are of questionable clinical relevance since the concentrations at which resistance was found were substantially lower than that of commercially available products. An additional disadvantage is the risk of immunoglobulin E–mediated allergic reactions to chlorhexidine.[7] Cases are likely underreported because of the difficulty identifying the source of anaphylactic reactions perioperatively. Chlorhexidine is present in a wide range of medical and community-based products, including wipes, impregnated central venous catheters, toothpaste, mouthwash, contact lens cleanser, and food preservatives. Therefore, potentially sensitizing exposures are common.

Iodine and iodophors (iodine with a polymer carrier) penetrate the cell wall and impair protein synthesis and cell membrane function.[6] They are bactericidal against gram-positive, gram-negative, and some spore-forming bacteria including clostridia and *Bacillus* species; they are inactive against spores. They also have activity against mycobacteria, viruses, and fungi. Their persistence is relatively poor. They cause more contact dermatitis than other commonly used agents, and allergies to this class of topical agent are common. Iodophors generally cause fewer side effects than iodine agents.

The choice of an antiseptic depends on the expected pathogens, acceptability by health care workers, and cost. In general,

Table 8-2 Indications for Hand Hygiene

When hands are visibly dirty or contaminated with proteinaceous material or are visibly soiled with blood or other body fluids, wash hands with either a nonantimicrobial soap and water or an antimicrobial soap and water.
If hands are not visibly soiled, use an alcohol-based hand rub for routinely decontaminating hands. Alternatively, wash hands with an antimicrobial soap and water.
Decontaminate hands before having direct contact with patients.
Decontaminate hands before donning sterile gloves when inserting a central intravascular catheter.
Decontaminate hands before inserting indwelling urinary catheters, peripheral vascular catheters, or other invasive devices that do not require a surgical procedure.
Decontaminate hands after contact with a patient's intact skin (e.g., applying monitors, moving patient).
Decontaminate hands after contact with body fluids or excretions, mucous membranes, nonintact skin, and wound dressings if hands are not visibly soiled.
Decontaminate hands if moving from a contaminated-body site (e.g., mouth during tracheal intubation) to a clean-body site (e.g., adjusting gas flow, turning on ventilator, starting IV) during patient care.
Decontaminate hands after contact with inanimate objects (including medical equipment) in the immediate vicinity of the patient. Take care to reduce contamination of the anesthesia machine (e.g., after tracheal intubation) as well!
Decontaminate hands after removing gloves.
Before eating and after using a restroom, wash hands with a nonantimicrobial soap and water or with an antimicrobial soap and water.
Antimicrobial-impregnated wipes (i.e., towelettes) may be considered as an alternative to washing hands with nonantimicrobial soap and water. Because they are not as effective as alcohol-based hand rubs or washing hands with an antimicrobial soap and water for reducing bacterial counts on the hands of HCWs, they are not a substitute for using an alcohol-based hand rub or antimicrobial soap.

IV, intravenous (tube); HCW, health care worker.

Modified from Boyce JM, Pittet D; Healthcare Infection Control Practices Advisory Committee, HICPAC/SHEA/APIC/IDSA Hand Hygiene Task Force. Guideline for Hand Hygiene in Health-Care Settings. Recommendations of the Healthcare Infection Control Practices Advisory Committee and the HIPAC/SHEA/APIC/IDSA Hand Hygiene Task Force. *Am J Infect Control.* 2002;30:S1–S46.

antiseptics cost about $1 per patient day, far less than the cost of health care–associated infections. In nine studies that examined the effect of improved hand hygiene adherence on health care–associated infections, the majority demonstrated that as hand hygiene practices improved, infection rates decreased.[6]

Barriers to hand hygiene include skin irritation and fear of skin irritation, inaccessibility, time, and health care worker acceptance (largely related to the other factors mentioned). Although alcohol-based agents have long been believed to cause more skin irritation, several recent trials have demonstrated less skin irritation and better acceptance with emollient-containing, alcohol-based hand rubs compared with either antimicrobial or nonantimicrobial soaps. The use of appropriate (glove-compatible) lotions twice a day also reduces skin irritation, leading to a 50% increase in hand hygiene frequency in one study.[6] Alcohol-based gels and foams are also generally more accessible than antiseptic soap and water, as the dispenser may be pocket-sized or placed conveniently near sites of patient care. It has been estimated that alcohol-based gels and foams require only about 25% of the time of going to a sink to wash one's hands. However, soap and water should be used to remove particulate matter including blood and other body fluids or after 5 to 10 applications of an alcohol-based agent.

Adherence to hand hygiene guidelines (Tables 8-2 to 8-4) generally decreases as the frequency of indicated hand washing increases, as the workload increases, and as staffing decreases. CDC guidelines for health care providers traditionally focused

Table 8-3 Hand Hygiene Technique

When decontaminating hands with an alcohol-based hand rub, apply the recommended volume of product to the palm of one hand and rub hands together, covering all surfaces of hands and fingers, until hands are dry.
When washing hands with soap and water, wet hands first with water, apply an amount of the product recommended by the manufacturer to hands, and rub hands together vigorously for at least 15 s, covering all surfaces of the hands and fingers. Rinse hands with water and dry thoroughly with a disposable towel. Use towel to turn off the faucet. Avoid using hot water because repeated exposure to hot water may increase the risk of dermatitis.
Liquid, bar, leaflet, or powdered forms of plain soap are acceptable when washing hands with a nonantimicrobial soap and water. When bar soap is used, soap racks that facilitate drainage and small bars of soap should be used.

Modified from Boyce JM, Pittet D; Healthcare Infection Control Practices Advisory Committee, HICPAC/SHEA/APIC/IDSA Hand Hygiene Task Force. Guideline for Hand Hygiene in Health-Care Settings. Recommendations of the Healthcare Infection Control Practices Advisory Committee and the HIPAC/SHEA/APIC/IDSA Hand Hygiene Task Force. *Am J Infect Control.* 2002;30:S1–S46.

Table 8-4 Skin Care

Provide health care workers with hand lotions or creams to minimize the occurrence of irritant contact dermatitis associated with hand antisepsis or hand washing.
Solicit information from manufacturers regarding any effects that hand lotions, creams, or alcohol-based hand antiseptics may have on the persistent effects of antimicrobial soaps being used in the institution, as well as on glove integrity. Select a combination of products that minimizes these effects.

Modified from Boyce JM, Pittet D; Healthcare Infection Control Practices Advisory Committee, HICPAC/SHEA/APIC/IDSA Hand Hygiene Task Force. Guideline for Hand Hygiene in Health-Care Settings. Recommendations of the Healthcare Infection Control Practices Advisory Committee and the HIPAC/SHEA/APIC/IDSA Hand Hygiene Task Force. *Am J Infect Control*. 2002;30:S1–S46.

on hand hygiene prior to entering and after leaving a patient room. More recently, the World Health Organization has developed a campaign highlighting the "5 Moments" of hand hygiene (Fig. 8-1AB). The campaign emphasizes the need to perform hand hygiene after each contact with a patient or their immediate environment.[8]

In an intensive care unit (ICU), hand hygiene for nurses is generally indicated about 20 times per hour, as compared with lower acuity units, where this number decreases to 8 times per hour.[6] In the OR, frequent patient contact by the anesthesiologist requires frequent hand hygiene, probably at about the level of nurses in the ICU, while accessibility to the resources necessary to perform hand hygiene is often quite limited. Sinks are available only outside the OR. Therefore, alcohol-based agents should be available within hand's reach of the anesthesia machine.

Patients, anesthetists, and environmental reservoirs (e.g., anesthesia work area), all contribute to cross-transmission of pathogens responsible for health care–associated infections.[9] Hand hygiene by anesthetists and attention to bacterial decontamination of the anesthesia work area (e.g., during and after induction) are central to preventing SSI and other perioperative health care–associated infections.[9] Koff et al.[5] demonstrated that increased hand hygiene episodes (7 to 9 per hour compared to <0.5 per hour during the control period) triggered by an alarm and encouraged by education decreased work area contamination, decreased intravenous stopcock contamination from 32% to 8%, and decreased health care–associated infections significantly, even though opportunities were not measured and hand hygiene episodes were not necessarily coordinated with one of the 5 Moments. Implementation of a bundle that included patient decolonization, hand hygiene, segregation of contaminated equipment and wiping down the anesthesia workspace after induction, clean handling of syringes, and disinfection of intravenous ports before injection reduced cross-transmission and health care–associated infections.[9] Thus, transmission of bacterial contamination by the anesthesia provider appears to be common, a potential source of nosocomial infections, and largely preventable.

Wearing gloves does not reduce the need for hand hygiene. Although gloves provide protection, bacterial flora from patients may be cultured from up to 30% of health care workers who wear gloves during patient contact.[6] Therefore, hand hygiene should be practiced both before putting on gloves and immediately after their removal. Moreover, gloves should be removed or changed immediately after each procedure, including vascular access, intubation, and neuraxial anesthesia, because gloves become contaminated by patient contact just as hands do. Balancing hand hygiene with close attention to the patient during critical portions of the case (e.g., securing the airway) can be challenging. Double gloving and providing a convenient location for contaminated equipment have been suggested as effective approaches.[10,11] During high-acuity care, another approach is to apply hand hygiene directly to the gloves, which is substantially faster than changing gloves, but protects the workspace and patient environment from cross-contamination.[12]

Artificial and long fingernails, as well as chipped fingernail polish, are associated with higher concentrations of bacteria on the hands of health care workers. Artificial nails have been identified as a source in several hospital-associated outbreaks of infection with gram-negative bacilli and yeast. CDC guidelines discourage the wearing of artificial nails by health care workers in high-risk settings (e.g., the OR), and many hospitals have banned the wearing of artificial nails by any employee who has direct patient contact.[6] It may also be appropriate to counsel patients scheduled for surgery that artificial nails may increase their risk of infection, although this has not been investigated. Large quantities of bacteria are typically trapped under the fingernails. The 2002 CDC guidelines recommend that health care workers keep their nail tips trimmed to less than ¼ inch.[6]

Bacteria may be cultured at higher concentrations from the skin beneath a ring. On the other hand, wearing a ring does not increase overall bacterial levels measured on the hands of health care workers. Therefore, it remains unclear whether transmission of infection could be reduced by prohibiting health care workers from wearing rings.[6]

Antisepsis

Masks have long been advocated as preventing SSIs and are used almost universally in ORs in the United States. Tunevall[13] studied the rate of wound infections in 3,088 patients over 115 weeks. In alternating weeks, OR personnel either wore masks or did not (personnel with active respiratory infections continued to wear masks). There was no difference in the rate of surgical wound infections (4.7% vs. 3.5%, respectively) in the two groups, nor in bacterial species cultured from the wounds. Friberg et al.[14] demonstrated comparable air and surface contamination during sham surgery in a simluated OR with horizontal laminar flow air exchange, whether OR personnel wore a nonsterile hood and mask or a sterilized helmet aspirator system. However, when the head cover, but not the mask, was omitted, contamination increased three- to fivefold. These data suggest that wearing a head cover is useful for preventing SSI, while wearing a mask is not. Nonetheless, the study by Tunevall is a small one, and most hospitals continue to require a mask in the OR while surgical instruments are open. Moreover, the mask does serve the purpose of protecting the health care provider, particularly when combined with eye protection, and thus should most likely be used during tracheal intubation, emergence from anesthesia, and at other times when exposure to body fluids is likely. The value of masks (especially respirator masks like N95s) in protecting health care workers has been highlighted during the SARS-CoV-2 pandemic.

Although the preponderance of postoperative surgical infections is caused by flora that are endogenous to the patient, environmental and airborne contaminants may also play a causative role. An important, but frequently overlooked, consideration is the role that traffic patterns into an OR can play in patient exposure to airborne organisms, although the importance of this factor may have been reduced by improved ventilation and a higher requirement for air changes in the OR in recent years. Current recommended practices are to limit the flow of people through an OR that is in use, and that no more people than necessary should

Your 5 moments for HAND HYGIENE

Design: mondofragilis network

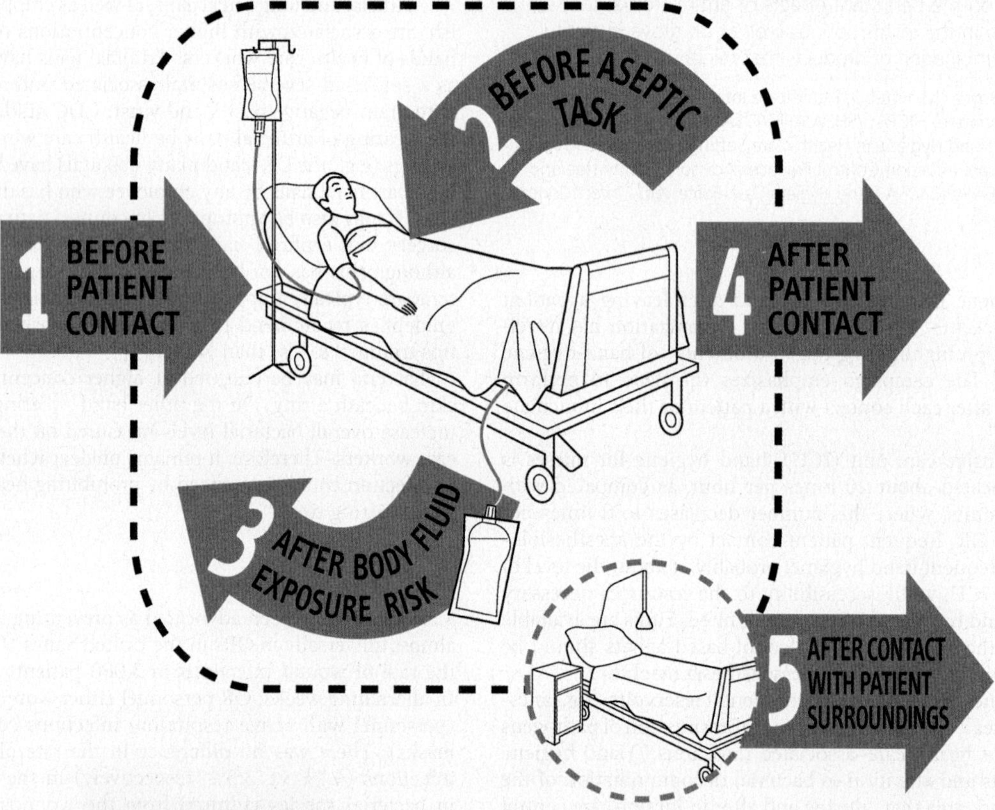

1 BEFORE PATIENT CONTACT	WHEN? Clean your hands before touching a patient when approaching him or her WHY? To protect the patient against harmful germs carried on your hands
2 BEFORE AN ASEPTIC TASK	WHEN? Clean your hands immediately before any aseptic task WHY? To protect the patient against harmful germs, including the patient's own germs, entering his or her body
3 AFTER BODY FLUID EXPOSURE RISK	WHEN? Clean your hands immediately after an exposure risk to body fluids (and after glove removal) WHY? To protect yourself and the health care environment from harmful patient germs
4 AFTER PATIENT CONTACT	WHEN? Clean your hands after touching a patient and his or her immediate surroundings when leaving WHY? To protect yourself and the health care environment from harmful patient germs
5 AFTER CONTACT WITH PATIENT SURROUNDINGS	WHEN? Clean your hands after touching any object or furniture in the patient's immediate surroundings, when leaving - even without touching the patient WHY? To protect yourself and the health care environment from harmful patient germs

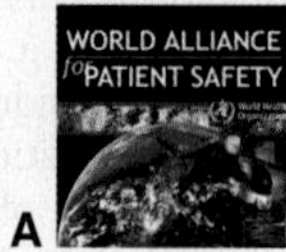

WHO acknowledges the Hôpitaux Universitaires de Genève (HUG), in particular the members of the Infection Control Programme, for their active participation in developing this material.

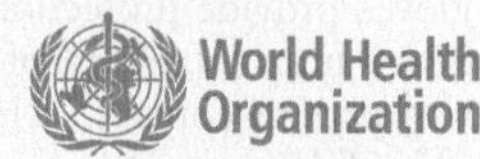

October 2006, version 1.

A

Figure 8-1 A: World Health Organization (WHO) schematic of the 5 Moments for hand hygiene. (*continued*)

5 MOMENTS FOR HAND HYGIENE

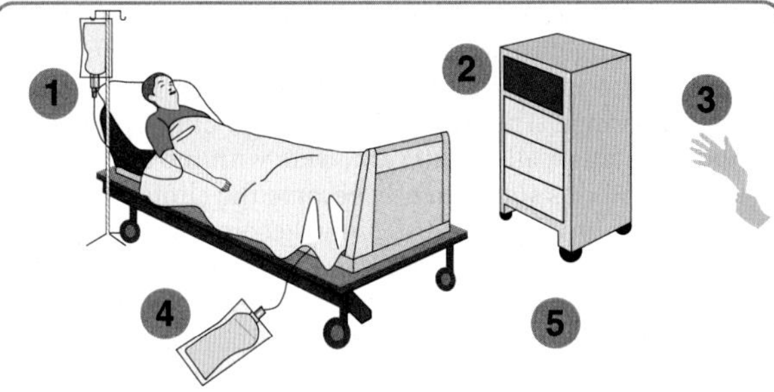

Ensure hand sanitizer is easily available on the anesthesia cart & use frequently, particularly:

1. Before & after touching patient
2. Before & after touching equipment & carts
3. Before clean/aseptic tasks
4. When hands are soiled, including after removing gloves
5. Upon entering or exiting room

B

Figure 8-1 *(continued)* **B:** WHO 5 Moments adapted for the operating room environment. (Courtesy of Harriet W. Hopf and Beca Chacin.)

be in an OR during a procedure.[2] The anesthesiologist is clearly in a position to play a leadership role in controlling human traffic through the OR.

Central venous lines placed by the anesthesiologist in the OR have been shown to become infected more often than those placed by surgeons or other providers, whether in or out of the OR. Contributing factors appeared to be site of placement and the stringency of aseptic technique. Infection risk is significantly higher with femoral or jugular site selection as compared to subclavian placement; however, subclavian placement does have a higher associated rate of pneumothorax. Chlorhexidine–alcohol skin preparation results in a lower rate of central venous catheter–associated bloodstream infection than povidone–iodine with alcohol and should be used preferentially. Use of a maximal sterile barrier technique versus sterile gloves and small sterile drapes significantly reduces central venous catheter–related infection. Therefore, gowning and gloving, careful aseptic technique, and use of a wide sterile field should be routine. Use of ultrasound guidance for placement is not associated with an increased infection rate, and therefore is recommended since it decreases mechanical complications during placement. In anesthetized patients, the central line is ideally placed before the surgical site is draped in order to avoid contamination of the wire on the underside of the surgical drape.[15]

Epidural abscess formation is an extremely rare but potentially catastrophic complication of neuraxial anesthesia and epidural catheter placement. Therefore, careful attention to aseptic technique and infection control is required. The most important consideration is to prevent contamination of the needle and catheter. Thus, hand washing, skin preparation, draping, and maintenance of a sterile field should be carefully observed. Gowning and wearing a mask likely play a smaller role but are reasonable, given the devastating consequences of infection. Finally, epidurals should probably be avoided in patients known or suspected to have bacteremia or deferred until after appropriate antibiotics are administered.

Role of Single-Use Disposables in Infection Control

Single-use disposable devices including noninvasive blood pressure cuffs, laryngoscopes, and textiles (e.g., gowns, drapes, scrub hats, and jackets) have proliferated in health care because of a misperception of reduced infection risk and reduced cost.

There is no compelling evidence that single-use disposables reduce infections, except where adequate disinfection is not (currently) possible (e.g., vascular catheters, duodenoscopes). While the cost of acquisition is lower for disposables, the per-use cost is almost always orders of magnitude greater. In addition, life-cycle analyses have shown that disposables and cause demonstrable public health harm (in the range of that caused by medical errors) by increasing waste, pollution, and greenhouse gas emissions, offsetting any theoretical protection from infection.[16] 3

The SARS-CoV-2 pandemic disrupted the supply chain for single-use disposables and provided opportunities to assess the impact of reusables on infection rates. Malhotra et al. compared SSI rates reported to the National Healthcare Safety Network[17] at a single institution in the 2 years preceding the pandemic with those in the first 12 months of the pandemic. Supply chain issues led to replacement of disposable shoe covers, head covers, and face masks with reusable versions. This change was associated with a reduction in SSI rate from 5.1% to 2.6%, despite a 14% *increase* in surgical volume and the number of higher-risk cases. Of particular note, at the same time, audited hand hygiene compliance increased from 71% to 85%. It is likely that the bulk of the benefit came from increased attention to infection prevention measures in general; nonetheless, the study is reassuring that reusable textiles do not increase the risk of infection.[17]

Antibiotic Prophylaxis

After antibiotics came into widespread use in the 1940s and 1950s, there was much debate over the possibility that antibiotic prophylaxis might prevent SSIs. In 1957, Miles et al.[18] used a guinea pig model for proof of the principle that administration of an antibiotic prior to contamination (incision) could reduce the risk of SSI. When appropriate antibiotics were given within 2 hours before or after intradermal injection of bacteria, they were effective in preventing invasive infection and necrosis. When given outside this window, they were not effective. This gave rise to the concept of a "decisive period" in which antibiotics will be effective, which remains a guiding principle of antibiotic prophylaxis. Miles et al. also demonstrated that injection of epinephrine intradermally prior to administration of antibiotics led to antibiotic failure, as demonstrated by an increased wound infection rate. This demonstrated the crucial role of local perfusion in delivering antibiotics to their target site. Using the same model, Knighton et al.[19] demonstrated that increased inspired oxygen was equally as effective as antibiotics in preventing infection, and that the two effects were additive (Fig. 8-2). Knighton et al.[20] also delayed the administration of oxygen for up to 6 hours after inoculation and demonstrated no reduction in effect. Thus, the decisive period for oxygen is considerably longer than that for antibiotics.

In 1964, two surgeons at Washington University in St. Louis, Harvey Bernard and William Cole,[21] reported on the first controlled clinical trial of the efficacy of antibiotic prophylaxis and demonstrated a benefit in abdominal operations. Thereafter, numerous clinical trials were performed with somewhat variable results. Eventually, these served to define the timing and population in which prophylactic antibiotics work. By the 1970s, antibiotic prophylaxis for high-risk surgery—meaning clean-contaminated and contaminated cases—was becoming well accepted and widely used, although some skeptics remained. In 1992, Classen et al.[22] published their prospective series including 2,847 patients undergoing clean or clean-contaminated surgical procedures at LDS Hospital in Salt Lake City, UT (Fig. 8-3). They demonstrated that the decisive period for SSIs in humans

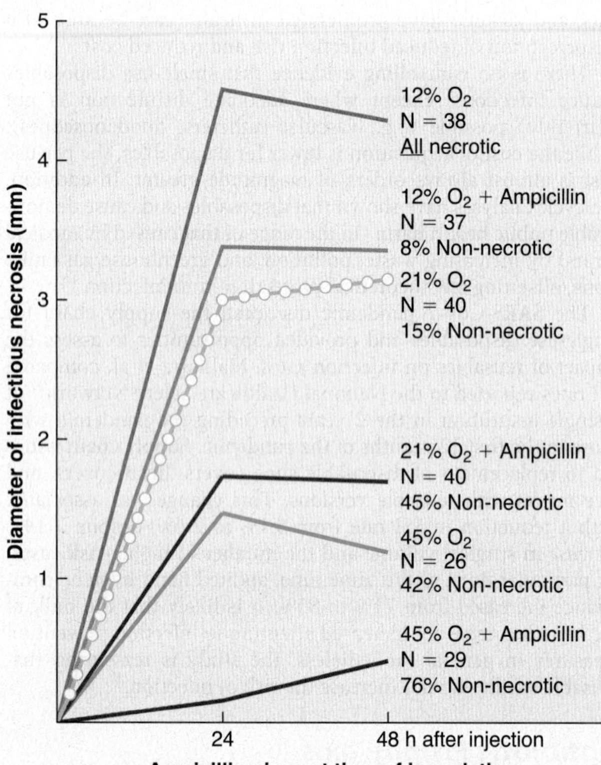

Figure 8-2 The effect of oxygen and/or antibiotics on lesion diameter after intradermal injection of bacteria into guinea pigs. Note that at every level, oxygen adds to the effect of antibiotics and that increasing oxygen in the breathing mixture from 12% to 20% or from 20% to 45% exerts an effect comparable to that of appropriately timed antibiotics. (Reprinted with permission from Rabkin J, Hunt TK. Infection and oxygen. In: Davis J, Hunt TK, eds. *Problem Wounds: The Role of Oxygen*. Elsevier; 1988:1.)

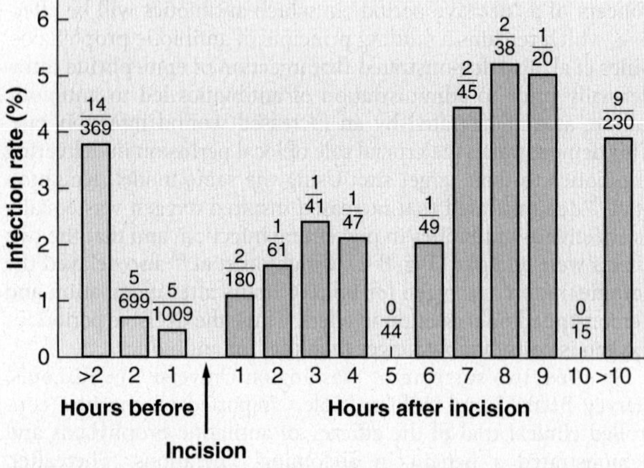

Figure 8-3 The figure demonstrates rates of surgical wound infection corresponding to the temporal relation between antibiotic administration and the start of surgery. The number of infections and the number of patients for each hourly interval appear as the numerator and denominator, respectively, of the fraction for that interval. The trend toward higher rates of infection for each hour that antibiotic administration was delayed after the surgical incision was significant (z score = 2.00; $p < .05$ by the Wilcoxon test). (Adapted from Classen DC, Evans RS, Pestotnik KS, et al. The timing of prophylactic administration of antibiotics and the risk of surgical-wound infection. *N Engl J Med*. 1992:326;281.)

undergoing surgery was essentially the same as for experimental infections in guinea pigs. That is, they found the lowest infection rate when antibiotics were given within 2 hours before or after incision, and a rapid increase in SSI rate when they were given outside that range. The best results, though only by a small margin and not statistically significant, were within 0 and 60 minutes of surgery, and this subsequently became the clinical standard.

Antibiotic prophylaxis has now become standard for surgeries in which there is more than a minimum risk of infection (NICV 8-1). Although not every surgery and situation has been studied, a strong rationale for the approach to prophylactic antibiotics has emerged. Ideally, the antimicrobial of choice for prophylaxis should prevent SSI, prevent SSI-related morbidity and mortality, be cost-effective, avoid adverse effects, and have no adverse consequences on the microbial flora of the patient or of the hospital.[23] The agent for antibiotic prophylaxis must cover the most likely spectrum of bacteria presented in the surgical field. The most common surgical-site pathogens in clean procedures are skin flora, including *Staphylococcus aureus* and coagulase-negative staphylococci (e.g., *Staphylococcus epidermidis*). In clean-contaminated procedures, the most common pathogens include gram-negative rods, and enterococci in addition to skin flora. Data from the National Nosocomial Infections Surveillance (NNIS) system for 2006 to 2007 indicate that the proportion of SSI caused by *S. aureus* has increased to 30%, with about half caused by MRSA. Infections caused by MRSA are associated with higher mortality rates, prolonged hospital stays, and higher hospital costs than infections caused by other agents. Nevertheless, vancomycin is not recommended for routine agent for surgical antimicrobial prophylaxis.[23]

Several groups separately developed guidelines for use of sur- 4
gical prophylactic antibiotics, culminating in recommendations published in 2004 by the National Surgical Infection Prevention Project and updated in 2013.[23] These guidelines emphasize timing and choice of appropriate agents; a number of agents are recommended as appropriate for each procedure, allowing for choices to be guided by local sensitivity patterns and providing for alternate agents in the case of drug sensitivity or allergy. (See Table 8-5 for general recommendations.) The most commonly used antibiotic for surgical prophylaxis is cefazolin, a first-generation cephalosporin. It has proven efficacy, safety, and desirable duration of action, and its spectrum of activity covers the organisms commonly encountered in SSIs.[23]

By definition, prophylactic antibiotics are given pre- or intraop- 5
eratively. The exact timing for the administration of the antibiotic depends on the pharmacology and half-life of the drug. It has been suggested that administration of prophylactic antibiotics is ideally within 30 minutes to 1 hour of incision.[22,23] Drugs given by bolus administration (e.g., cefazolin) achieve adequate tissue concentration rapidly, so giving these drugs within 0 to 30 minutes of incisions appears equally efficacious. Giving the antibiotics too early (so that the incision is more than 60 minutes after the dose) is a recurrent issue at many hospitals, especially in cases that require complex patient positioning. Giving the antibiotics closer to the incision time prevents this problem. Providing timely prophylactic antibiotics is relatively uncomplicated for antibiotics that can be given as a bolus dose (e.g., cephalosporins) or as an infusion over a few minutes (e.g., clindamycin) and thus provide tissue levels within minutes. For drugs like vancomycin that require infusion over an hour or more, coordination of administration is more complex. In general, it is considered acceptable if the infusion is started within 120 minutes before incision. Vancomycin is usually given in the context of known or suspected MRSA colonization; giving a dose of cefazolin in addition within an hour of incision is a way to ensure adequate antibiotic levels at the time of incision

Table 8-5 General Recommendations for Antibiotic Prophylaxis

- Antibiotic prophylaxis choice, dose, and timing should be determined by a hospital committee based on national guidelines,[24] local patterns of antibiotic sensitivity, and other considerations.
- Always confirm the antibiotic selection with surgeons at the time-out or earlier.
  - The surgeon may wish to delay antibiotics until after culture.
  - Antibiotics may not be indicated (e.g., low-risk, elective procedures such as laparoscopic cholecystectomy or breast biopsy where implants will not be used).
  - Make sure to record the reason for not giving antibiotics on the record.
- β-Lactam allergies.
  - Penicillin allergy is almost never a contraindication to cefazolin or other cephalosporin administration. A *documented* history of anaphylaxis or other serious reaction (angioedema, hives, bronchospasm, Stevens–Johnson syndrome, or toxic epidermal necrolysis) is the exception. Determine the severity of a patient's β-lactam allergy prior to choosing an alternative antimicrobial.
  - Lack of understanding of a true allergic reaction can lead to choosing an antimicrobial with reduced efficacy, increased cost, and greater risk of side effects.[24]
- Ideally, an antibiotic infusion should be completed before incision, but CMS guidelines consider starting the infusion before incision adequate. When possible, for drugs requiring slow (>30 min) infusion, the infusion should be initiated preoperatively.
- When a tourniquet is used, the dose should be completed at least 5 min before the tourniquet is inflated.
- Dosing schedules are more frequent than for therapeutic use to maintain wound tissue levels throughout surgery and ongoing contamination. Renal insufficiency may delay redosing, although initial dose is usually not affected.
- Additional intraoperative doses should be given when there is significant blood loss (~ half to one blood volume). Use the recommended second dose for this purpose.
- When *therapeutic* antibiotics are given preoperatively for an infection or presumed infection (e.g., acute appendicitis), prophylactic antibiotics are not required. Each situation should be examined individually: In some cases, coverage of skin flora may be appropriate prior to skin incision, but often continuation of the therapeutic antibiotics is all that is required.

CMS, The Centers for Medicare and Medicaid Services.
Used with permission from University of Utah Health.

while providing coverage for MRSA with the vancomycin. When a tourniquet is used, the infusion must be complete prior to inflation of the tourniquet. An appropriate dose based on body weight and volume of distribution should be given. Depending on the half-life, antibiotics should be repeated during long operations or operations with large blood loss.[23] For example, cefazolin is normally dosed every 8 hours but the dose should be repeated every 4 hours intraoperatively.[23] Finally, prophylactic antibiotics should be discontinued by 24 hours following surgery if postoperative dosing is selected at all. Prolonging the course of prophylactic antibiotics does not reduce the risk of infection but does increase the risk of adverse consequences of antibiotic administration,[23] including resistance, *C. difficile* infection, and sensitization.

Because they have access to the patient during the 60 minutes prior to incision and can optimize timing of administration, anesthesiologists should work in consultation with the surgeon to use guidelines determined by the local infection control committee to take initiative for administering prophylactic antibiotics (NICV 8-2). In this way, anesthesiologists can make a major contribution to preventing SSI. The Centers for Medicare and Medicaid Services has identified timely and appropriate antibiotic prophylaxis administration as a cornerstone of SSI prevention. Physician and hospital reimbursements are increasingly tied to such performance measures, meaning anesthesiologists also have an economic interest in ensuring adherence to guidelines.

Mechanisms of Wound Repair

Wound healing is a complex process, requiring a coordinated repair response including hemostasis, inflammation, matrix production, neovascularization, epithelialization, and remodeling. Many factors may impair wound healing. Systemic factors such as medical comorbidities, nutrition,[25] sympathetic nervous system activation,[26] and age[25] have a substantial effect on the repair process. Local environmental factors in and around the wound including bacterial load, degree of inflammation, moisture content, oxygen tension, and vascular perfusion also have a profound effect on healing.[25,27,28] Although all of these factors are important, perhaps the most critical element is oxygen supply to the wound. Wound hypoxia impairs each of the components of healing.[26]

Although the role of oxygen is usually thought of in terms of aerobic respiration and energy production via oxidative phosphorylation, in wound healing, oxygen is required as a cofactor for enzymatic processes and for cell-signaling mechanisms. Oxygen is a rate-limiting component in leukocyte-mediated bacterial killing and collagen formation because specific enzymes require oxygen at a partial pressure of at least 40 mmHg.[29] The mechanisms by which the other processes are oxygen dependent are less clear, but these processes also require oxygen at a concentration much above that required for cellular respiration.[30,31]

The Initial Response to Injury

A surgical incision disrupts the skin barrier, creating an acute wound. An effective initial response to injury depends on hemostasis and the ability to clean out foreign material and to resist infection. This response initiates a sequence of events that starts with any source of injury that disrupts homeostasis in the local environment and eventually leads to healing.

Wound healing is described in four overlapping phases: hemostasis, inflammation, proliferation, and remodeling.[32] Each phase is composed of complex interactions between host cells, contaminants, cytokines, and other chemical mediators that, when functioning properly, lead to repair of injury. These processes are highly conserved across species, indicating the critical importance of the inflammatory response that directs the process of cellular and tissue repair. When any component of healing is disturbed and interrupts the orderly progression of repair, wound failure may result.[25,32]

Injury damages the local circulation and causes platelets to aggregate and release a variety of substances, including

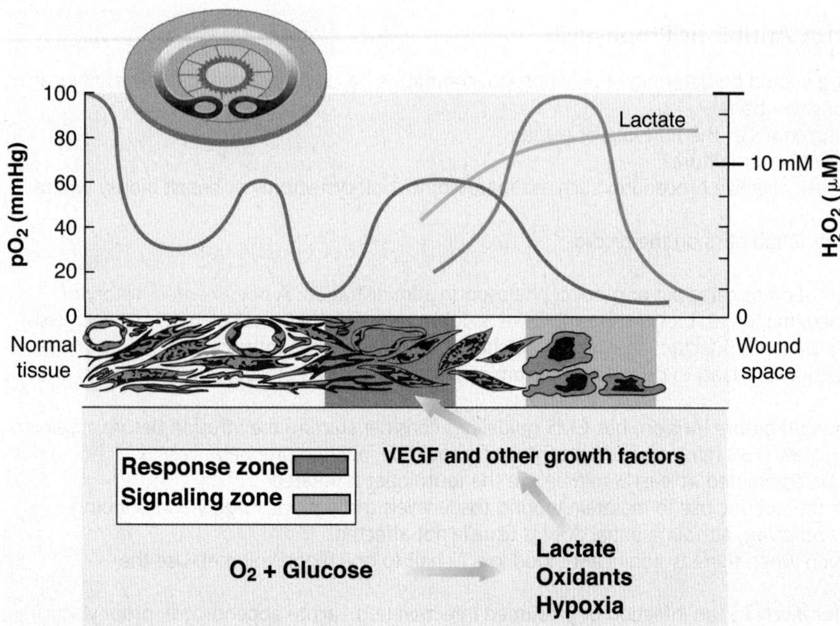

Figure 8-4 The varying oxygen tension in the wound module. Cross-section of the wound module in a rabbit ear chamber is in left upper corner of figure. PO_2, depicted graphically above the cross-section (*orange line*), is highest next to the vessels, with a gradient down to zero at the wound edge. Note also the lactate gradient (*green line*), high in the dead space and lower (but still above plasma) toward the vasculature. Hydrogen peroxide (H_2O_2) is present at fairly high concentrations (*blue line*) and is also a major stimulus to wound repair.[37] Growth factors such as VEGF are produced by inflammatory cells in the hypoxic, high lactate, high hydrogen peroxide "signaling zone" and then diffuse to the "response zone" where they act on fibroblasts and endothelial cells to promote healing. VEGF, vascular endothelial growth factor. (Modified from Silver IE. The physiology of wound healing. In: Hunt TK, Dunphy JE, eds. *Fundamentals of Wound Management*. Appleton-Century-Crofts, 1980:30.)

chemoattractants and growth factors.[32] The initial result is coagulation, which prevents exsanguination but also widens the area that is no longer perfused. Platelet degranulation releases platelet-derived growth factor, transforming growth factor beta (TGF-β), epidermal growth factor, and insulin-like growth factor-1 (IGF-1), which jointly initiate the inflammatory process.[32] Bradykinin, complement, and histamine released by mast cells cause vasodilation and increased vascular permeability. Polymorphonuclear leukocytes arrive at the wound almost immediately and are followed by macrophages within 24 to 48 hours. These inflammatory cells activate in response to endothelial integrins, selectins, cell adhesion molecules, cadherins, fibrin, lactate, hypoxia, foreign bodies, infectious agents, and growth factors.[32] In turn, macrophages and lymphocytes produce more lactate[33] and growth factors, including IGF-1, leukocyte growth factor, interleukins (ILs) 1 and 2, TGF-β, and vascular endothelial growth factor (VEGF).[32] This early inflammatory phase is characterized by erythema and edema of the wound edges.

Activated neutrophils and macrophages also release proteases, including neutrophil elastase, neutrophil collagenase, matrix metalloproteinase, and macrophage metalloelastase.[32] These proteases degrade damaged extracellular matrix components to allow their replacement. Proteases also degrade the basement membrane of capillaries to enable inflammatory cells to migrate into the wound.

In wounds, local blood supply is compromised at the same time that metabolic demand is increased. As a result, the wound environment becomes hypoxic and acidotic with high lactate levels.[34] This represents the sum of three effects: (1) decreased oxygen supply due to vascular damage and coagulation; (2) increased metabolic demand due to the heightened cellular response (anaerobic glycolysis); and (3) aerobic glycolysis by inflammatory cells.[35] Leukocytes contain few mitochondria and therefore acquire energy from glucose, primarily by production of lactate and even in the presence of adequate oxygen supply.[35] In activated neutrophils, the respiratory burst, in which oxygen and glucose are converted to superoxide, hydrogen ion, and lactate, accounts for up to 98% of oxygen consumption; in the setting of injury, this activity increases by up to 50-fold over baseline.[29]

Local hypoxia is a normal and inevitable result of tissue injury (1 Video 8-1).[36] Hypoxia acts as a stimulus to repair,[33] but also leads to poor healing and increased susceptibility to infection.[27] Numerous experimental models as well as human clinical experience have led to the conclusion that healing is delayed in hypoxic wounds. The partial pressure of oxygen in dermal wounds is heterogeneous, ranging from 0 to 10 mmHg in the central ("dead space") portion of the wound, to 80 to 100 mmHg (near arterial) adjacent to perfused arterioles and capillaries (Fig. 8-4). The PO_2 of a given area depends on diffusion of oxygen from perfused capillaries, and thus wound PO_2 depends on capillary density, arterial PO_2, and the metabolic activity of the cells, with some contribution from shifts in the oxyhemoglobin dissociation curve associated with wound pH and temperature.

Resistance to Infection

After a disruption of the normal skin barrier, successful wound healing requires the ability to clear foreign material and resist infection. Neutrophils provide nonspecific immunity and prevent infection. Leukocytes migrate in tissue toward the site of injury via chemotaxis, defined as locomotion oriented along a chemical gradient.[32] Chemical gradients can be produced both exogenously and endogenously. Exogenous gradients result from bacterial products present in contaminated tissues. Endogenous mediators include components of the complement system (C5a), products of lipoxygenase pathway (leukotriene B4), and cytokines (IL-1, 8), along with lactate.[38,39] Together, these chemical mediators help to organize and control leukocyte invasion, bacterial killing, necrotic tissue removal, and the initiation of neovascularization and matrix production. In the absence of infection, neutrophils disappear by about 48 hours. Nonspecific phagocytosis and intracellular killing are the major immune pathways activated in wounds.[29]

Neutrophils are the primary cells responsible for nonspecific immunity, and their function depends on a high partial pressure of oxygen.[29] This is because reactive oxygen species are the major component of the bactericidal defense against wound pathogens.[29] Phagocytosis of the pathogen activates the phagosomal oxidase

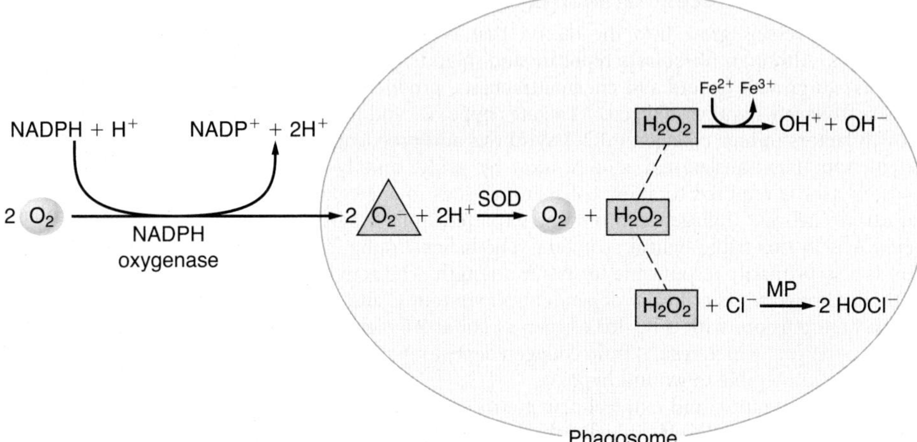

Figure 8-5 Schematic of superoxide and other oxidant production within the phagosome. NADPH, nicotinamide adenine dinucleotide phosphate-oxidase; NADP, nicotinamide adenine dinucleotide phosphate; SOD, superoxide dismutase; MP, myeloperoxidase. (Reprinted from Hunt TK, Hopf HW. Wound healing and wound infection. What surgeons and anesthesiologists can do. *Surg Clin North Am*. 1997;77(3):587–606. Copyright © 1997 Elsevier. With permission.)

(also known as the primary oxidase or nicotinamide adenine dinucleotide phosphate-oxidase [NADPH]-linked oxygenase), present in the phagocytic membrane, which uses oxygen as the substrate to catalyze the formation of superoxide. Superoxide itself is bactericidal, but more importantly, it initiates a series of cascades that produce other oxidants within the phagosome that increase bacterial-killing capacity (Fig. 8-5). For example, in the presence of superoxide dismutase, superoxide is reduced to hydrogen peroxide (H_2O_2). H_2O_2 combines with chloride and in the presence of myeloperoxidase forms the bactericidal hypochlorous acid, more commonly recognized as the active ingredient in bleach.[40] Since intraphagosomal oxidant production depends on conversion of oxygen to superoxide, the process is exquisitely sensitive to the partial pressure of oxygen in the tissue. The K_m (half-maximal velocity) for the phagosomal oxidase using oxygen as a substrate is 40 to 80 mmHg.[29] This means that resistance to infection is critically impaired by wound hypoxia and becomes more efficient as PO_2 increases even to very high levels (500 to 1,000 mmHg).[29] Such levels do not occur naturally in tissue, but can be achieved by the administration of hyperbaric oxygen.[41,42] This is one mechanism for the proposed benefit of hyperbaric oxygen therapy as an adjunctive treatment for necrotizing infections and chronic refractory osteomyelitis.[43]

Oxidants produced by inflammatory cells have a dual role in wound repair. Not only are they central to resistance to infection, but they also play a major role in initiating and directing the healing process. Oxidants, and in particular hydrogen peroxide produced via the respiratory burst, increase neovascularization and collagen deposition in vitro and in vivo.[40]

Proliferation

The proliferative phase normally begins approximately 4 days after injury, concurrent with a waning of the inflammatory phase. It consists of granulation tissue formation and epithelialization. Granulation involves neovascularization and synthesis of collagen and connective tissue proteins.

Neovascularization

New blood vessels must replace the injured microcirculation. Neovascularization in wounds proceeds both by angiogenesis and vasculogenesis. Angiogenesis is the phenomenon of new vessel growth via budding from existing vessels. In the setting of wounds, new vessels grow from mature vessels, usually intact postcapillary venules in the undamaged tissue immediately adjacent to the site of injury. Normally, the oxygen tension in adjacent tissue is sufficient to support this process. The new vessel growth extends and enters into the damaged areas that are typically high in lactate and have a low partial pressure of oxygen. Mature extracellular matrix is required for ingrowth of mature vessels.[44]

In vasculogenesis, bone marrow–derived endothelial precursor cells (EPCs) populate the tissue and differentiate and grow into new vessel tubules. In wounds, these tubules appear in the damaged area before any direct anastomosis with pre-existing vessels are made. These tubules must connect with existing vasculature to establish an intact blood supply in the wound. Angiogenesis has long been held as the primary mechanism for new blood vessel growth in granulation tissue. Recent research, however, has demonstrated that as many as 15% to 20% of new blood vessels in wounds are derived from hematopoietic stem cells.[44,45]

Angiogenesis and vasculogenesis both occur in response to similar stimuli, consisting of some combination of redox stress, hypoxia, and lactate. However, the specific mechanisms by which they proceed appear to differ somewhat. Angiogenesis involves the movement of endothelial cells in response to three waves of growth factors. The first wave of growth factors comes with the release by platelets of platelet-derived growth factor, TGF-β, IGF-1, and others during the inflammatory phase. The second wave comes from fibroblast growth factor released from normal binding sites on connective tissue molecules. The third and dominant wave comes from VEGF, delivered largely by macrophages stimulated by fibrinopeptides, hypoxia, and lactate.[32] Although it is usually present, hypoxia is not required for granulation because of constitutive (aerobic) lactate production by inflammatory cells and fibroblasts. Too little lactate leads to inadequate granulation, while levels in excess of about 15 mM—usually associated with inflammation or infection—delay granulation.[46] The capillary endothelial response to angiogenic agents requires oxygen so that angiogenesis progresses in proportion to blood perfusion and arterial PO_2.[47]

Vasculogenesis occurs in response to similar stressors as angiogenesis. EPCs are mobilized from the bone marrow into the circulation via a nitric oxide–mediated mechanism. Tissue hypoxia induces release of VEGF-A, which activates bone marrow stromal nitric oxide synthase. Increased bone marrow nitric oxide leads to release of EPCs into the circulation. These circulating EPCs home to the wound via tissue-hypoxia–induced upregulation of stromal cell-derived factor 1α. Within the wound, EPCs undergo differentiation and participate in the formation of new blood vessels.[45]

Collagen and Extracellular Matrix Deposition

New blood vessels grow into the matrix that is produced by fibroblasts. Although fibroblasts replicate and migrate mainly in response to growth factors and chemoattractants, production of mature collagen requires oxygen.[26] Lactate, hypoxia, and some growth factors induce collagen mRNA synthesis and procollagen production. Posttranslational modification by prolyl and lysyl hydroxylases is required to allow collagen peptides to aggregate into triple helices. Collagen can only be exported from the cell when it is in this triple helical structure. The helical configuration is also primarily responsible for tissue strength. The activity of the hydroxylases is critically dependent on vitamin C and tissue oxygen tension, with a K_m for oxygen of about 25 mmHg.[26] Wound strength, which results from collagen deposition, is therefore highly vulnerable to wound hypoxia.

Neovascularization and extracellular matrix (primarily collagen) production are closely linked. Fibroblasts cannot produce mature collagen in the absence of mature blood vessels that deliver oxygen to the site. New blood vessels cannot mature without a strong collagen matrix. Mice kept in a hypoxic environment of 13% inspired oxygen develop some new blood vessels in a test wound with the addition of exogenous VEGF or lactate, but these vessels are immature with little surrounding matrix and demonstrate frequent areas of hemorrhage.[30]

Epithelialization

Epithelialization is characterized by replication and migration of epithelial cells across the skin edges in response to growth factors. Cell migration may begin from any site that contains living keratinocytes, including remnants of hair follicles, sebaceous glands, islands of living epidermis, or the normal wound edge. In acute wounds that are primarily closed, epithelialization is normally completed in 1 to 3 days. In open wounds healing by secondary intention, epithelialization is the final phase of healing and cannot progress until the wound bed is fully granulated. Like immunity and granulation, epithelialization depends on growth factors and oxygen. Silver[48] and Medawar[49] demonstrated in vivo that the rate of epithelialization depends on local oxygen. Topical oxygen applied in a manner that does not dry out epithelial cells has been advocated as a method to increase the rate of epithelialization.[50] Ngo et al.[51] demonstrated oxygen-dependent differentiation and cell growth in human keratinocyte culture. In contrast, O'Toole et al.[52] demonstrated that hypoxia increases epithelial migration in vitro. This may be explained, at least in part, by the dependence of epithelialization on the presence of a bed of healthy granulation tissue, which is known to be oxygen dependent.

Maturation and Remodeling

The final phase of wound repair is maturation, which involves ongoing remodeling of the granulation tissue and increasing wound tensile strength. As the matrix becomes denser with thicker, stronger collagen fibrils, it becomes stiffer and less compliant. Fibroblasts are capable of adapting to changing mechanical stress and loading. Fibroblasts migrate throughout the matrix to help mold the wound to new stresses. Matrix metalloproteinases and other proteases help with fibroblast migration and continued matrix remodeling in response to mechanical stress. Some fibroblasts differentiate into myofibroblasts under the influence of TGF-β, resulting in contractile cells. As the myofibroblasts contract, the collagenous matrix cross-links in the shortened position. This helps to strengthen the matrix and minimize scar size. Contraction is inhibited by the use of high doses of corticosteroids.[25] Even steroids given several days after injury have this effect. In those wounds where contraction is detrimental, this effect can be used for benefit. Although there is little definitive evidence, one dose of dexamethasone intraoperatively to prevent postoperative nausea and vomiting does not appear to impair healing.

Net collagen synthesis continues for at least 6 weeks and up to 6 months after wounding. Over time, the initial collagen threads are reabsorbed and deposited along stress lines, conferring greater tensile strength. Collagen found in granulation tissue is biochemically different from collagen of uninjured skin, and a scar never achieves the tensile strength of uninjured skin. Hydroxylation and glycosylation of lysine residues in granulation tissue collagen lead to thinner collagen fibers. At 1 week, a wound closed by primary intention has only reached 3% of the tensile strength of normal skin. By 3 weeks it is at 30%, and it only reaches its maximum tensile strength of 80% after 3 to 6 months.

Some wounds heal to excess. Hypertrophic scar and keloid are common forms of abnormal scar due to aberrant responses to healing. Hypertrophic scarring may be thought of as "exuberant" scarring within the boundaries of the wound. The inflammatory process that allows wound healing remains excessively active, resulting in stiff, rubbery, nonmobile scar tissue. Hypertrophic scars are most commonly seen following burns and in incisions over areas of tension. They are thought to correlate with the length of time required to close the wound and opposing tension forces present in the wound, although other factors are also believed to play a role. Keloids are scars that outgrow the boundaries of the initial scar and are most typically seen following skin incisions. Keloid formation most likely has a genetic predisposition, although exogenous inflammatory factors may also play a role.

Wound Perfusion and Oxygenation

Complications of wounds include failure to heal, infection, and excessive scarring or contracture. Rapid repair has the least potential for infection and excess scarring. The perioperative physician's goals, therefore, are to avoid contamination, ensure rapid tissue synthesis, and optimize the immune response. All surgical procedures lead to some degree of contamination that must be controlled by local host defenses. The initial hours after contamination represent a decisive period during which inadequate local defenses may allow an infection to become established.

Normally, wounds on the extremities and trunk heal more slowly than those on the face. The major difference in these wounds is the degree of tissue perfusion and thus the wound tissue oxygen tension. As a rule, repair proceeds most rapidly and immunity is strongest when wound oxygen levels are high, and this is only achieved by maintaining perfusion of injured tissue.[26] Ischemic or hypoxic tissue, on the other hand, is highly susceptible to infection and heals poorly, if at all.[42] Wound tissue oxygenation is complex and depends on the interaction of blood perfusion, arterial oxygen tension, hemoglobin dissociation conditions, carrying capacity, mass transfer resistances, and local oxygen consumption. Wound oxygen delivery depends on vascular anatomy, the degree of vasoconstriction, and arterial PO_2.

The standard teaching that oxygen delivery depends more on hemoglobin-bound oxygen (oxygen content) than on arterial PO_2 may be true of working muscle, but it is not true of wound healing. In muscle, intercapillary distances are small and oxygen consumption is high. In contrast, intercapillary distances are large and oxygen consumption is relatively low in subcutaneous tissue.[31] In wounds, where the microvasculature is damaged, diffusion distances are substantially increased. Peripheral vasoconstriction further increases diffusion distance.[36] The driving force of diffusion is partial pressure. Hence, a high PO_2 is needed to force oxygen into injured and healing tissues, particularly in subcutaneous tissue, fascia, tendon, and bone, the tissues most at risk for poor healing.

6 Although oxygen consumption is relatively low in wounds, it is consumed by processes that require oxygen at a high concentration. Inflammatory cells use little oxygen for respiration, producing energy largely via the hexose monophosphate shunt.[29] Most of the oxygen consumed in wounds is used for oxidant production (bacterial killing), with a significant contribution as well for collagen synthesis, angiogenesis, and epithelialization. The rate constants (K_m) for oxygen for these components of repair fall within the physiologic range of 25 to 100 mmHg.[26,29]

Because of the high rate constants for oxygen substrate for the components of repair, the rate at which repair proceeds varies according to tissue PO_2 from 0 to at least 250 mmHg. In vitro fibroblast replication is optimal at a PO_2 of about 40 to 60 mmHg. Neutrophils lose their ability to kill bacteria in vitro below a PO_2 of about 40 mmHg.[26] These in vitro observations are clinically relevant. "Normal" subcutaneous PO_2, measured in test wounds in uninjured, euthermic, euvolemic volunteers breathing room air, is 65 ± 7 mmHg.[53] Thus, any reduction in wound PO_2 may impair immunity and repair. In surgical patients, the rate of wound infections is inversely proportional[27] and collagen deposition is directly proportional[26] to postoperative subcutaneous wound tissue oxygen tension.

High oxygen tensions (>100 mmHg) can be reached in wounds but only if perfusion is rapid and arterial PO_2 is high.[26] This is because subcutaneous tissue serves a reservoir function, so there is normally flow in excess of nutritional needs and wound cells consume relatively little oxygen, about 0.7/100 mL of blood flow at a normal perfusion rate.[31] When arterial oxygen tension (PaO_2) is high, this small volume can be carried by plasma alone. Contrary to popular belief, therefore, oxygen-carrying capacity—that is, hemoglobin concentration—is not particularly important to wound healing, provided that perfusion is normal.[54] Wound PO_2 and collagen synthesis remain normal in individuals who have hematocrit levels as low as 15% to 18% provided they can appropriately increase cardiac output, and vasoconstriction is prevented.[54]

7 Peripheral vasoconstriction, which results from central sympathetic control of subcutaneous vascular tone, is probably the most frequent and clinically the most important impediment to wound oxygenation. Subcutaneous tissue is both a reservoir to maintain central volume and a major site of thermoregulation. There is little local regulation of blood flow, except by local heating.[26] Therefore, subcutaneous tissue is particularly vulnerable to vasoconstriction. Sympathetically induced peripheral vasoconstriction is stimulated by cold, pain, fear, and blood volume deficit,[26] and by various pharmacologic agents including nicotine,[53] β-adrenergic antagonists, and α_1-agonists, all commonly present in the perioperative environment. Use of low doses of vasopressor agents to correct anesthesia (vasodilation)-induced hypotension, however, does not generally impair wound perfusion or free-flap survival.[55] Perioperative hypothermia is common and results from anesthetic drugs, exposure to cold, and redistribution of body heat from the core to the periphery.[56] Blood loss and increases in insensible losses increase fluid requirements in the perioperative period, thereby leaving the patient vulnerable to inadequate fluid replacement. Thus, vasomotor tone is, to a large degree, under the perioperative physician's control.

8 Prevention or correction of hypothermia[57] and blood volume deficits[58] have been shown to decrease wound infections and increase collagen deposition in patients undergoing major abdominal surgery. Preoperative systemic (forced air warmer) or local (warming bandage) warming have also been shown to decrease wound infections, even in clean, low-risk surgeries such as breast surgery and inguinal hernia repair.[59] Subcutaneous tissue oxygen tension is significantly higher in patients with good pain control than in those with poor pain control after arthroscopic knee surgery.[60] Stress also causes wound hypoxia and significantly impairs wound healing and resistance to infection.[25] These effects are clearly mediated, in large part, by changes in the partial pressure of oxygen in the injured tissue.

A number of groups have evaluated whether increasing inspired oxygen during surgery can reduce SSIs by increasing wound oxygen levels. A 2015 Cochrane systematic review of 28 randomized controlled trials did not demonstrate a benefit of 60% to 90% inspired oxygen during surgery (except in some models that supported a benefit for colorectal surgery), although heterogeneity and bias limited conclusions.[61] Given the above discussion, it is notable that few of the studies explicitly controlled for wound perfusion or oxygenation. Greif et al.,[62] in the only study in which wound oxygen was measured, demonstrated in a randomized, controlled, double-blind trial including 500 patients that in warm, volume-replete patients with good pain control undergoing major colon surgery, administration of 80% versus 30% oxygen intraoperatively and for the first 2 hours after surgery significantly reduced the wound infection rate by 50%. Wound oxygen levels were significantly higher (almost double) intraoperatively and in the postanesthesia care unit (PACU) in the 80% oxygen group. Belda et al.[63] replicated these results (significant 40% reduction in SSI) in a randomized, controlled, double-blind trial in 300 colon surgery patients randomized to 80% versus 30% oxygen intraoperatively and during the first 6 hours after surgery. Surgical and anesthetic management were standardized and intended to support optimal perfusion, although wound oxygen was not measured. Myles et al.[64] demonstrated a significant reduction in major postoperative complications, as well as specifically wound infections, in 2,050 major surgery patients randomized to 80% oxygen in 20% nitrogen versus 30% oxygen in 70% nitrous oxide intraoperatively.

On the other hand, Meyhoff et al.[37] found no difference in SSI rate (20.1% vs. 19.1%, $p = \text{NS}$) as a function of oxygen administration in 1,400 patients undergoing colon and gynecologic surgery. A major difference in design from the studies that demonstrated benefit was the use of a highly restricted volume replacement regimen. The stated aim was that patients were to gain no more than 1 kg by the second day after operation. Without data on wound oxygen (which was not measured), it is difficult to determine the reason for the difference in outcome compared to the Greif, Belda, and Myles studies, but wound vasoconstriction and a resulting lack of increase in wound oxygen tension is a strong possibility.

Although the preponderance of evidence indicates that use of high-inspired oxygen intraoperatively and providing supplemental oxygen postoperatively in *well-perfused* patients undergoing major abdominal surgery will reduce the risk of wound infection, there remains controversy about the benefits of high-inspired oxygen. One factor in the hesitation to adopt high-inspired oxygen is concern about potential side effects or toxicity of 80% oxygen. Two of the above studies examined this question in detail and found no difference in pulmonary complications or atelectasis.[37,65] A randomized controlled trial in patients at low risk for SSI ($n = 100$) found no difference in postoperative oxygen requirement in patients randomized to 30% oxygen intraoperatively versus those randomized to more than 90%.[66] The 2015 Cochrane analysis of studies of high perioperative inspired oxygen[61] found no significant effect on mortality, although the authors point out that the sample size is not sufficient to rule out the possibility of harm. Thus, high-inspired oxygen appears to be a low-risk approach to enhancing host defenses and reducing SSI, so long as the priority is maintaining peripheral perfusion.

Perfusion and oxygen also play a key role in the effectiveness of antibiotic prophylaxis. Delivery of antibiotics depends on perfusion. Parenteral antibiotics dosed so that high levels of antibiotic are present in the blood at the time of wounding (i.e., surgical prophylactic antibiotics) reduce wound infections, but do not eliminate them; other interventions beyond antisepsis and prophylactic antibiotics are required.[22] In about one-third of all wound infections, the bacteria cultured from the wound are sensitive to the prophylactic antibiotic given to the patient, even when the antibiotics were given according to standard procedure.[22] The vulnerable third of patients appear to be the hypoxic and vasoconstricted group. When antibiotics are present in the wound at the time of injury, they are trapped in the fibrin clot at the wound site where they may have efficacy against contaminating organisms. Antibiotics diffuse poorly into the fibrin clot, however, so that later administration, whether more than 2 hours after injury or in response to wound infection, will have little effect. On the other hand, oxygen diffuses easily through the fibrin clots and is effective even 6 hours after contamination.[19]

Bactericidal antibodies currently in use employ oxygen to kill organisms in much the same way as phagocytes. Kohanski[67] has demonstrated that quinolones, β-lactams, and aminoglycosides kill *S. aureus* and *Escherichia coli* by stimulating hydroxyl radical production from oxygen, even though all have different mechanisms for entering bacteria. Suller and Lloyd[68] observed a logarithmic reduction in bacterial cell counts in 10 to 15 hours in aerobic conditions compared with more than 60 hours to achieve the same result in an anaerobic environment for four facultative anaerobic staphylococcal strains exposed to vancomycin in air-equilibrated versus hypoxic conditions. Thus, maintaining conditions that optimize wound oxygen will also optimize the effectiveness of many commonly used antibiotics.

Patient Management

A recent meta-analysis of 16 randomized controlled trials, quasiexperimental studies, and cohort studies[69] demonstrated that the use of "bundles" of evidence-based care in patients undergoing colorectal surgery significantly reduced the risk of SSI. Unfortunately, as the authors note, there is currently "no consensus as to what comprises the optimal colorectal surgical care bundle." Standardization of care is likely responsible for some of the benefit. Further study is required to identify individual best practices. In the meantime, the following are approaches that anesthesiologists can take with the aim of improving wound healing and resistance to infection in their patients.

Preoperative Preparation

Given knowledge of the physiology of wound healing, what are the best strategies for an anesthesiologist to pursue to ensure optimal healing? SSIs result from a multitude of factors that include the health of the patient, the type of surgery, the number and type of organisms contaminating the surgical site, and surgical technique. To the degree they are predictable, interventions can be targeted to those patients most at risk (Table 8-6).

Modifiable or potentially modifiable risks include smoking, malnutrition, obesity, diabetes and hyperglycemia, chronic kidney disease, steroid use, anemia, hypercholesterolemia, and hypertension. When possible, these should be assessed and corrected prior to surgery. The decision to delay surgery must take into account both the urgency of the surgery and the severity of the risk.

Stress also predisposes to poor wound healing. Adverse psychosocial circumstances at the time of surgery may put patients at risk for poor wound healing. Kiecolt-Glaser et al.[70] studied the impact of hostile marital interactions on the healing of experimental blister wounds. High-hostile couples produced more proinflammatory cytokines and healed more slowly than low-hostile couples. Using a tape-stripping model, Muizzuddin et al.[71] investigated the effect of marital dissolution on skin barrier recovery and found that high stress was associated with slower recovery. Bosch et al.[72] studied the healing of a circular wound on the oral hard palate in subjects who varied in depression and/or dysphoria. High-dysphoric individuals had higher wound sizes from day 2 onward and depressive symptoms predicted slower wound healing. Collectively, these studies point to links between psychosocial distress, dysregulation at the system level, and impaired capacity for wound healing. It seems likely that stress-reduction techniques will reduce wound complications, and well-designed clinical trials are needed in this area.

Table 8-6 Preoperative Checklist
Assess and optimize cardiopulmonary function. Correct hypertension.
Assess wound risk in order to decide on the extent to which prophylactic measures should be taken.
Assess recent nutrition and treat as appropriate. Provide preoperative clear liquids until 2–3 h before scheduled surgery
Prevent peripheral vasoconstriction: attend to blood volume, thermoregulatory vasoconstriction, pain, and anxiety.
Improve or maintain blood sugar control.

Intraoperative Management

Careful surgical technique is fundamental to optimal wound healing (Table 8-7). Delicate handling of the tissue, adequate hemostasis, and surgeon experience leads to healthier wounds. Incisions should be planned with regard to blood supply, particularly when operating near or in old incisions. Mechanical retractors should be released from time to time to allow perfusion to the wound edges. Judicious antibiotic irrigation of contaminated areas may be effective. Because dried wounds lose perfusion, wounds should be kept moist, especially during long operations. Not all wounds can be anatomically closed. Edema, obesity, the possibility of unacceptable respiratory compromise, or the need to debride grossly contaminated or necrotic soft tissues can all interfere with closure of the wound.

As the operation proceeds, new wounds are made and contamination continues. All anesthetic agents tend to cause hypothermia—first, by causing vasodilation, which redistributes

Table 8-7 Intraoperative Management
Appropriate prophylactic antibiotics should be given at the start of any procedure in which infection is highly probable and/or has potentially disastrous consequences. Maintain antibiotic levels during long operations.
Keep patients normothermic.
Assess intravascular volume and optimize fluid management.
Consider increasing inspired oxygen in patients at high risk for infection.

heat from core to periphery in previously vasoconstricted patients, and second, by increasing heat loss and decreasing heat production.[56] Vasoconstriction is uncommon intraoperatively, as the threshold for thermoregulatory vasoconstriction is decreased, but may be severe in the immediate postoperative period when anesthesia is discontinued and the thermoregulatory threshold returns to normal in the face of core hypothermia. The onset of pain with emergence from anesthesia adds to this vasoconstriction because of the associated catecholamine release.[60] Maintenance of a high room temperature or active warming before, during, and after the operation is significantly more effective than other methods of warming such as application of warm blankets, circulating water blankets placed on the operating table surface, and humidification of the breathing circuit.[73]

Forced air warming was the first practical means of keeping patients warm intraoperatively. More recently, a number of other effective approaches have been introduced, including resistive warming, negative pressure warming, and thin, adhesive circulating water pads that are applied directly to the skin.[74]

Volume Management

Intravascular volume management during surgery has implications for tissue perfusion and, therefore, wound healing. Numerous factors, including patient comorbidities, medications such as diuretics, fever, preoperative volume state, surgical procedure, blood and insensible losses, and surgical stress, all influence fluid requirements during surgery. It is widely agreed that the goal of intraoperative fluid management is to ensure sufficient intravascular volume to maintain perfusion and maximize oxygen delivery to the tissues, while avoiding the ill effects of hypervolemia, namely interstitial edema; what is difficult to determine is how to achieve that goal. Patient monitoring, fluid choice, and fluid administration strategy are topics of much debate, with a poorly standardized and often contradictory literature. For a comprehensive review of fluid management, see Chapter 16.

Estimating preoperative volume status can be challenging, as there are many factors to consider. Preoperative fluid state may be reduced by fasting, mechanical bowel preparation, or medication use. Pre-existing medical conditions such as systolic and diastolic heart failure may cause hypervolemia and physiology that is exquisitely sensitive to fluid overload. While hemodialysis reliably induces hypovolemia, patients with end-stage renal disease are also susceptible to fluid overload, and intraoperative fluid replacement is complex. Patient history and physical examination, for more straightforward patients, and other tools such as preoperative echocardiography, for complex patients, can give the anesthesiologist an idea of presurgical patient's general volume status.

There are known serious complications of both hyper- and hypovolemia, particularly in the perioperative period. The major complications of hypovolemia, aside from hemodynamic instability, include decreased oxygenation of surgical wounds (which predisposes to wound infection),[26,27,75] decreased collagen formation,[58] impaired wound healing, and increased wound breakdown. The major complications associated with hypervolemia include pulmonary edema, congestive heart failure, edema of gut with prolonged ileus, and possibly an increase in cardiac arrhythmias.[76] Inappropriately high fluid administration may result in elevated atrial natriuretic peptide, inducing endothelial glycocalyx dysfunction, with resultant vascular permeability and extravascular fluid shifts.[81]

Patients appear to benefit from ingestion of high-carbohydrate, clear liquids 2 to 3 hours prior to surgery in order to achieve a euvolemic state at the start of surgery.[78] In addition to providing hydration, there is evidence that this is a safe practice with the additional benefits of increased patient satisfaction and decreased postoperative insulin resistance.

Intraoperative assessment of fluid status is necessary for optimization of intravascular volume. Estimates of blood loss, third-space fluid losses, and maintenance requirements are notoriously inaccurate and may lead to either over- or underreplacement if used as guides. Surgical stress can result in increased intravenous fluid requirements. The increased fluid requirement may be partly due to substances like IL-6, TNF, substance-P, and bradykinin, which are released in response to, and in proportion to, surgical stress.[79] These inflammatory mediators cause both vasodilation and an increase in vascular permeability.[80] However, the concept of third spacing as a cause of functional intravascular fluid depletion has been challenged.[81]

Optimizing the volume of perioperative fluid administration 9
to minimize morbidity and mortality remains a significant and controversial challenge. Currently, most practitioners rely on clinical acumen, vital signs such as heart rate and blood pressure, and urine output to manage perioperative fluids. Surgical patients can be markedly hypovolemic without a change in any one of these variables because of the compensatory action of peripheral vasoconstriction.[26] Unfortunately, this shunts blood away from skin, increases wound hypoxemia, and increases the risk of surgical wound infection. Static monitors such as heart rate, blood pressure, urine output, central venous pressure,[26,82] and pulmonary artery catheters have been shown to be limited. More dynamic monitors such as stroke volume assessment, pulse pressure variation, and systolic pressure variation can be predictive of fluid responsiveness[83]; however, these have limitations, including the requirements of a regular R to R interval, closed chest, and adequate tidal volumes. Echocardiography, including assessment of stroke volume and other indices for preload, afterload, and contractility, can be a helpful intraoperative guide,[84] but large-scale clinical trials are needed to validate its use as a dynamic modality for monitoring. Additional limitations include lack of available hardware and expertise, although newer technologies and increasing focus on training in perioperative point-of-care ultrasound are beginning to address these.

Intraoperative fluid optimization strategies have ranged from liberal, to restrictive (also known as zero balance), to goal directed (SV optimization). There is evidence that increased volume may be beneficial for skin perfusion. Arkilic et al.[75] randomized 56 patients to liberal (16 to 18 mL/kg/h) or conservative (8 mL/kg/h) intraoperative fluid therapy and measured tissue perfusion and oxygen tension as a surrogate for wound healing. The liberal fluid regimen was associated with significantly greater intraoperative subcutaneous oxygen tension as measured by a tissue oxygen sensor. The study was too small to evaluate the effect on wound complications. Kabon et al.[85] performed a randomized, controlled trial to compare standard- (8 mL/kg/h) versus high (16 to 18 mL/kg/h)-volume administration in 253 patients undergoing elective colon resection. The group that received high volume had a rate of 8.5% SSI; the rate was 11.3% in the group with standard volume which would be a clinically significant reduction, if real. Unfortunately, the study was terminated early, so it had inadequate power to detect a difference of that size. Patients at high risk for heart failure or with end-stage renal disease were excluded, so the study also has limited generalizability. On the other side, there is concern that liberal fluid administration may be excessive and may be detrimental to patients. In a systematic review, Holte et al.[81] found benefit in avoiding excessive fluid administration in major surgery.

The discussion of "liberal" and "restricted" fluids requires consideration of whether colloids or crystalloids are preferable for intraoperative fluid administration. Synthetic colloids have been associated with coagulopathy when large volumes are delivered, which appears to be in large part mediated by dilution of coagulation factors.[86] The intravascular half-life of colloids, either albumin or synthetic colloids, is much longer than that of crystalloids, allowing the total volume of fluid administered to be reduced by including colloids in surgical fluid resuscitation.[86] Edema formation may also be decreased. A number of studies[76,86–89] purport to evaluate intraoperative or postoperative fluid administration in terms of restrictive versus traditional fluid management. Virtually all have compared colloid ("restrictive" group) with crystalloid ("traditional" group) administration. Thus, the "restricted" volume group likely received a larger amount of effective intravascular volume than the traditional or "liberal" group. In general, these studies have demonstrated improved outcomes (reduction in SSI, earlier return of bowel function) for the colloid group. The mechanism for the benefit is unclear, however, as on the basis of effective intravascular volume delivered, the crystalloid groups might actually have been less well volume replaced than the colloid groups.

What is clear is that fluid overload to the point of interstitial edema is not beneficial for most organ function, including kidneys, liver, lungs, and heart. Interstitial edema can result in poor wound healing and infection due to decreased oxygen diffusion distance. Finding the balance between appropriate volume supplementation for adequate perfusion and avoiding tissue edema is the challenge. One of the difficulties in interpreting the literature on volume management is the lack of standardization of definitions such as "liberal" and "restricted," the amount and combinations of fluid used for replacement, and the lack of standardization of targets and outcomes. At this time, an individualized plan based on preoperative and intraoperative volume assessment, and appropriate monitoring, depending on the complexity of comorbidities and the surgical procedure, is required to attempt to find this balance for every patient. Goal-directed therapy, using stroke volume variation or echocardiography, holds promise, but much work remains to be done to define and implement reliable standards.

Current best recommendations include replacing fluid losses based on standard recommendations (Table 8-8) for the type of surgery, replacement of blood loss, and replacement of other ongoing fluid losses (e.g., high urine output due to diuretic or dye administration, hyperglycemia, or thermoregulatory vasoconstriction). Maintenance of normothermia is also critical to optimal volume management. Warm patients are unlikely to develop pulmonary edema with a high rate of fluid administration because they have excess capacitance due to vasodilation. Cold patients, on the other hand, are highly susceptible to pulmonary edema even after relatively small fluid boluses. Thermoregulatory vasoconstriction increases afterload, causing increased cardiac work. Moreover, administered fluid cannot open up constricted vessels until the hypothermic stimulus is removed; thus, there is virtually no excess capacitance in the system.

Pain control should be addressed intraoperatively so that patients do not have severe pain on emergence. Achieving the goal is more important than the technique used to do so. Although regional anesthesia and analgesia may provide superior pain relief, the effects of specific analgesic regimens on wound outcome have not yet adequately been studied.

Postoperative Management

Wounds are most vulnerable in the first few hours after surgery (Table 8-9). Although antibiotics lose their effectiveness after the first hours, oxygen-mediated natural wound immunity lasts longer.[19] Even a short period of vasoconstriction during the first day is sufficient to reduce oxygen supply and increase infection risk.[27] Correction and prevention of vasoconstriction in the first 24 to 48 hours after surgery will have significant beneficial effects.[27] Given the large number of diabetic patients who undergo surgery, along with the fact that the stress response frequently induces hyperglycemia intraoperatively even in nondiabetic patients, guidelines for controlling blood sugar in perioperative patients are critical to prevention of SSI. Unfortunately, balancing a narrow therapeutic window between hypoglycemia and hyperglycemia is a complex issue in blood sugar control. Clinical trials have provided conflicting results. A 2001 randomized controlled trial demonstrated a 25% reduction in risk of septicemia in critically ill surgical patients whose blood glucose levels were more tightly controlled than a comparison group.[90] On the other hand,

Table 8-8 Standard Volume Management Guidelines for Surgical Patients

Fluid requirement = deficit + maintenance (baseline plus replacement) + estimated blood loss and other sensible fluid losses
Deficit = maintenance (1.5 mL/kg/h) × hours NPO
Adjust for fever, high NG output, bowel preparation, and other sources of ongoing preoperative increased fluid loss
Use goal-directed therapy as available
Replace EBL 3:1 with crystalloid, 1:1 with colloid
Maintenance requirements for different surgeries: Superficial surgical trauma: 1–2 mL/kg/h Peripheral surgery Minimal surgical trauma: 3–4 mL/kg/h Head and neck, hernia, knee surgery Moderate surgical trauma: 5–6 mL/kg/h Major surgery without exposed abdominal contents Severe surgical trauma: 8–10 mL/kg/h Major abdominal, especially with exposed abdominal contents

EBL, estimated blood loss; NG, nasogastric; NPO, nothing by mouth.

Table 8-9 Postoperative Management

Keep patient warm.
Provide analgesia to keep patient comfortable, if not pain free. Patient report and the ability to move freely are the best signs of adequate pain relief.
Only one more dose of antibiotic unless an infection is present or contamination continues.
Keep up with third-space losses. Remember that fever increases fluid losses.
Assess perfusion and react to abnormalities.
Avoid diuresis until pain is gone and patient is warm.
Assess losses (including thermal losses) if wound is open.
Assess need for parenteral or enteral nutrition and respond.
Continue to control hypertension and hyperglycemia.

in 2007, Gandhi et al.[91] found no difference in SSI in 400 cardiac surgery patients comparing a target blood sugar of 80 to 100 versus less than 200 mg/dL. The NICE-SUGAR study in 6,104 ICU patients demonstrated excess mortality in the tight control (81 to 108 mg/dL) versus standard (<180 mg/dL) group.[92] The current recommendation is to keep glucose close to normal (e.g., 100 to 180 or 200 mg/dL).[93]

All vasoconstrictive stimuli must be corrected simultaneously to allow optimal healing. Volume is the last to be corrected because vasoconstriction for other reasons induces diuresis and renders the patient relatively hypovolemic (peripherally, not centrally). These measures are particularly important in any patients at high risk for wound complications for other reasons (e.g., malnutrition, steroid use, diabetes), or when vasoconstrictive drugs such as β-blockers and α-agonists are required for other reasons.

Local perfusion is not assured until patients have a normal blood volume, are warm and pain free, and are receiving no vasoconstrictive drugs; that is, until the sympathetic nervous system is inactivated. Warming should continue until patients are thoroughly awake and active and can maintain their own thermal balance. After major operations, warming may be useful for many hours or even days. The goal is to achieve warmth at the skin; wound vasoconstriction due to cold surroundings often coexists with core hyperthermia. Moderate hyperthermia is not, itself, a problem. When extensive wounds are left open, warmth should be continued, and heat losses due to evaporation should be prevented to avoid vasoconstriction and to minimize caloric losses.

Assessing perfusion, especially in the PACU, is critical. Unfortunately, urine output is a poor, often misleading guide to peripheral perfusion. Markedly low output may indicate decreased renal perfusion, but normal or even high urine output has little correlation to wound or tissue PO_2. Many factors commonly present in the perioperative period, including hyperglycemia, dye administration, thermoregulatory vasoconstriction, adrenal insufficiency, and various drugs, may cause inappropriate diuresis in the face of mild hypovolemia.

Physical examination of the patient is a better guide to hypovolemia and vasoconstriction. Assess vasoconstriction by a capillary return time of more than 2 to 3 seconds at the forehead and more than 5 seconds over the patella. Eye turgor is another good measure of volume status. Finally, patients can usually distinguish thirst from a dry mouth. Skin should be warm and dry.

After major abdominal surgery, third-space losses continue for about 12 to 24 hours, so increased fluid requirements continue. In general, for large abdominal cases, 2 to 3 mL/kg/h of IV fluids is sufficient for the first 12 to 24 postoperative hours. After that period, the IV rate should be decreased below calculated maintenance levels because edema fluid begins to be mobilized, thus increasing circulating intravascular volume.

When excessive tissue fluids have accumulated, diuresis should be undertaken gently so that transcapillary refill can maintain blood volume. This applies to patients who need renal dialysis as well. The average dialysis patient vasoconstricts sufficiently to lower tissue PO_2 by 30% or more during dialysis; it takes about 24 hours for vasomotor tone and wound and tissue PO_2 to return normal.[94] Fluid losses from the vascular system are not necessarily replaced from the tissues as rapidly as they are sustained. Tissue edema may be the price paid for adequate intravascular volume. Edema increases intracapillary distance, so that there may be a delicate balance between excessive edema and peripheral vasoconstriction (which worsens the hypoxia caused by edema).

Vasoconstrictive drugs should be avoided. The most common and most avoidable is nicotine in the form of cigarettes. High-dose α-adrenergic agonists or other vasopressors may cause harm by decreasing tissue PO_2, but lower doses have little or no effect on wound/tissue PO_2.[55] It is important to remember that decreasing cardiac output may also reduce wound perfusion. Thus, a balance must be maintained between minimizing use of vasopressors and maintaining adequate cardiac output.

Maintenance of tissue PO_2 requires attention to pulmonary 10
function postoperatively. Administration of supplemental oxygen via face mask or nasal cannula increases safety in patients receiving systemic opioids.[95] Pain control also appears important since it favorably influences both pulmonary function and vascular tone. This is particularly true in patients at high risk for pulmonary complications postoperatively, such as morbidly obese patients and those with pulmonary disease.

Summary

In patients with moderate to high risk of SSI, anesthesiologists 11
have the opportunity to enhance wound healing and reduce the incidence of wound infections by simple, inexpensive, and readily available means. Intraoperatively, appropriate antibiotic use, hand hygiene and attention to reducing workspace contamination, and prevention of vasoconstriction through appropriate volume administration and active warming clearly have benefit. In patients at high risk of SSI, maintenance of a high PaO_2 (300 to 500 mmHg) may also have benefit—and there is no evidence of harm from brief exposures of several hours. Postoperatively, the focus should remain on prevention of vasoconstriction through pain relief, warming, and adequate volume administration in the PACU. The addition of measures to reduce and prevent the stress response is likely to be effective as well, although further study is required.

For additional information please see NICV 8-3 in the eBook bundled with this text.

For further review and interactivities, please see the videos and narrative interactive clinical vignettes (NICVs) accessible in the complimentary eBook bundled with this text. Access instructions are located on the inside front cover.

REFERENCES

1. Centers for Disease Control National Healthcare Safety Network Surgical Site Infection Event (SSI) Procedure-Associated Module, January 2023. Accessed online 7 February, 2023. https://www.cdc.gov/nhsn/pdfs/pscmanual/9pscssicurrent.pdf
2. Berríos-Torres SI, Umscheid CA, Bratzler DW, et al; Healthcare Infection Control Practices Advisory Committee. Centers for Disease Control and Prevention guideline for the prevention of surgical site infection, 2017. *JAMA Surg*. 2017;152(8):784–791. doi: 10.1001/jamasurg.2017.0904
3. Lee JP, Hopf HW, Cannon-Albright LA. Empiric evidence for a genetic contribution to predisposition to surgical site infection. *Wound Rep Regen*. 2013;21:211–215. doi: 10.1111/wrr.12024
4. Noakes TD, Borresen J, Hew-Butler T, Lambert MI, Jordaan E. Semmelweis and the aetiology of puerperal sepsis 160 years on: an historical review. *Epidemiol Infect*. 2008;136(1):1–9. doi: 10.1017/S0950268807008746
5. Koff MD, Loftus RW, Burchman CC, et al. Reduction in intraoperative bacterial contamination of peripheral intravenous tubing through the use of a novel device. *Anesthesiology*. 2009;110:978–985. doi: 10.1097/ALN.0b013e3181a06ec3
6. Boyce JM, Pittet D; Healthcare Infection Control Practices Advisory Committee, HICPAC/SHEA/APIC/IDSA Hand Hygiene Task Force. Guideline for hand hygiene in health-care settings. Recommendations of the Healthcare Infection Control Practices Advisory Committee and the HIPAC/SHEA/APIC/IDSA Hand Hygiene Task Force. *Am J Infect Control*. 2002;30:S1–S46. doi: 10.1086/503164.
7. Sivathasan N, Goodfellow PB. Skin cleansers: the risks of chlorhexidine. *J Clin Pharmacol*. 2011;51:785–786. doi: 10.1177/0091270010372628
8. Sax H, Allegranzi B, Uçkay I, Larson E, Boyce J, Pittet D. 'My five moments for hand hygiene': a user-centered design approach to understand, train, monitor and report hand hygiene. *J Hosp Infect*. 2007;67:9–21. doi: 10.1016/j.jhin.2007.06.004

9. Sharma A, Fernandez PG, Rowlands JP, Koff MD, Loftus RW. Perioperative infection transmission: the role of the anesthesia provider in infection control and healthcare-associated infections. *Curr Anesthesiol Rep*. 2020;10(3):233–241. doi: 10.1007/s40140-020-00403-8
10. Mecham E, Hopf HW. A proposal to minimize work area contamination during induction. *Anesthesiology*. 2012;116:712. doi: 10.1097/ALN.0b013e318231fc3e
11. Birnbach DJ, Rosen LF, Fitzpatrick M, Carling P, Arheart KL, Munoz-Price LS. Double gloves: a randomized trial to evaluate a simple strategy to reduce contamination in the operating room. *Anesth Analg*. 2015 Apr;120(4):848–852. doi: 10.1213/ANE.00000see00000000230. PMID: 24836472.
12. Chang J, Jeong TD, Lee S, et al. Intactness of medical nonsterile gloves on use of alcohol disinfectants. *Ann Lab Med*. 2018;38(1):83–84. doi: 10.3343/alm.2018.38.1.83
13. Tunevall TG. Postoperative wound infections and surgical face masks: a controlled study. *World J Surg*. 1991;15:383–387.
14. Friberg B, Friberg S, Ostensson R, Burman LG. Surgical area contamination—comparable bacterial counts using disposable head and mask and helmet aspirator system, but dramatic increase upon omission of head-gear: an experimental study in horizontal laminar air-flow. *J Hosp Infect*. 2001;47:110–115. doi: 10.1053/jhin.2000.0909
15. Ling ML, Apisarnthanarak A, Jaggi N, et al. APSIC guide for prevention of central line associated bloodstream infections (CLABSI). *Antimicrob Resist Infect Control*. 2016;5:16. doi: 10.1186/s13756-016-0116-5
16. MacNeill AJ, Hopf H, Khanuja A, et al. Transforming the medical device industry: road map to a circular economy. *Health Aff (Millwood)*. 2020;39(12):2088-2097.
17. Malhotra GK, Tran T, Stewart C, et al. Pandemic operating room supply shortage and surgical site infection: considerations as we emerge from the coronavirus disease 2019 pandemic. *J Am Coll Surg*. 2022;234(4):571–578. doi: 10.1097/XCS.0000000000000087
18. Miles AA, Miles EM, Burke J. The value and duration of defence reactions of the skin to the primary lodgement of bacteria. *Br J Exp Pathol*. 1957;38:79–96.
19. Knighton DR, Halliday B, Hunt TK. Oxygen as an antibiotic: the effect of inspired oxygen on infection. *Arch Surg*. 1984;119:199–204. doi: 10.1001/archsurg.1984.01390140057010
20. Knighton DR, Halliday B, Hunt TK. Oxygen as an antibiotic: a comparison of the effects of inspired oxygen concentration and antibiotic administration on in vivo bacterial clearance. *Arch Surg*. 1986;121:191–195. doi: 10.1001/archsurg.1986.01400020077009
21. Bernard HR, Cole WR. The prophylaxis of surgical infection: the effect of prophylactic antimicrobial drugs on the incidence of infection following potentially contaminated operations. *Surgery*. 1964;56:151–157.
22. Classen DC, Evans RS, Pestotnik SL, Horn SD, Menlove RL, Burke JP. The timing of prophylactic administration of antibiotics and the risk of surgical-wound infection. *N Engl J Med*. 1992; 326:281–286. doi: 10.1056/NEJM199201303260501
23. Bratzler DW, Dellinger EP, Olsen KM, et al; American Society of Health-System Pharmacists, Infectious Disease Society of America, Surgical Infection Society, Society for Healthcare Epidemiology of America. Clinical practice guidelines for antimicrobial prophylaxis in surgery. *Am J Health Syst Pharm*. 2013;70:195–283. doi: 10.1056/NEJM199201303260501
24. Blumenthal KG, Ryan EE, Li Y, Lee H, Kuhlen JL, Shenoy ES. The impact of a reported penicillin allergy on surgical site infection risk. *Clin Infect Dis*. 2018;66(3):329–336. doi: 10.1093/cid/cix794
25. Guo S, Dipietro LA. Factors affecting wound healing. *J Dent Res*. 2010;89(3):219–229. doi: 10.1177/0022034509359125
26. Ueno C, Hunt TK, Hopf HW. Using physiology to improve surgical wound outcomes. *Plast Reconstr Surg*. 2006;117:59S–71S. doi: 10.1097/01.prs.0000225438.86758.21
27. Hopf HW, Hunt TK, West JM, et al. Wound tissue oxygen tension predicts the risk of wound infection in surgical patients. *Arch Surg*. 1997;132:997–1004. doi: 10.1001/archsurg.1997.01430330063010
28. Federman DG, Ladiiznski B, Dardik A, et al. Wound Healing Society 2014 update on guidelines for arterial ulcers. *Wound Repair Regen*. 2016;24(1):127–135. doi: 10.1111/wrr.12395
29. Allen DB, Maguire JJ, Mahdavian M, et al. Wound hypoxia and acidosis limit neutrophil bacterial killing mechanisms. *Arch Surg*. 1997;132:991–996. doi: 10.1001/archsurg.1997.01430330057009
30. Hopf HW, Gibson JJ, Angeles AP, et al. Hyperoxia and angiogenesis. *Wound Repair Regen*. 2005;13:558–564. doi: 10.1111/j.1524-475X.2005.00078.x
31. Evans NTS, Naylor PFD. Steady states of oxygen tension in human dermis. *Respir Physiol*. 1966;2:46–60.
32. Rodrigues M, Kosaric N, Bonham CA, Gurtner GC. Wound healing: a cellular perspective. *Physiol Rev*. 2019;99(1):665–706. doi: 10.1152/physrev.00067.2017
33. Constant J, Suh D, Hussain M, et al. Wound healing angiogenesis: the metabolic basis of repair. In: *Molecular, Cellular, and Clinical Aspects of Angiogenesis*. Plenum Press; 1996:151–159.
34. Zabel DD, Feng JJ, Scheuenstuhl H, Hunt TK, Hussain MZ. Lactate stimulation of macrophage-derived angiogenic activity is associated with inhibition of poly(ADP-ribose) synthesis. *Lab Invest*. 1996;74:644–649.
35. Trabold O, Wagner S, Wicke C, et al. Lactate and oxygen constitute a fundamental regulatory mechanism in wound healing. *Wound Repair Regen*. 2003;11:504–509. doi: 10.1046/j.1524-475x.2003.11621.x
36. Silver IA. Cellular microenvironment in healing and non-healing wounds. In: Hunt TK, Heppenstall RB, Pines E, eds. *Soft and Hard Tissue Repair*. Praeger; 1984:50–66.
37. Meyhoff C, Wetterslev J, Jorgensen LN, et al; PROXI Trial Group. Effect of high perioperative oxygen fraction on surgical site infection and pulmonary complications after abdominal surgery: the PROXI randomized clinical trial. *JAMA*. 2009;302:1543–1550. doi: 10.1001/jama.2009.1452
38. Sen CK, Khanna S, Babior BM, Hunt TK, Ellison EC, Roy S. Oxidant-induced vascular endothelial growth factor expression in human keratinocytes and cutaneous wound healing. *J Biol Chem*. 2002;277:33284–33290. doi: 10.1074/jbc.M203391200
39. Beckert S, Farrahi F, Aslam RS, et al. Lactate stimulates endothelial cell migration. *Wound Repair Regen*. 2006;14:321–324. doi: 10.1111/j.1743-6109.2006.00127.x
40. Lam GY, Huang J, Brumell JH. The many roles of NOX2 NADPH oxidase-derived ROS in immunity. *Semin Immunopathol*. 2010;32:415–430. doi: 10.1007/s00281-010-0221-0
41. Rollins MD, Gibson JJ, Hunt TK, Hopf HW. Wound oxygen levels during hyperbaric oxygen treatment in healing wounds. *Undersea Hyperb Med*. 2006;33:17–25.
42. Fife CE, Smart DR, Sheffield PJ, Hopf HW, Hawkins G, Clarke D. Transcutaneous oximetry in clinical practice: consensus statements from an expert panel based on evidence. *Undersea Hyperb Med*. 2009;36(1):43–53.
43. Thom SR. Hyperbaric oxygen: its mechanisms and efficacy. *Plast Reconstr Surg*. 2011;127(Suppl 1): 131S–141S.
44. Hunt TK, Aslam RS, Beckert S, et al. Aerobically derived lactate stimulates revascularization and tissue repair via redox mechanisms. *Antioxid Redox Signal*. 2007;9:1115–1124. doi: 10.1089/ars.2007.1674
45. Velazquez OC. Angiogenesis and vasculogenesis: inducing the growth of new blood vessels and wound healing by stimulation of bone marrow–derived progenitor cell mobilization and homing. *J Vasc Surg*. 2007;45(Suppl A):A39–A47. doi: 10.1016/j.jvs.2007.02.068
46. Beckert S, Hierlemann H, Müschenborn N, Witte M, Ranke M, Coerper S. Experimental ischemic wounds: correlation of cell proliferation and insulin-like growth factor I expression and its modification by different local IGF-I release systems. *Wound Repair Regen*. 2005;13: 278–283. doi: 10.1111/j.1067-1927.2005.130310.x
47. Knighton DR, Silver IA, Hunt TK. Regulation of wound-healing angiogenesis-effect of oxygen gradients and inspired oxygen concentration. *Surgery*. 1981;90:262–270.
48. Silver IA. Oxygen tension and epithelialization. In: Maibach HI, Rovee DT, eds. *Epidermal Wound Healing*. Year Book Medical Publishers; 1972:291.
49. Medawar PS. The behavior of mammalian skin epithelium under strictly anaerobic conditions. *Q J Microsc Sci*. 1947;88:27.
50. Feldmeier JJ, Hopf HW, Warriner RA 3rd, Fife CE, Gesell LB, Bennett M. UHMS position statement: topical oxygen for chronic wounds. *Undersea Hyperb Med*. 2005;32:157–168.
51. Ngo MA, Sinitsyna NN, Qin Q, Rice RH. Oxygen-dependent differentiation of human keratinocytes. *J Invest Dermatol*. 2007;127:354–361.
52. O'Toole EA, Marinkovich MP, Peavey CL, et al. Hypoxia increases human keratinocyte motility on connective tissue. *J Clin Invest*. 1997;100:2881–2891. doi: 10.1172/JCI119837
53. Jensen JA, Goodson WH, Hopf HW, Hunt TK. Cigarette smoking decreases tissue oxygen. *Arch Surg*. 1991;126:1131–1134. doi: 10.1001/archsurg.1991.01410330093013
54. Hopf HW, Viele M, Watson JJ, et al. Subcutaneous perfusion and oxygen during acute severe isovolemic hemodilution in healthy volunteers. *Arch Surg*. 2000;135:1443–1449. doi: 10.1001/archsurg.135.12.1443
55. Motakef S, Mountziaris PM, Ismail IK, Agag RL, Patel A. Emerging paradigms in perioperative management for microsurgical free tissue transfer: review of the literature and evidence-based guidelines. *Plast Reconstr Surg*. 2015;135(1):290–299. doi: 10.1097/PRS.0000000000000839
56. Hopf HW. Perioperative temperature management: time for a new standard of care? *Anesthesiology*. 2015;122(2):229–230. doi: 10.1097/ALN.0000000000000552
57. Kurz A, Sessler DI, Lenhardt R. Perioperative normothermia to reduce the incidence of surgical-wound infection and shorten hospitalization: Study of Wound Infection and Temperature Group. *N Engl J Med*. 1996;334:1209–1215. doi: 10.1056/NEJM199605093341901
58. Hartmann M, Jönsson K, Zederfeldt B. Effect of tissue perfusion and oxygenation on accumulation of collagen in healing wounds. Randomized study in patients after major abdominal operations. *Eur J Surg*. 1992 Oct;158(10):521–526. PMID: 1360822.
59. Melling AC, Ali B, Scott EM, Leaper DJ. Effects of preoperative warming on the incidence of wound infection after clean surgery: a randomised controlled trial. *Lancet*. 2001;358:876–880.
60. Akça O, Melischek M, Scheck T, et al. Postoperative pain and subcutaneous oxygen tension [letter]. *Lancet*. 1999;354:41–42.
61. Wetterslev J, Meyhoff CS, Jørgensen LN, Gluud C, Lindschou J, Rasmussen LS. The effects of high perioperative inspiratory oxygen fraction for adult surgical patients. *Cochrane Database Syst Rev*. 2015;6:CD008884.
62. Greif R, Akça O, Horn EP, Kurz A, Sessler DI; Outcomes Research Group. Supplemental perioperative oxygen to reduce the incidence of surgical-wound infection. *N Engl J Med*. 2000;342:161–167. doi: 10.1056/NEJM200001203420303
63. Belda FJ, Aguilera L, García de la Asunción J, et al; Spanish Reduccion de la Tasa de Infeccion Quirurgica Group. Supplemental perioperative oxygen and the risk of surgical wound infection: a randomized controlled trial. *JAMA*. 2005;294:2035–2042. doi: 10.1001/jama.294.16.2035
64. Myles PS, Leslie K, Chan MT, et al; ENIGMA Trial Group. Avoidance of nitrous oxide for patients undergoing major surgery: a randomized controlled trial. *Anesthesiology*. 2007;107: 221–231. doi: 10.1097/01.anes.0000270723.30772.da

65. Akça O, Podolsky A, Eisenhuber E, et al. Comparable postoperative pulmonary atelectasis in patients given 30% or 80% oxygen during and 2 hours after colon resection. *Anesthesiology*. 1999;91:991–998. doi: 10.1097/00000542-199910000-00019
66. Mackintosh N, Gertsch MC, Hopf HW, et al. High intraoperative inspired oxygen does not increase postoperative supplemental oxygen requirements. *Anesthesiology*. 2012;117:271–279. doi: 10.1097/ALN.0b013e318259a7e8
67. Kohanski MA, Dwyer DJ, Hayete B, Lawrence CA, Collins JJ. A common mechanism of cellular death induced by bactericidal antibiotics. *Cell*. 2007;130:797–810. doi: 10.1016/j.cell.2007.06.049
68. Suller MT, Lloyd D. The antibacterial activity of vancomycin towards Staphylococcus aureus under aerobic and anaerobic conditions. *J Appl Microbiol*. 2002;92:866–872. doi: 10.1046/j.1365-2672.2002.01594.x
69. Tanner J, Padley W, Assadian O, Leaper D, Kiernan M, Edmiston C. Do surgical care bundles reduce the risk of surgical site infections in patients undergoing colorectal surgery? A systematic review and cohort meta-analysis of 8,515 patients. *Surgery*. 2015;158:66–77. doi: 10.1016/j.surg.2015.03.009
70. Kiecolt-Glaser JK, Loving TJ, Stowell JR, et al. Hostile marital interactions, proinflammatory cytokine production, and wound healing. *Arch Gen Psychiatry*. 2005;62:1377–1384.
71. Muizzuddin N, Matsui MS, Marenus KD, Maes DH. Impact of stress of marital dissolution on skin barrier recovery: tape stripping and measurement of trans-epidermal water loss (TEWL). *Skin Res Technol*. 2003;9:34–38. doi: 10.1034/j.1600-0846.2003.00354.x
72. Bosch JA, Engeland CG, Cacioppo JT, Marucha PT. Depressive symptoms predict mucosal wound healing. *Psychosom Med*. 2007;69:597–605. doi: 10.1097/PSY.0b013e318148c682
73. Kurz A, Kurz M, Poeschl G, Faryniak B, Redl G, Hackl W. Forced-air warming maintains intraoperative normothermia better than circulating water mattresses. *Anesth Analg*. 1993;77:89–95. doi: 10.1213/00000539-199307000-00018
74. Galvão CM, Marck PB, Sawada NO, Clark AM. A systematic review of the effectiveness of cutaneous warming systems to prevent hypothermia. *J Clin Nurs*. 2009;18:627–636. doi: 10.1111/j.1365-2702.2008.02668.x
75. Arkiliç CF, Taguchi A, Sharma N, et al. Supplemental perioperative fluid administration increases tissue oxygen pressure. *Surgery*. 2003;133:49–55. doi: 10.1067/msy.2003.80
76. Nisanevich V, Felsenstein I, Almogy G, Weissman C, Einav S, Matot I. Effect of intraoperative fluid management on outcome after intraabdominal surgery. *Anesthesiology*. 2005;103:25–32. doi: 10.1097/00000542-200507000-00008
77. Alphonsus CS, Rodseth RN. The endothelial glycocalyx: a review of the vascular barrier. *Anaesthesia*. 2014;69:777–784. doi: 10.1111/anae.12661
78. Gupta R, Gan TJ. Peri-operative fluid management to enhance recovery. *Anaesthesia*. 2016;71(Suppl 1):40–45. doi: 10.1111/anae.13309
79. Kehlet H. Surgical stress response: does endoscopic surgery confer an advantage? *World J Surg*. 1999;23:801–807. doi: 10.1007/s002689900583
80. Holte K, Sharrock NE, Kehlet H. Pathophysiology and clinical implications of perioperative fluid excess. *Br J Anaesth*. 2002;89:622–632. doi: 10.1093/bja/aef220
81. Chappell D, Jacob M, Hofmann-Kiefer K, Conzen P, Rehm M. A rational approach to perioperative fluid management. *Anesthesiology*. 2008;109:723–740. doi: 10.1097/ALN.0b013e3181863117
82. Marik PE, Baram M, Vahid B. Does central venous pressure predict fluid responsiveness? A systematic review of the literature and the tale of seven mares. *Chest*. 2008;134:172–178. doi: 10.1378/chest.07-2331
83. Marik PE, Cavallazzi R, Vasu T, Hirani A. Dynamic changes in arterial waveform derived variables and fluid responsiveness in mechanically ventilated patients: a systematic review of the literature. *Crit Care Med*. 2009;37:2642–2647. doi: 10.1097/CCM.0b013e3181a590da
84. Porter TR, Shillcutt SK, Adams MS, et al. Guidelines for the use of echocardiography as a monitor for therapeutic intervention in adults: a report from the American Society of Echocardiography. *J Am Soc Echocardiogr*. 2015;28:40–56. doi: 10.1016/j.echo.2014.09.009
85. Kabon B, Akca O, Taguchi A, et al. Supplemental intravenous crystalloid administration does not reduce the risk of surgical wound infection. *Anesth Analg*. 2005;101:1546–1553. doi: 10.1213/01.ANE.0000180217.57952.FE
86. Grocott MP, Mythen MG, Gan TJ. Perioperative fluid management and clinical outcomes in adults. *Anesth Analg*. 2005;100:1093–1106. doi: 10.1213/01.ANE.0000148691.33690.AC
87. Ruttmann TG, James MF, Aronson I. In vivo investigation into the effects of haemodilution with hydroxyethyl starch (200/0.5) and normal saline on coagulation. *Br J Anaesth*. 1998;80:612–616. doi: 10.1093/bja/80.5.612
88. Lobo DN, Bostock KA, Neal KR, Perkins AC, Rowlands BJ, Allison SP. Effect of salt and water balance on recovery of gastrointestinal function after elective colonic resection: a randomised controlled trial. *Lancet*. 2002;359:1812–1818. doi: 10.1016/S0140-6736(02)08711-1
89. Brandstrup B, Tønnesen H, Beier-Holgersen R, et al; Danish Study Group on Perioperative Fluid Therapy. Effects of intravenous fluid restriction on postoperative complications: comparison of two perioperative fluid regimens: a randomized assessor-blinded multicenter trial. *Ann Surg*. 2003;238:641–648. doi: 10.1097/01.sla.0000094387.50865.23
90. van den Berghe G, Wouters P, Weekers F, et al. Intensive insulin therapy in the critically ill patients. *N Engl J Med*. 2001;345:1359–1367. doi: 10.1056/NEJMoa011300
91. Gandhi GY, Nuttall GA, Abel MD, et al. Intensive intraoperative insulin therapy versus conventional glucose management during cardiac surgery: a randomized trial. *Ann Intern Med*. 2007;146:233–243. doi: 10.7326/0003-4819-146-4-200702200-00002
92. NICE-SUGAR Study Investigators; Finfer S, Chittock DR, Su SY, et al. Intensive versus conventional glucose control in critically ill patients. *N Engl J Med*. 2009;360:1283–1297. doi: 10.1056/NEJMoa0810625
93. Griesdale DE, de Souza RJ, van Dam RM, et al. Intensive insulin therapy and mortality among critically ill patients: a meta-analysis including NICE-SUGAR study data. *CMAJ*. 2009;180:821–827. doi: 10.1503/cmaj.090206
94. Jensen JA, Goodson WH 3rd, Omachi RS, Lindenfeld SM, Hunt TK. Subcutaneous tissue oxygen tension falls during hemodialysis. *Surgery*. 1987;101:416–421.
95. Stone JG, Cozine KA, Wald A. Nocturnal oxygenation during patient-controlled analgesia. *Anesth Analg*. 1999;89:104–110. doi: 10.1097/00000539-199907000-00018

9 The Allergic Response

JERROLD H. LEVY

KEY POINTS

1 Anesthesiologists routinely administer multiple parenteral agents in the perioperative period, including drugs (antibiotics, anesthetic agents, neuromuscular blocking agents [NMBAs]), polypeptides (i.e., protamine), and blood products, or patients are exposed to environmental antigens (i.e., latex) all of which can produce an allergic reaction.

2 Cytokines are inflammatory cell activators synthesized to act as secondary messengers and activate endothelial and white cells.

3 Antibodies are specific proteins called immunoglobulins that can recognize and bind to specific antigens, and usually, IgE or IgG is implicated in allergic reactions.

4 Immune competence during surgery can be affected by direct and hormonal effects of anesthetic drugs, immunologic effects of other drugs used, type of surgery, coincident infection, and transfused blood products.

5 Most of the allergic reactions evoked by intravenous drugs occur within 5 minutes of administration. In the anesthetized patient, the most common life-threatening manifestation of an allergic reaction is circulatory collapse, reflecting vasodilation, and decreasing venous return.

6 Some drugs administered perioperatively, such as vancomycin, can release histamine in a dose-dependent, nonimmunologic fashion.

7 A plan for treating anaphylactic reactions should be considered by clinicians that includes airway maintenance, 100% oxygen administration, intravascular volume expansion, and epinephrine, which are essential to treat the hypotension and hypoxia resulting from vasodilation, increased capillary permeability, and bronchospasm. Norepinephrine, vasopressin, and additional diagnostic monitoring should be considered for refractory shock.

8 After an anaphylactic reaction, it is important to attempt to identify the causative agent to prevent readministration.

9 Health care workers, children following multiple procedures, and individuals with specific food allergies have been recognized to be at increased risk for latex anaphylaxis. However, latex has been removed as an environmental antigen over the years.

10 NMBAs have several unique molecular features that make them potential antigens that can cause anaphylaxis.

Introduction

1 Allergic reactions represent an important cause of perioperative complications. Anesthesiologists routinely administer multiple drugs and blood products and manage patients during their perioperative medical care, where they are exposed to multiple agents, including drugs (i.e., antibiotics, anesthetic agents, neuromuscular blocking agents [NMBAs]), polypeptides (protamine), blood products, and environmental antigens (i.e., latex). Anesthesiologists must be able to rapidly recognize and treat anaphylaxis, the most life-threatening form of an allergic reaction.[1]

The allergic response represents just one aspect of the pathologic response that the immune system evolved to recognize foreign substances. As part of normal host surveillance mechanisms, a series of cellular and humoral elements oversees foreign surfaces of cell surfaces and molecular structures called *antigens* to provide host defense. These foreign substances (antigens) consist of molecular arrangements found on cells, bacteria, viruses, proteins, or complex macromolecules.[2,3] Immunologic mechanisms (1) involve antigen interaction with antibodies or specific effector cells; (2) are reproducible; and (3) are specific and adaptive, distinguishing foreign substances and amplifying reactivity through a series of inflammatory cells and proteins. The immune system serves to protect the body against external microorganisms and toxins, as well as internal threats from neoplastic cells; however, it can respond inappropriately to cause hypersensitive (allergic) reactions. Life-threatening allergic reactions to drugs and other foreign substances observed perioperatively may represent different expressions of the immune response.[2,3]

Basic Immunologic Principles

The immune system protects the body from invasion by organisms by recognizing and removing foreign substances called *antigens* that are molecular structures, usually proteins and/or carbohydrates. The body also has mechanisms to tolerate similar molecular configurations of the host (self-tolerance); however, problems arise when the immune system is dysfunctional, as in cases of autoimmunity that can give rise to serious diseases, including rheumatoid arthritis and lupus. The immune response includes both cell-mediated immunity and humoral immunity. Cell-mediated immunity involves immune cells directed at the elimination or destruction of pathogens or cells. Humoral immunity comprises antibodies and proteins (e.g., complement, cytokines, and signaling molecules) that can directly or in concert with cellular immunity orchestrate cell injury and destruction. The purpose is to provide host defense mechanisms.

2 As part of humoral immune responses, protein mediators called cytokines and chemokines are released initially by inflammatory responses to bring other immune cells to the site of the injury or infection, cause additional inflammatory responses and fever, and increase capillary permeability to allow other immune cells to migrate and translocate to the site of injury. This inflammatory response also causes hemostatic activation and produces pain, erythema, and edema locally and potentially systemically, depending on the extent of the injury. Cytokines have an extensive spectrum of inflammatory effects and have been extensively studied following acute infections.[4] The immune response can be variable in onset from immediate in anaphylaxis to days for cellular responses, and can remember antigens for many years, especially following immunization.

Although this is a simplified review of the immune system, it is important to consider individual aspects of the immune response and their importance.

Antigens

As mentioned, molecules stimulating an immune response (antibody production or lymphocyte stimulation) are called *antigens*.[5,6] Only a few drugs used by anesthesiologists, such as polypeptides (protamine) and other large macromolecules (dextrans), are complete antigens (Table 9-1). Most commonly used drugs are simple organic compounds of low molecular weight (around 1,000 Da). For most drugs that are small molecules, to become immunogenic, they must bind two circulating proteins or tissues to result in an antigen (hapten–macromolecular complex). Small molecular weight substances such as drugs or drug metabolites that bind to host proteins or cell membranes to sensitize patients are called *haptens*. Haptens are not antigenic by themselves. Often, a reactive drug metabolite (i.e., penicilloyl derivative of penicillin) is believed to bind with macromolecules to become antigens. Certain molecular structures in bacteria or fungi are immediately recognized as foreign by multiple aspects of the immune system.

Table 9-1 Agents Administered During Anesthesia That Act as Antigens

Haptens	Macromolecules
Penicillin and its derivatives	Aprotinin Blood Products
Anesthetic drugs	Chymopapain Colloid Volume Expanders Neuromuscular Blocking Agents Protamine Latex

Thymus-Derived (T-cell) and Bursa-Derived (B-cell) Lymphocytes

The thymus of the fetus differentiates immature lymphocytes into thymus-derived cells (T cells). T cells have receptors that are activated by binding with foreign antigens and secrete mediators that regulate the immune response. The subpopulations of T cells in humans include helper, suppressor, cytotoxic, and killer cells.[5,6] The two types of regulatory T cells are helper cells (OKT4) and suppressor cells (OKT8). Helper cells are important for key effector cell responses, whereas suppressor cells inhibit immune function. Infection of helper T cells with a retrovirus, the human immunodeficiency virus, produces a specific increase in the number of suppressor cells. Cytotoxic T cells destroy mycobacteria, fungi, and viruses. Other lymphocytes, called natural killer cells, do not need specific antigen stimulation to set up their role. Both the cytotoxic T cells and natural killer cells take part in defense against tumor cells and in transplant rejection. T cells produce mediators that influence the response of other cell types involved in the recognition and destruction of foreign substances.[5,6]

B cells represent a specific lymphocyte cell line that can differentiate into specific plasma cells that synthesize antibodies, a step controlled by both helper and suppressor T-cell lymphocytes. B cells are also called bursa-derived cells because, in birds, the bursa of Fabricius is important in producing cells responsible for antibody synthesis.

Antibodies

Antibodies are specific proteins called *immunoglobulins* that can 3
recognize and bind to a specific antigen. The basic structure of the antibody molecule is illustrated in Figure 9-1. Each antibody

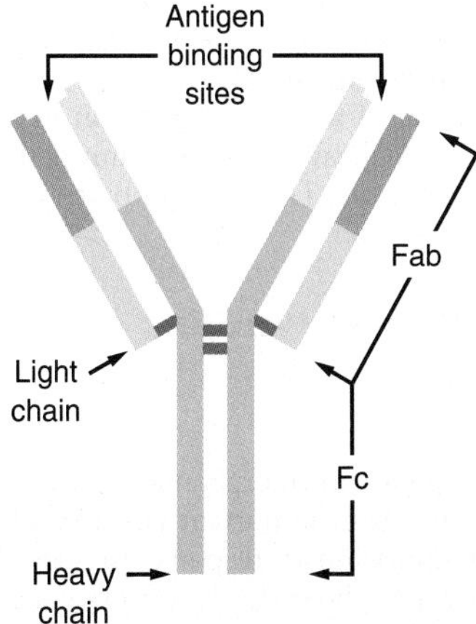

Figure 9-1 Basic structural configuration of the antibody molecule representing human immunoglobulin G (IgG). Immunoglobulins are composed of two heavy chains and two light chains bound by disulfide linkages (represented by *crossbars*). Papain cleaves the molecule into two Fab fragments and one Fc fragment. Antigen binding occurs on the Fab fragments, whereas the Fc segment is responsible for membrane binding or complement activation. (Reprinted from Levy JH. *Anaphylactic Reactions in Anesthesia and Intensive Care*. 2nd ed. Butterworth-Heinemann; 1992. Copyright © 1992 Elsevier. With permission.)

Table 9-2 Biologic Characteristics of Immunoglobulins

	IgG	IgM	IgA	IgE	IgD
Heavy chain	γ	μ	α	ε	δ
Molecular weight	160,000	900,000	170,000	188,000	184,000
Subclasses	1, 2, 3, 4	1, 2	1, 2		
Serum concentration (mg/dL)	6–14	0.5–1.5	1–3	<-0.5 × 10^3	<0.1
Complement activation	All but IgG_4	+	–	–	–
Placental transfer	+	–	–	–	–
Serum half-life (days)	23	5	6	1–5	2–8
Cell binding	Mast cells (IgG_4	Lymphocytes		Mast cells	Neutrophils
	Neutrophils			Basophils	Lymphocytes
	Lymphocytes				
	Mononuclear cells				
	Platelets				

has at least two heavy chains and two light chains that are bound together by disulfide bonds. The Fab fragment has the ability to bind antigen, and the Fc, or crystallizable, fragment is responsible for the unique biologic properties of the different classes of immunoglobulins (cell binding and complement activation). Antibodies function as specific receptor molecules for immune cells and proteins. When antigen binds covalently to the Fab fragments, the antibody undergoes conformational changes to activate the Fc receptor. The results of antigen–antibody binding depend on the cell type, which causes a specific type of activation (i.e., lymphocyte proliferation and differentiation into antibody-secreting cells, mast cell degranulation, and complement activation). Multiple therapeutic agents are based on Fab fragments that bind irreversibly to a specific molecular configuration or drug and include such agents as abciximab (a platelet inhibitor that binds the IIb/IIIa receptor) and idarucizumab (that binds to dabigatran to reverse its anticoagulant effect).

Five major classes of antibodies occur in humans: IgG, IgA, IgM, IgD, and IgE. The heavy chain determines the structure and function of each molecule. The basic properties of each antibody are listed in Table 9-2.

Effector Cells and Proteins of the Immune Response

Cells

Monocytes, neutrophils (polymorphonuclear leukocytes [PMNs]), and eosinophils represent important effector cells that migrate into areas of inflammation in response to specific chemotactic factors, including lymphokines, cytokines, and complement-derived mediators. The deposition of antibody or complement fragments on the surface of foreign cells is called *opsonization*, a process that promotes killing foreign cells by effector cells. In addition, lymphokines and cytokines produce chemotaxis of other inflammatory cells as described in the following sections.[5,6] Activation of this cellular process is orchestrated by multiple mechanisms as part of host defense systems that function to contain and remove invading organisms during acute infections.[4,7]

As part of this complex acute inflammatory response, host injury occurs, as we have seen during the pandemic due to COVID-19.[4,7]

Monocytes and Macrophages

Macrophages regulate immune responses by processing and presenting antigens to affect inflammatory, tumoricidal, and microbicidal functions. Macrophages arise from circulating monocytes or may be confined to specific organs such as the lung. They are recruited and activated in response to microorganisms or tissue injury. Macrophages ingest antigens before they interact with receptors on the lymphocyte surface to regulate their action. Macrophages synthesize mediators to facilitate both B-lymphocyte and T-lymphocyte responses.

Polymorphonuclear Leukocytes (Neutrophils)

The first cells to appear in an acute inflammatory reaction are neutrophils that contain acid hydrolases, neutral proteases, and lysosomes. Once activated, they produce hydroxyl radicals, superoxide, and hydrogen peroxide, which aid in microbial killing.

Eosinophils

The exact function of the eosinophil in host defense is unclear; however, inflammatory cells recruit eosinophils to collect at sites of parasitic infections, tumors, and allergic reactions.

Basophils

Basophils comprise 0.5% to 1% of circulating granulocytes in the blood. On the surface of basophils are IgE receptors, which function similarly to those on mast cells.

Mast Cells

Mast cells are important cells for immediate hypersensitivity responses. They are tissue fixed and located in the perivascular spaces of the skin, lung, and intestine. On the surface of mast cells are IgE receptors, which bind to specific antigens. Once activated, these cells release physiologically active mediators important to immediate hypersensitivity responses (see IgE-Mediated Pathophysiology section under Anaphylactic Reactions). Mast cells can be activated by a series of both immune and nonimmune stimuli.

Proteins

Cytokines/Interleukins

Cytokines are inflammatory cell activators synthesized by macrophages to act as secondary messengers and activate endothelial cells and white cells.[8] Interleukins, tumor necrosis factor, and interferon are examples of cytokines considered important mediators of the biologic responses to infection and other inflammatory reactions. Liberation of interleukin-1 and tumor necrosis factor produces fever, neuropeptide release, endothelial cell activation, increased adhesion molecule expression, neutrophil priming, hypotension, myocardial suppression, and a catabolic state.[8] The term *interleukin* was coined for a group of cytokines that promotes communication between and among ("inter") leukocytes ("leukin"). Interleukins are a group of different regulatory proteins that control many aspects of the immune and inflammatory responses. The interleukins are polypeptides synthesized in response to cellular activation; they produce their inflammatory effects by activating specific receptors on inflammatory cells and vasculature. T-cell lymphocytes influence the activity of other immunologic and nonimmunologic cells by producing an array of interleukins that they secrete. Different interleukins of this class have been isolated and characterized; they function as short-range or intracellular soluble mediators of the immune and inflammatory responses. The interleukin family of cytokines has been rapidly growing in number because of advances in gene cloning.

Complement

The primary humoral response to antigen and antibody binding is the activation of the complement system.[9,10] The complement system consists of around 20 different proteins that bind to activated antibodies, other complement proteins, and cell membranes. The complement system is an important effector system of inflammation. Complement activation can be initiated by IgG or IgM binding to antigen, by plasmin through the classic pathway, by endotoxin, or by drugs through the alternate (properdin) pathway (Fig. 9-2). Specific fragments released during complement activation include C3a, C4a, and C5a, which have important humoral and chemotactic properties (see Non–IgE-Mediated Reactions section). The major function of the complement system is to recognize bacteria both directly and indirectly by attracting phagocytes (chemotaxis), as well as the increased adhesion of phagocytes to antigens (opsonization), and cell lysis by activation of the complete cascade.[9,10]

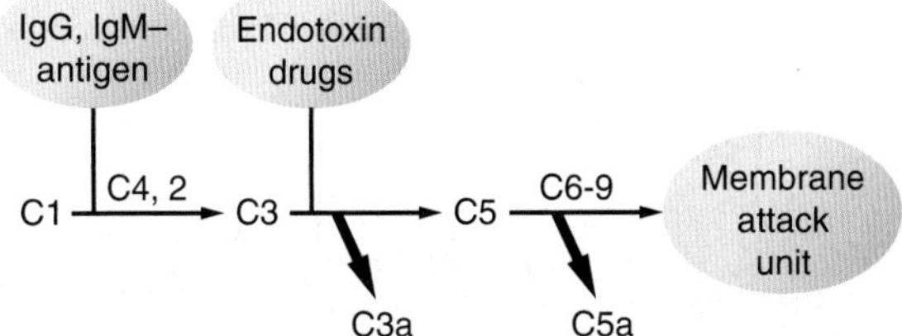

Figure 9-2 Diagram of complement activation. Complement system can be activated by either the classic pathway (IgG, IgM-antigen interaction) or the alternate pathway (endotoxin, drug interaction). Small peptide fragments of C3 and C5 called anaphylatoxins (C3a, C5a) that are released during activation are potent vasoactive mediators. Formation of the complete complement cascade produces a membrane attack unit that lyses cell walls and membranes. An inhibitor of the complement cascade, the C1 esterase inhibitor, ensures the complement system is turned off most of the time.

A series of inhibitors regulates activation to ensure regulation of the complement system. Hereditary (autosomal dominant) or acquired (associated with lymphoma, lymphosarcoma, chronic lymphatic leukemia, and macroglobulinemia) angioedema is an example of a deficiency in an inhibitor of the C1 complement system (C1 esterase deficiency). This syndrome is characterized by recurrent increased vascular permeability of specific subcutaneous and serosal tissues (angioedema), which produces laryngeal obstruction and respiratory and cardiovascular abnormalities after tissue trauma and surgery, or without any obvious precipitating factor.[11] One of the important pathologic manifestations of complement activation is acute pulmonary vasoconstriction associated with protamine administration.[1]

Effects of Anesthesia on Immune Function

4

Anesthesia and surgery depress nonspecific host resistance mechanisms, including lymphocyte activation and phagocytosis.[12] Immune competence during surgery can be affected by direct and hormonal effects of anesthetic drugs, immunologic effects of other drugs used, specific surgery, coincident infections, and transfused blood products. Blood represents a complex of humoral and cellular elements that may alter immunomodulation to various antigens. Although multiple studies demonstrate in vitro changes in immune function, no studies have ever proved their importance.[12] Besides, such changes are likely of minor importance compared with the hormonal aspects of stress responses.

Hypersensitivity Responses (Allergy)

Gell and Coombs first described a scheme for classifying immune responses to understand specific diseases mediated by immunologic processes. The immune pathway functions as a protective mechanism, but can also react inappropriately to produce hypersensitivity or allergic response. They defined four basic types of hypersensitivity, types I to IV. It is useful first to review all four mechanisms to understand the different immune reactions that occur in humans.

Type I Reactions

Type I reactions are anaphylactic or immediate-type hypersensitivity reactions (Fig. 9-3). Physiologically active mediators are released from mast cells and basophils after antigen binding to IgE

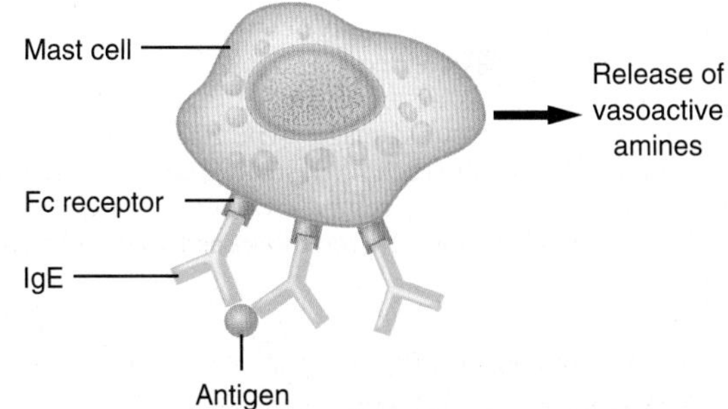

Figure 9-3 Type I immediate hypersensitivity reactions (anaphylaxis) involve IgE antibodies binding to mast cells or basophils by way of their Fc receptors. On encountering immunospecific antigens, the IgE becomes cross-linked, inducing degranulation, intracellular activation, and release of mediators. This reaction is independent of complement.

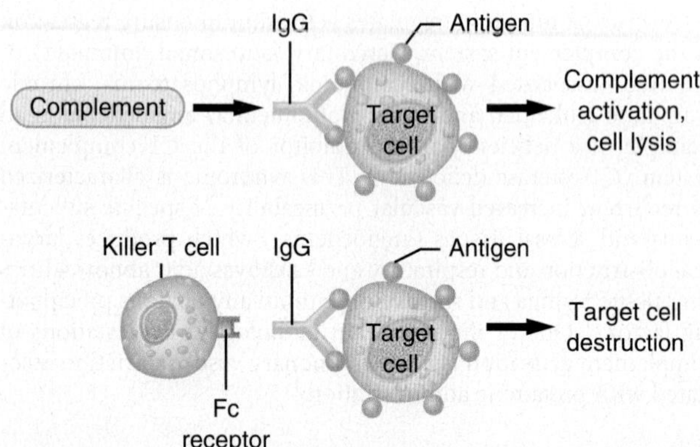

Figure 9-4 Type II or cytotoxic reactions. Antibody of an IgG or IgM class is directed against antigens on an individual's own cells (target cells). The antigens may be integral membrane components or foreign molecules that have been absorbed. This may lead to complement activation, including cell lysis (*upper figure*) or cytotoxic action by killer T-cell lymphocytes (*lower figure*).

antibodies on the membranes of these cells. Type I hypersensitivity reactions include anaphylaxis, extrinsic asthma, and allergic rhinitis.

Type II Reactions

Type II reactions are also known as antibody-dependent cell-mediated cytotoxic hypersensitivity or cytotoxic reactions (antibody-dependent cell-mediated cytotoxic) (NICV 9-1, Fig. 9-4). These reactions are mediated by either IgG or IgM antibodies directed against antigens on the surface of foreign cells. These antigens may be either integral cell membrane components (A or B blood group antigens in ABO incompatibility reactions) or haptens that absorb to the surface of a cell, stimulating the production of antihapten antibodies (autoimmune hemolytic anemia). The cell damage in type II reactions is produced by (1) direct cell lysis after complete complement cascade activation, (2) increased phagocytosis by macrophages, or (3) killer T-cell lymphocytes producing antibody-dependent cell-mediated cytotoxic effects. Examples of type II reactions in humans are ABO-incompatible transfusion reactions, drug-induced immune hemolytic anemia, and heparin-induced thrombocytopenia.

Type III Reactions (Immune Complex Reactions)

Type III reactions result from circulating soluble antigens and antibodies that bind to form insoluble complexes that deposit in the microvasculature (Video 9-1, Fig. 9-5). Complement is activated, and neutrophils are localized to the site of complement deposition to produce tissue damage. Type III reactions include classic serum sickness observed after snake antisera or antithymocyte globulin, and immune complex vascular injury, and may occur through mechanisms of protamine-mediated pulmonary vasoconstriction.[1]

Type IV Reactions (Delayed Hypersensitivity Reactions)

Type IV reactions result from the interactions of sensitized lymphocytes with specific antigens (Fig. 9-6). Delayed hypersensitivity reactions are mainly mononuclear, manifest in 18 to 24 hours, peak at 40 to 80 hours, and disappear in 72 to 96 hours.

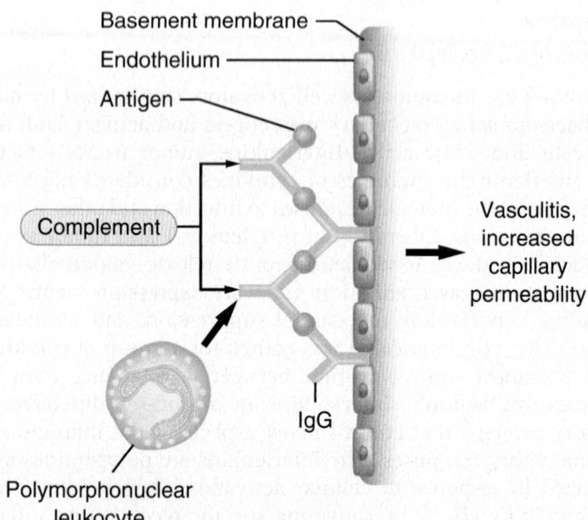

Figure 9-5 Type III immune complex reactions. Antibodies of an IgG or IgM type bind to the antigen in the soluble base and are subsequently deposited in the microvasculature. Complement is activated, resulting in chemotaxis and activation of polymorphonuclear leukocytes at the site of antigen–antibody complexes and subsequent tissue injury.

Antigen–lymphocyte binding produces lymphokine synthesis, lymphocyte proliferation, and generation of cytotoxic T cells, attracting macrophages and other inflammatory cells. Cytotoxic T cells are produced specifically to kill target cells that bear antigens identical to those that triggered the reaction. This form of immunity is important in tissue rejection, graft-versus-host reactions, contact dermatitis (e.g., poison ivy), and tuberculin immunity.

Intraoperative Allergic Reactions

Understanding perioperative anaphylaxis is important because of the potential for morbidity and mortality (NICV 9-2).[13] However, most estimates of the incidence are based on retrospective data, which may account for variability in the incidence. The risk of perioperative anaphylaxis is reported as between 1:3,500 and 1:20,000, with a mortality rate of 4% and an additional 2% surviving with severe brain damage.[13,14] More than 90% of the allergic reactions evoked by intravenous drugs occur within 5 minutes of administration. In the anesthetized patient, the most common life-threatening manifestation of an allergic reaction is circulatory collapse, reflecting vasodilation and decreased venous return (Table 9-3). The only manifestation of an allergic reaction may be refractory hypotension. Portier and Richet first used the word *anaphylaxis* (from *ana*, "against," and *prophylaxis*, "protection") to 5

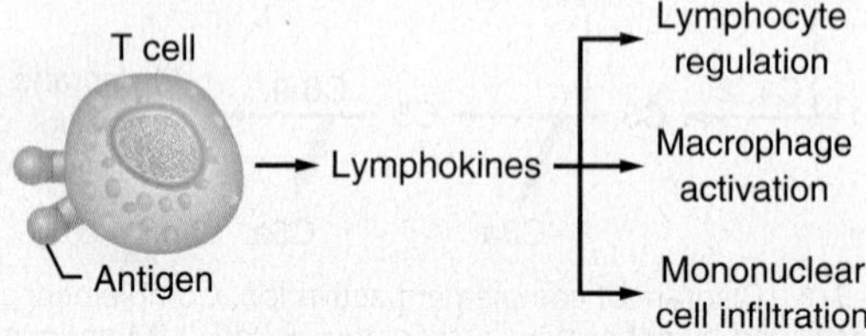

Figure 9-6 Type IV immune complex reactions (delayed hypersensitivity or cell-mediated immunity). Antigen binds to sensitized T-cell lymphocytes to release lymphokines after a second contact with the same antigen. This reaction is independent of circulating antibody or complement activation. Lymphokines induce inflammatory reactions and activate, as well as attract, macrophages and other mononuclear cells to produce delayed tissue injury.

Table 9-3 Recognition of Anaphylaxis During Regional and General Anesthesia

Systems	Symptoms	Signs
Respiratory	Dyspnea Chest discomfort	Coughing Wheezing Sneezing Laryngeal edema Decreased pulmonary compliance Fulminant pulmonary edema Acute respiratory failure
Cardiovascular	Dizziness Malaise Retrosternal oppression	Disorientation Diaphoresis Loss of consciousness Hypotension Tachycardia Dysrhythmias Decreased systemic vascular resistance Cardiac arrest Pulmonary hypertension
Cutaneous	Itching Burning Tingling	Urticaria (hives) Flushing Periorbital edema Perioral edema

Reprinted from Levy JH. *Anaphylactic Reactions in Anesthesia and Intensive Care*. 2nd ed. Butterworth-Heinemann; 1992. Copyright © 1992 Elsevier. With permission.

describe the profound shock and resulting death that sometimes occurred in dogs immediately after a second challenge with a foreign antigen.[15] When life-threatening allergic reactions mediated by antibodies occur, they are defined as anaphylactic. Although the term *anaphylactoid* has been used in the past to describe nonimmunologic reactions, this term is now rarely used.

Anaphylactic Reactions

IgE-Mediated Pathophysiology

Antigen binding to IgE antibodies initiates anaphylaxis (2 Video 9-2, Fig. 9-7). Prior exposure to the antigen or a substance of similar structure is needed to produce sensitization, although an allergic history may be unknown to the patient. On reexposure, binding of the antigen to bridge two immunospecific IgE antibodies found on the surfaces of mast cells and basophils releases stored mediators, including histamine, tryptase, and chemotactic factors.[13,16,17] Arachidonic acid metabolites (leukotrienes and prostaglandins), kinins, and cytokines are subsequently synthesized and released in response to cellular activation.[18] The released mediators produce a symptom complex of bronchospasm and upper airway edema in the respiratory system, vasodilation and increased capillary permeability in the cardiovascular system, and urticaria in the cutaneous system. Different mediators are released from mast cells and basophils after activation.

Molecular Mediators of Anaphylaxis

Histamine stimulates H_1, H_2, and H_3 receptors. H_1 receptor activation releases endothelium-derived relaxing factor (nitric oxide) from vascular endothelium, increases capillary permeability, and contracts airway and vascular smooth muscle.[16,19] H_2 receptor activation causes gastric secretion, inhibits mast cell activation, and contributes to vasodilation. When injected into the skin, histamine produces the classic wheal (increased capillary permeability producing tissue edema) and flare (cutaneous vasodilation) response in humans.[20,21] Histamine undergoes rapid metabolism in humans by the enzymes histamine *N*-methyltransferase and diamine oxidase found in endothelial cells.

Peptide Mediators of Anaphylaxis

Factors are released from mast cells and basophils that cause granulocyte migration (chemotaxis) and collection at the site of the inflammatory stimulus.[17,18] Eosinophilic chemotactic factor of anaphylaxis (ECF-A) is a small–molecular-weight peptide chemotactic for eosinophils.[22] Although the exact role of ECF-A or

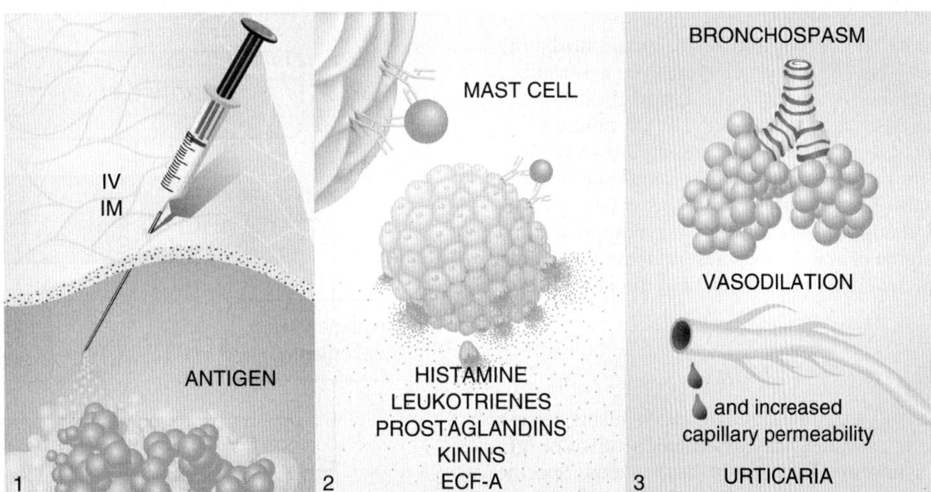

Figure 9-7 During anaphylaxis (type I immediate hypersensitivity reaction), (1) antigen enters a patient during anesthesia through a parenteral route. (2) It bridges two IgE antibodies on the surface of mast cells or basophils. In a calcium-dependent and energy-dependent process, cells release various substances—histamine, eosinophilic chemotactic factor of anaphylaxis, leukotrienes, prostaglandins, and kinins. (3) These released mediators produce the characteristic effects in the pulmonary, cardiovascular, and cutaneous systems. The most severe and life-threatening effects of the vasoactive mediators occur in the respiratory and cardiovascular systems. (Courtesy of Jerrold H. Levy. In: Levy JH. *Identification and Treatment of Anaphylaxis: Mechanisms of Action and Strategies for Treatment Under General Anesthesia*. Smith Laboratories; 1983.)

the eosinophil in acute allergic response is unclear, eosinophils release enzymes that can inactivate histamine and leukotrienes.[18] In addition, a neutrophilic chemotactic factor is released that causes chemotaxis and activation.[18,23] Neutrophil activation may be responsible for recurrent manifestations of anaphylaxis.

Arachidonic Acid Metabolites

Leukotrienes and prostaglandins are synthesized after mast cell activation from arachidonic acid metabolism of phospholipid cell membranes through either lipoxygenase or cyclooxygenase pathways.[22] The classic slow-reacting substance of anaphylaxis is a combination of leukotrienes C_4, D_4, and E_4. Leukotrienes produce bronchoconstriction (more intense than that produced by histamine), increased capillary permeability, vasodilation, coronary vasoconstriction, and myocardial depression.[24] Prostaglandins are potent mast cell mediators that produce vasodilation, bronchospasm, pulmonary hypertension, and increased capillary permeability. Prostaglandin D_2, the major metabolite of mast cells, produces bronchospasm and vasodilation. Elevated plasma levels of thromboxane B_2 (the metabolite of thromboxane A_2), also a prostaglandin synthesized by mast cells as well as by PMNs, have been demonstrated after protamine reactions associated with pulmonary hypertension.

Kinins

Small peptides called *kinins* are synthesized in mast cells and basophils to produce vasodilation, increased capillary permeability, and bronchoconstriction. Kinins can stimulate vascular endothelium to release vasoactive factors, including prostacyclin, and endothelial-derived relaxing factors such as nitric oxide.

Platelet-Activating Factor

Platelet-activating factor (PAF), an unstored lipid synthesized in activated human mast cells, is a potent biologic material. PAF aggregates and activates human platelets, and perhaps leukocytes, to release inflammatory products. PAF levels were significantly higher in patients with anaphylaxis than in controls, and were correlated with the severity of anaphylaxis.[23]

Recognition of Anaphylaxis

The onset and severity of the reaction relate to the mediator's specific end-organ effects. Antigenic challenge in a sensitized individual usually produces immediate clinical manifestations of anaphylaxis, but the onset may be delayed 2 to 20 minutes.[24–27] The reaction may include some or all of the symptoms and signs listed in Table 9-3. Individuals vary in their manifestations and course of anaphylaxis. A spectrum of reactions exists, ranging from minor clinical changes to the full-blown syndrome leading to death.[24,28] The enigma of anaphylaxis lies in the unpredictability of happening, the severity of the attack, and the lack of prior allergic history.

Non–IgE-Mediated Reactions

Other immunologic and nonimmunologic mechanisms release many of the mediators previously discussed independent of IgE, creating a clinical syndrome identical to anaphylaxis. Specific pathways important in producing the same clinical manifestations are considered later.

Complement Activation

Complement activation follows both immunologic (antibody mediated; i.e., classic pathway) or nonimmunologic (alternative) pathways to include a series of multimolecular, self-assembling proteins that release biologically active complement fragments of C3 and C5.[9,10] C3a and C5a are called *anaphylatoxins* because they release histamine from mast cells and basophils, contract smooth muscle, increase capillary permeability, and cause interleukin synthesis (Table 9-4). C5a interacts with specific high-affinity receptors on PMNs and platelets, causing leukocyte chemotaxis, aggregation, and activation.[9,10] Aggregated leukocytes embolize to various organs, producing microvascular occlusion and liberation of inflammatory products, such as arachidonic acid metabolites, oxygen free radicals, and lysosomal enzymes (Fig. 9-8). Antibodies of the IgG class directed against antigenic determinants or granulocyte surfaces can also produce leukocyte aggregation.[29] These antibodies are called *leukoagglutinins*. Investigators have associated complement activation and PMN aggregation in producing the clinical expression of transfusion reactions, pulmonary vasoconstriction after protamine reactions, adult respiratory distress syndrome, and septic shock.[1]

Table 9-4 Biologic Effects of Anaphylatoxins

Biologic Effects	C3a	C5a
Histamine release	+	+
Smooth muscle contraction	+	+
Increased vascular permeability	+	+
Chemotaxis	+	
Leukocyte and platelet aggregation	+	
Interleukin release	+	+

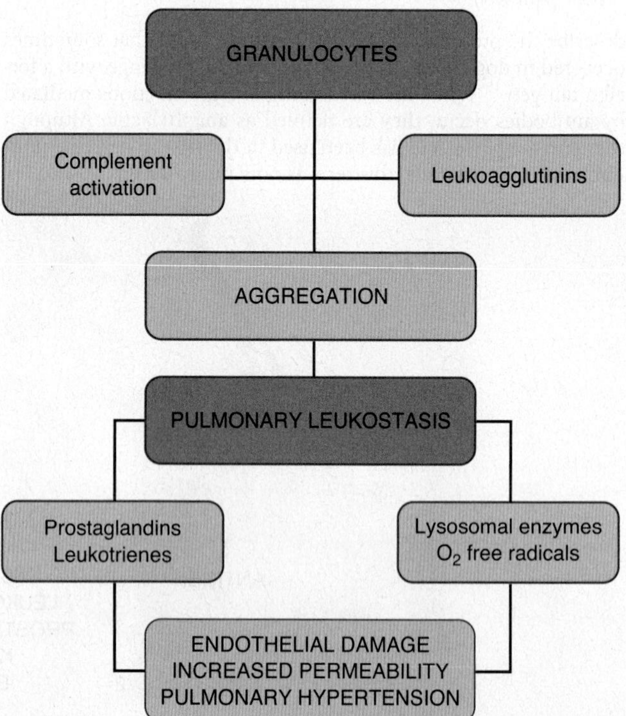

Figure 9-8 Sequence of events producing granulocyte aggregation, pulmonary leukostasis, and cardiopulmonary dysfunction. (Reprinted from Levy JH. *Anaphylactic Reactions in Anesthesia and Intensive Care.* 2nd ed. Butterworth-Heinemann; 1992. Copyright © 1992 Elsevier. With permission.)

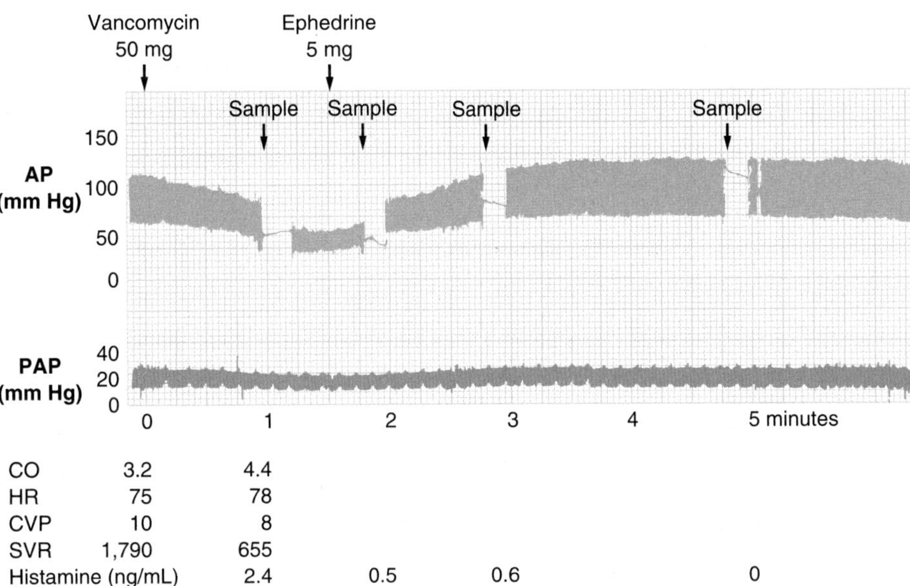

Figure 9-9 Example of an anaphylactic reaction after rapid vancomycin administration in a patient. Hypotension is associated with an increased cardiac output and decreased calculated systemic vascular resistance. Plasma histamine levels 1 minute after vancomycin administration were 2.4 ng/mL and subsequently decreased to zero. The patient was given ephedrine 5 mg, and blood pressure returned to baseline values. AP, arterial pressure; PAP, pulmonary artery pressure; CO, cardiac output; HR, heart rate; CVP, central venous pressure; SVR, systemic vascular resistance. (Reprinted with permission from Levy JH, Kettlekamp N, Goertz P, et al. Histamine release by vancomycin: A mechanism for hypotension in man. *Anesthesiology.* 1987;67:122.)

Angioedema can also occur from allergic reactions but also from complement deficiency states.[11] Hereditary angioedema (HAE) is an example of the complement deficiency state that can present with life-threatening episodes of airway edema and gastrointestinal edema/diarrhea requiring emergency or urgent interventions. Several variants of HAE exist that occur due to unopposed activation of multiple kinins and mediators, including kallikrein and bradykinin, causing increased vascular permeability and edema.[11] Older treatment was anabolic steroids and antifibrinolytics. C1 esterase inhibitor (C1-INH) concentrates are licensed in the United States for use in HAE patients, one for prophylaxis (Cinryze, ViroPharma, administered every 3 or 4 days for routine prophylaxis against angioedema attacks in HAE patients) and the other for treating acute abdominal and facial HAE attacks (Berinert P, CSL Behring).[11] Other novel agents including kinin pathway modulator, ecallantide (Kalbitor, Dyax), and bradykinin antagonists (Icatibant, Shire) are also licensed in the United States for treating HAE attacks.[11]

Nonimmunologic Release of Histamine

6 Many diverse molecules administered during the perioperative period release histamine in a dose-dependent, nonimmunologic fashion (Table 9-5 and Fig. 9-9).[1] The mechanisms involved in nonimmunologic histamine release are not well understood, but represent selective mast cell and not basophil activation (Fig. 9-10).[30,31] Human cutaneous mast cells are the only cell population that releases histamine in response to both drugs and endogenous stimuli (neuropeptides). Nonimmunologic histamine release may involve mast cell activation through specific cell-signaling activation (Fig. 9-11). Different molecular structures release histamine in humans, which suggests that different mechanisms are involved. Histamine release is not dependent on the μ-receptor because fentanyl and sufentanil, the most potent μ-receptor agonists clinically available, do not release histamine in human skin.[32] Although the newer muscle relaxants may be more potent at the neuromuscular junction, drugs that are mast cell degranulators are equally capable of releasing histamine.[33] On an equimolar basis, atracurium is as potent as *d*-tubocurarine or metocurine, in its ability to degranulate mast cells.[33] Although these agents are no longer used clinically, the aminosteroidal agents such as rocuronium and pancuronium at clinically recommended doses have minimal effects on histamine release.[34,35]

Table 9-5 Drugs Capable of Nonimmunologic Histamine Release

Antibiotics (vancomycin, pentamidine)
Basic compounds
Hyperosmotic agents
Muscle relaxants (*d*-tubocurarine, metocurine, atracurium, mivacurium, doxacurium)
Opioids (morphine, meperidine, codeine)

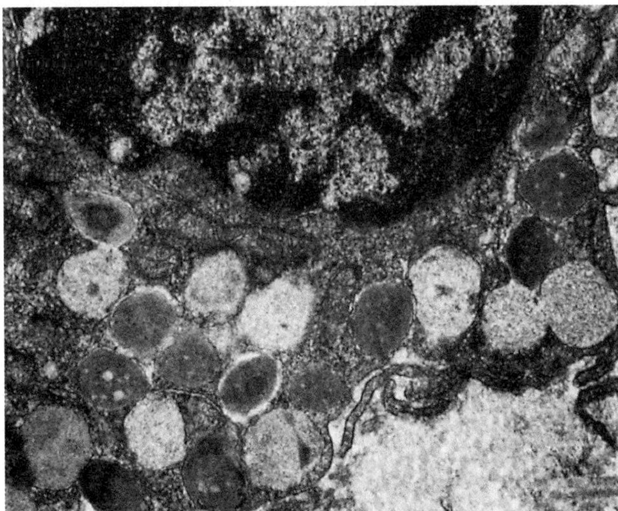

Figure 9-10 Electron micrograph of human cutaneous mast cell after injection of dynorphin, a κ-opioid agonist. The cell outline is rounded and most of the cytoplasmic granules are swollen, exhibiting varying degrees of decreased electron density and flocculence consistent with ongoing degranulation. The perigranular membranes of the adjacent granules at the periphery of the cell are fused to each other and to the plasma membrane. Original magnification × 72,000. (Reprinted from Casale TB, Bowman S, Kaliner M. Induction of human cutaneous mast cell degranulation by opiates and endogenous opioid peptides: Evidence for opiate and nonopiate receptor participation. *J Allergy Clin Immunol.* 1984;73(6):775–781. Copyright © 1984 Elsevier. With permission.)

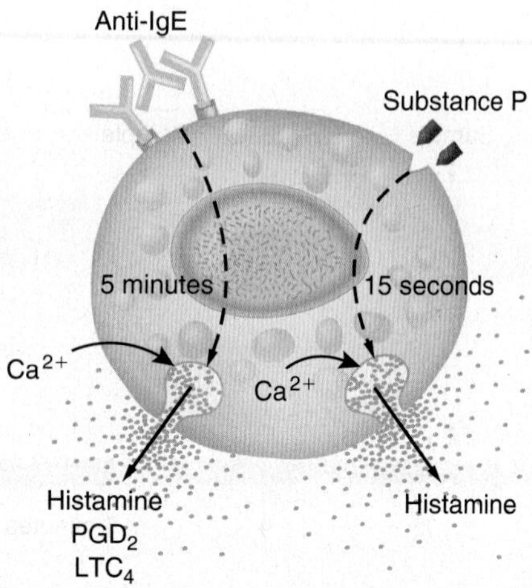

Figure 9-11 Different mechanisms of mediator release from human cutaneous mast cells stimulated immunologically by anti-IgE and by nonimmunologic stimuli with substance P. Anti-IgE stimulation, like antigen stimulation, initiates the release of histamine, prostaglandin D_2 (PGD_2), or leukotriene C_4 (LTC_4) by a mechanism that takes 5 minutes to reach completion and requires the influx of intracellular calcium. Nonimmunologic activation with drugs or substance P releases histamine but not PGD_2 or LTC_4 by a mechanism that is complete within 15 seconds and uses calcium mobilized from intracellular sources. (Adapted with permission from Springer: Caulfield JP, El-Lati S, Thomas G, et al. Dissociated human foreskin mast cells degranulate in response to anti-IgE and substance P. *Lab Invest*. 1990;63(4):502–510.)

Antihistamine pretreatment before administration of drugs known to release histamine in humans does not inhibit histamine release; rather, the antihistamines compete with histamine at the receptor and may attenuate decreases in systemic vascular resistance.[1] However, the effect of any drug on systemic vascular resistance may depend on other factors in addition to histamine release.

Treatment Plan

7 A plan for treating anaphylactic reactions must be established before the event. Airway maintenance, 100% oxygen administration, intravascular volume expansion, and epinephrine are essential to treat the hypotension and hypoxemia that result from vasodilation, increased capillary permeability, and bronchospasm.[1] Table 9-6 lists a protocol for managing anaphylaxis during general anesthesia, with representative doses for a 70-kg adult. Therapy must be titrated to cardiopulmonary stability with monitoring.[1] Severe reactions need aggressive therapy and may be protracted, with persistent hypotension, pulmonary hypertension, lower respiratory obstruction, or laryngeal obstruction that may persist 5 to 32 hours despite vigorous therapy. All patients who have experienced an anaphylactic reaction should be admitted to an intensive care unit for 24 hours of monitoring because manifestations may recur after successful treatment.

Initial Therapy

Although it may not be possible to stop antigen administration, limiting antigen administration may prevent further mast cell and basophil activation.

Maintain Airway and Administer 100% Oxygen

Profound ventilation–perfusion abnormalities producing hypoxemia can occur with anaphylactic reactions. Always administer 100% oxygen with ventilatory support as needed. Arterial blood gas values may be useful to follow during resuscitation.

Table 9-6 Management of Anaphylaxis During General Anesthesia

Initial Therapy
1. Stop administration of antigen
2. Maintain airway and administer 100% O_2
3. Discontinue all anesthetic agents
4. Start intravascular volume expansion (2–4 L of crystalloid/colloid with hypotension)
5. Give epinephrine (5–10 μg IV bolus with hypotension, titrate as needed; 0.1–1.0 mg IV with cardiovascular collapse)

Secondary Treatment
1. Antihistamines (0.5–1 mg/kg diphenhydramine)
2. Catecholamine infusions (starting doses: Epinephrine 4–8 μg/min; norepinephrine 4–8 μg/min; titrated to desired effects)
3. Bronchodilators: Inhaled albuterol, terbutaline, and/or anticholinergic agents with persistent bronchospasm)
4. Corticosteroids (0.25–1 g hydrocortisone; alternatively, 1–2 g methylprednisolone)[a]
5. Airway evaluation (before extubation)
6. Refractory shock: vasopressin and additional monitoring/echocardiography

[a]Methylprednisolone may be the drug of choice if the reaction is suspected to be mediated by complement.
IV, intravenous administration.
Reprinted from Levy JH. *Anaphylactic Reactions in Anesthesia and Intensive Care*. 2nd ed. Butterworth-Heinemann; 1992:162. Copyright © 1992 Elsevier. With permission.

Discontinue All Anesthetic Drugs

Inhalational anesthetic drugs are not the bronchodilators of choice in treating bronchospasm after anaphylaxis, especially during hypotension. These drugs interfere with the body's compensatory response to cardiovascular collapse.

Provide Volume Expansion

Hypovolemia rapidly follows during anaphylactic shock with up to 40% loss of intravascular fluid into the interstitial space during reactions. Therefore, volume expansion is important with epinephrine in correcting the acute hypotension. Initially, 2 to 4 L of lactated Ringer's solution, or colloid or normal saline, should be administered, considering that an additional 25 to 50 mL/kg may be necessary if hypotension persists. Refractory hypotension after volume and epinephrine administration requires additional hemodynamic monitoring. The use of transesophageal echocardiography for rapid assessment of intraventricular volume and ventricular function, and to determine other occult causes of acute cardiovascular dysfunction, can be important for accurate assessment of intravascular volume and guidance of rational therapeutic interventions.[1] Fulminant noncardiogenic pulmonary edema with loss of intravascular volume can occur after anaphylaxis. This condition requires intravascular volume repletion with careful hemodynamic monitoring until the capillary defect improves. Colloid volume expansion has not proved to be more effective than crystalloid volume expansion for treating anaphylactic shock.

Administer Epinephrine

Epinephrine is the drug of choice when resuscitating patients during anaphylactic shock. α-Adrenergic effects vasoconstrict to reverse hypotension; β_2-receptor stimulation bronchodilates and inhibits mediator release by increasing cyclic adenosine monophosphate (cAMP) in mast cells and basophils. The route of epinephrine administration and the dose depend on the patient's condition. Rapid and timely intervention is important when treating anaphylaxis. Furthermore, patients under general anesthesia may have altered sympathoadrenergic responses to acute anaphylactic shock, whereas the patient under spinal or epidural anesthesia may be partially sympathectomized and may need even larger doses of catecholamines.

In hypotensive patients, 5- to 10-μg boluses of epinephrine should be administered intravenously and incrementally titrated to restore blood pressure. (This dose of epinephrine can be obtained with 0.05 to 0.1 mL of a 1:10,000 dilution [100 μg/mL] or by mixing 2 mg epinephrine with 250 mL of fluid to yield an 8 μg/mL solution.) Additional volume and incrementally increased doses of epinephrine should be administered until hypotension is corrected. Although infusion is an ideal method of administering epinephrine, it is usually impossible to infuse the drug through peripheral intravenous access lines during acute volume resuscitation. With cardiovascular collapse, full intravenous cardiopulmonary resuscitative doses of epinephrine, 0.1 to 1.0 mg, should be administered and repeated until hemodynamic stability resumes. Patients with laryngeal edema without hypotension should receive subcutaneous epinephrine. Epinephrine should not be administered IV to patients with normal blood pressures.

Secondary Treatment

Antihistamines

Because H_1 receptors mediate many of the adverse effects of histamine, the intravenous administration of 0.5 to 1 mg/kg of an H_1 antagonist, such as diphenhydramine, may be useful in treating acute anaphylaxis. Antihistamines do not inhibit anaphylactic reactions or histamine release, but compete with histamine at receptor sites. H_1 antagonists are indicated in all forms of anaphylaxis. The H_1 antagonists available for parenteral administration may have antidopaminergic effects and should be given slowly to prevent precipitous hypotension in potentially hypovolemic patients.[1] The indications for administering an H_2 antagonist once anaphylaxis has occurred remain unclear.

Catecholamines

Epinephrine infusions may be useful in patients with persistent hypotension or bronchospasm after initial resuscitation.[1] Epinephrine infusions should be started at 0.05 to 0.1 μg/kg/min (5 to 10 μg/min) and titrated to correct hypotension. Norepinephrine infusions may be needed in patients with refractory hypotension due to decreased systemic vascular resistance. It may be started at 0.05 to 0.1 μg/kg/min (5 to 10 μg/min) and adjusted to correct hypotension.[1]

Bronchodilators

Inhaled β-adrenergic agents include inhaled albuterol or terbutaline if bronchospasm is a major feature.[36] Inhaled ipratropium may be especially useful for the treatment of bronchospasm in patients receiving β-adrenergic blockers.[36] Special adaptors allow administration of bronchodilators through the endotracheal tube.

Corticosteroids

Corticosteroids have anti-inflammatory effects mediated by multiple mechanisms, including altering the activation and migration of other inflammatory cells (i.e., PMNs) after an acute reaction. Consider infusing high-dose corticosteroids early in therapy, although beneficial effects are delayed at least 4 to 6 hours.[36] Despite their unproven usefulness in treating acute reactions, they are often administered as adjuncts to therapy when refractory bronchospasm or refractory shock occurs after resuscitative therapy. Although the exact corticosteroid dose and preparation are unclear, investigators have recommended 0.25 to 1 g intravenously of hydrocortisone in IgE-mediated reactions. Alternatively, 1 to 2 g of methylprednisolone (30 to 35 mg/kg) intravenously may be useful in reactions believed to be complement mediated, such as catastrophic pulmonary vasoconstriction after protamine transfusion reactions. Administering corticosteroids after an anaphylactic reaction may also be important in attenuating the late-phase reactions reported occurring 12 to 24 hours after anaphylaxis.

Airway Evaluation

Because profound laryngeal edema can occur, the airway should be evaluated before extubation of the trachea. Persistent facial edema suggests airway edema. The tracheas of these patients should remain intubated until the edema subsides. Developing a significant air leak after endotracheal tube cuff deflation and before extubation of the trachea is useful in assessing airway patency. If there is any question of airway edema, direct laryngoscopy should be performed before the trachea is extubated.

Refractory Hypotension

Vasopressin is an important drug for refractory shock, including vasodilatory shock associated with anaphylaxis. Vasodilatory shock is characterized by hypotension association with high cardiac output and is thought to be due to the multiple activation of vasodilator mechanisms and the inability of α-adrenergic mechanisms to compensate. Starting doses to consider are 0.01 units/min as an infusion. Vasopressin may attenuate pathologic-induced vasodilation and is used extensively in patients who are vasoplegia following mediator-induced septic shock. Further, additional monitoring, including echocardiography should be considered in patients with refractory hypotension to further evaluate cardiac function or hypovolemia.

Perioperative Management of the Patient with Allergies

Allergic drug reactions account for 6% to 10% of all adverse reactions, and the risk of an allergic drug reaction occurring is approximately 1% to 3% for most drugs, and around 5% of adults in the United States may be allergic to one or more drugs.[37–39] Unfortunately, patients often refer to adverse drug effects as being allergic in nature. For example, opioid administration can produce nausea, vomiting, or even local release of histamine along the vein of administration. Patients will say that they are "allergic" to a specific drug when their adverse reaction is independent of allergy. Nearly 15% of adults in the United States believe that they are allergic to specific medication(s) and may be denied treatment with an indicated drug. To understand allergic reactions, the spectrum of adverse reactions to drugs needs to be considered.

Predictable adverse drug reactions account for about 80% of adverse drug effects. They are often dose dependent, related to known pharmacologic actions of the drug, and typically occur in normal patients. Most serious, predictable adverse drug reactions are toxic and are directly related to the drug in the body (overdosage) or an unintentional route of administration (e.g., lidocaine-induced seizures or cardiovascular collapse). Side effects are the most common adverse drug reactions and are undesirable pharmacologic actions of the drugs occurring at usual prescribed dosages. Most anesthetic drugs present multiple side effects that can produce precipitous hypotension. For example, morphine dilates the venous capacitance bed, thereby decreasing preload; releases histamine from cutaneous mast cells, thereby producing arterial and venous dilation; slows the heart rate; and decreases sympathetic tone. However, the net effects of morphine on blood pressure and myocardial function depend on the patient's blood volume, sympathetic tone, and ventricular function. Hypotension rapidly develops in a volume-depleted trauma patient in pain who is given morphine. Drug interactions also represent important predictable adverse drug reactions. Intravenous fentanyl administration to a patient who has just received intravenous benzodiazepines or other sedative-hypnotic drugs may produce precipitous hypotension that results from decreased sympathetic tone or direct vasodilation from propofol administration.[40] This represents a dose-dependent, predictable adverse drug reaction independent of allergy.

Unpredictable adverse drug reactions are usually dose-independent and usually not related to the drug's pharmacologic actions, but are often related to the immunologic response (allergy) of the individual. On occasion, adverse reactions can be related to genetic differences (i.e., idiosyncratic) in a susceptible individual with an isolated genetic enzyme deficiency. In most allergic drug reactions, an immunologic mechanism is present or, more often, presumed. Determining whether the causing event involves a reaction between the drug or drug metabolites with drug-specific antibodies or sensitized T lymphocytes is often impractical. Without direct immunologic evidence, which may be helpful in distinguishing an allergic reaction from other adverse reactions, including allergic reactions that occur in only a small percentage of patients receiving the drug, the clinical manifestations do not resemble known pharmacologic actions. In the absence of prior drug exposure, allergic symptoms rarely appear after less than 1 week of continuous treatment. After sensitization, the reaction develops rapidly on reexposure to the drug. In general, drugs that have been administered without complications for several months or longer are rarely responsible for producing drug allergy. The time between exposure to the drug and noticed manifestations is often the most vital information in deciding which drugs administered were the cause of a suspected allergic reaction.

Although the reaction may produce a life-threatening response in the cardiopulmonary system (anaphylaxis), various cutaneous manifestations, fever, and pulmonary reactions have been attributed to drug hypersensitivity. Usually, the reaction may be reproduced by small doses of the suspected drug or other agents having similar or cross-reacting chemical structures. On occasion, drug-specific antibodies or lymphocytes have been identified that react with the suspected drug, although the relationship is seldom diagnostically useful in practice. Even when an immune response to a drug is demonstrated, it may not be associated with a clinical allergic reaction. As with adverse drug reactions in general, the reaction usually subsides within several days of discontinuation of the drug.

Immunologic Mechanisms of Drug Allergy

Different immunologic responses to any antigen can occur. Drugs have been associated with all the immunologic mechanisms proposed by Gell and Coombs. Although more than one mechanism may contribute to a particular reaction, any one can occur. Penicillin may produce different reactions in different patients or a spectrum of reactions in the same patient. In one patient, penicillin can produce anaphylaxis (type I reaction), hemolytic anemia (type II reaction), serum sickness (type III reaction), and contact dermatitis (type IV reaction).[5,6] Therefore, any one antigen has the ability to produce a diffuse spectrum of allergic responses in humans. Why some patients have localized rashes or angioedema in response to penicillin whereas others suffer complete cardiopulmonary collapse is unknown. Most anesthetic drugs and agents administered perioperatively have been reported to produce anaphylactic reactions (Table 9-7).[31,39] Muscle relaxants are the most common drugs responsible for evoking intraoperative allergic reactions. In this regard, there is cross-sensitivity between succinylcholine and the nondepolarizing muscle relaxants. Unexplained intraoperative cardiovascular collapse has been attributed to anaphylaxis triggered by latex (natural rubber).

Table 9-7 Agents Implicated in Allergic Reactions During Anesthesia

Anesthetic Agents
Induction agents (cremophor-solubilized drugs, barbiturates, etomidate, propofol)
Local anesthetics (para-aminobenzoic ester agents)
Muscle relaxants (succinylcholine, pancuronium, *d*-tubocurarine, metocurine, atracurium, vecuronium, mivacurium)
Opioids (meperidine, morphine, fentanyl)
Other Agents
Antibiotics (cephalosporins, penicillin, quinolones, sulfonamides, vancomycin)
Aprotinin
Blood products (whole blood, packed cells, plasma/fresh frozen plasma, platelets, cryoprecipitate, fibrin glue, immunoglobulins)
Bone cement
Chlorhexidine
Chymopapain
Corticosteroids
Cyclosporine (intravenous)
Drug additives (preservatives)
Furosemide
Heparin
Insulin
Isosulfan blue dye and other vital dyes
Mannitol
Nonsteroidal anti-inflammatory drugs
Protamine
Radiocontrast agents
Latex (natural rubber)
Streptokinase
Sugammadex
Vascular graft material
Colloid volume expanders (dextrans, protein fractions, albumin, hydroxyethyl starch)

Reprinted from Levy JH. *Anaphylactic Reactions in Anesthesia and Intensive Care*. 2nd ed. Butterworth-Heinemann; 1992. Copyright © 1992 Elsevier. With permission.

Life-threatening allergic reactions are potentially thought to occur more likely in patients with a history of allergy, atopy, or asthma, although this concept is also controversial and in part based on older data.[41] Nevertheless, because the incidence is low, the history is not a reliable predictor that an allergic reaction will occur and does not mandate that such patients should be investigated or pretreated or that specific drugs be selected or avoided. Although different mechanisms have been proposed, no one theory has been proved. The drugs and foreign substances listed in Table 9-7 may have both immunologic and nonimmunologic mechanisms for adverse drug reactions in humans.

Evaluation of Patients with Allergic Reactions

Identifying the drug responsible for a suspected allergic reaction depends on circumstantial evidence, suggesting the temporal sequence of drug administration. Conventional *in vivo* and *in vitro* methods of diagnosing allergic reactions to most anesthetic drugs are unavailable or not applicable. The most important factor in diagnosis is the awareness of the physician that an untoward event may be related to a drug the patient received. The physician must always be aware of the capacity of any drug to produce an allergic reaction. The history is important when evaluating whether an adverse drug reaction is allergic and whether the drug can be readministered. Although a prior allergic reaction to the drug in question is important, this is rarely the case. Direct challenge of a patient with a test dose of the drug is the only way to prove a reaction, but this is potentially dangerous and not recommended. Although anesthesiologists often administer small test doses of anesthetic drugs, these are pharmacologic test doses and have nothing to do with immunologic dosages. The demonstration of drug-specific IgE antibodies is accepted as evidence that the patient may be at risk for anaphylaxis if the drug is administered. Different clinical tests are of historical interest, and few of them are available to confirm or diagnose drug allergy, but these are considered in the following section.

Testing for Allergy

8 After an anaphylactic reaction, it is important to identify the causative agent to prevent readministration. When one particular drug has been administered, and there is a clear correlation between the time of administration and the occurrence of a reaction, testing may be unnecessary, and general avoidance of the drug should be instituted. However, when patients have simultaneously received multiple drugs (e.g., an opioid, muscle relaxant, hypnotic, and antibiotic), it is often difficult to prove which particular drug caused the reaction. Further, the reaction might have been caused by the vehicle or by one of the preservatives. For patients who want to know which drug was responsible and for patients scheduled for subsequent procedures, some degree of allergy evaluation should be undertaken to evaluate the drug at risk. Unfortunately, few *laboratory* tests exist for anesthetic drugs; therefore, the available allergy tests are discussed.

Leukocyte Histamine Release

Leukocyte histamine is performed by incubating the patient's leukocytes with the offending drug and measuring histamine release as a marker for basophil activation, although false-positive results can occur. This test is not easy to perform, although variations allow the use of whole blood instead of isolated PMNs, and is generally not available nor used.

In Vitro Immunologic Testing

The enzyme-linked immunosorbent assay (ELISA) measures antigen-specific antibodies. The ELISA evaluates immunospecific IgE directed against the antigen in question by adding an anti-IgE coupled to an enzyme such as peroxidase that acts as a chromogen. A colorless substrate is acted on by peroxidase to produce a colored byproduct. The ELISA has been used to prove IgE antibodies to proteins such as protamine, has been developed to screen for other antibodies to diverse agents, and has become the mainstay of immunologic testing. Although antibodies can occur, patients may be asymptomatic. An older test previously used was the radioallergosorbent test (RAST), which used radiolabeled antibodies directed against human IgE and was counted in a scintillation counter, and has been largely replaced by ELISA assays. Major limitations to in vitro immunologic testing too many anesthetic drugs include the commercial availability of the drug prepared as an antigen.

Intradermal Testing (Skin Testing)

Skin testing is the method most often used in patients after anaphylactic reaction to anesthetic drugs after the history has suggested the relevant antigens for testing.[42] Within minutes after antigen introduction, histamine released from cutaneous mast cells causes vasodilation (flare) and localized edema from increased vascular permeability (wheal). Fisher suggested that this is a simple, safe, and useful method of establishing a diagnosis in most cases of anaphylactic reactions occurring in the perioperative period. If the strict protocols established by Fisher are used, intradermal reactions are helpful.[42] Intradermal testing is of no value in reactions to contrast media or colloid volume expanders. Cross-sensitivity between drugs of similar structures can often be evaluated based on skin testing.

Agents Implicated in Allergic Reactions

Any drug or biologic agent can cause anaphylaxis in a patient. However, the agents most often implicated in the perioperative period include antibiotics, blood products, chlorhexidine, neuromuscular blocking drugs (NMBDs), polypeptides (aprotinin, latex, and protamine), and intravascular volume expanders. Most of the information about perioperative anaphylaxis is from Australia, Europe, the United Kingdom, and New Zealand, where centers have existed for many years to investigate perioperative anaphylaxis when it occurs.[43–48] In one of the largest reports, perioperative anaphylaxis was evaluated over an 8-year period from 1997 to 2004 in France. Among the 2,516 patients with anaphylaxis, IgE-mediated reactions occurred in 1,816 cases (72.2%). The most common causes for the IgE-mediated events were NMBDs in 58% (n = 1067), latex in 19.6% (n = 316), and antibiotics in 12.8% (n = 236).[49] One of the concerns regarding NMBA allergy is that if patients are allergic to a muscle relaxant, there is a potential for cross-reactivity because of the similarity of the active site, a quaternary ammonium molecule, among the different types of relaxants, and alternatives cannot be chosen without some degree of immunologic testing. Because of the different immune and nonimmune causes of reported anaphylactic reactions, the perioperative incidence varies worldwide, with reports of 1 in 1,250 to 1 in 18,600 procedures with inconsistency about the underlying agent responsible. As noted, NMBA reactions are common in France but not in Denmark or the United States.[50]

From the U.S./North American perspective, only a few reports note either the incidence or agents implicated for perioperative anaphylaxis. However, European reports suggest the most frequent agent reported for perioperative IgE-mediated anaphylaxis is NMBAs.[51] A report from 2011 in the United States examined a skin test database of 38 patients with perioperative anaphylaxis who were tested to medications implicated in the reactions.[52] The history obtained by an allergist, skin test results, and tryptase measurements were reported.[52] Of note, 40% of the surgical procedures were aborted, and 58% of events resulted in intensive care unit admissions, suggesting the severity of the responses.[52] Of the 38 patients, 18 were considered IgE-mediated reactions by skin testing, 6 were non–IgE-mediated anaphylactic reactions determined by elevated tryptase levels and negative skin testing, and 14 were probable non–IgE-mediated anaphylactic reactions because tryptase levels were normal or not obtained and skin testing was negative. Of the IgE-mediated anaphylactic reactions, antibiotics were the causative agents in half of the patients, while NMBAs were implicated solely as a likely causative agent in only one reaction. The authors noted causative agents could not be determined in the other half of the patients.[52] The authors identified only one true IgE-mediated reaction to an NMBA; however, another patient had positive skin tests to three agents, including vecuronium, propofol, and cefazolin, making the diagnosis uncertain. A previous Danish study reported 68 patients, of which 36 underwent complete investigations with in vitro testing and skin testing, and found that only one patient tested positive for NMBAs

(4.8%: 1/21). At the same time, chlorhexidine accounted for 19.1% of reactions and antibiotics, 14.3%.[53] In the current study, chlorhexidine was tested in only 4% of cases and may account for some of the undiagnosed reactions with elevated tryptase.[52]

Because of this information, antibiotics, latex, and NMBAs will be considered in more detail, along with local anesthetic (LA) agents.

Antibiotics

Most surgical patients receive an antibiotic that includes a cephalosporin or vancomycin for prophylaxis. Despite their widespread use, the incidence of antibiotic allergy and its reported prevalence varies widely, as cutaneous manifestations are often the presenting reaction.[39] The risk of anaphylaxis to penicillins is low, as most of the widely quoted data is based on older reports, and penicillin per se is rarely used.[38,39,54–57] Further, anaphylaxis to cephalosporins can occur independently without a penicillin allergy, and antibiotics are the most common agent implicated in perioperative anaphylaxis.[52,55] In surgical patients, vancomycin will often be used for prophylaxis in patients with a history of penicillin allergy, but vancomycin is a potent histamine-releasing agent that can cause severe hypotension and flushing on administration, especially with rapid infusion.[30,31]

As reviewed previously, managing the patient with a penicillin allergy history when the surgeon requests cephalosporin administration is still unclear based on reported data.[1,55–57] Although previous reports suggest cross-reactivity to cephalosporins among penicillin-allergic patients is high and suggest choosing another agent, a practice that developed from case reports of anaphylaxis following first-generation cephalosporins together with in vitro and skin testing, which showed extensive cross-reactivity between penicillins and first-generation cephalosporins. However, the risk of acute cephalosporin reactions among patients with positive penicillin skin tests is reported to be ~4.4%, compared with 0.6% among patients with negative penicillin skin tests.[56,57] Anaphylactic reactors were selectively omitted from these open studies. Further, an allergic reaction to a cephalosporin may occur independently of prior penicillin sensitization. Although most patients who have a history of penicillin allergy will tolerate cephalosporins, indiscriminate administration cannot be recommended, especially for patients who have had serious acute reactions to any β-lactam antibiotic.[1,39] Penicillin skin testing, when available, can be useful in identifying the 85% of patients with histories of penicillin allergy who no longer have (or never had) IgE antibodies to major and minor determinants and are therefore at negligible risk of cephalosporin reactions. For the remaining patients who are skin test positive, gradual escalation of the first dose of a cephalosporin under careful observation will further mitigate against uncommon but potentially serious acute reactions.

The risk versus benefit of specific antibiotic use should be considered with known antibiotic allergies. Often for surgical wound prophylaxis, there is flexibility in the choice of specific antibiotics compared to critically ill hospitalized patients who require specific antibiotic treatment. Potential management strategies suggest if a patient has a penicillin allergy history consistent with anaphylaxis and penicillin skin testing is unavailable, then cephalosporins should be used with caution, with graded dose escalation of the first dose. A patient who has experienced an allergic reaction to a specific cephalosporin should probably not receive that cephalosporin again. However, the risk of an acute reaction when a different cephalosporin is administered appears to be low, but systemic evaluations of reaction risks when administering other cephalosporins or β-lactam antibiotics to patients with IgE antibodies to a particular cephalosporin are not available. Unfortunately, patient histories are often unreliable in this circumstance.[1,38,39,54–57]

Latex Allergy

For the anesthesiologist, latex represents an environmental agent often implicated as an important cause of perioperative anaphylaxis (NICV 9-3). Latex is the milky sap derived from the tree *Hevea brasiliensis*, to which multiple agents, including preservatives, accelerators, and antioxidants, are added to make the final rubber product. Latex is present in a variety of different products. Latex allergy is an IgE-dependent immediate hypersensitivity reaction to latex proteins. The first case of an allergic reaction because of latex was reported in 1979 and was manifested by contact urticaria. In 1989, the first reports of intraoperative anaphylaxis because of latex were reported.

Health care workers and children with spina bifida, urogenital abnormalities, or certain food allergies have also been recognized as people at increased risk for anaphylaxis to latex. Brown and colleagues reported a 24% incidence of irritant or contact dermatitis and a 12.5% incidence of latex-specific IgE positivity in anesthesiologists. Of this group, 10% were clinically asymptomatic, although IgE positive.[58] A history of atopy was also a significant risk factor for latex sensitization. Brown and colleagues suggested that these people are in their early stages of sensitization, and perhaps, by avoiding latex exposure, their progression to symptomatic disease can be prevented.[58] Patients allergic to bananas, avocados, and kiwis have also been reported to have antibodies that cross-react with latex.[59,60] Multiple attempts are being made to reduce latex exposure to both health care workers and patients. If latex allergy occurs, there should be strict avoidance of latex from gloves and other sources, following recommendations as reported by Holzman.[61,62] Although latex was previously a common environmental antigen, ongoing effort by suppliers of hospital equipment has significantly reduced latex exposure in recent years.

More importantly, anesthesiologists must be prepared to treat the life-threatening cardiopulmonary collapse that occurs in anaphylaxis as previously discussed. The most important preventive therapy is to avoid antigen exposure; although clinicians have used pretreatment with antihistamine (diphenhydramine and cimetidine) and corticosteroids, there are no data in the literature to suggest that pretreatment prevents anaphylaxis or decreases its severity.[1] Patients in whom latex allergy is suspected should be referred to an allergist for proper evaluation and potential testing for definitive diagnosis. When this is not possible, patients should be treated as if they were latex allergic, and the antigen avoided. Patients with a documented history of latex allergy should wear Medic Alert bracelets.

Local Anesthetics

Skin testing to LAs is considered a direct challenge or provocative dose testing. LA drugs are injected in increasing quantities under controlled circumstances. This testing decides if the person can safely receive amide derivatives (e.g., lidocaine) and can also be used to decide if the person is sensitive to *para*-aminobenzoic ester agents (e.g., procaine, tetracaine). Because the immediate hypersensitivity reactions to LAs are unknown, they are commonly regarded as "pseudoallergic" or "nonimmune type" anaphylaxis, as immunologically mediated reactions have rarely been observed with positive skin-prick tests.[63] Other ingredients in LA preparations have to be considered as elicitors; for example, preservatives like benzoates or sulfites or latex contaminants in injection bottles. Practical management of patients with a history of LA reaction includes a careful allergy history and skin-prick and intradermal tests. Undiluted LA solutions may elicit false-positive intradermal test reactions. If prick and intradermal tests are negative, the procedure of subcutaneous provocation testing is applied in a placebo-controlled manner. When patients are constantly reacting to placebo, a regimen of "reverse placebo provocation" with injection of an LA (verum) is applied while the patient is informed about receiving placebo in order to "rule out psychosomatic involvement." With this regimen, it is possible to eliminate anxiousness and fear, and the patient has proof that he has tolerated the respective LA substance.[63]

However, the diagnostic evaluation of patients with suspected allergy to LAs who have experienced a reaction remains controversial. One of the largest reports of skin testing for LA allergy evaluation is a retrospective chart review of patients following LA skin testing who underwent prick and intradermal skin testing followed by incremental subcutaneous and open subcutaneous challenge.[64] A total of 178 patients underwent 227 LA skin tests, of which 220 (97%) were negative, and 214 (97%) had negative challenge or probable non–IgE-mediated events during challenge while three patients with six negative skin tests had a local reaction during the challenge. Only seven skin tests per five patients met the criteria for a positive skin test, and one patient had a skin reaction without systemic effects, three patients had a negative subcutaneous challenge, and one patient did not undergo a challenge. Overall, 98% of patients receiving Las after open subcutaneous challenge tolerated the medications. The negative predictive value of the LA skin test was 97% with few positive skin tests. Positive LA skin tests are uncommon and the LA skin tests have an excellent negative predictive value.[64]

Neuromuscular Blocking and Reversal Agents

10 NMBAs have several unique molecular features that make them potential antigens. All NMBAs are functionally divalent and are thus capable of cross-linking cell-surface IgE and causing mediator release from mast cells and basophils without binding or haptenating to larger carrier molecules. NMBAs have also been implicated in epidemiologic studies of anesthetic drug-induced anaphylaxis. Epidemiologic data from France suggest that NMBAs are responsible for 62% to 81% of reactions, depending on the time period evaluated. NMBA allergy is more frequently reported in females, with 75% of the reactions occurring in women.[3,33]

In more recent years, NMBAs, especially steroid-derived agents, have been reported as potential causative agents of anaphylactic reactions during anesthesia. The data associating NMBAs in the most recent reports from France are mainly based on skin testing; however, studies have previously reported that steroidal-derived NMBAs and other molecules produce false-positive skin tests (i.e., weal and flare). One of the major problems is that anaphylaxis to NMBAs is rare in the United States but has been reported more often in Europe. Although suggestions have been made that this is because of underreporting, the severity of anaphylaxis and its sequelae to produce adverse outcomes make this unlikely based on the current medicolegal climate that exists in the United States. One of the only ways to explain this widely divergent perspective is to understand how the diagnosis is made, because the recommended threshold test concentrations have not been defined, resulting in unreliable results.

We have previously reported that steroid-derived agents can induce positive weal and flare responses independent of mast cell degranulation, even at low concentrations, following intradermal injection. This effect is likely because of a direct effect on the cutaneous vasculature that occurs for most NMBAs at concentrations as low as 10^{-5} M, using intradermal skin tests in 30 volunteers. A positive cutaneous reaction without evidence of mast cell degranulation was noted at low concentrations (100 μg/mL) of rocuronium in almost all the volunteers. We have used intradermal injections to compare cutaneous effects of anesthetic and other agents.

Other investigators have also reported similar results. Because prick tests are often used for authenticating NMBAs as causative drugs, Dhonneur and colleagues evaluated 30 volunteers, using prick testing. Each subject received 10 prick tests (50 μL) on both forearms.[65] The investigators studied the weal and flare responses to prick tests with rocuronium and vecuronium, using four dilutions (1/1,000, 1/100, 1/10, and 1) and two controls, and measured weal and flare immediately after and at 15 minutes. They noted 50% and 40% of the subjects had a positive skin reaction to undiluted rocuronium and vecuronium, respectively. To avoid false-positive results, they suggested that prick testing with rocuronium and vecuronium should be performed in subjects who have experienced a hypersensitivity reaction during anesthesia, with concentrations below that commonly inducing positive reactions in anesthesia-naive, healthy subjects (i.e., for men in a dilution of 1/10 and for women in a dilution of 1/100).[65] Guidelines for prick testing that Have international agreement need to be established. Many of these differences may explain the various incidences of allergy to NMBAs among countries. Concentration–skin response curves to rocuronium and vecuronium suggest that prick tests should be performed with dilution of the commercially available preparation. Female volunteers significantly ($P < .01$) reacted to lower vecuronium and rocuronium concentrations more frequently than males. In female subjects, positive skin reactions were reported with dilutions of 1/100 of both relaxants. In male subjects, positive skin reactions were noted with the undiluted concentration, except for one volunteer who reacted to rocuronium (1/10 dilution).[65] Sugammadex, a novel cyclodextrin structure that binds NMBAs for reversal, has also been reported to produce anaphylaxis.[66]

Summary

Although the immune system functions to provide host defense, it can respond inappropriately to produce hypersensitivity or allergic reactions. A spectrum of life-threatening allergic reactions to any drug or agent can occur in the perioperative period. The enigma of these reactions lies in their unpredictable nature. Certain patients undergoing high-risk procedures with multiple blood product exposures are also at higher risk. However, a high index of suspicion, prompt recognition, and appropriate and aggressive therapy can help avoid a disastrous outcome.

For further review and interactivities, please see the videos and narrative interactive clinical vignettes (NICVs) accessible in the complimentary eBook bundled with this text. Access instructions are located on the inside front cover.

REFERENCES

1. Levy JH, Adkinson NF Jr. Anaphylaxis during cardiac surgery: implications for clinicians. *Anesth Analg*. 2008;106:392–403.
2. Kay AB. Allergy and allergic diseases. Two parts. *N Engl J Med*. 2001;344:30–37; 2001;344:109–113.
3. Muraro A, Worm M, Alviani C, et al. EAACI guidelines: anaphylaxis (2021 update). *Allergy*. 2022;77:357–377.
4. Iba T, Levy JH. Inflammation and thrombosis: roles of neutrophils, platelets and endothelial cells and their interactions in thrombus formation during sepsis. *J Thromb Haemost*. 2018;16:231–241.
5. Delves PJ, Roitt IM. The immune system. Two parts. *N Engl J Med*. 2000;343:37–49. *N Engl J Med*. 2000;343:108–117.
6. Reber LL, Hernandez JD, Galli SJ. The pathophysiology of anaphylaxis. *J Allergy Clin Immunol*. 2017;140:335–348.
7. Iba T, Connors JM, Levy JH. The coagulopathy, endotheliopathy, and vasculitis of COVID-19. *Inflamm Res*. 2020;69:1181–1189.

8. Levy JH, Iba T, Gardiner EE. Endothelial injury in COVID-19 and acute infections: putting the pieces of the puzzle together. *Arterioscler Thromb Vasc Biol*. 2021;41:1774–1776.
9. Cianferoni A. Non-IgE-mediated anaphylaxis. *J Allergy Clin Immunol*. 2021;147:1123–1131.
10. Walport MJ. Complement. Two parts. *N Engl J Med*. 2001;344:1058–1066, 1140–1144.
11. Levy JH, Freiberger DJ, Roback J. Hereditary angioedema: current and emerging treatment options. *Anesth Analg*. 2010;110:1271–1280.
12. Stevenson GW, Hall SC, Rudnick S, Seleny FL, Stevenson HC. The effect of anesthetic agents on the human immune response. *Anesthesiology*. 1990;72:542–552.
13. Sampson HA, Muñoz-Furlong A, Bock SA, et al. Symposium on the definition and management of anaphylaxis: summary report. *J Allergy Clin Immunol*. 2005;115:584–591.
14. Mertes PM, Laxenaire MC, Alla F; Groupe d'Etudes des Réactions Anaphylactoïdes Peranesthésiques. Anaphylactic and anaphylactoid reactions occurring during anesthesia in France in 1999–2000. *Anesthesiology*. 2003;99:536–545.
15. Portier P, Richet CR. De l'action anaphylactique de certains venins. *C R Soc Biol*. 1902;54: 170–172.
16. MacGlashan D Jr. Histamine: a mediator of inflammation. *J Allergy Clin Immunol*. 2003;112: S53–S59.
17. Kalesnikoff J, Galli SJ. Anaphylaxis: mechanisms of mast cell activation. *Chem Immunol Allergy*. 2011;95:45–66.
18. Lieberman P, Garvey LH. Mast cells and anaphylaxis. *Curr Allergy Asthma Rep*. 2016;16:20.
19. Marone G, Bova M, Detoraki A, Onorati AM, Rossi FW, Spadaro G. The human heart as a shock organ in anaphylaxis. *Novartis Found Symp*. 2004;257:133–149.
20. Majno G, Palade GE. Studies on inflammation. 1. The effect of histamine and serotonin on vascular permeability: an electron microscopic study. *J Biophys Biochem Cytol*. 1961;11:571–605.
21. Majno G, Palade GE, Schoefl GI. Studies on inflammation. II. The site of action of histamine and serotonin along the vascular tree: a topographic study. *J Biophys Biochem Cytol*. 1961;11:607–626.
22. Nguyen SMT, Rupprecht CP, Haque A, Pattanaik D, Yusin J, Krishnaswamy G. Mechanisms governing anaphylaxis: inflammatory cells, mediators, endothelial gap junctions and beyond. *Int J Mol Sci*. 2021;22:7785.
23. Vadas P, Gold M, Perelman B, et al. Platelet-activating factor, PAF acetylhydrolase, and severe anaphylaxis. *N Engl J Med*. 2008;358:28–35.
24. Pumphrey RS. Lessons for management of anaphylaxis from a study of fatal reactions. *Clin Exp Allergy*. 2000;30:1144–1150.
25. Pumphrey R. Anaphylaxis: can we tell who is at risk of a fatal reaction? *Curr Opin Allergy Clin Immunol*. 2004;4:285–290.
26. Pumphrey RSH. Fatal anaphylaxis in the UK, 1992–2001. *Novartis Found Symp*. 2004;257: 116–128.
27. Delage C, Irey NS. Anaphylactic deaths: a clinicopathologic study of 43 cases. *J Forensic Sci*. 1972;17:525–540.
28. Pumphrey RS, Roberts IS. Postmortem findings after fatal anaphylactic reactions. *J Clin Pathol*. 2000;53:273–276.
29. Sheppard CA, Lögdberg LE, Zimring JC, Hillyer CD. Transfusion-related acute lung injury. *Hematol Oncol Clin North Am*. 2007;21:163–176.
30. Veien M, Szlam F, Holden JT, Yamaguchi K, Denson DD, Levy JH. Mechanisms of nonimmunological histamine and tryptase release from human cutaneous mast cells. *Anesthesiology*. 2000;92:1074–1081.
31. Levy JH, Kettlekamp N, Goertz P, Hermens J, Hirshman CA. Histamine release by vancomycin: a mechanism for hypotension in man. *Anesthesiology*. 1987;67:122–125.
32. Levy JH, Brister NW, Shearin A, et al. Wheal and flare responses to opioids in humans. *Anesthesiology*. 1989;70:756–760.
33. Levy JH, Adelson D, Walker B. Wheal and flare responses to muscle relaxants in humans. *Agents Actions*. 1991;34:302–308.
34. Levy JH, Davis GK, Duggan J, Szlam F. Determination of the hemodynamics and histamine release of rocuronium (Org 9426) when administered in increased doses under N_2 O/O_2-sufentanil anesthesia. *Anesth Analg*. 1994;78:318–321.
35. Levy JH, Pitts M, Thanopoulos A, Szlam F, Bastian R, Kim J. The effects of rapacuronium on histamine release and hemodynamics in adult patients undergoing general anesthesia. *Anesth Analg*. 1999;89:290–295.
36. 2005 CARE AHAGFCRAEC. Part 10.6: anaphylaxis. *Circulation*. 2005;112:IV143–IV145.
37. DeSwarte RD. Drug allergy: problems and strategies. *J Allergy Clin Immunol*. 1984;74:209–224.
38. Gruchalla RS. Drug allergy. *J Allergy Clin Immunol*. 2003;111:S548–S559.
39. Gruchalla RS, Pirmohamed M. Clinical practice: antibiotic allergy. *N Engl J Med*. 2006;354: 601–609.
40. Reich DL, Hossain S, Krol M, et al. Predictors of hypotension after induction of general anesthesia. *Anesth Analg*. 2005;101:622–628.
41. Laforest M, More D, Fisher M. Predisposing factors in anaphylactoid reactions to anaesthetic drugs in an Australian population: the role of allergy, atopy and previous anaesthesia. *Anaesth Intensive Care*. 1980;8:454–459.
42. Fisher MM, Bowey CJ. Intradermal compared with prick testing in the diagnosis of anaesthetic allergy. *Br J Anaesth*. 1997;79:59–63.
43. Galletly DC, Treuren BC. Anaphylactoid reactions during anaesthesia: seven years' experience of intradermal testing. *Anaesthesia*. 1985;40:329–333.
44. Laxenaire MC. Drugs and other agents involved in anaphylactic shock occurring during anaesthesia: a French multicenter epidemiological inquiry. *Ann Fr Anesth Reanim*. 1993;12:91–96.
45. Laxenaire MC, Mertes PM; Groupe d'Etudes des Réactions Anaphylactoïdes Peranesthésiques. Anaphylaxis during anaesthesia. Results of a two-year survey in France. *Br J Anaesth*. 2001;87:549–558.
46. Harboe T, Guttormsen AB, Irgens A, Dybendal T, Florvaag E. Anaphylaxis during anesthesia in Norway: a 6-year single-center follow-up study. *Anesthesiology*. 2005;102:897–903.
47. Mertes PM. Anaphylactic reactions during anaesthesia: let us treat the problem rather than debating its existence. *Acta Anaesthesiol Scand*. 2005;49:431–433.
48. Fisher M, Baldo BA. Anaphylaxis during anaesthesia: current aspects of diagnosis and prevention. *Eur J Anaesthesiol*. 1994;11:263–284.
49. Mertes PM, Alla F, Tréchot P, Auroy Y, Jougla E; Groupe d'Etudes des Réactions Anaphylactoïdes Peranesthésiques. Anaphylaxis during anesthesia in France: an 8-year national survey. *J Allergy Clin Immunol*. 2011;128(2):366–367.
50. Moscicki RA, Sockin SM, Corsello BF, Ostro MG, Bloch KJ. Anaphylaxis during induction of general anesthesia: subsequent evaluation and management. *J Allergy Clin Immunol*. 1990;86:325–332.
51. Levy JH. Anaphylactic reactions to neuromuscular blocking drugs: are we making the correct diagnosis? *Anesth Analg*. 2004;98:881–882.
52. Gurrieri C, Weingarten TN, Martin DP, et al. Allergic reactions during anesthesia at a large United States referral center. *Anesth Analg*. 2011;113(5):1202–1212.
53. Garvey LH, Roed-Petersen J, Menné T, Husum B. Danish anaesthesia allergy centre: preliminary results. *Acta Anaesthesiol Scand*. 2001;45:1204–1209.
54. Castells M, Khan DA, Phillips EJ. Penicillin allergy. *N Engl J Med*. 2019;381:2338–2351
55. Kelkar PS, Li JT. Cephalosporin allergy. *N Engl J Med*. 2001;345:804–809.
56. Savic LC, Khan DA, Kopac P, et al. Management of a surgical patient with a label of penicillin allergy: narrative review and consensus recommendations. *Br J Anaesth*. 2019;123:e82–e94.
57. Pichichero ME. Cephalosporins can be prescribed safely for penicillin-allergic patients. *J Fam Pract*. 2006;55:106–112.
58. Brown RH, Schauble JF, Hamilton RG. Prevalence of latex allergy among anesthesiologists: identification of sensitized but asymptomatic individuals. *Anesthesiology*. 1998;89:292–299.
59. Lavaud F, Prevost A, Cossart C, Guerin L, Bernard J, Kochman S. Allergy to latex, avocado pear, and banana: evidence for a 30 kd antigen in immunoblotting. *J Allergy Clin Immunol*. 1995;95:557–564.
60. Blanco C, Carrillo T, Castillo R, Quiralte J, Cuevas M. Latex allergy: clinical features and cross-reactivity with fruits. *Ann Allergy*. 1994;73:309–314.
61. Holzman RS. Clinical management of latex-allergic children. *Anesth Analg*. 1997;85:529–533.
62. Parisi CAS, Kelly KJ, Ansotegui IJ, et al. Update on latex allergy: new insights into an old problem. *World Allergy Organ J*. 2021;14:100569.
63. Ring J, Franz R, Brockow K. Anaphylactic reactions to local anesthetics. *Chem Immunol Allergy*. 2010;95:190–200.
64. McClimon B, Rank M, Li J. The predictive value of skin testing in the diagnosis of local anesthetic allergy. *Allergy Asthma Proc*. 2011;32:95–98.
65. Dhonneur G, Combes X, Chassard D, Merle JC. Skin sensitivity to rocuronium and vecuronium: a randomized controlled prick-testing study in healthy volunteers. *Anesth Analg*. 2004;98:986–989.
66. Orihara M, Takazawa T, Horiuchi T, et al. Comparison of incidence of anaphylaxis between sugammadex and neostigmine: a retrospective multicentre observational study. *Br J Anaesth*. 2020;124:154–163.

10 Mechanisms of Anesthesia and Consciousness

C. MICHAEL CROWDER • BEN J. A. PALANCA • ALEX S. EVERS

KEY POINTS

1 The components of the anesthetic state include unconsciousness, amnesia, analgesia, immobility, and attenuation of autonomic responses to noxious stimulation.

2 Minimum alveolar concentration (MAC) remains the most robust measurement and the standard for determining the potency of volatile anesthetics (VAs).

3 Anesthetic interactions with membrane lipids may also contribute to anesthetic action. Emerging evidence indicates that anesthetic effects on lipid nanodomains may modify functionally important lipid–protein interactions.

4 Direct interactions of anesthetic molecules with specific binding pockets on membrane proteins can account for most of the observed cellular and behavioral effects of anesthetics. Protein interactions satisfy the Meyer–Overton rule and provide the simplest explanation for compounds that deviate from this rule.

5 While current data still support the prevailing view that neuronal excitability is only slightly affected by general anesthetics, this small effect may nevertheless contribute significantly to the clinical actions of VAs.

6 The synapse is generally thought to be the most likely relevant site of anesthetic action. Existing evidence indicates that even at this one site, anesthetics produce various effects, including presynaptic inhibition of neurotransmitter release, inhibition of excitatory neurotransmission, and enhancement of inhibitory neurotransmission. Furthermore, the effects of anesthetics on synaptic function differ among various anesthetic agents, neurotransmitters, and neuronal preparations.

7 The essential criteria for demonstrating a protein as an anesthetic target are (i) the function of the protein is affected by the anesthetic at relevant concentrations; (ii) the functional alteration of the protein could plausibly produce a component of anesthesia; (iii) genetic or pharmacologic manipulation of the protein alters sensitivity to the anesthetic; and (iv) the protein binds to the anesthetic.

8 $GABA_A$ receptors meet all the criteria as a target for certain anesthetics.

9 Hyperpolarization-activated cyclic nucleotide-gated channels are inhibited by volatile and some intravenous anesthetics and may contribute to their anesthetic effect.

10 Certain background K^+ channels have electrophysiologic, genetic, and biochemical evidence implicating them as relevant VA targets.

11 Some sodium and calcium channel subtypes are inhibited by VAs and these effects may be responsible in part for inhibition of neurotransmitter release and neuronal excitability.

12 The shaker potassium channel subtype (Kv1.2) is activated by VAs and has both genetic and biochemical evidence implicating it as a relevant target.

13 NMDA glutamate receptors are inhibited by nitrous oxide and ketamine but mammalian genetic data is currently insufficient to link this effect to anesthesia.

14 VA inhibition of mitochondria and synaptic vesicle release machinery may also contribute to anesthesia.

15 While anesthetic action to produce immobility occurs largely at the spinal cord, specific molecular targets for amnesia lie in the hippocampus.

16 Anesthetic-induced unconsciousness can be viewed as impairment of both arousal and awareness. These actions are mediated by targets distributed across the brain stem, hypothalamus, thalamus, and cerebral cortex.

17 Anesthetic ablation of arousal relies on disruption of redundant subcortical systems that regulate sleep and patterns of cortical activity.

18 Anesthetics alter the interaction of cortical networks responsible for cognitive functions and may thereby alter awareness by limiting the capacity to both represent and integrate information.

The introduction of general anesthetics into clinical practice over 150 years ago stands as one of the seminal innovations of medicine. This single discovery facilitated the development of modern surgery and spawned the specialty of anesthesiology. Despite the importance of general anesthetics and despite more than 100 years of active research, the molecular mechanisms responsible for anesthetic action are not fully understood.

Why have the mechanisms of anesthesia been so difficult to elucidate? Anesthetics, as a class of drugs, are challenging to study for three major reasons:

1. Anesthesia, by definition, is a change in the responses of an *intact animal* to external stimuli. Making a definitive link between anesthetic effects observed in vitro and the anesthetic state observed and defined in vivo has proven difficult.
2. No structure–activity relationships are apparent among anesthetics; a wide variety of structurally unrelated compounds, ranging from steroids to elemental xenon, are capable of producing clinical anesthesia. This suggests that there are multiple molecular mechanisms that can produce clinical anesthesia.
3. Anesthetics work at very high concentrations in comparison to drugs, neurotransmitters, and hormones that act at specific receptors. This implies that if anesthetics act by binding to specific receptor sites, they must bind with very low affinity and probably stay bound to the receptor for very short periods of time. Low-affinity binding is much more difficult to observe and characterize than high-affinity binding.

Despite these difficulties, molecular, structural, and genetic tools are now available that allow for major insights into anesthetic mechanisms. The aim of this chapter is to provide a conceptual framework for the reader to catalog current knowledge and integrate future developments about mechanisms of anesthesia. Five specific questions will be addressed in this chapter:

1. What is anesthesia and how do we measure it?
2. What are the molecular targets of anesthetics?
3. What are the cellular neurophysiologic mechanisms of anesthesia (e.g., effects on synaptic function vs. effects on neuronal excitability)?
4. What are the most likely anesthetic molecular targets responsible for anesthesia?
5. What are the anatomic sites of anesthetic action in the central nervous system (CNS)?

What Is Anesthesia?

General anesthesia can be broadly defined as a drug-induced reversible depression of the CNS resulting in the loss of response to and perception of all external stimuli. Unfortunately, such a broad definition is inadequate for two reasons. First, the definition is not actually broad enough. Anesthesia is not simply a deafferented state; amnesia and unconsciousness are important aspects of the anesthetic state. Second, the definition is too broad, as all general anesthetics do not produce equal depression of all sensory modalities. For example, barbiturates are considered to be anesthetics but produce minimal analgesia. These conflicting problems with the definition can be bypassed by a more practical description of the anesthetic state as a collection of "component" changes in behavior or perception. The components of the 1
anesthetic state include unconsciousness, amnesia, analgesia, immobility, and attenuation of autonomic responses to noxious stimulation.

Regardless of which definition of anesthesia is used, rapid and reversible drug-induced changes in behavior or perception are essential to anesthesia. As such, anesthesia can only be defined and measured in the intact organism. Changes in behavior such as unconsciousness or amnesia can be intuitively understood in higher organisms such as mammals, but become increasingly difficult to define as one descends the phylogenetic tree. Thus, while anesthetics have effects on organisms ranging from paramecium to man,[1] it is difficult to map with certainty the effects of anesthetics observed in lower organisms to any of our behavioral definitions of anesthesia. This contributes to the difficulty of using simple organisms as models to study the molecular mechanisms of anesthesia. Similarly, any cellular or molecular effects of anesthetics observed in higher organisms can be extremely difficult to link with the constellation of behaviors that constitute the anesthetic state. The absence of a simple and concise definition of anesthesia has clearly been one of the stumbling blocks to elucidating the mechanisms of anesthesia at a molecular and cellular level. Precise definitions for each of the component behaviors of the anesthetic state will be an important tool in dissecting the molecular and cellular mechanisms of each of the clinically important effects of anesthetic agents.

An additional difficulty in defining anesthesia is that our understanding of the mechanisms of consciousness is rather amorphous at present. One cannot easily define anesthesia when the neurobiologic phenomena ablated by anesthesia are not well understood. As discussed later in this chapter, the neural substrates for consciousness are beginning to be unraveled[2] and new theories[3,4] have incorporated this new anatomic knowledge, leading to identification of surrogate physiologic markers of consciousness.[5]

Finally, it has long been assumed that anesthesia is a state that is achieved when an anesthetic agent reaches a specific concentration at its effect site in brain. Surprisingly, it takes a higher anesthetic brain concentration to induce anesthesia than to maintain anesthesia (i.e., emergence occurs at a significantly lower concentration than induction).[6] This phenomenon, referred to as neural inertia, adds a wrinkle to the definition of anesthesia, suggesting that the mechanisms of anesthetic induction and emergence may be different. This suggestion is supported by the finding that the sedative component of anesthesia can be reversed by stimulation of specific arousal pathways in brain, even in the presence of "anesthetic" concentrations of inhalational agents.[7,8]

How Is Anesthesia Measured?

In order to study the pharmacology of anesthetic action, quantitative measurements of anesthetic potency are essential. To this end, Quasha and colleagues[9] have defined the concept of minimum alveolar concentration (MAC). MAC is defined as the alveolar partial pressure of a gas at which 50% of humans do not respond to a surgical incision. In animals, MAC is defined as the alveolar partial pressure of a gas at which 50% of animals do not respond to a noxious stimulus, such as tail clamp, or at which they lose their righting reflex. The use of MAC as a measure of anesthetic potency has two major advantages. First, it is an extremely reproducible measurement that is remarkably constant over a wide range of species.[9] Second, the use of end-tidal gas concentration provides an index of the "free" concentration of drug required to produce anesthesia since the end-tidal gas concentration is in equilibrium with the free concentration in plasma.

The MAC concept has several important limitations, particularly when trying to relate MAC values to anesthetic potency observed *in vitro*. First, the end point in a MAC determination is quantal: A subject is either anesthetized or unanesthetized; it cannot be partially anesthetized. Furthermore, MAC represents the average response of a whole population of subjects rather than the response of a single subject. The quantal nature of the MAC measurement makes it very difficult to compare MAC measurements to concentration–response curves obtained in vitro, where the graded response of a single preparation is measured as a function of anesthetic concentration. The second limitation of MAC measurements is that they can only be directly applied to anesthetic gases. Parenteral anesthetics (barbiturates, neurosteroids, propofol) cannot be assigned a MAC value, making it difficult to compare the potency of parenteral and volatile anesthetics (VAs). A MAC equivalent for parental anesthetics is the free concentration of the drug in plasma required to prevent response to a noxious stimulus in 50% of subjects; this value has been estimated for several parenteral anesthetics.[10] A third limitation of MAC is that it is highly dependent on the anesthetic end point used to define it. For example, if loss of response to a verbal command is used as an anesthetic end point, the MAC values obtained (MAC_{awake}) will be much lower than classic MAC values based on response to a noxious stimulus. Indeed, each behavioral component of the anesthetic state will likely have a
2 different MAC value. Despite its limitations, MAC remains the most robust measurement and the standard for determining the potency of VAs.

Because of the limitations of MAC, monitors that measure some correlate of anesthetic depth have been introduced into clinical practice.[11] The most popular of these monitors converts spontaneous electroencephalogram (EEG) waveforms into a single value that correlates with anesthetic depth for some general anesthetics. To date, these monitors have not been shown to be more effective at preventing awareness during anesthesia than simply maintaining an adequate end-tidal anesthetic concentration[12,13] or giving a standard dose of intravenous anesthetic. Nonetheless, different individuals likely have different sensitivities to anesthetics and measuring a surrogate end point such as a processed EEG value, an evoked potential,[14] or a functional neuroimaging signal indicative of integrated cortical activity may be a better indicator of anesthetic depth than merely measuring delivered concentration.

What Is the Chemical Nature of Anesthetic Target Sites?

The Meyer–Overton Rule

More than 100 years ago, Meyer and Overton independently observed that the potency of gases as anesthetics was strongly correlated with their solubility in olive oil (Fig. 10-1, 1 Video 10-1). Since a wide variety of structurally unrelated compounds obey the Meyer–Overton rule, it has been reasoned that all anesthetics are likely to act at the same molecular site. This idea is referred to as the *unitary theory of anesthesia*. It has also been argued that since solubility in a specific solvent strongly correlates with anesthetic potency, the solvent showing the strongest correlation between anesthetic solubility and potency is likely to most closely mimic the chemical and physical properties of the anesthetic target site in the CNS. On the basis of this reasoning, the anesthetic target site was assumed to be hydrophobic in nature. Since olive oil/gas partition coefficients can be determined for gases and volatile liquids, but not for liquid anesthetics, attempts have been made to correlate anesthetic potency with solvent/water partition coefficients. To date, the octanol/water partition coefficient best correlates with anesthetic potency. This correlation holds for a variety of classes of anesthetics and spans a 10,000-fold range of anesthetic potencies.[15] The properties of the solvent octanol suggest that anesthetics produce their effects by interacting with sites having both polar and nonpolar characteristics. Either membrane lipids or hydrophobic domains of proteins could satisfy these properties for a functionally relevant site for anesthetic interactions.

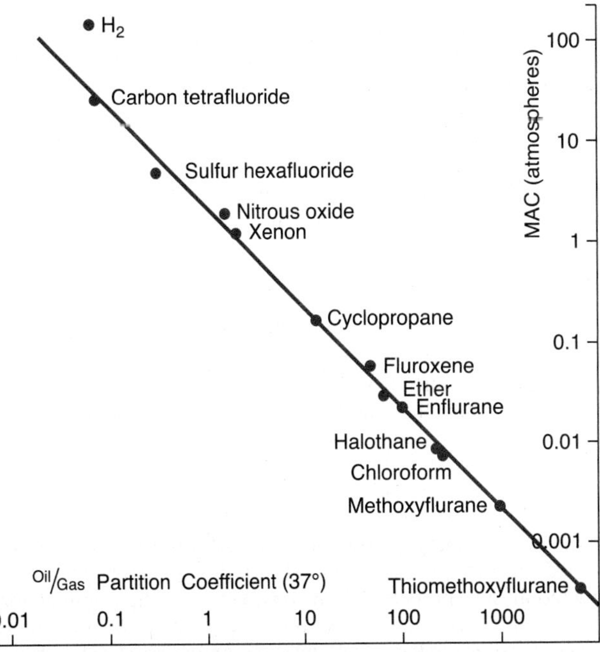

Figure 10-1 The Meyer–Overton rule. There is a linear relationship (on a log–log scale) between the oil/gas partition coefficient and the anesthetic potency (minimum alveolar concentration, MAC) of a number of gases. The correlation between lipid solubility and MAC extends over a 70,000-fold difference in anesthetic potency. (Reproduced with permission from Tanfiuji Y, Eger EI, Terrell RC. Some characteristics of an exceptionally potent inhaled anesthetic: thiomethoxyflurane. *Anesth Analg.* 1977;56:387.)

Exceptions to the Meyer–Overton Rule

While correlations of anesthetic activity with solvent solubility (olive oil/gas or octanol/water) can explain the potency of anesthetic agents, there are several exceptions to these correlations. First, halogenated ethers, barbiturates, and neurosteroids can be either convulsants or nonanesthetics despite predictions based on solvent solubility that they should produce anesthesia.[16] Interestingly, some of these polyhalogenated compounds do produce amnesia in animals[17] and are thus referred to as *nonimmobilizers* rather than as nonanesthetics. Second, several homologous series of anesthetics (*n*-alkanes, *n*-alkanols, cycloalkanemethanols, and perfluoroalkanes) show a *cutoff effect*, where long-chain compounds cease to have anesthetic properties despite increasing solubility predictive of increasing anesthetic potency.[18] A final deviation from the Meyer–Overton rule is the observation that enantiomers of anesthetics differ in their potency as anesthetics. Enantiomers (mirror-image compounds) are a class of stereoisomers that have identical physical properties, including identical solubility in solvents such as octanol or olive oil. Animal studies of barbiturate anesthetics, ketamine, neurosteroids, etomidate, and isoflurane all show enantioselective differences in anesthetic potency. These exceptions to the Meyer–Overton rule indicate that the properties of solvents such as octanol or olive oil describe some, but not all, of the properties of an anesthetic-binding site. Properties such as size and shape must also be important determinants of anesthetic sites of action.

Lipid versus Protein Targets

Anesthetics might interact with several possible molecular targets to produce their effects on the *function* of ion channels and other proteins. Anesthetics might dissolve in the *lipid* bilayer, causing physicochemical changes in membrane structure that alter the ability of embedded membrane proteins to undergo conformational changes important for their function. Alternatively, anesthetics could bind directly to *proteins* (e.g., an ion channel protein) interfering with either binding of a ligand (e.g., a neurotransmitter, a substrate, a second messenger molecule) or altering the equilibrium between functionally important conformations of the protein. The following section summarizes the arguments for and against lipid and protein theories of anesthesia.

Lipid Theories of Anesthesia

In its simplest incarnation, the lipid theory of anesthesia postulates that anesthetics dissolve in the lipid bilayers of biologic membranes, perturbing the bulk physical properties of the membrane and producing anesthesia when they reach a critical concentration. While perturbations of bulk membrane properties are produced by general anesthetics, the magnitude of the changes produced at clinical concentrations is quite small and is unlikely to disrupt nervous system function.[19] With the increased understanding that biologic membranes are composed of heterogeneous nanodomains composed of specific lipids and sterols with differing biophysical properties,[20] the possible role of lipid interactions in anesthetic action is being revisited. One provocative study showed that anesthetics can alter membrane protein localization to membrane nanodomains. This study examined the mechanism of VA activation of the ion channel TREK-1. The study found that VAs disrupt localization of the enzyme phospholipase D2 to lipid raft nanodomains, increasing the production of phosphatidic acid which then binds to and activates the ion channel, TREK-1.[21] While this result suggests a lipid-mediated mechanism of action, another recent study identified specific binding sites for isoflurane on TREK-1.[22] The effects of anesthetics (and other small hydrophobic 3
molecules) on the dynamics of lipid nanodomains is an emerging area of investigation and the interaction of anesthetics with lipids remains a plausible contributor to anesthetic action. Indeed, studies with model ion channels indicate that small hydrophobic molecules can alter channel function by a combination of membrane effects and protein binding.[23]

Protein Theories of Anesthesia

Over the past several decades, a strong body of evidence has been developed indicating that anesthetics can directly bind to specific hydrophobic sites on proteins and thus alter their function. Direct interaction of anesthetic molecules with proteins satisfies 4
the Meyer–Overton rule and also provides the simplest explanation for compounds that deviate from this rule. Anesthetic binding sites on proteins are likely to be defined by properties such as size, shape, and localized polarity in addition to their solvent properties. These additional properties could explain all of the exceptions to the Meyer–Overton rule.

Relevant anesthetic target proteins are likely to be intrinsic membrane proteins both because of their role in neuronal excitability and signaling and because anesthetics are concentrated in membranes (i.e., they have a large membrane:water partition coefficient). There are two likely kinds of anesthetic binding sites on membrane proteins:

1. Many membrane proteins have binding sites for endogenous hydrophobic ligands, (e.g., endocannabinoids, prostaglandins, steroids) through which these ligands act as either orthosteric or allosteric modulators of protein function. Anesthetics could compete with endogenous ligands for binding to such sites.
2. Hydrophobic amino acids are the major constituents of the α-helices that form the membrane-spanning regions of membrane proteins and constitute the protein surface that faces the membrane lipid. Anesthetic molecules could interact with pockets formed between the α-helices or with the hydrophobic surface of these membrane proteins, disrupting normal lipid–protein interactions, thus affecting protein conformation and function.

Evidence for Anesthetic Binding to Proteins

Several lines of experimental evidence indicate that anesthetics bind to specific sites on membrane proteins. First, site-directed mutagenesis of anesthetic-sensitive ion channels has identified amino acid residues that are crucial to anesthetic action. While the residues identified in these studies may contribute to anesthetic-binding sites, they may alternatively be sites that are essential for anesthetic-induced conformational changes in the protein. More direct approaches, including NMR spectroscopy and photoaffinity labeling, have identified anesthetic binding sites on ion channel proteins. Anesthetic analog photoaffinity labeling reagents have been developed for several parenteral anesthetics, including etomidate,[24] propofol,[25,26] barbiturates,[27] and neurosteroids[28,29] and used to identify putative anesthetic binding sites on the $GABA_A$ receptor, an important functional target of anesthetics (see section on GABA-Activated Ion Channels). The functional significance of these sites has been validated using site-directed mutagenesis, providing strong evidence that anesthetics modulate ion channel function by binding to specific sites on the channel protein. Photoaffinity labeling reagents have also been developed for inhalational anesthetics and have identified

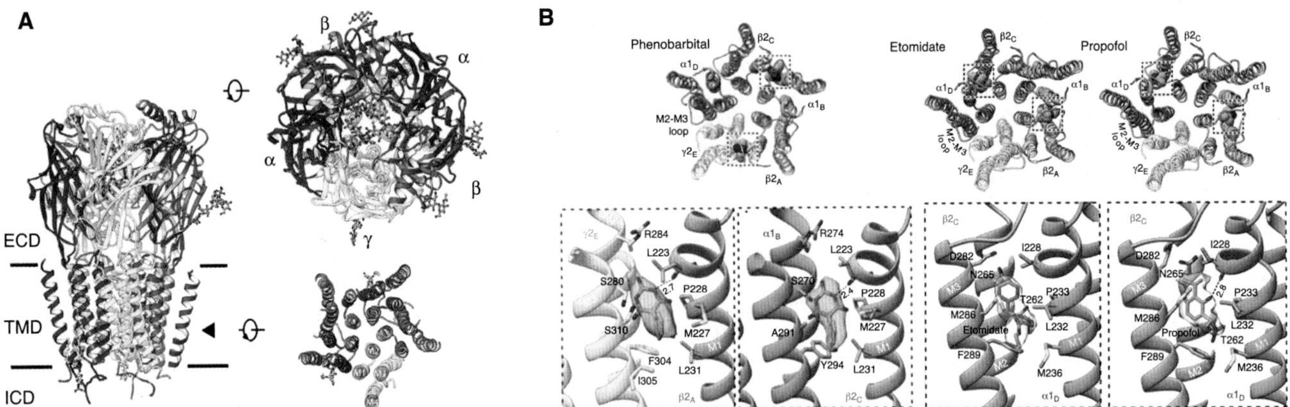

Figure 10-2 **Cryo-EM images of parenteral anesthetic binding to heteromeric GABA$_A$ receptors. A:** Structure of the GABA$_A$ receptor. **Left:** A side view of the receptor (from the plane of the membrane) shows the transmembrane domains (TMDs), extracellular domain (ECD where GABA binds), and the intracellular domain (ICD) which is poorly visualized by cryo-EM. Top right view from the ECD shows the five subunits (2α, 2β, and 1γ) arranged around a central ion-conducting pore. **Bottom right:** The receptor viewed from the ECD showing that each subunit is composed of 4 transmembrane helices with TM2 from each subunit lining the pore and TM1 from each subunit interacting with TM3 from an adjacent subunit. (From[38] with permission.) **B:** Top view from the ECD looking down through the pore. The barbiturate, phenobarbital, binds between adjacent subunits at the α(+)/β(–) and γ(+)/β(–) interfaces, whereas etomidate and propofol bind at the β(+)/α(–) interfaces. Bottom side view of the receptor shows atomic detail of the binding of (**left to right**) phenobarbital, etomidate, and propofol at the interfaces between adjacent subunits. (From[32] with permission.)

putative anesthetic binding sites on several ion channels, including GABA$_A$ receptors.[30]

GABA$_A$ receptors are composed of five subunits arranged in a ring with the outside facing the lipids of the plasma membrane and the center forming an ion-conducting pore (Fig. 10-2A). There are multiple subunit isoforms, but GABA$_A$ receptors are generally composed of two α, two β, and one either γ or δ subunits, with each subunit containing a transmembrane domain (TMD) composed of four membrane-spanning α-helices (TM1-TM4), an extracellular domain that binds GABA and a cytosolic intracellular domain. Photolabeling studies have consistently identified anesthetic binding sites between the TMDs of adjacent subunits (intersubunit sites) on the outside of the pentameric ring facing membrane lipid. Etomidate and propofol bind between TM3 (the "+" side) of a β-subunit and TM1 (the "–" side) of an α-subunit in the extracellular half of the TMDs. Anesthetic neurosteroids bind in the same β(+)–α(–) interface, but in the cytoplasmic half of the TMDs (not shown). Barbiturates bind in α(+)–β(–) interfaces (where propofol can also bind) as well as in γ(+)–β(–) interfaces. Mutagenesis of amino acids in these subunit interfaces strongly inhibits anesthetic potentiation of GABA-elicited currents, confirming the functional importance of these intersubunit sites. Photolabeling studies have also identified intrasubunit binding sites for propofol within the 4-TMD bundle of the β-subunit at the interface of the extracellular domain and the TMDs[25] and for neurosteroids at corresponding sites in both the α- and β-subunits.[28] Finally, VA analog photolabeling studies have also demonstrated putative-specific binding sites on GABA$_A$ receptors.[30] The combined results of these photoaffinity-labeling studies and associated site-directed mutagenesis studies provide definitive evidence that anesthetics bind to specific sites on the GABA$_A$ receptor and that these interactions are mechanistically responsible for modulation of channel function. Collectively, these data provide definitive evidence that anesthetics bind to membrane proteins.

Although photoaffinity-labeling techniques can provide extensive information about anesthetic-binding sites on proteins, they cannot reveal the details of the three-dimensional structure of these sites. x-ray diffraction crystallography and cryogenic electron microscopy (cryo-EM) can provide this kind of three-dimensional detail and have been used to study anesthetic interactions with membrane proteins. Initial crystallographic studies examined the interactions of anesthetics with the bacterial pentameric ligand-gated ion channel GLIC. GLIC is inhibited by clinical concentrations of anesthetics and the crystal structures of GLIC complexed with either desflurane or propofol have been solved.[31] These structures reveal a preformed "intrasubunit" binding cavity between the transmembrane α-helices within each subunit of the ion channel. In the past few years, the cryo-EM "resolution revolution" has enabled high-resolution structures of heteropentameric (αβγ) GABA$_A$ receptors complexed with parenteral anesthetics.[32] These structures visualize binding of etomidate and propofol in intersubunit sites between the β(+) and α(–) subunits and barbiturates between the α(+) and β(–) and the γ(+) and β(–) subunits (Fig. 10-2B), consistent with previous photolabeling studies. Structures of neurosteroids bound to GABA$_A$ receptors are not yet available. However, multiple structures of anesthetic neurosteroids bound to chimeric proteins, in which the TMDs of a GABA$_A$ receptor α-subunit are fused with the ECD of other pLGICs, have been solved.[33–35] All of these structures show the neurosteroid (either allopregnanolone, alphaxolone, or pregnanolone) bound in an intersubunit site (α(+)/α(–)) on the cytoplasmic end of the TMDs with the 3-OH group of the steroid forming a hydrogen bond with glutamine 241 of the α-subunit. Mutation of this glutamine to a leucine or tryptophan markedly reduces the efficacy of neurosteroids as potentiators of GABA$_A$ receptor currents.[36]

While x-ray crystallographic and cryo-EM structures provide exquisite detail about the atomic-level interactions of anesthetics with their binding sites on target proteins, they may not fully describe how and where anesthetics act. Photolabeling studies have identified sites for both propofol[25,26] and neurosteroids[28] on GABA$_A$ receptors that are not observed in cryo-EM images, raising the question as to whether all anesthetic binding sites are observed in structural studies. There are several possible reasons why a bound ligand may not be observed in an x-ray crystallographic or cryo-EM structure. First, ion channels fluctuate between multiple conformations (e.g., closed, open, desensitized), whereas x-ray and cryo-EM structures are static "snapshots" of just one conformation.

Each structure represents a single stable conformation of the protein, which may not be the preferred state to which a ligand binds in the "unobserved site." In addition, structures are obtained of proteins either in detergent solution or in nanodiscs, which may yield unnatural conformations[37,38] or conformations to which anesthetics do not bind. Finally, many anesthetics are very small molecules which are challenging to resolve. The currently available structures likely visualize anesthetic binding to the highest affinity sites on a protein; less tightly bound anesthetics may be difficult to visualize because the anesthetics are more mobile and thus less well resolved. The technology of cryo-EM structural analysis of protein structure is rapidly improving[39] and better and higher-resolution structures of anesthetics bound to $GABA_A$ receptors and other target proteins will become available in the near future. These structures should provide valuable insight into the full range of sites in which anesthetics bind, which conformation(s) they bind to and how they stabilize those conformations. This granular structural information will provide the basis for virtual drug screening which should enable identification of anesthetic agents with optimized specificity and affinity for their target sites.

Summary

Strong evidence demonstrates that anesthetics can bind to hydrophobic pockets on proteins and that anesthetic–protein interactions can account for the Meyer–Overton rule and deviations from it. Photoaffinity-labeling studies demonstrate that parenteral anesthetics, including etomidate, propofol, barbiturates, and neurosteroids, bind to hydrophobic pockets between the TMDs of $GABA_A$ receptor subunits. Mutagenesis of amino acids in these intersubunit sites dramatically reduces the anesthetic modulation of GABA-elicited ion currents, providing unequivocal evidence that anesthetics can directly alter protein function by binding to specific protein sites. Finally, recent cryo-EM studies of heteromeric ($\alpha_1\beta_x\gamma_2$) $GABA_A$ receptors have provided the first three-dimensional structures of anesthetic-binding sites on a relevant target protein. While the long-standing controversy between lipid and protein theories of anesthesia may be behind us, new evidence is emerging that anesthetic effects on membrane nanodomains may also contribute to the effects of anesthetics. There remain numerous unanswered questions about anesthetic–protein interactions, including the following:

1. Do anesthetics compete with endogenous ligands for binding to hydrophobic pockets on protein targets or do they bind to fortuitous cavities in the protein?
2. Do all anesthetics bind to the same pocket on a protein or are there multiple hydrophobic pockets for different anesthetics?
3. How many proteins have hydrophobic pockets in which anesthetics can bind at clinically used concentrations?
4. How does anesthetic binding stabilize specific conformations of a target protein?
5. Is it feasible to develop antagonists and/or inverse agonists for anesthetics that will reverse anesthesia or enhance cognition?

How Do Anesthetics Interfere with the Electrophysiologic Function of the Nervous System?

The functional unit of the CNS is the neuron and ultimately general anesthetics must disrupt the function of neurons mediating behavior, consciousness, and memory (NICV 10-1). In the simplest terms, anesthetics could accomplish this by altering the intrinsic firing rate of individual neurons, termed neuronal excitability, and/or by altering communication between neurons, generally occurring via synaptic transmission.

Neuronal Excitability

Neurons transmit information down their axons through action potentials. The propensity of a neuron to generate and propagate action potentials from the cell body to its nerve terminals is called its excitability. Intrinsic neuronal excitability is chiefly determined by three parameters: resting membrane potential, the threshold potential for action potential generation, and the size/propagation of the action potential. Anesthetics can hyperpolarize (i.e., create a more negative resting membrane potential) both spinal motor neurons and cortical neurons, and this ability to hyperpolarize neurons correlates with anesthetic potency. In general, the hyperpolarization produced by anesthetics is small in magnitude and is unlikely to alter *propagation* of an action potential down an axon. Small changes in resting potential may, however, inhibit the *initiation* of an action potential generated in response to synaptic excitation or in a spontaneously firing neuron. Indeed, isoflurane has been shown to hyperpolarize thalamic neurons, leading to an inhibition of tonic firing of action potentials. Anesthetics have not been shown to reliably alter the threshold potential of a neuron for action potential generation. However, the data are conflicting on whether the size of the action potential, once initiated, is diminished by general anesthetics. A classic article by Larabee and Posternak demonstrated that concentrations of ether and chloroform that completely block synaptic transmission in mammalian sympathetic ganglia have no effect on presynaptic action potential amplitude. Similar results have been obtained with fluorinated VAs in mammalian brain preparations. This dogma that the action potential is relatively resistant to general anesthetics has been challenged by reports that VAs at clinical concentrations produce a small but significant reduction in the size of the action potential in mammalian neurons. At a large synapse, amenable to direct measurement of the action potential and transmitter release in the same neuron, the slightly smaller action potential was shown to produce a substantial reduction in transmitter release due to the exponential relationship between the two.[40] Thus, while current data still support the prevailing view that neuronal excitability is only slightly affected by general anesthetics, this small effect may nevertheless contribute significantly to the clinical actions of VAs.

Synaptic Transmission

Synaptic transmission is widely considered to be the most likely subcellular site of general anesthetic action. Neurotransmission across both excitatory and inhibitory synapses is markedly altered by general anesthetics. General anesthetics inhibit excitatory synaptic transmission in a variety of preparations, including sympathetic ganglia, olfactory cortex, hippocampus, and spinal cord. However, not all excitatory synapses appear to be equally sensitive to anesthetics; indeed, transmission across some hippocampal excitatory synapses is enhanced by inhalational anesthetics. In a similar fashion, general anesthetics both enhance and depress inhibitory synaptic transmission in various preparations. In a classic study, Nicoll et al. showed that barbiturates enhanced inhibitory synaptic transmission by prolonging the decay of the GABAergic inhibitory postsynaptic current. Enhancement of inhibitory transmission has also been observed with many other general anesthetics including etomidate, propofol, inhalational anesthetics, and neurosteroids. As discussed below, a growing body of genetic experiments in mice demonstrate that the potentiation of GABAergic inhibitory postsynaptic currents mediates a significant portion of the behavioral effects of each of these classes of anesthetics.

Presynaptic Effects

Neurotransmitter release at glutamatergic synapses has consistently been found to be inhibited by clinical concentrations of VAs. For example, a study by Perouansky and colleagues[41] conducted in mouse hippocampal slices showed that halothane inhibited excitatory postsynaptic potentials elicited by presynaptic electrical stimulation, but not those elicited by direct application of glutamate. This indicates that halothane must be acting to prevent the release of glutamate. MacIver and colleagues extended these observations by finding that the inhibition of glutamate release from hippocampal neurons is not due to effects at GABAergic synapses that could indirectly decrease transmitter release from glutamatergic neurons.[42] Reduction of glutamate release by intravenous anesthetics has also been demonstrated, but the evidence is more limited and the effects potentially indirect.

The data for anesthetic effects on inhibitory neurotransmitter release is mixed. Inhibition, stimulation, and no effect on GABA release have been observed for both volatile and intravenous anesthetics. In a brain synaptosomal preparation where both GABA and glutamate release could be studied simultaneously, Westphalen and Hemmings[43] found that glutamate and, to a lesser degree, GABA release were inhibited by clinical concentrations of isoflurane. The same group has shown that release of norepinephrine, dopamine, and acetylcholine from synaptosomes is also inhibited by isoflurane although less potently compared to glutamatergic synaptosomes. The mechanism underlying anesthetic effects on transmitter release has not been established. The mechanism does not appear to involve reduced neurotransmitter synthesis or storage, but rather is a direct effect on neurosecretion. A variety of evidence argues that at some synapses, a substantial portion of the anesthetic effect is upstream of the transmitter release machinery, perhaps on presynaptic sodium channels or potassium leak channels (see later discussion). However, as discussed below, genetic data in *Caenorhabditis elegans* show that mutations in the transmitter-release machinery strongly influence VA sensitivity.[44] Evidence in rodent preparations suggests that this mechanism may be conserved in mammals.

Postsynaptic Effects

At a variety of synapses, anesthetics alter the postsynaptic response to released neurotransmitter. Anesthetic modulation of excitatory neurotransmitter receptor function varies depending on the receptor type, anesthetic agent, and preparation. In a classic study, Richards and Smaje examined the effects of several anesthetic agents on the response of olfactory cortical neurons to application of glutamate, the major excitatory neurotransmitter in the CNS. They found that while pentobarbital, diethyl ether, methoxyflurane, and alphaxalone depressed the electrical response to glutamate, halothane did not. In contrast, when acetylcholine was applied to the same olfactory cortical preparation, halothane and methoxyflurane enhanced the electrical response whereas pentobarbital had no effect; only alphaxalone depressed the electrical response to acetylcholine. Anesthetic modulation of neuronal responses to inhibitory neurotransmitters is more consistent. A wide variety of anesthetics, including barbiturates, etomidate, neurosteroids, propofol, and the fluorinated VAs, have been shown to potentiate the electrical response to exogenously applied GABA.

Summary

VAs alter the two fundamental determinants of neuronal communication, neuronal excitability, and synaptic transmission. Both volatile and parental anesthetics have powerful and widespread effects on synaptic transmission that would logically contribute to general anesthesia. Thus, the synapse is generally thought to be 6
the more relevant site of anesthetic action. Existing evidence indicates that even at the synapse, anesthetics have diverse actions, including presynaptic inhibition of neurotransmitter release, inhibition of excitatory neurotransmitter effect, and enhancement of inhibitory neurotransmitter effect. Furthermore, the synaptic effects of anesthetics differ among various anesthetic agents, neurotransmitters, and neuronal preparations.

Potential Anesthetic Targets

The functions of a large number and variety of proteins are altered by one or more general anesthetics (Table 10-1). However, demonstrating that any of them is a relevant anesthetic target requires more than the observation that anesthetics affect their function. The anesthetic effect must occur within a concentration range 7
at which anesthesia occurs. Second, the anesthetic effect should plausibly contribute to anesthesia; at the very least, the protein should function in the brain or spinal cord in a way where the perturbation of function might promote anesthesia. Third, anesthetics need to bind to the protein for it to be a direct anesthetic target. Finally, genetic or pharmacologic manipulation of the protein should alter anesthetic potency *in vivo*. A genetic mutation that alters anesthetic binding or the effect of binding without otherwise altering the function or expression of the protein provides the most definitive experimental test of the relevance of that binding to anesthesia. If such a mutation produces an anesthetic-resistant animal, this is very strong evidence that this protein is a functional anesthetic target. What follows is a review of the evidence for the proteins that best meet these criteria as anesthetic targets.

GABA-Activated Ion Channels

GABA is the most important inhibitory neurotransmitter in the mammalian CNS. GABA-activated ion channels ($GABA_A$ receptors) mediate the postsynaptic response to synaptically released GABA by selectively allowing chloride ions to enter and thereby hyperpolarize neurons. $GABA_A$ receptors are pentameric multisubunit proteins consisting of various combinations of α, β, γ, δ, and ε subunits with many subtypes for each of these subunits. The function of $GABA_A$ receptors is modulated by a wide variety of pharmacologic agents including convulsants, anticonvulsants, sedatives, anxiolytics, and anesthetics. The following section briefly reviews the effects of anesthetics on $GABA_A$ receptor function.

Barbiturates, anesthetic steroids, benzodiazepines, propofol, etomidate, and the VAs, all modulate $GABA_A$ receptor function. These drugs produce three kinds of effects on the electrophysiologic behavior of the $GABA_A$ receptor channels: potentiation, direct gating, and inhibition. *Potentiation* refers to the ability of an anesthetic to increase the current elicited by low concentrations of GABA at concentrations that produce no direct effect in the absence of GABA. Potentiation is illustrated in Figure 10-3, showing the effects of halothane on currents elicited by a range of GABA concentrations in dissociated cortical neurons. Anesthetic potentiation of $GABA_A$ currents generally occurs at concentrations of anesthetics within the clinical range. *Direct gating*

Table 10-1 Potential Anesthetic Targets

Protein	Anesthetics	Molecular Effects	Cellular Effects	Behavioral Effects[a]	Binding Sites
$GABA_A$ receptor	VAs, barbiturates, propofol, etomidate, neurosteroids	Potentiates GABA	Hyperpolarize neurons	Etomidate—hypnosis, immobility, amnesia; VAs—hypnosis, amnesia, immobility; propofol, barbiturates—hypnosis, immobility; neurosteroids—hypnosis	CryoEM: propofol, tomidate, phenobarbital—TMD; photoaffinity: propofol—TMD, x-ray crystal: alphaxalone—TMD
HCN1	VAs, propofol, ketamine	Inhibits channel	Decreases neuronal excitability	VAs—hypnosis, amnesia; ketamine—hypnosis; propofol—hypnosis	Undetermined
TREK-1	VAs, N_2O	Activates channel	Hyperpolarizes neurons	VAs—hypnosis, immobility	Indirect evidence for VA disruption of TREK-1–associated lipid rafts; photoaffinity: isoflurane—TMD
TASK-1, TASK-3	VAs	Activates channel	Hyperpolarizes neurons	Hypnosis, immobility	Undetermined
Sodium channels	VAs	Inhibits channel	Reduces action potentials, reduces transmitter release	Genetic data inconclusive	Undetermined
T-type calcium channel	VAs, neurosteroids	Inhibits channel	Decreases neuronal excitability	VAs—genetic data inconclusive, neurosteroids—hypnosis	Undetermined
Shaker-family potassium channels	Sevoflurane	Activates channel	Hyperpolarize neurons, inhibit action potential	Hypnosis in fly (genetic) and in mouse (pharmacologic)	Photoaffinity: sevoflurane—TM linker
NMDA receptor	Ketamine, nitrous oxide	Channel blocker	Blocks glutamate-gated depolarization	Mouse genetic data inconclusive, Nitrous oxide disrupts normal locomotion in worm	Ketamine—TMD
Mitochondrial complex 1	VAs	Reduces mitochondrial ATP production	Inhibits excitatory postsynaptic potentials	Worm, mouse, and human mutants hypersensitive to Immobility	Undetermined
Synaptic vesicle release machinery	VAs, propofol	Undetermined	Reduces transmitter release	VAs—unknown in mammals, slows emergence in fly, VAs—reduced locomotion in worm	NMR–VAs bind to syntaxin 1A, SNAP-25, ternary SNARE complex

[a]Behavioral effects by genetic or pharmacologic experiments in mouse unless otherwise stated.
VA, volatile anesthetics; TMD, transmembrane domain.

refers to the ability of anesthetics to activate $GABA_A$ channels in the absence of GABA. In general, direct gating of $GABA_A$ currents occurs at anesthetic concentrations higher than those used clinically, but the concentration–response curves for potentiation and for direct gating can overlap. It is not known whether direct gating of $GABA_A$ channels is either required for or contributes to the effects of anesthetics on GABA-mediated inhibitory synaptic transmission in vivo. In the case of anesthetic steroids, strong evidence indicates that potentiation, rather than direct gating of $GABA_A$ currents, is required for producing anesthesia. Anesthetics

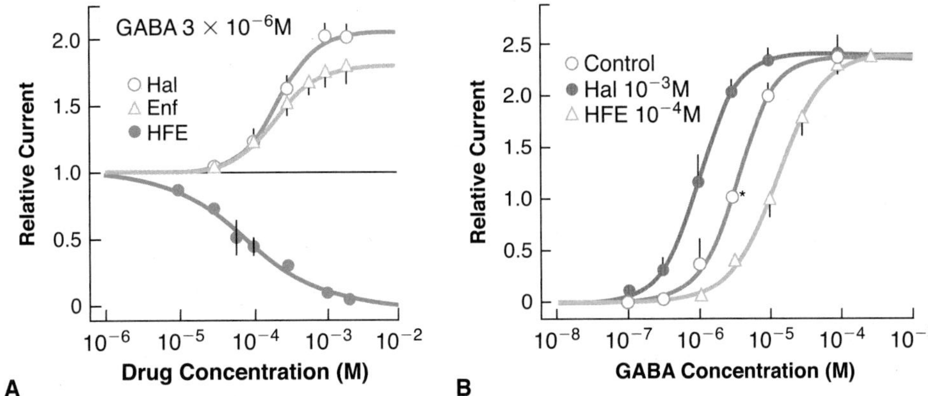

Figure 10-3 The effects of halothane (Hal), enflurane (Enf), and fluorothyl (HFE) on GABA-activated chloride currents in dissociated rat CNS neurons. **A:** Clinical concentrations of halothane and enflurane potentiate GABA-elicited chloride currents. The convulsant fluorothyl antagonizes the effects of γ-aminobutyric acid (GABA). **B:** GABA causes a concentration-dependent activation of a chloride current. Halothane shifts the GABA concentration–response curve to the left (increases the apparent affinity of the channel for GABA), whereas fluorothyl shifts the curve to the right (decreases the apparent affinity of the channel for GABA). (Reproduced with permission from Wakamori M, Ikemoto Y, Akaike N. Effects of two volatile anesthetics and a volatile convulsant on the excitatory and inhibitory amino acid responses in dissociated CNS neurons of the rat. *J Neurophysiol.* 1991;66(6):2014–2021. Copyright © American Physiological Society.)

can also inhibit GABA-activated currents. *Inhibition* refers to the ability of anesthetics to prevent GABA from initiating current flow through $GABA_A$ channels, and has generally been observed at high concentrations of both GABA and anesthetic. Inhibition of $GABA_A$ channels may help to explain why VAs have, in some cases, been observed to inhibit rather than facilitate inhibitory synaptic transmission.

Effects of anesthetics have also been observed on the function of single $GABA_A$ channels. These studies show that barbiturates, propofol, and VAs do not alter the conductance (rate at which ions traverse the open channel) of the channel; instead, they increase the frequency with which the channel opens and/or the average length of time that the channel remains open. Collectively, the whole cell and single channel data are most consistent with the idea that clinical concentrations of anesthetics produce a change in the conformation of $GABA_A$ receptors that increases the affinity of the receptor for GABA. This is consistent with the ability of anesthetics to increase the duration of inhibitory postsynaptic potentials since higher affinity binding of GABA would slow the dissociation of GABA from postsynaptic $GABA_A$ channels. Anesthetics would not be expected to increase the peak amplitude of a GABAergic inhibitory postsynaptic potential since synaptically released GABA probably reaches very high concentrations in the synapse.

Despite the similar effects of many anesthetics on $GABA_A$ receptor function, different anesthetics act on distinct subtypes of $GABA_A$ receptors. This is well illustrated for benzodiazepine sensitivity, which requires the presence of the γ2 subunit subtype. Sensitivity to etomidate has been shown to require the presence of a β2 or β3 subunit. The presence of a δ or ε subunit in a $GABA_A$ receptor has been shown to confer insensitivity to the potentiating effects of some anesthetics. Interestingly, $GABA_A$ receptors composed of ρ-type subunits (referred to as *$GABA_C$ receptors*) have been shown to be inhibited rather than potentiated by VAs. This property has been exploited to construct chimeric receptors composed of part of the ρ-receptor coupled to part of an α, β, or glycine receptor subunit. By screening these chimeras for anesthetic sensitivity, regions of the α, β, and glycine subunits responsible for anesthetic sensitivity have been identified, and subsequent site-directed mutagenesis studies were performed to identify the specific amino acids responsible for conferring anesthetic sensitivity. These studies revealed two critical amino acids near the extracellular regions of TMDs 2 and 3 (TM2, TM3) of the glycine and $GABA_A$ receptors that are required for VA potentiation.[45] One of the amino acids (TM3 site) has also been shown to be required (in the β_2/β_3 subunit) for the potentiating effects of etomidate.[46] In contrast, the TM2 and TM3 sites are not required for potentiation by propofol, barbiturates, or neurosteroids.[47] A distinct amino acid in the TM3 region of the β_1 subunit of the $GABA_A$ receptor has been shown to selectively modulate the ability of propofol to potentiate GABA agonist effects. Neurosteroid effects on $GABA_A$ receptors require specific sites within the transmembrane spanning regions of the α_1 and β_2 subunits, distinct from those for benzodiazepines and pentobarbital.[36] Collectively, these data provide strong evidence that anesthetics act on $GABA_A$ receptors at specific sites that are distinct for different anesthetics.

The role of the $GABA_A$ receptor in anesthesia has been extensively studied using mouse genetic techniques. Mice carrying mutations in α, β, and δ $GABA_A$ receptor subunits have been tested for their effects on anesthetic behavioral endpoints. α–Subunit knockout (KO) mutations (where the gene is fully inactivated) and knockin mutations (where a functional but altered gene product is produced) have been examined. KO of the α1 and α4 subunits produced similar phenotypes with a large reduction of the efficacy of isoflurane at blocking learning and memory tasks.[48] Similarly, an α5 KO mouse was strongly resistant to the amnestic effects of etomidate.[49] A knockin α1 mouse strain expressing a double mutated α1(S270H, L277A) subunit, has also been tested for its anesthetic sensitivity.[50–52] The α1(S270H) mutation had been shown to block GABA potentiation by VAs,[53] but the mutation also increased native sensitivity to GABA and α1(S270H) single-mutant mice are quite abnormal behaviorally, thus confounding interpretation of the data.[54] Thus, a second mutation, L277A, was introduced into the α1 subunit that compensated for the change in native gating properties.[50] The α1(S270H, L277A) mice are viable and behaviorally grossly normal. These mice are mildly resistant to the hypnotic effects of isoflurane, enflurane, and etomidate as well as the ataxic effects of etomidate; however, the potency of the drugs in MAC and fear-conditioning assays (a measure of learning) are not altered by the double-mutant α1 subunit.

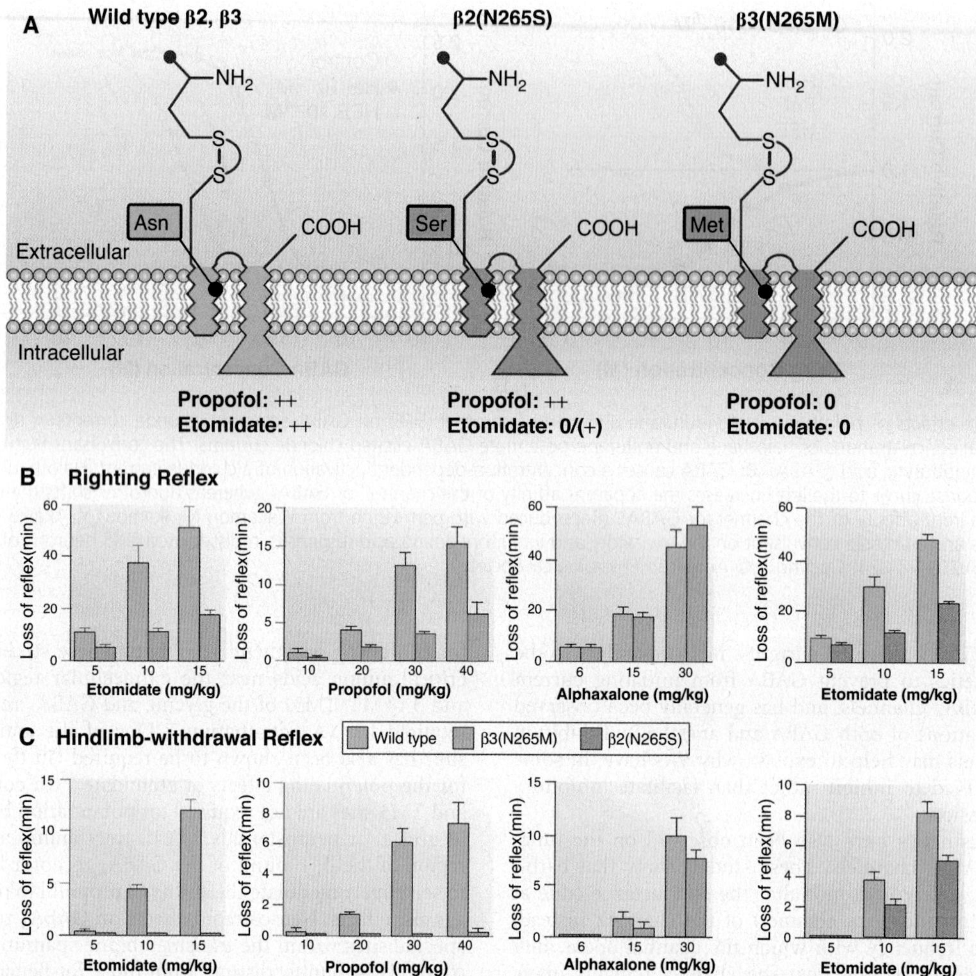

Figure 10-4 Mutations in the β2 and β3 subunits of the $GABA_A$ receptor reduce sensitivity to etomidate and propofol. A: Knockin transgenic mice were generated with mutation of a conserved asparagine (Asn) in the second transmembrane domain to a serine (Ser) in the β2 subunit or a methionine (Met) in the β3 subunit. **B:** The sensitivities of the wild type and the two knockin mice strains were measured in a loss of righting reflex assay, which is thought to model hypnosis. Mutant sensitivities to etomidate and propofol are highly significantly different compared to wild type. The neurosteroid alphaxalone is equally potent in wild type and in the β3(N265M) strain. **C:** The sensitivities of the wild type and the two knockin mice strains were measured in a hindlimb withdrawal reflex to a painful stimulus assay, which is thought to model immobility. Note the lack of significant sensitivities to either etomidate or propofol in the β3(N265M) strain. (Adapted with permission from Nature: Rudolph U, Antkowiak B. Molecular and neuronal substrates for general anaesthetics. *Nat Rev Neurosci.* 2004;5:709.)

While the anesthetic behavioral phenotypes of the α-subunit mutant mice are only incrementally different from wild-type mice, β subunit mutants have profound differences for the intravenous anesthetics etomidate and propofol. Based on its insensitivity to potentiation by etomidate and propofol in electrophysiologic experiments, a β3(N265M) knockin mutation mouse was generated and tested by Rudolph and colleagues, who showed that the strain was fully resistant to the immobilizing effects of etomidate, propofol, and pentobarbital (Fig. 10-4).[55,56] These results provided the first definitive link in mammals between an *in vitro* anesthetic action and an *in vivo* anesthetic behavioral endpoint. However, the β3(N265M) mice were not completely resistant to the hypnotic action of these anesthetics, indicating that other targets also contribute to their immobilization. Interestingly, the respiratory depressant effects of etomidate and propofol are also blocked by the β3(N265M) mutation, but the cardiovascular and hypothermic actions of the drugs are not.[57,58] The β3(N265M) mice also have a modest reduction in sensitivity to the immobilizing actions of VAs,[59] suggesting that the β3 subunit may play a minor role in their immobilizing effect, but the mutant has unaltered sensitivity to the amnestic effects of isoflurane and propofol.[57,60] Additional evidence for the importance of the β3 subunit comes from selective KO of β3 in mouse forebrain. In context fear-conditioning assays (a measure of hippocampal-dependent memory formation), β3(N265M) mice were found to be markedly resistant to isoflurane.[61] The β2 subunit has also been shown to be important for anesthetic sensitivity. A β2(N265S) mutant mouse has reduced sensitivity to etomidate although no anesthetic endpoint is fully blocked by this mutation (Fig. 10-4).[62,63] Finally, strains carrying a KO mutation of the δ subunit of the $GABA_A$ receptor have a shorter duration of neurosteroid-induced loss-of-righting reflex, whereas their sensitivity to other intravenous and VAs is unchanged.[64] Thus, the δ subunit may play a relatively specific role for neurosteroids.

As discussed in previous sections of this chapter, the evidence for binding of anesthetics to $GABA_A$ receptors is substantial, including cryo-EM evidence for binding of propofol, etomidate, and phenobarbital to a TMD pocket implicated by the genetic

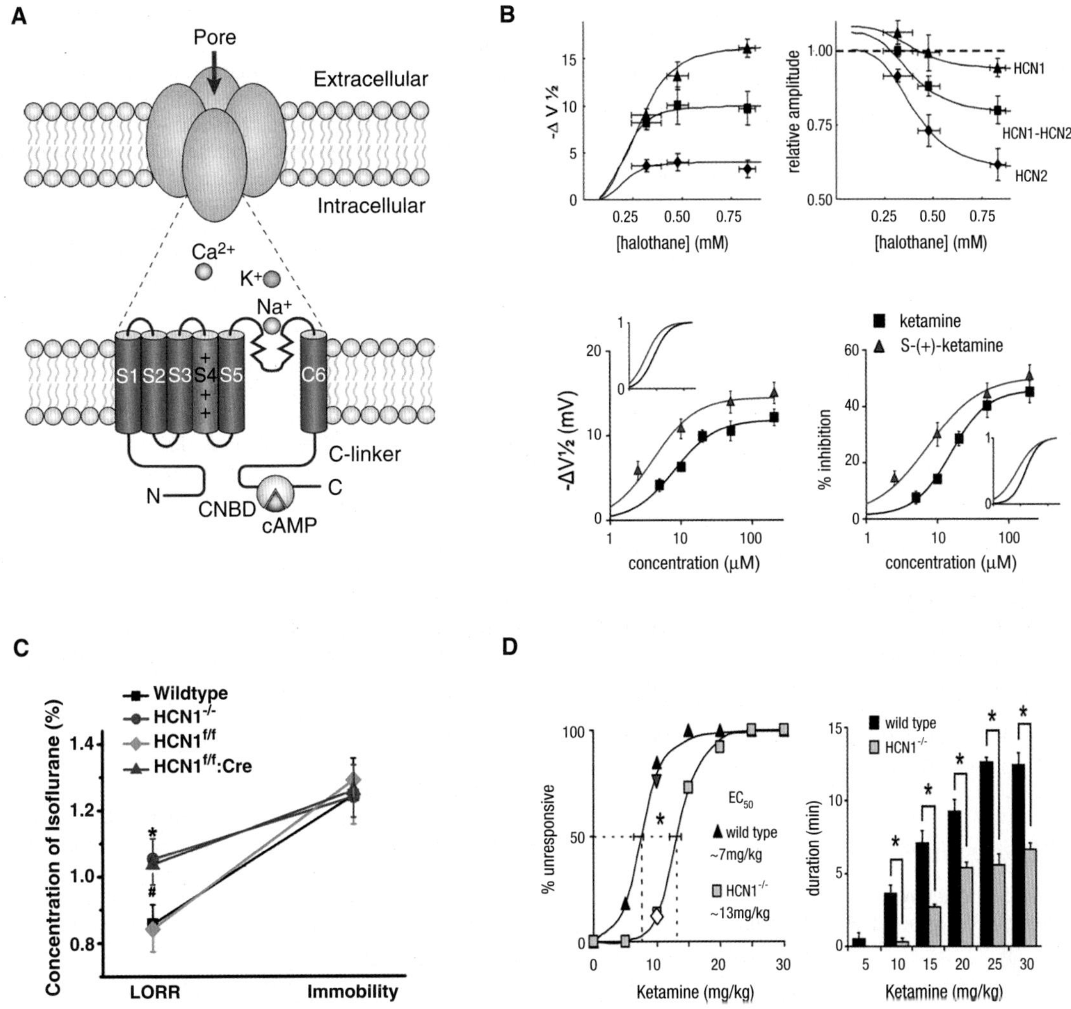

Figure 10-5 The HCN channel is inhibited by multiple anesthetics and is required *in vivo* for their potency. A: HCN channels are homomeric or heteromeric tetramers with each subunit composed of six transmembrane domains (S1–S6). The S4 domain is relatively positively charged and is the putative voltage sensor. The ion selectivity filter lies in an extracellular loop between S5 and S6 and is selective for Na^+ and K^+. A cyclic nucleotide binding domain (CNBD) lies in the C-terminal intracellular domain. (From[125].) **B:** Halothane and ketamine inhibit the mouse HCN channel by altering the voltage at which it is activated ($V_{1/2}$) and reducing maximum current amplitude. The effects depend in part on subunit composition. The ketamine data is for heteromeric HCN1–HCN2 channels. (From[65,66].) **C:** A global knockout of HCN1 ($HCN^{-/-}$) and a forebrain selective HCN1 knockout ($HCN^{f/f}$:cre) are partially resistant to isoflurane in a loss-of-righting reflex assay compared to wild type and the $HCN1^{f/f}$ without Cre control ($p < .05$). (from[67]). **D:** HCN1 knockout mice ($HCN1^{-/-}$) are resistant compared to the wild-type strain to the effects of ketamine in a loss-of-righting reflex assay with both a shift in the potency (**left**—dose/response curves) and reduced duration of LORR after a ketamine bolus (**right**—bar graph). (From[66].)

experiments.[32] Similarly, neurosteroids have been shown to bind to a specific site between the transmembrane domains of adjacent
8 subunits.[34] Thus, the $GABA_A$ receptor meets all of the criteria as a relevant anesthetic target for propofol, etomidate, barbiturates, and neurosteroids. For VAs, the genetic evidence is less definitive and no structural binding data has been published. Nevertheless, the $GABA_A$ receptor is likely a relevant but not exclusive target for VAs.

Hyperpolarization-Activated Cyclic Nucleotide-Gated Channels

9 *Hyperpolarization-activated cyclic nucleotide-gated channels* (HCN channels) are modulated by clinical concentrations of both volatile and some intravenous anesthetics. HCN channels pass a depolarizing current (termed I_h in the CNS) consisting of a mix of sodium and potassium ions and are activated by membrane hyperpolarization, the voltage dependence of which is shifted to a more depolarized range by the second messenger cyclic AMP (Fig. 10-5A). Therefore, cAMP activates HCN channels under most physiologic conditions. HCN channels are composed of homomeric and heteromeric combinations of four subunits—HCN1, 2, 3, and 4, all of which are expressed in both brain and heart. HCN channels have been shown to regulate resting membrane potential and rhythmic firing of the sinoatrial node and spontaneously spiking neurons and thereby are important for synchronous oscillations of neuronal networks.

VAs, propofol, and ketamine have been shown to inhibit HCN-mediated currents in both cell culture and native mouse neurons. The Bayliss group has shown that halothane shifts the voltage-dependent activation of the I_h current to more negative membrane potentials and inhibits its maximal amplitude.[65] Expression of HCN1 and HCN2 homomeric channels in cultured cells showed that halothane alters voltage dependence of activation of HCN1 channels while reducing the maximal amplitude of HCN2 currents (Fig. 10-5B). In isolated spinal motor neurons, halothane reduces the I_h current, consistent with inhibition of HCN channels. Similar inhibition of HCN1 channels was subsequently observed with clinical concentrations of propofol and ketamine. The inhibition of HCN1 by ketamine was stereoselective in the same manner as its stereoselectivity for general anesthesia (Fig. 10-5C).[66] Notably, in this same study, etomidate was not found to inhibit HCN1 channel activation. Thus, HCN1 channels may be important for the actions of both VAs and a subset of intravenous anesthetics. Genetic experiments described below argue that anesthetic inhibition of HCN1 and HCN2 channels may contribute to anesthesia.

Both global and forebrain-specific KO mouse strains of the HCN1 subunit and a global KO of the HCN2 subunit have been generated and tested for their anesthetic sensitivity. Both global and forebrain-specific HCN1 KO strains are mildly but significantly resistant to isoflurane and sevoflurane in assays of hypnosis and amnesia but similar to wild type for immobility (Fig. 10-5C).[67] The HCN1 global KO strain is strongly resistant to ketamine (85% increased ED_{50}) (Fig. 10-5D) and propofol (47% increased ED_{50}) and normally sensitive to etomidate.[66] The lack of effect of etomidate indicates that the increase is not due to some nonspecific increase in sensitivities to all hypnotics. An HCN2 global KO strain has reduced sensitivity to the effects of xenon on thalamic neuron currents, thalamocortical signaling, and on sedation.[68] Whether any anesthetic directly binds to HCN1 remains to be determined.

Two-Pore Potassium Channels

Background or *leak K⁺ channels* are activated by both volatile and gaseous anesthetics. Background or leak channels are so named because they tend to be open at all voltages including the resting membrane potential of neurons, producing a "leak current." Leak currents can significantly regulate the excitability of neurons in which they are expressed. Anesthetic activation of a leak channel was first observed in a ganglion of the pond snail, *Lymnea stagnalis*.[69] Clinical concentrations of halothane activated this channel called $I_{K(AN)}$, resulting in silencing of the spontaneous bursting of these neurons (Fig. 10-6A). A similar anesthetic-activated background potassium channel was subsequently found by Winegar and Yost in the marine mollusk *Aplysia*. The importance of VA activation of these invertebrate potassium channels became apparent with the discovery of a large family of background potassium channels in mammals. These mammalian potassium channels share a unique structure with two pore-forming domains in tandem plus four transmembrane segments (2P/4TM; Fig. 10-6,C). Patel et al.[70] have studied the effects of VAs on several members of the mammalian 2P/4TM family. They have shown that TREK-1 channels are activated by clinical concentrations of chloroform, diethyl ether, halothane, and isoflurane (Fig. 10-6B). In contrast, closely related TRAAK channels are insensitive to all the VAs, and TASK channels are activated by halothane and isoflurane, inhibited by diethyl ether, and unaffected by chloroform. These authors further showed that the C-terminal regions of TASK and TREK-1 contain amino acids essential for anesthetic action. TREK-1 but not TASK was found to be activated by clinical concentrations of the gaseous anesthetics: xenon, nitrous oxide, and cyclopropane. Thus, activation of background K⁺ channels in mammalian vertebrates could be a general mechanism through which inhalational and gaseous anesthetics regulate neuronal resting membrane potential and thereby excitability.

The roles in anesthetic sensitivity of several background potassium channels have been tested in limited mouse genetic studies. A TREK-1 KO mouse was found to be significantly, but not fully, resistant to multiple VAs for hypnotic and immobility endpoints (Fig. 10-7).[71] The VA resistance of the TREK-1 KO is

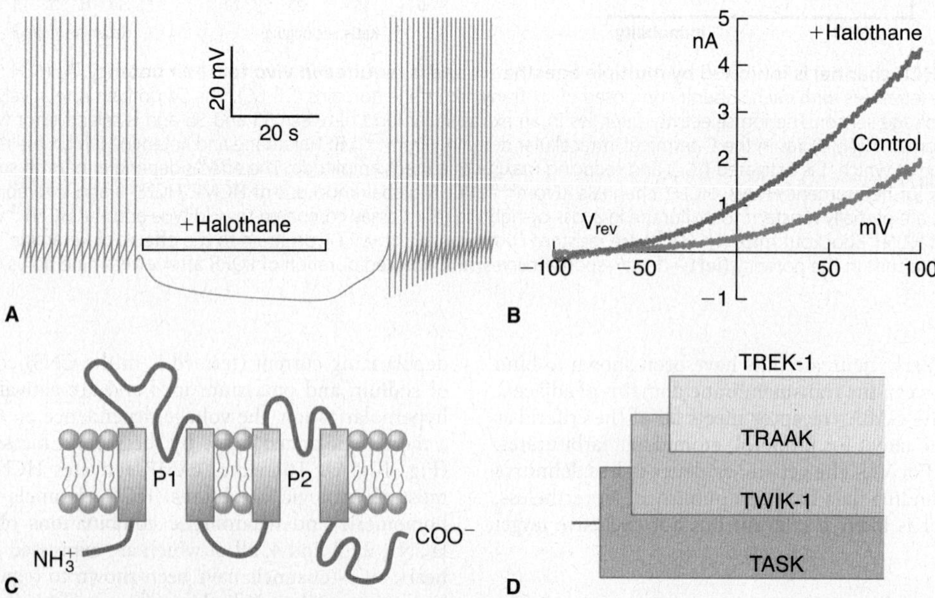

Figure 10-6 Volatile anesthetics activate background K⁺ channels. A: Halothane reversibly hyperpolarizes a pacemaker neuron from *Lymnaea stagnalis* (the pond snail) by activating a potassium current called I_{Kan}. **B:** Halothane (300 μM) activates human recombinant TREK-1 channels expressed in COS cells. The figure shows current–voltage relationships with reversal potential (V_{rev}) of −88 mV, indicative of a K⁺ channel. **C:** Predicted structure of a typical subunit of the mammalian background K⁺ channels. Note the four transmembrane spanning segments (orange rectangles) and the two pore-forming domains (P1 and P2). Some, but not all, of these 2P/4TM K⁺ channels are activated by volatile anesthetics. **D:** Phylogenetic tree for the 2P/4TM family. (Reproduced with permission from Nature: Franks NP, Lieb WR. Background K⁺ channels: An important target for anesthetics? *Nat Neurosci*. 1999;2:395.)

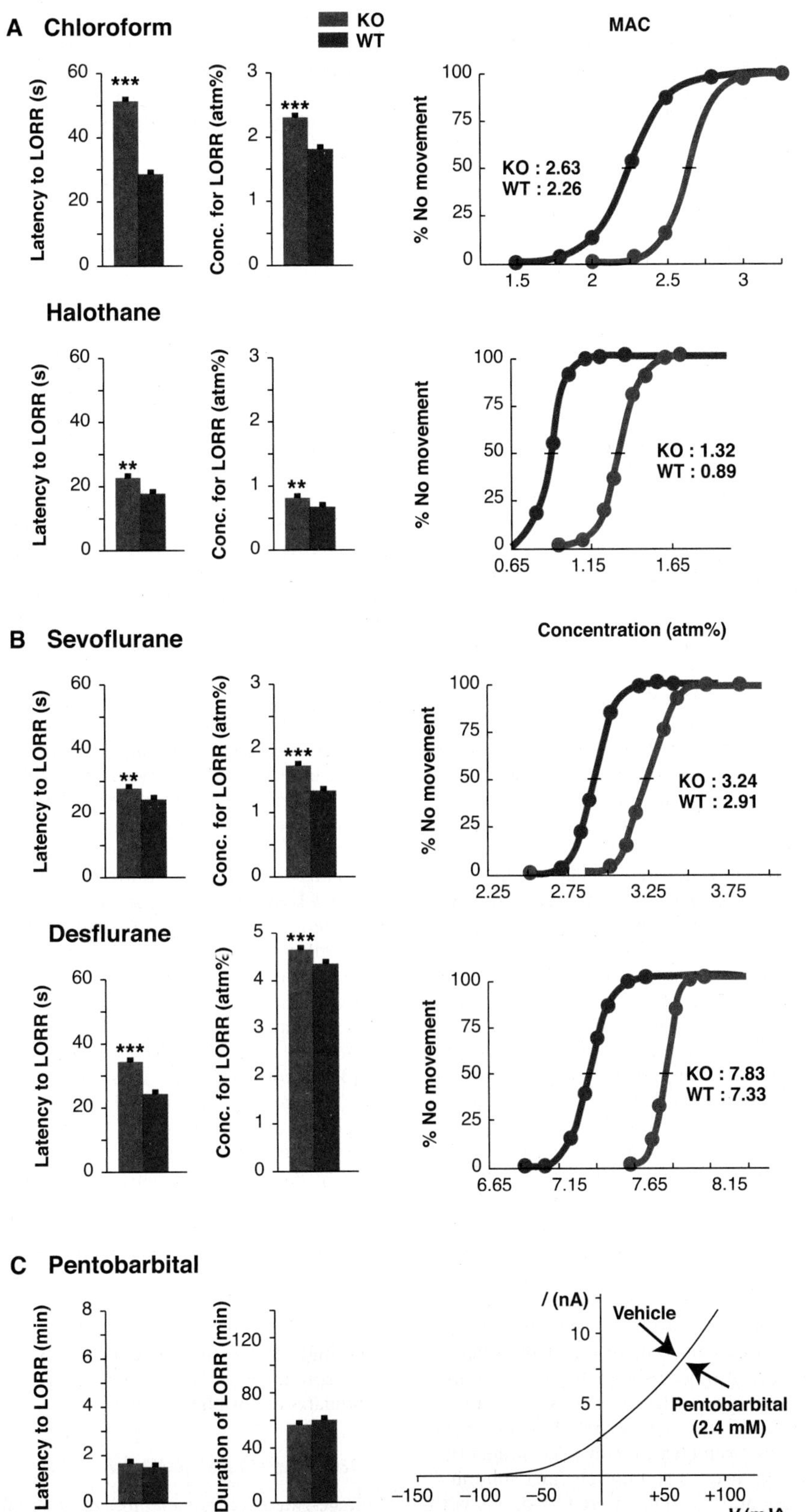

Figure 10-7 Mice without TREK-1 are resistant to volatile anesthetics. Mouse TREK-1 knockout (KO) and wild type (WT) strains were tested in a loss-of-righting reflex assay (LORR—**left**) and a tail clamp withdrawal reflex assay (MAC—**right**, EC_{50}s are noted) for sensitivities to the volatile anesthetics chloroform, halothane, sevoflurane, and desflurane (A,B) and the barbiturate pentobarbital (C). Bar graphs are mean +/– sem, $^{**}p < .001$, $^{***}p < .0001$, versus WT, t-test. (From[71].)

substantial, particularly for halothane where MAC was increased by 48%. Importantly, the TREK-1 KO mice have normal sensitivity to pentobarbital, consistent with electrophysiologic data, arguing against a nonspecific effect of the mutation. Westphalen et al. used the TREK-1 KO strain to test the hypothesis that TREK-1 mediates some of the presynaptic inhibitory effects of VAs.[72] Indeed, glutamate release from synaptosomes prepared from the TREK-1 KO strain is significantly resistant to inhibition by halothane compared to release from wild-type control synaptosomes. The role of TASK-2, another two-pore background potassium channel, has been tested by measuring the MAC of a TASK-2 KO mouse. Unlike the TREK-1 KO, the TASK-2 KO has MAC values similar to wild-type controls for desflurane, halothane, and isoflurane. This result is surprising given that TASK-2 is strongly activated by halothane and isoflurane and may be explained by the lower level of TASK-2 expression in the nervous system compared to TREK-1. KO strains for TASK-1 and TASK-3 exhibit modest but significant resistance to VA-induced hypnosis and immobility,[73] consistent with a role for these channels in anesthesia. As discussed above, recent evidence argues for binding of VAs directly to the TREK-1 protein and to nearby lipid rafts to
10 activate them.[21,22] Thus, although the evidence is not as extensive as for the $GABA_A$ receptor, TREK-1 meets each of the criteria for a relevant VA target.

Sodium Channels

Voltage-dependent sodium channels are largely involved in generating and shaping action potentials. The effects of anesthetics on these channels were studied by Haydon and Urban in the squid giant axon. These studies showed that these invertebrate sodium channels are remarkably insensitive to VAs. For example, 50% inhibition of the peak sodium channel current required halothane concentrations eight times those required to produce anesthesia. Similar results have been obtained in a mammalian cell line (GH_3 pituitary cells) where sodium currents were inhibited by halothane only at concentrations greater than five times those required to produce anesthesia. However, several studies with VAs have challenged the notion that all voltage-dependent sodium channels are insensitive to anesthetics. Rehberg and colleagues expressed rat brain IIA sodium channels in a mammalian cell line, and showed that clinically relevant concentrations of a variety of inhalational anesthetics suppressed voltage-elicited sodium currents. Ratnakumari and Hemmings showed that sodium flux mediated by rat brain sodium channels was significantly inhibited by clinical concentrations of halothane. Shiraishi and Harris documented the effects of isoflurane on a variety of sodium channel subtypes and found that several but not all subtypes are sensitive to clinical concentrations. As previously described, in a rat brainstem neuron, Wu and colleagues[40] found that a small inhibition of sodium currents by isoflurane resulted in a large inhibition of synaptic activity. Thus, sodium channel activity not only appears to be inhibited by VAs, but this inhibition results in a significant reduction in synaptic function, at least at some mammalian synapses. Intravenous anesthetics have also been shown to inhibit sodium channels, but the concentrations for this effect are supraclinical.

Genetic studies of sodium channels as relevant anesthetic targets are limited. Pal et al. examined mutant mice strains that have reduced activity of the Nav1.6 sodium channel subunit.[74] Two distinct Nav1.6 mouse mutant strains were tested, one with reduced protein expression and the other with reduced activity of the channel. Both mutants were hypersensitive to the hypnotic effects of VAs isoflurane and sevoflurane. Interestingly, the mice were hypersensitive to induction of anesthesia but not emergence. Both of these mutants have significant baseline neurologic disturbances; thus, the effects of the mutants on anesthetic sensitivity could well be indirect, thereby confounding determination of the role of these sodium channel subunits in anesthesia. At present, there is no experimental evidence that anesthetics bind to any of the sodium channel subtypes.

T-Type Calcium Channels

Voltage-dependent calcium channels (VDCCs) couple electrical activity to specific cellular functions. Six types of calcium channels (designated L, N, P, Q, R, and T) have been identified on the basis of electrophysiologic properties and amino acid sequence similarities. As a general rule, VAs inhibit most VDCCs (50% reduction in current) at concentrations two to five times those required to produce anesthesia in humans, with less than a 20% inhibition of calcium current at clinical concentrations. However, T-type calcium channels have been found to be quite sensitive to VAs and anesthetic neurosteroids. T-type calcium channels are widely expressed throughout the CNS, including the dorsal root ganglion and thalamus. These channels regulate neuronal excitability, bursting behavior, and network oscillations and have been implicated in epilepsy and neuropathic pain. Takenoshita and Steinbach reported a T-type calcium current in dorsal root ganglion neurons that was inhibited by subanesthetic concentrations of halothane. Similarly, T-type channels in the thalamus have been found to be inhibited by VAs.[75] T-type channels are also potently inhibited by anesthetic neurosteroids.

T-type channels have three isoforms ($Ca_v3.1$, 3.2, 3.3), each of which is inhibited by clinical concentrations of VAs.[75] KO mutations in the genes encoding all three isoforms have been tested for their anesthetic sensitivity. KO of the $Ca_v3.1$ isoform does not alter VA sensitivity for either hypnotic or immobility endpoints in mice; however, these mice required a longer induction time to produce hypnosis but not immobility.[76] For neurosteroids, compared to wild-type controls, a significantly smaller fraction of $Ca_v3.1$ KO mice lost consciousness with a single dose of an anesthetic neurosteroid.[77] A mouse strain with a KO of $Ca_v3.2$ similarly exhibited a delayed VA induction phenotype, but it was hypersensitive to immobilization by isoflurane and halothane.[78] On the other hand, $Ca_v3.3$ KO mice had a shortened VA induction time and had no change in sensitivities for either hypnosis or immobility endpoints.[79] The neurosteroid resistance phenotype of $Ca_v3.1$ is consistent with it as a relevant anesthetic target. However, for the VAs, whether the hypersensitive mutant phenotypes and alterations in the kinetics of induction indicate that T-type channels are volatile anesthetic targets is at this point unclear. Clearly, none of these channels are necessary for VA sensitivity because resistance would be observed. In addition, the mutants have effects on baseline behavior and CNS function that confound interpretation, and physiologic parameters such as cardiac output and minute ventilation that would impact speed of induction were not measured in the mutant strains. Finally, binding of anesthetics to any of the T-type channels has not been reported. Nevertheless, 11
their high level of anesthetic sensitivity and important function in nociception and CNS excitability make T-type channels appealing candidates as anesthetic targets.

Shaker Potassium Channels

Voltage-gated six transmembrane potassium channels (Kv channels) open in response to membrane depolarization and repolarize membranes, for example, after an action potential. Thus, Kv channels negatively regulate neuronal action potential duration and frequency and thereby control neuronal excitability and neurotransmitter release. High concentrations of both VAs and intravenous anesthetics are required to affect the function of most voltage-gated K^+ channels. However, members of the Shaker family of potassium channels (Kv1.x) are sensitive to clinically relevant concentrations of VAs. The Shaker family is named after a Drosophila mutant that exhibited a leg-shaking phenotype when anesthetized with ether as was routinely done to examine fly strains. The shaker gene was positionally cloned and found to encode a protein with features homologous to the previously identified sodium channel. Subsequently, electrophysiologic experiments with the cloned and expressed protein confirmed that the fly Shaker gene encoded a potassium channel. Kv1.1 and Kv1.2 are the mammalian versions of the fly Shaker protein. Sevoflurane at clinical concentrations increases current through both Kv1.1 and Kv1.2 channels.[80] Conductance through the closely related Kv1.3 channel was similarly increased by isoflurane and desflurane. Kv1.1 and Kv1.2 are expressed throughout the mammalian CNS and increased conductance through these channels by anesthetics should result in a widespread decrease in neuronal excitability.

Genetic experiments with Shaker-family mutants are limited to the flies in which the viable Shaker mutants were first isolated. Drosophila strains with loss-of-function mutations in the Shaker gene are strongly resistant to hypnosis by halothane or isoflurane,[81] providing support for their role in anesthesia in the fly. Interestingly, subsequent experiments by the Kelz group demonstrated that most of the anesthetic-resistant phenotype of the Shaker mutant could be accounted for by increased emergence from anesthesia and less so by reduced induction.[82] Thus, the Shaker channel may play a greater role in the transition from the hypnotic to awake state. While no genetic evidence is available in higher organisms, microinjection of a selective Kv1.1, 1.3, and 1.6 inhibitor into the thalamus restored the righting reflex in animals that were exposed to hypnotic concentrations of sevoflurane.[80] Similarly, thalamic microinjection of an antibody against Kv1.2 reversed sevoflurane hypnosis in a significant fraction of
12 rats.[83] These data are certainly consistent with the hypothesis that the Shaker family of channels contributes to the anesthetic state.

While there are no direct structural data visualizing anesthetic bound to a Shaker-family channel, a photoaffinity anesthetic ligand structurally related to sevoflurane labeled three amino acid residues in Kv1.2 that could be competed away with sevoflurane.[84] Mutation of one of these residues modestly reduced the conductance increases by sevoflurane, adding support to the hypothesis that this residue lines a relevant sevoflurane-binding pocket.

NMDA-Subtype Glutamate-Activated Ion Channels

Glutamate-activated ion channels have been classified into three categories based on selective agonists: AMPA receptors, kainate receptors, and NMDA receptors. AMPA and kainate receptors are relatively nonselective monovalent cation channels involved in fast excitatory synaptic transmission, whereas NMDA channels conduct not only Na^+ and K^+ but also Ca^{++} and are involved in long-term modulation of synaptic responses (long-term potentiation). The NMDA receptor is a four-subunit heteromeric complex composed of two obligate GluN1 subunits, encoded by a single gene, and two GluN2 subunits (GluN2A-D encoded by four genes). GluN3 subunits can also form complexes with GluN1 but the properties of this protein are unclear and may not form functional glutamate-gated channels.

NMDA-activated currents are sensitive to a subset of anesthetics. Electrophysiologic studies show minimal to no effects of clinical concentrations of VAs, neurosteroids, or barbiturates on NMDA-activated currents. On the other hand, ketamine is

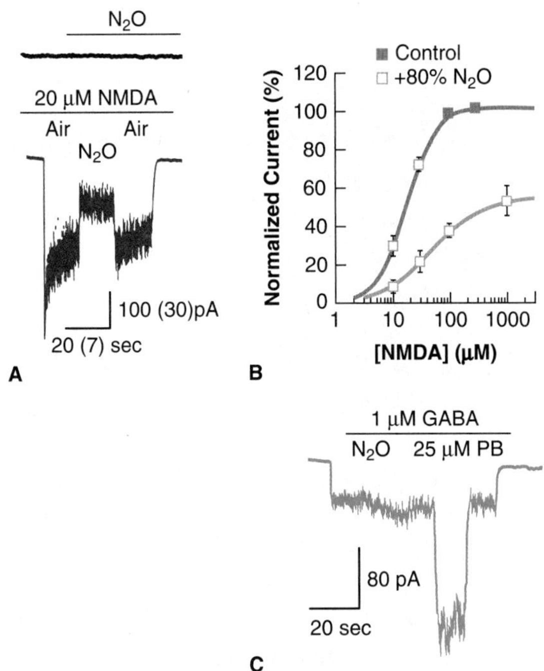

Figure 10-8 Nitrous oxide inhibits NMDA-elicited but not GABA-elicited currents in rat hippocampal neurons. A: Eighty percent N_2O has no effect on holding current (*upper trace*), but inhibits the current elicited by NMDA (*pink trace*). **B:** N_2O causes a rightward and downward shift of the NMDA concentration–response curve, indicating a mixed competitive/noncompetitive antagonism. **C:** Eighty percent N_2O has little effect on GABA-elicited currents. In contrast, an equipotent anesthetic concentration of pentobarbital markedly enhances the GABA-elicited current. (Reproduced with permission from Nature: Jevtovic-Todorovic V, Todorovic SM, Mennerick S, et al: Nitrous oxide (laughing gas) is an NMDA antagonist, neuroprotectant, and neurotoxin. *Nat Med.* 1998:4:460.)

a potent and stereoselective inhibitor of NMDA-activated currents. The anesthetic effects of ketamine in intact animals show the same stereoselectivity as that observed in vitro, consistent with the hypothesis that the NMDA receptor is a relevant molecular target for ketamine. The NMDA receptors may also be an important target for nitrous oxide and xenon. N_2O[85] and xenon[86] are potent and selective inhibitors of NMDA-activated currents (Fig. 10-8).

Mouse NMDA genetics experiments are hampered by the fact that a KO mutation of the obligate GluN1 subunit is lethal; mice die shortly after birth. Similarly, GluN2B subunit KO mice have severe behavioral abnormalities and die at birth. GluN2A, C, and D KO mice are able to develop into adults but do have milder behavioral and electrophysiologic phenotypes. The GluN2A KO mouse strain has been tested for anesthetic sensitivity. The GluN2A KO mice are partially resistant to the hypnotic effects of ketamine[87]; however, they are also significantly resistant to propofol, pentobarbital, midazolam, and diazepam, drugs that have no known effects on the electrophysiologic activity of the NMDA receptor. Thus, an indirect effect of the GluN2A mutation on ketamine sensitivity cannot be ruled out and is almost certainly the case for the other drugs. Similarly, the relevance of the partial resistance of the GluN2A mutants to nitrous oxide is unclear and may be due to secondary changes in monaminergic signaling in these animals. Overall, the limited mouse genetic experi- 13
ments are not sufficient to demonstrate that the NMDA receptor is essential to the action of ketamine or nitrous oxide. However,

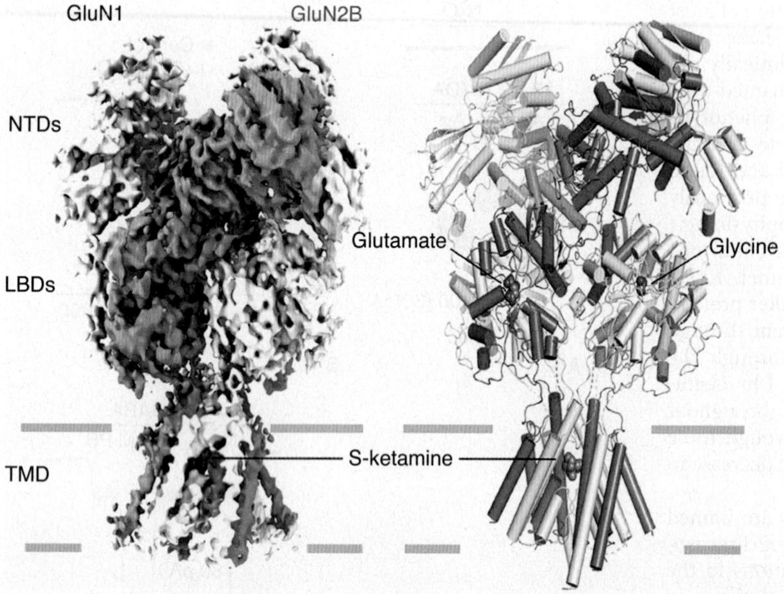

Figure 10-9 S-Ketamine binding site on the NMDA receptor. Cryo-EM densities (**left**) and structural models (**right**) of the human GluN1–GluN2B heterodimeric NMDA receptor bound with co-agonist glutamate and glycine visualized in their ligand binding domains (LBDs) and S-ketamine bound in a pocket within the transmembrane domains (TMDs); NTDs, N-terminal domain. (From[90].)

mutation of the essential NMDA receptor subunit in the nematode *C. elegans* was shown to completely abolish sensitivity to nitrous oxide while having no effect on VA sensitivity[88]; mutation of a distinct glutamate receptor subunit is required for the effects of Xenon in *C. elegans*.[89] Thus, in the simpler nematode nervous system, the NMDA receptor is required for the behavioral effects of nitrous oxide.

Recently, the structures of human GluN1::GluN2A and GluN1::GluN2B bound to the S enantiomer of ketamine, glutamate, and glycine were solved by cryo-EM methods.[90] S-ketamine was found bound in a TMD pocket near the channel gate (Fig. 10-9); this location is consistent with the electrophysiologic effects of ketamine as a channel blocker. Mutation of amino acid residues in the ketamine-binding pocket resulted in resistance of the mutant receptor to ketamine inhibition in electrophysiologic in vitro assays. In addition to demonstrating that NMDA receptors bind ketamine, these results also suggest a means to generate viable GluN1 mutant mice with selective mutations that will allow more definitive determination of the role of NMDA receptors in ketamine anesthesia.

Mitochondrial Complex I

The first true genetic screens for mutants with altered general anesthetic sensitivity were performed in the nematode *C. elegans* by Phil Morgan and Margaret Sedensky.[91] They screened for altered sensitivity to immobilization of C. elegans by supraclinical concentrations of halothane. One of the isolated mutants called *fc21* was markedly hypersensitive to not only halothane but also to isoflurane and enflurane. The *fc21* mutation was subsequently identified as a missense change in gene called *gas-1*, which encodes mitochondrial NADH:ubiquinone reductase, a subunit of complex 1 of the mitochondrial electron transport chain.[92] The Morgan and Sedensky group later showed that mice with a mutation in *Ndufs4*, another complex 1 protein, were hypersensitive to immobilization by isoflurane, halothane, and to hypnosis by propofol but resistant to hypnosis by ketamine.[93] The finding of ketamine resistance argues against generalized sickness or global nervous system dysfunction accounting for the increased sensitivity to the other anesthetics. Subsequently, Morgan and Sedensky demonstrated that mouse complex 1 function was inhibited by clinically relevant concentrations of isoflurane and that mitochondria from the *Ndufs4* mutant mice were hypersensitive to isoflurane.[94] Electrophysiologic recordings from hippocampal neurons showed that the *Ndufs4* mutant was hypersensitive to the effects of isoflurane on reducing synaptic vesicle recycling during high-frequency stimulation. Remarkably, pediatric patients with mitochondrial complex 1 defects likewise have been found to be exquisitely sensitive to VAs whereas patients with other mitochondrial defects are not reliably hypersensitive.[95] At present, no studies showing specific binding of anesthetics to mitochondrial complex 1 have been reported.

Synaptic Vesicle Release Machinery

Using behavioral endpoints in *C. elegans* that occur at concentrations of VAs in the clinical range, Crowder and colleagues screened for VA-resistant mutants and found mutations in proteins regulating neurotransmitter release.[44] The mutations with the largest effect were in syntaxin 1A, a neuronal protein highly conserved from *C. elegans* to humans and essential for fusion of neurotransmitter vesicles with the presynaptic membrane.[44] Although all of the mutations reduced the normal function of syntaxin, some mutations produced hypersensitivity to VAs while others conferred resistance. These allelic differences in anesthetic sensitivity could not be accounted for by effects on the process of transmitter release itself; rather, the genetic data argued that syntaxin interacts with a protein critical for VA action, perhaps an anesthetic target. Subsequent experiments in Drosophila found that the expression of the same syntaxin mutation also produced isoflurane resistance in the fly.[96] Interestingly, as with the shaker potassium mutants, the syntaxin mutant primarily enhanced emergence from anesthesia in Drosophila with less of an effect on induction.[96] In mammalian models, expression of the same mutant syntaxin in cultured rat neurons reduces the potency of isoflurane at inhibiting neurotransmitter release.[97] A highly evolutionarily conserved presynaptic protein called UNC-13 in *C. elegans* has been implicated in this syntaxin-regulated VA mechanism.[98] *C. elegans unc-13* mutants are fully resistant to the effects of clinical concentration of isoflurane, and isoflurane prevents the normal synaptic localization of UNC-13 in *C. elegans*.

Using NMR-based methods, Nagele et al. found that isoflurane and halothane bind to rat syntaxin *in vitro* at clinically relevant concentrations and to a protein complex composed of rat syntaxin and two other proteins that form what is called the SNARE complex.[99] In all metazoans, the SNARE complex mediates fusion of synaptic vesicles with the presynaptic membrane and thereby release of neurotransmitter into the synaptic cleft. The effect of this anesthetic binding on the function of syntaxin and the SNARE complex is unclear and may or may not relate to the anesthetic resistance of the syntaxin mutants.

Summary

Multiple proteins are likely to be bound by anesthetics and the function of many of these may be altered. Which of these anesthetic targets might actually contribute to anesthesia is the subject of the preceding section. Using the criteria as outlined above, $GABA_A$ receptors meet all criteria as the primary relevant target for etomidate and propofol. For VAs, the $GABA_A$ receptor and the TREK-1 channel are also likely targets but are unlikely to be the only targets. Eight other potential anesthetic targets are discussed, each of which has strong evidence for the protein as a probable relevant anesthetic target, but unlike for the $GABA_A$ receptor and to a lesser degree the TREK-1 channel, for none of these other potential targets is the evidence sufficient to declare it a target for any particular anesthetic. A major limitation in making a definitive assignment of a protein as a relevant mammalian anesthetic target is the lack of genetic reagents that specifically eliminate the anesthetic target entirely without otherwise producing secondary neurobiologic phenotypes that confound interpretation of the data or preclude testing entirely. More facile methods to make single point mutations in genes such as Crispr-Cas9–based strategies combined with structural anesthetic binding data from relatively recently developed cryo-EM methods should move some of these anesthetic targets from probable to definite in the future.

How and Where in the Central Nervous System Do Anesthetics Work?

Spinal Cord—Immobility

15 Several lines of evidence indicate that the spinal cord is the main site at which anesthetics inhibit motor responses to noxious stimulation. This is, of course, the end point used in most measurements of anesthetic potency. MAC values for fluorinated VAs are unaffected in the rat by either decerebration or cervical spinal cord transection. Isolation of the cerebral circulation of goats demonstrated that when isoflurane is administered only to the brain, MAC is 2.9%, whereas when it is administered to the body and brain, MAC is 1.2%. Surprisingly, when isoflurane was preferentially administered to the body and not to the brain, isoflurane MAC was reduced to 0.8%, suggesting that anesthetic action on the brain may actually sensitize the cord to noxious stimuli through neurons in the mesencephalic locomotor region.[100] Anesthetic action at the spinal cord underlies MAC through multiple targets. VAs directly reduce excitatory synaptic transmission of spinal neurons. Propofol depresses activity in ventral horn neurons via a GABAergic mechanism that can be blocked by the antagonist picrotoxin. In contrast, while isoflurane inhibits both dorsal horn neurons and motoneurons, the mechanism appears to be independent of GABA receptors. Isoflurane also suppresses interneurons of central pattern generators involved in coordinated movements. Thus, anesthetics can alter descending, afferent, efferent, and modulatory limbs of spinal cord reflex arcs for reacting to noxious stimulation.

Brainstem—Autonomic Control

Anesthetics exert profound effects on cardiopulmonary and thermoregulatory homeostatic circuitry within autonomic centers in the brainstem and hypothalamus. Inspiratory neurons in the medulla drive phrenic motor neurons to activate diaphragmatic contraction. Halothane suppresses the spontaneous activity of these neurons in dogs by reducing glutamatergic input. Anesthetics also perturb cardiovascular reflexes mediated by nuclei in the brainstem. For example, the nucleus ambiguous contains cardiac vagal neurons whose efferents are critical in the regulation of heart rate by the parasympathetic nervous system. In rats, both propofol and isoflurane augment the inhibitory potentials of cardiac vagal neurons in response to GABA. Similarly, neurons in the nucleus of the solitary tract receive sensory input from carotid and aortic body baroreceptors; in vitro studies demonstrate GABA-mediated inhibition of these neurons by propofol and isoflurane.

Mechanisms of Anesthesia—Lessons from Sleep

Anesthetic-induced unconsciousness and sleep share putative underlying circuits and EEG patterns; this relationship serves as a mechanistic basis for how different classes of anesthetic agents induce endpoints of unconsciousness and amnesia. The descent into deep sleep and induction of anesthesia are both accompanied by a shift toward lower frequencies of oscillatory EEG activity, "EEG slowing," with the emergence of θ band (4 to 8 Hz) and δ band (0.5 to 4 Hz) oscillations. In addition, occipital α (8 to 12 Hz) oscillations commonly present during wakefulness, known as the posterior dominant rhythm, are replaced by different EEG motifs. Natural sleep is classified into nonrapid eye movement (NREM) sleep and rapid eye movement (REM) sleep, each with distinct EEG, electrooculographic (EOG), and electromyographic (EMG) patterns relative to wakefulness. Within NREM, Stage N1 is a transitory state with mixed frequency EEG activity and vertex waves. N2 is defined by the emergence of sleep spindles—crescendo–decrescendo oscillatory motifs with fundamental frequencies in the 9- to 13-Hz range—and polyphasic large amplitude motifs known as K-complexes. N3 sleep, often described as slow wave sleep, is defined by the predominance of slow oscillations in the δ frequency band. The resemblance between the EEG patterns of N2 and N3 sleep and those of states of unconsciousness induced by dexmedetomidine, GABAergic sedative hypnotics (benzodiazepines, barbiturates, and propofol), or VAs suggest that sleep and anesthetics engage shared neural circuitry across cortical and subcortical structures. Dexmedetomidine is thought to promote biomimetic sleep, as transitions into states with EEG resembling N2 and N3 sleep are evoked in a dose-dependent manner.

The analogy of anesthetic-induced unconsciousness and sleep states has limitations. REM sleep is characterized by mixed EEG frequencies with similarities to the EEG frequency distribution observed in wakefulness superimposed with θ band "sawtooth waves," lack of EMG activity, and REMs. EEG patterns observed in REM sleep have some similarity, but also notable differences from, the patterns observed with ketamine, nitrous oxide, or xenon. Within this framework, the current state of elucidating endpoints of unconsciousness and amnesia is reviewed.

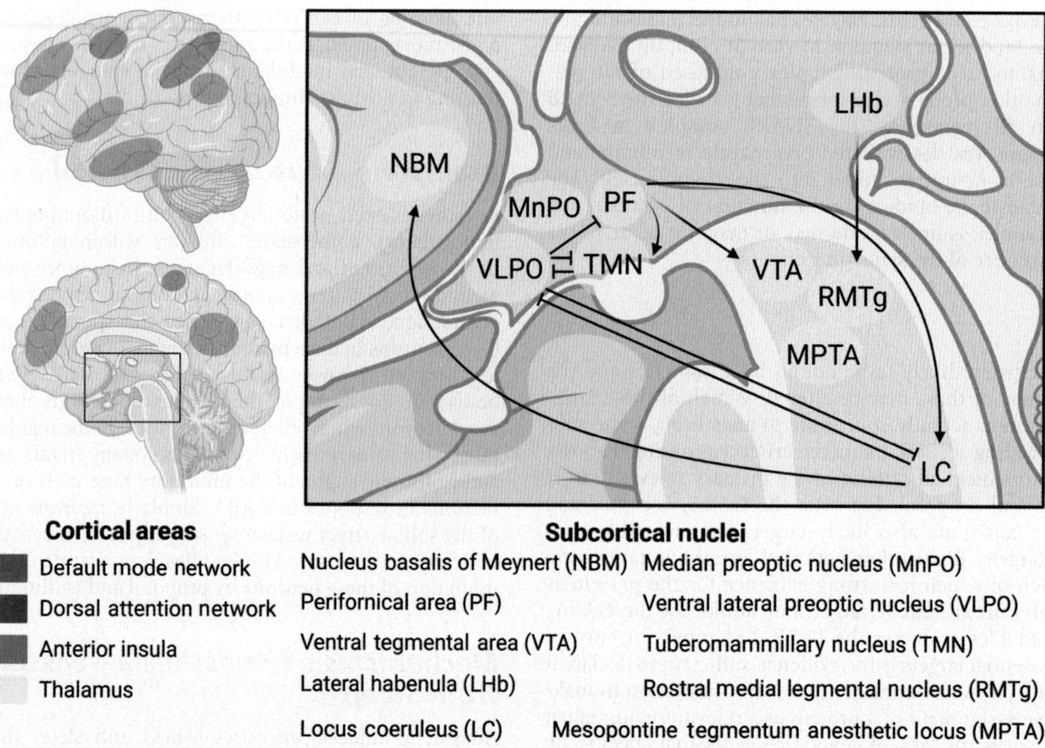

Figure 10-10 Cortical and subcortical areas implicated in anesthetic-induced unconsciousness. Regions implicated in anesthetic-induced unconsciousness include member nodes of the default mode and dorsal attention networks (DMN and DAN) that span lateral and medial cortical regions across different lobes of the brain. Fragmentation of DMN and DAN are potential mechanisms at the cortical level that disrupt awareness during anesthetic-induced unconsciousness. The anterior insula is another cortical area where anesthetic effects could result in impaired switching between internally directed attention (DMN) or externally directed attention (DAN). Disruptions in feedback and/or thalamocortical connectivity may underlie altered network interactions. Anesthetics also target neurons in subcortical circuits of nuclei distributed across the basal forebrain, thalamus, hippocampus, midbrain, and pons. These nuclei serve a critical function of regulating arousal through redundant excitatory and inhibitory interactions such that no single area has been substantiated as a unitary mechanism underlying anesthetic-induced unconsciousness. *Pointed arrows* indicate excitatory pathways while *flathead arrows* show inhibitory projections.

Subcortical and Cortical Structures—Unconsciousness

16 Consciousness is a complex state that can be operationally divided into the components of arousal and awareness that may have differential susceptibility to anesthetics.[101] *Awareness* is the ability to process and store information to interact with the internal or external environment. In contrast, *arousal* or *wakefulness* is the state of receptivity to the external environment and is likely mediated through subcortical structures such as the reticular activating system (RAS) and other arousal centers. From an operational standpoint, sedation implies easily arousable states in response to noxious stimuli, as with sleep, with alterations in level of arousal (drowsiness), and/or awareness (amnesia or altered perceptions of self or the world). In contrast, the unconsciousness of general anesthesia arises through robust impairment of both awareness and arousal, and encompasses the inability to easily rouse an individual despite painful stimuli. The number and distribution of arousal centers are consistent with the redundancy of neural structures devoted toward maintaining and stabilizing arousal and vigilance (Fig. 10-10).

Subcortical Structures—Regulation of Arousal and Sleep

17 The RAS is a diffuse collection of brainstem neurons that mediate arousal, such that electrical stimulation in this structure arouses anesthetized animals. The RAS includes the reticular formation (RF), the tuberomammillary nucleus (TMN), the ventral tegmental area (VTA), and the thalamic intralaminar nucleus.

The RF is a heterogeneous collection of neurons in the midbrain and pons involved in the regulation of arousal and sleep. Lesions of the midbrain RF can induce coma while electrical stimulation of the midbrain awakens sleeping animals. Similar stimulation paradigms induce EEG patterns of restored arousal in rats rendered unresponsive and anesthetized by halothane or isoflurane. GABA levels in the pontine RF are higher during wakefulness than in REM sleep or isoflurane-induced unconsciousness. As the manipulation of GABA levels in the pontine RF can prolong or shorten induction time, the pontine RF remains a plausible direct target for ablation of arousal by anesthetic agents.

Spanning the hypothalamus, the TMN, and areas within the preoptic area are putative loci for anesthetic action in suppressing arousal (Fig. 10-10). The TMN and ventral lateral preoptic nucleus (VLPO) form a bistable mutually inhibitory control circuit promoting wakefulness (TMN) or NREM sleep (VLPO).[102] The median preoptic nucleus (MnPO) is involved in stabilizing sleep and maintaining sleep homeostasis.

Activation of VLPO and the MnPO appears to contribute to sedation but not to the unconsciousness endpoint of general anesthesia. Propofol enhances excitatory transmission to VLPO neurons. In rodents, activation of VLPO neurons by dexmedetomidine induces sedation but not the loss of righting reflex[103] and can antagonize the sedative effects of isoflurane.[104] Ablation of sleep-active VLPO neurons confers resistance to isoflurane induction.[105] In contrast, isoflurane, but not halothane, may also activate MnPO neurons.[106] Stimulation of both sleep- or wake-promoting neurons in the VLPO and MnPO have shown that their role in modulating sleep architecture does not extend into altering the transition between wakefulness and isoflurane-induced unconsciousness.[107]

The TMN contains wake-active neurons and is the sole source of excitatory histaminergic efferents in the CNS. Rats that have had bilateral lesions of the TMN or been treated with intraventricular injections of histamine receptor antagonists manifest both shortened induction and prolonged emergence with isoflurane.[108] Application of a GABAergic antagonist directly onto the TMN diminished the efficacy of the anesthetics propofol and pentobarbital. β3(N265M) $GABA_A$ receptor mutant mice also implicate this nucleus as a target of propofol; the inhibitory postsynaptic potentials of their TMN neurons and the hypnotic effects of propofol are reduced. In addition to direct antagonism of the TMN, inhibitory afferents of the VLPO suppress the locus coeruleus (LC) and the perifornical area (PF).

The PF in the lateral hypothalamus (Fig. 10-10) appears to be critical in anesthetic emergence rather than induction of unconsciousness. It is the sole source of orexin, a neurotransmitter that stabilizes the flip-flopping of the VLPO/TMN sleep switch to favor activation of the arousal-promoting TMN. Orexin KO animals show frequent sleep/wake transitions akin to narcolepsy. In rodents anesthetized by isoflurane, intraventricular injections of orexin-A shift the EEG from burst-suppression to arousal-like patterns. Shortened emergence from propofol or dexmedetomidine can also be induced by orexin-A injections into CSF. Moreover, activation of orexin neurons expedites emergence from isoflurane anesthesia.[109] While ablation of arousal by either isoflurane or sevoflurane is not affected in orexin KO animals, recovery from anesthesia is delayed,[110] suggesting asymmetry in the neural mechanisms underlying induction and emergence.

The lateral habenula (LHb) is a glutamatergic nucleus that connects midbrain and limbic forebrain structures (Fig. 10-10) and regulates dopaminergic and serotoninergic tone. Blockage of excitatory output from this nucleus antagonizes the ability of propofol to induce sedation whereas stimulating output suppresses motor activity.[111] Isoflurane increases activity in glutamatergic LHb neurons. Ablation of these neurons confers resistance to the induction of general anesthesia.[112] GABAergic neurons in the rostral medial tegmental nucleus (RMTg) have been shown to be an important output of the LHb. Propofol promotes excitatory output from the LHb to the RMTg,[111] while activation of RMTg neurons confers sedation and lowers the dose of sevoflurane that induces loss of righting reflex.[113] Thus, this structure may be important in modulating anesthetic sedation but targeting of the RMTg is not sufficient to induce the unconsciousness of general anesthesia.

Within the midbrain, the mesopontine tegmentum anesthetic locus (MPTA) (Fig. 10-10) has been isolated as an important nucleus. Microinjections of pentobarbital and propofol at this site induced general anesthesia, suggesting a potential "switch" for anesthetic-induced unconsciousness.[114] This site is important in regulating sleep and wakefulness, with lesions conferring modestly reduced sensitivities to pentobarbital, etomidate, and propofol but with no effects on the potency of neurosteroids and non-GABAergic anesthetics.[115]

The VTA provides dopaminergic inputs to the prefrontal cortical areas, the hippocampus, and amygdala. In contrast, the LC within the pons is the primary adrenergic source to the cortex, thalamus, and hypothalamus. Dual inhibitors of these two pathways restore righting reflex in isoflurane-anesthetized rats.[8] The VTA and the dopamine D1 receptor play important roles in isoflurane, sevoflurane, and propofol anesthesia. LC activation prolongs induction, antagonizes cortical suppression during anesthetic maintenance, and facilitates emergence through α1 adrenergic receptor mechanisms.[116] These studies suggest that both the VTA and LC play important roles in anesthetic unconsciousness.

Suppression of the nucleus basalis of Meynert (NBM) in the basal forebrain is likely important in mediating anesthetic suppression of arousal and awareness. The NBM receives input from arousal centers and is the major source of excitatory cholinergic input to the thalamus, RAS, and the cerebral cortex. Norepinephrine infused into the NBM induces arousal in rats with righting reflexes ablated by desflurane. Activation of the NBM by histamine reverses EEG slowing and accelerates emergence from isoflurane but not intravenous anesthetics.[117]

Thalamus and Cerebral Cortex—Arousal and Content of Consciousness

The thalamus, as a key structure that regulates widespread cortical excitability and relays information to specialized cortical regions, is a likely target for anesthetic ablation of arousal and awareness.[118] Anesthetic agents do not appear to induce thalamic deafferentation in relay nuclei for vision (lateral geniculate nucleus) or other sensory modalities; peripheral sensory stimulation leads to activation of corresponding cortical areas during general anesthesia and even during burst suppression. In contrast, neurons in the thalamic reticular nuclei (TRN) and medial thalamic nuclei remain plausible potential anesthetic targets. TRN neurons process excitatory input from the cerebral cortex, dorsal thalamic nuclei, and the RAS. They are in a key position to dampen recurrent loops between thalamic and cortical neurons.[118] While TRN neurons are inhibited by etomidate and isoflurane, demonstration of their role in vivo has not been reported. Elsewhere in the thalamus, the stimulation or ablation of the centromedian nuclei alter attention and arousal. Microinfusions targeting Kv1.2 potassium channels[83] or nicotinic cholinergic receptors in these regions reverse VA hypnosis. Humans rendered unconscious by propofol or sevoflurane show weakened correlation between the neural activity in midline thalamic regions and the cortical regions involved in attention and introspection. Optogenetic and chemogenetic techniques should provide a method for testing whether anesthetics induce unconsciousness primarily at these thalamic nuclei, or through their recurrent interactions with specific cortical regions, or within the cerebral cortical regions mediating awareness of space and time.

The cerebral cortex is the major site for generating awareness of the external environment. Primary sensory areas provide focused feed-forward activity to association and "higher" cortical areas that provide reciprocal diffuse feedback. As such, alterations in distributed cortical activity can be viewed as a final common pathway toward anesthetic-induced unconsciousness. 18

The disruption of feedback connections by anesthetics may contribute to impaired consciousness by attenuating the integration of information distributed among cortical regions. The late components of rat visual neuron responses to flashed stimuli are attenuated by desflurane. These high-latency responses are associated with feedback activity and mediate contextual modulation from higher cortical areas. Electrode recordings in rats have also compared the directional bias of activity between frontal and parietal cortical areas in both awake and anesthetized states. While interactions are balanced during wakefulness, feedback interactions were preferentially diminished when rats were anesthetized by isoflurane. Human fMRI[119] and EEG studies have yielded similar findings of reduced feedback from frontal to posterior areas, with propofol, sevoflurane, or ketamine. At a molecular level, attenuation of intracortical feedback could occur between layer 1 apical dendrites and in layer 5 cell bodies, via anesthetic blockade of metabotropic glutamate and cholinergic receptors.

The effects of anesthetics on both cortical firing rates and the timing of action potentials may contribute to the ablation of awareness by limiting both the diversity of information that can be represented and the integration of neural information. Concurrent cortical and thalamic recordings in humans anesthetized with propofol revealed changes in correlated oscillatory activity linking these two structures.[120] Anesthetics alter the topology of distinct networks of distributed cortical areas that subserve attention and higher cognitive processes through patterns of correlated activity. With induction of propofol- or sevoflurane-induced unconsciousness, two such networks have shown weaker correlations among constituent cortical areas: the default mode network, associated with memory and consciousness, and the ventral attention network, linked with externally directed attention.[121,122] These networks represent potential cortical targets of anesthetic action. The weakening of correlated brain activity between regions of different networks suggests that the blurring of boundaries between specialized groups of cortical areas may contribute to impaired consciousness. Alternatively, anesthetics could confer a state of disconnected consciousness by targeting the key cortical regions that govern the switching of attention or conscious access to external stimuli. The anterior insula has become a candidate target, as a cortical region that governs switching between internally and externally directed attention.[123] Thus, anesthetics may induce unconsciousness through targeting key spatially distributed cortical regions (Fig. 10-10).

Hippocampus, Amygdala, and Cerebral Cortex—Amnesia

While the neurobiologic mechanisms underlying learning and memory remain unclear, the hippocampus is a plausible anesthetic target for the suppression of memory formation. Bilateral resection of these structures induces anterograde amnesia as demonstrated by the well-documented case of H.M. Similarly, anesthetics ablate the formation of new memories and substantially alter neural activity while leaving prior memories seemingly intact. Genetic and pharmacologic experiments support a crucial role for the hippocampus in the amnestic actions of anesthetics. The α5 subtype of the $GABA_A$ receptor is primarily expressed in the hippocampus and controls synaptic transmission within this structure. Hippocampal GABA receptors with α5 subunits show conductances that are exquisitely sensitivity to isoflurane and mediate memory deficits that persist after anesthetic exposure. Moreover, α5 $GABA_A$ receptor KO mice are resistant to the amnestic effects of etomidate.[49] The amnestic effects of both volatile and intravenous anesthetics have been localized to extrasynaptic α5 $GABA_A$ receptors. Computational modeling suggests that augmentation of neuronal inhibition by extrasynaptic α5 $GABA_A$ receptors could lead to downstream disruption of pools of synchronous hippocampal–cortical neuronal assemblies.[124] Thus, extrasynaptic α5 $GABA_A$ receptors in the hippocampus are a potential target of several anesthetic agents to induce amnesia.

Summary

Anesthetics suppress circuits in the spinal cord and brain stem to induce immobility and disrupt autonomic homeostasis. The hippocampus is a major site of anesthetic action for anterograde amnesia. As the neurobiologic underpinnings of arousal and awareness are distributed across brainstem, subcortical, and cortical structures, no single anatomic site is responsible for anesthetic-induced unconsciousness. Networks of subcortical and thalamic nuclei are altered in the ablation of arousal but a sole site that is necessary and specific for anesthetic-induced unconsciousness does not appear to exist. Cortical networks critical for cognitive processing of awareness are the tentative substrates for the extinction of subjective percepts, both noxious and otherwise. Network perturbations in frequency content and directionality are putative mechanisms for altered integration and neural representation.

Conclusions

In this chapter, evidence has been reviewed concerning the anatomic, physiologic, and molecular loci of anesthetic action. It is clear that all anesthetic effects cannot be localized to a specific anatomic site in the CNS; indeed, considerable evidence supports the conclusion that different components of the anesthetic state are mediated by actions at disparate anatomic sites. Likewise, the actions of anesthetics cannot be localized to a single neurophysiologic process. While there is consensus that anesthetics ultimately affect synaptic function as opposed to intrinsic neuronal excitability, their particular effects on pre- and postsynaptic function vary by agent and synapse. At a molecular level, VAs show some selectivity, but still affect the function of multiple ion channels and synaptic proteins. The intravenous anesthetics, etomidate, propofol, barbiturates, and neurosteroids are more specific with the $GABA_A$ receptor as their major target. Recent high-resolution structural studies demonstrate binding sites for etomidate, propofol, and a barbiturate on $GABA_A$ receptors. Genetic data plainly demonstrate that the unitary theory of anesthesia is not correct. No single mechanism is responsible for the effects of all general anesthetics, nor does a single mechanism account for all effects of a single anesthetic. The $GABA_A$ receptor, however, does meet all the criteria for an anesthetic target for propofol and etomidate.

Although the precise set of molecular interactions responsible for producing anesthesia has not been fully elucidated, anesthetics do act via selective effects on specific molecular targets. The technologic revolutions in molecular biology, genetics, neurophysiology, structural biology, and neuroimaging make it likely that the next decade will provide additional answers to the anesthetic mechanism puzzle.

Acknowledgments

The authors acknowledge generous ongoing funding support from National Institute of General Medical Sciences, National Institute of Neurological Disorders and Stroke, National Center for Research Resources, the National Center for Advancing Translational Sciences, National Institute for Mental Health, and the Taylor Institute for Innovative Psychiatry (ASE), for ASE-R01 GM108799, 1P50MH122379, CMC-1R01NS100350, 1R01NS109088, 1R01GM129034, and BJAP-1R01AG057901 and 1U01MH128483.

For further review and interactivities, please see the videos and narrative interactive clinical vignettes (NICVs) accessible in the complimentary eBook bundled with this text. Access instructions are located on the inside front cover.

REFERENCES

1. Kelz MB, Mashour GA. The biology of general anesthesia from paramecium to primate. *Curr Biol*. 2019;29(22):R1199–R1210.
2. Mashour GA. Top-down mechanisms of anesthetic-induced unconsciousness. *Front Syst Neurosci*. 2014;8:115.

3. Tononi G. Consciousness as integrated information: a provisional manifesto. *Biol Bull.* 2008;215(3):216–242.
4. Tononi G, Koch C. Consciousness: here, there and everywhere? *Philos Trans R Soc Lond B Biol Sci.* 2015;370(1668):20140167.
5. Akeju O, Loggia ML, Catana C, et al. Disruption of thalamic functional connectivity is a neural correlate of dexmedetomidine-induced unconsciousness. *Elife.* 2014;3:e04499.
6. Friedman EB, Sun Y, Moore JT, et al. A conserved behavioral state barrier impedes transitions between anesthetic-induced unconsciousness and wakefulness: evidence for neural inertia. *PLoS One.* 2010;5(7):e11903.
7. Kelz MB, García PS, Mashour GA, Solt K. Escape from oblivion: neural mechanisms of emergence from general anesthesia. *Anesth Analg.* 2019;128(4):726–736.
8. Solt K, Cotten JF, Cimenser A, Wong KF, Chemali JJ, Brown EN. Methylphenidate actively induces emergence from general anesthesia. *Anesthesiology.* 2011;115(4):791–803.
9. Quasha AL, Eger EI 2nd, Tinker JH, Determination and applications of MAC. *Anesthesiology,* 1980;53(4):315–334.
10. Franks NP, Lieb WR. Molecular and cellular mechanisms of general anaesthesia. *Nature.* 1994;367(6464):607–614.
11. Bowdle TA. Depth of anesthesia monitoring. *Anesthesiol Clin.* 2006;24(4):793–822.
12. Avidan MS, Jacobsohn E, Glick D, et al; BAG-RECALL Research Group. Prevention of intraoperative awareness in a high-risk surgical population. *N Engl J Med.* 2011;365(7):591–600.
13. Avidan MS, Zhang L, Burnside BA, et al. Anesthesia awareness and the bispectral index. *N Engl J Med.* 2008;358(11):1097–1108.
14. Bruhn J, Myles PS, Sneyd R, Struys MMRF. Depth of anaesthesia monitoring: what's available, what's validated and what's next? *Br J Anaesth.* 2006;97(1):85–94.
15. Franks NP, Lieb WR. Where do general anaesthetics act? *Nature.* 1978;274(5669):339–342.
16. Koblin DD, Chortkoff BS, Laster MJ, Eger EI 2nd, Halsey MJ, Ionescu P. Polyhalogenated and perfluorinated compounds that disobey the Meyer-Overton hypothesis. *Anesth Analg.* 1994;79(6):1043–1048.
17. Kandel L, Chortkoff BS, Sonner J, Laster MJ, Eger EI 2nd. Nonanesthetics can suppress learning. *Anesth Analg.* 1996;82(2):321–326.
18. Alifimoff JK, Firestone LL, Miller KW, Anaesthetic potencies of primary alkanols: implications for the molecular dimensions of the anaesthetic site. *Br J Pharmacol.* 1989;96(1):9–16.
19. Franks NP. Molecular targets underlying general anaesthesia. *Br J Pharmacol.* 2006;147 (Suppl 1):S72–S81.
20. Sezgin E, Levental I, Mayor S, Eggeling C. The mystery of membrane organization: composition, regulation and roles of lipid rafts. *Nat Rev Mol Cell Biol.* 2017;18(6):361–374.
21. Pavel MA, Petersen EN, Wang H, Lerner RA, Hansen SB. Studies on the mechanism of general anesthesia. *Proc Natl Acad Sci U S A.* 2020;117(24):13757–13766.
22. Wague A, Joseph TT, Woll KA, et al. Mechanistic insights into volatile anesthetic modulation of K2P channels. *Elife.* 2020;9:e59839.
23. Rusinova R, He C, Andersen OS. Mechanisms underlying drug-mediated regulation of membrane protein function. *Proc Natl Acad Sci U S A.* 2021;118(46):e2113229118.
24. Li GD, Chiara DC, Sawyer GW, Husain SS, Olsen RW, Cohen JB. Identification of a GABAA receptor anesthetic binding site at subunit interfaces by photolabeling with an etomidate analog. *J Neurosci.* 2006;26(45):11599–11605.
25. Yip GM, Chen ZW, Edge CJ, et al. A propofol binding site on mammalian GABAA receptors identified by photolabeling. *Nat Chem Biol.* 2013;9(11):715–720.
26. Jayakar SS, Zhou X, Chiara DC, et al. Multiple propofol-binding sites in a gamma-aminobutyric acid type A receptor (GABAAR) identified using a photoreactive propofol analog. *J Biol Chem.* 2014;289(40):27456–27468.
27. Chiara DC, Dostalova Z, Jayakar SS, Zhou X, Miller KW, Cohen JB. Mapping general anesthetic binding site(s) in human $\alpha 1\beta 3$ γ-aminobutyric acid type A receptors with [(3)H]TDBzl-etomidate, a photoreactive etomidate analogue. *Biochemistry.* 2012;51(4): 836–847.
28. Chen ZW, Bracamontes JR, Budelier MM, et al. Multiple functional neurosteroid binding sites on GABAA receptors. *PLoS Biol.* 2019;17(3):e3000157.
29. Jayakar SS, Chiara DC, Zhou X, et al. Photoaffinity labeling identifies an intersubunit steroid-binding site in heteromeric GABA type A (GABAA) receptors. *J Biol Chem.* 2020;295(33): 11495–11512.
30. Woll KA, Zhou X, Bhanu NV, et al. Identification of binding sites contributing to volatile anesthetic effects on GABA type A receptors. *FASEB J.* 2018;32(8):4172–4189.
31. Nury H, Bocquet N, Le Poupon C, et al. Crystal structure of the extracellular domain of a bacterial ligand-gated ion channel. *J Mol Biol.* 2010;395(5):1114–1127.
32. Kim JJ, Gharpure A, Teng J, et al. Shared structural mechanisms of general anaesthetics and benzodiazepines. *Nature.* 2020;585(7824):303–308.
33. Laverty D, Thomas P, Field M, et al. Crystal structures of a GABA(A)-receptor chimera reveal new endogenous neurosteroid-binding sites. *Nat Struct Mol Biol.* 2017;24(11):977–985.
34. Miller PS, Scott S, Masiulis S, et al. Structural basis for GABA(A) receptor potentiation by neurosteroids. *Nat Struct Mol Biol.* 2017;24(11):986–992.
35. Chen Q, Wells MM, Arjunan P, et al. Structural basis of neurosteroid anesthetic action on GABAA receptors. *Nat Commun.* 2018;9(1):3972.
36. Hosie AM, Wilkins ME, da Silva HMA, Smart TG. Endogenous neurosteroids regulate GABAA receptors through two discrete transmembrane sites. *Nature.* 2006;444(7118):486–489.
37. Zhu S, Noviello CM, Teng J, Walsh RM Jr, Kim JJ, Hibbs RE. Structure of a human synaptic GABA(A) receptor. *Nature.* 2018;559(7712):67–72.
38. Laverty D, Desai R, Uchański T, et al. Cryo-EM structure of the human $\alpha 1\beta 3\gamma 2$ GABA(A) receptor in a lipid bilayer. *Nature.* 2019;565(7740):516–520.
39. Nakane T, Kotecha A, Sente A, et al. Single-particle cryo-EM at atomic resolution. *Nature.* 2020;587(7832):152–156.
40. Wu XS, Sun JY, Evers AS, Crowder M, Wu LG. Isoflurane inhibits transmitter release and the presynaptic action potential. *Anesthesiology.* 2004;100(3):663–670.
41. Perouansky M, Baranov D, Salman M, Yaari Y. Effects of halothane on glutamate receptor-mediated excitatory post-synaptic currents. A patch-clamp study in adult mouse hippocampal slices. *Anesthesiology.* 1995;83(1):109–119.
42. MacIver MB, Roth SH. Inhalational anaesthetics exhibit pathway-specific and differential actions on hippocampal synaptic responses in vitro. *Br J Anaesth.* 1988;60:680–691.
43. Westphalen RI, Hemmings HC Jr. Selective depression by general anesthetics of glutamate versus GABA release from isolated cortical nerve terminals. *J Pharmacol Exp Ther.* 2003; 304(3):1188–1196.
44. van Swinderen B, Saifee O, Shebester L, Roberson R, Nonet ML, Crowder CM. A neomorphic syntaxin mutation blocks volatile-anesthetic action in Caenorhabditis elegans. *Proc Natl Acad Sci U S A.* 1999;96(5):2479–2484.
45. Mihic SJ, Ye Q, Wick MJ, et al. Sites of alcohol and volatile anaesthetic action on GABA(A) and glycine receptors. *Nature.* 1997;389(6649):385–389.
46. Belelli D, Lambert JJ, Peters JA, Wafford K, Whiting PJ. The interaction of the general anesthetic etomidate with the gamma-aminobutyric acid type A receptor is influenced by a single amino acid. *Proc Natl Acad Sci U S A.* 1997;94(20):11031–11036.
47. Krasowski MD, Koltchine VV, Rick CE, Ye Q, Finn SE, Harrison NL. Propofol and other intravenous anesthetics have sites of action on the gamma-aminobutyric acid type a receptor distinct from that for isoflurane. *Mol Pharmacol.* 1998;53(3):530–538.
48. Rau V, Iyer SV, Oh I, et al. Gamma-aminobutyric acid type A receptor alpha 4 subunit knockout mice are resistant to the amnestic effect of isoflurane. *Anesth Analg.* 2009;109(6):1816–1822.
49. Cheng VY, Martin LJ, Elliott EM, et al. Alpha5GABAA receptors mediate the amnestic but not sedative-hypnotic effects of the general anesthetic etomidate. *J Neurosci.* 2006;26(14):3713–3720.
50. Borghese CM, Werner DF, Topf N, et al. An isoflurane- and alcohol-insensitive mutant GABA(A) receptor alpha(1) subunit with near-normal apparent affinity for GABA: characterization in heterologous systems and production of knockin mice. *J Pharmacol Exp Ther.* 2006;319(1):208–218.
51. Sonner JM, Werner DF, Elsen FP, et al. Effect of isoflurane and other potent inhaled anesthetics on minimum alveolar concentration, learning, and the righting reflex in mice engineered to express alpha1 gamma-aminobutyric acid type A receptors unresponsive to isoflurane. *Anesthesiology.* 2007;106(1):107–113.
52. Werner DF, Blednov YA, Ariwodola OJ, et al. Knockin mice with ethanol-insensitive alpha1-containing gamma-aminobutyric acid type A receptors display selective alterations in behavioral responses to ethanol. *J Pharmacol Exp Ther.* 2006;319(1):219–227.
53. Nishikawa K, Jenkins A, Paraskevakis I, Harrison NL. Volatile anesthetic actions on the GABAA receptors: contrasting effects of alpha 1(S270) and beta 2(N265) point mutations. *Neuropharmacology.* 2002;42(3):337–345.
54. Homanics GE, Elsen FP, Ying SW, et al. A gain-of-function mutation in the GABA receptor produces synaptic and behavioral abnormalities in the mouse. *Genes Brain Behav.* 2005;4(1):10–19.
55. Jurd R, Arras M, Lambert S, et al. General anesthetic actions in vivo strongly attenuated by a point mutation in the GABA(A) receptor beta3 subunit. *FASEB J.* 2003;17(2):250–252.
56. Zeller A, Arras M, Jurd R, Rudolph U. Identification of a molecular target mediating the general anesthetic actions of pentobarbital. *Mol Pharmacol.* 2007;71(3):852–859.
57. Zeller A, Arras M, Jurd R, Rudolph U. Mapping the contribution of beta3-containing GABAA receptors to volatile and intravenous general anesthetic actions. *BMC Pharmacol.* 2007;7:2.
58. Zeller A, Arras M, Lazaris A, Jurd R, Rudolph U. Distinct molecular targets for the central respiratory and cardiac actions of the general anesthetics etomidate and propofol. *FASEB J.* 2005;19(12):1677–1679.
59. Lambert S, Arras M, Vogt KE, Rudolph U. Isoflurane-induced surgical tolerance mediated only in part by beta3-containing GABA(A) receptors. *Eur J Pharmacol.* 2005;516(1):23–27.
60. Liao M, Sonner JM, Jurd R, et al. Beta3-containing gamma-aminobutyric acidA receptors are not major targets for the amnesic and immobilizing actions of isoflurane. *Anesth Analg.* 2005;101(2):412–418, table of contents.
61. Rau V, Oh I, Liao M, et al. Gamma-aminobutyric acid type A receptor beta3 subunit forebrain-specific knockout mice are resistant to the amnestic effect of isoflurane. *Anesth Analg.* 2011;113(3):500–504.
62. Cirone J, Rosahl TW, Reynolds DS, et al. Gamma-aminobutyric acid type A receptor beta 2 subunit mediates the hypothermic effect of etomidate in mice. *Anesthesiology.* 2004;100(6):1438–1445.
63. Reynolds DS, Rosahl TW, Cirone J, et al. Sedation and anesthesia mediated by distinct GABA(A) receptor isoforms. *J Neurosci.* 2003;23(24):8608–8617.
64. Mihalek RM, Banerjee PK, Korpi ER, et al. Attenuated sensitivity to neuroactive steroids in gamma-aminobutyrate type A receptor delta subunit knockout mice. *Proc Natl Acad Sci U S A.* 1999;96(22):12905–12910.
65. Chen X, Sirois JE, Lei Q, Talley EM, Lynch C 3rd, Bayliss DA. HCN subunit-specific and cAMP-modulated effects of anesthetics on neuronal pacemaker currents. *J Neurosci.* 2005; 25(24):5803–5814.

66. Chen X, Shu S, Bayliss DA. HCN1 channel subunits are a molecular substrate for hypnotic actions of ketamine. *J Neurosci*. 2009;29(3):600–609.
67. Zhou C, Liang P, Liu J, et al. HCN1 channels contribute to the effects of amnesia and hypnosis but not immobility of volatile anesthetics. *Anesth Analg*. 2015;121(3):661–666.
68. Mattusch C, Kratzer S, Buerge M, et al. Impact of hyperpolarization-activated, cyclic nucleotide-gated cation channel type 2 for the xenon-mediated anesthetic effect: evidence from in vitro and in vivo experiments. *Anesthesiology*. 2015;122(5):1047–1059.
69. Franks NP, Lieb WR. Volatile general anaesthetics activate a novel neuronal K+ current. *Nature*. 1988;333(6174):662–664.
70. Patel AJ, Honoré E, Lesage F, Fink M, Romey G, Lazdunski M. Inhalational anesthetics activate two-pore-domain background K+channels. *Nat Neurosci*. 1999;2(5):422–426.
71. Heurteaux C, Guy N, Laigle C, et al. TREK-1, a K+ channel involved in neuroprotection and general anesthesia. *EMBO J*. 2004;23(13):2684–2695.
72. Westphalen RI, Krivitski M, Amarosa A, Guy N, Hemmings HC Jr. Reduced inhibition of cortical glutamate and GABA release by halothane in mice lacking the K+ channel, TREK-1. *Br J Pharmacol*. 2007;152(6):939–945.
73. Lazarenko RM, Willcox SC, Shu S, et al. Motoneuronal TASK channels contribute to immobilizing effects of inhalational general anesthetics. *J Neurosci*. 2010;30(22):7691–7704.
74. Pal D, Jones JM, Wisidagamage S, Meisler MH, Mashour GA. Reduced Nav1.6 sodium channel activity in mice increases in vivo sensitivity to volatile anesthetics. *PLoS One*. 2015;10(8): e0134960.
75. Timic Stamenic T, Todorovic SM. Thalamic T-type calcium channels as targets for hypnotics and general anesthetics. *Int J Mol Sci*. 2022;23(4).
76. Petrenko AB, Tsujita M, Kohno T, Sakimura K, Baba H. Mutation of alpha1G T-type calcium channels in mice does not change anesthetic requirements for loss of the righting reflex and minimum alveolar concentration but delays the onset of anesthetic induction. *Anesthesiology*. 2007;106(6):1177–1185.
77. Timic Stamenic T, Feseha S, Manzella FM, et al. The T-type calcium channel isoform Ca(v)3.1 is a target for the hypnotic effect of the anaesthetic neurosteroid (3β,5β,17β)-3-hydroxyandrostane-17-carbonitrile. *Br J Anaesth*. 2021;126(1):245–255.
78. Orestes P, Bojadzic D, Chow RM, Todorovic SM. Mechanisms and functional significance of inhibition of neuronal T-type calcium channels by isoflurane. *Mol Pharmacol*. 2009;75(3): 542–554.
79. Feseha S, Timic Stamenic T, Wallace D, et al. Global genetic deletion of Ca(V)3.3 channels facilitates anaesthetic induction and enhances isoflurane-sparing effects of T-type calcium channel blockers. *Sci Rep*. 2020;10(1):21510.
80. Lioudyno MI, Birch AM, Tanaka BS, et al. Shaker-related potassium channels in the central medial nucleus of the thalamus are important molecular targets for arousal suppression by volatile general anesthetics. *J Neurosci*. 2013;33(41):16310–16322.
81. Weber B, Schaper C, Bushey D, et al. Increased volatile anesthetic requirement in short-sleeping Drosophila mutants. *Anesthesiology*. 2009;110(2):313–316.
82. Joiner WJ, Friedman EB, Hung HT, et al. Genetic and anatomical basis of the barrier separating wakefulness and anesthetic-induced unresponsiveness. *PLoS Genet*. 2013;9(9):e1003605.
83. Alkire MT, Asher CD, Franciscus AM, Hahn EL. Thalamic microinfusion of antibody to a voltage-gated potassium channel restores consciousness during anesthesia. *Anesthesiology*. 2009;110(4):766–773.
84. Woll KA, Peng W, Liang Q, et al. Photoaffinity ligand for the inhalational anesthetic sevoflurane allows mechanistic insight into potassium channel modulation. *ACS Chem Biol*. 2017; 12(5):1353–1362.
85. Mennerick S, Jevtovic-Todorovic V, Todorovic SM, Shen W, Olney JW, Zorumski CF. Effect of nitrous oxide on excitatory and inhibitory synaptic transmission in hippocampal cultures. *J Neurosci*. 1998;18(23):9716–9726.
86. Franks NP, Dickinson R, de Sousa SL, Hall AC, Lieb WR. How does xenon produce anaesthesia? [letter]. *Nature*. 1998;396:324.
87. Sato Y, Kobayashi E, Murayama T, Mishina M, Seo N. Effect of N-methyl-D-aspartate receptor epsilon1 subunit gene disruption of the action of general anesthetic drugs in mice. *Anesthesiology*. 2005;102(3):557–561.
88. Nagele P, Metz LB, Crowder CM. Nitrous oxide (N(2)O) requires the N-methyl-D-aspartate receptor for its action in Caenorhabditis elegans. *Proc Natl Acad Sci U S A*. 2004;101(23):8791–8796.
89. Nagele P, Metz LB, Crowder CM. Xenon acts by inhibition of non-N-methyl-D-aspartate receptor-mediated glutamatergic neurotransmission in Caenorhabditis elegans. *Anesthesiology*. 2005;103(3):508–513.
90. Zhang Y, Ye F, Zhang T, et al. Structural basis of ketamine action on human NMDA receptors. *Nature*. 2021;596(7871):301–305.
91. Morgan PG, Cascorbi HF. Effect of anesthetics and a convulsant on normal and mutant Caenorhabditis elegans. *Anesthesiology*. 1985;62(6):738–744.
92. Kayser EB, Morgan PG, Sedensky MM. GAS-1: a mitochondrial protein controls sensitivity to volatile anesthetics in the nematode Caenorhabditis elegans. *Anesthesiology*. 1999;90(2):545–554.
93. Quintana A, Morgan PG, Kruse SE, Palmiter RD, Sedensky MM. Altered anesthetic sensitivity of mice lacking Ndufs4, a subunit of mitochondrial complex I. *PLoS One*. 2012;7(8): e42904.
94. Zimin PI, Woods CB, Kayser EB, Ramirez JM, Morgan PG, Sedensky MM. Isoflurane disrupts excitatory neurotransmitter dynamics via inhibition of mitochondrial complex I. *Br J Anaesth*. 2018;120(5):1019–1032.
95. Hsieh VC, Niezgoda J, Sedensky MM, Hoppel CL, Morgan PG. Anesthetic hypersensitivity in a case-controlled series of patients with mitochondrial disease. *Anesth Analg*. 2021;133(4):924–932.
96. Troup M, Zalucki OH, Kottler BD, Karunanithi S, Anggono V, van Swinderen B. Syntaxin1A neomorphic mutations promote rapid recovery from isoflurane anesthesia in drosophila melanogaster. *Anesthesiology*. 2019;131(3):555–568.
97. Herring BE, Xie Z, Marks J, Fox AP. Isoflurane inhibits the neurotransmitter release machinery. *J Neurophysiol*. 2009;102(2):1265–1273.
98. Metz LB, Dasgupta N, Liu C, Hunt SJ, Crowder CM. An evolutionarily conserved presynaptic protein is required for isoflurane sensitivity in Caenorhabditis elegans. *Anesthesiology*. 2007; 107(6):971–982.
99. Nagele P, Mendel JB, Placzek WJ, Scott BA, D'Avignon DA, Crowder CM. Volatile anesthetics bind rat synaptic snare proteins. *Anesthesiology*. 2005;103(4):768–778.
100. Jinks SL, Bravo M, Satter O, Chan YM. Brainstem regions affecting minimum alveolar concentration and movement pattern during isoflurane anesthesia. *Anesthesiology*. 2010;112(2):316–324.
101. Laureys S. The neural correlate of (un)awareness: lessons from the vegetative state. *Trends Cogn Sci*. 2005;9(12):556–559.
102. Saper CB, Chou TC, Scammell TE. The sleep switch: hypothalamic control of sleep and wakefulness. *Trends Neurosci*. 2001;24(12):726–731.
103. Zhang Z, Ferretti V, Güntan İ, et al. Neuronal ensembles sufficient for recovery sleep and the sedative actions of alpha2 adrenergic agonists. *Nat Neurosci*. 2015;18(4):553–561.
104. McCarren HS, Chalifoux MR, Han B, et al. α2-Adrenergic stimulation of the ventrolateral preoptic nucleus destabilizes the anesthetic state. *J Neurosci*. 2014;34(49):16385–16396.
105. Moore JT, Chen J, Han B, et al. Direct activation of sleep-promoting VLPO neurons by volatile anesthetics contributes to anesthetic hypnosis. *Curr Biol*. 2012;22(21):2008–2016.
106. Han B, McCarren HS, O'Neill D, Kelz MB, et al. Distinctive recruitment of endogenous sleep-promoting neurons by volatile anesthetics and a nonimmobilizer. *Anesthesiology*. 2014;121(5):999–1009.
107. Vanini G, Bassana M, Mast M, et al. Activation of preoptic GABAergic or glutamatergic neurons modulates sleep-wake architecture, but not anesthetic state transitions. *Curr Biol*. 2020;30(5):779–787.e4.
108. Luo T, Leung LS. Involvement of tuberomamillary histaminergic neurons in isoflurane anesthesia. *Anesthesiology*. 2011;115(1):36–43.
109. Zhou W, Cheung K, Kyu S, et al. Activation of orexin system facilitates anesthesia emergence and pain control. *Proc Natl Acad Sci U S A*. 2018;115(45):E10740–E10747.
110. Kelz MB, Sun Y, Chen J, et al. An essential role for orexins in emergence from general anesthesia. *Proc Natl Acad Sci U S A*. 2008;105(4):1309–1314.
111. Gelegen C, Miracca G, Ran MZ, et al. Excitatory pathways from the lateral habenula enable propofol-induced sedation. *Curr Biol*. 2018;28(4):580–587.e5.
112. Liu C, Liu J, Zhou L, et al. Lateral habenula glutamatergic neurons modulate isoflurane anesthesia in mice. *Front Mol Neurosci*. 2021;14:628996.
113. Vlasov K, Pei J, Nehs CJ, et al. Activation of GABAergic neurons in the rostromedial tegmental nucleus and other brainstem regions promotes sedation and facilitates sevoflurane anesthesia in mice. *Anesth Analg*. 2021;132(4):e50–e55.
114. Sukhotinsky I, Minert A, Soja P, Devor M. Mesopontine switch for the induction of general anesthesia by dedicated neural pathways. *Anesth Analg*. 2016;123(5):1274–1285.
115. Minert A, Baron M, Devor M. Reduced sensitivity to anesthetic agents upon lesioning the mesopontine tegmental anesthesia area in rats depends on anesthetic type. *Anesthesiology*. 2020; 132(3): 535–550.
116. Vazey EM, Aston-Jones G. Designer receptor manipulations reveal a role of the locus coeruleus noradrenergic system in isoflurane general anesthesia. *Proc Natl Acad Sci U S A*. 2014; 111(10):3859–3864.
117. Luo T, Leung LS. Basal forebrain histaminergic transmission modulates electroencephalographic activity and emergence from isoflurane anesthesia. *Anesthesiology*. 2009;111(4):725–733.
118. Alkire MT, Haier RJ, Fallon JH. Toward a unified theory of narcosis: brain imaging evidence for a thalamocortical switch as the neurophysiologic basis of anesthetic-induced unconsciousness. *Conscious Cogn*. 2000;9(3):370–386.
119. Jordan D, Ilg R, Riedl V, et al. Simultaneous electroencephalographic and functional magnetic resonance imaging indicate impaired cortical top-down processing in association with anesthetic-induced unconsciousness. *Anesthesiology*. 2013;119(5):1031–1042.
120. Malekmohammadi M, Price CM, Hudson AE, DiCesare JAT, Pouratian N. Propofol-induced loss of consciousness is associated with a decrease in thalamocortical connectivity in humans. *Brain*. 2019;142(8):2288–2302.
121. Boveroux P, Vanhaudenhuyse A, Bruno MA, et al. Breakdown of within- and between-network resting state functional magnetic resonance imaging connectivity during propofol-induced loss of consciousness. *Anesthesiology*. 2010;113(5):1038–1053.
122. Palanca BJA, Mitra A, Larson-Prior L, Snyder AZ, Avidan MS, Raichle ME. Resting-state functional magnetic resonance imaging correlates of sevoflurane-induced unconsciousness. *Anesthesiology*. 2015;123(2):346–356.
123. Huang Z, Tarnal V, Vlisides PE, et al. Anterior insula regulates brain network transitions that gate conscious access. *Cell Rep*. 2021;35(5):109081.
124. Storer KP, Reeke GN. γ-Aminobutyric acid type A receptor potentiation inhibits learning in a computational network model. *Anesthesiology*. 2018;129(1):106–117.
125. Postea O, Biel M. Exploring HCN channels as novel drug targets. *Nat Rev Drug Discov*. 2011;10(12):903–914.

11 Basic Principles of Clinical Pharmacology

JERRY INGRANDE • THOMAS K. HENTHORN

KEY POINTS

1. Most drugs must pass through cell membranes to reach their sites of action. Consequently, drugs tend to be relatively lipophilic, rather than hydrophilic.
2. The highly lipophilic anesthetic drugs have a rapid onset of action because they rapidly diffuse into well-perfused brain tissue. They have a very short duration of action because of redistribution of drug from the central nervous system to the blood.
3. The cytochrome P450 (CYP) superfamily is the most important group of enzymes involved in drug metabolism. It and other drug-metabolizing enzymes exhibit genetic polymorphism.
4. The kidneys eliminate hydrophilic drugs and relatively hydrophilic metabolites of lipophilic drugs. Renal elimination of lipophilic compounds is negligible.
5. The liver is the most important organ for metabolism of drugs. Hepatic drug clearance depends on three factors: the intrinsic ability of the liver to metabolize a drug, hepatic blood flow, and the extent of binding of the drug to blood components.
6. The volume of distribution quantifies the extent of drug distribution. The greater the affinity of tissues for a drug relative to blood, the greater its volume of distribution (i.e., lipophilic drugs have greater volumes of distribution).
7. Elimination clearance is the parameter that characterizes the ability of drug-eliminating tissues to irreversibly remove drugs from the body. The efficiency of the body in clearing drugs is proportional to the elimination clearance.
8. All else being equal, an increase in the volume of distribution of a drug will increase its elimination half-life; an increase in elimination clearance will decrease elimination half-life.
9. Most drugs bring about a pharmacologic effect by binding to a specific receptor that results in a change in cellular function.
10. Although most pharmacologic effects can be characterized by both dose–response curves and concentration–response curves, dose–response curves cannot be used to determine whether variations in pharmacologic response are caused by differences in pharmacokinetics, pharmacodynamics, or both.
11. Integrated pharmacokinetic–pharmacodynamic models allow temporal characterization of the relationship between dose, plasma concentration, and pharmacologic effect.
12. In vitro drug–drug interactions due to pharmaceutical (physiochemical) properties of drugs can significantly alter drug bioavailability and produce unintended toxic byproducts.
13. Novel approaches to antagonizing neuromuscular blockade have been developed that take advantage of in vivo physiochemical drug–drug interactions, thereby avoiding some of the systemic side effects associated with inhibition of plasma acetylcholinesterase.
14. Distribution clearance is influenced by changes in cardiac output and regional blood flow.
15. Inhibition of CYP isozyme activity can make it difficult to achieve adequate analgesia when using opioids such as codeine and tramadol that require CYP 2D6 activity for conversion to the biologically active opioid.

16 Serotonin syndrome can be precipitated by a wide array of drugs with serotonergic activity, including selective serotonin reuptake inhibitors (SSRIs), serotonin–norepinephrine reuptake inhibitors (SNRIs), and phenylpiperidine opioids.

17 Simulations of multicompartmental pharmacokinetic models that describe intravenous anesthetics demonstrate that for most anesthetic dosing regimens, the distribution of drug from the plasma to the inert peripheral tissues has a greater influence on the plasma concentration profile of the drug compared to the elimination of drug from the body.

18 Target-controlled infusions are achieved with computer-controlled infusion pumps worldwide (not yet approved by the Food and Drug Administration in the United States), and permit clinicians to make use of the drug concentration–effect relationship, optimally accounting for pharmacokinetics and predicting the offset of drug effect.

19 Classic pharmacokinetic models inaccurately describe the initial several minutes of drug distribution and, therefore, overestimate interindividual pharmacodynamic variability.

20 By understanding the interactions between the opioids and the sedative-hypnotics (e.g., response surface models), it is possible to select target concentration pairs of the two drugs that produce the desired clinical effect while minimizing unwanted side effects associated with high concentrations of either drug.

In 1943, Halford[1] labeled thiopental as "an ideal method of euthanasia" for war surgical patients but pronounced that "open drop ether still retains primacy!" Based on this recount of the experience with thiopental at Pearl Harbor, it is impressive that cooler heads prevailed; Adams and Gray[2] detailed a case of a civilian gunshot wound where they carefully titrated thiopental without any adverse respiratory or cardiovascular events. To highlight the importance of the quiet case report versus the animated condemnation of intravenous (IV) anesthesia for patients with hemorrhagic shock, an anonymous editorial appeared in the same issue of *Anesthesiology* that attempted to give some scientific justification for the discrepancy in opinions.[3] As the editorial detailed, thiopental has a small therapeutic index, and the tolerance to normal doses is decreased in extreme physical conditions (e.g., blood loss, sepsis). Therefore, just like with open drop ether, small doses of thiopental should be titrated to achieve the desired effects and avoid side effects associated with overdose. Fortuitously, the anesthesia community did not simply abandon the use of thiopental, and in 1960, Price[4] utilized mathematical models to describe the effects of hypovolemia on thiopental distribution.

Anesthetic drugs are administered with the goal of rapidly establishing and maintaining a therapeutic effect while minimizing undesired side effects. Although open drop ether and chloroform were administered using knowledge of a dose–effect relationship, the more potent volatile agents, along with the IV hypnotics, neuromuscular junction blocking agents, and IV opioids, all require a sound knowledge of pharmacokinetics and pharmacodynamics in order to accurately achieve the desired pharmacologic effect for the desired period of time without any drug toxicity.

This chapter attempts to guide the reader through the fundamental knowledge of what the body does to a drug (i.e., pharmacokinetics) and what a drug does to the body (i.e., pharmacodynamics). The initial section of this chapter discusses the biologic and pharmacologic factors that influence the absorption, distribution, and elimination of a drug from the body. Where necessary, quantitative analyses of these processes are discussed to give readers insight into the intricacies of pharmacokinetics that cannot be easily described by text alone. The second section concentrates on the factors that determine the relationship between drug concentration and pharmacologic effect. Once again, mathematical models are presented as needed in order to clarify pharmacodynamic concepts. The third section applies concepts from the first two sections in order to describe the clinically important drug–drug interactions that are encountered in the perioperative period. The final section builds on the reader's knowledge gained from the first two sections to apply the principles of pharmacokinetics and pharmacodynamics to determine the target concentration of IV anesthetics required and the dosing strategies necessary to produce an adequate anesthetic state. Understanding these concepts should allow the reader to integrate the anesthetic drugs of the future into a rational anesthetic regimen. Although specific drugs are utilized to illustrate pharmacokinetic and pharmacodynamic principles throughout this chapter, the principles discussed are universal. Detailed pharmacologic information of the anesthetic pharmacopeia are presented in subsequent chapters of this book.

Pharmacokinetic Principles

Drug Absorption and Routes of Administration

Transfer of Drugs across Membranes

Even drugs that are administered directly into the bloodstream 1
must move across at least one cell membrane to get to their site of action. Because biologic membranes are lipid bilayers composed of a lipophilic core sandwiched between two hydrophilic layers, only small lipophilic drugs can passively diffuse across the membrane down their concentration gradients. For water-soluble drugs to passively diffuse across the cell membrane down a concentration gradient, a hydrophilic channel formed from transmembrane proteins is required. Nonspecific hydrophilic channels are abundant in the capillary endothelium of all organs except for the central nervous system (CNS). As a result, *passive transport* of drugs from the intravascular space into the interstitium of various organs is limited by blood flow, not by the lipid solubility of the drug.[5]

In the CNS, the blood–brain barrier capillary endothelial cells have very limited numbers of transmembrane hydrophilic channels. Hydrophilic drugs can only enter the CNS after binding to drug-specific transmembrane proteins that actively transport the hydrophilic drug across the capillary endothelium into the CNS interstitium. When these transmembrane carrier proteins require energy to transport the drug across the membrane, they are able to shuttle compounds against their concentration gradients, a process called *active transport*. In contrast, when these carrier proteins do not require energy to shuttle drugs, they cannot overcome concentration gradients, a process called *facilitated diffusion*. Active transport is not limited to the CNS; it is also found in the organs related to drug elimination (e.g., hepatocytes, renal tubular cells, pulmonary capillary endothelium), where the ability to transport drugs against the concentration gradient has specific biologic advantages. Both active transport and facilitated diffusion of drugs are saturable processes that are primarily limited by the number of carrier proteins available to shuttle a specific drug.[5]

For lipophilic compounds, transporters are not needed for the drug to diffuse across the capillary wall into tissues, but the presence of transporters does affect the concentration gradients that exist. For instance, some lipophilic drugs are transported out of tissues by adenosine triphosphate (ATP)-dependent transporters such as p-glycoprotein (P-gp). The lipophilic potent μ-opioid agonist, loperamide, used for the treatment of diarrhea, has limited bioavailability because of P-gp transporters at the intestine-portal capillary interface. What does reach the circulation has its CNS penetrance limited by P-gp at the blood–brain barrier.[6] Conversely, lipophilic compounds can be transported into tissues, increasing the tissue concentration of the drug beyond what would be accomplished by passive diffusion. The class of transporters called organic anion polypeptide transporters (OATPs) is located in the microvascular endothelium of the brain and transports endogenous opioids into the brain.[7,8] These OATPs also transport drugs. The degree to which transporter proteins may account for intra- and interindividual responses to anesthetic drugs has not been well-studied to date.[9]

Intravenous Administration

In order for a drug to be delivered to the site of drug action, it must be absorbed into the systemic circulation. Therefore, IV administration results in immediate delivery of a drug with 100% bioavailability. This can lead to rapid overshoot of the desired plasma concentration which can potentially result in immediate and severe side effects for drugs that have a low *therapeutic index* (defined as the ratio of the blood concentration that produces a toxic effect in 50% of the population to the blood concentration that produces a therapeutic effect in 50% of the population). Except for IV administration, the absorption of a drug into the systemic circulation is an important determinant of the time course of drug action and the maximum drug effect produced. As the absorption of drug is slowed, the maximum plasma concentration achieved—and therefore the maximum drug effect achieved—is limited. However, as long as the plasma concentration is maintained at a level above the minimum effective plasma concentration, the drug will produce a drug effect.[10] Therefore, non-IV methods of drug administration can produce a sustained and significant drug effect that may be more advantageous than IV administration.[11]

Bioavailability is the *relative amount* of a drug dose that reaches the systemic circulation unchanged and the *rate* at which this occurs. For most intravenously administered drugs, the absolute bioavailability is close to unity and the rate is nearly instantaneous. However, the pulmonary endothelium can slow the rate at which intravenously administered drugs reach the systemic circulation if distribution into the alveolar endothelium is extensive, such as it is with fentanyl. The pulmonary endothelium also contains enzymes that may metabolize intravenously administered drugs (e.g., propofol) on first pass.[12]

Oral Administration

For almost all therapeutic agents, oral administration is the safest and most convenient method of administration. However, this route is not utilized significantly in anesthesia practice because of the limited and inconstant rate of bioavailability. The absorption rate in the gastrointestinal tract is highly variable because the main determinant of the timing of absorption is gastric emptying into the small intestines, where the surface area for absorption is several orders of magnitude greater than that of the stomach or large intestines. In addition, the active metabolism of drug by the small intestine mucosal epithelium, and the obligatory path through the portal circulation before entering the systemic circulation, contribute to decreased bioavailability of drugs administered via the oral route.[13] In fact, the metabolic capacity of the liver for drugs is so high that only a small fraction of most orally administered lipophilic drugs actually reach the systemic circulation. Because of this extensive *first-pass metabolism*, the oral dose of most drugs must be significantly higher than the IV dose to generate a therapeutic plasma concentration. In addition, time until peak concentration is prolonged and variable, making the oral route impractical to utilize in the perioperative setting.

Highly lipophilic drugs that can maintain a high contact time with nasal or oral (sublingual) mucosa can be absorbed without needing to traverse the gastrointestinal tract. Sublingual administration of drug has the additional advantage that absorbed drug directly enters the systemic venous circulation and therefore is able to bypass the metabolically active intestinal mucosa and hepatic first-pass metabolism. Therefore, small doses of drug can rapidly achieve high plasma concentration and therapeutic effect.[14] However, because of formulation limitations and the small surface area available for absorption, there are only a limited number of drugs that are available for sublingual administration (e.g., nitroglycerin, fentanyl).

Transcutaneous Administration

A few lipophilic drugs have been manufactured in formulations that are sufficient to allow penetration of intact skin. Although scopolamine, nitroglycerin, opioids, and clonidine all produce therapeutic systemic plasma concentrations when administered as "drug patches," the extended amount of time that it takes to achieve an effective therapeutic concentration limits practical application except in the context of maintenance therapy. The use of electric current to increase the speed of passive drug diffusion has been described for fentanyl but is still limited in practicality.[15]

Intramuscular and Subcutaneous Administration

Absorption of drugs from depots in subcutaneous or muscle tissue is directly dependent on the drug formulation and the blood flow to the depot. Blood flow to muscles is high in most physiologic states. Therefore, intramuscular drug absorption is relatively rapid and complete. As a result, some aqueous drugs can be administered as intramuscular injection with rapid and predictable effects (e.g., neuromuscular junction blocking agents). Drug absorption following subcutaneous administration is more unpredictable because of the variability of subcutaneous blood flow, especially in the context of certain disease pathologies; this is the primary reason that subcutaneous heparin and regular insulin administered perioperatively have variable times of onset and maximum effect.

Intrathecal, Epidural, and Perineural Injection

Because the spinal cord is the primary site of action of many anesthetic agents, direct injection of local anesthetics and opioids into the intrathecal space bypasses the limitations of drug absorption and drug distribution by any other route of administration. This is not the case for epidural and perineural administration of local anesthetics, because such administration still requires that drug be absorbed through the dura or nerve sheath in order to reach its site of action. The major downside to these routes of administration is the relative expertise required to perform them.

Inhalational Administration

Owing to the large surface area afforded by pulmonary alveoli and high volume of blood flow in the pulmonary capillaries, administration of drugs by inhalation is extremely desirable.[16] New technologies have been developed which can rapidly and predictably aerosolize a wide range of drugs and thus achieve pharmacokinetic effects comparable to IV administration.[17,18] These devices are currently in Phase II Food and Drug Administration (FDA) trials.

Drug Distribution

Once drug has entered the systemic circulation, it is transported through the circulation to all of the organs of the body. The relative distribution of cardiac output among organ vascular beds determines the speed at which organs are exposed to drug. The highly perfused core circulatory components—brain, lungs, heart, and kidneys—receive the highest relative distribution of cardiac output and therefore are the first organs to reach equilibrium with plasma drug concentrations.[4] Drug concentrations then equilibrate with the less well-perfused muscles and liver and then, finally, with the relatively poorly perfused splanchnic vasculature, adipose tissue, and bone.

Whether by passive diffusion or transporter mediation, drug transport at the capillaries is not usually saturable, so the amount of drug uptake by tissues and organs is limited by the blood flow they receive (i.e., flow-limited drug uptake).

Although the rate of initial drug delivery may be dependent on the relative blood flow to the organ, the rate of drug equilibration by the tissue is dependent on the ratio of blood flow to tissue content. Therefore, drug uptake rapidly approaches equilibrium in the highly perfused, but low-volume brain, kidneys, and lungs in minutes, whereas drug transfer to the less well-perfused, intermediate-volume muscle tissue may take hours to approach equilibrium, and drug transfer to the poorly perfused, large cellular volumes of adipose tissue does not equilibrate for days.[11]

Redistribution

2 Highly lipophilic drugs such as thiopental and propofol rapidly diffuse into the well-perfused brain tissue usually within a minute after IV injection. Because of the low tissue volume but high perfusion of the brain, the drug concentration in the cerebral arterial blood rapidly equilibrates with the concentration in the brain tissue (usually within 3 minutes). As drug continues to be taken up by other tissues with lower blood flows and higher tissue mass, the plasma concentration of the drug rapidly decreases. Once the drug concentration in the brain tissue is higher than the plasma concentration of drug, there is a reversal of the drug concentration gradient so that the lipophilic drug readily diffuses back into the blood and is *redistributed* to the other tissues that are still taking up drug.[4,19,20] This process continues for each of the organ beds; ultimately, the adipose tissue contains the majority of the lipophilic drug that has not been removed from the body by metabolism or excretion. However, after a single bolus of a highly lipophilic drug, the brain's tissue concentration rapidly decreases below therapeutic levels due to redistribution of drug to muscle tissue, which has a greater relative perfusion compared to adipose tissue.[4,20] Although single, moderate doses of highly lipophilic drugs have a very short CNS duration of action because of redistribution of drug from the CNS to the blood and less well-perfused tissues, repeated injections of a drug allow the rapid establishment of significant peripheral tissue concentrations. When the tissue concentrations of a drug are high enough, the decrease in plasma drug concentration below therapeutic threshold becomes solely dependent on drug elimination.[21]

Drug Elimination

Besides being excreted unchanged from the body, a drug can be biotransformed (metabolized) into one or more new compounds that are then eliminated from the body. Either mechanism of elimination will decrease the drug concentration such that the concentration will eventually be negligible and therefore unable to produce a drug effect. Elimination is the pharmacokinetic term that describes all the processes that remove a drug from the body. Although the liver and the kidneys are considered the major organs of drug elimination, drug metabolism can occur at many other locations that contain active drug-metabolizing enzymes (e.g., pulmonary vasculature, red blood cells), and drug can be excreted unchanged from other organs (e.g., lungs).

Elimination clearance (drug clearance) is the theoretical volume of blood from which drug is completely and irreversibly removed in a unit of time.[22] *Total* drug clearance can be calculated with pharmacokinetic models of blood concentration versus time data.

Biotransformation Reactions

Most drugs that are excreted unchanged from the body are hydrophilic and therefore readily pass into urine or stool. Drugs that are not sufficiently hydrophilic to be able to be excreted unchanged require modification into more hydrophilic, excretable compounds. Enzymatic reactions that metabolize drugs can be classified into Phase I and Phase II biotransformation reactions. Phase I reactions tend to transform a drug into one or more polar, and hence potentially excretable compounds. Phase II reactions transform the original drug by conjugating a variety of endogenous compounds to a polar functional group of the drug, making the drug more hydrophilic. Often drugs will undergo a Phase I reaction to produce a new compound with a polar functional group that will then undergo a Phase II reaction, making the new metabolite even more hydrophilic. However, it is possible for a drug to undergo either a Phase I or Phase II reaction alone.

Phase I Reactions

Phase I reactions may hydrolyze, oxidize, or reduce the parent compound. *Hydrolysis* is the insertion of a molecule of water into another molecule, which forms an unstable intermediate compound that subsequently splits apart. Thus, hydrolysis cleaves the original substance into two separate molecules. Hydrolytic reactions are the primary way amides (such as lidocaine and other amide local anesthetics) and esters (such as succinylcholine) are metabolized.

Many drugs are biotransformed by oxidative reactions. *Oxidations* are defined as reactions that remove electrons from a molecule. The common element of most, if not all, oxidations is an enzymatically mediated reaction that inserts a hydroxyl group (OH) into the drug molecule. In some instances, this produces a chemically stable, more polar hydroxylated metabolite. However, hydroxylation usually creates unstable compounds that spontaneously split into separate molecules. Many different biotransformations are affected by this basic mechanism. Dealkylation (removal of a carbon-containing group), deamination (removal of nitrogen-containing groups), oxidation of nitrogen-containing groups, desulfuration, dehalogenation, and dehydrogenation, all follow an initial hydroxylation. Hydrolysis and hydroxylation are comparable processes. Both have an initial, enzymatically mediated step that produces an unstable compound that rapidly dissociates into separate molecules.

Some drugs are metabolized by *reductive reactions,* that is, reactions that add electrons to a molecule. In contrast to oxidations, where electrons are transferred from NADPH to an oxygen atom, the electrons are transferred to the drug molecule. Oxidation of xenobiotics requires oxygen, but reductive biotransformation is inhibited by oxygen; there, these reactions are facilitated when intracellular oxygen tension is low.

Cytochrome P450 Enzymes

3 The cytochrome P450 (CYP) is the superfamily of constitutive and inducible enzymes that catalyze most Phase I biotransformations. CYP3A4 is the single most important enzyme, accounting for 40% to 45% of all CYP-mediated drug metabolism. CYPs are incorporated into the smooth endoplasmic reticulum of hepatocytes and the membranes of the upper intestinal enterocytes in high concentrations. CYPs are also found in the lungs, kidneys, and skin, but in much smaller numbers. CYP isoenzymes oxidize their substrates primarily by the insertion of an atom of oxygen in the form of a hydroxyl group, while another oxygen atom is reduced to water.

Several constitutive CYPs are involved in the production of endogenous compounds, such as cholesterol, steroid hormones, prostaglandins, and eicosanoids. In addition to the constitutive forms, production of CYPs can be induced by a variety of xenobiotics. CYP drug-metabolizing activity increases after exposure to various exogenous chemicals, including many drugs. The number and type of CYPs present at any time depends on exposure to different xenobiotics. The CYP system is able to protect the organism from the deleterious effects of accumulation of exogenous compounds because of its two fundamental characteristics—broad substrate specificity and the capability to adapt to exposure to different substances by induction of different CYP isoenzymes. Table 11-1 groups drugs encountered in anesthetic practice according to the CYP isoenzymes responsible for their biotransformation.

Biotransformations can be inhibited if different substrates compete for the drug-binding site on the same CYP member. The effect of two competing substrates on each other's metabolism depends on their relative affinities for the enzyme. Biotransformation of the compound with the lower affinity is inhibited to a greater degree. This is the mechanism by which the histamine-2 (H_2) receptor antagonist cimetidine inhibits the metabolism of many drugs, including meperidine, propranolol, and diazepam. The newer H_2 antagonist ranitidine has a different structure and causes fewer clinically significant drug interactions. Other drugs, notably calcium channel blockers and antidepressants, also inhibit oxidative drug metabolism in humans. This information allows clinicians to predict which combinations of drugs are more likely to lead to clinically significant interactions because of altered drug metabolism.

Table 11-1 Substrates for CYP Isoenzymes Encountered in Anesthesiology

CYP3A4	CYP2D6
Acetaminophen	Captopril
Alfentanil	Codeine
Alprazolam	Hydrocodone
Bupivacaine	Metoprolol
Cisapride	Ondansetron
Codeine	Oxycodone
Diazepam	Propranolol
Digitoxin	Timolol
Diltiazem	**CYP2A6**
	Dexmedetomidine
Fentanyl	**CYP2B6**
Lidocaine	Methadone
	Propofol
Midazolam	**CYP2C9**
Nicardipine	Diclofenac
Nifedipine	Ibuprofen
Omeprazole	Indomethacin
Ropivacaine	**CYP2C19**
Statins	Diazepam
Sufentanil	Omeprazole
Verapamil	Propranolol
Warfarin	Warfarin

Phase II Reactions

Phase II reactions are also known as *conjugation* or *synthetic reactions.* Many drugs do not have a polar chemical group suitable for conjugation, so conjugation occurs only after a Phase I reaction. Other drugs, such as morphine, already have a polar group that serves as a "handle" for conjugation, and they undergo these reactions directly. Various endogenous compounds can be attached to parent drugs or their Phase I metabolites to form conjugation products. These endogenous substrates include glucuronic acid, acetate, and amino acids. Mercapturic acid conjugates result from the binding of exogenous compounds to glutathione. Other conjugation reactions produce sulfated or methylated derivatives of drugs or their metabolites. Like the CYP system, the enzymes that catalyze Phase II reactions are inducible. Phase II reactions produce conjugates that are polar, water-soluble compounds. This facilitates the ultimate excretion of the drug via the kidneys or hepatobiliary secretion. Like CYP, there are different families and superfamilies of the enzymes that catalyze Phase II biotransformations.

Genetic Variations in Drug Metabolism

For most enzymes involved in Phase I and Phase II reactions, there are several biologically available isoforms. Drug metabolism varies among individuals because of variability in the genes controlling the numerous enzymes responsible for biotransformation. For most drugs, the population distribution of the rates of metabolism is unimodal. If there are genetic variants (polymorphisms) that affect the rate of drug metabolism, the population distribution of the rates of metabolism will be multimodal. More detailed analysis of this multimodal distribution will reveal subpopulations that have different rates of drug elimination, and the rates of drug metabolism in each of these subpopulations will be in a unimodal distribution. For example, different genotypes result in either normal, low, or (rarely) absent plasma pseudocholinesterase activity, accounting for the well-known differences in responses to succinylcholine. Many drug-metabolizing enzymes exhibit genetic polymorphism, including CYP and various transferases that catalyze phase II reactions.

Chronologic Variations in Drug Metabolism

The activity and capacity of the CYP enzymes increase from subnormal levels in the fetal and neonatal periods to normal levels by about 1 year of age. Although age is a covariate in mathematical models of drug elimination, it is not clear if these changes are related to chronologic changes in organ function (age-related organ dysfunction) or to a decrease in CYP levels with age. In contrast, although the neonate has a limited ability to perform phase II conjugation reactions, after 1 year, advanced age does not affect the capacity to perform phase II reactions.

Renal Drug Clearance

4 The primary role of the kidneys in drug elimination is to excrete into urine the unchanged, hydrophilic drugs, and the hepatically derived metabolites from Phase I and Phase II reactions of lipophilic drugs. The elimination of drugs by passive glomerular filtration is a very inefficient process—any significant degree of protein binding of the drug will decrease the renal drug clearance below the glomerular filtration rate. In order to make renal elimination more efficient, the proximal renal tubular cells contain active transporters for both organic acids and bases. Although these transporters are saturable, they allow for the rate of renal drug clearance to approach the renal blood flow.

In reality, renal drug clearance of actively secreted drugs can be inhibited by both passive tubular reabsorption of lipophilic drugs and active, carrier-mediated tubular reabsorption of hydrophilic drugs. Therefore, the small amount of filtered and secreted lipophilic drug is easily reabsorbed in the distal tubules, making the net renal clearance negligible. In contrast, the large amount of filtered and secreted hydrophilic drug can be passively reabsorbed if renal tubular flow decreases substantially (e.g., oliguria) and/or the urine pH favors the unionized form of the hydrophilic drug. Renal drug clearance, even for drugs eliminated primarily by tubular secretion, is dependent on renal function. Therefore, in patients with acute and chronic causes of decreased renal function, including age, low cardiac output states, and hepatorenal syndrome, drug dosing must be altered in order to avoid accumulation of parent compounds and potentially toxic metabolites (e.g., lidocaine, meperidine) (Table 11-2).

Hepatic Drug Clearance

5 Drug elimination by the liver depends on the intrinsic ability of the liver to metabolize the drug (intrinsic clearance, Cl_i), and the amount of drug available to diffuse into the liver. Many types of mathematical models have been developed to attempt to accurately describe the relationships among hepatic artery blood flow, portal artery blood flow, intrinsic clearance, and drug binding to plasma proteins.[23,24] According to these models, the unbound concentration of drug in the hepatic venous blood (C_v) is in equilibrium with the drug within the liver that is available for elimination. These models also make the assumption that all of the

Table 11-2 Drugs with Significant Renal Excretion Encountered in Anesthesiology

Aminoglycosides	Pancuronium
Atenolol	Penicillins
Cephalosporins	Procainamide
Digoxin	Pyridostigmine
Edrophonium	Quinolones
Nadolol	Rocuronium
Neostigmine	Sugammadex

drug delivered to the liver is available for elimination and that the elimination is a first-order process—a constant *fraction* of the available drug is eliminated per unit time. The fraction of the drug removed from the blood passing through the liver is the hepatic extraction ratio, *E*:

$$E = \frac{C_a - C_v}{C_a} \quad (11\text{-}1)$$

where C_a is the mixed hepatic arterial–portal venous drug concentration and C_v is the mixed hepatic venous drug concentration. The total hepatic drug clearance, Cl_H, is:

$$Cl_H = Q \cdot E \quad (11\text{-}2)$$

where *Q* is hepatic blood flow. Therefore, hepatic clearance is a function of hepatic blood flow and the ability of the liver to extract drug from the blood.

The ability to extract drug depends on the activity of drug-metabolizing enzymes and the capacity for hepatobiliary excretion—the intrinsic clearance of the liver (Cl_i).

Intrinsic clearance represents the ability of the liver to remove drug from the blood in the absence of any limitations imposed by blood flow or drug binding. The relationship of total hepatic drug clearance to the extraction ratio and intrinsic clearance, Cl_i, is:

$$Cl_H = Q \cdot E = Q\left(\frac{Cl_i}{Q + Cl_i}\right) \quad (11\text{-}3)$$

The right-hand side of Equation 11-3 indicates that if intrinsic clearance is very high (many times larger than hepatic blood flow, Cl_i WQ), total hepatic clearance approaches hepatic blood flow. On the other hand, if intrinsic clearance is very small ($Q + Cl_i \approx Q$), hepatic clearance will be nearly equivalent to intrinsic clearance.

Thus, hepatic drug clearance and extraction are determined by two independent variables, intrinsic clearance and hepatic blood flow. Changes in either will change hepatic clearance. However, the extent of the change depends on the initial relationship between intrinsic clearance and hepatic blood flow, according to the nonlinear relationship:

$$E = \frac{Cl_i}{Q + Cl_i} \quad (11\text{-}4)$$

If the initial intrinsic clearance is small relative to hepatic blood flow, then the extraction ratio is also small, and Equation 11-5 reduces to the following relationship:

$$E = \frac{Cl_i}{Q} \ll 1 \quad (11\text{-}5a)$$

Equation 11-5a indicates that doubling intrinsic clearance will produce an almost proportional increment in the extraction ratio, and, consequently, hepatic elimination clearance (Fig. 11-1, inset). However, if intrinsic clearance is much greater than hepatic blood flow, Equation 11-4 reduces to the following relationship:

$$E = \frac{Cl_i}{Cl_i} \approx 1 \quad (11\text{-}5b)$$

Equation 11-5b demonstrates that the extraction ratio is independent of intrinsic clearance and therefore, a change in intrinsic clearance has a negligible effect on the extraction ratio and hepatic drug clearance (Fig. 11-1). In nonmathematical terms, high intrinsic clearance indicates efficient hepatic elimination. It is hard to enhance an already efficient process, whereas it is relatively easy to improve on inefficient drug clearance because of low intrinsic clearance.

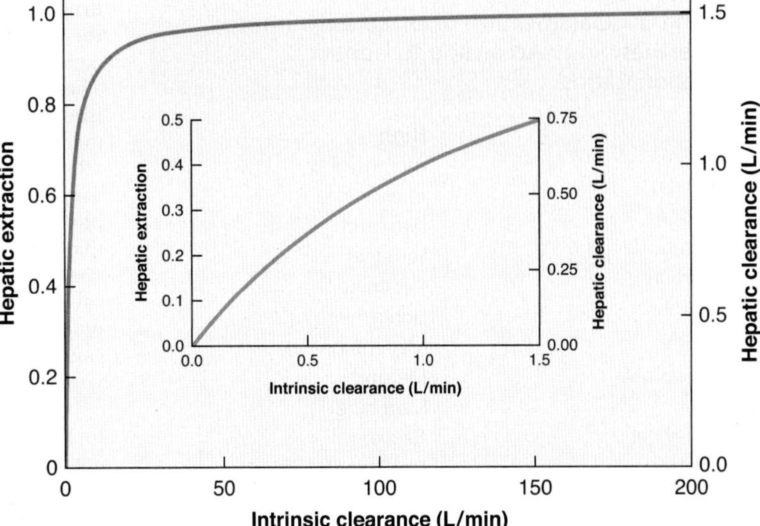

Figure 11-1 The relationship between hepatic extraction ratio (*E*, right *y*-axis), intrinsic clearance (Cl_i, *x*-axis), and hepatic clearance (Cl_H, left *y*-axis) at the normal hepatic blood flow (*Q*) of 1.5 L/min. For drugs with a high intrinsic clearance ($Cl_i >> Q$), increasing intrinsic, clearance has little effect on hepatic extraction, and total hepatic clearance approaches hepatic blood flow. In contrast, if the intrinsic clearance is small ($Cl_i \leq Q$), the extraction ratio is similar to the intrinsic clearance (inset). (Adapted from Wilkinson GR, Shand DG. A physiologic approach to hepatic drug clearance. *Clin Pharmacol Ther*. 1975;18:377. Copyright © 1975 American Society for Clinical Pharmacology and Therapeutics.)

For drugs with a high extraction ratio and a high intrinsic clearance, hepatic elimination clearance is directly proportional to hepatic blood flow. Therefore, any manipulation of hepatic blood flow will be directly reflected by a proportionate change in hepatic elimination clearance (Fig. 11-2). In contrast, when the intrinsic clearance is low, changes in hepatic blood flow produce inversely proportional changes in extraction ratio (Fig. 11-3); therefore, the hepatic elimination clearance is essentially independent of hepatic blood flow and exquisitely related to intrinsic clearance. Classifying drugs as having either low, intermediate, or high extraction ratios (Table 11-3) allows predictions to be made on how intrinsic hepatic clearance and hepatic blood flow affect hepatic elimination clearance. This allows gross adjustments to be made in hepatically metabolized drug dosing to avoid excess accumulation of drugs (decreased hepatic elimination without dose adjustment) or subtherapeutic dosing strategies (increased hepatic elimination without dose adjustment).

Pharmacologic and pathologic manipulations of cardiac output, with its consequences on hepatic/splanchnic blood flow and renal blood flow, are important covariates when designing drug-dosing strategies.[25] As detailed above, in states where cardiac output is decreased (e.g., heart failure, shock, spinal anesthesia), high–extraction ratio drugs will have a decrease in hepatic elimination, whereas low–extraction rate drugs will have minimal change in clearance.[26,27] Autoregulation of renal blood flow maintains a relatively constant renal elimination clearance across a wide range of cardiac outputs until low urine output states eventually allow increased reabsorption of drugs from the distal tubules.[28]

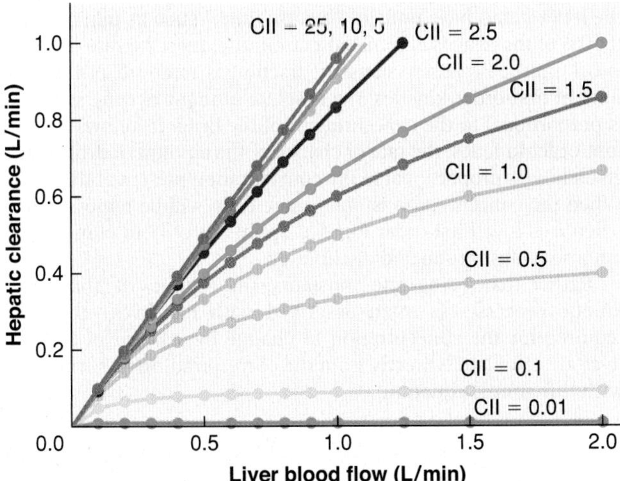

Figure 11-2 The relationship between liver blood flow (*Q*, *x*-axis) and hepatic clearance (Cl_H, *y*-axis) for different values of intrinsic clearance (Cl_i). When the intrinsic clearance is low, hepatic elimination clearance is independent of liver blood flow—the drug elimination is limited by the capacity of the liver to metabolize the drug (i.e., the intrinsic clearance). In contrast, as intrinsic clearance increases, the hepatic elimination becomes more dependent on hepatic blood flow—the liver is able to metabolize all of the drug that it is exposed to and therefore only limited by the amount of drug that is delivered to the liver (i.e., flow limited metabolism).

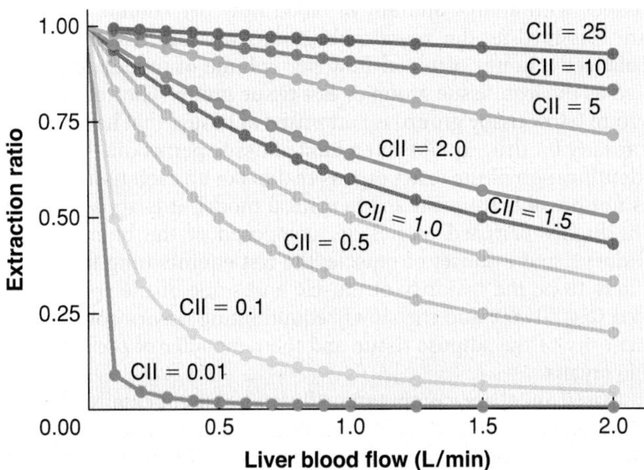

Figure 11-3 The relationship between liver blood flow (*Q*, *x*-axis) and hepatic extraction ratio (*E*, *y*-axis) for different values of intrinsic clearance (Cl_i). When the intrinsic clearance is low, increases in hepatic blood flows cause a decrease in the extraction ratio because the liver has limited metabolic capabilities. In contrast, when the intrinsic clearance is high, the extraction ratio is essentially independent of hepatic blood flow because the liver's ability to eliminate drug is well above the amount of drug provided by normal hepatic blood flow.

Table 11-3 Classification of Drugs Encountered in Anesthesiology According to Hepatic Extraction Ratios

Low	High
Diazepam	Alprenolol
Lorazepam	Bupivacaine
Methadone	Diltiazem
Phenytoin	Fentanyl
Rocuronium	Ketamine
Theophylline	Lidocaine
Thiopental	Meperidine
Intermediate	Metoprolol
Alfentanil	Morphine
Methohexital	Naloxone
Midazolam	Nifedipine
Vecuronium	Propofol
	Propranolol

Pharmacokinetic Models

The concentration of drug at its site or sites of action is the fundamental determinant of a drug's pharmacologic effects. Although the blood is rarely the site of action for a drug, the tissue drug concentration in any given organ is a function of the blood flow to that organ, the concentration of drug in the arterial inflow to the organ, the capacity of the organ to take up the drug, and the degree to which the drug diffuses between the blood and the organ.

Physiologic versus Compartment Models

Initial pharmacokinetic models of IV and inhalational anesthetics used physiologic or perfusion models.[4] In these models, body tissues are lumped into groups that have similar distribution of cardiac output and capacity for drug uptake. Highly perfused tissues with a large amount of blood flow per volume of tissue are classified as the vessel-rich group, whereas tissues with a balanced amount of blood flow per volume of tissue are classified as the lean tissue group or fast tissue group. The vessel-poor group (slow tissue group) is comprised of tissues that have a large capacity for drug uptake but a limited tissue perfusion. Although identification of the exact organs that make up each tissue group is not possible from the mathematical model, it is apparent that the highly perfused tissues are composed of the brain, lungs, kidneys, and a subset of muscle; the fast equilibrating tissue are likely to be the majority of muscle and some of the splanchnic bed (e.g., liver); and the slowly equilibrating tissues contain the majority of the adipose tissue and the remainder of the splanchnic organs.

Based on these computationally and experimentally intense physiologic models, Price[4,19] was able to demonstrate that awakening after a single dose of thiopental was primarily the result of redistribution of thiopental from the brain to the muscle with little contribution by distribution to less well-perfused tissues or drug metabolism. This fundamental concept of redistribution applies to all lipophilic drugs and was not delineated until an accurate pharmacokinetic model had been constructed.

Perfusion-based physiologic pharmacokinetic models have provided significant insights into how physiologic, pharmacologic, and pathologic distribution of cardiac output can affect drug distribution and elimination.[29,30] However, verification of the predictions of these models requires measurement of drug concentrations in many different tissues, which is impractical. Therefore, simpler mathematical models have been developed. In these models, the body is comprised of one or more compartments. Drug concentrations in the blood are used to define the relationship between dose and the time course of changes in the drug concentration. The compartments of the compartmental pharmacokinetic models cannot be equated with the tissue groups that make up physiologic pharmacokinetic models because the compartments are theoretical entities that are used to mathematically characterize the blood concentration profile of a drug. These models allow the derivation of pharmacokinetic parameters that can be used to quantify drug distribution and elimination—volume of distribution, clearance, and half-lives.

Although the simplicity of compartmental models, compared to physiologic pharmacokinetic models, has advantages, there are also some disadvantages. For example, cardiac output is not a parameter of compartmental models, and compartmental models therefore cannot be used to predict the effect of cardiac failure on drug disposition.[31] However, compartmental pharmacokinetic models can still quantify the effects of reduced cardiac output on the disposition of a drug if a group of patients with cardiac failure is compared to a group of healthy subjects.

The discipline of pharmacokinetics is—to the despair of many—mathematically based. In the succeeding sections, formulas are used to illustrate the concepts needed to understand and interpret pharmacokinetic studies. Readers are encouraged to concentrate on the concepts, not the formulas.

Pharmacokinetic Concepts

The disposition of most drugs follows *first-order* kinetics. A first-order kinetic process is one in which a constant fraction of the drug is removed during a finite period of time, regardless of the drug amount or concentration. This fraction is equivalent to the rate constant of the process. Rate constants are usually denoted by the letter k and have units of "inverse time," such as min^{-1} or h^{-1}. If 10% of the drug is eliminated per minute, then the rate constant is 0.1 min^{-1}. Because a constant fraction is removed per unit of time in first-order kinetics, the absolute amount of drug removed is proportional to the concentration of the drug. It follows that, in first-order kinetics, the rate of change of the amount of drug at any given time is proportional to the concentration present at that time. When the concentration is high, more drug will be removed than when it is low. First-order kinetics apply not only to elimination, but also to absorption and distribution.

Rather than using rate constants, the rapidity of pharmacokinetic processes is often described with half-lives—the time required for the concentration to change by a factor of 2. Half-lives are calculated directly from the corresponding rate constants with this simple equation:

$$t_{1/2} = \frac{\ln 2}{k} = \frac{0.693}{k} \tag{11-6}$$

Thus, a rate constant of 0.1 min^{-1} translates into a half-life of 6.93 minutes. The half-life of any first-order kinetic process, including drug absorption, distribution, and elimination, can be calculated. First-order processes asymptotically approach completion because a constant fraction of the drug, not an absolute amount, is removed per unit of time. However, after five half-lives, the process will be almost 97% complete (Table 11-4). For practical purposes, this is essentially 100%, and therefore, there is a negligible amount of drug remaining in the body.

Table 11-4 Half-Lives and Corresponding Percentage of Drug Removed

Number of Half-Lives	Percentage of Drug Remaining	Percentage of Drug Removed
0	100	0
1	50	50
2	25	75
3	12.5	87.5
4	6.25	93.75
5	3.125	96.875

Volume of Distribution

6 The volume of distribution quantifies the extent of drug distribution. The physiologic factor that governs the extent of drug distribution is the overall capacity of tissues versus the capacity of blood for that drug. Overall tissue capacity for uptake of a drug is in turn a function of the total mass of the tissues into which a drug distributes and their average affinity for the drug. In compartmental pharmacokinetic models, drugs are envisaged as distributed into one or more "boxes," or compartments. These compartments cannot be equated directly with specific tissues. Rather, they are hypothetical entities that permit analysis of drug distribution and elimination and description of the drug concentration versus time profile.

The volume of distribution is an "apparent" volume because it represents the size of these hypothetical boxes, or compartments, that are necessary to explain the concentration of drug in a reference compartment, usually called the *central* or *plasma compartment*. The volume of distribution, V_d, relates the total amount of drug present to the concentration observed in the central compartment:

$$V_d = \frac{\textit{amount of drug administered}}{\textit{initial drug plasma concentration}} \qquad (11\text{-}7)$$

If a drug is extensively distributed, then the concentration will be lower relative to the amount of drug present, which equates to a larger volume of distribution. For example, if a total of 10 mg of drug is present and the concentration is 2 mg/L, then the apparent volume of distribution is 5 L. On the other hand, if the concentration was 4 mg/L, then the volume of distribution would be 2.5 L.

Simply stated, the apparent volume of distribution is a numeric index of the extent of drug distribution that does not have any relationship to the actual volume of any tissue or group of tissues. It may be as small as plasma volume, or, if overall tissue uptake is extensive, the apparent volume of distribution may exceed the total volume of the body. In general, lipophilic drugs have larger volumes of distribution than hydrophilic drugs. Because the volume of distribution is a mathematical construct to model the distribution of a drug in the body, the volume of distribution cannot provide any information regarding the actual tissue concentration in any specific real organ in the body. However, this simple mathematical construct provides a useful summary of the behavior of the drug in the body. In fact, the loading dose of drug required to achieve a target plasma concentration can be easily calculated by rearranging Equation 11-7 as follows:

$$\textit{Loading Dose} = V_d \times \textit{Target Concentration} \qquad (11\text{-}8)$$

Based on this equation, it is clear that an increase in the volume of distribution means that a larger loading dose will be required to "fill up the box" and achieve the same concentration. Therefore, any change in state because of changes in physiologic and pathologic conditions can alter the volume of distribution, necessitating dosing adjustments.

Total Drug (Elimination) Clearance

Elimination clearance (drug clearance) is the theoretical volume of 7
blood from which drug is completely and irreversibly removed in a unit of time. Elimination clearance has the units of flow – volume per time. *Total* drug clearance can be calculated with pharmacokinetic models of blood concentration versus time data. Drug clearance is often corrected for weight or body surface area, in which case, the units are mL/min/kg or mL/min/m^2, respectively.

Elimination clearance, *Cl*, can be calculated from the declining blood levels observed after an IV injection, as follows:

$$Cl = \frac{\textit{dose of drug administered}}{\textit{area under the concentration versus time curve}} \qquad (11\text{-}9)$$

If a drug is rapidly removed from the plasma, its concentration will fall more quickly than the concentration of a drug that is less readily eliminated. This results in a smaller area under the concentration versus time curve, which equates to greater clearance (Fig. 11-4).

Without additional organ-specific data (e.g., urine drug concentration measurements, drug arterial inflow concentration) calculating elimination clearance from compartmental pharmacokinetic models usually does not specify the relative contribution of different organs to drug elimination. Nonetheless, estimation of drug clearance with these models has made important contributions to clinical pharmacology. In particular, these models have provided a great deal of clinically useful information regarding altered drug elimination in various pathologic conditions.

Elimination Half-Life

Although the elimination clearance is the pharmacokinetic parameter that best describes the physiologic process of drug elimination (i.e., drug delivery to organs of elimination coupled with the capacity of the organ to eliminate the drug), the pharmacokinetic variable most often reported in textbooks and literature is the ***elimination half-life*** of a drug ($t_{1/2\beta}$). The elimination half-life is the time during which the amount of drug in the body

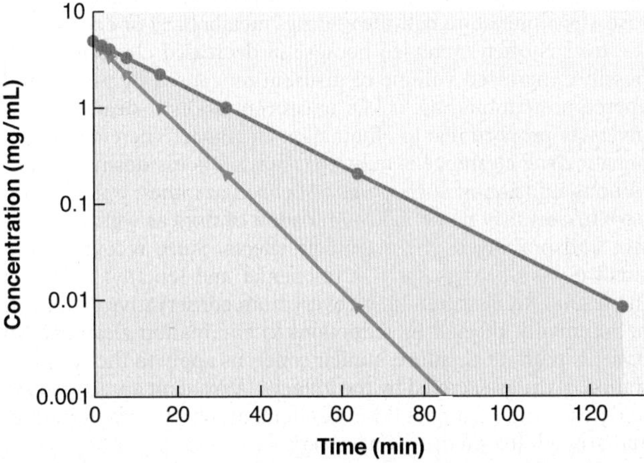

Figure 11-4 The plasma concentration (y-axis) versus time (x-axis) curve for two drugs which only differ in their elimination clearance. Notice that the areas under the curves are different, signifying that the drug that has the smaller area under the curve is more rapidly eliminated from the body than the drug that has the slower elimination clearance.

decreases by 50%. Although this parameter appears to be a simple summary of the physiology of drug elimination, it is actually a complex parameter, influenced by the distribution and the elimination of the drug, as follows:

$$t_{1/2_\beta} = \frac{\ln 2}{k_\beta} = 0.693 \times \frac{V_d}{Cl_E} \quad (11\text{-}10)$$

Therefore, when a physiologic or pathologic perturbation changes the elimination half-life of a drug, it is not a simple reflection of a change in the body's ability to metabolize or eliminate the drug. For example, the elimination half-life of thiopental is prolonged in the elderly; however, the elimination clearance is unchanged and the volume of distribution is increased.[32] Therefore, elderly patients need dosing strategies that accommodate for a change in the distribution of the drug rather than decreased metabolism of the drug. In contrast, in patients with renal insufficiency, the increase in the elimination half-life of pancuronium is due to a simple decrease in renal drug elimination, and the volume of distribution is unchanged.[33]

Aside from its inability to give insight into the mechanism by which a drug is retained in the body, the elimination half-life is unable to give insight into the time that it takes for a single dose or a series of repeated drug doses to terminate its effect. Although elimination of drug from the body begins the moment the drug is delivered to the organs of elimination, the rapid termination of effect of a bolus of an IV agent is due to redistribution of drug from the brain to the blood and subsequently other tissues (e.g., muscle). Therefore, the effects of most anesthetics have waned long before even one elimination half-life has been completed, making this measure of drug kinetics incapable of providing useful information regarding the duration of action following the administration of IV agents. Thus, the elimination half-life has limited utility in anesthetic practice.[10]

Effect of Hepatic or Renal Disease on Pharmacokinetic Parameters

Diverse pathophysiologic changes preclude precise prediction of the pharmacokinetics of a given drug in individual patients with hepatic or renal disease. In addition, liver function tests are unreliable predictors of the degree of liver function and the remaining metabolic capacity for drug elimination. However, some generalizations can be made. In patients with hepatic disease, the elimination half-life of drugs metabolized or excreted by the liver is often increased because of decreased clearance, and, possibly, increased volume of distribution caused by ascites and altered protein binding.[10,34] Drug concentration at steady state is inversely proportional to elimination clearance. Therefore, when hepatic drug clearance is reduced, repeated bolus dosing or continuous infusion of such drugs as benzodiazepines, opioids, and barbiturates may result in accumulation of drug as well as excessive and prolonged pharmacologic effects. Since recovery from small doses of drugs such as thiopental and fentanyl is largely the result of redistribution, recovery from conservative doses will be minimally affected by reductions in elimination clearance. In patients with renal failure, similar concerns apply to the administration of drugs excreted by the kidneys. A prudent approach is to underestimate a patient's dose requirement, observe the response, and give additional drug if necessary.

Nonlinear Pharmacokinetics

The physiologic and compartmental models thus far discussed are based on the assumption that drug distribution and elimination are first-order processes. Therefore, their parameters, such as clearance and elimination half-life, are independent of the dose or concentration of the drug. However, the rate of elimination of a few drugs is dose-dependent, or *nonlinear.*

Elimination of drugs involves interactions with either enzymes catalyzing biotransformation reactions or carrier proteins for transmembrane transport. If sufficient drug is present, the capacity of the drug-eliminating systems can be exceeded. When this occurs, it is no longer possible to excrete a constant fraction of the drug present, and a constant amount of drug is excreted per unit time. Phenytoin is a well-known example of a drug that exhibits nonlinear elimination at therapeutic concentrations;[35] however, when high doses of thiopental are utilized for cerebral protection, it can demonstrate zero-order elimination.[36] In theory, all drugs are cleared in a nonlinear fashion. In practice, the capacity to eliminate most drugs is so great that this is usually not evident, even with supratherapeutic concentrations.

Compartmental Pharmacokinetic Models

One-Compartment Model

Although for most drugs the one-compartment model is an oversimplification, it does serve to illustrate the basic relationships among clearance, volume of distribution, and the elimination half-life. In this model, the body is envisaged as a single homogeneous compartment. Drug distribution after injection is assumed to be instantaneous, so there are no concentration gradients within the compartment. The concentration can decrease only by elimination of drug from the system. The plasma concentration versus time curve for a hypothetical drug with one-compartment kinetics is shown in Figure 11-5. The decrease in plasma concentration (C) with time from the initial concentration (C_0) can be characterized by the simple monoexponential function:

$$C(t) = C_0 \times e^{-k_e \times t} \quad (11\text{-}11)$$

With the concentration plotted on a logarithmic scale, the concentration versus time curve becomes a straight line. The slope of the logarithm of concentration versus time is equal to the first-order elimination rate constant (k_e).

In the one-compartment model, drug clearance, Cl, is equal to the product of the elimination rate constant, k_e, and the volume of distribution:

$$Cl = k_e \cdot V_d \quad (11\text{-}12)$$

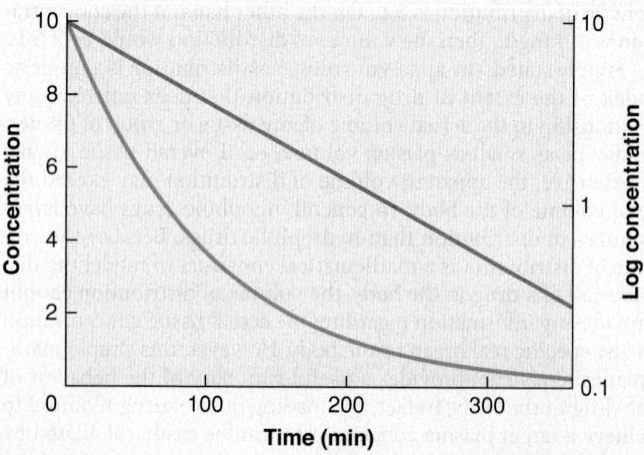

Figure 11-5 The plasma concentration versus time profile plotted on both linear (*blue line*, left *y*-axis) and logarithmic (*red line*, right *y*-axis) scales for a hypothetical drug exhibiting one-compartment, first-order pharmacokinetics. Note that the slope of the logarithmic concentration profile is equal to the elimination rate constant (k_e) and related to the elimination half-life ($t_{1/2\beta}$) as described in Equation 11-9.

Combining Equations 11-6 and 11-11 yields Equation 11-13 (where $k_e = k_\beta$):

$$t_{1/2_\beta} = \frac{\ln 2}{k_e} = 0.693 \times \frac{V_d}{Cl_E} \quad (11\text{-}13)$$

8 Therefore, when it is appropriate to make the simplifying assumption of instantaneous mixing of drug into a single compartment, the elimination half-life is inversely proportional to the slope of the concentration–time curve. For drugs that require consideration of their multicompartmental pharmacokinetics, the relationship among clearance, volume of distribution, and the elimination half-life is not a simple linear one such as Equation 11-13. Nevertheless, the same principles apply. All else being equal, the greater the clearance, the shorter the elimination half-life; the larger the volume of distribution, the longer the elimination half-life. Thus, the elimination half-life depends on two other variables, clearance and volume of distribution, that characterize, respectively, the extent of drug distribution and efficiency of drug elimination.

Two-Compartment Model

For many drugs, a graph of the logarithm of the plasma concentration versus time after an IV injection is similar to the schematic graph shown in Figure 11-6. There are two discrete phases in the decline of the plasma concentration. The first phase after injection is characterized by a very rapid decrease in concentration. The rapid decrease in concentration during this "distribution phase" is largely caused by passage of drug from the plasma into tissues. The distribution phase is followed by a slower decline of the concentration, owing to drug elimination. Elimination also begins immediately after injection, but its contribution to the drop in plasma concentration is initially much smaller than the fall in concentration because of drug distribution.

To account for this biphasic behavior, one must consider the body to be made up of two compartments: a central compartment, which includes the plasma, and a peripheral compartment (Fig. 11-7). This two-compartment model assumes that it is the central compartment into which the drug is injected and from which the blood samples for measurement of concentration are obtained, and that drug is eliminated only from the central compartment. Drug distribution within the central compartment is considered to be instantaneous. In reality, this cannot be true. However, drug uptake into some of the highly perfused tissues is so rapid that it cannot be detected as a discrete phase on the plasma concentration versus time curve.

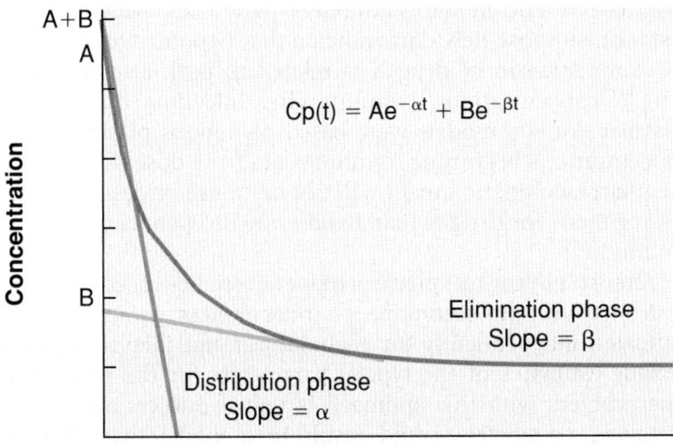

Figure 11-6 The logarithmic plasma concentration versus time profile for a hypothetical drug exhibiting two-compartment, first-order pharmacokinetics. Note that the distribution phase has a slope that is significantly larger than that of the elimination phase, indicating that the process of distribution is not only more rapid than elimination of the drug from the body, but also responsible for most of the decline in plasma concentration in the several minutes after drug administration.

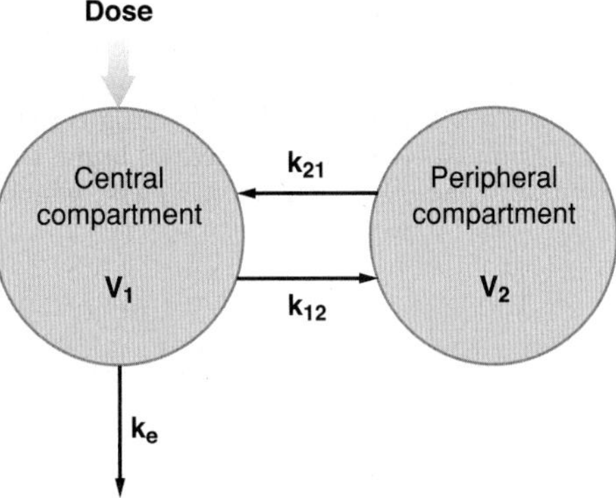

Figure 11-7 A schematic of a two-compartment pharmacokinetic model. See text for explanation.

The distribution and elimination phases can be characterized by graphic analysis of the plasma concentration versus time curve, as shown in Figure 11-6. The elimination phase line is extrapolated back to time zero (the time of injection). In Figure 11-6, the zero time intercepts of the distribution and elimination lines are points *A* and *B*, respectively. The *hybrid rate constants*, α and β, are equal to the slopes of the two lines, and are used to calculate the distribution and elimination half-lives; α and β are called hybrid rate constants because they depend on both distribution and elimination processes.

At any time after an IV injection, the plasma concentration of drugs with two-compartment kinetics is equal to the sum of two exponential terms:

$$C_p(t) = Ae^{-\alpha t} + Be^{-\beta t} \quad (11\text{-}14)$$

where t = time, $C_p(t)$ = plasma concentration at time t, A = y-axis intercept of the distribution phase line, α = hybrid rate constant of the distribution phase, B = y-axis intercept of the elimination phase line, and β = hybrid rate constant of the elimination phase. The first term characterizes the distribution phase and the second term characterizes the elimination phase. Immediately after injection, the first term represents a much larger fraction of the total plasma concentration than the second term. After several distribution half-lives, the value of the first term approaches zero, and the plasma concentration is essentially equal to the value of the second term (Fig. 11-6).

In multicompartmental models, the drug is initially distributed only within the central compartment. Therefore, the initial apparent volume of distribution is the volume of the central compartment. Immediately after injection, the amount of drug present is the dose, and the concentration is the extrapolated concentration at time t = 0, which is equal to the sum of the intercepts of the distribution and elimination lines. The volume of the central compartment, V_1, is calculated by modifying Equation 11-7:

$$V_1 = \frac{dose}{initial\ plasma\ concentration} = \frac{dose}{A + B} \quad (11\text{-}15)$$

The volume of the central compartment is important in clinical anesthesiology because it is the pharmacokinetic parameter that determines the peak plasma concentration after an IV bolus injection. Hypovolemia, for example, reduces the volume of the central compartment. If doses are not correspondingly reduced, the higher plasma concentrations will increase the incidence of adverse pharmacologic effects.

Immediately after IV injection, all of the drug is in the central compartment. Simultaneously, three processes begin. Drug moves from the central to the peripheral compartment, which also has a volume, V_2. This intercompartmental transfer is a first-order process, and its magnitude is quantified by the rate constant k_{12}. As soon as drug appears in the peripheral compartment, some pass back to the central compartment, a process characterized by the rate constant k_{21}. The transfer of drug between the central and peripheral compartments is quantified by the *distributional* or *intercompartmental clearance*:

$$\text{Intercompartmental Clearance} = Cl_{12} = Cl_{21} = V_1 \times k_{12} = V_2 \times k_{21} \quad (11\text{-}16)$$

The third process that begins immediately after administration of the drug is irreversible removal of drug from the system via the central compartment. As in the one-compartment model, the elimination rate constant is k_e, and *elimination clearance* is:

$$\text{Elimination Clearance} = Cl_E = V_1 \times k_e \quad (11\text{-}17)$$

The rapidity of the decrease in the central compartment concentration after IV injection depends on the magnitude of the compartmental volumes, the intercompartmental clearance, and the elimination clearance.

At equilibrium, the drug is distributed between the central and the peripheral compartments, and by definition, the drug concentrations in the compartments are equal. Therefore, the ultimate volume of distribution, termed the volume of distribution at steady state (V_{ss}), is the sum of V_1 and V_2. Extensive tissue uptake of a drug is reflected by a large volume of the peripheral compartment, which, in turn, results in a large V_{ss}. Consequently, V_{ss} can greatly exceed the actual volume of the body.

As in the single-compartment model, in multicompartment models, the elimination clearance is equal to the dose divided by the area under the concentration versus time curve. This area, as well as the compartmental volumes and intercompartmental clearances, can be calculated from the intercepts and hybrid rate constants, without having to reach steady-state conditions.

Three-Compartment Model

After IV injection of some drugs, the initial, rapid distribution phase is followed by a second, slower distribution phase before the elimination phase becomes evident. Therefore, the plasma concentration is the sum of three exponential terms:

$$C_p(t) = Ae^{-\alpha t} + Be^{-\beta t} + Ge^{-\gamma t} \quad (11\text{-}18)$$

where t = time, $C_p(t)$ = plasma concentration at time t, A = intercept of the rapid distribution phase line, α = hybrid rate constant of the rapid distribution phase, B = intercept of the slower distribution phase line, β = hybrid rate constant of the slower distribution phase, G = intercept of the elimination phase line, and γ = hybrid rate constant of the elimination phase. This triphasic behavior is explained by a three-compartment pharmacokinetic model (Fig. 11-8). As in the two-compartment model, the drug is injected into and eliminated from the central compartment. Drug is reversibly transferred between the central compartment and two peripheral compartments, which accounts for two distribution phases. Drug transfer between the central compartment and the more rapidly equilibrating, or "shallow," peripheral compartment is characterized by the first-order rate constants k_{12} and k_{21}. Transfer in and out of the more slowly equilibrating, "deep" compartment is characterized by the rate constants k_{13} and k_{31}. In this

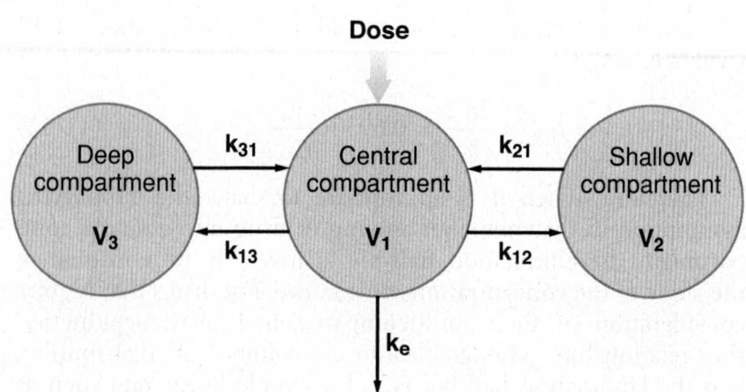

Figure 11-8 A schematic of a three-compartment pharmacokinetic model. See text for details.

model, there are three compartmental volumes: V_1, V_2, and V_3, whose sum equals V_{ss}; and three clearances: the rapid intercompartmental clearance, the slow intercompartmental clearance, and elimination clearance.

The pharmacokinetic parameters of interest to clinicians, such as clearance, volumes of distribution, and distribution and elimination half-lives, are determined by calculations analogous to those used in the two-compartment model. Accurate estimates of these parameters depend on accurate characterization of the measured plasma concentration versus time data. A frequently encountered problem is that the duration of sampling is not long enough to define accurately the elimination phase. Similar problems arise if the assay cannot detect low concentrations of the drug. Conversely, samples are sometimes obtained too infrequently following drug administration to be able to characterize the distribution phases.[37,38] Whether a drug exhibits two- or three-compartment kinetics is of no clinical consequence.[10] In fact, some drugs have two-compartment kinetics in some patients and three-compartment kinetics in others. In selecting a pharmacokinetic model, the most important factor is that it accurately characterizes the measured concentrations.

In general, the model with the smallest number of compartments or exponents that accurately reflects the data is used. However, it is good to consider that the data collected in a particular study may not be reflective of the clinical pharmacologic issues of concern in another situation, making published pharmacokinetic model parameters potentially irrelevant. For instance, suppose new data indicate that hypotension following IV administration of drug X is related to peak arterial plasma drug X concentrations 1 minute after injection, but previous pharmacokinetic models were based on venous plasma drug X concentrations beginning 5 minutes after the dose. In this case, the pharmacokinetic model will not be of use in designing dosing regimens for drug X that avoid toxic drug concentrations at 1 minute.[10,39,40]

Almost all earlier pharmacokinetic studies used *two-stage modeling*. With this technique, pharmacokinetic parameters were estimated independently for each subject and then averaged to provide estimates of the typical parameters for the population. One problem with this approach is that if outliers are present, averaging parameters could result in a model that does not accurately predict typical drug concentrations. Currently, most pharmacokinetic models are developed using *population pharmacokinetic modeling*, which has been made feasible because of advances in modeling software and increased computing power. With these techniques, the pharmacokinetic parameters are estimated using all the concentration versus time data from the entire group of subjects in a single stage, with the help of sophisticated nonlinear regression methods.

Noncompartmental (Stochastic) Pharmacokinetic Models

Often, investigators performing pharmacokinetic analyses of drugs want to avoid the experimental requirements of a physiologic model—data or empirical estimations of individual organ inflow and outflow concentration profiles and organ tissue drug concentrations are required in order to identify the components of the model.[41] Although compartmental models do not assume any physiologic or anatomic basis for the model structure, investigators often attribute anatomic and physiologic function to these empiric models.[42] Even if the disciplined clinical pharmacologist avoids overinterpretation of the meaning of compartment models, the simple fact that several competing models can provide equally good descriptions of the mathematical data, or that some subjects in a data set may better fit with a three-compartment model rather than the two-compartment model that provides the best fit for the other data set subjects, leads many to question whether there is a true best model architecture for any given drug. As a result, some investigators prefer to employ mathematical techniques to characterize pharmacokinetic data that attempt to avoid any preconceived notion of structure, and yet yield the pharmacokinetic parameters that summarize drug distribution and elimination. These techniques are classified as noncompartmental techniques or stochastic techniques and are similar to the methods utilized in process analysis of chemical engineering systems. Although these techniques are often called model independent, like any mathematical construct, assumptions must be made to simplify the mathematics. The basic assumptions of noncompartmental analysis are that (1) all of the elimination clearance occurs directly from the plasma; (2) the distribution and elimination of drug is a linear and first-order process, and (3) the pharmacokinetics of the system does not vary over the time of the data collection (time invariant). All of these assumptions are also made in the basic compartmental and most physiologic models. Therefore, the main advantage of noncompartmental pharmacokinetic methods is that a general description of drug absorption, distribution, and elimination can be made without resorting to more complex mathematical modeling techniques.[41]

Another appealing facet of noncompartmental analysis is that the parameters that describe drug distribution (volume of distribution at steady-state, Vd_{ss}) and drug elimination (elimination clearance, Cl_E) are analogous to parameters found in other pharmacokinetic techniques. In fact, when properly defined, the estimates of these parameters from the noncompartmental approach and a well-defined compartmental model yield similar values. The main unique parameter of noncompartmental analysis is the mean residence time (MRT), which is the average time a drug molecule spends in the body before being eliminated.[43] The MRT, unfortunately, suffers from the main failings of the elimination half-life derived from compartmental models—not only does it fail to capture the contribution of extensive distribution versus limited elimination to allow a drug to linger in the body, but both parameters also fail to describe the situation where the drug effect can dissipate by redistribution of drug from the site of action back into blood and then into other, less well-perfused tissues.[44]

Neural Networks and Artificial Intelligence

In 1943, neurophysiologist Warren McCulloch and mathematician Walter Pitts introduced the concept of the "nervous net".[45] This network—analogous to the network of synapses formed by neurons in the animal brain—allows the computation of a succeeding state from the description of a previous state. This sentinel manuscript formed the concept of neural networks. Only 7 years later, the concept of artificial intelligence was introduced by Alan Turing, who described a computer's ability to achieve human-level performance in cognitive tasks.[46]

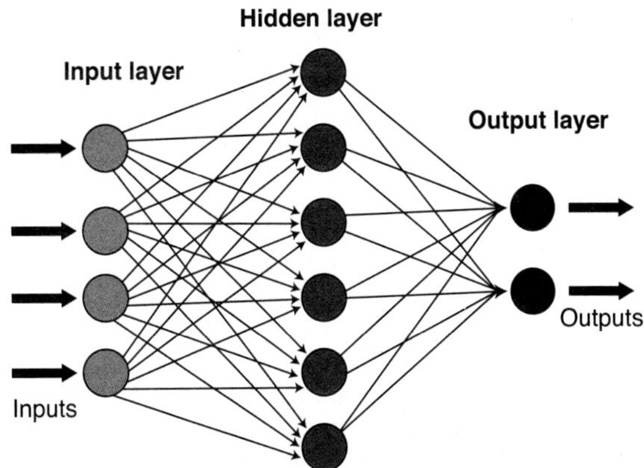

Figure 11-9 Schematic of a typical feed-forward multilayered neural network. (Adapted with permission from Ramesh AN, Kambhampati C, Monson JRT, et al. Artificial intelligence in medicine. *Ann R Coll Surg Engl.* 2004;86(5):334–338.)

Neural networks are the most popular type of artificial intelligence used in medicine[47] and are comprised of networks of interconnected computer processors that can perform computations in parallel. These networks are organized in a series of layers including an input layer, various hidden layers, and an output layer (Fig. 11-9). Neural networks can analyze complex, nonlinear data and are not limited to a preset model structure. In this regard, they are initially stochastic in nature.

It took nearly 50 years for neural networks to be applied toward modeling medical data.[48–52] At the same time, they were also being used to model pharmacokinetic data.[53–55] Neural networks were shown to be superior to a Bayesian approach when estimating the area under the curve.[53] Brier et al. used neural networks to model gentamicin steady-state concentrations with less prediction error compared to mixed effects models.[56] Since neural networks are not confined to a specific structural model, they are not as prone to model misspecification.[53]

Recently, Lee et al. demonstrated the superiority of neural networks compared to response surface models in predicting processed EEG values based on propofol and remifentanil target-controlled infusion (TCI) rates.[57] Their model incorporated over 2 million data points and remarkably, took less than 2 hours to complete—much shorter than what is required using mixed effects models—as neural networks, being parallel, can utilize a computer's graphical processing unit.

The success of neural networks at modeling pharmacometrics data—and medical data in general—has seen them being championed as potential replacements for other techniques currently in use.[58] However, though powerful in their ability to model complex, nonlinear data, neural networks have several limitations. Neural networks require large amounts of data to first train and subsequently validate the model. When training datasets are small, unacceptably high variance may result.[59] Therefore, the utility of neural networks to model prospectively acquired pharamacokinetic or pharmacodynamic data may be limited by the relative lack of data available to train the model.[60] Also, neural networks lack a conceptual basis and therefore require access to artificial intelligence computation.

Nevertheless, with large datasets, neural networks are reliable and valid.[57] Automated, closed-loop drug delivery using artificial intelligence and sensors monitoring depth of anesthesia and nociception has been touted as a possible means to improve patient safety and care.[61] Whether this prediction comes to fruition remains to be seen.

Pharmacodynamic Principles

Much of the clinical pharmacology efforts of the late 1980s and 1990s were devoted to applying the new computational power of desktop computers to deciphering the pharmacokinetics of IV anesthetics. However, the premise behind developing models to better characterize and understand the effects of various physiologic and pathologic states on drug distribution and elimination was that the relationship between a drug dose and its effect(s) had already been characterized. As computational power and drug assay technology grew, it became possible to characterize the relationship between a drug concentration and the associated pharmacologic effect. As a result, pharmacodynamic studies since the 1990s have focused on the quantitative analysis of the relationship between the drug concentration in the blood and the resultant effects of the drug on physiologic processes.

Drug–Receptor Interactions

9 Most pharmacologic agents produce their physiologic effects by binding to a specific receptor, which brings about a change in cellular function. The majority of pharmacologic receptors are cell membrane proteins, although some receptors are located in the cytoplasm or the nucleoplasm of the cell.

Binding of drugs to receptors, like the binding of drugs to plasma proteins, is usually reversible, and follows the law of mass action:

$$[drug] + [receptor] \leftrightarrow [drug - receptor\ complex] \quad (11\text{-}19)$$

This relationship demonstrates that the higher the concentration of free drug or unoccupied receptor, the greater the tendency to form the drug–receptor complex. Plotting the percentage of receptors occupied by a drug against the logarithm of the concentration of the drug yields a sigmoid curve, as shown in Figure 11-10.[62]

The percentage of receptors occupied by a drug is not equivalent to the percentage of maximal effect produced by the drug. In fact, most receptor systems have more receptors than required to obtain the maximum drug effect.[63] The presence of "extra" unoccupied receptors will promote the formation of the drug–receptor complex (Law of Mass Action, Equation 11-19); therefore, near-maximal drug effects can occur at very low drug concentrations. This not only allows extremely efficient responses to drugs, but it provides a large margin of safety—an extremely large number of a drug's receptors must be bound to an antagonist before the drug is unable to produce its pharmacologic effect. For example, at the neuromuscular junction, only 20% to 25% of the postjunctional nicotinic cholinergic receptors need to bind acetylcholine to produce contraction of all the fibers in the muscle, while 75% of the receptors must be blocked by a nondepolarizing neuromuscular antagonist to produce a significant drop in muscle strength. This accounts for the "margin of safety" of neuromuscular transmission.[63]

The binding of drugs to receptors and the resulting changes in cellular function are the last two steps in the complex series of events between administration of a drug and production of its pharmacologic effects. There are two primary schemes by which the binding of an agonist to a receptor changes cellular function: receptor-linked membrane ion channels called *ionophores,* and guanine nucleotide–binding proteins, referred to as *G-proteins*. The nicotinic cholinergic receptor in the neuromuscular postsynaptic membrane is one example of a receptor–ionophore complex. Binding of acetylcholine opens the cation ionophore, leading to an influx of Na^+ ions, propagation of an action potential, and, ultimately, muscle contraction. The γ-aminobutyric acid (GABA) receptor–chloride ionophore complex is another example of this type of effector mechanism. Binding of either endogenous neurotransmitters (GABA) or exogenous agonists (benzodiazepines and IV anesthetics) increases Cl^- conductance, which hyperpolarizes the neuron and decreases its excitability. Adrenergic receptors are the prototypical G-protein coupled receptors. G-proteins change the intracellular concentrations of various so-called *second messengers,* such as Ca^{2+} and cyclic adenosine monophosphate (AMP), in order to transduce their signal and produce modified cellular behavior.

Desensitization and Downregulation of Receptors

Receptors are not static entities. Rather, they are dynamic cellular components that adapt to their environment (1 Video 11-1). Prolonged exposure of a receptor to its agonist leads to desensitization—subsequent doses of the agonist will produce lower maximal effects. With sustained elevation of the cytosolic second messengers downstream of the G-proteins, pathways to prevent further G-protein signaling are activated. Phosphorylation by G-protein receptor kinases and arrestin-mediated blockade of the coupling site needed to form the active heterotrimeric G-protein complex prevents

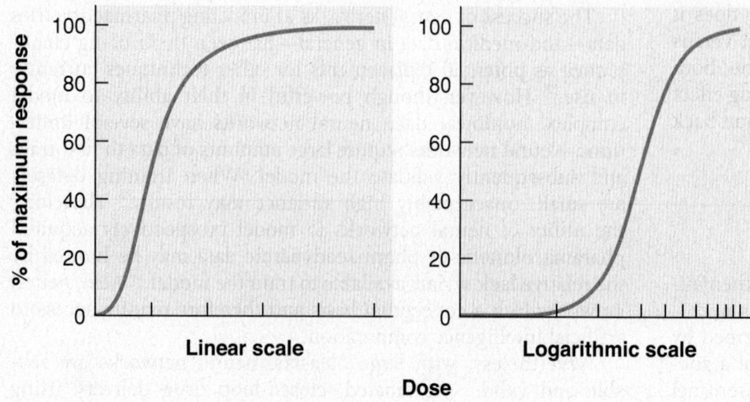

Figure 11-10 A schematic curve of the effect of a drug plotted against dose. In the left panel, the response data is plotted against the dose data on a linear scale. In the right panel, the same response data are plotted against the dose data on a logarithmic scale yielding a sigmoid dose–response curve that is linear between 20% and 80% of the maximal effect.

G-protein–coupled receptors from becoming active. Arrestins and other cell membrane proteins can tag receptors that have sustained activity, so that these non–G-protein receptors are internalized and sequestered so they are no longer accessible to agonists. Similar mechanisms will prevent the trafficking of stored receptors to the cell membrane. The combined increased rate of internalization and decreased rate of replenishing of receptor results in *downregulation*—a decrease in the total number of receptors. Signals that produce downregulation with sustained receptor activation are essentially reversed in the face of constant receptor inactivity. Therefore, chronically denervated neuromuscular junctions, just like cardiac tissue constantly bathed with adrenergic antagonists, will upregulate the specific receptors in an attempt to produce a signal in the face of lower concentrations of agonists.

Agonists, Partial Agonists, and Antagonists

Drugs that bind to receptors and produce an effect are called *agonists*. Different drugs that act on the same receptor may be capable of producing the same maximal effect (E_{max}), although they may differ in the concentration that produces the effect (i.e., potency). Agonists that differ in potency but bind to the same receptors will have parallel concentration–response curves (Fig. 11-11, curves *A* and *B*). Differences in potency of agonists reflect differences in affinity for the receptor. *Partial agonists* are drugs that are not capable of producing the maximal effect, even at very high concentrations (Fig. 11-11, curve *C*).

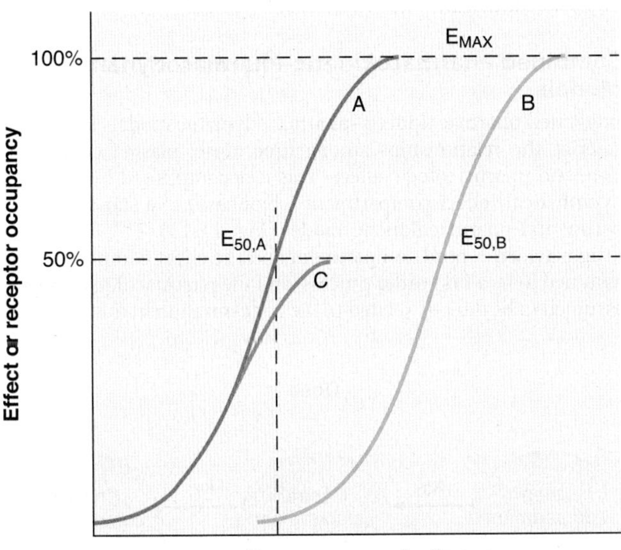

Figure 11-11 Schematic pharmacodynamic curves, with dose or concentration on the x-axis and effect or receptor occupancy on the y-axis, that illustrate agonism, partial agonism, and antagonism. Drug A produces a maximum effect, E_{max}, and a 50% of maximal effect at dose or concentration $E_{50,A}$. Drug B, a full agonist, can produce the maximum effect, E_{max}; however, it is less potent ($E_{50,B} > E_{50,A}$). Drug C, a partial agonist, can only produce a maximum effect of approximately 50% E_{max}. If a competitive antagonist is given to a patient, the dose response for the agonist would shift from curve A to curve B—although the receptors would have the same affinity for the agonist, the presence of the competitor would necessitate an increase in agonist in order to produce an effect. In fact, the agonist would still be able to produce a maximal effect, if a sufficient overdose was given to displace the competitive antagonist. However, the competitive antagonist would not change the binding characteristics of the receptor for the agonist and so curve B is simply shifted to the right but remains parallel to curve A. In contrast, if a noncompetitive antagonist binds to the receptor, the agonist would no longer be able to produce a maximal effect, no matter how much of an overdose is administered (curve C).

Compounds that bind to receptors without producing any changes in cellular function are referred to as *antagonists*—antagonists make it impossible for agonists to bind their receptors. *Competitive antagonists* bind reversibly to receptors, and their blocking effect can be overcome by high concentrations of an agonist (i.e., competition). Therefore, competitive antagonists produce a parallel shift in the dose–response curve, but the maximum effect is not altered (Fig. 11-11, curves *A* and *B*). *Noncompetitive antagonists* bind irreversibly to receptors. This has the same effect as reducing the number of receptors and shifting the dose–response curve downward and to the right, decreasing both the slope and the maximum effect (Fig. 11-11, curves *A* and *C*). The effect of noncompetitive antagonists is reversed only by synthesis of new receptor molecules.

Agonists produce a structural change in the receptor molecule that initiates changes in cellular function. Partial agonists may produce a qualitatively different change in the receptor, whereas antagonists bind without producing a change in the receptor that results in altered cellular function. The underlying mechanisms by which different compounds that bind to the same receptor act as agonists, partial agonists, or antagonists are not fully understood.

Dose–Response Relationships

Dose–response studies determine the relationship between increasing doses of a drug and the ensuing changes in pharmacologic effects. Schematic dose–response curves are shown in Figure 11-10, with the dose plotted on both linear and logarithmic scales. There is a curvilinear relationship between dose and the intensity of response. Low doses produce little pharmacologic effect. Once effects become evident, a small increase in dose produces a relatively large change in effect. At near-maximal response, large increases in dose produce little change in effect. Usually, the dose is plotted on a logarithmic scale (Fig. 11-10, right panel), which demonstrates the linear relationship between the logarithm of the dose and the intensity of the response between 20% and 80% of the maximum effect.

Acquiring the pharmacologic effect data from a population of subjects exposed to a variety of doses of a drug provides four key characteristics of the drug dose–response relationship—potency, drug-receptor affinity, efficacy, and population pharmacodynamic variability. The *potency* of the drug—the dose required to produce a given effect—is usually expressed as the dose required to produce a given effect in 50% of subjects, the *ED50*. The *slope* of the curve between 20% and 80% of the maximal effect indicates the rate of increase in effect as the dose is increased and is a reflection of the affinity of the receptor for the drug. The maximum effect is referred to as the *efficacy* of the drug. Finally, if curves from multiple subjects are generated, the *variability* in potency, efficacy, and the slope of the dose–response curve can be estimated.

The dose needed to produce a given pharmacologic effect var- 10
ies considerably, even in "normal" patients. The patient who is most resistant to a drug usually requires a dose two- to threefold greater than the patient who has the lowest dose requirement. This variability is caused by differences among individuals in the relationship between drug concentration and pharmacologic effect, superimposed on differences in pharmacokinetics. Dose–response studies have the disadvantage of not being able to determine whether variations in pharmacologic response are caused by differences in pharmacokinetics, pharmacodynamics, or both.

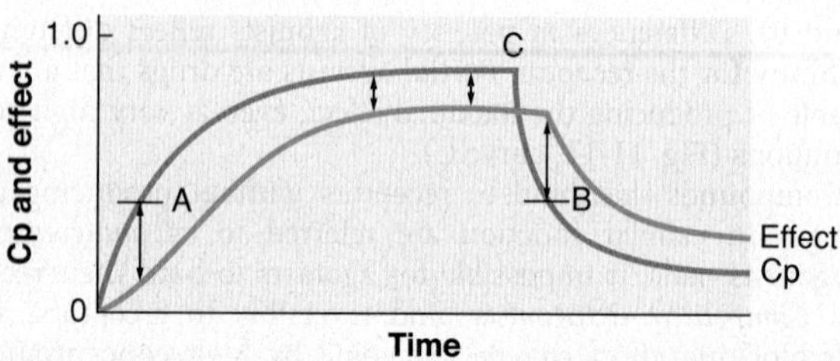

Figure 11-12 The changes in plasma drug concentration and pharmacologic effect during and after an intravenous infusion. See text for explanation. (Adapted with permission from Stanski DR, Sheiner LB. Pharmacokinetics and pharmacodynamics of muscle relaxants. *Anesthesiology*. 1979;51:103.)

Concentration–Response Relationships

The onset and duration of pharmacologic effects depend not only on pharmacokinetic factors but also on the pharmacodynamic factors governing the degree of temporal disequilibrium between changes in concentration and changes in effect. The magnitude of the pharmacologic effect is a function of the amount of drug present at the site of action, so increasing the dose increases the peak effect. Larger doses have a more rapid onset of action because pharmacologically active concentrations at the site of action occur sooner. Increasing the dose also increases the duration of action because pharmacologically effective concentrations are maintained for a longer time.

Ideally, the concentration of drug at its site of action should be used to define the concentration–response relationship (2 Video 11-2). Unfortunately, these data are rarely available, so the relationship between the concentration of drug in the blood and pharmacologic effect is studied instead. This relationship is easiest to understand if the changes in pharmacologic effect that occur during and after an IV infusion of a hypothetical drug are considered. If a drug is infused at a constant rate, the plasma concentration initially increases rapidly and asymptotically approaches a steady-state level after approximately five elimination half-lives have elapsed (Fig. 11-12). The effect of the drug initially increases very slowly, then more rapidly, and eventually also reaches a steady state. When the infusion is discontinued, indicated by point *C* in Figure 11-12, the plasma concentration immediately decreases because of drug distribution and elimination. However, the effect stays the same for a short period, and then also begins to decrease; there is always a time lag between changes in plasma concentration and changes in pharmacologic response. Figure 11-12 also demonstrates that the same plasma concentration is associated with different responses if the concentration is changing. At points *A* and *B* in Figure 11-12, the plasma concentrations are the same, but the effects at each time differ. When the concentration is increasing, there is a concentration gradient from blood to the site of action. When the infusion is discontinued, the concentration gradient is reversed. Therefore, at the same plasma concentration, the concentration at the site of action is higher after, compared to during, the infusion. This is associated with a correspondingly greater effect.

In theory, there must be some degree of temporal disequilibrium between plasma concentration and drug effect for all drugs with extravascular sites of action. However, for some drugs, the time lag may be so short that it cannot be demonstrated. The magnitude of this temporal disequilibrium depends on several factors:

- The perfusion of the organ on which the drug acts
- The tissue:blood partition coefficient of the drug
- The rate of diffusion or transport of the drug from the blood to the cellular site of action
- The rate and affinity of drug–receptor binding
- The time required for processes initiated by the drug–receptor interaction to produce changes in cellular function

The consequence of this time lag between changes in concentration and changes in effects is that the plasma concentration will have an unvarying relationship with pharmacologic effect only under steady-state conditions. At steady state, the plasma concentration is in equilibrium with the concentrations throughout the body and is thus directly proportional to the steady-state concentration at the site of action. Plotting the logarithm of the steady-state plasma concentration versus response generates a curve identical in appearance to the dose–response curve shown in the right panel of Figure 11-10. The $Cp_{ss}50$, the steady-state plasma concentration producing 50% of the maximal response, is determined from the concentration–response curve. Like the ED50, the $Cp_{ss}50$ is a measure of sensitivity to a drug, but the $Cp_{ss}50$ has the advantage of being unaffected by pharmacokinetic variability. Because it takes five elimination half-lives to approach steady-state conditions, it is not practical to determine the $Cp_{ss}50$ directly. For drugs with long elimination half-lives, the pseudoequilibrium during the elimination phase can be used to approximate steady-state conditions, because the concentrations in plasma and at the site of action are changing very slowly.

Combined Pharmacokinetic–Pharmacodynamic Models

Integrated pharmacokinetic–pharmacodynamic models fully characterize the relationships among time, dose, plasma concentration, and pharmacologic effect. This is accomplished by adding a hypothetical "effect compartment" (biophase) to a standard compartmental pharmacokinetic model (Fig. 11-13).[64–66] Transfer of drug between central compartment and the effect compartment is assumed to be a first-order process, and the pharmacologic effect is assumed to be directly related to the concentration in the biophase. 11

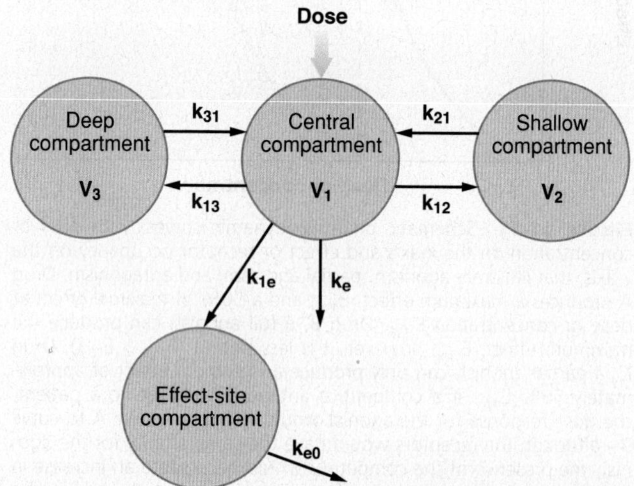

Figure 11-13 A schematic of a three-compartment pharmacokinetic model with the effect site linked to the central compartment. The rate constant for transfer between the plasma (central compartment) and the effect site, k_{1e}, and the volume of the effect site are both presumed to be negligible to ensure that the effect site does not influence the pharmacokinetic model. The rate constant for drug removal from the effect site, which relates the concentration in the central compartment to the pharmacologic effect is k_{e0}.

The biophase is a "virtual" compartment, although linked to the pharmacokinetic model, and does not actually receive or return drug to the model; therefore, the effect site processes do not influence the pharmacokinetic model. By simultaneously characterizing the pharmacokinetics of the drug and the time course of drug effect, the combined pharmacokinetic–pharmacodynamic model is able to quantify the temporal dissociation between the plasma (central compartment) concentration and effect with the rate constant for equilibration between the plasma and the biophase, k_{e0}. By quantifying the time lag between changes in plasma concentration and changes in pharmacologic effect, these models can also define the $Cp_{ss}50$, even without steady-state conditions. These models have contributed greatly to our understanding of factors influencing the response to IV anesthetics, opioids, and nondepolarizing muscle relaxants in humans.

The rate of equilibration between the plasma and the biophase, k_{e0}, can also be characterized by the half-life of effect site equilibration ($T_{1/2ke0}$) using the formula:

$$T_{1/2k_{e_0}} = \frac{\ln 2}{k_{e0}} = \frac{0.693}{k_{e0}} \qquad (11\text{-}20)$$

$T_{1/2ke0}$ is the time for the effect site concentration to reach 50% of the plasma concentration when the plasma concentration is held constant. For anesthetics with a short $T_{1/2ke0}$ (high k_{e0}), equilibration between the plasma and the biophase is rapid and therefore there is little delay before an effect is reached when a bolus of drug is administered or a drug infusion is initiated. However, because the decline in the effect site concentration will also depend on the concentration gradient between the effect site and the plasma, drugs that rapidly equilibrate with the biophase may take longer to redistribute.[67] Therefore, the offset of drug effect is more dependent on the pharmacokinetics of the body than on the rapidity of biophase–plasma equilibration.[21,67]

Population Pharmacokinetic–Pharmacodynamic Models

Population pharmacokinetic–pharmacodynamic (PK-PD) modeling has emerged as a nearly essential part of study design and data analysis in the clinical pharmacology of anesthetic drugs.[68] Despite the term "population," these techniques are designed to bring an individual's specific physiologic characteristics into dose regimen selection. These analyses were made possible through the combined efforts of a theoretical statistician, Stuart Beal, and a leading clinical pharmacologist, Lewis Sheiner, and found early adoption in anesthesiology.[69,70] Sheiner and Beal used nonlinear mixed effects (meaning both fixed and random effects) modeling and wrote a computer program (NONMEM) to fit PK-PD data from multiple individuals, and even from multiple studies, while building an overarching statistical description.[71] In this way, a typical (or median) value for each parameter (e.g., clearance, volume, EC_{50}) of the PK-PD model (called fixed effects, or thetas, θ, in NONMEM terminology) could be combined with a random effect variable (eta, η, in NONMEM) that described where on the distribution (e.g., Gaussian) of all ηs each individual η lies for each parameter, θ.[68]

With nonlinear mixed effects modeling, it is possible to include the interindividual variability of each parameter into a PK-PD model for the population(s) studied—an important concept when trying to predict the next dose administered to the next patient. Furthermore, the spread of the random effects (ηs) can be reduced by including in the model each individual's demographic (i.e., covariate) data, for example, genomic and physiologic factors, in the form of covariates that refine the model and enhance its ability to predict the next patient's response to a drug.

Allometric scaling has developed as a corollary to population PK-PD modeling. Allometry derives from an observation that interspecies metabolism varies by an animal's weight raised to the 0.75 power (instead of 1.0).[72] It has been widely applied to scale pharmacokinetic models across species. More recently, allometry has been applied to intraspecies (human) scaling when developing population mixed effects PK-PD models at the extremes of age (i.e., pediatric and geriatric) or size (i.e., morbid obesity).[73–75]

Population PK-PD models were developed to facilitate individualized medicine in drug therapy. However, dosing regimens are rapidly becoming calculation intensive, with the inclusion of increasing numbers of important covariates, especially with additional nonlinear allometric considerations. Thus, to allow precision dosing in the practice of anesthesiology, these complex calculations should ideally be incorporated into drug-specific infusion pumps (e.g., TCI pumps) or into applications the clinician can have on a personal digital assistant or similar aide at the bedside.

Therapeutic Thresholds and Therapeutic Window

The timing of the onset and the offset of drug action is not only dependent on the effect site's concentration profile (i.e., the drug's pharmacokinetics and pharmacodynamics), but also on the minimum concentration that produces a discernible drug effect—the therapeutic threshold of the drug. The therapeutic threshold of a drug depends on the magnitude of the desired effect or the intensity of the stimulus being treated. For example, superficial procedures (i.e., mastectomy, melanoma excision, etc) are not as painful (Fig. 11-14, dashed green line) as orthopedic procedures (i.e., long bone instrumentation, spine fusion, etc., dotted green line). Therefore, the dose of fentanyl that produces analgesia for superficial procedures (black solid concentration profile) does not produce clinically discernible analgesia for the orthopedic procedures (i.e., below the therapeutic threshold). In contrast, the dose of fentanyl that produces analgesia for orthopedic procedures (blue solid concentration profile) will not only provide analgesia for the superficial procedures, but it will also have a faster onset of effect because it reaches the therapeutic threshold faster. In addition, since the larger bolus of fentanyl results in concentrations of drug that are above the toxic threshold for the superficial procedures (red dashed line, Low toxic threshold), the patient will have significant ventilatory depression until the effect site concentration of fentanyl decreases below this toxic threshold. This profound ventilatory depression would start approximately 2 minutes after the larger bolus of fentanyl was administered and would last for about 18 minutes after administration. The therapeutic window that should be targeted to provide adequate analgesia after a superficial procedure is below the toxic threshold (red dashed line) and above the therapeutic threshold (green dashed line). The therapeutic window that should be targeted for orthopedic procedures has the entire window "shifted higher" (i.e., below the red dotted line and above the green dotted line).

Drug Interactions

Taking into account premedication, perioperative antibiotics, IV agents used for induction or maintenance, inhalational anesthetics, opioids, muscle relaxants, the drugs used to restore neuromuscular transmission, and postoperative analgesics, 10 or more drugs are frequently administered as part of a "routine" anesthetic. Consequently, thorough understanding of the mechanisms

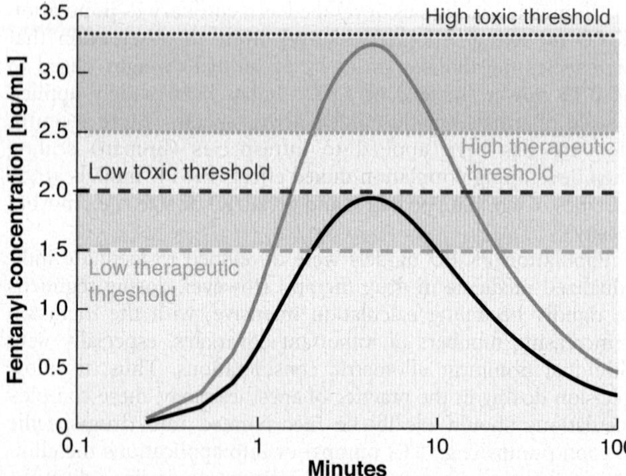

Figure 11-14 The effect-site concentration versus time profiles after a small intravenous bolus (*solid black line*) and a larger intravenous bolus (*solid blue line*) of fentanyl. Representative therapeutic thresholds (the minimum concentration required to produce clinically discernible analgesia), and toxic threshold (the concentration above which profound opioid-induced ventilatory depression occurs) are demonstrated superficial procedures, such as mastectomy (*green dashed line,* low therapeutic threshold), and for orthopedic procedures, such as long bone instrumentation (*dotted green line,* high therapeutic threshold). A given bolus of fentanyl only produces clinically discernible analgesia from the time it produces an effect site concentration above the therapeutic threshold concentration for a patient until the time when the effect site concentration decreases below the therapeutic threshold concentration. If the effect site concentration does not exceed the toxic threshold for a patient, then it does not produce profound opioid-induced ventilatory depression. In contrast, if the bolus does produce an effect site concentration above the toxic threshold concentration, it will produce profound ventilatory depression that is sustained until the effect site concentration decreases below the toxic threshold concentration. For example, after superficial surgery, a small dose of fentanyl (*solid black line*) will initially produce detectable analgesia approximately 2 minutes after administration (when it crosses the low therapeutic threshold, *dashed green line*) which will last until approximately 10 minutes after administration (when the concentration decreases below the low therapeutic threshold, *green dashed line*). Since the dose does not produce a concentration above the low toxic threshold (*dashed red line*), hypoventilation will not occur after this single bolus. In contrast, for the same superficial procedure, a larger bolus of fentanyl (*solid blue line*) will initially produce analgesia less than 1 minute after administration (when it crosses the low therapeutic threshold, *dashed green line*), which will last until approximately 30 minutes after administration (when the concentration decreases below the low therapeutic threshold, *green dashed line*). Since the dose produces an effect site concentration above the toxic threshold (*dashed red line*), it will produce profound hypoventilation from approximately 2 minutes until the effect site concentration decreases below the same toxic threshold at approximately 18 minutes. So, although the larger bolus produces a quicker onset of action and a longer duration of action, it produces toxicity for a portion of this time. After orthopedic procedures (*dotted green line* for high therapeutic threshold and *dotted red line* for high toxic threshold), a small bolus of fentanyl will be subtherapeutic and ineffective (*black solid line*) because it does not produce a concentration above the high therapeutic threshold (*dotted green line*). In contrast, a larger bolus of fentanyl produces clinically discernible analgesia from approximately 2 through 10 minutes after administration (time that *blue line* is above *green dotted line*).

of drug interactions and specific interactions with drugs used in anesthesia are essential to safe practice. Indeed, anesthesia providers often deliberately take advantage of drug interactions. For example, moderate to high doses of opioid are often utilized to decrease the amount of volatile anesthetic required to provide immobility and hemodynamic stability for surgical incision (e.g., MAC* and MAC_{BAR}), thereby avoiding the side effects of higher concentrations of inhaled anesthetics (e.g., vasodilation, prolonged recovery). In this section, we will examine the major classes of drug–drug interactions by detailing common examples encountered in the perioperative period.

Pharmaceutical (Physiochemical) Interactions

In Vitro Interactions

12

Anesthesia providers often overlook the drug interactions produced by pharmaceutical (physicochemical) properties because most perioperative drugs are administered intravenously or via inhalation and therefore have high bioavailability. However, in vitro drug–drug interactions due to physiochemical properties of drugs can significantly alter drug bioavailability and produce unintended toxic byproducts. Basic acid–base chemistry can predict many of the observed in vitro interactions. One classic example of a physiochemical drug–drug interaction that alters drug bioavailability is the formation of insoluble salts that precipitate when acidic drugs, such as thiopental, and basic drugs, such as opioids or muscle relaxants, are "mixed," such as when administered through IV tubing with an insufficient fluid flow rate.[76] Another example is the observation that commercial preparations of local anesthetic solutions that contain epinephrine have a lower pH than plain local anesthetic solutions to which epinephrine is added shortly prior to administration because of the high acidity of the antioxidant stabilizers used in commercial preparations (i.e., sodium bisulfite or sodium pyrosulfite).[77] The unintended consequence of this commercial formulation is that the local anesthetic appears less effective owing to the increased concentration of the less permeable ionized form of local anesthetic that exists in acidic environments.

Although physiochemical drug interactions that affect the bioavailability of drugs are relatively easy to avoid or, at least, overcome by increasing the drug dose, some physiochemical interactions can result in unintended toxic compounds. One chemical agent often overlooked by anesthesia providers is the soda lime or Baralyme that is used in modern anesthesia machines to remove carbon dioxide from exhaled gases. Although patients are not directly administered this agent, the gas that they inhale from the anesthesia machine often contains the byproducts of the interaction between the constituents of the exhaled gas and the carbon dioxide absorbent. While this allows the patient to receive a "heated and humidified" inhaled gas mixture, if conditions are correct, the halogenated volatile anesthetics can undergo degradation by the strong base (i.e., sodium and/or potassium hydroxide) contained in the carbon dioxide absorbent.[78] This chemical reaction led the FDA to recommend that sevoflurane exposure should not exceed 2 MAC-hours when fresh gas flow rates of 1 to less than 2 L/min were used, in order to minimize exposure to the potentially nephrotoxic haloalkene ("compound A") formed by dehydrofluorination of sevoflurane by soda lime or Barolyme.[79] Although the effects of compound A on human renal function are not of great clinical concern, the strong bases in the carbon dioxide can also degrade the difluoromethyl containing

***MAC: Minimum alveolar concentration is the pseudo–steady-state end-tidal alveolar concentration at which 50% of patients do not move in response to surgical incision or do not have an increase in heart rate or blood pressure in response to surgical incision (BAR: blocks autonomic responses).**

halogenated volatile anesthetics (i.e., desflurane and isoflurane) to carbon monoxide.[80] These patient safety concerns led to the development and the increased use of Amsorb, a carbon dioxide adsorbent that contains calcium hydroxide lime in place of sodium and/or potassium hydroxide, and causes minimal to no carbon monoxide or compound A formation.[81]

In Vivo Interactions

13 Whereas many of the in vitro physiochemical interactions can result in unintended toxicity due to exposure to either subtherapeutic drug concentrations or toxic degradation products, physiochemical interactions have been exploited to develop two novel approaches to antagonize neuromuscular junction blocking agents. The first approach, which was approved for use in the European Union in 2008 and in the United States in 2016, is the selective relaxant binding agent, sugammadex. Sugammadex is a synthetic cyclodextrin that encapsulates and electrostatically binds rocuronium. By essentially irreversibly binding plasma rocuronium, sugammadex acts as a chelator that not only rapidly decreases the free plasma rocuronium concentration but also promotes redistribution of rocuronium from the neuromuscular junction (extracellular space) to the intravascular space.[82] Therefore, if there is an excess of sugammadex molecules relative to rocuronium molecules, the neuromuscular blockade is antagonized. Although sugammadex was developed to antagonize neuromuscular blockade produced by rocuronium, it is also able to antagonize profound neuromuscular blockade produced by the other commonly used steroidal neuromuscular blocking agents, such as vecuronium and pipecuronium.[83,84] However, sugammadex is unable to antagonize neuromuscular blockade produced by the benzylisoquinoline neuromuscular blocking agent, cisatracurium. Molecules from the cucurbit[n]uril family can encapsulate both the steroidal and benzylisoquinoline family of neuromuscular blocking agents in preclinical models and may ultimately be a more comprehensive solution for antagonism of neuromuscular blockade via molecular encapsulation.[85–87] An alternative approach to neuromuscular blockade antagonism is to design a molecule that can be inactivated via nonbiologic routes. This approach has led to Phase 1 studies of a new class of nondepolarizing neuromuscular blocking drugs called the fumarates (olefinic diester isoquinolinium compounds). These molecules are rapidly inactivated by the nonenzymatic formation of cysteine adducts when combined with plasma cysteine.[88] Therefore, cysteine administration antagonizes the neuromuscular blockade. These two novel approaches to drug development could be used to develop designer drugs that can be readily antagonized via nonbiologic routes, if the important receptor targets for sedation and amnesia components of general anesthesia are identified.

Pharmacokinetic Interactions

Drugs can alter each other's absorption, distribution, and elimination. Understanding the basis for alterations in the pharmacokinetics allows anesthesiologists to not only avoid unintentional supratherapeutic or subtherapeutic concentrations of the perioperative medications, but also to strategically employ alterations in pharmacokinetics to achieve the desired concentration profile.

Absorption (Uptake)

Some drugs can alter the absorption of other drugs, by either altering the delivery of drug to site of drug absorption (uptake) or by altering the local blood flow to the site of drug administration. Although this type of drug–drug interaction will alter bioavailability, it should not alter any other pharmacokinetic parameter. Drugs like ranitidine, which alters gastric pH, and metoclopramide, which speeds gastric emptying, affect absorption from the gastrointestinal tract. Vasoconstrictors that decrease local blood flow and decrease systemic uptake of drug can be beneficial when added to local anesthetic solutions because they prolong the duration of action of the local anesthetic at the site of injection and can decrease the risk of systemic toxicity from rapid absorption. However, when systemically administered, vasoactive drugs can decrease blood flow to skin and muscle and decrease the systemic uptake of drugs given by subcutaneous or intramuscular injection. In a similar manner, vasoactive agents can alter the ventilation–perfusion ratio, thereby altering pulmonary uptake of volatile anesthetics, despite a constant inspired concentration. Because of the variability produced by vasoactive agents in drug uptake, careful thought must be given when choosing to administer drugs via the non-IV route in perioperative patients.

Distribution

Some drugs can alter the systemic distribution of other drugs. Alterations in drug distribution will change some or all of a pharmacokinetic model's volume parameters. It can also alter one or all of the *intercompartmental* clearance parameters of a multicompartmental pharmacokinetic model. There are two main mechanisms by which drug–drug interactions are purported to alter drug distribution: (1) changing the volume of tissue available for drug uptake and (2) changing the amount of drug available for tissue uptake. Since the drug dose required to achieve a desired drug concentration is intimately linked to systemic drug distribution, understanding what common drug–drug interactions produce real alterations in drug distribution can avoid unintentional exposure to subtherapeutic and supratherapeutic drug concentrations.

Although a drug cannot alter the actual volume of tissue avail- 14
able for drug uptake, changing the exposure of blood to different tissue beds changes a drug's apparent tissue volume of distribution. Therefore, drug-induced alterations of cardiac output and the distribution of cardiac output to tissues can change the distribution clearance of other drugs. Once again, vasoactive agents can alter tissue distribution by altering regional blood flow even if the total cardiac output is unchanged. Because the change in the plasma drug concentration produced by a prescribed dosing regimen is inversely related to the distribution clearance, the drug dose must be decreased when vasoactive drugs decrease cardiac output or the distribution of cardiac output; otherwise, the patient will be exposed to supratherapeutic drug concentrations.[89–91] In addition, the unintended cardiovascular effects of anesthetic drugs, such as the decrease in cardiac output with increasing doses of the direct myocardial depressant, halothane, or the direct arterial dilator, isoflurane, can lead to similar increases in the plasma drug concentration.[92,93]

There is an abundance of clinical pharmacology literature that examines the ability of one drug to displace another drug from its protein-binding site(s), thereby increasing the concentration of unbound drug in the blood that could cause supratherapeutic concentrations and potential toxicity. When examining specific pharmacokinetic parameters, an increase in the fraction of unbound drug in the plasma could theoretically increase the total apparent volume of distribution (V_{ss}), as more molecules of drug are available for distribution into the tissue. Although most changes in protein binding will not influence clinical drug exposure, analysis of the equations governing the steady-state pharmacokinetics suggests that drugs that are extensively protein bound, have a high hepatic extraction ratio, and have a low therapeutic index may be the exception that require dose adjustment.[94] However, the clinical importance of protein binding as it pertains to anesthetic drugs is based on several common misconceptions regarding drug distribution. First, the number of unoccupied binding sites is several orders of magnitude higher than the number of molecules of anesthetic drug administered in clinical practice. Therefore, it is hard to envision a scenario where a significant amount of displacement could occur. Even if a drug could displace a significant amount of another drug from its protein-binding site, the liver has the capacity available to metabolize this sudden influx of free drug, thereby returning the free drug concentration to the predisplacement concentrations (i.e., flow-limited metabolism). Finally, the theoretical argument supporting the importance of protein binding on highly lipophilic drugs ignores the fact that lipophilic drugs not only have flow-limited elimination clearance, but also flow-limited tissue distribution. Therefore, the equations supporting the negligible role of protein binding on flow-limited elimination clearance also generalize to include flow-limited tissue distribution.[94] Indirect proof of this is provided by the fact that there are no examples in the literature of drug–drug interactions that produce changes in protein binding of opioids and hypnotics that are clinically relevant.[95]

Metabolism

15 Drugs that alter hepatic blood flow (i.e., vasoactive drugs, volatile anesthetics) can proportionally alter hepatic metabolism of drugs with flow-limited clearance.[89,90–93] In addition, drugs that inhibit or induce the enzymes that catalyze biotransformation reactions can affect clearance of other concomitantly administered drugs (Table 11-5). The concomitant use of CYP isozyme inducers can usually be overcome by increasing the administered dose, especially if an easy measure of biologic activity is available or the therapeutic concentration range is known. For example, the anticonvulsant phenytoin shortens the duration of action of the nondepolarizing neuromuscular junction–blocking agents by inducing CYP3A4 and thereby increasing drug elimination clearance.[96] In contrast, when CYP isozyme inhibition is present, it is

Table 11-5 Inducers and Inhibitors of Hepatic Drug Metabolism
Inducers
Carbamazepine
Ethanol
Glucocorticoids
Phenobarbital
Phenytoin
Rifampin
St John's wort
Tamoxifen
Inhibitors
Azole antifungal drugs (i.e., ketoconazole, itraconazole)
Cimetidine
Disulfiram
Grapefruit juice
Macrolide antibiotics (i.e., clarithromycin, erythromycin)
Protease inhibitors (i.e., ritonavir, indinavir, saquinavir)
Quinidine
Selective serotonin reuptake inhibitors (i.e., fluoxetine, sertraline)

more difficult to adjust the drug dose without achieving supratherapeutic, and possibly toxic drug concentrations, unless a suitable rapidly responsive measure of biologic activity is available. For example, it may be possible to safely administer opioids in the presence of a drug that inhibits CYP such as the protease inhibitor ritonavir, because opioids can be titrated in small doses to clinical effect; however, it is more difficult to titrate warfarin or glyburide when instituting short-term therapy with a CYP inhibiting drug such as an antifungal agent. Furthermore, prodrugs that require CYP isozyme activity for conversion to active moieties may be difficult to titrate to adequate clinical effect if there are other sources of interindividual variability in drug dose–response. The opioid prodrugs codeine, oxycodone, hydrocodone, and tramadol all require CYP2D6 for conversion to the biologically active opioid.[95] Because CYP2D6 is highly polymorphic, it is difficult to determine whether a patient who is taking a drug that inhibits CYP2D6 activity (such as selective serotonin reuptake inhibitors) will receive adequate analgesia from these opioids.

Pharmacodynamic Interactions

Pharmacodynamic interactions fall into two broad classifications. Drugs can interact either directly or indirectly at the same receptor. For example, opioid antagonists directly displace opioids from opiate receptors. On the other hand, cholinesterase inhibitors indirectly antagonize the effects of neuromuscular blockers by increasing acetylcholine, which displaces the blocking drug from nicotinic receptors. Pharmacodynamic interactions can also occur if two drugs affect a physiologic system at different sites.[97,98] For example, μ-opioid receptor–mediated ventilatory depression can be selectively antagonized by ampakines that potentiate α-amino-3-hydroxy-5-methyl-4-isoxazolepropionic acid (AMPA) receptor-mediated glutamatergic excitation without mitigating opioid-induced analgesia.[99]

The synergistic pharmacodynamic interaction between hypnotics and opioids each acting at its own receptor, is one of the most advantangeous to clinical anesthesia practice.[100] The pharmacodynamic interaction between two drugs can be characterized by utilizing response surface models.[101–106] The three-dimensional models are useful in delineating the concentration pairs of a hypnotic (e.g., volatile anesthetic, propofol, midazolam) and an opioid (e.g., remifentanil, alfentanil, fentanyl) that produce adequate anesthesia, while minimizing undesired side effects.[107] (See Response Surface Models, below.)

Serotonin Syndrome

One pharmacodynamic interaction that has become more common with the widespread use of medications that modulate the serotonergic pathway is the potentially fatal serotonin syndrome (NICV 11-1).[108,109] High CNS concentrations of serotonin can produce mental status changes (confusion, hyperactivity, memory problems), muscle twitching, excessive sweating, shivering, and fever. Classically, unusually high CNS serotonin levels have been associated with drugs that inhibit monoamine oxidase (MAOIs), an enzyme responsible for metabolizing serotonin in the brain. However, serotonin excess has also been associated with other antidepressant medications, including serotonin reuptake inhibitors and serotonin–norepinephrine reuptake inhibitors (Table 11-6). The interaction of meperidine with MAOIs is the most classic drug–drug interaction associated with serotonin syndrome. Other common perioperative medications, such as methylene blue, which is a potent reversible MAOI, and the phenylpiperidine series of opioids (i.e, fentanyl and its congeners, methadone, meperidine, tramadol), which act as weak serotonin 16

Table 11-6 Serotonergic Psychiatric Drugs Implicated in the Cases of Serotonin Syndrome with Methylene Blue[a]

Class	Generic	Brand Name(s)
Selective serotonin reuptake inhibitors (SSRIs)	Paroxetine	Paxil, Paxil CR, Pexeva
	Fluvoxamine	Luvox, Luvox CR
	Fluoxetine	Prozac, Sarafem, Symbyax
	Sertraline	Zoloft
	Citalopram	Celexa
	Escitalopram	Lexapro
	Vilazodone	Viibryd
Serotonin–norepinephrine reuptake inhibitors (SNRIs)	Venlafaxine	Effexor, Effexor XR
	Desvenlafaxine	Pristiq
	Duloxetine	Cymbalta
Tricyclic antidepressants (TCAs)	Amitriptyline	Amitid, Amitril, Elavil, Endep, Etrafon, Limbitrol, Triavil
	Desipramine	Norpramin, Pertofrane
	Clomipramine	Anafranil
	Imipramine	Tofranil, Tofranil PM, Janimine, Pramine, Presamine
	Nortriptyline	Pamelor, Aventyl hydrochloride
	Protriptyline	Vivactil
	Doxepin	Sinequan, Zonalon, Silenor
	Trimipramine	Surmontil
Monoamine oxidase inhibitors (MAOIs)	Isocarboxazid	Marplan
	Phenelzine	Nardil
	Selegiline	Emsam, Eldepryl, Zelapar
	Tranylcypromine	Parnate
Others	Amoxapine	Asendin
	Maprotiline	Ludiomil
	Nefazodone	Serzone
Trazodone	Desyrel, Oleptro, Trialodine	Wellbutrin, Wellbutrin SR, Wellbutrin XL, Zyban, Aplenzin
	Bupropion	Buspar
	Buspirone	Remeron, Remeron Soltab
	Mirtazapine	

[a]Adapted from U.S. Food & Drug Administration website, updated 11/08/2011 (http://www.fda.gov/Drugs/DrugSafety/ucm276119.htm).

reuptake inhibitors, have been reported to be associated with serotonin toxicity in case reports.[109,110–112] Ideally, serotonergic drugs would be held perioperatively until sufficient CNS drug washout could occur. However, many SSRIs have long elimination half-lives that would require greater than 4 weeks' cessation; in most cases, the risk of withholding these drugs (worsening depression or neuropathic pain) are considered to outweight the benefits. When adequate washout cannot be obtained and a drug such as methylene blue must be administered, the serotonergic drug should not reinstated for 24 hours after the last dose of methylene blue.[111] Furthermore, when methylene blue or phenylpiperidine opioids must be administered to patients taking serotonergic psychiatric medications, clinicians should have a high clinical suspicion for the development of serotonin syndrome. This is especially important in the perioperative period when other more common clinical states, such as postoperative delirium or perioperative fever, can mimic the symptoms of serotonin toxicity. Although cyproheptadine, a serotonin receptor antagonist, is the most common treatment for moderate to severe serotonin toxicity, it is only available as an oral formulation, thereby limiting its bioavailability in critically ill patients. IV chlorpromazine is an alternative serotonin receptor antagonist that has been used successfully with concomitant supportive care.

Clinical Applications of Pharmacokinetics and Pharmacodynamics to the Administration of Intravenous Anesthetics

While no new inhaled anesthetics have been synthesized since the 1960s, IV drugs that act on the CNS continue to be developed. Anesthesiologists have become accustomed to the exquisite control of anesthetic blood (and effect site) concentrations afforded by modern volatile anesthetic agents and their vaporizers, as well as end-tidal anesthetic gas monitoring. Although pharmacokinetic and pharmacodynamic principles and data have contributed greatly to our understanding of the behavior of IV anesthetics, their primary utility is to determine optimal dosing. In most pharmacotherapeutic scenarios outside of anesthesia care, the time scales for onset of drug effect, maintenance, and offset are measured in days, weeks, or even years. In such cases, global pharmacokinetic variables (and one-compartment models) such as total volume of distribution (V_d), elimination clearance (Cl_e), and half-life ($t_{1/2}$) are sufficient for calculating dose regimens. However, in the operating room and intensive care unit, the temporal tolerances for onset and offset of desired drug effects are measured in minutes.[39,40] Consequently, these global variables are insufficient to describe the details of kinetic behavior of drugs in the minutes following IV administration. This is particularly true of lipid-soluble hypnotics and opioids that rapidly and extensively distribute throughout the various tissues of the body because distribution processes dominate pharmacokinetic behavior during the time frame of most anesthetics. In addition, the therapeutic indices of many IV anesthetic drugs are small and two-tailed (e.g., an underdose, resulting in awareness, is just as "toxic" as an overdose). Optimal dosing in these situations requires use of all the variables of a multicompartmental pharmacokinetic model to account for drug distribution in blood and other tissues.

It is not easy to predict pharmacokinetic behavior in a multicompartmental system by simple examination of the kinetic variables.[10] Computer simulation is required to meaningfully interpret or accurately devise new dosing regimens. In addition, there are several pharmacokinetic concepts that are uniquely applicable to IV administration of drugs with multicompartmental kinetics and must be taken into account when administering IV infusions.

To achieve similar degrees of control of intravenously administered anesthetic drug concentrations in blood and in the CNS, new technologies and software to manage the daunting pharmacokinetic principles involved are needed. This section examines the current state of IV infusion devices and the pharmacokinetic and pharmacodynamic principles required for precise delivery of anesthetic agents.

Rise to Steady-State Concentration

The drug concentration versus time profile for the rise to steady state is the mirror image of its elimination profile. In a one-compartment model with a decline in concentration versus time that is monoexponential following a single dose, the rise of drug concentration to the steady-state concentration (C_{SS}) is likewise monoexponential during a continuous infusion. That is, in one elimination half-life, an infusion is halfway to its eventual steady-state concentration, in another half-life, it reaches half of what remains between halfway and steady state (i.e., 75% of the eventual steady state is reached in two elimination half-lives), and so on for each half-life increment. The equation describing this behavior is:

$$C_p(t) = C_{ss}[1 - e^{-kt}] \qquad (11\text{-}21)$$

where $C_p(t)$ = the concentration at time t, k is the rate constant related to the elimination half-life, and t is the time from the start of the infusion. This relationship can also be described by:

$$C_p(n) = C_{ss}[1 - (1/2)^n] \qquad (11\text{-}22)$$

in which $C_p(n)$ is the concentration at n half-lives. Equation 11-22 indicates that during a constant infusion, the concentration reaches 90% of C_{SS} after 3.3 half-lives, which is usually deemed close enough for clinical purposes.

However, for a drug such as propofol, which partitions extensively into pharmacologically inert body tissues (e.g., muscle, gut), a monoexponential equation, or single-compartment model, is insufficient to describe the time course of propofol concentrations in the first minutes and hours after drug administration is initiated. Instead, a multicompartmental or multiexponential model must be used. With such a model, the time course for the plasma drug concentration to rise toward steady state changes drastically. The rate of rise toward steady state is determined by the distribution rate constants to the degree that their respective exponential terms contribute to the total area under the concentration versus time curve. Thus, for the three-compartment model describing the pharmacokinetics of propofol, Equation 11-21 becomes:

$$C_P(t) = C_{SS}\left[\frac{A}{A+B+G}(1 - e^{-\alpha t}) + \frac{B}{A+B+G}(1 - e^{-\beta t}) + \frac{G}{A+B+G}(1 - e^{-\gamma t})\right] \qquad (11\text{-}23)$$

in which t = time; $C_p(t)$ = plasma concentration at time; A = coefficient of the rapid distribution phase and α = hybrid rate constant of the rapid distribution phase; B = coefficient of the slower distribution phase and β = hybrid rate constant of the slower distribution; and G = coefficient of elimination phase and γ = hybrid rate constant of the elimination phase. $A + B + G$ is the sum of the coefficients of all the exponential terms. For most lipophilic anesthetics and opioids, A is typically one order of magnitude greater than B, and B is in turn an order of magnitude greater than G. Therefore, distribution-phase kinetics for IV anesthetics have a much greater influence on the time to reach C_{SS} than do elimination-phase kinetics.[67]

For example, propofol has an elimination half-life of approximately 6 hours; using the simple one-compartment rule in Equation 11-22, it would take 6 hours from the start of a constant rate infusion to reach even 50% of the eventual steady-state propofol plasma concentration and 12 hours to reach 75%. In contrast, with a full three-compartment propofol kinetic model, Equation 11-23 accurately predicts that 50% of steady state is reached in less than 30 minutes and 75% will be reached in less than 4 hours. This example emphasizes the necessity of using multicompartment models to describe the clinical pharmacokinetics of IV anesthetics.

Manual Bolus and Infusion Dosing Schemes

Based on a one-compartment pharmacokinetic model, a stable steady-state plasma concentration ($C_{p,ss}$) can be maintained by administering an infusion at a rate (I) that is proportional to the elimination of drug from the body (Cl_E):

$$I = C_{p,SS} \times Cl_E \qquad (11\text{-}24)$$

However, if the drug was only administered by initiating and maintaining this infusion, it would take one elimination half-time to reach 50% of the target plasma concentration and three times that long to reach 90% of the target plasma concentration. To decrease the time until the target plasma concentration is achieved, an initial bolus (loading dose) of drug can be administered that would produce the target plasma concentration—

$$Bolus = C_{p,SS} \times V_{d,SS} \qquad (11\text{-}25)$$

Although this method is very efficient in achieving and maintaining the target plasma concentration of a drug that instantaneously mixes and equilibrates throughout the tissues of the body (e.g., drugs modeled with a one-compartment pharmacokinetic model), utilizing the steady-state elimination clearance and volume of distribution to calculate the loading dose and maintenance infusion rate will result in plasma drug concentrations that are higher throughout the initial distribution phase (Fig. 11-15).

Using Equations 11-24 and 11-25 and $V_{d,SS}$ = 262 L and Cl_E = 1.7 L/min (for a 50-year-old man who is 178 cm tall and weighs 70 kg, from Schnider et al.[170]), the loading dose and infusion rate of propofol that is needed to achieve a steady-state plasma concentration of 5 μg/mL is 1,300 mg (18 mg/kg) and 120 μg/kg/min.

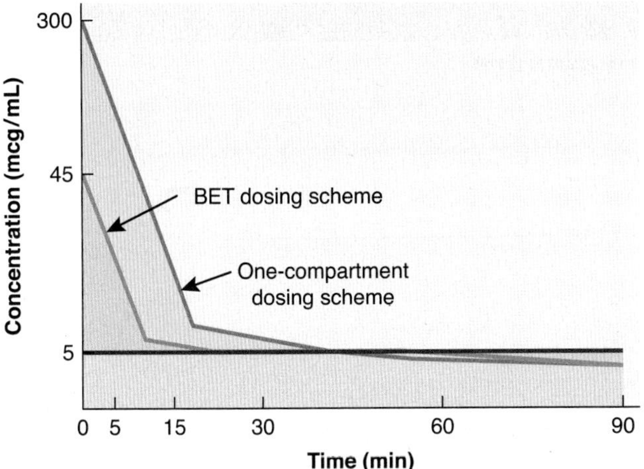

Figure 11-15 A computer simulation of the plasma propofol concentration profile during and after the administration of a single bolus and infusion scheme calculated using the steady-state, one-compartment pharmacokinetic parameters (*red line*) and the BET scheme from **Table 11-7** (*blue line*) to achieve a plasma concentration of 5 μg/mL. $V_{d,SS}$ = 262 L and Cl_E = 1.7 L/min for a 50-year-old male who is 178 cm tall and weighs 70 kg.

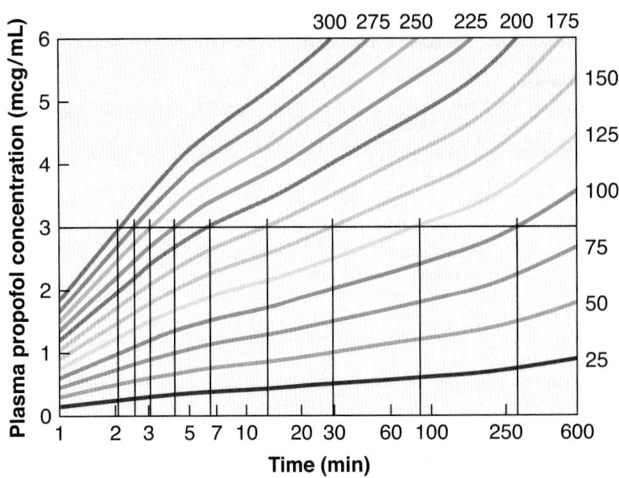

Figure 11-16 Isoconcentration nomogram for determining propofol infusion rates designed to maintain a desired plasma propofol concentration. This nomogram is based on the pharmacokinetics of Schnider et al. and is plotted on a log–log scale to better delineate the early time points. *Curved lines* represent the plasma propofol concentration versus time plots, resulting from the various continuous infusion rates indicated along the right and upper borders (units in μg/kg/min). A horizontal line is placed at the desired target plasma propofol concentration (3 μg/mL in this case) and vertical lines are placed at each intersection of a curved concentration–time plot. The *vertical lines* indicate the times that the infusion rate should be set to the one represented by the *next intersected curve* as one moves from left to right along the horizontal line drawn at 3 μg/mL. In this example, the infusion rate would be reduced from 300 μg/kg/min to 275 μg/kg/min at 2.5 minutes, to 250 μg/kg/min at 3 minutes, to 225 μg/kg/min at 4.5 minutes, and so on until it is turned to 100 μg/kg/min at 260 minutes.

Obviously, the loading dose of propofol is too high, compared to clinically utilized doses (1 to 2 mg/kg), while the infusion rate appears to be clinically reasonable. The erroneous estimate of the loading dose is due to the fact that the initial bolus of drug is not instantaneously mixed and equilibrated with the entire volume of tissue that will eventually take up drug. Therefore, manual dosing strategies for IV anesthetics need to be modified to account for the fact that when a bolus of drug is administered, it rapidly mixes and equilibrates with the blood and only a small volume of tissue (e.g., the central compartment); it then distributes over time into other tissues.

To design a manual bolus that more precisely achieves the desired target plasma concentration, it is necessary to choose a bolus that is based on the small, initial volume of distribution (V_c). To maintain the target plasma concentration, a series of infusions of decreasing rate can be used that match the elimination clearance and compensate for drug loss from the central to the peripheral compartments during the initial period of extensive drug distribution and the second period of moderate drug distribution. This manual dosing scheme has been termed the BET scheme, where B is the loading bolus dose, E is the infusion to replace drug removed by elimination clearance, and T is a continuously decreasing infusion that compensates for transfer of drug to the peripheral tissues (i.e., distribution).[113] An example of a BET scheme for propofol to achieve a target plasma concentration of 5 μg/mL is shown in Table 11-7.

Table 11-7 The Bolus–Elimination–Infusion (BET) Scheme to Achieve a Propofol Plasma Concentration of 5 μg/mL for 120 Minutes

Bolus	2.8 mg/kg	
Infusion	238 μg/kg/min	0–10 min
	187 μg/kg/min	10–20 min
	136 μg/kg/min	20–60 min
	112 μg/kg/min	60–120 min

Pharmacokinetic Simulation Software

One of the many challenges in disseminating pharmacokinetic information is that the concept of drug disposition is described in mathematical terms. Historically, bridging the connection between the mathematical language of pharmacometrics and a graphical interpretation of drug concentration versus time has been limited either to clinical pharmacologists with a background in mathematical modeling, or those with statistical coding skills and ready access to commercially available pharmacokinetic–pharmacodynamic modeling software.[114] These computational techniques are not taught in anesthesia training.

Not surprisingly, reported pharmacokinetic parameter estimates can be difficult to interpret and require translation or denumeration to guide clinical decision making and dosing recommendations.[115] The concept of denumeration of pharmacokinetics was described nearly 40 years ago.[116] However, only recently have software tools been introduced that make accessible user-friendly pharmacokinetic simulation, incorporating a graphical interface.[117] These programs allow for the conceptualization of pharmacokinetics by displaying a numerical and graphical interpretation of drug concentration versus time in response to user input of dose and dose interval.[117] There are numerous simulation programs available. These programs range from free, open-source web-based tools to commercially available desktop applications.[117,118]

Access to user-friendly pharmacokinetic simulation software is important for teaching clinical pharmacology principles. One of the sentinel programs designed specifically for the education and conceptualization of anesthetic pharmacology was created

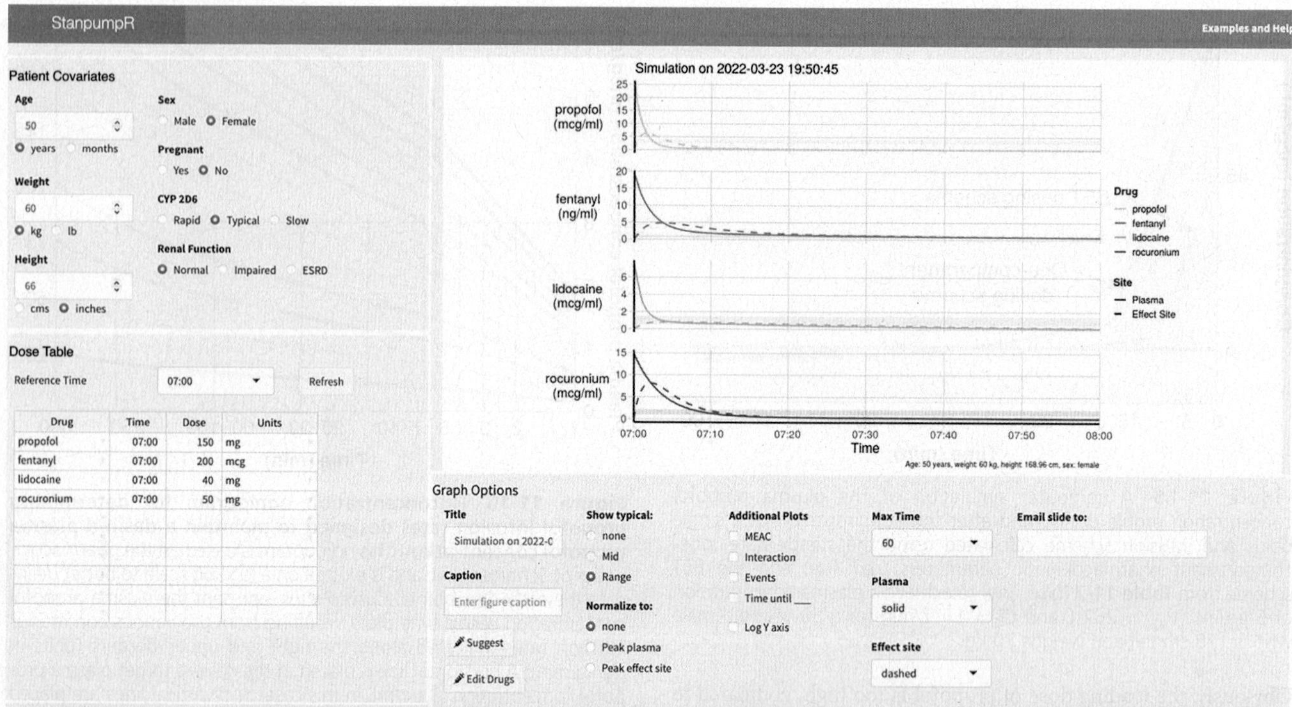

Figure 11-17 Screenshot of StanpumpR graphical user interface. (Used with permission from Dr. Steven L. Shafer. http://www.stanpumpr.io)

nearly 40 years ago. This program was created specifically to simulate inhalational anesthetic uptake and distribution.[119] Recently, Steven Shafer developed the StanpumpR program—an R language successor to Stanpump—which simulates plasma and effect site anesthetic concentrations. StanpumpR, like its precursor, is an open-source program with embedded pharmacokinetic–pharmacodynamic models of a large cache of commonly administered anesthetic drugs. However, unlike Stanpump, StanpumpR does not support drug delivery. Rather, StanpumpR serves as a web-based pharmacokinetic simulator designed to support teaching and research. The simulations are based on the pharmacokinetic–pharmacodynamic models published in peer-reviewed literature. StanpumpR is different from many other simulation programs in that it is free, widely available, and provides a user-friendly graphical interface in which drug inputs can be entered and computed plasma and effect-site concentration versus time curves will be displayed (Fig. 11-17). No prior expertise in modeling or statistical coding is required.

Context-Sensitive Decrement Time

17 During an infusion, drug is taken up by the inert, peripheral tissues.[19] Once drug delivery is terminated, recovery occurs when the effect site concentration decreases below a threshold concentration for producing a pharmacologic effect (e.g., MAC_{AWAKE}—the concentration where 50% of patients follow commands).[67,106] Although the rate of elimination of the drug from the body can give some indication for the time required to reach a subtherapeutic effect, site, drug concentration, and distribution to and from the peripheral tissues also contribute to the time course of decreasing drug concentrations of the central and the effect site. For drugs with multicompartmental kinetics, the elimination half-life will always overestimate the time to recovery from anesthetic drugs. The *context-sensitive half-time* is defined as the time required for the plasma drug concentration to decrease by 50%, where the context is the duration of the infusion.[120] The context-sensitive half-time for the common synthetic opioids fentanyl, alfentanil, sufentanil, and remifentanil are illustrated in Figure 11-18.

The context-sensitive half-time is not a pharmacokinetic parameter *per se*. It is calculated by simulating a TCI of a particular length (the length is the context) and then observing the time required for the plasma concentration to reach one-half of the target concentration from the time the infusion is terminated. As the length of the infusion increases, the value of the half-time increases and will eventually asymptotically approach a maximum half-time at steady state. In general, for multicompartmental pharmacokinetic models, the half-time will always be less than the elimination half-life.

When an infusion is terminated at steady state, input into the system's central compartment is lost and net transfer of drug is no longer zero. Instead, net drug distribution immediately begins moving toward the central compartment from the peripheral

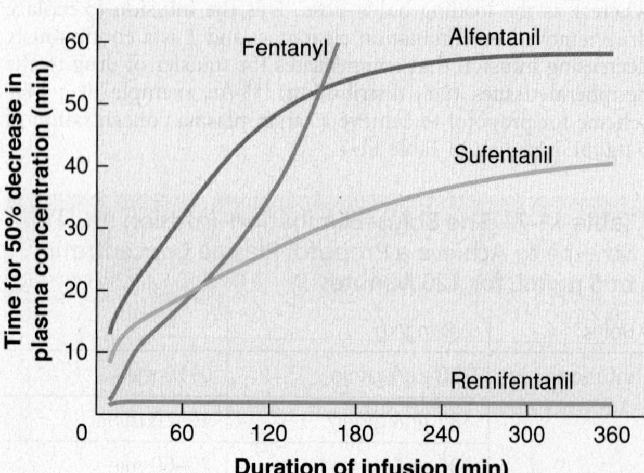

Figure 11-18 The context-sensitive plasma half-time for fentanyl, alfentanil, sufentanil, and remifentanil.

compartments rather than away, as was the case during infusion, and elimination from the central compartment continues unabated by the infusion's input. Plasma or central compartment concentrations will fall relatively rapidly compared to the elimination half-life, until set concentration ratios of central:fast and central:slow are achieved. These ratios with higher peripheral compartment drug concentrations will achieve the net drug distribution flux into the central compartment that will balance the elimination flux to create a constant elimination rate.

During the elimination phase, the multicompartmental system behaves kinetically as a single compartment, but only does so because there are (fixed) drug concentration ratios among the compartments. With a short infusion, the peripheral compartment drug concentrations will have only achieved low drug concentrations, and the plasma drug concentration will have to fall quite far to reach the central:peripheral drug concentration ratios needed to enter the constant elimination phase. Thus, the half-time is less with shorter infusion contexts. After a very long infusion with peripheral compartment drug concentrations reaching higher drug concentrations as they approach their steady state, plasma drug concentrations will not need to fall as much to reach the concentration ratios required for the elimination phase, and the rate of plasma drug decline will begin approaching the elimination half-life sooner, resulting in longer half-times.

The concept of context-sensitive half-times has limitations.[10,21] First, it is not a kinetic parameter; it only describes a specific simulation event. This means it cannot be extrapolated backward or, more importantly, forward to lesser or greater drug concentration decrements, as is possible with true kinetic parameters. Second, it cannot be directly calculated from other kinetic parameters. Rather, a model of the specific drug pharmacokinetics is programmed into a simulation with a set drug infusion regimen. Third, the most relevant concentration decrease may not be one-half. It could be less than one-half or, as is more likely in practice, more than one-half. Therefore, simulating both the specific infusion context as well as the required percentage decrease from the target concentration should be done to get the best estimate of when a drug's effect will reach the clinically desired end point.

Although a 50% decrease in plasma concentration is an appealing and comprehensible parameter, larger or smaller decreases in plasma concentrations may be required for recovery from the drug. Simulations show that the times for different percent decreases in plasma concentration are not linear.[10,21] Therefore, if a 25% or 75% decrease in plasma concentration is required, simulations must be performed to calculate the context-sensitive 25% decrement time or context-sensitive 75% decrement time (Fig. 11-19). In addition, if the concentration of interest is the effect site concentration rather than the plasma concentration,

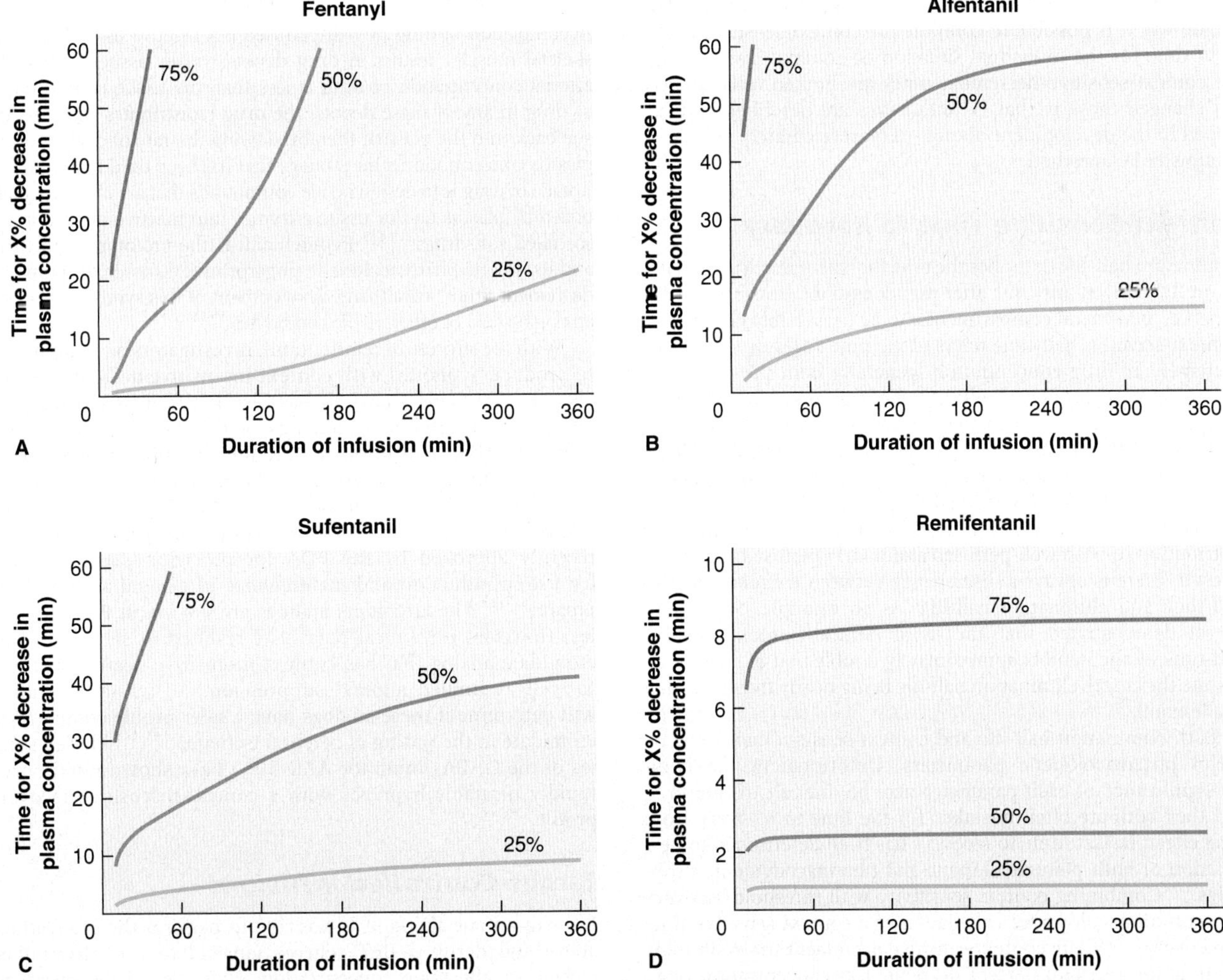

Figure 11-19 The context-sensitive 25%, 50%, and 75% plasma decrement times for fentanyl, alfentanil, sufentanil, and remifentanil.

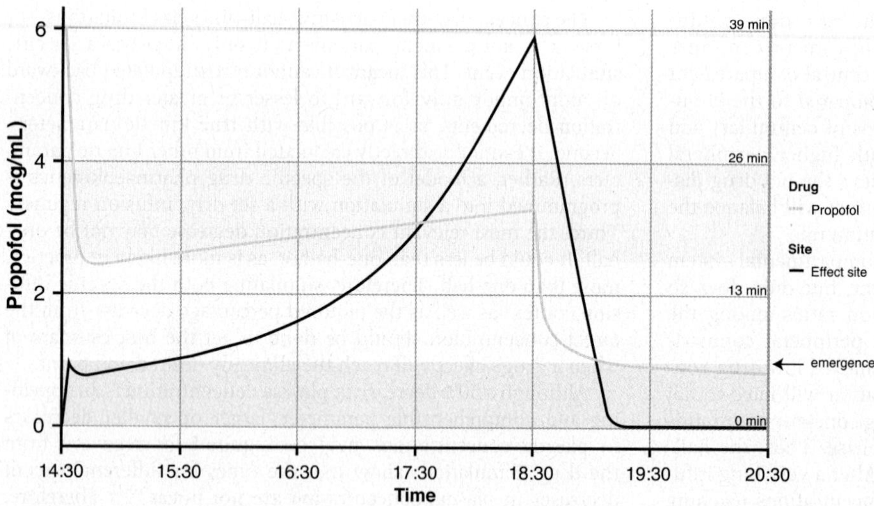

Figure 11-20 Simulation of effect-site concentration (*solid yellow line* and left y-axis) and context-sensitive time to emergence (*solid black line* and right y-axis) after propofol bolus (150 mg) and 4-hour infusion (150 mcg/kg/min). Time to emergence (i.e., reaching an effect site concentration of 1 mcg/mL) after a 4-hour infusion is approximately 38 minutes. (Used with permission from Dr. Steven L. Shafer. http://www.stanpumpr.io)

simulations can be performed to calculate the context-sensitive effect site decrement time. Finally, if a constant plasma or effect-site concentration is not maintained throughout the delivery of the drug (which is typically the case with manual bolus and infusion schemes), the context-sensitive decrement times are guidelines of recovery rather than an absolute prediction of the decay in drug concentration. If precise drug administration data are known, it is possible to compute the context-sensitive decrement time for the individual situation or context. Even though the context-sensitive decrement times are limited, this concept has changed the way that IV anesthetics are described and has helped in the development of tools to more accurately and safely administer IV anesthetics.

Context-Sensitive Time to Recovery

Elimination half-life describes the time for half of the drug remaining in the body at any time after pseudoequilibration with all tissues (i.e., peripheral compartments) to be irreversibly eliminated. Context-sensitive half-time refers to the time necessary for a 50% decrement of drug concentration (generally from the plasma or effect-site compartments) after immediate discontinuation of drug administration and in the context of varying durations of drug administration. Half-life and half-time are identical for drugs whose kinetics are described by a one-compartmental model. However, for IV and inhalational drug delivery, characterization of pharmacokinetic behavior requires models that account for distribution to both well-perfused and poorly perfused tissues; as a result, there is always a discrepancy between context-sensitive half-time and elimination half-life. As an example, Shafer and Varvel demonstrated that the usual clinical context-sensitive half-time of alfentanil is approximately double that of sufentanil, despite the latter's elimination half-life being nearly five times that of alfentanil.[121]

Both elimination half-life and context-sensitive half-time are useful pharmacokinetic parameters. Unfortunately, the clinical significance of each parameter may be difficult to interpret, and they both are often mistaken for the time to recovery from drug effect. In fact, time to recovery has been determined to be a function of both pharmacokinetic and pharmacodynamic properties.[122] Combining context sensitivity with threshold recovery concentrations allows for calculation of a context-sensitive time to recovery.[123] Where context-sensitive decrement times simulate the time for a certain percent decrement in concentration (e.g., half-time), context-sensitive recovery times simulate the time to reach a particular threshold concentration after terminating a drug infusion, resulting in dissipation of drug effect. Newer simulation software can simulate context-sensitive time to recovery (Fig. 11-20).

Soft Pharmacology and Anesthesiology

Accumulation of drug in well-perfused but inactive tissue beds (i.e., skeletal muscle) results in drug depots within tissues. When the arterial concentration of drug is less than the tissue concentration of drug in any of these depots, the drug redistributes from the tissue back into the plasma, thereby slowing the rate of decline of the plasma concentration. One strategy that has been used to limit tissue uptake of drug is to design active compounds that are rapidly metabolized by plasma and/or tissue enzymes into inactive metabolites—so-called soft drugs.[124,125] Remifentanil is the prototypic soft drug, and its unique pharmacokinetic fingerprint (i.e., context-insensitive decrement times) resulted in development of this synthetic fentanyl analog instead of other viable candidates.[66,126]

With the success of remifentanil, investigators have attempted to produce hypnotics with context-insensitive decrement times (Fig. 11-21). This approach has resulted in a new benzodiazepine, several etomidate analogs, and a novel hypnotic that inhibits $GABA_A$ receptors.[127–130] Remimazolam is a new benzodiazepine that is metabolized by plasma and tissue esterases. It has a chemical structure nearly identical to its parent compound midazolam with the addition of an ester linkage. The drug was recently approved by the FDA for procedural sedation, and for use in induction and maintenance of general anesthesia in Japan.[131–135] The etomidate analogs are not yet in Phase I studies. However, preclinical data have resulted in selection of an etomidate analog that has context-insensitive decrement times as well as limited adrenal suppression.[134–142] Further studies will determine if these analogs have a safer profile compared to etomidate in the setting of cerebral ischemia.[143–145] Phase I studies of the $GABA_A$ inhibitor AZD-3043 have shown rapid onset, rapidly titratable hypnosis with a context-insensitive recovery profile.[130,146–148]

Target-Controlled Infusions

Prior to an anesthetic, it is possible to perform the calculations above and derive a BET scheme targeted to a predetermined plasma or effect-site concentration. However, in the operating room, once the anesthetic has commenced, without the help of a

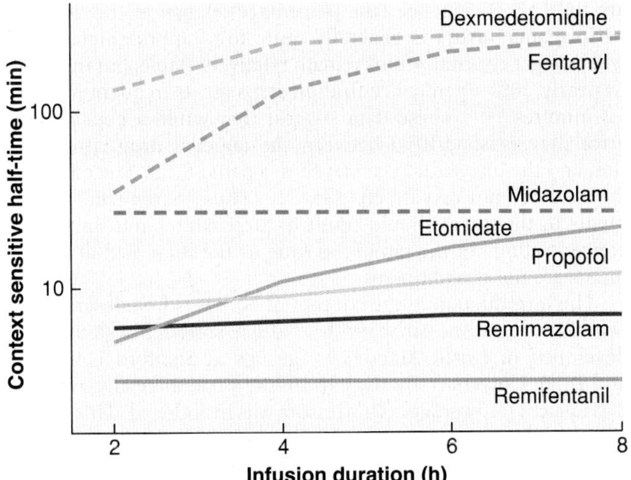

Figure 11-21 The effect site context-sensitive half-times (CSHTs) for the classic anesthetic drugs and their analogous soft drugs. Note that the *y*-axis is in a log scale in order to allow the drugs with the CSHTs more than 30 minutes (i.e., dexmedetomidine, fentanyl, midazolam, and etomidate) to be displayed with the drugs that have the short CSHTs (i.e., remifentanil, remimazolam, and propofol), which are almost context insensitive.

computer, software, and possibly an assistant, it is laborious and difficult to make calculations to determine how to adjust an infusion or to bolus a drug in order to manipulate the target plasma concentration.[149] By linking a computer with the appropriate pharmacokinetic model to an infusion pump, it is possible for the physician to enter the desired target plasma concentration of a drug, and for the computer to nearly instantaneously calculate the appropriate infusion scheme to quickly achieve this target.[150] Because drug accumulates at various rates among the tissues and organs in the body, the computer continually calculates the current drug concentration and adjusts the infusion pump in order to account for the current status of drug uptake, distribution, and elimination. In this way, the computer-driven BET scheme can in fact control the infusion pump to achieve a steady target concentration (Fig. 11-22).

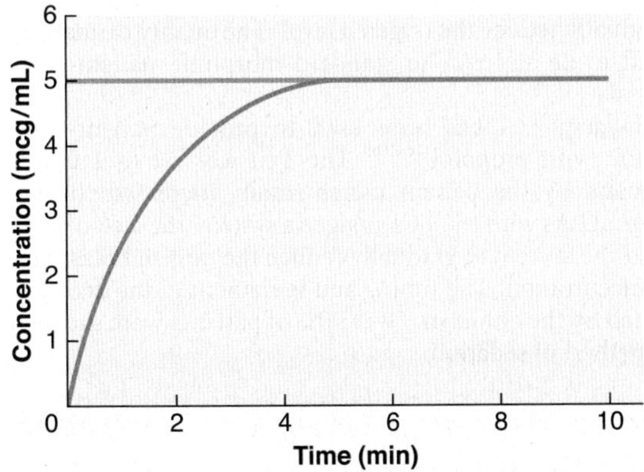

Figure 11-22 This is a simulation of a target-controlled infusion (TCI) in which the plasma concentration is targeted at 5 μg/mL. The *blue line* represents the predicted plasma propofol concentration of 5 μg/mL, which in theory is attained at time t = 0 and is then maintained by a variable rate infusion. The *red line* is the predicted effect site concentration under the conditions of a constant pseudo–steady-state plasma concentration. Note that 95% of the target concentration is reached in the effect site at approximately 4 minutes.

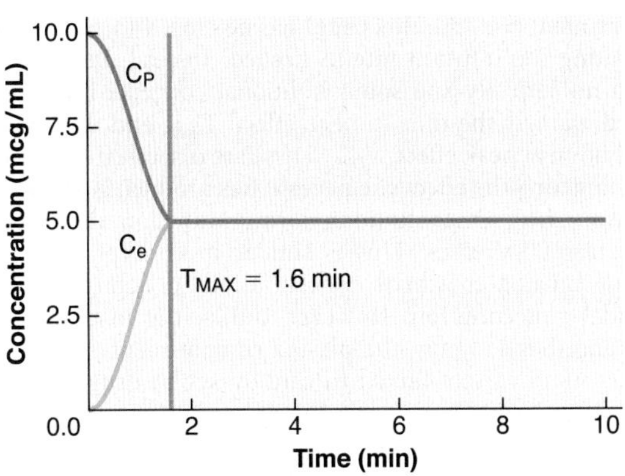

Figure 11-23 This is a simulation of a target-controlled infusion (TCI) in which the effect site concentration (C_e) is targeted at 5 μg/mL. The *orange line* represents the predicted plasma propofol concentration (C_p) that results from a bolus dose, given at time t = 0, that is predicted to purposely overshoot the plasma propofol concentration target until time t = T_{max} (1.6 minutes). At T_{max} pseudo-equilibration between the effect site and the plasma occurs and both concentrations are then predicted to be the same until the target is changed. Note that the effect site attains the target in less than half the time with effect site targeting compared to the plasma concentration targeting seen in Figure 11-22.

The success of this approach is influenced by the extent to which the drug pharmacokinetic and pharmacodynamic parameters programmed into the computer match those of the particular patient on whom the model is being applied. While this same limitation applies to the more rudimentary (non-TCI) dosing done routinely in every clinical setting, we must examine the special ramifications of pharmacokinetic–pharmacodynamic model misspecification with TCI in any discussion of its future importance in the clinical setting.

The mathematical principles governing TCI are actually quite simple. For a computer control pump to produce and maintain a plasma drug concentration, it must first administer a dose equal to the product of the central compartment, V_1, and the target concentration (Fig. 11-23). Then for each moment after that, the amount of drug to be administered into the central compartment to maintain the target concentration is equal to drug eliminated from the central compartment *plus* drug distributed from the central compartment to peripheral compartments *minus* drug returning to the central compartment from peripheral compartments. The software keeps track of the estimated drug in each compartment over time and applies the rate constants for intercompartmental drug transfer from the pharmacokinetic model to these amounts to determine drug movement at any given time. It then matches the estimated concentrations to the target concentration at any time to determine the amount of drug that should be infused. The software can also predict future concentrations, usually with the assumption that the infusion will be stopped so that emergence from anesthesia or the dissipation of drug effect will occur optimally according to the context-sensitive decrement time.

There is a delay or hysteresis between the attainment of a drug concentration in the plasma and the production of a drug effect, and it is advantageous to have the mathematics of this delay incorporated into TCI. By adding the kinetics of the effect site, it is possible to target effect-site concentrations as would be in keeping with the principle of working as closely to the relevant concentration–effect relationship as possible. A dose scheme that targets concentrations in a compartment remote from the central compartment (i.e., the effect site) has no closed-form solution for calculating the infusion rate(s) needed. Instead, the solution is solved numerically and some additional concepts must be considered, namely the time to peak effect, T_{max}, and the volume of distribution at peak effect, V_{DPE}. These are discussed later. In principle, targeting the effect site necessitates producing an overshoot in plasma drug concentrations during induction and for subsequent target increases. This is similar in concept to overpressurizing inhaled anesthetic concentrations to achieve a targeted end-tidal concentration. However, unlike the inspiratory limb of an anesthesia circuit, the plasma compartment concentration appears more closely linked to cardiovascular drug effects; as a result, large overshoots in plasma drug concentration may produce unwanted side effects.

The performance of TCI is influenced by the pharmacokinetic model chosen. Most modern TCI models, whether they target the plasma or the effect site, seem to be similar in performance, they all produce overshoot for 10 to 20 minutes when increasing the target concentration.[37] This is because the dose adjustments made are based on calculations that utilize a central compartment that ignores the complexity of intravascular mixing, thereby overestimating the central compartment's true volume (V_C), the rate of transfer to the fast peripheral tissue (Cl_F), and the size of the peripheral tissue compartment (V_F) (Fig. 11-24). The performance of TCI is also influenced by the variance between pharmacokinetic parameters determined from group or population studies and the individual patient. Median absolute performance errors for fentanyl,[151] alfentanil,[152] sufentanil,[153] midazolam,[154,155] and propofol[155,156] are in the range of ±30% when literature values for pharmacokinetic parameters are used to drive the TCI device; error rates fall to approximately ±7% when the average kinetics of the test subjects themselves are used.[152] Divergence (the percentage change of the absolute performance error) is generally quite low (approximately 1%) when target concentrations remain relatively stable, but increases to nearly 20% when concentration steps are as frequent as every 12 minutes.[37,156] These data suggest that while a considerable error may exist (±30%) between the targeted drug concentration and the one actually achieved in a patient, the concentration attained will not vary much over time. Thus, incremental adjustments in the target should result in incremental and stable new concentrations in the patient as long as the incremental adjustments are not too frequent.

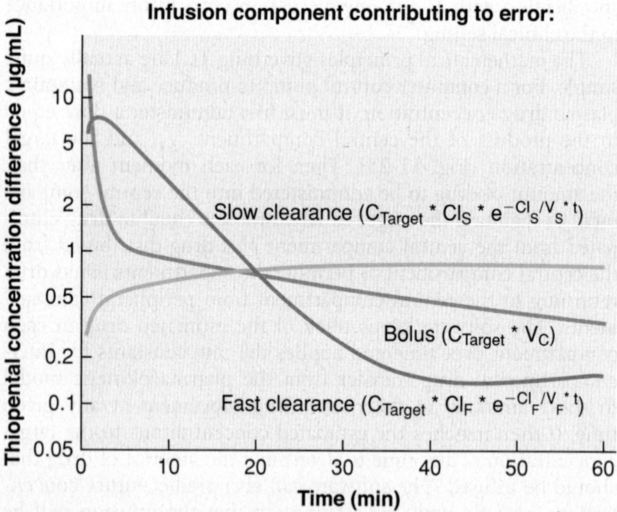

Figure 11-24 The influence of the misspecification of each of the components of the traditional three-compartment pharmacokinetic models on the prolonged discrepancy (overshoot) between predicted and targeted concentrations with target-controlled infusions. The error resulting from elimination clearance was negligible and therefore not illustrated. Notice that the loading dose (based on V_C) produces a large amount of error in the initial minutes; however, from 1 to 20 minutes, the deviation from the target concentration is largely due to the overestimation of Cl_F. The equations listed are for the respective BET infusions of the TCI system. (Reprinted with permission from Avram MJ, Krejcie TC. Using front-end kinetics to optimize target-controlled drug infusions. *Anesthesiology.* 2003;99:1078–1086.)

The introduction of the concept of TCI, was first described by 18
Schwilden et al. in early 1980s[157] Other software systems were developed in North America by groups at Stanford University and Duke University. By the late 1990s, a commercially available TCI system for propofol (Diprifusor) was introduced. This greatly increased both anesthesiologists' interest in this mode of delivery and their understanding of the concentration–effect relationships for hypnotics and opioids. In most of the world, devices for delivering propofol by TCI are commercially available from at least three companies (Graseby, Alaris, and Fresenius) with similar performance parameters.[158] In the United States, there are still no FDA-approved devices. For investigational purposes, Stanpump (developed by Steve Shafer at Stanford University) can be interfaced via an RS232 port to an infusion pump. Stanpump currently provides pharmacokinetic parameters for 19 different drugs but has the ability to accept any kinetic model for any drug provided by the user. RugLoop is TCI software (developed by Michel Struys of Ghent University) similar to STANPUMP but operates in Windows rather than DOS and is capable of controlling multiple drug infusions simultaneously. (Information regarding RugLoop is available at http://www.demed.be/index.html.)

While the pharmacologic principle of relating a concentration rather than a dose is scientifically sound, only a few limited studies have actually compared manual infusion control versus TCI. Some have shown better control and a more predictable emergence with TCI,[158,159] whereas others have shown no advantage.[160,161]

TCI principles continue to be developed beyond the scope of IV anesthesia techniques. TCI has been used to provide postoperative analgesia with alfentanil.[162,163] In this system, a desired target plasma alfentanil concentration was set in the range of 40 to 100 ng/mL. Demand by the patient automatically increased the target level by 5 ng/mL. Lack of a demand caused the system to gradually reduce the targeted level. The quality of analgesia was judged to be superior to standard morphine patient-controlled analgesia.

Similarly, TCI has been used to provide patient-controlled sedation with propofol.[164,165] The TCI was set to 1 µg/mL and a demand by the patient incrementally increased the level by 0.2 µg/mL. As with the TCI analgesia system, the lack of a demand caused the system to gradually reduce the targeted plasma propofol concentration. The timing and increment of the decrease were adjusted by the clinician. Over 90% of patients were satisfied with this method of sedation.

Time to Maximum Effect Compartment Concentration (T_{max})

Earlier in this chapter, the delay between attaining a plasma concentration and an effect-site concentration was described (Fig. 11-12). This delay, or hysteresis, is presumed to be a result of transfer of drug between the plasma compartment, V_C, and an effect compartment, V_e, as well as the time required for a cellular response. By simultaneously modeling the plasma drug concentration versus time data (pharmacokinetics) and the measured drug effect (pharmacodynamics), an estimate of the drug transfer rate constant, k_{e0}, between plasma and the putative effect site can be estimated.[65] However, estimates of k_{e0}, like all rate constants, are model specific.[166,167] That is, k_{e0} cannot be transported from one set of kinetic parameters determined in one specific pharmacokinetic–pharmacodynamic study to any other set of pharmacokinetic parameters. Likewise, it is not valid to compare estimates of k_{e0} among studies of the same drug or across different drugs and, therefore, one should not be surprised that reported values for k_{e0} for the same drug vary markedly in the literature. The model-independent parameter that characterizes the delay between the plasma and effect site is the time to maximal effect, or T_{max}.[167] Accordingly, if the T_{max} and the pharmacokinetics for a drug are known from independent studies, a k_{e0} can be estimated by numeric techniques for the independent kinetic set that would produce the known effect site T_{max}.

The concept of a transportable, model-independent parameter that characterizes the kinetics of the effect site is important for robust effect site–targeted, computer-controlled infusions. This is because there are many more pharmacokinetic studies characterizing a wider variety of patient types and groups in the literature than there are complete pharmacokinetic–pharmacodynamic studies. By making the generally valid assumption that interindividual differences are small in a drug's rate of effect site equilibration, it is possible with a known T_{max} to estimate effect site kinetics for a drug across a wide variety of patient groups where only the pharmacokinetics are known. This cannot be done in a valid manner using k_{E0} or $t½_{Ke0}$ alone.[166,167]

Volume of Distribution at Peak Effect (V_{DPE})

While the plasma concentration can be brought rapidly to the targeted drug concentration by administering a bolus dose to the central compartment ($C \times V_C$) and then held there by a computer-controlled infusion (Fig. 11-22), the time for the effect site to reach the target concentration will be much longer than T_{max} (4 minutes for the propofol effect site concentration to reach 95% of that targeted). It is possible to calculate a bolus dose that will attain the estimated effect site concentration at T_{max} without overshoot at the effect site. However, plasma drug concentration will be overshot (Fig. 11-21). Calculating this bolus dose is done using the concept that drug distributes into an expanding volume that starts at V_C and approaches V_β (the apparent volume of distribution during the elimination phase) over time and combining that information with the concept of T_{max}.[168,169]

Volume of distribution over time is calculated by dividing the total amount of drug remaining in the body by the plasma drug concentration at each time, *t*. The time-dependent volume at the time of peak effect (or T_{max}) is V_{DPE}. The product of the targeted effect site concentration and V_{DPE} plus the amount lost to elimination in the time to T_{max} becomes the proper bolus dose that will attain the target concentration at the effect site as rapidly as possible without overshoot. In practical terms, this bolus is given at time $t = 0$, after which the infusion stops until time $t = T_{max}$. It then resumes infusing drug in its normal "stop loss" manner.

Some software programs for controlling TCIs include this concept in their algorithms. Figure 11-16 illustrates an isoconcentration nomogram for propofol using the pharmacokinetic–pharmacodynamic parameters described in Schnider et al.[170]; in a 70-kg man, this model predicts a T_{max} of 1.6 minutes, a V_{DPE} of 16.62 L, and an elimination loss of 23.8% of the dose over 1.6 minutes. Thus, the proper propofol bolus for a targeted effect site concentration of 5 μg/mL is 109 mg. The computer-controlled infusion pump will deliver this dose as rapidly as possible and then begin a targeted infusion for 5 μg/mL at t = 1.6 minutes (Fig. 11-23).

Front-End Pharmacokinetics

Classic PK-PD models make the simplifying assumption that there 19
is instantaneous and complete mixing of drug in the intravascular space—a mathematical construct that disregards the physiology that drives drug disposition.[171–173] Therefore, classic PK models inaccurately describe the initial/central distribution volume (V_C); as a result, they incorrectly estimate intercompartmental clearances and are unable to characterize cardiac output and its distribution.[37,40,89,171,173–176] Misspecification of V_C also results in misspecification of the effect site kinetics and compensates by overestimating interindividual PD variability.[37,173,176] Physiologically based PK-PD models that can accurately estimate distribution volumes and clearances result in more realistic estimates of PD variability (Fig. 11-25).[176] Another source of PK and PD variability is cardiac output and its distribution.[89,173,174,176,177] Cardiac output and its distribution influences PK by modifying the distribution of drug to tissue compartments. In addition, cardiac output influences PD by changing the blood-effect site equilibration rate (Fig. 11-26).[176] Because they cannot characterize cardiac output and its distribution, classic PK-PD models will be unable to identify the changes in cardiac output and its distribution that are the result of alterations in physiology related to sex, age, body composition, or pathologic processes.[178,179] Therefore, classic PK-PD models will not identify factors that solely alter cardiac output and its distribution as a source of PK variability and will overestimate the true PD.[37,176,180,181]

The term *front-end pharmacokinetics* refers to the intravascular mixing, pulmonary uptake, and recirculation events that occur in the first few minutes during and after IV drug administration.[40] These kinetic events and the drug concentration versus time profile that results are important because the peak effect of rapidly

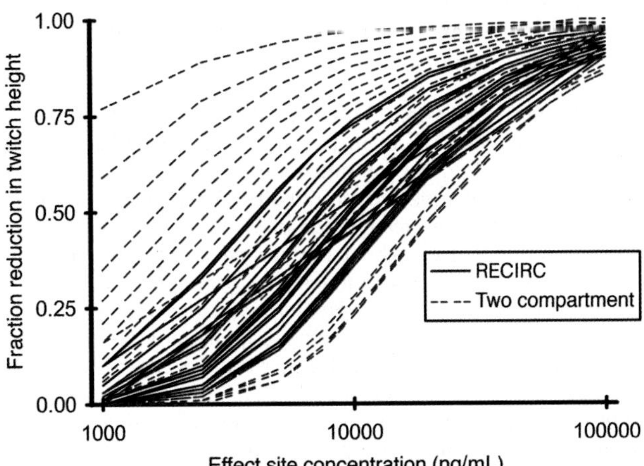

Figure 11-25 The misestimation of the central distribution volume (Vc) by a traditional compartmental PK-PD model results in more interindividual variability in pharmacodynamic estimates than pharmacodynamic estimates from a high-resolution, recirculatory PK-PD model. This figure uses Monte Carlo simulation of the effect site concentration–pharmacologic effect relationships to demonstrate the interindividual variability from a traditional compartmental PK-PD model (2 COMP, *blue dashed lines*) and a high-resolution recirculatory PK-PD model (RECIRC, *black solid lines*). (Adapted with permission from the rocuronium data of Kuipers JA, Boer F, Olofsen E, et al. Recirculatory pharmacokinetics and pharmacodynamics of rocuronium in patients: the influence of cardiac output. *Anesthesiology*. 2001;94:47–55.)

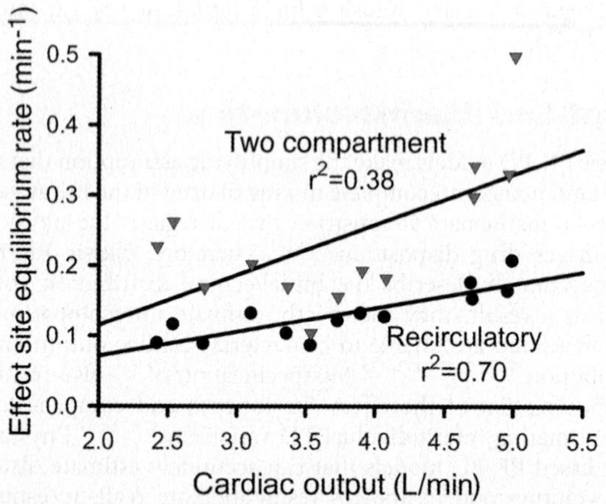

Figure 11-26 The effects of cardiac output on the blood–effect-site equilibration rate (k_{e0}) when the PK-PD model is a high-resolution "recirculatory" model (*black circles*) versus a traditional compartmental model (*triangles*). While the traditional model has a moderate correlation between measured cardiac output and k_{e0} and significant systematic error (*grey line*), the high-resolution recirculatory model has a very strong correlation between measured cardiac output and k_{e0} (*black line*). Therefore, for lipophilic drugs with flow-limited tissue distribution (i.e., opioids, hypnotics, etc.), a high-resolution PK-PD model provides a physiologic basis for transfer of drug from the blood to the effect site. In addition, these high-resolution PK-PD models can quantitate the effects of physiologic perturbations on the PK and PD of these drugs more accurately than the traditional compartmental models. (Adapted with permission from the rocuronium data of Kuipers JA, Boer F, Olofsen E, et al. Recirculatory pharmacokinetics and pharmacodynamics of rocuronium in patients: the influence of cardiac output. *Anesthesiology*. 2001;94:47–55.)

acting drugs occurs during this temporal window.[39,176,182,183] Although it has been suggested that front-end pharmacokinetics be used to guide drug dosing,[37] current TCI does not incorporate front-end kinetics into the models from which drug infusion rates are calculated. As described above, not doing so introduces further error.

TCI relies on pharmacokinetic models that are based on the simplifying assumption of instantaneous and complete mixing within V_C. However, the determination of V_C is routinely overestimated in most pharmacokinetic studies. When used to calculate TCI infusion rates, overestimation of V_C results in plasma drug concentrations that overshoot the desired target concentration, especially in the first few minutes after beginning the infusion. Furthermore, correct description of drug distribution to tissues is dependent on an accurate V_C estimate, so inaccuracies caused by not taking front-end pharmacokinetics into account may be persistent and result in undershoot as well as overshoot. Simulation indicates that pharmacokinetic parameters derived from studies in which the drug is administered in a short (approximately 2 minutes) infusion better estimate V_C and tissue-distribution kinetics than those administered in a rapid IV bolus infusion.[37,38] When the latter drug administration method is used, full characterization of the front-end recirculatory pharmacokinetics is required to obtain valid estimates of V_C for use in TCI.[37,38]

Closed-Loop Infusions

When a valid and nearly continuous measure of drug effect is available, drug delivery can be automatically titrated by feedback control. Such systems have been used experimentally for control of blood pressure,[184] oxygen delivery,[185] blood glucose,[186] neuromuscular blockade,[187] and depth of anesthesia.[188–194] A target value for the desired effect measure (the output of the system) is selected and the rate of drug delivery (the input into the system) is dependent on whether the effect measure is above, below, or at the target value. Thus, the output feeds back and controls the input. Standard controllers (referred to as *proportional-integral-derivative* [PID] *controllers*) adjust drug delivery based on both the integral, or magnitude, of the deviation from target and the rate of deviation, or the derivative.

Under a range of responses, standard PID controllers work quite well. However, they have been shown to develop unstable characteristics in situations where the output may vary rapidly and widely. Schwilden et al.[190] proposed a controller in which the output (measured response) controls not only the input (drug infusion rate), but also the pharmacokinetic model driving the infusion rate. This is known as a *model-driven* or *adaptive* closed-loop system. Such a system has performed well in clinical trials,[189] and in a simulation of extreme conditions, it was demonstrated to outperform a standard PID controller.[192]

Closed-loop systems for anesthesia are the most difficult to design and implement because the precise definition of "anesthesia" remains elusive, as does a robust monitor for "anesthetic depth."[106] Because modification of consciousness must accompany anesthesia, processed electroencephalogram (EEG) parameters that correlate with level of consciousness, such as the bispectral index (BIS), electroencephalographic entropy, and auditory evoked potentials, make it possible to undertake closed-loop control of anesthesia.[195] There is keen interest in further developing these tools to make them more reliable, because advances in pharmacokinetic modeling, including the effect compartment, the implementation of such models into drug delivery systems, and the creation of adaptive controllers based on these models, has made routine closed-loop delivery of anesthesia imaginable.[188] Over the past 10 years, clinical trials investigating closed-loop delivery of propofol or propofol and remifentanil have demonstrated superior efficiency in drug delivery and emergence from anesthesia with closed-loop devices compared to manual titration by experienced anesthesia providers.[196–201] So far, it has been difficult to bring a true closed-loop system to market in medical applications due to regulatory agency hurdles. From a regulatory point of view, an open-loop TCI system is much easier to attain and offers many of the benefits of actual closed-loop systems. Unless there is a regulatory or design "breakthrough," closed-loop systems for anesthesia will likely remain in the theoretical and experimental realms.[202,205]

Response Surface Models of Drug–Drug Interactions

During the course of an operation, the level of anesthetic drug administered is adjusted to ensure amnesia to ongoing events, provide immobility to noxious stimulation, and blunt the sympathetic response to painful stimuli. Although it is possible to achieve an adequate anesthetic state with a high dose of a sedative-hypnotic alone (i.e., a volatile anesthetic or propofol), the effect site drug concentration necessary is often associated with excessive hemodynamic depression,[98] and a deeper than necessary plane of hypnosis that may be associated with longstanding morbidity or mortality.[204,205] Therefore, to limit side effects, an opioid and a sedative-hypnotic are administered together. Although the administration of two volatile anesthetics or a volatile anesthetic and propofol produce a net-additive effect, the combination of an opioid and a sedative-hypnotic are synergistic for most pharmacologic effects. By understanding the interactions between the opioids and the sedative-hypnotics, it is possible to select target concentration pairs of the two drugs that produce the desired

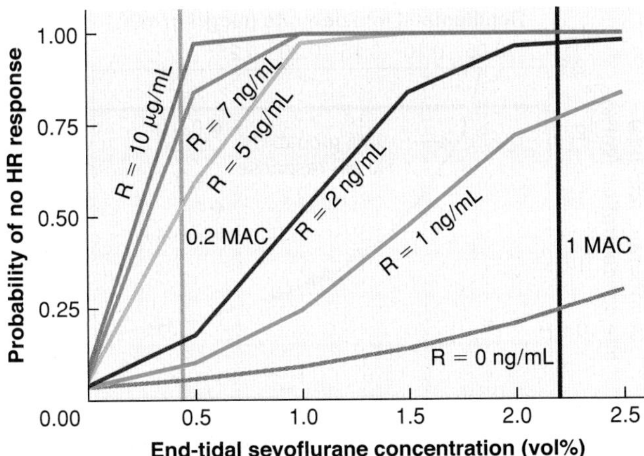

Figure 11-27 The effect of adding remifentanil on the concentration–effect curve for sevoflurane-induced analgesia (no hemodynamic response to a 5-second, 50-mA tetanic stimulation in volunteers). Each curve represents the concentration–effect relation for sevoflurane with a fixed effect site concentration of remifentanil. The leftward shift in the curves indicates that remifentanil decreases the amount of sevoflurane needed to produce adequate analgesia. The changes in the slopes of the concentration–response curves indicate that there is significant pharmacodynamic synergy between sevoflurane–remifentanil. Also note that there is a ceiling effect to this pharmacodynamic interaction—the magnitude of the leftward shift decreases as the remifentanil concentration increases. (Adapted with permission from Manyam SC, Gupta DK, Johnson KB, et al. Opioid-volatile anesthetic synergy: a response surface model with remifentanil and sevoflurane as prototypes. *Anesthesiology*. 2006;105:267–278.)

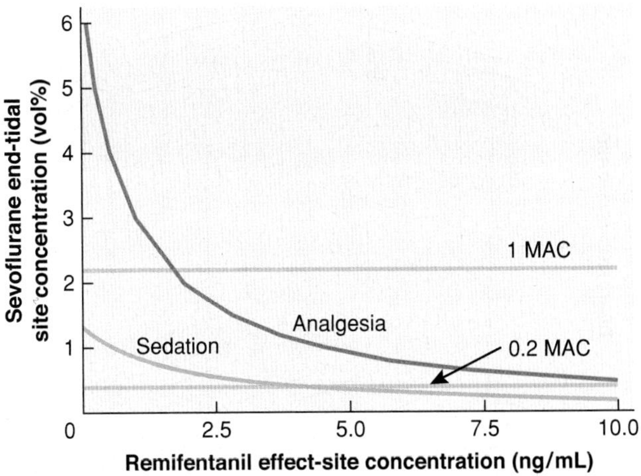

Figure 11-28 Remifentanil–sevoflurane interaction for sedation (*green line*) and analgesia to electrical tetanic stimulation (*red line*) for volunteers. The respective 95% isoboles demonstrate the myriad target concentration pairs of remifentanil and sevoflurane that have a 95% probability of producing the desired pharmacodynamic end point. (Adapted with permission from Manyam SC, Gupta DK, Johnson KB, et al. Opioid-volatile anesthetic synergy: a response surface model with remifentanil and sevoflurane as prototypes. *Anesthesiology*. 2006;105:267–278.)

clinical effect while minimizing unwanted side effects associated with higher concentrations of either drug.

Studies designed to evaluate the pharmacodynamic interactions between an opioid and a sedative-hypnotic have traditionally focused on the effects of adding one or two fixed doses or concentrations of the opioid to several defined concentrations or doses of the sedative-hypnotic.[97,98,206–213] Graphic demonstrations of these interaction data are most commonly performed by demonstrating a shift of parallel dose–response curves (Fig. 11-27). An alternative mathematical model is the isobologram—iso-effect curves that show dose combinations that result in equal effect (Fig. 11-28). Isobolographic analysis has the additional benefit of characterizing the interaction between the two drugs as additive, antagonistic, or synergistic (Fig. 11-29), whereas shifts of dose–response curves require more complex concentrations to determine if the interaction demonstrated by a leftward shift in the curve is more than additive.

An alternative mathematical model that can fully characterize the complete spectrum of interaction between two drugs for all possible concentrations and effects is the response surface model.[102,105] The surface morphology of a response surface not only demonstrates whether the interaction is additive, synergistic, or antagonistic, but the model itself can quantitatively describe the degree of interaction between the two drugs. Furthermore, isobolograms can be derived from the projection of the response surface onto the appropriate horizontal effect plane (Fig. 11-30), and concentration–response curves can be derived from taking a vertical slice through a response surface in the plane perpendicular to the fixed-opioid concentration of interest (Fig. 11-30).[102,105,106] Therefore, response surface models can be viewed as generalizations of the traditional pharmacodynamic methods of analysis. The major limitation of response surface models is that they require a large number of pharmacodynamic measurements across all possible concentration pairings to accurately characterize the entire surface.[214] This is most efficiently done in the laboratory setting utilizing volunteers who can be exposed to subtherapeutic and supratherapeutic drug concentration pairs. However, because response surface models characterize the drug concentration pairs that provide adequate anesthesia and also adequate recovery from anesthesia, these models provide information that is not normally available from studies that generate an isobologram from surgical patients.

Isobolograms and response surface models clearly dem- 20
onstrate that there are multiple target concentration pairs of an opioid and a sedative-hypnotic that can provide adequate anesthesia—a 95% probability of no hemodynamic response to a noxious stimulus and 95% probability of clinically adequate sedation.[103,104,107] Combining the response surface pharmacodynamic

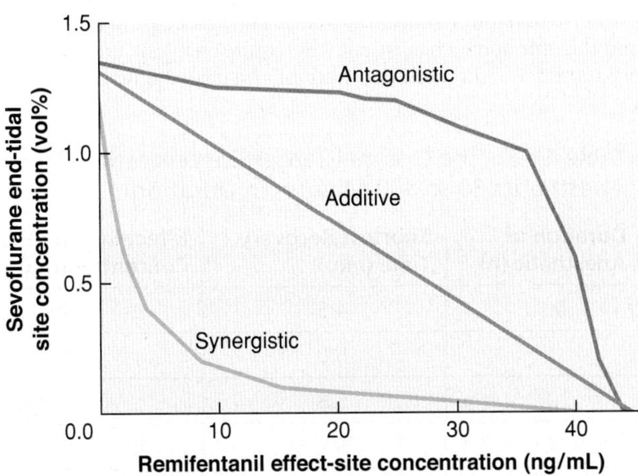

Figure 11-29 Isoboles to demonstrate additive (*blue line*), synergistic (*green line*), and antagonistic (*red line*) interactions between drug A and drug B.

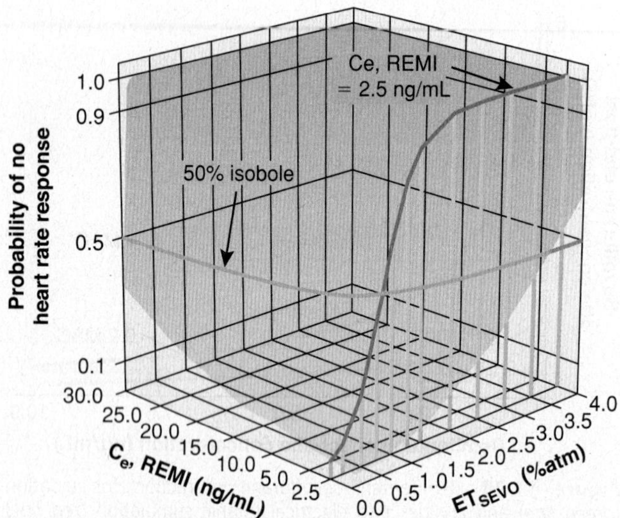

Figure 11-30 A response surface model characterizing the remifentanil–sevoflurane interaction for analgesia to electrical tetanic stimulation. The projection of the response surface onto the 50% probability horizontal plane results in the 50% effect isobole while the projection of the response surface onto the 2.5 ng/mL remifentanil effect site concentration vertical plane results in the sevoflurane concentration–response curve under 2.5 ng/mL of remifentanil. (Adapted with permission from Manyam SC, Gupta DK, Johnson KB, et al. Opioid-volatile anesthetic synergy: a response surface model with remifentanil and sevoflurane as prototypes. *Anesthesiology*. 2006;105:267–278.)

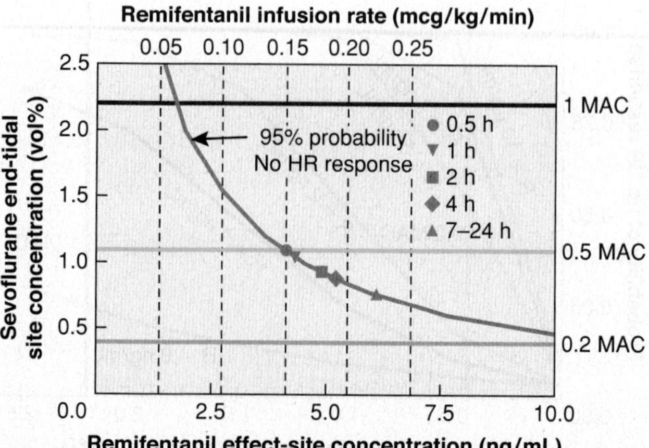

Figure 11-31 The optimal target concentration pairs of remifentanil and sevoflurane to maintain adequate analgesia (95% isobole for analgesia to electrical tetanic stimulation) and result in the most rapid emergence for anesthetics of various durations. For example, for a 2-hour anesthetic, target concentrations of 0.93 vol% sevoflurane, and 4.9 ng/mL remifentanil would result in a 5.8-minute time to awakening. As the duration of anesthesia increases, a minimum sevoflurane target concentration of 0.75 vol% is reached. (Adapted with permission from Manyam SC, Gupta DK, Johnson KB, et al. Opioid-volatile anesthetic synergy: a response surface model with remifentanil and sevoflurane as prototypes. *Anesthesiology*. 2006;105:267–278.)

models with pharmacokinetic models allows computer simulations to be performed to identify the target concentration pair of the opioid and the sedative-hypnotic that produces an adequate anesthetic and yet optimizes one or more pharmacodynamic end points, such as the speed of awakening from anesthesia, drug-induced respiratory depression, or drug acquisition costs.[100,104] For sevoflurane–remifentanil anesthetics, these types of PK-PD simulations demonstrate the benefit of minimizing the administered dose of even the low solubility volatile anesthetic sevoflurane to near 0.5 MAC to take advantage of the pharmacokinetic efficiency of remifentanil, especially as the duration of anesthesia increases (Fig. 11-31 and Table 11-8).[104] These response surface models can accurately predict loss of responsiveness and loss of response to painful stimuli as well as emergence from anesthesia and the time at which a patient will require analgesia in the recovery room.[215–218] In addition, these pharmacodynamic targets can be incorporated into closed-loop controllers to deliver closed-loop anesthesia.[198]

Conclusion

Since World War II, we have moved from describing anesthetics by a dose–response relationship to the development of sophisticated models that characterize the synergistic interaction between sedative-hypnotics and opioids. In addition, technology is now available to accurately administer a drug to achieve a desired concentration at the drug effect site. The rational selection of drug target concentrations required to achieve adequate anesthesia while minimizing side effects and the methods by which to efficiently achieve those concentration targets requires a solid understanding of the clinical pharmacology of anesthetics. As new drugs enter the anesthetic armamentarium, careful characterization of their pharmacokinetic and pharmacodynamic properties will allow them to be safely and appropriately utilized as part of a balanced anesthetic.[106]

Table 11-8 The Optimal Target Concentration Pairs of Sevoflurane and Remifentanil for Anesthetics 30 to 900 Minutes in Duration

Duration of Anesthetic (h)	Shortest Recovery Time (min)	Effect-Site Remifentanil Concentration (ng/mL)	Remifentanil Infusion Rate (μg/kg/min)	End-Tidal Sevoflurane Concentration (vol%)
0.5	4.5	4.1	0.15	1.1
1	5.0	4.3	0.16	1.05
2	5.8	4.9	0.18	093
4	6.7	5.2	0.19	0.88
7–24	7.2–7.7	6.1	0.22	0.75

Reprinted with permission from Jonkman K, Duma A, Olofsen E, et al. Pharmacokinetics and bioavailability of inhaled esketamine in healthy volunteers. *Anesthesiology*. 2017;127:675–683.

For further review and interactivities, please see the videos and narrative interactive clinical vignettes (NICVs) accessible in the complimentary eBook bundled with this text. Access instructions are located on the inside front cover.

REFERENCES

1. Halford FJ. A critique of intravenous anesthesia in war surgery. *Anesthesiology*. 1943;4:67–96.
2. Adams RC, Gray HK. Intravenous anesthesia with pentothal sodium in the case of gunshot wound associated with accompanying severe traumatic shock and loss of blood: report of a case. *Anesthesiology*. 1943;4:70–73.
3. The question of intravenous anesthesia in war surgery. *Anesthesiology*. 1943;4:74–77.
4. Price HL. A dynamic concept of the distribution of thiopental in the human body. *Anesthesiology*. 1960;21:40–45.
5. Pratt WB, Taylor P. *Principles of Drug Action: The Basis of Pharmacology*. 3rd ed. Churchill Livingstone; 1990.
6. Johnstone RW, Ruefli AA, Smyth MJ. Multiple physiological functions for multidrug transporter P-glycoprotein? *Trends Biochem Sci*. 2000;25:1–6.
7. Gao B, Hagenbuch B, Kullak-Ublick GA, Benke D, Aguzzi A, Meier PJ. Organic anion-transporting polypeptides mediate transport of opioid peptides across blood-brain barrier. *J Pharmacol Exp Ther*. 2000;294:73–79.
8. Hagenbuch B, Gao B, Meier PJ. Transport of xenobiotics across the blood-brain barrier. *News Physiol Sci*. 2002;17:231–234.
9. Upton RN. Cerebral uptake of drugs in humans. *Clin Exp Pharmacol Physiol*. 2007;34:695–701.
10. Shafer SL, Stanski DR. Improving the clinical utility of anesthetic drug pharmacokinetics. *Anesthesiology*. 1992;76:327–330.
11. Stanski DR, Greenblatt DJ, Lowenstein E. Kinetics of intravenous and intramuscular morphine. *Clin Pharmacol Ther*. 1978;24:52–59.
12. Kuipers JA, Boer F, Olieman W, Burm AG, Bovill JG. First-pass lung uptake and pulmonary clearance of propofol: assessment with a recirculatory indocyanine green pharmacokinetic model. *Anesthesiology*. 1999;91:1780–1787.
13. Ding X, Kaminsky LS. Human extrahepatic cytochromes P450: function in xenobiotic metabolism and tissue-selective chemical toxicity in the respiratory and gastrointestinal tracts. *Annu Rev Pharmacol Toxicol*. 2003;43:149–173.
14. Stanley TH, Hague B, Mock DL, et al. Oral transmucosal fentanyl citrate (lollipop) premedication in human volunteers. *Anesth Analg*. 1989;69:21–27.
15. Ashburn MA, Streisand J, Zhang J, et al. The iontophoresis of fentanyl citrate in humans. *Anesthesiology*. 1995;82:1146–1153.
16. Eger EI 2nd, Severinghaus JW. Effect of uneven pulmonary distribution of blood and gas on induction with inhalation anesthetics. *Anesthesiology*. 1964;25:620–626.
17. Avram MJ, Henthorn TK, Spyker DA, et al. Recirculatory pharmacokinetic model of the uptake, distribution, and bioavailability of prochlorperazine administered as a thermally generated aerosol in a single breath to dogs. *Drug Metab Dispos*. 2007;35:262–267.
18. Jonkman K, Duma A, Olofsen E, et al. Pharmacokinetics and bioavailability of inhaled esketamine in healthy volunteers. *Anesthesiology*. 2017;127:675–683.
19. Price HL, Kovnat PJ, Safer JN, et al. The uptake of thiopental by body tissues and its relationship to the duration of narcosis. *Clin Pharmacol Ther*. 1960;1:16.
20. Saidman LJ, Eger EI 2nd. The effect of thiopental metabolism on duration of anesthesia. *Anesthesiology*. 1966;27:118–126.
21. Shafer SL, Varvel JR. Pharmacokinetics, pharmacodynamics, and rational opioid selection. *Anesthesiology*. 1991;74:53–63.
22. Wilkinson GR. Clearance approaches in pharmacology. *Pharmacol Rev*. 1987;39:1–47.
23. Ahmad AB, Bennett PN, Rowland M. Models of hepatic drug clearance: discrimination between the 'well stirred' and 'parallel-tube' models. *J Pharm Pharmacol*. 1983;35:219–224.
24. Wilkinson GR, Shand DG. Commentary: a physiological approach to hepatic drug clearance. *Clin Pharmacol Ther*. 1975;18:377–390.
25. Weiss M, Krejcie TC, Avram MJ. Transit time dispersion in pulmonary and systemic circulation: effects of cardiac output and solute diffusivity. *Am J Physiol Heart Circ Physiol*. 2006;291:H861–H870.
26. Nies AS, Shand DG, Wilkinson GR. Altered hepatic blood flow and drug disposition. *Clin Pharmacokinet*. 1976;1:1351–1355.
27. Wilkinson GR. Pharmacokinetics of drug disposition: hemodynamic considerations. *Annu Rev Pharmacol*. 1975;15:11–27.
28. Rane A, Villeneuve JP, Stone WJ, Nies AS, Wilkinson GR, Branch RA. Plasma binding and disposition of furosemide in the nephrotic syndrome and in uremia. *Clin Pharmacol Ther*. 1978;24:199–207.
29. Ebling WF, Wada DR, Stanski DR. From piecewise to full physiologic pharmacokinetic modeling: applied to thiopental disposition in the rat. *J Pharmacokinet Biopharm*. 1994;22:259–292.
30. Wada DR, Björkman S, Ebling WF, Harashima H, Harapat SR, Stanski DR. Computer simulation of the effects of alterations in blood flows and body composition on thiopental pharmacokinetics in humans. *Anesthesiology*. 1997;87:884–899.
31. Henthorn TK, Avram MJ, Krejcie TC. Intravascular mixing and drug distribution: the concurrent disposition of thiopental and indocyanine green. *Clin Pharmacol Ther*. 1989;45:56–65.
32. Homer TD, Stanski DR. The effect of increasing age on thiopental disposition and anesthetic requirement. *Anesthesiology*. 1985;62:714–724.
33. Miller RD, Stevens WC, Way WL. The effect of renal failure and hyperkalemia on the duration of pancuronium neuromuscular blockade in man. *Anesth Analg*. 1973;52:661–666.
34. Patwardhan RV, Johnson RF, Hoyumpa A Jr, et al. Normal metabolism of morphine in cirrhosis. *Gastroenterology*. 1981;81:1006–1011.
35. Lund L, Alvan G, Berlin A, Alexanderson B. Pharmacokinetics of single and multiple doses of phenytoin in man. *Eur J Clin Pharmacol*. 1974;7:81–86.
36. Stanski DR, Mihm FG, Rosenthal MH, Kalman SM. Pharmacokinetics of high-dose thiopental used in cerebral resuscitation. *Anesthesiology*. 1980;53:169–171.
37. Avram MJ, Krejcie TC. Using front-end kinetics to optimize target-controlled drug infusions. *Anesthesiology*. 2003;99:1078–1086.
38. Chiou WL, Peng GW, Nation RL. Rapid estimation of volume of distribution after a short intravenous infusion and its application to dosing adjustments. *J Clin Pharmacol*. 1978;18:266–271.
39. Fisher DM. (Almost) everything you learned about pharmacokinetics was (somewhat) wrong! *Anesth Analg*. 1996;83:901 903.
40. Krejcie TC, Avram MJ. What determines anesthetic induction dose? It's the front-end kinetics, doctor! *Anesth Analg*. 1999;89:541–544.
41. Weiss M, Krejcie TC, Avram MJ. A minimal physiological model of thiopental distribution kinetics based on a multiple indicator approach. *Drug Metab Dispos*. 2007;35:1525–1532.
42. Hull CJ. How far can we go with compartmental models? *Anesthesiology*. 1990;72:399–402.
43. Kong AN, Jusko WJ. Definitions and applications of mean transit and residence times in reference to the two-compartment mammillary plasma clearance model. *J Pharm Sci*. 1988;77:157–165.
44. Jacobs JR, Shafer SL, Larsen JL, Hawkins ED. Two equally valid interpretations of the linear multicompartment mammillary pharmacokinetic model. *J Pharm Sci*. 1990;79:331–333.
45. McCulloch WS, Pitts W. A logical calculus of the ideas immanent in nervous activity. *The bulletin of mathematical biophysics*. 1943;5:115–133.
46. Turing AM, Haugeland J. Computing machinery and intelligence. *The Turing Test: Verbal Behavior as the Hallmark of Intelligence*. 1950:29–56.
47. Steimann F. On the use and usefulness of fuzzy sets in medical AI. *Artif Intell Med*. 2001;21:131–137.
48. Gunn AA. The diagnosis of acute abdominal pain with computer analysis. *J R Coll Surg Edinb*. 1976;21:170–172.
49. Baxt WG. Use of an artificial neural network for the diagnosis of myocardial infarction. *Ann Intern Med*. 1991;115:843–848.
50. Baxt WG, Skora J. Prospective validation of artificial neural network trained to identify acute myocardial infarction. *Lancet*. 1996;347:12–15.
51. Stamey T, Barnhill S, Zhang Z, et al. Effectiveness of ProstAsure in detecting prostate cancer (PCa) and benign prostatic hyperplasia (BPH) in men age 50 and older. *J Urol*. 1996;155:436A.
52. Pesonen E, Ohmann C, Eskelinen M, Juhola M. Diagnosis of acute appendicitis in two databases. Evaluation of different neighborhoods with an LVQ neural network. *Methods Inf Med*. 1998;37:59–63.
53. Ng CM. Comparison of neural network, Bayesian, and multiple stepwise regression-based limited sampling models to estimate area under the curve. *Pharmacotherapy*. 2003;23:1044–1051.
54. Chow HH, Tolle KM, Roe DJ, Elsberry V, Chen H. Application of neural networks to population pharmacokinetic data analysis. *J Pharm Sci*. 1997;86:840–845.
55. Brier ME, Aronoff GR. Application of artificial neural networks to clinical pharmacology. *Int J Clin Pharmacol Ther*. 1996;34:510–514.
56. Brier ME, Zurada JM, Aronoff GR. Neural network predicted peak and trough gentamicin concentrations. *Pharm Res*. 1995;12:406–412.
57. Lee HC, Ryu HG, Chung EJ, Jung CW. Prediction of bispectral index during target-controlled infusion of propofol and remifentanil: a deep learning approach. *Anesthesiology*. 2018;128:492–501.
58. Gambus P, Shafer SL. Artificial intelligence for everyone. *Anesthesiology*. 2018;128:431–433.
59. Geman S, Bienenstock E, Doursat R. Neural networks and the bias/variance dilemma. *Neural computation*. 1992;4:1–58.
60. Ingrande J, Gabriel RA, McAuley J, Krasinska K, Chien A, Lemmens HJM. The performance of an artificial neural network model in predicting the early distribution kinetics of propofol in morbidly obese and lean subjects. *Anesth Analg*. 2020;131:1500–1509.
61. Maheshwari K, Cywinski JB, Papay F, Khanna AK, Mathur P. Artificial intelligence for perioperative medicine: perioperative intelligence. *Anesth Analg*. 2022;10:1213.
62. Norman J. Drug-receptor reactions. *Br J Anaesth*. 1979;51:595–601.
63. Waud BE, Waud DR. The margin of safety of neuromuscular transmission in the muscle of the diaphragm. *Anesthesiology*. 1972;37:417–422.
64. Segre G. Kinetics of interaction between drugs and biological systems. *Farmaco Sci*. 1968;23:907–918.

65. Sheiner LB, Stanski DR, Vozeh S, Miller RD, Ham J. Simultaneous modeling of pharmacokinetics and pharmacodynamics: application to d-tubocurarine. *Clin Pharmacol Ther*. 1979;25:358–371.
66. Kern SE, Stanski DR. Pharmacokinetics and pharmacodynamics of intravenously administered anesthetic drugs: concepts and lessons for drug development. *Clin Pharmacol Ther*. 2008;84:153–157.
67. Jacobs JR, Reves JG. Effect site equilibration time is a determinant of induction dose requirement. *Anesth Analg*. 1993;76:1–6.
68. Olofsen E, Dahan A. Population pharmacokinetics/pharmacodynamics of anesthetics. *AAPS J*. 2005;7:E383–E389.
69. Sheiner LB, Beal SL. Evaluation of methods for estimating population pharmacokinetics parameters. I. Michaelis-Menten model: routine clinical pharmacokinetic data. *J Pharmacokinet Biopharm*. 1980;8:553–571.
70. Maitre PO, Vozeh S, Heykants J, Thomson DA, Stanski DR. Population pharmacokinetics of alfentanil: the average dose-plasma concentration relationship and interindividual variability in patients. *Anesthesiology*. 1987;66:3–12.
71. Group NP. *NONMEN User's Guide*. University of California; 1999.
72. West GB, Brown JH, Enquist BJ. A general model for the origin of allometric scaling laws in biology. *Science*. 1997;276:122–126.
73. Mahmood I. Dosing in children: a critical review of the pharmacokinetic allometric scaling and modelling approaches in paediatric drug development and clinical settings. *Clin Pharmacokinet*. 2014;53:327–346.
74. Cortinez LI, De la Fuente N, Eleveld DJ, et al. Performance of propofol target-controlled infusion models in the obese: pharmacokinetic and pharmacodynamic analysis. *Anesth Analg*. 2014;119:302–310.
75. Mahmood I. Prediction of drug clearance in premature and mature neonates, infants and children ≤2 years of age: a comparison of the predictive performance of 4 allometric models. *J Clin Pharmacol*. 2016;56(6):733–739.
76. Morton WD, Lerman J. The effect of pancuronium on the solubility of aqueous thiopentone. *Can J Anaesth*. 1987;34:87–89.
77. Dejong RH, Cullen SC. Buffer-demand and Ph of local anesthetic solutions containing epinephrine. *Anesthesiology*. 1963;24:801–807.
78. Anders MW. Formation and toxicity of anesthetic degradation products. *Annu Rev Pharmacol Toxicol*. 2005;45:147–176.
79. Kharasch ED. Adverse drug reactions with halogenated anesthetics. *Clin Pharmacol Ther*. 2008;84:158–162.
80. Baxter PJ, Garton K, Kharasch ED. Mechanistic aspects of carbon monoxide formation from volatile anesthetics. *Anesthesiology*. 1998;89:929–941.
81. Kharasch ED, Powers KM, Artru AA. Comparison of Amsorb, sodalime, and Baralyme degradation of volatile anesthetics and formation of carbon monoxide and compound a in swine in vivo. *Anesthesiology*. 2002;96:173–812.
82. Bom A, Bradley M, Cameron K, et al. A novel concept of reversing neuromuscular block: chemical encapsulation of rocuronium bromide by a cyclodextrin-based synthetic host. *Angew Chem Int Ed Engl*. 2002;41:266–270.
83. Suy K, Morias K, Cammu G, et al. Effective reversal of moderate rocuronium- or vecuronium-induced neuromuscular block with sugammadex, a selective relaxant binding agent. *Anesthesiology*. 2007;106:283–288.
84. Tassonyi E, Pongrácz A, Nemes R, Asztalos L, Lengyel S, Fülesdi B. Reversal of pipecuronium-induced moderate neuromuscular block with sugammadex in the presence of a sevoflurane anesthetic: a randomized trial. *Anesth Analg*. 2015;121:373–380.
85. Haerter F, Eikermann M. Reversing neuromuscular blockade: inhibitors of the acetylcholinesterase versus the encapsulating agents sugammadex and calabadion. *Exp Opin Pharmacother*. 2016;17:819–833.
86. Haerter F, Simons JCP, Foerster U, et al. Comparative effectiveness of calabadion and sugammadex to reverse non-depolarizing neuromuscular-blocking agents. *Anesthesiology*. 2015;123:1337–1349.
87. Hoffmann U, Grosse-Sundrup M, Eikermann-Haerter K, et al. Calabadion: a new agent to reverse the effects of benzylisoquinoline and steroidal neuromuscular-blocking agents. *Anesthesiology*. 2013;119:317–325.
88. Heerdt PM, Malhotra JK, Pan BY, Sunaga H, Savarese J. Pharmacodynamics and cardiopulmonary side effects of CW002, a cysteine-reversible neuromuscular blocking drug in dogs. *Anesthesiology*. 2010;112:910–916.
89. Avram MJ, Krejcie TC, Henthorn TK, Niemann CU. Beta-adrenergic blockade affects initial drug distribution due to decreased cardiac output and altered blood flow distribution. *J Pharmacol Exp Ther*. 2004;311:617–624.
90. Niemann CU, Henthorn TK, Krejcie TC, Shanks CA, Enders-Klein C, Avram MJ. Indocyanine green kinetics characterize blood volume and flow distribution and their alteration by propranolol. *Clin Pharmacol Ther*. 2000;67:342–350.
91. Krejcie TC, Wang Z, Avram MJ. Drug-induced hemodynamic perturbations alter the disposition of markers of blood volume, extracellular fluid, and total body water. *J Pharmacol Exp Ther*. 2001;296:922–930.
92. Avram MJ, Krejcie TC, Niemann CU, Enders-Klein C, Shanks CA, Henthorn TK. Isoflurane alters the recirculatory pharmacokinetics of physiologic markers. *Anesthesiology*. 2000;92:1757–1768.
93. Avram MJ, Krejcie TC, Niemann CU, et al. The effect of halothane on the recirculatory pharmacokinetics of physiologic markers. *Anesthesiology*. 1997;87:1381–1393.
94. Benet LZ, Hoener BA. Changes in plasma protein binding have little clinical relevance. *Clin Pharmacol Ther*. 2002;71:115–121.
95. Gupta DK, Krejcie TC, Avram MJ. Pharmacokinetics of opioids. In: Evers A, Maze M, Kharasch ED, eds. *Anesthetic Pharmacology: Physiologic Principles and Clinical Practice*. 2nd ed. Cambridge University Press; 2011:509–530.
96. Wright PM, McCarthy G, Szenohradszky J, Sharma ML, Caldwell JE. Influence of chronic phenytoin administration on the pharmacokinetics and pharmacodynamics of vecuronium. *Anesthesiology*. 2004;100:626–633.
97. Zbinden AM, Maggiorini M, Petersen-Felix S, Lauber R, Thomson DA, Minder CE. Anesthetic depth defined using multiple noxious stimuli during isoflurane/oxygen anesthesia. I. Motor reactions. *Anesthesiology*. 1994;80:253–260.
98. Zbinden AM, Petersen-Felix S, Thomson DA. Anesthetic depth defined using multiple noxious stimuli during isoflurane/oxygen anesthesia. II. Hemodynamic responses. *Anesthesiology*. 1994;80:261–267.
99. Oertel BG, Felden L, Tran PV, et al. Selective antagonism of opioid-induced ventilatory depression by an ampakine molecule in humans without loss of opioid analgesia. *Clin Pharmacol Ther*. 2010;87:204–211.
100. Vuyk J, Mertens MJ, Olofsen E, Burm AG, Bovill JG. Propofol anesthesia and rational opioid selection: determination of optimal EC50-EC95 propofol-opioid concentrations that assure adequate anesthesia and a rapid return of consciousness. *Anesthesiology*. 1997;87:1549–1562.
101. Bouillon TW, Bruhn J, Radulescu L, et al. Pharmacodynamic interaction between propofol and remifentanil regarding hypnosis, tolerance of laryngoscopy, bispectral index, and electroencephalographic approximate entropy. *Anesthesiology*. 2004;100:1353–1372.
102. Greco WR, Bravo G, Parsons JC. The search for synergy: a critical review from a response surface perspective. *Pharmacol Rev*. 1995;47:331–385.
103. Kern SE, Xie G, White JL, Egan TD. A response surface analysis of propofol-remifentanil pharmacodynamic interaction in volunteers. *Anesthesiology*. 2004;100:1373–1381.
104. Manyam SC, Gupta DK, Johnson KB, et al. Opioid-volatile anesthetic synergy: a response surface model with remifentanil and sevoflurane as prototypes. *Anesthesiology*. 2006;105:267–278.
105. Minto CF, Schnider TW, Short TG, Gregg KM, Gentilini A, Shafer SL. Response surface model for anesthetic drug interactions. *Anesthesiology*. 2000;92:1603–1616.
106. Shafer SL, Stanski DR. Defining depth of anesthesia. *Handb Exp Pharmacol*. 2008:409–423.
107. Manyam SC, Gupta DK, Johnson KB, et al. When is a bispectral index of 60 too low? Rational processed electroencephalographic targets are dependent on the sedative-opioid ratio. *Anesthesiology*. 2007;106:472–483.
108. Boyer EW, Shannon M. The serotonin syndrome. *N Engl J Med*. 2005;352:1112–1120.
109. Rastogi R, Swarm RA, Patel TA. Case scenario: opioid association with serotonin syndrome: implications to the practitioners. *Anesthesiology*. 2011;115:1291–1298.
110. Gillman PK. Monoamine oxidase inhibitors, opioid analgesics and serotonin toxicity. *Br J Anaesth*. 2005;95:434–441.
111. Gillman PK. CNS toxicity involving methylene blue: the exemplar for understanding and predicting drug interactions that precipitate serotonin toxicity. *J Psychopharmacol*. 2011;25:429–436.
112. Schwiebert C, Irving C, Gillman PK. Small doses of methylene blue, previously considered safe, can precipitate serotonin toxicity. *Anaesthesia*. 2009;64:924.
113. Schuttler J, Schwilden H, Stoekel H. Pharmacokinetics as applied to total intravenous anaesthesia: practical implications. *Anaesthesia*. 1983;38(Suppl):53–56.
114. Meineke I, Brockmöller J. Simulation of complex pharmacokinetic models in Microsoft Excel. *Comput Methods Programs Biomed*. 2007;88:239–245.
115. Hammer G, Shafer SL. Playing with dexmedetomidine pharmacokinetics! *Br J Anaesth*. 2020;124:238–240.
116. Bourne DW, Triggs EJ, Eadie M. *Pharmacokinetics for the non-mathematical*, Springer; 1986.
117. Charles BG, Duffull SB. Pharmacokinetic software for the health sciences: choosing the right package for teaching purposes. *Clin Pharmacokinet*. 2001;40:395–403.
118. Kantasiripitak W, Van Daele R, Gijsen M, Ferrante M, Spriet I, Dreesen E. Software tools for model-informed precision dosing: how well do they satisfy the needs? *Front Pharmacol*. 2020;11:620.
119. Philip JH. Gas man–an example of goal oriented computer-assisted teaching which results in learning. *Int J Clin Monit Comput*. 1986;3:165–173.
120. Hughes MA, Glass PS, Jacobs JR. Context-sensitive half-time in multicompartment pharmacokinetic models for intravenous anesthetic drugs. *Anesthesiology*. 1992;76:334–341.
121. Shafer SL, Varvel JR. Pharmacokinetics, pharmacodynamics, and rational opioid selection. *Anesthesiology*. 1991;74:53–63.
122. Schraag S, Mohl U, Hirsch M, Stolberg E, Georgieff M. Recovery from opioid anesthesia: the clinical implication of context-sensitive half-times. *Anesth Analg*. 1998;86:184–90.
123. Bailey JM. Context-sensitive half-times: what are they and how valuable are they in anaesthesiology? *Clin Pharmacokinet*. 2002;41:793–799.

124. Egan TD. Is anesthesiology going soft? Trends in fragile pharmacology. *Anesthesiology*. 2009;111:229–230.
125. Johnson KB. New horizons in sedative hypnotic drug development: fast, clean, and soft. *Anesth Analg*. 2012;115:220–222.
126. Egan TD, Muir KT, Hermann DJ, et al. The electroencephalogram (EEG) and clinical measures of opioid potency: defining the EEG-clinical potency relationship ('fingerprint') with application to remifentanil. *Int J Pharmaceutical Med*. 2001;15:11–19.
127. Kilpatrick GJ, McIntyre MS, Cox RF, et al. CNS 7056: a novel ultra-short-acting benzodiazepine. *Anesthesiology*. 2007;107:60–66.
128. Cotten JF, Husain SS, Forman SA, et al. Methoxycarbonyl-etomidate: a novel rapidly metabolized and ultra-short-acting etomidate analogue that does not produce prolonged adrenocortical suppression. *Anesthesiology*. 2009;111:240–249.
129. Jonsson Fagerlund M, Sjödin J, Dabrowski MA, Krupp J. Reduced efficacy of the intravenous anesthetic agent AZD3043 at GABA(A) receptors with beta2 (N289M) and beta3 (N290M) point-mutations. *Eur J Pharmacol*. 2012;694:13–19.
130. Egan TD, Obara S, Jenkins TE, et al. AZD-3043: a novel, metabolically labile sedative-hypnotic agent with rapid and predictable emergence from hypnosis. *Anesthesiology*. 2012;116: 1267–1277.
131. Antonik LJ, Goldwater DR, Kilpatrick GJ, Tilbrook GS, Borkett KM. A placebo- and midazolam-controlled phase I single ascending-dose study evaluating the safety, pharmacokinetics, and pharmacodynamics of remimazolam (CNS 7056). Part I. Safety, efficacy, and basic pharmacokinetics. *Anesth Analg*. 2012;115:274–283.
132. Wiltshire HR, Kilpatrick GJ, Tilbrook GS, Borkett KM. A placebo- and midazolam-controlled phase I single ascending-dose study evaluating the safety, pharmacokinetics, and pharmacodynamics of remimazolam (CNS 7056). Part II. Population pharmacokinetic and pharmacodynamic modeling and simulation. *Anesth Analg*. 2012;115:2842–2896.
133. Pambianco DJ, Borkett KM, Riff DS, et al. A phase IIb study comparing the safety and efficacy of remimazolam and midazolam in patients undergoing colonoscopy. *Gastrointest Endosc*. 2016;83:984–992.
134. Keam. SJ: Remimazolam: First Approval. *Drugs*. 2020;80:625–633.
135. Goudra B, Mason KP.: Emerging Approaches in Intravenous Moderate and Deep Sedation. *J Clin Med*. 2021;10.
136. Cotten JF, Forman SA, Laha JK, et al. Carboetomidate: a pyrrole analog of etomidate designed not to suppress adrenocortical function. *Anesthesiology*. 2010;112:637–644.
137. Cotten JF, Le Ge R, Banacos N, et al. Closed-loop continuous infusions of etomidate and etomidate analogs in rats: a comparative study of dosing and the impact on adrenocortical function. *Anesthesiology*. 2011;115:764–773.
138. Ge R, Pejo E, Husain SS, Cotten JF, Raines DE. Electroencephalographic and hypnotic recoveries after brief and prolonged infusions of etomidate and optimized soft etomidate analogs. *Anesthesiology*. 2012;117:1037–1043.
139. Husain SS, Pejo E, Ge R, Raines DE. Modifying methoxycarbonyl etomidate inter-ester spacer optimizes in vitro metabolic stability and in vivo hypnotic potency and duration of action. *Anesthesiology*. 2012;117:1027–1036.
140. Ge R, Pejo E, Cotten JF, Raines DE. Adrenocortical suppression and recovery after continuous hypnotic infusion: etomidate versus its soft analogue cyclopropyl-methoxycarbonyl metomidate. *Crit Care*. 2013;17:R20.
141. Pejo E, Santer P, Jeffrey S, Gallin H, Husain SS, Raines DE. Analogues of etomidate: modifications around etomidate's chiral carbon and the impact on in vitro and in vivo pharmacology. *Anesthesiology*. 2014;121:290–301.
142. Pejo E, Liu J, Lin X, Raines DE. Distinct hypnotic recoveries after infusions of methoxycarbonyl etomidate and cyclopropyl methoxycarbonyl metomidate: the role of the metabolite. *Anesth Analg*. 2016;122:1008–1014.
143. Edelman GJ, Hoffman WE, Charbel FT. Cerebral hypoxia after etomidate administration and temporary cerebral artery occlusion. *Anesth Analg*. 1997;85:821–825.
144. Hoffman WE, Charbel FT, Edelman G, Misra M, Ausman JI. Comparison of the effect of etomidate and desflurane on brain tissue gases and pH during prolonged middle cerebral artery occlusion. *Anesthesiology*. 1998;88:1188–1194.
145. Drummond JC, McKay LD, Cole DJ, Patel PM. The role of nitric oxide synthase inhibition in the adverse effects of etomidate in the setting of focal cerebral ischemia in rats. *Anesth Analg*. 2005;100:841–846.
146. Kalman S, Koch P, Ahlén K, et al. First human study of the investigational sedative and anesthetic drug AZD3043: a dose-escalation trial to assess the safety, pharmacokinetics, and efficacy of a 30-minute infusion in healthy male volunteers. *Anesth Analg*. 2015;121: 885–893.
147. Norberg A, Koch P, Kanes SJ, et al. A bolus and bolus followed by infusion study of AZD3043, an investigational intravenous drug for sedation and anesthesia: safety and pharmacodynamics in healthy male and female volunteers. *Anesth Analg*. 2015;121:894–903.
148. Bjornsson MA, Norberg Å, Kalman S, Simonsson USH. A recirculatory model for pharmacokinetics and the effects on bispectral index after intravenous infusion of the sedative and anesthetic AZD3043 in healthy volunteers. *Anesth Analg*. 2015;121:904–913.
149. Maitre PO, Shafer SL. A simple pocket calculator approach to predict anesthetic drug concentrations from pharmacokinetic data. *Anesthesiology*. 1990;73:332–336.
150. Egan TD. Target-controlled drug delivery: progress toward an intravenous "vaporizer" and automated anesthetic administration. *Anesthesiology*. 2003;99:1214–1219.
151. Shafer SL, Varvel JR, Aziz N, Scott JC. Pharmacokinetics of fentanyl administered by computer-controlled infusion pump. *Anesthesiology*. 1990;73:1091–1102.
152. Barvais L, Cantraine F, D'Hollander A, Coussaert E. Predictive accuracy of continuous alfentanil infusion in volunteers: variability of different pharmacokinetic sets. *Anesth Analg*. 1993;77:801–810.
153. Barvais L, Heitz D, Schmartz D, et al. Pharmacokinetic model-driven infusion of sufentanil and midazolam during cardiac surgery: assessment of the prospective predictive accuracy and the quality of anesthesia. *J Cardiothorac Vasc Anesth*. 2000;14:402–408.
154. Barvais L, D'Hollander AA, Cantraine F, Coussaert E, Diamon G. Predictive accuracy of midazolam in adult patients scheduled for coronary surgery. *J Clin Anesth*. 1994;6:297–302.
155. Veselis RA, Glass P, Dnistrian A, Reinsel R. Performance of computer-assisted continuous infusion at low concentrations of intravenous sedatives. *Anesth Analg*. 1997;84:1049–1057.
156. Vuyk J, Engbers FH, Burm AG, Vletter AA, Bovill JG. Performance of computer-controlled infusion of propofol: an evaluation of five pharmacokinetic parameter sets. *Anesth Analg*. 1995;81:1275–1282.
157. Schwilden H. A general method for calculating the dosage scheme in linear pharmacokinetics. *Eur J Clin Pharmacol*. 1981;20(5):379–386.
158. Schraag S, Flaschar J. Delivery performance of commercial target-controlled infusion devices with Diprifusor module. *Eur J Anaesthesiol*. 2002;19:357–360.
159. Passot S, Servin F, Allary R, et al. Target-controlled versus manually-controlled infusion of propofol for direct laryngoscopy and bronchoscopy. *Anesth Analg*. 2002;94:1212–1216.
160. Gale T, Leslie K, Kluger M. Propofol anaesthesia via target controlled infusion or manually controlled infusion: effects on the bispectral index as a measure of anaesthetic depth. *Anaesth Intensive Care*. 2001;29:579–584.
161. Suttner S, Boldt J, Schmidt C, Piper S, Kumle B. Cost analysis of target-controlled infusion-based anesthesia compared with standard anesthesia regimens. *Anesth Analg*. 1999;88:77–82.
162. Checketts MR, Gilhooly CJ, Kenny GN. Patient-maintained analgesia with target-controlled alfentanil infusion after cardiac surgery: a comparison with morphine PCA. *Br J Anaesth*. 1998;80:748–751.
163. van den Nieuwenhuyzen MC, Engbers FH, Burm AG, Vletter AA, van Kleef JW, Bovill JG. Target-controlled infusion of alfentanil for postoperative analgesia: contribution of plasma protein binding to intra-patient and inter-patient variability. *Br J Anaesth*. 1999;82: 580–585.
164. Campbell L, Imrie G, Doherty P, et al. Patient maintained sedation for colonoscopy using a target controlled infusion of propofol. *Anaesthesia*. 2004;59:127–132.
165. Irwin MG, Thompson N, Kenny GN. Patient-maintained propofol sedation: assessment of a target-controlled infusion system. *Anaesthesia*. 1997;52:525–530.
166. Gentry WB, Krejcie TC, Henthorn TK, et al. Effect of infusion rate on thiopental dose–response relationships: assessment of a pharmacokinetic-pharmacodynamic model. *Anesthesiology*. 1994;81:316–324.
167. Minto CF, Schnider TW, Gregg KM, Henthorn TK, Shafer SL. Using the time of maximum effect site concentration to combine pharmacokinetics and pharmacodynamics. *Anesthesiology*. 2003;99:324–333.
168. Henthorn TK, Krejcie TC, Shanks CA, Avram MJ. Time-dependent distribution volume and kinetics of the pharmacodynamic effector site. *J Pharm Sci*. 1992;81:1136–1138.
169. Shafer SL, Gregg KM. Algorithms to rapidly achieve and maintain stable drug concentrations at the site of drug effect with a computer-controlled infusion pump. *J Pharmacokinet Biopharm*. 1992;20:147–169.
170. Schnider TW, Minto CF, Gambus PL, et al. The influence of method of administration and covariates on the pharmacokinetics of propofol in adult volunteers. *Anesthesiology*. 1998;88: 1170–1182.
171. Chiou WL. Potential pitfalls in the conventional pharmacokinetic studies: effects of the initial mixing of drug in blood and the pulmonary first-pass elimination. *J Pharmacokinet Biopharm*. 1979;7:527–536.
172. Henthorn TK. The effect of altered physiological states on intravenous anesthetics. *Handb Exp Pharmacol*. 2008:363–377.
173. Henthorn TK, Krejcie TC, Avram MJ. Early drug distribution: a generally neglected aspect of pharmacokinetics of particular relevance to intravenously administered anesthetic agents. *Clin Pharmacol Ther*. 2008;84:18–22.
174. Krejcie TC, Henthorn TK, Gentry WB, et al. Modifications of blood volume alter the disposition of markers of blood volume, extracellular fluid, and total body water. *J Pharmacol Exp Ther*. 1999;291:1308–1316.
175. Krejcie TC, Henthorn TK, Niemann CU, et al. Recirculatory pharmacokinetic models of markers of blood, extracellular fluid and total body water administered concomitantly. *J Pharmacol Exp Ther*. 1996;278:1050–1057.
176. Kuipers JA, Boer F, Olofsen E, Bovill JG, Burm AG. Recirculatory pharmacokinetics and pharmacodynamics of rocuronium in patients: the influence of cardiac output. *Anesthesiology*. 2001;94:47–55.
177. Avram MJ, Sanghvi R, Henthorn TK, et al. Determinants of thiopental induction dose requirements. *Anesth Analg*. 1993;76:10–17.

178. Forbes GB, Hursh JB. Age and sex trends in lean body mass calculated from K40 measurements: with a note on the theoretical basis for the procedure. *Ann N Y Acad Sci*. 1963;110:255–263.
179. Sathyaprabha TN, Pradhan C, Rashmi G, Thennarasu K, Raju TR. Noninvasive cardiac output measurement by transthoracic electrical bioimpedence: influence of age and gender. *J Clin Monit Comput*. 2008;22:401–408.
180. Avram MJ, Henthorn TK, Spyker DA, et al. Recirculatory kinetic model of fentanyl administered as a thermally generated aerosol to volunteers. *Anesthesiology*. 2008;109:A815.
181. Avram MJ, Henthorn TK, Spyker DA, et al. Recirculatory pharmacokinetic model of fentanyl aerosol in volunteers. *Clin Pharmacol Ther*. 2008;83:PI-76.
182. Avram MJ, Krejcie TC, Henthorn TK. The concordance of early antipyrine and thiopental distribution kinetics. *J Pharmacol Exp Ther*. 2002;302:594–600.
183. Kuipers JA, Boer F, Olofsen E, et al. Recirculatory and compartmental pharmacokinetic modeling of alfentanil in pigs: the influence of cardiac output. *Anesthesiology*. 1999;90:1146–1157.
184. Woodruff EA, Martin JF, Omens M. A model for the design and evaluation of algorithms for closed-loop cardiovascular therapy. *IEEE Trans Biomed Eng*. 1997;44:694–705.
185. Tehrani F, Rogers M, Lo T, et al. Closed-loop control if the inspired fraction of oxygen in mechanical ventilation. *J Clin Monit Comput*. 2002;17:367–376.
186. Renard E. Implantable closed-loop glucose-sensing and insulin delivery: the future for insulin pump therapy. *Curr Opin Pharmacol*. 2002;2:708–716.
187. O'Hara DA, Hexem JG, Derbyshire GJ, et al. The use of a PID controller to model vecuronium pharmacokinetics and pharmacodynamics during liver transplantation: proportional-integral-derivative. *IEEE Trans Biomed Eng*. 1997;44:610–619.
188. De Smet T, Struys MMRF, Greenwald S, Mortier EP, Shafer SL. Estimation of optimal modeling weights for a Bayesian-based closed-loop system for propofol administration using the bispectral index as a controlled variable: a simulation study. *Anesth Analg*. 2007;105:1629–1638.
189. Mortier E, Struys M, De Smet T, Versichelen L, Rolly G. Closed-loop controlled administration of propofol using bispectral analysis. *Anaesthesia*. 1998;53:749–754.
190. Schwilden H, Schüttler J, Stoeckel H. Closed-loop feedback control of methohexital anesthesia by quantitative EEG analysis in humans. *Anesthesiology*. 1987;67:341–347.
191. Schwilden H, Stoeckel H. Effective therapeutic infusions produced by closed-loop feedback control of methohexital administration during total intravenous anesthesia with fentanyl. *Anesthesiology*. 1990;73:225–229.
192. Struys MMRF, De Smet T, Greenwald S, Absalom AR, Bingé S, Mortier EP. Performance evaluation of two published closed-loop control systems using bispectral index monitoring: a simulation study. *Anesthesiology*. 2004;100:640–647.
193. Struys MMRF, De Smet T, Mortier EP. Closed-loop control of anaesthesia. *Curr Opin Anaesthesiol*. 2002;15:421–425.
194. Struys MMRF, De Smet T, Versichelen LF, Van De Velde S, Van den Broecke R, Mortier EP. Comparison of closed-loop controlled administration of propofol using Bispectral Index as the controlled variable versus "standard practice" controlled administration. *Anesthesiology*. 2001;95:6–17.
195. Tzabazis A, Ihmsen H, Schywalsky M, Schwilden H. EEG-controlled closed-loop dosing of propofol in rats. *Br J Anaesth*. 2004;92:564–569.
196. Liu N, Chazot T, Genty A, et al. Titration of propofol for anesthetic induction and maintenance guided by the bispectral index: closed-loop versus manual control: a prospective, randomized, multicenter study. *Anesthesiology*. 2006;104:686–695.
197. Liu N, Chazot T, Hamada S, et al. Closed-loop coadministration of propofol and remifentanil guided by bispectral index: a randomized multicenter study. *Anesth Analg*. 2011;112:546–557.
198. Liu N, Lory C, Assenzo V, et al. Feasibility of closed-loop co-administration of propofol and remifentanil guided by the bispectral index in obese patients: a prospective cohort comparison. *Br J Anaesth*. 2015;114:605–614.
199. Orliaguet GA, Benabbes Lambert F, Chazot T, Glasman P, Fischler M, Liu N. Feasibility of closed-loop titration of propofol and remifentanil guided by the bispectral monitor in pediatric and adolescent patients: a prospective randomized study. *Anesthesiology*. 2015;122:759–767.
200. Puri GD, Mathew PJ, Biswas I, et al. A multicenter evaluation of a closed-loop anesthesia delivery system: a randomized controlled trial. *Anesth Analg*. 2016;122:106–114.
201. Short TG, Hannam JA, Laurent S, et al. Refining target-controlled infusion: an assessment of pharmacodynamic target-controlled infusion of propofol and remifentanil using a response surface model of their combined effects on bispectral index. *Anesth Analg*. 2016;122:90–97.
202. Manberg PJ, Vozella CM, Kelley SD. Regulatory challenges facing closed-loop anesthetic drug infusion devices. *Clin Pharmacol Ther*. 2008;84:166–169.
203. Liu N, Rinehart J. Closed-loop propofol administration: routine care or a research tool? What impact in the future? *Anesth Analg*. 2016;122:4–6.
204. Monk TG, Saini V, Weldon BC, Sigl JC. Anesthetic management and one-year mortality after noncardiac surgery. *Anesth Analg*. 2005;100:4–10.
205. Monk TG, Weldon BC, Garvan CW, et al. Predictors of cognitive dysfunction after major noncardiac surgery. *Anesthesiology*. 2008;108:18–30.
206. Katoh T, Ikeda K. The effects of fentanyl on sevoflurane requirements for loss of consciousness and skin incision. *Anesthesiology*. 1998;88:18–24.
207. Katoh T, Kobayashi S, Suzuki A, Iwamoto T, Bito H, Ikeda K. The effect of fentanyl on sevoflurane requirements for somatic and sympathetic responses to surgical incision. *Anesthesiology*. 1999;90:398–405.
208. Katoh T, Nakajima Y, Moriwaki G, et al. Sevoflurane requirements for tracheal intubation with and without fentanyl. *Br J Anaesth*. 1999;82:561–565.
209. Katoh T, Uchiyama T, Ikeda K. Effect of fentanyl on awakening concentration of sevoflurane. *Br J Anaesth*. 1994;73:322–325.
210. McEwan AI, Smith C, Dyar O, Goodman D, Smith LR, Glass PS. Isoflurane minimum alveolar concentration reduction by fentanyl. *Anesthesiology*. 1993;78:864–869.
211. Sebel PS, Glass PS, Fletcher JE, Murphy MR, Gallagher C, Quill T. Reduction of the MAC of desflurane with fentanyl. *Anesthesiology*. 1992;76:52–59.
212. Vuyk J, Lim T, Engbers FH, Burm AG, Vletter AA, Bovill JG. Pharmacodynamics of alfentanil as a supplement to propofol or nitrous oxide for lower abdominal surgery in female patients. *Anesthesiology*. 1993;78:1036–1045.
213. Vuyk J, Lim T, Engbers FH, Burm AG, Vletter AA, Bovill JG. The pharmacodynamic interaction of propofol and alfentanil during lower abdominal surgery in women. *Anesthesiology*. 1995;83:8–22.
214. Short TG, Ho TY, Minto CF, Schnider TW, Shafer SL. Efficient trial design for eliciting a pharmacokinetic-pharmacodynamic model-based response surface describing the interaction between two intravenous anesthetic drugs. *Anesthesiology*. 2002;96:400–408.
215. Johnson KB, Syroid ND, Gupta DK, et al. An evaluation of remifentanil propofol response surfaces for loss of responsiveness, loss of response to surrogates of painful stimuli and laryngoscopy in patients undergoing elective surgery. *Anesth Analg*. 2008;106:471–479.
216. Johnson KB, Syroid ND, Gupta DK, et al. An evaluation of remifentanil-sevoflurane response surface models in patients emerging from anesthesia: model improvement using effect-site sevoflurane concentrations. *Anesth Analg*. 2010;111:387–394.
217. Syroid ND, Johnson KB, Pace NL, et al. Response surface model predictions of emergence and response to pain in the recovery room: an evaluation of patients emerging from an isoflurane and fentanyl anesthetic. *Anesth Analg*. 2010;111:380–386.
218. Ting CK, Johnson KB, Teng WN, et al. Response surface model predictions of wake-up time during scoliosis surgery. *Anesth Analg*. 2014;118:546–553.

Section 3

CORE PRINCIPLES

12 Cardiac Anatomy and Physiology

PAUL S. PAGEL • DUSTIN HANG • BRENT T. BOETTCHER • JULIE K. FREED • DAVID F. STOWE

KEY POINTS

1. The cartilaginous skeleton, myocardial fiber orientation, valves, blood supply, and conduction system of the heart determine its functional capabilities and limitations.
2. The major determinants of coronary blood flow are Poiseuille's law, extravascular compression, metabolic regulation, pressure-flow autoregulation, and the autonomic nervous system.
3. Coronary blood flow reserve is substantial, but it may be reduced by flow-limiting stenoses, pressure-overload hypertrophy, or microvascular dysfunction.
4. Oxygen extraction by the left ventricle (LV) is nearly maximal under baseline conditions. As a result, increases in myocardial oxygen demand are dependent on proportional increases in coronary blood flow mediated by locally produced vasodilators.
5. Metabolic regulation is a "feed-forward" mechanism based on the action of carbon dioxide and reactive oxygen species produced by cardiac myocytes and involves endothelium-derived nitric oxide (NO) and adenosine triphosphate–sensitive potassium (K_{ATP}) channels in vascular smooth muscle.
6. The cardiac myocyte is engineered for contraction and relaxation, not protein synthesis.
7. Laplace's law describes the mechanism whereby alterations in muscle tension and length that occur during contraction and relaxation in the sarcomere are translated into phasic changes in pressure and volume that occur in the intact heart.
8. The cardiac cycle is a coordinated, temporally related series of electrical, mechanical, and valvular events.
9. A time-dependent, two-dimensional projection of continuous pressure and volume during the cardiac cycle provides a useful framework for the analysis of systolic and diastolic function.
10. Preload is the quantity of blood that a cardiac chamber contains immediately before contraction begins, whereas afterload is the external resistance to emptying to which the chamber is confronted after the onset of contraction.
11. Myocardial contractility is quantified using indices derived from pressure–volume relations, isovolumic contraction, or the ejection phase; these indices have limitations because contractile state and loading conditions are interrelated.
12. Diastolic function is defined as the ability of a cardiac chamber to effectively collect blood at a normal filling pressure.
13. The pericardium exerts important restraining forces on cardiac chamber filling and is a major determinant of ventricular interdependence.
14. The atria serve three mechanical functions: conduit, reservoir, and contractile chamber.
15. Heart failure occurs when the LV is unable to eject blood at a sufficient rate to meet metabolic demands or it cannot fill completely without elevated pressure; heart failure is classified based on LV ejection fraction (EF) less than or greater than 50%.
16. LV systolic dysfunction characterizes heart failure with reduced ejection fraction (HFrEF), whereas LV diastolic dysfunction, ventricular and arterial stiffening, left atrial (LA) dysfunction, pulmonary hypertension, and right ventricular (RV) dysfunction are common in heart failure with preserved ejection fraction (HFpEF).

Introduction

The heart is a phasic, electrically self-actuated, variable speed, hydraulic pump composed of two dual-component, elastic muscular chambers, each consisting of an atrium and a ventricle. These chambers simultaneously provide an equal quantity of blood to the pulmonary and systemic circulations. Myocardium in the atria and ventricles responds to stimulation rate and muscle stretch before (preload) and after (afterload) contraction begins. The heart provides its own energy supply through an intricate coronary circulation. The heart adapts to changing physiologic conditions by altering its intrinsic mechanical behavior (Frank–Starling principle) and by responding to neurohormonal signaling. The overall performance of the heart is determined by the contractile performance of its atria and ventricles and by the ability of its chambers to collect blood at normal filling pressures. This implies that heart failure may occur as a result of either systolic or diastolic dysfunction. A thorough knowledge of cardiac anatomy and physiology is essential for modern anesthesia practice.

Gross Anatomy

The gross anatomy of the heart determines its functional capabilities and limitations. The annuli of the valves, the aortic and pulmonary arterial roots, the central fibrous body, and the left
1 and right fibrous trigones form the heart's skeleton. This flexible cartilaginous structure is located at the superior aspect (known as the "base") of the heart and serves three primary functions: (1) support the translucent, macroscopically avascular valves; (2) resist the forces of developed pressure and blood flow within the chambers; and (3) provide a site of insertion for superficial subepicardial muscle. Most atrial and ventricular muscle is not directly connected to this central fibrous skeleton, but arises from and inserts within adjacent surrounding myocardium, an observation that is consistent with the heart's embryologic origin as an expanded artery.[1] An interstitial collagen fiber network also provides structural support to the myocardium. Elastin is interwoven within this collagen matrix, which provides flexibility and elasticity without compromising strength. Atrial and ventricular myocardium cannot be separated into distinct layers[*] using an "unwinding" dissection technique, as was originally proposed by William Harvey.[2] Instead, myocardium consists of a continuum of interconnecting cardiac muscle fibers. The left and right atria (LA and RA, respectively) are composed of two relatively thin sheets of myocardium that are oriented perpendicular to each other. The right ventricular (RV) and left ventricular (LV) walls are thicker (measuring approximately 5 and 10 mm, respectively) than those of the atria and consist of three muscle layers: the interdigitating deep sinospiral, the superficial sinospiral, and the superficial bulbospiral (Fig. 12-1). Well-ordered, differential alterations in fiber angle extending from the endocardium to the epicardium are spatially conserved in ventricular myocardium. Subendocardial and subepicardial muscle fibers of the LV follow orthogonal, oblique, and helical routes from the base to the apex (inferior aspect of the heart). The orientation of these interdigitating sheets of cardiac muscle reverses direction at the LV midpoint. This fiber structure resembles a flattened "figure of eight." Contraction of obliquely arranged subepicardial and subendocardial fibers shortens the LV chamber along its longitudinal axis and causes a torsional twisting motion (similar to wringing a wash cloth) that substantially increases the force applied to blood within the chamber. Loss of this torsional twist reduces ejection fraction (EF) and is a characteristic finding in patients with LV systolic dysfunction. Elastic recoil of systolic twist during LV relaxation is the major determinant of the diastolic suction mechanism, which enhances early LV filling during hypovolemia and exercise.[3] Midmyocardial fibers are circumferentially oriented around the LV cavity. The contraction of these fibers reduces chamber diameter.

The LV free walls are thickest near the base and gradually thin toward the apex because of a progressive decrease in the quantity of midmyocardial fibers. Subendocardial layers of both the LV and RV combine with LV midmyocardium extending from the LV free wall to create the interventricular septum.[4] Because most of the septum is derived from the LV, it normally thickens toward the LV chamber during contraction. The septum may move abnormally toward the RV chamber during systole when RV pressure overload is present. A gradual decrease in midmyocardial fibers produces a base-to-apex reduction in septal thickness. The LV apical free wall is composed of subendocardial and subepicardial fibers, but the apical septum contains only LV and RV subendocardial fibers. These regional differences in LV wall thickness and laminar myocardial fiber orientation contribute to load-dependent alterations in LV mechanics. Irregular ridges of subendocardium (known as "trabeculae carnae"; Latin for "meaty ridges") are present in the LV apex and RV. The physiologic implications of trabeculae carnae are unknown. Endocardial endothelium lines the subendocardium.

The LV apex and septum remain relatively fixed in space within the mediastinum, but the lateral and inferior walls move anteriorly and rightward during contraction. These actions displace the LV longitudinal axis from a plane oriented toward the mitral valve (which favors LV filling) to a position that is more parallel to the LV outflow tract (which facilitates ejection). This anterior-right movement also causes the point of maximum impulse, which is usually palpable on the anterior chest wall in the left fifth or sixth intercostal space in the midclavicular line. Subendocardial and subepicardial fiber shortening, papillary muscle contraction, and recoil resulting from ejection of blood into the aortic root cause the LV base to descend toward the apex during systole. Thus, LV contraction shortens its long axis, decreases its chamber diameter, and rotates its apex in an anterior-right direction toward the chest wall (Fig. 12-2). LV ejection is also associated with an apex-to-base gradient in wall tension, which creates an

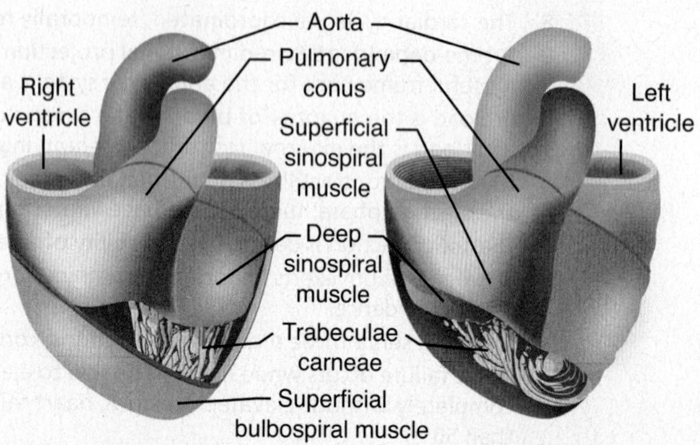

Figure 12-1 Illustration depicting the components of the myocardium. The outer muscle layers pull the apex of the heart toward the base. The inner circumferential layers constrict the lumen, particularly of the left ventricle (LV).

[*]The term "layer" will be used as a metaphor throughout this section.

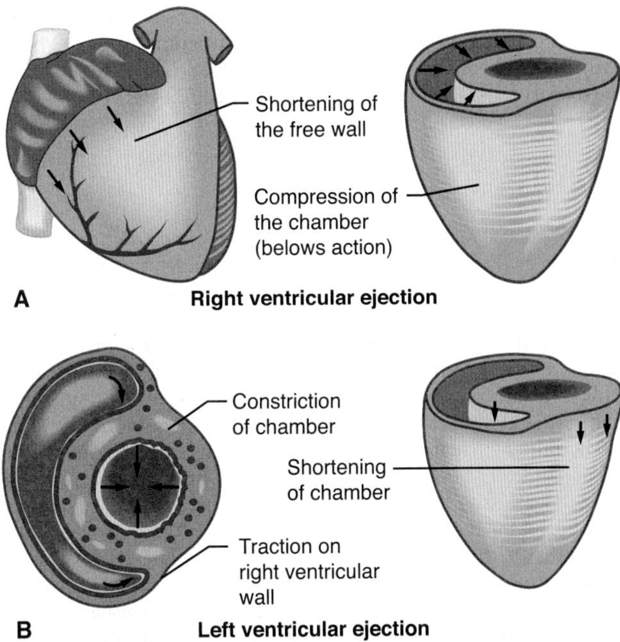

Figure 12-2 Illustration depicting the contraction characteristics and modes of emptying of the right ventricle (RV) and left ventricle (LV). The volumes ejected by each ventricle are equal, but the LV requires a more circumferential muscular wall to eject its volume at a pressure that is approximately four to five times greater than that in the RV.

intraventricular pressure gradient that efficiently transfers stroke volume (SV) from the LV into the aorta.

The RV is located anterior and to the right of the LV within the mediastinum. Unlike the thicker-walled, ellipsoidal-shaped LV that ejects oxygenated blood into the high-pressure arterial vasculature, the thinner-walled, crescent-shaped RV pumps deoxygenated blood into a lower pressure, more compliant pulmonary arterial tree. In contrast to the LV's temporally uniform activation sequence, the RV contracts in a more peristaltic manner, in part because it is composed of embryologically distinct inflow and outflow tracts. The RV moves toward the septum with a "bellows-like" action, with the septum and LV providing a "splint" against which the RV free wall shortens during contraction. LV contraction also makes an important contribution to RV systolic function. These features provide the less muscular RV with a mechanical advantage that allows it to eject an SV equivalent to that of the LV. However, the thinner RV is more vulnerable to acute increases in afterload because the thicker LV can generate pressure–volume work that is five- to seven-fold greater than that of the RV. Conversely, the RV is more compliant and can accommodate excess volume more easily than the LV. Nevertheless, RV compliance is limited by pericardial restraint.

Valves

Two pairs of valves ensure unidirectional blood flow through the right and left sides of the heart. The pulmonic and aortic valves are trileaflet structures located at RV and LV outlets, respectively, and operate passively with changes in hydraulic pressure resulting from ejection. The pulmonic valve leaflets are named based on their anatomic position (right, left, and anterior), whereas the name of each aortic valve leaflet is based on the presence or absence of an adjacent coronary ostium. The effective orifice area of each of these valves during peak ejection is nearly equal to the cross-sectional area of the respective annulus. The proximal aortic root contains dilated segments called sinuses of Valsalva located above each leaflet; they prevent the aortic valve leaflets from adhering to the aortic wall by facilitating the formation of hydraulic flow vortices (eddy currents) during ejection. This clever design assures that the right and left coronary leaflets do not occlude their coronary ostia. The eddy currents also assist with aortic valve closure when ejection ceases by assuring that the leaflets remain fully mobile during early diastole. The proximal pulmonary artery does not contain sinuses of Valsalva.

The thin, flexible, and strong mitral valve separates the LA from the LV. The mitral valve is an oval, saddle-shaped structure containing two leaflets, identified as anterior and posterior based on their anatomic location. The leaflets approximate in a central curve with the anterior mitral leaflet forming the convex border. The oval-shaped anterior mitral leaflet occupies a greater central diameter across the annulus, whereas the crescent-shaped posterior mitral leaflet extends further around the annular circumference. The area of each leaflet is similar. The leaflets join at anterior-lateral and posterior-medial commissures, which are located above the corresponding papillary muscles. The leaflets thicken slightly along the line of coaptation. The pressure gradient between the LA and LV chambers near the end of LV relaxation combined with LV elastic recoil causes the mitral valve to open, whereas retrograde blood flow toward the valve during LV contraction drives the leaflets in a superior direction to close them. Thin fibrous bands of tissue (chordae tendinae) are attached to the papillary muscles. Primary and secondary chordae tendinae insert into the edges and the bodies of the leaflets, respectively. Tertiary chordae tendinae extend from the posterior-medial papillary muscle and insert into the posterior mitral leaflet or the adjacent myocardium near the annulus. Each papillary muscle is an outpouching of subendocardial myocardium that provides chordae tendinae to both mitral valve leaflets and contracts synchronously with the LV. Papillary muscle contraction tightens the chordae tendinae, which inhibits excessive leaflet motion past the coaptation zone and prevents leaflet inversion. Chordal rupture is a common cause of severe mitral regurgitation because excessive leaflet motion occurs, which allows unobstructed retrograde blood flow from the pressurized LV into a low-pressure LA outlet. The mitral annular circumference also decreases modestly during LV contraction through a sphincter-like action of the surrounding subepicardial myocardium. This action reduces annular area and assists in valve closure. The mitral valve apparatus contributes to LV systolic function through papillary muscle contributions to LV apical contraction. Predictably, removal of chordae tendinae–papillary muscle attachments during mitral valve replacement surgery is associated with a reduction in LV EF. In addition to producing acute mitral regurgitation, papillary muscle ischemia or infarction may cause LV systolic dysfunction through a similar mechanism.

The anterior, posterior, and septal leaflets and their corresponding chordae tendinae and papillary muscles comprise the tricuspid valve. Identification of a septal papillary muscle can often be used to distinguish the morphologic RV from the LV in patients with complex congenital heart disease. A lateral band of myocardium (moderator band) connects the apical anterior and septal papillary muscles and demarcates the RV inflow and outflow tracts. The RV has coarse trabeculae carnae throughout the chamber, whereas finer trabeculations are present in the LV. Unlike the mitral valve, the tricuspid valve does not have a clearly defined cartilaginous annulus. Instead, the tricuspid leaflets originate from the atrioventricular (AV) groove that separates the RA from the RV. The right coronary artery lies within this groove and must be avoided during tricuspid valve surgery.

Conduction System

The mechanism by which the heart is electrically activated plays an essential role in its function. The sinoatrial (SA) node is the primary cardiac pacemaker so long as marked decreases in firing rate, conduction delays or blockade, or accelerated firing of secondary pacemakers are absent. The anterior, middle (Wenckebach), and posterior (Thorel) internodal pathways rapidly transmit the initial SA node depolarization through the RA myocardium to the AV node. Bachmann's bundle (an anterior internodal pathway branch) transmits the SA node depolarization from the RA to the LA across the atrial septum. Internodal pathways are clearly identified in the electrophysiology laboratory but are difficult to identify histologically. The cartilaginous skeleton of the heart isolates the atria from the ventricles by acting as an electrical insulator. As a result, atrial depolarization is directed to the ventricles through the AV node and is not indiscriminately transmitted throughout the heart. The electrical isolation between the atrial and ventricular chambers and the normal transmission delay through the slowly conducting AV node are responsible for establishing the sequential pattern of atrial followed by ventricular contraction. Pathologic direct accessory pathways (e.g., bundle of Kent) between the atria and ventricles that bypass the AV node often precipitate reentrant supraventricular tachyarrhythmias such as Wolff–Parkinson–White syndrome.

The His bundle pierces the connective tissue of the cartilaginous skeleton and transmits the AV depolarization signal along the right and left bundle branches to the RV and LV myocardium, respectively; this occurs through a conductive tissue complex called the Purkinje network located within the inner one-third of the ventricular walls. The fibers of the His bundle, the bundle branches, and the Purkinje network assure rapid, coordinated distribution of depolarization. This electrical configuration facilitates synchronous biventricular contraction and coordinated ejection. It is noteworthy that artificial cardiac pacing (e.g., epicardial RV pacing during cardiac surgery) bypasses this normal conduction system and produces dyssynchronous LV activation, resulting in uncoordinated contraction that may decrease LV EF or cause new regional wall motion abnormalities in the absence of acute myocardial ischemia. Such contractile dyssynchrony also occurs due to chronic RV apical pacing and is known to cause detrimental effects on LV chamber geometry and function. Recognition of the essential relationship between a normal electrical activation sequence and appropriately timed LV contraction forms the basis for the use of cardiac resynchronization therapy in some patients with heart failure with reduced ejection fraction (HFrEF).

Coronary Anatomy

The left anterior descending, left circumflex, and right coronary arteries (LAD, LCCA, and RCA, respectively) supply blood to the heart (Fig. 12-3). All three coronary arteries contribute to the LV's blood supply. Inadequate blood flow resulting from a critical stenosis or abrupt occlusion of a coronary artery causes acute myocardial ischemia accompanied by a regional wall motion abnormality. The LAD and its septal and diagonal branches supply the medial half of the LV anterior wall, the apex, and the anterior two-thirds of the interventricular septum in the majority of individuals. The LCCA and its obtuse marginal branches supply the anterior and inferior aspects of the lateral wall. The RCA and its distal branches supply the medial portions of the inferior wall and the posterior one-third of the interventricular septum. Despite these general anatomic observations, substantial variations in blood supply to the LV are observed between individuals. The coronary artery that supplies blood to the posterior descending coronary artery (PDA) defines the right or left dominance of the circulation. Right dominance (RCA supply) is observed in approximately 80% of patients, whereas left dominance (LCCA supply) occurs in the remainder. Direct connections between the distal coronary arteries or collateral blood vessels between the major coronary arteries may also be present. These vessels provide an alternative route of blood flow to myocardium, but their presence is variable. In most people, either the RCA or the LCCA provides the sole blood supply to the posterior-medial papillary muscle (ratio of RCA to LCCA of 2:1), which renders it vulnerable to ischemia. However, approximately one-third of individuals have a dual blood supply (RCA and LCCA) to the posterior papillary muscle, which makes them less susceptible to posterior-medial papillary muscle ischemia. The LAD and the LCCA usually provide a dual blood supply to the anterior-lateral papillary muscle. As a result, ischemic dysfunction of this papillary muscle is unusual.

The RCA and its branches supply most of the RV, but the anterior wall of the RV also receives blood supply from LAD branches.

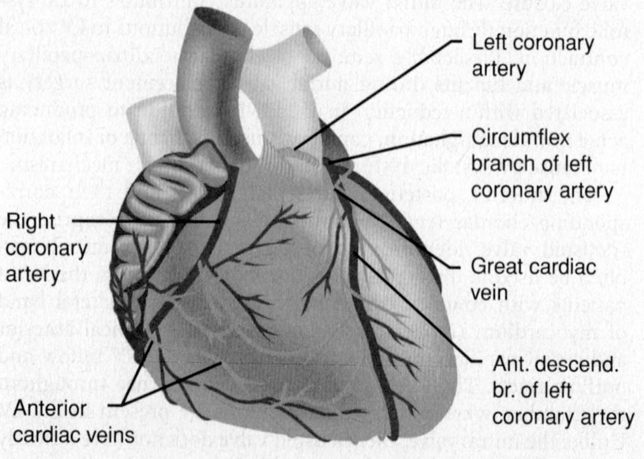

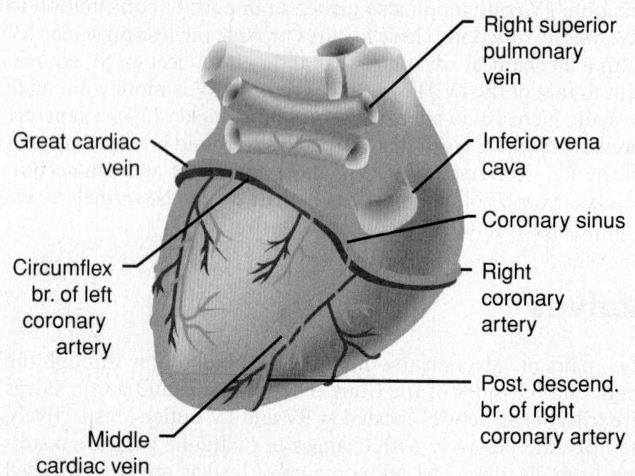

Figure 12-3 An anterior view of the heart (**left**) shows right coronary and left anterior descending coronary arteries. A posterior view (**right**) shows left circumflex and posterior descending coronary arteries. The anterior cardiac veins from the right ventricle (RV) and the coronary sinus, which drain primarily the left ventricle (LV), empty into the right atrium (RA).

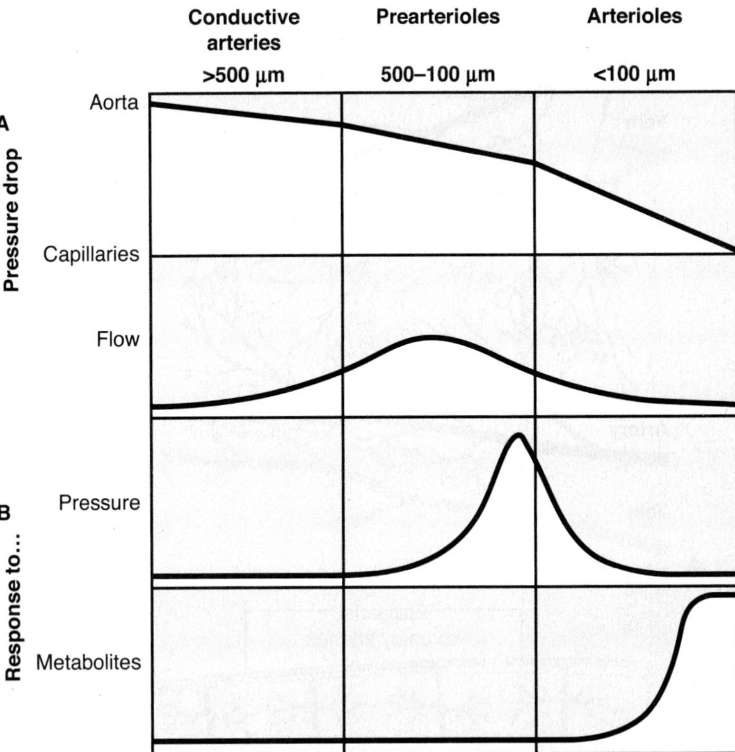

Figure 12-4 Functional anatomy of coronary arterial system. (Adapted from Camici PG, Crea F. Coronary microvascular dysfunction. *N Engl J Med*. 2007;356:830–840, Camici PG, Rimoldi OE. The clinical value of myocardial blood flow measurement. *J Nucl Med*. 2009 Jul;50(7):1076–87, and from Koo, BK, Lee, JM. Concept of Invasive Coronary Physiology: Focus on FFR. In: Hong MK, ed. *Coronary Imaging and Physiology*. Springer; 2018. Figure 20.2.)

As a result, RV dysfunction may occur because of either RCA or LAD occlusion. Coronary blood flow to the LA is derived from branches of the LCCA.[5] Enhanced LA contractility resulting from activation of the Frank–Starling principle occurs when LAD ischemia or infarction is present; however, this compensatory response may not be observed when LCCA blood flow is compromised because of LA ischemia.[6] Branches of the RCA and the LCCA provide coronary blood flow to the RA.[7] A nodal artery from the RCA (55% of patients) or the LCCA (45% of patients) supplies the SA node. Similarly, RCA branches, or less commonly branches from the LCCA, supply the AV node. Ischemia in either of these two perfusion territories may delay the transmission through the proximal conduction system and cause bradyarrhythmias.

The RCA, LCCA, and LAD and their proximal branches are located on the epicardial surface of the heart and give rise to intramural vessels that penetrate deep into the myocardium. Three functionally distinct compartments exist in the coronary circulation: large conductive arteries (proximal), prearterioles
2 (intermediate), and arterioles (distal) (Fig. 12-4). The large epicardial coronary arteries in the proximal compartment are 0.5 to 5 mm in diameter. These vessels act as conduits, respond to flow-mediated vasodilation, and usually do not exert meaningful resistance to coronary blood flow unless atherosclerosis is present. Prearterioles (100 to 500 µm in diameter) make up the intermediate compartment. A moderate pressure drop occurs along the length of these vessels, which make a relatively minor contribution to overall coronary vascular resistance. The primary function of prearterioles is to maintain pressure within a narrow range at the origin of the arterioles when changes in coronary perfusion pressure and blood flow occur. Prearteriole diameter is regulated through a myogenic mechanism, which refers to the tendency of vascular smooth muscle to contract or dilate in response to increases or decreases in pressure, respectively. Intramural arterioles (<100 µm in diameter) are the major component of the distal compartment and make the largest contribution to coronary vascular resistance. The intramural arterioles possess significant vasodilator reserve and are exquisitely sensitive to vasoactive metabolites produced by the myocardium in response to metabolic demand. A high density of capillaries is present in myocardium because of the heart's exceptionally high metabolic demand; the ratio of capillaries to muscle fibers is approximately one. Adjacent capillaries are usually separated by the diameter of a single myocyte. Capillary recruitment serves to maintain myocardial oxygen tension when demand increases. The capillary distribution is quite uniform throughout the atria and ventricles (3,000 and 4,000/mm^2) except in the AV node and interventricular septum, where capillary volume is less dense. This observation helps to explain why the proximal portion of the RV and LV conduction system seems to be more vulnerable to ischemia. Coronary capillaries are the sites for oxygen and carbon dioxide exchange and for the movement of larger molecules (e.g., glucose) across the endothelium.

Arterial branches with diameters between 50 and 500 µm form interconnecting anastomoses, whereas arterioles between 100 and 200 µm in diameter form a plexus within the subendocardium (Fig. 12-5). Collateral vessels between different branches of the same coronary artery or between branches of two different coronary arteries are also variably present. Blood flow through coronary collaterals is usually minimal because the driving pressure across the vessels is relatively equal. However, if blood flow supplying one branch of a collateral vessel is restricted by a stenosis or occlusion, a pressure gradient develops that diverts flow from the patent artery through the collateral vessel into the distribution of the artery with inadequate flow. The presence and extent of coronary collaterals often determines whether a patient with coronary artery disease will develop anginal symptoms in response to an increase in myocardial oxygen demand.

The coronary venous drainage of the heart retraces the course of the major coronary arteries along the AV and interventricular grooves. The great cardiac vein courses along the AV groove and

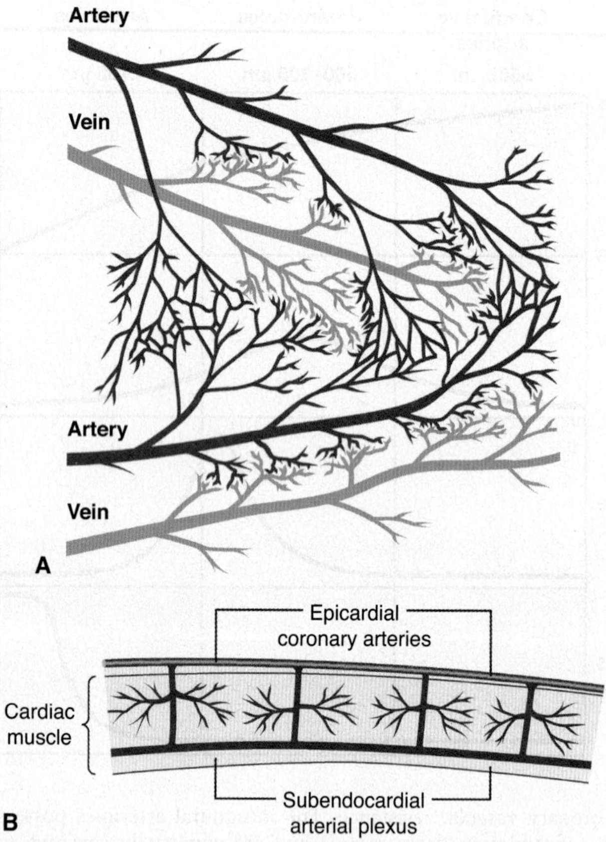

Figure 12-5 **A.** Diagram of the arterial-to-arterial and venous-to-venous anastomoses of the coronary arterial system, which allow diversion of flow if one distribution becomes blocked. **B.** Diagram of the epicardial coronary vessels lying on the cardiac muscle surface, the penetrating deep vessels, and the subendocardial arterial plexus connecting the deep vessels.

the LAD; the anterior cardiac vein is located adjacent to the RCA; and the middle cardiac vein is associated with PDA. Two coronary veins lie along either side of each major coronary artery branch. The coronary veins converge into the coronary sinus which empties into the posterior aspect of the RA immediately above the tricuspid valve. Venous blood flow into the coronary sinus peaks during late systole because the contracting LV compresses major venous drainage channels. Approximately 85% of total coronary blood flow returning from the LV empties into the coronary sinus, whereas the remaining flow drains directly into the atrial and ventricular cavities through the thebesian veins (RA > LA and LV). The RV veins drain into the anterior cardiac veins which in turn empty individually into the RA.

Coronary Physiology

Poiseuille's law governs blood flow. Originally formulated assuming continuous laminar flow of a Newtonian fluid through a rigid tube,[8] Poiseuille's law does not strictly apply to the intact circulation for several reasons: arterial pressure is phasic, the viscosity of blood varies with shear rate, and vessels are compliant. Despite its nonphysiologic assumptions, Poiseuille's law provides a useful model for understanding blood flow dynamics.[9] In general, blood flow through a vascular bed is directly proportional to the arterial–venous pressure gradient and is inversely related to resistance. In the coronary circulation, blood flow is driven almost entirely by coronary perfusion pressure, which is represented by the difference between aortic diastolic and LV end-diastolic pressures (coronary venous pressure is negligible), while arteriolar smooth muscle controls vascular resistance. Small changes in vessel caliber are associated with relatively large changes in resistance, which varies to the fourth power of the vessel radius in accordance with Poiseuille's law. This observation implies that regulation of coronary vascular resistance is exquisitely sensitive to the multitude of factors that affect arteriolar vasomotor tone. Coronary blood flow is also related to vessel length and blood viscosity. Vessel length remains essentially constant in the intact heart, and blood viscosity (governed mainly by hemoglobin concentration) usually plays a relatively minor role in determining flow unless marked polycythemia or profound hemodilution is present. Resting coronary blood flow in the adult is approximately 250 mL/min (1 mL/min/g), which represents approximately 5% of cardiac output (CO).

Coronary blood flow to the LV occurs almost entirely during diastole because extravascular compressive forces are exerted on the subendocardial intramural vessels during contraction.[10] Despite this subendocardial flow limitation during systole, preferential flow to the subendocardium occurs during diastole through a metabolically mediated reduction in arteriolar vasomotor tone. This action preserves uniform transmural LV perfusion (ratio of subepicardial to subendocardial blood flow is 1:1). An increase in heart rate shortens diastole, but subendocardial blood flow is usually maintained because coronary flow reserve is recruited.
However, tachycardia can compromise this reserve and cause sub- 3
endocardial ischemia when a flow-limiting coronary artery stenosis (decreased oxygen supply) or pressure-overload hypertrophy (increased demand) is present. In contrast to the LV, RV, LA, and RA, pressures remain lower than aortic pressure throughout the cardiac cycle. As a result, compressive forces do not impede coronary blood flow to these chambers, which is reflected in the contour of the aortic pressure waveform (Fig. 12-6).[11]

The heart depends almost entirely on aerobic metabolism to satisfy its energy requirements,[12] which are disproportionately high (7% of total body) based on weight (0.5% of total body). Almost all high-energy phosphates formed within the cardiac myocyte are derived from mitochondrial oxidative phosphorylation of fatty acids, glucose, and lactate. If oxygen supply is restricted, the cardiac myocyte depends on anaerobic conversion of glucose to lactate to generate ATP. However, this alternative pathway is quite limited in its ability to supply enough energy to sustain function because contraction will cease within 10 to 15 seconds after acute coronary artery occlusion unless the ischemic territory receives sufficient collateral blood flow from another vessel. As a result, myocardial oxygen supply must be closely matched to demand to maintain the heart's uninterrupted cycle of contraction and relaxation. This flow–metabolism coupling is achieved through an intrinsic regulatory mechanism in which the myocardium releases mediators that dilate coronary arterioles and enhance coronary blood flow in parallel with increases in oxygen demand.
The tight relationship between demand and supply is essential 4
because myocardial oxygen extraction is nearly maximal under baseline conditions. Indeed, approximately 75% of oxygen carried by hemoglobin is extracted from blood traversing the myocardial capillaries, an observation that explains why coronary sinus oxygen tension is only 20 mmHg. As a result, the LV has limited oxygen extraction reserve and is almost completely dependent on increases in blood flow to satisfy increased oxygen demand. These compensatory increases in flow occur through recruitment of coronary vasodilator reserve by metabolites produced in the myocardium.

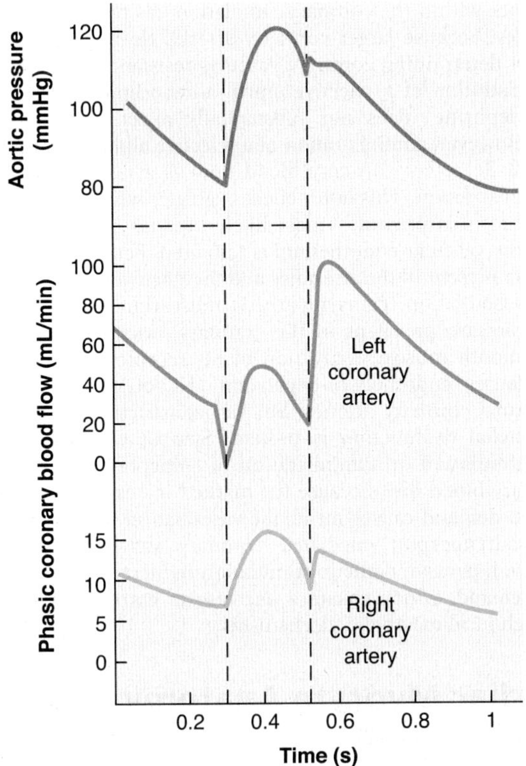

Figure 12-6 Schematic representation of blood flow in the left and right coronary arteries during phases of the cardiac cycle. Note that most left coronary flow occurs during diastole while right coronary flow (and coronary sinus flow) occurs mostly during late systole and early diastole.

5 Metabolic regulation is most likely a "feed-forward" phenomenon in which vasodilators including carbon dioxide (generated through Krebs cycle decarboxylation reactions) and reactive oxygen species (formed in the mitochondrial respiratory chain) are produced by the myocardium in proportion to energy utilization.[13] Nitric oxide (NO) and adenosine triphosphate–sensitive potassium (K_{ATP}) channels are the most likely downstream mediators of this flow response. The free radical NO is synthesized by the constitutively expressed enzyme endothelial NO synthase (eNOS). An increase in intracellular Ca^{2+} concentration within the vascular endothelium in response to receptor activation (e.g., bradykinin, acetylcholine) or wall shear stress stimulates eNOS to produce NO. This NO then diffuses into the underlying arteriolar smooth muscle, where it stimulates cyclic guanosine monophosphate (cGMP) to cause relaxation. NO has a very limited range of action and a short half-life because it is rapidly scavenged by hemoglobin. Atherosclerosis, diabetes, and hypercholesterolemia inhibit the release of NO from coronary vascular endothelium, which contributes to dysregulation of coronary blood flow and increases the risk of myocardial ischemia.[14] The K_{ATP} channel responds to metabolic status to modulate a cell's activity. K_{ATP} channels open when ATP concentrations decrease. This action causes vascular smooth muscle hyperpolarization by shifting the membrane potential toward the K^+ reversal potential. The hyperpolarization inhibits Ca^{2+} entry through voltage-dependent Ca^{2+} channels, which causes vasodilation. K_{ATP} channels mediate basal coronary vascular tone and regulate coronary vasodilation associated with reduced perfusion pressure, increased myocardial oxygen demand, and reactive hyperemia.

The endothelium produces several other metabolites that modulate coronary vasomotor tone. The ATP metabolite adenosine was previously thought to play an important role in regulation of coronary blood flow, but coronary vasodilation by adenosine is probably only relevant during tissue hypoxia (the condition under which it is formed and released). Prostaglandin I_2 (prostacyclin) is an arachidonic acid metabolite that inhibits platelet aggregation and causes arteriolar vasodilation by opening K_{ATP} channels through a receptor-activated mechanism. Prostaglandin I_2 most likely does not play a major role in local metabolic regulation of coronary blood flow. Endothelin-1 is an endogenous peptide produced by endothelium that binds to coronary vascular smooth muscle to cause intense vasoconstriction through endothelin subtype A and B receptors.[15] Endothelin-1 does not substantially affect the coronary circulation under normal conditions because its actions as a vasoconstrictor are probably counterbalanced by tonic release of NO, but a shift in this equilibrium resulting from impaired NO release or excessive endothelin-1 production may cause pathologic vasoconstriction in systemic or pulmonary hypertension, diabetes, and heart failure.

The ratio of maximum to baseline coronary blood flow defines coronary flow reserve, which can be determined by analysis of the transient increase in flow that occurs after a brief coronary artery occlusion (reactive hyperemia; Fig. 12-7) or by administration of a potent coronary vasodilator.[16] Coronary flow reserve is very large (between 500% and 600%) in normal coronary arteries that perfuse the LV and RV, but it is reduced by a coronary stenosis, pressure-overload hypertrophy, and microvascular dysfunction. A decline in coronary flow reserve renders the myocardium more susceptible to ischemia during an increase in oxygen demand. Reduced perfusion pressure is primarily responsible for the impaired reactive hyperemic response when a hemodynamically significant flow-limiting stenosis is present. Vasodilator reserve

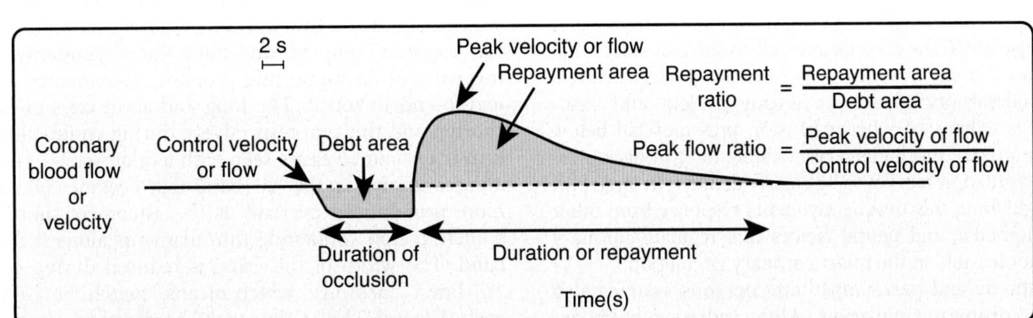

Figure 12-7 Schematic illustration of reactive hyperemia in response to a 10-second coronary artery occlusion. (Reproduced with permission from Kaplan JA, Augoustides JGT, Manecke Jr GR, et al. *Kaplan's Cardiac Anesthesia: For Cardiac and Noncardiac Anesthesia*. 7th ed. Elsevier; 2017:189; permission conveyed from Copyright Clearance Center, Inc. (Figure 7-10))

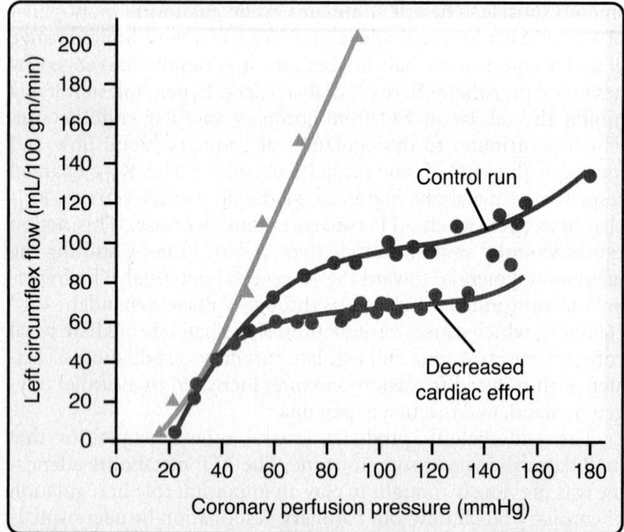

Figure 12-8 Autoregulation at two levels of myocardial oxygen demand. Pressure in the cannulated left circumflex coronary artery was varied independently of aortic pressure. When pressures were acutely raised or lowered from 40 mmHg, flow instantaneously increased with pressure (*steep line, triangles*). Flow decreased to the steady-state level determined by oxygen demand over time (*circles*). The distance between the steady-state (autoregulating) line and the acute pressure–flow line is coronary flow reserve. (Reproduced with permission from Kaplan JA, Augoustides JGT, Manecke Jr GR, et al. *Kaplan's Cardiac Anesthesia: For Cardiac and Noncardiac Anesthesia*, 7th ed. Elsevier; 2017:189; permission conveyed from Copyright Clearance Center, Inc. (Figure 7-9))

is recruited in response to the decrease in perfusion pressure to maintain coronary blood flow through pressure-flow autoregulation. A decrease in peak coronary hyperemic blood flow can first be appreciated when the diameter of the coronary artery lumen is decreased by 50%. Peak reactive hyperemia is abolished when luminal diameter is reduced by approximately 90%. This magnitude of narrowing is associated with anginal symptoms with minimal exertion and defines the threshold for the diagnosis of unstable angina in patients with coronary artery disease.

The ability of coronary circulation to maintain relatively constant blood flow across a wide range of perfusion pressures is known as pressure-flow autoregulation.[17] Compensatory adjustments in vasomotor tone are responsible for this intrinsic myogenic phenomenon: lower perfusion pressures produce vasodilation, whereas higher pressures cause vasoconstriction. This pressure-flow autoregulation is not dependent on autonomic nervous system activity or metabolic factors. The upper and lower pressure limits of pressure-flow autoregulation are approximately 140 and 60 mmHg, respectively (Fig. 12-8). Perfusion pressures greater than 140 mmHg distend the coronary vessels to such an extent that the ability of vascular smooth muscle to constrict is overwhelmed; conversely, maximal vasodilation is already present and vasodilator reserve is exhausted when perfusion pressures fall below 60 mmHg. The precise mechanism responsible for coronary pressure-flow autoregulation has yet to be clearly defined, in large part because distinguishing this unique myogenic response from other metabolic, endothelial, and neural factors that regulate coronary blood flow is not feasible in the intact coronary circulation.

The sympathetic and parasympathetic nervous systems also innervate the coronary circulation. Alpha$_1$-adrenoceptors are most prevalent in large- and intermediate-sized coronary vessels, whereas alpha$_2$-adrenoceptors are the predominant subtype in the arterioles. This distribution of alpha-adrenoceptor subtypes within the coronary circulation has predictable consequences. Because larger coronary arteries do not play a major role in determining coronary vascular resistance, intracoronary administration of a selective alpha$_1$-adrenoceptor agonist (e.g., phenylephrine) does not substantially affect coronary blood flow. However, administration of a selective alpha$_2$-adrenoceptor agonist decreases coronary blood flow as a result of arteriolar vasoconstriction. This latter effect is greater when coronary atherosclerosis is present,[18] most likely because basal NO release from the vascular endothelium is impaired. Beta$_1$-adrenoceptors are also present in the arterioles and their activation causes coronary vasodilation. Parasympathetic muscarinic subtype 3 (M_3) receptors are prevalent in the coronary vascular endothelium and smooth muscle. Activation of M_3 receptors by acetylcholine causes endothelium-dependent (NO-cGMP) vasodilation in normal coronary arteries, but vasoconstriction occurs when endothelial dysfunction is present. Sympathetic nervous system stimulation or administration of epinephrine increases LV coronary blood flow because the marked increase in myocardial oxygen demand causes metabolic vasodilation that overwhelms alpha-adrenoceptor$_2$–mediated coronary vasoconstriction. As expected, parasympathetic stimulation reduces myocardial oxygen demand, which causes a decrease in coronary blood flow through local metabolic mechanisms.

Cardiac Myocyte Anatomy and Function

Ultrastructure

The heart contracts and relaxes nearly 3 billion times during an average lifetime, based on an average heart rate of 70 beats per minute and a life expectancy of 75 years. A review of cardiac myocyte ultrastructure provides insights into how this remarkable feat is achieved. The sarcolemma is the external membrane of the cardiac muscle cell. This bilayer lipid membrane contains ion channels (e.g., Na^+, K^+, Ca^{2+}, Cl^-), active and passive ion transporters (e.g., Na^+-K^+ ATPase, Ca^{2+}-ATPase, Na^+-Ca^{2+} and Na^+-H^+ exchangers), receptors (e.g., beta$_1$-adrenergic, muscarinic cholinergic, adenosine, opioid), and transport enzymes (e.g., glucose) that modulate intracellular ion concentrations, regulate homeostasis of contraction and electrophysiology, mediate signal transduction, and provide substrates for metabolism. Sarcolemmal invaginations (transverse tubules) penetrate deeply into the myoplasm to facilitate rapid transmission of cellular depolarization. The myocyte is densely packed with mitochondria responsible for the generation of high-energy phosphates required for contraction and relaxation. The sarcomere is the contractile unit of the cardiac myocyte. Its myofilaments are arranged in parallel cross-striated bundles of thin fibers (containing actin, tropomyosin, and the troponin complex) and thick fibers (primarily composed of myosin and its supporting proteins). Sarcomeres are connected end-to-end in series. The long and short axes of each myocyte shorten and thicken, respectively, during contraction. Thick and thin fibers can be easily seen with a microscope. They interact in an area known as the "A" band that becomes wider (indicating more pronounced overlap) as the sarcomere shortens. The sarcomere region containing thin filaments alone is termed the "I" band. The width of this band is reduced during contraction. A "Z" line ("zuckung," which means "twitch" in German) bisects each "I" band. The "Z" line is the border of two sarcomeres. Thus, the "A" band and two split "I" bands (between the "Z" lines) define the length of each sarcomere. The "A" band also contains a central "M" band composed of thick filaments that are oriented in a cross-sectional hexagonal arrangement by myosin-binding protein C.

Each cardiac myocyte contains an extensive sarcoplasmic reticulum (SR) network that surrounds the contractile proteins. The SR is the primary Ca^{2+} reservoir of the cardiac myocyte, and its extensive distribution ensures almost homogenous dispersal and reuptake of Ca^{2+} throughout the myofilaments during contraction and relaxation. Subsarcolemmal cisternae within the SR are located adjacent to the sarcolemma and the transverse tubules. These cisternae contain ryanodine receptors that are the SR's primary Ca^{2+} release channel and stimulate Ca^{2+}-induced Ca^{2+} release from the SR when the sarcolemma depolarizes. The contractile apparatus and the mitochondria that supply its high-energy phosphates constitute more than 80% of the myocyte's total volume, whereas the cytosol and nucleus occupy less

than 15%. This observation underscores that contraction, and not protein synthesis, is the predominant function of the cardiac myocyte. Intercalated discs mechanically join adjacent myocytes through the fascia adherens (which links actin molecules at each "Z" line) and desmosomes. They also create electrical continuity between myocytes through gap junctions that allow diffusion of ions and small molecules.

Contractile Apparatus Proteins

The contractile apparatus is composed of six major proteins: myosin, actin, tropomyosin, and the three-protein troponin complex. Myosin contains a pair of intertwined alpha-helical proteins (tails), each with a globular head that binds the actin molecule, and two adjoining pairs of light chains. Enzymatic digestion of myosin reveals the presence of light meromyosin (composed of the tail sections) and heavy meromyosin (containing the globular heads and the light chains). The primary structural support of the myosin molecule is the elongated tail section (Fig. 12-9). The globular heads of the myosin dimer contain two hinges that are located at the distal light chain tail–double helix junction and are responsible for myofilament shortening during contraction. The binding of the myosin head to the actin molecule stimulates a cascade of events initiated by activation of a myosin ATPase that mediates hinge rotation and actin release during contraction and relaxation, respectively. The activity of this myosin ATPase is a major determinant of the maximum velocity of sarcomere shortening, which defines its contractile state. Myosin molecules are oriented in series along the length of the thick filament and are joined "tail to tail" in the filament's center at the "M" line. This orientation produces equivalent shortening of each half of the sarcomere as the actin molecules are pulled toward the center.

The four light chains in the myosin complex are considered regulatory or essential. Regulatory myosin light chains influence myosin–actin interaction by modulating Ca^{2+}-dependent protein kinase phosphorylation. The role of essential light chains is unclear, but genetic modification may form the basis of reduced contractile function in some disease states. Thick filaments are composed of myosin, its binding protein, and titin, which is a long elastic molecule that attaches myosin to the "Z" lines. Titin is an essential contributor to myocardial elasticity and acts as a length sensor (like a bidirectional spring) by creating progressively larger restoring forces as the sarcomere approaches its maximum or minimum length.[19] Thus, titin compression and stretching are observed during decreases and increases in load that serve to limit additional shortening and lengthening of the sarcomere. Titin's elasticity is an important regulator of the stress–strain behavior of cardiac muscle.

Actin is the major component of the thin filament and is composed of an oval-shaped, globular protein. Actin exists in a polymerized filamentous configuration wound in double-stranded helical chains of monomers that resemble two intertwined strands of pearls. A single helix of actin contains 14 monomers and is 77 nm in length. Actin does not directly hydrolyze high-energy phosphates. Instead, it binds adenosine diphosphate (ADP) and divalent cations including Ca^{2+} and Mg^{2+}. Actin functions as the *activ*ator of myosin ATPase through its reversible binding with myosin. The actin–myosin complex hydrolyzes ATP, supplying the energy needed to cause conformational changes in the myosin heads during contraction and relaxation. Tropomyosin is a major inhibitor of the interaction between actin and myosin. This protein contains a rigid double-stranded alpha-helix protein linked by a single disulfide bond. Human tropomyosin has alpha and beta isoforms.[20] A Ca^{2+}-dependent interaction of tropomyosin with the troponin complex is the mechanism by which excitation–contraction coupling occurs, that is, the relationship between sarcolemma depolarization and the resultant binding of actin and myosin responsible for contraction. Tropomyosin also stiffens the thin filament because of its position within the longitudinal cleft between the interwoven helices (Fig. 12-10). Cytoskeletal proteins (e.g., actinin, nebulette) anchor the thin filaments to the sarcomere's "Z" lines.

The troponin complex contains three proteins that regulate the contractile apparatus, each of which serves a distinct role. Troponin complexes are interspersed at 40-nm intervals along the thin filament. A highly conserved, single isoform of troponin C (named for its *Ca*$^{2+}$ binding ability) is present in cardiac muscle. Troponin C is composed of a central nine-turn alpha helix separating two globular regions that contain four discrete divalent cation-binding amino acid sequences, two of which are Ca^{2+}-specific. The troponin C molecule responds directly to the changes in intracellular Ca^{2+} concentration. Troponin I is the primary inhibitor of actin–myosin binding when combined with tropomyosin. This

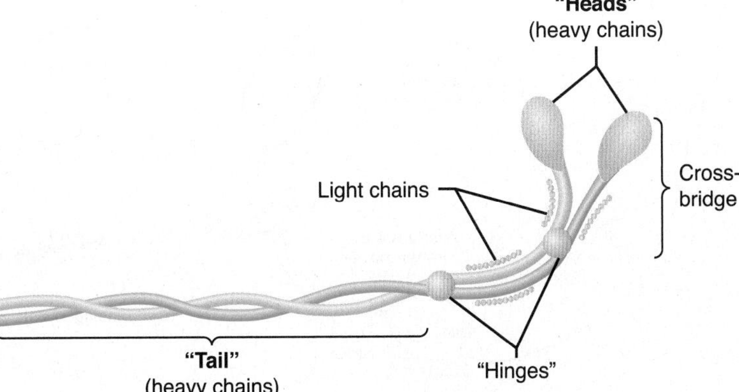

Figure 12-9 Schematic illustration of the myosin molecule demonstrating the double helix tail, globular heads that form cross-bridges with actin during contraction, two pairs of light chains, and "hinges" (cleavage sites of proteolytic enzymes) that divide the molecule into meromyosin fragments (see text).

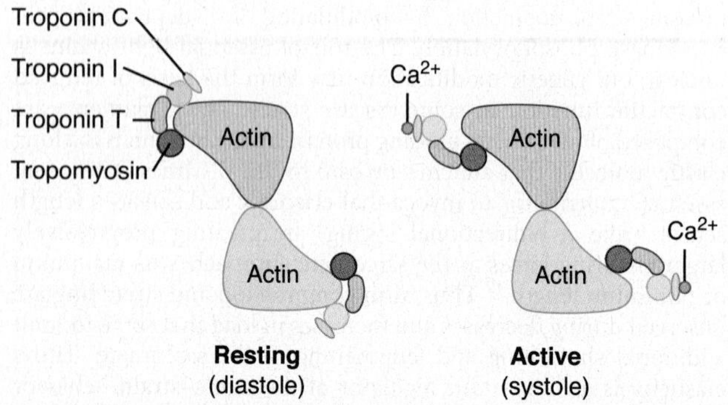

Figure 12-10 Cross-sectional schematic illustration demonstrating the structural relationship between the troponin-tropomyosin complex and actin under resting conditions (**left panel**) and after Ca^{2+} binding to troponin C (**right panel**, see text).

inhibition is responsive to receptor-operated signal transduction, as the troponin I molecule contains a serine residue that is susceptible to protein kinase A–mediated phosphorylation through cyclic adenosine monophosphate (cAMP). Phosphorylation of this serine residue reduces the ability of troponin C to bind Ca^{2+}, an action that facilitates relaxation during administration of a beta-adrenoceptor agonist or phosphodiesterase fraction III inhibitor. Troponin T (binds to other *t*roponin molecules and *t*ropomyosin) is the largest troponin protein. Troponin T is an anchor for the other troponin molecules and influences the relative Ca^{2+} sensitivity of troponin C.[21]

Ca^{2+}-Myofilament Interaction

Ca^{2+}-troponin C binding produces a series of conformational changes in the troponin–tropomyosin complex that expose the myosin-binding site on actin. Small amounts of Ca^{2+} are bound to troponin C when the intracellular Ca^{2+} concentration is low (10^{-7} M) during diastole. The troponin complex confines each tropomyosin molecule to the outer region of the groove between actin filaments and prevents myosin–actin interaction by inhibiting cross-bridge formation. This resting inhibitory state is reversed by the 100-fold increase in intracellular Ca^{2+} concentration (to 10^{-5} M) that results from sarcolemmal depolarization, which opens L- and T-type Ca^{2+} channels, allows Ca^{2+} influx from the extracellular space, and stimulates ryanodine receptor-mediated Ca^{2+}-induced Ca^{2+} release from the SR. The Ca^{2+} binding to troponin C that occurs during these conditions elongates the troponin C protein and enhances its interactions with troponin T and I. These allosteric modifications weaken the interaction between troponin I and actin, promote repositioning of the tropomyosin molecule relative to actin, and minimize the inhibition of actin–myosin binding by tropomyosin. As a result, the binding of Ca^{2+} to troponin C causes the myosin-binding site on the actin molecule to be exposed, which facilitates cross-bridge formation. Subsequent dissociation of Ca^{2+} from troponin C reverses this process, preventing further myosin–actin interaction by restoring of the original conformation of the troponin–tropomyosin complex on actin.

An energy-dependent ion pump located in the SR membrane (sarcoendoplasmic reticulum Ca^{2+}-ATPase; SERCA) removes the vast majority of Ca^{2+} ions from the myofilaments and the myoplasm when the sarcolemma repolarizes. This Ca^{2+} is stored in the SR at a concentration of approximately 10^{-3} M bound to calsequestrin and calreticulin until the next sarcolemma depolarization occurs. Another Ca^{2+}-ATPase and the Na^+/Ca^{2+} exchanger, each located in the sarcolemmal membrane, also play roles in the removal of Ca^{2+} from the myoplasm after repolarization. Phospholamban in the SR membrane modulates the activity of SERCA by partially inhibiting this Ca^{2+} pump. Phosphorylation of phospholamban by protein kinase A antagonizes this inhibition and enhances SERCA-mediated Ca^{2+} uptake into the SR.[22] Dobutamine and milrinone act by modifying protein kinase A–mediated signal transduction to enhance the rate and extent of relaxation by facilitating Ca^{2+} reuptake (lusitropic effect), while simultaneously increasing the amount of Ca^{2+} available for contraction (inotropic effect).

Myosin–Actin Interaction

The biochemistry of contraction is usually described using a four-component model (Fig. 12-11). Binding of ATP to the catalytic

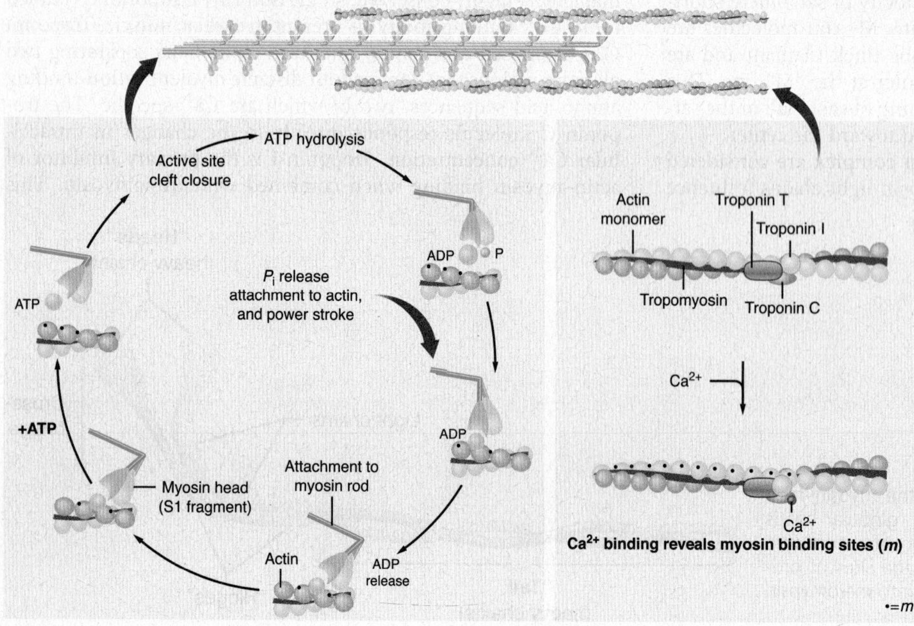

Figure 12-11 Schematic illustration of the actin filaments and their individual monomers and active myosin bindings sites (*m*; **left panel**). The myosin head is dissociated from actin by binding with adenosine triphosphate (ATP). Subsequent ATP hydrolysis and release of inorganic phosphate (P_i) "cocks" the head group into a tension-generating configuration. Attachment of the myosin head to actin allows the head to apply tension to the myosin rod and the actin filament. The **right panel** illustrates Ca^{2+} binding to troponin C, which causes troponin I to decrease its affinity for actin. As a result of the conformational shift in tropomyosin position (see text), seven sites on actin monomers are revealed.

domain of myosin starts a sequence of events that causes sarcomere shortening. Myosin ATPase hydrolyzes ATP into ADP and inorganic phosphate. These products remain bound to myosin, forming an active complex that retains the potential energy released by the hydrolysis reaction. In the absence of actin, ADP and phosphate eventually dissociate from myosin, and the muscle remains relaxed. However, when the myosin–ADP–phosphate complex is bound to actin, myosin ATPase activity is markedly enhanced, and the energy released by ATP hydrolysis is translated into mechanical work. First, myosin binding to actin releases the phosphate anion from the myosin head, producing a tension-inducing conformation within the cross-bridge. Next, release of ADP and potential energy from this activated orientation combine to rotate the cross-bridge at the hinge point separating the helical tail from the globular head of myosin (commonly known as the power stroke). Each cross-bridge rotation generates 3.5×10^{-12} newtons of force and moves myosin 11 nm along the actin molecule.[23] The myosin–actin complex does not immediately dissociate after rotation but remains in a low-energy bound (rigor) state. Finally, dissociation of the myosin and actin molecules occurs when a new ATP molecule binds to myosin. This process is then repeated, provided that ATP is present and the myosin-binding site on actin is not inhibited by the troponin–tropomyosin complex.

Several factors affect cross-bridge biochemistry and the sarcomere shortening that it produces. There is a direct relationship between the maximal velocity of unloaded muscle shortening (V_{max}) and myosin ATPase activity. The 100-fold increase in intracellular Ca^{2+} concentration associated with sarcolemmal depolarization enhances myosin ATPase activity by a factor of five before it interacts with actin, which increases V_{max}. The extent of sarcomere shortening during contraction is also dependent on sarcomere length before sarcolemmal depolarization. This length-dependent activation of the sarcomere forms the basis of the Frank–Starling principle in the intact heart and may be related to an increase in myofilament Ca^{2+} sensitivity, more optimal spacing between actin and myosin, or titin-induced elastic recoil. Abrupt increases in load during shortening (Anrep effect) or after an extended pause between contractions (Woodworth phenomenon) cause a transient rise in contractile force through this length-dependent activation mechanism. An increase in stimulation frequency also augments shortening through enhanced myofilament Ca^{2+} sensitivity and more pronounced release of Ca^{2+} from the SR.

Laplace's Law

The relationship between myocyte length and chamber volume (V) may be modeled as a pressurized, spherical shell, where volume is proportional to the cube of the radius (r): $V = 4\pi r^3/3$
7 (Fig. 12-12, Video 12-1). The relationship between wall stress (defined as tension exerted over a cross-sectional area) and pressure within a cardiac chamber is complex. Laplace's law relates wall stress to pressure and chamber geometry based on three fundamental assumptions[24]: (1) the chamber is spherical with a uniform wall thickness (h) and an internal radius (r); (2) the stress (σ) throughout the thickness of the chamber wall is constant; and (3) the chamber is in static equilibrium, that is, it is not actively contracting. Tension development within each sarcomere causes a corresponding increase in wall stress that is translated into the generation of pressure (P) within the chamber. The pressure is defined as a perpendicular distending force exerted against the chamber walls, whereas wall stress is the force exerted around the circumference of the chamber that resists this distention. Bisecting the chamber into two equal halves exposes the forces within it. The product of pressure and wall cross-sectional area (πr^2) represents the total force pushing chamber hemispheres apart. The force within the chamber walls resisting this distracting force is equal to σ times the cross-sectional wall area. The two forces must balance for the chamber to remain in equilibrium: $P\pi r^2 = \sigma[\pi(r + h)^2 - \pi r^2]$. Elimination of the redundant terms simplifies this equation: $Pr = \sigma h(2 + h/r)$. The chamber wall is thin relative to its internal radius. As a result, the h/r term may be neglected, and the remaining expression is easily rearranged to become: $\sigma = Pr/2h$. Thus, Laplace's law for a thin-walled, static sphere indicates that wall stress varies directly with internal pressure and radius and inversely with wall thickness.

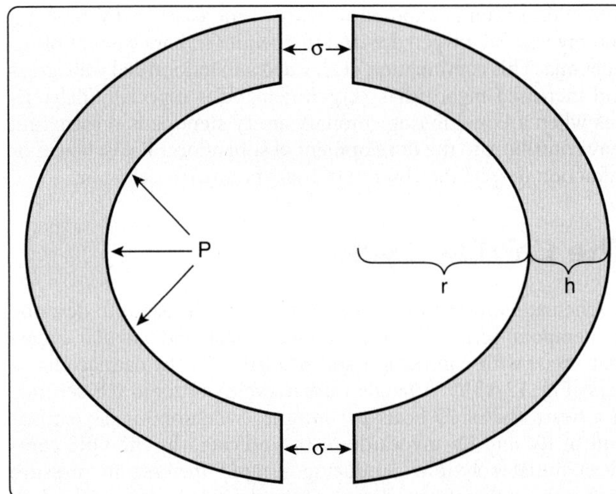

Figure 12-12 This schematic diagram depicts the opposing forces within a theoretical left ventricular (LV) sphere that determine the Law of Laplace. LV pressure (P) pushes the sphere apart, whereas wall stress (σ) holds the sphere together. R, LV radius; h, LV thickness. (Reproduced with permission from Kaplan JA, Augoustides JGT, Manecke Jr GR, et al. *Kaplan's Cardiac Anesthesia: For Cardiac and Noncardiac Anesthesia*. 7th ed. Elsevier; 2017:150; permission conveyed from Copyright Clearance Center, Inc. (Figure 6-6))

Laplace's law provides a powerful description of the factors that contribute to changes in LV stress, despite its simplifying assumptions. For example, LV dilation (increased r) associated with chronic aortic valve insufficiency increases diastolic LV wall stress and reflects greater tension on each sarcomere within the chamber wall. Analogously, the elevated LV pressure in severe aortic valve stenosis produces greater systolic LV wall stress. These increases in LV wall stress cause parallel increases in myocardial oxygen demand because the myofilaments require more energy to develop enhanced tension. Conversely, Laplace's law indicates that an increase in wall thickness will reduce wall stress and tension developed by individual sarcomeres. As a result, hypertrophy is an important compensatory adaptation to chronically altered chamber load that serves to reduce the tension and myocardial oxygen demand. Prolate ellipsoidal models of chamber geometry and those incorporating radial, circumferential, and meridional components of wall stress require more complex derivations of Laplace's law. Formal derivations of these models are available elsewhere.[25] Despite their complexity, the principles linking changes in length and tension in the sarcomere to pressure, volume, and wall thickness in the intact heart are consistently shown in these models.

It is noteworthy that wall stress is not uniformly distributed across LV thickness in the intact heart; it is greatest in the subendocardium and progressively declines toward the epicardial surface. Regional differences in wall stress are particularly important in LV pressure-overload hypertrophy, a condition in which the subendocardium is exposed to marked increases in LV pressure and myocardial oxygen demand that render it more susceptible to ischemia. This combination of elevated subendocardial wall stress and increased myocardial oxygen demand is especially deleterious when a flow-limiting coronary artery stenosis is present and may contribute to the development of subendocardial ischemia or infarction despite the absence of frank coronary occlusion.

The Cardiac Cycle

8 A schematic illustration of the cardiac cycle is useful to describe the temporal series of electrical, mechanical, and valvular events that occur with contraction and relaxation of the cardiac chambers (Fig. 12-13).[26] A single cardiac cycle occurs in 0.8 seconds at a heart rate of 75 beats per minute. Synchronous depolarization of RV and LV myocardium (as indicated by the QRS complex) initiates systole, producing a rapid increase in pressure within these chambers. Closure of the tricuspid and mitral valves occurs when RV and LV pressures exceed the corresponding atrial

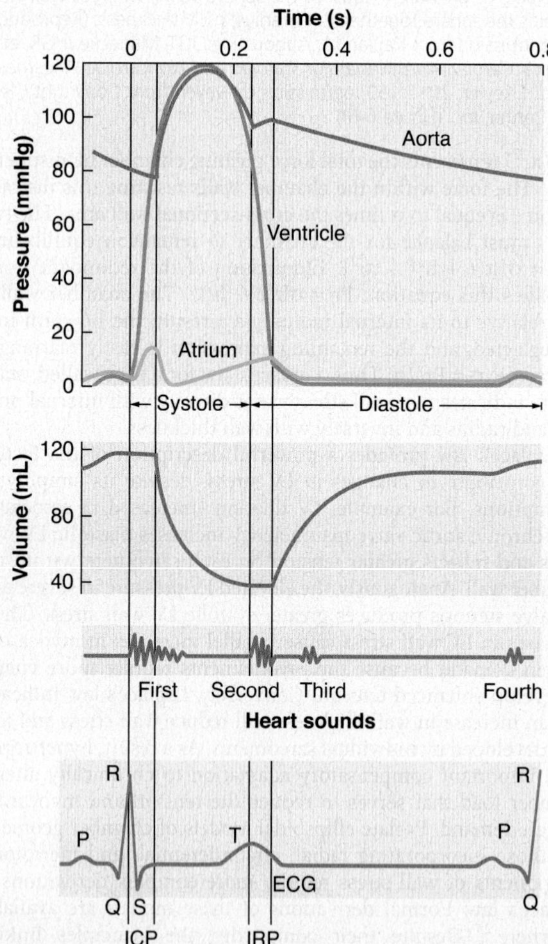

Figure 12-13 Mechanical and electrical events of the cardiac cycle showing also the left ventricular (LV) volume curve and the heart sounds. Note the LV isovolumic contraction (ICP) and the relaxation period (IRP) during which there is no change in LV volume because aortic and mitral valves are closed. The LV decreases in volume as it ejects its contents into the aorta. During the first third of systolic ejection (the rapid ejection period), the curve of emptying is steep. ECG, electrocardiogram.

pressures and causes the first heart sound (S_1). The first phase of LV systole is isovolumic contraction, which describes the time interval between mitral valve closure and aortic valve opening during which LV volume remains constant. This event is somewhat analogous to isometric (constant length) contraction of isolated cardiac muscle. The LV is transformed from an ellipsoidal shape at end diastole to a more spherical geometry during isovolumic contraction because the longitudinal axis shortens and LV wall thickness increases. The maximum rate of increase of LV pressure (dP/dt_{max}) occurs during LV isovolumic contraction and is an index of myocardial contractility. True isovolumic contraction does not occur in the RV because of the sequential nature of contraction of the inflow and outflow tracts. The pressure in the aortic root falls to its minimum value immediately before the aortic valve opens. Rapid ejection occurs when LV pressure exceeds aortic pressure. Approximately two-thirds of the LV end-diastolic volume is ejected during this rapid ejection phase. Dilation of the elastic aorta and proximal great vessels occurs with this rapid increase in volume as the kinetic energy of LV contraction is transferred to the aorta as potential energy. The compliance of the proximal arterial vessels determines the magnitude of this potential energy that is stored and subsequently released to its distal vascular bed during diastole. Further ejection of additional blood from the LV slows precipitously as the pressure within the aorta reaches its maximum. Ejection stops entirely when the LV begins to repolarize and the arterial force resisting further ejection is greater than the ventricular force continuing to propel blood forward. Similar events occur in the RV and pulmonary artery during systole. As the period of slower ejection comes to an end, aortic and pulmonary artery pressures exceed LV and RV pressures, respectively. These pressure gradients cause the aortic and pulmonic valves to shut, causing the second heart sound (S_2). This event signifies the beginning of diastole. The aortic valve closes slightly before the pulmonic valve during inspiration because RV ejection is modestly prolonged by augmented venous return. This temporal discrepancy between aortic and pulmonic valve closure produces a "split" S_2 heart sound. The normal end-diastolic and end-systolic volumes (V_{ed} and V_{es}) are approximately 120 and 40 mL, respectively. Thus, SV (the difference between V_{ed} and V_{es}) is 80 mL and EF (the ratio of SV to V_{ed}) is 67%.

LV diastole is divided into four phases: isovolumic relaxation, early ventricular filling, diastasis, and atrial systole. LV isovolumic relaxation defines the period between aortic valve closure and mitral valve opening during which LV volume remains constant. LV pressure falls very rapidly as the myofilaments relax. When LV pressure falls below LA pressure, the mitral valve opens, and blood volume stored in the LA enters the LV driven by the pressure gradient between the chambers (Fig. 12-14). LV pressure continues to fall below LA pressure after mitral valve opening as sarcomere relaxation is completed and myocardial elastic components recoil.[27] These factors contribute to the creation of a sustained pressure gradient between the LA and LV that extends from the base to the apex. The rate and extent of LV pressure decline together with the LA pressure when the mitral valve opens determine the magnitude and duration of the pressure gradient between the chambers. Early LV filling occurs rapidly, as indicated by the observation that the peak blood flow velocity across the mitral valve during this phase of diastole often exceeds the flow rate across the aortic valve during LV ejection.[28] Vortex formation created by the primary mitral blood flow jet also facilitates selective filling of the LV outflow tract.[29] A delay in LV relaxation may occur due to age or disease (e.g., myocardial ischemia, hypertrophy) and is a common cause of blunted early LV filling because the initial LA–LV pressure gradient is reduced. After the mitral valve opens, the pressure gradient between the LA and the LV

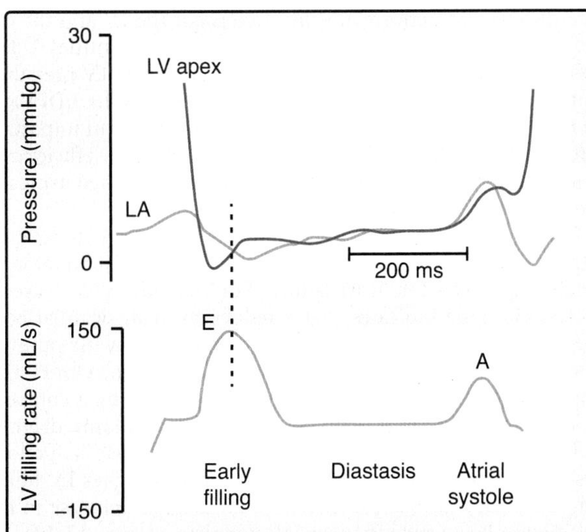

Figure 12-14 This diagram depicts the relationship between left ventricular (LV) and left atrial (LA) pressure (**top panel**) and the corresponding LV filling rate (**bottom panel**) during early filling (E), diastasis, and atrial systole (A). Note that LV pressure initially falls below LA pressure, thereby creating a pressure gradient between the chambers that causes early LV filling. (Reproduced with permission from Kaplan JA, Augoustides JGT, Manecke Jr GR, et al. *Kaplan's Cardiac Anesthesia: For Cardiac and Noncardiac Anesthesia*. 7th ed. Elsevier; 2017:151; permission conveyed from Copyright Clearance Center, Inc. (Figure 6-8))

is dependent on the relative pressure within each chamber. Most of the increase in LV volume observed during early ventricular filling occurs while LV pressure continues to fall. LV pressure will decrease to a subatmospheric level even if blood flow across the mitral valve is completely obstructed,[3] indicating that the LV continues to fill through this diastolic suction mechanism when LA pressure is zero.[30] Diastolic suction preserves early LV filling during profound hypovolemia and strenuous exercise. The early filling phase of diastole normally provides 70% to 75% of the total SV ejected during the next LV contraction. Early LV filling ends when LA and LV pressures equalize or the gradient between these chambers transiently reverses. The mitral valve then remains open and pulmonary venous blood flows directly through the LA into the LV. As a result, the LA is a conduit during diastasis. The small amount of blood flow from pulmonary veins occurring during diastasis usually adds less than 5% to the total LV stroke volume. Progressive increases in heart rate shorten and eventually eliminate diastasis.

Atrial systole is the final phase of diastole. LA contraction increases the pressure in this chamber, which creates a second positive pressure gradient for blood flow from the LA and the LV. The peristaltic pattern of LA contraction and the unique anatomy of the pulmonary venous–LA junction largely prevent retrograde blood flow into the pulmonary veins during atrial systole when LA pressures are not elevated. Atrial systole usually accounts for between 15% and 25% of total LV stroke volume. Atrial systole becomes more important to the maintenance of LV filling in pathologic states characterized by delayed LV relaxation or reduced LV compliance. Improperly timed LA contraction or atrial tachyarrhythmias may cause profound hemodynamic compromise in patients who are particularly dependent on atrial systole for LV filling (e.g., acute myocardial ischemia, pressure-overload hypertrophy). RV diastole has similar characteristics to LV diastole with the exception that true isovolumic relaxation does not occur in the RV.

The LA pressure waveform is composed of three major deflections during sinus rhythm. The LA contracts immediately after the P wave of atrial depolarization, producing the "a" wave of atrial systole. This "a" wave may be enhanced by an increase in LA preload or contractile state. The rate of decline of the "a" wave is an index of LA relaxation.[31] LV contraction with the onset of systole causes a pressure wave to be transmitted to the LA in retrograde fashion by closure of the mitral valve, resulting in a small increase in LA pressure ("c" wave). During late LV isovolumic contraction, LV ejection, and the majority of LV isovolumic relaxation, pulmonary venous blood progressively fills the LA and gradually increases LA pressure, resulting in the LA "v" wave. This "v" wave may be enhanced in the presence of mitral regurgitation or reductions in LA compliance. RA pressure waveform deflections are very similar to those observed in the LA. The RA "a-c-v" waveform morphology is transmitted to the jugular veins and may be observed in the neck during physical examination in the supine position. In contrast to the biphasic LA pressure waveform, the LA volume waveform is monophasic. Minimum LA volume occurs immediately after the completion of LA contraction and corresponds closely to the mitral valve closure, whereas maximal LA volume is observed immediately before the mitral valve opens.

Pressure–Volume Diagrams

9

A time-dependent, two-dimensional plot of continuous LV pressure and volume during a single cardiac cycle creates a phase space diagram that provides a useful framework for the analysis of LV systolic and diastolic function (Fig. 12-15). Otto Frank initially described the theoretical foundations of this technique at the end of the 19th century.[32,33] In the 1970s, Hiroyuki Suga and Kiichi Sagawa were the first to widely apply pressure–volume analysis after technologic advances enabled the measurement of high-fidelity LV pressure and continuous LV volume.[34–36] Temporal changes in LV pressure with respect to volume are projected in a counterclockwise fashion. The cardiac cycle begins at end diastole (point A, Fig. 12-15). An abrupt increase in LV pressure at constant LV volume occurs during isovolumic contraction. Opening of the aortic valve occurs when LV pressure exceeds aorta pressure (point B, Fig. 12-15) and ejection begins. LV volume decreases rapidly as blood is ejected from the LV into the aorta and proximal great vessels. When LV pressure declines below aortic pressure at the end of ejection, the aortic valve closes (point C, Fig. 12-15). This event is immediately followed by a rapid decline in LV pressure in the absence of changes in LV volume (isovolumic relaxation). The mitral valve opens when LV pressure falls below LA pressure (point D, Fig. 12-15), which initiates LV filling. The LV pressure–volume diagram is completed as the LV refills its volume for the next contraction in conjunction with modest increases in pressure during early filling, diastasis, and LA systole (2 Video 12-2).

The steady-state LV pressure–volume diagram provides advantages over plots of individual LV pressure and volume waveforms when identifying major cardiac events without electrocardiographic correlation (e.g., aortic or mitral valve opening or closure) or evaluating acute alterations in LV loading conditions. For example, the lower right (point A) and upper left (point C) corners of the diagram identify V_{ed} and V_{es}, respectively, allowing rapid calculation of SV and EF. Rightward movement of the right side of the pressure–volume diagram is characteristic of an increase in preload and greater SV, whereas an increase in afterload causes the pressure–volume diagram to become taller (greater LV pressure) and narrower (decreased SV). The area of

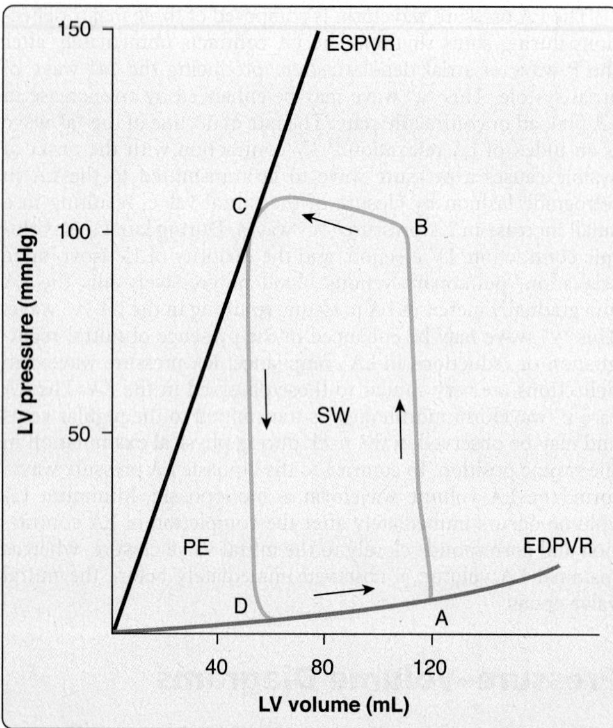

Figure 12-15 This illustration depicts the steady-state left ventricular (LV) pressure–volume diagram. The cardiac cycle proceeds in a time-dependent counterclockwise direction (*arrows*). Points A, B, C, and D correspond to LV end diastole (closure of the mitral valve), opening of the aortic valve, LV end systole (closure of the aortic valve), and opening of the mitral valve, respectively. Segments AB, BC, CD, and DA represent isovolumic contraction, ejection, isovolumic relaxation, and filling, respectively. The LV is constrained to operate within the boundaries of the end-systolic and end-diastolic pressure–volume relations (ESPVR and EDPVR, respectively). The area inscribed by the LV pressure–volume diagram is stroke work (SW) performed during the cardiac cycle. The area to the left of the LV pressure–volume diagram between ESPVR and EDPVR is the remaining potential energy (PE) of the system. (Reproduced with permission from Kaplan JA, Augoustides JGT, Manecke Jr GR, et al. *Kaplan's Cardiac Anesthesia: For Cardiac and Noncardiac Anesthesia*. 7th ed. Elsevier; 2017:152; permission conveyed from Copyright Clearance Center, Inc. (Figure 6-9))

the diagram defines the LV pressure–volume work (stroke work) for a single cardiac cycle. A series of differentially loaded LV pressure–volume diagrams can be produced by transient changes in preload or afterload with mechanical or pharmacologic interventions. This nested set of diagrams allows calculation of relatively heart rate- and load-insensitive estimates of myocardial contractility, including the slope of the end-systolic pressure-volume relation (ESPVR; the slope of this relation is termed end-systolic elastance, E_{es}) and the stroke work-end-diastolic volume relation (a linear Frank-Starling analog also known as "preload recruitable stroke work").[36,37] The family of pressure–volume diagrams also describes the end-diastolic pressure–volume relationship (EDPVR) that characterizes LV compliance, which is a major determinant of LV filling.[24] The LV operates within the constraints of these end-systolic and end-diastolic pressure–volume relations. The ESPVR and the EDPVR are determined by the intrinsic properties of the LV, but the relative positions of the end-diastolic and end-systolic points that lie along these lines for any given cardiac cycle are established primarily by venous return (preload) and arterial tone (afterload). The model emphasizes that analysis of cardiovascular performance must consider the LV and the circulation with which it interacts as interdependent entities.[38] The triangular-shaped area to the left of the steady-state LV pressure–volume diagram that lies between the ESPVR and the EDPVR is the remaining potential energy of the system and is an important factor in determining LV energetics and mechanical efficiency.[39] RV systolic and diastolic function also may be quantified using the principles of this pressure–volume theory.

Pressure–volume analysis also provides a useful illustration of the pathophysiology of LV systolic or diastolic dysfunction as underlying causes for heart failure. For example, a decrease in the ESPVR slope indicates that a reduction in myocardial contractility has occurred. This finding is consistent with pure LV systolic dysfunction and may be observed in patients with HFrEF (Fig. 12-16). Such an event is often accompanied by a compensatory LV dilation (movement of the pressure–volume diagram to the right) along a normal EDPVR. This increase in preload preserves SV and CO but occurs at the cost of higher LV filling and pulmonary venous pressures. In contrast, an increase in the EDPVR implies a reduction in LV compliance (Fig. 12-13). As a result, the LV cannot completely fill without higher LV end-diastolic pressure. This finding is indicative of diastolic dysfunction and is a characteristic feature of heart failure with preserved ejection fraction (HFpEF). Myocardial contractility may remain relatively normal in HFpEF, but LV filling pressures are elevated, which produces pulmonary venous congestion and clinical symptoms. Simultaneous depression of the ESPVR and elevation of the EDPVR indicate the presence of both LV systolic and diastolic dysfunction. These findings are often encountered in HFrEF. Stroke volume and CO may be severely reduced because compensatory changes in preload or afterload, represented by movement of the steady-state LV pressure–volume diagram within the ESPVR and the EDPVR boundaries, are limited.

The pressure–volume plane may be extrapolated to a single region or dimension of the LV. For example, ultrasonic transducers placed within the LV wall may be used to measure changes in segment length, LV diameter, or wall thickness. The time for ultrasound to be transmitted between a pair of these transducers is directly proportional to the length between them. Segment length or LV diameter normally increases during diastole and shortens during systole analogous to changes in continuous LV volume, whereas reciprocal changes in wall thickness are observed. Acute changes in LV loading conditions produce a set of diagrams for measurement of LV end-systolic and end-diastolic pressure-segment length, -diameter, or -wall thickness relationships. The use of regional versus global LV pressure–volume analysis is advantageous when studying the effects of myocardial ischemia. Acute coronary artery occlusion causes a time-dependent collapse of the steady-state LV pressure–length diagram in the central ischemic zone consistent with a rapid decline (hypokinesis) and eventual absence of regional stroke work (akinesis). The LV pressure–segment length diagram tilts to the right in a border zone surrounding a central ischemic region. Three regions in this diagram can be identified that correspond to systolic lengthening (paroxysmal systolic aneurysmal bulging of the ischemic zone), postsystolic shortening (shortening in the ischemic zone that occurs after ejection as a result of tethering to adjacent normal myocardium), and a variable area between the two that makes a contribution to regional stroke work (Fig. 12-17). These parameters can be used to quantify the relative severity of regional myocardial ischemia.[40]

Pressure–volume analysis also may be applied to the study of atrial function. The steady-state LA pressure–volume diagram is composed of two intersecting loops arranged in a horizontal "infinity" pattern that incorporates active ("A" loop) and passive

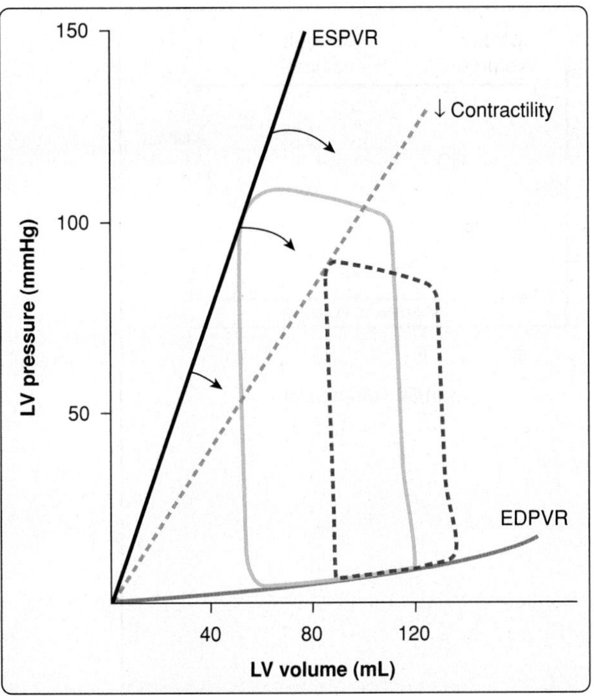

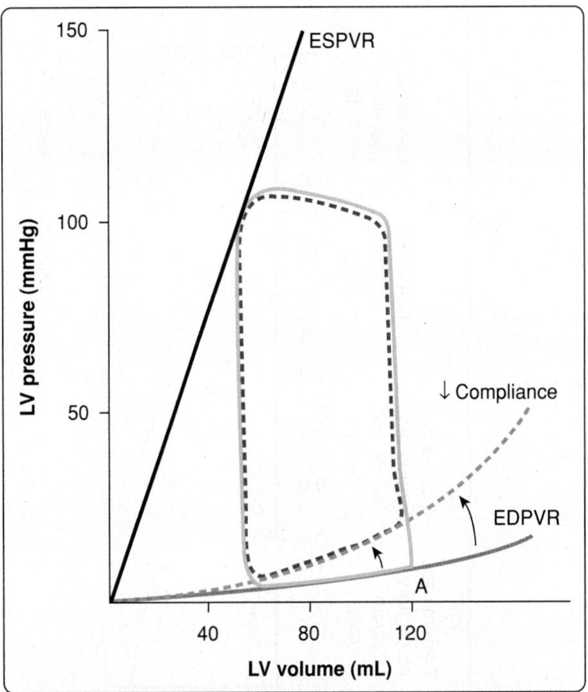

Figure 12-16 These schematic illustrations demonstrate alterations in the steady-state left ventricular (LV) pressure–volume diagram produced by a reduction in myocardial contractility as indicated by a decrease in the slope of the end-systolic pressure–volume relation (ESPVR; **left panel**) and a decrease in LV compliance as indicated by an increase in the position of the end-diastolic pressure–volume relation (EDPVR; **right panel**). These diagrams emphasize that heart failure may result from LV systolic or diastolic dysfunction independently. (Reproduced with permission from Kaplan JA, Augoustides JGT, Manecke Jr GR, et al. *Kaplan's Cardiac Anesthesia: For Cardiac and Noncardiac Anesthesia*. 7th ed. Elsevier; 2017:154; permission conveyed from Copyright Clearance Center, Inc. (Figure 6-11))

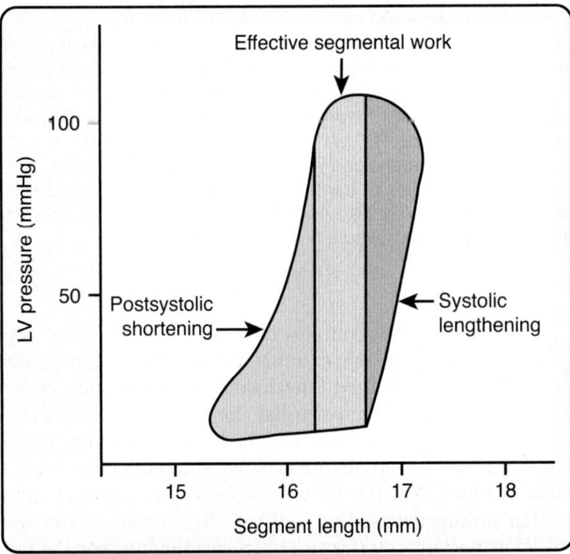

Figure 12-17 This figure depicts a steady-state left ventricular (LV) pressure–segment length diagram measured within the border zone of the central ischemia region during acute occlusion of the left anterior descending coronary artery. Areas of systolic lengthening (**right side of diagram**) and postsystolic shortening (**left side of diagram**) produced by partial ischemia and tethering to the central ischemia zone do not contribute to segmental work, but a small area of the diagram (**center**) demonstrates effective segment shortening that contributes to global LV stroke work. (Reproduced with permission from Kaplan JA, Augoustides JGT, Manecke Jr GR, et al. *Kaplan's Cardiac Anesthesia: For Cardiac and Noncardiac Anesthesia*. 7th ed. Elsevier; 2017:156; permission conveyed from Copyright Clearance Center, Inc. (Figure 6-13).)

("V" loop) components (Fig. 12-18).[41] The shape of the LA pressure–volume diagram derives from the biphasic morphology of the LA pressure waveform. Beginning at LA end diastole (corresponding to the end of LV diastasis), the active component of the diagram traces a counterclockwise outline as the LA ejects its contents into the LV. LA end systole (corresponding to LV end diastole) marks the end of atrial contraction and is defined by minimum LA volume. Identification of LA end diastole and end systole on the diagram facilitates calculation of LA emptying fraction (analogous to LV EF). After the mitral valve closes, LA filling occurs throughout LV systole and isovolumic relaxation. LA pressure and volume gradually increase during this reservoir phase, forming the bottom part of the "A" loop and the upper part of the "V" loop. The area of the "A" loop represents active LA stroke work. The passive component ("V" loop) of the LA pressure–volume diagram proceeds in a clockwise direction. Total LA reservoir volume is determined from the steady-state LA pressure–volume diagram as the difference between maximum and minimum LA volumes.[31] The "V" loop area represents the passive energy stored by the LA during the reservoir phase and is an index of reservoir function. The slope of the line between minimum LA pressure of the "A" loop and maximum LA pressure in the "V" loop is an index of LA compliance; regional myocardial ischemia[6] or severe LV dysfunction[42] increase the slope of this line. LA emptying after mitral valve opening causes a rapid decline in LA volume that forms the bottom part of the "V" loop. Additional pulmonary venous return also enters the LA during LV diastasis, but this blood flow does not alter LA volume because the mitral valve is open. Thus, the LA conduit phase is defined between mitral valve opening and LA end diastole, and LA conduit volume is calculated as the difference between maximum and end-diastolic volumes. The interrelationship among LA loading

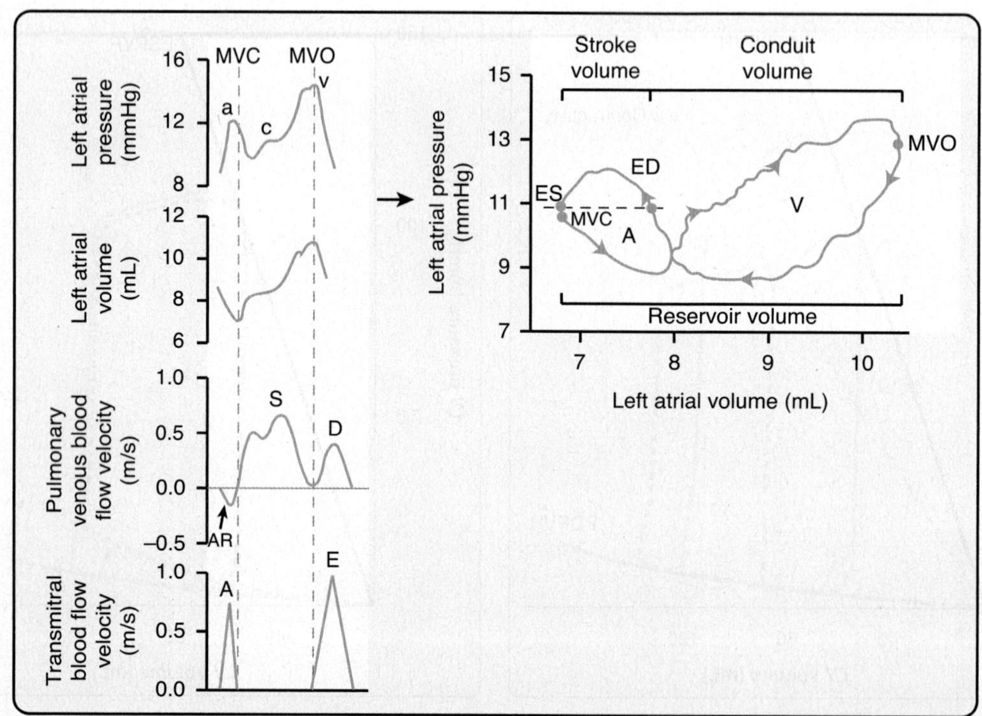

Figure 12-18 Left atrial (LA) pressure and volume waveforms (**left panel**) and the corresponding steady-state LA pressure–volume diagram (**right panel**) inscribed in phase space by these waveforms during a single cardiac cycle. The corresponding schematic pulmonary venous and transmitral blood flow velocity waveforms are also depicted (**left panels**). The "a" wave of LA pressure corresponds to atrial systole, the "c" wave represents the small increase in LA pressure that occurs during early left ventricular (LV) isovolumic contraction, and the "v" wave identifies the increase in LA pressure associated with LA filling. In contrast to this biphasic LA pressure waveform, the morphology of the LA volume waveform is monophasic. The resulting LA pressure–volume diagram is shaped in a horizontal figure-of-eight pattern. The arrows indicate the time-dependent direction of movement around the diagram. The "A" portion of the diagram (**left loop** of the figure of eight) incorporates active LA contraction and temporally proceeds in a counterclockwise fashion. The "V" portion of the diagram (**right loop**) represents passive LA reservoir function and proceeds in a clockwise manner over time. Mitral valve closure and opening (MVC and MVO, respectively) also are depicted on the individual waveforms and the LA pressure–volume diagram. Left atrial end-diastole (ED) is defined as the time point immediately before LA contraction at which LA pressure corresponds to LA end-systolic (ES) pressure (*horizontal dashed line*). LV isovolumic contraction, ejection, and the majority of isovolumic relaxation occur between MVC and MVO illustrated on the LA pressure–volume diagram. The pulmonary venous blood flow velocity waveform consists of an atrial reversal ("AR") wave, a biphasic "S" wave that occurs during LV systole, and a "D" wave that is observed with opening of the mitral valve (see text). The corresponding atrial systole (A) and early LV filling (E) waves of transmitral blood flow velocity are also illustrated. The AR and D waves of pulmonary venous blood flow velocity occur in conjunction with the A and E waves of transmitral blood flow velocity, respectively. (Reproduced with permission from Kaplan JA, Augoustides JGT, Manecke Jr GR, et al. *Kaplan's Cardiac Anesthesia: For Cardiac and Noncardiac Anesthesia*. 7th ed. Elsevier; 2017:157; permission conveyed from Copyright Clearance Center, Inc. (Figure 6-14).)

conditions, LA and LV contractile state, the rate and extent of LA relaxation, LA elastic properties, and pulmonary venous blood flow combine to determine the relative areas of the "A" and "V" loops and the point of intersection between them.[41] Acute alterations in LA loading conditions may be used to assess LA myocardial contractility and dynamic compliance using LA end-systolic and end-reservoir pressure–volume relations.[43]

Determinants of Cardiac Performance

The ability of each cardiac chamber to function as a hydraulic pump depends on how effectively it can collect and eject blood. The authors will focus here on the LV, but the principles that determine LV pump performance are equally applicable to the heart's other chambers. LV systolic function is most often clinically quantified using CO and EF. These variables are dependent on the intrinsic contractile properties of the LV myocardium, the quantity of blood it contains immediately before contraction begins (preload), and the external forces that resist emptying with which it is confronted (afterload). The interaction between preload, afterload, and myocardial contractility establishes the SV (Fig. 12-19). When combined with heart rate and rhythm, preload, afterload, and myocardial contractility determine the volume of blood that the LV is capable of pumping per minute assuming unimpeded venous return. The LV's structural integrity is an important determinant of its systolic function, as mitral or aortic valve disease (e.g., regurgitation) or the presence of an abnormal route of intracardiac blood flow (e.g., ventricular septal defect) reduces effective forward flow. These abnormalities limit the use of SV, CO, and EF as indices of LV systolic function. Pulmonary venous blood flow, LA function, mitral valve dynamics, pericardial restraint, and the active (relaxation) and passive (compliance) properties of the LV during diastole determine its ability to properly fill. LV diastolic function is normal when these factors combine to provide an LV preload that supplies sufficient CO to satisfy cellular metabolism without an elevation in LV end-diastolic pressure (approximately 10 mmHg). In contrast, LA

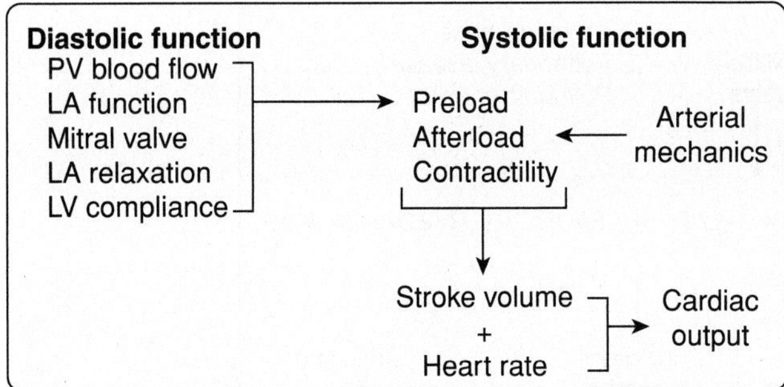

Figure 12-19 This illustration depicts the major factors that determine left ventricular (LV) diastolic (**left**) and systolic (**right**) function. Note that pulmonary venous (PV) blood flow, left atrial (LA) function, mitral valve integrity, LA relaxation, and LV compliance combine to determine LV preload. (Reproduced with permission from Kaplan JA, Augoustides JGT, Manecke Jr GR, et al. *Kaplan's Cardiac Anesthesia: For Cardiac and Noncardiac Anesthesia*. 7th ed. Elsevier; 2017:157; permission conveyed from Copyright Clearance Center, Inc. (Figure 6-15).)

or mitral valve dysfunction, delayed LV relaxation, reduced LV compliance, or increased pericardial pressure may substantially restrict the ability of the LV to properly fill unless LV filling pressures increase. Thus, LV diastolic dysfunction is invariably associated with higher pulmonary venous, LA, and LV end-diastolic pressures.

Heart Rate

An increase in the stimulation frequency of isolated cardiac muscle produces a parallel increase in myocardial contractility. The Bowditch, "staircase," or "treppe" (German for "stair") phenomenon or "force–frequency" relationship has been shown in the isolated and intact LV. Maximal contractile force occurs at 150 to 180 stimulations per minute during isometric contraction of isolated cardiac muscle. The "treppe"-induced increase in LV contractility is essential during strenuous exercise in highly trained athletes by matching CO to venous return at heart rates of approximately 175 beats/min. Contractility deteriorates above this heart rate because the intracellular processes responsible for diastolic Ca^{2+} removal from the contractile apparatus have insufficient time to occur.[44] As a result, hypotension can accompany tachyarrhythmias or rapid pacing. An increase in heart rate within the normal physiologic range has little effect on overall pump performance despite modestly increasing LV contractility; however, tachycardia and its resultant "treppe"-induced enhanced contractility are important compensatory mechanisms that maintain CO when LV filling is restricted (e.g., tamponade). Pressure- or volume-overload hypertrophy decreases the stimulation rate at which the peak "treppe" effect occurs. The phenomenon may be completely abolished in failing myocardium. The force–frequency relationship is also illustrated when a prolonged delay is observed between beats (e.g., AV conduction abnormality) or after an LV extrasystole because the force of the subsequent LV contraction is enhanced. This phenomenon is termed the "interval-strength" effect. A temporal increase in the amount of Ca^{2+} available for contractile activation and an increase in preload resulting from greater diastolic filling are most likely responsible for this effect.

Preload

Preload is conventionally defined as sarcomere length imme-
10 diately before the onset of myocyte contraction. Alternatively,
it may be described by the degree of muscle stretch applied to isolated cardiac muscle before it is stimulated to contract. These definitions may be adequate in the laboratory setting, however, in the intact heart, preload is more difficult to define because of the dynamic, three-dimensional changes in geometry that occur in each chamber throughout the cardiac cycle. As a result, preload is most often described as the volume of blood contained within each chamber at its end diastole[§]. This blood volume effectively determines the length of each myocyte immediately before isovolumic contraction and is related to LV end-diastolic wall stress. Precise real-time measurement of continuous LV volume throughout the cardiac cycle (including left ventricular volume at end diastole, LV V_{ed}) remains a technically challenging problem. Experimental methods used to measure LV V_{ed} (e.g., sonomicrometry, conductance catheter) are very precise but impractical because they require invasive instrumentation.[45] Noninvasive methods including radionuclide angiography or cardiac magnetic resonance imaging (MRI) may also be used to measure LV V_{ed}, but these imaging techniques cannot be used in the operating room or intensive care unit. Cardiac anesthesiologists usually rely on two- or three-dimensional transesophageal echocardiography (TEE) to facilitate real-time estimates of preload during surgery, but even these techniques may be difficult to apply during rapidly changing hemodynamic conditions. The transgastric LV midpapillary short-axis TEE view is particularly useful for measuring LV end-diastolic area or diameter as a surrogate marker of preload.

LV preload may be estimated using a variety of other methods, each of which has inherent limitations (Fig. 12-20). LV end-diastolic pressure may be measured invasively in the cardiac catheterization laboratory or during surgery by advancing a fluid-filled or pressure transducer–tipped catheter from the aorta across the aortic valve or through the LA across the mitral valve. LV end-diastolic pressure is related to V_{ed} based on the exponential EDPVR. Anesthesiologists most often use other estimates of LV V_{ed} that are dependent on measurements obtained "upstream" from the LV including mean LA, pulmonary capillary occlusion, pulmonary arterial diastolic, and RA (central venous) pressures. These estimates of LV V_{ed} are affected by functional integrity of the structures that separate each measurement location from the LV itself. For example, a correlation between RA and LV end-diastolic pressures assumes that the fluid column between the RA and LV has not been adversely influenced by pulmonary disease, airway pressure, RV or pulmonary vascular pathology, LA dysfunction, mitral valve abnormalities, or LV compliance. This assumption is reasonable in healthy subjects but may not be true in patients with significant pulmonary or cardiac disease. The correlation among LV V_{ed}, pulmonary capillary occlusion pressure, and RA pressure is notoriously poor in patients with LV systolic dysfunction, and measurement of such pressures "upstream" from the LV is of limited utility in the assessment of LV preload under such circumstances. In the remainder of this chapter, the terms "preload" and "end-diastolic volume" will be used synonymously.

Afterload

Afterload is the additional load to which myocardium is exposed immediately after contraction begins. This definition of afterload is clear and easily quantified in isolated cardiac muscle but is more difficult to conceptualize and measure in the intact cardiovascular system. Several methods have been used to quantify

§The authors will refer primarily to the LV for the purposes of this discussion of preload.

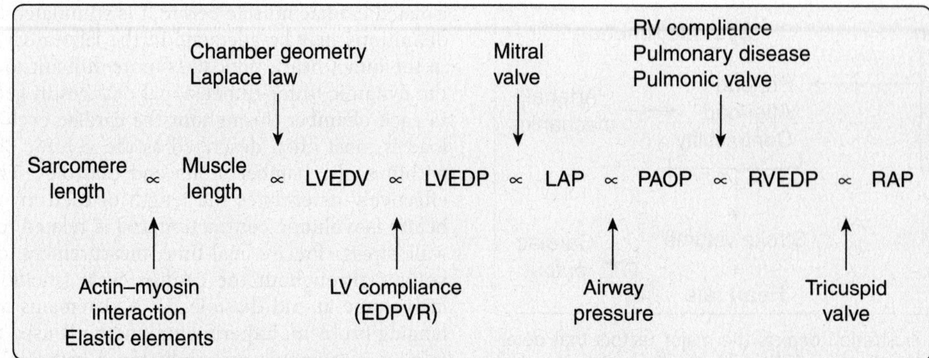

Figure 12-20 This schematic diagram depicts factors that influence experimental and clinical estimates of sarcomere length as a pure index of the preload of the contracting left ventricular (LV) myocyte. LVEDV and LVEDP, LV end-diastolic volume and end-diastolic pressure, respectively; EDPVR, end-diastolic pressure–volume relation; LAP, left atrial pressure; PAOP, pulmonary artery occlusion pressure; RV, right ventricle; RVEDP, RV end-diastolic pressure; RAP, right atrial pressure. (Reproduced with permission from Kaplan JA, Augoustides JGT, Manecke Jr GR, et al. *Kaplan's Cardiac Anesthesia: For Cardiac and Noncardiac Anesthesia*. 7th ed. Elsevier; 2017:158; permission conveyed from Copyright Clearance Center, Inc. (Figure 6-17).)

afterload (Table 12-1). Aortic input impedance [$Z_{in}(\omega)$] is defined as the ratio of aortic pressure (the forces acting on the blood) to blood flow (the resultant motion) and is derived from power spectral or Fourier series analysis of high-fidelity measurements of aortic pressure and blood flow. $Z_{in}(\omega)$ incorporates arterial viscoelasticity, frequency dependence, and wave reflection[46] and is characterized by modulus and phase angle spectra expressed in the frequency domain. $Z_{in}(\omega)$ is most often interpreted using an electrical three-element Windkessel model (Fig. 12-21),[47] which identifies three components: characteristic aortic impedance (Z_c), total arterial compliance (C), and total arterial resistance (R).[48] Z_c represents resistance to LV ejection produced by the aorta and great vessels; C is determined by the compliance of the proximal large arterial vasculature (its energy storage component); and R is the combined resistances of the remaining arterial circulation. The three-element Windkessel model closely approximates $Z_{in}(\omega)$ under a variety of physiologic conditions.[47] This methodology is quite useful from an engineering perspective but has limited practical applicability.

The forces to which the LV is subjected during ejection also may be used to define LV afterload. Increases in LV pressure and wall thickness occur during isovolumic contraction accompanied by a large decrease in LV volume after the aortic valve opens. These factors combine to cause a dramatic increase in LV systolic wall stress, which reaches a maximum during early LV ejection and then declines (Fig. 12-22). Peak LV systolic wall stress is a major stimulus for the development of pressure-overload hypertrophy in poorly controlled hypertension and aortic valve stenosis. The area beneath the LV systolic wall stress curve is an estimate of myocardial oxygen demand. At end systole, the forces driving further ejection and those resisting it are equal. As a result, LV end-systolic wall stress is a determinant of SV. However, assumptions about LV geometry, the nonlinear distribution of force between the subendocardium and subepicardium, and the nonuniformity of wall thickness throughout the LV complicate the use of LV end-systolic wall stress as a quantitative index of LV afterload. These potential confounding factors are particularly relevant when acute or chronic regional wall motion abnormalities (e.g., ischemia, LV remodeling after infarction) are present.

Afterload many also be approached from a mechanical systems perspective. Optimal transfer of energy from the LV to the arterial circulation during ejection requires that these two elastic chambers are coupled.[49,50] LV–arterial coupling is usually described with a series elastic chamber model in which LV elastance (E_{es}) and effective arterial elastance (E_a) are determined

Table 12-1 Indices of Left Ventricular Afterload

Aortic input impedance (magnitude and phase spectra)
Windkessel parameters Characteristic aortic impedance (Z_c) Total arterial compliance (C) Total arterial resistance (R)
End-systolic pressure
End-systolic wall stress
Effective arterial elastance (E_a)
Systemic vascular resistance

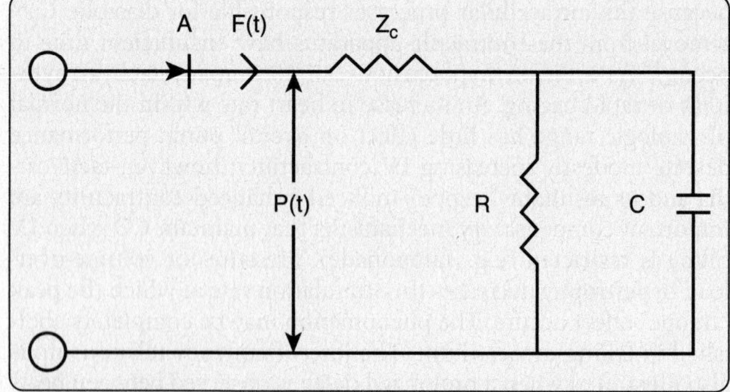

Figure 12-21 Electrical analog of the three-element Windkessel model of aortic input impedance [$Z_{in}(\omega)$]. The diode "A" represents the aortic valve. Time-dependent blood flow [F(t)] entering the arterial system from the left ventricle (LV) first encounters the resistance of the proximal aorta and great vessels [characteristic aortic impedance (Z_c)]. Total arterial resistance (R) and total arterial compliance (C; the energy storage component of the arterial vasculature) determine further arterial blood flow, which is associated with a time-dependent change in arterial pressure [P(t)] from the aortic root to the capillary bed. (Reproduced with permission from Kaplan JA, Augoustides JGT, Manecke Jr GR, et al. *Kaplan's Cardiac Anesthesia: For Cardiac and Noncardiac Anesthesia*. 7th ed. Elsevier; 2017:159; permission conveyed from Copyright Clearance Center, Inc. (Figure 6-19).)

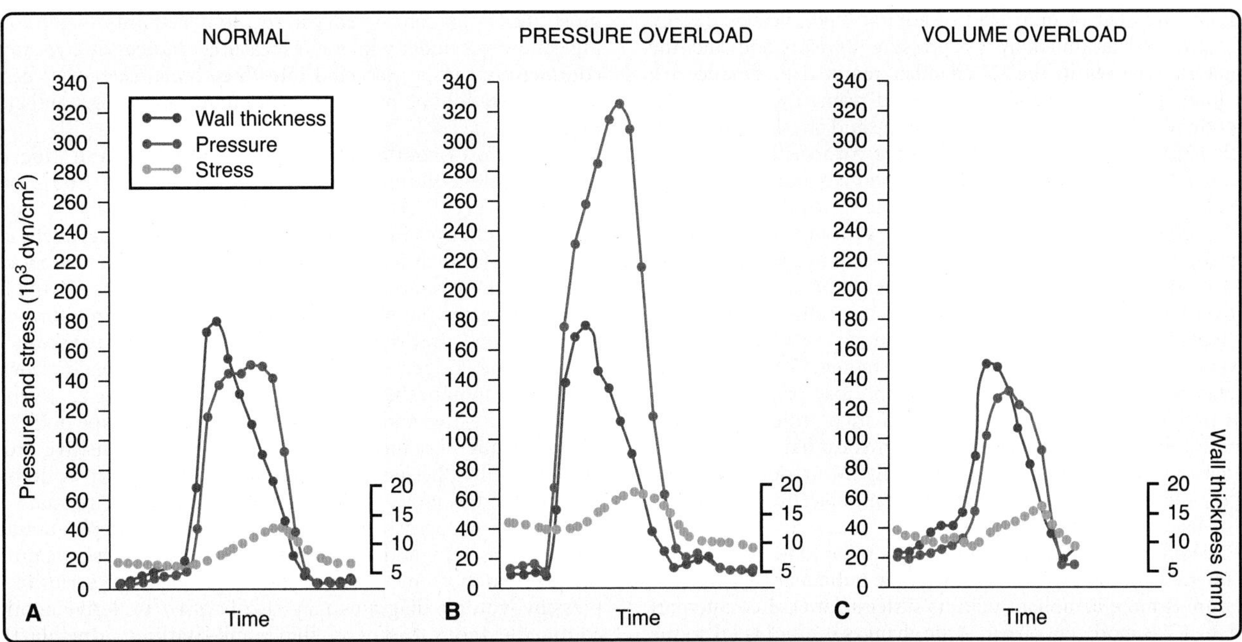

Figure 12-22 This illustration depicts left ventricular (LV) pressure (*red circles*), wall thickness (*purple circles*), and wall stress (*green circles*) during the cardiac cycle. Compared with the normal LV (**left panel**), LV pressure-overload hypertrophy (**middle panel**) occurs concomitant with dramatic increases in LV pressure, but compensatory increases in wall thickness maintain wall stress in the normal range and configuration. In contrast, end-diastolic stress is markedly elevated in LV volume-overload hypertrophy (**right panel**). (Reproduced with permission from Kaplan JA, Augoustides JGT, Manecke Jr GR, et al. *Kaplan's Cardiac Anesthesia: For Cardiac and Noncardiac Anesthesia*. 7th ed. Elsevier; 2017:161; permission conveyed from Copyright Clearance Center, Inc. (Figure 6-23).)

in the pressure–volume plane using the slopes of the LV ESPVR and the aortic end-systolic pressure–stroke volume relation, respectively (Fig. 12-23). The ratio of E_{es} to E_a defines coupling between the LV and the arterial circulation,[51] specifies the SV that may be transferred between them, and provides a foundation from which to study myocardial energetics and mechanical efficiency.[39] E_a may also be estimated as the ratio of end-systolic arterial pressure to SV and has been clinically applied to approximate LV afterload using this definition. Regardless of its derivation, E_a is a composite variable that is affected by arteriolar resistance and compliance of the proximal great vessels, but it does not consider arterial frequency dependence, nor does it include arterial wave reflection properties. Consequently, E_a is not a quantitative index of LV afterload.

The magnitude of $Z_{in}(\omega)$ is determined in large part by total arterial resistance (a property of terminal arterioles), which can be approximated by systemic vascular resistance (SVR) calculated using the familiar formula: (MAP-RAP)80/CO, where MAP and RAP are mean arterial and right atrial pressures, respectively, CO is cardiac output, and 80 is a constant that converts mmHg/min/L to dynes·sec·cm^{-5}. Similar to LV end-systolic wall stress and E_a, SVR is not a quantitative measure of LV afterload because it ignores the mechanical characteristics of the blood (e.g., viscosity, density) and arterial walls (e.g., compliance), fails to incorporate arterial wave reflection, and does not consider the frequency-dependent, phasic nature of arterial blood pressure and blood flow (SVR assumes constant blood flow). The phasic contributions to arterial load are especially important in elderly patients or when peripheral vascular atherosclerosis is present. As a result, SVR should not be used to quantify changes in LV afterload produced by vasoactive drugs or cardiovascular disease and is most appropriately applied as a nonparametric estimate.

Four components mediate LV afterload in the intact cardiovascular system: (1) the physical properties (e.g., diameter, length,

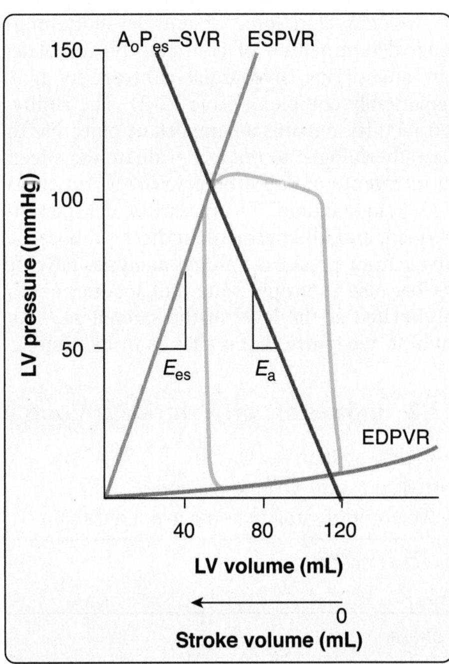

Figure 12-23 This schematic diagram illustrates the left ventricular (LV) end-systolic pressure–volume and aortic end-systolic pressure–stroke volume relations (ESPVR and A_oP_{es}-SVR, respectively) used to determine LV–arterial coupling as the ratio of end-systolic elastance (E_{es}; the slope of ESPVR) and effective arterial elastance (E_a; the slope of A_oP_{es}-SVR). EDPVR, end-diastolic pressure–volume relation. (Reproduced with permission from Kaplan JA, Augoustides JGT, Manecke Jr GR, et al. *Kaplan's Cardiac Anesthesia: For Cardiac and Noncardiac Anesthesia*, 7th ed. Elsevier; 2017:159; permission conveyed from Copyright Clearance Center, Inc. (Figure 6-20).)

elasticity, number of branches) of arterial blood vessels; (2) LV wall stress (determined by LV pressure development and the geometric changes in the LV chamber required to produce it); (3) total arterial resistance (determined primarily by arteriolar smooth muscle tone); and (4) the volume and physical properties of blood (e.g., rheology, viscosity, density). An acute increase in LV afterload is well tolerated in healthy individuals, but patients with HFrEF are exquisitely sensitive to an acute increase in afterload,[52] and severe LV systolic dysfunction may occur in response. Reflex activation of the sympathetic nervous system occurs in response to LV systolic dysfunction, but this compensatory mechanism also inadvertently increases LV afterload and may further decrease CO. LV hypertrophy is also an important adaptive response to chronic elevations in LV afterload that serves to reduce LV wall stress by increasing wall thickness. This adaptation may preserve LV systolic function, but the greater mass of LV myocardium makes the hypertrophied LV more susceptible to myocardial ischemia and LV diastolic dysfunction. Thus, decreasing LV afterload by reducing the inciting stress is the most important objective in the clinical management of HFrEF.

Descriptions of RV afterload are very similar to those described for the LV with two major differences: the pulmonary arterial vasculature is more compliant than its systemic arterial counterpart and the RV is more sensitive to acute changes in afterload than the LV. The ability of the atrial–ventricular valves to open freely and the compliance of the LV and RV are the primary determinants of LA and RA afterload, respectively.

Myocardial Contractility

11 Rigid control of loading conditions and measurement of the magnitude, velocity, and force of muscle shortening facilitate experimental determination of contractility in isolated cardiac muscle but quantifying myocardial contractility in the intact heart is remarkably complex (Table 12-2). The ability to quantify LV contractility remains an important objective that would allow an anesthesiologist to reliably evaluate the effects of pharmacologic interventions or pathologic processes on LV systolic function. A "gold standard" of myocardial contractility has not been developed, and all contractile indices proposed, including those derived from pressure–volume analysis, have substantial limitations because inotropic state and loading conditions are inseparably related at the level of the sarcomere.[53] As a result, it is essential to recognize that a change in LV systolic function must always be considered within the constraints of the loading conditions under which it is measured. Indices of myocardial contractility can be classified into three broad categories based on pressure–volume relations, isovolumic contraction, and ejection phase.

Table 12-2 Indices of Left Ventricular Contractility

Pressure-volume analysis
End-systolic pressure–volume relation (E_{es})
Stroke work-end-diastolic volume relation (M_{sw})
Isovolumic contraction
dP/dt_{max}
Ejection phase
Stroke volume
Cardiac output
Ejection fraction
Fractional area change
Fractional shortening
Wall thickening

dP/dt_{max}, maximum rate of increase of left ventricular pressure; E_{es}, end-systolic elastance; M_{sw}, slope of the stroke work—end-diastolic volume relation.

The ratio of continuous LV pressure-to-volume during the cardiac cycle is termed "time-varying elastance" [E(t)], such that $E(t) = P(t)/[V(t) - V_0]$, where P(t) and V(t) are the time-dependent changes in LV pressure and volume, respectively, and V_0 is LV volume at 0 mmHg of LV pressure.[34,35] In this model, maximum LV elastance (E_{max}) occurs at or very close to the left upper corner of the steady-state LV pressure–volume diagram. As mentioned previously, a nested set of LV pressure–volume diagrams may be generated by an acute change in loading conditions; each loop in this set has a distinct E_{max}. These E_{max} values are linearly related and establish the ESPVR. The slope of ESPVR ("end-systolic elastance"; E_{es}) is an afterload-insensitive index of contractility because the analysis from which it is derived is performed at end systole. Alterations in contractile state are reflected in changes in E_{es} (Fig. 12-24). For example, dobutamine increases E_{es} and the magnitude of this increase quantifies the positive inotropic effect of the drug. The same series of LV pressure–volume diagrams may also be used to derive another contractile index based on the Frank–Starling principle that relates preload to CO. The area of each LV pressure–volume diagram (stroke work; SW) in this nested set of loops and its corresponding V_{ed} are linearly related, such that $SW = M_{sw}(V_{ed} - V_{sw})$, where M_{sw} and V_{sw} are the slope and volume intercept of the relation. The slope of this "preload recruitable stroke work" relation has been shown to quantify changes in contractility in a relatively load-independent manner.[37] E_{es} and M_{sw} are not used on a routine basis in clinical anesthesiology because invasive measurements of LV pressure and volume are generally required for their derivation and extensive offline analysis must be performed. Nevertheless, both indices of inotropic state are useful conceptual tools with which to understand LV, RV, and atrial contractility in the intact heart.

Indices of global myocardial contractility may also be derived during isovolumic contraction using the LV pressure waveform. The most used isovolumic index of contractility is dP/dt_{max}. This index requires invasive measurement of continuous LV pressure and is most often recorded in the cardiac catheterization laboratory, but it may also be estimated noninvasively using TEE. LV dP/dt_{max} sensitively indicates changes in contractile state, but its absolute value is less important than the magnitude of its change in response to an intervention such as administration of an inotropic drug (e.g., epinephrine). LV dP/dt_{max} is generally considered to be afterload independent because the aortic valve opens after the maximal rate of rise of LV pressure occurs. However, dP/dt_{max} is highly dependent on preload, and another index of contractility based on LV pressure–volume analysis that accounts for this preload dependence has been developed and applied in laboratory and clinical settings.[54] LV mass, chamber geometry, and valve disease also influence dP/dt_{max}. Decreases in global LV inotropic state caused by regional myocardial ischemia also may not be accurately quantified with dP/dt_{max} because compensatory increases in contractility occur in the surrounding nonischemic myocardium, which effectively normalizes overall function.

EF is the most commonly used clinical index of LV contractility. EF is usually measured with two- or three-dimensional echocardiography, but other methods, including radionuclide angiography and cardiac MRI, also provide reliable estimates of this ejection phase index of inotropic state. In the operating room, two-dimensional TEE midesophageal four or two chamber windows obtained at end systole and end diastole are analyzed using

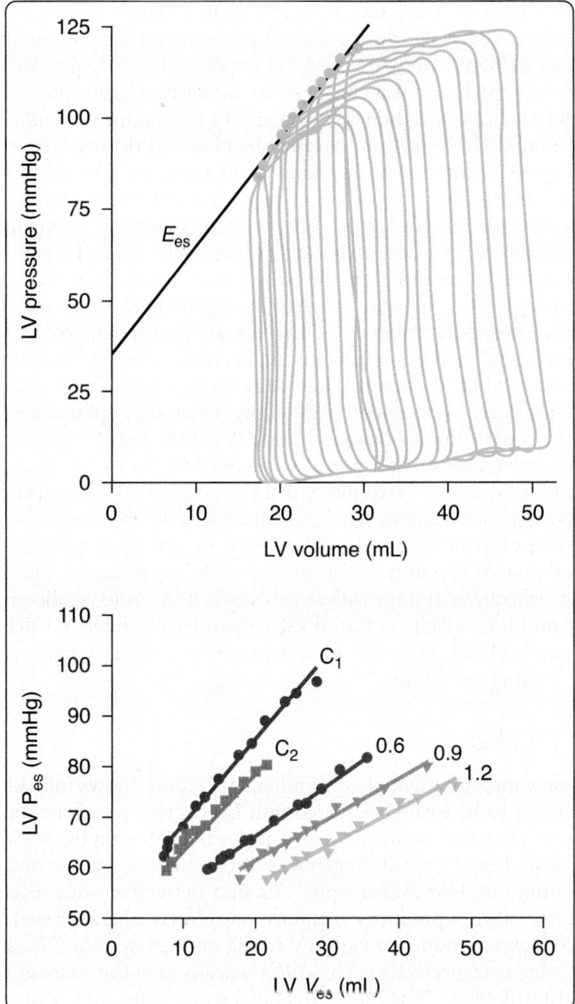

Figure 12-24 This illustration depicts the method used to derive the left ventricular (LV) end-systolic pressure–volume relation (ESPVR) from a series of differentially loaded LV pressure–volume diagrams generated by abrupt occlusion of the inferior vena cava in a canine heart *in vivo*. The maximal elastance (E_{max}; pressure/volume ratio) for each pressure–volume diagram is identified as its left upper corner, and a linear regression analysis is used to define the slope (E_{es}; end-systolic elastance) and volume intercept of the ESPVR (**top panel**). The effects of isoflurane (0.6, 0.9, and 1.2 minimum alveolar concentration) on the ESPVR are illustrated in the **bottom panel**. C_1, control 1 (before isoflurane); C_2, control 2 (after isoflurane). (Reproduced with permission from Kaplan JA, Augoustides JGT, Manecke Jr GR, et al. *Kaplan's Cardiac Anesthesia: For Cardiac and Noncardiac Anesthesia*. 7th ed. Elsevier; 2017:162; permission conveyed from Copyright Clearance Center, Inc. (Figure 6-24))

Simpson's rule of discs to determine EF. However, this technique is time-consuming and impractical to perform in the presence of unstable hemodynamics. Regional approximations of EF, such as fractional shortening and fractional area change (FAC), are often used by examining midpapillary short-axis diameter and area, respectively, at end systole and end diastole. For example, FAC is determined as EDA-ESA/EDA, where EDA and ESA are end-diastolic and end-systolic areas, respectively, measured by tracing the LV's endocardial borders. All ejection phase indices of contractility are dependent on loading conditions and inotropic state. Thus, interpretation of EF, FAC, or fractional shortening must be considered within the context under which the data were obtained. For example, profoundly depressed EF in a patient with severe hypertension may occur because afterload is markedly increased and not because myocardial contractility is grossly impaired. Ejection phase indices may also be inaccurate in the presence of mitral or aortic valve disease or a ventricular septal defect. Indeed, EF may be greater than normal during acute mitral regurgitation because a substantial portion of blood flow from the LV is diverted into a low-pressure outlet (the LA) during systole and not because the LV is inherently "hyperdynamic."

Evaluation of Diastolic Function

The ability of each chamber to efficiently fill with normal pressure is essential to cardiac performance. LV diastolic function has been studied most extensively, but the relaxation, filling, and distensibility characteristics of the more compliant RV and the atrial chambers have also been described in detail. This section will focus mainly on invasive evaluation of LV diastolic function, as noninvasive assessment of diastolic function using echocardiography is covered elsewhere. As previously discussed, LV diastole encompasses a complicated sequence of temporally related, heterogeneous events (Table 12-3). No single index of LV diastolic function comprehensively describes this period of the cardiac cycle or is able to selectively identify patients at highest risk of developing clinical signs and symptoms of heart failure (Table 12-4).[55] The majority of indices of LV diastolic function are highly dependent on heart rate, loading conditions, and myocardial contractility and alterations in these variables require careful interpretation within the constraints of these limitations.

Table 12-3 Determinants of Left Ventricular Diastolic Function
Heart rate and rhythm
LV systolic function
Wall thickness
Chamber geometry
Duration, rate, and extent of myocyte relaxation
LV untwisting and elastic recoil
Magnitude of diastolic suction
LA–LV pressure gradient
Passive elastic properties of LV myocardium
Viscoelastic effects (rapid LV filling and atrial systole)
LA structure and function
Mitral valve structure and function
Pulmonary venous blood flow
Pericardial restraint
RV loading conditions and function
Ventricular interdependence
Coronary blood flow and vascular engorgement
Compression by mediastinal masses

LA, left atrium; LV, left ventricle; RV, right ventricle.

Table 12-4 Common Causes of Left Ventricular Diastolic Dysfunction

Age >60 y
Acute myocardial ischemia (supply or demand)
Myocardial stunning, hibernation, or infarction
Ventricular remodeling after infarction
Pressure-overload hypertrophy (e.g., aortic stenosis, hypertension)
Volume-overload hypertrophy (e.g., aortic or mitral regurgitation)
Hypertrophic obstructive cardiomyopathy
Dilated cardiomyopathy
Restrictive cardiomyopathy (e.g., amyloidosis, hemochromatosis)
Pericardial diseases (e.g., tamponade, constrictive pericarditis)

Relaxation

Relaxation of the cardiac myocyte is an energy-dependent process that requires active removal of Ca^{2+} from the myoplasm. Relaxation is associated with rapid dissociation of the contractile proteins and recoil of elastic elements compressed during contraction. Delays in relaxation can be considered a form of "active elasticity" because failure of actin–myosin cross bridges to dissociate occurs when energy supply is inadequate or intracellular Ca^{2+} homeostasis is abnormal. A delay in relaxation may substantially blunt early LV filling and render overall LV filling more dependent on the contribution of LA contraction. The loss of LA contraction that occurs with the onset of a new atrial tachyarrhythmia may cause acute heart failure in patients with diseases in which delayed LV relaxation is prominent. Delayed LV relaxation resulting from hypoxemia or regional myocardial ischemia in a relatively large perfusion territory may also reduce LV compliance (upward-leftward shift of the EDPVR).[56] A delay in LV relaxation compromises coronary blood flow because incomplete actin–myosin dissociation prolongs the extravascular compression of subendocardial arterioles. Evaluation of LV isovolumic relaxation provides essential information about early diastolic behavior that directly influences subsequent events during filling.

An invasively implanted, high-fidelity pressure transducer is required to precisely determine the rate and extent of LV pressure decline during isovolumic relaxation. Analogous to the use of LV dP/dt_{max} as an index of inotropic state during isovolumic contraction, the peak rate of LV pressure decrease (dP/dt_{min}) has been used to quantify relaxation. Unfortunately, LV dP/dt_{min} is unreliable because the parameter is highly dependent on the magnitude of LV end-systolic pressure.[57] LV pressure decline during relaxation follows an exponential time course between the periods of aortic valve closure and mitral valve opening. As a result, LV relaxation can be quantified using a time constant (τ) derived from the equation: $P(t) = P_0e^{-t/\tau}$, where P(t) is time-dependent LV pressure, P_0 is LV pressure at end systole, e is the natural exponent, and t is time (ms) after LV end systole. While conceptually useful, this model is flawed because it mathematically constrains LV pressure to fall to 0 mmHg. However, LV pressure may drop to a subatmospheric pressure during marked hypovolemia or exercise[58]; conversely, it may remain greater than 0 mmHg when forces outside the LV are acting on it (e.g., tamponade). A more physiologically relevant model of isovolumic relaxation derives the time constant assuming a non-zero value of LV pressure decay.[59] Despite the limitations of the model, increases in τ signify delays in LV relaxation that occur during disease processes such as acute myocardial ischemia, pressure-overload hypertrophy, or hypertrophic cardiomyopathy, or as a consequence of negative inotropic drugs such as volatile anesthetics.[60] Conversely, reductions in τ indicate more rapid LV relaxation that may be observed during tachycardia, sympathetic nervous system stimulation, or administration of positive inotropic medications (e.g., dobutamine, milrinone).

Interpretation of changes in τ produced by disease or medications requires qualification because τ is also affected by LV loading conditions.[24] Similarly, τ is linearly related to afterload because afterload affects the duration, rate, and extent of LV ejection.[24] This afterload-dependence of LV relaxation is enhanced in the failing heart[61] and has important implications; afterload reduction not only enhances forward flow but also facilitates LV relaxation and indirectly improves early LV filling dynamics in patients with HFrEF.[52] Isovolumic relaxation time (IVRT; the duration between aortic valve closure and mitral valve opening) is the most commonly used noninvasive index of LV relaxation. IVRT is usually measured with Doppler echocardiography as the interval between the cessation of aortic blood flow and the onset of transmitral blood flow. When mitral or aortic valve disease is absent, the rate of LV relaxation and the difference between LV end-systolic pressure and LA pressure at mitral valve opening are the major determinants of IVRT. Like τ, IVRT is dependent on both LV relaxation and loading conditions.

LV Filling

Invasive measurement of continuous LV volume allows indices of LV filling to be easily calculated, but LV volume waveforms also may be obtained noninvasively using echocardiography, angiography, and cardiac MRI. Regardless of the method used to obtain a continuous LV volume signal, its first derivative with respect to time (dV/dt) produces a biphasic waveform characterized by peaks corresponding to early LV filling and LA systole ("E" and "A" waves, respectively). The dV/dt waveform is the basis of the transmitral blood flow profile obtained using pulse wave Doppler echocardiography and the pattern of mitral annulus motion seen in tissue Doppler imaging. A wide variety of filling parameters may be determined using the dV/dt waveform, including E and A wave peak filling rates, the deceleration rate and half-time of the E wave, E/A ratio, the areas obtained by integration of the E and A waves (corresponding to early LV filling and LA systole blood volumes, respectively), the ratio of early LV filling to total LV end-diastolic volumes (percentage of early LV filling), and measurements of the time intervals of these events. Progressive development of HFrEF produces similar changes in the dV/dt morphology compared with the transmitral blood flow velocity waveform, as indicated by transition of "delayed relaxation" (grade 1 diastolic dysfunction) through "pseudonormal" (grade 2) and "restrictive" (grade 3) filling patterns (Fig. 12-25).[62] An analogous set of parameters may be derived from continuous measurement of LV dimension (e.g., segment length, diameter, wall thickness), but how well these variables can be extrapolated to describe global LV filling are dependent on geometric assumptions, the LV region examined, and the absence of regional wall motion abnormalities.[55]

Compliance

Derived from a series of differentially loaded LV pressure–volume diagrams, the EDPVR describes LV compliance (Fig. 12-13). This relationship between end-diastolic pressure (P_{ed}) and V_{ed} is exponential: $P_{ed} = Ae^{KV_{ed}} + B$, where K is the modulus of chamber

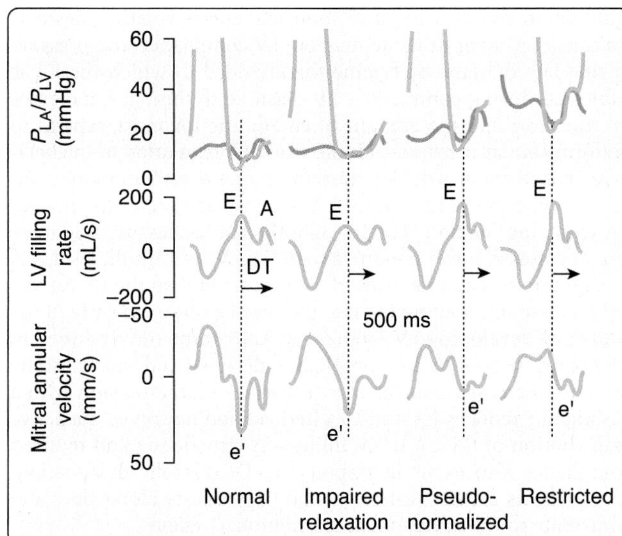

Figure 12-25 This illustration depicts the simultaneous relationships between left atrial (LA) and left ventricular (LV) pressures (P_{LA} and P_{LV}, respectively; **top panels**), LV filling rate during early filling (E) and atrial systole (A; **middle panels**), and early mitral annular velocity (e'; **bottom panels**) under normal conditions and during evolving diastolic dysfunction (impaired relaxation, pseudonormal, and restrictive). Note the initial lengthening of E wave deceleration time (DT) during impaired relaxation and the subsequent shortening of DT as diastolic function worsens. (Reproduced with permission from Kaplan JA, Augoustides JGT, Manecke Jr GR, et al. *Kaplan's Cardiac Anesthesia: For Cardiac and Noncardiac Anesthesia*. 7th ed. Elsevier; 2017:168; permission conveyed from Copyright Clearance Center, Inc. (Figure 6-30).)

stiffness (end-diastolic elastance) and A and B are curve-fitting constants. An increase in K produced by a disease process such as pressure-overload hypertrophy indicates that the LV chamber is stiffer and implies that a higher LV P_{ed} is required to achieve normal V_{ed}. The EDPVR provides a simple model of LV compliance that is easy to visualize but has limitations. LV geometry, mass, and wall thickness influence the modulus of chamber stiffness. Because the relationship between P_{ed} and V_{ed} is exponential, comparisons of K between patients or interventions should be made using a similar range of pressure and volume. Measurements of the modulus of chamber stiffness do not consider parallel shifts in the EDPVR.[24] For example, tamponade causes a parallel upward shift of the EDPVR, which indicates that LV pressure is greater at each LV volume. Thus, both the relative position of the EDPVR and the magnitude of the modulus of chamber stiffness are important in determining LV compliance because a shift in the relation up or to the left indicates that a higher LV pressure is required to distend the LV to a given volume.

The material properties of the myocardium (independent of LV size, geometry, and external forces) may also be derived from stress–strain relations. Hooke's law describes the elastic behavior of myocardium, which develops a resisting force (stress; σ) as its length (strain; ε) increases. As a result, the forces resisting further increases in myocardial length are enhanced as the muscle is stretched. In the intact heart, this process occurs during LV filling and atrial systole. Strain is defined as the percent change in muscle length (L) from unstressed muscle length (L_0; estimated at an LV pressure of 0 mmHg). Lagrangian $[\varepsilon = (L - L_0)/L_0]$ or natural $(\varepsilon = L/L_0)$ strain is most often used to normalize muscle length. The stress–strain relation is exponential: $\sigma = \alpha(e^{\beta\varepsilon} - 1)$, where α is the coefficient of gain and β is the modulus of myocardial stiffness.[63] A shift of the stress–strain relationship up and to the left is consistent with an increase in β, which is known to occur during acute myocardial ischemia, pressure-overload hypertrophy, and hypertrophic cardiomyopathy. Myocardium also demonstrates viscous properties. Viscoelasticity occurs when the forces resisting further alterations in length are dependent on the magnitude of the change in length and rate at which this change occurs. Viscoelastic effects are most evident during early LV filling when the rate of change of LV volume is greatest. An increase in viscous effects may modestly attenuate early LV filling in the normal heart.

Pericardial Restraint

The pericardium encloses the heart, proximal great vessels, distal inferior and superior vena cava, and main pulmonary veins. The smooth surface of the visceral pericardium, surfactant phospholipids, and pericardial fluid (15 to 35 mL), which is composed of plasma ultrafiltrate, myocardial interstitial fluid, and a small quantity of lymph, facilitate cardiac movement. The pericardium also acts as a physical barrier separating the heart from other mediastinal structures and constrains the heart within its inferior (diaphragmatic) and superior (great vessels) attachments. The fibrous layer of the parietal pericardium determines the "J"-shaped pericardial pressure–volume relationship (Fig. 12-26). The pericardium is much less compliant than LV myocardium. This lack of elasticity implies the pericardium has very limited volume reserve and is only capable of accommodating a small increase in volume without a large increase in pressure occurs.[64] Pericardial pressure is normally subatmospheric (between −5 and 0 mmHg), varies with changes in intrathoracic pressure, and has a negligible effect in a normal heart under euvolemic conditions. The pericardium exerts a restraining force on the filling of all four cardiac

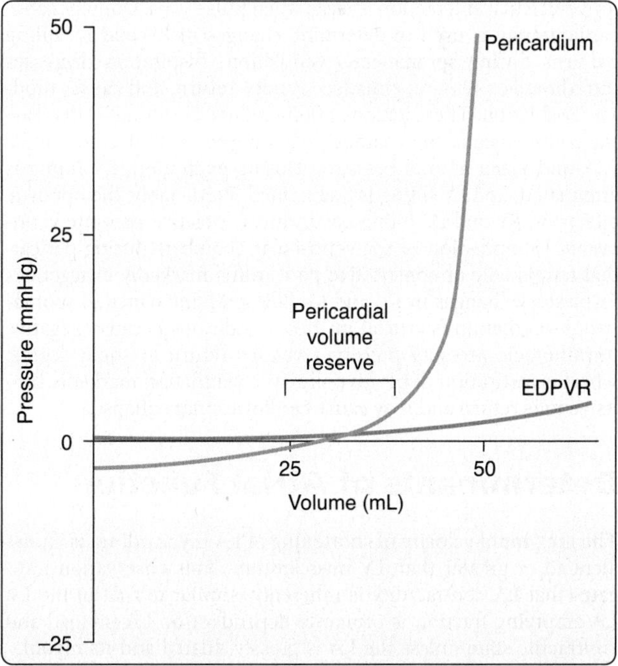

Figure 12-26 Pressure-volume relation of the pericardium (*solid line*) compared with the left ventricular (LV) end-diastolic pressure–volume relation (EDPVR; *dashed line*). Note that large increases in pericardial occur after reserve volume is exceeded. (Reproduced with permission from Kaplan JA, Augoustides JGT, Manecke Jr GR, et al. *Kaplan's Cardiac Anesthesia: For Cardiac and Noncardiac Anesthesia*, 7th ed. Elsevier; 2017:173; permission conveyed from Copyright Clearance Center, Inc. (Figure 6-36).)

chambers. This effect is exaggerated during pericardial compression (e.g., tamponade) or acute increases in chamber dimension during volume loading. Pericardial restraint is most apparent in the thinner-walled atria and RV and is a major determinant of the diastolic pressure–volume relationship of these chambers. The pericardium resists further increases in atrial and RV chamber size during volume loading, and pressure within these chambers rises more rapidly than predicted based on their elasticity alone. The pericardium also plays an important role in LV filling, as an acute increase in pericardial pressure causes a parallel upward shift of the LV EDPVR, as previously discussed. This elevation of the EDPVR combined with greater ventricular interdependence is responsible for the severely restricted LV filling observed with tamponade. After pericardiectomy, atrial volume, RV and LV end-diastolic volumes, stroke volume, and CO increase because pericardial restraining forces are no longer present, and the myocardium alone determines the compliance of each chamber. In contrast to the effects of an acute increase in pericardial or cardiac chamber volume, chronic pericardial effusion or chamber enlargement gradually stretches the pericardium, increasing its compliance and attenuating or abolishing its restraining characteristics. This compensatory response to a chronic increase in pericardial load explains why hemodynamic instability usually does not occur in the presence of a very large (>500 mL) pericardial effusion or profound atrial or ventricular dilatation.

The pericardium plays an essential role in ventricular interdependence (the influence of the pressure and volume of one ventricle on the other). The pericardium restrains both the RV and the LV equally despite the differences in compliance between the chambers. An increase in RV size (e.g., volume overload) causes pericardial pressure to increase, which reduces LV compliance and restricts LV filling. Similarly, LV distention encroaches on the RV, shifts its EDPVR up and to the left, and limits RV filling. Evidence for ventricular interaction is clear when pulse wave Doppler echocardiography is used to determine changes in RV and LV filling patterns during spontaneous ventilation. Inspiration decreases intrathoracic pressure, enhances venous return, and causes modest RV dilation. These actions mildly reduce LV filling by decreasing compliance of the chamber, resulting in small declines in SV, CO, and mean arterial pressure. During expiration, RV filling is attenuated, and LV filling is augmented. Predictably, the opposite effects on RV and LV filling occur during positive-pressure ventilation. Compression of the ventricular chambers during pericardial tamponade or constrictive pericarditis markedly exaggerates respiratory changes in RV and LV filling. Maintenance of spontaneous ventilation is crucial in these conditions because negative intrathoracic pressure preserves venous return to some degree, whereas institution of positive-pressure ventilation markedly limits venous return and may cause cardiovascular collapse.

Determinants of Atrial Function

The maximum velocity of shortening of LA myocardium is equivalent to or greater than LV myocardium. This observation indicates that LA contractility is inherently similar to that of the LV. LA emptying fraction is primarily dependent on LA preload and contractile state unless the LA is grossly dilated and its myofilaments are extended beyond optimal operating length. When this situation occurs, emptying fraction decreases precipitously and LA contraction no longer makes a meaningful contribution to LV V_{ed}. Alterations in the activity of the autonomic nervous system produce similar changes in LA compared with LV contractile state. Sympathetic nervous system activation increases LA emptying fraction and the LA contribution to LV filling; parasympathetic stimulation causes a negative inotropic effect. Volatile anesthetics cause LA myocardial depression. LV compliance and pressure during late diastasis determine the afterload to which the LA is subjected during contraction. LV diastolic dysfunction increases LA afterload and the amount of energy the LA must expend to perform similar pressure–volume work. Upregulation of the beta-myosin isoform in atrial myocardium serves as an important compensatory response to elevated LA afterload and serves to preserve LA emptying fraction. The LA, like the RV, has less muscle mass and operates at lower pressures than the LV. As a result, the LA is much more susceptible to afterload mismatch than the LV. An initial increase in LA emptying fraction may be observed early in the course of developing LV failure, but LA contractile dysfunction eventually occurs as LV compliance declines and end-diastolic pressure increases. Conversely, treatment of hypertension with a vasodilator reduces LA and LV afterload and improves the active contribution of the LA to LV filling. LA remodeling and reduced compliance also occur in response to LV diastolic dysfunction. These effects further restrict pulmonary venous blood flow and contribute to the development of pulmonary edema.

Several factors determine LA reservoir and conduit function. LA relaxation after contraction facilitates forward flow from the 14
pulmonary veins during early LV isovolumic contraction,[65] but relaxation abnormalities produced by LA ischemia, hypertrophy, or dilation attenuate the chamber's ability to function as a reservoir. Descent of the LV base toward the apex during LV systole is also an important determinant of LA reservoir function. This action is attenuated in the presence of severe LV systolic dysfunction, which decreases LA reservoir function because pulmonary venous return is markedly reduced or entirely absent.[66] Transmission of RV stroke volume through the pulmonary circulation to the LA occurs during the late reservoir phase. As a result, RV systolic dysfunction also adversely affects LA reservoir function. In addition to these factors, LA compliance plays a vital role in the ability of the chamber to act as a reservoir and a conduit; a decrease in compliance is associated with impaired LA filling. The LA appendage is more compliant than the main body of the chamber[67] and plays an essential role in LA filling. LA appendage exclusion, clipping, or resection reduces the compliance of the remaining LA. This action attenuates reservoir function and blunts subsequent early LV filling. These effects are especially pronounced when LA dilation or hypertension is present. The pericardium also limits LA filling. Pericardiectomy increases LA compliance and augments reservoir and conduit function.

Exercise and age produce characteristic changes in LA function. LA contractility and reservoir function are enhanced during exercise. The increase in reservoir capacity contributes to the formation of a larger LA–LV pressure gradient during early LV filling, which results in greater SV and CO. An increase in conduit function also has been observed in endurance athletes compared with normal subjects. In contrast, LA dilation and declines in passive emptying occur in elderly individuals. These changes are associated with a compensatory increase in LA ejection force, which enhances the LA contribution to LV V_{ed}. LA dilation also increases storage fraction (ratio of LA reservoir to LV SV), but this dilation may contribute to a further increase in LA wall stress and contractile dysfunction.

Pathophysiology of Heart Failure

Heart failure occurs when the LV is unable to eject blood at a suf- 15
ficient rate to meet metabolic demands or it cannot completely fill without elevated pressure. The notion that abnormal LV diastolic function contributes to or is an independent cause of heart failure

Table 12-5 Comparison of Major Features of Heart Failure with Reduced versus Preserved Ejection Fraction

	HFrEF	HFpEF
Clinical Features		
Age	Younger	Older
Sex	Men > women	Women > men
Medical comorbidities[a]	CAD CABG/PCI Tobacco abuse HLD PVD	CAD HTN Atrial fibrillation DM Obesity Metabolic syndrome COPD CKD Anemia Deconditioning
Physical findings	S_3 gallop	PND Peripheral edema JVD Elevated PCWP
Pathophysiology		
Myocardial contractility	Markedly depressed	Depressed
LV ESPVR	Reduced E_{es}	Elevated E_{es} (systolic stiffening)
LV end-diastolic pressure	Increased	Increased
LV relaxation	Delayed	Delayed
Myocardial stiffness	Normal to increased	Markedly increased
Extracellular matrix	Less interstitial fibrosis	Greater interstitial fibrosis
LV afterload	Increased secondary to neurohormonal activation	Prominent arterial stiffening (increased E_a)
LV–arterial coupling	$E_{es}/E_a < 1$	$E_{es}/E_a > 1$
PAH/RV dysfunction	Common	Common
Chronotropic incompetence	Less common	More common

[a]These comorbidities are not mutually exclusive.

CABG, coronary artery bypass graft; CAD, coronary artery disease; CKD, chronic kidney; COPD, chronic obstructive pulmonary disease; DM, diabetes mellitus; E_a, effective arterial elastance; E_{es}, slope of the LV ESPVR; ESPVR, end-systolic pressure–volume relationship; HLD, hyperlipidemia; HTN, hypertension; JVD, jugular venous distension; LV, left ventricle; LV, left ventricle; PCI, percutaneous coronary intervention; PCWP, pulmonary capillary wedge pressure; PND, paroxysmal nocturnal dyspnea; PVD, peripheral vascular disease.

emerged several decades ago based on studies of LV mechanics in experimental models of heart failure and transthoracic echocardiography was first widely applied in clinical cardiology.[62,68,69] It is now well recognized that more than half of all patients who present with heart failure have an LV EF that is relatively normal (≥50%).[70–73] One survey reported that about half of all patients with heart failure were classified as HFpEF (previously termed "diastolic heart failure"), whereas 33% had HFrEF (EF <40%; formerly known as "systolic heart failure") and 16% had modestly
16 depressed LV EF (EF 40% to 49%).[74,75] The distinction between these two types of heart failure based solely on a LV EF of 50% seems rather arbitrary, but this classification system is now firmly entrenched in the literature because EF is easily measured using echocardiography and because the risk factors, mechanisms, treatment, and outcomes of HFrEF and HFpEF have been established based on this definition.[71] The proportion of patients with HFpEF and their hospitalization rates are steadily increasing. The prevalence of conditions with which HFpEF is closely associated, including hypertension, diabetes mellitus, obesity, metabolic syndrome, chronic kidney disease, atrial fibrillation, sedentary lifestyle, and generalized deconditioning, continues to rise as the population ages and most likely accounts for the disproportionate increase in HFpEF compared with HFrEF (Table 12-5).

Presentation

It is now widely appreciated that HFrEF and HFpEF are distinct clinical phenotypes.[71] Several observations support this contention. HFpEF rarely becomes HFrEF in long-term survivors.[76] Many risk factors for HFpEF (e.g., obesity, metabolic syndrome, physical inactivity, deconditioning) are not associated with HFrEF.[77] HFpEF is a heterogeneous clinical syndrome in which comorbid conditions such as diabetes, obesity, and metabolic syndrome conspire to produce a sustained low-grade proinflammatory state that further exacerbates preexisting LV and arterial stiffening, causes coronary microvascular dysregulation, and impairs skeletal muscle oxygen utilization.[78] These actions accelerate disease progression beyond what is anticipated based on the comorbidities alone. They also demonstrate a higher prevalence of coronary atherosclerosis, myocardial ischemia or infarction, previous percutaneous coronary intervention or coronary artery bypass graft surgery, and peripheral vascular disease than their counterparts with HFpEF. In addition, myocardial necrosis, apoptosis, eccentric LV remodeling, and compensatory neurohormonal activation for depressed myocardial contractility and reduced CO are characteristic features of HFrEF but not HFpEF.

The diagnosis of HFrEF is generally easy to make based on clinical presentation alone.[74,79] In contrast, HFpEF is often more difficult to recognize because patients may initially be asymptomatic or mildly symptomatic at rest and only display symptoms during exercise. Indeed, provocative testing may be required to definitively establish the diagnosis of HFpEF in its early stages.[75] Whereas patients with HFrEF respond positively to renin-angiotensin-aldosterone axis inhibitors, beta-adrenoceptor antagonists, neprilysin inhibitors, nitrates, and digitalis glycosides,[79] these approaches to medical therapy are ineffective in patients with HFpEF as documented by many large-scale randomized controlled trials. To date, the only medications with any documented efficacy in the management of HFpEF are sodium-glucose cotransport protein 2 inhibitors (SGLT2), which appear to reduce the risk of cardiovascular-related death and hospitalization for heart failure independent of diabetes.[80,81] With the exception of SGLT2 inhibitors, treatment of HFpEF is restricted to mitigation of symptoms, lifestyle modifications (e.g., exercise training, weight loss), and management of chronic comorbid conditions. The reader should refer to recent reviews for further details about the management of HFpEF.[71–73] Suffice it to say, the heterogeneous pathophysiology of HFpEF is probably an important reason why HFpEF does not positively respond to interventions that are used to successfully treat HFrEF.

The demographics of HFrEF and HFpEF differ substantially. In contrast to the male predominance of HFrEF, women are more likely to be affected by HFpEF than men, and this gender difference widens with age.[82] Racial disparities in the prevalence, hospitalization rates, and outcomes of HFpEF also exist, black women are disproportionately affected by HFpEF, whereas black men are at greater risk of HFrEF.[83] Diastolic dysfunction resulting from LV and arterial stiffening is a predominant characteristic of HFpEF, whereas abnormal LV filling dynamics in HFrEF usually occur as a result of LV systolic dysfunction. Despite a relatively normal LV EF, intrinsic myocardial contractility can be shown to be modestly reduced in HFpEF when quantified using more sensitive indices (e.g., E_{es}), whereas LV systolic function is more profoundly depressed in HFrEF. LV remodeling and geometry (concentric versus eccentric hypertrophy) were once presumed to be key features that allowed a distinction between HFpEF and HFrEF, but it is now clear that the LV does not follow such a consistent pattern of remodeling. Death from a primary cardiovascular cause is more common in patients with HFrEF, but hospital admission and readmission for noncardiac causes occur more frequently in those with HFpEF.

Diagnosis

The diagnosis of HFrEF is usually straightforward based on clinical presentation alone.[74,79] Common symptoms and signs include fatigue, tachypnea, dyspnea at rest or on exertion, paroxysmal nocturnal dyspnea, orthopnea, a S_3 gallop, jugular venous distention, peripheral edema, and evidence of reduced tissue perfusion. When LV ejection fraction is decreased, these symptoms allow the clinician to make the diagnosis of HFrEF using established guidelines,[84] provided that other causes (e.g., pericardial or valve disease) are excluded. In contrast, HFpEF is often more difficult to recognize because patients may be asymptomatic or only symptomatic during exercise. As a result, provocative testing may be required to establish the diagnosis of HFpEF.[75] The American College of Cardiology Foundation/American Heart Association (ACCF/AHA) and the European Society of Cardiology (ESC) have published guidelines for the diagnosis of HFpEF.[74,79] The ACCF/ACA guidelines focus on three diagnostic features: heart failure symptoms, EF ≥50%, and evidence of LV diastolic dysfunction detected using transthoracic echocardiography.[79] This approach is useful for patients with clear symptomatology but may be less reliable when subclinical HFpEF is present. The ESC criteria are more detailed and include several echocardiographic indices based on two-dimensional echocardiographic measurements (LV size, wall thickness, and mass; LA size), transmitral blood flow velocity (early LV filling peak velocity [E]), tissue Doppler imaging (lateral mitral annulus velocity [e'], E/e' ratio), and plasma natriuretic peptide concentrations.[74] Both the ACCF/AHA and the ESC guidelines rely entirely on resting assessment and do not incorporate provocative testing. Cardiopulmonary exercise testing is now recognized to be important for identifying HFpEF in patients who display minimal symptoms at rest. These individuals usually develop severe symptoms resulting from exaggerated increases in LV filling pressures during exercise.[85] Cardiopulmonary exercise testing evaluates symptoms, continuous systemic and pulmonary arterial pressures, and peak oxygen consumption during stepwise increases in workload. Patients with HFpEF report greater dyspnea earlier during graded exercise, achieve lower maximum workloads, and develop marked increases in respiratory rate, mean pulmonary artery pressure, and pulmonary capillary wedge pressure compared to healthy individuals (Fig. 12-27).

Functional Characteristics

The defining characteristic of HFrEF is a reduction in myocardial contractility, most often resulting from ischemia, infarction, or cardiomyopathy. Pressure–volume analysis provides a useful illustration of the pathophysiology of reduced myocardial contractility as an underlying cause for HFrEF. A shallow slope of the LV end-systolic pressure–volume relationship (E_{es}) indicates that contractility is reduced compared with the normal heart. This depression of myocardial contractility is usually accompanied by compensatory LV dilation (movement of the pressure–volume diagram to the right) along the LV EDPVR. The increase in LV end-diastolic volume preserves SV and CO, but at the cost of higher LV filling pressures and pulmonary venous congestion. Neurohormonal activation (e.g., sympathetic predominance of autonomic nervous system tone, stimulation of the renin–angiotensin–aldosterone axis) serves to mitigate the decreases in CO and mean arterial pressure observed in HFrEF. However, this response also causes deleterious increases in heart rate, LV afterload, and myocardial oxygen demand that further compromise forward flow.

LV diastolic dysfunction is the primary determinant of elevated LV filling pressures in HFpEF. The LV EDPVR consistently demonstrates that increased LV filling pressures are required to achieve normal LV V_{ed}. The steeper rise of the EDPVR curve results from delays in LV relaxation and increases in myocardial stiffness. Taken together, these abnormalities restrict LV filling, increase LV diastolic pressure, and predispose the patient with HFpEF to developing LA hypertension, LA systolic and diastolic

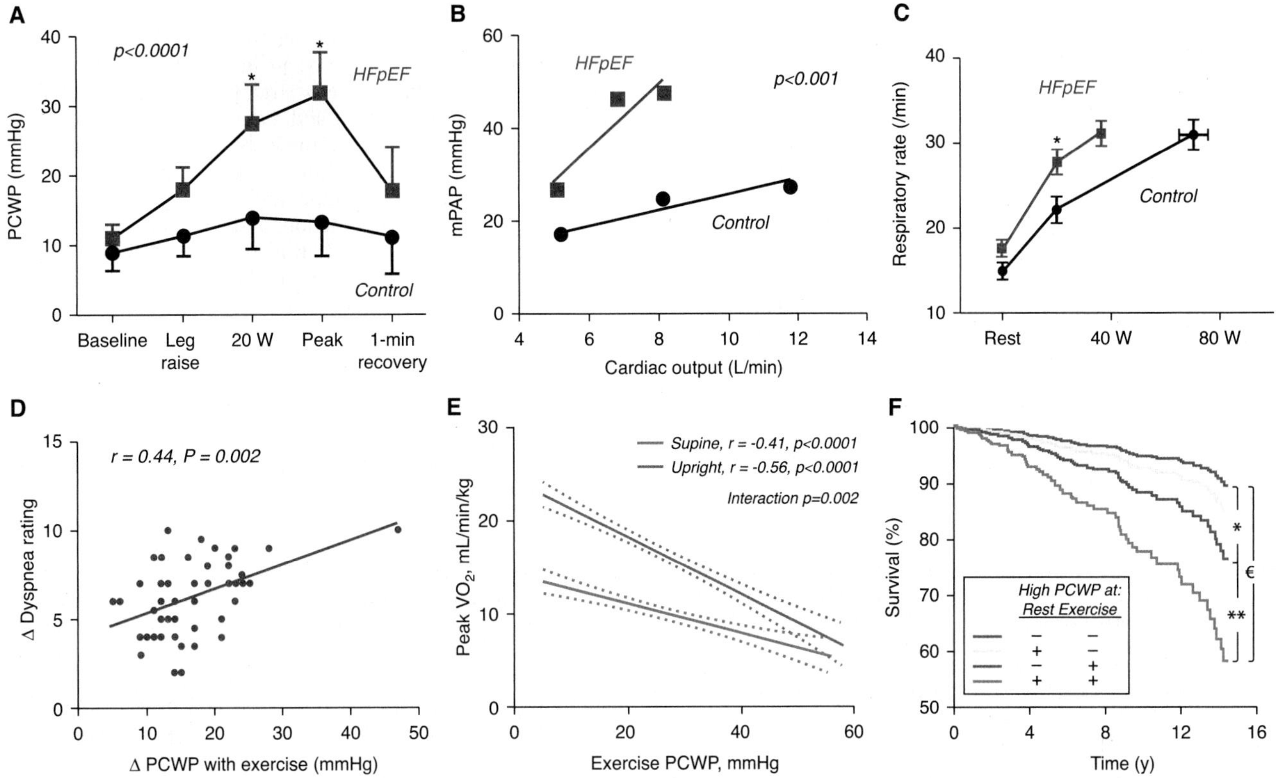

Figure 12-27 Exercise hemodynamics, symptoms, peak O_2 consumption, and survival in heart failure with preserved ejection fraction (HFpEF). Patients with HFpEF (*red*) have greater increases in pulmonary capillary wedge pressure (PCWP), mean pulmonary arterial pressure, and respiratory rate (panels A, B, and C, respectively) than controls (*black*) during exercise. The perception of dyspnea and peak O_2 consumption are directly and inversely correlated with PCWP (panel D and E, respectively). Elevated PCWP is associated with mortality (panel F). (Reproduced with permission from Pfeffer MA, Shah AM, Borlaug BA. Heart failure with preserved ejection fraction. In perspective. *Circ Res*. 2019;124:1598–1617.)

dysfunction, pulmonary venous congestion, dyspnea, pulmonary hypertension, and RV dilation and dysfunction. The afterload sensitivity of LV relaxation is especially prominent in HFpEF because hypertension and arterial stiffening are almost invariably present. These abnormalities incite further delays in LV relaxation, compromising early LV filling by attenuating the LA–LV pressure gradient, blunting torsional recoil, inhibiting the diastolic suction mechanism, and raising LV diastolic pressure.[86] In patients with HFpEF, LV relaxation does not shorten in response to tachycardia.[87] This factor contributes to the exercise intolerance commonly observed in these patients.

A chronic proinflammatory state characterized by elevated nitrosative–oxidative stress contributes to the interstitial fibrosis and cardiac myocyte stiffening observed in patients with HFpEF.[88] An increase in inflammatory markers is a predictor of the development of HFpEF in elderly patients; the intensity and pattern of this inflammatory response makes HFpEF quite distinct from HFrEF. Cardiac myocyte diameter, myofibrillar density, and collagen volume are greater in endomyocardial biopsies obtained from patients with HFpEF compared to those with HFrEF. Coronary microvascular density is reduced and endothelial dysfunction is present in HFpEF. These findings correlate with the extent of myocardial fibrosis and result in a limitation in coronary blood flow reserve.[89] Dysregulation of NO metabolism also adversely modifies specific isoforms of titin. These changes which are linked to increases in myocardial stiffness in HFpEF.

Cardiac catheterization is required to measure EDPVR in patients with HFpEF, but this approach is impractical for most patients. Instead, echocardiography is used to estimate LV compliance with established algorithms based on two-dimensional imaging and Doppler measurement of blood flow and mitral annular velocities.[90] Impaired LV filling, attenuated systolic pulmonary venous blood flow, reduced tissue Doppler velocities, enlarged LA size, and increased LV wall thickness with relatively normal chamber dimensions are the most common echocardiographic findings in HFpEF. Without clinical symptoms, the presence of LV diastolic dysfunction alone does not establish the diagnosis of HFpEF, as approximately 70% of patients over the age of 75 years have some echocardiographic evidence of LV diastolic dysfunction. However, moderate or severe LV diastolic dysfunction in patients without heart failure is often predictive of the subsequent development of HFpEF.

In contrast to the findings in HFrEF, a steep slope of the ESPVR (consistent with systolic stiffening) and smaller LV chamber size are characteristic of HFpEF.[91] Despite the increase in baseline E_{es}, myocardial contractility is abnormal in patients with HFpEF. The reduction of myocardial contractility is substantially less in patients with HFpEF versus HFrEF, but the ability to augment contractility and raise CO in response to exercise or physiologic stress is attenuated. This limitation of systolic reserve is another cause of exercise intolerance in patients with HFpEF. The systolic stiffening of HFpEF also has implications for vasodilator therapy. Afterload reduction substantially improves SV with only modest declines in arterial pressure in HFrEF because of the shallow slope of the LV ESPVR. This beneficial effect is not observed when systolic stiffening is present, as vasodilation causes substantial hypotension with only a modest increase in SV. As a result, vasodilator therapy is a mainstay in the treatment of HFrEF but not HFpEF.

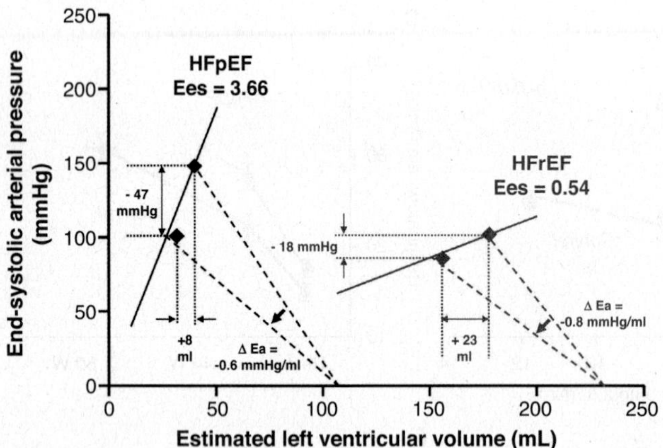

Figure 12-28 Contractility is severely depressed (low E_{es}) and the end-systolic pressure–volume relationship (*solid line*) is very shallow in heart failure with reduced ejection fraction (HFrEF) (*red*). Under these circumstances, a reduction in left ventricular (LV) afterload (E_a) produces a relatively minor decrease in arterial pressure, but a large increase in stroke volume. In contrast, E_{es} is high in heart failure with preserved ejection fraction (HFpEF) (*black*), indicative of systolic stiffening and a similar reduction in LV afterload causes a prominent decline in arterial pressure concomitant with a small increase in stroke volume. (Reproduced from Reddy YNV, Borlaug BA. Heart failure with preserved ejection fraction. *Curr Prob Cardiol* 2016;41(4):145–188. Copyright © 2015 Elsevier. With permission.)

A reduction in compliance of the aorta and proximal great vessels is another cardinal feature of HFpEF. That increases in arterial pulse pressure, LV afterload, and myocardial oxygen demand. The degree of arterial stiffening observed in HFpEF exceeds that predicted on the basis of preexisting hypertension or advanced age alone. This increase in arterial stiffness is an important contributing factor to the lability in arterial pressure and afterload mismatch that commonly occur in patients with HFpEF.[92] Endothelial dysfunction resulting from impaired NO metabolism probably plays a role in arterial stiffening because flow-mediated vasodilation is markedly attenuated in patients with HFpEF. A series elastic chamber model helps illustrate the interaction between arterial and LV systolic stiffening in HFpEF. Both LV end-systolic elastance (E_{es}) and effective arterial elastance (E_a) are increased in patients with HFpEF (reflecting LV systolic and arterial stiffening, respectively), assuring near-optimal transfer of SV from the LV to the great vessels at rest. However, the steep slopes of E_{es} and E_a imply that even modest reductions in loading conditions produced by a diuretic, an arterial vasodilator, or exercise may cause a large decline in arterial pressure (Fig. 12-28).[93] In contrast, LV–arterial coupling is abnormal ($E_{es}/E_a < 1$) at rest in HFrEF, primarily because myocardial contractility is depressed (reduced E_{es}) while arterial stiffness is less affected. A decrease in LV afterload (represented by E_a) produced by a vasodilator is beneficial under these conditions because matching between the LV and arterial circulation results in greater forward flow without pronounced hypotension.

The LA progressively dilates in response to reductions in LV compliance and increases in LV diastolic pressures in HFpEF. As emphasized previously, this LA dilation initially increases the chamber's systolic contribution to LV filling and buffers retrograde transmission of elevated LV diastolic pressures to the pulmonary circulation and the RV.[94] However, the compensatory augmentation of LA contractility declines as HFpEF worsens because LA afterload continues to increase and the LA dilates further. These actions attenuate the LA's pumping ability, rendering it less able to contribute to LV preload during atrial systole. LA dilation resulting from chronic increases in LA pressure also reduces its compliance and ability to collect pulmonary venous blood.[41] Indeed, remodeling and reduced compliance occur in response to LV diastolic dysfunction, effects that further restrict pulmonary venous blood flow into the LA.[41] LA systolic and diastolic dysfunction occur in both forms of heart failure, but these abnormalities are especially prominent in HFpEF. LA dysfunction in HFpEF is yet another factor that limits exercise tolerance and is associated with pulmonary hypertension, RV dysfunction, and mortality.[94] LA dilation is also a primary cause of atrial fibrillation, which is present in as many as two-thirds of patients with HFpEF and is a major cause of morbidity.[95]

Pulmonary hypertension is common in both HFrEF and HFpEF because elevated LV filling pressures are transmitted through the LA to the pulmonary venous circulation. The resulting chronic pulmonary venous hypertension combined with temporal remodeling of pulmonary venules and arterioles increases pulmonary vascular resistance and reduces pulmonary arterial compliance.[96] Pulmonary hypertension is observed in more than three-quarters of patients with HFpEF and is linked to the severity of LV diastolic dysfunction. It is also directly associated with mortality. Pulmonary vasodilation in response to exercise is attenuated in patients with HFpEF regardless of pulmonary vascular resistance under resting conditions, and peak pulmonary vascular resistance during exercise is a predictor of heart failure–related hospitalization and mortality in HFpEF.[97] Pulmonary hypertension contributes to the development of RV dysfunction in approximately one-third of patients with HFpEF. Patients with HFpEF and RV dysfunction are more likely to develop tricuspid regurgitation, atrial fibrillation, renal insufficiency, and LV dysfunction. RV dysfunction can also occur in HFpEF, independent of pulmonary hypertension. Distention of the RV reduces LV filling through ventricular interdependence, despite increased LV filling pressures. Like pulmonary hypertension, RV dysfunction is associated with substantially increased mortality in patients with HFpEF.

Heart rate is the major determinant of increased CO during exercise. CO reserve does not reach its predicted maximum in patients with HFpEF because the peak heart rate that can be achieved during exercise is limited.[98] This "chronotropic incompetence" probably results from beta-adrenoceptor desensitization rather than dysfunctional sympathetic nervous system outflow.[99] The development of new chronotropic incompetence may predict the onset of symptoms or indicate further decompensation in patients with HFpEF. The ability to enhance SV during exercise is also blunted in HFpEF because LV diastolic stiffening and chronically elevated LV end-diastolic pressures limit further LV filling, effectively eliminating the Frank-Starling mechanism.

For additional information please see NICV 12-1, NICV 12-2, and Video 12-3 in the eBook bundled with this text.

For further review and interactivities, please see the videos and narrative interactive clinical vignettes (NICVs) accessible in the complimentary eBook bundled with this text. Access instructions are located on the inside front cover.

REFERENCES

1. Keith A. Harveian lecture on the functional anatomy of the heart. *Br J Med.* 1918;1:361–363.
2. Mall FP. On the muscular architecture of the ventricles of the human heart. *Am J Anat.* 1911; 11:211–278.
3. Yellin EL, Hori M, Yoran C, Sonnenblick EH, Gabbay S, Frater RW. Left ventricular relaxation in the filling and nonfilling intact canine heart. *Am J Physiol.* 1986;250:H620–H629.
4. Greenbaum RA, Ho SY, Gibson DG, Becker AE, Anderson RH. Left ventricular fibre architecture in man. *Br Heart J.* 1981;45:248–263.

5. Porter WT. The influence of the heart-beat on the flow of blood through the walls of the heart. *Am J Physiol*. 1898;1:145–163.
6. Stefanadis C, Dernellis J, Tsiamis E, Toutouzas P. Effects of pacing-induced and balloon coronary occlusion ischemia on left atrial function in patients with coronary artery disease. *J Am Coll Cardiol*. 1999;33:687–696.
7. James TN, Burch GE. The atrial coronary arteries in man. *Circulation*. 1958;17:90–98.
8. Poiseuille JLM. Recherches experimentales sur le mouvement des liquides dans les tubes de tres petits diametres. *Mem Acad Sci (Paris)*. 1846;9:433–544.
9. Crystal GJ, Pagel PS. The physiology of oxygen transport by the cardiovascular system: evolution of knowledge. *J Cardiothoracic Vasc Anesth*. 2020;34:1142–1151.
10. Feigl EO. Coronary physiology. *Physiol Rev*. 1983;63:1–205.
11. Crystal GJ, Pagel PS. Right ventricular perfusion: physiology and clinical implications. *Anesthesiology*. 2018;128:202–218.
12. Stanley WC, Recchia FA, Lopaschuk GD. Myocardial substrate metabolism in the normal and failing heart. *Physiol Rev*. 2005;85:1093–1129.
13. Deussen A, Ohanyan V, Jannasch A, Yin L, Chilian W. Mechanisms of metabolic coronary flow regulation. *J Mol Cell Cardiol*. 2012;52:794–801.
14. Moncada S, Palmer RM, Higgs EA. Nitric oxide: physiology, pathophysiology, and pharmacology. *Pharmacol Res*. 1991;43:109–142.
15. Barton M, Yanagisawa M. Endothelin: 30 years from discovery to therapy. *Hypertension*. 2019; 74:1232–1265.
16. Coffman JD, Gregg DE. Reactive hyperemia characteristics of the myocardium. *Am J Physiol*. 1960;199:1143–1149.
17. Goodwill AG, Dick GM, Kiel AM, Tune JD. Regulation of coronary blood flow. *Compr Physiol*. 2017;7:321–382.
18. Baumgart D, Haude M, Gorge G, et al. Augmented alpha-adrenergic constriction of atherosclerotic human coronary arteries. *Circulation*. 1999;99:2090–2097.
19. Cazorla O, Vassort G, Garnier D, Le Guennec JY. Length modulation of active force in rat cardiac myocytes: is titin the sensor? *J Mol Cell Cardiol*. 1999;31:1215–1227.
20. Schiaffino S, Reggiani C. Molecular diversity of myofibrillar proteins: gene regulation and molecular significance. *Physiol Rev*. 1996;76:371–423.
21. Tobacman LS. Thin filament-mediated regulation of cardiac contraction. *Annu Rev Physiol*. 1996;58:447–481.
22. Luo W, Grupp IL, Harrer J, et al. Targeted ablation of the phospholamban gene is associated with markedly enhanced myocardial contractility and loss of b-agonist stimulation. *Circ Res*. 1994; 75:401–409.
23. Finer JT, Simmons RM, Spudich JA. Single myosin molecule mechanics: piconewton forces and nanometer steps. *Nature*. 1994;368:113–119.
24. Gilbert JC, Glantz SA. Determinants of left ventricular filling and of the diastolic pressure-volume relation. *Circ Res*. 1989;64:827–852.
25. Regen DM. Calculation of left ventricular wall stress. *Circ Res*. 1990;67:245–252.
26. Wiggers CJ. The Henry Jackson Memorial Lecture: dynamics of ventricular contraction under abnormal conditions. *Circulation*. 1952;5:321–348.
27. Cheng CP, Freeman GL, Santamore WP, Constantinescu MS, Little WC. Effect of loading conditions, contractile state, and heart rate on early diastolic left ventricular filling in conscious dogs. *Circ Res*. 1990;66:814–823.
28. Little WC, Oh JK. Echocardiographic evaluation of diastolic function can be used to guide clinical care. *Circulation*. 2009;120:802–809.
29. Kheradvar A, Gharib M. On mitral valve dynamics and its connection to early diastolic flow. *Ann Biomed Eng*. 2009;37:1–13.
30. Suga H, Goto Y, Igarashi Y, Yamada O, Nozawa T, Yasumura Y. Ventricular suction under zero source pressure for filling. *Am J Physiol*. 1986;251:H47–H55.
31. Barbier P, Solomon SB, Schiller NB, Glantz SA. Left atrial relaxation and left ventricular systolic function determine left atrial reservoir function. *Circulation*. 1999;100:427–436.
32. Frank O. Zur dynamik des herzmuskels. *Z Biol*. 1895;32:370–437.
33. Frank O. Die grundform des arteriellen pulses. *Z Biol*. 1898;39:483–526.
34. Suga H, Sagawa K. Instantaneous pressure-volume relationships and their ratio in the excised, supported canine left ventricle. *Circ Res*. 1974;35:117–126.
35. Suga H, Sagawa K, Shoukas AA. Load-independence of the instantaneous pressure-volume ratio of the canine left ventricle and effects of epinephrine and heart rate on the ratio. *Circ Res*. 1973; 32:314–322.
36. Sagawa K. The end-systolic pressure-volume relation of the ventricle: Definition, modifications and clinical use. *Circulation*. 1981;63:1223–1227.
37. Glower DD, Spratt JA, Snow ND, et al. Linearity of the Frank-Starling relationship in the intact heart: the concept of preload recruitable stroke work. *Circulation*. 1985;71:994–1009.
38. Kass DA, Maughan WL, Guo ZM, Kono A, Sunagawa K, Sagawa K. Comparative influence of load versus inotropic states on indexes of ventricular contractility: Experimental and theoretical analysis based on pressure-volume relationships. *Circulation*. 1987;76: 1422–1436.
39. Suga H. Ventricular energetics. *Physiol Rev*. 1990;70:247–277.
40. Glower DD, Spratt JA, Kabas JS, Davis JW, Rankin JS. Quantification of regional myocardial dysfunction after acute ischemic injury. *Am J Physiol*. 1988;255:H85–H93.
41. Pagel PS, Kehl F, Gare M, Hettrick DA, Kersten JR, Warltier DC. Mechanical function of the left atrium: New insights based on analysis of pressure-volume relations and Doppler echocardiography. *Anesthesiology*. 2003;98:975–994.
42. Dernellis JM, Stefanadis CI, Zacharoulis AA, Toutouzas PK. Left atrial mechanical adaptation to long-standing hemodynamic loads based on pressure-volume relations. *Am J Cardiol*. 1998; 81:1138–1143.
43. Hoit BD, Shao Y, Gabel M, Walsh RA. In vivo assessment of left atrial contractile performance in normal and pathological conditions using a time-varying elastance model. *Circulation*. 1994; 89:1829–1838.
44. Mitchell JH, Wallace AG, Skinner Jr NS. Intrinsic effects of heart rate on left ventricular performance. *Am J Physiol*. 1963;205:41–48.
45. Little WC, Freeman GL, O'Rourke RA. Simultaneous determination of left ventricular end-systolic pressure-volume and pressure-dimension relationships in closed-chest dogs. *Circulation*. 1985;71:1301–1308.
46. Milnor WR. Arterial impedance as ventricular afterload. *Circ Res*. 1975;36:565–570.
47. Burkhoff D, Alexander J Jr, Schipke J. Assessment of Windkessel as a model of aortic input impedance. *Am J Physiol*. 1988;255:H742–H753.
48. Wesseling KH, Jansen JRC, Settels JJ, Schreuder JJ. Computation of aortic flow from pressure in humans using a nonlinear, three element model. *J Appl Physiol*. 1993;74:2566–2573.
49. Sunagawa K, Maughan WL, Burkhoff D, Sagawa K. Left ventricular interaction with arterial load studied in isolated canine ventricle. *Am J Physiol*. 1983;245:H773–H780.
50. Sunagawa K, Maughan WL, Sagawa K. Optimal arterial resistance for the maximal stroke work studied in isolated canine left ventricle. *Circ Res*. 1985;56:586–595.
51. Little WC, Cheng CP. Left ventricular-arterial coupling in conscious dogs. *Am J Physiol*. 1991; 261:H70–H76.
52. Little WC. Enhanced load dependence of relaxation in heart failure. Clinical implications. *Circulation*. 1992;85:2326–2328.
53. Kass DA, Maughan WL. From 'Emax' to pressure-volume relations: a broader view. *Circulation*. 1988;77:1203–1212.
54. Little WC. The left ventricular dP/dt_{max}-end-diastolic volume relation in closed-chest dogs. *Circ Res*. 1985;56:808–815.
55. Yew WY. Evaluation of left ventricular diastolic function. *Circulation*. 1989;79:1393–1397.
56. Aroesty JM, McKay RG, Heller GV, Royal HD, Als AV, Grossman W. Simultaneous assessment of left ventricular systolic and diastolic dysfunction during pacing-induced ischemia. *Circulation*. 1985;71:889–900.
57. Weisfeldt ML, Scully HE, Frederiksen J, et al. Hemodynamic determinants of maximum negative dP/dt and periods of diastole. *Am J Physiol*. 1974;227:613–621.
58. Yellin EL, Nikolic S, Frater RWM. Left ventricular filling dynamics and diastolic function. *Prog Cardiovasc Dis*. 1990;32:247–271.
59. Raff GL, Glantz SA. Volume loading slows left ventricular isovolumic relaxation rate: evidence of load-dependent relaxation in the intact dog heart. *Circ Res*. 1981;48:813–824.
60. Pagel PS, Kampine JP, Schmeling WT, Warltier DC. Alteration of left ventricular diastolic function by desflurane, isoflurane, and halothane in the chronically instrumented dog with autonomic nervous system blockade. *Anesthesiology*. 1991;74:1103–1114.
61. Eichhorn EJ, Willard JE, Alvarez L, et al. Are contraction and relaxation coupled in patients with and without congestive heart failure? *Circulation*. 1992;85:2132–2139.
62. Ohno M, Cheng C-P, Little WC. Mechanism of altered patterns of left ventricular filling during the development of congestive heart failure. *Circulation*. 1994;89:2241–2250.
63. Mirsky I. Assessment of diastolic function: Suggested methods and future considerations. *Circulation*. 1984;69:836–841.
64. Watkins MW, LeWinter MM. Physiologic role of the normal pericardium. *Annu Rev Med*. 1993;44:171–180.
65. Keren G, Bier A, Sherez J, Miura D, Keefe D, LeJemtel T. Atrial contraction is an important determinant of pulmonary venous flow. *J Am Coll Cardiol*. 1986;7:693–695.
66. Keren G, Sonnenblick EH, LeJemtel TH. Mitral anulus motion. Relation to pulmonary venous and transmitral flows in normal subjects and in patients with dilated cardiomyopathy. *Circulation*. 1988;78:621–629.
67. Hoit BD, Shao Y, Tsai LM, Patel R, Gabel M, Walsh RA. Altered left atrial compliance after atrial appendectomy. Influence on left atrial and ventricular filling. *Circ Res*. 1993;72:167–175.
68. Grossman W. Diastolic dysfunction in congestive heart failure. *N Engl J Med*. 1991;325: 1557–1564.
69. Cheng C-P, Noda T, Nozawa T, Little WC. Effect of heart failure on the mechanism of exercise-induced augmentation of mitral valve flow. *Circ Res*. 1993;72:795–806.
70. Reddy YNV, Borlaug BA. Heart failure with preserved ejection fraction. *Curr Prob Cardiol*. 2016;41:145–188.
71. Borlaug BA. Evaluation and management of heart failure with preserved ejection fraction. *Nat Rev Cardiol*. 2020;17:559–573.
72. Pfeffer MA, Shah AM, Borlaug BA. Heart failure with preserved ejection fraction in perspective. *Circ Res*. 2019;124:1598–1617.
73. Pagel PS, Tawil JN, Boettcher BT, et al. Heart failure with preserved ejection fraction: a comprehensive review and update of diagnosis, pathophysiology, treatment, and perioperative implications. *J Cardiothorac Vasc Anesth*. 2021;35:1839–1859.

74. Ponikowski P, Voors AA, Anker SD, et al; ESC Scientific Document Group. 2016 ESC Guidelines for the diagnosis and treatment of acute and chronic heart failure: The Task Force for the diagnosis and treatment of acute and chronic heart failure of the European Society of Cardiology (ESC) developed with the special contribution of the Heart Failure Association (HFA) of the ESC. *Eur Heart J*. 2016;37:2129–2200.
75. Pieske B, Tschope C, de Boer RA, et al. How to diagnose heart failure with preserved ejection fraction: the HFA-PEFF diagnostic algorithm: a consensus recommendation from the Heart Failure Association (HFA) of the European Society of Cardiology (ESC). *Eur Heart J*. 2019;40:3297–3317.
76. Lupón J, Gavidia-Bovadilla G, Ferrer E, et al. Heart failure with preserved ejection fraction infrequently evolves toward a reduced phenotype in long-term survivors. *Circ Heart Fail*. 2019;12:e005652.
77. Pandey A, Patel KV, Vadugnathan M, et al. Physical activity, fitness, and obesity in heart failure with preserved ejection fraction. *JACC Heart Fail*. 2018;6:975–982.
78. Dhakal BP, Malhotra R, Murphy RM, et al. Mechanisms of exercise intolerance in heart failure with preserved ejection fraction: the role of abnormal peripheral oxygen extraction. *Circ Heart Fail*. 2015;8:286–294.
79. Yancy CW, Jessup M, Bozkurt B, et al; American College of Cardiology Foundation; American Heart Association Task Force on Practice Guidelines. 2013 ACCF/AHA guideline for the management of heart failure: a report of the American College of Cardiology Foundation/American Heart Association Task Force on Practice Guidelines. *J Am Coll Cardiol*. 2013;62:e147–e239.
80. Butler J, Handelsman Y, Bakris G, Verma S. Use of sodium-glucose co-transporter-2 inhibitors in patients with and without type 2 diabetes: implications for incident and prevalent heart failure. *Eur J Heart Fail*. 2020;22:604–617.
81. Anker SD, Butler J, Filippatos G, et al; EMPEROR-Preserved Trial Investigators. Empagliflozin in heart failure with a preserved ejection fraction. *N Engl J Med*. 2021;385:1451–1461.
82. Beale AL, Meyer P, Marwick TH, Lam CSP, Kaye DM. Sex differences in cardiovascular pathophysiology: why women are overrepresented in heart failure with preserved ejection fraction. *Circulation*. 2018;138:198–205.
83. Chang PP, Wruck LM, Shahar E, et al. Trends in hospitalization and survival of acute decompensated heart failure in four US communities (2005–2014): ARIC study community surveillance. *Circulation*. 2018;138:12–24.
84. McKee PA, Castelli WP, McNamara PM, Kannel WB. The natural history of congestive heart failure: the Framingham study. *N Engl J Med*. 1971;285:1441–1446.
85. Reddy YNV, Olson TP, Obokata M, Melenovsky V, Borlaug BA. Hemodynamic correlates and diagnostic role of cardiopulmonary exercise testing in heart failure with preserved ejection fraction. *JACC Heart Fail*. 2018;6:665–675.
86. Sharma K, Kass DA. Heart failure with preserved ejection fraction: mechanisms, clinical features, and therapies. *Circ Res*. 2014;115:79–96.
87. Hay I, Rich J, Ferber P, Burkhoff D, Maurer MS. Role of impaired myocardial relaxation in the production of elevated left ventricular filling pressure. *Am J Physiol Heart Circ Physiol*. 2005;288:H1203–H1208.
88. Sanderson JE. Factors related to outcome in heart failure with a preserved (or normal) left ventricular ejection fraction. *Eur Heart J Qual Care Clin Outcomes*. 2016;2:153–163.
89. Shah SJ, Lam CSP, Svenlund S, et al. Prevalence and correlates of coronary microvascular dysfunction in heart failure with preserved ejection fraction: PROMIS-HFpEF. *Eur Heart J*. 2018;39:3439–3450.
90. Nagueh SF, Smiseth OA, Appleton CP, et al. Recommendations for the evaluation of left ventricular diastolic function by echocardiography: an update from the American Society of Echocardiography and the European Association of Cardiovascular Imaging. *J Am Soc Echocardiogr*. 2016;29:277–314.
91. Kawaguchi M, Hay I, Fetics B, Kass DA. Combined ventricular systolic and arterial stiffening in patients with heart failure and preserved ejection fraction: implications for systolic and diastolic reserve limitations. *Circulation*. 2003;107:714–720.
92. Reddy YNV, Andersen MJ, Obokata M, et al. Arterial stiffening with exercise in patients with heart failure and preserved ejection fraction. *J Am Coll Cardiol*. 2017;70:136–148.
93. Borlaug BA, Kass DA. Ventricular-vascular interaction in heart failure. *Heart Fail Clin*. 2008;4:23–26.
94. Melenovsky V, Hwang SJ, Redfield MM, Zakeri R, Lin G, Borlaug BA. Left atrial remodeling and function in advanced heart failure with preserved or reduced ejection fraction. *Circ Heart Fail*. 2015;8:295–303.
95. Zakeri R, Chamberlain AM, Roger VL, Redfield MM. Temporal relationship and prognostic significance of atrial fibrillation in heart failure patients with preserved ejection fraction: a community-based study. *Circulation*. 2013;128:1085–1093.
96. Fayyaz AU, Edwards WD, Maleszewski JJ, et al. Global pulmonary vascular remodeling in pulmonary hypertension associated with heart failure and preserved or reduced ejection fraction. *Circulation*. 2018;137:1796–1810.
97. Huang W, Oliveira RKF, Lei H, Systrom DM, Waxman AB. Pulmonary vascular resistance during exercise predicts long-term outcomes in heart failure with preserved ejection fraction. *J Card Fail*. 2018;24:169–176.
98. Brubaker PH, Kitzman DW. Chronotropic incompetence: causes, consequences, and management. *Circulation*. 2011;123:1010–1020.
99. Borlaug BA, Melenovsky V, Russell SD, et al. Impaired chronotropic and vasodilator reserves limit exercise capacity in patients with heart failure and a preserved ejection fraction. *Circulation*. 2006;114:2138–2147.

13 Autonomic and Cardiovascular Pharmacology

PAUL S. PAGEL • DUSTIN HANG • BRENT T. BOETTCHER • JULIE K. FREED

KEY POINTS

1 Drugs that mimic the effects of acetylcholine are most commonly used in ophthalmology.

2 Anticholinesterases prolong the actions of acetylcholine by preventing its metabolism; these drugs are used for reversal of neuromuscular blockade and treatment of central anticholinergic syndrome.

3 Muscarinic antagonists inhibit the effects of acetylcholine mediated through the parasympathetic nervous system.

4 The cardiovascular effects of endogenous and synthetic catecholamines are dependent on their specificity for alpha- and beta-adrenoceptor subtypes.

5 Catecholamines have well-documented utility in the treatment of acute left ventricular dysfunction, but may cause arrhythmias, hypertension, and myocardial ischemia.

6 Alpha$_1$-adrenoceptor antagonists reduce arterial pressure but also produce reflex tachycardia and orthostatic hypotension, especially in patients with hypovolemia.

7 The alpha$_2$-adrenoceptor agonists clonidine and dexmedetomidine are used extensively for sedation, anxiolysis, and analgesia.

8 Milrinone and levosimendan are important medications for the management of acute left ventricular dysfunction and cause synergistic positive inotropic effects when administered with catecholamines by enhancing the intracellular cAMP-mediated signaling.

9 Vasopressin is the most potent arterial vasoconstrictor currently available and is useful for treatment of vasoplegia associated with sepsis or cardiac surgery.

10 Beta-blockers play major roles in the treatment of hypertension, coronary artery disease, myocardial infarction, and heart failure with reduced ejection fraction (HFrEF).

11 Calcium channel blockers reduce arterial pressure and dilate coronary arteries, but some of these drugs also affect sinoatrial node automaticity and atrioventricular node conduction, actions which are beneficial in the presence of supraventricular tachyarrhythmias.

12 Angiotensin converting enzyme inhibitors and angiotensin receptor blockers are useful for the treatment of hypertension and HFrEF.

From the Anesthesia Service, the Clement J. Zablocki Veterans Affairs Medical Center (PSP), Milwaukee, Wisconsin and the Department of Anesthesiology, Medical College of Wisconsin (DH, BTB, JKF), Milwaukee, Wisconsin. This work was supported entirely by departmental funds. The authors have no conflicts of interest pursuant to this work.

Introduction

This chapter discusses the pharmacology of medications that affect the autonomic nervous and cardiovascular systems, including cholinergic and anticholinergic drugs, endogenous and synthetic catecholamines, sympathomimetics, alpha$_1$-antagonists, alpha$_2$-agonists, beta-blockers, phosphodiesterase inhibitors, digitalis glycosides, vasopressin, and antihypertensive drugs (nitrates, calcium [Ca^{2+}] channel blockers, and angiotensin converting enzyme [ACE] inhibitors). These drug classifications will be reviewed in detail with primary emphasis on their cardiovascular actions. A thorough working knowledge of this subject matter is essential for the anesthesiologist.

Cholinergic Drugs

There are relatively few drugs in current clinical use that influence the function of parasympathetic nervous system by modulating actions or metabolism of the neurotransmitter acetylcholine (Ach). Cholinergic drugs mimic, enhance, or block the actions of Ach in autonomic ganglia and skeletal muscle at nicotinic receptors or in parasympathetic postganglionic neurons through muscarinic receptors. In general, cholinergic drugs have greater site specificity and exert more prolonged effects than the primary neurotransmitter. Ach itself has virtually no therapeutic applications because of its diffuse action, extensive side effect profile, and rapid hydrolysis by acetylcholinesterase and butyrylcholinesterase
(also known as pseudocholinesterase). Topical ACh eye drops are 1
occasionally used when acute miosis is required during ophthalmologic surgery or for the treatment of glaucoma, but systemic cholinergic effects are usually not observed because little ACh uptake occurs and ACh is quickly metabolized.

Cholinergic Agonists

Synthetic cholinergic agonists are not used in anesthesia practice, but an understanding of their pharmacology remains important because anesthesiologists often encounter patients who receive them (Fig. 13-1; Table 13-1). Ach is a quaternary ammonium compound that causes changes in membrane conformation when it interacts with postsynaptic receptors, increasing the permeability to Na^+, K^+, and Cl^- ions down their respective electrochemical gradients to cause membrane depolarization. Two important binding sites on the postsynaptic ACh receptor are essential for this process to occur: an "ester" site that binds the ester part of the molecule, and an "ion" site that binds the quaternary amine. Subtle modifications in the chemical structure of ACh are capable of producing more selective muscarinic activity while simultaneously reducing the rate of metabolism. Two major classes of cholinergic agonists currently exist: choline esters and alkaloids. Beta-methylation of choline produces methacholine, a synthetic muscarinic agonist that is highly resistant to hydrolysis by cholinesterase. Methacholine is used almost exclusively as a provocative agent for identifying the presence

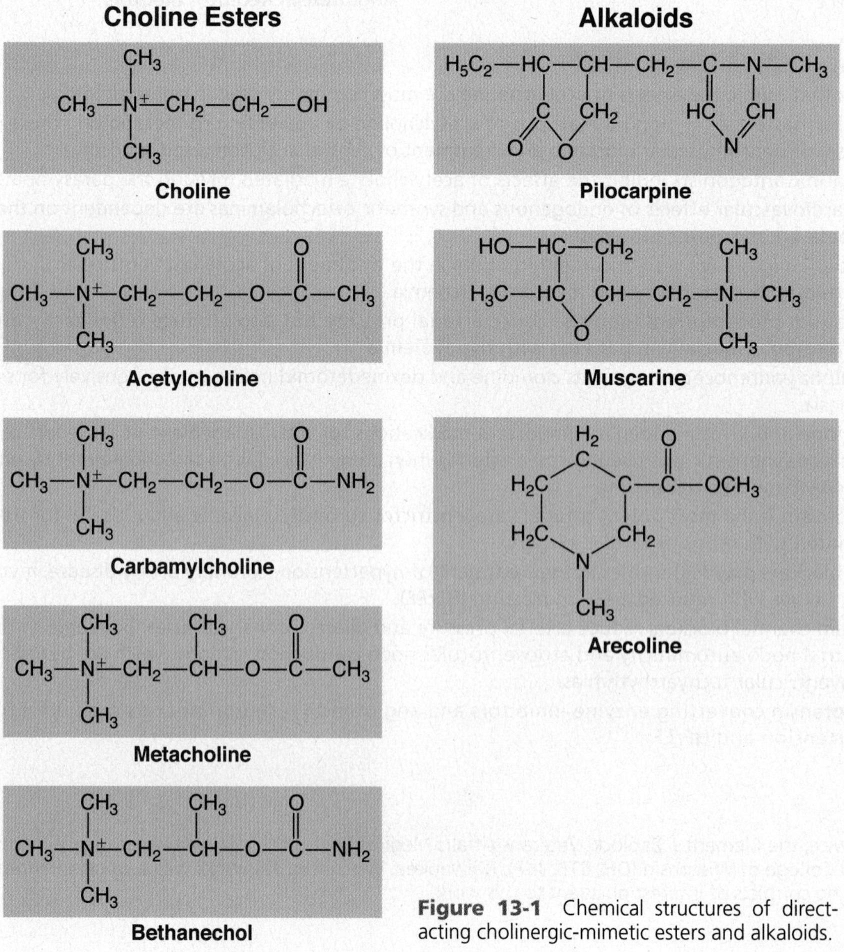

Choline Esters

Choline

Acetylcholine

Carbamylcholine

Metacholine

Bethanechol

Alkaloids

Pilocarpine

Muscarine

Arecoline

Figure 13-1 Chemical structures of direct-acting cholinergic-mimetic esters and alkaloids.

Table 13-1 Comparative Muscarinic Actions of Direct Cholinomimetic Agents

	Systemic				
	Acetylcholine	*Methacholine*	*Carbamylcholine*	*Bethanechol*	*Pilocarpine*
Esterase hydrolysis	+++	+	0	0	0
Eye (topical)					
Iris	++	++	+++	+++	+++
Ciliary	++	++	+++	+++	++
Heart					
Rate	–	–	–	–	
Contractility	–	–	–	–	
Conduction	–	–	–	–	
Smooth muscle					
Vascular	–	–	–		–
Bronchial	++	++	+	+	++
Gastrointestinal motility	++	++	+++	+++	++
Gastrointestinal sphincters	–	–	–	–	++
Biliary	++	++	+++	+++	++
Bladder					
Detrusor	++	++	+++	+++	++
Sphincter	–	–	–	–	–
Exocrine glands					
Respiratory	+++	++	+++	++	++++
Salivary	++	++	++	++	+++++
Pharyngeal	++	++	++	++	++++
Lacrimal	++	++	++	++	++++
Sweat	++	++	++	++	+++++
Gastrointestinal acid and secretions	++	++	++	++	++++
Nicotinic actions	+++	+	+++	–	+++

+, stimulation; –, inhibition.

of reactive airway disease by causing bronchoconstriction, an increase in airway secretions, and a reduction in peak expiratory flow rate through activation of bronchial muscarinic M_3 receptors.[1] Predictably, methacholine may also produce bradycardia and hypotension as a result of M_3 receptor activation in myocardium and vascular endothelium, respectively. Methacholine-induced stimulation of M_3 receptors activates the pertussis toxin-insensitive $G_{q/11}$ protein coupled-phospholipase C-inositol triphosphate-mediated signaling cascade, culminating in endothelial nitric oxide (NO) synthase activation, NO production, and dilation of vascular smooth muscle.[2] Use of methacholine is relatively contraindicated in patients with documented asthma or chronic obstructive pulmonary disease because marked bronchospasm may occur. Emergency airway equipment, supplemental oxygen, inhaled beta$_2$-adrenoceptor agonists, and resuscitative medications should be readily available when conducting methacholine provocative testing.

Bethanechol is a choline ester (a carbamate derivative of methacholine) that is relatively selective for the M_3 receptors in the urinary and gastrointestinal tracts. Bethanechol may be useful for treatment of nonobstructive urinary retention during the postoperative period or in some cases of neurogenic bladder as an alternative to chronic catheterization.[3] Bethanechol also increases gastrointestinal motility and stimulates peristalsis. Carbamylcholine is a choline ester derivative that is used topically to produce miosis in patients with wide-angle glaucoma. Pilocarpine is an alkaloid cholinergic agonist used as a topical miotic agent to reduce intraocular pressure in patients with glaucoma. Oral pilocarpine may also be used to increase salivary and lacrimal gland production in patients with xerostomia after head and neck irradiation or in those with Sjögren syndrome[4]. Finally, muscarinic agonists that stimulate central nervous system receptors may also be useful for treatment of patients with Alzheimer disease.[5]

Cholinesterase Inhibitors

2 Cholinesterase inhibitors (anticholinesterases) have been used for decades to produce the sustained cholinergic effect necessary to overcome nondepolarizing neuromuscular blockade. The development and widespread use of the steroidal neuromuscular blocker-chelator sugammadex now provides an alternative approach to rapid reversal of neuromuscular blockade.[6] Nevertheless, cholinesterase inhibitors are still commonly used in practice. Cholinesterase inhibitors are also used for treatment of myasthenia gravis, glaucoma, and Alzheimer disease. These medications have important anesthetic implications. The pharmacology of anticholinesterases as neuromuscular blockade reversal medications is described in detail in another chapter; the current discussion will focus solely on the actions of these drugs as cholinergic mimetics. In contrast to organophosphate compounds (e.g., pesticides, nerve toxins) that irreversibly inhibit acetylcholinesterase and butyrylcholinesterase, clinically used cholinesterase inhibitors (e.g., neostigmine) reversibly inhibit these enzymes, which very rapidly hydrolyze ACh (half-life of microseconds) into acetate and choline under normal conditions, thereby inactivating the neurotransmitter. This inhibition of acetylcholinesterase and butyrylcholinesterase enhances the actions of ACh at postganglionic muscarinic receptors, resulting in intense parasympathetic nervous system activity similar to those produced by direct cholinergic agonists. The accumulation of ACh also causes dual actions on autonomic nervous system ganglia and skeletal muscle, initially stimulating but subsequently depressing neurotransmission through their nicotinic receptors. Similar initial stimulation followed by depression of central nervous system cholinergic receptors also occurs with exposure to a lethal dose of an anticholinesterase, for example, when an organophosphate overdose occurs during its use as a pesticide or when a nerve toxin is used as a weapon of mass destruction.[7] Organophosphates are especially insidious toxins because they are often odorless, are rapidly absorbed through the skin, are highly lipid soluble, and move easily across the blood–brain barrier into the central nervous system.

Clinically used cholinesterase inhibitors are either carbamoyl esters (including neostigmine, physostigmine, and pyridostigmine) or quaternary ammonium alcohols (edrophonium; Fig. 13-2). Three areas on the acetylcholinesterase molecule are capable of binding inhibitory ligands: two are located in the enzyme's active center (the acyl pocket and a choline subsite, referred to collectively as the "esteratic" site), whereas the third is a peripheral "anionic" site. The specificity and duration of action of cholinesterase inhibitors depend on their specific binding site, affinity, and rate of hydrolysis. For example, edrophonium reversibly binds to the choline subsite, but its chemical structure facilitates rapid renal excretion and relatively short duration of action (approximately one hour). The carbamate cholinesterase inhibitors also bind to acetylcholinesterase's "esteratic" site, but these drugs are more slowly metabolized because their carbamoyl ester linkage is less susceptible to hydrolysis. As a result, their duration of action is approximately 4 hours. In contrast, organophosphates bind irreversibly to the active center of anticholinesterase and require stimulated hydrolysis of the phosphate-enzyme complex to restore the enzyme's activity with drugs such as pralidoxime.

The most prominent pharmacologic effects of the cholinesterase inhibitors are their actions on muscarinic receptors, but when used to reverse nondepolarizing neuromuscular blockade, the intended target of these drugs are the nicotinic receptors at the motor end-plate of skeletal muscle. Higher concentrations of ACh are required to activate nicotinic than muscarinic receptors. As a result, the relative excess of ACh needed to overcome nondepolarizing neuromuscular blockade of nicotinic receptors also stimulates muscarinic receptors and causes pronounced cholinergic side effects. Administration of a muscarinic antagonist (e.g., atropine, glycopyrrolate) is most often required to block the adverse effects of cholinesterase inhibitors (e.g., bradycardia, hypotension, bronchospasm, sialorrhea, miosis, increased intestinal motility, sphincter relaxation) while sparing the actions of these medications at the nicotinic receptors. Unlike neostigmine, pyridostigmine and edrophonium, physostigmine is a tertiary amine that readily crosses the blood–brain barrier and inhibits acetylcholinesterase in the central nervous system. As a result, physostigmine is effective for the treatment of atropine or scopolamine overdose (muscarinic antagonists that also penetrate the blood–brain barrier) and central anticholinergic syndrome. Other centrally acting cholinesterase inhibitors (e.g., donepezil) are a mainstay in the treatment Alzheimer disease[8] and have been reported to affect the duration of action of succinylcholine.[9]

Echothiophate is the only clinically used organophosphate cholinesterase inhibitor, which is applied topically for the treatment of glaucoma. The drug's primary advantage over other topical glaucoma medications is its prolonged duration of action, as it may remain effective for several weeks after cessation of therapy. Topical absorption of echothiophate is highly variable, but it can be considerable. As a result, succinylcholine may have a prolonged duration of action in patients who are receiving it. Nevertheless,

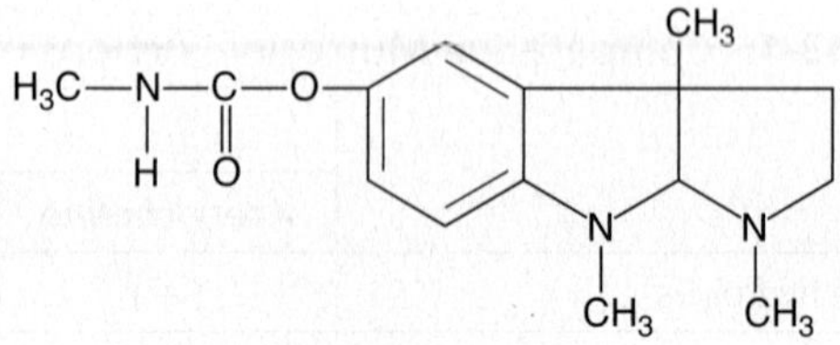

Physostigmine

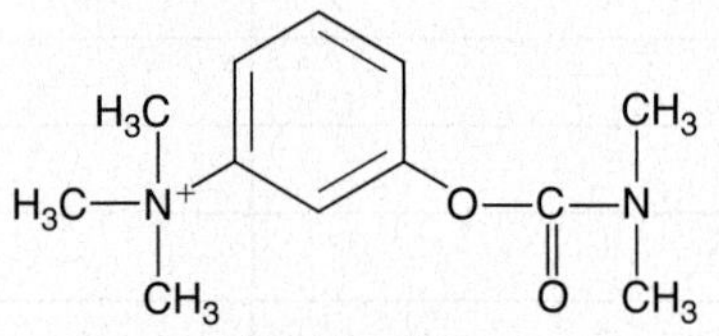

Neostigmine

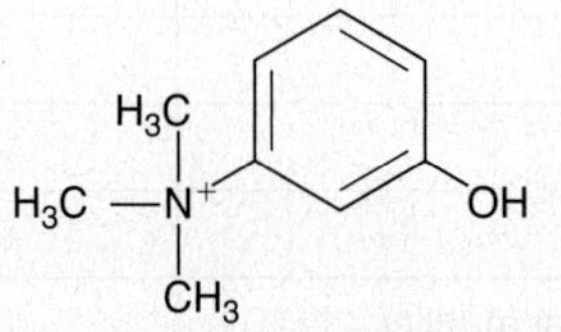

Edrophonium

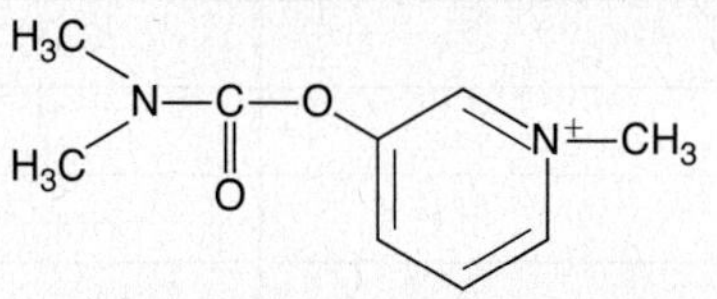

Pyridostigmine

Figure 13-2 Chemical structures of clinical anticholinesterases.

succinylcholine is not strictly contraindicated when the depolarizing neuromuscular blocker is needed.

Muscarinic Antagonists

3 The muscarinic antagonists atropine, scopolamine, and glycopyrrolate are commonly used in anesthesia practice (Table 13-2). Atropine and scopolamine are belladonna alkaloids that are derived from plants including deadly nightshade, jimson weed, and henbane. These drugs have been used for millennia as toxins and therapeutic agents. Atropine, scopolamine, and glycopyrrolate are competitive inhibitors of ACh at the parasympathetic muscarinic receptor and act to increase heart rate; inhibit salivary, bronchial, and gastrointestinal secretions; attenuate gastric acid production; reduce gastrointestinal motility; cause bronchodilation; and antagonize the muscarinic side effects of anticholinesterases during reversal of nondepolarizing neuromuscular blockade. They also bind to presynaptic muscarinic receptors on norepinephrine-secreting postganglionic neurons. This action may enhance sympathetic nervous system activity because ACh-induced stimulation of these presynaptic receptors normally inhibits norepinephrine release. Anesthesiologists first used atropine to reduce salivation and vagal-mediated bradycardia during open-drop ether or chloroform anesthesia. The antisialagogue effect of a muscarinic antagonist such as glycopyrrolate during fiberoptic intubation is a major clinical indication for its use. The potencies of atropine, scopolamine, and glycopyrrolate are quite different, but the drugs have little or no muscarinic receptor subtype specificity, and as a result, they exert similar anticholinergic effects in most target organs except for the heart and central nervous system (see below). Selective muscarinic subtype receptor antagonists are used extensively for treatment of overactive bladder conditions without causing pronounced adverse systemic anticholinergic effects.[10]

Atropine and scopolamine are tertiary amines that easily penetrate the blood–brain barrier and produce central nervous system effects. Scopolamine is a central nervous system depressant that causes sedation, amnesia, and euphoria. These properties made scopolamine useful for premedication in patients undergoing cardiac or major noncardiac surgery before midazolam was first introduced into clinical practice in the 1980s. Transdermal scopolamine is currently used for prophylaxis against kinetosis (motion sickness) and is also effective for the treatment of postoperative nausea and vomiting, but it may be associated with anticholinergic side effects. Lower doses of atropine are relatively devoid of central nervous system effects, but higher doses (greater than 2 mg; used most often in combination with an anticholinesterase inhibitor to reverse neuromuscular blockade or for the treatment of symptomatic bradyarrhythmias) often produce central nervous system effects including restlessness, disorientation, hallucinations, and delirium. In contrast to atropine and scopolamine, glycopyrrolate is a quaternary amine that does not cross the blood–brain barrier and is devoid of actions in the central nervous system. When combined with its more prolonged duration of action, this latter property makes glycopyrrolate more attractive for routine use in anesthesiology than atropine.

Atropine, and to a lesser extent glycopyrrolate, increase heart rate when sinus bradycardia occurs as a result of vagal stimulation (e.g., peritoneal traction) or inhibition of cardiac sympathetic nerve traffic (e.g., high spinal anesthesia). Atropine is also a treatment of choice for symptomatic bradyarrhythmias. Conversely, atropine must be used with extreme caution when tachycardia is deleterious (e.g., coronary artery stenosis, aortic valve stenosis, hypertrophic cardiomyopathy, pheochromocytoma, thyroid storm). Paradoxically, very low doses of atropine (<0.1 mg) may decrease heart rate through blockade of presynaptic parasympathetic neuron M_1 receptors.[11] Scopolamine usually produces little change in heart rate when administered through by an intramuscular route for premedication. Atropine and scopolamine cause mydriasis and cycloplegia because they exert muscarinic antagonist effects on ACh-mediated cranial nerve II (afferent) and III (efferent) control of pupillary reactivity and ocular accommodation, respectively. Indeed, atropine derivatives are widely used in ophthalmology because pupillary dilation facilitates visual inspection of the posterior chamber and retina. Muscarinic antagonists are relatively contraindicated in patients with narrow-angle glaucoma because pupillary dilation thickens the peripheral iris and narrows the

Table 13-2 Comparative Effects of Muscarinic Antagonists

Name	Chemical Structure	Duration IV (h)	Duration IM (h)	CNS	Heart Rate	Antisialagogue Effect	Mydriasis Cycloplegia
Atropine		0.25–0.5	2–4	Stimulation	+++	+	+
Scopolamine		0.5–1	4–6	Sedation	0	++	+
Glycopyrrolate		2–4	6–8	0	+	++	0

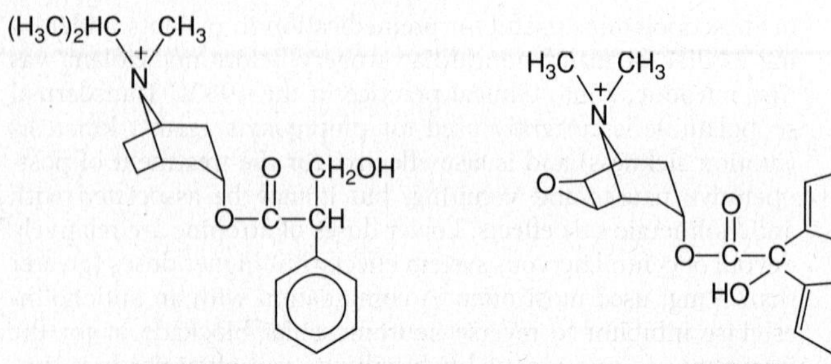

Ipratropium Tiotropium

Figure 13-3 Chemical structures of inhaled muscarinic antagonists.

iridocorneal angle. These actions impair aqueous humor drainage and increase intraocular pressure. Muscarinic antagonists inhibit sympathetic nervous system innervation of sweat glands because ACh is the neurotransmitter in these postganglionic neurons. Children may develop hyperthermia when treated with these drugs because they are more reliant on sweating to maintain normal body temperature than adults. Muscarinic antagonists are also relatively contraindicated in febrile patients for similar reasons.

Ipratropium and tiotropium are muscarinic antagonists that resemble atropine and are used for the treatment of chronic obstructive pulmonary disease (Fig. 13-3).[12] These drugs are bronchial smooth muscle dilators that are administered using metered-dose inhalers. The bronchodilation produced by ipratropium and tiotropium is less pronounced than that observed with beta$_2$-adrenoceptor agonists. Ipratropium and tiotropium effectively inhibit airway reactivity induced by provocative substances including methacholine, histamine, prostaglandin F_{2a}, but they are ineffective against leukotriene-induced bronchoconstriction. Neither drug substantially affects mucociliary clearance. Because of their quaternary ammonium structures, ipratropium and tiotropium are poorly absorbed into the systemic circulation and do not produce adverse anticholinergic side effects with the exception of xerostomia. The inhaled muscarinic antagonists are more efficacious in patients with chronic obstructive pulmonary disease than in those suffering from asthma.

Muscarinic Antagonist Toxicity

Atropine and other muscarinic antagonists cause symptoms associated with blockade of ACh at parasympathetic and sympathetic postganglionic neurons (Table 13-3). The familiar medical school phrase "dry as a bone; red as a beet; blind as a bat; hot as a hare; mad as a hatter" summarizes these effects. The central nervous system effects of muscarinic antagonists are particularly noteworthy because muscarinic ACh receptors are abundant in the brain and their blockade causes psychoactive effects including excitation, restlessness, sedation, confusion, hallucinations, stupor, delirium, psychosis, seizures, and coma. These alterations in sensorium are characteristic features of central anticholinergic syndrome, which may persist beyond the expected duration of the offending drug's metabolism. Antihistamines, tricyclic antidepressants, phenothiazines, benzodiazepines, and a variety of other medications are also associated with central anticholinergic syndrome (Table 13-4). Physostigmine is the treatment of choice for central anticholinergic syndrome because it crosses the blood–brain barrier and increases ACh concentrations in the central nervous system, as previously discussed. Physostigmine is most often administered in 1 or 2 mg doses to avoid producing peripheral cholinergic agonist activity. Notably, the duration of action of physostigmine action may be shorter than that of the muscarinic antagonist, and repeat treatment may be required if symptoms recur. The drug must be used with caution in the absence of a muscarinic antagonist because of unopposed cholinergic agonist effects.

Table 13-3 Atropine Toxicity

Dose Range (mg)	Muscarinic Antagonist Effects
0.5–1.0	Increased heart rate; xerostomia (dry mouth); thirst; lack of sweating; mild pupillary dilation
2–5	Tachycardia; palpitations; mydriasis; cycloplegia; restlessness or confusion; inability to swallow, urinate, defecate, or sweat; hot skin
10 or greater	Profound tachycardia, mydriasis, and cycloplegia; hot, red skin; fever; hallucinations; delirium; coma; death

Adapted from Brown JA, Laiken N. Muscarinic receptor agonists and antagonists. In: Brunton LL, Chabner BA, Knollmann BC, eds. *Goodman & Gilman's The Pharmacological Basis of Therapeutics*. 12th ed. McGraw-Hill Medical; 2011:226.

Fundamentals of Catecholamine Pharmacology

Alpha, beta, and dopamine adrenergic receptor subtypes mediate 4
the cardiovascular effects of endogenous (epinephrine, norepinephrine, dopamine) and synthetic (dobutamine, isoproterenol) catecholamines (Table 13-5, NICV 13-1). These substances stimulate beta$_1$-adrenoceptors located on the sarcolemmal membrane of atrial and ventricular myocytes to varying degrees. Activation of beta$_1$-adrenoceptors causes positive chronotropic (heart rate), dromotropic (conduction velocity), inotropic (contractility), and lusitropic (relaxation) effects. A stimulatory guanine nucleotide-binding (G_s) protein couples the beta$_1$-adrenoceptor to the intracellular enzyme adenylyl cyclase (Fig. 13-4). Activation of the beta$_1$-adrenoceptor by an agonist increases the rate of formation of the second messenger cyclic adenosine monophosphate (cAMP) from adenosine triphosphate (ATP). This signaling mechanism has three major consequences for myocardial calcium (Ca^{2+}) homeostasis: (1) greater Ca^{2+} availability for contractile activation; (2) increased efficacy of activator Ca^{2+} at troponin C (TnC) of the contractile apparatus; and (3) faster removal of Ca^{2+} from the contractile apparatus and the sarcoplasm after contraction. The first two of these actions directly increase contractility, whereas the third facilitates more rapid myocardial relaxation
during early diastole. Predictably, treatment of acute left or right 5
ventricular (RV or LV, respectively) dysfunction is the major perioperative indication for the use of catecholamines. The relative

Table 13-4 Antimuscarinic Compounds Associated with Central Anticholinergic Syndrome

Belladonna Alkaloids	**Over-the-Counter**
Atropine sulfate	Asthmador—atropine like
Scopolamine hydrobromide	Compoz—scopolamine sedation
Synthetic and Natural Tertiary Amine Compounds	Sleep Eze—scopolamine sedation
Dicyclomine antispasmodic with local anesthetic activity	Sominex—scopolamine sedation
Thiphenamil antispasmodic with local anesthetic activity	**Antiparkinson Drugs**
Procaine	Benztropine
Cocaine	Trihexyphenidyl
Cyclopentolate mydriatic	Biperiden
Quaternary Derivatives of Belladonna Alkaloids	Ethopropazine
Methscopolamine bromide—antispasmodic	Procyclidine
Homatropine methylbromide—sedative, antispasmodic	**Antipsychotic Drugs**
Homatropine hydrobromide—ophthalmic solution—mydriatic	Chlorpromazine
Synthetic Quaternary Compounds	Thioridazine
Methantheline bromide	Haloperidol
Propantheline bromide	Droperidol
Antihistamines	Promethazine
Chlorpheniramine	**Tricyclic Antidepressants**
Diphenhydramine	Amitriptyline
Plants	Imipramine
Deadly nightshade (atropine)	Desipramine
Bittersweet	**Synthetic Opioids**
Potato leaves and sprouts	Meperidine
Jimson or loco weed	Methadone
Coca plant (cocaine)	

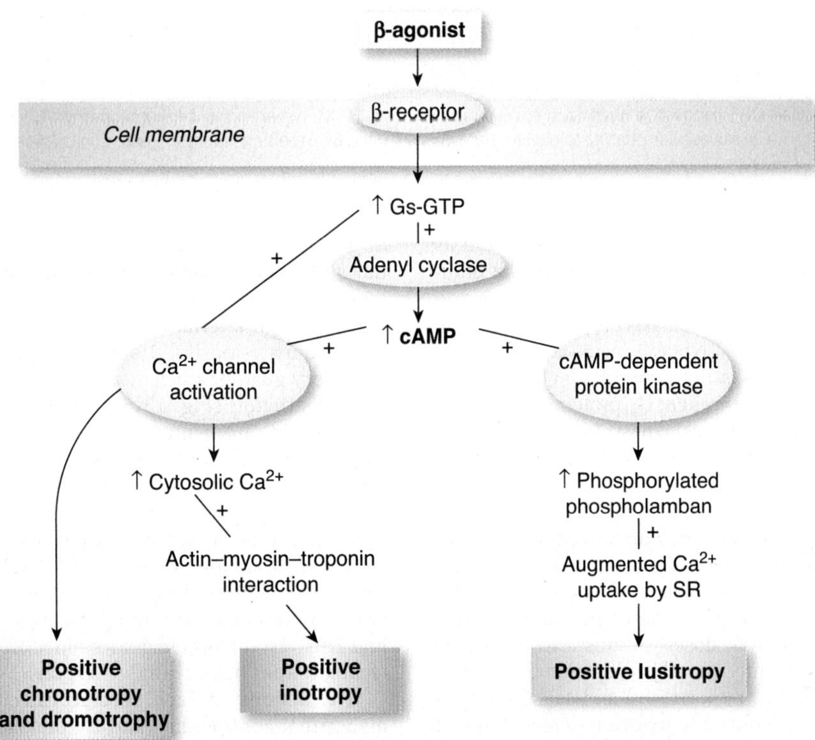

Figure 13-4 Schematic illustration of beta-adrenoceptor agonist mechanism of action in myocardium. (Adapted with permission from Springer: Gillies M, Bellomo R, Doolan L, et al. Bench-to-bedside review: Inotropic drug therapy after adult cardiac surgery—a systematic literature review. *Crit Care.* 2005;9:266–279.)

Table 13-5 Comparative Effects of Endogenous and Synthetic Catecholamines

Name	Chemical Structure	β_1	β_2	α_1	Dopamine$_1$
Epinephrine	HO, HO, OH, H, N	++++	+++	+++++	0
Norepinephrine	HO, HO, OH, NH_2	+++	+	+++++	0
Dopamine	HO, HO, NH_2	++++	++	+++	+++++
Dobutamine	HO, HO, H, N, OH	+++++	+++	+	0
Isoproterenol	HO, HO, OH, H, N	+++++	+++++	0	0
Phenylephrine	HO, OH, H, N	0	0	+++++	0

IV, intravenous; IM, intramuscular; CHF, congestive heart failure; AS, aortic stenosis; HCM, hypertrophic cardiomyopathy.
Modified from Linn KA, Pagel PS. Cardiovascular pharmacology. In: Barash PG, Cullen BF, Stoelting RK, et al., eds. *Clinical Anesthesia Fundamentals.* Wolters Kluwer; 2015:234–235.

density and functional integrity of the beta$_1$-adrenoceptor and its downstream signaling cascade substantially influence the clinical efficacy of catecholamines because receptor downregulation and abnormal intracellular Ca^{2+} homeostasis commonly occur in the presence of LV dysfunction.[13,14] Notably, beta$_2$-adrenoceptors are also present in myocardium (atrial > ventricular), which are also linked to adenylyl cyclase through G_s proteins and act to partially preserve myocardial responsiveness to catecholamine stimulation in the presence of beta$_1$-adrenoceptor dysfunction or downregulation.

The tissue-specific distribution of alpha- and beta-adrenoceptor subtypes and differences in each catecholamine's relative selectivity for adrenoceptors determine their actions in other perfusion beds. This selectivity is often dose related. Dopamine provides a particular useful (but not strictly accurate) pedagogical illustration of this principle. Lower doses of this catecholamine (<3 $\mu g \cdot kg^{-1} \cdot min^{-1}$) predominantly stimulate dopamine subtype 1 and 2 receptors (DA_1 and DA_2, respectively) and cause splanchnic and renal arterial vasodilation. Progressively larger doses of dopamine sequentially activate beta$_1$- (5 to 10 $\mu g \cdot kg^{-1} \cdot min^{-1}$) and alpha$_1$-adrenoceptors (>10 $\mu g \cdot kg^{-1} \cdot min^{-1}$), enhancing contractility and causing arterial vasoconstriction, respectively. Alpha$_1$-adrenoceptors are major regulators of vasomotor tone in arteries, arterioles, and veins. Catecholamines with substantial alpha$_1$-adrenoceptor agonist activity (e.g., norepinephrine) increase systemic vascular resistance and reduce venous capacitance through arterial and venous vasoconstriction, respectively. Phospholipase-inositol 1,4,5-triphosphate signaling through an inhibitory guanine nucleotide-binding (G_i) protein mediates this vasoconstriction (Fig. 13-5). The cascade opens Ca^{2+} channels, releases Ca^{2+} from intracellular stores (endoplasmic reticulum and calmodulin), and activates several Ca^{2+}-dependent protein kinases. These actions increase intracellular Ca^{2+} concentration and cause vascular smooth muscle to contract. Alpha$_1$-adrenoceptors predominate in many vascular beds, but beta$_2$-adrenoceptors are the most common adrenoceptor subtype in skeletal muscle. Activation of beta$_2$-adrenoceptors by catecholamines produces arteriolar vasodilation through adenylyl cyclase-mediated signaling. This vasodilation increases blood flow to skeletal muscle and facilitates the "fight-or-flight" response.

The actions of each specific catecholamine on heart rate, myocardial contractility, and LV preload and afterload combine to determine its overall effect on arterial pressure. For example, if a catecholamine acts primarily through the alpha$_1$-adrenoceptor, an increase in arterial pressure occurs because enhanced arterial and venous vasomotor tone increases systemic vascular resistance

Dose Range	Clinical Indications	Major Side Effects
IV: 0.01–0.2 µg/kg/min Bolus: 1 mg IV q3–5 min IM (1:1,000): 0.1–0.5 mg	Shock (cardiogenic, vasodilatory) Bronchospasm Anaphylaxis Symptomatic bradycardia unresponsive to atropine/pacing	Arrhythmias Myocardial Ischemia Sudden cardiac death Hypertension Stroke
IV: 0.01–0.2 µg/kg/min	Shock (cardiogenic, vasodilatory)	Arrhythmias Bradycardia Peripheral ischemia Hypertension Tissue necrosis with extravasation
IV: 2–20 µg/kg/min	Shock (cardiogenic, vasodilatory) Symptomatic bradycardia unresponsive to atropine/pacing	Hypertension Arrhythmias Myocardial ischemia Peripheral ischemia (high doses)
IV: 2–20 µg/kg/min	Low cardiac output (CHF, cardiogenic shock, sepsis-induced myocardial dysfunction) Symptomatic bradycardia unresponsive to atropine/pacing	Tachycardia Arrhythmias Myocardial ischemia Hypertension Hypotension
IV: 2–10 µg/kg/min	Bradyarrhythmias Denervated heart	Arrhythmias Myocardial ischemia Hypertension Hypotension
IV: 0.15–0.75 µg/kg/min Bolus: 0.1–0.5 mg	Hypotension with tachycardia Hypotension in AS or HCM	Reflex bradycardia Hypertension Peripheral and visceral vasoconstriction Tissue necrosis with extravasation

(greater afterload) and facilitates venous return (increased preload), respectively. Alternatively, a catecholamine with primarily beta-adrenoceptor activity and little or no effect on the alpha$_1$-adrenoceptor modestly decreases arterial pressure because reductions in systemic vascular resistance (through beta$_2$-adrenoceptor activation) offset increases in cardiac output caused by tachycardia and enhanced myocardial contractility (beta$_1$-adrenoceptor effects). It is noteworthy that all catecholamines have the potential to cause detrimental increases in myocardial oxygen demand in patients with flow-limiting coronary artery stenoses and may contribute to the development of acute myocardial ischemia. As a result, the use of a catecholamine to treat acute LV systolic dysfunction in a patient with coronary artery disease requires caution. For this reason, afterload reduction is usually a more prudent approach to improve cardiac output and reduce congestive symptoms in a patient with coronary artery disease complicated by heart failure with reduced ejection fraction (HFrEF).

Epinephrine

Methylation of norepinephrine by phenylethanolamine *N*-methyltransferase converts the norepinephrine into epinephrine in adrenal medullary chromaffin cells. Epinephrine is stored in and released from specific chromaffin cells that differ from those that store norepinephrine. These chromaffin cell types appear to release their respective catecholamines somewhat selectively to differing stimuli. For example, chromaffin cells may release the epinephrine in response to histamine exposure, whereas norepinephrine is primarily released by nicotinic agonists.[15] Epinephrine exerts its major cardiovascular effects through activation of alpha$_1$-, beta$_1$-, and beta$_2$-adrenoceptors. Epinephrine stimulates beta$_1$-adrenoceptors located on the cell membranes of sinoatrial (SA) node cells and cardiac myocytes to increase heart rate and myocardial contractility, respectively. Epinephrine-induced activation of beta$_1$-adrenoceptors also enhances the rate and extent of myocardial relaxation. This action improves LV filling dynamics during early diastole. The combination of these actions on heart rate and LV systolic and diastolic function markedly increases cardiac output: increases in cardiac index of 0.1, 0.7, and 1.2 $L \cdot min^{-1} \cdot m^2$ were observed during intravenous infusion of epinephrine (0.01, 0.02, and 0.04 $\mu g \cdot kg^{-1} \cdot min^{-1}$, respectively) in humans.[16] The initial tachycardia that occurs during administration of an intravenous infusion of epinephrine is partially attenuated over time as baroreceptor reflexes are activated. Epinephrine is particularly useful for the treatment of acute biventricular failure during cardiac surgery because it predictably increases cardiac output. Epinephrine (0.01 to 0.03 $\mu g \cdot kg^{-1} \cdot min^{-1}$) caused similar

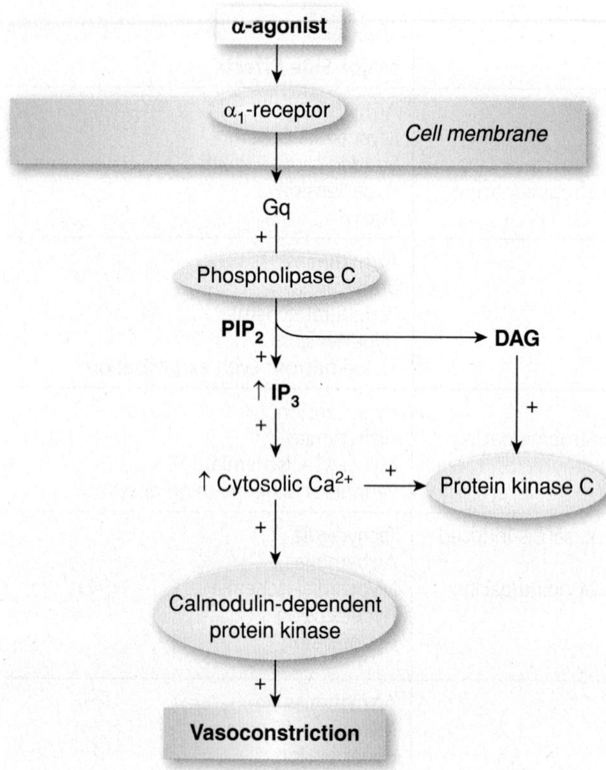

Figure 13-5 Schematic illustration of alpha-adrenoceptor agonist mechanism of action in vascular smooth muscle. (Adapted with permission from Springer: Gillies M, Bellomo R, Doolan L, et al. Bench-to-bedside review: Inotropic drug therapy after adult cardiac surgery—a systematic literature review. *Crit Care*. 2005;9:266–279.)

hemodynamic effects with less pronounced tachycardia compared with dobutamine (2.5 to 5.0 $\mu g \cdot kg^{-1} \cdot min^{-1}$) in patients after coronary artery bypass graft surgery.[17] The current authors recommend epinephrine as the primary inotropic drug for the treatment of acute LV dysfunction after cardiopulmonary bypass because it causes very predictable increases in cardiac output compared with its synthetic derivatives. Data suggesting that routine use of dobutamine in cardiac surgery adversely affects outcome supports this contention.[18] Epinephrine also enhances cardiac output and oxygen delivery without producing deleterious tachycardia in patients with sepsis. Epinephrine's efficacy as a positive inotropic drug may be limited by its propensity to cause atrial or ventricular tachyarrhythmias. Epinephrine increases conduction velocity and reduces refractory period in the AV node, His bundle, Purkinje fibers, and ventricular muscle. The positive dromotropic effect of epinephrine on AV nodal conduction may stimulate supraventricular tachyarrhythmias or cause pronounced increases in ventricular rate when atrial flutter or fibrillation is present. Either of these clinical conditions may inadvertently cause hypotension because profound tachycardia compromises LV filling and coronary perfusion. Epinephrine may increase the automaticity of latent pacemakers because spontaneous depolarization is enhanced. Irritability in other parts of the conduction system may also precipitate ventricular arrhythmias including premature ventricular contractions, ventricular tachycardia, and ventricular fibrillation, especially in the presence of an arrhythmogenic substrate (e.g., regional myocardial ischemia).

Epinephrine's overall effects on blood flow are dependent on the organ-specific distribution of $alpha_1$- and $beta_2$-adrenoceptors. Epinephrine causes vasoconstriction in cutaneous, mesenteric, splenic, and renal vascular beds because it is an $alpha_1$-adrenoceptor agonist, but the catecholamine also simultaneously vasodilates arterial blood vessels supplying skeletal muscle as a result of $beta_2$-adrenoceptor activation. These actions are dose dependent: lower doses (<0.02 $\mu g \cdot kg^{-1} \cdot min^{-1}$) of epinephrine primarily stimulate $beta_2$-adrenoceptors to cause vasodilation and modest declines in arterial pressure, whereas higher doses (>0.1 $\mu g \cdot kg^{-1} \cdot min^{-1}$) activate $alpha_1$-adrenoceptors to increase systemic vascular resistance and arterial pressure. Higher doses of epinephrine also cause intense renal arterial vasoconstriction resulting from a combination of $alpha_1$-adrenoceptor agonist effects and facilitation of renin release. The increase in arterial pressure associated with a large bolus dose (e.g., 1 mg in adults) of epinephrine improves coronary blood flow and survival during cardiopulmonary resuscitation. As a result, epinephrine is the drug of choice in the American Heart Association Adult Advanced Cardiac Life Support protocols for malignant ventricular arrhythmias, pulseless electrical activity, and asystole.[19]

Epinephrine produces venoconstriction and enhances venous return because the venous circulation also contains a high density of $alpha_1$-adrenoceptors. Epinephrine also causes vasoconstriction of the pulmonary arterial vascular smooth muscle and increases pulmonary arterial pressures through $alpha_1$-adrenoceptor stimulation. These actions may be especially pronounced in patients with preexisting pulmonary hypertension. $Alpha_1$- and $beta_2$-adrenoceptors are present in the coronary circulation, but selective activation of either of these receptor subtypes does not represent the major mechanism by which epinephrine affects coronary blood flow. Instead, increases in coronary blood flow observed during administration of epinephrine occur almost entirely as a result of metabolic autoregulation. Nevertheless, epinephrine may directly constrict epicardial coronary arteries and reduce coronary blood flow when maximal coronary vasodilation is present through direct $alpha_1$-adrenoceptor stimulation.

The vasoconstriction produced by epinephrine makes it useful for several other clinical applications. Subcutaneous infiltration of epinephrine is used to substantially reduce bleeding during dental, otolaryngology, plastic surgery, and orthopedic surgery procedures. The mixture of lidocaine with a dilute concentration of epinephrine reduces blood loss during tumescent anesthesia for liposuction. The vasoconstriction produced by epinephrine also substantially decreases the risk of adverse cardiovascular side effects (e.g., hypertension, arrhythmias) because the catecholamine is slowly absorbed under these circumstances. Anesthesiologists routinely use epinephrine as a vasoconstrictor to prolong the duration of neuraxial or regional anesthesia by delaying the absorption of local anesthetics. A secondary benefit of epinephrine-induced vasoconstriction is a decrease in plasma local anesthetic concentration, which reduces the risk of systemic toxicity. Mucosal vasoconstriction resulting from inhalation of aerosolized racemic epinephrine (containing a mixture of the levo- and dextrorotary optical isomers) is used to treat airway edema associated with prolonged endotracheal intubation, airway trauma, or croup. Intramuscular injection of epinephrine may be preferred to inhalation in children with severe croup because rebound edema may occur when using inhalation because the half-life of inhaled epinephrine is relatively short.[20] Epinephrine-induced activation of $beta_2$-adrenoceptors in airway smooth muscle causes bronchodilation in patients with reactive airway disease. Finally, epinephrine also decreases antigen-mediated release of histamine and leukotrienes from mast cells, which makes it useful for the treatment of bronchospasm caused by anaphylaxis.[21]

Prior administration of an alpha- or a beta-adrenoceptor antagonist affects epinephrine's cardiovascular effects. For example, epinephrine causes greater increases in systemic vascular resistance and arterial pressure when administered in the presence of a nonselective beta-blocker because $beta_2$-adrenoceptor–mediated arterial vasodilation no longer opposes $alpha_1$-adrenoceptor–induced vasoconstriction. Beta blockade also competitively inhibits epinephrine's activation of myocardial $beta_1$-adrenoceptors, which attenuates its positive chronotropic and inotropic effects. As a result, the hemodynamic effects of epinephrine may be quite similar to those of the synthetic $alpha_1$-adrenoceptor agonist phenylephrine (see below) in the presence of complete $beta_1$- and $beta_2$-adrenoceptor blockade. Conversely, epinephrine's $beta_2$-adrenoceptor–mediated vasodilation is unmasked in the presence of $alpha_1$-adrenoceptor blockade, and it may produce hypotension under these conditions. $Alpha_2$-adrenoceptor antagonists (e.g., cocaine) enhance the intensity and duration of action of the epinephrine's cardiovascular effects by inhibiting its reuptake.

Norepinephrine

Norepinephrine is the endogenous neurotransmitter released from postganglionic sympathetic nervous system nerve terminals. Norepinephrine activates $alpha_1$-, $alpha_2$-, and $beta_1$-adrenoceptors, but it has little effect on $beta_2$-adrenoceptors, unlike epinephrine. As a result of its adrenoceptor selectivity, norepinephrine enhances myocardial contractility and causes intense arterial vasoconstriction. These actions increase arterial pressure while cardiac output remains relatively unchanged. In contrast, administration of a pure $alpha_1$-adrenoceptor agonist produces dose-related declines in cardiac output in normal and failing myocardium by increasing LV afterload because $beta_1$-adrenoceptors are not stimulated and resulting increases in contractility do not occur. Unlike epinephrine, norepinephrine usually does not cause tachycardia because elevated arterial pressure activates baroreceptor reflexes, effectively negating the direct positive chronotropic effects of $beta_1$-adrenoceptor stimulation. In general, greater increases in diastolic arterial pressure and systemic vascular resistance occur during administration of norepinephrine compared with epinephrine. Norepinephrine constricts venous capacitance vessels through $alpha_1$-adrenoceptor stimulation. This action increases venous return, and combined with a $beta_1$-adrenoceptor–mediated positive inotropic effect, modestly augments stroke volume despite simultaneous increases in LV afterload.

Norepinephrine is most often used for treatment of refractory hypotension resulting from pronounced vasodilation. Norepinephrine is an established treatment in patients with septic shock that is unresponsive to volume administration or other vasoactive medications because it increases arterial pressure, cardiac index, and urine output.[22] The combination of norepinephrine and the gasotransmitter-scavengers methylene blue or hydroxocobalamin is also useful for the treatment of vasoplegic syndrome, a hypotensive state characterized by low systemic vascular resistance resulting from excessive production of NO and hydrogen sulfide that sometimes occurs during or after prolonged cardiopulmonary bypass in patients undergoing cardiac surgery.[23] Norepinephrine increases coronary perfusion pressure in patients with severe coronary artery disease, but the catecholamine also dramatically increases myocardial oxygen demand and may produce acute myocardial ischemia in the presence of flow-limiting coronary stenoses despite an improvement in coronary perfusion pressure. Norepinephrine may also cause spasm of internal mammary or radial artery grafts used during coronary artery surgery as a result of activation of $alpha_1$-adrenoceptors. Ventricular and supraventricular arrhythmias are sometimes observed during administration of norepinephrine, but the arrhythmogenic potential of norepinephrine is less than that of epinephrine. As a result, substitution of norepinephrine for epinephrine may be appropriate when hemodynamically significant atrial or ventricular arrhythmias are present.

Norepinephrine stimulates $alpha_1$-adrenoceptors in pulmonary arterial vascular smooth muscle and causes dose-related increases in pressures that may precipitate RV dysfunction or failure. An inhaled selective pulmonary vasodilator (e.g., NO, prostacyclin) may help to attenuate norepinephrine's direct pulmonary vasoconstrictor effects when the catecholamine is used in patients with pulmonary hypertension and depressed myocardial contractility. When systemic arterial pressure is normal or modestly reduced, norepinephrine causes dose-dependent decreases in hepatic, skeletal muscle, splanchnic, and renal blood flow through $alpha_1$-adrenoceptor–mediated vasoconstriction. However, norepinephrine increases perfusion pressure and blood flow to these vascular beds when arterial pressure is profoundly reduced, but sustained reductions in renal, mesenteric, and peripheral vascular blood flow represent a major limitation of prolonged use of norepinephrine. Activation of renal dopamine receptors with low-dose dopamine or the selective DA_1 agonist fenoldopam to partially counteract the deleterious actions of norepinephrine on renal blood flow may preserve renal perfusion and urine output but does not reduce the incidence or severity of acute kidney injury in patients with hypotension. Norepinephrine is typically administered through a central venous catheter to avoid the possibility of tissue necrosis from extravasation, but a recent large retrospective observational study suggests that dilute norepinephrine solutions (20 $\mu g\ ml^{-1}$ or less) can be administered safely through peripheral access.[24]

Dopamine

Dopamine is the biochemical precursor of norepinephrine (NICV 13-2). The catecholamine activates several adrenergic and dopaminergic receptor subtypes in a dose-related fashion. Lower doses (below 3 $\mu g{\cdot}kg^{-1}{\cdot}min^{-1}$) selectively activate DA_1 receptors to dilate renal, mesenteric, and splenic arterial blood vessels and increase renal and splanchnic blood flow. Lower doses of dopamine also reduce norepinephrine release from pre- and postganglionic sympathetic neurons through a DA_2 receptor-mediated mechanism. As a result of these actions, lower doses of dopamine modestly decrease arterial pressure. Moderate doses (3 to 8 $\mu g{\cdot}kg^{-1}{\cdot}min^{-1}$) of dopamine activate both $alpha_1$- and $beta_1$-adrenoceptors, resulting in elevated arterial pressure and positive inotropic effects. In contrast, high doses (in excess of 10 $\mu g{\cdot}kg^{-1}{\cdot}min^{-1}$) of dopamine act primarily on $alpha_1$-adrenoceptors to increase arterial pressure through arteriolar vasoconstriction. Unfortunately, this dose–response description of dopamine pharmacodynamics is overly simplistic because differences in receptor density and regulation, drug interactions, and patient variability cause a wide, often unpredictable range of clinical responses.[25] It was once presumed that low doses of dopamine provided renal protective effects through DA_1 receptor–mediated increases in renal blood flow, but this hypothesis was debunked because even low doses of dopamine are capable of producing simultaneous $alpha_1$- and $beta_1$-adrenoceptor activation that may attenuate or abolish the catecholamine's intended renal dopaminergic effect. Conversely, renal blood flow and urine output may be relatively preserved during administration of higher doses of dopamine because DA_1 receptors continue to be activated despite a predominant $alpha_1$-adrenoceptor agonist effect. Varied responses such as these may explain why the results of several clinical trials indicated that dopamine does not consistently provide renal protective effects despite improvements in renal perfusion and urine output. For example, a large meta-analysis of 61 clinical trials involving 3,359 patients demonstrated that low-dose dopamine transiently increased urine output, but the catecholamine did not reduce the incidence or severity of renal dysfunction or prevent mortality.[26] As a result, the use of low-dose dopamine to maintain or enhance renal function and prevent acute kidney injury is not recommended.

Dopamine is still occasionally used as a positive inotropic medication in patients with acute LV dysfunction by some practitioners, but the current authors prefer to use more potent catecholamines that have more predictable pharmacodynamic profiles (e.g., epinephrine, norepinephrine) with or without a cardiac phosphodiesterase fraction III inhibitor (e.g., milrinone) for this purpose. Dopamine increases myocardial contractility through activation of beta$_1$-adrenoceptors. Dopamine also stimulates arterial and venous alpha$_1$-adrenoceptors, increasing LV afterload and enhancing venous return, respectively. As a result of these combined actions on alpha$_1$- and beta$_1$-adrenoceptors, dopamine increases arterial pressure and cardiac output. The use of dopamine for the treatment of hypotension in the presence of depressed contractility is limited to some degree in patients with pulmonary hypertension or when LV filling pressures are elevated. Right atrial, mean pulmonary arterial, and pulmonary capillary occlusion pressures were greater in patients undergoing cardiac surgery receiving dopamine compared with dobutamine despite similar increases in cardiac output. Dopamine may also cause more pronounced tachycardia than epinephrine in cardiac surgery patients. An arterial vasodilator (e.g., sodium nitroprusside) may be used to blunt dopamine-induced increases in LV afterload and further enhance cardiac output. However, inotrope-vasodilators (e.g., milrinone, levosimendan) are more commonly used for this purpose in modern anesthesia practice. Like epinephrine and norepinephrine, dopamine directly increases myocardial oxygen demand and may precipitate myocardial ischemia when hemodynamically significant coronary stenoses are present.

Dobutamine

Commercial preparations of the synthetic catecholamine dobutamine contain two stereoisomers (– and +), both of which stimulate beta-adrenoceptors. These stereoisomers cause opposing effects on alpha$_1$-adrenoceptors. Dobutamine is a potent stimulator of beta-adrenoceptors, but the drug has no effect on alpha$_1$-adrenoceptors when it is administered at infusion rates less than 5 $\mu g \cdot kg^{-1} \cdot min^{-1}$. As a result, dobutamine enhances myocardial contractility and reduces arterial vasomotor tone through beta$_1$- and beta$_2$-adrenoceptor activation, respectively. These actions combine to markedly improve LV-arterial coupling, enhance myocardial efficiency, and increase cardiac output in the presence or absence of LV systolic dysfunction. The beneficial effect of dobutamine on mechanical matching between the LV and the arterial vasculature contributes to a decrease in the severity of mitral regurgitation observed when it is administered to patients with dilated cardiomyopathy and increased LV filling pressures. The dobutamine (–) isomer progressively stimulates the alpha$_1$-adrenoceptor as infusion rates increase above 5 $\mu g \cdot kg^{-1} \cdot min^{-1}$, which attenuates the degree of vasodilation resulting from beta$_2$-adrenoceptor activation. The alpha$_1$-adrenoceptor agonist effect of higher doses of dobutamine not only maintains LV preload, afterload, and arterial pressure, but also blunts the baroreceptor-mediated tachycardia that might otherwise occur. Nevertheless, dobutamine often increases heart rate by direct beta$_1$-adrenoceptor–mediated positive chronotropic and dromotropic effects. Indeed, dobutamine causes more pronounced tachycardia than epinephrine at equivalent values of cardiac index in patients after coronary artery surgery. Dobutamine directly increases myocardial oxygen demand and may cause acute myocardial ischemia in patients with coronary artery disease. This principle is the basis of dobutamine stress echocardiography as a diagnostic tool for the detection of a flow-limiting coronary stenosis because a regional wall motion abnormality will be observed in the affected coronary perfusion territory in response to the myocardial oxygen supply–demand mismatch.[27] Conversely, dobutamine often reduces heart rate in patients with acute LV systolic function or HFrEF because increases in cardiac output and oxygen delivery improve tissue perfusion and reduce elevated sympathetic nervous system tone. Dobutamine may also favorably decrease myocardial oxygen demand in the failing heart because stimulation of beta$_2$-adrenoceptors decreases LV preload and afterload, and consequently decreases LV end-diastolic and end-systolic wall stress, respectively.

Dobutamine modestly decreases pulmonary arterial pressures and pulmonary vascular resistance through beta$_2$-adrenoceptor stimulation. Thus, dobutamine is a useful positive inotropic drug for patients with pulmonary arterial hypertension, in contrast to dopamine.[28] Dobutamine is also preferred to dopamine in heart failure patients with elevated pulmonary vascular resistance and LV filling pressures. Nevertheless, dobutamine-induced pulmonary vasodilation has the potential to exacerbate ventilation–perfusion mismatch, increase transpulmonary shunt, and contribute to relative hypoxemia. Dobutamine indirectly improves renal perfusion by increasing cardiac output, but it does not directly activate DA$_1$ receptors to cause renal arterial vasodilation, unlike dopamine. Despite its theoretical beneficial cardiovascular effects, the results of several clinical trials indicated that use of dobutamine was linked to an increased incidence of major adverse cardiac events including mortality in patients with decompensated heart failure.[29] Dobutamine was also associated with adverse sequelae in cardiac surgery patients.[18] As a result of these and other compelling data, the current authors no longer use dobutamine for positive inotropic support in their cardiac anesthesiology practices. Dobutamine is efficacious for the treatment of depressed myocardial contractility in patients with sepsis.[30]

Isoproterenol

Isoproterenol is a synthetic catecholamine derived from dopamine that is a nonselective beta-adrenoceptor agonist with low affinity for the alpha-adrenoceptor. As a result, isoproterenol increases heart rate and myocardial contractility and decreases arterial pressure through beta$_1$- and beta$_2$-adrenoceptor agonist effects, respectively. Historically, isoproterenol was used for "pharmacologic pacing" in patients with symptomatic bradyarrhythmias or AV conduction block because of the drug's positive chronotropic effects. Isoproterenol was also used during cardiac transplantation to increase heart rate and enhance myocardial contractility in the denervated donor heart. Transcutaneous or transvenous pacing has largely replaced isoproterenol for treatment of bradyarrhythmias because of the drug's propensity to precipitate adverse supraventricular and ventricular tachyarrhythmias. Isoproterenol was previously used to treat RV dysfunction resulting from severe pulmonary hypertension because it causes pulmonary vasodilation by stimulating beta$_2$-adrenoceptors in pulmonary arterial vascular smooth muscle. However, isoproterenol has been replaced by selective inhaled pulmonary vasodilators (e.g., NO, prostaglandin I_2) for this purpose because these medications are more effective and have fewer adverse side effects. The current clinical applicability of isoproterenol is limited, but comparison of the pharmacology of isoproterenol with other catecholamines merits continued discussion because of its unique adrenoceptor profile.

Isoproterenol causes $beta_2$-adrenoceptor-mediated arteriolar vasodilation in renal, mesenteric, splenic, and skeletal muscle circulations. These actions reduce systemic vascular resistance and decrease arterial pressure. Isoproterenol causes direct positive chronotropic and dromotropic effects and increases heart rate because of $beta_1$-adrenoceptor activation. Tachycardia also occurs because hypotension stimulates baroreceptor-mediated increases in heart rate. Isoproterenol is a positive inotropic drug, but anticipated increases in cardiac output may not occur because profound tachycardia attenuates LV filling and $beta_2$-adrenoceptor–mediated venodilation decreases LV preload. As a result, isoproterenol does not increase cardiac output in patients undergoing coronary artery or valve replacement surgery, unlike dobutamine. Predictably, the hemodynamic effects of isoproterenol cause dose-related increases in myocardial oxygen demand. Isoproterenol also reduces coronary perfusion pressure and decreases diastolic filling time. These unfavorable changes in myocardial oxygen supply–demand relations may contribute to the development of acute myocardial ischemia or cause subendocardial necrosis, even in the absence of flow-limiting coronary stenoses.

Selective $Beta_2$-Adrenoceptor Agonists

Several short- and long-acting selective $beta_2$-adrenoceptor agonists, including metaproterenol, albuterol, salmeterol, and fenoterol, are currently in clinical use for treatment of asthma and chronic obstructive pulmonary disease. A hydroxyl substitution on the phenyl ring or addition of a large moiety to the amino group of a catecholamine's structure increases the new molecule's relative $beta_2$-adrenoceptor affinity. These drugs stimulate $beta_2$-adrenoceptors in bronchial smooth muscle to produce bronchodilation, reduce airway resistance, and improve obstructive symptoms. Reductions in histamine and leukotriene release from pulmonary mast cells and improvements in mucociliary function also contribute to the beneficial effects of selective $beta_2$-adrenoceptor agonists in patients with reactive airway disease. To minimize the systemic side effects of $beta_2$-adrenoceptor activation (e.g., tremor, anxiety, restlessness), the drugs are typically administered using a hand-held nebulizer or a metered-dose inhaler. However, the $beta_2$-adrenoceptor selectivity of these drugs progressively decreases and $beta_1$-adrenoceptor-mediated adverse effects (e.g., tachycardia, arrhythmias) become more apparent as larger doses are used. Terbutaline is another $beta_2$-adrenoceptor agonist that is administered subcutaneously or intramuscularly and may be useful in the management of status asthmaticus.

Fenoldopam

Fenoldopam mesylate is a selective DA_1-receptor agonist that does not exert activity at alpha- or beta-adrenoceptors.[31] The drug dilates mesenteric, splenic, and renal arterioles, increases renal blood flow, decreases renal vascular resistance, reduces systemic vascular resistance, improves creatinine clearance, and promotes both natriuresis and diuresis. Fenoldopam was initially developed as an antihypertensive medication because of its actions as a vasodilator. Some initial evidence suggested that fenoldopam protects the kidney against nephropathy produced by angiographic contrast, presumably by virtue of enhanced renal blood flow. This potential to attenuate renal injury, particularly in the presence of hypotension or preexisting kidney damage, prompted intense investigation of fenoldopam as a possible renal protective agent.[32] Unfortunately, large randomized controlled clinical trials failed to support the early results. Fenoldopam did not protect against contrast-induced nephropathy, nor decrease the need for dialysis in patients with early acute tubular necrosis, nor reduce the requirement for renal replacement therapy or 30-day mortality in patients with acute kidney injury undergoing cardiac surgery.[33] Thus, despite the fact that fenoldopam is a potent direct renal vasodilator and promotes increased urine output, the drug does not exert protection against kidney injury. Fenoldopam has a rapid onset of action as an antihypertensive medication. The drug undergoes hepatic metabolism and is excreted in the urine. The elimination half-life of fenoldopam is approximately 5 minutes. Unlike the findings with intravenous vasodilators (see below), tolerance to fenoldopam's antihypertensive effects is uncommon and rebound hypertension after abrupt discontinuation of the drug does not usually occur. The most common adverse effects of fenoldopam are related to its effects as a vasodilator and include hypotension, tachycardia, flushing, dizziness, headache, and nausea.

Sympathomimetics

Ephedrine

Ephedrine exerts direct and indirect pharmacologic actions on adrenergic receptors, but its predominant effect is indirect. Endocytosis of ephedrine into $alpha_1$- and $beta_1$-adrenoceptor presynaptic postganglionic nerve terminals displaces norepinephrine from the synaptic vesicles. The displaced norepinephrine is then released to activate the corresponding postsynaptic receptors to cause arterial and venous vasoconstriction and increased myocardial contractility. Ephedrine's initial cardiovascular effects resemble those of epinephrine because dose-related increases in heart rate, cardiac output, and systemic vascular resistance are observed. Ephedrine is less potent than epinephrine, but its duration of action is longer than that of the direct-acting endogenous catecholamine. Ephedrine also directly stimulates $beta_2$-adrenoceptors, which limits the increases in arterial pressure that occur as a result of $alpha_1$-adrenoceptor activation. Tachyphylaxis to ephedrine's hemodynamic effects occurs with repetitive administration of the drug because presynaptic norepinephrine stores are rapidly depleted and ephedrine is then released from synaptic vesicles as a false neurotransmitter. In contrast, tachyphylaxis does not occur with epinephrine because it directly stimulates alpha- and beta-adrenoceptors independent of a displacement and release mechanism. Predictably, drugs that block the ephedrine uptake into adrenergic nerves (e.g., cocaine) and those that deplete norepinephrine reserves (e.g., reserpine) attenuate its cardiovascular effects. The most common clinical use of ephedrine during anesthesia is treatment of acute decreases in arterial pressure accompanied by bradycardia.

Phenylephrine

The structure of phenylephrine is similar to epinephrine, but phenylephrine does not have a hydroxyl group attached to the phenyl ring. As a result of this minor difference in chemistry, phenylephrine almost exclusively stimulates alpha$_1$-adrenoceptors to increase venous and arterial vasomotor tone while exerting almost no effect on beta-adrenoceptors. Phenylephrine acts directly on the alpha$_1$-adrenoceptor and is not dependent on presynaptic norepinephrine displacement to produce its cardiovascular effects, unlike ephedrine. Phenylephrine constricts venous capacitance vessels and causes cutaneous, skeletal muscle, mesenteric, splenic, and renal vasoconstriction. These actions increase LV preload and afterload and cause dose-related increases in arterial pressure. Predictably, baroreceptor-mediated decreases in heart rate also occur. Cardiac output usually remains relatively constant when LV function is normal, but cardiac output may decline when HFrEF is present because failing myocardium is more sensitive to acute increases in afterload.[34] Phenylephrine also increases pulmonary artery pressures through pulmonary arterial vasoconstriction and greater venous return. Unlike endogenous or synthetic catecholamines, phenylephrine is not arrhythmogenic. Intravenous boluses or infusions of phenylephrine are most often used for treatment of hypotension in the presence of normal or elevated heart rate, such as is observed during acute hypovolemia.

Alpha$_1$-adrenoceptor Antagonists

Blockade of alpha$_1$-adrenoceptors in arterial and venous vascular smooth muscle causes vasodilation by inhibiting the actions of endogenous catecholamines (and other sympathomimetic amines) at this receptor subtype. For this reason, alpha$_1$-adrenoceptor blockers were previously used for the treatment of essential hypertension, but beta-blockers, ACE inhibitors, angiotensin II receptor blockers, Ca^{2+} channel blockers, diuretics, and nitrates have largely replaced these drugs for this clinical
6 indication in modern practice. Alpha$_1$-adrenoceptor antagonists (e.g., prazosin) are certainly very effective antihypertensive medications, but many patients complained that the side effect profile, which includes debilitating orthostatic hypotension, baroreceptor-mediated tachycardia with or without palpitations, nasal congestion, and fluid retention, was intolerable during chronic use of these drugs. The presence of alpha$_1$-adrenoceptor blockade also has the potential to cause unopposed beta$_1$- and beta$_2$-adrenoceptor activity. For example, epinephrine will activate only beta$_1$- and beta$_2$-adrenoceptors because its alpha$_1$-adrenoceptor agonist effects are inhibited. As a result, epinephrine produces pronounced tachycardia (a beta$_1$ effect) and severe hypotension (activation of beta$_2$ receptors causing arterial and venous vasodilation) when administered in the presence of an alpha$_1$-adrenoceptor blocker. Similarly, norepinephrine and ephedrine will only activate beta$_1$-adrenoceptors because their alpha$_1$-adrenoceptor agonist actions are inhibited. The pure alpha$_1$-agonist phenylephrine also has no effect as a vasoconstrictor under these conditions. The response of a given vascular bed to an alpha$_1$-adrenoceptor antagonist is dependent on its intrinsic level of vasomotor tone, as blood vessels with higher resting vascular smooth muscle tone will generally be more responsive to alpha$_1$-adrenoceptor blockade.

Phenoxybenzamine is an orally administered, relatively nonselective alpha-adrenoceptor antagonist that binds irreversibly to alpha$_1$- and alpha$_2$-adrenoceptors at a ratio of selectivity of approximately 100:1. Because phenoxybenzamine's actions at alpha-adrenoceptors are irreversible, synthesis of new receptors is required to reverse its effects as a vasodilator. Phenoxybenzamine has a prolonged half-life, which also contributes to its sustained actions at the alpha-adrenoceptor. Phenoxybenzamine is used almost exclusively to normalize arterial pressure before surgery in patients with pheochromocytoma.[35,36] The onset of alpha-adrenoceptor blockade produced by phenoxybenzamine is typically slow because it requires structural modification in situ to become pharmacologically active. Several weeks of treatment is commonly needed to bring hypertension under control in patients with pheochromocytoma. Restoration of intravascular volume status is also an important goal of phenoxybenzamine therapy, as chronic hypertension resulting from elevated serum catecholamine concentrations cause relative hypovolemia, which often contributes to hemodynamic lability during tumor resection. Addition of a beta-adrenoceptor antagonist after phenoxybenzamine therapy has been initiated is also useful as an antihypertensive medication and further serves to protect the myocardium from the adverse effects of chronic catecholamine stimulation. However, beta-blockade should not be started first because unopposed alpha-adrenoceptor stimulation by circulating catecholamines will worsen hypertension and may contribute to the development of acute myocardial ischemia or infarction or cause hemorrhagic stroke. When properly combined, alpha- and beta-adrenoceptor antagonists facilitate greater cardiovascular stability during pheochromocytoma resection, which is usually associated with additional release of norepinephrine and epinephrine during tumor manipulation. The most prominent side effect of phenoxybenzamine is orthostatic hypotension. Vasopressin is often needed to effectively manage refractory hypotension associated with phenoxybenzamine overdose.

The competitive intravenous alpha$_1$- and alpha$_2$-adrenoceptor antagonist phentolamine is also used in patients with pheochromocytoma. In contrast to phenoxybenzamine, the effects of phentolamine are reversible (half-life of less than 10 minutes). Phentolamine is a potent vasodilator that rapidly decreases arterial pressure, but in so doing, also causes marked baroreceptor-mediated tachycardia. Blockade of cardiac alpha$_2$-adrenoceptors by phentolamine may contribute to the development of arrhythmias. Moreover, phentolamine exerts antihistamine and cholinergic activity, the latter of which may produce abdominal cramping and diarrhea. Because the drug causes hypotension and tachycardia, phentolamine should only be used with caution in patients with flow-limiting coronary artery stenoses because acute myocardial ischemia or infarction may occur as a result of myocardial oxygen supply–demand mismatch. Phentolamine is occasionally used as a local vasodilator to prevent tissue necrosis after iatrogenic extravasation of a vasoconstrictor (e.g., norepinephrine). The alpha-adrenoceptor antagonist may also be effective when treating refractory hypertension associated with clonidine withdrawal or tyramine exposure in patients receiving a monoamine oxidase inhibitor.

Unlike phenoxybenzamine and phentolamine, prazosin is a relatively selective antagonist of alpha$_1$-adrenoceptors (alpha$_1$ to alpha$_2$ ratio of approximately 1,000:1) that causes arterial and venous vasodilation. Because of prazosin's relative alpha$_1$-adrenergic selectivity, alpha$_2$-adrenoceptor modulation of norepinephrine release from postganglionic sympathetic neurons remains intact. As a result, baroreceptor-mediated tachycardia is substantially attenuated when prazosin is administered. Orthostatic hypotension is the most important clinical side effect of prazosin when it is used for the treatment of hypertension. Prazosin undergoes hepatic metabolism. The drug also increases the ratio of high- to low-density lipoproteins. In contrast with ACE inhibitors, prazosin does not improve survival in patients with HFrEF; the drug is no longer recommended for this indication. Other alpha$_1$-adrenoceptor antagonists (e.g., terazosin, doxazosin, tamsulosin) are used for the treatment of benign prostatic hyperplasia because the prostate contains a large number of alpha$_{1A}$-adrenoceptors.[37] Anesthesiologists should be aware that anesthetic-induced vasodilation might be exacerbated in the presence of these urologic alpha$_1$-adrenoceptor antagonists.

Alpha$_2$-adrenoceptor Agonists: Clonidine and Dexmedetomidine

7 The alpha$_2$-adrenoceptor agonists clonidine and dexmedetomidine are commonly used for sedation, anxiolysis, and analgesia.[38,39] Clonidine is a partial alpha$_2$-adrenoceptor agonist with relative selectivity for alpha$_2$- versus alpha$_1$-receptors of approximately 200:1. Clonidine binds to alpha$_2$-adrenoceptors and inhibits norepinephrine release from presynaptic postganglionic sympathetic neurons, blocks sympathetic nerve traffic through pre- and postsynaptic mechanisms in the central nervous system, and attenuates spinal presynaptic sympathetic nerve transmission. Because of its sympatholytic effects, clonidine was originally used for the treatment of hypertension. Clonidine blunts centrally mediated sympathetic nervous system tone, decreases serum norepinephrine and norepinephrine concentrations, and reduces activation of the renin–angiotensin–aldosterone axis. In addition, clonidine stimulates parasympathetic nervous system activity to cause bradycardia. Unlike other vasodilating antihypertensive medications, clonidine does not affect baroreceptor-mediated reflex control of heart rate. The alpha$_2$-adrenoceptor agonist usually does not cause orthostatic hypotension, unlike alpha$_1$-antagonists or ACE inhibitors. However, hypotension and bradycardia may occur when large doses of the drug are administered. These effects may be reversed with vasoactive medications.

Clonidine reduces volatile and intravenous anesthetic requirements, blunts the hemodynamic responses to laryngoscopy and endotracheal intubation, promotes intraoperative cardiovascular stability, partially attenuates the sympathetic stress response associated with surgery, and decreases postoperative tissue oxygen requirements. A large meta-analysis of 23 controlled trials with 3,395 patients showed that clonidine and other alpha$_2$-adrenoceptor agonists reduce the risk of perioperative myocardial ischemia and infarction and decrease mortality in patients undergoing major vascular or cardiac surgery.[40] These anti-ischemic actions were presumably related to the drug's sympatholytic effects, which reduce myocardial oxygen demand. Clonidine augments the effects of local anesthetics and opioids and increases their duration of action when used for neuraxial and regional anesthesia.[41] As a result, clonidine indirectly decreases local anesthetic and opioid toxicity because lower amounts of these drugs are needed for anesthesia and analgesia. Clonidine is an effective postoperative analgesic and has well-documented utility in the treatment of complex regional pain syndrome and neuropathic pain. The sedative and anxiolytic effects of clonidine are attributed to activation of alpha$_2$-adrenoceptors in the locus coeruleus. It is noteworthy that clonidine does not substantially inhibit respiratory drive despite its sedative effect. As a result, clonidine's sedative-analgesic effects are particularly useful in patients with compromised respiratory function. Hyperglycemia may occur in patients treated with clonidine because it inhibits insulin release in patients with or without diabetes mellitus. Clonidine is also used to mitigate withdrawal symptoms during treatment of substance abuse disorders.

Discontinuation of clonidine may be necessary during the perioperative period if a patient is unable to ingest oral medications. Abrupt withdrawal of the alpha$_2$-adrenoceptor agonist often causes severe rebound hypertension associated with tachycardia, headache, anxiety, tremor, and diaphoresis. Invasive monitoring of arterial pressure in an intensive care unit setting and treatment of hypertension with other medications may be necessary until symptoms are controlled or oral clonidine therapy is resumed. Beta-blockers should not be used alone under such circumstances because unopposed alpha$_1$-adrenoceptor stimulation causes profound vasoconstriction, thereby worsening hypertension. Alternatively, transdermal clonidine may be used to attenuate withdrawal rebound hypertension in those patients who are unable to consume it. However, transdermal clonidine requires approximately 48 hours after its initial application to achieve therapeutic plasma concentrations.

Dexmedetomidine is approximately sevenfold more selective for the alpha$_2$-adrenoceptor (alpha$_2$ to alpha$_1$ ratio of 1,600:1) and has a substantially shorter context-sensitive half-life than clonidine (NICV 13-3). These characteristics make an intravenous infusion of dexmedetomidine useful for sedation, amnesia, and analgesia in the operating room and intensive care unit.[42] Like clonidine, dexmedetomidine reduces anesthetic requirements during general, neuraxial, and regional anesthesia; decreases heart rate, arterial pressure, and plasma catecholamine concentrations; attenuates intraoperative cardiovascular lability; and does not cause clinically significant respiratory depression. This latter feature is especially beneficial in the setting of elective fiberoptic intubation or weaning from mechanical ventilation. Dexmedetomidine's relative preservation of respiratory drive and its lack of effects on electrophysiologic monitoring also make it useful for functional neurosurgery.[43] Dexmedetomidine facilitates perioperative care of obese patients with obstructive sleep apnea and those undergoing bariatric surgery because the drug provides analgesia, reduces opioid requirements, and does not substantially depress respiration.[44] Dexmedetomidine reduces the incidence of delirium compared with other sedatives including propofol in elderly patients undergoing cardiac[45] or noncardiac surgery.[46] Dexmedetomidine may be associated with hypothermia because the drug lowers the threshold body temperature at which compensatory thermoregulation mechanisms are activated.

Like clonidine, dexmedetomidine produces a biphasic arterial pressor–depressor response. The initial hypertension occurs as a result of direct stimulation of postsynaptic alpha$_2$-adrenoceptors in arterial vascular smooth muscle, an action which results in an increase in systemic vascular resistance. Subsequent declines in arterial pressure occur because activation of medullary alpha$_2$-adrenergic or imidazoline receptors by the drug alters the balance between centrally mediated sympathetic and parasympathetic nervous system tone. Dexmedetomidine causes an initial bradycardia that results from increased vagal tone mediated by a baroreceptor response to hypertension. This bradycardia is subsequently reinforced by central sympathetic withdrawal.[47] The hemodynamic effects of dexmedetomidine contribute to reductions in major adverse cardiovascular events including mortality in patients undergoing cardiac surgery.[48]

Beta-Adrenoceptor Antagonists (Beta-Blockers)

Many of the cardiovascular effects of beta-adrenoceptor antagonists (more commonly known as "beta-blockers") may be anticipated based on the previous discussion of catecholamines. Beta-blockers are a first-line treatment for patients with ST- and non-ST-segment elevation myocardial infarction in the absence of cardiogenic shock, hemodynamically significant bradyarrhythmias, or reactive airway disease. These medications have been repeatedly shown to reduce morbidity and mortality associated with myocardial infarction in many large-scale randomized controlled trials. Beta-blockers bind to beta$_1$-adrenoceptors and inhibit the actions of circulating catecholamines and norepinephrine released from postganglionic sympathetic neurons. As a result, heart rate and myocardial contractility are reduced. The decrease in heart rate prolongs diastole, increases coronary blood flow to the left ventricle (LV), enhances coronary collateral perfusion to ischemic myocardium, and improves oxygen delivery to the coronary microcirculation. These actions reduce myocardial oxygen demand and increase supply. Beta-blockers have also been shown to inhibit platelet aggregation, which is important during acute myocardial ischemia or evolving myocardial infarction because platelet aggregation at the site of an atherosclerotic plaque may worsen a coronary stenosis or produce acute occlusion of the vessel. Beta-blockers are very effective for the treatment of essential hypertension, produce antiarrhythmic effects through negative chronotropic actions, and have well-established roles in the treatment of HFrEF, hypertrophic cardiomyopathy, acute aortic dissection, thyrotoxicosis, pheochromocytoma, and migraine headache prophylaxis. Topical beta-blockers are also used for treatment of open-angle glaucoma. Beta-blockers have been shown to reduce the incidence of myocardial infarction in patients undergoing noncardiac surgery.[49,50] These drugs are strongly recommended for patients with documented or multiple risk factors for myocardial ischemia, but not for those who do not have clear evidence of coronary artery disease.

Propranolol is the prototypical beta-blocker against which all other medications in this pharmacologic class are compared (Table 13-6). Propranolol and other beta-blockers are chemically related to isoproterenol. They contain an aromatic ring linked to ethanolamine group, the latter of which allows interaction with the beta-adrenoceptor. Additions to the molecule's aromatic group determine the degree of beta$_1$-adrenoceptor specificity. All beta-blockers have a chiral center; the negative enantiomer of each drug is biologically active. The relative selectively of beta-blockers for beta$_1$- and beta$_2$-adrenoceptors, their lipid solubility, and the presence or absence of intrinsic sympathomimetic ability (e.g., partial stimulation of the beta$_1$-adrenoceptor), myocardial membrane stabilizing activity, and additional cardiovascular actions combine with each drug's pharmacokinetic effects to distinguish individual beta-blockers from one another. The ability to prevent isoproterenol-induced increases in heart rate defines each beta-blocker's potency. Propranolol is a "first-generation" (nonselective) beta-blocker that competitively inhibits both beta$_1$- and beta$_2$-adrenoceptors, whereas metoprolol, atenolol, and esmolol are classified as "second-generation" beta-blockers because these drugs are more selective for the beta$_1$-adrenoceptor. However, this selectivity is relative because larger doses of second-generation beta-blockers inhibit both receptor subtypes. "Third-generation" beta-blockers exert other cardiovascular effects besides their actions at beta-adrenoceptors. Labetalol blocks alpha$_1$-adrenoceptors. Carvedilol exerts antioxidant and anti-inflammatory actions. Bucindolol has intrinsic sympathomimetic effects because it is a partial agonist of beta$_1$-adrenoceptors. Nebivolol produces NO-mediated vasodilation through its actions on vascular endothelium.

The reductions in heart rate and myocardial contractility produced by beta-blockers are more pronounced in the presence of increased sympathetic nervous system tone (e.g., surgical stimulation, exercise, HFrEF). Nonselective beta-blockers initially reduce cardiac output as a result of negative chronotropic and inotropic effects concomitant with arterial vasoconstriction mediated through blockade of vascular smooth muscle beta$_2$-adrenoceptors and compensatory sympathetic stimulation of alpha$_1$-adrenoceptors. This transient increase in systemic vascular resistance gradually dissipates during long-term use. Selective beta$_1$-blockers with or without alpha$_1$-adrenoceptor antagonist activity and those with direct vasodilator effects generally reduce systemic vascular resistance and preserve cardiac output to varying degrees despite their inherent negative inotropic effect. Beta-blockers are used extensively for the treatment of hypertension, but the precise mechanisms by which beta-blockers without specific additional vasodilating properties reduce arterial blood pressure remain to be clearly defined (Fig. 13-6). Stimulation of beta$_1$-adrenoceptors in renal juxtaglomerular cells by the sympathetic postganglionic neurons causes renin secretion and activates the renin–angiotensin–aldosterone axis (see below). Many beta-blockers inhibit this renin release, but their antihypertensive effects usually occur before plasma renin concentrations decline. Similarly, some beta-blockers do not substantially affect renin metabolism and yet are quite effective at reducing arterial pressure in patients with hypertension. It is also unlikely that beta-blockers cause antihypertensive effects through a decrease in centrally mediated sympathetic nervous system tone because drugs with markedly different lipid solubility are equally effective at decreasing arterial pressure. Beta-blockers most likely do not favorably modulate postganglionic sympathetic neuron norepinephrine release despite the presence of presynaptic beta-adrenoceptors that are known to stimulate the neurotransmitter's release. Selective beta-blockers that do not affect beta$_2$-adrenoceptor viability ("second-generation") and those than inhibit alpha$_1$-adrenoceptors or produce vasodilation through other mechanisms also decrease arterial pressure. Nevertheless, nonselective beta-blockers such as propranolol continue to be very efficacious antihypertensive medications independent of any alternative vasodilating characteristics.

Beta-blockers have been a mainstay in the pharmacologic treatment of acute myocardial ischemia and infarction since they were first introduced into clinical practice in the 1960s. As mentioned previously, beta-blockers directly reduce the hemodynamic determinants of myocardial oxygen demand and improve coronary perfusion. These actions favorably alter myocardial oxygen supply–demand balance and reduce ischemic burden, thereby minimizing the severity of myocardial necrosis, preserving LV systolic function, attenuating the development of malignant ventricular arrhythmias, improving long-term functional capacity, and decreasing mortality. The results supporting the use of beta-blockers in acute myocardial infarction are among the most convincing data ever published in the medical literature. Many randomized controlled trials demonstrated unequivocally that beta-blockers are not only effective for treatment of acute myocardial infarction but also substantially decrease the risk of developing a subsequent infarction in patients with coronary artery disease.[51] Indeed, the estimated overall reduction in mortality associated with use of beta-blockers in myocardial infarction is approximately 25%. Beta-blockers also have well-established efficacy for the treatment of HFrEF. The use of beta-blockers in HFrEF was initially viewed with skepticism because administration of a drug that further depresses myocardial contractility would appear to be counterintuitive. However, sympathetic nervous system tone is chronically elevated in HFrEF, and this excessive sympathetic activity produces a series of alterations in beta$_1$-adrenoceptor density and function, intracellular signal transduction, contractile protein expression, and Ca^{2+} homeostasis that promote mitochondrial dysfunction, stimulate myocyte apoptosis (programmed cell death), cause pathologic ventricular remodeling, and accelerate disease progression. Clinical trials demonstrated that beta-blockers significantly decrease mortality in patients with HFrEF independent of disease severity. In fact, some large randomized studies were halted before completion because patients with moderate to severe heart HFrEF receiving beta-blockers had markedly improved mortality compared with those treated with placebo. Beta-blockers mitigate clinical

Table 13-6 Comparative Effects of β-blockers

Name	Chemical Structure	β_1	Selectivity β_2	α_1	Plasma Half-Life (h)	Intrinsic Sympathomimetic Activity	Membrane Stabilizing Activity	Lipid Solubility	Metabolism
Propranolol	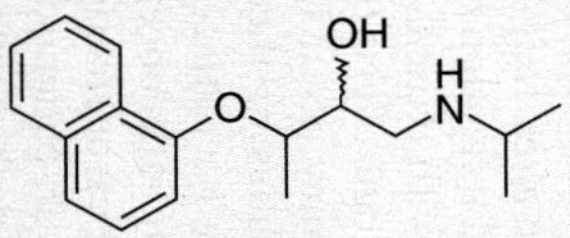 O, OH, H N	+	+	0	3–4	0	+	+++	Liver
Metoprolol	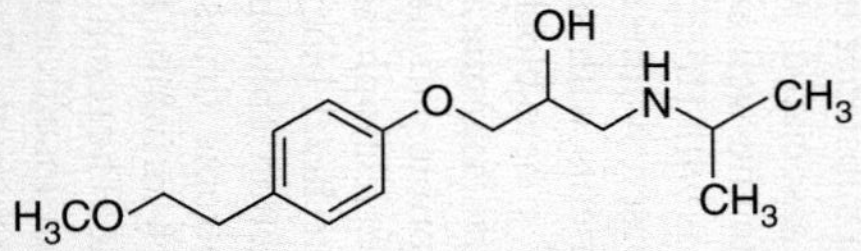 H_3CO, O, OH, H N, CH_3, CH_3	+	0	0	3–4	0	0	++	Liver
Atenolol	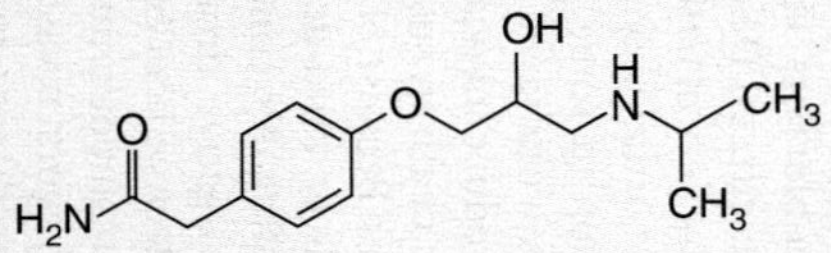 H_2N, O, O, OH, H N, CH_3, CH_3	+	0	0	6–9	0	0	+	Renal
Esmolol	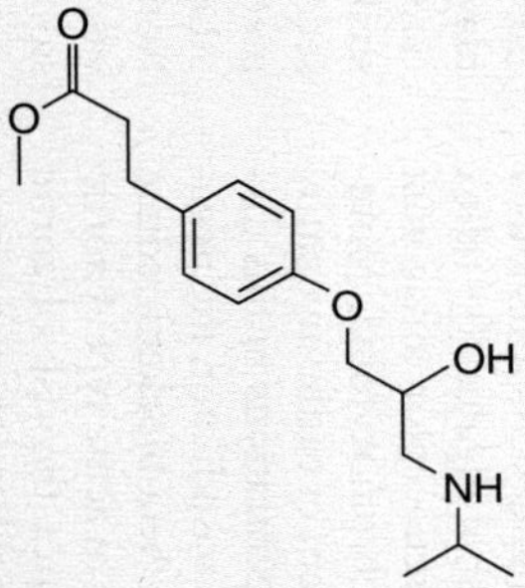 O, O, O, OH, NH	+	0	0	0.15	0	0	+	RBC esterase
Labetalol	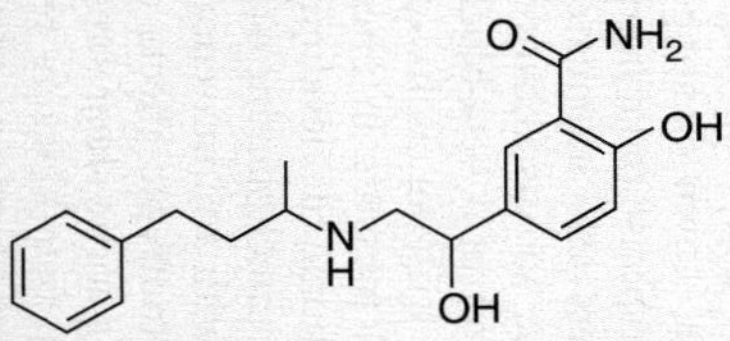 N H, OH, O, NH_2, OH	+	+	+	6	+	0	+	Liver
Carvedilol	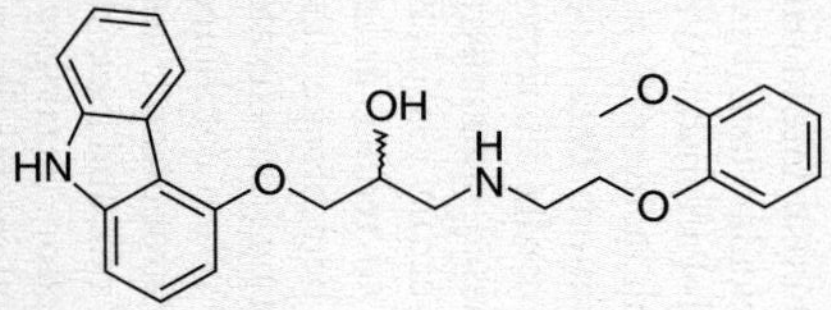 HN, O, OH, H N, O, O	+	+	+	2–8	0	+	+++	Liver

RBC, red blood cell.

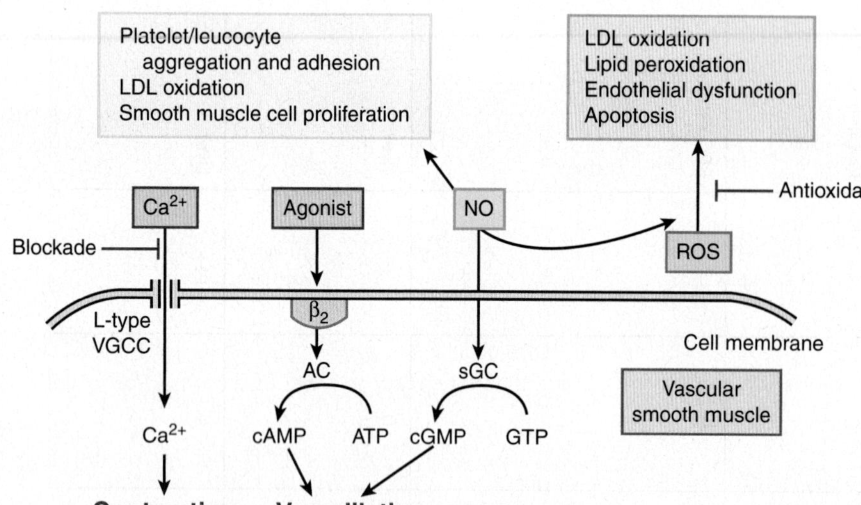

Figure 13-6 Schematic illustration of potential mechanism by which beta-blockers produce vasodilation. VGCC, voltage-gated Ca^{2+} channel; AC, adenylyl cyclase; NO, nitric oxide; sGC, soluble guanylyl cyclase; ROS, reactive oxygen species; LDL, low-density lipoprotein. (Modified from Toda N. Vasodilating β-adrenoceptor blockers as cardiovascular therapeutics. *Pharmacol Ther.* 2003;100(3):215–234. Copyright 2003 Elsevier. With permission.)

symptoms, improve exercise tolerance, reduce the need for and duration of subsequent hospitalization, and decrease the risk of sudden cardiac death in patients with HFrEF. Thus, beta-blockers are clearly beneficial for the treatment of HFrEF[52] and are strongly recommended for this indication in the current American College of Cardiology Foundation/American Heart Association and European Society of Cardiology guidelines.[53,54] Nevertheless, the relative utility of beta-blockers in patients with heart failure with preserved ejection fraction (HFpEF) has not been confirmed in many studies that addressed this hypothesis.[55,56]

The electrophysiologic effects of beta-blockers make these drugs quite useful for the treatment of tachyarrhythmias. Beta-blockers reduce SA node automaticity, inhibit the activity of subsidiary ectopic pacemakers, decrease impulse conduction velocity through atrial conduction pathways, prolong conduction time through the atrioventricular (AV) node, and increase the AV node's refractory period. Both $beta_1$- and $beta_2$-adrenoceptors mediate these negative chronotropic and dromotropic effects. Some beta-blockers also exert membrane-stabilizing activity that may theoretically contribute to their antiarrhythmic efficacy, but these "quinidine-like" actions are most likely only of clinical relevance when an overdose has occurred. Beta-blockers are used to reduce ventricular rate in patients with atrial fibrillation or flutter, supraventricular tachycardia, and reentrant tachyarrhythmias (e.g., Wolff–Parkinson–White, Lown–Ganong–Levine). Beta-blockers inhibit tachycardia in response to laryngoscopy and endotracheal intubation. Beta-blockers also attenuate baroreceptor-mediated tachycardia in response to vasodilator therapy. As previously discussed, administration of a beta-blocker mitigates the reflex tachycardia associated with an $alpha_1$-adrenoceptor antagonist used to reduce arterial pressure in pheochromocytoma. Moreover, beta-blockers attenuate the development of cardiomyopathy resulting from elevated catecholamine concentrations in this disease. When combined with an intravenous vasodilator, the negative chronotropic and inotropic effects of beta-blockers reduce heart rate and ascending aortic shear stress in acute type A aortic dissection. Analogously, beta-blockers reduce the risk of aortic dissection and the rate of ascending aortic dilatation in patients with Marfan syndrome by decreasing pulsatile hydraulic forces on the aortic root.[57] Beta-blockers decrease heart rate and inhibit the development of tachyarrhythmias in hyperthyroidism and thyroid storm, in part by preventing the peripheral conversion of thyroxine to its more active triiodothyronine form. As a result, beta-blockers are useful adjuncts to propylthiouracil in the treatment of hyperthyroidism. Beta-blocker–induced declines in heart rate concomitant with depression of myocardial contractility substantially reduce dynamic LV outflow tract pressure gradient and the magnitude of associated mitral regurgitation while improving symptoms in patients with hypertrophic cardiomyopathy.[58]

Topical beta-blockers (e.g., timolol, betaxolol) are used for the treatment of open-angle glaucoma. These drugs reduce aqueous humor production but do not affect pupil size or accommodation, unlike anticholinergic medications. Topical beta-blockers may be systemically absorbed and may exert adverse cardiovascular or pulmonary side effects. As a result, topical beta-blockers may be relatively contraindicated in patients with symptomatic bradyarrhythmias or reactive airway disease. A role for beta-blockers in prophylaxis against migraine headache is well established, but the mechanism for this beneficial effect remains unclear.[59] Beta-blockers may also be useful for reducing sympathetically mediated symptoms, including palpitations, tachycardia, and tremor, associated with high-pressure performance situations that provoke anxiety (e.g., public speaking, oral examinations). Similarly, beta-blockers may also be helpful in controlling sympathetic nervous system activation that occurs with alcohol or drug withdrawal in patients with substance use disorders.

Beta-blockers are associated with a number of important adverse effects. Despite the well-established beneficial effects of beta-blockers in patients with HFrEF, the negative inotropic effects of these drugs may worsen symptoms and lead to further decompensation in some patients with severe LV systolic dysfunction. Abrupt withdrawal of a beta-blocker after long-term treatment may produce myocardial ischemia and infarction or cause sudden cardiac death in susceptible patients with critical coronary artery stenoses. Because of the electrophysiologic effects of beta-blockers, second- or third-degree heart block may occur in patients with preexisting AV conduction abnormalities or those treated with other negative dromotropic drugs (e.g., diltiazem, verapamil). Nonselective beta-blockers inhibit $beta_2$-adrenoceptors in arterial vascular smooth muscle. The resulting vasoconstriction may occasionally worsen vascular insufficiency in patients with peripheral vascular disease or precipitate Raynaud's phenomenon in susceptible individuals. Nevertheless, beta-blockers remain a mainstay in the treatment of patients with peripheral vascular disease because the vast majority of these patients also have flow-limiting coronary stenoses that substantially increase their risk of myocardial ischemia, infarction, malignant ventricular arrhythmias, and mortality. Propranolol and other first-generation beta-blockers inhibit bronchial beta$_2$-adrenoceptors and may cause severe bronchoconstriction in patients with asthma or chronic obstructive pulmonary disease. Long-term use of beta$_1$-blockers (e.g., atenolol) for the treatment of hypertension, myocardial ischemia and infarction, or HFrEF must be approached with caution in patients with reactive airway disease because the beta$_1$-selectivity of these drugs is relative and suitable alternatives are available (e.g., Ca^{2+} channel blockers, nitrates, ACE inhibitors). Nevertheless, a selective beta$_1$-adrenoceptor antagonist may be advantageous in some patients with coronary artery disease and chronic obstructive pulmonary disease.[60] Beta-blockers interfere with carbohydrate and lipid metabolism. Endogenous catecholamines stimulate glycogenolysis, lipolysis, and gluconeogenesis, promoting the release of glucose into the circulation. Nonselective beta-blockers may inhibit this physiologic response to hypoglycemia, especially in patients with diabetes mellitus. Nonselective beta-blockers also attenuate the sympathetically mediated tremor, tachycardia, and anxiety associated with hypoglycemia. Thus, nonselective beta-blockers may be relatively contraindicated in patients with poorly controlled diabetes who often develop hypoglycemic episodes. Beta$_1$-adrenoceptor selective medications may be preferable in this setting.

Propranolol

Propranolol inhibits beta$_1$- and beta$_2$- but not alpha$_1$-adrenoceptors and possesses some degree of membrane stabilization activity at higher doses, but does not exert intrinsic sympathetic activity. It is available in oral and intravenous forms, is highly lipophilic, is easily absorbed, and undergoes extensive first-pass hepatic metabolism. A high degree of variability is observed in propranolol metabolism between patients. Liver disease delays the drug's metabolism and requires that the dose be adjusted accordingly. However, renal insufficiency does not substantially affect propranolol's pharmacokinetics. Propranolol is used for treatment of hypertension and coronary artery disease. Despite its relatively short half-life (approximately 4 hours), propranolol can most often be administered using a twice-per-day dosing regimen because its antihypertensive effect persists beyond what is expected based on its metabolism. Several weeks of propranolol treatment are often required to achieve optimal reduction in arterial pressure. Attenuation of maximal heart rate achieved in response to exercise suggests that beta-blockade is adequate. Intravenous propranolol was initially used for treatment of atrial tachyarrhythmias, but esmolol is now preferred for this indication in clinical practice because of its short half-life. The landmark β-Blocker Heart Attack Trial (BHAT) demonstrated that propranolol therapy substantially decreases mortality (7.2% compared with 9.8%) in patients with acute myocardial infarction.[61] Use of propranolol has gradually decreased because of the development and widespread application of second and third of other generation beta-blockers with other cardiovascular effects.

Metoprolol

Metoprolol is relatively selective for beta$_1$-adrenoceptors but has no intrinsic sympathetic or membrane stabilization activity. The drug is available in oral and intravenous formulations. Like propranolol, oral metoprolol is rapid absorbed. The drug undergoes first-pass hepatic metabolism by cytochrome P450 2D6 that limits its initial availability. The kidney excretes less than 10% of the drug in its original form. Metoprolol's half-life of 3 to 4 hours allows twice-per-day dosing in patients with normal metabolism, but an extended-release form is also available that allows once-daily administration. The half-life of metoprolol is doubled in patients with limited cytochrome P450 2D6 metabolism; these individuals are approximately fivefold more likely to develop adverse side effects after oral metoprolol administration. Metoprolol is commonly used for treatment of hypertension, angina pectoris, acute myocardial infarction, and HFrEF.[62]

Atenolol

Like metoprolol, atenolol is a selective inhibitor of beta$_1$-adrenoceptors and does not possess intrinsic sympathetic or membrane stabilization activity. The drug has a longer half-life (5 to 8 hours) than metoprolol that facilitates a daily dosing regimen. Atenolol is excreted in its original form by the kidney and is not metabolized by the liver. As a result, the dose of atenolol must be reduced in patients with renal insufficiency. The lack of first-pass hepatic metabolism reduces variability in plasma atenolol concentrations between patients after oral administration.[63] The clinical indications for atenolol are similar to those for other beta-blockers. 8

Esmolol

Esmolol is a relatively selective beta$_1$-adrenoceptor blocker. The chemical structure of esmolol is similar to that of propranolol and metoprolol, but esmolol contains an additional methylester group that facilitates the drug's hydrolysis by red blood cell esterase. The elimination half-life of esmolol is approximately 9 minutes. The rapid onset and metabolism of esmolol makes the drug very useful for the treatment of acute tachycardia and hypertension during surgery. Esmolol is most often administered as an intravenous bolus, which causes almost immediate dose-related decreases in heart rate and myocardial contractility. Arterial pressure decreases in response to these negative chronotropic and inotropic effects. Esmolol is often used to attenuate the sympathetic nervous system response to laryngoscopy, endotracheal intubation, or surgical stimulation, particularly in patients with coronary artery disease who are at risk for acute myocardial ischemia. Esmolol is also useful for rapid control of heart rate in patients with supraventricular tachyarrhythmias (e.g., atrial fibrillation, atrial flutter). Esmolol effectively blunts the sympathetically mediated tachycardia and hypertension that occur shortly after the onset of seizure activity during electroconvulsive therapy. Because esmolol has little effect on beta$_2$-adrenoceptors, hypotension is more commonly observed after its administration compared with nonselective beta-blockers.

Labetalol

Labetalol is composed of four stereoisomers that inhibit alpha- and beta-adrenoceptors to varying degrees. One of the four stereoisomers is an alpha$_1$-adrenoceptor antagonist, another is a nonselective beta-blocker, and the remaining two do not appreciably affect adrenergic receptors. The net effect of this mixture is a drug that selectively inhibits alpha$_1$-adrenoceptors while simultaneously blocking beta$_1$- and beta$_2$-adrenoceptors in a nonselective manner. The intravenous formulation of labetalol contains a ratio of alpha$_1$- to beta-blockade of approximately 1:7. As expected, blockade of the alpha$_1$-adrenoceptor causes arteriolar vasodilation and decreases arterial pressure through a reduction in systemic vascular resistance. This property makes the drug very useful for the treatment of perioperative hypertension. Despite its nonselective beta-blocking properties, labetalol is also a partial beta$_2$-adrenoceptor agonist. This latter characteristic also contributes to vasodilation. Labetalol-induced inhibition of beta$_1$-adrenoceptors decreases heart rate and myocardial contractility, but stroke volume and cardiac output are essentially unchanged because vasodilation also occurs. Unlike other vasodilators, labetalol does not trigger baroreceptor-mediated tachycardia. This latter action is beneficial for the treatment of hypertension in the setting of acute myocardial ischemia. Labetalol is also useful for controlling arterial pressure without producing tachycardia in patients with hypertensive emergencies and those with acute aortic dissection. Labetalol has been shown to attenuate the sympathetic nervous system response to laryngoscopy and endotracheal intubation, although the drug's relatively long elimination half-life (approximately 6 hours) limits its utility in this setting.

Carvedilol

Carvedilol is another third-generation beta-blocker that inhibits $beta_1$-, $beta_2$-, and $alpha_1$-adrenoceptors.[64] Like labetalol, the drug causes arterial vasodilation because it is an $alpha_1$-adrenoceptor antagonist. The drug is a membrane stabilizer but lacks intrinsic sympathomimetic activity. Carvedilol exerts antioxidant and anti-inflammatory effects: it suppresses production of reactive oxygen species and is a scavenger of free radical intermediates. These actions inhibit the uptake of deleterious low-density lipoproteins into coronary vascular endothelium and protect myocardium against ischemia-reperfusion injury, in part by attenuating recruitment, chemotaxis, and activation of cytotoxic neutrophils. Carvedilol is commonly used in the treatment of hypertension, stable angina pectoris, and acute myocardial infarction, but the drug has been shown to be particularly efficacious in patients with HFrEF. Several large clinical trials provided convincing evidence that carvedilol improves LV function, reverses or slows the progression of pathologic LV remodeling, decreases the need for and the duration of hospitalization, and substantially reduces mortality in HFrEF resulting from a variety of underlying causes including coronary artery disease. Indeed, the beneficial effects of carvedilol appear to be greater than those of metoprolol in HFrEF. Carvedilol is now recommended as the preferred therapeutic option in this setting. Carvedilol is highly lipophilic, is almost entirely absorbed after oral administration, and undergoes extensive first-pass hepatic oxidative metabolism through cytochrome P450 2D6, similar to propranolol and metoprolol.

Phosphodiesterase Inhibitors

The phosphodiesterases are structurally related enzymes that hydrolyze the second messengers cAMP and cGMP to terminate their physiologic effects.[65] At least seven different phosphodiesterase isoform subtypes have been identified. Inhibitors of these enzymes enhance the intracellular effects of cAMP and cGMP by preventing their metabolism. The phosphodiesterase inhibitors currently in clinical use are somewhat isoenzyme selective at lower doses, but this selectivity is lost when higher doses are administered. Myocardium and vascular smooth muscle contain the type III phosphodiesterase isoenzyme (PDE III), which is bound to the sarcoplasmic reticulum and cleaves cAMP to adenosine monophosphate (AMP). Selective inhibition of cardiac PDE III by bipyridine compounds alters intracellular Ca^{2+} regulation to enhance myocardial contractility without affecting catecholamine release or activating $beta_1$ adrenoceptors. Milrinone is currently the only PDE III inhibitor in clinical use. PDE III inhibitors cause increases in cAMP concentration, enhance protein kinase A activity, and phosphorylate voltage-dependent Ca^{2+} channels. These actions combine to increase transsarcolemmal Ca^{2+} influx into the cardiac myocyte and promote Ca^{2+}-induced Ca^{2+} release from its sarcoplasmic reticulum, which exerts a positive inotropic effect as larger quantities of Ca^{2+} become available for contractile activation. Inhibition of cAMP metabolism also stimulates greater Ca^{2+} reuptake by phosphorylating phospholamban, the major sarcoplasmic reticulum Ca^{2+}-ATPase regulatory protein. As a result, PDE III inhibitors enhance the rate and extent of myocardial relaxation.

PDE III inhibitors cause pronounced arterial and venous vasodilation by blocking cGMP metabolism and facilitating its actions in vascular smooth muscle. The proclivity of PDE III inhibitors to enhance contractility and cause vasodilation simultaneously defines these medications as "inodilators." PDE III inhibitors cause greater vasodilation than $beta_2$ adrenoceptor agonists. The reduction in LV afterload leads to an increase in cardiac output, improves LV-arterial coupling, and enhances mechanical efficiency. Intravenous or inhalational administration of PDE III inhibitors also reduces pulmonary vascular resistance, an action that may be particularly helpful in patients with pulmonary hypertension and RV dysfunction.[66,67] However, this pulmonary vasodilation is capable of adversely increasing intrapulmonary shunt and producing hypoxemia. PDE III inhibitors dilate venous capacitance vessels and reduce preload. Notably, these decreases in preload and afterload resulting from administration of a PDE III inhibitor reduce myocardial oxygen demand in patients with HFrEF despite simultaneous positive inotropic, lusitropic, and chronotropic effects. In general, mean arterial pressure is either maintained or may be modestly reduced during administration of PDE III inhibitors, provided that intravascular volume is adequately supplemented, because increases in cardiac output are capable of compensating for reductions in afterload.

PDE III inhibitors cause less pronounced increases in heart rate than those observed during administration of catecholamines. Indeed, a selective $beta_1$ adrenoceptor antagonist may abolish the increase in heart rate produced by a PDE III inhibitor without affecting its positive inotropic effect. PDE III inhibitors may precipitate the development of malignant ventricular arrhythmias because these drugs increase intracellular cAMP and Ca^{2+} concentrations. PDE III inhibitors block platelet aggregation, suppress neointimal hyperplasia associated with endothelial injury, and attenuate the proinflammatory effects of cardiopulmonary bypass. These drugs also dilate native epicardial coronary arteries and arterial bypass conduits. As a result, PDE III inhibitors have the potential to exert anti-ischemic effects in patients undergoing coronary artery surgery. The efficacy of PDE III inhibitors is reduced in HFrEF, but not to the degree observed with $beta_1$ adrenoceptor agonists. These pharmacologic properties stimulated a number of large randomized controlled trials designed to evaluate the efficacy of orally administered PDE III inhibitors for the treatment of chronic severe HFrEF. The PDE III inhibitors tested in these trials enhanced cardiac performance and improved functional capacity but, unfortunately, the drugs also significantly increased mortality resulting from ventricular arrhythmias and sudden cardiac death. As a result, PDE III inhibitors are contraindicated for the treatment of chronic HFrEF. However, these medications remain very useful for the treatment of acute LV systolic dysfunction. The authors often use the combination of a PDE III inhibitor and a $beta_1$-adrenoceptor agonist when weaning patients with preexisting LV systolic dysfunction from cardiopulmonary bypass because these drugs produce synergistic positive inotropic effects on the basis of their actions on cAMP-mediated intracellular signaling.

Milrinone (Table 13-7) has been used extensively for inotropic support during and after cardiac surgery. Milrinone is 15 to 20-fold more potent than the chemically similar compound inamrinone. The latter drug was the first clinically used PDE III inhibitor and exerted cardiovascular effects that were almost identical to those of milrinone, but use of inamrinone was abandoned because of its propensity to cause profound thrombocytopenia during prolonged administration. Milrinone enhances myocardial

Table 13-7 Comparative Effects of Milrinone, Levosimendan, and Vasopressin

Name	Chemical Structure	Mechanism of Action	Dose Range	Clinical Indications	Major Side Effects
Milrinone	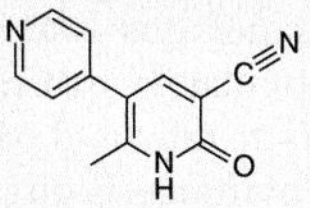	PDE III inhibition	Load: 25–50 μg/kg IV: 0.375–0.75 μg/kg/min	Acute LV dysfunction	Arrhythmias Myocardial ischemia Sudden cardiac death Hypertension Stroke
Levosimendan	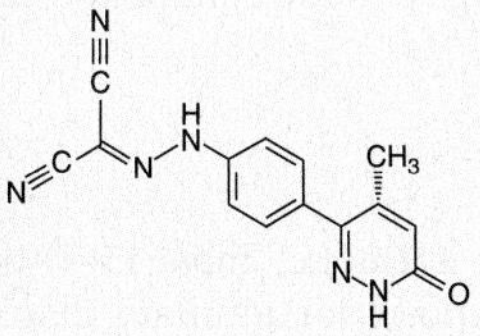	Myofilament Ca^{2+} sensitization PDE III Inhibition K_{ATP} channel opener	Load: 12–24 μg/kg IV: 0.05–0.2 μg/kg/min	Acute LV dysfunction Heart failure	Tachycardia Hypotension
Vasopressin	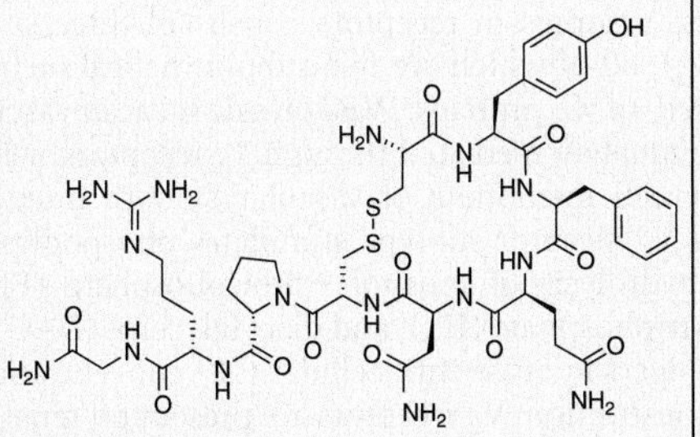	V_1 (vascular smooth muscle) and V_2 (renal collecting tubules) agonist	IV: 0.01–0.1 U/min	Shock (vasodilatory, cardiogenic) Cardiac arrest	Arrhythmias Hypertension Myocardial ischemia Reduced cardiac output Peripheral ischemia Splanchnic vasoconstriction

IV, intravenous; LV, left ventricular; Ca^{2+}, calcium; PDE, phosphodiesterase; K_{ATP}, adenosine triphosphate-sensitive potassium channel.
Modified from Linn KA, Pagel PS. Cardiovascular pharmacology. In: Barash PG, Cullen BF, Stoelting RK, et al., eds. *Clinical Anesthesia Fundamentals*. Wolters Kluwer; 2015:234–235.

contractility and causes arterial and venous vasodilation, thereby improving the likelihood of successful weaning of patients with LV systolic dysfunction from cardiopulmonary bypass. The pharmacokinetics and pharmacodynamics of milrinone were extensively studied in patients undergoing cardiac surgery and those in the intensive care unit. Milrinone loading doses of 25 or 50 $\mu g \cdot kg^{-1}$ and infusion rates ranging between 0.375 and 0.75 $\mu g \cdot kg^{-1} \cdot min^{-1}$ are useful for increasing cardiac output and oxygen delivery in these settings.

Levosimendan

Myofilament Ca^{2+} sensitizers are positively inotropic, vasodilating drugs that enhance myocardial contractility by increasing the Ca^{2+} sensitivity of the contractile apparatus.[68] Levosimendan (Table 13-7) is the only drug in this class that is currently available, although a number of other myofilament Ca^{2+} sensitizers were previously tested in clinical trials. Levosimendan is used extensively in Europe for short-term treatment of HFrEF and for inotropic support in patients undergoing cardiac surgery.[69] However, use of the drug in the United States is relatively limited because it remains unclear whether levosimendan provides unique advantages over conventional therapy. Levosimendan was initially touted as a treatment for acute decompensation of chronic HFrEF that would decrease morbidity and mortality, but the myofilament Ca^{2+} sensitizer did not reduce the incidence of death or major adverse cardiac events compared with dobutamine. Intermittent ambulatory treatment with levosimendan also did not improve functional capacity or quality of life in patients with advanced HRrEF.[70] Levosimendan produced rapid improvement of symptoms in patients with acutely decompensated heart failure, but the drug also increased the risk of cardiovascular-related complications. As a result of these and other recent clinical trials, the future of levosimendan as a treatment for heart failure is uncertain.

Levosimendan exerts its positive inotropic and vasodilator actions through three major mechanisms. First, the drug binds to TnC and stabilizes the Ca^{2+}-bound conformation of the regulatory protein in a Ca^{2+}-dependent manner. This action prolongs the interaction between actin and myosin filaments and enhances the rate and extent of myocyte contraction to increase myocardial contractility. The Ca^{2+}-dependence of levosimendan-TnC binding prevents relaxation abnormalities that would otherwise be expected to occur. Second, levosimendan is a potent PDE III inhibitor that produces positive inotropic and lusitropic effects and causes systemic, pulmonary, and coronary vasodilation. Finally, levosimendan opens ATP-dependent K^+ (K_{ATP}) channels, which contributes to the drug's vasodilator properties and may also produce the additional benefit of myocardial protection against ischemic injury. Levosimendan decreases LV filling pressures, mean arterial pressure, and pulmonary and systemic vascular resistances and increases cardiac output in patients with HFrEF. The modest reductions in arterial pressure observed with levosimendan are similar to those produced by milrinone and usually respond to volume administration. Levosimendan also improves LV-arterial coupling and mechanical efficiency, while causing only minimal increases in heart rate and myocardial oxygen demand. Similar to the findings in the setting of heart failure, levosimendan also improves cardiac performance concomitant with reductions in pulmonary capillary occlusion pressure and systemic vascular resistance in patients with normal and depressed LV systolic function undergoing cardiac surgery.[71] Levosimendan has a biologically active metabolite that most likely contributes to the parent drug's more prolonged hemodynamic effects compared with catecholamines or PDE III inhibitors.

Digitalis Glycosides

The search for new drugs that chronically enhance myocardial contractility in the failing heart has been remarkably disappointing. Digitalis glycosides continue to be the only currently available class of positive inotropic drugs for oral treatment of mild to moderate HFrEF, and these medications have been used for centuries. Digitalis glycosides are naturally occurring substances that are found in several plant species including "foxglove" (*Digitalis purpurea*). The most commonly prescribed digitalis glycosides are digoxin and digitoxin, but a number of related compounds are also used. Digitalis glycosides enhance contractile function, but this positive inotropic effect is relatively minor when compared with other drugs used for the treatment of acute LV systolic dysfunction. Digitalis glycosides selectively bind to the alpha-subunit of the sarcolemmal Na^+-K^+ ATPase on its extracellular surface and reversibly inhibit the enzyme. An increase in extracellular K^+ concentration partially inhibits this digitalis-Na^+-K^+ ATPase binding. As a result, administration of K^+ is capable of reversing digitalis toxicity resulting from hypokalemia. Inhibition of sarcolemmal Na^+-K^+ ATPase indirectly increases Ca^{2+} availability, which enhances myocardial contractility. The Na^+-K^+ ATPase enzyme normally trades three Na^+ (intracellular to extracellular) for two K^+ ions (extracellular to intracellular) against their concentration gradients. Inhibition of this ion exchange produces a modest increase in intracellular Na^+ concentration, which causes a reduction in the extrusion of Ca^{2+} from the myoplasm by the sarcolemmal Na^+-Ca^{2+} exchanger. This additional Ca^{2+} is stored in the sarcoplasmic reticulum and is then released during the subsequent contraction. The mechanism of action of digitalis glycosides is similar to that implicated for the Treppe ("staircase") physiologic phenomenon, in which a rapid increase in heart rate causes a delay in Na^+-K^+ ATPase activity, leading to a transient increase in intracellular Na^+ concentration and enhanced contractile force mediated by favorable Na^+-Ca^{2+} exchange. In contrast to other drugs that increase myocardial contractility, tachyphylaxis to the positive inotropic effects of digitalis glycosides does not occur.

The increase in myocardial contractility produced by digitalis glycosides is associated with declines in LV preload and afterload, LV wall tension, and myocardial oxygen demand in HFrEF. Heart rate remains unchanged. Because digitalis glycosides augment contractility and improve cardiac output, these drugs reduce the chronically elevated sympathetic nervous system activity that is a characteristic feature of heart failure. Reductions in norepinephrine concentrations with consequent declines in LV afterload also occur in response to this withdrawal of sympathetic tone. The decrease in sympathetic nervous system activity observed with digitalis glycosides is also related to the direct actions of these drugs on cardiac baroreceptors. These combined actions play important roles in reducing morbidity and mortality in patients with HFrEF. In contrast, digoxin did not affect cardiovascular mortality and heart failure hospitalizations in patients with HFpEF.[72] Digitalis-induced inhibition of Na^+-K^+ ATPase causes profound alterations in electrophysiology (e.g., SA and AV nodes, conduction pathways, His–Purkinje fibers) because this enzyme is responsible for maintaining resting membrane potential. The withdrawal of sympathetic nervous system activity and increases in parasympathetic nervous system activity further modulate the electrophysiologic effects of digitalis glycosides. As a result, digitalis glycosides have a propensity to cause arrhythmias including sinus bradycardia or arrest, AV conduction delays, and second- or third-degree heart block. It is noteworthy that toxic levels of digitalis glycosides may paradoxically increase sympathetic nervous system tone and precipitate the development of ventricular tachyarrhythmias. Digitalis glycosides have a low therapeutic ratio and narrow margin of safety. Mortality resulting from arrhythmias is directly related to a digitalis drug's plasma concentration. Digitalis glycosides are most often used for management of supraventricular tachyarrhythmias with rapid ventricular response during the perioperative period because the drugs prolong AV node conduction time.

Vasopressin

Vasopressin (antidiuretic hormone; Table 13-7) is a peptide hormone released from the posterior pituitary that regulates water reabsorption in the kidney and exerts potent hemodynamic effects. Vasopressin receptors consist of three subtypes (V_1, V_2, and V_3), all of which are five-subunit helical membrane proteins coupled to G proteins. Vasopressin's cardiovascular effects are predominately mediated through V_1 receptors, which are located in the cell membrane of vascular smooth muscle.[73] Activation of the V_1 receptor subtype stimulates phospholipase C and triggers hydrolysis of inositol 4,5-bisphosphate (PIP_2) to inositol 1,4,5-triphosphate (IP_3), and diacylglycerol (DAG). These second messengers increase intracellular Ca^{2+} concentration and produce vasoconstriction. V_2 receptors are present on renal collecting duct cells and, when activated, increase reabsorption of free water, whereas V_3 receptors are located in the pituitary itself and act as autocoid modulators.

Along with the sympathetic nervous system and renin–angiotensin–aldosterone axis, endogenous vasopressin plays an essential role in maintenance of arterial pressure. Exogenous administration of vasopressin does not substantially affect arterial pressure in healthy subjects because activation of central V_1 receptors in the area postrema enhances baroreceptor-mediated inhibition of efferent sympathetic nervous outflow. This action negates the elevated system vascular resistance resulting from V_1-mediated arterial vasoconstriction. In contrast, vasopressinergic mechanisms are essential for maintaining arterial pressure when sympathetic nervous system or renin-angiotensin-aldosterone axis dysfunction is present. Exogenous administration of vasopressin effectively supports arterial pressure when a relative vasopressin deficiency exists (e.g., catecholamine-refractory hypotension, vasodilatory shock). ACE inhibitors and angiotensin receptor blockers (ARBs) used to treat hypertension also affect autonomic nervous system and renin–angiotensin–aldosterone axis function. Intraoperative hypotension that is relatively refractory to administration of catecholamines or sympathomimetics is well-known in patients who are receiving these medications. General or neuraxial anesthesia also reduces sympathetic nervous system tone, resulting in decreased plasma stress hormone concentrations including vasopressin. Under these circumstances, administration of vasopressin activates V_1 vascular smooth muscle receptors and rapidly increases arterial pressure. Vasopressin therapy reduces mortality associated with acute vasodilatory states such as anaphylaxis. In addition, infusion of vasopressin is indicated for the treatment of vasoplegia during and after prolonged cardiopulmonary bypass in patients who are otherwise unresponsive to catecholamines.

Vasopressin is a useful drug for the treatment of sepsis and cardiac arrest. Vasodilation that is refractory to fluid resuscitation, combined with a relative deficiency of endogenous vasopressin, is a characteristic feature of sepsis. Inadequate sympathetic nervous system and renin–angiotensin–aldosterone axis responses to hypotension also occur. Under these circumstances, the administration of vasopressin stabilizes hemodynamics and improves survival. However, vasopressin must be used with caution because sustained administration of higher doses may produce mesenteric ischemia, peripheral vascular insufficiency, and cardiac arrest, as the drug causes pronounced vasoconstriction of cutaneous, skeletal muscle, splanchnic, and coronary vascular beds concomitant with reduced perfusion of and oxygen delivery to these tissues. The combined use of vasopressin with other vasoactive medications reduces the overall dose of vasopressin required to maintain arterial pressure and limits its adverse effects on organ perfusion. Bolus intravenous administration of vasopressin is also part of the American Heart Association Adult Advanced Cardiac Life Support algorithm for cardiac arrest resulting from ventricular fibrillation, pulseless electrical activity, or asystole.

Nitrovasodilators

Organic nitrates (e.g., nitroglycerin) and NO donors (e.g., sodium nitroprusside) are nitrovasodilators that release NO through either enzymatic sulfhydryl group reduction or a spontaneous mechanism that does not require metabolism, respectively. Exogenous NO stimulates guanylate cyclase within the vascular smooth muscle cell to convert guanosine triphosphate to cGMP, similar to endogenous NO produced by the vascular endothelium. This second messenger activates protein kinase G, which dephosphorylates myosin light chains and contributes to relaxation of vascular smooth muscle. NO stimulates Ca^{2+} reuptake into the endoplasmic reticulum by activating its Ca^{2+}-ATPase through a cGMP-independent mechanism. This action decreases intracellular Ca^{2+} concentration and causes relaxation. Moreover, NO causes K^+ efflux from the cell by opening the K^+ channel. This shift in K^+ balance produces cellular hyperpolarization, which, in turn, closes the voltage-gated Ca^{2+} channel and facilitates relaxation through a third mechanism.

Nitrovasodilators are often used to improve hemodynamics and myocardial oxygen supply–demand relations and are a mainstay in the treatment of patients with HFrEF. However, these medications do not improve outcome in patients with HFpEF.[74,75] Venodilation reduces venous return, which contributes to declines in LV and RV end-diastolic volume, pressure, and wall stress. Arterial vasodilation also reduces systemic and pulmonary arterial pressures, which decreases LV and RV end-systolic wall stress. These actions decrease myocardial oxygen demand. Nitrovasodilators increase myocardial oxygen supply by dilating epicardial coronary arteries. The reduction in LV end-diastolic pressure observed with nitrovasodilators, coupled with coronary vasodilation, substantially enhances subendocardial perfusion. The initial efficacy of nitrovasodilators is variable between patients, but the cardiovascular effects of these drugs inevitably decline with prolonged use. Some patients may be relatively resistant to the effects of organic nitrates in the presence of oxidative stress because superoxide anions scavenge NO, cause reversible oxidation of guanylate cyclase, and inhibit aldehyde dehydrogenase. This latter action prevents further release of NO. A progressive attenuation of the hemodynamic responses to nitrovasodilators may develop in other patients as a result of sympathetic nervous system and renin–angiotensin–aldosterone axis activation. This phenomenon, known as "pseudo-tolerance," accounts for the rebound hypertension that may be observed when nitrovasodilators are abruptly discontinued. Inhibition of guanylate cyclase activity is most likely responsible for true tolerance to organic nitrates. A daily "drug holiday" is a useful strategy for reversing this effect in patients requiring prolonged treatment. Administration of *N*-acetylcysteine, a sulfhydryl donor, may also be effective for reversing true tolerance. Prolonged use of organic nitrates may also cause methemoglobinemia, interfere with platelet aggregation, and produce heparin resistance. Organic nitrates should be used with caution in patients receiving phosphodiesterase type V inhibitors (e.g., sildenafil) because NO-induced vasodilation is enhanced and profound hypotension, myocardial ischemia or infarction, and death may result.

Nitroglycerin

Nitroglycerin dilates venules to a greater degree than arterioles. At lower doses, the drug produces venodilation without causing a significant decrease in systemic vascular resistance. Arterial pressure and cardiac output fall in response to the reduction in preload despite a modest baroreceptor-mediated increase in heart rate. Nitroglycerin also decreases pulmonary arterial pressures and vascular resistance. At higher doses, nitroglycerin dilates arterioles and reduces LV afterload. These effects cause more pronounced decreases in arterial pressure and stimulate greater reflex tachycardia. Overshoot hypotension and tachycardia is particularly common in the setting of hypovolemia, such as is often observed in patients with poorly controlled essential hypertension and parturients with pregnancy-induced hypertension.

Nitroglycerin improves the balance of myocardial oxygen supply to demand through its actions as a direct coronary vasodilator (which increase supply) and its systemic hemodynamic effects (which reduce demand). Nitroglycerin dilates both normal and poststenotic epicardial coronary arteries, enhances blood flow through coronary collateral vessels, and preferentially improves subendocardial perfusion. The drug also inhibits coronary vasospasm and dilates the arterial conduits (e.g., internal mammary artery, radial artery) that are used during coronary artery surgery. Nitroglycerin decreases myocardial oxygen demand by reducing LV preload and, to a lesser extent, afterload thereby producing corresponding reductions in LV end-diastolic and end-systolic wall stress. These effects are particularly important in patients with LV systolic dysfunction resulting from acute myocardial ischemia. Nevertheless, caution should be exercised when using nitroglycerin in patients with ischemia who are also hypovolemic because nitroglycerin may cause severe hypotension by further compromising coronary perfusion pressure.

Sodium Nitroprusside

Sodium nitroprusside is a short-acting direct NO donor (NICV 13-4). It is a potent venous and arterial vasodilator that rapidly reduces arterial pressure by decreasing LV preload and afterload, respectively. Sodium nitroprusside is a first line drug in the management of hypertensive emergencies. Sodium nitroprusside is also useful for the treatment of cardiogenic shock because arterial vasodilation improves forward flow by reducing impedance to LV ejection while venodilation decreases LV filling pressures. Unlike nitroglycerin, sodium nitroprusside is relatively contraindicated in patients with acute myocardial ischemia because the drug causes abnormal redistribution of coronary blood flow away from ischemic myocardium (a phenomenon known as coronary steal). This effect occurs because sodium nitroprusside produces greater coronary vasodilation in vessels that perfuse normal myocardium compared with those that supply the ischemic territory, the latter of which are already maximally vasodilated. Baroreceptor-mediated tachycardia is also more pronounced during administration of sodium nitroprusside because it is a more potent arteriolar vasodilator than nitroglycerin. This reflex tachycardia dramatically increases heart rate and myocardial oxygen demand. These consequences are detrimental when acute myocardial ischemia is present. Sodium nitroprusside is often combined with a beta$_1$-adrenoceptor antagonist such as esmolol to decrease arterial pressure, depress myocardial contractility, and reduce ascending aortic wall stress in patients with acute type A aortic dissection. Clinical use of sodium nitroprusside is limited by its toxic metabolites, which accumulate when administration is prolonged or relatively high doses are used. Metabolism of sodium nitroprusside produces cyanide, which binds with cytochrome oxidase to inhibit aerobic metabolism, with hemoglobin to form methemoglobin, and with sulfur to form thiocyanate. The latter metabolite may accumulate in patients with renal insufficiency and produce neurologic complications including delirium and seizures.

Hydralazine

Hydralazine is a direct vasodilator that reduces intracellular Ca^{2+} concentration in vascular smooth muscle in part by activating K_{ATP} channels in small arteries and arterioles in coronary, cerebral, splanchnic, and renal vascular beds. This action decreases systemic vascular resistance and arterial pressure. However, LV preload is relatively preserved because hydralazine does not dilate venous capacitance vessels. The reduction in afterload produced by hydralazine stimulates baroreceptor-mediated tachycardia and increases cardiac output. The magnitude of tachycardia observed after administration of hydralazine is often greater than expected based on baroreceptor reflexes alone and may reflect a direct effect of the drug on cardiovascular regulation in the central nervous system. Pronounced tachycardia has the potential to produce acute myocardial ischemia in patients with flow-limiting coronary stenoses based on increases in myocardial oxygen demand. Hydralazine-induced tachycardia does respond appropriately to beta$_1$-adrenoceptor antagonists, but caution should be exercised when combining these medications because hypotension may then result. Hydralazine is commonly used for management of sustained postoperative hypertension in the absence of tachycardia.

Calcium Channel Blockers

Ca^{2+} channels are asymmetric biochemical pores consisting of at least four subunits (alpha$_1$, alpha$_2$/delta, and beta with or without gamma) that traverse many biologic membranes. Ca^{2+} channels remain closed under quiescent conditions, but they open through a voltage-dependent or receptor-operated mechanism to allow Ca^{2+} entry into the cell or an organelle (e.g., mitochondria, sarcoplasmic reticulum). Myocardial and vascular smooth muscle cell membranes contain two types of voltage-dependent Ca^{2+} channels that are defined on the basis of their duration of opening: T (transient) and L (long). The L-type Ca^{2+} channel is the predominant target of the Ca^{2+} channel blockers in current use, which do not block the T-type Ca^{2+} channel. Ca^{2+} channel blockers may be divided into four chemical groups: 1,4-dihydropyridines (e.g., nifedipine, nicardipine, nimodipine, clevidipine), benzothiazepines (diltiazem), phenylalkylamines (verapamil), and diarylaminopropylamine ethers (bepridil). The first three of these groups are in current clinical use (Table 13-8), but bepridil has been withdrawn.

11 In general, Ca^{2+} channel blockers produce varying degrees of vasodilation, direct negative chronotropic, dromotropic, and inotropic effects, and baroreceptor-mediated increases in heart rate depending on each drug's selectivity for myocardial and vascular smooth muscle L-type Ca^{2+} channels. All Ca^{2+} channel blockers produce greater relaxation of arterial compared with venous vascular smooth muscle. As a result, LV afterload is reduced while preload is relatively preserved. Ca^{2+} channels blockers cause coronary vasodilation and inhibit coronary artery vasospasm. These actions increase coronary blood flow provided that coronary perfusion pressure is not substantially reduced as a result of concomitant arterial vasodilation. In addition to causing declines in LV afterload, some Ca^{2+} channel blockers (e.g., diltiazem, verapamil) also reduce myocardial oxygen demand by decreasing heart rate and myocardial contractility. In contrast, other Ca^{2+} channel blockers (e.g., dihydropyridines) may increase myocardial oxygen demand because of baroreceptor-induced tachycardia. As a result, larger doses of these Ca^{2+} channel blockers may be detrimental to patients with coronary artery disease.

Nifedipine

Nifedipine and related dihydropyridine Ca^{2+} channel blockers (e.g., amlodipine, felodipine, isradipine) are most often used for treatment of essential hypertension. Nifedipine is a relatively selective arterial vasodilator that does not substantially affect venous vasomotor tone. This effect decreases arterial pressure, but in so doing, it also activates the sympathetic nervous system and elicits baroreceptor-mediated increases in heart rate. Nifedipine produces direct myocardial depression in vitro, but this negative inotropic effect is not apparent when the drug is used clinically because arterial vasodilation occurs at plasma concentrations that are substantially less than those required for reductions in myocardial contractility to occur. Similarly, typical doses of nifedipine only minimally alter SA node automaticity and AV conduction. Maintenance of venous return and contractility combined with modest tachycardia and a decline in LV afterload result in small increases in cardiac output. Nifedipine can be safely used for treatment of hypertension in patients with coronary artery disease, most often in combination with a beta-blocker to attenuate the baroreceptor-mediated tachycardia.[76] Nifedipine is a direct epicardial coronary vasodilator. The drug is indicated for the treatment of variant angina (also known as Prinzmetal or vasospastic angina), a disease process in which reductions in coronary blood flow occur as a result of regional coronary vasoconstriction independent of coronary artery stenoses.[77] Nifedipine is probably more effective than nitrates for the treatment of variant angina because the Ca^{2+} channel blocker causes more profound, consistent coronary vasodilation. Vasospasm may occur in patients with unstable angina resulting from atherosclerosis, and nifedipine is also beneficial in this setting.[77] Despite these salutary effects, nifedipine does not improve and may worsen mortality when it is used in patients with acute myocardial infarction, in contrast to other Ca^{2+} channel blockers such as diltiazem and verapamil.[78] Nifedipine is also used to provide arterial vasodilation in patients with Raynaud phenomenon.

Nicardipine

Nicardipine is another dihydropyridine Ca^{2+} channel antagonist that is highly selective for vascular smooth muscle. Nicardipine produces cardiovascular effects that are similar to nifedipine, but it has a longer half-life. Like other dihydropyridine Ca^{2+} channel antagonists, nicardipine preferentially dilates arteriolar vessels, which decreases arterial pressure. In contrast to diltiazem and verapamil, nicardipine does not substantially depress myocardial contractility nor does the drug affect the rate of SA node firing. As a result, stroke volume and cardiac output are relatively

Table 13-8 Comparative Effects of Ca^{2+} Channel Blockers

Name	Chemical Structure	Myocardial Depression	Coronary Blood Flow	Suppression of SA Node (Automaticity)	Suppression of AV Node (Conduction)
Nifedipine	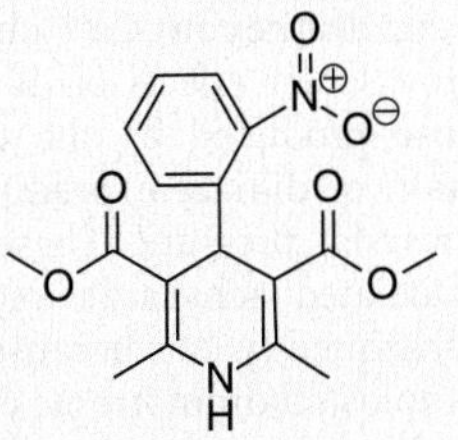	+	+++++	+	0
Nicardipine	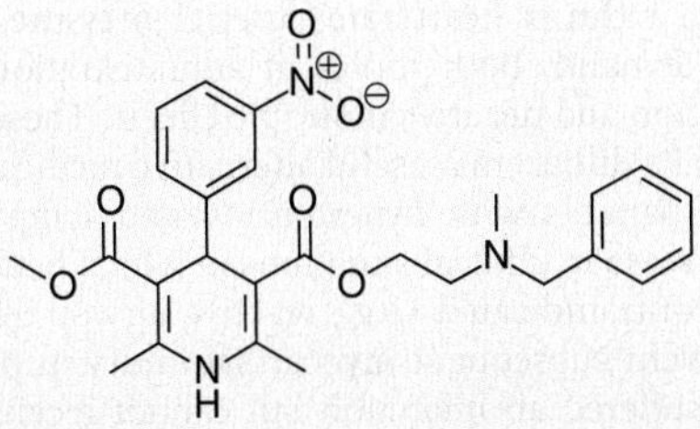	0	+++++	+	0
Clevidipine	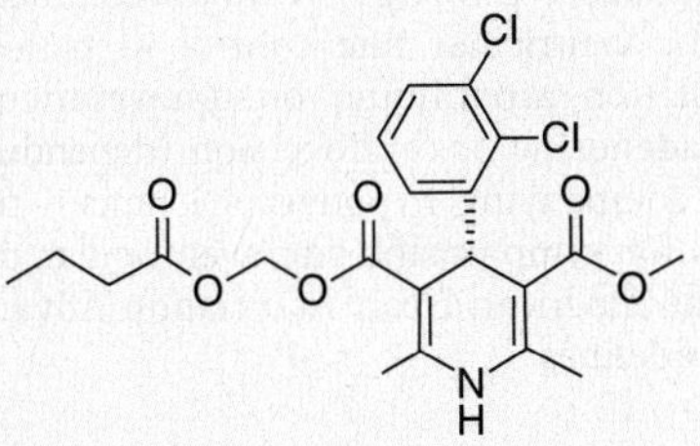	+	+++++	+	0
Nimodipine	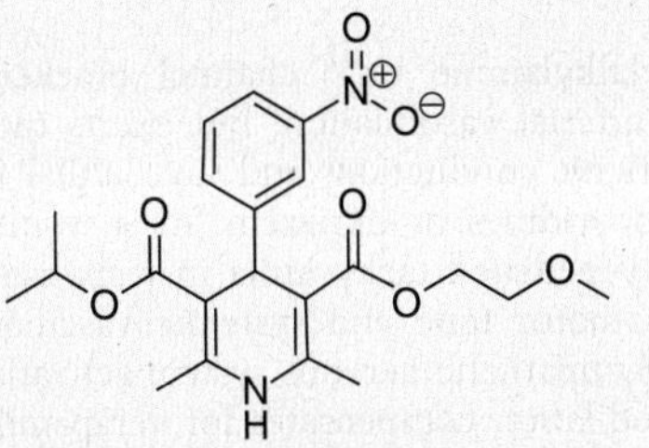	+	++++	+	0
Diltiazem	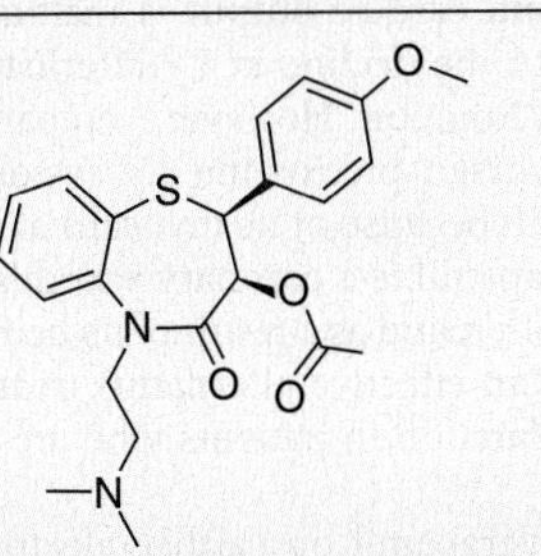	++	+++	+++++	++++
Verapamil	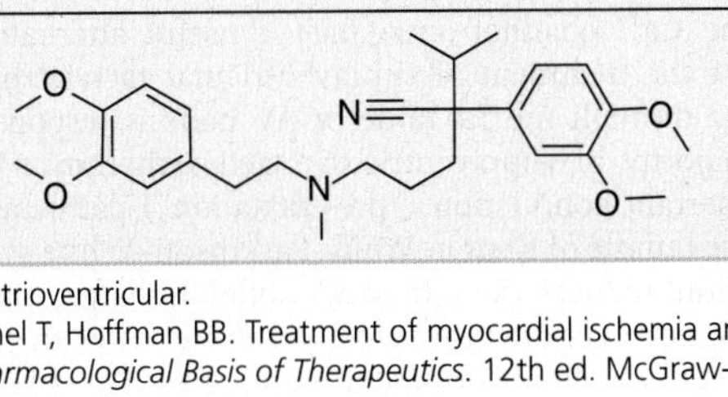	++++	++++	+++++	++++

SA, sinoatrial; AV, atrioventricular.

Adapted from Michel T, Hoffman BB. Treatment of myocardial ischemia and hypertension. In: Brunton LL, Chabner BA, Knollman BC, eds. *Goodman and Gilman's The Pharmacological Basis of Therapeutics*. 12th ed. McGraw-Hill Medical; 2011:756.

preserved or may increase. Nicardipine-induced decreases in arterial pressure trigger increases in heart rate through activation of baroreceptor reflexes, but the tachycardia observed during administration of nicardipine is less pronounced than typically occurs with sodium nitroprusside at comparable levels of arterial pressure. Nicardipine is a potent coronary vasodilator and is often used to dilate arterial conduits during coronary artery surgery. Nicardipine is primarily used for treatment of sustained perioperative hypertension and not for acute, often transient hypertensive episodes that are commonly observed during surgery because of its relatively long half-life.

Clevidipine

Clevidipine is an ultrashort-acting dihydropyridine Ca^{2+} channel antagonist with a plasma half-life of approximately 2 minutes.[79] Like nicardipine and nifedipine, clevidipine exerts pronounced effects at the less negative resting membrane potentials typically observed in vascular smooth muscle cells, but demonstrates lower potency in cardiac myocytes in which resting membrane potentials are substantially more negative. As a result of these differences in cellular electrophysiology, clevidipine is highly selective for arterial vascular smooth muscle and is nearly devoid of negative chronotropic or inotropic effects. This hemodynamic profile may be especially useful for the treatment of hypertension in patients with acute LV systolic dysfunction.[80] Clevidipine causes dose-related arteriolar vasodilation while sparing venous vasomotor tone, thereby reducing systemic vascular resistance and arterial pressure without affecting LV preload. Modest increases in heart rate may also occur during administration of clevidipine as a result of baroreceptor reflex activation. Unlike other short-acting antihypertensive drugs, clevidipine is not associated with the development of tachyphylaxis, and abrupt discontinuation of the drug does not usually cause rebound hypertension. Because tissue and plasma esterases are responsible for clevidipine metabolism, little to no accumulation of the drug occurs even in the setting of hepatic or renal insufficiency. Clevidipine compares favorably with nitroglycerin, sodium nitroprusside, and nicardipine for the management of acute hypertension in cardiac surgery patients.[81,82] Clevidipine has demonstrated efficacy for treatment of hypertension associated with pheochromocytoma[83] and acute intracerebral hemorrhage,[84] and is also useful for producing controlled hypotension during spine surgery.

Nimodipine

The dihydropyridine nimodipine is more lipophilic and crosses the blood barrier more easily than other drugs in this class of Ca^{2+} channel blockers. Consequently, nimodipine produces greater cerebral arterial vasodilation than other dihydropyridines. Nimodipine is currently the only medication approved by the United States Food and Drug Administration for treatment of cerebral vasospasm after aneurysmal subarachnoid hemorrhage.[85] Several clinical trials in patients with cerebral vasospasm demonstrated that nimodipine significantly reduces the severity of symptoms, the incidence of cerebral infarction, the occurrence of delayed neurologic deficits, and mortality while improving long-term neurologic functional status after the initial hemorrhage. However, nimodipine did not affect the incidence of recurrent hemorrhage or prevent other adverse reactions. Nimodipine does not reverse angiographic evidence of vasospasm, indicating that the mechanism by which the Ca^{2+} channel blocker improves outcome in this setting is most likely not related to dilation of large cerebral arteries. Instead, nimodipine appears to reduce cerebral arteriolar resistance and enhance blood flow through pia mater collateral vessels. Nimodipine also attenuates Ca^{2+}-mediated neurotoxicity and may exert clinically relevant neuroprotective effects.

Diltiazem

Diltiazem is the only benzothiazepine Ca^{2+} channel blocker in clinical use.[86] The cardiovascular effects of diltiazem are somewhat different than those produced by the dihydropyridines. Intravenous administration of diltiazem produces arterial vasodilation and decreases arterial pressure. These actions initially stimulate baroreceptor-mediated tachycardia and increase cardiac output, but heart rate subsequently falls because diltiazem exerts potent negative chronotropic and dromotropic effects on SA node automaticity and AV node conduction. Oral administration of diltiazem reduces heart rate, arterial pressure, and myocardial oxygen demand. Both routes of administration cause coronary vasodilation and negative inotropic effects. These combined properties make diltiazem a useful alternative medication for the treatment of patients with hypertension and symptomatic coronary artery disease in clinical situations in which beta-blockers are relatively contraindicated (e.g., reactive airway disease). Diltiazem may prevent subsequent myocardial injury in patients who have already suffered an infarction but cannot receive a beta-blocker. Because diltiazem prolongs AV node conduction, the drug is effective for ventricular rate control in patients with chronic atrial fibrillation, atrial flutter, or supraventricular tachycardia.[87] However, adenosine or cardioversion (depending on the magnitude of accompanying hypotension) remain the recommended treatments for symptomatic supraventricular tachycardia in the most recent American Heart Association Advanced Cardiac Life Support guidelines.[19]

Verapamil

The phenylalkylamine Ca^{2+} channel blocker verapamil produces less arterial vasodilation, but exerts more potent effects on automaticity, conduction, and myocardial contractility than the dihydropyridines or diltiazem. As a result, the anticipated baroreceptor-mediated tachycardia in response to reductions in arterial vasomotor tone and systemic vascular resistance does not occur. Sympathetic nervous system activation resulting from arterial vasodilation compensates for verapamil's direct negative inotropic effects, and cardiac output is maintained or modestly increases because of the decline in LV afterload in patients with normal LV systolic function. However, verapamil has the potential to markedly worsen preexisting LV systolic dysfunction in patients with HFpEF because of its myocardial depressant effects. Like diltiazem, verapamil is a coronary vasodilator and decreases myocardial oxygen demand as a result of its hemodynamic effects. Thus, verapamil is an effective alternative treatment for myocardial ischemia or infarction in patients who are unable to tolerate beta-blockers.

The actions of verapamil on cardiac electrophysiology make the Ca^{2+} channel antagonist a useful alternative to adenosine for the treatment of supraventricular tachyarrhythmias.[19] Reentry through the SA node or AV node is responsible for the vast majority of supraventricular tachyarrhythmias except when an aberrant conduction ("pre-excitation") pathway is present (e.g., the bundle of Kent in Wolff–Parkinson–White syndrome).[88] Verapamil reduces the rate of SA node discharge, markedly decreases AV node conduction velocity, and increases the refractory period of the AV node consistent with a class IV antiarrhythmic. These actions prolong PR interval and increase AV conduction time. Verapamil has been shown to significantly reduce the risk of supraventricular tachyarrhythmias in patients undergoing cardiac and noncardiac surgery because of these actions on the proximal cardiac conduction system. Verapamil is useful for the treatment of atrial fibrillation or flutter with rapid ventricular response because the drug substantially reduces ventricular rate. Verapamil may also facilitate conversion of atrial arrhythmia to sinus rhythm. Verapamil is contraindicated in the presence of an aberrant reentry supraventricular tachyarrhythmia because blockade of AV conduction leaves direct transmission from the atrium to the ventricle through the aberrant pathway unopposed, exposing the patient to the risk of malignant ventricular arrhythmias and sudden cardiac death.[89] Administration of verapamil in the presence of a beta-blocker may cause complete heart block or profound myocardial depression. Verapamil is contraindicated in patients with sick sinus syndrome or AV-node dysfunction.

Angiotensin Converting Enzyme Inhibitors

The renin–angiotensin–aldosterone system is a major regulator of cardiovascular homeostasis. Renal cortical juxtaglomerular cells secrete renin in response to three stimuli: (1) decreases in Na^+ reabsorption by the macula densa; (2) reduced perfusion pressure to preglomerular arterioles; and (3) sympathetic nervous system activation mediated through $beta_1$-adrenoceptors. Renin cleaves angiotensinogen into the 10 amino acid peptide angiotensin I (Fig. 13-7). Angiotensin converting enzyme is synthesized in pulmonary vascular endothelium. This enzyme cleaves the C-terminal histidine and leucine residues from the angiotensin I molecule to form the biologically active octapeptide angiotensin II. Angiotensin II is a potent vasoconstrictor of renal and mesenteric arterioles through its actions at the angiotensin subtype I (AT_1) receptor mediated through G_q protein-phospholipase C-inositol triphosphate-Ca^{2+} signaling.[90] Angiotensin II enhances the release of norepinephrine and epinephrine from the adrenal medulla and attenuates baroreceptor-mediated reductions in sympathetic nervous system tone that occur in response to compensatory increases in arterial pressure. Angiotensin II facilitates the release of norepinephrine from sympathetic postganglionic neurons and augments its actions in vascular smooth muscle. Angiotensin II further stimulates the synthesis and release of aldosterone from the zona glomerulosa of the adrenal cortex, and aldosterone then augments the actions of angiotensin II on renal tubular Na^+ retention and K^+ excretion. The renal tubular reabsorption of Na^+ is inhibited, thereby reducing Na^+ and water excretion and enhancing K^+ excretion. The net result is elevated arterial pressure and increased intravascular volume.

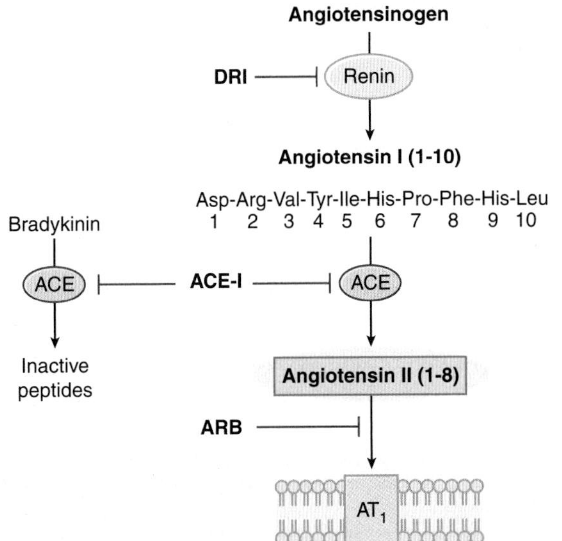

Figure 13-7 Schematic illustration of inhibitors of the renin-angiotensin system. DRI, direct renin inhibitor; ACE, angiotensin converting enzyme; ACE I, angiotensin converting enzyme inhibitor; ARB, angiotensin receptor blocker; AT_1, angiotensin subtype 1 receptor. (Used with permission of McGraw Hill Education, from Hilal-Dandan R. Renin and angiotensin. In: Brunton LL, Chabner BA, Knollman BC, ed. *Goodman and Gilman's The Pharmacological Basis of Therapeutics*, 12th ed. McGraw Hill Medical; 2011:731; permission conveyed through Copyright Clearance Center, Inc. (Fig. 26-8))

ACE inhibitors block the conversion of angiotensin I to angiotensin II. These drugs are used extensively for the treatment of hypertension and HFrEF. There are currently eleven ACE inhibitors in clinical use in the United States, which differ in potency, duration of action, metabolism and clearance, and whether hepatic esterase conversion of a prodrug form to a metabolite is required for activity (e.g., enalapril, quinapril, ramipril). Captopril was the first ACE inhibitor, but it is less commonly used in contemporary practice because the drug causes more side effects and drug interactions than other ACE inhibitors. Enalapril is the only ACE inhibitor available in an intravenous form (enalaprilat). Lisinopril is the only orally administered drug in this class with a prolonged half-life that does not require multiple daily dosing. ACE inhibitors reduce LV afterload and decrease arterial pressure through a reduction in arterial vasomotor tone in patients with essential or renal vascular hypertension, but not in those with primary aldosteronism. Cardiac output remains unchanged or modestly increases while LV preload is unaffected. Sympathetic nervous system tone does not change substantially despite the decrease in arterial pressure, and baroreceptor reflexes remain intact. As a result, patients do not develop orthostatic hypotension or limited exercise capacity when treated with an ACE inhibitor unless relative hypovolemia is present because of concomitant diuretic therapy. Orthostatic hypotension may occur if an ACE inhibitor is administered with another arterial vasodilator (e.g., Ca^{2+} channel blocker) or if elevated plasma renin concentrations are present.

ACE inhibitors decrease LV afterload, improve arterial compliance, reduce arterial pressure, enhance cardiac output, increase renal blood flow, and facilitate natriuresis. These hemodynamic effects reduce chronically elevated sympathetic nervous system tone and the renal actions favorably reduce in intravascular volume. ACE inhibitors have been shown to be very effective in the treatment of HRrEF.[53,54] Several large randomized controlled trials provided convincing evidence that ACE inhibitors halt or delay the progression and improve quality of life in patients with HFrEF. ACE inhibitors reduce the need for hospitalization, the incidence of myocardial infarction, and the risk of sudden cardiac death in these patients. Despite the well-documented efficacy of ACE inhibitors in HFrEF, these medications did not substantially affect outcome in patients with HFpEF, as several major randomized controlled trials failed to show that ACE inhibitors reduce mortality and hospitalization rates.[55,56] ACE inhibitors have well-documented beneficial effects in patients with acute myocardial infarction, especially those with diabetes mellitus and hypertension.[91] Moreover, ACE inhibitors substantially decreased the incidence of myocardial infarction, stroke, and mortality in patients with vascular disease or diabetes who are at high risk for major adverse cardiovascular events.[92] Finally, ACE inhibitors exert renal protective effects in diabetic patients and mitigate the progression of renal dysfunction in other forms of nephropathy.[93]

ACE inhibitors produce several side effects, the most common of which is a dry cough that affects as many as 20% of patients. Blockade of bradykinin degradation by ACE inhibitors exacerbates the pulmonary effects of this inflammatory mediator and is the cause of this complication. Nonsteroidal anti-inflammatory drugs attenuate the ability of ACE inhibitors to reduce arterial pressure in patients with hypertension. ACE inhibitors may cause hyperkalemia in patients with chronic renal insufficiency and in those with normal renal function who are treated with K^+-sparing diuretics (e.g., spironolactone, triamterene) or K^+ supplements. Conversely, ACE inhibitors blunt the hypokalemic effects of thiazide and loop diuretics. Acute renal failure, reversible neutropenia, fetal teratogenicity, and dermatitis are other adverse effects of ACE inhibitors. Angioedema is a rare (0.1 to 0.5% of patients) but potentially life-threatening complication of ACE inhibitors in which rapidly developing edema of the lips, nose, tongue, mouth, hypopharynx, and glottis may rapidly compromise airway integrity. Angioedema resulting from an ACE inhibitor usually occurs with the initial dose of the drug and may require emergent endotracheal intubation or a surgical airway to prevent death from asphyxia. It is noteworthy that African-Americans are approximately 4.5-fold more likely to develop this complication than Caucasians for reasons that are unclear. Perhaps of most relevance to the anesthesiologist, treatment with an ACE inhibitor may cause profound hypotension in the presence of vasodilating anesthetics that is resistant to treatment with catecholamines.[94] Two alternate metabolic pathways for angiotensin I and II may be at least partially responsible for this catecholamine-refractory hypotension. Neural and propyl-endopeptidases convert the excess angiotensin I that accumulates during ACE inhibition into the heptapeptide angiotensin 1–7. A second form of angiotensin converting enzyme (ACE2) that is not blocked by clinically used ACE inhibitors may also generate angiotensin 1–7. In contrast to the potent vasoconstriction produced by angiotensin II, angiotensin 1–7 is a vasodilator that exerts its effects through the endothelial Mas receptor.[95] Thus, it is likely that both the absence of angiotensin II-mediated vasoconstriction and the presence of the vasodilating metabolite angiotensin 1–7 contribute to the development of severe hypotension during anesthesia in some patients. Vasopressin or V_1 agonists (e.g., terlipressin) are indicated for treatment of this form of intraoperative hypotension.[96] This complication can be avoided by discontinuing ACE inhibitor therapy before elective surgery, but this decision must be weighed against the potential adverse risks associated with unmasked hypertension.

Angiotensin Receptor Blockers

12 ARBs inhibit the AT_1 receptor with high affinity. This action markedly attenuates the cardiovascular, endocrine, and renal effects of angiotensin II. All ARBs are potent antihypertensive medications that more effectively inhibit the actions of angiotensin II at AT_1 receptors than ACE inhibitors and also have a greater margin of safety.[97] ARBs do not affect angiotensin II-induced activation of angiotensin subtype 2 (AT_2) receptors, in contrast to ACE inhibitors. The clinical implications of these differences in pharmacodynamics between ARBs and ACE inhibitors remain unclear. Similar to ACE inhibitors, ARBs (e.g., losartan, candesartan, valsartan) improved functional capacity and reduced morbidity and mortality in patients with HFrEF[98] and acute myocardial infarction complicated by LV dysfunction,[99] but not in those with HFpEF.[55,56] Whether the combination of an ARB and an ACE inhibitor provides any added benefits in these settings has not been resolved. ARBs are most often used in patients with HFrEF who are unable to tolerate the side effects of ACE inhibitors. Like ACE inhibitors, ARBs provide renal protection in patients with diabetes mellitus independently of the effects of these drugs on arterial pressure. ARBs reduce the risk of stroke in patients with hypertension, maintain sinus rhythm after cardioversion in patients with long-term atrial fibrillation, and improve symptoms in patients with portal hypertension. As predicted by their pharmacologic mechanism of action, ARBs are less likely to cause cough, dermatitis, or angioedema than ACE inhibitors. However, ARBs are teratogenic and may cause hyperkalemia in patients treated with K^+-sparing diuretics or those with renal insufficiency, similar to ACE inhibitors.

Acknowledgments

The authors gratefully acknowledge the contributions of previous edition author, Loreta Grecu, as portions of those chapters have been retained in this revision.

For further review and interactivities, please see the videos and narrative interactive clinical vignettes (NICVs) accessible in the complimentary eBook bundled with this text. Access instructions are located on the inside front cover.

REFERENCES

1. Cockcroft DW, Davis BE, Blais CM. Direct bronchoprovocation test methods: history 1945–2018. *Expert Rev Respir Med*. 2019;13:279–289.
2. Edwards JM, McCarthy CG, Wenceslau CF. The obligatory role of acetylcholine-induced endothelium-dependent contraction in hypertension: Can arachidonic acid resolve this inflammation? *Curr Pharm Des*. 2020;26:3723–3732.
3. Moro C, Phelps C, Veer V, et al. The effectiveness of parasympathomimetics for treating underactive bladder: A systematic review and meta-analysis. *Neurourol Urodyn*. 2022;41:127–139.
4. Mercadante V, Al Hamad A, Lodi G, Porter S, Fedele S. Interventions for management of radiotherapy-induced xerostomia and hyposalivation: A systemic review and meta-analysis. *Oral Oncol*. 2017;66:64–74.
5. Scarpa M, Hesse S, Bradley SJ. M1 muscarinic acetylcholine receptors: A therapeutic strategy for symptomatic and disease-modifying effects in Alzheimer's disease? *Adv Pharmcol*. 2020; 88:277–310.
6. Keating GM. Sugammadex: A review of neuromuscular blockade reversal. *Drugs*. 2016;76: 1041–1052.
7. Amend N, Niessen KV, Seeger T, Wille T, Worek F, Thiermann H. Diagnostics and treatment of nerve agent poisoning–current status and future developments. *Ann N Y Acad Sci*. 2020; 1479:13–28.
8. Sharma K. Cholinesterase inhibitors as Alzheimer's therapeutics. *Mol Med Rep*. 2019;20: 1479–1487.
9. Crowe S, Collins L. Suxamethonium and donepezil: A cause of prolonged paralysis. *Anesthesiology*. 2003;98:574–575.
10. Chapple CR, Khullar V, Gabriel Z, Muston D, Bitoun CE, Weinstein D. The effects of antimuscarinic treatments in overactive bladder: An update of a systematic review and meta-analysis. *Eur Urol*. 2008;54:543–562.
11. Wellstein A, Pitschner HF. Complex dose-response curves of atropine in man explained by different functions of M1- and M2 cholinoceptors. *Naunyn Schmiedebergs Arch Pharmacol*. 1988;338:19–27.
12. Cheyne L, Irvin-Sellers MJ, White J. Tiotropium versus ipratropium bromide for chronic obstructive pulmonary disease. *Cochrane Database Syst Rev*. 2015;2015:CD009552.
13. Wang J, Gareri C, Rockman HA. G-protein-coupled receptors in heart disease. *Circ Res*. 2018;123:716–735.
14. Steinberg SF. Beta$_1$-adrenergic receptor regulation revisited. *Circ Res*. 2018;123:1199–1201.
15. Lymperopoulos A, Brill A, McCrink KA. GPCRs of adrenal chromaffin cells and catecholamines: The plot thickens. *Int J Biochem Cell Biol*. 2016;77(Pt B):213–219.
16. Leenen FH, Chan YK, Smith DL, Reeves RA. Epinephrine and left ventricular function in humans: effects of beta-1 vs nonselective beta-blockade. *Clin Pharmacol Ther*. 1988;43:519–528.
17. Butterworth JF 4th, Prielipp RC, Royster RL, et al. Dobutamine increases heart rate more than epinephrine in patients recovering from aortocoronary bypass surgery. *J Cardiothoracic Vasc Anesth*. 1992;6:535–541.
18. Fellahi J-L, Parienti J-J, Hanouz J-L, Plaud B, Riou B, Ouattara A. Perioperative use of dobutamine in cardiac surgery and adverse cardiac outcome: Propensity-adjusted analyses. *Anesthesiology*. 2008;108:979–987.

19. Panchal AR, Bartos JA, Cabanas JG, et al. Part 3: Adult basic and advanced life support: 2020 American Heart Association guidelines for cardiopulmonary resuscitation and emergency cardiovascular care. *Circulation.* 2020;142(16_suppl_2):S366–S468.
20. Walker DM. Update on epinephrine (adrenaline) for pediatric emergencies. *Curr Opin Pediatr.* 2009;21:313–319.
21. Bochner BS, Lichtenstein LM. Anaphylaxis. *N Engl J Med.* 1991;324:1785–1790.
22. Russell JA, Rush B, Boyd J. Pathophysiology of septic shock. *Crit Care Clin.* 2018;34:43–61.
23. Ortoleva J, Shapeton A, Vanneman M, Dalia AA. Vasoplegia during cardiopulmonary bypass: Current literature and rescue therapy options. *J Cardiothorac Vasc Anesth.* 2020;34:2766–2775.
24. Pancaro C, Shah N, Pasma W, et al. Risk of Major Complications After Perioperative Norepinephrine Infusion Through Peripheral Intravenous Lines in a Multicenter Study. *Anesth Analg.* 2020;131:1060–1065.
25. MacGregor DA, Smith TE, Prielipp RC, Butterworth JF, James RL, Scuderi PE. Pharmacokinetics of dopamine in healthy male subjects. *Anesthesiology.* 2000;92:338–346.
26. Friedrich JO, Adhikari N, Herridge MS, Beyene J. Meta-analysis: Low-dose dopamine increases urine output but does not prevent renal dysfunction or death. *Ann Intern Med.* 2005;142:510–524.
27. Aronson S, Dupont F, Savage R, Drum M, Gunnar W, Jeevanandam V. Changes in regional myocardial function after coronary artery bypass graft surgery are predicted by intraoperative low-dose dobutamine echocardiography. *Anesthesiology.* 2000;93:685–692.
28. Zamanian RT, Haddad F, Doyle RL, Weinacker AB. Management strategies for patients with pulmonary hypertension in the intensive care unit. *Crit Care Med.* 2007;35:2037–2050.
29. Abraham WT, Adams KF, Fonarow GC, et al; ADHERE Scientific Advisory Committee and Investigators; ADHERE Study Group. In-hospital mortality in patients with acute decompensated heart failure requiring intravenous vasoactive medications: An analysis from the Acute Decompensated Heart Failure National Registry (ADHERE). *J Am Coll Cardiol.* 2005;46:57–64.
30. Evans L, Rhodes A, Alhazzani W, et al. Surviving sepsis campaign: International Guidelines for Management of Sepsis and Septic Shock 2021. *Crit Care Med.* 2021;49:e1063–e1143.
31. Noce A, Marrone G, Rovella V, et al. Fenoldopam mesylate: A narrative review of its use in acute kidney injury. *Curr Pharm Biotechnol.* 2019;20:366–375.
32. Landoni G, Biondi-Zoccai GGL, Tumlin JA, et al. Beneficial impact of fenoldopam in critically ill patients with or at risk for acute renal failure: a meta-analysis of randomized clinical trials. *Am J Kidney Dis.* 2007;49:56–68.
33. Bove T, Zangrillo A, Guarracino F, et al. Effect of fenoldopam on use of renal replacement therapy among patients with acute kidney injury after cardiac surgery: A randomized clinical trial. *JAMA.* 2014;312:2244–2253.
34. Little WC. Enhanced load dependence of relaxation in heart failure. Clinical implications. *Circulation.* 1992;85:2326–2328.
35. Patel D, Phay JE, Yen TWF, et al. Update on pheochromocytoma and paraganglioma from the SSO Endocrine/Head and Neck-Site Work Group. Part 1 of 2: Advances in pathogenesis and diagnosis of pheochromocytoma and paraganglioma. *Ann Surg Oncol.* 2020;27:1329–1337.
36. Patel D, Phay JE, Yen TWF, et al. Update on pheochromocytoma and paraganglioma from the SSO Endocrine/Head and Neck-Site Work Group. Part 2 of 2: perioperative management and outcomes of pheochromocytoma and paraganglioma. *Ann Surg Oncol.* 2020;27:1338–1347.
37. Zitoun OA, Farhat AM, Mohamed MA, Hamad MR, Aramini B, Haider KH. Management of benign prostatic hyperplasia (BPH) by combinatorial approach using alpha-1-adrenergic antagonists and 5-alpha-reductase inhibitors. *Eur J Pharmacol.* 2020;883:173301.
38. Nguyen V, Tieman D, Park E, Salehi A. Alpha-2 agonists. *Anesthesiol Clin.* 2017;35:233–245.
39. Weerink MAS, Struys MMRF, Hannivoort LN, Barends CRM, Absalom AR, Colin P. Clinical pharmacokinetics and pharmacodynamics of dexmedetomidine. *Clin Pharmacokinet.* 2017;56:893–913.
40. Wijeysundera DN, Naik JS, Beattie WS. Alpha-2 adrenergic agonists to prevent perioperative cardiovascular complications: A meta-analysis. *Am J Med.* 2003;114:742–752.
41. Eisenach JC, De Kock M, Klimscha W. Alpha(2)-adrenergic agonists for regional anesthesia. A clinical review of clonidine (1984–1995). *Anesthesiology.* 1996;85:655–674.
42. Keating GM. Dexmedetomidine: A review of its use for sedation in the intensive care setting. *Drugs.* 2015;75:1119–1130.
43. Rozet I. Anesthesia for functional neurosurgery: The role of dexmedetomidine. *Curr Opin Anaesthesiol.* 2008;21:537–543.
44. Carollo DS, Nossaman BD, Ramadhyani U. Dexmedetomidine: A review of clinical applications. *Curr Opin Anaesthesiol.* 2008;21:457–461.
45. Djaiani G, Silverton N, Fedorko L, et al. Dexmedetomidine versus propofol sedation reduces delirium after cardiac surgery: A randomized controlled trial. *Anesthesiology.* 2016;124:362–368.
46. Shen Q-H, Li H-F, Zhou X-Y, Yuan X-Z. Dexmedetomidine in the prevention of postoperative delirium in elderly patients following non-cardiac surgery: A systematic review and meta-analysis. *Clin Exp Pharmacol Physiol.* 2020;47:1333–1341.
47. Penttila J, Helminen A, Anttila M, Hinkka S, Scheinin H. Cardiovascular and parasympathetic effects of dexmedetomidine in healthy subjects. *Can J Physiol Pharmacol.* 2004;82:359–362.
48. Ji F, Li Z, Nguyen H, et al. Perioperative dexmedetomidine improves outcomes of cardiac surgery. *Circulation.* 2013;127:1576–1584.
49. Fleisher LA, Fleischmann KE, Auerbach AD, et al. 2014 ACC/AHA guideline on perioperative cardiovascular and management of patients undergoing noncardiac surgery: A report of the American College of Cardiology/American Heart Association Task Force on Practice Guidelines. *Circulation.* 2014;130:e278–e333.
50. Wijeysundera DN, Duncan D, Nkonde-Price C, et al. Perioperative beta blockade in noncardiac surgery: A systemic review for the 2014 ACC/AHA guideline on perioperative cardiovascular evaluation and management of patients undergoing noncardiac surgery: A report of the American College of Cardiology/American Heart Association Task Force on practice guidelines. *J Am Coll Cardiol.* 2014;64:2406–2425.
51. Writing Committee Members; Gulati M, Levy PD, Amsterdam E, et al. 2021 AHA/ACC/ASE/CHEST/SAEM/SCCT/SCMR guideline for the evaluation and diagnosis of chest pain: A report of the American College of Cardiology/American Heart Association Joint Committee on Clinical Practice Guidelines. *J Am Coll Cardiol.* 2021;78:e187–e285.
52. Hjalmarson A, Goldstein S, Fagerberg B, et al. Effects of controlled-release metoprolol on total mortality, hospitalizations, and well-being of patients with heart failure: the Metoprolol CR/XL Randomized Intervention Trial in congestive heart failure (MERIT-HT). MERIT-HF Study Group. *JAMA.* 2000;283:1295–1302.
53. Yancy CW, Jessup M, Bozkurt B, et al. 2013 ACCF/AHA guideline for the management of heart failure: A report of the American College of Cardiology Foundation/American Heart Association Task Force on Practice Guidelines. *J Am Coll Cardiol.* 2013;62:e147–e239.
54. Ponikowski P, Voors AA, Anker SD, et al. 2016 ESC Guidelines for the diagnosis and treatment of acute and chronic heart failure: the Task Force for the diagnosis and treatment of acute and chronic heart failure of the European Society of Cardiology (ESC) developed with the special contribution of the Heart Failure Association (HFA) of the ESC. *Eur Heart J.* 2016;37:2129–2200.
55. Borlaug BA. Evaluation and management of heart failure with preserved ejection fraction. *Nat Rev Cardiol.* 2020;17:559–573.
56. Pagel PS, Tawil JN, Boettcher BT, et al. Heart failure with preserved ejection fraction: a comprehensive review and update of diagnosis, pathophysiology, treatment, and perioperative implications. *J Cardiothorac Vasc Anesth.* 2021;35:1839–1859.
57. Lacro RV, Dietz HC, Sleeper LA, et al. Atenolol versus losartan in children and young adults with Marfan's syndrome. *N Engl J Med.* 2014;371:2061–2071.
58. Maron BJ, Desai MY, Nishimura RA, et al. Management of hypertrophic cardiomyopathy: JACC state-of-the-art review. *J Am Coll Cardiol.* 2022;79:390–414.
59. Urits I, Gress K, Charipova K, et al. Pharmacological options for treatment of chronic migraine pain. *Best Pract Res Clin Anaesthesiol.* 2020;34:383–407.
60. Filho FSL, Choi L, Sin DD. Beta-blockers in chronic obstructive pulmonary disease: the good, the bad and the ugly. *Curr Opin Pulm Med.* 2021;27:125–131.
61. National Heart Lung and Blood Institute. A randomized trial of propranolol in patients with acute myocardial infarction. I. Mortality results. *JAMA.* 1982;247:1707–1714.
62. Grassi G. Metoprolol in the treatment of cardiovascular disease: a critical reappraisal. *Curr Med Res Opin.* 2018;34:1635–1643.
63. Feldman RD, Hussain Y, Kuyper LM, McAlister FA, Padwal RS, Tobe SW. Intraclass differences among antihypertensive drugs. *Annu Rev Pharmacol Toxicol.* 2015;55:333–352.
64. DiNicolantonio JJ, Hackam DG. Carvedilol: A third-generation beta-blocker should be a first-choice beta-blocker. *Expert Rev Cardiovasc Ther.* 2012;10:13–25.
65. Nandkeolyar S, Rye R, Mohammed A, et al. A review of inotropes and inopressors for effective utilization in patients with acute decompensated heart failure. *J Cardiovasc Pharmacol.* 2021;78:336–345.
66. Sabato LA, Salerno DM, Moretz JD, Jennings DL. Inhaled pulmonary vasodilator therapy for management of right ventricular dysfunction after left ventricular assist device placement and cardiac transplantation. *Pharmacotherapy.* 2017;37:944–955.
67. Liu K, Wang H, Yu S-J, Tu G-W, Luo Z. Inhaled pulmonary vasodilators: A narrative review. *Ann Transl Med.* 2021;9:597.
68. Conti N, Gatti M, Raschi E, Diemberger I, Potena L. Evidence and current use of levosimendan in the treatment of heart failure: filling the gap. *Drug Des Devel Ther.* 2021;15:3391–3409.
69. Toller W, Heringlake M, Guarracino F, et al. Preoperative and perioperative use of levosimendan in cardiac surgery: European expert opinion. *Int J Cardiol.* 2015;184:323–336.
70. Altenberger J, Parissis JT, Costard-Jaeckle A, et al. Efficacy and safety of the pulsed infusions of levosimendan in outpatients with advanced heart failure (LevoRep) study: a multicentre randomized trial. *Eur J Heart Fail.* 2014;16:898–906.
71. De Hert SG, Lorsomradee S, Cromheecke S, Van der Linden PJ. The effects of levosimendan in cardiac surgery patients with poor left ventricular function. *Anesth Analg.* 2007;104:766–773.
72. Ahmed A, Rich MW, Fleg JL, et al. Effects of digoxin on morbidity and mortality in diastolic heart failure: the ancillary digitalis investigation group trial. *Circulation.* 2006;114:397–403.
73. Treschan TA, Peters J. The vasopressin system: physiology and clinical strategies. *Anesthesiology.* 2006;105:599–612.
74. Redfield MM, Anstrom KJ, Levine JA, et al. Isosorbide mononitrate in heart failure with preserved ejection fraction. *N Engl J Med.* 2015;373:2314–2324.
75. Borlaug BA, Anstrom KJ, Lewis GD, et al. Effect of inorganic nitrite vs placebo on exercise capacity among patients with heart failure with preserved ejection fraction: the INDIE-HRpEF randomized clinical trial. *JAMA.* 2018;320:1764–1773.
76. Fihn SD, Blankenship JC, Alexandder KP, et al. 2014 ACC/AHA/AATS/PCNA/SCAI/STS focused update of the guideline for the diagnosis and management of patients with stable ischemic heart disease: a report of the American College of Cardiology/American Heart

Association Task Force on Practice Guidelines, and the American Association for Thoracic Surgery, Preventive Cardiovascular Nurses Association, Society for Cardiovascular Angiography and Interventions, and Society of Thoracic Surgeons. *Circulation*. 2014;130:1749–1767.
77. Harris JR, Hale GM, Dasari TW, Schwier NC. Pharmacotherapy of vasospastic angina. *J Cardiovasc Pharmacol Ther*. 2016;21:439–451.
78. Opie LH, Yusuf S, Kubler W. Current status of safety and efficacy of calcium channel blockers in cardiovascular diseases: a critical analysis based on 100 studies. *Prog Cardiovasc Dis*. 2000; 43:171–196.
79. Keating GM. Clevidipine: a review of its use for managing blood pressure in perioperative and intensive care settings. *Drugs*. 2014;74:1947–1960.
80. Peacock WF, Chandra A, Char D, et al. Clevidipine in acute heart failure: results of the A Study of Blood Pressure Control in Acute Heart Failure-A Pilot Study (PRONTO). *Am Heart J*. 2014; 167:529–536.
81. Singla N, Warltier DC, Gandhi SD, et al. Treatment of acute postoperative hypertension in cardiac surgery patients: an efficacy study of clevidipine assessing its postoperative antihypertensive effect in cardiac surgery-2 (ESCAPE-2), a randomized, double-blind, placebo-controlled trial. *Anesth Analg*. 2008;107:59–67.
82. Aronson S, Dyke CM, Stierer KA, et al. The ECLIPSE trials: comparative studies of clevidipine to nitroglycerin, sodium nitroprusside, and nicardipine for acute hypertension treatment in cardiac surgery patients. *Anesth Analg*. 2008;107:1110–1121.
83. Lord MS, Augoustidis JGT. Perioperative management of pheochromocytoma: focus on magnesium, clevidipine, and vasopressin. *J Cardiothorac Vasc Anesth*. 2012;26:526–531.
84. Saldana S, Breslin J 2nd, Hanify J, et al. Comparison of clevidipine and nicardipine for acute blood pressure reduction in hemorrhagic stroke. *Neurocrit Care*. 2021;(In Press).
85. Carlson AP, Hanggi D, Macdonald RL, Shuttleworth CW. Nimodipine reappraised: an old drug with a future. *Curr Neuropharmacol*. 2020;18:65–82.
86. Grossman E, Messerli FH. Calcium antagonists. *Prog Cardiovasc Dis*. 2004;47:34–57.
87. Lim SH, Anantharaman V, Teo WS, Chan YH. Slow infusion of calcium channel blockers compared with intravenous adenosine in the emergency treatment of superventricular tachycardia. *Resuscitation*. 2009;80:523–528.
88. Al-Khatib SM, Arshad A, Balk EM, et al. Risk stratification for arrhythmic events in patients with asymptomatic pre-excitation: a systematic review for the 2015 ACC/AHA/HRS guideline for the management of adult patients with supraventricular tachycardia: a report of the American College of Cardiology/American Heart Association Task Force on Clinical Practice Guidelines and the Heart Rhythm Society. *J Am Coll Cardiol*. 2016;67:1624–1638.
89. Redfearn DP, Krahn AD, Skanes AC, Yee R, Klein GJ. Use of medications in Wolff-Parkinson-White syndrome. *Expert Opin Pharmacother*. 2005;6:955–963.
90. Mehta PK, Griendling KK. Angiotensin II cell signaling: physiological and pathological effects in the cardiovascular system. *Am J Physiol Cell Physiol*. 2007;292:C82–C97.
91. ACE Inhibitor Myocardial Infarction Collaborative Group. Indications for ACE inhibitors in the early treatment of acute myocardial infarction: systemic overview of individual data from 100,000 patients in randomized controlled trials. *Circulation*. 1998;97:2202–2212.
92. Yusuf S, Sleight P, Pogue J, et al. Effects of an angiotensin-converting-enzyme inhibitor, ramipril, on cardiovascular events in high-risk patients. *N Engl J Med*. 2000;342:145–153.
93. Ruggenenti P, Cravedi P, Remuzzi G. The RAAS in the pathogenesis and treatment of diabetic nephropathy. *Nat Rev Nephrol*. 2010;6:319–330.
94. Kheterpal S, Khodaparast O, Shanks A, O'Reilly M, Tremper KK. Chronic angiotensin-converting enzyme inhibitor or angiotensin receptor blocker therapy combined with diuretic therapy is associated with increased episodes of hypotension in noncardiac surgery. *J Cardiothoracic Vasc Anesth*. 2008;22:180–186.
95. Schnizari F, Tesauro M, Veneziani A, Mores N, Di Daniele N, Cardillo C. Favorable vascular actions of angiotensin-(1–7) in human obesity. *Hypertension*. 2018;71:185–191.
96. Morelli A, Tritapepe L, Rocco M, et al. Terlipressin versus norepinephrine to counteract anesthesia-induced hypotension in patients treated with renin-angiotensin system inhibitors: effects on systemic and regional hemodynamics. *Anesthesiology*. 2005;102:12–19.
97. Chen R, Suchard MA, Krumholz HM, et al. Comparative first-line effectiveness and safety of ACE (angiotensin-converting enzyme) inhibitors and angiotensin receptor blockers. A multinational cohort study. *Hypertension*. 2021;78:591–603.
98. Maggioni AP, Anand I, Gottlieb SO, et al. Effects of valsartan on morbidity and mortality in patients with heart failure not receiving angiotensin-converting enzyme inhibitors. *J Am Coll Cardiol*. 2002;40:1414–1421.
99. Pfeffer MA, McMurray JJ, Velazquez EJ, et al. Valsartan, captopril, or both in myocardial infarction complicated by heart failure, left ventricular dysfunction, or both. *N Engl J Med*. 2003;349: 1893–1906.

14 Autonomic Nervous System Anatomy and Physiology

LORETA GRECU

KEY POINTS

1 The autonomic nervous system (ANS) includes that part of the central nervous system (CNS) and peripheral nervous system concerned with the involuntary regulation of cardiac muscle, smooth muscle, and glandular and visceral functions.

2 The sympathetic and parasympathetic nervous systems (SNS, PNS) affect cardiac pump function in three ways: (1) by changing the rate (chronotropism), (2) by changing the strength of contraction (inotropism), and (3) by modulating coronary blood flow.

3 SNS nerves are by far the most important regulators of peripheral circulation.

4 The ANS can be pharmacologically subdivided by the neurotransmitter secreted at the effector cell: acetylcholine (ACh) released by the PNS, and the catecholamines: epinephrine (EPI) and norepinephrine (NE), which are the mediators of peripheral SNS activity.

5 An agonist is a substance that interacts with a receptor to evoke a biologic response. An antagonist is a substance that at the receptor site stops the response produced by an agonist (counteracts an agonist).

6 The SNS receptors (adrenoreceptors or adrenergic receptors) are G-protein–coupled receptors named adrenergic or noradrenergic, depending on their responsiveness to EPI and NE.

7 The numbers and sensitivity of adrenoreceptors can be influenced by normal, genetic, and developmental factors

8 The ANS reflex comprises (1) sensors, (2) afferent pathways, (3) CNS integration, and (4) efferent pathways to the receptors and efferent organs.

9 The clinical application of ANS pharmacology is based on knowledge of ANS anatomy, physiology, and molecular pharmacology.

10 Clinically, anticholinesterase drugs may be divided into two types: reversible and nonreversible cholinesterase inhibitors.

Anesthesia and the Autonomic Nervous System

Anesthesiology is the practice of autonomic medicine. Drugs that produce anesthesia may also have potent autonomic side effects. The greater part of anesthesia training and practice is spent acquiring skills in utilizing or averting the autonomic nervous system (ANS) side effects of anesthetic drugs under a variety of pathophysiologic conditions. The success of any anesthetic depends on how well homeostasis is maintained. The anesthetic record reflects ANS function.

1 The ANS includes that part of the central and peripheral nervous systems concerned with the involuntary regulation of cardiac muscle, smooth muscle, and glandular and visceral functions. ANS activity refers to visceral reflexes that function below the conscious level. The ANS is also responsive to changes in the somatic motor and sensory activities of the body. The physiologic evidence of visceral reflexes that result from somatic events is abundantly clear. The ANS is therefore not as distinct an entity as the term suggests. Neither somatic nor ANS activity occurs in isolation.[1] The ANS organizes visceral support for somatic behavior and adjusts body states in anticipation of emotional behavior or responses to the stress of disease. In brief, it determines "fight-or-flight" responses.[2,3]

Afferent fibers from visceral structures are the first link in the reflex arcs of the ANS and may relay visceral pain or changes in vessel stretch. Most ANS efferent fibers are accompanied by sensory fibers that are now commonly recognized as components of the ANS. However, the afferent components of the ANS cannot be as distinctively divided as can the efferent nerves. ANS visceral sensory nerves are anatomically indistinguishable from somatic sensory nerves. The clinical importance of visceral afferent fibers is closely implicated in the management of chronic pain states.

Functional Anatomy

The ANS is organized into two divisions based on anatomy, physiology, and pharmacology. Langley divided this nervous system into two parts in 1921. He retained the term *sympathetic* (sympathetic nervous system [SNS]) introduced by Willis in 1665 for the first part and introduced the term "parasympathetic" (parasympathetic nervous system [PNS]) for the second. The term ANS was adopted to encompass both components. Table 14-1 lists the complementary effects of SNS (adrenergic, sympathetic) and PNS (cholinergic, parasympathetic) activity of organ systems.

Central Autonomic Organization

Pure central ANS versus somatic centers are not known. Integration of ANS activity occurs at all levels of the cerebrospinal axis. Efferent ANS activity can be initiated locally and by centers located in the spinal cord, brainstem, and hypothalamus. The cerebral cortex is the highest level of ANS integration. Fainting at the sight of blood is an example of this higher level of somatic and ANS integration. ANS function has also been successfully modulated through conscious, intentional efforts, demonstrating that somatic responses are always accompanied by visceral responses, and vice versa.

Table 14-1 Homeostatic Balance between Adrenergic and Cholinergic Effects

	Response	
Organ System	***Adrenergic***	***Cholinergic***
Heart		
Sinoatrial node	Tachycardia	Bradycardia
Atrioventricular node	Increased conduction	Decreased conduction
His–Purkinje	Increased automaticity and conduction velocity	Minimal
Myocardium	Increased contractility, conduction velocity, automaticity	Minimal decrease in contractility
Coronary vessels	Constriction (α_1) and dilation (β_1)	Dilation and constriction
Blood Vessels		
Skin and mucosa	Constriction	Dilation
Skeletal muscle	Constriction (α_1) > dilation (β_2)	Dilation
Pulmonary	Constriction	Dilation
Bronchial Smooth Muscle	Relaxation	Contraction
Gastrointestinal Tract		
Gallbladder and ducts	Relaxation	Contraction
Gut motility	Decreased	Increased
Secretions	Decreased	Increased
Sphincters	Constriction	Relaxation
Bladder		
Detrusor	Relaxation	Contraction
Trigone	Constriction	Relaxation
Glands		
Nasal Lacrimal Parotid Submandibular Gastric Pancreatic	Vasoconstriction and reduced secretion	Stimulation of secretions
Sweat Glands	Diaphoresis (cholinergic)	None
Apocrine Glands	Thick, odiferous secretion	None
Eye		
Pupil	Mydriasis	Miosis
Ciliary muscle	Relaxation for far vision	Contraction for near vision

The principal site of ANS organization is the *hypothalamus*. SNS functions are controlled by nuclei in the posterolateral hypothalamus. Stimulation of these nuclei results in a massive discharge of the sympathoadrenal system. PNS functions are governed by nuclei in the midline and some anterior nuclei of the hypothalamus. The anterior hypothalamus is involved with the regulation of temperature. The supraoptic hypothalamic nuclei regulate water metabolism and are anatomically and functionally associated with the posterior lobe of the pituitary (see Interaction of Autonomic Nervous System Receptors). This hypothalamic–neurohypophyseal connection represents a central ANS mechanism that affects the kidney using antidiuretic hormone (ADH). Long-term blood pressure control, reactions to physical and emotional stress, sleep, and sexual reflexes are regulated by the hypothalamus.

The *medulla oblongata* and *pons* are vital centers of acute ANS organization. Together, they integrate momentary hemodynamic adjustments and maintain the sequence and automaticity of ventilation. Integration of afferent and efferent ANS impulses at this central nervous system (CNS) level is responsible for the tonic activity exhibited by the ANS. Tonicity holds visceral organs in a state of intermediate activity that can be either diminished or augmented by altering the rate of nerve firing. The nucleus tractus solitarius, located within the medulla, is the primary area for the relay of afferent chemoreceptor and baroreceptor information from the glossopharyngeal and vagus nerves. Increased afferent impulses from these two nerves inhibit peripheral SNS vascular tone, producing vasodilation; they also increase vagal tone, producing bradycardia. Studies of patients with high spinal cord lesions show that a number of reflex changes are mediated at the spinal or segmental level. ANS hyperreflexia is an example of spinal cord mediation of ANS reflexes without integration of function from higher inhibitory centers.[1]

Peripheral Autonomic Nervous System Organization

The peripheral ANS is the efferent (motor) component of the ANS and consists of the same two complementary parts: the SNS and the PNS. Most organs receive fibers from both divisions (Fig. 14-1). In general, activities of the two systems produce opposite but complementary effects (Table 14-1). A few tissues, such as sweat glands and the spleen, are innervated by only SNS fibers. Although the anatomy of the somatic and ANS sensory pathways is identical, the motor pathways are characteristically different. The efferent somatic motor system, like somatic afferents, is composed of a single (unipolar) neuron with its cell body in the ventral gray matter of the spinal cord. Its myelinated axon extends directly to the voluntary striated muscle unit. In contrast, the efferent (motor) ANS is a two-neuron (bipolar) chain from the CNS to the effector

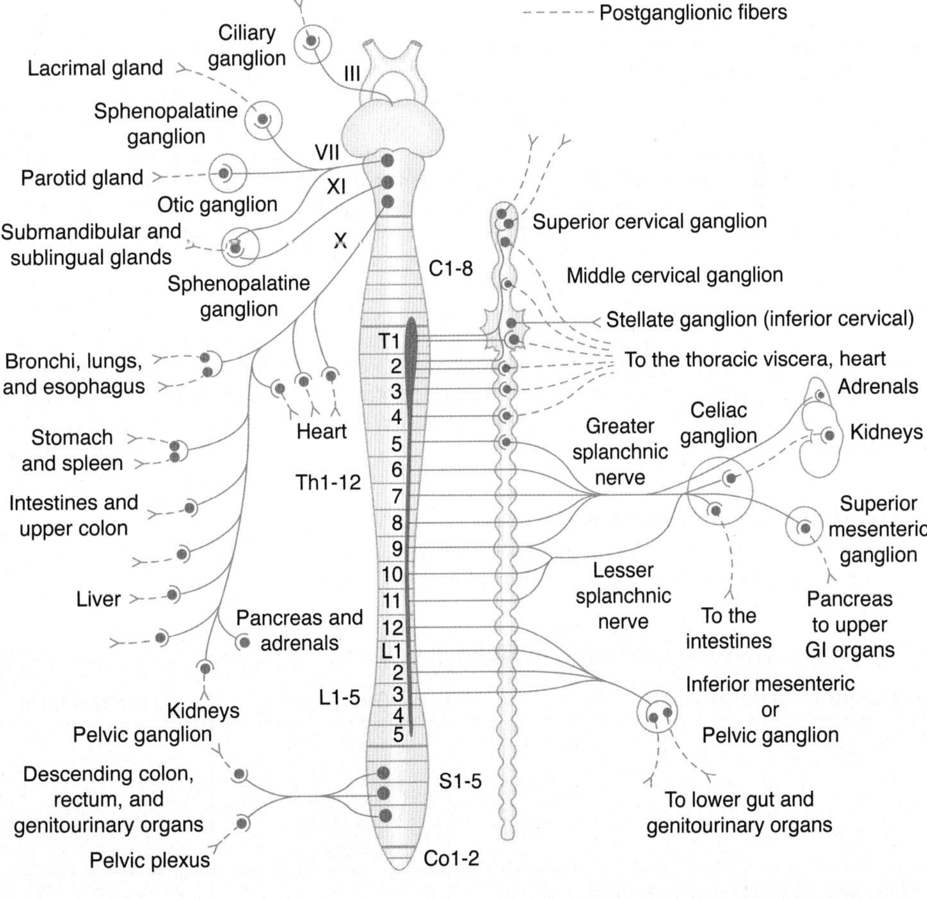

Figure 14-1 Schematic distribution of the craniosacral (parasympathetic) and thoracolumbar (sympathetic) nervous systems. Parasympathetic preganglionic fibers pass directly to the organ that is innervated. Their postganglionic cell bodies are situated near or within the innervated viscera. This limited distribution of parasympathetic postganglionic fibers is consistent with the discrete and limited effect of parasympathetic function. The postganglionic sympathetic neurons originate in either the paired sympathetic ganglia or one of the unpaired collateral plexuses. One preganglionic fiber influences many postganglionic neurons. Activation of the SNS produces a more diffuse physiologic response rather than a discrete, localized effect. GI, gastrointestinal.

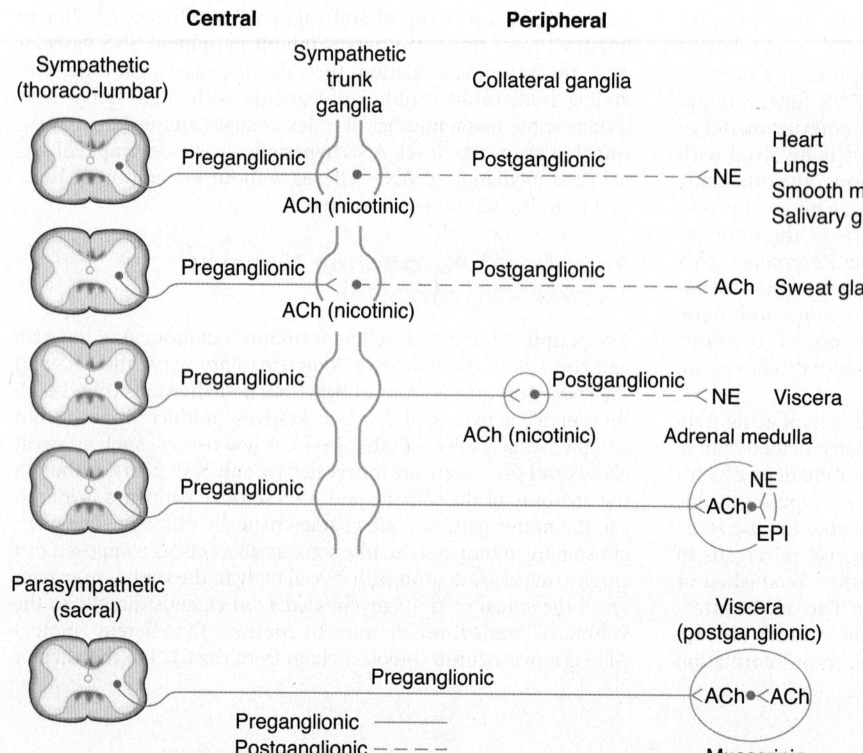

Figure 14-2 Schematic diagram of the efferent ANS. Efferent impulses are integrated centrally and sent reflexively to the adrenergic and cholinergic receptors. Sympathetic fibers ending in the adrenal medulla are preganglionic, and acetylcholine (ACh) is the neurotransmitter. Stimulation of the chromaffin cells, acting as postganglionic neurons, releases epinephrine (EPI) and norepinephrine (NE).

organ. The first neuron of both the SNS and PNS originates within the CNS but does not make direct contact with the effector organ. Instead, it relays the impulse to a second station known as an *ANS ganglion,* which contains the cell body of the second ANS (postganglionic) neuron. Its axon contacts the effector organ. Thus, the motor pathways of both divisions of the ANS are schematically a serial two-neuron chain consisting of a preganglionic neuron and a postganglionic effector neuron (Fig. 14-2).

Preganglionic fibers of both subdivisions are myelinated with diameters of less than 3 mm.[1] Impulses are conducted at a speed of 3 to 15 m/s. The postganglionic fibers are unmyelinated and conduct impulses at slower speeds of less than 2 m/s. They are similar to unmyelinated visceral and somatic afferent C fibers (Table 14-2). Compared with the myelinated somatic nerves, the ANS conducts impulses at speeds that preclude its participation in the immediate phase of a somatic response.

Sympathetic Nervous System

The efferent SNS is referred to as the thoracolumbar nervous system. Figure 14-1 demonstrates the distribution of the SNS and its innervation of visceral organs. The preganglionic fibers of the SNS (thoracolumbar division) originate in the intermediolateral gray column of the 12 thoracic (T1–T12) and the first three lumbar segments (L1–L3) of the spinal cord. The myelinated axons of these nerve cells leave the spinal cord with the motor fibers to form the white (myelinated) communicating rami (Fig. 14-3). The rami enter one of the paired 22 sympathetic ganglia at their respective segmental levels. Upon entering the paravertebral ganglia of the lateral sympathetic chain, the preganglionic fiber may follow one of three courses: (1) synapse with postganglionic fibers in ganglia at the level of exit; (2) course upward or downward in the trunk of the SNS chain to synapse in ganglia at other levels; or (3) track for variable distances through the sympathetic chain and exit without synapsing to terminate in an outlying, unpaired, SNS collateral ganglion. The adrenal gland is an exception to the rule. Preganglionic fibers pass directly into the adrenal medulla without synapsing in a ganglion (Fig. 14-2). The cells of the medulla are derived from neuronal tissue and are analogous to postganglionic neurons.

The sympathetic postganglionic neuronal cell bodies are located in ganglia of the paired lateral SNS chain or unpaired collateral ganglia in more peripheral plexuses. Collateral ganglia,

Table 14-2 Classification of Nerve Fibers

Description of Nerve Fibers	Group	Diameter (μm)	Conduction Velocity (m/s)
Myelinated somatic	A alpha (α)	20	120
	A beta (β)		
	A gamma (γ)		5–40 (pain fibers)
	A delta (δ)	3–4	5–40 (pain fibers)
	A epsilon (ε)	2	5
Myelinated visceral (preganglionic autonomic)	B	<3	3–15
Unmyelinated somatic	C	<2	0.5–2.0 (pain fibers)

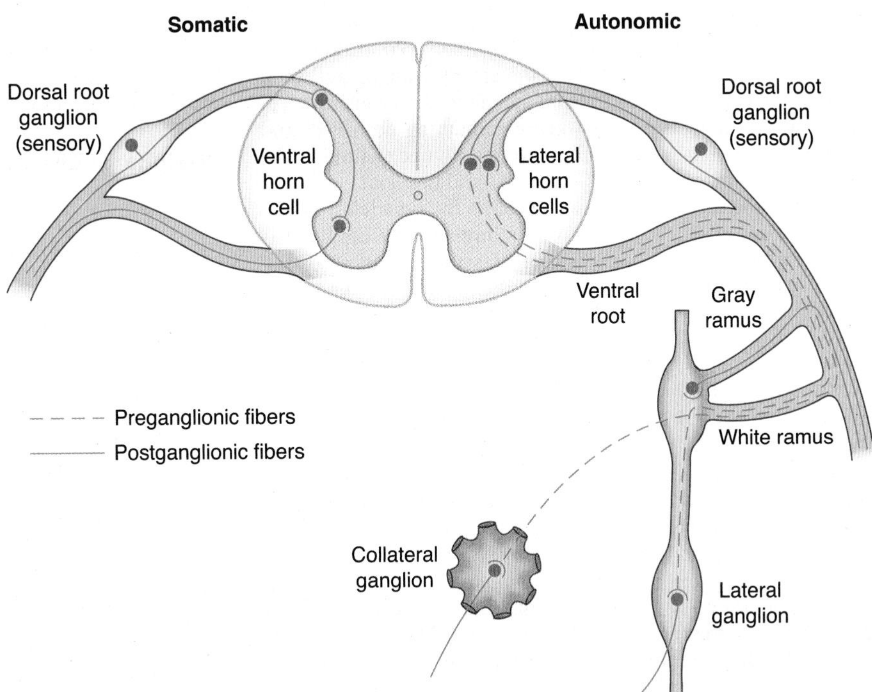

Figure 14-3 The spinal reflex arc of the somatic nerves is shown on the left. The different arrangements of neurons in the sympathetic system are shown on the right. Preganglionic fibers coming out through white rami may make synaptic connections following one of three courses: (1) synapse in ganglia at the level of exit, (2) course up or down the sympathetic chain to synapse at another level, or (3) exit the chain without synapsing to an outlying collateral ganglion.

such as the celiac and inferior mesenteric ganglia (plexus), are formed by the convergence of preganglionic fibers with many postganglionic neuronal bodies. SNS ganglia are almost always located closer to the spinal cord than to the organs they innervate. The sympathetic postganglionic neurons can therefore originate in either the paired lateral paravertebral SNS ganglia or one of the unpaired collateral plexuses. The unmyelinated postganglionic fibers then proceed from the ganglia to terminate within the organs they innervate. Many of the postganglionic fibers pass from the lateral SNS chain back into the spinal nerves, forming the gray (unmyelinated) communicating rami at all levels of the spinal cord (Fig. 14-2). They are distributed distally to sweat glands, pilomotor muscle, and blood vessels of the skin and muscle. These nerves are unmyelinated C-type fibers (Table 14-2) and are carried within the somatic nerves. Approximately 8% of the fibers in the average somatic nerve are sympathetic.

The first four or five thoracic spinal segments generate preganglionic fibers that ascend in the neck to form three special paired ganglia. These are the superior cervical, middle cervical, and cervicothoracic ganglia. The last is known as the stellate ganglion and is actually formed by the fusion of the inferior cervical and first thoracic SNS ganglia. These ganglia provide sympathetic innervation of the head, neck, upper extremities, heart, and lungs. Afferent pain fibers also travel with these nerves, accounting for chest, neck, or upper extremity pain with myocardial ischemia.

Activation of the SNS produces a diffuse physiologic response (mass reflex) rather than discrete effects. Historically, SNS postganglionic neurons have been thought to outnumber the preganglionic neurons in an average ratio of 20:1 to 30:1, however, more recent evidence suggests this ratio is closer to 1:4.[4–6] One preganglionic fiber influences a larger number of postganglionic neurons, which are dispersed to many organs.

Parasympathetic Nervous System

The PNS, like the SNS, has both pre- and postganglionic neurons. The preganglionic cell bodies originate in the brainstem and sacral segments of the spinal cord. PNS preganglionic fibers are found in cranial nerves III (oculomotor), VII (facial), IX (glossopharyngeal), and X (vagus). The sacral outflow originates in the intermediolateral gray horns of the second, third, and fourth sacral nerves. Figure 14-1 shows the distribution of the PNS division and its innervation of visceral organs.

The vagus (cranial nerve X) nerve has the most extensive distribution of all the PNS, accounting for more than 75% of PNS activity. The paired vagus nerves supply PNS innervation to the heart, lungs, esophagus, stomach, small intestine, proximal half of the colon, liver, gallbladder, pancreas, and upper portions of the ureters. The sacral fibers form the pelvic visceral nerves, or nervi erigentes. These nerves supply the remainder of the viscera that are not innervated by the vagus. They supply the descending colon, rectum, uterus, bladder, and lower portions of the ureters and are primarily concerned with emptying. Various sexual reactions are also governed by the sacral PNS. The PNS is responsible for penile erection, but SNS stimulation governs ejaculation.

In contrast to the SNS division, PNS preganglionic fibers pass directly to the organ that is innervated. The postganglionic cell bodies are situated near or within the innervated viscera and generally are not visible. The proximity of PNS ganglia to or within the viscera provides a limited distribution of postganglionic fibers. The ratio of postganglionic to preganglionic fibers in many organs appears to be 1:1 to 3:1 compared with the 20:1 found in the SNS system. The Auerbach plexus in the distal colon is the exception, with a ratio of 8,000:1. The fact that PNS preganglionic fibers synapse with only a few postganglionic neurons is consistent with the discrete and limited effect of PNS function. For example, vagal bradycardia can occur without a concomitant change in intestinal motility or salivation. Mass reflex action is not a characteristic of the PNS. The effects of organ response to PNS stimulation are outlined in Table 14-1.

Autonomic Innervation

Heart

The heart is well supplied by the SNS and PNS. These nerves affect cardiac pump function in three ways: (1) by changing the 2 rate (chronotropism), (2) by changing the strength of contraction (inotropism), and (3) by modulating coronary blood flow. The PNS cardiac vagal fibers approach the stellate ganglia and then join the efferent cardiac SNS fibers; therefore, the vagus nerve to the heart and lungs is a mixed nerve containing both PNS and SNS efferent fibers. The PNS fibers are distributed mainly to the sinoatrial and atrioventricular (AV) nodes and to a lesser extent to the atria. There is little or no distribution to the ventricles. Therefore, the main effect of vagal cardiac stimulation to the heart is chronotropic. Vagal stimulation decreases the rate of sinoatrial node discharge and decreases excitability of the AV junctional fibers, slowing impulse conduction to the ventricles. A strong vagal discharge can completely arrest sinoatrial node firing and block impulse conduction to the ventricles.[7–9]

The physiologic importance of the PNS on myocardial contractility is not as well understood as that of the SNS. Cholinergic blockade can double the heart rate (HR) without altering contractility of the left ventricle. Vagal stimulation of the heart can reduce left ventricular maximum rate of tension development (dP/dT) and decrease contractile force by as much as 10% to 20%. However, PNS stimulation is relatively unimportant in this regard compared with its predominant effect on HR. The SNS has the same supraventricular distribution as the PNS, but with stronger representation to the ventricles. SNS efferents to the myocardium funnel through the paired stellate ganglia. The right stellate ganglion distributes primarily to the anterior epicardial surface and the interventricular septum. Right stellate stimulation decreases systolic duration and increases HR. The left stellate ganglion supplies the posterior and lateral surfaces of both ventricles. Left stellate stimulation increases mean arterial pressure and left ventricular contractility without causing a substantial change in HR. Normal SNS tone maintains contractility approximately 20% above that in the absence of any SNS stimulation.[1,8] Therefore, the dominant effect of the ANS on myocardial contractility is mediated primarily through the SNS. Intrinsic mechanisms of the myocardium, however, can maintain circulation quite well without the ANS, as evidenced by the success of cardiac transplants (see Chapter 52). The heart and ANS are in perfect symbiosis. The ANS via its components imprints the cardiac electrophysiology by potentially inducing significant dysrhythmias or electrocardiographic abnormalities, which in the end may lead to global cardiac dysfunction. The precise role of the ANS is unknown, specifically whether it is an active component or just an accompaniment. Future research interests concern the modification of autonomic cardiac innervation through pharmacology or alternative approaches.[5] Early investigations, performed in anesthetized, open-chest animals, demonstrated that cardiac ANS nerves exert only slight effects on the coronary vascular bed; however, more recent studies on chronically instrumented, intact, conscious animals show considerable evidence for a strong SNS regulation of the small coronary resistance and larger conductance vessels (see below, Adrenergic Receptors).[6,7,9,10]

Different segments of the coronary arterial tree react differently to various stimuli and drugs. Normally, the large conductance vessels contribute little to overall coronary vascular resistance (see Chapter 12). Fluctuations in resistance reflect changes in the lumen size of the small, precapillary vessels. Blood flow through the resistance vessels is regulated primarily by the local metabolic requirements of the myocardium. The larger conductance vessels, however, can constrict markedly due to neurogenic stimulation. Neurogenic influence also assumes a greater role in the resistance vessels when they become hypoxic and lose autoregulation. Recent studies emphasize the possibility that a sympathetic stimulus that increases contractility, HR, and oxygen consumption is similarly responsible for increasing oxygen delivery. In clinical circumstances where only a mild coronary stenosis exists, a sympathetic stimulus will induce compensatory vasodilation. In contrast, when a critical stenosis is present, there is profound vasoconstriction induced by to α_2 adrenoceptor activation.[11]

Peripheral Circulation

The SNS nerves are by far the most important regulators of 3
peripheral circulation. The PNS nerves play only a minor role in this regard. The PNS dilates vessels, but only in limited areas such as the genitalia. SNS stimulation produces both vasodilation and vasoconstriction, with vasoconstrictor effects predominating. The SNS effect on the vascular bed is determined by the type of receptors on which the SNS fiber terminates (see below, Adrenergic Receptors). SNS constrictor receptors are distributed to all segments of the circulation. Blood vessels in the skin, kidneys, spleen, and mesentery have an extensive SNS distribution, whereas those in the heart, brain, and muscle have less SNS innervation.

Basal vasomotor tone is maintained by impulses from the lateral portion of the vasomotor center in the medulla oblongata that continually transmits impulses through the SNS, maintaining partial arteriolar and venular constriction. Circulating epinephrine (EPI) from the adrenal medulla has additive effects. This basal ANS tone maintains arteriolar constriction at an intermediate diameter. The arteriole, therefore, has the potential for either further constriction or dilation. If the basal tones were not present, the SNS could only affect vasoconstriction and not vasodilation.[8] The SNS tone in the venules produces little resistance to flow compared with the arterioles and the arteries. The importance of SNS stimulation of veins is to reduce or increase their capacity. By functioning as a reservoir for approximately 80% of the total blood volume, small changes in venous capacitance produce large changes in venous return and thus, cardiac preload.

Lungs

The lungs are innervated by both the SNS and PNS. Postganglionic SNS fibers from the upper thoracic ganglia (stellate) pass to the lungs to innervate the smooth muscles of the bronchi and pulmonary blood vessels. PNS innervation of these structures is via the vagus nerve. SNS stimulation produces bronchodilation and pulmonary vasoconstriction.[12] Little else has been proven about the vasomotor control of the pulmonary vessels other than that they adjust to accommodate the output of the right ventricle. The effect of stimulation of the pulmonary SNS nerves on pulmonary vascular resistance is not ideal but may be important in maintaining hemodynamic stability during stress and exercise by balancing right and left ventricular output. Stimulation of the vagus nerve produces almost no vasodilation of the pulmonary circulation. Hypoxic pulmonary vasoconstriction is a local phenomenon capable of providing a faster adjustment to the requirements of the organism.

Both the SNS and the vagus nerve provide active bronchomotor control. SNS stimulation causes bronchodilation, whereas vagal stimulation produces constriction. PNS stimulation may also increase secretions of the bronchial glands. Vagal receptor endings in the alveolar ducts also play an important role in the reflex regulation of the ventilation cycle. The lung has important nonventilatory activity as well. It serves as a metabolic organ that removes local mediators such as norepinephrine (NE) from the circulation and converts others, such as angiotensin 1, to active compounds (see below, Interaction with Other Regulatory Systems).[10]

Autonomic Nervous System Transmission

Transmission of excitation across the terminal junctional sites (synaptic clefts) of the peripheral ANS occurs through the

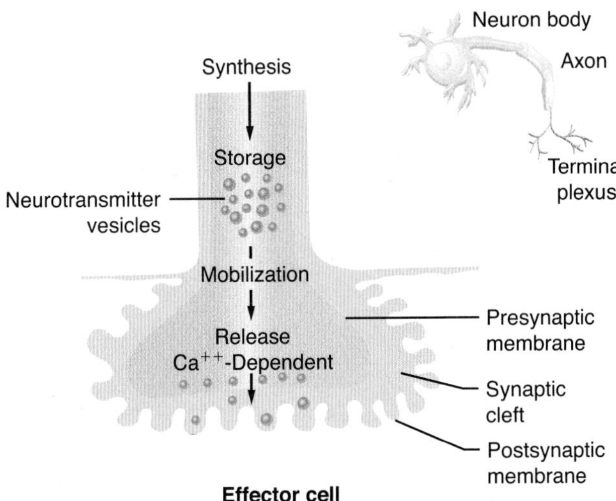

Figure 14-4 The anatomy and physiology of the terminal postganglionic sympathetic and parasympathetic fibers are similar.

mediation of released chemicals (Fig. 14-4). Transmitters interact with receptors on the end organ to evoke a biologic response.

The ANS can be pharmacologically subdivided by the neurotransmitter secreted at the effector cell. Pharmacologic parlance designates the SNS and PNS as adrenergic and cholinergic, respectively. The terminals of the PNS postganglionic fibers release acetylcholine (ACh). Except sweat glands, NE is the principal neurotransmitter released at the terminals of the sympathetic postganglionic fibers (see Fig. 14-2). Cotransmission of adenosine triphosphate (ATP), neuropeptide Y (NPY), and NE has been demonstrated at vascular sympathetic nerve terminals in a number of different tissues including muscle, intestine, kidney, and skin. The preganglionic neurons of both systems secrete ACh.

The terminations of the postganglionic fibers of both ANS subdivisions are anatomically and physiologically similar. The terminations are characterized by multiple branchings called *terminal effector plexuses* or *reticulae*. These filaments surround the elements of the effector unit "like a mesh stocking."[13] Thus, for example, one SNS postganglionic neuron can innervate approximately 25,000 effector vascular smooth muscle cells. The terminal filaments end in presynaptic enlargements called varicosities. Each varicosity contains vesicles, approximately 500 Å in diameter, in which the neurotransmitters are stored (Fig. 14-4). The rate of synthesis depends on the level of ANS activity and is regulated by local feedback. The distance between the varicosity and the effector cell (synaptic or junctional cleft) varies from 100 Å in ganglia and arterioles to as much as 20,000 Å in large arteries. The time for diffusion is directly proportional to the width of the synaptic gap. Depolarization on the nerve releases the vesicular contents into the synaptic cleft by exocytosis.

Parasympathetic Nervous System Transmission

Synthesis

ACh is considered the primary neurotransmitter of the PNS. ACh is formed in the presynaptic terminal by acetylation of choline with acetyl coenzyme A. This step is catalyzed by choline acetyltransferase (Fig. 14-5). ACh is then stored in a concentrated form in presynaptic vesicles. A continual release of small amounts of ACh, called quanta, occurs during the resting state. Each quantum results in small changes in the electrical potential of the synaptic end plate without producing depolarization. These are known as miniature end-plate potentials. Arrival of an action potential causes a synchronous release of hundreds of quanta, resulting in depolarization of the end plate. Release of ACh from the vesicles is dependent on the influx of calcium (Ca^{2+}) from the interstitial space. ACh is not reused like NE; therefore, it must be synthesized constantly.

Metabolism

The ability of a receptor to modulate function of an effector organ is dependent on rapid recovery to its baseline state after stimulation. For this to occur, the neurotransmitter must be quickly removed from the vicinity of the receptor. ACh removal occurs by rapid hydrolysis by acetylcholinesterase (Fig. 14-5). This enzyme is found in neurons, at the neuromuscular junction, and in various other tissues of the body. A similar enzyme, pseudocholinesterase or plasma cholinesterase, is also found throughout the body but only to a limited extent in neural tissue. It does not appear to be physiologically important in the termination of the action of ACh. Both acetylcholinesterase and pseudocholinesterase hydrolyze ACh as well as other esters (such as the ester-type local anesthetics), and they may be distinguished by specific biochemical tests.[14]

Sympathetic Nervous System Transmission

Traditionally, the catecholamines EPI and NE were considered the main mediators of peripheral SNS activity (see NICV 13-1). NE is released from localized presynaptic vesicles of nearly all postganglionic sympathetic nerves. Vascular SNS nerve terminals, however, also release ATP. Thus, ATP and NE are co-neurotransmitters.

ACETYL-CoA + CHOLINE —Choline acetyl Transferase→ ACETYLCHOLINE

$$CH_3-\overset{\displaystyle O}{\overset{\|}{C}}-O-CH_2-CH_2-\overset{+}{N}(CH_3)_3$$

ACETYLCHOLINE —Cholinesterase→ CHOLINE + ACETIC ACID

$$OH-CH_2-CH_2-\overset{+}{N}(CH_3)_3 \qquad CH_3COOH$$

Figure 14-5 Synthesis and metabolism of acetylcholine.

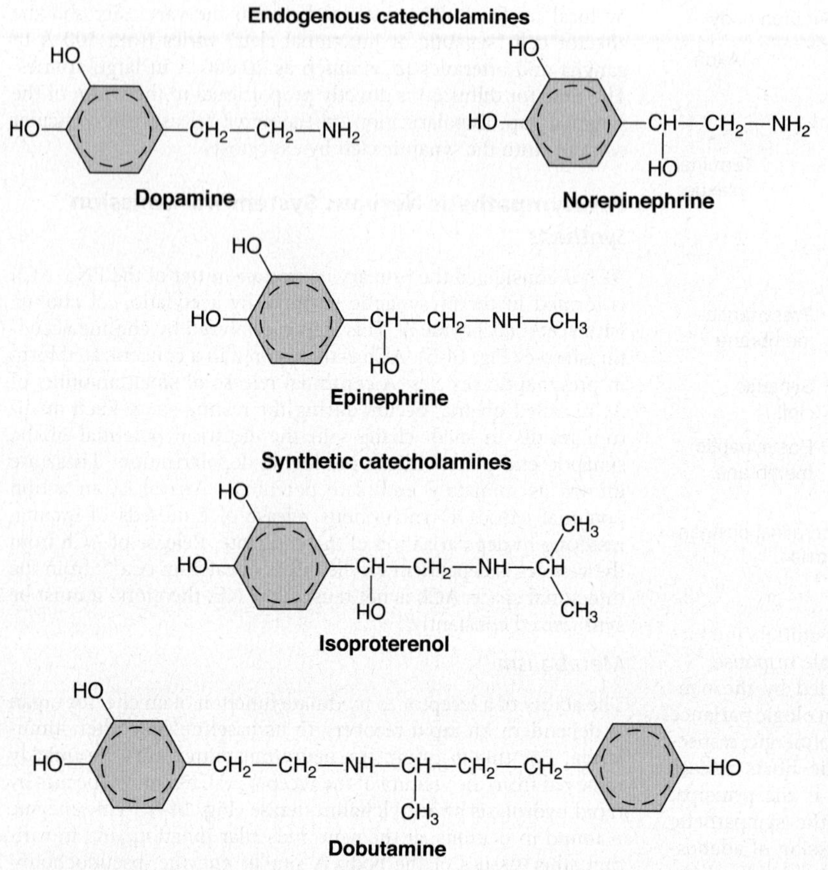

Endogenous catecholamines

Dopamine

Norepinephrine

Epinephrine

Synthetic catecholamines

Isoproterenol

Dobutamine

Figure 14-6 The chemical configurations of three endogenous catecholamines are compared with those of three synthetic catecholamines. Sympathomimetic drugs differ in their hemodynamic effects largely because of differences in substitution of the amine group on the catechol nucleus.

They are released directly to their site of action. Their postjunctional effects appear to be synergistic in tissues.

The SNS fibers ending in the adrenal medulla are preganglionic, and ACh is the neurotransmitter (Fig. 14-2). It interacts with the chromaffin cells in the adrenal medulla, causing the release of EPI and NE. The chromaffin cells take the place of the postganglionic neurons. Stimulation of the sympathetic nerves innervating the adrenal medulla, however, causes the release of large quantities of a mixture of EPI and NE into the circulation. Normally, the greater portion of this hormonal surge is EPI. EPI and NE, when released into the circulation, are classified as hormones in that they are synthesized, stored, and released from the adrenal medulla to act at distant sites.

Hormonal EPI and NE have essentially the same effects on effector cells as those caused by local direct sympathetic stimulation. The hormonal effects, although brief, last about 10 times as long as those caused by direct stimulation. EPI has a greater metabolic effect than NE. It can increase the metabolic rate of the body as much as 100%. It also increases glycogenolysis in the liver and muscle, leading to glucose release into the blood. These functions are all necessary to prepare the body for fight or flight.

Catecholamines: The First Messenger

A catecholamine is any compound with a catechol nucleus (a benzene ring with two adjacent hydroxyl groups) and an amine-containing side chain (1 Video 14-1). The chemical configuration of five of the more common catecholamines in clinical use is demonstrated in Figure 14-6. In humans, the endogenous catecholamines are dopamine (DA), NE, and EPI. Dopamine is a neurotransmitter present in the CNS, primarily involved in coordinating motor activity in the brain. It is the precursor of NE. NE is synthesized and stored in nerve endings of postganglionic SNS neurons. It is also synthesized in the adrenal medulla and is the chemical precursor of EPI. Stored EPI is located chiefly in chromaffin cells of the adrenal medulla. About 80% to 85% of the catecholamine content of the adrenal medulla is EPI and 15% to 20% is NE. The brain contains both noradrenergic and dopaminergic receptors. Circulating catecholamines do not cross the blood–brain barrier; the catecholamines present in the brain are synthesized locally.

Catecholamines are often referred to as adrenergic drugs because their effector actions are mediated through receptors specific to the SNS. Sympathomimetics can activate these same receptors because of their structural similarity. For example, clonidine is an α_2-receptor agonist that does not possess a catechol nucleus and has two ring systems that are aplanar. However, clonidine enjoys a remarkable spatial similarity to NE that allows it to activate the α receptor.[15] Drugs that produce sympathetic-like effects but lack basic catecholamine structure are called sympathomimetics. All clinically useful catecholamines are sympathomimetics, but not all sympathomimetics are catecholamines. The effects of endogenous or synthetic catecholamines on adrenergic receptors can be direct or indirect. Indirect-acting catecholamines (i.e., ephedrine) have little intrinsic effect on adrenergic receptors but produce their effects by stimulating release of the stored neurotransmitter from SNS nerve terminals. Some synthetic and endogenous catecholamines stimulate adrenergic receptor sites directly (e.g., phenylephrine), whereas others have a mixed mode of action. The actions of direct-acting catecholamines are independent of endogenous NE stores; however, the indirect-acting catecholamines are entirely dependent on adequate neuronal stores of endogenous NE.

Phenylalanine
Tyrosine
Tyrosine hydroxylase
DOPA
DOPA decarboxylase
Dopamine
Dopamine β-hydroxylase
Norepinephrine
Phenylethanolamine N-methyltransferase
Epinephrine
Feedback inhibition

Figure 14-7 Schematic of the synthesis of catecholamines. The conversion of tyrosine to DOPA by tyrosine hydroxylase is inhibited by increased NE synthesis. Epinephrine is shown in these steps but is primarily synthesized in the adrenal medulla. DOPA, dihydroxyphenylalanine.

Synthesis

The main site of NE synthesis is in or near the postganglionic nerve endings. Some synthesis does occur in vesicles near the cell body that pass to the nerve endings. Phenylalanine or tyrosine is taken up into the axoplasm of the nerve terminal and modified into either NE or EPI. Figure 14-7 demonstrates this synthesis cascade. Tyrosine hydroxylase catalyzes the conversion of tyrosine to dihydroxyphenylalanine. This is the rate-limiting step at which NE synthesis is controlled through feedback inhibition. Dopamine (DA) synthesis occurs in the cytoplasm of the neuron. The vesicles of peripheral postganglionic neurons contain the enzyme dopamine-β-hydroxylase, which converts dopamine to NE. The adrenal medulla additionally contains phenylethanolamine-N-methyltransferase, which converts NE to EPI. This reaction takes place outside the medullary vesicles, and the newly formed EPI then enters the vesicle for storage (Fig. 14-8). All the endogenous catecholamines are stored in presynaptic vesicles and are released on arrival of an action potential. Excitation–secretion coupling in sympathetic neurons is Ca^{2+} dependent.

Regulation

Increased SNS activity, as in congestive heart failure or chronic stress, stimulates the synthesis of catecholamines. Glucocorticoids from the adrenal cortex stimulate an increase in phenylethanolamine-N-methyltransferase that methylates NE to EPI.

The release of NE is dependent on depolarization of the nerve and an increase in calcium ion permeability. This release is inhibited by colchicine and prostaglandin E_2, suggesting a contractile mechanism. NE inhibits its own release by stimulating presynaptic (prejunctional) α_2 receptors. Phenoxybenzamine and phentolamine, α-receptor antagonists, increase the release of NE by blocking inhibitory presynaptic α_2 receptors (Fig. 14-9). Other receptors are also important in NE regulation (see section that follows, *Other Receptors*).

Inactivation

The catecholamines are removed from the synaptic cleft by three mechanisms (Fig. 14-8). These are reuptake into the presynaptic terminals, extraneuronal uptake, and diffusion. Termination of NE action at the effector site is almost entirely by reuptake of NE into the terminals of the presynaptic neuron. This is an active, energy-requiring, and temperature-dependent process. The reuptake of NE in the presynaptic terminals is also a stereospecific process. Structurally similar compounds (guanethidine, metaraminol) may enter the vesicles and displace the neurotransmitter. Tricyclic antidepressants and cocaine inhibit the reuptake of NE, resulting in high synaptic NE concentrations and accentuated receptor response. In addition, evidence suggests that NE reuptake is mediated by a presynaptic β-adrenergic mechanism because β-blockade causes marked elevations of EPI and NE (Figs. 14-8 and 14-9).[16] Extraneuronal uptake is a minor pathway for inactivating NE. Effector cells and other extraneuronal tissues take up NE. The NE that is taken up by the extraneuronal tissue is metabolized by monoamine oxidase (MAO) and by catechol-O-methyltransferase (COMT) to form vanillylmandelic acid. The minute amount of catecholamine that escapes these two mechanisms diffuses into the circulation, where it is metabolized by the liver and kidney. The same enzymes inactivate EPI. Reuptake is the predominant pathway for inactivation of the endogenous catecholamines, while metabolism by the liver and kidney is the

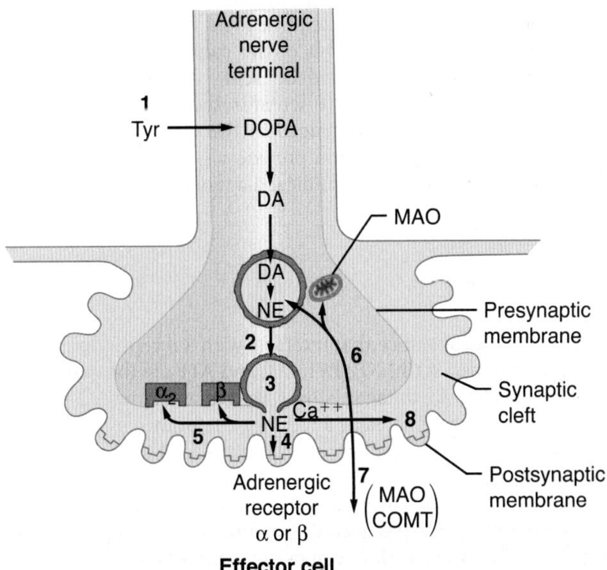

Figure 14-8 Schematic of the synthesis and disposition of NE in adrenergic neurotransmission. (1) Synthesis and storage in neuronal vesicles; (2) Action potential permits calcium entry with (3) exocytosis of NE into synaptic gap. (4) Released NE reacts with receptors on effector cell. NE (5) may react with presynaptic α_2 receptor to inhibit further NE release or with presynaptic β-receptor to enhance reuptake of NE (6) (uptake 1). Extraneuronal uptake (uptake 2) absorbs NE into effector cell (7) with overflow occurring systemically (8). MAO, monoamine oxidase; COMT, catechol-O-methyltransferase; Tyr, tyrosine; DOPA, dihydroxyphenylalanine; NE, norepinephrine.

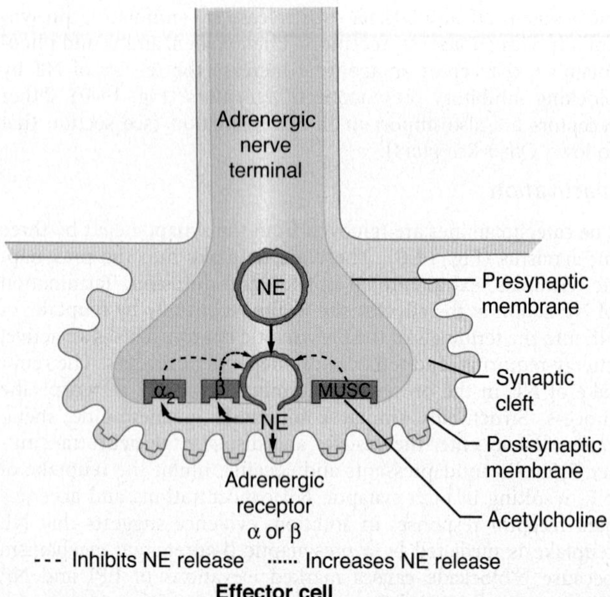

Figure 14-9 This schematic demonstrates just a few of the presynaptic adrenergic receptors thought to exist. Agonist and antagonist drugs are clinically available for these receptors (Table 14-5). The α_2 receptors serve as a negative feedback mechanism whereby NE stimulation inhibits its own release. Presynaptic β-stimulation increases NE uptake, augmenting its availability. Presynaptic muscarinic (MUSC) receptors respond to ACh diffusing from nearby cholinergic terminals. They inhibit NE release and can be blocked by atropine. NE, norepinephrine.

predominant pathway for catecholamines given exogenously. This accounts for the longer duration of action of the exogenous catecholamines than that noted at the local synapse.

The final metabolic product of the catecholamines is vanillylmandelic acid. Vanillylmandelic acid constitutes the major metabolite (80% to 90%) of NE found in the urine. Less than 5% of released NE appears unchanged in the urine. The metabolic products excreted in the urine provide a gross estimate of SNS activity and can facilitate the clinical diagnosis of pheochromocytoma (see Chapter 47).

Receptors

5 An agonist is a substance that interacts with a receptor to evoke a biologic response. ACh, NE, EPI, DA, and ATP are the major agonists of the ANS. An antagonist is a substance that interferes with the evocation of a response at a receptor site by an agonist. Receptors are therefore target sites that lead to a response by the effector cell when activated by an agonist. Receptors are protein macromolecules; they are located in the plasma membrane. Several thousand receptors have been demonstrated in a single cell. The enormity of this network becomes apparent when one considers that ~25,000 single cells can be innervated by a single neuron.

Cholinergic Receptors

ACh is the neurotransmitter for three distinct classes of receptors. These receptors can be differentiated by their anatomic location and their affinity for various agonists and antagonists. ACh mediates the "first messenger" function of transmitting impulses within the PNS, the ganglia of the SNS, and the neuroeffector junction of striated, voluntary muscle (Fig. 14-2). Cholinergic receptors are further subdivided into muscarinic and nicotinic receptors because muscarine and nicotine stimulate them selectively. However, both muscarinic and nicotinic receptors respond to ACh (see section that follows, *Cholinergic Drugs*). Muscarine activates cholinergic receptors at the postganglionic PNS junctions of cardiac and smooth muscle. Muscarinic stimulation is characterized by bradycardia, decreased inotropism, bronchoconstriction, miosis, salivation, gastrointestinal hypermotility, and increased gastric acid secretion (Table 14-1). Muscarinic receptors can be blocked by atropine without effect on nicotinic receptors (see *Cholinergic Drugs*). Muscarinic receptors are known to exist in sites other than PNS postganglionic junctions. They are found on the presynaptic membrane of sympathetic nerve terminals in the myocardium, coronary vessels, and peripheral vasculature (Fig. 14-9). These are referred to as adrenergic muscarinic receptors because of their location; however, ACh stimulates them also. Stimulation of these receptors inhibits release of NE in a manner similar to α_2-receptor stimulation. Muscarinic blockade removes the inhibition of NE release, augmenting SNS activity. Atropine, the prototypical muscarinic blocker, may produce sympathomimetic activity in this manner as well as vagal blockade. Neuromuscular blocking drugs that cause tachycardia are thought to have a similar mechanism of action. ACh acting on presynaptic adrenergic muscarinic receptors is a potent inhibitor of NE release.[17] The prejunctional muscarinic receptor may play an important physiologic role because several autonomically innervated tissues (e.g., the heart) possess ANS plexi in which the SNS and PNS nerve terminals are closely associated. In these plexuses, ACh, released from the nearby PNS nerve terminals (vagus nerve), can inhibit NE release by activation of presynaptic adrenergic muscarinic receptors.

Nicotinic receptors are found at the synaptic junctions of both SNS and PNS ganglia. Because both junctions are cholinergic, ACh or ACh-like substances such as nicotine will excite postganglionic fibers of both systems (Fig. 14-2). Low doses of nicotine produce stimulation of ANS ganglia whereas high doses produce blockade. This dualism is referred to as the nicotinic effect (see section that follows, *Ganglionic Drugs*). Nicotinic stimulation of the SNS ganglia produces hypertension and tachycardia by causing the release of EPI and NE from the adrenal medulla. Adrenal hormone release is mediated by ACh in the chromaffin cells, which are analogous to postganglionic neurons. A further increase in nicotine concentration produces hypotension and neuromuscular weakness, as it becomes a ganglionic blocker. The cholinergic neuroeffector junction of skeletal muscle also contains nicotinic receptors, although they are not identical to the nicotinic receptors in ANS ganglia.

Adrenergic Receptors

The adrenergic receptors are termed adrenergic or noradrenergic, depending on their responsiveness to EPI or NE. The dissimilarities of these two drugs led Ahlquist in 1948 to propose two types of opposing adrenergic receptors, termed alpha (α) and beta (β). The development of new agonists and antagonists with relatively selective activity allowed subdivision of the β-receptors into β_1 and β_2, and more recently, β_3, responsible for increased lipolysis; α-receptors were subsequently divided into α_1, and α_2, that are further subdivided into α_{1A}, α_{1B}, and α_{1D}, and respectively α_{2A}, α_{2B}, and α_{2C}. These were later further subdivided using molecular cloning. The sympathomimetic adrenergic drugs in current use differ from one another in their effects, largely because of differences in substitution on the amine group, which influences the relative α or β effect (Fig. 14-6).[18] 6

Another major peripheral adrenergic receptor specific for dopamine is termed the dopaminergic or dopamine (DA) receptor. Further studies have revealed not only subsets of the α and

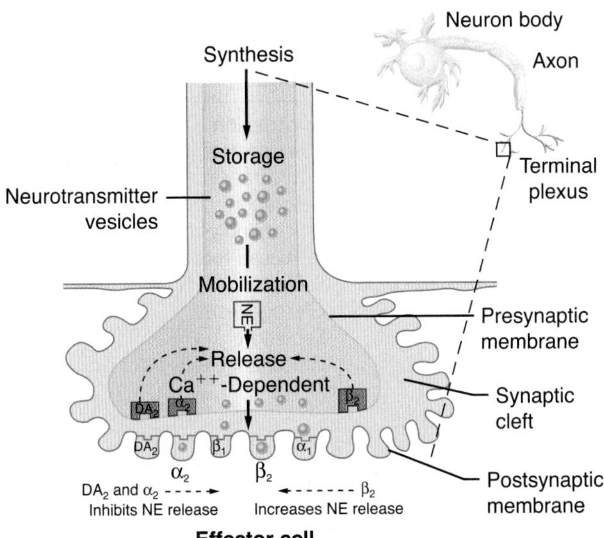

Figure 14-10 Location of several known adrenergic receptors. The presynaptic α_2 and DA receptors serve as a negative feedback mechanism, whereby stimulation of NE inhibits its own release. Presynaptic β_2 stimulation increases NE uptake, augmenting its availability. Postsynaptic α_2 and β_2 receptors are extrasynaptic and are considered noninnervated hormonal receptors. DA, dopamine; NE, norepinephrine.

β receptors but also the DA receptor: DA_1 and DA_2. These DA receptors have been identified in the CNS and in renal, mesenteric, and coronary vessels. The physiologic importance of these receptors is a matter of controversy because there are no identifiable peripheral DA neurons. Dopamine measured in the circulation is assumed to result from spillover from the brain.

The function of dopamine in the CNS has long been known, but the peripheral dopamine receptor has been elucidated only within the past 25 years. The presence of the peripheral DA receptor was obscured because dopamine does not affect the DA receptor exclusively. It also stimulates α and β receptors in a dose-related manner. However, DA receptors function independently of α or β blockade and are modified by DA antagonists such as haloperidol, droperidol, and phenothiazines.

The distribution of adrenergic receptors in organs and tissues is not uniform and their function differs not only by their location but also in their numbers and/or distribution. Adrenergic receptors are found in two loci in the sympathetic neuroeffector junction. They are found in both pre- (prejunctional) and postsynaptic (postjunctional) sites as well as extrasynaptic sites (Fig. 14-10). Table 14-3 is a review of the function and synaptic location of some of the clinically important receptors and their subtypes.

α-Adrenergic Receptors

The α-adrenergic (α) receptors have been further subdivided into two classes, α_1 and α_2. This classification is based on their response to the α-antagonists yohimbine and prazosin. Prazosin is a more potent antagonist of α_1 receptors, whereas α_2 receptors are more sensitive to yohimbine. Recently, pharmacologic experiments have demonstrated the existence of two subtypes within the α_1 group, namely α_{1A} and α_{1B}, and at least two subtypes within the α_2 group, α_{2A} and α_{2B}. The importance of these subsets is still emerging, with evidence that the spleen and liver contain mainly α_{1B} receptors, and the heart, neocortex, kidney, vas deferens, and hippocampus contain equal amounts of α_{1A} and α_{1B} receptors. The α_1-adrenergic receptors are found in the smooth muscle cells of the peripheral vasculature, coronary arteries, skin, uterus, intestinal mucosa, and splanchnic beds (Table 14-4).[18] The α_1 receptors serve as postsynaptic activators of vascular and intestinal smooth muscle as well as endocrine glands. Their activation results in either decreased or increased tone, depending on the effector organ. The response in resistance and capacitance vessels is constriction, whereas in the intestinal tract it is relaxation. There is now a large body of evidence documenting the presence of postjunctional α_1 adrenoceptors in the mammalian heart. α_1-Adrenergic receptors have been shown to have a positive inotropic effect on cardiac tissues in most mammals studied, including humans. Experimental work strongly supports the concept that enhanced myocardial α_1 responsiveness plays a primary role in the genesis of malignant arrhythmias induced by catecholamines during myocardial ischemia and reperfusion. Drugs possessing potent α_1-antagonist activity such as prazosin and phentolamine provide significant antiarrhythmic activity. The clinical mechanism and significance of these findings are not yet clear. However, there is no doubt that α_1-adrenergic antagonists prevent catecholamine-induced ventricular arrhythmias.[19] In contrast, studies of the effects of β-antagonists in experimental and clinical myocardial infarction have provided conflicting results.

The discovery of presynaptic α-adrenoceptors and their role in the modulation of NE transmission provided the stimulus for the subclassification of α receptors into α_1 and α_2 subtypes. Presynaptic α_1 receptors have not been identified; receptors appear confined only to the postsynaptic membrane. On the other hand, α_2 receptors are found on both pre- and postsynaptic membranes of the adrenergic neuroeffector junction. Table 14-4 reviews these sites. Postsynaptic membranes contain a near equal mix of α_1 and α_2 receptors.

The α_2 adrenoceptors may be subdivided even further into as many as four subtypes. The postsynaptic α_2 receptors have many actions, which include arterial and venous vasoconstriction, platelet aggregation, inhibition of insulin release, inhibition of bowel motility, stimulation of growth hormone release, and inhibition of ADH release.

α_2 Receptors can be found in cholinergic pathways as well as in adrenergic pathways. They can also significantly modulate parasympathetic activity. Current research implies that α_2 stimulation of the parasympathetic pathways plays a role in the modulation of the baroreceptor reflex (increased sensitivity), vagal mediation of HR (bradycardia), bronchoconstriction, and salivation (dry mouth). However, cholinergic receptors can also be found in adrenergic pathways; thus, muscarinic and nicotinic receptors have been found in pre- and postsynaptic locations, where in turn they modulate sympathetic activity (Fig. 14-9). There is speculation that the features that are desirable to the anesthesiologist, such as sedation, anxiolysis, analgesia, and hypnosis, are mediated through this site.

Stimulation of presynaptic α_2 receptors mediates inhibition of NE release into the synaptic cleft, serving as a negative feedback mechanism. The central effects are primarily related to a reduction in sympathetic outflow with a concomitantly enhanced parasympathetic outflow (e.g., enhanced baroreceptor activity). This results in decreased systemic vascular resistance, decreased cardiac output (CO), decreased inotropic state in the myocardium, and decreased HR. The peripheral presynaptic α_2 effects are similar, and NE release is inhibited in postganglionic neurons. However, stimulation of postsynaptic α_2 receptors, like the α_1 postsynaptic receptor, affects vasoconstriction. NE acts on both α_1 and α_2 receptors. Thus, NE not only activates smooth muscle vasoconstriction (postsynaptic α_1 and α_2 receptors) but also stimulates presynaptic α_2 receptors and inhibits its own release. Selective stimulation of the presynaptic α_2 receptor could produce a beneficial reduction in peripheral vascular resistance.

Table 14-3 Adrenergic Receptors: Order of Potency of Agonists and Antagonists

Receptor		Agonists[a]	Antagonists	Location	Action
α_1	++++	Norepinephrine	Phenoxybenzamine[b]	Smooth muscle (vascular, iris, radial, ureter, pilomotor, uterus, trigone, gastrointestinal, and bladder sphincters)	Contraction
	+++	Epinephrine	Phentolamine[b]		Vasoconstriction
	++	Dopamine	Ergot alkaloids[b]		Neurotransmission
	+	Isoproterenol	Prazosin		Relaxation
			Tolazoline[b]		Glycogenolysis
			Labetalol[b]	Brain	Increased force,[c] glycolysis
				Smooth muscle (gastrointestinal)	Secretion (K^+, H_2O)
					Glycogenesis
				Heart	Secretion
				Salivary glands	Gluconeogenesis Na^+ reabsorption
				Adipose tissue	
				Sweat glands (localized)	
				Kidney (proximal tubule)	
α_2	++++	Clonidine	Yohimbine	Adrenergic nerve endings	Inhibition norepinephrine release
	+++	Norepinephrine	Piperoxan	Presynaptic—CNS	
	++	Epinephrine	Phentolamine[b]		
	++	Norepinephrine	Phenoxybenzamine[b]	Platelets	Aggregation, granule release
	+	Phenylephrine	Tolazoline[b]		
			Labetalol[b]	Adipose tissue	Inhibition lipolysis
				Endocrine pancreas	Inhibition insulin release
				Vascular smooth muscle—?	Contraction
				Kidney	Inhibition renin disease
				Brain	Neurotransmission
β_1	++++	Isoproterenol[b]	Acebutolol	Heart	Increased rate, contractility, conduction velocity
	+++	Epinephrine	Practolol		
	++	Norepinephrine	Propranolol[b]		Coronary vasodilation
	+	Dopamine	Alprenolol[b]	Adipose tissue	Lipolysis
			Metoprolol		
			Esmolol		
β_2	++++	Isoproterenol[a]	Propranolol[b]	Liver	Glycogenolysis, gluconeogenesis
	+++	Epinephrine	Butoxamine		
	++	Norepinephrine	Alprenolol		
	+	Dopamine	Esmolol	Skeletal muscle	Glycogenolysis, lactate release
			Nadolol		
			Timolol	Smooth muscle (bronchi, uterus, vascular, gastrointestinal, detrusor, spleen capsule)	Relaxation
			Labetalol		
				Endocrine pancreas	Insulin secretion
				Salivary glands	Amylase secretion
DA_1	++++	Fenoldopam	Vascular smooth muscle	Vasodilation	
	++	Dopamine	Haloperidol	Renal and mesentery	
	+	Epinephrine	Droperidol		
	+	Metoclopramide	Phenothiazines		
DA_2	++	Dopamine			
	+	Bromocriptine	Domperidone	Presynaptic—adrenergic nerve endings	Inhibits norepinephrine release

CNS, central nervous system; DA, dopamine.
[a]Listed in decreasing order of potency.
[b]Nonselective.
[c]β_1-Adrenergic responses are greater.
Pluses indicate potency.

Table 14-4 Adrenergic Receptors

Receptor	Synaptic Site	Anatomic Site	Action	LV Function and Stroke Volume
α_1	Postsynaptic	Peripheral vascular smooth muscle	Constriction	Decreased
		Renal vascular smooth muscle	Constriction	
		Coronary arteries, epicardial	Constriction	
		Myocardium	Positive inotropism	Improved
		30–40% of resting tone		
		Renal tubules	Antidiuresis	
α_2	Presynaptic	Peripheral vascular smooth muscle release	Inhibit NE	
			Secondary vasodilation	Improved
		Coronaries		
		CNS	Inhibition of CNS activity	
			Sedation	
			Decrease MAC	
	Postsynaptic	Coronaries, endocardial	Constriction	Decreased
		CNS	Inhibition of insulin release	
			Decreased bowel motility	
			Inhibition of antidiuretic hormone	
			Analgesia	
		Renal tubule	Promotes Na^{2+} and H_2O excretion	
β_1	Postsynaptic NE sensitive	Myocardium	Positive inotropism and chronotropism	Improved
		Sinoatrial (SA) node		
		Ventricular conduction		
		Kidney	Renin release	
		Coronaries	Relaxation	
β_2	Presynaptic NE sensitive	Myocardium	Accelerates NE release	Improved
		SA node ventricular conduction vessels	Opposite action to presynaptic α_2 agonism	
			Constriction	
	Postsynaptic (extrasynaptic) (EPI sensitive)	Myocardium	Positive inotropism and chronotropism	Improved
		Vascular smooth muscle	Relaxation	Improved
		Bronchial smooth muscle	Relaxation	Improved
		Renal vessels	Relaxation	
DA_1	Postsynaptic	Blood vessels (renal, mesentery, coronary)	Vasodilation	Improved
		Renal tubules	Natriuresis	
			Diuresis	
		Juxtaglomerular cells	Renin release (modulates diuresis)	
		Sympathetic ganglia	Minor inhibition	
DA_2	Presynaptic	Postganglionic sympathetic nerves	Inhibit NE release	Improved
			Secondary vasodilation	
	Postsynaptic	Renal and mesenteric vasculature	? Vasoconstriction	

CNS, central nervous system; DA, dopamine; EPI, epinephrine; LV, left ventricular; MAC, minimum alveolar concentration; NE, norepinephrine.

Unfortunately, most known presynaptic α_2 agonists also stimulate the postsynaptic α_2 receptors, causing vasoconstriction. Blockade of α_2 presynaptic receptors, however, ablates normal inhibition of NE, causing vasoconstriction. Vasodilation occurs with the blockade of postsynaptic α_1 and α_2 receptors.

α-Adrenergic Receptors in the Cardiovascular System

Postsynaptic α_1 and α_2 receptors in the mammalian myocardium and coronary arteries mediate several responses.

Coronary Arteries

The presence of postsynaptic α_1 and α_2 receptors in mammalian models has been demonstrated. Sympathetic nerves cause coronary vasoconstriction, which is mediated predominately by postsynaptic α_2. The larger epicardial arteries possess mainly α_1 receptors, whereas α_2 receptors and some α_1 receptors are present in the small coronary artery resistance vessels.[20] Epicardial vessels contribute only 5% to the total resistance of the coronary circulation; therefore, α_1 agonists such as phenylephrine have little influence on coronary resistance.[21] Myocardial ischemia has been shown to increase α_2 receptor density in the coronary arteries. Ischemia has also been shown to cause a reflex increase in sympathetic activity mediated by α mechanisms. This cascade may further increase coronary constriction. Postsynaptic α_1 receptors do not rely on extracellular Ca^{2+} to constrict the vessel, whereas the α_2-constrictor response is highly dependent on extracellular influx and exquisitely sensitive to calcium channel inhibitors. Aging is associated with an upregulation of the adrenergic response, similar to that seen in heart failure, which results in an increased risk of arrhythmias and left ventricular dysfunction.[22]

Myocardium

The role of β receptors in mediating catecholamine-induced inotropism and arrhythmogenesis is well known (see below, β-Adrenergic Receptors). Studies have shown the presence of postsynaptic myocardial α_1 receptors, which also exert a major, faciliatory, positive inotropic effect on the myocardium of several species of mammals including humans. Their contribution to malignant reperfusion arrhythmogenesis has also been recognized.

Phenylephrine, an α_1 agonist, can increase myocardial contractility two- to threefold compared with a six- to sevenfold increase produced by isoproterenol, a pure β agonist. Myocardial postsynaptic α_1 receptors mediate perhaps as much as 30% to 50% of the basal inotropic tone of the normal heart.

Postsynaptic myocardial α_1 receptors play a more prominent inotropic role in the failing heart by serving as a reserve to the normally predominant β_1 receptors. Although the response to both α_1 and β_1 agonists is reduced in the failing myocardium, the interaction between the two receptors is more apparent. Chronic heart failure is known to produce a reduced density (downregulation) of myocardial β_1 receptors as a result of high levels of circulating catecholamines. However, there is no evidence of downregulation of either α_1 or β_2 receptors in cardiac failure. The increase in density of myocardial α_1 adrenoreceptors is more pronounced with failure and myocardial ischemia.[18] Thus, enhanced myocardial α_1-receptor numbers and sensitivity may contribute to the positive inotropism seen during ischemia as well as to the malignant arrhythmias that occur with reperfusion. Intracellular mobilization of cytosolic Ca^{2+} by the activated α_1-myocardial receptors during ischemia appears to contribute to these arrhythmias. The α_1 receptor also increases the sensitivity of the contractile elements to Ca^{2+}. Drugs possessing potent α_1 antagonism such as prazosin and phentolamine have been shown to possess significant antiarrhythmic activity but are of limited usefulness because of hypotension. Enhanced α_1 activity in the setting of myocardial ischemia may explain why the antiarrhythmic benefits of β antagonists in patients with acute myocardial infarction are unpredictable. The contribution of β receptors to positive inotropism and arrhythmogenesis during ischemia and reperfusion may be overshadowed by α receptor activation during acute heart failure and ischemia.

Peripheral Vessels

Activation of the presynaptic α_2-vascular receptors produces vasodilation, whereas the postsynaptic α_1- and α_2-vascular receptors result in vasoconstriction. Presynaptic vascular α_2 receptors inhibit NE release. This represents a negative feedback mechanism by which NE inhibits its own release via the prejunctional receptor. Presynaptic α_2 agonists, such as clonidine, inhibit NE release at the neurosympathetic junction, producing vasodilatation. The effect of selective presynaptic α_2-receptor agonists to ameliorate coronary vasoconstriction in humans is unclear. Excitation of the inhibitory presynaptic α_2 receptors by endogenous or synthetic catecholamines also inhibits NE release. However, most sympathomimetics are nonselective α agonists that will excite equally presynaptic α_2 vasodilating receptors and vasoconstrictive postsynaptic α_1 and α_2 receptors. Postsynaptic α_1 and α_2 receptors coexist in both the arterial and venous sides of the circulation with the relative distribution of α_2 receptors being greater on the venous side.[21] This may explain why pure α_1 agonists, such as methoxamine, produce little venoconstriction, whereas many nonselective agonists such as phenylephrine produce significant venoconstriction. NE is the most potent venoconstrictor of all catecholamines. Clinically, venoconstriction would have the effect of preloading by shifting venous capacitance centrally, whereas stimulation of arterial postsynaptic α_1 and α_2 receptors would affect afterloading by increasing arterial resistance.

α-Adrenergic Receptors in the Central Nervous System

All subtypes of the α, β, and DA receptors have been found in various regions of the brain and spinal cord. The functional role of the cerebral α and β receptors suggests a close association with blood pressure and HR control. Cerebral and spinal cord presynaptic α_2 receptors are also involved in inhibition of presynaptic NE release. Although the brain contains adrenergic and dopaminergic receptors, circulating catecholamines do not cross the blood–brain barrier. The catecholamines in the brain are synthesized there. Many actions have been attributed to the cerebral postsynaptic α_2 receptor. These include inhibition of insulin release, inhibition of bowel motility, stimulation of growth hormone release, and inhibition of ADH release. Central neuraxial injections of α_2 agonists, such as clonidine, induce analgesia, sedation, and cardiovascular depression. This mechanism may explain the increased duration of epidural or intrathecal anesthesia observed with the addition of nonselective α agonists to local anesthetic.

Dexmedetomidine is an α_2 receptor agonist with a growing role in anesthesia practice as well as in the intensive care units due to its analgesic and sedative properties. It also tends to decrease the risk of delirium while preserving respiratory function. The most common side effects are hypotension and bradycardia.[23]

α Receptors in the Kidney

The kidney has an extensive and exclusive adrenergic innervation of the afferent and efferent glomerular arterioles, proximal and distal renal tubules, ascending loop of Henle, and juxtaglomerular apparatus. The greatest density of innervation is in the thick ascending loop of Henle, followed by the distal convoluted tubules and proximal tubule. Both α_1 and α_2 subtypes are found in the kidney, with the α_2 receptor dominating. The α_1 receptor is predominant in the renal vasculature and elicits vasoconstriction, which modulates renal blood flow. Tubular α_1 receptors enhance sodium and water reabsorption, leading to antinatriuresis, whereas tubular α_2 receptors promote sodium and water excretion.

β-Adrenergic Receptors

The β-adrenergic receptors, like the α receptor, have been divided into subtypes. They are designated as the β_1 and β_2 subtypes. Recently, molecular cloning has demonstrated the existence of a third subtype, namely the β_3 receptor. Activation of all these receptor subtypes induces the activation of adenylyl cyclase and increased conversion of ATP to cyclic adenosine-3′,5′-monophosphate (cAMP). β_1 Receptors predominate in the myocardium, the sinoatrial node, and the ventricular conduction system. The β_1 receptors also mediate the effects of the catecholamines on the myocardium. These receptors are equally sensitive to EPI and NE, which distinguishes them from the β_2 receptors. Effects of β_1 stimulation are outlined in Table 14-4.

The β_2 receptors are located in the smooth muscles of the blood vessels in the skin, muscle, mesentery, and bronchial smooth muscle. Stimulation produces vasodilation and bronchial relaxation. β_2 receptors are more sensitive to EPI than NE. β Receptors are found in both pre- and postsynaptic membranes of the adrenergic neuroeffector junction. β_1 Receptors are distributed to postsynaptic sites and have not been identified on the presynaptic membrane. Presynaptic β receptors are of the β_2 subtype. The effects of activation of the presynaptic β_2 receptor are diametrically opposed to those of the presynaptic α_2 receptor. The presynaptic β_2 receptor accelerates endogenous NE release, whereas blockade of this receptor inhibits NE release. Antagonism of the presynaptic β_2 receptors produces a physiologic result similar to activation of the presynaptic α_2 receptor. The postsynaptic β_1 receptors are located on the synaptic membrane and respond primarily to neuronal NE. The postsynaptic β_2 receptor, like the postsynaptic α_2 receptor, responds primarily to circulating EPI.

β Receptors in the Cardiovascular System

Myocardium

Myocardial β receptors were originally classified as β_1 receptors. Those in the vascular and bronchial smooth muscle were called the β_2 subtype. However, studies have confirmed the coexistence of β_1 and β_2 receptors in the myocardium.[24] Both β_1 and β_2 receptors are functionally coupled to adenylate cyclase, suggesting a similar involvement in the regulation of inotropism and chronotropism. Postsynaptic β_1 receptors are distributed predominantly to the myocardium, the sinoatrial node, and the ventricular conduction system. The β_2 receptors have the same distribution but are presynaptic. Activation of the presynaptic β_2 receptor accelerates the release of NE into the synaptic cleft. The β_2 receptor comprises 20% to 30% of the β receptors in the ventricular myocardium and up to 40% of the β receptors in the atrium.

The effect of NE on inotropism in the normal heart is mediated entirely through the postsynaptic β_1 receptor, whereas the inotropic effects of EPI are mediated through both the β_1- and β_2-myocardial receptors. The β_2 receptors may also mediate the chronotropic responses to EPI which explains why selective β_1 antagonists are less effective in suppressing induced tachycardia than the nonselective β_1 antagonist propranolol.[25]

Peripheral Vessels

The postsynaptic vascular β receptors are virtually all of the β_2 subtype. The β_2 receptors are located in the smooth muscle of the blood vessels of the skin, muscle, mesentery, and bronchi. Stimulation of the postsynaptic β_2 receptor produces vasodilation and bronchial relaxation. Modest vasoconstriction occurs when subjected to blockade because the actions of the vascular postsynaptic β_2 receptors no longer oppose the actions of the α_1- and α_2-postsynaptic receptors.

β Receptors in the Kidney

The kidney contains both β_1 and β_2 receptors, with the β_1 being predominant. Renin release from the juxtaglomerular apparatus is enhanced by β stimulation. The β_1 receptor evokes renin release in humans. Renal β_2 receptors also appear to regulate renal blood flow at the vascular level. They have been identified pharmacologically and mediate a vasodilatory response.

Dopaminergic Receptors

Dopamine, synthesized in 1910, was recognized in 1959 not only as a vasopressor and the precursor of NE and EPI, but also as an important central and peripheral neurotransmitter. Dopamine receptors (DA) are localized in the CNS, on blood vessels and postganglionic sympathetic nerves (Table 14-4). Two clinically important types of DA receptors have been recognized: DA_1 and DA_2; other subtypes such as DA_4 and DA_5 are still being investigated. The DA_1 receptors are postsynaptic, whereas the DA_2 receptors are both pre- and postsynaptic. The presynaptic DA_2 receptor, like the presynaptic α_2 receptor, inhibits NE release and can produce vasodilatation. Like the postsynaptic α_2 receptor, the postsynaptic DA_2 receptor may promote vasoconstriction. This effect is opposite to that of the postsynaptic DA_1 renal vascular receptor. The zona glomerulosa of the adrenal cortex also contains DA_2 receptors, which inhibit the release of aldosterone.

Myocardium

Defining specific dopaminergic receptors has been difficult because dopamine also exerts effects on the α and β receptors. DA receptors have not been described in the myocardium. Effects of dopamine are those related to the activation of β_1 receptors, which promote positive inotropism and chronotropism. β_2 Activation may produce some systemic vasodilatation.

Peripheral Vessels

The greatest numbers of DA_1 postsynaptic receptors are found on vascular smooth muscle cells of the kidney and mesentery, but they are also found in other systemic arteries including coronary, cerebral, and cutaneous arteries. The vascular receptors are, like the β_2 receptors, linked to adenylate cyclase and mediate smooth muscle relaxation. Activation of these receptors produces vasodilatation, increasing blood flow to these organs. Concurrent activation of vascular presynaptic DA_2 receptors also inhibits NE release at presynaptic α_2 receptors, which may also contribute to peripheral vasodilatation. Higher doses of dopamine can mediate vasoconstriction via the postsynaptic α_1 and α_2 receptors. The constrictive effect is relatively weak in the cardiovascular system, where the action of dopamine on adrenergic receptors is 1/35 and 1/50 as potent as that of EPI and NE, respectively.[26]

Central Nervous System

DA receptors have been identified in the hypothalamus, where they are involved in prolactin release. They are also found in the basal ganglia, where they coordinate motor function. Degeneration of dopaminergic neurons in the substantia nigra is the cause of Parkinson disease. Another central action of dopamine is to stimulate the chemoreceptor trigger zone of the medulla, producing nausea and vomiting. Dopamine antagonists such as haloperidol and droperidol are clinically effective in countering this action.[27]

Kidney and Mesentery

Apart from their effect on the vessels of the kidney and mesentery, DA receptors on the smooth muscle of the esophagus, stomach, and small intestine enhance secretion production and reduce intestinal motility.[28] Metoclopramide, a dopamine antagonist, is useful for aspiration prophylaxis by promoting gastric emptying. The distribution of DA receptors in the renal vasculature is well known, but DA receptors have other functions within the kidney. DA_1 receptors are located on renal tubules, where they inhibit sodium reabsorption, resulting in natriuresis and diuresis. The natriuresis may be the result of a combination of renal vasodilatation, improved CO, and DA_1 receptor activation on the renal tubules. Juxtaglomerular cells also contain DA_1 receptors, which increase renin release when activated. This action modulates the diuresis produced by DA_1 activation of the tubules.

Dopamine has unique autonomic effects by activating specific peripheral dopaminergic receptors, which promote natriuresis and reduce afterload via dilatation of the renal and mesenteric arterial beds. Peripheral dopaminergic activity serves as a natural antihypertensive mechanism. Its actions are overshadowed by the opposite effect of its main biologic partner, NE. Plasma NE levels are known to increase with aging, likely the result of reduced clearance, while peripheral dopaminergic activity is known to diminish. Subtle changes in the DA–NE balance with aging may account for the diminished ability of the aged kidney to excrete a salt load.

Other Receptors

Adenosine Receptors

Adenosine produces inhibition of NE release. The effect of adenosine is blocked by caffeine and other methylxanthines. The physiologic function of these receptors may be the reduction of sympathetic tone under hypoxic conditions when adenosine production is enhanced. As a consequence of reduced NE release, cardiac work is decreased, and oxygen demand is reduced. Adenosine has been effectively used to produce controlled hypotension, short-term bradycardia, and coronary vasodilation.[29]

Serotonin

Serotonin (5-hydroxytryptamine [5-HT]) depresses the response of isolated blood vessels to SNS stimulation and decreases the release of labeled NE in these preparations. Raising the external calcium ion concentration antagonizes this inhibitory action of serotonin. Thus, serotonin may inhibit neuronal NE release by a mechanism that limits the availability of calcium ions at the nerve terminal.

Prostaglandin E2, Histamine, and Opioids

Prostaglandin E2, histamine, and several opioids have been reported to act on prejunctional receptor sites to inhibit NE release in certain sympathetically innervated tissue. However, these inhibitory receptors are unlikely to play a physiologic role in limiting NE release since their direct antagonists, compounds such as inhibitors of cyclooxygenase, histamine antagonists, and naloxone do not increase NE release.

Histamine acts in a manner similar to the neurotransmitters of the SNS. The cell membrane has specific receptors for histamine, with the individual response being determined by the type of cell being stimulated (see Chapter 9). Two receptors for histamine have been identified; these have been designated H_1 and H_2. Stimulation of H_1 receptors produces bronchoconstriction and intestinal contraction. The major role of the H_2 receptors is related to acid production by the parietal cells of the stomach; however, histamine is also present in relatively high concentrations in the myocardium and cardiac conducting tissue, where it exerts positive inotropic and chronotropic effects while depressing dromotropism. The positive inotropic and chronotropic effects of histamine at H_2 receptors are not blocked by β antagonism. These effects are blocked by H_2 antagonists, such as cimetidine, which accounts for the occasional report of cardiovascular collapse following the use of cimetidine. Negative dromotropism and coronary spasm are caused by histamine effects at H_1 receptors.

Adrenergic Receptor Numbers and Sensitivity

Receptors, once thought to be static entities, are now believed to be dynamically regulated by a variety of conditions and to be in a constant state of flux. Receptors are synthesized in the sarcoplasmic reticulum (SR) of the parent cell, where they may remain extrasynaptic or externalize to the synaptic membranes. Membrane receptors may be removed or internalized to intracellular sites for either degradation or recycling.

The number and sensitivity of adrenergic receptors can be 7
influenced by normal, genetic, and developmental factors. Changes in the number of receptors alter the response to catecholamines. Alteration in the number or density of receptors is referred to as either up- or downregulation. As a rule, the number of receptors is inversely proportional to the ambient concentration of the catecholamines. Extended exposure of receptors to their agonists markedly reduces, but does not ablate, the biologic response to catecholamines. For example, increased adrenergic activity occurs in response to reduced perfusion as a result of acute or chronic myocardial dysfunction. Plasma catecholamines are increased. Subsequently, the myocardial postsynaptic β_1 receptors are "downregulated" (see Chapter 11). This is thought to explain the diminished inotropic and chronotropic response to β_1 agonists and exercise in patients with chronic heart failure. However, calcium-induced inotropism is not impaired because extrasynaptic β_2-receptor numbers remain relatively intact. The β_2 receptors may account for up to 40% of the inotropism of the failing heart compared with 20% in the normal heart.[20,30] Tachyphylaxis to infused catecholamines is also thought to be the result of acute downregulation of receptors. There appears to be a reduction in numbers or sensitivity of β receptors in hypertensive patients who also have elevated plasma catecholamines. Downregulation is the presumptive explanation for the lack of correlation between plasma catecholamine levels and the blood pressure elevation observed in patients with pheochromocytoma. Chronic use of β agonists such as terbutaline, isoproterenol, or EPI for the treatment of asthma can result in tachyphylaxis because of downregulation. Even short-term use (1 to 6 hours) of β agonists may cause downregulation of receptor numbers. Downregulation is reversible on termination of the agonist. Chronic treatment of animals with nonselective β blockade causes a 100% increase in the number of β receptors. This accounts for the propranolol withdrawal syndrome in which the acute discontinuation of the β antagonist leaves the α receptors unopposed, in addition to an increased number of β receptors. Clonidine withdrawal can be explained by the same mechanism. Up- or downregulation of receptor numbers may not alter sensitivity of the receptor. Likewise, sensitivity may be increased or decreased in the presence of normal numbers of receptors. The pharmacologic factors affecting up- or downregulation of the α and β receptors are similar.

Autonomic Nervous System Reflexes and Interactions

The ANS reflex has been compared to a computer circuit. This 8
control system, as in all reflex systems, has (1) sensors, (2) afferent pathways, (3) CNS integration, and (4) efferent pathways to the receptors and efferent organs. Fine adjustments are made at the local level through positive and negative feedback mechanisms. The baroreceptor is an example. The variable to be controlled (blood pressure) is sensed (carotid sinus), integrated (medullary vasomotor center), and adjusted through specific effector–receptor sites. Drugs or diseases can interrupt this circuit at any point. β-Blockers may attenuate the effector response, whereas an α agonist such as clonidine may alter both the effector and the integrator functions of blood pressure control.

Baroreceptors

Several reflexes in the cardiovascular system help control arterial blood pressure, CO, and HR. The aim of the circulation is

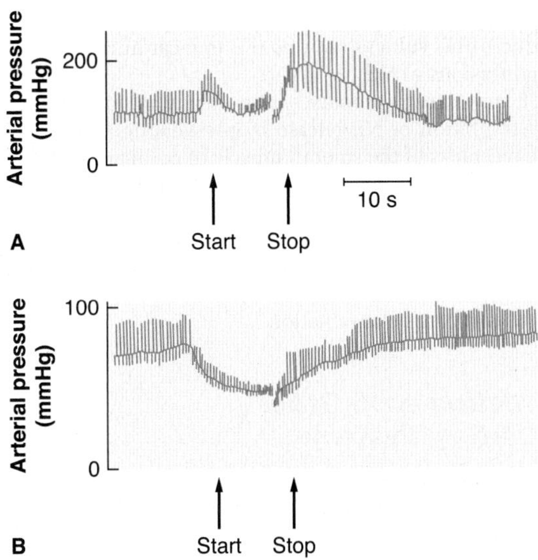

Figure 14-11 **A:** The normal blood pressure response to the Valsalva maneuver is demonstrated. Pulse rate moves in a reciprocal direction according to Marey law of the heart. **B:** An abnormal Valsalva response is shown in a patient with C5 quadriplegia.

to provide blood flow to all the body organs (see Chapter 12). Yet, the most important controlled variable to which the sensors are attuned is blood pressure, a product of blood flow and vascular resistance. Étienne Marey noted in 1859 that the pulse rate is inversely proportional to the blood pressure, and this is known as the Marey law. Subsequently, Hering, Koch, and others demonstrated that the alterations in HR evoked by changes in blood pressure are dependent on baroreceptors located in the aortic arch and carotid sinuses. These pressure sensors react to alterations in stretch caused by blood pressure. Impulses from the carotid sinus and aortic arch reach the medullary vasomotor center by the glossopharyngeal and vagus nerves, respectively. Increased sensory traffic from the baroreceptors, caused by increased blood pressure, inhibits SNS effector traffic. The relative increase in vagal tone produces vasodilation, slowing of the HR, and a lowering of blood pressure. Real increases in vagal tone occur when blood pressure exceeds normal limits. The Valsalva maneuver can best demonstrate the arterial baroreceptor reflex (Fig. 14-11). The Valsalva maneuver raises the intrathoracic pressure by forced expiration against a closed glottis. The arterial blood pressure rises momentarily as the intrathoracic blood is forced into the heart (increased preload). Sustained intrathoracic pressure diminishes venous return, reduces the CO, and drops the blood pressure. Reflex vasoconstriction and tachycardia ensue. Blood pressure returns to normal with release of the forced expiration, but then briefly "overshoots" because of the vasoconstriction and increased venous return. A slowing of the HR accompanies the overshoot in pressure. The cardiovascular responses to the Valsalva maneuver require an intact ANS circuit from peripheral sensor to peripheral adrenergic receptors. The Valsalva maneuver has been used to identify patients at risk for ANS instability during anesthesia. This was once a major concern in patients receiving drugs that depleted catecholamines, such as reserpine. Dysfunction of the SNS is implicated if exaggerated and prolonged hypotension develops during the forced expiration phase (50% from resting mean arterial pressure). In addition, the overshoot at the end of the Valsalva maneuver is absent. Dysfunction of the PNS can be assumed if the HR does not respond appropriately to the blood pressure changes.

Venous baroreceptors may be more dominant in the moment-to-moment regulation of CO. Baroreceptors in the right atrium and great veins produce an increase in HR when stretched by increased right atrial pressure. Reduced venous pressure decreases HR. Unlike the arterial baroreceptors, venous sensors are not thought to alter vascular tone; however, venoconstriction is postulated to occur when atrial pressures decline. Stretch of the venous receptors produces changes in HR opposite to those produced when the arterial pressure sensors are stimulated. The arterial and venous pressure receptors separately monitor two of the four major determinants of CO: afterload and preload, respectively. Venous baroreceptors sample preload by stretch of the atrium. Arterial baroreceptors survey resistance, or afterload, as reflected in the mean arterial pressure. Afterload and preload produce opposite effects on CO; thus, one should not be surprised that the venous and arterial baroreceptors produce opposing effects after a similar stretch stimulus—pressure.

Bainbridge described the venous baroreceptor reflex and demonstrated that it can be abolished by vagal resection. Numerous investigators have confirmed the acceleration of HR in response to volume. However, the magnitude and direction of the HR response are dependent on the prevailing HR at the time of stimulation. The denervated, transplanted mammalian heart also accelerates in response to volume loading. HR, like CO, can apparently be adjusted to the quantity of blood entering the heart. The Bainbridge reflex relates to the characteristic but paradoxical slowing of the heart seen with spinal anesthesia. Blockade of the SNS levels of T1–T4 ablates the efferent limb of the cardiac accelerator nerves. This source of cardiac deceleration is obvious, as the vagus nerve is unopposed. However, bradycardia during spinal anesthesia is more related to the development of arterial hypotension than to the height of the block. The primary defect in the development of spinal hypotension is a decrease in venous return. Theoretically, arterial hypotension should reflexively produce tachycardia through the arterial baroreceptors. Instead, bradycardia is more common. Greene suggests that in the unmedicated person, the venous baroreceptors are dominant over the arterial. A reduced venous pressure, therefore, slows HR.[31] In contrast, humorally mediated tachycardia is the usual response to hypotension or acidosis from other causes. In patients with difficult-to-control blood pressure, decreasing the sympathetic outflow seems to be beneficial in better regulating the blood pressure. Therefore, surgical interruption of the renal efferent sympathetic outflow with radiofrequency ablation through femoral artery catheterization increases natriuresis and diuresis and reduces renin production. Also, baroreflex sensitization through an implantable carotid sinus stimulator seems to be extremely promising in patients with refractory hypertension.[32]

Denervated Heart

Reflex modulation of the adrenergic agonists is best seen in the denervated transplant heart, which retains the recipient's innervated sinoatrial node and the donor's denervated sinoatrial node (see Chapter 52). NE infusion in the transplanted heart produces a slowing of the recipient's atrial rate through vagal feedback as the blood pressure rises. In the unmodulated donor heart, atrial rate increases. The baroreceptors are therefore not operant in the transplanted heart. Isoproterenol, a pure β agonist, increases the discharge rate of both the recipient and donor node by direct action, with the donor rate near doubling that of the recipient node. Atropine accelerates the recipient's atrial rate, whereas no effect is seen on the donor rate, which now controls HR.

β-Blockade produces a comparable slowing of the sinoatrial node of both recipient and donor. The exercise capability of the denervated heart is conspicuously reduced by β blockade, presumably because of its reliance on circulating catecholamines. Propranolol has also been demonstrated to reduce the β response to the chronotropic effects of NE and isoproterenol in the transplanted heart. The CO of the transplanted heart varies appropriately with changes in preload and afterload. There is new evidence that over time, months to years, the process of cardiac reinnervation does occur, albeit limited in extent and distribution, and perhaps predominantly involving sympathetic fibers that may affect the HR as well as responses to stimuli.[33]

Interaction of Autonomic Nervous System Receptors

Strong interactions have been noted between SNS and PNS nerves in organs that receive dual, antagonistic innervation. Release of NE at the presynaptic terminal is modified by the PNS. For example, vagal inhibition of left ventricular contractility is accentuated as the level of SNS activity is raised. This interaction is termed "accentuated antagonism" and is mediated by a combination of pre- and postsynaptic mechanisms. The coronary arteries present an example of this phenomenon and deserve special attention.

The myocardium and coronary vessels are abundantly supplied with adrenergic and cholinergic fibers. Strong activity of both α and β receptors has been demonstrated in the coronary vascular bed. Selective stimulation of both the α_1 and postsynaptic α_2 receptors increases coronary vascular resistance, whereas selective α-blockade eliminates this effect. Therefore, both β_1 and α_1 adrenoreceptors are present in coronary arteries and accessible to NE released by sympathetic nerves.[11,20,24]

The presynaptic adrenergic terminals of the myocardium and coronary vessels, like all blood vessels studied, contain muscarinic receptors.[34] Recent observations confirm that muscarinic agents and vagal stimulation, acting on the presynaptic, SNS muscarinic receptor, inhibit the release of NE in a manner similar to that of the presynaptic α_2 and DA_2 receptors (Fig. 14-9). Conversely, blockade of the muscarinic receptors with atropine markedly augments the positive inotropic response to catecholamines.[35] Suppression of NE release explains, in part, vagal-induced attenuation of the inotropic response to strong SNS stimulation (accentuated antagonism) and only a weak negative inotropic effect of vagal stimulation when there is low background SNS activity. This may also explain why vagal activity reduces the vulnerability of the myocardium to fibrillation during infusions of NE.

ACh may cause coronary spasm during periods of high SNS tone.[35] Inhibition of NE release by presynaptic adrenergic muscarinic receptors of the smooth muscle of coronary vessels would lessen the coronary relaxation normally produced by NE on the β_1 receptor (Fig. 14-9). In anesthetized dogs, the rate of NE outflow into the coronary sinus blood evoked by cardiac SNS stimulation is markedly diminished by simultaneous vagal efferent stimulation.[36] This action is known to be prevented by atropine, which also causes coronary vasodilation.

Interaction with Other Regulatory Systems

The ANS is integrally related to several endocrine systems that ultimately summate to control blood pressure and regulate homeostasis (2 Video 14-2). These include the renin–angiotensin system, ADH, glucocorticoids, and insulin (see Chapter 47). Both α and β receptors have been found in the endocrine pancreas and modulate insulin release (Table 14-4). β Stimulation increases insulin release, whereas α stimulation decreases it. The overall importance of this interaction is not entirely clear, but decreased tolerance to glucose and potassium has been noted in subjects taking β-blocking drugs. The renin–angiotensin system 2 is a complex endocrine system that modulates both blood pressure and water–electrolyte homeostasis (Fig. 14-12). Renin is a proteolytic enzyme released by the cells of the juxtaglomerular apparatus of the renal cortex. Renin acts on plasma angiotensinogen to form angiotensin I. Angiotensin I is then converted to angiotensin II by a converting enzyme in the lung. Angiotensin II is a powerful angiotensin direct arterial vasoconstrictor. It also acts on the adrenal cortex to release aldosterone and on the adrenal medulla to release EPI. In addition to its direct effects on vascular smooth muscle, angiotensin II augments NE release via presynaptic receptors, thus enhancing peripheral SNS tone. Captopril, enalapril, and lisinopril inhibit the action of angiotensin-converting enzyme, thus preventing the conversion of angiotensin I to angiotensin II. Renin is released in response to hyponatremia, decreased renal perfusion pressure, and ANS stimulation via β receptors on juxtaglomerular cells. Changes in sympathetic tone may thus alter renin release and affect homeostasis in a variety of ways.

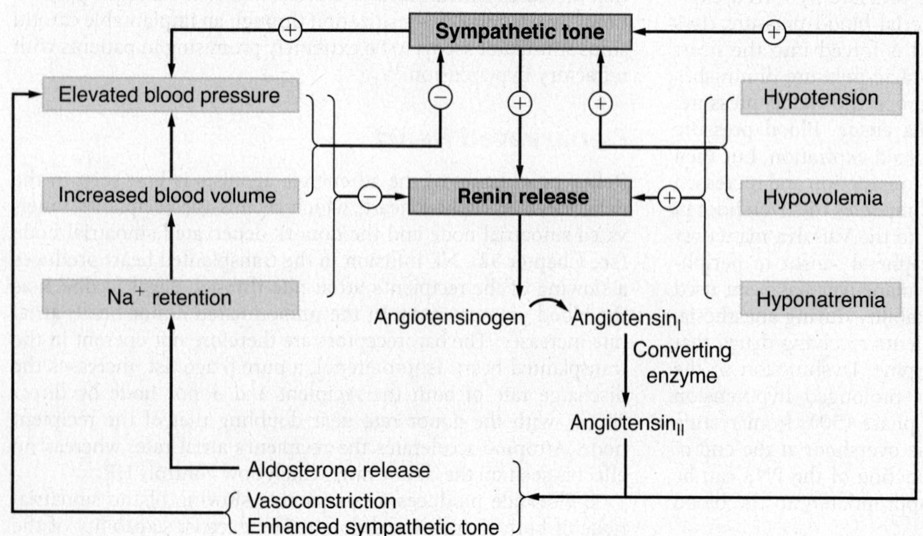

Figure 14-12 The interactions of the renin–angiotensin and SNS in regulating homeostasis are shown schematically along with the physiologic variables that modulate their function. Arrows with a plus sign (+) represent stimulation, and those with a minus sign (–) represent inhibition.

The ANS is also intimately related to adrenocortical function. As outlined above, glucocorticoid release modulates phenylethanolamine-N-methyltransferase formation and thus synthesis of EPI. Glucocorticoids are also important in regulating the response of peripheral tissues to changes in SNS tone. Thus, the ANS is important to other homeostatic mechanisms.

Clinical Autonomic Nervous System Pharmacology

9 The clinical application of ANS pharmacology is based on the knowledge of ANS anatomy, physiology, and molecular pharmacology. Drugs that modify ANS activity can be classified by their site of action, mechanism of action, or the pathophysiology for which they are most commonly used. Antihypertensive drugs are an example of the third category. This classification is a matter of degree because there exists considerable functional overlap. An example of classification by site relates to the ganglionic agonists or blocking agents. ANS drugs can be further categorized as those that act at the prejunctional membrane and those acting postjunctionally. They can then be more specifically classified by the predominant receptor or receptors on which they act.

Mode of Action

ANS drugs may be broadly classified by mode of action according to their mimetic or lytic actions. This may also be termed agonist or antagonist. A sympathomimetic, such as ephedrine, mimics SNS activity by stimulation of adrenergic receptor sites both directly and indirectly. Sympatholytic drugs cause dissolution of SNS activity at these same receptor sites. β Receptor blockers are examples of sympatholytic drugs. Several modes of ANS drug action become evident when following the cascade of neurotransmission. Drugs that act on prejunctional membranes may (1) interfere with transmitter synthesis (α-methyl paratyrosine), (2) disrupt transmitter storage (reserpine), (3) block transmitter release (clonidine), (4) stimulate transmitter release (ephedrine), or (5) interfere with transmitter reuptake (cocaine). Drugs may also (6) modify metabolism of the neurotransmitter in the synaptic cleft (anticholinesterase). Drugs acting at postjunctional sites may (7) directly stimulate postjunctional receptors, or (8) interfere with the transmitter agonist at the postjunctional receptor.

The ultimate response of an effector organ to an agonist or antagonist depends on (1) the drug, (2) its plasma concentration, (3) the number of receptors in the effector organ, (4) binding by the receptor, (5) the concurrent activities of other drugs and hormones, (6) the cellular metabolic status, and (7) reflex adjustments by the organism.

Ganglionic Drugs

SNS and PNS ganglia are pharmacologically similar in that the transmission through these ANS ganglia is mediated by ACh (Fig. 14-2). Most ganglionic agonists and antagonists are not selective and affect SNS and PNS ganglia equally. This nonselective property creates many undesirable and unpredictable side effects, which have limited the clinical utility of this category of drug.

Agonists

There are essentially no clinically useful ganglionic agonists. Nicotine is the prototypical ganglionic agonist. In low doses, it stimulates ANS ganglia and the neuromuscular junction of striated muscle. High doses produce ganglionic and neuromuscular blockade. The protean side effects of nicotinic stimulation render it useful only as an investigative tool.

Antagonists

Drugs that interfere with neurotransmission at ANS ganglia are known as ganglionic blocking agents. Nicotine, in high doses, is the prototypical ganglionic blocking agent; however, early stimulatory nicotinic activity can be blocked both at the ganglia and at the muscle end plates with other ganglionic blockers and muscle relaxants, respectively, without blocking muscarinic effects. Ganglionic blockers produce their nicotinic effects by competing, mimicking, or interfering with ACh metabolism. Hexamethonium, trimethaphan, and pentolinium produce a selective nondepolarizing blockade of neurotransmission at ANS ganglia without producing nicotinic neuromuscular blockade. They compete with ACh in the ganglia without stimulating the receptors. The introduction of drugs that produce vasodilation directly or by action on the SNS vasomotor center has made the ganglionic blockers obsolete. D-Tubocurare (dTC) produces a competitive nondepolarizing block of both motor end plates and ANS ganglia. The action of motor paralysis predominates, but the concomitant ganglionic blockade at higher doses explains part of the hypotensive effect often seen with the use of dTC for muscle relaxation. Anticholinesterase drugs may produce nicotinic-type ganglionic blockade by competition with ACh as well as by persistent depolarization via accumulated ACh.

Trimethaphan produces blockade by competition with ACh for receptors, thus stabilizing the postsynaptic membrane. However, side effects and rapid-onset tachyphylaxis have markedly reduced its use in anesthesia.[37] The patient's pupils become fixed and dilated during administration, which obscures eye signs, an important consideration for neurosurgery. In this regard, it is distinctly inferior to nitroprusside. The major advantage of trimethaphan is its short duration of action, which is the result of hydrolysis by pseudocholinesterase.

Cholinergic Drugs

Muscarinic Agonists

The cholinomimetic muscarinic drugs act at sites in the body where ACh is the transmitter of the nerve impulse. These drugs may be divided into three groups, the first two of which are direct muscarinic agonists. The third group acts indirectly. These groups are choline esters (ACh, methacholine, carbamylcholine, bethanechol), alkaloids (pilocarpine, muscarine), and anticholinesterases (physostigmine, neostigmine, pyridostigmine, edrophonium, echothiophate).

Direct Cholinomimetics

ACh has virtually no therapeutic applications because of its diffuse action and rapid hydrolysis by cholinesterase (Fig. 14-5). One may encounter the use of topical ACh (1%) drops during cataract extraction when rapid miosis is desired. Systemic effects are not usually seen because of the rapidity of ACh hydrolysis. Other choline esters, derivatives of ACh, have been synthesized, which possess more selective muscarinic activity than ACh. They differ from ACh in being more resistant to inactivation by cholinesterase and thus having a more prolonged and useful action. They also differ from ACh in their relative muscarinic and nicotinic activities. The best studied of these drugs are methacholine, bethanechol, and carbamylcholine. The chemical structures of ACh and these

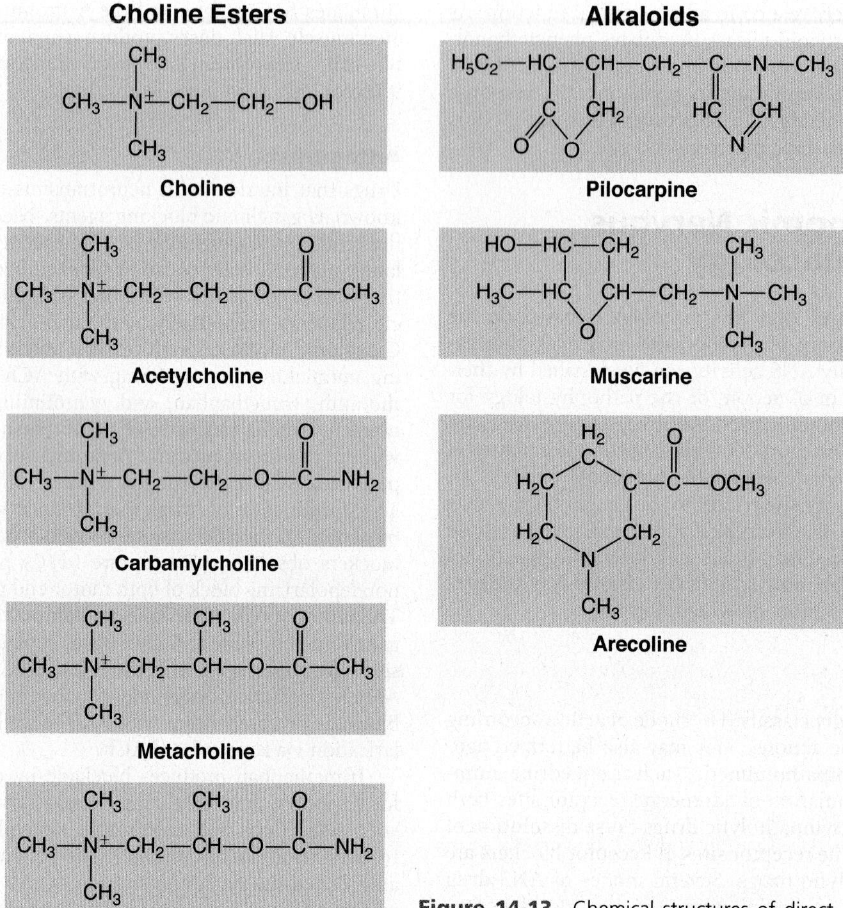

Figure 14-13 Chemical structures of direct-acting cholinomimetic esters and alkaloids.

choline esters are shown in Figure 14-13. Their pharmacologic actions are compared with those of ACh in Table 14-5.

ACh is a quaternary ammonium compound that interacts with postsynaptic receptors, causing conformational membrane changes. This results in increased permeability to small ions and, thus, depolarization. All the receptors translate the reversible binding of ACh into openings of discrete channels in excitable membranes, allowing Na^+ and K^+ ions to flow along their electrochemical gradients. Structure–activity relationships point to the presence of two important binding sites on the receptor, an esteratic site that binds the ester end of the molecule and an ionic site that binds the quaternary amine portion (Fig. 14-5). Subtle changes in the structure of the compound can markedly alter the response among different tissue groups. The degree of muscarinic activity falls if the acetyl group is replaced, but this confers a resistance to enzymatic hydrolysis. Bethanechol is resistant to hydrolysis but possesses mainly muscarinic activity. β-Methyl substitution produces methacholine, which is less resistant to hydrolysis and is primarily a muscarinic agonist. Methacholine slows the heart and dilates peripheral blood vessels. It is used to terminate supraventricular tachydysrhythmias, especially paroxysmal tachycardia, when other measures have failed. It also increases intestinal tone. Methacholine should not be given to patients with asthma. Hypertensive patients may also develop marked hypotension. Side effects are those of PNS stimulation such as nausea, vomiting, and flushed sweating. Overdose is treated with atropine. Bethanechol is relatively selective for the gastrointestinal and urinary tracts. In usual doses, it does not slow the heart or lower the blood pressure. Bethanechol is of value in treating postoperative abdominal distention (nonobstructive paralytic ileus), gastric atony following bilateral vagotomy, congenital megacolon, nonobstructive urinary retention, and some cases of neurogenic bladder.

Direct-acting cholinomimetic alkaloids include muscarine and pilocarpine. They act at the same sites as ACh, and their effects are similar to those of Ach, as described in Table 14-5. Pilocarpine is the only drug of this group used therapeutically in the United States. It is used as a topical miotic drug in ophthalmologic practice to reduce intraocular pressure in glaucoma.

Muscarinic agonists are particularly dangerous in patients with myasthenia gravis (who are receiving anticholinesterases), bulbar palsy, cardiac disease, asthma, peptic ulcer, progressive muscular atrophy, or mechanical intestinal obstruction or urinary retention because they exacerbate these conditions.

Indirect Cholinomimetics

Indirect-acting cholinomimetic drugs produce their effects as a result of inhibition or inactivation of the enzyme acetylcholinesterase, which normally destroys ACh by hydrolysis. They are referred to as cholinesterase inhibitors or anticholinesterases. Most of these drugs inhibit both acetylcholinesterase and pseudocholinesterase. Inhibition of acetylcholinesterase permits the accumulation of ACh transmitter in the synapse, resulting in intense PNS activity similar to that of the direct cholinomimetic

Table 14-5 Comparative Muscarinic Actions of Direct Cholinomimetic Agents

			Systemic		
	Acetylcholine	***Methacholine***	***Carbamylcholine***	***Bethanechol***	***Pilocarpine***
Esterase hydrolysis	+++	+	0	0	0
Eye (topical)					
Iris	++	++	+++	+++	+++
Ciliary	++	++	+++	+++	++
Heart					
Rate	–	–	–	–	
Contractility	–	–	–	–	
Conduction	–	–	–	–	
Smooth muscle					
Vascular	–	–	–	–	–
Bronchial	++	++	+	+	++
Gastrointestinal motility	++	++	+++	+++	++
Gastrointestinal sphincters	–	–	–	–	++
Biliary	++	++	+++	+++	++
Bladder					
Detrusor	++	++	+++	+++	++
Sphincter	–	–	–	–	–
Exocrine glands					
Respiratory	+++	++	+++	++	++++
Salivary	++	++	++	++	+++++
Pharyngeal	++	++	++	++	++++
Lacrimal	++	++	++	++	++++
Sweat	++	++	++	++	+++++
Gastrointestinal acid and secretions	++	++	++	++	++++
Nicotinic actions	+++	+	+++	–	+++

+, stimulation; –, inhibition.

agents. The accumulation of ACh by the anticholinesterases potentially can produce all of the following: (1) stimulation of muscarinic receptors at ANS-effect organs, (2) stimulation followed by depression of all ANS ganglia and skeletal muscle (nicotinic), and (3) stimulation with later depression of cholinergic receptor sites in the CNS. All of these effects may be seen with lethal doses of anticholinesterase drugs, but therapeutic doses only produce the first two.

Anticholinesterase drugs are used routinely in anesthesia to reverse nondepolarizing neuromuscular block. The most prominent pharmacologic effects of the anticholinesterase drugs are muscarinic. Their most useful actions are their nicotinic effects. Muscarinic activity is evoked by lower concentrations of ACh than are necessary to produce the desired nicotinic effect. For example, the anticholinesterase neostigmine reverses neuromuscular blockade by increasing ACh concentration at the muscle end plate, a nicotinic receptor. Nicotinic reversal of neuromuscular blockade can usually be produced safely only when the patient has been protected by atropine or other muscarinic blockers. This prevents the untoward muscarinic effects of bradycardia, hypotension, bronchospasm, or intestinal spasm. Reversal of neuromuscular blockade in patients who have had bowel anastomosis was at one time a major controversy. Some thought that the muscarinic effects of anticholinesterase drugs (hypermotility) increased the risk of anastomotic leakage whereas others found no association between their use and subsequent breakdown. National experience has favored the latter opinion.

Clinically, anticholinesterase drugs may be divided into two 10
types: the reversible and nonreversible cholinesterase inhibitors.[38] Reversible cholinesterase inhibitors delay the hydrolysis of ACh from 1 to 8 hours. Nonreversible drugs are so named because their inhibitory effects may last from days to weeks. The differences in duration of various anticholinesterases likely depend on whether they inhibit the anionic or esteratic site of acetylcholinesterase. Therefore, the anticholinesterase drugs have also been pharmacologically subdivided. Drugs that inhibit the anionic site are called competitive inhibitors. Their action is due to competition between the anticholinesterase and ACh for the anionic site. These drugs tend to be short acting. Edrophonium is an example. Drugs that inhibit the esteratic site are called acid-transferring inhibitors. These drugs include the longer-acting neostigmine, pyridostigmine, and physostigmine.

Most of the reversible cholinesterase inhibitors are quaternary ammonium compounds and do not cross the blood–brain barrier (3 Video 14-3 and 4 Video 14-4). Physostigmine is a tertiary amine that readily passes into the CNS (Fig. 14-14). It produces central muscarinic stimulation and, thus, is not used to reverse neuromuscular blockade but can be used to treat atropine poisoning. Conversely, atropine is used to treat physostigmine poisoning. Physostigmine has also been found to be a specific antidote in

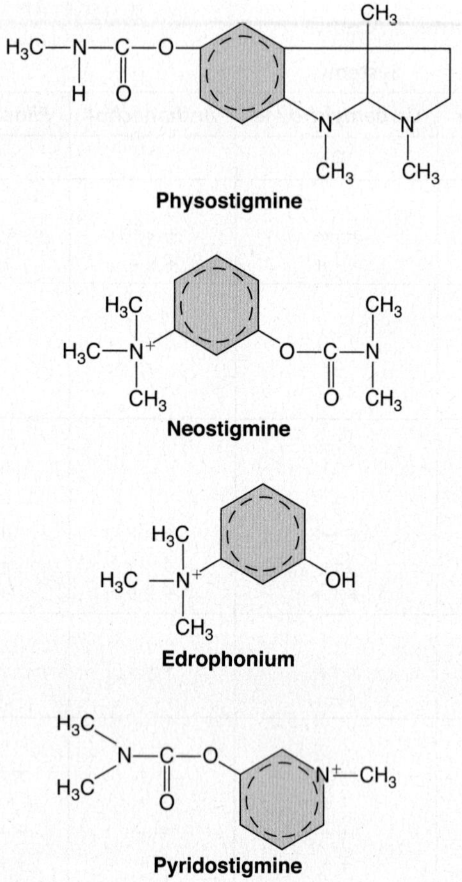

Physostigmine

Neostigmine

Edrophonium

Pyridostigmine

Figure 14-14 Structural formulas of clinically useful reversible anticholinesterase drugs. Physostigmine is a tertiary amine and crosses the blood–brain barrier. It is useful in treating the central anticholinergic syndrome.

the treatment of postoperative delirium (see below, Central Anticholinergic Syndrome).[39]

The irreversible cholinesterase inhibitors are mostly organophosphate compounds. The organophosphate compounds are highly lipid-soluble, readily pass into the CNS, and are rapidly absorbed through the skin. They are used as the active ingredient in potent insecticides and chemical warfare agents known as nerve gases (see Chapter 53). The only therapeutic drug of this group is echothiophate, which is available in the form of topical drops for the treatment of glaucoma. Its primary advantage is its prolonged duration of action. Topical absorption is variable but considerable. However, echothiophate can remain effective for 2 or 3 weeks following cessation of therapy. A patient history of echothiophate use increases the risk of prolonged action of succinylcholine, which requires pseudocholinesterase for its hydrolysis. Organophosphate poisoning manifests all the signs and symptoms of excess Ach. The antidote cartridges dispensed to troops to counter the effects of anticholinesterase nerve gases contain only atropine, which would effectively counter the muscarinic effects of the gas; however, atropine does little to counter the high-dose nicotinic muscle paralysis or the central ventilatory depression that contributes to death from nerve gases. Treatment requires high doses of atropine, 35 to 70 mcg/kg IV every 3 to 10 minutes until muscarinic symptoms abate. Lower doses at less frequent intervals may be required for several days. Central ventilatory depression and weakness require respiratory support and specific therapy. Pralidoxime has been reported to reactivate cholinesterase activity by hydrolysis of the phosphate enzyme complex. It is particularly effective with parathion poisoning and is the only cholinesterase reactivator available in the United States.[40]

Muscarinic Antagonists

Muscarinic antagonist refers to a specific drug action for which the term anticholinergic is widely used. Any drug that interferes with the action of Ach as a transmitter can be considered an anticholinergic agent. The term anticholinergic refers to a broader classification that also includes the nicotinic antagonists.

Atropine-Like Drugs

Atropine, scopolamine, and glycopyrrolate are the most commonly used muscarinic antagonists used in anesthesia (Fig. 14-15). The actions of these drugs include inhibition of salivary, bronchial, pancreatic, and gastrointestinal secretions; as such, they antagonize the muscarinic side effects of anticholinesterases during the reversal of muscle relaxants. Historically, atropine was introduced to anesthesia practice to prevent excessive secretions during ether anesthesia and to prevent vagal bradycardia during the administration of chloroform.[41] Antimuscarinic agents do not inhibit transmission equally, and there are marked variations in sensitivity at different muscarinic sites owing to differences in penetration and affinities of the various receptors. Differences in relative potency between the different antimuscarinics are outlined in Table 14-6. Atropine and scopolamine are tertiary amines (Fig. 14-15) and easily penetrate the blood–brain barrier and placenta. Glycopyrrolate is a quaternary amine that, like the reversible anticholinesterase drugs, does not easily penetrate these barriers. Glycopyrrolate, a synthetic antimuscarinic, has gained popularity because it avoids the central effects of the other two drugs. Clinical observations suggested that bradycardia associated with spinal anesthesia is refractory to the administration of glycopyrrolate, and that atropine and ephedrine are the drugs of choice in order to prevent a possible cardiac arrest. Nevertheless, recent data (69 parturients) demonstrated that prophylactic administration of glycopyrrolate does prevent bradycardia associated with spinal anesthesia for cesarean delivery; however, it does not affect

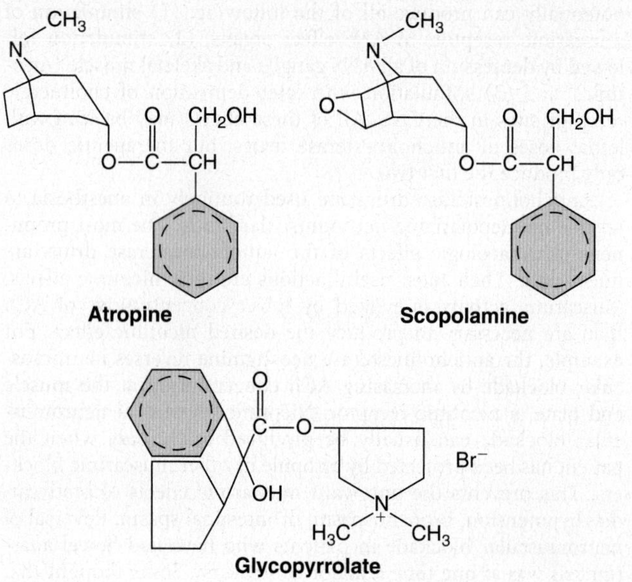

Atropine

Scopolamine

Glycopyrrolate

Figure 14-15 Structural formulas of the clinically useful antimuscarinic drugs.

Table 14-6 Comparison of Antimuscarinic Drugs

	Duration				
	IV	*IM*	CNS Effects[a]	Antisialogogue Effects	Heart Rate
Atropine	15–30 min	2–4 h	++	+	+++[b]
Scopolamine	30–60 min	4–6 h	+++[c]	+++	+
Glycopyrrolate	2–4 h	6–8 h	0	++	+

CNS, central nervous system; GI, gastrointestinal; IM, intramuscular; IV, intravenous.
[a]CNS effects includes sedation, amnesia, mydriasis, and cycloplegia.
[b]May cause an initial decrease in heart rate.
[c]Initial sedation may be followed by excitation.

the vasopressor dose required for the management of hypotension.[42] Atropine and scopolamine have notable CNS effects that are dissimilar. Scopolamine differs from atropine mainly in its central depressant effects, which produce sedation, amnesia, and euphoria. Such properties are widely used for premedication for cardiac patients in combination with morphine and a major tranquilizer. Scopolamine also has been used to induce amnesia in patients who have a high risk for intraoperative awareness, such as trauma victims who are hemodynamically unstable and cannot receive adequate inhalational anesthesia. As a premedication, atropine has minimal effects on the CNS, including mild stimulation. Higher doses such as those given for reversal of muscle relaxants (1 to 2 mg) may produce restlessness, disorientation, hallucinations, and delirium (see below, Central Anticholinergic Syndrome).

Atropine is useful in increasing CO when sinus bradycardia due to vagal stimulation is present. Atropine and scopolamine are noted to produce paradoxical bradycardia when given in low doses. Scopolamine (0.1 to 0.2 mg) usually causes more HR slowing than atropine but also produces less cardiac acceleration at higher doses. The usual intramuscular premedication doses of scopolamine cause either a decrease or no change in HR. Atropine may also produce sympathomimetic effects by blocking presynaptic muscarinic receptors found on adrenergic nerve terminals.[43] Ach stimulation of these receptors inhibits NE release, and blockade by atropine releases this inhibition (see Cholinergic Receptors: Muscarinic). Atropine-like drugs that cross the blood–brain barrier also produce dilation of the pupil (mydriasis) and paralysis of accommodation (cycloplegia). Atropine-like drugs are widely used in ophthalmology as mydriatics and cycloplegics.[44] Atropine is contraindicated in patients with narrow-angle glaucoma (see Chapter 49). Pupillary dilation thickens the peripheral part of the iris, which narrows the iridocorneal angle. This leads to impaired drainage of aqueous humor and an increase in intraocular pressure. Doses of atropine used for premedication have little effect in this regard, whereas comparable doses of scopolamine cause mydriasis. Prudence would dictate avoidance of either agent in patients with narrow-angle glaucoma.

Atropine and scopolamine also possess antiemetic action, and they act as 5-HT_3 receptor antagonists.[43] Atropine, however, reduces the opening pressure of the lower esophageal sphincter, which theoretically increases the risk of passive regurgitation. The belladonna alkaloids (atropine and scopolamine) also block Ach transmission to sweat glands, which, although they are cholinergic, are innervated by the SNS. Antimuscarinic agents produce antinicotinic actions at higher doses and result in important actions on CNS transmission that are pharmacologically similar to the postganglionic cholinergic functions. Atropine is best avoided where tachycardia would be harmful or is already present, as in thyrotoxicosis, pheochromocytoma, or obstructive coronary artery disease. Atropine should be avoided in febrile patients because it inhibits sweating.

Central Anticholinergic Syndrome[45]

The belladonna alkaloids have long been known to produce undesirable side effects ranging from stupor (scopolamine) to delirium (atropine) (NICV 14-1). This syndrome has been called postoperative delirium, atropine toxicity, and central anticholinergic syndrome. Biochemical studies have demonstrated abundant muscarinic ACh receptors in the brain that can be affected by any drug possessing antimuscarinic activity and capable of crossing the blood–brain barrier. Hundreds of drugs exist that meet these criteria and with which this syndrome has been associated. Table 14-7 lists some of those drugs.[46] High doses of atropinic alkaloids rapidly produce dryness of the mouth, blurred vision with photophobia (mydriasis), hot and dry skin (flushed), and fever. Mental symptoms range from sedation, stupor, and coma to anxiety, restlessness, disorientation, hallucinations, and delirium. Convulsions may occur if lethal poisoning has occurred. Although an alarming reaction may occur, fatalities are rare. Intoxication is usually short lived and followed by amnesia. These reactions can be controlled by the intravenous injection of physostigmine. Physostigmine is an anticholinesterase that, by virtue of being a tertiary amine, readily passes into the CNS to counter antimuscarinic activity. It should be given slowly in 1-mg increments, not to exceed 3 mg, to avoid producing peripheral cholinergic activity. Neostigmine, pyridostigmine, and edrophonium are not effective because they cannot pass into the CNS. The duration of physostigmine action may be shorter than that of the offending antimuscarinic agent and therefore repeat dosing may be necessary. Physostigmine appears safe when used within dose recommendations and when indications are established. Central disorientation alone does not establish a diagnosis. Peripheral signs of antimuscarinic activity should be present in addition to central anticholinergic syndrome.

Physostigmine has been reported to reverse the CNS effects of many of the drugs listed in Table 14-7, including antihistamines, tricyclic antidepressants, and tranquilizers. Reversal of the sedative effects of opioids and benzodiazepines has also been described.[39] Anticholinesterase agents potentiate cholinergic synaptic transmission and increase neuronal activity, even if no receptor antagonist is present. Thus, arousal may not be a function independent of its cholinesterase activity and claims that physostigmine is a nonspecific CNS stimulant may not be warranted. These considerations, in association with the risk of significant bradycardia, have limited the clinical utility of physostigmine.

Table 14-7 Antimuscarinic Compounds Associated with Central Anticholinergic Syndrome

Belladonna Alkaloids Atropine sulfate Scopolamine hydrobromide	**Over the Counter** Asthmador—atropine like Sleep-Eze (diphenhydramine)—scopolamine sedation Sominex (diphenhydramine)—scopolamine sedation
Synthetic and Natural Tertiary Amine Compounds Dicyclomine antispasmodic with local anesthetic activity Thiphenamil antispasmodic with local anesthetic activity Procaine Cocaine Cyclopentolate mydriatic	**Antiparkinson Drugs** Benztropine Trihexphenidyl Biperiden Ethopropazine Procyclidine
Quaternary Derivatives of Belladonna Alkaloids Methscopolamine bromide—antispasmodic Homatropine methylbromide—sedative, antispasmodic Homatropine hydrobromide—ophthalmic solution—mydriatic	**Antipsychotic Drugs** Chlorpromazine Thioridazine Haloperidol Droperidol Promethazine
Synthetic Quaternary Compounds Methantheline bromide Propantheline bromide	**Tricyclic Antidepressants** Amitriptyline Imipramine Desipramine
Antihistamines Chlorpheniramine Diphenhydramine	**Synthetic Opioids** Meperidine Methadone
Plants Deadly nightshade (atropine) Bittersweet Potato leaves and sprouts Jimson or loco weed Coca plant (cocaine)	

Autonomic Syndromes and Autonomic Regulation

Recent research in different clinical fields seems to connect the autonomic system and its regulation with the course of various diseases, demonstrating its importance beyond the classical role of fight or flight.

The autonomic system plays a role in balancing inflammatory processes and the immune response; release of ACh, may be a mechanism by which an anti-inflammatory action occurs. Autonomic dysregulation is observed in chronic pain conditions, such as fibromyalgia. Knowledge of the role of neurotransmitters in the pathophysiology of these conditions may ultimately lead to novel treatment interventions, especially since vagal activity may be manipulated by behavioral, surgical, and pharmacologic interventions, including the use of β-blockers.[47]

At the onset of temporal seizures, there appears to be a decrease in parasympathetic tone, which returns slowly to normal at the end of the seizure episode. This phenomenon is inversely correlated with the patient's age and duration of the seizure episode, and also with postictal hypoxemia, which in extreme cases may increase the risk of patient death.[48,49]

Even more importantly, cardiac autonomic dysregulation plays a central role in the evolution of several cardiovascular syndromes such as hypertension, arrhythmias, heart failure, and even myocardial infarction.[50,51] Therefore, addressing the ANS and specifically the upregulation of the SNS may have a great impact on the treatment of these conditions.

Elevated sympathetic tone may precipitate malignant arrhythmias, including atrial fibrillation, ventricular tachyarrhythmias due to ischemia, cardiomyopathy, heart failure, prolonged QT syndrome, Brugada syndrome, and idiopathic ventricular fibrillation.[51] Autonomic testing may be useful to predict which patients are at greatest risk and subsequently guide management decisions. Cardiac autonomic testing includes HR variability, baroreflex sensitivity, HR turbulence, HR deceleration capacity, and T-wave alternans. Vagal nerve stimulation is a possible avenue for the management of some of these arrhythmias as well as heart failure.[52]

Some authors suggest that atrial fibrillation may be due to simultaneous and thus imbalanced discharge of both sympathetic and parasympathetic discharges, with the stellate ganglion and vagus nerve playing essential roles in this process. Renal denervation has been proposed as an adjunct therapy for hypertension, atrial fibrillation, and ventricular arrhythmias, since it appears to lead to a reduction in HR, AV conduction, and secretion of NE. Acupuncture has been proposed as a useful, albeit less traditional tool for atrial fibrillation management. Other possible therapeutic interventions include low-level vagus nerve stimulation, spinal cord stimulation, left cardiac sympathetic denervation, ganglionated plexus ablation, and cutaneous stimulation, which may prove to be a better alternative in patients who cannot tolerate pharmacologic treatment; some of these techniques may also be effective for patients with chronic heart failure.[10,53,54] Patients with resistant hypertension may benefit from bilateral renal nerve ablation by catheters delivering high-frequency ultrasound, as well as bilateral, and more recently unilateral carotid baroreceptor stimulation via an implanted stimulator. However, study results have been mixed and more research is needed to elucidate the role of these therapies in clinical practice.[55]

Autonomic impairment may be used to predict outcomes in patients with serious medical conditions. In a cohort of patients admitted to the emergency department, short-term mortality was associated with deceleration capacity, a factor assessed using HR

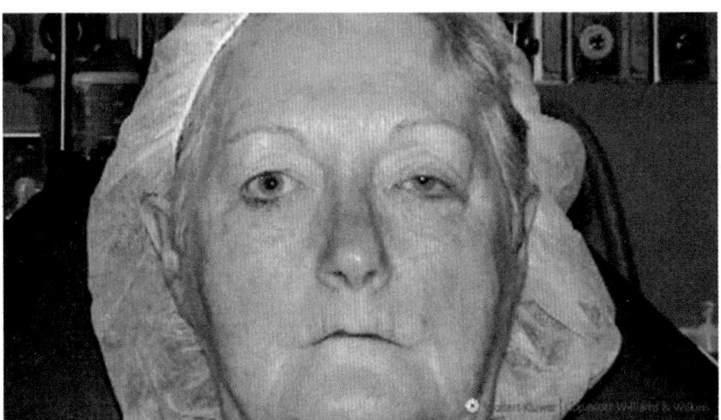

Figure 14-16 Horner syndrome (left eye). Note miosis and ptosis. Loss of sweating not shown.

and R-R interval, which was significantly lower in nonsurvivors compared survivors.[56] In addition, autonomic impairment in patients with traumatic brain injury, which is measured by HR variability and baroreflex sensitivity, appears to increase the risk of death in these patients.[57,58] The ANS seems to be implicated as a cause of sudden cardiac death in epilepsy by several possible mechanisms.[59]

Modulation of autonomic function may also be helpful in treating certain chronic disease. For example, obese patients with insulin resistance may benefit from sympathetic blockade, either with pharmacologic methods or through renal denervation, but results are controversial regarding the efficacy of these methods.[60,61]

Horner Syndrome

Horner syndrome, also known as oculosympathetic paresis, classically manifests as miosis, ptosis, and anhidrosis (Fig. 14-16). Its occurrence is the result of a lesion anywhere along a three-neuron adrenergic pathway from the hypothalamus, through the brachial plexus to the superior cervical ganglion, and then through the cavernous sinus within the adventitia of the internal carotid artery toward the eye. There, the oculosympathetic pathway converges with the ophthalmic division of the trigeminal nerve and innervates the iris dilator muscle (Muller muscle), which causes lower lid retraction and a portion of upper lid elevation.

The causes of Horner syndrome are stroke, tumor, trauma, demyelinating diseases, dissections, or aneurysms of the internal carotid artery, as well as idiopathic events.

It is essential to differentiate more precisely the location of the injury along the sympathetic tract, such as first-, second-, or third-order neuron in order to facilitate more specific testing, which will lead to a more accurate diagnosis. For example, injuries along the first-order neuron include commonly lateral medullary infarction, as well as strokes, tumors, and demyelinating afflictions, and usually are associated with other neurologic signs such as weakness, sensory deficits, hoarseness, and possible vertigo. Second-order neuron injuries include apical pulmonary tumors and thyroid malignancies. Several regional anesthesia procedures such as epidural nerve blocks may produce Horner syndrome symptoms due to the effect of local anesthetics on the preganglionic neuron. Third-order neuron syndromes include diseases of the carotid artery, such as aneurysm, dissection, thrombosis, and even carotid endarterectomy. In these cases, common symptoms are face and neck pain.[62]

Pharmacologic confirmation of the diagnosis can be performing utilizing either cocaine or apraclonidine eye drops. Cocaine blocks the reuptake of NE and induces pupillary dilatation more in the normal eye than in the Horner pupil. Apraclonidine, a direct α-adrenergic receptor agonist, causes pupillary dilatation in the Horner pupil and constriction in the normal pupil.

In order to determine the location of the lesion along the sympathetic tract, one can utilize a few drops of hydroxyamphetamine, or its derivative pholedrine, which release NE. In cases of first- or second-order Horner, the pupil will dilate, while in third-order Horner's, the pupil will not dilate. Neuroimaging with CT scanning, and even MRI, are required for a more precise diagnosis.

Treatment is mainly supportive and based on the cause and location of the offending lesion.[62]

Diabetic Neuropathy

Diabetic neuropathy is probably the best-known affliction caused by ANS dysfunction. There is a progression of the symptoms with sensory loss initially and motor weakness as the disease progresses. The first symptoms relate to a deficiency in vibratory sensation, as well as impairment of sensation to pain, light touch, and temperature, classically characterized as a "stocking-glove" sensory deficit. These symptoms are associated with depressed ankle reflexes, and a gradual evolution toward more generalized motor weakness and loss of reflexes. This is not an uncommon occurrence in adult-onset diabetes, with a prevalence of approximately 41.9% to 26.4%, in a more recent study.[63–65] Diabetic neuropathy can predispose patients to the development of foot ulcers, either acute or chronic, as well as muscle and joint pathology, including muscle atrophy, arthropathies, and stress fractures.

There are several methods of assessing the severity of neuropathy, which can be mild, moderate, or severe. Electrodiagnostic testing is necessary for atypical presentations, as well as for classification in clinical and epidemiologic studies. A combination of large and small fiber dysfunction is important for the diagnosis of diabetic neuropathy.[66,67]

Orthostatic Hypotension

Orthostatic hypotension is characterized by a decrease in blood pressure after standing or eating, and can be manifested by dizziness and syncope, which may progress to angina and, in rare cases, even to death. In normal circumstances, upon standing, a certain volume of blood is pooled by gravity toward the splanchnic vessels and lower extremities, which leads to a decrease in venous return and subsequently a drop in blood pressure. The normal response is a compensatory mechanism that involves the central and peripheral nervous system and consists of an increase in sympathetic outflow that instead raises the peripheral vascular resistance, venous return, and CO and maintains blood pressure within normal limits. The main conditions that lead to orthostatic hypotension are autonomic dysfunction and significant hypovolemia, and they appear to be more common in the elderly population.

These conditions are different from short-lived reflex syncope, which includes vasovagal, situational, and carotid sinus syncope; reflex syncope manifests with vasodilation and bradycardia instead of expected tachycardia, which subsequently causes hypotension followed by cerebral hypoperfusion, and thus causes the main symptom of temporary loss of consciousness.[68]

This condition may be due to neurodegenerative diseases whose common denominator is inappropriately low release of NE from the postganglionic sympathetic neurons, followed by inadequate vasoconstriction, reduced intravascular volume, and orthostatic hypotension. These diseases include Parkinson disease, dementia with Lewy bodies, multiple system atrophy, and pure autonomic failure. In addition, there are peripheral neuropathies, as well as autoimmune blockade of ganglionic transmission, that produce the same manifestations, including diabetes mellitus, Guillain–Barré, paraneoplastic autonomic neuropathy, and familial dysautonomia. Orthostatic hypotension is among the side effects of several medications including alcohol, α-blockers, antidepressants, sympathetic nervous system blockers, antiparkinsonism drugs, β-blockers, diuretics, muscle relaxants, morphine, phosphodiesterase inhibitors, sedatives, and vasodilators. Aging contributes to a decrease in baroreceptor sensitivity, and it may be the cause of milder forms of orthostatic hypotension.

Symptoms, which vary in intensity, consist of dizziness, lightheadedness, weakness, blurred vision, and in severe cases syncope, angina, or even stroke. Less specific symptoms may include generalized weakness, fatigue, cognitive slowing, neck pain, and localized headache in the posterior cervical and shoulder region, also called coat hanger headache.

Diagnosis is made when there is at least a 20 mmHg drop in systolic blood pressure and/or 10 mmHg decrease in diastolic blood pressure, associated commonly with increase in HR within 2 to 5 minutes after changing posture from supine to standing.[68]

Treatment is symptomatic, starting with removal of medications that may possibly induce this pathology, lifestyle modification, avoiding dehydration, exercise, physical maneuvers such as crossing legs when standing, increasing the salt and water intake, avoiding large meals, and drinking water with meals. Medications that can be used to alleviate symptoms include fludrocortisone, sympathetic agents such as ephedrine, phenylephrine, midodrine, other supplements such as pyridostigmine, nonsteroidal agents, caffeine, and erythropoietin. Other experimental agents including vasopressin analogs, yohimbine, somatostatin, dihydroergotamine, dihydroxyphenylserine, dopamine antagonists such as metoclopramide, atomoxetine, and even ambulatory NE infusion have been attempted with some positive results.[69,70]

Monoamine Oxidase Inhibitors

Monoamine oxidase inhibitors (MAOIs) and tricyclic antidepressants are used to treat psychotic depression.[71,72] These drugs are not used in the practice of anesthesia but are a source of potentially serious anesthetic interactions in patients who take them chronically. Their use is rapidly declining, as nontricyclic antidepressants are more efficacious and produce fewer side effects. Few of the MAOIs or tricyclic antidepressants will be encountered in anesthesia practice today, with the exceptions of phenelzine (Nardil) and amitriptyline (Amitril, Elavil). Their pharmacologic actions and side effects are the direct result of their effect on the cascade of catecholamine metabolism. MAOIs block the oxidative deamination of endogenous catecholamines into inactive vanillylmandelic acid. They do not inhibit synthesis. Thus, blockade of MAO would produce an accumulation of NE, EPI, dopamine, and 5-HT in adrenergically active tissues, including the brain. The action of sympathomimetic amines is potentiated in patients taking MAOIs. Indirect-acting sympathomimetics (ephedrine, tyramine) produce an exaggerated response as they trigger the release of accumulated catecholamines. Foods containing a high tyramine content such as cheese, red Italian wine, and pickled herring can also precipitate hypertensive crises.[73] Meperidine has been reported to produce hypertensive crisis, convulsions, and coma in patients with MAOIs. Hepatotoxicity has been reported that does not seem to be related to dosage or duration of treatment. Its incidence is low but remains a factor in selecting anesthesia.

The anesthetic management of patients taking MAOIs remains controversial. Currently, recommendations for management include discontinuation of the drugs for at least 2 weeks before surgery; however, this recommendation is not based on controlled studies but rather limited case reports that suggest potent drug interactions.

Tricyclic Antidepressants

On the basis of their chemical structure, this group of antidepressant drugs is referred to as tricyclic antidepressants. These drugs have almost replaced MAOIs, since they have fewer side effects, and they are used for other indications including neuropathic pain.[74] All of these agents block uptake of NE into adrenergic nerve endings. Just as with MAOIs, high doses of tricyclic antidepressants can induce seizure activity that is responsive to diazepam. Neuroleptic drugs may potentiate the effects of tricyclic antidepressants by competition with metabolism in the liver. Chronic barbiturate use increases metabolism of tricyclic antidepressants by microsomal enzyme induction. Other sedatives, however, potentiate the tricyclic antidepressants in a manner similar to that occurring with MAOIs. Atropine also has an exaggerated effect because of the anticholinergic effect of tricyclic antidepressants. Prolonged sedation from thiopental has been reported. Ketamine may also be dangerous in patients taking tricyclic antidepressants by producing acute hypertension and cardiac dysrhythmias. The latency of onset of tricyclic antidepressants is from 2 to 5 weeks Despite potentially serious interactions, discontinuation of these drugs before surgery is probably not necessary. A thorough knowledge of the possible drug interactions and autonomic countermeasures now available obviates the need for treatment interruption.

Selective Serotonin Reuptake Inhibitors

The mechanism of action of the selective serotonin reuptake inhibitors (SSRIs) appears to be the selective inhibition of neuronal uptake of serotonin. This potentiates the behavioral changes induced by the serotonin precursor 5-hydroxytryptophan.[75–77] The availability of sympathetic antagonists for treatment of possible side effects during anesthesia weighs in favor of continuation of therapy versus the risk of exacerbation of a severe depression. Prozac (fluoxetine) is a popular oral nontricyclic antidepressant. The elimination half-life of Prozac is 1 to 3 days and can lead to significant accumulation of the drug. Prozac's metabolism, like that of other compounds, including tricyclic antidepressants, phenobarbital, ethanol, and pentothal, involves the P450 II D6 system; concomitant therapy with drugs also metabolized by this enzyme system may lead to drug interactions and prolongation of effect of the benzodiazepines. Bupropion hydrochloride is available in a both a regular (Wellbutrin) and sustained-release (Zyban) form. Wellbutrin is used as an antidepressant, whereas Zyban is marketed as a nonnicotine aid to smoking cessation. The neurochemical mechanism of the antidepressant effect of bupropion is not known. It does not inhibit MAO and is a weak blocker of the neuronal uptake of serotonin and NE. It also inhibits the neuronal uptake of dopamine to some extent. No systematic data have been collected on the interactions of bupropion and other drugs. Patients with heart disease have emerged as a special category due to the finding that depression significantly affects cardiovascular health. Several studies support the safety of SSRIs in these patients due to their association with a decrease in morbidity and mortality, and the need for continuous treatment, especially in the elderly. Nevertheless, there is some evidence, although small, that these drugs may increase the risk of bleeding. Since these patients may concomitantly use other antiplatelet/anticoagulation therapies, increased vigilance is mandatory.[78]

For further review and interactivities, please see the videos and narrative interactive clinical vignettes (NICVs) accessible in the complimentary eBook bundled with this text. Access instructions are located on the inside front cover.

REFERENCES

1. Hall JE, Hall ME. The autonomic nervous system and the adrenal medulla. In: Hall JE, Hall ME eds. *Guyton and Hall Textbook of Medical Physiology*. 14th ed. Elsevier; 2020.
2. Gibbons CH. Basics of autonomic nervous system function. *Handb Clin Neurol*. 2019;160: 407–418.
3. Waxenbaum JA, Reddy V, Varacallo M. Anatomy, Autonomic Nervous System. [Updated 2022 Jul 25]. In: *StatPearls [Internet]*. Treasure Island (FL): StatPearls Publishing; 2023 Jan. Available from: https://www.ncbi.nlm.nih.gov/books/NBK539845/
4. Brooks-Fournier R, Coggeshall RE. The ratio of preganglionic axons to postganglionic cells in the sympathetic nervous system of the rat. *J Comp Neurol*. 1981;197:207–216.
5. Gibbins I. Functional organization of autonomic neural pathways. *Organogenesis*. 2013;9:169–175.
6. Wolf Jr GA. The ratio of preganglionic neurons to postganglionic neurons in the visceral nervous system. *J Comp Neurol*. 1941;75:235–243.
7. Armstrong R, Wheen P, Brandon L, Maree A, Kenny RA. Heart rate: control mechanisms, pathophysiology and assessment of the neurocardiac system in health and disease. *QJM*. 2022;115:806–812.
8. Kishi T. Heart failure as an autonomic nervous system dysfunction. *J Cardiol*. 2012;59:117–122.
9. Zhang DY, Anderson AS. The sympathetic nervous system and heart failure. *Cardiol Clin*. 2014; 32:33–45, vii.
10. Florea VG, Cohn JN. The autonomic nervous system and heart failure. *Circ Res*. 2014;114: 1815–1826.
11. Goodwill AG, Dick GM, Kiel AM, Tune JD. Regulation of coronary blood flow. *Compr Physiol*. 2017;7:321–382.
12. Bruno RM, Ghiadoni L, Seravalle G, Dell'oro R, Taddei S, Grassi G. Sympathetic regulation of vascular function in health and disease. *Front Physiol*. 2012;3:284.
13. McCorry LK. Physiology of the autonomic nervous system. *Am J Pharm Educ*. 2007;71:78.
14. Becker DE. Basic and clinical pharmacology of autonomic drugs. *Anesth Prog*. 2012;59: 159–168; quiz 169.
15. Giovannitti JA Jr, Thoms SM, Crawford JJ. Alpha-2 adrenergic receptor agonists: a review of current clinical applications. *Anesth Prog*. 2015;62:31–39.
16. Stanford SC, Heal DJ. Catecholamines: knowledge and understanding in the 1960s, now, and in the future. *Brain Neurosci Adv*. 2019;3:2398212818810682.
17. Martyn JAJ, Fagerlund MJ, Eriksson LI. Basic principles of neuromuscular transmission. *Anaesthesia*. 2009;64:1–9.
18. Bylund DB. Adrenergic receptors. In: Perez DM, ed. *The Adrenergic Receptors: In the 21st Century*. Humana Press, 2006: 3–21.
19. Richer LP, Vinet A, Kus T, Cardinal R, Ardell JL, Armour JA. Alpha-adrenoceptor blockade modifies neurally induced atrial arrhythmias. *Am J Physiol Regul Integr Comp Physiol*. 2008; 295:R1175–R1180.
20. Motiejunaite J, Amar L, Vidal-Petiot E. Adrenergic receptors and cardiovascular effects of catecholamines. *Ann Endocrinol (Paris)*. 2021;82:193–197.
21. Jensen BC, O'Connell TD, Simpson PC. Alpha-1-adrenergic receptors: targets for agonist drugs to treat heart failure. *J Mol Cell Cardiol*. 2011;51:518–528
22. Santulli G, Iaccarino G. Adrenergic signaling in heart failure and cardiovascular aging. *Maturitas*. 2016;93:65–72.
23. Naaz S, Ozair E. Dexmedetomidine in current anaesthesia practice- a review. *J Clin Diagn Res*. 2014;8:Ge01–Ge04.
24. Wang Y, Yuan J, Qian Z, et al. β2 adrenergic receptor activation governs cardiac repolarization and arrhythmogenesis in a guinea pig model of heart failure. *Sci Rep*. 2015;5:7681.
25. Woo AYH, Xiao RP. β-Adrenergic receptor subtype signaling in heart: From bench to bedside. *Acta Pharmacol Sin*. 2012;33:335–341.
26. De Backer D, Biston P, Devriendt J, et al; SOAP II Investigators. Comparison of dopamine and norepinephrine in the treatment of shock. *N Engl J Med*. 2010;362:779–789.
27. Juárez Olguín H, Calderón Guzmán D, Hernández García E, Barragán Mejía G. The role of dopamine and its dysfunction as a consequence of oxidative stress. *Oxid Med Cell Longev*. 2016;2016:9730467.
28. Channer B, Matt SM, Nickoloff-Bybel EA, et al. Dopamine, Immunity, and Disease. *Pharmacol Rev*. 2023;75:62–158.
29. Guieu R, Deharo JC, Maille B, et al. Adenosine and the cardiovascular system: the good and the bad. *J Clin Med*. 2020;9(5):1366.
30. Lohse MJ, Engelhardt S, Eschenhagen T. What is the role of β-adrenergic signaling in heart failure? *Circ Res*. 2003;93:896–906.
31. Kougias P, Weakley SM, Yao Q, Lin PH, Chen C. Arterial baroreceptors in the management of systemic hypertension. *Med Sci Monit*. 2010;16:Ra1–Ra8.
32. Zhang J, Zhou S, Xu G. Carotid baroreceptor stimulation: a potential solution for resistant hypertension. *Interv Neurol*. 2014;2:118–122.
33. Awad M, Czer LSC, Hou M, et al. Early denervation and later reinnervation of the heart following cardiac transplantation: a review. *J Am Heart Assoc*. 2016;5:e004070.
34. Kruse AC, Kobilka BK, Gautam D, Sexton PM, Christopoulos A, Wess J. Muscarinic acetylcholine receptors: novel opportunities for drug development. *Nat Rev Drug Discov*. 2014;13: 549–560.
35. Yasue H, Mizuno Y, Harada E. Coronary artery spasm – clinical features, pathogenesis and treatment. *Proc Jpn Acad Ser B Phys Biol Sci*. 2019;95:53–66.
36. Miyamoto T, Kawada T, Takaki H, et al. High plasma norepinephrine attenuates the dynamic heart rate response to vagal stimulation. *Am J Physiol Heart Circ Physiol*. 2003;284:H2412–H2418.
37. Wilkins BW, Hesse C, Charkoudian N, et al. Autonomic cardiovascular control during a novel pharmacologic alternative to ganglionic blockade. *Clin Pharmacol Ther*. 2008;83:692–701.
38. Colović MB, Krstić DZ, Lazarević-Pašti TD, Bondžić AM, Vasić VM. Acetylcholinesterase inhibitors: pharmacology and toxicology. *Curr Neuropharmacol*. 2013;11:315–335.
39. Arens AM, Shah K, Al-Abri S, Olson KR, Kearney T. Safety and effectiveness of physostigmine: a 10-year retrospective review. *Clin Toxicol (Phila)*. 2018;56:101–107.
40. Kassa J. Review of oximes in the antidotal treatment of poisoning by organophosphorus nerve agents. *J Toxicol Clin Toxicol*. 2002;40:803–816.
41. Poterman M, Scheeren TWL, van der Velde MI, et al. Prophylactic atropine administration attenuates the negative haemodynamic effects of induction of anaesthesia with propofol and high-dose remifentanil: a randomised controlled trial. *Eur J Anaesthesiol*. 2017;34:695–701.
42. Deshar R, Subedi A, Pokharel K, Sah BP, Prasad JN. Effect of glycopyrrolate on vasopressor requirements for non-elective cesarean section under spinal anesthesia: a randomized, double-blind, placebo-controlled trial. *BMC Anesthesiol*. 2022;22:327.
43. Lochner M, Thompson AJ. The muscarinic antagonists scopolamine and atropine are competitive antagonists at 5-HT3 receptors. *Neuropharmacology*. 2016;108:220–228.
44. Zhao C, Cai C, Ding Q, Dai H. Efficacy and safety of atropine to control myopia progression: a systematic review and meta-analysis. *BMC Ophthalmol*. 2020;20:478.
45. Cook B, Spence AA. Post-operative central anticholinergic syndrome. *Eur J Anaesthesiol*. 1997;14:1–2.
46. Lott EL, Jones EB. Cholinergic Toxicity. [Updated 2022 Dec 5.] In: *StatPearls [Internet]*. Treasure Island (FL): StatPearls Publishing; 2023 Jan. Available from: https://www.ncbi.nlm.nih.gov/books/NBK539783/.
47. Martins DF, Viseux FJF, Salm DC, et al. The role of the vagus nerve in fibromyalgia syndrome. *Neurosci Biobehav Rev*. 2021;131:1136–1149.
48. Yuen AWC, Sander JW. Can natural ways to stimulate the vagus nerve improve seizure control? *Epilepsy Behav*. 2017;67:105–110.
49. Szurhaj W, Troussière AC, Logier R, et al. Ictal changes in parasympathetic tone: prediction of postictal oxygen desaturation. *Neurology*. 2015;85:1233–1239.
50. Khemani P, Mehdirad AA. Cardiovascular disorders mediated by autonomic nervous system dysfunction. *Cardiol Rev*. 2020;28:65–72.
51. Huang WA, Boyle NG, Vaseghi M. Cardiac innervation and the autonomic nervous system in sudden cardiac death. *Card Electrophysiol Clin*. 2017;9:665–679.
52. Nasi-Er BG, Wenhui Z, HuaXin S, et al. Vagus nerve stimulation reduces ventricular arrhythmias and increases ventricular electrical stability. *Pacing Clin Electrophysiol*. 2019;42:247–256.
53. Wu P, Vaseghi M. The autonomic nervous system and ventricular arrhythmias in myocardial infarction and heart failure. *Pacing Clin Electrophysiol*. 2020;43:172–180.
54. Shen MJ, Zipes DP. Role of the autonomic nervous system in modulating cardiac arrhythmias. *Circ Res*. 2014;114:1004–1021.
55. Mancia G, Grassi G. The autonomic nervous system and hypertension. *Circ Res*. 2014;114: 1804–1814.
56. Eick C, Rizas KD, Meyer-Zürn CS, et al. Autonomic nervous system activity as risk predictor in the medical emergency department: a prospective cohort study. *Crit Care Med*. 2015;43: 1079–1086.
57. Thijs RD, Ryvlin P, Surges R. Autonomic manifestations of epilepsy: emerging pathways to sudden death? *Nat Rev Neurol*. 2021;17:774–788.
58. Bermeo-Ovalle AC, Kennedy JD, Schuele SU. Cardiac and autonomic mechanisms contributing to SUDEP. *J Clin Neurophysiol*. 2015;32:21–29.
59. Purkayastha S, Stokes M, Bell KR. Autonomic nervous system dysfunction in mild traumatic brain injury: a review of related pathophysiology and symptoms. *Brain Inj*. 2019;33:1129–1136.
60. Miroslawska AK, Gjessing PF, Solbu MD, Fuskevåg OM, Jenssen TG, Steigen TK. Renal denervation for resistant hypertension fails to improve insulin resistance as assessed by hyperinsulinemic-euglycemic step clamp. *Diabetes*. 2016;65:2164–2168.
61. Gamboa A, Okamoto LE, Arnold AC, et al. Autonomic blockade improves insulin sensitivity in obese subjects. *Hypertension*. 2014;64:867–874.
62. Martin TJ, Horner syndrome: a clinical review. *ACS Chem Neurosci*. 2018;9:177–186.
63. Feldman EL, Callaghan BC, Pop-Busui R, et al. Diabetic neuropathy. *Nat Rev Dis Primers*. 2019;5:42.
64. Vinik AI, Nevoret ML, Casellini C, Parson H. Diabetic neuropathy. *Endocrinol Metab Clin North Am*. 2013;42:747–787.
65. Rosenberger DC, Blechschmidt V, Timmerman H, Wolff A, Treede RD. Challenges of neuropathic pain: focus on diabetic neuropathy. *J Neural Transm (Vienna)*. 2020;127:589–624.

66. Selvarajah D, Kar D, Khunti K, et al. Diabetic peripheral neuropathy: advances in diagnosis and strategies for screening and early intervention. *Lancet Diabetes Endocrinol*. 2019;7:938–948.
67. Carmichael J, Fadavi H, Ishibashi F, Shore AC, Tavakoli M. Advances in screening, early diagnosis and accurate staging of diabetic neuropathy. *Front Endocrinol (Lausanne)*. 2021;12:671257.
68. Wieling W, Kaufmann H, Claydon VE, et al. Diagnosis and treatment of orthostatic hypotension. *Lancet Neurol*. 2022;21:735–746.
69. Palma JA, Kaufmann H. Management of orthostatic hypotension. *Continuum (Minneap Minn)*. 2020;26:154–177.
70. Santer P, Anstey MH, Patrocínio MD, et al; MIDAS Study Group. Effect of midodrine versus placebo on time to vasopressor discontinuation in patients with persistent hypotension in the intensive care unit (MIDAS): an international randomised clinical trial. *Intensive Care Med*. 2020;46:1884–1893.
71. Thase ME. The role of monoamine oxidase inhibitors in depression treatment guidelines. *J Clin Psychiatry*. 2012;73(Suppl 1):10–16.
72. Saraghi M, Golden LR, Hersh EV. Anesthetic considerations for patients on antidepressant therapy-part I. *Anesth Prog*. 2017;64:253–261.
73. Burns C, Kidron A. Biochemistry, Tyramine. [Updated 2022 Oct 10]. In: *StatPearls [Internet]*. Treasure Island (FL): StatPearls Publishing; 2023 Jan. Available from: https://www.ncbi.nlm.nih.gov/books/NBK563197/.63197/
74. Schneider J, Patterson M, Jimenez XF. Beyond depression: other uses for tricyclic antidepressants. *Cleve Clin J Med*. 2019;86:807–814.
75. Patetsos E, Horjales-Araujo E. Treating chronic pain with SSRIs: what do we know? *Pain Res Manag*. 2016;2016:2020915.
76. Hofmann SG, Curtiss J, Carpenter JK, Kind S. Effect of treatments for depression on quality of life: a meta-analysis. *Cogn Behav Ther*. 2017;46:265–286.
77. Joshi A. Selective serotonin re-uptake inhibitors: an overview. *Psychiatr Danub*. 2018;30:605–609.
78. Laporte S, Chapelle C, Caillet P, et al. Bleeding risk under selective serotonin reuptake inhibitor (SSRI) antidepressants: a meta-analysis of observational studies. *Pharmacol Res*. 2017;118:19–32.

15 Respiratory Function in Anesthesia

TIMOTHY G. GAULTON • MAURIZIO CEREDA

KEY POINTS

1. Elastic and restrictive forces are the major impedances to the delivery of air into the lungs.
2. Functional residual capacity has a key role in determining oxygen reserves, propensity to atelectasis, and biologic effects of mechanical ventilation.
3. Driving pressure is a surrogate for global lung strain. Higher values are associated with increased risk of postoperative pulmonary complications.
4. Anesthesia results in smaller and stiffer lungs, primarily due to atelectasis. Trendelenburg position, obesity, and pneumoperitoneum further reduce respiratory system compliance.
5. Ventilation and perfusion mismatch is common during anesthesia. Shunt physiology, due to atelectasis, is the primary etiology of hypoxemia and can be addressed with restoration of end-expiratory lung volume.
6. As the amount of shunt increases, oxygen content in pulmonary venous blood has a greater contribution to arterial oxygenation and delivery.
7. Dead space volume increases during anesthesia. Instrumental dead space from breathing devices can be significant when alveolar ventilation is already maximized.
8. Anesthetics disrupt different aspects of ventilator control in a dose-dependent manner and cause alveolar hypoventilation.
9. There is no compelling evidence that defines rules for ordering preoperative pulmonary function tests. Rather, they should only be obtained to ascertain the presence of reversible pulmonary dysfunction (bronchospasm) or to define the severity of advanced pulmonary disease.
10. Individuals with morbid obesity are at high risk of postoperative pulmonary complications. Use of continuous positive airway pressure after tracheal extubation can improve their end-expiratory lung volumes.
11. Multidisciplinary perioperative pulmonary rehabilitation improves pulmonary outcomes in individuals at high risk of complications.

Introduction

Whether in delivery of oxygen via simple nasal cannula or insertion of a breathing tube and initiation of invasive mechanical ventilation, anesthesiologists support respiratory function for millions of individuals undergoing procedures each year. Adverse respiratory events are common during anesthesia and can be catastrophic. Therefore, a thorough understanding of the physiology of respiratory system and how anesthesia affects breathing is fundamental to safe and effective practice in our specialty. Within this chapter, we provide a focused and practical overview of respiratory mechanics and gas exchange for the anesthesia provider.

Respiratory Mechanics

Equation of Motion

The movement of air into and out of the lungs requires there to 1
be a pressure difference between proximal (e.g., mouth) and distal (e.g., alveoli) parts of the lung. The pressure difference generates the flow of air that moves into airways and increases the volume of gas in the lungs during inflation. In unassisted breathing, the contraction of the respiratory muscles, namely the diaphragm, generates a decrease in pleural pressure in relation to atmospheric pressure, with subsequent air entry and lung expansion. In controlled breathing, proximal pressure is driven by an

artificial device such as a mechanical ventilator. In assisted breathing, a combination of the patient and the ventilator contributes to the needed pressure difference. The movement of air into the lungs however does not occur unimpeded. Two major forces of physical impedance can challenge the flow of air into the lungs—(1) the resistance of the airways and tissue, and (2) the elastance, or stiffness, of the respiratory system. The higher the resistance and/or the stiffer the lungs or chest wall, the lower the flow of gas that enters the lung. Higher airway or pleural pressures are therefore required to maintain appropriate lung volume.

The equation of motion allows for the mathematical description of the total airway pressure (P_{aw}) needed for air movement during inflation and reflects resistive (P_{res}) and elastic forces (P_{el}):

$$P_{aw} = P_{res} + P_{el} + PEEP \quad (15\text{-}1)$$

$$P_{aw} = P_{vent} + P_{musc} = V_t \times E_{RC} + R_{aw} \times \dot{V}_I + PEEP + PEEP_i \quad (15\text{-}2)$$

where P_{vent} is the airway pressure applied by the ventilator, P_{mus} is the pressure generated from patient inspiratory muscles, V_t is tidal volume, E_{RS} is respiratory system elastance, R_{aw} is airway resistance, $\dot{V}_I$ is inspiratory flow, PEEP is the positive end-expiratory pressure, and $PEEP_i$ is intrinsic PEEP. The equation above is the most basic model of the respiratory system. All these variables—resistance, elastance, pressure, flow, and volume—are interdependent. More complex models do exist that account for the complexity of these relationships, including how resistance and elastance change with different volumes and flow.[1] Moreover, there are frictional impediments to gas flow within the airway and lung tissue, in addition to inertia. For the sake of practical simplicity, we will focus on the elastic and resistive forces of the respiratory system, as these are major determinants of airway pressure most disrupted—and modifiable—by anesthesia.

Work and Power of Breathing

With each breath, energy is required to generate change in airway pressure and move a volume of air into the lungs. Work of breathing is the product of pressure and volume. Work is expressed in joules per liter of ventilation with 1 J representing the energy needed to move 1 L of gas across a 10 cmH_2O pressure difference. A higher pressure for each breath requires more work. Mechanical power, in contrast, represents the work applied to the lung per unit of time in joules per minute. Mechanical power incorporates respiratory rate and inspiratory flow. Studies suggest that mechanical power determines lung injury during mechanical ventilation, via energy transfer to the tissues.[2] A key goal of mechanical ventilation is to both reduce work of breathing and minimize the mechanical power applied to the lung. A key goal of the anesthesiologists is to understand and optimize elastic and resistive forces that may otherwise become excessive and cause harm.

Elastic Forces

The stiffness of an elastic body can be described by compliance—the change in volume per unit change in the pressure difference across the elastic body (i.e., transmural pressure). Compliance has become a term far more verbalized in clinical practice as opposed to its reciprocal, elastance. For the respiratory system, the compliance of the lungs (C_L) and chest wall (C_{cw}) contribute to the total compliance of the respiratory system (C_{RS}) in series, similar to electrical capacitances.

$$1/C_L + 1/C_{cw} = 1/C_{RS} \quad (15\text{-}3)$$

2 For the lung, transmural pressure is termed transpulmonary pressure (P_L) and represents the difference between pressure in the alveolus (P_{alv}) and pressure in the pleural space (P_{pl}). P_{alv} is often estimated by airway pressure, whereas P_{pl} is often estimated by esophageal pressure, as discussed below. P_L is a marker of deforming lung stress, defined as the force applied over an area of lung. For the chest wall, transmural pressure is between atmospheric pressure and P_{pl}. In healthy individuals, the compliance of the chest wall and the lung are equal, and the ratio of C_L/C_{RS} is ~0.5. However, C_{RS} is nonlinear and varies across a range of lung volume as shown in Figure 15-1. Peak compliance typically occurs near functional residual capacity (FRC) when the inherent recoil of the lungs is equally balanced by the inherent expansion of the chest wall. FRC has a key role in determining oxygen reserves, propensity to atelectasis, and biologic effects of mechanical ventilation. As lung volume increases or decreases beyond FRC, compliance may worsen, illustrating the nonlinear pressure–volume relationship of the lung.

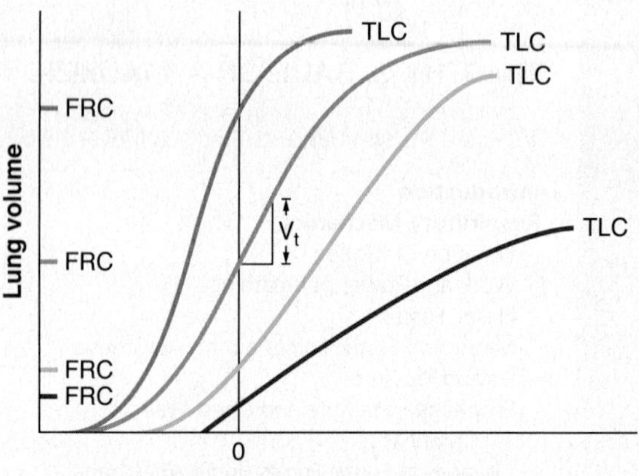

Figure 15-1 Pulmonary pressure–volume relationships at different values of total lung capacity (TLC), ignoring hysteresis. The *blue* depicts the normal pulmonary pressure–volume relationships. Humans normally breathe on the linear, steep part of this sigmoidal curve, where the slope (equal to compliance) is greatest. The *black vertical line* at zero defines functional residual capacity (FRC), regardless of the position of the curve on the graph. Mild restrictive lung disease, indicated by the *green* line, shifts the curve to the right with little change in slope. However, with restrictive disease, the patient breathes on a lower FRC, at a point on the curve where the slope is less. Severe restrictive pulmonary disease profoundly depresses the FRC and diminishes the slope of the entire curve (*red line*). Obstructive disease (*orange line*) elevates both FRC and compliance.

Forces other than transmural pressure also dictate lung expansion and collapse. For example, the lung has an inherent architecture that contains bronchioles and alveolar walls tethered together in a tissue matrix.[3] Major divisions of the right and left lung are listed in Table 15-1. Pressure applied to one part of the lung will undoubtably transmit within its architecture to other regions in a very interdependent process. Surface tension tends to cause alveoli to collapse as their size decreases; however, this is mitigated by the life-saving effect of pulmonary surfactant. For a bubble to remain inflated, the gas pressure within the bubble is contained by surface tension and must be higher than the surrounding gas pressure. Alveoli resemble bubbles in this respect, but unlike a bubble, alveolar gas communicates with the atmosphere via the airways. The Laplace equation describes this phenomenon: $P = 2T/R$, where P is the pressure within the bubble ($dyn \times cm^{-2}$), T is the surface tension of the liquid ($dyn \times cm^{-1}$), and R is the radius of the bubble (cm).

During inspiration, the surface tension of the liquid in the lung increases to 40 mN/m, a value close to that of plasma. During

Table 15-1 Major Divisions of the Lung

Lung Side/Lobe	Bronchopulmonary Segment
Right	
Upper	Apical Anterior Posterior
Middle	Medial Lateral
Lower	Superior Medial basal Lateral basal Anterior basal Posterior basal
Left	
Upper	Apical posterior Anterior
Lingula	Superior Inferior
Lower	Superior Posterior basal Anteromedial basal Lateral basal

expiration, this surface tension falls to 19 mN/m, a value lower than that of most other fluids. This change in surface tension creates hysteresis of the alveoli—the phenomenon of different pressure–volume relationships of the alveoli during inspiration versus expiration (Fig. 15-2). Unlike a bubble, the pressure within an alveolus decreases as the radius of curvature decreases, creating gas flow from larger to smaller alveoli that maintains structural stability and prevents lung collapse.

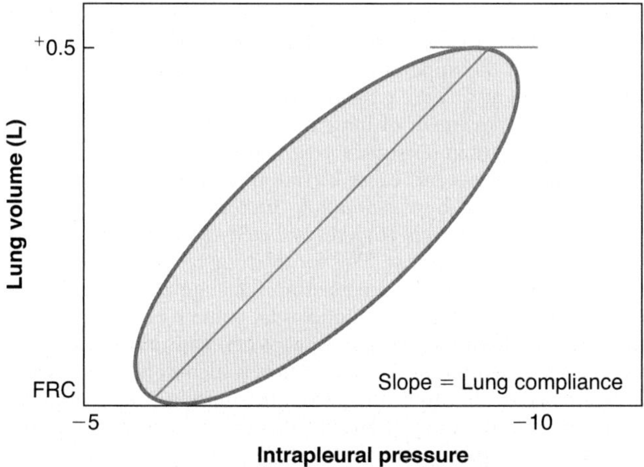

Figure 15-2 Dynamic pressure–volume loop of resting tidal volume. Quiet, normal breathing is characterized by hysteresis of the pressure–volume loop. The lung is more resistant to deformation than expected and returns to its original configuration less easily than expected. The slope of the line connecting the zenith and nadir lung volumes is lung compliance, about 500 mL/3 cm H_2O = 167 mL/cm H_2O.

Measuring Elastic Forces during Anesthesia

When a volume of air fills the lung, subsequent pressure can be measured to calculate compliance. Ideally, compliance is measured during a prolonged inspiratory pause (at least 3 seconds). The pressure measured after inflation with a certain volume is termed the plateau pressure. C_{rs} can then be measured from the following formula:

$$C_{RS} = \Delta V_t/\Delta P \text{ where } \Delta P = \text{Plateau} - \text{PEEP} \qquad (15\text{-}4)$$

Absence of flow never truly occurs, however. Passive expiration results in an immediate decrease in airway pressure. When preocclusion flow is defined, this pressure can be used to quantify airway resistance. A second and slower change then occurs that reflects equilibration of pressure across compartments of the lung.[4] Gas redistribution in the absence tidal volume change can occur between regions of the lung with different regional mechanics and time constants known as *pendelluft*.[5,6] Decreases in pressure after interruption of flow may also occur due to recovery of lung tissue from a state of stress.[7,8] In a normal lung with homogeneous time constants, pendelluft is minimal. Regardless, most anesthesia machine ventilators do not allow for a long enough inspiratory pause to achieve a static condition. Instead, plateau pressure can be approximated through the addition of a brief (0.2 to 1 second) end-inspiratory pause. In this setting, flow remains present, resulting in higher pressures and lower calculated respiratory system compliance when compared to truly static conditions.

Driving Pressure

3

Driving pressure represents the change in volume of the lung above FRC and is a surrogate for global lung strain, a marker of ventilator-induced injury and a predictor of mortality in acute respiratory distress syndrome (ARDS).[9] It is defined as plateau pressure minus PEEP or, with rearrangement of Equation 15-4, the ratio of V_t to respiratory system compliance. As compared to tidal volume, driving pressure accounts for pre-existing characteristics of the lung. Lower driving pressures during anesthesia appear to correlate with lower odds of postoperative pulmonary complications, more so than other ventilatory parameters.[10] The association, however, may be mediated through factors related to (1) inherent characteristics of the lung and (2) severity of pre-existing lung injury. Intraoperative ventilation during thoracic surgery targeted to minimizing driving pressure has been shown to lower postoperative pulmonary complications compared to a standard ventilation parameters (e.g., V_t 6 mL/kg, PEEP 5 cmH_2O) and recruitment.[11] It is critical to note that any adjustment of tidal volume needs to be done with an understanding of FRC. When driving pressure and strain are already low, further reduction in tidal volumes to meet arbitrary weight-based guidelines may be unnecessary and can result in both atelectasis and ventilator dyssynchrony in nonparalyzed individuals. In fact, lowering V_t (to 6 cc/kg or less) may increase mortality when respiratory system compliance is high, as seen in patients with acute respiratory distress syndrome.[12]

Esophageal Pressure and Chest Wall Compliance

While not a standard measurement in clinical practice, pleural pressure can allow for separate determination of C_L and C_{Cw}. Esophageal pressure (P_{es}) has been suggested as a more easily measurable surrogate for pleural pressure.[13] The most common technique for measuring P_{es} involves insertion of a balloon-catheter filled with air into the esophagus and connected to a pressure transducer. Expanding on Equation 15-2, the required pressure needed for inflation (ΔP_{aw}) can be divided into components that (1) moves the lungs—the change in transpulmonary pressure (ΔP_L) and (2) moves the chest wall—the change in pleural pressure (ΔP_{pl}). From here, the C_L and C_{cw} may be calculated based on the following formulas, respectively, to determine the relative ratio of C_L and C_{cw} to C_{rs}.

$$C_L = \Delta V_t/[P_{L,\ end\text{-}inspiration} - P_{L,\ end\text{-}expiration}] \quad (15\text{-}5)$$

$$C_{cw} = \Delta V_t/[P_{pl,\ end\text{-}inspiration} - P_{pl,\ end\text{-}expiration}] \quad (15\text{-}6)$$

In addition, transpulmonary pressure can be used to set (1) PEEP to achieve a positive P_L at the end of expiration of 0 to 5 cmH_2O and (2) tidal volumes to achieve a P_L at the end of inspiration of <20 cmH_2O in a noninjured lung.[13,14]

Changes in Elastic Forces under Anesthesia

4 Several changes to the chest wall and lung occur during anesthesia that impact respiratory system compliance and FRC. Overall, the lungs become smaller and relatively stiffer during anesthesia. The main reason for the decrease in the size of the lung is due to its deaeration, termed atelectasis. Atelectasis under anesthesia is universal and occurs with any anesthetic—intravenous or inhalational, whether breathing is spontaneous or controlled, and whether the lungs are healthy or sick.[15] Up to one-fifth of normally aerated lung can become collapsed or poorly aerated under anesthesia, as visualized with computed tomography.[16] Of concern, atelectasis is still present in most patients during recovery from anesthesia, and results in prolonged hypoxemia and the potential need for invasive ventilation in certain susceptible populations.[17] Application of continuous airway pressure through a noninvasive interface, such as a face-mask following tracheal extubation, may prevent atelectasis and help restore lung function in patients with morbid obesity.[18] More dramatically, atelectasis and decreased inspiratory strength persists weeks to months after median sternotomy for cardiac operations.[19] The principal cause of atelectasis is likely from compressive forces due to an increase in regional pleural pressure (P_{pl}). Without a positive distending pressure, alveolar collapse occurs. P_{pl} is partially dependent on gravity, becoming more positive in dependent areas of the lung. P_{pl} increases during anesthesia as the diaphragm shifts further into the thorax when relaxed, and becomes less capable of preventing pressure transmission from abdomen. The loss of tone in respiratory muscles, exacerbated with neuromuscular paralysis, decreases the overall cross-sectional area of the chest wall and limits its outward expansion. Pressure transmission across the diaphragm can be minimized with upright positioning.

It is not surprising that compliance is even lower in certain clinical scenarios that increase the weight in the abdomen and the force applied across the diaphragm and chest wall (e.g., Trendelenburg position, obesity, or when inappropriate low tidal ventilation is applied). When pleural pressure is elevated, high airway pressure is required to maintain positive transpulmonary pressure and limit alveolar collapse during exhalation. Airway pressure can be applied without either excessive lung stress and significant adverse hemodynamic compromise in this setting. Even with physiology in mind, the PROBESE trial comparing PEEP of 4 cmH_2O to a PEEP of 12 cmH_2O with recruitment maneuvers in obese patients under general anesthesia did not demonstrate a meaningful difference in the incidence of postoperative pulmonary complications (e.g., pneumonia).[20] However, obese patients in the higher PEEP and recruitment group displayed lower driving pressures and rates of hypoxemia intraoperatively, suggesting improvement in end-expiratory lung volumes. Moreover, postoperative pulmonary complications are influenced by several factors unrelated to intraoperative ventilator management. Finally, the technique of recruitment is impactful. A recruitment approach found to be beneficial in obese individuals with ARDS can be applied,[21] whereby the ventilator can be set to pressure control ventilation with driving pressure of 10 cmH_2O, I:E ratio 1:1, respiratory rate 10 and a stepwise increase in PEEP by 5 cmH_2O every 30 seconds up to a maximal plateau pressure of 50 cmH_2O and maintained for 1 minute.

Notably, pneumoperitoneum has a different effect on respiratory system compliance than obesity. Obesity shifts the pressure–volume curve of the chest wall to right without a change of shape. Lung compliance is therefore more negatively affected.[22] In pneumoperitoneum, the thoracic cavity changes shape, resulting in reduced chest wall compliance with relative preservation of lung compliance.[23] A higher proportion of applied airway pressure then goes into moving the chest wall rather than lungs.

Another key mechanism of atelectasis during anesthesia is resorption. Resorption occurs when the rate of gas flow out of alveoli into blood exceeds the rate of gas flow into alveoli (as distal airways close). Significant airway closure has been seen in obese individuals under general anesthesia with pneumoperitoneum.[24] If delivered airway pressure does not exceed the pressure required to open these proximal airways, no ventilation occurs and gas remains trapped. Airway closure is exacerbated during Trendelenburg positioning. Resorption atelectasis may occur even in the absence of distal airway occlusion with (1) alveoli that have low ventilation/perfusion (V/Q) ratios and (2) when the rate of gas leaving the alveoli is increased such as when high concentrations of inspired oxygen are used or mixed venous oxygen content is low.

Resistive Forces

Increases in resistance to gas flow are common during anesthesia and alter both gas exchange and cardiovascular function. Air entering the lung must overcome the resistance of two major components before it can reach the alveoli. First, there is resistance to gas flow in the upper airways, trachea, bronchi and—if present—artificial airways (e.g., endotracheal tube). Second, there is resistance to movement of lung and chest wall tissue at a given volume. Increases in resistance during inspiration are well known to anesthesiologists and cause elevation in airway pressure, ventilator alarms, and hypoventilation. Increased airway resistance affects expiration as well. High resistance lengthens the expiratory time constant—the time it takes for the lung to empty. Mild expiratory resistance can be overcome through augmentation of inspiratory work and achieving a higher tidal volume, which increases the pressure driving expiratory flow. When expiratory resistance becomes excessive, however, expiration is incomplete and hyperinflation occurs. In this setting, accessory muscles are recruited to expel air from the lungs; however, this does not occur in deeply anesthetized or paralyzed individuals.[25]

Anatomy of the Airways

The trachea is a fibromuscular tube 10 to 12 cm long in adults with an outer diameter of approximately 20 mm. Structural support is provided by U-shaped structures composed of hyaline cartilage, with the opening of the U facing posteriorly. The cricoid membrane tethers the trachea to the cricoid cartilage at the level of the sixth cervical vertebral body. The trachea enters the superior mediastinum and bifurcates at the sternal angle. Normally, half of the trachea is intrathoracic and half is extrathoracic. Because both ends of the trachea are attached to mobile structures, the adult carina can move superiorly as much as 5 cm from its normal resting position. Following tracheal intubation, the distal end of the endotracheal tube moves an average of 3.8 cm with flexion (toward the carina) and extension (away from the carina) of the neck.[26] In infants and children, small movements of the endotracheal tube movement may result in mainstem intubation or unplanned extubation.

The airway below the carina consists of right and left main stem bronchi. The diameter of the right bronchus is generally greater than that of the left. In the adult, the right bronchus leaves the trachea at approximately 25 degrees from the vertical tracheal axis, whereas the angle of the left bronchus is about 45 degrees. Thus, unintentional endobronchial intubation or aspiration of foreign material is more likely to occur on the right than on the left. Furthermore, the right upper lobe bronchus dives almost directly posterior at approximately 90 degrees from the right main bronchus. In children younger than 3 years of age, the angles created by the right and left main stem bronchi are approximately equal, with takeoff angles of ~55 degrees.

The adult right main bronchus is about 2.5 cm long before it initially branches into lobar bronchi. However, in 10% of adults, the right upper lobe bronchus departs from the right main stem bronchus less than 2.5 cm from the carina. Furthermore, in 2% to 3% of adults, the right upper lobe bronchus opens into the trachea, superior to the carina. Patients with these anomalies require special consideration when placing double-lumen endotracheal tubes, particularly if one contemplates inserting a right-sided endobronchial tube. After the right upper and middle lobe bronchi divide from the right main bronchus, the main channel becomes the right lower lobe bronchus. The left main bronchus is about 5 cm long before its initial branching point to the left upper lobe and the lingula; it then continues as the left lower lobe bronchus.

The bronchioles, typically 1 mm in diameter, are devoid of cartilaginous support and have the highest proportion of smooth muscle in their walls. Of the three to four bronchiolar generations, the final generation is the terminal bronchiole, which is the last airway component incapable of gas exchange.

Airway Resistance

Resistance in the airways (e.g., mouth, pharynx, trachea, main and peripheral bronchi) is a primary concern in anesthesia. T\As the total cross-sectional area of the tracheobronchial tree increases from central to peripheral airways, airway resistance drops.

Resistance is dependent on the flow of gas per unit of time and the type of flow. Two different types of flow that often occur together are relevant to the respiratory system.[27] The first is laminar flow. Laminar flow is directly proportional to airway driving pressure—the higher the driving pressure, the higher the flow. Resistance in laminar flow is inversely proportional to the rate of flow and can be calculated by the Hagen–Poiseuille equation where

$$R = [8 \times \text{length} \times (\text{viscosity})]/[\pi \times (\text{radius})^4] \quad (15\text{-}7)$$

Laminar flow assumes that airways are straight and unbranched. The second type of flow is turbulent flow, where flow is less ordered. Turbulent flow occurs with high-flow rates, at branch points and angles and when airway diameter changes. Flow is proportional to the square of airway driving pressure. Resistance increases in proportion to the rate of flow, but is not amenable to such an intuitive equation as laminar flow. Frictional forces between gas and airway are more prominent in turbulent flow. Whether flow will be turbulent or laminar can be described using Reynold number.

$$\text{Reynold's number} = V \times d \times \text{gas density/gas viscosity} \quad (15\text{-}8)$$

Where V is the velocity of gas flow and d is the diameter of the airway. Laminar flow predominates at Reynold numbers under 2,000, turbulent flow predominates over 4,000, and intermediate values are transitional. As an example of the effect of gas density, helium has a lower density than air and increases the likelihood of laminar flow when airways narrow such as when upper airway edema is present.

Tissue Resistance

During inflation and deflation, tissue (lung and chest wall) resists deformation. This resistance can contribute up to half of total airway resistance. The chest wall may contribute an even higher proportion of resistance when its expansion is limited by intra-abdominal pressure as in obesity and in pneumoperitoneum. As mentioned previously, the slower change in airway pressure after airway occlusion likely reflects the recovery of the lung from a state of expansion and stress, particularly in normal lungs.[4,7]

Measurement of Resistance

Resistance is the change in pressure per unit of flow, typically in cmH_2O per liter per second.

$$R_{rs} = \Delta P/\text{Flow rate of inflation} \quad (15\text{-}9)$$

Resistance can be measured on ventilator with an inspiratory pause and visualization of the pressure–time waveform. For airway resistance, ΔP is the difference between peak airway pressure to the first pressure drop (P_1) (Fig. 15-3). For tissue resistance, ΔP is the difference between P_1 and P_2, a more gradual pressure decline. To make a simpler calculation, inspiratory flow can be set to 60 L/min or 1 L/sec. Measurements are most accurate with paralysis. Measurement during spontaneous breathing can be performed with the interrupter resistance technique involving transient airway occlusion during expiration.[28]

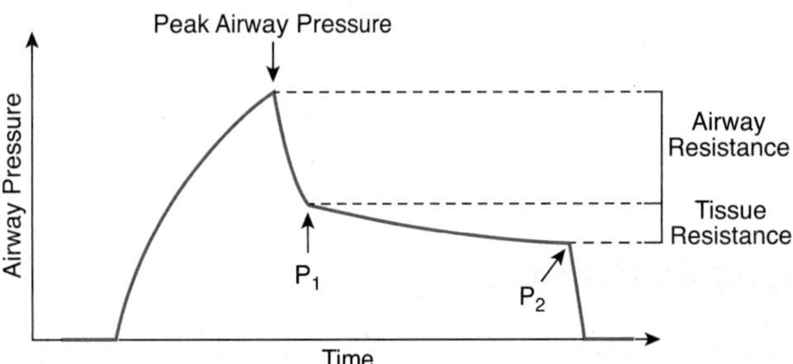

Figure 15-3 Representation of a pressure-time ventilator waveform in a paralyzed, healthy individual. Airway occlusion during constant flow inspiration allows for visualization and measurement of respiratory system resistance. P_1 is the pressure after immediate airway occlusion, representing the pressure contributing to the resistance of the airway tree. P_2 is the pressure after a more gradually decline following occlusion, representing the viscoelastic properties of the respiratory system tissue as pendelluft under these conditions is minimal.

Changes in Resistance during Anesthesia

Anesthesia influences resistance through three mechanisms: (1) changes in airway diameter, (2) changes in lung volume, and (3) changes in gas flow. Factors that reduce airway diameters throughout the tracheobronchial tree will increase resistance—for example, upper airways collapse during propofol anesthesia due to inhibition of genioglossus muscle activity[29]; the glottis can narrow in laryngospasm or with edema; bronchial smooth muscle tone increases during airway stimulation. Endotracheal tubes add additional resistance, more so if kinked or obstructed. The work of breathing related to the endotracheal tube may not differ significantly due to glottic narrowing, however.[30] Lung volume also influences airway resistance. When lung volume decreases, radial stress applied to bronchioles is altered and airways can narrow. Airway resistance will then increase if bronchomotor tone remains constant. Normal inverse associations between lung volume and resistance will differ in individuals with chronic obstructive pulmonary disease (COPD) where hyperinflation compresses small airways.[31] Of note, dependent airways have a higher propensity for collapse than other areas of the lung. The volume at which these airways collapse is known as closing capacity and increases linearly with age. Finally, high levels of flow during expiration will result in reduced airway pressure based on the Bernoulli principle. If intrathoracic pressure is high enough (e.g., obesity, pneumothorax), flow-related collapse will occur.

Intrinsic PEEP

Intrinsic PEEP involves elements of elastance and resistance. Intrinsic PEEP is any additional end-expiratory pressure beyond what is applied to the patient.[32] It occurs when exhalation is not completed due to flow limitation or airway closure. The time needed for exhalation is dependent on the product of resistance and compliance—the expiratory time constant—and the volume at the end of inspiration. Cases of high resistance (e.g., asthma) and high compliance (e.g., COPD) require more time for the lung to empty completely. For example, if resistance is 10 cmH_2O per liters per sec and compliance is 0.05 liters per cmH_2O, the time constant is 0.5 seconds. Approximately three time constants are required for the lung to empty. If exhalation is interrupted before this time, higher than expected volume and pressure remain in the alveoli. Intrinsic PEEP may also occur due to expiratory flow limitation, even when sufficient time is given for exhalation.[33] Here, exhalation is biphasic with quick empty following by stagnation of flow due to airway collapse (as described previously with obesity) or internal obstruction related to mucous plugging. Intrinsic PEEP can be detected from review of the ventilator flow-time curve demonstrating that flow does not return to zero prior to the next breath. It may also manifest as unexpected decrease in respiratory system compliance, higher airway pressures, or at latter stages, systemic hypotension.

Gas Exchange

To support life, the lungs must inhale oxygen and exhale carbon dioxide, although gas exchange can be replaced with extracorporeal membrane oxygenation for short periods of time. The alveolus and surrounding capillaries represent the functional unit for gas exchange. For efficient and effective gas exchange, two systems must co-exist—(1) ventilation (V)—the inflow and outflow of gas transport in the alveolar space, and (2) perfusion (Q)—the inflow and outflow of gas transport in the capillary. Matching of ventilation and perfusion is described with the V/Q ratio. Overall, the V/Q ratio is 0.8 where normal ventilation in

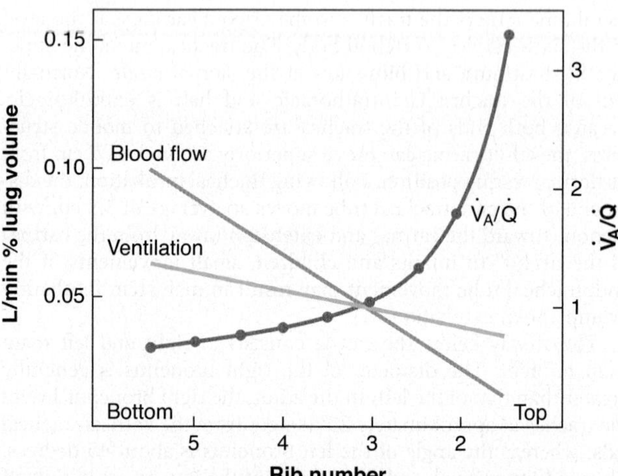

Figure 15-4 Distribution of ventilation, blood flow, and ventilation–perfusion ratio in the normal, upright lung. Straight lines have been drawn through the ventilation and blood flow data. Because blood flow falls more rapidly than ventilation with distance up the lung, ventilation–perfusion ratio rises, slowly at first, then rapidly. (Reprinted with permission from West JB. *Ventilation/Blood Flow and Gas Exchange*. 4th ed. Blackwell Scientific; 1985. Copyright © 1985 John Wiley & Sons.)

the alveoli is 4 L/min and normal cardiac output is 5 L/min. As heterogeneity in the lung is the norm, V/Q varies widely across alveoli (Fig. 15-4). Alveoli that receive more perfusion than ventilation and have V/Q ratios that approach zero are termed shunt. Alveoli that receive more ventilation than perfusion and have V/Q ratios that approach infinity are termed dead space. Silent units are alveoli with both minimal perfusion and ventilation (Fig. 15-5) (1 Video 15-1). In healthy individuals, the

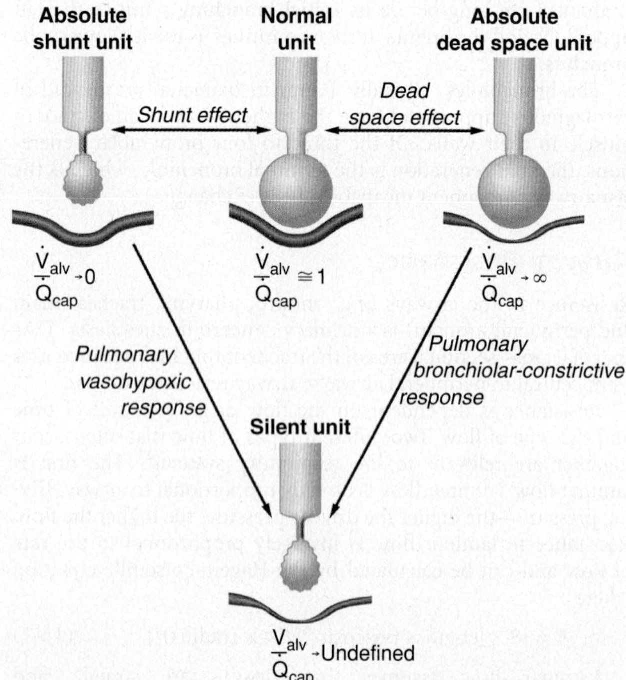

Figure 15-5 Continuum of ventilation–perfusion relationships. Gas exchange is maximally effective in normal lung units and only partially effective in shunt and dead space effect units. It is totally absent in silent units, absolute shunt, and dead space units.

majority of alveoli are more evenly matched with values between 1 and 0.8. A simplified model by Riley and Cournand describes alveolar gas exchange based on these three compartments.[34] Local V/Q ratios dependent on gravity, the inherent structure of lung and capillaries, regional differences in lung mechanics, and presence of lung injury. The dependent lung receives greater proportions of ventilation and perfusion than nondependent areas of the lung. Part of this distribution is secondary to gravity. As we previously mentioned, pleural pressure is higher (and transpulmonary pressure lower) in dependent areas of the lung. Inspiration therefore starts at more favorable compliance for inflation. In regard to perfusion, a hydrostatic pressure difference exists across the pulmonary arterial vasculature. Taken together, John West described a gravitational model for the relationship between pulmonary arterial, venous, and alveolar pressures as shown in Figure 15-6 (see also 2 Video 15-2). In uppermost lung regions (e.g., lung apex when standing or upright), alveolar pressure is higher than pulmonary artery and venous pressure (Zone 1) and these alveoli receive little blood flow. In middle lung regions, pulmonary artery pressure exceeds alveolar pressure (Zone 2) and in the lower lung regions, alveolar pressure is less than both pulmonary artery and venous pressure (Zone 3).[35] Later work has demonstrated variability in pulmonary blood flow at the same vertical height.[36] Nongravitational mechanisms, such as from inherent architecture of the pulmonary vasculature and prior blood flow, likely have a more prominent effect than gravity.[37]

Real-time measurement and visualization of V/Q ratios and their distributions across the lung are not currently integrated to clinical practice due to these complexities. Historically, V/Q distribution has been measured using the multiple inert gas elimination technique (MIGET). MIGET is a technique that infuses solutions of six different inert gases intravenously and measures their retention in arterial blood and expired air.[38,39] Newer techniques may be more practical. Electrical impendence tomography is a noninvasive, bedside imaging technique that measures impedance changes related to the thoracic content of air and blood, and has been used to characterize ventilation and perfusion distributions in acute respiratory distress syndrome.[40]

Impairments in Gas Exchange during Anesthesia

5

Overall, anesthesia results in more pronounced mismatch between ventilation and perfusion and gas exchange impairment compared to the awake state.[41] Below, we describe in depth how this relates to oxygen and carbon dioxide.

Oxygen

The lung interacts with the heart and peripheral vasculature to ensure adequate delivery of oxygen in response to metabolic demands. Along with cardiac output and the oxygen carrying capacity of blood (e.g., hemoglobin content and quality), the arterial PO_2 (P_aO_2) determines oxygen delivery. P_aO_2 is determined from the concentration of oxygen in alveoli (P_AO_2), which is estimated by the alveolar gas equation:

$$P_AO_2 = F_iO_2 \times (P_{atm} - PH_2O) - P_aCO_2 \times (VO_2/VCO_2) \quad (15\text{-}10)$$

where F_iO_2 is the inspired oxygen concentration, P_{atm} is the barometric pressure, PH_2O is the water vapor pressure (usually 47 cmH_2O), P_aCO_2 is the concentration CO_2 in the blood, and VO_2/VCO_2 is the inverse of respiratory quotient (the ratio between carbon dioxide production and oxygen consumption with a normal ratio of 0.8 depending on individual's diet). The alveolar gas equation is best illustrated in altitude physiology. At the top of Mount Everest (8,400 m), atmospheric pressure is 272 mmHg and P_aO_2 without supplemental oxygen is 30 mmHg. Survival requires hyperventilation to achieve P_aCO_2 near 13 mmHg.[42]

Transfer of oxygen into the blood occurs at full equilibrium in healthy lungs and the normal difference between P_AO_2 and P_aO_2 is fairly minimal—about 5 to 10 mmHg due to physiologic shunt.[43] The alveolar–arterial oxygen gradient widens with impairments in gas exchange. A more commonly used measure of gas exchange is the P_aO_2 to F_iO_2 ratio (P/F). The P/F ratio is a key component of the definition of acute respiratory distress syndrome, but does have limitations.[44] Varying F_iO_2 will change the P/F ratio depending on the amount of shunt present and caution is needed to prevent misinterpretation of these values.

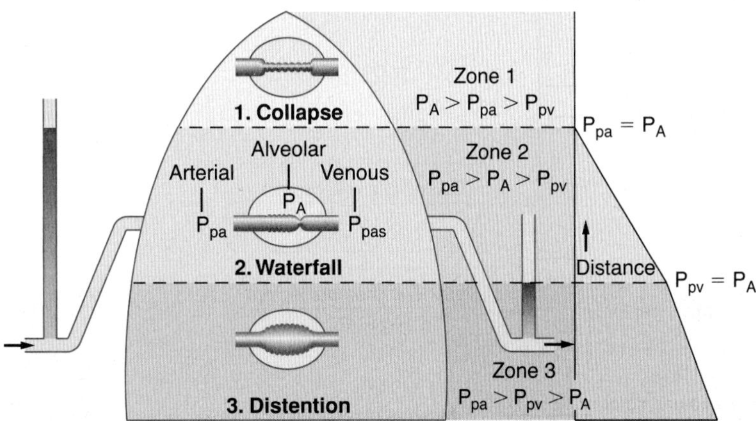

Figure 15-6 Distribution of blood flow in the isolated lung. In Zone 1, alveolar pressure (P_A) exceeds pulmonary artery pressure (P_{pa}), and no flow occurs because the vessels are collapsed. In Zone 2, arterial pressure exceeds alveolar pressure, but alveolar pressure exceeds pulmonary venous pressure (P_{pv}). Flow in Zone 2 is determined by the arterial–alveolar pressure difference ($P_{pa} - P_A$), which steadily increases down the zone. In Zone 3, pulmonary venous pressure exceeds alveolar pressure, and flow is determined by the arterial–venous pressure difference ($P_{pa} - P_{pv}$), which is constant down this pulmonary zone. However, the pressure across the vessel walls increases down the zone so their caliber increases, as does flow. (Adapted from West JB, Dollery CT, Naimark A. Distribution of blood flow in isolated lung: Relation to vascular and alveolar pressures. *J Appl Physiol.* 1964;19:713–724. Copyright © American Physiological Society.)

6 Hypoxemia is the main consequence of ventilation and perfusion mismatch. During anesthesia, hypoxemia primarily occurs due to shunt from atelectasis.[41] In shunt, venous blood either does not participate or participates very little in gas exchange, and directly mixes in with arterial blood. The proportion of venous admixture (or shunt fraction) can be calculated using mixed venous and arterial blood gases in the following formula:

$$Q_s/Q_t = (CCO_2 - CaO_2)/(CCO_2 - CVO_2) \quad (15\text{-}11)$$

where CaO_2 is the arterial blood oxygen content, CVO_2 is the mixed venous blood oxygen content, and CCO_2 is the end-capillary blood oxygen content. P_AO_2 from the alveolar gas equation can be substituted for CCO_2. With higher shunt, arterial oxygenation is more impacted by the concentration of oxygen in the pulmonary venous blood (P_VO_2). When shunt is unable to be reversed, consideration to mixed venous oxygenation needs to be considered. Efforts to increase cardiac output may further increase shunt yet improve overall arterial oxygenation and oxygen delivery through an increase in mixed venous oxygenation.

In response to alveolar hypoxia, as well as low P_VO_2, pulmonary arteries will vasoconstrict to maintain V/Q matching and preserve P_aO_2. This intrinsic response is termed hypoxic pulmonary vasoconstriction (HPV).[45] HPV is most evident during one-lung ventilation where flow through the nonventilated lung is reduced by 50%. HPV is inhibited by inhalational anesthetics and high concentrations of inspired oxygen.

Carbon Dioxide

Exhalation of carbon dioxide is another critical function of pulmonary gas exchange. It is the principal reason why we breathe. Alveolar CO_2 concentration (P_ACO_2) is determined by cellular metabolism, CO_2 production (VCO_2), and alveolar ventilation (V_A).

$$P_ACO_2 = VCO_2/V_A \times K \text{ where K is a constant.} \quad (15\text{-}12)$$

P_ACO_2 is closely linked to alveolar ventilation. Alveolar ventilation is not the same as minute ventilation. Minute ventilation is the product of respiratory rate and tidal volume, and encompasses alveolar ventilation and dead space ventilation. The volume of lung involved in dead space ventilation includes three components: (1) anatomic dead space—nose, pharynx, and conducting airways, (2) alveolar dead space where alveolar blood flow is minimal (e.g., decrease cardiac output, venous air embolism), and (3) instrumental dead space—masks, ventilator components distal to the Y-piece such as an endotracheal tube, connectors, heat and moisture exchanger. Instrumental dead space is sometimes overlooked, yet can be easily modified.[46] It can account for significant volume when minute ventilation is already maximized and tidal volumes are low. Dead space can be quantified from the Enghoff modification of Bohr equation: 7

$$V_d/V_t = (P_aCO_2 - P_ECO_2)/P_aCO_2 \quad (15\text{-}13)$$

where P_aCO_2 is assumed to be similar to P_ACO_2 and P_ECO_2 is the partial pressure of CO_2 in mixed expired gas. P_ECO_2 can be approximated from the midpoint of phase III of expired capnogram waveform. V_d/V_t is approximately 0.33 in spontaneously breathing individuals and up to 0.5 in healthy individuals receiving positive-pressure ventilation.

Control of Breathing

Control of breathing centers in a network of neurons in the pons and medulla that integrate neural signals for spontaneous ventilation. The continual output from neural respiratory centers regulates the respiratory cycle. The main rhythm generator for inspiration appears to be in the PreBotzinger Complex in the ventrolateral medulla.[47] Output transmits further along a pathway to spinal motor neurons at the level of the cervical spine to the neuromuscular junction of the diaphragm. The main inputs to the respiratory centers are through cortical, chemical, and reflexive feedback (Fig. 15-7).

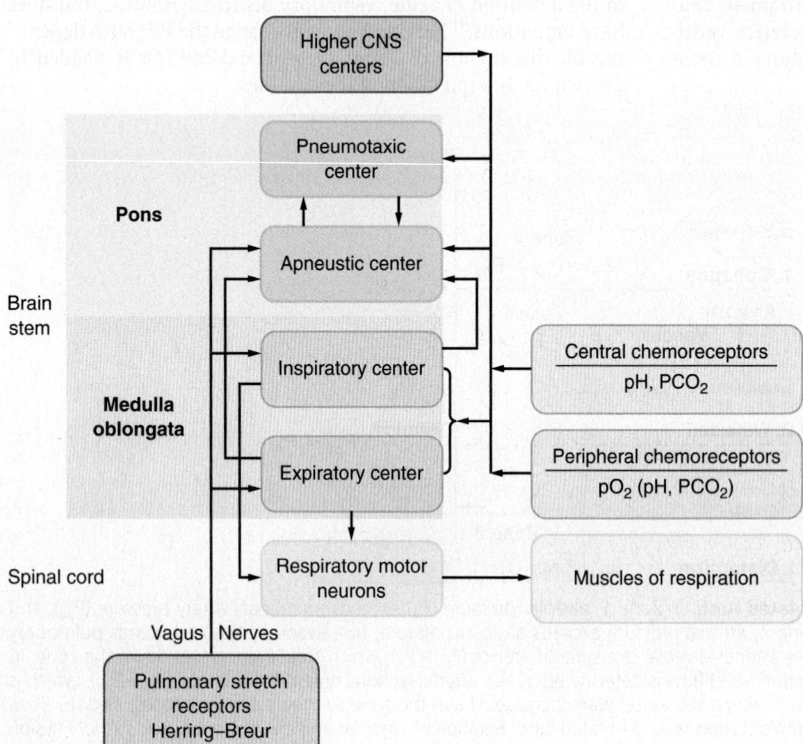

Figure 15-7 Classic central nervous system (CNS) respiratory centers. Diagram illustrates major respiratory centers, neurofeedback circuits, primary neurohumoral sensory inputs, and mechanical outputs.

Chemical Feedback of Breathing

Peripheral and central chemoreceptors sense changes in P_aCO_2, pH, and P_aO_2, and modulate respiratory center output and alveolar ventilation. CO_2 is the main stimulant for respiratory drive. Change in P_aO_2 is a weaker modulator sensed by peripheral chemoreceptors at the carotid bifurcation. Response to P_aCO_2 occurs in central chemoreceptors located on the ventrolateral surface of the medulla. CO_2 crosses the brain blood barrier and increases local hydrogen ion concentrations in the cerebrospinal fluid, resulting in a rapid increase in respiratory drive. Minute ventilation increases linearly, on average 2 to 3 liters per minute per mmHg of P_aCO_2 in healthy individuals (Fig. 15-8). P_aCO_2 at steady state resting conditions is determined by the intersection of the P_aCO_2–ventilation response curve and the metabolic hyperbola. The metabolic hyperbola is determined by CO_2 production and dead space fraction.[48] Below a certain P_aCO_2, termed the apneic threshold, minute ventilation is reduced and may cease in individuals who are asleep or sedated. When awake, individuals continue to breathe below this threshold, as the sensation of apnea is disturbing. A rise in minute ventilation from hypercarbia first occurs via an increase in V_t with elevation of respiratory rate occurring only later after respiratory drive has become significantly elevated above resting ventilation.[49] Changes in respiratory rate may occur sooner in individuals with constraints on V_t, such as those with neuromuscular weakness or with high dead space. Over time, the ventilatory response to elevated CO_2 declines as cerebrospinal pH normalizes through transport of bicarbonate. This is seen in individuals with chronic CO_2 retention.

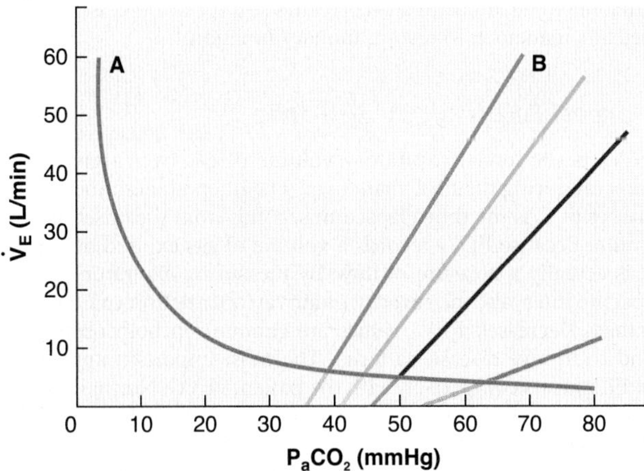

Figure 15-8 Carbon dioxide–ventilatory response curve. The metabolic hyperbola, curve A, is generated by varying minute ventilation (V_E) and measuring changes in carbon dioxide concentration. The hyperbolic configuration makes it cumbersome for clinical use. The carbon dioxide–ventilatory response curve, B, is linear between approximately 20 and 80 mmHg. It is generated by varying P_aCO_2 (usually by controlling inspired carbon dioxide concentration) and measuring the resultant V_E. This is the most commonly used test of ventilatory response. The slope defines "sensitivity"; the setpoint, or resting P_aCO_2, occurs at the intersection of the metabolic hyperbola and the carbon dioxide–ventilatory response curve; and the apneic threshold can be obtained by extrapolating the carbon dioxide–ventilatory response curve to the *x*-intercept. In the absence of surgical stimulation, increasing doses of potent inhaled anesthesia or opioids will shift the curve to the right and eventually depress the slope (*green, red, and brown lines*). Painful stimulation will reverse these changes to varying and unpredictable degrees.

Reflexive Control of Breathing

Reflexes that directly influence ventilatory pattern usually do so to prevent airway obstruction. Deglutition, or swallowing, involves the glossopharyngeal and vagus nerves. Stimulation of the anterior and posterior pharyngeal pillars of the posterior pharynx induces swallowing. During swallowing, inspiration ceases momentarily, is usually followed by a single large breath, and briefly increases ventilation.

Vomiting significantly modifies normal ventilatory activity.[50] Swallowing, salivation, gastrointestinal reflexes, rhythmic spasmodic ventilatory movements, and significant diaphragmatic and abdominal muscular activity must be coordinated over a very brief interval. Because of the risk of aspirating gastric contents, it is advantageous to inhibit inspiration during vomiting. Input into the respiratory centers occurs from both cranial and spinal cord nerves.

Coughing results from stimulation of the tracheal subepithelium, especially along the posterior tracheal wall and carina.[51] Coughing also requires coordination of both airway and ventilatory muscle activity. An effective cough requires deep inspiration and then forced exhalation against a momentarily closed glottis to increase intrathoracic pressure, thus allowing an expulsive expiratory maneuver.

Proprioception in the pulmonary system, the qualitative knowledge of the gas volume within the lungs, probably arises from smooth muscle spindle receptors. These proprioceptors, which are located within the smooth muscle of all airways, are sensitive to pressure changes. Airway stretch reflexes can be demonstrated during distention of isolated airways. Airway pressure, rather than volume distention, appears to be the primary stimulation.[52] Clinical conditions in which pulmonary airway stretch receptors are stimulated include pulmonary edema and atelectasis.

Golgi tendon organs (tendon spindles), which are arranged in series within ventilatory muscles, facilitate proprioception. The intercostal muscles are rich in tendon spindles, whereas the diaphragm has a limited number. Thus, the pulmonary stretch reflex primarily involves the intercostal muscles, but not the diaphragm. When the lungs are full and the chest wall is stretched, these receptors send signals to the brainstem that inhibit further inspiration.

Finally, the Hering–Breuer reflex has been shown in lower-order mammals to cease or decrease ventilatory effort during sustained lung distention and is blocked by bilateral vagotomy.[53] In healthy adults, however, the reflex may only be weakly present.

CO_2 Exchange under Anesthesia

Under anesthesia, impairments in CO_2 occur through three mechanisms:

1. Changes in alveolar ventilation. Drugs administered during 8
   anesthesia—volatile anesthetics, opioids, hypnotics (e.g., propofol)—all disrupt different aspects of ventilator control in a dose-dependent manner and cause alveolar hypoventilation. Volatile anesthetics appear to preserve respiratory drive via activation of respiratory centers.[54] During apnea, P_aCO_2 increases ~10 mmHg in the first minute and 3.5 mmHg per minute afterward. High concentrations of inhaled anesthetics and hypnotics may depress both the ventilator response to hypoxemia and hypercarbia. Opiates result in a right-shift of the P_aCO_2 –ventilation response curve and a higher resting P_aCO_2.
2. V/Q mismatch after 2. As discussed with oxygen, mismatch between perfusion and ventilation worsens with anesthesia. In

particular, the volume of dead space increases. The addition of breathing devices and connectors adds instrumental dead space. Alveolar dead space is higher, yet the mechanisms and degree across individuals is variable. Regional inhomogeneity in ventilation may result in overventilation of areas of lung that receive lower relative pulmonary blood flow. It becomes more evident with hypovolemia, pulmonary vasodilation, and obstruction of pulmonary vessels with emboli or microthrombosis. High inspiratory pressure and PEEP can cause alveolar overdistention, particularly in nondependent areas of the lung, further widening alveolar–arterial CO_2 gradient. As it does for oxygen, shunt will widen the gradient. However, the effect of shunt on P_aCO_2 is less significant because there is a much lower difference between venous and arterial carbon dioxide compared to oxygen.
3. CO_2 production (VCO_2). In general, metabolic rate and CO_2 production during anesthesia are significantly less than during ambulatory wakefulness. However, CO_2 can increase under hypermetabolic states such as shivering, fever, and malignant hyperthermia. Administration of sodium bicarbonate to correct metabolic acidemia will increase VCO_2.

Lung Volumes and Capacities

Finally, a comment on lung volumes and pulmonary function tests is needed. Lung volumes and related capacities are schematically illustrated in Figure 15-9 (see also 3 Video 15-3).

Tidal volume is the volume of gas that moves in and out of the lungs during quiet breathing and is about 6 to 8 mL/kg. Tidal volume falls with decreased lung compliance or when the patient has reduced ventilatory muscle strength.

Vital capacity is usually around 60 mL/kg but may vary as much as 20% from normal in healthy individuals. Vital capacity correlates well with deep breathing and effective coughing. It is decreased by restrictive pulmonary disease such as pulmonary edema or atelectasis. Vital capacity may also be reduced by

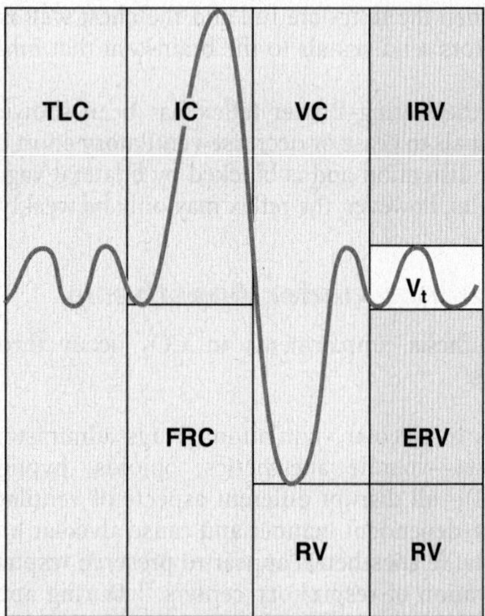

Figure 15-9 Lung volumes and capacities. The *darkest shaded bar* on the far right depicts the four basic lung volumes that sum to create TLC. Other lung capacities are composed of two or more lung volumes. The overlying spirographic tracing orients the reader to the relationship between the lung volumes and capacities and the spirogram. ERV, expiratory reserve volume; FRC, functional residual capacity; IC, inspiratory capacity; IRV, inspiratory reserve volume; RV, residual volume; TLC, total lung capacity; VC, vital capacity; V_t, tidal volume.

extrapulmonary restriction seen in pleural effusion, pneumothorax, pregnancy, large ascites, or ventilatory muscle weakness.

The *inspiratory capacity* is the largest volume of gas that can be inspired from the resting expiratory level and is frequently decreased in the presence of significant extrathoracic airway obstruction. This measurement is one of the few simple tests that can detect extrathoracic airway obstruction. Most routine pulmonary function tests measure only exhaled flows and volumes, which may be relatively unaffected by extrathoracic obstruction until it is severe. Changes in the absolute volume of inspiratory capacity usually parallel changes in vital capacity.

Expiratory reserve volume is not of great diagnostic value. Residual volume is the gas remaining within the lungs at the end of forced maximal expiration.

Pulmonary Function Tests

9

Forced Vital Capacity

The forced vital capacity (FVC) is the largest volume of gas that an individual can expire after maximal inspiration. It is a global measure of respiratory capacity as it accounts for inspiratory and expiratory muscle strength. Measurement requires patient cooperation. Since forced expiration significantly increases intrapleural pressures yet changes airway pressure minimally, bronchiolar collapse, obstructive lesions, and gas trapping are exaggerated. Thus, FVC may be reduced in chronic obstructive diseases even when the vital capacity appears near normal. FVC is nearly always decreased by restrictive diseases. FVC values lower than 15 mL/kg are associated with an increased incidence of PPCs.[55] FVC reduced to this level represents a profound defect, most commonly seen in quadriplegics or severe neuromuscular disease. Single breath count—how many numbers an individual can count after maximal inhalation—correlates with FVC and is a simple bedside maneuver to test pulmonary function.[56]

Forced Expiratory Volume

FEV_T is the forced expiratory volume of gas over a given time interval during the FVC maneuver. The interval, described by the subscript T, is the time elapsed in seconds from the onset of expiration. Because FEV_T records a volume of gas expired over time, it is actually a measure of flow. By measuring expiratory flow at specific intervals, the severity of airway obstruction can be ascertained. Decreased FEV_T values are common in both obstructive and restrictive disease patterns. The most important application of FEV_T is its comparison with the patient's FVC. Normal subjects can expire at least three-fourths of FVC within the first second of the forced expiratory maneuver. The FEV_1, the most frequently employed value, is normally greater than or equal to 75% of the FVC, or $FEV_1/FVC \geq 0.75$.

Normally, an individual can expire 50% to 60% of FVC in 0.5 second, 75% to 85% in 1 second, 94% in 2 seconds, and 97% in 3 seconds. Cooperative patients with obstructive disease will exhibit a reduced FEV_1/FVC in most cases. However, patients with restrictive disease usually have normal FEV_1/FVC ratios. The validity of the evaluation of the FEV_1/FVC is highly dependent on patient cooperation and effort. It is possible to deliberately produce an artificially low FEV_1/FVC.

Forced Expiratory Flow

$FEF_{25\%-75\%}$ is the average forced expiratory flow during the middle half of the FEV maneuver. This test is also called maximum midexpiratory flow rate. The length of time required for a subject to

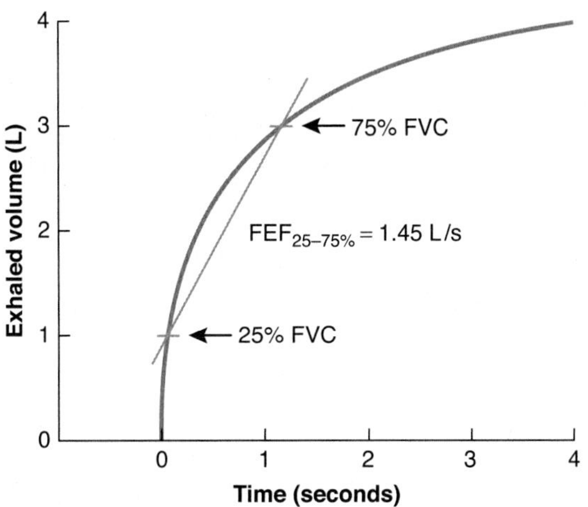

Figure 15-10 $FEF_{25\%-75\%}$. The spirogram depicts a 4 L FVC on which the points representing 25% and 75% FVC are marked. The slope of the line connecting these points is the $FEF_{25\%-75\%}$.

expire the middle half of the FVC is divided into 50% of the FVC. The spirogram in Figure 15-10 marks the place from 25% to 75% of FVC, constituting the middle 50% of FVC. The straight line connecting the 25% and 75% volumes has a slope approximately equal to average flow. A normal value for a healthy 70-kg man is approximately 4.7 L/sec (or 280 L/min). Normally, both the absolute value and the percentage of predicted value for the individual being studied are recorded. A normal value is 100 ± 25% of predicted. Decreased flow rates from this middle 50% of FVC are indicative of obstructive disease of medium size airways. This value is typically normal in restrictive diseases. This test is fairly sensitive in the early stages of obstructive airway disease. Decreased $FEV_{25\%-75\%}$ frequently will be observed before other obstructive manifestations occur. Although somewhat effort dependent, the test is much more reliable and reproducible than FEV_1/FVC.

Flow–Volume Loops

A flow–volume loop graphically demonstrates the flow generated during the respiratory cycle over the volume of gas expired (Fig. 15-11, 4 Video 15-4). In spontaneously breathing individuals, forced expiration occurs followed by inhalation to vital capacity. Although various numbers can be generated from the flow–volume loop, the configuration of the loop itself is probably the most informative part of the test. In mechanical ventilation, the flow volume loop is usually inverted.

Flow–volume loops were formerly useful in the diagnosis of large airway and extrathoracic airway obstruction prior to the availability of precise imaging techniques. Imaging techniques such as CT and MRI provide more precise and useful information in the diagnosis of upper airway and extrathoracic obstruction, and have replaced the use of flow–volume loops for diagnosis of these conditions. Therefore, it is rare that flow–volume loops are useful for preoperative pulmonary evaluation in the modern era of imaging.

Carbon Monoxide Diffusing Capacity

Since PO_2 in the pulmonary capillary blood varies with time as it moves through the pulmonary microvasculature, oxygen cannot be used to assess diffusing capacity. Instead, a gas mixture containing carbon monoxide is traditionally used to measure diffusing capacity. The partial pressure of carbon monoxide in the blood

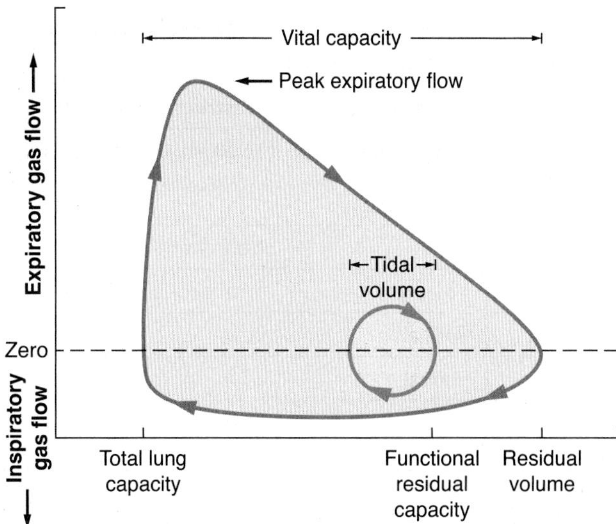

Figure 15-11 Flow–volume loop. The figure depicts a normally configured adult flow–volume loop. The slope of the loop after the subject reaches peak expiratory flow is nearly linear.

is nearly zero, and its affinity for hemoglobin is 200 times that of oxygen.[57] Carbon monoxide diffusing capacity (DLCO) collectively measures all the factors that affect diffusion across the alveolar–capillary membrane. The DLCO is recorded in mL CO/min/mmHg at standard atmospheric conditions. In persons with normal hemoglobin concentrations and normal V/Q matching, the main factor limiting diffusion is the alveolar–capillary membrane. The average value for resting subjects when the single-breath method is used is 25 mL CO/min/mmHg. DLCO values can increase to two or three times normal during exercise. The DLO_2 may be estimated from the DLCO by multiplying DLCO by 1.23, although the DLCO is usually the reported value. DLCO can be divided by the lung volume at which the measurement was made to obtain an expression of diffusing capacity per unit lung volume. Some of the other factors that can influence DLCO are as follows:

1. Hemoglobin concentration: decreased hemoglobin concentration decreases the DLCO
2. Alveolar PCO_2: an increased P_aCO_2 raises DLCO
3. Body position: the supine position increases DLCO
4. Pulmonary capillary blood volume

Diffusing capacity is decreased in alveolar fibrosis associated with sarcoidosis, asbestosis, berylliosis, oxygen toxicity, and pulmonary edema. These states are frequently categorized as diffusion defects, but low DLCO is probably more closely related to loss of lung volume or capillary bed perfusion. DLCO is decreased in obstructive disease because of the decreased alveolar surface area, loss of capillary bed, the increased distance from the terminal bronchiole to the alveolar–capillary membrane, and V/Q mismatching. In short, few disease states truly inhibit oxygen diffusion across the alveolar–capillary membrane.

Practical Application of Pulmonary Function Tests

Of the many pulmonary function tests, spirometry is the most useful, cost-effective, and commonly used test.[58] Screening spirometry yields VC, FVC, and FEV_1. From these values, two basic types of pulmonary dysfunction can be identified and quantitated: obstructive defects and restrictive defects. The primary criterion

Table 15-2 Pulmonary Function Tests in Restrictive and Obstructive Lung Disease

Value	Restrictive Disease	Obstructive Disease
Definition	Proportional decreases in all lung volumes	Small airway obstruction to expiratory flow
FVC	↓↓↓	Normal or slightly ↑
FEV_1	↓↓↓	Normal or slightly ↓
FEV_1/FVC	Normal	↓↓↓
$FEF_{25-75\%}$	Normal	↓↓↓
FRC	↓↓↓	Normal or ↑ if gas trapping
TLC	↓↓↓	Normal or ↑ if gas trapping

FEV, forced expiratory volume; FRC, functional residual capacity; FVC, forced vital capacity; TLC, total lung capacity; ↓↓↓, ↑↑↑ = large decrease or increase, respectively; ↓, ↑ = small/moderate decrease or increase, respectively.

for airflow obstruction is decreased FEV_1/FVC ratio. Other measurements, such as $FEF_{25\%-75\%}$, can be used to support the diagnosis of an obstructive defect or to assist in management (e.g., use of bronchodilators). A restrictive defect is a proportional decrease in all lung volumes (VC, FVC, and FEV_1), but FEV_1/FVC remains normal. When there is a question about whether a decreased VC is due to restriction, TLC should be measured. Reduced TLC defines a restrictive defect, but is not necessary unless VC on screening spirometry is reduced. The American Thoracic Society published an expert consensus on standardization of pulmonary function tests and values in 2019.[59] Table 15-2 summarizes the distinctions between results from those with restrictive versus obstructive defects.

Summary

10 In ending the chapter, we highlight the goal of anesthesia—as it
11 relates to respiratory function—to maintain optimal pulmonary
function and prevent pulmonary complications and resultant morbidity and mortality. Within the chapter, we have discussed how certain approaches such as alveolar recruitment and continuous positive airway pressure can be applied to restore lung volumes and maintain optimal gas exchange. Yet, we recognize that to minimize pulmonary complications (NICV 15-1), attention and diligence is needed across the entire perioperative setting, starting at the time of preoperative surgical assessment and ending far after a patient has left the hospital. Optimal respiratory care must therefore extend beyond the operating room or immediate recovery area, a point even more salient for several populations known to be at a high risk for pulmonary complications after surgery (see Table 15-3).[60] For example, pulmonary rehabilitation done prior to surgery—in the form of inspiratory muscle training, breathing exercises—has reduced certain pulmonary complications in these high-risk populations.[61] Postoperative interventions focused on lung expansion and early mobilization are also effective. These interventions require a multidisciplinary team involving anesthesiology, surgery, respiratory therapy, physical and occupational therapy, and nursing staff, among many others.

Table 15-3 Populations at Elevated Risk of Postoperative Pulmonary Complications

Demographic Factors and Pre-existing Conditions	Morbid obesity Current smoking Chronic lung disease Older age Dependent functional status Recent respiratory infection (~4 wks prior to surgery) Malignancy Male sex Anemia (<10 g/dL)
Procedure Factors	Intrathoracic surgery Longer duration of surgery (>3 hrs) Emergency procedure

For further review and interactivities, please see the videos and narrative interactive clinical vignettes (NICVs) accessible in the complimentary eBook bundled with this text. Access instructions are located on the inside front cover.

REFERENCES

1. Carvalho AR, Zin WA. Respiratory system dynamical mechanical properties: modeling in time and frequency domain. *Biophys Rev.* 2011;3(2):71.
2. Gattinoni L, Tonetti T, Cressoni M, et al. Ventilator-related causes of lung injury: the mechanical power. *Intensive Care Med.* 2016;42(10):1567–1575.
3. Zeng C, Lagier D, Lee JW, et al. Perioperative pulmonary atelectasis: Part I. Biology and mechanisms. *Anesthesiology*. 2022;136(1):181–205.
4. Bates JH, Baconnier P, Milic-Emili J. A theoretical analysis of interrupter technique for measuring respiratory mechanics. *J Appl Physiol (1985)*. 1988;64(5):2204–2214.
5. Otis AB, McKerrow CB, Bartlett RA, et al. Mechanical factors in distribution of pulmonary ventilation. *J Appl Physiol.* 1956;8(4):427–443.
6. Yoshida T, Torsani V, Gomes S, et al. Spontaneous effort causes occult pendelluft during mechanical ventilation. *Am J Respir Crit Care Med.* 2013;188(12):1420–1427.
7. D'Angelo E, Calderini E, Torri G, Robatto FM, Bono D, Milic-Emili J. Respiratory mechanics in anesthetized paralyzed humans: effects of flow, volume, and time. *J Appl Physiol (1985)*. 1989; 67(6):2556–2564.
8. Bates JH, Ludwig MS, Sly PD, Brown K, Martin JG, Fredberg JJ. Interrupter resistance elucidated by alveolar pressure measurement in open-chest normal dogs. *J Appl Physiol (1985)*. 1988;65(1):408–414.
9. Amato MB, Meade MO, Slutsky AS, et al. Driving pressure and survival in the acute respiratory distress syndrome. *N Engl J Med.* 2015;372(8):747–755.
10. Neto AS, Hemmes SN, Barbas CS, et al. Association between driving pressure and development of postoperative pulmonary complications in patients undergoing mechanical ventilation for general anaesthesia: a meta-analysis of individual patient data. *Lancet Respir Med.* 2016; 4(4):272–280.
11. Park M, Ahn HJ, Kim JA, et al. Driving pressure during thoracic surgery: a randomized clinical trial. *Anesthesiology.* 2019;130(3):385–393.
12. Goligher EC, Costa ELV, Yarnell CJ, et al. Effect of lowering Vt on mortality in acute respiratory distress syndrome varies with respiratory system elastance. *Am J Respir Crit Care Med.* 2021; 203(11):1378–1385.
13. Mauri T, Yoshida T, Bellani G, et al. Esophageal and transpulmonary pressure in the clinical setting: meaning, usefulness and perspectives. *Intensive Care Med.* 2016;42(9):1360–1373.
14. Beitler JR, Sarge T, Banner-Goodspeed VM, et al. Effect of titrating positive end-expiratory pressure (PEEP) with an esophageal pressure-guided strategy vs an empirical high PEEP-FiO_2 strategy on death and days free from mechanical ventilation among patients with acute respiratory distress syndrome: a randomized clinical trial. *JAMA.* 2019;321(9):846–857.
15. Duggan M, Kavanagh BP. Pulmonary atelectasis: a pathogenic perioperative entity. *Anesthesiology.* 2005;102(4):838–854.
16. Reber A, Engberg G, Sporre B, et al. Volumetric analysis of aeration in the lungs during general anaesthesia. *Br J Anaesth.* 1996;76(6):760–766.
17. Akca O, Podolsky A, Eisenhuber E, et al. Comparable postoperative pulmonary atelectasis in patients given 30% or 80% oxygen during and 2 hours after colon resection. *Anesthesiology.* 1999;91(4):991–998.

18. Neligan PJ, Malhotra G, Fraser M, et al. Continuous positive airway pressure via the Boussignac system immediately after extubation improves lung function in morbidly obese patients with obstructive sleep apnea undergoing laparoscopic bariatric surgery. *Anesthesiology*. 2009; 110(4):878–884.
19. Johnson D, Hurst T, Thomson D, et al. Respiratory function after cardiac surgery. *J Cardiothorac Vasc Anesth*. 1996;10(5):571–577.
20. Writing Committee for the PCGotPVNftCTNotESoA, Bluth T, Serpa Neto A, et al. Effect of intraoperative high positive end-expiratory pressure (PEEP) with recruitment maneuvers vs low PEEP on postoperative pulmonary complications in obese patients: a randomized clinical trial. *JAMA*. 2019;321(23):2292–2305.
21. Fumagalli J, Santiago RRS, Teggia Droghi M, et al. Lung recruitment in obese patients with acute respiratory distress syndrome. *Anesthesiology*. 2019;130(5):791–803.
22. Sharp JT, Henry JP, Sweany SK, Meadows WR, Pietras RJ. Effects of mass loading the respiratory system in man. *J Appl Physiol*. 1964;19:959–966.
23. Loring SH, Behazin N, Novero A, et al. Respiratory mechanical effects of surgical pneumoperitoneum in humans. *J Appl Physiol (1985)*. 2014;117(9):1074–1079.
24. Grieco DL, Anzellotti GM, Russo A, et al. Airway closure during surgical pneumoperitoneum in obese patients. *Anesthesiology*. 2019;131(1):58–73.
25. Campbell EJ. The effects of increased resistance to expiration on the respiratory behaviour of the abdominal muscles and intra-abdominal pressure. *J Physiol*. 1957;136(3):556–562.
26. Conrardy PA, Goodman LR, Lainge F, Singer MM. Alteration of endotracheal tube position. Flexion and extension of the neck. *Crit Care Med*. 1976;4(1):8–12.
27. Lumb AB, Thomas, CR. *Nunn's Applied Respiratory Physiology*, 9th ed.: Elsevier Limited; 2021, 27–30.
28. Beydon N. Interrupter resistance: what's feasible? *Paediatr Respir Rev*. 2006;7(Suppl 1):S5–S7.
29. Eastwood PR, Platt PR, Shepherd K, Maddison K, Hillman DR. Collapsibility of the upper airway at different concentrations of propofol anesthesia. *Anesthesiology*. 2005;103(3): 470–477.
30. Thille AW, Richard JC, Brochard L. The decision to extubate in the intensive care unit. *Am J Respir Crit Care Med*. 2013;187(12):1294–1302.
31. Nakagawa M, Hattori N, Haruta Y, et al. Effect of increasing respiratory rate on airway resistance and reactance in COPD patients. *Respirology*. 2015;20(1):87–94.
32. Marini JJ. Dynamic hyperinflation and auto-positive end-expiratory pressure: lessons learned over 30 years. *Am J Respir Crit Care Med*. 2011;184(7):756–762.
33. Junhasavasdikul D, Telias I, Grieco DL, et al. Expiratory flow limitation during mechanical ventilation. *Chest*. 2018;154(4):948–962.
34. Riley RL, Cournand A. Ideal alveolar air and the analysis of ventilation-perfusion relationships in the lungs. *J Appl Physiol*. 1949;1(12):825–847.
35. West JB. Ventilation-perfusion inequality and overall gas exchange in computer models of the lung. *Respir Physiol*. 1969;7(1):88–110.
36. Glenny RW, Bernard S, Robertson HT, Hlastala MP. Gravity is an important but secondary determinant of regional pulmonary blood flow in upright primates. *J Appl Physiol (1985)*. 1999; 86(2):623–632.
37. Galvin I, Drummond GB, Nirmalan M. Distribution of blood flow and ventilation in the lung: gravity is not the only factor. *Br J Anaesth*. 2007;98(4):420–428.
38. Riley RL, Cournand A. Analysis of factors affecting partial pressures of oxygen and carbon dioxide in gas and blood of lungs; theory. *J Appl Physiol*. 1951;4(2):77–101.
39. Wagner PD. The multiple inert gas elimination technique (MIGET). *Intensive Care Med*. 2008; 34(6):994–1001.
40. Spinelli E, Kircher M, Stender B, et al. Unmatched ventilation and perfusion measured by electrical impedance tomography predicts the outcome of ARDS. *Crit Care*. 2021;25(1):192.
41. Tokics L, Hedenstierna G, Svensson L, et al. V/Q distribution and correlation to atelectasis in anesthetized paralyzed humans. *J Appl Physiol (1985)*. 1996;81(4):1822–1833.
42. Grocott MP, Martin DS, Levett DZ, et al. Arterial blood gases and oxygen content in climbers on Mount Everest. *N Engl J Med*. 2009;360(2):140–149.
43. Bigatello L, Pesenti A. Respiratory physiology for the anesthesiologist. *Anesthesiology*. 2019; 130(6):1064–1077.
44. Force ADT, Ranieri VM, Rubenfeld GD, et al. Acute respiratory distress syndrome: the Berlin Definition. *JAMA*. 2012;307(23):2526–2533.
45. Moudgil R, Michelakis ED, Archer SL. Hypoxic pulmonary vasoconstriction. *J Appl Physiol (1985)*. 2005;98(1):390–403.
46. Lellouche F, Delorme M, Brochard L. Impact of respiratory rate and dead space in the current era of lung protective mechanical ventilation. *Chest*. 2020;158(1):45–47.
47. Alheid GF, McCrimmon DR. The chemical neuroanatomy of breathing. *Respir Physiol Neurobiol*. 2008;164(1–2):3–11.
48. Vaporidi K, Akoumianaki E, Telias I, Goligher EC, Brochard L, Georgopoulos D. Respiratory drive in critically ill patients. Pathophysiology and clinical implications. *Am J Respir Crit Care Med*. 2020;201(1):20–32.
49. Duffin J, Mohan RM, Vasiliou P, Stephenson R, Mahamed S. A model of the chemoreflex control of breathing in humans: model parameters measurement. *Respir Physiol*. 2000;120(1):13–26.
50. Wang SC, Borison HL. The vomiting center; a critical experimental analysis. *Arch Neurol Psychiatry*. 1950;63(6):928–941.
51. Canning BJ, Chang AB, Bolser DC, et al. Anatomy and neurophysiology of cough: CHEST Guideline and Expert Panel report. *Chest*. 2014;146(6):1633–1648.
52. Davis HL, Fowler WS, Lambert EH. Effect of volume and rate of inflation and deflation on transpulmonary pressure and response of pulmonary stretch receptors. *Am J Physiol*. 1956;187(3): 558–566.
53. Clark FJ, von Euler C. On the regulation of depth and rate of breathing. *J Physiol*. 1972; 222(2):267–295.
54. Czick ME WJ, Gross JB. Sources of inspiration: a neurophysiologic framework for understanding anesthetic effects on ventilatory control. *Curr Anesthesiol Rep*. 2014(4):67–75.
55. Oh TK, Park IS, Ji E, Na HS. Value of preoperative spirometry test in predicting postoperative pulmonary complications in high-risk patients after laparoscopic abdominal surgery. *PLoS One*. 2018;13(12):e0209347.
56. Elsheikh B, Arnold WD, Gharibshahi S, Reynolds J, Freimer M, Kissel JT. Correlation of single-breath count test and neck flexor muscle strength with spirometry in myasthenia gravis. *Muscle Nerve*. 2016;53(1):134–136.
57. Apthorp GH, Marshall R. Pulmonary diffusing capacity: a comparison of breath-holding and steady state methods using carbon monoxide. *J Clin Invest*. 1961;40:1775–1784.
58. Crapo RO. Pulmonary-function testing. *N Engl J Med*. 1994;331(1):25–30. doi: 10.1056/NEJM199407073310107
59. Graham BL, Steenbruggen I, Miller MR, et al. Standardization of Spirometry 2019 Update. An Official American Thoracic Society and European Respiratory Society Technical Statement. *Am J Respir Crit Care Med*. 2019;200(8):e70–e88.
60. Canet J, Gallart L, Gomar C, et al. Prediction of postoperative pulmonary complications in a population-based surgical cohort. *Anesthesiology*. 2010;113(6):1338–1350.
61. Morano MT, Araujo AS, Nascimento FB, et al. Preoperative pulmonary rehabilitation versus chest physical therapy in patients undergoing lung cancer resection: a pilot randomized controlled trial. *Arch Phys Med Rehabil*. 2013;94(1):53–58.

16 Acid–Base, Fluids, and Electrolytes

TREFAN ARCHIBALD • DASUN S. PERAMUNAGE • CHRISTOPHER R. BARNES

KEY POINTS

1. Nearly half of all hospitalized patients will develop an acid–base disorder during their hospitalization.
2. Accurate diagnosis of acid–base disturbances requires a systematic, stepwise approach.
3. While control of blood glucose in the critically ill is associated with improved clinical outcomes, it is clear that tight, conservative control targeting glucose ranges of 81 to 108 mg/dL is associated with higher mortality than compared with targeting blood glucoses below 180 mg/dL.
4. In healthy ASA I–II patients undergoing minor procedures, liberal fluid administration is associated with decreased risks of postoperative nausea and vomiting (PONV). However, in higher-risk patients, or those undergoing major operations, restrictive, goal-directed therapy (GDT) is associated decreased risks of postoperative ileus, pneumonia, and increased length of stay.
5. While the use of albumin has failed to show clinical differences in primary outcomes in septic shock, there may be benefit to its use in the acute burns resuscitation.
6. In both non-critically and critically ill patients, the use of balanced crystalloids in comparison to 0.9% saline is associated with fewer metabolic derangements, notably hyperchloremic metabolic acidosis, as well as acute kidney injury.
7. Dynamic assessments for determining volume responsiveness are more sensitive and specific in determining if patients will respond well to ongoing fluid challenges.
8. New oral potassium-binding agents are effective at quickly lower [K^+] by increasing total body K^+ elimination.
9. Ca^{2+} is essential to achieve proper hemostasis given its role in platelet activation and propagation as well as a critical co-factor in the activation of the coagulation cascade.
10. The diamond of death—Hypocalcemia is now recognized as fourth component to the formerly known lethal triad of hypothermia, acidosis, and coagulopathy.
11. Magnesium has demonstrated analgesic properties as a result of *N*-methyl-D-aspartate (NMDA) receptor antagonism.

Patient comorbidities, in addition to the complex changes in acid–base and volume status, or electrolyte derangements they undergo during the perioperative period require a thorough understanding of these essential principles of physiology. Care based on a comprehensive knowledge of these fundamentals–acid–base physiology, fluids and volume status, and electrolytes–allows the vigilant anesthesiologist to have a greater impact on reducing perioperative morbidity and mortality.

Acid–Base Equilibrium

Acid–Base Interpretation and Treatment

Over the course of a day, the average individual generates approximately 10,000 to 15,000 mmol of volatile acid and about 50 to 100 mEq of nonvolatile acid. To maintain homeostasis, these acids are buffered in the cells and extracellular fluid (ECF) before being excreted by the lungs and kidneys, respectively. Normally the pH of ECF is roughly 7.4, but the normal range in clinical practice is between 7.35 and 7.45. Acid–base disturbances occur when the body's normal pH is altered either by acid or base loads that overwhelm the buffering and excretion capacity of the body or by the presence of abnormal renal and pulmonary function. The terms **acidemia** and **alkalemia** are used to describe either a decrease or increase in blood pH respectively from the normal range, and the terms **acidosis** and **alkalosis** are used to describe the physiologic processes that can lead to an increase of decrease in pH. Tables 16-1 and 16-2 outline the physiologic consequences of severe acidemia and alkalemia.[1] Broadly speaking there are four main categories of acid–base disturbances: metabolic acidosis, metabolic alkalosis, respiratory acidosis, respiratory alkalosis (Table 16-3). In studies of hospitalized patients, 1
acid–base disorders were found in roughly 51% to 56% of hospitalized patients; of this population, the overall prevalence of metabolic acidosis was 10% to 12%, metabolic alkalosis was 16% to 28%, respiratory acidosis 27% to 26%, respiratory alkalosis 29% to 42% and 6% were mixed disorders.[2,3] In this section we will explore the diagnosis and treatment of these acid–base derangements.

The three methods used to quantify acid–base disturbance are the base excess approach, physiologic approach, and the

Table 16-1 Physiologic Consequences of Severe Acidemia (pH < 7.2)

Cardiovascular
- Impaired myocardial contractility with reduction in cardiac output
- Increased pulmonary vascular resistance
- Decreases the threshold to trigger malignant arrhythmias
- Reduced responsiveness to catecholamines

Respiratory
- Hyperventilation
- Dyspnea
- Decreased respiratory muscle strength leading to respiratory fatigue

Metabolic
- Insulin resistance
- Reduction in ATP synthesis
- Hyperkalemia
- Increase in protein degradation

Cerebral
- Changes in mental status/coma
- Inhibition of cellular metabolism and cell-volume regulation

Modified from Adrogué HJ, Madias NE. Management of life-threatening acid–base disorders. *N Engl J Med*. 1998;338(2):107–111.

physiochemical approach. The base excess and physiologic approaches are the two main approaches used in clinical practice. Both the base excess and physiologic approach use the Henderson–Hasselbalch equation:

$$pH = 6.1 + \log_{10}\left(\frac{[HCO_3^-]}{0.3 \times (PaCO_2)}\right) \quad (16\text{-}1)$$

Where 6.1 is the pKa of carbonic acid and 0.3 is the blood solubility coefficient of carbon dioxide at 37°C. In the Henderson–Hasselbalch approach to acid–base disorders, plasma pH is directly determined by the concentration of carbon dioxide and bicarbonate buffer. Base excess was introduced by Siggaard-Andersen in an effort to separate the metabolic and respiratory components of pH, while Schwartz and Relman developed an approach based on the in vivo relationship between bicarbonate and the partial pressure of carbon dioxide.[4,5] Modern blood gas analyzers report both base excess and bicarbonate concentrations.

Table 16-2 Physiologic Consequences of Severe Alkalemia (pH > 7.6)

Cardiovascular
- Arteriolar constriction
- Reduction in coronary blood flow
- Decreases the threshold to trigger malignant arrhythmias
- Left shift of the oxygen dissociation curve

Respiratory
- Hypoventilation

Metabolic
- Hypokalemia
- Decrease in serum ionized calcium, magnesium, and phosphate

Cerebral
- Decreased cerebral blood flow
- Tetany, seizure, fatigue, delirium, and coma

Modified from Adrogué HJ, Madias NE. Management of life-threatening acid–base disorders. *N Engl J Med*. 1998;338(2):107–111.

Table 16-3 Primary Acid–Base Disturbances with Expected Compensation

Metabolic Acidosis:
- Compensatory respiratory alkalosis within 12–24 hours
- *Winter's formula:* $PaCO_2 = 1.5 \times [HCO_3^-] + 8 \pm 2$ mmHg, or
- $\downarrow\Delta PaCO_2 = 1.1 \times \downarrow\Delta[HCO_3^-]$

Metabolic Alkalosis:
- Compensatory respiratory acidosis within 24–48 hours
- $PaCO_2 = 0.7 \times [HCO_3^-] + 20 \pm 5$ mmHg, or
- $\uparrow\Delta PaCO_2 = 0.75 \times \uparrow\Delta[HCO_3^-]$

Respiratory Acidosis:
- Compensatory metabolic alkalosis over 48–96 hours
- *Acute:* $\downarrow\Delta$ pH = $0.008 \times (PaCO_2 - 40)^a$; $\uparrow\Delta[HCO_3^-] = 0.1 \times \uparrow\Delta PaCO_2$, or $\Delta[HCO_3]$ = +1 mEq/L for each increase in $PaCO_2$ of 10 mmHg
- *Chronic:* $\downarrow\Delta$ pH = $0.003 \times (PaCO_2 - 40)^*$; $\uparrow\Delta[HCO_3^-] = 0.35 \times \uparrow\Delta PaCO_2$, or $\Delta[HCO_3]$ = +4 mEq/L for each increase in $PaCO_2$ of 10 mmHg

Respiratory Alkalosis:
- Compensatory metabolic acidosis over 48–96 hours
- *Acute:* $\downarrow\Delta[HCO_3^-] = 0.2 \times \downarrow\Delta PaCO_2$, or $\Delta[HCO_3]$ = −2 mEq/L for each decrease in $PaCO_2$ of 10 mmHg
- *Chronic:* $\downarrow\Delta[HCO_3^-] = 0.4 \times \downarrow\Delta PaCO_2$, or $\Delta[HCO_3]$ = −5 mEq/L for each decrease in $PaCO_2$ of 10 mmHg

[a]40 is used to represent the normal physiologic $PaCO_2$.

In the Stewart approach to acid–base interpretation, three independent variables: $PaCO_2$; strong ion difference; and concentration of weak acids determine plasma pH and bicarbonate concentration.[6] This approach incorporates the laws of mass action, conservation of mass, and electric neutrality. The plasma strong ions in the Stewart approach are completely dissociated and include sodium, potassium, chloride, and lactate. Unlike the Henderson–Hasselbalch approach, the Stewart approach to acid–base disturbances provides insight into the mechanisms underlying an acid–base disturbance. However, it is unclear if the Stewart approach is better than the traditional methods used to diagnose and manage acid–base disorders nor is it a better approach for prognostication of disease.[7,8]

Metabolic Acidosis

Metabolic acidosis is characterized by acidemia (pH < 7.35), decrease serum bicarbonate ($[HCO_3]$ <21 mEq/L), and a compensatory decrease in $PaCO_2$. Depending on the clinical circumstance, it can be benign or reflect a life-threatening emergency. The physiologic consequences of severe metabolic acidosis are listed in Table 16-1. The etiology of metabolic acidosis can be due to increased bicarbonate loss, decreased renal excretion of acid, an imbalance between production and consumption of endogenous acids, or administration of exogenous acid. This metabolic disorder can be categorized into either anion gap or non-anion gap metabolic acidosis. The balance of anions and cations maintain plasma neutrality. Serum sodium represents the predominant cation and is in balance with the sum of measured serum anions, such as chloride and bicarbonate, and unmeasured anions. A rise in unmeasured anions creates a gap that is referred to as the anion gap, which is represented by the following equation:

$$\textit{Anion Gap} = [Na^+] - ([Cl^-] + [HCO_3]) \quad (16\text{-}2)$$

Table 16-4 Etiologies of Metabolic Acidosis

Anion Gap Metabolic Acidosis	Non-Anion Gap Metabolic Acidosis
• Advanced chronic kidney disease • Ketoacidosis ▪ Diabetic ▪ Alcoholic ▪ Starvation • Lactic acidosis • Uremia • Metformin • Toxins ▪ Methanol ▪ Ethylene glycol ▪ Salicylates ▪ Paraldehyde ▪ Propylene glycol	• Renal tubular acidosis • Diarrhea • Carbonic anhydrase inhibitors • Early chronic kidney disease • Fluid resuscitation with saline • HCL administration • Ureteral diversion • Biliary fistula

An anion gap < 13 mEq/L is indicative of a non-anion gap metabolic acidosis and is seen in conditions where serum bicarbonate is excreted or in resuscitation with 0.9% saline.[9,10] An anion gap > 13 mEq/L makes the diagnosis of an anion gap acidosis. Common causes of anion gap and non-anion gap metabolic acidosis are listed in Table 16-4. It is important to correct for serum albumin levels as albumin is a major serum anion and its serum concentration can have an impact of the calculated anion gap.

The treatment of metabolic acidosis involves addressing the underlying cause of the acidosis. If a metabolic acidosis is recognized while the patient is mechanically ventilated, then every effort should be made to maintain ventilatory compensation. In a spontaneously ventilating patient, the normal compensatory response to a metabolic acidosis is hyperventilation. If shock is the underlying cause of the metabolic acidosis, then careful consideration of the patient's volume status should be determined in efforts to treat the underlying cause.

In critically ill patients, there is no strong clinical evidence to suggest that the acidemia induced by metabolic acidosis should be treated with sodium bicarbonate buffer, though there is an associated increase in mortality with a pH < 7.2 in septic and hypovolemic shock.[11,12] The BICAR-ICU trial was a multicenter open label trial that investigated the benefits of bicarbonate therapy in severe metabolic acidemia and found no difference in a composite score of mortality in 28 days and at least one organ failure at day 7 between the group treated with bicarbonate therapy and placebo; but a secondary analysis suggested that patients with acute kidney injury (AKI) had better mortality outcomes with bicarbonate therapy and were less likely to receive renal replacement therapy.[11] Nevertheless, many clinicians continue to administer sodium-bicarbonate therapy in clinically deteriorating patients with severe metabolic acidosis caused by persistent lactic acidosis. In contrast to sodium-bicarbonate, the buffer tris-hydroxymethyl aminomethane (THAM) effectively reduces [H+], without increasing plasma sodium or generate carbon dioxide as a byproduct of buffering.[13] Despite its advantages over bicarbonate, there are no clinical trials supporting the use to THAM.

Metabolic Alkalosis

Metabolic alkalosis is characterized by an alkalemia (pH > 7.45) with a concomitant elevated serum bicarbonate ($[HCO_3]$ > 27 mEq/L) and a compensatory rise in $PaCO_2$ due to hypoventilation. Metabolic alkalosis can be categorized as chloride responsive or chloride resistant (Table 16-5) and can be caused by intracellular shifts of hydrogen ions secondary to hypokalemia; gastrointestinal or renal loss of hydrogen ions; administration of exogenous bicarbonate ions; or volume contraction. Normally the kidney can compensate by excreting excess bicarbonate in the urine, but a metabolic alkalosis develops when renal clearance of bicarbonate ion is impaired. Physiologic consequences of severe metabolic alkalosis are listed in Table 16-2.

Table 16-5 Etiologies of Metabolic Alkalosis

Chloride Responsive	Chloride Resistant
• Vomiting/Nasogastric suctioning • Chloride wasting diarrhea • Villous adenoma • Diuretic therapy • Posthypercapnia • Bicarbonate therapy for organic acidosis	• Hyperaldosteronism • Cushing syndrome • Milk-alkali syndrome • Exogenous steroid use • Barter syndrome • Refeeding alkalosis • Renal artery stenosis • Severe hypokalemia

Once the diagnosis of metabolic alkalosis is made, its etiology can often be determined by the patient's clinical history; the three most common causes are emesis, diuretic use, and excess of mineralocorticoids. If the etiology is unknown, checking a urine [Cl-] can assist in determining if the cause of the metabolic alkalosis will reverse with the administration of saline. The urine [Cl-] is always low (<20 mEq/L) in a saline responsive metabolic alkalosis as it represents a hypovolemic state and the activation of the normal renin–angiotensin–aldosterone system. The administration of saline will replenish the intravascular volume, which decreases the release of aldosterone and allows the excess bicarbonate to be renally excreted. Patients with metabolic alkalosis due to excess mineralocorticoid, hypokalemia, or renal insufficiency are chloride resistant, and their metabolic alkalosis will not correct with saline. It is important to recognize the presence of a metabolic alkalosis in the perioperative setting, as a severe alkalemia can be induced by an iatrogenic respiratory alkalosis from over ventilation.

The treatment of a metabolic alkalosis is entirely dependent on its etiology. If volume contraction is the cause, then expansion of intravascular volume with 0.9% saline and repletion of potassium with KCL will cause the alkalosis to resolve. In patients with excessive mineralocorticoid production, spironolactone can be used to inhibit the effects of excessive aldosterone/corticosteroids. Potassium sparing diuretics can be used in patients with severe hypokalemia. Hypokalemia can promote metabolic alkalosis by increasing H^+ excretion, ammonia production, and chloride wasting by the kidneys. Potassium repletion or potassium sparing diuretics can correct this finding. In critically ill patients with metabolic alkalosis, acetazolamide is often used to correct the alkalemia and promote further diaresis.[14,15] Hydrochloric acid given through a central line has also been utilized to correct severe metabolic alkalosis refractory to acetazolamide therapy.[16] In patients with renal failure, dialysis against a high chloride/low bicarbonate dialysate can be used to correct the alkalemia.

Respiratory Alkalosis

Primary respiratory alkalosis is an acid–base disorder characterized by alkalemia (pH > 7.45), hypocarbia ($PaCO_2$ < 36 mmHg) and decrease in serum bicarbonate concentrations. The mechanism is due to a disproportionately high minute ventilation that exceeds what is necessary to remove the volatile acids (CO_2) generated by cellular metabolism. Broadly speaking the etiology of respiratory alkalosis can be categorized into central, hypoxemic, pulmonary,

Table 16-6 Etiologies of Respiratory Alkalosis

Hypoxia	CNS Disorders
Ventilator induced	Pregnancy
Pulmonary embolism	Liver failure
Pneumonia	Salicylate overdose
Early restrictive lung disease	Analeptic overdose
Mild pulmonary edema	Sepsis
Anxiety	Hyperthyroidism
Pain	Hyperventilation syndrome

and iatrogenic causes. Common etiologies of respiratory alkalosis are listed in (Table 16-6). Hyperventilation syndrome, which can cause a primary respiratory alkalosis, is a diagnosis of exclusion and not commonly seen in the perioperative setting; there is a lack of consensus regarding the diagnosis of this disorder, but there is an association with anxiety and panic attacks.[17]

Severe respiratory alkalosis may lead to hypocalcemia, hypokalemia, vasoconstriction, bronchoconstriction, and cardiac arrhythmias. Cerebral blood flow and cerebral pH are closely regulated by $PaCO_2$. Deliberate hypocapnia is often utilized in neurosurgical procedures to relax the brain and facilitate surgical exposure. Furthermore, it is often utilized to decrease cerebral blood flow, which reduces an acutely elevated intracranial pressure (ICP) by decreasing the overall cerebral blood volume. It is important to note that the effect of hypocarbia on reducing ICP is a temporary measure and cerebral blood flow will return to previous levels as central nervous system (CNS) bicarbonate levels normalize with time. There is growing evidence that the cerebral vasoconstriction caused by hyperventilation leads to worse outcomes in traumatic brain injury (TBI) and hemorrhagic stroke due to induced ischemia.[18,19]

Respiratory alkalosis will resolve with treatment of the underlying disease process. However, it is important to recognize hyperventilation in the perioperative setting and maintain a similar intraoperative $PaCO_2$. This may necessitate placement of an arterial line for serial blood gas measurements. Excretion of bicarbonate in the urine is the renal compensatory response to chronic respiratory alkalosis and happens over a period of hours to days.

Respiratory Acidosis

Primary respiratory acidosis is characterized by acidemia (pH < 7.35), hypercarbia ($PaCO_2$ > 44 mmHg) and increase in serum bicarbonate concentrations. The hypercarbia and acidosis found in this disorder is due an increase in metabolic CO_2 production or reduction in alveolar minute ventilation. Normally, an increase in $PaCO_2$ stimulates central chemoreceptors in the brainstem to increase minute ventilation (increasing the ventilatory rate and tidal volumes) to match CO_2 production. Sedatives can impair this central regulation of respiration. Increases in airflow resistance as seen in COPD or asthma, lung and chest wall stiffness, and neuromuscular weakness can impair alveolar ventilation and lead to hypercarbia. Hypermetabolic states such as sepsis, carbohydrate rich diets, malignant hyperthermia, and fever can increase production of volatile acids. Chronic respiratory acidosis leads to renal compensation which involves excretion of H^+ and ammonium in the urine and reabsorption of bicarbonate; this compensatory metabolic alkalosis counters the acidosis over the course of several days. Common etiologies of respiratory acidosis are listed in Table 16-7. The use of lung protective ventilation (LPV) strategies to reduce ventilator induced lung injury has been shown to decrease mortality in patients with acute respiratory distress syndrome (ARDS); however, the clinician should anticipate a resultant respiratory acidosis secondary to the intentional alveolar hypoventilation associated with LPV.[20,21]

Table 16-7 Etiologies of Respiratory Acidosis

CNS depressants	Thoracic cage limitations
Neuromuscular disorders	Pneumothorax
Ventilator induced	Pleural effusion
Cardiopulmonary arrest	Obstructive lung disorders
Obesity	• COPD
	• Asthma

The physiologic consequences of severe acidemia have been reported above in Table 16-1. However, respiratory acidosis incurs some beneficial effects such as: increased catecholamine release leading to an increase in cardiac output (CO) and blood pressure (BP); and an increase in perfusion to organs such as the brain, heart, and kidneys.[22] Furthermore, it shifts the oxygen dissociation curve of hemoglobin to the right, as described by the Bohr effect, which increases oxygen unloading to the tissues. The utilization of bicarbonate therapy to treat a severe respiratory acidosis is controversial and there is a lack of clinical evidence supporting its use; though use of extracorporeal membrane oxygenation may be considered.[23–25]

The chronicity of the disorder dictates the therapy for respiratory acidosis. An acute respiratory acidosis may require noninvasive or mechanical ventilation to address the symptoms unless there is a known reversible cause (e.g., residual neuromuscular blockade, opiate or sedative overdose). Chronic respiratory acidosis is usually treated with efforts to improve the underlying pulmonary function rather than mechanical ventilation. The chronicity can be ascertained by assessing the patient's arterial blood gases as seen in Table 16-8. In the perioperative setting, it is important not to hyperventilate patients with a compensated chronic respiratory acidosis and target a normal pH intraoperatively. Normalizing ventilation in these patients runs the risk of inducing a profound respiratory alkalosis. Careful titration of opioids or sedatives is necessary so as not to worsen the underlying acidosis with further depression of the central respiratory drive. Multimodal analgesia or regional anesthetics should be considered in these patients to minimize the use of opiate medications. However, the choice of regional technique matters, upper brachial plexus blocks, such as interscalene or supraclavicular blocks, will elicit varying degrees of phrenic nerve palsy and further impair ventilation.[26]

Diagnosis of Acid–Base Disorders and Interpretation of Arterial Blood Gas

Accurate diagnosis of acid–base disturbances requires a systematic, 2
stepwise approach seen in Table 16-9.[27] A thorough clinical history and physical examination will often provide clues regarding the underlying acid–base disorder. If such a disorder is suspected, then an ABG and venous electrolyte panel should be drawn simultaneously. The calculated bicarbonate level in the ABG and the measured serum bicarbonate level should be within 2 to 3 mEq/L.[28] A discrepancy indicates a lab error or that the samples were not drawn simultaneously. The plasma electrolytes, pH, and $PaCO_2$ will be utilized to determine the underlying acid–base disorder. The first step is to use the arterial pH to determine if the patient has an acidemia or alkalemia. Once the underlying disorder is determined, the second step involves analysis of the $PaCO_2$ and plasma $[HCO_3]$ to categorize the primary process as *respiratory* or *metabolic*. If the patient is acidemic with an elevated $PaCO_2$ then the primary disorder is a respiratory acidosis. Acidemia with concurrent decrease in serum bicarbonate concentrations represents a metabolic acidosis. Alkalemia with an increased plasma bicarbonate is consistent with a metabolic alkalosis, while respiratory alkalosis is represented

Table 16-8 Stepwise Approach to Arterial Blood Gas Interpretation

Step 1	Identify if the patient is academic or alkalemic • pH < 7.35 = acidemia • pH >7.45 = alkalemia
Step 2	Determine if there reflects a primary respiratory or metabolic process • pH ↓, $PaCO_2$ ↑ = respiratory acidosis • pH ↓, $PaCO_2$ ↓ = metabolic acidosis • pH ↑, $PaCO_2$ ↓ = respiratory alkalosis • pH ↑, $PaCO_2$ ↑ = metabolic alkalosis
Step 3	Assess if there has been an appropriate compensation
Step 4	Calculate the serum anion gap (AG); normal <13 mEq/L • Serum AG = $[Na^+] - ([Cl^-] + [HCO_3^-])$ or, • 2.5 × [albumin]
Step 5	If a non-anion gap acidosis is identified, calculate urine anion gap: • Urine AG (mEq/L) = Urine $(Na^+ + K^+ - Cl^-)$ • *Positive urine AG = gastrointestinal HCO_3^- losses, i.e., diarrhea* • *Negative urine AG = renal HCO_3^- losses, i.e., RTA.*
Step 6	Calculate the *delta-delta* (ΔΔ) = ΔAG/Δ HCO_3^- • ΔΔ < 1.0 = mixed anion gap + non-anion gap metabolic acidosis • ΔΔ 1–2 = pure anion gap metabolic acidosis • ΔΔ >2.0 = mixed anion gap metabolic acidosis + metabolic alkalosis, or a well-compensated chronic respiratory acidosis

RTA, renal tubular acidosis.

by alkalemia with a decrease in $PaCO_2$. If the primary disorder is respiratory in nature, then Table 16-8 can be used to determine if the change in bicarbonate concentration represents a chronic or acute process. The fourth step is to determine the anion gap, which should be adjusted for serum albumin concentration. To account for serum albumin, which is a major anion, the observed anion gap is corrected by adding a correction factor 2.5 × ([*normal albumin*] – [*observed albumin*]) to the observed anion gap.[29] The anion gap should always be calculated even if a primary metabolic acidosis is not initially identified or the pH and $PaCO_2$ are within the normal ranges as this could indicate the presence of a mixed acid–base disorder. A high anion-gap should warrant further ancillary testing to identify the etiology. A non-anion gap acidosis should prompt a urine anion gap study to determine if the cause is secondary to gastrointestinal losses or renal losses of bicarbonate. The presence of a metabolic acidosis or alkalosis should warrant a determination if there is a concurrent respiratory compensation. Winter's formula ($PaCO_2 = (1.5 \times HCO_3) + 8 \pm 2$) is used to determine if there is appropriate respiratory compensation for a metabolic acidosis, and the expected respiratory compensation for a primary metabolic alkalosis is determine by ($PaCO_2 = 40 + 0.7 \times (HCO_{3measured} - HCO_{3normal}) \pm 5$.[30] If an anion gap is present, then the sixth and final step is to calculate the delta delta ratio (Δ/Δ). The Δ/Δ compares the change in anion gap to the change in bicarbonate. A ratio between 1 and 2 indicates a pure anion gap acidosis, <1.0 indicates the presence of a concurrent non-anion gap metabolic acidosis, and >2.0 indicates either a concurrent metabolic alkalosis or a compensated chronic respiratory acidosis.

Table 16-9 Arterial Blood Gas Example 1: Stat Laboratory Findings

Parameter	Result
Arterial Blood Gas	
• pH	7.14
• $PaCO_2$	73 mmHg
• HCO_3^-	21 mEq/L
Electrolytes	
• $[Na^+]$	138 mEq/L
• $[Cl^-]$	105 mEq/L
• $[HCO_3^-]$	23 mEq/L
• [Cr]	1.8 mg/dL

Examples

The following clinical cases illustrate the stepwise approach to identifying acid–base disturbances discussed above.

Example 1

An 84-year-old female is admitted to the intensive care unit (ICU) following a mechanical fall during a recent snowstorm with resultant displaced, right-sided ribs 4–9 fractures as well as an AKI. She recently received scheduled acetaminophen and ketorolac, and break-through intravenous morphine, which she has received since her admission 24 hours ago. You are paged to assess her given concerns for progressive somnolence. You request a stat arterial blood gas and chemistry profile be drawn on your way to the bedside, which are notable for the following (Table 16-10). Working through our stepwise approach to her acid–base derangement is as follows:

1. The patient is acidemic.
2. The $PaCO_2$ is severely elevated, indicative of a primary respiratory acidosis.
3. There appears to be no metabolic compensation, thus representing an acute process.
4. The serum anion gap is normal.

Table 16-10 Arterial Blood Gas Example 2: Stat Laboratory Findings

Parameter	Result
Arterial Blood Gas	
• pH	7.18
• $PaCO_2$	22 mmHg
• HCO_3^-	11 mEq/L
Electrolytes, Serum	
• $[Na^+]$	132 mEq/L
• $[Cl^-]$	98 mEq/L
• $[HCO_3^-]$	12 mEq/L
• [Glucose]	398 mg/dL
Urinalysis	
• $[Na^+]$	28 mEq/L
• $[K^+]$	3 mEq/L
• $[Cl^-]$	41 mEq/L
• Ketones	3+
• Glucose	4+

5. No anion gap acidosis identified, thus urine anion gap is not warranted.
6. As this is an acute respiratory acidosis without metabolic compensation with a normal serum anion gap, a *delta-delta* is not needed.

Given her ongoing intravenous morphine doses, this case likely represents opioid induced respiratory depression. This situation is likely further complicated by her advanced age and the buildup of active morphine metabolites in the setting of her concurrent AKI. Recall that for every 1 mmHg increase in $PaCO_2$ there is a corresponding decrease in pH of 0.008; thus, in this case an increase of 33 mmHg $PaCO_2$ from a normal base line of 40, would result in a decrease in serum pH of 0.264 to 7.14. As these data solely reflect an acute respiratory acidosis resulting from opioid induced respiratory depression, it should appropriately be reversed by the administration of the opioid antagonist, naloxone.

Example 2

A previously healthy 15-year-old male presents to the emergency department with several days of nausea, vomiting, non-bloody diarrhea, confusion, and progressing polydipsia with polyuria following a recent trip to South America with his family. He is afebrile, tachypneic with a respiratory rate of 32, with a normal BP, but mildly tachycardic with a heart rate of 112. Urinalysis is notable for 4+ glucose, 3+ ketones, Urine $[Na^+]$ 28, $[K^+]$ 3, and $[Cl^-]$ of 41. Notable electrolytes and arterial blood gas are shown in Table 16-10. A stepwise approach his acid–base derangement is as follows:

1. The patient is acidemic.
2. The $PaCO_2$ and $[HCO_3^-]$ are both decreased, reflecting an ongoing metabolic acidosis
3. *Winter's formula* can be used to assess for appropriate respiratory alkalosis compensation in the setting of a metabolic acidosis. Predicted $PaCO_2 = 1.5 \times [HCO_3^-] + 8 \pm 2$; or 24–28 mmHg. The measured $PaCO_2$ is 20, suggesting a mixed acid–base disorder is present.
4. The serum anion gap is 22, reflecting an elevated anion gap metabolic acidosis.
5. The Δ/Δ, [(measured anion gap – normal anion gap)/(normal $[HCO_3^-]$ – measured $[HCO_3^-]$)], or in this case [(22-13)/(24-12)], equals 0.75. As the (Δ/Δ) is <1.0 it suggests a concomitant anion gap acidosis as well as a non-anion gap acidosis is present.
6. When a non-anion gap is present, a urine anion gap can be calculated, in this case urine ($[Na^+] + [K^+] - [Cl^-]$) is (28 + 3 – 41) equals –10; a negative urine anion gap indicates ongoing gastrointestinal $[HCO_3^-]$ losses.

Thus, reflecting a mixed elevated anion gap and non-anion gap metabolic acidoses without an appropriate compensatory respiratory alkalosis. Given his overall clinical picture, the clinician should be most concerned for the presence of diabetic ketoacidosis (DKA), further worsened by a non-anion gap acidosis resulting for ongoing gastrointestinal losses from vomiting and diarrhea. Despite his tachypnea and elevated minute ventilation, suspicious for Kussmaul respirations, he is unable to appropriately compensate for this severe, concurrent metabolic acidoses.

Fluid Management

Physiology

Body Fluid Compartments

Assessment of fluid losses and correctly replacing those losses is predicated on understanding the body's different compartments and the volumes of distribution for water, important solutes, and colloids within those compartments. Water comprises the majority of the human body by weight, averaging approximately 60% in adult males and 50% in adult females. Total body water (TBW) is distributed between the intracellular and extracellular compartments. Intracellular fluid (ICF) comprises 55% to 65% of TBW while ECF accounts for the remaining 35% to 45%. ECF is found in two distinct spaces, the interstitial and intravascular. Most of the ECF is in the interstitial space, approximately 75%, leaving the remaining 25% of the ECF in the intravascular space. Notably, red cell volume is considered intracellular and not intravascular fluid. In a 70-kg male contains approximately 42 L of TBW, 25.2 L being ICF and 16.8 L being ECF. His ECF is further divided into interstitial fluid and intravascular fluid, 12.6 L and 4.2 L, respectively.

Water freely diffuses across cellular membranes to move between the intracellular space and extracellular space. The diffusion of water is a response to the gradient in effective osmolarity between the compartments. Effective osmolarity in determined by the solute concentration and the solute reflection coefficient on the cellular membrane. Large sodium cation (Na^+) and potassium cation (K^+) gradients are maintained between the spaces through Na-K-ATPase pumps. This pump leads the major solute to differ extracellularly and intracellularly, which are Na^+ and K^+, respectively. The ECF concentration of Na^+ ($[Na^+]$) is approximately 140 mEq/L and the ICF concentration of K^+ ($[K^+]$) is approximately 150 mEq/L. The result of these gradients is that ECF volume is largely determined by sodium content of the body, which is highly regulated through salt intake and renal excretion. Importantly, ECF volume is necessary for circulation and thereby influences vital organ functions.

Water movement between intracellular and intravascular spaces is not determined by effective osmolarity, as between ICF and ECF, but rather Starling forces (hydrostatic and osmotic pressure gradients). The difference in determinants of water movement is explained by the differences in the barriers separating compartments. Intracellular and intravascular spaces are separated by capillary membranes which, unlike cellular membranes, are highly permeable to small solutes such as Na^+ and K^+ and therefore do not generate any driving force for the movement of water. However, capillary membranes are less permeable to larger molecules, such as albumin, which can exert oncotic (osmotic pressure from colloids) across the barrier. Albumin is the most important oncotically active colloid in the ECF.

Distribution of Infused Fluids

Infusion of intravenous fluids (IVFs) is done for many reasons: correction of ECF or ICF deficit, temporizing treatment for increased ICP, correction of deranged electrolytes, etc. Given the sundry goals a clinician may have for fluid infusion and the potential for infusions to cause derangement of electrolytes, volume status, and osmotic gradients, it is important to be able to predict the effect of said intervention.

Classically, these predictions have assumed that body fluid spaces are static, as opposed to a kinetic model where the body fluid spaces are considered dynamic. For example, a static prediction of plasma volume (PV) expansion from fluid infusion may assume an 80-kg patient has suffered an acute blood loss of 2 L, 40% of his predicted 5 L blood volume. The mathematical prediction describing the effects of replacement with 5% dextrose in water (D_5W), lactated Ringer solution, or 5% or 25% human serum albumin is as follows:

$$\text{Expected PV increment} = \text{volume infused} \times \text{normal PV/distribution volume} \quad (16\text{-}3)$$

By rearranging the above equation, the volume of a given fluid required to produce a certain PV incremental change can be calculated:

$$\text{Volume infused} = \text{expected PV increment} \times \text{distribution volume/normal PV} \quad (16\text{-}4)$$

To restore blood volume using D_5W, assuming a distribution volume for sodium-free water of TBW, requires 32 L:

$$32\ \text{L} = 2\ \text{L} \times 48\ \text{L}/3\ \text{L} \quad (16\text{-}5)$$

where 2 L is the desired PV increment, 48 L = TBW in an 80-kg person, and 3 L is the normal estimated PV.

Alternatively, to restore blood volume using lactated Ringer solution requires 12 L:

$$12\ \text{L} = 2\ \text{L} \times 18\ \text{L}/3\ \text{L} \quad (16\text{-}6)$$

where 18 L = ECV in an 80-kg person.

Although these numbers are simplified for convenience, one can see the application of principles. If 5% albumin were infused, the infused volume initially would remain in the PV because the colloid osmotic pressure exerted by the infused fluid is similar to plasma, and may even attract additional interstitial fluid intravascularly. Twenty-five percent human serum albumin is a concentrated colloid which can expand PV by approximately 400 mL for each 100 mL infused.

The static body fluid spaces assumed by the preceding predictions is now thought to be overly simplistic. The static assumption disregards the complex systems in place to regulate intravascular, interstitial, and intracellular volumes, osmolarity, etc. Svensén and Hahn proposed a more comprehensive kinetic prediction model which allow more accurate estimation of the time course of volume changes produced by infusion of a fluid of particular composition. This estimate permits estimation of peak volume expansion and clearance of infused fluid and aids analysis of effects such as changes in cardiac filling pressure or CO.[31]

Kinetic analysis also allows examination of the effects of common physiologic and pharmacologic influences on fluid distribution in experimental animals or humans. Connolly et al.[32] demonstrated that in chronically instrumented sheep, fluid infusion during an isoflurane anesthetic was associated with greater expansion of extravascular volume than in the conscious state. They additionally found that despite similar kinetics of expansion of PV after fluid infusion between conscious and anesthetized sheep, the anesthetized state was associated with reduced urinary output and greater expansion of extravascular volume which was attributable to isoflurane and not to mechanical ventilation.[32] A study in volunteers suggested that the effects of anesthesia on fluid kinetics could be mediated through lower mean arterial pressures and activation of the renin/angiotensin/aldosterone system.[33] Administration of catecholamine infusions before and during fluid infusions in sheep was found to profoundly altered intravascular fluid retention, with phenylephrine diminishing and isoproterenol enhancing intravascular fluid retention (Fig. 16-1).[34] More recent studies show the effect of rapid infusion on the integrity of the endothelial glycocalyx may potentially confound volume kinetic assessment of PV by potentially releasing noncirculating fluid volume (FV) that is trapped within the endothelial glycocalyx resulting in apparent rather than actual plasma dilution.[35] There is likely much that we currently do not understand about how infusions and body fluids behave, however, each additional experimental study is certain to improve our understanding of the subject.

Regulation of Osmolarity and Circulating Volume

Simplistically, TBW is determined by water intake and output. In an average adult, intake includes ingested liquid plus approximate

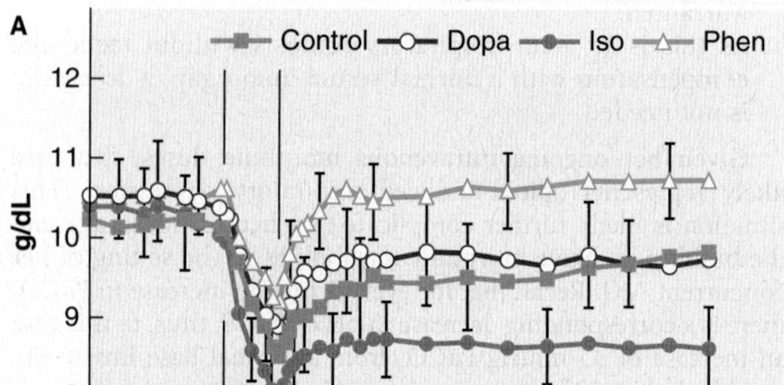

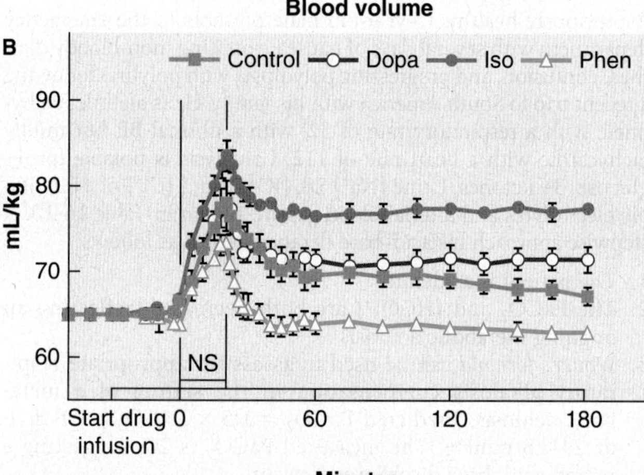

Figure 16-1 **A:** Blood hemoglobin (mean ± SEM) sampled at three baseline periods during a 30-minute catecholamine infusion and for 3 hours after starting a 20-minute 0.9% NaCl bolus of 24 mL/kg. Catecholamine protocols are dopamine (Dopa, *open diamonds*), isoproterenol (Iso, *closed circles*), phenylephrine (Phen, *open triangles*), and no-drug control (Control, *closed squares*). The 0.9% NaCl bolus decreased hemoglobin in all protocols at the end of the 20-minute 0.9% NaCl infusion and in all protocols except the Phen protocol thereafter. Postinfusion protocol differences were Phen ≥ Dopa = Control ≥ Iso. **B:** Calculated blood volume (mean ± SEM) at three baseline periods during a catecholamine infusion and for 3 hours after starting a 20-minute 0.9% NaCl bolus of 24 mL/kg. The 0.9% NaCl bolus increased blood volume in all protocols at T_{20} and in all protocols except the Phen protocol thereafter. Postinfusion protocol differences were Iso ≥ Dopa = Control ≥ Phen. NS, normal saline bolus. (Adapted with permission from Vane LA, Prough DS, Kinsky MA, et al. Effects of different catecholamines on the dynamics of volume expansion of crystalloid infusion. *Anesthesiology*. 2004;101:1136–1144.)

750 mL of water ingested as solid food and 350 mL generated metabolically. Average output includes urinary output plus gastrointestinal losses of about 100 to 150 mL and insensible losses 1,000 mL/day. The homeostasis of TBW is controlled by numerous feedback mechanisms where a sensed change in an afferent limb causes an adjustment in an effector limbs that works to balance intake and output of water and sodium in the body. If either limb of the mechanism is deranged, the body cannot adjust its handling of water or sodium and a positive or negative balance of either can ensue.

Intake of water is regulated through thirst. This fact has very important implications for patients that cannot access water, such as those with altered mental status, are infants, or those that have obligate intake through IV fluids or parenteral therapies. Thirst is caused by increased plasma tonicity, as little as 2%, or by decreased effective circulating volume (ECV). Increased osmolarity draws water from cells into the blood dehydrating hypothalamic osmoreceptors that stimulate drinking. Decrease in ECV stimulates vascular receptors that signal brain centers to initiate thirst. Lastly, baroreceptors/volume receptors in the kidney release renin, thus activating the renin that leads to production angiotensin II also initiates thirst.

Although the body loses water in many different ways, the body has little control of most losses outside of urine. Therefore, control of output of water is primarily mediated through the management of water and sodium in the kidney. Renal management of water and sodium is regulated by changes in blood flow and by the renin–angiotensin–aldosterone system, antidiuretic hormone (ADH), and natriuretic peptides.

Decreased stretch in the baroreceptors of the aortic arch and carotid body and stretch receptors in the great veins, pulmonary vasculature, and atria result in increased sympathetic tone. This increased sympathetic tone, in combination with sensing decreased ECV, prompt the juxtaglomerular apparatus (JGA) to secrete the hormone renin. Renin converts angiotensinogen to angiotensin I (Ang I), which is then converted to angiotensin II (Ang II) by angiotensin-converting enzyme (ACE). Ang II subsequently has many actions to maintain mean arterial pressure in the face of decreased ECV. Ang II is a vasoconstrictor, stimulates sodium retention, and stimulates aldosterone release. When ECV is low Ang II also preferentially increases renal efferent arteriolar tone, which tends to preserve GFR and increases the filtration fraction by altering Starling forces in the glomerulus leading to enhanced proximal sodium and water retention. In addition, Ang II enhances sodium absorption through its effect on secretion of aldosterone and volume reabsorption by activating apical membrane sodium-hydrogen (Na^+-H^+) exchangers in the proximal tubule.[36]

Aldosterone acts primarily in the distal tubules, causing sodium reabsorption which can reduce urinary excretion of sodium nearly to zero.[37] In addition to its ability to provoke renin secretion as noted above, sympathetic nervous system indirectly stimulates proximal tubular sodium reabsorption by influencing filtration fraction through altering preglomerular and postglomerular arteriolar tone and directly stimulate proximal tubular fluid reabsorption through receptors on the basolateral membrane of the proximal convoluted tubule cells.[38]

Natriuretic peptides are powerful hormones that help regulate total body sodium. Atrial natriuretic peptide (ANP), brain natriuretic peptide (BNP), and C-type natriuretic peptide, stimulate natriuresis, diuresis, and vasodilation.[39] Atrial distention and a sodium load cause release of ANP by atrial myocytes. BNP is released from the ventricular myocardium in response to increase in ventricular diastolic pressure. C-type natriuretic peptide is synthesized and secreted from endothelium in response to many stimuli, sheer stress, and inflammatory cytokines being examples.[40]

Arginine vasopressin (AVP), also known as antidiuretic hormone (ADH), leads to increased water reabsorption in the collecting ducts. ADH is synthesized in the hypothalamus and secreted by the posterior pituitary gland primarily in response to hypertonicity, and also to severely decreased ECV. Congestive heart failure, cirrhosis, nephrotic syndrome, adrenal insufficiency, certain cancers, nausea, pain, and medications, including opiates have all been shown to lead to increased ADH.[41] ADH release is suppressed in response to hypotonicity and ECF volume overload sensed by arterial baroreceptors and atrial receptors. In addition to its antidiuretic effect, at higher concentrations, ADH can lead to systemic vasoconstriction through the V_1 receptors.[42] The antidiuretic action results from activation of the V_2 receptor (G-protein–coupled receptor) on the principal cell of the collecting duct. This receptor activation leads to increased cAMP levels and subsequent increased synthesis and insertion of aquaporin-2 water channels into the luminal membrane, leading to increase water reabsorption.[43,44] ADH also appears to have synergistic effects with aldosterone on sodium transport in the cortical collecting duct (CCD).[45] This effect can lead to variation in urine osmolarity from 50 to 1,200 mOsm/kg and urinary volume from 0.4 to 20 L/day (Figs. 16-2 and 16-3), Video 16-1).[46]

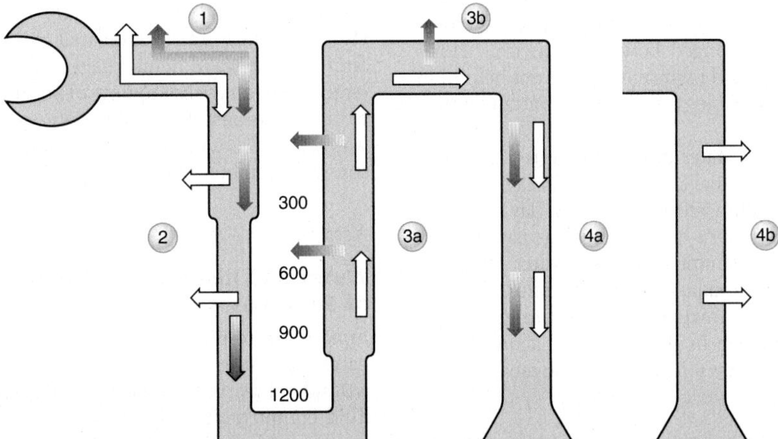

Figure 16-2 Renal filtration, reabsorption, and excretion of water. *Open arrows* represent water and *solid arrows* represent electrolytes. Water and electrolytes are filtered by the glomerulus. In the proximal tubule *(1)*, water and electrolytes are absorbed isotonically. In the descending loop of Henle *(2)*, water is absorbed to achieve osmotic equilibrium with the interstitium while electrolytes are retained. The numbers (300, 600, 900, and 1,200) between the descending and ascending limbs represent the osmolality of the interstitium in milliosmoles per kilogram. The delivery of solute and fluid to the distal nephron is a function of proximal tubular reabsorption; as proximal tubular reabsorption increases, delivery of solute to the medullary *(3a)* and cortical *(3b)* diluting sites decreases. In the diluting sites, electrolyte-free water is generated through selective reabsorption of electrolytes while water is retained in the tubular lumen, generating a dilute tubular fluid. In the absence of vasopressin, the collecting duct *(4a)* remains relatively impermeable to water and diluted urine is excreted. When vasopressin acts on the collecting ducts *(4b)*, water is reabsorbed from these vasopressin-responsive nephron segments, allowing the excretion of concentrated urine. (Adapted from Fried LF, Palevsky PM. Hyponatremia and hypernatremia. *Med Clin North Am*. 1997;81(3):585–609. Copyright © 1997 Elsevier. With permission.)

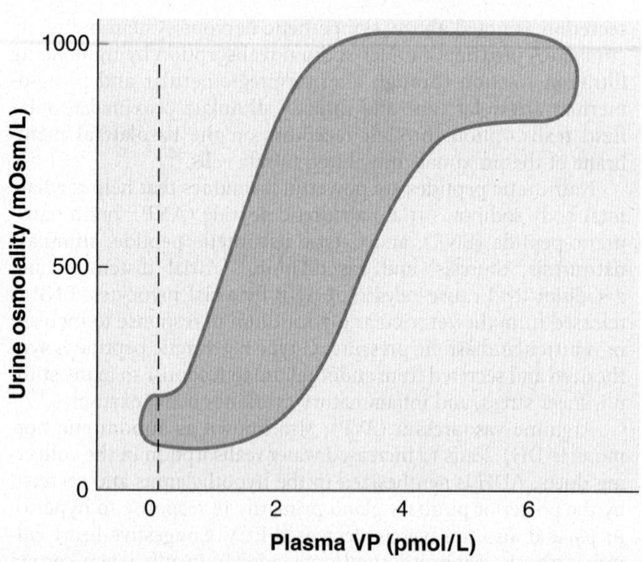

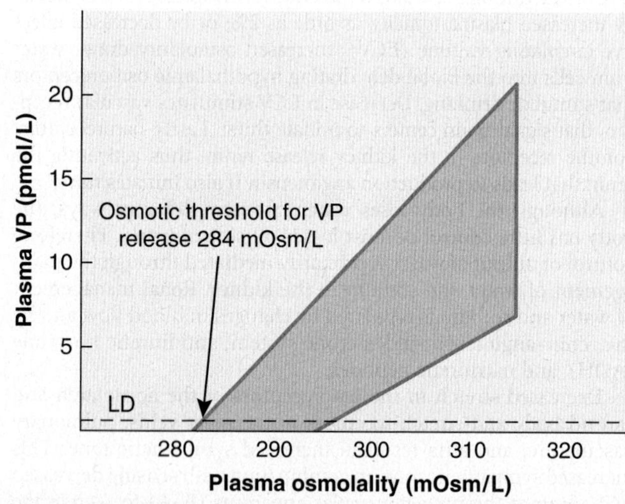

Figure 16-3 Left: The sigmoid relationship between plasma vasopressin (VP) and urinary osmolality. Data were obtained during water loading and fluid restriction in a group of healthy adults. Maximum urinary concentration is achieved by plasma VP values of 3 to 4 pmol/L. **Right:** The linear relationship between plasma osmolality and plasma VP. Increases in VP in response to hypertonicity induced by infusion of 855 mmol/L saline in a group of healthy adults. The *shaded area* represents the reference range response. LD represents the limit of detection of the VP assay, 0.3 pmol/L. (Adapted with permission from Ball SG. Vasopressin and disorders of water balance: the physiology and pathophysiology of vasopressin. *Ann Clin Biochem*. 2007;44(5):417–431.)

Fluid Replacement Therapy

Maintenance Requirements for Water, Sodium, and Potassium

Patients who cannot take in adequate oral intake or have increased fluid losses are at risk of developing hypovolemia and electrolyte disturbances (NICV 16-1). The concept of maintenance fluid is useful in that it seeks to prevent this deficit of fluid and electrolyte. Classically, calculation of maintenance fluid requirements (Table 16-11) has been based on weight alone. These calculations may be useful in those without acute change in physiology and who have restricted oral intake, such as a preoperative patient or postoperative patient with prolonged bowel dysfunction. However, calculated maintenance fluid requirements are not helpful in those with acutely altered physiology, such as the intraoperative or acutely ill patient.

In healthy adults, sufficient water intake is required to negate the fluid losses from gastrointestinal (100 to 200 mL/day), urinary (1,000 mL/day), and insensible (500 to 1,000 mL/day) sources. Losses exceeding these estimates may represent pathophysiologic states that should be examined. As with water, there are daily requirements for sodium and potassium, which for a healthy adult in equilibrium are approximately 75 and 40 mEq, respectively, however this may change in the setting of acute illness. Wider ranges of sodium intake are tolerated because renal sodium conservation and elimination are efficient. The same is true of potassium, though to a lesser extent.

Table 16-11 Hourly and Daily Maintenance Water Requirements

Weight (kg)	Water (mL/kg/hr)	Water (mL/kg/day)
1–10	4	100
11–20	2	50
21–n+	1	20

Dextrose

Traditionally, glucose-containing IVFs have been given perioperatively to prevent hypoglycemia and limit protein catabolism. This practice is now limited to patients who are at particular risk of hypoglycemia, such as infants or patients receiving insulin, because of the risk for hyperglycemic from surgical stress. Iatrogenic hyperglycemia can induce an osmotic diuresis impairing resuscitation and may aggravate ischemic neurologic injury.[47] Hyperglycemia is also associated with worsened clinical outcome after subarachnoid hemorrhage and TBI.[48,49] Multiple studies and larger meta-analyses support of studies performed in critically ill patients demonstrated a blood glucose target of 180 mg/dL or less was associated with reduced mortality and morbidity in comparison with a tighter control target of 81 to 108 mg/dL.[50,51]

3

Surgical Fluid Requirements

Water and Electrolyte Composition of Fluid Losses

In addition to replacing obligate losses discussed above, surgical patients require replacement of PV and ECV losses secondary to wound or burn edema, ascites, and gastrointestinal secretions. The fluid composition of losses should be considered when deciding how to replace them. Wound, burn, and ascitic fluid is protein-rich, with electrolyte concentrations similar to plasma. Gastrointestinal secretions vary greatly in composition. The fluid to match GI losses need not be closely matched if ECV is adequate and renal and cardiovascular functions are normal. However, substantial loss of gastrointestinal fluids requires more accurate replacement of electrolytes. Substantial GI losses can also produce acid–base disturbances. Gastric fluid is acidic and contains substantial chloride so it's loss may produce hypochloremic metabolic alkalosis which can be corrected with 0.9% saline. Conversely, diarrhea may result in bicarbonate loss and subsequent hyperchloremic metabolic acidosis that may be prevented or corrected by infusion of fluid containing bicarbonate or bicarbonate equivalent (e.g., lactate). If there is cardiovascular or renal dysfunction, close laboratory monitoring and more precise replacement may be required.

Influences of Perioperative and Intraoperative Fluid Infusion Rates on Clinical Outcomes

Traditional intraoperative fluid management included replacement of fluid thought to accumulate extravascularly in surgically manipulated tissue (the "third space") in addition to blood loss as well as other sensible and insensible losses.[52] Depending on how traumatic the surgery was considered to be, it was commonplace to administer 4 to 6 mL/kg/hr for surgeries causing minimal trauma and up to 8 to 12 mL/kg/hr for those causing severe trauma. However, recent evidence has demonstrated no benefit and perhaps even morbidity with replacing "third space" losses.[52]

Numerous clinical trials have been undertaken to determine the best method of intraoperative fluid management. Although we are far from having an agreed upon gold-standard method for intraoperative fluid management, individual studies and focused meta-analyses have found strong links between perioperative fluid management and important outcomes. Furthermore, these findings regarding perioperative fluid volume and composition appear to be specific to the type of surgery and patient population.

Assessing the adequacy of intravascular volume and targeting a goal related to intravascular volume are now commonplace with Enhanced Recovery After Surgery (ERAS) protocols.[53] Several clinical studies have shown that goal-directed hemodynamic therapy during high-risk surgery, including cardiac, hip, and major bowel surgery, is associated with improved postoperative outcome.[53] In general, monitoring techniques are used to estimate whether additional fluid administration will improve CO, hopefully while avoiding excessive fluid administration.

Maharaj et al.[54] randomized 80 American Society of Anesthesiologist (ASA) class I or II patients scheduled for gynecologic laparoscopy to receive preoperative fluid boluses with either large volume(defined as 2 mL/kg/hr) or fasting or small volume (defined as total fluid of 3 mL/kg). In patients receiving the higher dose, postoperative nausea (PON) and postoperative vomiting (POV), and pain were significantly reduced (Fig. 16-4). Holte et al.[55] in 2007 randomized 48 ASA class I–II patients undergoing laparoscopic cholecystectomy to receive either 15 or 40 mL/kg of lactated Ringer solution intraoperatively. The higher dose was associated with improved postoperative pulmonary function and exercise capacity, reduced neurohumoral stress response, nausea, general sense of well-being, thirst, dizziness, drowsiness, fatigue, and balance function. Another 2007 study from Holte et al.[56] randomized 48 ASA class I–III patients undergoing fast-track elective knee arthroplasty under intraoperative neuraxial anesthesia and postoperative epidural analgesia to either liberal or restricted fluids. Median lactated Ringer's administered perioperatively in the restrictive group was 1,740 mL (range, 1,100 to 2,165 mL) and in the liberal group was 3,275 mL (range, 2,400 to 4,000 mL). Restrictive fluid administration was associated with a higher incidence of vomiting but less hypercoagulability and no difference in short-term postoperative mobility or ileus. A larger Cochrane[57] review of 41 studies with 4,224 participants, predominantly ASA class I or II, who underwent ambulatory or short length of stay surgical procedures to determine the effect of supplemental IV crystalloid on PON and POV. Supplemental intravenous crystalloid administration of 15 to 30 mL/kg was found to likely reduce the risk of PON (RR 0.62, 95% confidence interval [CI] 0.51–0.75) and POV (RR 0.50, 95% CI 0.40–0.63). There was also likely a decreased need for pharmacologic for nausea or vomiting or differences in readmission or adverse events observed. Therefore, in patients undergoing surgery of limited scope, fluid restriction appears to be less well tolerated than more liberal fluid therapy.

In patients undergoing major invasive surgery the data are mixed with respect to benefits of different fluid strategies. Brandstrup et al.[58] randomized 172 elective colon surgery patients to restrictive perioperative fluid management or standard perioperative fluid management, with the primary goal of maintaining preoperative body weight in the fluid-restricted group. The fluid-restricted group received less perioperative fluid and gained less than 1 kg as opposed to more than 3 kg in the standard therapy group. Cardiopulmonary complications, tissue-healing

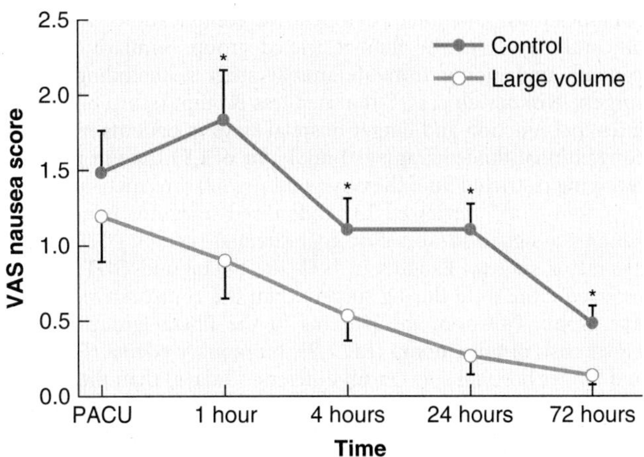

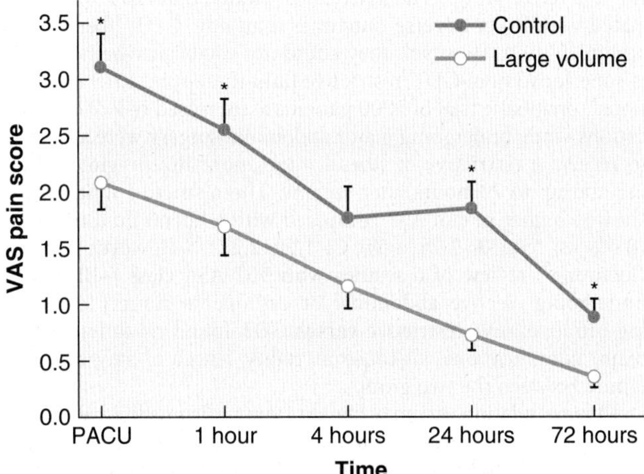

Figure 16-4 Top: Mean postoperative verbal analog scale (VAS) nausea scores in each group over the first 72 postoperative hours. Mean VAS nausea scores were significantly lower in the group that received the large-volume intravenous fluid infusion compared with the control group at 1, 4, 24, and 72 hours postoperatively. **Bottom:** Mean postoperative VAS pain scores in each group over the first 72 postoperative hours. Mean VAS pain scores were significantly lower in the group that received the large-volume intravenous fluid infusion compared with the control group at 0, 1, 24, and 72 hours postoperatively. *Significantly higher ($p < 0.05$, *t*-test postanalysis of variance) VAS score compared with the large volume group. PACU, postanesthesia care unit. (Adapted with permission from Maharaj CH, Kallam SR, Malik A, et al. Preoperative intravenous fluid therapy decreases postoperative nausea and pain in high risk patients. *Anesth Analg*. 2005;100:675–682.)

complications, and total postoperative complications were significantly fewer in the fluid-restricted group. Similarly, in 152 patients undergoing intra-abdominal surgery, including colon surgery, Nisanevich et al.[59] reported less prompt return of gastrointestinal function and longer hospital stays in patients receiving conventional fluid therapy (10 mL/kg/hr of LR) than in patients receiving restricted fluid therapy (4 mL/kg/hr). In a meta-analysis, Corcoran et al.[60] reviewed 23 randomized trials involving 3,861 patients assigned to liberal or goal-directed therapy (GDT) during major surgery. Patients in both the liberal and GDT groups received more fluid during surgery than the comparative restrictive group. However, the patients in the liberal groups had a higher risk of pneumonia (RR 2.2), pulmonary edema (RR 3.8), and longer hospital stay (mean difference 2 days) than their com-
4 parative groups. The patients in the GDT groups had a lower risk of pneumonia and renal complications (RR 0.7), and shorter hospital stay (mean difference 2 days) compared to the patients in the non–GDT group. The authors concluded that GDT was associated with fewer adverse outcomes than non–GDT, liberal fluid administration. However, they could not establish whether GDT is superior to non–GDT, restrictive fluid therapy. A 2018 international, pragmatic trial of 3000 patients at increased risk of complications while undergoing major abdominal surgery were assigned to receive a restrictive or liberal intravenous-fluid regimen during and up to 24 hours after surgery. The restrictive fluid group showed higher rate of AKI compared with a liberal fluid regimen (8.6% vs. 5%; RR 1.71, 95% CI 1.29–2.27).[61] However, a 2019 Cochrane[62] review of 6 studies with 562 ASA class I–III adults undergoing elective abdominal or orthopedic surgery examining intraoperative restrictive versus GDT found no difference in major complications, all-cause mortality, length of stay, or renal failure between the two groups.

One population that may benefit from judicious fluid administration is the critically ill with acute lung injury (ALI). The ARDS Clinical Trials Network[63] randomized 1,000 patients with ALI to a 7-day trial comparing a conservative fluid strategy with a liberal fluid strategy. The conservative strategy group had a slightly negative cumulative net fluid balance in comparison to nearly 7 L positive balance in the liberal group. Overall mortality was no different in the two groups, however the conservative fluid group had better oxygenation, fewer ventilator and ICU days, and had no greater incidence of acute renal failure.

Colloids, Crystalloids, and Hypertonic Solutions

Physiology and Pharmacology

Osmosis is the spontaneous movement of solvent (e.g., water) across a selectively permeable membrane from an area of low solute concentration to an area of high solute concentration until an equilibrium is reached. *Osmolarity* and *osmolality* are both units of osmotically active solute concentration in a solvent; the first being solute per *liter* of solvent and the latter being solute per *kilogram* of solvent. For dilute solutions, such as serum, the difference is insignificant and the two terms are sometimes used interchangeably. Serum osmolarity can be estimated as follows:

$$\text{Osmolarity} = ([\text{Na}^+] \times 2) + (\text{Glucose}/18) + \left(\tfrac{\text{BUN}}{2.8}\right) \quad (16\text{-}7)$$

osmolarity is expressed in mmol/kg, $[Na^+]$ is expressed in mEq/L, serum glucose is expressed in mg/dL, and BUN is blood urea nitrogen expressed in mg/dL. There are other osmoles that are not part of this calculation that form the "osmolar gap," or the difference between directly measured and calculated osmolarity, which is usually less than 10. Sugars, alcohols, and radiographic dyes increase measured osmolarity and can contribute to an elevated osmolar gap.

Serum osmolarity is normally 275 to 290 mmol/kg. Elevated osmolarity is due to high concentrations of osmotically active particles. Uremia and hypernatremia increase serum osmolarity. A different term, *tonicity*, is used when discussing plasma. Tonicity is different from osmolarity is that plasma tonicity reflects the concentration of solutes that do not easily cross cell membranes rather than total solutes, and therefore affect the distribution of water between the cells and the ECV. Tonicity is predominantly determined by $[Na^+]$. For example, urea is an osmole but it distributes throughout TBW and therefore an increase in BUN does not cause *hypertonicity*. Sodium is largely restricted to the ECV and, therefore, causes hypertonicity and drives osmotically mediated redistribution of water from ICV to ECV. The term *tonicity* is also used colloquially to compare the osmotic pressure of a parenteral solution to that of plasma.

Proteins, although a small proportion of the osmotically active particles in blood, are essential in determining the equilibrium of fluid between the interstitial and plasma compartments of ECV. The osmotic activity of a protein (also referred to as *colloid osmotic pressure* or *oncotic pressure*) is determined by the concentration differential across a capillary bed and the permeability of capillary membranes to the protein, which is termed its reflection coefficient (σ). A σ of 0 represents free permeability and 1 represents complete impermeability. The σ for albumin ranges from 0.6 to 0.9 in various capillary beds. The oncotic pressure exerted by plasma proteins is higher than interstitial oncotic pressure and tends to preserve PV. The filtration rate of fluid from the capillaries into the interstitial space is the net result of a combination of forces, traditionally referred to as Starling forces, including the gradient of oncotic pressures and the hydrostatic pressures between intravascular and interstitial spaces. The movement of fluid across any capillary system can be approximated by Starling law of capillary filtration, as expressed in the equation:

$$Q = kA\,[(P_c - P_i) + \sigma(\pi_i - \pi_c)] \quad (16\text{-}8)$$

where Q = fluid filtration, k = capillary filtration coefficient (conductivity of water), A = area of the capillary membrane, P_c = capillary hydrostatic pressure, P_i = interstitial hydrostatic pressure, σ = the reflection coefficient for albumin, π_i = interstitial oncotic pressure, and π_c = capillary oncotic pressure. This estimation is oversimplified as the Starling law does not account for the important role capillary glycocalyx performs in fluid filtration, which is strongly influenced by disease processes and fluid administration.[64] An important part of this phenomena is the attachment of albumin to the endothelial glycocalyx which results in the oncotic pressure gradient actually being the difference between π_c and the oncotic pressure in the space between the endothelial glycocalyx and the capillary wall.[65] The glycocalyx usually causes actual filtration rates from the capillary to the interstitial space to be much less that theoretical rates.[65]

The interstitial fluid volume (IFV) is determined by capillary filtration and lymphatic drainage. Capillary hydrostatic pressure is the most powerful factor promoting fluid movement into the IFV and is determined by capillary flow, arterial resistance, venous resistance, and venous pressure. Water and sodium filtration normally exceed protein filtration, resulting in relative increase of π_c and dilution of π_i, increasing the oncotic pressure gradient, the most powerful factor opposing fluid movement into the IFV. Lymphatic drainage works with oncotic pressure to limit the accumulation of fluid in the interstitium. If P_c overwhelms oncotic pressure and lymphatic drainage, then IFV accumulates and creates edema.

Clinical Implications of Choice between Alternative Fluids

Crystalloid versus Colloid

If capillary membrane permeability is intact, the volume of distribution of colloid molecules such as albumin or hydroxyethyl starch (HES) is essentially limited to PV. This distribution leads colloid-containing fluids to preferentially expand PV rather than IFV. Approximately 70% of the infused volume of 5% albumin will stay intravascular as opposed to 20% of NS. Notably, colloid fluids come suspended in a carrier solution that has crystalloid solutes of varying tonicity. Some concentrated colloid-containing solutions can be isotonic or hypertonic and exert sufficient oncotic pressure to completely stay intravascularly or to even translocate substantial volumes of IFV into the PV, thereby expanding PV by a volume greater that infused volume. Minimizing IFV expansion offers some advantages: lower volume fluid administration, less peripheral and pulmonary edema, and reduced cardiopulmonary consequences of later fluid mobilization (Table 16-12). Despite these theoretical advantages of colloids, however, exhaustive research failed to demonstrate the superiority of either colloid or crystalloid fluids for intraoperative or postoperative use. The lack of evidence and the higher cost of colloid, especially albumin, should give the clinician pause when considering its use.

A 2018 Cochrane[66] review of 69 studies (65 RCTs, 4 quasi-RCTs) with 30,020 participants examined effects of crystalloid *versus* colloid resuscitation in critically ill patients in the hospital and emergency out-of-hospital setting. Twenty-eight studies investigated starch solutions, 20 dextrans, 7 gelatins, and 22 albumin or fresh frozen plasma (FFP). The authors concluded that colloid *versus* crystalloid probably makes little or no difference to mortality; however, starches probably slightly increase the need for blood transfusion and RRT. Another Cochrane[67] review from 2012 of 86 trials, with a total of 5,484 critically ill and surgical patients requiring resuscitation, examined the outcomes associated with different types of colloid (albumin, plasma, HES, dextran, and gelatin). The authors concluded that was no detectable differences in mortality between colloids, although confidence intervals were wide. Notably, there were only reports of adverse events related to gelatin and HES. Individual studies subsequent to the above meta-analysis point to more effective volume expansion, lower overall fluid administration, and less vasopressor requirements,[68,69] although there are studies show conflicting results regarding mortality and morbidity.[70,71]

The use of albumin in particular has persisted despite the lack of conclusive evidence of efficacy.[72] In patients with sepsis or septic shock, the Early Albumin Resuscitation during Septic Shock (EARSS) study[73] and the Albumin Italian Outcome Sepsis (ALBIOS) trial[74] failed to find any difference in their primary outcomes of 28-day mortality. However, in ALBIOS, the time to discontinue vasoactive agents (one of the trials numerous secondary outcomes) was shorter in the albumin group (3 vs. 4 days) and, in a post hoc analysis, the subgroup of patients presenting with septic shock had a significantly reduced 90-day mortality if they received albumin. This benefit remained after adjustment of confounding variables.[75] Meta-analyses conclusions regarding albumin administration are conflicting. Burns patients administered albumin appear to enjoy decreased mortality and incidence of abdominal compartment syndrome.[76] In a meta-analysis of ARDS patients, albumin was associated with improved oxygenation but no increase in survival.[77] Overall, these studies and meta-analyses are difficult to interpret as a body of literature. However, the evidence for albumin resuscitation can be said to demonstrate minor, transient benefits of uncertain clinical importance without clear signal for improvement of mortality or morbidity at a significant increase cost compared to crystalloid resuscitation.

Cirrhotic patients may represent a specific subset of patients in whom albumin infusion could be beneficial. Albumin may prevent hemodynamic changes and worsening renal function after large volume paracentesis (>5 L) in cirrhotic patients with diuretic-resistant ascites, although these findings are still controversial.[78,79] Patients with cirrhosis who develop spontaneous bacterial peritonitis likely benefit from a decrease in risk of renal impairment and mortality with albumin as well.[80,81] Although albumin has traditionally been a part of medical therapy for patients with cirrhosis who develop hepatorenal syndrome, its benefit is now debatable.[82]

Hydroxy ethyl starch (HES), a once commonly used synthetic colloid, fell out of favor due to its association in the critically ill to increased mortality and morbidity such as coagulopathy, pruritus, nephrotoxicity, and acute renal failure.[83] In the "6S Trial," HES was associated with an increased risk of death and end-stage renal failure in comparison to Ringer acetate.[84] A 2013 Cochrane[85] review of 42 studies with 11,399 patients demonstrated a significant increase in the need for renal replacement therapy (RRT) in those who received HES *versus* other fluid therapies (RR 1.31, 95% CI 1.16–1.49) and the number with kidney failure (RR 1.59, 95% CI 1.26–2.00). There were no differences in subgroup analyses based on type of HES, amount of substitution, or septic *versus* nonseptic patients. Consequently, the Surviving Sepsis Campaign recommended that HES be eliminated from treatment of septic patients.[86] Overall, the evidence suggests that HES lacks any significant clinical benefit in any patient population, but is associated with significant harm, especially kidney failure.

Table 16-12 Claimed Advantages and Disadvantages of Colloid versus Crystalloid Intravenous Fluids

Solution	Advantages	Disadvantages
Colloid	Smaller infused volume Prolonged increase in plasma volume Less peripheral edema	Greater cost Coagulopathy (dextran > HES) Pulmonary edema (capillary leak states) Decreased GFR Osmotic diuresis (low–molecular-weight dextran) Greater duration of excessive volume expansion
Crystalloid	Lower cost Greater urinary flow Interstitial fluid replacement	Transient increase in intravascular volume Transient hemodynamic improvement Peripheral edema (protein dilution) Pulmonary edema (protein dilution plus high PAOP)

HES, hydroxyethyl starch; GFR, glomerular filtration rate; PAOP, pulmonary arterial occlusion pressure.

Table 16-13 Hypertonic Resuscitation Fluids: Advantages and Disadvantages

Solution	Advantages	Disadvantages
Hypertonic crystalloid	Inexpensive Promotes urinary flow Small initial volume Arteriolar dilation Reduced peripheral edema Lower intracranial pressure	Hypertonicity Subdural hemorrhage Transient effect Potential rebound intracranial hypertension
Hypertonic crystalloid plus colloid (in comparison to hypertonic crystalloid alone)	Sustained hemodynamic response Reduced subsequent volume requirements	Added expense Osmotic diuresis Hypertonicity

Reprinted with permission from Prough DS, Johnston WE. Fluid resuscitation in septic shock: no solution yet. *Anesth Analg.* 1989;69:699–704.

Implications of Crystalloid and Colloid Infusions on Intracranial Pressure

The blood–brain barrier is highly impermeable to sodium, thus abrupt changes in serum osmolarity due to changes in serum sodium produce reciprocal changes in brain water content and thereby brain volume. Given that the cranium has a fixed volume, a change in brain volume affects the volume of intracranial blood and CSF as well as ICP. The effects of acute changes in colloid osmotic pressure are less clear. In anesthetized rabbits, reducing plasma osmolarity from 295 to 282 mOsm/kg (~250 mmHg of osmotic pressure) increased cortical water content and ICP; in contrast, reducing colloid osmotic pressure from 20 to 7 mmHg produced no significant change.[87] In anesthetized rats subjected to TBI followed by hemorrhage of 20 mL/kg, resuscitation with 90 mL/kg of isotonic lactated Ringer solution was associated with equivalent blood volume expansion to 20 mL/kg of 5% albumin, but at the expense of higher brain water.[88] In the Saline *versus* Albumin for Fluid Resuscitation in Patients with Traumatic Brain Injury (SAFE) Trial, 2-year follow-up of 460 patients with TBI (Glasgow Coma Scale score ≤13) demonstrated a nearly twofold increased risk of death in patients receiving colloid.[89] Secondary analysis of the SAFE trial data suggested that patients receiving 4% albumin had a higher incidence of refractory intracranial hypertension, which may be the mechanism of increased mortality.[90] However, Van Aken et al.[91] pointed out that the 4% albumin solution used in the SAFE trial was suspended in a hypo-osmolar carrier solution, so it is still debated whether the albumin, the reduced osmolarity, or perhaps both were at fault (NICV 16-2).

Notably, in the experimental animal studies above, 5% albumin was suspended in a slightly hyperosmolar solution in contrast to the hypo-osmolar 4% solution used in the SAFE clinical trial.[91] Although the role of colloid in resuscitation of brain-injured patients remains unclear, it is appropriate to avoid large volumes of hypo-osmotic or hypo-oncotic fluids.[92]

Buffered versus Nonbuffered Crystalloid

6 There has been much interest recently in the differences in effect between infusions of buffered and nonbuffered crystalloid solutions. Individual studies reported metabolic derangements, particularly hyperchloremic metabolic acidosis, and more importantly AKI.[93,94] However, data collected prior to these studies included in a 2017 Cochrane[95] review of 18 randomized controlled trials with a total of 1,096 patients examining the effects on buffered *versus* nonbuffered crystalloid IV fluids on adult surgical patients. They found insufficient evidence on the effects of fluid therapies on mortality and postoperative organ dysfunction, or renal insufficiency. There were differences in postoperative pH of at least 0.05 units (95% CI 0.04–0.07; I^2 = 61%), although this difference resolved by postoperative day 1. They also observed higher postoperative serum chloride with nonbuffered fluids (MD 6.77 mmol/L, 95% CI 3.38–10.17) which persisted until postoperative day 1. The clinical significance of any of these positive findings is questionable. Similarly, a 2016 Cochrane[96] review examined the effects of normal saline *versus* low chloride solution for adult kidney transplant patients which demonstrated similar outcomes.

Clinical Implications of Hypertonic Fluid Administration

An ideal alternative to conventional crystalloid and colloid fluids would be inexpensive, produce minimal peripheral or pulmonary edema, generate sustained hemodynamic effects, and be effective even if administered in small volumes. Hypertonic, hypernatremic solutions, with or without added colloid, appear to fulfill some of these criteria (Table 16-13).

Hypertonic solutions exert favorable effects on cerebral hemodynamics, in part because of the reciprocal relationship between plasma osmolarity and brain water.[87] Resuscitation from hemorrhagic shock with lactated Ringer solution has been shown to increase ICP, but resuscitation with 7.5% saline did not.[97] However, in a dog model with hemorrhagic shock and an intracranial mass, hypertonic resuscitation demonstrated a delayed increase in ICP.[98] Despite concerns about hypertonicity and hypernatremia, acute increases in serum sodium to 155 to 160 mEq/L produced no apparent harm in hypovolemic trauma patients resuscitated with hypertonic saline (HS).[99]

The theoretical advantages of hypertonic fluids appear most attractive in the acute resuscitation of hypovolemic patients who have decreased intracranial compliance. Hypertonic solutions are also used to reduce brain water and intracranial volume during neurosurgery and episodes of increased ICP. Although reduced brain water can be accomplished with mannitol, some clinicians prefer HS solutions.[100] HS and mannitol of similar osmolarity have similar effects on brain water, intracranial volume, and ICP. The most salient difference between the two is that infusion of HS increases intravascular volume, while diuresis secondary to mannitol decreases intravascular volume. While few complications relate specifically to osmotic therapy, acute severe hyperosmolarity could, theoretically, precipitate blood–brain barrier opening. Clinical use of HS is associated, as is 0.9% saline, with hyperchloremic acidosis, which usually requires no treatment, but must be differentiated from other causes of metabolic acidosis. Although there are plenty of theoretical benefits of HS in resuscitation of patients with TBI, a randomized trial failed to demonstrate an improvement in outcome.[101]

The theoretical benefits of hypertonic fluid administration have also been examined perioperatively. A 2016 Cochrane[102] review including 18 studies with 1087 adult perioperative patients ASA class I–III who received some amount of HS *versus* solely isotonic saline (IS) solution. Most participants were in positive fluid balance postoperatively (4.4 L IS and 2.5 L HS), with the excess significantly less in HS participants (MD –1.92 L, 95% CI –2.61 to –1.22 L; $P < .00001$). IS participants received a mean volume of 2.4 L and HS participants received 1.49 L (MD –0.91 L, 95% CI –1.24 to –0.59 L; $P < .00001$). The maximum average serum sodium ranged 138.5 to 159 mEq/L in HS groups compared to 136 to 143 mEq/L in the IS groups (MD 7.73, 95% CI 5.84–9.62; $P < .00001$. Notably, there were no reports of serious adverse events. Differences in in morbidity or mortality could not be determined.

Fluid Status: Assessment and Monitoring

For most surgical patients, conventional clinical assessment of intravascular volume is the appropriate. For high-risk patients, goal-directed hemodynamic management may be superior.

Conventional Clinical Assessment

Assessment of blood volume and ECV begins with identification of factors predisposing one to hypovolemia (e.g., preoperative bowel preparation, diuretic, sepsis, burns, trauma) or hypervolemia (e.g., renal disease, heart failure, high obligate IV fluid). Assessment of hypovolemia is mainly based on physical signs that include oliguria, supine hypotension, and a positive tilt test. In general, oliguria implies hypovolemia, however the presence of diuretics, renal disease, or endocrine disease can obscure the clinical picture. Supine hypotension suggests a blood volume deficit greater than 30%, although many medical conditions, such as chronic hypertension, sympathomimetic use, agitated delirium, may lead to a normal arterial BP representing relative hypotension from hypovolemia as well as many conditions that can lead to hypotension despite adequate intravascular volume, such as heart failure, cirrhosis, endocrine disease.

A positive tilt test, defined as an increase in heart rate of at least 20 beats/min and a decrease in systolic BP of 20 mmHg or more when the subject assumes the upright position, can be falsely negative or positive. Young, healthy subjects can withstand acute loss of 20% of blood volume while exhibiting only postural tachycardia. In contrast, orthostasis occurs in up to 30% of the elderly despite normal blood volume. Wong et al.[103] demonstrated that, in volunteers, phlebotomy of 500 mL of blood was associated with a greater increase in heart rate on standing than prior to blood loss, but with no significant difference in the differences in BP or cardiac index.

Many laboratory markers are suggestive of hypovolemia or low ECV and include azotemia, low urinary sodium, metabolic alkalosis (mild hypovolemia), and metabolic acidosis (severe hypovolemia). The sensitivities and specificities of laboratory measurement for hypovolemia are poor as numerous conditions can affect these measurements. For example, BUN can increase with high-protein intake, gastrointestinal bleeding, or accelerated catabolism. Conversely, severe liver dysfunction can lower BUN. Serum creatinine (SCr) is poor marker of AKI given its delay in raising and an insensitive indicator of chronic kidney dysfunction as 40% to 50% of nephrons must become dysfunctional before normal range is exceeded. SCr may also be misleadingly low in elderly, female, or sarcopenic patients. In contrast, in muscular or acutely catabolic patients, SCr can exceed the normal range without hypovolemia. A ratio of BUN to SCr exceeding normal (10 to 20) suggests dehydration. In prerenal oliguria, enhanced sodium reabsorption should reduce urinary [Na^+] to 20 mEq/L or less and enhanced water reabsorption should increase urinary concentration (i.e., urinary osmolarity >400 mOsm/kg, urine/plasma creatinine ratio >40:1). These urinary changes also make the fractional excretion of sodium (FENa) less than 1%, although results can be misleading with diuretic use, chronic renal disease, urinary tract obstruction, and acute glomerulonephritis. Severe hypovolemia may result in systemic hypoperfusion and subsequent lactic acidosis.

Intraoperative Clinical Assessment

The goal of fluid resuscitation is maintenance of adequate intravascular volume and, subsequently, tissue perfusion. Many challenges exist for the anesthesiologist to estimate intravascular volume status including: unknown preoperative fluid status; difficulty estimating blood loss, insensible loss, and "third space" loss; inability to assess for symptoms; and anesthetic effects on hemodynamics. These unknowns lead the anesthesiologist to infer adequacy of intraoperative fluid resuscitation by integrating multiple clinical variables (i.e., hemodynamics and labs). However, clinical variables are error prone and often difficult to interpret, leading to the need to integrate numerous points of clinical data.

Assessing the adequacy of intravascular volume and targeting a goal related to intravascular volume are common components of ERAS protocols as discussed above. Several studies demonstrate outcome benefits with goal-directed hemodynamic therapy during high-risk surgery, including cardiac, hip, and major bowel surgery.[53,104] The premise is that monitoring techniques will help guide fluid administration with the goal to improve CO while avoiding excessive fluid administration. Traditionally static parameters have been used but recently there have been increased examination of dynamic parameters.

Static Parameters

Static parameters are the ones traditionally used: BP, heart rate, urine output (UOP), central venous pressure (CVP), and labs. Ability to maintain normal BP in the setting of potent vasodilators (i.e., volatile inhalational anesthetics) suggests adequate intravascular volume. However, in a study of patients undergoing major abdominal surgery, there was not relationship found between BP and CO which is a measure of gross perfusion.[105] In severe hypovolemia, the accuracy of indirect measurements of BP is diminished and direct arterial pressure measurements should be considered. Tachycardia lacks sensitivity and specificity as an indicator of hypovolemia, especially during anesthesia. In the setting of normal renal function and absence of diuretics, UOP usually declines precipitously during moderate-to-severe hypovolemia. Therefore, appropriate UOP (0.5 to 1.0 mL/kg/hr) suggests adequate renal perfusion. The converse is not true, inhalational anesthetic and surgical stress can cause oliguria in the setting of euvolemia. This notion may be why UOP is not predictive of AKI.[106] CVP of 6 to 12 mmHg was previously thought to suggest adequate intravascular volume, however it is now considered to be a poor surrogate of cardiac preload, fluid responsiveness, or impending pulmonary edema.[107] CO can be normal despite severely reduced regional blood flow and perioperative oxygen consumption is extremely variable. These issues limit the usefulness of mixed venous oxygen saturation.[108,109] Lactic acidosis and acidemia occur only when tissue hypoperfusion becomes severe. Given the issues with static parameters, it is no wonder that even with continuous monitoring of them, poor perfusion can go unrecognized.

Dynamic Parameters

Dynamic parameters are hemodynamic indices that are used to assess fluid responsiveness and guide goal-directed fluid management. These include intra-arterial pressure waveform analysis, esophageal Doppler, echocardiography, and noninvasive monitors. These are often used to supplement traditional static parameters for those undergoing major invasive surgery or significantly comorbid patients. However, a 2016 Cochrane[110] review failed to demonstrate any difference in outcomes with advanced hemodynamic monitoring *versus* usual care in patients undergoing proximal femur surgery.

Intra-arterial pressure waveform analysis can be done with a number of different measurements, including pulse pressure variation (PPVar), stroke volume variation (SVV), and systolic BP variation (SPV). The analysis detects hemodynamic changes due to the intrathoracic pressure changes with mechanical ventilation. During inspiration with mechanical ventilation the intrathoracic pressure is increased which reduces venous return and subsequently right ventricle filling and stroke volume. This change in stroke volume causes systemic BP variation with the respiratory cycle. The variations in these parameters are normally less than 10%, however can be greater with hypovolemia.[110] To be useful these measurements have many requisites: stable vasomotor and cardiac function; mechanically ventilated patient without dyssynchrony; tidal volume of 8 cc/kg or more; PEEP <15 cmH_2O (including auto-PEEP); intact thoracic cavity; no evidence of atrial fibrillation, and no venous obstruction (e.g., cardiac tamponade, abdominal compartment syndrome).[111–113] Measurements are also
7 limited by their marginal sensitivity and specificity. A 2018 systematic review and meta-analysis showed PPVar had a sensitivity of 80% and specificity of 83%, with an area under curve (AUC) of 0.86 while SVV had a sensitivity of 82% and specificity of 77%, with an AUC of 0.87.[113] Further measurement can be obtained from intra-arterial pressure waveform analysis by assessing the effect of passive leg raise or a 250 mL bolus challenge. After either of those maneuvers, if a PPVar of over 13% decreases below that threshold (or CO increases over 15%), an increase in cardiac preload will be associated with an increase in CO.[114] passive leg raise cannot be used in patients with abdominal hypertension or in patients with TBI because passive leg raise may increase ICP.

Esophageal Doppler uses a flexible Doppler probe to measure flow velocity in the descending aorta and allows assessment of corrected flow time (FT_c) and descending aortic stroke volume.[114] In general, an FT_c less than 0.35 second suggests that volume expansion should improve CO, while an FT_c greater than 0.4 second suggests that further volume expansion will be ineffective.[115] Using the esophageal Doppler to guide administration of colloid boluses, Venn et al.[116] and Gan et al.[104] reported decreased length of hospital stay after hip surgery and major surgery, respectively. However, Horowitz and Kumar[117] speculated that the infusion of colloid rather than the monitor-driven algorithm was responsible for the improved results. Large multicenter trials are needed to determine the true benefit of esophageal Doppler. However, its use should be considered if intra-arterial waveform analysis cannot be accomplished.

Formal transthoracic echocardiography (TTE) and transesophageal echocardiography (TEE) as well as point-of-care ultrasound (PCUS) are very powerful hemodynamic and volume monitoring tools. Although an in-depth review of these modalities for volume assessment is beyond the scope of this chapter, there are a few principles worth noting. First, whenever possible it is useful to assess a patient at their baseline or euvolemia before surgery or other acute illness. Hypovolemia can manifest as decrease LV cavity size, hyperdynamic systolic function, and small, collapsible inferior vena cava. Per American Society of Echocardiography Guidelines,[118] LV internal diameter measurements are taken at the end of diastole as end-systolic LV size can be decreased by low systemic vascular resistance or increased inotropy in addition to hypovolemia. A small, collapsible inferior vena cava is also indicative of hypovolemia, however this is of most use with spontaneously breathing patients so its diagnostic value is decreased with anesthesia and mechanical ventilation.[119] See Chapter 27 Echocardiography and Point-of-Care Ultrasound for a detailed discussion.

Recently, several types of noninvasive commercially available proprietary technologies that estimate CO and/or assess fluid responsiveness have been studied (e.g., pleth variability index, pulse wave transit time or contour analysis, carbon dioxide rebreathing, and thoracic electrical bioimpedance or bioreactance devices). A 2017 meta-analysis demonstrated that the percentage error of these devices for measurements of CO can be significant compared with standard thermodilution techniques.[120]

Electrolytes

Sodium

Physiologic Role

Sodium (Na^+) is the principal cation in the ECF with a serum concentration of 135 to 145 mEq/mL, and the largest determinant of serum osmolarity, that typically ranges from 275 to 290 mOsm/kg H_2O. The concentration gradient between ECF and ICF is maintained by the ubiquitous Na-K-ATPase pump that actively exports three Na^+ cations into the ECF while importing two K^+ cations into the cell at the cost of a single adenosine triphosphate (ATP) molecule. These cation exchanges occur against their respected concentration gradient, establishing very potent resting action potentials. As previously discussed, and often confused for osmolarity, tonicity refers to the amount of osmoles that cannot freely cross cellular membranes. Tonicity is predominantly determined by ECF [Na^+] and drives the movement of water via transmembrane aquaporins, into the ECF or ICF, to achieve osmotic equilibrium.[121–123] Hypertonic plasma results in net water efflux out of cells and into the ECF, causing cellular shrinkage. Conversely, hypotonic plasma results in net influx of water into cells and resultant cellular swelling. Extracellular Na^+ and TBW therefore have an intimate relationship, and clinical sodium disorders such as hyponatremia and hypernatremia should be thought of as abnormalities in TBW. Beyond sodium's crucial roles in maintaining ECF volume, it is also essential in establishing action potentials, as well as functioning in cellular signaling transduction, and membrane transportation.

Total body sodium regulation is primarily a reflection of one's thirst drive, and interactions between the renal and endocrine systems (Table 16-14). ADH, also known as AVP, is synthesized in the hypothalamus, then stored and released from the posterior pituitary. Hypertonic ECF results in hypothalamic cell shrinkage, osmoreceptors in response trigger the release ADH which downstream binds to V_2-receptors in the nephron's collecting duct, promoting water reabsorption to lower overall serum tonicity.[121,122] This mechanism is one of the major ways that the nephron concentrates urine. Amazingly, the healthy kidney can concentrate or dilute urine over an incredibly wide range of 50 to 1,200 mOsm/kg H_2O in response to varying ECF tonicity.[122–125] Similarly, hypotension sensed in carotid and aortic arch baroreceptors will trigger the release of ADH to promote water retention in an effort to correct a perceived hypovolemic state at the expense of serum

Table 16-14 Regulation of the Total Body Electrolyte Mass and Plasma Concentrations

Electrolyte	Regulated by
Sodium	Total body sodium regulated by aldosterone, ANP, [Na^+] altered by ADH
Potassium	Total body potassium regulated by aldosterone, intrinsic renal mechanisms; [K^+] regulated by epinephrine, insulin
Calcium	Both total body calcium and [Ca^{2+}] regulated by PTH, vitamin D
Phosphate	Both total body phosphate and [HPO_4^-] regulated primarily by renal mechanisms with a minor contribution from PTH
Magnesium	Both total body magnesium and [Mg^{++}] regulated primarily by renal mechanisms with a minor contribution from PTH and vitamin D

ANP, atrial natriuretic peptide; [Na^+], sodium concentration; ADH, antidiuretic hormone; PTH, parathyroid hormone.

hypotonicity.[122] This mechanism requires an appropriate production of ADH in the hypothalamus, release from the posterior pituitary gland, and renal response to maintain tight homeostasis of serum osmolarity between 275 and 290 mOsm/kg. While ADH acts to alter overall ECF tonicity and therefore the serum [Na^+], aldosterone and ANP secretion have bigger impacts on overall total body sodium as they function to promote Na^+ excretion (natriuresis) as discussed above.

Hyponatremia

Hyponatremia is defined as a serum [Na^+] of <135 mEq/L, severe being [Na^+] <125 mEq/L. It affects approximately 5% of all adults, and 15% to 30% of all hospitalized patients, nearly a quarter of all critically ill patients, and is associated with severe systemic disease.[124–127] With regard to the perioperative patient, a retrospective analysis of the American College of Surgeons National Surgical Quality Improvement Program (NSQIP) database demonstrated that preoperative hyponatremia was associated with greater risks for major adverse coronary events (1.8% vs. 0.7%), surgical site infections (7.4% vs. 4.6%), pneumonia, overall increased length of stay and increased risk for 30-day mortality.[128]

Simply put, hyponatremia is predominantly a disorder of water balance as a result of an excess TBW relative to total body sodium. Given this complex interplay, there are a multitude of mechanisms and physiologic states that can lead to the development of hyponatremia. Some common conditions encountered by the anesthesiologist include: acute stress response in postoperative care, medication-induced, the syndrome of inappropriate ADH (SIADH), malignancy, cerebral salt wasting or more broadly intracranial pathologies. Clinical manifestations are generally CNS-related, and reflect on both the degree of severity and pace of onset.[124,125,127,129] Acute presentations (occurring within <48 hours) are more likely to be symptomatic, as more chronic presentations are associated with adaptive compensatory measures. CNS symptomatology reflects cellular cerebral edema from osmotic, intracellular H_2O shifts across the tightly maintained blood brain barrier as a result of ECF hypotonicity.[123,129] Mild presentations include headache, confusion, or nausea without vomiting.[129] On the other hand, severe and life-threatening cases may demonstrate vomiting, somnolence, seizures, cardiorespiratory distress, or ultimately brain herniation[123,125,127] (NICV 16-3).

The majority of hyponatremic patients are hypotonic with a serum osmolarity of <270 mOsm/kg H_2O. However, there are several pathologic states that lead to increased serum osmoles (glucose, protein, glycine) that increase osmolarity and H_2O influx into the ECF with resultant decreased serum [Na^+]. These reflect isotonic or even hypertonic, hyponatremic states.[124] In addition, pseudohyponatremia can be seen with highly elevated serum lipids or proteins that interfere with how sodium is measured, but does not reflect a change in osmolarity *per se*. Historically, high volumes of nonconductive, glycine-containing irrigation solutions used in transurethral resection of the prostate (TURP) was associated with an acute iso- or hypertonic, hyponatremic state in the perioperative period.[124,129] The most common etiology of hypertonic hyponatremia is secondary to hyperglycemia. For each 100 mg/dL increase in serum glucose, there is an approximate reduction in [Na^+] of 1.6 to 2.4 mEq/dL.

As the differential for hyponatremia is so broad, and can reflect changes in serum osmolarity, as well as ECF volume status, it is important to follow a regimented algorithmic approach to determine the underlying etiology. While assessments of fluid volume status is essential in clinic practice, it has low sensitivity and specificity with regard to the etiology of hyponatremia, and if done early in the evaluation, may lead to the misclassification of the hyponatremic etiology.[124] Instead The European guideline for the diagnostic evaluation of hyponatremia begins with quantifiable laboratory value assessments, with fluid volume assessment occurring at the end of the overall algorithm (Fig. 16-5).[124,129] Beginning with the measurement of serum osmolarity, hypertonic and pseudohyponatremic etiologies can be quickly identified. When serum osmolarity is hypotonic (<270 mOsm/kg H_2O), the next step is to assess urine osmolarity, to gauge vasopressin (ADH) activity. In pathologic states where hyponatremia results from excessive water intake, vasopressin release will be maximally suppressed resulting in dilute urine with an osmolarity of <100 mOsm/kg. This phenomenon can be seen in primary polydipsia, beer potomania, or a low solute intake state such as the "Tea and Toast" diet.[124,129] Conversely when vasopressin activity is present, urine concentration will occur with urine osmolarity >100 mOsm/kg. Urinary [Na^+] excretion should then be assessed as a surrogate marker for intravascular volume status. A urine [Na^+] <30 mEq/L is indicative of hypovolemia or other low effective arterial volume states and reflects physiologic attempts to maximally retain both Na^+ and water.[124] There are important caveats to highlight: patients with low sodium diets, rare in the United States, will have relatively low urine [N^+], inversely patients taking diuretics or those with chronic kidney disease (CKD) will likely have elevated urine [Na^+] as a result of increased Na^+ excretion, or impaired Na^+ reabsorption, respectively.

With regard to the low effective arterial volume state, the differential can be narrowed to patients with ECF expansion or contraction; or hyper- *versus* hypovolemic states, respectively. Classic examples of pathophysiologic ECF expansion and hyponatremia, or *hypervolemic hyponatremia*, include congestive heart failure, cirrhosis, or nephrotic syndrome. ECF contraction, or *hypovolemic hyponatremia*, on the other hand can be seen in trauma or prolonged exposure, diarrhea, or vomiting. Therefore, when the etiology is suggestive of a low effective arterial volume state, the clinical assessment of the patient's volume status becomes one in differentiating between the two ends of the physiologic spectrum: volume overloaded or hypovolemic.[124]

The remaining etiologies on the differential diagnosis will have urine [Na^+] >30 mEq/L, which outside of diuretic use and CKD, should coincide with an underlying euvolemic state.

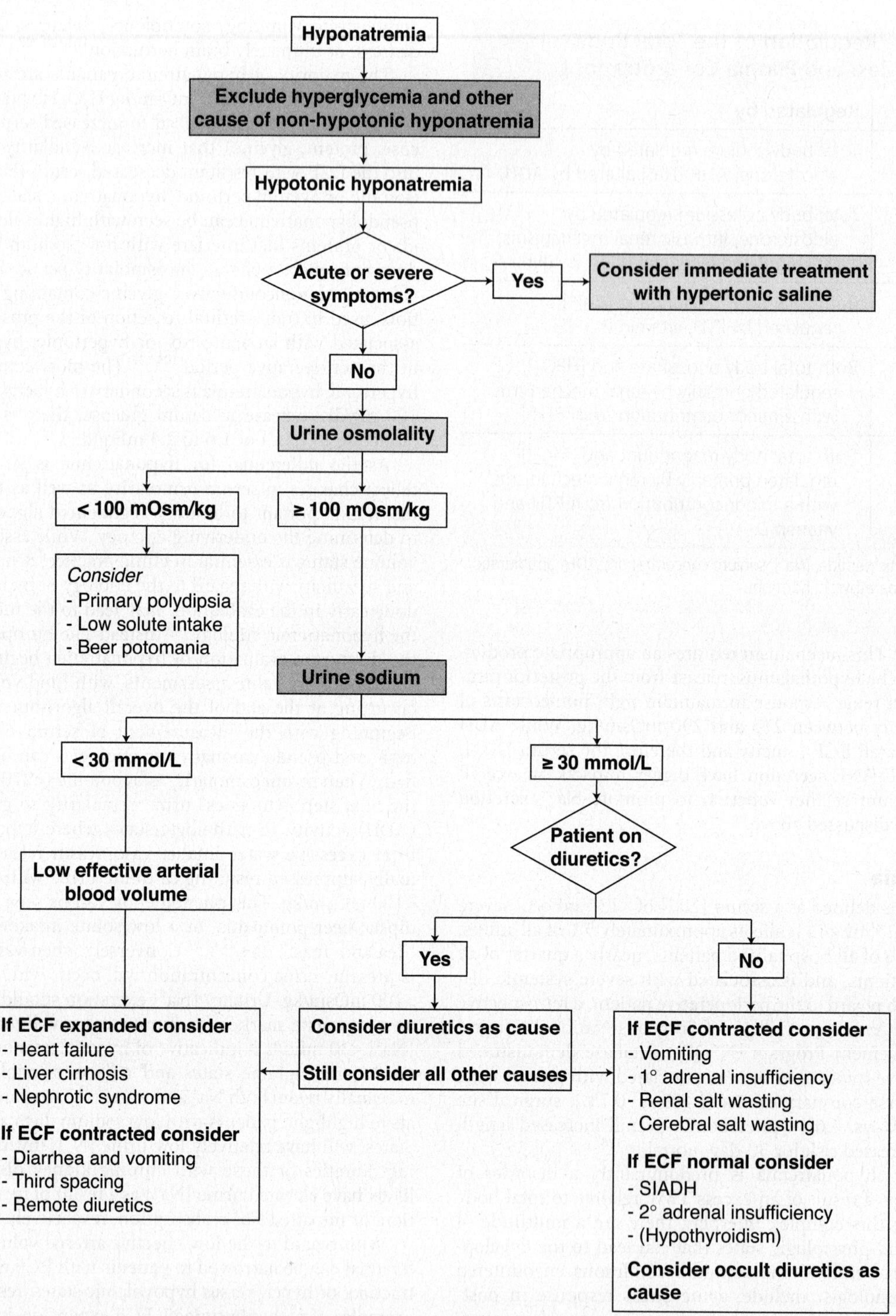

Figure 16-5 The European Guideline Diagnostic Algorithm for Hyponatremia. (Reprinted with permission from Hoorn EJ, Zietse R. Diagnosis and treatment of hyponatremia: compilation of the guidelines. *J Am Soc Nephrol.* 2017;28(5):1340–1349 and modified from Spasovski G, Vanholder R, Allolio B, Annane D, Ball S, Bichet D, et al. Clinical practice guideline on diagnosis and treatment of hyponatraemia. *Eur J Endocrinol.* 2014;170(3):G1–47.)

While the differential diagnosis remains broad, it can be narrowed down to SIADH, hypothyroidism, adrenal insufficiency, and ongoing diuretic use, notably thiazide or potassium sparing diuretics.[124]

It is worth highlighting the diagnosis of SIADH as it is frequently seen in the perioperative period, but remains a diagnosis of exclusion. Conditions that are frequently associated with SIADH are listed in Table 16-15. Paraneoplastic syndromes, intrathoracic and intracranial pathologies, as well as medication-induced, and the, "reset osmostat" are all commonplace. The diagnostic criteria for SIADH can be found in Table 16-16. The pathophysiologic mechanism of SIADH is a disconnection of ADH secretion from normal osmotic stimuli. The increased secretion of ADH results in TBW overexpansion with resultant serum [Na^+] dilution.

Table 16-15 Common Associations with the Syndrome of Inappropriate Antidiuretic Hormone (SIADH)

Neoplastic Disease
Carcinoma (e.g., lung)
Thymoma
Mesothelioma
Lymphoma, leukemia
Ewing sarcoma
Carcinoid
Bronchial adenoma
Neurologic Disorders
Head injury, neurosurgery
Brain abscess or tumor
Meningitis, encephalitis
Cerebral hemorrhage
Guillain–Barré syndrome
Hydrocephalus
Alcohol withdrawal
Peripheral neuropathy
Seizures
Subdural hematoma
Chest Disorders
Pneumonia
Tuberculosis
Empyema
Cystic fibrosis
Pneumothorax
Aspergillosis
Drugs
Sulfonylureas
Opiates
Thiazides and loop diuretics
Dopamine antaqonists
Anticonvulsants
Tricyclic antidepressants
SSRIs
Miscellaneous
Idiopathic
Psychosis
Porphyria

SSRI, selective serotonin reuptake inhibitor.

Modified with permission from Ball SG. Vasopressin and disorders of water balance: the physiology and pathophysiology of vasopressin. *Ann Clin Biochem*. 2007;44(5):417–431.

Compensatory mechanisms aimed at maintaining ECF are then elicited to prevent systemic hypervolemia, namely increased secretion of ANP and suppression of the renin–angiotensin–aldosterone system, both leading to increased natriuresis.[127]

Cerebral salt wasting (CSW) is a phenomenon commonly associated with subarachnoid hemorrhage, TBIs, and other intracranial pathologies that have a very similar clinical presentation, and as a result, is often confused for SIADH.[130] The key difference separating the two syndromes is the underlying effective arterial volume state. SIADH as previously discussed, is seen in the euvolemic patient whereas CSW ultimately leads to hypovolemia and a low effective arterial volume state. Thus, the treatment strategies for the two should differ. The treatment of SIADH focuses on free water restriction, decreasing TBW by 0.5 to 1.0 L/day. In comparison, the treatment for CSW is based on: (a) volume expansion and (b) hypertonic solutions such as 3% saline to overcome ongoing [Na^+] excretion.[130] In practice, this debate remains mostly academic in patients with underlying neurologic pathologies. The fear is from worsening hypovolemia and compromising cerebral perfusion in vulnerable patients by restricting access to free water in patients with CSW misdiagnosed as SIADH. Likewise, for those with SIADH misdiagnosed as CSW progressive cerebral edema may result from attempts at volume expansion with isotonic solutions, which only serves to increase the amount of free water that can be reabsorbed, further diluting serum [Na^+]. Thus, the prudent approach to treating hyponatremia in the setting of underlying neurologic pathologies is administering 3.0% saline for symptomatic patients, or vigilant serum [Na^+] monitoring and oral sodium chloride tablets for the stable, asymptomatic patient.[123]

Table 16-16 The Diagnostic Criteria for the Syndrome of Inappropriate Antidiuretic Hormone

Essential Criteria
• Serum osmolality < 275 mOsm/kg
• Urine osmolality > 100 mOsm/kg
• Urine [Na^+] > 30 mEq/L
• Euvolemic on examination
• No history of diuretic use
• Absence of adrenal insufficiency, hypothyroidism, or CKD
Supplemental Criteria
• Fractional uric acid excretion >12%
• Failure to increase serum [Na^+] following 0.9% saline infusion
• Increase in serum [Na^+] through fluid restriction

CKD, chronic kidney disease.

Modified from Spasovski G, Vanholder R, Allolio B, et al. Clinical practice guideline on diagnosis and treatment of hyponatraemia. *Eur J Endocrinol.* 2014;170(3):G1–47, Hoorn EJ, Zietse R. Diagnosis and treatment of hyponatremia: compilation of the guidelines. *J Am Soc Nephrol.* 2017; 28(5):1340–1349.

Vaptans function by blocking vasopressin (ADH) V_2-receptor activation in the renal collecting duct and therefore result in urine dilution and water excretion. In simple, non-neurologic pathology-associated SIADH, vaptans can also be considered. Similarly, in the low effective arterial volume state with ECF expansion, or *hypervolemic hyponatremia*, such as cirrhosis or heart failure, vaptans have been safely used to increase serum [Na^+].[124]

Overall treatment strategies should focus on severity of symptoms and the chronicity of hyponatremia, shown in Table 16-17 (see also 2 Video 16-2). Even in severe, symptomatic hyponatremia, an increase in serum [Na^+] by 4 to 6 mEq/L should be enough to reduce cerebral edema and impending herniation, as well as abate hyponatremia-related seizures.[123] This change can reliably be achieved with the administration of 100 mL 3% saline infused over 10 minutes. The concern for overzealous hyponatremia correction is the development of osmotic demyelination syndrome (Fig. 16-6), notably central pontine myelinolysis.[121,123,125,126] Symptoms typically present several days after rapid [Na^+] correction and may include pseudobulbar palsy, quadriparesis, movement disorders, or seizures.[121] The pathophysiology of osmotic demyelination syndromes is the destruction of myelin shafts and oligodendrocytes, possibly through apoptosis as a stress response to rapid changes in intracellular tonicity and decreased cellular volume.[121,127] Patients at greatest risk for

Table 16-17 Treatment Guidelines in the Management of Hyponatremia

Presentation	Management
Acute or symptomatic hyponatremia	• Severe symptoms: Bolus 3% saline, 100 mL over 10 min, repeat ×3 as needed • Moderate symptoms: 3 saline infusion 0.5–2 mL/kg per hour
Chronic hyponatremia • SIADH	• 1st line: Free water restriction • 2nd line: Vaptans
• Hypovolemic hyponatremia	• Volume expansion with isotonic saline
• Hypervolemic hyponatremia	• Fluid restriction • Vaptans • Treatment of underlying hypervolemic state
Recommended serum [Na⁺] correction rates	• Minimum: [Na^+] 4–8 mEq/L per day • Maximum: [Na^+] 8–10 mEq/L per day[a]
Recommend serum [Na^+] assessments	• Every 4–6 hours over the first 24 hours • After any bolus of 3% saline

[a]Maximal [Na^+] correction of 10–12 mEq/L per day should only be done in acute, or severely symptomatic patients.

Modified from Spasovski G, Vanholder R, Allolio B, et al. Clinical practice guideline on diagnosis and treatment of hyponatraemia. *Eur J Endocrinol.* 2014;170(3):G1–47, Hoorn EJ, Zietse R. Diagnosis and treatment of hyponatremia: compilation of the guidelines. *J Am Soc Nephrol.* 2017;28(5):1340–1349.

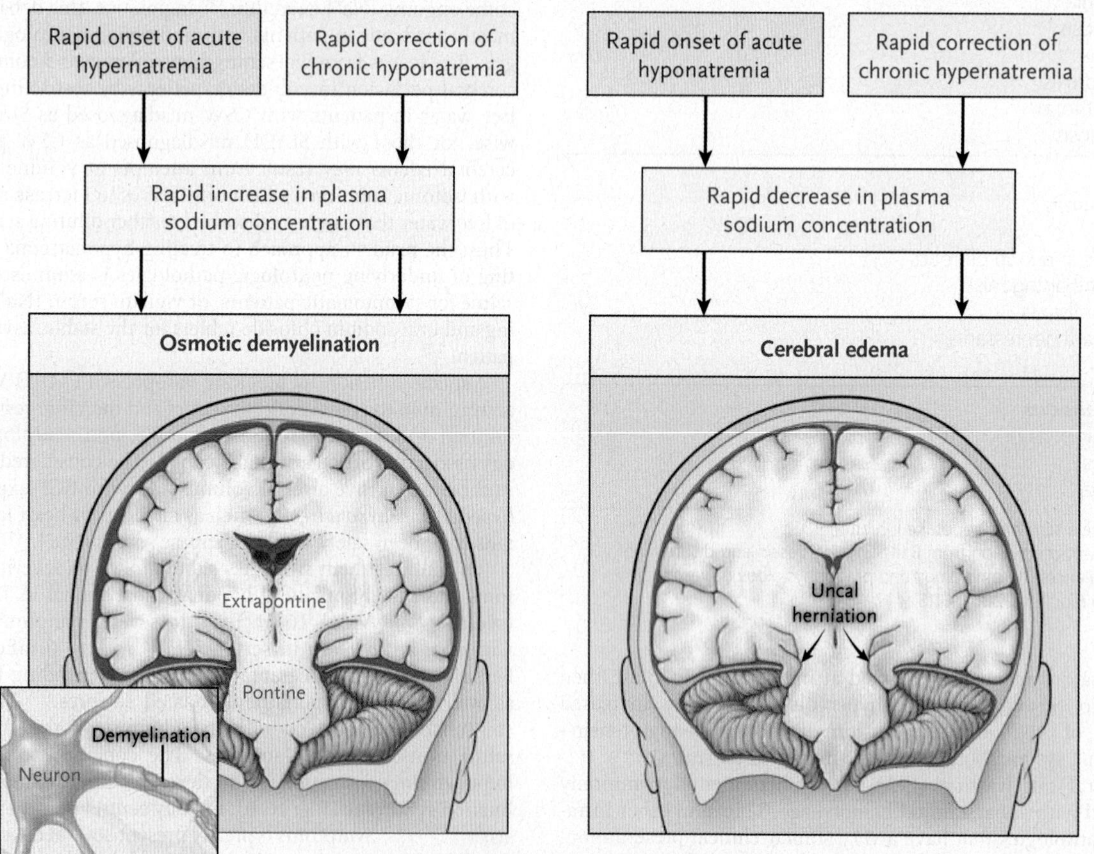

Figure 16-6 Consequences of rapid changes in plasma sodium concentration. From Sterns RH. Disorders of plasma sodium–causes, consequences, and correction. *N Engl J Med.* 2015;372(1):55–65. Figure 3.

developing osmotic demyelination syndrome are those with critically low hyponatremia with serum [Na^+] <105 mEq/L, those with underlying chronic malnutrition, chronic alcohol dependence, chronic liver disease, or concurrent hypokalemia.[131] In the event that rapid overcorrection does occur, HS should be discontinued and replaced with hypotonic solutions. In addition, 2 to 4 mcg intravenous desmopressin every 6 to 8 hours can be administered to promote water reabsorption in the collecting duct with a downstream reduction in serum [Na^+].[122,124,125,127,129]

Hypernatremia

Hypernatremia is defined as a serum [Na^+] >145 mEq/L and results from TBW depletion. It is relatively uncommon in the hospitalized patient with less than 1% presenting with hypernatremia on admission. Between 6% and 26% of patients develop hypernatremia in the ICU however.[132] Hypernatremia is associated with increased ICU length of stay and a 40% to 60% increase in mortality rates. The severity of hypernatremia, rather than duration of, is of greater concern.[133] Most commonly hypernatremia results from an impaired thirst mechanism, or restricted access to free water.

Similar to hyponatremia, symptoms of hypernatremia may be nonspecific in nature, but are most commonly CNS related. This observation is secondary to cerebral cellular shrinkage (rather than expansion seen with hyponatremia) with free water influx into ECF in response to hypertonic serum. Symptoms may manifest as lethargy, irritability or agitation, hyperreflexia, increased tone or nuchal rigidity, myoclonus,or asterixis. If left untreated hypernatremia can progress to seizures, intracranial hemorrhage, coma, or death.[121,126,132–134] In addition, there is a poorly understood association with hypernatremia and congestive heart failure.[133] The pathophysiology of hypernatremia can be categorized into three major mechanisms: (1) increased renal losses; (2) extrarenal losses; or (3) excessive sodium intake.

Increased renal water losses can be brought on by diabetes insipidus (DI), renal dysfunction, or can be medication-induced. Central DI reflects a reduction in either the production of, or release of ADH and is frequently observed in patients with TBIs, pineal gland or pituitary gland adenomas, or following surgical removal of pituitary adenomas, Sheehan's syndrome, and inflammatory granulomatous diseases (sarcoidosis, tuberculosis).[133] Nephrogenic DI on the other hand, occurs in the setting of appropriate ADH secretion, but a failure of the kidneys to respond accordingly, which may occur secondary to renal dysfunction, concurrent electrolyte disturbances such as hypokalemia or hypercalcemia, or commonly induced by medications such as lithium.[133] Other common medications that are associated with the development of hypernatremia can be found in Table 16-18. In addition, excessive renal water loss can be induced by the administration of loop and osmotic diuretics as well as corticosteroids.[132–134]

Extrarenal water losses account for more than half of all hypernatremia seen in the critically ill.[132] Impaired thirst drive (hypodipsia or adipsia) is common in patients with altered mental status, sepsis, or those with damage to hypothalamic osmoreceptors that drives thirst as a response to increased plasma osmolarity.[123,126,133,134] Osmoreceptor sensitivity declines with age, and likely explains why impaired thirst and hypernatremia are more commonly seen in the elderly.[123,134] Increased insensible losses are more likely to be seen as the underlying etiology of increased extrarenal losses. Insensible losses account for a net free water loss of approximately 14 mL/kg per day. Fever can increase insensible losses by as much as 3 to 5 mL/kg per day, per 1°C above euthermia.[132] In addition, cutaneous losses can be seen with excessive sweating, burns, trauma, or large open wounds. Similarly, tachypnea or increased minute ventilation will result in increased insensible losses from the respiratory tract. Further, gastrointestinal losses seen in vomiting, diarrhea, nasogastric suctioning, or large enterocutaneous fistulas can also result in hypernatremia.

Table 16-18 Common Medications Associated with Hypernatremia

Drug	Main Mechanism (s)
Lithium	(i) Hypercalcemia leading to nephrogenic diabetes insipidus and causing water loss (ii) Central diabetes insipidus
Hypervitaminosis A and D	Hypokalemia leading to nephrogenic diabetes insipidus
Cisplatin	Hypokalemia leading to nephrogenic diabetes insipidus
Aminoglycosides	Hypokalemia leading to nephrogenic diabetes insipidus
Demeclocycline	Nephrogenic diabetes insipidus
Amphotericin B	Nephrogenic diabetes insipidus
Phenytoin	Central diabetes insipidus
Ethanol	Central diabetes insipidus
Loop diuretics	Water loss
Manitol	Osmotic diuresis
Corticosteroids	Urea increase
Vasopressin receptor inhibitors (vaptans)	Water diuresis
Lactulose/sorbitol	Hypotonic gastrointestinal losses
Hypertonic $NaHCO_3$ or NaCl solution	Increased Na^+ administration

Reprinted with permission from Liamis G, Filippatos TD, Elisaf MS. Evaluation and treatment of hypernatremia: a practical guide for physicians. *Postgrad Med.* 2016;128(3):299–306.

Lastly increased sodium intake can result from conditions that lead to inappropriately elevated renal [Na^+] reabsorption such as primary hyperaldosteronism or Cushing syndrome.[133] Increased sodium administration can occur iatrogenically as well, commonly seen in patients receiving HS, or that received ampules of 8.4% sodium bicarbonate as an emergency measure, common in pre-hospital or emergency department care. For example, a standard 50-mL 8.4% sodium bicarbonate ampule contains 1 mEq/mL of Na^+, or 1,000 mEq/L. Excessive salt intake can also occur iatrogenically in patients receiving total parenteral nutrition as well as concentrated enteral tube feeding. In the infant presenting with hypernatremia, errors in diluting powdered formulas should be considered.[126,134] Toxic ingestions of salt or sea water, or the use of salt water emetics can lead to hypernatremia.

The evaluation of hypernatremia should begin with a thorough history and physical examination, attempting to determine the onset and underlying volume status (Table 16-19). Similar to hyponatremia, presentations within 48 hours of onset are acute in nature, while those with symptoms for greater than 48 hours, or unknown durations are considered chronic.

Assessment of urine osmolarity is particularly helpful in discriminating between renal or extrarenal sources. Hypernatremia

Table 16-19 Hypernatremia: Underlying Etiologies, Examination, and Laboratory Findings

Category	Mechanism	Supportive Findings
Inadequate H_2O intake	Lack of access or thirst drive	• Signs of hypovolemia on examination • U_{Osm} > 600 mOsm/kg • AMS • Extremes of age (infants and the elderly)
Extrarenal H_2O losses	Increased: GI, fever, cutaneous, insensible losses	• Signs of hypovolemia on examination • History of: fever, diarrhea, burns, open wounds, nasogastric suctioning, enterocutaneous fistula • U_{Osm} > 600 mOsm/kg
Increased renal H_2O losses	Diuretics Osmotic diuresis Central DI	• Loop diuretics • Hyperglycemia with glucosuria • History of TBI, recent neurosurgical procedure, granulomatous disease • U_{Osm} <300 mOsm/kg • U_{Osm} ↑ with DDAVP
	Nephrogenic DI	• Lithium administration • Hypercalcemia or hypokalemia • U_{Osm} < 300 mOsm/DDAVP • No response to DDAVP
Excessive salt intake		• Signs of hypervolemia on examination • Signs of mineralocorticoid excess on examination • U_{Osm} > 600 mOsm/kg • U_{Na} > 100 mEq/L • History of hypertonic saline, or emergent $NaHCO_3$ administration • TPN or concentrated enteral tube feeds • Formula-fed infant

AMS, altered mental status; DDAVP, desmopressin; DI, diabetes insipidus; GI, gastrointestinal; TBI, traumatic brain injury; TPN, total parenteral nutrition.
Modified from Seay NW, Lehrich RW, Greenberg A. Diagnosis and management of disorders of body tonicity-hyponatremia and hypernatremia: core curriculum 2020. *Am J Kidney Dis*. 2020;75(2):272–286. Copyright © 2020 Elsevier. With permission.

with urine osmolarity <300 mOsm/kg, (or less than serum osmolarity), is suggestive of DI and the administration of desmopressin (DDAVP) can be used to differentiate between the central or nephrogenic DI. Central DI will respond by increasing urine osmolarity, whereas nephrogenic DI is the result of ADH resistance, and therefore will not change urine osmolarity following DDAVP administration.[133] In comparison, patients with urine osmolarity >600 mOsm/kg suggests an appropriate secretion and response to ADH resulting in preserved renal concentrating abilities. Hypernatremia with elevated urine osmolarity suggests extrarenal water losses, or excessive sodium intake.

Treatment strategies for hypernatremia are based on both identifying the underlying etiology as well as duration from onset. Acute presentations within 48 hours can be more rapidly corrected, especially if symptomatic. Chronic presentations require a more controlled $[Na^+]$ correction to avoid inducing cerebral edema (**NaFg2**). The mainstay of managing hypernatremia is repleting the TBW deficit that has resulted in the underlying hypertonic state. TBW deficit can be calculated using the following equation:

$$\text{TBW deficit} = 0.6 \times \text{body weight (kg)} \times \frac{[Na^+]}{140} - 140 \quad (16\text{-}9)$$

Note: $[Na^+]$ the current serum Na^+ concentration.

With regard to the pace of correction, a reduction in serum $[Na^+]$ <10 mEq/L in 24 hours should be targeted to avoid the risk of causing cerebral edema.[133] This rate can be achieved with the administration of dextrose 5% water, increased enteral access to free water, or both.

When eunatremia is achieved, focus should then be placed on addressing the underlying etiology of hypernatremia. For instance, patients with central DI should be started on 10 to 20 mcg intranasal DDAVP. In the setting of nephrogenic DI, the administration of thiazide diuretics and NSAIDs can be trialed, especially if secondary to toxicity, as COX2 inhibition has been shown to reduce lithium-induced polyuria.[133] Patients with hypovolemia in the setting of hypernatremia should receive appropriate volume repletion with isotonic solutions in addition to the hypotonic dextrose 5% water aimed at correcting hypernatremia. Obviously in the setting of medication-induced hypernatremia, any offending agent should be discontinued. Lastly, patients with severe, symptomatic hypernatremia, especially with underlying CKD, those who failed to correct appropriately with hypotonic fluid administration or those with concerns for concurrent decompensated congestive heart failure, hemodialysis, or continuous renal replacement therapy should be considered.[133]

Potassium

Physiologic Role

Potassium (K^+) is an essential dietary electrolyte and is the most abundant intracellular cation. Potassium is critical for maintaining cell membrane potentials, protein synthesis, and action potentials seen in excitable cells such as muscle, neurons, and cardiac tissue.[135–138] The ubiquitous Na-K-ATPase pump drives these processes and preserves a steep gradient between extracellular and intracellular $[K^+]$ that ultimately serves as a source of potential

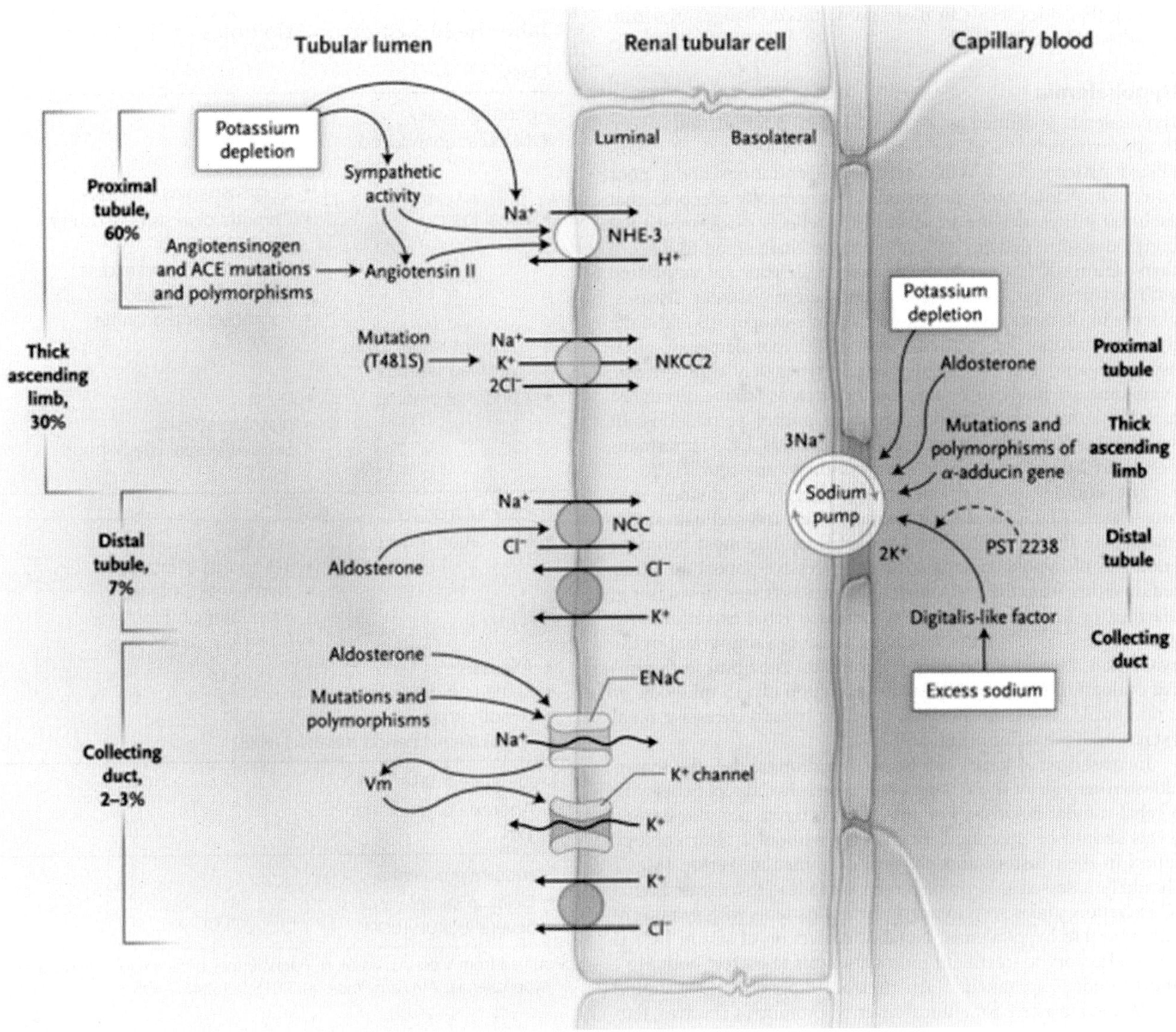

Figure 16-7 Renal cellular mechanism of potassium excretion. From Adrogue HJ, Madias NE. Sodium and potassium in the pathogenesis of hypertension. *N Engl J Med*. 2007;356(19):1966–1978.

energy within the cell. Extracellular [K^+] is therefore tightly regulated within a relatively narrow range of 3.5 to 5.0 mEq/L, making up less than 2% of total body potassium.[135] In comparison, the intracellular compartment [K^+] is typically around 150 mEq/L, making up the remaining 98% of total body potassium.[135,138] On an average, approximately only 3% of adult Americans have an adequate potassium intake with the typical dietary intake of 2,600 mg/day; less than the 4,700 mg/day recommended by the Food and Nutrition Board of Institute of Medicine or 3,150 mg/day recommended by the World Health Organization (WHO). Mediterranean diets, or those rich in fruits, vegetables, legumes, dairy, and seafood are associated with far greater daily potassium intake.

Approximately 90% of potassium ingested each day is renally excreted, with a smaller portion being excreted in stool.[135] Potassium is freely filtered in the glomerulus and mostly reabsorbed in the proximal tubule and loop of Henle.[138] The remaining filtered K^+ enters the distal convoluted tubule and the CCD, the primary sites where potassium excretion occurs. The major determinants of potassium excretion are regulated by aldosterone and serum [K^+], and to a lesser extent, acid–base status, filtered [Na^+]concentrations, and nephron flow rates (Fig. 16-7).[135,136] Aldosterone is the major mineralocorticoid in humans and stimulates increased luminal Na^+ reabsorption, which results in downstream K^+ secretion into the CCD lumen, that then leads to K^+ excretion. Similarly, increased serum [K^+] (hyperkalemia), as well as alkalemia, results in net increase in Na^+ delivery to the CCD, allowing for increased Na^+ reabsorption, and therefore K^+ excretion. Notably a circadian rhythm to K^+ excretion is also seen with the majority of excretion occurring in the afternoon and evening.[135,136,138]

Other notable physiologic conditions can greatly impact serum [K^+]. Acidemia resulting from either a metabolic or respiratory acidosis will result in extracellular K^+ shifts, increasing serum [K^+], whereas alkalotic states are associated with intracellular K^+ shifts and a decrease in serum [K^+]. Intracellular K^+ shifts can also be induced with the administration of β_2-agonists and insulin. With these conditions, K^+ shifts are transient and do not alter total body [K^+]. There are pathologic states associated with intracellular K^+

shifting that does result in more pronounced changes in serum [K+] discussed below.[139,140]

Hypokalemia

Hypokalemia is defined as serum [K+] of <3.5 mEq/L and is seen in approximately 3% of the total population and 20% of hospitalized patients.[140,141] While serum concentrations are a poor reflection of total body potassium, it is generally accepted that each 1.0 mEq/L decline in serum [K+] reflects a 300-mEq total body potassium deficit.[140,141] While more challenging to discern than serum [K+], total body potassium deficits are associated with hypertension, cardiovascular and cerebrovascular diseases, glucose intolerance, and increased risk for osteoporosis and bone demineralization.[142,143] Patients with mild hypokalemia are often asymptomatic, and as the degree of hypokalemia progresses, symptoms are likely to be nonspecific such as fatigue, myalgias, malaise, lethargy, constipation, dyspnea, and or palpitations. In severe cases of hypokalemis, ascending paralysis, ECG abnormalities, heart failure, and even lethal arrythmias can occur.[141,144]

The etiology of hypokalemia can largely be divided into four classes (Table 16-20): abnormal losses, transcellular shifts, inadequate intake, or pseudo-hypokalemia. The most common etiologies of hypokalemia result from excessive potassium elimination either from the gastrointestinal tract as is seen in vomiting, diarrhea or laxative use, or from increased renal excretion with diuretic use.[140,141,144] Thus, a thorough history is important in the evaluation. Measuring urinary K^+ excretion is helpful in the initial evaluation with a total 24-hour excretion of >15 mEq/day, or a random U_K:U_{Cr} ratio of > 1.5, pointing toward excessive renal excretion of potassium (Fig. 16-8).[140,144]

Increased renal losses can be seen in diuretic use, the hyperaldosterone state or those taking corticosteroids, and patients with a renal-tubular acidosis. For this reason, renin and aldosterone levels should be measured for patients without a clear etiology found in their history and physical examination. Serum [Mg^{2+}] should be assessed as hypomagnesemia can lead to increased renal K^+ excretion, and is seen in nearly 50% of patients with symptomatic or severe hypokalemia. Notably, correction of serum [K+] is often refractory to treatment unless attempts to correct both Mg^{2+} and K^+ deficits are taken.[144] An electrocardiogram (ECG) should be obtained to assess for clinical severity; prominent U waves, flattened or inverted T waves, and ST elevation can all be observed in otherwise asymptomatic patients.[141,144]

The management of hypokalemia is twofold: (1) potassium repletion; and (2) identification and treatment of the underlying cause. [K+] should be urgently corrected to >4 mEq/L in patients with underlying heart failure or coronary arterial disease; otherwise mild-to-moderate cases with [K+] of 3.0 to 3.5 mEq/L can be corrected safely over time with oral repletion by administering up to 100 to 150 mEq/day.[135,141] With peripheral intravenous repletion, no more than 10 to 20 mEq/hr should be administered, and continuous ECG monitoring should be in place to assess for the development of unstable cardiac arrhythmias secondary to iatrogenic hyperkalemia.[140,141] Patients with central venous access can safely receive up to 40 mEq/hr intravenous potassium repletion. In life-threatening hypokalemia (unstable arrhythmias) rapid administration of potassium can be considered, giving 2 mEq/min over 10 minutes, followed by 10 mEq over an additional 10 minutes.[145,146]

Table 16-20 Common Etiologies of Hypokalemia

Class	
Abnormal losses	
• Medication induced	• Diuretics • Laxatives • Corticosteroids
• Renal losses	• Osmotic diuresis (glucosuria; proteinuria) • Mineralocorticoid excess • Renal tubular acidosis • Polydipsia and polyuria
• Gastrointestinal losses	
• Hypomagnesemia	
• Abnormal binding	• Dialysis • plasmapheresis • Extracorporeal Life Support (ECLS)
Transcellular shifts	
• Medication induced	• Insulin • Β-Agonists (Albuterol) • Xanthines (Caffeine) • Amphotericin B • Aminoglycosides
• Alkalosis	
• Refeeding syndrome	
• Hypothermia	
• Hypokalemic period paralysis (HPP)	
Inadequate intake	
• Anorexia or starvation	
• TPN	
Pseudo-hypokalemia	
• Delay in sample analysis	
• Severe leukocytosis	

Modified from Viera AJ, Wouk N. Potassium disorders: hypokalemia and hyperkalemia. *Am Fam Physician*. 2015;92(6):487–495.

Hyperkalemia

Hyperkalemia is generally defined as a serum [K+] of > 5.0 mEq/L, and ranges from mild cases between 5.0 and 5.5 mEq/L, moderate 5.5 and 6.0 mEq/L, and severe >6.0 mEq/L[145,147] (NICV 16-4). Hyperkalemia is uncommon with a likely incidence of 2.5% to 3.5% in the hospitalized patients, and higher in patients with underlying CKD.[139,148,149] Clinical manifestations can range from weakness, paresthesias, or heart palpitations, to dyspnea, flaccid paralysis, or malignant cardiac arrhythmias including cardiac arrest.[145] An ECG should be obtained for all patients found to have hyperkalemia to assess for cardiac conduction abnormalities. ECG changes are unlikely to be seen with [K+] <5.5 mEq/L, but when [K+] reaches the 5.5 to 6.5 mEq/L range, the characteristic peaked T waves can be seen (Fig. 16-9).[145,149,150] At [K+] >6.5 mEq/L, increased cardiac myocyte excitability and a shortened repolarization phase can also result in PR-segment prolongation. With [K+] >7.0 to 8.0 mEq/L, the p wave can be lost, and eventually progresses to QRS widening, or conduction velocity slowing causing symptomatic bradycardia or complete heart block.[145,149–151] If left untreated this pattern can further deteriorate to ventricular tachycardia, ventricular fibrillation, or asystole. Unfortunately, ECG changes are not always seen in hyperkalemia, and equally as important, life-threatening cardiac conductions manifestations can be seen in even moderate hyperkalemia with [K+] <6.0 mEq/L[149,152] (3 Video 16.3).

There are four main mechanisms that can lead to hyperkalemia: (1) impaired renal K^+ excretion, (2) excessive intake,

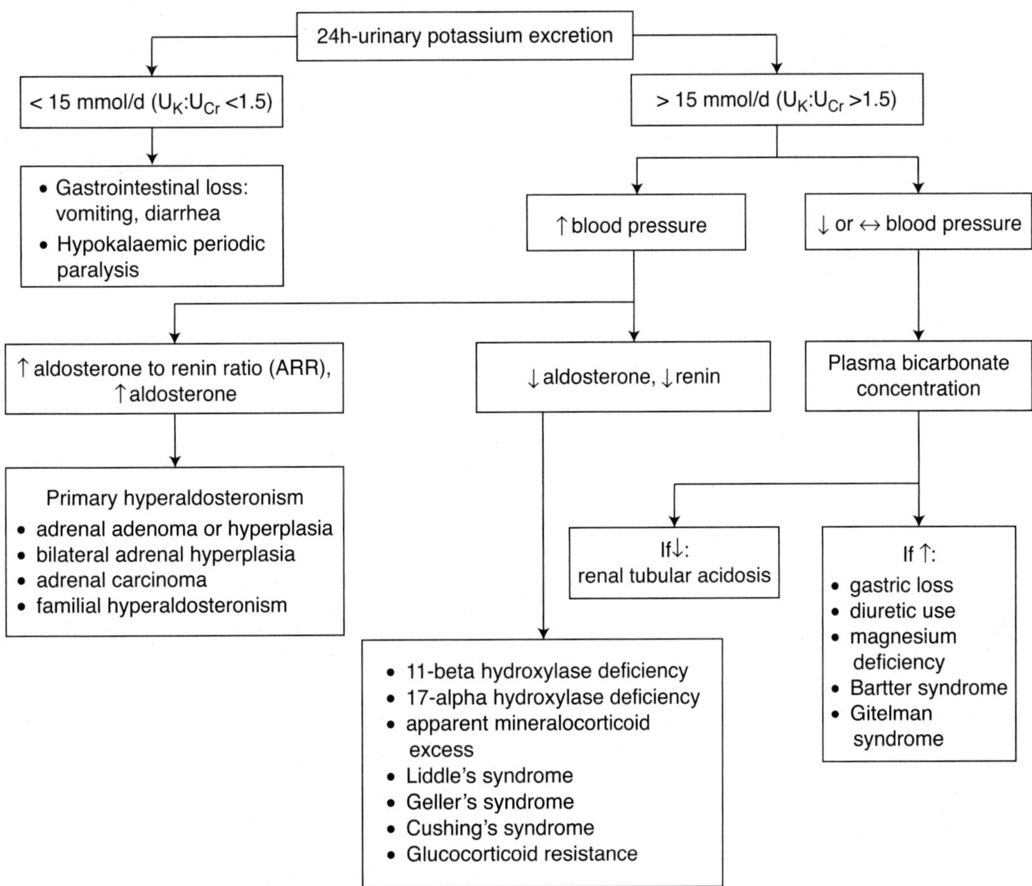

Figure 16-8 A diagnostic algorithm for the evaluation of hypokalemia. (Used with permission of BioScientifica, from Kardalas E, Paschou SA, Anagnostis P, et al. Hypokalemia: a clinical update. *Endocr Connect*. 2018;7(4):R135–R46; permission conveyed from Copyright Clearance Center, Inc.)

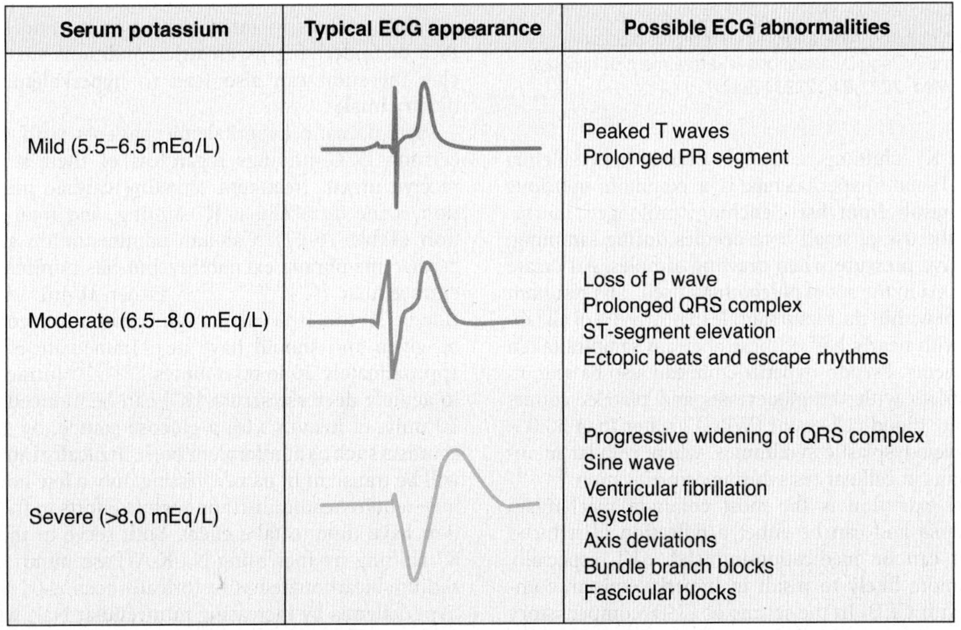

Serum potassium	Typical ECG appearance	Possible ECG abnormalities
Mild (5.5–6.5 mEq/L)		Peaked T waves Prolonged PR segment
Moderate (6.5–8.0 mEq/L)		Loss of P wave Prolonged QRS complex ST-segment elevation Ectopic beats and escape rhythms
Severe (>8.0 mEq/L)		Progressive widening of QRS complex Sine wave Ventricular fibrillation Asystole Axis deviations Bundle branch blocks Fascicular blocks

Figure 16-9 Electrocardiographic (ECG) manifestations of hyperkalemia. Derived from Viera AJ, Wouk N. Potassium disorders: hypokalemia and hyperkalemia. Am Fam Physician. 2015;92(6):487–495; Sood MM, Sood AR, Richardson R. Emergency management and commonly encountered outpatient scenarios in patients with hyperkalemia. *Mayo Clin Proc*. 2007;82(12):1553–1561.

Table 16-21 Common Causes of Hyperkalemia

Impaired Renal Excretion • Reduced renal function: ▪ Oilguric renal failure ▪ Defect in cortical collecting tubule ▪ Hypoaldosteronism • Drug induced: ▪ NSAIDs ▪ ACE-i, ARBs ▪ Triamterene, amiloride ▪ Cyclosporine; tacrolimus ▪ Potassium sparing diuretics
Extracellular K⁺ Shifts • Acidosis, metabolic or respiratory • Hypertonic states: ▪ DKA ▪ Toxic alcohol ingestions ▪ Hemolysis ▪ Hyperosmolar therapy ▪ Hypertriglyceridemia ▪ Hyperproteinemia • Succinylcholine • β-Blockers • Insulin deficiency • Hyperkalemic periodic paralysis • Cellular injury or lysis: ▪ Tumor lysis syndrome ▪ Rhabdomyolysis ▪ Malignant hyperthermia
Pseudohyperkalemia • Phlebotomy technique • Thrombocytosis >500 x 10^9/L • Leukocytosis >50 x 10^9/L • Myelodysplastic disorders
Excessive Intake

NSAIDs, nonsteroidal anti-inflammatory drugs; ACE-I, angiotensin-converting enzyme inhibitor; ARB, angiotensin receptor blocker.
Modified from Palmer BF, Clegg DJ. Diagnosis and treatment of hyperkalemia. *Cleve Clin J Med*. 2017;84(12):934–942.

(3) extracellular K^+ shifting, and (4) pseudo-hyperkalemia (Table 16-21).[153] Pseudo-hyperkalemia is a common, spurious finding that can result from fist clenching, prolonged tourniquet application, the use of small bore needles during sampling, or excessive negative pressure when drawing samples. All create pseudo-hyperkalemia in the act of phlebotomy itself. The resultant hemolysis is present within the blood sample in nearly 4% of all laboratory samples, with nearly half of these aberrant samples taken from newborn patients. Pseudo-hyperkalemia can also be seen in hematologic disorders with thrombocytosis and platelet counts >500 × 10^9/L, white blood cell count (WBC) greater than 50.0 × 10^9/L, or other myelodysplastic syndromes, where cellular membrane fragility results in cellular lysis during centrifugation.[153–155]

Impaired renal excretion is the most common mechanism of true hyperkalemia and can be either a reflection of reduced renal function or can be medication-induced. AKI, especially with oliguria, is more likely to result in hyperkalemia in comparison to those with CKD. In the setting of CKD, compensatory increases in Na-K-ATPase within the remaining nephrons maximize renal potassium excretion. In addition, adaptive increases in gastrointestinal excretion function to maintain normal potassium homeostasis.[153] Glomerular filtration rate (GFR) needs to fall below 10 to 15 mL/min before renal excretion is impaired enough to result in hyperkalemia in CKD, and if present in the setting of higher GFRs, a concurrent aldosterone deficiency, or tubule defect should be suspected.[153]

More commonly, medications are the underlying etiology of hyperkalemia, especially renin–angiotensin–aldosterone system inhibitors such as angiotensin-converting enzyme inhibitors (ACE-I), angiotensin II receptor blockers (ARBs), mineralocorticoid receptor antagonists such as spironolactone, and nonsteroidal anti-inflammatory drugs (NSAIDs). Renin–angiotensin–aldosterone system inhibitors result in hyperkalemia by decreasing overall mineralocorticoid activity, similar to what is seen with hypoaldosteronism. Interestingly, heparin can induce hypoaldosteronism by decreasing adrenal synthesis of aldosterone.[153] Hyperkalemia can also frequently be seen in patients with diabetes mellitus as it is associated with a chronic hyporeninemic, hypoaldosterone state.[156]

Extracellular [K^+] shifting as an etiology of hyperkalemia is commonly seen in the hospitalized or critically ill patients. Given how tightly potassium hemostasis is regulated, even small shifts in total body potassium can result in drastic increases in serum [K^+]. Shifts can be transient in nature, as seen in metabolic or respiratory acidoses, and result from a compensatory extracellular K^+ efflux due to increased intracellular [H^+]. Transient extracellular K^+ is also seen following the administration of succinylcholine, as postjunctional membrane depolarization results in the efflux of K^+ ions into the ECF, resulting in increases serum [K^+] of 0.5 to 1.0 mEq/L.[156] Upregulation of extrajunctional fetal acetylcholine receptors (AChR) results from pathologic states such as chronic immobilization, or major burns. With induced spontaneous AChR depolarization following succinylcholine administration, severe and catastrophic extracellular K^+ shift can occur. Cellular lysis will also result in extracellular K^+ shifts during hemolysis, tumor lysis syndrome, rhabdomyolysis, and malignant hyperthermia.

Lastly, excessive potassium intake can result in hyperkalemia, but usually requires some level of impaired renal excretion concurrently given how tightly potassium homeostasis is typically maintained.[153] Common foods rich in potassium include bananas, melons, potatoes, citrus fruits, and salt substitutes.[153] Pica or underlying psychiatric conditions that result in chronic clay ingestion can also lead to hyperkalemia from excessive dietary intake.

Symptomatic hyperkalemic patients with weakness or concerning ECG findings regardless of their serum [K^+] should receive urgent treatment targeting cardiac membrane stabilization, acute intracellular K^+ shifting, and total body K^+ elimination (Table 16-22). Calcium administration serves to decrease cardiac membrane excitability, but has minimal to no effects on extracellular [K^+].[139,141,152,153] Either 10-mL 10% calcium chloride or 30-mL 10% calcium gluconate intravenous solutions can be given and should have near immediate effects that last for approximately 30 to 60 minutes.[141,145,152] Intracellular K^+ shifting to acutely decrease serum [K^+] can be induced by administering 10 units of insulin with a glucose source, by giving inhaled β_2-agonists such as albuterol, or both. Typically intracellular K^+ shifts will be transient in nature, lasting only a few hours, and therefore may require readministration while efforts to increase K^+ elimination have time to take effect. Both serve to induce intracellular K^+ shifting by increasing Na-K-ATPase pump activity. Similarly, sodium bicarbonate has historically been used in the treatment of hyperkalemia by increasing intracellular Na^+, which downstream facilitates intracellular K^{+s} shifting via the Na-K-ATPase, but there is limited clinical evidence to support its efficacy unless treating hyperkalemia with a concurrent metabolic acidosis.[145,152,153]

Table 16-22 The Emergent Management of Hyperkalemia

Monitoring
• Continuous telemetry monitoring • Serial ECG as needed • Serial serum [K^+] level
Cardiac Membrane Stabilization
• IV Calcium chloride (10 mL) 10% solution over 10 min; OR • IV Calcium gluconate (30 mL) 10% solution over 10 min
Induce Intracellular [K^+] Shifting
• 10 units regular insulin with 25–50 g glucose • β_2-Agonists (Albuterol) • Sodium bicarbonate (50–100 mEq over 5–10 min)[a]
Total Body [K^+] Elimination
• Loop diuretic • Potassium-binding agents (Patiromer, SZC) • Emergent hemodialysis

ECG, electrocardiogram; IV, intravenous; SZC, sodium zirconium cyclosilicate.
[a]Sodium bicarbonate should only be considered in patients with hyperkalemia and a concurrent metabolic acidosis.

Lastly, steps must be taken to promote total body K^+ elimination. Both thiazide and loop diuretics promote renal K^+ excretion and even in the setting of oliguric AKI, can be given in efforts increase K^+ elimination. In the past, cation exchange resins, typically sodium polystyrene sulfonate, under the trade name *Kayexalate*, was given to promote gastrointestinal K^+ losses; however there are no clinical trials that demonstrate its efficacy in promoting gastrointestinal K^+ elimination and serious complications such as colonic necrosis have been reported with its use, thus it is no longer recommended in emergent management of hyperkale-
8 mia.[139,152] Fortunately there are two new oral potassium-binding agents, patiromer sorbitex calcium (*Patiromer*), and sodium zirconium cyclosilicate under the trade name *Lokelma*, have been approved in the United States and European Union in the past several years.[139,152] In recent phase II and III clinical trials, a subgroup analysis of patients with [K^+] >6.0 mEq/mL, the median time to a serum [K^+] <5.5 mEq/L was just 4 hours.[139,152,157] Lastly, emergency hemodialysis should be considered for the unstable patient, or those with anuric kidney injury or chronic renal failure where renal K^+ elimination is not reliable.

Calcium

Physiologic Role

A thorough understanding of the physiologic role of Calcium is essential to the anesthesiologist. Calcium (Ca^{2+}) is a divalent cation that is predominantly (99%) stored in bone the form of hydroxyapatite crystals with the remainder being found in the ECF.[158,159] Within the serum, calcium is near evenly divided (45% to 55%) between being protein bound, largely to albumin, or in the active ionized form of Ca^{2+}.[158–160] A small portion of free calcium exists in serum as salts such as calcium phosphate or calcium citrate. Standard calcium serum concentrations range from 8.5 to 10.5 mg/dL, but as the free ionized Ca^{2+} form is biologically active, it best to clinically follow ionized [Ca^{2+}] that ranges from 1.0 to 1.25 mmol/L.[160–162] Historically formulas have been used to "correct" total calcium concentrations with regard to serum albumin level, but these have proven to be unreliable clinically, especially in the critically ill.[158] Importantly, intracellular [Ca^{2+}] levels are at least 1,000-fold lower than ECF allowing for a significant gradient that is critical for driving key physiologic processes such as certain action potentials as well as many cellular signaling pathways discussed below.[163]

Ca^{2+} homeostasis (Fig. 16-10) is maintained by three major calciotropic hormones: (1) parathyroid hormone (PTH) increases serum [Ca^{2+}] by promoting increased skeletal bone resorption and calcium release as well as renal reabsorption; (2) vitamin D (1,25-dihydroxycholecalciferol) increases [Ca^{2+}] by increasing intestinal absorption; and lastly; (3) calcitonin which ultimately lowers [Ca^{2+}] by promoting Ca^{2+} losses via renal excretion and the

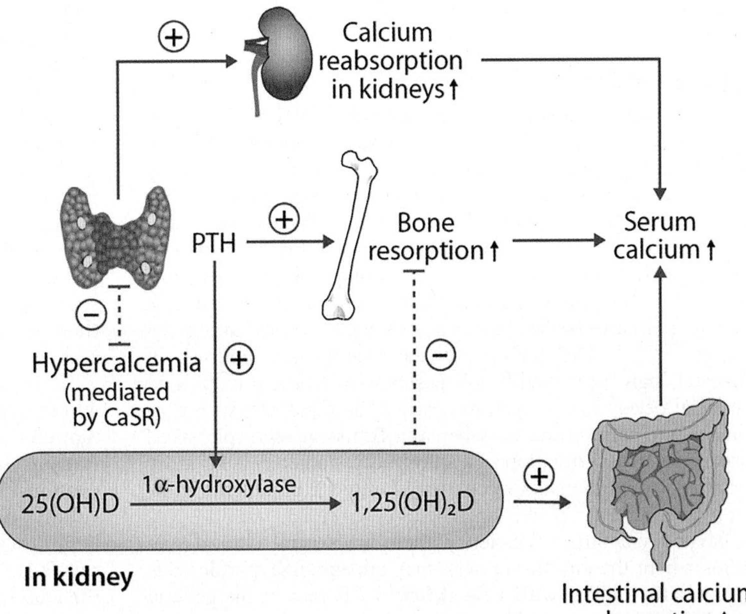

Figure 16-10 Maintaining calcium homeostasis. (Reprinted from Matikainen N, Pekkarinen T, Ryhanen EM, et al. Physiology of calcium homeostasis: an overview. *Endocrinol Metab Clin North Am.* 2021;50(4): 575–590. Copyright © 2021 Elsevier. With permission.)

inhibition of osteoclastic bone resorption.[158,163] Even in periods of prolonged starvation without adequate dietary calcium intake, PTH and vitamin D can maintain appropriate calcium concentrations by promoting osteoclast activity that serves to transfer calcium deposits from bone to serum. The main sources of dietary calcium come from dairy products, green vegetables, and nuts and seeds.[164]

The physiologic importance of calcium cannot be overemphasized. Intracellularly, Ca^{2+} serves as the principal signaling cation necessary for muscle contraction, synapse transmission, cellular proliferation, and ATP metabolism, cyclic adenosine monophosphate (cAMP) secondary messaging, and technically serves as a hormone and ligand for calcium-sensing receptors.[164,165]

It is important to highlight several of the physiologic roles that calcium plays which are integral to practice of anesthesiology. The importance of calcium in the cardiovascular system is well understood. Calcium is essential to cardiac myocyte contractility, driven by calcium-induced calcium release (CICR) at the sarcoplasmic reticulum.[160,165] Likewise cardiac contractility and pace-making in myocardial cells is driven by Ca^{2+} L- and T-type channels, respectively. Class IV antiarrhythmics such as diltiazem or verapamil target myocardial Ca^{2+} channels, blocking Ca^{2+} action potentials at SA and AV nodes, thus slowing the heart rate.[165] As a result, hypocalcemia is associated with prolonged QTc intervals and cardiac arrhythmias.[160] Equally as important, smooth muscle and vascular tone are highly dependent on calcium concentrations, also driven by CICR.[160,163] In other words, $[Ca^{2+}]$ depletion can result in decreased cardiac contractility and vascular tone.

From a hematologic standpoint, calcium plays several key roles. Influx of intracellular platelet Ca^{2+} triggered by thromboxane-A2 released by nearby activated platelets, leads to the conformational changes and further activation of local platelets allowing for both platelet adhesion to damaged endothelium, and further amplification of surrounding platelet activation.[160,163,166] Ca^{2+} serves as a cofactor necessary for activation of coagulation factor XII in the intrinsic pathway, factor VII, IX, and X in the extrinsic pathway, and ultimately factor II (thrombin) which serves to activate fibrinogen to fibrin sheaths that are fundamental in platelet plug formation and clot propagation.[160,163] In addition, within the coagulation cascade, Ca^{2+} is required for protein C and S activation.

Hypocalcemia

Hypocalcemia is defined as a serum ionized $[Ca^{2+}]$ <1.0 mmol/L and is seen in nearly 20% of hospitalized patients, and as high as 85% of those that are critically ill.[167] Vitamin D deficiency is the most common etiology, especially at more northern latitudes. It is not uncommon for patients to be asymptomatic, especially in mild or chronic presentations. While patients can present with symptoms involving a number of organ systems (Table 16-23), neuromuscular irritability such as skeletal muscle twitching or paresthesias, but it classically presents as carpopedal spasms.[158,167,168] The classic physical examination findings of Chvostek sign (provoked facial spasms with repeated tapping of the facial nerve) can be seen in nearly 25% of patients with normal calcium concentrations, whereas a Trousseau sign (provoked carpal spasm after inflation of a sphygmomanometer) is far more specific tor hypocalcemia, occurring in only 1% of patients without hypocalcemia.[158,167,168]

Beyond vitamin D deficiency, there are several clinical scenarios where the anesthesiologist may encounter hypocalcemia. Hypoparathyroidism with PTH deficiency is rare in the general population but is seen in 3% to 8% of post thyroidectomy patients as a result of surgical removal or injury to the parathyroid glands, and can be transient or permanent in nature. Acute postoperative patients with symptomatic hypocalcemia can present with dysphonia, aphonia, or more concerningly, as stridor and or airway obstruction.

Table 16-23 Clinical Manifestations of Hypocalcemia

Organ System	Symptom
Neurologic	• Paresthesias • Tetany • Chvostek and Trousseau signs • Seizures • Coma
Cardiovascular	• Prolonged QTc interval • 2:1 AV blockade • Cardiomyopathy or heart failure • hypotension
Respiratory	• Laryngeal stridor • Bronchospasm
Musculoskeletal	• Fatigue • Myalgias • Muscle twitching or spasms • cramps
Renal	• Hypercalciuria • Nephrocalcinosis • Reduced GFR
Dermatologic	• Alopecia
Psychiatric	• Extrapyramidal disorders • Anxiety or depression • Dementia • Bipolar disorder • Psychosis

AV, atrioventricular nodal; GFR, glomerular filtration rate.
Modified from Aguilera IM, Vaughan RS. Calcium and the anaesthetist. *Anaesthesia*. 2000;55(8):779–790, Pepe J, Colangelo L, Biamonte F, et al. Diagnosis and management of hypocalcemia. *Endocrine*. 2020;69(3):485–495.

Hypomagnesemia or hyperphosphatemia especially in the setting of CKD are associated with hypocalcemia and discussed in depth elsewhere in this chapter. Sepsis, pancreatitis, rhabdomyolysis and tumor lysis syndrome, major burns and or polytraumatic injuries are also common etiologies of hypocalcemia in critically ill patients. Several common medications can also induce hypocalcemia, notably loop diuretics; antiepileptic drugs such as phenytoin carbamazepine, and phenobarbital; chemotherapy agents; gadolinium contrast cinacalcet; and the drug additive EDTA.[168]

It is important to highlight two other common scenarios where hypocalcemia is prominent in the operative setting: cardiopulmonary bypass (CPB) and patients requiring massive transfusion as seen in liver transplantation or major trauma resuscitations. Components of the bypass machine such as the large volume, acidity, and protein content of priming fluid, as well as large doses of heparin necessary for CPB are associated with hypocalcemia.[163] Massive transfusion historically has been defined by the administration of ≥10 units of pack red blood cells (pRBCs), or the transfusion of more than the patient's blood volume in a

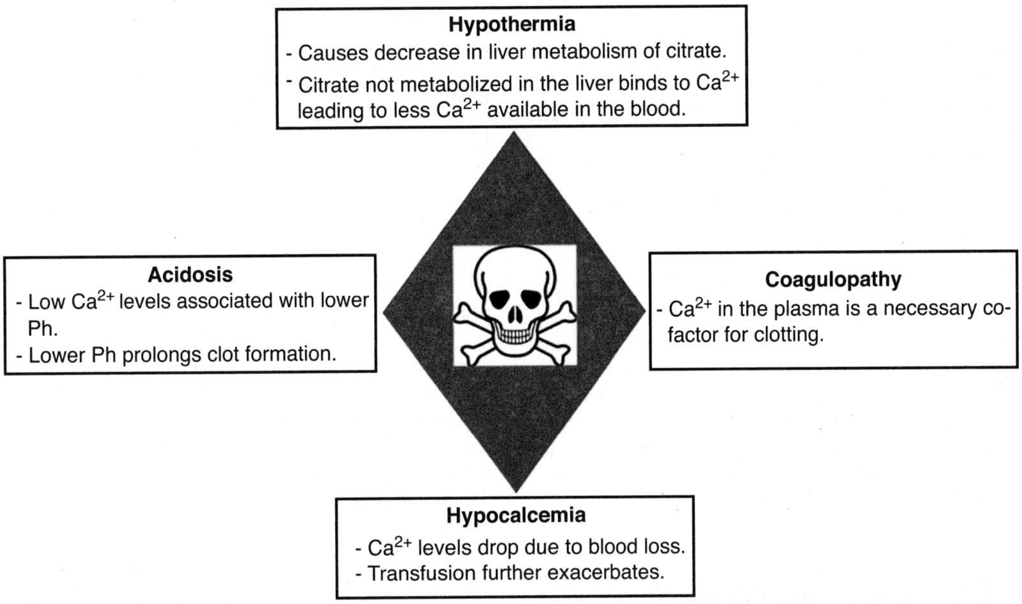

Hypothermia
- Causes decrease in liver metabolism of citrate.
- Citrate not metabolized in the liver binds to Ca^{2+} leading to less Ca^{2+} available in the blood.

Acidosis
- Low Ca^{2+} levels associated with lower Ph.
- Lower Ph prolongs clot formation.

Coagulopathy
- Ca^{2+} in the plasma is a necessary co-factor for clotting.

Hypocalcemia
- Ca^{2+} levels drop due to blood loss.
- Transfusion further exacerbates.

Figure 16-11 The Diamond of death. The clinical significance of hypocalcemia's contribution to caring for patients with acute trauma requiring massive transfusions. The "Lethal Triad" is now expanded to the, "Diamond of Death."From Wray JP, Bridwell RE, Schauer SG, et al. The diamond of death: Hypocalcemia in trauma and resuscitation. *Am J Emerg Med.* 2021;41:104–109, Napolitano L. Hemostatic defects in massive transfusion: an update and treatment recommendation. *Expert Rev Hematol.* 2021;14(2):219–239.

24-hour period.[166] While approximately 55% of patients with traumatic injuries are found to have hypocalcemia on arrival, the main driving force for the development of hypocalcemia is blood product administration, with hypocalcemia occurring in 70% to 97% of patients requiring massive transfusion.[161] The mechanism is driven by calcium sequestration in the setting of large citrate loads. A unit of pRBC is stored in 3 g of citrate, similarly fresh whole blood being stored in 1.66-g citrate; with the citrate serving as an anticoagulant to prevent coagulation during storage. In normal physiologic circumstances the liver can metabolize 3 g of citrate every 5 minutes, but unfortunately in times of systemic stressors such as major trauma, especially with concurrent acidosis or hypothermia, hepatic citrate metabolism is greatly reduced. In the setting of ongoing massive transfusion the citrate load from blood product administration can exceed hepatic metabolism, allowing for increased circulating citrate concentrations to freely bind with ionized Ca^{2+} resulting in progressive hypocalcemia. Given the implications of progressively worsening hypocalcemia, the classical "lethal triad of trauma"—hypothermia, acidosis,
10 and coagulopathy—is now better described as the, "Diamond of Death" (Fig. 16-11) and includes hypocalcemia into the aforementioned, "Lethal Triad".[160,166]

In asymptomatic patients with ionized [Ca^{2+}] <1.0 mmol/L or those with symptoms, calcium should be repleted intravenously. Calcium gluconate 10% is most commonly used for repletion for the hospitalized patient and contains 90 mg of elemental calcium. Compared with calcium chloride 10% which contains 272 mg of elemental calcium and is more commonly used intraoperatively and for emergency repletion.[158,162,163] Calcium chloride is associated with vein sclerosis and thus should be administered through a central venous catheter I possible.

Bolus doses of intravenous calcium will only result in transient rises in serum ionized [Ca^{2+}] and therefore should be followed by continuous infusions of elemental calcium at 0.5 to 1.5 mg/kg per hour[158,168] (Table 16-24). In patients with concurrent hypomagnesemia, magnesium should a repleted as a necessary cofactor in PTH production, and blunts the PTH responsiveness that ultimately leads to secondary hypocalcemia. Vitamin D supplementation can further be added to patients with persistent hypocalcemia despite ongoing efforts of repletion.[158,163,168] During calcium repletion, patients should be closely monitored for the development of hypercalciuria which ultimately puts them at risk for developing nephrocalcinosis and nephrolithiasis. Patients are at greater risk if calcium-phosphate levels are greater than 55 mg/dL, and thiazide diuretics should then be considered to reduce renal calcium reabsorption.[158,168] In patients with hyperphosphatemia in addition to their hypocalcemia, as frequently seen in CKD, it is imperative to correct hyperphosphatemia prior to calcium repletion, otherwise one risks inducing calcium-phosphate precipitation, calcification, and or calciphylaxis.

Table 16-24 The Management of Hypocalcemia

Calcium Repletion: • IV: 10 mL of 10% calcium gluconate over 5–10 min, followed by an infusion at 0.5–1.5 mg/kg/hr • PO: 500–1,000-mg calcium carbonate every 6–8 hrs
Magnesium Repletion[a]: • IV: Magnesium sulfate 1–2 g/hr over 3–6 hrs, followed by an infusion at 0.5–1 g/hr
Vitamin D Repletion: • PO: Calcitriol 0.25–2.0 mcg/day
Monitor for: • Electrocardiogram (ECG) changes • Hypercalcemia • Hypercalciuria

[a]If concurrent hypomagnesemia is present, magnesium should also be repleted.

Hypercalcemia

Hypercalcemia is commonly defined as a total serum Ca^{2+} concentration >10.5 mg/dL, but free ionized Ca^{2+} is clinically more accurate and defined as an ionized [Ca^{2+}] >1.5 mmol/L with moderate cases being >2.0 mmol/L, and severe cases > 2.5 mmol/L[162] (NICV 16-5). Patients can present with a variety of symptoms affecting numerous organ systems (Table 16-25). The predominate etiologies of hypercalcemia are the result of primary hyperparathyroidism or malignancy, which together make up nearly 80% of total cases.[162,169] With regard to primary hyperparathyroidism, 80% to 85% of cases are the result of benign hyperplasia (adenoma) of a singular parathyroid gland, with the remainder being adenomas of multiple glands and less than 1% of cases are the result of malignant parathyroid cancer.[162,169,170] Hyperparathyroidism results in the overzealous production of PTH leading to increased bone resorption and renal Ca^{2+} reabsorption, ultimately resulting in hypercalcemia. Malignancy can be associated with the paraneoplastic production of PTH-related protein (PTHrp) which results in a similar physiologic responses to PTH. In addition, malignancy with bone metastasis and/or destruction can lead to hypercalcemia.

Secondary and tertiary hyperparathyroidism are discussed below. Secondary hyperparathyroidism is the result of generalized parathyroid hyperplasia as a response to chronic hypocalcemia, hyperphosphatemia, or both. Over time, secondary hyperparathyroidism can progress to tertiary hyperparathyroidism and is commonly seen in CKD and end-stage renal disease (ESRD). Tertiary hyperparathyroidism, similar to primary hyperparathyroidism, eventually results in hypercalcemia, but the mechanism is the result of the development of autonomous parathyroid function that is PTH-signaling independent.[159,169,170]

There are multiple non-PTH or malignancy-associated etiologies of hypercalcemia as well (Table 16-26). Drug-induced hypercalcemia can be seen with excessive administration of calcium carbonate (Milk-alkali syndrome), vitamin D supplementation, thiazide diuretics, and lithium toxicity.[169] In addition, granulomatous diseases such as sarcoidosis, tuberculosis, and Hanson disease are linked to hypercalcemia as a result of excessive granuloma macrophage production of 1-α-hydroxylase, which converts 25-hydroxy vitamin D to 1,25-dihydroxy vitamin D (calcitriol), the active form of vitamin D, that increases intestinal calcium absorption.[159,169]

The management of hypercalcemia depends largely on the severity of symptoms as well as treating the underlying cause. In general, the first step is to focus on volume expansion. Hypercalcemia, especially with polyuria, will result in decreased renal reabsorption of water leading to hypovolemia, which is frequently

Table 16-25 The Clinical Manifestations of Hypercalcemia

Cardiovascular: • Hypertension • Shortened QTc interval • Arrhythmias or heart block • Digitalis sensitivity
Neurologic: • Confusion • Somnolence • Lethargy • Depression or anxiety • Psychosis or hallucinations • Hypotonicity • Seizures • Coma
Renal: • Polyuria and polydipsia • Nephrocalcinosis or nephrolithiasis • Nephrogenic diabetes insipidus • Renal failure
Gastrointestinal: • Nausea and vomiting • Constipation • Abdominal pain • Peptic ulcer disease • Anorexia • Pancreatitis
Musculoskeletal: • Myalgias • Fatigue or weakness • Osteoporosis • Bone pain • Pathologic fractures

Modified from Maier JD, Levine SN. Hypercalcemia in the intensive Ccare unit: a review of pathophysiology, diagnosis, and modern therapy. *J Intensive Care Med.* 2015;30(5):235–252; Chang WT, Radin B, McCurdy MT. Calcium, magnesium, and phosphate abnormalities in the emergency department. *Emerg Med Clin North Am.* 2014;32(2):349–366.

Table 16-26 Etiologies of Hypercalcemia

Hyperparathyroidism • Primary hyperparathyroidism • Tertiary hyperparathyroidism
Malignancy • Parathyroid hormone-related protein (PTHrp) production • Bone metastasis or osteolysis
Medication Induced • Calcium carbonate; antacids (Milk-alkali syndrome) • Vitamin D and A supplementation • Thiazide diuretics • Lithium toxicity
Granulomatous Diseases • Sarcoidosis • Tuberculosis • Hanson disease • Coccidioidomycosis
Renal Failure • CKD or ESRD • Rhabdomyolysis with acute renal failure
Endocrinopathies • Thyrotoxicosis • Pheochromocytoma • Adrenal insufficiency
Other • Chronic immobilization • Pancreatitis

Modified with permission from Maier JD, Levine SN. Hypercalcemia in the intensive care unit: a review of pathophysiology, diagnosis, and modern therapy. *J Intensive Care Med.* 2015;30(5):235–252.

further compounded by poor oral intake secondary to hypercalcemia induced anorexia and/or nausea and vomiting.[159,168–170] Saline 0.9% repletion is recommended given the sodium-linked calcium diuresis that occurs in the proximal tubule because of the higher [Na^+] of 0.9% saline compared to balanced crystalloids solutions.[168–170] One to 2 L 0.9% saline should be bolused with the intent of volume expansion, followed by infusion of 75 to 300 mL/hr to promote calciuresis, ideally targeting 100 to 150 mL/hr urinary output.[159,168,169] Historically when euvolemia was reached, loop diuretics were added to further aid in calcium excretion, but loop diuretics are no longer recommended given the concern for further iatrogenic electrolyte derangements, nor is it supported by evidence-based medicine, and therefore should be used with caution unless there are concurrent concerns for volume overload.

While volume expansion alone may correct mild cases of hypocalcemia, bisphosphonates (pamidronate or zoledronic acid) should be added for patients with moderate-to-severe hypercalcemia. Bisphosphonates are pyrophosphates that function by binding to hydroxyapatite in bone and inhibit osteoclastic bone resorption.[159,162] As a result, bisphosphonates have become the cornerstone in the management of malignancy-induced osteolysis and hypercalcemia. When treating primary hyperparathyroidism, the calcimimetic, cinacalcet, should be initiated and can normalize calcium levels in nearly 70% of cases, and is now generally accepted as an acceptable alternative when parathyroidectomy is not feasible or is contraindicated.[159,168,170] Calcitonin can be further added to the regimen in managing hypercalcemia, especially if rapid correction is needed. As stated above, calcitonin functions to both increase Ca^{2+} renal excretion, and inhibits osteoclastic bone resorption. Of note, calcitonin administration is associated with tachyphylaxis after 48 hours of use, so its clinical utility is time limited.[159,168,169]

Glucocorticoids have been used in cases of severe hypercalcemia to lower serum [Ca^{2+}] by decreasing intestinal absorption of the active form of vitamin D, calcitriol, and should be considered when treating hypercalcemia secondary to granulomatous diseases, vitamin D toxicity, and malignancies such as multiple myeloma or lymphoma.[159,168,169] Denosumab, a monoclonal antibody targeting RANK-Ligand (RANK-L) activity was initially studied as a therapeutic agent for osteoporosis, but is now accepted as an additional agent in the treatment of malignancy-induced hypercalcemia that is refractory to bisphosphonate therapy.[159,168,169] Inhibiting RANK-L prevents osteoclast maturation and function. Lastly, in true life-threatening or refractory hypercalcemia, hemodialysis should be considered until the underlying etiology can be appropriately treated.

Magnesium

Physiologic Role

Magnesium (Mg^{2+}), a divalent cation, is the fourth most common element in the human body, and the second most abundant intracellular cation.[171] Magnesium is largely stored in mineralized bone (50% to 65%) with the remainder found in skeletal muscle (~30%) and soft tissue and organs (20%).[172,173] Serum [Mg^{2+}] is less than 1% of total body magnesium, with the majority being in the free ionized state (70%), with the remaining 30% being protein bound, predominately to albumin.[172,174] Normal serum [Mg^{2+}] ranges from 1.7 to 2.1 mg/dL (0.75 to 1.10 mmol/L).[173]

While widely available in many types of foods, and especially abundant in leafy green vegetables, it is estimated that 60% of Americans do not consume the recommended daily intake of Mg^{2+} of 420 and 320 mg for men and women, respectively,[171] with diets consisting of predominately processed foods as a culprit. Approximately 80% to 90% of Mg^{2+} is lost during food processing.[171,174] Magnesium is absorbed in the gastrointestinal tract via a complex and poorly understood process relying on PTH, calcitonin, insulin, and vasoactive intestinal peptides.[174] The majority of serum [Mg^{2+}] (70%) is filtered through renal glomerulus with approximately 30% being reabsorbed, mostly in the thick ascending limb of the loop of Henle, with the remainder being renally excreted.[173] The loop of Henle is therefore where the majority of malabsorption can occur, as seen with chronic loop diuretic use.[174]

Physiologically, Mg^{2+} serves as an essential cofactor (Fig. 16-12) in over 600 enzymatic reactions for cellular metabolism as is required in all reactions that utilize ATP, and DNA and RNA polymerases; hormone receptor binding; skeletal muscle contraction and smooth muscle tone; cardiac excitability; neurotransmitter release and neuronal conduction activity.[172–174] Importantly, Mg^{2+} serves as a Ca^{2+} *antagonist,* given the ability to compete with Ca^{2+} in ion-gated channels or with binding sites of Ca^{2+} transporters.[173] This competitive antagonism has multiple clinically relevant implications. Within neurons, Mg^{2+} downregulates the NMDA receptor excitability by occupying Ca^{2+} channels within the NMDA receptor, thus preventing glutamatergic excitatory signaling.[173] In the cardiovascular systems, Mg^{2+} plays a crucial role in an inhibitory role in the L-type Ca^{2+} channels in phase II of the cardiac action potential.[173] In addition, Mg^{2+} in increased concentrations results in vascular smooth muscle relaxation and vasodilation, acting as an endogenous calcium channel blocker and increasing nitric oxide (NO) release.[173,174] Skeletal muscle is also highly impacted by Mg^{2+} concentrations given muscle contraction dependence on CICR from sarcoplasmic reticulum.[171]

Magnesium, predominantly magnesium sulfate ($MgSO_4$), has several clinical uses that can be applied in the perioperative setting (Table 16-27). Serum Mg^{2+} may decrease anesthetic requirements by competitive antagonism of presynaptic Ca^{2+} channels within the hippocampus, reducing CNS neurotransmitter release.[175] In addition, magnesium has analgesic properties when administered intravenously, likely as a result of NMDA receptor antagonism secondary to its ability to compete and therefore inhibit Ca^{2+} influx necessary for activation.[175] Magnesium sulfate has also long been used in obstetric care for the management of preeclampsia and eclampsia. It is also used as a tocolytic agent in preterm labor, by inducing systemic smooth muscle relaxation, systemic vasodilation, and uterine tone relaxation.[172,175] The use of $MgSO_4$ injected perineurally as an adjunct in regional anesthetic techniques has also been demonstrated to promote superior analgesia as well as prolonged duration of both sensory and motor blockade.[172,176,177]

Building on its clinical use, $MgSO_4$ has long been used in the management of cardiac dysrhythmias, notably as a first-line agent for *torsades de pointes*. Further, $MgSO_4$ has been used in the management of supraventricular, ventricular, and digoxin toxicity-induced arrhythmias. In addition, $MgSO_4$ is useful to treat post-CPB atrial fibrillation because of its ability to function as a calcium channel antagonist, thus slowing L-type Ca^{2+} channel polarization and resulting in slower and more stabilized cardiac conduction.[171,172,175]

Intravenous $MgSO_4$ administration is also an effective strategy for maintaining hemodynamic stability during pheochromocytoma resection as well as pheochromocytoma crisis due to vascular smooth muscle relaxation with resultant arteriolar vasodilation as well as direct inhibition of catecholamine release from the adrenal medulla.[175,181] Beyond unstable arrhythmias and pheochromocytoma crises, $MgSO_4$ has also been used clinically in obstructive lung disease crises such as severe asthma or COPD exacerbations by inhibiting the release of bronchoconstrictors (histamine and acetylcholine,) resulting in bronchodilation, as well as having anti-inflammatory properties.[171,173,175]

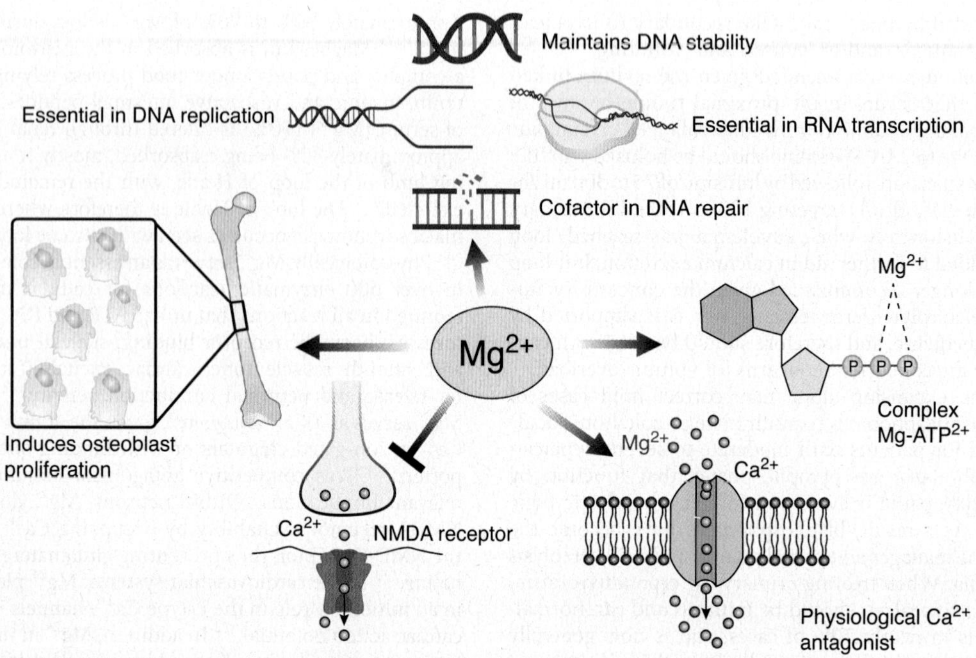

Figure 16-12 Magnesium as an enzymatic co-factor. A representation of the critical roles that Mg^{2+} serves throughout the body. (From Fiorentini D, Cappadone C, Farruggia G, et al. Magnesium: biochemistry, nutrition, detection, and social impact of diseases linked to Its deficiency. *Nutrients*. 2021;13(4). Copyright © 2021 by the authors. https://creativecommons.org/licenses/by/4.0/.)

Table 16-27 Common Indication and Dosages for the Perioperative Use of Magnesium Sulfate

Multimodal Analgesia, adjuvant	30–50 mg/kg loading dose + 6–20 mg/kg/hr[175,178]
Regional Anesthetic, perineural adjuvant	150–600 mg $MgSO_4$ + primary local anesthetic.[177]
Obstetrics: • Preeclampsia; eclampsia • Tocolytic agent	• 4–6 g IV loading dose + 1–2g IV continuous infusion; or 4–5 g IM, repeated every 4 hrs • 6 g IV loading dose +2 g/hr[179]
Cardiovascular: • Torsades de pointes	• Pulseless: 1–2 g IV over 5–20 min • With a pulse: 1–2 g IV over 5–60 min
Pheochromocytoma: • Intraoperative management	• 40–60 mg/kg loading dose prior to intubation + 1–2 g/hr[175,180]
Pulmonary: • Asthma/COPD exacerbation	• 2 g IV load over 30–60 min
Hypomagnesemia, severe (<1.2 mg/dL)	• 1–2 g/hr IV over 3–6 hrs + 0.5–1 g/hr as needed thereafter

One gram $MgSO_4$ equates to approximately 4-mmol, 8-mEq, or 98-mg elemental magnesium.

Modified from Herroeder S, Schönherr ME, De Hert SG, et al. Magnesium–essentials for anesthesiologists. *Anesthesiology*. 2011;114(4):971–993.

Hypomagnesemia

Defined as serum [Mg^{2+}] levels of <1.8 mg/dL, hypomagnesemia is seen in approximately 10% of hospitalized patients; however, it is far more common in the critically will, with an incidence as high as 65%.[175] For mild-to-moderate deficiencies (Table 16-28) patients are often asymptomatic but when present symptoms are nonspecific in nature such as fatigue, muscle weakness or spasms, depression, or nausea and vomiting. With profound hypomagnesemia (serum [Mg^{2+}] <1.2 mg/dL) symptoms can be more severe, such as cardiac conduction abnormalities or dysrhythmias, tetany, seizures, or coma.[171]

While dietary intake has decreased drastically over the past several decades, Mg^{2+} remains abundant enough that hypomagnesemia is rarely the result of inadequate intake.[171,173] Rather, hypomagnesemia is more likely to reflect poor gastrointestinal absorption or an excess in renal excretion. Notably patients taking a proton pump inhibitor (PPI) chronically can develop hypomagnesemia as a result of decreased Mg^{2+} absorption from PPI-induced inhibition of the transient receptor potential melastatin-6 and 7 (TRPM6/7) channels that are critical for Mg^{2+} absorption.[182] In the hospitalized patient, excessive gastrointestinal losses should be considered as nausea and vomiting, diarrhea or steatorrhea, pancreatitis, high-output gastrointestinal fistula or drains, or simple nasogastric suctioning, can all lead to hypomagnesemia. Renal losses typically reflect ongoing diuretic use.[182] Lastly, it is important to highlight that hypomagnesemia is particularly common in patients with chronic alcohol dependence and is multifactorial in nature: excessive renal Mg^{2+} excretion, chronic vomiting and or diarrhea, and a reduced serum PTH levels.[171,182]

In the patient where the etiology of hypomagnesemia remains unclear, measuring a 24-hour urine collection can be considered. Urine Mg^{2+} of ≥10 to 30 mg/day in a patient with normal renal function is indicative of excessive renal wasting. Urine Mg^{2+} <10 mg/day is suggestive of either inadequate gastrointestinal absorption or excessive losses.[182]

Table 16-28 Serum Magnesium Levels and Associated Symptoms

Magnesium Level			Presentation
mg/dL	*mEq/L*	*Mmol/L*	
<1.2	<1.0	<0.5	• Tetany • Seizures • Arrhythmias
1.2–1.8	1–1.5	0.5–0.75	• Neuromuscular irritability • Electrolyte derangements: Hypocalcemia; hypokalemia
1.8–2.5	***1.5–2.1***	***0.75–1.05***	***Normal***
2.5–5	2.1–4.2	1.05–2.1	Asymptomatic
5–7	4.2–5.8	2.1–2.9	• Flushing • Nausea and vomiting • Lethargy or drowsiness • Decreased DTR
7–12	5.8–10	2.9–5.0	• Somnolence • Loss of DTR • Hypotension • ECG abnormalities
>12	>10	>5.0	• Complete heart block or cardiac arrest • Comatose • Paralysis; apnea

DTR, deep tendon reflex; ECG, electrocardiogram.
Note: this is a copy with modifications from previous version of this chapter.
Reprinted with permission from Springer: Topf JM, Murray PT. Hypomagnesemia and hypermagnesemia. *Rev Endocr Metab Disord.* 2003;4: 195–206.

Fortunately Mg^{2+} deficits can be corrected easily with oral supplementation, and for mild cases, dietary corrections alone will suffice. Oral repletion can be accomplished with 60 to 90 mEq/day magnesium oxide. For symptomatic or severe cases, repletion should occur intravenously with 1 to 2 g/hr over 3 to 6 hours, with further repletion guided by serum [Mg^{2+}] (Table 16-27). Sufficient repletion typically takes 3 to 4 days.[171] With the exception of pulseless *torsades de pointes*, more rapid repletion should not be considered given the theoretic risk of inducing cardiac conduction abnormalities. In addition to heart rate and rhythm and BP monitoring, patients should also have deep tendon reflexes (DTR) assessed frequently during ongoing repletion, as loss of DTR may reflect a transition to hypermagnesemia.

Hypermagnesemia

Hypermagnesemia defined as serum [Mg^{2+}] >2.5 mg/dL, is far less common. It occurs mainly in patients with renal failure who are unable excrete Mg^{2+} appropriately. It also occurs iatrogenically as a result of excessive magnesium administration as in treatment of preeclampsia or eclampsia, or due to magnesium containing laxatives and enemas such as magnesium citrate.[171,175] Table 16-28 displays the clinical manifestations of dysregulated [Mg^{2+}]. Mild cases are often asymptomatic, or may present with flushing, nausea and vomiting, or lethargy. As Mg^{2+} acts as an endogenous Ca^{2+} antagonist, increasing serum [Mg^{2+}] will mimic hypocalcemia. Fatigue, lethargy or somnolence, and reduced DTRs progresses to cardiac conduction abnormalities or complete heart block, coma, apnea, or even cardiac arrest.[171,173,175] In severe cases of hypermagnesemia where neuromuscular or cardiac toxicity is observed, the immediate administration of intravenous Ca^{2+} (5 to 10 mEq) should be used to antagonize Mg^{2+} as a temporizing measure, in addition to ongoing supportive care.[162] All magnesium supplementations must be stopped, and care should be focused on promoting maximal renal excretion, either by volume expansion, administering loop diuretics, or both. In emergency situations, hemodialysis should also be considered for rapid Mg^{2+} removal.[162,171,175]

Phosphorus

Physiologic Role

Elemental phosphorus is vital for all cellular life, in the form of inorganic phosphate (Pi), notably as the anions HPO_4^{2-} and $H_2PO_4^-$.[183,184] Beyond the role in cellular metabolism via ATP and nicotinamide adenine dinucleotide phosphate ($NADP^+$), Pi is used in other cellular energy stores such as creatine phosphate, the phosphodiesters that make up nucleic acids in DNA and RNA, and is used in the enzymatic process of glycolysis as well as many intracellular signaling pathways such as cyclic-AMP (cAMP) and phospholipase-C. Pi is also essential in the regulation of hemoglobin's oxygen-carrying capacity as red blood cell production of 2,3-diphosphoglycerate (2,3-DPG) will result in shifts of the oxygen dissociation curve, with increased 2,3-DPG resulting in a rightward shift, and decreased 2,3-DPG in a leftward shift, respectively.[183]

The vast majority (85% to 90%) of phosphate in the human body is in the form calcium phosphate crystals (apatite), with 10% to 15% found in soft tissues and organs, leaving less than 1% present in the ECF. Within serum, phosphate is further divided 85% in the Pi anion (HPO_4^{2-} or PO_4^-) form, with approximately 10% being protein bound, and the remainder 5% in salt complexes.[183,184] Serum concentrations range from 2.5 to 4.5 mg/dL. Dietary intake of phosphorus is found most abundantly in protein with approximately 15 mg of phosphorus per gram of ingested protein, and intake generally exceeds daily estimated average requirements (EARs) by twofold.[184] Pi is absorbed throughout the small intestine. Average daily net neutral Pi balances between deposition and resorption within bone. Pi reabsorption and excretion primarily occurs within the kidneys. Pi is filtered freely at the glomeruli and reabsorbed in the proximal tubule. Reabsorption is further regulated by fibroblast growth factor-23 (FGF-23), PTH, and the active form of vitamin D, calcitriol.[184]

Hypophosphatemia

Defined as serum [Pi] <2.5 mg/dL, is common in postoperative patients, or those with major traumatic injuries, and can be seen in 10% to 20% of critically ill patients.[185] In severe cases with [Pi] <1.0 mg/dL life-threatening organ failure can be seen. Patients can present with symptoms from nearly every organ system (Table 16-29), though in severe cases, encephalopathy, seizures, respiratory failure, or cardiovascular collapse can be seen. There are three major mechanisms that can lead to hypophosphatemia: (1) poor intestinal absorption such as chronic

Table 16-29 Clinical Manifestations of Hypophosphatemia

Cardiovascular • Congestive heart failure • Arrhythmias
Respiratory • Dyspnea • Respiratory failure • Difficulty with ventilator liberation
Gastrointestinal • Re-feeding syndrome
Neurologic • Paresthesias • Delirium • Encephalopathy • Seizures • Coma
Hematologic • Hemolysis • Platelet dysfunction
Musculoskeletal • Weakness • Myopathy or myalgias • Rhabdomyolysis

Modified from Gaasbeek A, Meinders AE. Hypophosphatemia: an update on its etiology and treatment. *Am J Med*. 2005;118(10):1094–1101.

diarrhea or steatorrhea, chronic phosphate-binding antacid use, or vitamin D deficiency; (2) increased urinary excretion as a result of hyperparathyroidism, diuretic use, Fanconi syndrome, or chronic alcoholism; and (3) most commonly seen internal redistribution such as refeeding syndrome, recovery from DKA, or respiratory alkalosis.[185] Certain chemotherapy classes, notably ones with renal toxicity, such as alkylating agents such as cyclophosphamide, tyrosine kinase inhibitors, or high-dose estrogen therapy, have also been associated with induced hypophosphatemia.

Patients with symptomatic or severe hypophosphatemia ([Pi] <1.0 mg/dL) require close monitoring and prompt intravenous phosphorus repletion (Table 16-30) in the form of potassium phosphate or sodium phosphate. Administration should be done slowly and not exceed 1 to 3 mEq/hr given the risk for induced hypocalcemia from calcium phosphate precipitation, or in severe cases calciphylaxis.[162,185,186] Oral repletion is therefore more favorable and typically takes place over the course of 3 to 10 days depending on the severity of hypophosphatemia, and Pi, K^+, and Ca^{2+} levels should be monitored closely to assess for iatrogenic electrolyte imbalances resulting from Pi repletion.[185]

Table 16-30 Hypophosphatemia: Acute Treatment

Parenteral phosphate, 0.2 mM–0.68 mM/kg (5–16 mg/kg) over 12 hrs
Potassium phosphate (93 mg/mL of phosphate)
Sodium phosphate (93 mg/mL of phosphate)

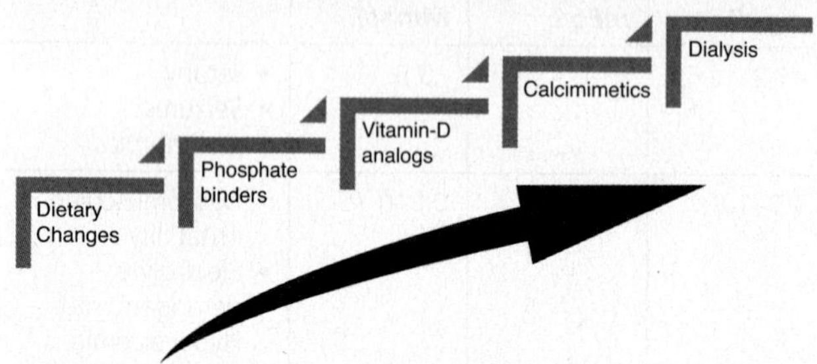

Figure 16-13 The Conventional Approach to managing Hyperphosphatemia. Dietary changes are the first line management in hyperphosphatemia. Medications can be added stepwise or simultaneously depending on the patient's underlying pathology or coexisting existing electrolyte abnormalities.

Hyperphosphatemia

The incidence of hyperphosphatemia varies widely from 20% to 45% of patients and is more commonly associated with patients with ongoing critical illness and is associated with an increased all-cause mortality.[187] Severe hyperphosphatemia, defined as a serum [Pi] > 4.5 mg/dL, is most commonly seen in patients with CKD as a result of reduced GFR and the inability to appropriately excrete Pi.

Hyperphosphatemia may also result from two other major mechanisms: (1) increased intestinal absorption via dietary or supplemental intake; or (2) pathologic redistribution from intracellular stores such as cell lysis as seen in tumor lysis syndrome, hemolysis, trauma, sepsis, or rhabdomyolysis.[162,187]

The estimated average requirement of dietary Pi intake is approximately 600 mg, and the average American diet provides 800 to 1,500 mg, of which nearly 80% to 90% is eventually reabsorbed in proximal tubules.[184] As GFR declines in CKD, Pi excretion declines as well, thus without a necessary change in dietary Pi intake, patients will ultimately progress toward developing hyperphosphatemia.[184,186,188,189] Hyperphosphatemia with concurrent hypocalcemia should trigger the clinician to evaluate for hypoparathyroidism, especially in the postoperative setting following total thyroidectomy as briefly discussed earlier in this chapter.

The treatment of hyperphosphatemia is highly dependent on the patient's underlying renal function (Fig. 16-13). With a normal GFR, dietary restrictions of Pi should suffice in correcting hyperphosphatemia.[162,188] However, given the prevalence of hyperphosphatemia in CKD, treatment strategies should have three main objectives: (1) identifying and treating the underlying cause, (2) decreasing intake and absorption, and (3) increasing Pi excretion. Beyond dietary restrictions, decreasing intake and absorption can be aided with the addition of phosphate-binders taken with meals, such as calcium carbonate, sevelamer, or more historically, aluminum hydroxide.[162,186,188,189] Increased Pi excretion can be promoted by volume expansion of the ECF, the administration of loop or thiazide diuretics, or carbonic anhydrase inhibitors.[162] For chronic hyperparathyroidism associated with ESRD, vitamin D and calcimimetics are further added to indirectly decrease Pi by decreasing PTH, and any further bone resorption.[189] Ultimately, in patients with severe symptomatic hyperphosphatemia, or those with anuric renal disease, hemodialysis or peritoneal dialysis should be considered. The colloquial triad has been referred to as the, "3D's of hyperphosphatemia management: diet, drugs, and dialysis."

For additional information please see NICV 16-6 in the eBook bundled with this text.

For further review and interactivities, please see the videos and narrative interactive clinical vignettes (NICVs) accessible in the complimentary eBook bundled with this text. Access instructions are located on the inside front cover.

REFERENCES

1. Adrogué HJ, Madias NE. Management of life-threatening acid–base disorders. *N Engl J Med.* 1998;338(2):107–111.
2. Palange P, Carlone S, Galassetti P, Felli A, Serra P. Incidence of acid-base and electrolyte disturbances in a general hospital: a study of 110 consecutive admissions. *Recenti Prog Med.* 1990;81(12):788–791.
3. Hodgkin JE, Soeprono FF, Chan DM. Incidence of metabolic alkalemia in hospitalized patients. *Crit Care Med.* 1980;8(12):725–728.
4. Schwartz WB, Relman AS. A critique of the parameters used in the evaluation of acid-base disorders. "Whole-blood buffer base" and "standard bicarbonate" compared with blood pH and plasma bicarbonate concentration. *N Engl J Med.* 1963;268:1382–1388.
5. Andersen OS, Engel K, Jorgensen K, Astrup P. A Micro method for determination of pH, carbon dioxide tension, base excess and standard bicarbonate in capillary blood. *Scand J Clin Lab Invest.* 1960;12:172–176.
6. Stewart PA. Independent and dependent variables of acid-base control. *Respir Physiol.* 1978; 33(1):9–26.
7. Rastegar A. Clinical utility of Stewart's method in diagnosis and management of acid-base disorders. *Clin J Am Soc Nephrol.* 2009;4(7):1267–1274.
8. Ho KM, Lan NS, Williams TA, et al. A comparison of prognostic significance of strong ion gap (SIG) with other acid-base markers in the critically ill: a cohort study. *J Intensive Care.* 2016;4:43.
9. Waters JH, Miller LR, Clack S, Kim JV. Cause of metabolic acidosis in prolonged surgery. *Crit Care Med.* 1999;27(10):2142–2146.
10. Prough DS, Bidani A. Hyperchloremic Metabolic Acidosis Is a Predictable Consequence of Intraoperative Infusion of 0.9% Saline. *Anesthesiology.* 1999;90(5):1247–1249.
11. Jaber S, Paugam C, Futier E, et al. Sodium bicarbonate therapy for patients with severe metabolic acidaemia in the intensive care unit (BICAR-ICU): a multicentre, open-label, randomised controlled, phase 3 trial. *Lancet.* 2018;392(10141):31–40.
12. Forsythe SM, Schmidt GA. Sodium bicarbonate for the treatment of lactic acidosis. *Chest.* 2000;117(1):260–267.
13. Holmdahl MHS, Wiklund L, Wetterberg T, et al. The place of THAM in the management of acidemia in clinical practice. *Acta Anaesthesiol Scand.* 2000;44(5):524–527.
14. Dickinson GE, Myers ML, Goldbach M, Sibbald W. Acetazolamide in the treatment of ventilatory failure complicating acute metabolic alkalosis. *Anesth Analg.* 1981;60(8):608–610.
15. Moviat M, Pickkers P, van der Voort PH, van der Hoeven JG. Acetazolamide-mediated decrease in strong ion difference accounts for the correction of metabolic alkalosis in critically ill patients. *Crit Care.* 2006;10(1):R14.
16. Guffey JD, Haas CE, Crowley A, Connor KA, Kaufman DC. Hydrochloric acid infusion for the treatment of metabolic alkalosis in surgical intensive care unit patients. *Ann Pharmacother.* 2018;52(6):522–526.
17. Lewis RA, Howell JB. Definition of the hyperventilation syndrome. *Bull Eur Physiopathol Respir.* 1986;22(2):201–205.
18. Fortune JB, Feustel PJ, deLuna C, Graca L, Hasselbarth J, Kupinski AM. Cerebral blood flow and blood volume in response to O2 and CO2 changes in normal humans. *J Trauma.* 1995;39(3):463–471; discussion 71–72.
19. Zhang Z, Guo Q, Wang E. Hyperventilation in neurological patients: from physiology to outcome evidence. *Curr Opin Anaesthesiol.* 2019;32(5):568–573.
20. Laffey JG, O'Croinin D, McLoughlin P, Kavanagh BP. Permissive hypercapnia–role in protective lung ventilatory strategies. *Intensive Care Med.* 2004;30(3):347–356.
21. Hickling KG, Walsh J, Henderson S, Jackson R. Low mortality rate in adult respiratory distress syndrome using low-volume, pressure-limited ventilation with permissive hypercapnia: a prospective study. *Crit Care Med.* 1994;22(10):1568–1578.
22. Yaster M, Gross JB. CO2 is Good for You! *Anesth Analg.* 2021;132(1):e13.
23. Chand R, Swenson ER, Goldfarb DS. Sodium bicarbonate therapy for acute respiratory acidosis. *Curr Opin Nephrol Hypertens.* 2021;30(2):223–230.
24. Combes A, Hajage D, Capellier G, et al. Extracorporeal membrane oxygenation for severe acute respiratory distress syndrome. *N Engl J Med.* 2018;378(21):1965–1975.
25. Adrogué HJ, Madias NE. Alkali therapy for respiratory acidosis: a medical controversy. *Am J Kidney Dis.* 2020;75(2):265–271.
26. El-Boghdadly K, Chin KJ, Chan VWS. Phrenic nerve palsy and regional anesthesia for shoulder surgery: anatomical, physiologic, and clinical considerations. *Anesthesiology.* 2017;127(1): 173–191.
27. Berend K, de Vries AP, Gans RO. Physiological approach to assessment of acid-base disturbances. *N Engl J Med.* 2014;371(15):1434–1445.
28. Kumar V, Karon BS. Comparison of measured and calculated bicarbonate values. *Clin Chem.* 2008;54(9):1586–1587.
29. Figge J, Jabor A, Kazda A, Fencl V. Anion gap and hypoalbuminemia. *Crit Care Med.* 1998; 26(11):1807–1810.
30. Adrogué HJ, Madias NE. Secondary responses to altered acid-base status: the rules of engagement. *J Am Soc Nephrol.* 2010;21(6):920–923.
31. Svensen CH, Rodhe PM, Prough DS. Pharmacokinetic aspects of fluid therapy. *Best Pract Res Clin Anaesthesiol.* 2009;23(2):213–224.
32. Connolly Cara M, Kramer George C, Hahn Robert G, et al. Isoflurane but not mechanical ventilation promotes extravascular fluid accumulation during crystalloid volume loading. *Anesthesiology.* 2003;98(3):670–681.
33. Norberg Å, Hahn RG, Li H, et al. Population volume kinetics predicts retention of 0.9% saline infused in awake and isoflurane-anesthetized volunteers. *Anesthesiology.* 2007;107(1):24–32.
34. Vane Luiz A, Prough Donald S, Kinsky Michael A, Williams Chad A, Grady James J, Kramer George C. Effects of different catecholamines on the dynamics of volume expansion of crystalloid infusion. *Anesthesiology.* 2004;101(5):1136–1144.
35. Chappell D, Dörfler N, Jacob M, et al. Glycocalyx protection reduces leukocyte adhesion after ischemia/reperfusion. *Shock.* 2010;34(2):133–139.
36. Anders H-J, Davis JM, Thurau K. Nephron protection in diabetic kidney disease. *N Engl J Med.* 2016;375(21):2096–2098.
37. von Lueder TG, Sangaralingham SJ, Wang BH, et al. Renin-angiotensin blockade combined with natriuretic peptide system augmentation: novel therapeutic concepts to combat heart failure. *Circ Heart Fail.* 2013;6(3):594–605.
38. DiBona GF. Physiology in perspective: the wisdom of the body. Neural control of the kidney. *Am J Physiol Regul Integr Comp Physiol.* 2005;289(3):R633–R641.
39. Potter LR, Yoder AR, Flora DR, Antos LK, Dickey DM. Natriuretic peptides: their structures, receptors, physiologic functions and therapeutic applications. *Handb Exp Pharmacol.* 2009(191):341–366.
40. Lumsden NG, Khambata RS, Hobbs AJ. C-type natriuretic peptide (CNP): cardiovascular roles and potential as a therapeutic target. *Curr Pharm Des.* 2010;16(37):4080–4088.
41. Schrier RW. Body water homeostasis: clinical disorders of urinary dilution and concentration. *J Am Soc Nephrol.* 2006;17(7):1820–1832.
42. Goldsmith SR. Vasopressin as vasopressor. *Am J Med.* 1987;82(6):1213–1219.
43. Schrier RW. The sea within us: disorders of body water homeostasis. *Curr Opin Investig Drugs.* 2007;8(4):304–311.
44. Nielsen S, Chou CL, Marples D, Christensen EI, Kishore BK, Knepper MA. Vasopressin increases water permeability of kidney collecting duct by inducing translocation of aquaporin-CD water channels to plasma membrane. *Proc Natl Acad Sci U S A.* 1995;92(4): 1013–1017.
45. Schafer JA, Hawk CT. Regulation of Na+ channels in the cortical collecting duct by AVP and mineralocorticoids. *Kidney Int.* 1992;41(2):255–268.
46. Ball SG. Vasopressin and disorders of water balance: the physiology and pathophysiology of vasopressin. *Ann Clin Biochem.* 2007;44(5):417–431.
47. Baughman VL. Brain protection during neurosurgery. *Anesthesiol Clin North Am.* 2002;20(2): 315–327.
48. Lanzino G, Kassell NF, Germanson T, Truskowski L, Alves W. Plasma glucose levels and outcome after aneurysmal subarachnoid hemorrhage. *J Neurosurg.* 1993;79(6):885–891.
49. Rovlias A, Kotsou S. The influence of hyperglycemia on neurological outcome in patients with severe head injury. *Neurosurgery.* 2000;46(2):335–342.
50. Griesdale DEG, de Souza RJ, van Dam RM, et al. Intensive insulin therapy and mortality among critically ill patients: a meta-analysis including NICE-SUGAR study data. *CMAJ.* 2009; 180(8):821–827.
51. Kansagara D, Fu R, Freeman M, Wolf F, Helfand M. Intensive insulin therapy in hospitalized patients: a systematic review. *Ann Intern Med.* 2011;154(4):268–282.
52. Jacob M, Chappell D, Rehm M. The 'third space' – fact or fiction? *Best Pract Res Clin Anaesthesiol.* 2009;23(2):145–157.
53. Thiele RH, Bartels K, Gan T-J. Inter-device differences in monitoring for goal-directed fluid therapy. *Can J Anaesth.* 2015;62(2):169–181.
54. Maharaj CH, Kallam SR, Malik A, Hassett P, Grady D, Laffey JG. Preoperative intravenous fluid therapy decreases postoperative nausea and pain in high risk patients. *Anesth Analg.* 2005;100(3):675–682.
55. Holte K, Klarskov B, Christensen DS, et al. Liberal versus restrictive fluid administration to improve recovery after laparoscopic cholecystectomy: a randomized, double-blind study. *Ann Surg.* 2004;240(5):892–899.
56. Holte K, Kristensen BB, Valentiner L, Foss NB, Husted H, Kehlet H. Liberal versus restrictive fluid management in knee arthroplasty: a randomized, double-blind study. *Anesth Analg.* 2007;105(2):465–474.
57. Jewer JK, Wong MJ, Bird SJ, Habib AS, Parker R, George RB. Supplemental perioperative intravenous crystalloids for postoperative nausea and vomiting. *Cochrane Database Syst Rev.* 2019;3(3):CD012212.

58. Brandstrup B, Tønnesen H, Beier-Holgersen R, et al. Effects of intravenous fluid restriction on postoperative complications: comparison of two perioperative fluid regimens: a randomized assessor-blinded multicenter trial. *Ann Surg*. 2003;238(5):641–648.
59. Nisanevich V, Felsenstein I, Almogy G, Weissman C, Einav S, Matot I. Effect of intraoperative fluid management on outcome after intraabdominal surgery. *Anesthesiology*. 2005;103(1): 25–32.
60. Corcoran T, Emma Joy Rhodes J, Clarke S, Myles PS, Ho KM. Perioperative fluid management strategies in major surgery. *Anesth Analg*. 2012;114(3):640–651.
61. Myles PS, Bellomo R, Corcoran T, et al. Restrictive versus liberal fluid therapy for major abdominal surgery. *N Engl J Med*. 2018;378(24):2263–2274.
62. Wrzosek A, Jakowicka-Wordliczek J, Zajaczkowska R, et al. Perioperative restrictive versus goal-directed fluid therapy for adults undergoing major non-cardiac surgery. *Cochrane Database Syst Rev*. 2019;12(12):CD012767.
63. National Heart, Lung, Blood Institute Acute Respiratory Distress Syndrome (ARDS) Clinical Trials Network, et al. Comparison of two fluid-management strategies in acute lung injury. *N Engl J Med*. 2006;354(24):2564–2575.
64. Collins SR, Blank RS, Deatherage LS, Dull RO. Special article: the endothelial glycocalyx: emerging concepts in pulmonary edema and acute lung injury. *Anesth Analg*. 2013;117(3): 664–674.
65. Alphonsus CS, Rodseth RN. The endothelial glycocalyx: a review of the vascular barrier. *Anaesthesia*. 2014;69(7):777–784.
66. Lewis SR, Pritchard MW, Evans DJ, et al. Colloids versus crystalloids for fluid resuscitation in critically ill people. *Cochrane Database Syst Rev*. 2018;8(8):CD000567.
67. Bunn F, Trivedi D. Colloid solutions for fluid resuscitation. *Cochrane Database of System Reviews*: John Wiley & Sons, Ltd; 2012.
68. He H, Liu D, Ince C. Colloids and the microcirculation. *Anesth Analg*. 2018;126(5): 1747–1754.
69. Wigmore GJ, Anstey JR, St. John A, et al. 20% human albumin solution fluid bolus administration therapy in patients after cardiac surgery (the HAS FLAIR study). *J Cardiothorac Vasc Anesth*. 2019;33(11):2920–2927.
70. Heming N, Lamothe L, Jaber S, et al. Morbidity and mortality of crystalloids compared to colloids in critically ill surgical patients. *Anesthesiology*. 2018;129(6):1149–1158.
71. Reiterer C, Kabon B, Halvorson S, Sessler DI, Mascha EJ, Kurz A. Hemodynamic responses to crystalloid and colloid fluid boluses during noncardiac surgery. *Anesthesiology*. 2021;136(1): 127–137.
72. Vincent J-L, Russell JA, Jacob M, et al. Albumin administration in the acutely ill: what is new and where next? *Crit Care*. 2014;18(4):231-.
73. Charpentier J, Mira J-P, EARSS Study Group. Efficacy and tolerance of hyperoncotic albumin administration in septic shock patients: The EARSS study [abstract]. *Intensive Care Med*. 2011;37:S115–S0438.
74. Caironi P, Tognoni G, Masson S, et al. Albumin replacement in patients with severe sepsis or septic shock. *N Engl J Med*. 2014;370(15):1412–1421.
75. Caironi P, Gattinoni L. Proposed benefits of albumin from the ALBIOS trial: a dose of insane belief. *Crit Care*. 2014;18(5):510.
76. Navickis RJ, Greenhalgh DG, Wilkes MM. Albumin in burn shock resuscitation: a meta-analysis of controlled clinical studies. *J Burn Care Res*. 2016;37(3):e268–e278.
77. Uhlig C, Silva PL, Deckert S, Schmitt J, de Abreu MG. Albumin versus crystalloid solutions in patients with the acute respiratory distress syndrome: a systematic review and meta-analysis. *Crit Care*. 2014;18(1):R10-R.
78. Bernardi M, Caraceni P, Navickis RJ, Wilkes MM. Albumin infusion in patients undergoing large-volume paracentesis: a meta-analysis of randomized trials. *Hepatology*. 2012;55(4): 1172–1181.
79. Singh V, Dheerendra PC, Singh B, et al. Midodrine versus albumin in the prevention of paracentesis-induced circulatory dysfunction in cirrhotics: a randomized pilot study. *Am J Gastroenterol*. 2008;103(6):1399–1405.
80. Sigal SH, Stanca CM, Fernandez J, Arroyo V, Navasa M. Restricted use of albumin for spontaneous bacterial peritonitis. *Gut*. 2007;56(4):597–599.
81. Salerno F, Navickis RJ, Wilkes MM. Albumin infusion improves outcomes of patients with spontaneous bacterial peritonitis: a meta-analysis of randomized trials. *Clin Gastroenterol Hepatol*. 2013;11(2):123–130.e1.
82. Best LMJ, Freeman S, Sutton AJ, et al. Treatment for hepatorenal syndrome in people with decompensated liver cirrhosis: a network meta-analysis. *Cochrane Database Syst Rev*. 2019; 9(9):CD013103.
83. Hartog C, Reinhart K. CONTRA: Hydroxyethyl starch solutions are unsafe in critically ill patients. *Intensive Care Med*. 2009;35(8):1337–1342.
84. Perner A, Haase N, Guttormsen AB. Hydroxyethyl starch 130/0.4 versus ringer's acetate in severe sepsis. *N Engl J Med*. 2012;367(2):124–134.
85. Mutter TC, Ruth CA, Dart AB. Hydroxyethyl starch (HES) versus other fluid therapies: effects on kidney function. *Cochrane Database Syst Rev*. 2013;23;(7):CD007594.
86. Executive Summary: Surviving Sepsis Campaign, International guidelines for the management of sepsis and septic shock 2021: Erratum. *Crit Care Med*. 2022;50(4):e413–e414.
87. Zornow Mark H, Todd Michael M, Moore Suzanne S. The acute cerebral effects of changes in plasma osmolality and oncotic pressure. *Anesthesiology*. 1987;67(6):936–941.
88. Jungner M, Grände P-O, Mattiasson G, Bentzer P. Effects on brain edema of crystalloid and albumin Fluid Resuscitation after Brain Trauma and Hemorrhage in the Rat. *Anesthesiology*. 2010;112(5):1194–1203.
89. Saline or albumin for fluid resuscitation in patients with traumatic brain injury. *N Engl J Med*. 2007;357(9):874–884.
90. Cooper DJ, Myburgh J, Heritier S, et al. Albumin resuscitation for traumatic brain injury: is intracranial hypertension the cause of increased mortality? *J Neurotrauma*. 2013;30(7):512–518.
91. Van Aken HK, Kampmeier TG, Ertmer C, Westphal M. Fluid resuscitation in patients with traumatic brain injury. *Curr Opin Anaesthesiol*. 2012;25(5):563–565.
92. Lira A, Pinsky MR. Choices in fluid type and volume during resuscitation: impact on patient outcomes. *Ann Intensive Care*. 2014;4:38.
93. Semler MW, Self WH, Rice TW. Balanced crystalloids versus saline in critically ill adults. *N Engl J Med*. 2018;378(20):1951.
94. Self WH, Semler MW, Wanderer JP, et al. Balanced crystalloids versus saline in noncritically ill adults. *N Engl J Med*. 2018;378(9):819–828.
95. Bampoe S, Odor PM, Dushianthan A, et al. Perioperative administration of buffered versus non-buffered crystalloid intravenous fluid to improve outcomes following adult surgical procedures. *Cochrane Database Syst Rev*. 2017;9(9):CD004089.
96. Wan S, Roberts MA, Mount P. Normal saline versus lower-chloride solutions for kidney transplantation. *Cochrane Database Syst Rev*. 2016;2016(8):CD010741.
97. Prough Donald S, Whitley John M, Taylor Carol L, Deal Dwight D, DeWitt Douglas S. Regional cerebral blood flow following resuscitation from hemorrhagic shock with hypertonic saline influence of a subdural mass. *Anesthesiology*. 1991;75(2):319–327.
98. Prough DS, Whitley JM, Taylor CL, Deal DD, DeWitt DS. Rebound intracranial hypertension in dogs after resuscitation with hypertonic solutions from hemorrhagic shock accompanied by an intracranial mass lesion. *J Neurosurg Anesthesiol*. 1999;11(2):102–111.
99. Vassar MJ. A multicenter trial for resuscitation of injured patients with 7.5% sodium chloride. *Arch Surg*. 1993;128(9):1003.
100. Thongrong C, Kong N, Govindarajan B, Allen D, Mendel E, Bergese SD. Current purpose and practice of hypertonic saline in neurosurgery: a review of the literature. *World Neurosurg*. 2014;82(6):1307–1318.
101. Cooper DJ, Myles PS, McDermott FT, et al. Prehospital hypertonic saline resuscitation of patients with hypotension and severe traumatic brain injury. *JAMA*. 2004;291(11):1350.
102. Shrum B, Church B, McArthur E, Burns KEA, Znajda T, McAlister V. Hypertonic salt solution for peri-operative fluid management. *Cochrane Database Syst Rev*. 2016;2016(6):CD005576.
103. Wong DH, O'Connor D, Tremper KK, Zaccari J, Thompson P, Hill D. Changes in cardiac output after acute blood loss and position change in man. *Crit Care Med*. 1989;17(10):979–983.
104. Gan Tong J, Soppitt A, Maroof M, et al. Goal-directed intraoperative fluid administration reduces length of hospital stay after major surgery. *Anesthesiology*. 2002;97(4):820–826.
105. Kouz K, Bergholz A, Timmermann LM, et al. The relation between mean arterial pressure and cardiac index in major abdominal surgery patients: a prospective observational cohort study. *Anesth Analg*. 2021;134(2):322–329.
106. Myles PS, McIlroy DR, Bellomo R, Wallace S. Importance of intraoperative oliguria during major abdominal surgery: findings of the Restrictive versus Liberal Fluid Therapy in Major Abdominal Surgery trial. *Br J Anaesth*. 2019;122(6):726–733.
107. Eskesen TG, Wetterslev M, Perner A. Systematic review including re-analyses of 1148 individual data sets of central venous pressure as a predictor of fluid responsiveness. *Intensive Care Med*. 2016;42(3):324–332.
108. Renner J, Scholz J, Bein B. Monitoring fluid therapy. *Best Pract Res Clin Anaesthesiol*. 2009;23(2):159–171.
109. Knotzer H, Hasibeder WR. Microcirculatory function monitoring at the bedside—a view from the intensive care. *Physiol Meas*. 2007;28(9):R65–R86.
110. Lewis SR, Butler AR, Brammar A, Nicholson A, Smith AF. Perioperative fluid volume optimization following proximal femoral fracture. *Cochrane Database Syst Rev*. 2016;3(3):CD003004.
111. Perel A. Using dynamic variables to guide perioperative fluid management. *Anesthesiology*. 2020;133(4):929–935.
112. Yang SY, Shim JK, Song Y, Seo SJ, Kwak YL. Validation of pulse pressure variation and corrected flow time as predictors of fluid responsiveness in patients in the prone position. *Br J Anaesth*. 2013;110(5):713–720.
113. Messina A, Pelaia C, Bruni A, et al. Fluid challenge during anesthesia. *Anesth Analg*. 2018; 127(6):1353–1364.
114. Carsetti A, Cecconi M, Rhodes A. Fluid bolus therapy. *Curr Opin Crit Care*. 2015;21(5):388–394.
115. DiCorte CJ, Latham P, Greilich PE, Cooley MV, Grayburn PA, Jessen ME. Esophageal Doppler monitor determinations of cardiac output and preload during cardiac operations. *Ann Thorac Surg*. 2000;69(6):1782–1786.
116. Venn R, Steele A, Richardson P, Poloniecki J, Grounds M, Newman P. Randomized controlled trial to investigate influence of the fluid challenge on duration of hospital stay and perioperative morbidity in patients with hip fractures. *Br J Anaesth*. 2002;88(1):65–71.
117. Horowitz Peter E, Kumar A. It's the Colloid, Not the Esophageal Doppler Monitor. *Anesthesiology*. 2003;99(1):238–239.
118. Porter TR, Shillcutt SK, Adams MS, et al. Guidelines for the use of echocardiography as a monitor for therapeutic intervention in adults: a report from the american society of echocardiography. *J Am Soc Echocardiogr*. 2015;28(1):40–56.

119. Bendjelid K, Romand J-A, Walder B, Suter PM, Fournier G. Correlation between measured inferior vena cava diameter and right atrial pressure depends on the echocardiographic method used in patients who are mechanically ventilated. *J Am Soc Echocardiogr*. 2002;15(9):944–949.
120. Joosten A, Desebbe O, Suehiro K, et al. Accuracy and precision of non-invasive cardiac output monitoring devices in perioperative medicine: a systematic review and meta-analysis. *Br J Anaesth*. 2017;118(3):298–310.
121. Kraft MD, Btaiche IF, Sacks GS, Kudsk KA. Treatment of electrolyte disorders in adult patients in the intensive care unit. *Am J Health Syst Pharm*. 2005;62(16):1663–1682.
122. Seay NW, Lehrich RW, Greenberg A. Diagnosis and management of disorders of body tonicity-hyponatremia and hypernatremia: core curriculum 2020. *Am J Kidney Dis*. 2020;75(2):272–286.
123. Sterns RH. Disorders of plasma sodium–causes, consequences, and correction. *N Engl J Med*. 2015;372(1):55–65.
124. Spasovski G, Vanholder R, Allolio B, et al. Clinical practice guideline on diagnosis and treatment of hyponatraemia. *Eur J Endocrinol*. 2014;170(3):G1–G47.
125. Adrogue HJ, Tucker BM, Madias NE. Diagnosis and management of hyponatremia: a review. *JAMA*. 2022;328(3):280–291.
126. Harring TR, Deal NS, Kuo DC. Disorders of sodium and water balance. *Emerg Med Clin North Am*. 2014;32(2):379–401.
127. Rafat C, Flamant M, Gaudry S, Vidal-Petiot E, Ricard JD, Dreyfuss D. Hyponatremia in the intensive care unit: how to avoid a Zugzwang situation? *Ann Intensive Care*. 2015;5(1):39.
128. Leung AA, McAlister FA, Rogers SO Jr., Pazo V, Wright A, Bates DW. Preoperative hyponatremia and perioperative complications. *Arch Intern Med*. 2012;172(19):1474–1481.
129. Hoorn EJ, Zietse R. Diagnosis and treatment of hyponatremia: compilation of the guidelines. *J Am Soc Nephrol*. 2017;28(5):1340–1349.
130. Sterns RH, Silver SM. Cerebral salt wasting versus SIADH: what difference? *J Am Soc Nephrol*. 2008;19(2):194–196.
131. Tandukar S, Sterns RH, Rondon-Berrios H. Osmotic demyelination syndrome following correction of hyponatremia by </= 10 mEq/L per day. *Kidney360*. 2021;2(9):1415–1423.
132. Lindner G, Funk GC. Hypernatremia in critically ill patients. *J Crit Care*. 2013;28(2):216 e11-220.
133. Muhsin SA, Mount DB. Diagnosis and treatment of hypernatremia. *Best Pract Res Clin Endocrinol Metab*. 2016;30(2):189–203.
134. Liamis G, Filippatos TD, Elisaf MS. Evaluation and treatment of hypernatremia: a practical guide for physicians. *Postgrad Med*. 2016;128(3):299–306.
135. Palmer BF, Clegg DJ. Physiology and pathophysiology of potassium homeostasis: Core curriculum 2019. *Am J Kidney Dis*. 2019;74(5):682–695.
136. McDonough AA, Youn JH. Potassium homeostasis: The knowns, the unknowns, and the health benefits. *Physiology (Bethesda)*. 2017;32(2):100–111.
137. Lomivorotov VV, Leonova EA, Belletti A, Shmyrev VA, Landoni G. Calcium administration during weaning from ccardiopulmonary bypass: a narrative literature review. *J Cardiothorac Vasc Anesth*. 2020;34(1):235–244.
138. Gumz ML, Rabinowitz L, Wingo CS. An integrated view of potassium homeostasis. *N Engl J Med*. 2015;373(1):60–72.
139. Palmer BF, Carrero JJ, Clegg DJ, et al. Clinical management of hyperkalemia. *Mayo Clin Proc*. 2021;96(3):744–762.
140. Unwin RJ, Luft FC, Shirley DG. Pathophysiology and management of hypokalemia: a clinical perspective. *Nat Rev Nephrol*. 2011;7(2):75–84.
141. Viera AJ, Wouk N. Potassium disorders: hypokalemia and hyperkalemia. *Am Fam Physician*. 2015;92(6):487–495.
142. Adrogue HJ, Madias NE. Sodium and potassium in the pathogenesis of hypertension. *N Engl J Med*. 2007;356(19):1966–1978.
143. Weaver CM. Potassium and health. *Adv Nutr*. 2013;4(3):368S–377S.
144. Kardalas E, Paschou SA, Anagnostis P, Muscogiuri G, Siasos G, Vryonidou A. Hypokalemia: a clinical update. *Endocr Connect*. 2018;7(4):R135–R146.
145. Alfonzo AV, Isles C, Geddes C, Deighan C. Potassium disorders–clinical spectrum and emergency management. *Resuscitation*. 2006;70(1):10–25.
146. Lott C, Truhlar A, Alfonzo A, et al. European resuscitation council guidelines 2021: Cardiac arrest in special circumstances. *Resuscitation*. 2021;161:152–219.
147. Lopes MB, Rocha PN, Pecoits-Filho R. Updates on medical management of hyperkalemia. *Curr Opin Nephrol Hypertens*. 2019;28(5):417–423.
148. Kovesdy CP. Updates in hyperkalemia: Outcomes and therapeutic strategies. *Rev Endocr Metab Disord*. 2017;18(1):41–47.
149. Gupta AA, Self M, Mueller M, Wardi G, Tainter C. Dispelling myths and misconceptions about the treatment of acute hyperkalemia. *Am J Emerg Med*. 2022;52:85–91.
150. Sood MM, Sood AR, Richardson R. Emergency management and commonly encountered outpatient scenarios in patients with hyperkalemia. *Mayo Clin Proc*. 2007;82(12):1553–1561.
151. Weiss JN, Qu Z, Shivkumar K. Electrophysiology of hypokalemia and hyperkalemia. *Circ Arrhythm Electrophysiol*. 2017;10(3):e004667.
152. Depret F, Peacock WF, Liu KD, Rafique Z, Rossignol P, Legrand M. Management of hyperkalemia in the acutely ill patient. *Ann Intensive Care*. 2019;9(1):32.
153. Palmer BF, Clegg DJ. Diagnosis and treatment of hyperkalemia. *Cleve Clin J Med*. 2017;84(12):934–942.
154. Bnaya A, Ruchlemer R, Itzkowitz E, Gabbay E, Mosenkis A, Shavit L. Incidence, risk factors, and recognition of pseudohyperkalemia in patients with chronic lymphocytic leukemia. *Int J Hematol*. 2021;114(1):102–108.
155. Saleh-Anaraki K, Jain A, Wilcox CS, Pourafshar N. Pseudohyperkalemia: three cases and a review of literature. *Am J Med*. 2022;135(7):e150–e154.
156. Hunter RW, Bailey MA. Hyperkalemia: pathophysiology, risk factors and consequences. *Nephrol Dial Transplant*. 2019;34(Suppl 3):iii2–iii11.
157. Kosiborod M, Peacock WF, Packham DK. Sodium zirconium cyclosilicate for urgent therapy of severe hyperkalemia. *N Engl J Med*. 2015;372(16):1577–1578.
158. Kelly A, Levine MA. Hypocalcemia in the critically ill patient. *J Intensive Care Med*. 2013;28(3):166–177.
159. Maier JD, Levine SN. Hypercalcemia in the intensive care unit: a review of pathophysiology, diagnosis, and modern therapy. *J Intensive Care Med*. 2015;30(5):235–252.
160. Wray JP, Bridwell RE, Schauer SG, et al. The diamond of death: Hypocalcemia in trauma and resuscitation. *Am J Emerg Med*. 2021;41:104–109.
161. MacKay EJ, Stubna MD, Holena DN, et al. Abnormal calcium levels during trauma resuscitation are associated with increased mortality, increased blood product use, and greater hospital resource consumption: a pilot investigation. *Anesth Analg*. 2017;125(3):895–901.
162. Chang WT, Radin B, McCurdy MT. Calcium, magnesium, and phosphate abnormalities in the emergency department. *Emerg Med Clin North Am*. 2014;32(2):349–366.
163. Aguilera IM, Vaughan RS. Calcium and the anaesthetist. *Anaesthesia*. 2000;55(8):779–790.
164. Matikainen N, Pekkarinen T, Ryhanen EM, Schalin-Jantti C. Physiology of calcium homeostasis: an overview. *Endocrinol Metab Clin North Am*. 2021;50(4):575–590.
165. Grant AO. Cardiac ion channels. *Circ Arrhythm Electrophysiol*. 2009;2(2):185–194.
166. Napolitano L. Hemostatic defects in massive transfusion: an update and treatment recommendation. *Expert Rev Hematol*. 2021;14(2):219–239.
167. Cooper MS, Gittoes NJ. Diagnosis and management of hypocalcaemia. *BMJ*. 2008;336(7656):1298–1302.
168. Pepe J, Colangelo L, Biamonte F, et al. Diagnosis and management of hypocalcemia. *Endocrine*. 2020;69(3):485–495.
169. Tonon CR, Silva T, Pereira FWL, et al. A review of current clinical concepts in the pathophysiology, etiology, diagnosis, and management of hypercalcemia. *Med Sci Monit*. 2022;28:e935821.
170. Turner JJO. Hypercalcaemia – presentation and management. *Clin Med (Lond)*. 2017;17(3):270–273.
171. de Baaij JH, Hoenderop JG, Bindels RJ. Magnesium in man: implications for health and disease. *Physical Rev*. 2015:95(1):1–46.
172. Fawcett WJ, Haxby EJ, Male DA. Magnesium: physiology and pharmacology. *Br J Anaesth*. 1999;83(2):302–320.
173. Fiorentini D, Cappadone C, Farruggia G, Prata C. Magnesium: biochemistry, nutrition, detection, and social impact of diseases linked to its deficiency. *Nutrients*. 2021;13(4):1136.
174. Laurant P, Touyz RM. Physiological and pathophysiological role of magnesium in the cardiovascular system: implications in hypertension. *J Hypertens*. 2000;18(9).1177–1191.
175. Herroeder S, Schönherr ME, De Hert SG, Hollmann MW. Magnesium–essentials for anesthesiologists. *Anesthesiology*. 2011;114(4):971–993.
176. Desai N. Albrecht E, El-Boghdadly K. Perineural adjuncts for peripheral nerve block. *BJA Educ*. 2019;19(9):276–282.
177. Li M, Jin S, Zhao X et al. Does magnesium sulfate as an adjuvant of local anesthetics facilitate better effect of perineural nerve blocks?: A meta-analysis of randomized controlled trials. *Clin J Pain*. 2016;32(12):1053–1061.
178. Do S-H. Magnesium: a versatile drug for anesthesiologists. *Korean J Anesthesiol*. 2013;65(1):4–8.
179. Elliott JP, Lewis DF, Morrison JC, Garite TJ. In defense of magnesium sulfate. *Obstet Gynecol*. 2009;113(6):1341–1348.
180. Connor D, Boumphrey S. *Perioperative Care of Phaeochromocytoma*. BJA Education; 2016; 153–8.
181. James MF, Cronjé L. Pheochromocytoma crisis: the use of magnesium sulfate. *Anesth Analg*. 2004;99(3):680–686.
182. Agus ZS. Mechanisms and causes of hypomagnesemia. *Curr Opin Nephrol Hypertens*. 2016;25(4):301–307.
183. Kritmetapak K, Kumar R. Phosphate as a Signaling Molecule. *Calcif Tissue Int*. 2021;108(1):16–31.
184. Peacock M. Phosphate metabolism in health and disease. *Calcif Tissue Int*. 2021;108(1):3–15.
185. Gaasbeek A, Meinders AE. Hypophosphatemia: an update on its etiology and treatment. *Am J Med*. 2005;118(10):1094–101.
186. Friedman EA. Consequences and management of hyperphosphatemia in patients with renal insufficiency. *Kidney Int Suppl*. 2005(95):S1–S7.
187. Zheng WH, Yao Y, Zhou H, Xu Y, Huang HB. Hyperphosphatemia and outcomes in critically ill patients: a systematic review and meta-analysis. *Front Med (Lausanne)*. 2022;9:870637.
188. Vervloet MG, Sezer S, Massy ZA, et al. The role of phosphate in kidney disease. *Nat Rev Nephrol*. 2017;13(1):27–38.
189. Rastogi A, Bhatt N, Rossetti S, Beto J. Management of hyperphosphatemia in end-stage renal disease: a new paradigm. *J Ren Nutr*. 2021;31(1):21–34.

17 Hemostasis and Transfusion Medicine

LOUANNE M. CARABINI • GLENN RAMSEY

KEY POINTS

1 Modern transfusion medicine focuses on patient-centered blood component therapy.

2 Blood must not only be maintained as a fluid in normal circulation, but also be capable of forming a solid clot to stanch leaks in the vascular wall, yet can be subsequently dismantled once the vascular endothelium is repaired.

3 Clotting factors in the plasma are activated at sites of endothelial injury and assemble in enzymatic complexes to activate thrombin.

4 All of the clotting factors are primarily produced in the liver, except for VIII, which is also released by endothelial cells and is well maintained in liver disease.

5 Fibrin clots must be broken down after their job is done, and fibrinolysis is a complex process with checks and balances.

6 The first screening test for hemostatic problems should always be the patient's medical history.

7 A general oversight of plasma clotting factor activity is obtained by the prothrombin time (PT) for the extrinsic (tissue) pathway and the activated partial thromboplastin time (aPTT) for the intrinsic (contact) pathway.

8 Disseminated intravascular coagulation (DIC) describes unchecked coagulation initiated by pathologic systemic activation of the intrinsic clotting pathway.

9 The risk for venous thromboembolism is increased by intercurrent factors such as physical inactivity or immobilization, malignancy, hormone therapy, trauma, and pregnancy.

10 Most anticoagulant therapies need ongoing or selective testing for assessment of therapeutic effect.

11 Leukoreduction (LR) to remove WBCs from red blood cells (RBCs) and platelets reduces the risk of HLA alloimmunization, febrile nonhemolytic transfusion reactions (FNHTRs), and CMV transmission in patients who require these precautions.

12 Plasma derivatives are proteins processed from plasma for therapeutic infusions.

13 Many years of effort have gone into the search for an oxygen-carrying substitute for RBCs.

14 Routine RBC compatibility testing includes ABO and RhD typing, an antibody screen for IgG non-ABO RBC antibodies, and an RBC cross-match.

15 Over the past decade, transfusion practices for medical and surgical patients shifted from a liberal strategy to more restrictive management with lower thresholds and careful consideration of the balance between transfusion risks and the physiologic consequences of anemia.

16 Oxygen delivery to the tissues (DO_2) is dependent on cardiac output (CO), regional blood flow, and oxygen-carrying capacity, also known as the oxygen content (CaO_2) of blood.

17 Numerous recommendations provide guidance for the transfusion management of thrombocytopenia and acquired or inherited platelet disorders.

18 Cryoprecipitate is created by a controlled thaw of frozen plasma, which allows for precipitation of large molecules, most notably fibrinogen and vWF.

19 Over the past few decades, the risk–benefit ratio of blood product transfusion has been the subject of several studies and review articles.

20 Given the extensive use of more sensitive methods for screening and controlling the infectious risks of blood product transfusion, noninfectious complications have emerged as the major source of transfusion-related morbidity and mortality.

21 Transfusion-related acute lung injury (TRALI) is a clinical diagnosis that can be clouded by confounding comorbidities or patient acuity; therefore, TRALI tends to be underreported in the literature and is extremely difficult, if not impossible, to study with randomized prospective clinical trials.

22 Preoperative autologous donation programs are most effective when double units are donated with ample time for erythrogenesis prior to the date of surgery.

23 Over the past decade, RBC salvage techniques have improved drastically and now offer an efficient, cost-effective, and safe method for perioperative blood conservation.

24 Disorders of hemostasis can be classified as those that cause a propensity for hemorrhage and those that facilitate inappropriate thrombosis.

25 Symptomatically, disorders of primary hemostasis often present with superficial signs of bleeding on the skin or mucosa.

26 Von Willebrand disease (vWD) is the most common hereditary bleeding disorder, with a prevalence of approximately 1% in the general population.

27 Hemophilia is a genetic disease that results from deficiencies or dysfunction of specific clotting factors.

28 Antiplatelet therapy is indicated for patients at risk for cerebral vascular accident, myocardial infarction, or other vascular thrombosis complications.

29 Heparin-induced thrombocytopenia (HIT) is a clinical disorder that develops after extended use of heparin therapy. It occurs in approximately 1% to 5% of patients receiving heparin and is associated with morbidity from thromboembolic complications.

30 Recombinant activated factor VII (rFVIIa) is only indicated for the treatment of hemophiliacs with inhibitors/antibodies and factor VII deficiency.

31 Prothrombin complex concentrates are now the drug of choice for emergent reversal of oral anticoagulants in place of fresh frozen plasma (FFP).

32 Antifibrinolytic agents have been used to prevent and treat surgical blood loss for several decades.

Introduction

1 The focus on quality, safety, and cost-effectiveness in health care extends to the practice of transfusion medicine. Patient-centered blood management emphasizes the use of evidence-based decisions and blood conservation strategies to balance the risks and benefits associated with blood component therapy. There continues to be significant variability in blood product transfusion practices despite guidelines from experts and task forces from the American Society of Anesthesiologists (ASA), the American Association of Blood Banks (AABB), the American Red Cross, the Society of Cardiac Anesthesiologists (SCA), and the British Society of Haematology (BSH) consistently advocating for restrictive transfusion practices. Lower hemoglobin thresholds continue to demonstrate improved outcomes with noninferior or reduced morbidity and mortality; however, it remains unclear which patient characteristics determine the appropriate transfusion goal for a given diagnosis or acute clinical situation. Therefore, it is imperative for the anesthesia provider to understand the treatment benefits, the rare and common adverse effects, and the specific therapeutic details of blood product preparation, conservation, and administration in order to best manage their patients.

This chapter begins with a review of primary and secondary hemostasis, fibrinolysis, and regulation of the coagulation pathway. We continue with a description of the most common coagulation profile tests, followed by the method for blood product collection and storage. The therapeutic indications and risks associated with blood component therapy are discussed at length. The chapter also includes extensive clinical sections discussing congenital and acquired deficiencies in hemostasis and coagulation, as well as an up-to-date presentation of available pharmacologic management strategies to maintain a balanced hemostatic mechanism.

Hemostasis and Coagulation

Primary Hemostasis

Blood must not only be maintained as a fluid in normal circulation, 2
but also be capable of forming a solid clot to stanch leaks in the vascular wall, yet can be subsequently dismantled once the vascular endothelium is repaired. This delicate equilibrium between anticoagulation and coagulation is maintained by a complex system of counterbalanced blood proteins and cells (platelets). Many congenital and acquired disorders can push the system toward either bleeding or thrombosis. The patient care team has a number of tests to evaluate the system, and many therapeutic modalities to correct identified problems.

Platelets adhere to sites of endothelial disruption, undergo activation to recruit more platelets and amplify the platelet response, and then cross-link with fibrin, the end product of the plasma clotting factor cascade, to form a platelet plug. *Primary hemostasis* (Fig. 17-1) describes the initiation of the platelet plug and clotting mechanism.

Adherence

When the endothelial lining is disrupted to expose the underlying matrix, platelets attach to collagen via surface integrin receptors—glycoproteins (GP) Ia/IIa and GP VI (Fig. 17-1A). Collagen adherence is favored in low-shear conditions such as venous circulation.[1] In high-shear arterial blood flow, von Willebrand factor (vWF) from endothelial cells and from pre-existing clot binds to integrin Ib/IX, the other major adherence anchor.[3] In capillary blood flow, platelets are pushed to the periphery by red blood cells (RBCs), so anemia lessens platelet contact and reduces platelet function.[4]

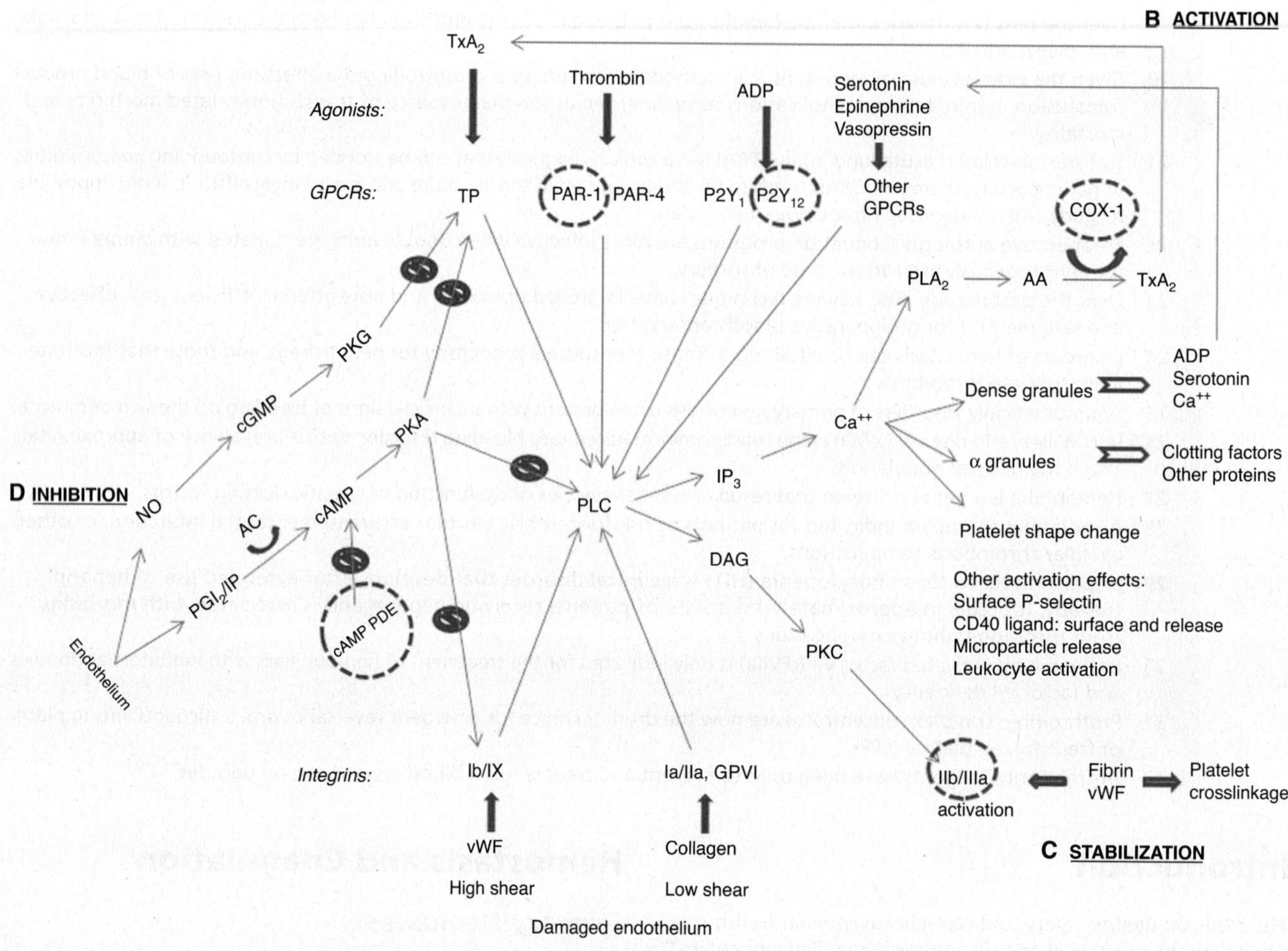

Figure 17-1 Overview of platelet pathways for adherence, activation, stabilization, and physiologic inhibition. Many pathway intermediaries and other elements are not shown, but are reviewed elsewhere.[1,2] *Thin arrows:* signaling pathways. *Thick arrows:* ligand binding. *Curved arrows:* catalysis. *Clear arrows:* secretion. *Slashed circles:* inhibitory signaling pathways. *Round circles:* antiplatelet drug targets. (**A**) Adherence. vWF, von Willebrand factor. Glycoproteins Ib/IX, Ia/IIa, and VI. (**B**) Activation. Agonists: TxA_2, thromboxane A_2; ADP, adenosine diphosphate. Receptors: GPCR, G-protein–coupled receptor; TP, thromboxane prostanoid; PAR, protease-activated receptor. Intermediaries: PLC, phospholipase C; IP_3, inositol-1,4,5–triphosphate; DAG, diacylglycerol; PKC, protein kinase C; Ca^{2+}, calcium; PLA_2, phospholipase A_2; AA, arachidonic acid; COX, cyclooxygenase. (**C**) Stabilization. Glycoprotein IIb/IIIa. (**D**) Inhibition. NO, nitric oxide; PGI_2, prostaglandin I_2 (prostacyclin); IP, PGI_2 receptor; AC, adenylate cyclase; cAMP, cyclic adenosine monophosphate; PDE, phosphodiesterase; cGMP, cyclic guanosine monophosphate; PKA, protein kinase A; PKG, protein kinase G. Targets of antiplatelet drugs. COX-1: aspirin, triflusal. $P2Y_{12}$: clopidogrel, prasugrel, ticlopidine, cangrelor, ticagrelor. cAMP PDE: dipyridamole, cilostazol. IIb/IIIa: abciximab, eptifibatide, tirofiban.

Activation

Platelet activation can be mediated by numerous signaling pathways from the platelet surface (Fig. 17-1B). In "outside-in" signaling, a central target is phospholipase C (PLC). The above adherence integrins trigger pathways to activate PLC. Another set of surface receptors, G-protein–coupled receptors (GPCRs), are activated by an array of corresponding agonists, including thrombin from the factor clotting cascade, adenosine diphosphate (ADP), thromboxane A_2 (TxA_2), serotonin, epinephrine, and vasopressin. Each of these agonist–GPCR pairings set off activation pathways for PLC as well.[4]

Activated PLC leads to several structural changes in the platelets. Via inositol-1,4,5–triphosphate (IP_3), calcium (Ca^{2+}) is released from storage tubules. Calcium ions catalyze release of dense granules and α-granules at the platelet surface. These granules contain ADP, serotonin, and more Ca^{2+}, all of which can activate more platelets. The α-granules contain numerous proteins, including platelet factor 4 (PF4), which promotes clotting by binding and neutralizing heparin-like compounds and heparin.[4] (This heparin–PF4 complex is the target antigen for the antibodies causing heparin-induced thrombocytopenia [HIT], discussed in depth later in this chapter.) Calcium also facilitates rearrangement of the platelet microskeleton to change the platelet shape from round and discoid to flat and spiky. Furthermore, the Ca^{2+} helps activate phospholipase A_2 (PLA_2), which releases arachidonic acid (AA) from the platelet membrane. AA, as catalyzed by cyclooxygenase-1 (COX-1), is modified to TxA_2, which can then activate more platelets. Activated platelets also have surface P-selectin and surface-bound and released CD40 ligand. They also release circulating microparticles and attract and activate leukocytes; these features further contribute to hemostasis and also play a role in inflammation.[4]

Stabilization

The activated PLC initiates "inside-out" signaling of GP IIb/IIIa via diacylglycerol (DAG) and protein kinase C (Fig. 17-1C). This changes the shape of GP IIb/IIIa, which permits it to better bind fibrin and vWF. These proteins can bridge to other activated platelets. The fibrin binding can also enmesh the platelets, contributing to the formation of the platelet plug in the convergence of the platelet and clotting factor systems.[5]

Inhibition

To maintain hemostatic balance, platelets are naturally inhibited in their endothelial environment. Endothelial cells secrete prostaglandin I_2 (PGI_2), which binds to a surface receptor to signal increased cyclic adenosine monophosphate (cAMP). Elevated cAMP activates protein kinase A (PKA), a multisite inhibitor of vWF adherence, TxA_2 activation, and PLC internal signaling. However, cAMP is metabolized by cAMP phosphodiesterase (PDE). Endothelial cells also secrete nitric oxide (NO), which at high levels initiates a signaling pathway leading to inhibition of the TxA_2 receptor.

Mechanisms of Antiplatelet Medications

Figure 17-1 shows the sites of action for current antiplatelet medications.[1,4] No drugs are available to counteract the first step, platelet adherence (Fig. 17-1A). Aspirin and triflusal dampen the secretion of TxA_2 by inhibiting COX-1, the enzyme which converts AA into TxA_2 (Fig. 17-1B). Another agonist, ADP, has its $P2Y_{12}$ receptor blocked by clopidogrel, ticagrelor, and several other drugs. The protease-activated receptor-1 (PAR-1) for thrombin activation is blocked by vorapaxar. Formation and stabilization of the platelet plug is blocked by abciximab, eptifibatide, and tirofiban, which act at GP IIb/IIIa (Fig. 17-1C). Finally, the major inhibitory pathway mediated by endothelial PGI_2 is upregulated by dipyridamole and cilostazol (Fig. 17-1D).[1] These medications are discussed later in this chapter.

Secondary Hemostasis

3 Clotting factors in the plasma are activated at sites of endothelial injury and assemble in enzymatic complexes to activate thrombin. This *initiates* secondary hemostasis. Thrombin then *amplifies* production of itself by activating other more efficient enzymes, which *propagate* a thrombin burst. Thrombin also converts fibrinogen to fibrin, which cross-links with activated platelets to form the platelet plug. Each of the three enzymatic complexes in the clotting process consists of four parts: an enzyme in the serine protease family, a cofactor, a plasma membrane phospholipid surface such as the platelet, and calcium ion (Ca^{2+}). The proteases convert other clotting factors from their inactive circulating configuration to an active form (termed [factor number] a).[1,3,5]

The extrinsic pathway (Fig. 17-2). The process begins when endothelial disruption exposes tissue factor (TF) on underlying cell membranes extrinsic to the circulation—hence the term "extrinsic pathway." TF binds both VII and VIIa, which circulate at low levels, and is a cofactor for the activation of factor VII. VIIa enzyme, TF cofactor, cell membrane phospholipid, and Ca^{2+} form the first complex, a low-efficiency extrinsic-pathway "tenase" that activates factor X and factor IX. Then Xa enzyme, its cofactor Va (derived in large part from factor V released from activated platelet α-granules), phospholipid, and Ca^{2+} assemble to form the second complex, a "prothrombinase," which converts prothrombin (II) to thrombin (IIa).[3]

The intrinsic pathway (Fig. 17-2). Thrombin has several central functions. It activates platelets via surface receptors PAR-1 and PAR-4 (see Primary Hemostasis), cleaves more V to Va, and initiates the "intrinsic" (intravascular) coagulation pathway by cleaving factors XI to XIa. XIa cleaves more IX to IXa. Thrombin also activates VIII to VIIIa. (VIII is carried and stabilized in the plasma by vWF until needed, so vWF deficiency also results in low plasma VIII levels.) The third complex is then formed: FIXa enzyme, FVIIa cofactor, phospholipid, and Ca^{2+}. This is a high-efficiency intrinsic-pathway "tenase," which provides many times more FXa for more prothrombinase complex. Ultimately, thrombin cleaves fibrinogen to fibrin monomers, which then polymerize extensively. Fibrin polymers are cross-linked by factor XIIIa (also activated by thrombin) to form the stable fibrin clot. Fibrin also cross-links activated platelets by their GP IIb/IIIa receptors to enmesh platelets and fibrin in the platelet plug (see Primary Hemostasis).[3,5]

All of the clotting factors are primarily produced in the liver, 4
except for FVIII, which is also released by endothelial cells and is well maintained in liver disease. The plasma half-life of most clotting factors is around 1.5 to 3 days, except for the initiating factor VII (6 hours) and the cofactors V and VIII (8 to 12 hours), which are much shorter. Four critical enzyme factors—VII in the

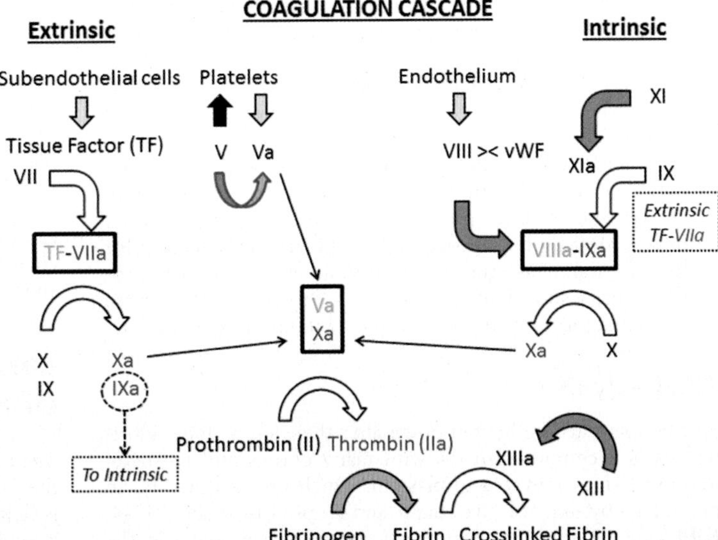

Figure 17-2 Schematic diagram of the coagulation cascade of clotting factors, with extrinsic, intrinsic, and common pathways. Von Willebrand factor (vWF) and factor VIII circulate together (><). *Gray arrows:* secretion. *Red:* vitamin K–dependent factors. *Green:* cofactors. *Purple arrows:* thrombin activation. *Black arrow:* uptake. *Dotted lines:* intrinsic–extrinsic crossover. *Solid boxes:* also Ca^{++} and platelet phospholipid.

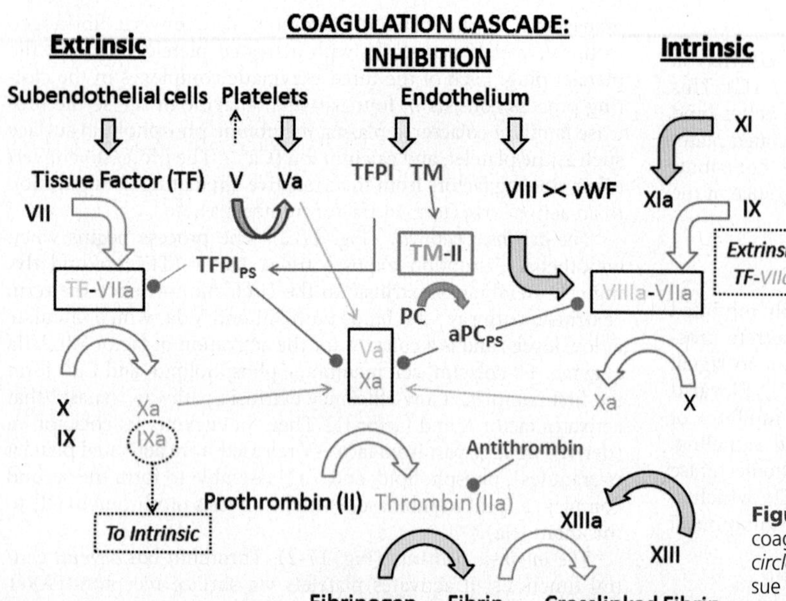

Figure 17-3 Schematic diagram of inhibitory control of the coagulation cascade. *Purple arrows:* thrombin activation. *Blue circle-head arrows:* inhibition. TM, thrombomodulin; TFPI, tissue factor pathway inhibitor. *Red:* vitamin K–dependent factors. *Green:* cofactor.

extrinsic tenase, IX in the intrinsic tenase, X in the prothrombinase, and prothrombin (II)—must be carboxylated at multiple glutamic acid residues after translation, in order to interact with phospholipid and Ca^{2+}. Vitamin K in its reduced form is the cofactor for the glutamyl-carboxylase enzyme, and thus these four factors (II, VII, IX, X) are vitamin K–dependent.[3]

Inhibition of Clotting Factors

The clotting pathways have three main regulatory inhibitors (Fig. 17-3)[3,5]:

1. TF pathway inhibitor (TFPI) inhibits the external tenase complex by binding to the VIIa protease and to its Xa product. TFPI is produced in endothelial cells, and its release is stimulated by heparin. Heparin in turn binds to and raises the inhibitory efficiency of TFPI.
2. Antithrombin-III (AT-III) is a serine protease inhibitor or serpin. Serpins disrupt the active sites and increase the clearance of their target proteases. AT-III inhibits proteases in all clotting pathways: VIIa in extrinsic tenase, Xa in prothrombinase, XIa and IXa in the intrinsic tenase pathway, and thrombin. AT-III's inhibitory function is greatly increased when bound to heparin.
3. Protein C-ase is an enzymatic complex with the same four-part structure as the coagulation complexes above: an enzyme, thrombin, its cofactor thrombomodulin, phospholipid, and Ca^{2+}. Thrombomodulin is expressed on endothelial cell membranes. In the protein C-ase complex, thrombin cleaves and activates protein C. Activated protein C (APC) brakes clotting by cleaving VIIIa and Va, the cofactors for the external tenase and the prothrombinase complexes. Protein C has a short half-life of 6 hours. Protein S is thought to be a cofactor for protein C; both are vitamin K–dependent.[3]

Fibrinolysis

5 Fibrin clots must be broken down after their job is done. Fibrinolysis is a complex process with many checks and balances. Plasminogen is activated to plasmin, which breaks down fibrin polymers, by one of two main serine proteases (Fig. 17-4, 1 Video 17-1).[5] The major activator of plasminogen in the blood is tissue plasminogen activator (tPA), which is secreted from endothelial cells and platelets. Both plasminogen and tPA bind to lysine sites on fibrin. When associated with cross-linked fibrin, tPA becomes much more efficient. Once some plasmin is formed, it cleaves tPA to a more active form. tPA also directly cleaves fibrin polymers.

In tissues, urokinase is the main plasminogen activator. Urokinase-type plasminogen activator is secreted from the endothelium, monocytes, macrophages, and urinary epithelium. These cells also bind plasminogen with two receptors, the annexin A2 complex and the urokinase receptor, which facilitate its conversion to plasmin. Plasmin also activates urokinase to a more active form. Urokinase and tPA can be administered as medications to lyse thrombi.

Inhibition of Fibrinolysis

Plasminogen activation inhibitor-1 (PAI-1) is a serpin which binds to tPA and urokinase and accelerates their clearance from plasma (Fig. 17-4, 2 Video 17-2). Activated platelets release PAI-1 from α-granules. PAI-2, which acts similarly to PAI-1, is secreted by the placenta and is prominent in pregnancy. Thrombin-activated fibrinolysis inhibitor (TAFI) is secreted from endothelial cells and is activated by the thrombin–thrombomodulin complex. TAFI cleaves fibrin and fibrin polymers in a fashion that inhibits the action of tPA, and TAFI also inhibits the action of plasmin on fibrin. α_2-Antiplasmin binds to plasmin and blocks its action, although this also slows the metabolism of plasmin.[5]

Fibrinolysis is inhibited pharmacologically by epsilon-aminocaproic acid (EACA) and tranexamic acid (TXA), which stabilize clots. These drugs are lysine analogs that block the lysine-binding sites of plasminogen, preventing it from acting on fibrin.

Laboratory Evaluation of Hemostasis

The first screening test for hemostatic problems should always be the patient's medical history. The nature of any abnormal bleeding is helpful; dermal or mucosal bleeding may suggest platelet dysfunction, whereas hemarthroses or soft tissue bleeding suggests 6

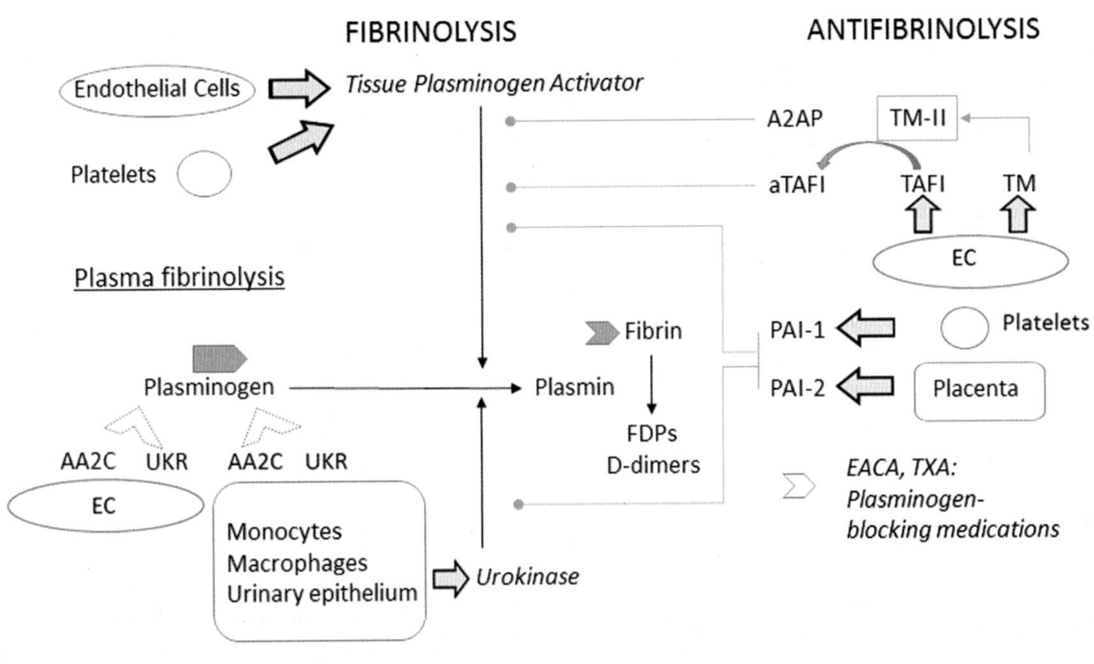

Figure 17-4 Fibrinolysis and antifibrinolysis pathways. AA2C, annexin A2 complex; A2AP, α-2–antiplasmin; EACA, epsilon-aminocaproic acid; EC, endothelial cells; FDPs, fibrin degradation products; PAI, plasminogen activator inhibitor; (a) TAFI, (activated) thrombin-activated fibrinolysis inhibitor; TM, thrombomodulin; II, factor II (thrombin); TXA, tranexamic acid; UKR, urokinase receptor. *Gray arrows:* secretion. *Black arrows:* enzyme activation. *Curved arrow:* thrombin activation. *Round-headed lines:* inhibition. *Dotted angles:* AA2C and UKR cell-membrane receptors binding to plasminogen. *Solid pentagon* on plasminogen: lysine-binding sites attaching to fibrin. *Solid chevron* on fibrin: lysines to which plasminogen binds. *Clear chevron:* antifibrinolytic medications blocking the lysine-binding sites on plasminogen. *Italics:* pharmacologic therapies promoting (tPA, urokinase) or inhibiting (EACA, TXA) fibrinolysis.

factor deficiencies. Besides any direct history of bleeding, thrombosis, or laboratory abnormalities, the patient's experience with hemostatic challenges such as surgery, dental procedures, and menstruation may help rule-out clinical problems or suggest a lifelong congenital or more recent acquired disorder. The family history is helpful in diagnosing a congenital problem and the possible pattern of inheritance. Anticoagulants and antiplatelet medications, including over-the-counter drugs, should always be reviewed before ordering laboratory studies.

Laboratory Evaluation of Primary Hemostasis

The normal automated platelet count in adults is approximately 150,000 to 400,000/μL. The peripheral blood smear should be examined in specimens with abnormal platelet counts. Microscopic review may reveal clotted specimens, artifactual platelet clumping in vitro, or abnormal platelet morphology. Large platelets are seen in some congenital disorders. More recently, the influence of platelet qualitative assessment over quantitative count drives further testing for platelet function in the clinical setting. One of the first platelet function tests (PFTs) was the template bleeding time, in which a standardized small cut is made on the subject's forearm and the bleeding duration timed. Bleeding time can identify disorders of both inherited and acquired etiologies, but it is invasive, labor-intensive, impractical to repeat frequently, poorly reproducible, and only modestly predictive for bleeding problems.[2]

In vitro PFTs use various platelet agonists to activate and aggregate the patient's platelets. For example, the IMPACT; Cone and Plate(let) Analyzer (DiaMed, Cressier, Switzerland), and the PFA-100 or updated Innovance PFA-200 device (Siemens, Munich, Germany) simulates capillary blood flow through a chamber after activation by collagen and either epinephrine or ADP. Prolonged "closure time" with collagen/epinephrine, but not collagen/ADP, suggests aspirin or other antiplatelet medications. In contrast, when both pairs are abnormal, other congenital or acquired platelet dysfunctions, such as von Willebrand Disease (vWD), Bernard–Soulier syndrome, or Glanzmann's thromboasthenia may be present. However, the sensitivity and specificity are low. False negatives are common and abnormal results can be caused by thrombocytopenia, uremia, or anemia.[2]

Platelet aggregation testing using platelet-rich plasma is the most detailed overall PFT and still considered the gold standard test for platelet function. Platelets are tested with multiple isolated agonists including ADP, AA, collagen, and EPI to assess their patterns of physical aggregation and, in turn, the platelets' own agonist release. Some uncommon congenital disorders lack responses to specific agonists in a characteristic fashion, and newer methods using whole blood aggregometry allow for more specific analysis of anticoagulated whole blood samples. For example, the VerifyNow system (ITC, Edison NJ, USA) tests for specific antiplatelet medication effects from aspirin or $P2Y_{12}$ inhibitors. The Plateletworks system (Helena Laboratories, Beaumont, TX, USA) provides both a quantitative assessment of platelet count as well as function.[2]

vWD is a factor deficiency with clinical features of platelet dysfunction, due to the central role of vWF in cross-linking activated platelets to form the platelet plug. Up to 1% of all patients have vWD, with a wide range of severity due to either quantitative or functional defects of vWF. Only about 1 in 1,000 patients have clinical symptoms of bleeding.[2,6] Diagnostic testing is integral to deciphering the specific defect and type of vWD to ensure the appropriate treatment. Since vWF is the carrier for factor VIII

(FVIII) in plasma, vWF protein levels usually correlate with FVIII levels. Initial testing for vWD should include the vWF antigen level, vWF activity level, and FVIII activity level for comparison with vWF.[6] Type 1 vWD is a quantitative deficiency, with decreased antigen and activity. Type 2 vWD may have normal antigen levels but decreased activity from a defective protein. Within type 2, there are several subtypes with different molecular defects, and specialized identification is needed to determine the best therapy. Type 3 vWD is a rare, very severe autosomal recessive deficiency.[7] Acquired vWD occurs through removal of vWF from the plasma by adsorption to paraproteins or high number of platelets (hematologic disorders such as Waldenstrom macroglobulinemia), autoantibodies to vWF, or depletion by turbulent blood flow in congenital heart disease, dysfunctional heart valves, and left ventricular assist devices.[7] The clinical features and management of vWD are discussed later in this chapter.

Laboratory Evaluation of Secondary Hemostasis and Coagulation

7 A general oversight of plasma clotting factor activity is obtained by the *prothrombin time (PT)* for the extrinsic (tissue) pathway and the *aPTT* for the intrinsic (contact) pathway (Fig. 17-2), with both tests relevant to the common pathway.[5] These clotting tests are performed in blood specimens collected in a chelator (3.2% citrate), which binds Ca^{2+} to prevent clotting in the tube. The in vitro clotting test is activated by TF in the PT, or by negatively charged surfaces in the aPTT, using phospholipid as a platform (substituting for platelets). Ca^{2+} is then added to overcome the specimen chelation, and the time until complete fibrin clotting is measured. Representative normal ranges are around 12 to 15 seconds for the PT and 25 to 35 seconds for the aPTT, but are defined by each laboratory using its own equipment, reagents, and normal specimens. Testing is routinely performed at 37°C because hypothermia in the patient impairs the enzymatic reactions of clot formation.

Clotting physiology is more complicated than the traditional diagrams of separate cascade pathways for these two tests. For example, thrombin from the extrinsic pathway can activate the intrinsic pathway. In vitro, the aPTT clotting test is activated by synthetic contact materials that initiate via factor XII, so deficiencies of XII and other related contact factors cause a prolonged aPTT. However, deficiencies of these contact factors do not cause bleeding and may be associated with impaired fibrinolysis and thrombosis. Fibrinogen activity is also a critical parameter. Most assays measure the functional conversion of fibrinogen to fibrin, although the fibrinogen protein level can also be measured for comparison to assess fibrinogen dysfunction. Normal fibrinogen levels are around 150 to 400 mg/dL.[5]

Mixing Studies

To investigate elevated PT or aPTT values, the test should be repeated after mixing the patient's plasma with equal volumes of normal plasma. Even in severe factor deficiencies, the PT or aPTT shows substantial correction toward normal in a mixing study. However, if the patient's plasma contains an inhibitor or an anticoagulant, the normal plasma will also be affected and the PT or aPTT will not correct after incubating with normal plasma.[8]

Individual factor level activities are determined by the degree of correction observed when patient plasma is mixed with factor-deficient plasma. The classic congenital factor deficiencies are FVIII deficiency (hemophilia A) and factor IX deficiency (hemophilia B). Both are X-linked and thus nearly always in males. Women are heterozygous carriers with reduced factor levels and only mild symptoms. Factor XI deficiency has previously been labeled as hemophilia C, but it is more appropriately classified as a rare bleeding disorder rather than a hemophilia.[9] Acquired factor deficiencies usually involve multiple factors. The vitamin K–dependent factors are II (thrombin), VII, IX, and X. In liver disease, all-factor synthesis is deficient except FVIII, which also comes from endothelium. However, FVIII and other factors can be low in disseminated intravascular coagulation (DIC). As noted, FVIII may be low as part of vWD. Isolated FX deficiency occurs in some patients with amyloidosis because the abnormal protein absorbs this factor. Assessing factors V (liver disease), VII (liver disease or vitamin K deficiency), and VIII (consumption) may suggest a pattern to aid in the diagnosis of specific clinical syndromes.

Coagulation inhibitors are substances, usually antibodies, that block one or more clotting factors. Most do not cause bleeding; the most common examples are lupus anticoagulants (LAs), a type of antiphospholipid antibodies (APLAs). However, factor-specific inhibitor antibodies can block clotting in vivo and cause bleeding.[8] They are identified by their effect on the plasma factor's activity and semiquantified by assessing how much interference the patient's plasma gives to factor level measurements in normal plasma. Some severe hemophiliacs and other factor-deficient patients develop alloantibodies to therapeutic clotting factors, interfering with treatment and necessitating alternative factor therapies or immunosuppression. Bovine thrombin used for topical hemostasis can induce cross-reacting antibodies to the patient's own FV. Autoantibodies to specific clotting factors, most commonly FVIII, can cause serious coagulopathy.

DIC describes unchecked coagulation initiated by pathologic 8
systemic activation of the intrinsic clotting pathway. The specific pathophysiology of DIC is discussed later in this chapter, but diagnostic criteria require an inciting condition such as extensive tissue injury or a systemic inflammatory response secondary to infection, obstetrical complication, or malignancy.[10] Intravascular platelet activation and fibrin formation lead to thrombocytopenia, hypofibrinogenemia, and RBCs sheared by fibrin strands (schistocytes). The results of coagulation testing vary, but often show prolonged PT and aPTT. In some patients, thrombosis is the most prominent clinical finding, but in most patients, the depletion of platelets and clotting factors with accompanying activation of fibrinolysis leads to diffuse consumptive coagulopathy. Fibrin formation followed by fibrinolysis generates the fibrin fragments called D-dimers, which when quantified in immunologic testing are a useful indicator of DIC.

Three other tests are performed during surgery with whole-blood specimens: the *activated clotting time (ACT)*, *ecarin clotting time (ECT*, sometimes referred to as *ecarin chromogenic assay*, *diluted thrombin time [dTT])*, and viscoelastic whole-blood clotting tests. The ACT, a point-of-care test, assesses the intrinsic clotting pathway and is used mainly to monitor heparin anticoagulation and protamine reversal during cardiopulmonary bypass or vascular surgery. The ECT also describes the intrinsic clotting function, but it is primarily used for measuring the clinical effects of direct thrombin inhibitors (DTIs) such as bivalirudin and argatroban. The ACT and aPTT also reflect the clinical efficacy of DTIs, but at high doses required for cardiopulmonary bypass, ECT or dTT is more accurate.[11] However, neither of these tests are widely available.

Viscoelastic Testing

Whole-blood clot formation, stabilization, and fibrinolysis can be assessed by viscoelastic testing with thromboelastography (TEG, Haemoscope Corp., Niles, IL, USA) or rotation

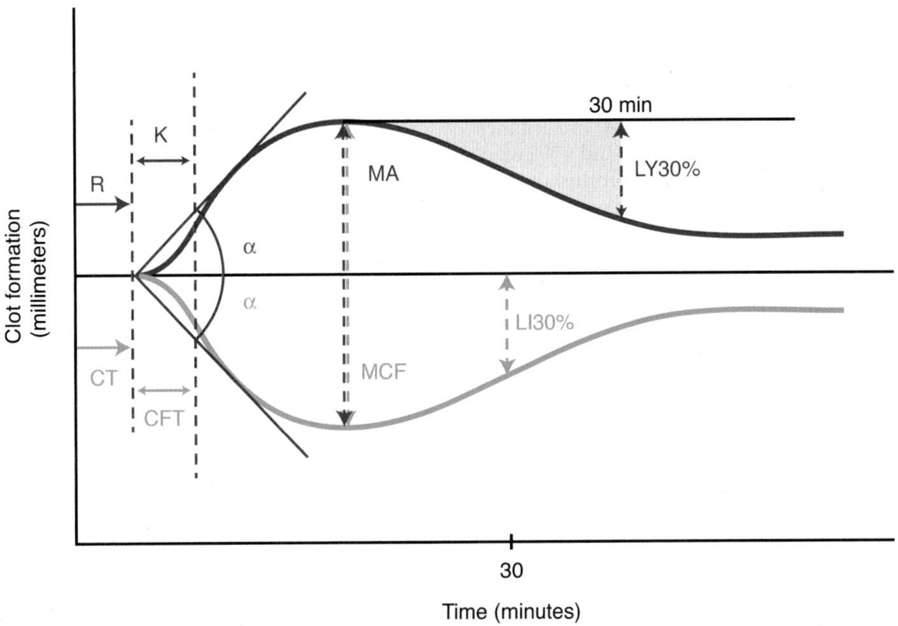

Figure 17-5 Pictorial representation of the different parameters measured by TEG versus ROTEM viscoelastic assays. TEG provides results in terms of R = reaction time and K = clot formation kinetics, α-angle = tangential angle to midline, MA = maximum amplitude indicating clot strength, and LY30 = percent lysis at 30 minutes. ROTEM measures similar metrics with different labels including CT = clot time, CFT = clot formation time, α-angle = tangential angle to midline, MCF = maximum clot formation, and CLI30 = clot lysis index at 30 minutes.

thromboelastometry (ROTEM, Pentapharm GmBH, Munich, Germany).[12] These tests measure the rate of clot initiation, maximum clot strength, and time to lysis using citrated whole blood samples with the potential for point-of-care testing. As opposed to standard coagulation assays such as PT, aPTT, and INR studies, visoelastography provides a more complete assessment of coagulation in vivo, as it assesses the primary and secondary hemostatic pathways in a cell-based format. There are minor differences in the mechanisms and terminology for TEG versus ROTEM (Fig. 17-5); however, both involve the use of whole blood in a heated cup with the addition of a sensor pin. The cup or the pin oscillates while the blood clots. The increasing resistance to oscillation is transmitted through the sensor pin, resulting in a graphic depiction of clot formation. The patterns obtained can implicate defects in factor levels, platelet function, fibrinogen concentration, and/or the presence of abnormal fibrinolysis, the last of which is difficult to measure rapidly otherwise.[12]

Both testing platforms require an activator to initiate clot formation. TEG uses kaolin for standard testing and TF for the rapid TEG point-of-care test. Testing can be performed in the presence of inhibitors of heparin or fibrinolysis to help judge whether these medications would be effective therapies. The ROTEM platform offers several different activators to focus on the extrinsic hemostatic factors (EXTEM test activated by TF and phospholipids), the intrinsic factors (INTEM test activated by ellagic acid), or to differentiate the influence of platelets from fibrinogen with the FIBTEM test (activated with TF accompanied by a platelet inhibitor). These test formats also assess antiplatelet therapy and monitor the effects of anticoagulants including heparin (HEPTEM ROTEM test using a heparinase with ellagic acid), DTIs, and DOACs.[12] Viscoelastic testing is helpful in determining the appropriate therapy, including platelets, plasma, fibrinogen replacement, or antifibrinolytics (APTEM test in ROTEM platform that includes the use of aprotinin), for particularly complex bleeding syndromes such as massive hemorrhage with consumptive or dilutional coagulopathy. Transfusion algorithms using TEG and ROTEM for special circumstances such as trauma-induced coagulopathy are discussed later in this chapter.

Diagnosis of Thromboembolic Disorders

The risk for deep venous thrombosis (DVT), pulmonary embolism (PE), venous thromboembolism (VTE), and other thromboses is increased by intercurrent factors such as physical inactivity or immobilization, malignancy, oral contraceptives, estrogen therapy, and pregnancy. However, in addition to or especially in the absence of such factors, laboratory testing often identifies an underlying congenital or acquired predisposing abnormality that tips the hemostatic systems toward thrombosis. Discovery of one or more risk factors may influence the course of therapy and suggest the benefit of genetic studies.

Congenital Risk Factors for Thrombosis

The most commonly tested congenital problems discussed below increase the risk of VTE.[13] Although arterial thrombosis may involve a few of these factors, platelets are more directly involved on the arterial side, and congenital contributions are less well defined. Some investigators have described a "sticky platelet syndrome," with hyperactive platelet aggregometry. Although severe congenital problems may present in childhood, they are rare; most thrombotic presentations are in adulthood over a lifetime of potential risk. Congenital problems are mostly categorized as deficiencies in antithrombotic pathways or hypercoagulable clotting factors.

Several congenital factors involve the protein C-ase complex and its function. The most common hypercoagulable mutation is factor V Leiden (FVL), in about 5% of Caucasians. FV is the cofactor for FX when the latter activates prothrombin to thrombin. Activated protein C is the natural brake on FV, by cleaving it at Arg506. FVL carries the autosomal dominant mutation

Arg506Gln, rendering FV fairly resistant to APC. Thus, FV is overactive and thrombin formation is favored. The FVL polymorphism is readily identified genetically.[13]

Protein C itself is functionally deficient in up to 0.5% of the population, with autosomal dominant inheritance (NICV 17-1). This leads to overactive FVIII and FV cofactors in their respective intrinsic tenase and prothrombinase complexes. Most have low activity and antigen levels (type I), but some have low activity with normal antigen levels (type II). Homozygous protein C deficiency is a very severe thrombotic disorder beginning in infancy. Protein S deficiency can lead to thrombosis because of its cofactor role to protein C. Around 1 in 700 persons has autosomal dominant deficiency. Protein S circulates partly bound to the complement C4-binding protein and partly as the unbound (free) active form. Nearly all cases of protein S deficiency can be identified by assaying the free antigen and then categorized as to whether the total antigen is low (type I) or normal (type II). Type II is rare.[13] Both protein C and protein S are vitamin K–dependent, and therefore vitamin K deficiency or warfarin interferes with laboratory assessment of their activities. Warfarin-induced skin necrosis in protein C or S deficiencies is discussed in antithrombotic therapy testing below. In AT-III deficiency, the relative lack of its normal blocking function on the key enzymes VIIa, IXa, Xa, and XIa leads to thrombosis risk. Testing for AT-III activity will detect both quantitative (type I) and qualitative defects (type II).[13]

Acquired Risk Factors for Thrombosis

Several factors increase the risk of thrombosis. APLAs are associated with both arterial and venous thrombosis risk and are primarily responsible for the hypercoagulable state associated with antiphospholipid syndrome. These antibodies bind to circulating phospholipid–protein complexes to activate endothelial cells, which in turn may initiate coagulation and/or cause vascular injury. They also interfere with phospholipids in the protein C-ase enzyme complex, leading to diminution of protein C's regulatory function. The various antigenic targets and mechanisms of APLAs require multiple tests for detection. Diagnostic algorithms should include tests of clotting function, most notably LA tests, and studies of solid-phase binding to antigen targets, such as anticardiolipin antibodies (ACLAs) and anti–β_2-glycoprotein-1 (AβGP). AβGP is a protein often present in the phospholipid–protein complex targeted by these antibodies.[14]

LA antibodies are a common cause of prolonged aPTT that does not correct by mixing with normal plasma. It should be emphasized that the prolonged aPTT is a phenomenon of the in vitro test and is NOT associated with bleeding. However, not all LAs prolong the aPTT. Laboratories testing for LA should use at least two different tests to improve sensitivity and specificity, given that the clinical manifestation of antiphospholipid syndrome is varied in both symptom onset and severity of illness. Clinical suspicion should be raised in patients with evidence of venous or arterial thrombosis and a history of miscarriage. Additional clinical signs and symptoms include rash or skin ulcers, thrombocytopenia, hemolytic anemia, heart valve thickening or vegetations, and renal or neurologic complications of vaso-occlusive disease.[14]

ACLA and AβGP antibody tests usually employ enzyme immunoassays (EIAs). AβGP may be more specific for physiologic thrombotic effect, by presenting an actual target of in vivo antibodies, whereas ACLAs may develop in other conditions such as infections. For example, false-positive nontreponemal syphilis serology is sometimes seen with ACLAs.

Hyperhomocysteinemia is a risk factor for venous and possibly arterial thrombosis. This amino acid is made from methionine and is then either converted back or processed to cysteine. The mechanism for thrombosis risk is unclear, but endothelial cell injury has been proposed. Fasting total homocysteine is the initial screening test. Hyperhomocysteinemia can be due to various congenital mutations in homocysteine's metabolic pathways, or can be acquired via vitamin deficiencies affecting its metabolism (folate, B_{12}, B_6) or in many other medical conditions.

Monitoring Anticoagulation Therapeutic Agents

Most anticoagulant therapies need ongoing or selective testing for assessment of therapeutic effect. Appropriate monitoring ensures that these agents are maintained within the therapeutic range; otherwise, patients are at risk for thromboembolism and bleeding complications, which can have devastating consequences.

Warfarin Anticoagulation

Warfarin therapy must be monitored by the PT and its analog for this purpose, the international normalized ratio (INR), to avoid under- or overcoagulation. PT methods and reagents can widely differ between laboratories, yielding varying PT values for the same degree of factor deficiency. However, each PT test vendor supplies a conversion parameter to express the PT as the INR for patients on warfarin. The INR is a normalized value which is intended to compare results across laboratories for evaluating combined deficiencies of factors II, VII, IX, and X, the warfarin-dependent factors. The INR's therapeutic range for warfarin anticoagulation is generally 2.0 to 3.0, but treatment goals may vary depending on the indication for anticoagulation and the risk of bleeding specific to each patient.

When warfarin is started or stopped, the factors with the fastest plasma turnover (i.e., the shortest half-lives) decline or rise the fastest, respectively. Thus, the inhibitor protein C, with a 6-hour half-life, declines faster than most clotting factors as warfarin takes effect. This can cause an imbalance toward clotting during the initiation of warfarin therapy. Warfarin-induced skin necrosis is a thrombotic complication often occurring when previously unrecognized congenital protein C deficiency accentuates this imbalance.

Warfarin's pharmacology is affected by genetic variations in the metabolism of the drug (cytochrome P450, CYP2C9) or its counterbalancing vitamin K (vitamin K epoxide reductase complex subunit 1, VKORC1). The INR is not calibrated to evaluate nonwarfarin deficiencies such as liver disease, which affects most other clotting factors. Thus, the INR is not intended to be used in other conditions, including liver disease.

Heparin Anticoagulation Testing

The aPTT is used to assess heparin anticoagulation. Each laboratory determines its own therapeutic target range for heparin anticoagulation, typically of the order of 1.5 to 2.5 times the normal mean. The laboratory determines the exact range for their test system based on a functional enzymatic test for heparin action, the antifactor Xa activity (aFXa). (This is a different test than the clotting factor X activity level). Using the aFXa assay, therapeutic target heparin levels of 0.3 to 0.7 aFXa units/mL are correlated with aPTT results for that range. In recent years, preference has shifted to using the aFXa testing directly in lieu of aPTT to titrate heparin anticoagulation and assess for heparin resistance.

Low–molecular-weight heparin (LMWH) drugs and their analog, synthetic pentasaccharide (e.g., fondaparinux), do not affect the aPTT assay, and coagulation testing is usually not needed. However, if necessary, the drugs' plasma activity levels can be assessed by aFXa assays calibrated for each drug. This may be helpful in renal failure affecting drug excretion, or in pregnant women, obese patients, and neonates for whom drug levels are less certain after subcutaneous injection. Like heparin, these agents inhibit FXa indirectly via their enhancing effect on antithrombin.

Heparin (and to a lesser degree LMWH) can stimulate the production of antibodies against the heparin–PF4 complex. These heparin-PF4–IgG immune complexes can in turn cause thrombocytopenia and/or activation of platelets to induce thrombosis. Clinical suspicion for HIT should arise with thrombocytopenia or thrombosis after the initiation of heparin therapy. Diagnosis should be based on the clinical criteria established with the "4T-score system" which includes thrombocytopenia, timing of platelet count decline, evidence of thrombosis, and influence of other factors that may contribute to thrombocytopenia.[15] The 4T-score guides further testing for laboratory confirmation of the diagnosis. The specificity of this scoring system approaches 100% for patients with low scores, but its positive predictive value is not sufficient for diagnosis. Should a patient exhibit clinical signs consistent with intermediate or high pretest probability, the ELISA immunoassay and/or functional assays such as the serotonin release assay, should be ordered to identify heparin-PF4 antibodies. Patients with high suspicion of HIT should avoid heparin and heparin products even during the diagnostic process.[15]

Direct Acting Anticoagulant Testing

The direct oral anticoagulants have become widely used alternatives to warfarin. Dabigatran is a DTI, while the other agents in the "xaban" class, including rivaroxaban, edoxaban, apixaban, and betrixaban, directly inhibit factor Xa. Monitoring is not routinely needed for any of these drugs. If drug activity must be assessed, aFXa assays calibrated for each specific drug may be used or quantitative plasma drug concentrations. Dabigatran activity may also be assessed with the dTT or ECT coagulation assays. Although PT and/or PT may be prolonged, these coagulation studies are not reliable indicators of drug effect.[16]

DTIs also pose challenges for coagulation testing. These include hirudin from leeches, its recombinant "-rudin" mimicking molecules (intravenous bivalirudin, desirudin), and small synthetic molecules acting at the same site as hirudin on thrombin (intravenous argatroban, oral dabigatran). They all prolong the PT and aPTT and interfere with clot-based fibrinogen assays. There is no consensus on how to quantify the effect of these drugs. The ECT has been promulgated. In the ECT, ecarin, an enzyme in snake venom, cleaves prothrombin to a metabolic intermediate, which is inhibited by hirudin and its analogs. The dilute thrombin time has also been used. However, neither of these tests are widely available.

Blood Component Production

Blood Collection

The production of blood components is highly controlled by regulations and accreditation requirements in the interests of donor and recipient safety, as well as therapeutic efficacy. Blood donors are carefully screened and tested, and blood products are made in specialized laboratories and regulated facilities. Regional blood centers collect and provide most blood components for transfusion, although some hospitals collect blood or platelets to augment their supply. Virtually all blood components come from volunteer unpaid donors. Pharmaceutical companies process plasma into various derivatives or synthesize some desired proteins for infusion. The most recent publication from the National Blood Collection and Utilization Survey (NBCUS) reports the collection of 11,590,000 units of whole blood and apheresis RBCs in 2019, a 5.1% decline from 2017 collection rates. NBCUS also reports the transfusion rates for RBCs and component therapies with a 2.5% increase in 2019 (10,852,000 units) compared to 2017 (10,654,000 units) transfusion rates.[17] These rates of donor response, donor deferral, collection, and transfusion are closely monitored given the importance of patient blood management (PBM) to overall acute care and hemostasis therapy.

Blood donors undergo a confidential interview to screen for medical problems for their own donation safety, as well as for risks of disease transmission to their recipients. They are questioned about risk factors, exposure, or signs of human immunodeficiency virus (HIV), hepatitis, and other infections. There are geographically based deferral criteria for tropical exposure to malaria. The donor's pulse, blood pressure, and hemoglobin/hematocrit level (US minimum 12.5 g/dL or 38% for women and 13 g/dL or 39% for men) are checked. Phlebotomy is performed with validated antiseptic measures to reduce the risk of bacterial contamination in the blood bags. In the United States, donors are deferred for 8 weeks after a whole-blood donation to avoid iron deficiency.

Table 17-1 shows the contents and storage parameters for blood components. In whole-blood donations, 450 to 500 mL of

Table 17-1 Blood Components

Component	Average Volume	Storage Parameters
Packed red blood cells	300 mL	1°–6°C for 21–35 d or 42 d with additive solution
Red blood cells, frozen	300 mL	< −65°C for 10 yr
Platelets, whole-blood derived	50 mL per bag, usual dose 4–6 bags	20°–24°C for 5 d
Platelets, apheresis	300 mL	20°–24°C for 5 d
Plasma, fresh frozen	250 mL	< −18°C for 1 yr or < −65°C for 7 yr
Plasma, frozen within 24 h	250 mL	< −18°C for 1 yr
Cryoprecipitate	15 mL per bag, usual dose 4–6 bags	< −18°C for 1 yr

blood is collected into citrate anticoagulant and then separated by centrifugation into RBCs, platelets, and/or plasma. The RBC units usually have most plasma removed and replaced with preservative. In the United States, the plasma must be frozen within 6 hours of collection to be labeled fresh frozen plasma (FFP). A large proportion of plasma is now made as plasma frozen within 24 hours, with minimal effect on clotting factor content compared to FFP. Cryoprecipitate is made from barely thawed FFP, which yields a precipitate rich in fibrinogen; the precipitate is isolated by centrifugation and refrozen. Five bags of "cryo" comprise a typical adult dose. Whole-blood–derived platelets (sometimes called "random-donor platelets") are derived from platelet-rich plasma in the United States and from the buffy-coat centrifugation layer in other countries. Four to six units are pooled to yield one adult-sized dose of platelets. Traditionally, pooling was done at the hospital just before transfusion, but blood centers can now provide prepooled platelets to hospitals.

Blood components are also collected by apheresis, in which the donor's blood is processed by ex vivo centrifugation, the desired component(s) are siphoned off into citrate anticoagulant, and the remainder returned to the donor. Most platelets are produced by apheresis (sometimes called single-donor platelets). Plasma and RBCs can also be collected by apheresis, and if the donor's blood volume and cell counts permit, two doses of the desired component can be obtained in one collection session.[18]

All donors are checked against files of deferred donors, and all donations are tested for blood-borne infectious agents. Tests for HIV, hepatitis B virus (HBV), and hepatitis C virus (HCV) are universally required. The addition of sensitive nucleic acid testing (NAT; e.g., polymerase chain reaction) to routine serology shortens the window period in a recently infected donor down to 7 to 10 days for HIV and HCV and 1 month for HBV. The US FDA also requires testing for syphilis, human T-cell lymphotropic virus (HTLV), and West Nile virus (WNV). Also available for donors at risk is a test for *Trypanosoma cruzi* (Chagas disease). Cytomegalovirus (CMV) is found mainly in leukocytes (WBCs). Selected patients at risk for complications of infection from cellular components can receive either CMV-negative units or leukoreduced units.

At some centers, directed donations can be made by family or friends for a specific patient. These donations augment the overall supply of blood and donors, and potentially reduce the number of donor exposures by using the same donor(s) more than once. However, the infectious risk from these units is not considered any less than from community volunteer donors. Cellular components from blood relatives must be irradiated to prevent the risk of transfusion graft-versus-host disease (GVHD) from closely matched donor lymphocytes that are not rejected by the recipient.

Autologous donations by the patient can be made in advance of scheduled surgery, with physician approval. The usual minimum hemoglobin or hematocrit is 11 g/dL or 33%, respectively, which is lower than the minimum allowed for regular donors. Patients should be on erythropoietin or iron supplementation to support RBC replenishment. In order to achieve a net gain in RBC mass, donations should be scheduled with some lead time within the 6-week storage period to permit erythropoiesis before surgery. Erythropoietin assists with multiple donations. Autologous units are only used for the patient and cannot be given to anyone else, since they often have a lower RBC content than normal requirements, and surgical patients frequently have conditions disqualifying them for regular donation. Autologous donations often create iatrogenic anemia with limited efficacy; they are best reserved for patients with difficult crossmatch concerns.

Component Processing and Storage

Leukoreduction (LR) to remove WBCs from RBCs and platelets reduces the risk of several immune-mediated transfusion reactions including human leukocyte antigen (HLA) alloimmunization, febrile nonhemolytic reactions, and viral transmission from intracellular pathogens. The process involves filtration pre- or poststorage for whole blood RBC components or whole-blood–derived platelet packs, but it can also be completed at the time of collection with apheresis donations. Prestorage LR is considered most efficacious as it also minimizes the effects of product storage by reducing the amount of cellular breakdown products and cytokine release from cellular damage. Most whole blood components contain roughly 10^9 WBCs/unit, and LR is expected to reduce the number to less than 5×10^6 WBCs/unit.[19]

In addition to the routine indications above, LR has been studied for the prevention of transfusion-related acute lung injury (TRALI) and the so-called transfusion-related immunomodulation (TRIM)—possible immunosuppressive and proinflammatory effects mediated by donor WBCs. Based on the NBCUS from 2019, over 97% of all RBC, whole blood, and apheresis platelet units were leukoreduced. This treatment is credited with a significant decrease in the incidence of immunologic transfusion reactions.[18]

Washing cellular components with saline is indicated for patients with allergic transfusion reactions such as those who are IgA deficient, or those predisposed to the hyperkalemia associated with PRBC transfusion and not responsive to pretreatment.[19] It should remove >95% of the plasma and plasma proteins, but it does not affect the antigens on the cells and does not remove enough WBCs to prevent GVHD or HLA alloimmunization.

Irradiation of cellular components is performed to prevent transfusion GVHD from directed-donor units from blood relatives, or in highly immunosuppressed patients at risk for this complication because of leukemia, lymphoma, hematopoietic stem cell transplants, congenital cellular immunodeficiencies, and purine analogs such as fludarabine.[19] The units are exposed to gamma irradiation (2,500 cGy) to damage donor WBC DNA and prevent a cellular immune proliferative response to the recipient's tissues. The blood units do not come in contact with the radioisotope and are not radioactive.

Platelets are most commonly stored at room temperature to preserve clotting function, but this increases the risk of bacterial growth in contaminated units, compared to other blood components. Several safety measures were implemented to minimize the risk of contamination during the collection and storage process, including standardized donor skin disinfection, diversion of the first 30 to 40 mL, and more stringent donor screening questions. In addition to mitigation strategies, platelet components are either tested for bacterial contamination during storage to increase screening sensitivity or treated with pathogen reduction processes to inactivate bacteria.[20]

RBC preservation solutions use CPDA—Citrate for anticoagulation, Phosphate as a buffer, 1 to 2 g of Dextrose (D-glucose), and Adenine—to maintain adenosine triphosphate (ATP) levels and RBC membrane integrity. However, despite preservatives, several metabolic changes occur during RBC storage. 2,3–Diphosphoglycerate (2,3–DPG) is depleted in the first 2 weeks, and shifts the oxygen dissociation curve to the left, increasing hemoglobin binding of oxygen (although this reverses after transfusion). Furthermore, by the end of the 42-day shelf life of additive-solution RBCs, the pH is 6.5, the plasma K^+ is 50 mmol/L from RBC leakage and hemolysis, and 15% to 20% of the RBCs are nonviable. RBC storage lesions may be related to observations linking older units to adverse outcomes such as short-term mortality and multiple organ failure. However, randomized trials comparing outcomes with fresher RBCs versus routinely stored RBCs have not shown overall benefit for fresher units in large randomized controlled trials including high-risk critically ill patients.[21]

Plasma Derivatives

12 Plasma derivatives are proteins processed from plasma for therapeutic infusions. They include albumin, immunoglobulins (IGs), clotting factors, and other proteins. Donors for plasma derivatives are screened and tested similarly to blood component donors, and the separation techniques provide a degree of purification from microbial pathogens. However, the large number of donor units that must be pooled together for production of plasma derivatives introduces the possibility of contamination of an entire lot by a small number of infected donors. Such was the case in the early years of HIV when factor concentrates infected a large proportion of hemophiliacs before the risk was known. Because intact cells are not required, many derivatives can undergo purification and pathogen inactivation methods which are impractical for blood components.

Albumin is produced in large quantities for intravascular volume support and is pasteurized at 60°C for sterility. IGs are given for immune support or for immunomodulation to suppress native antibody production. IGs can also withstand robust pathogen inactivation processes, and in some cases are nanofiltered to remove viruses. To be given intravenously, IGs need extra processing to avoid reaction-provoking protein aggregates. Hyperimmune globulins are fractionated from the plasma of donors with high levels of antibody to specific antigens of interest, such as viruses (HBV, CMV, varicella zoster) or the Rh blood group D antigen (RhIG to prevent anti-D formation in RhD-negative women).

Factor concentrates for patients with congenital deficiencies are made with special techniques to ultrapurify factors VIII, IX, X, XIII, vWF, fibrinogen, and in some countries, factor XI, while also applying pathogen inactivation methods and viral filtration to remove microbes. However, recombinant factors VIII, IX, and vWF are also available to further allay concern about disease transmission, and recombinant activated factor VII (rFVIIa) is approved for rare VII-deficient patients. Some hemophiliacs develop inhibitory antibodies to the FVIII or factor IX they are missing. These inhibitor patients often need products that "bypass" their missing clotting step. The therapeutic potential of prothrombin complex concentrates (PCCs) containing multiple factors or rFVIIa to bypass secondary hemostasis and generate a thrombin burst is discussed later in this chapter. On the antithrombotic side of hemostasis, AT concentrate is available.

Other plasma proteins that are purified for selected deficiencies include complement C1 esterase inhibitor (for hereditary angioedema) and α_1-antitrypsin.

RBC and Platelet Substitutes

13 Many years of effort have gone into the search for an oxygen-carrying substitute for RBCs. Most potential substances still require hemoglobin derived from bovine or human sources. Oxygen-avid perfluorocarbon chemicals underwent international trials, but the initial studies demonstrated renal toxicity and immune system inhibition. Active research continues to investigate new derivations. The potential for these artificial oxygen-carrying formulations to eventually contribute to acute patient care remains possible.[22] Several hemoglobin solutions have been made from pools of human or bovine hemoglobin, or from recombinant hemoglobin, all of which were chemically modified to facilitate extracellular O_2 offloading. However, the potentially toxic effects of free hemoglobin, including nephrotoxicity and both systemic and pulmonary hypertension, remain a significant obstacle to ongoing product development. Genetically engineered recombinant hemoglobin affords more potential to replace RBC transfusion given these products offer cell-free functional hemoglobin molecules that do not act as oxygen scavengers, nor do they present any infectious risk for blood born pathogen transmission.[22] There is also active research on a product called "HemeAct" which offers hemoglobin bonded to albumin proteins.[23] This alternative seems to have potential as it has been tested in rats without the hypertensive or coagulopathic side effects commonly seen with other oxygen carriers. Although there are currently no clinically available RBC alternatives, it seems not only possible, but likely that a suitable blood substitute will be offered in the future.

Blood Products and Transfusion Practice

Compatibility Testing

Routine RBC compatibility testing includes ABO and RhD typing, an antibody screen for IgG non-ABO RBC antibodies, and an RBC cross-match (NICV 17-2).[24] RBCs must be ABO compatible to avoid intravascular hemolysis, and RhD-negative patients should receive D-negative RBCs to avoid anti-D alloimmunization. Rh, Kell, Kidd, Duffy, and some other non-ABO antibodies can also hemolyze transfused RBCs; 1% of all patients and 5% to 20% of heavily transfused patients have such antibodies. If no antibodies are present, the cross-match can be electronic; that is, RBC units are selected by the laboratory computer to be ABO and RhD compatible. But if hemolytic antibodies are detected or are on record, RBC units negative for the incompatible antigen(s) must be found, and a serologic cross-match of patient plasma versus donor RBCs is performed to confirm compatibility. Most hospitals have blood order schedules for their most common surgical procedures, which set forth a recommended number of RBC units to cover 80% to 90% of patients undergoing each procedure. 14

RBC compatibility testing takes 45 to 60 minutes, and much longer if antibodies are found. Hence, testing in advance of scheduled surgery is desirable. In emergencies, uncross-matched group O RBCs can be given, albeit with the risk of non-ABO antibody incompatibility. Group AB is the universal donor plasma and avoids transfusing anti-A or anti-B versus the patient's RBCs.

Red Blood Cells

Over the past decade, national and worldwide surveys reported consistent annual declines in blood product usage as the healthcare community embraced more restrictive transfusion strategies and conservative management protocols, with lower thresholds for transfusion and careful consideration of the balance between transfusion risks and the physiologic consequences of anemia. The most recent NBCUS data report the collection and use of blood products throughout the United States in 2019 and report confirm concerns regarding a growing imbalance between the blood supply and ongoing transfusion demands. 2019 showed a 2.5% increase in RBCs transfused since 2017 with a 5.1% decrease in whole blood and apheresis RBC collections.[17] Healthcare systems and blood banks continue to work with PBM programs to 15

Table 17-2 International Society Transfusion Guidelines[19,25–28]

Guideline Sponsoring Society	Asymptomatic ICU Patients	Cardiovascular Disease	Active Bleeding	Other
American Society of Anesthesiologists (ASA), *Anesthesiology 2015*				Restrictive goal: 6–10 g/dL
American Red Cross, *3rd Ed. 2017*	>7 g/dL	>8 g/dL	>7.0 g/dL for hemorrhagic shock	>6–7 g/dL for healthy patients
Pan-European Task Force for Advanced Bleeding Care in Trauma, 5th Ed., *Crit Care 2019*			7.0–9.0 g/dL for severely injured trauma patients	Lack of evidence to support liberal transfusion in TBI
AABB (Former American Association of Blood Banks), *JAMA 2016*	>7 g/dL	>8 g/dL	>8 g/dL for "major orthopedic surgery"	No supportive evidence for higher thresholds with acute neurologic injury
Society of Cardiovascular Anesthesiologists (SCA), *Anesth Analg 2019*		7.5–10.0 g/dL		Acute normovolemic hemodilution may reduce PRBC transfusion

ICU, intensive care unit; TBI, traumatic brain injury.

optimize the use and distribution of the blood supply. As significant users of blood component therapy and leaders in the perioperative management of surgical patients, it is the responsibility of our anesthesia community to learn best practice strategies to mitigate blood loss and transfuse responsibly based on professional guidelines and evidence-based recommendations.

The ASA's most recent publication on the *Practice Guidelines for Perioperative Blood Management* defines restrictive practices as "hemoglobin criteria for transfusion less than 8 g/dL and hematocrit values less than 25%." The ASA recommendations for RBC transfusion thresholds are consistent with the guidelines published by other national and international societies in perioperative management and acute care for trauma and bleeding conditions, whose goals for hemoglobin range between 7 and 10 g/dL (Table 17-2).[25]

There are countless studies comparing liberal versus restrictive transfusion practices for acute anemia; the historically relevant landmark trials include the Transfusion Requirements in Critical Care (TRICC), the Transfusion Requirements After Cardiac Surgery (TRACS) trial, the Functional Outcomes in Cardiovascular Patients Undergoing Surgical hip fracture repair (FOCUS) study, and a randomized controlled trial with patients suffering from acute upper gastrointestinal bleeding.[19] Unfortunately, there is still little evidence to support a clear recommendation for hemoglobin thresholds in patients at high risk of secondary injury and end-organ dysfunction in the setting of acute neurologic injury or traumatic brain injury (TBI) as often these patients are excluded from studies with restrictive transfusion practices. The most recent guidelines from the pan-European multidisciplinary Task Force for Advanced Bleeding Care in Trauma acknowledge the lack of evident to support more liberal transfusion targets specifically for TBI.[26] There are several active trials enrolling patients to answer this question more definitively.

The TRICC trial included critically ill, but euvolemic patients in a large multicenter randomized controlled trial. The investigators compared the survival of patients transfused to hemoglobin levels greater than 10 g/dL in the liberal group, with patients treated under a restrictive strategy with a goal hemoglobin greater than 7 g/dL. Overall survival for more than 800 patients did not differ between the groups. Subsequent subgroup analysis and several meta-analyses and systematic reviews confirmed these results, and established the risks associated with liberal transfusion management for various patient populations, including those less than 55 years old, trauma patients, and those with stable cardiovascular disease.

Historically, patients with cardiovascular disease and anemia were considered to be at significant risk of tissue ischemia and thought to benefit from higher hemoglobin goals in the perioperative and critical care settings. These recommendations were based on two observational studies in the 1990s that showed an association between anemia and mortality that improved with transfusion. Several subsequent studies and systematic reviews have since contradicted these findings by documenting the safety of hematocrits less than 24% during cardiac surgery with cardiopulmonary bypass. The TRACS trial randomized postcardiac surgery patients to restrictive (hematocrit >24%) versus liberal (hematocrit >30%) transfusion strategies and found no difference in 30-day mortality or severe morbidity. Furthermore, transfusion was found to be an independent risk factor for morbidity and mortality in cardiac surgery patients. Accordingly, the most recent guidelines published by the Society for Cardiovascular Anesthesiologists recognize that although cardiac surgery patients are at risk for tissue hypoxia with acute anemia, a restrictive transfusion practice is noninferior and may mitigate morbidity and mortality after cardiac surgery. These most recent guidelines specifically advocate for transfusion at hemoglobin levels between 7.5 and 10.0 g/dL, stating that "an RBC transfusion threshold of Hb ≤7.5 g/dL is clinically reasonable and practical in most cardiac surgery patients."[27]

The noninferiority of restrictive transfusion practice for at-risk patients was again confirmed with the FOCUS trial, which enrolled 2016 patients over 50 years old undergoing hip fracture repair with a history of cardiovascular disease, diabetes, peripheral vascular disease, or smoking. This trial is most influential for reporting functional outcomes in the form of a walking test, in addition to 30- and 60-day mortality and morbidity. The investigators found no difference in outcomes, despite the restrictive group receiving a third of the transfusions, compared to the liberal group, with 59% of patients receiving no RBCs compared to only 3% in the liberal group. Villanueva et al. demonstrated improved mortality and morbidity in the restrictive arm of a study involving patients with active upper gastrointestinal hemorrhage. These authors also showed an association in the liberal group between receiving more RBC transfusions and demonstrating progressive bleeding and poor hemostasis. These large trials in critically ill and perioperative patients confirm the recommendations of the ASA and SCA as well as the AABB, the American Red Cross, and the pan-European Task Force with representatives from multidisciplinary international societies representing anesthesiology, emergency medicine, hemostasis, and thrombosis, as well as the European Society of Intensive Care Medicine (Table 17-2).[19,25–28]

Patients with acute neurologic illness such as ischemic stroke, subarachnoid hemorrhage, and TBI are at significant risk for secondary injury from tissue hypoxia. Acute and chronic anemia both initiate physiologic compensatory mechanisms discussed below, as well as neuroprotective strategies for tolerating decreases in cerebral oxygen delivery at critically low hemoglobin levels between 4 and 5 g/dL, as demonstrated by studies in Jehovah's Witness patients who refuse blood transfusions.[29] The hemoglobin level at which anemia induces detrimental patient outcomes for those with acute neurologic injury remains unclear. Evidence indicates that both hemoglobin levels less than 9 g/dL and RBC transfusion are independently predictive of poor outcome in patients with stroke, cerebral hemorrhage, or TBI.[26] Clinicians have little guidance to decide when and who should be transfused with acute neurologic injury. There are several studies underway that may provide stronger evidence to support a clear transfusion target.

Physiologic Compensation for Anemia

16 There is ample evidence for the human tolerance of both acute and chronic anemia. Oxygen delivery to the tissues (DO_2) is dependent on cardiac output (CO), regional blood flow, and the blood's oxygen-carrying capacity (i.e., oxygen content [CaO_2]). The relationship between these variables and oxygen consumption (VO_2) is shown in Table 17-3. Hemoglobin plays an integral role in oxygen transport and delivery to the tissues. The clinical justification for RBC transfusion assumes that increasing the hemoglobin will improve oxygen-carrying capacity and therefore avoid tissue hypoxia. However, given the ability of the body to compensate for anemia, it is unclear whether increasing hemoglobin in a stable anemic patient improves tissue oxygenation. There are several compensatory mechanisms for anemia, most notably increased CO, altered microcirculatory blood flow, and improved tissue oxygen extraction from hemoglobin.[29] These physiologic changes, together with the detrimental impact of RBC storage limit the therapeutic effects of transfusion.

1. *Increased CO.* There are several mechanisms that increase CO as compensation for isovolemic hemodilution. First, the heart rate increases secondary to a sympathetic surge initiated by anemia and hypoxia. Second, higher stroke volume results from increased preload secondary to decreases in both systemic vascular resistance and afterload. Isovolemic hemodilution occurs when acute blood loss is resuscitated with crystalloid or colloid fluids, thereby maintaining blood volume with a lower hemoglobin. The resultant decrease in blood viscosity reduces shear stress in the microvasculature, which significantly increases flow and venous return. Furthermore, tissue acidosis induces arteriolar vasodilation, thereby decreasing overall afterload.
2. *Altered microcirculatory blood flow.* The decrease in blood viscosity associated with isovolemic hemodilution and chronic anemia improves blood flow through the microcirculation secondary to lower shear force in capillary beds. Furthermore, microcirculatory blood flow increases with dilation of arterioles secondary to the release of NO from endothelial cells in response to tissue hypoxia. NO also induces arteriovenous shunting and recruitment of new circulatory beds, thereby increasing blood flow to ischemic tissue. Patients with chronic anemia also increase angiogenesis and overall microcirculatory blood volume to compensate for the decreased oxygen-carrying capacity. These mechanisms are extremely efficient. In fact, studies in anemic critically ill patients fail to show additional improvements in tissue oxygenation measures after transfusion.
3. *Increased tissue oxygen extraction.* Anemia causes the oxyhemoglobin disassociation curve to shift to the right secondary to increased levels of 2,3–DPG in RBCs. This adaptive process is particularly influential for the physiologic compensation of chronic anemia, and often is the only mechanism necessary to maintain oxygen delivery. Isovolemic hemodilution to hematocrit levels less than 25% generates an increase in 2,3–DPG levels. Furthermore, acidemia associated with acute hemorrhage also shifts the oxygen dissociation curve to the right, thereby decreasing the affinity of oxygen for hemoglobin and improving the tissue oxygen extraction ratio.

There continues to be controversy about RBC transfusion given the lack of evidence to support a universal transfusion threshold. Despite the wealth of literature documenting its potential harm, transfusion continues to be the mainstay of treatment for acute and chronic anemia. Healthy patients are most often able to compensate for anemia and tolerate critically low hemoglobin levels; however, the risk of tissue hypoxia in acute situations or in patients who are unable to compensate remains unclear. As CO increases to compensate for anemia with increased heart rates

Table 17-3 Equations for Tissue Oxygenation

Parameter	Unit	Equation
Oxygen delivery (DO_2)	mL O_2/min	$DO_2 = CO\ (L/min) \times C_aO_2\ (mL/dL)$
Arterial oxygen content (C_aO_2) Venous oxygen content (C_vO_2)	mL O_2/dL	$C_aO_2 = 1.36 \times Hgb\ (g/dL) \times S_aO_2\ (\%) + [P_aO_2 \times 0.003]$ $C_vO_2 = 1.36 \times Hgb\ (g/dL) \times S_vO_2\ (\%) + [P_vO_2 \times 0.003]$
Blood flow, cardiac output (CO)	L/min	Flow = $\pi r^4 \Delta P / 8 \eta L$ (r = radius, ΔP = change in pressure, η = viscosity, and L = length of the vessel)
Oxygen consumption (VO_2)	mL O_2/min	$VO_2 = CO\ (L/min) \times [C_aO_2 - C_vO_2]$
Oxygen extraction ratio (O_2EF)	%	$O_2EF = [C_aO_2 - C_vO_2]/C_aO_2 \times 100\%$ or $= VO_2/DO_2 \times 100\%$

Hgb, hemoglobin; P_aO_2, partial pressure of oxygen in arterial blood; P_vO_2, partial pressure of oxygen in venous blood.

Table 17-4 Clinical Indications of Tissue Hypoxia

- Unstable vital signs
  - Tachycardia
  - Hypotension
  - Tachypnea or dyspnea
- Laboratory and invasive monitor indices
  - Mixed venous O_2 saturation (SV_mO_2) <50%
  - Central venous O_2 saturation (SV_cO_2) <60%
  - Increased O_2 extraction ratio (O_2ER) >50%
  - Lactic acidosis (metabolic acidemia with lactate >2 mmol/L)
- Signs of end-organ dysfunction
  - Electrocardiographic (ST changes, onset of arrhythmias) or echocardiographic indications of myocardial ischemia
  - Electroencephalographic indications of cerebral hypoperfusion
  - New-onset oliguria (less than 0.5 mL/kg/h for >6 h)

and a disproportionate increase in coronary blood flow, the critical hemoglobin level for each patient varies with their amount of cardiovascular reserve and the acute stress of their clinical situation.

Overall, each clinician must consider the patient's comorbidities, the acuity of anemia, and their ability to compensate adequately without signs or symptoms of tissue hypoxia (Table 17-4). Furthermore, it is important to measure the response to transfusion with follow-up hemoglobin levels in order to identify consumptive anemia, hemolysis, or ongoing bleeding as well as to guide further transfusions. In stable patients without ongoing bleeding, the hemoglobin should rise 1 g/dL (approximately 3% rise in hematocrit) for each unit of packed RBCs given.[28]

The above discussion focuses on isovolemic hemodilution secondary to chronic anemia or acute hemorrhage and fluid resuscitation when compensatory mechanisms allow adaptation to the detrimental effects of decreased hemoglobin levels. It is important to recognize that further transfusion may be necessary prior to the availability of measured hemoglobin and hematocrit levels during acute hemorrhage, intraoperative bleeding, or trauma resuscitation. In the case of uncompensated blood loss, hemoglobin levels may be normal or misleadingly high. In these situations, the clinician must estimate blood loss from the patient's hemodynamic picture and assessment of the operative field or severity of hemorrhage shock, in order to guide transfusion management. The AABB guidelines recommend a goal of hemoglobin over 8 g/dL, and the pan-European Task Force recommends a target hemoglobin between 7 and 9 g/dL for the patients with acute hemorrhage.[26,28]

Platelets

Platelet transfusions are indicated for the management of thrombocytopenia and acquired or inherited platelet disorders; with guidance from national and international guideline publications outlining transfusion thresholds and specific indications depending on both quantitative and qualitative measures of platelet activity and the clinical setting. Table 17-5 outlines typical platelet thresholds for transfusion based on the clinical situation and patient history. For stable patients with severe thrombocytopenia, transfusion can be held until counts fall below 10,000 μL, in the absence of signs or symptoms of bleeding.[30] Prophylactic platelet transfusion is necessary for patients with severe thrombocytopenia (below 50,000/μL) who are about to undergo major surgery. There are some minor procedures where the bleeding risk is low enough to tolerate more restrictive transfusion thresholds. For example, lumbar puncture may be performed if the platelet count is >40,000/ μL and central venous catheters can be placed when platelets exceed 20,000/μL.[30] Epidural catheter placement or removal should be supported with platelets >80,000/ μL, and surgery on the eye or the central nervous system requires platelets of at least 100,000/μL. This high platelet goal is also appropriate for critical blood loss with hemorrhage shock, poly-trauma, intracerebral hemorrhage, or TBI. Symptomatic bleeding that is not life-threatening may be managed conservatively with platelet goals of >30,000/ μL, but any patient with significant ongoing blood loss should have a higher transfusion trigger—in excess of 50,000/μL.[30]

Transfusion is not necessary for platelet counts over 100,000/μL in clinically stable patients without suspicion of platelet dysfunction, whereas most patients with counts below 50,000/μL and clinical bleeding require therapeutic transfusion. There are several relative indications for transfusion of platelet counts between 50,000 and 100,000/μL.[19] 17

Platelet transfusion should not be guided by platelet counts alone, but also by the clinical suspicion of platelet dysfunction that can be inherited or acquired. Qualitative dysfunction is often associated with systemic diseases such as uremia, liver failure, and disseminated intravascular coagulopathy (DIC). It also occurs with cardiopulmonary bypass, extracorporeal circulation such as dialysis or plasmapheresis, and as a result of medication side effects (Table 17-6). Regardless of the platelet count, if bleeding is out of proportion to the level of thrombocytopenia, qualitative deficiency should be investigated and treated.

The average dose of platelets is one concentrate from apheresis donation, or a random donor pool of four to six concentrates from whole-blood donations. These "units" generally contain about 5.5×10^{10} platelets in 40 to 70 mL of plasma.[19] Once platelets are given, a posttransfusion response should be followed to guide

Table 17-5 Indications for Platelet Transfusion

Stable patients without evidence of bleeding or coagulopathy	<10,000/μL
Prophylaxis for central venous catheterization	<20,000/μL
Prophylaxis for lumbar puncture	<40,000/μL
Prophylaxis for major surgery	<50,000/μL
Stable patients with clinical evidence of bleeding	<50,000/μL
Prophylaxis for insertion or removal of epidural catheter	<80,000/μL
Patients having surgery at critical sites such as the eye or central nervous system	<100,000/μL
Patients with critical blood loss, acute intracerebral hemorrhage or TBI	<100,000/μL
Microvascular bleeding attributed to platelet dysfunction such as uremia, liver disease, postcardiopulmonary bypass	Clinician judgment

TBI, traumatic brain injury.

Table 17-6 Causes of Acquired Platelet Dysfunction

Uremia
Liver disease
Paraproteinemia (multiple myeloma, Waldenström macroglobulinemia, monoclonal gammopathy, or polyclonal hypergammaglobulinemia)
Myeloproliferative disease
Myelodysplastic syndrome
Disseminated intravascular coagulopathy
Extracorporeal circulation (dialysis, cardiopulmonary bypass, ECMO, plasmapheresis)
Medications (aspirin, NSAIDs, thienopyridines, GPIIb/IIIa antagonists, β-lactam antibiotics, antidepressants, phenothiazines)
Herbal remedies (fish oil, flaxseed oil, ginger, *Ginkgo biloba*, garlic, grape seed extract, saw palmetto, feverfew, bilberry, bromelain)

ECMO, extracorporeal membrane oxygenation; NSAIDs, nonsteroidal anti-inflammatory drugs; GP, glycoprotein.

Table 17-7 Indications for the Use of Plasma Products

- Correction of inherited factor deficiencies when there is no specific factor concentrate (e.g., factor V) and when the PT or aPTT is >1.5 times the mean control or INR >2.0.
- Replacement of multifactor deficiencies with clinical bleeding after transfusion of more than one blood volume (>70 mL/kg) when PT, INR, or aPTT cannot be obtained immediately.
- Correction of acquired multifactor deficiencies with clinical evidence of bleeding or in anticipation of major surgery or an invasive procedure with PT or aPTT >1.5 times the control, or INR >2.0.
  - Liver dysfunction with clinical signs of bleeding.
  - DIC with clinical signs of bleeding.
  - Reversal of vitamin K antagonists (warfarin) *when PCCs are not available.*
  - Heparin resistance secondary to AT deficiency when AT concentrate is not available.
  - Treatment of thrombotic microangiopathies (thrombotic thrombocytopenic purpura, HELLP syndrome, or hemolytic uremic syndrome).
- Treatment of hereditary angioedema when C1–esterase inhibitor is not available.

DIC, disseminated intravascular coagulation; PT, prothrombin time; aPTT, activated partial thromboplastin time; PCCs, prothrombin complex concentrates; AT, antithrombin; HELLP, hemolytic anemia elevated liver enzymes and low platelet count.

further therapy and to rule-out ongoing consumptive pathophysiology. In an average 70-kg adult patient, one unit dose of platelets should increase the platelet count by approximately 25,000 to 60,000/μL.[19] Refractoriness at 20 to 24 hours is generally associated with older platelets or increased consumption secondary to fever, infection, bleeding, or medications. Adjunctive therapy for platelet dysfunction can be established with antifibrinolytics, DDAVP (1–deamino-8–D-arginine vasopressin, desmopressin), or PCCs as discussed later in this chapter.

Plasma Products

Plasma contains all the factors involved in hemostasis. Modern preparations of plasma now include fresh frozen within 8 hours of phlebotomy (FFP), plasma frozen within 24 hours of collection (PF24), or "thawed plasma," which includes units of frozen plasma that have been thawed for more than 24 hours yet remain usable for up to 4 additional days. The preparation and storage method for each formulation involves either separation from whole blood or apheresis; both maintain normal levels of stable factors and at least 70% normal levels of labile factors such as FVIII and FV. Prior to use, each unit must be thawed at 30° to 37°C, but can be stored at 4° ± 2°C for up to 24 hours as thawed FFP or 5 days as thawed plasma.[19] Throughout this chapter, the inclusive term, "plasma" will be used for FFP, PF24, and thawed plasma unless otherwise specified. During preparation and distribution, care must be taken to ensure ABO compatibility for plasma transfusion to avoid transfusion of donor anti-A and anti-B antibodies that may lead to hemolysis.[31]

Plasma is indicated for the treatment of coagulopathy secondary to congenital or acquired factor deficiencies. The specific indications for plasma products outlined in Table 17-7 are based on one of the most recent guidelines from the ASA, BSH, and the American Red Cross.[19,25,31] The initial therapeutic dose of plasma is 10 to 20 mL/kg in an effort to obtain at least 30% factor activity. Repeat dosing is guided by serial diagnostic coagulation tests such as the PT, INR, aPTT, and thromboelastography. Recent updates to these guidelines emphasize key practice points in their recommendations against the use of plasma prophylactically for patients with elevated clotting times, but without clinical evidence of bleeding. Systematic reviews fail to demonstrate the efficacy of prophylactic plasma to reduce RBC transfusion, morbidity, or mortality, especially when given to patients with mild derangements in PT, INR (1.5–1.9), or aPTT and no clinical signs of bleeding.[31] The administration of plasma carries risks of several transfusion reactions, most notably TRALI, allergic reactions, and transfusion-associated circulatory overload (TACO). Together with limited prophylactic benefits and ongoing risks for transfusion associated adverse events, plasma remains the product with the highest frequency of inappropriate use.

Over the past decade there has been continuous debate over "damage control" resuscitation protocols for trauma patients with major bleeding. Historically, trauma patients were resuscitated first with fluid and RBCs, and only received plasma based on the results of coagulation tests. This approach perpetuates dilutional coagulopathy, acute anemia, and prolonged microvascular bleeding, especially when long turn-around-time coagulation assays are used to assess hemostasis. Several observational studies originally showed improved outcomes with higher ratios of plasma to RBC units (more than 2:3) and with transfusion protocols that provide a balanced ratio of platelets, plasma coagulation factors, and RBCs. However, these retrospective studies limited the strength of their conclusions given the likelihood of results confounded by injury severity and "survivor bias" that occurs when patients die of massive hemorrhage before plasma can be thawed and transfused.

Two large prospective multicenter trials—the Prospective, Observational, Multicenter Major Trauma Transfusion

(PROMMTT) trial and the Pragmatic, Randomized Optimal Platelets, and Plasma Ratios (PROPPR)[32] trial—were both designed to definitively answer the question of whether fixed ratio transfusion protocols for trauma resuscitation can improve patient outcomes. Both trials demonstrated the feasibility of providing patients with thawed plasma in a timely manner, although this practice significantly increases the wastage rate. When plasma resuscitation is delayed, patients are at increased risk of hemorrhagic shock and death, supporting one trauma society's recommendations that Level I trauma centers have thawed universal donor plasma available. However, neither trial demonstrated a survival benefit at either 24 hours or 30 days for patients receiving a higher ratio of platelets to plasma to RBCs (1:1:1 vs. 1:1:2).[32] Those with the higher ratio of plasma were less likely to expire secondary to exsanguination at 6 hours; however, overall mortality at 24 hours and 30 days did not differ between groups and most commonly resulted from TBI, sepsis, and multiorgan system failure. Furthermore, the intervention group of the PROPPR trial that received higher ratios of plasma also received platelets as the first blood product immediately administered upon randomization. Post-hoc studies hypothesize this additional variable in the study design may have contributed to early hemostasis. Accordingly, the most recent update to the guidelines from the pan-European task force for Advanced Bleeding Care in Trauma recommend using fixed ratios of plasma:RBC of at least 1:2 for resuscitation of massive hemorrhage only until goal-directed PBM strategies can be prescribed based on coagulation profile assay results.[26]

Cryoprecipitate

18 Cryoprecipitate is created by a controlled thaw of FFP, which allows for precipitation of large molecules. It is then centrifuged, the supernatant removed, and the final product resuspended in 5 to 20 mL of plasma, containing concentrated doses of fibrinogen (at least 150 mg/unit), fibronectin, vWF, FVIII, and FXIII. Small concentrates from each FFP unit are typically combined for a single adult dose from five pools and refrozen at –18°C for up to 12 months.[19] Current use of cryoprecipitate is limited to a few countries (United States and Canada) and generally only indicated for critical bleeding with evidence of hypofibrinogenemia (Table 17-8).[19,25,26] Compared to plasma, cryoprecipitate contains more fibrinogen per volume and therefore functions as a low-volume alternative for fibrinogen replacement, especially during acquired hypofibrinogenemia states such as DIC and massive hemorrhage. Consensus from various guidelines recommends conservative goals with fibrinogen targets of only 50 to 80 mg/dL in nonbleeding patients, and the use of cryoprecipitate to achieve fibrinogen concentrations of at least 150 mg/dL in the setting of acute major bleeding. Critical blood loss associated with obstetric hemorrhage at the time of delivery should be treated more aggressively with target fibrinogen concentrations of 150 to 200 mg/dL.[5,25,26] It carries similar transfusion risks as plasma, and consequently has been replaced in several countries, including in Europe, with fibrinogen concentrates that can be virally inactivated.

Table 17-8 Indications for Fibrinogen Replacement

- Acute bleeding with hypofibrinogenemia
  - DIC with fibrinogen <150 mg/dL
  - Hemorrhage or massive transfusion with fibrinogen <150 mg/dL
  - Obstetric hemorrhage at the time of delivery with fibrinogen <150–200 mg/dL
- Prophylaxis for patients without acute bleeding with fibrinogen <50–80 mg/dL
- Prophylaxis in patients with hemophilia A and vWD (if specific factor concentrates are unavailable or ineffective due to inhibitors)
- Prophylaxis for patients with congenital dysfibrinogenemias

DIC, disseminated intravascular coagulation; vWD, von Willebrand disease.

Fibrinogen Concentrate

Fibrinogen concentrates are derived from plasma after several steps of viral inactivation that also minimize antibodies and antigens to produce a lyophilized powder formulation that can be stored at room temperature and reconstituted for administration in less than 10 minutes. They are used frequently around the world as a safe, low-volume alternative to cryoprecipitate, but are only approved by the FDA for the treatment of bleeding patients with congenital hypofibrinogenemia. Fibrinogen is primarily responsible for clot stabilization, but it also assists with platelet activation and aggregation and, at adequate concentrations, may compensate for low thrombin states.[5] With growing concern for the scarcity of the blood supply, many blood management protocols and transfusions experts consider fibrinogen concentrates an alternative to cryoprecipitate for treatment of critical bleeding and massive hemorrhage.[26]

Emerging Blood Products

Low-titer group O whole blood (LTOWB) can be used for emergency transfusions in bleeding patients, providing RBCs, plasma, and platelets in one product. It is stored at 1 to 6°C for up to 14 to 21 days to preserve some platelet function. To reduce the risk of hemolysis from the anti-A and anti-B in group O plasma, donors are screened to exclude those with high IgM anti-A and anti-B; titer cutoffs of 50 to 200 are used. Blood collection facilities also have varying practices regarding whether these units are leukoreduced (using filters which preserve platelets) and whether D-negative RBCs are available for women of childbearing age. Their short shelf-life makes inventory management challenging, but a growing number of trauma centers are using LTOWB.[33]

Cold-stored platelets (CSPs) are under investigation for bleeding patients. Cold temperatures activate platelets. Although they do not circulate very long, in vitro testing and early clinical evaluations suggest they may be useful for bleeding patients with low or dysfunctional platelets. Storage at 1° to 6°C for up to 10 to 14 days would provide a more flexible inventory for hospitals which maintain a small stock of platelets for emergency use. Interest in CSP has also been enhanced by concerns about bacterial growth in platelets stored at 20° to 24°C. Clinical trials in cardiac surgery and trauma are in progress.[34]

The Risks of Blood Product Administration

According to the 2019 update from the National Blood Collec- 19
tion and Utilization Survey, over 17 million blood products are transfused annually throughout the United States.[17] The Center for Disease Control and Prevention (CDC)-supported Hemovigilance Module of the National Healthcare Safety Network (NHSN) has growing participation from transfusion centers and hospitals nationwide. Data from fiscal years 2013 to 2018 published in the most recent report suggest that the overall risk of a transfusion reaction is approximately 220 per 100,000 components with 9%

of reactions, infectious and noninfectious, being severe or life-threatening.[35] This NHSN data use a representative sample from participating transfusion centers across the country. Similar rates of adverse events associated with transfusion were reported by the US FDA and the United Kingdom's Serious Hazards of Transfusion (SHOT) annual reports.[36,37] The SHOT report highlights a risk of death over the last decade to approximate 0.92/100,000 products transfused.[37] Advances in pathogen reduction techniques and safe storage strategies minimized the impact of transfusion transmitted infections and immune-mediated noninfectious adverse reactions. The most recent data report that human errors of clerical nature, miscommunication, delays in care, or overtransfusion are now the most common causes of serious adverse events associated with transfusion.[35–37]

National hemovigilance networks worldwide suspect both underreporting of transfusion reactions and avoidable morbidity and mortality secondary to clerical errors or inadequate clinical evaluation of patients with hemorrhage, or those undergoing blood product transfusion. Patients receiving blood component therapy should be continuously monitored for fever, hypotension, and cardiopulmonary complications. Mild fever with or without pruritus or rash is still the most common reaction, and can be treated symptomatically with antihistamines or antipyretics. In the event of a more severe fever (≥39°C, or ≥2°C rise in temperature) with constitutional symptoms (e.g., rigors, myalgia, nausea, vomiting, or diaphoresis), transfusion should be halted and the product returned to the blood bank for retesting of compatibility and antibodies. Sepsis (underlying or resulting from blood products) should be ruled out if fever is persistent. Pulmonary symptoms during or acutely related to transfusion should be investigated for transfusion-associated dyspnea (TAD), TRALI, TACO), or anaphylaxis. Typically, acute hemolytic reactions will involve hypotension, shock, and cardiopulmonary collapse. Transfusion should not be discontinued if shock symptoms are likely secondary to hemorrhage.

Infectious Risks of Blood Product Administration

In the mid-1980s, the realization of transfusion-transmissible infections such as HIV and hepatitis raised concerns about the infectious risks of blood product administration. Since the introduction of Nucleic Acid Amplification Testing (NAT) for major transfusion-transmittable viral infections (HCV in 2000, HIV in 2003, and HBV in 2006), the risk of infection from blood product transfusion has decreased substantially. Prior to the institution of NAT, the blood supply was simply tested for the presence of viral antibodies. This left a long window period when the blood was potentially infectious, but with insufficient time for the donor to mount an antibody response detectable by conventional testing. NAT increased the sensitivity of donor screening by testing for the presence of specific viral DNA or RNA. This significantly shortened the window period between when a donor gets infected and when the viral load is detectable. The residual risk of transfusion-transmitted infections now depends mostly on the length of this window period, relative to the reproductive rate of each virus and the prevalence of the disease. There are additional risks of false negatives NATs or the mistaken release of quarantined blood products; however, these events account for less than 0.5% of the residual risk of transfusion-transmitted viral infection.

The reported incidence of transfusion-transmittable infections is quite low, with <1% reported in the most recent published data from 2013 to 2018 NHSN data.[35] Transmission depends not only on the variability of donor response to pathogen inoculation, but also the immune state of the recipient. The residual risk can still be mathematically modeled from the prevalence of infection in donors and the known window period of each viral illness. The estimated residual risk of major viral infection and the viral-specific window periods are shown in Table 17-9, based on the reported incidence of infection in donors for the American Red Cross Blood Services. These residual risks are likely overestimates,

Table 17-9 Residual Risk of Transfusion-Transmitted Infections[36–39]

Infection	Residual Risk	Window Period and Comments
Viral Infections		
Human immunodeficiency virus (HIV)	1/2,300,000	7–10-d window
Hepatitis C (HCV)	1/2,600,000	7–8-d window
Hepatitis B (HBV)	1/1,500,000	18–38-d window
West Nile virus (WNV)	Rare	13 cases reported since 2003
Cytomegalovirus (CMV)—all donors	1–3%	
Leukoreduced products	0.023%	
Emerging infections	Rare	Incidence is too small to estimate
Chagas and malaria		Donor screening limits risk in the United States
Creutzfeldt–Jakob (vCJD)		Incubation for years
Babesia species		Testing required in states where endemic
Parvovirus (B19v)		May cause aplastic anemia in immunosuppressed patients
Bacterial Contamination—all types	1/3,000	
Packed red blood cells	1/250,000–1/10 million	Lower risk than platelet concentrates
Platelets	1/20,000	Apheresis decreases risk

since not all transfusions of known infected blood products result in recipient infection. The estimates assume 100% infectivity with even one infectious unit of viral particles per blood bag. It also presumes that the collection and storage process is harmless to viral reproduction. Furthermore, viral infectivity will vary depending on the acute phase of infection when an immunocompetent recipient could resist transmission or the chronic phase of infection when antibodies are present and reduce infectivity.[37]

Transfusion-transmitted viral infections traditionally receive the most attention from patients due to their associated morbidity and mortality. Despite increased awareness and public health initiatives, the prevalence of HIV and HCV in the donor population perseveres secondary to prolonged survival of patients, making the prevalence of HIV and HCV in the general population higher. Contrary to HIV and HCV, the prevalence of HBV has decreased since 1999 presumably due to high vaccination rates. Overall, the prevalence of disease in the general population is now the largest determinant of transfusion-transmittable infection risk. Many patients inquire about directed donations from family and friends. They should be made aware of the stringent processes for random donor screening for infectious risk factors, as well as the ongoing prevalence of viral infections—especially HCV and HBV—in directed donations.

Human Immunodeficiency Virus

As a retrovirus, HIV is transmitted as RNA and requires translation into DNA prior to replication. This virus was highly transmittable in the U.S. blood supply until sensitive NAT and donor screening became available. The incidence of transfusion transmission of HIV was as high as 1 in every 100 donations in the early 1980s, but only 1 in every 400,000 donations in 1997. The estimated residual risk of HIV has fallen to 0.04 per million blood product donations or 1:2.3 million donations.[38] The SHOT annual report form 2021 claims that with 1.9 million blood collections every year, the current screening and testing strategy may miss a potentially infectious donation once every 14 years.[37] However, despite a short window period of 8 to 10 days, the residual risk of HIV transmission via blood supply is expected to persist secondary to increased prevalence of HIV in the general population due to improved treatments and prolonged survival.[38]

Hepatitis C Virus

Although HCV is rarer than the other types of transmittable hepatitis and has a relatively benign acute phase, it progresses to chronic carrier state in up to 80% to 85% of infections and is associated with significant risk of fulminant hepatic failure, cirrhosis, hepatocellular carcinoma, and death.[4] Similar to HIV, the transfusion risk of HCV decreased drastically with the increased sensitivity of NAT testing and donor screening. However, the prevalence of donor HCV increased over the past 5 to 7 years due to increases in both incidence and prevalence in the general population. Furthermore, HCV infections become more aggressive and transmittable in patients coinfected with HIV due to the increased viral load that results from immunosuppression, but donor testing remains robust with a short window period of just 7 to 8 days to detect seroconversion in donors.[38] The latest data from SHOT report a prevalence of 0.02 per million collected donations, with a risk of possible transmission once every 22 years.[37] Data from the American Red Cross and the Transfusion Transmissible Infections Monitoring System (TTIMS) report a risk of 1:2.6 million donations.[38]

Hepatitis B Virus

HBV is a common blood-borne pathogen with fairly high incidence of infection in the general population and over 300 million carriers worldwide. The acute infection associated with HBV is asymptomatic in most patients, or limited to mild constitutional signs and jaundice. Rarely, however, it can progress to fulminant hepatic failure. The residual risk of transfusion-transmitted HBV remains high at an estimated rate of 0.81 per million donations according to the SHOT annual report and 1:1.5 million donors per the TTIMS.[38] This translates to a risk of transfusion-transmitted infection once every 6 months according to mathematical models.[37] Given the long window period for identifying donors with seroconversion or acute infection, transfusion risk will remain higher than other viral illnesses. However global health efforts to reduce HBV prevalence using the HBV vaccine have been highly successful.

Human T-Cell Lymphotropic Virus-1 and Virus-2

HTLV-1 causes T-cell leukemia and lymphoma, or HTLV-associated myelopathy in a small percentage of infected persons. HTLV-2 does not have any significant consequences for immunocompetent or even HIV-coinfected patients. Regardless of the relatively infrequent disease association with HTLV, the US blood supply is routinely tested for anti-HTLV antibodies indicative of previous infection as asymptomatic donors can transmit the virus.[39] Given that HTLV is cell associated, the transmission risk via transfusion may be eradicated with LR.

Cytomegalovirus

CMV is ubiquitous in the general population and thus, it was previously considered the most common transfusion-transmitted infection. In immunocompetent recipients the infection is often asymptomatic or mild and self-limited. However, in immunocompromised patients—in particular, neonates, patients with HIV, and transplant recipients—the disease can be associated with severe multiorgan system failure involving the liver, lungs, kidneys, hematologic system, gastrointestinal tract, and the central nervous system. The CMV virus is carried by white blood cells and transmitted via CMV-seropositive cellular components. LR decreases the infectivity of CMV-positive donor products, but has not completely eradicated the transfusion transmission of CMV. Therefore, it is recommended that patients at highest risk for CMV infection, continue to receive LR blood products from CMV-seronegative–only donors.[40]

Emerging Infections

HIV remains the most historically noteworthy microbe to infect the blood supply. Several pathogens have also emerged through changes in ecologic and geographic factors such as travel, climate change, or new insect and animal vectors. Other examples of a significant new transfusion-transmissible infection include the WNV, a mosquito-borne flavivirus that emerged in 1999. WNV causes only a mild febrile illness in healthy patients, but may progress to encephalitis or meningitis in immunosuppressed patients. The peak of the WNV epidemic occurred in 2002 to 2003, with 23 transfusion-transmitted illnesses that year. However, since the institution of donor screening with NAT testing in 2003, the incidence of transfusion-transmitted WNV has dropped to only 13 reported cases since 2003, 12 of which reported false-negative testing results and one transmission without donor unit testing.[39] Surveillance studies continue to investigate the virulence of various strains of WNV worldwide and the ability of the current NAT test to recognize seroconversion in donors.

A few other pathogens have been red flagged by the FDA as potential threats to the safety of the US blood supply. Most concerning are human vCJD, *Babesia* species, Chagas, parvovirus B19, and the *Plasmodium* species, which causes malaria.[39] vCJD is the human form of bovine spongiform encephalitis. It results in fatal degenerative neurologic disease secondary to prion proteins that precipitate an abnormal formation and structure of other proteins. It gained attention after an epidemic of cases in the 1980s to 1990s throughout the United Kingdom. Thus far, there have been three cases of confirmed transfusion-transmitted vCJD. There are no known effective treatments, and the incubation period is reported in years. Currently no testing regimens exist for diagnosis of prion disease in donors or collected blood. However, in the absence of any further transfusion cases for several years, the FDA recently rescinded donor deferrals for long-term residence in vCJD regions. The incidence and infectivity of other viral and parasitic pathogens is so rare that they do not warrant a careful discussion here. Thus far, the SARS-CoV-2 virus has not caused any known cases of transmission via blood product transfusion; it is important to remember that there may be emerging infections that are yet unrecognized, leaving the blood supply at constant risk. Western countries continue to evaluate the risk–benefit ratios and ethical cost considerations for screening tests and donor deferral questions, with the knowledge that testing to ensure 100% sensitivity is highly unlikely and adds significant costs.

Bacterial Contamination

Despite significant public concern for transfusion-transmitted viral disease, bacterial contamination of blood components poses the largest risk of transfusion-related infection and mortality outweighing the total risk from all known viruses combined.[39] Frequent pathogens implicated in bacterial contamination of blood products stem from skin flora, including *Staphylococcus* and *Bacillus* species, but gram-negative species such as *Escherichia coli*, *Enterobacter cloacae*, and especially *Yersinia enterocolitica* more frequently lead to sepsis given the higher tolerance for cold storage.[39] Platelet concentrates still carry the highest risk of bacterial contamination, since they are stored at 20° to 24°C, which provides a more suitable environment for the exponential bacterial replication to occur over 4 to 5 days in storage. The risks were as high as 1 in 1,000 to 2,000 platelet units possibly contaminated prior to the widespread implementation of pathogen reduction techniques. More recent estimates approximate the risk of bacterial contamination to be 1 in every 20,000 platelet units transfused.[39]

Some of the methods aimed at reducing the risk of transfusion-transmitted bacterial infections include apheresis collections, which are associated with less contamination than platelet concentrates from pooled units, likely due to fewer venipunctures and exposures to skin flora, and to collection processes. Secondly, it is now standard practice to divert the first 20 to 40 mL of collected blood into a separate collection chamber to avoid contaminating the whole donation with blood and epidermal tissue from the initial venipuncture. Standards for skin preparation prior to blood donation and sterile techniques for collection and processing procedures have also decreased contaminants. Furthermore, all apheresis platelets are culture tested prior to storage.[41] Traditional testing of platelet products in the United States relied on indirect testing of pH, glucose, and platelet morphology. As new methodologies such as automated cultures and rapid immunoassays become more widely implemented, the sensitivity for detecting contamination increases; however, a residual risk of bacterial transmission remains. New techniques for pathogen reduction have become widely implemented at blood centers around the world with the goal of extending safe platelet storage while mitigating the risks of contamination.[41]

Noninfectious Risks of Blood Product Administration

20 Given the extensive use of more sensitive methods for screening and controlling the infectious risks of blood product transfusion, noninfectious complications have emerged as the major source of transfusion-related morbidity and mortality. Table 17-10 summarizes the relative incidences and main features of the most common and concerning noninfectious risks of blood product administration.

Immune-Mediated Transfusion Reactions

Febrile Nonhemolytic Transfusion Reactions

Allergic and febrile reactions are the most common complications of transfused blood products, although the incidence of both has decreased with widespread use of LR products. FNHTRs classically present within 4 hours of transfusion with fever (documented at ≥38°C or an increase in temperature of ≥1°C) and may be associated with chills, rigors, and headache. They are typically self-limited, but can be prevented or treated with anti-inflammatory or antipyretic medications. The pathophysiology of FNHTRs involves recipient alloimmunization to HLAs from donor WBCs and the release of leukocyte-derived cytokines accumulated in the donor product during storage.[39] As a result, the risk of febrile reactions increases with repetitive transfusions. Prior to the widespread institution of LR, the incidence of FNHTR was as high as 30%, but currently it is between 0.01% and 1%.[39] Although these reactions are common, more serious adverse effects of transfusion, such as sepsis, anaphylaxis, and hemolysis may also present with fever, and should be ruled out prior to diagnosing an FNHTR.

Allergic Reactions

Minor allergic reactions, a relatively common type of transfusion reaction, occur in about 2% of transfusions, although the risk is much higher with platelet and plasma components. Symptoms are most commonly described as urticaria, hives with or without pruritus, and angioedema. The specific cause of allergic reactions is unclear, but likely involves an immune response to recipient WBC antigens or transfused plasma proteins. Prophylaxis with antihistamines is common practice for patients with a history of allergic reactions to blood products, but several studies have demonstrated no symptom reduction with pretreatment.[39] Best practice should be to reduce the rate of transfusion and treat supportively when symptoms arise. If symptoms become severe with recurrent or frequent transfusion needs, cellular products can be washed.

Major allergic reactions present as anaphylactoid or anaphylactic reactions with hemodynamic instability, bronchospasm, rash, flushing, and/or angioedema. These reactions are rare, but the reaction can be fatal if unrecognized. Pathophysiologically, the recipient—typically patients who are IgA deficient with anti-IgA antibodies or with anti-haptoglobulin or anti-C4 antibodies—mounts an immediate immune response to transfused plasma proteins or cellular antigens.[39] Classically, anaphylaxis requires an immediate type I hypersensitivity IgE-mediated reaction; however, most major allergic responses to blood transfusions do not show laboratory evidence of IgE antibodies, and are therefore anaphylactoid reactions. These transfusion complications can be mitigated in patients with known IgA deficiency or history of allergic reaction by washing blood products prior to transfusion or by using products obtained from IgA-deficient donors.

Acute hemolytic transfusion reactions (AHTRs) are rare, but carry a significant risk of mortality when they occur. They result from the transfusion of incompatible blood products when preexisting IgM or IgG antibodies in recipients form complexes with donor RBC antigens, causing complement activation and immediate intravascular hemolysis. Classically, AHTRs result from ABO incompatibility secondary to native anti-A or anti-B IgM. Careful

Table 17-10 Noninfectious Transfusion Reactions[24,36,37,39]

Adverse Reaction	Incidence	Notes
Immune-mediated Reactions		
Febrile nonhemolytic transfusion reaction	0.1–1%	Most common type of transfusion reaction
Minor allergic reactions (urticaria, flushing)	1–3%	
Anaphylactic/toid reactions		IgA deficiency increases risk
Packed red blood cells	0.5/100,000	Washing may avoid reaction
Fresh frozen plasma and platelets	2–3/100,000	More prevalent with plasma-containing products
Acute hemolytic transfusion reaction (AHTR)	1/70,000	
Delayed hemolytic transfusion reaction (DHTR)	1/2,500	Associated with alloantibodies to minor RBC antigens, Kidd, or Rh; one-third have clinical reaction
Transfusion-related immunomodulation (TRIM)	100%	
Alloimmunization	2–4%	For all patients, risk increases to 35–80% for patients who require chronic transfusion
Transfusion-related acute lung injury (TRALI)	1/10,000	Varies with blood product component and patient population
Graft-versus-host disease (TA-GVHD)	Rare	high fatality rate; reduced risk with irradiation
Posttransfusion purpura (PTP)	Rare	Attributed to antihuman platelet antigen-1a
Reactions Related to Patient Comorbidities or Transfusion Practice		
Transfusion-associated circulatory overload (TACO)	1–2.7%	Higher in patients with CHF and CRI
Transfusion Associate Dyspnea (TAD) Hyperkalemia Citrate toxicity Iron overload Hypothermia		

Frequencies are presented as percentages when >0.1% and otherwise as ratios.
IgA, immunoglobulin A; CHF, congestive heart failure; CRI, chronic renal insufficiency.

adherence to protocols for specimen phlebotomy and blood component administration is vital for prevention. However, growing evidence exists for the implication of other RBC antigens such as Kidd, Kell, and Duffy, causing acute hemolytic reactions in patients with a history of transfusion exposure and alloimmunization. Rarely, the transfusion of incompatible platelets or plasma (type O plasma or whole blood to a patient with type A, B, or AB blood) has resulted in AHTRs as well.[39] These reactions are rare and have become less frequent with the institution of safety measures to reduce clerical error and improve the availability of crossmatched blood products, but AHTR still accounted for 4% of transfusion-associated mortality in the most recent national surveillance database describing incidence from 2013 to 2018, and 7% to 9% of transfusion-related fatalities in the FDA report for fiscal years FY16–FY20.[35,36] Fortunately, less than half of patients transfused with incompatible blood products become symptomatic. The overall fatality rate from incompatible transfusion is high, but is significantly dependent on the volume transfused

AHTRs occur secondary to IgM-mediated antibody–antigen complexes that activate complement and result in intravascular and extravascular hemolysis in the spleen and liver. The release of bradykinin causes fever, hypotension, and hemodynamic instability, while histamine release from mast cells leads to bronchospasm and urticaria, as well as symptoms of dyspnea, flushing, and severe anxiety. Hemolysis results in the release of free hemoglobin that is bound by haptoglobin and plasma proteins, but will also be eliminated by the kidney when these proteins are unavailable. Severe hemolysis may lead to renal failure, DIC, and death. General anesthesia can mask several of the presenting symptoms of AHTRs such as back or flank pain, fever and chills; therefore, vigilance during transfusion of an anesthetized patient must remain high, as survival depends on discontinuing the transfusion.[39]

The diagnosis of hemolytic reactions is confirmed with laboratory findings of elevated lactate dehydrogenase, low haptoglobin, bilirubin increases, a positive direct antiglobulin (Coombs) test, and hematuria. Suspicion of a transfusion reaction should prompt immediate discontinuation of the transfusion, and investigation into the donor and recipient blood types and antigen–antibody components. Treatment of AHTR involves supportive care for hemodynamic instability and microvascular bleeding, as well as maintenance of adequate urine output to avoid renal failure associated with hemaglobinuria.[39]

Delayed hemolytic transfusion reactions (DHTRs) result from passive transfusion of RBC antibodies to native antigens in the recipient, or more commonly, alloantibodies in the recipient to minor RBC antigens in the Rh, Kell, Kidd, Duffy, MNSs, and other blood groups. DHTRs generally present 3 to 10 days after transfusion of an apparently "compatible" blood component. Typically, the recipient has IgG alloantibodies to a particular RBC antigen, and will mount an amnestic immune response; however, the pretransfusion antibody levels are too low for serologic detection. Symptoms of DHTRs are much milder than AHTRs and rarely result in major morbidity or mortality because the hemolysis occurs extravascularly in the reticuloendothelial system, liver, and spleen. Patients experience mild constitutional symptoms, with laboratory signs of hemolysis such as jaundice, hemaglobinuria, low haptoglobin, positive direct Coombs test, and acute anemia. The incidence of DHTRs is likely underreported as symptoms are subtle and may be attributed to the patient's underlying systemic illness. The reported incidence estimates 1 in 2,500 product transfusions may cause DHTR, with risks much higher in patients who require frequent transfusion (e.g., 11% of transfusions in patients with sickle cell disease).[39] Symptoms are generally self-limited and treated supportively with hydration to protect the renal tubules during hemolysis, and further compatible transfusions to support anemia as indicated.

Transfusion-Related Immunomodulation

In the 1970s, transfusion-related immunomodulation (TRIM) was discovered from improved survival of renal allografts in patients who had received a transfusion pretransplant. This highlighted the potential immunosuppressant effects of stored allogeneic blood products. However, these beneficial effects are patient-specific. Immunosuppression also proved to increase the recurrence of malignancies for patients undergoing cancer surgery and the incidence of serious health-care–associated infections after perioperative allogenic blood transfusions.[42]

Recent studies clarified the multifactorial mechanisms for immunomodulation after allogenic blood transfusion, implicating transfused WBCs, donor plasma HLA class 1 peptides, cytokines, and immune mediators released during blood product storage leading to an increase in CD4 cells, a decrease in the overall CD4/CD8 T cell ratio, and inhibition of natural killer cells and lymphocytes.[42] Several experts have also proposed a "two-insult" model for TRIM. Presumably, most patients requiring blood products are suffering from a precondition that "primes" both the immune system and vascular endothelium (e.g., trauma, surgery, or acute illness). This constitutes the first insult and causes active neutrophils to adhere to vascular endothelial cells and become hypersensitive to blood-borne immune mediators. The second insult occurs with the infusion of transfused blood products that contain WBCs with HLA class I antigens, as well as soluble immune response modifiers in the form of cytokines, complement factors, and the breakdown products of lipid membranes. Several studies demonstrate a decrease in T-cell responsiveness and the inhibition of monocyte and lymphocyte function after transfusion of RBCs.[42]

The degree of TRIM-induced injury has been attributed to progressive storage lesions thought to be related to the age of RBC products at the time of transfusion. However, several controlled trials, including the ARIPI trial in premature infants, the ABLE and TRANSFUSE trials in critically ill patients, the RECESS trial in cardiac surgery, and the TOTAL trial in children with hemorrhagic shock, consistently report no significant association between RBC storage duration and mortality or other adverse transfusion outcomes. Nevertheless, evidence collected over the past 30 years from clinical trials and animal studies supports the hypothesis that TRIM involves both proinflammatory mechanisms and systemic immunosuppression.

Alloimmunization

Alloimmunization refers to the induction of an immune response to allogenic antigen exposure. This process occurs occasionally through pregnancy, but the majority of alloimmunization results from transfusion of blood products containing immunogenic antigens on the surface of RBCs. Unlike classic ABO antigens, which consist of carbohydrate chains, most of the non-ABO alloantigens (Kell, Kidd, Duffy, etc.) result from single amino acid polymorphisms between the recipient and donor. AHTRs result from the immediate IgM-mediated immune response to ABO incompatibility with naturally occurring anti-A or anti-B antibodies. In contrast, alloimmunization prompts an amnestic IgG-mediated humoral immunity to foreign proteins and does not result in RBC destruction until the second antigen exposure, which may cause complement activation and delayed extravascular hemolysis.[43] Thus, the clinical consequences of alloimmunization are rarely immediate or fatal, but the generation of antibodies may cause DHTRs and adds difficulty to subsequent cross-matching.

The incidence of alloimmunization is estimated between 2% and 4% of the overall patient population transfused, but up to 35% to 80% in chronically transfused patients such as those with sickle cell disease, hematologic malignancy, or thalassemia, with the range of incidence dependent on the prevalence of the minor blood antigen in the donor population.[43] This is especially evident for patients who require frequent platelet transfusions. Platelets carry significant levels of multiple human platelet antigens (HPA 1 to 15) and other polymorphisms that can result in the destruction of transfused platelets and refractory thrombocytopenia. The use of single-donor apheresis units may limit the exposure to HPA and HLA. Furthermore, early studies demonstrate that preemptive matching of RBC units beyond just ABO blood groups significantly reduces the risk of alloimmunization. This practice could alter the long-term prognosis for chronic transfusion patients.

Transfusion-Associated Dyspnea

As noted above, TAD is a relatively new diagnosis for mild respiratory symptoms that develop within 24 hours of blood product administration. It is a diagnosis of exclusion established for patients with tachypnea, mild hypoxemia, and shortness of breath. The symptoms are generally self-limited and rarely require more than minimal supportive care with supplemental oxygen. Patients who exhibit respiratory distress with blood products should be immediately evaluated for more serious transfusion associated adverse reactions including TRALI, anaphylaxis, and TACO. The risk of TAD can be mitigated by slowing the rate of transfusions in patient with pre-existing pulmonary disease or previous history of dyspnea with blood product administration.[39]

Transfusion-Related Acute Lung Injury

21

For at least the past decade, TRALI has been internationally recognized as a significant cause of transfusion-associated mortality, with an incidence that approximates 1:10,000 transfused products, yet accounting for 13% to 27% of transfusion related fatality in national data published by the FDA for 2016–2020.[24,36,39] Over the past decade, the National Healthcare Safety Network Hemovigilance Module established consistent criteria for clear diagnosis of TRALI, including acute onset dyspnea within 6 hours of transfusion, hypoxemia ($PaO_2/FiO_2 \leq 300$ mmHg or oxygen saturation ≤90% on room air), bilateral infiltrates on chest radiography, and no evidence of left atrial hypertension.[24,39] Historically, patients with risk factors for acute lung injury or ARDS prior to transfusion such as trauma or sepsis were diagnosed as having possible or probable TRALI. Current diagnostic criteria more clearly differentiate TRALI type I as definitive diagnosis and TRALI type II in patients with risk factors for ARDS.[24]

The pathophysiology of TRALI is complex and not fully understood. The clinical picture involves low-pressure noncardiogenic pulmonary edema secondary to neutrophil activation and sequestration in the lungs. This results in endothelial injury and capillary leakage of proteinaceous fluid into the interstitium and intra-alveolar spaces. There are two leading theories on the mechanism of lung injury, both with sound experimental and clinical evidence. The antibody-mediated model stems from evidence of antibody–antigen complexes in the plasma of transfusion recipients who suffered from TRALI. These antibodies are mostly against HLAs (class I and II) and human neutrophil antigens (HNAs). Antibodies form in the donor plasma after alloimmunization from pregnancy, prior transfusion, or prior transplantation. Accordingly, plasma donation from multiparous women has been implicated as one of the highest risks associated with TRALI. Once the antibodies are transfused into the recipient, they complex with native WBC antigens on the surface of monocytes (HLA class II), endothelial cells (HLA class I), and neutrophils (HNAs and HLA class I), thereby activating the neutrophils to facilitate aggregation and release of cytotoxic mediators. Subsequently, the endothelial lining of capillaries in the lung is damaged, resulting in extravasation of WBCs and leakage of edema fluid.[24,39]

The second proposed mechanism of TRALI was termed the "Two-Hit Model" in the late 1990s by Silliman et al., when they discovered the role of biologic response modifiers in its pathophysiology. Stored blood components accumulate lipid degradation products (mostly phosphatidylcholine derivatives) that function to activate neutrophils primed and sequestered on the endothelial vascular lining of lung tissue. Acute illness causes the immune system to be hyperreactive, with neutrophils poised on the microvasculature endothelium and "primed" to be activated by various biologic response modifiers, including cytokines, complement, and leukotrienes. The transfusion of stored blood products and associated reactive lipid particles marks the second "hit," which activates primed neutrophils and results in the destruction of the capillary lining of lung microvasculature.[24] The overall pathophysiology of TRALI likely involves both of these mechanisms.

The management of TRALI focuses on supportive measures to limit lung injury and optimize oxygenation. This includes maximizing positive end-expiratory pressures, avoiding volume overload, and using low tidal volume lung protective strategies during mechanical ventilation. Several studies have demonstrated decreased incidence of TRALI with deferral of high risk alloimmunization donors such as those with history of pregnancy, transfusion, or high antibody titers. Laboratory testing for antibody titers is time-consuming and inefficient; however, forcing many blood management services to use male-only donors for platelet and plasma products.[39] Additional strategies including prestorage LR and the use of solvent detergent-treated plasma products have also been employed to minimize the incidence and severity of TRALI, and likely have a significant clinical benefit for patients at high risk with critical illness or immunosuppression.[24] Overall, prevention is the best treatment for TRALI, and is currently a major focus of clinical and experimental study, with emphasis on blood conservation strategies and restrictive transfusion practices.

Transfusion-Associated Graft-Versus-Host Disease

Transfusion-associated GVHD (TA-GVHD) is a rare but fulminant and fatal complication of blood products containing cellular components (platelets and RBCs). Although its incidence is decreasing secondary to preventative γ irradiation and LR, mortality is more than 90%. It occurs when donor T-cell lymphocytes engraft in the recipient and attack host cells they recognize as foreign. Patients at risk for TA-GVHD include those immunocompromised from stem cell transplants, B-cell malignancies (e.g., multiple myeloma, non-Hodgkin lymphoma) or acute lymphocytic leukemia, or with Hodgkin disease or congenital immunodeficiency syndromes.[39] Immunocompetent patients may also be at risk when transfused with directed donations from blood relations with similar HLA types because transfused donor lymphocytes are not recognized as foreign, yet still reject the recipient's tissue. TA-GVHD classically presents 8 to 10 days after transfusion, but clinical suspicion should exist for up to 6 weeks. Symptoms progress rapidly and generally affect the skin, hepatic, digestive, and hematopoietic organ systems causing fever, maculopapular rash, liver dysfunction, watery diarrhea, and pancytopenia. There are no known curative treatments at this time, thus emphasis focuses on prevention using irradiated blood products or components subjected to pathogen inactivation techniques for T-cell destruction.[39]

Posttransfusion Purpura

Defined as severe thrombocytopenia with purpura occurring 5 to 10 days posttransfusion, posttransfusion purpura (PTP) is a very rare complication of transfusion, but associated with high morbidity and mortality as platelet counts can fall <10,000/L or <25% of pretransfusion levels. Most patients are female and have platelet-specific alloantibodies such as anti–HPA-1a. These antibodies are almost exclusively found in previously pregnant women and cause platelet destruction of both transfused and autologous platelets. Intravenous IG is the first line of treatment, but plasmapheresis may be necessary to remove antibody and avoid bleeding complications.[39]

Nonimmune-Mediated Transfusion Reactions

Transfusion-Associated Circulatory Overload

With consistent and defined criteria for the diagnosis of TACO, reported rates have increased and revealed significant morbidity and mortality associated with this class of transfusion reaction. TACO occurs with 1% of platelet transfusion and and up to 2.7% of RBCs administered and was reported to be the leading cause of transfusion-associated fatalities in the resent SHOT annual report as well as FDA data from 2016 through 2020.[36,39] The signs and symptoms of TACO can be confused with TAD and TRALI, but it differs from TRALI in that it is not immune mediated or associated with increased capillary permeability, and it responds rapidly to diuretic therapy and afterload reduction. In 2018 the CDC updated their definition to require at least three of the following findings including evidence of acute respiratory distress within 6 hours of transfusion, increased central venous pressure, increased brain natriuretic peptide, clinical signs of volume overload, and radiographic evidence of bilateral acute pulmonary edema.[24] Similar to TRALI, TACO can be difficult to diagnose despite the improved clarity of definitions. Thus, the true incidence of TACO is unknown, especially in at risk and critically ill patients with a history of heart failure, chronic diuretic dependence, and underlining renal insufficiency.

Preventative measures to mitigate the risk of TACO include slowing the rate of transfusion when appropriate, administering one blood product at a time, frequent assessment of vital signs, symptoms, and pulmonary status, and rapid treatment of volume overload with diuretics.[24] The symptoms of respiratory distress and volume overload associated with TACO typically respond well to diuretics such as furosemide because the pathophysiology involves high-pressure pulmonary edema and not immunogenic acute lung injury.

Metabolic Derangements

The metabolic derangements from transfusion are usually not evident unless patients received a large-volume transfusion or rapid infusion rates, but often include hyperkalemia, citrate toxicity, and hypothermia. As storage time for blood products increases, the cellular components leak potassium and metabolize glucose into lactate, resulting in hyperkalemia and/or acidemia in the transfused product. The acidosis is quickly cleared by physiologic buffers, as citrate preservative in blood products is metabolized to bicarbonate; therefore, ongoing acidosis in patients undergoing massive transfusion is likely secondary to tissue hypoxia and not to transfusion of acidemic blood products. However, hyperkalemia results from high-volume transfusion, especially when infusion rates exceed 100 to 150 mL/hr. Packed RBCs can contain over 7 mEq/dL of potassium depending on the storage age and can produce consequences of hyperkalemia, such as ventricular arrhythmia or sudden cardiac arrest, particularly in neonates and patients with renal insufficiency.[19]

Citrate is a common anticoagulant used in stored blood products and is readily metabolized by the liver and quickly eliminated. However, with rapid infusion rates, massive transfusion, or in patients with liver dysfunction, citrate accumulates in the plasma and chelates calcium, resulting in hypocalcemia. Severe hypocalcemia leads to muscle weakness, tetany, arrhythmias, myocardial dysfunction, and acquired coagulopathy.[19]

Blood product transfusion can also lead to hypothermia, especially during rapid infusion of previously cold or recently thawed blood products. Coagulation factor activity decreases by 10% for every 1°C decrease in core body temperature. Fluid warmers are standard of care for rapid transfusion; nevertheless, hypothermia is commonly associated with massive transfusion and can result in platelet and coagulation factor dysfunction, arrhythmias, hepatic dysfunction, decreased citrate and drug metabolism, and myocardial depression. Additional preventative measures include warming the surrounding environment, surface warming, heated and humidified inspired gases, and fluid warmers for all infusion lines.[19]

Iron Overload

Packed RBCs carry increasing concentrations of iron as a result of hemolysis during storage and transfusion. Each unit of RBCs contains an average of 200 to 250 mg of iron which accumulates in patients who require frequent transfusions for chronic anemia or hemoglobinopathies. Increased mortality has been demonstrated for patients who receive more than 20 units of PRBCs as the iron deposits in the liver, heart, and endocrine systems, resulting in organ dysfunction. Stored iron is not directly detrimental to organ systems; however, iron metabolism produces harmful intracellular free radicals, which in turn cause cellular dysfunction and organ failure. Patients who require chronic transfusions often suffer from cardiomyopathy and cirrhosis. Furthermore, iron availability for microorganisms increases the risk of recurrent infections in these at-risk patients. Chelation therapy with agents such as deferoxamine or deferasirox are the first line of treatment, but difficult to administer secondary to their bioavailability and side effects. Plasma exchange transfusion therapy decreases the iron load better than traditional transfusion, but it is expensive and associated with complications from central venous access and a larger amount of blood products.[39]

Patient Blood Management

The past few years highlighted the scarcity of the blood supply and the unpredictable impact of healthcare administration policies on transfusion practices. Blood centers and hospitals investing in PBM programs provided leadership and direction for blood conservation strategies and distribution of limited blood product resources. The World Health Organization defines PBM as a "patient-focused, evidence-based and systematic approach to optimize the management of patients and transfusion of blood products for quality and effective patient care."[44,45] There are several techniques that will be discussed in this section to optimize PBM in the surgical patient population including preoperative anemia management, perioperative autologous blood transfusion (ABT), and pharmacologic adjuvant therapies (Table 17-11). PBM should be a multimodal approach to patient care with inclusion of several, if not all of these techniques when appropriate for the specific patient situation. The recent meta-analysis by Althoff demonstrated a 39% reduction in RBC transfusion rates and an average decrease of 0.43 RBC units per patient for healthcare systems that endorse a multimodal approach to PBM.[25,45]

Table 17-11 Perioperative Blood Conservation Strategies

Technique	Comments
Preoperative anemia management	Diagnosis and treatment of iron-deficiency anemia improves patient tolerance for acute surgical blood loss
Preoperative autologous donation (PAD)	Increased overall transfusion requirement; lower preoperative hemoglobin
Acute normovolemic hemodilution (ANH)	Limited benefit; contains clotting factors and platelets
Intraoperative blood salvage (IOBS)	Cost-effective, low risk, and highly efficacious
Postoperative blood salvage (POBS)	Efficacious for high-risk orthopedic surgery
Pharmacologic Agents	
Stimulants of erythropoiesis	Erythropoietin, vitamin B_{12}, folate
Prohemostatic agents	Vitamin K, DDAVP, antifibrinolytics, factor concentrates

DDAVP, 1-deamino-8-D-arginine vasopressin.

Preoperative Anemia Management

Several outcome trials have shown that preoperative anemia is associated with in-hospital and 30-day mortality, as well as acute myocardial infarction, acute ischemic stroke, and acute renal failure. Furthermore, healthcare systems with an organized clinical care program to diagnosis and treat anemia demonstrated improved perioperative outcomes with reduced transfusion requirements. Thus, the most recent PBM recommendations from the 2018 Frankfurt Consensus Conference endorsed by several international societies including the AABB, the European Blood Alliance, and the International Society of Blood Transfusion, recommended preoperative anemia be diagnosed and managed with administration of iron supplementation. These guidelines did not recommend the routine use of ESA for patients with preoperative anemia.[44] The prevalence of preoperative anemia ranges from 10% to 48% in published observational trials, with iron deficiency being the most common etiology. Randomized controlled trials concluded that appropriate iron supplementation significantly improves preoperative hemoglobin concentrations despite the limited evidence proving it can reduce perioperative transfusion requirements.[44–46]

Perioperative Iron Supplementation

Several perioperative guidelines and expert opinions endorse the use of iron supplementation for management of iron-deficiency anemia.[19,25,44] However, there are few written recommendations specifying the route and dosing protocols for its administration. Oral iron will increase hemoglobin but takes 2 to 4 weeks to be effective. It is also associated with poor bioavailability and significant side effects limiting patient compliance with long-term use. Parenteral iron produces a more robust increase in hemoglobin concentrations when compared to placebo and when compared to oral iron regimens. Furthermore, intravenous iron is effective in the short term for treatment of preoperative anemia when surgery is more urgent and cannot be delayed weeks to months for anemia management. Historically, there was significant concern for anaphylaxis with parenteral iron supplementation, however, the more recently use formulations of iron sucrose and iron gluconate are well tolerated and proven to be safe and efficacious.[19]

Perioperative Erythropoietin

Erythropoietin is the primary regulator of erythropoiesis. Its endogenous release is stimulated by anemia or physiologic hypoxia. It is FDA approved for treatment of anemia in oncology patients with chemotherapy-induced anemia and patients with chronic renal failure. It has also been used to optimize patients with preoperative anemia undergoing surgery with significant risk of transfusion and patients undergoing preoperative autologous donation (PAD), because conventional PAD programs maintain hematocrit levels well above the threshold for endogenous erythropoietin release, causing insufficient native stimulation of erythropoiesis. However, there is ongoing concern for increased risk of thromboembolic events and overall safety issues when erythropoietin is used routinely. For these reasons, its routine use is not recommended at this time, but it is specifically recommended for in conjunction with iron supplementation in anemic patients with hemoglobin levels <13.0 g/dL anticipating major orthopedic surgery.[45]

Autologous Blood Transfusion

Most healthy patients undergoing routine surgery will not require allogenic blood transfusion. However, there are some elective procedures such as liver resection, orthopedic surgery, cardiac surgery, and spinal instrumentation where the risk of blood transfusion is clinically significant and can impact patient outcomes. As discussed in detail earlier, blood component therapy is associated with significant morbidity and mortality for all patient populations. It is also a scarce and costly resource. ABT as a strategy for blood conservation first gained popularity because of the rising risk of transfusion-transmitted viral infections in the 1980s. All forms of ABTC reduce the need for allogenic blood components; however, now that the incidence of infectious risks with allogenic blood has declined substantially, the utility and cost-effectiveness of ABT is not as certain, especially when the process involves blood storage. ABT encompasses three separate processes: (1) preoperative autologous blood donation; (2) acute normovolemic hemodilution (ANH); and (3) perioperative blood cell salvage.

PAD summarizes the process of patients donating their own whole blood in the weeks preceding a planned surgical procedure to ensure that they receive autologous blood, should red cell replacement be necessary on the day of surgery. PAD was initially popular in the 1980s, when concern for transfusion-transmitted HIV was high; however, it has since become less frequently used given the reduced risk of viral infections and new concerns about the risks and adverse effects of postdonation anemia as well as the inflammatory risks associated with stored blood. PAD eliminates the risk of transfusion-transmitted infection and alloimmunization, and it may also decrease the risk of TRALI. However, recipients of stored autologous blood remain at risk for clerical error, TACO, bacterial infection, metabolic derangements, and TRIM. PAD reduces the need for allogenic blood transfusion when performed with appropriate protocols that include early donation and use of iron supplementation and erythrocyte-stimulating agents (ESAs) to allow for sufficient erythrogenesis. However, given the general acceptance for restrictive transfusion practices, the increased wastage of PAD units (up to 45%), diminishes the utility and cost-effectiveness of its routine use, especially since intraoperative blood salvage (IOBS) is clinically efficacious.[19]

PAD is currently indicated for use in patients in whom it 22
would be difficult to find compatible blood products due to multiple antibodies or rare blood types, and those who refuse to receive allogenic transfusion. Typically, each donation session collects a single or double unit of whole blood and can technically be repeated weekly until 72 hours prior to the scheduled procedure. Patients are rarely able to donate more than four units because of the limited storage time, and hemoglobin must remain above 11 g/dL before donation.[19] However, the earlier the donation, the more time a patient has to recover from iatrogenic anemia. Despite the ability to donate up until 72 hours before surgery, it is not recommended to undergo donation within 28 days of planned surgery as PAD rapidly loses its effectiveness when donation occurs in proximity to surgery and patients present with preoperative anemia. PAD is most effective when used in conjunction with erythropoietin, which increases the tolerance for repeat donations. Iron supplementation is not indicated and generally not helpful in patients who are already iron replete; however, oral iron should be administered to patients known to be iron deficient prior to autologous donation and surgery.

PAD should be avoided if the scheduled procedure is at risk of postponement because autologous donated units may become outdated if surgery does not proceed on time. Furthermore, directed donations are not subjected to the same testing or deferral procedures as allogenic blood collection, and therefore cannot be used by the general population if they are not transfused into the patient. Transfusion of autologous blood should still be guided by the same indications for transfusion of allogenic RBCs—avoiding wastage is not an appropriate reason to transfuse autologous units. In other words, patients should not be overtransfused simply because they have stored autologous blood. In large retrospective studies comparing PAD to IOBS techniques, PAD is less effective at reducing allogenic transfusion rates and presents several risks such as symptomatic donation, preoperative anemia (average preoperative hemoglobin level 1.1 g/dL below controls), increased rates of overall transfusion, and higher costs. As with any perioperative management plan, the advantages and disadvantages should be individually considered in the context of the patient's history, planned procedure, and physical status before blood donation.

ANH is the process of extracting multiple units of blood immediately before surgical incision while maintaining euvolemia with crystalloid or colloid supplementation. The withdrawn blood is high in hematocrit and contains clotting factors and functional platelets. After ANH, the patient loses blood with lower hemoglobin and fewer red cells. This process reduces the oxygen-carrying capacity of blood, but healthy patients maintain oxygen delivery with intact compensatory mechanisms such as increased CO and oxygen extraction. At the end of surgery, the autologous units are reinfused, thereby replacing RBCs, platelets, and plasma proteins active in hemostasis. This process eliminates the infectious and alloimmunization risks of allogenic transfusion, as well as the immunomodulatory risks of blood storage.[19] ANH was first introduced in the 1970s and gained popularity in the 1990s, when transfusion-transmitted infectious risks were high. In the last 20 years, however, large meta-analyses documented only modest decreases in the risk of allogenic transfusion rates, and highlighted limitations and controversy associated with publication bias for ANH trials.[47] Furthermore, most comparative studies demonstrated ANH to be inferior to high-efficiency IOBS and protocolized PAD for non-cardiac surgery.

Procedurally, ANH involves the removal of a predetermined volume of blood after the induction of anesthesia, but prior to surgical incision. Target hematocrit nadirs will vary based on individual patient history and baseline physiologic state; however, these usually range from 25% to 30%.[47] The simple formula for allowable blood loss is used to calculate the volume to be removed. Volume to be removed = EBV × $[(Hct_i - Hct_t)/Hct_{ave}]$ where EBV is the estimated blood volume; Hct_i, the starting hematocrit; Hct_t, the target low hematocrit; Hct_{ave}, the average of Hct. Euvolemia should be maintained with either crystalloids or colloids administered based on dynamic volume assessment parameters.

Given the limited evidence of benefit, ANH is not recommended for routine use. However, it may be considered for patients with multiple antibodies or a rare blood type that creates difficulty with finding compatible products, or for patients who refuse allogenic transfusion or stored blood component therapy such as Jehovah's Witnesses. ANH is most effective in patients with high preoperative hemoglobin levels, minimal cardiovascular comorbidities that allow intraoperative anemia, and a surgical risk for large-volume blood loss. This technique of autologous transfusion is favorable compared to PAD in selected patient populations.

Perioperative Blood Salvage

23 RBC salvage was first attempted in the early 19th century for patients with postpartum hemorrhage. Not surprisingly, it was fraught with complications throughout its early development. It was not until the 1970s that commercial cell salvage devices became available for clinical use, yet there were still frequent complications such as hemolysis, air embolism, and coagulopathy.[48] Over the past decade RBC salvage techniques have improved significantly and now offer an efficient, cost-effective, and safe method for perioperative blood conservation. In general, cell salvage involves the collection of shed surgical blood, which is filtered and washed prior to reinfusion. This process is most often carried out intraoperatively with direct suction of the surgical field, or postoperatively in the case of orthopedic, cardiac, and thoracic surgery using the blood from wound drainage.

IOBS uses a double-lumen suction catheter with one port for aspiration from the surgical field and the other for the addition of an anticoagulant solution, usually heparin or citrate. Suctioned blood is collected in a reservoir, filtered to remove large debris, and centrifuged to produce RBC concentrates. The final step of washing clears the product of residual contaminants such as plasma, platelets, free hemoglobin, cellular fragments, WBCs, and the remaining heparin or citrate. The resultant red cells are resuspended in saline and ready for reinfusion.[48] This is usually reinfused to the patient immediately through standard blood filters, but may be stored at 4°C for up to 6 hours with careful patient and product identification. On average, IOBS yields a hematocrit ranging from 55% to 70%.[48] The efficiency depends on several factors including the volume of blood processed at a time, the length of time that blood remains in the wound, and the rate and precision of suctioning, since increased turbulence from the surgical field adds shear stress, which damages RBCs. Most modern-day cell savers, when used appropriately, provide RBC concentrates with a hematocrit equivalent to that of stored PRBC.[48]

IOBS is demonstrated to reduce allogenic blood transfusion in major orthopedic surgery, particularly multilevel spine fusions, and vascular or cardiac surgery. However, recent studies and a meta-analysis on the use of cell salvage in routine knee and hip arthroplasty demonstrate reduced efficacy and cost-effectiveness for IOBS. This is likely secondary to more restrictive transfusion practices, better preoperative optimization of hemoglobin levels, and the use of antifibrinolytics, all of which reduce overall blood loss and the need for RBC transfusion.[48] However, IOBS continues to be indicated for patients with low preoperative hemoglobin who cannot tolerate PAD or ANH, those unwilling to consent to allogenic transfusion, and patients with pre-existing bleeding risks or multiple alloantibodies. Evidence shows that salvaged blood has better oxygen-carrying capacity and tissue oxygenation than stored blood, secondary to retention of red cell's biconcave disc shape and increased levels of 2,3–DPG and ATP.[48] Overall, IOBS is cost-effective, convenient, and advantageous for emergency procedures and surgeries with high risk of significant perioperative blood loss.

The complications of IOBS are rare and are mostly associated with either the method of suctioning or contamination from the surgical field. Risks include nonimmunogenic hemolysis, fever, and contamination with various substances such as topical anticoagulants, urine, amniotic fluid, or bacteria. Washing the salvaged blood clears most contaminants, and variable suction devices limit the sheer stress that causes hemolysis. Reinfusion of salvaged blood in volumes greater than 50% of the estimated blood volume can result in dilutional coagulopathy similar to massive transfusion of allogenic RBCs, since neither contains clotting factors or platelets. Lastly, IOBS can cause gas embolism if the reinfusion bag is connected in a continuous circuit with the patient.[48] Careful adherence to the recommended application of modern cell-saver devices effectively eliminates many of these concerns.

Traditionally, cell salvage was contraindicated in cancer surgery and operations where blood loss is contaminated by urine, anticoagulants, or amniotic fluid (NICV 17-3). However, several studies now demonstrate the safety of cell salvage when blood is processed, washed, and administered through a leukodepletion filter. Use in surgery for prostate cancer and gynecologic oncology, which often involves urine and malignant cells contaminating the field, has not shown significant increases in morbidity, mortality, or cancer recurrence. However, it is recommended that IOBS be filtered and irradiated when there is concern for malignancy, and avoided completely when the tumor is ruptured causing an overwhelming concentration of cancer cells in shed blood.[48] The use of IOBS for obstetric cases raises concerns about inducing alloimmunization or amniotic fluid embolism, recently termed "anaphylactoid syndrome of pregnancy." Because this syndrome is very rare, it is difficult to establish the safety of a new technique. However, leukodepletion filters remove most of the amniotic fluid, immune mediators, and debris. Although fetal RBCs cannot be differentiated from maternal red cells and may potentiate alloimmunization, this risk is already present during delivery and not exacerbated by the use of IOBS. Cell salvage does not reduce risk for allogenic PRBCs when used routinely for caesarean deliveries, but should be considered for high-risk obstetric patients such as those undergoing planned cesarean hysterectomy or those with placenta accreta.[48] The only absolute contraindications to IOBS are microbial contamination of the surgical field, and cancer surgery where tumor rupture or direct manipulation is likely.

Postoperative blood salvage (POBS) involves the collection and reinfusion of blood shed into surgical wound drains in the immediate postoperative period. The recovered blood product can be processed in one of the two ways: "washed" POBS is centrifuged, washed, and resuspended as RBC concentrates, whereas "unwashed" POBS is simply filtered before reinfusion. The resultant hematocrit of unwashed POBS ranges from 20% to 30% and should not be expected to increase the patient's hemoglobin level. Rather, it will aid in avoidance of dilutional anemia associated with the fluid resuscitation for postoperative bleeding. There are advantages and disadvantages to both techniques, resulting in continued controversies over the safety and efficacy of POBS.

POBS studies are limited, but meta-analyses demonstrate efficacy in orthopedic procedures such as knee and hip arthroplasty. Unwashed POBS is most commonly used in orthopedics, as it is highly efficacious, cost-effective, and requires little additional training in comparison to use of washed POBS. POBS has also been studied in postcardiac surgery patients and shown to be efficacious at reducing the need for allogenic blood transfusion.[48] However, shed blood from surgical wounds, involving the thorax and mediastinum, contains inflammatory mediators, activated clotting factors, fibrin and fibrin split products, and the products of hemolysis such as free hemoglobin. These substances can precipitate renal damage, lung injury, or coagulopathy. POBS for cardiac surgery should be washed prior to reinfusion in accordance with the most recent guidelines from the SCA.

POBS continues to be part of the multimodal approach to perioperative PBM especially for routine orthopedic and cardiac surgeries. Complications include concern for hemolysis and immunomodulation, and its overall efficacy and cost-effectiveness remain unclear. It is contraindicated for patients with preexisting hemoglobinopathies such as sickle cell disease and thalassemia. Furthermore, similar to IOBS, blood should not be reinfused if it has been contaminated with microbials or drugs used topically in the surgical field that are not indicated for systemic use (e.g., betadine, chlorhexidine, and topical antibiotics).

Jehovah's Witnesses belong to an international and well-established religious society with over 7.8 million followers who believe in a literal translation of the Bible (NICV 17-4). Passages such as Genesis 9, verse 4 ("But you shall not eat flesh with its life, that is, its blood") and Leviticus 17, verse 10 ("If any one of the house of Israel…eats any blood, I will … cut him off from among his people") lead to a proscription against receiving blood product transfusions. Followers believe that once blood has left the body it should not be consumed in any way. Receipt of a blood transfusion is believed to cause irreversible death to a member's soul without hope of eternal life. Most Jehovah's Witnesses understand and accept the threat of death as a possible result of refusing therapeutic transfusion. Clearly this is challenging for treating physicians, especially in the case of trauma or unexpected critical bleeding. The best management for Jehovah's Witnesses is to have a well-prescribed perioperative care plan to maximize blood conservation strategies and a clear conversation about the patient's individual concerns and beliefs. Some patients consent to blood component therapy, factor concentrates derived from blood (e.g., albumin or PCCs), or extracorporeal circulation, which may include cardiopulmonary bypass, ANH, and IOBS if left in continuous circulation with the body. These decisions are made based on a patient's review of their conscience and their own interpretation of religious scripture.[49]

Jehovah's Witnesses are fully aware of how their belief system affects medical management with routine life-sustaining treatments. Accordingly, there are over 1,700 Hospital Liaison Committees worldwide designed to assist with personal healthcare management plans that provide both patient autonomy and the best medical care available. Some of the most challenging questions arise with minors, emergencies, and unconscious patients, when the physician is unable to have a clear conversation about the patient's specific beliefs. There is a great deal of individual variability within the religion that can lead to drastically different management plans for bleeding and acute anemia. Often adult Jehovah's Witnesses will carry cards with an advance directive; however, if questions arise, physicians should seek the guidance of their hospital ethics committees and legal advisors. An urgent application to the court system is appropriate in the case of minors or unconscious patients without decision-making capacity.

In preparation for elective surgery for a Jehovah's Witness patient, the use of prohemostatic medications such as ESAs, antifibrinolytics, vitamin K, factor concentrates, and desmopressin should be considered, and should be available. In addition, the patient's preoperative hemoglobin should be optimized by stimulating erythropoiesis with high-dose recombinant erythropoietin, intravenous iron, and supplemental vitamin B_{12} and folate.[49] There is ongoing research into the clinical use of hemoglobin-based oxygen carriers that could revolutionize the treatment not only of Jehovah's Witnesses, but have yet to be approved in the United States.

Disorders of Hemostasis: Diagnosis and Treatment

As discussed previously, hemostasis is a complex mechanism of 24
checks and balances that aims to control bleeding from sites of vascular injury while maintaining blood flow throughout the rest of the body. It involves countless proteins, enzymes, ligands, and molecules to serve as activators, cofactors, regulators, and inhibitors in hemostasis. When the equilibrium of this process is disrupted, it results in abnormal bleeding or clotting, depending on the specific dysfunction or deficiency. Accordingly, disorders of hemostasis can be classified as those that facilitate hemorrhage and those that facilitate inappropriate thrombosis. The disorders are further separated by the involvement in primary hemostasis (the initial platelet plug) or secondary hemostasis (the clotting cascade and fibrin cross-linkage). Finally, hemostatic disorders are caused by either inherited genetic disease or acquired deficiencies.

Symptomatic disorders of primary hemostasis often present 25
with superficial signs of bleeding on the skin or mucosa. Patients complain of petechiae, mucosal bleeding, and easy bruising. They often suffer from prolonged bleeding from minor injury, frequent epistaxis, and menorrhagia secondary to deficient or dysfunctional platelet activity. In contrast, disorders of secondary hemostasis involve qualitative or quantitative dysfunction of clotting factors and cause more severe and deep tissue bleeding. These patients present with spontaneous hemarthroses, hematomas, and excessive hemorrhage after traumatic injuries. Treatments depend on the specific cause of the disorder and often involve blood component therapy or pharmacologic agents that enhance, inhibit, or bypass specific sites in the hemostatic process.

Disorders of Primary Hemostasis

Primary hemostasis involves the initial recruitment of platelets at the site of vascular injury to form a fragile platelet plug. Once platelets bind to the injured subendothelium, they become activated, thereby exposing additional receptor sites and releasing factors involved in further platelet recruitment, activation, aggregation, and the initiation of secondary hemostasis.

Hereditary disorders of platelets are rare and usually associated with defective receptor binding. Bernard–Soulier syndrome is an autosomal recessive disorder that results from an abnormality of the GP Ib receptor. This qualitative and quantitative dysfunction

Table 17-12 Classification of Inherited Von Willebrand Disease

Type	Pathophysiology	Comments
1	Partial quantitative deficiency of vWF	Mildest; most common; responds to DDAVP
2A	Dysfunction in platelet adhesion	May respond to DDAVP
2M	Dysfunction in platelet adhesion	May respond to DDAVP
2B	Increased platelet-binding affinity	Thrombocytopenia with DDAVP
2N	Decreased FVIII-binding affinity	Often confused with hemophilia A
3	Severe quantitative deficiency of vWF	Rarest; most severe; usually requires factor concentrates

vWF, von Willebrand factor; DDAVP, desmopressin; FVIII, factor VIII.

impairs platelet adhesion to exposed vWF at the site of vascular injury. Glanzmann thrombasthenia is an autosomal recessive genetic disorder that results from a defect in the platelet integrin αIIbβ3 receptor which, under normal circumstances, allows fibrinogen and other ligands to bind and facilitate platelet aggregation. Other inherited disorders of platelets involve ligand receptors or defects in the signaling cascade for molecules involved in platelet activation (e.g., thromboxane and adenine diphosphate).

26 *vWD* is the most common hereditary bleeding disorder, with a prevalence of approximately 1% in the general population, although it is only reportedly symptomatic in 0.1% (NICV 17-5).[6] The clinical features and severity of vWD vary immensely, since it has several different types and classifications depending on the nature of the genetic mutation and its effect on the functionality of vWF (Table 17-12). Although the most common type of vWD has an autosomal dominant inheritance pattern and thus affect both woman and men, women often present earlier with significant bleeding during menstruation and peripartum. Different genetic mutations affect various domains of vWF, causing different quantitative and functional deficiencies, and in fact there are several complex laboratory evaluations necessary to classify the exact type of disease. It is important to reach the correct diagnosis, since appropriate treatment and prophylaxis differs for each class of the disorder.[6]

vWF is produced in endothelial cells and megakaryocytes, and functions in primary platelet adhesion and aggregation at the site of vascular injury through interaction with the GP Ib receptor on the platelet surface. Once exposed, vWF facilitates the interaction of platelets with collagen within the subendothelium as well as platelet–platelet interactions. Both of these result in the initial platelet plug and subsequent platelet activation. Furthermore, vWF circulates as a complex with FVIII, providing stability to the otherwise labile clotting factor until vWF binds to activated platelets via the GP IIb/IIIa receptor. This localizes FVIII to the site of injury. The clinical features of vWD vary with differing levels of functionality that result from inherited disorders in protein synthesis, structure, function, and clearance. Most types of vWD result from decreased levels or deficient function of vWF in primary hemostasis. Patients typically present with mucocutaneous bleeding (e.g., epistaxis), menorrhagia, and prolonged bleeding from minor wounds and dental extractions. Frequently, patients are not aware of the disorder until they undergo a bleeding questionnaire in anticipation of surgery.

There are three types of vWD. Types 1 and 3 result from quantitative deficiencies of vWF, whereas type 2 occurs with various mutations causing qualitative dysfunction. Type 2 is further classified (A, B, M, and N) depending on the domain of the protein that is affected and the functional defect (Table 17-12).[6] Type 1 has an autosomal dominant inheritance pattern and results from a partial quantitative deficiency in vWF levels either from decreased synthesis and secretion or from accelerated proteolysis and clearance. It is the most common and mildest type of vWD. Type 3 is the most severe, but also the rarest; it has a recessive pattern of inheritance and results in significantly depressed levels of vWF. This is the only type likely to cause spontaneous hemorrhage in joints and soft tissues. Types 2A and 2M result in deficiencies in platelet adhesion and decreased activity of vWF relative to the factor levels within the plasma. Type 2B involves increased affinity of vWF for the GP Ib receptor on the platelet surface. This causes spontaneous binding of vWF to circulating platelets, thereby increasing the cleavage and clearance of vWF. This type of vWD can be associated with thrombocytopenia. DDAVP treatment is commonly used to increase cleavage from FVIII and overall availability. Lastly, type 2N is characterized by decreased affinity for FVIII and deficiencies in secondary hemostasis.[6] This type is often confused with hemophilia A, given the depressed levels of FVIII associated with significantly decreased factor half-life.

The three primary criteria for diagnosis of vWD are (1) a history of mucosal bleeding or prolonged bleeding after dental extractions, surgical procedures, or postpartum hemorrhage; (2) a family history of bleeding disorders (understanding this can be unreliable or unavailable); and (3) reduced activity of vWF demonstrated by various assays designed to test platelet adhesion, aggregation, and levels of vWF or FVIII complexes (e.g., vWF:factor antigen, vWF:ristocetin cofactor activity, vWF:collagen-binding activity, and vWF:GP 1b binding activity).[6] The laboratory diagnosis and classification of vWD is complex and often requires a hematologist to correctly specify the type of disorder, and to prescribe the appropriate prophylaxis and treatment options. Overall, it is important to recognize that traditional coagulation profile tests such as PT and aPTT are often normal in patients with vWD.

There are two primary treatment options for patients with vWD—DDAVP and factor concentrates. DDAVP promotes the cleavage of vWF from FVIII and increases the availability of both. This is beneficial for most patients with type I partial deficiency and some type 2 subclassifications of vWD (with the exception of type 2B as discussed above). DDAVP may not be therapeutic by itself for patients with type 3 and severely depressed levels of vWF. Often these patients require treatment with additional hemostatic medications such as antifibrinolytics and/or factor replacement with plasma-derived vWF/FVIII concentrates (Heamate P/Humate P). These concentrates are only needed in approximately 20% of patients with vWD who do not respond to DDAVP, and may vary in efficacy. Accordingly, it is important to obtain the correct diagnosis in order to best manage each patient prophylactically before surgery and therapeutically in the event of uncontrolled bleeding.[6]

On rare occasions, vWD may be acquired in association with various disease processes such as lymphoproliferative or myeloproliferative disorders; autoimmune disease; cardiac dysfunction (e.g., aortic stenosis, ventricular assist devices), or medication-induced from quinolones, valproic acid, and hydroxyl ethyl starches. The pathophysiology of acquired vWD is multifactorial and may involve various mechanisms including immune-mediated clearance by ADAMTS-13–mediated cleavage of high–molecular-weight vWF, binding or absorption with large molecules such as the starches, or enhanced proteolysis secondary to shear stress.[50] Treatment starts with discontinuation of the offending agent or management of the underlying condition; however, adjunctive treatment with DDAVP and/or antifibrinolytics is helpful.

Disorders of Secondary Hemostasis

The Hemophilias

27 Hemophilia is a genetic disease that results from deficiencies or dysfunction of specific clotting factors. The most common form is hemophilia A, which accounts for about 85% of the disease and stems from deficiencies of FVIII. Hemophilia B (Christmas disease) involves a defect in the production of FIX, and is the second most common type of hemophilia. Both hemophilia A and B are X-linked recessive disorders and are found almost exclusively in male patients, although new mutations are common and account for about a third of hemophilias in male and female patients without family history.[9,51] Hemophilia was originally called the "royal disease," since Queen Victoria of England was a carrier of hemophilia B and passed the disorder to the royal families of Spain, Germany, and Russia. Lastly, hemophilia C is very rare (1% of all hemophiliacs), and results from genetic mutations in FXI, and is the only form that has an autosomal recessive inheritance pattern.

Hemophilia A affects approximately 1 in 5,000 males worldwide. Clinically, these patients suffer from spontaneous bleeding into their joints and muscles, rarely internal organs. Patients often require orthopedic surgery for long-term complications of hemarthroses. Central nervous system bleeding is rare, but can lead to severe disability and death.[9] Normal plasma concentrations of FVIII range between 100 and 200 ng/mL, and the severity of disease varies depending on the residual factor activity. Patients with mild disease maintain factor levels between 5% and 40% of normal, and account for about 50% of patients with hemophilia A. Approximately 10% of patients have moderate disease, with only 1% to 5% of residual FVIII activity. The most severely affected patients account for about 40% of the disease prevalence and have less than 1% of normal factor activity.[51] Carrier females generally maintain about 50% of FVIII activity with no clinical signs of bleeding. Homozygous females may present with hemophilia, but this is rare and often associated with Turner syndrome or X-chromosomal mosaicism. Diagnosis starts with patients reporting a personal and/or family history of bleeding disorders among male relations. Confirmatory laboratory evidence includes prolonged aPTT and low factor activity levels. Typically, the PT and bleeding times will be normal.

Treatment for all hemophilia patients involves replacement of coagulation factor deficiencies and is accomplished with plasma transfusion or factor concentrates. Historically, hemophiliacs were exposed to several transfusion-related infectious risks prior to the availability of recombinant and virally inactivated factor concentrates. In the 1980s, a significant percentage of patients with hemophilia contracted AIDS from transfusion-transmitted HIV. Frequent transfusions for these patients are clearly associated with numerous infectious and noninfectious transfusion risks, including the development of factor inhibitors and alloantibodies. Approximately 30% of patients with severe hemophilia A and 10% of those with FIX deficiency develop inhibitor antibodies to FVIII by the time they reach adulthood, making them less responsive to factor concentrates. Patients with severe hemophilia are at highest risk for developing inhibitors, since they require frequent high-dose treatment and primary prophylaxis starting at younger ages.

The goals of managing hemophilia focus on prophylaxis against spontaneous bleeding, as well as aggressive blood conservation strategies for anticipated invasive procedures. Antifibrinolytic agents such as tranexamic acid and epsilon aminocaproic acid are good adjuncts to use during minor procedures and perioperatively. Patients with mild hemophilia A and hemophilia C also benefit from treatment with DDAVP, to raise the circulating availability of FVIII by increasing dissociation from vWF.[51] However, those with more severe disease require treatment of spontaneous and traumatic bleeding episodes, as well as prophylaxis to avoid the long-term complications of hemarthroses. This is accomplished with nonreplacement substitution therapy with emicizumab, or transfusion of specific factor concentrates derived from virally inactivated plasma-derived or recombinant products. Emicizumab is a relatively new therapeutic option approved for routine prophylaxis use in hemophilia A. It is a synthetic antibody that binds to factors IX and X to mimic the role of FVIII in the tenase complex. Of note, this agent is not indicated for treatment of bleeding, and only used as prophylaxis. Patients with clinical signs of bleeding should be treated with factor-replacement products.[9,51] Those who have a known or suspected history of inhibitors to FVIII or FIX often respond to bypass agents such as rFVIIa or PCCs. Factor concentrates are given in anticipation of surgery or invasive procedures, and are dosed individually depending on severity of illness and risk of bleeding. The appropriate dosing regimen for prophylaxis is highly variable among patients, due to differing levels of disease severity and the impact of factor inhibitors. Titration of the dose of factor concentrates to trough levels of no less than 1 IU/dL (1% of normal) is recommended during long-term prophylaxis.[51]

Hemophilia B is clinically and pathophysiologically similar to hemophilia A, except it involves FIX and is much less common worldwide, affecting roughly 1 in 25,000 males. This form of hemophilia is treated with recombinant FIX concentrates, but requires less frequent dosing regimens than FVIII concentrates due to a longer half-life (18 hours as opposed to 12 hours). Fortunately, the development of factor inhibitors is much less prevalent in patients with hemophilia B than in patients with hemophilia A. These patients are also generally responsive to bypass treatment with PCCs or rFVIIa in the case of urgent bleeding.[9,51]

Acquired hemophilia is a rare disease that usually develops in association with connective tissue disorders, pregnancy, or malignancy. It rarely occurs in young patients and stems from the development of antibodies to FVIII. The clinical symptoms of acquired hemophilia typically include subcutaneous bleeding episodes and soft tissue hematomas, as opposed to the hemarthroses common to congenital hemophilia. Diagnostically, the aPTT is prolonged in conjunction and low FVIII levels do not correct in a mixing study due to the presence of inhibitors. The treatment for acquired hemophilia with acute bleeding depends on bypass agents such as rFVIIa or PCCs, although some patients with mild disease will respond to adjunctive therapies such as DDAVP and antifibrinolytics. Once hemostasis is achieved, long-term management involves immunosuppression with steroids or cytotoxic agents.

Hereditary Hypercoagulability

The *FVL* genetic mutation causes resistance to the anticoagulant effects of APC on clotting FV. It is the most common hereditary risk factor for hypercoagulability. Heterozygous patients have a fivefold increase in the risk of VTE. This rises to 10-fold increased risk in homozygotes. Treatment involves lifelong therapeutic anticoagulation. The prevalence among Caucasians is approximately 3% to 7% throughout North America and Europe. Some investigators propose that the high prevalence in Caucasians stems from a protective genetic interplay against bleeding and mortality risk associated with hemophilia.[13]

Protein C and S deficiencies are autosomal dominant genetic diseases that result in increased risk of VTE. Protein C inactivates FVa and FVIIIa to curb the clotting cascade, and depends on protein S as a cofactor for appropriate function. Accordingly, deficiencies (quantitative type I) or dysfunction (qualitative type II) in either protein C or S result in a prothrombotic state. For the prevalence of protein C and protein S deficiency is estimated to be approximately 0.3% and 0.1%, respectively. Clinically, patients present with VTE in early adulthood, but arterial thrombosis is rare. Treatment of acute thrombosis requires therapeutic anticoagulation. Anticoagulation is indicated for long-term management, but warfarin should be started slowly once the patient is therapeutic on heparin, to avoid the risk of warfarin limb necrosis.[13]

Acquired Disorders of Hemostasis

Vitamin K Deficiency

Vitamin K is one of the essential fat-soluble vitamins required for the synthesis and final processing of several hemostatic factors, including factors II, VII, IX, X, and proteins C and S. Without vitamin K, these proteins do not undergo carboxylation and therefore cannot actively bind to the phospholipid membrane of platelets during secondary hemostasis. There are two sources of vitamin K—phylloquinone (K_1) is available in a number of foods such as leafy greens, whereas menaquinone (K_2) is synthesized in the GI tract by intestinal bacteria and accounts for the bulk of vitamin K stored in the liver. The absorption of both types occurs in the small intestine and depends on the availability of bile salts. Accordingly, liver insufficiency, the sterile gut in newborns, and oral antibiotic treatments are some of the leading causes of vitamin K deficiency. Other causes include chronic kidney disease, total parenteral nutrition, intestinal obstruction, or hyperperistalsis.

Vitamin K deficiency presents with prolonged PT and aPTT, but can also be diagnosed by low vitamin K levels or measures of noncarboxylated prothrombin. It is treated with vitamin K replacement, which can be administered parenterally, orally, or subcutaneously. Oral administration has the best bioavailability, but can take 24 hours for full effect. When rapid correction for a bleeding patient is needed, improvements in PT can be seen within 6 to 8 hours of intravenous administration, especially with high doses of 5 to 10 mg.[52]

Liver Disease

Patients with severe liver disease often present with bleeding complications, including central nervous system hemorrhage or gastrointestinal bleeding. They were traditionally managed with prophylactic transfusions and adjunctive hemostatic medications prior to surgical procedures or in response to a prolonged PT. However, new guidelines recommend against prophylaxis without clinical symptoms of bleeding. There are several etiologies of bleeding diathesis associated with liver disease, including endothelial dysfunction, portal hypertension, thrombocytopenia, and the procoagulant imbalance discussed in the following section. However, the hemostatic system in chronic liver disease often remains in balance, although fragile. Conventional laboratory tests such as the PT and aPTT overestimate the bleeding tendency of patients with liver disease and should not be used as the sole method for titrating plasma transfusion or treatment with hemostatic agents.[53]

Primary hemostasis was typically thought to be inefficient in chronic liver disease because of thrombocytopenia secondary to decreased production of thrombopoietin in the liver. However, the low platelet count is balanced with increased circulating levels of vWF that result from a reduced presence of ADAMTS-13, the protease that regulates plasma concentrations of vWF. This balance remains fragile, given that patients with severe liver disease and acute illness are also prone to endothelial and platelet dysfunction.

Secondary hemostasis is also affected because liver disease results in deficiencies of factors II, V, VII, IX, X, and XI that will prolong the PT and aPTT in vitro. However, the liver is also responsible for the synthesis of protein C, protein S, and AT, which are integral anticoagulant factors. Furthermore, these patients have increased circulating levels of FVIII in association with the increases in vWF mentioned above. Thus, the decreased levels of procoagulant factors are offset by deficient amounts of anticoagulant factors and increased FVIII activity, maintaining secondary hemostasis.[53]

Although hemostatic equilibrium is generally maintained with chronic liver disease, the balance is not stable and can be tipped toward either hemorrhage or thrombosis by acute illness, malnutrition, renal injury, infection, or medications. Laboratory testing difficult because conventional PT and aPTT conducted in vitro do not mimic the in vivo compensation mechanisms associated with chronic liver disease. Thrombin generation by procoagulant factors is regulated in vivo by the anticoagulant activity of protein C and its main activator, thrombomodulin. In contrast, in vitro thrombin generation only assesses activation by procoagulant factors and will misrepresent the actual bleeding tendency of the patient.[53]

Lastly, fibrinolysis is maintained in chronic liver disease. Although these patients are plasminogen deficient, they have higher than normal levels of tPA secondary to lower levels of TAFI. This maintains the normal ratio of plasminogen to plasmin. However, the balance of fibrinolysis and antifibrinolysis can be disrupted by infection, trauma, surgery, and medications common to chronic liver patients.

As mentioned above, conventional hemostatic tests such as PT and aPTT assays do not reflect the bleeding or thrombotic tendencies of chronic liver disease. Patients with normal coagulation profiles can present with catastrophic gastrointestinal bleeding or prolonged PTs, yet develop venous, arterial, and portal thrombosis. The overall hemostatic state can be evaluated with viscoelastography, or by measuring thrombin generation in the presence and absence of thrombomodulin. The circumstances of these tests are more akin to the in vivo state of patients with liver disease than conventional PT and aPTT tests. Accordingly, it is no longer recommended to prophylactically transfuse plasma in response to PT times, elevated INR, or prior to minor procedures in such patients without clinical signs of bleeding. Furthermore, despite prolonged coagulation tests, patients with liver disease are still at significant risk for venous and arterial thrombosis and should be treated with appropriate prophylactic anticoagulation.[53]

Disseminated Intravascular Coagulation (DIC)

DIC is a disorder characterized by systemic activation of coagulation. It is always associated with a comorbid condition such as infection, inflammation, or malignancy, which causes widespread activation of the coagulation cascade. Table 17-13 lists the medical diseases and syndromes known to cause DIC. Supportive care and treatment of the underlining disorder are the mainstays of DIC management. There are two types of DIC, one characterized by coagulation factor consumption, fibrinolysis, and critical bleeding, and the second represented by microthrombi and fibrin disposition causing multiorgan system failure. In severe cases of major hemorrhage or ischemic organ failure, DIC is treated with factor and fibrinogen replacement, anticoagulation, or pharmacologic therapies.[10]

Table 17-13 Common Disorders Associated With Disseminated Intravascular Coagulation

Disorder	Average Incidence of DIC	Comments
Sepsis	30–50%	Highest with gram-negative bacilli
Trauma and burns	Rare	Associated with the degree of tissue injury
Malignancy	Up to 20%	Highest with adenocarcinoma or leukemia and lymphoma
Vascular disease	Rare	Higher with giant hemangiomas
Obstetric complication	Up to 50%	Including preeclampsia, placental abruption, or amniotic fluid embolism
Hemolysis	Rare	Higher with intravascular hemolysis
Severe organ dysfunction	Rare	Including pancreatitis, hepatitis, and end-stage renal failure

The exact pathophysiology of DIC depends on the causative condition, but primarily involves uncontrolled activation of hemostatic mechanisms for thrombin generation with simultaneous inhibition of fibrinolysis. Thrombin generation in DIC is initiated by TF and activated factor VII in the extrinsic pathway for coagulation. The exposure of TF is facilitated by extensive vascular injury, expression on neoplastic cells, or the release of proinflammatory cytokines such as interleukin-6. DIC progresses as the regulation of thrombin generation is impaired secondary to decreased levels of naturally occurring anticoagulants including AT-III, protein C, and TFPI. Finally, impaired fibrinolysis from an inappropriate increase in circulating levels of PAI-1 facilitates the progression of vascular microthrombi.[10]

DIC is a catastrophic complication for many hospitalized patients with both chronic and acute illness. The clinical presentation of DIC ranges from thromboembolism and organ dysfunction to consumptive coagulopathy and major bleeding. The kidneys and lungs are particularly vulnerable to ischemia from microthrombi and may progress to acute renal failure and acute respiratory distress syndrome, especially in patients with DIC secondary to obstetric complications or sepsis. The bleeding type of DIC results from widespread activation of hemostasis with consumption of coagulation factors and platelets. The primary diagnosis for these patients is often trauma or hematopoietic malignancy, who present with bleeding from sites of vascular injury, or spontaneous intracranial or intraperitoneal hemorrhage. DIC with features of microthrombi, organ dysfunction, and consumption results in severe thrombocytopenia and often leads to massive hemorrhage with a poor overall prognosis. However, major bleeding is rather infrequent with DIC and usually occurs only with platelets less than 50,000/μL or patients undergoing procedures.

The diagnosis of DIC must consider the underlying disorder in conjunction with an abnormal hemostasis profile. Unfortunately, there is not a single laboratory finding indicative of DIC. High levels of fibrin split products are a sensitive marker, but carry very low specificity. Rather, the compilation of prolonged PT and aPTT, thrombocytopenia, hypofibrinogenemia, and increasing fibrin degradation products in a patient with an associated condition leads to the clinical diagnosis of DIC. The International Society of Thrombosis and Hemostasis developed a scoring algorithm for the diagnosis of overt DIC that depends on these four laboratory findings (Table 17-14).[10] This algorithm is only one of several clinically used scoring systems worldwide, but was prospectively validated and found to have a sensitivity of 91% and a specificity of 97%. Overall, DIC is a dynamic condition and most accurately diagnosed with repeated measures of coagulation tests showing progression of thrombocytopenia and hypofibrinogenemia, with increasing prolongation of PT and levels of fibrin degradation products.

The management for DIC primarily involves treatment of the causative condition and supportive measures to control progressive thrombosis and hemorrhage. Consumptive coagulopathy and thrombocytopenia with clinical signs of bleeding are treated with transfusion of plasma and platelets, respectively. There is no evidence for improved outcomes with transfusion of plasma or platelets unless thrombocytopenia is severe (platelet counts <10,000 to 20,000/μL) or moderate (<50,000/μL), with clinical signs of bleeding, or in preparation for invasive procedures.

Plasma is the mainstay of replacement therapy for consumption of clotting factors in DIC; however, it often requires large volumes (10 to 15 mL/kg) to correct the coagulopathy. In the past, rFVIIa and PCCs have been used for patients with active bleeding and consumptive coagulopathy; however, the administration of active factor concentrates in the preparations of rFVIIa and PCCs can lead to progressive thrombosis in patients with overt DIC and is not recommended. Rather, the use of specific factor concentrate is preferred for measured factor deficiencies in patients with active bleeding. Cryoprecipitate is the product of choice for treatment of overt DIC with consumptive coagulopathy and major bleeding,

Table 17-14 Scoring Algorithm for the Diagnosis of Disseminated Intravascular Coagulation

Diagnostic Test	Score
Platelet count	>100,000/mm³ = 0 <100,000/mm³ = 1 <50,000/mm³ = 2
Prothrombin time prolongation	<3 s = 0 >3 s but <6 s = 1 >6 s = 2
Fibrin degradation products	No increase = 0 Moderate increase = 2 Strong increase = 3
Fibrinogen level	>1 g/L = 0 <1 g/L = 1
Score calculation: If ≥5, consistent with overt DIC. If <5, not likely overt DIC; repeat tests in 1–2 days.	

Algorithm developed by the International Society of Thrombosis and Hemostasis.

because it contains FVIII and fibrinogen with a low overall volume of transfusion.

Arterial and venous thromboembolisms are more concerning than hemorrhage in patients with DIC and evidence of acute organ dysfunction. Anticoagulation is indicated to inhibit further activation of hemostasis in patients with signs of microthrombi such as organ failure or diagnosed thromboembolism. Studies of patients with DIC in sepsis proved the efficacy of heparin to halt thrombin generation, improve the coagulation profile, and reduce the risk of thrombosis. It is understandably difficult to initiate therapeutic anticoagulation on a patient with signs or risks of bleeding; however, maintaining chemoprophylaxis against VTE is of utmost importance, especially early in the course of DIC in the absence of major bleeding.[10] Literature support is limited, but LMWH alternatives to unfractionated heparin (UFH) may provide better efficacy with lower bleeding risks.[8]

In research trials investigating the therapeutic benefits of recombinant activated protein C specifically for DIC associated with septic shock, the adverse bleeding risk mitigated any mortality benefits. Current efforts are studying the efficacy of recombinant thrombomodulin and ADAMST13 supplementation for patients with low levels of the protease and unbalanced platelet activation with microthrombi.[10] Overall, the best therapy for overt DIC of any cause is to treat the underlying condition, continue to support organ function, and maintain control of hemostasis.

Anticoagulation and Pharmacologic Therapy

Anticoagulation Regimens and Associated Anesthetic Concerns

28 *Antiplatelet therapy* is indicated for patients at risk for cerebral vascular accident, myocardial infarction, or other vascular thrombosis complications. There are several mechanisms to induce platelet dysfunction including COX inhibition, PDE inhibition, ADP receptor antagonism, and GP IIb/IIIa receptor antagonism.

Cyclooxygenase Inhibitors

Aspirin and nonsteroidal anti-inflammatory drugs (NSAIDs) are the most notable members of this class. There are two forms of the COX enzyme with variable distribution throughout the body. COX-1 plays an integral part in maintaining the integrity of the gastric lining, renal blood flow, and initiating the formation of TxA_2, an important molecule for platelet aggregation. Inhibition of COX-1 puts the patient at risk for bleeding, as well as for gastrointestinal and renal morbidity. COX-2 is primarily responsible for synthesizing the prostaglandin mediators of pain and inflammation. Aspirin is a noncompetitive and irreversible inhibitor of both COX enzymes. Consequently, the effects of aspirin therapy last the lifetime of the affected platelets and can only be fully reversed with platelet transfusion, although DDAVP is frequently used to improve platelet function in the presence of aspirin.[52]

NSAIDs are competitive antagonists whose effects last only as long as the drug's time to elimination. Most NSAIDs (naprosyn and ibuprofen) are nonselective COX inhibitors. However, the development of selective COX-2 antagonists such as celecoxib aimed to provide pain relief without the gastrointestinal bleeding complications. Unfortunately, the initial benefits of COX-2 inhibitors were not sustained in long-term outcome studies, and the decreased incidence of gastrotoxicity is clinically insignificant when patients are simultaneously taking aspirin. Postmarket clinical trials with selective COX-2 antagonists reported increased risks for cardiovascular complications likely secondary to impaired vascular endothelial function.[54] The mechanism for cardiovascular risk is unchecked inhibition of PGI_2 without antagonizing the synthesis of TxA_2 from COX-1 within platelets. This tips the balance in favor of a prothrombotic state.[54] In 2007, the American Heart Association (AHA) recommended a stepwise approach to prescribing NSAIDs in patients with cardiovascular disease, emphasizing the use of nonselective or partially selective COX inhibitors first. If selective COX-2 inhibitors (e.g., celecoxib) are needed, they recommend the lowest effective dose for the shortest duration of treatment in conjunction with a proton pump inhibitor and low-dose aspirin.

Phosphodiesterase Inhibitors

PDE inhibitors are primarily used for stroke prophylaxis, since they increase the production of cAMP, an active inhibitor of platelet aggregation. These medications are rarely the drug of choice for patients with cerebrovascular disease, but rather used in conjunction with aspirin therapy. Dipyridamole is a reversible ADP reuptake inhibitor and the prime therapeutic agent in this class, but caffeine, aminophylline, and theophylline also result in reversible platelet dysfunction.[52]

ADP Receptor Antagonists

$P2Y_{12}$ ADP receptor antagonists, such as clopidogrel, prasugrel, and ticagrelor, prevent the expression of GP IIb/IIIa on the surface of activated platelets, thereby inhibiting platelet adhesion and aggregation. These drugs are indicated for patients with coronary artery disease to prevent myocardial infarction and in-stent thrombosis, or for patients with cerebrovascular or peripheral artery disease to inhibit thromboembolism. Clopidogrel is the most commonly prescribed agent in the class of thienopyridines and is a noncompetitive and irreversible antagonist. It is an inactive prodrug that requires oxidation to its active metabolite. Recently, a genetic polymorphism was discovered that results in the inability to metabolize clopidogrel, making it ineffective and putting patients at risk for cardiovascular morbidity and mortality.[55] The FDA put a black box warning on the medication to remind clinicians to monitor the activity. Platelet function studies are insensitive and unreliable for clopidogrel, but tests are now available to measure the inhibition of the $P2Y_{12}$ ADP receptor. Patients who are resistant to clopidogrel may be converted to prasugrel or a non-thienopyridines such as ticagrelor for increased antiplatelet effects.[55] Prasugrel is also an irreversible $P2Y_{12}$ ADP inhibitor indicated for primary prevention of acute coronary syndrome, but not recommended by the AHA for immediate use in patients presenting with acute myocardial ischemia. Ticagrelor is a reversible inhibitor that binds the P2Y12 receptor causing a confirmational change and inactivation. It does not require bioactivation, but it is metabolized by the CYP3A4 system with active metabolites.[55] Both ticagrelor and prasugrel are associated with higher bleeding risk than clopidogrel and should be used with caution in conjunction with high-dose aspirin or anticoagulants.

GP IIb/IIIa Receptor Antagonists

GP IIb/IIIa receptor blockers inhibit the cross-linkage of fibrinogen, the final step in the common hemostatic pathway for platelet aggregation. They include the monoclonal antibody abciximab, and two other molecules which simulate the binding sight of fibrinogen, tirofiban, and eptifibatide. These agents are administered intravenously and primarily used for management of acute coronary syndrome. Their effects are monitored with ACTs and reversed by clearance of the drug. Most of these agents are renally excreted, with half-lives around 20 to 40 minutes, except for abciximab which has a significantly longer context-sensitive half-time secondary to protein binding (24 to 48 hours).[52] All of these drugs cause thrombocytopenia, but the effect is strongest with abciximab with an incidence of about 2.5%, as opposed to 0.5% with the other receptor antagonists.[52]

Protease-Activated Receptor (PAR)-1 Antagonist

Vorapaxar is in a separate class of antithrombotic agents. It functions by inhibiting the protease-activated receptor (PAR)-1, which in turn antagonizes thrombin-induced platelet activation. The indications for vorapaxar are limited due to the clinical effectiveness of ADP receptor antagonists, but of consideration for patients with severe cardiovascular or peripheral artery disease unresponsive to standard regimens of DAPT, and those with chronic renal insufficiency.[52,56]

Vitamin K Antagonists

Warfarin is an oral anticoagulant therapy previously used as the drug of choice for management of hypercoagulable disorders, VTE, and stroke prophylaxis. However, with the significant increase in DOAC administration for similar indications, warfarin use dropped from 77% of overall anticoagulants prescribed to 12% over the last 10 years. Currently it is used in specific circumstances including stoke prevention in patients with mechanical heart valves, mitral valve stenosis or hypertrophic cardiomyopathy, and for those with a history of antiphospholipid antibody syndrome. Warfarin may also be preferred for obese patients with a BMI > 40 kg/m^2 and in those with severe chronic renal disease.[57] Mechanistically, it competes with vitamin K for carboxylation-binding sites and inhibits the synthesis of vitamin K–dependent clotting factors II, VII, IX, and X. Proteins C and S are also dependent on vitamin K, and are also inhibited with warfarin therapy. In fact, patients may be hypercoagulable during the initial phase of treatment, since proteins C and S have shorter half-lives than most clotting factors and thus inhibited first, thereby leaving thrombin generation unregulated. Patients at high risk for thromboembolism must be bridged with another anticoagulation regimen until the target INR is achieved. Warfarin therapy is monitored with the INR (see section on laboratory interpretation). Therapeutic targets generally range between 2.0 and 3.0, and will vary depending on the disease and the patient's bleeding risk.

There is a significant risk of bleeding with any anticoagulation regimen, which demands appropriate protocols for reversal of the specific drug effects. The management protocol for warfarin reversal depends on the patient's symptoms and the urgency. Because warfarin inhibits the synthesis of vitamin K–dependent clotting factors II, VII, IX, and X, the most logical and appropriate reversal agent is replacement of vitamin K. For patients with INR higher than 5.0 and no signs or symptoms of bleeding, warfarin administration should be held for one to two doses. Oral vitamin K should be administered if the INR is over 8.0. Patients who present with high INR and nonmajor bleeding should be reversed with 1 to 3 mg of intravenous vitamin K; this usually corrects the INR within 6 to 8 hours.[58] Emergency reversal for patients with major bleeding or those who require immediate surgery can be achieved with PCCs. Four-factor PCCs (II, VII, IX, X) are generally preferred to three-factor PCCs because the three-factor formulations lack sufficient amounts of factor VII to reliably reverse the effects of warfarin. When three-factor PCCs are used in this setting, factor VII can be supplemented with the addition of plasma.[58] Furthermore, patient-centered protocols that include weight-based dosing and/or consideration for the initial INR, the target INR, and clinical bleeding risks are preferred. The half-life of most PCCs is short, and vitamin K should be given simultaneously for sustained results.[58] Historically, emergency reversal of warfarin was achieved with plasma; however, this requires large volumes of transfusion (10 to 30 mL/kg) and provides unreliable results with inherent delay in treatment secondary to the time needed to type and screen the patient, thaw, prepare, and administer multiple units of plasma. Plasma transfusion is also associated with significant risks for adverse reactions and transfusion-associated infections, especially with the volume of plasma required to reverse therapeutic warfarin.[58] rFVIIa has also been used to reverse warfarin, but the supporting literature is retrospective. Although it reliably corrects the INR, it does not consistently correct clinical bleeding likely secondary to the ongoing inhibition of other vitamin K–dependent clotting factors. Thus, rFVIIa is no longer considered an appropriate reversal agent for warfarin toxicity. Consequently, the BCSH, SCCM, and Neurocritical Care Society recommend the use of plasma only when PCCs are not available, especially for patients with warfarin-related intracranial hemorrhage.[58]

Anticoagulation regimens using oral vitamin K antagonists can be difficult to regulate within the target range. Warfarin has a long onset and offset of action that puts patients at risk for thrombosis and bleeding, especially in the perioperative period. It also has many food and drug interactions, and its metabolism is subject to pharmacogenomics that make dosing highly variable. Warfarin is hepatically metabolized by the P450 CYP2 enzymes and will interact with other commonly used medications such as antibiotics, barbiturates, phenytoin, and proton pump inhibitors. Alterations in dietary intake of vitamin K will also vary the clinical effect of maintenance dosages. Furthermore, there are genetic polymorphisms for the CYP2 enzymes that decrease the metabolism of warfarin and increase bleeding risk.[57] For these reasons, alternative oral anticoagulant agents have been pursued for many years, with a new focus on oral DTIs and FXa inhibitors.

New Oral Anticoagulants

Dabigatran (a DTI), and the FXa inhibitors, rivaroxaban, apixaban, and edoxaban are all FDA approved for stroke prophylaxis in patients with nonvalvular atrial fibrillation, and therapeutic anticoagulation for patients with history of VTE.[59] Thrombin and factor X are at the end of the common pathway for clot formation and stabilization, and play an integral part in secondary hemostasis. Consequently, they are highly desirable targets for antagonism of anticoagulation. These agents are significantly easier to manage than warfarin. They have short half-lives and rapid onsets of action that negate the need for bridging therapy. They are also reliably bioavailable and have little interindividual variability. Thus, coagulation monitoring is unnecessary, although efficacy can be measured with diluted thrombin times or agent-specific anti-Xa assays. Lastly, DOACs have few drug or dietary interactions. All of these agents have a wide therapeutic window, making dosing simple and universal with the exception of patients with significant renal insufficiency. Dabigatran and rivaroxaban, in particular, rely on renal excretion for clearance. Dabigatran may be cleared with dialysis; however, both carry FDA warnings against use in patients with end-stage renal disease (Table 17-15).

The Re-Ly investigators, the ARISTOTLE group, and the EINSTEIN, ENGAGE-AF, and ROCKET-AF trials, all compared dabigatran, apixaban, rivaroxaban, and edoxaban to warfarin, in large, multicenter, randomized controlled trials.[59] These trials were mostly noninferiority studies documenting the efficacy of DOACs compared to warfarin for treatment of VTE, and stroke prevention in valvular and nonvalvular atrial fibrillation. Recent trials demonstrate their usefulness for prevention of VTE in perioperative orthopedic patients undergoing knee and hip arthroplasty. Their full clinical potential has yet to be determined, especially in the perioperative setting. Unfortunately, there is no

Table 17-15 Oral Anticoagulation Medications

	Warfarin	Dabigatran	Apixaban	Rivaroxaban	Edoxaban
Target	Vitamin K	Thrombin	Factor Xa	Factor Xa	Factor Xa
Time to peak (h)	72–96	0.5–2	3–4	2–4	1.5
Half-life (h)	36–42	13–22	12–13	7–113	10–14
Protein binding (%)	35	87	95	55	
Monitoring test	INR	Thrombin time	Anti-Xa	Anti-Xa	Anti-Xa
Renal excretion (%)	None	85	54	73	56
Metabolism	CYP2C9	minimal	CYP3A4	CYP3A4	CYP3A4

reliable coagulation test to monitor the clinical effects or more importantly the bleeding risks associated with these agents. They may prolong the aPTT, PT, or thrombin time, but these are not sensitive monitors for increased risk of bleeding and should not be used to gauge drug levels in the perioperative setting.[59] Rather, perioperative planning for discontinuing DOACs should be based on holding the specific agent 2 to 4 days prior to surgery depending on the bleeding risks and renal function.[59]

In an emergency, there is limited evidence to guide therapeutic reversal of the DOACs. Various societies drafted recommendations for the use of PCCs, either inactive four-factor PCCs, or activated PCCs which contain factors II, IX, X, and various concentrations of activated FVII depending on the formulation. A monoclonal antibody (idarucizumab) was recently FDA approved for reversal of dabigatran after favorable results were published in the interim analysis of the RE-VERSE AD study. Furthermore, dabigatran can be cleared with dialysis.[59] There is no specific antidotes for the direct FXa inhibitors at this time, but new recommendations from expert panels suggest the use of andexanet alfa for patients with major bleeding or to reverse the effects of DOACs before emergency invasive procedures.

Andexanet alfa is a synthetic variant of FXa engineered to bind FXa inhibitors with high affinity, thereby neutralizing their inhibitory action.[59] Guidelines from the SCCM and the Neurocritical Care Society recommend PCCs to reverse the clinical bleeding risks associated with direct FXa inhibitors, and idarucizumab for reversal of dabigatran.[52] However, these recommendations were published prior to the widespread investigation of andexanet alfa and may not recognize its therapeutic potential for emergency reversal of critical bleeding associated with DOACs. There are special circumstances when andexanet alfa would not be the best agent for reversal, however (e.g., cardiac surgery patients who are expected to require heparinization therapy for cardiopulmonary bypass). The mechanism of action of andexanet alfa is not consistent with preoperative goals of care for cardiac surgery; therefore, PCCs are preferable for reversal of DOACs prior to heparinization.[59] Furthermore, the cost of andexanet alfa averages $30,000 to $60,000 and may be prohibitively expensive in many healthcare systems. Perioperatively, DOACs should be discontinued 48 to 72 hours before major surgery. The half-lives of these agents are approximately 12 hours; thus, assuming normal hepatic and renal function, more than four half-lives ensure significant drug clearance.

Heparin Therapy

Heparin therapy is one of the oldest and most common anticoagulation regimens. There are two main forms of heparin, UFH, and LMWH. UFH indirectly inhibits thrombin and FXa by binding to AT-III, causing a conformational shape change which significantly increases its activity. Although the use of UFH for prophylaxis against VTE has decreased in favor of LMWH and DOACs, it is still used for immediate anticoagulation with acute coronary syndrome, PE, and during cardiopulmonary bypass or vascular surgery. The clinical effects of heparin therapy are monitored with an anti-factor Xa assay, aPTT, or ACT. Patients may be resistant to UFH if they have a hereditary insufficiency of AT-III or an acquired deficiency from prolonged heparin administration. AT-III can be replenished with plasma transfusion or administration of AT-III concentrate. Therapeutic UFH is administered parenterally and its clinical effects are fully reversible with protamine.[52] The main complication is HIT, discussed later in this section.

LMWH is a fractionated form of heparin with similar mechanism of action, but with more specific inhibition of FXa. Several agents are currently available, including enoxaparin, dalteparin, and reviparin. LMWH is preferred over UFH for both DVT prophylaxis and treatment because laboratory monitoring is unnecessary, and its longer half-life allows for once- or twice-daily dosing. Treatment can be monitored with FXa levels, but this is only necessary for obese patients and those with renal insufficiency, which prolongs elimination. Reversal with protamine is unpredictable and not likely to completely resolve bleeding tendencies.[52]

Indirect Factor Xa Antagonists

Fondaparinux is the principal agent used in this class. It is a highly specific antagonist for free FXa that also acts via binding with AT-III. Like LMWH, it is popular for DVT treatment and prophylaxis because it has a long half-life and requires only once-daily dosing, and highly reliable absorption that negates the need for coagulation monitoring. However, fondaparinux undergoes renal elimination, necessitating a lower dose or coagulation monitoring with FXa levels in patients with renal insufficiency. There is no available antidote in the event of bleeding or the need for emergency procedures. Fortunately, the incidence of HIT is relatively low; and although they are not approved for use in patients with a history of HIT, fondaparinux is likely safe and efficacious in patients with concern for HIT. Given the expanding use of DOACs for anticoagulation and secondary prevention in venous thromboembolic disease, the indications for fondaparinux are limited. It is considered appropriate for use in pregnancy.[15]

Heparin-Induced Thrombocytopenia

HIT is a clinical disorder that develops after extended heparin therapy (NICV 17-6). It occurs in approximately 1 in 5,000 hospitalized patients, with higher risk in postoperative patients and women.[15] It is associated with significant organ failure, 29 vascular compromise, and mortality from thromboembolic complications. There are two types: HIT1 describes mild thrombocytopenia, is benign and does not involve immune complexes. HIT2 is an immune-mediated response and carries a significant risk of thrombosis. IgG antibodies bind to heparin–PF4 complexes on the surface of platelets, thereby initiating primary hemostasis and thrombin generation. HIT2 can occur in any patient receiving heparin therapy. Typically, 5 to 10 days are required to mount a significant immune response, but patients who have recent exposure to heparin or a history of HIT can present with clinical symptoms immediately. Any form of heparin therapy can initiate HIT; however, UFH is more likely than LMWH to lead to immune complexes because the fractionated form is less antigenic with a weaker bond to heparin–PF4.[15]

There are no specific laboratory tests for the clear diagnosis of HIT, and clinical signs can be clouded by alternative causes of thrombocytopenia and thrombosis. Guidelines from the American College of Chest Physicians and the national European guidelines recommend a diagnostic scoring algorithm, the 4T-score, to determine the pretest probability of clinical HIT. Variables to consider include the degree of thrombocytopenia (defined as a fall in platelet count of 30% to 50%), the timing of platelet decrease (typically day 5 to 10 of heparin therapy), any thromboembolic complications, and the likelihood of alternative diagnoses. Intermediate to high clinical suspicion of HIT is then confirmed with laboratory tests. The enzyme-linked immunosorbent assay (ELISA) for heparin–PF4 IgG antibodies is sensitive, but not as specific as the serotonin release functional assay, which is currently the gold standard test.[15] Patients suspected of having HIT should be managed with therapeutic anticoagulation and immediate discontinuation of all heparin therapy including heparin-coated indwelling catheters. The most commonly used agents are the parenteral DTIs such as bivalirudin and argatroban. Oral vitamin K antagonists are contraindicated for HIT treatment because the decreased synthesis of proteins C and S enhances the patient's prothrombotic state. Furthermore, warfarin has been shown to cause gangrenous thrombosis of the limbs in patients with HIT. Platelet transfusion should also be held unless the patient is severely thrombocytopenic (<20,000/μL) with signs of bleeding.

Parenteral Direct Thrombin Inhibitors

Argatroban and bivalirudin are synthetic agents that directly inhibit thrombin in its free and fibrin-bound states. They are not immunogenic and there is no risk of HIT. The half-lives of these agents vary. Furthermore, there are currently no known antidotes to the DTIs; therefore, reversal depends upon clearance. Clinical effects can be monitored with ACT or aPTT measurements. They are both approved for use in the United States for treatment of HIT. Argatroban is metabolized by the liver, with variable clearance in patients with hepatic dysfunction. It is commonly used for patients with HIT, who suffer from concurrent renal failure. Argatroban will prolong the INR as well as the aPTT, which can complicate clinical titration of warfarin therapy for long-term anticoagulation. Bivalirudin is a short-acting DTI with rapid onset of action and renal excretion. It is the drug of choice for patients with both renal and hepatic dysfunction, and its clinical versatility makes it a good agent for use during cardiopulmonary bypass in patients with HIT.[15]

Recombinant Activated Factor VII

30 Recombinant activated factor VII (rFVIIa) was originally FDA approved for prophylaxis and treatment of patients with hemophilia A or B complicated by inhibitors to FVIII and factor IX concentrates. It is now also indicated for the treatment of acquired hemophilia and FVII deficiency.[60] However, most of its use is off-label for the prevention and treatment of coagulopathy and major blood loss in patients with postpartum hemorrhage, trauma, reversal of various anticoagulants, and high-risk cardiac surgery. The supporting data for these uses stem from retrospective reports, observational studies, and case series. There are few randomized controlled trials showing improved clinical outcomes and no trials that report definitive mortality benefits. In fact, a meta-analysis demonstrated an increased risk of arterial thromboembolism, especially in elderly patients with use of high doses of rFVIIa (>120 μg/kg).[60] The current guidelines for the reversal of DOACs recommend PCCs as the drugs of choice; however, if activated PCCs are not available, low-dose rFVIIa (15 to 20 μg/kg) should be considered for life-threatening hemorrhage. Overall, the lack of consistent dosing protocols and definitive evidence leaves one without clear indications for the use of rFVIIa for critical bleeding.

The mechanism for rFVIIa remains unclear, but likely involves more than the physiologic role of factor VII in secondary hemostasis. Theoretically, rFVIIa will only act with TF exposed from the vascular endothelial lining at a site of injury. However, certain hemorrhagic disorders such as DIC or polytrauma can initiate systemic release of TF. Furthermore, rFVIIa can directly activate FX and platelets, generating a thrombin burst for procoagulant activity. These mechanisms explain why arterial and venous thromboembolisms are the major adverse effects of rFVIIa, and why DIC and high thromboembolism risk are the main contraindications.[60]

Prothrombin Complex Concentrates

PCCs have been available for treatment of patients with hemophilia B for several decades. They were first used as a source of FIX in the 1970s prior to the advent of specific factor concentrates. Subsequently they provided bypass treatment for hemophiliacs with factor inhibitors. Over the years, the safety and efficacy of PCCs have improved dramatically, and they are now FDA approved for use in hemophilia and reversal of vitamin K antagonists. PCCs are also indicated for rescue therapy of trauma induced coagulopathy, control of critical bleeding, and reversal of DOACs, although evidence is limited and their use for these indications remain off label.

There are several commercially available formulations of PCCs, containing varying amounts of three to four coagulation factors, as well as one or more type of anticoagulant. The compositions include the vitamin K–dependent factors (II, VII, IX, and X), although not all products contain significant concentrations of FVII. Some PCCs are "three-factor" concentrates lacking FVII, but most formulations contain all four factors, with the addition of a natural anticoagulant such as heparin or AT to decrease the thrombogenic risks. Activated PCCs such as the Factor Eight Inhibitor Bypass Agent (FEIBA), contain activated FVIIa and FXa, and may be administered for bypass therapy in hemophilia patients with inhibitors, or for reversal of direct anti-factor Xa antagonists.[61]

PCCs are the drug of choice for immediate reversal of warfa- 31
rin in place of rFVIIa and plasma. They are preferred for several reasons. First, they correct coagulopathy much faster than the time required to thaw and administer plasma. Furthermore, PCCs stem from human plasma, but they are treated with at least one viral reduction process, whereas transfusion of several units of plasma (10 to 15 mL/kg required to reverse warfarin) carries a significant risk of infectious and noninfectious transfusion reactions. It is important to remember that although PCCs provide factor

replacement for thrombin generation, their action still depends on adequate concentrations of platelets and fibrinogen.

The potential for PCCs to generate a significant thrombin burst puts patients at risk for thrombotic complications. The exact pathogenesis for thrombosis remains unclear, but animal models indicate that the accumulation of prothrombin, inactive factor II, and/or factor X after PCC administration correlates with thrombogenesis. Furthermore, this risk is associated with patients having thrombotic tendencies, such as those on anticoagulation and elderly patients who have a history of stroke. There are very few outcome studies evaluating their safety, but thus far no significant thrombotic complications have been reported with PCCs for critical bleeding.[61]

The thromboembolic risk can be minimized by avoiding repeat dosing. The factors within PCCs have varied half-lives, with prothrombin remaining active in plasma for up to 60 hours and factor X present for 30 hours. This is in contrast to labile FVII, whose half-life is only approximately 6 hours. Consequently, factors II and X, which are thought to be primarily responsible for thrombotic complications, have the potential to accumulate with repeat doses of PCCs. The need for repeat dosing can be avoided by the coadministration of vitamin K in patients treated for oral anticoagulant toxicity. This allows for increased synthesis of coagulation factors. Furthermore, PCC dosing should be guided by the appropriate coagulation profile test. PT and INR only measure the procoagulant half of the hemostatic mechanism, and ignore the presence of anticoagulant activity such as heparin, AT or proteins C and S. In patients with severe liver disease or dilutional coagulopathy, the PT and INR times may be prolonged, but the concentrations of anticoagulants are also decreased, leaving hemostasis balanced. Thrombin generation times or thromboelastography are more appropriate measures of the patient's risk of bleeding and better indicators of the efficacy of PCC. These tests should be considered before redosing, since these patients may require simultaneous treatment with AT, platelets, or fibrinogen. The only absolute contraindications to PCC administration are in patients at high risk for thrombosis, such as those in DIC or with active HIT.

Desmopressin

Desmopressin (DDAVP) is a synthetic analog for the endogenous antidiuretic hormone, vasopressin. It acts at the V2 receptor found in the nephron and within endothelial cells. DDAVP was originally introduced for treatment of diabetes insipidus, but it was also found to improve hemostasis and platelet function. Consequently, it is one of the drugs of choice for treatment of mild bleeding in patients with vWD and mild hemophilia A, as discussed earlier.[62] Mechanistically, it causes the release of FVIII and vWF from within vascular endothelial cells, thereby improving platelet function. The appropriate dose for hemostasis is 0.3 µg/kg intravenously over 20 to 30 minutes, with therapeutic effects lasting for approximately 6 to 8 hours. Clinical benefits have been demonstrated for high-risk surgery, especially in patients with aspirin-induced platelet dysfunction. Hypotension is the most commonly reported side effect, presumably secondary to arterial vasodilation from the release of NO; it is best avoided with slower infusion rates. Hyponatremia and water retention are rare complications, but have been reported in pediatric patients. As with all prothrombotic agents, DDAVP should be avoided in patients at high risk for thromboembolism, although the most recent meta-analysis did not report a significant incidence of thromboembolic complications.[62]

The hemostatic potential for DDAVP has been carefully studied for patients with critical bleeding from cardiac or spine surgery, uremia, antiplatelet agents, and liver disease. Several meta-analyses of randomized controlled trials report mild decreases in blood loss (80 mL per patient) but fail to translate into significant outcome improvements. There is no apparent effect on the number of patients transfused or the incidence of postoperative complications (including reoperation). The only consistent clinical benefit of DDAVP is improved bleeding times for patients with congenital or acquired platelet dysfunction from cardiopulmonary bypass, chronic renal failure, or aspirin therapy.

Antifibrinolytic Therapy

Antifibrinolytic agents have been used to prevent and treat surgical blood loss for several decades. There are two types—the lysine analogs EACA and TXA, and a serine protease inhibitor, aprotinin. Aprotinin was reported to have superior efficacy for reducing blood loss, minimizing transfusions, and preventing reoperations in cardiac surgery. However, it was removed from the market after observational studies raised concern for relative risk of renal failure, myocardial infarction, and death. These findings were confirmed by the Blood Conservation Using Antifibrinolytics in a Randomized Trial (BART), which was stopped early due to significantly higher mortality associated with aprotinin when compared to EACA and TXA. However, the risks may have been exaggerated with methodologic concerns with the BART trial. Aprotinin is currently available in Canada and worldwide. Both the lysine derivatives are widely used throughout the United States.[63] Today, they are commonly administered as part of a multimodal approach to perioperative blood conservation strategies with established efficacy to reduce mortality due to bleeding in trauma, postpartum hemorrhage, and TBI, and cardiac surgery.[64,65] 32

Aprotinin is a nonspecific serine protease inhibitor. It prevents the action of several proteins involved in coagulation and fibrinolysis, including trypsin, plasmin, and kallikrein. It may also have an indirect effect on platelets to preserve their function, especially during extracorporeal circulation specifically cardiopulmonary bypass. The clinical efficacy of aprotinin to reduce perioperative blood loss, transfusions, and reoperations is clear; however, there is also evidence reporting the negative association with renal failure and mortality.[63] Overall, aprotinin remains an option for perioperative blood conservation, but it is not currently the antifibrinolytic agent of choice in the United States.

Lysine Analog

EACA and TXA are synthetic derivatives of the amino acid, lysine (NICV 17-7). They competitively inhibit the binding site on plasminogen, thereby preventing cleavage to plasmin and the resultant fibrinolysis. Both agents are excreted by the kidney and may be administered intravenously or topically. Although there is more evidence to support the use of TXA, these agents appear to have equivalent efficacy and have been shown to moderately decrease perioperative blood loss in cardiac surgery, as well as liver transplantation, orthopedic operations, and spine fusions.[63,66] They are also known to improve survival after trauma (CRASH II), TBI (CRASH III), and postpartum hemorrhage (WOMAN trial), when administered early in the course of critical bleeding.[64,65] Active research continues to focus on clarifying the appropriate dosing regimens and patient population to determine effects on rates of transfusion, reoperation, length of stay, morbidity, and mortality. The lysine analogs are inexpensive compared to aprotinin, and there have been no reports of increased risk of thrombotic complications or renal failure. The only documented adverse effect is seizure risk associated with TXA at high doses.[63,66] Overall, the lysine analogs are inexpensive and low-risk adjunctive agents that should be included in blood management protocols for major surgery, trauma, or critical bleeding as part of a multimodal approach to blood conservation.

Conclusions

Clinical anesthesiology is a perioperative specialty that aims to maintain the patient's health and wellness throughout the course of surgery. This requires a clear understanding of how a person's pre-existing comorbid status and anticipated surgical procedure can best be managed to gain the most therapeutic benefits from interventions with the least incurred risk. The anesthesiologist must remain vigilant and anticipate the possibility of derangements to coagulation and hemostasis that may occur with surgery, trauma, or critical illness. They must also know the best methods for avoiding and treating hemorrhagic or thrombotic complications of surgery while limiting the risks of transfusion therapy and hemostatic pharmacologic agents.

Overall, understanding the hemostatic mechanisms and the specifics of transfusion therapy is integral to the practice of anesthesia.

For further review and interactivities, please see the videos and narrative interactive clinical vignettes (NICVs) accessible in the complimentary eBook bundled with this text. Access instructions are located on the inside front cover.

REFERENCES

1. Depta JP, Bhatt DL. New approaches to inhibiting platelets and coagulation. *Annu Rev Pharmacol Toxicol*. 2015;55:373–397.
2. Paniccia R, Priora R, Liotta AA, Abbate R. Platelet function tests: A comparative review. *Vasc Health Risk Manag*. 2015;11:133–148.
3. Mann KG. Thrombin generation in hemorrhage control and vascular occlusion. *Circulation*. 2011;124(2):225–235.
4. Koupenova M, Clancy L, Corkrey HA, Freedman JE. Circulating platelets as mediators of immunity, inflammation, and thrombosis. *Circ Res*. 2018;122(2):337–351.
5. May JE, Wolberg AS, Lim MY. Disorders of fibrinogen and fibrinolysis. *Hematol Oncol Clin North Am*. 2021;35(6):1197–1217.
6. Weyand AC, Flood VH. Von willebrand disease: Current status of diagnosis and management. *Hematol Oncol Clin North Am*. 2021;35(6):1085–1101.
7. Connell NT, Flood VH, Brignardello-Petersen R, et al. ASH ISTH NHF WFH 2021 guidelines on the management of von Willebrand disease. *Blood Adv*. 2021;5(1):301–325.
8. Sborov DW, Rodgers GM. How I manage patients with acquired haemophilia A. *Br J Haematol*. 2013;161(2):157–165.
9. Berntorp E, Fischer K, Hart DP, et al. Haemophilia. *Nat Rev Dis Primers*. 2021;7(1):45.
10. Levi M, Sivapalaratnam S. Disseminated intravascular coagulation: An update on pathogenesis and diagnosis. *Expert Rev Hematol*. 2018;11(8):663–672.
11. Beyer JT, Lind SE, Fisher S, Trujillo TC, Wempe MF, Kiser TH. Evaluation of intravenous direct thrombin inhibitor monitoring tests: Correlation with plasma concentrations and clinical outcomes in hospitalized patients. *J Thromb Thrombolysis*. 2020;49(2):259–267.
12. Schmidt AE, Israel AK, Refaai MA. The utility of thromboelastography to guide blood product transfusion. *Am J Clin Pathol*. 2019;152(4):407–422.
13. MacCallum P, Bowles L, Keeling D. Diagnosis and management of heritable thrombophilias. *BMJ*. 2014;349:g4387.
14. Sammaritano LR. Antiphospholipid syndrome. *Best Pract Res Clin Rheumatol*. 2020;34(1): 101463.
15. Marcucci R, Berteotti M, Gori AM, et al. Heparin induced thrombocytopenia: Position paper from the Italian society on thrombosis and haemostasis (SISET). *Blood Transfus*. 2021;19(1): 14–23.
16. Chen A, Stecker E, Warden BA. Direct oral anticoagulant use: A practical guide to common clinical challenges. *J Am Heart Assoc*. 2020;9(13):e017559.
17. Jones JM, Sapiano MRP, Mowla S, Bota D, Berger JJ, Basavaraju SV. Has the trend of declining blood transfusions in the United States ended? Findings of the 2019 national blood collection and utilization survey. *Transfusion*. 2021;61 Suppl 2:S1–S10.
18. Mowla SJ, Sapiano MRP, Jones JM, Berger JJ, Basavaraju SV. Supplemental findings of the 2019 national blood collection and utilization survey. *Transfusion*. 2021;61 Suppl 2:S11–S35.
19. *A Compendium of Transfusion Practice Guidelines*. 3rd ed. American Red Cross; 2017.
20. Cloutier M, De Korte D, ISBT Transfusion-Transmitted Infectious Diseases Working Party SoB. Residual risks of bacterial contamination for pathogen-reduced platelet components. *Vox Sang*. 2022;117(7):879–886.
21. Irving A, Higgins A, Ady B, et al. Fresh red cells for transfusion in critically ill adults: An economic evaluation of the standard issue transfusion versus fresher red-cell use in intensive care (TRANSFUSE) clinical trial. *Crit Care Med*. 2019;47(7):e572–e579.
22. Charbe NB, Castillo F, Tambuwala MM, et al. A new era in oxygen therapeutics? From perfluorocarbon systems to haemoglobin-based oxygen carriers. *Blood Rev*. 2022;54:100927.
23. Haruki R, Kimura T, Iwasaki H, et al. Safety evaluation of hemoglobin-albumin cluster "HemoAct" as a red blood cell substitute. *Sci Rep*. 2015;5:12778.
24. van den Akker TA, Grimes ZM, Friedman MT. Transfusion-associated circulatory overload and transfusion-related acute lung injury. *Am J Clin Pathol*. 2021;156(4):529–539.
25. American Society of Anesthesiologists Task Force on Perioperative Blood Management. Practice guidelines for perioperative blood management: An updated report by the American Society of Anesthesiologists Task Force on perioperative blood management*. *Anesthesiology*. 2015;122(2):241–275.
26. Spahn DR, Bouillon B, Cerny V, et al. The European guideline on management of major bleeding and coagulopathy following trauma: Fifth edition. *Crit Care*. 2019;23(1):98.
27. Raphael J, Mazer CD, Subramani S, et al. Society of cardiovascular anesthesiologists clinical practice improvement advisory for management of perioperative bleeding and hemostasis in cardiac surgery patients. *Anesth Analg*. 2019;129(5):1209–1221.
28. Carson JL, Guyatt G, Heddle NM, et al. Clinical practice guidelines from the AABB: Red blood cell transfusion thresholds and storage. *JAMA*. 2016;316:2025–2035.
29. Hare GM. Tolerance of anemia: Understanding the adaptive physiological mechanisms which promote survival. *Transfus Apher Sci*. 2014;50(1):10–12.
30. Estcourt LJ, Birchall J, Allard S, et al. Guidelines for the use of platelet transfusions. *Br J Haematol*. 2017;176(3):365–394.
31. Green L, Bolton-Maggs P, Beattie C, et al. British society of haematology guidelines on the spectrum of fresh frozen plasma and cryoprecipitate products: Their handling and use in various patient groups in the absence of major bleeding. *Br J Haematol*. 2018;181(1):54–67.
32. Holcomb JB, Tilley BC, Baraniuk S, et al. Transfusion of plasma, platelets, and red blood cells in a 1:1:1 vs a 1:1:2 ratio and mortality in patients with severe trauma: The PROPPR randomized clinical trial. *JAMA*. 2015;313(5):471–482.
33. Dishong D, Cap AP, Holcomb JB, Triulzi DJ, Yazer MH. The rebirth of the cool: A narrative review of the clinical outcomes of cold stored low titer group O whole blood recipients compared to conventional component recipients in trauma. *Hematology*. 2021;26(1):601–611.
34. Zhao H, Devine DV. The missing pieces to the cold-stored platelet puzzle. *Int J Mol Sci*. 2022;23(3):1100.
35. Kracalik I, Mowla S, Basavaraju SV, Sapiano MRP. Transfusion-related adverse reactions: Data from the national healthcare safety network hemovigilance module – united states, 2013–2018. *Transfusion*. 2021;61(5):1424–1434.
36. Fatalities reported to FDA following blood collection and transfusion annual summary for FY 2020 (FDA's center for biologics evaluation and research). 1–18.
37. *The 2021 Annual SHOT Report*. 25. 2022:1–258. Serious Hazards of Transfusion (SHOT). https://www.shotuk.org/wp-content/uploads/myimages/SHOT-REPORT-2021-FINAL-bookmarked.pdf
38. Dodd RY, Crowder LA, Haynes JM, Notari EP, Stramer SL, Steele WR. Screening blood donors for HIV, HCV, and HBV at the american red cross: 10-year trends in prevalence, incidence, and residual risk, 2007 to 2016. *Transfus Med Rev*. 2020;34(2):81–93.
39. Abdallah R, Rai H, Panch SR. Transfusion reactions and adverse events. *Clin Lab Med*. 2021; 41(4):669–696.
40. AABB Clinical Transfusion Medicine Committee, Heddle NM, Boeckh M, Grossman B, et al. AABB committee report: Reducing transfusion-transmitted cytomegalovirus infections. *Transfusion*. 2016;56(6 Pt 2):1581–1587.
41. Schmidt M, Ramirez-Arcos S, Stiller L, McDonald C, ISBT Transfusion-Transmitted Infectious Diseases Working Party SoB. Current status of rapid bacterial detection methods for platelet components: A 20-year review by the ISBT transfusion-transmitted infectious diseases working party subgroup on bacteria. *Vox Sang*. 2022;117(8):983–988.
42. Aguilar-Nascimento JE, Zampieri-Filho JP, Bordin JO. Implications of perioperative allogeneic red blood cell transfusion on the immune-inflammatory response. *Hematol Transfus Cell Ther*. 2021;43(1):58–64.
43. Tormey CA, Hendrickson JE. Transfusion-related red blood cell alloantibodies: Induction and consequences. *Blood*. 2019;133(17):1821–1830.
44. Mueller MM, Van Remoortel H, Meybohm P, et al. Patient blood management: recommendations from the 2018 Frankfurt Consensus Conference. *JAMA*. 2019;321(10):983–997.
45. Althoff FC, Neb H, Herrmann E, et al. Multimodal patient blood management program based on a three-pillar strategy: a systematic review and meta-analysis. *Ann Surg*. 2019;269(5): 794–804.
46. Ng O, Keeler BD, Mishra A, et al. Iron therapy for preoperative anaemia. *Cochrane Database Syst Rev*. 2019;12:CD011588.

47. Zhou X, Zhang C, Wang Y, Yu L, Yan M. Preoperative acute normovolemic hemodilution for minimizing allogeneic blood transfusion: A meta-analysis. *Anesth Analg*. 2015;121(6): 1443–1455.
48. Frank SM, Sikorski RA, Konig G, et al. Clinical utility of autologous salvaged blood: A review. *J Gastrointest Surg*. 2020;24(2):464–472.
49. Crowe EP, DeSimone RA. Transfusion support and alternatives for Jehovah's witness patients. *Curr Opin Hematol*. 2019;26(6):473–479.
50. Jilma-Stohlawetz P, Quehenberger P, Schima H, et al. Acquired von willebrand factor deficiency caused by LVAD is ADAMTS-13 and platelet dependent. *Thromb Res*. 2016;137: 196–201.
51. Srivastava A, Santagostino E, Dougall A, et al. WFH guidelines for the management of hemophilia, 3rd edition. *Haemophilia*. 2020;26 Suppl 6:1–158.
52. Frontera JA, Lewin JJ 3rd, Rabinstein AA, et al. Guideline for reversal of antithrombotics in intracranial hemorrhage: Executive summary. A statement for healthcare professionals from the neurocritical care society and the society of critical care medicine. *Crit Care Med*. 2016;44(12):2251–2257.
53. O'Leary JG, Greenberg CS, Patton HM, Caldwell SH. AGA clinical practice update: Coagulation in cirrhosis. *Gastroenterology*. 2019;157(1):34–43 e1.
54. El-Malah AA, Gineinah MM, Deb PK, et al. Selective COX-2 inhibitors: Road from success to controversy and the quest for repurposing. *Pharmaceuticals (Basel)*. 2022;15(7):827,
55. Al-Abcha A, Radwan Y, Blais D, et al. Genotype-guided use of P2Y12 inhibitors: A review of current state of the art. *Front Cardiovasc Med*. 2022;9:850028.
56. Kamran H, Jneid H, Kayani WT, et al. Oral antiplatelet therapy after acute coronary syndrome: A review. *JAMA*. 2021;325(15):1545–1555.
57. Fahmi AM, Elewa H, El Jilany I. Warfarin dosing strategies evolution and its progress in the era of precision medicine, a narrative review. *Int J Clin Pharm*. 2022;44(3):599–607.
58. Tran HA, Chunilal SD, Harper PL, Tran H, Wood EM, Gallus AS; Australasian Society of Thrombosis and Haemostasis (ASTH). An update of consensus guidelines for warfarin reversal. *Med J Aust*. 2013;198(4):198–199.
59. Budd AN, Wood B, Zheng W, Rong LQ. Perioperative management of direct oral anticoagulants in cardiac surgery: Practice recommendations based on current evidence. *J Cardiothorac Vasc Anesth*. 2022;36:4141–4149.
60. Levi M, Levy JH, Andersen HF, Truloff D. Safety of recombinant activated factor VII in randomized clinical trials. *N Engl J Med*. 2010;363(19):1791–800.
61. Tanaka KA, Shettar S, Vandyck K, Shea SM, Abuelkasem E. Roles of four-factor prothrombin complex concentrate in the management of critical bleeding. *Transfus Med Rev*. 2021;35(4):96–103.
62. Sreeraman S, McKinlay S, Li A, Crowther M, Motalo O. Efficacy of parenteral formulations of desmopressin in the treatment of bleeding disorders: A systematic review. *Thromb Res*. 2022; 213:16–26.
63. Klein A, Agarwal S, Cholley B, et al. A review of European guidelines for patient blood management with a particular emphasis on antifibrinolytic drug administration for cardiac surgery. *J Clin Anesth*. 2022;78:110654.
64. CRASH-trial Collaborators. Effects of tranexamic acid on death, disability, vascular occlusive events and other morbidities in patients with acute traumatic brain injury (CRASH-3): A randomised, placebo-controlled trial. *Lancet*. 2019;394(10210):1713–1723.
65. WOMAN Trial Collaborators. Effect of early tranexamic acid administration on mortality, hysterectomy, and other morbidities in women with post-partum haemorrhage (WOMAN): An international, randomised, double-blind, placebo-controlled trial. *Lancet*. 2017;389(10084): 2105–2116.
66. Taeuber I, Weibel S, Herrmann E, et al. Association of intravenous tranexamic acid with thromboembolic events and mortality: A systematic review, meta-analysis, and meta-regression. *JAMA Surg*. 2021;156:e210884.

Section 4

ANESTHETIC DRUGS AND ADJUVANTS

18 Inhaled Anesthetics

THOMAS J. EBERT

KEY POINTS

1. At equilibrium, the partial pressure of inhaled anesthetics in the brain equals the arterial partial pressure, which in turn equals the alveolar partial pressure if cardiopulmonary function is normal.
2. The inspired concentration and the blood:gas solubility of an inhaled anesthetic are the major determinants of the speed of induction. Solubility alone determines the rate of elimination, provided there is normal cardiopulmonary function.
3. Isoflurane is the most potent of the volatile anesthetics in clinical use, desflurane is the least soluble in blood, and sevoflurane is the least irritating to the airways.
4. Nitrous oxide (N_2O) can expand a pneumothorax to double or triple its size in 10 to 30 minutes. Abrupt discontinuation of N_2O inhalation can transiently lower alveolar concentrations of oxygen and carbon dioxide, a phenomenon called *diffusion hypoxia*.
5. Minimum alveolar concentration (MAC) is the alveolar concentration of an inhaled anesthetic at one atmosphere that prevents movement in response to a surgical stimulus in 50% of patients. Concentrations of inhaled anesthetics that provide loss of awareness and recall are about 0.4 to 0.5 MAC.
6. MAC decreases approximately 6% per decade of patient age.
7. Volatile anesthetics depress cerebral metabolic rate in a dose-dependent manner and at higher concentrations will increase cerebral blood flow. The latter effect may increase intracranial pressure in patients with a mass-occupying lesion of the brain.
8. Hypocapnia may blunt or abolish volatile anesthetic-induced increases in cerebral blood flow depending on when the hypocapnia is induced and the nature of the cerebral disease process.

9 Volatile anesthetics produce dose-dependent depression of the electroencephalogram, sensory-evoked potentials, and motor-evoked potentials.

10 Volatile anesthetics in current use decrease arterial blood pressure, systemic vascular resistance, and myocardial function comparably and in a dose-dependent fashion.

11 Volatile anesthetics decrease tidal volume, decrease ventilatory response to hypercarbia and hypoxia, increase respiratory rate, and relax airway smooth muscle in a dose-dependent fashion.

12 Unlike halothane, volatile anesthetics in current use have minimal adverse effects on the liver and might afford some protection for hepatocytes from ischemic and/or hypoxic injury.

13 Volatile anesthetics are potent triggers for malignant hyperthermia in genetically susceptible patients.

14 CO_2 absorbents degrade sevoflurane, desflurane, and isoflurane to carbon monoxide when the normal water content of the absorbent (13% to 15%) is markedly decreased (<5%).

15 Volatile anesthetics have a global warming potential far greater than CO_2 and should be delivered with a lower fresh gas flow to reduce their impact.

Introduction

Inhalation anesthetics are the most common drugs used for the provision of general anesthesia. Adding only a fraction of a volatile anesthetic to the inspired oxygen results in a state of unconsciousness and amnesia. When combined with intravenous adjuvants, such as opioids and benzodiazepines, a balanced technique is achieved that results in analgesia, further sedation/hypnosis, and amnesia. Inhaled anesthetics for surgical procedures are popular because of their ease of administration and the clinician's ability to reliably monitor their effects with both clinical signs and end-tidal concentrations of exhaled gases. In addition, the volatile anesthetic gases are relatively inexpensive in terms of overall cost.

Sevoflurane, desflurane, and isoflurane are the most popular potent inhaled anesthetics used in adult surgical procedures (Fig. 18-1). Although there are many similarities in terms of the overall effects of the volatile anesthetics (e.g., they all have a dose-dependent effect to decrease blood pressure [BP]), there are some unique differences that might influence the clinician's selection process depending on the patient's age, health, and the surgical procedure. For example, sevoflurane is the most common anesthetic used for children because of its relative lack of pungency when inhaled and its speed of emergence. These beneficial attributes outweigh the emergence agitation often associated with the use of sevoflurane in children. Discussion of the attributes of the three most popular inhaled anesthetics provides the major emphasis of this chapter. For the sake of completeness and for historical perspective related to metabolism and toxicity, comments on halothane and enflurane are also included.

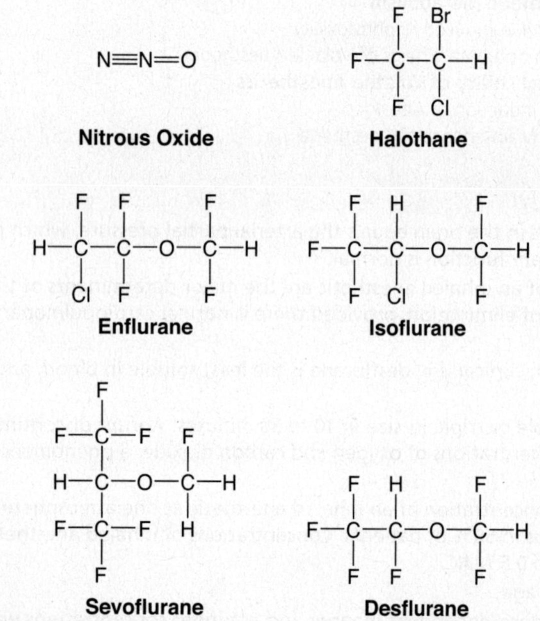

Figure 18-1 Chemical structure of inhaled anesthetics. Halothane is an alkane, a halogen-substituted ethane derivative. It is no longer available commercially. Isoflurane and enflurane are isomers that are methyl ethyl ethers. Desflurane differs from isoflurane in the substitution of a fluorine for a chlorine atom and sevoflurane is a methyl isopropyl ether.

Pharmacokinetic Principles

Kety[1] in 1950 was the first to examine the pharmacokinetics of inhaled agents in a systematic fashion. Eger[2] accomplished much of the early research in the field, leading to his landmark text on the subject in 1974. The inhaled anesthetics differ substantially from nearly all other therapeutic drugs because they are gases given via inhalation. Drug pharmacology is classically divided into two disciplines, pharmacodynamics and pharmacokinetics. *Pharmacodynamics* can be defined as what drugs do to the body. It describes the desired and undesired effects of drugs, as well as the cellular and molecular changes leading to these effects. *Pharmacokinetics* can be defined as how the body handles drugs. It describes where drugs are distributed, how they are transformed, and the cellular and molecular mechanisms underlying these processes.

Tissues are often grouped into hypothetical *compartments* based on perfusion. An important implication of different compartments and perfusion rates is the concept of redistribution. After a given amount of drug is administered, it reaches highly perfused tissue compartments first, where it can equilibrate rapidly and exert its effects. With time, however, compartments with lower perfusion rates receive sufficient drug to reach equilibrium between blood and tissue. As the tissues with lower perfusion rates absorb the drug, maintenance of equilibria throughout the body requires drug transfer from highly perfused compartments back into the bloodstream. This lowering of drug concentration in one compartment by delivery into another compartment is called *redistribution*.

In discussions of the inhaled anesthetics, the absorption phase is usually called *uptake*, the metabolic phase is usually called *biotransformation*, and the excretion phase is usually called *elimination*.

Unique Features of Inhaled Anesthetics

Speed, Gas State, and Route of Administration

The inhaled anesthetics are among the most rapidly acting drugs in existence, and when used for general anesthesia, this speed provides a margin of safety. The ability to quickly increase or decrease anesthetic levels as necessary can mean the difference between an anesthetic state and an anesthetic misadventure. Speed also means efficiency. Rapid induction and recovery may lead to faster operating room (OR) turnover times, shorter recovery room stays, and earlier discharge times to home. Only N_2O and xenon are true gases, while the so-called *potent anesthetics* are the vapors of volatile liquids. But for simplicity, all of them are referred to as gases because they are all in the gas phase when administered via the lungs. As gases, none deviate significantly from ideal gas behavior. These anesthetics are all nonionized and have low molecular weights. This allows them to diffuse rapidly without the need for facilitated diffusion or active transport from bloodstream to tissues. The other advantage of gases is that they can be delivered to the bloodstream via a unique route available in all patients: the lungs.

Speed, gaseous state, and route of administration combine to form the major beneficial feature of the inhaled anesthetics: the ability to decrease plasma concentrations as easily and as rapidly as they are increased (1 Video 18-1).

Physical Characteristics of Inhaled Anesthetics

1 The physical characteristics of inhaled anesthetics are shown in Table 18-1. The goal of delivering inhaled anesthetics is to produce the anesthetic state by establishing a specific concentration of anesthetic molecules in the central nervous system (CNS), which is done by establishing the specific partial pressure of the agent in the lungs that ultimately equilibrates with the brain and spinal cord.[1] At equilibrium, CNS partial pressure equals blood partial pressure, which in turn equals alveolar partial pressure:

$$P_{CNS} = P_{blood} = P_{alveoli} \qquad (18\text{-}1)$$

where *P* is partial pressure. Equilibration is a result of three factors:

1. Inhaled anesthetics are gases rapidly transferred bidirectionally via the lungs to and from the bloodstream and subsequently to and from CNS tissues as partial pressures equilibrate.
2. Plasma and tissues have a low capacity to absorb the inhaled anesthetics relative to the amount that can be delivered to the lungs, allowing quick establishment or reduction of anesthetizing concentrations of anesthetic in the bloodstream and ultimately the CNS.
3. Metabolism, excretion, and redistribution of the inhaled anesthetics are minimal relative to the rate at which they are delivered or removed from the lungs. This permits easy maintenance of blood and CNS concentrations.

The so-called permanent gases, such as oxygen and nitrogen, exist only as gases at ambient temperatures. Gases such as N_2O can be compressed into liquids under high pressure at ambient temperature. *Potent volatile anesthetics* with the exception of desflurane are liquids at ambient temperature and pressure. If volatile liquids reside in a closed container, molecules of the substance will equilibrate between the liquid and gas phases. At equilibrium, the pressure exerted by molecular collisions of the gas against the container walls is the *vapor pressure.* One important property of vapor pressure is that as long as *any* liquid remains in the container, the vapor pressure is independent of the volume of that liquid. As with any gas, however, vapor pressure is proportional to temperature.

Table 18-1 Physiochemical Properties of Volatile Anesthetics

Property	Sevoflurane	Desflurane	Isoflurane	Enflurane	Halothane	N_2O
Boiling point (°C)	59	24	49	57	50	−88
Vapor pressure at 20 °C (mmHg)	157	669	238	172	243	38,770
Molecular weight (g)	200	168	184	184	197	44
Oil:gas partition coefficient	47	19	91	97	224	1.4
Blood:gas partition coefficient	0.65	0.42	1.46	1.9	2.50	0.46
Brain:blood solubility	1.7	1.3	1.6	1.4	1.9	1.1
Fat:blood solubility	47.5	27.2	44.9	36	51.1	2.3
Muscle:blood solubility	3.1	2.0	2.9	1.7	3.4	1.2
MAC in O_2 30–60 y, at 37 °C P_B 760 (%)	1.8	6.6	1.17	1.63	0.75	104
MAC in 60–70% N_2O (%)	0.66	2.38	0.56	0.57	0.29	—
MAC, >65 y (%)	1.45	5.17	1.0	1.55	0.64	—
Preservative	No	No	No	No	Thymol	No
Stable in moist CO_2 absorber	No	Yes	Yes	Yes	No	Yes
Flammability (%) (in 70% N_2O/30% O_2)	10	17	7	5.8	4.8	
Recovered as metabolites (%)	2–5	0.02	0.2	2.4	20	

MAC, minimum alveolar concentration; N_2O, nitrous oxide.

At room temperature, most of the potent agents have a vapor pressure that is below atmospheric pressure. If the temperature is raised, the vapor pressure increases. The *boiling point* of a liquid is the temperature at which its vapor pressure exceeds atmospheric pressure in an open container. Desflurane is bottled in a special container because its boiling point of 23.5 °C makes it boil at typical room temperatures. Boiling does not occur within the bottle because it is countered by buildup of vapor pressure within the bottle, but once opened to air, the desflurane would quickly boil away.

Gases in Mixtures

For any mixture of gases in a closed container, each gas exerts a pressure proportional to its *fractional mass*. This is its *partial pressure*. The sum of the partial pressures of each gas in a mixture of gases equals the total pressure of the entire mixture (Dalton's law):

$$P_{total} = P_{gas1} + P_{gas2} + \cdots + P_{gasN} \quad (18\text{-}2)$$

Another way to state this is that each gas in a mixture of gases at a given volume and temperature has a partial pressure, that is, the pressure it would have *if it alone* occupied the volume. The entire mixture behaves just as if it were a single gas according to the ideal gas law.

Gases in Solution

Partial pressure of a gas in solution is a bit complex because pressure can only be measured in the gas phase, while in solution the amount of gas is measured as a concentration. Partial pressure of a gas in solution refers to the pressure of the gas in the gas phase (if it were present) in equilibrium with the liquid. However, it is important to talk of partial pressures, because gases equilibrate based on partial pressures, not concentrations.

Gas molecules within a liquid interact with solvent molecules to a much larger extent than do molecules in the gas phase. *Solubility* is the term used to describe the tendency of a gas to equilibrate with a solution, hence determining its concentration in solution. Henry's law expresses the relationship of concentration of a gas in solution to the partial pressure of the gas with which the solution is in equilibrium:

$$C_g = kP_g \quad (18\text{-}3)$$

where C_g is concentration of gas in solution, k is a solubility constant, and P_g is the partial pressure of the gas. From Equation 18-3, one can see that doubling the pressure of a gas doubles its concentration in solution. A more clinically useful expression of solubility is the solubility coefficient, λ:

$$\lambda = V_{dissolved\ gas} / V_{liquid} \text{ at } 37\ °C \quad (18\text{-}4)$$

where V = volume. This equation states that for any gas in equilibrium with a liquid, a certain volume of that gas dissolves in a given volume of liquid.

The principles of partial pressures and solubility apply in mixtures of gases in solution. That is, the concentration of any one gas in a mixture of gases in solution depends on two factors: (1) its partial pressure in the gas phase in equilibrium with the solution, and (2) its solubility within that solution.

The implications of these properties are that anesthetic gases administered via the lungs diffuse into blood until the partial pressures in alveoli and blood are equal. The concentration of anesthetic in the blood depends on the partial pressure at equilibrium and the anesthetic solubility in blood. Likewise, transfer of anesthetic from blood to target tissues also proceeds toward equalizing partial pressures, but at this interface, there is no gas phase. A partial pressure still exists to force anesthetic molecules out of solution and into a gas phase but there is no gas phase because blood (outside the lungs) and tissues are like closed, liquid-filled containers. Remember the principle: The partial pressure of a gas in solution represents the pressure that the gas in equilibrium with the liquid *would have* if a gas phase existed in contact with the liquid phase.

The concentration of anesthetic in target tissue depends on the partial pressure at equilibrium and the target tissue solubility. Because inhaled anesthetics are gases, and because partial pressures of gases equilibrate throughout a system, *monitoring the alveolar concentration of inhaled anesthetics provides an index of their effects in the brain.*

In summary:

1. Inhaled anesthetics equilibrate based on their partial pressures in each tissue (or tissue compartment), *not* based on their concentrations.
2. The partial pressure of a gas in solution is defined by the partial pressure in the gas phase with which it is in equilibrium. Where there is no gas phase, the partial pressure reflects a force to move out of solution.
3. The concentration of anesthetic in a tissue depends on its partial pressure and the tissue solubility of the anesthetic.

Finally, the particular terminology used when referring to gases in the gas phase or absorbed in plasma or tissues is important. Inspired concentrations or fractional volumes of inhaled anesthetic are typically used rather than partial pressure. Partial pressure is expressed in millimeters of mercury (mmHg) or Torr (1 Torr = 1 mmHg) or kilopascals (kPa). For most drugs, concentration is expressed as mass (milligram [mg]) per volume (milliliter [mL]), but it can also be expressed in percent by weight or volume. Since volume of a gas in the gas phase is directly proportional to mass according to the ideal gas law, it is easier to express this fractional concentration as a percent by volume. In the gas phase, fractional concentration is equal to the partial pressure divided by ambient pressure, usually atmospheric, or:

$$\text{Fractional volume} = P_{anesthetic}/P_{barometric} \quad (18\text{-}5)$$

Anesthetic Transfer: Machine to Central Nervous System

When the fresh gas flow (FGF) and the vaporizer are turned on, fresh gas with a fixed fractional concentration of anesthetic leaves the fresh gas outlet and mixes with the gas in the circuit—the bag, tubing, absorbent canister, and piping. It is immediately diluted to a lower fractional concentration, then slowly rises as this compartment equilibrates with the delivered flow. With spontaneous patient ventilation by mask, the anesthetic gas passes from circuit to airways. The fractional concentration of anesthetic leaving the circuit is designated as F_I (fraction inspired). In the lungs, the gas comprising the dead space in the airways (trachea, bronchi) and the alveoli further dilutes the circuit gas. The fractional concentration of anesthetic present in the alveoli is F_A (fraction alveolar). The anesthetic then passes across the alveolar–capillary membrane and dissolves in pulmonary blood according to the partial pressure of the gas and its blood solubility. It is further diluted and travels via bulk blood flow throughout the vascular tree. The anesthetic then passes via simple diffusion from blood to tissues as well as between tissues.

The vascular system delivers blood to three physiologic tissue groups: the vessel-rich group (VRG), the muscle group, and the

Table 18-2 Distribution of Cardiac Output by Tissue Group

Group	% Body Mass	% Cardiac Output	Perfusion (mL/min/100 g)
Vessel-rich	10	75	55–500
Muscle	50	19	3
Fat	20	6	1

fat group. The VRG includes the brain, heart, kidney, liver, digestive tract, and glandular tissues. The percent of body mass and perfusion of each group are shown in Table 18-2. The CNS tissues of the VRG are referred to as *tissues of desired effect*. The other tissues of the VRG that comprise the compartment are referred to as *tissues of undesired effects*. The tissues of the muscle and fat groups comprise the *tissues of accumulation*.

Anesthetic is delivered most rapidly to the VRG because of high blood flow. Here it diffuses according to partial pressure gradients. CNS tissue takes in the anesthetic according to the tissue solubility, and at a high enough tissue concentration, unconsciousness and anesthesia are achieved. Increasing CNS tissue concentrations cause progressively deeper stages of anesthesia. As this is occurring, anesthetic is also being distributed to other VRG tissues. Also coincident with delivery to the CNS, anesthetic is being delivered—albeit more slowly because of lower perfusion—to muscle and fat, where it accumulates and may affect the speed of emergence from the anesthetic. In reality, the fat solubilities provide little influence on emergence in cases lasting more than 4 hours since the delivery of anesthetic to fat tissue is extremely slow as a result of low blood flow. The concentration of inhaled anesthetic in a given tissue at a particular time during the administration depends not only on tissue blood flow, but also on tissue solubility, which governs how the inhaled anesthetics partition themselves between blood and tissue. Partitioning depends on the relative solubilities of the anesthetic for each compartment. These relative solubilities are expressed by a partition coefficient, δ, which is the ratio of dissolved gas (by volume) in two-tissue compartments at equilibrium. Some of the partition coefficients for the inhaled anesthetics are shown in Table 18-1.

Uptake and Distribution

F_A/F_I

A simple, common way to assess anesthetic uptake is to follow the ratio of fractional concentration of alveolar anesthetic to inspired anesthetic (F_A/F_I) over time (2 Video 18-2). Data from human studies for F_A/F_I versus time during induction are shown in Figure 18-2. The faster F_A rises relative to F_I, the faster the speed of induction since F_A is proportional to P_A ($F_A = P_A/P_{barometric}$) and $P_A = P_{blood} = P_{CNS}$; that is, the alveolar fraction is directly proportional to the partial pressure of anesthetic in the CNS.

2 As fresh gas carrying anesthetic begins to flow into the air-filled circuit (assuming complete mixing), the concentration in the circuit (F_I) will rise according to first-order kinetics:

$$F_I = F_{FGO}(1 - e^{-T/\tau}) \quad (18\text{-}6)$$

F_{FGO} is the fraction of inspired anesthetic in the gas leaving the fresh gas outlet (i.e., the vaporizer setting), T is time, and τ is a time constant. The time constant is simply the volume or "capacity" of the circuit (V_C) divided by the FGF or $\tau = V_C/\text{FGF}$. For example, if the bag, tubing, absorbent canister, and piping

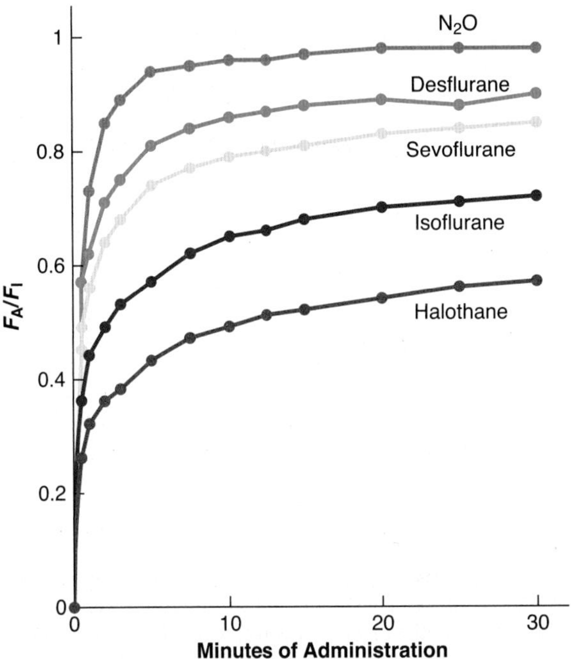

Figure 18-2 The rise in alveolar (F_A) anesthetic concentration toward the inspired (F_I) concentration is most rapid with the least soluble anesthetics, (nitrous oxide, desflurane, and sevoflurane) and slow with the more soluble anesthetics (halothane). All data are from human studies. (Adapted with permission from Yasuda N, Lockhart SH, Eger II EI, et al. Comparison of kinetics of sevoflurane and isoflurane in humans. *Anesth Analg*. 1991;72(3):316–324; and Yasuda N, Lockhart SH, Eger II EI, et al. Kinetics of desflurane, isoflurane, and halothane in humans. *Anesthesiology*. 1991;74(3):489–498.)

comprise 8 L, and the FGF is 2 L, the time constant $\tau = 8/2 = 4$. One of the characteristics of first-order kinetics is that 95% of maximum is reached after three time constants—in this case, $3 \times 4 = 12$ minutes.

Since 12 minutes is relatively long, starting with a higher F_{FGO} can increase the rate of rise of F_I. Using the earlier example with $\tau = 4$, by first-order kinetics, 63% of maximum is reached after one time constant, or 4 minutes. To attain an F_I of 2% at 4 instead of 12 minutes, the F_{FGO} can be set to 3.2% (2% divided by 0.63) and then lowered to 2% at the 4-minute mark.

Other ways to speed the increase in F_I include increasing the FGF, thus decreasing τ. Furthermore, the rebreathing bag can be collapsed prior to starting the FGF, such that the capacity in the circuit (V_C) is less, which also decreases τ. Finally, at high flows, (>4 L/min) there is far less mixing because fresh gas pushes "old" gas out of the circuit via the pop-off valve before complete mixing occurs, causing F_I to increase at a greater rate; this is the most important factor in rapidly increasing F_I to the desired concentration.

One factor that can delay the rate of rise of F_I is that CO_2 absorbent can decompose the inhaled anesthetics. However, from a practical standpoint, this does not affect the rate of rise in F_I to a significant extent compared with other factors. Another factor that can delay the rate of rise of F_I is solubility of the inhaled anesthetics in some of the plastic and rubber parts of the anesthesia circuit. Again, this absorption plays only a small role in decreasing the rate of rise of F_I.

Rise in F_A in the Absence of Uptake

The rate of rise in F_I discussed earlier assumes that no anesthetic is mixing with gas in the patient's lungs. In reality, circuit gas mixes with exhaled gases from the lung with each breath, thus lowering F_I within the circuit. If high FGFs (>4 L/min), which produce a high volume of gas at the desired concentration, are used, little mixing with exhaled air occurs and F_I is relatively fixed. In this situation, circuit gas enters the lungs where it mixes with alveolar gas. If there were no blood flow to the lungs, F_A would rise in a fashion analogous to F_I; that is:

$$F_A = F_I(1 - e^{-T/\tau}) \tag{18-7}$$

In this equation, τ is the time constant for alveolar rise in anesthetic concentration and equals the functional residual capacity (FRC) of the patient's lungs divided by minute ventilation ($\dot{V}_A$). There are two ways to speed the equilibration of F_A with F_I, that is, to decrease τ. One way is to increase minute ventilation, and the other is to decrease FRC. Both of these methods can be used to speed induction by mask; the patient can exhale deeply before applying the mask (to decrease the initial FRC), and the patient can breathe deeply and rapidly (to increase) after the mask is applied. Importantly, high alveolar ventilation relative to uptake from the lungs to the bloodstream generates the initial high slope to the curves shown in Figure 18-2.

One of the reasons that pediatric inductions by spontaneous breathing of inhaled anesthetics are so much quicker than adult inductions is that the low FRC relative to $\dot{V}_A$ of children makes for a low time constant, and hence a more rapid increase in F_A/F_I. One important caveat about the relationship of F_A to FRC is that FRC includes airway dead space; thus, in reality, F_A by Equation 18-7 is not just the concentration of inhaled anesthetic in the alveoli but also the concentration in the entire lung. However, it is simply called the alveolar concentration because the dead space in the airways is relatively insignificant and only the alveolar gas is exchanging anesthetic with the blood.

Rise in F_A in the Presence of Uptake

Anesthetics *are* soluble in tissues, thus uptake of anesthetic from alveoli to blood is again characterized by first-order kinetics:

$$P_{bl}\ (\text{blood}) = P_A\ (\text{alveoli}) \times (1 - e^{-T/\tau}),$$

where

$$P_A = F_A \times P_B\ (\text{barometric}) \tag{18-8}$$

Here, P_B is the barometric pressure and the time constant, τ, equals "capacity" (volume of anesthetic dissolved in blood at the desired alveolar partial pressure) divided by flow (volume of anesthetic delivered per unit time). For any given flow of anesthetic into the system, this capacity for the more soluble halothane is greater than the capacity for the less soluble desflurane; thus, τ for halothane is greater than that for desflurane. The more soluble the inhaled anesthetic, the larger the capacity of the blood and tissues for that anesthetic, and the longer it takes to saturate at any given delivery rate.

The most important factor in the rate of rise of F_A/F_I is uptake of anesthetic from the alveoli into the bloodstream. The rate of rise of F_A/F_I (especially the position of the "knees" in the curves of Fig. 18-2) reflects the speed at which alveolar anesthetic (F_A) equilibrates with that being delivered to the lungs (F_I). Since there is uptake from alveoli to blood, F_A is not solely a function of F_I and time. The greater the uptake, the slower the rate of rise of F_A/F_I, and vice versa. Since uptake is proportional to tissue solubility, the less soluble the anesthetic (such as desflurane), the lesser its uptake and the faster it reaches equilibrium, $P_A = P_{blood} = P_{CNS}$.

Consider a hypothetical example. Suppose that halothane and desflurane are soluble in blood, but insoluble in all other tissues. Suppose further that total lung capacity and blood volume were both 5 L. If a fixed volume of anesthetic is delivered to the lungs (by asking the patient to take one deep breath and hold it), according to the blood:gas partition coefficients for halothane (2.5) and desflurane (0.42), 71.4% of the delivered halothane will be transferred to the blood while 28.6% remains in the alveoli (71.4/28.6 = 2.5). In contrast, 29.6% of the desflurane will be transferred to the blood while 70.4% remains in the alveoli (29.6/70.4 = 0.42). Therefore, 2.4 times (71.4/29.6) more halothane than desflurane (by volume or number of molecules) will be transferred from alveoli to bloodstream before partial pressures equilibrate. At equilibrium, the alveolar partial pressures of halothane and desflurane are 28.6% and 70.4% of their inhaled values, respectively. This means that F_A rises faster with desflurane than halothane, as does F_A/F_I.

Blood uptake of anesthetic is expressed by the equation:

$$\dot{V}_B = \delta^{b}/_{g} * Q \times (P_A - P_V)/P_B \tag{18-9}$$

where $\dot{V}_B$ is blood uptake, $\delta_{b/g}$ is the blood:gas partition coefficient, Q is cardiac output, P_A is alveolar partial pressure of anesthetic, P_v is mixed venous partial pressure of anesthetic, and P_B is barometric pressure. This is the Fick equation applied to blood uptake of inhaled anesthetics. *The greater the value of $\dot{V}_B$, the greater the uptake from alveoli to blood, and the slower the rise in F_A/F_I.* These factors influencing the rate of rise of *Fa/Fi* are shown in Figure 18-4.

From the preceding paragraphs, the parameters that increase or decrease the rate of rise in F_A/F_I during induction can now be clearly delineated and these important factors have been substantiated in experimental models.

Distribution (Tissue Uptake)

The maximum F_A/F_I at a given inspired concentration of anesthetic, cardiac output, and minute ventilation depends entirely on the solubility of that drug in the blood as characterized by the blood:gas partition coefficient $\delta_{b/g}$. This can be seen in the time curves for the rise in F_A/F_I during induction for the various inhalation anesthetics shown in Figure 18-2. The first "knee" in each curve in Figure 18-2 represents the point at which the rapid rise in P_v begins to taper off; that is, when significant inhaled anesthetic concentrations begin to buildup in the bloodstream because of distribution to and equilibration with the various tissue compartments.

As blood is equilibrating with alveolar gas, it also begins to equilibrate with the VRG, muscle, and, more gradually, the fat compartments based on perfusion. Muscle is not that different from the VRG, having partition coefficients that range from 1.2 (N_2O) to 3.4 (halothane), just under a threefold difference; and for each anesthetic except N_2O, the muscle partition coefficient is approximately double that for the VRG. Although both VRG and muscle are lean tissues, the muscle compartment equilibrates far more slowly than the VRG. The explanation comes in part due to the mass of the compartments relative to perfusion. The perfusion of the VRG is about 75 mL/min/100 g of tissue, whereas it is only 3 mL/min/100 g of tissue in the muscle (Table 18-2). This 25-fold difference in perfusion between VRG (especially brain) and muscle means that even if the partition coefficients were equal, the muscle would still take 25 times longer to equilibrate with blood.

Fat is perfused to a lesser extent than muscle and its time for equilibration with blood is considerably slower because the partition coefficients are so much greater. All of the potent agents are highly lipid-soluble. Partition coefficients range from 27 (desflurane) to 51 (halothane). On average, the solubility for these agents is about 25 times greater in fat than in the VRG group. Thus, fat equilibrates far more slowly with the blood and does not play a significant role in determining speed of induction. After long anesthetic exposures (>4 hours), the high saturation of fat tissue may play a role in delaying emergence.

Nitrous oxide represents an exception. Its partition coefficients are similar in each tissue: It does not accumulate to any great extent and is not a very potent anesthetic. Its utility lies as an adjunct to the potent agents, and as a vehicle to speed induction.

Metabolism

Data suggest that enzymes responsible for biotransformation of inhaled anesthetics become saturated at less than anesthetizing doses of these drugs, such that metabolism plays little role in opposing induction. It may, however, have some significance to recovery from anesthesia, as discussed later.

Overpressurization and the Concentration Effect

There are several ways to speed uptake and induction of anesthesia with the inhaled anesthetics. The first is *overpressurization*, which is analogous to an intravenous bolus. This is the administration of a higher partial pressure of anesthetic than the alveolar concentration (F_A) targeted for the patient. Inspired anesthetic concentration (F_I) can influence both F_A and the *rate of rise* of F_A/F_I. The greater the inspired concentration of an inhaled anesthetic, the greater the rate of rise. This concentration effect has two components: the concentrating effect and an augmented gas inflow effect.

For example, consider the administration of 10% anesthetic (10 parts anesthetic and 90 parts other gas) to a patient in whom 50% of the anesthetic in the alveoli is absorbed by the blood. In this case, 5 parts (0.5 × 10) anesthetic remain in the alveoli, 5 parts enter the blood, and 90 parts remain as other alveolar gas. The alveolar concentration is now 5/(90 + 5) = 5.3%. Consider next administering 50% anesthetic with the same 50% uptake. Now 25 parts anesthetic remain in alveoli, 25 parts pass into blood, and 50 parts remain as other alveolar gas. The alveolar concentration becomes 25/(50 + 25) = 33%. Giving five times as much anesthetic will lead to a 33%/5.3% = 6.2 times greater alveolar concentration. The higher the F_I, the greater the effect. Thus N_2O, typically given in concentrations of 50% to 70%, has the greatest concentrating effect. This is why the F_A/F_I versus time curve in Figure 18-2 rises the most quickly with N_2O, even though desflurane has a slightly lower blood:gas solubility.

This is not the complete picture; there is yet another factor to consider. As gas is leaving the alveoli for the blood, new gas at the original F_I is entering the lungs to replace that which is taken up by the blood. This other aspect of the concentration effect has been called *augmented gas inflow*. Again, take the example of 10% anesthetic delivered with 50% uptake into the bloodstream. The five parts anesthetic absorbed by the bloodstream are replaced by gas in the circuit that is still 10% anesthetic. The 5 parts anesthetic and 90 parts other gas left in the lungs mix with 5 parts replacement gas, or 5 × 0.10 = 0.5 parts anesthetic. Now the alveolar concentration is (5 + 0.5)/(100) = 5.5% (as compared to 5.3% without augmented inflow). For 50% anesthetic and 50% uptake, 25 parts of anesthetic removed from the alveoli are replaced with 25 parts of 50% anesthetic, giving a new alveolar concentration of (25 + 12.5)/(100) = 37.5% (as compared to 33% without augmented inflow). Thus, 5 times the F_I leads to 37.5/5.5 = 6.8 times greater F_A (compared to 6.2 times without augmented gas inflow). Of course, this cycle of absorbed gas being replaced by fresh gas inflow is continuous and has a finite rate, so our example is a simplification.

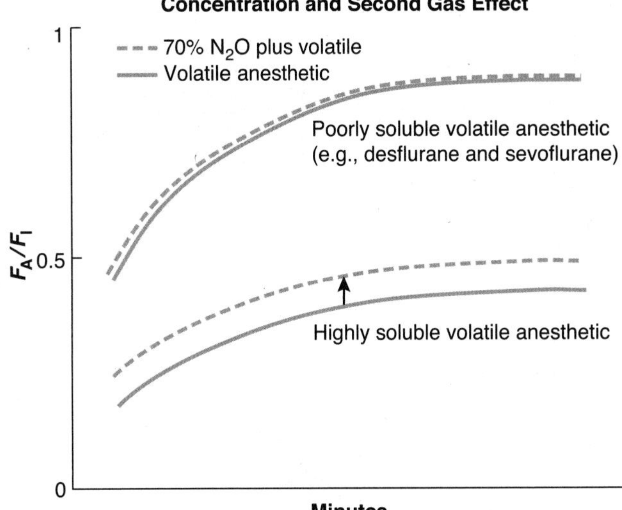

Figure 18-3 The second gas effect is demonstrated in the graphs. The F_A/F_I ratio for a more soluble gas such as halothane rises more rapidly when given with 70% N_2O than when given with 10% N_2O. This effect is less with less soluble gases. (Adapted with permission from Epstein RM, Rackow H, Salanitre E, et al. Influence of the concentration effect on the uptake of anesthetic mixtures: the second gas effect. *Anesthesiology*. 1964;25:364.)

Second Gas Effect

A special case of concentration effect applies to administration of a potent anesthetic with N_2O, that is, two gases simultaneously. Along with the concentration of potent agent in the alveoli via its uptake, there is further concentration via the uptake of N_2O, a process called the *second gas effect*. The principle is simple (Fig. 18-3). Consider, for example, administering 2% of a potent anesthetic in 70% N_2O and 28% oxygen. In this case, N_2O, with its extremely high partial pressure (despite low solubility), partitions into the blood more rapidly than the potent anesthetic, decreasing the alveolar N_2O concentration by some amount (e.g., by 50%). Ignoring uptake of the potent anesthetic, the uptake of N_2O is 35 parts, leaving 35 parts N_2O, 28 parts O_2, and 2 parts potent agent in the alveoli. The anesthetic gas is now present in the alveoli at a concentration of 2/(2 + 35 + 28) = 3.1%. The potent agent has been concentrated and F_A is increased. Clinically, the second gas effect acts minimally to speed induction.

Ventilation Effects

As indicated by Figure 18-2, inhaled anesthetics with very low tissue solubility have an extremely rapid rise in F_A/F_I with induction. This suggests that there is very little room to improve this rate by increasing or decreasing ventilation, which is demonstrated in Figure 18-4. The greater the solubility of an inhaled anesthetic, the more rapidly it is absorbed by the bloodstream, such that anesthetic delivery to the lungs may be rate limiting to the rise in F_A/F_I. Therefore, for more soluble anesthetics, augmentation of anesthetic delivery by increasing minute ventilation also increases the rate of rise in F_A/F_I.

However, spontaneous minute ventilation is not static, and to the extent that the inhaled anesthetics depress spontaneous ventilation with increasing inspired concentration, $\dot{V}_A$ will decrease and so will the rate of rise of F_A/F_I. This negative feedback should not be considered a drawback of the inhaled anesthetics because

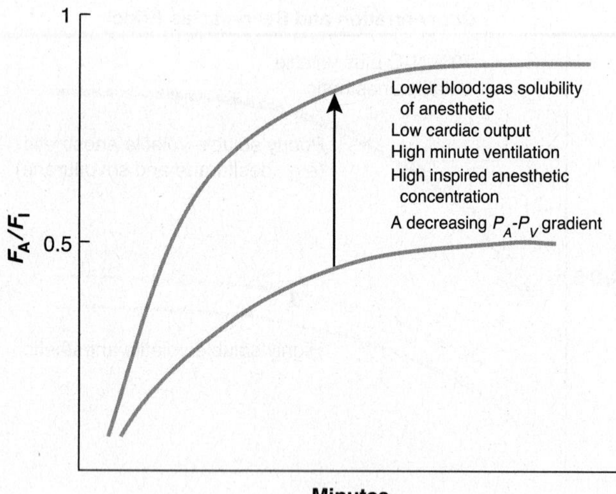

Figure 18-4 The F_A/F_I ratio rises more rapidly if ventilation and the anesthetic concentration are increased. A decreasing P_A-P_V gradient that occurs shortly after anesthetic induction, slows anesthetic uptake and increases the rate of rise of F_A/F_I. A low CO and low blood:gas solubility slow anesthetic uptake (Equation 18-9) and increases the rate of rise of F_A/F_I. The influence of CO and ventilation on F_A/F_I are magnified for the more soluble anesthetics.

the respiratory depression produced at high anesthetic concentrations essentially slows the rise in F_A/F_I. This might arguably add a margin of safety in preventing an overdose. Controlled ventilation does not offer this margin of safety.

Perfusion Effects

A low cardiac output will accelerate the rise of F_A/F_I. As with ventilation, cardiac output is not static during the course of induction. For the less soluble agents, changes in cardiac output do not affect the rate of rise of F_A/F_I to a great extent, but for the more soluble agents the effect is noticeable (Fig. 18-4). However, as inspired concentration increases, greater cardiovascular depression reduces anesthetic uptake and actually increases the rate of rise of F_A/F_I. This positive feedback can rapidly lead to profound cardiovascular depression.

Ventilation–Perfusion Mismatching

Ventilation and perfusion are normally fairly well matched in healthy patients, such that P_A (alveolar partial pressure)/P_I and P_a (arterial partial pressure)/P_I are the same curve. However, if significant intrapulmonary shunt occurs, as in the case of inadvertent bronchial intubation, the rate of rise of alveolar and arterial anesthetic partial pressures can be affected (Fig. 18-5). Ventilation of the intubated lung is dramatically increased while perfusion increases slightly. The nonintubated lung receives no ventilation, while perfusion decreases slightly. For the less-soluble anesthetics, increased ventilation of the intubated lung cannot appreciably increase alveolar partial pressure relative to inspired concentration on that side, but alveolar partial pressure on the nonintubated side is essentially zero. Pulmonary mixed venous blood, therefore, comprises nearly equal parts of blood containing normal amounts of anesthetic and blood containing no anesthetic; that is, diluted relative to normal. Thus, the rate of rise in P_a (arterial) relative to P_I is significantly reduced. There is less total anesthetic uptake, so the rate of rise of P_A (alveolar) relative to P_I increases even though induction of anesthesia is slowed because CNS partial pressure equilibrates with P_a. For the more soluble anesthetics, increased ventilation of the intubated lung *does* increase the alveolar partial pressure relative to inspired concentration on that side. Pulmonary venous blood from the intubated side contains a higher concentration of anesthetic that lessens the dilution by blood from the nonintubated side. Thus, the rate of rise of P_a/P_I is not as reduced and induction of anesthesia is less delayed relative to normal.

Elimination

Percutaneous and Visceral Loss

Although the loss of inhaled anesthetics via the skin is very small, it does occur and the loss is the greatest for N_2O. Inhaled anesthetics also pass across gastrointestinal viscera and the pleura. During open abdominal or thoracic surgery, there is some anesthetic loss via these routes. N_2O must be used with caution if there are enclosed air spaces in a patient (e.g., pneumothorax, pneumoperitoneum, intracranial, middle ear, intraocular) as it will diffuse into the space and elevate the pressure.

Diffusion between Tissues

Using more elaborate mathematical modeling of inhaled anesthetic pharmacokinetics than presented here, several laboratories have derived a five-compartment model that best describes tissue compartments. These compartments are the alveoli, the VRG, the muscle, the fat, and one additional compartment. Current opinion is that this fifth compartment represents adipose tissue adjacent to lean tissue that receives anesthetic via intertissue diffusion. This transfer of anesthetic is significant and may account for up to one-third of uptake during long administration.

Exhalation and Recovery

Recovery from anesthesia, like induction, depends on anesthetic solubility, cardiac output, and minute ventilation. Solubility is

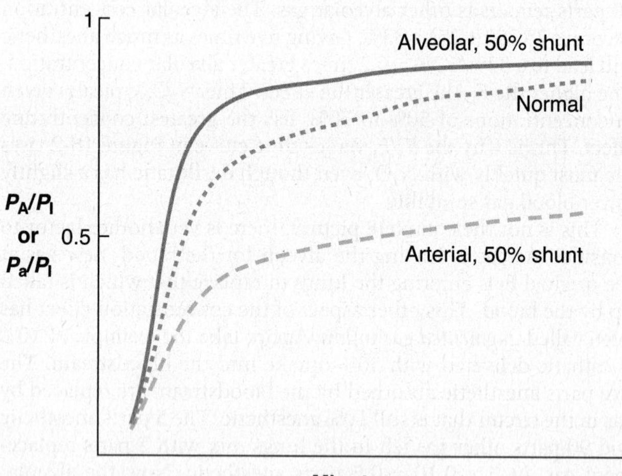

Figure 18-5 When no ventilation/perfusion abnormalities exist, the alveolar (P_A) and arterial (P_a) anesthetic partial pressures rise together (*dotted blue lines*) toward the inspired partial pressure (P_I). When 50% of the cardiac output is shunted through the lungs, such as with a mainstem intubation, the rate of rise of the alveolar partial pressure, P_A (*orange lines*) is accelerated while the rate of rise of the arterial partial pressure, P_a (*dotted green lines*) is slowed, resulting in a slower induction of anesthesia. The greatest effect of shunting is found with the least soluble anesthetics, for example, sevoflurane and desflurane.

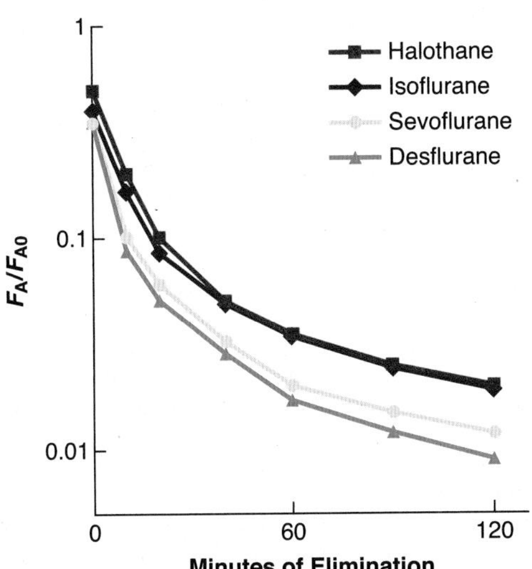

Figure 18-6 Elimination of anesthetic gases is defined as the ratio of end-tidal anesthetic concentration (F_A) to the last F_A during administration and immediately before the beginning of elimination (F_{A0}). During the 120-minute period after ending the anesthetic delivery, the elimination of sevoflurane and desflurane is 2 to 2.5 times faster than isoflurane or halothane (note logarithmic scale for the ordinate). (Adapted with permission from Yasuda N, Lockhart SH, Eger II EI, et al. Comparison of kinetics of sevoflurane and isoflurane in humans. *Anesth Analg*. 1991;72(3):316–324; and Yasuda N, Lockhart SH, Eger II EI, et al. Kinetics of desflurane, isoflurane, and halothane in humans. *Anesthesiology*. 1991;74(3):489–498.)

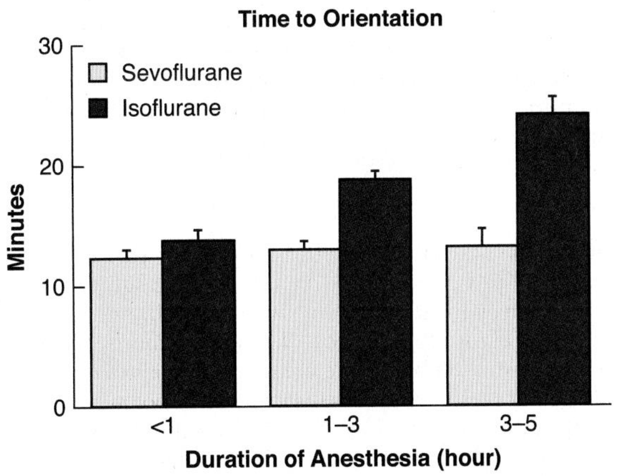

Figure 18-7 The recovery times to orientation after anesthesia of varying durations. With the less soluble anesthetic sevoflurane, the time to orientation was independent of the anesthetic duration. In contrast, long anesthetic durations with isoflurane were associated with delayed times to orientation. (Adapted with permission from Ebert TJ, Robinson BJ, Uhrich TD, et al. Recovery from sevoflurane anesthesia: a comparison to isoflurane and propofol anesthesia. *Anesthesiology*. 1998;89:1524.)

the primary determinant of the rate of fall of F_A (Fig. 18-6). The greater the solubility of inhaled anesthetic, the larger the capacity for absorption in the bloodstream and tissues. The "reservoir" of anesthetic in the body at the end of administration depends on tissue solubility (which determines the capacity) and the dose and duration of anesthetic (which determine how much of that capacity is filled). Recovery from anesthesia, or "washout," is usually expressed as the ratio of expired fractional concentration of anesthetic (F_A) to the expired concentration at time zero (F_{A0}) when the anesthetic was discontinued (or F_A/F_{A0}). One of the arguments for using sevoflurane and desflurane has been their relative speed in terms of emergence from anesthesia. This argument has been tempered somewhat by the basic knowledge that downward titration of volatile anesthetics can speed emergence times. Even the more soluble drug, isoflurane, can be titrated downward guided by clinical experience and/or a processed EEG monitor, permitting fast wake-ups. However, in general, the use of the less-soluble drugs in the longest surgical cases makes awakening a simpler and expedient process (Fig. 18-7).[3]

There are two major pharmacokinetic differences between recovery and induction. First, whereas overpressurization can increase the speed of induction, there is no "underpressurization." Both induction and recovery rates depend on the P_A to P_v gradient, and P_A can never fall below zero. Second, whereas all tissues begin induction with zero anesthetic, each begins recovery with quite different anesthetic concentrations. The VRG tissues begin recovery with the same anesthetic partial pressure as that in alveoli, since $P_{CNS} = P_{blood} = P_{alveoli}$. The partial pressures in muscle and fat depend on the inspired concentration during anesthesia, the duration of administration, and the anesthetic tissue solubilities. As long as an arterial-to-tissue partial pressure gradient exists, these tissues will absorb anesthetic—especially fat, since it is a huge potential reservoir whose anesthetic partial pressures are typically minimal after hours of anesthesia. After discontinuation of anesthesia, muscle and fat may continue to absorb anesthetic, even hours later. The redistribution continues until blood/alveolar anesthetic partial pressure falls below tissue partial pressure. This redistribution causes the early rate of decline in alveolar anesthetic concentration during recovery to exceed its early rate of increase during induction.

Because VRG tissues are highly perfused and washout of anesthetic is mostly via elimination from these tissues early in recovery, all anesthetics, regardless of duration of administration, have approximately the same rate of elimination to 50% of F_{A0}. Unfortunately, halving the CNS concentration of anesthetic is rarely sufficient for waking the patient. More commonly, 80% to 90% of inhaled anesthetic must be eliminated before emergence. At these amounts of washout, the more soluble anesthetics are eliminated more slowly than less soluble agents.

Diffusion Hypoxia

During recovery from anesthesia, washout of high concentrations of N_2O from blood can lower alveolar concentrations of O_2 and CO_2, a phenomenon called *diffusion hypoxia*. The resulting alveolar hypoxia can cause hypoxemia, and alveolar hypocarbia can depress respiratory drive, which may exacerbate hypoxemia. It is therefore appropriate when utilizing N_2O to briefly administer 100% O_2 prior to administration of a lower concentration of O_2 or room air.

Clinical Overview of Current Inhaled Anesthetics

Isoflurane

Isoflurane is a halogenated methyl ethyl ether that is a clear, nonflammable liquid at room temperature and has a high degree of pungency. It is the most potent of the volatile anesthetics in clinical use, has great physical stability, and undergoes essentially no deterioration during storage for up to 5 years or on exposure to sunlight. It has become the "gold standard" anesthetic since its introduction in the 1970s. There was a brief period of 3 controversy concerning the use of isoflurane in patients with coronary disease because of the possibility for coronary "steal" arising from the potent effects of isoflurane on coronary vasodilation. In clinical use, however, this has been, at most, a rare occurrence.

Desflurane

Desflurane is a fluorinated methyl ethyl ether that differs from isoflurane by just one atom: A fluorine atom is substituted for a chlorine atom on the α-ethyl component of isoflurane (Fig. 18-1). Fluorination of the ether molecule has several effects. It decreases blood and tissue solubility (the blood:gas solubility of desflurane equals that of N_2O), which results in a loss of potency (the minimum alveolar concentration [MAC] of desflurane is five times higher than isoflurane). It also results in a high vapor pressure owing to decreased intermolecular attraction, requiring an electrically driven, heated, pressurized vaporizer to deliver a regulated concentration of desflurane as a gas. The strong carbon–fluorine bond lessens the degradation in the atmosphere resulting in a long atmospheric lifetime, making it a potent greenhouse gas. Desflurane is resistant to metabolism to serum trifluoroacetate. This makes immune-mediated hepatitis a rare occurrence. Desflurane is the most pungent of MAC-equivalent volatile anesthetics and, if administered via the facemask, may result in coughing, salivation, breath holding, and laryngospasm. Desflurane has the lowest blood:gas solubility of the potent volatile anesthetics; moreover, its fat solubility is roughly half that of the other volatile anesthetics. Thus, desflurane requires less downward titration toward the end of long surgical procedures to achieve a rapid emergence by virtue of decreased tissue saturation. This may be particularly advantageous in the morbidly obese patient.[4] Desflurane has been associated with tachycardia and hypertension when used with minimal opioids and, in select cases, myocardial ischemia when used in high concentrations or when rapidly increasing the inspired concentration.

Sevoflurane

Sevoflurane is a sweet-smelling, completely fluorinated methyl isopropyl ether (Fig. 18-1). Its vapor pressure is roughly one-fourth that of desflurane, and it can be used in a conventional vaporizer. The blood:gas solubility of sevoflurane is second only to desflurane in terms of potent volatile anesthetics. Sevoflurane is approximately half as potent as isoflurane, and some of the preservation of potency, despite fluorination, is because of the bulky propyl side chain on the ether molecule. Its pleasant odor, lack of pungency, and potent bronchodilating characteristics make sevoflurane administration via the facemask for induction of anesthesia in both children and adults a reasonable alternative to intravenous anesthetics. Sevoflurane is half as potent a coronary vasodilator as isoflurane but is 10 to 20 times more vulnerable to metabolism than isoflurane. The metabolism of sevoflurane results in inorganic fluoride but has not been associated with renal-concentrating defects. Unlike other potent volatile anesthetics, sevoflurane is not metabolized to trifluoroacetate; rather, it is metabolized to an acyl halide (hexafluoroisopropanol). This does not stimulate formation of antibodies associated with hepatitis.

Sevoflurane also breaks down in the presence of the carbon dioxide absorber to form a vinyl halide called *compound A*. Compound A has been shown to be a dose-dependent nephrotoxin in rats but has not been associated with renal injury in human volunteers or patients, with or without renal impairment, even when FGFs are 1 L/min or less. Sevoflurane has 130 times the potency of CO_2 as a greenhouse gas, far less than desflurane, but it still should be used in a low FGF system to minimize atmospheric contamination.

Xenon

Xenon is an inert gas occurring naturally in air at 0.05 parts per million (ppm) (NICV 18-1). Xenon has received considerable interest in the last few years because it has many characteristics approaching those of an "ideal" inhaled anesthetic.[5] It has a quick onset and offset, minimal effects on the cardiovascular and neural systems, and it is not a trigger for malignant hyperthermia (MH). It is not a pollutant or an occupational hazard, and it does not add to global warming or the greenhouse gas effect. Its blood:gas partition coefficient is 0.115, and unlike the other potent volatile anesthetics (except methoxyflurane), xenon provides some degree of analgesia. This action is likely due to N-methyl-D-aspartate (NMDA) receptor inhibition. The MAC of xenon in humans is 71%, which might prove to be a limitation. It is nonexplosive, nonpungent, and odorless, and thus can be inhaled with ease. In addition, it does not produce significant myocardial depression or alter coronary blood flow.[6] Because of its scarcity and high cost related to extraction by fractional distillation of the atmosphere, its role as a replacement for current lower-cost anesthetics remains uncertain. It may have potential for neuroprotection in select settings via its inhibitory action of the NMDA receptor glycine site.

Nitrous Oxide

Nitrous oxide is a sweet-smelling, nonflammable gas of low potency (MAC = 104%) and is relatively insoluble in blood. It is most commonly administered as an anesthetic adjuvant in combination with opioids or volatile anesthetics during the conduct of general anesthesia. At room temperature, it is a gas; its boiling point is –88.48 °C (Table 18-1). It is stored in cylinders and condensed to 50 atmospheres, leading to a pressure of 745 psi. Only cylinder weight is a reliable indicator of the volume of N_2O in storage tanks since a steady psi is maintained until no liquid remains. Although not flammable, N_2O will support combustion. It is both a greenhouse gas and is destructive to the ozone layer. Unlike the potent volatile anesthetics in clinical use, N_2O does not produce significant skeletal muscle relaxation, but it does have modest analgesic effects. Despite a long track record of use, controversy has surrounded N_2O in four areas:[7] its role in postoperative nausea and vomiting (PONV), its potential toxic effects on cell function via inactivation of vitamin B_{12}, its adverse effects related to absorption and expansion into air-filled structures and bubbles, and lastly, its effect on embryonic development. The most valid and clinically relevant concern is the ability of N_2O to expand air-filled spaces because of its greater solubility in blood compared to nitrogen. This might explain the increased PONV associated with N_2O use since closed gas spaces reside in the middle ear and bowel. Since nitrogen in air-filled spaces cannot be removed readily via the bloodstream, N_2O delivered to a patient diffuses from the blood into these closed gas spaces quite easily until the partial pressure equals that of the blood and alveoli. Compliant spaces will continue to expand until sufficient pressure is generated to oppose further N_2O flow into the space.

Seventy-five percent N_2O can expand a pneumothorax to double or triple its size in 10 and 30 minutes, respectively. Air-filled cuffs of pulmonary artery catheters and endotracheal tubes also expand with the use of N_2O, possibly causing tissue damage via increased pressure in the pulmonary artery or trachea, respectively. Accumulation of N_2O in the middle ear can diminish hearing postoperatively[8] and is contraindicated for tympanoplasty because the increased pressure can dislodge a tympanic graft.

Neuropharmacology of Inhaled Anesthetics

Minimum Alveolar Concentration

5 Pharmacodynamic effects of anesthetics are based on their dosing. In the case of inhaled agents, we describe dose as the *minimum alveolar concentration* or MAC. MAC is the alveolar concentration of an anesthetic at one atmosphere (in volume%) that prevents movement in response to a surgical stimulus in 50% of patients. It is analogous to the ED_{50} expressed for intravenous drugs and can be used to compare anesthetic potency, that is, the lower the MAC the more potent the agent. Movement to a surgical stimulus, commonly abdominal incision, has been used to establish the MAC in humans for each inhaled anesthetic (Table 18-1).

The 95% confidence ranges for MAC are approximately ±25% of the listed MAC values. Manufacturer's recommendations and clinical experience establish 1.2 to 1.3 times MAC as a dose that will often prevent patient movement during a surgical stimulus. Loss of consciousness typically precedes the absence of stimulus-induced movement by a wide margin.

Concentrations of inhaled anesthetics that provide loss of self-awareness and recall are about 0.4 to 0.5 MAC barring other conditions that increase MAC in a given patient (Table 18-3). Several lines of reasoning support the assertion. First, most patients receiving only 50% N_2O (approximately 0.4 to 0.5 MAC), as in a typical dentist's office, will have no recall of their procedure during N_2O administration. Second, studies in primates have shown that a shift in EEG dominance to the anterior leads, that is, the shift from self-aware to non–self-aware, accompanies loss of consciousness occur at 0.5 MAC.[9] Third, in dogs, loss of consciousness accompanies a sudden nonlinear fall in cerebral metabolic rate ($CMRO_2$) at approximately 0.5 MAC (Fig. 18-8).

MAC values can be established for any measurable response. For example, MAC awake is the alveolar concentration of anesthetic at which a patient opens their eyes to command, and it varies from 0.15 to 0.5 MAC. Interestingly, transition from awake to unconscious and back typically shows some hysteresis in that it quite consistently takes 0.4 to 0.5 MAC to lose consciousness, but less than that (as low as 0.15 MAC) to regain it. This may be because of the speed of alveolar wash-in versus wash-out.[10] MAC-BAR is the alveolar concentration of anesthetic that blunts adrenergic responses to noxious stimuli. It has been approximated at 50% higher than standard MAC.[11] MAC values also have been established for discreet levels of EEG activity, such as onset of burst suppression or isoelectricity.

Standard MAC values are roughly additive. Administering 0.5 MAC of a potent agent and 0.5 MAC of N_2O is equivalent to 1 MAC of potent agent in terms of preventing *patient movement*,

Table 18-3 Factors that Increase Minimum Alveolar Concentration

Increased central neurotransmitter levels (monoamine oxidase inhibitors, acute dextroamphetamine administration, cocaine, ephedrine, levodopa)
Hyperthermia
Chronic ethanol abuse (determined in humans)
Hypernatremia

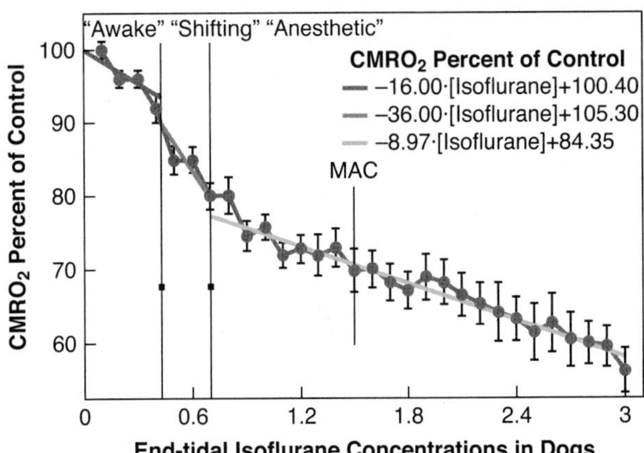

Figure 18-8 The effects of isoflurane on cerebral metabolic rate of oxygen consumption ($CMRO_2$) as a percentage of control ("awake"). $CMRO_2$ is plotted versus end-tidal isoflurane concentration. Regression lines for changes in $CMRO_2$ are drawn for each electroencephalogram-determined area. The pattern depicted here is characteristic of all of the anesthetics examined (enflurane, halothane, and isoflurane). MAC, minimum alveolar concentration. (Adapted with permission from Stullken EH Jr, Milde JH, Michenfelder JD, et al. The nonlinear responses of cerebral metabolism to low concentrations of halothane, enflurane, isoflurane and thiopental. *Anesthesiology.* 1977;46:28.)

although this does not hold over the entire range of N_2O doses. MAC effects for other response parameters, such as cardiovascular or respiratory measures, are not necessarily additive. For example, combining 0.6 MAC of N_2O with 0.6 MAC of isoflurane produces less hypotension than 1.2 MAC of isoflurane alone because isoflurane is a more potent vasodilator and myocardial depressant at equivalent MAC than N_2O.

Various factors increase (Table 18-3) or decrease (Table 18-4) MAC. Unfortunately, no single mechanism explains these alterations, supporting the view that anesthesia is the net result of numerous and widely varying physiologic alterations. In general, those factors that increase CNS metabolic activity, neurotransmission, and CNS neurotransmitter levels increase MAC; upregulated CNS responses to chronically depressed neurotransmitter levels (as in chronic alcoholism) also seem to increase MAC. Conversely, those factors that decrease CNS metabolic activity, neurotransmission, and CNS neurotransmitter levels, as well as downregulated CNS responses to chronically elevated neurotransmitter levels, all seem to decrease MAC. Many notable factors do not alter MAC, including duration of administration, gender, type of surgical stimulation, thyroid function, hypo- or hypercarbia, metabolic alkalosis, hyperkalemia, and magnesium levels. However, there may be a genetic component influencing MAC. Red-haired females may have altered pain thresholds, perhaps explaining the 19% increase in MAC compared with dark-haired females.[12] Studies suggest involvement of mutations of the melanocyte-stimulating hormone receptor (*MC1R*) allele. MAC also can vary in relationship to genotype and chromosomal substitutions as shown in rats.[13]

The Effect of Age on MAC

The MAC for each of the potent anesthetic gases shows a clear, age-related change (Fig. 18-9). MAC decreases with age and there are similarities between agents in the decline in MAC and age. There is a linear model that describes a change in MAC of approximately 6% per decade, a 22% decrease in MAC from 6

Table 18-4 Factors that Decrease Minimum Alveolar Concentration

Increasing age
Metabolic acidosis
Hypoxia (PaO_2, 38 mmHg)
Induced hypotension (mean arterial pressure <50 mmHg)
Decreased central neurotransmitter levels (α-methyldopa, reserpine, chronic dextroamphetamine administration, levodopa)
α_2-agonists
Hypothermia
Hyponatremia
Lithium
Hypo-osmolality
Pregnancy
Acute ethanol administration[a]
Ketamine
Pancuronium[a]
Physostigmine (10 times clinical doses)
Neostigmine (10 times clinical doses)
Lidocaine
Opioids
Opioid agonist–antagonist analgesics
Barbiturates[a]
Chlorpromazine[a]
Diazepam[a]
Hydroxyzine[a]
Δ-9-Tetrahydrocannabinol
Verapamil
Anemia (<4.3 mL O_2/dL blood)

[a]Determined in humans.

age 40 to 80 years, and a 27% decrease in MAC from age 1 to 40 years.[14]

Other Alterations in Neurophysiology

The modern potent anesthetics, isoflurane, desflurane, and sevoflurane, all have reasonably similar effects on a wide range of parameters including $CMRO_2$, the EEG, cerebral blood flow (CBF), and flow–metabolism coupling. There are notable differences in effects on intracerebral pressure (ICP), CO_2 vasoreactivity, CBF autoregulation, and cerebral protection. Nitrous oxide departs from the potent agents in several important ways and is therefore discussed separately.

Although neuroprotection from volatile anesthetics is a well-defined concept, the volatile anesthetics can cause injury in certain conditions via cerebral vasodilation and increases in intracranial pressure. A full understanding of the anesthetic effects on cerebral physiology helps prevent adverse cerebral events in clinical practice.

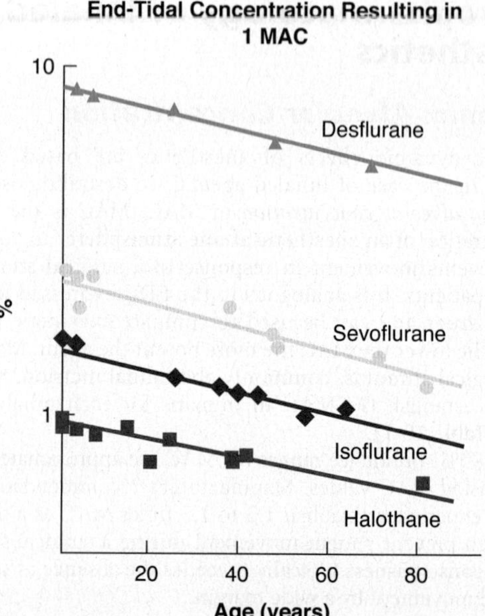

Figure 18-9 Effect of age on minimum alveolar concentration (MAC) is plotted. Regression lines are fitted to published values from separate studies. Data are from patients aged 1 to 80 years. (Adapted from Mapleson WW. Effect of age on MAC in humans: a meta-analysis. *Br J Anaesth*. 1996;76(2):179–185. Copyright © 1996 Elsevier. With permission.)

Cerebral Metabolic Rate and Electroencephalogram

For most of the potent agents, $CMRO_2$ (cerebral metabolic rate) is decreased only to the extent that spontaneous cortical neuronal activity (as reflected on the EEG) is decreased. Once this activity is absent (an isoelectric EEG), no further decreases in $CMRO_2$ are generated. Isoflurane causes a larger MAC-dependent depression of $CMRO_2$ than halothane, and because of this, can abolish EEG activity at clinical doses that are usually well tolerated from a hemodynamic standpoint.[15] Desflurane and sevoflurane both cause decreases in $CMRO_2$ similar to isoflurane.[16,17] Interestingly, while both desflurane and sevoflurane depress the EEG and abolish activity at clinically tolerated doses of approximately 2 MAC[16,17] in *dogs*, desflurane-induced isoelectric EEG reverts to continuous activity with time despite an unchanging MAC, a property unique to desflurane.[16]

Sevoflurane has no noteworthy adverse effects on cerebral physiology at normal CO_2 and BP.[18] During sevoflurane use combined with extreme hyperventilation to decrease CBF by half, brain lactate levels can increase. High, long-lasting concentrations of sevoflurane (1.5 to 2.0 MAC), a sudden increase in cerebral sevoflurane concentrations, especially in females, and/or hypocapnia can trigger EEG abnormalities that have resulted in increases in HR in both adults and children.[19,20] These data question the appropriateness of sevoflurane in patients with epilepsy,[21] but it remains uncertain if sevoflurane truly has a proconvulsant effect.

Cerebral Blood Flow, Flow–Metabolism Coupling, and Autoregulation

All the potent agents increase CBF in a dose-related manner. Isoflurane, sevoflurane, and desflurane cause far less cerebral vasodilation per MAC-multiple than halothane (Fig. 18-10). Desflurane and sevoflurane both influence CBF in a manner similar to isoflurane, with minimal changes in CBF at concentrations less than 1.5 MAC.[16,17,22] An initial increase in CBF with isoflurane

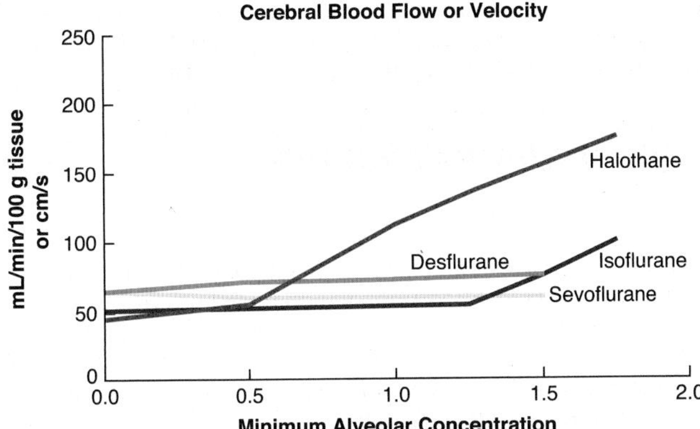

Figure 18-10 Cerebral blood flow (and velocity) measured in the presence of normocapnia and in the absence of surgical stimulation in volunteers receiving halothane or isoflurane. At light levels of anesthesia, halothane (but not isoflurane) increased cerebral blood flow. At 1.6 minimum alveolar concentration (MAC), isoflurane also increased cerebral blood flow. Cerebral blood flow velocity measured before and during sevoflurane and desflurane anesthesia up to 1.5 MAC showed no change in cerebral blood flow and velocity. (Adapted from: Eger EI 2nd. Isoflurane (Forane): A compendium and reference. Madison, Ohio Medical Products, 1985 and *Anesth Analg*. 2000;91:152.)

administration to animals subsequently recovers to preinduction levels in approximately 2 to 5 hours. The mechanism of this recovery is unclear.

7 The increase in CBF with increasing anesthetic dose occurs despite decreases in $CMRO_2$. This phenomenon has been called *uncoupling*, but from a mechanistic standpoint, true uncoupling of flow from metabolism may not occur. That is, as $CMRO_2$ is depressed by the volatile anesthetics, there still is a coupled decline in CBF opposed by a coincident direct vasodilatory effect on the cerebral blood vessels. The net effect on the cerebral vessels depends on the sum of indirect vasoconstricting and direct vasodilating influences.

Autoregulation is the intrinsic myogenic regulation of vascular tone. In normal brain, the mechanisms of autoregulation of CBF over a range of mean arterial pressures from 50 to 150 mmHg are incompletely understood. Because the volatile anesthetics are direct vasodilators, all are considered to diminish autoregulation in a dose-dependent fashion such that at high anesthetic doses, CBF is essentially pressure passive. Sevoflurane preserves autoregulation up to approximately 1 MAC.[17] At 1.5 MAC, the dynamic rate of autoregulation (change in middle cerebral artery blood flow after a rapid transient decrease in BP) is better preserved with sevoflurane than isoflurane.[23] This may result in a lesser direct vasodilator effect of sevoflurane, preserving the ability of the vessel to respond to changes in BP at 1.5 MAC. Based on a similar model but a separate study of dynamic autoregulation of CBF, both desflurane and isoflurane reduced autoregulation in a dose-dependent manner.[24]

Intracerebral Pressure

For most anesthesiologists, an area of great clinical interest is the effect of volatile anesthetics on ICP. In general, ICP will increase or decrease in proportion to changes in CBF. Isoflurane increases ICP minimally in animals both with and without brain pathology, including those with an already elevated ICP.[25] In human studies, there usually are mild increases in ICP with isoflurane administration that are blocked or blunted by hyperventilation or barbiturate coadministration.[26] However, there are some contradictory data. In one human study, hypocapnia did not prevent elevations in ICP with isoflurane administration in patients with space-occupying brain lesions.[27]

Like isoflurane, both sevoflurane and desflurane greater than 1 MAC produce mild increases in ICP, paralleling their mild increases in CBF.[16,17,28,29] One potential advantage of sevoflurane is that its lower pungency and airway irritation may lessen the risk of coughing and bucking and the associated rise in ICP as compared with desflurane or isoflurane. In fact, introduction of desflurane after propofol induction of anesthesia has led to significant increases in HR, mean arterial pressure, and middle cerebral artery blood flow velocity.[30] This may relate to the airway irritant effects of desflurane rather than a specific alteration in neurophysiology. However, several studies in both children and adults suggest that increases in ICP from desflurane are slightly greater than from either isoflurane or sevoflurane.[30,31] CSF production and resorption are modestly and variably affected by volatile anesthetics and are clinically far less important than anesthetic effects on CBF. The bottom line is that all three potent agents may be used at appropriate doses, especially with adjunctive and compensatory therapies, in nearly any neurosurgical procedure.

Cerebral Blood Flow Response to Hypercapnia and Hypocapnia

Significant hypercapnia is associated with dramatic increases 
in CBF whether or not volatile anesthetics are administered. As discussed earlier, hypocapnia can blunt or abolish volatile anesthetic-induced increases in CBF depending on when the hypocapnia is produced. This vasoreactivity to CO_2 may be somewhat altered by the volatile anesthetics as compared with normal. Isoflurane does not abolish hypocapnic vasoconstriction.[32] Similarly, CO_2 vasoreactivity under desflurane anesthesia is normal up to 1.5 MAC,[25] and CO_2 vasoreactivity for sevoflurane is preserved at 1 MAC.[33]

Cerebral Protection

When isoflurane is used to lower BP and cerebral perfusion, tissue oxygen content is improved as compared to a similar BP effect created by other pharmacologic means. The improvement is most likely due to the beneficial effect of isoflurane to decrease $CMRO_2$.[34] Both sevoflurane and desflurane have been shown to improve neurologic outcome after incomplete cerebral ischemia in a rat model.[35,36] In piglets undergoing low-flow cardiopulmonary bypass, desflurane improved neurologic outcome compared with a fentanyl/droperidol-based anesthetic.[37]

In humans, desflurane has been shown to increase brain tissue PO_2 during administration, and to maintain PO_2 to a greater extent than thiopental during temporary cerebral artery occlusion during cerebrovascular surgery.[38] Neuroprotection and clinical outcome studies for sevoflurane and desflurane have not been published.

Postoperative Cognitive Dysfunction

A direct link between volatile anesthetics and short- and long-term neurocognitive decline after surgery in adults has been difficult to establish (NICV 18-2). In animal models, a causal relationship between anesthetic gases and cognitive decline has been linked to neuroinflammation, a neurotransmitter imbalance and decreased brain-derived neurotrophic factor concentration.[39] In studies of patients undergoing general anesthesia for surgery, reducing the concentration of volatile anesthetics using a processed EEG monitor can reduce, but not eliminate postoperative delirium in the first 5 days after surgery and seems to lessen cognitive impairment at 1 year.[40]

But a number of well-conducted studies challenge the belief that general anesthetics have a causal role in the etiology of postoperative delirium and adverse long-term neurocognitive outcomes. These randomized trials did not find differences in cognitive outcomes after regional versus general anesthesia for surgical interventions in high-risk older adults.[41–43] It is worth noting that N_2O does not seem to alter short-term postoperative delirium or the progression of cognitive decline after surgery based upon evaluations of cognitive outcomes in patients receiving a potent volatile anesthetic with or without the addition of N_2O.[44,45]

Processed Electroencephalograms and Neuromonitoring

9 All of the volatile anesthetics produce dose-dependent effects on the EEG, sensory-evoked potentials (SEPs), and motor-evoked potentials (MEPs). EEGs recorded on the scalp can be processed to quantify the amount of activity in each of four frequency bands: δ (0 to 3 Hz), θ (4 to 7 Hz), α (8 to 13 Hz), and β (>13 Hz). All three currently used agents at greater than 1 MAC and N_2O at 30% to 70% can produce shifts to increasing frequencies. Between 1 and 2 MAC, the potent agents produce shifts to decreasing frequencies and increases in amplitude. At greater than 2 MAC, all of the potent agents can produce burst suppression or electrical silence. These are important factors to remember because EEG changes during administration of general anesthesia can also be caused by hypoxia, hypercarbia, and hypothermia. The EEG must always be interpreted within the appropriate clinical context.

All of the volatile agents cause a dose-dependent increase in latency and decrease in amplitude in all cortical SEP modalities. In subcortical modalities, such as brainstem auditory-evoked potentials, these agents are associated with negligible effects. In general, visual-evoked potentials are somewhat more sensitive to the effects of the volatile anesthetics than somatosensory-evoked potentials. Like EEGs, these effects from anesthetics must be kept in mind when changes during SEPs occur, and appropriate doses of the volatile agents must be used. Sudden changes in the anesthetic regimen (>0.5 MAC) also seem to have greater effects on SEPs than more gradual changes.

MEPs evaluate the functional integrity of descending motor pathways. The evoked response is most commonly recorded as a muscle potential or a peripheral nerve signal. The trigger is typically transosseous activation via electrical or magnetic stimulation. MEPs are exquisitely sensitive to depression by volatile anesthetics, which are usually avoided in these cases.

Nitrous Oxide

The effects of N_2O on cerebral physiology are not clear. Both the MAC for N_2O and its effects on $CMRO_2$ vary widely depending on species. In human studies, N_2O administration preserved CBF but decreased $CMRO_2$.[15]

Another complexity comes from the use of N_2O as a coanesthetic with potent agents where the $CMRO_2$ effects may differ depending on the presence or absence of potent agent as well as the particular agent and dose. Addition of N_2O to 1 MAC isoflurane does not alter $CMRO_2$, but it does increase CBF.

Barbiturates, narcotics, or a combination of the two appear to decrease or eliminate the changes in $CMRO_2$ and CBF produced by N_2O. N_2O administration increases ICP, but as is the case for $CMRO_2$ and CBF, changes in ICP are decreased or eliminated by a variety of coanesthetics and, more importantly, by hypocapnia.

Nitrous oxide may be neuroprotective in rat models of cerebral ischemia, but other work suggests it is neurotoxic.[46] Given the conflicting data on the effects of N_2O on $CMRO_2$, CBF, ICP, and neuroprotection during ischemia, avoidance or discontinuation of its use should be considered in surgical cases with a high likelihood of elevated ICP or significant cerebral ischemia.

The Circulatory System

Hemodynamics

The cardiac, vascular, and autonomic effects of the volatile anesthetics have been defined through several studies carried out in human volunteers not undergoing surgery.[47–50] In general, the information from these volunteer studies has translated well to the patient population commonly exposed to these anesthetics during elective and emergent surgeries.

A common effect of the potent volatile anesthetics has been to decrease BP in a dose-related fashion with essentially no differences noted between the volatile anesthetics at equianesthetic concentrations (Fig. 18-11). Their primary mechanism to decrease BP is via a potent effect to relax vascular smooth muscle leading to decreases in regional and systemic vascular resistance (Fig. 18-12). They have only minimal effects on cardiac output. 10

In volunteers, sevoflurane up to about 1 MAC does not change HR while isoflurane and desflurane result in 5% to 10% increases in HR from baseline (Fig. 18-12). Both desflurane and, to a lesser extent, isoflurane have been associated with transient and significant increases in HR during rapid increases in the inspired concentration of either anesthetic.[51,52] The mechanism(s) underlying

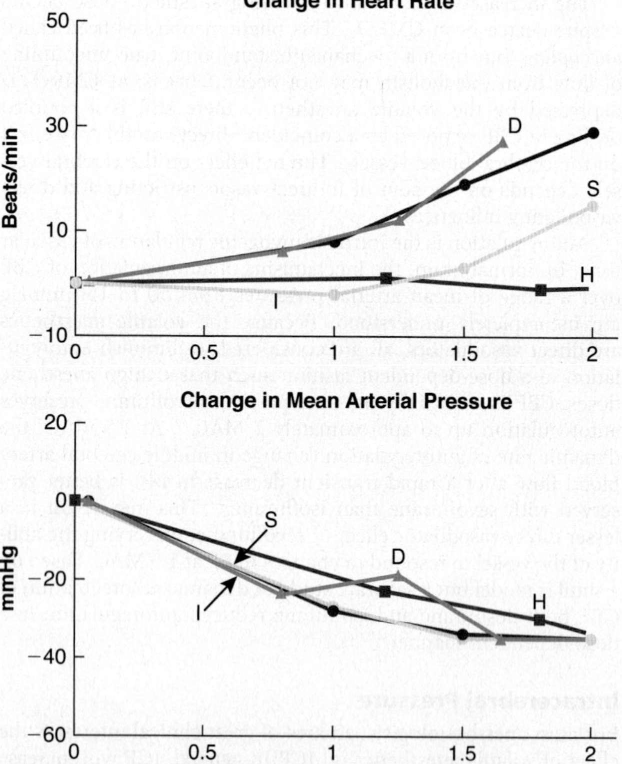

Figure 18-11 Heart rate and blood pressure changes (from awake baseline) in volunteers receiving general anesthesia with isoflurane (I), desflurane (D), or sevoflurane (S). Sevoflurane produced little or no change in heart rate below 1.5 minimum alveolar concentration.[48,60] All anesthetics caused similar decreases in blood pressure. Halothane (H) is presented for historical perspective.

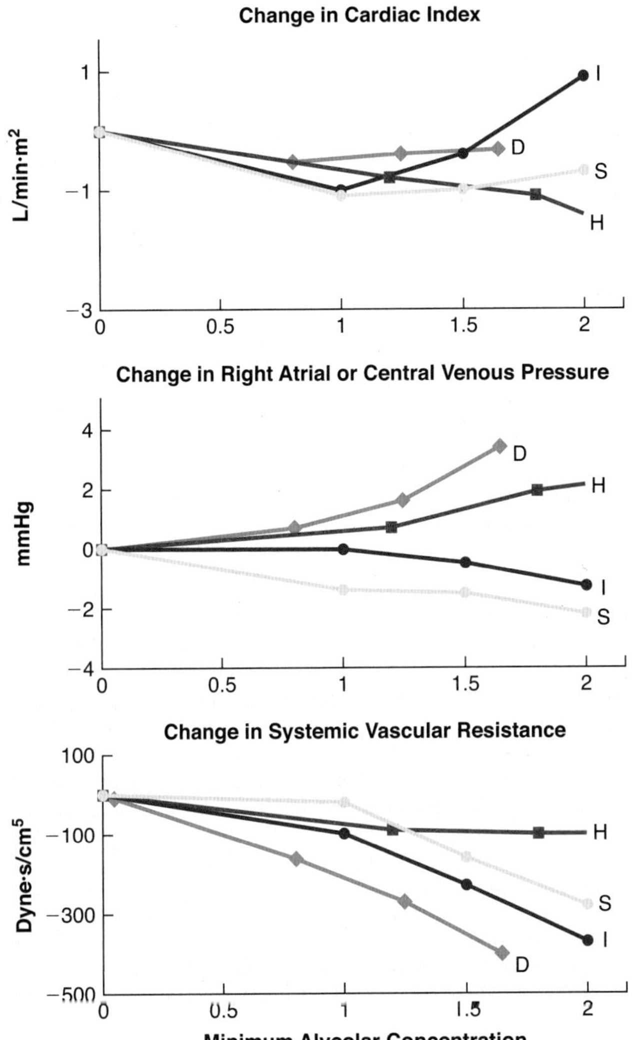

Figure 18-12 Cardiac index, central venous pressure (or right atrial pressure), and systemic vascular resistance changes (from awake baseline) in volunteers receiving general anesthesia with isoflurane (I), desflurane (D), or sevoflurane (S).[48,60] Increases in central venous pressure from desflurane might be due to venoconstriction. Halothane (H) is presented for historical perspective.

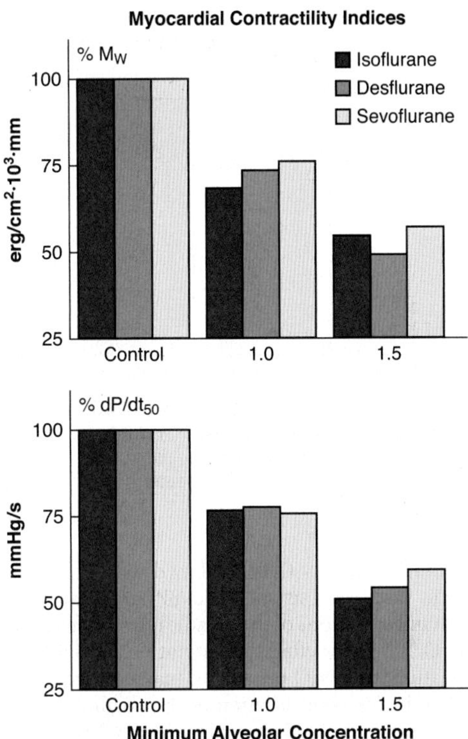

Figure 18-13 Myocardial contractility indices from chronically instrumented dogs. For these measurements, pharmacologic blockade of the autonomic nervous system was established to eliminate neural or circulating humoral influences on the inotropic state of the heart. The conscious control data were assigned 100%, and subsequent reductions in the inotropic state are depicted for both 1 and 1.5 minimum alveolar anesthetic concentrations of sevoflurane, desflurane, and isoflurane. There were no differences between these three volatile anesthetics. M_w, slope of the regional preload recruitable stroke work relationship; dP/dt_{50}, change in pressure per unit of time. (Adapted with permission from Pagel PS, Kampine JP, Schmeling WT, et al. Influence of Volatile Anesthetics on Myocardial Contractility In Vivo: Desflurane versus Isoflurane. *Anesthesiology*. 1991;74:900–907; and Harkin CP, Pagel PS, Kersten JR, et al. Direct negative inotropic and lusitropic effects of sevoflurane. *Anesthesiology*. 1994;81:156–167.)

these transient HR surges is likely due to the relative pungency of these anesthetics, which stimulates airway receptors to elicit a reflex tachycardia.[53] The tachycardia can be lessened with opioid or α_2-agonist pretreatment.[54–56]

Myocardial Contractility

Myocardial contractility indices have been directly evaluated in animals (Fig. 18-13) and indirectly evaluated in human volunteers during the administration of each of the volatile anesthetics. Isoflurane, desflurane, and sevoflurane produced similar dose-dependent reductions in indices of myocardial function.[48–50] Despite small reductions in baseline contractility, the anesthetics did not impair the functional reserve of the heart, even if baseline ventricular function was compromised as determined by the preserved ability of the myocardium to respond to an acute increase in cardiac preload.[57,58] Volatile anesthetics do not have any clinically relevant negative effect on early diastolic relaxation in patients with diastolic dysfunction although decreases in global atrial function may impact late diastolic left ventricular filling.[59]

Other Circulatory Effects

Most of the volatile anesthetics have been studied during both controlled and spontaneous ventilation.[48,49,60] The process of spontaneous ventilation reduces the high intrathoracic pressures from positive pressure ventilation. The negative intrathoracic pressure during the inspiratory phase of spontaneous ventilation augments venous return and cardiac filling and improves cardiac output and BP. Spontaneous ventilation is associated with higher $PaCO_2$, causing cerebral and systemic vascular relaxation. This contributes to an improved cardiac output via afterload reduction. Spontaneous ventilation in theory would improve the safety of volatile anesthetic administration because the anesthetic concentration that produces cardiovascular collapse exceeds the concentration that results in apnea.

Nitrous oxide is commonly combined with potent volatile anesthetics to maintain general anesthesia. Nitrous oxide has unique cardiovascular actions. It increases sympathetic nervous system activity and vascular resistance when given in a 40%

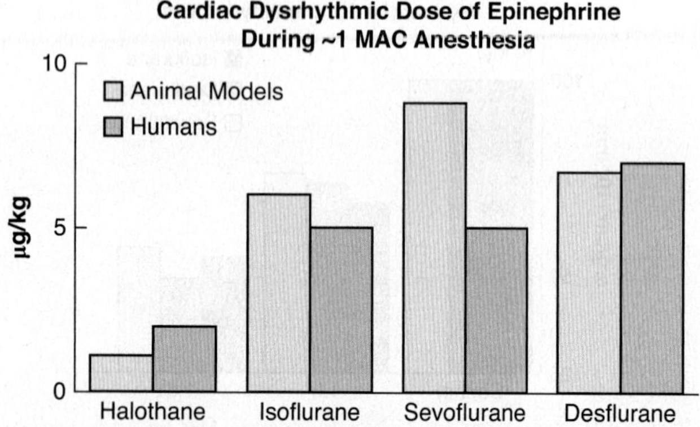

Figure 18-14 The dose of epinephrine associated with cardiac dysrythmias in animal and human models was least with halothane. The ether-based anesthetics—isoflurane, desflurane, and sevoflurane—required three- to sixfold greater doses of epinephrine to cause arrhythmias.

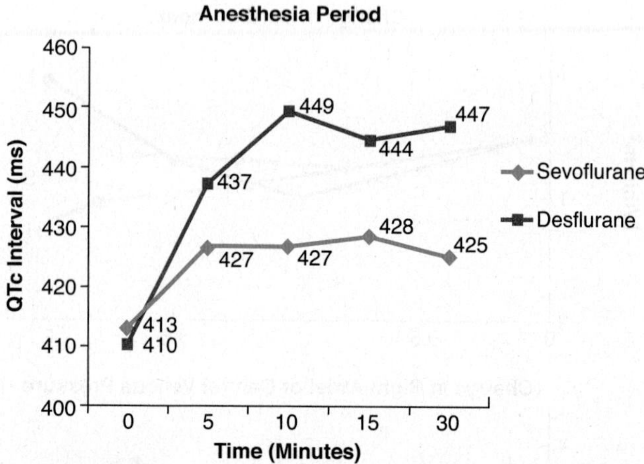

Figure 18-15 Mean QTc intervals in children, aged 1 to 14 years, after inhalation of 2% sevoflurane or 6% desflurane, both in 66% N_2O/O_2. (Adapted from Aypar E, Karagoz AH, Ozer S, et al. The effects of sevoflurane and desflurane anesthesia on QTc interval and cardiac rhythm in children. *Pediatr Anaesth*. 2007;17:563–567. Copyright © 2007 John Wiley & Sons.)

concentration.[61] When N_2O is combined with volatile anesthetics, systemic vascular resistance and BP are greater than when equipotent concentrations of the volatile anesthetics are evaluated without N_2O.[48,62] These effects might not be due solely to sympathetic activation from N_2O per se, but may be partially attributed to a decrease in the concentration of the coadministered potent volatile anesthetic required to achieve a MAC equivalent when using N_2O.

Oxygen consumption is decreased approximately 10% to 15% during general anesthesia.[63] The distribution of cardiac output also is altered by anesthesia. Blood flow to liver, kidneys, and gut is decreased, particularly at deep levels of anesthesia. In contrast, blood flow to the brain, muscle, and skin is increased or not changed during general anesthesia.[64] In humans, increases in muscle blood flow are noted with isoflurane, desflurane, and sevoflurane with minimal differences between anesthetics at equipotent concentrations.[65]

Isoflurane, sevoflurane, and desflurane do not sensitize the heart to the arrhythmogenic effects of epinephrine (Fig. 18-14). Volatile anesthetics have direct effects on cardiac pacemaker cells and conduction pathways.[66] Sinoatrial node discharge rate is slowed by the volatile anesthetics and conduction in the His–Purkinje system, and conduction pathways in the ventricle also are prolonged by the volatile anesthetics. The volatile anesthetics prolong QT_c interval, and in theory, especially with a baseline prolongation in myocardial repolarization, may predispose to ventricular tachyarrhythmias including *torsade de pointes*. Such an effect has been noted in a child with congenital prolonged QT syndrome.[67] In children studied at steady state 1 MAC, QT_c was more prolonged with desflurane than sevoflurane (Fig. 18-15).[68] When the effects of sevoflurane, propofol, and desflurane on QT interval dispersion and p dispersion were evaluated in adults, only desflurane prolonged intervals, although no increase in cardiac dysrhythmias was noted.[69]

Coronary Steal, Myocardial Ischemia, and Cardiac Outcome

Isoflurane (and most other potent volatile anesthetics) increases coronary blood flow beyond that of the myocardial oxygen demand, thereby creating potential for "steal." Steal is the diversion of blood from a myocardial bed with limited or inadequate perfusion to a bed with more adequate perfusion, especially one that has a remaining element of autoregulation.

Despite early worries that the potent vasodilation from isoflurane might cause coronary steal, clinical outcome studies have been unable to find an association between the use of isoflurane in patients undergoing coronary artery bypass graft (CABG) operations with an increased incidence of myocardial infarction or perioperative death.[70] This is in agreement with findings in a chronically instrumented dog model of multivessel coronary artery obstruction where neither isoflurane, sevoflurane, or desflurane at concentrations up to 1.5 MAC resulted in abnormal collateral coronary blood flow redistribution (steal); whereas adenosine, a potent coronary vasodilator, clearly resulted in abnormal flow distribution.[71–73]

Several studies in patients with coronary artery disease undergoing either noncardiac or CABG surgery have demonstrated that myocardial ischemia and outcome from sevoflurane were no different from isoflurane.[74,75] Desflurane also appears to result in similar outcome effects as isoflurane in cardiac patients having CABG[76] with one exception. In a study in which desflurane was given without opioids to patients with coronary artery disease requiring CABG surgery, significant ischemia mandating the use of β-blockers was noted.[77] Most studies would suggest that determinants of myocardial oxygen supply and demand, rather than the anesthetic, are of far greater importance to patient outcomes.

Cardioprotection from Volatile Anesthetics

A preconditioning stimulus such as brief coronary occlusion and ischemia initiates a signaling cascade of intracellular events that helps protect the cardiac myocyte and reduce reperfusion myocardial injury following subsequent ischemic episodes. The volatile anesthetics given before (preconditioning) or immediately after (postconditioning) mimic ischemic preconditioning and trigger a similar cascade of intracellular events resulting in reduced myocardial injury and myocardial protection that lasts beyond the elimination of the anesthetic.[78–80] Volatile anesthetics diffuse through myocardial cell membranes and alter mitochondrial electron transport such that reactive oxygen species are formed.[81] This may be the trigger for preconditioning via protein kinase C activation of K_{ATP} channel opening.[82,83] Approximately 30% to 40% of the cardioprotection from the volatile anesthetics appears

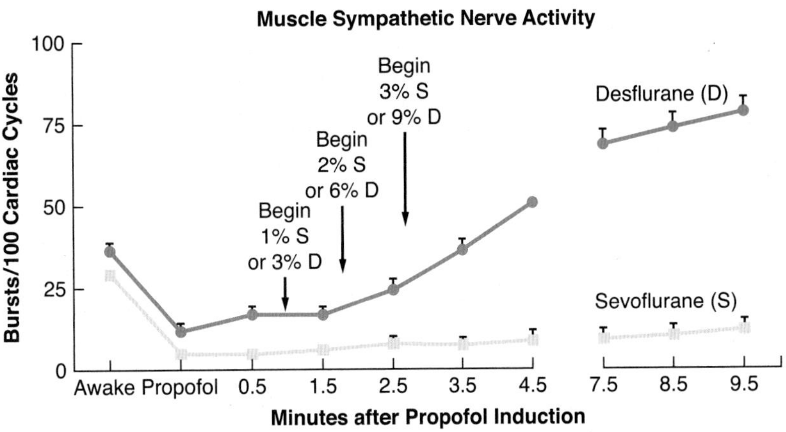

Figure 18-16 Consecutive measurements of sympathetic nerve activity (SNA; mean ± SE) from human volunteers during induction of anesthesia with propofol and the subsequent mask administration of sevoflurane or desflurane for a 10-minute period. The inspired concentration of these anesthetics was increased at 1-minute intervals beginning after propofol administration (0.41 MAC of sevoflurane and desflurane). In both groups, propofol reduced SNA and mean arterial pressure. Desflurane resulted in significant increases in SNA that persisted throughout the 10-minute mask administration period. (Adapted with permission from Ebert TJ, Muzi M, Lopatka CW. Neurocirculatory responses to sevoflurane in humans: a comparison to desflurane. *Anesthesiology*. 1995;83:88.)

to be related to a reduced loading of calcium into the myocardial cells during ischemia. This reduction in calcium accumulation improves the recovery of contractile function following reperfusion and makes the mitochondrial membrane more permeable to ATP precursors.

These findings may or may not translate to high-risk patients having cardiac or noncardiac surgery.[84] Meta-analyses have found that anesthetic cardioprotection can reduce myocardial damage and can improve cardiac outcomes during "on- and off-pump" cardiac surgery.[85–87] However, a 2019 pragmatic, multicenter trial did not find reduced myocardial ischemia or 1-year survival from using volatile anesthetics in elective CABG patients[88] and a retrospective cohort study with a 3-year follow-up found total intravenous anesthesia was associated with better survival outcomes after coronary artery bypass grafting when compared to volatile anesthetic based care.[89]

Worth noting are studies suggesting volatile anesthetics as well as xenon may protect other organs from ischemic injury, including kidney, liver, and brain.[90–93]

Autonomic Nervous System

The autonomic nervous system is modulated by baroreceptor reflex mechanisms. Studies have examined the behavior of the arterial baroreflex system during a hypotensive or hypertensive stimulus by evaluating changes in HR and sympathetic nerve activity in humans. Anesthetic-mediated, dose-dependent decreases in reflex control of sympathetic output are most prominent at the 1 MAC or greater of the volatile anesthetics.[93–96] At these concentrations, there is a greater reduction in the reflex compensation to hypovolemia than at normovolemia. This may lead to earlier recognition of blood loss intraoperatively, as there is less masking of hypovolemia by sympathetic regulation of vasoconstriction and tachycardia.

Desflurane has a unique and prominent effect on sympathetic outflow in humans, which is not apparent in animal models. With increasing steady-state concentrations of desflurane, there is a progressive increase in resting sympathetic nervous system activity (Fig. 18-16) and plasma norepinephrine levels.[95] Despite this increase in tonic sympathetic outflow, BP decreases similarly to sevoflurane and isoflurane as shown in Figure 18-11. This raises the question as to whether desflurane has the ability to uncouple neuroeffector responses. In addition, when the inspired concentration of desflurane is increased, especially to concentrations above 5% to 6%, it can cause substantial activation of the sympathetic nervous system leading to hypertension and tachycardia[51,97] Furthermore, the endocrine axis is activated as evidenced by 15- to 20-fold increases in plasma antidiuretic hormone, epinephrine, and norepinephrine (Fig. 18-17). The hemodynamic response persists for 4 to 5 minutes, and the endocrine

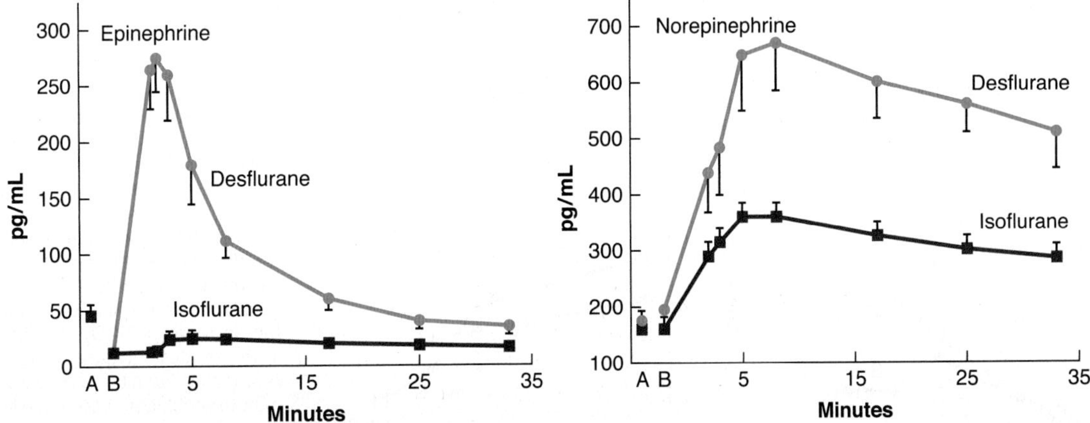

Figure 18-17 Stress hormone responses to a rapid increase in anesthetic concentration, from 4% to 12% inspired. Volunteers given desflurane showed a larger increase in plasma epinephrine and norepinephrine concentrations than when given isoflurane. Data are mean ± SE. A, awake value; B, value after 32 minutes of 0.55 minimum alveolar concentration; time represents minutes after the first breath of increased anesthetic concentration. (Adapted with permission from Weiskopf RB, Moore MA, Eger EI II, et al. Rapid increase in desflurane concentration is associated with greater transient cardiovascular stimulation than with rapid increase in isoflurane concentration in humans. *Anesthesiology*. 1994;80:1035.)

response persists for up to 30 minutes.[47,51,52] Adequate concentrations of opioids or an α_2 agonist given prior to increasing the concentration of desflurane can attenuate these responses.[54–56] The source of the neuroendocrine activation is likely from receptors in both the upper and lower airways that initiate the sympathetic activation.[53]

The Pulmonary System

General Ventilatory Effects

11 All volatile anesthetics decrease tidal volume and increase respiratory rate such that the decrease in minute ventilation at low inspired concentrations is relatively minor (Fig. 18-18). The ventilatory depressant effects of volatile anesthetics at higher concentrations are dose dependent, with higher concentrations of volatile anesthetics resulting in greater decreases in tidal volume and greater increases in respiratory rate. Isoflurane is an exception in that it does not increase respiratory rate above 1 MAC. The net effect of a gradual decrease in minute ventilation is an associated increase in resting $PaCO_2$. The respiratory depression of volatile anesthetics can be partially antagonized by the "pain" of surgical stimulation. Nitrous oxide increases respiratory rate as much or more than the volatile anesthetics. When N_2O is added to inhaled volatile anesthetics $PaCO_2$ increases in a degree similar to equi-MAC concentrations of the volatile anesthetic in O_2.

Ventilatory Mechanics

FRC is decreased during general anesthesia; this has been explained by a number of mechanisms including a decrease in the intercostal muscle tone, alteration in diaphragm position, changes in thoracic blood volume, and the onset of phasic expiratory activity of respiratory muscles. About 40% of the muscular work of breathing is via intercostal muscles and about 60% is from the diaphragm. During anesthesia, the diaphragmatic muscle function is relatively spared when contrasted to the parasternal intercostal muscles. However, inspiratory rib cage expansion is reasonably well maintained during anesthesia because of preserved activity of the scalene muscles. Expiration is generally considered a passive function mediated by the elastic recoil of the lung. The process of applying a resistance or load to expiration typically results in a slowing of respiration, but under anesthesia, further responses include a substantial asynchrony of the thoracic movements with respiration. This suggests that in patients with pulmonary disease associated with increased expiratory resistance, spontaneous ventilation during general anesthesia might be poorly tolerated.

Response to Carbon Dioxide and Hypoxemia

In conscious humans, the central chemoreceptors respond vigorously to changes in arterial carbon dioxide tension such that minute ventilation increases 3 L/min per a 1 mmHg increase in $PaCO_2$. All the inhaled anesthetics produce a dose-dependent

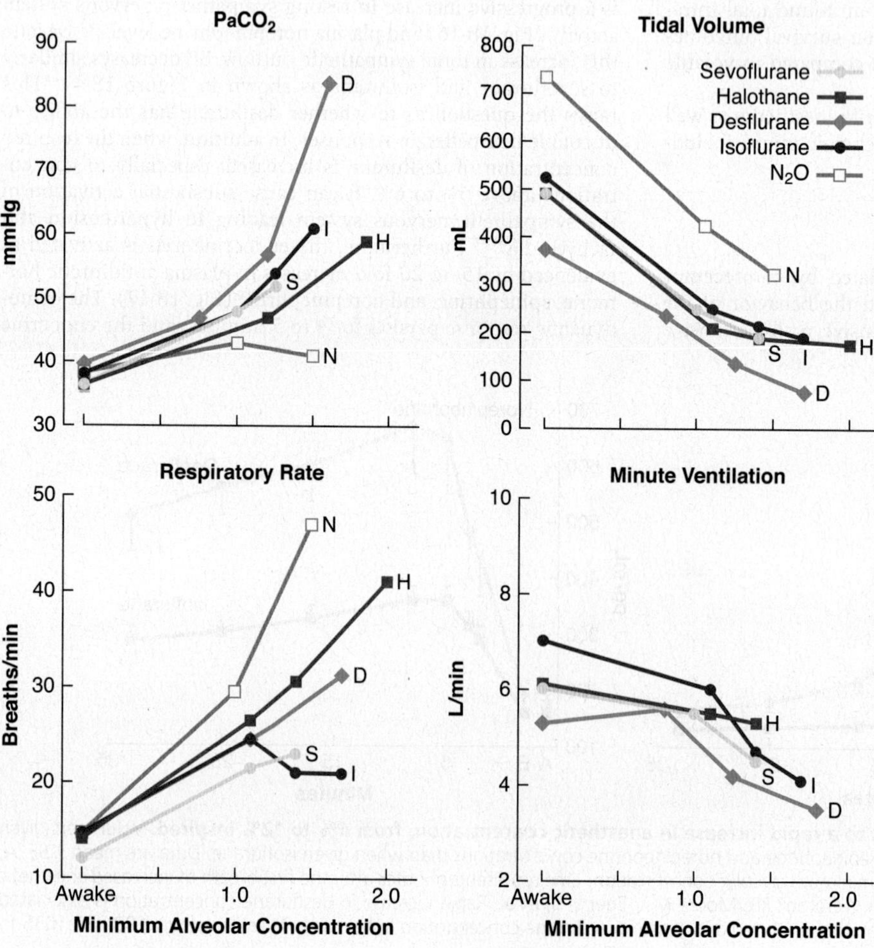

Figure 18-18 Comparison of mean changes in resting $PaCO_2$, tidal volume, respiratory rate, and minute ventilation in patients anesthetized with isoflurane, sevoflurane, desflurane, or N_2O(N). Anesthetic-induced tachypnea compensates in part for the ventilatory depression caused by all volatile anesthetics (decrease in minute ventilation and tidal volume, and concomitant increase in $PaCO_2$). Desflurane results in the greatest increase in $PaCO_2$ with corresponding reductions in tidal volume and minute ventilation. Isoflurane, like all other inhaled agents, increases respiratory rate, but does not result in dose-dependent tachypnea. (Adapted from *Anesthesiology*. 1991;74:484, *Anesthesiology*. 1971;35:26, *Anesth Analg*. 1987;66:241, Anesth Analg. 1978;57:610.)

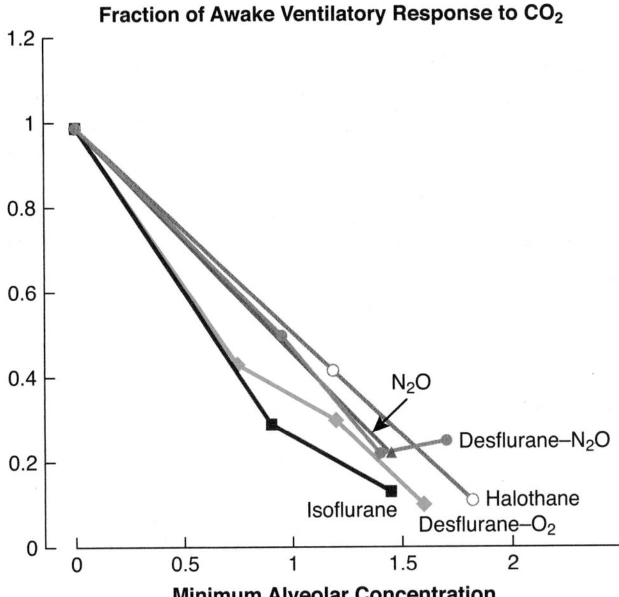

Figure 18-19 All inhaled anesthetics produce similar dose-dependent decreases in the ventilatory response to carbon dioxide (CO_2). N_2O, nitrous oxide. (Adapted from Eger EI 2nd. Desflurane. *Anesth Rev.* 1993;20:87.)

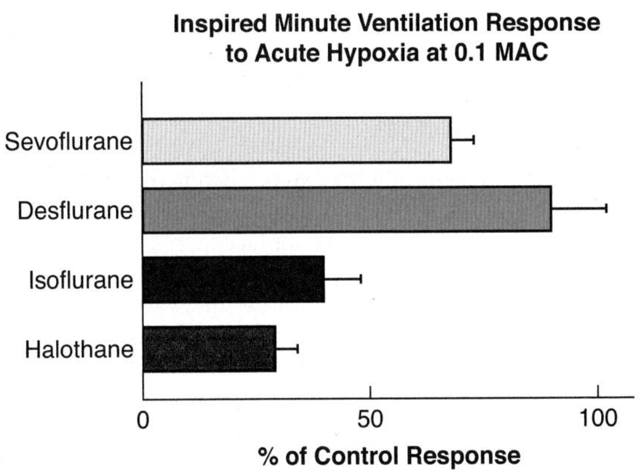

Figure 18-20 Influence of 0.1 minimum alveolar concentration (MAC) of four volatile anesthetic agents on the ventilatory response to a step decrease in end-tidal oxygen concentration. Values are mean ± SD. Subanesthetic concentrations of the volatile anesthetics, except desflurane and sevoflurane, profoundly depress the response to hypoxia. (Adapted with permission from Sarton E, Dahan A, Teppema L, et al. Acute pain and central nervous system arousal do not restore impaired hypoxic ventilatory responses during sevoflurane sedation. *Anesthesiology.* 1996;85:295.)

depression of the ventilatory response to hypercarbia (Fig. 18-19). The addition of N_2O to a volatile anesthetic can lessen this effect. The threshold where respiratory drive ceases is called the apneic threshold. It is generally 4 to 5 mmHg below the prevailing resting $PaCO_2$ in a spontaneously breathing patient. It is unrelated to the slope of the CO_2 response curves or to the level of the resting $PaCO_2$. The clinical relevance of this threshold may be realized when assisting ventilation in an anesthetized patient who is breathing spontaneously. This only serves to lower the $PaCO_2$ to approach that of the apneic threshold, therefore mandating more control of ventilation.

Inhaled anesthetics, including N_2O, also produce a dose-dependent attenuation of the ventilatory response to hypoxia. This action appears to depend on the peripheral chemoreceptors. In fact, even subanesthetic concentrations of volatile anesthetics (0.1 MAC) elicit anywhere from a 25% to 75% depression of the ventilatory drive to hypoxia (Fig. 18-20). The extreme sensitivity of the volatile anesthetics to inhibit ventilatory responses to hypoxia has important clinical implications, especially in patients who depend on hypoxic drive to set their level of ventilation, such as those with chronic respiratory failure or patients with obstructive sleep apnea. Residual effects of volatile anesthetics would be unwanted in the recovery room. In this regard, the short-acting anesthetics (sevoflurane and desflurane) may prove advantageous because of their more rapid washout and their minimal effect on hypoxic sensitivity at subanesthetic concentrations.

Bronchiolar Smooth Muscle Tone

Bronchoconstriction under anesthesia can result (1) from direct stimulation of the laryngeal and tracheal areas, (2) from the administration of adjuvant drugs that cause histamine release, and (3) from noxious stimuli-activating vagal afferent nerves. The reflex response to these stimuli will be greater in lightly versus deeply anesthetized patients.[98] The response also is enhanced in patients with known reactive airway disease, including those requiring bronchodilator therapy or those with chronic smoking histories.

Airway smooth muscle extends as far distally as the terminal bronchioles and is under the influence of both parasympathetic and sympathetic nerves. The volatile anesthetics relax airway smooth muscle primarily by directly reducing smooth muscle tone and indirectly by inhibiting the reflex neural pathways.[99] Direct effects of the volatile anesthetics partially depend on an intact bronchial epithelium, suggesting that epithelial damage or inflammation secondary to asthma or a respiratory virus may lessen their bronchodilating effect.[100] In animal models studying fourth-order bronchi, desflurane and sevoflurane were better bronchodilators than isoflurane.[100] The dilation was epithelium dependent and mediated in part by a cyclooxygenase product and nitric oxide. In humans, early administration of desflurane after tracheal intubation and high concentrations (1.5 MAC) at steady state will transiently increase airway resistance (Fig. 18-21).[101,102] This may be attributed to a direct effect on bronchial smooth muscle from the pungency of desflurane. Volatile anesthetics have been used effectively to treat status asthmaticus when other

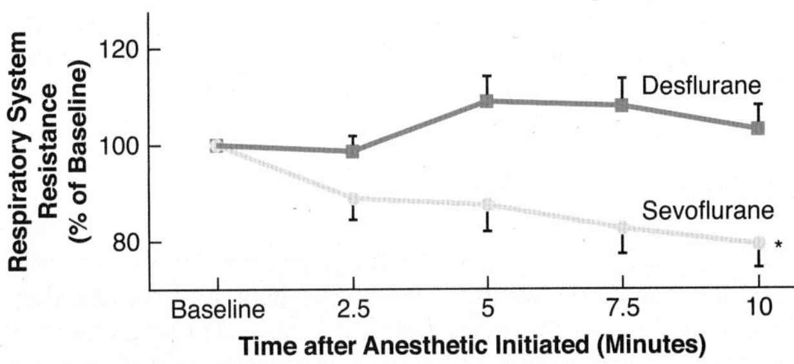

Figure 18-21 Changes in respiratory system resistance expressed as a percentage of the baseline recorded after tracheal intubation but prior to administration of sevoflurane or desflurane to the inspired gas mixture. Airway resistance responses to sevoflurane were significantly different from desflurane (*$p < .05$). (Adapted with permission from Goff MJ, Arain SR, Ficke DJ, et al. Absence of bronchodilation during desflurane anesthesia: a comparison to sevoflurane and thiopental. *Anesthesiology.* 2000;93:404.)

conventional treatments have failed and also appear to cause beneficial bronchodilation in patients with COPD.[103,104]

Mucociliary Function

Ciliated respiratory epithelium extends from the trachea to the terminal bronchioles. Cells and glands in the tracheobronchial tree secrete mucus that captures surface particles for transport via ciliary action. There are several factors involved in diminished mucociliary function, particularly in the mechanically ventilated patient where dried, inspired gases impair ciliary movement, thicken the protective mucus, and reduce the ability of mucociliary function to transport surface particles out of the airway. Volatile anesthetics and N_2O reduce ciliary movement and alter the characteristics of mucus.[105] Smokers have impaired mucociliary function, and the combination of a volatile anesthetic in a smoker who is mechanically ventilated sets up a scenario for inadequate clearing of secretions, mucus plugging, atelectasis, and hypoxemia.

Pulmonary Vascular Resistance

Although systemic vascular smooth muscle is notably affected by the volatile anesthetics, the pulmonary vascular relaxation from clinically relevant concentrations of inhaled anesthetics is minimal. The small amount of pulmonary vasodilation from volatile anesthetics is offset by anesthetic-related decreases in cardiac output, resulting in little or no change in pulmonary artery pressures and pulmonary blood flow.[106]

Perhaps more important in terms of volatile anesthetics and pulmonary blood flow is their potential to attenuate hypoxic pulmonary vasoconstriction (HPV). During periods of hypoxemia, HPV reduces pulmonary blood flow to underventilated areas of the lung, thereby diverting blood flow to areas of the lung with greater ventilation. The net effect is to improve the ventilation/perfusion (V/Q) matching, resulting in a reduced amount of venous admixture and improved arterial oxygenation. Although all of the modern inhaled anesthetics in high concentrations have been shown to attenuate HPV in animal models, the situation is less clear in patients. This may reflect the multifactorial effects of the volatile anesthetics on factors involved in pulmonary blood flow, including their cardiovascular, autonomic, and humoral actions. Furthermore, nonpharmacologic variables impair HPV, including surgical trauma, temperature, pH, $PaCO_2$, size of the hypoxic segment, and intensity of the hypoxic stimulus. One-lung ventilation (OLV) serves as a model where HPV should lessen the expected decrease in Pao_2 and intrapulmonary shunt fraction (Qs/Qt). In patients undergoing OLV during thoracic surgery, volatile anesthetics have had minimal effects on Pao_2 and Qs/Qt when changing from two-lung ventilation to OLV.[107]

Hepatic Effects

12 Unlike most intravenous anesthetic drugs, modern-day volatile anesthetics undergo minimal liver metabolism, and because they are excreted primarily via the lungs, it is not surprising that they minimally affect hepatic function. The various factors that are known to affect drug metabolism, such as age, disease, genetics, and enzyme-inducing agents, have minor effects on the elimination of volatile anesthetics.

Historically, considerable concern was raised that halothane could damage the liver—so-called "halothane hepatitis." However, this has not been an issue of concern with volatile anesthetics in current use. This subject is discussed in greater detail in Chapter 46.

In addition, there is convincing evidence that volatile anesthetics can infer organ protection from ischemic injury (discussed earlier in the chapter). For example, in CABG surgery, postoperative biochemical markers of hepatic dysfunction were lower after asevoflurane-based anesthetic than a propofol-based anesthetic.[92]

Neuromuscular System and Malignant Hyperthermia

The inhaled anesthetics have two important actions on neuromuscular function: (1) they directly relax skeletal muscle through a dose-dependent effect and (2) they potentiate the action of neuromuscular blocking drugs.[108,109] Relaxation of skeletal muscle is most prominent for potent volatile anesthetics above 1.0 MAC, with an effect enhanced by 40% in patients with myasthenia gravis.[110] Nitrous oxide does not affect skeletal muscle relaxation.

The amount of rocuronium or cisatracurium to maintain a set level of neuromuscular block is reduced by 30% to 40% during isoflurane, desflurane, and sevoflurane administration.[109,111] While the mechanism of volatile anesthetic potentiation of the neuromuscular blocking drugs is not entirely clear, it appears to be largely because of a postsynaptic effect at the nicotinic acetylcholine receptor located at the neuromuscular junction.[112,113]

MH is a clinical syndrome of acute, uncontrolled, increased 13
skeletal muscle metabolism resulting in heightened oxygen consumption, lactate formation, heat production, and rhabdomyolysis. The hallmark findings of MH are a rapidly rising temperature, increasing up to 1 °C every 5 minutes along with increasing end-tidal CO_2, arrhythmias, mixed respiratory/metabolic acidosis, and skeletal muscle rigidity.[114] Susceptibility to MH is an inherited autosomal-dominant genetic disorder with reduced penetrance and variable expression. While N_2O and xenon are considered safe in MH-susceptible patients, all volatile anesthetics serve as triggers for MH in these patients.[115,116] See Chapter 24 for additional information on MH.

Uterine Tone, Genetic Markers, Fetal Development, and Neonatal Neurobehavioral Outcomes

Uterine smooth muscle tone is diminished by volatile anesthetics in similar fashion to the effects of volatile anesthetics on vascular smooth muscle. There is a dose-dependent decrease in spontaneous myometrial contractility that is consistent among the volatile anesthetics. Desflurane and sevoflurane also inhibit the frequency and amplitude of myometrial contractions induced by oxytocin in a dose-dependent manner.[117] Uterine relaxation/atony can become problematic at concentrations of volatile anesthesia greater than 1 MAC and might delay the onset time of newborn respiration.[118] Consequently, a common technique used to provide general anesthesia for urgent cesarean sections is to administer low concentrations of the volatile anesthetic, such as 0.5 to 0.75 MAC, combined with N_2O. This decreases the likelihood of uterine atony and blood loss, especially at a time after delivery when oxytocin responsiveness of the uterus is essential. In some situations, uterine relaxation may be desirable, such as to remove a retained placenta. In this case, a brief, high concentration of a volatile anesthetic may be advantageous.

The possibility of a health risk from brief but chronic exposures to volatile anesthetics directly or as waste gases has been sought for several decades, and the cumulative data suggests the risk is likely minimal or nonexistent. The Ames test has been applied as a test for mutagenicity or carcinogenicity and has been negative for isoflurane, desflurane, sevoflurane, and N_2O. Genotoxicity can be inferred by demonstrating sister chromatid exchanges (SCEs) in lymphocytes from peripheral blood where desflurane but not sevoflurane transiently increased the frequency of SCE.[119,120] Anesthesiologists compared to nonanesthesiologists have more SCE in lymphocytes.[121,122] Although the clinical implications of these findings are not clear, the National Institute for Occupational Safety and Health has set exposure limits of 25 ppm for N_2O and 2 ppm for volatile anesthetics. Scavenging systems are important in limiting exposure to anesthesia and other OR personnel.

Volatile anesthetics can be teratogenic in animals,[123] but do not cause teratogenicity in humans. The reproductive outcomes in 5,405 surgeries in 2 million patients have been evaluated and no increase in teratogenicity was found.[124] Nitrous oxide decreases the activity of vitamin B_{12}-dependent enzymes, methionine synthetase, and thymidylate synthetase via an irreversible oxidation of the cobalt atom of vitamin B_{12}. This action might affect the rapidly developing embryo/fetus because methionine and thymidylate synthetase are involved in the formation of myelin and the formation of DNA, respectively. Based on animal studies that include 24-hour exposures to varying concentration of N_2O in a rat model, there appears to be no contraindication to the use of N_2O in the OR or other non-OR sites (e.g., radiology, dental operatories), or using it when necessary in pregnant surgical patients.[125] However, scavenging of N_20 is highly recommended.

There has been a historical concern about the incidence of spontaneous abortions in OR personnel chronically exposed to trace concentrations of inhaled anesthetics.[126] Early epidemiologic studies suggested that OR personnel had an increased incidence of spontaneous abortions and congenital abnormalities in offspring. However, subsequent analysis of the data suggests that inaccurate study design, confounding variables, and nonresponders might have led to flawed conclusions.[127] In prospective studies, no causal relationship has been shown between exposure to waste anesthetic gases and adverse health effects, regardless of the presence or absence of scavenging systems. Despite this, concerns for an adverse influence have resulted in the use of scavenging systems to remove anesthetic gases from operating and recovery rooms and have led to the establishment of standards for waste gas exposure.

In terms of neonatal effects from brief exposure to general anesthesia for cesarean section, Apgar scores and acid–base balance are not affected by anesthetic technique, such as spinal versus general.[128] More sensitive measures of short-term neurologic and behavioral function, such as the Scanlon Early Neonatal Neurobehavioral Scale and the Neurologic and Adaptive Capacities Score (NACS) indicate some transient depression of scores following general anesthesia for cesarean section that resolves at 24 hours after delivery.[128,129]

The potential for the potent volatile anesthetics to cause a more permanent effect via neurotoxicity in the rapidly developing brain of the neonate undergoing surgery is one of the more worrisome problems facing the pediatric anesthesia community. Neonatal brain development is a complicated, yet intricate process of excess neuron generation followed by apoptosis. The "threshold effect" for neurotoxicity has been established in in vivo neonatal murine models, with accelerated neuronal apoptosis and degenerative effects noted in the temporal/somatosensory cortices, frontal cortex, and hippocampus related to increasing anesthetic exposure.[130,131] Observed cognitive and behavioral deficits in these models have been associated with disturbances in neuronal circuitry, mitochondrial morphology, and dendritic spine development. It is unclear if the findings in rodents can be extrapolated to humans, as the period of peak vulnerability with rapid synaptogenesis in rodents is very brief and easily exposed to an anesthetic. The equivalent period in humans extends from midgestation to several years after birth. Retrospective observational studies in humans have demonstrated more learning disorders and behavioral impairment among children with multiple exposures to anesthesia.[132,133] Prospective studies suggest that a single anesthetic exposure of relatively brief duration (<4 hours) is not associated with an increased incidence of adverse neurobehavioral effects in later childhood.[134–136] Recent meta-analysis of prospectively assessed neurodevelopmental outcomes after a single anesthetic exposure in early childhood found a significant increase in parent reports of behavioral problems with no difference in general intelligence.[137] Interpretation of these studies is challenged by the difficulty to distinguish between anesthetic-induced neurotoxicity and confounders such as comorbidities, pre-existing but undiagnosed behavioral problems, and other periprocedural factors.

Anesthetic Degradation by Carbon Dioxide Absorbers

Compound A

Sevoflurane undergoes base-catalyzed degradation in carbon dioxide absorbents to form a vinyl ether called *compound A*. The production of compound A is enhanced in low-flow or closed-circuit breathing systems and by warm or very dry CO_2 absorbents.[138,139] Desiccated barium hydroxide lime produces more compound A than soda lime, and this can be attributed to slightly higher absorbent temperature during CO_2 extraction.[140] Desiccated barium hydroxide lime also has been implicated in the heat and fires associated with sevoflurane. This absorbent has been removed from the U.S. market.

In patients and volunteers receiving sevoflurane in closed-circuit or low-flow delivery systems, inspired compound A concentrations averaged 8 to 24 ppm and 20 to 32 ppm with soda lime and barium hydroxide lime, respectively.[141–144] Total exposures as high as 320 to 400 ppm/h have had no clear effect on clinical markers of renal function.[145–147] In randomized and prospective volunteer and patient studies, no adverse renal effects from low-flow (0.5 to 1.0 L/min) or closed-circuit sevoflurane anesthesia were detected using both standard clinical markers of renal function (serum creatinine and blood urea nitrogen concentrations) and experimental markers of renal function and structural integrity (proteinuria, glucosuria, and enzymuria).[142–144,146,148–150] In a prospective, multicenter, randomized study in patients with pre-existing renal disease, there were no adverse renal effects of long-duration, low-flow sevoflurane.[151,152] One explanation for the lack of human renal toxicity from compound A is the relative absence of a renal enzymatic pathway to breakdown compound A to a toxic thiol.[153] Based on the absence of adverse findings, most countries have no FGF restrictions. Clinical experience over the past decades since sevoflurane was introduced and a careful review by the FDA adverse events reporting system supports the science that sevoflurane does not cause renal injury in patients.

Carbon Monoxide and Heat

Carbon dioxide (CO_2) absorbents containing strong bases will degrade sevoflurane, desflurane, and isoflurane to carbon monoxide (CO) when the normal water content of the absorbent 14

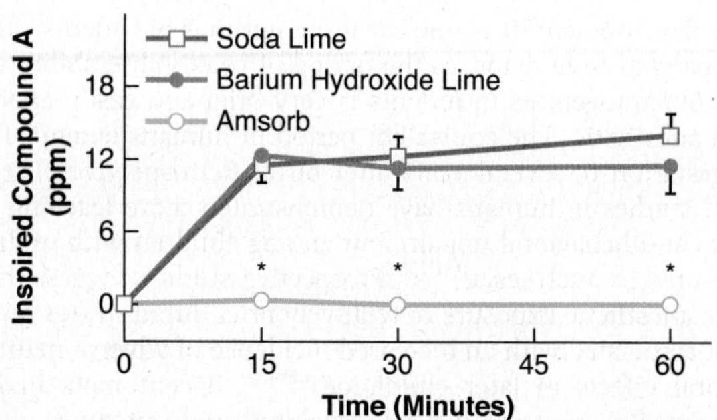

Figure 18-22 Compound A levels produced from three nondessicated carbon dioxide absorbents during 1 minimum alveolar concentration sevoflurane anesthesia delivered to volunteers at 1 L/min fresh gas flow (mean ± SE). Gas samples were taken from the inspired limb of the anesthesia circuit. *Different from barium hydroxide lime or soda lime ($p < .05$). (Adapted with permission from Mchaourab A, Arain SR, Ebert TJ. Lack of degradation of sevoflurane by a new carbon dioxide absorbent in humans. *Anesthesiology*. 2001;94:1007.)

(typically 13% to 15%) is low (less than 5%).[154–156] The degradation is the result of an exothermic reaction of the anesthetics with the absorbent. There are no clinically useful humidification detectors in current anesthetic workstations that house CO_2 absorbents. Formation of CO is dependent on both the anesthetic molecular structure and the presence of a strong base in the carbon dioxide absorbent.[155] Desflurane and isoflurane contain a difluoromethoxy moiety that is essential for the formation of CO. When studies are conducted with dry CO_2 absorbents maintained at or just above room temperature, desflurane given at just under 1 MAC produced up to 8,000 ppm of CO versus 79 ppm with nearly 2 MAC sevoflurane.[156] Instances of CO poisoning of patients have been reported in situations where the CO_2 absorbent presumably has been desiccated because an anesthetic machine had been left on with a high FGF passing through the CO_2 absorbent over an extended period of time.[157,158]

Higher temperatures of the CO_2 absorbents can promote CO formation. Lower FGFs increase the normal (25 to 45 °C) canister temperature. Although desflurane produces the most CO with desiccated CO_2 absorbers, the reaction with sevoflurane produces the most heat.[159] The strong exothermic reaction with significant heat production has caused fires and patient injuries.[160–162] An important safety initiative in the United States has led to the removal of barium hydroxide as a CO_2 absorbent from the anesthesia marketplace thereby lessening the chance of CO and heat production in clinical practice.

There are newer CO_2 absorbents primarily composed of calcium hydroxide (NICV 18-3). This change in absorbent content eliminates degradation of anesthetics (to either compound A or CO, Fig. 18-22) and will reduce exothermic reactions.[163]

Anesthetic Metabolism

Fluoride-Induced Nephrotoxicity

The metabolism of anesthetic gases has the potential to adversely affect organs via toxicity from the metabolite. The outdated anesthetics methoxyflurane and enflurane are well known for causing renal injury. The nephrotoxicity has been attributed to an increase in plasma fluoride and presents as a renal concentrating defect that is unresponsive to vasopressin and is characterized by dilute polyuria, dehydration, serum hypernatremia, hyperosmolality, elevated blood urea nitrogen, and creatinine.[164] The traditional "fluoride toxicity" hypothesis stated that both the duration of the high systemic fluoride concentrations (area under the fluoride–time curve) and the peak fluoride concentration (peaks above 50 μM appear to represent the toxic threshold) were related to nephrotoxicity. Sevoflurane undergoes 5% metabolism leading to transient increases in serum fluoride concentrations without a renal-concentrating defect. The safety of sevoflurane may be the result of a rapid decline in plasma fluoride concentrations because of less availability of the anesthetic for metabolism from a fast elimination compared with enflurane.[165] In addition, renal defluorination of sevoflurane is minimal and may add to the absence of an adverse renal-concentrating effect.[166]

Environmental Effects of Volatile Anesthetics

The environmental cost of volatile anesthetics is now well recognized,[167–169] and strategies to reduce their effect are being reported.[170–172] Volatile anesthetic wastage to the environment is estimated to account for up to 1% of the U.S. health care industry's greenhouse gas emissions.[169] Each volatile anesthetic has a greater global warming potential (GWP) than CO_2, the quintessential greenhouse gas.[173] As a reference, GWP measures how much energy (i.e., heat) is absorbed in the atmosphere by the emissions of 1 ton of gas over a specified period of time, compared to the emissions of 1 ton of CO_2. When looking at a 100-year time frame, desflurane has a GWP of 2,540 compared to isoflurane at 510, sevoflurane at 130, N_2O at 265, and CO_2 the reference point at 1.[168,173] Nitrous Oxide is not only a greenhouse gas but is also destructive to the ozone layer.[168,174] When comparing volatile anesthetics use at an FGF of 1 L/min to gasoline-consuming cars, 1 MAC-hour of desflurane is equivalent to driving 190 car miles while for sevoflurane and isoflurane, the distances are 4 and 8 miles, respectively.[170] Extending this calculation for desflurane to a typical OR day with varying use of FGF for induction and maintenance phases of anesthesia, it is not difficult to exceed 1,000 miles a day of CO_2 emissions from a driving equivalency perspective. The American Society of Anesthesiologists has called upon anesthesiologists to reduce their own emission footprint and has created the *Anesthesiology Sustainability Checklist* (Table 18-5).[175]

15

Table 18-5 Strategies to Lessen the Environmental Impact of Potent Volatile Anesthetics

1. Reduce the period of high fresh gas flow (FGF) during induction of general anesthesia
   - Determine a minimum FGF during mask ventilation
   - Turn off the FGF during the intubation phase
2. Lower the FGF to a minimum during the maintenance phase of the procedure
   - Estimate patient oxygen consumption as 5 mL/kg/min
     - 100-kg patient requires a minimum of 500 mL/min
     - Circuit leaks and side-stream analyzer will add to FGF needs
   - Target ~0.7–1 L/min FGF
   - Monitor exhaled anesthetic concentration to avoid awareness
3. Consider less use of desflurane and N_2O
4. Employ other strategies to lower volatile anesthetic requirements
   - Use adjuvants such as opioids, α_2 agonists
   - Neuraxial/regional blocks or local anesthetic infiltration at surgical site

Clinical Utility of Volatile Anesthetics

For Induction of Anesthesia

Induction of anesthesia by inhalation via a mask, as opposed to use of an intravenous agent, can be very useful in children and in adults who are uncooperative or who have a compromised airway.[176–178] Sevoflurane is potent, poorly soluble in blood, nonpungent, and therefore inhaled easily. Spontaneous ventilation is preserved with a gas induction since patients essentially regulate their own depth of anesthesia (too much sevoflurane would suppress ventilation). Clinical studies indicate that stage two excitation is avoided with high concentrations of sevoflurane. The typical time to loss of consciousness is 60 seconds when delivering 8% sevoflurane via the face mask. Sevoflurane also has been administered by mask as an approach to the difficult adult airway because it preserves spontaneous ventilation and does not cause salivation.[179] Laryngeal mask placement can be successfully achieved 2 minutes after administering 7% sevoflurane via the face mask.[179] The addition of N_2O to the inspired gas mixture does not add significantly to the induction sequence. The gas induction technique is improved by pretreatment with benzodiazepines and worsened with opioid pretreatment because of apnea.[177] Patient acceptance of this technique has been high, exceeding 90%.[176]

For Maintenance of Anesthesia

The volatile anesthetics are clearly the most popular drug used to maintain anesthesia. They are easily administered via inhalation, readily titrated, have a high safety ratio in terms of preventing recall, and the depth of anesthesia can be quickly adjusted in a predictable way while monitoring tissue levels via end-tidal concentrations. They are effective regardless of age or body habitus. They have some properties that prove beneficial in the operating room, including relaxation of skeletal muscle, preservation of cardiac output and CBF, relatively predictable recovery profiles, and organ protection from ischemic injury. Some of the drawbacks to the use of the current volatile anesthetics are their absence of analgesic effects, association with PONV, their concern for causing neurobehavioral changes in neonates, and their greenhouse gas effects promoting global warming.

Acknowledgments

We gratefully acknowledge the contributions of previous edition author, Sawyer A. Naze, as portions of their chapter have been retained in this revision.

For further review and interactivities, please see the videos and narrative interactive clinical vignettes (NICVs) accessible in the complimentary eBook bundled with this text. Access instructions are located on the inside front cover.

REFERENCES

1. Kety SS. The physiological and physical factors governing the uptake of anesthetic gases by the body. *Anesthesiology*. 1950;11:517.
2. Eger EI. *Anesthetic Uptake and Action*. Williams & Wilkins; 1974.
3. Ebert TJ, Robinson BJ, Uhrich TD, Mackenthun A, Pichotta PJ. Recovery from sevoflurane anesthesia: a comparison to isoflurane and propofol anesthesia. *Anesthesiology*. 1998; 89:1524–1531.
4. McKay RE, Malhotra A, Cakmakkaya OS, Hall KT, McKay WR, Apfel CC. Effect of increased body mass index and anaesthetic duration on recovery of protective airway reflexes after sevoflurane vs desflurane. *Br J Anaesth*. 2010;104:175–182.
5. Law LSC, Lo EAG, Gan TJ. Xenon anesthesia: a systematic review and meta-analysis of randomized controlled trials. *Anesth Analg*. 2016;122:678–697.
6. Schaefer W, Meyer PT, Rossaint R, et al. Myocardial blood flow during general anesthesia with xenon in humans: a positron emission tomography study. *Anesthesiology*. 2011;114: 1373–1379.
7. Schallner N, Goebel U. The perioperative use of nitrous oxide: renaissance of an old gas or funeral of an ancient relic? *Curr Opin Anaesthesiol*. 2013;26:354–360.
8. Waun JE, Sweitzer RS, Hamilton WK. Effect of nitrous oxide on middle ear mechanics and hearing acuity. *Anesthesiology*. 1967;28:846–850.
9. Tinker JH, Sharbrough FW, Michenfelder JD. Anterior shift of the dominant EEG rhythm during anesthesia in the Java monkey: correlation with anesthetic potency. *Anesthesiology*. 1977;46:252–259.
10. Katoh T, Suguro Y, Kimura T, Ikeda K. Cerebral awakening concentration of sevoflurane and isoflurane predicted during slow and fast alveolar washout. *Anesth Analg*. 1993;77:1012–1017.
11. Roizen MF, Horrigan RW, Frazer BM. Anesthetic doses blocking adrenergic (stress) and cardiovascular responses to incision–MAC BAR. *Anesthesiology*. 1981;54:390–398.
12. Liem EB, Lin CM, Suleman MI, et al. Anesthetic requirement is increased in redheads. *Anesthesiology*. 2004;101:279–283.
13. Stekiel TA, Contney SJ, Bosnjak ZJ, Kampine JP, Roman RJ, Stekiel WJ. Reversal of minimum alveolar concentrations of volatile anesthetics by chromosomal substitution. *Anesthesiology*. 2004; 101:796–798.
14. Mapleson WW. Effect of age on MAC in humans: a meta-analysis. *Br J Anaesth*. 1996;76: 179–185.
15. Smith AL, Wollman H. Cerebral blood flow and metabolism: effects of anesthetic drugs and techniques. *Anesthesiology*. 1972;36:378–400.
16. Lutz LJ, Milde JH, Milde LN. The cerebral functional, metabolic, and hemodynamic effects of desflurane in dogs. *Anesthesiology*. 1990;73:125–131.
17. Scheller MS, Nakakimura K, Fleischer JE, Zornow MH. Cerebral effects of sevoflurane in the dog: comparison with isoflurane and enflurane. *Br J Anaesth*. 1990;65:388–392.
18. Fujibayashi T, Sugiura Y, Yanagimoto M, Harada J, Goto Y. Brain energy metabolism and blood flow during sevoflurane and halothane anesthesia: effects of hypocapnia and blood pressure fluctuations. *Acta Anaesthesiol Scand*. 1994;38:413–418.
19. Yli-Hankala A, Vakkuri A, Särkelä M, Lindgren L, Korttila K, Jäntti V. Epileptiform electroencephalogram during mask induction of anesthesia with sevoflurane. *Anesthesiology*. 1999;91:1596–1603.
20. Julliac B, Guehl D, Chopin F, et al. Risk factors for the occurrence of electroencephalogram abnormalities during induction of anesthesia with sevoflurane in nonepileptic patients. *Anesthesiology*. 2007;106:243–251.
21. Hisada K, Morioka T, Fukui K, et al. Effects of sevoflurane and isoflurane on electrocorticographic activities in patients with temporal lobe epilepsy. *J Neurosurg Anesthesiol*. 2001;13: 333–337.
22. Algotsson L, Messeter K, Nordström CH, Ryding E. Cerebral blood flow and oxygen consumption during isoflurane and halothane anesthesia in man. *Acta Anaesthesiol Scand*. 1988; 32:15–20.
23. Summors AC, Gupta AK, Matta BF. Dynamic cerebral autoregulation during sevoflurane anesthesia: a comparison with isoflurane. *Anesth Analg*. 1999;88:341–345.
24. Strebel S, Lam AM, Matta B, Mayberg TS, Aaslid R, Newell DW. Dynamic and static cerebral autoregulation during isoflurane, desflurane, and propofol anesthesia. *Anesthesiology*. 1995;83:66–76.
25. Lutz LJ, Milde JH, Milde LN. The response of the canine cerebral circulation to hyperventilation during anesthesia with desflurane. *Anesthesiology*. 1991;74:504–507.
26. Adams RW, Cucchiara RF, Gronert GA, Messick JM, Michenfelder JD. Isoflurane and cerebrospinal fluid pressure in neurosurgical patients. *Anesthesiology*. 1981;54:97–99.
27. Grosslight K, Foster R, Colohan AR, Bedford RF. Isoflurane for neuroanesthesia: risk factors for increases in intracranial pressure. *Anesthesiology*. 1985;63:533–536.
28. Talke P, Caldwell JE, Richardson CA. Sevoflurane increases lumbar cerebrospinal fluid pressure in normocapnic patients undergoing transsphenoidal hypophysectomy. *Anesthesiology*. 1999;91:127–130.
29. Talke P, Caldwell J, Dodsont B, Richardson CA. Desflurane and isoflurane increase lumbar cerebrospinal fluid pressure in normocapnic patients undergoing transsphenoidal hypophysectomy. *Anesthesiology*. 1996;85:999–1004.
30. Muzzi DA, Losasso TJ, Dietz NM, Faust RJ, Cucchiara RF, Milde LN. The effect of desflurane and isoflurane on cerebrospinal fluid pressure in humans with supratentorial mass lesions. *Anesthesiology*. 1992;76:720–724.
31. Sponheim S, Skraastad Ø, Helseth E, Due-Tønnesen B, Aamodt G, Breivik H. Effects of 0.5 and 1.0 MAC isoflurane, sevoflurane and desflurane on intracranial and cerebral perfusion pressures in children. *Acta Anaesthesiol Scand*. 2003;47:932–938.
32. Drummond JC, Todd MM, Toutant SM, Shapiro HM. Brain surface protrusion during enflurane, halothane, and isoflurane anesthesia in cats. *Anesthesiology*. 1983;59:288–293.
33. Bundgaard H, von Oettingen G, Larsen KM, et al. Effects of sevoflurane on intracranial pressure, cerebral blood flow and cerebral metabolism. A dose-response study in patients subjected to craniotomy for cerebral tumours. *Acta Anaesthesiol Scand*. 1998;42:621–627.

34. Seyde WC, Longnecker DE. Cerebral oxygen tension in rats during deliberate hypotension with sodium nitroprusside, 2-chloroadenosine, or deep isoflurane anesthesia. *Anesthesiology*. 1986;64:480–485.
35. Engelhard K, Werner C, Reeker W, et al. Desflurane and isoflurane improve neurological outcome after incomplete cerebral ischaemia in rats. *Br J Anaesth*. 1999;83:415–421.
36. Werner C, Möllenberg O, Kochs E, Schulte J am Esch. Sevoflurane improves neurological outcome after incomplete cerebral ischaemia in rats. *Br J Anaesth*. 1995;75:756–760.
37. Loepke AW, Priestley MA, Schultz SE, McCann J, Golden J, Kurth CD. Desflurane improves neurologic outcome after low-flow cardiopulmonary bypass in newborn pigs. *Anesthesiology*. 2002;97:1521–1527.
38. Hoffman WE, Charbel FT, Edelman G, Ausman JI. Thiopental and desflurane treatment for brain protection. *Neurosurgery*. 1998;43:1050–1053.
39. Wang CM, Chen WC, Zhang Y, Lin S, He HF. Update on the mechanism and treatment of sevoflurane-induced postoperative cognitive dysfunction. *Front Aging Neurosci*. 2021;13: 702231.
40. Evered LA, Chan MTV, Han R, et al. Anaesthetic depth and delirium after major surgery: a randomised clinical trial. *Br J Anaesth*. 2021;127:704–712.
41. Li T, Li J, Yuan L, et al; RAGA Study Investigators. Effect of regional vs general anesthesia on incidence of postoperative delirium in older patients undergoing hip fracture surgery: the RAGA randomized trial. *JAMA*. 2022;327:50–58.
42. Whitlock EL, Diaz-Ramirez LG, Smith AK, et al. Association of coronary artery bypass grafting vs percutaneous coronary intervention with memory decline in older adults undergoing coronary revascularization. *JAMA*. 2021;325:1955–1964.
43. Neuman MD, Feng R, Carson JL, et al; REGAIN Investigators. Spinal anesthesia or general anesthesia for hip surgery in older adults. *N Engl J Med*. 2021;385:2025–2035.
44. Leung JM, Sands LP, Vaurio LE, Wang Y. Nitrous oxide does not change the incidence of postoperative delirium or cognitive decline in elderly surgical patients. *Br J Anaesth*. 2006;96:754–760.
45. Sprung J, Abcejo ASA, Knopman DS, et al. Anesthesia with and without nitrous oxide and long-term cognitive trajectories in older adults. *Anesth Analg*. 2020;131:594–604.
46. Bracco D, Hemmerling TM. Nitrous oxide: from neurotoxicity to neuroprotection? *Crit Care Med*. 2008;36:2705–2706.
47. Ebert TJ, Muzi M, Lopatka CW. Neurocirculatory responses to sevoflurane in humans: a comparison to desflurane. *Anesthesiology*. 1995;83:88–95.
48. Malan TP Jr, DiNardo JA, Isner RJ, et al. Cardiovascular effects of sevoflurane compared with those of isoflurane in volunteers. *Anesthesiology*. 1995;83:918–928.
49. Weiskopf RB, Cahalan MK, Eger EI 2nd, et al. Cardiovascular actions of desflurane in normocarbic volunteers. *Anesth Analg*. 1991;73:143–156.
50. Stevens WC, Cromwell TH, Halsey MJ, Eger EI 2nd, Shakespeare TF, Bahlman SH. The cardiovascular effects of a new inhalation anesthetic, Forane, in human volunteers at a constant arterial carbon dioxide tension. *Anesthesiology*. 1971;35:8–16.
51. Ebert TJ, Muzi M. Sympathetic hyperactivity during desflurane anesthesia in healthy volunteers: a comparison with isoflurane. *Anesthesiology*. 1993;79:444–453.
52. Weiskopf RB, Moore MA, Eger EI 2nd, et al. Rapid increase in desflurane concentration is associated with greater transient cardiovascular stimulation than with rapid increase in isoflurane concentration in humans. *Anesthesiology*. 1994;80:1035–1045.
53. Muzi M, Ebert TJ, Hope WG, Robinson BJ, Bell LB. Site(s) mediating sympathetic activation with desflurane. *Anesthesiology*. 1996;85:737–747.
54. Yonker-Sell AE, Muzi M, Hope WG, Ebert TJ. Alfentanil modifies the neurocirculatory responses to desflurane. *Anesth Analg*. 1996;82:162–166.
55. Pacentine GG, Muzi M, Ebert TJ. Effects of fentanyl on sympathetic activation associated with the administration of desflurane. *Anesthesiology*. 1995;82:823–831.
56. Devcic A, Muzi M, Ebert TJ. The effects of clonidine on desflurane-mediated sympathoexcitation in humans. *Anesth Analg*. 1995;80:773–779.
57. De Hert SG, Van der Linden PJ, ten Broecke PW, Vermeylen KT, Rodrigus IE, Stockman BA. Effects of desflurane and sevoflurane on length-dependent regulation of myocardial function in coronary surgery patients. *Anesthesiology*. 2001;95:357–363.
58. De Hert SG, Cromheecke S, ten Broecke PW, et al. Effects of propofol, desflurane, and sevoflurane on recovery of myocardial function after coronary surgery in elderly high-risk patients. *Anesthesiology*. 2003;99:314–323.
59. Bolliger D, Seeberger MD, Kasper J, et al. Different effects of sevoflurane, desflurane, and isoflurane on early and late left ventricular diastolic function in young healthy adults. *Br J Anaesth*. 2010;104:547–554.
60. Weiskopf RB, Cahalan MK, Ionescu P, et al. Cardiovascular actions of desflurane with and without nitrous oxide during spontaneous ventilation in humans. *Anesth Analg*. 1991;73: 165–174.
61. Ebert TJ, Kampine JP. Nitrous oxide augments sympathetic outflow: direct evidence from human peroneal nerve recordings. *Anesth Analg*. 1989;69:444–449.
62. Cahalan MK, Weiskopf RB, Eger EI 2nd, et al. Hemodynamic effects of desflurane/nitrous oxide anesthesia in volunteers. *Anesth Analg*. 1991;73:157–164.
63. Theye RA, Michenfelder JD. Whole-body and organ VO_2 changes with enflurane, isoflurane, and halothane. *Br J Anaesth*. 1975;47:813–817.
64. Crawford MW, Lerman J, Pilato M, Orrego H, Saldivia V, Carmichael FJ. Haemodynamic and organ blood flow responses to sevoflurane during spontaneous ventilation in the rat: a dose-response study. *Can J Anaesth*. 1992;39:270–276.
65. Ebert TJ, Harkin CP, Muzi M. Cardiovascular responses to sevoflurane: a review. *Anesth Analg*. 1995;81(6 suppl):S11–S22.
66. Atlee JL 3rd, Bosnjak ZJ. Mechanisms for cardiac dysrhythmias during anesthesia. *Anesthesiology*. 1990;72:347–374.
67. Saussine M, Massad I, Raczka F, Davy JM, Frapier JM. Torsade de pointes during sevoflurane anesthesia in a child with congenital long QT syndrome. *Paediatr Anaesth*. 2006;16:63–65.
68. Aypar E, Karagoz AH, Ozer S, Celiker A, Ocal T. The effects of sevoflurane and desflurane anesthesia on QTc interval and cardiac rhythm in children. *Paediatr Anaesth*. 2007;17: 563–567.
69. Kazanci D, Unver S, Karadeniz U, et al. A comparison of the effects of desflurane, sevoflurane and propofol on QT, QTc, and P dispersion on ECG. *Ann Card Anaesth*. 2009;12:107–112.
70. Slogoff S, Keats AS, Dear WE, et al. Steal-prone coronary anatomy and myocardial ischemia associated with four primary anesthetic agents in humans. *Anesth Analg*. 1991;72:22–27.
71. Hartman JC, Pagel PS, Kampine JP, Schmeling WT, Warltier DC. Influence of desflurane on regional distribution of coronary blood flow in a chronically instrumented canine model of multivessel coronary artery obstruction. *Anesth Analg*. 1991;72:289–299.
72. Hartman JC, Kampine JP, Schmeling WT, Warltier DC. Steal-prone coronary circulation in chronically instrumented dogs: isoflurane versus adenosine. *Anesthesiology*. 1991;74:744–756.
73. Kersten JR, Brayer AP, Pagel PS, Tessmer JP, Warltier DC. Perfusion of ischemic myocardium during anesthesia with sevoflurane. *Anesthesiology*. 1994;81:995–1004.
74. Ebert TJ, Kharasch ED, Rooke GA, Shroff A, Muzi M. Myocardial ischemia and adverse cardiac outcomes in cardiac patients undergoing noncardiac surgery with sevoflurane and isoflurane. *Anesth Analg*. 1997;85:993–999.
75. Searle NR, Martineau RJ, Conzen P, et al. Comparison of sevoflurane/fentanyl and isoflurane/fentanyl during elective coronary artery bypass surgery. *Can J Anaesth*. 1996;43:890–899.
76. Thomson IR, Bowering JB, Hudson RJ, Frais MA, Rosenbloom M. A comparison of desflurane and isoflurane in patients undergoing coronary artery surgery. *Anesthesiology*. 1991;75: 776–781.
77. Helman JD, Leung JM, Bellows WH, et al. The risk of myocardial ischemia in patients receiving desflurane versus sufentanil anesthesia for coronary artery bypass graft surgery. *Anesthesiology*. 1992;77:47–62.
78. Swyers T, Redford D, Larson DF. Volatile anesthetic-induced preconditioning. *Perfusion*. 2014;29:10–15.
79. Lotz C, Kehl F. Volatile anesthetic-induced cardiac protection: molecular mechanisms, clinical aspects, and interactions with nonvolatile agents. *J Cardiothorac Vasc Anesth*. 2015;29: 749–760.
80. Riess ML, Stowe DF, Warltier DC. Cardiac pharmacological preconditioning with volatile anesthetics: from bench to bedside? *Am J Physiol Heart Circ Physiol*. 2004;286:H1603–H1607.
81. Stowe DF, Kevin LG. Cardiac preconditioning by volatile anesthetic agents: a defining role for altered mitochondrial bioenergetics. *Antioxid Redox Signal*. 2004;6:439–448.
82. Novalija E, Kevin LG, Camara AK, Bosnjak ZJ, Kampine JP, Stowe DF. Reactive oxygen species precede the epsilon isoform of protein kinase C in the anesthetic preconditioning signaling cascade. *Anesthesiology*. 2003;99: 421–428.
83. Kwok WM, Martinelli AT, Fujimoto K, Suzuki A, Stadnicka A, Bosnjak ZJ. Differential modulation of the cardiac adenosine triphosphate-sensitive potassium channel by isoflurane and halothane. *Anesthesiology*. 2002;97:50–56.
84. Sellers D, Fedorko L, Djaiani G. Myocardial preconditioning with volatile anesthetics: goodbye to all that? *J Cardiothorac Vasc Anesth*. 2020;34:3257–3258.
85. Uhlig C, Bluth T, Schwarz K, et al. Effects of volatile anesthetics on mortality and postoperative pulmonary and other complications in patients undergoing surgery: a systematic review and meta-analysis. *Anesthesiology*. 2016;124:1230–1245.
86. Yu CH, Beattie WS. The effects of volatile anesthetics on cardiac ischemic complications and mortality in CABG: a meta-analysis. *Can J Anaesth*. 2006;53:906–918.
87. Landoni G, Biondi-Zoccai GGL, Zangrillo A, et al. Desflurane and sevoflurane in cardiac surgery: a meta-analysis of randomized clinical trials. *J Cardiothorac Vasc Anesth*. 2007;21: 502–511.
88. Landoni G, Lomivorotov VV, Neto CN, et al; MYRIAD Study Group. Volatile anesthetics versus total intravenous anesthesia for cardiac surgery. *N Engl J Med*. 2019;380:1214–1225.
89. Oh TK, Song IA. Total intravenous anesthesia was associated with better survival outcomes after coronary artery bypass grafting: a retrospective cohort study with three-year follow-up in South Korea. *J Cardiothorac Vasc Anesth*. 2020;34:3250–3256.
90. Clarkson AN. Anesthetic-mediated protection/preconditioning during cerebral ischemia. *Life Sci*. 2007;80:1157–1175.
91. Lee HT, Ota-Setlik A, Fu Y, Nasr SH, Emala CW. Differential protective effects of volatile anesthetics against renal ischemia-reperfusion injury in vivo. *Anesthesiology*. 2004;101: 1313–1324.
92. Lorsomradee S, Cromheecke S, Lorsomradee S, De Hert SG. Effects of sevoflurane on biomechanical markers of hepatic and renal dysfunction after coronary artery surgery. *J Cardiothorac Vasc Anesth*. 2006;20:684–690.

93. Ma D, Lim T, Xu J, et al. Xenon preconditioning protects against renal ischemic-reperfusion injury via HIF-1alpha activation. *J Am Soc Nephrol*. 2009;20:713–720.
94. Muzi M, Ebert TJ. A randomized, prospective comparison of halothane, sevoflurane and enflurane on baroreflex control of heart rate in humans. In: Bosnjak Z, Kampine JP, eds. *Advances in Pharmacology. Vol. 31: Anesthesia and Cardiovascular Disease*. Academic Press; 1994:379–387.
95. Muzi M, Ebert TJ. A comparison of baroreflex sensitivity during isoflurane and desflurane anesthesia in humans. *Anesthesiology*. 1995;82:919–925.
96. Ebert TJ, Perez F, Uhrich TD, Deshur MA. Desflurane-mediated sympathetic activation occurs in humans despite preventing hypotension and baroreceptor unloading. *Anesthesiology*. 1998; 88:1227–1232.
97. Muzi M, Lopatka CW, Ebert TJ. Desflurane-mediated neurocirculatory activation in humans: effects of concentration and rate of change on responses. *Anesthesiology*. 1996;84:1035–1042.
98. Hirshman CA, Bergman NA. Factors influencing intrapulmonary airway calibre during anaesthesia. *Br J Anaesth*. 1990;65:30–42.
99. Hirshman CA, Edelstein G, Peetz S, Wayne R, Downes H. Mechanism of action of inhalational anesthesia on airways. *Anesthesiology*. 1982;56:107–111.
100. Park KW, Dai HB, Lowenstein E, Sellke FW. Epithelial dependence of the bronchodilatory effect of sevoflurane and desflurane in rat distal bronchi. *Anesth Analg*. 1998;86:646–651.
101. Goff MJ, Arain SR, Ficke DJ, Uhrich TD, Ebert TJ. Absence of bronchodilation during desflurane anesthesia: a comparison to sevoflurane and thiopental. *Anesthesiology*. 2000;93: 404–408.
102. Nyktari V, Papaioannou A, Volakakis N, Lappa A, Margaritsanaki P, Askitopoulou H. Respiratory resistance during anaesthesia with isoflurane, sevoflurane, and desflurane: a randomized clinical trial. *Br J Anaesth*. 2011;107:454–461.
103. Ng D, Fahimi J, Hern HG. Sevoflurane administration initiated out of the ED for life-threatening status asthmaticus. *Am J Emerg Med*. 2015;33:1110.e3–1110.e6.
104. Volta CA, Alvisi V, Petrini S, et al. The effect of volatile anesthetics on respiratory system resistance in patients with chronic obstructive pulmonary disease. *Anesth Analg*. 2005;100: 348–353.
105. Ledowski T, Manopas A, Lauer S. Bronchial mucus transport velocity in patients receiving desflurane and fentanyl vs. sevoflurane and fentanyl. *Eur J Anaesthesiol*. 2008;25:752–755.
106. Reiz S. Nitrous oxide augments the systemic and coronary haemodynamic effects of isoflurane in patients with ischaemic heart disease. *Acta Anaesthesiol Scand*. 1983;27:464–469.
107. Pagel PS, Fu JL, Damask MC, et al. Desflurane and isoflurane produce similar alterations in systemic and pulmonary hemodynamics and arterial oxygenation in patients undergoing one-lung ventilation during thoracotomy. *Anesth Analg*. 1998;87:800–807.
108. Kurahashi K, Maruta H. The effect of sevoflurane and isoflurane on the neuromuscular block produced by vecuronium continuous infusion. *Anesth Analg*. 1996;82:942–947.
109. Wulf H, Kahl M, Ledowski T. Augmentation of the neuromuscular blocking effects of cisatracurium during desflurane, sevoflurane, isoflurane or total i.v. anaesthesia. *Br J Anaesth*. 1998; 80:308–1302.
110. Nitahara K, Sugi Y, Higa K, Shono S, Hamada T. Neuromuscular effects of sevoflurane in myasthenia gravis patients. *Br J Anaesth*. 2007;98:337–341.
111. Bock M, Klippel K, Nitsche B, Bach A, Martin E, Motsch J. Rocuronium potency and recovery characteristics during steady-state desflurane, sevoflurane, isoflurane or propofol anaesthesia. *Br J Anaesth*. 2000;84:43–47.
112. Paul M, Fokt RM, Kindler CH, Dipp NC, Yost CS. Characterization of the interactions between volatile anesthetics and neuromuscular blockers at the muscle nicotinic acetylcholine receptor. *Anesth Analg*. 2002;95:362–367.
113. Wright PM, Hart P, Lau M, et al. The magnitude and time course of vecuronium potentiation by desflurane versus isoflurane. *Anesthesiology*. 1995;82:404–411.
114. Rosenberg H, Pollock N, Schiemann A, Bulger T, Stowell K. Malignant hyperthermia: a review. *Orphanet J Rare Dis*. 2015;10:93.
115. Wappler F. Anesthesia for patients with a history of malignant hyperthermia. *Curr Opin Anaesthesiol*. 2010;23:417–422.
116. Carlomagno M, Esposito C, Marra A, Vargas M, Corcione A. Xenon anaesthesia in a patient with susceptibility to malignant hyperthermia: a case report. *Eur J Anaesthesiol*. 2016;33:147–150.
117. Yildiz K, Dogru K, Dalgic H, et al. Inhibitory effects of desflurane and sevoflurane on oxytocin-induced contractions of isolated pregnant human myometrium. *Acta Anaesthesiol Scand*. 2005;49:1355–1359.
118. Abboud TK, Zhu J, Richardson M, Peres da Silva E, Donovan M. Desflurane: a new volatile anesthetic for cesarean section: maternal and neonatal effects. *Acta Anaesthesiol Scand*. 1995;39:723–726.
119. Krause T, Scholz J, Jansen L, et al. Sevoflurane anaesthesia does not induce the formation of sister chromatid exchanges in peripheral blood lymphocytes of children. *Br J Anaesth*. 2003;90:233–235.
120. Akin A, Ugur F, Ozkul Y, Esmaoglu A, Gunes I, Ergul H. Desflurane anaesthesia increases sister chromatid exchanges in human lymphocytes. *Acta Anaesthesiol Scand*. 2005;49: 1559–1561.
121. Eroglu A, Celep F, Erciyes N. A comparison of sister chromatid exchanges in lymphocytes of anesthesiologists to nonanesthesiologists in the same hospital. *Anesth Analg*. 2006;102: 1573–1577.
122. Wiesner G, Schiewe-Langgartner F, Lindner R, Gruber M. Increased formation of sister chromatid exchanges, but not of micronuclei, in anaesthetists exposed to low levels of sevoflurane. *Anaesthesia*. 2008;63:861–864.
123. Mazze RI, Wilson AI, Rice SA, Baden JM. Fetal development in mice exposed to isoflurane. *Teratology*. 1985;32:339–345.
124. Mazze RI, Källén B. Reproductive outcome after anesthesia and operation during pregnancy: a registry study of 5405 cases. *Am J Obstet Gynecol*. 1989;161:1178–1185.
125. Mazze RI, Wilson AI, Rice SA, Baden JM. Reproduction and fetal development in rats exposed to nitrous oxide. *Teratology*. 1984;30:259–265.
126. Lane GA, Nahrwold ML, Tait AR, Taylor-Busch M, Cohen PJ, Beaudoin AR. Anesthetics as teratogens: nitrous oxide is fetotoxic, xenon is not. *Science*. 1980;210:899–901.
127. McGregor DG. Occupational exposure to trace concentrations of waste anesthetic gases. *Mayo Clin Proc*. 2000;75:273–277.
128. Abboud TK, Nagappala S, Murakawa K, et al. Comparison of the effects of general and regional anesthesia for cesarean section on neonatal neurologic and adaptive capacity scores. *Anesth Analg*. 1985;64:996–1000.
129. Warren TM, Datta S, Ostheimer GW, Naulty JS, Weiss JB, Morrison JA. Comparison of the maternal and neonatal effects of halothane, enflurane, and isoflurane for cesarean delivery. *Anesth Analg*. 1983;62:516–520.
130. Liang G, Ward C, Peng J, Zhao Y, Huang B, Wei H. Isoflurane causes greater neurodegeneration than an equivalent exposure of sevoflurane in the developing brain of neonatal mice. *Anesthesiology*. 2010;112:1325–1334.
131. Amrock LG, Starner ML, Murphy KL, Baxter MG. Long-term effects of single or multiple neonatal sevoflurane exposures on rat hippocampal ultrastructure. *Anesthesiology*. 2015;122:87–95.
132. Gano D, Andersen SK, Glass HC, et al. Impaired cognitive performance in premature newborns with two or more surgeries prior to term-equivalent age. *Pediatr Res*. 2015;78:323–329.
133. Wilder RT, Flick RP, Sprung J, et al. Early exposure to anesthesia and learning disabilities in a population-based birth cohort. *Anesthesiology*. 2009;110:796–804.
134. Davidson AJ, Disma NM de Graaff JC, et al; GAS consortium. Neurodevelopmental outcome at 2 years of age after general anaesthesia and awake-regional anaesthesia in infancy (GS): an international multicentre, randomized controlled trial. *Lancet*. 2016;387:239–250.
135. Sun LS, Li G, Miller TLK, et al. Association between a single general anesthesia exposure before age 36 months and neurocognitive outcomes in later childhood. *JAMA* 2016;315:2312–2320.
136. McCann ME, de Graff JC, Dorris L, et al; GAS consortium. Neurodevelopmental outcome at 5 years of age after general anaesthesia or awake-regional anaesthesia in infancy (GAS): an international, multicentre, randomized, controlled equivalence trial. *Lancet* 2019;393:664–677.
137. Ing C, Jackson WM, Zaccariello MJ, et al. Prospectively assessed neurodevelopmental outcomes in studies of anaesthetic neurotoxicity in children: a systematic review and meta-analysis. *Brit J Anaesth*. 2021;126:433–444.
138. Ruzicka JA, Hidalgo JC, Tinker JH, Baker MT. Inhibition of volatile sevoflurane degradation product formation in an anesthesia circuit by a reduction in soda lime temperature. *Anesthesiology*. 1994;81:238–244.
139. Fang ZX, Kandel L, Laster MJ, Ionescu P, Eger EI. Factors affecting production of compound A from the interaction of sevoflurane with Baralyme and soda lime. *Anesth Analg*. 1996;82:775–781.
140. Frink EJ Jr, Malan TP, Morgan SE, Brown EA, Malcomson M, Brown BR Jr. Quantification of the degradation products of sevoflurane in two CO_2 absorbents during low-flow anesthesia in surgical patients. *Anesthesiology*. 1992;77:1064–1069.
141. Ebert TJ, Arain SR. Renal responses to low-flow desflurane, sevoflurane, and propofol in patients. *Anesthesiology*. 2000;93:1401–1406.
142. Kharasch ED, Frink EJ Jr, Zager R, Bowdle TA, Artru A, Nogami WM. Assessment of low-flow sevoflurane and isoflurane effects on renal function using sensitive markers of tubular toxicity. *Anesthesiology*. 1997;86:1238–1253.
143. Bito H, Ikeuchi Y, Ikeda K. Effects of low-flow sevoflurane anesthesia on renal function: comparison with high-flow sevoflurane anesthesia and low-flow isoflurane anesthesia. *Anesthesiology*. 1997;86:1231–1237.
144. Bito H, Ikeda K. Closed-circuit anesthesia with sevoflurane in humans. Effects on renal and hepatic function and concentrations of breakdown products with soda lime in the circuit. *Anesthesiology*. 1994;80:71–76.
145. Eger EI 2nd, Koblin DD, Bowland T, et al. Nephrotoxicity of sevoflurane versus desflurane anesthesia in volunteers. *Anesth Analg*. 1997;84:160–168.
146. Ebert TJ, Messana LD, Uhrich TD, Staacke TS. Absence of renal and hepatic toxicity after four hours of 1.25 minimum alveolar concentration sevoflurane anesthesia in volunteers. *Anesth Analg*. 1998;86:662–667.
147. Eger EI 2nd, Gong D, Koblin DD, et al. Dose-related biochemical markers of renal injury after sevoflurane versus desflurane anesthesia in volunteers. *Anesth Analg*. 1997;85:1154–1163.
148. Ebert TJ, Frink EJ Jr, Kharasch ED. Absence of biochemical evidence for renal and hepatic dysfunction after 8 hours of 1.25 minimum alveolar concentration sevoflurane anesthesia in volunteers. *Anesthesiology*. 1998;88:601–610.
149. Groudine SB, Fragen RJ, Kharasch ED, Eisenman TS, Frink EJ, McConnell S. Comparison of renal function following anesthesia with low-flow sevoflurane and isoflurane. *J Clin Anesth*. 1999;11:201–207.

150. Bito H, Ikeda K. Renal and hepatic function in surgical patients after low-flow sevoflurane or isoflurane anesthesia. *Anesth Analg*. 1996;82:173-176.
151. Conzen PF, Kharasch ED, Czerner SFA, et al. Low-flow sevoflurane compared with low-flow isoflurane anesthesia in patients with stable renal insufficiency. *Anesthesiology*. 2002;97:578–584.
152. Litz RJ, Hübler M, Lorenz W, Meier VK, Albrecht DM. Renal responses to desflurane and isoflurane in patients with renal insufficiency. *Anesthesiology*. 2002;97:1133–1136.
153. Spracklin D, Kharasch ED. Evidence for the metabolism of fluoromethyl 2,2-difluoro-1-(trifluoromethyl)vinyl ether (compound A), a sevoflurane degradation product, by cysteine conjugate beta-lyase. *Chem Res Toxicol*. 1996;9:696–702.
154. Holak EJ, Mei DA, Dunning MB 3rd, et al. Carbon monoxide production from sevoflurane breakdown: modeling of exposures under clinical conditions. *Anesth Analg*. 2003;96:757–764.
155. Baxter PJ, Garton K, Kharasch ED. Mechanistic aspects of carbon monoxide formation from volatile anesthetics. *Anesthesiology*. 1998;89:929–941.
156. Fang ZX, Eger EI 2nd, Laster MJ, Chortkoff BS, Kandel L, Ionescu P. Carbon monoxide production from degradation of desflurane, enflurane, isoflurane, halothane, and sevoflurane by soda lime and Baralyme. *Anesth Analg*. 1995;80:1187–1193.
157. Berry PD, Sessler DI, Larson MD. Severe carbon monoxide poisoning during desflurane anesthesia. *Anesthesiology*. 1999;90:613–616.
158. Woehlck HJ, Dunning M 3rd, Connolly LA. Reduction in the incidence of carbon monoxide exposures in humans undergoing general anesthesia. *Anesthesiology*. 1997;87:228–234.
159. Woehlck HJ, Dunning M 3rd, Raza T, Ruiz F, Bolla B, Zink W. Physical factors affecting the production of carbon monoxide from anesthetic breakdown. *Anesthesiology*. 2001;94:453–456.
160. Castro BA, Freedman LA, Craig WL, Lynch C 3rd. Explosion within an anesthesia machine: Baralyme, high fresh gas flows and sevoflurane concentration. *Anesthesiology*. 2004;101:537–539.
161. Wu J, Previte JP, Adler E, Myers T, Ball J, Gunter JB. Spontaneous ignition, explosion, and fire with sevoflurane and barium hydroxide lime. *Anesthesiology*. 2004;101:534–537.
162. Fatheree RS, Leighton BL. Acute respiratory distress syndrome after an exothermic Baralyme-sevoflurane reaction. *Anesthesiology*. 2004;101:531–533.
163. Kharasch ED. Putting the brakes on anesthetic breakdown. *Anesthesiology*. 1999;91:1192–1194.
164. Frink EJ Jr, Malan TP Jr, Isner RJ, Brown EA, Morgan SE, Brown BR Jr. Renal concentrating function with prolonged sevoflurane or enflurane anesthesia in volunteers. *Anesthesiology*. 1994;80:1019–1025.
165. Mazze RI. The safety of sevoflurane in humans. *Anesthesiology*. 1992;77:1062–1063.
166. Kharasch ED, Hankins DC, Thummel KE. Human kidney methoxyflurane and sevoflurane metabolism. Intrarenal fluoride production as a possible mechanism of methoxyflurane nephrotoxicity. *Anesthesiology*. 1995;82:689–699.
167. Sherman J, Le C, Lamers V, Eckelman M. Life cycle greenhouse gas emissions of anesthetic drugs. *Anesth Analg*. 2012;114:1086–1090.
168. McGain F, Muret J, Lawson C, Sherman JD. Environmental sustainability in anaesthesia and critical care. *Br J Anaesth*. 2020;125:680–692.
169. Varughese S, Ahmed R. Environmental and occupational considerations of anesthesia: a narrative review and update. *Anesth Analg*. 2021;133:826–835.
170. Mostad D, Klepstad P, Follestad T, Pleym H. Desflurane consumption with automated vapour control systems in two different anaesthesia machines. A randomized controlled study. *Acta Anaesthesiol Scand*. 2021;65:895–901.
171. Kennedy RR, French RA, Vesto G, Hanrahan J, Page J. The effect of fresh gas flow during induction of anaesthesia on sevoflurane usage: a quality improvement study. *Anaesthesia*. 2019;74:875–882.
172. Zuegge KL, Bunsen SK, Volz LM, et al. Provider education and vaporizer labeling lead to reduced anesthetic agent purchasing with cost savings and reduced greenhouse gas emissions. *Anesth Analg*. 2019;128:e97–e99.
173. Sulbaek Andersen MP, Nielsen OJ, Karpichev B, Wallington TJ, Sander SP. Atmospheric chemistry of isoflurane, desflurane, and sevoflurane: kinetics and mechanisms of reactions with chlorine atoms and OH radicals and global warming potentials. *J Phys Chem A*. 2012;116:5806–5820.
174. Ravishankara AR, Daniel JS, Portmann RW. Nitrous Oxide (N2O): the dominant ozone-depleting substance emitted in the 21st century. *Science*. 2009;326:123–125.
175. American Society of Anesthesiologists Task Force on Environmental Sustainability Committee on Equipment and Facilities. Greening the operating room and perioperative arena: environmental sustainability for anesthesia practice. 2017. Accessed May 11, 2022. https://www.asahq.org/about-asa/governance-and-committees/asa-committees/environmental-sustainability/greening-the-operating-room
176. Thwaites A, Edmends S, Smith I. Inhalation induction with sevoflurane: a double-blind comparison with propofol. *Br J Anaesth*. 1997;78:356–361.
177. Muzi M, Colinco MD, Robinson BJ, Ebert TJ. The effects of premedication on inhaled induction of anesthesia with sevoflurane. *Anesth Analg*. 1997;85:1143–1148.
178. Muzi M, Robinson BJ, Ebert TJ, O'Brien TJ. Induction of anesthesia and tracheal intubation with sevoflurane in adults. *Anesthesiology*. 1996;85:536–543.
179. Mostafa SM, Atherton AM. Sevoflurane for difficult tracheal intubation. *Br J Anaesth*. 1997;79:392–393.

19 Intravenous Anesthetics

RAMON E. ABOLA • SOFIA GERALEMOU • MARTIN SZAFRAN • TONG JOO (TJ) GAN

KEY POINTS

1 The ideal intravenous anesthetic would cause hypnosis and amnesia with a rapid onset, minimal cardiovascular and respiratory effects, and rapid metabolism.

2 Context-sensitive half-time (i.e., half-life) is defined as the time to achieve a 50% reduction in concentration after stopping a continuous infusion. Context-sensitive half-time demonstrates the influence of the distributive process in governing drug disposition.

3 The mechanism by which the unconscious state is attained by propofol is complicated, but primarily occurs via enhancement of gamma-aminobutyric acid (GABA) inhibitory pathways.

4 The rapid and smooth induction and emergence from anesthesia helped transform propofol into an intravenous sedative–hypnotic that is a viable alternative to standard inhalational agents and other intravenous drugs.

5 Etomidate is a hemodynamically stable induction medication with a relatively large safety margin. Adrenocortical suppression is a recognized adverse effect of etomidate.

6 Ketamine causes "dissociative anesthesia" acting through the N-methyl-D-aspartate (NMDA) receptor, and is associated with nystagmus, significant analgesia, and unconsciousness.

7 Dexmedetomidine, an alpha-2 agonist, has been used for intensive care unit (ICU) sedation in mechanically ventilated patients, procedural sedation, and as an adjunct to general anesthesia. Dexmedetomidine is unique as a sedative in that it has limited respiratory depressant effects.

8 Benzodiazepines are frequently used to produce several clinically desirable effects: anxiolysis, anterograde amnesia, sedation, and hypnosis.

9 The mechanism of action of barbiturates involves cortical and brainstem GABA inhibitory pathways, leading to loss of consciousness, as well as respiratory and cardiovascular depression.

10 New drugs are being developed in an effort to achieve the ideal intravenous anesthetic with a short duration of action, a short context-sensitive half-time that allows for infusion administration, and minimal adverse effects.

Pharmacokinetics: General Principles for Intravenous Anesthetics

Traditionally, intravenous anesthetics have been utilized for the induction of anesthesia. Thiopental was introduced into clinical practice in 1934 and was the "gold standard" for intravenous anesthetics for 50 years. Thiopental had a rapid, smooth onset of sedative and hypnotic effects, predictable pharmacokinetics, and a rapid and smooth emergence. However, thiopental has a long context-sensitive half-time that made it less ideal for use as an infusion. A review article from 1989 stated that the use of intravenous anesthetics for maintenance was unpopular because bolus administration resulted in swings in hemodynamics and anesthetic level.[1] The introductions of anesthetics with shorter durations (midazolam, propofol, remifentanil) and the development of variable rate infusion pumps allowed for routine use of intravenous anesthetics for maintenance. Combination of these modalities with a depth of anesthesia monitor has been utilized to create a closed-loop automated anesthesia delivery system. Intravenous anesthetics are now a key component of modern anesthesia practice.

Table 19-1 Properties of the Ideal Intravenous Anesthetic Agent

Pharmacodynamic/Pharmacokinetic Properties
Hypnosis and amnesia
Rapid onset (time of one arm-brain circulation)
Rapid metabolism to inactive metabolites
Minimal cardiovascular and respiratory depression
No histamine release or hypersensitivity reactions
Nontoxic, nonmutagenic, noncarcinogenic
No untoward neurological effects, such as seizures, myoclonus, antanalgesia, neurotoxicity
Other beneficial effects: analgesia, antiemetic, neuroprotection, cardioprotection
Pharmacokinetic-based models to guide accurate dosing
Ability to continuously monitor delivery
Physiochemical Properties
Water-soluble
Stable formulation, nonpyrogenic
Nonirritating: painless on intravenous injection
Small volume needed for induction
Inexpensive to prepare and formulate
Antimicrobial preparation

1 No single anesthetic agent is perfect. The characteristics of the ideal intravenous anesthetic agent were described by Hemmings and are outlined in Table 19-1.[2] The ideal intravenous anesthetic would cause hypnosis and amnesia with a rapid onset (time of one arm–brain circulation), minimal cardiovascular and respiratory effects, and rapid metabolism. Propofol has become the new "gold standard" in anesthesia practice with a rapid onset, rapid recovery after bolus administration from redistribution, and its utility as a continuous infusion. Propofol is unique with patients awake and oriented after administration with lack of "hangover" effect that was associated with older anesthetics. Added benefits of propofol include its antiemetic properties. Propofol has been used in multiple different settings: (1) induction of anesthesia, (2) maintenance of anesthesia, either with volatile anesthetics or as a sole anesthetic agent in total intravenous anesthesia (TIVA), and (3) monitored anesthesia care (MAC) sedation for minor procedures. Propofol is not without its problems. It causes hypotension, respiratory depression, pain with injection, and has a prolonged duration with continuous infusion. Prolonged infusion can cause propofol infusion syndrome (PRIS) (association with doses of 4 mg/kg/h for greater than 48 hours).[3] Future medications will likely improve on our currently available anesthetics.

Intravenous anesthetics have a rapid onset after administration. They rapidly distribute to higher perfused and vessel-rich tissues. Their lipophilicity allows for rapid crossing of the blood–brain barrier. The slight delay between target blood concentration and effect organ (brain) response is known as hysteresis. This delay occurs because of differences between peak plasma concentration and peak drug concentration in the brain. The action of a single bolus injection is terminated by redistribution of the anesthetic to lean tissues such as muscle. This property of intravenous anesthetics is key to understanding their pharmacokinetics in relation to continuous infusion and maintenance. An initial bolus or loading dose of an anesthetic establishes the desired blood concentration of the drug. Redistribution of intravenous anesthetics to nonactive tissues accounts for part of their initial clearance; however, this becomes less important as those tissues equilibrate with the blood. Therefore, the rate of infusion of an intravenous anesthetic for maintenance of anesthesia decreases over the duration of an infusion to maintain the desired blood concentration.

An understanding of the pharmacokinetics of intravenous anesthetics is important to their administration. Following a bolus of an intravenous drug, the plasma concentration over time resembles the curve in Figure 19-1. This graph shows the blood concentration of an intravenous anesthetic (i.e., propofol) after bolus injection. The curve can be explained by a triexponential equation. Essentially, there are three phases that occur after a bolus injection of propofol.[4] The first phase is a rapid distribution

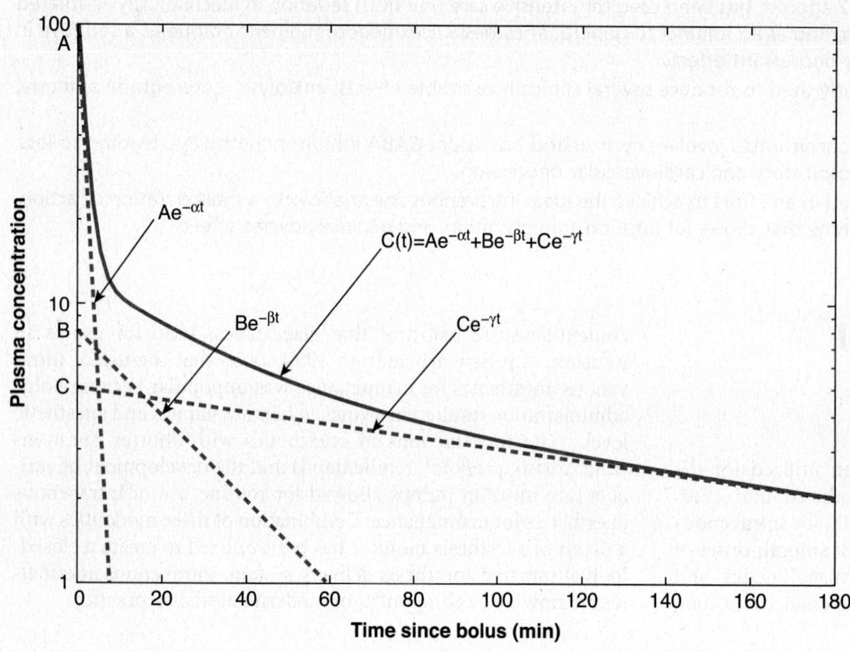

Figure 19-1 Plasma concentration after bolus injection of an intravenous anesthetic. Decreases in blood concentration occur in three components corresponding to rapid distribution (*A*), slow distribution (*B*), and elimination (*C*). The individual lines associated with each component term are also shown. The triexponential curve represents the algebraic sum of the individual exponential functions. The intercepts of the curve peel are shown as A, B, and C. These are present as coefficients of the triexponential equation. (Adapted with permission from Struys MMRF, De Smet T, Glen JB, et al. The history of target-controlled infusion. *Anesth Analg*. 2016;122(1):56–69.)

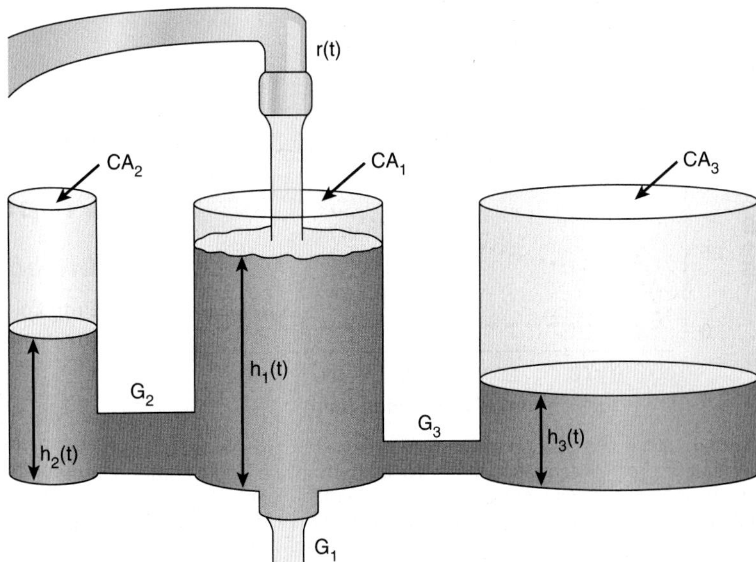

Figure 19-2 Hydraulic depiction of a three-compartment model. r(t) represented a drug infusion via a syringe pump adding drug to the blood. CA1 represents the central compartment (blood). Administered medication will distribute to the peripheral compartments (CA2, CA3) which affects the drug's concentration in the blood. Ultimately the drug is eliminated by the body depicted as G1. (Reprinted with permission from Hughes MA, Glass PS, Jacobs JR. Context-sensitive half time in multicompartment pharmacokinetic models for intravenous anesthetic drugs. *Anesthesiology*. 1992;76:334–341.)

phase; propofol rapidly distributes from the plasma to peripheral tissues. The second phase is a slow distribution phase; propofol continues to distribute to other tissues concurrent with return of the drug to the plasma from the rapid distribution tissue. The last phase is the terminal phase, or elimination phase, where propofol is removed from the body.

The three-compartment model is used to describe the behavior of an intravenous anesthetic. Figure 19-2 depicts a hydraulic version of the three-compartment model. We will use this model to understand the behavior of a propofol infusion. When propofol is first administered, it fills the central compartment (blood, CA1). The propofol then distributes to peripheral compartments (CA2, CA3), one rapid and the other slow. The distribution of drug to the peripheral compartments and the elimination of propofol (G1) can be matched with an appropriate infusion rate (r[T]) that would then allow for maintaining a desired target blood concentration. However, over time, the propofol will begin to accumulate in the peripheral compartments. Less propofol is removed from central circulation by redistribution to these peripheral compartments. With prolonged infusion, the contributions of propofol from the peripheral compartments become greater, thus requiring less drug to be infused to maintain target blood concentration. This also leads to a longer time to awakening, and to the concept of context-sensitive half-time.

A concept most are familiar with is elimination half-time ($t_{1/2}$). It is the time it takes for the plasma concentration of a drug to decrease to 50% of its original concentration. This concept works well to describe a one-compartment model for a drug distributed only to the blood, or if the drug is administered only once. In contrast, pharmacokinetic modeling that describes intravenous anesthetics administered by infusion needs to account for multiple compartments, phases of distribution, and elimination.

Context-sensitive half-time is defined as the time to achieve 2
a 50% reduction in concentration after stopping a continuous infusion. Context-sensitive half-time demonstrates the influence of the distributive process in governing drug disposition. This refers to both the transfer of drug out of the plasma into peripheral compartments and the reverse process when there is a net transfer of drug back to the central compartment. Figure 19-3 shows the context-sensitive half-time of several anesthetics drugs.

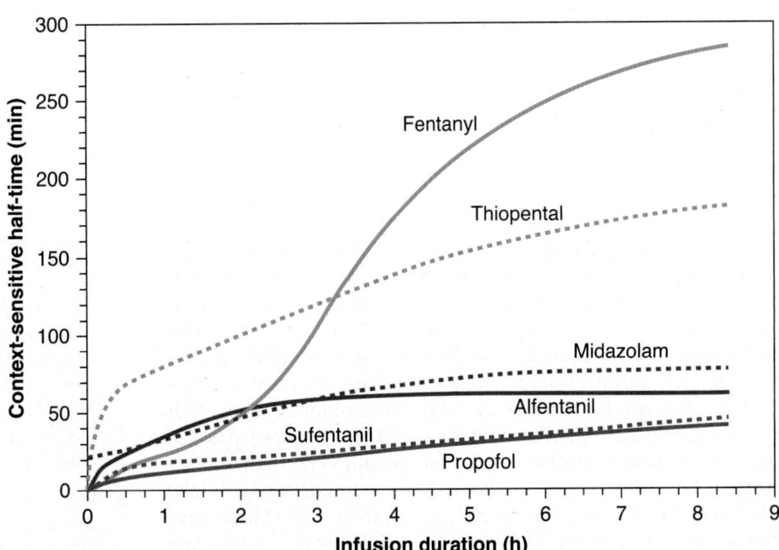

Figure 19-3 Context-sensitive half-time of intravenous anesthetics. (Reprinted with permission from Hughes MA, Glass PS, Jacobs JR. Context-sensitive half time in multicompartment pharmacokinetic models for intravenous anesthetic drugs. *Anesthesiology*. 1992;76:334–341.)

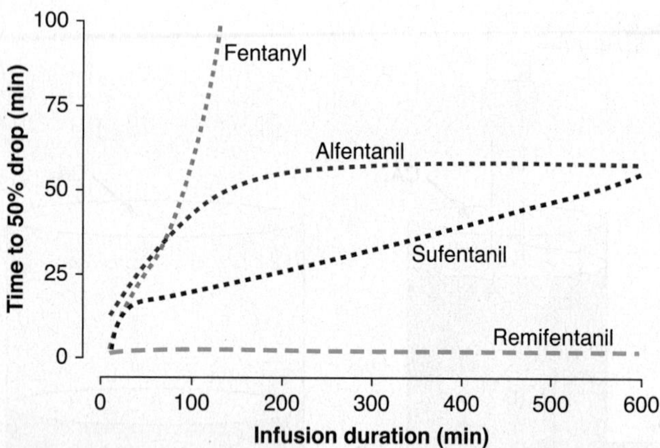

Figure 19-4 A simulation of the time necessary to achieve a 50% decrease in drug concentration in the blood after variable-length intravenous infusions of remifentanil, fentanyl, alfentanil, and sufentanil. Note that the context-sensitive half-time for remifentanil is independent of infusion duration. (Reprinted with permission from Egan TD, Lemmens HJM, Fiset P, et al. The pharmacokinetics of the new short-acting opioid remifentanil (GI87084B) in healthy adult male volunteers. *Anesthesiology*. 1993;79:881–892.)

In comparison to thiopental, propofol has a much lower context-sensitive half-time. Although, the elimination of propofol is prolonged with longer infusions, it is not to the same magnitude as with thiopental. It is the low context-sensitive half-time that allows for propofol to be used as a continuous infusion. Thiopental by comparison has a much longer context-sensitive half-time and is a poor choice to be used for continuous infusion.

The medication that best illustrates the concept of context-sensitive half-time is remifentanil. Remifentanil is an ultrashort opioid agonist. It has an ester component in its chemical structure and is eliminated rapidly because of metabolism by nonspecific plasma esterases. Because of these properties, remifentanil has a context-sensitive half-time that is essentially independent of the duration of the infusion (Fig. 19-4). The brevity of action allows for easy titration and optimal intraoperative analgesia with a quick recovery time. Elimination time of remifentanil is the same for a 1-hour infusion as it is for a 10-hour infusion (3 minutes for both). The future may yield intravenous anesthetics with similar pharmacokinetic properties to remifentanil that may allow for the so-called "anesthesia off" switch that our surgical colleagues believe we possess.

These pharmacokinetic principles of intravenous anesthesia are incorporated into target-controlled infusion (TCI) devices (see Video 11-2). The anesthesiologist sets the target blood or brain concentration on a TCI. This idea is intuitive to an anesthesiologist as this is how we administer inhaled anesthetics because end-tidal concentrations of inhaled anesthetics reflect brain concentration after equilibrium. TCI devices incorporate patient factors (age, sex, height, weight), the amount of drug that has been delivered, and the amount of drug that has accumulated in the tissues to determine the appropriate infusion rate.[4] The appropriate infusion rate is calculated using these pharmacokinetic models of intravenous anesthetics. The accuracy of these devices relies on the accuracy of the pharmacokinetic model that is used. Because of pharmacokinetic variability between patents, the actual plasma concentration may be different than the set target concentration. The Food and Drug Administration (FDA) cited this lack of precision as an unacceptable risk. These concerns were raised despite extensive use of TCI systems outside the United States with a good safety record.[5]

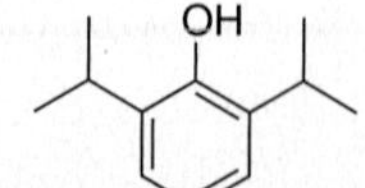

Figure 19-5 Propofol. 2,6-diisopropylphenol.

Propofol

Introduction

Propofol (2,6-diisopropylphenol) has become one of the most frequently used intravenous anesthetics on the market today. Its pharmacokinetic profile presents a desirable rapid onset, a predictable context-sensitive half-time, and a rapid emergence from anesthesia. In addition, a favorable side-effect profile and its antiemetic property allow for a wide spectrum of uses, including induction and maintenance of general anesthesia, intensive care unit (ICU) sedation, and as a sedative–hypnotic in a variety of outpatient procedures (Fig. 19-5, Table 19-2).

Derivation of the appropriate propofol formulation has always centered around the challenge of managing its lipophilicity and relative insolubility in aqueous solutions. After its introduction in the 1970s in Cremphor EL formulation,[6] it was rapidly withdrawn from the market due to concern for anaphylactic reactions.[7] Nearly a decade later, it was reintroduced in its more current form consisting of 1% propofol, 10% soybean oil, 2.25% glycerol, and 1.2% egg phospholipid emulsifier. In the 1990s,

Table 19-2 Propofol

Key Pharmacology	Key Clinical Uses
Primary mechanism: GABA-A receptor agonist	General anesthesia induction and maintenance
Predictable context-sensitive half-time across various comorbidities	Commonly used for TIVA
CNS depressant, neuroprotective, anticonvulsant, decreases CMRO2, CBF, and ICP	Conscious and deep sedation, including out-of-operative-room settings
Can be used for EEG burst suppression	Intensive care unit sedation
Cardiovascular: Significant decreases in systemic vascular resistance, stroke volume, and cardiac output	Postoperative nausea and vomiting prophylaxis
Pulmonary: Respiratory depressant and potent bronchodilator	Safe for use in patients with malignant hyperthermia
Addiction potential: May elicit feelings of well-being or euphoria during emergence	
Side effects: Associated pain with injection, propofol infusion syndrome	

CBF, cerebral blood flow; CMRO2, cerebral metabolic oxygen consumption rate; CNS, central nervous system; EEG, electroencephalogram; GABA-A, gamma-aminobutyric acid-A; ICP, intracranial pressure; TIVA, total intravenous anesthesia.

ethylenediamenetetraacetic acid (EDTA) was added to this formulation to deter microbial growth within the emulsion. The lipid emulsion comes in a familiar milky white consistency, and can be stored at room temperature without any significant degradation.

Pharmacokinetics

Propofol is primarily metabolized by the liver, and subsequently, its inactive and water-soluble metabolites are excreted by the kidneys. A small amount of unmetabolized propofol is excreted in both urine and feces, but that is considered negligible (less than 3%). Despite the primary mechanism of metabolism, liver and kidney disease have not been noted to alter pharmacokinetics of propofol significantly. Also, the clearance rate for propofol has been reported to be 20 to 30 mL/kg/min (approximately 1.5 L/min), exceeding average hepatic blood flow (15 mL/kg/min), suggesting that other forms of metabolism and elimination play a significant role. The most common extrahepatic sites of metabolism are the kidneys and lungs, both responsible for up to 30% of the common propofol metabolites, explaining why pharmacokinetics of propofol are relatively consistent across patient populations with different comorbid states.

To truly understand the kinetic properties of propofol, evaluation of multicompartment models is crucial. The distribution of propofol after an initial bolus dose has been described in a variety of kinetic models. In a simple two-compartment model, the blood concentration of propofol drops rapidly with the initial distribution half-life of propofol estimated to be 2 to 4 minutes. In a three-compartment model, propofol has the initial distribution half-life estimated to be 1 to 8 minutes and the secondary slow distribution half-life at 30 to 70 minutes. Elimination half-lives for both models are significantly slower, reported in a wider range of 2 to 24 hours. As noted in Figure 19-3, infusion duration of up to 8 hours maintains a reliable context-sensitive half-life of 40 minutes or less, allowing clinicians to take advantage of the predictable kinetic properties that yield a rapid recovery after initial bolus administration and continuous infusion.

Pharmacodynamics

3

The mechanism by which the unconscious state is attained by induction doses of propofol is complicated and not fully understood. Primarily, it occurs via enhancement of gamma-aminobutyric acid-A (GABA-A) inhibitory pathways.[7] Other neuroreceptors have been linked to propofol activity, including alpha-adrenergic receptors and N-methyl-D-aspartate (NMDA) receptors. Alteration of the central cholinergic transmission by propofol may also play a role in achieving a state of unconsciousness.[8] The neurotransmission target is the vast array of interneurons involved within the cerebral cortex, brain stem, and thalamus that ultimately play a critical role in arousal.[9,10]

Initial low doses of propofol produce sedation, but at increased doses, a state of paradoxical excitation may occur, where a patient is disinhibited, has unpredictable movement, broken speech, and is not readily arousable.[11] A further increase in dose of propofol leads to loss of consciousness, apnea, relative relaxation of muscles, loss of brainstem reflexes, and subsequently necessitates airway support (Fig. 19-6).

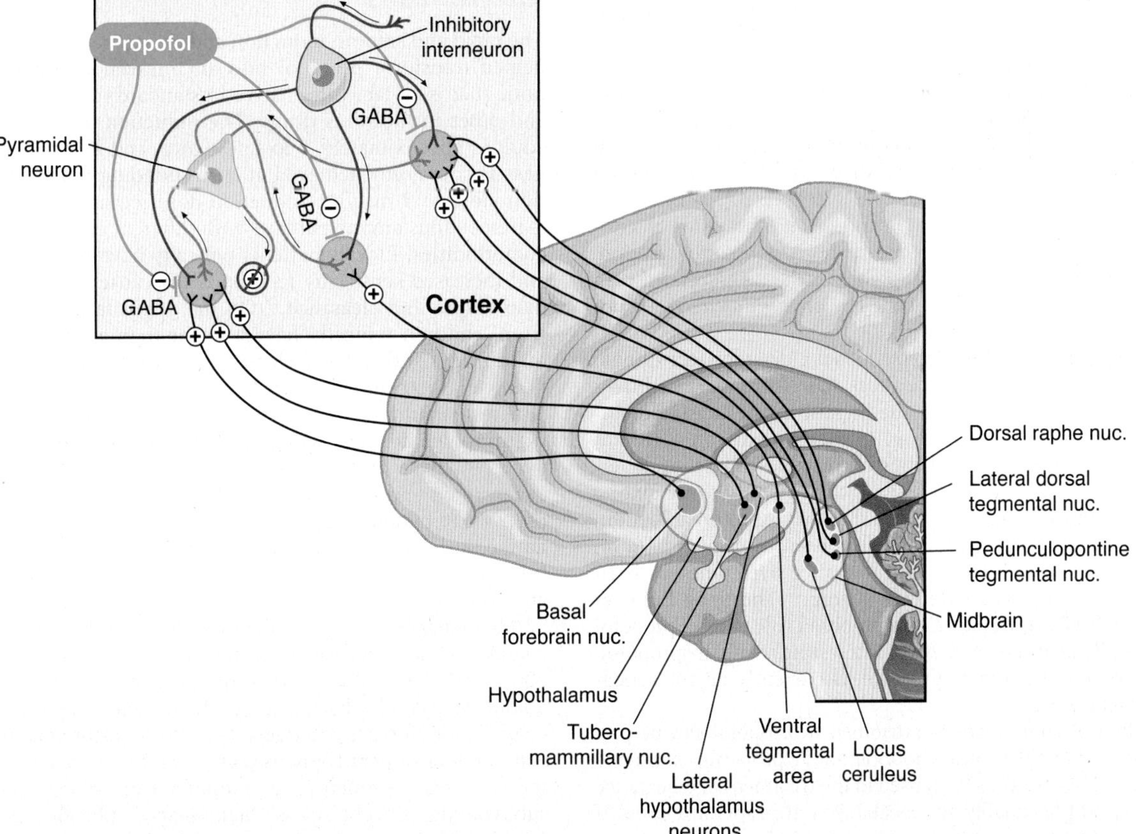

Figure 19-6 Propofol's proposed mechanism of action in the central nervous system. Ascending arousal pathways arise from both the thalamus and the midbrain to send excitatory inputs to a pyramidal neuron (*orange*). A GABAergic inhibitory interneuron (*purple*) synapses onto this pyramidal neuron. Propofol binds postsynaptically and enhances GABAergic inhibition. Unconsciousness occurs as this enhanced GABAergic inhibition counteracts ascending arousal inputs to the pyramidal neuron and decreases excitatory activity.

Central Nervous System Effects

Similar to other intravenous anesthetics, the changes in electroencephalogram (EEG) pattern with propofol are dependent on the depth of anesthesia achieved. At lower sedative doses, a characteristic increase in beta-wave activity is common. After an induction dose, initial stages of general anesthesia are reached, and the EEG pattern often resembles that of deep non-rapid eye movement (non-REM) sleep, with progressively increased low-frequency and high-amplitude activity. This ultimately means that beta-wave activity decreases, with a simultaneous increase in alpha and delta activity.[12] Burst suppression is marked by periods of electrical inactivity with alternating higher frequency activity, and is commonly employed as a neuroprotective measure prior to aneurysm clipping. It can be attained at higher doses of plasma propofol concentration (8 mcg/mL) that are significantly higher than the plasma concentrations needed to reach the initial stages of general anesthesia (3 mcg/mL). A further increase in propofol concentration will lead to an isoelectric EEG pattern.

Neuroprotective effects of propofol are likely multifactorial. It lowers cerebral metabolic oxygen consumption (CMRO2) and decreases intracranial pressure (ICP) primarily by lowering cerebral blood flow (CBF). At the same time, cerebral perfusion pressures (CPP) may also be lowered, thus this benefit is not without limitations and should be employed carefully. Propofol has specific antioxidant properties, and its function as a free radical scavenger has been hypothesized to play a role in preventing injury during neurodegenerative processes such as stroke and trauma.[13] Other protective mechanisms have been hypothesized, including attenuation of excitotoxic glutamate pathways[14] that lower the likelihood of programmed neuronal apoptosis,[15] and its overall anti-inflammatory effects (e.g., decreasing TNF-alpha).[16]

Propofol is generally considered an anticonvulsant. At induction doses that reached burst suppression, EEG epileptiform activity is limited.[17] These results have not been reproduced in patients with epilepsy at lower sedative doses.[18] It has also been used successfully to treat status epilepticus, thus it is rarely the anesthetic of choice during induction of anesthesia for electroconvulsive therapy (ECT) because it shortens seizure duration. Contradictory case reports of propofol anesthetics associated with grand-mal seizures do exist, but the proconvulsant effects are not well elucidated.

Although not traditionally considered a drug for recreational use, the incidence of propofol abuse has likely increased over the last 10 years, and is by far the highest in anesthesia providers with easy access to the drug. In the United States, 18% of academic institutions have reported propofol abuse or diversion in the last decade, with a significant mortality rate among residents.[19] Propofol has properties that may result in addiction; emergence from propofol sedation has been associated with an overall feeling of well-being, and tolerance over time has been documented in the intensive care setting.[20] The Drug Enforcement Agency (DEA) did develop a proposed rule to label propofol as a controlled substance in 2010. Interestingly only fospropofol, a water-soluble prodrug of propofol, is currently on the scheduled substance list.[21]

The loss of consciousness attributed to propofol can be partially reversed by the central cholinomimetic properties of physostigmine.[22] This drug has been used in the treatment of emergence delirium, and presumably, the mechanism of propofol reversal is similar. Activation of central cholinergic pathways leads to an overall state of arousal, and likely alters propofol-induced state of unconsciousness.

Cardiovascular Effects

The hemodynamic effects of propofol are dose dependent and more significant after an induction dose than during a continuous infusion. There is a characteristic drop in systolic and diastolic blood pressure without the expected increase in heart rate. The observed blood pressure drop results from a decrease in cardiac output, stroke volume, and systemic vascular resistance (SVR). Propofol decreases sympathetic activity and leads to indirect arterial vasodilation and venodilation. This effect is enhanced by direct effects on smooth muscle and depressant effects on the myocardium, affecting intracellular calcium balance and influx.[23] The decreased sympathetic tone is also coupled with direct inhibition of the baroreceptor response, leading to a diminished reflex increase in heart rate and a more pronounced hemodynamic effect. Suppression of supraventricular tachycardia has also been reported, and may be a direct result of propofol effects on the heart conduction system.[24]

Respiratory System Effects

The respiratory depressant effects of propofol are also dose dependent. Apnea is relatively common with a higher induction dose, while a typical maintenance dose of propofol results in diminished tidal volumes and increased respiratory rate. There is also a blunted response to hypoxia that may be a direct effect on chemoreceptors, as well as a decreased respiratory response to hypercarbia. Propofol is a potent bronchodilator, primarily because of its direct effects on intracellular calcium homeostasis.

Clinical Uses

The rapid and smooth induction and emergence from anesthesia helped transform propofol into an intravenous sedative–hypnotic that is a viable alternative to standard inhalational agents and other intravenous drugs. The induction dose in a healthy adult is approximately 1 to 2.5 mg/kg, and loss of consciousness is commonly achieved at corresponding blood concentration close to 3 mcg/kg. Induction dose requirement variability is tremendous among patients with different characteristics and comorbidities. Elderly patients typically have prolonged effects and increased sensitivity to propofol because of decreased cardiac output and clearance.[25] On the opposite end of the spectrum, children typically have a larger than average volume of distribution and quicker clearance, resulting in increased propofol requirement on a per-kilogram basis.[26] Morbidly obese patients should have lean body weight used when calculating propofol dosing.[27] Patients with chronic alcohol abuse, as expected, have an increased induction dose requirement. An exaggerated hemodynamic response is likely after induction of propofol in patients with cardiovascular disease. Thus, determination of the appropriate propofol induction dose requires careful assessment of premedication administration, patient history, and comorbidity.

Maintenance of general anesthesia with propofol can commonly be achieved with infusions rate between 100 to 200 mcg/kg/min. TIVA with propofol alone—or together with opioids as part of a balanced anesthetic—has been utilized successfully for all types of surgery. One of the major benefits is prevention of postoperative nausea and vomiting (PONV), although the antiemetic properties of propofol can be replicated with subhypnotic concentrations. Maintenance infusions as low as 10 mcg/kg/min and blood concentration levels as low as 350 ng/mL have been noted to result in significant decreases in PONV.[28] These levels can be reached after recovery from general anesthesia leading only to minimal sedation, but more commonly intraoperative infusion of propofol is employed as a nausea-sparing technique. Propofol can also be used as the anesthetic of choice in patients with malignant hyperthermia (MH), as it is not a trigger for MH. Maintenance infusion of propofol is also commonly employed when inhalational anesthetics are avoided intentionally or are difficult to administer. One example includes surgery with a shared airway such as rigid bronchoscopy during which administration of inhaled anesthetics may be less predictable. Office-based anesthesia is another example where an anesthesia machine may not be readily available.

Sedation with propofol is employed commonly for minor procedures, outpatient surgery, and off-site anesthetics, as well as ICU sedation of mechanically ventilated patients. Typical infusion doses range between 25 to 75 mcg/kg/min. Clinical effects of propofol are dose dependent, and apnea can be avoided with careful titration of infusion rate.

Side Effects

Pain on injection occurs in approximately 60% to 70% patients when propofol is administered in a peripheral vein without additives. Numerous interventions have been tested to minimize this common side effect, with varying levels of success. The most efficacious technique is pretreatment with a local anesthetic such as lidocaine in conjunction with venous occlusion using a tourniquet, or in essence a modified Bier block.[29] Using the antecubital vein as an alternative to smaller peripheral vein sites (e.g., hand) has proved to be the most effective nondrug technique for minimizing pain on injection.[30] Addition of lidocaine to propofol, or pretreatment with lidocaine without the use of a tourniquet has also been shown to be beneficial. Pretreatment with opioids is commonly performed prior to induction with propofol, and it decreases pain on injection. Techniques to lower free propofol concentration, such as diluting the emulsion and changing the lipid solvent have shown some improvement. Pretreatment with other drugs has shown limited success, including nonsteroidal anti-inflammatory drugs (NSAIDs), ketamine, steroids, and beta-blockers.[30]

PRIS is an extremely rare, but potentially deadly side effect of propofol that was first described in children in the 1990s and subsequently in adults after its use for sedation in the ICU setting.[31,32] The key clinical characteristics include unexplained metabolic acidosis, hyperkalemia, hyperlipidemia, rhabdomyolysis, hepatomegaly, renal failure, and most importantly electrocardiogram (ECG) changes, arrhythmias, and progression to cardiac failure. The pathophysiology of PRIS is not well understood, but may involve mitochondrial toxicity and uncoupling of the intracellular respiration chain, although other hypotheses such as inhibition of fatty acid oxidation have been suggested. Development of clinical symptoms of PRIS is likely dependent on both the infusion dose and duration, but even short-duration infusions have been associated with cardiac failure. In 2006, the FDA altered the recommended maximum propofol infusion dose to 4 mg/kg/h, but it is unclear if the recommendations have altered the frequency of PRIS. Currently, the rate of mortality from PRIS is still close to 50%.[33]

Prolonged infusion of propofol, especially in the ICU setting, has yielded several case reports of production of green urine as a side effect. The likely etiology may be due to increased extrahepatic metabolism of propofol, and subsequent excretion of these metabolites in urine. Case reports of single-dose propofol causing green urine do exist, but are less common than the typically reported 6 to 64 hours after infusion has started.[34]

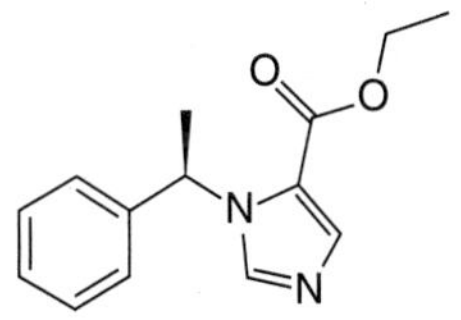

Figure 19-7 Etomidate. Ethyl 3-[(1R)-1-phenylethel)]-imidazole-5-carboxylate.

Etomidate

Introduction

In 1972, etomidate made its way into anesthetic practice as an induction agent (NICV 19-1). It subsequently gained much popularity because of its stable hemodynamic profile. However, it lost some proponents with increased reports of adrenal suppression, pain on injection, thrombophlebitis, PONV, myoclonus, and hiccups. Like most other decisions regarding drug selection, the choice of etomidate involves a risk/benefit analysis. If hemodynamic stability is of paramount importance, one may choose to induce with etomidate and prepare to manage these unwanted side effects (Fig. 19-7, Table 19-3).

Pharmacokinetics

Etomidate is an imidazole derivative (the D [+] enantiomer) and is not stable in neutral pH solutions. The solvents in its formulation, namely propylene glycol, contribute to the venoirritation and phlebitis that occur frequently. Similar to other induction agents, etomidate has a quick onset of action ("vein to brain"), fast resolution of effect secondary to redistribution, and follows the three-compartment kinetic model. Etomidate's use as a continuous infusion is limited by its association with adrenal suppression. Etomidate is metabolized in the liver and excreted predominantly by the kidney (approximately 80%) and in bile (approximately 20%). It is largely protein bound (approximately 75%) and thus affected by pathologic conditions and/or drugs that alter serum proteins. Other pharmacokinetic values of etomidate are found in the Table 19-4.

Pharmacodynamics and Clinical Uses

Etomidate binds as an agonist to the GABA-A receptor and thus has an inhibitory influence on the brain. It is a potent vasoconstrictor that reduces CBF, ICP, and CMRO2. Because of etomidate's minimal effect on the mean arterial pressure (MAP), CPP is either maintained or increased. Unlike benzodiazepines, etomidate can achieve burst suppression with a concomitant decrease in ICP.

Table 19-3 Etomidate

Key Pharmacology	Key Clinical Uses
GABA-A receptor agonist	Hemodynamically stable induction
Hemodynamically stable	Cardiac, trauma, and hypovolemic patients
Adrenocortical suppression	
Postoperative nausea and vomiting	

GABA-A, gamma-aminobutyric acid-A.

Table 19-4 Etomidate Pharmacokinetics

Initial distribution half-life	2.7 min
Redistribution half-life	29 min
Elimination half-life	2.9–5.3 h
Volume of distribution	2.5–4.5 L/kg
Induction dose	0.2–0.3 mg/kg

However, despite its neurodepressant properties at high doses, etomidate is often associated with epileptogenic activity (excitatory spikes) on EEG. This alone may render etomidate an undesirable induction agent for patient's undergoing neurosurgical procedures. The epileptogenic EEG activity is not to be confused with the observable seizure-like, myoclonic movements that often follow an induction dose of etomidate (although, excitatory EEG spikes may also be present during this time). Similar to other maintenance intravenous anesthetics, etomidate will increase the latency intervals measured on somatosensory-evoked potentials (SSEPs). Paradoxically, etomidate increases the amplitude of SSEPs, in contrast to the typical effect of other anesthetics. Etomidate is used frequently for ECT. Similar to barbiturates, etomidate is proconvulsant and lowers the seizure threshold.

5 Etomidate is often touted as a hemodynamically stable induction medication with a relatively large safety margin. Etomidate has a minimal or nonexistent effect on MAP, pulmonary artery (PA) pressure, PA wedge pressure, central venous pressure (CVP), stroke volume, cardiac index, SVR, and pulmonary vascular resistance (PVR).[35] Etomidate is frequently used for induction of anesthesia in cardiac operating rooms. Etomidate is also used for trauma patients who are hemodynamically unstable and are often hypovolemic.

There are mixed data regarding etomidate's effect on the respiratory system. It is widely believed that etomidate depresses airway reflexes less than propofol (unless co-administered with another sedative/analgesic agent). Etomidate also relaxes the smooth musculature of the pulmonary vasculature system to a similar degree as propofol.

Etomidate is a reasonable choice for MAC sedation because of the preservation of airway reflexes.

Side Effects

Adrenocortical suppression may be the most significant adverse effect of etomidate. Etomidate inhibits the activity of the enzyme 11-beta-hydroxylase and prevents the conversion of cholesterol to cortisol. It has been postulated that one dose is sufficient to transiently suppress the adrenocortical axis. Some suggest pretreatment with dexamethasone to curtail this effect.[36] Although many studies conclude that there are no direct adverse outcomes following a bolus of etomidate, even in the septic population,[37] other studies propose the opposite.[38] However, most practitioners, in an effort to limit this possibility, will not administer repeat doses or continuous infusions.

Ketamine

Introduction

6 Phencyclidine (PCP, angel dust) was long ago noted to have remarkable analgesics and anesthetic effects (NICV 19-2). Ketamine was discovered in the search for a phencyclidine derivative with similar anesthetic and analgesics properties, but with fewer psychomimetic effects. Ketamine was described as causing "dissociative anesthesia" in human volunteers in 1965, acting through the NMDA receptor.[39] Key features associated with ketamine administration included marked nystagmus, significant analgesia, and unconsciousness. Emergence from ketamine anesthesia was associated with emergence delirium, hallucinations, and alterations in mood and affect. The use of ketamine as an anesthetic has been limited by its cardiovascular stimulating properties and the disturbing emergence reactions. Interestingly, the NMDA receptor has been found to play a key role in nociception, and low-dose ketamine has an opiate-sparing effect in the management of acute pain. The effects of ketamine related to pain can be best described as antihyperalgesic, antiallodynic, or tolerance protective.[40] More recently, ketamine has gained interest in the treatment of major depression and post-traumatic stress disorder, however, its clinical effects are of short duration (Fig. 19-8, Table 19-5).[41]

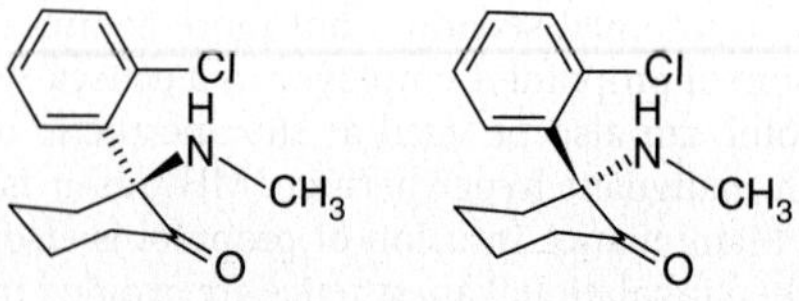

R-(−)-Ketamine *S*-(+)-Ketamine

Figure 19-8 Ketamine. (RS)-2-2-chlorophenyl-2-(methylamino) cyclohexanone.

Pharmacokinetics

Ketamine is an analog of phencyclidine that is a chiral compound and is a racemic mixture of S and R enantiomers. The S(+) enantiomer of ketamine is three to four times more potent than the R enantiomer. The S enantiomer has a shorter duration of action and is cleared more rapidly.[42] Ketamine is bioavailable by multiple routes of administration. Intramuscular (IM) administration has a 93% bioavailability, transnasal has 25% to 50% bioavailability, and rectal or oral administration has 16% bioavailability.[43] The

Table 19-5 Ketamine

Key Pharmacology	Key Clinical Uses
NMDA receptor antagonist	Anesthesia—intravenous and intramuscular induction
Cardiovascular stability; increases heart rate and blood pressure	Analgesia
Mild respiratory depression	Chronic pain
Side effects: Emergence delirium, hallucinations, nystagmus, increased salivation	Depression
Trance-like cataleptic unconscious state ("dissociative anesthesia")	Bronchodilator
	Procedural sedation, especially in pediatric and burn patients

NMDA, N-methyl-D-aspartate.

high lipid solubility and low protein binding (20%) allow for a rapid uptake of ketamine in the brain, as well as a fairly rapid redistribution. The onset of anesthesia after intravenous administration of ketamine is 30 to 60 seconds, with duration of 10 to 15 minutes. The induction dose of ketamine is 0.5 to 2 mg/kg for intravenous administration and 4 to 6 mg/kg for IM administration. Peak plasma levels averaged 0.75 mg/mL and cerebrospinal fluid (CSF) levels were about 0.2 mg/mL 1 hour after dosing.[44]

After intravenous bolus administration, ketamine shows a bi- or triexponential pattern of elimination. The alpha-elimination phase (redistribution of ketamine from the central nervous system [CNS] to peripheral tissues) is 11 minutes, and the beta-elimination phase is 2.5 hours.[45] Ketamine is metabolized primarily in the liver by cytochrome P-450 enzymes (CYP 3A4 > CYP 2C9 > CYP 2B6). The liver extensively metabolizes ketamine by demethylation to its principle metabolite norketamine. Norketamine is biologically active but only has 20% to 30% the activity of racemic ketamine. Norketamine is eliminated by renal excretion. Due to its lipophilicity, ketamine is only partially removed by dialysis.

Pharmacodynamics

The neuropharmacology of ketamine is complex. Antagonism of the NMDA receptor is primarily responsible for ketamine-specific clinical effects. However, ketamine also has clinical effects at opioid, noradrenergic, cholinergic, nicotinic, and muscarinic receptors.

Ketamine binds preferentially to the NMDA receptors on inhibitory interneurons in the cortex, limbic system and hippocampus. This binding promotes uncoordinated increases in neuronal activity, produces an active EEG pattern and causes unconsciousness.[46] Ketamine has been shown to increase the bispectral index (BIS) from 40 to 63 with higher doses of ketamine (0.5 mg/kg) under general anesthesia with propofol and fentanyl.[47]

There are NMDA receptors present on nearly all CNS cells, and especially those cells involved with nociception such as primary afferent nociceptors in the spinal dorsal horn. Ketamine binds to an interchannel site of the NMDA receptor called the PCP binding site and decreases channel opening time. Ketamine decreases the amplification of repeated stimulation of the NMDA receptor ("wind up") that is considered an elementary form of CNS sensitization. Antagonism of the channel is more profound if the NMDA channel has been previously opened by glutamate.[48]

Functional magnetic resonance imaging (MRI) has provided some insight into the analgesic pharmacodynamics of ketamine. Volunteers who were subjected to painful heat stimulation showed a typical pattern of pain activation from the thalamus to the insula, to the cingulate, and ultimately to the prefrontal cortex. There was a dose-dependent reduction in these cerebral activation pathways when volunteers were given ketamine. Ketamine has also been found to block signals from the spinoretiular pathway. Activity of the medial thalamic nuclei and medial reticular formation—important relays in nociceptive transmission between the spinal and supraspinal levels—are both depressed.[48]

Ketamine has been found to bind to opioid, noradrenergic, and cholinergic receptors. Ketamine binds to mu, delta, and kappa opioid receptors; however, this does not account for its analgesics effects.[48] The primary analgesic mechanism of ketamine is believed to be in the prevention of developing hyperalgesia.[49] Ketamine causes stimulation of CNS noradrenergic neurons and inhibition of catecholamine uptake, which provokes a hyperadrenergic state (with increased release of norepinephrine, dopamine, and serotonin). Ketamine's effect on noradrenergic neurons is partly responsible for the hypnotic, psychic, and analgesic effects observed. Ketamine also affects CNS cholinergic neurons, and anticholinergic physostigmine can antagonize the hypnotic effects of ketamine (Fig. 19-9).

Clinical Uses

Anesthesia

Ketamine administration has been described as causing a dissociative amnestic state. Patients are unconscious with eyes open, maintain spontaneous respiration, and do not react to painful or noxious stimuli.[39] EEG shows a depression of the thalamocortical pathways and concomitant activation of the limbic system. Despite this increased epileptiform activity, there is no clinical evidence of seizure activity or spread of the epileptiform activity to cortical areas. Therefore, ketamine is less likely to cause a seizure and may in fact have CNS protective properties. Ketamine anesthesia is associated with profound analgesia that occurs at subanesthetic levels.

Induction doses of ketamine are 1 to 2 mg/kg, with an onset of 1 minute and a duration of 10 to 20 minutes. Ketamine administration is associated with an increase in heart rate and blood pressure. Ketamine is therefore a good choice for anesthetic induction in the hemodynamically unstable patient. Ketamine has been compared to etomidate in the unstable patient and has the advantage of not causing adrenal suppression.[50] The increased blood pressure and heart rate associated with ketamine may make it unsuitable for some cardiac patients (critical coronary artery disease). An increase in PVR associated with ketamine may make it an unsuitable choice in patients with severe right heart dysfunction.

Sedation

Ketamine has been used to provide sedation to burn patients during wound care. Benefits of ketamine in this patient population include analgesia, as well as maintenance of spontaneous respiration and airway reflexes. Ketamine can be administered via IM injection and has been used to provide sedation or anesthesia in uncooperative or hostile patients, including those with acute behavioral disturbance from various etiologies in the prehospital setting. Ketamine has also been used in pediatric patients for painful procedures such as fixation of bones after a fracture in the emergency department, as an example of its broad use for procedural sedation in this setting.[43]

Analgesia

Ketamine has been extensively studied for its role as an analgesic in the management of acute postoperative pain. Ketamine has been shown to lower pain scores and decrease opiate requirements in postoperative patients. Administration of both a ketamine bolus prior to surgical incision and a ketamine infusion postoperatively has been found to be the most effective use of ketamine for acute pain. The analgesic effects of ketamine are achieved at subanesthetic blood concentrations. Ketamine reduces opiate requirements for postsurgical pain, but it cannot replace opiates altogether. Ketamine is useful in patients who will require high doses of opiates, such as patients on chronic opiate therapy or patients with a history of opiate abuse.[51]

The exact mechanism of analgesia provided by ketamine is unclear. The NMDA receptor has been found to be associated with central sensitization and wind up at the spinal cord associated with chronic pain. Studies have suggested that ketamine analgesia occurs by the prevention of both hyperalgesia and decreases in CNS sensitization that occurs with acute pain.[40]

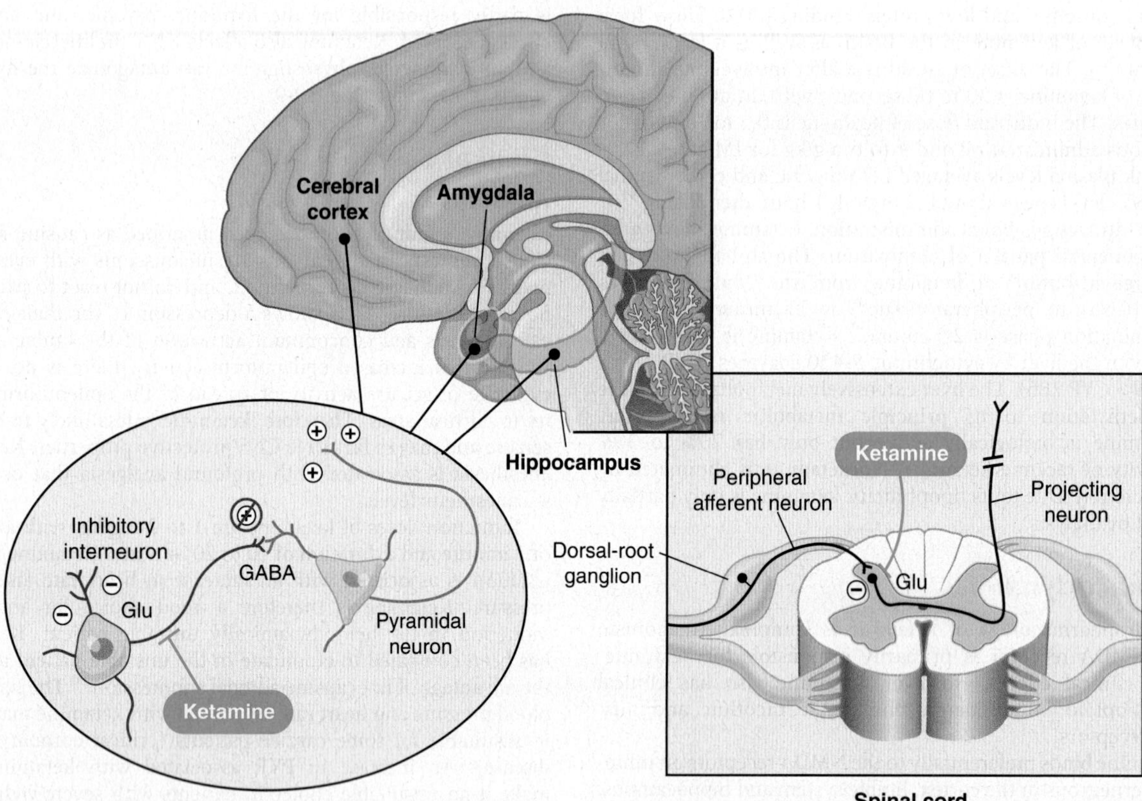

Figure 19-9 Ketamine's mechanism of action in the central nervous system. Ketamine binds preferentially to the N-methyl-D-aspartate (NMDA) receptors on inhibitory interneurons in the cortex, amygdala, and hippocampus. Unconsciousness results from an uncoordinated increase in neural activity. In the spinal cord, ketamine decreases arousal by blocking NMDA glutamate–mediated nociceptive signals from peripheral afferent neurons in the dorsal root ganglion to projecting neurons.

Chronic Pain

Due to its NMDA receptor role in preventing hyperalgesia, ketamine has also been investigated for the management of chronic pain. Ketamine has been most extensively studied in patients with complex regional pain syndrome (CRPS). Ketamine administration to patient with CRPS yields a decrease in both pain scores and opiate consumption.[52] Unfortunately, these effects are only of limited duration after ketamine administration. Future studies are required to determine the most effective regimen for ketamine administration in patients with chronic pain. Ketamine has also been used for cancer patients with severe pain. Ketamine is associated with a decrease, but not elimination of opiate requirements. Unfortunately, the CNS side effects and lack of reliable oral administration limit the application of ketamine in patients with chronic pain.

Intranasal ketamine has been investigated for the use in chronic pain and was found to significantly lower the intensity of breakthrough pain in patients with chronic pain when compared to placebo.[52,53] Intranasal ketamine also decreased pain scores in patients with chronic neuropathic pain.[54] Both studies reported no serious side effects. Intranasal ketamine, in combination with intranasal midazolam, has been used in the management of acute postoperative pain showing similar efficacy to morphine patient-controlled analgesia (PCA) after spine surgery.[55] Further studies are needed to determine the utility of intranasal ketamine.

Depression

Ketamine has been evaluated as a possible treatment for major depression. Ketamine has a rapid effect on depression with decreased depression symptoms and suicidal ideation within 1 hour of administration.[56,57] Ketamine as an antidepressant represents a possible novel treatment, and has generated excitement because of variable results with current treatments of depression (slow onset, poor efficacy). The duration of ketamine's antidepressant effect may last from a couple of days to approximately 2 weeks following a single injection. For treatment of depression, ketamine is typically infused intravenously over 40 minutes at a subanesthetic dose of 0.5 mg/kg.[58] Further investigation is required to determine the best regimen to use ketamine as an antidepressant.[42] The mechanism of ketamine's antidepressant effects remains unclear. Investigations using memantine, also an NMDA antagonist, failed to improve depressive symptoms.[59] Therefore, the antidepressant effects of ketamine may not be related to its NMDA antagonism, but rather its effect on other CNS receptors (dopamine, adrenergic). Understanding the mechanism of action of ketamine in depression may yield new targets for the treatment of major depression.

Side Effects

CNS: The major side effect of ketamine is the psychogenic reactions seen with its administration. Patients can experience hallucinations and out-of-body experiences that have been described as frightening. Studies have shown that these symptoms can be reduced with co-administration of benzodiazepines. Ketamine will also cause patients to have a lateral gaze nystagmus.[39]

Cardiovascular: Administration of ketamine is associated with increased heart rate and increased blood pressure. The exact mechanism is unclear but it is hypothesized that ketamine causes activation of the sympathetic nervous system. Ketamine is one of the few intravenous anesthetics that increase SVR, and therefore is an attractive option for the induction of anesthesia in patients who are hemodynamically unstable. That said, ketamine has also been found to cause direct myocardial depression. There are reports of ketamine causing cardiovascular collapse in patients who have been sympathetically depleted.[60] Theoretically, this cardiovascular collapse is due to ketamine's myocardial depression in the absence of sympathetic vasoconstriction due to depleted catecholamines.

Respiratory: Ketamine maintains spontaneous respiration. Hypoxia can occur, but it is easily treated with supplemental oxygen. Ketamine is also a bronchodilator, although it is not effective as a sole agent for the treatment of bronchospasm.[61] Rather, it is a secondary agent to consider for the management of severe bronchospasm or status asthmaticus. Ketamine increases salivation that may result in laryngospasm.

ICP/seizure issues: Historically, ketamine was not recommended in patients with elevated ICP. The excitatory CNS effects of ketamine would increase CMRO2 and increase CBF. However, studies have found that ICP typically remains normal with ketamine administration in neurosurgical patients with controlled ventilation. In fact, ketamine may be neuroprotective.[62] Ketamine is associated with epileptiform activity on EEG; however, these excitement waveforms are not seen in the cortex, and therefore ketamine seems unlikely to precipitate a seizure.

Dexmedetomidine

Introduction

Dexmedetomidine is an alpha-2-adrenergic agonist similar to clonidine (see NICV 13-3). It has seven to eight times greater affinity for the alpha-2-adrenergic receptor than clonidine. Introduced into clinical practice in 1999, dexmedetomidine has been used for ICU sedation in mechanically ventilated patients, procedural sedation, and as a component of general anesthesia. Dexmedetomidine is unique as a sedative in that it has limited respiratory depressant effects (Fig. 19-10, Table 19-6).

Table 19-6 Dexmedetomidine

Key Pharmacology	Key Clinical Uses
Alpha-2-adrenergic agonist	Intensive care unit sedation in mechanically ventilated patients
Sedation with minimal respiratory depression	Procedural sedation
Mimics normal sleep pattern on EEG	Pediatrics: preoperative anxiolysis and emergence delirium
Provides analgesia at the spinal cord level	
Administration: bolus 0.5–1 mcg/kg over 15 min, followed by 0.3–0.7 mcg/kg/h infusion	
Side effects: bradycardia and hypotension	

EEG, electroencephalogram.

Pharmacokinetics

Following intravenous administration, dexmedetomidine exhibits the following pharmacokinetic parameters: a rapid distribution phase with a distribution half-life of approximately 6 minutes; a terminal elimination half-life of approximately 2 hours, and a steady-state volume of distributions of approximately 118 L. Dexmedetomidine exhibits linear pharmacokinetics in the dose range of 0.2 to 0.7 mcg/kg/h when administered by intravenous infusion for up to 24 hours.[63] The average protein binding is 94% and constant across different plasma concentrations. The fraction of dexmedetomidine bound to plasma protein is significantly decreased in subjects with hepatic impairment compared to healthy subjects.

Dexmedetomidine undergoes almost complete biotransformation with very little unchanged dexmedetomidine in the urine and feces. Biotransformation involves both direct glucuronidation and cytochrome P450–mediated metabolism. The terminal elimination half-life is approximately 2 hours and clearance is estimated to be approximately 39 L/h. Clearance values for dexmedetomidine are lower in patients with varying degrees of hepatic impairment. Dexmedetomidine pharmacokinetics are not significantly different in patients with severe renal impairment compared to healthy subjects.[64]

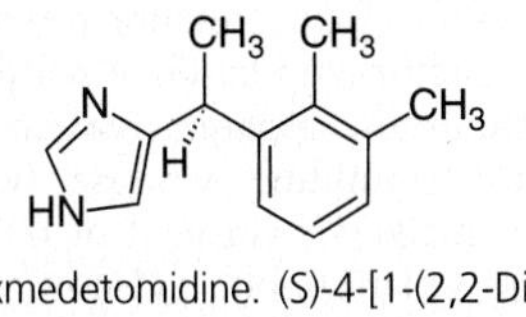

Figure 19-10 Dexmedetomidine. (S)-4-[1-(2,2-Dimethylphenyl)ethyl]-3-H-imidazole

Pharmacodynamics

Dexmedetomidine acts on the alpha-2-adrenergic receptors in the spinal cord and brain. Its effects are primarily at the locus coeruleus that activates sleep centers in the brain. Interestingly, the EEG pattern observed in patients receiving dexmedetomidine resembles that of non-REM sleep. Clinically, patients are sedated but easily arousable, and able to follow commands with minimal respiratory depression (Fig. 19-11).[65]

The cardiovascular effects of dexmedetomidine are as expected for an alpha-2 agonist: bradycardia and hypotension. Compared to placebo, dexmedetomidine causes a 7 mmHg decrease in systolic blood pressure and a decrease in mean heart rate of 1 to 8 beats per minute.[63]

Clinical Uses

7

Dexmedetomidine has been used to provide sedation for mechanically ventilated patients in the ICU. Patients receiving dexmedetomidine required less rescue sedation with midazolam or morphine versus placebo.[63] Maintenance of spontaneous respiration allows for ICU patients to be extubated while receiving a dexmedetomidine infusion. Dexmedetomidine is also attractive for ICU sedation in neurosurgery as patients can participate in neurologic examinations while receiving this medication. Dexmedetomidine has been found to have analgesic properties, and can reduce opiate requirements in ICU patients who are mechanically ventilated. However, a systematic review of controlled trials failed to find sedation superiority when comparing dexmedetomidine to midazolam for ICU sedation.[66]

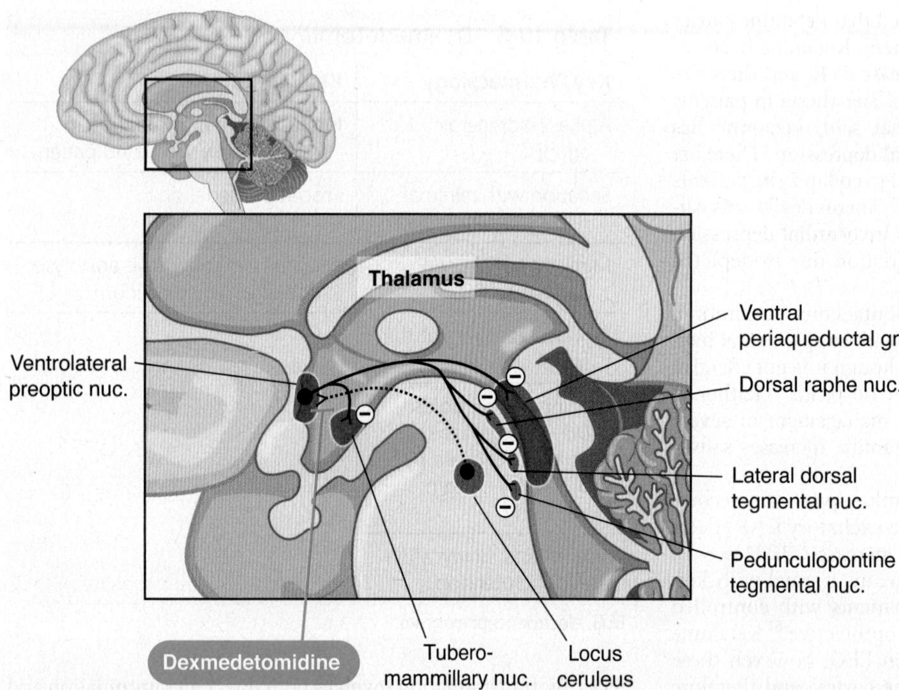

Figure 19-11 Dexmedetomidine's mechanism of action in the central nervous system. Dexmedetomidine activates the sleep centers in the brain. Dexmedetomidine binds to alpha-2 receptors on neurons from the locus coeruleus, inhibiting norepinephrine release (*dashed line*) in the ventrolateral preoptic nucleus. The disinhibited ventrolateral preoptic nucleus reduces arousal of the midbrain, hypothalamic, and pontine arousal nuclei.

Dexmedetomidine can also be used for procedural sedation. Dexmedetomidine has been studied as an agent for sedation during awake fiberoptic intubation.[63] Maintenance of spontaneous ventilation makes this drug useful for this very purpose. Dexmedetomidine can also be used to provide MAC sedation alone or in combination with other medications. Typical administration involves at 0.5 to 1 mcg/kg loading dose over 15 minutes, followed by an infusion of 0.3 to 0.7 mcg/kg/h.

Several studies have compared the efficacy of dexmedetomidine to propofol for procedural sedation. In the operating room, dexmedetomidine provided adequate sedation compared to propofol with less hypotension, and better pain scores in the postanesthesia care unit (PACU). However, the onset of sedation was longer with dexmedetomidine, and patients had prolonged sedation and more hypotension in the PACU when compared to propofol.[67,68] Two studies found dexmedetomidine to be inferior to propofol for sedation for upper endoscopy procedures.[69,70]

Although not approved for use in pediatrics, many investigators have evaluated its off-label use in children.[64] Intranasal dexmedetomidine (1 mcg/kg) has been used for preoperative anxiolysis, with an onset of 25 minutes and duration of 85 minutes. Dexmedetomidine was found to be superior to oral midazolam in ensuring satisfactory levels of sedation; however, its long onset time limits this application. Because it preserves spontaneous respiration, dexmedetomidine has been used in airway procedures such as rigid bronchoscopy. Dexmedetomidine has been used as an adjunct to TIVA during posterior spine fusion surgery, and lowers both propofol and sevoflurane requirements. Dexmedetomidine has been found to have minimal effect on SSEPs and motor-evoked potentials (MEPs) during spine surgery.[71]

Dexmedetomidine has been investigated for the prevention of emergence delirium. A meta-analysis found that alpha-2 agonists (clonidine or dexmedetomidine) decrease emergence delirium when given via the oral, intravenous, or caudal route. Dexmedetomidine given by intravenous bolus or infusion has been shown to decrease emergence delirium, but the optimal dose is unknown. Compared to placebo, dexmedetomidine (0.5 to 1 mcg/kg) decreases the incidence of emergence delirium from 47% to 2.8% with slightly prolonged emergence time.[72]

Dexmedetomidine has been investigated as a local anesthetic adjuvant for regional anesthesia. Dexmedetomidine was found to prolong both motor and sensory blocks when administered intrathecally in combination with local anesthetic. Perineural injection of dexmedetomidine as part of a brachial plexus block did extend the duration of the block, but this was not found to be statistically significant. Further studies are needed to define the potential benefit of dexmedetomidine as a local anesthesia adjuvant.[73]

Side Effects

The main adverse reactions of dexmedetomidine are hypotension, bradycardia, dry mouth, nausea, and hypertension. The incidence of bradycardia is reported as high as 40%, and can be managed with atropine, ephedrine, or volume administration.[74] There are case reports of patients who have developed severe bradycardia and cardiac arrest with dexmedetomidine administration.[75] However, in these reports, dexmedetomidine is unlikely to be the only causative agent of these cardiac arrests. Therefore, care should be taken in using dexmedetomidine in patients who will not tolerate bradycardia, or patients who are receiving medications that cause bradycardia. The bradycardia associated with dexmedetomidine typically occurs after a loading dose. Omitting the loading dose decreases the incidence of bradycardia.[74]

Dexmedetomidine is associated with hypotension that is expected with an alpha-2-adrenergic agonist. In healthy volunteers, after a 1 mcg/kg bolus, blood pressure decreased 23% compared to baseline. Infusions of 0.2 to 0.7 mcg/kg/h were associated with larger decreases in blood pressure when compared to placebo. Blood pressure returns to baseline within 6 hours of treatment cessation without any apparent rebound effects. There are case reports of dexmedetomidine overdose. Two patients received infusions of 2 or 4 mcg/kg/h (instead of 0.2 to 0.4 mcg/kg/h) which caused excess sedation, but had minimal effect on hemodynamics.[76] In a 3-year-old child who received an unintentional

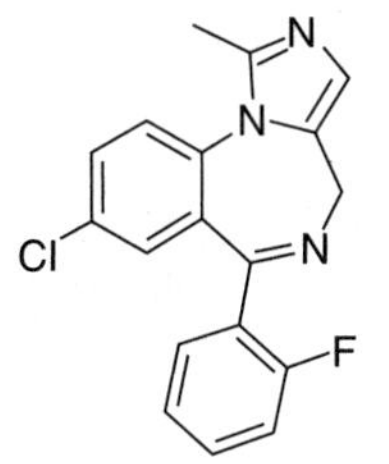

Figure 19-12 Midazolam. 8-chloro-6-(2-fluorophenyl)-1-methyl-4*H*-imidazo[1,5-a][1,4]benzodiazepine.

bolus of 9 mcg/kg of dexmedetomidine, the heart rate, blood pressure, and oxygen saturation were all decreased. However, the child was managed with supplemental oxygen, fluid bolus, and epinephrine infusion, and recovered to baseline after 7 hours.[77]

Benzodiazepines

Introduction

8 Benzodiazepines—midazolam in particular—are frequently used by anesthesiologists to produce several clinically desirable effects: anxiolysis, anterograde amnesia, sedation, and hypnosis. They can also be used as muscle relaxants and anticonvulsants. Benzodiazepines have a favorable safety profile and can be reversed by flumazenil to manage excessive sedation or respiratory depression.

Midazolam was first discovered in 1976 and is the most widely used benzodiazepine in the perioperative period. Its use as a premedication and anesthetic is largely due to its quick onset, short elimination half-life, anterograde amnestic effect, and minimal side-effect profile.[78] Midazolam can be administered intravenously, intranasally, orally, rectally, and intramuscularly. This flexibility in route of administration also contributes to its popularity. A 0.5 mg/kg dose of oral midazolam given 30 minutes preoperatively in children yields a reliable anxiolytic and sedative effect without delayed emergence.[79] Some studies have even found a positive behavioral effect 1 week postoperatively in pediatric patients premedicated with oral midazolam.[80] Midazolam is also used as an infusion in the ICU setting. One meta-analysis reported that "infusions of both midazolam and propofol appear to provide similar quality sedation, that extubation time and recovery time is shorter in patients sedated with propofol, and that hemodynamic complications related to either drug regimen are not usually clinically significant" (Fig. 19-12, Table 19-7).[81]

Pharmacokinetics

Benzodiazepines are highly protein bound and highly lipophilic. High protein binding renders a smaller free fraction of the drug available to cross the blood–brain barrier, and high lipophilicity results in a larger volume of distribution. Clinically, less drug

Table 19-7 Benzodiazepines

Key Pharmacology	Key Clinical Uses
GABA-A receptor agonist	Anxiolysis
Minimal respiratory depression	Anterograde amnesia
Minimal cardiovascular depression	Sedation
Large therapeutic window	Induction of anesthesia, hemodynamically stable
Reversible with flumazenil	Anticonvulsant

GABA-A, gamma-aminobutyric acid-A.

is free to cross the blood–brain barrier, but the high lipophilicity results in a rapid onset of action (the peak effect of intravenous midazolam is within 2 to 3 minutes).[82] Only a fraction of the available CNS binding sites need to be occupied to produce clinical effects. Midazolam's high lipid solubility, short duration of action, and short context-sensitive half-time allow this drug to be administered as a continuous infusion, unlike other benzodiazepines (Table 19-8, Table 19-9).[83]

Metabolism of benzodiazepines occurs largely in the hepatic cytochrome P450 system via oxidation and glucuronic conjugation. The metabolized drug is then renally excreted. Some drugs, such as diazepam, have pharmacologically active metabolites (i.e., desmethyldiazepam, 3-hydroxydiazepam) with long elimination half-lives that lead to a prolonged duration of action, especially in patients with renal failure. Drugs that inhibit the cytochrome P450 system can result in prolonged duration of benzodiazepines.

Favorable properties of midazolam are its high rate of hepatic clearance and relatively short elimination half-life. Midazolam has a volume of distribution of 1 to 3.1 L/kg after a single bolus dose, an elimination half-life of 1.8 to 2.6 hours (mean approximately 3 hours), and a total clearance of 6.4 to 11 mL/kg/min.[84] Midazolam's active metabolite (1-hydroxymidazolam) contributes minimally to its clinical effects (approximately 20% of midazolam's potency). These properties are influenced by the patient's age and comorbidities, particularly kidney and liver dysfunction. With continuous infusions of midazolam, the metabolite will accumulate and exert a more pronounced and prolonged effect. Rather than metabolism, redistribution of midazolam results in the termination of its effects.

Pharmacodynamics and Clinical Uses

The three most commonly used parenteral benzodiazepines are lorazepam, diazepam, and midazolam. Lorazepam and diazepam are not soluble in water and often cause vein irritation due to the propylene glycol admixture. Alternative formulations are available as a lipid emulsion, but with a decrease in bioavailability.

Table 19-8 Benzodiazepine Metabolism and Clearance

Drug	Duration	Metabolites	Hepatic Clearance
Midazolam	Short	1-hydroxymidazolam (mild CNS depressant)	High
Diazepam	Intermediate	Oxazepam and desmethyldiazepam	Slow
Lorazepam	Long	Inactive	Intermediate

CNS, central nervous system.

Table 19-9 Benzodiazepine Pharmacokinetics

Drug	Induction Dose (mg/kg)	Duration of Action (min)	Redistribution Half-Life (min)	Protein Binding (%)	Volume of Distribution (L/kg)	Clearance (mL/kg/min)	Elimination Half-Life (h)
Midazolam	0.1–0.3	15–20	7–15	94	1–3.1	6.4–11	1.8–2.6
Diazepam	0.3–0.6	15–30	10–15	98	0.7–1.7	0.2–0.5	20–50
Lorazepam	0.03–0.1	60–120	3–10	98	0.8–1.3	0.8–1.8	11–22

Midazolam is water-soluble and undergoes conformational change in the bloodstream, becoming more lipophilic. Midazolam is manufactured as an acidic formulation that may produce mild local tissue and vein irritation.

Benzodiazepines bind to specific receptor sites that are part of the GABA-A receptor complex. This binding augments the effect of the GABA-A receptor/chloride channel coupling, resulting in increased frequency of chloride channel opening. The resultant hyperpolarization of the cell ultimately leads to neural inhibition. It is this enhanced affinity of the GABA-A receptor for the GABA molecule, and subsequent decreased unbinding that produces the so-called "ceiling effect."[85] Benzodiazepines thus have a dose-dependent CNS depressant effect (Table 19-10). For example, at 30% to 50% receptor occupancy, sedation is often produced, while at 20% occupancy, one usually only achieves anxiolysis.[86]

The high density of GABA-A receptors in the cerebral cortex helps explain the sedative/hypnotic, anxiolytic, and amnestic capabilities of these drugs. Benzodiazepines also decrease both the CMRO2 and CBF, while maintaining carbon dioxide responsiveness. They exert little if any effect on ICP. Because of the ceiling effect of benzodiazepines, an isoelectric EEG or burst suppression is not attained. This is in direct contrast to propofol and thiopental, each of which can achieve burst suppression. Thus, the neuroprotectant effect of benzodiazepines is quite limited, but likely not entirely absent. Some investigators have demonstrated that activation of GABA-A receptors, including the specific binding subunits for propofol and midazolam, play a role in the inhibition of neuronal death induced by brain ischemia.

In addition, benzodiazepines are anticonvulsants and are a first-line therapy in the management of seizures. They can also be used as muscle relaxants, but this spinal cord–mediated response typically requires supratherapeutic doses.

Benzodiazepines can also have a profound effect on the respiratory system. Upper airway reflexes may be decreased and central respiratory drive is depressed. In the usual premedication dosage, respiratory depression is rarely an issue; however, if the patient has other comorbidities and/or concurrent opioid use, then adverse respiratory events are more likely to occur.

Table 19-10 Midazolam Dosing by Clinical Use

Clinical Use	Dose
Premedication: (anxiolysis/ anterograde amnesia)	0.02–0.04 mg/kg IV/IM; 0.4–0.8 mg/kg PO
Induction: (hypnosis/amnesia/ sedation)	0.1–0.2 mg/kg IV
Infusion (in conjunction with volatile anesthetics): (hypnosis/ amnesia)	0.25–1 mcg/kg/min

IM, intramuscular; IV, intravenous; PO, oral.

Benzodiazepines, especially in induction doses, depress the SVR and decrease blood pressure. This effect is quite minimal as there is some preservation of homeostatic reflexes. This response may be more pronounced in the hypovolemic patient. Benzodiazepines are overall regarded as hemodynamically stable induction agents.

Remimazolam: This new drug is a benzodiazepine with a structure and onset time similar to midazolam, and binds as an agonist to the GABA-A receptor. It has a rapid offset that follows first-order kinetics at the recommended doses due to metabolism by tissue esterases (similar to remifentanil), and thus does not result in accumulation of drug. In addition to organ-independent metabolism, this drug is reversible with flumazenil, further adding to the safety profile. The quick onset and offset offer the potential for use as an infusion. Remimazolam is initially being developed for procedural sedation during procedures such as colonoscopy.[87] It is also being considered for ICU sedation, as many critically ill patients have end-organ dysfunction and would benefit from the organ-independent metabolism of this drug. This drug provides a sedation alternative to propofol by avoiding PRIS and accumulation of drug leading to prolonged sedation, Remimazolam takes advantage of the hypnotic and amnestic effects of midazolam with a speed and mode of metabolism similar to remifentanil.[88]

A meta-analysis of randomized controlled trials for procedural sedation found that compared to midzaolam, remimazolam resulted in an improved procedure success rate, a reduction in the need for rescue medication, a decrease in time to recovery and a better cognitive recovery. The number of adverse events was similar for both drugs. Therefore, remimazolam may be a better choice for procedural sedation than midazolam.[89] Remiazolam has also been compared to propofol for the maintenance of general anesthesia. Time to loss of consciousness was slightly longer for remimazolam when compared to propofol. The incidence of hypotension and the need for vasopressor support was lower in patients who received remimazolam compared to propofol.[90] An additional attractive feature of remimazolam is the ability to provide medication reversal with flumazenil. Further studies are needed to define the clinical uses of remimazolam, given these early positive findings.

Side Effects

Aside from their previously discussed systemic effects (e.g., hypotension in hypovolemic patients, respiratory depression—particularly when combined with opioids), benzodiazepines are associated with limited adverse events. Anaphylaxis is extremely rare following the administration of a benzodiazepine. More frequently described is pain or thrombophlebitis that ensues following intravenous injection, especially diazepam. As noted previously, propylene glycol is the organic solvent for diazepam and causes the pain associated with injection. In contrast, midazolam is water-soluble, but may also cause burning with injection secondary to its acidic formulation.

Barbiturates

Introduction

Thiopental is one of the earliest intravenous anesthetics used, discovered in the 1930s and first used on human patients in 1934, and has withstood the test of time as an induction agent because of its favorable pharmacokinetic profile. In 2011, production of thiopental in the United States ceased, leading to a drastic decrease in its intraoperative use; however, it is still a commonly used induction agent outside the country, particularly in low- and middle-income countries. Two major classes of barbiturates, oxybarbiturates and thiobarbiturates, are of anesthetic clinical and historical relevance. Both classes contain a pyrimidine center, and either an oxygen or sulfur molecule at position 2. Those used in clinical practice are the thiobarbiturates thiopental (2.5%) and thiamylal (2%), and the oxybarbiturate methohexital (1%). The thiobarbiturate solutions are produced as racemic mixtures, despite unequal potency between their two stereoisomers. Methohexital has two chiral centers and four potential stereoisomers, but not all isomers are included in the final product. Barbiturate solutions are highly alkaline, allowing for formation of water-soluble salts. Addition or reconstitution in acidic solutions (e.g., vecuronium) leads to precipitation of these salts, hampering intravenous use. Unlike propofol, barbiturates cannot be stored for an extended period of time at room temperature after reconstitution in solvent. In alkaline solution, thiobarbiturates can be stored up to 2 weeks, and methohexital up to 6 weeks (Fig. 19-13, Table 19-11).

Table 19-11 Barbiturates

Key Pharmacology	Key Clinical Uses
GABA-A receptor agonist	Induction of general anesthesia
Prolonged context-sensitive half-time	Methohexital used for sedation, premedication and electroconvulsive therapy
CNS depressant, neuroprotective, anti-convulsant, decreases CMRO2, CBF, and ICP	Barbiturate coma (thiopental)
EEG burst suppression (thiopental)	Thiopental intra-arterial injection can lead to tissue necrosis
Cardiovascular: decreases mean arterial pressure, venous vascular tone, and cardiac output	
Pulmonary: dose-dependent respiratory depression, does not cause bronchodilation	

CBF, cerebral blood flow; CMRO2, cerebral metabolic oxygen consumption rate; EEG, electroencephalogram; GABA-A, gamma-aminobutyric acid-A; ICP, intracranial pressure.

Pharmacokinetics

Primary metabolism of both barbiturates classes is hepatic, yielding water-soluble inactive metabolites that are subsequently eliminated in urine and bile. Oxidation of thiopental and methohexital to their respective hydroxyl derivatives is the most common form of metabolism.[91] Thiopental has a relatively long elimination half-life (12 hours), and its clearance rate (3 mL/kg/min) is 10-fold longer than that of propofol. Methohexital elimination half-life (4 hours) is also shorter than thiopental, secondary to a more efficient hepatic extraction of the drug (clearance rate 11 mL/kg/min). A negligible percentage of barbiturates is eliminated without metabolism in the urine.

Multicompartment pharmacokinetic models of barbiturates after administration of an induction dose have been described. Similar to other intravenous agents, rapid redistribution into highly perfused compartments accounts for the rapid termination of drug action after a single induction dose. After an extended infusion of thiopental, accumulation in poorly perfused compartments and elimination play larger pharmacokinetic roles, resulting in a prolonged context-sensitive half-time and delayed recovery. The long context-sensitive half-time of thiopental after high doses is explained by the drug exhibiting zero-order kinetics. The elimination of thiopental then becomes independent of both drug plasma concentration and level of compartmental saturation, and remains constant and defined by the slow rate of clearance.

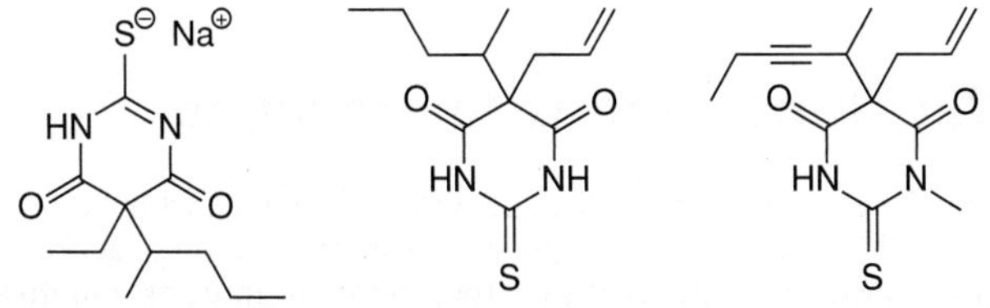

Thiopental Thiamylal Methohexital

Figure 19-13 Thiopental. (*RS*)-[5-ethyl-4,6-dioxo-5-(pentan-2-yl)-1,4,5,6-tetrahydropyrimidin-2-yl]sulfanide sodium. Thiamylalal. 5-Allyl-5-(1-methylbutyl)-2-thioxodihydropyrimidine-4,6(1*H*,5*H*)-dione. Methohexital. 5-hex-3-yn-2-yl-1- methyl-5-prop-2-enyl-1, 3-diazinane-2,4,6-trione.

Pharmacodynamics

The mechanism of action of barbiturates involves cortical and brainstem GABA inhibitory pathways, leading to loss of consciousness, as well as respiratory and cardiovascular depression. Hypnotic effects of barbiturates are likely enhanced by the inhibition of central excitatory pathways, specifically those mediated by glutamate via NMDA receptors and acetylcholine.

Central Nervous System Effects

The progression of EEG changes after administration of barbiturates is dose dependent. Initial low doses can generate a light level of anesthesia often associated with a high-frequency and low-amplitude EEG pattern. With higher doses, both burst suppression and an isoelectric EEG can be attained.[92] Thiopental is generally considered an anticonvulsant, having been used successfully for treatment of status epilepticus. At smaller concentrations, thiopental has been noted to have proconvulsant properties. Methohexital is considered to have significant proconvulsant effects in patients with epilepsy, and is often the agent of choice for induction of anesthesia prior to ECT.[93] The excitatory effects of methohexital are commonly apparent in muscle twitches that occur after an induction dose of the drug.

Barbiturates cause a decrease in CMRO2 that is dose dependent, eventually leading to an isoelectric EEG that is associated with up to a 50% decrease in oxygen consumption.[94] A concomitant increase in cerebral vascular resistance leads to decreased CBF and ICP. CPP is often unchanged or even improved, as the decrease in MAP is typically less than the decrease in ICP. Barbiturate-induced CNS effects are considered neuroprotective and in part explained by the decrease in CMRO2, although CMRO2 decreases are not directly proportional to levels of ischemic neuroprotection.[95] Other neuroprotective mechanisms likely play a role, including barbiturate anticonvulsant properties, improved blood flow to ischemic parts of the brain (reverse steal effect), free-radical scavenging, attenuation of excitatory neurotransmitter release and pathways, and membrane stabilization. The reverse steal effect is a result of flow-metabolism coupling. At higher doses, the reduction in oxygen consumption in well-perfused areas of the brain leads to decreased flow, with subsequent diversion of blood flow to ischemic areas.

Historically, barbiturate-induced "brain relaxation" has been utilized as a protective strategy during neurosurgery and after head trauma. The clinical benefit after barbiturate administration has been reproduced by other techniques, including cooling (to lower CMRO2) and antihypertensive strategies. Barbiturate neuroprotection is generally considered more effective for focal and incomplete ischemia, rather than global injury. In the setting of comatose cardiac arrest survivors, thiopental loading after arrest has not been shown to significantly improve outcome.[96] In contrast, thiopental-induced burst suppression and isoelectric EEG prior to potential focal ischemic insult during cardiopulmonary bypass and carotid surgery has been shown to have clinical benefit.

Cardiovascular Effects

The most prominent cardiovascular changes after an induction dose of thiopental are decreases in both MAP and cardiac output. The primary mechanism is reduction of venous vascular tone, followed by peripheral pooling of venous blood and a decrease in venous return.[97] Thiopental also has negative inotropic effects, directly by altering intracellular calcium homeostasis and indirectly by diminishing sympathetic tone. Baroreceptor-mediated heart rate increase may be impaired by thiopental administration, but a reflex elevation in heart rate of 10% to 30% is still typically present. The negative hemodynamic effects after a thiopental bolus are more pronounced in patients with underlying cardiovascular disease or hypovolemia. Induction doses of methohexital are typically associated with a smaller decrease in MAP and larger increase in heart rate than what is described for thiopental.[98]

Respiratory System Effects

Barbiturates cause respiratory depression in a dose-dependent manner, leading to central apnea at deeper stages of anesthesia. After a typical induction dose, apnea is commonly noted after 1 to 1.5 minutes, with ventilatory response to carbon dioxide returning to baseline in approximately 6 minutes. The time course to recovery from respiratory depression is shorter with thiopental than with propofol.[99] Thiopental does not cause as much bronchodilation as propofol or inhalational anesthetics.[100,101] Case reports of laryngospasm and bronchospasm after induction of anesthesia with thiopental exist, although airway reflexes are generally considered to be more preserved compared to induction with propofol.

Clinical Uses

Rapid onset and emergence from a bolus dose of thiopental have made it an ideal induction agent. The typical induction dose is 2.5 to 5 mg/kg, resulting in light stages of anesthesia in 15 to 30 seconds, and deeper stages in 30 to 40 seconds that last for approximately 1 minute. Premedication may decrease the required induction dose by as much as 50%, and nitrous oxide may decrease the plasma concentration of thiopental required for hypnosis by 67%.[102] Patient variability will affect the required induction dose. Unpremedicated healthy children may require a 5 to 6 mg/kg induction dose, and infants may have an even higher requirement.[79] Elderly patients have a lower induction dose requirement, although no significant age-specific difference in plasma concentrations of thiopental were noted to achieve a given hypnotic effect.[102] The necessary reduction in dose is likely due to variation in pharmacokinetic profile of elderly patients, including decreased volume of distribution and slower redistribution times. Obesity also has been noted to lower thiopental induction requirement on a per kilogram basis,[103] but similar to propofol, the use of lean body mass to determine induction dose corrects the difference. Numerous comorbid states have been associated with a decrease in induction dose requirement—if not relative contraindication—including liver disease, heart failure, shock, and severe anemia. Methohexital can also be used for induction of anesthesia, with the typical intravenous induction dose 1 to 2 mg/kg. It has also historically been administered rectally in solution form as a sedative in the pediatric population, with the recommended dose of 25 mg/kg.[104]

Thiopental is rarely used as an intravenous infusion for maintenance of general anesthesia because higher doses lead to zero-order kinetics and a slow plasma clearance. The context-sensitive half-time of thiopental is relatively high and results in unpredictable and prolonged recovery from infusion. Methohexital has a shorter elimination half-life than thiopental, and at infusion doses of 50 to 150 mcg/kg/min has been used for maintenance of sedation and general anesthesia. Concern for seizure activity after prolonged infusions in susceptible patient populations has minimized this utility. As noted, thiopental infusion for maintenance of barbiturate coma has been utilized in patients with elevated ICP after acute brain injury, but the efficacy of thiopental in preventing long-term brain injury and improving outcomes has been questioned.

Side Effects

Intravenous administration of thiopental is typically not irritating or painful, but if injected outside the vein into subcutaneous tissue, it can cause discomfort. Methohexital-induced pain on injection is much more prevalent. Inadvertent arterial administration of thiopental has to be managed promptly, as formation of crystals can lead to decreased flow due to vasospasm and thrombus formation, pain at the arterial site, and possible tissue necrosis. Management includes arterial administration of papaverine, heparinization, and potential arteriodilation by appropriate regional anesthetic technique. Barbiturates are contraindicated in patients with acute intermittent porphyria, as an exacerbation of symptoms may be augmented by their direct effects on hepatic enzymes.

New Intravenous Anesthetics

New drugs are constantly being developed in an effort to achieve 10
the ideal intravenous anesthetic with a short duration of action, a short context-sensitive half-time that allows for infusion administration, and minimal adverse effects (Fig. 19-14).

Propofol Formulations

Propofol is a hydrophobic oil that requires a lipid emulsion as a vehicle of administration. This emulsion, comprised largely of egg

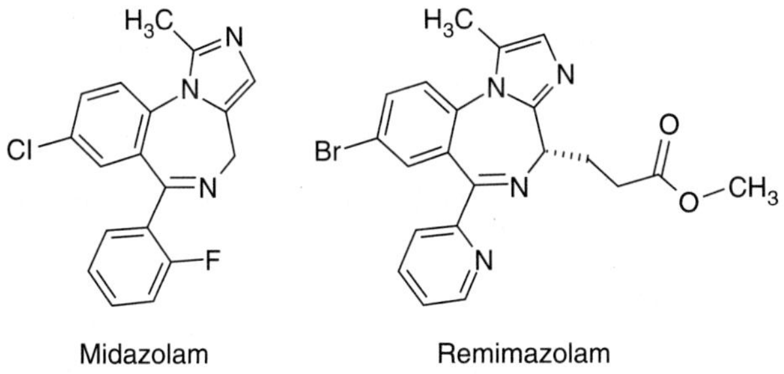

Midazolam Remimazolam

Figure 19-14 Structural comparison between midazolam and remimazolam.

Etomidate CPMM

Etomidate metabolite CPMM metabolite

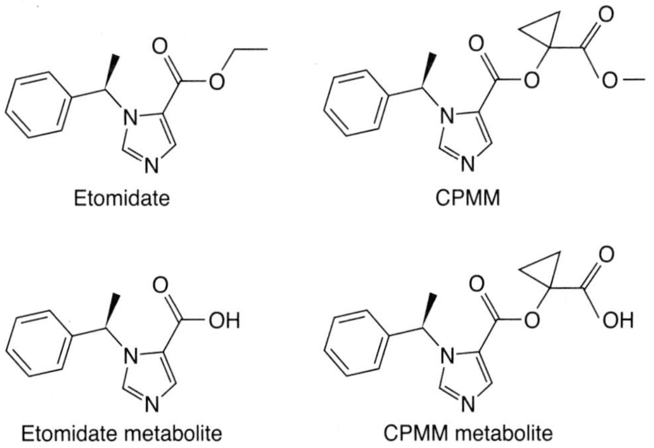

Figure 19-15 Etomidate, cyclopropyl–methoxycarbonyl metomidate (CPMM), and their metabolites.

yolk lecithin, soybean oil, and glycerol, has several drawbacks. The most common complaint is pain on injection. More serious adverse effects include anaphylaxis, sepsis secondary to microbial contamination of an open vial (despite antimicrobial additives), and PRIS.[105] Many attempts have been made to develop a formulation of propofol that reduces these problems, including (1) to reduce the percentage of lipid in the emulsion; (2) to eliminate the lipid; and (3) to create a prodrug. One major challenge with tailoring the current formulation is that the drug's well-described pharmacokinetics may also be altered.

Fospropofol: Fospropofol is a prodrug of propofol that designed to reduce or eliminate the adverse effects of the current propofol emulsion. Fospropofol is a water-based solution that yields less pain on injection, less hyperlipidemia, and less risk for bacteremia. Its clinical application as a sedative–hypnotic has been approved for MAC sedation, but not for general anesthesia. A major deterrent to its use is its delayed onset time and longer elimination time. Although hypotension and respiratory depression may occur less frequently, these reactions still do occur. Fospropofol is also associated with an increase in pruritus and paresthesias.[106] Fospropofol was initially developed as a drug to be used by nonanesthesia medical providers. However, fospropofol is associated with similar respiratory depression as propofol, and practitioners must be able to rescue patients from unintended deep sedation or general anesthesia. Fospropofol is currently not approved for use in the United States. Possible reasons for this includes its delayed onset of effect, slower recovery compared to propofol, and significant associated perineal paresthesia and pruritus.

Cyclopropyl-methoxycarbonyl metomidate (CPMM). CPMM, also known as AB700, is an analog of etomidate that has shown promise in animal studies. It causes less adrenal suppression compared with etomidate. It also is less potent and has a shorter duration of action than etomidate. The investigators of this drug purport its use as a bolus or infusion medication for both sedation and general anesthesia.[107] Although its structure is a derivative of etomidate, its clinical application seems to be more consistent with that of propofol. Some studies have even demonstrated that compared to propofol, CPMM has less drug accumulation and therefore more rapid recovery after prolonged infusion (Fig. 19-15).[107]

THRX-918661/AZD-3043. The search for a sedative/hypnotic agent whose effects are terminated in a predictable and consistent time frame regardless of dose or duration of infusion has led to the development of THRX-918661/AZD-3043. This medication is a metabolically labile, positive allosteric modulator of the GABA-A receptor. This investigational drug is water-soluble and rapidly hydrolyzed by blood and tissue esterases to an inactive carboxylate metabolite.[108] A phase I clinical trial showed no serious adverse events and a rapid recovery after infusion administration. Further studies will be required to evaluate the potential of THRX-918661/AZD-3043 to provide rapid recovery regardless of duration of anesthesia.[109]

SEDASYS. In May 2013, the FDA approved Sedasys, a computer-assisted patient-controlled sedation system that administers propofol for colonoscopies/endoscopies. Patients are monitored with ECG, pulse oximetry, noninvasive blood pressure, and end-tidal carbon dioxide. Sedation is also further monitored via an earpiece through which the computer tells the patient to squeeze a handset. Based on these parameters, Sedasys will algorithmically adjust the infusion rate of propofol.

An early study of 1,000 ASA class 1 to 3 patients, who used the Sedasys system reported fewer episodes of desaturation and improved patient and physician satisfaction.[110] Sedasys affords nonanesthesia providers the ability to conduct procedures that require minimal to moderate sedation with propofol. Health care cost savings might theoretically result from removing the anesthesiologist from the cost of the procedure. However, many physicians, especially anesthesiologists, are skeptical of the safety of this patient-controlled system. For example, there are times when deeper planes of anesthesia are needed, yet cannot be provided by Sedasys. Patients may cough or buck or obstruct their airway during the procedure, and nonanesthesia providers may not be sufficiently trained or skilled in airway management. Furthermore, sampling of the end-tidal carbon dioxide may not be accurate secondary to the endoscope physically being near the airway.[111] Sedasys failed to gain popularity and adoption for the following reasons: (1) the device was programmed only to decrease, but not increase depth of sedation, (2) its dosing algorithm was not sufficiently efficient for the fast pace and turnover of most diagnostic upper GI endoscopic procedures, and (3) the device failed to satisfy both patients and providers, limited by the FDA approval for no more than moderate sedation.[112] As of 2016, the device is no longer marketed.

For further review and interactivities, please see the videos and narrative interactive clinical vignettes (NICVs) accessible in the complimentary eBook bundled with this text. Access instructions are located on the inside front cover.

REFERENCES

1. White PF. Clinical uses of intravenous anesthetic and analgesic infusions. *Anesth Analg.* 1989;68(2):161–171.
2. Perouanski MA, Hemmings HC. Intravenous anesthetic agents. In Hemmings HC, Hopkins PM, eds. *Foundations of Anesthesia.* 2nd Edn. Philadelphia: Mosby Elsevier; 2006:295–310.

3. Kam PCA, Cardone D. Propofol infusion syndrome. *Anaesthesia*. 2007;62(7):690–701.
4. Gepts E. Pharmacokinetic concepts for TCI anaesthesia. *Anaesthesia*. 1998;53(Suppl 1):4–12.
5. Struys MMRF, De Smet T, Glen JIB, Vereecke HEM, Absalom AR, Schnider TW. The history of target-controlled infusion. *Anesth Analg*. 2016;122(1):56–69.
6. Kay B, Rolly G.I.C.I. 35868, a new intravenous induction agent. *Acta Anaesthesiol Belg*. 1977;28(4):303–316.
7. Krasowski MD, Koltchine VV, Rick CE, Ye Q, Finn SE, Harrison NL. Propofol and other intravenous anesthetics have sites of action on the gamma-aminobutyric acid type a receptor distinct from that for isoflurane. *Mol Pharmacol*. 1998;53(3):530–538.
8. Kikuchi T, Wang Y, Sato K, Okumura F. In vivo effects of propofol on acetylcholine release from the frontal cortex, hippocampus and striatum studied by intracerebral microdialysis in freely moving rats. *Br J Anaesth*. 1998;80(5):644–648.
9. Alkire MT, Hudetz AG, Tononi G. Consciousness and anesthesia. *Science*. 2008;322(5903): 876–880.
10. Fiset P, Paus T, Daloze T, et al. Brain mechanisms of propofol-induced loss of consciousness in humans: a positron emission tomographic study. *J Neurosci*. 1999;19(13):5506–5513.
11. Bevan JC, Veall GR, Macnab AJ, Ries CR, Marsland C. Midazolam premedication delays recovery after propofol without modifying involuntary movements. *Anesth Analg*. 1997;85(1):50–54.
12. Feshchenko VA, Veselis RA, Reinsel RA. Propofol-induced alpha rhythm. *Neuropsychobiology*. 2004;50(3):257–266.
13. Murphy PG, Myers DS, Davies MJ, Webster NR, Jones JG. The antioxidant potential of propofol (2,6-diisopropylphenol). *Br J Anaesth*. 1992;68(6):613–618.
14. Lingamaneni R, Birch ML, Hemmings HC Jr. Widespread inhibition of sodium channel-dependent glutamate release from isolated nerve terminals by isoflurane and propofol. *Anesthesiology*. 2001;95(6):1460–1466.
15. Engelhard K, Werner C, Eberspächer E, et al. Influence of propofol on neuronal damage and apoptotic factors after incomplete cerebral ischemia and reperfusion in rats: a long-term observation. *Anesthesiology*. 2004;101(4):912–917.
16. Liu J, Gao XF, Ni W, Li JB. Effects of propofol on P2X7 receptors and the secretion of tumor necrosis factor-α in cultured astrocytes. *Clin Exp Med*. 2012;12(1):31–37.
17. Ebrahim ZY, Schubert A, Van Ness P, Wolgamuth B, Awad I. The effect of propofol on the electroencephalogram of patients with epilepsy. *Anesth Analg*. 1994;78(2):275–279.
18. Samra SK, Sneyd JR, Ross DA, Henry TR. Effects of propofol sedation on seizures and intracranially recorded epileptiform activity in patients with partial epilepsy. *Anesthesiology*. 1995; 82(4):843–851.
19. Wischmeyer PE, Johnson BR, Wilson JE, et al. A survey of propofol abuse in academic anesthesia programs. *Anesth Analg*. 2007;105(4):1066–1071.
20. Fulton B, Sorkin EM. Propofol: an overview of its pharmacology and a review of its clinical efficacy in intensive care sedation. *Drugs*. 1995;50(4):636–657.
21. Drug Enforcement Agency USDoJ. Drugs of Abuse, A Resource Guide. 2020. Accessed July 26, 2022. https://www.dea.gov/sites/default/files/2020-04/Drugs%20of%20Abuse%20 2020-Web%20Version-508%20compliant-4-24-20_0.pdf
22. Meuret P, Backman SB, Bonhomme V, Plourde G, Fiset P. Physostigmine reverses propofol-induced unconsciousness and attenuation of the auditory steady state response and bispectral index in human volunteers. *Anesthesiology*. 2000;93(3):708–717.
23. Samain E, Bouillier H, Marty J, Safar M, Dagher G. The effect of propofol on angiotensin II-induced Ca(2+) mobilization in aortic smooth muscle cells from normotensive and hypertensive rats. *Anesth Analg*. 2000;90(3):546–552.
24. Pires LA, Huang SK, Wagshal AB, Kulkarni RS. Electrophysiological effects of propofol on the normal cardiac conduction system. *Cardiology*. 1996;87(4):319–324.
25. Kirkpatrick T, Cockshott ID, Douglas EJ, Nimmo WS. Pharmacokinetics of propofol (diprivan) in elderly patients. *Br J Anaesth*. 1988;60(2):146–150.
26. Marsh B, White M, Morton N, Kenny GN. Pharmacokinetic model driven infusion of propofol in children. *Br J Anaesth*. 1991;67(1):41–48.
27. Ingrande J, Brodsky JB, Lemmens HJM. Lean body weight scalar for the anesthetic induction dose of propofol in morbidly obese subjects. *Anesth Analg*. 2011;113(1):57–62.
28. Gan TJ, Glass PS, Howell ST, Canada AT, Grant AP, Ginsberg B. Determination of plasma concentrations of propofol associated with 50% reduction in postoperative nausea. *Anesthesiology*. 1997;87(4):779–784.
29. Picard P, Tramèr MR. Prevention of pain on injection with propofol: a quantitative systematic review. *Anesth Analg*. 2000;90(4):963–969.
30. Jalota L, Kalira V, George E, et al; Perioperative Clinical Research Core. Prevention of pain on injection of propofol: systematic review and meta-analysis. *BMJ*. 2011;342:d1110.
31. Parke TJ, Stevens JE, Rice AS, et al. Metabolic acidosis and fatal myocardial failure after propofol infusion in children: five case reports. *BMJ*. 1992;305(6854):613–616.
32. Cremer OL, Moons KG, Bouman EA, Kruijswijk JE, de Smet AM, Kalkman CJ. Long-term propofol infusion and cardiac failure in adult head-injured patients. *Lancet*. 2001;357(9250):117–118.
33. Krajčová A, Waldauf P, Anděl M, Duška F. Propofol infusion syndrome: a structured review of experimental studies and 153 published case reports. *Crit Care*. 2015;19:398.
34. Tan CK, Lai CC, Cheng KC. Propofol-related green urine. *Kidney Int*. 2008;74(7):978.
35. Gooding JM, Corssen G. Effect of etomidate on the cardiovascular system. *Anesth Analg*. 1977;56(5):717–719.
36. Meyancı Köksal G, Erbabacan E, Tunalı Y, Karaören G, Vehid S, Öz H. The effect of single dose etomidate during emergency intubation on hemodynamics and adrenal cortex. *Ulus Travma Acil Cerrahi Derg*. 2015;21(5):358–365.
37. Gu WJ, Wang F, Tang L, Liu JC. Single-dose etomidate does not increase mortality in patients with sepsis: a systematic review and meta-analysis of randomized controlled trials and observational studies. *Chest*. 2015;147(2):335–346.
38. Chan CM, Mitchell AL, Shorr AF. Etomidate is associated with mortality and adrenal insufficiency in sepsis: a meta-analysis*. *Crit Care Med*. 2012;40(11):2945–2953.
39. Domino EF, Chodoff P, Corssen G. Pharmacologic effects of CI-581, a new dissociative anesthetic, in man. *Clin Pharmacol Ther*. 1965;6:279–291.
40. Visser E, Schug SA. The role of ketamine in pain management. *Biomed Pharmacother*. 2006;60(7):341–348.
41. Fond G, Loundou A, Rabu C, et al. Ketamine administration in depressive disorders: a systematic review and meta-analysis. *Psychopharmacology (Berl)*. 2014;231(18):3663–3676.
42. Potter DE, Choudhury M. Ketamine: repurposing and redefining a multifaceted drug. *Drug Discov Today*. 2014;19(12):1848–1854.
43. Marland S, Ellerton J, Andolfatto G, et al. Ketamine: use in anesthesia. *CNS Neurosci Ther*. 2013;19(6):381–389.
44. Clements JA, Nimmo WS, Grant IS. Bioavailability, pharmacokinetics, and analgesic activity of ketamine in humans. *J Pharm Sci*. 1982;71(5):539–542.
45. Clements JA, Nimmo WS. Pharmacokinetics and analgesic effect of ketamine in man. *Br J Anaesth*. 1981;53(1):27–30.
46. Brown EN, Lydic R, Schiff ND. General anesthesia, sleep, and coma. *N Engl J Med*. 2010; 363(27):2638–2650.
47. Sengupta S, Ghosh S, Rudra A, Kumar P, Maitra G, Das T. Effect of ketamine on bispectral index during propofol–fentanyl anesthesia: a randomized controlled study. *Middle East J Anaesthesiol*. 2011;21(3):391–395.
48. Mion G, Villevieille T. Ketamine pharmacology: an update (pharmacodynamics and molecular aspects, recent findings). *CNS Neurosci Ther*. 2013;19(6):370–380.
49. Hirota K, Lambert DG. Ketamine: new uses for an old drug? *Br J Anaesth*. 2011;107(2):123–126.
50. Jabre P, Combes X, Lapostolle F, et al; KETASED Collaborative Study Group. Etomidate versus ketamine for rapid sequence intubation in acutely ill patients: a multicentre randomised controlled trial. *Lancet*. 2009;374(9686):293–300.
51. Schmid RL, Sandler AN, Katz J. Use and efficacy of low-dose ketamine in the management of acute postoperative pain: a review of current techniques and outcomes. *Pain*. 1999;82(2): 111–125.
52. Niesters M, Martini C, Dahan A. Ketamine for chronic pain: risks and benefits. *Br J Clin Pharmacol*. 2014;77(2):357–367.
53. Carr DB, Goudas LC, Denman WT, et al. Safety and efficacy of intranasal ketamine for the treatment of breakthrough pain in patients with chronic pain: a randomized, double-blind, placebo-controlled, crossover study. *Pain*. 2004;108(1-2):17–27.
54. Huge V, Lauchart M, Magerl W, et al. Effects of low-dose intranasal (S)-ketamine in patients with neuropathic pain. *Eur J Pain*. 2010;14(4):387–394.
55. Riediger C, Haschke M, Bitter C, et al. The analgesic effect of combined treatment with intranasal S-ketamine and intranasal midazolam compared with morphine patient-controlled analgesia in spinal surgery patients: a pilot study. *J Pain Res*. 2015;8:87–94.
56. Newport DJ, Carpenter LL, McDonald WM, Potash JB, Tohen M, Nemeroff CB; APA Council of Research Task Force on Novel Biomarkers and Treatments. Ketamine and other NMDA antagonists: early clinical trials and possible mechanisms in depression. *Am J Psychiatry*. 2015;172(10):950–966.
57. Murrough JW, Iosifescu DV, Chang LC, et al. Antidepressant efficacy of ketamine in treatment-resistant major depression: a two-site randomized controlled trial. *Am J Psychiatry*. 2013;170(10):1134–1142.
58. Kohtala S. Ketamine-50 years in use: from anesthesia to rapid antidepressant effects and neurobiological mechanisms. *Pharmacol Rep*. 2021;73(2):323–345.
59. Zarate CA Jr, Singh JB, Quiroz JA, et al. A double-blind, placebo-controlled study of memantine in the treatment of major depression. *Am J Psychiatry*. 2006;163(1):153–155.
60. Lippmann M, Appel PL, Mok MS, Shoemaker WC. Sequential cardiorespiratory patterns of anesthetic induction with ketamine in critically ill patients. *Crit Care Med*. 1983;11(9): 730–734.
61. Allen JY, Macias CG. The efficacy of ketamine in pediatric emergency department patients who present with acute severe asthma. *Ann Emerg Med*. 2005;46(1):43–50.
62. Mayberg TS, Lam AM, Matta BF, Domino KB, Winn HR. Ketamine does not increase cerebral blood flow velocity or intracranial pressure during isoflurane/nitrous oxide anesthesia in patients undergoing craniotomy. *Anesth Analg*. 1995;81(1):84–89.
63. Hoy SM, Keating GM. Dexmedetomidine: a review of its use for sedation in mechanically ventilated patients in an intensive care setting and for procedural sedation. *Drugs*. 2011; 71(11):1481–1501.
64. Tobias JD. Dexmedetomidine: applications in pediatric critical care and pediatric anesthesiology. *Pediatr Crit Care Med*. 2007;8(2):115–131.
65. Gertler R, Brown HC, Mitchell DH, Silvius EN. Dexmedetomidine: a novel sedative-analgesic agent. *Proc (Bayl Univ Med Cent)*. 2001;14(1):13–21.

66. Adams R, Brown GT, Davidson M, et al. Efficacy of dexmedetomidine compared with midazolam for sedation in adult intensive care patients: a systematic review. *Br J Anaesth.* 2013;111(5):703–710.
67. Arain SR, Ebert TJ. The efficacy, side effects, and recovery characteristics of dexmedetomidine versus propofol when used for intraoperative sedation. *Anesth Analg.* 2002;95(2):461–466, table of contents.
68. Kaygusuz K, Gokce G, Gursoy S, Ayan S, Mimaroglu C, Gultekin Y. A comparison of sedation with dexmedetomidine or propofol during shockwave lithotripsy: a randomized controlled trial. *Anesth Analg.* 2008;106(1):114–119, table of contents.
69. Muller S, Borowics SM, Fortis EAF, et al. Clinical efficacy of dexmedetomidine alone is less than propofol for conscious sedation during ERCP. *Gastrointest Endosc.* 2008;67(4):651–659.
70. Eberl S, Preckel B, Bergman JJ, van Dieren S, Hollmann MW. Satisfaction and safety using dexmedetomidine or propofol sedation during endoscopic oesophageal procedures: A randomised controlled trial. *Eur J Anaesthesiol.* 2016;33(9):631–637.
71. Mahmoud M, Mason KP. Dexmedetomidine: review, update, and future considerations of paediatric perioperative and periprocedural applications and limitations. *Br J Anaesth.* 2015; 115(2):171–182.
72. Pickard A, Davies P, Birnie K, Beringer R. Systematic review and meta-analysis of the effect of intraoperative α_2-adrenergic agonists on postoperative behaviour in children. *Br J Anaesth.* 2014;112(6):982–990.
73. Abdallah FW, Brull R. Facilitatory effects of perineural dexmedetomidine on neuraxial and peripheral nerve block: a systematic review and meta-analysis. *Br J Anaesth.* 2013;110(6): 915–925.
74. Piao G, Wu J. Systematic assessment of dexmedetomidine as an anesthetic agent: a meta-analysis of randomized controlled trials. *Arch Med Sci.* 2014;10(1):19–24.
75. Ingersoll-Weng E, Manecke GR Jr, Thistlethwaite PA. Dexmedetomidine and cardiac arrest. *Anesthesiology.* 2004;100(3):738–739.
76. Jorden VSB, Pousman RM, Sanford MM, Thorborg PAJ, Hutchens MP. Dexmedetomidine overdose in the perioperative setting. *Ann Pharmacother.* 2004;38(5):803–807.
77. Nath SS, Singh S, Pawar ST. Dexmedetomidine overdosage: an unusual presentation. *Indian J Anaesth.* 2013;57(3):289–291.
78. Kanto J, Allonen H. Pharmacokinetics and the sedative effect of midazolam. *Int J Clin Pharmacol Ther Toxicol.* 1983;21(9):460–463.
79. Coté CJ, Goudsouzian NG, Liu LM, Dedrick DF, Rosow CE. The dose response of intravenous thiopental for the induction of general anesthesia in unpremedicated children. *Anesthesiology.* 1981;55(6):703–705.
80. Kain ZN, Mayes LC, Wang SM, Hofstadter MB. Postoperative behavioral outcomes in children: effects of sedative premedication. *Anesthesiology.* 1999;90(3):758–765.
81. Magarey JM. Propofol or midazolam–which is best for the sedation of adult ventilated patients in intensive care units? A systematic review. *Aust Crit Care.* 2001;14(4):147–154.
82. Fragen RJ. Pharmacokinetics and pharmacodynamics of midazolam given via continuous intravenous infusion in intensive care units. *Clin Ther.* 1997;19(3):405–419; discussion 367–368.
83. Hughes MA, Glass PS, Jacobs JR. Context-sensitive half-time in multicompartment pharmacokinetic models for intravenous anesthetic drugs. *Anesthesiology.* 1992;76(3):334–341.
84. Cunha J. Midazolam Injection 2015. 2015. Accessed June 29, 2022. https://www.rxlist.com/midazolam-injection-drug.htm
85. Bianchi MT, Botzolakis EJ, Lagrange AH, Macdonald RL. Benzodiazepine modulation of GABA(A) receptor opening frequency depends on activation context: a patch clamp and simulation study. *Epilepsy Res.* 2009;85(2-3):212–220.
86. Amrein R, Hetzel W, Hartmann D, Lorscheid T. Clinical pharmacology of flumazenil. *Eur J Anaesthesiol Suppl.* 1988;2:65–80.
87. Agency EM. Byfavo (remimazolam). 2021. Accessed June 29, 2022. https://www.ema.europa.eu/en/medicines/human/EPAR/byfavo
88. Goudra BG, Singh PM. Remimazolam: the future of its sedative potential. *Saudi J Anaesth.* 2014;8(3):388–391.
89. Jhuang BJ, Yeh BH, Huang YT, Lai PC. Efficacy and safety of remimazolam for procedural sedation: a meta-analysis of randomized controlled trials with trial sequential analysis. *Front Med (Lausanne).* 2021;8:641866.
90. Kilpatrick GJ. Remimazolam: non-clinical and clinical profile of a new sedative/anesthetic agent. *Front Pharmacol.* 2021;12:690875.
91. Dundee JW. Biotransformation of thiopental and other thiobarbiturates. *Int Anesthesiol Clin.* 1974;12(2):121–133.
92. Paul R, Harris R. A comparison of methohexitone and thiopentone in electrocorticography. *J Neurol Neurosurg Psychiatry.* 1970;33(1):100–104.
93. Rampton AJ, Griffin RM, Stuart CS, Durcan JJ, Huddy NC, Abbott MA. Comparison of methohexital and propofol for electroconvulsive therapy: effects on hemodynamic responses and seizure duration. *Anesthesiology.* 1989;70(3):412–417.
94. Baughman VL. Brain protection during neurosurgery. *Anesthesiol Clin North Am.* 2002; 20(2):315–327, vi.
95. Warner DS, Takaoka S, Wu B, et al. Electroencephalographic burst suppression is not required to elicit maximal neuroprotection from pentobarbital in a rat model of focal cerebral ischemia. *Anesthesiology.* 1996;84(6):1475–1484.
96. Brain Resuscitation Clinical Trial I Study Group. Randomized clinical study of thiopental loading in comatose survivors of cardiac arrest. *N Engl J Med.* 1986;314(7):397–403.
97. Chamberlain JH, Seed RG, Chung DC. Effect of thiopentone on myocardial function. *Br J Anaesth.* 1977;49(9):865–870.
98. Bernhoff A, Eklund B, Kaijser L. Cardiovascular effects of short-term anaesthesia with methohexitone and propanidid in normal subjects. *Br J Anaesth.* 1972;44(1):2–7.
99. Blouin RT, Conard PF, Gross JB. Time course of ventilatory depression following induction doses of propofol and thiopental. *Anesthesiology.* 1991;75(6):940–944.
100. Goff MJ, Arain SR, Ficke DJ, Uhrich TD, Ebert TJ. Absence of bronchodilation during desflurane anesthesia: a comparison to sevoflurane and thiopental. *Anesthesiology.* 2000; 93(2):404–408.
101. Wu RS, Wu KC, Sum DC, Bishop MJ. Comparative effects of thiopentone and propofol on respiratory resistance after tracheal intubation. *Br J Anaesth.* 1996;77(6):735–738.
102. Becker KE Jr, Tonnesen AS. Cardiovascular effects of plasma levels of thiopental necessary for anesthesia. *Anesthesiology.* 1978;49(3):197–200.
103. Jung D, Mayersohn M, Perrier D, Calkins J, Saunders R. Thiopental disposition in lean and obese patients undergoing surgery. *Anesthesiology.* 1982;56(4):269–274.
104. Rodriguez E, Jordan R. Contemporary trends in pediatric sedation and analgesia. *Emerg Med Clin North Am.* 2002;20(1):199–222.
105. Egan TD. Exploring the frontiers of propofol formulation strategy: is there life beyond the milky way? *Br J Anaesth.* 2010;104(5):533–535.
106. Bengalorkar GM, Bhuvana K, Sarala N, Kumar T. Fospropofol: clinical pharmacology. *J Anaesthesiol Clin Pharmacol.* 2011;27(1):79–83.
107. Campagna JA, Pojasek K, Grayzel D, Randle J, Raines DE. Advancing novel anesthetics: pharmacodynamic and pharmacokinetic studies of cyclopropyl-methoxycarbonyl metomidate in dogs. *Anesthesiology.* 2014;121(6):1203–1216.
108. Egan TD, Shafer SL, Jenkins TE, et al. The pharmacokinetics and pharmacodynamics of THRX-918661, a novel sedative/hypnotic agent. *Anesthesiology.* 2003;99:A–516.
109. Norberg Å, Koch P, Kanes SJ, et al. A bolus and bolus followed by infusion study of AZD3043, an investigational intravenous drug for sedation and anesthesia: safety and pharmacodynamics in healthy male and female volunteers. *Anesth Analg.* 2015;121(4):894–903.
110. Pambianco DJ, Vargo JJ, Pruitt RE, Hardi R, Martin JF. Computer-assisted personalized sedation for upper endoscopy and colonoscopy: a comparative, multicenter randomized study. *Gastrointest Endosc.* 2011;73(4):765–772.
111. Goudra BG, Singh PM, Chandrasekhara V. SEDASYS(®), airway, oxygenation, and ventilation: anticipating and managing the challenges. *Dig Dis Sci.* 2014;59(5):920–927.
112. Goudra B, Singh PM. Failure of sedasys: destiny or poor design? *Anesth Analg.* 2017;124(2): 686–688.

20 Opioids

ALBERT DAHAN • MARIEKE NIESTERS • TERRY SMITH • FRANK J. OVERDYK

KEY POINTS

1 Opioids produce analgesia as well as serious side effects. All physicians who prescribe opioids for relief of acute or chronic pain need to know how to use these drugs safely. This requires an in-depth understanding of the pharmacokinetics and pharmacodynamics of opioids as well as the acquisition of sufficient clinical experience in their use.

2 Opioids can be classified according to strength or potency based on the plasma concentrations at which they exert their effects (C_{50} or the plasma concentration causing a 50% effect). Strong opioids include fentanyl, sufentanil, and remifentanil. Weak opioids include codeine and tramadol. An intermediate group includes morphine, methadone, oxycodone, and buprenorphine.

3 Opioids act through specific opioid receptors on neuronal tissues such as peripheral nerves and neurons in the spinal cord and brain. The most important receptors include the μ-opioid receptor (MOR), δ-opioid receptor (DOR), and κ-opioid receptor (KOR). For anesthesia and pain relief, the MOR is most important. Opioids also act through nonneuronal pathways, such as those affecting the immune system, which may be of relevance in the treatment of inflammatory pain.

4 Endogenous opioid pathways are activated in cases of stress-induced analgesia, placebo-induced analgesia, and conditioned pain modulation (CPM). CPM occurs when pain arising from one focus is decreased by application of a second painful stimulus (pain inhibits pain).

5 Opioid-induced hyperalgesia (OIH) is a paradoxical opioid effect whereby pain sensitivity increases during or following escalating opioid treatment. It is also observed postoperatively following the use of a remifentanil infusion during anesthesia. Greater and more frequent doses of morphine are required to treat postoperative pain. OIH may be treated and prevented by administration of a low dose of ketamine, an *N*-methyl-D-aspartate (NMDA) receptor antagonist.

6 Tolerance to opioid-induced respiratory depression develops more slowly than tolerance to pain relief. Tolerance is a dynamic process and after a long period of abstinence from opioids, the risk of opioid toxicity increases.

7 The pharmacokinetic characteristics of a drug determine its behavior in the body of a patient. One important pharmacokinetic concept for opioids is that of context-sensitive half-time (CSt½). This is the time needed for the opioid's plasma concentration to decrease by 50% from a steady-state concentration. This value is not a constant but is dependent on the duration of the infusion of the opioid. For example, the CSt½ of fentanyl increases rapidly with the infusion duration. In contrast, the CSt½ of remifentanil is independent of the infusion duration due to its rapid elimination from plasma by nonspecific plasma esterases in plasma.

8 Opioid metabolism is affected by drugs that interfere with metabolizing cytochrome P450 (CYP) enzymes, most importantly CYP3A4. Opioid metabolites can be active or inactive. Active metabolites need to be considered when treating patients. For example, the active metabolite of morphine, morphine-6-glucuronide, can accumulate in patients with renal impairment. Genetic variability in the CYP system can have important clinical implications, especially in case of variations in the copies of a gene coding for the metabolizing enzyme. An example is the enzyme CYP2D6, which catalyzes the conversion of codeine into morphine. Patients with multiple copies of the CYP2D6 gene and who receive codeine will have large plasma morphine concentrations with all related beneficial and adverse side effects.

9 Opioid effects are variable among patients. Dosing is optimum when opioids are titrated to the effect. It is also important to consider the delay between the administration of an opioid and its effect, which is defined as the blood–effect site equilibration half-life, or $t\frac{1}{2}k_{e0}$. This will allow proper and timely dosing, particularly when anticipating a stressful event (laryngoscopy, intubation, skin incision, etc.) and administering opioids to prevent the occurrence of a large hemodynamic response to these stimuli. Since the $t\frac{1}{2}k_{e0}$ of morphine is about 90 minutes, it is important to give an initial bolus dose or morphine at least 60 minutes before the end of surgery when using the drug for postoperative pain relief.

10 Opioids reduce the requirement of inhalational anesthetics and propofol during anesthesia, which makes rapid awakening from anesthesia possible. Using known pharmacokinetic and pharmacodynamic data, it can be determined what doses and plasma concentrations will permit the shortest time to awakening. For example, termination of drug infusions at plasma concentrations of propofol 1.5 µg/mL and remifentanil 9.0 ng/mL will lead to patient awakening within 6.5 minutes.

11 In the perioperative setting, careful, slow infusion of opioids allows the gradual accumulation of arterial CO_2, which serves as a respiratory stimulant at the chemoreceptors and lowers the probability of apnea.

12 Administration of opioids can potentially lead to life-threatening respiratory depression. The incidence of serious perioperative respiratory events is approximately 0.5% (1 in every 200 patients). In the acute setting, risk factors include sleep-disordered breathing, obesity, renal impairment, pulmonary disease, neurologic disorders, and CYP450 enzyme polymorphism. In the pediatric population, risk factors include morphine administration in patients with renal impairment, adenotonsillectomy for recurrent tonsillitis, and/or obstructive sleep apnea and codeine use in patients with CYP2D6 gene polymorphism associated with the ultrarapid metabolizer phenotype. In chronic pain patients, risk factors included renal failure, sensory deafferentation, and drug–drug interactions.

13 The risk of opioid-induced respiratory depression increases when opioids are consumed in combination with other centrally acting respiratory depressants such as alcohol, benzodiazepines, antidepressants, and antipsychotics. This is a serious cause of enhanced mortality, as a large number of patients that die from opioids also had sedatives in their system.

14 The nonspecific opioid receptor antagonist, naloxone, is currently the drug of choice to reverse opioid-induced respiratory depression. The required dose of naloxone depends on the pharmacokinetic and pharmacodynamic properties and the dose of the opioid that needs reversal. Postoperatively, when there is persistent apnea, opioid concentrations are often just above the threshold for respiratory depression. Intravenous administration of naloxone using incremental doses of 40 to 80 µg, to a cumulative dose of less than 400 µg, may be sufficient for breathing to resume.

15 New drugs are being developed that reverse or prevent opioid-induced respiratory depression without affecting analgesia. Drugs that stimulate opioid-depressed breathing include ketamine, nicotinic acetylcholine receptor agonists, ampakines, and potassium channel blockers acting at the carotid bodies.

16 Apart from respiratory depression, opioids cause a large number of side effects that require treatment: nausea, smooth muscle spasms, skeletal muscle rigidity, histamine release, pruritus (especially after spinal administration), miosis, sedation, and dizziness. The cardiovascular side effects of opioids include bradycardia and hypotension but are generally mild at usual clinical doses. However, when combined with anesthetics, even at usual clinical doses, or in severely ill patients, opioids may produce hemodynamic instability, which requires treatment.

Introduction

1 Modern medicine depends heavily on opioid analgesics for the management of moderate to severe pain. While opioids were initially intended for use in palliative care and for treatment of acute (perioperative) pain, in recent decades, there has been an exponential rise in the prescription of opioid analgesics for treatment of chronic noncancer pain, particularly oxycodone. This rise was encouraged in part by pain guidelines that emphasized aggressive treatment of any form of pain with opioids, lead to opioid dependence and addiction, encouraged illicit opioid uses (heroin, fentanyl), and spawned the opioid epidemic.[1,2] Consequently, a significant number of patients in developed countries are exposed to these potent drugs that not only produce pain relief but also cause a variety of side effects that range from orthostatic hypotension, nausea, and constipation to harmful and potentially lethal effects such as addiction and cardiorespiratory collapse. The large increase in opioid consumption leads to hundreds of thousands of opioid deaths worldwide from these lethal effects.[3] This inappropriate use of opioids has also resulted in increasingly complex postoperative pain management problems for surgical patients,[4,5] an increase in opioid-related complications for patients with pain in general, and opioid use disorder in hundreds of thousands of individuals worldwide that are without pain but were initially treated with oxycodone or other potent opioids.[1–4] Consequently, there is an urgent need for improved education and expertise in the use of opioids in the operating room, following surgery, and on the ward, and when caring for patients with chronic pain. This education should cover all aspects of opioid treatment, including pharmacokinetics (PK), pharmacodynamics (PD), side effect profile, serious adverse event profile, and the physical and psychological consequences of opioid dependence and abuse.

History

Opium is among the oldest drugs in the world. Fossilized opium poppies have been found in Neanderthal excavation sites dating back to 30,000 BC. Many old civilizations, including the Sumerians, Egyptians, Greeks, Romans, and Chinese, used opium for nutritional, medicinal, euphoric, spiritual, and religious purposes. Just over 210 years ago, the German pharmacist and chemist Friedrich Sertürner isolated a stable alkaloid crystal from the opium sap and named it morphine after the Greek god of dreams, Morpheus.[6,7] Morphine was 10-fold more potent than opium and

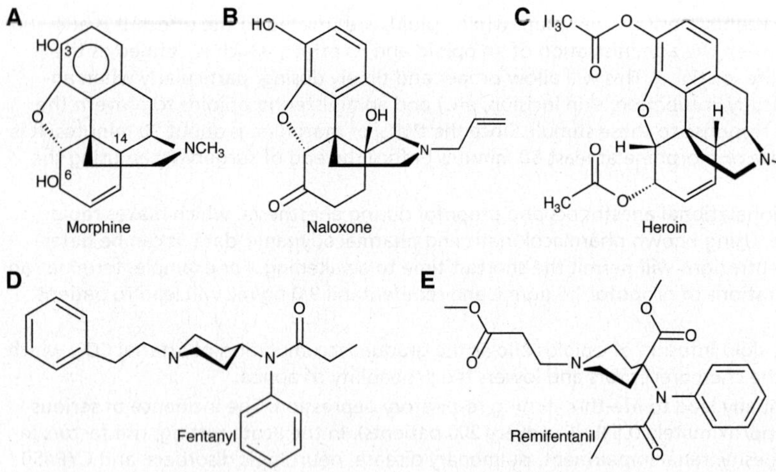

Figure 20-1 Chemical structure of commonly used opioids.

soon replaced it not only for the treatment of severe pain, but also for a myriad of other purposes such as cough and diarrhea. After the invention of the hypodermic syringe in 1853, the Englishman Alexander Wood was the first to inject morphine in a controlled fashion into a patient producing more than a day's sleep.[8] The first reported casualty from morphine occurred shortly thereafter when Wood injected his wife with morphine resulting in a fatal overdose from respiratory depression. Morphine revolutionized the treatment of the wounded in battlefield medicine, but euphoric and addictive properties led to the addiction of thousands of soldiers to morphine during the American Civil War. The synthesis of heroin in 1874 was based on the empirical finding that boiling morphine with specific acids caused the replacement of the two morphine –OH groups by –$OCOH_3$, producing diamorphine or heroin (Fig. 20-1).

Oxycodone was first synthesized in Germany during World War 1 (1916) from thebaine; in 1937, meperidine (or pethidine) became the first synthetic opioid synthesized on the basis of the central structure of morphine. Since then, many synthetic and semisynthetic opioids have been produced, including the clinically important opioid antagonists naloxone and naltrexone, by replacing the N-methyl substituent in morphine with allyl and cyclopropylmethyl groups, respectively (Fig. 20-1).[9]

2 For clinical use during anesthesia, the most important opioids are the fenylpiperidines: fentanyl, sufentanil, alfentanil, and remifentanil. These opioids produce potent analgesia and suppression of cardiovascular responses to noxious stimulation from surgery with predictable PK and PD.

Given the addictive nature of opioids and their serious cardiorespiratory depressant effects, novel opioids have recently been developed with specific characteristics intended to reduce the risk of serious side effects. For example, so-called multifunctional opioids are being developed (see below). These opioids act simultaneously at multiple receptor systems. One such opioid is tapentadol, a μ-opioid receptor (MOR) agonist that additionally inhibits the neuronal uptake of noradrenaline.[10] The adrenergic and MOR pathways behave synergistically in causing potent analgesia, with fewer side effects and less likability than oxycodone. Another novel development is the production of so-called "biased ligands" that preferentially activate the G-protein intracellular pathway, causing analgesia, at the expense of the β-arrestin pathway, which is responsible for the respiratory depressive effects of opioids. One example of a biased ligand is oliceridine.[11] The continued development of novel opioids is driven by concerns that the side effect profile of potent opioids, which presents a serious risk to patients, needs to be minimized.

The Endogenous Opioid System

A major breakthrough in the understanding of opioid pharmacol- 3
ogy came from a series of discoveries of opioid receptors, endogenous opioid peptides, their encoding genes, and endogenous opioid alkaloids. The endogenous opioid system is composed of a family of structurally related endogenous peptides that act at a four-member opioid receptor family consisting of the MOR, κ-opioid receptor (KOR), δ-opioid receptor (DOR), and nociception (NOP) receptor.[12,13] This opioid system is involved in a variety of regulatory functions including important roles in nociceptive, stress, emotional, and hedonic responses, as well as modulation of thermoregulation, breathing, neuroendocrine function, gastrointestinal (GI) motility, and immune responses.

In rodents, various subtypes of opioid receptors have also been identified, with different pharmacologic functions. For example, at least three MOR subtypes have been described: μ_1 is predominantly involved in opioid analgesia, μ_2 is involved in opioid-induced respiratory depression, and μ_3 is involved in opioid-induced immune suppression.[14,15] The functional validation of most opioid receptor subtypes awaits the development of antagonists with sufficient selectivity to allow a clear differentiation by effect. The endogenous opioid peptides include endorphins, enkephalins, and dynorphins, each of which displays different affinities for MOR, KOR, and DOR.[16] β-Endorphins have a high affinity for the MOR, met- and leu-enkephalins for the DOR, and Dynorphin A for the KOR. The recently discovered nociceptin has been identified as a selective endogenous ligand of the NOP receptor,[13] whereas endogenous morphine acts via the μ_3-receptor located on immune cells, such as human monocytes.[17]

Opioid receptors are members of the large G-protein-coupled receptor (GPCR) family.[18] GPCRs mediate a cascade of downstream signaling pathways leading to (1) the inhibition of adenyl cyclase and decreased cyclic adenosine monophosphate (cAMP), (2) activation of Ca^{2+} and K^+ channels, and (3) activation of mitogen-activated protein kinase/extracellular signal-regulated kinase, protein kinase C, and P13 K/Akt.[19] Interactions between opioid ligands and selective receptors have a number of important clinical effects. Morphine-induced analgesia and respiratory depression are both induced through activation of the MOR and subsequent activation of the adenylate cyclase/cyclic AMP pathway.[20]

Multifunctional Opioids

Most opioid analgesics act at multiple opioid receptors with different affinities.[21] For example, morphine acts with high affinity at the MOR and with lower affinities at the KOR and DOR. Some opioids act at opioid and nonopioid receptors. For example, methadone is an MOR agonist and relatively potent antagonist at the *N*-methyl-D-aspartate (NMDA) receptor.[22,23] Antagonism of the NMDA receptor is clinically useful in reducing opioid tolerance and opioid-induced hyperalgesia (OIH) and in chronic pain states leading to pain hypersensitivity.[24]

Cebranopadol is a single molecule acting at multiple receptor systems, most importantly the MOR and NOP receptors.[10] In various animal models of acute and chronic (neuropathic) pain, cebranopadol produces potent antinociception with a favorable side effect profile. Human studies are currently ongoing.

DPI-125 is an experimental drug opioid acting at MOR, KOR, and DORs. Studies in rodents suggest that this combination opioid produces less respiratory depression due to a negative effect on DOP activation and less addiction due to KOP activation.[25] Clinical studies are needed to confirm this finding.

Finally, nonopioids may also act at opioid receptors. An important example is ketamine, which is an NMDA receptor antagonist with affinity for multiple receptor systems including the opioid receptors.[26] Its anesthetic properties are related to its effect at the NMDA receptors while its analgesic effects are predominantly due to MOR activation.

Nociception and Pain

Whereas nociception is the neural process of encoding and processing of noxious stimuli that can potentially (or actually) damage tissue,[27] pain is the subjective translation of these stimuli into a perception or sensation. The International Association for the Study of Pain defines pain as an unpleasant sensory and emotional experience associated with actual or potential tissue damage, or described in terms of such damage.[28] In addition, they state[28]:

- Pain is always a personal experience that is influenced to varying degrees by biologic, psychological, and social factors.
- Pain and nociception are different phenomena. Pain cannot be inferred solely from activity in sensory neurons.
- Through their life experiences, individuals learn the concept of pain.
- A person's report of an experience as pain should be respected.
- Although pain usually serves an adaptive role, it may have adverse effects on function and social and psychological well-being.
- Verbal description is only one of several behaviors to express pain; inability to communicate does not negate the possibility that a human or a nonhuman animal experiences pain.

The Inaugural International Pain Summit in Montreal, Canada (2010) convened with the Declaration of Montreal, that stated "Access to pain management is a human right."

Opioids and Opioid Mechanisms

Classification of Exogenous Opioids

Opioids may be classified on the basis of their synthesis, chemical structure, potency, receptor binding, and effect at the opioid receptors. There are *natural* (opiates including morphine), *semisynthetic* (buprenorphine, codeine, etorphine, heroin, hydromorphone, oxycodone, and oxymorphone), and *synthetic* opioids (piperidines: loperamide, meperidine, alfentanil, fentanyl, sufentanil, remifentanil; methadones: methadone, dextropropoxyphene). Opioid potency ranges from *weak opioids* such as codeine, dextropropoxyphene, tramadol, and hydrocodone to *strong opioids*, which include etorphine, fentanyl, sufentanil, alfentanil, and remifentanil. Medium-potency opioids include morphine, methadone, oxycodone, hydromorphone, and buprenorphine. Irrespective of the "strength" of these agents, all of these agents may potentially produce serious and potentially life-threatening side effects including sedation and respiratory depression, hypotension, and bradycardia. During surgery, *strong* opioids are used in high doses, while in the postoperative phase, medium-strength opioids such as morphine or methadone are used for treatment of acute pain. In 1986, the World Health Organization designed a stepwise approach for treatment of chronic cancer pain in which *weak* opioids are prescribed before *strong* opioids (www.who.int/cancer/palliative/painladder/en/). Opioids may be *full agonists,* which cause the maximum possible effect when activating their receptors. Opioid full agonists at the MOR include morphine, piperidines, and methadone. Opioid *partial agonists*, such as buprenorphine and nalbuphine, activate their receptor but cause only a partial or reduced effect. Naloxone and naltrexone are opioid *antagonists*. It is more practical to classify opioids with a rapid onset and offset of action (e.g., remifentanil and alfentanil) versus agents with a slow onset/offset of action (e.g., morphine and buprenorphine). The concept of onset/offset of action will be discussed below.

Central Opioid Analgesia

Opioids modify both nociception and the perception of a noxious stimulus (emotional coloring of pain). Different types of peripheral sensory nociceptors, often free nerve endings, are stimulated by tissue damage. The resulting pain information is transmitted to the spinal cord by two types of small diameter peripheral afferent fibers: slow conducting, unmyelinated C-fibers (which cause a dull burning pain) and faster, thinly myelinated Aδ fibers (which cause sharp, pricking pain). Both types of primary afferent fibers enter the dorsal horn of the spinal cord and terminate in its superficial layers (lamina I-II). Projection neurons from these laminae give rise to the ascending pathways of the spinothalamic tract. Thalamic nuclei receive the nociceptive inputs and pass the information to key brain pain reception sites such as the periaqueductal gray (PAG), amygdala, and somatosensory cortex. Activation of the MORs extensively located in these higher brain centers stimulates analgesia by activating *descending modulatory pathways* from the PAG and rostroventral medulla (RVM) that inhibit (or excite) nociceptive dorsal horn neuron firing in the spinal cord (Fig. 20-2).[29,30] Opioids also exert actions in the cortex and limbic systems affecting cholinergic systems that lead to changes in arousal and pain perception.[31] Opioid receptors are further abundantly present in the spinal cord dorsal horn at pre- and postsynaptic locations. In the superficial laminae of the dorsal horn, local neuronal circuits process both ascending and descending pain pathways and are regulated by local endogenous opioid circuits.

MOR-induced analgesia and descending inhibitory pathways may be activated not only by exogenous opioids, but also by activation of endogenous opioid systems. Direct electrical stimulation of the PAG and RVM induces analgesia that is reversed by opioid antagonists.[32] The electrically stimulated sites overlap with the opioid receptor sites and with opioid-containing interneurons, linking together the actions of exogenously applied analgesic stimuli and endogenous opioid systems. Three major examples of analgesia driven by the endogenous opioid system are (1) stress-induced analgesia[33]; (2) placebo-induced analgesia[34]; and (3) conditioned pain modulation (CPM).[35]

1. *Stress-induced analgesia.* The endogenous opioid system is activated under stressful conditions, as demonstrated by the delayed onset of pain by soldiers wounded in battle.[36] The same

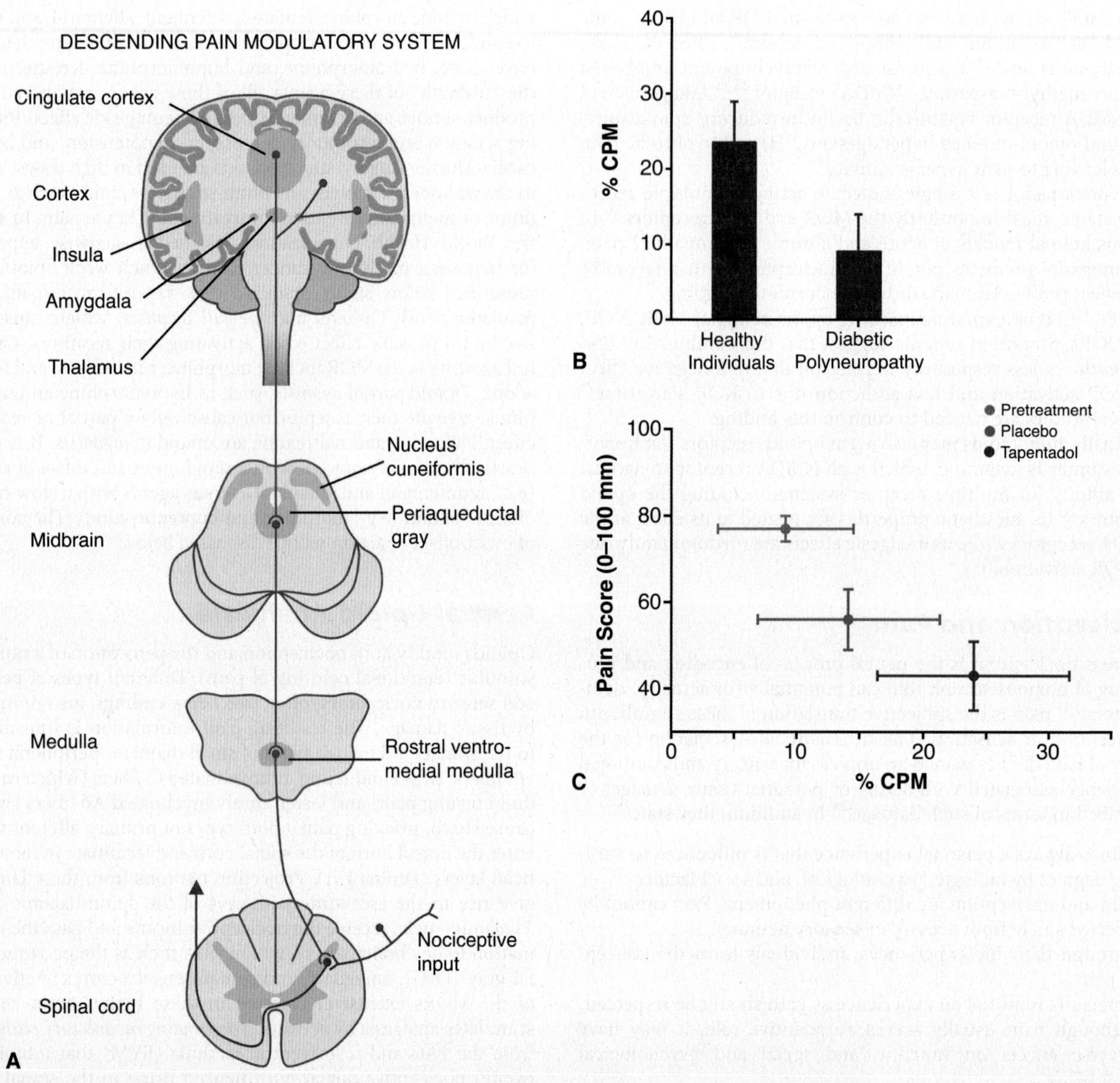

Figure 20-2 **A:** Simplified diagram of activated descending inhibitory pathways (*green lines*) in response to afferent nociceptive input (*red lines*). Descending inhibition is activated in various higher brain centers, including the rostral ventromedial medulla, periaqueductal gray, amygdala, cingulate cortex, insula, and orbitofrontal cortex. These same areas are involved in Conditioned Pain Modulation (CPM). (Reprinted from Dahan A, Niesters M, Sarton E. Endogenous modulation of pain is visible in the brain. *Clin Neurophysiol.* 2012;123(4):642–643. Copyright © 2011 International Federation of Clinical Neurophysiology. With permission.) **B:** Reduced or absent CPM responses are present in patients with diabetic polyneuropathy, reflecting inactive descending inhibitory pathways. **C:** Effect of 4-week treatment with the opioid/norepinephrine reuptake inhibitor tapentadol and placebo on CPM and pain scores in patients with diabetic polyneuropathy. (Data from Niesters M, Niesters M, Aarts L, et al. Tapentadol potentiates descending pain inhibition in chronic pain patients with diabetic polyneuropathy. *Br J Anaesth.* 2014;113:148–156.)

higher brain centers bearing MORs are involved in the implementation of stress-induced analgesia.

2. *Placebo-induced analgesia.* The endogenous opioid system also mediates placebo-induced analgesia, a reduction of pain resulting from an expectation of pain relief. Studies using functional magnetic resonance imaging (fMRI) and positive emmison tomography show activation of the endogenous opioid systems and MORs in the brains of subjects receiving placebo described as an analgesic.[37,38]
3. *CPM.* Formerly known as diffuse noxious inhibitory control, CPM is a condition in which pain arising from a noxious stimulus applied to one part of the body is decreased by application of a second remote noxious stimulus (pain inhibits pain).[39,40] CPM is due to activation of descending inhibitory pathways by higher brain centers. An example of CPM from animal physiology is the observation that an imposed nose twitch in a horse attenuates the increase in heart rate induced by painful stimuli.[41] Since naloxone blocks this effect, it is assumed that endogenous opioids are released during the nose twitch. In humans, tapentadol is an example of an opioid that induces analgesia through activation of descending pathways.[42]

Peripheral Opioid Analgesia

Opioids are also involved in peripheral analgesia by acting directly on sensory neurons (Aδ and C-fibers) to inhibit pain signal transmission. This is especially important in inflammatory pain.

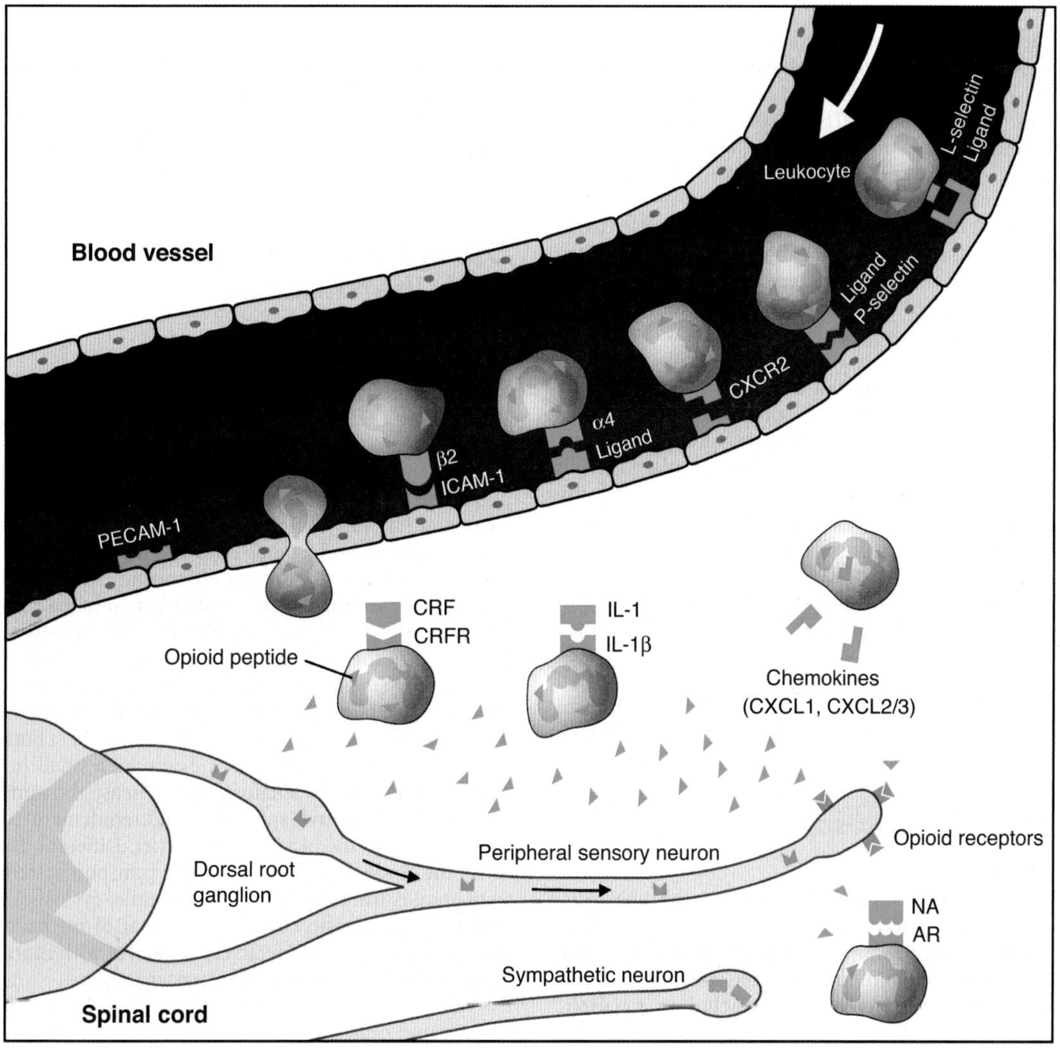

Figure 20-3 Schematic diagram illustrating the role of opioids in analgesia of peripheral inflammation. Opioid-containing leukocytes are attracted to inflamed tissue by various chemokines and cytokines. Specific upregulated protein facilitates leukocyte migration through the vascular endothelium. In the inflamed tissue, leukocytes interact with releasing agents such as corticotropin-releasing factor (CRF), interleukin-1 (IL-1), and norepinephrine (NA) derived from postganglionic sympathetic neurons, to secrete opioid peptides. These bind to peripheral opioid receptors, synthesized in the dorsal root ganglia and transported to peripheral endings of sensory neurons, to mediate analgesia. AR, adrenergic receptor; CRFR, corticotropin-releasing factor receptor; PECAM-1, platelet endothelial adhesion molecule 1; ICAM-1, intracellular adhesion molecule 1; CXCR2, chemokine (C-X-C motif) receptor 2; CXCL1, chemokine (C-X-C motif) ligand 1; CXCL2/3, chemokine (C-X-C motif) ligand 1/2.

However, the immune system is also widely involved in peripheral analgesia.[43] Opioid receptors are located not only on neurons but also on immune cells, such as human leukocytes.[44] An insult to a peripheral tissue triggers the local release of many proinflammatory mediators that generate an inflammatory cascade, induce spontaneous nociceptor activity, and sensitize sensory neurons to induce spontaneous pain, allodynia (a nonpainful stimulus is perceived as painful), and hyperalgesia (increased pain sensitivity). Early in the inflammatory process, there is an influx of leukocytes into the inflamed area and these cells are a major source of opioid peptides to inflamed sites. Opioid peptides released locally interact with the opioid neuronal receptors to induce analgesia (Fig. 20-3).[45] The inflammatory process also stimulates further opioid receptor upregulation and thereby increases the antinociceptive action of opioid peptides released by immune cells. In aggregate, the inflammatory process not only promotes inflammation and its painful sequelae, but also initiates and sustains a counteracting analgesia driven by endogenous opioids.[46]

Opioid-Induced Hyperalgesia and Opioid Tolerance

Opioids can induce the paradoxical effect of OIH or an increase in 5
pain sensitivity.[47] OIH may limit the analgesic effects of opioids. During long-term and/or high-dose opioid treatment, rapid opioid dose escalation, or administration of an opioid with rapid onset/offset (e.g., remifentanil), a paradoxical increase in pain accompanies the treatment escalation.[48,49] The MOR is not a prerequisite for OIH, because there is ample evidence from knockout mice studies (mice devoid of MORs) or studies in mice treated with naloxone or naltrexone that OIH develops in response to exposure to high-dose opioids.[50] There may be various mechanisms for OIH, including activation of the central glutaminergic system, central nitric oxide production, and facilitation of descending pronociceptive systems.

Postoperative patients who have received remifentanil infusions intraoperatively can have a higher incidence of OIH and need greater doses of morphine for control of postoperative pain than patients receiving nonremifentanil-based anesthesia. Although animal and human data indicate that all μ-opioids may cause OIH, there seems to be a gradual difference in prevalence, with most observation of OIH following administration of rapid-acting opioids, such as remifentanil. In addition, this high incidence of exaggerated pain in surgical patients following remifentanil infusions may be related to its rapid offset of analgesia. In order to prevent severe pain responses following remifentanil-based anesthesia, administration of morphine (0.1 to 0.25 mg/kg) 45 to 60 minutes before the end of surgery is advisable, and adding a low-dose ketamine infusion may prevent the development of OIH (dose range: 10 to 30 mg/h) due to ketamine's NMDA antagonistic properties.

OIH is not the same phenomenon as opioid tolerance. *Acute opioid tolerance* due to tachyphylaxis requires increasing doses of the opioid to reach a specific analgesic end point during the initial hours of opioid treatment. *Chronic tolerance*, often seen in opioid abusers, occurs over days and manifests as a decreasing analgesic effect, resulting in dose escalation and increasing the likelihood of OIH. In contrast to OIH, opioid receptor–related and postactivation intracellular processes play an important role in the development of tolerance (including β-arrestin–dependent receptor desensitization and internalization, and G-receptor uncoupling).[51,52] Finally, *pseudotolerance* is a phenomenon seen in chronic pain patients due to progression of disease with an increase in the level of nociception often due to destruction of nerves in the tumor region, resulting in neuropathic pain, which is poorly responsive to opioid dose escalation.

Opioid Tolerance to Respiratory Depression

6 Experimental studies indicate that tolerance to the analgesic, euphoric, and respiratory effects are dissociated. Development of tolerance to opioid-induced respiratory depression is slower than to other opioid effects. Opioid tolerance has pharmacokinetic and pharmacodynamic causal components including metabolic enzyme induction, upregulation of drug transporters causing efflux of the opioid from the brain compartment, opioid receptor desensitization due to protein kinase C upregulation, NMDA receptor activation, β-arrestin recruitment, and increased cAMP activity. Note that less protein kinase C is present in the respiratory network in the brainstem, which may be the reason of the much slower (and possibly lesser) opioid tolerance to respiratory depression. In a recent study, fentanyl potency and risk of fentanyl apnea were reduced four- to fivefold in individuals with an opioid use disorder compared to opioid-naive individuals (Fig. 20-4).[53] This is an important observation as tolerance is a dynamic process and a decline in tolerance after a period of abstinence (detoxification or incarceration) contributes to an increased risk of fatalities due to an unintended opioid overdose.

Opioid Pharmacokinetics and Pharmacodynamics

Opioid Pharmacokinetics

When injected intravascularly, opioids are rapidly transported to the heart and pulmonary vessels from where they disperse to the various organs and tissues. After a standard dose of opioid, the interpatient variability in plasma concentrations is at least 30-fold and related to various factors including weight-related parameters (lean and fat body mass), organ function (metabolic hepatic and renal function), and cardiac output. This variability is manifest in the distribution and elimination constants that describe the PK profile of these drugs, which is also related to their physicochemical properties, such as molecule size, pK_a (affects the degree of ionization of the molecule and depends on the plasma pH), protein binding (to albumin and α_1-acid glycoprotein), and lipid solubility. These factors affect the passage of the drug into the brain across the blood–brain barrier, and thereby affect both the opioid's PK and PD characteristics. For example, a small increase in pH seen with respiratory alkalosis will increase the nonionized form of morphine, fentanyl, sufentanil, and remifentanil, which subsequently crosses the blood–brain barrier. Different drugs may also affect the blood–brain barrier's active transport systems that eliminate opioids from the brain. For example, cyclosporine enhances morphine's analgesic effect but not that of methadone, suggesting that cyclosporine selectively interferes with morphine's efflux from the brain via specific transporter proteins.

When an opioid is injected into the venous system, there is an initial rapid peak in plasma concentration. Next, the drug rapidly enters multiple organ systems with high blood flow (such as the brain, liver, kidney) from which the plasma drug concentration rapidly drops followed by a slower drop due to redistribution to organs (such as the muscles and later tissues with high fat content) that are less well perfused. These concentration changes over time are often described by noncompartmental PK models.

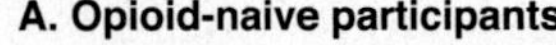

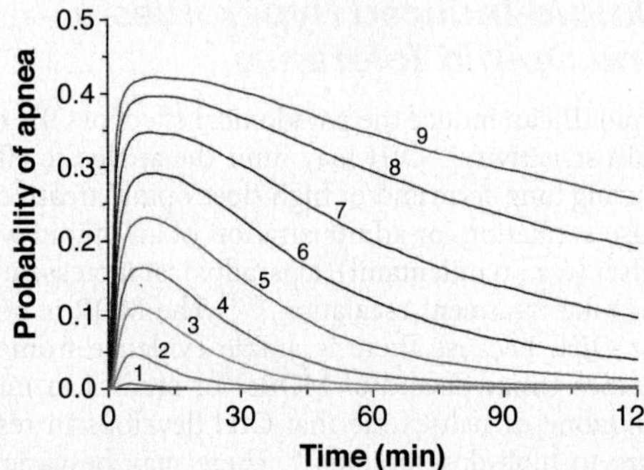

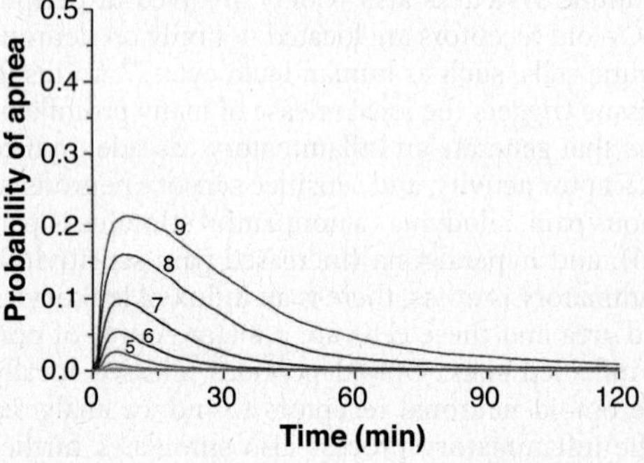

Figure 20-4 Risk of respiratory depression from an intravenous fentanyl administration in opioid-naive individuals (**A**) and individuals with an opioid use disorder (**B**). The fentanyl doses are (1) 75 μg/70 kg, (2) 150 μg/70 kg, (3) 250 μg/70 kg, (4) 350 μg/70 kg, (5) 500 μg/70 kg, (6) 700 μg/70 kg, (7) 1,000 μg/70 kg, (8) 1,500 μg/70 kg, and (9) 2,000 μg/70 kg. In chronic opioid users, the probability of apnea at doses <500 μg/70 kg is <1%. (Reprinted with permission from Algera M, Olofsen E, Moss L, et al. Tolerance to opioid-induced respiratory depression in chronic high-dose opioid users: a model-based comparison with opioid-naïve individuals. *Clin Pharmacol Ther*. 2020;109:637–645. Copyright © 2020 The Authors.)

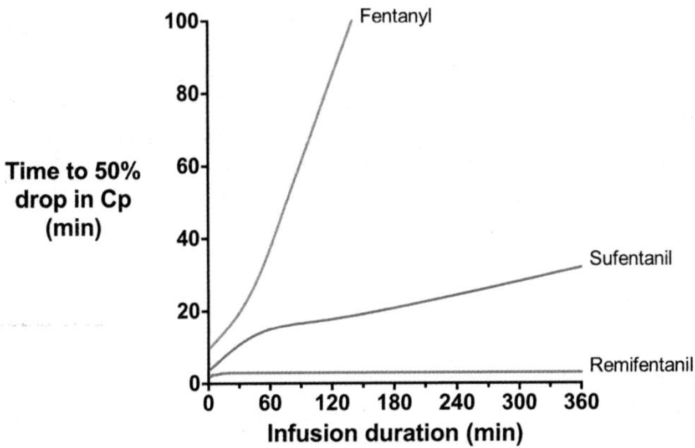

Figure 20-5 Context-sensitive half-times, or the time to a 50% drop in plasma concentration (Cp) versus infusion duration for remifentanil, fentanyl, and sufentanil.

Such models describe the drug's PK behavior in terms of volume of distribution (V_D = drug dose/steady-state plasma drug concentration), rapid and slow distribution half-lives, and elimination half-life ($t½_{elim}$). A high V_D is observed for lipophilic opioids with low protein-binding affinity such as fentanyl (V_D = 300 L), whereas a low V_D is observed for remifentanil and alfentanil, due to a high clearance (remifentanil) and/or high protein binding. When V_D is small, clearance is responsible for the fall in plasma concentration and consequently the loss of analgesia, whereas redistribution accounts for loss of analgesic effect in drugs with a high V_D.

7 The time needed for the drug's plasma concentration to decrease by 50%, from a steady-state plasma concentration after the drug infusion has stopped, is called the context-sensitive half-time (CSt½) (Fig. 20-5).[54,55] A drug has not just one, but many such half-times, depending on the duration of the infusion, which is the context to which the term applies. For fentanyl, the CSt½ increases with the duration of the infusion,[54] while for remifentanil the half-time is independent of the duration because of its rapid clearance (50% drop in plasma concentration is 2 minutes, 75% drop is 8 minutes).[55] In clinical practice, the time to the loss of analgesia depends on the opioid dose, neuronal and receptor kinetic processes, the transport of the opioids from brain to plasma, and the CSt½. The time course of a specific effect is difficult to predict for individual patients. For some side effects such as opioid-induced respiratory depression, the prediction of onset or offset of effect is even more complicated due to counteracting forces, such as the respiratory stimulant effects of increased arterial carbon dioxide (CO_2) and the presence of pain.[56]

Metabolism: Which Pathways and Metabolites Are Clinically Relevant?

8 Most opioids are metabolized in the liver through either phase I (oxidative and reductive reactions catalyzed by the cytochrome P450 enzyme system) or phase II reactions (conjugation to a specific substrate). Metabolism may occur at other sites as well, such as in the mucosa of the mouth, enterocytes of the GI tract, the kidney, or the brain. Excretion of the parent drug and/or metabolites occurs via the kidney and/or via the biliary tract into the gut where some opioids (morphine, buprenorphine) may undergo reuptake of the compound into the bloodstream.

Several aspects of opioid metabolism have clinical importance:

1. Medications that inhibit or induce the Cytochrome P450 system may increase or decrease the clinical effect of opioids, respectively, by interfering with their metabolism (Table 20-1).[57]
2. Opioid metabolites may be either active or inactive, which applies not only to their analgesic effect but also to their unwanted side effects.[58–60]
3. Genetic variability in the Cytochrome P450 system has clinical implications that are discussed in the pharmacogenetics section.

Table 20-1 Inhibitors and Inducers of CYP3A and Inhibitors of CYP2D6

CYP3A Inhibitors
Antibiotics
• Erythromycin
• Clarithromycin
Calcium channel blockers
• Diltiazem
• Verapamil
Anti-HIV agents
• Delavirdine
• Indinavir
• Ritonavir
• Saquinavir
Antifungal agents
• Itraconazole
• Ketoconazole
Other
• Grapefruit juice
CYP3A Inducers
Antibiotics
• Rifampicin
Anticonvulsants
• Carbamazepine
• Phenytoin
• Phenobarbital
Anti-HIV agents
• Efavirenz
• Nevirapine
Others
• St. John's wort
• Dexamethasone
CYP2D6 Inhibitors
Antidepressants
• Clomipramine
• Fluoxetine
• Paroxetine
Antipsychotics
• Haloperidol
Antidysrhythmics
• Quinidine
Other
• Cimetidine

Data from Wilkinson GR. Drug metabolism and variability among patients in drug response. *N Engl J Med*. 2005;352:2211–2221.

Morphine

Morphine undergoes rapid metabolism by a phase II reaction through UGT2B7 in the liver. Within minutes after its administration, the two most important hydrophilic metabolites appear in plasma: morphine-3-glucuronide (M3G) and

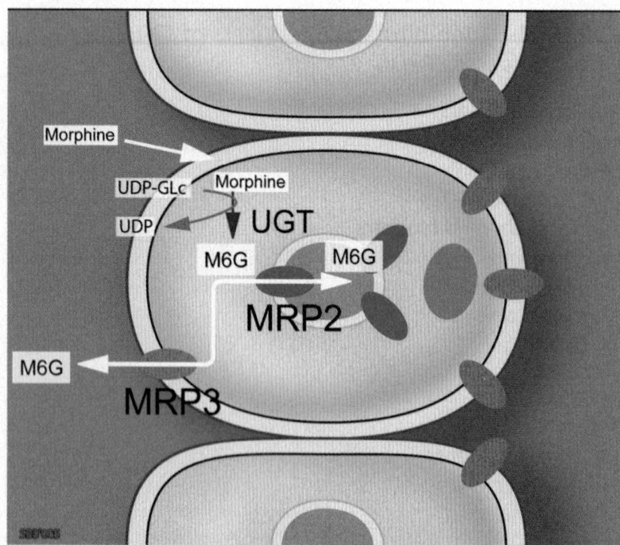

Figure 20-6 Morphine metabolism in the liver and transport of its metabolites into the bloodstream and bile system. Morphine enters the hepatocyte, where it undergoes metabolism by UGT2B7 (a phase II reaction) into morphine-3-glucuronide (not shown) and morphine-6-glucuronide (M6G). These two glucuronides are transported via transporter protein MRP3 (*red*) back into the systemic circulation and via transporter protein MRP2 (*blue*) back into the biliary duct system.

morphine-6-glucuronide (M6G).[58] M3G is the major metabolite and about 60% of morphine is converted into M3G, while just 5% to 10% is converted to M6G. In humans, M3G has no analgesic or antianalgesic action. M6G is a full MOR agonist, but at the concentrations observed following morphine administration in a patient with normal renal function, its contribution to the overall analgesic effect is minimal.[58] Due to its low lipophilicity, passage of M6G across the blood–brain barrier is slow and consequently limited. In the hepatocytes, both M3G and M6G are transported back into the bloodstream via transporter protein MRP3, while a small part is transported into the bile ducts via transporter protein MRP2 (Fig. 20-6).[58] In the gut, both glucuronides are deglucuronidated and the resultant morphine molecule is partly absorbed by the enterocytes. Enterocytes are able to metabolize morphine and transport the resultant M3G and M6G and remnant morphine to the bloodstream (the enterohepatic cycle).

Since the morphine-glucuronides are excreted via the kidney, patients with renal failure are at risk for M6G-related side effects.[58,59] Because M6G is a full MOR agonist, these side effects are typical of opioids and, most importantly, include sedation and respiratory depression. In patients with compromised renal function, morphine treatment causes M6G to accumulate in high concentrations that may cause loss of consciousness and severe respiratory depression.[58]

Piperidines

Fentanyl, alfentanil, sufentanil, and remifentanil are lipophilic opioids that rapidly cross the blood–brain barrier. Fentanyl, alfentanil, and sufentanil are metabolized by the liver, catalyzed by the cytochrome P450 enzyme system.[61,62] *Fentanyl* has a high hepatic extraction ratio with clearance approaching liver blood flow (1.5 L/min). The major metabolite of fentanyl is the inactive compound norfentanyl. *Sufentanil* also has a high hepatic extraction ratio with a clearance of 0.9 L/min. *Alfentanil* is metabolized by CYP3A4 and 3A5 forming the inactive compounds noralfentanil and *N*-phenylpropionamide. The polymorphic expression of the CYP3A5 gene accounts for the great variability in alfentanil metabolism and clearance.[62] *Remifentanil* contrasts with the other piperidines in that it is not metabolized in the liver.[63] Remifentanil contains a methyl ester side chain (Fig. 20-1) that is metabolized by blood (within the erythrocyte) and tissue nonspecific esterases. This causes a rapid clearance of the drug (context-sensitive half-life of 2 minutes) making it the most rapidly acting opioid currently available. Clearance of remifentanil is 3 to 5 L/min, which exceeds liver blood flow affirming its extrahepatic clearance. Remifentanil is usually administered as a continuous infusion since its plasma level decreases by 50% in as little as 40 seconds.[54,63]

Methadone

Methadone is extensively metabolized to an inactive form by CYP2B6, which is also affected by pharmacogenetic variability (NICV 20-1).[64] Methadone has a 60% to 95% oral bioavailability, high potency, and a long duration of action. Furthermore, there is considerable variation among recipients in their response to the drug. While methadone has characteristics that make it attractive for use intravenously as a perioperative analgesic, in a controlled and well-monitored environment, these same properties may prove hazardous when methadone is administered orally for treatment of patients with chronic pain. Large numbers of patient deaths have been attributed to the long, and often unpredictable, duration of action of methadone when administered orally.

Naloxone

Naloxone is the most valuable and popular nonspecific MOR antagonist (NICV 20-2).[65] Since it has a low and unpredictable bioavailability after oral intake due to an extensive (>95%) first-pass effect, naloxone is best given via the intravenous route. The most important metabolic pathway of naloxone is glucuronidation into the inactive naloxone-3-glucuronide. Its duration of effect is short, ranging from 15 to 45 minutes, which requires it to be redosed or administered as a continuous infusion when antagonism is required for long-acting opioids or for patients experiencing an opioid overdose.

Pharmacodynamics: Which End Point Serves the Clinician Best?

The PK of a drug describes the time course of dose to concentration; the PD describes the concentration-to-effect relationship; the effect can be any of the desired or undesired drug effects (Video 20-1 and Chapter 11, Video 11-2). Pharmacokinetic–pharmacodynamic (PKPD) models are constructed for each drug to enable the clinician to understand and predict the clinical implication of a given dose to a desired effect.[66] These models allow dosing regimens to be constructed on the basis of patient characteristics such as total or lean body weight, gender, age, and other characteristics, making them particularly helpful when treating individual patients. The PK part of such models describes the drug distribution kinetics. This relates to both the parent drug and the possible metabolites. In compartmental models, the concentration–time profiles are described by drug transfer between interconnected hypothetical compartments, mimicking drug absorption, distribution, elimination, and metabolism. The PD part of the model describes the drug concentration–effect relationship. This hypothetical effect compartment is made infinitely small so that it does not influence the drug's disposition (PK) and is located at the drug's target organ, such as the muscle endplate for muscle relaxants and the brain for hypnotic drugs. For most opioid effects, such as analgesia, sedation, and respiratory depression, the effect site is located within the central

9

nervous system (CNS) while the effect site for constipation is the GI tract. The delay between the peak drug concentration in the plasma and the peak concentration at the effect site is described by the plasma–effect site equilibration constant k_{e0} (or its half-life $t½k_{e0} = \ln 2/k_{e0}$),[67,68] which is commonly referred to as hysteresis. For the analgesic and respiratory depressive effects of opioids, the hysteresis is determined by the drug's passage across the blood–brain barrier (the more lipophilic an opioid, the faster the transfer into the brain compartment), receptor kinetics, and neuronal dynamics. The effect site concentration–effect relationship is described by a sigmoid E_{max} model[66–68]:

$$Effect = (C_E/C_{50})^{\gamma}/[1 + (C_E/C_{50})^{\gamma}]$$

where C_E is the drug concentration in the hypothetical effect site, C_{50} is the measure of drug potency or the effect site or steady-state concentration causing 50% of the effect, and γ is the Hill or steepness parameter. In summary, any PKPD analysis using the above-mentioned descriptions yields PK parameters (volumes of distribution and clearances), as well as PD parameters related to drug potency (C_{50}) and the onset/offset times of the drug ($t½k_{e0}$). It is important to understand that PK (volumes of distribution and rate constant) and PD (potency) values vary largely among patients. This is related to differences in physiology, underlying disease, age, weight, ethnicity, and other factors. Thus, the clinician should choose a PK/PD set derived from a population of subjects whose characteristics are most similar to the individual they are treating. For example, due to changes in PK and PD behavior, elderly patients display a greater opioid sensitivity[69]; patients with liver or renal insufficiency require adaptation to their dosing; and patients with certain genetic abnormalities may experience unusual responses to opioids (see below).

For most opioids, the target effect when constructing PKPD models has traditionally been the slowing of the frequency components of the electroencephalogram (EEG), quantified by a shift in the 95th percentile of the power spectrum (95% spectral edge frequency). The C_{50} and $t½k_{e0}$ derived from these studies are useful to compare the potency and onset/offset of opioids. However, since the C_{50} for EEG effects occurs beyond the normal clinical dose range of opioids, more clinically useful C_{50} values would include those for the analgesic, respiratory depressive, and sedative effect of opioids. For alfentanil and fentanyl, C_{50} values range from 75 and 1 ng/mL for sedation to 150 and 2 ng/mL for analgesia, respectively.[70,71] This indicates that these clinically relevant effects occur at lower doses than their effects on the EEG. For fentanyl, it is of further interest that $t½k_{e0}$ values for analgesia (20 to 40 minutes) and respiratory depression are much longer (15 minutes) than those observed for EEG slowing (5 to 6 minutes). In Table 20-2, values of $t½k_{e0}$ for the end points of pain relief and respiratory depression are given for various analgesics currently in use.

Table 20-2 Estimates of Analgesic $t½k_{e0}$ for Clinically Relevant End Points of Pain Relief and Respiratory Depression

Drug	$t½k_{e0}$	End Point Measured
Morphine	1.5 h	Postoperative analgesia
Ibuprofen	0.5 h	Postoperative analgesia
Acetaminophen	1 h	Postoperative analgesia
Morphine (men)	1.5 h	Relief of experimental pain
Morphine (women)	5 h	Relief of experimental pain
Fentanyl	20–40 min	Relief of experimental pain
Alfentanil	1–10 min	Relief of experimental pain
Remifentanil	1–1.5 min	Relief of experimental pain
Buprenorphine	2.5 h	Relief of experimental pain
S-ketamine	<1 min	Relief of experimental pain
Oliceridine	<1 min	Relief of experimental pain
Morphine	1.2 h	Respiratory depression
Buprenorphine	1.5 h	Respiratory depression
Fentanyl	15 min	Respiratory depression
Remifentanil	0.5 min	Respiratory depression
Naloxone	5–8 min	Relief of respiratory depression

Data from Martini C, Olofsen E, Yassen A, Aarts L, Dahan A. Pharmacokinetic-pharmacodynamic modeling in acute and chronic pain: an overview of the recent literature. *Exp Rev Pharmacother.* 2011;4:719–728.

Pharmacodynamics: Pain Relief

In postoperative patients following major orthopedic surgery under general anesthesia, it has been observed that some patients require a morphine dose of 0.02 mg/kg to obtain a visual analog pain score of 30 mm (on a scale from 0, no pain, to 100 mm, most intense pain) or less while others require a dose 40 times as large (0.8 mg/kg).[72] Younger (<40 years) healthy volunteers of normal weight (BMI <25 kg/m^2) had analgesic responses to a fixed dose of morphine that varied by a factor of 20.[73] This variability is not restricted to morphine, but is observed for all opioids used for treatment of acute, perioperative, and chronic pain, including strong opioids such as fentanyl and remifentanil. These data suggest that the variability in opioid effect is related to both variability in PK-related parameters (which in turn are attributable to differences in age, weight, body fat and muscle content, renal/liver function, cardiac output, genetic polymorphism in metabolic pathways, and co-medication) and variability in PD-related parameters. These PD differences of opioid sensitivity and pain perception most likely have a genetic origin. To date, no clear genetic basis for variability in morphine or any other opioid PD effect has been demonstrated (for exceptions, see the pharmacogenetics section). Recently, it was shown that the ability to score pain in a consistent and reliable fashion depends on various factors, including the presence of chronic pain and prior opioid administration (Fig. 20-7).[74,75] This may be related to changes in brain areas involved in the translation of nociceptive stimuli into a verbal numeric response (a complex cognitive process that requires many steps, including number sensing). In chronic pain patients, these changes may be due to neuroplastic changes in the frontal and parietal cortices. Opioids may cause transient effects on cognition and signal processing.[75]

These data indicate that the safest approach to opioid analgesia is one of careful titration to analgesic effect during surgery and in the postoperative period, with acute awareness of the undesirable dose-related side effects. This admonition to carefully titrate the administration of opioids is perhaps even more crucial when administering long-acting opioids orally for the treatment of chronic pain.

During surgery, opioids are titrated in doses sufficient to dampen and prevent exaggerated hemodynamic responses to painful surgical stimuli. In the postoperative period (and in

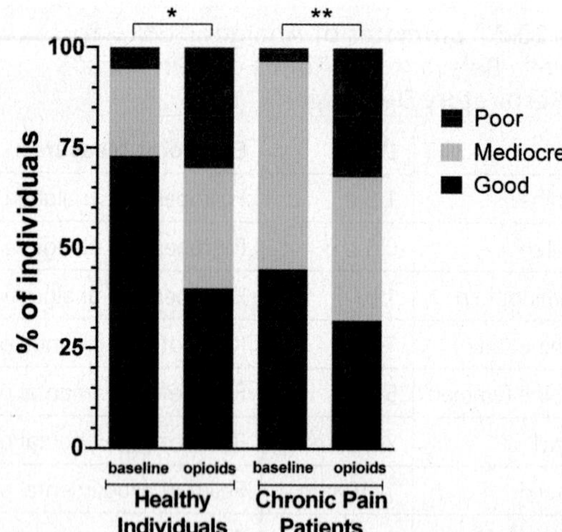

Figure 20-7 The ability to reliably translate a randomly applied nociceptive stimulus into a numerical pain score (between pain threshold and pain tolerance) is shown in healthy individuals and chronic pain patients, to demonstrate the effects of opioid treatment. Scores are divided into good, mediocre, and poor, reflecting the amount of deviation from an expected pain score. *p = .015, **p = .016. (Reprinted with permission from Oudejans LCJ, van Velzen M, Olofsen E, et al. Translation of random painful stimuli into numerical responses in fibromyalgia and perioperative patients. *Pain*. 2016;157:128–136.)

chronic pain patients), opioids are usually titrated to the patient's verbal response to pain. This distinction requires not only a difference in administration, but also a difference in vigilance with respect to opioid side effects. During surgery, potent high-dose piperidines (e.g., fentanyl, remifentanil) are the opioids of choice, while in the postoperative period, medium-strength opioids (morphine, methadone) are often chosen. During anesthesia, one should be aware of hypotension and bradycardia, a common side effect of strong opioids. In contrast, in the postoperative period, the most important side effects to avoid are respiratory depression and severe sedation, while other non–life-threatening side effects impacting patient satisfaction and health costs are nausea/vomiting and loss of bowel motility.

Morphine

In two studies on the postoperative effects of morphine following major surgery, the average intravenous dose of morphine to reach 50% pain relief was 20 mg. This dose resulted in a plasma concentration of 34 ng/mL and a $t^{1/2}k_{e0}$ of about 2 hours, although the initial onset of analgesia occurred between 15 and 30 minutes.[76,77] Thus, there is a 1- to 2-hour delay between peak plasma morphine concentration and peak analgesic effect (i.e., hysteresis). Surprisingly, these parameters are not influenced by the patient's age, weight, and gender. Given the long time to peak analgesia, a practical strategy for dosing morphine in adults is to give an initial morphine bolus dose (0.15 to 0.2 mg/kg) at least 60 minutes before the end of surgery. When the patient is in pain in the postanesthesia care unit (PACU), 2 mg bolus doses at 5- to 10-minute intervals may be given until visual analog pain scores decrease to 30 or less (on a scale from 0 to 100) (Fig. 20-8). At that point, the patient can be started on a patient-controlled analgesia (PCA) pump.

Two considerations must accompany every postoperative acute pain plan. First, the postoperative analgesic regimen should be multimodal with morphine (or any other opioid) and combined with opioid-sparing drugs such as acetaminophen and nonsteroidal anti-inflammatory drugs such as diclofenac. Second, some patients require large doses of morphine, yet their pain appears unresponsive to morphine. The cause of such reduced opioid sensitivity is unclear. Irrespective of the cause, it is wise not to continue dosing (see Opioid-Induced Respiratory Depression versus Opioid Analgesia) but to add an adjuvant such as the NMDA receptor antagonist ketamine (0.125 mg/kg), or an α_2-adrenergic receptor agonist, such as clonidine (75 μg). Both drugs are analgesics in their own right and enhance morphine's analgesic effect.[78,79] A practical morphine PCA regimen may consist of a 1-mg dose, a 5-minute lockout, and a maximum of 24 mg per 4 hours.

Fentanyl

Fentanyl is about 100 times more potent than morphine. Like all opioids, the analgesic response to intravenous fentanyl is highly variable. Fentanyl's lipophilic structure means it rapidly crosses the blood–brain barrier, as is evident from a characteristic δ-wave

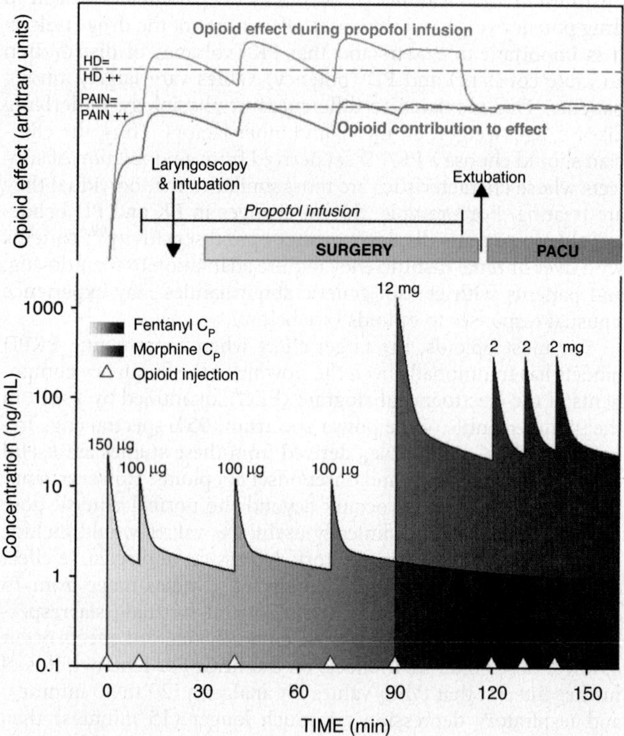

Figure 20-8 Simulated effect of multiple bolus doses of fentanyl (100 to 150 μg) during anesthesia, and morphine during and following anesthesia, on the analgesic and hemodynamic state of the patient. **Bottom:** An initial dose of morphine (12 mg) is given 30 minutes before the end of surgery followed by three 2-mg doses (at the end of this titration phase the patient can be set on PCA morphine). The *blue* and *red lines* are the simulated fentanyl and morphine plasma concentration (Cp). **Top:** The effect profile induced by the two opioids. During anesthesia, fentanyl dosing is based predominantly on hemodynamic and other autonomic parameters; in the PACU morphine dosing is based on pain rating. During anesthesia, the combination of fentanyl and propofol (*orange line*) provides greater analgesia than opioids alone (*green line*). When propofol infusion is terminated the analgesic profile reverts to a lower level (from *orange* via *orange-green* to *green* line). HD indicates that hemodynamic and other autonomic responses are in the normal range, HD++ indicates increased responses (such as high blood pressure, tachycardia, and sweating) due to the surgical stress; PAIN indicates adequate analgesia, PAIN++ indicates pain. The *dotted lines* are the arbitrary divisions between adequate anesthesia and inadequate anesthesia, and adequate analgesia and inadequate analgesia.

appearing on the EEG (t½k_{e0} 6.5 minutes). However, fentanyl's t½k_{e0} for analgesic effect is longer with values ranging between 10 and 20 minutes[70]; fentanyl's potency (C_{50}) for analgesia ranges from 1 to 2 ng/mL.[70] Fentanyl is used during anesthesia to dampen cardiovascular responses to noxious stimulation from laryngoscopy, intubation, skin incision, and surgical stress. On average, the requirements for inhalational anesthetics and propofol are reduced by about 50% when administering 1.5 to 3 µg/kg IV fentanyl.[80–82] In fact, by combining fentanyl (or any other potent opioid) with propofol, the requirement of both drugs to prevent movement and hemodynamic responses to laryngoscopy and surgical stress is reduced (Fig. 20-8).[81,82] Fentanyl dosing should be repeated at regular intervals in order to maintain a comfortable analgesic state (the dose and frequency are dependent on the patient's weight, dose, type of surgery, etc.). Be aware that a continuous infusion leads to the accumulation of the drug in the body as its 50% CSt½ increases rapidly with the duration of infusion (Fig. 20-5).[54,55] Similarly, frequent dosing of the drug may cause accumulation. Considering the drug's t½k_{e0} fentanyl should be administered 5 to 10 minutes prior to an anticipated painful/stressful event such as laryngoscopy or skin incision (Fig. 20-8).

In the 1980s, high-dose fentanyl was often used in combination with nitrous oxide to provide both analgesia and suppression of consciousness. Although this combination provided excellent hemodynamic stability, it could not assure amnesia. Hence, it is not surprising that this technique has been replaced by the technique of "balanced anesthesia" or total intravenous anesthesia (TIVA) where opioids are combined with sedatives, intravenous anesthetics, and muscle relaxants to assure amnesia, as well as analgesia.

Fentanyl is also used in the treatment of chronic pain. For example, the fentanyl patch is used in a large number of cancer and noncancer chronic pain patients. The transcutaneous delivery of fentanyl ranges from 12 to 100 µg/h, although absorption depends on a variety of factors such as skin thickness, subcutaneous fat layer, and subcutaneous perfusion. Peak analgesic effect is reached only after 10 to 12 hours and the effect of one patch lasts 3 to 4 days. Other methods of administration include intranasal fentanyl, sublingual fentanyl, fentanyl lozenges (a solid preparation in the form of a lollipop), mucosal patch—all four methods are used for treatment of breakthrough pain—and iontophoretic transdermal fentanyl applications. The home use of fentanyl in chronic pain patients comes with the danger of misuse and abuse by the patients or by family members or friends. This is a major concern as it leads to an increasing number of opioid fatalities.

Sufentanil

Sufentanil is a thienyl derivate of fentanyl and about 10 times more potent than fentanyl; its lipophilicity is 2 times greater than that of fentanyl. Sufentanil acts selectively at the MOR with a C_{50} for analgesia of 30 pg/mL and t½k_{e0} similar to that of fentanyl. Sufentanil is metabolized in the liver to various inactive and one active compound, desmethylsufentanil. The latter has 10% of the activity of sufentanil, and since it is produced in minute quantities has no clinical relevance. Sufentanil is used predominantly as an analgesic during anesthesia, as it produces stable hemodynamics and cardiac output. A sublingual sufentanil PCA system for postoperative pain relief has also been introduced. Compared to other clinically available opioids, sufentanil has a high therapeutic index (=LD_{50}/ED_{50} where LD_{50} is the lethal dose in 50% of animals tested, and ED_{50} the effective dose in 50% of animals tested).

Remifentanil

Remifentanil, the newest piperidine available for use in humans, differs from the other strong opioids in its rapid onset/offset for all clinical effects including respiration (Fig. 20-9).[83] Indications for its use include anesthesia/surgery, PCA analgesia and sedation in the ICU, diagnostic procedures, and the treatment of obstetric labor pain. The use of remifentanil in spontaneous breathing patients at relatively low infusion rates (<0.1 to 0.2 µg/kg/min) is feasible[56,83] but requires adequate monitoring and skilled personnel to detect and manage an adverse respiratory event.

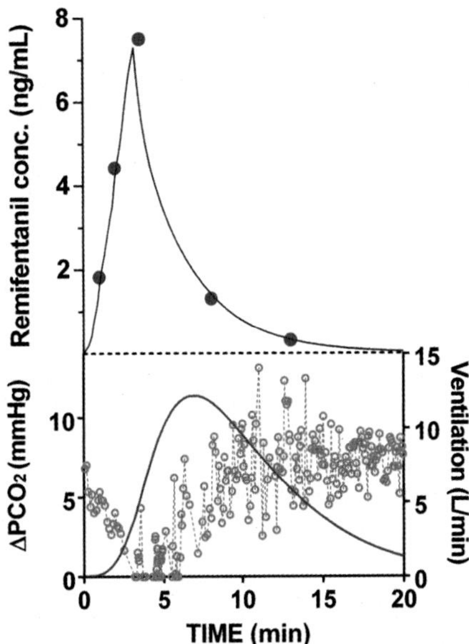

Figure 20-9 Effect of a short remifentanil infusion on breathing. Top: The measured remifentanil plasma concentration (*blue dots*) and the pharmacokinetic data fit (*blue line*). **Bottom:** The increase in end-tidal PCO_2 (ΔPCO_2, *green line*), the measured inspired ventilation (*orange dots*, each dot is one breath). Note the absence of a delay between the remifentanil plasma concentration and ventilation, and the short delay between changes in the plasma concentration and the end-tidal PCO_2. (Data from Olofsen E, Boom M, Nieuwenhuijs D, et al. Modeling the non-steady-state respiratory effects of remifentanil in awake and propofol sedated healthy volunteers. *Anesthesiology*. 2010;212:1382–1395.)

Remifentanil is 100 to 200 times more potent than morphine. 10
Like other opioids, remifentanil displays large variability in effect among patients. For example, Drover and Lemmens[84] showed that the remifentanil plasma concentration causing a 50% probability (C_{P50}) of no clinical response to stimulation (laryngoscopy, intubation, skin incision, and skin closures) varies 50-fold, from 1.5 to 79 ng/mL, during abdominal surgery in patients anesthetized with a nitrous oxide and remifentanil combination. In that study, a clear gender difference in potency of remifentanil was found (C_{P50} men 4.1 ng/mL, women 7.5 ng/mL). This difference can be accounted for by the difference in surgical stimulation of the prostatectomies versus hysterectomies. Different surgeries produce differences in nociception (i.e., pain) and hemodynamic stress responses, and hence require different dosages to suppress pain and stress. The C_{P50} varied from 3.8 ng/mL for prostatectomies, 5.6 ng/mL for nephrectomies, and 7.5 ng/mL for abdominal hysterectomies. Like fentanyl, remifentanil causes a reduction in both volatile anesthetic and propofol requirements. Vuyk et al.[85] showed that by increasing the remifentanil concentration from 0 to 2 ng/mL, the mean propofol concentration required to obtain C_{P50} for laryngoscopy was reduced from 7 to 3 µg/mL, more than 60% reduction in dose requirement. When combining remifentanil with propofol (TIVA), the remifentanil effect remains variable. When added to a constant propofol plasma concentration

of 2 μg/mL, the remifentanil concentration required for suppression of hemodynamic and movement responses during abdominal surgery varies from 3 to 15 ng/mL. Interestingly, at a higher propofol concentration of 4 μg/mL, the variability was reduced to 0 to 5 ng/mL. These data reinforce that opioid dosing requires titration to effect based on careful observation of the clinical response of the patient. Variations in remifentanil infusion rate should be based on an *a priori* knowledge of the PK and PD properties of the drug, patient characteristics, and, most importantly, hemodynamic responses and nociceptive input during surgery. Between intubation and surgical incision, when there is no stimulation, decreases of 30% to 40% in blood pressure and heart rate are not uncommon unless the remifentanil infusion dose is reduced during that period. Due to its rapid PK activity, the need for an initial remifentanil bolus is rather limited especially when there is ample time between the start of infusion and the first nociceptive stimulus (such as laryngoscopy). If a bolus is required, a slow infusion (given in 1 to 2 minutes) of 0.5 to 1 μg/kg can be used.

The minimum alveolar concentration (MAC) reduction observed with remifentanil use and its very short CSt½ (Fig. 20-5) make rapid awakening possible at the end of surgery.[86] For example, after a 3-hour infusion of propofol and remifentanil for abdominal surgery, the shortest time to awakening (≈7 minutes) was observed after constant propofol and remifentanil concentrations of 2.5 and 4.8 ng/mL, respectively (Fig. 20-10).[85] At higher propofol concentrations, but lower remifentanil concentrations, the time to awakening increases. The occurrence of postoperative pain following remifentanil "fast-track" anesthesia is frequently reported.[48,49]

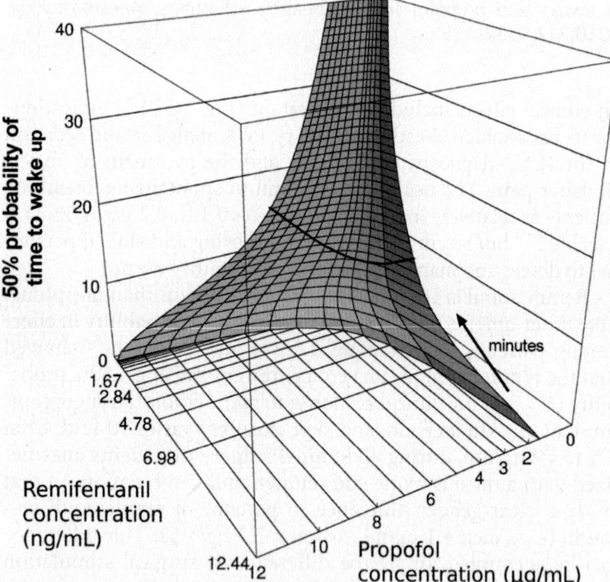

Figure 20-10 Propofol–remifentanil interaction on "time to wake up" following anesthesia. Remifentanil–propofol interaction causing 50% probability of no response to surgical stimulation is given at t = 0 minutes. Next, the infusion pumps are switched off causing the decreasing effect site concentrations. The *bold line* on top of the 3D surface represents the 50% probability of return of consciousness. The lowest point represents the optimal propofol–remifentanil concentration during surgery that gives the minimal recovery time after the pumps are switched off. Note that this occurs at steady-state concentrations of 4.78 ng/mL remifentanil and 2 μg/mL propofol, and 50% probability of waking up occurs after 7 minutes. (Reprinted with permission from Vuyk J, Mertens MJ, Olofsen E, et al. Propofol anesthesia and rational opioid selection. *Anesthesiology*. 1997;87:1549–1562.)

Postoperative pain scores are higher after a remifentanil-based anesthesia, and requirements for morphine are increased. This is due to the rapid decrease in opioid concentration causing a rapid decline in analgesic state, possibly combined with OIH. Strategies to counteract this problem include starting morphine administration 30 to 45 minutes before the end of surgery, or a single fentanyl bolus of 50 μg or ketamine 0.125 mg/kg at the end of surgery.[48]

Buprenorphine

Buprenorphine is a semisynthetic opioid analog derived from thebaine.[87] It is a partial high-affinity agonist at the MOR, antagonist at KOR and DOR, and an agonist at the nociceptin receptor. These properties give buprenorphine a unique activity profile, making it a valuable drug in the treatment of pain and opioid use disorder. For example, buprenorphine displays a ceiling effect to respiratory depression, but not to analgesia. Buprenorphine's high affinity at the MOR also makes it an excellent choice for treating opioid use disorder. Due to its high receptor affinity, abused and recreational opioids are unable to displace buprenorphine from its receptor; consequently, these opioids will not evoke the desired euphorigenic effects that opioid abusers seek.[87,88] Buprenorphine's safety was recently demonstrated in an isohypercapnic experiment, where buprenorphine effectively reduced the risk of apnea from up to 3 mg of intravenous fentanyl in subjects with an opioid use disorder.[89] A downside of buprenorphine's high affinity at the MORs, however, is that when serious respiratory depression does occur from buprenorphine, high doses and prolonged infusions of naloxone are required to reverse respiratory depression. In addition, when combined with a sedative, buprenorphine's advantages rapidly disappear, and the risk of respiratory and death is increased significantly.[90]

Oliceridine

The biased ligand, oliceridine, may have an advantage over other nonbiased ligands as they are associated with less respiratory depression.[11] The drug has recently been approved by the U.S. Food and Drug Administration (FDA) and is indicated for treatment of moderate to severe postoperative pain. In a recent reanalysis of volunteer data, it was observed that over the clinical dose range (10 to 30 ng/mL), oliceridine has a lower probability of respiratory depression at equianalgesic levels compared to morphine, as evident in the utility function analysis (Fig. 20-11).

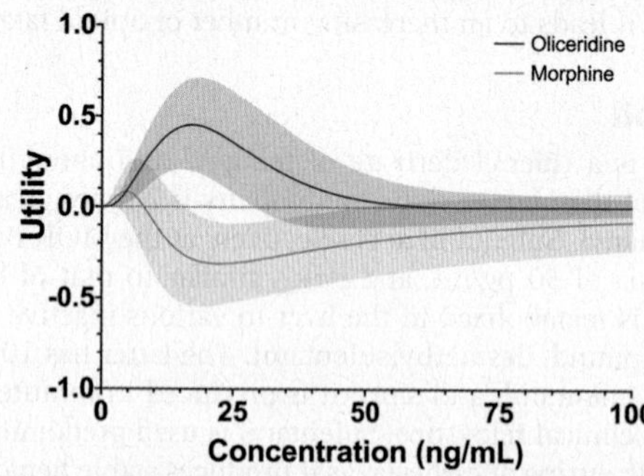

Figure 20-11 Utility functions constructed from the pharmacokinetic and pharmacodynamic volunteer data. Utility = the difference in probability of analgesia minus the probability of respiratory depression. The utility functions reflect the biophase oliceridine or morphine concentration. In *blue*, the oliceridine utility function (*blue continuous line* is the mean with *blue* 95% CI band). In orange, the morphine utility function (*continuous lines* are the mean with *orange* 95% CI band). (Reprinted with permission from Dahan A, van Dam J, Niesters M, et al. Benefit and risk evaluation of biased μ-receptor agonist oliceridine versus morphine. *Anesthesiology*. 2020;133:559–568.)

Reanalysis of the clinical data showed that respiratory events occurred at relatively low utility function (UFo) values (<0.2), which validates the concept of the UFos.[11] It's onset of action is rapid and similar to remifentanil and ketamine.

Pharmacogenetics

Pharmacogenetics describes the relationship between genetic variations and drug response. Variations occur in genes that code for components of the metabolic pathways and transport of the drug across the blood–brain barrier (affecting PK behavior), and in genes that code for the opioid receptor or proteins in downstream signaling pathways (affecting PD behavior). The existence of a pharmacogenetic effect on PK is well established in opioid pharmacology, whereas an effect of genetic makeup on PD is less certain. For example, the literature on the significance of a specific mutation in the gene coding for MOR, *OPRM1:c.118 A > G* (dbSNP1799971), is equivocal.[91] Some examples of pharmacogenetic variations that influence opioid analgesia are given below.

While most Cytochrome P450 (CYP) isoenzymes display polymorphisms, the genetic variability in the gene coding for CYP2D6 is clinically most important.[92,93] The CYP2D6 isoenzyme of the cytochrome P450 system is highly polymorphic with large variations between individuals in the number of gene copies in their DNA.[93] The rate of metabolism of opioids depends on the number of copies a subject expresses, ranging from ultrarapid metabolizing individuals with multiple copies of the *CYP2D6* gene to poor metabolizing individuals with two nonfunctional alleles of the gene. The more copies of the gene, the greater the metabolic power within the CYP2D6 pathway; the reverse is true for individuals without an active copy of the gene.[93] This is important for drugs that rely on CYP2D6 to convert an inactive precursor (prodrug), such as codeine, into the active component of pain therapy (for codeine, this is morphine).[94] Patients without an active gene will have no benefit from treatment with codeine. Dangerous circumstances may occur when a patient is an extensive metabolizer and produces large amounts of the active component. There are multiple case reports showing codeine intoxication due to ultrarapid CYP2D6 metabolism (see below). A tragic example reported by Koren et al.[95] describes a normal full-term breastfed neonate that developed lethargy on postnatal day 7 and was found dead 6 days later. His mother had been prescribed 30-mg codeine combined with 500-mg acetaminophen for episiotomy pain (two tablets every 12 hours, reduced to one tablet per 12 hours after day 2 because of somnolence and constipation). Postmortem morphine plasma concentrations were 70 ng/mL (normal values for children breastfed by mothers receiving codeine is 0.2 to 2 ng/mL). The mother's milk contained 87 ng/mL morphine (typical mother milk concentrations after repeated codeine dosing is 2 to 20 ng/mL). Genotype analysis revealed that the mother had a 2 × 2 CYP2D6 gene duplication and was classified as an ultrarapid CYP2D6 metabolizer. The clinical picture is that of death due to morphine-induced respiratory depression.

Variations in the *ABCB1* gene, the gene coding for P-glycoprotein, a protein involved in the efflux of xenobiotics from the brain, cause variations in the toxicity of fentanyl. Park et al.[96] monitored the clinical effects (respiration rate) of 2.5 μg/kg intravenous fentanyl in patients under spinal anesthesia and assessed the influence of three single nucleotide polymorphisms in *ABCB1*. They observed an effect of the different genotypes on respiratory depression with an increased risk for a reduction in respiratory rate in certain variant gene combinations. These data are best explained by a lesser efficacy of the variant P-glycoprotein to transport fentanyl away from the brain.

Opioid-Induced Respiratory Depression

Mechanisms of Opioid-Induced Respiratory Depression

The hundreds of thousands of deaths from the opioid epidemic have made most caregivers painfully aware of the lethal respiratory effects of opioids.[97] The cost of opioid respiratory morbidity and mortality is extremely high, both at the individual level and at socioeconomic level.

Although MORs are widely expressed within the respiratory network, the preBötzinger complex (the brainstem respiratory rhythm generator) and Kölliker-Fuse nucleus are two areas in the brainstem critical for development of opioid-induced respiratory depression.[98–100] Recent studies indicate that opioids have a dual mechanism of opioid-induced respiratory depression at the preBötzinger complex; namely, opioid-induced impairment of excitatory presynaptic neurotransmission, and opioid-induced intrinsic hyperpolarization of respiratory neurons.[100] Opioids may also affect the ventilatory control system at other sites, such as the carotid bodies, which are highly effective sensors of hypoxia and hypercapnia located at both the bifurcation of the common carotid artery and at respiratory neurons involved in CO_2-sensing in the brainstem. The balance between *stimulatory* inputs to the respiratory centers and *depressive* inputs from opioids of these same respiratory centers determine the *ventilatory drive* following opioid administration. During an opioid overdose, this ventilatory drive will transition from irregular breathing to cyclic breathing, gasping, and apnea. At that point, rhythmic respiratory activity is either restored, driven by high levels of arterial carbon dioxide at the central centers,[56] or respiratory activity collapses followed by severe hypoxia, bradycardia, and cardiopulmonary arrest.

When an opioid is administered to a patient and the injection rate is sufficiently slow (over minutes) that the depression of the respiratory neurons in the brainstem coincides with the accumulation of arterial CO_2, the stimulatory effect of the increased CO_2 at the peripheral and central chemoreceptors will offset the decrease in tidal volume and reduced respiratory rate.[56] When just monitoring respiratory rate and oxygen saturation, it appears that the opioid injected has no effect on the ventilatory system, but when also monitoring end-tidal (or arterial) CO_2, the opioid effect becomes visible. When a strong opioid that rapidly crosses the blood–brain barrier is injected, a rapid depression of respiratory neurons occurs and there will be no time for gradual CO_2 accumulation, resulting in an apneic patient. An example is given in Figure 20-9, which shows that a rapid short-term infusion of remifentanil causes apnea and hypercapnia.[56] Breathing is restored by a high arterial CO_2 level combined with the rapid drop in brain (effect site) remifentanil concentration. Slowing the speed of injection of this strong opioid allows the accumulation of arterial CO_2, and apnea will be prevented and the patient will continue to breathe, albeit at a higher arterial PCO_2.

Apart from their effect on brainstem respiratory neurons (causing central apnea), opioids may increase the collapsibility of the upper airways due to suppression of neurons in the brainstem involved in maintaining the upper airway muscle tone or from the loss of muscle tone related to sedation.[97] Opioids combined with anesthetics do not increase the incidence of upper airway obstruction but do increase the number of central apneic events.[101] However, any dose of opioid that produces a generalized state of sedation and/or reduced muscle tone will give rise to upper airway collapse, even when the patient is considered awake.[101] Furthermore, depression of the chemo- and arousal reflexes by opioids

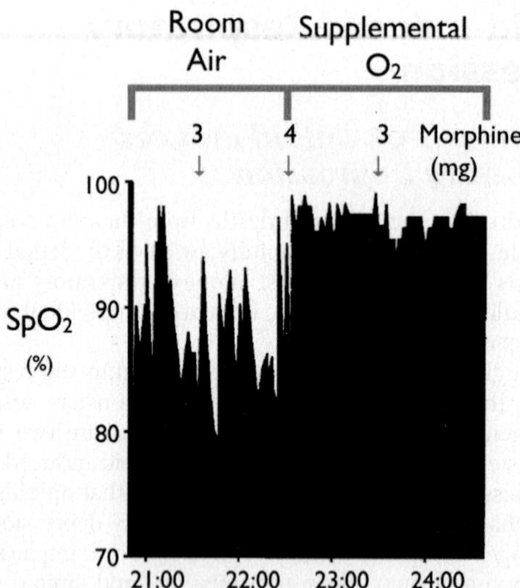

Figure 20-12 Effect of supplemental oxygen on pulse oximeter values in a postoperative patient on PCA morphine. (Reprinted with permission from Stone JG, Cozine KA, Wald A. Nocturnal oxygenation during patient-controlled analgesia. *Anesth Analg.* 1999;89:104–110.)

will cause a delayed and less forceful response to upper airway obstruction.[97] Most patients receiving opioids, whether diagnosed with obstructive sleep apnea syndrome or not, develop both central and obstructive apneic events resulting in recurrent hypoxemia during the first three to five nights postoperatively.[102–104] Stone et al.[104] showed that patients on PCA morphine without supplemental oxygen develop recurrent and deep hypoxic events during the first few postoperative nights (Fig. 20-12). While supplemental oxygen results in fewer hypoxic events, it has a serious disadvantage as it masks hypoventilation and early detection of an obstructive respiratory event because the lungs are primed with supplemental oxygen. Use of a pulse oximeter, especially in the presence of supplemental oxygen administration, is not a valid measure of the adequacy of ventilation. An example of the inability to detect an apneic event using pulse oximetry while on supplemental oxygen is given in Figure 20-13. A subject received a remifentanil bolus causing rapid respiratory depression and a reduction in respiratory rate, both during air and oxygen breathing. Desaturations were detected during air breathing only.[83]

Finally, strong, high-dose opioids, especially when given rapidly, cause skeletal muscle rigidity in thoracic, abdominal, and pharyngeal muscles (the rigid cage syndrome), all of which can contribute to respiratory insufficiency.[105,106] There are various strategies to reverse enhanced muscle tone such as administration of naloxone, the α_2-adrenergic receptor agonist dexmedetomidine, the α_1-adrenergic receptor agonist prazosine, and volatile anesthetics.[106]

Incidence and Risk Factors of Opioid-Induced Respiratory Depression

12 The incidence of respiratory depression from opioid treatment, acute or chronic, is poorly documented. The metrics in the older literature defining respiratory depression are inconsistent, the data are predominantly retrospective, and most studies rely on intermittent sampling of data.[97] Thus, a significant number of respiratory depression events from which the patient recovers spontaneously or is rescued by other means are likely missed. A systematic review of the literature on postoperative opioid-induced respiratory depression estimates an average incidence of 0.5% with a range of 0.2% to 2%.[97] This would suggest that only one in 200 patients develops a respiratory event from opioids that requires an intervention such as the administration of naloxone. In the case of randomized controlled trials where morphine is used as positive control, the incidence of morphine-induced respiratory depression is many times higher, with hypoventilation (a respiratory rate <8 breaths/min) occurring in as high as 30% of patients during PCA morphine treatment.[97,107] In a recent prospective multicenter multinational trial in over 1,300 opioid-treated postoperative patients that were monitored with continuous capnography (the PRODIGY trial), 1 in 2 patients developed at least one respiratory depression event, defined as respiratory rate ≤5 breaths/min, oxygen saturation ≤85%, or end-tidal carbon dioxide ≤15 or ≥60 mmHg for ≥3 minutes, an apnea episode lasting >30 seconds, or any respiratory opioid-related adverse event.[108] These data suggest that, in real life, the respiratory depression from opioids frequently goes undetected, and is therefore underreported. The same applies to opioid treatment for chronic pain. Accidental deaths from opioids in chronic cancer pain patients are often falsely attributed to the progression of the underlying disease.

Various patient groups are at higher risk for development of opioid-related respiratory depression. The PRODIGY trial developed a multivariable respiratory depression model using five independent variables: age ≥60 years, male sex, opioid naivety, sleep disorders, and chronic heart failure.[108] Patients in the high-risk groups had a sixfold higher risk of a respiratory event than low-risk group, and had on average 3-day longer hospital stays. Apart from the PRODIGY risk assessment, additional specific questionnaires, such as the STOP-BANG questionnaire for obstructive sleep apnea, should be part of the screening routine in the obese and aging patient population.[109]

Niesters et al.[110] published an analysis of all published cases of respiratory depression related to opioid administration in the pediatric population. They detected specific risk factors of opioid-induced respiratory depression: morphine administration in patients with renal impairment, causing accumulation of M6G; codeine use in patients with CYP2D6 gene polymorphism associated with the ultrarapid metabolizer phenotype, causing enhanced production of morphine; and opioid use in patients after adenotonsillectomy for recurrent tonsillitis and/or obstructive sleep apnea.

Opioid-Induced Respiratory Depression versus Opioid Analgesia

In general, when comparing opioid analgesics, it is important to not only anticipate their side effects (respiratory depression), but also assess side effects relative to their analgesic properties. One way to compare opioids in this respect is by constructing so-called safety or UFos.[111,112] UFos can be constructed by estimating *the difference* in probability of analgesia and respiratory depression from PKPD analyses. They can also be constructed based on measurements of clinical effects and side effects, without assumptions about the underlying PK and PD.[111–113] The UFo is defined based on one or more specific endpoints, such as <50% analgesia and <50% respiratory depression. A negative UFo value indicates that the probability for respiratory depression is larger than the probability for analgesic efficacy. In Figure 20-11, morphine and oliceridine UFos are compared.[11] Over the clinical concentration range of 10 to 30 ng/mL, the oliceridine UFo is positive, indicating that this drug has a higher probability of analgesia than respiratory depression, while the reverse is true for morphine. Overall, the

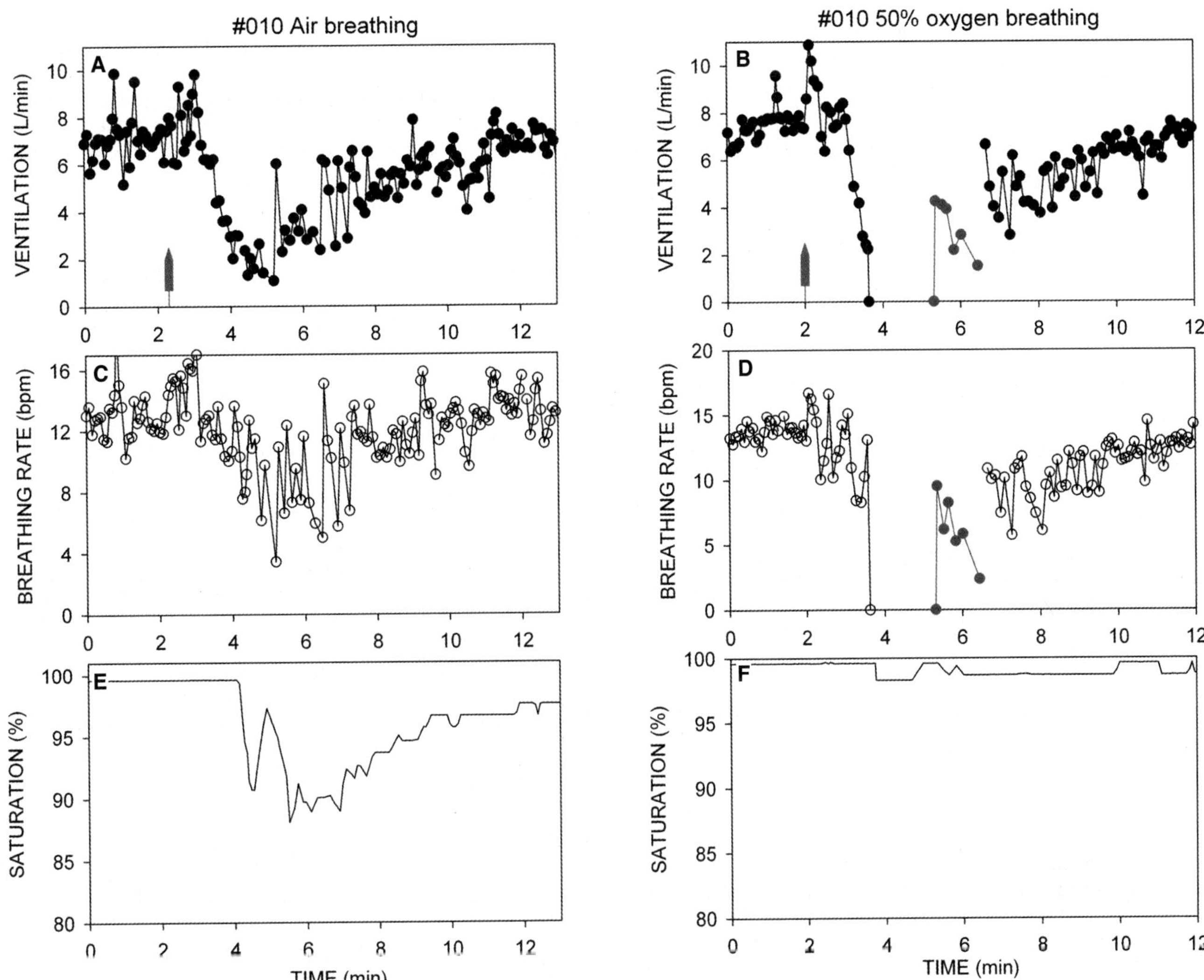

Figure 20-13 Effect of the administration of 50 µg remifentanil on ventilation in one subject during air breathing (**A, C,** and **E**) and during inhalation of 50% oxygen (**B, D,** and **F**). During air breathing, the depression in ventilation is apparent from the reduced oxygen saturation (apart from the reduction in ventilation and respiratory rate). During administration of supplemental oxygen, the pulse oximeter does not detect the apneic event. Mask ventilation is shown in red. The syringe indicates the time of remifentanil administration. (Reprinted from Niesters M, Mahajan RP, Aarts L, et al. High-inspired oxygen concentration further impairs opioid-induced respiratory depression. *Br J Anaesth*. 2013;110(5):837–841. Copyright © 2013 The Author(s). With permission.)

data analysis revealed similar analgesic potency of the two opioids but a lesser respiratory depression potential for oliceridine by a factor of 2.

The UFo curves of Figure 20-11 are constructed from data in healthy volunteers and later validated using real patient data. In patients, all respiratory events occurred at low UFo values (<0.2).[11] Since the UFo combines pain and respiratory responses into one function, the curves contructed from healthy volunteers are applicable to postoperative patients that are in pain and are treated with an opioid. Finally, it remains important to stress that a positive value of the UFo does not mean that the opioid does not cause respiratory depression.

Combining Opioids and Central Depressants

13 The risk of opioid-induced respiratory depression increases when opioids are administered in combination with other centrally acting respiratory depressants such as alcohol, benzodiazepines, antidepressants, and antipsychotics. This is a serious cause of enhanced mortality—a large fraction of patients suffering a cardiopulmonary arrest also have sedatives in their system, as determined at autopsy. One example is the combination of oxycodone and alcohol.[114] In both young and older (>65 years) individuals, the effect of 0.5 and 1 g/L ethanol (as measured in the expired air sample) was evaluated after 20-mg oral immediate-release oxycodone ingestion. Oxycodone by itself impaired breathing levels by 30%, rising to 50% when alcohol was added. Isohypercapnic ventilation was reduced by the opioid–ethanol combination by 50% (0.5 g/L) and 60% (1 g/L, see Fig. 20-14). Concomitant alcohol caused multiple apneic events that were more pronounced in the elderly population. Similar effects are expected from benzodiazepines and antidepressants, as well as for other opioids, including full agonists and partial agonists such as buprenorphine. We therefore strongly advise to restrict the use of alcohol and sedatives in patients receiving opioid therapy.

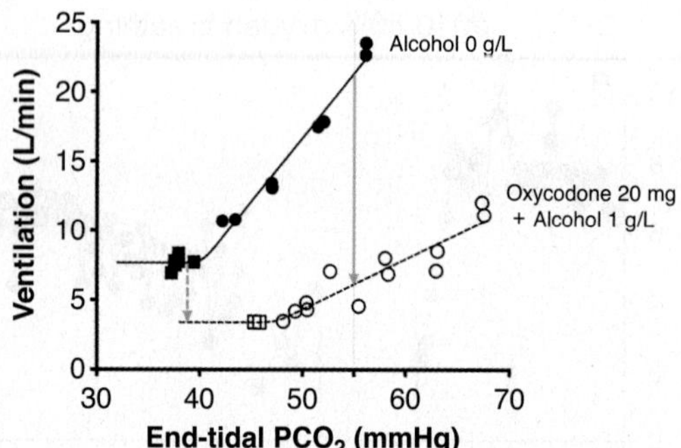

Figure 20-14 Ventilatory response to hypercapnia of an elderly participant under placebo conditions (breath ethanol concentration of 0 g/L) and during co-administration of ethanol (breath concentration of 1 g/L) combined with a 20-mg oxycodone immediate-release tablet. Squares are resting data points without added inspired carbon dioxide; circles are data at added inspired carbon dioxide. All data points are 1-minute median values obtained at steady-state ventilation. The line through the data is the "best" fit. The horizontal part of the data fit represents the estimate of resting ventilation, the linear ramp is the hypercapnic ventilatory response curve. The continuous *vertical gray line* depicts VE55 or the extrapolated minute ventilation at an end-tidal partial pressure of carbon dioxide (PCO2) of 55 mmHg. The *continuous gray arrow* is the decline in VE55 due to oxycodone and 1 g/L ethanol. The *broken gray arrow* is the decline in resting ventilation due to oxycodone and 1 g/L ethanol. (Reprinted with permission from van der Schrier R, Roozekrans M, Olofsen E, et al. Influence of ethanol on oxycodone-induced respiratory depression: a dose-escalating study in young and elderly volunteers. *Anesthesiology*. 2017;126:534–542.)

Reversal of Opioid-Induced Respiratory Depression

14 As noted above, the drug of choice in case of life-threatening respiratory depression or the inability to resume spontaneous breathing is naloxone.[65,115] Naloxone is a competitive MOR antagonist causing a parallel rightward shift of the opioid dose–response relationship. An oral MOR antagonist, naltrexone, is used in the treatment of alcoholism and opioid dependence.[65] Both antagonists are nonspecific, meaning that they antagonize all pharmacologic effects of opioids. The magnitude and duration of reversal of respiratory depression by naloxone depends on the PK and PD profile of the opioid that needs reversal and the administration mode of naloxone (bolus injections vs. continuous infusion).[115,116] Naloxone's onset time ($t½k_{e0}$) is 6.5 minutes, indicating that reversal is rapid. But the rate of decay of naloxone in plasma is relatively fast ($t½_{elim}$ 30 minutes), resulting in "renarcotization" when used to reverse effects from opioids with a longer plasma half-life than naloxone. However, opioid concentrations are often just above the threshold for respiratory depression, and intravenous titration of naloxone 40 to 80 μg bolus doses to cumulative doses of less than 400 μg is often sufficient to restore spontaneous breathing.[97] Respiratory depression from opioids occurs at higher receptor occupancy rates than analgesia. Therefore, analgesia is not compromised with careful titration of naloxone to respiratory effect. Large doses of naloxone, as commonly used in resuscitation, will reverse analgesia immediately and may predispose patients to pain- and catecholamine-associated hypertension and cardiac ischemia, if not monitored properly.[65]

The naloxone titration opioid reversal approach is adequate for most opioids, with the exception of opioids with a high affinity for the MOR, such as buprenorphine or carfentanil.[116] In that case, a continuous naloxone infusion (2 to 4 mg/h) will cause a slow but steady resumption of breathing activity. For remifentanil, the use of bolus naloxone doses in case of respiratory depression is unnecessary. The termination of the infusion will provide a rapid return of spontaneous breathing.

Recently, nasal naloxone spray became popular for treatment of an opioid overdose on the street, either by caretakers or by bystanders (take-home naloxone).[65] The dose is 2 to 4 mg, repeated every 2 to 3 minutes if the patient is unresponsive or relapses into respiratory depression.

Naloxone remains the mainstay of opioid respiratory depres- 

sion treatment. However, it has several drawbacks. It is not effective in reversing high-affinity or high-dose opioids, it has a short duration of action and therefore requires redosing to match opioid duration, and it may cause acute opioid withdrawal symptoms such as agitation and/or pain. Recently, various drugs have been developed to reverse opioid-induced respiratory depression without the drawbacks of naloxone. Development of respiratory stimulants without naloxone's unwanted effects is advantageous, particularly since opioids are often used or abused with other centrally acting agents where naloxone is not effective in reversing respiratory depression. Hence, nonopioid respiratory stimulants may be an important component of reversing respiratory depression from a variety of causes.

A variety of respiratory stimulants have been tested but none are currently ready for clinical use.[117] These stimulants include ketamine, nicotinic acetylcholine receptor agonists, ampakines, serotonin receptor agonists, potassium channel blockers acting at the carotid bodies[118,119] (Fig. 20-15), sequestration techniques, and partial opioid agonists/antagonists. Some reversal agents lack efficacy at deep respiratory depression. This may be related

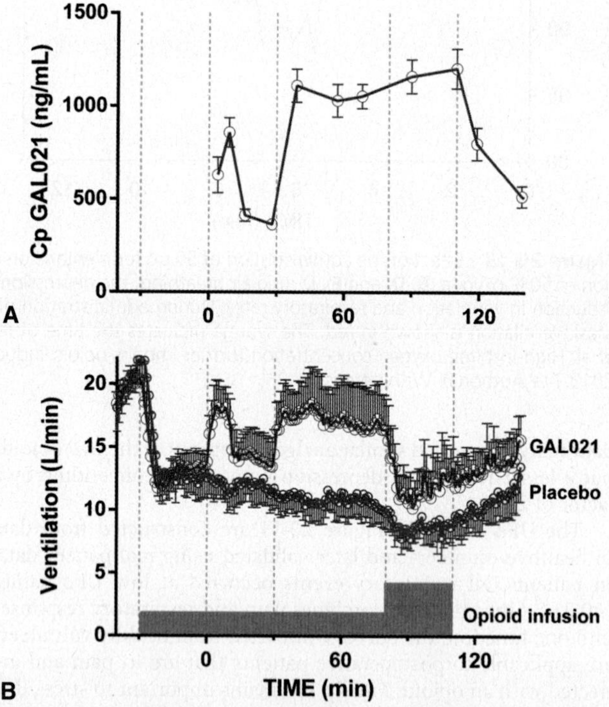

Figure 20-15 Influence of the BK_{Ca}-channel blocker GAL021 on opioid-induced respiratory depression. A: GAL021 plasma concentrations. **B:** The reduced ventilation induced by the opioid alfentanil (*orange*), along with the stimulatory effect of GAL021 are both clearly visible. (Data from Roozekrans M, Olofsen E, van der Schrier R, et al. Reversal of opioid-induced respiratory depression by BK-channel blocker GAL021: a pharmacokinetic-pharmacodynamic modelling study in healthy volunteers. *Clin Pharmacol Ther*. 2015;97:641–649.)

to ceiling effects or inability to be effective in case of apnea, as described by various pharmacodynamic models that may be used to simulate possible opioid-stimulant interactions.[120] Alternatively, combining these stimulants with low-dose naloxone is a more realistic scenario. So far, none of these reversal agents are viable alternatives to naloxone, which is still a critical therapy to restore and maintain normal ventilation.[117]

Monitoring

Monitoring of Nociception during Anesthesia and Surgery

Anesthesia care providers commonly use hemodynamic parameters to detect changes in nociception in patients under anesthesia. However, there is ample evidence that blood pressure and heart rate have low specificity as surrogates for nociception (i.e., other conditions that are unrelated to nociception cause changes in heart rate and blood pressure). To overcome this issue and give anesthesiologists an objective biomarker of nociception, several indices have been developed to detect nociceptive events.[121] These indices derive a numerical value either from single variables (such as heart rate variability, skin conductance, skin vasomotor reflex, the EEG, pupil diameter) or from a combination of these signals. The number of studies on these novel monitors is growing and their impact on clinical practice is hotly debated.[121] One monitor, the Nociception Level monitor or NOL, uses a machine learning technology to combine four signals (heart rate variability, heart rate, plethysmography, and skin conductance) and their derivatives to obtain an objective and quantifiable measure of nociception. The NOL ranges from 0 (absence of any nociception) to 100 (max. detectable nociception). A series of studies have validated the device and assessed its performance.[122–124] NOL-guided remifentanil dosing resulted in increased hemodynamic stability during anesthesia, while NOL-guided fentanyl dosing was associated with reduced pain in the PACU and lower stress hormone levels (Fig. 20-16).[123,124] Although further studies are needed in larger cohorts of patients, the future may see similar monitors being used to guide the response to nociceptive events and dose analgesic medication during and after surgery.

Monitoring on the Ward

On the ward, patients are monitored less comprehensively than in the operating room or PACU. On the ward, "spot" oxygen saturation measurements by regular nurse visits are insufficient to detect or predict the occurrence of life-threatening respiratory events.[125] A study in 833 patients recovering from noncardiac surgery in which continuous oxygen saturation was measured up to 48 hours after surgery showed that hypoxia was common and prolonged.[126] The saturation values recorded in medical records seriously underestimated the presence, duration, and severity of postoperative hypoxemia (21% of patients had oxygen saturation levels <90% for 10 minutes or more per hour; 8% had saturation levels <85% for 5 minutes or more per hour, Fig. 20-17).[126] Apart from cardiopulmonary causes such as ventilation–perfusion mismatch, significant drops in oxygen saturation and tachydysrhythmias do occur when the patient's breathing system has been compromised for an appreciable period by recurrent central or obstructive apneas (or both) and no arousal occurs. Arousal is a "wake-up" from a state of sleep

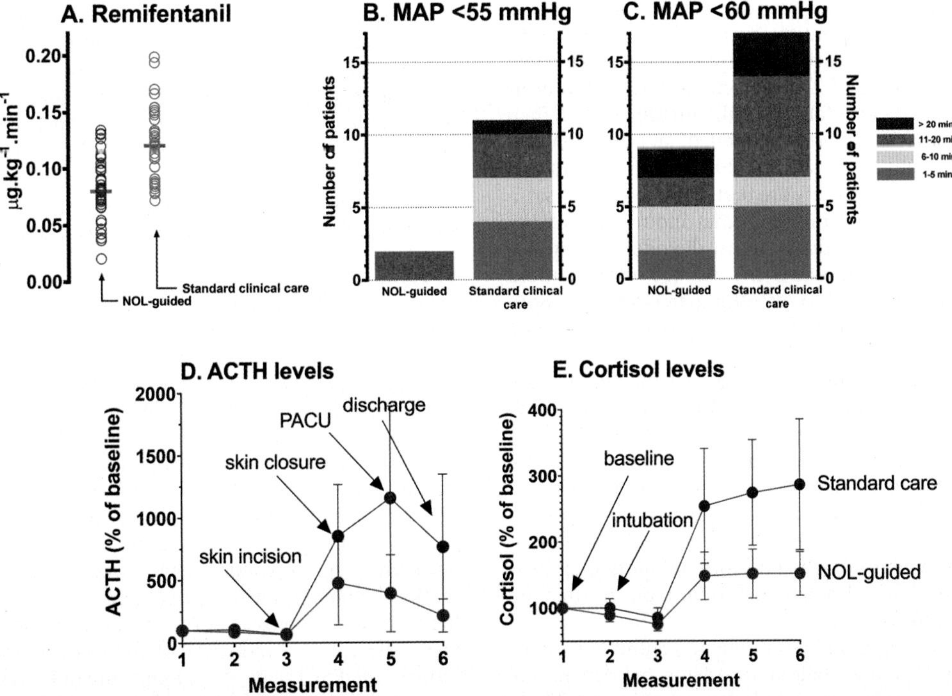

Figure 20-16 Nociception monitor-guided anesthesia. A: Effect of Nociception Level (NOL) monitor-guided remifentanil dosing on remifentanil consumption. **B:** Effect of NOL monitor-guided remifentanil dosing on severe hypotensive effects (mean arterial pressure, MAP <55 mmHg) and moderate hypotensice events (MAP <60 mmHg). (Reprinted with permission from Meijer F, Martini C, Broens S, et al. Nociception-guided versus standard care during remifentanil-propofol anesthesia: a randomized controlled trial. *Anesthesiology*. 2019;130:745–755.). **C** and **D:** Effect of NOL-guided fentanyl dosing on stress hormone levels during and following surgery. *Blue* = standard care, *red* = n + NOL monitor-guided care. (Reprinted from Meijer F, Honing M, Roor T, et al. Reduced postoperative pain in patients receiving Nociception Level-guided fentanyl-dosing during sevoflurane anesthesia—a randomized controlled trial. *Br J Anaesth*. 2020;125(6):1070-1078. Copyright © 2020 The Author(s). https://creativecommons.org/licenses/by/4.0/)

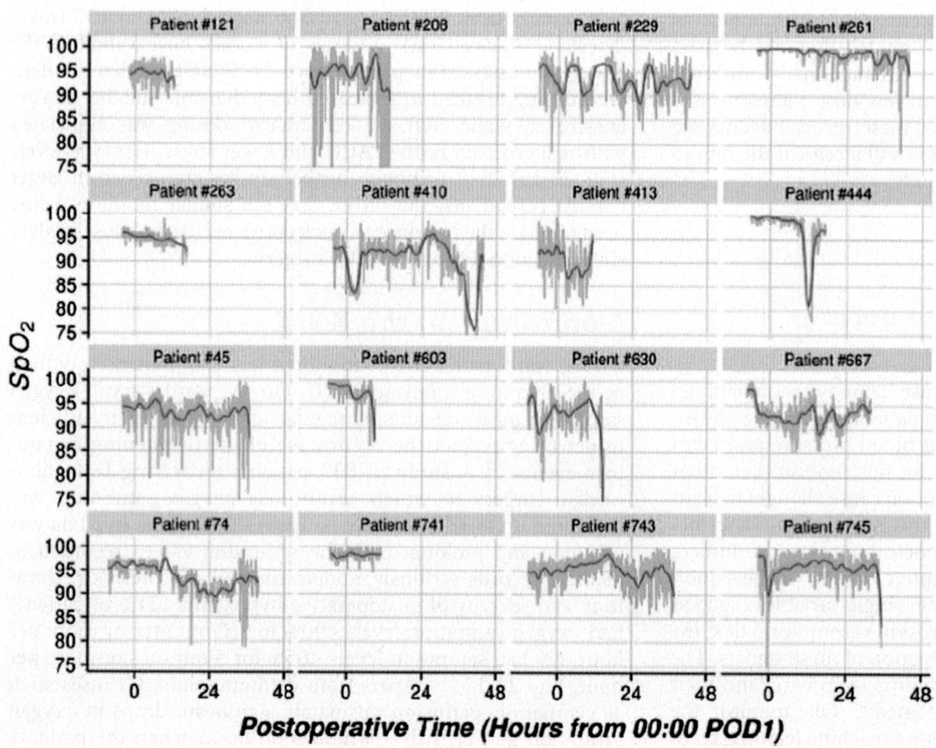

Figure 20-17 Oxygen saturation tracings of 16 patients following noncardiac surgery. The raw saturation data are shown (*light green*), along with the smoothed estimates (*black lines*). POD is postoperative day. (Reprinted with permission from Sun Z, Sessler DI, Dalton JE, et al. Postoperative hypoxemia is common and persistent: a prospective blinded observational study. *Anesth Analg.* 2014;121:709–715.)

or sedation, and allows the patient to open their throat and hyperventilate to overcome the preceding period of hypoxemia. Arousal is triggered by hypoxia, and depressed by opioids and sedatives. Postoperative respiratory events are often episodic, with arousals and hyperventilation in-between events. This will cause repetitive triggering of the oxygen saturation monitoring alarm and possibly alarm fatigue of the nursing staff. When the alarm is either inactivated or unattended, an arousal failure may occur and is potentially fatal (Fig. 20-18).[127] Monitors that directly indicate breathing activity are preferable to oxygen saturation monitoring, including monitors that indirectly measure expiratory flow, such as end-tidal carbon dioxide and humidity.[128,129] The latter device measures the exhaled water content and gives a reliable estimate of breathing frequency.[128] Both monitors will alarm in the event of airway obstruction (flow rate is zero) or reduced breathing rates.

A new development in monitoring is the integrated pulmonary index (IPI) that integrates four continuous measurements (end-tidal PCO_2, breathing rate, oxygen saturation, and heart rate) in real time into an index that reflects the respiratory state of the patient using a fuzzy-logic algorithm.[129] For example, patients with insufficient airflow at the mouth (as detected by low end-tidal PCO_2 and low respiratory rate) will have a low IPI score that deserves immediate attention. IPI and other monitors that measure flow at the mouth may become important tools in detecting serious opioid side effects.

The need for more ergonomic solutions to continuous monitoring of vital signs in hospitalized inpatients has led to the development of "wearable" or body-borne transducers. These transducers allow patients mobility while reducing false-positive alarms related to movement and disconnected cables that tethered the patient to a bedside monitor. This form factor, in combination with advanced signal processing techniques and machine learning algorithms, is making continuous inpatient monitoring—and eventually continuous home monitoring—a practical reality.[130]

Other Opioid-Related Side Effects

Apart from respiratory depression, opioids produce many other 16
side effects that can cause patient discomfort, as well as potentially serious consequences. Common side effects are nausea and vomiting, delayed gastric emptying, constipation, bowel distension, paralytic ileus, sphincter of Oddi spasm, urinary retention, histamine release, miosis, muscle rigidity, diffuse CNS effects (dizziness, light-headedness, sedation, drowsiness, euphoria, dysphoria), cognitive dysfunction (memory loss, inability to concentrate or focus attention), hallucinations, and cardiovascular effects.

Nausea and Vomiting

Postoperative nausea and vomiting (PONV) is a serious side effect from all opioids used in perioperative care (2 Video 20-2). Although inhalation anesthetics contribute significantly to this effect, opioids are the major cause of PONV with an incidence of greater than 50% following balanced anesthesia.[131] Female patients seem more sensitive to opioid-induced PONV (see below). Patient distress from PONV can be so severe that patients may prefer being in pain than being nauseated.[132] Furthermore, retching and vomiting will induce severe pain from the stress it places on recent surgical wounds. Opioids cause PONV by their effects on the chemoreceptor trigger zone (CTZ) in the area postrema of the brainstem, as well as by direct effects on the GI tract.[133] Movement effects (e.g., transport of the patient from the operating room to the PACU) may also contribute to PONV because opioids cause an increased sensitivity of the vestibular system. The CTZ contains opioid, serotonin ($5HT_3$), histamine, dopamine (D_2), and muscarinic acetylcholine receptors.[133] The CTZ, vagal nerve, and vestibular organs, all send neural projections to the vomiting center in the medulla. Drugs used in the treatment of PONV include dopamine antagonists (e.g., droperidol), 5HT-antagonists (e.g., ondansetron), and corticosteroids.[131,132] In patients with a

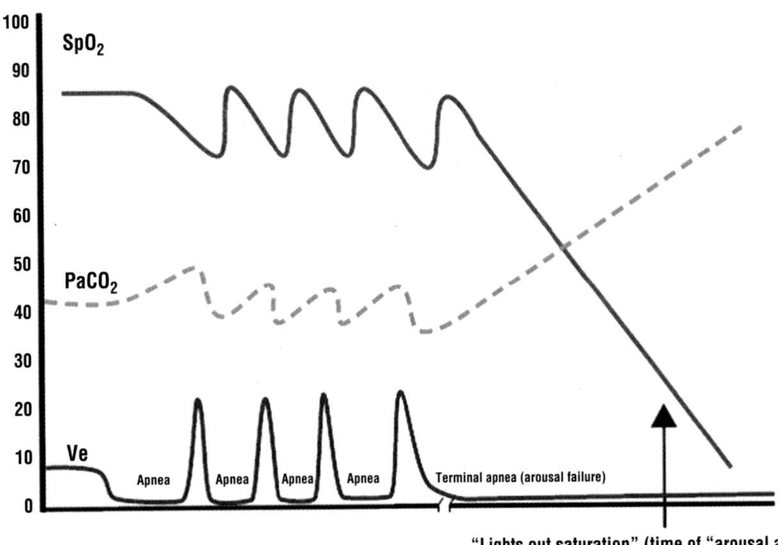

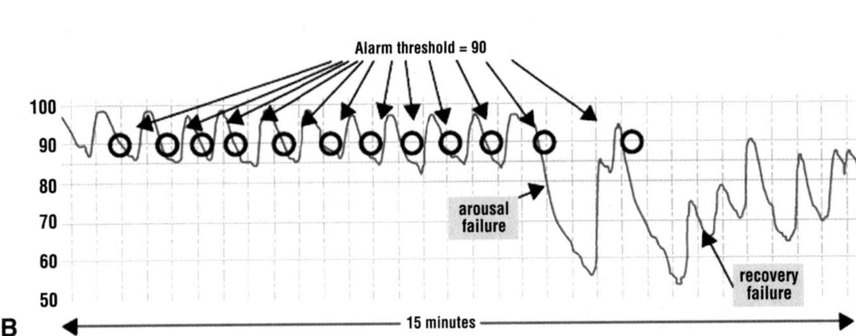

Figure 20-18 A: Episodic breathing pattern in a hypothetical patient with recurrent obstructive apneic events as might occur during sleep. SpO_2, oxygen saturation; $PaCO_2$, arterial carbon dioxide concentration; Ve, expired minute ventilation. **B:** Recurrent activation of the saturation alarm in a patient with sleep apnea (alarm threshold set at 90% oxygen saturation). This could possibly lead to alarm fatigue (y-axis = SpO_2). (Reprinted from Curry JP, Lynn LA. Threshold monitoring, alarm fatigue, and the patterns of unexpected hospital death. *APSF Newsletter Fall*. 2011;26:32. Copyright © 2011 Anesthesia Patient Safety Foundation.)

known history of PONV or those undergoing surgeries with a known high incidence of PONV, aggressive prevention strategies are used. Such strategies include the use of propofol rather than inhalation anesthetics, the use of regional postoperative analgesia rather than intravenous opioids, and multimodal pharmacologic therapy, including a 5HT-antagonist, a dopamine antagonist, and a steroid given prior to the end of surgery.

Smooth Muscle Effects

Opioid receptors are present in the enteric plexus within the smooth muscle layers of the GI tract. Opioids inhibit intestinal and pancreatic secretion, increase bowel tone, and decrease intestinal propulsive activity.[134] Consequently, opioids cause delayed gastric emptying, constipation, bowel distension, and paralytic ileus. Although opioids affect GI motility from central sites as well, blockade of opioid receptors with opioid antagonists that do not cross the blood–brain barrier (such as methylnaltrexone) will have a favorable effect on GI motility.[135]

Due to spasms of the sphincter of Oddi and common bile duct, opioids may cause acute upper abdominal pain and colic-like complaints.[136] Opioids may also contribute to misinterpretation of perioperative cholangiograms. Naloxone or glucagon can be used for treatment as both cause relaxation of the sphincter muscle.

Activated opioid receptors present in the wall of the bladder and ureters can cause acute urine retention.[137] It is most often seen after epidural or spinal opioid administration, with a higher incidence in men than in women. Urine retention is related to the inability of the urethral sphincter muscle to relax while the bladder tone increases. Opioid-induced bladder dysfunction can be treated with opioid antagonists.[138]

Cardiovascular Effects

Opioids affect the cardiovascular system at both central and peripheral sites.[139] Central effects include the activation of vagal nuclei and depression of vasomotor centers in the brainstem. Peripheral effects occur predominantly at high (supraclinical) doses and include direct myocardial depression and both arterial and venous dilatation. Morphine may cause additional cardiovascular effects via the release of histamine. The physiologic consequences are typically mild at clinical doses and include orthostatic hypotension, mild bradycardia, and a moderate reduction of systemic and pulmonary resistance. However, opioids at these doses can induce hemodynamic instability when combined with other drugs such as inhalation anesthetics, propofol, or benzodiazepines, and in severely ill patients (e.g., sepsis). Treatment of hemodynamic instability includes the administration of atropine and vasopressors and intravascular fluid therapy.

For further review and interactivities, please see the videos and narrative interactive clinical vignettes (NICVs) accessible in the complimentary eBook bundled with this text. Access instructions are located on the inside front cover.

REFERENCES

1. Jalal H, Buchanich JM, Roberts MS, Balmert LC, Zhang K, Burke DS. Changing dynamics of the drug overdose epidemic in the United States from 1979 through 2016. *Science*. 2018; 361:eaau1184
2. Bedene A, Lijfering WM, Niesters M, et al. Opioid prescription patterns and risk factors associated with opioid use in the netherlands. *JAMA Network Open*. 2019;2:e1910223.
3. Okie S. A flood of opioids, a rising tide of deaths. *N Engl J Med*. 2010;363:1981–1985.
4. Dunn KM, Saunders KW, Rutter CM, et al. Opioid prescriptions for chronic pain and overdose: a cohort study. *Ann Intern Med*. 2010;152:85–92.
5. Vila H Jr, Smith RA, Augustyniak MJ, et al. The efficacy of pain management before and after implementation of hospital-wide pain management standards: is patient safety compromised by treatment solely based on numerical pain ratings? *Anesth Analg*. 2005;101:474–480.
6. Sertürner F. Uber das Morphium, eine neue salzfühige Grundlage, und die Mekonsâure, als Hauptbestandtheile des Opiums. *Ann Physik*. 1917;5:56.
7. Huxtable RJ, Schwartz SK. The isolation of morphine. *Mol Interv*. 2001;1:189–191.
8. Bovill JG. Opium: a drug ancient and modern. In: Dahan A, van Kleef JW, eds. Advances in Anesthesia and Analgesia. University Medical Center; 2007;1:13.
9. Garfield E. The 1982 John Scott Award goes to Jack Fishman and Harold Blumberg for synthesis and investigation of naloxone. *Essays Inform Sci*. 1983;6:121.
10. Linz K, Christoph T, Tzschentke TM, et al. Cebranopadol: a novel potent analgesic nociception/orphanin FQ peptide and opioid receptor agonist. *J Pharmacol Exp Ther*. 2014; 349:535–548.
11. Dahan A, van Dam CJ, Niesters M, et al. Benefit and risk evaluation of biased μ-receptor agonist oliceridine versus morphine. *Anesthesiology*. 2020;133:559–568.
12. Kieffer BL, Gavériaux-Ruff C. Exploring the opioid system by gene knockout. *Prog Neurobiol*. 2002;66:285–306.
13. Chiou LC, Liao YY, Fan PC, et al. Nociceptin/orphanin FQ peptide receptors: pharmacology and clinical implications. *Curr Drug Targets*. 2007;8:117–135.
14. Pasternak GW. Pharmacological mechanisms of opioid analgesics. *Clin Neuropharmacol*. 1993;16:1–18.
15. Stefano GB. The μ_3 opiate receptor subtype. *Pain Forum*. 1999;8:206–209.
16. Alexander SPH, Mathie A, Peters JA. Guide to receptors and channels (GRAC), 4th ed. *Br J Pharmacol*. 2009;158(Suppl 1):S1–S254.
17. Standifer KM, Pasternak GW. G proteins and opioid receptor-mediated signaling. *Cell Signal*. 1997;9:237–248.
18. Waldhoer M, Bartlett SE, Whistler JL. Opioid receptors. *Annu Rev Biochem*. 2004;73:953–990.
19. Chen YL, Law PY, Loh HH. The other side of the opioid story: modulation of cell growth and survival signaling. *Curr Med Chem*. 2008;15:772–778.
20. Eguchi M. Recent advances in selective opioid receptor agonists and antagonists. *Med Res Rev*. 2004;24:182–212.
21. Bird MF, Lambert DG. Simultaneous targeting of multiple opioid receptor types. *Curr Opin Supprt Palliat Care*. 2015;9:98–102.
22. Callahan RJ, Au JD, Paul M, Liu C, Yost CS. Functional inhibition by methadone of N-methyl-D-aspartate receptors expressed in Xenopus oocytes: stereospecific and subunit effects. *Anesth Analg*. 2004;98:653–659.
23. Dykstra LA, Fischer BD, Balter RE, Henry FE, Schmidt KT, Miller LL. Opioid antinociception, tolerance and dependence: interactions with the N-methyl-D-aspartate system in mice. *Behav Pharmacol*. 2011;22:540–547.
24. Kissin I, Bright CA, Bradley EL Jr. The effect of ketamine on opioid-induced acute tolerance: can it explain reduction of opioid consumption with ketamine-opioid analgesic combinations? *Anesth Analg*. 2000;91:1483–1488.
25. Yi SP, Kong QH, Li YL, et al. The opioid receptor triple agonist DPI-125 produces analgesia with less respiratory depression and reduced abuse liability. *Acta Pharmacol Sin*. 2017;38:977–989.
26. Sarton E, Teppema LJ, Olievier C, et al. Involvement of μ-opioid receptor in ketamine-induced respiratory depression and antinociception. *Anesth Analg*. 2001;93:1495–1500.
27. Loeser JD, Treede RD. The Kyoto protocol of IASP Basic Pain Terminology. *Pain*. 2008;137: 473–477.
28. Raja SN, Carr DB, Cohen M, et al. The revised International Association for the Study of Pain definition of pain: concepts, challenges, and compromises. *Pain*. 2020;161:1976–1982.
29. Millan MJ. Descending control of pain. *Prog Neurobiol*. 2002;66:355–474.
30. Ossipov MH, Dussor GO, Porreca F. Central modulation of pain. *J Clin Invest*. 2010;120: 3779–3787.
31. Brown EN, Purdon PL, Van Dort CJ. General anesthesia and altered states of arousal: a systems neuroscience analysis. *Annu Rev Neurosci*. 2011;34:601–628.
32. Akil H, Mayer DJ, Liebeskind JC. Antagonism of stimulation-produced analgesia by naloxone, a narcotic antagonist. *Science*. 1976;191:961–962.
33. Butler RK, Finn DP. Stress-induced analgesia. *Prog Neurobiol*. 2009;88:184–202.
34. Eipert F, Bingel U, Schoell ED, et al. Activation of opioidergic descending pain control system underlies placebo analgesia. *Neuron*. 2009;63:533–543.
35. Pud D, Granovsky Y, Yarnitsky D. The methodology of experimentally-induced diffuse noxious inhibitory (DNIC)-line effects in humans. *Pain*. 2009;144:16–19.
36. Beecher HK. Pain in men wounded in battle. *Ann Surg*. 1946;123:96–105.
37. Zubieta JK, Bueller JA, Jackson LR, et al. Placebo effects mediated by endogenous opioid activity on μ-opioid receptors. *J Neurosci*. 2005;25:7754–7762.
38. Petrovic P, Kalso E, Petersson KM, Ingvar M. Placebo and opioid analgesia: imaging a shared neuronal network. *Science*. 2002;295:1737–1740.
39. Moont R, Pud D, Sprecher E, Sharvit G, Yarnitsky D. "Pain inhibits pain" mechanisms: is pain modulation simply due to distraction. *Pain*. 2010;150:113–120.
40. Niesters M, Dahan A, Swartjes M, et al. Effect of ketamine on endogenous pain modulation in healthy volunteers. *Pain*. 2010;152:656–663.
41. Lagerwij E, Nelis PC, Wiegant VM, van Ree JM. The twitch in horses: a variant of acupuncture. *Science*. 1984;225:1172–1174.
42. van de Donk T, van Velzen M, Dahan A, Niesters M. Cornea nerve fiber state determines analgesic response to tapentadol in fibromyalgia patients without effective descending pain modulation. *Eur J Pain*. 2019;23:1586–1595.
43. Scholz J, Woolf CJ. The neuropathic pain triad: neurons, immune cells and glia. *Nat Neurosci*. 2007;10:1361–1368.
44. Kapitzke D, Vetter I, Cabot PJ. Endogenous opioid analgesia in peripheral tissues and the implications for pain control. *Ther Clin Risk Manag*. 2005;1:279–297.
45. Stein S, Machelska H. Modulation of peripheral sensory information by the immune system: implication for pain therapy. *Pharmacol Rev*. 2011;63:860–881.
46. Busch-Dienstfertig M, Stein C. Opioid receptors and opioid peptide-producing leucocytes in inflammatory pain: basic and therapeutic aspects. *Brain Behav Immun*. 2010;24:683–694.
47. Bekhit MH. Opioid-induced hyperalgesia and tolerance. *Am J Ther*. 2010;17:498–510.
48. Bruno G, Bossard AE, Coste C, et al. Acute opioid tolerance: Intraoperative remifentanil increases postoperative pain and morphine requirement. *Anesthesiology*. 2000;93:409–417.
49. Joly V, Richebe P, Guignard B, et al. Remifentanil-induced postoperative hyperalgesia and its prevention with small-dose ketamine. *Anesthesiology*. 2005;103:147–155.
50. van Dorp EL, Kest B, Kowalczyk WJ, et al. Morphine-6β-glucuronide rapidly increases pain sensitivity independently of opioid receptors in mice and humans. *Anesthesiology*. 2009;110:1356–1363.
51. Bohn LM, Lefkowitz RJ, Gainetdinov RR, Peppel K, Caron MG, Lin FT. Enhanced morphine analgesia in mice lacking beta-arrestin 2. *Science*. 1999;286:2495–2498.
52. Zuo Z. The role of opioid receptor internalization and beta-arrestins in the development of opioid tolerance. *Anesth Analg*. 2005;101:728–734.
53. Algera H, Olofsen E, Moss L, et al. Tolerance to opioid-induced respiratory depression in chronic high-dose opioid users: a model-based comparison with opioid-naive individuals. *Clin Pharmacol Ther*. 2020;109:637–645.
54. Hughes MA, Glass PSA, Jacobs JR. Context-sensitive half-time in multicompartment: pharmacokinetic models for intravenous anesthetic drugs. *Anesthesiology*. 1992;76:334–341.
55. Kapila A, Glass PSA, Jacobes JR, et al. Measured context-sensitive half-times of remifentanil and alfentanil. *Anesthesiology*. 1995;83:968–975.
56. Olofsen E, Boom M, Nieuwenhuijs D, et al. Modeling the non-steady-state respiratory effects of remifentanil in awake and propofol sedated healthy volunteers. *Anesthesiology*. 2010;212:1382–1395.
57. Wilkinson GR. Drug metabolism and variability among patients in drug response. *N Engl J Med*. 2005;352:2211–2221.
58. van Dorp E, Romberg R, Sarton E, Bovill JG, Dahan A. Morphine-6-glucuronide: morphine's successor for postoperative pain relief? *Anesth Analg*. 2006;102:1789–1797.
59. Romberg R, Olofsen E, Sarton E, den Hartigh J, Taschner PEM, Dahan A. Pharmacokinetic/pharmacodynamic modeling of morphine-6-glucuronide-induced analgesia in healthy volunteers: absence of sex differences. *Anesthesiology*. 2004;100:120–133.
60. Dahan A, Lötsch J. Morphine is not a prodrug. *Br J Anaesth*. 2015;114:1005–1006.
61. Tateishi T, Krivoruk Y, Ueng YF, Wood AJ, Guengerich FP, Wood M. Identification of liver cytochrome P-450 3 A as the enzyme responsible for fentanyl and sufentanil N-dealkylation. *Anesth Analg*. 1996;82:167–172.
62. Smith HS. The metabolism of opioid agents and the clinical impact of their active metabolites. *Clin J Pain*. 2011;27:824–838.
63. Scott LJ, Perry CM. Spotlight on remifentanil for general anesthesia. *CNS Drugs*. 2005;19:1069–1074.
64. Kharasch ED. Intraoperative methadone: rediscovery, reappraisal and reinvigoration. *Anesth Analg*. 2011;112:13–16.
65. van Dorp ELA, Yassen A, Dahan A. Naloxone treatment in opioid addiction: the risks and benefits. *Expert Opin Drug Safe*. 2007;6:125–132.
66. Martini C, Olofsen E, Yassen A, Aarts L, Dahan A. Pharmacokinetic-pharmacodynamic modeling in acute and chronic pain: an overview of the recent literature. *Expert Rev Clin Pharmacol*. 2011;4:719–728.
67. Segre G. Kinetics of interaction between drugs and biological systems. *Farmaco Sci*. 1968;23:907–918.
68. Sheiner L, Stanski LB, Vozeh S, Miller RD, Ham J. Simultaneous modeling of pharmacokinetics and pharmacodynamics: application to d-tubocurarine. *Clin Pharmacol Ther*. 1979;25:358–371.
69. Aubrun F, Salvi N, Coriat P, Riou B. Sex- and age-related differences in morphine requirements for postoperative pain relief. *Anesthesiology*. 2005;103:156–160.

70. Dahan A, Boom M, Olofsen E. Differences in onset/offset times for different end-points: pain relief, pupil size and respiratory depression. *Anesthesiology*. 2011;A1569.
71. Olofsen E, Romberg R, Bijl H, et al. Alfentanil and placebo analgesia: absence of sex differences. *Anesthesiology*. 2005;103:130–139.
72. Aubrun F, Langeron O, Quesnel C, Coriat P, Riou B. Relationships between measurement of pain using visual analog score and morphine requirements during postoperative intravenous morphine titration. *Anesthesiology*. 2003;98:1415–1421.
73. Sarton E, Olofsen E, Romberg R, et al. Sex differences in morphine analgesia: an experimental study in healthy volunteers. *Anesthesiology*. 2000;93:1245–1254.
74. Wolrich J, Poots AJ, Kuehler BM, Rice ASC, Rahman A, Bantel C. Is number sense impaired in chronic pain patients? *Br J Anaesth*. 2014;113:1024–1031.
75. Oudejans L, van Velzen M, Olofsen E, Beun R, Dahan A, Niesters M. Translation of random painful stimuli into numerical responses in fibromyalgia and perioperative patients. *Pain*. 2016;157:128–136.
76. Abou Hammoud H, Simon N, Urien S, Riou B, Lechat P, Aubrun F. Intravenous morphine titration in immediate postoperative pain management: population kinetic-pharmacodynamic and logistic regression analysis. *Pain*. 2009;144:139–146.
77. Mazoit JX, Btscher K, Samii K. Morphine in postoperative patients: pharmacokinetics and pharmacodynamics of metabolites. *Anesth Analg*. 2007;105:70–78.
78. Tallarida RJ, Stone DJ Jr, McCary JD, Raffa RB. Response surface analysis of synergism between morphine and clonidine. *J Pharmacol Exp Ther*. 1999;289:8–13.
79. Schulte H, Sollevi A, Sgerdahl M. The synergistic effect of combined treatment with systematic ketamine and morphine on experimentally induced wind-up pain in humans. *Anesth Analg*. 2004;98:1574–1580.
80. Daniel M, Weiskopf RB, Noorani M, Eger EI 2nd. Fentanyl augments the blockade of the sympathetic response to incision (MAC-BAR) produced by desflurane and isoflurane: desflurane and isoflurane MAC-BAR without and with fentanyl. *Anesthesiology*. 1998;88:43–49.
81. Kazama T, Ikeda K, Morita K. The pharmacodynamic interaction between propofol and fentanyl with respect to suppression of somatic or hemodynamic responses to skin incision, peritoneum incision, and abdominal wall retraction. *Anesthesiology*. 1998;89:894–906.
82. Sebel PS, Glass PSA, Fletcher JE, Murphy MR, Gallagher C, Quill T. Reduction of the MAC of desflurane with fentanyl. *Anesthesiology*. 1992;88:52–59.
83. Niesters M, Mahajan RP, Aarts L, Dahan A. High-inspired oxygen concentration further impairs opioid-induced respiratory depression. *Br J Anaesth*. 2013;110:837–841.
84. Drover D, Lemmens HJM. Population pharmacodynamics and pharmacokinetics of remifentanil as a supplement to nitrous oxide anesthesia for elective abdominal surgery. *Anesthesiology*. 1998;89:869–877.
85. Vuyk J, Mertens MJ, Olofsen E, Burm AG, Bovill JG. Propofol anesthesia and rational opioid selection. *Anesthesiology*. 1997;87:1549–1562.
86. Lang E, Kapila A, Schlugman D, Hoke JF, Sebel PS, Glass PSA. Reduction of isoflurane minimal alveolar concentration by remifentanil. *Anesthesiology*. 1996;85:721–728.
87. Dahan A, van Lemmen M, Jansen S, Simons P, van der Schrier R. Buprenorphine: a treatment nd cause of respiratory depression. *Br J Anaesth* 2022;128:402–404.
88. Yassen A, Olofsen E, Romberg R, et al. Mechanism based PK/PD modeling of the respiratory depressant effect of buprenorphine and fentanyl in healthy volunteers. *Clin Pharmacol Ther*. 2007;81:50–58.
89. Wiest K, Algera MH, Moss L, van Velzen M, Dobbins R. High plasma buprenorphine concentrations decrease respiratory effects of intravenous fentanyl. American Society of Addiction Medicine. April 4, 2019. https://www.eventscribe.com/2019/posters/ASAM/SplitViewer.asp?PID=MzcwNzkzNTM2MDA
90. Vodovar D, Chevillard L, Caillé F, et al. Mechanisms of respiratory depression induced by the combination of buprenorphine and diazepam in rats. *Br J Anaesth*. 2022;128:584–595.
91. Klepstad P, Fladvad T, Skorpen F, et al; European Palliative Care Research Collaborative (EPCRC) and the European Association for Palliative Care Research Network. Influence from genetic variability on opioid use for cancer pain: a European genetic association study of 2294 pain patients. *Pain*. 2011;152:1139–1145.
92. Liem EB, Lin CM, Suleman MI, et al. Anesthetic requirement is increased in redheads. *Anesthesiology*. 2004;101:279–283.
93. Weinshiliboum R. Inheritance and drug response. *N Engl J Med*. 2003;348:529–537.
94. Ciszkowski C, Madadi P, Phillips MS, Lauwers AE, Koren G. Codeine, ultrarapid-metabolism genotype, and postoperative death. *N Engl J Med*. 2009;361:827–828.
95. Koren G, Cairns J, Chitayat D, Gaedigk A, Leeder SJ. Pharmacogenetics of morphine poisoning in a breastfed neonate of a codeine-prescribed mother. *Lancet*. 2006;368:704.
96. Park HJ, Shinn HK, Ryu SH, Lee HS, Park CS, Kang JH. Genetic polymorphism in the ABCB1 gene and the effects of fentanyl in Koreans. *Clin Pharmacol Ther*. 2007;81:539–546.
97. Dahan A, Aarts L, Smith TW. Incidence, reversal and prevention of opioid-induced respiratory depression. *Anesthesiology*. 2010;112:226–238.
98. Varga AG, Reid BT, Kieffer BL, Levitt ES. Differential input of two critical respiratory centers in opioid-induced respiratory depression in awake mice. *J Physiol*. 2020;598:189–205.
99. Palkovic B, Callison JJ, Marchenko V, Stuth EAE, Zuperku EJ, Stucke AG. Dose-dependent respiratory depression by remifentanil in the rabbit parabrachial nucleus/Kölliker-Fuse complex and preBötzinger complex. *Anesthesiology*. 2021;135:649–672.
100. Baertsch NA, Bush NE, Burgraff NJ, Ramirez JM. Dual mechanisms of opioid-induced respiratory depression in the inspiratory rhythm-generating network. *Elife*. 2021:10:e67523.
101. Bernards CM, Knowlton SL, Schmidt DF, et al. Respiratory and sleep effects of remifentanil in volunteers with moderate obstructive sleep apnea. *Anesthesiology*. 2009;110:41–49.
102. Wu A, Drummond GB. Sleep arousal after lower abdominal surgery and relation to recovery from respiratory obstruction. *Anesthesiology*. 2003;99:1295–1302.
103. Chung F, Liao P, Yang Y, et al. Postoperative sleep-disordered breathing in patients without preoperative sleep apnea. *Anesth Analg*. 2015;120:1214–1224.
104. Stone JG, Cozine KA, Wald A. Nocturnal oxygenation during patient-controlled analgesia. *Anesth Analg*. 1999;89:104–110.
105. Bennet JA, Abrams JT, Van Riper DF, Horrow JC. Difficult or impossible ventilation after sufentanil-induced anesthesia is caused primarily by vocal cord closure. *Anesthesiology*. 1997;87:1070–1074.
106. Weinger MB, Segal IS, Maze M. Dexmedetomidine, acting through central alpha-2 adrenoreceptors, prevents opiate-induced muscle rigidity in the rat. *Anesthesiology*. 1989;71:242–249.
107. Overdyk FJ, Carter R, Maddox RR, Callura J, Herrin AE, Henriquez C. Continuous oximetry/capnometry monitoring reveals frequent desaturations and bradypnea during patient-controlled analgesia. *Anesth Analg*. 2007;105:412–418.
108. Khanna AK, Bergese S, Jungquist C, et al; PRediction of Opioid-induced respiratory Depression In patients monitored by capnoGraphY (PRODIGY) Group Collaborators. Prediction of opioid-induced respiratory depression on inpatient wards using continuous capnography and oximetry: an international prospective, observational trial. *Anesth Analg*. 2020;131:1012–1020.
109. Chung F, Yegneswaran B, Liao P, et al. Stop questionnaire: a tool to screen for obstructive apnea. *Anesthesiology*. 2008;108:812–821.
110. Niesters M, Overdyk F, Smith T, Aarts L, Dahan A. Opioid-induced respiratory depression in peadiatrics: a review of case reports. *Br J Anaesth*. 2013;110:175–182.
111. Boom M, Olofsen E, Neukirchen M, et al. Fentanyl utility function: a risk-benefit composite of pain relief and breathing responses. *Anesthesiology*. 2013;119:663–674.
112. Dahan A, Olofsen E, Niesters M. Pharmacotherapy for pain: efficacy and safety issues examined by subgroup analyses. *Pain*. 2015;156:S119–S126.
113. Olesen AE, Broens S, Olesen SS, et al. A pragmatic utility function to describe the risk-benefit composite of opioid and non-opioid analgesic medication. *J Pharmacol Exp Ther*. 2019;371:416–421.
114. van der Schrier R, Roozekrans M, Olofsen E, et al. Influence of ethanol on oxycodone-induced respiratory depression: a dose-escalating study in young and elderly volunteers. *Anesthesiology*. 2017;126:534–542.
115. Olofsen E, van Dorp E, Teppema L, et al. Naloxone reversal of morphine and morphine-6-glucuronide-induced respiratory depression. *Anesthesiology*. 2010;112:1417–1427.
116. van Dorp E, Yassen A, Sarton E, et al. Naloxone-reversal of buprenorphine-induced respiratory depression. *Anesthesiology*. 2006;105:51–57.
117. van der Schrier R, Dahan JDC, Boon M, et al. Advances in reversal strategies of opioid-induced respiratory depression. *Anesthesiology*. 2022;136(4):618–632.
118. Roozekrans M, van der Schrier R, Okkerse P, Hay J, McLeod JF, Dahan A. Two studies on reversal of opioid-induced respiratory depression by BK-channel blocker GAL021 in human volunteers. *Anesthesiology*. 2014;121:459–468.
119. Roozekrans M, Olofsen E, van der Schrier R, et al. Reversal of opioid-induced respiratory depression by BK-channel blocker GAL021: a pharmacokinetic-pharmacodynamic modelling study in healthy volunteers. *Clin Pharmacol Ther*. 2015;97:641–649.
120. Algera MH, Kamp J, van der Schrier R, et al. Opioid-induced respiratory depression in humans: pharmacokinetic-pharmacodynamic modelling of reversal. *Br J Anaesth*. 2019;122:e168–e179.
121. Meijer FS, Niesters M, van Velzen M, et al. Does nociception monitor-guided anesthesia affect opioid consumption? A systematic review of randomized controlled trials. *J Clin Monit Comput*. 2020;34:629–641.
122. Martini CH, Boon M, Broens SJL, et al. Ability of the nociception level, a multiparameter composite of autonomic signals, to detect noxious stimuli during propofol-remifentanil anesthesia. *Anesthesiology*. 2015;123:524–534.
123. Meijer FS, Martini CH, Broens S, et al. Nociception-guided versus standard care during remifentanil-propofol anesthesia: a randomized controlled trial. *Anesthesiology*. 2019;130:745–755.
124. Meijer FS, Honing M, Roor T, et al. Reduced postoperative pain in patients receiving Nociception Level-guided fentanyl-dosing during sevoflurane anesthesia: a randomized controlled trial. *Br J Anaesth*. 2020;125:1070–1078.
125. Vincent JL, Einav S, Pearse R, et al. Improving detection of patient deterioration in the general hospital ward environment. *Eur J Anaesthesiol*. 2018;35:325–333.
126. Sun Z, Sessler DI, Dalton JE, et al. Postoperative hypoxemia is common and persistent: a prospective blinded observational study. *Anesth Analg*. 2015;121:709–715.
127. Curry JP, JungquistCR. A critical assessment of monitoring practices, patient deterioration, and alarm fatigue on inpatient wards: a review. *Patient Saf Surg*. 2014;8:29.
128. Niesters M, Mahajan R, Olofsen E, et al. Validation of a novel respiratory rate monitor based on exhaled humidity. *Br J Anaesth*. 2012;109:981–989.

129. Broens SJL, Prins SA, de Kleer D, Niesters M, Dahan A, van Velzen M. Postoperative respiratory state assessment using the Integrated Pulmonary Index (IPI) and resultant nurse interventions in the post-anesthesia care unit: a randomized controlled trial. *J Clin Monit Comp*. 2020; 35:1093–1102.
130. Michard F, Bellomo R, Taenzer A. The rise of ward monitoring: opportunities and challenges for critical care specialists. *Intensive Care Med*. 2019;45:671–673.
131. Apfel CC, Korttila K, Abdalla M, et al; IMPACT Investigators. A factorial trial of six interventions for the prevention of postoperative nausea and vomiting. *N Engl J Med*. 2004; 350:2441–2451.
132. Macario A, Weinger N, Truong P, Lee M. Which clinical anesthesia outcomes are both common and important to avoid? *Anesth Analg*. 1999;88:1085–1091.
133. Gan TJ. Mechanisms underlying postoperative nausea and vomiting and neurotransmitter receptor antagonist-based pharmacotherapy. *CNS Drugs*. 2007;21:813–833.
134. Panchal SJ, Müller-Schwefe P, Wurzelmann JI. Opioid-induced bowel dysfunction: prevalence, pathophysiology and burden. *Int J Clin Pract*. 2007;61:1181–1187.
135. Thomas J. Opioid-induced bowel dysfunction. *J Pain Symptom Manage*. 2008;35:103–113.
136. Thompson DR. Narcotic analgesic effects on the sphincter of Oddi: a review of the data and therapeutic implications in treating pancreatitis. *Am J Gastroenterol*. 2001;96: 1266–1272.
137. Verhamme KMC, Strurkenboom MCJM, Stricker BHC, Bosch R. Drug-induced urinary retention: incidence, management and prevention. *Drug Saf*. 2008;31:373–388.
138. Rosow CE, Gomery P, Chen TY, Stefanovich P, Stambler N, Israel R. Reversal of opioid-induced bladder dysfunction by intravenous naloxone and methylnaltrexone. *Clin Pharmacol Ther*. 2007;82:48–53.
139. DeSouza G, Lewis MC, TerRiet MF. Severe bradycardia after remifentanil. *Anesthesiology*. 1997;87:1019–1020.

21 Neuromuscular Blocking Drugs

WADE A. WEIGEL • STUART ALAN GRANT • STEPHAN R. THILEN

KEY POINTS

1 It should be recognized, from the outset, that neuromuscular blocking drugs do not alter consciousness or cause amnesia. For this reason, neuromuscular blocking drugs have been implicated in contributing to accidental awareness under anesthesia.

2 Depending on the specific drugs used for neuromuscular blockade and reversal, the occurrence of postoperative residual neuromuscular blocking drug effect (known as residual paralysis) has been estimated to occur in approximately 40% of patients.

3 Nondepolarizing neuromuscular blocking drugs bind and inhibit presynaptic $\alpha3\beta2$ acetylcholine receptors, leading to a reduction in muscle contraction with subsequent nerve signals.

4 Nondepolarizing neuromuscular blocking drugs bind to one or both alpha subunits of the nicotinic acetylcholine receptor without causing any activation of these ion receptor channels.

5 The four most common neuromuscular blocking drugs currently used in clinical practice have an ED_{95} of either 0.3 or 0.05 (succinylcholine and rocuronium ED_{95} 0.3, cisatracurium and vecuronium ED_{95} 0.05). There is a highly significant variation between patients in response to all neuromuscular blocking drugs.

6 Because of its molecular similarity to acetylcholine, succinylcholine depolarizes both postsynaptic and extrajunctional receptors.

7 A prolonged duration of succinylcholine blockade may occur when the concentration of normal pseudocholinesterase is very significantly reduced or when an atypical variant of pseudocholinesterase is present.

8 Nondepolarizing neuromuscular blocking drugs can be classified by their chemistry and molecular structure: aminosteroid (e.g., pancuronium, vecuronium, rocuronium) or benzylisoquinolinium (e.g., atracurium, cisatracurium, mivacurium). Clinically they are classified by their expected duration of action: long-, intermediate-, or short-acting.

9 Different classes of nondepolarizing neuromuscular blocking drugs should not be mixed in the same patient because this can lead to an unpredictable extended duration of muscle paralysis.

10 All clinical assessments (e.g., maximum inspiratory force, vital capacity, tidal volume, eye opening, handgrip, tongue protrusion, handgrip, leg lift, and head lift) are insensitive and thus render the clinician incapable of identifying the presence of residual paralysis.

11 In the absence of any tactile or visual recognition of fade with train-of-four subjective assessment, the train-of-four ratio can be as low as 0.3 to 0.4.

12 Quantitative monitoring is the only way to objectively measure train-of-four ratio, supporting expert recommendations for this technology to be used in clinical practice.

13 Blocking the breakdown of acetylcholine by acetylcholinesterase (with anticholinesterase drugs) results in an increase in the available pool of acetylcholine at the synaptic cleft and improves the chances of competing with a nondepolarizing neuromuscular blocking drug.

14 Only when the residual neuromuscular block is minimal (e.g., train-of-four count of 4 without fade or train-of-four ratio $\geq$0.4) is neostigmine a highly effective reversal agent.

15 For a train-of-four count 2 or more, a sugammadex dose of 2 mg/kg will reverse to a train-of-four ratio greater than 0.9 in 2 to 4 minutes.

Introduction

Neuromuscular blocking drugs have been incorporated into clinical medicine for many years since the introduction of curare in 1942 and succinylcholine in 1950. These medications serve to inhibit skeletal muscle function, thereby offering the potential to improve conditions for endotracheal intubation, as well as optimize operating conditions when muscle activity can be detrimental. Neuromuscular blocking drugs have also been used to facilitate mechanical ventilation in the intensive care unit (ICU), although published international guidelines cite weak evidence of improved outcomes and suggest only using intermittent
1 boluses rather than an infusion.[1] It should be recognized, from the outset, that these drugs do not alter consciousness or cause amnesia. For this reason, neuromuscular blocking drugs have been implicated in contributing to accidental awareness under anesthesia. There are only a few nondepolarizing neuromuscular blocking drugs in clinical practice today, which are limited to two classes (aminosteroid and benzylisoquinolinium). It is important to understand the clinical advantages and limitations, such as anaphylaxis, of each available drug. Proper neuromuscular blockade management also encompasses the particularly important process of drug regression and reversal, which research suggests has been
2 less than ideal in the past. Depending on the specific drugs used for neuromuscular blockade and reversal, the occurrence of postoperative residual neuromuscular blocking drug effect (known as residual paralysis) has been estimated to occur in approximately 40% of patients.[2] However, with proper understanding of neuromuscular blocking drugs, monitoring of depth of blockade, reversal with the proper drug at the proper time, and verification of return of strength, patients need not suffer from residual paralysis. One important focus of this chapter is to provide the insights needed to eliminate residual paralysis.

Physiology

Nerve Propagation and Nerve Terminal

The process of signal generation to muscle contraction begins with an electrical signal propagating down a nerve (presynaptic motor nerve), then transitions to a chemical signal via release of acetylcholine across the neuromuscular junction, and finally concludes with the mechanical response of a muscle contraction. The motor cortex of the brain starts the neuronal signal which then travels from the upper motor neurons to the lower motor neurons, whose cell bodies are in the ventral horn of the spinal cord. The lower motor neuron axons project outward via the ventral roots to the muscle fiber end-plate. These nerves are large in diameter, myelinated and fast-conducting until the terminal aspect of the nerve where they are unmyelinated. Each terminal fiber of a lower motor neuron supplies a single muscle fiber. The motor unit is an entity comprised of the motor neuron and muscle fiber. Nerves are comprised of many nerve axons which influence the strength of a muscle contraction by virtue of the number of motor units activated.

Presynaptic Events

In the lower motor neuron nerve terminal, presynaptic events take place that will allow chemical signaling. The primary signaling chemical is acetylcholine, whose formation is catalyzed by choline acetyltransferase from acetyl coenzyme A and choline. Acetylcholine is stored in vesicles that reside either in the active zone (ready for release into the synaptic cleft) or away from the active zone in a reserve pool. When the lower motor neuron electrical signal reaches the nerve terminal, voltage gated Ca^{2+} channels are activated leading to an influx of calcium. This calcium influx mobilizes the acetylcholine vesicles to the active zone via intracellular transport proteins. The active zone is where these vesicles will fuse with the nerve membrane and release their acetylcholine contents into the synaptic cleft (Fig. 21-1). Quanta, comprising of 5 to 10 thousand acetylcholine molecules, are released into the synaptic cleft spontaneously which does not result in any significant physiologic response. In contrast, when preceded by nerve conduction there is more coordinated release of acetylcholine leading to millions of molecules entering the synaptic cleft. Potassium channels regulate this process by limiting calcium influx, regulating acetylcholine quanta release, and initiating nerve membrane repolarization.

The process of acetylcholine mobilization and release utilizes calcium signaling; therefore, any impediment to that signaling (e.g., hypocalcemia) can cause weakness. Magnesium in high concentrations (hypermagnesemia) can also inhibit this process by binding to calcium channels, impeding Ca^{2+} influx signaling, and leading to weakness. Yet another mechanism of weakness is the targeting of these calcium channels by antibodies, which occurs in Eaton–Lambert syndrome. The intracellular proteins that facilitate the movement and fusion of acetylcholine vesicles (leading to acetylcholine release) are irreversibly inhibited by botulinum toxin, leading to weakness that can only be reversed by nerve regeneration.[3]

Acetylcholine released into the synaptic cleft may traverse to the muscle membrane, or alternatively, it may circle back and bind to acetylcholine receptors on the presynaptic motor nerve that have the pentameric chemical structure α3β2. This presynaptic motor nerve binding feedback loop promotes acetylcholine vesicle movement to the active zone in preparation for the next nerve signal and release of acetylcholine. Some neuromuscular blocking drugs (i.e., depolarizers) have no affinity for these presynaptic α3β2 acetylcholine receptors and thereby leave the next signal preparatory mechanism in place such that subsequent nerve signals result in equal muscle contractions. However, nondepolarizing neuromuscular 3 blocking drugs bind and inhibit presynaptic α3β2 acetylcholine receptors, leading to a reduction in muscle contraction with subsequent nerve signals. This phenomenon is known as fade and will be an important concept later when discussing the assessment of nondepolarizing neuromuscular blocking drug effects.

Neuromuscular Junction

Some of the acetylcholine released from the presynaptic nerve terminal will traverse the 50- to 70-nm synaptic cleft to the postjunctional muscle membrane. Within this cleft resides the enzyme acetylcholinesterase, which quickly and efficiently hydrolyzes acetylcholine into choline and acetic acid. Choline reenters the presynaptic nerve terminal to be reused in acetylcholine production. It is the acetylcholine that avoids breakdown that will bind to postjunctional nicotinic muscle type acetylcholine receptors present in high concentrations on the crests of the postjunctional muscle membrane folds (Fig. 21-1) and result in muscle contraction.

Post Synaptic Events

Located beyond the neuromuscular junction synapse at the muscle membrane are nicotinic muscle type acetylcholine receptors concentrated at the crests of the folds (Fig. 21-1). There are two types of nicotinic muscle type acetylcholine receptors, each made up of five proteins. The four proteins common to both are alpha(α)-alpha(α)-beta(β)-delta(δ). The immature nicotinic muscle type acetylcholine receptors also have a gamma (γ) subunit, whereas

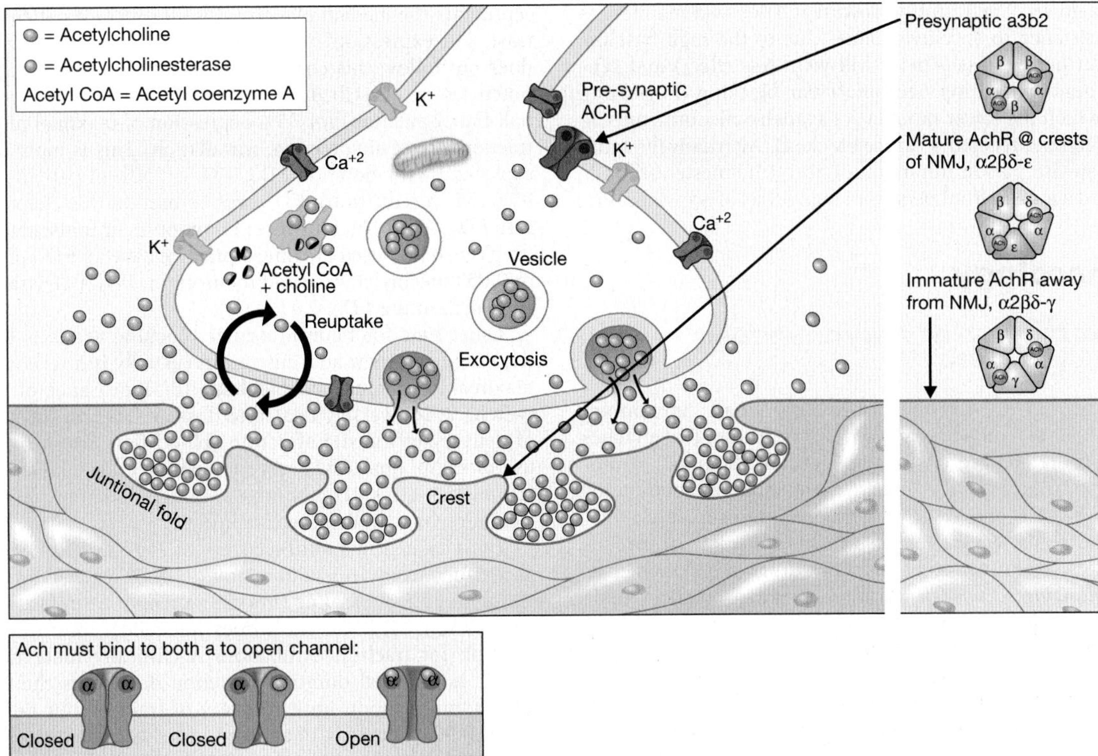

Figure 21-1 Schematic representation neuromuscular transmission across the neuromuscular junction (not drawn to scale). Acetylcholine is synthesized from choline and acetyl CoA by the enzyme choline acetyltransferase. acetyl CoA, acetyl coenzyme A; Ach, acetylcholine. (Modified from Thilen SR, Weigel WA. Neuromuscular Blocking Agents. In: Sharar SR, Cullen BF, Stock MC, Ortega R, Holt NF, Nathan N, Connor CW, eds. *Clinical Anesthesia Fundamentals*. 2nd ed. Wolters Kluwer; 2021:211–240. Figure 11.1.)

the mature nicotinic muscle type acetylcholine receptors have an epsilon (ε, think "Elderly" for the "ε") subunit. The fetal or immature five proteins (α α β δ γ) are arranged in a rosette that is closed in the resting state (Fig. 21-1). Compared to their mature counterparts, the immature nicotinic muscle type acetylcholine receptors have an opening time 10 times longer, a smaller channel, and may be spread out throughout the muscle. Immature nicotinic muscle type acetylcholine receptors are resistant to nondepolarizing drugs and sensitive to depolarizing drugs. In the normal adult state, mature nicotinic muscle type acetylcholine receptors predominate and are located almost exclusively (90%) at the neuromuscular synapse, which comprises only a small portion of the overall muscle surface area (0.1%). The same rosette structure occurs with mature nicotinic muscle type acetylcholine receptors utilizing the five proteins α α β δ ε, again creating a central pore that is closed in the resting state (Fig. 21-1). Compared to their immature counterparts, the mature nicotinic muscle type acetylcholine receptors have a shorter opening time and a larger central pore that allows higher ion conductance (Na^+, K^+, and Ca^{2+}). The opening of nicotinic muscle type acetylcholine receptors requires simultaneous acetylcholine binding to both alpha subunits; therefore, opening can be blocked by an antagonist at just one alpha subunit. Acetylcholine binding to both α subunits leads to a conformation change opening the central pore to allow muscle cell Na^+ influx, K^+ efflux, and depolarization of the cell. When this occurs spontaneously (not preceded by a nerve signal) then only small quanta of acetylcholine are released and the response is accordingly limited. This is categorized as a miniature end-plate potential (MEPP). In contrast, when a large quantity of acetylcholine is released and binds nicotinic muscle type acetylcholine receptors, there is sufficient end-plate depolarization, known as an end-plate potential (EPP), to trigger the excitation-contraction of muscle fibers. Voltage-gated Na^+ channels on the muscle membrane propagate this depolarization beyond the area of the neuromuscular junction. There are varying nerve:muscle fiber ratios depending on the level of coordination needed for the particular muscle. When fine coordination is required such as for eye and facial muscles, the nerve to muscle innervation ratio approaches 1:2. By contrast, in muscles responsible for powerful movements one nerve will be bulked together with many muscle fibers (back and thigh muscles have a nerve:muscle fiber ratio that approaches 1:2,000).

Receptor Up- and Downregulation

When upper or lower motor neuron disruption occurs over the course of days, the resultant decreased frequency of motor neuron activity will precipitate upregulation of immature nicotinic muscle type acetylcholine receptors throughout the associated muscles. Clinical scenarios where this is a concern include denervation injuries (e.g., spinal cord injury, Guillain–Barre), severe burns, crush injuries, prolong immobilization, or prolonged use of neuromuscular blockers in the ICU, cerebral vascular accident, and sepsis. The immature nicotinic muscle type acetylcholine receptor attributes of prolonged opening and sensitivity to depolarizing neuromuscular blockers combine to create the potential for a life-threatening hyperkalemic response if succinylcholine is administered 24 hours or longer after onset of the injury or disease process.

Downregulation of mature nicotinic muscle type acetylcholine receptors can occur in the context of continual agonism, which may occur with chronic administration of pyridostigmine or neostigmine (acetylcholinesterase enzyme inhibitors that increase synaptic acetylcholine concentration)—common treatments for myasthenia gravis. The resulting downregulation will manifest as extreme resistance to succinylcholine (due to the high baseline agonism, further agonist activity will yield less effect) and sensitivity to nondepolarizing neuromuscular blocking drugs (due to ease of which the lower numbers of available nicotinic muscle type acetylcholine receptors can be blocked). Alternatively, acute organophosphate poison inhibition of acetylcholinesterase leads to prolonged agonism from persistent high levels of acetylcholine.

Pharmacology

Characterization of Neuromuscular Blocking Drugs

Acetylcholine has a positively charged quaternary ammonium group with four carbon atoms and one nitrogen atom that attaches to the negatively charged cholinergic receptors. Similarly, neuromuscular blocking drugs are quaternary ammonium compounds that have at least one positively charged nitrogen atom that binds to the alpha subunit of postsynaptic nicotinic acetylcholine receptors. Neuromuscular blocking drugs are classified as either *depolarizing* or *nondepolarizing* depending on their mode of action. Succinylcholine, which is a depolarizing neuromuscular blocking drug, mimics the action of acetylcholine and depolarizes the postjunctional membrane. Compared with acetylcholine, the hydrolysis of succinylcholine is slow, resulting in sustained depolarization. Neuromuscular blockade develops because the depolarized postjunctional membrane cannot respond to a subsequent release of acetylcholine.

4 Nondepolarizing neuromuscular blocking drugs bind to one or both alpha subunits of the nicotinic acetylcholine receptor without causing any activation of these ion receptor channels. They act competitively with acetylcholine, but without causing a change in the configuration of the receptors. Nondepolarizing neuromuscular blocking drugs also act at prejunctional nicotinic acetylcholine receptors. Depending on their chemical structure, they can be further subclassified as either benzylisoquinolinium or aminosteroid compounds. Finally, neuromuscular blocking drugs are classified based on their duration of action as short-, intermediate-, or long-duration drugs.

Potency of a drug is determined by the dose required to produce a certain effect and is typically expressed in a dose versus response curve (Fig. 21-2). Commonly, drug potency is expressed as the effective dose for a percentage of patients. As such, ED_{95} represents the median effective dose for 95% of patients. In contrast, the expression of neuromuscular blocking drug potency does not follow this convention. Neuromuscular blocking drug potencies are described as the median dose (the dose required in half the population) for 95% depression of maximal muscle contraction after a single nerve stimulation. This is more accurately captured by the notation ED_{50} 95% (in 50% of patients there is a 95% twitch reduction). ED_{95} will be used in this chapter to indicate ED_{50} 95%. The four most common neuromuscular blocking drugs currently used in clinical practice have an ED_{95} of either 0.3 5
or 0.05 (succinylcholine and rocuronium ED_{95} 0.3, cisatracurium and vecuronium ED_{95} 0.05).

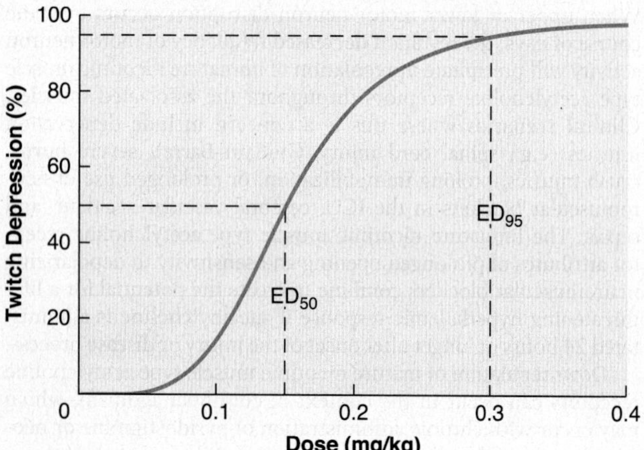

Figure 21-2 An example of a dose versus response curve.

Onset time for neuromuscular blocking drugs is defined as the time from their administration (usually intravenously) until maximal neuromuscular blockade (disappearance of the single twitch). It is inversely related to dose and can be affected by rate of delivery to the site of action (blood flow, speed of injection, use of saline flush, etc.), receptor affinity, mechanism of action (depolarizing vs. competitive nondepolarizing), and plasma clearance (metabolism, redistribution).

Duration of action until recovery to 25% (DUR 25%) is defined as the time from drug administration until recovery of the single twitch to 25% of baseline (normal) strength. Significant paralysis persists at DUR 25% and it does not reflect return of adequate strength for tracheal extubation. A clinically more meaningful metric is the total duration of action defined as the time from drug administration until recovery of train-of-four ratio to 0.90 (DUR 0.90). Duration of action is directly related to the dose of neuromuscular blocking drug administered, but varies significantly between patients (see below).

Recovery index is defined as the time of spontaneous recovery of the single twitch height from 25% to 75% of control, a period during which the spontaneous recovery is relatively linear and is not affected significantly by the total dose. It is a useful parameter for comparison of different neuromuscular blocking drugs.

Interpatient Variation

There is highly significant variation between patients in response to all neuromuscular blocking drugs, as demonstrated in a classic paper by Katz in 1967, where the effect of 0.1 mg/kg of curare on twitch height was determined in 100 patients.[4] In six patients there was no demonstrable depression of twitch height, whereas in seven patients the twitch was completely abolished. In the remaining patients there was a variable depression of twitch height. It was also determined that it was not possible to predict the response of a given patient to this dose of curare on the basis of age, sex, body build, or physical status (ASA classification). This extraordinary variation is not unique to curare but is typical for all neuromuscular blocking drugs. The duration of action is equally variable and unpredictable. Figure 21-3 demonstrates this well. It depicts the results for 526 patients who each received an equipotent dose of neuromuscular blocking drug at time zero (rocuronium, atracurium, or vecuronium). No patient received additional doses and none of them were pharmacologically reversed. The plots show the level of spontaneous recovery at time of arrival to the post anesthesia care unit. These data underscore the importance of adequate neuromuscular monitoring because it is not possible to use time to predict adequate recovery.

Depolarizing Neuromuscular Blocking NMB Drug: Succinylcholine

Succinylcholine is a depolarizing skeletal muscle relaxant consisting of two molecules of the endogenous neurotransmitter

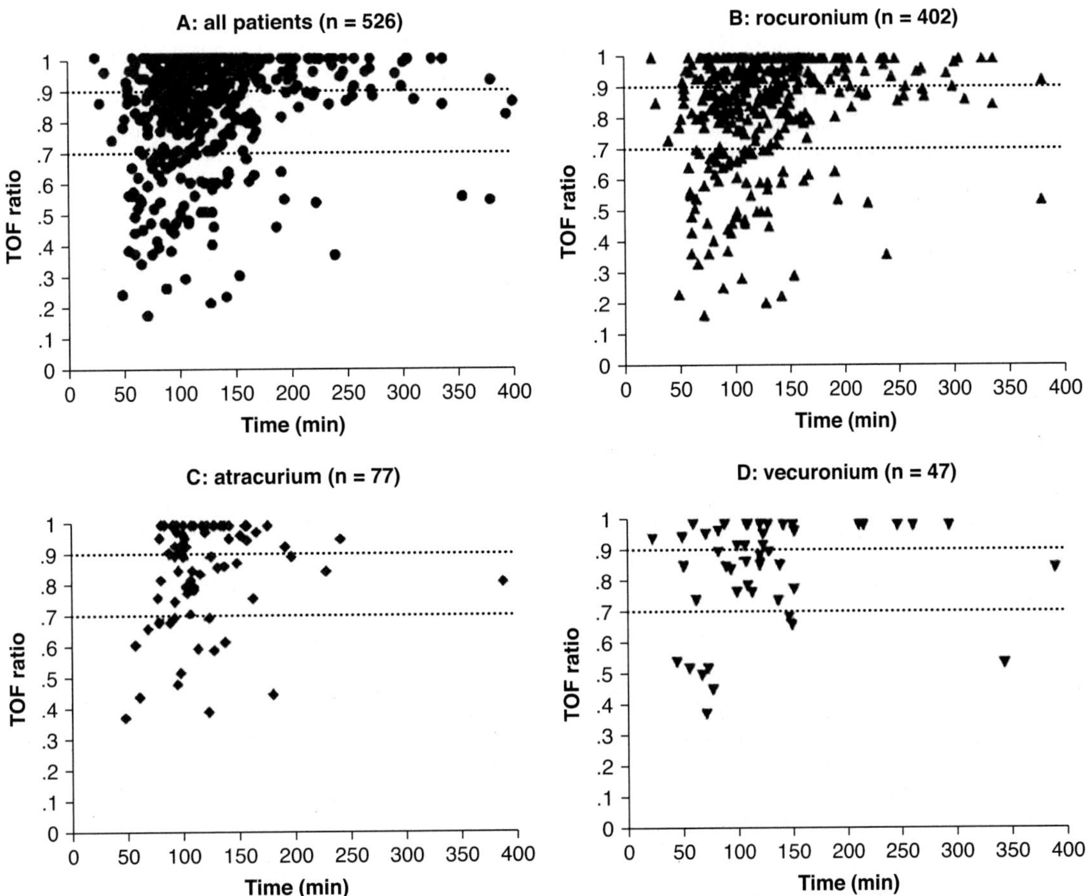

Figure 21-3 Train-of-four (TOF) ratio versus time interval between injection of drug and assessment. Each symbol represents one patient. Upper *dotted line* shows the 0.9 TOF ratio threshold; lower *dotted line* shows the 0.7 TOF ratio threshold. All the patients were presented on A, and patients receiving rocuronium, atracurium, and vecuronium were shown on B, C, and D, respectively. (Reprinted with permission from Debaene B, Plaud B, Dilly M-P. Residual Paralysis in the PACU after a single intubating dose of nondepolarizing muscle relaxant with an intermediate duration of action. *Anesthesiology*. 2003;98:1042–1048.)

acetylcholine linked by methyl groups. It is internationally known as suxamethonium and was first discovered by Hunt and Taveau in 1906.[5] It is currently the only clinically available depolarizing muscle relaxant. It was introduced into anesthesia practice in the early 1950s after Bovet had described its neuromuscular blocking properties.[6] It has the fastest onset and the shortest duration
6 of any neuromuscular blocking drug. Because of its molecular similarity to acetylcholine, succinylcholine depolarizes both postsynaptic and extrajunctional receptors. Unlike acetylcholine, succinylcholine is not metabolized by acetylcholinesterase, but instead metabolized by pseudocholinesterase (also known as plasma cholinesterase or butyrylcholinesterase). There is little or no pseudocholinesterase at the motor end-plate and succinylcholine depolarizes the muscle membrane for a longer period of time than acetylcholine. The initial receptor activation is manifested clinically as muscle fasciculations, followed by hyperpolarization and desensitization resulting in flaccid paralysis.

Depolarizing Blockade Characteristics

Depolarizing neuromuscular blockade has several characteristics that make it different from a nondepolarizing blockade. There is a lack of fade, both to train-of-four stimulation and tetanic stimulation, and absence of posttetanic potentiation. Anticholinesterase drugs potentiate the blockade and previous administration of a nondepolarizing neuromuscular blocking drug antagonizes the block. Finally, there are frequently fasciculations preceding the onset of the block.

A prolonged duration of succinylcholine blockade may occur 7
when the concentration of normal pseudocholinesterase is very significantly reduced or when an atypical variant of pseudocholinesterase is present. Under certain conditions, succinylcholine can induce a different type of blockade that is termed *phase II block*. In the past, it has also been referred to as "dual block" or "nondepolarization block." It has some features in common with the classic blockade induced by nondepolarizing neuromuscular blocking drugs, including fade to train-of-four and tetanic stimulation. A phase II block occurs after administration of a single large dose of succinylcholine ($\geq 10 \times ED_{95}$), repeated doses, or a prolonged continuous infusion.

Pharmacology of Succinylcholine

Following intravenous injection, succinylcholine induces maximum blockade within 1 minute and lasts for approximately 10 to 15 minutes. The ED_{95} is approximately 0.3 mg/kg and at doses of 1.0 to 1.5 mg/kg (3 to $5 \times ED_{95}$), the DUR 25% is 10 to 12 minutes but is prolonged beyond 15 minutes with larger doses. Despite paralysis at the adductor pollicis muscle, the diaphragm may start to contract, and spontaneous breathing may resume as fast as 5 minutes after 1 mg/kg has been administered. Succinylcholine is usually administered intravenously, but intraosseous, intralingual, and intramuscular routes have been reported when intravenous access is unavailable. Onset is delayed with intramuscular administration. The very short duration of succinylcholine is primarily due to its rapid hydrolysis by pseudocholinesterase. Pseudocholinesterase has a great capacity to hydrolyze succinylcholine and only a small fraction, approximately 10%, of the original intravenous dose reaches the neuromuscular junction.

Succinylcholine Side Effects

Succinylcholine can induce significant bradycardia and asystole. The risk is greater in children and with repeated administration. It is decreased by anticholinergic drug pretreatment. Myalgias are common 1 to 2 days postoperatively, occurring in 50% to 60% of patients. Fasciculations, which occur in 80% to 90% of patients, have been considered a possible mechanism for the myalgias, but uncertainty remains. A "defasciculating" dose of a nondepolarizing neuromuscular blocking drug (5% to 10% ED_{95}) can be used for pretreatment 3 to 5 minutes before succinylcholine to decrease fasciculations. The technique has become less common in recent years because of the concern for increased risk of regurgitation and pulmonary aspiration, especially in patients with increased sensitivity to nondepolarizing neuromuscular blocking drugs. If pretreatment is used, it is recommended to increase the dose of succinylcholine (up to 2 mg/kg). Fortunately, higher doses of succinylcholine have been associated with less myalgias. The most effective prophylaxis for myalgia is pretreatment with a nonsteroidal anti-inflammatory drug, with a number needed to treat of 2.5.[7] Lidocaine pretreatment also decreases the incidence of postoperative myalgias (lidocaine dose range 1 to 1.5 mg/kg).

Although succinylcholine may *increase intragastric pressure*, the lower esophageal sphincter tone is also increased, such that the intragastric-esophageal pressure gradient remains the same. Therefore, in patients with an intact and competent esophageal sphincter, there is not an increased risk of aspiration from the use of succinylcholine. Normal *intraocular pressure* is 12 to 20 mmHg with a diurnal variation of 2 to 3 mmHg, whereas changes in position may induce increases of up to 6 mmHg. Intraocular pressure increases up to 15 mmHg transiently (5 minutes duration) after administration of succinylcholine.[8] Succinylcholine is not considered contraindicated in cases of open-eye injury cases; however, it should be noted that increases in intraocular pressure can be significant in the context of inadequate anesthesia and neuromuscular blockade that allows the patient to cough and Valsalva during laryngoscopy and tracheal intubation.[9,10] Such events generate much larger increases in intraocular pressure than those associated with succinylcholine administration.

Elevation in intracranial pressure (ICP) after succinylcholine administration was first shown in cats and was reported in a classic 1983 paper.[11,12] The mechanism for the increase is not clear; however, significant increases in ICP have been confirmed in neurosurgical patients with reduced intracranial compliance. Importantly, a "defasciculating" dose of a nondepolarizing neuromuscular blocking drug administered prior to succinylcholine prevents the increase in the ICP.[13] Similar to the considerations concerning increased IOP, adequate anesthesia at the time of tracheal intubation is critical. In patients with traumatic brain injury (TBI), a hypertensive response to laryngoscopy and tracheal intubation can be associated with an increase in ICP of 100% or more.[14]

Succinylcholine administration is associated with an elevation of the serum potassium concentration. In normal patients, the increase is limited to approximately 0.5 mEq/L, however, in certain pathologic states *severe hyperkalemia* can occur. The mechanism is a proliferation of immature nicotinic acetylcholine receptors (see above, receptor up- and downregulation) that occurs with chronic denervation states (e.g., spinal cord injury, prolonged bed rest) and >24 hours after major burn injuries. Other settings in which the use of succinylcholine has been associated with hyperkalemia include acute renal failure, sepsis, encephalitis, and severe trauma.[15] Pretreatment with a small dose of a nondepolarizing neuromuscular blocking drug has not been shown to prevent this hyperkalemic response. Rapid treatment of hyperkalemia includes hyperventilation, intravenous calcium and bicarbonate, inhaled beta-2 agonists, and glucose with insulin to shift potassium into the intracellular space.

There have been rare reports of acute rhabdomyolysis with hyperkalemia followed by ventricular dysrhythmias, cardiac arrest, and death after the administration of succinylcholine to apparently healthy children who were subsequently found to have undiagnosed skeletal muscle myopathy, most frequently Duchenne muscular dystrophy (an X-linked recessive disorder most commonly seen in males). The U.S. Food and Drug Administration (FDA) has a "black box" warning against the use of succinylcholine in the pediatric population except for emergency tracheal intubation or instances where immediate securing of the airway is necessary (e.g., laryngospasm, or for intramuscular use when intravenous access is unavailable).

Succinylcholine may trigger *malignant hyperthermia* (MH), especially in patients anesthetized with volatile anesthetics. Some patients may exhibit *masseter muscle spasm* after succinylcholine, making intubating conditions difficult. In some cases, but not all, masseter spasm is associated with MH.

Succinylcholine is one of the perioperatively used drugs with the highest incidence of *anaphylaxis*, with an incidence of approximately 1:10,000.

Patients with an abnormal genetic variant of pseudocholinesterase can have a significantly prolonged effect of succinylcholine. The presence of atypical pseudocholinesterase is often recognized only after an otherwise healthy patient experiences prolonged paralysis. Registry data confirm that there is often a delay with identification of this important clinical problem. In addition, patients are at risk of unintended intraoperative awareness and recall if they are allowed to emerge from anesthesia while paralyzed.[16] Therefore, patients who are administered succinylcholine for the first time should be assessed using a peripheral nerve stimulator or a quantitative monitor. Patients with a prolonged effect of succinylcholine should be tested with determination of the *dibucaine number*. Dibucaine is an amide local anesthetic that inhibits normal plasma pseudocholinesterase by about 80% or greater. In contrast, the activity of homozygous atypical pseudocholinesterase enzyme is much less inhibited, only about 20%. The intermediate dibucaine inhibitions, 40% to 60%, represent the level seen in heterozygous atypical pseudocholinesterase patients. The most marked prolongation of succinylcholine block occurs in patients who are homozygous for the atypical enzyme (1/3,200) where the block can last for several hours. Patients who are heterozygous (1/480) will have a modest prolongation of the blockade (20 to 30 minutes). Management of patients with prolonged effect includes adequate sedation and neuromuscular monitoring until the blockade has regressed completely. There is no accepted intervention to reduce the time to recovery. Some have administered neostigmine (as a phase II block is commonly seen) or infused plasma, but this is not recommended (see also 1 Video 21-1).

Succinylcholine Clinical Uses

Succinylcholine is the "reference standard" drug for rapid attainment of optimal tracheal intubating conditions for rapid sequence induction (RSI). According to a survey in several European countries and the United States, the most desirable features of succinylcholine are rapid onset (88%), short duration (64%), and effective relaxation (61%).[17] Use of succinylcholine has decreased in recent years because of concerns over its side effects. While succinylcholine has a shorter duration, 5 to 10 minutes at 1 mg/kg dose, not all patients will resume some diaphragmatic function before developing severe hypoxemia. The alternative to succinylcholine for RSI is high-dose rocuronium (0.9 to 1.2 mg/kg). Rapid reversal with sugammadex (16 mg/kg administered 3 minutes after rocuronium 1.2 mg/kg) provides a means to shorten the duration of paralysis. A 2015 Cochrane systematic review found no statistically significant difference in intubation conditions between succinylcholine and rocuronium (1.2 mg/kg).[18] In obese patients who need RSI, the dose of succinylcholine should be calculated based on actual body weight rather than ideal body weight (which is used for nondepolarizing neuromuscular blocking drugs, though some use lean body weight). Children require a higher dose of succinylcholine than adults and the usual dose is 1.5 to 2.0 mg/kg (up to 3 mg/kg in infants).

Neostigmine, but not edrophonium, inhibits pseudocholinesterase (in addition to acetylcholinesterase) which leads to a prolonged effect of succinylcholine. Therefore, it is not recommended to administer succinylcholine in cases where surgical muscle relaxation is required immediately after neostigmine has been administered. It can be used for treatment of airway emergencies (e.g., laryngospasm) with the caveat that appropriate neuromuscular monitoring is used to ensure full recovery before tracheal extubation.

Succinylcholine Contraindications

Succinylcholine is contraindicated in patients (and their relatives) with a history of malignant hyperthermia. Other patients for whom succinylcholine is contraindicated are those with receptor upregulation (see above) because of the risk of severe hyperkalemia. In patients with renal failure, succinylcholine may be administered if the plasma potassium concentration is normal because they are not susceptible to exaggerated release of potassium, assuming they do not have uremic neuropathy. As already stated, the FDA has issued a black box warning for the use of succinylcholine in pediatric patients.

Nondepolarizing Neuromuscular Blocking Drugs

Curare use for anesthesia was first described in a case series in 1942.[19] The role of nondepolarizing neuromuscular blocking drugs is to facilitate tracheal intubation and to provide better operating conditions for surgery through relaxation of muscles. The search for the ideal nondepolarizing neuromuscular blocking drug with a quick onset, a quick offset, and no side effects continues.

Characteristics of Nondepolarizing Neuromuscular Blocking Drugs

Nondepolarizing neuromuscular blocking drugs are competitive antagonists at the neuromuscular junction. The drugs compete with acetylcholine and bind to one or both alpha subunits of nicotinic muscle type acetylcholine receptors. A characteristic of these drugs observed with partial nerve block is fade due to blocking of the presynaptic $\alpha 3\beta 2$ acetylcholine receptors as previously described. Fade is a muscle fatigue that develops with repeated stimulation between 0.1 and 2 Hz. The degree of fade is commonly determined clinically using a train-of-four stimuli delivered at 2 Hz. The train-of-four ratio is calculated by comparing the amplitude of the fourth response (T4) to the amplitude of the first response (T1) with a normal baseline or full recovery expressed as a train-of-four ratio (T4/T1) of 1.0 (see a more detailed train-of-four explanation in Peripheral Nerve Stimulators section). A second characteristic of these drugs is posttetanic facilitation (or potentiation). After a 5-second tetanic stimulation there is a transient amplification in the response that lasts 2 to 3 minutes (see a more detailed posttetanic count explanation in Peripheral Nerve Stimulators section). Nondepolarizing nerve block can be antagonized by the administration of an anticholinesterase drug or, in select instance, a gamma-cyclodextrin (see a more detailed explanation in Reversal of Neuromuscular Blockade section).

Drug Classification of Nondepolarizing Neuromuscular Blocking Drugs

Nondepolarizing neuromuscular blocking drugs can be classi- 8
fied by their chemistry and molecular structure: aminosteroid (e.g., pancuronium, vecuronium, rocuronium) or benzylisoquinolinium (e.g., atracurium, cisatracurium, mivacurium). Clinically they are classified by their expected duration of action: long-, intermediate-, or short-acting. The physicochemical properties of nondepolarizing neuromuscular blocking drugs are summarized in Table 21-1. Nondepolarizing neuromuscular blocking drugs are ionized hydrophilic compounds (because of their quaternary ammonium group) that also exhibit limited lipid solubility. Nondepolarizing neuromuscular blocking drugs do not easily cross lipid membranes, and hence do not cross the blood–brain barrier, placenta, gastrointestinal epithelium, or renal tubules. Renal tubule reabsorption is minimal, oral administration is ineffective and they do not adversely affect the fetus.

Onset of Action of Nondepolarizing Neuromuscular Blocking Drugs

Clinically, the onset of action of all nondepolarizing neuromuscular blocking drugs is similar and relatively slow compared to succinylcholine. The speed of onset can be shortened with rocuronium if a high dose is used. The speed of onset is inversely related to the potency, with the least potent neuromuscular blockers requiring the most molecules of drug at equipotent doses (Fig. 21-4). The low potency of rocuronium is leveraged to speed up the onset to around 1 minute when a large intubating dose is used (i.e., 1.2 mg/kg, 4× the rocuronium ED_{95} of 0.3 mg/kg). This higher intubating dose has implications for safe and complete recovery from paralysis. For all neuromuscular blockers the usual intubating dose is 2× or 3× the ED_{95} (i.e., 0.6 mg/kg for rocuronium). If intubation has already been achieved using succinylcholine prior to administering the nondepolarizing neuromuscular blocking drug, then only half of the intubating dose (a single multiple of the ED_{95}) is required to achieve clinically appropriate levels of paralysis (i.e., 0.3 mg/kg for rocuronium). Following an intubating dose of a nondepolarizing drug, and once a clinical neuromuscular block is established, only 10% to 25% of the intubating dose is required to re-establish a deeper block (i.e., 0.05 to 0.15 mg/kg for rocuronium).

Duration of Action of Nondepolarizing Neuromuscular Blocking Drugs

As previously mentioned, the duration of action of nondepolarizing neuromuscular blocking drugs is quite variable even in healthy
patients. Different classes of nondepolarizing neuromuscular block- 9
ing drugs should not be mixed in the same patient because this can lead to an unpredictable extended duration of muscle paralysis. Many physiologic disturbances and medications can extend the duration of nondepolarizing neuromuscular blocking drugs.

Table 21-1 Physiochemical Properties of Nondepolarizing Neuromuscular Blocking Drugs

	Vecuronium	Rocuronium	Pancuronium
Type duration	Intermediate	Intermediate	Long
Intubating dose (mg/kg)	0.1	0.6	0.1
ED_{95} Potency (mg/kg)	0.05	0.3	0.07
Redose for maintaining block % of intubating dose	10%	10%	10%
Infusion (µg/kg/min)	1–2	5–12	Not recommended
Onset time	3–4	1.5–3	2–4
Clinical duration	25–50	30–70	60–120
Elimination half-life Renal impairment Hepatic impairment	65–75 Mild increase Significant increase	100–250 Mild increase Significant increase	90–160 Significant increase Significant increase
Recovery index (RI 25–75) (minutes)	10–25	8–13	30–45
Volume of distribution (L/kg)	0.4	0.3–0.7	0.2–0.3
Elimination route	Renal 10–50% Hepatic 30–50%	Renal 30% Hepatic 70%	Renal 40–70% Hepatic 20%
Active metabolites	3-desacetyl-vecuronium (60% potency of vecuronium)	17-desacetyl-rocuronium (Minimal)	3-OH-pancuronium 17-OH-pancuronium
Side effect	Vagal block with large doses	Minimal	Vagal Block (Tachycardia)
Comments	Myopathy with prolonged ICU administration, T1/2 halved late pregnancy,	Prolonged T1/2 in ICU patients, metabolite only 20% activity	Significant accumulation, prone to residual block
	Atracurium	**Cisatracurium**	**Mivacurium**
Type duration	Intermediate	Intermediate	Short
Intubating dose (mg/kg)	0.5	0.15–0.2	0.2
ED95 Potency(mg/kg)	0.25	0.05	0.08
Redose for maintaining block % of intubating dose	10%	10%	10%
Infusion (µg/kg/min)	10–20	1–3	5–8
Onset time (min)	3–5	4–7	3–4
Clinical duration (min)	30–45	35–50	80–160
Elimination half-life Renal impairment Hepatic impairment	21 No change No change	23–30 Mild increase No change	2–2.5 Mild increase Mild increase
Recovery index (RI 25–75) (minutes)	10–15	12–15	7–9
Volume of distribution (L/kg)	0.14	0.12–0.26	0.05
Elimination route	Renal 10% Hoffman 30% Ester hydrolysis 60%	Hoffman 30% Ester hydrolysis 60%	Plasma cholinesterase (70% of succinylcholine rate)
Active metabolites	No active metabolites	No active metabolites	No active metabolites
Side effect	Histamine release; laudanosine and acrylates production	Histamine release at high doses	Histamine release
Comments	Organ independent elimination	Trivial histamine release; minimal laudanosine and acrylate levels	Reversal by cholinesterase inhibitors; mixture of 3 isomers; edrophonium for reversal more effective at deep block

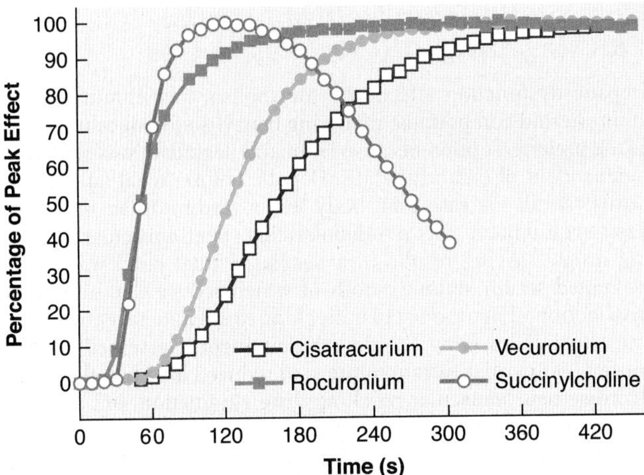

Figure 21-4 Neuromuscular blockade as a function of time for four neuromuscular blocking drugs. Onset is faster for the less potent succinylcholine and rocuronium than for the more potent vecuronium and cisatracurium. (Adapted with permission from Kopman AF, Klewicka MM, Kopman DJ, et al. Molar potency is predictive of the speed of onset of neuromuscular block for agents of intermediate, short, and ultrashort duration. *Anesthesiology*. 1999;90:425.)

Aminosteroids

Pancuronium is one of the oldest nondepolarizing neuromuscular blocker drugs with a long duration of action.[20] The long duration of action is, in part, due to its active metabolites (3-OH-pancuronium has half the potency). In addition, its action is prolonged in patients with renal and hepatic impairment or by repeated administration. Pancuronium produces tachycardia through a vagolytic mechanism, as well as by direct sympathomimetic actions. Anticholinesterase drug reversal is less successful than with newer drugs, but sugammadex can reverse shallow pancuronium block.[21] Pancuronium was historically used in longer operative cases and is still available in the United States, but is rarely used due to the increased risk of residual neuromuscular blockade.

Vecuronium is a quaternary aminosteroid with only one metabolite, 3-desacetylvecuronium, that exhibits 50% to 70% activity of the parent compound. Vecuronium is lipid soluble and undergoes biliary excretion. Renal failure has little effect on the duration of action except in repeat dosing. Vecuronium precipitates out of solution if administered concurrently with thiopental. There are case reports of prolonged duration of vecuronium in patients with diabetes.[22] Vecuronium is devoid of vagolytic effects and histamine release.

Rocuronium in an intermediate duration neuromuscular blocking drug of low potency. In patients with normal hepatic and renal function the plasma concentration after the initial bolus decreases rapidly due to redistribution, rather than elimination. There are minimal active metabolites. Rocuronium can be used in high dose (1.2 mg/kg) for rapid paralysis in approximately 90 seconds. This higher dose leads to a prolonged duration of action, however. The half-life of rocuronium is variable with wide ranges reported.[23] The drug is cleared in the bile unchanged and renal excretion accounts for elimination of 30% of the dose. Rocuronium and succinylcholine have the highest reported rates of anaphylaxis, in contrast to cisatracurium which has the lowest reported rate of IgE-mediated events.[24,25] Rocuronium-related IgE-mediated events have been described at a higher incidence in hairdressers, which may be due to repeated work exposure to quaternary ammonium compounds in hair products.[26] In pediatrics, pulmonary function changes are greater with rocuronium than with cisatracurium, although both reduce function.[27] In children, the onset and the duration of rocuronium are reduced, and the dose requirement is slightly higher. Abdominal insufflation reduces hepatic blood flow which may explain the 25% increased duration of rocuronium in laparoscopic cases.[28] The ED_{95} is 15% to 25% lower for women compared to men.[29] Both vecuronium and rocuronium have a significantly longer duration in elderly patients.[30] In patients with type II diabetes the duration is prolonged and residual paralysis risk is increased.[31]

Benzylisoquinolinium Drugs

The original, naturally occurring benzylisoquinolinium compound was d-tubocurarine. Modern benzylisoquinolinium compounds are synthetics: atracurium, cisatracurium, and mivacurium.

Atracurium has 10 isomers with varying potency. The chemical structure of atracurium permits competitive antagonism at the neuromuscular junction. Atracurium contains an ester group that undergoes hydrolysis during metabolism, as well as Hofmann elimination. During a Hofmann elimination reaction, quaternary ammonium groups are converted to tertiary amines by cleavage of a carbon nitrogen bond. The Hofmann reaction is both pH- and temperature-dependent, with higher pH and temperature favoring elimination. Atracurium causes histamine release. The ten atracurium isomers have been separated into three geometric groups (*cis-cis*, *cis-trans*, and *trans-trans*) and they are present in a ratio of 10:6:1. Atracurium at intubating doses ($2 \times ED_{95}$, 0.5 mg/kg) still has a relatively long onset of action (3 to 5 minutes). Increasing the dose to speed onset also increases the chance of histamine release, tachycardia, and hypotension.

Cisatracurium is the *cis-cis* isomer of atracurium and represents 15% of the atracurium mixture by weight but over 50% in potency. It is also metabolized by Hofmann elimination but, unlike atracurium, it does not release histamine. Metabolism is independent of liver function.

Mivacurium is a mixture of three stereoisomers, and it differs from other benzylisoquinolinium nondepolarizing neuromuscular blocking drugs by its longer central chain. Mivacurium is metabolized by pseudocholinesterase at around 80% of the rate of succinylcholine to an ester and dicarboxylic acid (and provides 15 to 20 minutes duration of action, defined as the time for T1 to return to 25% of baseline). Given mivacurium's low potency, large doses are required for intubation which leads to histamine release. To avoid large doses, one suggested technique has been to split initial dose, but this did not prevent side effects.[32] The duration of action of mivacurium is prolonged in patients with severely depleted pseudocholinesterase activity. Neostigmine also inhibits pseudocholinesterase (reducing mivacurium metabolism), but the prolongation effect is overridden by the acetylcholinesterase inhibition effect, resulting in the ability effectively reverse mivacurium.[33]

Adverse Effects of Nondepolarizing Neuromuscular Blocking Drugs

Neuromuscular blocking drugs may interact with nicotinic and muscarinic cholinergic receptors within the sympathetic and parasympathetic nervous systems. The dose responses are not reduced by slow injection, but instead are dose-related and additive over time. Newer drugs have less effect, but rocuronium weakly blocks cardiac muscarinic receptors. The autonomic effects of neuromuscular blockers manifest as hypotension (usually due to histamine release), tachycardia (pancuronium causes modest heart rate increases), bradycardia, and even asystole. Respiratory effects can vary depending on the affinity for M1–M3 airway receptors and have resulted in presynaptic M2 block with severe bronchospasm (as seen with the nondepolarizing neuromuscular blocking drug rapacuronium, which has been withdrawn from the market).

Nondepolarizing Neuromuscular Blocking Drug Interactions

Interactions among nondepolarizing neuromuscular blocking drugs can be complex and clinical use of combinations of nondepolarizing neuromuscular blocking drugs should be avoided. Interactions are considered additive or synergistic. Additive interactions have been demonstrated after administering chemically related drugs (e.g., atracurium and mivacurium). On the other hand, combining the chemically unrelated drugs rocuronium and cisatracurium produces a synergistic response.[34] The interaction not only depends on the group of drugs but also on the sequence the drugs are administered. Mivacurium recovery is prolonged if administered after atracurium in an additive manner. Because most receptors are occupied at the time of second drug administration the clinical picture is dominated by the kinetics of the first drug. As doses of the second drug are repeated, and more receptors are occupied by the second drug, the picture changes and is dominated by the kinetics of the second— now predominate—nondepolarizing neuromuscular blocking drug.

Inhalational anesthetic drugs extend the duration of nondepolarizing neuromuscular blocking drugs by effects on postjunctional receptors. Inhaled anesthetic drugs have different potentiating effects (desflurane > sevoflurane > isoflurane > nitrous oxide). There is an exaggeration of this prolongation effect for volatile drugs with a higher MAC, or when volatile drugs are administered over a longer period of time.[35] Propofol has minimal effect on neuromuscular transmission, but a propofol infusion will shorten the time to maximal rocuronium effect.[36]

Local anesthetics interact with depolarizing and nondepolarizing neuromuscular blocking drugs with pre- and postsynaptic effects.[37] Epidurally administered levobupivacaine significantly prolongs vecuronium recovery. In contrast, an intravenous lidocaine infusion has not demonstrated clinical effects on pharmacologic profile of rocuronium.[38,39]

Aminoglycoside antibiotics can influence neuromuscular blockers by potential involvement with acetylcholine release.[40] Two older antibiotics, streptomycin and neomycin, are known to depress neuromuscular function. Hypercarbia, acidosis, and hypothermia may potentiate effects of neuromuscular blocking drugs in critically ill patients. In the acute phase of anticonvulsant administration of phenytoin and carbamazepine, nondepolarizing neuromuscular blockade is potentiated. In contrast, after chronic anticonvulsant administration, the duration of action of aminosteroid compounds is significantly decreased, an effect that is present but negligible for benzylisoquinolinium compounds. Anticholinesterase drugs used for the treatment of Alzheimer disease (e.g., donepezil hydrochloride) can also act peripherally and increase the amount of acetylcholine. Case reports have described inadequate neuromuscular blocks with nondepolarizing neuromuscular blocking drugs and prolonged weakness with depolarizing neuromuscular blocking drugs. Beta-agonists delay the onset of rocuronium, while calcium channel antagonists have minimal clinical effect. Ephedrine hastens the onset of rocuronium, which is thought to be mediated by increased cardiac output. Corticosteroids, when administered chronically in critically ill ventilated patients for a prolonged period with vecuronium, will increase the incidence of myopathy.

Nondepolarizing Neuromuscular Blocking Drug Altered Responses

Hepatic dysfunction affects the metabolism and elimination of aminosteroid compounds, rendering benzylisoquinolinium drugs as the preferred option because Hofmann degradation is relatively independent of organ function. Hepatic failure, renal failure and burns can all increase total body water, leading to an increased dose requirement for nondepolarizing neuromuscular blocking drugs.[41] Aging results in a decreased total body water and decreased serum albumin, both of which reduce the volume of distribution of neuromuscular blocking drugs and have the opposite effect of lowering the dose requirement. Decreased cardiac output, glomerular filtration rate, and reduced liver blood flow all decrease neuromuscular blocking drug elimination, but to varying degrees depending on the drug class.

Hypothermia decreases receptor sensitivity and acetylcholine mobilization, decreases muscle contraction, reduces both renal and hepatic metabolism, and slows Hofmann degradation. Hypokalemia potentiates neuromuscular block and reduces the effectiveness of neostigmine antagonizing neuromuscular block. Hypermagnesemia inhibits pre- and postsynaptic Ca^{2+} channels, thereby potentiating neuromuscular blocking drug effect. Acidosis interferes with anticholinesterase drugs, reducing their ability to reverse nondepolarizing neuromuscular blocking drugs.[42] Hypercarbia produces acidosis and therefore also reduces antagonism.

Use of neuromuscular drugs in the ICU is common; however, prolonged use of neuromuscular blocking drugs should be avoided. Short-term infusions may facilitate ventilation in prone patients with acute respiratory distress, thereby reducing barotrauma and in-hospital mortality. This should be avoided, however, in patients who are diabetic or receiving steroids. Use of an appropriate dose of sedation to prevent unintended awareness is important in this setting.

Neuromuscular disease presents a variety of challenges depending on the type of disorder. In general, patients with neuromuscular diseases have increased sensitivity to depolarizing and variable sensitivity to nondepolarizing neuromuscular blocking drugs. In addition, because of the association with malignant hyperthermia and rhabdomyolysis in many common ICU conditions, succinylcholine should be avoided, and nondepolarizing neuromuscular blocking drugs use should be guided by objective monitoring.

Monitoring Neuromuscular Blockade

History and Clinical Significance of Monitoring Neuromuscular Blockade

Neuromuscular blocking drugs improve tracheal intubation and surgical conditions while also introducing drug-related complications including anaphylaxis. Even more dangerous has been the potentially devastating scenario of a paralyzed patient for whom an airway could not be secured. Over the years another insidious complication has increasingly been reported with a persistently high incidence–residual neuromuscular blockade after emergence from anesthesia. This complication occurs at different rates depending on the neuromuscular blocking drug, the reversal drugs chosen, and the type of monitoring employed. The problem, however, is not trivial, with as many as 30% to 40% of patients reversed with neostigmine demonstrating residual paralysis. The rate of residual paralysis is much lower with sugammadex reversal, but may still be as high as 5%. There are untoward patient outcomes resulting

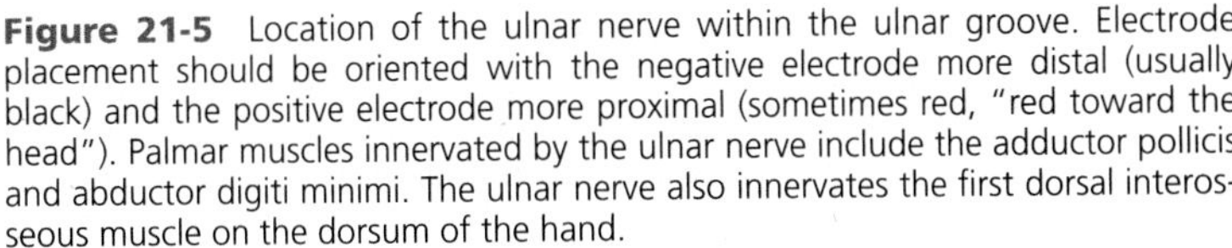

Figure 21-5 Location of the ulnar nerve within the ulnar groove. Electrode placement should be oriented with the negative electrode more distal (usually black) and the positive electrode more proximal (sometimes red, "red toward the head"). Palmar muscles innervated by the ulnar nerve include the adductor pollicis and abductor digiti minimi. The ulnar nerve also innervates the first dorsal interosseous muscle on the dorsum of the hand.

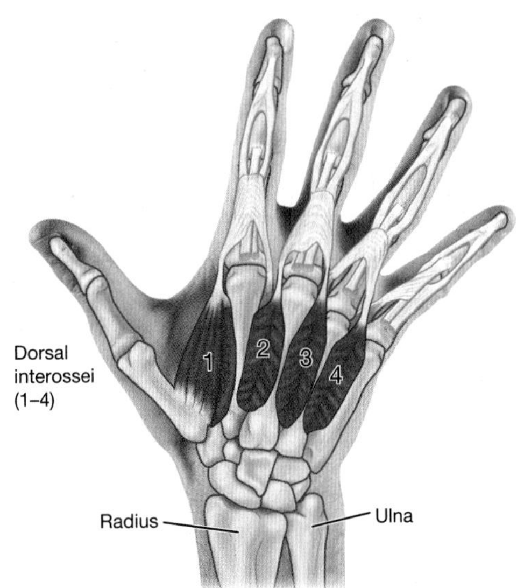

from residual paralysis that may impede the recovery process after surgery. Considering that worldwide there are 230 million surgical procedures performed each year, the total impact of residual paralysis is very significant. In contrast to residual paralysis, there is a paucity of complications associated with quantitative neuromuscular monitoring. This imbalance of clear benefit to limited harm is reflected in guidelines advocating for quantitative neuromuscular monitoring from Canada, France, Spain, Australian, New Zealand, the Czech Republic, Portugal, and Japan. A guideline from the United States has recently been published.[43]

See also 2 Video 21-2.

Time and Clinical Assessment of Neuromuscular Blockade

Clinicians around the world have historically used time from the last administration of neuromuscular blocking drug as the primary determinant for regression of paralysis despite the varia-
10 tion in offset for all neuromuscular blocking drugs.[44–46] Another approach has been to rely on physical assessments of muscle function, such as maximum inspiratory force, vital capacity, tidal volume, eye opening, tongue protrusion, handgrip, leg lift, and head lift.[2] Unfortunately, all these assessments are insensitive and thus render the clinician incapable of identifying the presence of residual paralysis. The most popular physical assessment is the five-second head lift, which in one study was accomplished by 11 out of 12 volunteers despite significant residual paralysis (i.e., train-of-four ratio ≤0.5, see below for explanation of train-of-four ratio).[47] Because of their insensitivity, neither time from last neuromuscular blocking drug administration nor physical assessments should be used to assess recovery from neuromuscular blockade.

Peripheral Nerve Stimulators

The next step in the evolution of neuromuscular blockade assessment was the use of a peripheral nerve stimulator and tactile or visual assessment of muscle movement. Peripheral nerve stimulators have been in use for over 65 years. They are generally battery operated, stand-alone devices that deliver a square wave current of 10 to 80 mA for 100 to 300 microseconds (greater than 300 microseconds may exceed the nerve refractory period). This delivered electrical impulse should have a square wave pattern (monophasic and rectangular) to assure constant current and avoid repetitious nerve stimulation that may occur with a biphasic impulse.[48] The intensity of the neurostimulation is the charge, measure in Coulombs, which equals the current multiplied by pulse width. Delivery of neurostimulation is most efficient if the negative electrode (usually white or black) is distal to the positive electrode (usually red) and in close proximity to a peripheral motor nerve.[49] This will result in a corresponding muscle contraction, often referred to as a twitch. To remember this configuration over the ulnar nerve at the wrist, think red (positive) is toward the head (more proximal, Fig. 21-5). To further improve electrical stimulus transfer to the nerve, proper skin preparation, including cleansing with alcohol and abrading with gauze, will reduce skin resistance (from 100,000 Ohms to <5,000 Ohms). Peripheral nerve stimulators use standard silver-silver chloride skin electrodes that should ideally have a diameter of 7 to 8 mm.

The muscle responses evaluated by tactile or visual human detection are subjective observations; therefore, inaccuracy and insensitivity are present in this technique. One pattern of nerve stimulation is the single repetitive twitch (ST, single twitch) which occurs at frequencies between 0.1 and 10 Hz (Fig. 21-6). If the frequency exceeds 0.1 Hz, then muscle fatigue may occur.

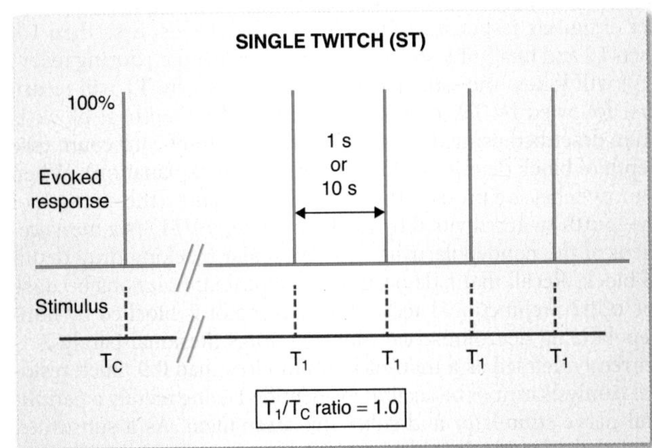

Figure 21-6 Single twitch nerve stimulation. If single twitches occur less than 2 seconds apart, there is some risk of physiologic fade with more than four subsequent twitches.

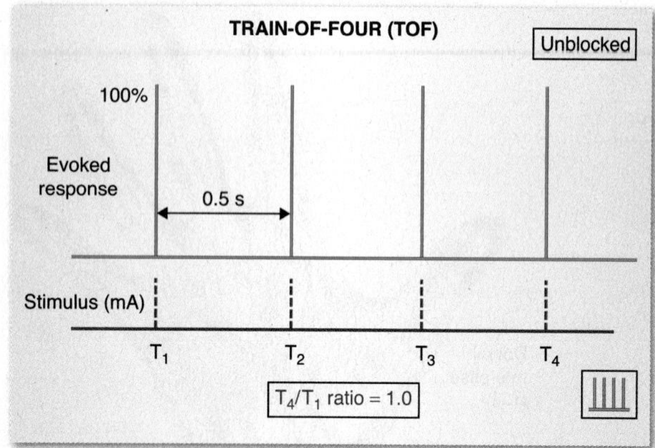

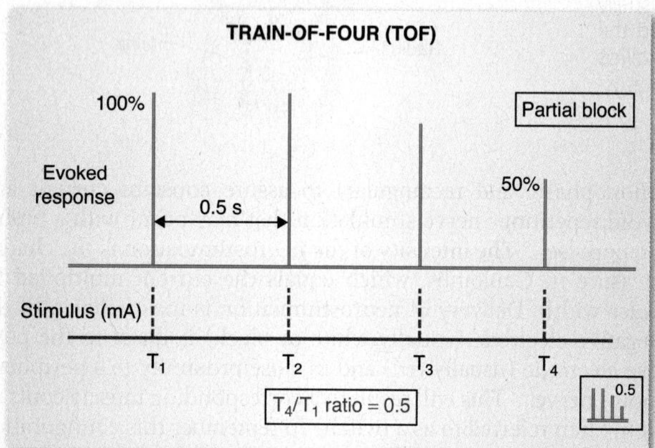

Figure 21-7 **A:** Following train-of-four (TOF) stimulation, the baseline T4/T1 ratio of 1 is observed. **B:** Following stimulation, depression of the T4/T1 to 0.5 is observed after administration of a nondepolarizing neuromuscular blocker.

Single twitch assessment is generally only used during the onset of neuromuscular blockade where reduction and subsequent loss of contraction can be appreciated.

Another pattern of stimulation, introduced in 1971, is the "train-of-four" which consists of four sequential stimuli (T1, T2, T3, and T4) delivered at 2 Hz frequency (Fig. 21-7). This should not be repeated more frequently than every 15 seconds to avoid potentiation or muscle contraction exaggeration. As the effects of a nondepolarizing neuromuscular blocking drug deepen, the number of muscle responses will decline, T4 will be lost first, then T3, then T2 and finally T1. Regression of drug effect (i.e., during recovery) will follow the same pattern in reverse, where T1 will return first followed by T2, then T3, and finally T4. Depth of block is often described using this twitch count, or train-of-four count (see depth of block definitions for a more detailed explanation). When four twitches are present, the "train-of-four ratio" (the strength of the fourth twitch divided by the first twitch, T4/T1) is a measurement of the nondepolarizing neuromuscular blocking drug depth of block. Recall that fade occurs with repeat stimulations because the α3β2 prejunctional acetylcholine receptor is blocked by nondepolarizing neuromuscular blocking drugs. Residual paralysis is currently defined as a train-of-four ratio less than 0.9. Such residual paralysis cannot be accurately identified using merely a peripheral nerve stimulator and subjective assessment. As a substitute, clinicians identify the presence of fade, or a noticeable reduction of T4 compared to T1 when utilizing the train-of-four stimulation.
11 Unfortunately, even in the absence of any tactile or visual recognition of fade, the train-of-four ratio can be as low as 0.3 to 0.4. Therefore, the limitation of subjective fade assessment by humans creates a blind zone of unknown train-of-four ratios between 0.4 and 0.9, leaving the patient at risk for residual paralysis.

Rapidly repeated stimulation at a high frequency (>30 Hz) fuse into one long sustained muscular tetanic contraction. The voluntary muscle contraction physiologic limit is 70 Hz, above which the muscle contraction may fade with sustained tetany. Tetanus mode can be used to assess fade from neuromuscular blockade with two settings available on most peripheral nerve stimulator units, 50 Hz and 100 Hz. The absence or presence of fade is assessed over 5 seconds of applied tetanus. This application of tetanus causes a large release of acetylcholine which potentiates further stimulations; therefore, tetany should not be repeated for 2 minutes after 50-Hz tetany and for 3 minutes after 100-Hz tetany. Detecting fade with 50 Hz translates to a train-of-four ratio less than approximately 0.4, making it as equally insensitive as train-of-four fade. If there is no subjectively appreciated fade with 100-Hz tetanus, that is the most sensitive means to utilize the peripheral nerve stimulator and subjective assessment, as it has been reported to correlate with a train-of-four ratio of approximately 0.85. The caveat, however, is that physiologic fade is possible with this high frequency; therefore, the occurrence of fade with 100-Hz tetanus may be misleading, as the patient may be partially paralyzed or may have returned to full strength, yet still displays physiologic fade.

"Double burst stimulation" was developed to address the difficulty with train-of-four in assessing the difference between two movements separated by two intervening movements (i.e., T1 compared to T4, trying to ignore T2 and T3). Double burst stimulation uses two short 50-Hz tetanic bursts, each appearing as one movement separated by 0.75 seconds (Fig. 21-8). There can be

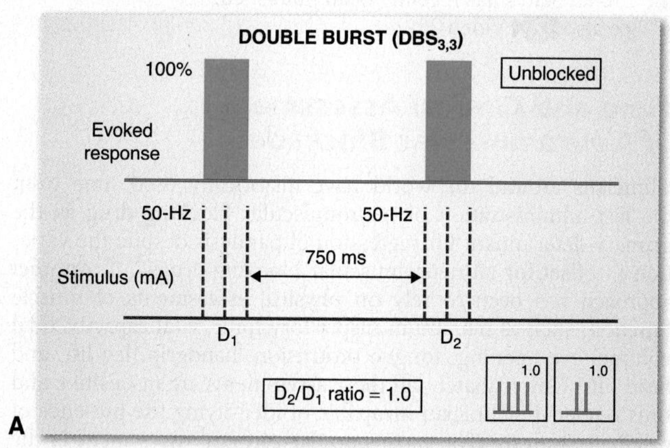

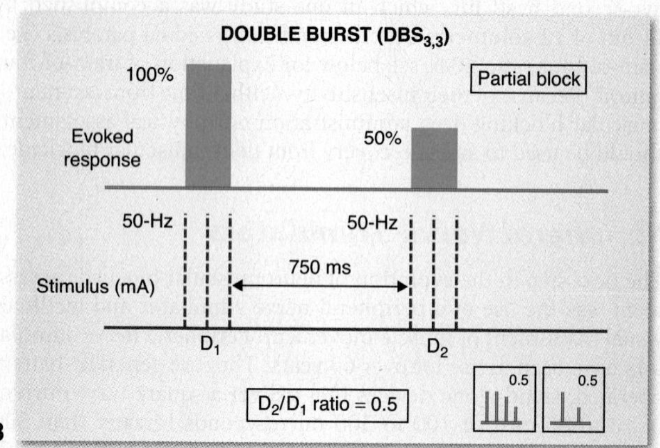

Figure 21-8 **A:** Double burst stimulation ($DBS_{3,3}$). **B:** Double burst stimulation ($DBS_{3,3}$) ratio 0.5.

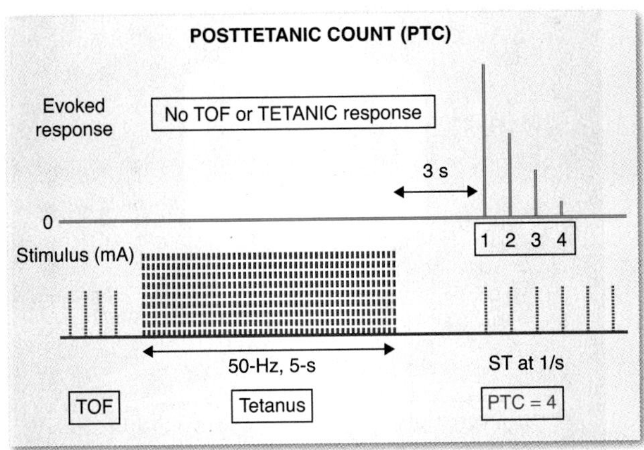

Figure 21-9 Posttetanic count. The number of single twitches observed (after 5 seconds of 50 Hz tetany) is inversely related to the depth of neuromuscular block.

either two bursts separated by 0.75 seconds of three stimuli at 50 Hz (DBS 3,3) or one burst of three stimuli followed by a burst of two stimuli (DBS 3,2). Twenty seconds recovery should be allowed between double burst stimulation assessments. Identifying fade with this pattern of stimuli has proved to be a slight improvement over train-of-four with fade, but even in the absence of any tactile or visual recognition of fade with double burst stimulation, the measured train-of-four ratio can still be as low as approximately 0.6. For these reasons, this subjective assessment cannot be used to accurately verify recovery from muscle paralysis.

The basis for posttetanic count stems from the substantial release of acetylcholine that occurs with tetanic stimulation—which floods the neuromuscular junction and presynaptic receptors with acetylcholine and serves to potentiate subsequent muscle responses for a brief period (Fig. 21-9). Using this technique, the depth of block at a train-of-four count of zero can be further defined. Posttetanic count uses 5 seconds of 50-Hz tetanus, followed by a three second pause, then 15 to 20 single stimuli delivered at one per second (1 Hz). The number of muscle contractions (twitches) observed after this flood of acetylcholine is known as the posttetanic count. To best use this technique, a zero train-of-four count should be confirmed before initiating the posttetanic testing sequence.

Quantitative Monitoring

12 Quantitative monitoring is the only way to objectively measure train-of-four ratio, which is why experts advocate for this technology to be used in clinical practice (Fig. 21-10).[50] This technique starts with the same delivery of current seen with the peripheral nerve stimulator (0- to 80-mA current, square wave, 100 to 300 microseconds), but also incorporates acceleromyography (AMG) and kinemyography. Proprietary, single-use electrodes are required for the commercially available electromyography (EMG) devices, as well as for the train-of-four ratio cuff. Many quantitative monitors include a mode that measures maximal current in order to set a supramaximal current. The sequence to determine maximal current starts with a very low current at which no response is detected, after which the current is sequentially increased (usually in 5 to 10 Hz increments) until muscle responses appear. The muscle responses strengthen as the current rises until a maximal muscle response eventually occurs that is not exceeded despite increased current. This inflection in the current response curve determines the maximal current. Supramaximal current is set at 20% higher than maximal current. Once the current is set, quantitative monitors can provide single twitch height (compared to baseline), double burst, or train-of-four ratio measurements. Supramaximal current is intended to provide reliable train-of-four measurements over time despite changes in skin resistance (e.g., from changing temperature). In addition, studies have shown that train-of-four ratios are consistent with current as low as 20 mA.[51,52] Regarding testing patients awake, there is less discomfort at 20 to 30 mA compared to 50 to 80 mA (with substantial between patient variability). Single twitch mode is used less commonly, as it requires a baseline measurement; however, it can be used to assess subsequent single twitch muscle responses compared to baseline. Unique to the single twitch modality is the ability to assess depolarizing blockade (no fade with repeat stimulations, recall $\alpha3\beta2$ prejunctional receptor is not blocked), as well as nondepolarizing blockade (where fade occurs with repeat stimulations due to $\alpha3\beta2$ prejunctional acetylcholine receptor blockade). Above all, the most advocated use of a quantitative monitor is to accurately measure the train-of-four ratio when measured at the adductor pollicis, ensuring that it reaches 0.9 before tracheal extubation.

There are multiple different technologies utilized in quantitative monitors. The reference standard is mechanomyography (MMG) which measures the isometric force created with thumb movement. Currently, MMG devices are not commercially available. EMG measures the compound action potential when contraction occurs in a muscle stimulated by an electrical impulse from the innervating nerve. A biphasic curve is generated. Muscle response (compound action potential) is calculated using the area under the biphasic curve, the peak-to-peak signal amplitude, or the peak to baseline signal amplitude. FDA-approved units have been commercially available for several years. AMG commercial units have been available for longer than the other technologies. This technology utilizes an accelerometer attached to the moving body part (thumb for ulnar nerve stimulation and resulting adductor pollicis muscle contraction). The acceleration is determined through its relationship to force by Newton's second law – Force = Mass * Acceleration – where the mass of the thumb is constant. This technology requires movement of the thumb (either free movement or movement with a set preload), which may be difficult to assess when the arms are tucked to the side during surgery. Kinemyography (KMG) is a technology in which a strip of isoelectric polymer material is placed in the space between the thumb and index finger and then deforms with thumb movement. The measured movement represents a thumb range of motion rather than force. The TOFcuff is a technology in which two electrodes are embedded within a blood pressure cuff. Nerve stimulation-induced muscular contractions are measured via a change in the internal pressure of the cuff. This is a volumetric measurement of muscle contraction rather than a measurement of force.

These various quantitative monitoring technologies provide slightly different muscle measurements; however, all are more accurate than any subjective assessment. The reference standard, as stated above, is MMG. EMG provides similar to lower values compared to MMG, while AMG provides slightly higher values compared to MMG that may be due to the thumb not returning to the original position prior to subsequent stimulations.[53] Preload can been applied to the thumb to mitigate this problem, but with limited success. Another solution to the exaggerated AMG values is normalization. Normalization involves taking a baseline (preneuromuscular blocking drug administration) AMG measurement and dividing all subsequent measurements by that number (thereby effectively making the maximum measured train-of-four ratio 1.0). As an example, if the baseline measurement train-of-four ratio is 1.1, then during recovery when

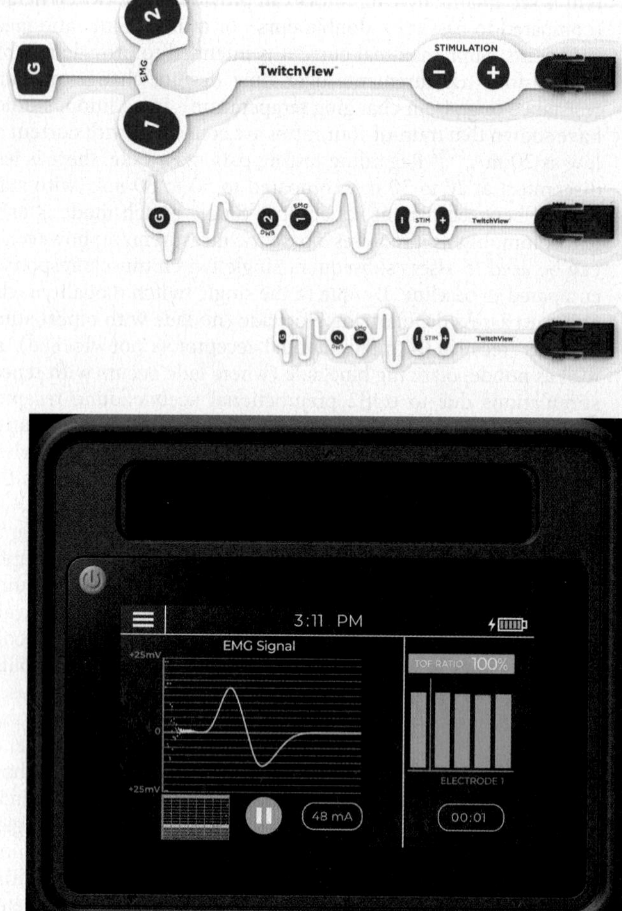

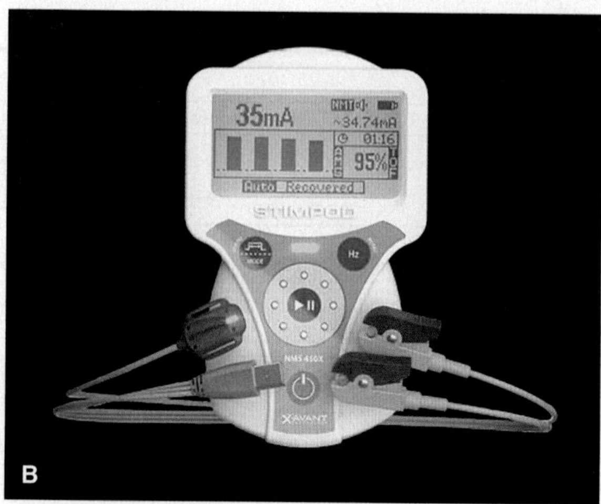

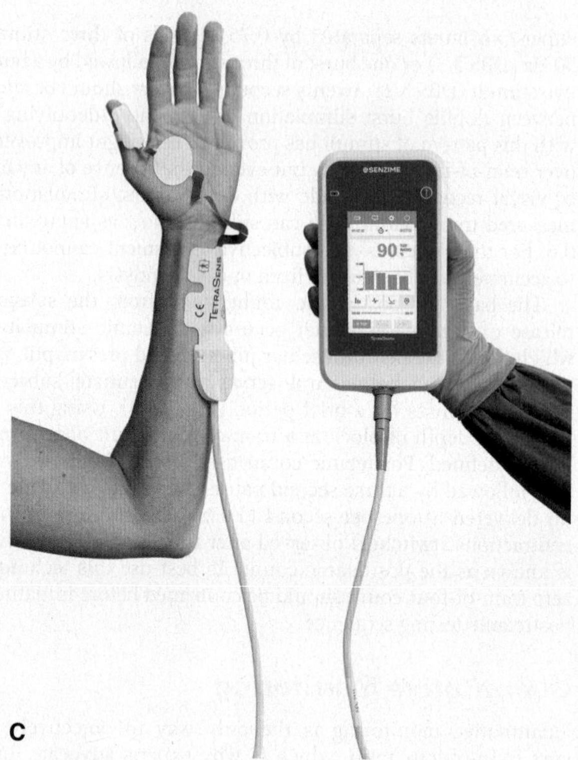

Figure 21-10 **A–C:** Modern electromyography and acceleromyography quantitative monitors. (**A:** Copyright © 2021 Blink Device Company. All rights reserved. **B:** Copyright © Xavant-Stimpod. **C:** Copyright © Senzime-Tetragaph.)

the monitor reads 0.95 this measurement would be normalized (0.95/1.1) to 0.85 (which is below the goal of train-of-four ratio of 0.9). Normalization usually yields lower train-of-four ratios; therefore, normalized observations are more likely than non-normalized observations to be classified as positive for residual neuromuscular blockade.

The measurement differences between these technologies suggest two types of bias inherent in quantitative monitoring. The first is a difference found when comparing response curves of different device when measuring a specific train-of-four ratio, usually between 0.7 and 0.9. There are no published concerns about inaccurately low train-of-four ratios, so in this context it is generally accepted that higher train-of-four ratios represent an overestimation that may falsely indicate adequate return of strength when partial paralysis persists. The second bias relates to the time required to attain a train-of-four ratio after pharmacologic reversal of neuromuscular blockade. In this context, the monitors that take a longer time to reach a given train-of-four ratio represent the safer option, again assuming the monitors that reach a given train-of-four ratio sooner are producing falsely elevated values. Tables 21-2 and 21-3 summarize the technology comparisons to the reference standard, MMG. There is only a small within-monitor bias for the reference standard technology, MMG. EMG and MMG produce similar values though there is a suggestion that EMG values might be lower than MMG. This data must be interpreted in the context of wide limits of agreement.

Table 21-2 Summary of Train-of-Four Ratio Differences (BIAS) at a Given Level of Neuromuscular Block (Derived from a Series of Measurements)[a]

Versus MMG	Measured $Bias^{TOFR}$	Biased Goal TOF Ratio
MMG (K-Nielsen, 1998)	$Bias^{TOFR}$ 2%	TOF ratio 0.92
EMG (Bowdle, 2020)	$Bias^{TOFR}$ −4.7%	TOF ratio 0.85
AMG (Capron, 2006)	$Bias^{TOFR}$ 5.3%	TOF ratio 0.95
AMG (Claudius, 2009)	$Bias^{TOFR}$ 0.11	TOF ratio 1.01
AMG (K-Nielsen, 1998)	$Bias^{TOFR}$ −8.1%	TOF ratio 0.82
AMG (Bowdle, 2020)	$Bias^{TOFR}$ 9.8%	TOF ratio 0.99
TOFcuff (Veiga Ruiz, 2017)	$Bias^{TOFR}$ 4.7%	TOF ratio 0.95

[a]The right column represents the train-of-four ratio approximation when mechanomyography train-of-four ratio is 0.9. The first row is a similar device comparison, mechanomyography versus mechanomyography. $Bias^{TOFR}$ refers to the train-of-four ratio of a monitoring modality when a specific train-of-four ratio was reached by the reference monitor, mechanomyography.

TOFR, train-of-four ratio; MMG, mechanomyography; EMG, electromyography; AMG, acceleromyography.

Table 21-3 Summary the Time Difference (BIAS) between Monitoring Modalities to Reach a Given Train-of-Four Ratio Compared to the Reference Standard, MMG

Versus MMG	Measured $Bias^{TIME}$
MMG (K-Nielsen, 1998)	$Bias^{TIME}$ 0.2%
AMG (K-Nielsen, 1998)	$Bias^{TIME}$ 0.8%
AMG (Claudius, 2009)	$Bias^{TIME}$ −11.5%
AMG (Claudius, 2009)	$Bias^{TIME}$ −17.8%
KMG (Dahaba, 2002)	$Bias^{TIME}$ −1.4%
KMG (Trager, 2006)	$Bias^{TIME}$ −0.6%

$Bias^{TIME}$ refers to difference in time to reach a specific train-of-four ratio of a monitoring modality versus the reference standard, mechanomyography.

MMG, mechanomyography; AMG, acceleromyography; KMG, kinemyography.

AMG train-of-four ratios appear to be higher than those of MMG at a given train-of-four ratio, although this was not found in all studies. The TOFcuff train-of-four ratio appears to be higher than MMG at a given train-of-four ratio (Table 21-2). Compared to MMG, the time for AMG to reach a given train-of-four ratio is shorter. The Kinemyography train-of-four ratio appears to be higher than MMG at a given train-of-four ratio by a small amount (Table 21-2). There are also comparisons between nonreference standard technologies. AMG train-of-four ratios appear to be higher than EMG at a given train-of-four ratio. Compared to AMG, the time for TOFcuff to reach a given train-of-four ratio is longer (Table 21-3). Compared to AMG, the time for kinemyography to reach a given train-of-four ratio was similar. To simplify these various train-of-four ratio bias reports, Table 21-2 provides a column that attempts to correlate the reference standard for adequate reversal (train-of-four ratio ≥ 0.9 using MMG) with a value that might be appropriate with the other technologies according to the cited studies. In summary, all technologies have inherent measurement inaccuracies. Nonetheless, the data suggest that EMG measurements more closely mimic MMG compared to AMG.

Although AMG values are higher than MMG or EMG, it is not clear whether AMG train-of-four ratio monitoring improves patient outcomes. The methodology employed in studies demonstrating patient harm with residual paralysis show a variety of technologies and train-of-four ratios (Table 21-4). There are 26 studies presented spanning 3 decades from 1992 to 2022. In 14 studies non-normalized AMG (train-of- four ratio of 0.9 or a range of train-of-four ratios) was used, 6 studies used MMG (train-of-four ratios ranged from 0.6 to 1), 5 studies used EMG (train-of-four ratio of 0.9 and train-of-four ratio not specified), 1 study used normalized AMG (train-of-four ratio of 0.9), and 1 study used kinemyography (train-of-four ratio of 0.9). A long list of patient harms were identified with either low train-of-four ratios or a train-of-four ratio below 0.9, including diplopia and impaired visual tracking, pharyngeal dysfunction, difficulty speaking, inability to seal a mouthpiece, swallowing dysfunction, impaired hypoxic ventilatory drive, reduced forced vital capacity and peak expiratory flow during recovery, hypoxia and oxygen support requirements during recovery, decreased upper pharyngeal sphincter tone, upper airway collapse and obstruction during transport and in recovery, increased need for airway support, increased critical respiratory events and respiratory failure during recovery, increased recovery room nursing visits, generalized weakness symptoms and lower quality of recovery, recovery room delayed discharge, prolonged ventilator weaning in the critical care unit, increased postoperative pulmonary complications, and longer hospital length of stay.

It is clear that AMG ratio values are exaggerated compared to MMG or EMG. It is important to anticipate this exaggeration and to raise the cutoff accordingly with an idealized AMG goal train-of-four ratio of 0.95 to 1.0. However, it remains the purview of the clinician, in context of a clinical scenario, to determine if tracheal extubation should occur at an AMG train-of-four ratio of 0.9 or higher. An alternative approach is to use a normalized train-of-four ratio threshold of 0.9.

Differential Muscle Sensitivity to Neuromuscular Blockade

There are differences in onset and return of function between various muscles in the body that may impact residual paralysis. Understanding that muscles differ in response to neuromuscular blocking drugs will aid neuromuscular blockade assessment and management. The reference standard location for assessing neuromuscular function is the adductor pollicis muscle, a site that has been extensively studied. However, muscles that influence intubating conditions include those innervating the vocal cords, abdominal muscles, and the diaphragm muscles—all of which are relatively resistant to neuromuscular blockade. Despite that fact, the preferential blood flow to these central muscles yields a faster onset of neuromuscular blockade. Therefore, although these muscles cannot be measured by commercial devices, a train-of-four count of zero may not be needed at the adductor pollicis before proceeding with tracheal intubation. The resistance to neuromuscular block seen in central muscles only becomes apparent in the steady state recovery profile, where movement returns sooner in these central muscles than in peripheral muscles (e.g., adductor pollicis). Because the highest degree of safety for tracheal

Table 21-4 Quantitative Monitoring Modality and Cutoff Showing Patient Harms when Residual Paralysis Was Present. 26 Studies[a]

AMG Non-normalized	**TOF Ratio 0.9**	**Lower TOF Ratio Patient Outcomes**
AMG (Butterly, 2010)	TOFR 0.9 Non-normalized	Longer PACU length of stay
AMG (Murphy, 2011)	TOFR 0.9 Non-normalized	More weakness, reduced quality of PACU recovery
AMG (Kumar, 2012)	TOFR 0.9 Non-normalized	Reduced forced vital capacity & peak expiratory flow in PACU
AMG (Pietraszewski, 2013)	TOFR 0.9 Non-normalized	More hypoxia in elderly
AMG (Norton, 2013)	TOFR 0.9 Non-normalized	More critical respiratory events and respiratory failure
AMG (Adembesa, 2018)	TOFR 0.9 Non-normalized	More upper airway obstruction in the PACU
AMG (Allenes, 2021)	TOFR 0.9 Non-normalized	More postoperative critical respiratory events
AMG (Weigel, 2022)	TOFR 0.9 Non-normalized	More pulmonary complications, longer PACU stay, longer hospital length of stay
AMG Non-Normalized	**TOF Ratio (Range)**	**Lower TOFR Patient Outcomes**
AMG (Blobner, 2020)	TOFR 0.92 Non-normalized	Increased postoperative pulmonary complications
AMG (Murphy, 2003)	TOFR 0.8 Non-normalized	In ICU post-CABG more visual disturbances/difficulty speaking, and generalized weakness. Prolonged weaning time.
AMG (Murphy, 2004)	TOFR 0.7-1 Non-normalized	In PACU more blurry vision, muscle weakness symptoms with TOFR<0.7, hypoxia and delayed PACU discharge more likely at TOFR<0.9
AMG (Murphy, 2008 Anesth)	TOFR <0.7, 0.98 Non-normalized	Increased upper AW obstruction during PACU transport, Increased critical respiratory events in PACU
AMG (Murphy, 2008 AA)	TOFR 0.62, 0.98 Non-normalized	Increased critical respiratory events in PACU with TOFR <0.7 versus TOFR 0.9, Increased p/o hypoxia
AMG (Eikermann, 2003)	TOFR 0.5–1 Non-normalized	Less able to seal mouthpiece & swallow, more airway obstruction
AMG Normalized	**TOF Ratio 0.9**	**Lower TOF Ratio Patient Outcomes**
AMG (Fortier, 2015)	TOFR 0.9 Normalized	More oxygen support and nurse visits required in PACU
MMG	**TOF Ratio (Range)**	**Lower TOF Ratio Patient Outcomes**
MMG (Eriksson, 1992)	TOFR 0.7	Impaired hypoxic ventilatory drive
MMG (Eriksson, 1993)	TOFR 0.7	Impaired hypoxic ventilatory drive
MMG (Eriksson, 1996)	TOFR 0.7 and 0.9	Impaired hypoxic ventilatory drive at TOFR 0.7, not impaired at TOFR 0.9
MMG (Eriksson, 1997)	TOFR 0.6–1.0	Upper pharyngeal sphincter resting tone decreased at TOFR<0.8, increased aspiration at TOFR<0.9
MMG (Berg, 1997)	TOFR 0.7	Increase postoperative pulmonary complications with TOFR<0.7 if given pancuronium
MMG (Sundman, 2000)	TOFR 0.6-0.9	Pharyngeal dysfunction at TOFR 0.7
EMG	**TOF Ratio 0.9**	**Lower TOFR Patient Outcomes**
EMG (Kopman, 1997)	TOFR 0.9	Diplopia and visual tracking difficulty
EMG (Eikermann, 2007)	TOFR 0.9	More upper airway collapse
EMG (Yip, 2010)	TOFR 0.9	Increased need for AW support in PACU
EMG (Weigel, 2022)	TOFR 0.9	More pulmonary complications, longer PACU stay, longer hospital length of stay
EMG	**TOFR Ratio (Unspecified)**	**Lower TOFR Patient Outcomes**
EMG (Todd, 2014)	Not specified	More PACU intubations before monitoring
KMG	**TOFR 0.9**	**Lower TOFR Patient Outcomes**
KMG (Alday, 2019)	TOFR 0.9	Atelectasis similar with neostigmine versus sugammadex when TOFR ≥0.9

[a]Distribution of monitoring technologies in the studies: acceleromyography 15 studies, mechanomyography 6 studies, electromyography 5 studies, kinemyography one study (acceleromyography and electromyography both used in one study). Among studies using acceleromyography, normalization was performed in one study, the other 14 used non-normalized acceleromyography. The train-of-four ratios specified in the studies were: train-of-four ratio 0.7 in 3 studies, train-of-four ratio 0.8 in 1 study, train-of-four ratio 0.9 in 15 studies, train-of-four ratio 0.95 in 1 study, and a range of train-of-four ratios were used for 7 studies. TOFR, train-of-four ratio; MMG, mechanomyography; EMG, electromyography; AMG, acceleromyography; KMG, kinemyography.

Table 21-5 Data Summary for Relative Muscle Sensitivity to Neuromuscular Block Compared to the Adductor Pollicis Muscle

Adductor Pollicis Muscle VERSUS...	Bias^{TIME}	Bias^{TOFR}	Residual Paralysis
First dorsal interosseous muscle		0.01 (Phillips, 2012)	
Masseter	Similar (Vega, 2016)		
Flexor hallucis brevis	Faster (Le Merrer, 2020) Similar (Le Merrer, 2020)		
Abductor digiti minimi muscle		0.1 (Phillips, 2012)	
Corrugator supercilii	Faster (Yamamoto, 2015; Thudium, 2020; Suzuki, 2009) Similar (Plaud, 2001)		
Orbicularis oculi	Faster (Abdulatif, 1997; Larsen, 2002)		Increased (Thilen, 2012)

Bias^{TIME} is the time to train-of-four ratio, longer times are preferable to avoid residual paralysis as measured at the adductor pollicis. Bias^{TOFR} reflects the difference when simultaneously measuring the train-of-four ratio at two sites, lower train-of-four are desired to ensure all muscles have recovered, the reference site is the adductor pollicis.
TOFR, train-of-four ratio.

extubation comes when recovery of all muscles has occurred, the most desirable sites of measurement are those most sensitive to neuromuscular blockade (e.g., adductor pollicis).

As with quantitative monitoring technologies, muscle sensitivity to neuromuscular block can be compared using time to train-of-four ratio by simultaneously measuring the train-of-four ratio at two anatomic sites. There are three muscles of interest in the hand (adductor pollicis, abductor digiti minimi, and first dorsal interosseous muscles) that will contract when electrodes are placed along the ulnar groove on the volar surface of the wrist and the ulnar nerve is stimulated (Fig. 21-5). Alternative sites that have been studied include muscles of the face (corrugator supercilii, orbicularis oculi, and masseter muscles), as well as one foot muscle (flexor hallucis brevis). Table 21-5 is a summary of muscle comparison data against the reference site, the adductor pollicis muscle. The table is organized top to bottom from most sensitive to most resistance to neuromuscular blockade. The first dorsal interosseous muscle most closely mimics the sensitivity of the adductor pollicis muscle and is located on the dorsum of the hand (Fig. 21-5). Table 21-6 is a summary of comparisons to the first dorsal interosseous muscle.

Table 21-6 Data Summary for Relative Muscle Sensitivity to Neuromuscular Block Compared to the First Dorsal Interosseous Muscle

First Dorsal Interosseous Muscle VERSUS...	Bias^{TIME}	Bias^{TOFR}
Flexor hallucis brevis	Faster (Sugi, 2013)	
Abductor digiti minimi muscle		0.09 (Philip, 2012)

Bias^{TIME} is the time to train-of-four ratio, longer times are preferable to avoid residual paralysis as measured at the adductor pollicis. Bias^{TOFR} reflects the difference when simultaneously measuring the train-of-four ratio at two sites, lower train-of-four are desired to ensure all muscles have recovered.
TOFR, train-of-four ratio.

Aggregating the available evidence, the two sites safest for making clinical patient care decisions are the adductor pollicis and the first dorsal interosseous site. The most resistant sites are the eye muscles, orbicularis oculi, and the corrugator supercilia; thus, monitoring at these sites should be avoided. One reason for this is that it may be difficult to avoid direct muscle stimulation (which bypasses the neuromuscular junction where neuromuscular blocking drugs have their effect) with facial nerve stimulation near the eye muscles. It has been reported that the FDA-approved dosage recommendations for sugammadex do not apply when train-of-four measurements are obtained from the corrugator supercilii.[54] Moreover, one study found that the incidence of residual paralysis was fivefold higher when intraoperative neuromuscular monitoring was conducted at the eye muscles instead of the adductor pollicis.[55] It is critical that if eye muscle monitoring is used intraoperatively, the monitoring site should be changed to the adductor pollicis before pharmacologic reversal.[56,57] Planning for effective reversal, which requires appropriate choice of drug and dose, must be based on a valid prereversal assessment and this can be obtained only at the adductor pollicis. The abductor digiti minimi and flexor hallucis brevis muscles appear to be resistant to neuromuscular blockade and therefore caution is warranted when measuring from these sites. The masseter muscle is a less common site of monitoring, but one small study showed it may yield similar train-of-four ratios as the adductor pollicis site.

Receptor Occupancy to Stimulation Response Relationship

Occupancy of nicotinic acetylcholine receptors is a concept that provides important insight regarding neuromuscular blocking drug dosing at various depths of block. It is estimated that only 25% to 30% of receptors need to be available (70% to 75% receptors occupied by neuromuscular blocking drug) for a normal train-of-four ratio.[58] As such, only a fraction of receptors needs to be blocked when redosing neuromuscular blocking drugs. Table 21-7 shows the various depths of block after a single intubating dose of nondepolarizing drug from complete block until adequate recovery with associated receptor occupancies.[59]

Adoption of Quantitative Monitoring into Clinical Practice

Incorporating quantitative monitoring into clinical practice has not yet occurred despite both accumulated evidence of benefit and numerous published recommendations. Likely the strongest deterrent to monitor use is a lack of education resulting in a belief among anesthesia providers that quantitative monitoring is unnecessary. If signs of severe weakness are not obvious in the immediate postoperative period, the perception is that no harm has been done. In addition, there is a strong belief among physicians that residual paralysis does not occur in their practice or that it is their partners' inferior management, rather than their own, that leads to residual paralysis rates well documented in the literature.[44,60,61] Education is the solution to breaking down this barrier.

Other barriers to using quantitative monitors for all patients include unreliable monitors and the need for training on how to use a monitor. Equipment development has resulted in more reliable equipment and is a trend that should continue. Even with these advancements in equipment, for a given practice to successfully adopt quantitative monitor use requires training, ongoing equipment support, and responsiveness to equipment issues (e.g., pole mounts, battery depletion, cable length, failed/broken cables or monitors, measurement reliability). There should also be protocols in place to use the equipment for ulnar nerve stimulation in cases when the arms are tucked or may have an obstructing peripheral IV or arterial line. In addition, there must be respect for the potential interruption in workflow that monitoring will impose. Workflow interruptions can be minimized with streamlined setup, as well as automatic electronic input of data into the anesthesia record.

The culture shift to quantitative monitoring has been accomplished in one practice with a systematic approach that included department-wide equipment trials to select the ideal equipment, a restructuring of the clinical environment by placing monitors in all anesthetizing location, and education about the clinical importance of residual paralysis. Instructions on equipment use should emphasize the twin goals that a train-of-four of 0.9 must be reached before tracheal extubation and that this must be documented in the anesthesia record. Postimplementation follow up with clinicians regarding individual performance, department performance education, establishment of practice performance metrics, and a policy linking quantitative monitoring use to credentialing have also proven useful.[62]

Quantitative neuromuscular monitoring should be thought of as similar to other critical measuring modalities of anesthesia practice such as blood pressure. For example, knowing the blood pressure may either prompt pharmacologic intervention or indicate that a pharmacologic intervention is not needed for hemodynamic support. Quantitative neuromuscular monitoring can play a similar role in managing neuromuscular blockade.

Table 21-7 Receptor Occupancy Estimates for the Six Levels of Neuromuscular Blockade

Depth of Neuromuscular Block	Receptor Occupancy	Quantitative Monitor
Pre	0%	TOF ratio 1.0
Complete	>95%	TOFC 0, PTC 0
Deep	90–95%	TOFC 0, PTC ≥ 1
Moderate	70–90%	TOFC 1–3
Shallow	60–70%	TOFC 4, TOF ratio <0.4
Minimal	60–70%	TOFC 4, TOF ratio 0.4–0.9
Recovered	<70%	TOFC 4, TOF ratio ≥0.9

TOF, train-of-four; PTC, posttetanic count; TOFC, train-of-four count.

Reversal of Neuromuscular Blockade

Depth of Block Definitions

Six levels of neuromuscular block have been described (Tables 21-7 and 21-8).[50] Three of these levels are refinements of the train-of-four count 4, which can only be accurately identified using quantitative monitoring. The most important level of block is "recovered," where the train-of-four count is 4 and the train-of-four ratio is ≥0.9. The next level of block is called "minimal," where the train-of-four count is 4 and the train-of-four ratio is 0.4 to 0.9. The lowest train-of-four count for depth of block is called "shallow," which is defined as a train-of-four count of 4 and train-of-four ratio <0.4. Of the three remaining more profound depths of block, two of them occur at a train-of-four count of zero. At the most profound depth of block no thumb twitch can be elicited, not even by posttetanic stimulation. This is called "complete" block, which is defined as a train-of-four count of zero and a posttetanic count of zero. The other, slightly less depth of block at a train-of-four count of zero occurs when one can elicit thumb movement only after applying tetany first. This is "deep" block, which is defined as a train-of-four count of zero and a posttetanic count ≥1. The sixth and final level of block encompasses all the train-of-four counts not yet mentioned (i.e., 1, 2, and 3). This is "moderate" block, which is defined as all train-of-four counts ranging from 1 to 3.

Anticholinesterase Drugs

Blocking the breakdown of acetylcholine by acetylcholinester- 13
ase results in an increase in the available pool of acetylcholine at the synaptic cleft and improves the chances of competing with a nondepolarizing neuromuscular blocking drug. The clinically available anticholinesterase drugs (also known as acetylcholinesterase inhibiting drugs or cholinesterase inhibiting drugs) are neostigmine, edrophonium, and pyridostigmine. Anticholinesterase drugs are quaternary compounds and do not cross the blood–brain barrier. Their duration of action at equivalent doses is similar (60 to 120 minutes), but onset of action is fastest for edrophonium, intermediate with neostigmine, and longest for pyridostigmine. Pyridostigmine's slow onset makes it unattractive for perioperative reversal of neuromuscular block; however, oral pyridostigmine is commonly used for treatment of myasthenia gravis. Neostigmine is the most frequently used anticholinesterase drug in current anesthesia practice. Neostigmine is most effective for reversal of minimal block, though its use is acceptable for shallow block in the context of quantitative monitoring.

Factors Affecting Neostigmine Reversal

It is important to consider that neostigmine results in two parallel processes that contribute to recovery from neuromuscular blockade. One is the inhibition of acetylcholinesterase that

Table 21-8 Recommendations for Pharmacologic Reversal of Intermediate Acting Nondepolarizing Neuromuscular Blocking Drugs

Reversal of Intermediate Duration Neuromuscular Blocking Drugs

Level of Block	Type of Monitoring		Reversal Agent			
	PNS + subjective evaluation	Quantitative monitoring	Neostigmine TIVA	Neostigmine volatile anesthesia	Edrophonium	Sugammadex[b]
Complete (intense)	No twitch PTC 0	PTC 0	Wait	Wait	Wait	Wait
Deep	TOFC 0 PTC ≥1	TOFC 0 PTC ≥1	Wait	Wait	Wait	4 mg/kg
Moderate	TOFC 1–3	TOFC 1–3	Wait	Wait	Wait	2 mg/kg
Shallow	TOFC 4 with fade	TOFR <0.4	40–50 mcg/kg	Wait[a]	Wait	2 mg/kg
Minimal	TOFC 4 without fade	TOFR 0.4–0.9	15–30 mcg/kg	15–30 mcg/kg	0.5 mg/kg	2 mg/kg
Acceptable recovery	Unable to assess	TOFR ≥0.9	None	None	None	None

[a]With quantitative monitoring, neostigmine reversal with 40 mcg/kg can be attempted, some patients can be successfully reversed from this level of block.
[b]Only for reversal of rocuronium or vecuronium induced block.
PNS, peripheral nerve stimulator; TIVA, total intravenous anesthesia; PTC, posttetanic count; TOFC, train-of-four count; TOFR, train-of-four ratio.

leads to an increased concentration of acetylcholine; the other is the continued metabolism and elimination of nondepolarizing neuromuscular blocking drug. When acetylcholinesterase is completely inhibited, the concentration of acetylcholine is limited by the amount released—this amount is not increased by further administration of neostigmine. Consequently, neostigmine effectiveness reaches a plateau (i.e., ceiling effect) when the dose exceeds that which is sufficient for complete inhibition of acetylcholinesterase. This also explains why the level of neuromuscular block is a major determinant of the effectiveness of neostigmine. These concepts were demonstrated in an in vitro study using a preparation of rat diaphragm.[63] Pancuronium was used to depress the single twitch to 40% of control, after which neostigmine was given at increasing concentrations. Neuromuscular function gradually improved; however, the highest attainable train-of-four ratio was 0.8, regardless of further neostigmine administration. When the block was deepened to a single twitch height of only 5% of control, the maximum attainable train-of-four ratio with increasing neostigmine was only 0.6. The threshold at which the ceiling effect is clinically significant has often been underestimated, such that neostigmine reversal has traditionally been attempted for moderate block (train-of-four count 1 to 3, Table 21-8). This practice was justified when the consensus threshold for adequate recovery was a train-of-four ratio of 0.7. However, the current consensus threshold train-of-four ratio for adequate recovery is ≥0.9, and as shown above, neostigmine cannot reliably antagonize a moderate block to a train-of-four ratio 0.9.[64] Even when the block is shallow (train-of-four count of 4 with subjective fade or a train-of-four ratio <0.4), there is no dose of neostigmine that can guarantee complete reversal to train-of-four ratio 0.9 within 10 minutes in 95% of patients.[65,66]
14 Only when the block is minimal (train-of-four count of 4 without fade or train-of-four ratio ≥0.4) is neostigmine highly effective.[67] Administration of neostigmine earlier than 10 to 15 minutes before anticipated tracheal extubation is not optimal because neostigmine has peak effect at approximately 10 minutes.[68,69] Therefore, if full recovery to a train-of-four ratio ≥0.9 is not accomplished by 10 minutes after neostigmine administration, the most likely explanation is that the block was too deep for reversal with neostigmine. In this case, spontaneous recovery will continue (while neostigmine's effect somewhat diminishes after its peak) and the patient will eventually reach full recovery. When, instead of quantitative devices, monitoring is performed by peripheral nerve stimulator and subjective evaluation, early administration of neostigmine for shallow block (or deeper levels) has a significant disadvantage, namely a longer and more unpredictable period of time during which the train-of-four ratio will be in the range 0.4 to 0.9.[70] This range has been referred to as *the zone of blind paralysis* because it is not possible to subjectively determine when the patient is fully recovered (i.e., there is no fade to train-of-four, yet no objective measure that the train-of-four ratio is ≥ 0.9).[2] When using quantitative monitoring it is acceptable to attempt neostigmine reversal for a block with a train-of-four count of 4 with fade, because some patients can be successfully reversed in a reasonable time. With quantitative monitoring the clinician will know when the recovered state has been attained and can therefor safely extubate. The approach of attempting neostigmine reversal at shallow block is more likely to be successful in the context of propofol total intravenous anesthesia and less likely to succeed with volatile anesthetics.[71]

Neostigmine Dosing

The FDA-approved dosage recommendations for neostigmine are based on whether the twitch height of a single twitch is close to, or substantially greater than, 10% of the baseline preparalysis single twitch (10% of the baseline value is equal to 90% twitch depression). Most often the clinical anesthesiologist does not have access to this baseline measurement. Moreover, studies of the correlation between a single twitch height and the train-of-four responses have reported highly variable results.[72,73] For these reasons, dosage recommendations based on the subjective or quantitative train-of-four response is more meaningful than single twitch response. A valid determination of the prereversal depth of block is essential to guide selection of antagonist drug and dose (Table 21-8) and should always be obtained at the adductor pollicis. If intraoperative monitoring is performed at the eye muscles, then a switch from facial nerve to ulnar nerve stimulation should be accomplished at the end of the surgical procedure, before the pharmacologic reversal drug is administered. For reversal of a shallow block (train-of-four count 4, train-of-four ratio <0.4) an appropriate dose of neostigmine is 40 to 50 mcg/kg. Doses higher than 50 mcg/kg are not recommended at any depth of block because higher doses have not been shown to increase effectiveness. For neostigmine reversal of minimal block (train-of-four count 4 without fade or train-of-four ratio ≥0.4), a dose of 15 to 30 mcg is recommended.[67,74] The shallower the block, the lower the dose of neostigmine that is required. When the train-of-four ratio exceeds 0.6, then a dose of 10 to 20 mcg/kg is adequate and higher doses do not bring further improvement in neuromuscular recovery.[75] There is no significant difference in the speed of recovery induced by neostigmine among the intermediate-acting nondepolarizing neuromuscular blocking drugs. When reversing minimal block with neostigmine, it is possible to hasten recovery to a train-of-four ratio ≥0.9 by increasing the dose from 8 to 40 mcg/kg. Schaller et al. studied neostigmine reversal of block with train-of-four ratio 0.5; doses of 8, 15, 25, and 40 mcg/kg induced recovery to train-of-four ratio ≥0.9 in less than 10 minutes in all subjects.[76] The median time to attain such recovery decreased with increasing dose—for 8 mcg/kg the median time was 5.3 minutes and for 40 mcg/kg it was 2.0 minutes. However, this also implies that if reversal is adequate within a few minutes, then a more than sufficient dose has been administered. Lower doses are recommended unless rapid reversal is a high priority because lower doses are associated with a decreased frequency and severity of side effects.

Age affects neostigmine-induced speed of reversal—it is faster in children compared to adults, and slower in the elderly. Most studies on neostigmine reversal have excluded obese patients so there are only limited data to guide weight adjusting dosages (ideal vs. lean vs. total body weight). It may be reasonable to use ideal body weight because neostigmine is a hydrophilic drug.[77,78] Finally, drugs and conditions that potentiate the effect of nondepolarizing neuromuscular blocking drugs will also prolong neostigmine-induced recovery time (e.g., volatile anesthetics, magnesium, and hypothermia).

Other Effects of Neostigmine

Neostigmine and edrophonium inhibit acetylcholinesterase at all cholinergic sites, including muscarinic receptors, and induce vagal stimulation. Therefore, anticholinergic drugs such as atropine or glycopyrrolate are coadministered with anticholinesterase drugs. Atropine is faster in onset than glycopyrrolate, produces more tachycardia, and crosses the blood–brain barrier. Glycopyrrolate has onset and offset times similar to neostigmine. For these reasons, glycopyrrolate is preferred with neostigmine (dose one-fifth that of neostigmine, 0.2-mg glycopyrrolate for every 1-mg neostigmine). Other side effects of neostigmine include increased salivation and bowel motility. Although anticholinergic drugs are effective in preventing salivation, their effects on bowel motility are limited; however, the clinical significance of this is uncertain. This is an additional reason to avoid higher doses of neostigmine beyond what is required for adequate reversal. A meta-analysis of the effects of neostigmine on postoperative nausea and vomiting have not supported an association. The current guideline for postoperative nausea and vomiting management advises against high-dose neostigmine.[79]

Neostigmine Weakness

Anticholinesterase drugs possess neuromuscular blocking drug properties in the absence of previously administered muscle relaxants. This has been known since the 1930s when experiments on cats found that neostigmine administered prior to curare caused depression of neuromuscular transmission, while small doses of curare abolished this neostigmine-induced depression.[80] This phenomenon was subsequently confirmed in anesthetized patients, finding that neostigmine administered alone, without previous administration of muscle relaxant, produced some characteristics of a depolarizing block.[81] Payne and Hughes confirmed that neostigmine in doses used for antagonism of muscle relaxants can produce weakness; however, the response to neostigmine was dependent on several factors, including the dose of neostigmine, exposure to a volatile drug, exposure to nondepolarizing neuromuscular blocking drugs, and mode of nerve stimulation (single twitch or 50-Hz tetanus).[82] These and several subsequent studies have made it clear that neostigmine must be used appropriately with carefully considered dosage. When a nondepolarizing neuromuscular blocking drug occupies a sufficient number of acetylcholine receptors, a protective effect from the depolarizing actions of excess acetylcholine occurs; patients are at highest risk for neostigmine-induced weakness if they have not received a muscle relaxant or if they have recovered completely from neuromuscular blockade. Healthy awake volunteers who were given neostigmine 35 mcg/kg showed signs of significant depolarizing block, including 20% reduction in hand grip strength compared to placebo control. When the dose was repeated 15 minutes later, this resulted in further weakness with a mean 41% reduction in hand grip strength (Fig. 21-11).[83] Pharmacologic reversal should therefore not be administered to patients who have an adequate spontaneous recovery to train-of-four ratio ≥0.9. However, as mentioned above, determination of whether adequate recovery has occurred is only possible with quantitative monitoring. Therefore, in the absence of quantitative monitoring and with a train-of-four response of 4 twitches without subjective fade, it is advisable to limit the neostigmine dose to 15 to 30 mcg/kg. The lower dose (15 mcg/kg) can be

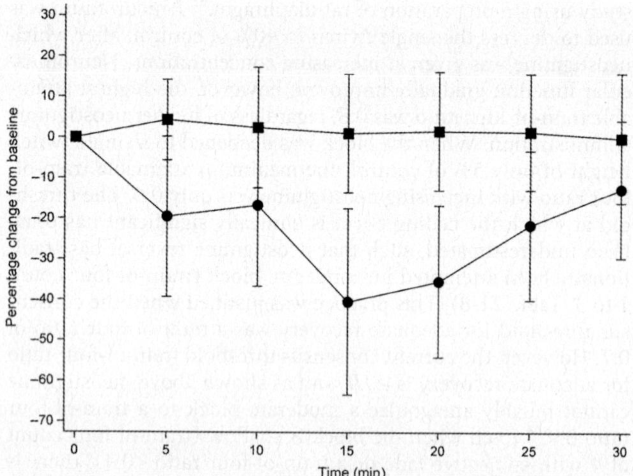

Figure 21-11 Hand grip strength mean percentage change from baseline in 14 healthy volunteers given neostigmine. (Reprinted from Kent NB, Liang SS, Phillips S, et al. Therapeutic doses of neostigmine, depolarising neuromuscular blockade and muscle weakness in awake volunteers: a double-blind, placebo-controlled, randomised volunteer study. *Anaesthesia* 2018;73:1079–1089. Copyright © 2018 Association of Anaesthetists.)

considered if it is known that subjective fade at the adductor pollicis has been absent for 30 minutes or more. There is controversy regarding what is the highest safe dose of neostigmine when the neuromuscular block may be fully recovered.[84,85] A study by Caldwell et al. of reversal of vecuronium-induced block compared neostigmine 40 to 20 mcg/kg. Only with the higher-dose and a prereversal train-of-four ratio ≥0.9 did some patients have a decrease in train-of-four ratio. Although in this study there was no evidence of weakness with 20 mcg/kg, the exact level of receptor occupancy was not known and it was unlikely to be zero.[84] Herbstreit et al. administered 30 mcg/kg to volunteers who had recovered from nondepolarizing blockade to an AMG-measured train-of-four ratio 1.0 and found an increased upper airway collapsibility and impaired genioglossus activation.[86] If sugammadex is used for rescue reversal after neostigmine has failed to induce adequate antagonism, there is the potential for complete removal of rocuronium and a zero receptor occupancy. If a large dose of neostigmine had been administered, it may induce significant weakness after reversal with sugammadex. This situation should be anticipated if there is a potential to use sugammadex after neostigmine, and is one more reason for reserving neostigmine for reversal of minimal block. Neostigmine-induced weakness is thought to be of relatively short duration (<30 minutes), but any weakness in the early postextubation period can have significant adverse consequences.

Neostigmine Cost Variation Over Time

The cost of neostigmine compared to sugammadex is an interesting and often misunderstood story.[87] When sugammadex was first FDA-approved in 2015, the cost of generic neostigmine was greater than that of sugammadex. This resulted from the FDA's 2011 "marketed unapproved drugs initiative" that targeted grandfathered drugs that were FDA-approved prior to the "new drug application" requirement. The FDA decided that these drugs—including neostigmine—should be subjected to the same standards as set out in a new drug application and that any company providing the safety and efficacy data would be granted sole-source status. Flamel Technologies provided the proper paperwork in 2013 and became the sole source manufacturer of neostigmine. This set off a series of price hikes which saw neostigmine cost increase from $4/vial in 2010 to $175/vial in February 2015. As more companies gained FDA approval to manufacture neostigmine the price declined slightly to $106/vial in 2015. This led to the unusual situation of a newly approved drug, sugammadex (~$90/vial) costing less than the generic drug combination of neostigmine plus glycopyrrolate (~$120). The price of neostigmine has since dropped, while that of sugammadex has remained relatively stable. Actual costs depend on hospital pharmacy purchasing agreements, but today neostigmine (10 mg vial) is 10% to 50% the cost of sugammadex (200 mg vial).

Edrophonium

Edrophonium is an anticholinesterase drug with an onset that is significantly faster than that of neostigmine. It produces peak antagonism in less than 2 minutes. It has traditionally been considered less effective than neostigmine for antagonism of moderate and deep neuromuscular blockade; however, antagonism of deep and moderate block is no longer recommended with any anticholinesterase drug (see above). Edrophonium's duration of antagonism is similar to that of neostigmine. Atropine is the antimuscarinic agent of choice for coadministration with edrophonium because of its faster onset. Edrophonium is the preferred antagonist of mivacurium-induced blockade because unlike neostigmine, it does not inhibit plasma cholinesterase that is required for metabolism of mivacurium. Edrophonium has not been available in the United States since 2018.

Selective Relaxant Binding Drugs: Sugammadex

Sugammadex is currently the only commercially available selective muscle relaxant binding drug.[88] Sugammadex is highly water-soluble and is a gamma-cyclodextrin—an eight membered ring with a central cavity that envelopes the steroid nuclease of steroidal neuromuscular blocking drugs (rocuronium > vecuronium >> pancuronium).[89] It has no affinity for depolarizing or nondepolarizing neuromuscular blocking drugs with other chemical structures. Binding to rocuronium is tight with no clinically relevant dissociation. Binding to vecuronium is only one-third as tight as rocuronium; therefore, assuming comparable depths of neuromuscular blockade and the same dose of sugammadex, the antagonism of rocuronium will be more rapid than the antagonism of vecuronium.[90] Following sugammadex administration, rapid binding of rocuronium and vecuronium occurs in the plasma. There is a subsequent reduction of free plasma neuromuscular blocking drug which changes the concentration gradient between the neuromuscular junction and the plasma. This results in a net movement of neuromuscular blocking drug into the plasma. This cycle continues (provided there is sufficient sugammadex in the plasma) culminating in a return of neuromuscular function. Sugammadex also combines with the active metabolite of vecuronium (3-desacetylvecuronium).

The speed of sugammadex reversal is dose-dependent—a larger dose will hasten recovery. The dosing depends on the depth of muscle relaxation at the time of reversal. For a train-of-four count 2 or more, a sugammadex dose of 2 mg/kg will reverse the majority of adult and pediatric patients to a train-of-four ratio ≥0.9 in 2 to 4 minutes.[91–93] Some patients—particularly the elderly—take significantly longer to attain such recovery. In one study of sugammadex dosing in 40 patients aged 75 or older, 1 patient required 9.9 minutes to attain a train-of-four ratio ≥0.9, and at least 5 patients required 5 to 6 minutes.[94] This is yet another reason for the recommendation to routinely use quantitative monitoring so that adequate recovery can be confirmed before tracheal extubation. For reversal from deeper levels of block, higher doses are required (sugammadex 4 mg/kg for train-of-four count 1 to posttetanic count of 1).[95] Importantly, the FDA notes that sugammadex reversal of neuromuscular block is not always successful and that objective monitoring to ensure complete reversal is advised. Reversal from profound blocks (e.g., failed intubation with inability to mask ventilate following an RSI dose of rocuronium up to 1.2 mg/kg) requires 16 mg/kg.[96]

Sugammadex distributes in the extracellular fluid, metabolism is limited, and it is eliminated primarily via renal excretion (with an elimination half-life of 100 minutes).[97] In patients with severe renal impairment, both sugammadex and the sugammadex/rocuronium complex can be removed using high-flux hemodialysis, but low-flux hemodialysis appears ineffective.[98]

Sugammadex is biologically inactive and does not combine with any known receptors. It has no hemodynamic side effects. Oral contraceptives can be affected (equivalent to missing a daily dose) and precautions should be taken by the patient for the remainder of that menstrual cycle. Sugammadex has been tested against many drugs for potential interactions and binding has only been reported for toremifene, flucloxacillin, and fusidic acid.[99] A review of allergic, hypersensitivity reactions to sugammadex reported that most cases occurred within 4 minutes of administration. When cardiovascular collapse followed administration

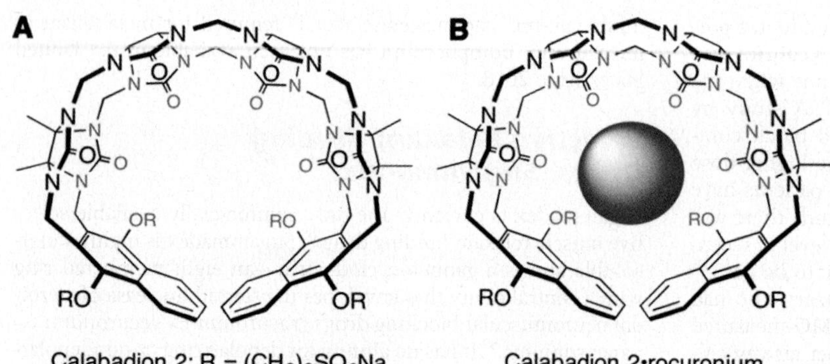

Figure 21-12 Calabadion 2 (**A**), the second-generation cucurbituril receptor, features a cavity with naphthalene walls and binds with high affinity to steroidal (**B**; Ka = 0.53–3.4 × 109 M-1) and benzylisoquinolinium (Ka = 4.8 × 106 M-1) neuromuscular blocking drugs. (Adapted with permission from Haerter F1, Simons JC, Foerster U, et al. Comparative effectiveness of calabadion and sugammadex to reverse nondepolarizing neuromuscular-blocking agents. *Anesthesiology*. 2015;123(6):1337–1349.)

it was successfully treated with high-dose epinephrine and fluid resuscitation.[100]

A 5.5% increase in activated partial thromboplastin time and a 3% increase in prothrombin time were observed 10 minutes following sugammadex dosing and returned to baseline within 60 minutes; however, there is no reported increase in postoperative bleeding.[101] There is no difference in bronchospasm and dosing in renal failure patients. Furthermore, the speed of sugammadex reversal at a train-of-four count 2 is equivalent to that of normal renal function patients. However, there is prolonged reversal with sugammadex (4 mg/kg) from deep neuromuscular block (posttetanic count 1 to 2) when compared to patients with normal renal function. The median time to reversal was 3.1 minutes in renal failure compared to 1.9 minutes in patients with normal renal function.[102,103] Mild hypothermia (34.5° C to 35° C) minimally prolongs sugammadex reversal time.[104]

For reversal of train-of-four count 2 or higher, 2 mg/kg dosing is recommended, although smaller doses have been used in clinical trials. In one trial, a dose of 1 mg/kg reversed rocuronium block from a train-of-four count 4 in 2 minutes, whereas a dose of 0.5 mg/kg reverses the same block in 8 minutes.[105] In morbidly obese patients debate exists whether sugammadex dosing should be based on ideal body weight, lean body weight (ideal body weight plus 40% difference between ideal and actual body weight), or actual body weight (currently recommended).[106,107] With the importance of full reversal in patients who are at higher risk for respiratory complications following surgery (including the obese), quantitative monitoring is again recommended to assess the adequacy of any reversal drug, including sugammadex. In pediatrics, a suboptimal dose administered based only on weight without objective monitoring in the operating room has resulted in residual paralysis in the PACU.[108,109] Although reversal to the recovered block level with sugammadex may be accomplished with low doses (0.5 to 1 mg/kg for deep block) there are case reports and studies showing this practice may lead to recurrent paralysis.[110–113] In one study of low-dose sugammadex reversal, a train-of-four ratio 0.9 was reached after initial reversal, but with one patient subsequently having a train-of-four ratio 0.72 one hour later.[113] Caution is warranted when lowering the dose of sugammadex, or titrating the dose to attain recovery, until further studies are performed establishing safe dosing guidelines. In the elderly, time to reversal with sugammadex can be delayed in patients with pulmonary, cardiac, or renal disease, or those with a BMI over 40.[114–116]

There are clinical settings where patients may require muscle relaxation immediately following reversal with sugammadex. The product insert recommends that at least 24 hours elapse before an aminosteroids neuromuscular blocker is administered in patients who have received sugammadex—a time that allows for renal elimination of the drug. Case reports have established that it is possible to re-establish neuromuscular blockade before this time; however, higher doses of rocuronium will be required. Of note, in these case reports sugammadex was readministered at the conclusion of surgery.[117,118] Careful use of quantitative monitoring of neuromuscular function remains essential in this setting. An alternative in this setting is to use succinylcholine or benzylisoquinolinium drugs to re-establish neuromuscular blockade.

See also NICV 21-1.

Selective Relaxant Binding Drugs: Future Drugs

Calabadion has been reported to encapsulate both steroidal and benzylisoquinolinium neuromuscular blocking drugs. Compared to sugammadex, the affinity of calabadion 1 for rocuronium is significantly lower. In contrast, calabadion 2 has an affinity for rocuronium 89 times greater than that of sugammadex (Fig 21-12).[119] Calabadion 2 also appears to have a high affinity for cisatracurium, as well as some affinity for other drugs (e.g., ketamine, etomidate). The complex is excreted unchanged in the urine and succinylcholine can be administered to re-establish neuromuscular blockade, if required.

For additional information please see NICV 21-2 in the eBook bundled with this text.

For further review and interactivities, please see the videos and narrative interactive clinical vignettes (NICVs) accessible in the complimentary eBook bundled with this text. Access instructions are located on the inside front cover.

REFERENCES

1. Evans L, Rhodes A, Alhazzani W, et al. Surviving sepsis campaign: international guidelines for management of sepsis and septic shock 2021. *Intensive Care Med*. 2021;47(11):1181–1247.
2. Plaud B, Debaene B, Donati F, Marty J. Residual paralysis after emergence from anesthesia. *Anesthesiology*. 2010;112(4):1013–1022.
3. Nigam PK, Nigam A. Botulinum toxin. *Indian J Dermatol*. 2010;55(1):8–14.
4. Katz RL. Neuromuscular effects of d-tubocurarine, edrophonium and neostigmine in man. *Anesthesiology*. 1967;28(2):327–336.
5. Hunt R, Taveau R. On the physiological action of certain cholin derivatives and new methods for detecting cholin. *BMJ*. 1906;2:1788–1791.
6. Bovet D. Some aspects of the relationship between chemical constitution and curare-like activity. *Ann N Y Acad Sci*. 1951;54(3):407–437.
7. Schreiber JU, Lysakowski C, Fuchs-Buder T, Tramèr MR. Prevention of succinylcholine-induced fasciculation and myalgia: a meta-analysis of randomized trials. *Anesthesiology*. 2005;103(4):877–884.

8. Kelly RE, Dinner M, Turner LS, Haik B, Abramson DH, Daines P. Succinylcholine increases intraocular pressure in the human eye with the extraocular muscles detached. *Anesthesiology*. 1993;79(5):948–952.
9. Libonati MM, Leahy JJ, Ellison N. The use of succinylcholine in open eye surgery. *Anesthesiology*. 1985;62(5):637–640.
10. Vachon CA, Warner DO, Bacon DR. Succinylcholine and the open globe. Tracing the teaching. *Anesthesiology*. 2003;99(1):220–223.
11. Cottrell JE, Hartung J, Giffin JP, Shwiry B. Intracranial and hemodynamic changes after succinylcholine administration in cats. *Anesth Analg*. 1983;62(11):1006–1009.
12. Cottrell JE. Succinylcholine and intracranial pressure. *Anesthesiology*. 2018;129(6):1159–1162.
13. Stirt JA, Grosslight KR, Bedford RF, Vollmer D. "Defasciculation" with metocurine prevents succinylcholine-induced increases in intracranial pressure. *Anesthesiology*. 1987;67(1):50–53.
14. Perkins ZB, Wittenberg MD, Nevin D, Lockey DJ, O'Brien B. The relationship between head injury severity and hemodynamic response to tracheal intubation. *J Trauma Acute Care Surg*. 2013;74(4):1074–1080.
15. Martyn JA, Richtsfeld M. Succinylcholine-induced hyperkalemia in acquired pathologic states: etiologic factors and molecular mechanisms. *Anesthesiology*. 2006;104(1):158–169.
16. Thomsen JL, Nielsen CV, Palmqvist DF, Gätke MR. Premature awakening and underuse of neuromuscular monitoring in a registry of patients with butyrylcholinesterase deficiency. *Br J Anaesth*. 2015;115(Suppl 1):i89–i94.
17. Karanović N, Carev M, Kardum G, et al. Succinylcholine use in adult anesthesia–A multinational questionnaire survey. *Coll Antropol*. 2011;35(Suppl 1):183–190.
18. Tran DTT, Newton EK, Mount VAH, et al. Rocuronium vs. succinylcholine for rapid sequence intubation: a Cochrane systematic review. *Anaesthesia*. 2017;72(6):765–777.
19. Griffith HR, Johnson GE. The use of curare in general anesthesia. *Anesthesiology*. 1942; 418–420.
20. Baird WL, Reid AM. The neuromuscular blocking properties of a new steroid compound, pancuronium bromide. A pilot study in man. *Br J Anaesth*. 1967;39(10):775–780.
21. Decoopman M, Cammu G, Suy K, Heeringa M, Demeyer I. Reversal of pancuronium-induced block by selective relaxant binding agent sugammadex. *Eur J Anaesth*. 2007;24:110.
22. Nitahara K, Sugi Y, Shigematsu K, Haraga I, Abe S, Higa K. Recovery of train-of-four ratio to 0.70 and 0.90 is delayed in type 2 diabetes with vecuronium-induced neuromuscular block. *Eur J Anaesthesiol*. 2013;30(2):80–84.
23. Andrews JI, Kumar N, van den Brom RH, Olkkola KT, Roest GJ, Wright PM. A large simple randomized trial of rocuronium versus succinylcholine in rapid-sequence induction of anaesthesia along with propofol. *Acta Anaesthesiol Scand*. 1999;43(1):4–8.
24. Sadleir PH, Clarke RC, Bunning DL, Platt PR. Anaphylaxis to neuromuscular blocking drugs: incidence and cross-reactivity in Western Australia from 2002 to 2011. *Br J Anaesth*. 2013; 110(6):981–987.
25. Reddy JI, Cooke PJ, van Schalkwyk JM, Hannam JA, Fitzharris P, Mitchell SJ. Anaphylaxis is more common with rocuronium and succinylcholine than with atracurium. *Anesthesiology*. 2015;122(1):39–45.
26. Dong S, Acouetey DS, Guéant-Rodriguez RM, et al. Prevalence of IgE against neuromuscular blocking agents in hairdressers and bakers. *Clin Exp Allergy*. 2013;43(11):1256–1262.
27. Yang CI, Fine GF, Jooste EH, Mutich R, Walczak SA, Motoyama EK. The effect of cisatracurium and rocuronium on lung function in anesthetized children. *Anesth Analg*. 2013; 117(6):1393–1400.
28. Wang T, Huang S, Geng G. Comparison of the duration of neuromuscular blockade following a single bolus dose of rocuronium during laparoscopic gynaecological surgery vs conventional open surgery. *Anaesthesia*. 2014;69(8):854–859.
29. Xue FS, Tong SY, Liao X, Liu JH, An G, Luo LK. Dose-response and time course of effect of rocuronium in male and female anesthetized patients. *Anesth Analg*. 1997;85(3):667–671.
30. Adamus M, Hrabalek L, Wanek T, Gabrhelik T, Zapletalova J. Influence of age and gender on the pharmacodynamic parameters of rocuronium during total intravenous anesthesia. *Biomed Pap Med Fac Univ Palacky Olomouc Czech Repub*. 2011;155(4):347–353.
31. Armendáriz-Buil I, Lobato-Solores F, Aguilera-Celorrio L, Morros-Díaz E, Fraile-Jiménez E, Vera-Bella J. Residual neuromuscular block in type II diabetes mellitus after rocuronium: a prospective observational study. *Eur J Anaesthesiol*. 2014;31(8):411–416.
32. Ali HH, Lien CA, Witkowski T, et al. Efficacy and safety of divided dose administration of mivacurium for a 90-second tracheal intubation. *J Clin Anesth*. 1996;8(4):276–281.
33. Cassel J, Staehr-Rye AK, Nielsen CV, Gätke MR. Use of neuromuscular monitoring to detect prolonged effect of succinylcholine or mivacurium: three case reports. *Acta Anaesthesiol Scand*. 2014;58(8):1040–1043.
34. Naguib M, Samarkandi AH, Ammar A, Elfaqih SR, Al-Zahrani S, Turkistani A. Comparative clinical pharmacology of rocuronium, cisatracurium, and their combination. *Anesthesiology*. 1998;89(5):1116–1124.
35. Reid JE, Breslin DS, Mirakhur RK, Hayes AH. Neostigmine antagonism of rocuronium block during anesthesia with sevoflurane, isoflurane or propofol. *Can J Anaesth*. 2001;48(4): 351–355.
36. Stäuble CG, Stäuble RB, Schaller SJ, Unterbuchner C, Fink H, Blobner M. Effects of single-shot and steady-state propofol anaesthesia on rocuronium dose-response relationship: a randomised trial. *Acta Anaesthesiol Scand*. 2015;59(7):902–911.
37. Braga Ade F, Carvalho VH, Braga FS, Rodrigues-Simioni L, Loyola YC, Potério GB. Influence of local anesthetics on the neuromuscular blockade produced by rocuronium: effects of lidocaine and 50% enantiomeric excess bupivacaine on the neuromuscular junction. *Rev Bras Anestesiol*. 2009;59(6):725–734.
38. Sahin SH, Colak A, Sezer A, et al. Effect of epidural levobupivacaine on recovery from vecuronium-induced neuromuscular block in patients undergoing lower abdominal surgery. *Anaesth Intensive Care*. 2011;39(4):607–610.
39. Czarnetzki C, Lysakowski C, Elia N, Tramèr MR. Intravenous lidocaine has no impact on rocuronium-induced neuromuscular block. Randomised study. *Acta Anaesthesiol Scand*. 2012; 56(4):474–481.
40. Paradelis AG, Triantaphyllidis C, Giala MM. Neuromuscular blocking activity of aminoglycoside antibiotics. *Methods Find Exp Clin Pharmacol*. 1980;2(1):45–51.
41. Vega-Villa KR, Kaneda K, Yamashita S, Woo S, Han TH. Vecuronium pharmacokinetics in patients with major burns. *Br J Anaesth*. 2014;112(2):304–310.
42. Miller RD, Roderick LL. Acid-base balance and neostigmine antagonism of pancuronium neuromuscular blockade. *Br J Anaesth*. 1978;50(4):317–324.
43. Thilen SR, Weigel WA, Todd MM, et al. 2023 American Society of Anesthesiologists practice guidelines for monitoring and antagonism of neuromuscular blockade: a report by the American Society of Anesthesiologists Task Force on Neuromuscular Blockade. *Anesthesiology*. 2023;138(1):13–41.
44. Videira RL, Vieira JE. What rules of thumb do clinicians use to decide whether to antagonize nondepolarizing neuromuscular blocking drugs? *Anesth Analg*. 2011;113(5):1192–1196.
45. Murphy GS, Szokol JW, Marymont JH, et al. Intraoperative acceleromyographic monitoring reduces the risk of residual neuromuscular blockade and adverse respiratory events in the postanesthesia care unit. *Anesthesiology*. 2008;109(3):389–398.
46. Debaene B, Plaud B, Dilly MP, Donati F. Residual paralysis in the PACU after a single intubating dose of nondepolarizing muscle relaxant with an intermediate duration of action. *Anesthesiology*. 2003;98(5):1042–1048.
47. Eikermann M, Groeben H, Hüsing J, Peters J. Accelerometry of adductor pollicis muscle predicts recovery of respiratory function from neuromuscular blockade. *Anesthesiology*. 2003;98(6): 1333–1337.
48. Kelly D, Brull SJ. Monitoring of neuromuscular function in the clinical setting. *Yale J Biol Med*. 1993;66(5):473–489.
49. Brull SJ, Silverman DG. Pulse width, stimulus intensity, electrode placement, and polarity during assessment of neuromuscular block. *Anesthesiology*. 1995;83(4):702–709.
50. Naguib M, Brull SJ, Kopman AF, et al. Consensus statement on perioperative use of neuromuscular monitoring. *Anesth Analg*. 2018;127(1):71–80.
51. Brull SJ, Ehrenwerth J, Connelly NR, Silverman DG. Assessment of residual curarization using low-current stimulation. *Can J Anaesth*. 1991;38(2):164–168.
52. Brull SJ, Ehrenwerth J, Silverman DG. Stimulation with submaximal current for train-of-four monitoring. *Anesthesiology*. 1990;72(4):629–632.
53. Silverman DG, Connelly NR, O'Connor TZ, Garcia R, Brull SJ. Accelographic train-of-four at near-threshold currents. *Anesthesiology*. 1992;76(1):34–38.
54. Yamamoto S, Yamamoto Y, Kitajima O, Maeda T, Suzuki T. Reversal of neuromuscular block with sugammadex: a comparison of the corrugator supercilii and adductor pollicis muscles in a randomized dose-response study. *Acta Anaesthesiol Scand*. 2015;59(7):892–901.
55. Thilen SR, Hansen BE, Ramaiah R, Kent CD, Treggiari MM, Bhananker SM. Intraoperative neuromuscular monitoring site and residual paralysis. *Anesthesiology*. 2012;117(5): 964–972.
56. Donati F. Neuromuscular monitoring: useless, optional or mandatory? *Can J Anaesth*. 1998; 45(5 Pt 2):R106–R116.
57. Donati F. Neuromuscular monitoring: more than meets the eye. *Anesthesiology*. 2012;117(5): 934–936.
58. Waud BE, Waud DR. The margin of safety of neuromuscular transmission in the muscle of the diaphragm. *Anesthesiology*. 1972;37(4):417–422.
59. O'Hara DA, Fragen RJ, Shanks CA. Comparison of visual and measured train-of-four recovery after vecuronium-induced neuromuscular blockade using two anaesthetic techniques. *Br J Anaesth*. 1986;58(11):1300–1302.
60. Thomsen JLD, Marty AP, Wakatsuki S, et al. Barriers and aids to routine neuromuscular monitoring and consistent reversal practice-A qualitative study. *Acta Anaesthesiol Scand*. 2020; 64(8):1089–1099.
61. Naguib M, Kopman AF, Lien CA, Hunter JM, Lopez A, Brull SJ. A survey of current management of neuromuscular block in the United States and Europe. *Anesth Analg*. 2010;111(1): 110–119.
62. Weigel WA, Williams BL, Hanson NA, et al. Quantitative neuromuscular monitoring in clinical practice: a professional practice change initiative. *Anesthesiology*. 2022;136(6):901–915.
63. Bartkowski RR. Incomplete reversal of pancuronium neuromuscular blockade by neostigmine, pyridostigmine, and edrophonium. *Anesth Analg*. 1987;66(7):594–598.
64. Kirkegaard H, Heier T, Caldwell J. Efficacy of tactile-guided reversal from cisatracurium-induced neuromuscular block. *Anesthesiology*. 2002;96(1):45–50.
65. Kopman A, Naguib M. Neostigmine-induced weakness after sugammadex – a reply. *Anaesthesia*. 2019;74(2):254.

66. Kaufhold N, Schaller SJ, Stäuble CG, et al. Sugammadex and neostigmine dose-finding study for reversal of residual neuromuscular block at a train-of-four ratio of 0.2 (SUNDRO20)†,. *Br J Anaesth.* 2016;116(2):233–240.
67. Fuchs-Buder T, Meistelman C, Alla F, Grandjean A, Wuthrich Y, Donati F. Antagonism of low degrees of atracurium-induced neuromuscular blockade: dose-effect relationship for neostigmine. *Anesthesiology.* 2010;112(1):34–40.
68. Miller R, Van Nyhuis L, Eger En, Vitez T, Way W. Comparative times to peak effect and durations of action of neostigmine and pyridostigmine. *Anesthesiology.* 1974;41(1):27–33.
69. Kirkegaard-Nielsen H, Helbo-Hansen HS, Lindholm P, Severinsen IK, Bülow K. Time to peak effect of neostigmine at antagonism of atracurium- or vecuronium-induced neuromuscular block. *J Clin Anesth.* 1995;7(8):635–639.
70. Donati F. Residual paralysis: a real problem or did we invent a new disease? *Can J Anaesth.* 2013;60(7):714–729.
71. Kim K, Cheong M, Lee H, Lee J. Tactile assessment for the reversibility of rocuronium-induced neuromuscular blockade during propofol or sevoflurane anesthesia. *Anesth Analg.* 2004;99(4):1080–1085.
72. Power SJ, Jones RM. Relationship between single twitch depression and train-of-four fade: influence of relaxant dose during onset and spontaneous offset of neuromuscular blockade. *Anesth Analg.* 1987;66(7):633–636.
73. Kopman AF, Klewicka MM, Neuman GG. The relationship between acceleromyographic train-of-four fade and single twitch depression. *Anesthesiology.* 2002;96(3):583–587.
74. Kopman AF, Eikermann M. Antagonism of non-depolarising neuromuscular block: current practice. *Anaesthesia.* 2009;64(Suppl 1):22–30.
75. Fuchs-Buder T, Baumann C, De Guis J, Guerci P, Meistelman C. Low-dose neostigmine to antagonise shallow atracurium neuromuscular block during inhalational anaesthesia: a randomised controlled trial. *Eur J Anaesthesiol.* 2013;30(10):594–598.
76. Schaller SJ, Fink H, Ulm K, Blobner M. Sugammadex and neostigmine dose-finding study for reversal of shallow residual neuromuscular block. *Anesthesiology.* 2010;113(5):1054–1060.
77. Aquilonius SM, Hartvig P. Clinical pharmacokinetics of cholinesterase inhibitors. *Clin Pharmacokinet.* 1986;11(3):236–249.
78. Thilen SR, Ng IC, Cain KC, Treggiari MM, Bhananker SM. Management of rocuronium neuromuscular block using a protocol for qualitative monitoring and reversal with neostigmine. *Br J Anaesth.* 2018;121(2):367–377.
79. Gan TJ, Belani KG, Bergese S, et al. Fourth consensus guidelines for the management of postoperative nausea and vomiting. *Anesth Analg.* 2020;131(2):411–448.
80. Briscoe G. The antagonism between curarine and acetylcholine. *J Physiol.* 1936;87(4):425–428.
81. Churchill-Davidson HC, Christie TH. The diagnosis of neuromuscular block in man. *Br J Anaesth.* 1959;31:290–301.
82. Payne JP, Hughes R, Al Azawi S. Neuromuscular blockade by neostigmine in anaesthetized man. *Br J Anaesth.* 1980;52(1):69–76.
83. Kent NB, Liang SS, Phillips S, et al. Therapeutic doses of neostigmine, depolarising neuromuscular blockade and muscle weakness in awake volunteers: a double-blind, placebo-controlled, randomised volunteer study. *Anaesthesia.* 2018;73(9):1079–1089.
84. Caldwell J. Reversal of residual neuromuscular block with neostigmine at one to four hours after a single intubating dose of vecuronium. *Anesth Analg.* 1995;80(6):1168–1174.
85. Murphy GS, Szokol JW, Avram MJ, et al. Neostigmine administration after spontaneous recovery to a train-of-four ratio of 0.9 to 1.0: a randomized controlled trial of the effect on neuromuscular and clinical recovery. *Anesthesiology.* 2018;128(1):27–37.
86. Herbstreit F, Zigrahn D, Ochterbeck C, Peters J, Eikermann M. Neostigmine/glycopyrrolate administered after recovery from neuromuscular block increases upper airway collapsibility by decreasing genioglossus muscle activity in response to negative pharyngeal pressure. *Anesthesiology.* 2010;113(6):1280–1288.
87. Almeter PJ, Labuhn JA, Morris PE, Hessel EA. US food and drug administration disruption of generic drug market increases hospital costs. *Anesth Analg.* 2018;127(6):1414–1420.
88. Schaller SJ, Fink H. Sugammadex as a reversal agent for neuromuscular block: an evidence-based review. *Core Evid.* 2013;8:57–67.
89. Tassonyi E, Pongrácz A, Nemes R, Asztalos L, Lengyel S, Fülesdi B. Reversal of pipecuronium-induced moderate neuromuscular block with sugammadex in the presence of a sevoflurane anesthetic: a randomized trial. *Anesth Analg.* 2015;121(2):373–380.
90. Suy K, Morias K, Cammu G, et al. Effective reversal of moderate rocuronium- or vecuronium-induced neuromuscular block with sugammadex, a selective relaxant binding agent. *Anesthesiology.* 2007;106(2):283–288.
91. Flockton EA, Mastronardi P, Hunter JM, et al. Reversal of rocuronium-induced neuromuscular block with sugammadex is faster than reversal of cisatracurium-induced block with neostigmine. *Br J Anaesth.* 2008;100(5):622–630.
92. Blobner M, Eriksson LI, Scholz J, Motsch J, Della Rocca G, Prins ME. Reversal of rocuronium-induced neuromuscular blockade with sugammadex compared with neostigmine during sevoflurane anaesthesia: results of a randomised, controlled trial. *Eur J Anaesthesiol.* 2010;27(10):874–881.
93. Khuenl-Brady KS, Wattwil M, Vanacker BF, Lora-Tamayo JI, Rietbergen H, Alvarez-Gómez JA. Sugammadex provides faster reversal of vecuronium-induced neuromuscular blockade compared with neostigmine: a multicenter, randomized, controlled trial. *Anesth Analg.* 2010;110(1):64–73.
94. McDonagh DL, Benedict PE, Kovac AL, et al. Efficacy, safety, and pharmacokinetics of sugammadex for the reversal of rocuronium-induced neuromuscular blockade in elderly patients. *Anesthesiology.* 2011;114(2):318–329.
95. Jones RK, Caldwell JE, Brull SJ, Soto RG. Reversal of profound rocuronium-induced blockade with sugammadex: a randomized comparison with neostigmine. *Anesthesiology.* 2008;109(5):816–824.
96. Lee C, Jahr JS, Candiotti KA, Warriner B, Zornow MH, Naguib M. Reversal of profound neuromuscular block by sugammadex administered three minutes after rocuronium: a comparison with spontaneous recovery from succinylcholine. *Anesthesiology.* 2009;110(5):1020–1025.
97. Peeters P, Passier P, Smeets J, et al. Sugammadex is cleared rapidly and primarily unchanged via renal excretion. *Biopharm Drug Dispos.* 2011;32(3):159–167.
98. Cammu G, Van Vlem B, van den Heuvel M, et al. Dialysability of sugammadex and its complex with rocuronium in intensive care patients with severe renal impairment. *Br J Anaesth.* 2012;109(3):382–390.
99. Zwiers A, van den Heuvel M, Smeets J, Rutherford S. Assessment of the potential for displacement interactions with sugammadex: a pharmacokinetic-pharmacodynamic modelling approach. *Clin Drug Investig.* 2011;31(2):101–111.
100. Tsur A, Kalansky A. Hypersensitivity associated with sugammadex administration: a systematic review. *Anaesthesia.* 2014;69(11):1251–1257.
101. Rahe-Meyer N, Fennema H, Schulman S, et al. Effect of reversal of neuromuscular blockade with sugammadex versus usual care on bleeding risk in a randomized study of surgical patients. *Anesthesiology.* 2014;121(5):969–977.
102. Staals LM, Snoeck MM, Driessen JJ, Flockton EA, Heeringa M, Hunter JM. Multicentre, parallel-group, comparative trial evaluating the efficacy and safety of sugammadex in patients with end-stage renal failure or normal renal function. *Br J Anaesth.* 2008;101(4):492–497.
103. Panhuizen IF, Gold SJ, Buerkle C, et al. Efficacy, safety and pharmacokinetics of sugammadex 4 mg kg-1 for reversal of deep neuromuscular blockade in patients with severe renal impairment. *Br J Anaesth.* 2015;114(5):777–784.
104. Lee HJ, Kim KS, Jeong JS, Kim KN, Lee BC. The influence of mild hypothermia on reversal of rocuronium-induced deep neuromuscular block with sugammadex. *BMC Anesthesiol.* 2015;15:7.
105. Pongrácz A, Szatmári S, Nemes R, Fülesdi B, Tassonyi E. Reversal of neuromuscular blockade with sugammadex at the reappearance of four twitches to train-of-four stimulation. *Anesthesiology.* 2013;119(1):36–42.
106. Monk TG, Rietbergen H, Woo T, Fennema H. Use of sugammadex in patients with obesity: a pooled analysis. *Am J Ther.* 2017;24(5):e507–e516.
107. Le Corre F, Nejmeddine S, Fatahine C, Tayar C, Marty J, Plaud B. Recurarization after sugammadex reversal in an obese patient. *Can J Anaesth.* 2011;58(10):944–947.
108. Iwasaki H, Takahoko K, Otomo S, Sasakawa T, Kunisawa T. A temporary decrease in twitch response following reversal of rocuronium-induced neuromuscular block with a small dose of sugammadex in a pediatric patient. *J Anesth.* 2014;28(2):288–290.
109. Van Gestel L, Cammu G. Is the effect of sugammadex always rapid in onset? *Acta Anaesthesiol Belg.* 2013;64(2):41–47.
110. Murata T, Kubodera T, Ohbayashi M, Murase K, Adachi YU, Matsuda N. Recurarization after sugammadex following a prolonged rocuronium infusion for induced hypothermia. *Can J Anaesth.* 2013;60(5):508–509.
111. Eleveld DJ, Kuizenga K, Proost JH, Wierda JM. A temporary decrease in twitch response during reversal of rocuronium-induced muscle relaxation with a small dose of sugammadex. *Anesth Analg.* 2007;104(3):582–584.
112. Drobnik L, Sparr HJ, Thörn SE, et al. A randomized simultaneous comparison of acceleromyography with a peripheral nerve stimulator for assessing reversal of rocuronium-induced neuromuscular blockade with sugammadex. *Eur J Anaesthesiol.* 2010;27(10):866–873.
113. Muramatsu T, Isono S, Ishikawa T, et al. Differences of recovery from rocuronium-induced deep paralysis in response to small doses of sugammadex between elderly and nonelderly patients. *Anesthesiology.* 2018;129(5):901–911.
114. Dahl V, Pendeville PE, Hollmann MW, Heier T, Abels EA, Blobner M. Safety and efficacy of sugammadex for the reversal of rocuronium-induced neuromuscular blockade in cardiac patients undergoing noncardiac surgery. *Eur J Anaesthesiol.* 2009;26(10):874–884.
115. Gaszynski T, Szewczyk T, Gaszynski W. Randomized comparison of sugammadex and neostigmine for reversal of rocuronium-induced muscle relaxation in morbidly obese undergoing general anaesthesia. *Br J Anaesth.* 2012;108(2):236–239.
116. Amao R, Zornow MH, Cowan RM, Cheng DC, Morte JB, Allard MW. Use of sugammadex in patients with a history of pulmonary disease. *J Clin Anesth.* 2012;24(4):289–297.
117. Cammu G, de Kam PJ, De Graeve K, et al. Repeat dosing of rocuronium 1.2 mg kg-1 after reversal of neuromuscular block by sugammadex 4.0 mg kg-1 in anaesthetized healthy volunteers: a modelling-based pilot study. *Br J Anaesth.* 2010;105(4):487–492.
118. Matsuki G, Takahata O, Iwasaki H. Repeat dosing of rocuronium after reversal of neuromuscular block by sugammadex. *Can J Anaesth.* 2011;58(8):769–770.
119. Haerter F, Simons JC, Foerster U, et al. Comparative effectiveness of calabadion and sugammadex to reverse non-depolarizing neuromuscular-blocking agents. *Anesthesiology.* 2015;123(6):1337–1349.

22 Local Anesthetics

WILLIAM P. QIAO • YI LIN

KEY POINTS

1. Local anesthetics provide anesthesia and analgesia by blocking the transmission of pain sensation along nerve fibers.
2. The key target of local anesthetics is the voltage-gated sodium channel. The binding is intracellular and is mediated by hydrophobic interactions.
3. The degree of nerve blockade depends on both drug concentration and volume.
4. Most clinically relevant agents contain a lipid-soluble benzene ring connected to an amide group and are categorized as either aminoesters or aminoamides based on their chemical linkage.
5. Potency is related to lipid solubility and physiochemical properties of the agent. In general, more potent agents are more lipid-soluble.
6. Clinical use of local anesthetics may be increased by addition of dexamethasone, epinephrine, opioids, and α_2-adrenergic agonists. The value of alkalinization of local anesthetics and liposomal bupivacaine appear to be debatable as a clinically useful tool to improve anesthesia.
7. The rate of local anesthetic system absorption depends on the site of injection, the dose, the drug's intrinsic pharmacokinetic properties, and the addition of a vasoactive agent.
8. Systemic toxicity from the clinical use of local anesthetics is an uncommon occurrence. Patients with cardiovascular collapse from bupivacaine, ropivacaine, and levobupivacaine may be especially difficult to resuscitate; however, intravenous lipid infusion is an effective new therapy.

1 Local anesthetics block the conduction of impulses in electrically excitable tissues. One of the important uses is to provide anesthesia and analgesia by blocking the transmission of pain sensation along nerve fibers. The molecular target of these agents is specific and the interaction has been extensively studied. Existing clinical applications are numerous and continue to expand. A comprehensive understanding of the mechanisms and the physiochemical properties of these agents will optimize the therapeutic potential and avoid complications associated with inadvertent systemic toxicity.

Mechanisms of Action of Local Anesthetics

Anatomy of Nerves

Local anesthetics are used to block nerves in the peripheral nervous system (PNS) and central nervous system (CNS) (1 Video 22-1). In the PNS, nerves contain both afferent and efferent fibers, which are bundled into one or more fascicles and organized within three tissue layers.[1] Individual nerve fibers within each fascicle are surrounded by the *endoneurium*, a loose connective tissue containing glial cells, fibroblasts, and blood capillaries. A dense layer of collagenous connective tissue called the *perineurium* surrounds each fascicle. A final layer of dense connective tissue, the *epineurium*, encases groups of fascicles into a cylindrical sheath (Fig. 22-1). These layers of tissue offer protection to the surrounded nerve fibers and act as barriers to passive diffusion of local anesthetics.[2]

Nerves in both the CNS and PNS are differentiated by the presence or absence of myelin sheath. Myelinated nerve fibers are surrounded by Schwann cells in the PNS and by oligodendrocytes in the CNS. The cells form a concentrically wrapped lipid bilayer sheath around the axons that cover the length of the nerve.[3] The myelin sheath is interrupted at short regular intervals by specialized regions called *nodes of Ranvier*, which contain densely clustered protein elements essential for transmission of neuronal signals (Fig. 22-2).[4] As electrical signals are renewed at each node, nerve impulses move in myelinated fibers by saltatory conduction. In contrast, there are no nodes of Ranvier in nonmyelinated nerve fibers. Although these nerve fibers are similarly encased in Schwann cells, the plasma membrane does not wrap around the axons concentrically. Several nerve fibers may be simultaneously embedded within a single Schwann cell (Fig. 22-3).[1]

Nerve fibers are commonly classified according to their size, conduction velocity, and function (Table 22-1). In general, nerve fibers with cross-sectional diameter greater than 1 mm are myelinated. Both a larger nerve size and the presence of myelin sheath are associated with faster conduction velocity.[5] Nerve fibers with large diameters have better intrinsic electric conductance. Myelin improves the electrical insulation of nerve fibers and permits more rapid impulse transmission via saltatory conduction. Large-diameter

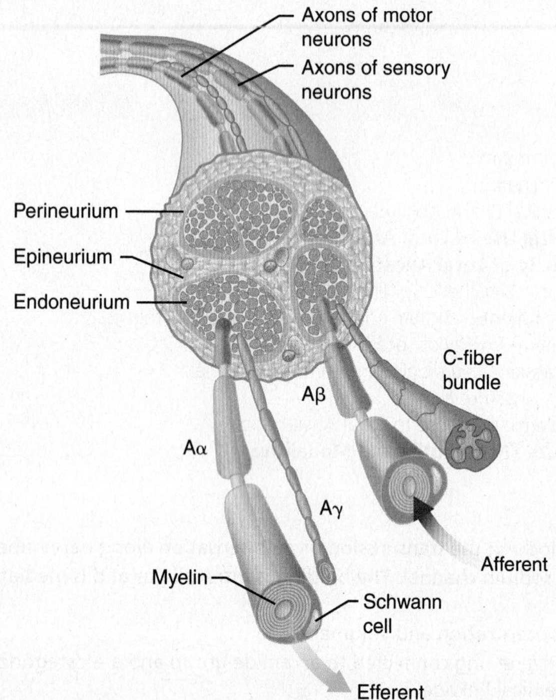

Figure 22-1 Schematic cross-section of a typical peripheral nerve. The epineurium, consisting of collagen fibers, is oriented along the long axis of the nerve. The perineurium is a discrete cell layer, whereas the endoneurium is a matrix of connective tissue. Both afferent and efferent axons are shown. Sympathetic axons (not shown) are also present in mixed peripheral nerves. (Adapted with permission from Strichartz GR. Neural physiology and local anesthetic action. In: Cousins MJ, Bridenbaugh PO, eds. *Neural Blockade in Clinical Anesthesia and Management of Pain*. Lippincott-Raven; 1998:35.)

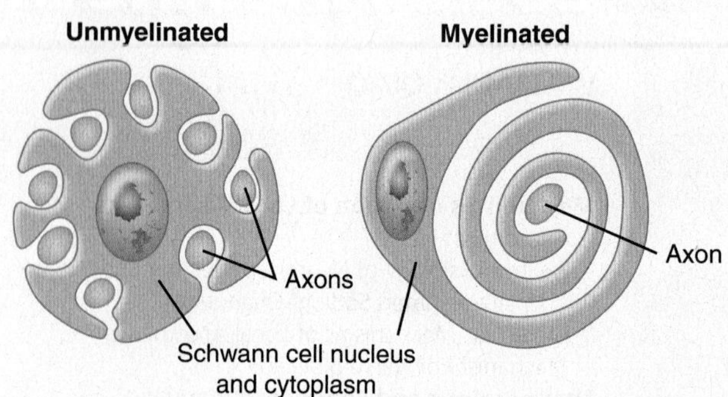

Figure 22-3 Schwann cells form myelin around one myelinated axon or encompass several unmyelinated axons. (Adapted with permission from Carpenter RL, Mackey DC. Local anesthetics. In: Barash PG, Cullen BF, Stoelting RF, eds. *Clinical Anesthesia*. 3rd ed. Lippincott-Raven; 1996:413.)

myelinated fibers, many of which are classified as A fibers, are typically involved in motor and sensory functions in which speed of nerve transmission is critical. In contrast, small-diameter nonmyelinated C fibers have slower conduction velocity and relay sensory information such as pain, temperature, and autonomic functions.

Electrophysiology of Neural Conduction and Voltage-Gated Sodium Channels

Transmission of electrical impulses along the cell membrane forms the basis of signal transduction along nerve fibers. Energy necessary for the propagation and maintenance of the electric potential is maintained on the cell surface by ionic disequilibria across the semipermeable cell membrane.[6] The resting membrane potential, approximately −60 to −70 mV in neurons (the extracellular electric potential is, by convention, defined as zero, and the intracellular potential is thus negative relative to it), is derived predominantly from a difference in the intracellular and extracellular concentrations of potassium and sodium ions. Neurons at rest are more permeable to potassium ions than sodium ions because of potassium leak channels; therefore, membrane potential is closer to the equilibrium potential of potassium (E_K −80 mV) than that of sodium (E_{Na} +60 mV). The ion gradient is continuously regenerated by protein pumps, cotransporters, and channels via an adenosine triphosphate-dependent process.

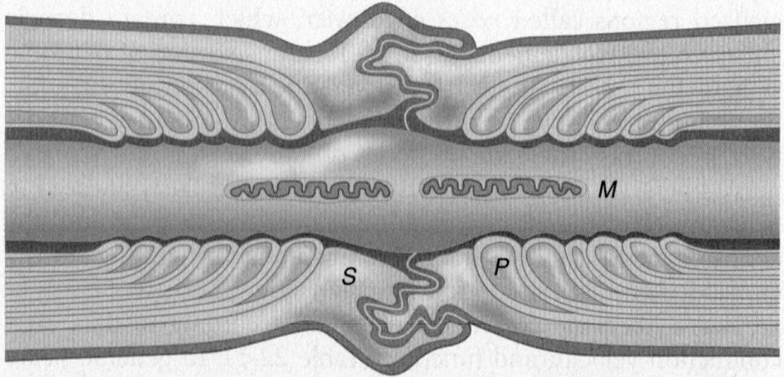

Figure 22-2 Diagram of node of Ranvier displaying mitochondria (*M*), tight junctions in paranodal area (*P*), and Schwann cell (*S*) surrounding node. (Adapted from Strichartz GR. Mechanisms of action of local anesthetic agents. In: Rogers MC, Tinker JH, Covino BG, et al., eds. Principles and Practice of Anesthesiology. Mosby Year Book; 1993:1197. Copyright © 1993 Elseiver. With permission.)

Electrical impulses are conducted along nerve fibers as action potentials. They are brief, localized spikes of positive charge, or depolarizations, on the cell membrane caused by rapid influx of sodium ions down its electrochemical gradient.[7] An action potential is initiated by local membrane depolarization, such as at the cell body or nerve terminal by a ligand–receptor complex. When a certain charge threshold is reached, an action potential is triggered and further depolarization occurs in an "all-or-none" fashion.[8] The spike in membrane potential peaks around +50 mV, at which point the influx of sodium is replaced with an efflux of potassium, causing a reversal of membrane potential, or repolarization. The passive diffusion of membrane depolarization triggers other action potentials in either adjacent cell membranes in *nonmyelinated* nerve fibers or adjacent nodes of Ranvier in *myelinated* nerve fibers, resulting in a wave of action potential being propagated along the nerve. A short *refractory period* that ensues after each action potential prevents the retrograde spread of action potential on previously activated membranes.[7]

The flow of ions responsible for action potentials is mediated by a variety of channels and pumps, the most important of which are the voltage-gated sodium channels. They are essential for the influx of sodium ions during the rapid depolarization phase of the action potential and belong to a family of channel proteins that also includes voltage-gated potassium and voltage-gated calcium channels. Each voltage-gated sodium channel is a complex made up of one principal α-subunit and one or more auxiliary β-subunits.[9] The α-subunit is a single-polypeptide transmembrane protein that contains most of the key components of the channel function. They include four homologous α-helical domains (D1 to D4) that form the channel pore and control ion selectivity, voltage-sensing regions that regulate gating function and inactivation, and phosphorylation sites for modulation by protein kinases. β-Subunits are short polypeptide proteins with a single transmembrane domain.

Table 22-1 Classification of Nerve Fibers

Classification	Diameter (mm)	Myelin	Conduction (m/s)	Location	Function
Aα, Aβ	6–22	+	30–120	Afferents/efferents for muscles and joints	Motor and proprioception
Aγ	3–6	+	15–35	Efferent to muscle spindle	Muscle tone
Aδ	1–4	+	5–25	Afferent sensory nerve	Pain Touch Temperature
B	<3	+	3–15	Preganglionic sympathetic	Autonomic function
C	0.3–1.3	–	0.7–1.3	Postganglionic sympathetic Afferent sensory nerve	Autonomic function Pain Temperature

They are linked to α-subunits by either noncovalent or disulfide bonds; although they are dispensable for channel activity, evidence suggests that they perhaps play a role in modulation of channel expression, localization, and function.

In the absence of a stimulus, voltage-gated sodium channels exist predominantly in the resting or closed state (Fig. 22-4). On membrane depolarization, positive charges on the membrane interact with charged amino acid residues in the voltage-sensing regions (S4).[10] This induces a conformational change in the channel, converting it to the open state. Sodium ions rush through the opened pore, which is lined with negatively charged residues. Ion selectivity is determined by these amino acid residues; changes in their composition can lead to increased permeability for other cations, such as potassium and calcium.[11] Within milliseconds after opening, channels undergo a transition to the inactivated state. Depending on the frequency and voltage of the initial depolarizing stimulus, the channel may undergo either fast or slow inactivation. Slow or fast inactivation refers to the duration in which the channel remains refractory to repeat depolarization before resetting to the closed state. Fast inactivation completes within a millisecond and is sensitive to the action of local anesthetics. It is mediated by a short mobile intracellular polypeptide loop connecting domains D3 and D4 that closes the channel from inside the cell via a hinge-lid mechanism.[12] A triad of highly hydrophobic amino acids (isoleucine, phenylalanine, and methionine [IFM]) appears to be an important structural determinant of fast activation; disrupting the loop or changing the hydrophobicity of the amino acids abrogates fast inactivation.[13,14] Slow activation, lasting seconds to minutes, is distinct from fast activation. It is resistant to the action of local anesthetics and its mechanism is less well understood. It often occurs after prolonged depolarization and is believed to be important in regulating membrane excitability.

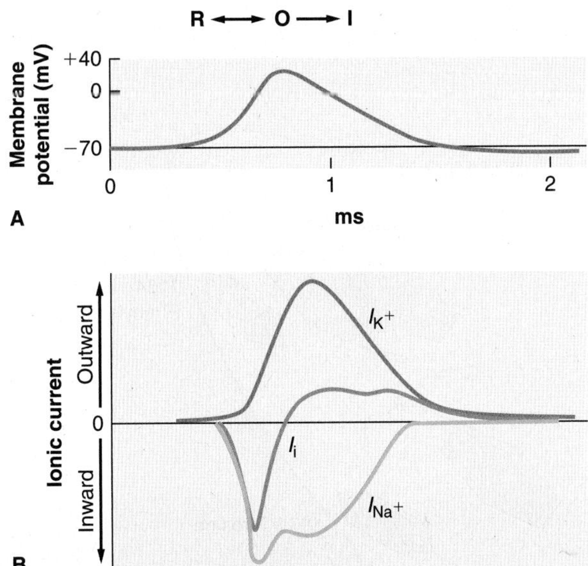

Figure 22-4 Illustration of dominant form of sodium channel during generation of an action potential. R, resting form; O, open form; I, inactive form. **A:** The concurrent generation of an action potential as the membrane depolarizes from resting potential. **B:** The concurrent changes in ion flux, as inward sodium current (I_{NA}+) and outward potassium current (I_K+) together yield the net ionic current across the membrane (I_i). (Adapted with permission from Strichartz GR. Neural physiology and local anesthetic action. In: Cousins MJ, Bridenbaugh PO, eds. *Neural Blockade in Clinical Anesthesia and Management of Pain*. Lippincott-Raven; 1998:35.)

Nine isoforms of voltage-gated sodium channels (Na_V 1.1 to Na_V 1.9) have been identified; each relates to a unique α-subunit subtype (Table 22-2). Each isoform varies slightly in its channel kinetics, such as threshold of activation and mode of inactivation, and its sensitivity to blocking agents like tetrodotoxins and local anesthetics. Cell and tissue expression of individual isoforms may be quite specific; for instance, Na_V 1.2 is found almost exclusively in the CNS, whereas Na_V 1.6 is restricted to nodes of Ranvier in both CNS and PNS.[15] Likewise, several isoforms could be present on a single cell type; both Na_V 1.8 and Na_V 1.9 have been found in small- to medium-sized neurons in dorsal root ganglia that are connected to Aδ and C fibers. Whether individual isoforms each have a separate and defined role remains to be seen; however, clues to their function may be inferred from studies of several inherited diseases that have been associated with sodium channelopathies. Hyperexcitability of Na_V 1.7 has been implicated in several painful disease states, such as primary erythromelalgia and paroxysmal extreme pain disorder.[16,17] Conversely the null mutation of Na_V 1.7 is linked to a rare genetic condition in which otherwise normal individuals have severely impaired perception to pain.[18,19]

Molecular Mechanisms of Local Anesthetics

Local anesthetics block the transmission of nerve impulses by targeting the function of voltage-gated sodium channels. Several local anesthetics can also bind to other receptors such as voltage-gated potassium channels and nicotinic acetylcholine receptors and their 2

Table 22-2 Voltage-Gated Sodium Channels

Name	Tissue Expression	Tetrodotoxin	Associated Channelopathies
Na_V 1.1	CNS, heart	Sensitive	Inherited febrile epilepsy
Na_V 1.2	CNS nonmyelinated axons	Sensitive	Inherited febrile epilepsy
Na_V 1.3	Fetal DRG	Sensitive	None known
Na_V 1.4	Skeletal muscle	Sensitive	Hyperkalemic periodic paralysis, paramyotonia congenital
Na_V 1.5	Heart, embryonic neurons	Insensitive	Brugada syndrome, long QT syndrome
Na_V 1.6	Nodes of Ranvier	Sensitive	None known
Na_V 1.7	CNS, DRG, sympathetic neurons	Sensitive	Erythromelalgia, paroxysmal extreme pain disorder, congenital insensitivity to pain
Na_V 1.8	Small DRG neurons	Insensitive	None known
Na_V 1.9	Small DRG neurons	Insensitive	None known

CNS, central nervous system; DRG, dorsal root ganglion.
Data adapted from Benarroch EE. Sodium channels and pain. *Neurology*. 2007:68:233; and Koopmann TT, Bezzina CR, Wilde AA. Voltage-gated sodium channels: Action players with many faces. *Ann Med*. 2006:38:472–482.

amphipathic nature may enable them to interact with plasma membranes. However, it is widely accepted that local anesthetics induce anesthesia and analgesia through direct interactions with the sodium channels. Other molecules with local anesthetic properties, such as tricyclic antidepressants and anticonvulsants, may likewise interact with voltage-gated sodium channels; however, it is unclear if they act through similar mechanisms. Therefore, the following discussion is limited to the "traditional" set of local anesthetic molecules.

Local anesthetics reversibly bind the intracellular portion of voltage-gated sodium channels (Fig. 22-5). Early experiments with giant squid axons demonstrated that a derivative of lidocaine with a permanent positive charge and that cannot cross the plasma membrane (QX-314) blocks ion current through voltage-gated sodium channels only with intra-axoplasmic injections, but not with external application.[20] Subsequent mutational analyses have supported this observation and identified specific sites on the channel involved in drug recognition.[21] Several hydrophobic aromatic residues (a phenylalanine at position 1,764 and a tyrosine at position 1,771 in Na_V 1.2) located within an α-helix (S6) of domains 1, 3, and 4 are essential for drug binding (Fig. 22-6).

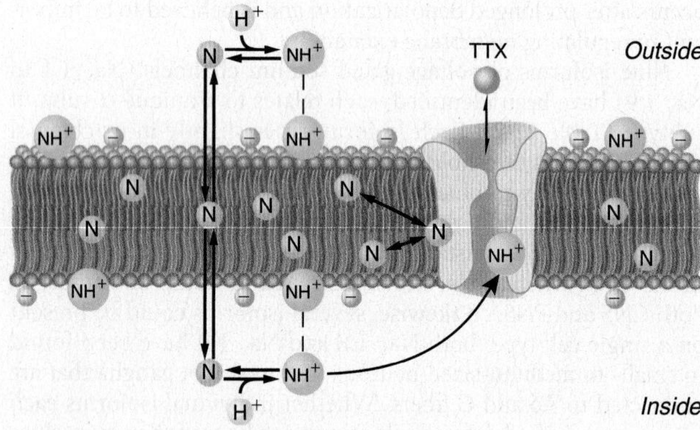

Figure 22-5 Diagram of the bilayer lipid membrane of conductive tissue with the sodium channel spanning the membrane. Tertiary amine local anesthetics exist as both neutral base (N) and protonated, charged form (NH⁺) in equilibrium. The neutral base (N) is more lipid soluble, preferentially partitions into the lipophilic membrane interior, and easily passes through the membrane. The charged form (NH⁺) is more water soluble and binds to the sodium channel at the negatively charged membrane surface. Both forms can affect the function of the sodium channel. The N form can cause membrane expansion and closure of the sodium channel. The NH⁺ form will directly inhibit the sodium channel by binding with a local anesthetic receptor. The natural "local anesthetic" tetrodotoxin (TTX) binds at the external surface of the sodium channel and has no interaction with the clinically used local anesthetics. (Adapted with permission from Strichartz GR. Neural physiology and local anesthetic action. In: Cousins MJ, Bridenbaugh PO, eds. *Neural Blockade in Clinical Anesthesia and Management of Pain*. Lippincott-Raven; 1998:35.)

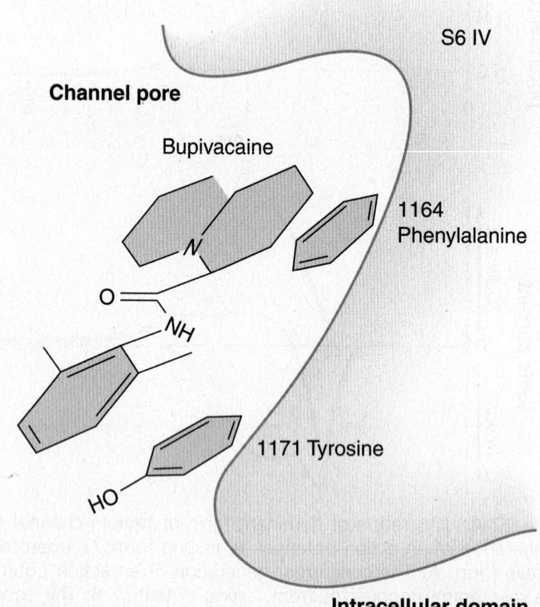

Figure 22-6 Diagram of the local anesthetic binding site, depicting a hydrophobic pocket within the sodium channel pore. (From Ragsdale DS, McPhee JC, Scheuer T, et al. Molecular determinants of state-dependent block of Na⁺ channels by local anesthetics. *Science*. 1994;265(5179):1724–1728. Adapted with permission from AAAS.)

They line an inner cavity within the intracellular portion of the channel pore and span a region about 11 Å apart, roughly the size of a local anesthetic molecule. Changes in either residue severely reduce the binding affinity. Another hydrophobic amino acid (an isoleucine at position 1,760), located near the outer pore opening, also influences the dissociation of local anesthetics from the channel by antagonizing the release of drugs through the channel pore.

Application of local anesthetics typically produces a concentration-dependent decrease in the peak sodium current.[22,23] Termed *tonic blockade*, this refers to the reduction in the number of sodium channels for a given drug concentration present in the open state at equilibrium. In contrast, repetitive stimulation of the sodium channels often leads to a shift in the steady-state equilibrium, resulting in a greater number of channels being blocked at the same drug concentration. This is termed *use-dependent blockade*—its exact mechanism is incompletely understood and has been the subject of many competing hypotheses. One popular theory, the *modulated-receptor theory*, proposes that local anesthetics bind to the open or the inactivated channels more avidly than the resting channels, suggesting that drug affinity is a function of a channel's conformational state. An alternate theory, the *guarded-receptor theory*, assumes that the intrinsic binding affinity remains essentially constant regardless of a channel's conformation; rather, the apparent affinity is associated with increased access to the recognition site resulting from channel gating. Experimental evidence so far has been inconclusive.

Mechanism of Nerve Blockade

Local anesthetics block peripheral nerves by disrupting the transmission of action potentials along nerve fibers. To get to its site of action, principally the voltage-gated sodium channels, local anesthetics have to reach the targeted nerve membrane. This entails the diffusion of drugs through tissues and the generation of a concentration gradient. Even with close proximity of deposition, only about 1% to 2% of injected local anesthetics ultimately penetrate into the nerve.[24] As discussed earlier, the perineural sheath encasing nerve fibers appears to be an important determinant; nerves that have been desheathed in vitro require about a 100-fold lower local anesthetic concentration (in 0.7 to 0.9 mM range for lidocaine) than nerves in vivo (the typical 2% lidocaine used clinically is equivalent to 75 mM concentration). Although it may vary with anatomic location and nerve physiology, functional block typically occurs within 5 minutes of injection in rat sciatic nerves, and this time course corresponds to the peak in the intraneural drug absorption.

3 The degree of nerve blockade depends on the local anesthetic concentration and volume. For a given drug, a minimal concentration is necessary to effect complete nerve blockade. It reflects the potency of the local anesthetics and the intrinsic conduction properties of nerve fibers, which in turn likely depend on the drug's binding affinity to the ion channels and the degree of drug saturation necessary to halt the transmission of action potentials. Accordingly, individual types of nerve fibers differ in their minimal blocking concentration, such that some A fibers are blocked by lower drug concentrations than C fibers.[25] Likewise, the pattern of stimulation (tonic vs. use-dependent blockade) influences the degree of conduction failure; repetitive stimulations, which can lead to a shift in steady-state equilibrium of blocked sodium channels, are associated with higher conduction failure than tonic stimulation at a given drug concentration.[26]

Of equal importance as drug concentration is the local anesthetic volume. A sufficient volume is needed to suppress the regeneration of nerve impulse over a critical length of nerve fiber.

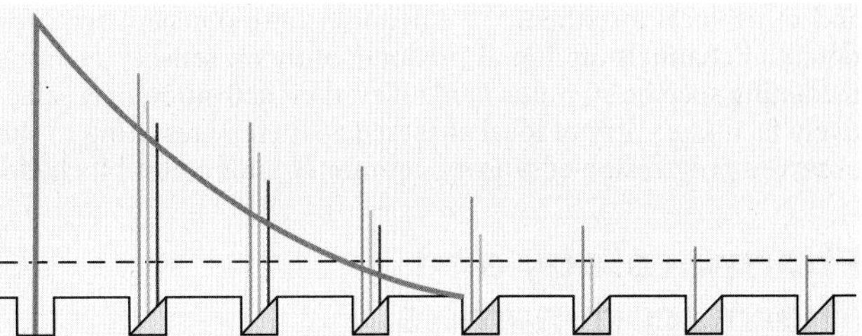

Figure 22-7 Diagram illustrating the principle of decremental conduction block by local anesthetic at a myelinated axon. The first node of Ranvier at left contains no local anesthetic and gives rise to a normal action potential (*solid curve*). If the nodes succeeding the first are occupied by a concentration of local anesthetic high enough to block 74% to 84% of the sodium conductance, then the action potential amplitudes decrease at successive nodes (amplitudes are indicated by *interrupted bars* representing three increasing concentrations of local anesthetic). Eventually, the impulse decays to below-threshold amplitude if the series of local anesthetic-containing nodes is long enough. Propagation of the impulse is then blocked by decremental conduction, even though none of the nodes are completely blocked. Concentrations of local anesthetics that block more than 84% of the sodium conductance at three successive nodes prevent any impulse propagation at all. (Adapted with permission from Fink BR. Mechanisms of differential axial blockade in epidural and spinal anesthesia. *Anesthesiology*. 1989;70:851.)

According to the model of decremental conduction (Fig. 22-7), as membrane depolarization from an action potential passively decays with distance along nerve fibers, the presence of local anesthetics decreases the ability of adjacent membrane or successive nodes of Ranvier to regenerate the impulse.[27] Transmission stops once the membrane depolarization falls below the threshold for action potential activation. If the exposure distance is inadequate, action potentials can "skip" over blocked segments and resume nerve conduction. In contrast, exposure over a long segment of nerve to even a relatively low drug concentration can still result in gradual extinction of impulse by decremental decay.

Not all sensory and motor modalities are blocked equally by local anesthetics. It has long been observed that application of local anesthetics produces an ordered progression of sensory and motor deficits, starting commonly with the disappearance of temperature sensation, followed in order by proprioception, motor function, sharp pain, and finally light touch. Termed *differential blockade*, historically this had been thought to be related simply to the diameter of the nerve fibers, with the smaller fibers inherently more susceptible to drug blockade than larger fibers.[28] However, although the "size principle" of differential blockade is consistent with many experimental findings, it is not universally true. Larger, myelinated Aδ fibers (believed to mediate sharp pain) are preferentially blocked over small, nonmyelinated C fibers (dull pain). Furthermore, within the C fibers are fast and slow components of impulse transmission, each with distinct susceptibilities to drug blockade.[29] These observations argue against a purely pharmacokinetic mechanism as the sole explanation for differential blockade.

More likely, explanations may additionally be found in the intrinsic excitatory properties of the nerve fibers, namely, the patterned expression of ion pores and channels on the cellular membrane. Indeed, sodium channel isoforms Na_v 1.7 and Na_v 1.8 are highly expressed on the dorsal root ganglia, and have been shown to have distinct sensitivities to lidocaine.[30] Similarly, experiments with large pore, nonspecific cation channels, the transient receptor potential channel subfamily V (TRPV1) and member A1 (TRPA1), suggest that they can be activated by lidocaine and other local anesthetics.[31,32] Because these transient receptor potential channels are found predominantly on sensory neurons mediating specific stimulus modalities, their activation may selectively facilitate entry of local anesthetics, thereby resulting in the observed progression of sensory, autonomic, and motor blockade.

Pharmacology and Pharmacodynamics

Chemical Properties and Relationship to Activity and Potency

4 Most clinically relevant local anesthetics consist of a lipid-soluble, aromatic benzene ring connected to an amide group via either an amide or an ester moiety. The type of linkage broadly defines them into two categories, the *aminoesters* and the *aminoamides*, and affects how they are metabolized. Aminoesters are hydrolyzed by plasma cholinesterases and aminoamides are degraded by hepatic carboxylesterases. Some metabolites of aminoesters, such as *para*-aminobenzoic acid, can induce immunologic reactions and are responsible for the slightly greater incidence of severe allergic reactions associated with aminoesters. Other than these characteristics, physiochemical properties of both aminoesters and aminoamides are similar and are mainly determined by their dissociative constant, lipophilic makeup, and spatial arrangement of the molecule.

The tertiary amide on local anesthetics can accept a proton at low affinity; thus, these compounds are classified as weak bases. In aqueous solution, local anesthetics are in constant equilibrium between the protonated cationic form and the lipid-soluble neutral form. The ratio of the two forms depends on the pK_a or the dissociation constant of the local anesthetics and the surrounding pH (Table 22-3). A ratio with high concentration of the lipid-soluble form favors intracellular entry, as the cellular membrane restricts passage of the cationic form, but not the lipid-soluble form.[2] Clinically, the proportion of the lipid-soluble form can be increased by alkalization of local anesthetic solution and thus accelerate the onset of action. Once inside the cell, equilibrium is reestablished between the cationic and the neutral forms, and experimental findings have shown that the cationic form is principally responsible for blockade of sodium channels.[33]

By far the most important physiochemical property of local anesthetics is their lipophilicity. Lipid solubility of local anesthetics is conferred by the composition of alkyl substitution on the amide and the benzene groups. In the laboratory, lipid solubility is measured by the partition coefficient in a hydrophobic solvent, octanol, and compounds with high octanol:buffer partition coefficient are more lipid soluble.[34] A positive correlation exists between the potency of the local anesthetics and their octanol:buffer partition coefficient; highly lipid-soluble agents are more potent and tend to have a longer duration of action than ones that are less lipid soluble.[35] The lipophilic property of local anesthetics may act at two levels. The first is at the level of cellular entry as greater lipid solubility facilitates passage through the lipid membrane barriers. The second is at the level of binding to the sodium channels. Detailed crystallographic findings show that local anesthetics bind to a hydrophobic pocket within the sodium channels and suggest that ligand binding may be mediated primarily by hydrophobic and van der Waals interactions (Fig. 22-6).[21]

The correlation between local anesthetic potency and lipophilicity is generally observed in vitro; however, it may be less exact in vivo. Compared with experimental setups using isolated nerves, many other factors may influence the potency of local anesthetics on nerves in situ.[36] Highly lipid-soluble agents may be sequestered into surrounding adipose cells and myelin sheaths. Local anesthetics cause vasodilation, which in turn could alter regional drug redistribution.[37,38] Finally, mounting evidence suggests that some local anesthetics can enter certain neurons via nonspecific cation channels, thereby circumventing the membrane barrier altogether.[31] Hence, relative potency of local anesthetics has been determined clinically for different applications, and these values are listed in Table 22-4. 5

Finally, anesthetic activity and potency are affected by the stereochemistry of the local anesthetic molecules. Many older drug preparations exist as racemic mixtures; that is, enantiomeric stereoisomers are in equal proportion. Newer agents, namely, ropivacaine and levobupivacaine, are available as specific enantiomers.

Table 22-3 Physicochemical Properties of Clinically Used Local Anesthetics

Local Anesthetic	pK_a	Percent Ionized (at pH 7.4)	Partition Coefficient (Lipid Solubility)	Percent Protein Binding
Amides				
Bupivacaine[a]	8.1	83	3,420	95
Etidocaine	7.7	66	7,317	94
Lidocaine	7.9	76	366	64
Mepivacaine	7.6	61	130	77
Prilocaine	7.9	76	129	55
Ropivacaine	8.1	83	775	94
Esters				
Chloroprocaine	8.7	95	810	N/A
Procaine	8.9	97	100	6
Tetracaine	8.5	93	5,822	94

[a]Levobupivacaine has same physicochemical properties as racemate.
N/A, not available.
Data from Liu SS. Local anesthetics and analgesia. In: Ashburn MA, Rice LJ, eds. *The Management of Pain*. Churchill Livingstone; 1997:141.

Table 22-4 Relative Potency of Local Anesthetics for Different Clinical Applications

	Bupivacaine	Chloroprocaine	Lidocaine	Mepivacaine	Prilocaine	Ropivacaine
Peripheral nerve	3.6	N/A	1	2.6	0.8	3.6
Spinal	9.6	1	1	1	1	N/A
Epidural	4	0.5	1	1	1	4

N/A, not available.

They were initially developed as less cardiotoxic alternatives to bupivacaine. Although the desired improvement in the safety index has been generally supported in clinical studies, this is at the expense of a slight decrease in potency overall and shorter duration of action compared with racemic mixtures.[39,40] The underlying mechanism has not been defined. Topographic features at the channel-binding site are likely to play a key role in stereoselectivity of local anesthetics.

6 Additives to Increase Local Anesthetic Activity

Epinephrine

Reported benefits of epinephrine include prolongation of local anesthetic block, increased intensity of block, and decreased systemic absorption of local anesthetic.[41] Epinephrine's vasoconstrictive effects augment local anesthetics by antagonizing inherent vasodilating effects of local anesthetics, decreasing systemic absorption and intraneural clearance, and perhaps by redistributing intraneural local anesthetic.[41,42]

Direct analgesic effects from epinephrine may also occur via interaction with α_2-adrenergic receptors in the brain and spinal cord,[43] especially because local anesthetics increase the vascular uptake of epinephrine.[44] The clinical effects of the use of epinephrine are listed in Table 22-5. The smallest dose is suggested because epinephrine combined with local anesthetics may have toxic effects on tissue,[45] the cardiovascular system,[46] peripheral nerves, and the spinal cord.[41]

Alkalinization of Local Anesthetic Solution

Local anesthetic solutions are alkalinized in order to hasten onset of neural block.[47] The pH of commercial preparations of local anesthetics ranges from 3.9 to 6.5 and is especially acidic if prepackaged with epinephrine.[48] Because the pK_a of commonly used local anesthetics ranges from 7.6 to 8.9 (Table 22-3), less than 3% of the commercially prepared local anesthetics exist as the lipid-soluble neutral form. As previously discussed, the neutral form is believed to be important for penetration into the neural cytoplasm, whereas the charged form primarily interacts with the local anesthetic receptor within the sodium channel. Therefore,

Table 22-5 Effects of Addition of Epinephrine to Local Anesthetics

	Increase Duration	Decrease Blood Levels (%)	Dose/Concentration of Epinephrine
Nerve Block			
Bupivacaine	+/–	10–20	1:200,000
Lidocaine	+ +	20–30	1:200,000
Mepivacaine	+ +	20–30	1:200,000
Ropivacaine	– –	0	1:200,000
Epidural			
Bupivacaine	+/–	10–20	1:300,000–1:200,000
Levobupivacaine	+/–	10	1:200,000–1:400,000
Chloroprocaine	+ +	1:200,000	
Lidocaine	+ +	20–30	1:600,000–1:200,000
Mepivacaine	+ +	20–30	1:200,000
Ropivacaine	– –	0	1:200,000
Spinal			
Bupivacaine	+/–	0.2 mg	
Lidocaine	+ +	0.2 mg	
Tetracaine	+ +	0.2 mg	

++, overall supported; —, overall not supported; +/–, inconsistent.

Data from Liu SS. Local anesthetics and analgesia. In: Ashburn MA, Rice LJ, eds. *The Management of Pain*. Churchill Livingstone; 1997:141; and Kopacz DJ. A comparison of epidural levobupivacaine 0.5% with or without epinephrine for lumbar spine surgery. *Anesth Analg*. 2001;93:755–760.

the rationale for alkalinization was to increase the ratio of local anesthetic existing as the lipid-soluble neutral form. However, clinically used local anesthetics cannot be alkalinized beyond a pH of 6.05 to 8 before precipitation occurs[48] and these pH values will only increase the neutral form to about 10%.

Clinical studies on the association between alkalinization of local anesthetics and hastening of block onset have shown an improvement of less than 5 minutes compared with commercial preparations.[47,49] Furthermore, results from a study in rats indicate that alkalinization of lidocaine may also decrease the duration of peripheral nerve blocks if the mixture contained no epinephrine.[50] Together, alkalinization of local anesthetics appears limited as a clinically useful adjuvant to improving anesthesia.

Opioids

Opioids have multiple central and peripheral mechanisms of analgesic action (see Chapter 20). Spinal administration of opioids provides analgesia primarily by attenuating C-fiber nociception[51] and is independent of supraspinal mechanisms.[52] Coadministration of opioids with central neuraxial local anesthetics results in synergistic analgesia.[53] An exception to this analgesic synergy is chloroprocaine, which appears to decrease the effectiveness of opioids coadministered epidurally.[54] The reason is unclear, but the mechanism does not seem to involve direct antagonism of opioid receptors.[55] Nonetheless, clinical studies support the practice of central neuraxial coadministration of local anesthetics and opioids for prolongation and intensification of analgesia and anesthesia.[53]

The discovery of peripheral opioid receptors initially generated much interest in the use of opioids as adjuvants to local anesthetics for peripheral nerve blockade.[56] However, although some studies have reported favorable outcomes for such coadministration, others have failed to demonstrate any increased efficacy.[57] A problem that has plagued many studies is the lack of adequate controls for differentiating the analgesic effects of opioids acting peripherally versus a more central mechanism resulting from systemically absorbed opioids. Nonetheless, recent carefully designed trials have shown that some opioids, namely, buprenorphine, may enhance and prolong postoperative analgesia better than either local anesthetics alone or local anesthetics administered with intramuscular buprenorphine.[58,59] Finally, cumulative evidence does not support the use of intra-articular coadministration of local anesthetic and opioid for postoperative analgesia.[60]

α_2-Adrenergic Agonists

α_2-Adrenergic agonists can be a useful adjuvant to local anesthetics. α_2-Specific agonists such as clonidine produce analgesia via supraspinal and spinal adrenergic receptors.[61] Clonidine also has direct inhibitory effects on peripheral nerve conduction (A and C nerve fibers).[62] Thus, addition of clonidine may have multiple mechanisms of action depending on the type of application. Preliminary evidence suggests that coadministration of an α_2-agonist and local anesthetic results in central neuraxial and peripheral nerve analgesic synergy,[63] whereas systemic (supraspinal) effects are additive.[64] On average, clonidine improves the duration of analgesia by about 2 hours, regardless of whether an intermediate- or long-acting local anesthetic is used.[65] Overall, results from clinical trials indicate that clonidine can enhance local anesthetic effects when used for intrathecal and epidural anesthesia and peripheral nerve blocks.[65,66]

Steroids

Potent glucocorticoid injections have been widely used for the treatment of chronic low back pain caused by radiculopathy. Experiments in animals with microsomal preparations of local anesthetics have found that addition of dexamethasone to the mixture prolongs the conduction block after peripheral nerve application.[67,68] In rodent models, the effects on block duration correlate with the potency of the glucocorticoid activity and appear to be steroid receptor dependent and locally mediated.[69]

Numerous clinical studies evaluating dexamethasone as an adjuvant to local anesthetics have shown prolongation of analgesic duration after peripheral nerve applications, including those to the brachial plexus,[70–72] sciatic,[73] and saphenous nerves (Fig. 22-8).[74,75] Compared with local anesthetics alone, addition of perineural dexamethasone extends the duration of analgesia by approximately 50% to 100%, depending on the specific techniques, the dose and characteristics of local anesthetics and the context of peripheral nerve targeted in the studies.[76,77] The optimal dose of steroids remains undefined; however, a dose–response relationship is seen between 1 to 4 mg of dexamethasone, with a possible ceiling effect observed for dosages greater than 4 mg.[72,78,79]

How steroids exert their effects on block duration is not known. As similar effects can be seen with systemic dose of dexamethasone, albeit to a lesser degree, an on-going debate centers on the uncertainty of whether the effects are perineurally mediated or as a part of generalized anti-inflammatory response to systemically absorbed steroids. The near-ubiquitous presence of steroid receptors makes differentiating the two models difficult.[80] High-dose, systemic dexamethasone is known to be associated with opiate-sparing properties and pain reduction after surgery[81]; this potential may also confound results in studies comparing opiate consumption or pain scores as primary endpoints.

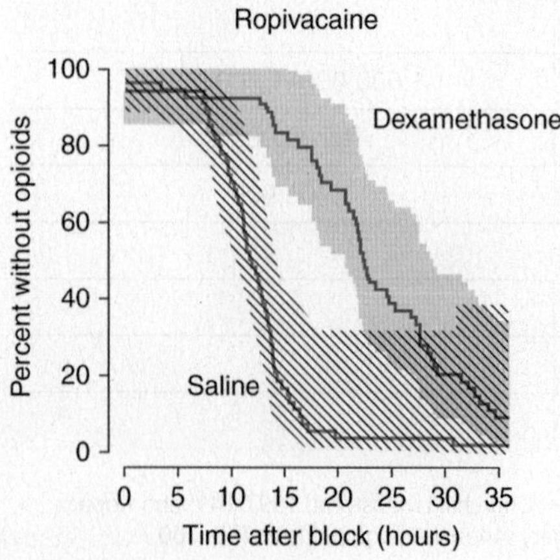

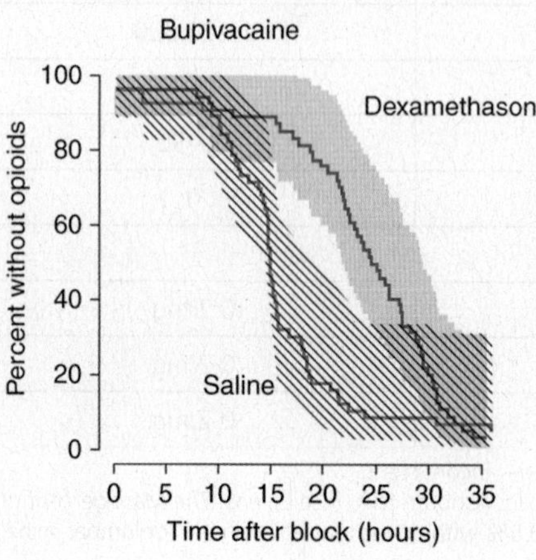

Figure 22-8 Addition of dexamethasone to either ropivacaine or bupivacaine increases the duration of analgesia after interscalene brachial plexus block. Data are shown as the Kaplan–Meier survival density estimates, with the shaded region representing the 95% confidence interval. (Reprinted with permission from Cummings KC, Napierkowski DE, Parra-Sanchez I, et al. Effect of dexamethasone on the duration of interscalene nerve blocks with ropivacaine or bupivacaine. *Br J Anaesth*. 2011;107(3):446–453.)

The emergence of reports claiming the absence of steroid-related effect on local anesthetics has led to challenges to the validity of steroids as an active adjuvant.[82] In these randomized, double- or triple-blinded, crossover trials on volunteers, neither perineural nor intravenous dexamethasone is seen to extend block duration of local anesthetics.[83,84] The reasons for the conflicting accounts are not apparent. It is possible that the small dose of local anesthetic used in these studies minimizes the benefit of steroids. Perhaps, an equally intriguing explanation may lie in differences between the study populations. In the volunteer trials, the subjects were enrolled solely for the study; they did not under any surgery or procedure. In contrast, in most reports that supported the positive pharmacodynamic effects of dexamethasone, the subjects were surgical patients. Could an active inflammatory response, such as following operative procedures, be required for steroid-associate effects? Consistent with this speculation, in the early animal experiments that identified dexamethasone as a potential adjuvant, the effect of dexamethasone was found to be dependent on concomitant presence of microsomes, which are known catalyst of localized inflammatory response.[69]

Liposomes

Commercially available preparations of liposomal bupivacaine are designed to provide extended duration of analgesia beyond currently achievable without catheters. Encapsulated local anesthetics are formulated to be released in a gradual, sustained fashion, ensuring continuous bioavailability at the site of action, and thereby prolonging the effects and decreasing risk of systemic spread and toxicity. Such preparations have been approved for a number of indications, including local infiltration of surgical wounds after bunionectomy and hemorrhoidectomy, transverse abdominis plane block and interscalene brachial plexus block for shoulder surgeries.[85]

The potential for reliably long-lasting analgesia has generated much initial enthusiasm and expectation for liposomal bupivacaine; however, coalesced clinical evidence is mixed and clouded with uncertainty. Many early trials were conducted against placebo controls. Surprisingly, even about half of these studies failed to discern any statistically significance for analgesic benefits.[86] In trials that show positive findings, the predominant use of cumulative pain score and opiate consumption over a block of time has hampered the clarity of actual analgesic duration.

As direct comparisons with equally large doses of unencapsulated bupivacaine may pose unacceptable risk and would be unethical, different local anesthetics at varying doses have been used as active comparators in trials against liposomal bupivacaine. Heterogeneous results aside,[85,86] most studies advocate comparators that lack the robustness to adequately address the raison d'etre to using liposomal bupivacaine, that is, to provide the most long-lasting analgesia after a single administration.

A recent investigation has confronted this question head on. Among the many adjuvants discussed previously, perineural dexamethasone has been shown to enhance analgesic duration by as much as 50% to 100% relative to plain bupivacaine, and thus, may be a worthy comparator to liposomal bupivacaine. In a prospective, double blinded, noninferiority trial with interscalene brachial plexus block for ambulatory shoulder surgery, liposomal bupivacaine was found not inferior to bupivacaine with dexamethasone in terms of average pain scores over 72 hours (mean 2.4 vs. 3.4), with no significant difference in the duration of analgesia, time to resolution of motor and sensory blockade, or opioid consumption.[87] Patient reported block duration was approximately 26 and 27 hours, respectively. Thus, in the setting of progressive multimodal analgesia regiment for shoulder surgeries, liposomal bupivacaine appears not unacceptably worse than bupivacaine with dexamethasone and may be equivalent in terms of analgesic duration and efficacy.

In animal models, perineural infiltration of liposomal bupivacaine was associated with tissue inflammation and myotoxicity.[88] The degree of myotoxicity was comparable to that of 0.5% bupivacaine, although the inflammation due to liposomal bupivacaine persisted for much longer duration. There was no evidence of local neurotoxicity or CNS or cardiac toxicity.[89] Clinically, most frequently reported untoward effects of liposomal bupivacaine were nausea and pyrexia.[90]

Pharmacokinetics of Local Anesthetics

Plasma concentration of local anesthetics is a function of the dose administered and the rates of systemic absorption, tissue distribution, and drug elimination. Elevated levels may produce unintended effects in other electric-sensitive systems, most importantly, the cardiovascular system and the CNS. Having a thorough understanding of the factors involved would enable one to maximize the local anesthetic potential while avoiding possible complications arising from systemic local anesthetic toxicity.

Systemic Absorption

Decreasing systemic absorption of local anesthetics increases their safety margin in clinical uses. The rate and extent of systemic absorption depends on the site of injection, the dose, the drug's intrinsic pharmacokinetic properties, and the addition of a vasoactive agent. The vascularity of the tissue markedly influences the rate of drug absorption, such that deposition of local anesthetics in vessel-rich tissues results in higher peak plasma levels in a shorter period of time. Accordingly, the rate of systemic absorption is greatest with intercostal nerve blocks, followed in decreasing order by caudal and epidural injections, brachial plexus block, and femoral and sciatic nerve blocks (Table 22-6). Thus, the same amount of local anesthetics injected would result in unequal peak plasma levels depending on the site of drug delivery.

For a given site of injection, the rate of systemic absorption and the peak plasma level are directly proportional to the dose of local anesthetic deposited. This relationship is nearly linear (Fig. 22-9) and independent of the drug concentration and the speed of injection.[91]

The rate of systemic absorption differs with individual local anesthetics. In general, more potent lipid-soluble agents are associated with a slower rate of absorption than less lipid-soluble compounds (Fig. 22-10). Sequestration into lipid-rich compartments may not be the only explanation. Local anesthetics exert direct effects on vascular smooth muscles in a concentration-dependent manner. At low concentrations, more potent agents appear to cause more vasoconstriction than less potent agents, thereby decreasing the rate of vascular absorption.[38] At high concentrations, vasodilatory effects seem to predominate for most local anesthetics.

Distribution

Systemic absorption of local anesthetics leads to rapid distribution throughout the body. The steady-state drug concentration in plasma can be readily derived from the apparent volume of

Table 22-6 Typical C_{max} after Regional Anesthesia with Commonly Used Local Anesthetics

Local Anesthetic	Technique	Dose (mg)	C_{max} (mg/mL)	T_{max} (min)	Toxic Plasma Concentration (mg/mL)
Bupivacaine	Brachial plexus	150	1.0	20	3
	Celiac plexus	100	1.50	17	
	Epidural	150	1.26	20	
	Intercostal	140	0.90	30	
	Lumbar sympathetic	52.5	0.49	24	
	Sciatic/femoral	400	1.89	15	
Levobupivacaine	Epidural	75	0.36	50	4
	Brachial plexus	250	1.2	55	
Lidocaine	Brachial plexus	400	4.00	25	5
	Epidural	400	4.27	20	
	Intercostal	400	6.8	15	
Mepivacaine	Brachial plexus	500	3.68	24	5
	Epidural	500	4.95	16	
	Intercostal	500	8.06	9	
	Sciatic/femoral	500	3.59	31	
Ropivacaine	Brachial plexus	190	1.3	53	4
	Epidural	150	1.07	40	
	Intercostal	140	1.10	21	

C_{max}, peak plasma levels; T_{max}, time until C_{max}.
Data from Liu SS. Local anesthetics and analgesia. In: Ashburn MA, Rice LJ, eds. *The Management of Pain*. Churchill Livingstone; 1997:141; Berrisford RG. Plasma concentrations of bupivacaine and its enantiomers during continuous extrapleural intercostal nerve block. *Br J Anaesth*. 1993;70:201–204; Kopacz DJ. A comparison of epidural levobupivacaine 0.5% with or without epinephrine for lumbar spine surgery. *Anesth Analg*. 2001;93:755–760; and Crews JC. Levobupivacaine for axillary brachial plexus block: a pharmacokinetic and clinical comparison in patients with normal renal function or renal disease. *Anesth Analg*. 2002;95:219–223.

distribution (VD_{ss}; Table 22-7); however, regional differences in local anesthetic concentrations are seen among individual organ systems. The pattern of distribution is largely dependent on organ perfusion, the partition coefficient between compartments, and plasma protein binding.[92] Organs that are well perfused, such as the heart and the brain, have higher drug concentrations. Unfortunately, they are also the organs most seriously affected by local anesthetic toxicity.

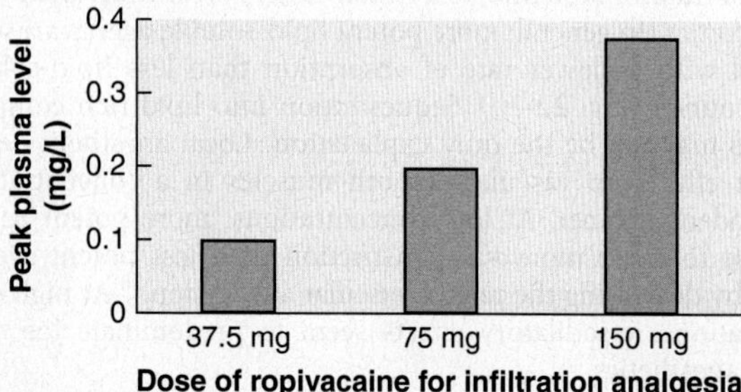

Figure 22-9 Increasing doses of ropivacaine used for wound infiltration result in linearly increasing maximal plasma concentrations (C_{max}). (Reproduced from Mulroy MF, Burgess FW, Emanuelsson B-M. Ropivacaine 0.25% and 0.5%, but not 0.125%, provide effective wound infiltration analgesia after outpatient hernia repair, but with sustained plasma drug levels. *Reg Anesth Pain Med*. 1999;24:136–141, with permission from BMJ Publishing Group Ltd.)

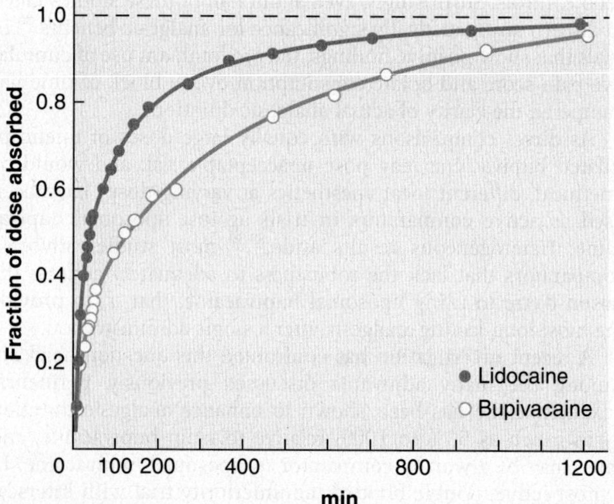

Figure 22-10 Fraction of dose absorbed into the systemic circulation over time from epidural injection of lidocaine or bupivacaine. Bupivacaine is a more lipid-soluble and more potent agent with less systemic absorption over time. (Adapted with permission from Tucker GT, Mather LE. Properties, absorption, and disposition of local anesthetic agents. In: Cousins MJ, Bridenbaugh PO, eds. *Neural Blockade in Clinical Anesthesia and Management of Pain*: Lippincott-Raven; 1998:55.)

Table 22-7 Pharmacokinetic Parameters of Clinically Used Local Anesthetics

Local Anesthetic	VD_{ss} (L/kg)	CL (L/kg/hr)	$T_{1/2}$ (hours)
Bupivacaine	1.02	0.41	3.5
Levobupivacaine	0.78	0.32	2.6
Chloroprocaine	0.50	2.96	0.11
Etidocaine	1.9	1.05	2.6
Lidocaine	1.3	0.85	1.6
Mepivacaine	1.2	0.67	1.9
Prilocaine	2.73	2.03	1.6
Procaine	0.93	5.62	0.14
Ropivacaine	0.84	0.63	1.9

VD_{ss}, volume of distribution at steady state; CL, total body clearance; $T_{1/2}$, terminal elimination half-life.

Data from Denson DD. Physiology and pharmacology of local anesthetics. In: Sinatra RS, Hord AH, Ginsberg B, et al., eds. *Acute Pain: Mechanisms and Management*. Mosby Year Book; 1992:124; and Burm AG, van der Meer AD, van Kleef JW, Zeijlmans PW, Groen K. Pharmacokinetics of the enantiomers of bupivacaine following intravenous administration of the racemate. *Br J Clin Pharmacol*. 1994;38:125–129.

Table 22-8 Relative Potency for Systemic Central Nervous System Toxicity by Local Anesthetics and Ratio of Dosage Needed for Cardiovascular System: Central Nervous System (CVS:CNS) Toxicity

Agent	Relative Potency for CNS Toxicity	CVS:CNS
Bupivacaine	4.0	2.0
Levobupivacaine	2.9	2.0
Chloroprocaine	0.3	3.7
Etidocaine	2.0	4.4
Lidocaine	1.0	7.1
Mepivacaine	1.4	7.1
Prilocaine	1.2	3.1
Procaine	0.3	3.7
Ropivacaine	2.9	2.0
Tetracaine	2.0	

Data from Liu SS. Local anesthetics and analgesia. In: Ashburn MA, Rice LJ, eds. *The Management of Pain*. Churchill Livingstone; 1997:141; and Groban L. Central nervous system and cardiac effects from long-acting amide local anesthetic toxicity in the intact animal model. *Reg Anesth Pain Med*. 2003;28:3–11.

Elimination

The metabolic pathway for clearance of local anesthetics is primarily determined by their chemical linkage. Aminoesters are hydrolyzed by plasma cholinesterases and aminoamides are transformed by hepatic carboxylesterases and cytochrome P450 enzymes. Severe liver disease may slow the clearance of aminoamide local anesthetics and significant drug levels may therefore accumulate.[93]

Clinical Pharmacokinetics

The primary benefit of understanding the systemic pharmacokinetics of local anesthetics is the ability to predict the peak plasma level (C_{max}) after the agents are administered, thereby avoiding the administration of toxic doses (Tables 22-6, 22-8, and 22-9). Nonetheless, pharmacokinetics are difficult to predict in any given circumstance because both physical and pathophysiologic characteristics will affect the individual pharmacokinetics. There is some evidence for increased systemic plasma levels of local anesthetics in the very young and in the elderly owing to decreased clearance and increased absorption;[94] however, the correlation of systemic blood levels between the dose of local anesthetic and weight is often inconsistent (Fig. 22-11).[95] Effects of gender on clinical pharmacokinetics of local anesthetics have not been well defined,[96] although pregnancy may decrease clearance.[97] Pathophysiologic states such as cardiac and hepatic disease will alter expected pharmacokinetic parameters (Table 22-10), and lower doses of local anesthetics should be used for these patients. As expected, renal disease has little effect on pharmacokinetic parameters of local anesthetics (Table 22-10). All of these factors should be considered when using local anesthetics and minimizing systemic toxicity, the commonly accepted maximal dosages (Table 22-9) notwithstanding.

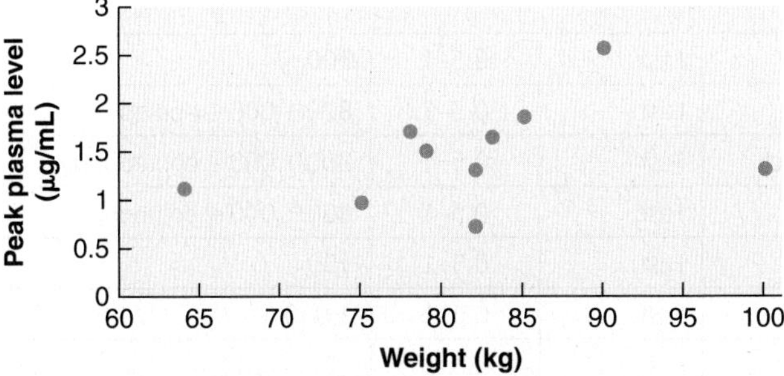

Figure 22-11 Lack of correlation between patient weight and peak plasma concentration after epidural administration of 150 mg of bupivacaine. (Data from Sharrock NE, Mather LE, Go G, Sculco TP. Arterial and pulmonary concentrations of the enantiomers of bupivacaine after epidural injection in elderly patients. *Anesth Analg*. 1998;86:812–817.)

Clinical Use of Local Anesthetics

There are a myriad of uses of local anesthetics in the modern practice of anesthesia. They all take advantage of their ability to attenuate or block pain and other noxious stimuli. When applied topically to the skin, a eutectic mixture of lidocaine and prilocaine reduces the sharp, painful sensation associated with needle insertion and intravenous catheter placement, particularly in the pediatric population. In the awake patient, aerosolized benzocaine and viscous lidocaine directed at the mucosal surface can help blunt the protective reflex responses associated with airway instrumentation (see Chapter 28). In addition, lidocaine can be given intravenously to decrease the incidence and the severity of pain associated with propofol administration (see Chapters 19 and 31). Likewise, intravenous lidocaine may also help to reduce the hemodynamic response to tracheal intubation and extubation.[98,99]

By far the most common application, local infiltration of the dermis, provides quick onset of anesthesia suitable for a broad variety of minor superficial procedures (2 Video 22-2). The clinical profile of some commonly used agents is listed in

Table 22-9 Clinical Profile of Local Anesthetics

Local Anesthetic	Concentration (%)	Clinical Use	Onset	Duration (hours)	Recommended Maximum Single Dose (mg)
Amides					
Bupivacaine	0.25	Infiltration	Fast	2–8	175/225 + epinephrine
Levobupivacaine	0.25–0.5	Peripheral nerve block	Slow	4–12	150
	0.5–0.75	Epidural anesthesia	Moderate	2–5	150
	0.03–0.25	Epidural analgesia	N/A	N/A	N/A
	0.5–0.75	Spinal anesthesia	Fast	1–4	20
Etidocaine	0.5	Infiltration	Fast	2–8	300/400 + epinephrine
	0.5–1	Peripheral nerve block	Fast	3–12	300/400 + epinephrine
	1–1.5	Epidural anesthesia	Fast	2–4	300/400 + epinephrine
Lidocaine	0.5–1	Infiltration	Fast	1–4	300/500 + epinephrine
	0.25–0.5	IV regional anesthesia	Fast	0.5–1	300
	1–1.5	Peripheral nerve block	Fast	1–3	300/500 + epinephrine
	1.5–2	Epidural anesthesia	Fast	1–2	300/500 + epinephrine
	1.5–5	Spinal anesthesia	Fast	0.5–1	100
	4	Topical	Fast	0.5–1	300
Mepivacaine	0.5–1	Infiltration	Fast	1–4	400/500 + epinephrine
	1–1.5	Peripheral nerve block	Fast	2–4	400/500 + epinephrine
	1.5–2	Epidural anesthesia	Fast	1–3	400/500 + epinephrine
	2–4	Spinal anesthesia	Fast	1–2	100
Prilocaine	0.5–1	Infiltration	Fast	1–2	600
	0.25–0.5	IV regional anesthesia	Fast	0.5–1	600
	1.5–2	Peripheral nerve block	Fast	1.5–3	600
	2–3	Epidural	Fast	1–3	600
Ropivacaine	0.2–0.5	Infiltration	Fast	2–6	200
	0.5–1	Peripheral nerve block	Slow	5–8	250
	0.5–1	Epidural anesthesia	Moderate	2–6	200
	0.05–0.2	Epidural analgesia	N/A	N/A	N/A
Mixture					
Lidocaine + prilocaine	2.5/2.5	Skin topical	Slow	3–5	20 g
Esters					
Benzocaine	Up to 20	Topical	Fast	0.5–1	200
Chloroprocaine	1	Infiltration	Fast	0.5–1	800/1,000 + epinephrine
	2	Peripheral nerve block	Fast	0.5–1	800/1,000 + epinephrine
	2–3	Epidural anesthesia	Fast	0.5–1	800/1,000 + epinephrine
Cocaine	4–10	Topical	Fast	0.5–1	150
Procaine	10	Spinal anesthesia	Fast	0.5–1	1,000
Tetracaine	2	Topical	Fast	0.5–1	20
	0.5	Spinal anesthesia	Fast	2–6	20

IV, intravenous; N/A, not available.

Adapted from Covino BG, Wildsmith JAW. Clinical pharmacology of local anesthetic agents. In: Cousins MJ, Bridenbaugh PO, eds. *Neural Blockade in Clinical Anesthesia and Management of Pain*. Lippincott-Raven; 1998:97.

Table 22-10 Effects of Cardiac, Hepatic, and Renal Disease on Lidocaine Pharmacokinetics

	VD_{ss} (L/kg)	CL (mL/kg/min)	$T_{1/2}$ (hours)
Normal	1.32	10.0	1.8
Cardiac failure	0.88	6.3	1.9
Hepatic disease	2.31	6.0	4.9
Renal disease	1.2	13.7	1.3

VD_{ss}, volume of distribution at steady state; CL, total body clearance; $T_{1/2}$, terminal elimination half-life.

Data from Thomson PD. Lidocaine pharmacokinetics in advanced heart failure, liver disease, and renal failure in humans. *Ann Intern Med.* 1973; 78:499–508.

Table 22-11 Dose-Dependent Systemic Effects of Lidocaine

Plasma Concentration (mg/mL)	Effect
1–5	Analgesia
5–10	Lightheadedness Tinnitus Numbness of tongue
10–15	Seizures Unconsciousness
15–25	Coma Respiratory arrest
>25	Cardiovascular depression

Table 22-9. For a wider and greater area of coverage, a regional anatomic approach to anesthesia and analgesia can be used. This can be accomplished either by intravenous administration of local anesthetics to a limb under pneumatic compression (Bier block) or by direct application of local anesthetics to individual peripheral nerves (nerve blocks). Local anesthetics can be deposited centrally near the nerve roots, either intrathecally in the lumbar cistern or epidurally in the thoracic, lumbar, and caudal regions of the spine (see Chapter 35). Alternatively, injections can be made peripherally at the plexus, such as at the brachial or lumbar plexus block or on the nerve fibers (see Chapter 36). The duration of the anesthesia and analgesia is dependent on the type of local anesthetics used, though it can be extended with continuous infusion through an indwelling catheter.

Toxicity of Local Anesthetics

Local Anesthetic Systemic Toxicity (LAST)

Local anesthetics are generally safe, but they are not without potential for harm. Accumulation of local anesthetics in the systemic circulation, as a result of either inadvertent injection or unanticipated rapid absorption into the blood stream, can result in toxic levels with serious and devastating consequences. Termed local anesthetic systemic toxicity or LAST, the effects can follow the use of any local anesthetics and via a variety of routes of administration. While local anesthetics can perturb a wide range of tissues, both the CNS and the cardiovascular system appear especially vulnerable to the deleterious effects of LAST, possibly a reflection of the sensitive and integral function of membrane potentials and channels to both systems.

Central Nervous System Toxicity

Local anesthetics readily cross the blood–brain barrier and, as a result, CNS toxicity can arise quickly after intravascular injections (NICV 22-1). The effects on the CNS are determined by the plasma concentration of the local anesthetics (Table 22-11). At low plasma concentration, mild disturbances to the sensory systems appear. As the plasma concentration increases, CNS excitation and seizure activities predominate. If the plasma concentration is sufficiently large or the increase is rapid, the CNS excitation may progress to generalized CNS depression and coma, leading to respiratory depression and arrest.[100]

The potential for CNS toxicity correlates directly with the potency of local anesthetics[100] (Tables 22-4 and 22-8). Highly potent lipid-soluble agents such as bupivacaine can cause CNS toxicity at doses that are a fraction of those of less potent agents. The potential for CNS toxicity is further modified by other factors. For example, a decrease in protein binding and clearance of local anesthetics, systemic acidosis, hypercapnia, and hypercarbia can all increase the risk for CNS toxicity. Conversely, coadministration of CNS depressive agents, such as barbiturates and benzodiazepines, may decrease the likelihood for seizures.[101]

Cardiovascular Toxicity

In general, cardiovascular toxicity is seen at a plasma concentration far greater than that for CNS toxicity. The potential for cardiovascular toxicity, like that for CNS toxicity, correlates closely with the potency, or lipid solubility, of local anesthetics (Tables 22-4 and 22-8). However, although all local anesthetics can give rise to hypotension, dysrhythmias, and myocardial depression, more potent agents such as bupivacaine, ropivacaine, and levobupivacaine are more likely to be associated with life threatening outcomes, such as cardiovascular collapse and complete heart block[102] (Fig. 22-12).

8

Among the potent long-acting agents, ropivacaine and levobupivacaine may offer a safer cardiovascular toxicity profile than bupivacaine. In animal models, both ropivacaine and levobupivacaine appear to exhibit 30% to 40% less cardiovascular toxicity than bupivacaine on a milligram-to-milligram basis (Fig. 22-13)[34,100,103]; however, in human studies, that difference appears less striking (Fig. 22-14).[104,105] Detailed electrophysiologic studies with isolated heart muscles and cultured cardiomyocytes support the view that *S*(-)-bupivacaine (levobupivacaine) is generally less potent than *R*(+)-bupivacaine both in blocking the cardiac action potential[106] and in binding of voltage-gated sodium channels during the inactivated stage.[107] Likewise for ropivacaine, evidence suggests that the propyl side chain renders it less cardiodepressive than the larger butyl side chain of bupivacaine.[108]

The underlying pathophysiology responsible for local anesthetic-induced cardiovascular collapse has not been fully established. Although local anesthetics can directly cause major disturbances to the heart, their effects on other components of cardiovascular systems may be just as important. For example, systemic bupivacaine has been shown to impair regulation by the CNS on the cardiovascular system. Disruption to the arterial baroreflex in the brainstem by bupivacaine can lead to attenuation of the heart rhythm response to changes in blood pressure.[109,110] Local anesthetics also act on smooth muscle endothelium surrounding blood vessels. In the periphery, vasoconstriction occurs

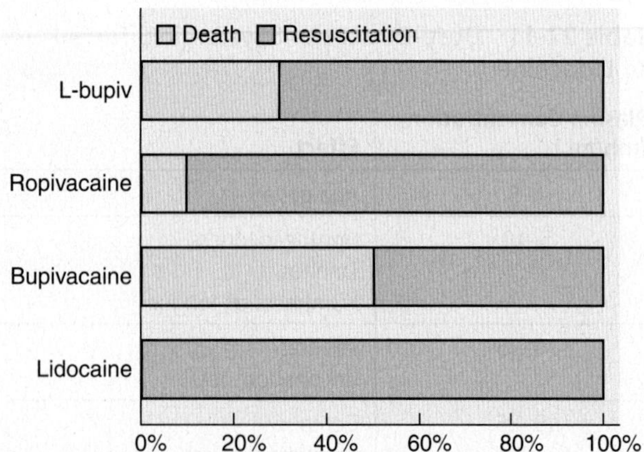

Figure 22-12 Success of resuscitation of dogs after cardiovascular collapse from intravenous infusions of lidocaine, bupivacaine, levobupivacaine (L-bupiv), and ropivacaine. Success rates were greater for lidocaine (100%) compared to ropivacaine (90%), levobupivacaine (70%), and bupivacaine (50%). Required doses to induce cardiovascular collapse were greater for lidocaine (127 mg/kg) compared to ropivacaine (42 mg/kg), levobupivacaine (27 mg/kg), and bupivacaine (22 mg/kg). (Data from Groban L, Deal DD, Vernon JC, James RL, Butterworth J. Cardiac resuscitation after incremental overdosage with lidocaine, bupivacaine, levobupivacaine, and ropivacaine in anesthetized dogs. *Anesth Analg*. 2001;92:37–43.)

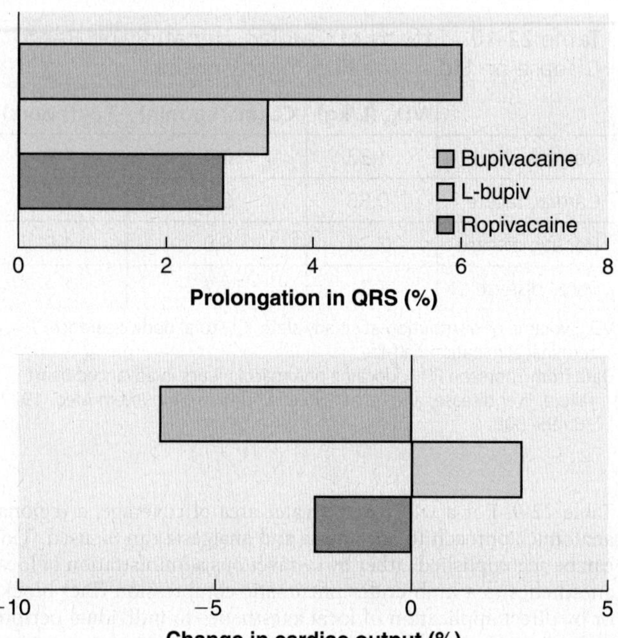

Figure 22-14 Mild prolongation in QRS interval and change in cardiac output after intravenous infusions of bupivacaine (103 mg), levobupivacaine (L-bupiv; 37 mg), and ropivacaine (115 mg) in healthy volunteers. (Data from Knudsen K, Beckman Suurkula M, Blomberg S, Sjövall J, Edvardsson N. Central nervous and cardiovascular effects of i.v. infusions of ropivacaine, bupivacaine and placebo in volunteers. *Br Anaesth*. 1997;78:507–514; and Stewart J, Kellett N, Castro D. The central nervous system and cardiovascular effects of levobupivacaine and ropivacaine in healthy volunteers. *Anesth Analg*. 2003;97: 412–416.)

at subclinical doses but vasodilation at higher doses.[111] In the pulmonary vasculature, however, increasing local anesthetic concentrations produce marked pulmonary artery hypertension.[112] The increase in the pulmonary vascular resistance occurs prior to any significant decrease in the cardiac output, suggesting that the result is primarily an effect of local anesthetic intoxication, rather than secondarily to a decline in cardiac contractility.

Elevated concentrations of local anesthetics have been shown to slow cardiac electrical conductivity and decrease cardiac contractility. Although all local anesthetics disturb the cardiac conduction system via a dose-dependent block of sodium channels (seen clinically as a prolongation of the PR interval and duration of the QRS complex), several features unique to bupivacaine seem to potentiate its cardiotoxicity. First, bupivacaine has an inherently greater affinity for binding sodium channels in the inactive or resting state than lidocaine.[113] Second, although all local anesthetics bind sodium channels during cardiac systole and dissociate in diastole (Fig. 22-15), the dissociation of bupivacaine during diastole occurs more slowly than lidocaine. This slow rate of dissociation prevents a complete recovery of the channels at the end of each cardiac cycle (at the physiologic heart rate of 60 to 80 beats/min), thereby leading to more blocked channels and worsening of the conduction defect. In contrast, lidocaine fully dissociates from the channels during diastole, resulting in fewer channels being blocked and less conduction delay (Fig. 22-16).[113,114] Finally, bupivacaine exerts a greater degree of direct myocardial depression than less potent agents (Fig. 22-17).[100,108]

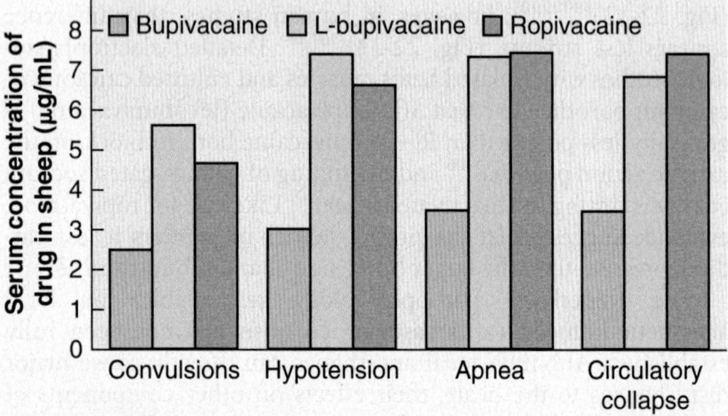

Figure 22-13 Serum concentrations in sheep at each toxic manifestation for bupivacaine, levo (L)-bupivacaine, and ropivacaine. Both levobupivacaine and ropivacaine required significantly greater serum concentrations than bupivacaine. (Data from Santos AC, DeArmas PI. Systemic toxicity of levobupivacaine, bupivacaine, and ropivacaine during continuous intravenous infusion to nonpregnant and pregnant ewes. *Anesthesiology*. 2001;95:1256–1264.)

Current understanding of the molecular mechanisms underlying local anesthetic cardiac toxicity is limited. It is widely accepted that local anesthetics bind and disrupt the normal function of the heart-specific voltage-gated sodium channel, Na_v 1.5, in cardiac myocytes; however, there may be other intracellular targets as well. Local anesthetics have been shown to antagonize the currents of other cations, primarily calcium and potassium.[113] The degree of antagonism between bupivacaine and less potent agents appears to differ, and may account for the differences observed in the severity of the disturbance on the cardiac membrane potentials. Lastly, in individuals with and animal models for L-carnitine deficiency, the effects of local anesthetics on cardiac toxicity are enhanced, possibly implicating the involvement of mitochondrial function and fatty acid metabolism in LAST.[115,116]

Clinical Presentation of LAST

CNS disturbances are prominent in about 80% to 90% of reported cases of LAST.[117,118] The most frequent CNS manifestations are seizures, agitation, and loss of consciousness, which are commonly preceded by prodromal sensory alterations, such as

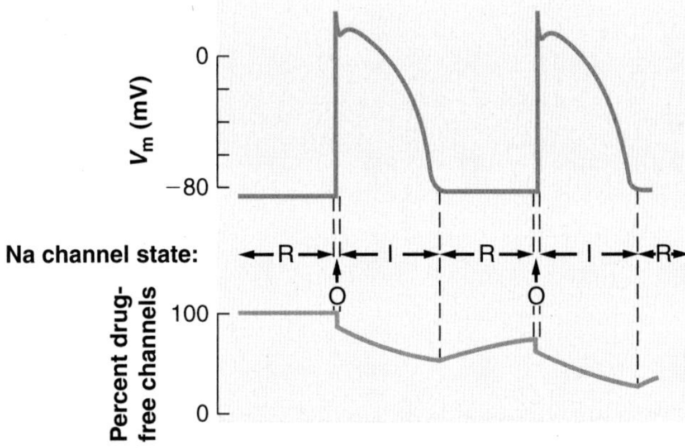

Figure 22-15 Diagram illustrating the relationship between cardiac action potential (*top*), sodium channel state (*middle*), and block of sodium channels by bupivacaine (*bottom*). Sodium channels are predominantly in the resting form during diastole, open transiently during the action potential upstroke, and are in the inactive form during the action potential plateau. Block of sodium channels by bupivacaine accumulates during the action potential (systole), with recovery occurring during diastole. Recovery of sodium channels results from dissociation of bupivacaine and is time-dependent. Recovery during each diastolic interval is incomplete and results in accumulation of sodium channel block with successive heartbeats. R, resting form; O, open form; I, inactive form. (Adapted with permission from Clarkson CW, Hondeghem LM. Mechanisms for bupivacaine depression of cardiac conduction: fast block of sodium channels during the action potential with slow recovery from block during diastole. *Anesthesiology*. 1985;62:396–405.)

perageusia and perioral parasthesia[117] (Fig. 22-18). Concomitant cardiovascular derangements occur in about half of these cases, with refractory hypotension and bradycardia being common presenting signs. Further deterioration leads to a spectrum of dysrhythmias, ranging from supraventricular tachyarrhythmia and wide complex dysrhythmias to complete heart block or asystole[117] (Fig. 22-19). The latter can be severe and profound, and often resistant to intervention. Finally, about 10% to 20% of cases

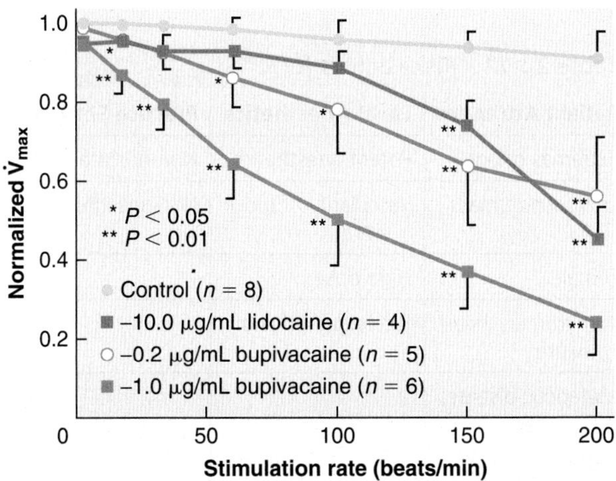

Figure 22-16 Heart rate–dependent effects of lidocaine and bupivacaine on velocity of the cardiac action potential (V_{max}). Bupivacaine progressively decreases V_{max} at heart rates above 10 beats/min because of accumulation of sodium channel block, whereas lidocaine does not decrease V_{max} until heart rate exceeds 150 beats/min. (Adapted with permission from Clarkson CW, Hondegham LM. Mechanisms for bupivacaine depression of cardiac conduction: Fast block of sodium channels during the action potential with slow recovery from block during diastole. *Anesthesiology*. 1985;62:396–405.)

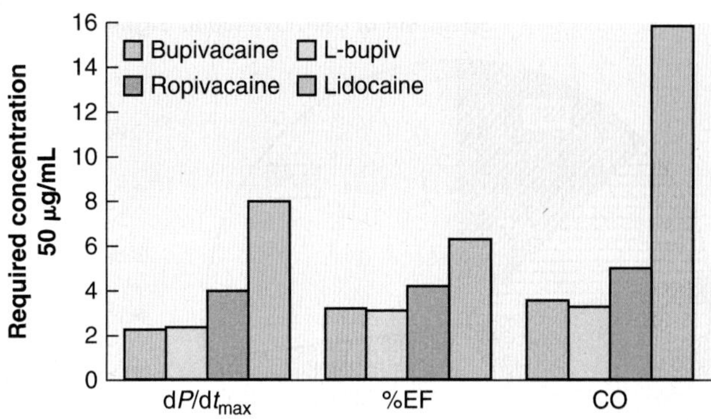

Figure 22-17 Plasma concentrations required to induce myocardial depression in dogs administered bupivacaine, levobupivacaine (L-bupiv), ropivacaine, and lidocaine. d*P*/dt_{max}, 35% reduction of inotropy from baseline measure; %EF, 35% reduction in ejection fraction from baseline measure; CO, 25% reduction in cardiac output from baseline measure. (Data from Groban L, Deal DD, Vernon JC, James RL, Butterworth J. Does local anesthetic stereoselectivity or structure predict myocardial depression in anesthetized canines? *Reg Anesth Pain Med*. 2002;27:460–468.)

of LAST do not have antecedent neurologic symptoms and present solely with cardiovascular findings; therefore, it behooves the practitioner to remain vigilant and maintain a high level of suspicion for any isolated disturbances of cardiovascular systems as potential manifestation of LAST.

The onset of LAST is typically very rapid following local anesthetic administration. A majority of cases occur less than a minute after the inciting event, with three-quarters of all cases noted within 5 minutes.[117] The few cases reported to present hours later are usually associated with use of continuous infusion catheters. More recent studies revealed a shift of cases toward more delayed onset. The reason for the shift is unclear; it may be due to a general increased awareness and practice of avoiding direct intravascular injections and a greater utilization of indwelling catheters to obviate the need for single large volume local anesthetic injection.

Incidence of LAST

Epidemiologic evidence indicates that the incidence of major CNS or cardiovascular toxicity associated with the use of local anesthetics in regional anesthesia is relatively uncommon.[119] The

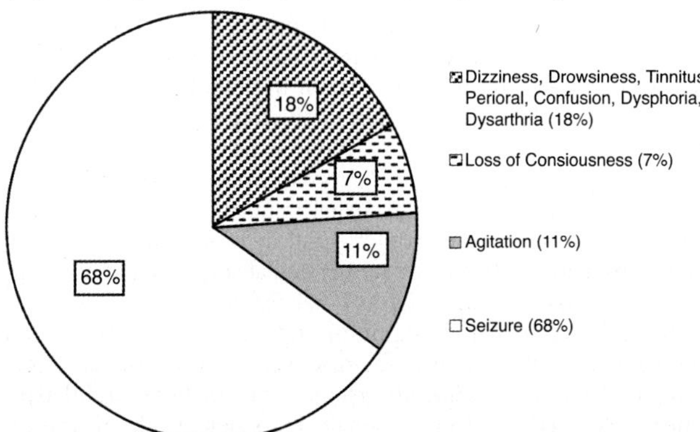

Figure 22-18 Reported frequency of signs of central nervous toxicity reported among published cases of LAST. (Reprinted with Di Gregorio G, Neal JM, Rosenquist RW, et al. Clinical presentation of local anesthetic systemic toxicity: a review of published cases, 1979–2009. *Reg Anesth Pain Med*. 2010;35:181–1817, with permission from BMJ Publishing Group Ltd.)

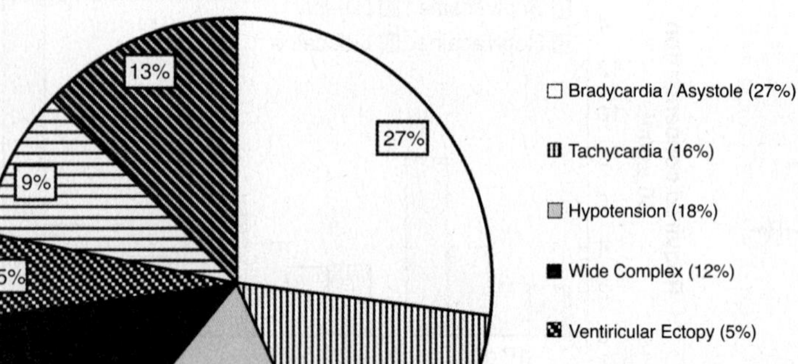

Figure 22-19 Reported frequency of signs of cardiovascular toxicity among published cases of LAST. (Reprinted with Di Gregorio G, Neal JM, Rosenquist RW, et al. Clinical presentation of local anesthetic systemic toxicity: a review of published cases, 1979–2009. *Reg Anesth Pain Med.* 2010;35:181–187, with permission from BMJ Publishing Group Ltd.)

overall incidence of LAST ranges broadly from 0.004% to 0.18%, depending on the database or case series used and the methodology deployed.[118,120–122] Nonetheless, many investigations observe an encouraging trend of gradual decrease in the yearly reported incidence of LAST over the study period.[121,122] Among the arthroplasty literatures, the odds of LAST following upper extremity blocks are greater than that for lower extremity blocks; however, in a wider series, penile blocks and local tissue infiltrations are responsible for a preponderance of reported LAST events. Although individuals of all ages and with various comorbid conditions are uniformly affected, those in extremes of age and baseline cardiac conditions appear to be at an increased odds of LAST; thus, it may be prudent be remain cautious and judicious in the use of local anesthetics in these populations.

Prevention and Treatment of LAST

The best management for LAST starts with prevention and risk reduction. An understanding of the pharmacokinetics of local anesthetics and the various factors that influence their systemic spread, such as absorption, distribution, metabolism and elimination, is crucial to maintaining safe practices. As described in previous sections, tissue vascularity is an important determinant of the rate of systemic absorption; the anatomic target and location should be among the considerations for the choice and doses of local anesthetic. Likewise, judicious dosing of local anesthetics is advisable in individuals at extremes of age, as decreased levels of plasma binding proteins may result in potentially greater fraction of unbound local anesthetics circulating systemically. Infants younger than 6 months of age are found to be at sixfold greater risk for LAST than older children.[119] Pregnant women are also likely at an increased risk, owing to the change in hormonal milieu, relative decreased plasma protein binding, and increased cardiac output, all which likely contribute to accelerated absorption and distribution.[123,124] Table 22-12 highlights other risk factors for LAST.

In addition to risk recognition and dose reduction, several practices may help minimize the risk of direct intravascular injection and decrease systemic absorption. They include careful aspiration before each injection; small, incremental administration (3 to 5 mL) with continuous heart rate monitoring; direct visualization and confirmation of the local anesthetic deposit with ultrasonographic guidance; and finally, incorporation of a vasoactive agent such as epinephrine to both decrease the rate of systemic absorption and serve an intravascular reporter.[119] No outcome studies have demonstrated efficacies of these measures in the prevention of LAST; nonetheless, together with broader awareness and education, they may partly be responsible for the gradual decline of yearly incidence of LAST observed over the last decade.

Treatment of Systemic Toxicity from Local Anesthetics

Effective treatment of LAST depends on early recognition and rapid intervention to prevent worsening outcomes. At the first sign of toxicity, administration of local anesthetic should cease and assistance be alerted. With impending loss of sensorium and possible development of epileptic activity, airway, and ventilation should be secured and supported in order to prevent exacerbation of LAST due to hypoxia, hypercapnia, and acidosis.[101]

Seizures should be promptly treated and suppressed, as generalized and uncontrolled muscular contractions can vastly increase the body's metabolic demand and the resultant metabolic acidosis may make resuscitation more difficult. Benzodiazepines, such

Table 22-12 Risk Factors for LAST

Patient Attributes	Local Anesthetics	Practice Setting
Extremes of age	Potent anesthetics	Non-hospital setting
Low muscle mass	Vascularity of block site	Non-anesthesiologist
Female	High dose	
Arrhythmias, heart failure	Prolonged infusion	
Metabolic disease, diabetes		
Hepatic insufficiencies		
CNS disease		
Low plasma protein binding		

Adapted from Neal JM, Barrington MJ, Fettiplace MR, et al. The Third American Society of Regional Anesthesia and Pain Medicine practice advisory on local anesthetic systemic toxicity: Executive summary 2017. *Reg Anesth Pain Med.* 2018;43:113–123.

as midazolam or diazepam, are the preferred agents for preventing and terminating seizures. If benzodiazepines are not available, small doses of hypnotic agents such as propofol and thiopental, may be administered with caution, as they can further accentuate cardiovascular dysfunction associated with LAST.[125] If seizure activity is prolonged, succinylcholine or other neuromuscular blockers can be administered, not only to facilitate pulmonary ventilation but also to disrupt muscular activity and reduce metabolic load. However, muscle relaxants do not reduce the electrical excitation in the CNS, and cerebral metabolic stress may continue unabated.

Hemodynamic management is guided by principles of advanced cardiac life support, with some exceptions. Mild myocardial depression and systemic vasodilation can be corrected with sympathomimetic agents such as ephedrine or epinephrine. However, results from animal experiments suggest that initial bolus of epinephrine should be limited to less than 1 mcg/kg to avoid possible transformation to malignant arrhythmias.[126] Vasopressin, calcium channel blockers, and beta blockers have all been associated with possible worse hemodynamic outcome and therefore, should not be used.[125] Ventricular dysrhythmias can be managed with amiodarone; however, other classes of antiarrhythmics, especially those involving sodium and calcium channel blockades, should be avoided altogether.

Cardiovascular collapse from severe cardiac dysrhythmias is the dreaded complication associated with LAST. Historically, emergent cardiopulmonary bypass was the only effective life-saving measure for this otherwise fatal outcome[127,128]; lack of timely access and availability made resuscitation effort difficult, if not impossible. Fortunately, the introduction of lipid resuscitation therapy has largely supplanted that need. Laboratory evidence[129,130] and successive clinical reports of dramatic rescues[131,132] have supported the use of intravenous lipid emulsion in hastening the return of normal cardiac function and improving survival after local anesthetic-induced cardiotoxicity. With emphasis on timing of administration over exact dosing, current society practice advisories unequivocally recommend initiation of lipid resuscitation therapy at the first sign of dysrhythmia from suspected LAST.[119] A guide to lipid emulsion administration and summary of the American Society of Regional Anesthesia and Pain Medicine (ASRA) practice advisory on treatment of local anesthetic systemic toxicity is listed in Table 22-13.[133] A concise cognitive checklist of the practice advisory is also available from ASRA.[134]

Much remains to be understood about how lipid emulsion rapidly reverses the course of cardiovascular dysfunction related to LAST. Several mechanisms have been postulated, including the "shuttle" effect, by which lipid particles may simply act as scavenger to remove tissue-bound local anesthetics via partition principles[135] and redistribute them away from electrically sensitive organs.[136] Others assert that lipid emulsion may exert a more direct, cardiotonic function in restoring vascular tone and improving cardiac contractility, perhaps by acting as an alternative mitochondrial energy source[137] or modifying intracellular signal cascades downstream of sodium channel inhibition. These mechanisms are neither necessarily exclusive nor likely the only explanations of how lipid emulsion restore cardiac function. Multiple pathways may ultimately be involved, a testament of the broad and complicated role of sodium channel dysfunction in LAST.

Table 22-13 Practice Advisory on Treatment of Local Anesthetic Systemic Toxicity

For Patients Experiencing Signs or Symptoms of Local Anesthetic Systemic Toxicity

1. Get help at the first signs of LAST
2. Airway management
   - **Secure airway** and ventilate with 100% oxygen
   - Prevent further exacerbation by avoiding hypoxia, hypercapnia, and acidosis
3. Administer **20% Lipid Emulsion**
   - **Bolus** over 2–3 min **100 mL** for patients over 70 kg or **12 mL/kg** for less than 70 kg
   - Follow by **infusion** over 15–20 min **200–250 mL** for patients over 70 kg or **0.25 mL/kg/min** for patients less than 70 kg
   - Consider repeating bolus and increasing the infusion to 0.5 mL/kg/min if cardiovascular instability continuous
   - Maintain infusion for at least 10 min after restoration of circulatory stability
   - Recommend 12 mL/kg lipid emulsion as the upper limit for initial dosing
4. Seizure management
   - Halt seizures with **benzodiazepines**
   - Consider small dose of succinylcholine for intractable seizures to minimize acidosis and hypoxemia
5. Cardiovascular resuscitations with modified advanced cardiac life support algorithm
   - Administer small initial doses of epinephrine (less than 1 μg/kg)
   - Recommend amariodarone for ventricular arrhythmias
   - Avoid vasopressin, calcium channel blockers, beta blockers, or local anesthetics
6. Alert the nearest facility having cardiopulmonary bypass capability if cardiac instability persists
7. Continue to monitor for at least 2–6 h after the resolution of symptoms, especially for patients with significant cardiovascular morbidities

Adapted from Neal JM, Barrington MJ, Fettiplace MR, et al. The Third American Society of Regional Anesthesia and Pain Medicine practice advisory on local anesthetic systemic toxicity: Executive summary 2017. *Reg Anesth Pain Med*. 2018;43:113–123.

Neural Toxicity of Local Anesthetics

In addition to their systemic effects, direct application of local anesthetics can result in histopathologic changes consistent with neuronal injury. The causative mechanisms remain speculative, but studies in animals and tissue cultures show evidence of demyelination, Wallerian degeneration, dysregulation of axonal transport, disruption of the blood–nerve barrier, decreased blood flow to the vasanervorum, and loss of cell membrane integrity.[138,139] The degree of neural injury appears to correlate with possible intraneural placement of local anesthetic, as well as the drug concentration and the duration of exposure to the local anesthetics. Intrafascicular injections result in more histologic changes than either extrafascicular or extraneural placement, with the latter associated with the mildest damage.[140] In large concentrations, all clinically important local anesthetics can produce dose-dependent abnormalities in nerve fibers; however, in clinically relevant concentrations, they appear generally safe.[141,142]

The significance of these experimental findings is unclear, because clinical injury is rare. A systematic review of approximately 2.7 million centrally administered local anesthetic neuraxial blocks determined an occurrence of radiculopathy at approximately 0.03% and of paraplegia at approximately 0.0008%.[143] Furthermore, direct intraneural injections of local anesthetics per se do not invariably lead to detectable neurologic symptoms.[144] Nonetheless, there have been clinical scenarios in which a greater propensity for nerve injury has been described. The use of microcatheters with a high concentration of lidocaine for continuous spinal anesthesia has been associated with an increased incidence of radiculopathy and cauda equina syndrome.[145] Likewise, chloroprocaine, used until the early 1980s for epidural and intrathecal injections, has been linked to prolonged sensory and motor deficits, possibly due to toxic effects of the preservative, sodium bisulfite.[146] Although the clinical use of local anesthetics appears to be safe, it behooves the practitioner to be mindful of their potential deleterious effects on nerves.

Transient Neurologic Symptoms after Spinal Anesthesia

Prospective randomized studies reveal a 4% to 40% incidence of transient neurologic symptoms (TNSs), including pain or sensory abnormalities in the lower back, buttocks, or lower extremities, after lidocaine spinal anesthesia[147,148] (see Chapter 35). These symptoms have been reported with other local anesthetics as well (Table 22-14), but have not resulted in permanent neurologic injury.[147] Increased risk of TNSs is associated with lidocaine, the lithotomy position, and ambulatory anesthesia, but not with baricity of solution or dose of local anesthetic.[147,148] The potential neurologic etiology of this syndrome coupled with known concentration-dependent toxicity of lidocaine led to concerns over a neurotoxic etiology for TNSs from spinal lidocaine.

However, evidence for a direct linear relation between nerve toxicity and symptoms is scant. Although the concentration of local anesthetics may be a strong factor for determining nerve injury, such as with cauda equina syndrome, there does not appear to be a dose relation in TNSs. The incidence of TNSs is similar when there is a 10-fold difference in the concentration of lidocaine utilized (0.5% and 5%).[149] Furthermore, a study comparing volunteers with and without TNSs after lidocaine spinal anesthesia shows no abnormalities detectable by routine electrophysiologic testing, such as electromyography, nerve conduction, or somatosensory-evoked potentials. Finally, effective treatment for TNS includes nonsteroidal anti-inflammatory agents and trigger point injections. These are regimens more effective for alleviating myofascial pain than for neuropathic pain.[147] Overall, there is little evidence to support a neurotoxic etiology for TNSs.[128] Other potential etiologies for TNSs include patient positioning, sciatic nerve stretch, muscle spasm, and myofascial strain.[147]

Myotoxicity of Local Anesthetics

As with neural toxicity, local anesthetics can also cause histopathologic changes in skeletal muscle. Myotoxicity can result from most local anesthetic agents in clinically relevant concentrations[150] and manifest clinically as muscle pain and dysfunction. Histopathologic studies show hypercontracted myofibrils, followed by lytic degeneration of striated muscle sarcoplasmic reticulum, and diffuse myonecrosis (Fig. 22-20). The changes are drug-specific (tetracaine and procaine produce the least injury; bupivacaine the most) and both dose- and duration-dependent,[151] and seem to affect the young more than the old.[152] Experimental evidence points to disturbances in the oxidative function of mitochondria and dysregulation of intracellular calcium homeostasis as possible subcellular pathologic mechanisms.[153] In cell cultures, these disruptions appear to be diminished with coapplication with erythropoietin or *N*-acetylcysteine.[154,155] It remains to be seen if these agents may become clinically useful or necessary, because most myotoxic injuries are subclinical and appear entirely reversible.[151]

Allergic Reactions to Local Anesthetics

Untoward reactions to local anesthetics are relatively common, but true immunologic reactions are rare. The immune-mediated hypersensitivity reaction may be type I (immunoglobulin E) or type IV (cellular immunity). Type I hypersensitivity reactions can result in anaphylaxis and potentially be life-threatening, but fortunately, the incidence is estimated to be less than 1% of all reported cases. Type IV hypersensitivity reactions are delayed-type reactions mediated by T lymphocytes.[156,157] The symptoms can manifest within 12 to 48 hours of exposure and most commonly present as contact dermatitis (dermal erythema, pruritus, papules, and vesicles). The vast majority of reported hypersensitivity reactions have been associated with aminoester agents, likely due to their metabolism to *para*-aminobenzoic acid, which is a recognized allergen. Preservatives, such as methylparaben and metabisulfite that are present in many local anesthetic preparations, may also trigger allergic responses. Evaluation with skin-pricks, intradermal injections, or subcutaneous provocative dose challenges are recommended for individuals with suspected local anesthetic allergy (see also Chapter 9).[158]

Table 22-14 The Incidence of Transient Neurologic Symptoms (TNSs) Varies with Type of Spinal Local Anesthetic and Surgery

Local Anesthetic	Concentration (%)	Type of Surgery	Approximate Incidence of TNSs (%)
Lidocaine	2–5	Lithotomy position	30–36
	2–5	Knee arthroscopy	18–22
	0.5	Knee arthroscopy	17
	2–5	Mixed supine position	4–8
Mepivacaine	1.5–4	Mixed	23
Procaine	10	Knee arthroscopy	6
Bupivacaine	0.5–0.75	Mixed	1
Levobupivacaine	0.5	Mixed	1
Prilocaine	2–5	Mixed	1
Ropivacaine	0.5–0.75	Mixed	1

Data from Pollock JE. Transient neurologic symptoms: Etiology, risk factors, and management. *Reg Anesth Pain Med.* 2002;27:581–586; and Breebaart MB. Urinary bladder scanning after day-case arthroscopy under spinal anaesthesia: Comparison between lidocaine, ropivacaine, and levobupivacaine. *Br J Anaesth.* 2003;90:309–313.

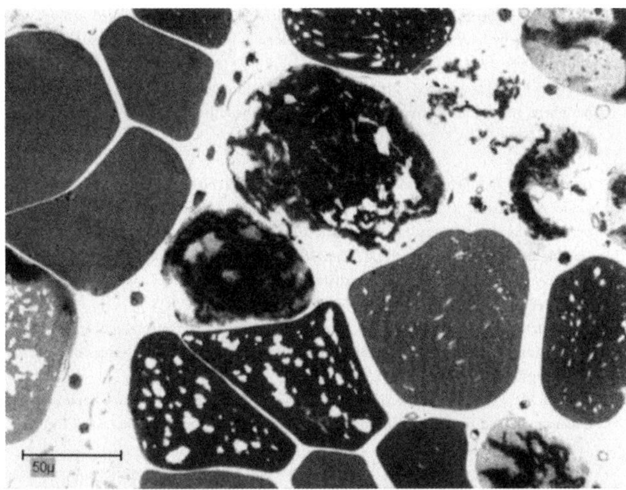

Figure 22-20 Skeletal muscle cross-section with characteristic histologic changes after continuous exposure to bupivacaine for 6 hours. A spectrum of necrobiotic changes can be encountered, ranging from slightly damaged vacuolated fibers and fibers with condensed myofibrils to entirely disintegrated and necrotic cells. The majority of the myocytes are morphologically affected. In addition, marked interstitial and myoseptal edema appears within the sections. However, scattered fibers remain intact. (Reprinted with Zink W, Graf B. Local anesthetic myotoxicity. *Reg Anesth Pain Med*. 2004;29:333–340, with permission from BMJ Publishing Group Ltd.)

Future Therapeutics and Modalities

Properties of ideal local anesthetics include selectivity for nociception, long duration of action, and absence of systemic and local tissue toxicities. Efforts to improve local anesthetics have benefitted from a better understanding of the molecular nature of pain. The identification of sodium channel isoforms and their associated channelopathies have focused much attention to developing molecules with specific channel selectivity.[159]

One of the new classes of molecules is the site 1 sodium channel blockers. They belong to a group of potent paralytic neurotoxins that reversibly antagonize voltage-gated sodium channels. In contrast to local anesthetics, they bind to the channel α-subunit extracellularly and have select affinity for channel isoforms.[160] Neosaxitoxin is a well-characterized member of this group and shares the same binding region on the channel outer pore (designated as site 1) as tetrodotoxin. Injected subcutaneously, neosaxitoxin produced hypoesthesia of a modest duration.[161] However, in combination with bupivacaine and epinephrine, neosaxitoxin extended the duration of hypoesthesia almost fivefold compared to bupivacaine alone (median duration 50 vs. 10 hours, respectively, $P = .007$).[162] Systemic adsorption can result in a dose-dependent decrease in respiratory and skeletal muscle strength[146]; however, due to its relatively poor affinity for the cardiac sodium channel (Na_v 1.5), cardiac outputs were maintained and no significant cardiac arrhythmias or arrests were seen with systemic infusion.[163] Finally, there was scant evidence of either myotoxicity or neurotoxicity with local injections.[164]

Another promising development toward long-lasting, selective analgesia focuses on modulating large-pore TRPV1 and TRPA1 to facilitate entry of impermeant sodium channel blocker into nociceptor neurons.[165] As discussed previously, TRPV1 and TRPA1 are membrane channels belonging to the transient receptor potential family. In response to heat, capsaicins, or other noxious stimuli, these channels permit passage of large, nonspecific cationic molecules into the cell. The strategy exploits the finding that their presence is restricted to primary sensory nociceptor neurons. Application of membrane impermeable local anesthetic, such as the permanently charged lidocaine QX-314, results in selective blockade of those sensory, but not motor or autonomic, neurons.[166] In animal studies, coadministration of capsaicin and QX-314 on sciatic nerves produced a long-lasting sensory block with minimal motor deficit.[166] The addition of lidocaine further prolonged the duration of the block at the expense of an initial short and concomitant period of nonselective motor block.[167] However, the duration of the sensory block was much longer than the motor block, leading to a differential blockade of approximately 16 hours (Fig. 22-21). Many questions remain to

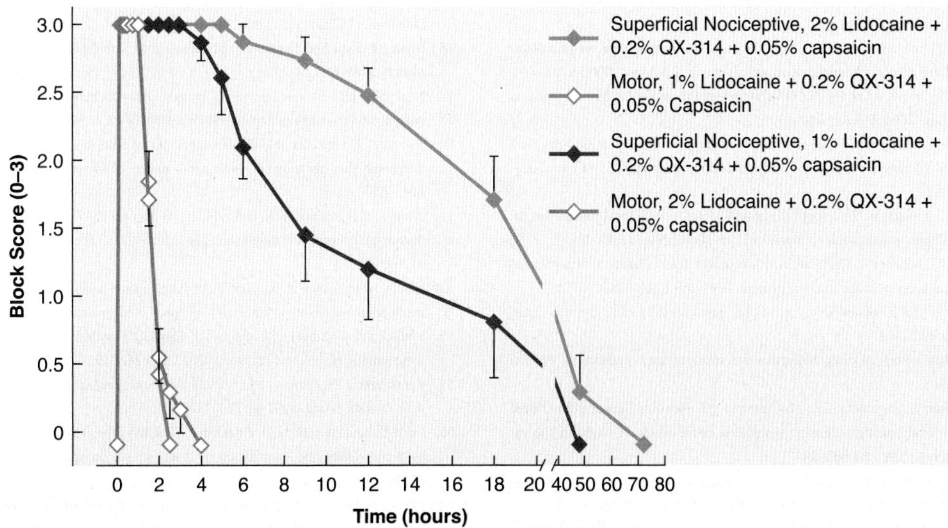

Figure 22-21 Comparison of the duration of nociceptive (*blue closed diamonds*) and motor (*blue open diamonds*) blockade produced by triple application of 1% lidocaine/capsaicin/QX-314 (*red diamonds*) or 2% lidocaine/capsaicin/QX-314 (*orange open diamonds*). Grading was as follows: 3, complete block; 2, partial block; 1, minimal block; 0, baseline. (Reprinted with permission from Binshtok AM, Gerner P, Oh SB, et al. Coapplication of lidocaine and the permanently charged sodium channel blocker QX-314 produces a long-lasting nociceptive blockade in rodents. *Anesthesiology*. 2009;111:127–137.)

be addressed before proceeding to volunteer studies. Nonetheless, if the laboratory findings are validated clinically, such combinations will be an invaluable addition to the use of local anesthetics for anesthesia and analgesia.

For further review and interactivities, please see the videos and narrative interactive clinical vignettes (NICVs) accessible in the complimentary eBook bundled with this text. Access instructions are located on the inside front cover.

REFERENCES

1. Wheater PR, Burkitt HG, Daniels VG. *Functional Histology*. 2nd ed. Churchill Livingstone; 1987:95.
2. Ritchie JM, Ritchie B, Greengard P. The effect of the nerve sheath on the action of local anesthetics. *J Pharmacol Exp Ther*. 1965;150:160–164.
3. Coggeshall RE. A fine structural analysis of the myelin sheath in rat spinal roots. *Anat Rec*. 1979;194:201–211.
4. Waxman SG, Ritchie JM. Organization of ion channels in the myelinated nerve fiber. *Science*. 1985;228:1502–1507.
5. Koester J. Passive membrane properties of the neuron. In: Kandel ER, Schwartz JH, Jessell TM. *Principles of Neuroscience*. 3rd ed. Elsevier Science; 1991.
6. Hodgkin AL, Katz B. The effect of sodium ions on the electrical activity of the giant axon of the squid. *J Physiol*. 1949;108:37–77.
7. Hodgkin AL, Huxley AF. A quantitative description of membrane current and its application to conduction and excitation in nerve. *J Physiol*. 1952;117:500–544.
8. Sigworth FJ, Neher E. Single Na+ channel currents observed in cultured rat muscle cells. *Nature*. 1980;287:447–449.
9. Catterall WA. From ionic currents to molecular mechanisms: The structure and function of voltage-gated sodium channels. *Neuron*. 2000;26:13–25.
10. Hirschberg B, Rovner A, Lieberman M, Patlak J. Transfer of twelve charges is needed to open skeletal muscle Na^+ channels. *J Gen Physiol*. 1995;106:1053–1068.
11. Heinemann SH, Terlau H, Stühmer W, Imoto K, Numa S. Calcium channel characteristics conferred on the sodium channel by single mutations. *Nature*. 1992;356:441–443.
12. Armstrong CM. Sodium channels and gating currents. *Physiol Rev*. 1981;61:644–683.
13. Stühmer W, Conti F, Suzuki H, et al. Structural parts involved in activation and inactivation of the sodium channel. *Nature*. 1989;339:597–603.
14. West JW, Patton DE, Scheuer T, Wang Y, Goldin AL, Catterall WA. A cluster of hydrophobic amino acid residues required for fast Na(+)-channel inactivation. *Proc Natl Acad Sci USA*. 1992;89:10910–10914.
15. Woods JN, Boorman JP, Okuse K, Baker MD. Voltage-gated sodium channels and pain pathways. *J Neurobiol*. 2004;61:55–71.
16. Drenth JPH, te Morsche RHM, Guillet G, Taieb A, Kirby RL, Jansen JBMJ. SCN9A mutations define primary erythermalgia as a neuropathic disorder of voltage gated sodium channels. *J Invest Dermatol*. 2005;124:1333–1338.
17. Fertleman CR, Baker MD, Parker KA, et al. SCN9A mutations in paroxysmal extreme pain disorder: Allelic variants underlie distinct channel defects and phenotypes. *Neuron*. 2006;52:767–774.
18. Cox JJ, Reimann F, Nicholas AK, et al. An SCN9A channelopathy causes congenital inability to experience pain. *Nature*. 2006;444:894–898.
19. Goldberg Y, Macfarlane J, Macdonald M, et al. Loss-of-function mutations in the Na(v) 1.7 gene underlie congenital indifference to pain in multiple human populations. *Clin Genet*. 2007;71:311–319.
20. Frazier DT, Narahashi T, Yamada M. The site of action and active form of local anesthetics. II. Experiments with quaternary compounds. *J Pharmacol Exp Ther*. 1970;171:45–51.
21. Ragsdale DS, McPhee JC, Scheuer T, Catterall WA. Molecular determinants of state-dependent block of Na^+ channels by local anesthetics. *Science*. 1994;265:1724–1728.
22. Scholz A. Mechanisms of (local) anaesthetics on voltage-gated sodium and other ion channels. *Br J Anaesth*. 2002;89:52–61.
23. Ulbricht W. Sodium channel inactivation: Molecular determinants and modulation. *Physiol Rev*. 2005;85:1271–1301.
24. Popitz-Bergez FA, Leeson S, Strichartz GR, Thalhammer JG. Relation between functional deficit and intraneural local anesthetic during peripheral nerve block. A study in the rat sciatic nerve. *Anesthesiology*. 1995;83:583–592.
25. Fink BR, Cairns AM. Differential slowing and block of conduction by lidocaine in individual afferent myelinated and unmyelinated axons. *Anesthesiology*. 1984;60:111–120.
26. Fink BR, Cairns AM. Differential use-dependent (frequency-dependent) effects in single mammalian axons: Data and clinical considerations. *Anesthesiology*. 1987;67:477–484.
27. Fink BR. Mechanisms of differential axial blockade in epidural and subarachnoid anesthesia. *Anesthesiology*. 1989;70:851–858.
28. Gasser HS, Erlanger J. The role of fiber size in the establishment of a nerve block by pressure or cocaine. *Am J Physiol*. 1929;88:581–591.
29. Gokin AP, Philip B, Strichartz GR. Preferential block of small myelinated sensory and motor fibers by lidocaine: In vivo electrophysiology in the rat sciatic nerve. *Anesthesiology*. 2001;95:1441–1454.
30. Chevrier P, Vijayaragavan K, Chahine M. Differential modulation of Nav 1.7 and Nav 1.8 peripheral nerve sodium channels by the local anesthetic lidocaine. *Br J Pharmacol*. 2004;142:576–584.
31. Leffler A, Fischer MJ, Rehner D, et al. The vanilloid receptor TRPV1 is activated and sensitized by local anesthetics in rodent sensory neurons. *J Clin Invest*. 2008;118:763–776.
32. Leffler A, Lattrell A, Kronewald S, Niedermirtl F, Nau C. Activation of TRPA1 by membrane permeable local anesthetics. *Molecular Pain*. 2011;7:62.
33. Narahashi T, Frazier DT, Yamada M. The site of action and active form of local anesthetics. I. Theory and pH experiments with tertiary compounds. *J Pharmacol and Exp Therap*. 1970;171:32–44.
34. Strichartz GR, Sanchez V, Arthur GR, Chafetz R, Martin D. Fundamental properties of local anesthetics. II. Measured octanol: Buffer partition coefficients and pK_a values of clinically used drugs. *Anesth Analg*. 1990;71:158–170.
35. Bokesch PM, Post C, Strichartz G. Structure-activity relationship of lidocaine homologs producing tonic and frequency-dependent impulse blockade in nerve. *J Pharmacol Exp Ther*. 1986;237:773–781.
36. Gissen AJ, Covino BG, Gregus J. Differential sensitivity of fast and slow fibers in mammalian nerve. III. Effect of etidocaine and bupivacaine on fast/slow fibers. *Anesth Analg*. 1982;61:570–575.
37. Johns RA, DiFazio CA, Longnecker DE. Lidocaine constricts or dilates rat arterioles in a dose-dependent manner. *Anesthesiology*. 1985;62:141–144.
38. Johns RA, Seyde WC, DiFazio CA, Longnecker DE. Dose-dependent effects of bupivacaine on rat muscle arterioles. *Anesthesiology*. 1986;65:186–191.
39. Foster RH, Markham A. Levobupivacaine: A review of its pharmacology and use as a local anaesthetic. *Drugs*. 2000;59:551–579.
40. McClellan KJ, Faulds D. Ropivacaine: An update of its use in regional anaesthesia. *Drugs*. 2000;60:1065–1093.
41. Neal JM. Effects of epinephrine in local anesthetics on the central and peripheral nervous systems: Neurotoxicity and neural blood flow. *Reg Anesth Pain Med*. 2003;28:124–134.
42. Sinnott CJ, Cogswell III LP, Johnson A, Strichartz GR. On the mechanism by which epinephrine potentiates lidocaine's peripheral nerve block. *Anesthesiology*. 2003;98:181–188.
43. Curatolo M, Petersen-Felix S, Arendt-Nielsen L, Zbinden AM. Epidural epinephrine and clonidine: Segmental analgesia and effects on different pain modalities. *Anesthesiology*. 1997;87:785–794.
44. Ueda W, Hirakawa M, Mori K. Acceleration of epinephrine absorption by lidocaine. *Anesthesiology*. 1985;63:717–720.
45. Magee C, Rodeheaver GT, Edgerton MT, Golden GT, Haury B, Edlich RF. Studies of the mechanisms by which epinephrine damages tissue defenses. *J Surg Res*. 1977;23:126–131.
46. Hall JA, Ferro A. Myocardial ischaemia and ventricular arrhythmias precipitated by physiological concentrations of adrenaline in patients with coronary artery disease. *Br Heart J*. 1992;67:419.
47. Lambert DH. Clinical value of adding sodium bicarbonate to local anesthetics. *Reg Anesth Pain Med*. 2002;27:328–329.
48. Ikuta PT, Raza SM, Durrani Z. pH adjustment schedule for the amide local anesthetics. *Reg Anesth*. 1989;14:229–235.
49. Neal JM, Hebl JR, Gerancher JC, Hogan QH. Brachial plexus anesthesia: essentials of our current understanding. *Reg Anesth Pain Med*. 2002;27:402–428.
50. Sinnott CJ, Garfield JM, Thalhammer JG. Addition of sodium bicarbonate to lidocaine decreases the duration of peripheral nerve block in the rat. *Anesthesiology*. 2000;93:1045–1052.
51. Wang C, Chakrabarti MK, Galletly DC, Whitwam JG. Relative effects of intrathecal administration of fentanyl and midazolam on A delta and C fibre reflexes. *Neuropharmacology*. 1992;31:439–444.
52. Niv D, Nemirovsky A, Rudick V. Antinociception induced by simultaneous intrathecal and intraperitoneal administration of low doses of morphine. *Anesth Analg*. 1995;80:886–889.
53. Walker SM, Goudas LC, Cousins MJ, Carr DB. Combination spinal analgesic chemotherapy: A systematic review. *Anesth Analg*. 2002;95:674–715.
54. Karambelkar DJ, Ramanathan S. 2-chloroprocaine antagonism of epidural morphine analgesia. *Acta Anaesth Scand*. 1997;41:774–778.
55. Coda B, Bausch S, Haas M, Chavkin C. The hypothesis that antagonism of fentanyl analgesia by 2-chloroprocaine is mediated by direct action on opioid receptors. *Reg Anesth*. 1997;22:43–52.
56. Janson W, Stein C. Peripheral opioid analgesia. *Curr Pharm Biotechnol*. 2003;4:270–274.
57. Picard PR, Tramer MR, McQuay HJ, Moore RA. Analgesic efficacy of peripheral opioids (all except intra-articular): A qualitative systematic review of randomised controlled trials. *Pain*. 1997;72:309–318.
58. Candido KD, Winnie AP, Ghaleb AH, Fattouh MW, Franco CD. Buprenorphine added to the local anesthetic for axillary brachial plexus block prolongs postoperative analgesia. *Reg Anesth Pain Med*. 2002;27:162–167.

59. Candido KD, Hennes J, Gonzalez S, et al. Buprenorphine enhances and prolongs the postoperative analgesic effect of bupivacaine in patients receiving infragluteal sciatic nerve block. *Anesthesiology*. 2010;113:1419–1426.
60. Rosseland LA. No evidence for analgesic effect of intra-articular morphine after knee arthroscopy: A qualitative systematic review. *Reg Anesth Pain Med*. 2005;30:83–98.
61. Eisenach JC, De Kock M, Klimscha W. Alpha(2)-adrenergic agonists for regional anesthesia: A clinical review of clonidine (1984–1995). *Anesthesiology*. 1996;85:655–674.
62. Butterworth JF, Strichartz GR. The α_2-adrenergic agonists clonidine and guanfacine produce tonic and phasic block of conduction in rat sciatic nerve fibers. *Anesth Analg*. 1993;76:295–301.
63. Gaumann DM, Brunet PC, Jirounek P. Clonidine enhances the effects of lidocaine on C fiber action potential. *Anesth Analg*. 1992;74:719–725.
64. Pertovaara A, Hamalainen MM. Spinal potentiation and supraspinal additivity in the antinociceptive interaction between systemically administered α_2-adrenoreceptor agonist and cocaine in the rat. *Anesth Analg*. 1994;79:261–266.
65. Popping DM, Elia N, Marret E, Wenk M, Tramèr MR. Clonidine as an adjuvant to local anesthetics for peripheral nerve and plexus blocks. *Anesthesiology*. 2009;111:406–415.
66. Colin JL, McCartney ED, Apatu E. Should we add clonidine to local anesthetic for peripheral nerve blockade? A qualitative systematic review of the literature. *Reg Anesth Pain Med*. 2007;32:330–338.
67. Curley J, Castillo J, Hotz J, et al. Prolonged regional nerve blockade: Injectable biodegradable bupivacaine/polyester microspheres. *Anesthesiology*. 1996;84:1401–1410.
68. Drager C, Benziger D, Gao F, Berde CB. Prolonged intercostal nerve blockade in sheep using controlled-release of bupivacaine and dexamethasone from polymer microspheres. *Anesthesiology*. 1998;89:969–979.
69. Castillo J, Curley J, Hotz J, et al. Glucocorticoids prolong rat sciatic nerve blockade in vivo from bupivacaine microspheres. *Anesthesiology*. 1996;85:1157–1166.
70. Parrington SJ, O'Donnell D, Chan VWS, et al. Dexamethasone added to mepivacaine prolongs the duration of analgesia after supraclavicular brachial plexus blockade. *Reg Anesth Pain Med*. 2010;35:422–426.
71. Cummings 3rd KC, Napierkowski DE, Parra-Sanchez I, et al. Effect of dexamethasone on the duration of interscalene nerve blocks with ropivacaine or bupivacaine. *Br J Anaesth*. 2011;107:446–453.
72. Liu J, Richman KA, Grodofsky SR, et al. Is there a dose response of dexamethasone as adjuvant for supraclavicular brachial plexus nerve block? A prospective randomized double-blinded clinical study. *J Clin Anesth*. 2015;27:237–242.
73. Rahangdale R, Kendall MC, McCarthy RJ, et al. The effects of perineural versus intravenous dexamethasone on sciatic nerve blockade outcomes: a randomized, double-blind, placebo-controlled study. *Anesth Analg*. 2014;118:1113–1119.
74. Hauritz RW, Hannig KE, Henriksen CW, Børglum J, Bjørn S, Bendtsen TF. The effect of perineural dexamethasone on duration of sciatic nerve blockade: a randomized, double-blinded study. *Acta Anaesthesiol Scand*. 2018;62:548–557.
75. Bjorn S, Linde F, Nielsen KK, Børglum J, Hauritz RW, Bendtsen TF. Effect of perineural dexamethasone on the duration of single injection saphenous nerve block for analgesia after major ankle surgery: a randomized, controlled study. *Reg Anesth Pain Med*. 2017;42:210–216.
76. Albrecht E, Kern C, Kirkham KR. A systematic review and meta-analysis of perineural dexamethasone for peripheral nerve blocks. *Anaesthesia*. 2015;70:71–83.
77. Tan ESJ, Tan YR, Liu CWY. Efficacy of perineural versus intravenous dexamethasone in prolonging the duration of analgesia when administered with peripheral nerve blocks: a systemic review and meta-analysis. *Korean J Anesthesiol*. 2022;75:255–265.
78. Albrecht E, Reynvoet M, Fournier N, Desmet M. Dose-response relationship of perineural dexamethasone for interscalene brachial plexus block: a randomized, controlled, triple-blind trial. *Anaesthesia*. 2019;74:1001–1008.
79. Kirkham KR, Jacot-Guillarmod A, Albrecht E. Optimal dose of perineural dexamethasone to prolong analgesia after brachial plexus blockade: a systematic review and meta-analysis. *Reg Anesth Pain Med*. 2018;126:270–279.
80. Rousseau GG, Baxter JD. Glucocorticoid receptors. *Monogr Endocrinol*. 1979;12:49–77.
81. De Oliverira GS Jr, Almeida MD, Benzon HT, McCarthy RJ. Perioperative single dose systemic dexamethasone for postoperative pain: a meta-analysis of randomized controlled trials. *Anesthesiology*. 2011;115:575–588.
82. Marhofer P, Columb M, Hopkins PM. Perineural dexamethasone: the dilemma of systemic reviews and meta-analysis. *Br J Anaesth*. 2018;120:201–203.
83. Short A, El-Boghdadly K, Clark H, et al. Effect of intravenous dexamethasone on the anaesthetic characteristics of peripheral nerve block: a double-blind, randomized controlled, dose-response volunteer study. *Br J Anaesth*. 2020;124:92–100.
84. Marhofer P, Columb M, Hopkins PM, et al. Dexamethasone as an adjuvant for peripheral nerve blockade: a randomized, triple-blinded crossover study in volunteers. *Br J Anaesth*. 2019;122:525–531.
85. Hussain N, Brull R, Sheehy BT, et al. Perineural liposomal bupivacaine is not superior to nonliposomal bupivacaine for peripheral nerve block analgesia. *Anesthesiology*. 2021:134;147–164.
86. Ilfeld BM, Eisenach JC, Gabriel RA. Clinical effectiveness of liposomal bupivacaine administered by infiltration or peripheral nerve block to treat postoperative pain: a narrative revew. *Anesthesiology*. 2021;134:283–244.
87. Kim DH, Liu JB, Beathe JC, et al. Interscalene brachial plexus block with liposomal bupivacaine versus standard bupivacaine with perineural dexamethasone: a noninferiority trial. *Anesthesiology*. 2022;136:434–447.
88. McAlvin JB, Padera RF, Shankarappa SA, et al. Multivesicular liposomal bupivacaine at the sciatic nerve. *Biomaterials*. 2014;35:4557–4564.
89. Viscusi ER, Candiotti KA, Onel E, Morren M, Ludbrook GL. The pharmacokinetics and pharmacodynamics of liposome bupivacaine administered via a single epidural injection to healthy volunteers. *Reg Anesth Pain Med*. 2012;37:616–622.
90. Ilfeld BM, Viscusi ER, Hadzic A, et al. Safety and side effect profile of liposome bupivacaine (Exparel) in peripheral nerve blocks. *Reg Anesth Pain Med*. 2015;40:572–582.
91. Morrison LM, Emanuelsson BM, McClure JH, et al. Efficacy and kinetics of extradural ropivacaine: comparison with bupivacaine. *Br J Anaesth*. 1994;72:164–169.
92. Tucker GT, Mather LE. Pharmacology of local anaesthetic agents: Pharmacokinetics of local anaesthetic agents. *Br J Anaesth*. 1975;47(suppl):213–224.
93. Thomson PD, Melmon KL, Richardson JA, et al. Lidocaine pharmacokinetics in advanced heart failure, liver disease, and renal failure in humans. *Ann Intern Med*. 1973;78:499–508.
94. Rosenberg PR, Veering BT, Urmey WF. Maximum recommended doses of local anesthetics: A multifactorial concept. *Reg Anesth Pain Med*. 2004;29:564–575.
95. Braid DP, Scott DB. Dosage of lignocaine in epidural block in relation to toxicity. *Br J Anaesth*. 1996;38:596.
96. Adinoff B, Devous Sr MD, Best SE, et al. Gender differences in limbic responsiveness, by SPECT, following pharmacologic challenge in healthy subjects. *Neuroimage*. 2003;18:697–706.
97. Tucker GT, Mather LE. Properties, absorption, and disposition of local anesthetic agents. In: Cousins MJ, Bridenbaugh PO, eds. *Neural Blockade in Clinical Anesthesia and Management of Pain*. 3rd ed. Lippincott- Raven Publishers; 1998:55.
98. Ugur B, Ogurlu M, Gezer E, Aydin ON, Gürsoy F. Effects of esmolol, lidocaine and fentanyl on haemodynamic responses to endotracheal intubation: a comparative study. *Clin Drug Investig*. 2007;27:269–277.
99. Adamzik M, Groeben H, Farahani R, Lehmann N, Peters J. Intravenous lidocaine after tracheal intubation mitigates bronchoconstriction in patients with asthma. *Anesth Analg*. 2007;104:168–172.
100. Groban L. Central nervous system and cardiac effects from long-acting amide local anesthetic toxicity in the intact animal model. *Reg Anesth Pain Med*. 2003;28:3–11.
101. Weinberg GL. Current concepts in resuscitation of patients with local anesthetic cardiac toxicity. *Reg Anesth Pain Med*. 2002;27:568–575.
102. Butterworth JF. Models and mechanisms of local anesthetic cardiac toxicity. *Reg Anesth Pain Med*. 2010;35:167–176.
103. Mather LE, Copeland SE, Ladd LA. Acute toxicity of local anesthetics: underlying pharmacokinetic and pharmacodynamic concepts. *Reg Anesth Pain Med*. 2005;30:553–566.
104. Knudsen K, Beckman Suurkula M, Blomberg S, Sjövall J, Edvardsson N. Central nervous and cardiovascular effects of i.v. infusions of ropivacaine, bupivacaine and placebo in volunteers. *Br J Anaesth*. 1997;78:507–514.
105. Stewart J, Kellett N, Castro D. The central nervous system and cardiovascular effects of levobupivacaine and ropivacaine in healthy volunteers. *Anesth Analg*. 2002;97:412–416.
106. Vanhoutte F, Vereecke J, Verbeke N, Carmeliet E. Stereoselective effects of the enantiomers of bupivacaine on the electrophysiological properties of the guinea-pig papillary muscle. *Br J Pharmacol*. 1991;103:1275–1281.
107. Valenzuela C, Snyders DJ, Bennett PB, Tamargo J, Hondeghem LM. Stereoselective block of sodium channels by bupivacaine in guinea pig ventricular myocytes. *Circulation*. 1995;92:3014–3024.
108. Groban L, Deal DD, Vernon JC, James RL, Butterworth J. Does local anesthetic stereoselectivity or structure predict myocardial depression in anesthetized canines? *Reg Anesth Pain Med*. 2002;27:460–468.
109. Pickering AE, Waki H, Headley PM, Paton JFR. Investigation of systemic bupivacaine toxicity using the in situ perfused working heart-brainstem preparation of the rat. *Anesthesiology*. 2002;97:1550–1556.
110. Chang KSK, Yang M, Andresen MC. Clinically relevant concentrations of bupivacaine inhibit rat aortic baroreceptors. *Anesth Analg*. 1994;78:501–506.
111. Newton DJ, McLeod GA, Khan F, Belch JJF. Vasoactive characteristics of bupivacaine and levobupivacaine with and without adjuvant epinephrine in peripheral human skin. *Br J Anaesth*. 2005;94:662–667.
112. Liu P, Feldman HS, Covina BM, Giasi R, Covino BG. Acute cardiovascular toxicity of intravenous amide local anesthetics in anesthetized ventilated dogs. *Anesth Analg*. 1982;61:317–322.
113. Guo XT, Castle NA, Chernoff DM, Strichartz GR. Comparative inhibition of voltage-gated cation channels by local anesthetics. *Ann N Y Acad Sci*. 1991;625:181–199.
114. Clarkson CW, Hondegham LM. Mechanisms for bupivacaine depression of cardiac conduction: fast block of sodium channels during the action potential with slow recovery from block during diastole. *Anesthesiology*. 1985;62:396–405.

115. Nouette-Gaulain K, Forestier F, Malgat M, Marthan R, Mazat J-P, Sztark F. Effects of bupivacaine on mitochondrial energy metabolism in heart of rats following exposure to chronic hypoxia. *Anesthesiology*. 2002;97:1507–1511.
116. Wong GK, Crawford MW. Carnitine deficiency increases susceptibility to bupivacaine-induced cardiotoxicity in rats. *Anesthesiology*. 2011;114:1417–1424.
117. Di Gregorio G, Neal JM, Rosenquist RW, Weinberg GL. Clinical presentation of local anesthetic systemic toxicity. A review of published cases, 1979–2009. *Reg Anesth Pain Med*. 2010;35:181–187.
118. Gitman M, Barrington MJ. Local anesthetic systemic toxicity: a review of recent case reports and registries. *Reg Anesth Pain Med*. 2018;43:124–130.
119. Neal JM, Bernards CM, Butterworth JF, et al. ASRA practice advisory on local anesthetic systemic toxicity. *Reg Anesth Pain Med*. 2010;35:152–161.
120. Morwald EE, Zubizarreta N, Cozowicx C, Poeran J, Memtsoudis SG. Incidence of local anesthetic systemic toxicity in orthopedic patients receiving peripheral nerve blocks. *Reg Anesth Pain Med*. 2017;42:442–445.
121. Rubin DS, Matsumoto MM, Weinberg G, Roth S. Local anesthetic systemic toxicity in total joint arthroplasty: incidence and risk factors in the United States from the national inpatient sample 1998–2013. *Reg Anesth Pain Med*. 2018;43:131–137.
122. Liu SS, Ortolan S, Vizarreta Sandoval M, et al. Cardiac arrest and seizures caused by local anesthetic systemic toxicity after peripheral nerve blocks: should we still fear the reaper? *Reg Anesth Pain Med*. 2016;41:5–21.
123. Moller RA, Datta S, Fox J, Johnson M, Covino BG. Effects of progesterone on the cardiac electrophysiologic action of bupivacaine and lidocaine. *Anesthesiology*. 1992;76:604–608.
124. Tsen LC, Tarshis J, Denson DD, Osathanondh R, Datta S, Bader AM. Measurements of maternal protein binding of bupivacaine throughout pregnancy. *Anesth Analg*, 1999;89:965–968.
125. Weinberg GL. Treatment of local anesthetic systemic toxicity (LAST). *Reg Anesth Pain Med*. 2010;35:188.
126. Wang QG, Wu C, Xia Y, et al. Epinephrine deteriorates pulmonary gas exchange in a rat model of bupivacaine-induced cardiotoxicity: a threshold dose of epinephrine. *Reg Anesth Pain Med*. 2017;42:342–350.
127. Long WB, Rosenblum S, Grady IP. Successful resuscitation of bupivacaine-induced cardiac arrest using cardiopulmonary bypass. *Anesth Analg*. 1989;79:403–406.
128. Soltesz EG, van Pelt F, Byrne JG. Emergent cardiopulmonary bypass for bupivacaine cardiotoxicity. *J Cardiothorac Vasc Anesth*. 2003;17:357–358.
129. Weinberg GL, VadeBoncouer T, Ramaraju GA, Garcia-Amaro MF, Cwik MJ. Pretreatment or resuscitation with a lipid infusion shifts the dose-response to bupivacaine-induced asystole in rats. *Anesthesiology*. 1998;99:1071–1075.
130. Weinberg G, Ripper R, Feinstein DL, Hoffman W. Lipid emulsion infusion rescues dogs from bupivacaine-induced cardiac toxicity. *Reg Anesth Pain Med*. 2003;28:198–202.
131. Rosenblatt MA, Abel M, Fischer GW, Itzkovich CJ, Eisenkraft JB. Successful use of a 20% lipid emulsion to resuscitate a patient after a presumed bupivacaine-related cardiac arrest. *Anesthesiology*. 2006;105:217–218.
132. Litz RJ, Popp M, Stehr SN, Koch T. Successful resuscitation of a patient with ropivacaine-induced asystole after axillary plexus block using lipid infusion. *Anaesthesia*. 2006;61:800–801.
133. Neal JM, Barrington MJ, Fettiplace MR, et al. The Third American Society of Regional Anesthesia and Pain Medicine practice advisory on local anesthetic systemic toxicity: Executive summary 2017. *Reg Anesth Pain Med*. 2018;43:113–123.
134. Neal JM, Neal EJ, Weinberg GL. American society of regional anesthesia and pain medicine local anesthetic systemic toxicity checklist: 2020 version. *Reg Anesth Pain Med*. 2021;46:81–82.
135. Weinberg GL, Ripper R, Murphy P, et al. Lipid infusion accelerates removal of bupivacaine and recovery from bupivacaine toxicity in the isolated rat heart. *Reg Anesth Pain Med*. 2006;31:296–303.
136. Fettiplace MR, Weinberg G. The mechanisms underlying lipid resuscitation therapy. *Reg Anesth Pain Med*. 2018;43:138–149.
137. Weinberg GL, Palmer JW, VadeBoncouer TR, Zuechner MB, Edelman G, Hoppel CL. Bupivacaine inhibits acylcarnitine exchange in cardiac mitochondria. *Anesthesiology*. 2000;92:523–528.
138. Kitagawa N, Oda M, Totoki T. Possible mechanism of irreversible nerve injury caused by local anesthetics and membrane disruption. *Anesthesiology*. 2004;100:962–967.
139. Kalichman MW. Physiologic mechanisms by which local anesthetics may cause injury to nerve and spinal cord. *Reg Anesth*. 1993;18:448–452.
140. Whitlock EL, Brenner MJ, Fox IK, Moradzadeh A, Hunter DA, Mackinnon SE. Ropivacaine-induced peripheral nerve injection injury in the rodent model. *Anesth Analg*. 2010;111:214–220.
141. Selander D. Neurotoxicity of local anesthetics: animal data. *Reg Anesth*. 1993;18:461–468.
142. Kroin JS, Buvanendran A, Williams DK, et al. Local anesthetic sciatic nerve block and nerve fiber damage in diabetic rats. *Reg Anesth Pain Med*. 2010;35:343–350.
143. Brull R, McCartney CJL, Chan VWS, El-Beheiry H. Neurological complications after regional anesthesia: contemporary estimates of risk. *Anesth Analg*. 2007;104:965–974.
144. Bigeleisen PE. Nerve puncture and apparent intraneural injection during ultrasound-guided axillary block does not invariably result in neurologic injury. *Anesthesiology*. 2006;105:779–783.
145. Rigler M, Drasner K, Krejcie T, et al. Cauda equina syndrome after continuous spinal anesthesia. *Anesth Analg*. 1991;72:275–281.
146. Reisner L, Hochman B, Plumer M. Persistent neurologic deficit and adhesive arachnoiditis following intrathecal 2-chloroprocaine injection. *Anesth Analg*. 1980;58:452–454.
147. Pollock JE. Transient neurologic symptoms: etiology, risk factors, and management. *Reg Anesth Pain Med*. 2002;27:581–586.
148. Zaric D, Christiansen C, Pace NL, Punjasawadwong Y. Transient neurologic symptoms after spinal anesthesia with lidocaine versus other local anesthetics: a systematic review of randomized, controlled trials. *Anesth Analg*. 2005;100:1811–1816.
149. Pollock JE, Liu SS, Neal JM, Stephenson CA. Dilution of lidocaine does not decrease the incidence of transient neurologic symptoms. *Anesthesiology*. 1999;90:445–450.
150. Hogan Q, Dotson R, Erickson S, Kettler R, Hogan K. Local anesthetic myotoxicity: a case and review. *Anesthesiology*. 1994;80:942–947.
151. Zink W, Bohl JRE, Hacke N, Sinner B, Martin E, Graf BM. The long-term myotoxic effects of bupivacaine and ropivacaine after continuous peripheral nerve blocks. *Anesth Analg*. 2005;101:548–554.
152. Nouette-Gaulain K, Dadure C, Morau D, et al. Age-dependent bupivacaine-induced muscle toxicity during continuous peripheral nerve block in rats. *Anesthesiology*. 2009;111:1120–1127.
153. Nouette-Gaulain K, Sirvent P, Canal-Raffin M, et al. Effects of intermittent femoral nerve injections of bupivacaine, levobupivacaine, and ropivacaine on mitochondrial energy metabolism and intracellular calcium homeostasis in rat psoas muscle. *Anesthesiology*. 2007;106:1026–1034.
154. Nouette-Gaulain K, Bellance N, Prevost B, et al. Erythropoietin protects against local anesthetic myotoxicity during continuous regional anesthesia. *Anesthesiology*. 2009;110:648–659.
155. Galbes O, Bourret A, Nouette-Gaulain K, et al. N-Acetylcysteine protects against bupivacaine-induced myotoxicity caused by oxidative and sarcoplasmic reticulum stress in human skeletal myotubes. *Anesthesiology*. 2010;113:560–569.
156. Boren E, Teuber SS, Naguwa SM, Gershwin ME. A critical review of local anesthetic sensitivity. *Clin Rev Allergy Immunol*. 2007;32:119–128.
157. Phillips JF, Yates AB, Deshazo RD. Approach to patients with suspected hypersensitivity to local anesthetics. *Am J Med Sci*. 2007;334:190–196.
158. McClimon B, Rank M, Li J. The predictive value of skin testing in the diagnosis of local anesthetic allergy. *Allergy Asthma Proc*. 2011;32:95–98.
159. Kwong K, Carr MJ. Voltage-gated sodium channels. *Curr Opin Pharmacol*. 2015;22:131.
160. Catterall WA. Neurotoxins that act on voltage-sensitive sodium channels in excitable membranes. *Annu Rev Pharmacol Toxicol*. 1980;20:15–43.
161. Rodriguez-Navarro AJ, Lagos N, Lagos M, et al. Neosaxitoxin as a local anesthetic: preliminary observations from a first human trial. *Anesthesiology*. 2007;106:339–345.
162. Lobo K, Donado C, Cornelissen L, et al. A phase 1, dose-escalation, double-blind, block-randomized, controlled trial of safety and efficacy of neosaxitoxin alone and in combination with 0.2% bupivacaine, with and without epinephrine for cutaneous anesthesia. *Anesthesiology*. 2015;123;873–885.
163. Wylie MC, Johnson VM, Carpino E, et al. Respiratory, neuromuscular, and cardiovascular effects of neosaxitoxin in isoflurane-anesthetized sheep. *Reg Anesth Pain Med*. 2012;37:152–158.
164. Templin JS, Wylie MC, Kim JD, et al. Improved therapeutic index using combinations with bupivacaine, with and without epinephrine. *Anesthesiology*. 2015;123;886–898.
165. Roberson DP, Binshtok AM, Blasl F, Bean BP, Woolf CJ. Targeting of sodium channel blockers into nociceptors to produce long-duration analgesia: a systemic study and review. *Br J Pharmacol*. 2011;164:48–58.
166. Binshtok AM, Bean BP, Woolf CJ. Inhibition of nociceptors by TRPV1-mediated entry of impermeant sodium channel blockers. *Nature*. 2007;449;607–610.
167. Binshtok AM, Gerner P, Oh SB, et al. Coapplication of lidocaine and the permanently charged sodium channel blocker QX-314 produces a long-lasting nociceptive blockade in rodents. *Anesthesiology*. 2009;111:127–137.

Section 5

PREOPERATIVE ASSESSMENT AND PERIOPERATIVE MONITORING

23 Preoperative Patient Assessment and Management

TARA M. HATA • LAUREN KEMP LICINA • DANIEL J. WYLER

KEY POINTS

1. The goals of a preoperative evaluation are to reduce patient risk and morbidity associated with surgery and anesthesia, prepare the patient medically and psychologically, and also promote efficiency and reduce costs.
2. The anesthesiologist is responsible for assessing the medical condition of the patient and developing the anesthesia plan of care. The American Society of Anesthesiologists (ASA) published basic standards for preoperative care, as well as an updated practice advisory for preanesthesia evaluation that details evidence-supported recommendations.
3. It is important for the evaluation to be complete, accurate, and clear, not only to allow the information to be relayed to others who may care for the patient perioperatively but also for medicolegal purposes.
4. The preoperative evaluation serves as a screening tool to anticipate and avoid airway difficulties or problems with anesthetic drugs. In addition to the history and physical examination, previous anesthetic records should be reviewed and contraindications to specific drugs, such as succinylcholine, nitrous oxide, or volatile agents, should be sought.
5. A review of the patient's medication list, including over-the-counter and herbal preparations, should investigate potential drug interactions and potential indications for stress dose steroid coverage. The anesthesiologist should be aware of the patient's allergies and previous drug reactions, including the possibility of latex allergy.
6. When evaluating the patient with hypertension, diabetes mellitus, or obesity, it is important to determine the presence of end-organ damage, such as cardiovascular disease.
7. Exercise tolerance is a significant predictor of cardiac risk. Multiple specialty groups have contributed to formal guidelines for the perioperative cardiovascular evaluation and management of patients undergoing noncardiac procedures. The algorithms provide useful guides for further testing and evaluation.
8. Preoperative laboratory tests should be ordered on the basis of positive findings from the history and physical examination or from anticipated physiologic disturbances during surgery, such as blood loss.
9. Optimization of the patient's health status prior to surgery includes clear instruction regarding fasting times as well as which medications to continue until the time of surgery. In general, most medications for hypertension or cardiac disease should be continued, and consideration should be given to initiating β-blocker therapy before the day of surgery in appropriate patients who are at risk for cardiac adverse events. The need for subacute bacterial endocarditis prophylaxis should be anticipated. Likewise, drugs for asthma or chronic obstructive pulmonary disease should be continued or administered prophylactically. Medications taken for the treatment of esophageal reflux should be continued or initiated for those patients with untreated symptoms. For diabetic patients, oral hypoglycemic agents should often be held, but patients requiring insulin will need to continue to take adjusted doses.
10. Although preoperative sedation is generally limited to drugs given immediately prior to anesthesia, the administration must be carefully planned to allow optimal effect and avoid operating room delays.

Introduction

1 The goals of a preoperative evaluation are to reduce patient risk and morbidity associated with surgery and anesthesia, prepare the patient medically and psychologically, and promote efficiency
2 and cost-consciousness. As we continue to expand our care at the extremes of age, we are held accountable for high-quality standards while we work to reduce costs. The Joint Commission on Accreditation of Healthcare Organizations (JCAHO) requires all patients undergo a preoperative anesthetic evaluation. The American Society of Anesthesiologists (ASA) website contains the ASA Basic Standards for Preanesthetic Care that outline the minimum requirements for a preoperative evaluation, as well as the updated Practice Advisory for Preanesthesia Evaluation.[1] The most recent ASA Practice Guidelines can be found at https://www.asahq.org/standards-and-guidelines. Conducting a preoperative evaluation is based on the premise that it will modify patient care and improve outcomes by allowing the anesthesiologist to prepare the patient and formulate an anesthetic plan that avoids dangers inherent in various disease states. Furthermore, preoperative evaluations may reduce both costs and surgery cancellation rates, increasing resource utilization in the operating room (OR).[2] This notion assumes that evaluations are done by anesthesiologists or other health care providers familiar with anesthesia, surgery, and perioperative events.

The preoperative evaluation has several components. It should include a review of the medical record and a history and physical examination pertinent to the patient and planned procedure. Based on this information, the appropriate diagnostic tests and preoperative consultations should be obtained. Through these, the anesthesiologist determines how best to optimize the patient's condition prior to surgery and develops the appropriate anesthetic care plan. Finally, the process is used to educate the patient about anesthesia and the perioperative period, answer all questions, and obtain informed consent.

The first part of this chapter outlines clinical risk factors pertinent to patients scheduled for anesthesia and surgery as well as the use of various tests to assess comorbid conditions. The second part discusses preoperative preparation. This chapter provides only an overview of the preoperative management process; for more details, the reader should refer to chapters focusing on specific organ systems.

Changing Concepts in Preoperative Evaluation

The practice of medicine has changed over the years and the majority of patients present to surgery from home. Consequently, the first time they meet their anesthesiologist is often immediately prior to surgery. This leaves little time to develop the doctor–patient relationship, engender trust, and answer questions. Under such conditions, it is often impossible to investigate coexisting diseases or alter medical therapy. However, preoperative screening clinics are becoming more effective and clinical practice guidelines are becoming more prevalent. The electronic medical record (EMR) aids the anesthesiologist in reviewing medical history, and preoperative questionnaires and computer-driven programs have become alternatives to traditional information retrieval. Finally, when anesthesiologists take responsibility for ordering preoperative laboratory tests, cost savings occur and cancellations of planned surgical procedures become less likely. In this setting, clear and efficient communication between the preoperative evaluation clinic and the anesthesiologist performing the anesthesia are critical.

Approach to the Healthy Patient

The preoperative evaluation form can serve as the basis for formulat- 3
ing the best anesthetic plan tailored to the patient. It should aid the anesthesiologist in identifying potential complications, increase consistency in best-care practices, and serve as a medicolegal document. Because it is more common today for the preoperative evaluation to be completed in a clinic by another physician or health professional who may not personally perform the anesthesia and because regulatory agencies such as JCAHO demand better documentation, the form's design must ensure that the information obtained is complete, concise, and legible. In hospitals with electronic medical records, legibility is rarely an issue; however, one must be wary of "copy forward" and entraining dated or incorrect information into the note. Table 23-1 offers one example of the pertinent areas of focus for a preoperative evaluation organized in a systems format.

Patient Identification, Diagnosis, and Planned Procedure

Identifying the patient is the first step when evaluating a patient preoperatively, typically done with legal name, date of birth, and medical record number. This also includes documenting the patient's sex assigned at birth, gender identity, preferred name, and preferred pronouns. Although EMRs may not have a clear format to display this information, it is important for the anesthesiologist to respectfully address their patient in the manner which they prefer. Assessment of vital signs, height, weight, and body mass index (BMI) provides information regarding physical characteristics, which will be necessary for planning anesthetic dosages, positioning, and evaluation of coexisting diseases as well as airway management. It is also important to ascertain the nature of the illness or injury necessitating surgery, as it will determine both the clinical urgency of the proposed operation and influence the available time and depth of the preoperative evaluation. True emergency procedures require a more abbreviated evaluation and are associated with higher anesthetic morbidity and mortality. The approach to urgent procedures is less well defined. The anesthesiologist and surgeon must weigh the risk of morbidity of operative delay against the benefits of establishing associated diagnoses that can influence patient management. Table 23-2 shows one classification of operative urgency, though individual hospitals may have their own definitions. The indication for the surgical procedure may also have implications for other aspects of perioperative management. For example, the presence of a small bowel obstruction has implications regarding the risk of aspiration and the need for a rapid sequence induction. Similarly, the extent of a lung resection will dictate the need for further pulmonary testing and perioperative monitoring. Patients undergoing carotid endarterectomy may require a more extensive neurologic examination as well as additional testing to rule out coronary artery disease (CAD). The planned procedure also dictates patient positioning and whether blood products will be necessary. Frequently, obtaining such information will require communication with the surgeon and the OR team, enhancing both patient safety and OR efficiency. A patient's advanced directive should be reviewed and addressed directly with the patient or family, especially when the surgery is for palliation of a terminal illness. While "do not resuscitate or intubate" orders are frequently rescinded for procedures, patients or families should be able to express their wishes or engage in a conversation regarding cardiopulmonary resuscitation and administration of life saving efforts.

Response to Previous Anesthetics

The ability to review previous anesthetic records is particularly 4
helpful for detecting the presence of a difficult airway, a history

Table 23-1 Preanesthetic Evaluation Screen

Diagnosis/Procedure
Age, Sex, Gender preference
Advance directives
Height/Weight/Vital signs/NPO status
Indwelling vascular lines/airways
Medications
Including OTCs, herbals, illicit drugs
Allergies/adverse reactions
Anesthetic/surgical history
MH/adverse reactions/airway difficulty
Airway
Difficult airway history, OSA
Teeth, Mallampati class, mouth opening, chin length, neck size/mobility, ability to prognath
Pulmonary
URI, pneumonia, asthma, COPD, cough, dyspnea, OSA, pneumothorax, tobacco, bronchodilator/steroid use, oxygen/CPAP/ventilator settings, endotracheal tube size/depth
Cardiovascular
CHD, hypertension, coronary artery/valvular disease, congestive heart failure, pulmonary hypertension, dysrhythmia/pacemaker, vascular disease, dyspnea orthopnea, angina, syncope, exercise intolerance
Central Nervous System
Stroke, seizures, ↑intracranial pressure, altered mental status psychiatric disorder, neuromuscular disease, spinal cord injury
Headaches, weakness, paresthesias, syncope
GI/Hepatic
Liver disease, hepatitis, bowel obstruction
Nausea/vomiting, reflux, ethanol use
Renal
Insufficiency, failure, dialysis
Hematology
Anemia, coagulopathy, sickle cell, chemotherapy, transfusions
Endocrine/Metabolic
Diabetes, thyroid disease, rheumatoid arthritis, steroid use
Infectious
Viral/bacterial/Tuberculosis/foreign travel
Contact/droplet/airborne precautions, antibiotic resistance
Other
Pregnancy, gestational age, trauma history

MH, malignant hyperthermia; NPO, nothing by mouth; URI, upper respiratory infection; COPD, chronic obstructive pulmonary disease; OSA, obstructive sleep apnea; CPAP, continuous positive airway pressure; CHD, congenital heart disease

of malignant hyperthermia (MH), and the individual's response to surgical stress and specific anesthetics. The patient should be questioned regarding any previous personal or familial difficulties with anesthesia. A patient's report of an "allergy" to anesthesia should raise suspicion for MH. A diagnosis of MH susceptibility will affect the anesthetic regimen and bring into question the appropriateness of outpatient surgery.

Although not life threatening, persistent nausea and vomiting after a previous surgery may be the patient's most negative and lasting memory. It also has the potential to cause a prolonged recovery room stay or an unplanned hospital admission. There are multiple predictors of postoperative nausea and vomiting (PONV), including type of surgical procedure, anesthetic agents, and patient factors (Table 23-3). One report predicting postoperative nausea and vomiting after *inhalation* anesthesia identified four risk factors: female gender, prior history of motion sickness or postoperative nausea, nonsmoking, and the use of postoperative opioids. The Apfel simplified risk score predicts PONV with 0, 1, 2, 3, or 4 risk factors as 10%, 20%, 40%, 60%, and 80%, respectively.[3] Society guidelines propose dual prophylactic antiemetic therapy when 1 to 2 risk factors are present and use of 3 to 4 agents for patients with more than 2 risk factors.[4,5] However, armed with this knowledge preoperatively, the anesthesiologist is also able to tailor the anesthetic or possibly avoid the most likely causes of PONV: volatile anesthetics, nitrous oxide, postoperative opioids, and an unnecessarily prolonged NPO time altogether.[5]

In children, Eberhart et al.[6] identified four independent predictors of postoperative vomiting (POV): duration of surgery longer than 30 minutes, age above 3 years, history of POV in patient or family, and strabismus surgery. Based on the presence of 0, 1, 2, 3, and 4 factors, the risk of POV was 9%, 10%, 30%, 55%, and

Table 23-2 Classification of Urgency of Surgical Procedures

Classification of Operation	Description	Optimal Timing	Example
Emergency	Life, limb, or organ-saving	<6 h	Ruptured aortic aneurysm Major trauma to thorax, abdomen Acute increase in intracranial pressure
Urgent	Conditions threaten life, limb, or organ	6–24 h	Perforated bowel Compound fracture Eye injury
Time sensitive	Stable, but requires intervention	Days to weeks	Tendon, nerve injuries Cancer procedures
Elective	Procedure planned at patient or surgeon convenience	Up to 1 yr	All other procedures that can be planned in advance

Adapted from Fleisher LA, Fleischmann KE, Auerbach AD, et al. ACC/AHA Guideline on perioperative cardiovascular evaluation and management of patients undergoing noncardiac surgery. *Circulation*. 2014;130:e278–e333.

Table 23-3 Risk Factors for PONV in Adults

Risk Factors With Positive Overall Evidence
Female sex
History of PONV or motion sickness
Nonsmoking
Younger age (<50 yr)
General versus regional anesthesia
Volatile anesthetics, nitrous oxide
Postoperative opioids
Duration of anesthesia
Type of surgery: cholecystectomy, laparoscopic, gynecologic

PONV, postoperative nausea and vomiting; ASA, American Society of Anesthesiologists.
Adapted with permission from Gan TJ, Belani KG, Bergese S, et al. Fourth consensus guidelines for the management of postoperative nausea and vomiting. *Anesth Analg*. 2020; 131(2):411–448.

70%, respectively. Most recent guidelines list eight risk factors for pediatric PONV and suggest pediatric patients with 1 to 2 risk factors receive dual antiemetic therapy with a 5HT3 antagonist and dexamethasone, while those with 3 or more risk factors should receive dual antiemetic therapy as well as consideration for TIVA (Table 23-4).

Medications/Allergies

The history should include a complete list of medications, including over-the-counter and herbal products (NICV 23-1, Table 23-5), to define a preoperative medication regimen, anticipate potential drug interactions, and provide clues to underlying disease. A complete list of drug allergies or reactions should be obtained, as well as any history of reaction to latex.

For the patient who presents on the day of surgery, the anesthesiologist should determine when the patient last ate solids and drank clear liquids. Once the general issues are completed, the preoperative history and physical examination can focus on specific systems.

Screening Patients Using a Systems Approach

Airway

One of the most critical aspects of the preoperative evaluation is the ability of the anesthesiologist to recognize the potential for difficulty in maintaining a patent airway with a mask, a laryngeal mask airway, or placement of an endotracheal tube when the patient is under general anesthesia. A review of previous anesthetic records is especially useful in uncovering an unsuspected "difficult airway" or to confirm previous uneventful tracheal intubations, noting whether the patient's body habitus or airway anatomy has changed in the interim. Patients should be questioned about their ability to breathe through their nose, whether there is suspected or diagnosed obstructive sleep apnea (OSA), and whether they have orthopnea. Evaluation of the airway involves examination of the oral cavity, including dentition, determination of the thyromental distance, assessment of the size of the patient's neck and potential tracheal deviation or masses, as well as evaluation of their ability to flex the base of the neck and extend the head. For trauma patients or patients with severe rheumatoid arthritis (RA) or Down syndrome, assessment for signs or symptoms of cervical cord compression is critical. In some instances, radiographic examination may also be required.

Table 23-4 Risk Factors for Pediatric Postoperative Nausea Vomiting (PONV)

Age ≥3 years
Strabismus surgery, adenotonsillectomy, otoplasty
History of PONV/motion sickness
Surgery duration ≥30 min
Family history of PONV
Volatile anesthetics
Post-pubertal female
Anticholinesterases
Long-acting opioids

Adapted with permission from Gan TJ, Belani KG, Bergese S, et al. Fourth Consensus Guidelines for the Management of Postoperative Nausea and Vomiting. *Anesth Analg*. 2020;131(2):411–448.

The Mallampati classification is the standard for assessing the relationship of the tongue size relative to the oral cavity (Table 23-6),[7] although by itself the Mallampati classification has a low positive predictive value in identifying patients who are difficult to intubate.[8,9] Intubation involves multiple steps: flexion of the lower neck, extension of the head on the neck, opening the mouth to insert the laryngoscope, and displacing the tongue forward and down into the submandibular space to expose the glottis. Therefore, a multifactorial approach to predicting intubation difficulty, as shown in Table 23-7, has proven to be more helpful. One must distinguish factors that predict a difficult intubation and factors that predict a difficult mask airway. For example, the absence of teeth clearly makes laryngoscopy less difficult, but at the same time can make mask ventilation more challenging.

Pulmonary System

A screening evaluation should include questions regarding the history of tobacco use, dyspnea, exercise tolerance, cough, wheezing, bronchodilator or steroid use, recent upper respiratory tract infection, stridor, and snoring or sleep apnea (NICV 23-2). Physical examination should assess respiratory rate, chest excursion, use of accessory muscles, nail color, and the patient's ability to carry on a conversation or to walk without dyspnea. Auscultation can detect decreased breath sounds, wheezing, stridor, or crackles. For the patient with positive findings, see the section on the evaluation of the patient with known pulmonary disease.

Cardiovascular System

When screening a patient for cardiovascular disease prior to surgery, the anesthesiologist is most interested in recognizing signs and symptoms of uncontrolled hypertension and unstable cardiac disease such as myocardial ischemia, congestive heart failure, valvular heart disease, and significant cardiac dysrhythmias. One should assess for symptoms of dyspnea, chest pain, syncope, or decreased exercise tolerance that would require further evaluation. Certain populations of patients, such as the elderly, women, or diabetics, may present with more atypical features. The presence of unstable angina has been associated with a high perioperative risk of myocardial infarction (MI).[10] The perioperative period is associated with a hypercoagulable state and surges in endogenous catecholamines, both of which may exacerbate the underlying process in unstable angina, increasing the risk of acute infarction. The patient should be questioned about symptoms of clinically important valvular disease, such as angina, dyspnea, syncope, or congestive heart failure, that would require further evaluation. Importantly, the anesthesiologist must identify patients who have undergone placement of a coronary artery stent, have an implantable cardiac device, or are taking an antiplatelet or anticoagulant

Table 23-5 Herbal/Dietary Supplements and Drug Interactions

Supplement	Common Uses	Pharmacologic Effects and Drug Interactions	Continue/Hold
Cannabinoids	Anxiolytic Sleep aid Antiemetic Epilepsy treatment	Sympathetic hyperactivity Impaired temperature regulation Airway irritability Increased risk of coronary vasospasm Interaction with anesthesia drugs	Discontinue at least 3 days but ideally 2 wk Does not apply to FDA approved uses: chemotherapy induced nausea
Ephedra	Weight loss aid Bacteriostatic Antitussive	Increased HR and BP, enhanced sympathomimetic effects with other sympathomimetics Potential arrhythmias with digoxin or halothane, hypertension with oxytocin	Discontinue, not a recommended supplement to use
Feverfew	Migraine prophylaxis Antipyretic	Inhibits platelet activity and increases bleeding Rebound headache with sudden cessation	Hold 2 wk
GBL, BD, GHB (γ-butyrolactone)	Bodybuilding Weight loss aid Sleep aid	Illegally distributed drugs Death, seizures, unconsciousness Bradycardia, slowed respirations	Discontinue
Garlic	Lower cholesterol, BP Antioxidant	Inhibition of platelet aggregation, potential for increased bleeding	Hold 2 wk
Ginger	Antinausea Antispasmodic	Potent inhibitor of thromboxane synthetase; may increase bleeding time	Hold 2 wk
Ginkgo	Blood thinner	May enhance bleeding in patients on anticoagulant or antithrombotic therapy	Hold 2 wk
Ginseng	Energy level enhancer Antioxidant	May inhibit platelet aggregation and increase bleeding Decreased blood glucose	Hold 1 wk
Goldenseal	Diuretic Anti-inflammatory Laxative	Functions as an oxytocic May worsen edema and/or hypertension High potential for drug interactions	Hold 2 wk
Kava-kava	Anxiolytic	Potentiates sedative effects of anesthetics May cause hepatotoxicity	Hold 2 wk
Licorice	Treats gastritis/ulcer	Glycyrrhetinic acid in licorice may cause mineralocorticoid effects: high blood pressure, hypokalemia, edema	Hold 2 wk
Melatonin	Sleep aid	May reduce anxiety May decrease delirium in hospitalized elderly patients	Continue
St. John's Wort	Treats depression and anxiety	May prolong effects of anesthesia	Hold 2 wk
Valerian	Mild sedative, anxiolytic	Considered safe	Continue
Vitamin E	Slows aging Promotes wound healing	May increase bleeding, especially with other anticoagulants	Hold 2 wk

Adapted from the ASA Physician Brochure: What You Should Know about your patient's use of herbal medicines and other dietary supplements, 2003.
Cummings KC 3rd, Keshock M, Ganesh R. Preoperative Management of Surgical Patients Using Dietary Supplements: Society for Perioperative Assessment and Quality Improvement (SPAQI) Consensus Statement. *Mayo Clin Proc.* 2021;96(5):1342–1355.

regimen. The perioperative care of these patients should be coordinated with a cardiologist (see the section on cardiovascular disease).

The anesthesiologist should be familiar with the American Heart Association (AHA) website (http://www.heart.org/) and its links to the latest AHA statements and guidelines for health professionals (NICV 23-3). Here one can find the most recent recommendations regarding specific patients and procedures that require subacute bacterial endocarditis prophylaxis.[11]

The examination of the cardiovascular system should include blood pressure evaluation, measuring both arms when appropriate. The anesthesiologist should consider the effects of preoperative anxiety and review resting blood pressure measurements. During auscultation of the heart, one should specifically listen

Table 23-6 Modified Mallampati Airway Classification System

Class	Direct Visualization, Patient Seated
I	Full view of soft palate, uvula, tonsillar pillars
II	Soft palate and upper portion of uvula
III	Soft palate
IV	Hard palate only

Modified with permission from Springer: Mallampati RS, Gatt SP, Gugino LD, et al. A clinical sign to predict difficult tracheal intubation: A prospective study. *Can Anaesth Soc J*. 1985;32:429–434.

for a murmur radiating to the carotids suggestive of aortic stenosis, abnormal rhythms, or a gallop suggestive of heart failure. The presence of bruits over the carotid arteries warrants further workup to determine the risk of stroke. The extremities should be examined for peripheral pulses to exclude peripheral vascular disease or congenital cardiovascular disease.

Neurologic System

Neurologic assessment in the apparently healthy patient can be accomplished through simple observation. The patient's ability to answer health history questions practically indicates a normal mental status. Questions can be directed regarding a history of stroke, symptoms of cerebrovascular disease, seizures, preexisting neuromuscular disease, or nerve injuries. The neurologic examination may be cursory in healthy patients or extensive in patients with coexisting disease. Testing of strength, reflexes, and sensation may be important in patients for whom the anesthetic plan or surgical procedure may result in a change in condition.

Endocrine System

Each patient should be questioned for a history or symptoms of endocrine diseases that may affect the perioperative course: diabetes mellitus, thyroid disease, parathyroid disease, endocrine-secreting tumors, and adrenal cortical suppression. For patients with known disease, a more in-depth evaluation will be covered in subsequent sections.

Table 23-7 Components of the Airway Examination That Suggest Difficult Tracheal Intubation

1. Long upper incisors
2. Prominent "overbite"
3. Inability to protrude the mandibular incisors anterior to maxillary incisors
4. Distance between incisors is <3 cm when mouth is fully opened
5. Uvula not visible when tongue is protruded with patient sitting
6. Shape of palate highly arched or very narrow
7. Mandibular space noncompliant
8. Thyromental distance <3 fingerbreadths
9. Neck short or thick
10. Limited range of motion of head and neck

Clinical context and judgment determine which of the components apply to a particular patient.

Modified with permission from Apfelbaum JL, Hagberg CA, Connis RT. 2022 American Society of Anesthesiologists Practice Guidelines for Management of the Difficult Airway. *Anesthesiology*. 2022;136(1):31–81.

Evaluation of the Patient With Known Systemic Disease

Cardiovascular Disease

Globally, more than 300 million surgical procedures are performed annually.[12] With an aging population, the incidence of comorbid conditions in patients undergoing noncardiac surgery has risen. Nearly half of patients over 45 years of age undergoing noncardiac surgery have multiple cardiovascular risk factors such as hypertension, hyperlipidemia, diabetes mellitus, obesity, and chronic kidney disease. Almost 25% of these patients have a history of atherosclerotic cardiovascular disease.[13] These risk factors place them at higher risk of perioperative cardiovascular complications such as death, MI, and stroke, which are a major source of morbidity and mortality, and occur at a rate of 3% for noncardiac surgeries.[14] The incidence of major adverse cardiovascular events (MACEs) is related to the risk factors present in each individual patient prior to surgery, as well as the risk-profile of the surgery itself.

The preoperative evaluation of the patient with known or suspected cardiovascular disease is focused on two areas: identification of clinical risk factors and preoperative cardiac testing. The goals are to define risk, identify which patients will benefit from further testing, determine whether perioperative β-blockade, interventional therapy, or even surgery would be beneficial before the planned procedure, and form an appropriate anesthetic plan.

Identifying Clinical Risk Factors

A focused history and cardiovascular physical examination is the first step in estimating perioperative cardiovascular risk. Comorbid conditions associated with MACE should be identified. These include a history of ischemic heart disease, presence of coronary stents, heart failure, dysrhythmias, valvular heart disease, systemic and pulmonary hypertension, chronic kidney disease, and diabetes.

7

Exercise tolerance remains one of the most important predictors of perioperative risk for noncardiac surgery and helps define the need for further testing and invasive monitoring. An excellent exercise tolerance, even in patients with stable angina, suggests that the myocardium can be stressed without failing. Alternatively, if patients experience dyspnea associated with chest pain during minimal exertion, the probability of extensive CAD is high, and is associated with greater perioperative risk. In addition, these patients are at risk for developing hypotension with ischemia and, therefore, may benefit from preoperative coronary intervention therapy, revascularization, or more intensive intraoperative monitoring.[15] Exercise tolerance can be assessed with formal treadmill testing or with a questionnaire that assesses activities of daily living (Table 23-8). Patient-reported poor exercise tolerance (i.e., inability to walk four blocks or climb two flights of stairs) is independently associated with a twofold risk of serious perioperative complications.[16] The likelihood of a serious adverse event is inversely related to the number of blocks that can be walked. Therefore, there is good evidence to suggest that minimal additional testing is necessary if the patient is able to describe a good exercise tolerance.

In virtually all studies, the preoperative presence of active congestive heart failure is a major risk factor for increased perioperative cardiac morbidity. Clinical evidence of heart failure includes symptoms of dyspnea, limited exercise tolerance, and orthopnea, as well as physical signs of jugular venous distention, crackles, third heart sound, and peripheral edema. A chest x-ray can reveal pulmonary edema or vascular redistribution. Significantly reduced left ventricular ejection fraction (e.g., <30%) appears to be an independent risk factor for adverse perioperative

Table 23-8 Estimated Energy Requirement for Various Activities

1 MET	Daily self-care Eat, dress, or use the toilet Walk indoors around the house Walk a block or two on level ground at 2–3 mph or 3.2–4.8 km/h Do light work around the house, like dusting or washing dishes
4 METs	Climb a flight of stairs or walk up a hill Walk on level ground at 4 mph or 6.4 km/h Run a short distance Do heavy work around the house, like scrubbing floors or lifting or moving heavy furniture Participate in moderate recreational activities like golf, bowling, dancing, doubles tennis, or throwing a baseball or football
>10 METs	Participate in strenuous sports like swimming, singles tennis, football, basketball, or skiing

MET, metabolic equivalent.
Adapted from the Duke Activity Status Index and American Heart Association Exercise Standards. Reproduced from Eagle K, Brundage B, Chaitman B, et al. Guidelines for perioperative cardiovascular evaluation of the noncardiac surgery. A report of the American Heart Association/American College of Cardiology Task Force on Assessment of Diagnostic and Therapeutic Cardiovascular Procedures. *Circulation*. 1996;93:1278.

outcome and long-term mortality.[17] Another study suggests that asymptomatic systolic or diastolic dysfunction is associated with increased 30-day cardiovascular perioperative risk.[18] Optimization of ventricular function and treatment of pulmonary edema are both important prior to elective surgery. Identifying the cause of heart failure is important (e.g., nonischemic cardiomyopathy or cardiac valvular insufficiency and/or stenosis) as it may alter the plan for perioperative monitoring and treatment.

Patients with known valvular heart disease can be effectively managed during the perioperative period to limit morbidity. The 2020 AHA/ACC guideline for the management of patients with valvular disease supports the use of preoperative echocardiography in patients with moderate or severe valvular stenosis or regurgitation with no echocardiography studies within 1 year, or worsening clinical status.[19] Valvular interventions (e.g., repair or replacement) may be indicated before elective noncardiac surgery depending on the symptoms or severity of disease and the urgency of the noncardiac surgery. Understanding the severity of stenotic or regurgitant valvular disease, coupled with an intraoperative monitoring and management plan, may reduce the risk of perioperative congestive heart failure and respiratory failure.

Adults with a prior MI almost always have CAD. Traditionally, risk assessment for noncardiac surgery was based on the time interval between the MI and surgery, which was based on older data that demonstrated an increased incidence of reinfarction if the MI was within 6 months of surgery.[20] The importance of the intervening time interval may no longer be valid in the current era of interventional therapy and improvements in perioperative care. Although many patients with an MI may continue to have myocardium at risk for subsequent ischemia and infarction, other patients may have their critical coronary stenoses either totally occluded or widely patent, with no such risk. For example, the use of percutaneous transluminal coronary angioplasty, thrombolysis, and early coronary artery bypass grafting (CABG) has changed the natural history of the disease. Therefore, patients should be individually evaluated from the perspective of their risk for ongoing ischemia.

Identifying Patients at Risk for Atherosclerotic Cardiac Disease

For those patients without overt cardiac symptoms, the probability of CAD varies with the type and number of atherosclerotic risk factors present. Peripheral arterial disease has been shown to be associated with CAD in multiple studies.[21] In patients with symptomatic coronary disease, the preoperative evaluation may reveal a change in the frequency or pattern of anginal symptoms. Certain populations of patients—for example, the elderly, women, or diabetics—may present with more atypical features and must be carefully assessed. The presence of unstable angina has been associated with a high perioperative risk of MI.[10]

Diabetes Mellitus

Diabetes mellitus is a common disease with a pathophysiology that affects multiple organ systems. Complications of diabetes mellitus are frequently the cause of urgent or emergent surgery, especially in the elderly. Diabetes accelerates the progression of atherosclerosis, so it is not surprising that diabetics have a higher incidence of CAD than nondiabetics as well as a high incidence of both silent MI and myocardial ischemia.[22] Eagle et al.[23] demonstrated that diabetes is an independent risk factor for perioperative cardiac morbidity. The duration of the disease and presence of associated end-organ dysfunction may also alter the overall cardiac risk. Autonomic neuropathy has been reported as the best predictor of silent ischemia.[24] Because these patients are at very high risk for a silent MI, a preoperative electrocardiogram (ECG) should be obtained to examine for the presence of Q waves.

Hypertension

Hypertension has also been associated with an increased incidence of silent myocardial ischemia and infarction.[22] Hypertensive patients who have left ventricular hypertrophy and are undergoing noncardiac surgery are at a higher perioperative risk than nonhypertensive patients.[25] Investigators have suggested that the presence of a strain pattern on ECG suggests a chronic ischemic state.[26]

Aggressive treatment of blood pressure is associated with reduction in long-term MI risk. The 2017 ACC/AHA guideline for the detection and management of high blood pressure, which defines normal blood pressure as less than 120 systolic and less than 80 diastolic, recommends treatment of confirmed hypertension through lifestyle or pharmacologic methods with a target BP less than 130/80.[27] However, there are no such guidelines to suggest a safe upper blood pressure limit when a patient presents for surgery with significant hypertension. There is little association reported between elevated blood pressures (up to 180 mmHg systolic or up to 110 mmHg diastolic) and postoperative outcomes. However, such patients are prone to perioperative myocardial ischemia, ventricular dysrhythmias, and lability in blood pressure. It is less clear in patients with blood pressures above 180/110 mmHg, as no absolute evidence exists that postponing surgery will reduce risk.[28,29] Although the literature suggests that elective surgery should be delayed if the diastolic pressure is above 110 mmHg, this study demonstrated no major morbidity in that small group of patients.[30] Thus, in the absence of end-organ changes, such as renal insufficiency or left ventricular hypertrophy with strain, the benefits of optimizing blood pressure must be weighed against the risks of delaying surgery.

Metabolic Syndrome/Tobacco

Metabolic syndrome and tobacco use are also associated with atherosclerotic cardiac disease. Metabolic syndrome is a disorder comprising a group of risk factors that includes high blood pressure, atherogenic dyslipidemia, high fasting glucose concentrations, and central obesity. Metabolic syndrome has been associated with higher rates of cardiovascular, pulmonary, and renal perioperative events, as well as wound infections.[31]

Importance of Surgical Procedure

The surgical procedure influences the scope of the preoperative evaluation by suggesting the range of physiologic changes that may occur during the perioperative period. Peripheral procedures are associated with an extremely low incidence of morbidity and mortality,[32] whereas major open vascular procedures are associated with the highest incidence of complications. Eagle et al.[33] published data from the Coronary Artery Surgery Study (CASS) on the incidence of perioperative MI and mortality by procedure for patients with known CAD and found that high-risk procedures included major vascular, abdominal, thoracic, and orthopedic surgery. Contemporary surgical techniques such as endovascular or minimally invasive surgery may decrease MACE in otherwise high-risk procedures.[34]

Calculation of Risk to Predict Perioperative Morbidity

Validated risk-prediction tools can help predict perioperative MACE in patients undergoing noncardiac surgery. Historically, these have included the ASA physical status index (Table 23-9) and the Goldman Cardiac Risk Index. The ASA classification system is independently associated with postoperative outcomes. In a prospective study of 6,301 surgical patients, healthy ASA I patients had a significantly lower risk of cardiac complications and mortality (0.1% and 0.1%), compared to ASA IV patients (18% and 18.3%).[35]

The Revised Cardiac Risk Index (RCRI) is an update of the Goldman Cardiac Risk Index, and is a validated method to assign perioperative risk using readily available clinical variables.[36] In a population of 4,315 patients aged 50 years and older undergoing elective, major noncardiac procedures, 6 independent predictors of complications were identified and included in the RCRI: high-risk type of surgery, history of ischemic heart disease, history of congestive heart failure, history of cerebrovascular disease, insulin-dependent diabetes, and chronic kidney disease (serum creatinine >2 mg/dL). Cardiac complications rose with an increase in the number of risk factors present. In patients with an RCRI score of 0, the risk of perioperative cardiovascular complications is 0.4% compared to approximately 11% in patients with a score of 3 or more (Table 23-10). Figure 23-1 shows the rate of major cardiac complications for patients in each RCRI class 1–4 according to the type of procedure performed. Other validated risk-prediction tools developed by the American College of Surgeons (ACS) include the National Surgical Quality Improvement Program (NSQIP) and the Myocardial Infarction and Cardiac Arrest (MICA).[37] The ACS NSQIP Surgical Risk Calculator uses current procedural terminology codes and 21 patient-specific variables for prediction of several groups of outcomes.[38] This may provide better predictive discrimination than the RCRI, although may not be practical in a busy preoperative clinic as the calculation takes more time and is more complex.

Preoperative Cardiac Testing

Multiple algorithms have been proposed to determine which patients require further cardiovascular testing. As described previously, the risk associated with the proposed surgical procedure influences the decision to perform further diagnostic testing and interventions. With the reduction in perioperative morbidity, it has been suggested that extensive cardiovascular testing is not always necessary.

The algorithm to determine the need for testing in a patient at risk for CAD proposed by the 2014 ACC/AHA Task Force is based on available evidence and expert opinion that integrates clinical history, surgery-specific risk, and exercise tolerance (Fig. 23-2). In the first step, the clinician evaluates the urgency of the surgery and the appropriateness of a formal preoperative assessment. Next, one determines if the patient has undergone a recent revascularization procedure or coronary evaluation. Those patients with unstable coronary syndromes should be identified, have appropriate consultations made, and treatment instituted. Finally, the decision to perform further testing depends on the interaction of the clinical risk factors, surgery-specific risk, and functional capacity. For patients at high risk, both exercise tolerance and the extent of the surgery are taken into account to determine the need for further testing. Most importantly, no preoperative cardiovascular testing should be performed if the results will not change perioperative management.

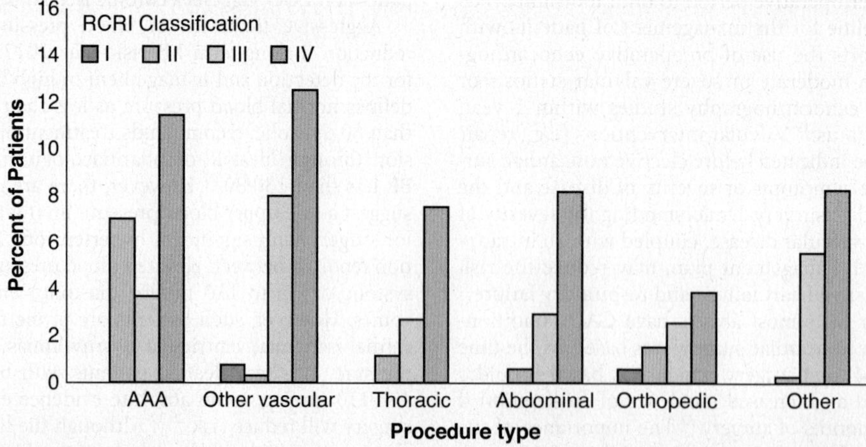

Figure 23-1 Cardiac risk (percent of patients expected to have major cardiac complications) by Revised Cardiac Risk Index (RCRI) class and type of surgical procedure. Bars represent rate of major cardiac complications in RCRI classes I to IV (based on patients with 0, 1, 2, or more risk factors, respectively) according to the type of procedure performed. Note that, by definition, patients undergoing abdominal aortic aneurysm (AAA), thoracic, and abdominal procedures were excluded from class I. In all subsets except patients undergoing AAA, there was a statistically significant trend toward greater risk with higher-risk class. See text for details. (Reproduced with permission from Lee TH, Marcantonio ER, Mangione CM, et al. Derivation and prospective validation of a simple index for prediction of cardiac risk of major noncardiac surgery. *Circulation*. 1999;100:1043–1049.)

Table 23-9 American Society of Anesthesiologists Physical Status Classification System

ASA PS Classification	Definition	Adult Examples, Including, but not Limited to:	Pediatric Examples, Including but not Limited to:	Obstetric Examples, Including but not Limited to:
ASA I	A normal healthy patient	Healthy, non-smoking, no or minimal alcohol use	Healthy (no acute or chronic disease), normal BMI percentile for age	
ASA II	A patient with mild systemic disease	Mild diseases only without substantive functional limitations. Current smoker, social alcohol drinker, pregnancy, obesity (30<BMI<40), well-controlled DM/HTN, mild lung disease	Asymptomatic congenital cardiac disease, well controlled dysrhythmias, asthma without exacerbation, well controlled epilepsy, non-insulin dependent diabetes mellitus, abnormal BMI percentile for age, mild/moderate OSA, oncologic state in remission, autism with mild limitations	Normal pregnancy*, well controlled gestational HTN, controlled pre-eclampsia without severe features, diet-controlled gestational DM.
ASA III	A patient with severe systemic disease	Substantive functional limitations; One or more moderate to severe diseases. Poorly controlled DM or HTN, COPD, morbid obesity (BMI ≥40), active hepatitis, alcohol dependence or abuse, implanted pacemaker, moderate reduction of ejection fraction, ESRD undergoing regularly scheduled dialysis, history (>3 months) of MI, CVA, TIA, or CAD/stents.	Uncorrected stable congenital cardiac abnormality, asthma with exacerbation, poorly controlled epilepsy, insulin dependent diabetes mellitus, morbid obesity, malnutrition, severe OSA, oncologic state, renal failure, muscular dystrophy, cystic fibrosis, history of organ transplantation, brain/spinal cord malformation, symptomatic hydrocephalus, premature infant PCA <60 weeks, autism with severe limitations, metabolic disease, difficult airway, long term parenteral nutrition. Full term infants <6 weeks of age.	Preeclampsia with severe features, gestational DM with complications or high insulin requirements, a thrombophilic disease requiring anticoagulation.
ASA IV	A patient with severe systemic disease that is a constant threat to life	Recent (<3 months) MI, CVA, TIA or CAD/stents, ongoing cardiac ischemia or severe valve dysfunction, severe reduction of ejection fraction, shock, sepsis, DIC, ARD or ESRD not undergoing regularly scheduled dialysis	Symptomatic congenital cardiac abnormality, congestive heart failure, active sequelae of prematurity, acute hypoxic-ischemic encephalopathy, shock, sepsis, disseminated intravascular coagulation, automatic implantable cardioverter-defibrillator, ventilator dependence, endocrinopathy, severe trauma, severe respiratory distress, advanced oncologic state.	Preeclampsia with severe features complicated by HELLP or other adverse event, peripartum cardiomyopathy with EF <40, uncorrected/decompensated heart disease, acquired or congenital.
ASA V	A moribund patient who is not expected to survive without the operation	Ruptured abdominal/thoracic aneurysm, massive trauma, intracranial bleed with mass effect, ischemic bowel in the face of significant cardiac pathology or multiple organ/system dysfunction	Massive trauma, intracranial hemorrhage with mass effect, patient requiring ECMO, respiratory failure or arrest, malignant hypertension, decompensated congestive heart failure, hepatic encephalopathy, ischemic bowel or multiple organ/system dysfunction.	Uterine rupture.
ASA VI	A declared brain-dead patient whose organs are being removed for donor purposes			

*Although pregnancy is not a disease, the parturient's physiologic state is significantly altered from when the woman is not pregnant, hence the assignment of ASA 2 for a woman with uncomplicated pregnancy.

**The addition of "E" denotes Emergency surgery: (An emergency is defined as existing when delay in treatment of the patient would lead to a significant increase in the threat to life or body part)

Table 23-10 Revised Cardiac Risk Index (RCRI)

Risk Factors	Points
Ischemic heart disease	1
Congestive heart failure	1
Cerebrovascular disease	1
Insulin dependent diabetes mellitus	1
Serum creatinine >2 mg/dL	1
High-risk surgery (intraperitoneal, intrathoracic, or suprainguinal vascular)	1
Points	**Risk % (95% confidence interval)**
0	0.4 (0.05–1.5)
1	0.9 (0.3–21)
2	6.6 (3.9–10.3)
≥3	11.0 (5.8–18.4)

Modified with permission from Lee TH, Marcantonio ER, Mangione CM, et al. Derivation and prospective evaluation of a simple index for prediction of cardiac risk of major noncardiac surgery. *Circulation*. 1999;100: 1043–1049.

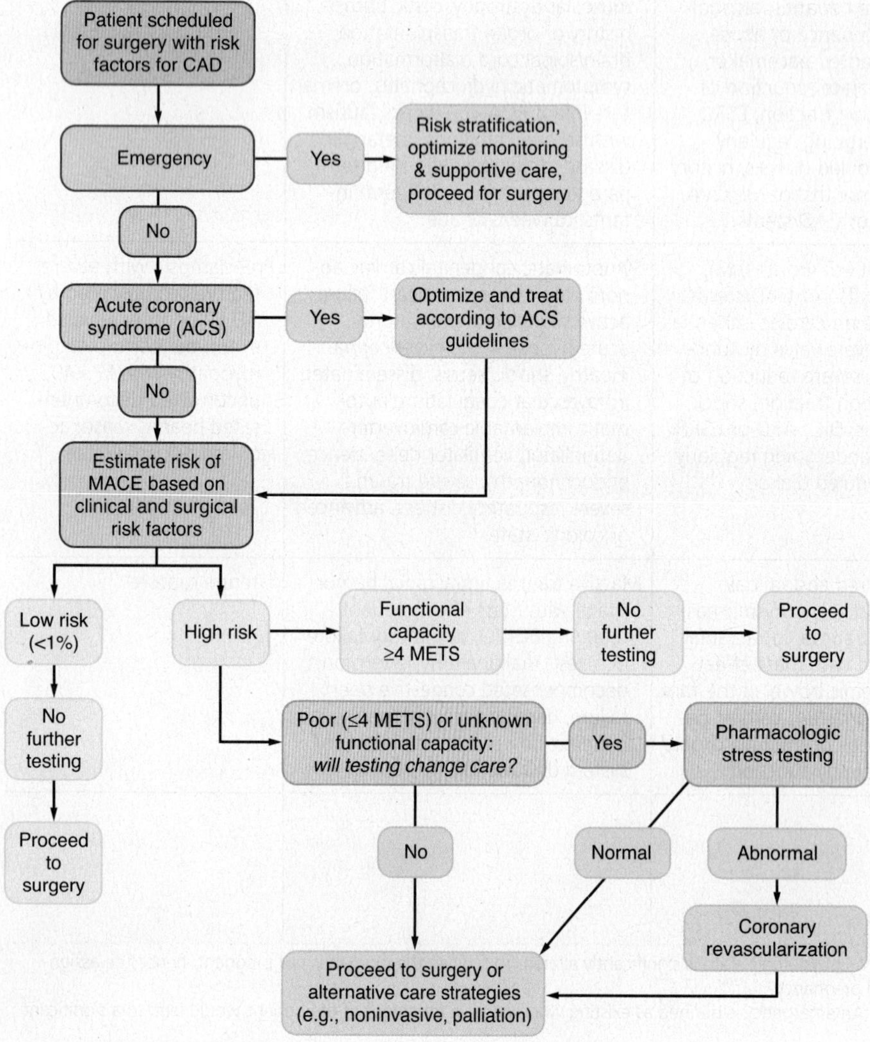

Figure 23-2 Approach to perioperative cardiac assessment for patients with coronary artery disease (CAD). (Modified from Fleisher LA, Fleischmann KE, Auerbach AD, et al. ACC/AHA guideline on perioperative cardiovascular evaluation and management of patients undergoing noncardiac surgery. *Circulation*. 2014;130:e278–e333. http://circ.ahajournals.org)

Electrocardiogram

A preoperative 12-lead ECG can establish the patient's baseline cardiac rhythm, identify clinically silent cardiac disease (e.g., prior MI and left ventricular hypertrophy), and serve as a baseline for changes in the postoperative period. Abnormal Q waves in high-risk patients are highly suggestive of a past MI. It has been estimated that approximately 30% of MIs occur without symptoms ("silent infarctions") and can only be detected on screening ECGs, with the highest incidence occurring in patients with either diabetes or hypertension. The Framingham Study showed that long-term prognosis after MI is not improved by lack of symptoms at the time of MI.[22] The absence of Q waves on the ECG, however, does not exclude the occurrence of a Q-wave MI in the past.[39] Those patients in whom the ECG reverts to normal have improved survival compared to those with consistent abnormalities, with or without Q waves. The presence of Q waves on a preoperative ECG in a high-risk patient, regardless of symptoms, should alert the anesthesiologist to the increased perioperative risk and the potential for active ischemia.

The 2014 ACC/AHA Clinical Practice Guideline recommends a preoperative resting 12-lead ECG only for patients with known CAD or other structural heart disease (except for low-risk surgical procedures) and consideration in asymptomatic patients with clinical risk factors.[34]

Transthoracic Echocardiography

Transthoracic echocardiography is a noninvasive method of evaluating cardiac ventricular function and valvular heart disease. There is an association between decreased LV ejection fraction and incidence of MACE, with the highest-risk patients having resting LVEF <35%.[34] The ACC/AHA endorses those with dyspnea of unknown origin and for those with current or prior heart failure with worsening dyspnea or other change in clinical status to have preoperative evaluations of left ventricular function. Otherwise, routine preoperative evaluation of LVEF is not recommended.

Echocardiography has the added advantage of assessing valvular function, which may have important implications for noncardiac surgery. Aortic stenosis has been associated with a poor prognosis in noncardiac surgical patients, and knowledge of valvular lesions may modify perioperative hemodynamic goals and therapy. The 2020 ACC/AHA guideline for the management of patients with valvular disease endorses preoperative echocardiography testing for moderate or severe degrees of valvular stenosis or regurgitation with no echocardiography studies within 1 year, or worsening clinical status.[19]

Assessment of Functional Capacity and Stress Testing for Myocardial Ischemia

The exercise ECG stress test has been the traditional method for evaluating patients with suspected CAD. It represents the most cost-effective and least invasive method for detecting ischemia, with a sensitivity of 70% to 80% and a specificity of 60% to 75% for identifying CAD. A positive exercise stress test alerts the anesthesiologist that the patient is at risk for ischemia associated with increased heart rate, with the greatest risk in those who develop ischemia after only mild exercise. As noted earlier, exercise tolerance remains one of the most important predictors of perioperative risk for noncardiac surgery. Therefore, the ability to exercise without symptoms of ischemia suggests that no further testing is necessary, and exercise ECG stress testing is infrequently indicated.

Noninvasive pharmacologic stress testing before surgery can be used in high-risk patients who either are unable to exercise or have contraindications to exercise (e.g., claudication). These tests offer value in assessing risk in patients who have poor or indeterminate functional capacity (<4 METs), but should be performed only if their results will change management.[34] Testing options include the dobutamine stress echocardiogram (DSE), in which dobutamine is used to increase myocardial oxygen demand by increasing heart rate and blood pressure. The appearance of either new or more severe regional wall motion abnormalities on the echocardiogram represents areas at risk for myocardial ischemia and is considered a positive test. The advantage of a stress echo is that it is a dynamic assessment of ventricular function. It is generally accepted that those at greatest risk demonstrate regional wall motion abnormalities at low heart rates.

Another noninvasive stress test is dipyridamole/adenosine/regadenoson myocardial perfusion imaging (MPI) with thallium-201 and/or technetium-99m and rubidium-82. Dipyridamole, adenosine, or regadenoson is administered as a coronary vasodilator to assess flow heterogeneity and the presence of a redistribution defect. The 2014 ACC/AHA Clinical Practice Guideline suggests that (1) a normal DSE or MPI supports a high negative predictive value for perioperative MI and/or cardiac death and (2) moderate to large areas of ischemia are associated with increased risk of perioperative MI and/or cardiac death. Findings of a fixed perfusion defect by MPI support a prior MI but offer limited predictive value, although this patient subset is at increased risk for long-term cardiac risk.[34]

Current recommendations are that patients with active cardiac conditions such as unstable angina, congestive heart failure, significant dysrhythmias, and severe valvular disease should undergo noninvasive stress testing before noncardiac surgery. For patients who require vascular or other high-risk surgery, and have multiple clinical risk factors and poor functional capacity, it is reasonable to undergo noninvasive stress testing if it will change management. Routine screening with noninvasive stress testing is not recommended for patients undergoing noncardiac surgery who are at low risk for perioperative MACE.[34]

Coronary Angiography and Revascularization

Coronary angiography remains the best method for defining coronary anatomy and also assesses ventricular and valvular function. Hemodynamic indices can be determined, such as atrial and ventricular pressures, as well as pressure gradients across valves. Although a critical coronary stenosis delineates an area of risk for developing myocardial ischemia, the functional response of that ischemia cannot be assessed by angiography alone. A critical stenosis may or may not be the underlying cause for a perioperative MI that occurs. In the ambulatory population, many infarctions are the result of acute thrombosis of a noncritical stenosis. The 2014 ACC/AHA Clinical Practice Guidelines do not recommend routine preoperative coronary angiography prior to noncardiac surgery without specific clinical indications.[34] Angiography is typically utilized in patients with signs or symptoms of unstable angina or a positive stress test, but only when the results of angiography would alter perioperative management. In patients with CAD, there are little data to support the use of coronary revascularization solely for the purpose of improving perioperative outcome, although it is true that for some patients scheduled for high-risk surgery, long-term survival may be enhanced by revascularization. The Coronary Artery Revascularization Prophylaxis trial randomized 510 patients with CAD to undergo coronary artery revascularization prior to vascular surgery.[40] This trial failed to show a difference in the rates of perioperative MI or long-term mortality between the two groups, although it was noted that high-risk patients with left main disease, LVEF <20%, or severe aortic stenosis were excluded from the trial. Based on this data, the ACC/AHA Clinical Practice Guidelines do not endorse routine coronary revascularization prior to noncardiac surgery for the sole purpose of reducing perioperative MACE.[34] After reviewing all available data, most clinicians believe the indication for CABG prior to noncardiac surgery remains the same as in other settings and is independent of the proposed noncardiac surgery.

Biomarker Measurement

There is a growing body of evidence for the use of biomarkers to aid in perioperative risk assessment. Laboratory measurement of biomarkers such as brain natriuretic peptide (BNP), N-terminal brain natriuretic peptide (NT-proBNP) may increase prediction accuracy.[41] However, due to significant variations in biomarker collection, and lack of control arms, routine biomarker measurements are not currently endorsed by the AHA/ACC as part of the routine perioperative risk evaluation.[34]

Cardiac troponin is a sensitive marker of myocardial injury, and should be measured along with an ECG if the patient is displaying signs and symptoms of myocardial ischemia or infarction in the perioperative period.[34]

Special Patient Populations

The Elderly

An aging population combined with advances in cardiovascular care has led to an increase in the incidence and prevalence of elderly patients presenting for noncardiac surgery with cardiovascular disease. Consistently, advanced age is independently associated with an increased risk of MACE.[34,42] The Perioperative Ischemic Evaluation-2 (POISE-2) Trial showed that age over 75 years old was an independent risk factor for postoperative MI (adjusted HR [95% CI] 1.89 [1.6–2.23]; $P < .001$). Elderly patients have age-related changes in cardiovascular physiology such as decreased sympathetic response to stress, reduced vascular compliance, impaired baroreceptor responses. This may place them at risk for blood pressure lability and susceptibility to hypotension in the perioperative period.[43] Elderly patients are an underrepresented population in clinical trials, and there are few guidelines which specifically address perioperative risk stratification and management. In addition to conventional outcomes, future studies should incorporate important outcomes such as functional status, maintenance of independence, and quality of life.[44]

Patients With Coronary Artery Stents

A history of prior MI is associated with both perioperative MI and 30-day mortality.[45] Recent clinical practice guidelines support delaying noncardiac surgery at least 60 days after an MI in the absence of coronary intervention. Importantly, recent MI within 6 months of noncardiac surgery appears to be a risk factor for perioperative stroke.[34] Early surgery after coronary stent placement is also associated with adverse cardiac events. Coronary stent placement within 1-year of noncardiac surgery is an independent risk factor for perioperative MACE and bleeding in patients with bare metal (BMS) or drug-eluting stents (DES).[46] The current 2014 ACC/AHA Clinical Practice Guideline supports the delay of elective noncardiac surgery for 14 days after coronary balloon angioplasty and 30 days after BMS placement. The optimal waiting period for elective noncardiac surgery after DES placement is 12 months; however, elective noncardiac surgery may be considered after 6 months based on comparative benefits of surgery compared with risk of stent thrombosis and myocardial ischemia.[34] This difference is because the incidence of stent thrombosis for DESs has been found to be similar to that of BMSs in the early phase after placement but is less well defined over a longer period of time. Dual antiplatelet therapy, for example, aspirin and clopidogrel, is often used after stent placement. A thienopyridine (ticlopidine or clopidogrel) is generally continued with aspirin for 1 month after BMS placement and for 12 months after DES placement (Fig. 23-3). Perioperative management must weigh the risk of bleeding versus stent thrombosis. The decision must involve the anesthesiologist, surgeon, cardiologist, and intensivist. For those patients who have a high risk for stent thrombosis, many advocate that at least aspirin be continued in the perioperative period. Also, the anesthesiologist must weigh the risk of regional versus general anesthesia when these patients are taking antiplatelet therapy. Surgery in patients with recent stent placement should probably only be considered in centers where interventional cardiologists are available.

Patients With Cardiovascular Implantable Electronic Devices

With the increasing prevalence of patients treated with pacemakers and implantable defibrillators, preoperative evaluation must address the management of cardiovascular implantable electronic devices (CIEDs) during the perioperative period (NICV 23-4). The function of these devices can be impaired by electromagnetic interference during surgery and it is imperative that the surgical team is aware of the best placement for the electrocautery pad, and understands when bipolar rather than unipolar cautery is the safest for the patient. It is important to understand the type of device, its programming, and its underlying clinical need. The cardiologist often needs to be involved in programming the CIED before and after surgery. In 2020 the ASA published updated clinical practice guidelines for perioperative management of patients with implantable defibrillators, pacemakers, and arrhythmia monitors (see Appendix 4: American Society of Anesthesiologists Standards, Guidelines, and Statements).[47]

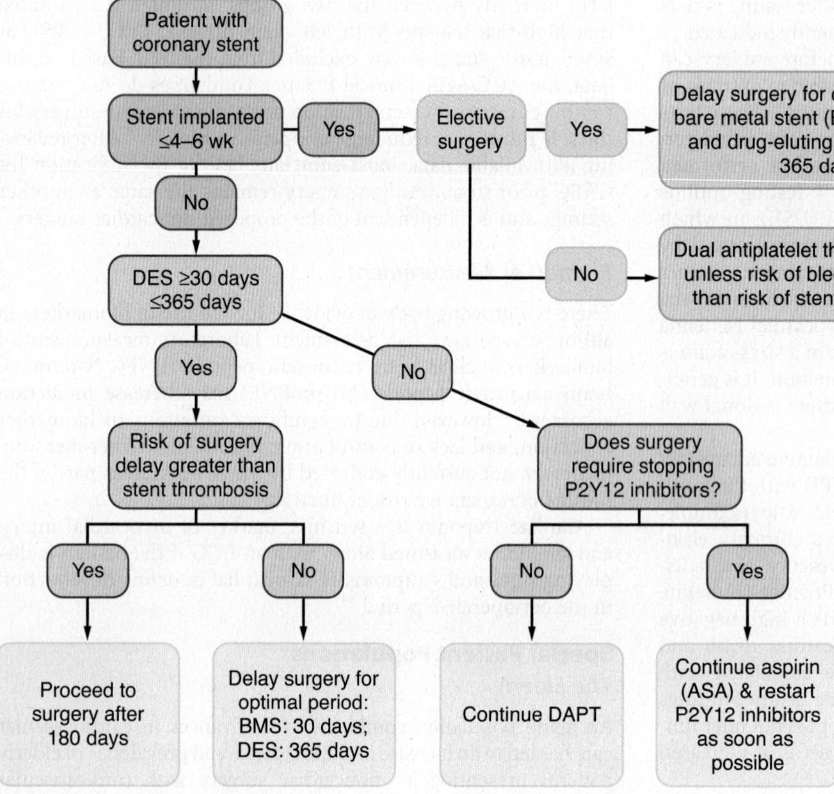

Figure 23-3 Approach to perioperative cardiac assessment for patients with coronary artery stent. P2Y12, Platelet receptor inhibitor (e.g., clopidogrel). (Modified from Fleisher LA, Fleischmann KE, Auerbach AD, et al. ACC/AHA guideline on perioperative cardiovascular evaluation and management of patients undergoing noncardiac surgery. *Circulation*. 2014;130:e278–e333. http://circ.ahajournals.org.)

Pulmonary Disease

Postoperative respiratory complications defined by the European Perioperative Clinical Outcome consensus statement included (1) respiratory infection, (2) respiratory failure, (3) pleural effusion, (4) atelectasis, (5) pneumothorax, (6) bronchospasm, and (7) aspiration pneumonitis.[48] During the perioperative period postoperative respiratory complications occur more frequently than cardiac complications in patients having major noncardiac surgeries. These are major causes of morbidity and mortality with increased length of hospital stay and substantial economic cost. The incidence of postoperative respiratory failure, defined as greater or equal to 48 hours of mechanical ventilation or reintubation after surgery, has been estimated at 3% in vascular and general surgery patients.[49] Notably, the risk of mortality with respiratory failure appears substantially higher than the risk after a perioperative MI. Analyses of large clinical databases have substantially increased the understanding of clinical risk factors.[49,50] Clinical guidelines from the American College of Physicians have estimated preoperative risk and recommend prevention strategies.[51] Preoperative pulmonary function testing and chest radiographs, although important diagnostic tools, appear to offer limited benefit in predicting perioperative respiratory failure and complication rates. Although chest x-rays identify structural lung abnormalities, these are not frequently associated with significant changes in management for the general population. In contrast, laboratory studies identifying a reduction in serum albumin levels and increased levels of blood urea nitrogen (BUN) appear associated with an increased risk of perioperative pulmonary morbidity.[49,50]

Epidemiologic studies support the relationship of the anatomic location of surgery and pulmonary risk.[49,50] Open aortic, thoracic, and upper abdominal surgeries are associated with the highest risk for postoperative pulmonary morbidity. Furthermore, cranial procedures, vascular, and neck surgeries are associated with increased risk.[49,52] The pathophysiology of decreased postoperative vital capacity and functional residual capacity with diaphragmatic dysfunction contribute to hypoxemia and atelectasis. Changes in functional residual capacity may take weeks to return to baseline. Diaphragmatic dysfunction can develop despite adequate analgesia related to phrenic nerve dysfunction. Neurosurgery and neck surgery are associated with perioperative aspiration pneumonia, related to an altered sensorium or cranial nerve dysfunction.

Emergency surgery and general anesthesia are consistent factors associated with increased risk. Not only can the surgery affect pulmonary function, but general anesthesia also results in mechanical changes, such as a decrease in the functional residual capacity and reduced diaphragmatic function, leading to ventilation/perfusion abnormalities and atelectasis. Volatile anesthetics inhibit mucociliary clearance, can increase alveolar–capillary permeability, inhibit surfactant production, increase nitric oxide synthetase, and increase sensitivity of the pulmonary vasculature to neurohumoral mediators. Subanesthetic levels of intravenous or volatile agents can blunt ventilatory response to hypoxemia and hypercarbia. Prolonged anesthesia is a well-established risk factor for postoperative pulmonary complications with morbidity rates increasing after 2 to 3 hours.[53] However, laparoscopic surgery, often longer in duration, is associated with decreased pulmonary complications compared with an open procedure despite increased anesthesia duration.[54]

ASA class 3 or greater, emergency surgery, high-risk surgical procedure (vascular, transplant, neurosurgery, thoracic, general, and burn surgery), history of congestive heart failure, and chronic pulmonary disease are the most common independent predictors for reintubation.[55]

The preoperative evaluation can identify pre-existing pulmonary disease, with a goal to maximize the patient's health status by working with the patient and consultants. Collaboration with the surgeon can support specific risk reduction strategies, such as operative approach, epidural or regional analgesia when appropriate, lung expansion methods, and deep venous thrombosis prophylaxis. Intraoperative measures to limit the risk of hospital-acquired pneumonia have been proposed, largely focused on reducing the risk of bacterial contamination of the lung during the perioperative period. For high-risk patient groups, studies support preoperative oral antiseptic decontamination before tracheal intubation to decrease the risk of nosocomial pneumonia.[56,57]

Smoking

Smoking is an important risk factor for perioperative respiratory complications (NICV 23-5). Smokers without chronic lung disease show increased carboxyhemoglobin levels, decreased tracheal ciliary function, and increased sputum production, with nicotine-induced stimulation of the cardiovascular system. Although cessation of smoking for 2 days can decrease carboxyhemoglobin levels, abolish nicotine effects, and improve mucous clearance, smoking cessation for 4 to 8 weeks appears necessary to reduce the rate of postoperative pulmonary complications.[58] Nicotine transdermal patches and nicotine e-cigarettes during the perioperative period remain controversial.[59] Patients who smoke can show increased airway reactivity under general anesthesia and may benefit from preoperative inhaled bronchodilators.

Recently, vaping has become popular among young adults. While no large studies are available at this time, there are reports of increased airway reactivity and complications under anesthesia due to pulmonary interstitial changes from e-cigarette use.[60]

Asthma

Asthma is one of the most common coexisting diseases that confront the anesthesiologist (NICV 23-6). The patient interview can elicit information regarding inciting factors, severity, reversibility, and current status. Frequent use of bronchodilators, hospitalizations for asthma, and requirement for systemic steroids are all indicators of more severe disease. After an acute exacerbation of asthma, airway hyperreactivity may persist for several weeks.[61] In addition to bronchodilators, perioperative steroids may benefit the severe asthmatic. Steroid-induced adrenal insufficiency is a concern in patients who have received more than a "burst and taper" of steroids in the previous 6 months. This group of patients should be considered for "stress doses" of steroids perioperatively. The complication rate for asthmatics treated with short-term steroids undergoing surgery is low, with no evidence for impaired wound healing or infections.[62] Patients using chronic inhaled steroids should continue regular use during the perioperative period.

Obstructive Sleep Apnea (OSA)

OSA is a syndrome defined by periodic obstruction of the upper airway during sleep, leading to episodic oxygen desaturation and hypercarbia (NICV 23-7). This episodic desaturation, in turn, causes episodic sleep arousal, leads to chronic sleep deprivation with daytime hypersomnolence and behavioral changes. It can result in chronic pulmonary hypertension and right heart failure. It afflicts 26% of U.S. adults between 30 and 70 years of age, exacerbated by the obesity epidemic.[63] Because of airway collapse and sleep deprivation, patients with OSA are susceptible to respiratory depression and airway obstruction after sedatives, opioids, and inhaled anesthetics both intraoperatively and postoperatively.

In 2014, the ASA published practice guidelines for the perioperative management of patients with OSA.[64] Preoperative identification of those patients at risk is critical to formulate a safe perioperative plan. Preoperative polysomnography is the standard diagnostic method for OSA. For the preoperative assessment, screening questionnaires can support the diagnosis of OSA. For example,

Table 23-11 Use of the STOP-Bang Questionnaire to Identify Surgical Patients at Risk for OSA

S – **S**nore loudly	**B** – **B**MI > 35 kg/m^2
T – **T**ired in the daytime	**A** – **A**ge > 50 yr
O – **O**bserved apnea, choking/gasping during sleep	**N** – **N**eck size large Male: >17 in; Female >16 in
P – high blood **P**ressure	**G** – **G**ender male
3–4 positive answers = intermediate risk for moderate to severe OSA	
>5 positive answers = high risk for moderate to severe OSA	

Adapted from Pivetta B, Chen L, Nagappa M, et al. Use and Performance of the STOP-Bang Questionnaire for Obstructive Sleep Apnea Screening Across Geographic Regions: A Systematic Review and Meta-Analysis. *JAMA Netw Open*. 2021;4(3):e211009. /jamanetworkopen.2021. PMID: 33683333

the STOP-Bang questionnaire (snoring, tiredness, observed apnea, blood pressure, body mass index, age, neck size, gender) accurately identifies moderate to severe OSA.[65] See Table 23-11.

The risk of perioperative complications in patients with OSA increases with the severity of sleep apnea, the invasiveness of surgery, and required postoperative opioids.[54] There is general consensus that preoperative initiation of nasal mask continuous positive airway pressure (CPAP) reduces perioperative risk, by decreasing sleep deprivation and secondary hypersomnolence. Importantly, OSA is associated with difficult airway management, making it even more important to examine previous anesthesia records and to perform a thorough airway examination. Emergency airway equipment should be readily available at the surgical center.

There are multiple management decisions to make in coordination with the surgeon with respect to the OSA patient: (1) consider a less invasive procedure to limit opioid need, (2) evaluate the feasibility of neuraxial, regional, or local anesthesia, decreasing the total amount of anesthesia or opioids, (3) review the benefit to risks of nonsteroidal anti-inflammatory agents, (4) evaluate safety of outpatient surgery, (5) plan for perioperative CPAP support, and (6) plan for postoperative ICU or monitored unit.

The ASA practice guidelines for OSA recommend hospitalization after uvulopalatoplasty surgery and after tonsillectomy for OSA in children younger than 3 years. Postoperative hospitalization is also recommended for those OSA patients with other coexisting diseases.[64]

Endocrine Disease

Diabetes Mellitus

Diabetes mellitus is the most common endocrinopathy, and according to the Centers for Disease Control and Prevention (CDC). Americans have an incidence of approximately 11% (>20% in those 65 years and older), with the highest rates in Native Americans, followed by Hispanics, Blacks, Asian Americans, then Whites (http://www.cdc.gov/diabetes). The incidence is expected to rise significantly for Americans born after 2000, largely because of the rise in obesity. Critical illness–induced hyperglycemia, defined as a blood glucose above 200 mg/dL in the absence of known diabetes, occurs most frequently in the elderly.[66] Diabetes mellitus has acute and chronic disease manifestations, making it more likely for diabetics to require surgery. The majority of diabetics develop secondary disease in one or more organ systems, which must be identified preoperatively so that an appropriate plan can be developed for perioperative management. Although long-term close control of glucose may limit some of the microvascular effects of diabetes (retinopathy, neuropathy, and nephropathy), macrovascular events such as myocardial ischemia, MI, or stroke may not be decreased. Diabetics have an increased risk of CAD, hypertension, congestive heart failure, and perioperative MI, with the incidence of silent ischemia increased due to associated autonomic neuropathy. The 2014 ACC/AHA Clinical Practice Guideline places diabetics, especially those receiving insulin, at an elevated risk.[34]

Diabetics are also more likely than the general population to have cerebral vascular, peripheral vascular, and renal vascular disease (1 Video 23-1). Diabetes mellitus is the leading cause of renal failure requiring dialysis. Peripheral neuropathies and vascular disease make these patients more susceptible to positioning injuries both during and after surgery. Autonomic neuropathy may predispose the patient to hemodynamic instability during anesthesia and theoretically increase the risk of pulmonary aspiration because of the associated gastroparesis. These deficits should be documented prior to anesthesia and the anesthetic plan adjusted accordingly. Stiff joint syndrome due to glycosylation of proteins and abnormal collagen cross-linking may significantly affect the temporomandibular, atlanto-occipital, and cervical spine joints in patients with longstanding type 1 diabetes, resulting in difficulty with tracheal intubation. A thorough airway examination should be performed prior to anesthesia and a high index of suspicion maintained for a potentially difficult airway. Some suggest using the "prayer sign" as an additional evaluation tool; patients who are unable to completely oppose their hands (with no space between) should be suspected of also having changes in other joints potentially impacting airway manipulation.

Regimens for perioperative glycemic control vary enormously, not only between type 1 and type 2 diabetics but also within each group. Patients with type 1 diabetes have an absolute insulin deficiency usually due to destruction of pancreatic β-cells. These patients must receive insulin to prevent diabetic ketoacidosis. Home glucose management most often relies on some combination of short, intermediate, and long-acting insulin regimens. Insulin pumps are increasingly common and are used to administer a continuous subcutaneous infusion of short-acting insulin, supplemented by boluses dictated by glucose levels, diet, and exercise. Type 2 diabetes accounts for the great majority of diabetics and is defined by variable degrees of insulin deficiency and resistance. Although most commonly associated with obesity, it may also be induced by corticosteroids or pregnancy. Ketoacidosis is uncommon in type 2 diabetics and the stress of severe infection or illness is more likely to provoke a nonketotic hyperosmolar state, which is characterized by severe dehydration, hyperglycemia, and hyperosmolarity. In type 2 diabetics, glucose control is most commonly achieved with diet, exercise, and oral hypoglycemic drugs. These agents primarily work by increasing endogenous insulin release, increasing insulin sensitivity, and/or decreasing hepatic gluconeogenesis. These drugs fall under the main categories of sulfonylureas, biguanides, thiazolidinediones, and meglitinides. If glycemic control is unsuccessful, then insulin is generally added to the regimen.

Ideally, both types 1 and 2 diabetic patients should be evaluated in the preoperative clinic as well as by the patient's endocrinologist 1 to 2 weeks before elective surgery. Questions should address the type, dose, and time of antidiabetic therapy as well as the frequency and manifestations of hypoglycemia and level at which symptoms occur.

In addition to a thorough history and physical examination, a judicious laboratory investigation should include determination of blood glucose, hemoglobin A1c, serum electrolytes, creatinine, and an ECG. If the results reveal inadequate glycemic control based on a hemoglobin A1c above the target range (<8% for type 1 diabetics and <7% for type 2 diabetics, as recommended by the American Diabetic Association), abnormal electrolytes, or ketonuria, then elective surgery should be delayed to allow optimization of preoperative glycemic control. Of note, there is no consensus in the literature determining an HbA1c indicative of adequate glycemic control for pediatric patients.[67] Initiation of β-blockers prior to the day of surgery should be considered in diabetic patients with at least two other risk factors for an adverse cardiac event, as there is no evidence that β-blockers will worsen glucose intolerance or mask hypoglycemic symptoms.[34]

Perioperative Glucose Management

Anesthesia and surgery interrupt the regular meal and insulin administration schedules of patients with diabetes mellitus. Perioperative stress may increase serum glucose concentrations secondary to the release of cortisol and catecholamines. The majority of available literature suggests that better glycemic control may limit morbidity (length of hospital/intensive care unit stay, infection rate, wound healing, outcomes after strokes/MIs) and mortality, particularly in cardiac surgery patients, carotid endarterectomy patients, and the critically ill.[66] It is hypothesized that elevated blood glucose (BG) levels impair neutrophil function and cause an overproduction of reactive oxygen species, free fatty acids (FFAs), and inflammatory mediators. These pathophysiologic changes contribute to direct cellular damage and vascular and immune dysfunction.[68]

More studies are needed to more closely define the target level for glucose control, and societies do vary on their recommendations. There is general consensus that an attempt should be made to control the upper limit of glucose to less than 200 mg/dL, although some will argue that even tighter control is warranted. For example, the Society for Ambulatory Anesthesia recommends glucose levels <180 mg/dL, the American Diabetic Association recommends 140 to 180 mg/dL, the Society of Critical Care Medicine recommends <150 mg/dL, and the American College of Physicians recommends 140 to 200 mg/dL.[68]

Guide for Perioperative Glucose Control

The following recommendations can serve as a general guide.[67,68]

- Plan with the surgeon to schedule the surgery as the first case of the day to prevent prolonged fasting.
- As a general rule, oral hypoglycemic agents are held on the day of surgery to avoid reactive hypoglycemia until oral intake is restarted.
- Insulin therapy should balance adequate glucose control with the avoidance of hypoglycemia. Insulin is usually continued through the evening before surgery.
- Schedule the patient to arrive in the early morning and check blood glucose on arrival and every hour if delayed.
- If patients develop symptoms or measurable hypoglycemia, they should be counseled to take a glucose tablet or clear juice if an IV is not in place to deliver a fluid with glucose.
- Type 1 diabetics should be continued on basal insulin administration even during preoperative fasting to prevent ketoacidosis. Hold the usual dose of rapid- or short-acting insulin, unless patient has hyperglycemia that requires correction.
- Use the patient's own sliding scale to administer short-acting insulin subcutaneously prior to the scheduled surgery and during short operations.
- Patients on insulin pumps may be managed by continuing the pump for short operations or changing over to an intravenous insulin infusion for longer or major operations.

This strategy, along with blood glucose determinations every 1 to 2 hours, may be all that is necessary for well-controlled diabetics undergoing short, noninvasive outpatient operations. In addition, it is important to prevent postoperative nausea and vomiting and to encourage the early resumption of diet, allowing return to their previous insulin regimen. For type 1 or 2 diabetics undergoing longer or major surgery, consultation with the patient's endocrinologist is recommended as insulin is generally administered in the form of an intravenous infusion of regular insulin rather than continuing a long-acting subcutaneous insulin or insulin pump. There are several methods of administering an insulin infusion, none of which has proved superior. Concurrent separate infusions of insulin and glucose are more easily adjusted and may provide better glycemic control than combined glucose/insulin/potassium infusions. To increase safety, the insulin infusion is added via a side port to the same line delivering the glucose infusion. A separate non glucose isotonic solution should be used to replace deficits and intraoperative fluid losses. All protocols rely on the frequent determination of a plasma glucose level at least every 1 to 2 hours to allow titration of insulin. For more in-depth information on diabetes mellitus, therapies, and perioperative management, please see the chapter on Endocrine Function.

Thyroid and Parathyroid Diseases

Thyroid and parathyroid diseases have clinical manifestations that are pertinent to the perioperative care of the patient. Although thyroid function tests are more sensitive, thyroid disease is usually adequately evaluated by clinical history, which should screen for signs and symptoms of hypothyroidism and hyperthyroidism. Hypothyroidism can lead to the development of hypothermia, hypoglycemia, hypoventilation, hyponatremia, and heart failure, as well as a susceptibility to anesthetics. Anesthesiologists should be alert to the possibility of the hypermetabolic state of thyroid storm in patients with hyperthyroidism. A large thyroid mass may distort the upper airway, producing inspiratory stridor or wheezing, especially evident in the supine position. In these cases, a chest x-ray should be obtained looking for evidence of tracheal deviation or narrowing. A CT scan of the upper airway and trachea will provide better detail of any airway compromise. Patients with hyperparathyroidism often have hypercalcemia, and a preoperative determination of a serum calcium level is warranted. Additional clinical manifestations of these conditions are shown in Table 23-12. For a more in-depth review, refer to the chapter on Endocrine Function.

Adrenal Disorders

The classic clinical presentation of a patient with pheochromocytoma includes intermittent hypertension, headache, diaphoresis, and tachycardia. Patients with endocrine tumors have a higher incidence of multiple endocrine neoplasia syndrome and pheochromocytoma should be ruled out as the cause of unexplained hypertension. Over time, the mortality for surgical resection of a pheochromocytoma has decreased because of improvements in perioperative therapy for these patients. A more important issue is that patients with a possible pheochromocytoma be identified before they are scheduled for other types of surgery.

Adrenal–cortical suppression (or *secondary adrenal insufficiency*) results from exogenous steroid use producing negative feedback on the hypothalamic pituitary adrenal axis (HPAA) resulting in impaired cortisol production. If additional corticosteroids are not administered, vasodilation and profound hypotension may result. Awake patients may exhibit altered mental status, weakness, nausea, vomiting, and abdominal pain. Preoperative preparation for patients with adrenal suppression includes correction of any fluid and electrolyte abnormalities, as well as steroid supplementation, although there is not clear guidance on this practice. Many anesthesiologists weigh the risk for HPAA suppression based upon dose and duration of previous steroid treatment, and the expected stress from surgery. Typically, patients taking steroids for less than 3 weeks or using prednisone 5 mg/day or less are considered low risk and may not warrant a perioperative stress dose. One must

Table 23-12 Clinical Manifestations of Thyroid and Parathyroid Diseases

	Hyperthyroidism	Hypothyroidism	Hyperparathyroidism
General	Weight loss; heat intolerance; warm, moist skin	Cold intolerance	Weight loss, polydipsia
Cardiovascular	Tachycardia, atrial fibrillation, congestive heart failure	Bradycardia, congestive heart failure, cardiomegaly, pericardial or pleural effusion	Hypertension, heart block
Neurologic	Nervousness, tremor, hyperactive reflexes	Slow mental function, minimal reflexes	Weakness, lethargy, headache, insomnia, apathy, depression
Musculoskeletal	Muscle weakness, bone resorption	Large tongue, amyloidosis	Bone pains, arthritis, pathologic fractures
Gastrointestinal	Diarrhea	Delayed gastric emptying	Anorexia, nausea, vomiting, constipation, epigastric pain
Hematologic	Anemia, thrombocytopenia		
Renal		Impaired free water clearance	Polyuria, hematuria

Adapted from Roizen MF. Anesthesia for the patient with endocrine disease, part 1. *Curr Rev Clin Anesth*. 1987;6:43.

be wary as the addition of supraphysiologic doses of steroids can increase the risk of acute side effects, such as hyperglycemia, hypertension, fluid retention, and an increased risk of infection. If a patient has Cushing syndrome, which is the most obvious manifestation of long-term high-dose steroid treatment (moon facies, striations of the skin, truncal obesity, hypertension, easy bruisability, and hypovolemia), then stress dose steroids should be administered. Hydrocortisone is the replacement drug of choice with doses ranging from 50 to 100 mg prior to incision followed by 25 to 50 mg every 8 hours for 24 hours.[69] There is a lack of solid evidence for these recommendations and practice varies. However, experts do agree that patients should continue to receive their usual daily glucocorticoid dose. Exogenous glucocorticoid administration should be considered in any patient who develops perioperative hypotension that is not responsive to standard resuscitative fluid administration or vasopressor therapy, and cannot be explained by other mechanisms, suggesting adrenal insufficiency.

Renal Disease

Renal disease has important implications for fluid and electrolyte management, as well as metabolism of drugs. The cause of renal failure has considerable impact on clinical management. Patients with primary renal disease are likely to be younger and have good cardiopulmonary reserve, whereas a significant percentage of older patients with renal failure secondary to diabetes mellitus or hypertension will also have diffuse atherosclerosis and heart disease. Chronic renal disease secondary to sickle cell disease, systemic lupus erythematosus, or vasculitis implies multisystem involvement and dysfunction.[70] In patients with renal failure, the timing of their most recent dialysis will determine whether they are hyper- or hypovolemic and hyper- or hypokalemic. It is important to assess the patient's electrolytes prior to surgery and to ensure they are euvolemic prior to induction of anesthesia. Some patients will require dialysis before surgery. Because renal failure is also associated with anemia and qualitatively deficient platelets, there should be a lower threshold for assessing these laboratory results preoperatively.

Liver Disease

Liver disease is associated with decreased plasma protein production, thereby affecting drug binding, volume of distribution, metabolism, and clearance. Coagulopathy accompanies liver failure and the etiology can be multifactorial; it can result from malnutrition (poor absorption of nutrients as a consequence of cholestasis), impaired synthesis of coagulation factors, or thrombocytopenia. The history should identify specific risk factors for liver disease, such as previous blood transfusions, illicit drug use, or excessive alcohol intake. The anesthesiologist should inquire about bruising, bleeding, or history of esophageal varices, the latter to potentially avoid esophageal instrumentation. Coagulation disorders may discourage the choice of regional anesthesia. The physical examination should screen for signs of underlying liver disease, such as jaundice, spider nevi, ascites, hepatosplenomegaly, or palmar erythema. Ascites, a more obvious physical finding of liver failure, may significantly affect the patient's respiratory mechanics and make it difficult to lie flat. In patients with chronic liver disease, perioperative risk increases with worsening severity of hepatic dysfunction as assessed by the Model for End-Stage Liver Disease (MELD) score. The MELD assigns the patient a score of 8 to 40 that is derived from a complex formula that incorporates three biochemical variables—the serum total bilirubin concentration, serum creatinine concentration, and international normalized ratio (INR). The MELD score has been prospectively validated as a prognostic marker of mortality in patients with cirrhosis, acute variceal bleeding, or acute alcoholic hepatitis.[71]

Infectious Disease

The anesthesiologist should inquire about infectious diseases, including questions about foreign travel, that will dictate the need for increased protective measures for OR personnel and equipment. The COVID-19 pandemic has led to many changing guidelines and practice standards. Due to the fluid nature of these circumstances, specific guidelines regarding tests, protective equipment and timing of surgery should be obtained from local hospital policies as well as recent information on the ASA website:https://www.asahq.org/in-the-spotlight/coronavirus-covid-19-information.

Other Diseases

Arthritis is becoming more prevalent in our aging population, worsened by our sedentary lifestyle. Osteoarthritis may result in difficulty positioning the head to facilitate tracheal intubation or difficulty in positioning for regional anesthesia. These are likewise problems in patients with RA; however, of particular importance is the potential for atlantoaxial instability or superior migration of the odontoid causing spinal cord compression. Involvement of the cervical spine in RA patients typically parallels the extent of peripheral disease and may warrant preoperative radiologic screening.[72] Although not as common, RA of the temporomandibular joint may impede mouth opening for tracheal intubation. RA is a multisystem disease, potentially leading to derangements in other organ systems, causing restrictive lung disease, pleural effusions, pericarditis, and anemia.

Preoperative Laboratory Testing

Defining Normal Values

In attempting to determine the optimal choice of preoperative tests, it is important to understand the interpretation of the results. Ideally, tests would either confirm or exclude the presence of a disease; however, most tests only increase or decrease the probability of disease. In determining reference ranges for diagnostic tests, values that fall outside the 95% confidence intervals for normal individuals are considered abnormal. Therefore, up to 5% of normal individuals can have "abnormal" test results. To determine its clinical relevance, a test must be interpreted within the context of the clinical situation. Performing tests in patients with no risk for having the pathophysiologic process of interest is likely to yield a high number of false-positive results. Interpreting these results as abnormal, and initiating treatment, could lead to harm without any benefit.

Risks and Costs versus Benefits

8 The 2012 ASA Practice Advisory for Preanesthesia Evaluation[1] states that routine preoperative tests do not make an important contribution to preanesthetic evaluation of an asymptomatic patient. Selective preoperative tests should be ordered only after consideration of specific information obtained from the medical record, history and physical, and the type or invasiveness of the planned procedure and anesthesia. Consideration should also be given to whether the results will affect the plan for the patient's perioperative course.

Medical testing is associated with significant cost, both in real dollars and in potential harm. Routine preoperative testing has been estimated to cost billions of dollars annually in the United States. An "abnormal" test that is later determined to be a false result can lead to significant cost and real harm. For example, a positive exercise ECG stress test in a healthy 40-year-old woman may lead to coronary angiography. Coronary angiography is not a benign procedure and can lead to vascular injuries. On the basis of Bayesian analysis, a positive ECG stress test result in this patient would most likely be a false positive, and hence it would be inappropriate to order this test. No additional information would be obtained, thousands of dollars in medical costs would accrue, and the patient may sustain iatrogenic injury.

Routine laboratory screening tests produce only minimal benefits in healthy patients,[73] and routine testing is not indicated.[74] The following protocol for laboratory testing is modified from a risk–benefit analysis[75] and the 2012 ASA Practice Advisory for Preanesthetic Evaluation.[1]

Clinical Considerations for Laboratory Testing

Blood count
Extremes of age
Liver or kidney disease
Anticoagulant use
Bleeding/hematologic disorder
Malignancy
Type and invasiveness of procedure

Coagulation studies
Liver or kidney disease
Bleeding disorder
Anticoagulant use
Chemotherapy

Serum chemistries (glucose, electrolytes, renal and liver function)
Liver or renal disease, or perioperative risk of dysfunction
Diabetes
Diuretic, digoxin, or steroid use
Central nervous system disease
Endocrine disorders
Elderly
Malnutrition
Type and invasiveness of procedure

Chest x-ray
Pulmonary disease or clinical manifestations
Unstable cardiovascular disease
Type and invasiveness of procedure

ECG
Cardiovascular disease or clinical risk factors
Pulmonary disease
Type and invasiveness of procedure

Pregnancy test
Possible pregnancy

Complete Blood Count and Hemoglobin Concentration

A preoperative hemoglobin or hematocrit value has been suggested as the only test necessary in many patients prior to elective surgery; however, even this minimal standard has been questioned. In only 1.1% of the records of 1,863 pediatric patients scheduled for elective outpatient procedures was the hematocrit found to be abnormal, and in none of these patients was the procedure canceled or the anesthetic plan modified.[76] However, a baseline hematocrit is still indicated in any procedure with a risk of significant blood loss.

Both the standard for the lowest acceptable perioperative hematocrit and the indication for a preoperative transfusion have changed. The current recommendations of the National Blood Resource Education Committee are that a hemoglobin level of 7 g/dL is acceptable in patients without systemic disease. In patients with systemic disease, signs of inadequate systemic oxygen delivery (tachycardia, tachypnea) are an indication for transfusion.

Coagulation Studies

Coagulation disorders can have a significant impact on the surgical procedure and perioperative management. In patients with hemophilia or von Willebrand disease, abnormal laboratory studies even in the absence of clinical abnormalities require preoperative preparation of the patient. Abnormal coagulation values may delay the surgery depending on the degree of abnormality and the procedure planned. For example, neurosurgery has little tolerance for values outside of the normal range due to the serious consequences if uncontrolled bleeding were to occur perioperatively. Surgery may be delayed for hours if fresh-frozen plasma or platelets are needed to acutely correct a coagulopathy, or for days if vitamin K is administered for correction.

Pregnancy Testing

Routine pregnancy testing in women of childbearing potential is a subject of considerable debate. Surgery itself may cause harm to the fetus or expose the fetus to potential teratogens, such as x-rays or certain medications. Thus, knowledge of pregnancy status may change the timing of surgery or anesthetic technique. Point-of-care urine β-hCG testing is easily and rapidly performed by nursing staff with high sensitivity and specificity; however, rare circumstances may lead to false negatives or positives such as low levels of β-hCG or hormone-secreting tumors. There are also ethical issues regarding privacy and autonomy, especially for the minor patient accompanied by parents. The ASA Practice Advisory for Preanesthesia Evaluation recommends that females of childbearing age be offered pregnancy testing if the result would change medical management, but it is not mandatory. Informed consent or assent should be obtained through shared decision making between the patient and provider (https://www.asahq.org/standards-and-guidelines/pregnancy-testing-prior-to-anesthesia-and-surgery)

Chest X-Rays

A preoperative chest x-ray can identify abnormalities that may lead to either delay or cancellation of the planned surgical procedure or modification of perioperative care. For example, identification of pneumonia, pulmonary edema, pulmonary nodules, or a mediastinal mass could all lead to modification of care. However, routine testing in the population without risk factors can lead to more harm than benefit and morbidity from additional, unwarranted follow-up procedures.[75]

The American College of Physicians suggests that a chest x-ray is indicated in the presence of active chest disease or an intrathoracic procedure but not on the basis of advanced age alone.[77] In a meta-analysis, a review of published reports from 1966 to 1992 in the English, French, and Spanish literature showed that abnormalities were reported in 10% of routine preoperative chest x-rays, of which only 1.3% were unexpected.[78] These findings resulted in modification in management in only 0.1% of patients, with unknown influence on outcome. The authors estimated a cost of $23,000 for each finding that influenced management, and concluded that routine chest x-rays without a clinical indication were not justified.

Pulmonary Function Tests

Consensus guidelines do not support the routine use of pulmonary function studies to predict perioperative respiratory complications. Pulmonary function tests can be divided into two categories: spirometry and arterial blood gas analysis. Spirometry can provide information on forced vital capacity (FVC), forced expiratory volume in 1 second (FEV_1), ratio of FEV_1/FVC, and average forced expiratory flow from 25% to 75% (FEF 25% to 75%). Although each of these measures has a sound physiologic basis, their practical assessment can vary greatly among healthy persons and the tests rarely provide additional information beyond that obtained from history. For those patients considered for pulmonary resection, evaluation using spirometry, diffusion capacity measurements, radionucleotide lung perfusion scanning, and cardiopulmonary exercise testing may help to define those patients at high risk.[79]

With the ubiquitous availability of pulse oximetry, the use of preoperative arterial blood gas sampling has become less important. It may still be indicated in those with poor pulmonary function, since determining the baseline CO_2 is useful in managing perioperative ventilator settings, and resting hypercapnia is associated with increased perioperative risk. One method of assessing the probability of CO_2 retention is evaluation of the serum bicarbonate. A normal serum bicarbonate value will virtually exclude the diagnosis of chronic CO_2 retention.

Summary of the Preoperative Evaluation

There are multiple factors that are associated with increased perioperative risk, as discussed within this chapter. Clinical judgment is necessary and requires addressing the following fundamental questions:

1. Are the risk factors modifiable?
2. Will delaying the procedure add to perioperative risk or patient morbidity?
3. What interventions during the preoperative period can be implemented to reduce risk?
4. Has the patient been provided enough information to make an informed decision?

An effective preoperative evaluation will address these concerns and recommend therapeutic interventions to limit risk. Finally, the anesthesiologist can play an important role in reducing inappropriate utilization of medical technology and in helping to coordinate the patient's care among the multiple physician specialties often required for patients with complex illnesses who require surgery.

Preparation

Smoking Cessation

Surgery provides an opportunity for intervention to promote smoking cessation, as the patient may be open to making changes to better their health. Hence, the ASA is encouraging anesthesiologists to use the preoperative evaluation as a teachable moment to discuss smoking cessation and provide educational resources available on the ASA website. Because patients will be unable to smoke in the hospital, such timing may help give them more incentive to quit. It should be explained to patients who smoke that they are at increased risk for pulmonary and cardiac complications as well as impaired wound healing and infection. The longer they are tobacco free before surgery the better, as their bodies will have more time for repair. Even only 12 hours of smoking cessation will reduce levels of nicotine and carbon monoxide, improving blood flow. The long-term benefits of quitting smoking include: addition of 6 to 8 years to their life, reduction in risk of lung cancer and heart disease, savings of at least $1,400 per year (not including health care costs), and reduced exposure of the family to secondhand smoke. Offer patients additional help to quit by referring them to 1-800-QUIT-NOW, a free and confidential counseling service (https://www.asahq.org/standards-and-guidelines/statement-on-smoking-cessation).

Continuing Current Medications/ Treatment of Coexisting Diseases

It is the responsibility of the anesthesiologist to instruct patients regarding which medications to take or not take preoperatively (NICV 23-8). Occasionally, new medications will be prescribed or doses increased, such as steroids for adrenal insufficiency. Prescribed and over-the-counter medications may affect the anesthetic; anesthesiologists must be knowledgeable about their actions. As a general rule, patients should take their prescription medications with water on the day of surgery. However, important exceptions exist, particularly for the management of diabetes.

β-Blockers

The role of β-blockers during the perioperative period has evolved over time, based on clinical studies evaluating both effectiveness and the potential for risk. Historically, β-blockers have been felt to reduce the incidence of mortality and nonfatal MIs after surgery. Current guidelines recommend that β-blockers be continued in those already receiving β-blockers to treat angina pectoris, symptomatic arrhythmias, and hypertension. Recent clinical studies, however, have questioned the decision to initiate perioperative β-blockers and have suggested that the decision be based on clinical judgment in evaluating the patient's risk factors for cardiovascular complications together with the type of surgery. The POISE trial (a large, multicenter, randomized controlled trial) compared preoperative β-blocker therapy with placebo.[80] Patients receiving β-blocker therapy had a lower risk of perioperative MI, but were at significantly increased risk for mortality and stroke. As potential mechanisms for enhanced risk, perioperative hypotension and bradycardia were significantly increased in patients receiving β-blockers. A meta-analysis evaluating perioperative β-blockade in noncardiac surgery in 33 randomized controlled trials with 12,306 patients found no difference in overall mortality, but decreased risk of perioperative MI.[81] Similar to the POISE trial, the risk of nonfatal stroke was increased with β-blockade. Recognizing these results, updated guidelines from the ACC/AHA support, as a class I recommendation, the perioperative continuation of β-blockers for patients already receiving β-blocker for appropriate conditions, and they support a role for β-blocker therapy titrated to heart rate and blood pressure during vascular or intermediate-risk surgeries in patients with CAD, cardiac ischemia identified by preoperative testing, or more than one RCRI risk factor.[34,82] Importantly, the ACC/AHA guidelines stress uncertainty for the role of β-blockade for vascular or intermediate-risk surgery in patients with only one risk factor without ischemic heart disease or in patients without risk factors who have not taken β-blocker therapy previously. A review of current literature shows a decreased risk of nonfatal MI at the expense of increased perioperative risk of stroke, death, hypotension, and bradycardia associated with fixed, high-dose β-blocker therapy begun on the day of surgery.[82] Initiation and titration of β-blockade 2 or more days prior to the day of surgery may offer a role in the reduction of risk for perioperative MI, but there is insufficient data to recommend this practice, and it remains controversial. This is acknowledged by the ACC/AHA and further multicenter RCTs are needed to address this knowledge gap.

Anticoagulation

The perioperative management of patients receiving chronic anticoagulation can be challenging, as it requires a balance between reducing the risk of thromboembolic events versus excessive bleeding and hemorrhagic complications. The ACC/AHA states that the risk of bleeding must be weighed against the benefit of remaining on anticoagulation on a case-by-case basis, considering the specific patient, medication, and procedure. Oral anticoagulation is often prescribed for patients with atrial fibrillation for stroke prevention, as well as patients with a history of venous thromboembolism and valvular heart disease. Depending on the pharmacokinetics of the oral anticoagulant, therapy is often interrupted 2 to 5 days prior to noncardiac surgery. In a randomized controlled trial, the effect of bridging anticoagulation in 1,884 patients with atrial fibrillation who had their warfarin interrupted prior to noncardiac surgery was evaluated. No difference was found in the rates of arterial thromboembolism, but the incidence of major bleeding was found to be significantly higher in the bridging group.[83] Interrupting anticoagulation therapy in patients with atrial fibrillation therefore appears to be safe, and perioperative bridging is typically unnecessary. In contrast, bridging anticoagulation may be appropriate in patients at high risk of arterial thromboembolism, such as patients with mechanical aortic or mitral valves.[34]

Aspirin

Aspirin is an irreversible inhibitor of platelet cyclooxygenase-1, which decreases platelet aggregation and thrombotic risk, but may increase intraoperative blood loss and hemorrhagic complications. POISE-2 Trial randomized over 10,000 patients undergoing noncardiac surgery at risk for vascular complications to aspirin 200 mg or placebo.[42] No protective effect on the incidence of MACE or death was seen in the aspirin group, however aspirin use was associated with an increased risk of major bleeding. Notably, patients within 6 weeks of placement of a bare metal cardiac stent or 12 months of a drug eluting stent placement were excluded, as well as patients undergoing carotid endarterectomy. The ACC/AHA does not recommend routine aspirin use prior to noncardiac surgery, although aspirin therapy may be appropriate for certain patient populations (e.g., high-risk CAD, cerebrovascular disease) if ischemic risks outweigh the risk of bleeding.[34]

Statins

There is growing evidence in the literature to suggest that perioperative statin therapy is safe and beneficial in reducing morbidity and mortality in the perioperative period. Statins work via several mechanisms: lowering lipids, enhancing nitric oxide–mediated pathways, reducing expression of cytokines and adhesion molecules, and lowering C-reactive protein levels with associated vasodilatory, anti-inflammatory, and antithrombotic effects. The greatest benefit occurs in patients at higher risk for cardiovascular complications. There is good evidence that the perioperative withdrawal of statins increases morbidity; both the ACC/AHA and the European Society of Cardiology (ESC) have made a class 1 recommendation that patients who are on a statin preoperatively should be restarted on a statin postoperatively as soon as possible. Patients with noncoronary atherosclerosis should be treated with statin therapy for secondary prevention, independent of noncardiac surgery. The ESC also recommends that statins be started in high-risk surgery patients, optimally between 30 days and at least 1 week before surgery. Guidelines from the ACC/AHA state that statin use is reasonable for patients undergoing vascular surgery with or without clinical risk factors, and statins may be considered for patients with at least one clinical risk factor who are undergoing intermediate-risk procedures.[34,84]

Angiotensin-Converting Enzyme Inhibitors and Angiotensin Receptor Blockers

The perioperative management of angiotensin-converting enzyme inhibitors (ACEIs) and angiotensin II receptor blockers (ARBs) is controversial. Intraoperative hypotension secondary to the continuation of ACEI/ARBs has led to many clinicians withholding therapy on the day of surgery, although outcomes data is inconsistent. A recent meta-analysis evaluated 9 studies with over 6,000 patients on chronic ACEI/ARB therapy before noncardiac surgery and showed that withholding ACEI/ARB treatment the day of surgery was associated with significantly less intraoperative hypotension (OR, 0.63; 95% CI, 0.47–0.85).[85] There was, however, no difference in mortality (OR 0.97; 95% CI 0.62–1.52) or in the occurrence of MACE (OR 1.12; 95% CI 0.82–1.52). The ACC/AHA acknowledges that there is a paucity of data regarding whether specific surgeries or patient subgroups are most likely to benefit from holding ACEI/ARB therapy preoperatively. Their recommendations are that continuation of ACEI/ARB therapy in the perioperative period is reasonable, however, if they are held prior to surgery, they should be restarted as soon as clinically feasible.[34]

Prevention of Perioperative Pulmonary Aspiration

Extrapolation from a primate study led to the statement in 1974 that patients who had a 25-mL residual gastric volume with a pH lower than 2.5 were at risk of aspiration, which might imply that some 40% to 80% of patients scheduled for elective surgery may be at risk.[86,87] However, clinically significant pulmonary aspiration is actually very rare today in healthy patients undergoing general anesthesia, quoted as occurring in 1 in 3,000 to 1 in 6,000 anesthetics, though increasing to 1 in 600 for emergency anesthesia. Some patients who present for anesthesia are at increased risk for aspiration—the Australian Anesthetic Incident Monitoring Study[88] found 133 cases of aspiration in 5,000 incidents reported, with the top 10 risk factors for aspiration shown in Table 23-13. However, almost 25% of the patients who aspirated had no risk factors. Errors in judgment, faults in airway management technique, and inadequate patient preparation were felt to be the most common factors contributing to these events.

ASA Fasting Guidelines

The ASA published updated Practice Guidelines for Preoperative Fasting and Pharmacologic Intervention for the Prevention of Perioperative Aspiration in 2017.[89] The guidelines specifically address healthy patients of all ages scheduled for elective procedures in which general anesthesia, regional anesthesia, or sedation will be administered. The purpose of the guidelines is not only to minimize the risk of pulmonary aspiration but also to avoid case delays as well as prolonged fasting leading to dehydration, hypoglycemia, and patient dissatisfaction. More conservative fasting intervals may be clinically appropriate in patients with comorbidities that impact gastric emptying such as pregnancy, obesity, hiatal hernia, ileus or bowel obstruction, or patients with a known or anticipated difficult airway, or gastroesophageal reflux disease.

Recommendations for Clear Liquids: At Least 2 Hours

The primary support for the task force recommendations comes from a meta-analysis of randomized controlled trials comparing fasting times for clear liquids of 2 to 4 hours versus more than 4 hours. Adult patients fasting for 2 to 4 hours had smaller gastric volumes and higher gastric pH values compared to those fasting more than 4 hours. The differences in gastric volumes were equivocal in children. Therefore, the task force recommendations are unchanged for healthy patients. Examples of clear liquids include, but are not limited to, water, fruit juices without pulp, carbonated beverages, clear tea, and black coffee. Clear liquids do not include alcohol. Of note, several European anesthesia societies and the Canadian Pediatric Anesthesia Society recommend a 1-hour clear fluid policy for healthy pediatric patients, as they feel evidence shows no increased risk of pulmonary aspiration and equivocal gastric emptying compared to 2-hour fasting.[90,91]

Table 23-13 Top 10 Factors Predisposing to Aspiration

1	Emergency surgery
2	Inadequate anesthesia
3	Abdominal pathology
4	Obesity
5	Opioid medication
6	Neurologic deficit
7	Lithotomy
8	Difficult intubation/airway
9	Reflux
10	Hiatal hernia

Adapted from Kluger MT, Short TG. Aspiration during anaesthesia: A review of 133 cases from the Australian Anaesthetic Incident Monitoring Study (AIMS). *Anaesthesia*. 1999;54:19–26. Copyright © 2018 Association of Anaesthetists.

Recommendations for Breast Milk: At Least 4 Hours

The fasting recommendations for breast milk are also unchanged, as the task force found only equivocal findings regarding gastric fluid volume and pH from observational studies in infants.[89]

Recommendations for Infant Formula, Nonhuman Milk, and Light Meal: At Least 6 Hours

Again, among the observational and randomized control studies, the task force found no evidence to support any change in the previous recommendations for at least a 6-hour fast before elective procedures.[89] They noted that the amount and type of food must be considered, and recommended at least 8 hours before elective procedures for fried or fatty food that typically delays gastric emptying time.

For a summary of the fasting guidelines, see Table 23-14.

Pharmacologic Agents to Reduce the Risk of Pulmonary Aspiration

Many different pharmacologic approaches have been used to decrease the volume and increase the pH of gastric fluid in an effort to reduce the risk of aspiration pneumonitis, such as histamine-2 (H-2) receptor antagonists, proton pump inhibitors (PPIs), antacids, antiemetics, and gastrokinetic agents. The ASA task force reviewed the literature and surveyed both experts and ASA members to arrive at their 2017 recommendations for pharmacologic

Table 23-14 Summary of Fasting Recommendations for all Ages to Reduce the Risk of Pulmonary Aspiration

Ingested Material	Minimum Fasting Period in Hours
Clear liquids	2 h
Breast milk	4 h
Infant formula	6 h
Nonhuman milk	6 h
Light meal	6 h
Fatty or Fried Foods	8 h

This summary applies only to healthy patients who are undergoing elective procedures and is not intended for women in labor. Following the guidelines does not guarantee complete gastric emptying. Examples of clear liquids are water, fruit juices without pulp, carbonated beverages, clear tea, and black coffee.

Adapted with permission from Practice guidelines for preoperative fasting and the use of pharmacologic agents to reduce the risk of pulmonary aspiration: Application to healthy patients undergoing elective procedures: An updated report by the American Society of Anesthesiologists Committee on Standards and Practice Parameters. *Anesthesiology*. 2011;114:495–511.

agents. They found that the literature is insufficient to evaluate or support the effect of administering any of these classes of drugs on the perioperative incidence of emesis/reflux or pulmonary aspiration. Therefore, they could not recommend the routine preoperative use of such drugs for patients who have no apparent increased risk for pulmonary aspiration.[89] However, the drugs were found to be effective for their intended use and are more cost-effective when prescribed for patients who have risk factors for pulmonary aspiration.

Histamine-2 (H-2) Receptor Antagonists

Meta-analyses of randomized placebo-controlled trials support the efficacy of the H-2 receptor antagonists cimetidine, ranitidine, and famotidine in reducing gastric volume and acidity.[89] They block the ability of histamine to induce secretion of gastric fluid with a high hydrogen ion concentration. Multiple-dose regimens may be more effective in increasing gastric pH than a single dose before operation on the day of surgery.

Cimetidine

Cimetidine is usually administered in 150 to 300 mg doses orally or parenterally. The gastric effects of cimetidine last as long as 3 or 4 hours; thus, this drug is suitable for operations of that duration.[89] Side effects of cimetidine include inhibition of the hepatic mixed-function oxidase enzyme system. More seriously, life-threatening cardiac dysrhythmias, hypotension, cardiac arrest, and central nervous system depression have been reported after cimetidine administration. These side effects may be especially likely to occur in critically ill patients after rapid intravenous administration.

Ranitidine

Ranitidine is more potent, specific, and longer acting than cimetidine. The usual oral dose of 150 mg or 50 mg given parenterally will increase gastric fluid pH within 1 hour. It is as effective as cimetidine and produces fewer cardiovascular or central nervous system side effects. The effects of ranitidine last up to 9 hours. Thus, it may be superior to cimetidine at the conclusion of lengthy procedures in reducing the risk of aspiration pneumonitis during emergence from anesthesia and extubation.

Famotidine

Famotidine is another H-2 receptor blocker that is given preoperatively to raise gastric fluid pH, typically administered as 40 mg orally 1.5 to 3 hours preoperatively. The pharmacokinetics are similar to those of cimetidine and ranitidine, with the exception of having a longer serum elimination half-life than the other two drugs.

Proton Pump Inhibitors (PPIs)

PPIs suppress gastric acid secretion in a dose-dependent manner by binding to the proton pump of the parietal cell. Meta-analysis of placebo controlled RCTs support their efficacy in reducing gastric volume and acidity.[89,92] For adult patients, oral doses of 40 mg to 80 mg must be given 2 to 4 hours before surgery to be effective, or omeprazole 40 mg intravenously 30 minutes before induction has been used. The effect on gastric pH may last as long as 24 hours.

Antacids

Antacids are used to neutralize the acid already present in gastric contents. Placebo controlled RCTs demonstrate their effectiveness.[89] A single dose of antacid given 15 to 30 minutes before induction of anesthesia is almost 100% effective in increasing gastric fluid pH above 2.5. Although colloid antacid suspensions may be more effective in increasing gastric fluid pH, aspiration of particulate antacids may cause significant and persistent pulmonary damage. Nonparticulate antacids do not produce pulmonary damage themselves if aspiration should occur. Consequently, the nonparticulate antacid, 0.3 M sodium citrate, is commonly used.

Withholding antacids because of concern about increasing gastric volume is not warranted, as it is more important to raise the pH. Animal evidence showed increased mortality after aspiration of low volumes of acidic gastric fluid (0.3 mL/kg, pH 1) compared to aspiration of large volumes of buffered gastric fluid (1 to 2 mL/kg, pH > 1.8).[93]

Gastrokinetic Agents: Metoclopramide

Metoclopramide is a dopamine antagonist with antiemetic properties that stimulates upper gastrointestinal motility, increases gastroesophageal sphincter tone, and relaxes the pylorus and duodenum to reduce gastric volume. A meta-analysis of randomized placebo-controlled trials supports the efficacy of metoclopramide to reduce gastric volume, but is equivocal regarding its effect on gastric acidity during the perioperative period.[89] Thus it is helpful in patients with large gastric fluid volumes, such as parturients, patients scheduled for emergency surgery, obese patients, trauma patients, and those with gastroparesis secondary to diabetes mellitus. It is not recommended for patients diagnosed with bowel obstruction. It may be administered orally or parenterally. A parenteral dose of 5 mg to 10 mg is usually given 30 minutes before induction. Administration intravenously over 3 to 5 minutes usually prevents the abdominal cramping that can occur from more rapid administration. An oral dose of 10 mg achieves onset within 30 to 60 minutes. The elimination half-life of metoclopramide is approximately 2 to 4 hours.

The combination of metoclopramide with an H-2 receptor antagonist does not decrease the effect of either drug, and the effects may be additive.[89]

As reviewed earlier, the drugs used to decrease gastric fluid volume and acidity are effective and relatively free of side effects. The use of these agents is warranted in patients with decreased gastric emptying, reflux, and those presenting for emergency procedures. However, none of the drugs or combination of drugs is absolutely reliable in preventing the risk of aspiration in all patients all of the time. Therefore, one must still employ anesthetic techniques to protect the airway during induction, maintenance, and emergence from anesthesia.

Psychological Preparation/ Premedication

Anesthetic management for patients begins with preoperative psychological preparation and, if necessary, preoperative medication. The anesthesiologist should assess the patient's mental and physical condition during the preoperative visit. Because it is actually the beginning of the anesthetic, the decision to administer preoperative medication, and which one, should be based on the same considerations as the choice of anesthesia, including considerations of the patient's medical problems, requirements of the surgery, and recovery goals. Satisfactory preparation lessens the patient's (and family's) anxiety and smooths the anesthetic induction. No consensus exists on the choice of preoperative medications and, historically, their use was dominated by tradition. However, the ever-increasing number of outpatient procedures has led to a significant decrease in preoperative sedation to facilitate rapid recovery from anesthesia.

Psychological Preparation

Psychological preparation of the patient involves a preoperative visit and interview with the patient and family members. The anesthesiologist should explain anticipated events and the proposed anesthetic management in an effort to reduce anxiety. A growing number of patients receive their preanesthetic evaluations by others in preoperative evaluation clinics, such that their initial encounter with the anesthesiologist may be in the immediate preoperative period outside of the OR. Preoperative visits must be conducted efficiently, but they must also be informative and reassuring. Most of the anesthesiologist's time is spent with the patient unconscious or sedated; therefore, time must be taken before the operation to earn the trust and confidence of that patient.

Studies show that, depending on the intensity of inquiry, 40% to 85% of patients are apprehensive before surgery. Most patients expect their apprehension to be relieved before they arrive in the OR, but an informative and comforting preoperative visit may replace many milligrams of a sedative medication. For example, more patients were adequately prepared for surgery after a preoperative interview than after 2 mg/kg of pentobarbital given intramuscularly 1 hour before surgery.[94] After the patient interview, the use of preoperative medication in selected patients serves to achieve sedation or amnesia as well as provide any needed analgesia. Preoperative depressant drugs though, should not be used as a substitute for a comforting and tactful preoperative visit.

Premedication

The ideal drug or combination of drugs for preoperative pharmacologic preparation is as elusive as is the ideal anesthetic technique and is not based on comprehensive or definitive data. In selecting the appropriate drug and dose for preoperative medication, the patient's psychological condition, physical status, age, and prior response to depressant drugs must be considered. Some patients should not receive depressant drugs before surgery. For example, those with little physiologic reserve, head injury, hypovolemia, or at the extremes of age may receive more harm than benefit from premedication. Finally, the surgical procedure, expected duration, and postoperative discharge plan are important factors as well.

The goals to be achieved for each patient with preoperative medication should be tailored to the individual. Some goals, such as relief of anxiety, apply to almost every patient, whereas a goal to dry airway secretions may be reserved for the patient with a potentially difficult airway who may require fiberoptic tracheal intubation.

10 The timing and route of administration of the preoperative medications are important. Every attempt should be made to time the administration so that the premedication achieves its full effect before the patient's arrival in the OR. As a general rule, oral tablets should be given to the patient 60 minutes before arrival in the OR. Intravenous agents, on the other hand, produce effects after a few circulation times. The drug(s), doses, route of administration, and effects should be recorded on the anesthetic record. A list of common preoperative medications is presented in Table 23-15.

Table 23-15 Common Preoperative Medications, Doses, and Administration Routes

Medication	Administration Route	Dose
Lorazepam	Oral, IV	0.5–4 mg
Midazolam	IV	1.0–2.5 mg doses
Fentanyl	IV	25–50 μg doses
Morphine	IV	1.0–2.5 mg doses
Meperidine	IV	10–25 mg doses
Cimetidine	Oral, IV	150–300 mg
Ranitidine	Oral IV	150 mg 50 mg
Metoclopramide	IV	5–10 mg
Atropine	IV	0.2–0.4 mg
Glycopyrrolate	IV	0.1–0.2 mg

IV, Intravenous.

Modified from Stoelting RK, Miller RD, eds. Basics of Anesthesia. New York: Churchill Livingstone; 1984. Copyright © 1984 Elsevier. With permission.

Benzodiazepines

Benzodiazepines are among the most popular preoperative medications because they produce anxiolysis, amnesia, and sedation (Table 23-16). Because the site of action of benzodiazepines is located on the GABA receptor in the central nervous system, there is relatively little depression of the ventilatory or cardiovascular systems with dosages used for premedication. Benzodiazepines have a wide therapeutic index and a low incidence of toxicity. Other than central nervous system depression, these drugs lack the side effects common to opioids, such as nausea and vomiting. However, benzodiazepines may not always produce a calming effect, but occasionally cause a paradoxical agitation manifested as restlessness and delirium. Benzodiazepines are not analgesic agents.

Midazolam

Midazolam has predominantly replaced lorazepam and diazepam for preoperative medication and moderate sedation (Fig. 23-4). It is common to administer sedative doses intravenously just prior to transfer to the OR. As with other benzodiazepines, midazolam produces anxiolysis, sedation, and amnesia. It is two to three times more potent than diazepam because of its increased affinity for the GABA receptor. The usual incremental dose is 1 mg to 2 mg titrated intravenously. There is no irritation or phlebitis with injection of midazolam, as opposed to diazepam. The incidence of side effects after administration is low, although depression of ventilation and sedation may be greater than expected, especially in elderly patients or when the drug is combined with other central nervous system depressants. Compared to diazepam, intravenous midazolam has a rapid onset of 1 to 2 minutes, and more rapid recovery due to its lipid solubility, rapid redistribution to the peripheral tissues, and metabolic biotransformation. For these reasons, midazolam should usually be given within 1 hour of induction. The elimination half-life of midazolam is approximately 1 to 4 hours and may be extended in the elderly. Tests show

Table 23-16 Comparison of Pharmacologic Variables of Benzodiazepines

	Diazepam	Lorazepam	Midazolam
Dose equivalent (mg)	10	1–2	3–5
Time to peak effect after oral dose (h)	1–1.5	2–4	0.5–1
Elimination half-time (h)	20–40	10–20	1–4
Clearance (mL/kg/min)	0.2–0.5	0.7–1.0	6.4–11.1

Adapted from Reves JG, Fragen RJ, Vinick HR, et al. Midazolam: Pharmacology and uses. *Anesthesiology*. 1985;62:310–324; and Stoelting RK. *Pharmacology and Physiology in Anesthetic Practice*. JB Lippincott; 1987.

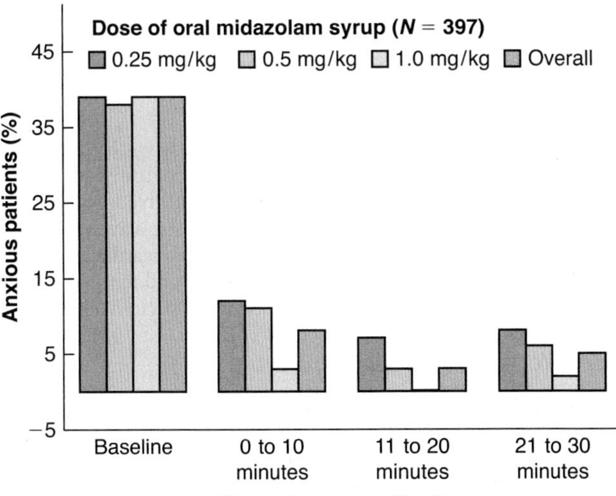

Figure 23-4 Percentage of patients exhibiting anxiety from baseline to time after oral midazolam. There was a positive association between dose and onset of anxiolysis ($p = .01$); a larger proportion of children achieved satisfactory anxiolysis within 10 minutes at the higher doses. (Reprinted with permission from Coté CJ, Cohen IT, Suresh S, et al. A comparison of three doses of a commercially prepared oral midazolam syrup in children. *Anesth Analg*. 2002;94:37.)

that mental function usually returns to normal within 4 hours of administration, and amnesia may only last 20 to 30 minutes.[95] These properties make midazolam ideal for shorter procedures.

Lorazepam and Diazepam

Lorazepam is 5 to 10 times more potent than diazepam and can produce profound amnesia, anxiolysis, and sedation.[96] Like diazepam, it has an extremely long half-life, but an even longer duration because of its affinity for the receptor.[97] Because of their duration, lorazepam and diazepam are not useful in instances in which rapid awakening is necessary, such as outpatient anesthesia. Their use may be more suited for those patients already taking chronic benzodiazepines for anxiety and who may need anxiolysis prior to arrival in the preoperative area.

Lorazepam intravenous administration is not associated with pain on injection or phlebitis. In addition to the intravenous route, lorazepam is reliably absorbed orally with demonstrated clinical effects 30 to 60 minutes after oral administration.[98] Peak plasma concentrations may not occur until 2 to 4 hours after oral administration, so oral lorazepam must be given well before surgery so that the drug has time to be effective. With recommended doses, anterograde amnesia may be produced for as long as 4 to 6 hours without excessive sedation. Higher doses lead to prolonged and excessive sedation without more amnesia. There are no active metabolites of lorazepam and because its metabolism is not dependent on microsomal enzymes, there is less influence from age or liver disease. As with diazepam, little cardiorespiratory depression occurs with lorazepam.

Diphenhydramine

Diphenhydramine is a histamine-1 receptor antagonist, which blocks the peripheral effects of histamine. It also has sedative, anticholinergic, and antiemetic activity. A dose of 50 mg will last 3 to 6 hours in an adult. Diphenhydramine is not often used for preoperative sedation, but it is often used in combination with histamine-2 blockers and steroids for prophylaxis in patients with latex allergy as well as for prophylaxis before chemotherapy and radiologic studies using contrast.

Opioids

Morphine and meperidine were commonly used opioids in the past for intramuscular preoperative medication during a time when the majority of patients were admitted the night before surgery. Currently, when analgesia is needed preoperatively, the administration of intravenous fentanyl, with its rapid onset and shorter duration, has become much more common. In patients not experiencing pain, opioids may produce dysphoria. Opioids given in premedication dosages do not produce sedation or amnesia and are often combined with a benzodiazepine for these effects. Opioids are also useful to ameliorate the discomfort during regional anesthesia procedures or during the insertion of invasive monitoring catheters or large intravenous lines. The analgesic properties and respiratory depressant effects of opioids usually go hand in hand, and the decrease in the CO_2 drive at the medullary respiratory center may be prolonged. Furthermore, there is a decrease in the responsiveness to hypoxia at the carotid body after injection of even low doses of opioids.[99] The anesthesiologist may consider supplemental oxygen for the patient receiving opioid premedication. A common side effect of all opioids is nausea and vomiting, due to effects on both the chemoreceptor trigger zone and the vestibular system.

Fentanyl is a synthetic opioid agonist structurally similar to meperidine. It is approximately 100 times more potent than morphine in its analgesia. The lipid solubility of fentanyl is greater than that of morphine, which contributes to its rapid onset of action. Peak plasma concentrations occur within 6 to 7 minutes following intravenous administration and its elimination half-time is 3 to 6 hours. The drug's much shorter duration of action is attributed to redistribution to inactive tissues, such as the lungs, fat, and skeletal muscle. Metabolism occurs primarily by N-demethylation to norfentanyl, which is a less potent analgesic. In doses of 1 to 2 μg/kg intravenously, fentanyl may be used to provide preoperative analgesia. Fentanyl causes neither myocardial depression nor histamine release, but may be associated with ventilatory depression and profound bradycardia. Elderly and debilitated patients can have an increased sensitivity to its effects. Synergistic effects with benzodiazepines warrant close observation when this combination is given in the preoperative period.

Opioid-Dependent Patients and the Opioid Epidemic

Opioid overdose has been a leading cause of death for Americans, and many people who ultimately abuse heroin or fentanyl started with prescription oral opioids. Many addicts state their abuse began with their personal or an acquaintance's prescription, emphasizing the importance in avoiding overprescribing and identifying at-risk individuals. Risk factors for opioid misuse include current opioid use, history of opioid use, current or past substance abuse, smoking, psychiatric illness such as anxiety or depression, chronic pain, younger age, and higher medical comorbidities. For these individuals, a multimodal pain treatment program is beneficial, such as nonopioid medications, regional anesthesia and counseling. The anesthesiologist can play a key role in setting expectations for analgesia postoperatively. Those individuals who are opioid dependent or have a past history of abuse require special consideration and planning which can start with the preoperative visit.[100] Working with the patient's pain or addiction medicine specialist can help formulate a safe plan to avoid relapse. Withdrawal symptoms produced by drug cessation preoperatively are an issue for the patient who is opioid dependent. There should be an attempt to maintain opioid use at the usual level by continuing methadone or substituting other appropriate agents for methadone. The anesthesiologist should be cautioned about using agonist–antagonist drugs in these patients for fear of precipitating withdrawal.

Dexmedetomidine

Dexmedetomidine is a highly selective alpha-2 adrenoreceptor agonist acting in the locus ceruleus that produces sedation similar to natural sleep and anxiolysis. Unlike opiates and benzodiazepines, it does so without respiratory depression. It is thought to be neuroprotective and to provide analgesic and antiemetic effects. However, it can lead to hypotension and bradycardia due to its inhibition of norepinephrine release and sympathetic activity. It can be given in a variety of ways: oral, intranasal, intramuscular, and intravenously. Intranasal doses range from 1 to 3 mcg/kg, and intravenous doses start at 0.5 to 1 mcg/kg given over 10 minutes. It is not as fast acting as midazolam or fentanyl; when given intranasally it requires 30 minutes for effect and 15 minutes for intravenous administration, thus appropriate planning and timing are necessary. Dexmedetomidine is eliminated through hepatic biotransformation with an elimination half-life of 2 to 3 hours, potentially delaying recovery for short procedures.[101]

Anticholinergics

Historically, anticholinergic drugs were widely used when inhalation anesthetics produced copious respiratory tract secretions and intraoperative bradycardia was a frequent danger. The advent of newer inhalation agents has markedly decreased the routine use of anticholinergic drugs for preoperative medication. Specific indications for an anticholinergic before surgery are (1) antisialagogue effect, (2) sedation and amnesia, and (3) vagolytic effect (Table 23-17).

Antisialagogue Effect

Anticholinergics have been prescribed in a selective fashion when drying of the upper airway is desirable. For example, when awake fiberoptic tracheal intubation or bronchoscopic examination is planned, conditions will be more satisfactory for visualization when an anticholinergic drug has been administered.[102] Anticholinergics are also felt to increase the effectiveness of topical anesthesia in the airway by preventing a dilutional effect from secretions and facilitating contact of the local anesthetic with the mucosa. Glycopyrrolate is the most potent antisialagogue, with less likelihood of increasing heart rate than atropine. Because glycopyrrolate is a quaternary amine, it does not easily cross the blood–brain barrier and does not produce sedation or amnesia as seen with scopolamine, a tertiary amine. Glycopyrrolate can be useful for counteracting the increased secretions caused by ketamine, or for producing a drier surgical field for intraoral surgery.

Sedation and Amnesia

Although midazolam has largely taken over as the preoperative sedative of choice, historically, scopolamine was often given intramuscularly in combination with an opioid. Scopolamine may not be as effective as lorazepam or diazepam in preventing recall and causing amnesia, but it does have an additive amnestic effect when combined with benzodiazepines. The combination of diazepam and scopolamine produces amnesia more reliably than diazepam alone.[103] This additive amnestic effect may be useful for the unstable patient who cannot tolerate general anesthesia.

Table 23-17 Comparison of Effects of Three Anticholinergic Drugs

	Atropine	Glycopyrrolate	Scopolamine
Increased heart rate	+++	++	+
Antisialagogue	+	++	+
Sedation	+	0	+++

0, no effect; +, small effect; ++, moderate effect; +++, large effect.
Adapted from Stoelting RK. *Pharmacology and Physiology in Anesthetic Practice*. JB Lippincott; 1991.

Vagolytic Action

The vagolytic action of the anticholinergic drugs is produced through the blockade of acetylcholine at the sinoatrial node. Atropine given intravenously is more potent than glycopyrrolate in increasing heart rate. The vagolytic action of the anticholinergic drugs is useful in the prevention of reflex bradycardia that may result from traction on extraocular muscles or abdominal viscera, carotid sinus stimulation, or repeated doses of succinylcholine.

Side Effects of Anticholinergic Drugs

Central Nervous System Toxicity

Scopolamine and atropine (tertiary amines) may cause central nervous system toxicity, known as central anticholinergic syndrome. This syndrome is most likely to occur after the administration of scopolamine, but can be seen after high doses of atropine and may include symptoms such as delirium, restlessness, confusion, and obtundation. Elderly patients and patients with pain appear to be particularly susceptible; the syndrome has been noted to be potentiated by inhalation anesthetics. The administration of 1 to 2 mg of physostigmine intravenously can successfully treat the syndrome.

Intraocular Pressure

Mydriasis and cycloplegia from anticholinergic drugs may place patients with glaucoma at risk for increased intraocular pressure. Atropine and glycopyrrolate may be less likely to increase intraocular pressure than scopolamine. In patients with glaucoma, it is generally safe to continue most glaucoma medications up until the time of surgery or use atropine or glycopyrrolate when necessary.

Hyperthermia

The sweat glands of the body are innervated by the sympathetic nervous system, but use cholinergic transmission. Therefore, administration of anticholinergic agents interferes with the sweating mechanism which may cause body temperature to increase, especially when using active warming devices in the OR. The patient typically appears hot and dry. In children, the subsequent increase in temperature may exacerbate tachycardia.

Antibiotic Prophylaxis

The goal of surgical antibiotic prophylaxis is to prevent surgical site infections and the direct consequences stemming from them such as morbidity and mortality, health care resource utilization and cost. At the same time, antimicrobial prophylaxis should have minimal adverse drug effects and impact on the patient's microbial flora. Antimicrobial prophylaxis has become an important outcome measure such that properly timed and dosed administration impacts hospital reimbursement or even accreditation status. Anesthesiologists frequently administer antibiotics to patients prior to surgery for contaminated and clean-contaminated procedures or for clean surgical procedures when infection would be catastrophic, such as for device implants. Other indications for the use of prophylactic antibiotics include the prevention of endocarditis and the prevention of infection in immunocompromised patients.

Cephalosporins, such as cefazolin, are the most popular antibiotics because they cover common skin microbes. However, for intestinal surgery anaerobic and gram-negative coverage is needed, and those colonized with methicillin-resistant *Staphylococcus aureus* require decolonization protocols and intraoperative vancomycin. The National Surgical Infection Project recommends that antibiotics be administered within 1 hour prior to incision.[104]

There are two exceptions to this policy: (1) vancomycin should be given 2 hours prior to incision and (2) when a tourniquet is used, the antibiotics should be administered prior to its inflation. Furthermore, if the surgical procedure is prolonged, it is recommended that the antibiotic be redosed when two half-lives have elapsed. For example, cefazolin has a half-life of 2 hours and should be redosed if the surgical procedure extends past 4 hours. Research on morbidly obese patients has shown that the dose required to achieve adequate tissue levels is twice that for normal-weight patients.[105] Those with a proven allergy to penicillin, cephalosporins, and related compounds (β-lactam allergy) may receive either vancomycin or clindamycin.

Summary of Patient Preparation

The anesthesiologist who invests time to adequately prepare the patient medically and psychologically for anesthesia and surgery will find that their job of caring for the patient intraoperatively becomes easier and is more likely to result in both a positive clinical outcome and a satisfied patient.

For additional information please see 2 *Video 23-2 in the eBook bundled with this text.*

For further review and interactivities, please see the videos and narrative interactive clinical vignettes (NICVs) accessible in the complimentary eBook bundled with this text. Access instructions are located on the inside front cover.

REFERENCES

1. Practice advisory for preanesthesia evaluation: An updated report by the American Society of Anesthesiologists Task Force on Preanesthesia Evaluation. *Anesthesiology*. 2012; 116(3):522–538. https://www.asahq.org/quality-and-practice-management/standards-and-guidelines.
2. Kash B, Cline K, Menser T, Zhang Y. *The Perioperative Surgical Home, A Comprehensive Literature Review for the American Society of Anesthesiologists*. 2014. https://www.asahq.org/psh
3. Apfel CC, Läärä E, Koivuranta M, Greim CA, Roewer N. A simplified risk score for predicting postoperative nausea and vomiting. *Anesthesiology*. 1999;91:693–700.
4. Apfel CC, Korttila K, Abdalla M, et al. A factorial trial of six interventions for the prevention of postoperative nausea and vomiting. *N Engl J Med*. 2004;350:2441–2451.
5. Gan TJ, Belani KG, Bergese S. Fourth Consensus Guidelines for the management of postoperative nausea and vomiting. *Anesth Analg*. 2020;131(2):411–448.
6. Eberhart LH, Geldner G, Kranke P, et al. The development and validation of a risk score to predict the probability of postoperative vomiting in pediatric patients. *Anesth Analg*. 2004;99: 1630–1637.
7. Mallampati RS, Gatt SP, Gugino LD, et al. A clinical sign to predict difficult tracheal intubation: A prospective study. *Can Anaesth Soc J*. 1985;32:429–434.
8. Frerk CM. Predicting difficult intubation. *Anaesthesia*. 1991;46:1005–1008.
9. Savva D. Prediction of difficult tracheal intubation. *Br J Anaesth*. 1994;73:149–153.
10. Shah KB, Kleinman BS, Rao T, Jacobs HK, Mestan K, Schaafsma M. Angina and other risk factors in patients with cardiac diseases undergoing noncardiac operations. *Anesth Analg*. 1990;70:240–247.
11. Wilson WR, Gewitz M, Lockhart PB, et al. Prevention of Viridans Group Streptococcal Infective Endocarditis: A Scientific Statement from the American Heart Association. *Circulation*. 2021;143(20):e963–e978. Erratum in: Circulation. 2022 Apr 26;145(17):e868.
12. Weiser TG, Haynes AB, Molina G, et al. Estimate of the global volume of surgery in 2012: an assessment supporting improved health outcomes. *Lancet*. 2015;385.
13. Smilowitz NR, Gupta N, Guo Y, et al. Trends in cardiovascular risk factor and disease prevalence in patients undergoing non-cardiac surgery. *Heart*. 2018;104(14):1180–1186.
14. Smilowitz NR, Gupta N, Ramakrishna H, Guo Y, Berger JS, Bangalore S. Perioperative major adverse cardiovascular and cerebrovascular events associated with noncardiac surgery. *JAMA Cardiol*. 2017;2(2):181–187.
15. Eagle K, Brundage B, Chaitman B, et al. Guidelines for perioperative cardiovascular evaluation of the noncardiac surgery. A report of the American Heart Association/American College of Cardiology Task Force on Assessment of Diagnostic and Therapeutic Cardiovascular Procedures. *Circulation*. 1996;93:1278–1317.
16. Reilly DF, McNeely MJ, Doerner D, et al. Self-reported exercise tolerance and the risk of serious perioperative complications. *Arch Intern Med*. 1999;159:2185–2192.
17. Healy KO, Waksmonski WA, Altman RK, Stetson PD, Reyentovich A, Maurer MS. Perioperative outcome and long-term mortality for heart failure patients undergoing intermediate and high-risk noncardiac surgery: Impact of left ventricular ejection fraction. *Congest Heart Fail*. 2010;16:45–49.
18. Flu WJ, Van Kuijk JP, Hoeks SE, et al. Prognostic implications of asymptomatic left ventricular dysfunction in patients undergoing vascular surgery. *Anesthesiology*. 2010;112:1316–1324.
19. Otto CM, Nishimura RA, Bonow RO, et al. 2020 ACC/AHA guideline for the management of patients with valvular heart disease: executive summary: a report of the American College of Cardiology/American Heart Association Joint Committee on Clinical Practice Guidelines. *Circulation*. 2021;143:e35–e71.
20. Shah KB, Kleinman BS, Sami H, Patel J, Rao TL. Reevaluation of perioperative myocardial infarction in patients with prior myocardial infarction undergoing noncardiac operations. *Anesth Analg*. 1990;71:231–235.
21. Hertzer NR, Bevan EG, Young JR, et al. Coronary artery disease in peripheral vascular patients: A classification of 1000 coronary angiograms and results of surgical management. *Ann Surg*. 1984;199:223–233.
22. Kannel W, Abbott R. Incidence and prognosis of unrecognized myocardial infarction: An update on the Framingham study. *N Engl J Med*. 1984;311:1144–1147.
23. Eagle KA, Coley CM, Newell JB, et al. Combining clinical and thallium data optimizes preoperative assessment of cardiac risk before major vascular surgery. *Ann Intern Med*. 1989; 110:859–866.
24. Acharya DU, Shekhar YC, Aggarwal A, Anand IS. Lack of pain during myocardial infarction in diabetics: is autonomic dysfunction responsible? *Am J Cardiol*. 1991;68:793–796.
25. Hollenberg M, Mangano DT, Browner WS, London MJ, Tubau JF, Tateo IM. Predictors of postoperative myocardial ischemia in patients undergoing noncardiac surgery. The study of perioperative ischemia research. *JAMA*. 1992;268:205–209.
26. Pringle SD, MacFarlane PW, McKillop JH, Lorimer AR, Dunn FG. Pathophysiologic assessment of left ventricular hypertrophy and strain in asymptomatic patients with essential hypertension. *J Am Coll Cardiol*. 1989;13:1377–1381.
27. Whelton P, Carey R, Aronow W, et al. 2017 ACC/AHA/AAPA/ABC/ACPM/AGS/APhA/ASH/ASPC/NMA/PCNA Guideline for the prevention, detection, evaluation, and management of high blood pressure in adults. *J Am Coll Cardiol*. 2018:71(19):e127–e248.
28. Howell SJ, Sear JW, Foex P. Hypertension, hypertensive heart disease and perioperative cardiac risk. *Br J Anaesth*. 2004;92:570–583.
29. Wesker N, Klien M, Szendro G. The dilemma of immediate preoperative hypertension. *J Clin Anesth*. 2003;15:179–183.
30. Goldman L, Caldera DL. Risks of general anesthesia and elective operation in the hypertensive patient. *Anesthesiology*. 1979;50:285–292.
31. Tzimas P, Petrou A, Laou E, Milionis H, Mikhailidis DP, Papadopoulos G. Impact of metabolic syndrome in surgical patients. *Br J Anaesth*. 2015;115(2):194–202.
32. Warner MA, Shields SE, Chute CG. Major morbidity and mortality within 1 month of ambulatory surgery and anesthesia. *JAMA*. 1993;270:1437–1441.
33. Eagle KA, Rihal CS, Mickel MC, Holmes DR, Foster ED, Gersh BJ. Cardiac risk of noncardiac surgery: Influence of coronary disease and type of surgery in 3368 operations. CASS Investigators and University of Michigan Heart Care Program. *Circulation*. 1997;96:1882–1887.
34. Fleisher LA, Fleischmann KE, Auerbach AD, et al. ACC/AHA Guideline on perioperative cardiovascular evaluation and management of patients undergoing noncardiac surgery. *Circulation*. 2014;130:e278–e333. http://circ.ahajournals.org.
35. Wolters U, Wolf T, Stützer H, Schröder T. ASA classification and perioperative variables as predictors of postoperative outcome. *Br J Anaesth*. 1996;77(2):217–222.
36. Lee TH, Marcantonio ER, Mangione CM, et al. Derivation and prospective validation of a simple index for prediction of cardiac risk of major noncardiac surgery. *Circulation*. 1999; 100:1043–1049.
37. Gupta PK, Gupta H, Sundaram A, et al. Development and validation of a risk calculator for prediction of cardiac risk after surgery. *Circulation*. 2011;124:381–387.
38. Cohen ME, Ko CY, Bilimoria KY, et al. Optimizing ACS NSQIP modeling for evaluation of surgical quality and risk: patient risk adjustment, procedure mix adjustment, shrinkage adjustment, and surgical focus. *J Am Coll Surg*. 2013;217:336–346.
39. Kalbfleisch JM, Shudaksharappa KS, Conrad LL, Sarkar NK. Disappearance of the Q deflection following myocardial infarction. *Am Heart J*. 1968;76:193–198.
40. McFalls EO, Ward HB, Moritz TE, et al. Coronary-artery revascularization before elective major vascular surgery. *N Engl J Med*. 2004;351(27):2795–2804.
41. Rodseth RN, Biccard BM, Le Manach Y, et al. The prognostic value of pre-operative and post-operative B-type natriuretic peptides in patients undergoing noncardiac surgery: B-type natriuretic peptide and N-terminal fragment of pro-B-type natriuretic peptide: a systematic review and individual patient data meta-analysis. *J Am Coll Cardiol*. 2014;63(2):170–180.
42. Devereaux PJ, Mrkobrada M, Sessler DI, et al. POISE-2 Investigators. Aspirin in patients undergoing noncardiac surgery. *N Engl J Med*. 2014;370(16):1494–1503.
43. Smilowitz NR, Berger JS. Perioperative cardiovascular risk assessment and management for noncardiac surgery: a review. *JAMA*. 2020;324(3):279–290.
44. Rich MW, Chyun DA, Skolnick AH, et al. American Heart Association Older Populations Committee of the Council on Clinical Cardiology, Council on Cardiovascular and Stroke Nursing, Council on Cardiovascular Surgery and Anesthesia, and Stroke Council; American College of Cardiology; and American Geriatrics Society. Knowledge gaps in cardiovascular care of the older adult population: A Scientific Statement from the American Heart Association, American College of Cardiology, and American Geriatrics Society. *Circulation*. 2016;133(21):2103–2122.
45. Livhits M, Ko CY, Leonardi MJ, et al. Risk of surgery following recent myocardial infarction. *Ann Surg*. 2011;253:857–864.

46. Mahmoud KD, Sanon S, Habermann EB, et al. Perioperative cardiovascular risk of prior coronary stent implantation among patients undergoing noncardiac surgery. *J Am Coll Cardiol.* 2016;67(9):1038–1049.
47. Practice Advisory for the Perioperative Management of Patients with Cardiac Implantable Electronic Devices: Pacemakers and Implantable Cardioverter–Defibrillators 2020: An Updated Report by the American Society of Anesthesiologists Task Force on Perioperative Management of Patients with Cardiac Implantable Electronic Devices. *Anesthesiology* 2020;132: 225–252. doi:https://doi.org/10.1097/ALN.0000000000002821
48. Jammer I, Wickboldt N, Sander M, et al. European Society of Anaesthesiology (ESA) and the European Society of Intensive Care Medicine (ESICM); European Society of Anaesthesiology; European Society of Intensive Care Medicine. Standards for definitions and use of outcome measures for clinical effectiveness research in perioperative medicine: European Perioperative Clinical Outcome (EPCO) definitions: a statement from the ESA-ESICM joint taskforce on perioperative outcome measures. *Eur J Anaesthesiol.* 2015;32(2):88–105.
49. Johnson RG, Arozullah AM, Neumayer L, Henderson WG, Hosokawa P, Khuri SF. Multivariable predictors of postoperative respiratory failure after general and vascular surgery: Results from the patient safety in surgery study. *J Am Coll Surg.* 2007;204(6):1188–1198.
50. Arozullah AM, Daley J, Henderson WG, Khuri SF. Multifactorial risk index for predicting postoperative respiratory failure in men after major noncardiac surgery. The National Veterans Administration Surgical Quality Improvement Program. *Ann Surg.* 2000;232(2):242–253.
51. Qaseem A, Snow V, Fitterman N, et al. Risk assessment for and strategies to reduce perioperative pulmonary complications for patients undergoing noncardiothoracic surgery: A guideline from the American College of Physicians. *Ann Intern Med.* 2006;144(8):575–580.
52. Arozullah AM, Khuri SF, Henderson WG, Daley J, Participants in the National Veterans Affairs Surgical Quality Improvement Program. Development and validation of a multifactorial risk index for predicting postoperative pneumonia after major noncardiac surgery. *Ann Intern Med.* 2001;135:847–857.
53. Fisher BW, Majumdar SR, McAlistar FA. Predicting pulmonary complications after nonthoracic surgery: A systematic review of blinded studies. *Am J Med.* 2002;112:219–225.
54. Hall JC, Tarala RA, Hall JL. A case-control study of postoperative pulmonary complications after laparoscopic and open cholecystectomy. *J Laparoendosc Surg.* 1996;6:87–92.
55. Brueckmann B, Villa-Uribe JL, Brian T, et al. Development and validation of a score for prediction of postoperative respiratory complications. *Anesthesiology.* 2013;118:1276–1285.
56. Collard HR, Saint S, Matthay MA. Prevention of ventilator-associated pneumonia: An evidence-based systematic review. *Ann Intern Med.* 2003;138(6):494–501.
57. Houston S, Hougland P, Anderson JJ, LaRocco M, Kennedy V, Gentry LO. Effectiveness of 0.12% chlorhexidine gluconate oral rinse in reducing prevalence of nosocomial pneumonia in patients undergoing heart surgery. *Am J Crit Care.* 2002;11(6):567–570.
58. Warner MA, Divertie MB, Tinker JH. Preoperative cessation of smoking and pulmonary complications in coronary artery bypass patients. *Anesthesiology.* 1984;60:609–616.
59. Paciullo CA, Short MR, Steinke DT, Jennings HR. Impact of nicotine replacement therapy on postoperative mortality following coronary artery bypass graft surgery. *Ann Pharmacother.* 2009;43(7):1197–1202.
60. Feinstein MM, Katz D. Sparking the discussion about vaping and anesthesia. *Anesthesiology.* 2020;132(3):599.
61. Whyte MK, Choudry NB, Ind PW. Bronchial hyperresponsiveness in patients recovering from acute severe asthma. *Respir Med.* 1993;87:29–35.
62. Kabalin CS, Yarnold PR, Grammer LC. Low complication rate of corticosteroid-treated asthmatics undergoing surgical procedures. *Arch Intern Med.* 1995;155:1379–1384.
63. Peppard PE, Young T, Barnet JH, Palta M, Hagen EW, Hla KM. Increased prevalence of sleep-disordered breathing in adults. *Am J Epidemiol.* 2013;177(9):1006–1014.
64. ASA Practice Guidelines for the Perioperative Management of Patients with Obstructive Sleep Apnea. Practice guidelines for the preoperative management of patients with obstructive sleep apnea: An updated report by the ASA task force on perioperative management of patients with obstructive sleep apnea. *Anesthesiology.* 2014;120(2):268–286.
65. Pivetta B, Chen L, Nagappa M, et al. Use and performance of the STOP-Bang questionnaire for obstructive sleep apnea screening across geographic regions: a systematic review and meta-analysis. *JAMA Netw Open.* 2021;4(3):e211009. /jamanetworkopen.2021.
66. Gandhi GY, Murad MH, Flynn DN, et al. Effect of perioperative insulin infusion on surgical morbidity and mortality: Systematic review and meta-analysis of randomized trials. *Mayo Clin Proc.* 2008;83(4):418–430.
67. Martin LD, Hoagland MA, Rhodes ET, Wolfsdorf JI, Hamrick JL, Society for Pediatric Anesthesia Quality and Safety Committee Diabetes Workgroup; Society for Pediatric Anesthesia Diabetes Workgroup members. Perioperative Management of Pediatric Patients with Type 1 Diabetes Mellitus, Updated Recommendations for Anesthesiologists. *Anesth Analg.* 2020;130(4):821–827.
68. Duggan EW, Carlson K, Umpierrez GE. Perioperative hyperglycemia management: an update. *Anesthesiology* 2017;126:547–560.
69. Liu MM, Reidy AB, Saatee S, Collard CD. Perioperative steroid management: approaches based on current evidence. *Anesthesiology.* 2017;127(1):166–172.
70. Sladen R. Anesthetic considerations for the patient with renal failure. *Anesthesiol Clin North America.* 2000;18(4):863–882.
71. Hanje AJ, Patel T. Preoperative evaluation of patients with liver disease. *Nat Clin Pract Gastroenterol Hepatol.* 2007;4(5):266–276.
72. Oda T, Fujiwara K, Yonenobu K, Azuma B, Ochi T. Natural course of cervical spine lesions in rheumatoid arthritis. *Spine.* 1995;20(10):1128–1135.
73. Narr BJ, Hansen TR, Warner MA. Preoperative laboratory screening in healthy Mayo patients: Cost-effective elimination of tests and unchanged outcomes. *Mayo Clin Proc.* 1991;66:155–159.
74. Narr BJ, Warner ME, Schroeder DR, Warner MA. Outcomes of patients with no laboratory assessment before anesthesia and a surgical procedure. *Mayo Clin Proc.* 1997;72:505–509.
75. Roizen MF, Cohn S. Preoperative evaluation for elective surgery: What laboratory tests are needed? In: Stoelting RK, ed. *Advances in Anesthesia.* Mosby Year Book;1993:25.
76. Baron MJ, Gunter J, White P. Is the pediatric preoperative hematocrit determination necessary? *South Med J.* 1992;85:1187–1189.
77. Sox HCJ. *Common Diagnostic Tests: Use and Interpretation.* American College of Physicians; 1990.
78. Archer C, Levy AR, McGregor M. Value of routine preoperative chest x-rays: A meta-analysis. *Can J Anaesth.* 1993;40:1022–1027.
79. Colice GL, Shafazand S, Griffin JP, Keenan R, Bolliger CT, American College of Chest Physicians. Physiologic evaluation of the patient with lung cancer being considered for resectional surgery: ACCP evidenced-based clinical practice guidelines (2nd edition). *Chest.* 2007; 132(3 Suppl):161S–177S.
80. Devereaux PJ, Yang H, Yusuf S, et al. Effects of extended-release metoprolol succinate in patients undergoing non-cardiac surgery (POISE trial): A randomized controlled trial. *Lancet.* 2008;371(9627):1839–1847.
81. Bangalore S, Wetterslev J, Pranesh S, Sawhney S, Gluud C, Messerli FH. Perioperative beta blockers in patients having non-cardiac surgery: A meta-analysis. *Lancet.* 2008;372(9654): 1962–1976.
82. Wijeysundera DN, Duncan D, Nkonde-Price C, et al. ACC/AHA Task Force Members. Perioperative beta blockade in noncardiac surgery: a systematic review for the 2014 ACC/AHA guideline on perioperative cardiovascular evaluation and management of patients undergoing noncardiac surgery: a report of the American College of Cardiology/American Heart Association Task Force on Practice Guidelines. *Circulation.* 2014;130(24):2246–2264.
83. Douketis JD, Spyropoulos AC, Kaatz S, et al. BRIDGE Investigators. Perioperative bridging anticoagulation in patients with atrial fibrillation. *N Engl J Med.* 2015;373(9):823–833.
84. Skrlin S, Hou V. A review of perioperative statin therapy for noncardiac surgery. *Semin Cardiothorac Vasc Anesth.* 2010;14(4):283–290.
85. Hollmann C, Fernandes NL, Biccard BM. A systematic review of outcomes associated with withholding or continuing angiotensin-converting enzyme inhibitors and angiotensin receptor blockers before noncardiac surgery. *Anesth Analg.* 2018;127(3):678–687.
86. Stoelting RK. Responses to atropine, glycopyrrolate and Riopan on gastric fluid pH and volume in adult patients. *Anesthesiology.* 1978;48:367–369.
87. Manchikanti L, Roush JR. The effect of preanesthetic glycopyrrolate and cimetidine in gastric fluid pH and volume in outpatients. *Anesth Analg.* 1984;63:40–46.
88. Kluger MT, Short TG. Aspiration during anaesthesia: A review of 133 cases from the Australian Anaesthetic Incident Monitoring Study (AIMS). *Anaesthesia.* 1999;54:19–26.
89. Practice guidelines for preoperative fasting and the use of pharmacologic agents to reduce the risk of pulmonary aspiration: application to healthy patients undergoing elective procedures. *Anesthesiology.* 2017;126:376–393.
90. Thomas M., Morrison C, Newton R, Schindler E. Consensus Statement on clear fluids fasting for elective pediatric general anesthesia. *Paediatric Anaesthesia.* 2018;28 (5):411–414.
91. Rosen, D. Canadian Pediatric Anesthesia Society statement on clear fluid fasting for elective pediatric anesthesia. *Canadian Journal of Anesthesia.* 2019;66:991–992.
92. Haskins DA, Jahr JS, Texidor M, Ramadhyani U. Single-dose oral omeprazole for reduction of gastric residual acidity in adults for outpatient surgery. *Acta Anaesthesiol Scand.* 1992;36:513–515.
93. James CF, Modell JH, Gibbs CP, Kuck EJ, Ruiz BC. Pulmonary aspiration: Effects of volume and pH in the rat. *Anesth Analg.* 1984;63:665–668.
94. Egbert LD, Battit GE, Turndorf H, Beecher HK. The value of the preoperative visit by the anesthetist. *JAMA.* 1963;185:553–555.
95. Reves JG, Fragen RJ, Vinick HR, Greenblatt DJ. Midazolam: Pharmacology and uses. *Anesthesiology.* 1985;62:310–324.
96. Fragen RJ, Caldwell N. Lorazepam premedication: Lack of recall and relief of anxiety. *Anesth Analg.* 1976;55:792–796.
97. White PF. Pharmacologic and clinical aspects of preoperative medication. *Anesth Analg.* 1986; 65:963–974.
98. Bradshaw EG, Ali AA, Mulley BA, Rye RM. Plasma concentrations and clinical effects of lorazepam after oral administration. *Br J Anaesth.* 1981;53:517–522.
99. Weil JV, McCullough RE, Kline JS. Diminished ventilatory response to hypoxia and hypercapnia after morphine in man. *N Engl J Med.* 1975;292:1103–1106.
100. Larach DB, Hah JM, Brummett CM. Perioperative opioids, the opioid crisis, and the anesthesiologist. *Anesthesiology.* 2022;136(4):594–608.
101. Gertler R, Brown HC, Mitchell DH, Silvius EN. Dexmedetomidine: a novel sedative-analgesic agent. Proc (Bayl Univ Med Cent). 2001;14(1):13–21
102. Falick YS, Smiler BG. Is anticholinergic premedication necessary? Anesthesiology. 1975; 43:472–473.
103. Frumin MJ, Herekar VR, Jarvik ME. Amnesic actions of diazepam and scopolamine in man. Anesthesiology. 1976;45:406–412.
104. Ban KA, Minei JP, Laronga C, et al. American College of Surgeons and Surgical Infection Society: Surgical Site Infection Guidelines, 2016 Update. J Am Coll Surg. 2017;224(1):59–74.
105. Gorden SM. Antibiotic prophylaxis against postoperative wound infections. *Cleve Clin J Med.* 2006;73:S42–S45.

24 Rare Coexisting Diseases

ANDREW F. STASIC • CHRISTOPHER L. HEINE • GABRIELLE FISHER • SUNG-WOOK CHOI • JENNIFER SMITH

KEY POINTS

1. The cytoskeleton of the muscle membrane in patients with muscular dystrophy is fragile. In these patients, succinylcholine and/or halogenated anesthetics can cause the massive release of intracellular contents resulting in hyperkalemic cardiac arrest.
2. Myotonic dystrophy produces cardiac conduction delay that can manifest as third-degree atrioventricular block.
3. Patients with myasthenia gravis are exquisitely sensitive to nondepolarizing muscle relaxants. Short-acting muscle relaxants and objective monitoring of neuromuscular function are indicated.
4. Small-cell carcinoma of the lung and other cancers are associated with the development myasthenic syndrome; in some cases, the syndrome is diagnosed before the cancer is discovered.
5. Patients with multiple sclerosis can have an exacerbation of their neurologic symptoms despite a well-managed anesthetic.
6. An unexpected increase in end-tidal carbon dioxide is the most sensitive sign of malignant hyperthermia.
7. Hypoglycemia and metabolic acidosis are constant risks to patients with glycogen storage diseases.
8. The deposition of mucopolysaccharides in the upper airway of patients with mucopolysaccharidoses often complicates airway management during anesthesia.
9. Repeated episodes of sickling in patients with sickle cell disease cause pulmonary hypertension that increases perioperative risks.
10. Rheumatoid arthritis is a multisystem disease that causes subclinical cardiac and pulmonary dysfunction.
11. Patients with rheumatoid arthritis can have significant degeneration of the cervical spine with few neurologic symptoms. Cervical manipulation during laryngoscopy and tracheal intubation requires special precautions.
12. Esophageal dysfunction in patients with scleroderma and dermatomyositis increases the risk of aspiration pneumonitis.
13. Patients with epidermolysis bullosa can have undiagnosed dilated cardiomyopathy.

Musculoskeletal Diseases

Muscular Dystrophy and Congenital Myopathy

Muscular dystrophies are a heterogeneous group of progressive muscle disorders that vary based on location of skeletal muscle weakness, severity, and age of onset (Table 24-1). Cardiac and smooth muscle of the gastrointestinal tract are also affected. These conditions are the result of insufficient or abnormal proteins such as dystrophin and sarcoglycans, which make up the cytoskeleton of the muscle membrane (Fig. 24-1). Skeletal muscle in the extremities, torso, and face may also be affected, along with the respiratory system. The classification of muscular dystrophies is complicated, as similar phenotypes are sometimes the result of mutations in different proteins; conversely, allelic disorders on the same protein can result in different disorders[1] (Fig. 24-2). As causative gene mutations have been identified, earlier diagnosis has become possible, which facilitates the implementation of disease-specific care.

Table 24-1 Types of Muscular Dystrophy and Congenital Myopathies

Muscular Dystrophies
Duchenne (DMD)
Becker (BMD)
Emery–Dreifuss
Limb-girdle (LGMD)
Facioscapulohumeral
Oculopharyngeal
Congenital muscular dystrophy
Congenital Myopathies
Nemaline myopathy
Central core disease
Minicore disease
Centronuaclear myopathy

Duchenne Muscular Dystrophy

Duchenne muscular dystrophy (DMD) is caused by the absence of dystrophin, a large protein that plays a major role in stabilization of the muscle membrane and signaling between the cytoskeleton and extracellular matrix (1 Video 24-1 and NICV 24-1). DMD is inherited as an X-linked recessive trait and is the most common inherited muscle disease of childhood. Patients with DMD suffer from progressive proximal muscle weakness and wasting that produces symptoms in early childhood. The severity is significant, resulting in loss of ambulation by 12 years of age. Although DMD patients have elevated creatine kinase (CK) levels early in life, these levels decrease as the patient ages, commensurate with the continued muscle atrophy. Most patients with DMD die before their fourth decade of life. Cardiac and respiratory complications are the most common causes of death. Typical electrocardiogram (ECG) abnormalities include an R:S ratio >1 in lead V1, deep Q-waves in leads I, aVL, V5, and V6, right axis deviation or a right bundle branch block, and may precede other signs of cardiac dysfunction. Echocardiography can reveal progressive left ventricle expansion and impaired systolic and diastolic function. Contrast-enhanced cardiac magnetic resonance imaging (MRI) now allows clinicians to identify early signs of myocardial damage and pending failure despite normal ventricular size and function. Cardiac evaluation is recommended every 2 years after diagnosis up until the age of 10, and every year thereafter. Early utilization of angiotensin-converting enzyme inhibitors, diuretics, and β-adrenergic blockers may result in ventricular remodeling and functional improvement. Female carriers of the DMD gene defect should also be evaluated every 5 years, as they too are prone to cardiomyopathy.[2,3]

Current treatment remains supportive and is aimed at improving cardiorespiratory function. Noninvasive ventilation and cough assist techniques (manual and mechanical) can improve pulmonary function and reduce the risk of aspiration pneumonia. Glucocorticoids are a standard of treatment and have been shown to result in improved time to loss of mobility and lifespan.[4] More recent therapeutic approaches using gene or antisense oligonucleotide therapy, aimed at restoring dystrophin production or dealing with the consequences of dystrophin deficiency, are in varying stages of utilization and investigation.

Becker Muscular Dystrophy

A reduction in normal amounts of dystrophin results in Becker muscular dystrophy (BMD). Patients with BMD have a similar, but milder disease course than patients with DMD. The onset of BMD is typically at adolescence although some patients will not be symptomatic until later in life. Causes of mortality are like that of DMD, but death does not usually occur until the fifth or sixth decade. It is recommended that asymptomatic patients with BMD have a cardiac evaluation every 5 years. More frequent evaluation is indicated if symptoms of cardiac disease develop. As with DMD, female carriers can also have cardiac abnormalities.

Emery–Dreifuss Muscular Dystrophy

Emery–Dreifuss muscular dystrophy may be caused by mutations in two different proteins that follow different inheritance patterns. The X-linked form results from a mutation in the emerin gene, whereas the autosomal dominant form is the result of mutation in the genes that code for the lamins A and C proteins. Although typical onset is in the early teens, the autosomal dominant form can present significantly earlier. Both forms characteristically present with contractures of the ankles, elbows, and neck, with accompanying development of progressive weakness of humeral, peroneal, and limb-girdle muscles. Cardiomyopathy and cardiac conduction abnormalities often manifest by the age 30.[5]

Limb-Girdle Muscular Dystrophy

Limb-Girdle muscular dystrophy (LGMD) is a progressive dystrophy subclassified further by inheritance pattern and the

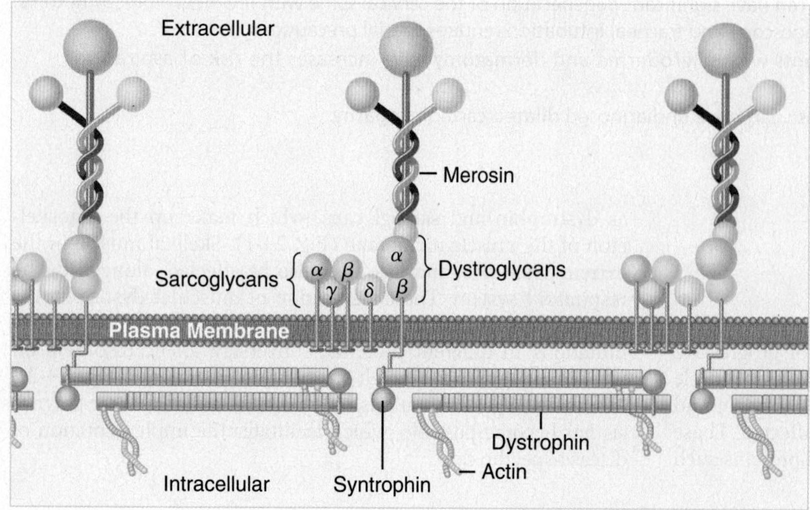

Figure 24-1 Muscle cell cytoskeleton. (Adapted and redrawn from Duggan DJ, Gorospe JR, Fanin M, et al. Mutations in the sarcoglycan genes in patients with myopathy. *N Engl J Med*. 1997;336:618–624.)

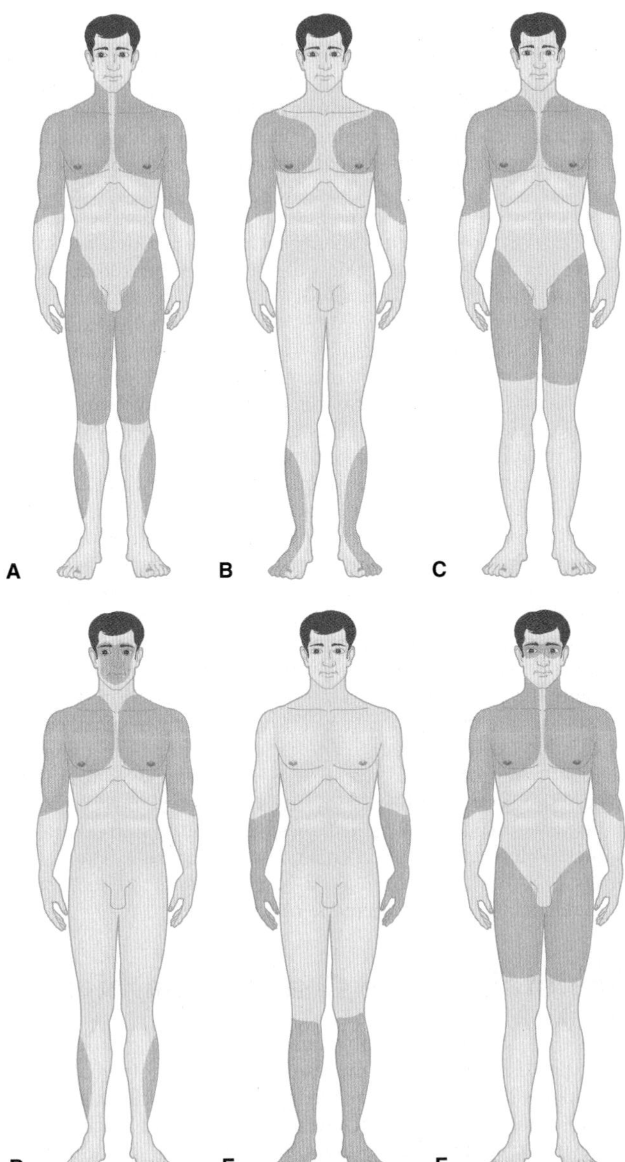

Figure 24-2 Distribution of predominant muscle weakness in different types of muscular dystrophy. **A:** Duchenne-type and Becker type. **B:** Emery–Dreifuss. **C:** Limb-girdle. **D:** Facioscapulohumeral. **E:** Distal. **F:** Oculopharyngeal. (Adapted from Emery AE. The muscular dystrophies. *BMJ*. 1998;317:991–995.)

responsible mutated protein. The autosomal dominant form tends to be less severe. CK can either be normal, mildly elevated, or elevated. These patients suffer from shoulder and pelvic muscle weakness and can also have significant cardiac involvement.

Facioscapulohumeral Muscular Dystrophy

This autosomal dominant dystrophy presents with weakness—frequently asymmetrical—in the facial and shoulder muscles that later extends to the foot and pelvic girdle muscles. Retinal vascular disease and hearing loss may occur. Cardiac conduction abnormalities can develop, but cardiac muscle involvement does not usually occur.

Oculopharyngeal Muscular Dystrophy

Weakness in the extraocular, upper facial, neck, and proximal limb muscles characterizes oculopharyngeal muscular dystrophy. Ptosis and dysphagia are the usual presenting symptoms in the third decade of life and the reasons for seeking surgical therapy.

Congenital Muscular Dystrophy and Myopathy

Congenital muscular dystrophy (CMD) is characterized by onset of hypotonia during infancy, developmental delay, feeding difficulties, and respiratory dysfunction. There are three groups of diseases: (1) collagenopathies (Ulrich CMD, Bethlem myopathy); (2) merosinopathies; and (3) dystroglycanopathies (Fukuyama CMD, muscle-eye-drain disease, Walker–Warburg syndrome). The congenital myopathies, now recognized as a class of diseases different than CMD, include nemaline myopathy, central core disease, and multiminicore disease, and centronuclear myopathy. Although respiratory muscle dysfunction can be severe, cardiac involvement is not as prominent as in Duchenne or Becker muscular dystrophy. Patients with congenital myopathies may be susceptible to malignant hyperthermia (MH).[6,7]

Management of Anesthesia

The perioperative management of patients with muscular dystrophy is dependent on the specific disease and its progression. The complications of greatest concern are cardiac involvement and respiratory muscle weakness. Preoperative review of cardiac echocardiograms and/or cardiac MRI will assist in planning for anesthesia. Some patients with muscular dystrophy have very poor left ventricular function and will require advanced cardiac monitoring in the perioperative period.

Premedication can be administered for anxiolysis, unless there is a significant risk of respiratory dysfunction or aspiration. Although muscular dystrophy was previously believed to be associated with an increased risk of MH, there is no evidence that the risk is greater than the general population. However, patients with congenital myopathies, such as central core disease or multiminicore disease, should be considered at increased risk for MH.

Patients with muscular dystrophy, especially DMD, are at risk 1
for rhabdomyolysis and severe hyperkalemia following succinylcholine administration, and possibly, halogenated inhaled anesthetics. The use of halogenated, inhaled anesthetics in patients with DMD is controversial.[8] A prudent approach would be to use these anesthetics only when necessary and for as brief a period of time as possible. Succinylcholine should be avoided.

Patients with muscular dystrophy are sensitive to nondepolarizing muscle relaxants, and neuromuscular function should be objectively monitored. Dysfunction of gastrointestinal smooth muscle predisposes muscular dystrophy patients to impaired swallowing, delayed gastric emptying, and increased risk of aspiration pneumonia. Muscular dystrophy patients with preoperative muscle weakness may require postoperative mechanical ventilation.

Myotonic Dystrophy

Myotonic Dystrophy, the most common and severe of the myotonic syndromes, is a progressive multisystem disorder characterized by the delayed relaxation of skeletal muscle after voluntary contraction. There are two types: myotonic dystrophy type 1 (DM-1), also known as steinert muscular dystrophy, and myotonic dystrophy type 2 (DM-2). DM-1 is the more common and severe form, with a wide phenotype ranging from asymptomatic to life threatening. Both DM-1 and DM-2 are autosomal dominant disorders, but the result of different unstable nucleotide repeat expansions in untranslated deoxyribonucleic acid (DNA). They both lead to errors in messenger ribonucleic acid (mRNA) splicing that cause widespread cellular abnormalities.[9]

Table 24-2 Classification of Myotonic Dystrophy

Muscular Dystrophy Type 1
Congenital
Childhood-onset
Adult-onset
Late-onset
Muscular Dystrophy Type 2
Proximal myotonic dystrophy
Proximal myotonic myopathy
Proximal myotonic myopathy syndrome

Myotonic Dystrophy Type 1

DM-1 is the result of a trinucleotide expansion (CTG) on chromosome 19q. It has effects on virtually any organ system, but most seriously the musculoskeletal, cardiovascular, gastrointestinal, respiratory, central nervous, and endocrine systems. DM-1 is subdivided by age of onset (Table 24-2). Its presentation is that of a dystrophic process, beginning distally and progressing proximally. An error in muscle membrane excitability results in myotonia, and a myotonic grip often precedes weakness. Respiratory muscle weakness can diminish the effectiveness of coughing, putting patients at risk for pneumonia, while myotonia of the respiratory muscles can result in severe dyspnea. Gastric atony and pharyngeal muscle weakness place patients at risk for aspiration.

2 Conduction disturbances and tachyarrhythmias are common heart problems in patients with DM-1 and result in 30% of deaths.[10] Ischemic heart disease and ventricular dysfunction play roles as well. ECG abnormalities—most commonly, prolonged PR interval and QRS duration—are good predictors of sudden death. Therefore, it is recommended that patients receive yearly ECGs. Echocardiogram and cardiac MRI may identify subclinical ventricular dysfunction.[11]

In addition, patients with DM-1 can suffer from cataracts, psychosocial problems, diabetes mellitus, thyroid dysfunction, adrenal insufficiency, and gonadal atrophy. Pregnancy can exacerbate myotonia and precipitate congestive heart failure. Pregnant patients are at risk for spontaneous abortion, prolonged labor, and postpartum hemorrhage. Their newborns are also at risk if they are congenitally affected, which can manifest as difficulty feeding and/or respiratory failure.

Myotonic Dystrophy Type 2

DM-2 is caused by a quadnucleotide expansion (CCTG) on chromosome 3q. Overall, the clinical course of DM-2 is milder than DM-1, although they may have similar features. Most commonly, patients present with mild proximal muscle weakness in the third decade of life or later. Compared to patients with DM-1, patients with DM-2 more often complain of myalgia and fatigue, and weakness is usually mild. Their chronic pain is often misdiagnosed as fibromyalgia and can lead to associated problems such as poor sleep. They can also suffer from cataracts, insulin insensitivity, and cardiac conduction defects, although sudden death is rare. Annual ECGs are still recommended as part of routine follow-up.

There is currently no cure for DM-1 or DM-2. Myotonia can be treated with multiple agents that target skeletal muscle sodium channels, most commonly mexiletine. Mobility aids, such as walkers, wheelchairs, and ankle-foot orthoses are commonly utilized, and physical and occupational therapy play major roles in maintaining activities of daily living.[12] Any changes noted on ECG should prompt an evaluation by a cardiologist who may consider the potential benefit of an implantable pacemaker defibrillator.

Management of Anesthesia

Patients with DM-1 are more likely to have perioperative complications compared to those with DM-2. The preoperative evaluation should include an assessment of disease severity and review of cardiac and respiratory testing.[13] Patients should be considered as having an increased risk of aspiration. Succinylcholine should be avoided, as patients have an exaggerated contracture response to succinylcholine that can potentially make ventilation and tracheal intubation difficult. Patients with DM are also sensitive to the respiratory depressant effects of opiates and benzodiazepines. If neuromuscular blockade (NMB) is necessary, a short-acting NMB is preferred, and dosage of NMB should be adjusted in proportion to the degree of muscle wasting. Neuromuscular monitoring can underestimate the degree of blockade, as a myotonic response to stimulation can mimic sustained tetany. Neostigmine has been safely used, despite the theory that it can provoke myotonia. Sugammadex can also be used for NMB reversal.[14]

No specific anesthetic technique has been shown to be superior in the management of patients with DM. Sevoflurane and propofol have been used successfully. Etomidate should be used with care given its potential to cause pain on injection and myotonic movements that may induce myotonia. Shorter-acting opiates and sedatives are preferred to reduce the need for postoperative ventilation. Close monitoring for cardiac arrythmias is advised. Extubation should be done when the patient is fully awake, and patients should be monitored for a prolonged period in the postanesthesia care unit or intensive care unit until the residual effects of anesthetics are eliminated. These patients often have a blunted ventilatory response to hypercarbia, relying on hypoxemia as their main respiratory stimulus; therefore, supplemental oxygen should be used with caution. Regional anesthesia and multimodal techniques with acetaminophen and nonsteroidal anti-inflammatory drugs (NSAIDs) have been used successfully to reduce opioid requirements in the perioperative period.

Skeletal Muscle Channelopathies

Skeletal muscle channelopathies are a group of rare genetic neuromuscular disorders that are the result of mutations of sarcolemmal ion channels that are responsible for skeletal muscle excitability. The ion channels affected include chloride, sodium, calcium, and potassium channels. Depending on the disorder, they can have varying effects on skeletal muscle, including weakness or myotonia. Pain is also common.[15] Symptoms tend to be episodic and may lead to an acute disability. Episodes can be precipitated by sudden movement (potentially leading to falls), prolonged rest, or change in temperature. The fear of precipitating an episode, coupled with pain, often results in patients preferring to lead sedentary lives. They are categorized into two groups, based on their predominant symptom: periodic paralyses and nondystrophic myotonias (Table 24-3). Historically, the nondystrophic myotonias were considered a myotonic dystrophy, but advances in molecular biology have better elucidated their underlying cause, resulting in reclassification.

Hyperkalemic Periodic Paralysis

Hyperkalemic periodic paralysis (hyperPP) is an autosomal dominant channelopathy caused by a mutation of the sodium channel. Most often, the condition manifests as varying degrees of flaccid paralysis brought on by an increase in serum potassium that can last minutes to hours. Myotonia may also be present.[16] The muscles responsible for respiration are usually spared. Episodes are most often brought on by exposure to cold, rest

Table 24-3 Skeletal Muscle Channelopathies

Periodic Paralysis
Hyperkalemic periodic paralysis
Hypokalemic periodic paralysis
Thyrotoxic periodic paralysis
Andersen–Tawil syndrome
Nondystrophic Myotonia
Sodium channel myotonia
Myotonia congenita
Paramyotonia congenita

after exertion, and potassium loading (Table 24-4). The use of potassium-wasting drugs such as thiazide diuretics or carbonic anhydrase inhibitors, along with maintaining a diet of carbohydrate-rich meals, can help prevent episodes. In the event of severe attacks, insulin and glucose can be used to reduce the serum potassium concentration.

Hypokalemic Periodic Paralysis

Hypokalemic periodic paralysis (hypoPP) is also autosomal dominant and is the result of mutations in both calcium ion (most common) and sodium ion channels. Patients begin having episodes of weakness, usually in their teenage years; these episodes last hours to days and are the result of a low serum potassium concentration. Proximal muscles are most often affected, while the diaphragm and muscles supplied by the cranial nerves are spared. Episodes often occur in the morning, but can also be brought on by stress, during rest after exercise, or meals rich in carbohydrates.

There is a form of hypoPP that is associated with symptoms of hyperthyroidism, known as thyrotoxic periodic paralysis. Patients suffer paralytic episodes along with suppressed thyroid stimulating hormone (TSH) and increased thyroid hormone. Most commonly, this condition is seen in Asian males. Treatment of the hypokalemia abates acute episodes, while control of the hyperthyroidism prevents future episodes.[17]

Table 24-4 Clinical Features of Familial Periodic Paralysis

Hyperkalemic
Sodium channel defect
Potassium >5.5 mEq/L during symptoms
Precipitating factors
Rest after exercise
Potassium infusions
Metabolic acidosis
Hypothermia
Skeletal muscle weakness may be localized to tongue and eyelids
Hypokalemic
Calcium channel defect
Potassium level <3 mEq/L during symptoms
Precipitating factors
High glucose meals
Strenuous exercise
Glucose-insulin infusions
Stress
Hypothermia
Chronic myopathy with aging

Andersen–Tawil Syndrome

Andersen–Tawil syndrome (ATS) is caused by a mutation in the potassium ion channel of skeletal muscle. This results in a periodic flaccid paralysis similar in presentation to hypoPP. Unlike the other channelopathies, ATS affects organ systems other than skeletal muscle; cardiac muscle involvement results in arrythmias, and bone development anomalies result in dysmorphic features. A long QT interval or U-waves are commonly seen on ECG. There is often an increased risk of ventricular arrythmias and sudden cardiac arrest, so many ATS patients become candidates for an implantable cardiac defibrillator.[18]

Management of Anesthesia

Due to the wide variety of clinical features, it is important that the team caring for a patient with a skeletal muscle channelopathy has a clear understanding of the patient's diagnosis and perioperative management goals. In the case of hyperPP and hypoPP, knowing the patient's baseline and preoperative serum potassium is important, as most adverse events are related to changes in potassium concentration. In general, metabolic changes (acidosis, alkalosis) and medications that affect serum potassium levels (diuretics, insulin) may precipitate paralytic events and should be used with caution. Serial serum potassium monitoring is ideal, particularly if the surgery will result in large fluid and electrolyte shifts. Normothermia and normocapnia should be maintained. Glucose loading should be avoided. Short-acting NMBs and objective monitoring should be used if paralysis is necessary.

Succinylcholine should not be administered, both due to its tendency to increase serum potassium levels and the risk of exaggerated contractures in patients with nondystrophic myotonias. These contractures have at times been misdiagnosed as signs of MH. MH precautions are not necessary for all patients with a channelopathy.[19] However, some forms of hypoPP caused by mutations in the RYR1 and CACNA1S genes do carry a strong association with MH. Patients who are known to have one of these variants should be deemed MH-susceptible until proven otherwise.

Myasthenia Gravis

Myasthenia gravis (MG) is the most common disorder affecting the neuromuscular junction, with an annual incidence of 8 to 10 cases per 1 million persons and a prevalence of 150 to 250 cases per 1 million (NICV 24-2).[20] It is an autoimmune disease characterized by antibodies against acetylcholine receptors or other proteins in the postsynaptic neuromuscular junction, such as muscle-specific tyrosine kinase or lipoprotein receptor-related protein 4 (LRP4). The antibodies trigger complement-mediated damage to the postsynaptic membrane, resulting in lysis of junctional folds. Patients with detectable antibodies on standard assay are considered to have seropositive MG, while those lacking these antibodies are classified as having seronegative MG. Although it is unclear whether the thymus' role in the pathogenesis of MG is primary or secondary, 90% of patients have a thymoma, thymic hyperplasia, or thymic atrophy.

The clinical hallmark and primary manifestation of MG is weakness of skeletal muscles that worsens with activity or repetitive use. MG can affect varying combinations of bulbar, limb,

3

Table 24-5 Clinical Presentations of Myasthenia Gravis

Type	Etiology	Onset	Sex	Thymus	Course
Neonatal myasthenia	Passage of antibodies from myasthenic mothers across the placenta	Neonatal	Both sexes	Normal	Transient
Congenital myasthenia	Congenital endplate pathology, genetic autosomal recessive pattern of inheritance	0–2 yrs	Male > female	Normal	Non-fluctuating, compatible with long survival
Juvenile myasthenia	Autoimmune disorder	2–20 yrs	Female > male (4:1)	Hyperplasia	Slowly progressive, tendency to relapse and remission
Adult myasthenia	Autoimmune disorder	20–40 yrs	Female > male	Hyperplasia > thymoma	Maximum severity with 3–5 yrs
Elderly myasthenia	Autoimmune disorder	>40 yrs	Male > female	Thymoma (benign or locally invasive)	Rapid progress, higher mortality

Reproduced with permission from Springer: Baraka A. Anesthesia and myasthenia gravis. *Can J Anaesth*. 1992; 39:476.

ocular, and respiratory muscles; those muscles innervated by cranial nerves are most affected, explaining why individuals with MG often present with diplopia, dysarthria, dysphagia, and ptosis early in their disease course. Up to 30% will experience a myasthenic crisis during their lifetime. Characterized by profound muscular weakness and respiratory failure, myasthenic crises may be triggered by physical or emotional stress, suboptimal pharmacologic management, hyperthermia, pregnancy, or systemic illness. MG can also present with cardiac abnormalities, including atrial fibrillation, atrioventricular (AV) conduction delay, and diastolic dysfunction.

Historically, women were more commonly affected than men, with a bimodal distribution of age at symptom onset—an early peak in the second to third decade of life in females and in the seventh to eight decades in males. This distribution remains true, but males are now more often affected, with the average onset of symptoms over 50 years. MG can occur in children (juvenile MG), representing 10% to 15% of cases.[21] Up to 20% of neonates born to mothers with MG will have neonatal MG, occurring because of the transplacental passage of maternal antibodies that interfere with function of the neuromuscular junction for up to several weeks (Table 24-5).

In 1997, a task force called the Myasthenia Gravis Foundation of America (MGFA) met to address the need for globally accepted classifications, grading systems, and methods of analysis for patients undergoing therapy for MG. The product of this work was the MGMA Clinical Classification Scale (Table 24-6), which identifies patients by skeletal muscle groups affected and disease severity.[22]

The efficacy of pyridostigmine may be incomplete or dissipate over time, after which patients should be prescribed corticosteroids and/or nonsteroidal immunosuppressive drugs such as azathioprine, cyclosporine, mycophenolate, methotrexate, or tacrolimus. These agents target the underlying immune dysregulation and decrease binding of acetylcholine receptors by antibodies. Patients with refractory MG may see transient benefits from plasmapheresis, intravenous immunoglobulin, or monoclonal antibodies, though these therapies do not alter the circulating concentrations of receptor antibodies.[23]

Surgical treatment via thymectomy may benefit both patients with and without thymomatous MG, and either prevent the need or decrease the duration of immunotherapy. Because the full effect may not be apparent for months after surgery, thymectomy is considered an elective procedure for which patients with generalized MG should be medically optimized.

Management of Anesthesia

The major perioperative concern in patients with MG is postoperative weakness requiring prolonged mechanical ventilation. The interactions between disease severity, medications, and anesthetic agents are unpredictable. Chronic use of anticholinesterases impairs the effect of plasma cholinesterase, which may result in prolonged NMB by succinylcholine. At the same time, reduced numbers of acetylcholine receptors at the postsynaptic junction are thought to contribute to the succinylcholine resistance observed in clinical practice. Conversely, MG patients are extremely sensitive to the effects of nondepolarizing muscle relaxants (Fig. 24-3).

Due to their variable response, NMBs should be avoided; if necessary, doses should be one-half to two-thirds of normal.

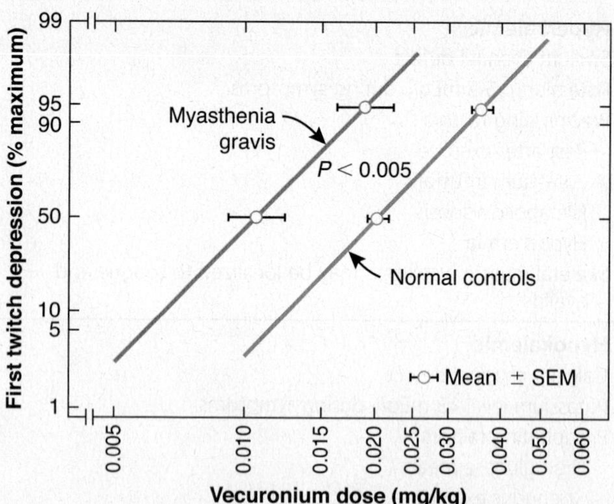

Figure 24-3 Dose–response for vecuronium in normal patients and patients with myasthenia gravis (MG). (Adapted with permission from Springer: Eisenkraft JB, Book WJ, Papatestas AE. Sensitivity to vecuronium in myasthenia gravis: a dose-response study. *Can J Anaesth*. 1990;37:301–306.)

Table 24-6 Myasthenia Gravis Foundation of America Clinical Classification

Class	Clinical Symptoms
I	Any ocular muscle weakness May have weakness of eye closure All other muscle strength is normal
II	Mild weakness affecting other than ocular muscles May also have ocular muscle weakness of any severity
IIA	Predominantly affecting limb, axial muscles, or both May also have lesser involvement of oropharyngeal muscles
IIB	Predominantly affecting oropharyngeal, respiratory muscles, or both May also have lesser or equal involvement of limb, axial muscles, or both
III	Moderate weakness affecting other than ocular muscles May also have ocular muscle weakness of any severity
IIIA	Predominantly affecting limb, axial muscles, or both May also have lesser involvement of oropharyngeal muscles
IIIB	Predominantly affecting oropharyngeal, respiratory muscles, or both May also have lesser or equal involvement of limb, axial muscles, or both
IV	Severe weakness affecting other than ocular muscles May also have ocular muscle weakness of any severity
IVA	Predominantly affecting limb and/or axial muscles May also have lesser involvement of oropharyngeal muscles
IVB	Predominantly affecting oropharyngeal, respiratory muscles, or both May also have lesser or equal involvement of limb, axial muscles, or both
V	Defined by intubation, with or without mechanical ventilation, except when employed during routine postoperative management. The use of a feeding tube without intubation places the patient in class IV B.

Adapted from Jaretzki A III, Barohn RJ, Ernstoff RM, et al. Myasthenia gravis: Recommendations for clinical research standards. *Neurology*. 2000;55(1):16–23.

Volatile inhalational agents can facilitate tracheal intubation and maintenance of relaxation, eliminating the need for paralytics. Opioids should be used sparingly, and any applicable regional anesthetic techniques may greatly reduce the incidence of postoperative respiratory depression.

MG criteria that have historically correlated with postoperative mechanical ventilation include duration of disease greater than 6 years, presence of pulmonary disease, pyridostigmine dose greater than 750 mg/day, and preoperative vital capacity less than 2.9 L.[24] Prior to extubation, patients should be fully awake, have a return to a "train of four," if muscle relaxants were employed, and a negative inspiratory force greater than 30 cm H_2O.

Myasthenic Syndrome

Myasthenic syndrome (Lambert–Eaton myasthenic syndrome or LEMS) is another autoimmune disorder of the neuromuscular junction, first described in 1956 as a paraneoplastic syndrome in patients with small cell lung carcinoma. Since then, it has been observed in patients without a coexisting without malignancy. LEMS is an acquired disorder secondary to IgG antibodies against P/Q-type voltage-sensitive calcium channels. The decreased calcium entering nerve endings and reduced release of acetylcholine from the neuromuscular junction.[25] 4

The skeletal weakness associated with LEMS usually affects the proximal lower limb muscles, causing diminished or absent tendon reflexes, while sparing the extraocular and bulbar muscles. Unlike MG, muscle strength typically improves transiently following activity. Patients also have autonomic symptoms such as dry mouth, orthostatic hypotension, hyperhidrosis, and a reduced pupillary light reflex (Table 24-7).

Therapy with cholinesterases alone is usually minimally effective. Muscle strength and autonomic function can be improved with 3,4-diaminopyridine (DAP) therapy, which blocks potassium channels, prolonging presynaptic nerve terminal membrane depolarization and increasing calcium entry and acetylcholine release. DAP may cause perioral and extremity paresthesias, headache, nausea, diarrhea, and rarely, seizures. Guanidine hydrochloride was previously the first-line therapy for LEMS, though its use has been limited due to more severe side effects, including bone marrow depression, renal tubular necrosis, cardiac arrhythmias, liver failure, and ataxia. Patients with refractory weakness may be on regimens that include intravenous immunoglobulin, plasmapheresis, and immunosuppressive agents such as steroids.

Patients are sensitive to both depolarizing and nondepolarizing muscle relaxants. Complete reversal of NMB at the end of a

Table 24-7 Comparison of Myasthenic Syndrome and Myasthenia Gravis

	Myasthenic Syndrome	Myasthenia Gravis
Manifestations	Proximal limb weakness (arms > legs)	Extraocular, bulbar, and facial muscle weakness
	Strength improves with exercise	Strength worsens with exercise
	Muscle pain common	Muscle pain uncommon
	Reflexes absent or decreased	Reflexes normal
Gender	Male > female	Female > male
Coexisting pathology	Small-cell carcinoma of lung	Thymoma
Response to muscle relaxants	Sensitive to succinylcholine and nondepolarizing muscle relaxants	Resistant to succinylcholine Sensitive to nondepolarizing muscle relaxants
Response to anticholinesterases	Poor response to anticholinesterases	Good response to anticholinesterases

Reprinted from Stoelting RK, Dierdorf SF, eds. *Anesthesia and co-existing disease*. 3rd ed. Churchill Livingstone; 1993. Copyright © 1993 Elsevier. With permission.

procedure may be challenging in the setting of pyridostigmine and DAP therapy. Like patients with MG, these patients have reduced respiratory reserve and anesthetic planning should include the possibility of postoperative mechanical ventilation.

Guillain–Barré Syndrome

The Guillain–Barré syndrome (GBS) is the most common cause of acute flaccid paralysis worldwide. GBS encompasses several peripheral nerve disorders that can be differentiated by the affected limbs or cranial nerves: acute inflammatory demyelinating polyneuropathy, acute motor axonal neuropathy, and Miller Fisher syndrome. Patients can suffer from multiple variants simultaneously, complicating diagnosis.[26] Severe neurologic disability will chronically affect 20% of patients, while GBS is fatal in 5%, despite appropriate treatment.

GBS is an autoimmune disease, usually triggered by a viral or bacterial infection. These infections result in the creation of autoantibodies to gangliosides, important components of peripheral nerves. The autoantibodies erroneously attack the patient's nervous system. There is good evidence that this is an example of molecular mimicry, as lipo-oligosaccharides that are structurally similar to gangliosides have been identified as the most common infectious causes of GBS. In addition to postinfectious causes, there are reports linking GBS to trauma, surgery,[27] and some vaccinations. Diagnosis is clinical but supported by the finding of increased protein and normal cell counts in cerebrospinal fluid.

The typical course of GBS is the onset of neurologic symptoms within 1 to 6 weeks of a respiratory or gastrointestinal infection. Some of the most common infectious sources are *Campylobacter jejuni*, *Haemophilus influenzae*, *Mycoplasma pneumoniae*, Epstein–Barr virus, and cytomegalovirus. Early symptoms include a combination of numbness, paresthesias, weakness, hyporeflexia, and pain in the lower limbs. In the subsequent 1 to 3 weeks, symptoms progress caudally, eventually resulting in an inability to walk independently in two-thirds of patients and respiratory difficulty in one-quarter. Autonomic dysfunction, including labile blood pressure, orthostatic hypotension, and life-threatening arrhythmias are seen in 20% of patients. Return of function is often but not always complete.

Immunotherapy with plasma exchange or intravenous immunoglobulin, initiated within two weeks of the onset of symptoms, is the most effective therapy. Other treatments are supportive and may include pain management, thromboprophylaxis, if the patient is immobile, and ventilatory support in the event of respiratory failure.

Management of Anesthesia

Impaired ability to swallow and cough can put patients with GBS at risk for aspiration. Succinylcholine should be avoided due to the danger of hyperkalemia, a risk that can persist after recovery from GBS.[28] If NMB is needed for surgical exposure, then a short-acting NMB should be used. Depending on the phase of the disease, patients may be resistant or sensitive to these drugs, so objective nerve function monitoring is important.[29] Profound hypotension can be seen following changes in intravascular volume, due to the lack of a compensatory cardiovascular response. On the other hand, sympathetic stimulation, like that seen during laryngoscopy or surgical incision, can result in exaggerated heart rate and blood pressure responses due to autonomic dysfunction. Mechanical ventilation may be required postoperatively depending on the patient's extent of disease. There are case reports of epidural anesthesia resulting in GBS,[30] but neuraxial anesthesia is still commonly used for patients with GBS in the operating room and for labor and delivery.

Central Nervous System Disease

Multiple Sclerosis

The features of multiple sclerosis (MS) are inflammation, demyelination, immune dysregulation, and failure of cell repair in the central nervous system (CNS) (NICV 24-3). There is a complex interaction between genetics and environmental factors that lead to demyelination of CNS cells and peripheral nerves. An antigen-presenting dendritic cell crosses the blood-brain barrier and converts T-cells into inflammatory cells. These T-cells induce macrophages that produce cytokines and oxygen radicals that cause demyelination and axonal decay. Demyelination interferes with neural transmission and CNS dysfunction ensues. As the disease progresses, there is loss of brain volume and gray matter.[31]

The symptoms of MS depend on the sites of demyelination. Brainstem involvement can produce nystagmus, diplopia, ataxia, autonomic dysfunction, and alterations in ventilation that lead to respiratory failure. Lesions of the spinal cord produce weakness and paresthesias. The legs are affected more than the arms. Bowel retention and urinary incontinence are frequent complaints. Many patients with MS develop central neuropathic pain, trigeminal neuralgia, spasticity, and tonic seizures. The course of MS is characterized by exacerbation of symptoms at unpredictable intervals over years. Patients are classified during the early stages of the disease as relapsing-remitting (85%) or primary progressive MS (15%). Many patients with relapsing-remitting MS develop neurodegeneration and are then categorized as having secondary progressive MS.

Clinical criteria for the diagnosis of MS include onset between 10 and 50 years of age, signs, and symptoms of CNS white matter disease, two or more attacks separated by a month or more, and involvement of two or more noncontiguous anatomic areas. Elevated levels of IgG and albumin in the cerebrospinal fluid are characteristic of MS. MRI is a sensitive diagnostic tool for MS and provides direct evidence of demyelinated plaques in the CNS. Pregnancy is generally associated with reduced risk of exacerbations while the postpartum period is notable for an increased risk of relapse.

Treatment of MS is directed at modulating the immunologic and inflammatory responses that damage the CNS. Interferon preparations and glatiramer are self-injectable drugs with good safety profiles. Mitoxantrone is a general immunosuppressant that has limited use because of cardiotoxicity and treatment-related leukemia. Natalizumab has limited use because of the development of progressive multifocal leukoencephalopathy. Most of the immunomodulating drugs increase the patient's risk of infection and malignancy.

There are three oral disease-modifying drugs currently used for the treatment of relapsing MS: fingolimod, terifunomide, and dimethyl fumarate. Side effects of fingolimod include bradycardia, macular edema, hypertension, and liver dysfunction. Terifunomide can cause lymphopenia, hepatotoxicity, hypertension, and peripheral neuropathy. Dimethyl fumarate causes flushing, nausea, abdominal pain, and diarrhea. Several monoclonal antibodies are under investigation for the treatment of MS.[32]

Management of Anesthesia

The effect of surgery and anesthesia on the course of MS is controversial. Some reports have suggested that general or regional anesthesia can exacerbate MS. Most reports, however, have found no influence of anesthesia on the course of the disease. It is likely that other factors such as infection, hyperpyrexia, and emotional stress are more likely contributors to perioperative exacerbations.

Preoperatively, the patient should be advised that surgery and anesthesia could produce a relapse despite a well-managed anesthetic. Several studies support the safe use of regional and neuraxial anesthesia in patients with MS.[33] There is no evidence that exposure to inhaled anesthetics, including nitrous oxide, increases the risk of MS to anesthesia providers.

The chronic effects of the neurologic dysfunction caused by MS and potent therapeutic drugs can be manifest during the perioperative period as autonomic dysfunction, myopathy, cardiotoxicity, and sensitivity or resistance to muscle relaxants. Succinylcholine can produce an exaggerated release of potassium. Respiratory muscle weakness increases the likelihood that postoperative ventilatory support will be needed.

Epilepsy

Epilepsy is a neurologic disorder marked by sudden recurrent episodes of sensory disturbance, loss of consciousness, or convulsions, associated with abnormal electrical activity in the brain. If untreated, they can recur at unpredictable intervals. Seizures are a common manifestation of many CNS diseases. A seizure is the result of an excessive discharge of large numbers of neurons. The onset of seizures may indicate focal brain disease (e.g., tumor) or be the result of cerebrovascular disease, head injury, infection, or metabolic abnormalities. Thus, a complete workup by a neurologist is required for a new-onset seizure. If no cause is found, then the patient has epilepsy.

Classification

Seizure classification begins with whether the initial manifestations are focal or centralized. Focal seizures are classified according to the patient's level of awareness, the most prominent motor or nonmotor features of the seizure, and whether a focal seizure evolves into a bilateral tonic–clonic seizure. Generalized seizures are classified according to motor or nonmotor manifestations. Motor seizures are either tonic–clonic or other motor seizures. Nonmotor generalized seizures are primarily absence seizures. Seizures can be classified as focal or generalized (as identified on electroencephalogram [EEG]).

The 2017 the International League Against Epilepsy (ILAE) introduced a new classification system for seizures and epilepsies that added two new categories: combined generalized and focal epilepsy, and unknown epilepsy. Up to one-third of patients are diagnosed as unknown. In addition, the term "epilepsy syndrome" has been introduced and refers to a cluster of features incorporating seizure type, EEG, neural imaging, and other features including genetics. This classification was proposed to emphasize the etiology of seizures and epilepsies. Epilepsies may have the following underlying causes: structural, genetic, infectious, metabolic, immune, or unknown. See Pack[34] for a complete discussion of the most recent classification.[34]

The most frequently encountered types of seizures are as follows:

1. *Grand mal seizures* are characterized by generalized tonic–clonic activity. All respiratory effort ceases and arterial hypoxemia ensues. The tonic phase lasts 20 to 40 seconds and is followed by the clonic phase. In the postictal period, the patient is lethargic and confused.
2. *Focal cortical seizures* may be motor or sensory depending on the site of neuronal discharge. There is usually no loss of consciousness, although the focal seizure may induce a grand mal seizure.
3. *Absence seizures* (petit mal) are a sudden, brief loss of awareness (30 seconds). Additional features include staring, blinking, and rolling of the eyes. These seizures typically occur in children and young adults.
4. *Akinetic seizures* are a sudden loss of consciousness and postural tone. These types of seizures usually occur in children and can cause head injury from the fall.
5. *Status epilepticus* is defined as two consecutive tonic–clonic seizures without regaining consciousness or seizure activity that is unabated for 30 minutes. Grand mal status epilepticus can last for 48 hours with 4 to 5 seizures per hour; the mortality can be up to 20%.[35]

As the seizure progresses, skeletal muscle activity diminishes, and seizure activity may only be evident on EEG. Respiratory effects of status epilepticus include respiratory center inhibition, impaired ventilation from uncoordinated skeletal muscle activity, and bronchoconstriction.

Treatment

The goal of antiepileptic drug (AED) therapy is to ensure the best possible quality of life for the patient by maximizing seizure control and minimizing drug toxicity.[36] There are many AEDs available (Table 24-8). Most AEDs affect ion transfer, increase inhibitory neurotransmitters (GABA), or decrease levels of excitatory neurotransmitters. AEDs can be divided into two general categories: broad and narrow spectrum. Broad-spectrum AEDs such as valproate, lamotrigine, topiramate, levetiracetam, and zonisamide are useful for generalized seizures. Narrow-spectrum

Table 24-8 Antiepileptic Drugs Classified by Mechanism of Action

Enhance GABAergic System
Barbiturates
Valproic acid
Tiagabine
Benzodiazepines
Primidone
Vigabatrin
Affect Cation Channels
Sodium channels
Carbamazepine
Felbamate
Lamotrigine
Phenytoin
Toprimate
Oxycarbazepine
Calcium channels
Gabapentin
Pregabalin
Ethosuximide
Potassium channels
Retigabine
Antagonists of Excitatory Amino Acids
Lacosamide
Talampanel
Levetiracetam
Unknown Mechanism of Action
Acetazolamide
Sulthiame

AEDs such as carbamazepine, phenytoin, gabapentin, tiagabine, oxycarbazepine, and pregabalin are more appropriate for focal seizures.[37] Vagal nerve stimulators are often implanted for the treatment of medically refractory epilepsy. Perucca et al. provide updated information on the pharmacologic management of epilepsy.[37]

The treatment of patients with status epilepticus requires airway protection and appropriate ventilatory assistance. Drug therapy for status epilepticus may include combinations of lorazepam, midazolam, phenytoin, fosphenytoin, phenobarbital, pentobarbital, and propofol. On rare occasion, general anesthesia may be required.

Management of Anesthesia

Many anesthetics, including halogenated inhaled anesthetics, nitrous oxide, etomidate, ketamine, and opioids, have been reported to produce seizure activity. The clinical significance of these reports is unclear.[38] The degree of preoperative seizure control may be more important than the anesthetic agents used intraoperatively. Interruption of the patient's AED therapy should be minimized during the perioperative period. Side effects of AEDs include leukopenia, anemia, hepatic dysfunction, pancreatitis, cardiotoxicity, hypothyroidism, and skin rash.[39] Vagal nerve stimulators can cause vocal cord paralysis, facial palsy, bradycardia/asystole, and airway obstruction.[40] AEDs can stimulate hepatic enzymes (cytochrome P450), which can accelerate the metabolism of other drugs.[41] In contrast, AEDs that are highly protein-bound may increase blood concentrations of drugs that normally bind to serum proteins.

Alzheimer Disease

Alzheimer disease (AD) is characterized by loss of cognition, poor decision making, language deterioration, gait disturbances, seizures, agitation, and psychosis.

AD is the major cause of dementia in the United States. The incidence of AD increases progressively after 65 years of age and may be as high as 30% in persons over 85 years of age. Ninety-five percent of AD cases are sporadic and 5% have a genetic basis. The pathogenesis of AD is complex but appears to start with the build-up of amyloid-β protein (Aβ), possibly years before clinical manifestations develop. Aβ protein most likely begins a cascade of events culminating in deposition of amyloid plaques, neurofibrillary tangles, and neuronal apoptosis (amyloid cascade). These changes cause a loss of cholinergic activity and a loss of glutamatergic neurons. Diagnostic Imaging studies show hippocampal atrophy (by MRI) and glucose hypometabolism (by positron emission tomography [PET] scan).[42] A more invasive test involves examination of the CSF for Aβ42, a hyperphosphorylated *tau* peptide (p-*tau*), and total *tau* protein content. MRI and PET scanning have shown no difference in diagnostic accuracy.[43]

Medications currently approved for the treatment of AD include three acetylcholinesterase inhibitors (donepezil, rivastigmine, galantamine) and one N-methyl-D-aspartate (NMDA) inhibitor (memantine).[45] Cholinesterase inhibitors improve the patient's ability to perform activities of daily living and may improve cognition. Side effects of cholinesterase inhibitors include nausea, emesis, bradycardia, syncope, and fatigue. Memantine, a noncompetitive NMDA receptor antagonist and a dopamine agonist, is used in patients with moderate to severe AD and impaired attention span or alertness. Antidepressants, anticonvulsants, and antipsychotics are used as adjuncts to treat neuropsychiatric symptoms.

Therapies under investigation are directed at early interruption of the amyloid cascade.[44] Future treatments of AD involve targeting purported etiologic pathologies, including neurofibrillary tangles which are composed of hyperphosphorylated-*tau* (p-*tau*) protein tangles and senile plaques (Aβ).[45]

Management of Anesthesia

There is considerable concern that general anesthesia may cause postoperative cognitive dysfunction (POCD) and accelerate symptom progression in patients with AD.[46] POCD is well known to occur with more frequency in elderly patients, but causality remains elusive.[47] Eckenhoff found that the solubility of Aβ protein decreased when exposed to inhalational agents (desflurane and isoflurane) as well as intravenous propofol.[48] Current research supports the hypotheses that anesthesia induces AD pathophysiology through oligomerization of Aβ and p-*tau*.[49] Thus, patients and their families should be advised that POCD is likely and may worsen AD symptoms.

The selection of anesthetics in patients with AD will be influenced by the patient's physiologic condition and the degree of neurologic impairment. The patient's preoperative drug list should be reviewed for the possibility of interactions with anesthetics. Patients may be confused and uncooperative because of dementia. Sedative premedication should be used with caution, if at all, as it may worsen mental confusion. If an anticholinergic is required, glycopyrrolate, which does not cross the blood–brain barrier, is preferred rather than atropine or scopolamine. Patients on chronic cholinesterase inhibitor therapy may have a prolonged response to succinylcholine.

Parkinson Disease

Parkinson disease (PD) is a degenerative CNS condition caused by a loss of dopaminergic cells in the basal ganglia. The etiology of PD is a complex interaction between genetic predisposition and environmental factors such as pesticide exposure, agricultural occupation, rural living, prior head injury, and β-adrenergic blocker use.

The diagnosis of PD is clinical. The most characteristic signs of PD are resting tremor, cog-wheel rigidity of the upper extremities, bradykinesia, shuffling gait, stooped posture, and facial immobility. These features are secondary to diminished inhibition of the extrapyramidal motor system due to dopamine deficiency. Other clinical manifestations include seborrhea, sialorrhea, constipation, orthostatic hypotension, bladder dysfunction, diaphragmatic spasm, oculogyric crises, dementia, and depression.[50]

The characteristic pathologic feature is the presence of Lewy bodies in the neurons of the substantia nigra. Lewy bodies are cytoplasmic inclusions consisting of α-synuclein, a nonsoluble, aggregated, fibrillar form. Lewy bodies and Lewy neurites are the pathologic hallmark of PD. In addition, recent studies have demonstrated neuroinflammation to be a significant and essential upstream contributor to α-synuclein aggregation and the neurodegenerative process.[51]

Braak and colleagues proposed six stages of Lewy pathology in PD.[52] They have suggested that the disease spreads stereotypically from the vagal dorsal motor nucleus progressing on to the substantia nigra and then to the cerebral hemispheres in the terminal phase. These findings have only been demonstrated in animals, however, they are believed to be the same in humans

Current therapies for PD are intended to ameliorate symptoms. Levodopa is the most effective treatment available for PD. Levodopa is used in combination with drugs such as carbidopa (peripheral decarboxylase inhibitor) and entacapone (catechol-o-methyltransferase inhibitor), which prevent the adverse peripheral effects of dopamine. Other drugs that may improve function in patients with PD are the monoamine oxidase-B inhibitors, selegiline, and rasagiline. Dopamine agonists such as bromocriptine, pramipexole, ropinirole, pergolide, and cabergoline may also be effective. Pergolide and cabergoline are ergot-derived drugs that are not routinely used because they may cause cardiac valvular fibrosis and insufficiency. Implantation of deep-brain stimulators may be effective for patients with advanced PD as well as younger patients with PD. The therapeutic regimen for PD is complex and requires the expertise of a skilled neurologist.[53] Ongoing treatment research is aimed at prevention of underlying neurodegeneration.

Management of Anesthesia

Patients with PD often have fluctuating symptoms and are usually on several medications, which makes perioperative management difficult.[54,55] One major preoperative challenge in anesthetizing patients with PD is the administration of dopaminergic medications during the *nil per os* (NPO) period. The half-life of levodopa is short, and interruption of therapy for more than 6 to 12 hours can result in skeletal muscle rigidity that may interfere with ventilation. Consultation with the patient's neurologist is advised; continuation of the patient's drug regimen may avert complications. Apomorphine is a dopamine agonist that can be administered subcutaneously or intravenously if oral levodopa cannot be given.

The major intraoperative challenges include (1) choice of appropriate anesthetic technique, (2) managing respiratory issues, and (3) managing dysautonomia. Dopamine antagonists such as phenothiazines, droperidol, and metoclopramide should be avoided. Alfentanil and fentanyl may produce dystonic reactions when administered rapidly. The incidence of side effects from propofol is low. Although ketamine may theoretically produce an exaggerated sympathetic nervous system response with tachycardia and hypertension, it has been used without difficulty in patients with PD. There are no reports of adverse responses to isoflurane, sevoflurane, or desflurane. The likelihood of coexisting heart disease in elderly patients with PD will influence the selection of anesthetics and monitoring techniques.[56]

In the postoperative period, problems that may occur include (1) timely reinitiation of dopaminergic medications, (2) adequate management of pain, nausea, and vomiting, (3) prevention of postoperative infections, and (4) management of delirium.[56] Anesthetics administered to patients who are receiving monoamine-B-oxidase inhibitors are generally uneventful. However, there are reports of agitation, muscle rigidity, and hyperthermia in patients receiving selegiline and meperidine. Patients being treated with dopamine agonists may be at increased risk for neuroleptic malignant syndrome.

Autonomic dysfunction is common. The most consistent cardiovascular effect is orthostatic hypotension which may be aggravated by the vasodilatory effects of anti-Parkinson drugs and inhaled anesthetics. Excessive salivation and esophageal dysfunction are common and increase the risk of aspiration pneumonitis. Perioperative respiratory complications are also common.[57] Upper airway obstruction may be a result of poor coordination of upper airway muscles secondary to neurotransmitter imbalance. Upper airway obstruction may respond favorably to anti-Parkinson drugs. Patients with PD are susceptible to postoperative confusion and hallucinations. These changes in mental function may not occur for 24 to 72 hours after surgery.

Anesthesia for PD patients undergoing implantation of deep brain stimulators can be challenging. During placement, the electrode passes through the thalamus, zona incerta, subthalamic nucleus, and substantia nigra. Positioning is confirmed by characteristic microelectrode stimulation as the probe is passed through these regions. In awake patients, this is accomplished by macrostimulation testing and passive movement in the contralateral limb.

However, agitated, and uncooperative patients require general anesthesia. Tsai et al. demonstrated that although general anesthesia using sevoflurane-induced changes in electrical oscillations in the basal ganglia, correct electrode placement for clinically effective subthalamic brain stimulation was achieved.[57] No significant differences during intraoperative testing of the stimulator were reported. No differences were seen in placement accuracy or clinical outcome.[58] Nevertheless, hypertension, seizures, and electrical interference with other devices can occur.[59]

Huntington Disease

Huntington disease (HD) is an autosomal dominant, progressive neurodegenerative disease caused by a trinucleotide (CAG) repeat on chromosome 4. The Huntingtin protein is expressed in all cell types but has a higher affinity in the brain. This CAG repeat expansion causes mutant Huntingtin protein development which results in neuronal dysfunction and apoptosis. The length of the trinucleotide repeat affects variability and penetrance in age of symptom onset and symptom progression. HD causes diffuse atrophy and neuronal loss in the caudate and putamen grey matter, as well as thalamic, cerebellar, and cortical white matter.

Clinical manifestations of HD commonly begin in middle age with choreiform movements, cognitive impairment, and neuropsychiatric disturbances. Diagnosis is confirmed by family history or positive genetic testing. The motor component, which is most characteristic, begins with a rapid phase of chorea that then evolves to bradykinesia with disease progression. Motor symptoms are accompanied by progressive dementia and mood-altering states marked by apathy and depression. Onset to end of life is approximately 20 years, and death is usually from malnutrition, aspiration pneumonitis, or suicide. Hypothalamic atrophy causes endocrine abnormalities including elevated cortisol, reduced testosterone, and diabetes. Skeletal muscle wasting and hepatic dysfunction are common.

There are few treatments for HD, and therapies remain palliative. Tetrabenazine, a high-affinity mono-amine uptake inhibitor, is the only approved drug for the treatment of chorea. Antiepileptics and antidepressants are commonly used for neuropsychiatric symptoms. There is promising research targeting the Huntington gene, which could alter the course of this disease.[60]

Management of Anesthesia

Many of the anesthetic concerns in patients with HD arise from the bulbar symptoms which cause pharyngeal muscle weakness and impaired gastric emptying; this increases aspiration risk and the risk of prolonged weakness from muscle relaxants. Delayed emergence and increased risk of respiratory complications should be anticipated.

Inhaled, intravenous, and neuraxial anesthetics have been used in patients with HD. Propofol is favored for its short half-life. There is some data to suggest decreased plasma pseudocholinesterase (PCE) activity that might prolong the duration of effects of succinylcholine.[61]

Amyotrophic Lateral Sclerosis

Amyotrophic lateral sclerosis (ALS, Lou Gehrig disease) is a fatal, progressive degenerative motor neuron disease. There are many proposed mechanisms explaining the cause of ALS, with leading theories focused on glutamate excitotoxicity and oxidative stress. The result is destruction of the neuromuscular junction and cell death of both upper and lower motor neurons. Most cases are sporadic with only 10% having a familial component. The progression of the disease is aggressive, with at least 50% mortality within 3 years of symptom onset. The most common cause of death is respiratory failure.

The clinical presentation of ALS is highly variable in age, constellation of symptoms, and progression of disease. Classically, ALS begins in middle age with unilateral distal limb muscle weakness that progresses to muscle atrophy, fasciculations, and slowed muscle movements. Bulbar onset presents with dysarthria and dysphagia. Diagnosis is mainly clinical, with the use of electromyelogram (EMG) and neuroimaging as diagnostic adjuncts. With disease progression, patients can have autonomic dysfunction, marked by resting tachycardia, orthostatic hypotension, and elevated circulating catecholamines. Respiratory muscles are affected and cause a decrease in pulmonary function, eventually leading to respiratory failure and the need for mechanical ventilatory support.[62]

There are only two approved pharmaceuticals for ALS. Riluzole, a glutamate-release inhibitor, is associated with a modest increase in survival (3 to 6 months). Newly approved is edaravone, a free radical scavenger; this drug is especially indicated in early ALS. The mainstays of treatment remain palliative and include antispasmodics and antisialagogues. Noninvasive mechanical ventilation is preferred for respiratory support. Treatments to avoid mechanical ventilatory support such as diaphragmatic pacing are under investigation.[63]

Management of Anesthesia

Patients with ALS often come to the operating room for supportive therapies such as gastrostomy tube or tracheostomy tube placement. Preoperative evaluation should focus on the presence and degree of dysphagia and respiratory compromise. Short-acting agents are preferred. Succinylcholine should be avoided, as it may cause life-threatening hyperkalemia. Nondepolarizing muscular blockers have been used, best at reduced doses and with complete proven reversal. Patients are at increased aspiration risk and are likely to require postoperative ventilatory support.[64]

Creutzfeldt–Jakob Disease

Creutzfeldt–Jakob disease (CJD) is a rare fatal neurodegenerative disease that is part of the transmissible spongiform encephalopathies or prion diseases. Normal prion protein, PrP^{sc} is found in all human cells but concentrated in neurons. CJD is an infection caused by a pathologic conformational change in the prion protein, PrP^{sc}. The accumulation of abnormal prion protein leads to neuronal degeneration and a characteristic vacuolation in brain cells, which leads to neuronal cell death. The structure of PrP^{SC} renders the protein resistant to conventional decontamination methods. There are four subtypes of CJD: familial (fCJD), sporadic (sCJD), iatrogenic (iCJD), and variant (vCJD). Sporadic CJD is the most common. Variant CJD thrust CJD into the international spotlight with the discovery of transmission of prion disease from cow to humans (Mad cow disease) in the mid-1990s.[65]

Clinical manifestations of CJD vary by subtype; however, all are uniformly fatal. Sporadic CJD is most common in the sixth to seventh decade of life and has a very rapid time course, with 90% mortality within 6 months. Rapid onset subacute dementia, ataxia, myoclonus, and a characteristic EEG pattern of diffuse slow activity and periodic complexes are seen. This leads to rapid cognitive and neurologic function loss. Variant CJD is contracted by ingestion of contaminated animal products. These patients first present with psychiatric changes in mood and behavior. Neurologic sequelae develop within a few months. Iatrogenic CJD has been linked to contaminated surgical instruments, contaminated dural graft materials, corneal transplants, and blood products including derivatives such as pooled growth hormones (GH). The gold standard for diagnosis is brain biopsy. Research is centered on therapies aimed at preventing prion transmission from the periphery into the CNS.[66]

Management of Anesthesia

CJD is highly transmissible. Appropriate precautions should be observed when administering anesthesia. Tissue with a high likelihood of transmission includes brain, spinal cord, cerebrospinal fluid, lymphatic tissue, and blood. Disposable single-use anesthesia supplies, including face masks, breathing circuits, laryngoscopes, and endotracheal tubes offer the highest degree of protection.[67]

Patients with CJD are prone to aspiration because of impaired swallowing function and decreased laryngeal reflexes. Succinylcholine should be avoided secondary to lower motor neuron dysfunction. Autonomic and peripheral nervous system dysfunction may cause abnormal cardiovascular responses to anesthesia and vasoactive drugs.

Other Inherited Disorders

Malignant Hyperthermia

MH is a pharmacogenetic disorder of skeletal muscle that, when triggered, results in a hypermetabolic process associated with significant morbidity and mortality (NICV 24-4). MH is commonly triggered by succinylcholine or halogenated, inhaled anesthetics. It has also been associated with extreme physiologic stress or heat exhaustion. Individuals susceptible to MH have a mutation of the ryanodine or dihydropyridine receptor that permits the uncontrolled release of calcium (Ca^{2+}) from the sarcoplasmic reticulum. This leads to sustained muscle contraction/rigidity, metabolic and respiratory acidosis, hypercarbia, tachycardia, hyperthermia, rhabdomyolysis, and hemodynamic instability.[68] Other mechanisms of calcium control may also be defective in patients with MH (Fig. 24-4).[69] The incidence of MH in adults varies from 1:40,000 to 1:250,000 but may be as high as 1:15,000 in children. Although the knowledge of the pathophysiology of MH has increased, mortality may still be as high as 9.5%.[70]

Management of the Acute Malignant Hyperthermia Episode

The earlier an episode of MH is identified and treated, the better the outcome. The first sign of an MH reaction is usually an increase in the end-tidal CO_2 ($ETCO_2$) that does not respond to an appropriate increase in ventilation. Tachycardia, tachypnea (spontaneous ventilation), and hypertension—although nonspecific—may be present. Muscle rigidity, masseter spasm, and a mixed respiratory and metabolic acidosis also support the diagnosis of MH. Hyperthermia may occur early or late in the episode. The initial symptoms are variable depending on the age of the patient.[71] Other conditions that may mimic MH are sepsis, hyperthyroidism, and neuroleptic malignant syndrome. A scoring system has been developed to assist the clinician with the diagnosis of a true MH reaction (Table 24-9).[72] If the presumptive diagnosis is an MH episode, any halogenated, inhaled anesthetic should be discontinued and hyperventilation with 100% oxygen should be initiated. The surgical team should be informed, and the procedure aborted or terminated as quickly as possible under intravenous anesthesia. Charcoal filters placed in the anesthesia

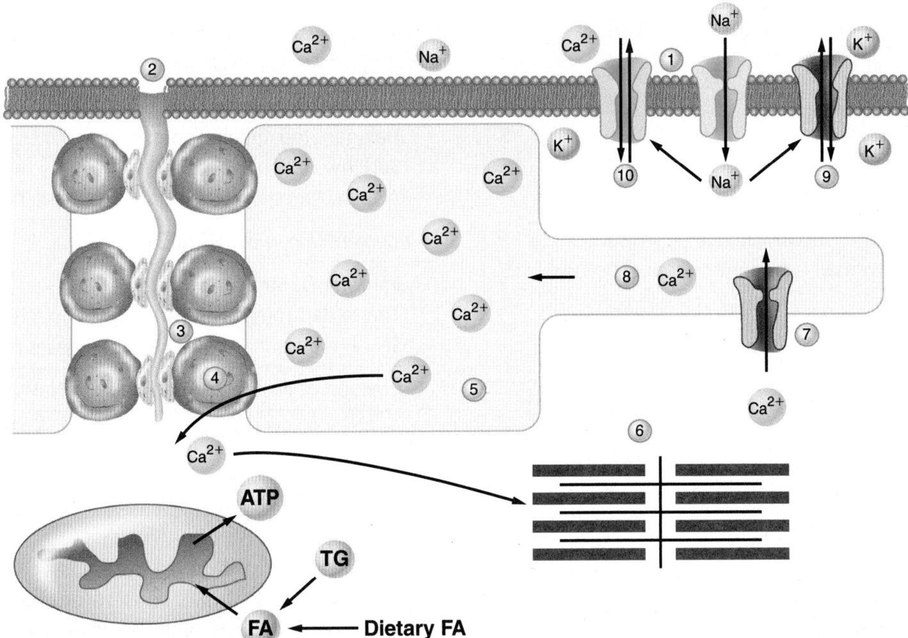

Figure 24-4 Excitation–contraction coupling and malignant hyperthermia (MH). The action potential generated at the endplate region of the neuromuscular junction is propagated down the sarcolemma (muscle plasma membrane) by the opening of voltage-dependent Na^+ channels. (*1*) The action potential continues down into the T-tubules (*2*) to the dihydropyridine receptors. (*3*) The dihydropyridine receptors in skeletal muscle function as voltage sensors and are coupled to the Ca^{2+} release channels. (*4*) Through this coupled signaling process, the Ca^{2+} release channels are opened, some of the available terminal cisternae Ca^{2+} stores (*5*) are released, and the levels of myoplasmic Ca^{2+} are elevated. The Ca^{2+} then diffuses to the myofibrils (*6*) and interacts with the troponin/tropomyosin complex associated with actin (*thin lines*) and allows interaction of actin with myosin (*thick lines*) for mechanical movement. The Ca^{2+} diffuses away from the myofibrils and this Ca^{2+} signal is terminated by an adenosine triphosphate (ATP)-driven Ca^{2+} pump (*7*), which pumps Ca^{2+} into the longitudinal sarcoplasmic reticulum (*8*). The Ca^{2+} diffuses from the longitudinal sarcoplasmic reticulum to the terminal cisternae, where it is concentrated for release by Ca^{2+} binding proteins. Na^+ entering during the action potential is subsequently extruded from the cell by the Na^+/K^+-ATPase (*9*) and possibly through Na^+/Ca^{2+} exchange (*10*). This latter process would elevate intracellular Ca^{2+} and could result from delayed inactivation of Na^+ currents. A major form of energy for supplying cellular ATP for the ion pumps and numerous other energy-consuming processes is fatty acids (FA) derived from the serum (dietary FA), or from intramuscular triglyceride (TG) stores. Therefore, a defect in the intracellular Ca^{2+} regulating processes (increased Ca^{2+} release or decreased Ca^{2+} uptake), or a defect in the sarcolemma could account for an increase in myoplasmic Ca^{2+}.

breathing system will rapidly purge the system of any halogenated anesthetic. The most definitive treatment for MH is dantrolene, a hydantoin derivative that inhibits the pathologic release of Ca^{2+}. The initial intravenous dose of dantrolene is 2.5 mg/kg, and this dose should be repeated until the MH reaction has subsided. If a cumulative dose of 10 mg/kg has been given without symptom improvement, the differential diagnosis should be revisited. However, some MH events have required 20 to 30 mg/kg of dantrolene before resolution of symptoms. A newer formulation of dantrolene (Ryanodex, Eagle Pharmaceuticals, Woodcliff, NJ) requires significantly less time for reconstitution than the older preparation.[73] Serial arterial blood gas measurements are helpful for tracking the response to therapy. Supportive measures include hyperventilation, treatment of acidosis and hyperkalemia, active cooling, and maintenance of an adequate urinary output (Table 24-10).[74]

Management of the Malignant Hyperthermia Susceptible Patient

The most definitive test for MH susceptibility is the caffeine-halothane contracture test, but this test must be performed at an experienced center. Supplemental genetic testing may detect an identifiable receptor mutation that can assist with diagnosis in relatives.[75,76] Patients who have a history of recurrent rhabdomyolysis or unknown congenital myopathies should be considered for genetic testing prior to receiving a triggering anesthetic.

Avoidance of known triggering agents is central to the anesthetic plan for an MH-susceptible patient. Most intravenous agents such as propofol, benzodiazepines, opioids, nondepolarizing muscle relaxants, and nitrous oxide are safe for these patients (Table 24-11). Preparation of the anesthesia machine includes removal or closure of vaporizers, change of all disposable components, and flushing the machine with 100% oxygen. Charcoal filters attached to both limbs of the anesthesia breathing circuit before and during the procedure are effective at reducing halogenated anesthetics to less than trace amounts and are an alternative to prolonged machine flushing.[77] Preoperative administration of prophylactic dantrolene is not recommended. Dantrolene should, however, be readily available. The Malignant Hyperthermia Association of the United States (MHAUS) has detailed recommendations for management of MH-susceptible patients.

Porphyrias

Porphyrias are a group of metabolic disorders that result from a deficiency of a specific enzyme involved in porphyrin synthesis. These compounds, of which heme is the most important in human physiology, play vital roles in oxygen storage, transport, and utilization. A defect of any of the eight enzymes along this

Table 24-9 Malignant Hyperthermia Clinical Grading Scale

Process I: Muscle Rigidity	
Generalized rigidity	15
Masseter rigidity	15
Process II: Myonecrosis	
Elevated CK >20,000 (after succinylcholine administration)	15
Elevated CK >10,000 (without exposure to succinylcholine)	15
Cola-colored urine	10
Myoglobin in urine >60 mg/L	5
Blood/plasma/serum K+ >6 mEq/L	3
Process III: Respiratory Acidosis	
$PETCO_2$ >55 with controlled ventilation	15
$PaCO_2$ >60 with controlled ventilation	15
$PETCO_2$ >60 with spontaneous ventilation	15
Inappropriate hypercarbia	15
Inappropriate tachypnea	10
Process IV: Temperature Increase	
Rapid increase in temperature	15
Inappropriate temperature >38.8°C in perioperative period	10
Process V: Cardiac Involvement	
Inappropriate tachycardia	3
Ventricular tachycardia or fibrillation	3

CK, creatine kinase; $PETCO_2$, end-tidal carbon dioxide; $PaCO_2$, arterial partial pressure of carbon dioxide.

See Larach, et al.[72] for full details of this scoring system. Briefly, a case may receive 15 points for the worst presentation in five of the first six categories. A sum of more than 50 points is termed *D6*, almost certainly a case of malignant hyperthermia (MH). A sum of 35 to 49 points is *D5*, very likely to be a case of MH.

Table 24-10 Treatment of an Acute Episode of Malignant Hyperthermia

Discontinue Triggering Agents Halogenated, inhaled anesthetics Succinylcholine Attach charcoal filters to the anesthesia breathing circuit
Hyperventilate with 100% Oxygen
Administer Dantrolene 2.5 mg/kg Titrate dantrolene to heart rate, temperature, and $PaCO_2$ Serial monitoring of arterial blood gases
Correction of Metabolic Acidosis with $NaHCO_3$
Control of Dysrhythmias Lidocaine Avoid calcium channel blockers
Active Cooling Surface ice packs, body cavity lavage Cardiopulmonary bypass for severe cases Cease cooling when temperature decreases to 38°C
Correction of Hyperkalemia Glucose, insulin, bicarbonate, hyperventilation Calcium if hyperkalemia causes cardiac dysfunction
After Acute Episode, monitor for recrudescence of MH, disseminated intravascular coagulation (DIC), myoglobinuria

complex synthetic pathway leads to the accumulation of porphyrin precursors that have toxic effects.

Porphyrias are classified by the major site of abnormal porphyrin accumulation (hepatic vs. erythropoietic) and by the specific enzymatic defect; functionally, they are divided into acute versus nonacute presentations (NICV 24-5 and Table 24-12).[78] Acute porphyrias are the most concerning because medications commonly administered in the perioperative setting may precipitate life-threatening reactions. These are: acute intermittent porphyria (AIP, most common), hereditary coproporphyria (HCP), variegate porphyria (VP), and ALA-dehydratase deficiency porphyria (ADP, the rarest). Erythropoietic porphyrias are not associated with drug-induced crises but manifest with skin photosensitivity and fragility, which may have significant implications when securing airway devices and during patient positioning.

When presenting as an acute porphyric crisis, it is difficult to identify a patient's specific disorder. Characteristic signs and symptoms of a porphyric crisis include parasympathetic and sympathetic nervous system dysfunction, severe abdominal pain, vomiting, anxiety, confusion, hypertension and tachycardia, and electrolyte abnormalities including hyponatremia, hypokalemia, and hypocalcemia. Both motor and sensory peripheral neuropathy may be present. Seizures and respiratory failure due to skeletal weakness may be life threatening (Table 24-13).[79] Conditions known to exacerbate or trigger acute crises include fever, prolonged fasting, physiologic or psychological stress, infections, and pregnancy.

Management of Anesthesia

Safe anesthetic management for patients with porphyria includes identifying susceptible individuals and avoiding potentially porphyrinogenic medications. Identification of an acute crisis, if it occurs, is also critical. Timely laboratory identification is often not practical, and only the presence of a strong

Table 24-11 Safe versus Unsafe Drugs in Malignant Hyperthermia

Safe Drugs	Unsafe Drugs
Antibiotics	Halothane
Antihistamines	Isoflurane
Barbiturates	Enflurane
Benzodiazepines	Sevoflurane
Dexmedetomidine	Desflurane
Droperidol	Succinylcholine
Ketamine	
Local anesthetics	
Nitrous oxide	
Nondepolarizing muscle relaxants	
Opioids	
Propofol	
Propranolol	
Vasoactive drugs	

Table 24-12 Classification of Porphyrias

Acute Porphyrias
Acute intermittent porphyria (AIP)
Hereditary coprophyria (HCP)
Variegate porphyria (VP)
ALA dehydratase deficiency porphyria (ADP)
Nonacute Porphyrias
Porphyria cutanea tarda (PCT)
Familial
Acquired
Erythropoietic
Uroporphyria
Protoporphyria

From Moore et al.[78]

family history typically triggers the search for a definitive diagnosis. Patients with AIP will exhibit increased δ-aminolevulinic acid (ALA) levels, increased urine porphyrin levels, normal or slightly increased plasma porphyrin, and fecal porphyrin levels. Erythrocyte porphobilinogen deaminase levels will decrease by about 50%.

Identification of drugs safe for a patient with porphyria is not straightforward, given that case reports of reactions may be based on anecdotal events and the presence of multiple confounding factors such as duration of exposure, concomitant illness, and absolute dose of a potentially triggering agent. In general, opioids, propofol, volatile anesthetics, and neuromuscular-blocking drugs are considered safe. Regional anesthesia with local anesthetics may be performed, though caution is warranted in the presence of neuropathy. Etomidate, ketamine, and thiopental are to be avoided, as are certain anticonvulsants. The American Porphyria Foundation maintains an up-to-date database that can be consulted and help identify any potential medications that should be avoided: (https://porphyriafoundation.org/drugdatabase/drug-safety-database-search/).

Optimal perioperative care includes aggressively treating pain, nausea, vomiting, dehydration, active infections, as well as anxiety. Treatment of an acute crisis should focus on supportive measures to ensure hemodynamic stability and adequate oxygenation and ventilation. Intravenous heme arginate therapy, which suppresses hepatic production of porphyrin precursors, may facilitate recovery.[80]

Cholinesterase Disorders

Pseudocholinesterase (PCE, also called plasma cholinesterase or butyrylcholinesterase) is an enzyme synthesized in the liver that facilitates hydrolysis of choline esters, which include succinylcholine, mivacurium, and the ester local anesthetics procaine, chloroprocaine, tetracaine, and cocaine (NICV 24-6). PCE deficiency results in delayed metabolism of these drugs; total absence of PCE is still compatible with life, and the diagnosis might not be evident unless the patient requires an anesthetic. The most significant anesthetic implication is prolonged apnea after succinylcholine or mivacurium administration. The molecular genetics of cholinesterase inheritance is complex and over 50 variants have been described.[81] Some variants produce cholinesterase with very little activity and succinylcholine-induced paralysis may last for up to 8 hours; in others, the variant may result in only a negligible increase in duration of NMB. A few genetic variants produce a cholinesterase that accelerates the hydrolysis of succinylcholine, shortening the duration of succinylcholine-induced muscle paralysis.

PCE deficiency can be both acquired and inherited. Acquired deficiencies of cholinesterase are associated with pregnancy, hepatic disease, and renal failure. Drugs known to decrease cholinesterase activity include but are not limited to cholinesterase inhibitors such as neostigmine and pyridostigmine, echothiophate, monoamine oxidase inhibitors (phenelzine), cyclophosphamides, esmolol, glucocorticoids, and oral contraceptives agents.[82]

Genetically, mutations in the cholinesterase gene can affect one or both alleles. Heterozygous patients with one abnormal gene may have a slightly prolonged block following succinylcholine administration, while homozygous individuals will experience a more prolonged blockade. The dibucaine-resistant variant, which produces an enzyme with 1/100 of normal affinity for succinylcholine, is the most common of the abnormal alleles.

Dibucaine, a local anesthetic, inhibits normal PCE activity by 80% but inhibits atypical enzyme activity by only 20% (Table 24-14). Laboratory tests utilize this property to help diagnose and qualitatively characterize PCE deficiency. The "dibucaine number" reflects the percentage inhibition of PCE under standardized conditions and temperature. A patient with normal PCE has a dibucaine number of 70 to 80, a homozygote for the most common abnormal allele will have a dibucaine number below 30, and a heterozygote will have a dibucaine number ranging from 40 to 60. A quantitative diagnosis can be made using electrophoretic measurement of PCE concentrations in a patient's plasma.

Management of Anesthesia

Preoperative knowledge of a plasma cholinesterase abnormality allows the anesthesiologist to avoid the use of drugs that are hydrolyzed by cholinesterase, and the course of anesthesia will be uneventful. However, the diagnosis is often unknown prior to surgery. In these cases, the usual clinical presentation is prolonged apnea after succinylcholine administration. Apnea can be very prolonged if additional succinylcholine is administered after tracheal intubation, or a nondepolarizing muscle relaxant is given followed by reversal with neostigmine. A prudent clinical practice is to be certain that recovery from the initial dose of succinylcholine has occurred before administering more muscle relaxant. Mechanical ventilation and adequate sedation should be continued until full recovery of neuromuscular function is assured.

If prolonged apnea after succinylcholine administration occurs, laboratory testing for DN and fluoride number (FN—a confirmatory test also decreased in the setting of cholinesterase deficiency) should be performed after the patient has fully recovered.

Glycogen Storage Diseases

The glycogen storage diseases (GSD) are inherited disorders caused 7
by abnormal enzymes that regulate glycogen synthesis and breakdown (Fig. 24-5).[83,96] These diseases have various manifestations and organ involvement (Table 24-15). There are, however, three common critical components: (1) acidosis related to fat and protein metabolism in metabolically active glycogen stores; (2) increased risk of hypoglycemia due to failure to metabolize glycogen to glucose; and (3) cardiac and hepatic dysfunction secondary to destruction and replacement of normal tissue by accumulated glycogen.

Many of the enzymes involved in glycogen metabolism have different isoforms controlled by several different genes. The clinical features vary markedly within each type of GSD.

Table 24-13 Presentation of an Acute Crisis of Acute Porphyria

Symptoms/Signs	Features	Misdiagnosed as:
Abdominal Pain	Recurrent, severe, poorly localized Assoc. nausea/vomiting Absence of fever or Leucocytosis	Other cause of acute abdomen Endometriosis Pelvic inflammatory disease Irritable bowel syndrome
Cardiovascular	Tachycardia Tachydysrhytmias Hypertension	Opioid addiction
Weakness	Proximal > distal Upper limbs > lower Up to 20% develop respiratory failure May progress to bulbar paresis in severe cases	Guillain–Barré syndrome Poliomyelitis Acute lead poisoning Vasculitis
Psychiatric features	Mood disturbance Confusion Psychosis	Anxiety disorder Somatization disorder Acute psychosis Acute confusional state
Pain and sensory disturbance	Back, thigh, or extremity pain Sensory neuropathy over the trunk	Chronic fatigue syndrome pain Fibromyalgia Chronic pain syndrome
Seizures	CNS manifestation of porphyria Secondary to hyponatremia	Epilepsy
Other autonomic features	Constipation Gastroparesis Postural hypotension	
Cutaneous lesions	Only in VP and HCP Vesicular rash Photosensitivity	Porphyria cutanea tarda Bullous skin disease
Hyponatremia and other electrolyte disturbance	Low serum sodium Low serum magnesium	Other disorders of sodium and water balance

AIP, acute intermittent porphyria; VP, variegate porphyria; HCP, hereditary coproporphyria.

Adapted with permission from Findley H, Philip A, Cole D, et al. Porphyrias: implications for anaesthesia, critical care, and pain medicine. *Anaesth Crit Care Pain Med*. 2012;12(3):128–133.

Management of Anesthesia

Type I (Von Gierke Disease; Glucose-6-phosphatase Deficiency)

Von Gierke disease is inherited as an autosomal recessive trait. Many patients survive to adulthood. Short stature and hepatomegaly are characteristic. Hypoglycemia, acidosis, and seizures are common. Prolonged bleeding due to platelet dysfunction has been described. These patients do not tolerate fasting and should have preoperative intravenous glucose-containing fluid therapy during any NPO periods. Preoperative hyperalimentation is often used to increase liver glycogen stores. Anesthesia and surgery cause a release of counterregulatory hormones (epinephrine, norepinephrine) that can result in severe lactic acidosis. Cardiac dysrhythmias and cardiac arrest have occurred during anesthesia when acidosis develops. Preoperative intravenous glucose should be administered at 1.5 times the estimated hepatic production rate of glucose. This will reduce insulin secretion and minimize the effects of the stress response. If acidosis develops, a continuous infusion of bicarbonate should be administered. Portocaval shunting has been performed with limited success in patients with hepatic cirrhosis.

Type II (Pompe Disease; Lysosomal Acid Glucosidase Deficiency)

The infantile form of Pompe disease is a devastating disease with a very poor prognosis. There is a deficiency of lysosomal acid glucosidase with an accumulation of glycogen in heart, liver, muscle, and CNS.[84] Infants present with generalized weakness, hypotonia, and massive cardiomegaly. Glycogen infiltration of cardiac muscle leads to concentric hypertrophic cardiomyopathy.[85] These patients are prone to tachydysrhythmias.[86] Enzyme replacement therapy (ERT), if started by 9 months of age, can decrease cardiac glycogen accumulation. Late-onset Pompe disease has a milder clinical course.[87] The late-onset form is characterized by a slow progressive myopathy culminating in respiratory failure. Preoperative evaluation should include an ECG, echocardiogram, and

Table 24-14 Classic Cholinesterase Genotypes

Genotype	Cholinesterase Activity	Dibucaine Number	Succinylcholine Apnea (min)
Normal (EuEu)	++++	78–86	5
Heterozygote (EuEa)	++	51–70	15
Homozygote (EaEa)	+	18–26	120–300

liver function tests. There are a significant number of reported cases of cardiac arrest during anesthesia in patients with the infantile form of Pompe disease, and mortality is high.[88] Induction of anesthesia with sevoflurane or high-dose propofol is more likely to result in adverse cardiac events, especially in patients with a left ventricular mass index >350 g/m^2. A preoperative echocardiogram is highly recommended. If feasible, surgery should be performed with local or regional anesthesia. If general anesthesia is required, a carefully monitored induction with ketamine is recommended.

Type III (Forbes or Cori Disease)

Type III GSD is due to a deficiency of amylo-1,6-glucosidase (glycogen debrancher). Symptoms result from defective catabolism of glycogen and excessive glycogen deposition in the liver. Hepatomegaly and short stature are common. Mild hyperlipidemia and elevated serum transaminase concentrations are characteristic. Fasting induces ketotic hypoglycemia. Cirrhosis develops in the third and fourth decades of life. The enzyme deficiency in skeletal and cardiac muscle leads to weakness and cardiomyopathy. There are subgroups based on skeletal muscle involvement. Anesthetic concerns include macroglossia, hypotonia, sensitivity to nondepolarizing muscle relaxants, hypertrophic cardiomyopathy, and tachydysrhythmias. Hypoglycemia is a particular risk as it may occur within 4 to 6 hours of fasting. Continuous administration of intravenous glucose should be performed in the preoperative period. Metabolic ketoacidosis may occur, even with careful management of anesthesia. Administration of lactate-containing intravenous fluids is generally avoided. Succinylcholine should also be avoided because of the potential for rhabdomyolysis. Postoperative respiratory complications may occur due to respiratory muscle weakness, ineffective cough, poor clearance of secretions, and residual effects of anesthetics.[89,90]

Type IV (Andersen Disease, Amylopectinosis)

Andersen disease is a very rare disorder caused by a deficiency of glycogen-branching enzyme (GBE). This leads to an accumulation of glycogen in liver, muscle, nerves, and cardiac muscle. Clinical manifestations are diverse depending on the affected tissues.[91] The severest form of the disease presents in infancy with hepatosplenomegaly, failure to thrive, and hypotonia. Esophageal varices, portal hypertension, and cirrhosis are common by two years of age. Muscle weakness with exercise intolerance and exertional dyspnea occur. Cardiac effects include dilated cardiomyopathy and congestive heart failure. The only effective treatment is liver transplantation. A neuromuscular variant presents in adults with sensory loss in the legs, gait disturbances, difficulty with urination, and cognitive dysfunction.

Type V (McArdle Disease)

McArdle disease is an autosomal recessive disorder due to a deficiency of glycogen phosphorylase in muscle. Skeletal muscle is

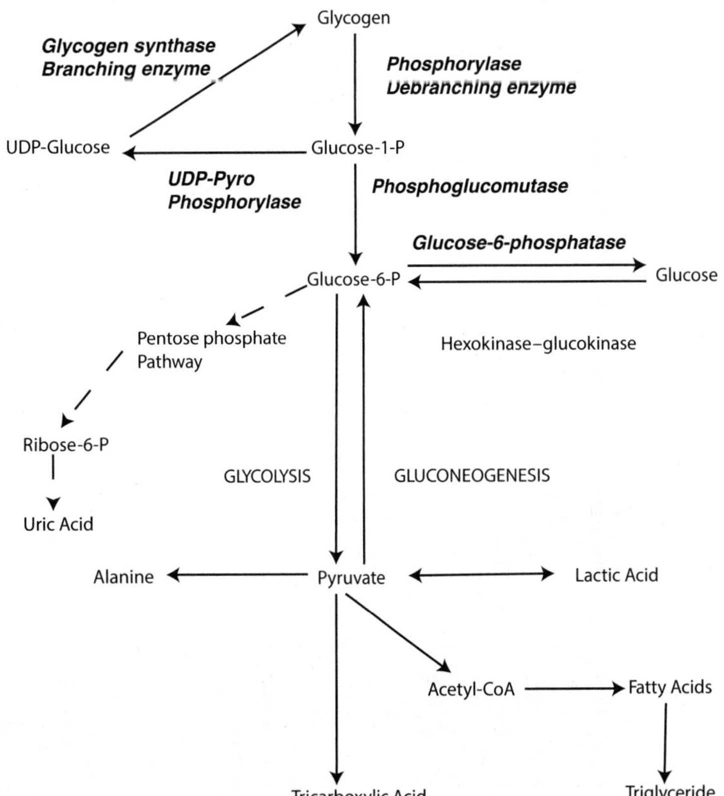

Figure 24-5 Simplified pathway of glycogen synthesis and degradation. (Adapted from Ozen H. Glycogen storage diseases: new perspectives. *World J Gastroenterol.* 2007;13: 2541–2553.)

Table 24-15 Classification of Glycogen Storage Diseases

(Type) MPS Eponym	Prevalence	Enzyme Defect	Main Clinical Features	Laboratory Abnormalities	Progressive Skeletal Muscle Deformities	Progressive Cardiac Involvement
Type I Von Gierke	1:200,000	Glucose-6-phophatase	Short stature, hepatomegaly, hepatic adenomas, seizures, dev. delay, failure to thrive, vomiting, xanthomata, nephromegaly, osteoporosis, inflammatory bowel disease	Symptomatic hypoglycemia, lactic acidosis, elevated triglycerides, platelet dysfunction, elevated uric acid, glucosuria, high urinary calcium	Muscle cramping, exercise intolerance	Severe cardiac arrhythmias, sudden death with fasting
Type II Pompe Early Onset	1:400,000	Lysosomal acid glucosidase (acid maltase)	Growth delay, devel. delay, hepatomegaly, macroglossia, progressive hypotonia death <1 yr of age	Markedly elevated creatinine kinase (CK) elevated AST, ALT, LDH	Progressive cardiac, respiratory, skeletal muscle weakness	Massive cardiomegaly, concentric LV hypertrophy, outflow tract obstruction, cardiomyopathy, CHF, SVT, VT, VF, ***Cardioresp. Arrest with Anesthesia***
Type II Pompe Late Onset	1:400,000	Lysosomal acid Glucosidase (acid maltase)	Onset 2nd–7th decade of life, progressive respiratory failure	Markedly elevated creatinine kinase CK I Elevated AST, ALT, LDH	Slow progressive myopathy	None
Type IIIa1 Forbes Cori	1:400,000	Amylo-1,6-glucosidase (glycogen debrancher)	Childhood-onset Muscle weakness, hepatic dysfunction	Fasting hypoglycemia Mild to moderate elevation of hepatic enzymes (ALT, AST) Elevation of creatinine kinase (CK), hyperlipidemia	Slowly progressive muscle weakness, gross motor delay	Concentric LV hypertrophy, rare cardiac dysfunction or arrhythmias
Type IIIa2 Forbes	1:400,000	Amylo-1, 6-glucosidase (glycogen debrancher)	Hepatic dysfunction onset in childhood persistence in adulthood and adult onset of muscle weakness	Fasting hypoglycemia, mild to moderate elevation of hepatic enzymes (ALT, AST) Elevation of creatinine kinase (CK), hyperlipidemia	Slowly progressive muscle weakness, gross motor delay	Concentric LV hypertrophy, rare cardiac dysfunction or arrhythmias
Type IIIa Forbes	1:400,000	Amylo-1, 6-glucosidase (glycogen debrancher)	Hepatic dysfunction onset in childhood & resolution in adulthood and adult-onset muscle weakness	Fasting hypoglycemia, mild to moderate elevation of hepatic enzymes (ALT, AST) Elevation of creatinine kinase (CK), hyperlipidemia	Slowly progressive muscle weakness, gross motor delay	Concentric LV hypertrophy, rare cardiac dysfunction or arrhythmias
Type IIIa Forbes	1:400,000	Amylo-1, 6-glucosidase (glycogen debrancher)	Adult-onset skeletal muscle symptoms	Fasting hypoglycemia mild to moderate elevation of hepatic enzymes (ALT, AST) Elevation of creatinine kinase (CK), hyperlipidemia	Slowly progressive muscle weakness, gross motor delay	Concentric LV hypertrophy, rare cardiac dysfunction or arrhythmias

Type IIIb Forbes	1:400,000	Amylo-1, 6-glucosidase (glycogen debrancher)	Hepatic dysfunction	Fasting hypoglycemia Mild to moderate elevation of hepatic enzymes (ALT, AST) Elevation of creatinine kinase (CK), hyperlipidemia	None	Rare cardiac dysfunction or arrhythmias
Type IV Andersen	1:1,000,000	Glycogen branching enzyme	Failure to thrive, hepatosplenomegaly, hypotonia, esophageal varices, portal hypertension. late hepatic cirrhosis/failure, neuropathy	Elevated creatinine kinase (CK), moderate elevation of hepatic enzymes (AST, ALT)	Two forms: ***stable* or *progressive*** myopathy, muscle weakness, exercise intolerance, exertional dyspnea, neuronal involvement	Dilated cardiomyopathy, CHF
Type V McArdle	1:100,000	Muscle glycogen phosphorylase	Muscle glycogenoses, exercise intolerance, NO hepatic involvement	Episodic myoglobinuria	Muscle cramps	None
Type VI Hers	Very rare	Hepatic glycogen phosphorylase	Mild symptomatology, short stature, hepatomegaly	Fasting Ketotic hypoglycemia, mild hyperlipdemia, myoglobinuria, increased AST, ALT Rarely proximal renal tubular acidosis	Hypotonia, muscle cramps	Usually none, rare cardiac failure with enzyme variant
Type VII Tarui	Very rare	Muscle phosphofructo-kinase	Muscle glycogenoses, exercise intolerance, NO hepatic involvement	Episodic myoglobinuria, hemolytic anemia	Muscle cramps	None
Type IX	Very rare	Glycogen phosphorylase kinase	Mild symptomatology, short stature, hepatomegaly X-linked variant	Fasting ketotic hypoglycemia, mild hyperlipidemia, myoglobinuria, increased AST, ALT Rarely proximal renal tubular acidosis	Hypotonia, muscle cramps	Usually none, rare cardiac failure with enzyme variant
Type XI Fanconi–Bickel	Very rare	Glucose transporter	Hepatic glycogenosis, Fanconi renal syndrome	Short stature, hepatic glycogenosis, Fanconi renal syndrome	None	None
Type 0	Unknown	Hepatic glycogen synthase	Short stature developmental delay (22%) seizures	Postprandial hyperglycemia and hyperlactatemia, recurring ketotic hypoglycemia, metabolic acidosis, fasting ketonuria	NO skeletal muscle involvement	None

Adapted from: Weinstein DA, Wolfsdorf JI. Glycogen storages diseases: a primer for clinicians. *Endocrin*. 2002;12:531–538.

Ozen H. Glycogen storage diseases: new Perspectives. *World J Gatroenterol*. 2007;13:2541–2533.

Chen M. Glycogen storage diseases. In: Monga SPS, ed. *Molecular Pathology of Liver Diseases*. Springer; 2011:677–681.

Santer R, Schneppenheim R, Suter D, Schaub J, Steinmann J. Fanconi-Bickell syndrome – the original patient and his natural history, historical steps leading to the primary defect, and a review of the literature. *Eur J Pediatr*. 1998;157:783–797.

unable to mobilize glycogen stores for sustained exercise and cramping with exercise is characteristic of this disorder. GSD Type V is a multisystem disease that presents in adolescence with progressive muscle weakness, myalgia, and lack of endurance. Episodes of myoglobinuria with overexertion are due to rhabdomyolysis and may also occur after administration of succinylcholine. Acute renal failure with rhabdomyolysis has been reported after cardiac surgery.[92] Tourniquets should not be employed, and frequent automated measurements of blood pressure should be performed with caution. Whether patients with McArdle disease are susceptible to MH is controversial. Dantrolene may, however, have a beneficial effect on non-MH rhabdomyolysis, should it occur. Cardiac muscle is typically not affected in patients with McArdle disease.

Type VI (Hers Disease)

Hers disease relatively benign disorder is caused by deficiency of a regulatory enzyme that controls hepatic glycogen phosphorylase. Symptoms include hepatomegaly, mild hypoglycemia, hyperlipidemia, and ketosis. A mild cardiomyopathy may develop with aging.[93] Symptoms usually improve with age. Fever and acidosis after an anesthetic with ketamine, halothane, and succinylcholine have been reported. Liver transplantation has been performed in patients with more severe forms of Hers disease.

Type VII (Tarui Disease)

Tarui disease is caused by a deficiency of muscle phosphofructokinase. This condition is comparable to McArdle disease and is characterized by muscle cramping. Patients with Tarui disease present with exercise intolerance and episodic myoglobinuria. There is usually no cardiac or hepatic involvement. The same enzyme defect in erythrocytes causes chronic hemolytic anemia. There are four forms of the disease: classic, late-onset, infantile (usually fatal), and hemolytic.[94]

Type IX

GSD type IX is caused by a deficiency of hepatic glycogen phosphorylase kinase and is clinically similar to Hers disease (type VI). There are several isoforms of the enzyme controlled by many genes. The clinical presentation can be very heterogeneous. Most patients have short stature, hypotonia, muscle cramps, exertional myoglobinuria, and hyperlipidemia.

Type XI (Fanconi–Bickel Syndrome)

Fanconi–Bickel syndrome is a rare autosomal recessive disorder caused by mutations of the glucose-transporting enzyme (Glut-2). These patients have short stature, hepatomegaly, glucose and galactose intolerance, fasting hypoglycemia, and a characteristic proximal renal tubular acidosis. They usually survive to adulthood.[95]

Type 0

Type 0 GSD is caused by a deficiency of the hepatic form of glycogen synthase that causes a decrease in liver glycogen. Consequently, hepatomegaly does not occur. Clinical features include fasting ketotic hypoglycemia, short status, and osteopenia. Many patients are asymptomatic and the disease is often diagnosed by the unsuspected discovery of hypoglycemia. As preoperative fasting may cause hypoglycemia, intravenous administration of glucose-containing solution may be necessary.

Mucopolysaccharidoses

The mucopolysaccharidoses (MPS) are rare familial diseases inherited as autosomal recessive disorders. The disorders are a result of a deficiency of a specific lysosomal enzyme that cleaves mucopolysaccharides. The result is an accumulation of mucopolysaccharides in the brain, heart, bone, liver, cornea, and tracheobronchial tree.[97]

There are eight types of MPS and several subtypes (Table 24-16). All forms of MPS are characterized by progressive craniofacial deformities, joint and skeletal anomalies, cardiac involvement, and early death from pulmonary infection or cardiac failure. The upper airway is characterized by a depressed nasal bridge, short neck, macroglossia, and tongue protrusion secondary to infiltration of mucopolysaccharides. Chronic rhinitis enlarged tonsils and adenoids, and obstructive sleep apnea are typical. Clinical phenotypes within each MPS type range from severe to attenuated variants with longer life expectancy.

Hunter and Hurler syndromes are the best known of the MPS diseases. Respiratory infection and cardiac disease (valvular and ischemic) lead to death at an early age. MPS type IV (Morquio syndrome) is associated with the most significant skeletal deformities. Respiratory insufficiency with marked chest wall deformity is common. Severe dysplasia or absence of the odontoid process frequently leads to chronic or acute myelopathy. Neurologic manifestations such as developmental delay and hydrocephalus are due to MPS depositions in the CNS. Cardiac involvement occurs in most forms of MPS except the San Filippo variants (Type III). MPS infiltration of the myocardium, cardiac valves, and conducting system often lead to myocardial ischemia, cardiomyopathy, and dysrhythmias.

Patients with MPS have coarse facial features (gargoylism), lumbar lordosis, stiff joints, chest deformities, small stature, corneal opacities, hepatomegaly, and splenomegaly. The diagnosis of MPS is based on detection of urinary glycosaminoglycans and measurement of enzyme activity in the serum, leukocytes, and fibroblasts. No definitive therapy exists for MPS. Depending on the specific enzyme defect, however, ERT may lessen the effects of the disease. ERT, however, does little to ameliorate the cardiac or neurologic effects of MPS.[98] The role of human stem cell transplantation (HSCT) for the treatment of MPS is controversial.

Management of Anesthesia

MPS patients have significant deformities of the upper airway and cardiorespiratory dysfunction, and the risks of perioperative management must not be underestimated. The variability of clinical abnormalities in patients with MPS requires individualized planning for each patient. Some types of MPS produce severe airway and cardiac effects, while other types have only mild dysfunction.

Airway management can be extremely challenging. Several 8
tools for airway management, including oropharyngeal airways, supraglottic airways, video laryngoscopes, and flexible fiberscopes should be readily available prior to induction of anesthesia. Careful positioning of the head and neck is required to minimize the risk of spinal cord damage. A slow, controlled inhalation induction with sevoflurane in oxygen is preferred. Mask ventilation, however, can become difficult and a supraglottic airway may be helpful during induction. Laryngoscopy is complicated by thick, noncompressible tissue of the upper airway, macroglossia, copious airway secretions, and bony deformities of the head and neck. Muscle relaxants should be avoided until the airway has been secured.[99,100] Postoperative respiratory complications are common.[101]

Careful preoperative evaluation with echocardiography is indicated for some types of MPS (e.g., Hurler syndrome). The presence of cardiac dysfunction will certainly influence the type of anesthesia and intraoperative monitoring.

Table 24-16 Mucopolysaccharidoses

(Type) MPS Eponym	Main Clinical Features	Prevalence	Enzyme Defect	Urinary Mucopolysaccharides	Progressive Cranio-Facial Deformities	Progressive Joint/ Skeletal Deformities	Progressive Cardiac Involvement
Type I (H) Hurler	Severe Hurler phenotype, mental retardation, corneal clouding, death <14 yrs	1:100,000	α–L-Idronidase	Dermatan sulfate Heparan sulfate	Macrocephaly coarse facies macroglossia hydrocephalus	Stiff Joints thoraco-lumbar kyphosis possible odontoid hypoplasia, short neck, short stature	Coronary intimal & valvular thickening mitral regurgitation cardiomegaly
Type I (S) Scheie	Corneal clouding, NL intelligence survival to adulthood	1:500,000	α-L-Idronidase	Dermatan sulfate	Mild to coarse facies mac-roglossia prognathia	Short neck normal stature	Aortic regurgitation
Type I (H/S) Hurler–Scheie	Intermediate phenotype	1:111,000	α-L-Idronidase	Dermatan sulfate Heparan sulfate	Macrocephaly coarse facies macroglossia micrognathia	Diffuse joint limitation short neck short stature	Mitral & aortic val-vular thickening/ regurgitation
Type II Hunter	Variable course severe to mild, survival to adulthood, w or w/o mental retardation	1:162,000	Iduronidate-2-sulfatase	Dermatan sulfate	Macrocephaly coarse facies hydrocephalus	Diffuse joint limitation short neck short stature	Coronary intimal thickening Ischemic cardio-myopathy
Type III A San Filippo	Behavioral problems, aggression	1:114,000	Heparan-*N*-sulfatasee	Heparan sulfate	Mild coarse facies	Mild stiff joints, lum-bar vertebral dys-plasia short stature	Minimal to none
Type III B San Filippo	Progressive dementia, seizures, survival: 2nd to 3rd decade	1:211,000	α-*N*-acetyl-glucose-am dase	Heparan sulfate	Mild coarse facies	Stiff joints that may not extend fully, ambulation difficulties	Minimal to none
Type III C San Filippo	Intrafamilial variability mild dysmorphism	1:1,407,000	α-*N*-acetyl-glucose-amidase, *N*-acetyltransferase	Heparan sulfate	Mild coarse facies	Stiff joints that may not extend fully, walking difficulty	Minimal to none
Type III D San Filippo	Coarse hair clear cornea NL height	1:1,056,000	*N*-acetyl-glucose-amine-6-su fatase	Heparan sulfate	Mild coarse facies	Stiff joints that may not extend fully walking problems	Minimal to none

(continued)

Table 24-16 Mucopolysaccharidoses (CONTINUED)

(Type) MPS Eponym	Main Clinical Features	Prevalence	Enzyme Defect	Urinary Mucopolysaccharides	Progressive Cranio-Facial Deformities	Progressive Joint/ Skeletal Deformities	Progressive Cardiac Involvement
Type IV A Morquio	Short trunk type of dwarfism, fine corneal opacities, skeletal dysplasia spondyl-epiphyseal dysplasia, final height <125 cm	1:1201,000	*N*-acetyl-Galactos-amine-6-sulfatase	Keratan sulfate	Mild coarse facies	Joint laxity severe kyphoscoliosis odontoid hypo-plasia short neck C1–C2 subluxation possible short stature	Aortic regurgitation
Type IV B Morquio	Same as MPS IV A but milder adult height >120 cm	1:248,000	β Galactosidase	Keratan sulfate	Mild to coarse facies	Joint laxity severe kypho-scoliosis, odontoid hypo-plasia short neck C1–C2 subluxation possible short stature	Aortic regurgitation
Type VI Maroteaux–Lamy	Hurler phenotype with marked corneal clouding, normal intelligence	1:100,000	*N*-acetyl-galactos-amine-4-sulfatase	Dermatan sulfate	Macrocephaly, coarse facies, macroglossia	Mild joint stiffness kyphoscoliosis odontoid hypopla-sia short stature	Mitral & aortic val-vular thickening/ regurgitation
Type VII Sly	Highly variable, dense inclusions in granulocytes	1:2,111,000	β–Glucuron-idase	Dermatan sulfate	Macrocephaly, coarse facies	Mild joint stiffness kyphoscoliosis odontoid hypopla-sia short stature	Mitral & aortic val-vular thickening/ regurgitation aortic dissection

Adapted from Diaz JH, Belani KG. Perioperative management of children with mucopolysaccharidoses. *Anesth Analg*. 1993;77:1261–1270; Yeung AH, Cowan MJ, Horn B, et al. Airway management in children with mucopolysaccharidoses. *Arch Oto*. 2009;135:73–79; and Meikle PJ, Hopwood JJ, Clague AE, et al. Prevalence of lysosomal storage diseases. *JAMA*. 2011;281:249–254.

Table 24-17 Anesthetic Considerations in Osteogenesis Imperfecta

Type	Clinical Severity	Inheritance	Mutant Gene	Manifestations	Anesthetic Considerations	Lifespan
I	Mild, nondeforming	Autosomal dominant	Col1A/2	Increased frequency of fractures; short stature; blue sclera; progressive hearing impairment	A: Normal dentition B: Dentinogenesis imperfecta	Long-term survival[a]
II	Perinatally lethal	Autosomal dominant	COL1A/2	Multiple fractures in utero; micromelia; bowed LEs; small thorax; respiratory failure	Death in utero or within first month of life	
III	Progressively deforming	Autosomal dominant	COL1A/2	Growth retardation; multiple fractures; progressive kyphoscoliosis; vertebral compression; blue sclera; dentinogenesis imperfecta	Airway anomalies	Death in second to fourth decade
IV	Moderately deforming	Autosomal dominant	COL1A/2	In utero fractures; fractures with minor trauma; LE bowing with weight bearing	A: Normal dentition B: Dentinogenesis imperfecta; midface or mandibular deformity	Long-term survival[a]
V	Moderately deforming	Autosomal dominant	Unknown	In utero fractures; fractures with minor trauma; LE bowing with weight bearing	Potential for midface or mandibular deformity	Long-term survival[a]
VI	Moderately to severely deforming	Autosomal recessive	Unknown	In utero fractures; fractures with minor trauma; bowing of LEs with weight bearing	Potential for midface or mandibular deformity	Long-term survival[a]

[a]With appropriate medical care.
LEs, lower extremities.
Adapted from Van Dijk FS, Pals G, Van Rijn RR, et al. Classification of osteogenesis imperfecta revisited. *Eur J Med Genet*. 2010;53(1):1–5. Copyright © 2010 Elsevier. With permission; and from Stynnowick GA, Tobias JD. Perioperative care of the patient with osteogenesis imperfect. *Orthopedics*. 2007;30(12):1043–1049, with permission.

Osteogenesis Imperfecta

Osteogenesis imperfecta (OI) is a heterogeneous group of diseases characterized by susceptibility to bone fractures due to a defect in collagen type I. OI is classified into subtypes depending on its genetic, radiographic, and clinical manifestations (Table 24-17).[102]

The triple-helix molecule of type 1 collagen is composed of two α1 chains and one α2 chain, encoded by COL1A1 and COL1A2, respectively. In 85% of cases, OI is caused by mutations in one of these two genes that encode type I collagen.[103,104] Type I collagen is the primary component of the extracellular matrix of bone and skin. Inheritance is autosomal dominant for most forms (type VI, autosomal recessive) and the incidence is 1 in 20,000 to 50,000 live births. OI is a multisystem disease characterized by brittle bones, short stature, osteoporosis, joint laxity, tendon weakness, muscle weakness, cardiac anomalies, blue sclera, platelet dysfunction, abnormal airway anatomy, and abnormal dentition. Vertebral fractures occur in 70% of patients with OI.[105] Pectus deformities of the chest, kyphoscoliosis, and rib fractures may lead to restrictive pulmonary disease and respiratory failure.[106]

The most common cardiac lesion is aortic insufficiency. Aortic root dilation may lead to aortic dissection. Mitral valve prolapse and insufficiency can occur.[107] Central nervous manifestations include craniovertebral instability and atlantoaxial subluxation that can lead to quadriparesis. Hydrocephalus is common.

Treatment

Treatment should be based on clinical presentation and severity. The main goals of treatment are to prevent fractures and correct alignment. Multidisciplinary care should be provided including medical genetics, orthopedic surgery, physical therapy, and dentistry.

Pharmacologic management may include growth hormone, bisphosphonates, and denosumab, a monoclonal antibody that targets the receptor activator of nuclear factor kappa-B ligand, a cytokine that mediates osteoclastogenesis and osteoclast survival. Osteo-anabolic therapy (teriparatide-parathyroid hormone) is utilized to increase osteoblastic activity and bone formation. Sclerostin-inhibitory antibodies target sclerosin, a glycoprotein that inhabits bone formation via inhibition of the Wnt signaling pathway in osteoblasts.

Management of Anesthesia

Operative intervention in indicated in patients with long bone deformities, acute or recurrent fractures, progressive deformity, and pain. Surgery is often performed on patients with the most severe types of OI, types III and IV.[108] Patients with OI need to be positioned carefully, as minor trauma can cause fractures. The upper airway should be carefully examined and cervical range of motion evaluated. Megalocephaly and a short neck can make direct laryngoscopy difficult, and alternative intubation techniques should be available in the operating room. A preoperative echocardiogram may be beneficial if there is a history of valvular heart disease.

Induction of anesthesia can be performed with inhalation or intravenous techniques. Regional anesthesia is generally avoided because of the risk of trauma to the spine and the potential for coagulopathy due to platelet dysfunction. Caudal analgesia has been used in selected patients.[109] A recent report documents the successful use of ultrasound guided combined spinal/epidural anesthesia.[110] Another report describes a patient with severe OI successfully undergoing scoliosis surgery.[110]

Mild intraoperative temperature elevation can occur in patients with OI. There is no evidence that OI patients are at increased risk for MH.[111]

Anemias

Anemia is commonly defined as a blood hemoglobin level below 13.0 g/dL. Regardless of cause, preoperative anemia has been linked to poor outcomes in patients undergoing major surgery. Anesthetic management of a patient with anemia should include knowledge of the disease process behind the reduction in hemoglobin, how to optimize the patient for surgery if time allows, and how the disease process may affect choice of anesthetic type or medications. The most common anemias are listed in Table 24-18. Identification and treatment of preoperative anemia with the aim of avoiding the need for blood transfusion has become the target of several blood management programs (e.g., ERAS). Intraoperatively, patients with anemia may exhibit compensatory physiologic responses to anemia, including increased cardiac output, increased plasma volume, decreased blood viscosity, and increased levels of 2,3-diphosphoglycerate (Table 24-19).

Table 24-18 Types of Anemia

Types of Anemia
Nutritional Deficiency
Iron
Vitamin B12
Folate
Anemia of chronic illness
Hemolytic
Spherocytosis
Glucose-6-phosphate dehydrogenase deficiency
Pyruvate kinase deficiency
Immune-mediated
Drug-induced ABO incompatibility
Hemoglobinopathies
Hemoglobin S (Sickle cell)
Thalassemia major (Cooley anemia)
Thalassemia intermedia
Thalassemia minor

Table 24-19 Compensatory Mechanisms to Increase Oxygen Delivery with Chronic Anemia

Compensatory Mechanisms
Increased cardiac output
Increased RBC 2,3-diphophoglycerate
Increased P50
Increased plasma volume
Decreased blood viscosity

P50, oxygen tension at which hemoglobin is 50% saturated.

Nutritional Deficiency Anemias

Anemia can be caused by nutritional deficit or impaired absorption of iron, vitamin B12, or folate. Preoperative optimization of patients with these deficiencies may help reduce the need for intra- and/or postoperative transfusion.[112]

Iron Deficiency Anemia

Iron deficiency is the most common cause of anemia and can be caused by low nutritional intake of iron or chronic blood loss. Preoperative anemia has been found in up to one-third of patients undergoing major elective surgery, with two-thirds of those patients having an iron deficiency that may have benefited from preoperative iron supplementation.[112] Lab work in patients with iron deficiency anemia shows normal or low mean corpuscular volume (MCV) (microcytosis), low mean corpuscular hemoglobin (MCH) (hypochromia), and low reticulocyte count. Options for treatment of iron deficiency anemia include iron supplementation, which is available in oral and intravenous forms, and treatment of any ongoing blood loss.

Folate and Vitamin B12 Deficiency Anemia

Deficiencies of folate (vitamin B9) or vitamin B12 are the most common causes of megaloblastic anemia, which is a form of macrocytic anemia (high MCV). These vitamins play critical roles in cell division within the bone marrow; deficiencies lead to decreased maturation of red blood cells (RBCs).

Vitamin B12 deficiency can be caused by decreased nutritional intake, pernicious anemia (autoimmune inhibition of vitamin B12 uptake), or disruptions in its complex absorption and storage pathways. Conditions that affect these pathways include gastric and small bowel pathology, pancreatic insufficiency, and medications that block or impair absorption (e.g., metformin, proton pump inhibitors, histamine 2 receptor antagonists). Nitrous oxide blocks an important step in vitamin B12 metabolism, though short exposure during a routine anesthetic is unlikely to cause measurable effects in an otherwise healthy patient.[113]

Folate deficiency can be caused by severe nutritional deficits, malabsorption, medications (e.g., methotrexate, antibiotics, antiepileptics), and increased requirements, such as in pregnancy or chronic hemolytic disease. In resource-rich countries, nutritional folate deficiency is rate, as many foods are fortified with folate.

Clinical presentation of vitamin B12 and folate deficiencies are similar and include macrocytic anemia, jaundice, and neurologic abnormalities (more common with vitamin B12 deficiency).[114] Neurologic changes with vitamin B12 deficiency include cognitive slowing and neuropathy caused by spinal cord demyelination (which may be a relative contraindication to neuraxial and regional anesthesia). Supplements containing vitamin B12 and folic acid are widely available.

Anemia of Chronic Disease

While not specifically the result of a nutritional deficiency, anemia of chronic disease (ACD) is often discussed in tandem with nutritional anemias, as dysregulation of iron is part of its pathophysiology. ACD is the second most common cause of anemia after iron deficiency and has been associated with a variety of conditions including infections, malignancies, and autoimmune processes.[115] The pathophysiology of ACD is a decrease in circulating iron due to dysregulated storage, which in turn inhibits erythropoiesis.

Management of ACD is targeted at treating the underlying condition; iron supplementation is useful if a patient also has an underlying iron deficiency.

Hemolytic Anemias

Hemolysis is the premature destruction of RBCs before their typical lifespan of 120 days. Hemolytic anemia may occur through multiple pathways, including intravascular or extravascular destruction, antibody or complement activation, and direct cellular damage or overwhelming oxidative stress. Patients with hemolytic anemia may present with jaundice, dyspnea, tachycardia, and hypotension. Identifying the underlying cause is imperative in the perioperative period as each has a different management (see below).[116]

Hereditary Spherocytosis

Hereditary spherocytosis (HS) is a disease affecting RBC membranes and one of the congenital hemolytic anemias. Characteristic features of HS include anemia, jaundice, splenomegaly, and in most cases, a family history. The degree of splenomegaly is usually the predictor of the severity of anemia and hemolysis. Seventy percent of all HS patients have an autosomal dominant inheritance, while 15% have autosomal recessive inheritance. Moderate to severe disease usually presents in infancy with hyperbilirubinemia.

The human RBC membrane is composed of an outer lipid bilayer and an inner layer of cytoplasmic spectrin-based cytoskeleton. Five membrane proteins that are in proximity with each other anchor the cytoskeleton. These include: α-spectrin, β-spectrin, ankyrin, Band 3, and Protein 4.2.[117] The α- and β-spectrin proteins form the αβ helical heterodimer which surrounds 65% of the RBC membrane. Band 3 resides in the lipid bilayer as a trimer. Further, the Band 3-trimer and ankyrin form a tetramer complex that binds to the ab spectrin heterodimer, thus anchoring the bilayer to the cytoskeleton. Protein 4.2 solidifies the connection of Band 3 and ankyrin. Because of this complex arrangement, defects in any of these component proteins result in decreased RBC life and cellular fragility.[118]

Diagnosis is made based on physical examination, complete blood count, reticulocyte count, and various other specific tests. However, no single laboratory test identifies all forms of HS. Most hematologists will add tests such as the acidified glycerol lysis test (AGLT) and the eosin-5′-maleimide binding test (EMABT) to discern if the patient has HS. Finally, if the diagnosis is still uncertain, genetic testing may be employed. All these tests have only moderate sensitivity and specificity make definitive diagnosis difficult. Thus, HS is included in the differential diagnosis of thalassemia, autoimmune hemolytic anemia (AIHA), and Glucose-6-phosphate deficiency. An updated protocol for diagnosis of HS has been by Wu et al.[119] Complications of HS include cholelithiasis and aplastic crisis following parvovirus 19 infection.[120]

Splenectomy is the standard treatment for moderate and severe forms of HS. Indications include patients with recurrent hemolytic crises, significant splenomegaly, severe aplastic crisis, cholelithiasis, and developmental delay. Splenomegaly should be accompanied by cholecystectomy in patients with symptomatic cholelithiasis with ultrasound-diagnosed presence of gall stones.

Although splenomegaly is effective at reducing hemolysis, splenectomy exposes patients to life-long risk of overwhelming postsplenectomy infection (OPSI) from encapsulated organisms, *Streptococcus pneumoniae, Haemophilus influenzae, and Neisseria meningitides*. This risk occurs despite immunizations against encapsulated bacteria and postoperative antibiotic prophylaxis. Thus, the risk is *never* eliminated. In addition, splenectomy does not correct the cytoskeletal defects of HS. RBCs are still spheroidal in shape with a disorganized membrane ultrastructure. They are also larger than normal RBC's.

Laparoscopic splenectomy, although technically difficult, is the method of choice for splenectomy. Due to the lifelong sepsis risk, many centers now advocate a partial splenectomy leaving about 15% of the spleen behind to carry out its vital immunologic and phagocytic functions. Partial splenectomy, particularly in pediatric patients, has been shown to retain splenic immunologic function, while decreasing hemolysis.

Management of Anesthesia

Anesthetic management of the patient with HS requires use of all routine physiologic monitors and careful postoperative pain management planning. Although controversial, it may also be wise to have packed RBCs in the ready for significant hemorrhage during surgery. Regional anesthesia is recommended to facilitate postoperative pain relief and reduce length of hospital stay.

Glucose-6-Phosphate Dehydrogenase Deficiency

Glucose-6-phosphate dehydrogenase (G6PD) is an enzyme involved in NADPH production, which provides reducing power and therefore a defense against oxidative damage (NICV 24-7).[121] G6PD deficiency, the most common human enzyme defect, therefore, causes a decrease in cells' ability to tolerate oxidative stress. As RBCs contain no mitochondria, they are particularly susceptible to deficiencies in NADPH production. Patients with G6PD deficiency are often asymptomatic until an episode of acute hemolytic anemia is triggered by an increase in oxidative stress; this can be brought about by medications (listed in Table 24-20), infection, or ingestion of fava beans.

Anesthetic management in patients with G6PD deficiency centers around avoidance of triggering medications. In patients with unexplained acute hemolysis in the setting of a known trigger, G6PD deficiency should be considered. Treatment of the acute hemolytic event is supportive with blood transfusion if necessary.

Pyruvate Kinase Deficiency

Pyruvate kinase is an enzyme that catalyzes a key step in glycolysis, which generates adenosine triphosphate (ATP) in RBCs.[122] Patients with pyruvate kinase deficiency may exhibit hemolytic anemia, splenomegaly, jaundice, and gallstones. Iron overload with or without blood transfusion may occur, and splenectomy is often performed. Anesthetic care should focus on the degree of anemia as well as potential comorbidities including osteopenia, endocrinopathies, and pulmonary hypertension.

Immune Hemolytic Anemias

AIHA, drug-induced immune hemolytic anemia, and hemolytic transfusion reactions are often discussed together under the category of immune hemolytic anemias. While the triggers differ, the pathophysiology of immune hemolytic anemia involves

Table 24-20 Drugs That Can Produce Hemolysis in Patients with Glucose-6-Phosphate Dehydrogenase Deficiency

Aspirin (high doses)
Chloramphenicol
Dapsone
Doxorubicin
Furazolidone
Isoniazid
Methylene blue
Nalidixic acid
Naphthalene
Niridazole
Nitrofurantoin
Penicillin
Phenacetin
Phenazopyridine
Primaquine
Quinidine
Quinine
Streptomycin
Sulfacetamide
Sulfanilamide
Sulfapyridine

antibody-mediated destruction of RBCs, and the primary goal of treatment is withdrawal of the offending agent.

AIHA is typically categorized into cold and warm, based on binding temperature, and can be caused by infections, autoimmune disease, connective tissue disorders, malignancy, blood transfusions, and organ transplantation[123]

Drug-induced hemolytic anemia results from drug-induced antibodies and has been shown to occur after administration of methyldopa, penicillin, cefotetan, ceftriaxone, piperacillin, and nonsteroidal anti-inflammatory medications.[116]

Hemolytic transfusion reactions occur because of antibodies reacting with donor RBCs. They can occur acutely or be delayed. Under anesthesia, administration of incompatible blood products may manifest as hypotension, tachycardia, fever, rash, bronchospasm, and hematuria. When a transfusion reaction is suspected, the transfusion should be discontinued, and crystalloid solution should be given to maintain circulating volume. Patients may also benefit from diuresis and alkalinization of the urine with sodium bicarbonate to prevent heme-mediated renal and vascular injury.

Hemoglobinopathies

Hemoglobinopathies are caused by genetic miscoding in the amino acid sequence of hemoglobin, which result in anemia and multiple effects on end-organ systems. The predominant adult hemoglobin is HbA, which consists of two alpha (α) and two beta (β) subunits or chains. The α subunits are coded on chromosome 16, while the non-α subunits, β, embryonic (ε), minor Hb A2 (δ), or fetal (HbF or γ) are coded on 11. Normal adult RBCs have three different types of hemoglobin: HbA (α2β2) ~95%; HbA2(α2δ2) ~2.5%; and HbF (α2γ2) 2.5%. The spatial arrangement of these subunits determines oxygen affinity, solubility, and stability.[120] Normal and variant hemoglobins are listed in Table 24-21. Hemoglobinopathies are commonly found in areas of the world that are endemic for malaria such as Africa and southwest Asia, as individuals who are heterozygous for a hemoglobinopathy are suspected of having increased resistance to malaria. Those who are homozygous, however, have a broad spectrum of illnesses due to anemia, accumulation of excessive iron and hemoglobin precursors, immunocompromise, tissue ischemia, and inflammation. The most common hemoglobinopathies are sickle cell disease (SCD) and thalassemia, both of which are among the most debilitating genetically inherited disorders in the world.

Table 24-21 Hemoglobin Variants

Hemoglobin	Globin Chains	Type
A	α2β2	Normal adult
A2	α2δ2	Normal adult (minor)
F	α2γ2	Normal fetal
S	α2βS2	Sickle (HbS)
C	α2βC2	HbC (clinical illness)
E	α2βE2	HbE (clinical illness)
Bart's	γ4	α-Thalassemia (fetal demise)
H	β4	α-Thalassemia major

Sickle Cell Disease

SCD is transmitted in an autosomal recessive pattern with an asymptomatic carrier state (NICV 24-8). In the United States, 1 in 500 African Americans have SCD, 1 in 12 African Americans carry the autosomal recessive mutation, and approximately 300,000 infants are born with sickle cell anemia annually worldwide.[124]

SCD is caused by a single amino acid substitution in the β-globin molecule. Valine is substituted for glutamine at the sixth amino acid position. The valine changes the physical characteristics of the affected hemoglobin under conditions of oxygen desaturation. When exposed to low oxygen tension, HbS polymerizes into fiber-like chains called tactoids that distort the normal biconcave shape into the characteristic crescent or "sickle cell" shape. These RBCs are relatively inflexible and have difficulty moving through capillaries. The spleen removes these abnormal cells from the circulation, reducing their lifespan to 12 to 17 days (normal = 120 days) and causing hemolytic anemia. The pathophysiology of SCD occurs because of microvascular obstruction and tissue ischemia. Vaso-occlusive episodes cause severe pain and progressive organ damage. Less evident and insidious mechanisms cause other detrimental effects (Table 24-22).

The propensity of RBCs in SCD patients to sickle depends on the proportion of hemoglobin S compared to normal hemoglobin. The heterozygous carrier state or sickle cell trait results

Table 24-22 Mechanisms of Cellular and Tissue Injury in Sickle Cell Disease

Capillary obstruction with tissue ischemia
RBC and platelet adhesion to the endothelium
Activation of coagulation with thrombosis and/or embolism
Reperfusion injury
Hemolysis and release of free hemoglobin
Leukocytosis and immune system activation
Free radical injury due to leukocyte superoxide release
Nitric oxide depletion due to superoxide release and uptake by free Hgb
Release of cytokines and inflammatory mediators
Endothelial injury
Iron accumulation

RBC, red blood cell; HgB, hemoglobin.

in the production of both hemoglobin A and S (usually 30% to 40% HbS); this condition has a relatively benign clinical picture as the cells only sickle when oxygen saturations approach 40%. This contrasts with the homozygous state (with near 100% HbS), which is a debilitating disease characterized by chronic hemolytic anemia, recurrent intermittent vaso-occlusion crises, severe pain, progressive organ damage, and early death. Sickling occurs at oxygen saturations as high as 85%. Many of these patients die before the age of 50. The clinical manifestations of SCD affect almost all organ systems (Table 24-23).

9 Several recurrent problems that cause significant morbidity and mortality afflict SCD patients. Vaso-occlusive crises (VOC) are often the first and most frequent manifestation of SCD and are secondary to musculoskeletal ischemia. The pain of VOC ranges from mild to excruciating. Mild cases can be managed with oral analgesics, rest, and hydration. Severe VOC requires hospitalization, parenteral narcotics, intravenous hydration, supplemental oxygen, RBC transfusion, and in some cases regional analgesia. Acute chest syndrome (ACS) has a mortality of 1% to 20% and represents the single greatest threat to patients with SCD. Clinical manifestations of ACS are chest pain, dyspnea, cough, wheezing, hypoxemia, and chest infiltrates (radiography). It may be caused by thrombosis, embolism (clot, fat), or infection. The treatment of ACS is supplemental oxygen, hydration, analgesia, and respiratory support. Antibiotics may be empirically administered pending the results of sputum culture. Severe ACS or ACS unresponsive to usual therapies may require RBC transfusion. The incidence of ACS after abdominal surgery is 10% to 20%. Factors that may contribute to postoperative ACS are pain, splinting, narcotics, and hypoventilation. The risk of postoperative ACS can be reduced by preoperative RBC transfusion and postoperative incentive spirometry. Sequestration crisis occurs when the splenic rate of RBC removal exceeds the rate of RBC production.

Complications of SCD include severe anemia and hemodynamic instability which occurs rapidly (Table 24-23). Sequestration may be an indication for splenectomy. Patients with SCD require a high and continuous rate of RBC production. Mild bone marrow suppression triggered by a viral infection (parvovirus B19) can precipitate an aplastic crisis. Asthma occurs in 50% of SCD patients and pulmonary hypertension occurs in 10% of SCD patients. Mortality is increased when either condition is present.[125]

Table 24-23 Complications of Sickle Cell Disease

Hematologic: hemolytic anemia, aplastic anemia, leukocytosis
Spleen: autoinfarction, hyposplenism, splenic sequestration
Central nervous system: stroke, hemorrhage, aneurysm, meningitis
Musculoskeletal: painful crisis, bone marrow hyperplasia, avascular necrosis, osteomyelitis, bone infarction, skeletal deformity, growth retardation, cutaneous ulceration
Cardiac: cardiomegaly, pulmonary hypertension, cor pulmonale, diastolic dysfunction, cardiomyopathy
Pulmonary: acute chest syndrome, asthma, fibrosis, pulmonary infarction, sleep apnea, pneumonia, hypoxemia, thromboembolism
Renal: papillary necrosis, glomerular sclerosis, renal failure
Genitourinary: priapism, infection
Hepatobiliary: jaundice, hepatitis, cirrhosis, cholelithiasis, cholestasis
Eye: retinopathy, hemorrhage, vision loss
Immune: immunosuppression, leukocytosis
Psychosocial: depression, anxiety, substance abuse, narcotic dependence

Preventive treatment of SCD patients includes oral hydroxyurea to increase HbF production, which has been shown to reduce transfusion requirements, as well as the frequency and severity of symptoms of VOC. Those with splenic involvement receive pneumococcal, *Hemophilus influenza* type B, and meningitis vaccinations to reduce the risk of sepsis. Transfusion of RBCs is performed when anemia is severe or as a preventive measure to reduce the amount of HbS. Bone marrow transplantation can be curative and is an option for severe SCD. Removal and genetic manipulation of the SCD patient's own bone marrow to increase HbF production is currently being investigated.[126]Acute crises require treatment of pain and dehydration. Severe pain and anemia may require hospitalization and blood transfusions.

Management of Anesthesia

Patients with SCD frequently require anesthesia and surgery. Patients enrolled in comprehensive sickle cell clinics are likely to have current surveillance evaluations by experienced hematologists. The clinic notes may provide important information. Preoperative evaluation is directed at identification of underlying organ dysfunction. Patients with a history of respiratory dysfunction, ECG abnormalities, functional limitations, or indicators of cor pulmonale should have a preoperative echocardiogram. Common findings include left ventricular hypertrophy, right ventricular dilation, atrial enlargement, and pulmonary hypertension. Fasting periods should be minimized to prevent dehydration, and patients are often admitted the day before surgery.

The goal of preoperative RBC transfusion is to achieve a hemoglobin level of at least 10 g/dL. When performed, it may reduce the likelihood of sickle cell complications such as ACS and VOC. There is a high incidence of alloimmunization among

SCD patients and obtaining cross-matched RBCs can be time-consuming. This fact, combined with the possibility of significant adverse effects associated with allogeneic blood products, preclude more aggressive transfusion thresholds except in the most invasive of procedures.

Active measures to maintain normothermia and normovolemia should be employed in the perioperative period. Extremity tourniquets can be used in situations where the success of the surgery is dependent on their use. The use of regional analgesia to improve analgesia and blood flow may be beneficial, though epinephrine should generally be avoided in local anesthetic solutions. Spinal anesthesia for Cesarean section has been shown to decrease perioperative blood loss and reduce the need for postoperative narcotics, though hypotension and hypoperfusion need to be treated quickly if they occur.[127] If opioids are required, careful monitoring of oxygenation and sedation should be performed. NSAIDs should be avoided in the presence of renal dysfunction.

Venous stasis should be minimized by careful positioning, avoidance of vena caval compression, and high-risk positions such as the prone position or the supine position in the pregnant patient. In general, the technique used is less important than meticulous attention to detail regarding perfusion, temperature control, and oxygenation.[128]

Thalassemia

Thalassemia is the result of deficient production of either the α- or β-globin components of hemoglobin. α-Thalassemia is caused by underproduction of α-globin and β-thalassemia from a deficit of β-globin. Anemia is caused by an inadequate amount of normal hemoglobin. The underproduction of one of the globin chains is not balanced by underproduction of the other globin chain. Thus, the globin that can be produced in normal amounts is in relative excess. These excess globin chains are ineffective as they are not paired with the correct globin to form a functional tetramer. The excess unpaired globin chains cause cellular and tissue injury. Ineffective erythropoiesis causes severe bone marrow hyperplasia, skeletal deformity, and skeletal fragility. Multisystem injury is caused by many of the mechanisms that cause systemic injury in SCD.

The terms thalassemia major, intermedia, and minor reflect the severity of the anemia that correlates with underproduction of the globin chain. Many patients with thalassemia minor do not require RBC transfusion. Routine transfusion of RBCs maintains an adequate hemoglobin level and suppresses bone marrow hyperplasia and extramedullary erythropoiesis. Routine transfusion, however, inevitably results in iron overload. Iron overload causes cardiac, hepatic, immune, and endocrine system dysfunction. Chelation therapy may reduce the amount of iron overload. Bone marrow transplantation may be considered for severely affected individuals.

Management of Anesthesia

Patients with thalassemia often require anesthesia for cholecystectomy, splenectomy, vascular access, and correction of skeletal abnormalities. The preoperative evaluation should include measurement of hemoglobin and the search for evidence of cardiac, hepatic, and endocrine dysfunction from iron overload. There is a high incidence of alloimmunization, and cross-matching blood can require considerable time.

Facial dysmorphisms can cause difficulties with airway management.[129] Spontaneous hemorrhage from extramedullary bone marrow deposits has been reported. Although spinal anesthesia has been successfully used for Cesarean section, bone marrow deposits in the spinal canal can be considered a relative contraindication to neuraxial anesthesia.

Connective Tissue Diseases

Rheumatoid arthritis (RA), systemic lupus erythematosus (SLE), systemic sclerosis (SSc), and inflammatory myopathies (dermatomyositis [DM]/polymyositis [PM]) are among the most common connective tissue diseases seen in the perioperative setting. While the etiologies of these diseases are not fully known, they share immune-mediated events which result in effects on the connective tissues of joints and muscles as well as more widespread systemic effects. Anesthetic considerations for patients with these disease processes require careful preoperative examination, careful intraoperative positioning, and management of systemic disease.

Rheumatoid Arthritis

Rheumatoid arthritis (RA) is an autoimmune disorder that causes inflammatory arthritis (NICV 24-9). This arthritis most commonly affects joints of the hands and feet but may be present in synovial joints throughout the body. Systemic effects are wide-ranging and important to note before developing an anesthetic plan for a patient with RA (Table 24-24).[130]

Management of Anesthesia

Preoperative evaluation of a patient with RA should focus on distribution and severity of joint disease, extra-articular symptoms, a thorough airway examination, and a review of the patient's current medication regimen. Joint pain and range of motion is important to note preoperatively, keeping in mind ideal surgical positioning and any modifications necessary to avoid excess joint motion or strain.

Extra-articular manifestations of RA may be subtle or undiagnosed; therefore, preoperative cardiac, respiratory, and hematologic testing may be prudent on all patients with RA. Cardiac disease is the main contributor to excess mortality in patients with RA, though presenting signs and symptoms are not always typical.[131] An ECG is useful to screen for left ventricular hypertrophy and conduction abnormalities. In any patient with recent cardiac symptomatology, an echocardiogram may be ordered to evaluate diastolic dysfunction, valvulopathy, and myocardial function. Respiratory evaluation may include chest radiography, pulmonary function testing, or room air arterial blood gas to assess for pulmonary fibrosis, effusions, or altered lung mechanics due 10

Table 24-24 Extra-articular Manifestations of Rheumatoid Arthritis

Cardiovascular	Pericarditis Valvular incompetence Vasculitis Conduction abnormalities
Hematologic	Anemia
Hepatic	Fibrosis
Integumentary	Fragile skin Sjogren syndrome
Renal	Glomerulonephritis Tubulointerstitial nephritis
Respiratory	Pleural effusion Pulmonary fibrosis Respiratory myopathy

Adapted from Samanta.[130]

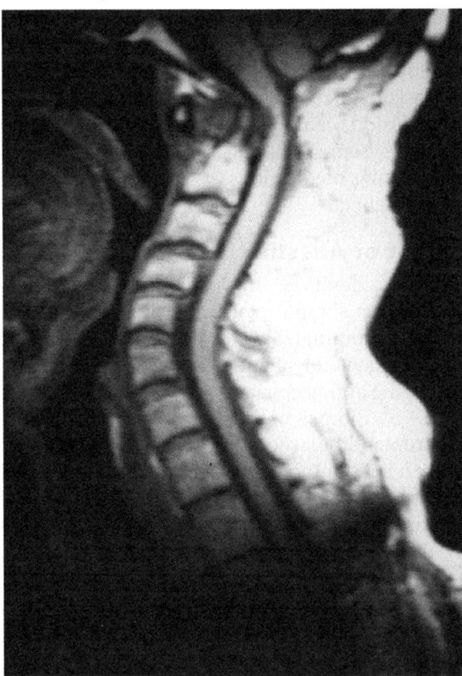

Figure 24-6 Magnetic resonance imaging of a cervical spine in a patient with rheumatoid arthritis (RA). Although the patient had no neurologic symptoms, there was severe spinal stenosis in the upper cervical spine.

to respiratory myopathy. A baseline complete blood count should be performed, as patients with RA are more likely to require perioperative blood transfusion due to ACD as well as medication side effects.[132]

11 Intraoperative management of patients with RA is determined by the extent of disease as well as the surgical procedure being performed. When general endotracheal anesthesia is required, particular care must be taken during intubation. Even in the absence of symptoms, patients with RA may have atlantoaxial subluxation and are at risk of neurologic injury from excessive neck movement (Fig. 24-6). Manual in-line stabilization is recommended during laryngoscopy even in patients without known cervical spine instability. With arthritic changes of the temporomandibular and cricoarytenoid joints, as well as a smaller-than-expected tracheal diameter, the presence of backup airway equipment including laryngeal mask airways, video laryngoscopy, and flexible fiberoptic bronchoscopy is also advised.

When possible, regional and neuraxial anesthesia are excellent options as they avoid airway and neck manipulation and allow for patient feedback during positioning. Peripheral nerve blocks are safe in patients with RA, acknowledging potential difficulty with positioning and anatomical changes from contractures or joint deformities. Neuraxial anesthesia provides similar benefits, though a higher-than-expected block should be expected in a patient with RA.[128]

The medication regimen of a patient with RA should be carefully examined preoperatively, with particular attention to corticosteroids, methotrexate, and disease-modifying antirheumatic drugs (DMARDs). Some adverse effects of these medications are listed in Table 24-25. For patients on greater than 10 mg of prednisone per day, stress dose hydrocortisone should be given intraoperatively in addition to their typical morning dose. The use of nitrous oxide in patients taking methotrexate has been a point of debate, as there is a theoretical potential for folate depletion. DMARDs have the potential to increase risk of infection, though

Table 24-25 Adverse Effects of Drugs Used to Treat Connective Tissue Diseases

Class of Drug	Adverse Effects
Corticosteroids	Hypertension, osteoporosis, hyperglycemia
Immunosuppressants	
Methotrexate	Hepatotoxicity, anemia, leukopenia
Azathioprine	Biliary stasis, leucopenia
Cyclosporine	Nephrotoxicity, hypertension, hypomagnesemia
Cyclophosphamide	Hemorrhagic cystitis, cholinesterase inhibition
Leflunomide	Hepatotoxicity, weight loss, hypertension
Mycophenolate mofetil	Nausea, emesis, diarrhea
TNF Antagonists	
Etanercept	Infections, tuberculosis
Infliximab	Lymphoma, heart failure
Adalimumab	infection, T-cell lymphoma, fatigue
Golimumab	Infection, lymphoma
Certolizumab	Infection, lymphoma
Interleukin Antagonists	
Anakinra	Infection, skin irritation
Tocilizumab	Infection, headache, stomatitis, fever
T-cell Inhibitors	
Abatacept	Infection
CD20 Monoclonal Antibody	
Rituximab	Infection, infusion reaction
Janus Kinase Inhibitors	
Tofacitinib	Infection, anemia, leucopenia
Antimalarials	
Hydroxychloroquine	Myopathy, retinopathy
Antibiotics	
Sulfasalazine	Nausea, neutropenia, hepatotoxicity
Heavy Metal Chelators	
Penicillamine	Autoimmune dermatoses, glomerulonephritis
Aspirin	Platelet dysfunction, peptic ulcers, sensitivity
NSAIDs	Peptic ulcers, leucopenia, coronary artery disease
COX-2 Inhibitors	Nephrotoxicity, cardiovascular dysfunction
Gold	Aplastic anemia, dermatitis, nephritis

TNF, tumor necrosis factor

changes to perioperative antibiotic therapy have not been recommended. As always, strict aseptic technique should be used for any invasive procedure.

Postoperatively, patients with RA should be monitored for possible respiratory compromise given a higher risk of respiratory myopathy or pulmonary manifestations of RA. It is also prudent to ensure full reversal of NMB, if used, as well as proof of return of good ventilatory function before extubation. Another important consideration is to assess whether a patient has the hand dexterity needed to utilize a patient-controlled analgesia (PCA) device, if indicated.

Systemic Lupus Erythematosus

Systemtic lupus erythematosus (SLE) is a chronic connective tissue disorder caused by both autoimmune damage and deposition of immune complexes in affected tissues. Several susceptibility genes have been implicated in the inheritance of SLE, particularly in major histocompatibility complexes. Triggering factors may also play a role, and include smoking, hormones, viruses, and exposure to certain drugs.

Management of Anesthesia

Preoperatively, a patient with SLE should be examined regarding recent or ongoing flares, organ involvement, and medication regimen. Elective procedures should be delayed if a patient is in an acute flare. The most common manifestations of SLE include nephritis, pericarditis, pleuritis, malar rash, and arthritis.[133]

Cardiovascular manifestations include pericarditis, myocarditis, noninfectious endocarditis (Libman–Sacks), valvular dysfunction, and dysrhythmias or conduction abnormalities. Importantly, pericarditis is typically chronic and rarely causes tamponade, though it has been reported. Preoperative echocardiography is warranted if there are findings suggestive of endocarditis (e.g., new murmur, fever, dyspnea, petechiae) or a decrease in exercise tolerance. Patients with SLE are at increased risk for thromboembolic events, particularly if they are positive for lupus anticoagulant or antiphospholipid antibodies. This subset of patients is at a higher risk for myocardial ischemia, and a baseline 12-lead ECG may be indicated.

Pulmonary effects of SLE include pleuritis, pleural effusion, interstitial lung disease (ILD), and diffuse alveolar hemorrhage. Pulmonary function tests of patients with pulmonary SLE most often show a deficit in diffusion capacity.

Lupus nephritis occurs in 60% of patients with SLE due to deposition of immune complexes, complement activation, and direct autoantibody effects in the kidneys.[134] Abnormalities in preoperative lab work, most commonly urinalysis or creatinine, are an indicator to avoid nephrotoxic medications. Overall, patients with SLE are at a 33% increase in odds of postoperative renal complications compared with controls.[135]

Anemia is also common in patients with SLE, due to ACD, AIHA, anemia of renal failure, and/or drug toxicity.

Medications used to treat the symptoms of SLE can have a wide range of adverse effects. Patients on long-term steroids may require stress dosing in the perioperative period. Cyclophosphamide and hydroxychloroquine may cause cardiac toxicity, Hepatotoxicity may occur with azathioprine and methotrexate use; methotrexate may also cause pulmonary toxicity.

Systemic Sclerosis (Scleroderma)

Scleroderma is a connective tissue disease characterized by changes in the microvasculature that cause inflammation and fibrosis of the skin and blood vessels (2 Video 24-2). SSc is a form of scleroderma where the inflammation and fibrosis affect internal organs. The pathophysiology of SSc involves a complex interaction of genetic susceptibility and environmental triggers that cause small-vessel vasculopathy, recurrent ischemia-reperfusion injury, and eventual fibrosis in affected organs.[131] Commonly involved organ systems are the skin, cardiovascular, respiratory, gastrointestinal, and neurologic systems. Patients with SSc often are prescribed immunomodulating medications, which should be reviewed for possible adverse effects (Table 24-25).

Management of Anesthesia

Preoperative considerations for patients with SSc undergoing surgical procedures should focus on risk stratification for optimal anesthetic planning. Skin manifestations, including skin thickening and Raynaud phenomenon may render intravenous access challenging and necessitate the use of ultrasound guidance (3 Video 24-3). Fibrosis of the skin around the mouth as well as of the temporomandibular joint can cause a restriction of mouth opening, which in conjunction with limited neck range of motion can pose significant challenges to securing an airway device.

Lung involvement in SSc, consisting mainly of ILD and less commonly, pulmonary arterial hypertension (PAH), causes most of the mortality in patients with SSc.[135] In patients with SSc-associated ILD, pulmonary function testing will show diminished diffusion capacity (DLCO) and a reduced forced vital capacity. Other testing that may be performed includes 6-minute walk tests and computed tomography. Patients with ILD are at increased risk for complications from mechanical ventilation. If necessary for the procedure being performed, lung-protective ventilatory strategies should be implemented.

Patients with SSc are prone to develop cardiac disease including congestive heart failure, diastolic dysfunction, and dysrhythmias which may be exacerbated by anesthetic medications. In patients with ILD, there is also a risk for impaired right ventricular function which may be exacerbated with intraoperative derangements caused by fluid administration and acidosis.

Renal dysfunction is common in patients with SSc due to renal vasculopathy. This can present as a scleroderma renal crisis, marked by hypertension, retinopathy, and acute deterioration of renal function.

Gastroesophageal reflux disease (GERD) occurs in 70% of 12
patients with SSc, and esophageal dysmotility combined with a hypotonic lower esophageal sphincter poses a significant aspiration risk. Aspiration chemoprophylaxis with histamine-2 antagonists, antacids, or proton pump inhibitors should be considered before general endotracheal anesthesia.

Given the high risk of general endotracheal anesthesia due to the combination of airway concerns, pulmonary disease, and aspiration risk, peripheral and neuraxial anesthesia may be safer when feasible for the procedure being performed.[136] Peripheral nerve blocks have been safely performed, though the effect of local anesthetic may be prolonged due to poor tissue perfusion and delayed clearance. Neuraxial anesthesia has also been shown to be successful in patients with SSc, though profound hypotension may occur after single-shot spinal injection due to autonomic dysregulation. Slow titration of epidural or intrathecal medications may mitigate the risk of severe hemodynamic changes.

Postoperatively, patients with SSc should be monitored closely for possible pulmonary, cardiac, renal, and thromboembolic complications.

Inflammatory Myopathies

The inflammatory myopathies are a group of diseases including dermatomyositis (DM), polymyositis (PM), necrotizing autoimmune myositis (NAM), inclusion-body myositis (IBM), and overlap myositis.[137] They share in common the presence of severe muscle weakness due to inflammation, often in the presence of autoantibodies.

Management of Anesthesia

Most inflammatory myopathies first affect proximal muscles, with distal effects occurring in advanced disease.[138] Neck and pharyngeal muscles may be involved, which has implications for airway management, including upper airway obstruction and altered laryngoscopic views. Respiratory myopathy occurs in advanced disease, and pulmonary function tests may be beneficial to determine postoperative risk and guide extubation criteria. Muscle atrophy occurs with chronic weakness, and succinylcholine should be avoided. Interestingly, rocuronium has been used in patients with DM at standard dosing (0.6 mg/kg) and has achieved complete blockade; however, the time to blockade was significantly longer than in patients without DM.[138] In the same patient, sugammadex was also effective but required a longer reversal time. It is believed that intramuscular fibrosis slows diffusion of rocuronium from the plasma to and from the neuromuscular junction, thus, increasing its time-to-peak effect. Conversely, intramuscular fibrosis slows diffusion back into the plasma when sugammadex is administered and also slows reversal. Treatment often includes corticosteroids and immunosuppressants.

Skin Disorders

Most skin disorders are localized and cause few systemic symptoms or complications within the perioperative period. Epidermolysis bullosa (EB) and pemphigus, are the exceptions; these skin blistering diseases can have perioperative significance and resultant complication.

Epidermolysis Bullosa

Epidermolysis bullosa (EB) is a heterogeneous group of acquired and inherited skin disorders that cause extreme skin fragility (4 Video 24-4).[139] The underlying cause has been tied to numerous genetic components that result in an abnormal functional protein at the dermo-epidermal junction. The acquired forms involve autoantibodies that destroy the basement membrane between the skin and mucosa. There is loss of intracellular bridges that results in skin layer separation, fluid accumulation, followed by blister formation. There have been numerous genetic mutations associated with inherited EB with up to 30 subtypes identified. Clinically, the most relevant subtypes are distinguished based on where the skin separation occurs. Epidermolysis simplex (EBS) is the most common for EB. In EBS, separation occurs within the epidermis; this condition has the fewest extracutaneous manifestations and usually has mild clinical symptoms. Junctional epidermolysis bullosa (JEB) is the separation of the lamina lucida and upper epidermis. Epidermolysis bullosa dystrophica (DEB) occurs when separation occurs underneath lamina densa (see Fig. 24-7). These subtypes can have severe extracutaneous involvement including the airway. JEB is so severe that usually it is lethal within the first few years of life.

Dystrophic EB is the most severe but survivable subtype of EB, that is caused by a defect in type VII collagen. These patients are typically diagnosed at birth, as lesions are present from delivery. Any frictional force causes sloughing of the skin which results in blistering that develops into scars and contractures. These patients commonly develop a mitten-like pseudosyndactyly (Figure 24-8). The mucosal surfaces and esophageal tissue contractures result in dysphagia, strictures, and malnutrition. With repetitive actions, such as chewing or oral care, these patients develop scarring of the mouth and become microstomic. This leads to poor dental care and hypoplasia of the tooth enamel. Anemia often develops because of malnutrition and recurrent secondary skin infections. These patients are also at risk of cardiac complications including dilated cardiomyopathy, ventricular dysfunction, aortic root dilation, and intracardiac thrombi formation. The most common cause of death is secondary to skin cancer, usually in the third to fourth decades of life.[140] 13

There are no therapies specifically for DEB and most care is supportive with good wound care, infection prevention, and pain management. Surgical procedures usually center around

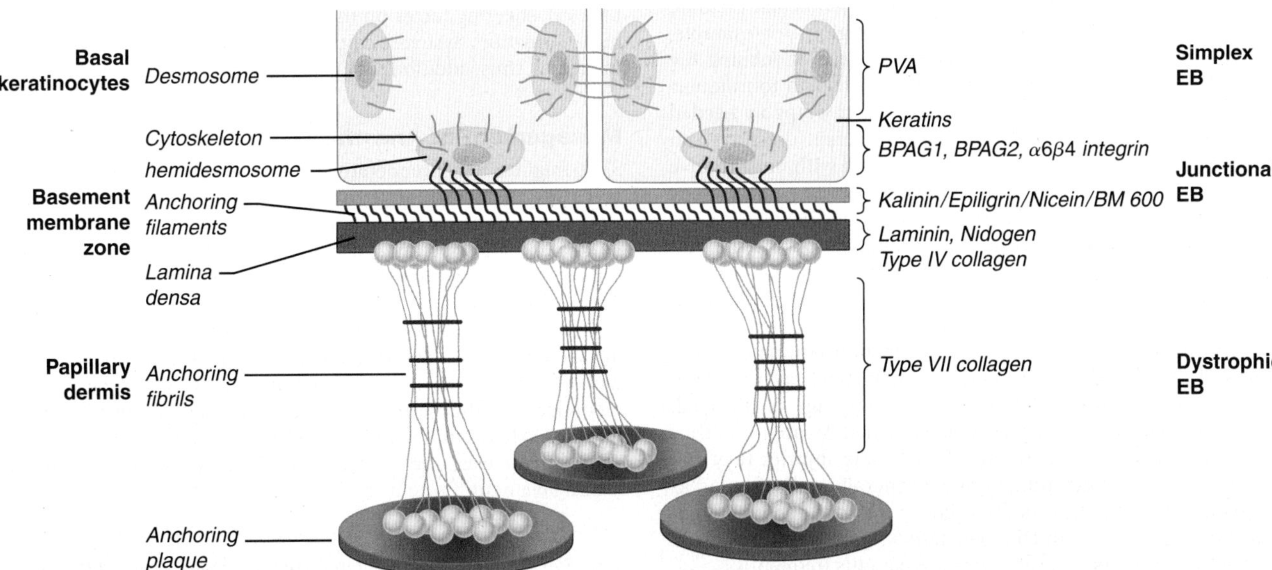

Figure 24-7 The ultrastructure of the zones of the skin. The diagram demonstrates where skin separation occurs in different types of epidermolysis bullosa (EB). (Adapted with permission from American Society for Clinical Investigation, from Uitto J, Christiano AM. Molecular genetics of the cutaneous basement membrane zone. *J Clin Invest*. 1992;90:687–692; permission conveyed from Copyright Clearance Center, Inc.)

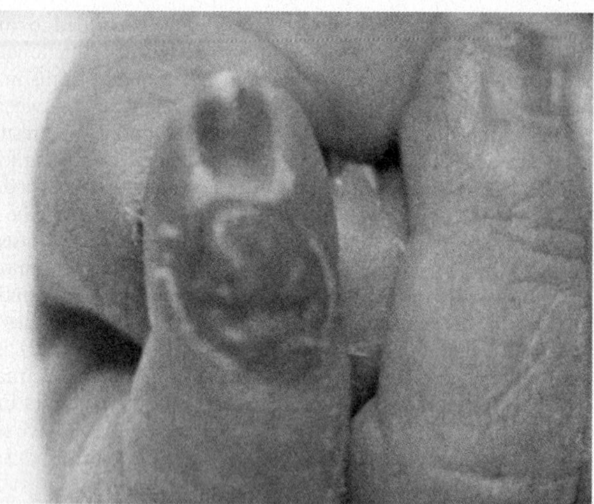

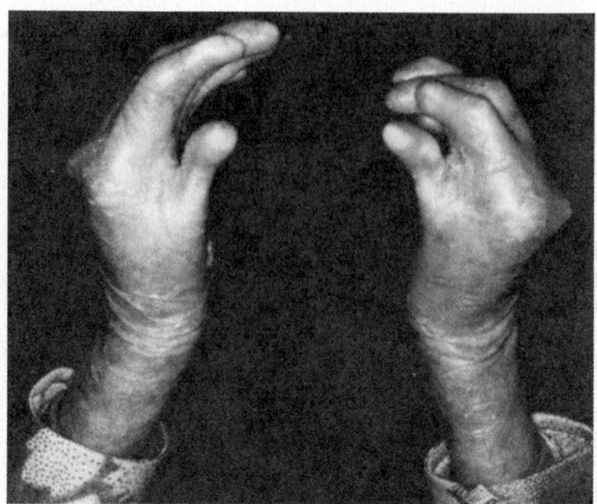

Figure 24-8 EB. **A:** Bullous lesion of the finger in a neonate with EB. **B:** Hands of an older child with epidermolysis progression to produce severe scarring and pseudosyndactyly. (Courtesy of James E B. *Division of Plastic Surgery*. Indiana University School of Medicine.)

amelioration of symptoms for improved function, pseudosyndactyly repair and esophageal dilations or gastrostomy tube for nutritional improvement.

Management of Anesthesia

A complete and thorough preoperative evaluation and planning are essential for preventing injury in these patients. All care team members interacting with the patient need to be aware of the diagnosis. During the preoperative evaluation, patients should be questioned to uncover symptoms of unrecognized cardiomyopathy. These patients often have decreased physical activity secondary to contractures, which makes evaluation of cardiac status difficult.

Minimizing damage to the skin requires alterations from normal anesthesia practice. Unnecessary patient movement should be avoided; it may be best to allow patients to position themselves. Frictional shearing forces must be avoided as this causes skin shearing and blister formation. Direct perpendicular pressure to the skin is better tolerated and less damaging (for example, dabbing the alcohol pad over the IV site instead of rubbing the skin). Padding underneath blood pressure cuffs and tourniquets is recommended. Silicone-based tapes, ties, and wraps are needed as adhesives from ECG leads, tape, and adherent dressings can be damaging. Intravenous lines can be secured with nonadhesive materials or sutures if longer-term access is needed.

Both intravenous and inhalational inductions have been used successfully for patients with DEB.[141] Preparation for difficult intravenous access and difficult airway is essential. Often these patients have microstomia with small mouth opening. Minimizing trauma to the face and pharyngeal structures with nonwater-based lubrication of the facemask, intubation equipment, and gloves of the provider are essential. Careful tracheal intubation without causing intraoral trauma or hemorrhage is the goal. Laryngeal mask airways are generally avoided because of shearing forces during placement and the pressure injuries they can cause. Nasal fiberoptic intubations are generally well tolerated as the nasal mucosa is less likely to blister. Despite the complexities in care, patients with DEB generally tolerate anesthesia well, especially in centers that care for these patients frequently.

For cases in which airway manipulation is not necessary, regional anesthesia, including neuraxial and peripheral blocks are well tolerated by DEB patients.

Pemphigus

Pemphigus is a group of autoimmune-mediated blistering skin diseases that involves the skin and mucous membranes (5 Video 24-5). Autoantibodies bind to desmoglein 1 and 3 proteins which leads to a loss of cell adhesion in the epithelial layers. There are multiple types, with pemphigus vulgaris (PV) being the most common. Other subtypes include pemphigus foliaceous, pemphigus erythematosus, paraneoplastic pemphigus, and drug-induced pemphigoid disease. Many drugs have been implicated as causing pemphigus.

PV is of utmost concern to the anesthesiologist related to the significant oral ulcerations and lesions. Often, the disease presents as oral lesions and almost all patients develop oral sequela during the disease process. Other locations of disease are larynx, esophagus, urethra, conjunctiva, and anus. Skin destruction and blister formation increase the risk of secondary infection and loss of fluids and proteins. All combine for poor wound healing and malnutrition. Like EB, sheering forces on the skin cause significant damage and bulla formation. Systemic corticosteroids are the mainstay of treatment and, thus, additional supplementation may be necessary.[142]

Management of Anesthesia

Skin fragility and preoperative drug therapy are the main concerns for the anesthesiologist. The high burden of oral disease puts these patients at high airway risk. Preparing for potentially poor oral opening, bleeding, and edema of the airway is important. Similar care should be performed as described for the patients with EB.[143]

While no anesthetic technique is contraindicated in terms of intravenous or inhalation agents, avoiding airway manipulation with use of neuraxial or regional anesthesia would be prudent secondary to the severe oropharyngeal and laryngeal disease burden. When employing neuraxial or regional anesthesia care should involve aseptic technique and avoidance of areas with bullae involvement.[143]

For further review and interactivities, please see the videos and narrative interactive clinical vignettes (NICVs) accessible in the complimentary eBook bundled with this text. Access instructions are located on the inside front cover.

REFERENCES

1. Mercuri E, Bönneman C, Muntoni F. Muscular dystrophies. *Lancet*. 2019;394:2025–2038.
2. Yilmaz A, Sechtem U. Cardiac involvement in muscular dystrophy: advances in diagnosis and therapy. *Heart*. 2012;98:420–429.
3. Amario D, Amodeo A, Adorisio R, et al. A current approach to heart failure in Duchenne muscular dystrophy. *Heart*. 2017;103:1770–1779.
4. McDonald C, Henricson E, Abresch R, et al. Long-term effects of glucocorticoids on function, quality of life, and survival in patients with Duchenne muscular dystrophy: a prospective cohort study. *Lancet*. 2018;391:451–461.
5. Emery A. The muscular dystrophies. *Lancet*. 2002;359:687–695.
6. Butterfield R. Congenital muscular dystrophy and congenital myopathy. *Continuum*. 2019; 25(6):1640–1661.
7. Taylor A, Lachlan K, Manners RM, Lotery AJ. A study of a family with the skeletal muscle RYR1 mutation (c.7354C>T) associated with central core myopathy and malignant hyperthermia susceptibility. *J Clin Neurosci*. 2012;19:65–70.
8. Veyckemans F. Can inhalation agents be used in the presence of a child with myopathy? *Curr Opin Anaesthesiol*. 2010;23:348–355.
9. Turner C, Hilton-Jones D. Myotonic dystrophy: diagnosis, management, and new therapies. *Curr Opin Neurol*. 2014, 27:599–606
10. Mathieu J, Allard P, Potvin L, Prévost C, Bégin P. A 10-year study of mortality in a cohort of patients with myotonic dystrophy. *Neurology*. 1999;52:1658–1662.
11. Lau J, Sy R, Corbett A, Kritharides L. Myotonic dystrophy and the heart: a systematic review of evaluation and management. *Int J Cardiol*. 2015;184:600–608.
12. Johnson N. Myotonic muscular dystrophies. *Continuum*. 2019;25(6):1682–1695.
13. Mangla C, Bais K, Yarmush J. Myotonic dystrophy and anesthetic challenges: a case report and review. *Case Rep Anesthesiol*. 2019;2019:4282305.
14. Veyckemans F, Scholtes JL. Myotonic dystrophies type 1 and 2: anesthetic care. *Paediatr Anaesth*. 2013;23:794–803.
15. Matthews E, Holmes S, Fialho D. Skeletal muscle channelopathies: a guide to diagnosis and management. *Pract Neurol*. 2021;21:196–205.
16. Bandschapp O, Iaizzo P. Pathophysiologic and anesthetic considerations for the patients with myotonia congenita or periodic paralyses. *Pediatr Anesth*. 2013;23:824–833.
17. Patel M, Ladak K. Thyrotoxic periodic paralysis: a case report and literature review. *Clin Med Res*. 2021;19(3):148–151.
18. Mazzanti A, Guz D, Trancuccio A, et al. Natural history and risk stratification in Andersen-Tawil Syndrome Type 1. *J Am Coll Cardiol*. 2020;75(15):1772–1784.
19. Litman R, Griggs S, Dowling J, Riazi S. Malignant hyperthermia susceptibility and related diseases. *Anesthesiology*. 2018;128(1):159–167.
20. Carr AS, Cardwell CR, McCarron PO, McConville J. A systematic review of population based epidemiological studies in myasthenia gravis. *BMC Neurol*. 2010;10:46.
21. Grob D, Brunner N, Nam T, Pagala M. Lifetime course of myasthenia gravis. *Muscle Nerve*. 2008;37(2):141–149.
22. Jaretzki A III, Barohn RJ, Ernstoff RM, et al. Myasthenia gravis: Recommendations for clinical research standards. *Neurology*. 2000;55(1):16–23.
23. Sanders DB, Wolfe GI, Benatar M, et al. International consensus guidance for management of myasthenia gravis: executive summary. *Neurology*. 2016;87:419–425.
24. Dillon FX. Anesthesia issues in the perioperative management of myasthenia gravis. *Semin Neurol*. 2004;1:83–94.
25. Lennon VA, Kryzer TJ, Griesmann GE, et al. Calcium-channel antibodies in the Lambert-Eaton syndrome and other paraneoplastic syndromes. *N Engl J Med*. 1995;332:1467–1474
26. Hocker S, Nagarajan E, Rubin M, Wijdicks E. Clinical factors associated with Guillain-Barré syndrome following surgery. *Neurol Clin Pract*. 2018;8(3):201–206.
27. Feldman JM. Cardiac arrest after succinylcholine in a pregnant patient recovered from Guillain-Barre syndrome. *Anesthesiology*. 1990;72:942–944.
28. Hypo and hypersensitivity to vecuronium in a patient with Guillain-Barre syndrome. *Anesth Analg*. 1994;78:187–189.
29. Mangar D, Sprenker C, Karinoski R, Puri S, Decker D, Camporesi E. Rapid onset of Guillain-Barre syndrome after an obstetric epidural block. *Anes Analg Case Rep*. 2013;1:19–22.
30. Yuki N, Hartung HP. Guillain-Barré syndrome. *N Engl J Med*. 2012;366:2294–2304.
31. Grigoriadis N, van Pesch V. A basic overview of multiple sclerosis immunopathology. *Eur J Neurol*. 2015;22(Suppl 2):3–13.
32. Wingerchuk DM, Carter JL. Multiple sclerosis: current and emerging disease-modifying therapies and treatment strategies. *Mayo Clin Proc*. 2014;89:225–240.
33. McSwain JR, Doty JW, Wilson SH. Regional anesthesia in patients with pre-existing neurologic disease. *Curr Opin Anesthesiol*. 2014;27:538–543.
34. Pack AM. Epilepsy overview and revised classification of seizures and epilepsies. *Continuum (Minneap Minn)*. 2019;25(2):306–321.
35. Betjemann JP, Lowenstein DH. Status epilepticus in adults. *Lancet Neurol*. 2015;14:615–624.
36. French JA, Pedley TA. Initial management of epilepsy. *N Engl J Med*. 2008;359:166–176.
37. Perucca P, Scheffer IE, Kiley M. The management of epilepsy in children and adults. *Med J Aust*. 2018;208:226–233.
38. Kofke WA. Anesthetic management of the patient with epilepsy or prior seizures. *Curr Opin Anesthesiol*. 2010;23:391–399.
39. Bates K. Epilepsy. *Prim Care*. 2015;42:217–232.
40. Ramani R. Vagus nerve stimulator therapy for seizures. *J Neurosurg Anesthesiol*. 2008;20:29–35.
41. Perks A, Cheema S, Mohanraj R. Anaesthesia and epilepsy. *Br J Anaesth*. 2012;108:562–571.
42. Weller J, Budson A. Current understanding of Alzheimer's disease and treatment. *F1000Research*. 2018;7:1161–1170.
43. Palmqvist S, Zetterberg H, Mattsson N, et al. Detailed comparison of amyloid PET and CSF biomarkers for identifying early Alzheimer's disease. *Neurology*. 2015;85:1240–1249.
44. Aisen P, Touchon J, Amariglio R, et al. EU/US/CTAD Task Force: lessons learned from recent and current Alzheimer's prevention trials. *J Prev Alzheimers Dis*. 2017;4(2):116–124.
45. Ehret MJ, Chamberlain KW. Current practices in the treatment of Alzheimer disease: where is the evidence after the phase III trials? *Clin Ther*. 2015;37:1604–1616.
46. Atri A. Current and future treatments in Alzheimer's disease. *Semin Neurol*. 2019;39:227–240.
47. Chen CW, Lin CC, Chen KB, Kuo YC, Li CY, Chung CJ. Increased risk of dementia in people with previous exposure to general anesthesia: a nationwide population-based case-control study. *Alzheimers Dement*. 2014;10:196–204.
48. Berger M, Burke J, Eckenhoff R, Mathew J. Alzheimer's disease, anesthesia, and surgery: a clinically focused review. *J Cardiothor Vasc Anesth*. 2014;28:1609–1623.
49. Carnini A, Lear JD, Eckenhoff RG. Inhaled anesthetic modulation of amyloid beta (1–40) assembly and growth. *Curr Alzheimer Res*. 2007;4:233–241.
50. Kalia LV, Lang AE. Parkinson's disease. *Lancet*. 2015;386:896–912.
51. Simon DK, Tanner CM, Brundin P. Parkinson disease epidemiology, pathology, genetics and pathophysiology. *Clin Geriatric Med*. 202;36:1–12.
52. Braak H, Del Tredici K. Neuropathological staging of brain pathology is sporadic Parkinson's disease. *Neurobiol Aging*. 2003;24:197–211.
53. Hickey P, Stacy M. Available and emerging treatments for Parkinson's disease: a review. *Drug Des Devel Ther*. 2011;5:241–254.
54. Kalenka A, Schwartz A. Anaesthesia and Parkinson's disease: how to manage with new therapies? *Curr Opin Anesthesiol*. 2009;22:419–424.
55. Lenka A, Om Mitral S, Lamotte G, Pagan FL. A pragmatic approach to the perioperative management of Parkinson's disease. *Can J Neurol Sci*. 2021;48:299–307.
56. Galvez-Jimenez N, Lang AE. The perioperative management of Parkinson's revisited. *Neurol Clin*. 2004;22:367–377.
57. Tsai ST, Tseng GF, Kuo CC, Chen TY, Chen SY. Sevoflurane and Parkinson's disease. *Anesthesiology*. 2020;132(5):1034–1044.
58. Liu Z, He S, Li L. General anesthesia versus local anesthesia for deep brain stimulation in Parkinson's disease: a meta-analysis. *Stereotact Funct Neurosurg*. 2019;97:381–390.
59. Poon CC, Irwin MG. Anaesthesia for deep brain stimulation and in patients with implanted neurostimulator devices. *Br J Anaesth*. 2009;103:152–165.
60. McColgan P, Tabrizi SJ. Huntington's disease: a clinical review. *Eur J Neurol*. 2018;25(1):24–34.
61. Nguyen PT, Meeks D, Liotiri D. Anaesthesia, and orphan disease: airway and anaesthetic management in Huntington's disease. *BMJ Case Rep*. 2017;2017:bcr2017221354.
62. Hoeper AM, Barbara DW, Watson JC, Sprung J, Weingarten TN. Amyotrophic lateral sclerosis and anesthesia: a case series and review of the literature. *J Anesth*. 2019;33(2):257–265.
63. Masrori P, Van Damme P. Amyotrophic lateral sclerosis: a clinical review. *Eur J Neurol*. 2020;27:1918–1929.
64. Prabhakar A, Owen CP, Kaye AD. Anesthetic management of the patient with amyotrophic lateral sclerosis. *J Anesth*. 2013;27(6):909–918.
65. Mackenzie G, Will R. Creutzfeldt-Jakob disease: recent developments. *F1000Res*. 2017;6: 2053.
66. Manix M, Kalakoti P, Henry M, et al. Creutzfeldt-Jakob disease: updated diagnostic criteria, treatment algorithm, and the utility of brain biopsy. *Neurosurg Focus*. 2015;39(5):E2.
67. Telfer JM. Creutzfeldt-Jakob disease–implications for anaesthetists in New Zealand. *Anaesth Intensive Care*. 2009;37(3):386–391.
68. Van Petegem F. Ryanodine receptors: allosteric ion channel giants. *J Mol Biol*. 2015;427:31–53.
69. Hirshey Dirksen SJ, Larach MG, Rosenberg H, et al. Special article: future directions in malignant hyperthermia research and patient care. *Anesth Analg*. 2011;113:1108–1119.
70. Larach MG, Brandom BW, Allen GC, Gronert GA, Lehman EB. Malignant hyperthermia deaths related to inadequate temperature monitoring, 2007–2012: a report from the North American malignant hyperthermia registry of the malignant hyperthermia association of the United States. *Anesth Analg*. 2014;119:1359–1366.
71. Otsuki S, Miyoshi H, Mukaida K, Yasuda T, Nakamura R, Tsutsumi YM. Age-specific clinical features of pediatric malignant hyperthermia: a review of 187 cases over 60 years in Japan. *Anesth Analg*. 2021;135(1):128–135.
72. Larach MG, Localio AR, Allen GC, et al. A clinical grading scale to predict malignant hyperthermia susceptibility. *Anesthesiology*. 1994;80:771–779.
73. Krause T, Gerbershagen MU, Fiege M, Weisshorn R, Wappler F. Dantrolene-a review of its pharmacology, therapeutic use, and new developments. *Anaesthesia*. 2004;59:364–373.
74. Schutte JK, Becker S, Starosse A, et al. Comparison of the therapeutic effectiveness of a dantrolene sodium solution and a novel nanocrystalline suspension of dantrolene sodium in malignant hyperthermia normal and susceptible pigs. *Eur J Anaesthesiol*. 2011;28:256–264.

75. Glahn KP, Ellis FR, Halsall PJ, et al. Recognizing and managing a malignant hyperthermia crisis. *Br J Anaesth*. 2010;105:417–420.
76. Riazi S, Kraeva N, Hopkins P. Malignant hyperthermia in the post genomics era. *Anesthesiology*. 2018;128(1):168–180.
77. Birgenheier N, Stoker R, Westenkow D, Orr J. Activated charcoal effectively removes inhaled anesthetics from modern anesthesia machines. *Anesth Analg*. 2011;112:1363–1370.
78. Moore MR, McColl KEL, Remington C, Goldberg A. *Disorders of Porphyrin Metabolism*. Plenum Medical Book Company; 1987.
79. Jensen NF, Fiddler DS, Striepe V. Anesthetic considerations in porphyrias. *Anesth Analg*. 1995;80:591–599.
80. Findley H, Philip A, Cole D, Nair A. Porphyrias: implications for anaesthesia, critical care, and pain medicine. *Anaesth Crit Care Pain Med*. 2012;12(3):128–133.
81. Wichmann S, Færk G, Bundgaard JR, Gätke MR. Patients with prolonged effect of succinylcholine or mivacurium had novel mutations in the butyrylcholinesterase gene. *Pharmacogenet Genomics*. 2016;26:351–356.
82. Lang JB, Kunsman SA, Hartman MT. Acquired pseudocholinesterase deficiency. *Curr Anaesth Crit Care*. 2010;21:297–298.
83. Weinstein DA, Wolfsdorf JI. Glycogen storages diseases: a primer for clinicians. *The Endocrin*. 2002;12:531–538.
84. Dasouki M, Jawdat O, Almadhoun O, et al. Pompe disease. *Neurol Clin*. 2014;32:751–776.
85. DeSena HC, Brumund MR, Superneau D, Snyder CS. Ventricular fibrillation in a patient with Pompe disease: a cautionary tale. *Congenit Heart Dis*. 2011;6:397–401.
86. Wang LJ, Ross AK, Li JS, et al. Cardiac arrhythmias following anesthesia induction in infantile-onset Pompe disease: a case series. *Paediatr Anaesth*. 2007;17:738–748.
87. Walker RW, Briggs G, Bruce J, Fletcher J, Wraith ED. Regional anesthetic techniques are an alternative to general anesthesia for infants with Pompe's disease. *Paediatr Anaesth*. 2007;17:697–702.
88. Kishnani PS, Austin SL, Arn P, et al. Glycogen storage type III diagnosis and management guidelines. *Genet Med*. 2010;12:446–463.
89. Mohart D, Russo P, Tobias JD. Perioperative management of a child with glycogen storage type III undergoing cardiopulmonary bypass and repair of an atrial septal defect. *Paediatr Anaesth*. 2002;12:649–654.
90. Ozen H. Glycogen storage diseases: new perspectives. *World J Gatroenterol*. 2007;13:2541–2533.
91. Lobato EB, Janelle GM, Urdaneta F, Malias MA. Noncardiogenic pulmonary edema and rhabdomyolysis after protamine administration in a patient with unrecognized McArdle's disease. *Anesthesiology*. 1999;91:303–305.
92. Bollig G. McArdle's disease (glycogen storage disease type V) and anesthesia-a case report and review of the literature. *Paediatr Anaesth*. 2013;23:817–823.
93. Roscher A, Patel J, Hewson S, et al. The natural history of glycogen storage disease type VI and IX: long term outcome from the largest metabolic center in Canada. *Mol Genet Metab*. 2014;113:171–176.
94. Wu PL, Yang YN, Tey SL, Yang CH, Yang SN, Lin CS. Infantile form of muscle phosphofructokinase deficiency in a premature neonate. *Pediatr Int*. 2015;57:746–749.
95. Al-Hagar M. Fanconi-Bickel syndrome as an example of marked allelic heterogeneity. *World J Nephol*. 2012;1:63–68.
96. Chen M. Glycogen storage diseases. In: Monga SPS, ed. *Molecular Pathology of Liver Diseases*. Springer; 2011:677–681.
97. Muenzer J. Overview of the mucopolysaccharidoses. *Rheumatology (Oxford)*. 2011;50:v4–v12.
98. Muenzer J. Early initiation of enzyme replacement therapy for mucopolysaccharidoses. *Mol Gen Metab*. 2014;115:63–72.
99. Walker R, Belani KG, Braunlin EA, et al. Anaesthesia and airway management in mucopolysaccharidoses. *J Inherit Metab Dis*. 2013;36:211–219.
100. Frawley G, Fuenzalida D, Donath S, Yaplito-Lee J, Peters H. A retrospective audit of anesthetic techniques and complications in children with mucopolysaccharidoses. *Paediatr Anaesth*. 2012;22:737–744.
101. Megens JH, de Wit M, van Hasselt PM, Boelens JJ, van der Werff DBM, de Graaff JC. Perioperative complications in patients diagnosed with mucopolysaccharidosis and the impact of enzyme replacement followed by hematopoietic stem cell transplantation at early age. *Paediatr Anaesth*. 2014;24:521–527.
102. Beesley OR, Lau K, Stacey S. Anesthetic considerations for thoracic surgery in a patient with osteogenesis imperfecta. *J Cardio Vasc Anes*. 2021;35:3727–3729.
103. Palomo T, Vilaca T, Lazaretti-Castro M. Osteogenesis imperfecta: diagnosis and diagnosis. *Curr Opin Endocrinol Diabetes Obes*. 2017;24:381–388.
104. Perea SH, Green DW. Osteogenesis imperfecta: treatment and surgical management. *Curr Opin Peds*. 2021;33:74–78.
105. Rossi V, Lee B, Marom R. Osteogenesis imperfecta: advancements in genetics and treatment. *Curr Opin Peds*. 2019;31:708–715.
106. Forlino A, Marini JC. Osteogenesis imperfecta. *Genetics of Bone Biology and Skeletal Disease*. 2nd ed. Academic Press; 2018:397–420.
107. Ashourina H, Johansen FT, Folkestad L, Diedrichsen ACP, Brixen K. Heart disease in patients with osteogenesis imperfecta-a systematic review. *Int J Cardiol*. 2015;196:149–157.
108. Stynowick GA, Tobias JD. Perioperative care of the patient with osteogenesis imperfecta. *Orthopedics*. 2007;30:1043–1049.
109. Gupta A, Kamal G, Gupta N, Aggarwal A. Combined spinal-epidural anesthesia with dexmedetomidine-based sedation for multiple corrective osteotomies in a child with osteogenesis imperfecta type III: a case report. *Anes Analg*. 2017;9(2):60–63.
110. Chin JWE, Stuart GM. Anesthetic considerations for scoliosis surgery in a patient with recessive severe/lethal form of osteogenesis imperfecta. *Ped Anesth*. 2018;28:817–818.
111. Bojanic K, Kivela JE, Gurrieri C, et al. Perioperative course and intraoperative temperatures in patients with osteogenesis imperfecta. *Eur J Anaesthesiol*. 2011;28:370–375.
112. Munoz M, Gomez-Ramirez S, Kozek-Langeneker S. Pre-operative haematological assessment in patients scheduled for major surgery. *Anaesthesia*. 2016;71(Suppl 1):19–28.
113. Duma A, Cartmill C, Blood J, Sharma A, Kharasch ED, Nagele P. The hematological effects of nitrous oxide anesthesia in pediatric patients. *Anesth Analg*. 2015;120:1325–1330.
114. Reynolds EH. The neurology of folic acid deficiency. *Handb Clin Neurol*. 2014;120:927.
115. Weiss G, Goodnough LT. Anemia of chronic disease. *N Engl J Med*. 2005;352(10): 1011–1023.
116. Phillips J, Henderson AC. Hemolytic anemia: evaluation and differential diagnosis. *Am Fam Physician*. 2018;98(6):354–361.
117. He BJ, Liao L, Tao YF, et al. Molecluar genetic mechanisms of hereditary spherocytosis: current perspectives. *Acta Haematol*. 2018;139:60–66.
118. Bolton-Maggs PHB, Langer JC, Tittensor P, King MJ. Guidelines for the diagnosis and management of Hereditary Spherocytosis–2011 update. *Br J Haematol*. 2011;156:37–49.
119. Wu Y, Liao L, Lin F. The diagnostic protocol for hereditay spherocytosis-2021. 2021; 35:e24034.
120. Manciu S, Matei E, Trandafir B. Hereditary spherocytosis – diagnosis, surgical treatment and outcomes. A literature review. *Chirurgia*. 2017;2:110–116.
121. Cappellini MD, Fiorelli G. Glucose-6-phosphate dehydrogenase deficiency. *Lancet*. 2008; 371:64–74.
122. Grace RF, Layton DM, Barcellini W. How we manage patients with pyruvate kinase deficiency. *Br J Haematol*. 2019;184:721–734.
123. Panch SR, Montemayor-Garcia C, Klein HG. Hemolytic transfusion reactions. *N Engl J Med*. 2019;381(2):150–162.
124. Wilson M, Forsyth P, Whiteside J. Haemoglobinopathy and sickle cell disease. Continuing education in Anaesthesia, *Critical Care & Pain*. 2010;10:24–28.
125. Abman SH, Hansmann G, Archer SL, et al. Pediatric pulmonary hypertension: guidelines from the American Heart Association and American Thoracic Society. *Circulation*. 2015;132: 2037–2099.
126. Eridani S, Mosca A. Fetal hemoglobin reactivation and cell engineering in the treatment of sickle cell anemia. *J Blood Med*. 2011;2:23–30.
127. Bakri MH, Ismail EA, Ghanem G, Shokry M. Spinal versus general anesthesia for cesarean section in patients with sickle cell anemia. *Korean J Anesthesiol*. 2015;68:469–475.
128. Firth PG. Anaesthesia for peculiar cells—a century of sickle cell disease. *Br J Anaesth*. 2005;95:287–299.
129. Staikou C, Stavroulakis E, Karmanaiolu I. A narrative review of peri-operative management of patients with thalassemia. *Anaesthesia*. 2014;69:494–510.
130. Samanta R, Shoukrey K, Griffiths R. Rheumatoid arthritis, and anaesthesia. *Anaesthesia*. 2011;66:1146–1159.
131. Turesson C, Janrenros A, Jacobsson L. Increased incidence of cardiovascular disease in patients with rheumatoid arthritis: results from a community-based study. *Ann Rheum Dis*. 2004;63:952–955.
132. Leino KA, Kuusniemi KS, Pälve HG, Korpelainen JT, Tiusanen HT, Tuppurainen TT. Spread of spinal block in patients with rheumatoid arthritis. *Acta Anaesthesiol Scand*. 2010; 54:65–69.
133. Ben-Menachem E. Systemic lupus erythematosus: a review for anesthesiologists. *Anesth Analg*. 2010;111:665–676.
134. Babazade R, Yilmaz HO, Leunig SM, Zimmerman NM, Turan A. Systemic lupus erythematosus is associated with increased adverse postoperative renal outcomes and mortality: a historical cohort study using administrative health data. *Anesth Analg*. 2017;124(4):1118–1126.
135. Carr ZJ, Klick J, McDowell BJ, Charchaflieh JG, Karamchandani K. An update on systemic sclerosis and its perioperative management. *Curr Anesthesiol Rep*. 2020;10(4):512–521.
136. Dempsey ZS, Rowell S, McRobert R. The role of regional and neuraxial anesthesia in patients with systemic sclerosis. *Local Reg Anesth*. 2011;4:47–56.
137. Suzuki T, Nameki H, Shimizu H, Shimizu Y, Nakamura R, Ogawa S. Efficacy of rocuronium and sugammadex in a patient with dermatomyositis. *Br J Anaesth*. 2012;108(4):703.
138. Bardhan A, Bruckner-Tuderman L, Chapple ILC, et al. Epidermolysis bullosa. *Nat Rev Dis Primers*. 2020;6(1):78.
139. Dalakas M. Inflammatory muscle diseases. *N Engl J Med*. 2015;372:1734–1747.
140. Mittal BM, Goodnough CL, Bushell E, Turkmani-Bazzi S, Sheppard K. Anesthetic management of adults with epidermolysis bullosa. *Anesth Analg*. 2022;134(1):90–101.
141. Brooks Peterson M, Strupp KM, Brockel MA, et al. Anesthetic management and outcomes of patients with epidermolysis bullosa: experience at a tertiary referral center. *Anesth Analg*. 2022;134(4):810–821.
142. Schmidt E, Kasperkiewicz M, Joly P. Pemphigus. *Lancet*. 2019;394(10201):882–894.
143. Bansal A, Tewari A, Garg S, Kanwal A. Anesthetic considerations in pemphigus vulgaris: case series and review of literature. *Saudi J Anaesth*. 2012;6:165–168.

25 The Anesthesia Workstation and Delivery Systems for Inhaled Anesthetics

BENJAMIN F. GRUENBAUM • KEVIN T. RIUTORT • KLAUS D. TORP • JAMES B. EISENKRAFT

KEY POINTS

1. The oxygen failure cutoff valves (previously known as "fail-safe" valves, "hypoxic guards," or "proportioning systems") minimize the likelihood of delivery of a hypoxic gas mixture, but they are not foolproof. Delivery of a hypoxic mixture may still result from (1) the wrong supply gas, either in the cylinder or in the main pipeline; (2) a defective or broken safety device; (3) leaks downstream from the safety devices; (4) inert gas administration (e.g., helium); and (5) dilution of the inspired oxygen concentration by high concentrations of inhaled anesthetics.
2. In the event of a gas pipeline crossover, two actions must be taken. The backup oxygen cylinder must be turned on (since the tank valve should always be turned off when not in use), and the wall/pipeline supply sources must be disconnected.
3. Because of desflurane's low boiling point (22.8°C) and high vapor pressure (669 mmHg at 20°C), delivery of desflurane requires specially designed vaporizers, such as the GE Healthcare Tec 6, the Dräger D-Vapor, and the GE Healthcare Aladin cassette vaporizing system.
4. Erroneous filling of an empty variable bypass vaporizer with desflurane could theoretically be catastrophic, resulting in delivery of a hypoxic mixture and a massive overdose of inhaled desflurane.
5. Inhaled anesthetics can interact with CO_2 absorbents and produce toxic compounds. During sevoflurane-only anesthesia, compound A can be formed, particularly at low fresh gas flow (FGF) rates. Carbon monoxide may be produced when volatile anesthetics are utilized, particularly with desiccated absorbents.
6. Desiccated strong base absorbents (particularly barium hydroxide lime, known as Baralyme) can react with sevoflurane, producing extremely high absorber temperatures and combustible decomposition products. These, in combination with the oxygen- or nitrous oxide–enriched environment of the circle system, have produced very high temperatures and fires within the breathing system. For this reason, Baralyme is no longer available in the United States. Lithium-based absorbents are nonreactive.

7 With older design machines, use of the oxygen flush valve during the inspiratory phase of mechanical ventilation could cause barotrauma, particularly in pediatric patients. The newer workstations have fresh-gas decouplers or peak-inspiratory pressure limiters that were designed to prevent these complications. Ventilators that use fresh gas decoupling (FGD) technology virtually eliminate the possibility of barotrauma by oxygen flushing during the inspiratory phase because FGF and oxygen flush flow are diverted to the reservoir bag. However, if the reservoir bag has a large leak or is missing, patient awareness under anesthesia and delivery of a lower-than-expected oxygen concentration could occur due to entrainment of room air.

8 Anesthesia ventilators with ascending bellows (bellows that ascend during the expiratory phase) were initially thought to be safer than descending bellows. This is because a breathing system disconnection would be obvious since the ascending bellows would not refill and rise during exhalation. Contemporary machines with descending bellows, however, have been carefully redesigned to address their initial limitations. Currently used descending bellows ventilators have featherlight bellows, an electric eye at the bottom of the bellows housing to detect bellows movement, and the bellows housing is subjected to positive end-expiratory pressure (PEEP), such that in case of a disconnect, the bellows would rise and stay up.

9 Modern ventilators compensate for the changes in FGF, respiratory rate, and I:E (inspiratory to expiratory) ratio so that the delivered tidal volume does not change from that set to be delivered. This compensation is achieved either by "fresh gas decoupling" (in Dräger Fabius, Tiro, and Apollo workstations) or by "fresh gas compensation" (in GE Healthcare workstations).

10 Two vital but often overlooked items in the preuse checkout of the anesthesia workstation are a readily available functioning self-inflating resuscitation bag (SIRB) and a full auxiliary tank of oxygen.

11 The low-pressure circuit (LPC) is the "vulnerable area" of the anesthesia workstation because it is most subject to breakage and leaks. The LPC is located downstream from all anesthesia machine safety features except the oxygen analyzer (or the ratio controller in some machines), and it is the portion of the machine where a leak is most likely to go unrecognized if an inappropriate LPC leak test is performed. Leaks in the LPC can cause delivery of a hypoxic or subanesthetic mixture, leading to hypoxic injury or awareness during anesthesia.

12 Because some GE Healthcare anesthesia machines have a one-way check valve in the LPC, a negative-pressure leak test is required to detect leaks in the LPC. A positive-pressure leak test will not detect leaks in the LPC of a machine with an outlet check valve.

13 Before administering an anesthetic, the circle breathing system must be checked for leaks and for correct flow. To test for leaks, the circle system is pressurized to 30-cm water pressure, and the circle system airway pressure gauge is observed (static test). To check for appropriate flow to rule out obstructions and faulty valves, the ventilator and a test lung (breathing bag) are used (dynamic test). In addition, the manual/bag circuit must be actuated by compressing the reservoir bag, in order to rule out obstructions to flow in the manual/bag mode.

14 Internal vaporizer leaks can only be detected with the vaporizer turned to the "on" position. In the "off" position, the vaporizer is excluded from the LPC.

15 Many new anesthesia workstation self-tests do not detect internal vaporizer leaks unless each vaporizer is individually turned on during repeated self-tests.

The anesthesia gas delivery system is the anesthesiologist's constant companion wherever inhaled anesthetics are delivered. A basic understanding of its anatomy and functions is essential for the safe practice of anesthesia.

Several studies have demonstrated that anesthesia practitioners' knowledge about the delivery system is often lacking, and that critical incidents related to use of the system are most commonly due to use error.[1] As the anesthesia delivery system evolves, advances in design and technology are continuously incorporated to improve patient safety and decrease the likelihood of use error. Ultimately, however, the anesthesiologist is responsible for the safety of the patient, and this responsibility requires optimal use and understanding of the safety features that are available, as well as having a backup plan in the event of a system failure.

While contemporary delivery systems may appear to differ among manufacturers, the systems for delivery of inhaled anesthetics all perform the same basic functions, have the same basic functional components, and have similar layouts. The evolution of each delivery system, even in recent years, has involved the integration of many of these similar functional components.

The basic configuration of the delivery system is as follows (Fig. 25-1):

1. The anesthesia **machine** receives gases (O_2/N_2O, air) from their sites of storage (central supply, tanks) and creates a gas mixture of known composition and flow rate that is delivered to the concentration-calibrated vaporizer which contains a potent inhaled anesthetic in liquid form.
2. The **vaporizer** converts the liquid anesthetic to a gas and adds the agent in a controlled concentration to the gas mixture, together forming the fresh gas mixture of known flow rate and composition, termed the fresh gas flow.
3. The fresh gas flow is delivered to the **patient breathing circuit**. This is an isolated environment from which the patient makes respiratory exchange. By controlling the composition of the inspired gas and ventilatory parameters, the patient's PaO_2, $PaCO_2$, and Pagent can be controlled. The partial pressure of the inspired (and thereby arterial) agent (Pagent) determines the depth of anesthesia.
4. **Ventilatory exchange** with the breathing circuit may be spontaneous, assisted, or controlled by a mechanical ventilator (bellows, piston, impeller, jet).
5. Since fresh gas flow into the circuit is continuous, a similar flow of gas leaves the circuit and is collected in the **waste gas scavenging system.** The only instance when this does not occur is when the fresh gas that is delivered is just

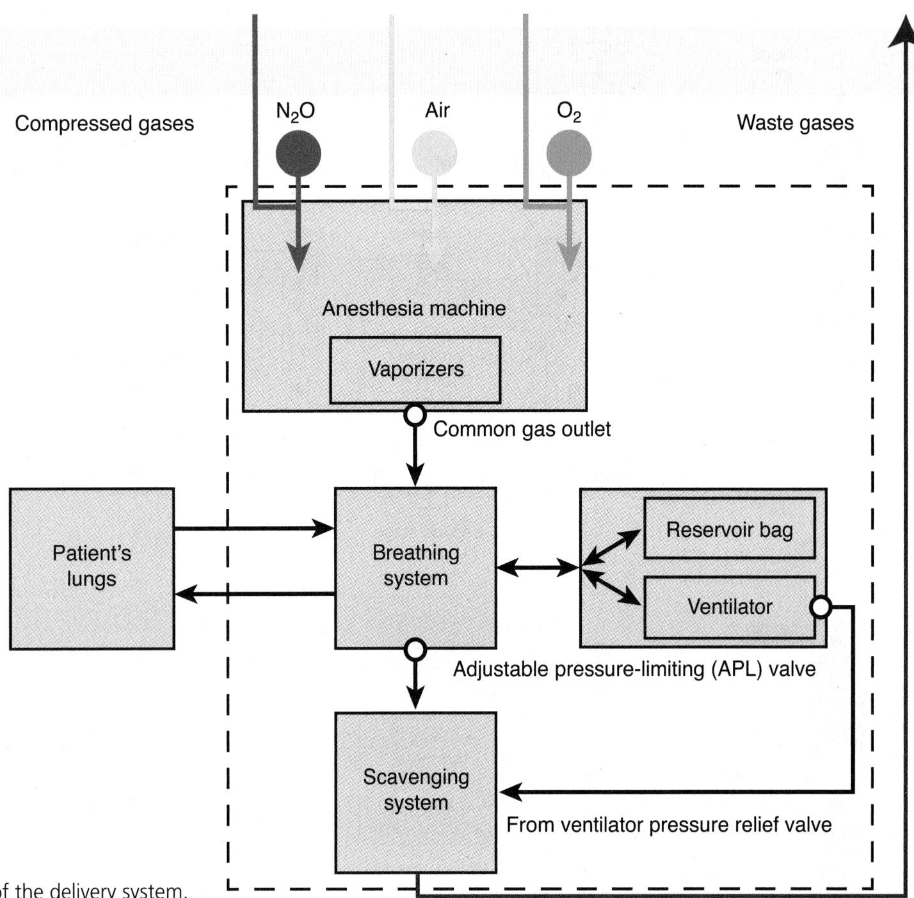

Figure 25-1 The basic configuration of the delivery system.

sufficient to meet the patient's oxygen and anesthetic gas requirements.

The term "anesthesia machine" was often used to describe the combination of the above components, but as they are now integrated, the term "workstation" is preferred. The anesthesia workstation, as defined by the International Standards Organization, is a system for administering anesthetics to patients consisting of an anesthesia gas delivery system, an anesthetic breathing system, required monitoring equipment, alarm systems, and protection devices.[2] The protection devices are designed to protect the patient from hazardous output due to incorrect delivery of energy (i.e., pressure) or substances (agent or gases).

In this chapter, the anesthesia workstation is examined piece by piece. The normal operation, function, and integration of major anesthesia workstation subsystems are described. In addition, the potential problems and hazards associated with the various components of the anesthesia delivery system, and the appropriate preoperative checks that may help to detect and prevent such problems, are presented.

The Anatomy of an Anesthesia Workstation

A schematic of a generic two-gas anesthesia machine is shown in Figure 25-2. The pressures within the anesthesia machine can be divided into three circuits: a high-, an intermediate-, and a low-pressure circuit (LPC). The *high-pressure circuit* is confined to the cylinders and the cylinder primary pressure regulators. For oxygen, the pressure range of the high-pressure circuit extends from a high of 2,200 pounds per square inch gauge pressure (psig) to 45 psig, which is the regulated cylinder pressure.* For nitrous oxide in the high-pressure circuit, pressures range from a high of 750 psig in the cylinder to a low of 45 psig. The *intermediate-pressure circuit* begins at the regulated cylinder supply sources at a pressure of 45 psig, includes the pipeline sources at 50 to 55 psig, and extends to the gas flow control valves. Depending on the manufacturer and specific machine design, second-stage pressure regulators may be used to decrease pipeline supply pressures to the flow control valves to even lower pressures such as 14 psig or 26 psig within the intermediate-pressure circuit.[3,4] Finally, the LPC extends from the flow control valves to the common gas outlet. The LPC includes the flow tubes (rotameters) or other flow control system, vaporizer manifold, vaporizers, and the one-way outlet check valve used on some GE Healthcare workstations.

Oxygen, nitrous oxide, and medical air can be supplied to the workstation from two sources: a pipeline supply source and a cylinder supply source (1 Video 25-1). In most operating rooms, the pipeline supply source is the primary gas source for the workstation. The hospital pipeline supplies gases at approximately 50 psig, which is the normal working pressure of most workstations. The cylinder supply source serves as a backup if the pipeline supply fails or acts as the primary supply if the

*Gauge pressure is the pressure above atmospheric pressure. Atmospheric pressure at sea level is 14.7 pounds per square inch absolute (psia). Thus, in absolute pressure terms, 45 psig would be 59.7 psia.

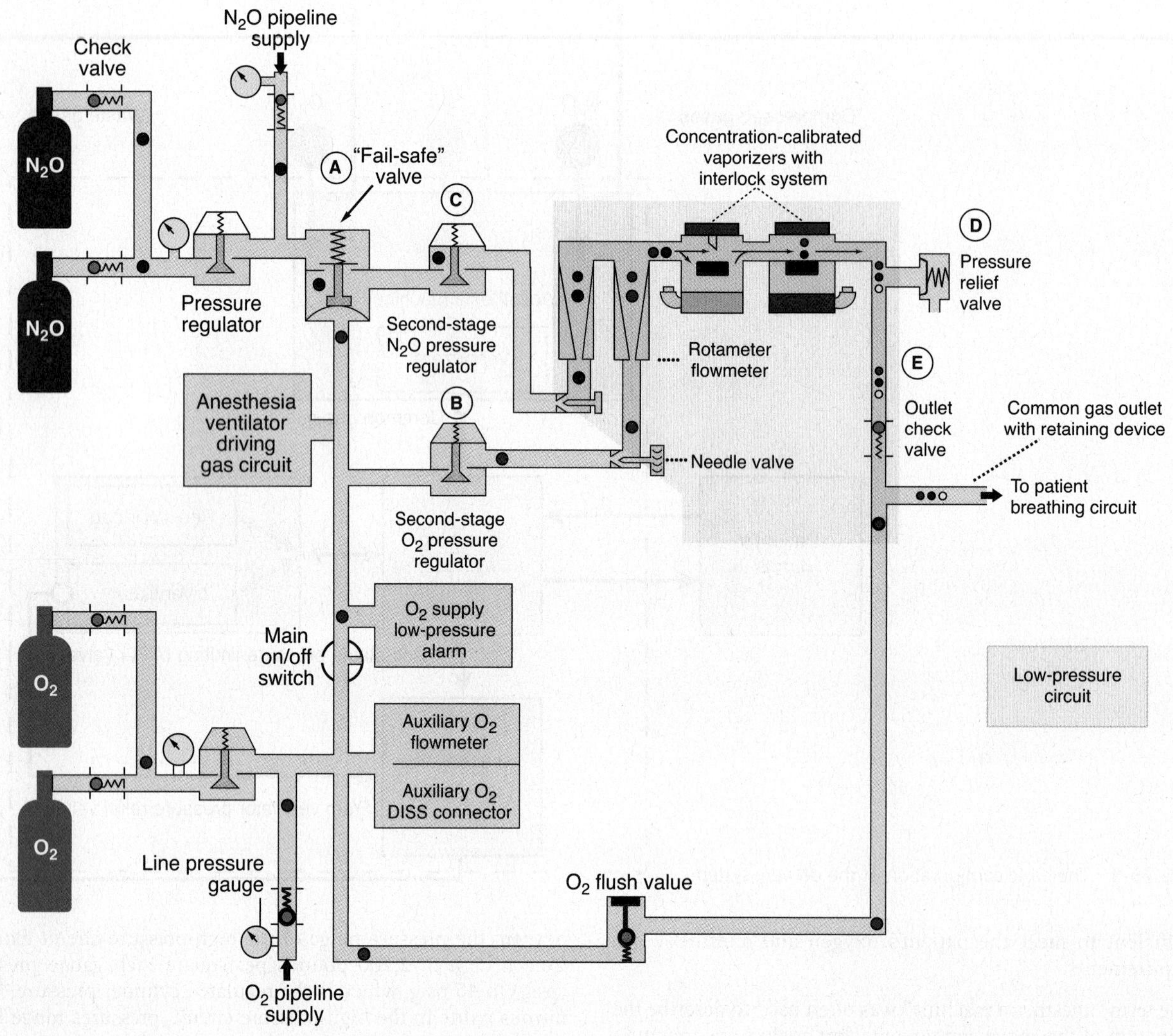

Figure 25-2 Diagram of a generic two-gas anesthesia machine. (Adapted from Check-Out, *A Guide for Preoperative Inspection of an Anesthesia Machine*. American Society of Anesthesiologists; 1987.)

workstation is used in a location that lacks pipeline-supplied gases. As previously described, the oxygen cylinder source is regulated from 2,200 psig to approximately 45 psig, and the nitrous oxide cylinder source is regulated from 745 psig to approximately 45 psig.[5]

A safety device traditionally referred to as the *fail-safe* valve (and currently more appropriately termed the "*oxygen failure cutoff valve*") is located downstream from the nitrous oxide supply source. It serves as an interface between the oxygen and nitrous oxide supply sources. This valve shuts off, or proportionally decreases, the supply of nitrous oxide if the oxygen supply pressure decreases. Contemporary workstations have a device to monitor the oxygen supply pressure. A high-priority alarm is actuated when a decreasing oxygen supply pressure reaches a predetermined threshold, such as 30 psig.

Some GE Healthcare workstations have a second-stage pressure regulator for oxygen that is located downstream from the oxygen supply source in the intermediate-pressure circuit. It is adjusted to a precise pressure level, such as 14 psig. This regulator supplies a constant pressure to the oxygen flow control valve regardless of fluctuating oxygen pipeline pressures. The flow from the oxygen flow control valve will be maintained at a constant, provided that its oxygen supply pressure is greater than 14 psig.

The flow control valves represent an important anatomic landmark within the anesthesia workstation because they separate the intermediate-pressure circuit from the LPC (2 Video 25-2). The LPC is the part of the machine that lies downstream from the flow control valves. The operator regulates flow entering the LPC by adjusting the flow control valves. The oxygen and nitrous oxide flow control valves are linked mechanically or pneumatically by a proportioning system to prevent unintended delivery of a hypoxic mixture. After leaving the rotameter tubes or other gas flow control system, the mixture of gases enters a common manifold and may be directed to a concentration-calibrated vaporizer. Precise amounts of potent inhaled volatile anesthetic can be added, depending on vaporizer concentration control setting. The total fresh gas flow (FGF) plus the anesthetic vapor then flow toward the common gas outlet. Some GE machines have a one-way check valve located in the mixed-gas line between the vaporizers and the common gas outlet. Its purpose is to prevent back flow into the vaporizer during positive-pressure ventilation, therefore minimizing the effects of downstream intermittent pressure fluctuations on inhaled anesthetic concentration 1 (see Vaporizers: Intermittent Back Pressure). The presence or absence of this check valve profoundly influences which preoperative leak test (i.e., positive vs. negative pressure) is indicated (see Checkout of the Anesthesia Workstation). The oxygen flush connection joins the mixed-gas line between the one-way check valve (when present) and the machine common gas outlet. When the oxygen flush valve is activated, oxygen (without any other gases) flows directly to the common gas outlet at a rate of 35 to 75 L/min and, in the absence of a dedicated pressure regulator, potentially at a pressure of 55 psig.

Pipeline Supply Source

Most hospitals have a central piping system to deliver medical gases including oxygen, nitrous oxide, air, and carbon dioxide to outlets in the operating room (NICV 25-1). The central piping system must supply the correct gases at the appropriate pressure for the anesthesia workstation to function properly. Unfortunately, this does not always occur. In 2002, a large medical center with a huge cryogenic bulk oxygen storage system was not immune to component failures that contributed to a critical oxygen pipeline supply failure.[6] In this case, a faulty joint ruptured at the bottom of the primary cryogenic oxygen storage tank, releasing 8,000 gallons of liquid oxygen to flood the surrounding area, and compromised oxygen delivery to the medical center.

In a survey of approximately 200 hospitals in 1976, 31% reported difficulties with pipeline systems.[7] The most common problem was inadequate oxygen pressure, followed by excessive pipeline pressures. The most devastating reported hazard, however, was accidental crossing of oxygen and nitrous oxide pipelines, which has led to many deaths. This problem caused 23 deaths in a newly constructed wing of a general hospital in Sudbury, Ontario, during a 5-month period,[8] and in 2002, 2 hypoxic deaths were reported in New Haven, Connecticut, that were attributed to an altered oxygen flowmeter that was connected to a wall supply source for nitrous oxide.[9]

2 In the event that a pipeline crossover is suspected, the workstation user must immediately take two corrective actions. First, the backup oxygen cylinder should be turned on. Then, the pipeline supply must be disconnected. This second step is mandatory because the machine will preferentially use the potentially inappropriate (i.e., wrong gas) 50 psig pipeline supply source instead of the lower-pressure (45 psig) oxygen cylinder source if the wall supply is not disconnected. It has been reported that the importance of these actions may often not be appreciated.[10,11]

Wall Outlets

The wall outlet connections for pipeline gases are gas specific (Fig. 25-3). If they are "quick connect" fittings, then they are gas specific *within the same manufacturer*. For example, a wall oxygen outlet made by Ohmeda will not accept an oxygen connector made by Chemetron, even though the gas is the same. This can create problems if outlets and connectors by more than one manufacturer exist in the same facility.[12] Many institutions seeking to create uniformity use nationally standardized Diameter Index Safety System (DISS) threaded connections. The DISS provides threaded, noninterchangeable connections for medical gas lines, which minimizes the risk of misconnection. Regardless of which type of gas-specific connector (DISS or "quick connect") exists at the wall end of the hose conducting gas to the anesthesia machine, the gas enters the anesthesia machine through DISS inlet connections (Fig. 25-4). A pressure gauge measures the pipeline gas pressure when the machine is connected to a pipeline supply. A check valve is located downstream from the inlet to prevent reverse flow of gases from the machine to the pipeline or the atmosphere.

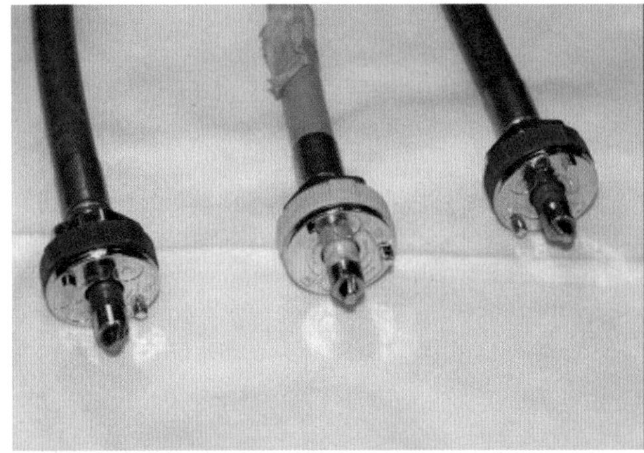

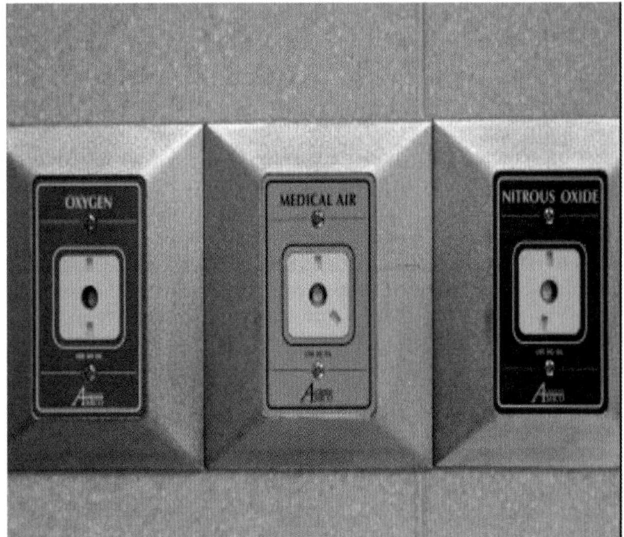

Figure 25-3 Gas-specific wall outlet connections for pipeline gases.

Cylinder Supply Source

Anesthesia workstations have backup E-cylinders for use when a pipeline supply source is not available or if the pipeline system fails. Anesthesia providers can easily become complacent and falsely assume that backup gas cylinders are, in fact, present on the anesthesia workstation, and further, if present, that they contain an adequate supply of compressed gas. The preuse checklist should contain steps that confirm both their presence and their status.

Medical gases supplied in E-cylinders are attached to the anesthesia machine via the hanger yoke assembly (Fig. 25-5). The hanger yoke assembly orients and supports the cylinder, provides a gas-tight seal (using a washer called a Bodok seal between tank and hanger yoke), and ensures a unidirectional flow of gases into the machine. Each hanger yoke is equipped with the Pin Index Safety System (PISS). The PISS is a safeguard introduced to eliminate cylinder interchanging and the possibility of accidentally placing the incorrect gas on a yoke designed to accommodate another gas. Two metal pins on the yoke assembly are arranged so that they project into corresponding holes in the cylinder valve (Fig. 25-5). Each gas or combination of gases has a specific and unique pin arrangement.[13] It is generally assumed that in the United States, all

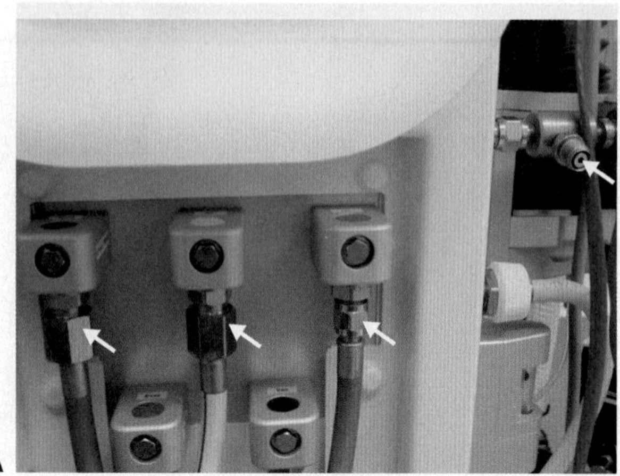

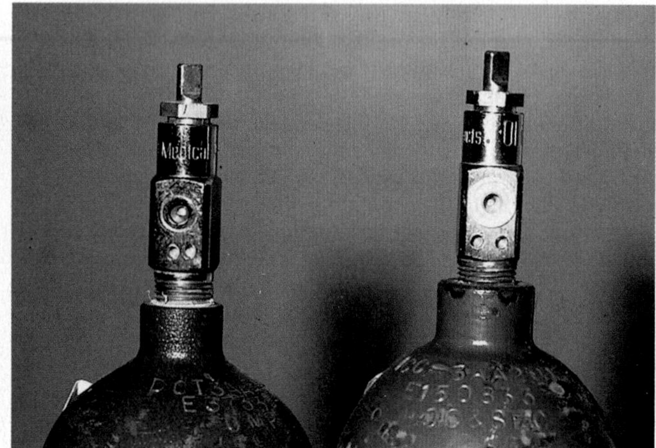

Figure 25-4 **A:** DISS connectors (*white arrows*). **B:** Note difference in PISS connectors for oxygen and nitrous oxide.

oxygen tanks are green in color and that the medical gas PISS will ensure that only an oxygen tank can be mounted in the hanger yoke for oxygen. However, there is no U.S. Food and Drug Administration standard for cylinder colors, so it is important to read the tank label.[14] A failure of the PISS, and failure of medical staff to properly identify E-cylinder contents, was the cause of an intraoperative fire during laparoscopy.[15] A mixture of CO_2 (14%) and oxygen (86%) was utilized rather than 100% CO_2. The wrong tank was able to be connected despite the PISS because all tanks containing more than 7% CO_2 have the same pin configuration.

Once the cylinders are turned on, compressed gases may pass from their respective high-pressure cylinder sources into the anesthesia workstation (Fig. 25-2). A check valve is located downstream from each cylinder if a double-yoke assembly is used. This check valve serves several functions. First, it minimizes gas transfer from a cylinder at high pressure to one with a lower pressure. Second, it allows an empty cylinder to be exchanged for a full one while gas flow continues from the other cylinder into the machine with minimal loss of gas or supply pressure. Third, it minimizes leakage from an open cylinder to the atmosphere if one cylinder is absent. A cylinder supply pressure gauge is located downstream from the check valves. The gauge indicates the pressure in the cylinder with the higher pressure when two reserve cylinders of the same gas are opened at the same time. In contemporary electronic workstations, gas pressures are measured by transducers and displayed on the checkout screen.

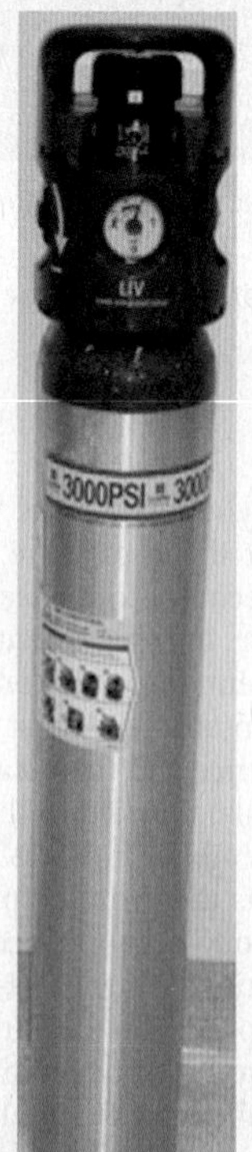

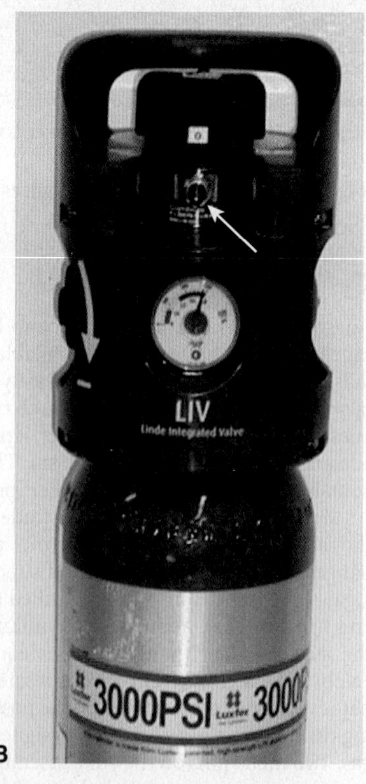

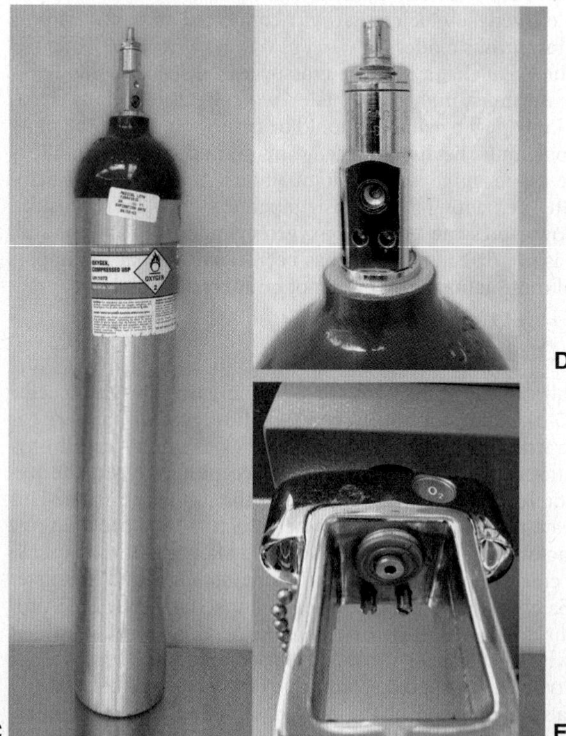

Figure 25-5 **A:** 3,000 psig E-cylinder with Linde Integrated Valve, LIV (Linde Gas North America LLC). **B:** The LIV permits adjustable flows of ¼ to 25 L/min from the low-pressure nozzle (*straight white arrow*). There is also a high-pressure regulator that can supply oxygen at 50 psig via a DISS connector (see Figure 25-6A). **C:** Standard E-cylinder. **D:** Pin-index safety system (PISS) in oxygen tank valve. **E:** Hanger yoke for oxygen tank.

Each cylinder supply source has a pressure-reducing valve known as the cylinder pressure regulator. It reduces the high and variable storage pressure present in a cylinder to a lower, more constant pressure suitable for use in the anesthesia workstation. The oxygen cylinder pressure regulator reduces the oxygen cylinder pressure from approximately 2,000 psig to approximately 45 psig. The nitrous oxide cylinder pressure regulator receives pressure of up to 745 psig and reduces it to approximately 45 psig.

The gas supply cylinder valves should be turned off when not in use, except during the preoperative machine preuse checkout. If the cylinder supply valves are left open, the reserve cylinder supply can be silently depleted whenever the pressure inside the machine decreases to a value lower than the regulated cylinder pressure. For example, oxygen pressure within the machine can decrease below 45 psig with oxygen flushing or possibly even during the use of a pneumatically driven ventilator, particularly at high inspiratory flow rates. In addition, the pipeline supply pressures of all gases can fall to less than 45 psig if problems exist in the central piping system. If the cylinders are left open when this occurs, they will eventually become depleted and no reserve supply may be available if a complete central pipeline failure were to occur.

The amount of time that an anesthesia machine can operate from the E-cylinder supply is important knowledge. This is particularly true now that anesthesia is being provided more frequently in office-based and in remote hospital settings (outside the operating room) where pipeline oxygen may not be available. Oxygen can exist only in gaseous form at room temperature. It obeys Boyle's law, which states that for a fixed mass of gas at constant temperature, the product of pressure times volume is constant ($P1 \times V1 = P2 \times V2$).[16] The volume of oxygen available from the cylinder is directly proportional to the cylinder pressure.

An E-cylinder has an internal volume of 4.8 L, and, when "full," is pressurized to approximately 2,000 psig. Since psig is the pressure measured in excess of atmospheric pressure (14.7 psia, pounds per square inch absolute pressure), the cylinder pressure is 2,014.7 psia. Applying Boyle's Law (3 Video 25-3):

$$2{,}014.7 \times 4.8 = 14.7 \times V2$$

Therefore, V2, the volume of oxygen available from a "full" E-cylinder at 1 atm is:

$$(2{,}014.7 \times 4.8)/14.7 = 658\,\text{L}.$$

The following equation has been proposed to help estimate the remaining time that oxygen can be delivered at a given flow rate[17]:

$$\text{Approx. remaining time (hrs)} = \text{Oxygen cylinder pressure (psig)}/(200 \times \text{oxygen flow rate [L/min]})$$

For example, an E-cylinder of oxygen with a pressure of 1,000 psig, used at an oxygen flow rate of 5 L/min would be depleted in

$$[1{,}000/(200 \times 5)] \approx 1 \text{ hour}$$

It should be noted that this calculation will provide only a gross estimate of remaining time and may not be exact. Furthermore, users should be cautioned that use of a pneumatically driven mechanical ventilator will dramatically increase oxygen utilization rates and decrease the remaining time until the cylinder is depleted.[18,19] Use of spontaneous or manual ventilation, with low FGF rates in a circle system with CO_2 absorption, will significantly reduce oxygen consumption from an E-cylinder if this is the only source of oxygen available. Because electrically powered piston-type anesthesia ventilators, such as those found in the Dräger Fabius and Apollo workstations, do not impact oxygen usage rates, they may be preferable to conventional gas-driven ventilators in practice settings where the supply of compressed gas cylinders may be limited.

An integrated valve and regulator for E-cylinders of oxygen is available that permits controlled delivery of oxygen via a nozzle at flows of 25 L/min or less for patient transport (Figs. 25-5 and 25-6). The tank regulator also permits delivery of oxygen at 50 psig from a DISS connection (Fig. 25-5B). If the oxygen hose from the anesthesia machine is connected to a central source (e.g., at the wall) via a DISS connector, and that central source becomes unavailable, then the machine hose can be easily connected to the tank's DISS connector and provide a backup supply of oxygen (Fig. 25-6). E-cylinders for oxygen and nitrous oxide with their distinct PISS are shown in Figure 25-4.

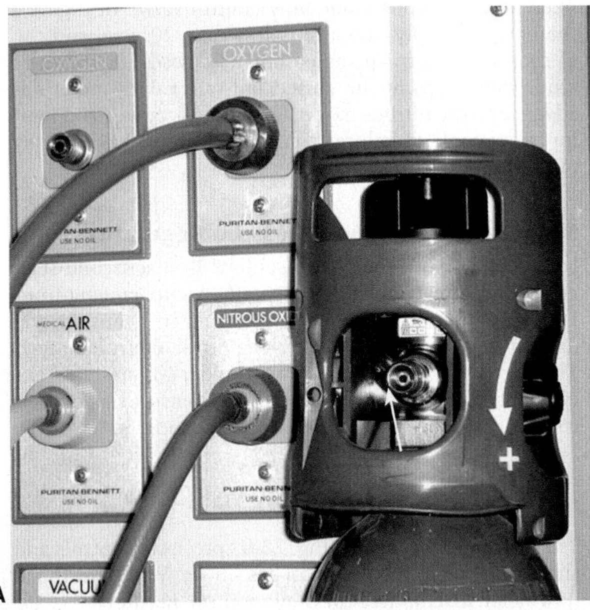

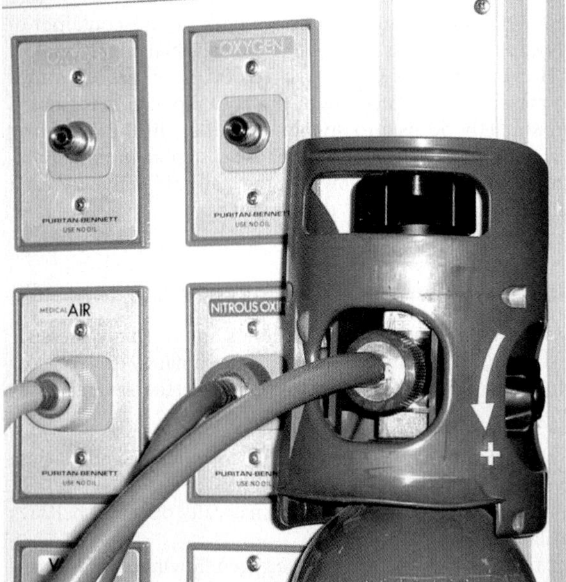

Figure 25-6 3,000 psig E-cylinder valve showing 50 psig DISS connection (*arrow*) (**A**) that could be connected to the machine oxygen hose if wall oxygen supply fails (**B**).

Nitrous Oxide

Nitrous oxide (N_2O) can be supplied to the anesthesia machine from the pipeline system at a pressure of approximately 50 psig or from a backup E-cylinder in the N_2O hanger yoke. N_2O has a molecular weight of 44 atomic mass units (AMU) and a boiling point of −88°C at 760 mmHg (14.7 psia) pressure.[20] The critical temperature (CT) is the highest temperature at which a gas can exist in liquid form. The CT of N_2O is 36.5°C (critical pressure: 1,054 psig); therefore, N_2O can exist as a liquid at room temperature (20°C). E-cylinders of N_2O are factory filled to 90% to 95% capacity with liquid N_2O. Above the liquid in the tank is N_2O vapor. Because the liquid agent is in equilibrium with its vapor or gas phase, the pressure exerted by the gaseous N_2O is its *saturated vapor pressure* (SVP) at the ambient temperature. At 20°C, the SVP of N_2O is 750 psig.

A full E-tank of N_2O generates approximately 1,600 L of gas at 1 atm pressure at sea level (14.7 psia). As long as some liquid N_2O is present in the tank and the ambient temperature remains at 20°C, the pressure in the N_2O tank will remain at 750 psig, which is the SVP of N_2O at 20°C. The volume of N_2O gas available from a tank therefore *cannot* be determined by reference to the N_2O tank pressure gauge. It must be determined by weighing the tank and subtracting the weight of the empty tank (44 g of N_2O equates to 24 L of gas at 1 atm pressure). Once all the liquid N_2O has been used and the tank contains only vapor, the pressure in the tank will begin to decrease as nitrous oxide is used. However, because N_2O is a vapor and not a gas, it *does not* obey Boyle's law and the volume of nitrous oxide remaining in the tank cannot be calculated from the tank pressure gauge. When the last drop of liquid N_2O has just evaporated, nearly one-quarter of a full cylinder remains (i.e., ~400 L).[21] From then on, as N_2O continues to be utilized, the tank pressure gauge reading will fall.

Nitrous oxide from the tank supply enters the N_2O hanger yoke at pressures of up to 750 psig (at 20°C) and then passes through a regulator that reduces this pressure to 40 to 45 psig (Fig. 25-2). The PISS is designed to ensure that only an N_2O tank may hang in an N_2O hanger yoke. As with oxygen, a check valve in each yoke prevents the back leakage of N_2O if no tank is hanging in the yoke.

The N_2O pipeline is supplied from a bulk storage container of liquid N_2O or from banks of large N_2O tanks, usually H-cylinders. (Each H-cylinder of N_2O evolves 16,000 L of gas at atmospheric pressure.) The pressure in the N_2O pipeline is regulated to approximately 50 psig to supply the outlets in the operating room. Having entered the anesthesia workstation intermediate-pressure system, N_2O must flow past the "fail-safe" valve to reach the N_2O flow control system.

Machine Intermediate-Pressure System

Having entered the anesthesia machine's intermediate-pressure system from the pipeline supply at approximately 50 psig, or from the tank supply at 45 psig, oxygen can take several paths (Fig. 25-2):

1. To the DISS auxiliary oxygen takeoff, to which a Sanders-type jet ventilating system can be connected
2. To supply the drive gas for a pneumatically powered bellows ventilator
3. Via a regulator and an auxiliary oxygen flowmeter to be connected to a nasal cannula, self-inflating manual resuscitation device, or other appropriate devices
4. To the oxygen low-pressure alarm sensor
5. To the pressure-sensitive shutoff ("fail-safe") valve
6. To the oxygen flush control valve
7. To the oxygen flowmeter (in some machines via a second-stage regulator)

Oxygen Supply Pressure Failure Safety Devices

Contemporary anesthesia machines have a number of safety devices that act together in a cascade manner to minimize the risk of delivery of a hypoxic gas mixture as oxygen pressure decreases. Several of these devices are described in the following sections.

Pneumatic and Electronic Alarm Devices

Some older anesthesia machines have a pneumatic alarm device that provides an audible warning when the oxygen supply pressure decreases to a predetermined threshold value such as 30 psig. Contemporary workstations use pressure transducers and electronic alarms.

Oxygen Failure Cutoff ("Fail-Safe") Valves

An oxygen failure cutoff valve is present in the gas line supplying each of the flowmeters except oxygen. Controlled by oxygen supply pressure, the valve shuts off (or proportionally decreases) the supply pressure of all other gases (nitrous oxide, and in some machines air) as the oxygen supply pressure decreases. Unfortunately, the misnomer "fail-safe" has led to the misconception that the valve prevents administration of a hypoxic mixture. This is not the case.

GE machines are equipped with a fail-safe valve known as the pressure-sensor shutoff valve. On older machines, this valve operates in a threshold manner and is either open or closed. Oxygen supply pressure opens the valve, and the valve return spring closes the valve. Figure 25-7 shows a nitrous oxide pressure-sensor shutoff valve with a threshold pressure of 20 psig. In Figure 25-7A, an oxygen supply pressure greater than 20 psig is exerted on the mobile diaphragm. This pressure moves the piston and pin upward and the valve opens. Nitrous oxide flows freely to the nitrous oxide flow control valve. In Figure 25-7B, the oxygen supply pressure is less than 20 psig, and the force of the valve return spring completely closes the valve. Nitrous oxide flow stops at the closed fail-safe valve, and it does not advance to the nitrous oxide flow control valve. See Figure 25-8 for an example of failure of fail-safe valve to prevent a hypoxic mixture.

Second-Stage Oxygen Pressure Regulator

Some contemporary GE workstations have a second-stage oxygen pressure regulator set at a specific value, ranging from 12 to 19 psig. Output from the oxygen flowmeter is constant when the oxygen supply pressure exceeds the threshold (minimum) value. The pressure-sensor shutoff valve of older GE machines is set at a higher threshold value (20 to 30 psig) to ensure that oxygen is the last gas flowing if oxygen pressure failure occurs.

Flowmeter Assemblies

The flowmeter assembly (Fig. 25-9) precisely controls and measures gas flow to the common gas outlet. With traditional glass flowmeter assemblies, the flow control needle valve regulates the amount of flow that enters a tapered, transparent flow tube known as a Thorpe tube. The tube is tapered such that it has

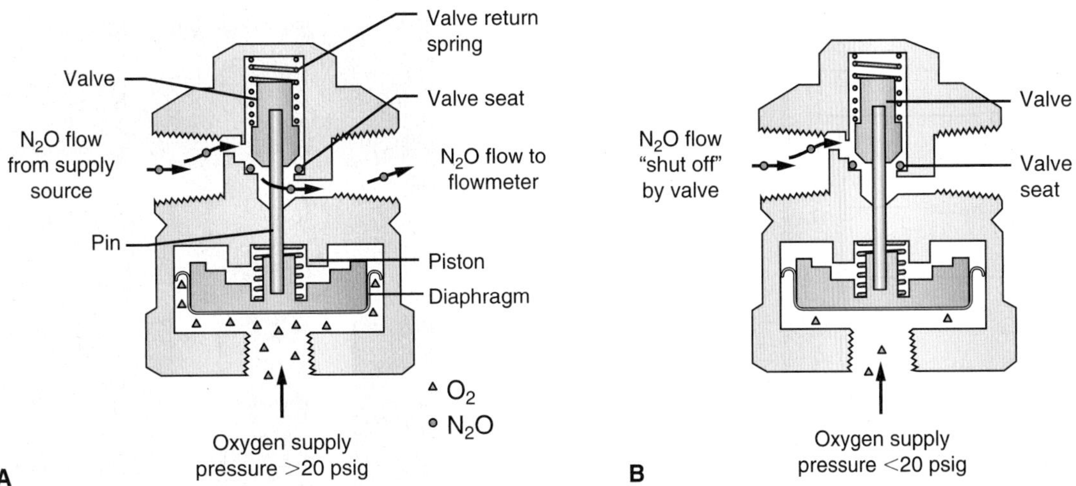

Figure 25-7 Pressure-sensor shutoff valve. **A:** The valve is open because the oxygen supply pressure is greater than the threshold value of 20 psig. **B:** The valve is closed because of inadequate oxygen pressure. (Adapted from Bowie E, Huffman LM. *The Anesthesia Machine: Essentials for Understanding*. Ohmeda, a division of BOC Healthcare, Inc.; 1985.)

a small cross-sectional area at its lower (low flow) end, and a larger cross-sectional area at its upper (high flow) end. A mobile indicator float inside the flow tube indicates the amount of flow passing through the associated flow control valve. The quantity of flow is indicated on a scale associated with the flow tube. Many contemporary workstations have replaced the conventional glass flow tubes with electronic flow sensors that measure the flow of the individual gases and display flows on a computer screen as virtual flowmeters. The flow rate data are then presented in numerical format, graphical format, or a combination of the two on the workstation screen (Fig. 25-10). The integration of these "electronic flowmeters" is an essential step in the evolution of the anesthesia workstation to becoming fully integrated with anesthesia information management systems (AIMS).

Operating Principles of Conventional Flowmeters

Opening the flow control needle valve allows gas to travel through the space between the float and the flow tube. This space is known as the annular space (Fig. 25-11). The indicator float hovers freely in an equilibrium position where the upward force resulting from gas flow equals the downward force on the float resulting from gravity at a given flow rate. The float moves to a new equilibrium position in the tube when flow is changed. These flowmeters are

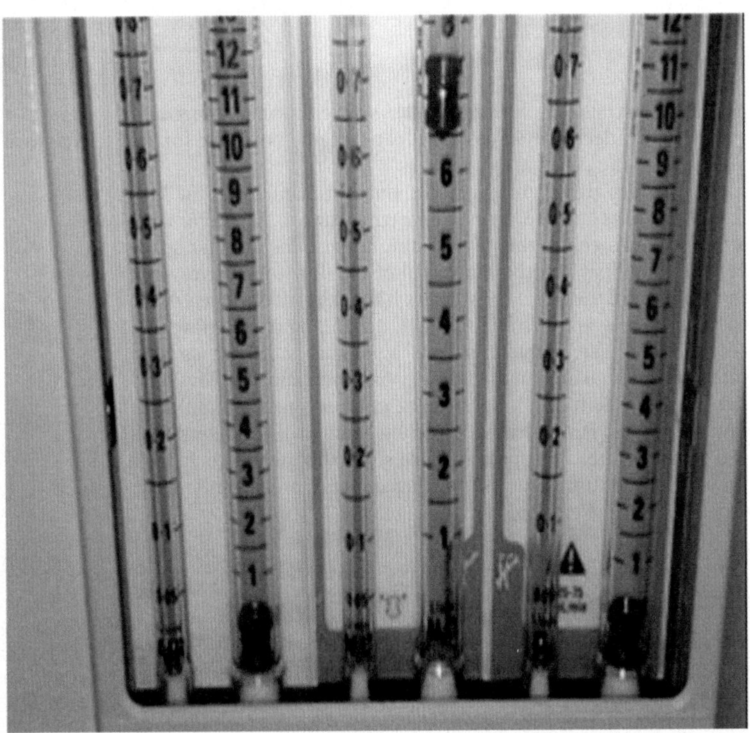

Figure 25-8 Failure of fail-safe valve to prevent a hypoxic mixture.

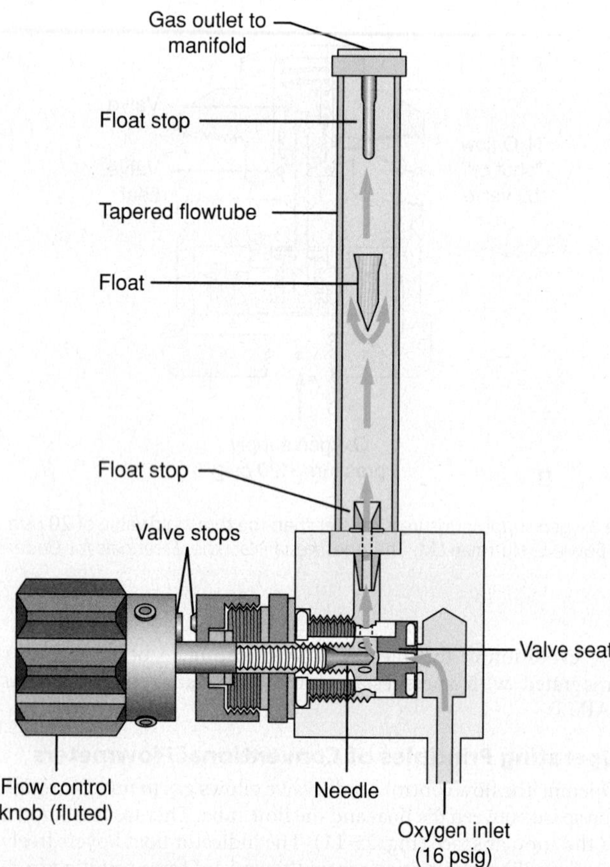

Figure 25-9 Oxygen flowmeter assembly. The oxygen flowmeter assembly is composed of the flow control valve assembly plus the flowmeter subassembly. Note that this is a GE Datex-Ohmeda design because in this figure oxygen is supplied to the flowmeter at 16 psig from a second-stage regulator. (Adapted from Bowie E, Huffman LM. *The Anesthesia Machine: Essentials for Understanding*. Ohmeda, a division of BOC Healthcare, Inc.; 1985.)

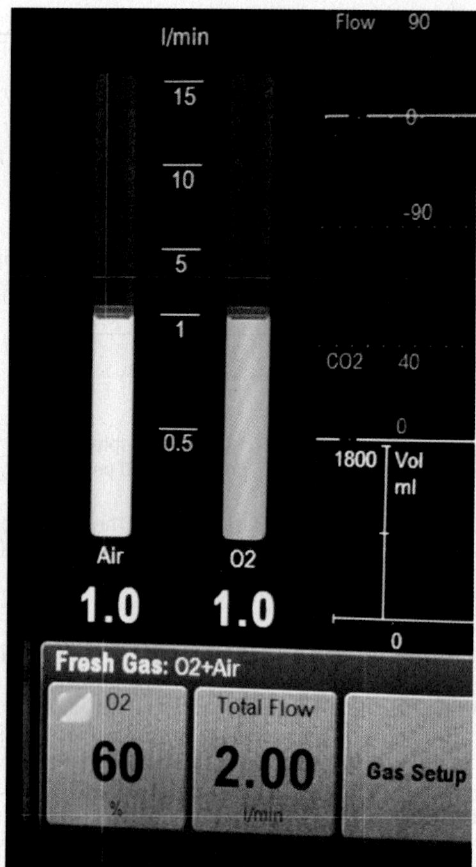

Figure 25-10 Electronic presentation of the flow rate.

described as *constant-pressure variable-orifice* flowmeters because the pressure decrease across the float remains constant for all positions in the tube.[21,22]

Flow tubes are tapered, with the smallest diameter at the bottom of the tube and the largest diameter at the top. The term *variable orifice* designates this type of unit because the annular space between the float and the inner wall of the flow tube varies with the position of the float. Flow through the constriction created by the float can be laminar or turbulent, depending on the flow rate (Fig. 25-12). The characteristics of a gas that influence its flow rate through a given constriction are viscosity (laminar flow) and density (turbulent flow). Because the annular space is tubular, at low flow rates, laminar flow is present, and *viscosity* determines the gas flow rate. The annular space simulates an orifice at high flow rates, and turbulent gas flow then depends predominantly on the *density* of the gas.

Components of the Flowmeter Assembly

Flow Control Valve Assembly

The flow control valve assembly (Fig. 25-9) consists of a flow control knob, a needle valve, a valve seat, and a pair of valve stops. The assembly can receive its pneumatic input either directly from the pipeline source (50 psig) or from a second-stage pressure regulator. The location of the needle valve in the valve seat changes to establish different orifices when the flow control valve is adjusted. Gas flow increases when the flow control valve is turned counterclockwise, and it decreases when the valve is turned clockwise. Extreme clockwise rotation may result in damage to the needle valve and valve seat; therefore, flow control valves are equipped with valve "stops" to prevent this occurrence.

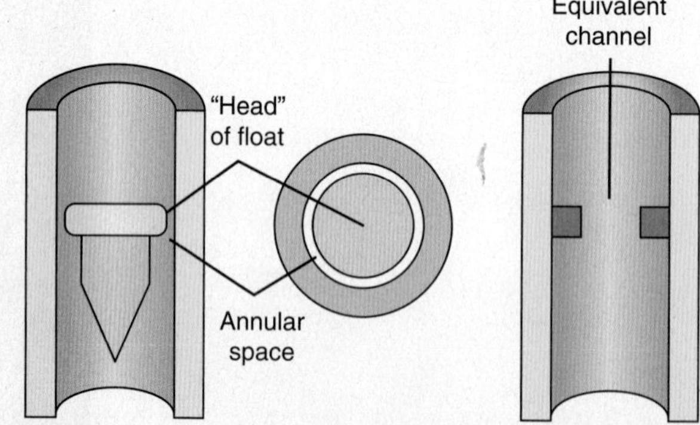

Figure 25-11 The annular space. The clearance between the head of the float and the flow tube is known as the annular space. It can be considered equivalent to a circular channel of the same cross-sectional area. (Adapted from Macintosh R, Mushin WW, Epstein HG. *Physics for the Anaesthetist*. 3rd ed. Blackwell Scientific Publications; 1963.)

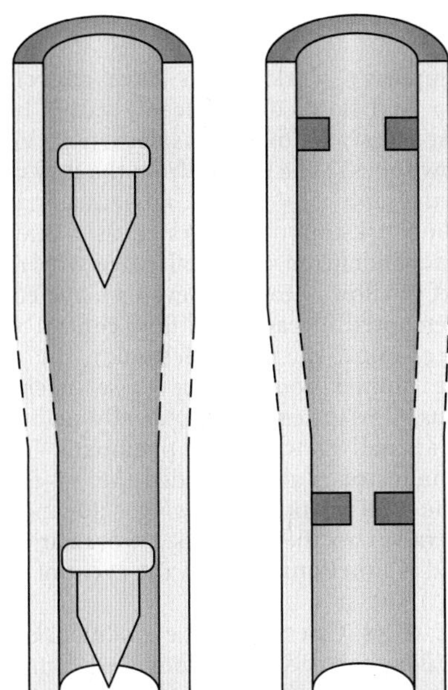

Figure 25-12 Flow tube constriction. The lower half of illustration represents the lower portion of a flow tube. The clearance between the head of the float and the flow tube is narrow. The equivalent channel is tubular because its diameter is less than its length. Viscosity is dominant in determining gas flow rate through this tubular constriction. The upper half of illustration represents the upper portion of a flow tube. The equivalent channel is orificial because its length is less than its width. Density is dominant in determining gas flow rate through this orificial constriction. (Adapted from Macintosh R, Mushin WW, Epstein HG. *Physics for the Anaesthetist*. 3rd ed. Blackwell Scientific Publications; 1963.)

Safety Features. Flow control valve assemblies have numerous safety features. The oxygen flow control knob is physically distinguishable from other gas knobs. It is distinctively fluted, projects beyond the control knobs of the other gases, and is larger in diameter than the flow control knobs of other gases. All knobs are color coded for the appropriate gas, and the chemical formula or name of the gas is permanently marked on each. Flow control knobs are recessed or protected with a shield or barrier to minimize accidental change from a preset position. If a single gas has two flow tubes, the tubes are arranged in series and are controlled by a single flow control needle valve.

In many contemporary workstations, the flowmeters have been replaced by electronic control panels that contain "soft keys" (Fig. 25-13). To adjust any gas flow, the operator must perform the following steps: (1) select and press the "soft key" to identify the gas and anesthetic agent selected; (2) turn the selector knob to adjust the desired flow level; and (3) press the selector knob again to confirm the selected flow level and anesthetic agent (see Electronic Gas Flow Control section).

Flowmeter Subassembly

The flowmeter subassembly (Fig. 25-9) consists of the flow tube, the indicator float with float stops, and the indicator scale.

Flow Tubes. Contemporary flow tubes are made of glass. Most have a single taper in which the inner diameter of the flow tube increases uniformly from bottom to top. Manufacturers provide double-flow tubes for oxygen and nitrous oxide to provide better visual discrimination at low flow rates. A fine flow tube indicates flow from approximately 200 mL/min to 1 L/min, and a coarse flow tube indicates flow from approximately 1 mL/min to 10 or

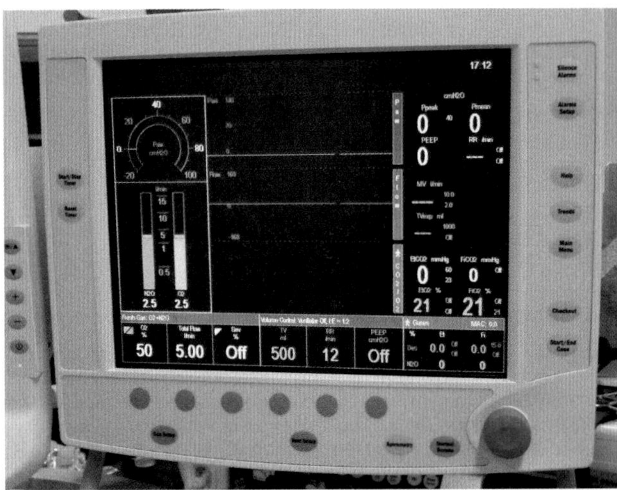

Figure 25-13 Example of an electronic control panel with "soft keys."

12 L/min. The two tubes are connected in series and supplied from a single flow control valve.

Indicator Floats and Float Stops. Anesthesia workstations with traditional flowmeters use several different types of bobbins or floats, including plumb-bob floats, rotating skirted floats, and ball floats. Flow is read at the top of plumb-bob and skirted floats and at the center of the ball on the ball-type floats. Flow tubes are equipped with float stops at the top and bottom of the tube. The upper stop prevents the float from ascending to the top of the tube and plugging the outlet. It also ensures that the float will be visible at maximum flows instead of being hidden in the manifold. The bottom float stop provides a central foundation for the indicator when the flow control valve is turned off.

Scale. The flowmeter scale can be marked directly on the flow tube or located to the right of the tube. Gradations corresponding to equal increments in flow rate are closer together at the top of the scale because the annular space increases more rapidly than does the internal diameter from bottom to top of the tube. Rib guides are used in some flow tubes with ball-type indicators to minimize this compression effect. They are tapered glass ridges that run the length of the tube. There are usually three rib guides that are equally spaced around the inner circumference of the tube. In the presence of rib guides, the annular space from the bottom to the top of the tube increases almost proportionally with the internal diameter. This results in a nearly linear scale. Rib guides are employed on many Dräger Medical flow tubes.

Problems with Flowmeters

Leaks

Flowmeter leaks are a significant hazard because the flowmeters are located downstream from all machine safety devices except the oxygen analyzer.[23] Leaks can occur at the O-ring junctions between the glass flow tubes and the metal manifold or in cracked or broken glass flow tubes, the most fragile pneumatic component of the anesthesia machine. Even though gross damage to conventional glass flow tubes is usually apparent, subtle cracks and chips may be overlooked, resulting in errors of delivered flows.[24]

Eger et al.[25] demonstrated that, in the presence of a flowmeter leak, a hypoxic mixture is less likely to occur if the oxygen flowmeter is located downstream from all other flowmeters.

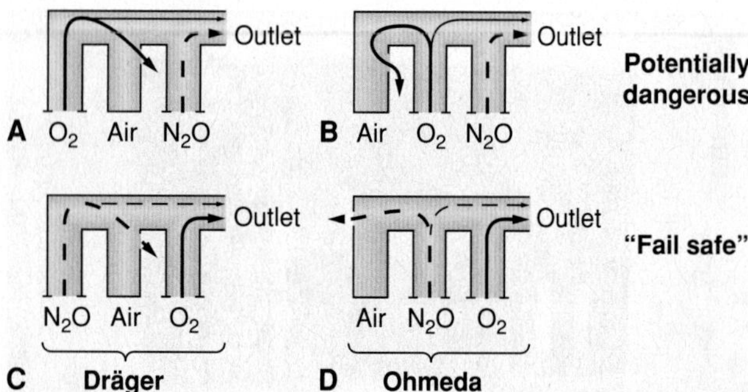

Figure 25-14 Flowmeter sequence—a potential cause of hypoxia. In the event of a flowmeter leak (in this example, air), a potentially dangerous arrangement exists when nitrous oxide is located in the downstream position (**A, B**). The safest configuration exists when oxygen is located in the downstream position (**C, D**). See text for details. (Adapted with permission from Eger EI 2nd, Hylton RR, Irwin RH, et al. Anesthetic flowmeter sequence—a cause for hypoxia. *Anesthesiology.* 1963;24:396.)

Figure 25-14 is an updated version of the figure from Eger's original publication. The unused air flow tube has a large leak. Nitrous oxide and oxygen flow rates are set at a ratio of 3:1. A potentially dangerous arrangement is shown in Figure 25-14A and B because the nitrous oxide flowmeter is located in the downstream position. A hypoxic mixture can result because a substantial portion of oxygen flow passes through the leak, and all nitrous oxide is directed to the common gas outlet. Safer configurations are shown in Figure 25-14C and D, where the oxygen flowmeter is located in the downstream position.

The above preferred arrangement is not infallible. A leak in the oxygen flow tube may result in creation of a hypoxic mixture even when oxygen is located in the downstream position (Fig. 25-15). Oxygen escapes through the leak and nitrous oxide continues to flow toward the common outlet, particularly at high ratios of nitrous oxide to oxygen flow.

Inaccuracy

Flow measurement error can occur even when flowmeters are assembled properly with appropriate components. Dirt or static electricity can cause a float to stick, and the actual flow may be higher or lower than that indicated. Sticking of the indicator float is more common in the low flow ranges because the annular space is smaller. A damaged float can cause inaccurate readings because the precise relationship between the float and the flow tube is altered. Back pressure from the breathing circuit can cause a float to drop so that it reads less than the actual flow. Finally, if flowmeters are not aligned properly in the vertical position (plumb), readings can be inaccurate because tilting distorts the annular space.

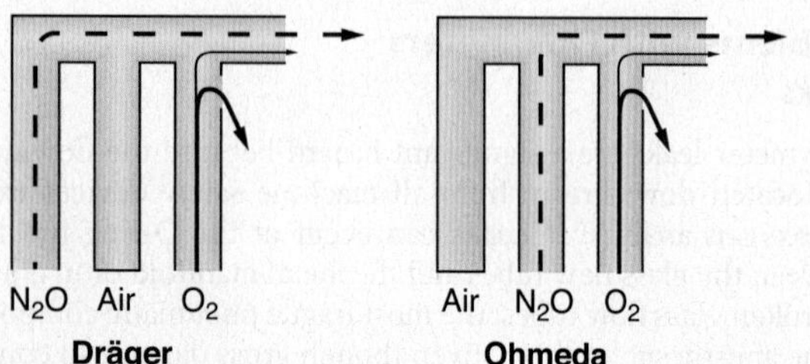

Figure 25-17 Oxygen flow tube leak. An oxygen flow tube leak can produce a hypoxic mixture regardless of flow tube arrangement. (Adapted from Brockwell RC. Inhaled anesthetic delivery systems. In: Miller RD, ed. *Anesthesia*. 6th ed. Churchill Livingstone; 2004:281. Copyright © 2004 Elsevier. With permission.)

Electronic Gas Flow Control

Many contemporary workstations have conventional flow control knobs and flow control needle valves but use electronic flow sensors and digital displays (i.e., virtual rather than glass flow tubes). The output from the flow control valve is represented graphically and/or numerically in liters per minute on the workstation's integrated user interface. These systems are dependent on electrical power to provide a precise display of gas flows. However, even when electrical power is totally interrupted, because the flow control valves themselves are mechanical (i.e., nonelectronic), the set gas flows will continue uninterrupted. Since these machines do not have individual flow tubes that physically quantify the flow of each gas, a small conventional pneumatic "fresh gas" or "total flow" indicator is also provided that gives the user an estimate of the total quantity of fresh gas flowing from all gas flow control valves to the anesthesia workstation's common gas outlet, and is functional even in the event of a total power failure (Fig. 25-16).

In the GE Aisys Carestation, the traditional manual needle valve gas flow controls and color-coded control knobs are replaced by an electronic flow control system housed in a gas mixer. Within the gas mixer are solenoid-controlled needle valves that control the flow of each gas. When a gas mixture and flows are set, the workstation computer controls the opening of each needle valve by adjusting the current flowing through each solenoid coil. Gas flows are measured downstream of the flow control valves using two separate flow sensors, the outputs of which are continuously fed back to the computer to maintain the gas flows as set by the operator.

In the GE Aisys Carestation, the controls to increase or decrease flows or agent concentration represent a departure from the traditional. The traditional needle valve gas flow controls were designed by mechanical engineers so that one turns the flow control knob counterclockwise to increase flow, by opening the valve wider. The same mechanism applies for increasing agent concentration on a variable bypass vaporizer. The Aisys Carestation controls are designed by electrical engineers where the standard is to increase the output by rotating the dial in a clockwise direction. Thus, when using the Aisys Carestation workstation, the operator must adapt to "clockwise to increase" and remember to confirm new settings; otherwise, they are not implemented. In the event the gas mixer fails, the Aisys Carestation will switch to a backup system that permits delivery of oxygen to the breathing system via an alternate oxygen flowmeter, which is a traditional mechanical needle valve and rotameter flow tube (Fig. 25-17).

Automated Fresh Gas Flow Optimization

Anesthetic gas cost and environmental impact of excessive waste anesthetic gas are important concerns.[26] The Dräger Apollo anesthesia workstation has an FGF optimization tool called the Low Flow Wizard (LFW). The LFW gives the user an indication of whether there is too much, too little, or the correct amount of FGF. It is important to understand how this tool works and to understand its limitations. Figure 25-18 shows three possible recommendations from the LFW.

The LFW determines minimum FGF by calculating the difference between inspiratory and expiratory minute volume. In addition, anesthetic uptake is calculated using inspired and expired anesthetic gas concentrations as well as N_2O and CO_2 concentrations. This algorithm is designed to err on the side of overestimation of uptake. Oxygen uptake is calculated using

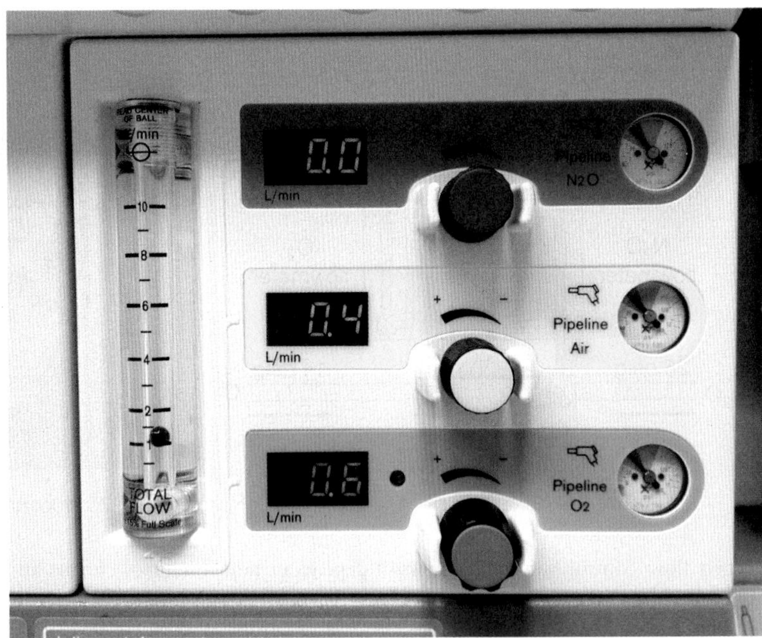

Figure 25-16 Note needle valve controls and graphical and digital flow displays on the workstation. The total gas flow rotameter continues to function if electrical power is lost.

CO_2 uptake because the gas analysis system is able to determine CO_2 concentrations with greater precision than oxygen concentrations. During laparoscopic surgery with CO_2 insufflation, if end-tidal CO_2 is increased, the calculated oxygen uptake will increase and thus the LFW will recommend higher FGF. In addition, application or removal of PEEP will transiently affect LFW calculations until gas flow dynamics reach a state of equilibrium. A simulator-based study demonstrated that use of the LFW reduced isoflurane consumption by 53% during the maintenance phase of anesthesia.[27]

GE has an optional software tool, called "ecoFLOW," to determine approximate minimum flow of O_2 required to maintain a preset FIO_2. This system (available on the Aisys CS^2 and Avance CS^2 models) also shows the approximate amount of agent used and its cost per hour. The minimum O_2 flow is calculated using patient O_2 uptake, the dilution effect of the delivered anesthetic agent, and the effects of the circle breathing system.

Proportioning Systems

Manufacturers equip anesthesia workstations with N_2O/O_2 proportioning systems designed to prevent creation and delivery of a hypoxic mixture when nitrous oxide is administered (4 Video 25-4). Nitrous oxide and oxygen are interfaced mechanically and/or pneumatically, or electronically (on the GE Aisys Carestation), so that the minimum oxygen concentration at the common gas outlet is between 23% and 25% depending on the manufacturer.

GE-Datex-Ohmeda Link-25 Proportion-Limiting Control System

Traditional GE machines use the Link-25 System. The heart of the system is the mechanical integration of the nitrous oxide and

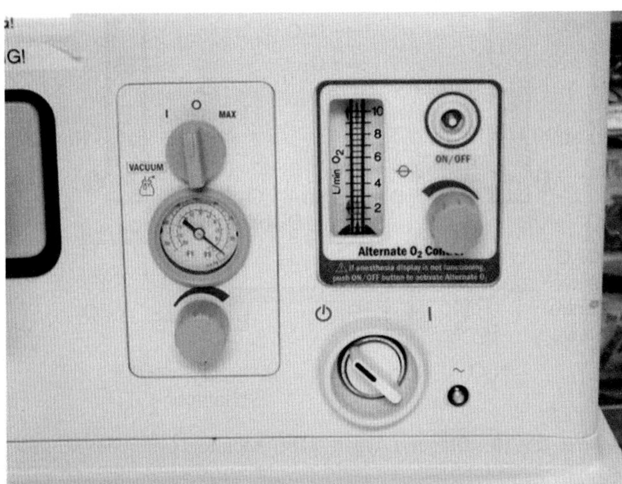

Figure 25-17 Alternate oxygen flowmeter backup system.

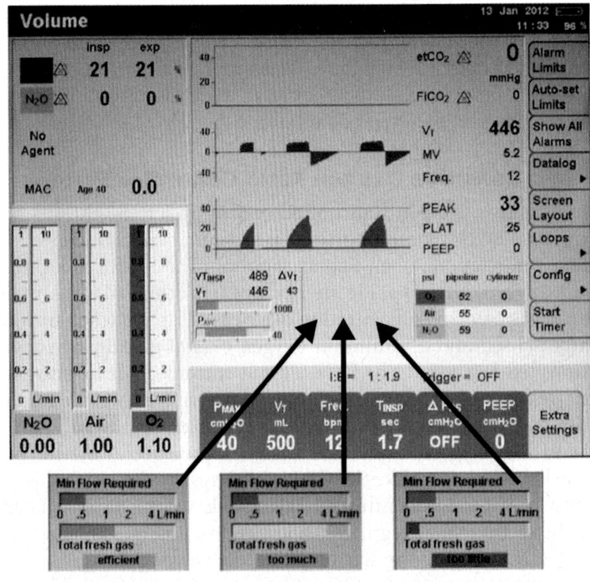

Figure 25-18 Low-flow wizard of a workstation.

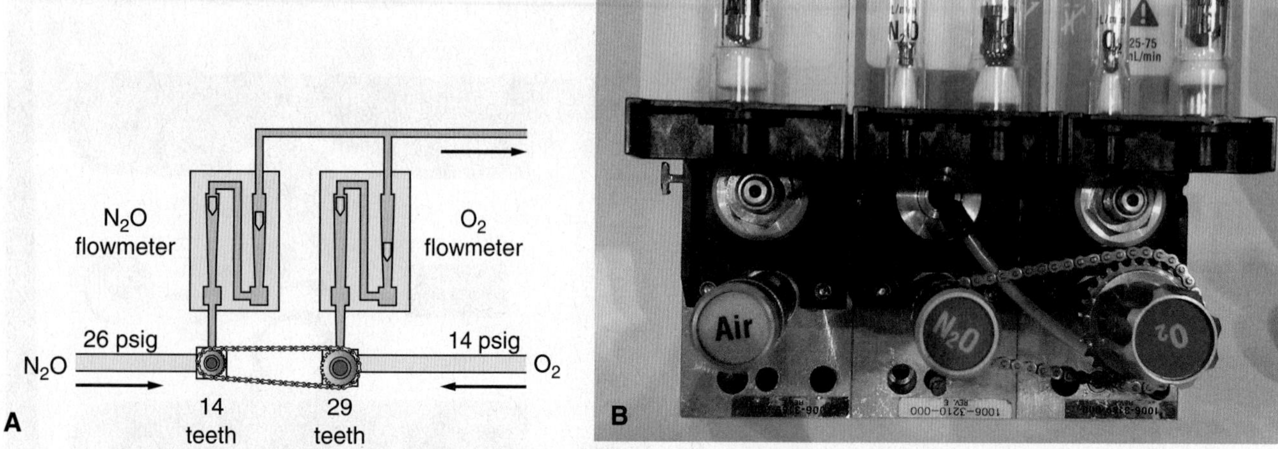

Figure 25-19 Schematic (**A**) and photo (**B**) of Ohmeda Link-25 Proportion-Limiting Control System. See text for details.

oxygen flow control valves. It allows independent adjustment of either valve, yet automatically intercedes to maintain a minimum 25% oxygen concentration with a maximum nitrous oxide–oxygen flow ratio of 3:1. The Link-25 automatically increases oxygen flow to prevent delivery of a hypoxic mixture.

Figure 25-20 illustrates the GE Link-25 System. A 14-tooth sprocket is attached to the nitrous oxide flow control valve, and a 29-tooth sprocket is attached to the oxygen flow control valve. A stainless-steel chain physically links the sprockets. When the nitrous oxide flow control valve is turned 2.09 revolutions, the oxygen flow control valve will revolve one time because of the gear ratio. The final 3:1 flow ratio occurs because the nitrous oxide flow control valve is supplied with nitrous oxide at a pressure of approximately 26 psig from a second-stage N_2O regulator, whereas the oxygen flow control valve is supplied by a second-stage regulator at 14 psig. The combination of the mechanical and pneumatic aspects of the system yields the final minimum 25% oxygen concentration. The GE Link-25 proportioning system increases oxygen flow when nitrous oxide flow would be excessive by opening the O_2 needle valve more. Conversely, if the oxygen flow is decreased such that the nitrous oxide flow would be excessive, it acts to decrease the flow of N_2O by physically decreasing the opening of the nitrous oxide needle valve. Failures of the Link-25 system have been reported that either resulted in an inability to administer oxygen without nitrous oxide or allowed creation of a hypoxic mixture.[28–31]

Dräger Sensitive Oxygen Ratio Controller System

The Sensitive Oxygen Ratio Monitor Controller (S-ORC) is the nitrous oxide:oxygen proportioning system used in Dräger anesthesia workstations (e.g., Fabius, Apollo). The S-ORC is a pneumatic oxygen–nitrous oxide interlock system designed to maintain a fresh gas oxygen concentration of at least 25 ± 3% when nitrous oxide is used and a minimum oxygen of 200 ml/min whenever nitrous oxide is used. The S-ORC limits nitrous oxide flow to prevent delivery of a hypoxic mixture by applying an opening force to the N_2O slave control valve which depends on the back-pressure of the oxygen flow versus the back pressure of the nitrous oxide flow. This is unlike the GE Link-25 system, in which the gas supply pressure to the nitrous oxide needle valve is held constant (by the second-stage regulator) and gas flow changes are made by physically changing the size of the needle valve opening.

A schematic of the S-ORC is shown in Figure 25-20. The figure shows an older version. In modern Dräger devices the S-ORC forms an autonomous compact block which also integrates the resistors which in the old versions were integrated in the flowmeters. It consists of an oxygen chamber, a nitrous oxide chamber, and a nitrous oxide slave control valve. All are interconnected by a mobile horizontal shaft. The pneumatic input into the device is from the oxygen and the nitrous oxide flowmeters. When nitrous oxide and oxygen are flowing, the resistors of the S-ORC create back pressures directed to the oxygen and nitrous oxide chambers. The value of the oxygen flow resistor is three to four times that of the nitrous oxide flow resistor, and the relative value of these resistors determines the value of the controlled fresh gas oxygen concentration. The back pressures in the oxygen and nitrous oxide chambers are applied against rubber diaphragms attached to the mobile horizontal shaft. Movement of the shaft adjusts the opening of the nitrous oxide slave control valve, which in turn adjusts the flow of the nitrous oxide.

If the oxygen flow, and therefore back pressure, is proportionally higher than the nitrous oxide back pressure, the nitrous oxide slave control valve opens more widely which results in an increase in nitrous oxide flow. As the nitrous oxide flow is increased manually, the nitrous oxide back pressure forces the shaft rightward toward the oxygen chamber. The nitrous oxide

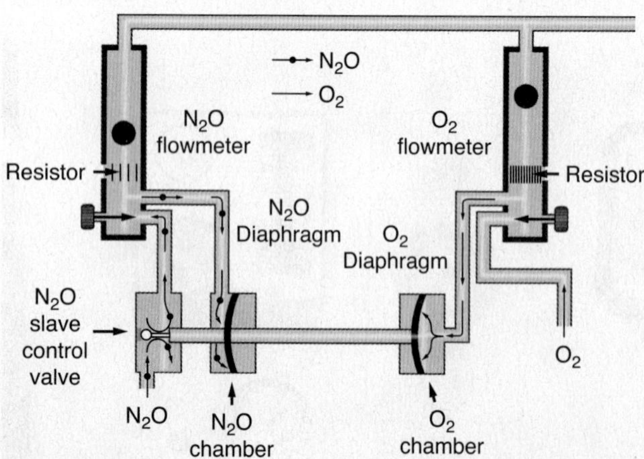

Figure 25-20 Dräger Oxygen Ratio Monitor Controller/Sensitive Oxygen Ratio Controller. See text for details. (Adapted from Schreiber P. *Safety Guidelines for Anesthesia Systems*. Telford, PA: North American Dräger; 1984.)

slave control valve opening becomes more restrictive and limits the nitrous oxide feed pressure to the flowmeter, which decreases the nitrous oxide flow. When the oxygen flow is less than 200 mL/min, the slave control valve closes completely, preventing any flow of nitrous oxide.

Figure 25-20 illustrates the action of a single S-ORC under different sets of circumstances. The back pressure exerted on the oxygen diaphragm in the upper configuration is greater than that exerted on the nitrous oxide diaphragm. This causes the horizontal shaft to move to the left, opening the nitrous oxide slave control valve. Nitrous oxide is then able to proceed to its flow control valve and out through the flowmeter. In the lower configuration, the nitrous oxide slave control valve is closed because of inadequate oxygen back pressure. To summarize, in contrast to the GE Link-25 System, which actively increases oxygen flow to maintain a fresh gas oxygen concentration 25% or higher, the Dräger S-ORC system limits nitrous oxide flow to prevent delivery of a fresh gas mixture with an oxygen concentration no higher than 25%.

Limitations

N_2O/O_2 proportioning systems are not foolproof. Workstations equipped with these systems can still deliver a hypoxic mixture under certain conditions. The following is a description of some of the situations in which this may occur.

Wrong Supply Gas

The efficacy of both the GE Link-25 and the Dräger S-ORC will be compromised if a gas other than oxygen is present in the oxygen pipeline and the machines will allow delivery of hypoxic gas mixtures. In the Link-25 System, the nitrous oxide and oxygen flow control valves will continue to be mechanically linked. Nevertheless, a hypoxic mixture can proceed to the common gas outlet. In the case of the Dräger S-ORC, the rubber diaphragm for oxygen will reflect adequate supply pressure on the oxygen side even though the incorrect gas is present, and flow of both the wrong gas plus nitrous oxide will result. The oxygen analyzer is the only workstation monitor besides an integrated multigas analyzer that would detect this condition in either system.

Defective Pneumatics or Mechanics

Normal operation of the GE Link-25 and the Dräger S-ORC is contingent on pneumatic and mechanical integrity.[32] Pneumatic integrity in the GE Link-25 system requires properly functioning second-stage regulators. A nitrous oxide:oxygen ratio other than 3:1 may result if the regulators are not precise. The chain connecting the two sprockets must be intact—if the chain is cut or broken, a 97% nitrous oxide concentration can result (Fig. 25-19).[33] In the Dräger System, a functional OFPD is necessary to supply appropriate pressure to the S-ORC. The mechanical aspects of the S-ORC, such as the rubber diaphragms, the flow tube resistors, and the nitrous oxide slave control valve, must likewise be intact.

Leaks Downstream

The S-ORC and the Link-25 function at the level of the flow control valves. A leak downstream from these devices, such as a broken oxygen flow tube (Fig. 25-15), can result in delivery of a hypoxic mixture to the common gas outlet. In this situation, oxygen escapes through the leak and the predominant gas delivered is nitrous oxide. The oxygen monitor and/or integrated multigas analyzer are the only machine safety devices that can detect this problem. For the majority of anesthesia workstations, a preuse positive- or negative-pressure leak test (depending on the manufacturer) is recommended to detect such a leak (see Checking Your Anesthesia Workstation section).

Inert Gas Administration

Administration of a third inert gas, such as helium, nitrogen, or carbon dioxide, can cause a hypoxic mixture because contemporary proportioning systems link only nitrous oxide and oxygen.[34] Use of an oxygen analyzer, or a multigas analyzer when available, to monitor the inspired oxygen concentration is mandatory if the operator uses a third gas.

Dilution of Inspired Oxygen Concentration by Potent Inhaled Volatile Anesthetics

Volatile inhaled anesthetics are added to the mixed gases downstream from both the flowmeters and the proportioning system. High concentrations of the less-potent inhaled anesthetic desflurane (MAC ~7%) may inadvertently be added downstream of the proportioning system, with a resulting gas/vapor mixture that may contain an inspired oxygen concentration that is below 21%. Awareness of this possibility, particularly when high concentrations of desflurane are used, is essential.

Oxygen Flush Valve

The oxygen flush valve allows direct communication between the oxygen intermediate-pressure circuit and the low-pressure system (Fig. 25-2, 5 Video 25-5). Flow from the oxygen flush valve enters the LPC downstream from the vaporizers and, most importantly, downstream from any outlet check valve, if present. The spring-loaded oxygen flush valve remains closed until the operator opens it by pressing the oxygen flush button. Actuation of the valve delivers 100% oxygen at a flow of 35 to 75 L/min to the breathing circuit.

Vaporizers

Rapid evolution of the anesthesia workstation in recent years has caused significant changes to vaporizers, from their early stages as rudimentary ether inhalers and the "Copper Kettle" to the temperature-compensated, computer-controlled, and flow-sensing devices in use today. In 1993, with the introduction of desflurane into clinical use, an even more sophisticated vaporizer was introduced to handle the unique physical properties of this agent. A new generation of anesthesia vaporizers blending traditional technology and "new" computerized control technology has emerged in the GE Aladin cassette vaporizer system and, more recently, injection vaporizers have become available in which controlled amounts of liquid agent are vaporized into the fresh gas stream. It is important to review certain physical principles to facilitate understanding of the operating principles, construction, and design of contemporary volatile anesthetic vaporizers.

Physics

The physical properties of potent inhaled volatile anesthetic agents that are pertinent to a discussion of vaporizers and vaporization are shown in Table 25-1.

Vapor Pressure

Contemporary potent inhaled volatile anesthetics exist in the liquid state at temperatures below 20°C. When a volatile liquid is in a closed container, molecules escape from the liquid phase into the vapor phase until the number of molecules in the vapor 3

Table 25-1 Physical Properties of Potent Inhaled Volatile Anesthetic Agents

Parameter/Agent	Halothane	Enflurane	Isoflurane	Sevoflurane	Desflurane
Structure	$CHBrClCF_3$	$CHFClCF_2OCHF_2$	$CF_2HOCHClCF_3$	$CH_2FOCH(CF_3)_2$	$CH_2HOCFHCF_3$
Molecular weight	197.4	184.5	184.5	200	168
Boiling point at 769 mmHg (°C)	50.2	56.5	48.5	58.5	22.8
SVP at 20°C (mmHg)	243	175	238	160	669
Saturated vapor concentration at 20°C and 1 atmosphere absolute (vol%)	32	23	31	21	87
MAC at 1 atmosphere absolute (vol%)	0.75	1.68	1.15	1.7	6.0–7.25[a]
P_{MAC1} (mmHg)	5.7	12.8	8.7	12.9	46–55[a]
Specific gravity of liquid at 20°C	123	130	130	120	143
Vapor (mL) per mL liquid at 20°C	226	196	195	182	207

SVP, Saturated Vapor Pressure.
[a]Age-related.

phase is constant and in equilibrium with the liquid phase. These molecules in the vapor phase bombard the walls of the container and create the saturated vapor pressure (SVP). As the temperature increases, more molecules enter the vapor phase, and the SVP also increases (Fig. 25-21). Vapor pressure is independent of atmospheric pressure and is dependent only on the temperature and physical characteristics of the liquid.

The *boiling point* of a liquid is defined as that temperature at which the vapor pressure equals atmospheric pressure. At 760 mmHg, the boiling points for desflurane, isoflurane, and sevoflurane are approximately 22.8°C, 48.5°C, and 58.5°C, respectively. Unlike other contemporary inhaled anesthetics, desflurane boils at temperatures that may be encountered in particularly warm clinical settings such as pediatric and burn operating rooms. This unique physical characteristic alone mandates a special vaporizer design to control the delivery of desflurane. If an agent-specific vaporizer is accidentally filled with an incorrect liquid anesthetic agent, the resulting mixture of volatile agents may demonstrate properties that differ from those of the individual component agents and may alter the anticipated output of the vaporizer (see Variable Bypass Vaporizers: Misfilling section).[35]

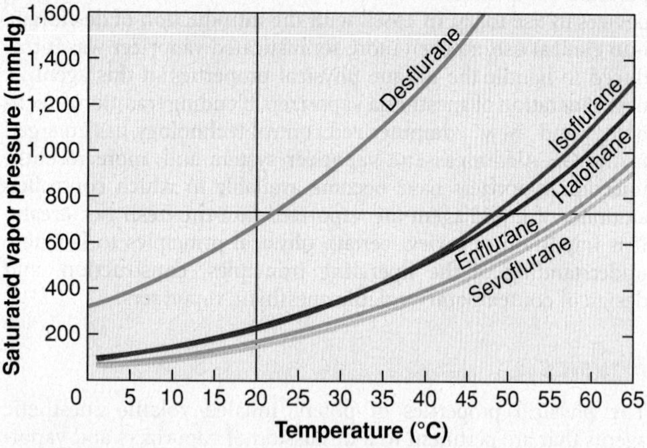

Figure 25-21 Saturated vapor pressure versus temperature curves for desflurane, isoflurane, halothane, enflurane, and sevoflurane. The vapor pressure curve for desflurane is both steeper and shifted to higher vapor pressures when compared with the curves for other contemporary inhaled anesthetics. (Adapted with permission from Inhaled anesthetic package insert equations and from Susay SR, Smith MA, Lockwood GG. The saturated vapor pressure of desflurane at various temperatures. *Anesth Analg*. 1996;83:864.)

Latent Heat of Vaporization

When a molecule is converted from a liquid to the gaseous phase, energy is consumed because the molecules of a liquid tend to cohere. The amount of energy that is consumed by a given liquid as it is converted to a vapor is referred to as the *latent heat of vaporization*. It is more precisely defined as the number of calories required to change 1 g of liquid into vapor without a temperature change. The thermal energy for vaporization is derived from the liquid itself or from an external source. In the absence of an external energy source, the temperature of the liquid itself will decrease during vaporization. This energy loss can lead to significant decreases in temperature of the remaining liquid and can greatly decrease subsequent vaporization.[36]

Specific Heat

The *specific heat* of a substance is the number of calories required to increase the temperature of 1 g of a substance (a solid, liquid, or gas) by 1°C. The concept of specific heat is important to the design, operation, and construction of vaporizers because it is applicable in two ways. First, the specific heat value for an inhaled anesthetic is important because it indicates how much heat must be supplied to the liquid to maintain a constant temperature when heat is being lost during vaporization. Second, manufacturers select vaporizer component materials that have a high specific heat to minimize temperature changes associated with vaporization.

Thermal Conductivity

Thermal conductivity is a measure of the rate at which heat flows through a substance. The higher the thermal conductivity, the better the substance conducts heat. Vaporizers are constructed of metals that have relatively high thermal conductivity, thus maintaining a uniform internal temperature.

Ambient Pressure Effects

These are discussed in the section titled (see The Tec 6 and D-Vapor Vaporizers for Desflurane).

Variable Bypass Vaporizers

The GE Tec 5, Tec 7, and 850 vaporizers, and the Dräger Vapor 2000 and 3000 series vaporizers, are classified as variable bypass, flow-over, temperature-compensated, agent-specific, out-of-breathing circuit vaporizers. *Variable bypass* refers to the method for regulating the anesthetic agent concentration output from the vaporizer. As fresh gas from the anesthesia machine flowmeters enters the vaporizer inlet, the concentration control dial setting determines the ratio of incoming gas that flows through the bypass chamber to that *exiting* the vaporizing chamber (sump). The gas channeled through the vaporizing chamber flows over a wick system saturated with the liquid anesthetic and subsequently also becomes saturated with vapor. Thus, *flow over* refers to the method of vaporization and is in contrast to a *bubble-through* system that was used in now-obsolete measured flow vaporizers (such as the Copper Kettle or Verni-Trol).

The GE Tec 5 and Tec 7, and the Dräger Vapor 2000 and 3000 series are further classified as *temperature compensated*. Each is equipped with an automated temperature-compensating device that helps maintain a constant vapor concentration output for a given concentration dial setting, and over a wide range of operating temperatures. These vaporizers are *agent specific* because each is designed to accommodate a single anesthetic agent, and are *out of circuit,* that is, located outside of the breathing circuit. Variable bypass vaporizers are used to deliver all potent inhaled agents except for desflurane.

Basic Operating Principles

A diagram of a generic, variable bypass vaporizer is shown in Figure 25-22. In principle, it creates a saturated vapor concentration of the liquid agent in the vaporizing chamber and dilutes this to clinically usable concentrations by mixing it with fresh gas from the vaporizer bypass. For example, the SVP of sevoflurane is 160 mmHg at 20°C, at sea level. This corresponds to a vapor concentration of 160 mmHg/760 mmHg × 100 = 21%, which is too high for clinical use. Therefore, the vaporizer must dilute this 21% concentration to a clinically desirable value indicated on the vaporizer dial. Vaporizer components include the concentration control dial, the bypass chamber, the vaporizing chamber, the filler port, and the filler cap. Using the filler port, the operator fills the vaporizing chamber with liquid anesthetic. The maximum safe fill level is predetermined by the position of the filler port, which is designed to minimize the likelihood of overfilling. Importantly, if a vaporizer is overfilled or tilted, liquid anesthetic can spill into the bypass via the inlet and outlet chambers. If this were to happen, both the vaporizing chamber flow and the bypass flow could potentially be carrying saturated anesthetic vapor, and an overdose would result. The concentration control dial is a variable restrictor, which proportions gas flow through the bypass with agent at its saturated vapor concentration leaving the vaporizing chamber.[37]

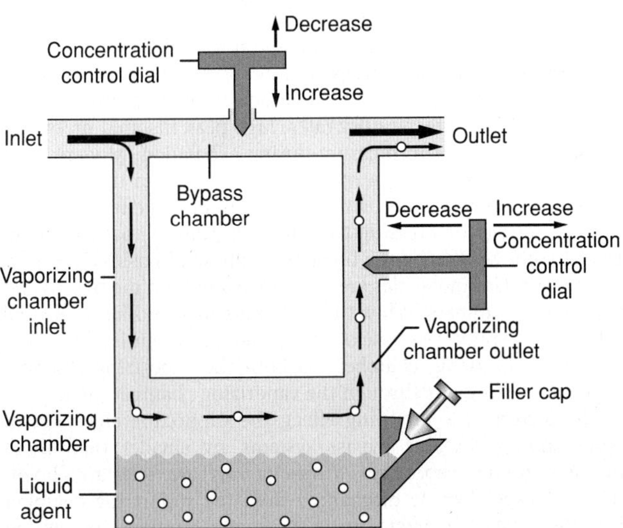

Figure 25-22 Generic variable bypass vaporizer. See text for details.

FGF from the machine's flowmeters enters the inlet of the vaporizer. Most of the flow passes straight through the bypass chamber to the vaporizer outlet. A smaller fraction of the fresh gas inflow enters the vaporizing chamber. Depending on the temperature and vapor pressure of the particular inhaled anesthetic, the fresh gas entering the vaporizing chamber entrains a specific flow of the anesthetic agent-saturated vapor. The mixture that exits the vaporizer outlet comprises flow through the bypass chamber, flow through the vaporizing chamber, and flow of entrained anesthetic vapor. The final concentration of inhaled anesthetic (in volumes percent) is the ratio of the flow of the entrained anesthetic vapor to the total gas flow.[38] The quantity (mL) of liquid volatile anesthetic agent used by a typical vaporizer is proportional to the FGF rate and the concentration set on the dial. It can be approximated from the following formula:

$$3 \times \text{FGF (L/min)} \times \text{vol\%} = \text{mL liquid volatile anesthetic/hr}$$

Figure 25-22 shows that the agent concentration emerging from the vaporizer is controlled by proportioning the vaporizing chamber outflow to the bypass flow. For example, assume that the vaporizing chamber outflow is 100 mL/min. The SVP of sevoflurane is 160 mmHg at 20°C (Table 25-1), and the saturated vapor concentration of sevoflurane is 21% (i.e., 160/760); therefore, each 100 mL of gas exiting the vaporizing chamber contains 21 mL of sevoflurane vapor, the other 79 mL consisting of the gas that entered the vaporizing chamber. If the vaporizer dial is set to deliver 1% sevoflurane, the bypass flow will be 2,000 mL/min because 21 mL of sevoflurane vapor will be diluted in a total volume of 2,100 mL (21 + 79 + 2,000), or 21/2,100 = 1% by volume. To achieve this, the vaporizer concentration dial has created a flow ratio of 2,000:100 or 20:1 between the bypass flow and the flow exiting the vaporizing chamber. When the dial is set to deliver 2% sevoflurane, the vaporizer concentration dial creates a ratio of 950:100, or 9.5:1; that is, 21 mL of sevoflurane vapor is diluted in a total volume of (21 + 79 + 950) 1,050 mL (21/1,050 = 2%).

In the case of an isoflurane vaporizer set to deliver 1% isoflurane, the concentration of isoflurane vapor in the vaporizing chamber will be 238/760 = 31% at 20°C (Table 25-1). Each 100 mL of gas leaving the vaporizing chamber includes 31 mL of isoflurane vapor, the other 69 mL consisting of the gas that entered the vaporizing chamber. The bypass flow must be 3,000 mL because now 31 mL of isoflurane vapor is diluted in a total volume of 3,100 (31 + 69 + 3,000). The vaporizer concentration dial has created a flow ratio of 30:1 between the bypass flow and the flow exiting the vaporizing chamber. For 2% isoflurane, the flow ratio would be 14.5:1 (i.e., 31 mL isoflurane vapor diluted in a total volume of [31 + 69 + 1,450] 1,550 mL). These examples demonstrate why *variable bypass vaporizers are agent specific*.

The SVP of a potent volatile anesthetic depends on the ambient temperature (Fig. 25-21). For example, at 20°C the SVP of isoflurane is 238 mmHg, whereas at 35°C the SVP is almost double, at 450 mmHg. Variable bypass vaporizers incorporate a mechanism to compensate for variations in ambient temperature. The temperature-compensating valve of the GE Tec-type vaporizers is shown in Figure 25-23. At relatively high ambient temperatures, such as those commonly seen in operating rooms designated for

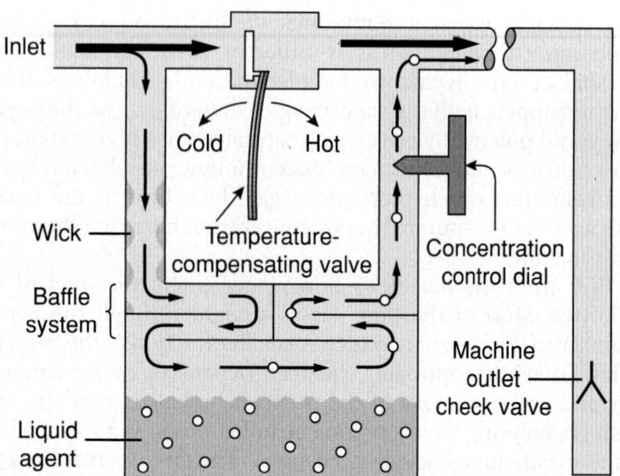

Figure 25-23 Simplified schematic of the GE Tec Type Vaporizer. Note bimetallic strip temperature-compensating mechanism in the bypass chamber. See text for details.

the care of pediatric or burn patients, the SVP in the vaporizing chamber is high. To compensate for this, the bimetallic strip of the temperature-compensating valve leans to the right, decreasing the resistance to gas flow through the bypass chamber. This allows more flow to pass through the bypass chamber and less flow to pass through the vaporizing chamber. In contrast, in a cold environment, the SVP of the agent in the vaporizing chamber is decreased. To compensate for this decrease in SVP, the bimetallic strip leans to the left. This increases the resistance to flow through the bypass chamber, causing relatively more flow to the vaporizing chamber and less flow to the bypass chamber. The net effect in both situations is maintenance of relatively constant vapor output concentration despite large swings in ambient temperature. Dräger Vapor vaporizers use an expansion element to achieve temperature compensation (Fig. 25-24).

Factors that Influence Vaporizer Output

If an ideal vaporizer existed, its output would be constant for a given concentration dial setting, regardless of changes in FGF rate, temperature, back pressure, and fresh gas mixture composition and ambient pressure. Designing such a vaporizer is difficult because as ambient conditions change, the physical properties of gases and of the vaporizers themselves can change. Contemporary vaporizers approach this ideal but still have some limitations. Even though some of the most sophisticated vaporizing systems now available use computer-controlled components and multiple sensors, they have yet to become significantly more accurate than conventional mechanical flow-proportioning (variable bypass) vaporizers. Several factors that affect vaporizer performance in general are described below.

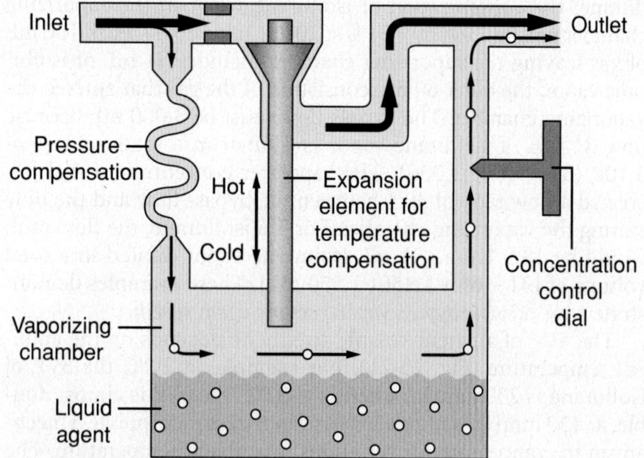

Figure 25-24 Simplified schematic of an expansion element in a vaporizer. Here an expansion element performs the same function as the bimetallic strip in the previous figure. See text for details.

Fresh Gas Flow Rate

With a fixed dial setting, vaporizer output can vary with the rate of gas flowing through the vaporizer. This variation is particularly notable at extremes of flow rates. The output of all variable bypass vaporizers is less than the dial setting at low flow rates (<250 mL/min). This results from the relatively high density of volatile inhaled anesthetic vapors. At low flow rates, insufficient turbulence is generated in the vaporizing chamber to advance the vapor molecules upwardly. At extremely high flow rates, such as 15 L/min, the output of most variable bypass vaporizers is less than that set on the dial. This discrepancy is attributed to incomplete mixing and failure to saturate the carrier gas in the vaporizing chamber. In addition, the resistance characteristics of the bypass chamber and the vaporizing chamber can vary as flow increases.

Temperature

As a result of improvements in design, the output of contemporary temperature-compensated vaporizers is almost linear over a wide range of temperatures. Automatic temperature-compensating mechanisms in the bypass chamber maintain a constant concentration output with varying temperatures. A bimetallic strip (Fig. 25-23), or an expansion element in Dräger Vapor vaporizers (Fig. 25-24), directs a greater proportion of gas flow through the bypass chamber as temperature increases. In addition, the wick systems are placed in direct contact with the metal wall of the vaporizer to help replace energy (heat) consumed during vaporization.

The materials from which vaporizers are constructed are chosen because they have a relatively high specific heat and high thermal conductivity. These factors help minimize the effect of cooling of the liquid anesthetic during vaporization. In addition, they should not react chemically with the liquid anesthetic agent.[39]

Intermittent Back Pressure

Intermittent back pressure that results from either positive-pressure ventilation or use of the oxygen flush valve may result in higher-than-expected vaporizer output. This phenomenon, known as the *pumping effect,* is more pronounced at low FGF rates, low concentration dial settings, and low levels of liquid anesthetic in the vaporizing chamber.[40,41] In addition, the pumping effect is increased by rapid respiratory rates, high peak inspired pressures, and rapid decreases in pressure during exhalation. Modern variable bypass vaporizers are relatively immune from the pumping effect. One proposed mechanism for the pumping effect is dependent on retrograde pressure transmission from the patient circuit to the vaporizer during the inspiratory phase of positive-pressure ventilation. Gas molecules are compressed in both the bypass and vaporizing chambers. When the back pressure is suddenly released during the expiratory phase of positive-pressure ventilation, vapor exits the vaporizing chamber via both the vaporizing chamber outlet and retrograde through the vaporizing chamber inlet.

To decrease the pumping effect, the vaporizing chambers of contemporary variable bypass systems are smaller than those of older model vaporizers. Consequently, no substantial volumes of vapor can be discharged from the vaporizing chamber into the bypass chamber during the expiratory phase of ventilation. The Dräger Vapor vaporizers (Fig. 25-24) have a long spiral

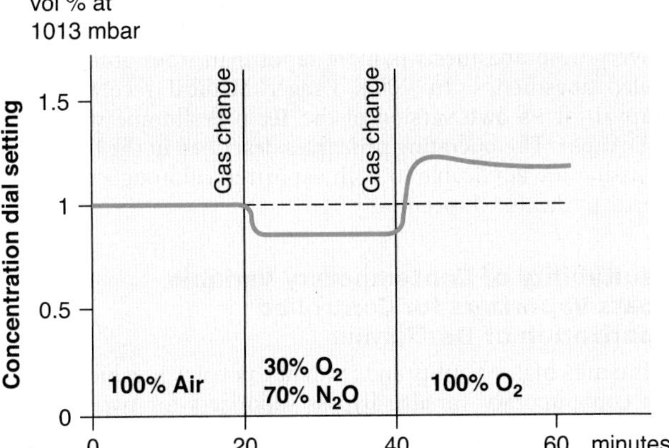

Figure 25-25 Influence of gas composition on delivered anesthetic concentration. A Dräger Vapor 2000 vaporizer is initially set at 1 vol% and 100% air. The concentration falls by 10% (not more than 0.4 vol%) of the set value after switching to a mixture of 30% O_2 and 70% N_2O. When 100% O_2 is used, the concentration rises by 10% of the set value (not more than 0.4 vol%). (Adapted from Schreiber P. *Anaesthetic Equipment: Performance, Classification, and Safety*. Springer; 1972.)

tube that serves as the inlet to the vaporizing chamber. When the pressure in the vaporizing chamber is released, some of the vapor enters this tube but does not enter the bypass chamber because of the tube's length.

Fresh Gas Composition

Although of minimal clinical importance, vaporizer output can be influenced by the composition of the gas that flows through the vaporizer.[42] Under experimental conditions, when the carrier gas is rapidly changed from 100% air to 30% oxygen/70% nitrous oxide, a sudden transient decrease in vaporizer output occurs, followed by a slow increase to a new steady-state value (Fig. 25-25).[43] Because nitrous oxide is more soluble than oxygen in the anesthetic liquid in the vaporizer sump, when this change occurs, the output from the vaporizing chamber is transiently decreased.[44] Once the anesthetic liquid is totally saturated with nitrous oxide, vaporizing chamber output increases somewhat, and a new steady state is established.

Safety Features

Contemporary vaporizers incorporate safety features that have minimized or eliminated many of the hazards once associated with variable bypass vaporizers (6 Video 25-6). Agent-specific, keyed filling devices help prevent filling a vaporizer with the wrong agent. Overfilling of vaporizers is minimized because the filler port is located at the maximum safe liquid level. Vaporizers are firmly secured to a vaporizer manifold on the anesthesia workstation and have antispill protection designs (such as the "Transport" setting on Dräger Vapor 2000 series vaporizers) so that problems associated with vaporizer tipping are prevented. Contemporary interlock systems prevent simultaneous administration of more than one inhaled volatile anesthetic.

Hazards

Despite many safety features, some hazards continue to be associated with contemporary variable bypass vaporizers.

Misfilling

Vaporizers not equipped with keyed fillers have been occasionally misfilled with the wrong anesthetic liquid. A potential for misfilling exists even on contemporary vaporizers equipped with keyed fillers.[45–47] When a vaporizer misfilling occurs, patients can be rendered inadequately or excessively anesthetized depending on which "incorrect" agent is in the vaporizer.[48] The use of an anesthetic agent analyzer should alert the user to such a problem. In principle, if a vaporizer designed for an agent with a relatively low SVP (e.g., sevoflurane-160 mmHg at 20°C) is erroneously filled with an agent that has a relatively high SVP (e.g., isoflurane-238 mmHg at 20°C), the output concentration of isoflurane (in vol%) will be greater than that set on the concentration dial of the sevoflurane vaporizer. Conversely, an isoflurane vaporizer misfilled with sevoflurane will deliver a lower concentration of sevoflurane than that set on the concentration dial. In addition to considering the agent concentration output of a misfilled vaporizer, one must also consider the potency output. Thus, a sevoflurane vaporizer set to deliver 2% sevoflurane [1 minimum alveolar anesthetic concentration (MAC)] that is misfilled with isoflurane will deliver about 3% isoflurane which would be more than double the potency (MAC multiple) expected.

Understanding the principles of operation of a variable bypass vaporizer (i.e., how gas flows are proportioned between bypass and vaporizing chamber) makes it possible to predict the output of an erroneously filled vaporizer. In certain situations (e.g., remote locations or impoverished countries with limited resources), deliberate mismatch has been safely used.[49] But caution is required. Mismatching of inhaled agent and vaporizer is a dangerous practice and should not be performed unless absolutely necessary.

Tipping

Tipping of a vaporizer can occur when it is incorrectly "switched out" or moved. However, tipping is unlikely when a vaporizer is secured to the anesthesia workstation manifold, short of the entire machine being turned over. Excessive tipping can cause the liquid agent to enter the bypass chamber and can result in an output with extremely high agent vapor concentration.[50]

One milliliter of liquid anesthetic produces approximately 200 mL of anesthetic vapor at 20°C and 1 atm pressure so that even a small quantity of liquid anesthetic in the bypass or elements of the breathing circle can produce a large amount of vapor (Table 25-1). If a vaporizer has been tipped, it should be withdrawn from clinical use until it has been purged for 20 to 30 minutes using a high FGF rate from the machine's flowmeters. As mentioned above, the Dräger Vapor 2000 and 3000 series vaporizers have a transport ("T") dial setting that prevents tipping-related problems. When the dial is set to this position, the vaporizer sump is isolated from the bypass chamber, thereby reducing the likelihood of spillage (and a possible accidental overdose). In order to remove a Vapor 2000 or 3000 from the anesthesia workstation, the control dial must be set to the "T" position.

The design of the GE Tec 6 and the Aladin cassette vaporizer systems has essentially eliminated the dangers of tipping. Since the Aladin vaporizer's bypass chamber is physically separated from the "cassette," and permanently resides in the anesthesia workstation, the possibility of tipping is virtually eliminated. Tipping of the Aladin cassettes themselves when they are not installed in the vaporizer is not problematic. Similarly, Dräger's D-Vapor (desflurane) vaporizer is hermetically tight and can be transported in any position.

Improper Filling

Overfilling of a vaporizer combined with failure of the vaporizer sight glass can cause an anesthetic overdose. When liquid anesthetic enters the bypass chamber, up to 10 times the intended vapor concentration can be delivered to the common gas outlet.[51,52] Most modern vaporizers are now relatively immune to overfilling because of side-fill rather than top-fill designs.

Just as with overfilling, underfilling of anesthetic vaporizers may also be problematic. When a Tec 5 sevoflurane vaporizer is in a low-fill state and used under conditions of high FGF rates (>7.5 L/min) and high dial setting (such as seen during inhalational inductions), the vaporizer output may abruptly decrease to less than 2%. The causes of this problem are likely multifactorial. However, the combination of low vaporizer fill state (<25% full) in combination with the high vaporizing chamber flow can result in a clinically significant and reproducible decrease in vapor output.[53]

Leaks

Vaporizer leaks do occur and can potentially result in patient awareness during anesthesia[54] or in contamination of the operating room environment. A loose filler cap is the most common source of vaporizer leaks. Leaks can also occur at the O-ring junctions between the vaporizer and its manifold. To detect a leak within a vaporizer, the concentration control dial must be in the "on" position. Even though vaporizer leaks in Dräger anesthesia systems can potentially be detected with a conventional positive-pressure low-pressure system leak test (because of the absence of an outlet check valve), a negative-pressure leak test is probably more sensitive. GE recommends a negative-pressure leak testing device, a suction bulb, to detect vaporizer leaks because of the check valve located just upstream of each machine's fresh gas outlet (see Checking The Anesthesia Workstation section).

Many newer anesthesia workstations are capable of performing self-testing procedures that, in some cases, may eliminate the need for the conventional negative-pressure leak testing. However, it is of vital importance that anesthesia providers understand that these self-tests may not detect internal vaporizer leaks in systems with add-on vaporizers. For the self-tests to determine if an internal vaporizer leak is present, the leak test must be repeated for each vaporizer sequentially, while its concentration control dial is turned to the "on" position. Recall that when a vaporizer's concentration control dial is set in the "off" position, it may not be possible to detect even major internal leaks such as an absent or loose filler cap.

Vaporizers in the MRI Suite

The presence of a powerful magnetic field, the significant noise pollution, and limited access to the patient during an MRI procedure all complicate care in this setting. It is imperative that only nonferrous, MRI-compatible equipment be used. Some anesthesia vaporizers, although they may appear nonferrous by testing with a horseshoe magnet, may indeed contain substantial internal ferrous components. Inappropriate use of such a device in an MRI suite may potentially turn it into a dangerous missile if left unsecured.[55]

Vaporizers for Desflurane

Because of its unique physical properties, the controlled vaporization of desflurane requires a novel approach to vaporizer design (7 Video 25-7). Ohmeda (now GE) developed the Tec 6 vaporizer, the first such system, and introduced it into clinical use in the early 1990s. The Tec 6 vaporizer is an electrically heated, pressurized device specifically designed to deliver desflurane.[56,57] The vapor pressure of desflurane is three to four times that of other contemporary inhaled anesthetics, and it boils at 22.8°C which is slightly above normal room temperature (Fig. 25-21). Desflurane has a minimum alveolar anesthetic concentration (MAC) value of 6% to 7%.[58] It is valuable because it has a low blood:gas partition coefficient of 0.45 at 37°C, and recovery from anesthesia is more rapid than from other potent inhaled anesthetics. In 2004, Dräger Medical received FDA approval for its own version of the Tec 6 desflurane vaporizer, the D-Vapor. The operating principles described in the following discussion are applicable to both vaporizers, although reference is made to the Tec 6 specifically.

Unsuitability of Contemporary Variable Bypass Vaporizers for Controlled Vaporization of Desflurane

Desflurane's high volatility and moderate potency preclude its use with contemporary variable bypass vaporizers for two primary reasons (Table 25-1):

1. At 20°C, the SVP of desflurane is 669 mmHg (almost 1 atm pressure at sea level). At temperatures of 22.8°C or higher at 1 atm, desflurane will boil. The amount of vapor produced would be uncontrolled and limited only by the heat energy available from the vaporizer.[45]
2. Contemporary variable bypass vaporizers lack an external heat source. The latent heat of vaporization for desflurane is approximately equal to those of the other potent agents but its MAC is four to nine times higher. Thus, the absolute amount of desflurane liquid vaporized over a given time period is considerably greater than that of the other anesthetic agents. To deliver desflurane via a conventional vaporizer in higher (equivalent MAC) concentrations would lead to excessive cooling of the vaporizer and would significantly reduce its output. In the absence of an external heat source, temperature compensation using traditional mechanical devices would be almost impossible. Because of the broad range of temperatures seen in the clinical setting, and because of desflurane's steep SVP versus temperature curve (Fig. 25-21), the delivery of desflurane in a conventional anesthetic vaporizer would be unpredictable.

Operating Principles of the Tec 6 and D-Vapor

The physical appearance and operation of the Tec 6 are similar to other vaporizers, but some aspects of the internal design and operating principles are radically different. Functionally, the Tec 6's operation is more accurately described as a dual-gas blender than as a vaporizer. A simplified schematic of the Tec 6 is shown in Figure 25-26. The vaporizer has two independent gas circuits arranged in parallel. The fresh gas circuit is shown in darker gray, and the vapor circuit in light gray. The FGF from the machine's flowmeters enters at the fresh gas inlet, passes through a fixed restrictor (R1), and exits at the vaporizer gas outlet. The vapor circuit originates at the desflurane sump, which is electrically heated and thermostatically controlled to 39°C, a temperature well above desflurane's boiling point at 1 atm. The heated sump assembly creates a reservoir of desflurane vapor. At 39°C, the vapor pressure in the sump is approximately 1,500 mmHg, or 2 atm absolute (Fig. 25-21). Just downstream from the sump is the shutoff valve. After the vaporizer has warmed up to working temperature, the shutoff valve fully opens when the concentration control valve is turned to the "on" position. A pressure-regulating valve located downstream from the shutoff valve regulates the pressure downward to approximately 1.1 atm absolute (74 mmHg gauge) at an FGF rate of 10 L/min. The operator controls desflurane output by adjusting the concentration control valve (R2), which is a variable restrictor. The vapor flow through R2 joins the FGF

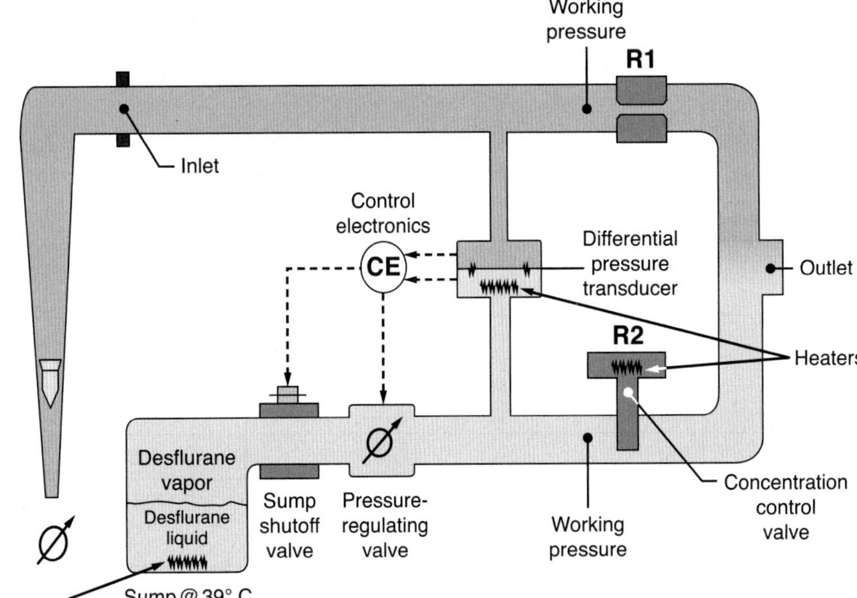

Figure 25-26 Simplified schematic of the Tec 6 desflurane vaporizer. (Modified from Andrews JJ. *Operating Principles of the Ohmeda Tec 6 Desflurane Vaporizer: A Collection of Twelve Color Illustrations.* Library of Congress; 1996.)

through R1 at a point downstream from the restrictors. Until this point, the two circuits are physically separated. They are interfaced pneumatically and electronically, however, through differential pressure transducers, a control electronics system, and a pressure-regulating valve. When a constant FGF encounters the fixed restrictor, R1, a specific back pressure, proportional to the FGF rate, pushes against the diaphragm of the control differential pressure transducer. The differential pressure transducer conveys the pressure difference between the fresh gas circuit and the vapor circuit to the control electronics system. The control electronics system adjusts the pressure-regulating valve so that the pressure in the vapor circuit equals the pressure in the fresh gas circuit. This equalized pressure supplying R1 and R2 is the working pressure and is constant at a fixed FGF rate. If the operator increases the FGF rate, more back pressure is exerted upon the diaphragm of the control pressure transducer, and the working pressure of the vaporizer increases.

Table 25-2 shows the approximate correlation between FGF rate and working pressure for a typical vaporizer. At an FGF rate of 1 L/min, the working pressure is 10 millibars, or 7.4 mmHg gauge. At an FGF rate of 10 L/min, the working pressure is 100 millibars, or 74 mmHg gauge. Therefore, there is a linear relationship between FGF rate and working pressure. When the FGF rate is increased 10-fold, the working pressure increases 10-fold.[56]

The following are two examples to demonstrate the operating principles of the Tec 6 (and D-Vapor).

Example A: Constant FGF rate of 1 L/min, with an increase in the dial setting. At a FGF rate of 1 L/min, the working pressure of the vaporizer is 7.4 mmHg. That is, the pressure supplying R1 and R2 is 7.4 mmHg. As the operator increases the dial setting, the opening at R2 becomes larger, allowing more vapor to pass through R2. Specific vapor flow rates at different dial settings are shown in Table 25-3.

Example B: Constant dial setting with an increase in FGF from 1 to 10 L/min. At a FGF rate of 1 L/min, the working pressure is 7.4 mmHg, and at a dial setting of 6%, the vapor flow rate through R2 is 64 mL/min (Tables 25-2 and 25-3). With a 10-fold increase in the FGF rate, there is a concomitant 10-fold increase in the working pressure to 74 mmHg. The ratio of resistances of R2 to R1 is constant at a fixed dial setting of 6%. Because R2 is supplied by 10 times more pressure, the vapor flow rate through R2 increases 10-fold to 640 mL/min. Vaporizer output in volumes percent is constant because both the FGF and the vapor flow increase proportionally.

Table 25-2 Fresh Gas Flow Rate versus Working Pressure

Fresh Gas Flow Rate (L/min)	Working Pressure at R1 and R2 (Gauge) (Gas Inlet Pressure)		
	mbar	*cm Water*	*mmHg*
1	10	10.2	7.4
5	50	51.0	37.0
10	100	102.0	74.0

Reprinted with permission from Andrews JJ, Johnston RV Jr. The new Tec 6 desflurane vaporizer. *Anesth Analg.* 1993;76(6):13386–1341.

Table 25-3 Dial Setting versus Flow through Restrictor R2

Dial Setting (vol%)[a]	Fresh Gas Flow Rate (L/min)	Approximate Vapor Flow Rate Through R2 (mL/min)
1	1	10
6	1	64
12	1	136
18	1	220

[a]vol% = [(vapor flow rate)/(fresh gas flow rate + vapor flow rate)] × 100%.
Reprinted with permission from Andrews JJ, Johnston RV Jr. The new Tec 6 desflurane vaporizer. *Anesth Analg.* 1993;76(6):13386–1341.

Table 25-4 Performance of OLDER[a] Tec Type Vaporizers versus the Tec 6 Desflurane Vaporizer at Varying Ambient Pressures

		Isoflurane Vaporizer with a Dial Setting of 0.89%			Tec 6 Desflurane Vaporizer with a Dial Setting of 6%
Atmospheres	**Ambient Pressure (mmHg)**	***Isoflurane Vapor Entrained by 100 cc O_2***	***Output Concentration (%)***	***Partial Pressure Output (mmHg)***	***Partial Pressure Output of Desflurane (mmHg)***
0.66 (2/3)	500 (10,000 ft)	91	1.753	8.77	30
0.74	560	74	1.429	8.0	33.6
0.80	608 (6,564 ft)	64.32	1.25	7.6	36.5
1.0	760	46	0.89	6.8	45.6
1.5	1,140	26.4	0.515	5.87	68.4
2	1,520	19	0.36	5.5	91.2
3	2,280	11.65	0.228	5.198	136

The following were assumed: 5,000 cc bypass chamber flow, 10 cc vaporizing chamber flow—equivalent to an isoflurane dial setting of 0.89%.
[a]Variable bypass vaporizers in which the incoming gas flow is split before gas enters the vaporizing chamber.

Altitude Can Influence Vaporizer Output

Changes in ambient pressure may significantly affect the output of older Tec-type vaporizers (i.e., those in which gas flow splitting occurs at the entrance to the vaporizing chamber rather than at the exit) in terms of volumes percent (i.e., concentration), but the effect on anesthetic potency (i.e., partial pressure of agent) is minimal. This effect is illustrated using the example of isoflurane shown in Table 25-4. With a constant dial setting of 0.89%, at 1 atm (760 mmHg), if perfectly calibrated, the volumes percent delivered would be 0.89% and the partial pressure of isoflurane would be 6.8 mmHg. Maintaining the same dial setting and lowering ambient pressure to 0.66 atm (roughly equivalent to 10,000 ft elevation) would result in an increase in the concentration output to 1.75% (almost double), but the partial pressure only increases to 8.77 mmHg (a 29% increase) because of the proportionate decrease in ambient pressure (Fig. 25-27).

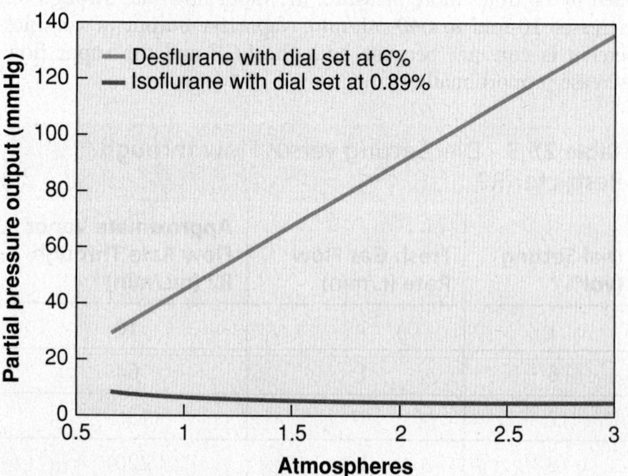

Figure 25-27 Performance of Tec type vaporizer versus the Tec 6 desflurane vaporizer at varying ambient atmospheric pressures (1 atm = 760 mmHg).

It is generally understood that the partial pressure of the anesthetic agent in the central nervous system, not its concentration in volumes percent, is responsible for the anesthetic effect. To obtain a consistent depth of anesthesia when gross changes in barometric pressure occur, the concentration in volumes percent must be changed in inverse proportion to the barometric pressure.

In contemporary variable bypass vaporizers (e.g., GE Tec 5, Tec 7, Dräger Vapor 2000), the flow proportioning occurs as gas leaves the vaporizing chamber, so that for any given dial setting and FGF, the volume of gas saturated with vapor that leaves the vaporizing chamber remains constant, to be diluted by the bypass flow. For example, assume that gas leaves the vaporizing chamber of an isoflurane vaporizer at 100 mL/min. At 1 atm (760 mmHg) that gas would be 31.3% isoflurane by volume (238/760) and the partial pressure would be 31.3% × 760 = 238 mmHg. At a barometric pressure of 500 mmHg, the gas exiting the vaporizing chamber would be 47.6% isoflurane by volume (238/500) and the partial pressure would be 47.6% × 500 = 238 mmHg. By proportioning flow as gas leaves the vaporizing chamber, these vaporizers essentially become ambient pressure compensated.

The above examples should be considered in stark contrast to the response of the Tec 6 desflurane vaporizer at varied altitudes (Fig. 25-27 and Table 25-4). One must remember this device is more accurately described as a dual gas "blender" than a vaporizer. Regardless of the ambient pressure, the Tec 6 will maintain a constant concentration of vapor output (in vol%), not a constant partial pressure. This means that at high altitudes, the partial pressure of desflurane for any given dial setting will be decreased in proportion to the atmospheric pressure divided by the calibration pressure (normally 760 mmHg) according to the following formula:

Required dial setting = normal dial setting (v/v × 760 mmHg)/ ambient pressure (mmHg)

Consider a Tec 6 vaporizer that is set to deliver 10% desflurane at 1 atmosphere. The partial pressure of desflurane delivered from the vaporizer (Pdes) is 76 mmHg (i.e., $10\% \times 760$). If used at an altitude at which the ambient pressure is 500 mmHg, the Tec 6 dial setting must be increased to 15% to maintain the same anesthetic potency ($15\% \times 500 =$ Pdes 75 mmHg). Conversely, the Tec 6's maintenance of a constant vol% output under hyperbaric conditions could produce significant increases in partial pressure output and, if not accounted for, the potential for anesthetic overdose. Therefore, in hyperbaric situations, the Tec 6 dial setting would need to be decreased to maintain the desired partial pressure output of desflurane.

Carrier Gas Composition Can Influence Vaporizer Output

Vaporizer output approximates the dial setting when oxygen is the carrier gas because the Tec 6 vaporizer is calibrated by the manufacturer using 100% oxygen. At low flow rates when a carrier gas other than 100% oxygen is used, however, a clear trend toward reduction in vaporizer output emerges. This reduction parallels the proportional decrease in viscosity of the carrier gas. Nitrous oxide has a lower viscosity than oxygen, so the back pressure generated by resistor R1 (Fig. 25-26) is less when nitrous oxide is the carrier gas, and the working pressure is reduced. At low flow rates using nitrous oxide as the carrier gas, vaporizer output is approximately 20% less than the dial setting. This suggests that, at clinically useful FGF rates, the gas flow across resistor R1 is laminar, and the working pressure is proportional to both the FGF rate and the viscosity of the carrier gas.[59]

Safety Features

4 Because desflurane's SVP at room temperature is near 1 atm, misfilling contemporary vaporizers with desflurane could theoretically result in both desflurane overdose and creation of a hypoxic gas mixture.[60] A unique, anesthetic-specific filling system was designed to minimize occurrence of this potential hazard. The agent-specific filler of the desflurane bottle known as the "Saf-T-Fill" adapter is intended to prevent its use with traditional vaporizers. The filling system also minimizes spillage of liquid or vapor anesthetic by maintaining a "closed system" during the filling process. Each desflurane bottle has a spring-loaded filler cap with an O-ring on the tip. The spring seals the bottle until it is engaged in the filler port of the vaporizer. Thus, this anesthetic-specific filling system interlocks the vaporizer and the dispensing bottle, preventing loss of anesthetic to the atmosphere. Despite these safety features designed to minimize filling errors, a case report described the misfilling of a Tec 6 desflurane vaporizer with sevoflurane. This error was possible because of similarities between a new type of keyed filler for sevoflurane and the desflurane Saf-T-Fill adapter. In that case, however, the desflurane vaporizer detected this error and automatically shut itself off.[45] Major vaporizer faults cause the shutoff valve located just downstream from the desflurane sump (Fig. 25-26) to close, producing a no-output situation. The valve is closed and a "no-output" alarm is activated immediately if any of the following conditions occur: (1) the anesthetic level decreases to <20 mL; (2) the vaporizer is tilted; (3) a power failure occurs; or (4) there is a disparity between the pressure in the vapor circuit versus the pressure in the fresh gas circuit exceeding a specified tolerance. Note the alarm panel on the front of the Tec 6 vaporizer (Fig. 25-28A) showing "no output," "low agent," "warm up," and "alarm battery low" indicators.

The Dräger D-Vapor vaporizer has similar alarms (Fig. 25-28B). The "no output" alarm (flashes red) indicates that the vaporizer is unable to deliver anesthetic (i.e., the vaporizer is warming up) or there is a device failure. The "delivery low" alarm (flashes red) triggers when the vaporizer is unable to supply the output set by the concentration dial (only with FGF >1.5 L/min), the reservoir is empty, or if there is a fault in the apparatus. The amber-colored glow "fill up" alarm indicates the reservoir level has dropped below the refill mark (the reservoir contains <40 mL). The "battery" alarm will indicate (1) *amber glow* if the vaporizer is not able to operate without power, (2) *amber flashing* if the vaporizer is currently operating on battery backup, (3) *flashing amber plus "no output" flashing red* if the vaporizer battery is depleted after operating on battery backup and another method of anesthesia is required. The vaporizer will also provide an audible alarm along with visual alarms. Medium-priority alarms (amber glowing and flashing) may be silenced; high-priority alarms (red flashing) cannot be silenced.

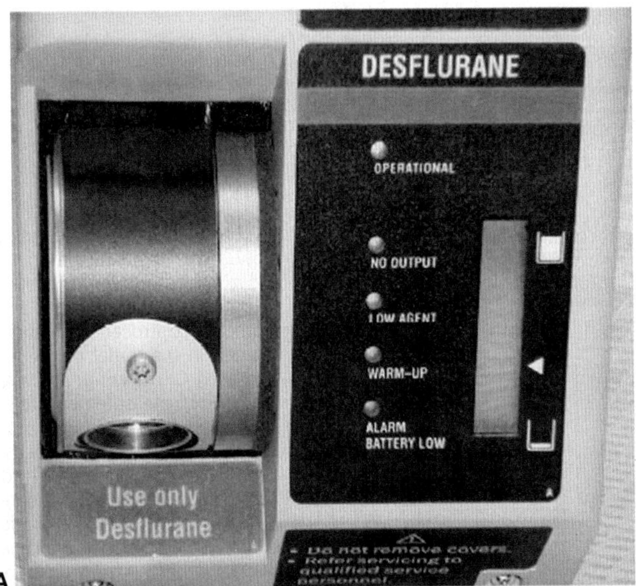

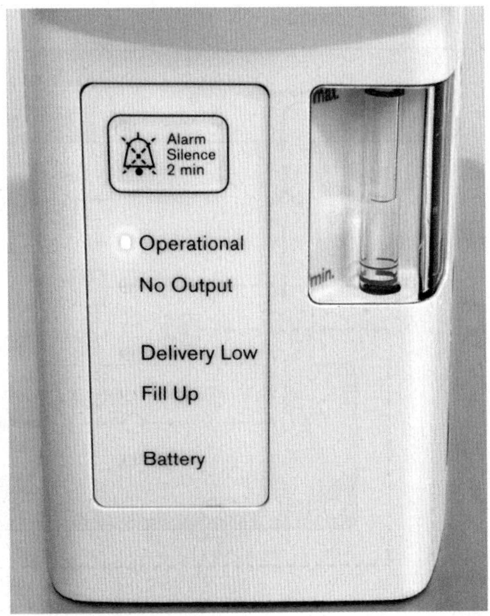

Figure 25-28 **A, B:** Desflurane alarm indicators.

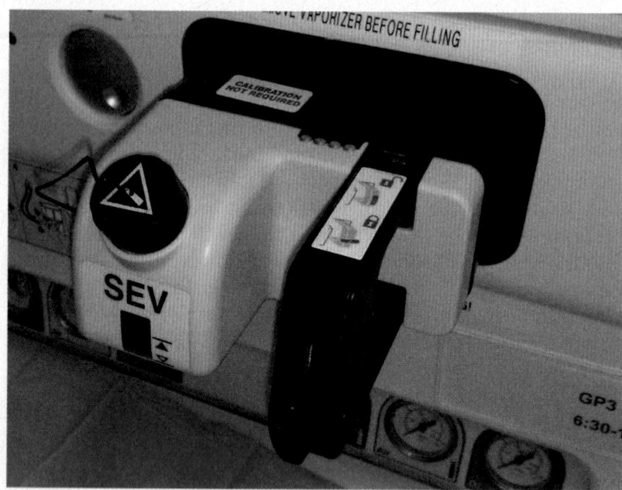

Figure 25-29 Aladin vaporizer sevoflurane cassette (courtesy of GE Healthcare).

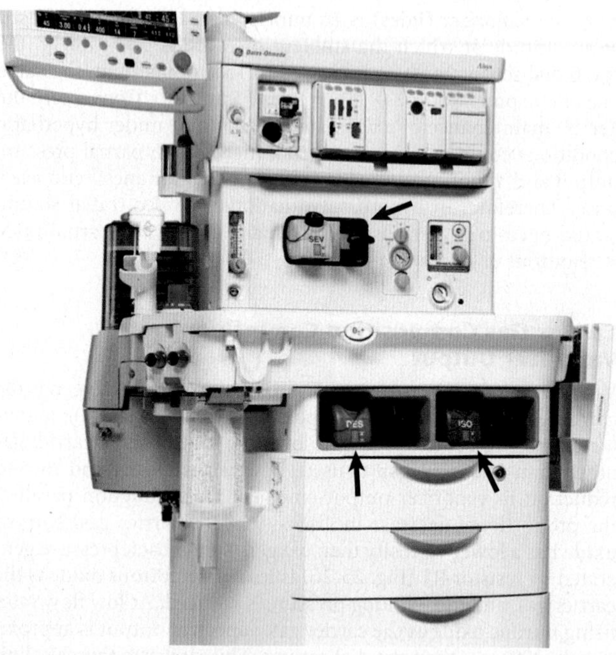

Figure 25-30 Aladin cassette vaporizers (*arrows*) on a GE Aisys Carestation. Upper cassette is in use, lower cassettes are stored on workstation.

The GE-Datex-Ohmeda Aladin Cassette Vaporizer

The vaporizer system used in the GE Aisys and Avance Carestations is unique in that the single electronically controlled vaporizer is designed to deliver five different inhaled anesthetics including halothane, isoflurane, enflurane, sevoflurane, and desflurane (Figs. 25-29 and 25-30). The vaporizer consists of a permanent internal control unit housed within the workstation and an interchangeable Aladin agent-specific cassette that contains anesthetic liquid. The Aladin agent cassettes are color coded for each anesthetic agent, and they are also magnetically coded so that the workstation can identify which anesthetic cassette has been inserted. The cassettes are filled using agent-specific fillers.

Though very different in external appearance, the functional anatomy of the Aladin cassette vaporizer (Fig. 25-31) is very similar to that of the traditional variable bypass vaporizers because it is also made up of a bypass chamber and vaporizing chamber. A fixed restrictor is located in the bypass chamber, and flow measurement sensors are located both in the bypass chamber and in the outlet of the vaporizing chamber. The heart of the Aladin vaporizer is the electronically regulated flow control valve located in the vaporizing chamber outlet. This valve is controlled by a central processing unit (CPU). The CPU receives input from multiple sources including the concentration control

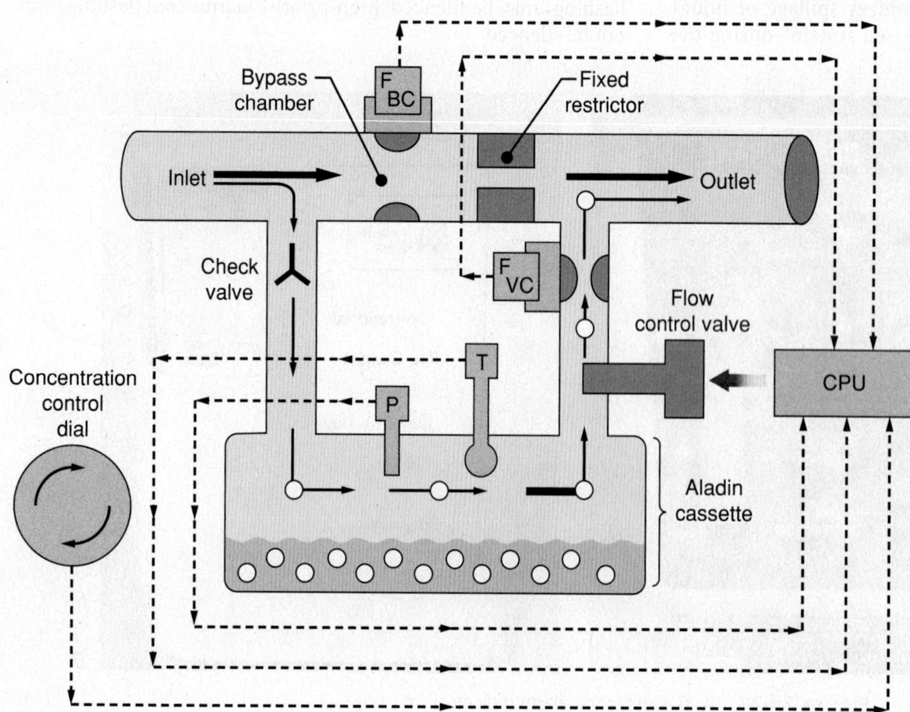

Figure 25-31 Simplified schematic of GE-Datex-Ohmeda Aladin Cassette Vaporizer. The *black arrows* represent flow from the flowmeters, and the *white circles* represent anesthetic vapor. The heart of the vaporizer is the electronically controlled flow control valve located in the outlet of the vaporizing chamber. CPU, central processing unit; FBC, flow measurement unit, which measures flow through the bypass chamber; FVC, flow measurement unit, which measures flow through the vaporizing chamber; P, pressure sensor; T, temperature sensor. (Modified from Andrews JJ. *Operating Principles of the Datex-Ohmeda Aladin Cassette Vaporizer: A Collection of Color Illustrations*. Library of Congress; 2000.)

dial, a pressure sensor located inside the vaporizing chamber (cassette), a temperature sensor located inside the vaporizing chamber, a flow measurement unit located in the bypass chamber, and a flow measurement unit located in the outlet of the vaporizing chamber. The CPU also receives input from the machine's flowmeters regarding the composition of the carrier gas. Using data from these multiple sources, the CPU is able to regulate precisely the flow control valve to attain the desired vapor concentration output. Appropriate electronic control of the flow control valve is essential to the proper functioning of this vaporizer.[61]

A fixed restrictor is located in the bypass chamber, and it causes flow from the vaporizer inlet to be split into two flow streams (Fig. 25-24). One stream passes through the bypass chamber, and the other portion enters the inlet of the vaporizing chamber and passes through a one-way check valve. The presence of this check valve is unique to the Aladin system. This one-way valve prevents retrograde flow of the anesthetic vapor back into the bypass chamber, and its presence is crucial when delivering desflurane if the room temperature is greater than the boiling point for desflurane (22.8°C). A precise amount of vapor-saturated carrier gas passes through the flow control valve, which is regulated by the CPU. This flow then joins the bypass flow and is directed to the outlet of the vaporizer.

As with the Tec 6, the controlled vaporization of desflurane presents a unique challenge, particularly when the room temperature is greater than the boiling point of desflurane (22.8°C). At higher temperatures, the pressure inside the vaporizer sump increases, and the sump becomes pressurized. When the sump pressure exceeds the pressure in the bypass chamber, the one-way check valve located in the vaporizing chamber inlet closes, preventing carrier gas from entering the vaporizing chamber. At this point, the carrier gas passes straight through the bypass chamber and its flow sensor. Under these conditions, the electronically regulated flow control valve simply meters in the appropriate flow of pure desflurane vapor needed to achieve the desired final concentration selected by the user.

During operating conditions in which high FGF rates and/or high dial settings are used, large quantities of anesthetic liquid are rapidly vaporized. The temperature of the remaining liquid anesthetic and the vaporizer itself decreases as a result of energy consumption of the latent heat of vaporization. To offset this cooling effect, the workstation (GE Aisys) is equipped with a fan that forces warmed air from an "agent heating resistor" across the cassette (vaporizer sump) to raise its temperature when necessary. The fan is activated during two common clinical scenarios: (1) desflurane induction and maintenance and (2) sevoflurane induction. A summary of the characteristics of various vaporizer models currently in use is found in Table 25-5.

Table 25-5 Vaporizer Models and Characteristics

Type of Vaporizer	Tec 4, Tec 5, SevoTec, Vapor 19.n, Vapor 2000, Aladin	Tec 6 (Desflurane), D-Vapor (Desflurane)
Carrier gas flow	Variable bypass	Dual circuit
Vaporization method	Flow-over	Gas/vapor blender
Temperature compensation	Automatic	Thermostatically controlled at 39°C
Calibration	Agent specific	Agent specific
Position	Out of circuit	Out of circuit
Fill capacity	Tec 4: 125 mL Tec 5: 300 mL Vapor 19.n: 200 mL Vapor 2000: 360 mL (dry wick) Aladin: 250 mL	Tec 6: 425 mL D-Vapor: 300 mL

Electronic Injector Vaporizers

The preparation of a standard vapor concentration, that is, volume of vapor produced per mL of liquid agent (Table 25-1), is applied in the vaporizing system of the Maquet FLOW-i workstation. In principle, and somewhat analogous to fuel injection in an automobile engine, measured amounts of liquid anesthetic are injected and evaporated into the FGF stream. An electronically controlled valve in the injector controls the quantity of anesthetic that is delivered. The fresh gas flows through a chamber into which the anesthetic is injected. Various electronic controls and feedback mechanisms as well as continuous gas analysis ensure that the desired concentration of inhaled anesthetic is delivered in the fresh gas flowing to the patient. The Dräger DIVA (Direct Injection of Volatile Anesthetic) vaporizer operates on a similar principle.

Anesthesia Breathing Systems

The Circle System

As the prescribed mixture of gases from the flowmeters and vaporizer exits the anesthesia workstation at the common gas outlet, it then enters an anesthetic breathing circuit. The function of the anesthesia breathing circuit is not only to deliver oxygen and anesthetic gases to the patient, but also to eliminate CO_2. Carbon dioxide can be removed either by washout with adequate fresh gas inflow or by the use of CO_2 absorbent media (e.g., soda lime absorption). For many years, the overall design of the circle breathing system underwent few changes. The individual components and the order in which they appear in the circle system were consistent across major platforms. More recently, however, with the increasing technologic complexity of the anesthesia workstation, the circle system has gone through significant changes. These changes have resulted in part from an effort to improve patient safety (as in the integration of fresh gas decoupling [FGD] and inspiratory pressure limiters) but have also allowed the deployment of new technologic advances. Examples of major new technologies include (1) a return to the application of single-circuit piston-type ventilators and (2) use of new spirometry devices that are located at the Y-connector instead of at the traditional location in the expiratory limb of the circuit. The following discussion first focuses on the traditional circle breathing system, and then is followed by a brief discussion of some variations in the designs of newer circle systems.

The Traditional Circle Breathing System

The circle system remains the most popular breathing system in the United States. It is so named because its components are arranged in a circular manner (Fig. 25-32). A coaxial version of the traditional circle system, referred to as either a "Universal F" (King Systems, Noblesville, IN) or a "single limb circuit," has increased in popularity over recent years. Although these systems

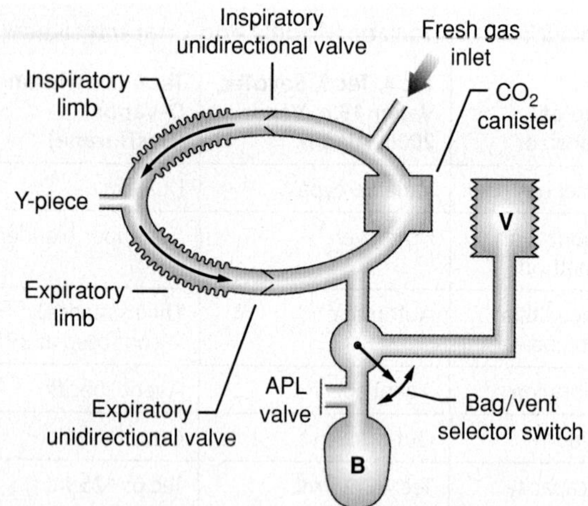

Figure 25-32 Components of the circle breathing system. B, reservoir bag; V, ventilator; APL, adjustable pressure-limiting (pop-off) valve. (Adapted from Brockwell RC. Inhaled anesthetic delivery systems. In: Miller RD, ed. *Anesthesia*. 6th ed. Churchill Livingstone; 2004:295. Copyright © 2004 Elsevier. With permission.)

appear very different externally, they have the same overall functional layout as the traditional circle system and the following discussion is applicable to both the traditional circle system and the coaxial Universal F system.

The circle system prevents rebreathing of CO_2 by use of CO_2 absorbents, but allows partial rebreathing of other exhaled gases. The extent of rebreathing of the other exhaled gases depends on breathing circuit component arrangement and the FGF rate. A circle system can be semiopen, semiclosed, or closed, depending on the amount of FGF.[62] A *semiopen* system has no rebreathing and requires a very high FGF. A *semiclosed* system is associated with some rebreathing of exhaled gases and is the system that is most commonly used in the United States. A *closed* system is one in which the FGF exactly matches what is taken up, or consumed, by the patient. In a closed system, there is complete rebreathing of exhaled gases after absorption of CO_2, and the overflow valve or ventilator pressure relief valve remains closed.

The circle system (Fig. 25-32) consists of seven primary components: (1) a fresh gas inflow source; (2) inspiratory and expiratory unidirectional valves; (3) inspiratory and expiratory corrugated tubes; (4) a Y-piece connector; (5) an overflow or pop-off valve, referred to as the adjustable pressure-limiting valve (APL) valve; (6) a reservoir bag; and (7) a canister containing CO_2 absorbent. The inspiratory and expiratory valves that are placed in the system to ensure gas flow through the corrugated hoses remain unidirectional. The fresh gas inflow enters the circle by a connection from the common gas outlet of the anesthesia workstation.

Numerous variations of the circle arrangement are possible, depending on the relative positions of the unidirectional valves, the APL valve, the reservoir bag, the CO_2 absorber, and the site of fresh gas entry. However, to prevent rebreathing of CO_2 in a traditional circle system, three rules must be followed:[63]

1. A unidirectional valve must be located between the patient and the reservoir bag on both the inspiratory and the expiratory limbs of the circuit.
2. The fresh gas inflow cannot enter the circuit between the expiratory valve and the patient.
3. The overflow (pop-off) valve cannot be located between the patient and the inspiratory valve.

If these rules are followed, any arrangement of the other components will prevent rebreathing of CO_2. Some newer anesthesia workstations now employ less traditional circle breathing systems. Two of these systems (the Datex-Ohmeda S/5 ADU breathing system and the Dräger Apollo and Fabius workstations breathing system) are discussed in greater detail (see below).

The most efficient circle system arrangement with the highest conservation of fresh gases is one in which the unidirectional valves are near the patient and the pop-off valve is located just downstream from the expiratory valve. This arrangement minimizes dead space gas and preferentially eliminates exhaled alveolar gases. A more practical arrangement, the one used on most conventional anesthesia machines (Fig. 25-32), is somewhat less efficient because it allows alveolar and dead space gases to mix before they are vented.[64]

The main advantages of the circle system over other breathing systems include its (1) maintenance of relatively stable inspired gas concentrations; (2) conservation of respiratory moisture and heat; and (3) prevention of operating room atmosphere contamination by waste gases. In addition, the circle system can be used as a semiclosed system or as a closed system with very low FGFs.

Hazards of the Circle System

The major disadvantage of the circle system stems from its complex design. Commonly, the circle system may have 10 or more different connections. These multiple connection sites leave room for misconnections, disconnections, obstructions, and leaks. In the American Society of Anesthesiologists (ASA) closed claims analysis of adverse anesthetic outcomes arising from gas delivery equipment in 1997, 25 out of 72 malpractice claims resulted from breathing circuit misconnections or disconnections.[65]

Malfunction of the circle system's unidirectional valves can result in life-threatening problems. Rebreathing can occur if the valves stick in the open position, and total occlusion of the circuit can occur if they are stuck shut. If the expiratory valve is stuck in the closed position, breath stacking and barotrauma or volutrauma can result. Obstructed filters located in the expiratory limb of the circle breathing system have caused increased airway pressures, hemodynamic collapse, and bilateral tension pneumothorax. Causes of circle system obstruction and failure include manufacturing defects, debris, patient secretions, and particulate obstruction from other sources such as albuterol nebulization.[66–69] Some systems, such as the GE 7900 SmartVent, use flow transducers located on both the inspiratory and the expiratory limbs of the circle system. In one report, cracks in the flow transducer tubing used by this system produced a leak in the circle system that was difficult to detect.[70]

Variations in Design: Coaxial

In the breathing circuit, corrugated tubes carry gases from the machine to the patient and are available in various configurations. The expiratory and inspiratory limbs may be configured as separate "dual-limb" branches or as a coaxial "tube-within-a-tube" arrangement. In the coaxial configuration, the inner tube is connected to the inspiratory port and the outer tube is connected to the expiratory port. The coaxial design eliminates twisting of inspiratory limbs, provides higher heat and moisture conservation,[71] and removes clutter from the work area. In the dual-limb design, damage to the circuit or a kink in the tubing is easier to detect. While corrugation helps reduce kinks in breathing circuit tubing, the anesthesia provider should consider the possibility of kinked tubing if a patient is difficult to ventilate. A kinked inner coaxial tube has been reported to mimic bronchospasm,[72] presenting with wheezing, elevated peak airway pressures, and patient desaturation. Increasing the length of breathing circuit tubing does not affect dead space or rebreathing. However, longer tubing does increase heat loss and moisture loss, increased circuit breathing resistance, and reduces system breathing system compliance.

CO_2 Absorbents: Canister, Chemistry, Interactions, Indicators

In the early 2000s, there were several reports of adverse chemical reactions between CO_2-absorbent materials and anesthetic agents. Some of these undesirable interactions were quite dramatic, such as sevoflurane interacting with desiccated Baralyme, resulting in fires within the breathing system and severe patient injury.[73,74] Although other sources of ignition and fire in the breathing system continue to be described, the Baralyme–sevoflurane problem is somewhat unique in that nothing "unusual" was added to or removed from the breathing system for this to occur.[75] In August 2004, the manufacturer of Baralyme (Allied Healthcare Products) discontinued the sale of this absorbent. Other reactions between agents such as desflurane or sevoflurane and desiccated strong base absorbents can produce more insidious patient morbidity and potentially even death from the release of byproducts such as carbon monoxide or compound A.[76] Although absorbent materials may be problematic, they still represent an important component of the circle breathing system.

Different anesthesia breathing systems eliminate CO_2 with varying degrees of efficiency. The closed and semiclosed circle systems both require that CO_2 be absorbed from the exhaled gases to avoid hypercapnia. If one could design an ideal CO_2 absorbent, its characteristics would include lack of reactivity with common anesthetics, lack of toxicity, low resistance to gas flow, low cost, ease of handling, and efficiency in CO_2 absorption.

The Absorber Canister

On many anesthesia machines, the absorber canister (Fig. 25-32) is composed of two clear plastic canisters arranged in series. The canisters can be filled either with loose bulk absorbent or with absorbent supplied by the factory in prefilled plastic disposable cartridges called prepacks. Free granules from bulk absorbent can create a clinically significant leak if they lodge between the clear plastic canister and the O-ring gasket of the absorber, or between other joints in the circuit.[77] Leaks have also been caused by defective prepacks, which were larger than factory specifications.[78] Prepacks can also cause total obstruction of the circle system if the clear plastic shipping wrapper is not removed prior to use.[79] Contemporary workstations from GE Healthcare and Dräger use proprietary CO_2 absorbent canisters that allow exchange of the canisters while maintaining the breathing circuit integrity.

The Chemistry of Absorbents

Several formulations of CO_2 absorbents are available today, including soda lime (the most commonly used agent) and calcium hydroxide lime (Amsorb).[80] All serve to remove CO_2 from the breathing circuit with varying degrees of efficiency.

By weight, the approximate composition of "high-moisture" soda lime is 80% calcium hydroxide, 15% water, 4% sodium hydroxide, and 1% potassium hydroxide (an activator). Small amounts of silica are added to produce calcium and sodium silicate. This addition produces a harder and more stable pellet and thereby reduces dust formation. The efficiency of the soda lime absorption varies inversely with the hardness; therefore, little silicate is used in contemporary soda lime.[81] Sodium hydroxide is the catalyst for the CO_2-absorptive properties of soda lime. Calcium hydroxide lime is one of the newer clinically available CO_2 absorbents. It consists primarily of calcium hydroxide and calcium chloride and contains two setting agents: calcium sulfate and polyvinylpyrrolidone. The latter two agents serve to enhance the hardness and porosity of the agent.[82] The most significant advantage of calcium hydroxide lime over other agents is its lack of the strong bases, sodium and potassium hydroxide. The absence of these chemicals eliminates the undesirable production of carbon monoxide, the potentially nephrotoxic substance known as compound A, and may reduce or eliminate the possibility of a fire in the breathing circuit.[83] The most significant disadvantages of calcium hydroxide lime are less absorptive capacity, about 50% less than strong-base–containing absorbents, and generally higher cost per unit than other absorbents.[84,85]

The size of the actual absorptive granules has been determined over time by trial and error. The current size particles represent a compromise between resistance to gas flow and absorptive efficiency. The smaller the granule size, the greater the surface area that is available for absorption. However, as particle size decreases, resistance to gas flow increases. The granular size of soda lime used in clinical practice is between 4 and 8 mesh, a size at which absorptive surface area and resistance to flow are optimized. Mesh size refers to the number of openings per linear inch in a sieve through which the granular particles can pass. The absorption of CO_2 by absorbents such as soda lime occurs by a series of chemical reactions; it is not a physical process like soaking water into a sponge. CO_2 combines with water to form carbonic acid. Carbonic acid reacts with the hydroxides to form sodium (or potassium) carbonate and water. Calcium hydroxide accepts the carbonate to form calcium carbonate and sodium (or potassium) hydroxide. The equations for the reactions are as follows:

1. $CO_2 + H_2O \Leftrightarrow H_2CO_3$
2. $H_2CO_3 + 2NaOH(KOH) \Leftrightarrow Na_2CO_3(K_2CO_3) + 2H_2O + Heat$
3. $Na_2CO_3(K_2CO_3) + Ca(OH)_2 \Leftrightarrow CaCO_3 + 2NaOH(KOH)$

Some CO_2 may react directly with $Ca(OH)_2$, but this reaction is much slower.

Absorptive Capacity

The maximum amount of CO_2 that can be absorbed by soda lime is 26 L of CO_2 per 100 g of absorbent. The absorptive capacity of calcium hydroxide lime is significantly less and has been reported at 10.2 L per 100 g of absorbent. However, as previously mentioned, absorptive capacity is the product of both available chemical reactivity and physical (granule) availability. As the absorbent granules stack up in the absorber canisters, small passageways inevitably form. These small passages channel gases preferentially through low-resistance areas. Because of this phenomenon, functional absorptive capacity of either soda lime or calcium hydroxide lime may be substantially decreased.[86]

Indicators

Ethyl violet is the pH indicator added to soda lime to help assess the functional integrity of the absorbent (8 Video 25-8). This compound is a substituted triphenylmethane dye with a critical pH of 10.3.[83] Ethyl violet changes from colorless to violet in color when the pH of the absorbent decreases as a result of CO_2 absorption. When the absorbent is fresh, the pH exceeds the critical pH of the indicator dye, and it exists in its colorless form. However, as absorbent becomes exhausted, the pH decreases below 10.3, and ethyl violet changes to its violet form because of alcohol dehydration. This change in color indicates that the absorptive capacity of the material has been consumed. Unfortunately, in some circumstances, ethyl violet may not always be a reliable indicator of the functional status of absorbent. For example, prolonged exposure of ethyl violet to fluorescent lights can produce photodeactivation of this dye.[87] When this occurs, the absorbent appears white even though it may have a reduced pH and its absorptive capacity has been exhausted. Even in the absence of color changes, evidence of CO_2 absorbent exhaustion includes the patient exhibiting clinical signs of hypercapnia such as hyperventilation, hypertension, and tachycardia. Ultimately, the patient may exhibit acidosis on blood gas analysis.

Although a diagnosis of depletion of CO_2 absorbent capability can be made by observation of clinical signs, the most sensitive indicator of this problem is capnography (CO_2 monitoring) (9 Video 25-9). If the end-expiratory level of exhaled CO_2 is increased, and the inspiratory level is greater than zero, then exhaustion of the CO_2 absorbent must be pursued as a possible cause.

Interactions of Inhaled Anesthetics with Absorbents

5 It is important and desirable to have CO_2 absorbents that neither release toxic particles or fumes nor produce toxic compounds when exposed to common anesthetics. Soda lime and Amsorb generally fit this description, but inhaled anesthetics do interact with all absorbents to some extent.

Sevoflurane has been shown to produce degradation products upon interaction with CO_2 absorbents.[88,89] The major degradation product produced is an olefin compound known as fluoromethyl-2, 2-difluoro-1-(trifluoromethyl) vinyl ether, or *compound A*. During sevoflurane anesthesia, factors apparently leading to an increase in the concentration of compound A include (1) low flow or closed circuit anesthetic techniques; (2) the use of Baralyme (now no longer available); (3) higher concentrations of sevoflurane in the anesthetic circuit; (4) higher absorbent temperatures; and (5) fresh absorbent.[90,91] Interestingly, the dehydration of Baralyme increased the concentration of compound A, but the dehydration of soda lime decreases the concentration of compound A.[92,93] Apparently, the degradation products released during clinical conditions do not commonly result in adverse effects in humans even during low-flow anesthesia.[94–96]

Hepatorenal function biomarkers using sevoflurane are unchanged in patients during low-flow anesthesia when compared to high-flow anesthesia.[97] Desiccated strong-base absorbents can also degrade contemporary inhaled anesthetics to clinically significant concentrations of carbon monoxide as well as trifluoromethane, which can interfere with anesthetic gas monitoring. Under certain conditions, this process can produce very high carboxyhemoglobin concentrations, reaching 35% or more.[98] Higher levels of carbon monoxide are more likely after prolonged contact between absorbent and anesthetics, and after disuse of an absorber for at least 2 days, especially over a weekend.[99] Thus, case reports describing carbon monoxide poisoning have been most common in patients anesthetized on Monday morning, presumably because continuous flow from the unused anesthesia machine desiccated the absorbents over the weekend. FGF rates of 5 L/min or more through the breathing system and absorbent (without connection to a patient) are sufficient to cause critical drying of the absorbent material. This is even worse when the reservoir bag is left off the breathing circuit. Absence of the reservoir bag facilitates retrograde flow through the circle system (Fig. 25-32).

Several factors appear to increase the production of carbon monoxide and result in increased carboxyhemoglobin levels. They include (1) the inhaled anesthetic used (for a given MAC multiple, the magnitude of CO production from greatest to least is desflurane ≥ enflurane > isoflurane >> halothane = sevoflurane); (2) the absorbent dryness (completely dry absorbent produces more CO than hydrated absorbent); (3) the type of absorbent (at a given water content, Baralyme produced more CO than does soda lime); (4) the temperature (increased temperature increases CO production); (5) the anesthetic concentration (more CO is produced from higher anesthetic concentrations)[92]; (6) low FGF rates; and (7) reduced experimental animal (patient) size per 100 g of absorbent.[100]

Several interventions have been suggested to reduce the incidence of carbon monoxide exposure in patients undergoing general anesthesia. These interventions include (1) educating anesthesia personnel regarding the etiology of CO production; (2) turning off the anesthesia machine at the conclusion of the last case of the day to eliminate FGF that dries the absorbent; (3) changing CO_2 absorbent if fresh gas was found flowing during the morning machine preuse check; (4) rehydrating desiccated absorbent by adding water; (5) changing the chemical composition of soda lime to reduce or eliminate potassium hydroxide (products now available include Drägersorb 800 plus, Sofnolime, and Spherasorb); and (6) using absorbent materials such as calcium hydroxide lime that are free of both sodium and potassium hydroxides. The elimination of sodium and potassium hydroxides from desiccated soda lime diminishes or eliminates degradation of desflurane to carbon monoxide and sevoflurane to compound A, but does not compromise CO_2 absorption.[101]

As a result of the increasing evidence that exposure of volatile anesthetics to desiccated CO_2 absorbents could be hazardous (Table 25-6), the Anesthesia Patient Safety Foundation (APSF) convened in 2005 a conference on CO_2 absorption safety considerations. The conference experts agreed with the following recommendations[80]:

1. Turn off all gas flow when the machine is not in use
2. Change absorbents regularly (on Monday mornings, since the absorbent may become desiccated over the weekend)
3. Change absorbent whenever the color change indicates exhaustion
4. Change BOTH canisters in a two-canister system
5. Change absorbent whenever the FGF has been left on for an extensive or indeterminate period of time
6. If compact canisters are used, consider changing them more frequently

One extremely rare but potentially life-threatening compli- 6
cation related to CO_2 absorbent use is the development of fires within the breathing system. Specifically, this can occur as the result of interactions between the strong-base absorbents (particularly with the now-obsolete Baralyme) and the inhaled anesthetic sevoflurane. When desiccated strong-base absorbents are exposed to sevoflurane, absorber temperatures of several hundred degrees may result from their interaction. The buildup of very high temperatures, the formation of combustible degradation by-products (formaldehyde, methanol, and formic acid), and the oxygen- or nitrous oxide–enriched environment provide all the substrates necessary for a fire to occur.

Modern absorbent formulations that limit or eliminate strong base (NaOH or KOH) have made it possible to safely decrease FGF to closed-circuit conditions without concern for toxic byproducts. For example, Litholyme contains a lithium catalyst to facilitate CO_2 absorption and does not use strong bases. Litholyme contains a lithium catalyst. The lithium catalyst does not react with common inhaled anesthetic agents and therefore eliminates the potential for generation of CO or compound A. Absorption of CO_2 is minimally exothermic. The indicator color change from off-white to violet is permanent and profound, indicating both

Table 25-6 Absorbent Comparisons[80a]

Company	Product Name	H_2O%	NaOH%	KOH%	$Ca(OH)_2$%	Significant Other	U.S. Availability
Allied Healthcare/Chemetron	Baralyme	11.0–16.0	0.0	<5	73	$Ba(OH)_2$	No longer
Allied Healthcare	Carbolime[b]	12.0–19.0	3	0.0	>75	—	Yes
W.R. Grace and Company	Sodasorb	15.0–17.0	3.7	—	50–100	—	Yes
Intersurgical Ltd.	Intersorb Plus	13.5–17.5	2.6	0.0	81	—	Yes
Intersurgical Ltd.	Spherasorb	13.5–17.5	1.3	0.0	78	4% Zeolite	Yes
Intersurgical Ltd.	LoFloSorb	13.5–17.5	0.0	0.0	78	6.5% Silica	Yes
Armstrong Medical Ltd.	Amsorb	13.5–16.5	0.0	0.0	79–82	$CaCl_2$	No longer
Armstrong Medical Ltd.	Amsorb Plus	13.0–18.0	0.0	0.0	>80	$CaCl_2$	Yes
Dräger Medical, Inc.	Drägersorb 800	—	~2	~3	—	—	No longer
Dräger Medical, Inc.	Drägersorb 800 Plus	~16	1–3	NA	75–83	—	Yes
Dräger Medical, Inc.	Drägersorb Free	14–18	0.5–2	NA	74–82	$CaCl_2$	Yes
Airgas/Molecular Products	Sodalime	—	<3.5	2.6	>80	—	Yes
Molecular Products	Sofnolime	12–19	<3.5	0.0	—	—	No[d]
GE Medical[c]/Molecular Products	Medisorb	—	<3.5	0.0	—	—	Yes

[a]This table was formulated based on information supplied by the various manufacturers. The APSF assumes no responsibility for variations in, or deviations from, the formulations that are represented in this table. The table is supplied for educational and conceptual purposes.
[b]Manufactured by Molecular Products.
[c]Distributor of product manufactured by Molecular Products.
[d]Not available in US market as a medical product, although diving and military grades are available in the United States. Medical grade is available outside the United States.
More than one manufacturer reported variable absorption capacity based on canister design, shape, volume FGF, hydration, and carbon dioxide concentration. Nearly all reported price variability dependent upon marketing and type of fill.
Reproduced from Olympio MA. Carbon dioxide absorbent desiccation safety conference convened by APSF. *APSF Newsletter*. 2005;20:256–29. Copyright © 2005 Anesthesia Patient Safety Foundation.

exhaustion and/or desiccation and eliminating the possibility for unintentional use of expended absorbent.

SpiraLith Ca (Micropore Inc., Elkton, MD) is supplied on a polymer matrix base and rolled up as a fixed spiral in a cylinder. It does not use lithium or an indicator to show exhaustion so that the anesthesiologist must monitor inspired CO_2. An advantage is that the exhausted absorbent can be recycled by the manufacturer.

Mapleson Circuits

In 1954, William Mapleson described the elimination of carbon dioxide in five different semiclosed breathing systems. These five systems are now classically referred to as the Mapleson systems and are designated with letters A through E (Fig. 25-33).[103] Subsequently, Willis et al.[104] described the F system that was added to the original five. The Mapleson systems consist of several common components: a facemask, an expiratory valve, corrugated reservoir tubing (not present in the C circuit), fresh gas inflow tubing, and a reservoir bag (not present in the E-circuit). Within the Mapleson systems, three distinct functional groups can be seen: the A group; the B and C group; and the D, E, and F group.

Although its components and component arrangements are simple, functional analysis of the Mapleson systems can be complex. Mapleson wanted to examine how much FGF from the anesthesia machine was necessary relative to a patient's minute ventilation in order to adequately prevent rebreathing during spontaneous ventilation. The amount of CO_2 rebreathing associated with each system is multifactorial, and variables that dictate the ultimate CO_2 concentration include (1) the fresh gas inflow rate, (2) the patient's minute ventilation, (3) the mode of ventilation (spontaneous or controlled), (4) the tidal volume, (5) the respiratory rate, (6) the I:E ratio, (7) the duration of the expiratory pause, (8) the peak inspiratory flow rate, (9) the volume of the reservoir tube, (10) the volume of the breathing bag, (11) ventilation by mask, (12) ventilation through an endotracheal tube, and (13) the CO_2 sampling site.

The performance of the Mapleson systems is best understood by studying the expiratory phase of the respiratory cycle.[105] Illustrations of the various Mapleson system component arrangements are shown in Figure 25-33. Figure 25-34 shows gas exchange during spontaneous and during controlled ventilation with Mapleson A and D circuits. During spontaneous ventilation, the Mapleson A has the best efficiency of the six systems requiring a fresh gas inflow rate of only 1 times the patient's minute ventilation to prevent rebreathing of exhaled CO_2. However, it has the least efficiency during controlled ventilation, requiring an FGF as high as 20 L/min to prevent rebreathing. Systems D, E, and F are slightly more efficient than systems B and C. To prevent rebreathing of CO_2, the D, E, and F systems require an FGF rate of approximately 2.5 times the minute ventilation, whereas the FGF rates required for B and C systems are somewhat higher.[106] The Mapleson A, B, and C systems are rarely used today, but the D, E, F systems are still commonly employed. In the United

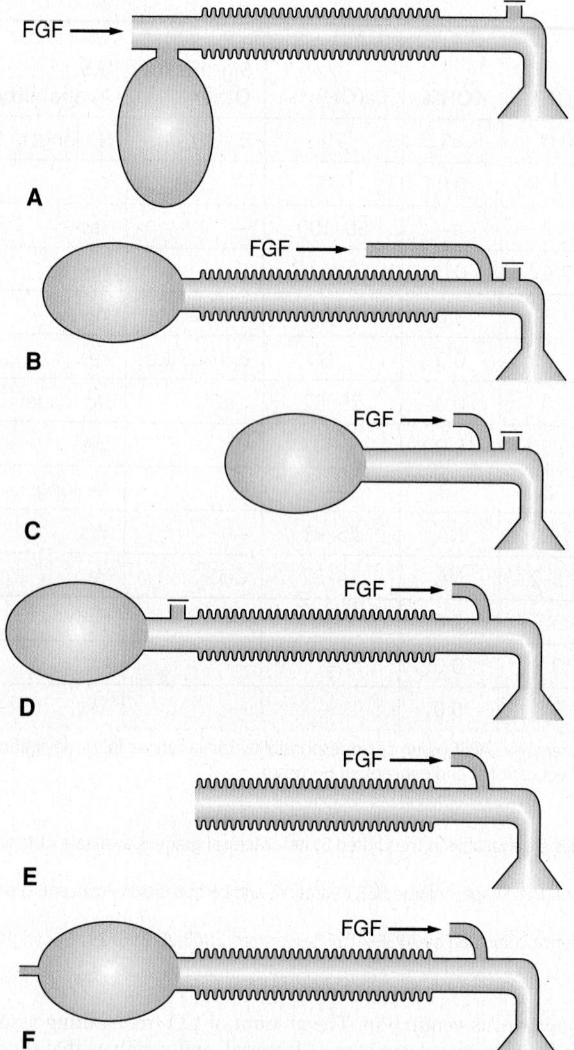

Figure 25-33 Mapleson breathing systems (**A–F**). (Adapted from Willis BA, Pender JW, Mapleson WW. Rebreathing in a T-piece: volunteer and theoretical studies of the Jackson-Rees modification of Ayre's T-piece during spontaneous respiration. *Br J Anaesth.* 1975;47:1239. Copyright © 1975 Elseiver. With permission.)

States, the most popular iteration of the D, E, F group is the Bain circuit.

The Bain Circuit

The Bain circuit is a coaxial circuit and a modification of the Mapleson D system. The fresh gas flows through a narrow inner tube within the outer corrugated tubing. The inner fresh gas tubing enters the outer corrugated hose near the reservoir bag, but the fresh gas actually empties into the circuit at the patient end (Fig. 25-35). Exhaled gases enter the corrugated tubing and are vented through the expiratory valve near the reservoir bag. The Bain circuit may be used for both spontaneous and controlled ventilation. The fresh gas inflow rate necessary to prevent rebreathing is 2.5 times the patient's minute ventilation.

The Bain circuit has many advantages over other systems. It is lightweight, convenient, and disposable. Scavenging of the waste gases from the "pop-off" valve is facilitated because the valve is located away from the patient. Exhaled gases in the outer reservoir tubing add warmth by countercurrent heat exchange to inspired fresh gases. The main hazards related to the use of the Bain circuit are either an unrecognized disconnection or kinking of the inner fresh gas hose. These problems can cause hypercapnia from inadequate gas flow or increased respiratory resistance. As with other circuits, an obstructed antimicrobial filter positioned between the Bain circuit and the tracheal tube can result in increased resistance in the circuit and may mimic the signs and symptoms of severe bronchospasm.[107]

The outer corrugated tube is transparent to allow ongoing inspection of the inner tube. The integrity of the inner tube can be assessed as described by Pethick.[108] With his technique, high-flow oxygen is fed into the circuit while the patient end is occluded until the reservoir bag is filled. The patient end is opened, and oxygen is flushed into the circuit. If the inner tube is intact, the Venturi effect occurs at the patient end. This causes a decrease in pressure within the circuit, and as a result, the reservoir bag deflates. Conversely, a leak in the inner tube allows the fresh gas to escape into the expiratory limb, and the reservoir bag will remain inflated. Testing for this is recommended as a part of the preanesthesia check if a Bain circuit is used.

The Jackson-Rees (Mapleson F) Circuit

The Jackson-Rees circuit is a Mapleson F system commonly used in pediatrics. Its primary advantage is low resistance and minimal dead space. The FGF required to prevent rebreathing is similar to the Mapleson D circuit (approximately 2.5 times minute ventilation). A valve to vent excess gases is employed. This mechanism may also be used to control circuit pressure for hand ventilation or opened for spontaneous ventilation. Compared to a pediatric circle system, the Jackson-Rees may offer less difficulty in breathing (though this appears to be negligible in most cases), as well as less gastric insufflation.[109]

The Self-Inflating Resuscitation Bag

Perhaps the two most important but often overlooked items in the preuse checkout of the anesthesia workstation are a functioning (tested) self-inflating resuscitation bag (SIRB) (Fig. 25-37) and a readily available full auxiliary tank of oxygen. This is "plan B"—the backup plan. Many of the adverse outcomes associated with anesthesia equipment mishaps could have been averted if the SIRB had been used or used sooner. Unfortunately, the SIRB is an item frequently missed in the preanesthesia setup.[110] SIRB devices are designed to be lightweight, usually with a textured bag for secure handling. They often have a clear valve housing with a 360-degree swivel connector that provides an unobstructed view of the valve operation and optimal device positioning. The oxygen tubing includes a universal connector. Common accessories include a manometer, PEEP valve, CO_2 detector, expiratory filter, and masks.

Anesthesia Ventilators

The ventilator on anesthesia workstations generates positive pressure to facilitate gas flow from the anesthesia machine into the patient's lungs and can be seen as a mechanized substitute for the manual squeezing of the reservoir bag of the circle system. While they started out as simple bellows devices to free up the hands of the anesthesia provider, they now have become sophisticated ventilation devices that can rival modern intensive care ventilators. While many similarities exist between today's anesthesia ventilator and ICU ventilator, some fundamental differences in ventilation parameters and control systems remain, such as the integration of a circle system into the anesthesia ventilators to conserve volatile anesthetics, whereas the ICU ventilators vent

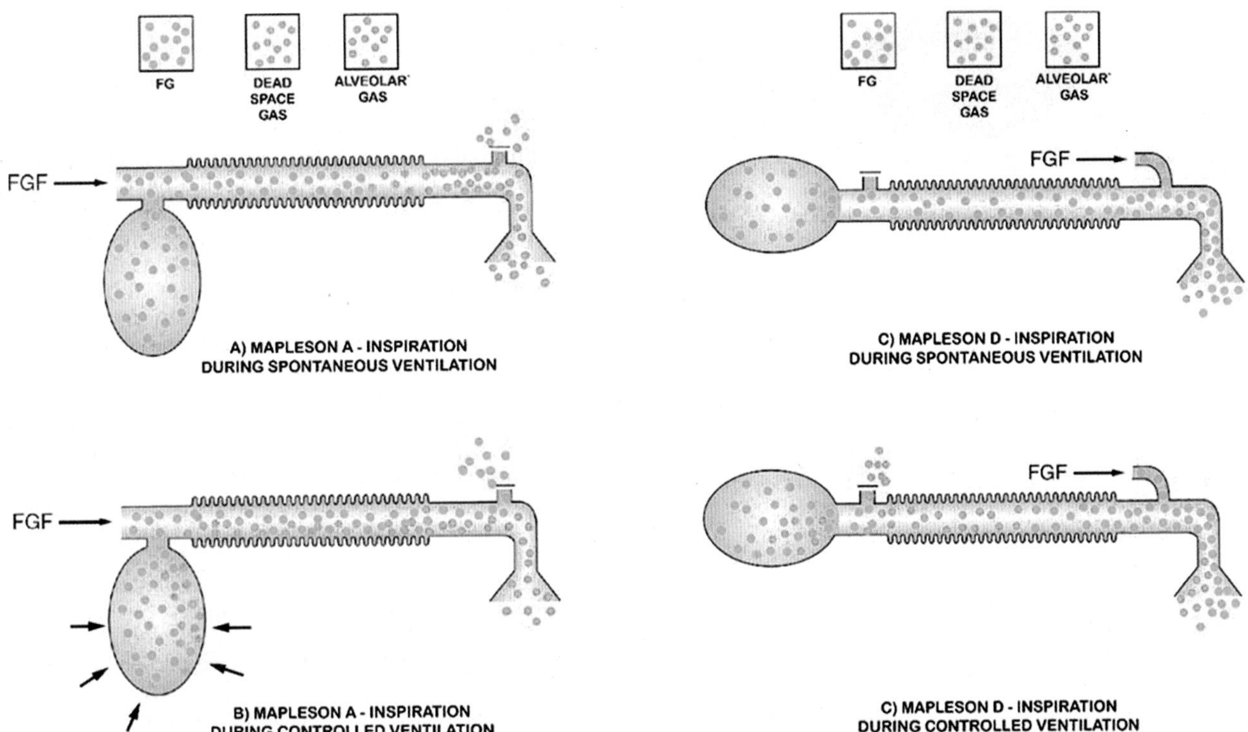

Figure 25-34 Illustration of gas exchange during spontaneous and controlled ventilation with Mapleson A and D circuits. The Mapleson A is the most efficient circuit for spontaneous ventilation. The Mapleson D is the most efficient during controlled ventilation.

the exhaled gas directly into the hospital room. The energy for modern anesthesia ventilators to provide flow to the lungs comes from either electricity or compressed gas. They are electronically controlled, and flow is directed through unidirectional flow and pressure relief valves.

Four different technologies are currently used to generate positive pressure gas flows in anesthesia ventilators:

1. Pneumatic-driven bellows using compressed gas from the wall outlet or cylinder that during expiration are either
   a. ascending (General Electric, Mindray up to A7, Spacelabs, and older Dräger machines), or
   b. descending (early generation anesthesia machines and Mindray Anestar)
2. Electric piston pumps (Dräger, Fabius, Apollo, and Atlan)
3. Electric turbines (Dräger Perseus, Zeus)
4. Volume exchangers using compressed medical gas straight from the wall outlet or cylinder (Maquet/Getinge and Mindray A8/A9)

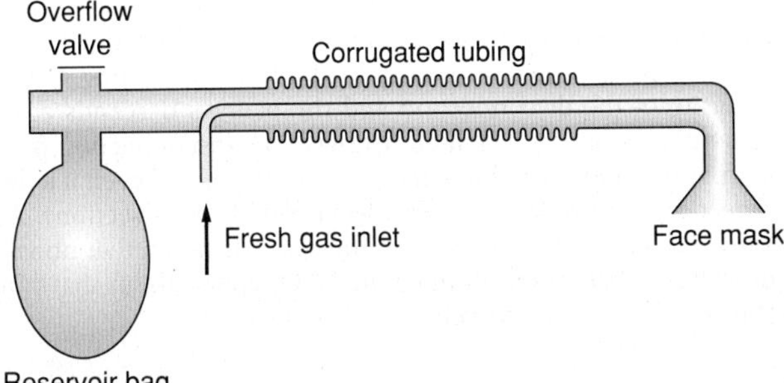

Figure 25-35 The Bain circuit (Coaxial version of Mapleson D). (Adapted with permission from Springer: Bain JA, Spoerel WE. A streamlined anaesthetic system. *Can Anaesth Soc J.* 1972;19(4):426–435.)

The different technologies not only differ in the way they provide gas flow to the lungs, but also how they accept the patient's exhalation, as well as providing for manual and spontaneous ventilation. A good understanding of the different technologies will help not only with troubleshooting in case of a malfunction but may also influence purchasing decisions according to their intended uses, such as for military and civilian environments, or other situations with limited availability of compressed gas.

Pneumatically Driven Bellows Ventilators

Traditionally, anesthesia ventilators were pneumatically driven bellows circle systems (Fig. 25-37) that are classified as a double-circuit ventilator. In this type of system, the patient circuit gas is inside the bellows, which is contained in a rigid plastic housing (called the bellows housing or chamber). The driving gas circuit consists of compressed gas connected to the rigid housing containing the bellows. The driving gas can be oxygen, air, or a mixture of both, through a machine setting provided by the manufacturer or biomedical engineering department, while the respired gas composition inside the bellows is a user setting adjusted by the anesthesia provider. While the old basic concept remains the same, modern anesthesia workstations have incorporated more safety features and are electronically controlled.

During the inspiratory phase (Fig. 25-37A), the driving gas enters the bellows chamber, causing the pressure within it to increase. This increase in pressure is responsible for two events. First, the ventilator relief valve closes, preventing gas from escaping into the scavenging system. Second, the bellows is compressed, and the respired gas within the bellows is delivered to the patient's lungs. This compression action is analogous to the hand of the anesthesiologist squeezing the breathing bag, leading to the machine's moniker of a "bag-in-a-bottle" ventilator.

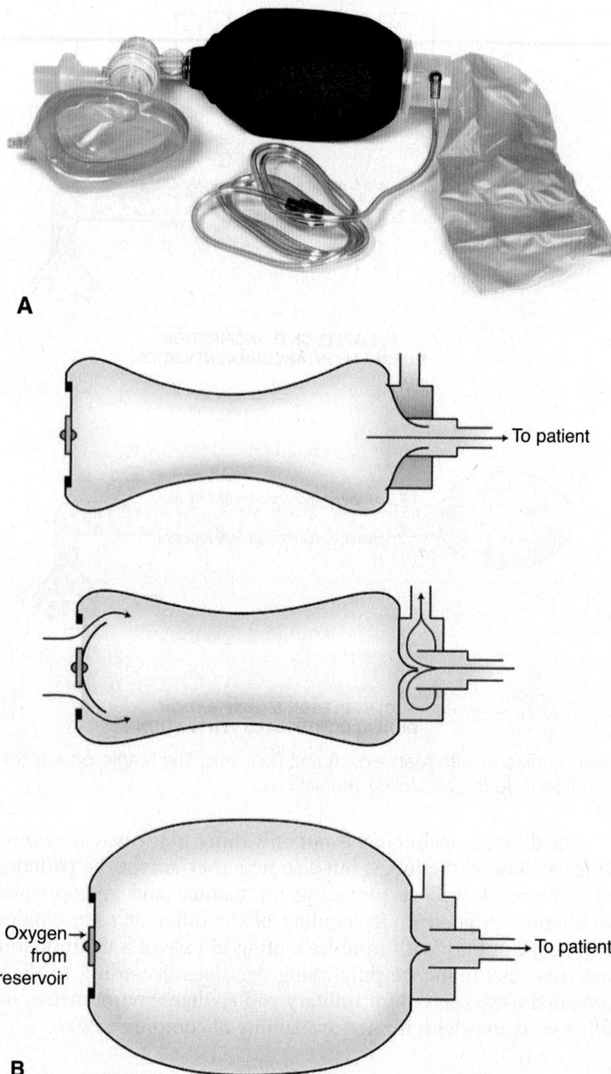

Figure 25-36 **A:** Self-inflating resuscitation bag (SIRB). **B:** Schematics of SIRB: a. Bag squeezed = inflation of lungs as the fishmouth valve opens to patient and closes exhalation path. b. Bag released = exhalation as fishmouth valve closes to patient and opens exhalation pathway. Bag re-expands and fills with oxygen from reservoir via one-way valve. c. Between breaths.

At the end of inspiration, the drive gas circuit inlet valve closes at the chosen tidal volume or pressure, providing an inspiratory pause.

During the expiratory phase (Fig. 25-37B), the driving gas exits the bellows housing through the outlet valve. This produces a decrease to atmospheric pressure within both the bellows housing and the pilot line controlling the ventilator relief valve. The decrease in pressure to the ventilator relief valve causes the "mushroom valve" portion of the assembly to open. Exhaled patient gases refill the bellows before any scavenging can begin. The bellows refills first because a weighted ball (like those used in ball-type PEEP valves) or similar device is incorporated into the base of the ventilator relief valve. This ball produces 2 to 3 cm H_2O of back pressure; therefore, flow to scavenging occurs only after the bellows fills completely and the pressure inside the bellows exceeds the pressure threshold of the "ball valve." This design causes all ascending bellows ventilators to produce 2 to 3 cm water pressure of PEEP within the breathing circuit when the ventilator is in use. Scavenging occurs only during the expiratory phase, as the ventilator relief valve is open only during expiration.

Contemporary electronic ventilators use a solid-state electronic timing device to cycle between inhalation and exhalation and are thus classified as time cycled and electronically controlled. More advanced ventilation modes such as synchronized intermittent mandatory ventilation (SIMV), pressure-controlled ventilation (PCV), and modes that utilize a pressure-support option have an adjustable threshold pressure trigger as well. In these modes, pressure sensors provide feedback to the ventilator control system to allow it to determine when to initiate and/or terminate the respiratory cycle. It is important to understand that on most older anesthesia workstations, gas flow from the anesthesia machine flowmeter tubes into the breathing circuit is continuous and independent of ventilator activity. During the inspiratory phase of mechanical ventilation, the ventilator relief valve is closed (Fig. 25-37A), and the breathing system's APL (pop-off) valve is most commonly out of circuit. Therefore, the patient's lungs receive the volume from the bellows in addition to that entering the circuit from the flowmeters during the inspiratory phase.

Factors that influence the relationship between set tidal volume and exhaled tidal volume are the FGF settings, the inspiratory time, the compliance of the breathing circuit, external leakage, and the location of the tidal volume sensor. Usually, the volume gained from the flowmeters during inspiration is offset by the volume lost to compliance of the breathing circuit, and set tidal volume generally approximates the exhaled tidal volume. However, certain conditions such as inappropriate activation of the oxygen flush valve during the inspiratory phase can result in barotrauma and/or volutrauma to the patient's lungs because excess pressure and volume may not be able to be vented from the circle system.[111] Pressure and flow sensors serve as feedback loops to adjust the bellows excursion, taking into account the amount of FGF used to maintain the predetermined ventilator settings, as the FGF usually enters the breathing circuit on the patient side of the ventilator downstream from the bellows. 7

During mechanical ventilation, the manual reservoir bag and the APL valve are separated from the active breathing circuit through a selector switch.

The direction of the bellows movement during the expiratory phase determines the bellows classification (10 Video 25-10, 11 Video 25-11). *Ascending (standing) bellows* ascend during the expiratory phase (Fig. 25-37B), whereas *descending (hanging) bellows* descend during the expiratory phase. Of the two configurations, the ascending bellows is generally thought to be safer. An ascending bellows will not fill if a total disconnection occurs. However, the bellows of a descending bellows ventilator will continue its upward and downward movement despite a patient disconnection, because the driving gas pushes the descending bellows upward during the inspiratory phase. Then during the expiratory phase, room air is entrained into the breathing system at the site of the disconnection and the bellows descends again as gravity acts on the weighted bellows. The disconnection pressure monitor and the volume monitor may be fooled even if a disconnection is complete (see Problems and Hazards section). An essential safety feature on any anesthesia workstation that utilizes a descending bellows is an integrated CO_2 apnea alarm that cannot be disabled while the ventilator is in use. 8

Electric Piston Pump Ventilators

More recently, with the introduction of circle breathing systems that integrate FGD, mechanically driven anesthesia ventilators

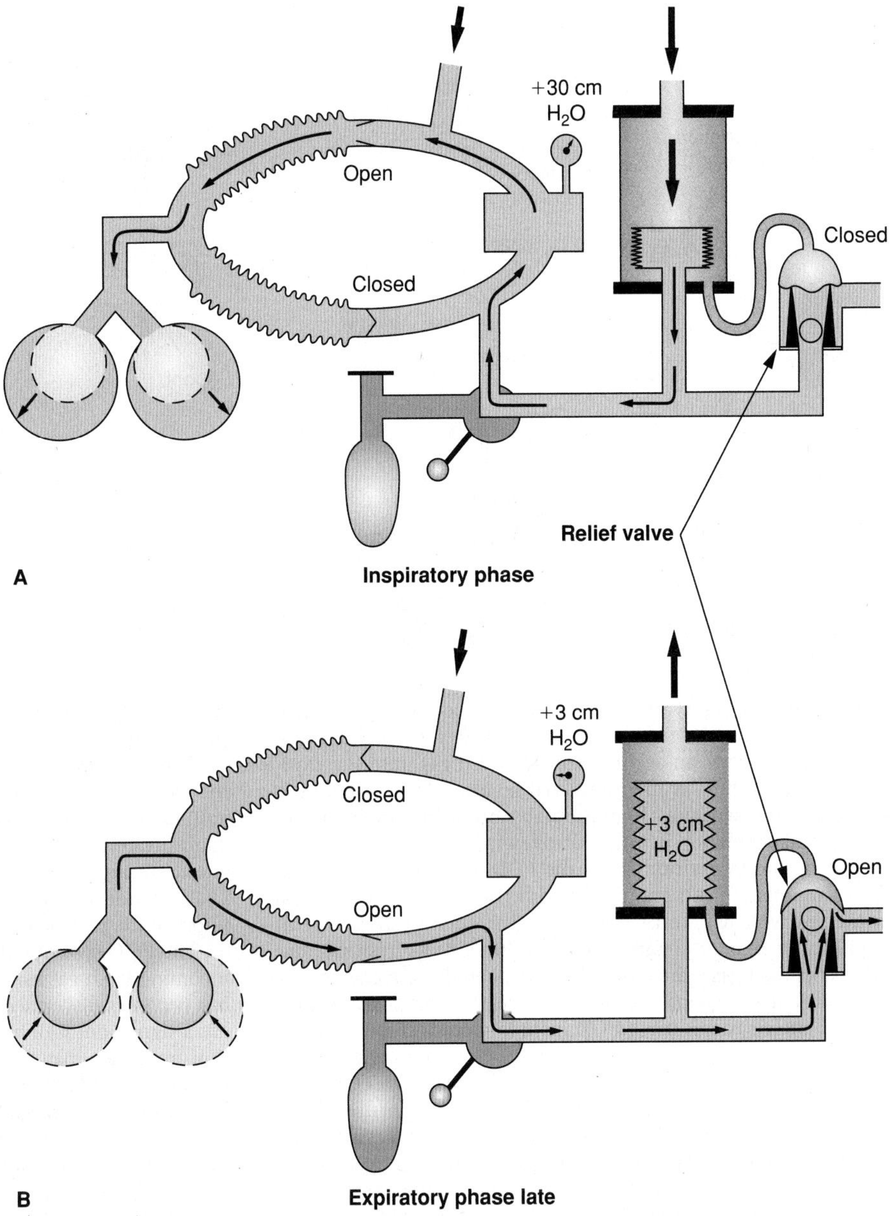

Figure 25-37 Inspiratory (**A**) and expiratory (**B**) phases of gas flow in a traditional circle system with an ascending bellows ventilator. The bellows physically separates the driving gas circuit from the patient gas circuit. The driving gas circuit is located outside the bellows, and the patient gas circuit is inside the bellows. During inspiratory phase (**A**), the driving gas enters the bellows chamber, causing the pressure within it to increase. This causes the ventilator relief valve to close, preventing anesthetic gas from escaping into the scavenging system, and the bellows to compress, delivering anesthetic gas within the bellows to the patient's lungs. During expiratory phase (**B**), pressure within the bellows chamber and the pilot line decreases to zero, causing the mushroom portion of the ventilator relief valve to open. Gas exhaled by the patient refills the bellows before any scavenging occurs, because a weighted ball is incorporated into the base of the ventilator relief valve. Scavenging occurs only during the expiratory phase, because the ventilator relief valve is only open during expiration. (Adapted from Andrews JJ. *The Circle System. A Collection of 30 Color Illustrations*. Library of Congress; 1998.)

have surged in popularity. These "piston"-type ventilators use a computer-controlled stepper motor instead of compressed drive gas to actuate gas movement in the breathing system. Thus, they are classified as electrically powered, piston driven, single circuit, and electronically controlled with FGD. In these systems, the piston operates much like the plunger of a syringe to deliver the desired tidal volume or airway pressure to the patient breathing circuit. Thus, it is able to deliver very accurate tidal volumes.

Sophisticated computerized controls are able to provide advanced types of ventilatory support such as SIMV, PCV, and pressure support–assisted ventilation, in addition to the conventional volume and pressure control. Since the patient's mechanical breath is delivered without the use of compressed gas to squeeze a bellows, these systems consume dramatically less compressed gas during ventilator operation than traditional pneumatic ventilators. This improvement in efficiency may have clinical significance when the anesthesia workstation is used in a setting where no pipeline gas supply is available.

The incorporation of this patient safety–enhancing technology 9
has required a significant redesign of the traditional circle system. A functional schematic of a circle system similar to the one used by the Dräger Fabius, Apollo, and Atlan series mechanical ventilation can be seen in Figure 25-38. To understand the operating principles of FGD, it is important to have a good understanding of gas flows in a traditional circle system during both inspiratory and expiratory phases of mechanical ventilation covered earlier in this section. The key concept of the FGD breathing system can be illustrated during the inspiratory phase of mechanical ventilation. During the inspiratory phase (Fig. 25-38), the piston pushes its volume into the lungs through the open inspiratory unidirectional valve with excess pressure vented through the Pmax/PEEP valve located on the patient side of the expiratory unidirectional valve. The fresh gas entering the breathing circuit from the anesthesia workstation flowmeters via the fresh gas inlet is diverted into the reservoir bag by a decoupling valve that is located between the fresh gas source and the ventilator circuit and is closed during

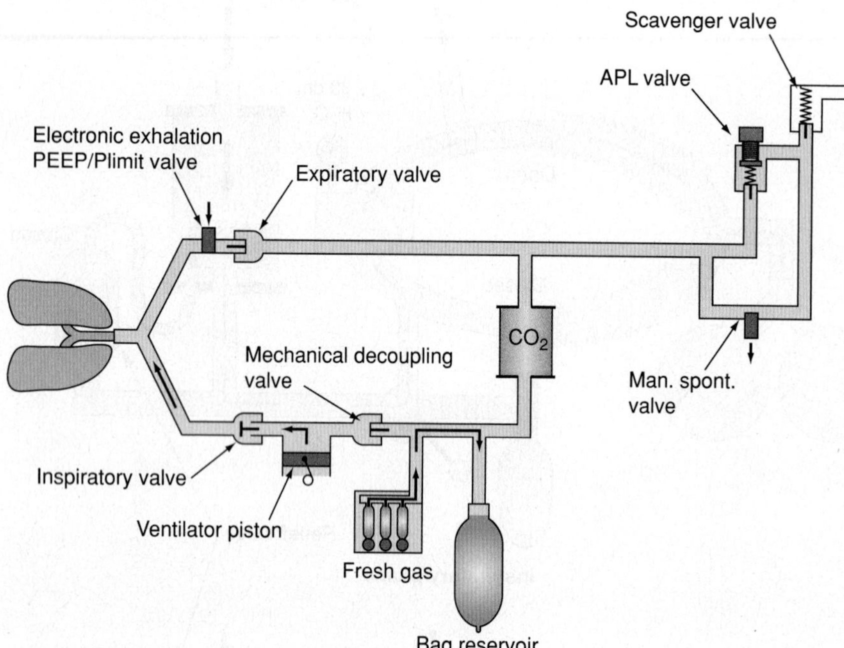

Figure 25-38 Fresh gas decoupled (FDG) breathing system during inspiratory phase of mechanical ventilation. The figure demonstrates the path of fresh gas (and O_2 flush) into the reservoir bag during upstroke of the ventilator piston. Note the requirement here for a mechanical decoupling valve and electronic exhalation/PEEP/Plimit valve. A man./spont. valve is electronically opened during CMV, so that excess gas can escape through the low-pressure scavenger valve, which also allows preferential filling of the reservoir bag during the inspiratory phase. (Adapted from Olympio MA. Modern anesthesia machines offer new safety features. *APSF Newsletter*. 2003;18:17. Copyright © 2003 Anesthesia Patient Safety Foundation.)

inspiration. The reservoir bag is always connected to the active breathing circuit as it serves as the reservoir for the patient's exhalation and serves as an accumulator for fresh gas until the expiratory phase begins; in the traditional bellows circle system, the reservoir bag is separated from the active breathing circuit during mechanical ventilation by the selector switch.

During the expiratory phase, the FGD valve opens, allowing the accumulated fresh gas, mixed with the patient's exhaled gas in the reservoir bag, to be drawn into the circle system to refill the piston ventilator chamber (Fig. 25-38). Excess fresh gas and exhaled patient gases are allowed to escape to the scavenging system through the open APL bypass valve. The proposed advantages of circle systems using FGD include more accurate delivery of the set tidal volume and decreased risk of barotrauma and volutrauma. With a traditional circle system, increases in FGF from the flowmeters or from inappropriate use of the oxygen flush valve may contribute directly to tidal volume, which, if excessive, may result in pneumothorax or other injuries. Since the FGD valve isolates fresh gas entering the system from reaching the patient during inhalation, the risk of barotrauma is greatly reduced.

Problems and Hazards with Piston Ventilators

In the FGD system, the retracting piston causes the piston chamber to refill under negative pressure. If the volume of gas contained in the reservoir bag plus the returning volume of gas exhaled from the patient's lungs is inadequate to refill the piston chamber, the reservoir bag collapses, and negative patient airway pressures could develop. To prevent this, an air entrainment valve is incorporated into the breathing system which opens below a preset value, such as –2 cm H_2O, drawing ambient air into the patient gas circuit. If this goes undetected, the entrained atmospheric gases could lead to a slow dilution of the inhaled anesthetic agents, the enriched oxygen mixture, or both. If unnoticed, this dilution of respired gases could lead to intraoperative patient awareness or hypoxia. High-priority alarms with both audible and visual alerts should notify the user that FGF is inadequate and room air is being entrained. The oxygen and anesthetic gas analyzers will also alert the anesthesia provider in those scenarios.

The delivery of FGF to the exhalation side and mixing with the exhaled gas, combined with a large internal breathing circuit volume, will delay the effects of adjustments to the different FGF concentrations and requires a more accurate anticipation of the anesthetic requirements during the different surgical stages. Newer Dräger models have smaller internal breathing circuit volumes to improve the responsiveness to changes in FGF composition.

The FGD system relies on the reservoir bag to accumulate the incoming fresh gas as well as patient-exhaled gas. If the reservoir bag becomes disconnected during mechanical ventilation, or if it has a significant leak from poor fit on the bag mount or a perforation, room air may enter the breathing circuit as the ventilator piston unit refills during expiratory phase[112] and may also result in dilution of the inhaled anesthetic agents, the enriched oxygen mixture, or both. Furthermore, this type of a disruption could lead to significant contamination of the operating room atmosphere with anesthetic gases as fresh gases and patient-exhaled gases would be allowed to escape into the room atmosphere. Incompetence of the FGD valve leads to inability to ventilate the patient's lungs using the ventilator, but the ability to ventilate using the reservoir bag in the circuit is maintained.[113]

An advantage of the FGD system is the ability to deliver a mechanical positive-pressure breath if there is a leak in the low-pressure system of the workstation upstream from the FGD valve (either in the reservoir bag or CO_2 absorber) that permits air entry as the piston "sucks" gas in, where manual positive-pressure ventilation would not be possible.[114] The ventilator would continue to deliver the tidal volume as air–FGF mix but at least it would deliver positive pressure until someone can troubleshoot the problem. In bellows circle systems, a leak or malposition of the CO_2 absorber cartridge would result in the inability (depending on the size of the leak) to provide positive pressure with manual or with mechanical ventilation. If the expiratory unidirectional valve is missing or incompetent, mechanical ventilation is possible, as the FGD valve will act as an expiratory valve for the mechanical ventilator, but manual ventilation is not possible.[115]

Electric Turbine Ventilators

Another mechanically driven ventilator technology uses a turbine to generate gas flow. It is single circuit, electrically powered, and electronically controlled with a turbine that constantly turns at variable speeds according to the chosen settings. Like with the piston ventilators, the reservoir bag is always part of the active breathing circuit to receive the patient's exhalation. In mechanical ventilation, during the inspiratory phase, the turbine increases its speed and draws the contents of the reservoir bag (containing the patient's exhalation and FGF) through the CO_2 absorber, pushing it through the inspiratory valve toward the patient's lungs. The manual APL valve is bypassed during mechanical ventilation through the APL-bypass valve, allowing excess gas to be released into the scavenging system. As with the piston-driven ventilator, FGF is continuously injected into the breathing system on the machine side of the inspiratory valve and will flow toward the reservoir bag through the turbine when the inspiratory valve is closed. However, it is not a mechanical FGF decoupling valve. The Pmax/PEEP valve is only active during mechanical ventilation and limits the pressure during inspiration and provides PEEP during exhalation. Since the turbine draws from the reservoir bag during inspiration (like the piston drawing from the bag), this breathing circuit also uses an air entrainment valve for negative-pressure relief to protect the patient's lungs against negative pressure by drawing in room air if the bag fully collapses.

In manual/spontaneous ventilation mode, the APL-bypass valve is closed, making the manual APL valve active. Closing the valve to the desired pressure level will allow positive-pressure ventilation by squeezing the bag as in all other anesthesia ventilators. However, the turbine can assist spontaneous efforts when it senses negative pressure, thereby considerably reducing the resistance in the breathing system and allowing the patient to breathe at a stable pressure that can be set higher than ambient pressure to provide CPAP. In addition, compared to all the other modern anesthesia ventilator modes, the turbine ventilator alone is able to provide airway pressure release ventilation (APRV), which was previously available only in ICU ventilators.

Volume Reflectors

The Maquet/Getinge FLOW-i, and Mindray A8/A9 workstations use a novel breathing system that dispenses with the need for a bellows, turbine, or piston to provide positive-pressure ventilation, similar to modern ICU ventilators but with an added circle system (Fig. 25-38). The system incorporates a volume reflector (a 3.6-m–long plastic coil with an internal volume of 1.2 L) located between the circle system, the reservoir bag, and APL/PEEP valve (Fig. 25-39). Also connected directly to the volume reflector is

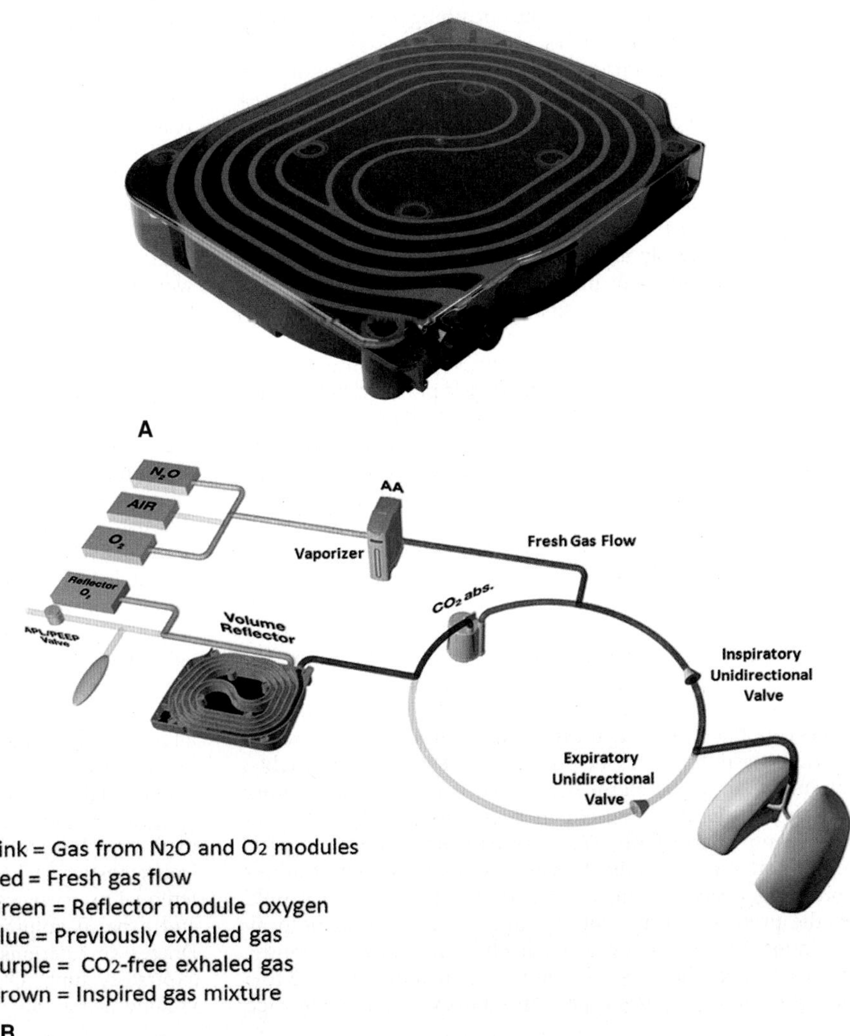

Figure 25-39 **A:** Maquet Flow-i volume reflector. **B:** Maquet FLOW-I breathing and ventilator circuit during positive-pressure inspiration. See text for details.

the reflector oxygen module that provides oxygen as the driving gas during positive-pressure ventilation. It is classified as gas powered, single circuit, and electronically controlled. During mechanical ventilation, the APL and the PEEP valve close. FGF is provided during inspiration for each selected gas (O_2/air/N_2O) by a compressed gas module, which then pass through an electronic vaporizer before being added to the inspiratory side of the circle system combining with the oxygen flow from the reflector gas module to achieve the set FiO_2 and anesthetic agent concentration.

Additional driving gas is added to the volume reflector from a separate oxygen gas module to make up the difference between the set tidal volume and the FGF, pushing the stored exhaled gas in the volume exchanger through the CO_2 absorber into the patient's lung, mixing with the FGF along the way. Even though there is no barrier between the oxygen drive gas and the exhaled gas, there is minimal mixing of the gases.

During exhalation, the PEEP valve opens to a set PEEP value, releasing the pressure in the breathing circuit. The patient exhales into the volume reflector with excess gas vented through the PEEP valve at the end of the volume reflector into the scavenging system.

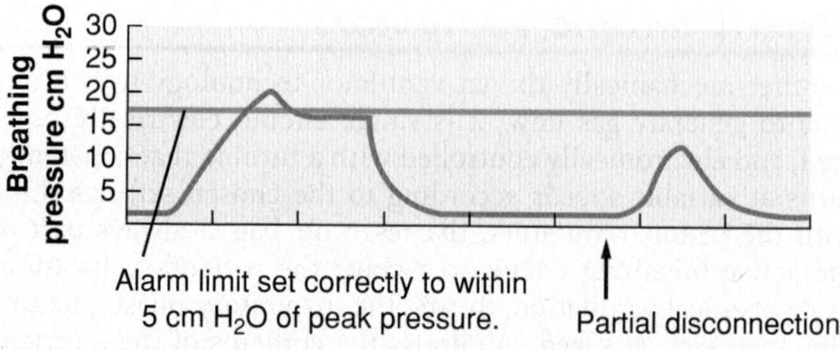

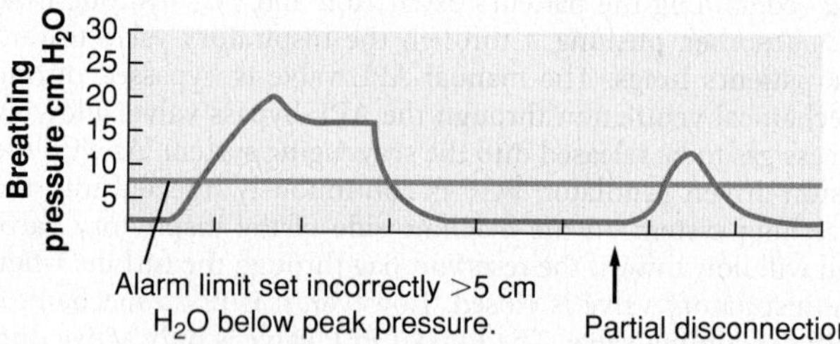

Figure 25-40 Threshold pressure alarm limit. **Top:** The threshold pressure alarm limit (*dotted line*) has been set appropriately. An alarm is actuated when a partial disconnection occurs (*arrow*) because the threshold pressure alarm limit is not exceeded by the breathing circuit pressure. **Bottom:** A partial disconnection is unrecognized by the pressure monitor because the threshold pressure alarm limit has been set too low. (Adapted from Baromed Breathing Pressure Monitor: *Operator's Instruction Manual*. Telford, PA: North American Dräger; 1986.)

Problems and Hazards

Numerous hazards are associated with anesthesia ventilators. These include problems with the breathing circuits, bellows assembly, and control assemblies.

Breathing circuit misconnections and disconnections are a leading cause of critical incidents in anesthesia.[116] The most common disconnection site is at the Y-piece. Disconnections can be complete or partial, with leaks. Preexisting undetected leaks can exist in compressed, corrugated, and/or disposable anesthetic circuits. To detect such a leak preoperatively, the collapsible circuit must be fully expanded before it is checked for leaks.[117] As previously mentioned, disconnections and leaks are made more obvious with the ascending bellows ventilator systems because they result in a situation in which the bellows will not refill.

Several breathing system disconnection monitors exist, although none should replace the anesthesia provider's own observation. Observation of chest wall excursion and/or monitoring of breath sounds is of value but because it is intermittent recognition of a disconnect may be delayed. Despite use of mechanical (spirometers and pressure sensors) and/or physiologic monitors, recognition of a disconnect requires continuous vigilance.

Pneumatic and electronic pressure monitors are helpful in detecting disconnections. Factors that influence monitor effectiveness include the disconnection site, the pressure sensor location, the threshold pressure alarm limit, the inspiratory flow rate, and the resistance of the disconnected breathing circuit.[118–120] Various anesthesia workstations and ventilators have different locations for the airway pressure sensor and different values for the threshold pressure alarm limit. The threshold pressure alarm limit may be preset at the factory or adjustable. An audible or visual alarm is actuated if the peak inspiratory pressure of the breathing circuit does not exceed the threshold pressure alarm limit. When an adjustable threshold pressure alarm limit is available, such as on many workstations from Dräger Medical and GE Healthcare, the operator should set the pressure alarm limit to within 5 cm H_2O of the peak inspiratory pressure. On systems that have an "auto-set" feature, when activated, the threshold limit is automatically set at 3 to 5 cm H_2O below the current peak inspiratory pressure. On such systems, failure to reset the threshold pressure alarm limit may result in either an "apnea pressure" or "threshold low" alert. Figure 25-40 illustrates how a partial disconnection, that is, a leak, may be unrecognized by the low-pressure monitor if the threshold pressure alarm limit is set too low or if the factory preset value is relatively low. Ventilators should be reset to default values for each new patient in order to avoid alarm limits that were set for a previous patient.

Respiratory volume monitors are also useful in detecting disconnections. Volume monitors may sense exhaled tidal volume, inhaled tidal volume, minute volume, or all three. The user should bracket the high and low threshold volumes slightly above and below the exhaled volumes. For example, if the exhaled minute volume of a patient is 10 L/min, reasonable alarm limits would be 8 to 12 L/min. Many of the older Datex-Ohmeda ventilators are equipped with volume monitor sensors that use infrared light/turbine technology. These volume sensors are usually located in the expiratory limb of the breathing circuit and thus measure exhaled tidal volume. In the case of the Datex-Ohmeda S/5 ADU, and later GE workstations that use a respired gas module, a special attachment known as the D-Lite spirometry connector is placed in the breathing circuit between the Y-piece and the patient's airway (i.e., tracheal tube connector, LMA). This device permits measurement of both inhaled and exhaled volumes and pressures. With the older infrared-type sensors, exposure to a direct beam of light from the overhead surgical lighting could cause erroneous volume readings as the surgical beam interferes with the infrared sensor. Other types of expiratory volume sensors can be seen in systems such as the GE Datex Aestiva, Aespire, and other workstations that utilize differential pressure transduction technology to determine inhaled and exhaled volumes and to measure airway pressures. Some Dräger workstations use an ultrasonic flow sensor located in the expiratory limb. Other systems from Dräger measure exhaled volume using "hot wire" sensor technology. With this type of sensor, a tiny array of two platinum wires is electrically heated to a high temperature. As gas flows past the heated wires, they tend to cool. The amount of energy required to maintain the temperature of the wire is proportional to the volume of gas flowing past it. This system, however, has been associated in at least one report of accidental fire in the breathing circuit likely due to lack of regular cleaning where lint inside may have been allowed to build up.

Capnographs (CO_2 monitors) are probably the best devices for revealing circuit disconnections. CO_2 concentration is measured near the Y-piece either directly (mainstream) or by continuous aspiration of a gas sample to the analyzer instrument (side stream). A sudden change in the differences between the inspiratory and end-tidal CO_2 concentrations or the acute absence of measured CO_2 indicates a disconnection, a nonventilated patient, or other problems. Importantly, an absence or decrease of exhaled CO_2 can also be an indication of low (or no) cardiac output such as might occur with a cardiac arrest, rather than a mechanical equipment problem.

Misconnections of the breathing system are unfortunately relatively common. Despite the efforts of standards committees to eliminate this problem by assigning different diameters to various hoses and hose terminals, they continue to occur. Anesthesia workstations, breathing systems, ventilators, and scavenging systems incorporate many of these diameter-specific connections. The misguided attempts of anesthesia providers to outwit these "foolproof" systems have led to various hoses being wrongly adapted or forcefully fitted to inappropriate terminals and even to various other solid cylindrically shaped protrusions of the anesthesia machine. In general, anesthesia machine connections should never be altered, as safety mechanisms that may not be immediately obvious could be compromised.

Occlusion of the breathing circuit may occur. Tracheal tubes can become kinked unnoticed under the drapes, and hoses throughout the breathing circuit are subject to occlusion by internal obstruction or external mechanical forces, which can impinge flow and have severe consequences. For example, blockage of a bacterial filter in the expiratory limb of the circle system has resulted in bilateral tension pneumothorax.[67] Incorrect insertion of flow direction–sensitive components can result in a no-flow state. Examples of these components include some PEEP valves and cascade humidifiers. Depending on the location of the occlusion relative to the pressure sensor, a high-pressure alarm may or may not alert the practitioner to the problem.

Excess inflow to the breathing circuit from the anesthesia machine during the inspiratory phase can cause barotrauma. The best example of this phenomenon is oxygen flushing. Excess volume cannot be vented from bellows systems during inspiration because the ventilator relief valve is closed, and the APL valve is out of circuit. A high-pressure alarm, if present, may be activated when the pressure becomes excessive. With many Dräger Medical systems, both audible and visual alarms are actuated when the high-pressure threshold is exceeded. The GE ventilators automatically switch from the inspiratory to the expiratory phase when the adjustable peak pressure threshold is exceeded.

On workstations equipped with adjustable inspiratory pressure limiters (such as the GE Aestiva and Aisys, and Dräger Medical's Fabius, Tiro, Apollo, and Atlan) the maximum inspiratory pressure may be set by the user to a desired peak airway pressure. An adjustable pressure relief valve will open when the predetermined user-selected pressure threshold is exceeded. This should prevent generation of excessive airway pressure. Unfortunately, this feature is dependent on the user having preset the appropriate "relief" pressure. If the setting is too low, insufficient pressure for ventilation may be generated, resulting in inadequate minute ventilation; if set too high, the excessive airway pressure may still occur and result in barotrauma. The piston-driven ventilator in the Dräger Fabius, Tiro, Apollo, Atlan and others includes a factory preset peak inspiratory pressure safety valve that opens at a preset airway pressure such as 75 cm H_2O to reduce the risk of barotrauma.

Bellows Assembly Problems

Leaks can occur in the bellows assembly. Improper seating of the plastic bellows housing can result in inadequate ventilation because a portion of the driving gas leaks to the atmosphere. A hole in the bellows can lead to alveolar hyperinflation and possibly barotrauma in some ventilators because high-pressure driving gas can enter the patient circuit. The oxygen concentration of the patient's respired gas may increase when the driving gas is 100% oxygen, or it may decrease if the driving gas is composed of air or an air–oxygen mixture.[121]

The ventilator relief valve can also cause problems. Hypoventilation occurs if the valve is incompetent because the anesthetic gases are delivered to the scavenging system instead of to the patient during the inspiratory phase. Gas molecules preferentially exit into the scavenging system because it represents the path of least resistance, and the pressure within the scavenging system can be subatmospheric. Ventilator relief valve incompetency can result from a disconnected pilot line, a ruptured valve, or from a damaged flapper valve.[122,123] A ventilator relief valve stuck in the closed or partially closed position can produce either barotrauma or undesired PEEP.[124] Excessive suction from the scavenging system can draw the ventilator relief valve to its seat and close the valve during both the inspiratory and expiratory phases. In this case, breathing circuit pressure increases because excess anesthetic gas cannot be vented.

It is worthwhile to note that during the expiratory phase, some newer machines from GE-Datex-Ohmeda (7100 and 7900 SmartVent) scavenge both excess patient gases and the exhausted ventilator driving gas. That is, when the ventilator relief valve opens, and waste anesthetic gases are vented from the breathing circuit, the driving gas from the bellows housing joins with it to enter the scavenging system.

Under certain conditions, the large volume of exhaust gases could overwhelm the scavenging system, resulting in contamination of the operating room atmosphere with waste anesthetic gases (see Scavenging Systems section). Other mechanical problems that can occur include leaks within the system, faulty pressure regulators, and faulty valves.

Control Assembly and Power Supply Problems

The control assembly can be the source of both electrical and mechanical problems. Electrical failure can be total or partial; the former is, of course, easier to notice. As anesthesia workstations are becoming increasingly dependent on integrated computer-controlled systems, power supply interruptions become more significant. Battery backup systems are designed to continue operation of essential electronics during brief outages. However, even with these systems, in the event of a failure, significant time may be required to reboot a computerized system after an electrical outage has occurred. During this time, the availability of certain workstation features such as manual or mechanical ventilation can be variable. One cluster of electrical failures that could have resulted in operating room fires was attributed to the workstation's power supply printed circuit boards.[125]

Future Technologies

Just like target-controlled intravenous anesthesia systems that are available outside the United States, new anesthesia machine developments have focused on more automation to provide end-tidal target-controlled concentration of volatile anesthetics and fraction of oxygen. In these machines, the anesthesia provider sets a target goal for each parameter and the anesthesia machine will adjust the FGF and the volatile anesthetic concentration to achieve those values. This has been shown to reduce the time to achieving the set goal without adverse events compared to standard manual adjustment, although saving of less volatile anesthetics is less clear and may depend on the type of volatile anesthetic used.[126] This optional feature requires changes to gas analysis hardware and machine software as well as electronic vaporizers. While this is already available outside the United States by various manufacturers including in Europe and Canada, there is currently only one manufacturer (GE) that has approval by the Food and Drug Administration, though others are likely to follow.

Waste Gas Scavenging Systems

Scavenging is the collection and the subsequent removal of waste anesthetic gases from the operating room (12 Video 25-12).[127] In most cases, the amount of gas used to anesthetize a patient for a given anesthetic far exceeds the minimum amount needed. Therefore, scavenging minimizes operating room contamination by removing this excess of gases.

In 1977, the National Institute for Occupational Safety and Health (NIOSH) published a document entitled "Criteria for a Recommended Standard: Occupational Exposure to Waste Anesthetic Gases and Vapors."[128] Although a minimum safe level of exposure could not be defined, NIOSH made the recommendations shown in Table 25-7. The recommended ceiling for volatile anesthetics was established before desflurane and sevoflurane were introduced into clinical practice. However, this limit is likely to be similarly applicable for the newer volatile anesthetics.[129] The NIOSH recommendations have never promulgated into law and therefore are not enforceable. For a more in-depth discussion of this topic, refer to the Chapter 3 (Occupational Health and Well Being).

Table 25-7 NIOSH Recommendations for Maximum Levels for Exposure of Personnel to Trace Anesthesia Gases and Vapors

Anesthetic Gas	Maximum TWA[a] Concentration (ppm)
Halogenated agent alone	2
Nitrous oxide	25
Combination of halogenated agent plus nitrous oxide	—
Halogenated agent	0.5
Nitrous oxide	25
Dental facilities (nitrous oxide alone)	50

Reprinted from US Department of Health, Education, and Welfare. *Criteria for a recommended standard: occupational exposure to waste anesthetic gases and vapors*. March ed., Washington, DC; 1977.

Note: Despite being in clinical use for more than 15 years, isoflurane, desflurane, and sevoflurane have not been tested for maximum recommended trace gas levels.

[a]TWA, time-weighted average. Time-weighted average sampling, also known as time-integrated sampling, is a sampling method that evaluates the average concentration of anesthetic gas over a prolonged period of time, such as 1 to 8 hours.

In 1991, the ASTM released the ASTM F1343–91 standard titled "Standard Specification for Anesthetic Equipment–Scavenging Systems for Anesthetic Gases."[130] The document provided guidelines for devices that safely and effectively scavenge waste anesthetic gases to reduce contamination in anesthetizing areas. Because of lack of safety data on exposure to the newer halogenated anesthetic agents, in 2006, NIOSH requested comments and information relevant to the evaluation of health risks associated with occupational exposure to these agents in order to establish recommended maximum exposure levels (REL).[131] The ASA Task Force on Trace Anesthetic Gases developed a booklet entitled "Waste Anesthetic Gases: Information for Management in Anesthetizing Areas and the Postanesthesia Care Unit." This ASA publication addresses analysis of the literature, the role of regulatory agencies, scavenging and monitoring equipment, and recommendations.[132]

The two major causes of waste gas contamination in the operating room are the anesthetic technique and equipment issues.[132] Regarding the anesthetic technique, the following factors cause operating room atmosphere contamination: (1) failure to turn off gas flow control valves at the end of an anesthetic; (2) poorly fitting masks; (3) flushing the circuit; (4) filling anesthetic vaporizers; (5) use of uncuffed tracheal tubes; and (6) use of breathing circuits such as the Jackson-Rees, which are difficult to scavenge. Equipment failure or lack of understanding of proper equipment use can also contribute to operating room contamination. Leaks can occur in the high-pressure hoses, the nitrous oxide tank mounting, the high-pressure circuit and LPC of the anesthesia machine, or in the circle system, particularly at the CO_2 absorber assembly. The anesthesia provider must be certain that the scavenging system is operational and adjusted properly to ensure adequate scavenging. If side-stream CO_2 or multigas analyzers are used, the analyzed gas (withdrawn from the circuit at a rate of 50 to 250 cc/min) must be directed to the scavenging system or returned to the breathing system to prevent contamination of the operating room atmosphere.

Components

Scavenging systems generally consist of five components (Fig. 25-41): (1) the gas-collecting assembly, (2) the transfer means, (3) the scavenging interface, (4) the gas-disposal assembly tubing, and (5) an active or passive gas-disposal assembly. An "active system" uses a central vacuum system to remove waste gases. The "weight" or pressure of the waste gas itself produces flow through a "passive system."

Gas-Collecting Assembly

The gas-collecting assembly captures excess anesthetic gas and delivers it to the transfer tubing. Waste anesthetic gases that do not escape into the room from a poor face mask fit or endotracheal tube leak are vented from the anesthesia system either through the APL valve or through the ventilator relief valve. Gas passing through these valves accumulates in the gas-collecting assembly and is directed to the transfer means. In some GE Healthcare workstations and others that incorporate either the 7100 or 7900 ventilators, the ventilator driving gas is also exhausted into the scavenging system. This is significant, because under conditions of high FGFs and high minute ventilation, the gases flowing into the scavenging interface may overwhelm the evacuation system.

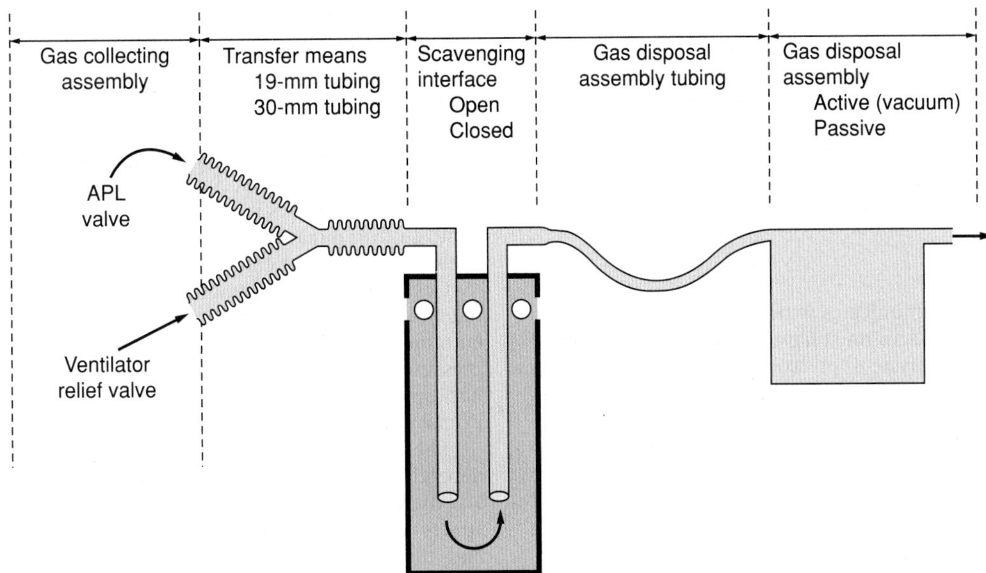

Figure 25-41 Components of a scavenging system. APL, adjustable pressure-limiting valve.

If this occurs, waste anesthetic gases may overflow the system via the positive-pressure relief valve (closed systems) or through the atmospheric vents (open systems) into the operating room atmosphere. In contrast, most other pneumatic ventilators from both GE Datex-Ohmeda and Dräger Narkomed with AV-E ventilators exhaust their driving gas (oxygen or an oxygen/air mixture) into the operating room through a small vent on the back of the ventilator control housing.

Transfer Means

The transfer means carries excess gas from the gas-collecting assembly to the scavenging interface. The tubing diameter must be either 19 or 30 mm, as specified by the ASTM F1343–91 standard.[130] The tubing should be sufficiently rigid to prevent kinking and as short as possible to minimize the chance of occlusion. Some manufacturers color code the transfer tubing with yellow bands to distinguish it from 22-mm diameter breathing system tubing. Many machines have separate transfer tubes for the APL valve and for the ventilator relief valve. The two tubes usually merge into a single hose before they enter the scavenging interface. Occlusion of the transfer means can be particularly problematic since it is upstream from the pressure-buffering features of the scavenging interface. If the transfer means is occluded, baseline breathing circuit pressure will increase and barotrauma can occur.

Scavenging Interface

The scavenging interface is the most critical component of the system because it protects the breathing circuit or ventilator from excessive positive or negative pressures. The interface should limit the pressures immediately downstream from the gas-collecting assembly to between –0.5 and +10 cm H_2O within normal working conditions. Positive-pressure relief is mandatory, irrespective of the type of disposal system used, to vent excess gas in case of occlusion downstream from the interface. If the disposal system is an "active system," negative-pressure relief is necessary to protect the breathing circuit or ventilator from excessive subatmospheric pressure. A reservoir is highly desirable with active systems since it stores waste gases until the evacuation system can remove them. Interfaces can be open or closed, depending on the method used to provide positive- and negative-pressure relief.

Open Interfaces

An open interface contains no valves and is open to the atmosphere, allowing both positive- and negative-pressure relief. Open interfaces should be used only with active disposal systems that use a central evacuation system and require a reservoir because waste gases are intermittently discharged in surges, whereas flow from the evacuation system is continuous.

Many contemporary anesthesia machines are equipped with open interfaces like those in Figures 25-42A and B.[133] An open canister provides reservoir capacity. The canister volume should be large enough to accommodate a variety of waste gas flow rates. Gas enters the system at the top of the canister and travels through a narrow inner tube to the canister base. Gases are stored in the reservoir between breaths. Positive- and negative-pressure relief is provided by holes in the top of the canister. The open interface shown in Figure 25-43A differs somewhat from the one shown in Figure 25-43B. The operator can regulate the vacuum

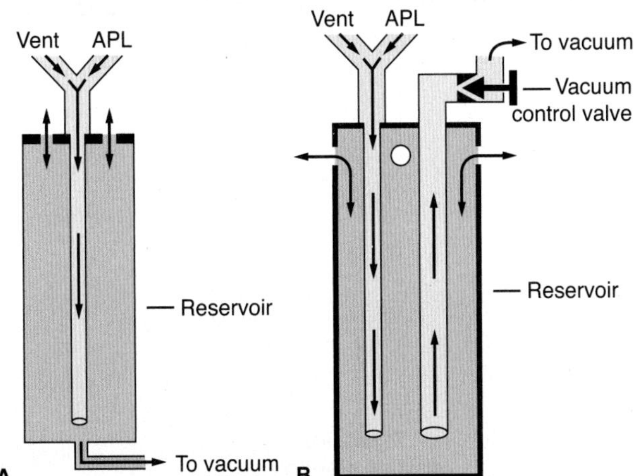

Figure 25-42 **A, B:** Two open reservoir scavenging interfaces. Each requires an active disposal system. APL, adjustable pressure-limiting valve. See text for details. (Adapted with permission from Dorsch JA, Dorsch SE. Controlling trace gas levels. In: Dorsch JA, Dorsch SE, eds. *Understanding Anesthesia Equipment*. 4th ed. Williams & Wilkins; 1999:355.)

by adjusting the vacuum control valve shown in Figure 25-42B. The efficiency of an open interface depends on several factors. The vacuum flow rate per minute must equal or exceed the volume of excess gases to prevent spillage. Spillage will occur if the volume of a single exhaled breath exceeds the capacity of the reservoir. The flow characteristics of the system are also critical because gas leakage can occur long before the volume of waste gas equals the reservoir volume if significant turbulence occurs within the interface.[134]

Closed Interfaces

A closed interface communicates with the atmosphere through valves. All closed interfaces must have a positive-pressure relief valve to vent excess system pressure if obstruction occurs downstream from the interface. A negative-pressure relief valve is mandatory to protect the breathing system from subatmospheric pressure if an active disposal system is used. Two types of closed interfaces are commercially available. One has positive-pressure relief only; the other has both positive- and negative-pressure relief. Each type is discussed in the following sections.

Positive-Pressure Relief Only. This interface (Fig. 25-43, left) has a single positive-pressure relief valve and is designed to be used only with passive disposal systems. Waste gas enters the interface at the waste gas inlets. Transfer of the waste gas from the interface to the disposal system relies on the "weight" or pressure of the waste gas itself since a negative-pressure evacuation system is not used. The positive-pressure relief valve opens at a preset value such as 5 cm water if an obstruction between the interface and the disposal system occurs.[135,136] On this type of system, a reservoir bag is not required.

Positive- and Negative-Pressure Relief. This interface has a positive-pressure relief valve, and at least one negative-pressure relief valve, in addition to a reservoir bag. It is used with active disposal systems. Figure 25-43 (right) is a schematic of a closed interface for suction systems. A variable volume of waste gas intermittently enters the interface through the waste gas inlets, and the reservoir intermittently accumulates excess gas until the evacuation system eliminates it. The operator should adjust the vacuum control valve so that the reservoir bag is properly inflated (A), not overdistended (B), or completely deflated (C).

Gas is vented to the atmosphere through the positive-pressure relief valve if the system pressure exceeds 5 cm water. Room air is entrained through the negative-pressure relief valve if the system pressure is more negative than –0.5 cm H_2O. On some systems, a backup negative-pressure relief valve opens at –1.8 cm H_2O if the primary negative-pressure relief valve becomes occluded.

The effectiveness of a closed system in preventing spillage depends on the rate of waste gas inflow, the evacuation flow rate, and the size of the reservoir. Leakage of waste gases into the atmosphere occurs only when the reservoir bag becomes fully inflated, and the pressure increases sufficiently to open the positive-pressure relief valve. In contrast, the effectiveness of an open system to prevent spillage depends not only on the volume of the reservoir but also on the flow characteristics within the interface.

Gas-Disposal Assembly Conduit

The gas-disposal assembly conduit, or disposal assembly tubing (Fig. 25-41), conducts waste gas from the scavenging interface to the gas-disposal assembly. It should be collapse proof and should run overhead, if possible, to minimize the chances of accidental occlusion.

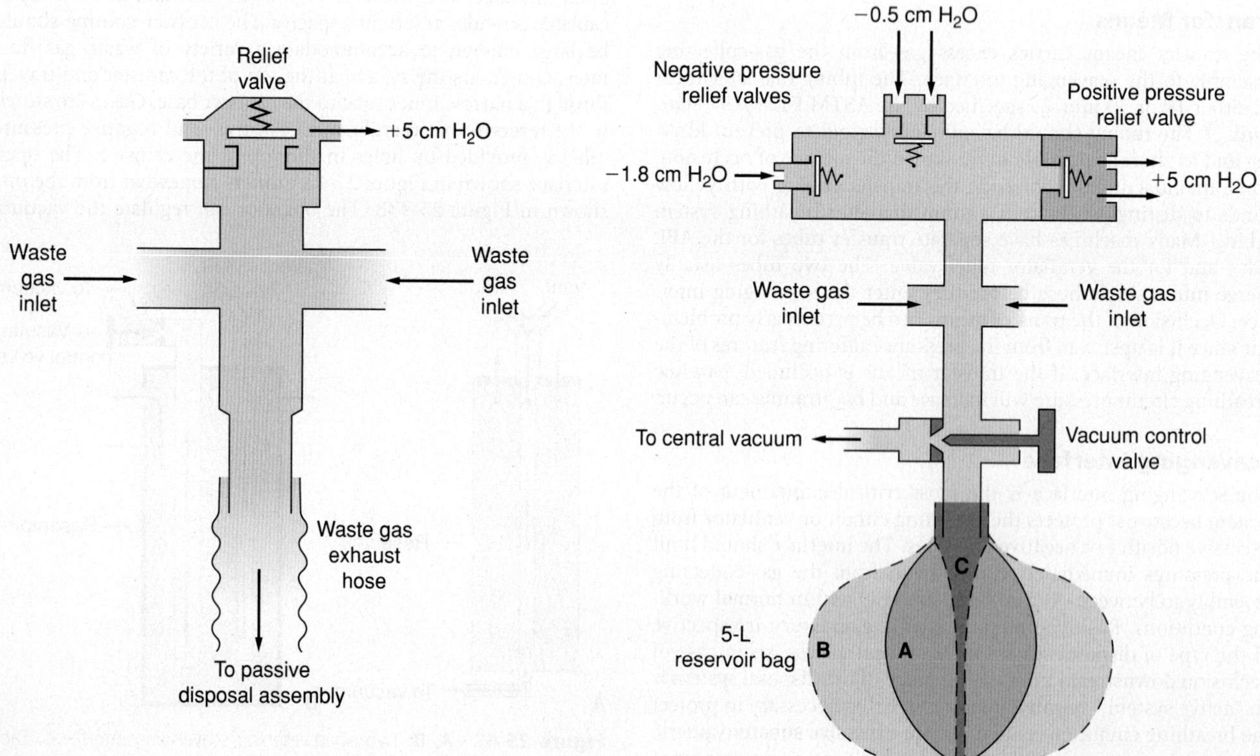

Figure 25-43 Closed scavenging interfaces. **Left:** Interface used with a passive disposal system. (Adapted from *Scavenger Interface for Air Conditioning: Instruction Manual*. Telford, PA: North American Dräger; 1984, obsolete.) **Right:** Interface used with an active system. (Adapted from Narkomed 2A *Anesthesia System: Technical Service Manual*. Telford, PA: North American Dräger; 1985, obsolete.)

Gas-Disposal Assembly

The gas-disposal assembly ultimately eliminates excess waste gas (Fig. 25-41). There are two types of disposal systems: active and passive.

Active assembly. The most common method of gas disposal is the active assembly, which uses a central evacuation system. A vacuum pump serves as the mechanical flow-inducing device that removes the waste gases, usually to the outside of the building. An interface with a negative-pressure relief valve is mandatory because the pressure within the system is negative. A reservoir is very desirable, and the larger the reservoir, the lower the suction flow rate needed.

Passive assembly. A passive disposal system does not use a mechanical flow-inducing device. Instead, the "weight" or pressure from the heavier-than-air anesthetic gases produces flow through the system. Positive-pressure relief is mandatory, but negative-pressure relief and a reservoir are unnecessary. Excess waste gases can be eliminated from the surgical suite in a number of ways. Some include venting through the wall, ceiling, or floor, or to the room exhaust grill of a nonrecirculating air conditioning system.

Problems and Hazards

Scavenging systems minimize operating room atmosphere contamination, yet they add complexity to the anesthesia system. A scavenging system functionally extends the anesthesia circuit all the way from the anesthesia machine to the ultimate disposal site. This extension increases the potential for problems. Obstruction of scavenging pathways can cause excessive positive pressure in the breathing circuit, and barotrauma can occur. Excessive vacuum applied to a scavenging system can result in undesirable negative pressures within the breathing system. For most contemporary anesthesia workstations, preuse checkout of the scavenging system is a function that must be performed manually by the operator according to the manufacturer's instructions.

Another unusual problem is a report of fires in engineering equipment rooms that house the vacuum pumps used for waste anesthetic gas evacuation.[137] In some hospitals, waste gases are not directly vented outside, but are vented into machine rooms that have vents open to the outside. Since certain anesthesia machines are designed such that ventilator driving gas (oxygen) is also scavenged, the environment in these machine rooms into which the scavenged gas is vented may become highly enriched with oxygen. These sites may contain equipment or materials such as petroleum distillates (pumps/oil/grease) that, in the presence of an oxygen-enriched atmosphere, could be excessively combustible and present a severe fire hazard.

Low-Flow Scavenging Systems

Active waste gas scavenging systems draw large volumes of gas—anesthetic waste plus entrained air in the range of 25 to 75 L/min—from each operating room. This requires large and costly vacuum pumps that operate continuously, incurring a high-energy cost. In an effort to reduce the carbon footprint associated with running these pumps, a more efficient, low-flow scavenger interface has been designed and evaluated.[138]

The Dynamic Gas Scavenging System (DGSS; Anesthetic Gas Reclamation, Nashville, TN) interface is a gas-tight metal container with a 3-L reservoir bag attached to ensure compliance with Occupational Safety and Health Administration (OSHA) recommendations (Fig. 25-44). The design is such that scavenging outflow to the vacuum system remains closed until a pressure of 0.5 cm H_2O from the anesthesia workstation exhaust, via the APL or ventilator pressure relief valve, is sensed in the interface enclosure by a sensitive pressure transducer. A solenoid valve then opens and remains open until the internal pressure reaches −0.5 cm H_2O, thus emptying the interface reservoir bag. In this way, the flow to the vacuum system is continuously titrated as needed. An additional benefit is that by producing a more concentrated flow of waste gases, technologies designed to recover potent inhaled anesthetic agents from the waste gas flow are facilitated. Such technologies are likely to become more critical because inhaled anesthetics are greenhouse gases with the potential to increase global warming.[139,140]

Failure of Anesthesia Equipment

According to a decade-long study of 1,000 anesthesia incidents, the most common failure of anesthesia equipment was due to an equipment leak (61 out of 1,000).[141] The authors propose that the most likely underlying cause of system leaks was due to "design weakness," for example, when push-on tapers in breathing circuits become disconnected. The second most prevalent causes of equipment failure included poor equipment maintenance and setup. Most often, the pulse oximeter alarm alerted the anesthesiologist to an equipment problem.[141]

In addition, ventilation of equipment is important for proper function and may be hindered by entrapped cables. This can be mitigated by careful attention to organization and tidiness of the anesthesia workstation environment.[142,143]

In a 1997 review of the ASA "Closed Claims" database, Caplan et al.[65] found that claims related to the medical gas-delivery system were rare, but tended to be severe, with 76% resulting in death or permanent brain injury. Authors identified the most common malfunctions in the breathing circuit (39%), followed by vaporizers (21%), ventilators (17%), gas tanks or gas lines (11%), and the anesthesia machine itself (7%). Use error was determined to be the cause of 75% out of the 72 gas delivery equipment claims in the review, and equipment failure was considered the cause in the remainder.[65] In 2013, Mehta et al.[1] published an update of the 1997 study. The review included the 40 most recent claims in the database for incidents between 1990 and 2011 and concluded that provider error occurred in 68% of incidents, equipment failure only in 13% of incidents, and both in 18% of cases. Of the 40 incidents, 35% were considered to have been avoidable if a proper preanesthesia checkout had been performed. Similarly, a more recent study from 2017 of 130 anesthesia machines found that results from the machines did not accord with requirements in nearly 14% of cases.[144] It is recommended to keep track of device performance to ensure that the machines are properly maintained or replaced if necessary.

Safety Features of Newer Anesthesia Workstations

Older conventional anesthesia machines have design limitations that impede their safety. Some machines lack features to prevent barotrauma during oxygen flush, cannot perform automated preuse checkout, have multiple external connections, or contain gas-driven ventilator bellows that do not fully empty and that may allow "breath stacking" as well as inaccurate tidal volume delivery.[145]

Modern workstations are designed to incorporate additional safety features such as FGD to prevent barotrauma during oxygen

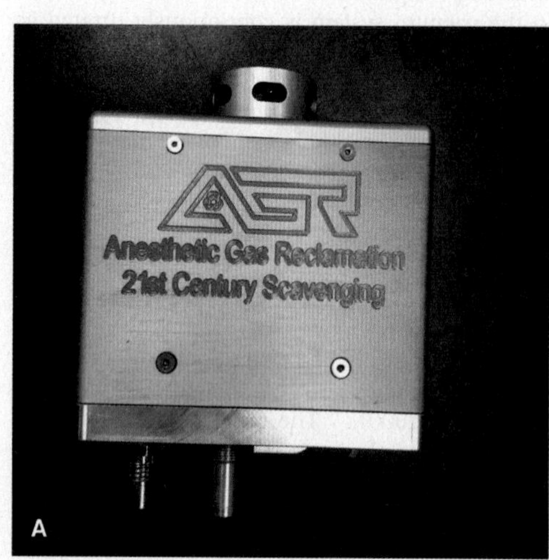

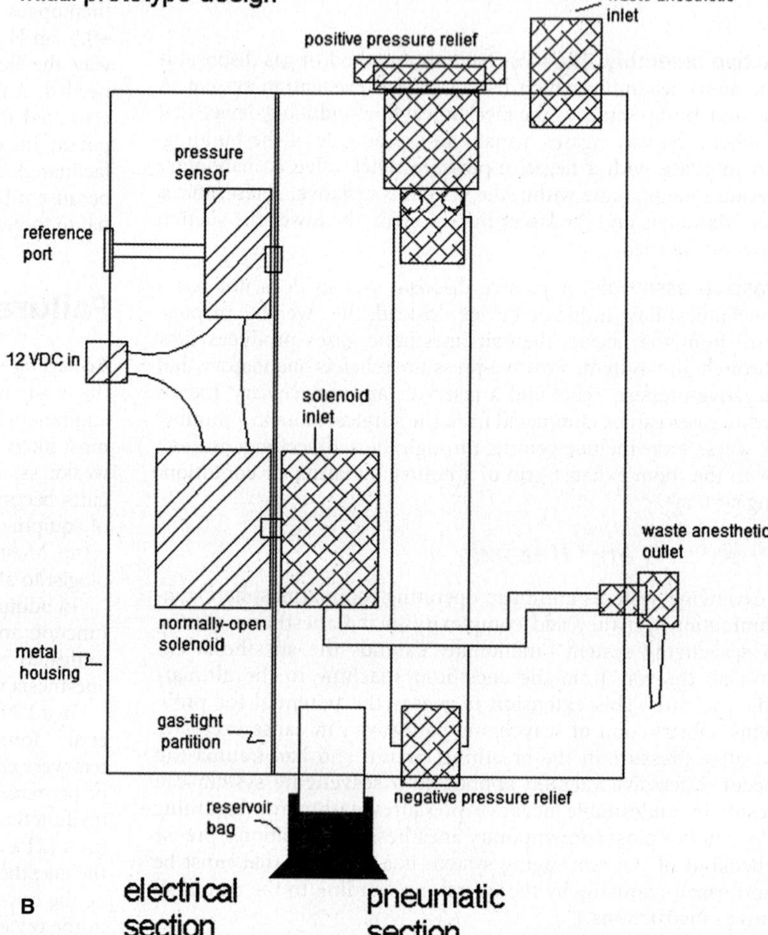

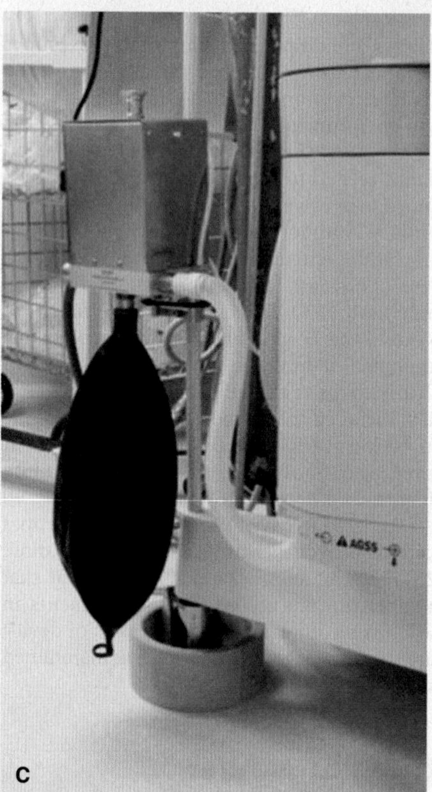

Figure 25-44 The Dynamic Gas Scavenging System (DGSS). (**A**) External view. (**B**) Schematic view. Waste gas enters the gas-tight chamber, while the solenoid valve remains closed, preventing gas from entering the waste gas outlet. When a positive pressure of +0.5 cm H_2O is detected by the pressure sensor, the solenoid valve opens, releasing gas to the waste gas outlet. The solenoid valve remains open until the pressure in the chamber decreases to –0.5 cm H_2O. In this way the waste gas flow into the hospital vacuum system is titrated according to the waste gas flowing from the anesthesia breathing circuit. *V DC*, volts, direct current. (**C**) DGSS mounted on an anesthesia workstation. (Courtesy Berry JM. Anesthesia Gas Reclamation, Dallas, TX.)

flush; integrated, software-driven self-checkout routines; limited external connections; and electronic, piston-driven ventilators that deliver accurate tidal volumes. Unfortunately, as new and more complex delivery systems are introduced, users become less and less able to troubleshoot problems. And increased training of anesthesia equipment maintenance personnel is required. In the event of workstation failure, having immediately available manual resuscitation equipment (portable oxygen tank, self-inflating bag, mask [Fig. 25-36]) becomes increasingly important.

Checkout of the Anesthesia Workstation

A complete anesthesia apparatus checkout procedure must be performed each day prior to the first use of the anesthesia workstation (NICV 25-2). An abbreviated checkout procedure should be performed before each subsequent case. The 1993 FDA Anesthesia Apparatus Checkout Recommendations (reproduced in Appendix A) remain applicable to the majority of older anesthesia machines in use worldwide.[146,147]

In 2008, the ASA published recommendations for preanesthesia checkout of machines, taking into consideration newer workstations that perform automated checkout.[148] Since the design of newer workstations varies considerably, no single preuse procedure is applicable. These guidelines present a template for individual departments and practitioners to design preanesthesia checkout procedures specific to their own needs and equipment (Appendix B).

Sample checkout procedures are published on the ASA website (www.asahq.org), and they encompass adult as well as pediatric equipment from major equipment manufacturers in the United States. The reader is strongly encouraged to review the checkout procedures reproduced in Appendices A and B at the end of this chapter and to understand the rationale for and importance of each step.

Since 2008, other recommended items for the checklist have emerged. One recommendation involves ensuring that the anesthesia machine is devoid of any residual inhaled anesthetic, especially for patients for whom this is contraindicated.[149]

10 Two critical items to include in the checkout of the anesthesia workstation are a functioning, tested SIRB (Fig. 25-36) and a full auxiliary tank of oxygen that should be readily available. This is "plan B," the backup plan. Many of the adverse outcomes associated with anesthesia equipment malfunction could have been averted if the SIRB had been used or used sooner. The SIRB is an item frequently missed in the preanesthesia setup.[110]

The next three most important preoperative checks are (1) oxygen analyzer calibration, (2) the LPC leak test, and (3) the circle system test. These are discussed in the following sections. Additional details regarding these systems are presented briefly in subsections describing the anatomy of the anesthesia workstation; for a more comprehensive review, the reader is encouraged to consult the operator's manual of their own equipment. For a simplified diagram of a two-gas anesthesia machine and the components described in the following discussion, please refer to Figure 25-2. A comprehensive discussion of Figure 25-2 can also be found in the Anatomy of an Anesthesia Workstation section.

Oxygen Analyzer Calibration

The oxygen analyzer is one of the most important monitors on the anesthesia workstation. It is the only machine safety device that continually evaluates the integrity of the LPC. Other machine safety devices, such as the oxygen supply pressure failure cutoff ("fail-safe") valve, the oxygen supply pressure failure alarm, and the N_2O/O_2 proportioning system, are all upstream from the flow control valves. The oxygen analyzer is the only monitor that detects problems downstream from the flow control valves. Calibration of this monitor is described in Step 9 of Appendix A (Anesthesia Apparatus Checkout Recommendations, 1993). The actual procedure for calibrating the oxygen analyzer has remained reasonably similar over the last several generations of the anesthesia workstations (Guideline for Designing Preanesthesia Checkout Procedures, 2008, Item 10 in Appendix B).

In general, the oxygen concentration–sensing element (usually a fuel cell on traditional machines) must be exposed to room air, at sea level, for calibration to 21%. This may require manually setting a dial on older machines, but on newer ones, it usually only involves temporarily removing the sensor, selecting and then confirming that the oxygen calibration is to be performed from a set of menus on the workstation's display screen, and finally reinstalling the sensor. The function of the low–oxygen concentration alarm should be verified by setting the alarm to trigger above the current oxygen reading. Some newer workstations use a sidestream sampling multigas monitoring module that incorporates a fast, paramagnetic oxygen analyzer. These analyzers undergo automatic periodic oxygen calibration.[120] It should be noted that both the fuel cell and the paramagnetic oxygen analyzers actually measure PO_2 and express it as a percentage of 1 atmosphere at sea level. Thus, if a fuel cell were calibrated to 21% O_2 at sea level and then used at an altitude where the total air pressure is reduced, it would read less than 21% even though the composition of the atmosphere had not changed.

Low-Pressure Circuit Leak Test

The LPC leak test checks the integrity of the anesthesia machine 11 from the flow control valves to the common gas outlet. It evaluates the portion of the machine that is downstream from all safety devices except the oxygen analyzer. The components located within this area are the ones most susceptible to breakage and leaks. Leaks in the LPC can cause hypoxia or patient awareness.[150] Flow tubes, the most delicate pneumatic component of the machine, can crack or break. A typical three-gas anesthesia machine has 16 O-rings in the LPC. Leaks can occur at the interface between the glass flow tubes[151] and the manifold, and at the O-ring junctions between the vaporizer and its manifold. Loose filler caps on vaporizers are a common source of leaks, and these leaks can lead to delivery of subanesthetic doses of inhaled agents, causing patient awareness during general anesthesia.[152]

Several different methods have been used to check the LPC for leaks. They include the oxygen flush test, the common gas outlet occlusion test, the traditional positive-pressure leak test, the North American Dräger positive-pressure leak test, internal positive-pressure leak test, the GE Datex-Ohmeda negative-pressure leak test, the 1993 FDA universal negative-pressure leak test, and others. One reason for the large number of methods is that the internal design of various machines differs considerably. The most notable example is that many GE Healthcare/Datex-Ohmeda (GE) machines and workstations have a check valve near the common gas outlet, unlike Dräger Medical workstations. The presence or absence of the outlet check valve can change which preuse check is indicated.

Several errors have resulted from application of the wrong leak 12 test to the wrong machine. Therefore, it is mandatory to perform the appropriate low-pressure system leak test each day. To do this, it is essential to understand the exact location and operating principles of the Datex-Ohmeda check valve. Many Datex-Ohmeda anesthesia workstations have a machine outlet check valve located in the LPS. The check valve is located downstream from the vaporizers and upstream from the oxygen flush valve (Fig. 25-2) and is open in the absence of back pressure. Gas flow from the manifold moves the rubber flapper valve off its seat and allows gas to proceed freely to the common gas outlet. The valve closes when back pressure is exerted. Back pressure sufficient to close the check valve may occur with the following conditions: use of the oxygen flush, peak breathing circuit pressures generated during positive-pressure ventilation or use of a positive-pressure leak test.

In general, the LPC of anesthesia workstations without an outlet check valve can be tested using a positive-pressure leak test, and machines with outlet check valves must be tested using a negative-pressure leak test. When performing a positive-pressure leak test, the operator generates positive pressure in the LPS using flow from the anesthesia machine or from a positive-pressure squeeze bulb to detect a leak. When performing a negative-pressure leak test, the operator creates negative pressure in the LPS using a suction bulb to detect leaks. Two different LPS leak tests are described below.

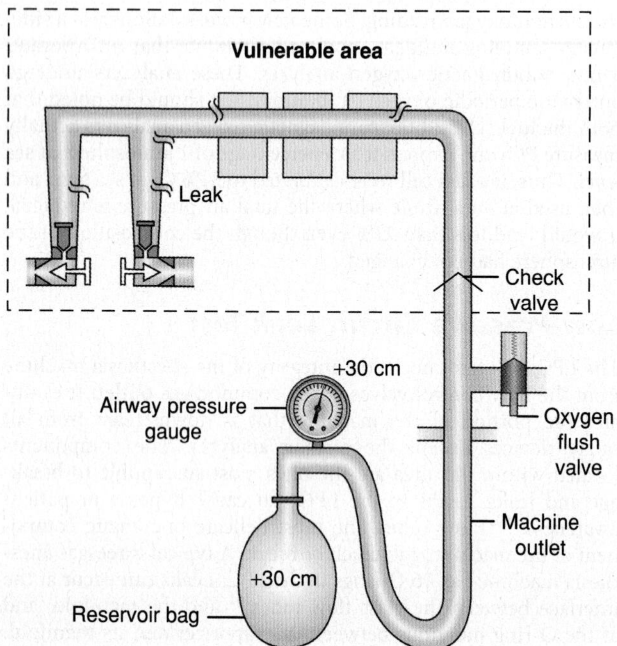

Figure 25-45 Inappropriate use of the oxygen flush valve to check the low-pressure circuit of a Datex-Ohmeda machine equipped with a check valve. The area within the rectangle is not checked by the inappropriate use of the oxygen flush valve. The components located within this area are precisely the ones most subject to breakage and leaks. Positive pressure within the patient circuit closes the check valve, and the value on the airway pressure gauge does not decrease despite leaks in the low-pressure circuit.

Oxygen Flush Positive-Pressure Leak Test

Older anesthesia machines did not usually have check valves in the LPC. Therefore, it was common practice to pressurize the breathing circuit and the LPC with the oxygen flush valve to test internally by observing the breathing system pressure gauge. Because some modern GE-Datex-Ohmeda machines have check valves in the LPC, application of a positive-pressure leak test on these machines can be misleading or even dangerous (Fig. 25-45). Inappropriate use of the oxygen flush valve or the presence of a leaking flush valve may lead to inadequate evaluation of the LPC for leaks. In turn, this can lead the workstation user into a false sense of security despite the presence of large leaks.[153] Positive pressure from the breathing circuit results in closure of the outlet check valve, and the value on the breathing system pressure gauge will fail to decrease. The system appears to be gas tight, but in actuality, only the circuitry downstream from the outlet check valve is leak free.[4] Thus, a vulnerable area exists from the check valve back to the flow control valves because this area is not tested by a positive-pressure leak test.

Verifying the Integrity of the Gas Supply Lines between the Flowmeters and the Common Gas Outlet

The 1993 FDA Universal negative-pressure leak test (Appendix A, Step 5) was named "universal" because at that time it could be used to check all contemporary anesthesia machines regardless of the presence or absence of an outlet check valve in the LPC. It remains applicable for many older anesthesia machines, but for many newer machines, this test is not applicable. Leaks in the gas supply lines between the flowmeters and the common gas outlet should be checked daily or whenever a vaporizer is changed (Appendix B, Item 8). The most thorough technique to check each vaporizer individually is by turning it on and then evaluating the low-pressure system for leaks. It is important to note that automated checkout procedures may not necessarily detect leaks at the vaporizer if the vaporizer is turned off during testing. In addition, vaporizers should be adequately filled, and filler ports should be tightly closed (Appendix B, Item 7). As mentioned previously, the ASA now recommends that individual institutions develop internal guidelines specific to their own equipment and needs.[154] 13

The 1993 FDA low-pressure system leak check is based on the Datex-Ohmeda negative-pressure leak test (Fig. 25-46). It is performed using a negative-pressure leak testing device, which is a simple suction 15-cc volume bulb that when evacuated generates a negative pressure of 65 mmHg. The machine's main ON/OFF switch, the flow control valves, and the vaporizers are all turned off. The suction bulb is connected to the common gas outlet and squeezed repeatedly until it is fully collapsed. This action creates a vacuum in the low-pressure system circuitry. The machine is considered leak free if the suction bulb remains collapsed for at least 10 seconds. A leak is present if the bulb reinflates during this period. The test is repeated with each vaporizer individually turned to the "on" position because internal vaporizer leaks can 14

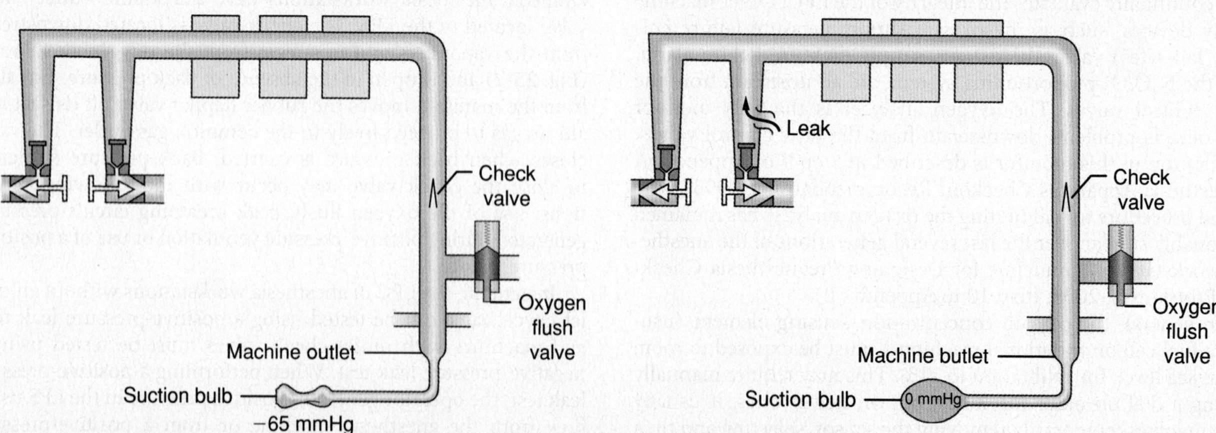

Figure 25-46 FDA negative-pressure leak test. A negative-pressure leak testing device is attached directly to the machine common gas outlet. Squeezing the bulb creates a vacuum in the low-pressure circuit and opens the check valve (**left**). When a leak is present in the low-pressure circuit, room air is entrained through the leak and the suction bulb inflates (**right**). (Adapted from Andrews JJ. Understanding anesthesia machines. In: 1988 Review Course Lectures. Cleveland: International Anesthesia Research Society; 1988:78. With permission.)

be detected only when the vaporizer is turned on and becomes part of the low-pressure system. Again, if the bulb reinflates in less than 10 seconds, a leak is present somewhere in the LPC.

Evaluation of the Circle System

The circle system tests (Appendix B, Items 12 and 13, 13 Video 25-13) evaluate the integrity of the circle breathing system, which spans from the machine common gas outlet to the Y-piece (Fig. 25-32). The test has two components: (1) breathing system pressure and leak testing, and (2) verification that gas flows properly through the breathing circuit during both inspiration and exhalation. To thoroughly check the circle system for leaks, valve integrity, and obstruction, both tests must be performed preoperatively. The ASA 2008 recommendations call for performing the breathing system test and leak test before starting each case, so that pressure can be developed in the system during both manual/bag and automatic/mechanical ventilation.[148] Automated leak testing routines are implemented in modern workstations; system compliance is also calculated and used to adjust volume delivery during mechanical ventilation (Appendix B, Item 12). Because pressure and leak testing cannot identify all obstructions in the breathing circuit or confirm the function of the inspiratory and expiratory unidirectional valves, a test lung or second reservoir bag connected at the Y-piece can be used to confirm circuit integrity and function.[155] Visual inspection of the unidirectional valves should be performed daily, although subtle damage to these valves may be difficult to determine. Older 1993 FDA checkout procedures to identify valve incompetence that may not be visually obvious can be implemented, but are typically too complex for daily testing (Appendix B, Item 13).[156]

In the 1993 FDA Anesthesia Apparatus Checkout Recommendations, a *leak test* is performed by closing the APL (or pop-off) valve, occluding the Y-piece, and pressurizing the circuit to 30 cm H_2O pressure using the oxygen flush valve. The value on the pressure gauge will not decrease if the circle system is leak-free, but this does not assure unidirectional valve integrity or function. The value on the pressure gauge will read 30 cm H_2O even if the unidirectional valves are stuck shut or are inadequate.

In addition, a *flow test* checks the integrity of the unidirectional valves, and it detects obstruction in the circle system. Although it violates the sterility of the disposable anesthesia circuit, it can be performed by removing the Y-piece from the circle system and breathing through the two corrugated hoses individually. The unidirectional valve leaflets should be present and should move appropriately. The operator should be able to inhale but not exhale through the inspiratory limb and to be able to exhale but not inhale through the expiratory limb. Before performing this test, the operator must ensure there is no anesthetic gas in the circuit. Perhaps more safely, the flow test can also be performed by using the ventilator and a reservoir bag connected to the Y-piece as described in the 1993 FDA Anesthesia Apparatus Checkout Recommendations (Appendix A, Steps 11 and 12).[147]

Workstation Self-Tests

Many new anesthesia workstations now incorporate technology that allows the machine to either automatically or manually guide the user through a series of integrated tests to check for functionality of electronic, mechanical, and pneumatic components. Components able to be tested commonly include the gas supply system, flow control valves, the circle system, ventilator, and integrated vaporizers. The comprehensiveness of these self-diagnostic tests varies from one model and manufacturer to another, and users must be certain to read and strictly follow all manufacturer

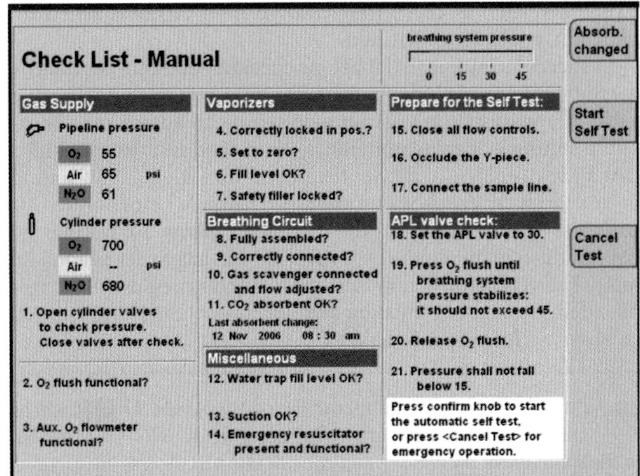

Figure 25-47 Manual checklist screen.

recommendations in performing these tests. Each workstation's self-testing program may be difficult to understand and may vary greatly among devices. None of the preuse checkouts are fully automated; therefore, the user must perform certain functions for the checkout to be complete. It is important for the user to know what is included in the automated checkout and even more important to know what is not included. Figures 25-47 and 25-48 show screen shots from the manual and automated workstation checkout procedures.

One particularly important point of caution with self-tests 15
should be noted on systems that have manifold-mounted vaporizers such as the Dräger Apollo and Dräger Fabius workstations. A manifold-mounted vaporizer does not become a part of an anesthesia workstation's low-pressure system until its concentration control dial is turned to the "on" position. Therefore, to detect internal vaporizer leaks in this type of system, the "leak test" portion of the self-diagnostic must be repeated with each individual vaporizer turned to the "on" position. If this precaution is not taken, large leaks that could potentially result in patient

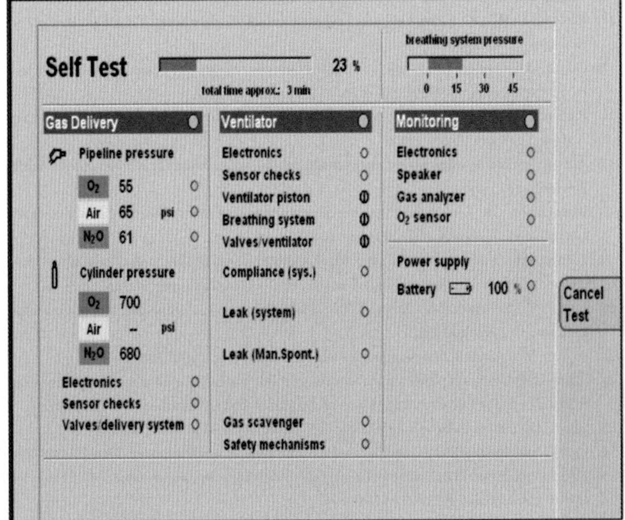

Figure 25-48 Automated self-test screen.

awareness, such as those from a loose filler cap or cracked fill indicator, could go undetected.

A successful automated machine checkout does not necessarily preclude machine failure. In one example, a leak in an APL bypass valve of a workstation was not detected by an automated checkout, resulting in a ventilator failure alarm. The authors concluded that a *functional test* of the ventilator and breathing circuit should be added to the checkout procedure. This may be performed by connecting a breathing bag to the circuit elbow. Activating the oxygen flush to inflate the bag will allow the bag to act as a model lung. The ventilator is now activated. Circuit pressure, tidal volume delivery, and bag inflation and deflation of the "lung" should be observed for proper function.[155]

For further review and interactivities, please see the videos and narrative interactive clinical vignettes (NICVs) accessible in the complimentary eBook bundled with this text. Access instructions are located on the inside front cover.

REFERENCES

1. Mehta SP, Eisenkraft JB, Posner KL, Domino KB. Patient injuries from anesthesia gas delivery equipment: a closed claims update. *Anesthesiology*. 2013;119:788–795.
2. Osborn DG, Jaffe MB. Standards and Regulatory Considerations. In: Ehrenwerth J, Eisenkraft JB, Berry JM, eds. *Anesthesia Equipment: Principles and Applications*. 3rd ed. Elsevier; 2021:593–613.
3. Bowie E, Huffman LM. *The Anesthesia Machine: Essentials for Understanding*. Madison, WI, Ohmeda, The BOC Group; 1985.
4. Dorsch JA, Dorsch SE. *A Practical Approach to Anesthesia Equipment*. Lippincott Williams & Wilkins; 2011.
5. Malayaman SN, Mychaskiw II G, Berry JM, Ehrenwerth J. Medical gases: Storage and supply. In: Ehrenwerth J, Eisenkraft JB, Berry JM, eds. *Anesthesia Equipment: Principles and Applications*. 3rd ed. Elsevier; 2021:3–24.
6. Schumacher SD, Brockwell RC, Andrews JJ, Ogles D. Bulk liquid oxygen supply failure. *Anesthesiology*. 2004;100:186–189.
7. Feeley TW, Hedley-Whyte J. Bulk oxygen and nitrous oxide delivery systems: design and dangers. *Anesthesiology*. 1976;44:301–305.
8. Pelton DA. *Non-Flammable Medical Gas Pipeline Systems*. University of Toronto Press; 1978.
9. Surgery mix-up causes 2 deaths. New Haven Register. January 20, 2002.
10. Mudumbai SC, Fanning R, Howard SK, Davies MF, Gaba DM. Use of medical simulation to explore equipment failures and human-machine interactions in anesthesia machine pipeline supply crossover. *Anesth Analg*. 2010;110:1292–1296.
11. Lorraway PG, Savoldelli GL, Joo HS, Chandra DB, Chow R, Naik VN. Management of simulated oxygen supply failure: is there a gap in the curriculum? *Anesth Analg*. 2006;102:865–867.
12. Ellett AE, Shields JC, Ifune C, Roa N, Vannucci A. A near miss: a nitrous oxide-carbon dioxide mix-up despite current safety standards. *Anesthesiology*. 2009;110:1429–1431.
13. Adriani J. Clinical application of physical principles concerning gases and vapor to anesthesiology. *The Chemistry and Physics of Anesthesia*. 2nd ed. Charles C Thomas; 1962:58.
14. Rose G, Durbin K, Eichhorn J. Gas cylinder colors ARE NOT an FDA Standard. *APSF Newsletter*. 2010;25:16.
15. Greilich PE, Greilich NB, Froelich EG. Intraabdominal fire during laparoscopic cholecystectomy. *Anesthesiology*. 1995;83:871–874.
16. Parbrook GD, Davis PD, Parbrook EO. *Basic Physics and Measurement in Anesthesia*. 2nd ed. Appleton Century Crofts; 1986.
17. Atlas G. A method to quickly estimate remaining time for an oxygen E-cylinder. *Anesth Analg*. 2004;98:1190.
18. Klemenzson GK, Perouansky M. Contemporary anesthesia ventilators incur a significant "oxygen cost." *Can J Anaesth*. 2004;51:616–620.
19. Taenzer AH, Kovatsis PG, Raessler KL. E-cylinder-powered mechanical ventilation may adversely impact anesthetic management and efficiency. *Anesth Analg*. 2002;95:148–150.
20. Davis PD, Parbrook GD, Kenny GNC. *Basic Physics and Measurement in Anaesthesia*. Butterworth-Heinemann; 2015.
21. Mushin WW, Jones PL. *Physics for the Anaesthetist*. Blackwell; 1987:1987.
22. Adriani J. Principles of physics and chemistry of solids and fluids applicable to anesthesiology. Adriani J, ed. *The Chemistry and Physics of Anesthesia*. 2nd ed. Charles C Thomas; 1962:7.
23. Schreiber P. *Safety Guidelines for Anesthesia Systems*. North American Dräger; 1985.
24. Eger EI 2nd, Epstein RM. Hazards of anesthetic equipment. *Anesthesiology*. 1964;25:490–504.
25. Eger EI 2nd, Hylton RR, Irwin RH, Guadagni N. Anesthetic flow meter sequence—a cause for hypoxia. *Anesthesiology*. 1963;24:396–396.
26. Wormer BA, Augenstein VA, Carpenter CL, et al. The green operating room: simple changes to reduce cost and our carbon footprint. *Am Surg*. 2013;79:666–671.
27. Luria I, Lampotang S, Schwab W, Cooper LA, Lizdas D, Gravenstein N. Automated, real-time fresh gas flow recommendations alter isoflurane consumption during the maintenance phase of anesthesia in a simulator-based study. *Anesth Analg*. 2013;117:1139–1147.
28. Mazze RI. Therapeutic misadventures with oxygen delivery systems: the need for continuous in-line oxygen monitors. *Anesth Analg*. 1972;51:787–790.
29. Cheng CJC, Garewal DS. A failure of the chain-link mechanism on the Ohmeda Excel 210 anesthetic machine. *Anesth Analg*. 2001;92:913–914.
30. Kidd AG, Hall I. Fault with an Ohmeda Excel 210 anaesthetic machine. *Anaesthesia*. 1994; 49:83–83.
31. Lohmann G. Fault with an Ohmeda Excel 410 machine. *Anaesthesia*. 1991;46:695–695.
32. Richards C. Failure of a nitrous oxide-oxygen proportioning device. *Anesthesiology*. 1989;71: 997–998.
33. Abraham ZA, Basagoitia J, Lowenstein E. A potentially lethal anesthesia machine failure. *Anesthesiology*. 1987;66:589–590.
34. Neubarth J. Another hazardous gas supply misconnection. *Anesth Analg*. 1995;80:206.
35. Korman B, Ritchie IM. Chemistry of halothane-enflurane mixtures applied to anesthesia. *Anesthesiology*. 1985;63:152–156.
36. Macintosh RR. Physics for the anaesthetist. *Physics for the anaesthetist*. 1946.
37. Schreiber P. *Anaesthesia Equipment: Performance, Classification and Safety*. Springer Science & Business Media; 2013.
38. Eisenkraft JB. Anesthesia vaporizers. In: Ehrenwerth J, Eisenkraft JB, Berry JM, eds. *Anesthesia equipment: principles and applications*. 3rd Ed. Elsevier; 2021:66–99.
39. Kharasch ED, Subbarao GN, Cromack KR, Stephens DA, Saltarelli MD. Sevoflurane formulation water content influences degradation by Lewis acids in vaporizers. *Anesth Analg*. 2009; 108:1796–1802.
40. Hill DW. The design and calibration of vaporizers for volatile anaesthetic agents. *Br J Anaesth*. 1968;40:648–659.
41. Hill DW, Lowe HJ. Comparison of concentration of halothane in closed and semiclosed circuits during controlled ventilation. *Anesthesiology*. 1962;23:291–298.
42. Diaz PM. The influence of carrier gas on the output of automatic plenum vaporizers. *BJA: Brit J Anaesthesia*. 1976;48:387–391.
43. Palayiwa E, Sanderson MH, Hahn CEW. Effects of carrier gas composition on the output of six anaesthetic vaporizers. *Br J Anaesth*. 1983;55:1025–1038.
44. Gould DB, Lampert BA, MacKrell TN. Effect of nitrous oxide solubility on vaporizer aberrance. *Anesth Analg*. 1982;61:938–940.
45. Broka SM, Gourdange PA, Joucken KL. Sevoflurane and desflurane confusion. *Anesth Analg*. 1999;88:1194.
46. George TM. Failure of keyed agent-specific filling devices. *Anesthesiology*. 1984;61: 228–229.
47. Riegle EV, Desertspring D. Failure of the agent-specific filling device. *Anesthesiology*. 1990; 73:353–354.
48. Abel M, Eisenkraft JB. Performance of erroneously filled sevoflurane, enflurane and other agent-specific vaporizers. *J Clin Monit*. 1996;12:119–125.
49. Adler AC, Connelly NR, Ankam A, Raghunathan K. Technical communication: inhaled anesthetic agent-vaporizer mismatch: management in settings with limited resources: don't try this at home. *Anesth Analg*. 2013;116:1272–1275.
50. Munson MW. Cardiac arrest: hazard of tipping a vaporizer. *Anesthesiology*. 1965;26:235–235.
51. Sinclair A, van Bergen J. Vaporizer overfilling. *Can J Anaesth*. 1993;40:77–78.
52. Craig DB. Vaporizer overfilling. *Can J Anaesth*. 1993;40:1005–1006.
53. Seropian MA, Robins B. Smaller-than-expected sevoflurane concentrations using the Sevotec 5® vaporizer at low fill states and high fresh gas flows. *Anesth Analg*. 2000;91:834–836.
54. Meister GC, Becker KE Jr. Potential fresh gas flow leak through Dräger vapor 19.1 vaporizer with key-index fill port. *Anesthesiology*. 1993;78:211–212.
55. Zimmer C, Janssen MN, Treschan TA, Peters J. Near-miss accident during magnetic resonance imaging by a "flying sevoflurane vaporizer" due to ferromagnetism undetectable by handheld magnet. *Anesthesiology*. 2004;100:1329–1330.
56. Andrews JJ, Johnston RV Jr. The new Tec6 desflurane vaporizer. *Anesth Analg*. 1993;76: 1338–1341.
57. Weiskopf RB, Sampson D, Moore MA. The desflurane (Tec 6) vaporizer: design, design considerations and performance evaluation. *Br J Anaesth*. 1994;72:474–479.
58. Eger EI 2nd. New inhaled anesthetics. *Anesthesiology*. 1994;80:906–922.
59. Johnston RV Jr, Andrews JJ, Deyo DJ, et al. The effects of carrier gas composition on the performance of the Tec 6 desflurane vaporizer. *Anesth Analg*. 1994;79:548–552.
60. Andrews JJ, Johnston RV Jr, Kramer GC. Consequences of misfilling contemporary vaporizers with desflurane. *Can J Anaesth*. 1993;40:71–76.
61. Hendrickx JFA, Carette RM, Deloof T, De Wolf AM. Severe ADU desflurane vaporizing unit malfunction. *Anesthesiology*. 2003;99:1459–1460.
62. Moyers J. A nomenclature for methods of inhalation anesthesia. *Anesthesiology*. 1953;14:609–611.
63. Eger EI 2nd. *Anesthetic Systems: Construction and Function*. Williams and Wilkins; 1974.
64. Eger EI 2nd, Ethans CT. The effects of inflow, overflow and valve placement on economy of the circle system. *Anesthesiology*. 1968;29:93–100.

65. Caplan RA, Vistica MF, Posner KL, Cheney FW. Adverse anesthetic outcomes arising from gas delivery equipment: a closed claims analysis. *Anesthesiology*. 1997;87:741–748.
66. Chacon AC, Kuczkowski KM, Sanchez RA. Unusual case of breathing circuit obstruction: plastic packaging revisited. *Anesthesiology*. 2004;100:753.
67. McEwan AI, Dowell AL, Karis JH. Bilateral tension pneumothorax caused by a blocked bacterial filter in an anesthesia breathing circuit. *Anesth Analg*. 1993;76:440–442.
68. Smith CE, Otworth JR, Kaluszyk P. Bilateral tension pneumothorax due to a defective anesthesia breathing circuit filter. *J Clin Anesth*. 1991;3:229–234.
69. Walton JS, Fears R, Burt N, Dorman BH. Intraoperative breathing circuit obstruction caused by albuterol nebulization. *Anesth Analg*. 1999;89:650.
70. Dhar P, George I, Mankad A, Sloan P. Flow transducer gas leak detected after induction. *Anesth Analg*. 1999;89:1587.
71. Mizrak A, Bilgi M, Koruk S, et al. Comparison of the coaxial circle circuit with the conventional circle circuit. *Eurasian J Med*. 2011;43:92.
72. Cohen JB, Chaudhry T. Kinked Inspiratory Limb of Coaxial Circuit Mimics Bronchospasm. *Anesth Patient Saf Found Newsletter*. 2012;27:234c.
73. Aso Kanno T, Aso C, Saito S, Yoshikawa D, Goto F. A combustive Destruction of expiration valve in an anesthetic circuit. *Anesthesiology*. 2003;98:577–579.
74. Laster M, Roth P, Eger EI 2nd. Fires from the interaction of anesthetics with desiccated absorbent. *Anesth Analg*. 2004;99:769–774.
75. Laudanski K, Schwab WK, Bakuzonis CW, Paulus DA. Thermal damage of the humidified ventilator circuit in the operating room: an analysis of plausible causes. *Anesth Analg*. 2010;111:1433–1436.
76. Holak EJ, Mei DA, Dunning MB 3rd, et al. Carbon monoxide production from sevoflurane breakdown: modeling of exposures under clinical conditions. *Anesth Analg*. 2003;96:757–764.
77. Kummar P, Korula G, Kumar S, Saravanan PA. Unusual cause of leak in Datex Aisys. *Anesth Analg*. 2009;109:1350–1351.
78. Kshatri AM, Kingsley CP. Defective carbon dioxide absorber as a cause for a leak in a breathing circuit. *Anesthesiology*. 1996;84:475–476.
79. Norman PH, Daley MD, Walker JR, Fusetti S. Obstruction due to retained carbon dioxide absorber canister wrapping. *Anesth Analg*. 1996;83:425–426.
80. Olympio MA. Carbon dioxide absorbent desiccation safety conference convened by APSF. *Anesth Patient Saf Found (APSF) Newsletter*. 2005;20:25–29.
81. Adriani J. *The chemistry and physics of anesthesia*. 2nd Ed. Thomas; 1977.
82. Murray JM, Renfrew CW, Bedi A, McCrystal CB, Jones DS, Fee JP. Amsorb: a new carbon dioxide absorbent for use in anesthetic breathing systems. *Anesthesiology*. 1999;91:1342–1348.
83. Versichelen LFM, Bouche MPLA, Rolly G, et al. Only carbon dioxide absorbents free of both NaOH and KOH do not generate compound A during in vitro closed-system sevoflurane: evaluation of five absorbents. *Anesthesiology*. 2001;95:750–755.
84. Higuchi H, Adachi Y, Arimura S, Kanno M, Satoh T. The carbon dioxide absorption capacity of Amsorb® is half that of soda lime. *Anesth Analg*. 2001;93:221–225.
85. Sosis MB. Why not use Amsorb alone as the CO2 absorbent and avoid any risk of CO production? *Anesthesiology*. 2003;98:1299; author reply 1299-1299; author reply 1299.
86. Carbon Dioxide Absorption During Inhalation Anesthesia: A Modern Practice. Feldman JM, Hendrickx J, Ross Kennedy R. *Anesth Analg*. 2021;132:993–1002.
87. Andrews JJ, Johnston RV Jr, Bee DE, Arens JF. Photodeactivation of ethyl violet: a potential hazard of Sodasorb. *Anesthesiology*. 1990;72:59–64.
88. Kharasch ED, Powers KM, Artru AA. Comparison of Amsorb, sodalime, and Baralyme degradation of volatile anesthetics and formation of carbon monoxide and compound A in swine in vivo. *Anesthesiology*. 2002;96:173–182.
89. Morio M, Fujii K, Satoh N, et al. Reaction of sevoflurane and its degradation products with soda lime. Toxicity of the byproducts. *Anesthesiology*. 1992;77:1155–1164.
90. Fang ZX, Kandel L, Laster MJ, Ionescu P, Eger EI 2nd. Factors affecting production of Compound A from the interaction of sevoflurane with Baralyme Registered Trademark and soda lime. *Anesth Analg*. 1996;82:775–781.
91. Frink EJ Jr, Malan TP, Morgan SE, Brown EA, Malcomson M, Brown BR Jr. Quantification of the degradation products of sevoflurane in two CO2 absorbants during low-flow anesthesia in surgical patients. *Anesthesiology*. 1992;77:1064–1069.
92. Eger EI 2nd, Ionescu P, Laster MJ, Weiskopf RB. Baralyme dehydration increases and soda lime dehydration decreases the concentration of compound A resulting from sevoflurane degradation in a standard anesthetic circuit. *Anesth Analg*. 1997;85:892–898.
93. Steffey EP, Laster MJ, Ionescu P, Eger EI 2nd, Gong D, Weiskopf RB. Dehydration of Baralyme increases compound A resulting from sevoflurane degradation in a standard anesthetic circuit used to anesthetize swine. *Anesth Analg*. 1997;85:1382–1386.
94. Bito H, Ikeuchi Y, Ikeda K. Effects of low-flow sevoflurane anesthesia on renal function: comparison with high-flow sevoflurane anesthesia and low-flow isoflurane anesthesia. *Anesthesiology*. 1997;86:1231–1237.
95. Eger EI 2nd, Koblin DD, Bowland T, et al. Nephrotoxicity of sevoflurane versus desflurane anesthesia in volunteers. *Anesth Analg*. 1997;84:160–168.
96. Kharasch ED, Frink EJ Jr, Zager R, Bowdle TA, Artru A, Nogami WM. Assessment of low-flow sevoflurane and isoflurane effects on renal function using sensitive markers of tubular toxicity. *Anesthesiology*. 1997;86:1238–1253.
97. Fukuda H, Kawamoto M, Yuge O, Fujii K. A comparison of the effects of prolonged (>10 hour) low-flow sevoflurane, high-flow sevoflurane, and low-flow isoflurane anaesthesia on hepatorenal function in orthopaedic patients. *Anaesth Intensive Care*. 2004;32:210–218.
98. Berry PD, Sessler DI, Larson MD. Severe carbon monoxide poisoning during desflurane anesthesia. *Anesthesiology*. 1999;90:613–616.
99. Woehlck HJ, Dunning M 3rd, Connolly LA. Reduction in the incidence of carbon monoxide exposures in humans undergoing general anesthesia. *Anesthesiology*. 1997;87:228–234.
100. Bonome C, Belda J, Alvarez-Refojo F, Soro M, Fernández-Goti C, Cortés A. Low-flow anesthesia and reduced animal size increase carboxyhemoglobin levels in swine during desflurane and isoflurane breakdown in dried soda lime. *Anesth Analg*. 1999;89:909.
101. Neumann MA, Laster MJ, Weiskopf RB, et al. The elimination of sodium and potassium hydroxides from desiccated soda lime diminishes degradation of desflurane to carbon monoxide and sevoflurane to compound A but does not compromise carbon dioxide absorption. *Anesth Analg*. 1999;89:768.
102. Zilberman P. The CO 2 Absorber Based on LiOH. *Acta Medica Marisiensis*. 2015;61.
103. Mapleson WW. The elimination of rebreathing in various semi-closed anaesthetic systems.*Br J Anaesth*. 1954;26:323–332.
104. Willis BA, Pender JW, Mapleson WW. Rebreathing in a T-piece: volunteer and theoretical studies of the Jackson-Rees modification of Ayre's T-piece during spontaneous respiration. *Br J Anaesth*. 1975;47:1239–1246.
105. Sykes MK. Rebreathing circuits. *Br J Anaesth*. 1968;40:666–674.
106. Froese AB, Rose DK. A detailed analysis of T-piece systems. In: Steward DJ, ed. *Some Aspects of Paediatric Anaesthesia*. Excerpta Medica; 1982:101.
107. Aarhus D, Søreide E, Holst-Larsen H. Mechanical obstruction in the anaesthesia delivery-system mimicking severe bronchospasm. *Anaesthesia*. 1997;52:992–994.
108. Pethick S. Untitled Letter to the Editor. *Can Anaesth Soc J*. 1975;22:115.
109. Von Ungern-Sternberg BS, Saudan S, Regli A, Schaub E, Erb TO, Habre W; SWISS PEDIATRIC RESPIRATORY RESEARCH GROUP. Should the use of modified Jackson Rees T-piece breathing system be abandoned in preschool children? *Pediatric Anesthesia*. 2007;17:654–660.
110. Demaria S Jr, Blasius K, Neustein SM. Missed steps in the preanesthetic set-up. *Anesth Analg*. 2011;113:84–88.
111. Scheller MS, Jones BR, Benumof JL. The influence of fresh gas flow and inspiratory/expiratory ratio on tidal volume and arterial CO2 tension in mechanically ventilated surgical patients. *J Cardiothorac Anesth*. 1989;3:564–567.
112. Sandberg WS, Kaiser S. Novel breathing circuit architecture: new consequences of old problems. *Anesthesiology*. 2004;100:755–756.
113. Ortega RA, Zambricki ER. Fresh gas decoupling valve failure precludes mechanical ventilation in a Draeger Fabius GS anesthesia machine. *Anesth Analg*. 2007;104:1000–1001.
114. Pai SL, Robards CB, Riutort KT, Torp KD. Oxygen delivery failure due to improper installation of carbon dioxide absorbent canister: a case report. *Braz J Anesth*. 2021;71:443–446.
115. Sims C. Absent expiratory valve missed by automated check in Dräger Primus anaesthesia workstation. *Anaesth Intensive Care*. 2013;41:681.
116. Cooper JB, Newbower RS, Kitz RJ. An analysis of major errors and equipment failures in anesthesia management: considerations for prevention and detection. *Anesthesiology*. 1984;60:34–42.
117. Reinhart DJ, Friz R. Undetected leak in corrugated circuit tubing in compressed configuration. *Anesthesiology*. 1993;78:218–218.
118. Raphael DT, Weller RS, Doran DJ. A response algorithm for the low-pressure alarm condition. *Anesth Analg*. 1988;67:876–883.
119. Slee TA, Pavlin EG. Failure of low pressure alarm associated with the use of a humidifier. *Anesthesiology*. 1988;69:791–793.
120. Jaffe MB, Eisenkraft JB, Orr J. Respiratory gas monitoring. In: Ehrenwerth J, Eisenkraft JB, Berry JM, eds. *Anesthesia Equipment: Principles and Application*. 3rd ed. Elsevier; 2021:195–217.
121. Feeley TW, Bancroft ML. Problems with mechanical ventilators. *Int Anesthesiol Clin*. 1982;20:83–93.
122. Khalil SN, Gholston TK, Binderman J, Antosh S. Flapper valve malfunction in an Ohio closed scavenging system. *Anesth Analg*. 1987;66:1334–1336.
123. Sommer RM, Bhalla GS, Jackson JM, Cohen MI. Hypoventilation caused by ventilator valve rupture. *Anesth Analg*. 1988;67:999–1001.
124. Bourke DL, Tolentino D. Inadvertent positive end-expiratory pressure caused by a malfunctioning ventilator relief valve. *Anesth Analg*. 2003;97:492–493.
125. Usher AG, Cave DA, Finegan BA. Critical incident with Narkomed 6000 Anesthesia System. *Anesthesiology*. 2003;99:762; discussion 762-762; discussion 762.
126. Wetz AJ, Mueller MM, Walliser K, et al. End-tidal control vs. manually controlled minimal-flow anesthesia: a prospective comparative trial. *Acta Anaesthesiol Scand*. 2017;61:1262–1269.
127. Eisenkraft JB, Loftus KM. Waste anesthetic gases and scavenging systems. In: Ehrenwerth J, Eisenkraft JB, Berry JM, eds. *Anesthesia Equipment: Principles and Application*. 3rd ed. Elsevier; 2021:125–148.
128. National Institute for Occupational Safety and Health (NIOSH). *Occupational exposure to waste anesthetic gases and vapors*. U.S. Department of Health, Education, and Welfare, Public Health Service, Centers for Disease Control; 1977.

129. Sessler DI, Badgwell JM. Exposure of postoperative nurses to exhaled anesthetic gases. *Anesth Analg*. 1998;87:1083–1088.
130. American Society for Testing and Materials (ASTM). Standard Specification for Anesthetic Equipment-Scavenging Systems for Anesthetic Gases (ASTM F1343–91). 1991.
131. A Notice by the Centers for Disease Control and Prevention on 02/21/2006. Request for information on waste halogenated anesthetic agents: isoflurane, desflurane, and sevoflurane. *Fed Regist*. 2006;71:8859–8860.
132. McGregor D, Baden J, Banniste C, et al. Waste anesthetic gases-information for management in anesthezising areas and the posanesthesia care unit (PACU). *Park Ridge, IL: Amer Soc Anesthesiol*. 1999;63:22.
133. Kanmura Y, Sakai J, Yoshinaka H, Shirao K. Causes of nitrous oxide contamination in operating rooms. *Anesthesiology*. 1999;90:693–696.
134. Scavenger OR. Operator's instruction manual. *Telford, PA, North Amer Dräger*. 1986.
135. Gray WM. Symposium on anaesthetic equipment. Scavenging equipment. *Br J Anaesth*. 1985;57:685–695.
136. Brockwell RC, Andrews JJ. Understanding your anesthesia machine. *ASA Refresher Courses Anesthesiol*. 2002;30:41–59.
137. Allen M, Lees DE. Fires in medical vacuum pumps: do you need to be concerned? *ASA Monitor*. 2004;68:22–23.
138. Barwise JA, Lancaster LJ, Michaels D, Pope JE, Berry JM. An initial evaluation of a novel anesthetic scavenging interface. *Anesth Analg*. 2011;113:1064–1067.
139. Ryan SM, Nielsen CJ. Global warming potential of inhaled anesthetics: application to clinical use. *Anesth Analg*. 2010;111:92–98.
140. Feldman JM. Managing fresh gas flow to reduce environmental contamination. *Anesth Analg*. 2012;114:1093–1101.
141. James RH. 1000 anaesthetic incidents: experience to date. *Anaesthesia*. 2003;58:856–863.
142. Robards C, Corda D. A potential hazard involving the gas sampling line and the adjustable pressure limiting valve on the Drager Apollo® Anesthesia Workstation. *Anesth Analg*. 2010; 111:578–579.
143. Kibelbek MJ. Cable trapped under Dräger Fabius automatic pressure limiting valve causes inability to ventilate. *Anesthesiology*. 2007;106:639–640.
144. Gurbeta L, Dzemic Z, Bego T, Sejdic E, Badnjevic A. Testing of anesthesia machines and defibrillators in healthcare institutions. *J Med Syst*. 2017;41:133.
145. Olympio MA. Modern anesthesia machines offer new safety features. *Anesth Patient Saf Found Newsletter*. 2003;18:24–27.
146. Brockwell RC, Andrews JJ. Anesthesia apparatus checkout recommendations. In: Miller RD, ed. *Miller's Anesthesia*. 6th ed. Elsevier Churchill Livingstone, Inc.; 2005:315–316.
147. US Food, Drug Administration (FDA). Anesthesia apparatus checkout recommendations, 1993. Rockville, MD: Food and Drug Administration. 1993.
148. Feldman JM, Olympio MA, Martin D, Striker A. New guidelines available for pre-anesthesia checkout. *Anesth Patient Saf Found (APSF) Newsletter*. 2008;23:1.
149. Zheng J, Du L, Zhang L. Seizure-like movements caused by residual sevoflurane inside the anesthesia machine: a case report. *Medicine (Baltimore)*. 2021;100:e24495.
150. Myers JA, Good ML, Andrews JJ. Comparison of tests for detecting leaks in the low-pressure system of anesthesia gas machines. *Anesth Analg*. 1997;84:179–184.
151. Eng TS, Durieux ME. Automated machine checkout leaves an internal gas leak undetected: the need for complete checkout procedures. *Anesth Analg*. 2012;114:144–146.
152. Eisenkraft JB, Jaffe MB. Hazards of the anesthesia workstation. In: Ehrenwerth J, Eisenkraft JB, Berry JM, eds. *Anesthesia Equipment: Principles and Applications*. 3rd Ed. Elsevier; 2021: 489–525.
153. Mann DP, Der Ananian J, Alston TA. Oxygen flush valve booby trap. *Anesthesiology*. 2004; 101:558–558.
154. Goyal VK, Venticinque SG. *Machine Checkout and Quality Assurance*. In: *Anesthesia Equipment: Principles and Applications*. 3rd Ed. Elsevier; 2021:559–583.
155. Dosch MP. Automated checkout routines in anesthesia workstations vary in detection and management of breathing circuit obstruction. *Anesth Analg*. 2014;118:1254–1257.
156. Weigel WA, Murray WB. Detecting unidirectional valve incompetence by the modified pressure decline method. *Anesth Analg*. 2005;100:1723–1727.

Appendix A

FDA 1993 Anesthesia Apparatus Checkout Recommendations

This checklist was developed several years ago and since then most anesthesia workstations are newer and more sophisticated. Nevertheless, this checkout, or a reasonable equivalent, represents a good generic list of steps that should be conducted before administration of anesthesia. These recommendations are only valid for an anesthesia system that conforms to current and relevant standards and includes an ascending bellows ventilator and at least the following monitors: Capnograph, pulse oximeter, oxygen analyzer, respiratory volume monitor (spirometer), and breathing system pressure monitor with high- and low-pressure alarms. This is a guideline that users are encouraged to modify to accommodate differences in equipment design and variations in local clinical practice. Such local modifications should have appropriate peer review. Users should refer to the operator's manual for the manufacturer's specific procedures and precautions, especially the manufacturer's low-pressure leak test (Step 5).

Emergency Ventilation Equipment

1. ***Verify Backup Ventilation Equipment is Available and Functioning**

High-Pressure System

2. ***Check Oxygen Cylinder Supply**
   a. Open O_2 cylinder and verify at least half full (about 1,000 psi)
   b. Close cylinder
3. ***Check Central Pipeline Supplies**
   a. Check that hoses are connected and pipeline gauges read about 50 psi

Low-Pressure System

4. ***Check Initial Status of Low-Pressure System**
   a. Close flow control valves and turn vaporizers off
   b. Check fill level and tighten vaporizers' filler caps
5. ***Perform Leak Check of Machine Low-Pressure System**
   a. Verify that the machine master switch and flow control valves are OFF
   b. Attach "suction bulb" to common (fresh) gas outlet
   c. Squeeze bulb repeatedly until fully collapsed
   d. Verify bulb stays fully collapsed for at least 10 seconds
   e. Open one vaporizer at a time and repeat "c" and "d" as above
   f. Remove suction bulb and reconnect fresh gas hose
6. ***Turn on Machine Master Switch and All Other Necessary Electrical Equipment**
7. ***Test Flowmeters**
   a. Adjust flow of all gases through their full range, checking for smooth operation of floats and undamaged flow tubes
   b. Attempt to create a hypoxic O_2/N_2O mixture and verify correct changes in flow and/or alarm

Scavenging System

8. ***Adjust and Check Scavenging System**
   a. Ensure proper connections between the scavenging system and both APL (pop-off) valve and ventilator relief valve
   b. Adjust waste gas vacuum (if possible)
   c. Fully open APL valve and occlude Y-piece
   d. With minimum O_2 flow, allow scavenger reservoir bag to collapse completely and verify that absorber pressure gauge reads about zero
   e. With the O_2 flush activated, allow the scavenger reservoir bag to distend fully and then verify that absorber pressure gauge reads <10 cm H_2O

Breathing System

9. ***Calibrate O_2 Monitor**
   a. Ensure monitor reads 21% in room air
   b. Verify low O_2 alarm is enabled and functioning
   c. Reinstall sensor in circuit and flush breathing system with O_2
   d. Verify that monitor now reads greater than 90%
10. **Check Initial Status of Breathing System**
   a. Set selector switch to "Bag" mode
   b. Check that breathing circuit is complete, undamaged, and unobstructed
   c. Verify that CO_2 absorbent is adequate
   d. Install the breathing circuit accessory equipment (e.g., humidifier, PEEP valve) to be used during the case
11. **Perform Leak Check of the Breathing System**
   a. Set all gas flows to zero (or minimum)
   b. Close APL (pop-off) valve and occlude Y-piece
   c. Pressurize breathing system to about 30 cm H_2O with O_2 flush
   d. Ensure that pressure remains fixed for at least 10 seconds
   e. Open APL (pop-off) valve and ensure that pressure decreases

Manual and Automatic Ventilation Systems

12. **Test Ventilation Systems and Unidirectional Valves**
   a. Place a second breathing bag on Y-piece
   b. Set appropriate ventilator parameters for next patient
   c. Switch to automatic ventilation (ventilator) mode
   d. Turn ventilator ON and fill bellows and breathing bag with O_2 flush
   e. Set O_2 flow to minimum, other gas flows to zero
   f. Verify that during inspiration, bellows deliver appropriate tidal volume and that during expiration bellows fill completely
   g. Set fresh gas flow to about 5 L/min
   h. Verify that the ventilator bellows and simulated lungs fill and empty appropriately without sustained pressure at end expiration
   i. Check for proper action of unidirectional valves
   j. Exercise breathing circuit accessories to ensure proper function
   k. Turn ventilator OFF and switch to manual ventilation (bag/APL) mode
   l. Ventilate manually and assure inflation and deflation of artificial lungs and appropriate feel of system resistance and compliance
   m. Remove second breathing bag from Y-piece

Monitors

13. **Check, Calibrate, and/or Set Alarm Limits of All Monitors**
   a. Capnometer
   b. Oxygen analyzer
   c. Pressure monitor with high- and low-airway pressure alarms
   d. Pulse oximeter
   e. Respiratory volume monitor (spirometer)

Final Position

14. **Check Final Status of Machine**
   a. Vaporizers off
   b. APL valve open
   c. Selector switch to "bag"
   d. All flowmeters to zero (or minimum)
   e. Patient suction level adequate
   f. Breathing system ready to use

*From Food and Drug Administration. Anesthesia Apparatus Checkout Recommendations. Rockville, MD: Food and Drug Administration; 1993.

Appendix B

Recommendations for Preanesthesia Checkout Procedures

Background

Improperly checking anesthesia equipment prior to use can lead to patient injury and has also been associated with an increased risk of severe postoperative morbidity and mortality.[1,2] In 1993, a PAC was developed and widely accepted to be an important step in the process of preparing to deliver anesthesia care.[3] Despite the accepted importance of the PAC, available evidence suggests that the current version is neither well understood nor reliably utilized by anesthesia providers.[4–6] Furthermore, anesthesia delivery systems have evolved to the point that one checkout procedure is not applicable to all anesthesia delivery systems currently on the market. For these reasons, a new approach to the PAC has been developed. The goal was to provide guidelines applicable to all anesthesia delivery systems so that individual departments can develop a PAC that can be performed consistently and expeditiously.

General Considerations

The following document is intended to serve not as a PAC itself, but rather as a template for developing checkout procedures that are appropriate for each individual anesthesia machine design. When using this template to develop a checkout procedure for systems that incorporate automated checkout features, items that are not evaluated by the automated checkout need to be identified, and supplemental manual checkout procedures included as needed.

Simply because an automated checkout procedure exists does not mean it can completely replace a manual checkout procedure or that it can be performed safely without adequate training and a thorough understanding of what the automated checkout accomplishes. An automated checkout procedure can be incomplete and/or misleading. For example, the leak test performed by some current automated checkouts does not test for leaks at the vaporizers. As a result, a loose vaporizer filler cap, or a leak at the vaporizer mount, could easily be missed.

Ideally, automated checkout procedures should clearly reveal to the user the functions that are being checked, any deficient function that is found, and recommendations to correct the problem. Documentation of the automated checkout process should preferably be in a manner that can be recorded on the anesthesia record.

Operator's manuals, which accompany anesthesia delivery systems, include extensive recommendations for equipment checkout. Although these recommendations are quite extensive and typically not utilized by anesthesia providers, they are nevertheless important references for developing machine-specific and institution-specific checkout procedures.

Personnel Performing the PAC

The previously accepted Anesthesia Apparatus Checkout Recommendation placed all of the responsibility for preuse checkout on the anesthesia provider. Sole reliance on one individual to complete the checkout process may increase the likelihood that one or more steps will be omitted or performed improperly. This guideline identifies those aspects of the PAC that could be completed by a qualified anesthesia and/or biomedical technician. Utilizing technicians to perform some aspects of the PAC may improve compliance with the PAC. Steps completed by a technician may be part of the morning preuse check or part of a procedure performed at the end of each day. Critical checkout steps (e.g., availability of backup ventilation equipment) will benefit from intentional redundancy (i.e., having more than one individual responsible for checking the equipment). *Regardless of the level of training and support by technicians, the anesthesia care provider is ultimately responsible for proper function of all equipment used to provide anesthesia care.*

Adaptation of the PAC to local needs, assignment of responsibility for the checkout procedures, and training are the responsibilities of the individual anesthesia department. Training procedures should be documented. Proper documentation should include records of completed coursework (e.g., a manufacturer course) or for in-house training, a listing of the competency items taught and records of successful completion by trainees.

Objectives for a New PAC

- Outline the essential items that need to be available and functioning properly prior to delivering every anesthetic.
- Identify the frequency with which each of the items needs to be checked.
- Suggest which items may be checked by a qualified anesthesia technician, biomedical technician, or a manufacturer-certified service technician.

Basic Principles

- The anesthesia care provider is ultimately responsible for ensuring that the anesthesia equipment is safe and ready for use. This responsibility includes adequate familiarity with the equipment, following relevant local policies for performing and documenting the PAC and being knowledgeable about those procedures.
- Depending upon the staffing resources in a particular institution, anesthesia technicians and/or biomedical technicians can participate in the PAC. Biomedical technicians are often trained and certified by manufacturers to perform on-site maintenance of anesthesia delivery systems and therefore can be a useful resource for completing regular checkout procedures. Anesthesia technicians are not commonly trained to perform checkout procedures. Involving the anesthesia technicians is intended to enhance compliance with

the PAC. Each department should decide whether the available technicians can or should be trained to assist with checkout procedures. Formal certification of anesthesia technicians by the American Society of Anesthesia Technicians and Technologists (ASATT) is encouraged but does not necessarily guarantee familiarity with checkout procedures.

- Critical items will benefit from redundant checks to avoid errors and omissions.
- When more than one person is responsible for checking an item, all parties should perform the check if intentional redundancy is deemed important, or either party may be acceptable, depending upon the available resources.
- Whoever conducts the PAC should provide documentation of successful performance. The anesthesia provider should include this documentation on the patient chart.
- Whenever an anesthesia machine is moved to a new location, a complete beginning-of-the-day checkout should be performed.
- Automated checks should clearly distinguish the components of the delivery system that are checked automatically from those which require manual checkout.
- Ideally, the date, time, and outcome of the most recent check(s) should be recorded and the information made accessible to the user.
- Specific procedures for preuse checkout cannot be prescribed in this document since they vary with the delivery systems. Clinicians must learn how to effectively perform the necessary preuse check for each piece of equipment they use.
- Each department or health care facility should work with the manufacturer(s) of their equipment to develop preuse checkout procedures that satisfy both the following guidelines and the needs of the local department.
- Default settings for ventilators, monitors, and alarms should be checked to determine if they are appropriate.
- These checkout recommendations are intended to replace the preexisting FDA-Approved Anesthesia Apparatus Checkout Recommendations. They are not intended to be a replacement for required preventive maintenance.
- The PAC is essential to safe care but should not delay initiating care if the patient needs are so urgent that time taken to complete the PAC could worsen the patient's outcome.

Guidelines for Developing Institution-Specific Checkout Procedures Prior to Anesthesia Delivery

These guidelines describe a basic approach to checkout procedures and rationale that will ensure that these priorities are satisfied. They should be used to develop institution-specific checkout procedures designed for the equipment and resources available. (Example of institution-specific procedures for current anesthesia delivery systems are published on the same website as this document.)

Requirements for Safe Delivery of Anesthesia Care

- Reliable delivery of oxygen at any appropriate concentration up to 100%.
- Reliable means of positive-pressure ventilation.
- Backup ventilation equipment available and functioning.
- Controlled release of positive pressure from the breathing circuit.
- Anesthesia vapor delivery (if intended as part of the anesthetic plan).
- Adequate suction.
- Means to conform to standards for patient monitoring.[7,8]

Specific Items

The following items need to be checked as part of a complete PAC. The intent is to identify what to check, the recommended frequency of checking and the individual(s) who could be responsible for the item. For these guidelines, the responsible party would fall into one of four categories: provider, technician, technician or provider, or technician and provider. The designation "technician and provider" means that the provider must perform the check whether or not it has been completed by a technician. It is not intended to make the use of technician checks mandatory. The intent is not to specify how an item needs to be checked, as the specific checkout procedure will depend upon the equipment being used.

Item 1: Verify whether auxiliary oxygen cylinder and self-inflating manual ventilation device are available and functioning.
Frequency: Daily
Responsible parties: Provider and technician
Rationale: Failure to be able to ventilate is a major cause of morbidity and mortality related to anesthesia care. Because equipment failure with resulting inability to ventilate the patient can occur at any time, a self-inflating manual ventilation device (e.g., AMBU bag) should be present at every anesthetizing location for every case and should be checked for proper function. In addition, a source of oxygen separate from the anesthesia machine and pipeline supply, specifically an oxygen cylinder with regulator and a means to open the cylinder valve, should be immediately available and checked. After checking the cylinder pressure, it is recommended that the main cylinder valve be closed to avoid inadvertent emptying of the cylinder through a leaky or open regulator.

Item 2: Verify patient suction is adequate to clear the airway.
Frequency: Prior to each use
Responsible parties: Provider and technician
Rationale: Safe anesthetic care requires the immediate availability of suction to clear the airway if needed.

Item 3: Turn on anesthesia delivery system and confirm that AC power is available.

Frequency: Daily

Responsible parties: Provider or technician

Rationale: Anesthesia delivery systems typically function with backup battery power if AC power fails. Unless the presence of AC power is confirmed, the first obvious sign of power failure can be a complete system shutdown when the batteries can no longer power the system. Many anesthesia delivery systems have visual indicators of the power source showing the presence of both AC and battery power. These indicators should be checked and connection of the power cord to a functional AC power source should be confirmed.

Desflurane vaporizers require electrical power and recommendations for checking power to these vaporizers should also be followed.

Item 4: Verify availability of required monitors and check alarms.

Frequency: Prior to each use

Responsible parties: Provider or technician

Rationale: Standards for patient monitoring during anesthesia are clearly defined.[7,8] The ability to conform to these standards should be confirmed for every anesthetic. The first step is to visually verify that the appropriate monitoring supplies (BP cuffs, oximetry probes, etc.) are available. All monitors should be turned on and proper completion of power-up self-tests confirmed. Given the importance of pulse oximetry and capnography to patient safety, verifying proper function of these devices before anesthetizing the patient is essential. Capnometer function can be verified by exhaling through the breathing circuit or gas sensor to generate a capnogram, or verifying that the patient's breathing efforts generate a capnogram before the patient is anesthetized. Visual and audible alarm signals should be generated when this is discontinued. Pulse oximeter function, including an audible alarm, can be verified by placing the sensor on a finger and observing for a proper recording. The pulse oximeter alarm can be tested by introducing motion artifact or removing the sensor.

Audible alarms have also been reconfirmed as essential to patient safety by the ASA, American Association of Nurse Anesthetists (AANA), APSF, and Joint Commission on the Accreditation of Healthcare Organizations (JCAHO). Proper monitor functioning includes visual and audible alarm signals that function as designed.

Item 5: Verify that pressure is adequate on the spare oxygen cylinder mounted on the anesthesia machine.

Frequency: Daily

Responsible parties: Provider and technician

Rationale: Anesthesia delivery systems rely on a supply of oxygen for various machine functions. At a minimum, the oxygen supply is used to provide oxygen to the patient. Pneumatically powered ventilators also rely on a gas supply. Oxygen cylinder(s) should be mounted on the anesthesia delivery system and determined to have an acceptable minimum pressure. The acceptable pressure depends on the intended use, the design of the anesthesia delivery system and the availability of piped oxygen.

- Typically, an oxygen cylinder will be used if the central oxygen supply fails.
- If the cylinder is intended to be the primary source of oxygen (e.g., remote site anesthesia), then a cylinder supply sufficient to last for the entire anesthetic is required. If a pneumatically powered ventilator that uses oxygen as its driving gas will be used, a full "E" oxygen cylinder may provide only 30 minutes of oxygen. In that case, the maximum duration of oxygen supply can be obtained from an oxygen cylinder if it is used only to provide fresh gas to the patient in conjunction with manual or spontaneous ventilation. Mechanical ventilators will consume the oxygen supply if pneumatically powered ventilators that require oxygen to power the ventilator are used. Electrically powered ventilators do not consume oxygen so that the duration of a cylinder supply will depend only on total fresh gas flow.
- The oxygen cylinder valve should be closed after it has been verified that adequate pressure is present, unless the cylinder is to be the primary source of oxygen (i.e., piped oxygen is not available). If the valve remains open and the pipeline supply should fail, the oxygen cylinder can become depleted while the anesthesia provider is unaware of the oxygen supply problem.
- Other gas supply cylinders (e.g., Heliox, CO_2, air, N_2O) need to be checked only if that gas is required to provide anesthetic care.

Item 6: Verify that piped gas pressures are 50 psig or higher.

Frequency: Daily

Responsible parties: Provider and technician

Rationale: A minimum gas supply pressure is required for proper function of the anesthesia delivery system. Gas supplied from a central source can fail for a variety of reasons. Therefore, the pressure in the piped gas supply should be checked at least once daily.

Item 7: Verify that vaporizers are adequately filled and, if applicable, that the filler ports are tightly closed.

Frequency: Prior to each use

Responsible parties: Provider. Technician if redundancy desired.

Rationale: If anesthetic vapor delivery is planned, an adequate supply is essential to reduce the risk of light anesthesia or recall. This is especially true if an anesthetic agent monitor with a low agent alarm is not being used. Partially open filler ports are a common cause of leaks that may not be detected if the vaporizer control dial is not open when a leak test is performed. This leak source can be minimized by tightly closing filler ports. Newer vaporizer designs have filling systems that automatically close the filler port when filling is completed.

High and low anesthetic agent alarms are useful to help prevent over- or underdosage of anesthetic vapor. Use of these alarms is encouraged and they should be set to the appropriate limits and enabled.

Item 8: Verify that there are no leaks in the gas supply lines between the flowmeters and the common gas outlet.

Frequency: Daily and whenever a vaporizer is changed

Responsible parties: Provider or technician

Rationale: The gas supply in this part of the anesthesia delivery system passes through the anesthetic vaporizer(s) on most anesthesia delivery systems. In order to perform a thorough leak test, each vaporizer must be turned on individually to check for leaks at the vaporizer mount(s) or inside the vaporizer. Furthermore, some machines have a check valve between the flowmeters and the common gas outlet, requiring a negative-pressure test to adequately check for leaks. Automated checkout procedures typically include a leak test but may not evaluate leaks at the vaporizer especially if the vaporizer is not turned on during the leak test. When relying upon automated testing to evaluate the system for leaks, the automated leak test would need to be repeated for each vaporizer in place. This test should also be completed whenever a vaporizer is changed. The risk of a leak at the vaporizer depends upon the vaporizer design. Vaporizer designs where the filler port closes automatically after filling can reduce the risk of leaks.

Technicians can provide useful assistance with this aspect of the machine checkout since it can be time-consuming.

Item 9: Test scavenging system function.

Frequency: Daily

Responsible parties: Provider or technician

Rationale: A properly functioning scavenging system prevents room contamination by anesthetic gases. Proper function depends upon correct connections between the scavenging system and the anesthesia delivery system. These connections should be checked daily by a provider or technician. Depending upon the scavenging system design, proper function may also require that the vacuum level is adequate, which should also be confirmed daily. Some scavenging systems have mechanical positive- and negative-pressure relief valves. Positive- and negative-pressure relief is important to protect the patient circuit from pressure fluctuations related to the scavenging system. Proper checkout of the scavenging system should ensure that positive- and negative-pressure relief is functioning properly. Due to the complexity of checking for effective positive- and negative-pressure relief, and the variations in scavenging system design, a properly trained technician can facilitate this aspect of the checkout process.

Item 10: Calibrate, or verify calibration of, the oxygen monitor and check the low-oxygen alarm.

Frequency: Daily

Responsible parties: Provider or technician.

Rationale: Continuous monitoring of the inspired oxygen concentration is the last line of defense against delivering hypoxic gas concentrations to the patient. The oxygen monitor is essential for detecting adulteration of the oxygen supply. Most oxygen monitors require calibration once daily, although some are self-calibrating. For self-calibrating oxygen monitors, they should be verified to read 21% when sampling room air. This is a step that is easily completed by a trained technician. When more than one oxygen monitor is present, the primary sensor that will be relied upon for oxygen monitoring should be checked.

The low oxygen concentration alarm should also be checked at this time by setting the alarm above the measured oxygen concentration and confirming that an audible alarm signal is generated.

Item 11: Verify carbon dioxide absorbent is not exhausted.

Frequency: Prior to each use

Responsible parties: Provider or technician

Rationale: Proper function of a circle anesthesia system relies on the absorbent to remove carbon dioxide from rebreathed gas. Exhausted absorbent as indicated by the characteristic color change should be replaced. It is possible for absorbent material to lose the ability to absorb CO_2 yet the characteristic color change may be absent or difficult to see. Some newer absorbents do change color when desiccated. Capnography should be utilized for every anesthetic and, when using a circle anesthesia system, rebreathing carbon dioxide as indicated by an inspired CO_2 concentration above 0 can also indicate exhausted absorbent. (See Additional Note 2, below.)

Item 12: Breathing system pressure and leak testing.

Frequency: Prior to each use

Responsible parties: Provider and technician

Rationale: The breathing system pressure and leak test should be performed with the circuit configuration to be used during anesthetic delivery. If any components of the circuit are changed after this test is completed, the test should be performed again. Although the anesthesia provider should perform this test before each use, anesthesia technicians who replace and assemble circuits can also perform this check and add redundancy to this important checkout procedure. Proper testing will demonstrate that pressure can be developed in the breathing system during both manual and mechanical ventilation and that pressure can be relieved during manual ventilation by opening the APL valve.

Automated testing is often implemented in the newer anesthesia delivery systems to evaluate the system for leaks and also to determine the compliance of the breathing system. The compliance value determined during this testing will be used to automatically adjust the volume delivered by the ventilator to maintain a constant volume delivery to the patient. It is important that the circuit configuration that is to be used be in place during the test.

Item 13: Verify that gas flows properly through the breathing circuit during both inspiration and exhalation.

Frequency: Prior to each use

Responsible parties: Provider and technician

Rationale: Pressure and leak testing does not identify all obstructions in the breathing circuit or confirm proper function of the inspiratory and expiratory unidirectional valves. A test lung or second reservoir bag can be used to confirm that flow through the circuit is unimpeded. Complete testing includes both manual and mechanical ventilation. The presence of the unidirectional valves can be assessed visually during the PAC. Proper function of these valves cannot be visually assessed since subtle valve incompetence may not be detected. Checkout procedures to identify valve incompetence that may not be visually obvious can be implemented but are typically too complex for daily testing. A trained technician can perform regular valve competence tests. (See Note 4 in Appendix.) Capnography should be used during every anesthetic and the presence of carbon dioxide in the inspired gases can help to detect an incompetent valve.

Item 14: Document completion of checkout procedures.

Frequency: Prior to each use

Responsible parties: Provider and technician

Rationale: Each individual responsible for checkout procedures should document completion of these procedures. Documentation gives credit for completing the job and can be helpful if an adverse event should occur. Some automated checkout systems maintain an audit trail of completed checkout procedures that are dated and timed.

Item 15: Confirm ventilator settings and evaluate readiness to deliver anesthesia care (ANESTHESIA TIME OUT).

Frequency: Immediately prior to initiating the anesthetic

Responsible parties: Provider

Rationale: This step is intended to avoid errors due to production pressure or other sources of haste. The goal is to confirm that appropriate checks have been completed and that essential equipment is indeed available. The concept is analogous to the "time out" used to confirm patient identity and surgical site prior to incision. Improper ventilator settings can be harmful especially if a small patient is following a much larger patient or vice versa. Pressure limit settings (when available) should be used to prevent excessive volume delivery from improper ventilator settings.

Items to check:

- Monitors functional?
- Capnogram present?
- Oxygen saturation by pulse oximetry measured?
- Flowmeter and ventilator settings proper?
- Manual/ventilator switch set to manual?
- Vaporizer(s) adequately filled?

Additional Notes

1. *Testing the flowmeters:* This step is present in the 1993 Checkout Recommendation and is intended to check the oxygen/nitrous oxide proportioning system. It has been eliminated from the preanesthesia checkout in these guidelines because proper function is verified during the preventive maintenance and failures of this system in a properly maintained delivery system are rare.
2. *Desiccated carbon dioxide absorbent:* Carbon dioxide absorbents which contain sodium, potassium, or barium hydroxide may become dangerous when desiccated, producing carbon monoxide and/or excessive heat leading to fires. Unfortunately, it is not possible to reliably identify when the absorbent material has been desiccated. Some departments elect to change all absorbent material on Monday morning to eliminate the possibility of using absorbent exposed to continuous fresh gas flow throughout the weekend. Other departments elect to use absorbent materials that do not pose a risk when desiccated. It is important to have a strategy to prevent the hazards related to using absorbents containing the problematic hydroxides that have desiccated. There are no steps that could be included in the checkout recommendation that can reliably identify desiccated absorbent. If a department uses absorbent that may be hazardous when desiccated, it may be prudent to change the absorbent material whenever the duration of time exposure to high fresh gas flow cannot be determined and is likely to have been prolonged. A protocol for preventing absorbent hazards should be part of every department's risk management strategy.
3. *Anesthesia information systems and automated record keepers:* These systems are being adopted by an increasing number of anesthesia departments and are the mainstay of the recordkeeping process in those departments. Reliably functioning systems is therefore important to the conduct of an anesthetic, although not essential to patient safety in the same fashion as the anesthesia delivery system and patient monitors. For departments that rely upon these systems, it would be prudent to have a protocol for checking connections and the proper functioning of the associated computers, displays, and network function.
4. *Testing circle system valve competence:* As part of the test Item 13 (verify that gas flows properly through the breathing circuit during both inspiration and exhalation), the inspiratory and expiratory valves are visually observed for proper cycling (opening and closing fully). Visual inspection will also detect a missing valve leaflet. Ascertaining full closure of the valve is subjective. Incompetence of the valve may also be detected during test item 13 through spirometry at the expiratory limb. For expiratory valve malfunction, a spirometer with reverse flow detection will alarm when gas flows retrograde in the expiratory limb. For inspiratory valve malfunction, the measured exhaled tidal volume will be less than the expected value. Capnography may also help to detect incompetence of the unidirectional valves. Intraoperatively, an inspiratory valve malfunction may not be indicated by an elevation of the inspired CO_2 baseline. If the delivered tidal volume exceeds the volume of gas in the inspiratory limb containing CO_2, rebreathing will appear on the capnogram as a gradual, instead of sharp, downstroke. An expiratory valve malfunction is indicated by an elevated CO_2 baseline as there is typically a large volume of exhaled gas containing CO_2 that can return to the patient.

SUMMARY OF CHECKOUT RECOMMENDATIONS BY FREQUENCY AND RESPONSIBLE PARTY

To Be Completed Daily

Item to Be Completed	Responsible Party
Item 1: Verify whether auxiliary oxygen cylinder and self-inflating manual ventilation device are available and functioning.	Provider and tech
Item 2: Verify patient suction is adequate to clear the airway.	Provider and tech
Item 3: Turn on anesthesia delivery system and confirm that AC power is available.	Provider or tech
Item 4: Verify availability of required monitors, including alarms.	Provider or tech
Item 5: Verify that pressure is adequate on the spare oxygen cylinder mounted on the anesthesia machine.	Provider and tech
Item 6: Verify that the piped gas pressures are ≥50 psig.	Provider and tech
Item 7: Verify that vaporizers are adequately filled and, if applicable, that the filler ports are tightly closed.	Provider or tech
Item 8: Verify that there are no leaks in the gas supply lines between the flowmeters and the common gas outlet.	Provider or tech
Item 9: Test scavenging system function.	Provider or tech
Item 10: Calibrate, or verify calibration of, the oxygen monitor and check the low-oxygen alarm.	Provider or tech
Item 11: Verify carbon dioxide absorbent is not exhausted.	Provider or tech
Item 12: Breathing system pressure and leak testing.	Provider and tech
Item 13: Verify that gas flows properly through the breathing circuit during both inspiration and exhalation.	Provider and tech
Item 14: Document completion of checkout procedures.	Provider and tech
Item 15: Confirm ventilator settings and evaluate readiness to deliver anesthesia care. (ANESTHESIA TIME OUT)	Provider

To Be Completed Prior to Each Procedure

Item to Be Completed	Responsible Party
Item 2: Verify patient suction is adequate to clear the airway.	Provider and tech
Item 4: Verify availability of required monitors, including alarms.	Provider or tech
Item 7: Verify that vaporizers are adequately filled and if applicable that the filler ports are tightly closed.	Provider
Item 11: Verify carbon dioxide absorbent is not exhausted	Provider or tech
Item 12: Breathing system pressure and leak testing.	Provider and tech
Item 13: Verify that gas flows properly through the breathing circuit during both inspiration and exhalation.	Provider and tech
Item 14: Document completion of checkout procedures.	Provider and tech
Item 15: Confirm ventilator settings and evaluate readiness to deliver anesthesia care. (ANESTHESIA TIME OUT)	Provider

REFERENCES TO APPENDIX B

1. Cooper JB, Newbower RS, Kitz RJ. An analysis of major errors and equipment failures in anesthesia management: considerations for prevention and detection. *Anesthesiology*. 1984;60:34–42.
2. Arbous MS, Meursing AE, van Kleef JW, et al. Impact of anesthesia management characteristics on severe morbidity and mortality. *Anesthesiology*. 2005;102:257–268.
3. Anesthesia Apparatus Checkout Recommendations, 1993. http://vam.anest.ufl.edu/fda-checklist4fold.doc
4. March MG, Crowley JJ. An evaluation of anesthesiologists' present checkout methods and the validity of the FDA checklist. *Anesthesiology*. 1991;75:724–729.
5. Lampotang S, Moon S, Lizdas DE, et al. Anesthesia machine pre-use check survey: preliminary results. *(abstracted) Anesthesiology*. 2005:A1195. http://www.asaabstracts.com/strands/asaabstracts/abstract.htm?year=2005&index=14&absnum=1619
6. Larson ER, Nuttall GA, Ogren BD, et al. A prospective study on anesthesia machine fault identification. *Anesth Analg*. 2007;104(1):154–156.
7. American Society of Anesthesiologists. Standards for Basic Anesthetic Monitoring. Last affirmed December 13, 2020. https://www.asahq.org/standards-and-guidelines/standards-for-basic-anesthetic-monitoring
8. Scope and Standards for Nurse Anesthesia Practice, In: *The Professional Practice Manual for the Certified Registered Nurse Anesthetist*. American Association of Nurse Anesthetists; 2006. https://www.aana.com/practice/practice-manual

26 Commonly Used Monitoring Techniques

CHRISTOPHER W. CONNOR • CHRISTOPHER M. CONLEY

KEY POINTS

1 The purpose of monitoring equipment is to augment the situational awareness of the anesthesiologist by providing clinical data either more rapidly than can be achieved manually or more precisely than can be achieved by direct examination of the patient. The value of any particular monitoring technique lies in its ability to inform the anesthesiologist so that the patient's physiologic condition can be maintained within satisfactory parameters. No monitoring technique, however sophisticated, can substitute for the judgment of the anesthesiologist.

2 It is mandatory to measure inspired oxygen concentration for patients receiving general anesthesia to prevent the inadvertent administration of a hypoxic gas mixture. However, inspired oxygen concentration monitoring cannot reliably detect disconnection of the circuit nor does it guarantee adequate arterial oxygenation.

3 Pulse oximetry provides a noninvasive means to detect the onset of hypoxemia rapidly. Modern pulse oximeters are noninvasive, continuous, auto-calibrating, have quick response times, and are suitable for use during transport. However, pulse oximetry is a poor indicator of adequate ventilation; desaturation is a late sign of apnea or respiratory insufficiency.

4 Monitoring of expired carbon dioxide is now recommended for procedures involving moderate to deep sedation in addition to procedures performed under general anesthesia. Advances in infrared absorption spectroscopy have led to the production of conveniently portable devices for expired gas analysis.

5 During direct invasive arterial pressure monitoring, the fidelity of the system is optimized when the catheter and tubing are stiff, the mass of the fluid is small, and the length of the connecting tubing is not excessive.

6 Automated noninvasive blood pressure monitors use the oscillometric method to estimate arterial blood pressure. Pulsatile flow generates oscillations in the internal pressure of an inflated blood pressure cuff; these oscillations are greatest when the cuff is inflated to mean arterial pressure. During prolonged surgical cases, it may be prudent to relocate the blood pressure cuff every few hours to reduce the risk of neurapraxia or cutaneous injury.

7 On the basis of available evidence, it is difficult to draw meaningful conclusions regarding the effectiveness of pulmonary artery catheter (PAC) monitoring in reducing morbidity and mortality in critically ill patients. Expert opinion suggests that perioperative complications may be reduced if PACs are used in the appropriate patients and settings and if clinicians interpret and apply the data provided by the PAC correctly.

8 New noninvasive devices have been developed to generate similar cardiac output (CO) parameters to the PAC as well as potentially to be able to predict fluid responsiveness. However, certain common comorbidities can impair the accuracy of these devices; the PAC thermodilution technique remains the clinical gold standard for measuring CO.

9 Clinical studies have demonstrated that patients in whom intraoperative hypothermia develops are at a higher risk for development of postoperative myocardial ischemia and wound infection compared with patients who are normothermic in the perioperative period. Although liquid crystal skin temperature strips are convenient to apply, they do not correlate well with core temperature measurements.

10 Although the algorithms used by processed electroencephalogram (EEG) monitors are proprietary, the general features of the EEG that they use are well described. Processed EEG monitors have not been demonstrated to be superior to end-tidal agent concentration monitoring in the prevention of awareness under anesthesia, although neither technique is sufficient to avoid awareness with complete reliability.

11 The advent of "smarter" and more technically sophisticated monitoring devices does not relieve anesthesiologists of their obligation to employ their clinical judgment wisely. On the contrary, it requires anesthesiologists to understand the operation of these devices intimately so that they can be used safely, accurately, and appropriately.

Introduction

Historically, the foundation of anesthetic practice has been vigilance and ongoing clinical examination of the patient. The development of modern monitoring equipment does not replace these responsibilities. Automated monitoring equipment provides the anesthesiologist with the ability to acquire clinical information either more rapidly or more frequently than can be achieved through manual techniques or in a more quantitatively precise manner than can be achieved by physical examination alone. The
1 purpose of monitoring equipment, then, is to augment the situational awareness of the anesthesiologist so that clinical problems can be recognized and addressed in a timely manner and to guide treatment. The value of any particular monitoring technique lies in its ability to inform the practice of the anesthesiologist so that the patient's physiologic condition can be maintained within satisfactory parameters. The term itself is derived from *monere*, which in Latin means to warn, remind, or admonish.

This chapter discusses the methods and biomedical devices through which anesthesiologists monitor the physiologic state of the patient during anesthesia care. The principles of operation for each of these devices are explained. These explanations are, by necessity, simplified, as the actual design of a biomedical device involves significant engineering complexity. However, the explanations are intended to be sufficient to allow the anesthesiologist to understand how the device acquires its clinical data and how that process might be compromised and the data made erroneous as well as to understand how the device works and how it may fail. There is little high-grade evidence that electronic monitors, by themselves, reduce morbidity and mortality. There is also controversy regarding the need for specific monitors in certain clinical situations, particularly in which use of the monitor in question may add significant cost or where the invasiveness of the monitoring technique may place the patient at risk of iatrogenic complications. Against these costs and risks, the anesthesiologist must balance the likely benefit from a particular monitoring technique when used and interpreted correctly. Therefore, alongside the science and engineering aspects of monitoring, there is also the clinical art of choosing how a patient should best be monitored intraoperatively. For each of the monitoring techniques, relative indications, contraindications, and common technical problems are discussed.

Standards for basic anesthetic monitoring have been established by the American Society of Anesthesiologists (ASA). Since 1986, these standards have emphasized the evolution of technology and practice. The current standards (which became effective on July 1, 2011) emphasize the importance of regular and frequent measurements, integration of clinical judgment and experience, and the potential for extenuating circumstances that can influence the applicability or accuracy of monitoring systems.[1]

Standard I requires qualified personnel to be present in the operating room during general anesthesia, regional anesthesia, and monitored anesthesia care to monitor the patient continuously and to modify anesthesia care based on clinical observations and the responses of the patient to dynamic changes resulting from surgery or drug therapy. Standard II focuses attention on continually evaluating the patient's oxygenation, ventilation, circulation, and temperature. Standard II specifically mandates the following:

1. Use of an inspired oxygen analyzer with a low concentration-limit alarm during general anesthesia.
2. Quantitative assessment of blood oxygenation during any anesthesia care.
3. Continuously ensuring the adequacy of ventilation by physical diagnostic techniques during all anesthesia care. Continual identification of expired carbon dioxide is performed unless precluded by the type of patient, procedure, or equipment.
4. Quantitative monitoring of tidal volume and capnography is strongly encouraged in patients undergoing general anesthesia.
5. When administering regional anesthesia or local anesthesia, ventilation sufficiency should be assessed by qualitative clinical signs. During moderate or deep sedation, ventilation shall be evaluated by continual evaluation of qualitative clinical signs as well as monitoring for the presence of exhaled carbon dioxide unless precluded by the type of patient, procedure, or equipment.

6. Ensuring correct placement of an endotracheal tube or laryngeal mask airway requires clinical assessment and qualitative identification of carbon dioxide in the expired gas.
7. When using a mechanical ventilator, use of a device that can detect a disconnection of any part of the breathing system.
8. The adequacy of circulation should be monitored by the continuous display of the electrocardiogram, and by determining the arterial blood pressure and heart rate (HR) at least every 5 minutes. During general anesthesia, circulatory function is to be continually evaluated by at least one of the following: palpation of a pulse, auscultation of heart sounds, monitoring of a tracing of intra-arterial pressure, ultrasound peripheral pulse monitoring, or pulse plethysmography or oximetry.
9. During all anesthetics, the means for continuously measuring the patient's temperature must be available. Every patient receiving anesthesia shall have temperature monitored when clinically significant changes in body temperature are intended, anticipated, or suspected.

Monitoring of Inspired Oxygen Concentration

Principles of Operation

Oxygen is a highly reactive chemical species, providing many chemical and physical opportunities to detect its presence. Three main types of oxygen analyzer are seen in clinical practice: paramagnetic oxygen analyzers, galvanic cell analyzers, and polarographic oxygen analyzers.

Paramagnetic gases are attracted to magnetic energy because of unpaired electrons in their outer shell orbits (1 Video 26-1). Oxygen is a highly paramagnetic gas. Differential paramagnetic oximetry has been incorporated into a variety of operating room monitors. These instruments detect the change in sample line pressure resulting from the attraction of oxygen by switched magnetic fields. Signal changes during electromagnetic switching correlate with the oxygen concentration in the sample line.[2]

Galvanic cell analyzers meet the performance criteria necessary for operative monitoring. These analyzers measure the current produced when oxygen diffuses across a membrane and is reduced to molecular oxygen at the anode of an electrical circuit.[3] The electron flow (current) is proportional to the partial pressure of oxygen in the fuel cell. Galvanic cell analyzers require regular replacement of the galvanic sensor capsule.

Polarographic oxygen analyzers are commonly used in anesthesia monitoring (2 Video 26-2). In this electrochemical system, oxygen diffuses through an oxygen-permeable polymeric membrane and participates in the following reaction: $O_2 + 2H_2O + 4e^- \rightarrow 4OH^-$. The current change is proportional to the number of oxygen molecules surrounding the electrode. Polarographic oxygen sensors are versatile and are important components of gas machine oxygen analyzers, blood gas analyzers, and transcutaneous oxygen analyzers.

Proper Use and Interpretation

The concentration of oxygen in the anesthetic circuit must be measured. Anesthesia machine manufacturers place oxygen sensors on the inspired limb of the anesthesia circuit to detect and alarm if hypoxic gas mixtures are delivered to the patient. Carbon dioxide may reduce the usable lifetime of a galvanic oxygen sensor, so it is preferable to place the oxygen sensor on the inspired limb. Oxygen monitors require a fast response time (2 to 10 seconds), accuracy (±2% of the actual level), and stability when exposed to humidity and inhalation agents.

The removable external oxygen sensors seen commonly on anesthesia machines, such as the Dräger Narkomed and Dräger Fabius (Dräger, Inc., Telford, PA) are of the galvanic type. These devices should be calibrated against room air (21% FiO_2) daily, and also after 8 hours of use. These devices may also infrequently require calibration against 100% FiO_2. As part of the preoperative checkout of the anesthesia machine, the clinician must confirm that the alarm limits of the inspired oxygen analyzer are set appropriately to alert to the presence of hypoxic mixtures. Inspired oxygen alarms cannot be relied upon to detect disconnection of the circuit.

Indications

According to the ASA Standards for Basic Anesthesia Monitoring,[1] 2
Standard 2.2.1 states, "During every administration of general anesthesia using an anesthesia machine, the concentration of oxygen in the patient breathing system shall be measured by an oxygen analyzer with a low oxygen concentration limit alarm in use."

The careful monitoring of the inspired oxygen concentration is of particular significance during low-flow anesthesia, in which the anesthesiologist attempts to minimize the fresh gas flow to the amount of oxygen necessary to replace the patient's metabolic utilization. The gas mixture within the breathing circuit may become hypoxic if insufficient fresh gas flow is supplied, even if the fresh gas flow itself comprises pure oxygen.

Contraindications

The requirement to monitor inspired oxygen concentration may be waived by the responsible anesthesiologist under extenuating circumstances. There are no clinical contraindications to monitoring inspired oxygen concentration.

Common Problems and Limitations

Adequate inspiratory oxygen concentration does not guarantee adequate arterial oxygen concentration.[4] Consequently, ASA Standard 2.2.2 mandates additional monitoring for blood oxygenation, including the provision of adequate lighting and exposure to assess the patient's color by direct observation. The practice of pediatric anesthesia merits additional vigilance to monitoring inspired oxygen concentration. Indications for altering inspired oxygen concentrations to facilitate anesthetics in children are common; for example, using a nitrous oxide–oxygen blend to facilitate inhalation inductions of anesthesia. Increased awareness of fire hazards in the operating room environment further reinforces the need for careful monitoring of FiO_2 in pediatric anesthesia. Tonsillectomy and adenoidectomy, among the most common of surgical procedures in the pediatric anesthesia population, carry an increased risk of airway fire. In addition to using of cuffed endotracheal tubes, careful monitoring and maintenance of a decreased inspired oxygen concentration whenever electrosurgical equipment is in use may decrease airway fire risk in these patients.[5,6]

Monitoring of Arterial Oxygenation by Pulse Oximetry

Principles of Operation

Pulse oximeters measure pulse rate and estimate the oxygen saturation of hemoglobin (SPO_2) on a noninvasive, continuous basis

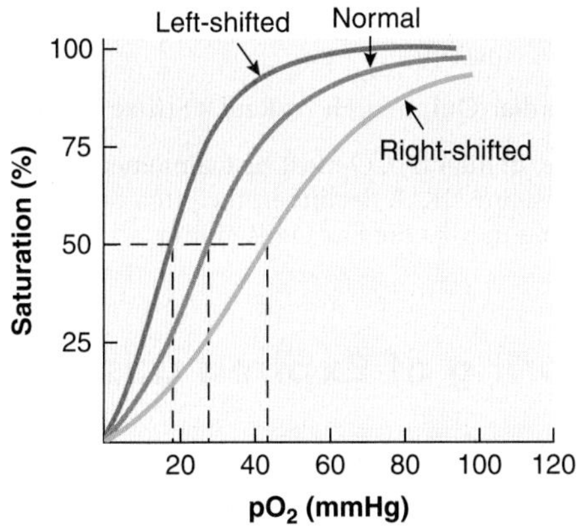

Figure 26-1 The oxyhemoglobin dissociation curve. The relationship between arterial saturation of hemoglobin and oxygen tension is represented by the sigmoid-shaped oxyhemoglobin dissociation curve. When the curve is left-shifted, the hemoglobin molecule binds oxygen more tightly. (Adapted from Brown M, Vender JS. Noninvasive oxygen monitoring. *Crit Care Clin*. 1988;4:493–509. Copyright © 1988 Elsevier. With permission.)

(NICV 26-1).[7] The oxygen saturation (SaO_2) of hemoglobin (as a percentage) is related to the oxygen tension (as a partial pressure, mmHg) by the oxyhemoglobin dissociation curve. On the steep part of the curve, a predictable correlation exists between SaO_2 and partial pressure of oxygen (PaO_2). In this range, the SaO_2 is a good reflection of the extent of hypoxemia and the changing status of arterial oxygenation. For $PaO_2 > 75$ mmHg, the SaO_2 reaches a plateau and no longer reflects changes in PaO_2. Coexisting medical conditions, such as hypercapnia, acidosis, and hyperthermia, cause the oxyhemoglobin dissociation curve to shift to the right and decrease the affinity of hemoglobin for oxygen. This change favors the unloading of oxygen from hemoglobin to peripheral tissues, as shown in Figure 26-1.

Pulse oximetry is based on the following premises:

1. The color of blood is a function of oxygen saturation.
2. The change in color results from the optical properties of hemoglobin and its interaction with oxygen.
3. The ratio of oxyhemoglobin (HbO_2) and hemoglobin (Hb) can be determined by absorption spectrophotometry.

Oxygen saturation is determined by spectrophotometry, which is based on the Beer–Lambert law. At a constant light intensity and hemoglobin concentration, the intensity of light transmitted through a tissue is a logarithmic function of the oxygen saturation of Hb. Two wavelengths of light are required to distinguish HbO_2 from Hb. Light-emitting diodes in the pulse sensor emit red (660 nm) and near infrared (940 nm) light. The percentage of HbO_2 is determined by measuring the ratio of infrared and red light sensed by a photodetector. Pulse oximeters perform a plethysmographic analysis to differentiate the pulsatile "arterial" signal from the nonpulsatile signal resulting from "venous" absorption and other tissues, such as skin, muscle, and bone. The absence of a pulsatile waveform during extreme hypothermia or hypoperfusion can limit the ability of a pulse oximeter to calculate the SPO_2.

The SPO_2 measured by pulse oximetry is not the same as the arterial saturation (SaO_2) measured by a laboratory co-oximeter. Pulse oximetry measures the "functional" saturation, which is defined by the following equation:

$$SPO_2 = \frac{HbO_2}{HbO_2 + Hb} \times 100\%$$

Laboratory co-oximeters use multiple wavelengths to distinguish other types of Hb, such as carboxyhemoglobin (COHb) and methemoglobin (MetHb) by their characteristic absorption. Co-oximeters measure the "fractional" saturation, which is defined by the following equation:

$$SaO_2 = \frac{HbO_2}{HbO_2 + Hb + COHb + MetHb} \times 100\%$$

In clinical circumstances in which other Hb moieties are present, the SPO_2 measurement may not correlate with the actual SaO_2 reported by the blood gas laboratory. For example, MetHb absorbs red and infrared wavelengths of light in a 1:1 ratio corresponding to an SPO_2 of approximately 85%. Therefore, increases in MetHb produce an underestimation when $SPO_2 > 70\%$ and an overestimation when $SPO_2 < 70\%$. Similarly, COHb also produces artificially high and misleading results; one study showed that at 70% COHb, the SPO_2 still measured 90%. In most patients, MetHb and COHb are present in low concentrations so that the functional saturation approximates the fractional value.[8]

Proper Use and Interpretation

The assessment of arterial oxygenation is an integral part of anesthesia practice. Early detection and prompt intervention may limit serious sequelae of hypoxemia. The clinical signs associated with hypoxemia (e.g., tachycardia, altered mental status, cyanosis) are often masked or difficult to appreciate during anesthesia.

The appropriate use of pulse oximetry necessitates an appreciation of both physiologic and technical limitations. Despite the numerous clinical benefits of pulse oximetry, other factors affect its accuracy and reliability. Factors that may be present during anesthesia care and that affect the accuracy and reliability of pulse oximetry include dyshemoglobins, dyes (methylene blue, indocyanine green, and indigo carmine), nail polish, ambient light, light-emitting diode variability, motion artifact, and background noise. Electrocautery can interfere with pulse oximetry if the radiofrequency emissions are sensed by the photodetector. Surgical stereotactic positioning systems that make use of infrared position sensors may interfere with the infrared signals used by the pulse oximeter. Reports of burns or pressure necrosis exist but are infrequent. Inspecting the digits during monitoring can reduce these complications.

Recent developments in pulse oximetry technology reportedly may permit more accurate measurements of SPO_2 during patient movement, low-perfusion conditions, and in the presence of dyshemoglobins. Some of these instruments use complex signal processing of the two wavelengths of light to improve the signal-to-noise ratio and reject artifacts. Studies in volunteers suggest that the performance of pulse oximeters incorporating this technology is superior to conventional oximetry during motion of the hand, hypoperfusion, and hypothermia.[9,10] Other pulse oximetry devices incorporate further wavelengths of light to more accurately measure COHb and MetHb.[8]

Indications

Pulse oximetry has been used in all patient age groups to detect and prevent hypoxemia. The clinical benefits of pulse oximetry are enhanced by its simplicity. Modern pulse oximeters are noninvasive, continuous, and auto-calibrating. They have quick response times and their battery backup provides monitoring during transport. The clinical accuracy is typically reported to be within ±2% to 3% at 70% to 100% saturation and ±3% at 50% to 70% saturation. Published data from numerous investigations support the accuracy and precision reported by instrument manufacturers. Quantitative assessment of arterial oxygen saturation is mandated by the ASA monitoring standards,[1] and the convenience and safety of pulse oximetry has now completely replaced earlier techniques such as heated transcutaneous pO_2 electrodes.

Pulse oximetry has wide medical applicability. Curiously, there are no definitive data to demonstrate a reduction in morbidity or mortality associated with the advent of pulse oximetry. However, a reduction in anesthesia mortality, as well as fewer malpractice claims from respiratory events, coincident with the introduction of pulse oximeters suggests that the routine use of these devices may have been a contributing factor.

Contraindications

There are no clinical contraindications to monitoring arterial oxygen saturation with pulse oximetry.

Common Problems and Limitations

Arterial oxygen monitors do not ensure adequacy of oxygen delivery to, or utilization by, peripheral tissues and should not be considered a replacement for arterial blood gas measurements or mixed central venous oxygen saturation when more definitive information regarding oxygen supply and utilization is required. Pulse oximeters do require a pulsatile waveform in order to distinguish the absorption of light by hemoglobin from absorption by other tissues, and therefore pulse oximeters do not function during cardiopulmonary bypass when blood flow is continuous rather than pulsatile. In recent years, there has been a notable increase in the number of patients in the community with implanted ventricular assist devices (VADs), either as a bridge to cardiac transplantation or as destination therapy. Such patients may present for urgent medical care that is unrelated to their cardiac pathology. However, the VAD provides a continuous rather than pulsatile cardiac output (CO), and so the satisfactory operation of the pulse oximeter will depend on the degree to which the patient's residual cardiac function still produces pulsatility. In such patients, it may be necessary to try placing the pulse oximeter on several different vascular beds until a location with satisfactory pulsatile perfusion is found.

3 Pulse oximetry is a poor indicator of adequate ventilation; patients who have been breathing supplemental oxygen may be apneic for several minutes before desaturation is detected by the pulse oximeter. Once the PaO_2 has fallen sufficiently to cause a detectable decrease in SPO_2, further desaturation may occur precipitously as the steep part of the oxyhemoglobin dissociation curve is reached.

Placing and obtaining reliable data from blood pressure cuffs and electrocardiogram leads may be challenging in an awake and vigorous child prior to inhalation induction. However, children will generally tolerate pulse oximetry and therefore, at a minimum, efforts should be made to place a pulse oximetry device on the child or infant prior to induction of anesthesia. Pulse oximetry has been shown to be a more sensitive monitor than capnography for unrecognized main stem/endobronchial intubation in pediatric anesthesia.[11] Respiratory events leading to inadequate ventilation and oxygenation represent the majority of perianesthetic morbidity in the pediatric anesthesia population. In conjunction with vigilant clinical assessment of the child's airway and oxygenation, the pulse oximeter usually provides the most important indicator of patient well-being during pediatric anesthesia.[12] Stress caused by hypoxemia and respiratory acidosis in infants and young children triggers a vagal response and subsequent systemic hypoperfusion. Infants cannot adequately increase their cardiac stroke volume (SV) in compensation and so, according to the CO equation:

$$\text{Cardiac Output} = \text{Heart Rate} \times \text{Stroke Volume}$$

Therefore, in infants, CO must be maintained with an increase over their baseline HR. A decline in the pitch or rapidity of pulse oximetry tones may be the first signs of impending cardiovascular collapse.

Monitoring of Expired Gases

Principles of Operation

The patient's expired gas is likely to be composed of a mixture of oxygen (O_2), nitrogen (N_2), carbon dioxide (CO_2), and anesthetic gases such as nitrous oxide (N_2O) and highly potent halogenated agents (sevoflurane, isoflurane, or desflurane). Measuring the composition of expired gases noninvasively and in real time can provide vital information regarding the patient's respiratory condition and assist in the titration of volatile anesthetic agents. Early anesthetic gas detectors were based simply on the change in elastance of rubber strips exposed to the circulating gas. Later methods made use of Raman scattering or multiplexed mass spectrometry, in which a single gas analyzer was shared between multiple operating rooms.

These techniques have now all been supplanted in clinical practice by infrared absorption spectrophotometry (IRAS). Asymmetric, polyatomic molecules such as CO_2 absorb infrared light at specific wavelengths. By transmitting light through a pure sample of a known gas over the range of infrared frequencies, a unique infrared transmission spectrum (like a fingerprint) can be created for the gas. CO_2, for example, strongly absorbs infrared light with a wavelength of 4.3 microns, as shown in Figure 26-2. At this wavelength, there is minimal interference from other gases that may also be present, such as water vapor, O_2, N_2O, and inhaled anesthetic agents. Infrared light at this wavelength can be passed through a sample of gas to an infrared detector. As the concentration of CO_2 increases, the intensity of the light that reaches the detector decreases in accordance with the Beer–Lambert law.

IRAS devices have five components: a multiple-wavelength 4
infrared light source, a gas sampler, an optical path, a detection

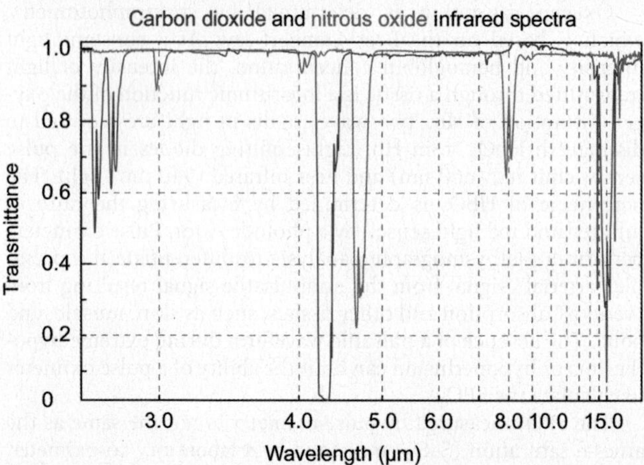

Figure 26-2 Gaseous-phase infrared transmission spectrum for carbon dioxide and nitrous oxide. (Modified from the National Institute of Standards and Technology (http://www.nist.gov); and Craver CD, Coblentz Society. *The Coblentz Society Desk Book of Infrared Spectra.* 2nd ed. The Society; 1982.)

system, and a signal processor. Operating room IRAS devices can detect CO_2, N_2O, and the potent inhaled anesthetic agents as mixed together in a sample of the patient's expired gas. The gas mixture is passed through the optical path of multiple infrared beams whose wavelengths are chosen to correspond to key features in the transmission spectra of the gases of interest. By analyzing the combination of absorption of infrared light at these wavelengths, the presence and concentrations of all of these gases can be determined simultaneously.[13] The use of multiple wavelengths allows the gases to be identified automatically. Older IRAS devices used a hot electrical element to generate radiant infrared light over a broad range of wavelengths, and an optical filter wheel was then used to cut out all but the desired wavelengths. Modern devices make use of small, lightweight lasers and filters, designed to emit only at the desired wavelengths. These consume much less electrical power, which has led to the development of convenient, portable handheld gas analyzers.[14]

Proper Use and Interpretation

Expired gas analysis allows the clinician to monitor inspired and expired concentrations of CO_2 and anesthetic gases simultaneously. These measurements require separate clinical interpretation. Critical events that can be detected by the analysis of respiratory gases and anesthetic vapors are listed in Table 26-1.

Interpretation of Inspired and Expired Carbon Dioxide Concentrations

Capnometry is the measurement and numeric representation of the CO_2 concentration during inspiration and expiration (3 Video 26-3). A capnogram is a continuous concentration–time display of the CO_2 concentration sampled at a patient's airway during ventilation. The capnogram is divided into four distinct phases, as shown in Figure 26-3.

Table 26-1 Detection of Critical Events by Implementing Gas Analysis

Event	Gas Measured by Analyzer
Error in gas delivery	O_2, N_2, CO_2, agent analysis
Anesthesia machine malfunction	O_2, N_2, CO_2, agent
Disconnection	CO_2, O_2, agent analysis
Vaporizer malfunction or contamination	Agent analysis
Anesthesia circuit leaks	N_2, CO_2 analysis
Endotracheal cuff leaks	N_2, CO_2
Poor mask or LMA fit	N_2, CO_2
Hypoventilation	CO_2 analysis
Malignant hyperthermia	CO_2
Airway obstruction	CO_2
Air embolism	CO_2, N_2
Circuit hypoxia	O_2 analysis
Vaporizer overdose	Agent analysis

LMA, laryngeal mask airway.

Modified from Knopes KD, Hecker BR. Monitoring anesthetic gases. In: Lake CL, ed. *Clinical Monitoring*. WB Saunders; 1990:24. Copyright © 1990 Elsevier. With permission.

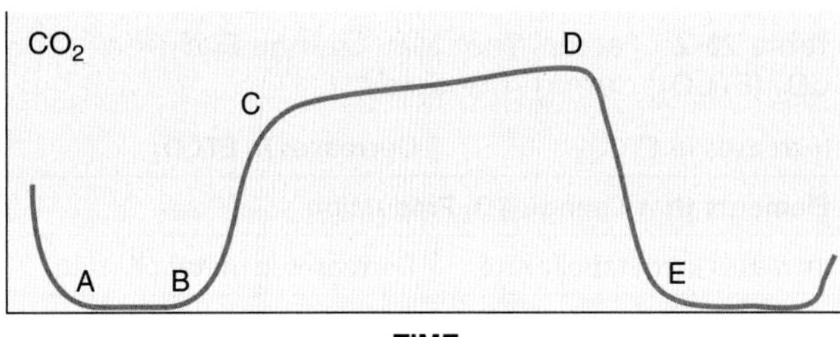

Figure 26-3 The normal capnogram. Point D delineates the end-tidal CO_2 ($ETCO_2$). $ETCO_2$ is the best reflection of the alveolar CO_2 partial pressure.

The first phase (A–B) represents the initial stage of expiration. Gas sampled during this phase occupies the anatomic dead space and is normally devoid of CO_2. At point B, CO_2-containing gas presents itself at the sampling site and a sharp upstroke (B–C) is seen in the capnogram. The slope of this upstroke is determined by the evenness of expiratory ventilation and alveolar emptying. Phase C–D represents the alveolar or expiratory plateau. At this phase of the capnogram, alveolar gas is being sampled. Normally, this part of the waveform is almost horizontal. However, when ventilation and perfusion are mismatched, Phase C–D may take an upward slope. Point D is the highest CO_2 value and is called the end-tidal CO_2 ($ETCO_2$). $ETCO_2$ is the best reflection of the alveolar CO_2 (P_ACO_2). As the patient begins to inspire, fresh gas is entrained and there is a steep downstroke (D–E) back to baseline. Unless rebreathing of CO_2 occurs, the baseline approaches zero. If the $PACO_2$–$PaCO_2$ gradient is constant and small, capnography provides a noninvasive, continuous, real-time reflection of ventilation. The $ETCO_2$–$PaCO_2$ gradient typically is around 5 mmHg during routine general anesthesia in otherwise healthy supine patients.

The size and shape of the capnogram waveform can provide additional clinical information. A slow rate of rise of the second phase (B–C) is suggestive of either chronic obstructive pulmonary disease or acute airway obstruction as from bronchoconstriction (asthma) secondary to mismatch in alveolar ventilation and alveolar perfusion. A normally shaped capnogram with an increase in $ETCO_2$ suggests alveolar hypoventilation or an increase in CO_2 production. Transient increases in $ETCO_2$ are often observed during tourniquet release, aortic unclamping, or the administration of bicarbonate.

Capnography is an essential element in determining the appropriate placement of endotracheal tubes. The presence of a stable $ETCO_2$ for three successive breaths indicates that the tube is not in the esophagus. A continuous stable CO_2 waveform ensures the presence of alveolar ventilation but does not necessarily indicate that the endotracheal tube is properly positioned in the trachea. An endobronchial intubation, in which the tip of the tube is located in a main stem bronchus, cannot be ruled out until breath sounds are auscultated bilaterally. A continuous CO_2 tracing also does not guarantee that the endotracheal tube is placed securely; an endotracheal tube placed proximally to the vocal cords may still produce an otherwise satisfactory tracing until it becomes dislodged.

A sudden drop in $ETCO_2$ to near zero followed by the absence of a CO_2 waveform heralds a potentially life-threatening problem that could indicate malposition of an endotracheal tube into the pharynx or esophagus, sudden severe hypotension, massive pulmonary embolism, a cardiac arrest, or a disconnection or disruption of sampling lines. When a sudden drop of the $ETCO_2$ occurs,

Table 26-2 Factors That May Change End-Tidal CO_2 ($ETCO_2$) during Anesthesia

Increases in $ETCO_2$	Decreases in $ETCO_2$
Elements that Change CO_2 Production	
Increases in metabolic rate	**Decreases in metabolic rate**
Hyperthermia	Hypothermia
Sepsis	Hypothyroidism
Malignant hyperthermia	
Shivering	
Hyperthyroidism	
Elements that Change CO_2 Elimination	
Hypoventilation	Hyperventilation
Rebreathing	Hypoperfusion
	Pulmonary embolism

it is essential to quickly verify that there is pulmonary ventilation and to identify physiologic and mechanical factors that might account for the $ETCO_2$ of zero. During life-saving cardiopulmonary resuscitation, the generation of adequate circulation can be assessed by the restoration of the CO_2 waveform.

Whereas abrupt decreases in the $ETCO_2$ are often associated with an altered cardiopulmonary status (e.g., embolism or hypoperfusion), gradual reductions in $ETCO_2$ more often reflect decreases in $PaCO_2$ that occur when there exists an imbalance between minute ventilation and metabolic rate (i.e., CO_2 production), as commonly occurs during anesthesia at a fixed minute ventilation. Increases in $ETCO_2$ can be expected when CO_2 production exceeds ventilation, such as in hyperthermia or when an exogenous source of CO_2 is present. Capnographic waveforms that do not return to zero during inspiration indicate rebreathing of CO_2. This non-zero inspiration phase can occur if the CO_2 absorber in an anesthesia machine is chemically exhausted, if a valve in the ventilator circuit is not functioning properly, or if the flow of fresh gas is insufficient. An elevated baseline can also be seen if the device is calibrated incorrectly.

Alterations in ventilation, CO, distribution of pulmonary blood flow, and metabolic activity influence $ETCO_2$ concentration and the capnogram obtained during quantitative expired gas analysis. Table 26-2 summarizes the common elements that may be reflected by changes in $ETCO_2$ during anesthesia care.

Interpretation of Inspired and Expired Anesthetic Gas Concentrations

Monitoring the concentration of expired anesthetic gases assists the anesthesiologist in titrating those gases to the clinical circumstances of the patient. At high fresh-gas flow rates, the concentration of an anesthetic gas in a circle breathing system will approximate the concentration set on the vaporizer. However, high fresh-gas flow rates lead to wasteful use of anesthetic vapor. As the fresh-gas flow rate is lowered, the concentration within the circuit and the concentration set at the vaporizer can become more decoupled. Inspired and expired gas concentration monitoring allows the anesthesiologist to maintain satisfactory and well-controlled agent levels in the circuit even when extremely low fresh-gas flows are used. In an ideal, leak-free anesthesia system, the fresh-gas flow can be minimized to only the amount of pure oxygen necessary to replace the patient's metabolic utilization—a practice known as "closed-circuit anesthesia." This practice makes the most economic use of potent anesthetic vapor, and also reduces the volume of these fluorocarbons released into the environment.[15]

Anesthetic gases have differing potencies; thus, their concentrations are often normalized against the concentration of that agent required to produce a predetermined clinical end point. The most commonly used end point is the MAC value, defined as the end-tidal gas concentration that when maintained constant for 15 minutes at a pressure of one atmosphere, inhibits movement in response to a midline laparotomy incision in 50% of patients.[16] Historically, MAC is an acronym for minimum alveolar concentration, though this is a misnomer. It is more accurately a median constant end-tidal partial pressure.[17] Monitoring of end-tidal gas concentrations performed with reference to MAC values helps to prevent the occurrence of intraoperative awareness and in some studies was superior to the use of processed electroencephalogram (EEG) monitors.[18]

Indications

Monitoring of the partial pressure of expiratory CO_2 has evolved into an important physiologic and safety monitor. Capnography is the standard of care for monitoring the adequacy of ventilation in patients receiving general anesthesia. It is also now mandated for use in monitoring ventilation during procedures performed while the patient is under moderate or deep sedation.[1]

Contraindications

There are no contraindications to the use of capnography, provided that the data obtained are evaluated in the context of the patient's clinical circumstances. It is generally safe to use capnography for the monitoring of all patients.

Monitoring of expired anesthetic gases is only informative if detectable gases are used to maintain anesthesia. Infrared spectroscopy cannot detect Xenon, and is not informative if anesthesia is maintained using a total intravenous technique.

Common Problems and Limitations

The sampling lines or water traps of expired gas analyzers may become occluded with condensed water vapor during prolonged use (4 Video 26-4). Disconnecting the sampling line and flushing it with air from a syringe can sometimes clear it, but it may be necessary to replace these components. Elevating the sidestream sampling line above the ventilator circuit helps prevent the entry of condensed water. A humidity barrier is also useful, although this will increase the response time of the capnogram.

Although mass spectroscopy and Raman scattering are no longer seen in clinical practice, these technologies are able to detect the concentration of N_2 directly. Nitrogen monitoring provides quantification of washout during preoxygenation. A sudden rise in N_2 in the exhaled gas indicates either introduction of air from leaks in the anesthesia delivery system or venous air embolism. Infrared gas analyzers do not detect N_2 directly and its concentration must be inferred as the amount remaining after other measurable gases are accounted for.

Although capnography provides a quantitative measurement of $ETCO_2$, it is not as accurate as blood gas analysis for the assessment of the partial pressure of arterial carbon dioxide ($PaCO_2$). A gradient exists between the $PaCO_2$ and $ETCO_2$; this gradient increases as the dead-space volume increases. In disease states characterized by increased dead space and ventilation–perfusion mismatch, such as emphysema or pulmonary embolism, or in iatrogenic single-lung ventilation or in very low CO states, an arterial blood gas analysis is necessary for an accurate determination of the $PaCO_2$.

Younger children desaturate rapidly following apnea, largely due to increased oxygen consumption and a smaller ratio of functional residual capacity (FRC) to closing volume.[19] Hypoxemia may precipitate a hypoperfusing bradycardic state, especially in neonates. Capnography's role in early recognition of apnea via a sudden drop or newly absent CO_2 signal makes it particularly valuable in pediatric anesthesia. Endotracheally intubated neonates, particularly very-low-birth weight infants in neonatal intensive care units, present unique challenges to accurate measurement of exhaled CO_2. These infants are typically intubated with cuffless endotracheal tubes. A cuffless tube permits a larger internal diameter, which reduces resistance to flow and work-of-breathing, but also allows leakage of expired gases. Capnography measurements therefore become more likely to underestimate actual end-tidal CO_2 levels.[20]

Sidestream capnography systems are the most commonly utilized in the operating room. Sidestream sampling units suction up to 200 mL/min of expired gas out of the breathing circuit, diverting this to a remote sensor where the gas is analyzed. Given that the neonatal minute ventilation is normally 200 to 300 mL/kg/min, sidestream sampling rates can approach and even surpass the minute ventilation of premature infants. In neonates, sidestream capnography systems may report erroneously low end-tidal CO_2 levels since the capnography system may be sampling gas that never actually participated in ventilation,[21] causing the true $ETCO_2$ to be erroneously diluted by fresh gas. Newer, low-flow sidestream capnography systems have since been developed to address this problem.[22] Because most anesthesia machines in the operating room are used with common higher-flow sidestream capnography devices, additional care must be taken when providing general endotracheal anesthesia for infants. In a neonate, an apparently normal $ETCO_2$ on the monitor may in fact represent inadequate ventilation, which would predispose the patient to respiratory acidemia.

Invasive Monitoring of Systemic Blood Pressure

Principles of Operation

Indwelling arterial cannulation permits the opportunity to monitor arterial blood pressure continuously and to have vascular access for arterial blood sampling (5 Video 26-5). Intra-arterial blood pressure monitoring uses fluid-filled tubing to transmit the force of the pressure pulse wave to a pressure transducer that converts the displacement of a silicon crystal into voltage changes. These electrical signals are amplified, filtered, and displayed as the arterial pressure trace. Intra-arterial pressure-transducing systems are subject to many potential errors based on the physical properties of fluid motion and the performance of the catheter–transducer–amplification system used to sense, process, and display the pressure pulse wave.

The behavior of transducers, fluid couplings, signal amplification, and display systems can be described by a complex second-order differential equation. Solving the equation predicts the output and characterizes the fidelity of the system's ability to faithfully display and estimate the arterial pressure over time. The fidelity of fluid-coupled transducing systems is constrained by two properties: *damping* (ζ) and *natural frequency* (f_n). Zeta (ζ) describes the tendency for fluid in the measuring system to extinguish motion and f_n describes the frequency at which the measuring system is most prone to resonance. The fidelity of the transduced pressure depends on optimizing ζ and f_n so that the system can respond appropriately to the range of frequencies contained in the pressure pulse wave. Analysis of high-fidelity recordings of arterial blood pressure indicates that the pressure trace contains frequencies from 1 to 30 Hz. The "fast flush" test is a method used at the bedside to determine the natural frequency and damping characteristics of the transducing system.[23]

Proper Use and Interpretation

Multiple arteries can be used for direct measurement of blood pressure, including the radial, brachial, axillary, femoral, and dorsalis pedis arteries (Table 26-3). The radial artery remains the most popular site for cannulation because of its accessibility and the presence of the collateral ulnar blood supply to the hand. In the past, it had been recommended to assess the patency of the ulnar circulation by performing an Allen test. This test is performed by compressing both radial and ulnar arteries; releasing the pressure on each artery in turn determines the dominant vessel supplying blood to the hand. However, the prognostic value of the Allen test in assessing the adequacy of the collateral circulation has not been confirmed and it is arguable that routine use of this test is no longer worthwhile.[24] Even a satisfactory Allen test does not rule out the possibility of formation of thrombus on the catheter itself and subsequent distal embolic complications. Although an intact palmar arch will provide some collateralization of arterial blood supply to the hand, this does not protect against emboli to the distal digital arteries.

Table 26-3 Arterial Cannulation and Direct Blood Pressure Monitoring

Arterial Cannulation Site	Clinical Points of Interest
Radial artery	Preferred site for monitoring Nontapered catheters preferred
Ulnar artery	Complication similar to radial Primary source of hand blood flow
Brachial artery	Insertion site medial to biceps tendon Median nerve damage is potential hazard Can accommodate 18-gauge cannula
Axillary artery	Insertion site at junction of pectoralis and deltoid muscles Specialized kits available
Femoral artery	Easy access in low-flow states Potential for local and retroperitoneal hemorrhage Longer catheters preferred
Dorsalis pedis artery	Collateral circulation = posterior tibial artery Higher systolic pressure estimates

Three techniques for cannulation are common: direct arterial puncture, guidewire-assisted cannulation (Seldinger technique), and the transfixion–withdrawal method (6 Videos 26-6 and 7 26-7).[25] A necessary condition for percutaneous placement is identification of the arterial pulse. Ultrasound imaging with Doppler color flowmetry can provide valuable assistance when the pulse is difficult to locate or the caliber of the vessel is small.[26]

Arterial blood pressure transduction systems must be "zeroed" before use (8 Video 26-8). The transducer is positioned at the same level as the right atrium, the stopcock is opened to the atmosphere so that the pressure-sensing crystal senses only atmospheric pressure, and the "Zero Sensor" (or equivalent) option is selected on the monitoring equipment. This procedure establishes the calibration of the sensor and establishes the level of the right atrium as the datum reference point. For neurosurgical procedures in which the patient may be positioned in an upright or beach-chair position, it is common practice to zero the transducer at the level of the circle of Willis so that the arterial pressure tracing provides a reading that is adjusted for the height of the fluid column between the heart and the brain; it represents the arterial pressure at the base of the brain.

Direct arterial pressure monitoring requires constant vigilance. The data displayed must correlate with clinical conditions before therapeutic interventions are initiated. Sudden increases in the transduced blood pressure may represent a hydrostatic error because the position of the transducer was not adjusted after change in the operating room table's height. Sudden decreases often result from kinking of the catheter or tubing. Before initiating therapy, the transducer system should be examined quickly and the patency of the arterial cannula verified. This check ensures the accuracy of the measurement and avoids the initiation of a potentially dangerous medication error.

Traumatic cannulation has been associated with hematoma formation, thrombosis, and damage to adjacent nerves (9 Video 26-9). Abnormal radial artery blood flow after catheter removal occurs frequently. Studies suggest that blood flow normalizes in 3 to 70 days. Radial artery thrombosis can be minimized by using small catheters, avoiding polypropylene-tapered catheters, and reducing the duration of arterial cannulation. Flexible guidewires may reduce the potential trauma associated with catheters negotiating tortuous vessels. After arterial cannulation has been performed, the tissues that are perfused by that artery should be examined intermittently for signs of thromboembolism or ischemia. During cannula removal, the potential for thromboembolism may be diminished by compressing the proximal and distal arterial segment while aspirating the cannula during withdrawal.

Indications

The standards for basic monitoring[1] stipulate that arterial blood pressure shall be determined and recorded at least every 5 minutes. This standard is usually met by intermittent, noninvasive blood pressure monitoring. However, continuous monitoring may be indicated by patient comorbidities or by the nature of the surgery to be performed.

Arterial catheters provide continuous monitoring of blood pressure and convenient vascular access to obtain blood samples for laboratory assays, including blood gas analysis to assess respiratory function. Placement of an arterial catheter can therefore be indicated by the need for any of these capabilities:

1. **Rapid changes in blood pressure or extremes of blood pressure are anticipated.**
   High-risk vascular surgeries, trauma surgeries, neurosurgical procedures, and intrathoracic and cardiac procedures are associated with the risk of sudden blood loss and rapid changes in blood pressure. These procedures may also involve periods of deliberate hypotension or hypertension.
2. **The ability of the patient to tolerate hemodynamic instability is impaired.**
   Patients with clinically significant cardiac disease, such as coronary artery disease, valvular disease, or heart failure, may require continuous monitoring in order to allow treatment for hypotension to be implemented rapidly and minimize the risk of coronary ischemia. Similar concerns apply to patients with a history of cerebrovascular disease. Procedures that involve potential compromise to the vascular supply of the spinal cord indicate the use of an arterial catheter to maintain adequate perfusion and decrease the risk of postoperative paraplegia from spinal cord infarction.
   Critically ill patients may already be hemodynamically unstable at the time of presentation and require the administration of inotropes and vasopressors. Continuous blood pressure monitoring is indicated to manage the titration of these agents.
3. **Compromise of the patient's respiratory function, oxygenation, or ventilation is anticipated.**
   Mismatch between pulmonary ventilation and perfusion will impair the ability of $ETCO_2$ to predict P_ACO_2. This variance may arise iatrogenically during procedures that require single-lung ventilation. Patients may present with pulmonary comorbidities, such as ARDS, pulmonary embolism, and pulmonary hypertension with consequent ventilation–perfusion mismatch and impaired alveolar diffusion. Arterial catheters provide a means to obtain arterial blood gas samples frequently to assess changes in respiratory function.
4. **Metabolic derangements are anticipated.**
   Surgical procedures that are anticipated to produce large-volume fluid shifts may indicate the placement of an arterial catheter to enable laboratory samples to be drawn frequently and to allow electrolyte and acid–base disturbances to be detected and corrected.

Contraindications

Arterial cannulation is regarded as an invasive procedure with documented morbidity (10 Video 26-10). Ischemia after radial artery cannulation resulting from thrombosis, proximal emboli, or prolonged shock has been described.[27] Contributing factors include severe atherosclerosis, diabetes, low CO, and intense peripheral vasoconstriction. Ischemia, hemorrhage, thrombosis, embolism, cerebral air embolism (retrograde flow associated with flushing), aneurysm formation, arteriovenous fistula formation, skin necrosis, and infection have reportedly occurred as the direct result of arterial cannulation, arterial blood sampling, or high-pressure flushing. Patients with compromised collateral arterial supply, such as those with Reynaud phenomenon or thromboangiitis obliterans (Buerger disease), are at increased risk for ischemic complications.[25]

Common Problems and Limitations

The fidelity of the transducer system is optimized when catheters and tubing are stiff, the mass of the fluid is small, the number of stopcocks is limited, and the connecting tubing is not excessive. Figure 26-4 demonstrates the effect of damping on the character of the arterial pressure trace. In clinical practice, underdamped transducer systems tend to overestimate the systolic pressure (SP) by 15 to 30 mmHg and amplify artifacts. Likewise, excessive increases in ζ reduce fidelity and underestimate SP. Due to heightened risk of thromboembolism, blood removed in the process of

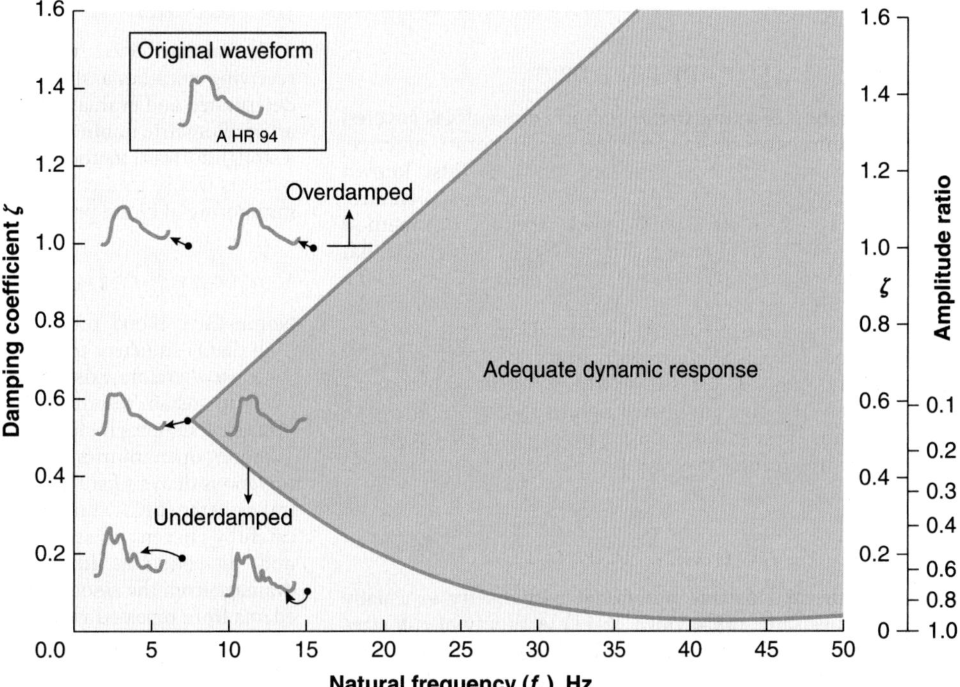

Figure 26-4 The relationship between the frequency of fluid-filled transducing systems and damping. The *shaded area* represents the appropriate range of damping for a given natural frequency (f_n). The size of the wedge also depends on the steepness of the arterial pressure trace and heart rate. (Adapted with permission from Gardner RM. Direct blood pressure measurement–dynamic response requirements. *Anesthesiology*. 1981;54:227–236.)

arterial line sampling should only be returned to the patient intravenously (not arterially). Meticulous care must be taken to ensure that all arterial line tubing is tightened securely to prevent hemorrhage from line disconnection.

Continuous-flush devices are incorporated into disposable transducer kits and infuse at 3 to 6 mL/hr. In neonates, the infusion volume may contribute to fluid overload. Continuous-flush devices have little effect on the blood pressure measurement. However, pressurized flush systems may serve as a source of an air embolism. Removing air from the pressurized infusion bag, stopcocks, and tubing minimizes the potential for air embolism.

Invasive blood pressure monitoring in the pediatric population presents unique challenges for the anesthesiologist. Smaller-caliber arteries, lower circulating blood volume, and a closer anatomic proximity of peripheral vessels to the great vessels, the heart, and the cerebral circulation combine to make line placement more technically difficult and make line maintenance more hazardous. Three of the more common sites of arterial blood pressure monitoring in pediatric and neonatal anesthesia are the umbilical artery, the radial artery, and the femoral artery.

In critically ill newborn infants, the umbilical artery represents a convenient site for catheterization in order to measure arterial blood pressure and for blood sampling for laboratory values although attaining access may require a cutdown procedure. Arterial catheters at this site carry a risk of aortic thrombosis and have been implicated in the development of other aortic complications, including coarctation; thus, these should be removed as soon as they are no longer necessary for patient care.[28]

The use of smaller catheters (i.e., 22 g, or even 24 g) for radial arterial catheterization in pediatric patients has been established as safe for invasive blood pressure monitoring in young patients, including children under 1 year of age. Preemptive use of ultrasound in radial artery cannulation may increase first-pass success and decrease iatrogenic injury in children.[29]

Femoral arterial lines have also been used extensively in critically ill infants and children, with high rates of success and low complication rates.[30] Though rare, complications including hematoma, minor bleeding, and AV fistula formation may occur. Young children (age <3 years) are at increased risk of pediatric groin line complications requiring surgical intervention. Routine use of ultrasound guidance in pediatric groin line placement decreases these risks.[31]

Practices that are commonly accepted in arterial line management and maintenance in adults may prove hazardous in pediatric patients. Flushing of the arterial line should be kept to a minimum, particularly in the care of smaller children and infants, to reduce the risk of volume overload and inadvertent hemodilution. High-pressure flushing should not be attempted in efforts to restore function to an apparently occluded indwelling arterial catheter. It is best instead to clear the line by hand with a small syringe, using the minimum pressure and volume necessary, as even small-volume flushes (0.5 to 1 mL) injected into the radial arteries of small infants using automated pressurizing systems may cause retrograde flow into the cerebral vessels.[32]

Intermittent Noninvasive Monitoring of Systemic Blood Pressure

Principles of Operation

The simplest method of blood pressure determination estimates systolic blood pressure by palpating the return of an arterial pulse while a more proximal occluding cuff is deflated. Modifications of this technique include the observance of the return of Doppler sounds, the transduced arterial pressure trace, or a photoplethysmographic pulse wave as produced by a pulse oximeter.

Auscultation of the Korotkoff sounds permits estimation of both systolic (SP) and diastolic (DP) blood pressures. Korotkoff sounds result from turbulent flow within an artery created by the mechanical deformation from the blood pressure cuff. SP is signaled by the appearance of the first Korotkoff sound. Disappearance of the sound or a muffled tone signals the DP. The mean arterial pressure (MAP) can be calculated using an estimating equation:

$$MAP = DP + (SP - DP)/3$$

6 The operation of automated blood pressure cuffs is covered by US and international standards. In contemporary practice, automated noninvasive blood pressure monitors (also known as automated sphygmomanometers) employ the oscillometric method[33] to estimate the arterial blood pressure. The method uses an occluding cuff to measure the pressure fluctuations that occur due to arterial pulsations. The SP is estimated using the maximum cuff pressure at which pressure oscillations can be perceived. The MAP is estimated by the cuff pressure at which the amplitude of the oscillations is greatest. The DP is estimated using the minimum cuff pressure at which pressure fluctuations can be perceived. Some automated noninvasive blood pressure monitors refine these estimates using proprietary, empirical formulae, and thus results may not be consistent from device to device.

Proper Use and Interpretation

In the anesthetized patient, automated oscillometry is usually accurate and versatile (Video 26-11). A variety of cuff sizes makes it possible to use oscillometry in all age groups. Different strategies of cuff inflation and deflation may be used to obtain blood pressure measurements. A common approach, as shown in Figure 26-5, is for the cuff to be rapidly inflated to a predetermined initial pressure expected to be above SP. A sensor checks to ensure that pressure fluctuations are not present. The cuff is then gradually deflated in small decremental intervals. At each interval, the sensor measures the magnitude of oscillations that are present in the cuff pressure. Once the cuff pressure falls below the point at which oscillations can be detected, the cuff is rapidly and completely deflated.

Another common strategy involves the opposite approach of incrementally inflating the cuff. Once the cuff pressure has increased above the SP, the sensor no longer perceives oscillations, and the cuff is rapidly and completely deflated.

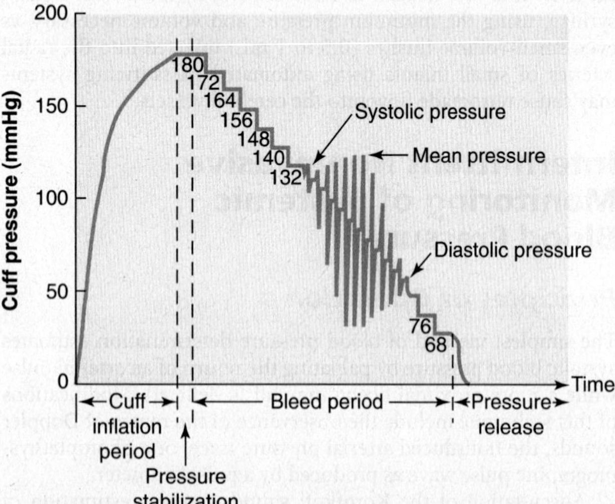

Figure 26-5 Sequence of oscillometric blood pressure determination. The pressure oscillations increase in magnitude, then decrease. The oscillations are analyzed to determine systolic, mean, and diastolic pressures as shown. (Adapted with permission from Dorsch JA, Dorsch SE. *Understanding Anesthesia Equipment.* 4th ed. Williams & Wilkins; 1999.)

Indications

ASA Standard 4.2.2 mandates the following: "Every patient receiving anesthesia shall have arterial blood pressure and HR determined and evaluated at least every five minutes." The use of an oscillometric noninvasive blood pressure cuff usually provides a straightforward method for satisfying this requirement for those patients whose medical comorbidities do not require continuous monitoring of blood pressure.

Contraindications

Noninvasive blood pressure cuffs apply force to the encircled limb that is sufficient to occlude blood flow. Contraindications to their use therefore exist in circumstances in which the patient is likely to sustain traumatic injury from this repeated mechanical process. Examples include local bone fracture (such as a humeral fracture), open injuries to the extremity, local presence of an arteriovenous dialysis fistula, or indwelling peripherally inserted central catheter (PICC) line. The site of measurement should also be carefully chosen in patients who have undergone axillary lymph node dissection, as these patients may have impaired lymphatic drainage from the associated limb and may be susceptible to limb edema from repeated vascular occlusion.

Noninvasive blood pressure cuffs can potentially become a source of iatrogenic injury even in normal use on a healthy limb. The repeated cycling of the blood pressure cuff during very prolonged surgical cases may lead to local skin abrasion or contusion; applying a light dressing underneath the cuff may mitigate these side effects. The radial nerve describes a spiraling path around the humerus and is also potentially susceptible to neurapraxia from mechanical compression.[34] During very prolonged surgical cases, it may be prudent to relocate the blood pressure cuff every few hours.

Common Problems and Limitations

The American Heart Association recommends that the bladder width for indirect blood pressure monitoring should approximate 40% of the circumference of the extremity. Bladder length should be sufficient to encircle at least 80% of the extremity. Falsely high estimates result when cuffs are too small, when cuffs are applied too loosely, or when the extremity is below heart level. Falsely low estimates result when cuffs are too large, when the extremity is above heart level, or after quick deflations.[35]

The detection of changes in Korotkoff sounds is subjective and prone to errors based on deficiencies in sound transmission or hearing. Cuff deflation rate also influences accuracy; quick deflations underestimate blood pressure. Noninvasive blood pressure cuffs are also subject to significant wear-and-tear from repeated use in the operating room. The development of a small air leak in the hose or cuff will often prevent the device from following its inflation strategy and render it inoperative.

Palpation, auscultatory, and oscillometric techniques require pulsatile blood flow and may be unreliable during conditions of low flow or if the arterial walls are sufficiently sclerotic or stiffened such that pulsations are not readily transmitted. This is particularly relevant given the increasing prevalence of patients with implanted VADs in the setting of heart failure.[36] As above, VADs generate a continuous, rather than pulsatile, CO and consequently the satisfactory operation of a noninvasive blood pressure cuff will depend on whatever residual pulsatile output is produced by the patient's impaired cardiac function.

Automated oscillometry has been demonstrated to correlate well with direct intra-arterial measurement of MAP and DP.[37] Oscillometry does require additional signal processing to smooth out pronounced respiratory variations or motion artifacts, but these events tend to occur at frequencies that are distinct from pulsatile variations in pressure. Cuff movement, erratic pulse transmission, arrhythmias, extrinsic force on the cuff, and inadvertent occlusion of the pressure tubing may influence accuracy. Periods of significant hemodynamic variability may require more frequent measurement of blood pressure to guide optimal intraoperative management. This problem can be approached statistically by assessing the ability of a blood pressure measurement to predict the next blood pressure measurement, and hence the ability of the anesthesiologist to infer and intervene upon unacceptable trends in the blood pressure. Although Standard 4.2.2 mandates that blood pressure be measured only every 5 minutes, some evidence exists that this predictive ability may begin to decline for measurement intervals of greater than 3 minutes.[38]

Automated noninvasive blood pressure cuffs are usually placed around the upper arm, but it is usually acceptable to place the cuff around the forearm, wrist, or ankle if the upper arm is inaccessible or if the patient's body habitus is otherwise unfavorable. As the site of measurement is moved more peripherally, the measured SP tends to increase, and the DP tends to decrease.[39–41] An exception is the parturient undergoing cesarean section; the correlation between calf and upper arm blood pressures was found to be poor in this patient population.[42]

In pediatric patients, the upper extremity is generally the preferred site for blood pressure monitoring as it more closely correlates with cerebral perfusion. Premature infants, particularly those with pulmonary hypertension or respiratory distress, are at higher risk for having patent ductus arteriosus. Placing the blood pressure cuff on the right arm (preductal) gives the best approximation of cerebral perfusion in this patient population. The greatest disparity between blood pressures measured in the upper versus lower extremity is found in patients weighing less than 1,000 g.[43]

Monitoring of Central Venous and Right-Heart Pressures

Principles of Operation

Central venous cannulas are important portals for intraoperative vascular access and for the assessment of changes in vascular volume (12 Video 26-12). Central venous cannulas permit the rapid administration of fluids, insertion of pulmonary artery catheters (PACs) or central venous oximetry catheters, insertion of transvenous electrodes, monitoring of central venous pressure (CVP), and a site for observation and treatment of venous air embolism. The main value of monitoring central venous and right-heart pressures lies in their ability to approximate or trend in conjunction with the left ventricular end-diastolic pressure (LVEDP). The LVEDP predicts left-ventricular filling (i.e., left ventricular end-diastolic volume, LVEDV) through the Frank–Starling mechanism.

Figure 26-6 demonstrates the progression of pressures from CVP through LVEDP (13 Video 26-13). Ideally, all proximal pressures reflect changes in LVEDP. The CVP is the easiest to measure as it does not require that any portion of the catheter to be placed within the heart. The CVP is essentially equivalent to right atrial pressure and serves as a reflection of right ventricular preload. The output of the right ventricle and the output of the left ventricle must be approximately the same in a structurally normal cardiopulmonary system, notwithstanding a small amount of physiologic shunt. However, it has been well demonstrated that right-sided pressures in the heart often are poor indicators of left ventricular filling, either as absolute numbers or in terms of the direction of change in response to therapy. The correlation of these pressures as estimates of LVEDP (and, by extension, LVEDV) is directly related to their proximity to the left ventricle and the status of ventricular compliance. PACs therefore provide more clinical information than central venous monitoring alone: PACs are able to separate the behavior of the right side of the heart, the lung parenchyma, and the left side of the heart. Pulsatile pressures in the pulmonary artery provide an assessment of right ventricular function. The *pulmonary capillary wedge pressure* (PCWP) provides the closest approximation to LVEDP. The PAC is allowed to wedge, with the balloon inflated, in the pulmonary vasculature. During end-diastole, there is cessation of forward blood flow and a static fluid column is presumed to exist from the left ventricle to the PAC tip with no pressure drop.

The measurement of right-heart pressures can therefore indirectly assess left ventricular preload, diagnose the existence of pulmonary hypertension, or differentiate cardiac and noncardiac causes of pulmonary edema.

Proper Use and Interpretation

Careful leveling and zeroing of the pressure transducers is essential, as described earlier for invasive arterial pressure monitoring

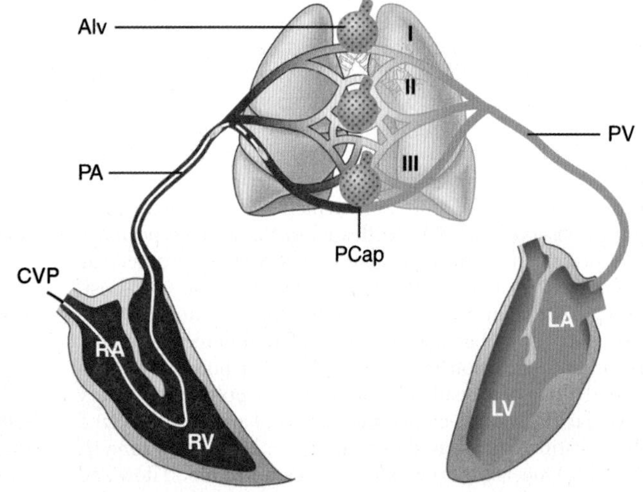

Figure 26-6 The progression of intracardiac pressures from central venous pressure to end-diastolic left ventricular pressure. The anatomic position of a pulmonary artery catheter in the pulmonary artery is shown. The *dashed line* shows the position of the inflated pulmonary artery catheter balloon in the "wedged" position. CVP, central venous pressure; RA, right atrium; RV, right ventricle; PA, pulmonary artery; Alv, alveolus; PCap, pulmonary capillary; PV, pulmonary vein; LA, left atrium; LV, left ventricle. I, II, and III characterize the relationship of $P_{alveolar}$, $P_{arterial}$, and P_{venous} as described by West et al.[44] The bottom of the figure shows a progressive correlation of vascular pressures. (Adapted from Vender JS. Invasive cardiac monitoring. *Crit Care Clin.* 1988;4(3):455–477. Copyright © 1988 Elsevier. With permission.)

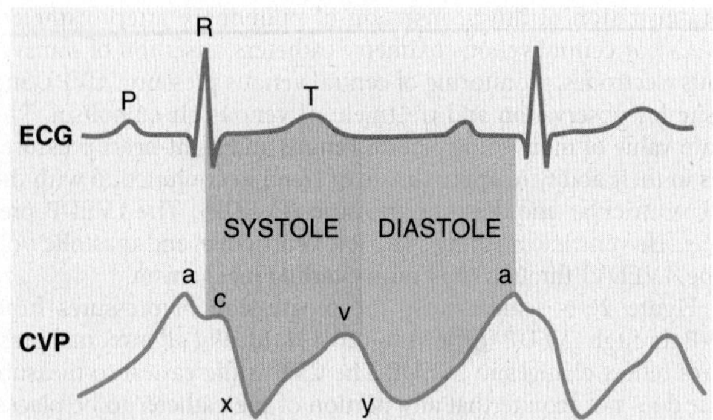

Figure 26-7 The normal central venous pressure (CVP) trace. ECG, electrocardiogram. (Adapted from Mark JB. Central venous pressure monitoring: Clinical insights beyond the numbers. *J Cardiothorac Vasc Anesth.* 1991;5:163–173. Copyright © 1991 Elsevier. With permission.)

(14 Video 26-14). The normal CVP waveform, as shown in Figure 26-7, consists of three peaks (*a*, *c*, and *v* waves) and two descents (*x*, *y*), each resulting from the ebb and flow of blood in the right atrium. The character of the CVP trace depends on many factors, including HR, conduction disturbances, tricuspid valve function, normal or abnormal intrathoracic pressure changes, and changes in right ventricular compliance. In patients with atrial fibrillation, *a* waves are absent. When resistance to the emptying of the right atrium is present, large *a* waves are often observed. Examples include tricuspid stenosis, right ventricular hypertrophy as a result of pulmonic stenosis, or acute or chronic lung disease associated with pulmonary hypertension. Large *a* waves may also be observed when right ventricular compliance is impaired.

Tricuspid regurgitation typically produces giant *v* waves that begin immediately after the QRS complex. Large *v* waves are often observed when right ventricular ischemia or failure is present or when ventricular compliance is impaired by constrictive pericarditis or cardiac tamponade. A prominent *v* wave during CVP monitoring may suggest right ventricular papillary muscle ischemia and tricuspid regurgitation. When right ventricular compliance decreases, the CVP often increases with prominent *a* and *v* waves fusing to form an *m* or *w* configuration.

CVP monitoring can be unreliable for estimating left ventricular filling pressures, especially when cardiac or pulmonary parenchymal disease processes alter the normal cardiovascular pressure–volume relationships. However, CVP monitoring is less invasive and less costly than pulmonary artery monitoring and offers an understanding of right-sided hemodynamic events and the status of vascular volume. The validity of PAC monitoring depends on a properly functioning pressure monitoring system, correctly identifying the "true" PCWP and integration of the various factors that affect the relationship of PCWP, and the other cardiac pressures and volumes that are determinants of ventricular function. Figure 26-8 depicts the transduced pressure waves observed as a PAC is floated to the wedged position. Catheter placement is most commonly performed by observing the pressure waves as the catheter is floated from the CVP position through the right heart chambers into the pulmonary artery.

West et al.[44] described a gravity-dependent difference between ventilation and perfusion in the lung. The variability in pulmonary blood flow is a result of differences in pulmonary artery (P_A), alveolar (P_{alv}), and venous pressures (P_V) and is categorized into three distinct zones, as shown in Figure 26-6. Only zone III ($P_A > P_V > P_{alv}$) meets the criteria for uninterrupted blood flow and for continuous communication via a static fluid column with distal intracardiac pressures. Flow-directed PACs usually advance to

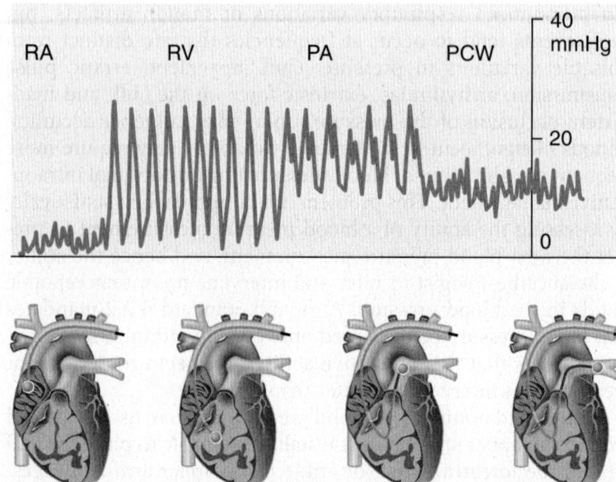

Figure 26-8 Pressure tracing observed during the flotation of a pulmonary artery catheter. RA, right atrium; RV, right ventricle; PA, pulmonary artery; PCW, pulmonary capillary wedge pressure. (Adapted from Dizon CT, Barash PG. The value of monitoring pulmonary artery pressure in clinical practice. *Conn Med.* 1977;41:622–625.)

gravity-dependent areas of highest blood flow. However, increases in alveolar pressure, decreases in perfusion, or changes in the position of the patient can convert areas of zone III into either zone II or I. The following characteristics suggest that the PAC tip is not in zone III: PCWP > pulmonary artery end-diastolic pressure (PAEDP), nonphasic PCWP tracing, and inability to aspirate blood from the distal port when the catheter is wedged.

Indications

Even without the monitoring of pressures, central venous access may be indicated to provide a route of administration for vasoactive drugs, parenteral nutrition, higher-concentration electrolyte solutions, prolonged vascular access, or a temporary pacemaker.

CVPs correlate well with right ventricular preload and so provide a quantitative, direct means of assessing the volumetric status of a patient. CVP monitoring may be indicated in cases in which there are expected to be rapid or large shifts in intravascular volume. CVP monitoring may also be useful in assessing volumetric status when other clinical signs of volumetric status, such as urine output, may be inaccurate or unavailable due either to the procedure or to the patient's comorbidities.

PACs have not been shown to improve outcomes.[45] The decision to place a PAC therefore requires careful individualization of patient care. There must be a specific question regarding the patient's management that can only be addressed with the data that the catheter will provide. This question should be of sufficient importance that the plan of management will potentially be altered depending on the results of PAC monitoring. The information that PACs provide may be particularly informative in the management of patients with severe pulmonary hypertension or to help differentiate noncardiogenic and cardiogenic shock. 7

Contraindications

Obstruction at the mitral valve from mitral stenosis, atrial myxoma, or clot can interfere with the ability of left atrial pressure to reflect LVEDP. Similarly, mitral regurgitation, a noncompliant left atrium, or left-to-right intracardiac shunting often is associated with large v waves. Decreases in left ventricular compliance, aortic regurgitation, or premature closure of the mitral valve may reverse the left atrial pressure–LVEDP pressure gradient. When these comorbidities occur, PCWP is not a valid reflection of LVEDP.

Central venous access represents an invasive process with inherent risks, some of which are rare but are potentially life-threatening. Adverse effects from CVP or PAC monitoring can be a result of accessing the central venous circulation, the catheterization procedure, or from use or presence of the catheter after placement. Unintentional puncture of nearby arteries, bleeding, neuropathy, and pneumothorax may result from needle insertion into adjacent structures. Air embolism may occur if a cannula is open to the atmosphere and air is entrained during or after catheter placement. Dysrhythmias are common during the catheterization procedure, with a reported incidence of 4.7% to 68.9%. Ventricular tachycardia or fibrillation may be induced during catheter advancement. Catheter advancement has been associated with right bundle-branch block and may precipitate complete heart block in patients with pre-existing left bundle-branch block. The most dreaded complication associated with PAC monitoring is pulmonary artery rupture. Pulmonary hypertension, coagulopathy, and heparinization are often present in patients who have died of pulmonary artery rupture. Perforations and subsequent hemorrhage can be avoided by restricting "overwedging," minimizing the number of balloon inflations, and using proper technique during balloon inflations. Table 26-4 summarizes the adverse effects as reported by the ASA Task Force on pulmonary artery catheterization.

Table 26-4 Adverse Effects Associated with Pulmonary Artery Monitoring

Complication	Reported Incidence (%)
Central venous access	
Arterial puncture	0.1–13
Postoperative neuropathy	0.3–1.1
Pneumothorax	0.3–4.5
Air embolism	0.5
Flotation of pulmonary artery catheter	
Minor dysrhythmias	4–68.9
Ventricular tachycardia or fibrillation	0.3–62.7
Right bundle-branch block	0.1–4.3
Complete heart block (prior left bundle-branch block)	0–8.5
Complications associated with catheter residence	
Pulmonary artery rupture	0.03–1.5
Positive cultures from catheter tip	1.4–34.8
Sepsis secondary to catheter residence	0.7–11.4
Thrombophlebitis	6.5
Venous thrombosis	0.5–66.7
Pulmonary infarction	0.1–5.6
Mural thrombus	28–61
Valvular or endocardial vegetations	2.2–100
Deaths attributed to pulmonary artery catheter	0.02–1.5

Reprinted with permission from American Society of Anesthesiologists Task Force on Pulmonary Artery Catheter. Practice guidelines for pulmonary artery catheterization: an updated report by the American Society of Anesthesiologists Task Force on Pulmonary Artery Catheterization. *Anesthesiology*. 2003;99(4):988–1014.

Common Problems and Limitations

The right internal jugular vein is the most common site for cannulation by anesthesiologists because it is accessible from the head of the operating table, has a predictable anatomy, and has a high success rate in both adults and children (15 Video 26-15).[46] The left-sided internal jugular vein is also available but is less desirable because of the potential for damaging the thoracic duct or difficulty in maneuvering catheters through the jugular–subclavian junction. Accidental carotid artery puncture is a potential problem with either location. Use of an ultrasound-guided technique is now strongly recommended by all relevant professional societies to reduce complications and improve first-attempt success rates when accessing the internal jugular veins.[47]

Alternatives to the internal jugular vein include the external jugular, subclavian, antecubital, and femoral veins. Although the Centers for Disease Control and Prevention suggests that the preferred site for central venous cannulation should be the subclavian site to potentially reduce bloodstream infections, this recommendation must be taken in the context of the particular clinical situation. The internal jugular approach may be superior in those patients with coagulopathies (in whom bleeding at the subclavian site may be more difficult to stop) or patients with severe acute lung injury (for whom the risk of pneumothorax may be heightened). When comparing the subclavian approach with the femoral approach, the reported reduction in infection risk favors subclavian. However, there is a paucity of prospective randomized data when comparing the subclavian to the internal jugular. Infection is a potential complication of the continued use of CVP catheters and PACs, although this complication may be preventable with scrupulous attention to sterile technique.[48]

Femoral, subclavian, and internal jugular veins are all utilized for central venous access in infants and children. Physician experience and comfort is the primary determinant of insertion site and has the greatest impact on complication rates, although the routine use of ultrasound for central venous catheter placement may decrease risk of iatrogenic vascular injury.[31,49] Subclavian venous catheters in pediatric patients may have a lower risk of dislodgement as well as being less restrictive to patients' range of motion, but the femoral vein may be the preferred site of central venous access in critically ill pediatric patients. Disadvantages of subclavian lines include lower success rates of placement and increased rates of catheter malposition, inadvertent arterial puncture, and pneumothorax. Femoral venous lines in children do not appear to carry an increased risk of infection compared with subclavian and jugular venous catheters,[50] although there is a higher risk of line maintenance-related complications, particularly catheter thrombosis, and accidental dislodgement. Internal jugular catheterizations appear to have the highest placement success rate, though they may cause increased patient discomfort, as site dressings may limit neck mobility.

Monitoring of Cardiac Output by Pulmonary Arterial Catheter

Principles of Operation

Provided that the heart is structurally normal, without septal defects and without a patent ductus so that no intracardiac recirculation or shunting of blood can occur, the time-averaged flow of blood through the right ventricular outflow tract (RVOT) will accurately approximate the CO. A small amount of venous return to the left side of the heart from the bronchial circulation and thebesian veins is neglected. Time averaging suppresses the effects of beat-to-beat pulsatility.

A properly positioned PAC passes through the RVOT (16 Video 26-16). CO monitoring using a pulmonary arterial catheter therefore depends on assessing the rate of blood flow through the right side of the heart and using this as a measure of CO. Techniques to measure the flow rate are based upon the idea of measuring the dilution of some known quantity of an indicator by the passing blood flow. Historically, this indicator could have been some sort of dye, but in modern clinical practice the most commonly used technique is based upon thermodilution. Thermodilution cardiac output (TCO) depends on the measurement of temperature near the tip of the PAC using a thermistor.

CO can be assessed intermittently by using a bolus injection of room-temperature or chilled fluid as the indicator. The thermistor on the pulmonary arterial catheter records the fall in temperature as this bolus is injected via a more proximal port on the PAC and mixes with the surrounding blood flow. The total flow through the RVOT, and hence the CO, can be estimated from the area under this blood temperature curve, combined with knowledge of the specific heat capacity and gravity of blood and the injectate, the volume of the injectate, and the size of the catheter. When performed properly, TCO measurements correlate well with direct Fick or dye dilution estimates of CO.[51]

Continuous CO monitoring offers the potential to identify acute changes in ventricular performance as they occur. A coiled filament creates a pulsed, low-power heating signal within the right atrium and ventricle in a cyclical manner based on a proprietary pseudorandom sequence. The thermistor at the tip of the PAC detects these changes in blood temperature and sends the temperature information to a microcomputer that creates a thermodilution curve based on the pulsed inputs and the measured temperatures. CO is then computed in a similar fashion to the bolus technique, using a conservation of heat equation, although effectively using a warmed bolus rather than a chilled bolus.[52] Although a time lag can exist, continuous CO monitoring compares favorably with bolus CO measurements, even under conditions of varying patient temperature and CO.

Proper Use and Interpretation

TCO measurements depend on the assumption that changes in thermal energy are carried forward to the thermistor; thus, the measurements depend on the correct positioning of the catheter. If the catheter is insufficiently advanced such that the port through which a bolus injectate is administered is still within the introducer sheath, then there will be reflux of the injectate within the introducer sheath. This will result in some of the change in thermal energy being "lost" into the sheath. A smaller-than-expected change in temperature will then be seen at the thermistor, appearing as if the injectate had been injected into a larger volume of blood flow. The TCO computer will interpret and present this as an erroneously high CO. Similarly erroneous readings may be produced if the catheter is advanced too far, such that the heating filament of a continuous TCO catheter lies beyond the pulmonic valve. Hypothermia and the rapid concurrent administration of unwarmed intravenous fluids may affect the accuracy of TCO measurements.

Indications

Measurement of CO is required to determine physiologic factors such as the rate of oxygen delivery to peripheral tissues. Possible clinical indications include severe sepsis, cardiogenic shock, and dependence on inotropes. An additional technologic refinement of the pulmonary arterial catheter is the *oximetric* PAC, which uses reflectance spectrophotometry to identify the saturation of the mixed venous blood ($S\bar{v}O_2$) surrounding the tip of the PAC. Knowledge of the $S\bar{v}O_2$ allows the rate of extraction of oxygen by peripheral tissues (ψo_2) to be calculated. Neglecting the small amount of oxygen dissolved in blood:

$$\psi o_2 = 13.8 \times [\text{Hgb}] \times \text{CO} \times (SaO_2 - S\bar{v}O_2)$$

where [Hgb] is the concentration of hemoglobin, 13.8 is a conversion factor for the oxygen-carrying capacity of hemoglobin, CO is the cardiac output in L/min, and ($SaO_2 - S\bar{v}O_2$) is the difference between the arterial and mixed venous oxygen saturations.

The use of PACs in practice has diminished over the last two decades.[53] This decline may be due to improvements in the availability of techniques such as transesophageal echocardiography (TEE) and arterial waveform analysis that can estimate CO in a less-invasive manner. However, thermodilution via a PAC remains the clinical gold standard for the determination of CO and should be considered when knowledge of the CO is necessary for the patient's management and when other comorbidities would render less invasive techniques inaccurate.

Contraindications

Measurement of CO requires a PAC that is designed for the purpose. Contraindications for this measurement are reflective of the contraindications to placing a pulmonary arterial catheter, including right-sided endocarditis, tumors, or masses. A risk-to-benefit analysis should be performed prior to PAC placement in severely coagulopathic and thrombocytopenic patients, as well as patients with left bundle-branch block.[54]

Common Problems and Limitations

The intermittent TCO technique assumes that there is adequate mixing of the cooled injectate with the surrounding blood flow (NICV 26-2). It is necessary that the temperature of the injectate be distinct from the temperature of the blood in order to generate a change in the distal temperature measurement. Improved measurements can be obtained by using a cooler injectate, producing a greater temperature change to detect and hence an improved signal-to-noise ratio.[55]

The presence of intracardiac shunts or significant tricuspid regurgitation can invalidate the assumptions underlying TCO. Intracardiac shunts allow accessory blood flow paths, such that flow through the RVOT may no longer approximate CO accurately. Significant tricuspid regurgitation can compromise thermodilution methods by permitting retrograde blood flow, invalidating the assumption that all changes in thermal energy caused by the indicator are carried forward to the detecting thermistor.

Clinicians are unable to estimate the cardiac index in pediatric patients reliably, even using associated clinical indicators such as SV variation, blood pressure, and HR (17 Video 26-17).[56] Nevertheless, continuous CO monitoring is rarely used in the perioperative management of pediatric patients. Femoral arterial thermodilution (FATD) has been validated as an alternative to pulmonary arterial thermodilution techniques in patients ranging from infancy to adolescence. FATD correlates closely with Fick-based calculations while only minimally overestimating cardiac index.[57] When compared to pulmonary-arterial sampling methods, FATD monitoring systems are less hazardous to place, as they avoid the potential for pneumothorax and pulmonary arterial injury.

Monitoring of Cardiac Output by Arterial Waveform Analysis

Principles of Operation

The use of a PAC remains the gold standard for the determination of CO, but the use of PACs in the management of patients requiring intensive care has not been demonstrated to be associated with reduced mortality. PACs are also associated with a high rate of iatrogenic complications,[58] and the ASA recommends that only clinicians with regular ongoing experience with the procedure should place PACs.[59] Nevertheless, the determination of CO allows more accurate assessment of the hemodynamic status of a critically ill patient than can be obtained by clinical assessment alone. This conundrum created increasing interest in biomedical devices that can estimate CO in a less invasive manner. Arterial waveform analysis is one such technique.[60]

There are three arterial waveform CO devices on the market that are based on peripheral arterial pressure readings from an invasive arterial cannula: FloTrac, PiCCO, and LiDCOrapid. These devices directly measure the fluctuations in arterial pressure and the HR, from which they estimate the beat-to-beat SV. The CO is given by the product of the HR and SV (CO = HR × SV).

A more recent device, ClearSight (Edwards Lifesciences, Irvine, CA) does not use an invasive arterial cannula, but instead uses a noninvasive finger blood-pressure cuff that is dynamically inflated and deflated to attempt to track the blood pressure in the brachial artery. This means of inferring arterial blood pressure relies on a method originally described by Peňáz,[61] in which the fingertip is compressed by a pressure cuff while simultaneously being transilluminated by infrared light. Arterial pulsations cause the volume of blood within the fingertip to increase, increasing the absorption of infrared light by hemoglobin. The system rapidly changes the inflation pressure of the cuff to attempt to hold the absorption of infrared light constant. Because the infrared absorption is held constant (according to the underlying assumptions of the method), the volume of blood within the fingertip must also be constant, which thus implies that the pressures applied to the fingertip are exactly equal and opposed to the arterial pulsation. Consequently, the finger cuff pressures must represent the arterial pressures. This simple model has been subsequently refined to include compensation for pressure reflection in the vascular tree between the fingertip and brachial artery and to reflect the variable vertical fluid column between the fingertip and the heart.[62] This noninvasive reconstruction of an arterial waveform then also allows CO to be estimated by arterial waveform analysis.

It is a straightforward matter to measure HR from an arterial waveform tracing; it is the estimation of beat-to-beat SV that presents the technical challenge. The first modern mathematical description of the shape of the arterial waveform was described by Otto Frank and gave rise to the "Windkessel" (German: *air chamber*) model for arterial behavior. When considering the flow of an incompressible fluid (such as blood) through a section of tube, the assumption is made that the volume of the fluid entering the tube is the same as the volume of the fluid leaving the tube. This assumption allows a *continuity equation* to be created from which models of fluid flow can be derived. The basis of the Windkessel model is the realization that although blood is incompressible, the artery itself is distensible, and so the volumes of blood entering and leaving an arterial segment at any given moment may be different. There is distension of the artery and storage of blood and during systole, followed by relaxation of the artery and ejection of blood during diastole. The volumes of blood entering and leaving are only the same when averaged over the cardiac cycle, as shown in Figure 26-9.

This behavior is mathematically similar to that seen in the modeling of a compressible fluid, such as air, when flowing in rigid vessels, hence the name of the "Windkessel" model. The air may store and release energy through changes in pressure and compression. In arterial waveform analysis, it is the fluid that is incompressible, and it is the nonrigid arterial vessel that may store and release energy by elastic deformation. The behavior of the artery depends on its resistance to flow *R* and its compliance *C*. These values are known to be predictable from patient demographics by cadaveric studies of the human aorta.[63]

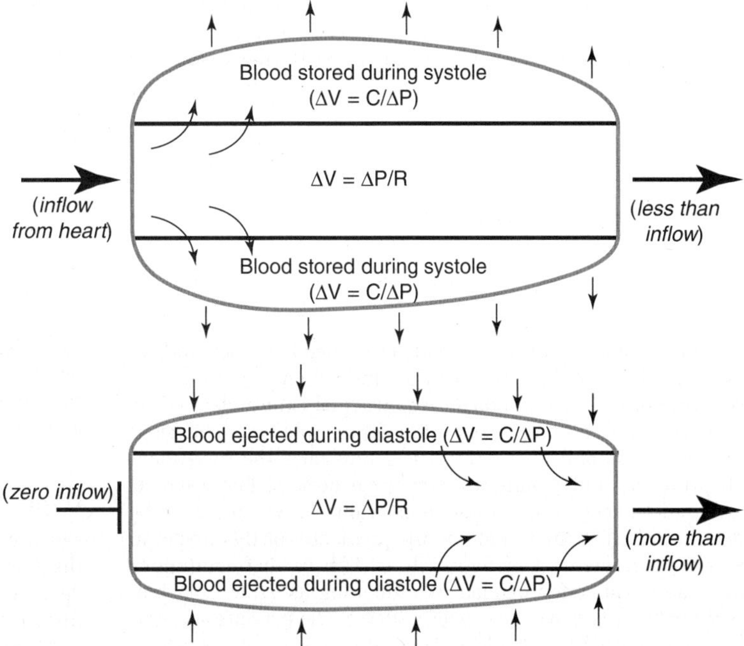

Figure 26-9 Depiction of blood flow into and out of a prototypical "Windkessel artery." Several points are to be noted: first, during systole, inflow into the artery is less than outflow because some of the blood is stored in the expanding compliant vessel. Second, during diastole, inflow into the artery is zero and outflow is enhanced by the contracting vessel. C, compliance; P, pressure; R, resistance; V, volume. (Adapted with permission from Thiele RH, Durieux ME. Arterial waveform analysis for the anesthesiologist: Past, present, and future concepts. *Anesth Analg.* 2011;113(4):766–776.)

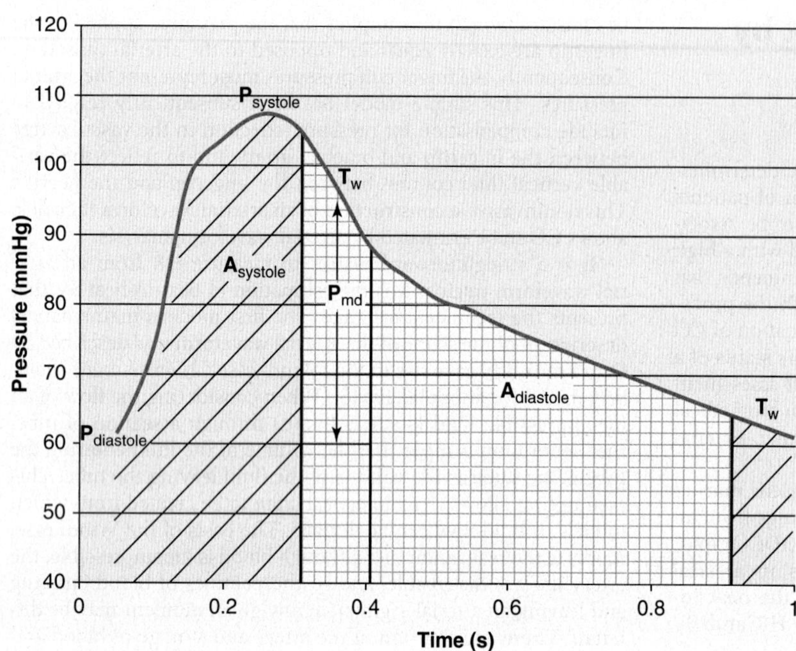

Figure 26-10 A graphical depiction of the components of the arterial waveform used by the Windkessel-based area under the curve method. Note that P_{md} represents the increment in mean pressure over the whole arterial bed at the end of systole and that T_w represents the transmission time (from the aorta to the periphery). (Adapted with permission from Thiele RH, Durieux ME. Arterial waveform analysis for the anesthesiologist: Past, present, and future concepts. *Anesth Analg.* 2011;113(4):766–776.)

The total SV must be equal to the volume of blood flowing forward in systole Q_s plus the volume of blood flowing forward in diastole Q_d, assuming the aortic valve is competent.

$$SV = Q_s + Q_d$$

At the beginning of diastole, there is no further inflow into the aorta, and so Q_d is proportional to the difference between the pressure in the aorta and the pressure in the arterial beds. This is described as the end-systolic mean distending pressure P_{md}, equivalent to the idea of a "pressure head." Therefore,

$$Q_d = k \times P_{md}$$

where k is a constant of proportionality dependent on the properties of resistance and compliance, as described earlier. As the peripheral vascular resistance should not change over a single cardiac cycle, the values of Q_s and Q_d should be proportional to A_s and A_d, the areas under the pressure curve during systole and diastole, respectively, as shown in Figure 26-10. Therefore,

$$Q_s/A_s = Q_d/A_d \quad \text{or, alternatively,} \quad Q_s = Q_d \frac{A_s}{A_d}$$

Rearranging these model equations:

$$SV = Q_d\left(1 + \frac{A_s}{A_d}\right) \quad \text{and so} \quad SV = kP_{md}\left(1 + \frac{A_s}{A_d}\right)$$

This model demonstrates how, in principle, a beat-to-beat estimate of SV can be generated from measurements of the arterial waveform. The algorithms used by actual clinical devices are more complex and proprietary. Although the previous analysis is necessarily simplified, it nevertheless illustrates the fundamental principles and requirements of these devices. For instance, the model depends on an additional value k, which has to be determined either by calibrating the prediction of this model to another measurement of SV (such as TEE or thermodilution) or in an uncalibrated manner by estimating its value from biophysical models based on variables such as the patient's age, sex, height, and weight.[64] The PiCCO device makes use of an external calibration reading, whereas the FloTrac and LiDCOrapid devices use an uncalibrated biophysical model approach.

Proper Use and Interpretation

Arterial waveform CO monitors make use of standard equipment for arterial cannulation. A stiff arterial line, flushed from a pressurized fluid source, is attached to the arterial cannula and zeroed in the usual fashion. However, in place of the usual piezoelectric pressure sensor with a single electrical connection, a specialized sensor is used with two connectors so that pressure information can be supplied simultaneously to the anesthesia monitor and to the CO monitor. The display of arterial pressures by the anesthesia monitor is unaffected by the presence of the CO monitor. It is possible to transduce arterial pressures alone without connecting the CO monitor. Uncalibrated devices, such as the FloTrac and LiDCOrapid, require information about the patient such as age, height, weight, and sex in order to estimate the physiologic properties of the patient's arterial system and estimated body surface area. The device may require a brief interval of time to gather initial arterial pressure data, but will shortly begin to report CO and other indices such as cardiac index, SV, stroke volume variation (SVV), and SV index. These indices represent various combinations of SV, HR, and body surface area. Further user intervention is not generally required. These values, in the manner estimated by the device, are most useful for assessing relative volume status and for assessing the response to fluid resuscitation.[65,66] The ability of the device to respond to changes in CO caused by inotropes or vasopressors[67,68] is uncertain; the limits of its reliability, accuracy, and utility in this setting are the subject of ongoing research and algorithmic refinement.

Indications

The use of an arterial waveform CO monitor is not mandated so the indications for use are at the discretion of the practitioner. The device is likely to be most helpful to the clinician in cases in which there are expected to be large fluid shifts and in which the patient's intravascular volume status may become difficult to determine by clinical assessment and usual monitoring techniques. It may be preferable, and less invasive, to guide fluid resuscitation with arterial waveform CO measurements rather than placing a central venous catheter or a PAC. This approach is particularly attractive if the patient already requires an arterial line for other indications or if the patient's comorbidities relatively contraindicate the placement of a central line or PAC. It is possible to extract other indices from analysis of the arterial waveform, and measurements such as systolic pulse variation (SPV) and SVV may also be useful in predicting responsiveness to fluid resuscitation.

Contraindications

Devices such as the FloTrac and LiDCOrapid that do not require additional calibration are no more invasive than the arterial line to which they are attached. The same contraindications that apply to arterial lines, such as poor or absent collateralization of arterial supply to the extremity, also apply to these devices.

Devices that estimate CO from the arterial waveform do so based upon a number of physiologic assumptions that were touched upon during the derivation of the simplified model. There are many disease states, some common, which violate these assumptions and can significantly compromise the accuracy of the device; these are discussed later.

Common Problems and Limitations

All arterial waveform CO monitors depend on accurate, high-fidelity measurement of arterial pressures. Satisfactory operation depends upon good arterial perfusion to the site of measurement and good peripheral arterial cannulation. The pressure transducer system must use appropriate tubing and be flushed and zeroed correctly so that bias, signal dampening, or flail are not seen in the arterial waveform. These artifacts corrupt the frequency spectrum of the arterial waveform and impair accurate measurement. The use of an intra-aortic balloon pump may distort the arterial waveform to such an extent that the resulting waveform is uninterpretable, rendering the device inoperative.[69]

The simplified model of arterial waveform analysis made use of information obtained from only a single cardiac cycle. In contrast, all of the current monitors make use of algorithms that depend on information obtained over many cardiac cycles. The FloTrac monitor is reported to depend, for example, upon the standard deviation, skewness, and kurtosis of the statistical distribution of arterial pressures obtained over the preceding 20 seconds.[64] This implicitly assumes that the CO remains relatively constant beat-to-beat over the sampling interval. This assumption can be violated in the presence of irregular heart rhythms, in which the preload of the left ventricle and hence the SV can demonstrate significant beat-to-beat variability. Arterial waveform CO monitors can therefore be prone to inaccuracy in the setting of atrial fibrillation.

In the simplified model, the properties of systemic vascular resistance (SVR) and arterial compliance (C) were subsumed into the parameter k, and it was proposed that k might be obtained from a population-based biophysical model. However, in the presence of sepsis[68,70] or some other high-output state, such as liver transplantation surgery,[71] the deviation of these values from the expected population norms can cause inaccuracy when compared to the measurement of CO by PAC. A similar problem applies to the iatrogenic reduction of the compliance of arterial vessels through the administration of vasopressors. Arterial waveform CO devices appear to be reliable at assessing changes in CO caused by fluid resuscitation, of some utility at detecting changes caused by inotropes, but poor at assessing changes caused by alteration in vascular tone by agents such as phenylephrine or norepinephrine.[66]

Finally, arterial waveform analysis depends on the assumption that there is no further inflow into the arterial system at the end of systole, as used in the analysis based on the parameter P_{md}. This assumption is violated in the setting of aortic insufficiency, in which there is negative regurgitant flow to the left ventricle. Arterial waveform analysis is expected to demonstrate inaccuracy in this presentation.[69] Conversely, aortic stenosis does not appear to impair the accuracy of measurement of CO.

In summary, arterial waveform analysis has been demonstrated in many studies to provide a reasonable estimate of CO and a reasonable approximation to more invasive techniques. The degree to which a new monitoring technique must agree with the gold standard to be clinically useful is a matter of clinical judgment and not a question that can be definitively addressed by statistics alone. Presently, these devices appear to be most useful as guides to fluid resuscitation and for trend monitoring rather than as guides to the administration of inotropes or vasopressors. There are a number of relatively common clinical scenarios in which the accuracy of these devices can be anticipated to be impaired based upon violation of the underlying physiologic assumptions on which their algorithms depend. The clinician must exercise caution in interpreting the measurements of CO obtained under those circumstances.

In the pediatric population, estimation of CO via arterial waveform analysis has proven more challenging. A technique called pressure recording analytical method (PRAM) has had only mixed results in its ability to reliably estimate pediatric CO despite the use of more advanced algorithms and higher sampling frequencies. Moreover, pediatric studies of this technology have excluded children with hemodynamic instability, arguably the clinical circumstance in which CO monitoring would be most useful to the anesthesiologist.[72,73]

Monitoring of Body Temperature

Principles of Operation

Heat is produced as a consequence of cellular metabolism. In adults, thermoregulation involves the control of basal metabolic rate, muscular activity, sympathetic arousal, vascular tone, and hormone activation balanced against exogenous factors that determine the need for the body to create heat or to adjust the transfer of heat to the environment. Both general and regional anesthesia inhibit afferent and efferent control of thermoregulation.

Heat losses may result from radiation, conduction, convection, and evaporation. Radiation refers to the infrared rays emanating from all objects above absolute temperature. Conduction refers to the transfer of heat from contact with objects. Convection refers to the transfer of heat from air passing by objects. Evaporation represents the heat loss that results when water vaporizes. For every gram of water evaporated, 0.58 kcal of heat is lost. Perioperative hypothermia predisposes patients to increases in metabolic rate (shivering) and cardiac work, decreases in drug metabolism and cutaneous blood flow, and creates impairments of coagulation. Anesthesiologists frequently monitor temperature and attempt to maintain central core temperature at near-normal values in all patients undergoing anesthesia. Clinical studies have demonstrated that patients in whom intraoperative hypothermia develops are at a higher risk for development of postoperative myocardial ischemia and wound infection compared with patients who are normothermic in the perioperative period.[74,75]

Proper Use and Interpretation

Central core temperatures can be estimated using probes that can be placed into the bladder, distal esophagus, ear canal, trachea, nasopharynx, or rectum. Pulmonary artery blood temperature is also a good estimate of central core temperature. Thermoregulatory responses are based on a physiologically weighted average reflecting changes in the mean body temperature. Mean body temperature is estimated by the following equation:

$$T_{mean\ body} = 0.85\ T_{core} + 0.15\ T_{skin}$$

Indications

The ability to monitor body temperature is a standard of anesthesia care. The continual observation of temperature changes in anesthetized patients allows for the detection of accidental heat loss or malignant hyperthermia.

Contraindications

There are no absolute contraindications to temperature monitoring. In patients whose thermoregulatory responses are intact, such as conscious patients or patients receiving light or moderate sedation, continuous temperature monitoring is usually uninformative.

Common Problems and Limitations

Skin temperature monitoring has been advocated to identify peripheral vasoconstriction but is not adequate to determine alterations in mean body temperature that may occur during surgery. Core temperature sites have been established as reliable indicators of changes in mean temperature. During routine noncardiac surgery, temperature differences between these sites are small. When anesthetized patients are being cooled, changes in rectal temperature often lag behind those of other probe locations, and the adequacy of rewarming is best judged by measuring temperature at several locations. Although liquid crystal skin temperature strips are convenient to apply, they do not correlate with core temperature measurements.[76]

Monitoring of Processed EEG Signals

Principles of Operation

EEG monitoring initially entered anesthetic practice as a highly sensitive and moderately specific means of monitoring for cerebral ischemia, and as such found use in carotid surgery (NICV 26-3). Occlusion of one of the carotid arteries for surgery makes the ipsilateral side of the brain dependent on perfusion from the contralateral carotid artery via the circle of Willis, creating a risk of ipsilateral ischemia. In this form, a dedicated technician usually performs intraoperative EEG monitoring.

More recently, EEG monitoring has begun to gain acceptance as a means of estimating depth of anesthesia. Statistical signal-processing techniques have been developed and embodied as biomedical devices that are able to take an ensemble of EEG data and, in real time, display an estimate of "anesthetic depth." The two most commonly used processed EEG monitors are the bispectral index (BIS) (Medtronic, Minneapolis, MN) and SedLine (Masimo, Irvine, CA). The operation of these devices is similar. After first cleaning the patient's forehead, a single-use set of small adhesive electrical sensors are applied. The sensors are positioned to enable the device to detect EEG activity in the frontal lobes of the brain. The sensors are attached to the main device via a single connector. The device checks the quality of the electrical connection to the sensors, and checks that each of the sensors has made a good electrical contact with the patient's forehead and that the sensors are not in inadvertent electrical connection with each other. In the event that the configuration of the sensors is unacceptable, the device displays a pictorial indication of the problem so that the clinician can attempt to remedy the problem. If the electrical connection between the sensor and the skin is poor, signal reception will be impaired and the device will warn that the sensor impedance (i.e., its electrical resistance) is too high. The sensors make use of a conductive electrical gel; poor connections can often be remedied by applying firm but careful pressure to the affected sensor to produce a better electrical contact. However, too much pressure may cause the gel to leak out from under the sensor and cause a "gel bridge," an inadvertent direct electrical connection to a neighboring electrode. In this case, the surplus gel may be wiped away or a new set of sensors may be required. When all the electrical connections are satisfactory, the device will begin to acquire and process EEG data.

Although the algorithms used by processed EEG monitors are proprietary, some general features of the EEG that they use have previously been described.[77] More recently, forensic examination of the devices has allowed open versions of EEG processing algorithms to be produced.[78,79] The most important EEG features appear to be:

- Beta (β)-Power Ratio: The β-power ratio describes the relative amount of low gamma band activity in the EEG signal (i.e., signal power between 30 and 47 Hz) compared to the amount of β-wave activity (signal power between 11 and 20 Hz). Changes in this ratio appear to correlate clinically with sedation.
- Power Concentration in the Gamma Band (40 to 47 Hz). There is a prevailing thalamocortical rhythm in the gamma EEG band at around 40 Hz, and the frequency of this particular peak of activity appears to be progressively lowered by the action of inhibitory agents.[80,81] Changes in the distribution of this peak of signal power compared to the whole EEG power spectrogram can be used to estimate depths of anesthesia in the range of general anesthesia. This gamma frequency band overlaps the frequency response of the EMG, and this most likely explains the well-known clinical observation that neuromuscular blockade tends to decrease the BIS score,[82] even in fully awake experimental volunteers.[83]
- Burst Suppression Ratio (BSR). During periods of deep anesthesia, the EEG may demonstrate periods of low voltage or even zero (isoelectric) voltage, and bursts of higher-voltage activity are no longer seen. Suppressed states are defined as those periods for which the EEG demonstrates a voltage of less than 5 mV for a period of at least 0.5 seconds, and the BSR is defined as the ratio of that time fraction to the overall EEG recording. Profoundly burst suppressed (isoelectric) states are sometimes induced as part of neuroanesthesia,[84] as they may provide some protection against cerebral ischemia by reducing cellular metabolic demand. Burst suppression is also seen in unanesthetized comatose patients, although in these patients it carries a grave prognosis.[85]

Proper Use and Interpretation

Both the BIS and SedLine devices display a unitless number in the range of 0 to 100, which is derived from the measured EEG data by the device's proprietary algorithms. A value of 0 corresponds to an absence of any discernible electrical activity. A value of 100 corresponds to the EEG activity seen in a fully awake and alert individual. The algorithms used in the devices specify a differing "optimal range" for general anesthesia: for the BIS it is defined as between 40 and 60, for the SedLine it is 25 to 50.

The algorithms used in the devices appear to correlate best with clinical assessment of the depth of anesthesia when anesthetic agents such as volatile gases or propofol are used, as shown in Figure 26-11, although increasing concentrations of these agents do not always reliably lower the reported number further[86,87] if the patient is already deeply anesthetized. This relationship between concentration and effect is not seen for all anesthetic agents.

Dissociative intravenous agents such as ketamine can actively confound processed EEG monitors through paradoxical cortical excitation; the monitor tends to misread the increased cortical

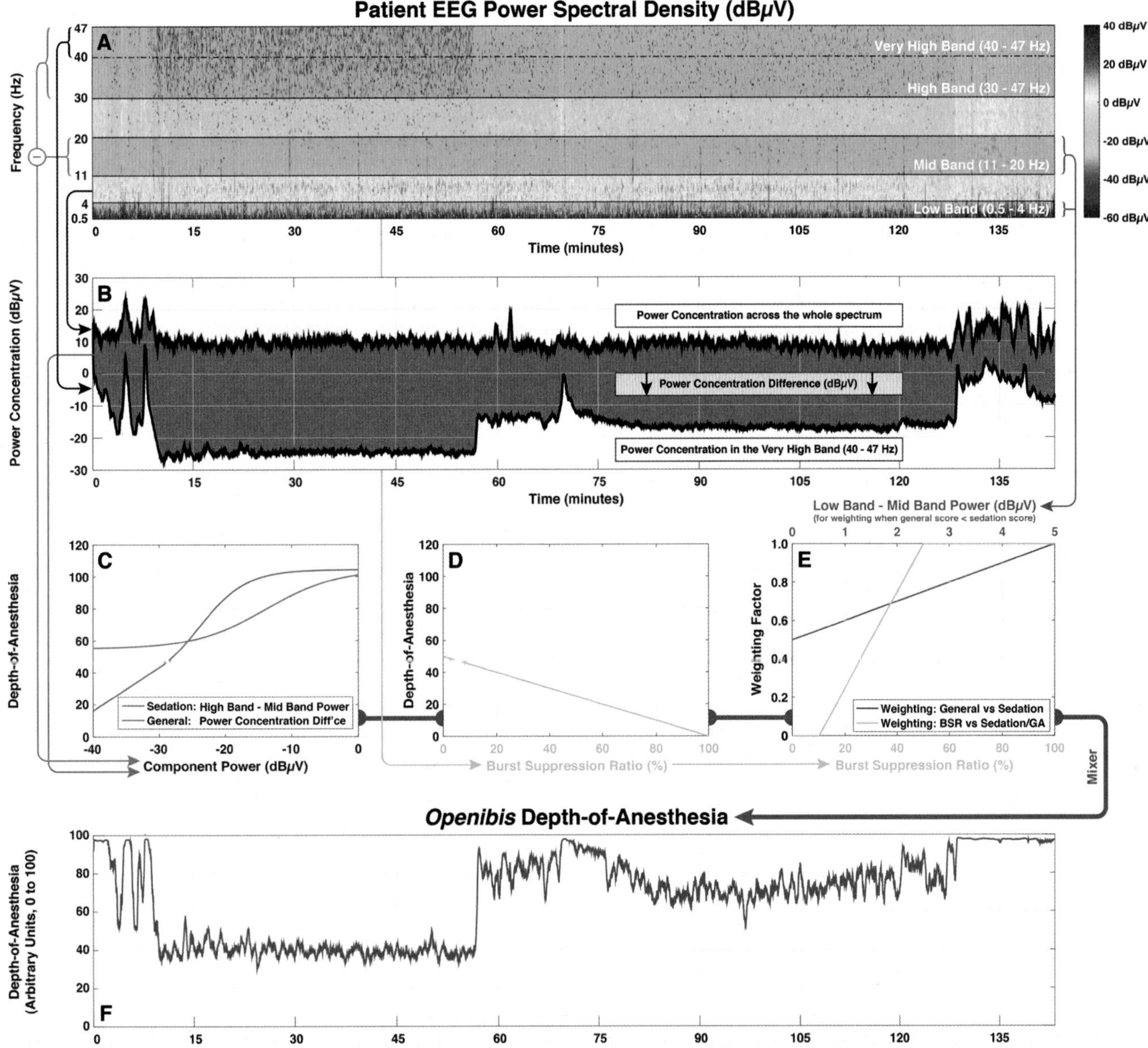

Figure 26-11 A graphical roadmap of an open algorithm for EEG processing for depth of anesthesia. (**A**) EEG epochs are converted into a power spectral density by Fourier transform. Subsequent calculations depend upon the relative power distributions across the whole frequency range, and across sub-bands spanning 0.5 to 4 Hz (low), 11 to 20 Hz (mid), 30 to 47 Hz (high), and 40 to 47 Hz (very high). (**B**) A component related to general anesthesia is derived from the difference in power concentration between the very high band and the spectrum as a whole. (**C**) The components related to sedation and general anesthesia are converted into depth-of-anesthesia scores using curvilinear logistic response functions. (**D**) The burst suppression rate (BSR) is converted linearly into a depth-of-anesthesia score. (**E**) The lower value of the sedation and general anesthesia scores predominates. Some transitional averaging between sedation and general occurs if the general score is lower and the difference between the low and mid band power is equivocal (≤5 dBμV). This score, representing the combination of sedation and general, is then weighted against the BSR score to produce a provisional final score. (**F**) Extreme values in the provisional score (≤10 or ≥97) are compressed into the allowable range of 0 to 100 to produce the final score. (Adapted from Connor CW. Open reimplementation of the BIS algorithms for depth of anesthesia. *Anesth Analg.* 2022;135(4):855–864.)

activity as a sign of lessened anesthesia.[88] Low doses of ketamine may be desirable as part of an overall anesthetic plan to reduce opioid administration; appropriate quantities of ketamine can be infused more slowly without apparently affecting the processed EEG reading.[89] Propofol and remifentanil are often used in combination for total intravenous anesthesia (TIVA), but processed EEG monitors can be insensitive to the administration of even high concentrations of opioids.[90] The monitor may therefore reflect mostly the action of the propofol on the anesthetic state.

Indications

The use of processed EEG monitors is not mandated; thus, the indications for use are at the discretion of the practitioner. Processed EEG monitors have not been demonstrated to be superior to end-tidal agent concentration monitoring in the prevention of awareness under anesthesia. However, the use of end-tidal agent concentration monitoring assumes that volatile anesthetic gases are used and that their end-tidal concentrations provide a reasonable surrogate for their action on consciousness. Processed EEG monitoring may be useful as a guide when a TIVA approach is planned, since it can provide some degree of feedback on the current pharmacodynamics effects of the administered agents when there is no end-tidal agent concentration to measure.

Patients with pre-existing cognitive deficits, sensory impairment, or known risk of postoperative delirium may benefit from the administration of less anesthesia than would be indicated by end-tidal agent monitoring alone.[91] Processed EEG monitoring may be useful in satisfactorily titrating their anesthetic plan to permit faster recovery from anesthesia.

For types of emergency surgery, such as cesarean sections under general anesthesia, trauma laparotomies, or surgery in the critically ill hemodynamically unstable patient, it may not be physiologically possible to administer the usual quantities of anesthesia, placing these patients at a greater risk of intraoperative awareness. Processed EEG monitoring may provide some assistance in titrating anesthesia in these vulnerable patients and some reassurance that explicit recall will be unlikely. A prior history of intraoperative awareness may therefore also be an indication.

Mechanically ventilated patients in the intensive care unit are usually assessed clinically for their level of sedation, but the use of the standard Sedation-Agitation Scale or the Richmond Agitation-Sedation Scale may be impossible in some patients due to therapeutic neuromuscular paralysis. Processed EEG monitors may provide some guidance to sedation management under these circumstances.

Contraindications

Use of a processed EEG device may be contraindicated in a patient with significant craniofacial trauma, such that the physical pressure required to place the sensors cannot be safely applied. Placement may also be relatively contraindicated in patients with existing superficial injury to the forehead in the region where the sensors will be applied.

The use of processed EEG sensors for patients who will be in the prone position for surgery is controversial and may be a relative contraindication. When prone, the patient's head may rest such that excessive continuous contact pressure is applied to the skin underneath the sensors. Disfiguring injury to the forehead has been reported,[92] perhaps related to a combination of pressure and irritation from the conductive gel on the sensors. This can lead to a dilemma: prolonged spinal surgery performed using somatosensory or motor-evoked potential monitoring can relatively contraindicate the use of volatile gases and neuromuscular blockers, and make a propofol–remifentanil TIVA technique attractive. This anesthetic technique provides an indication for processed EEG monitoring, but the prolonged prone positioning provides a relative contraindication. Prone positioning requires vigilant attention to facial features, such as the eyes and nose, to avoid injury by pressure and impingement. Therefore, if it is determined that processed EEG monitoring is to be applied to a prone patient, it is recommended that equally vigilant attention be paid to the condition of the forehead.

Common Problems and Limitations

It has been suggested that processed EEG monitoring devices may reduce the risk of intraoperative awareness.[93] However, subsequent studies have either failed to demonstrate a reduction in intraoperative awareness[94] or even, conversely, have found an increase in intraoperative awareness when compared to anesthetic practice guided by the end-tidal agent concentrations of anesthetic gases.[18]

Cases of intraoperative awareness were found when using either end-tidal agent concentration monitoring or processed EEG monitoring; neither technique was sufficient to avoid awareness with complete reliability. This difficulty may relate to our lack of understanding of what "anesthetic depth" even means. Intraoperative awareness as a phenomenon is dependent on the interaction of consciousness, memory, and the biologic action of anesthetic agents. These, even taken individually, are complex and incompletely understood processes. It should not therefore be surprising that any device or algorithm that seeks to reduce these processes to a single numerical readout may prove to be fallible.

Compared to adults, pediatric patients have more than three times greater incidence of awareness under anesthesia.[95,96] At the same time, there is a conflicting pressure to reduce exposure to anesthetic agents in young children. An increasing body of evidence suggests that anesthetic agents harm early brain development, with their potential to cause dose dependent neurodegeneration and neuroapoptosis.[97,98] The downstream neurocognitive impacts of exposing children to these agents are less clear; with results ranging from no difference to a measurable decline in listening comprehension and performance IQ in young children following surgery with anesthesia.[99] In the studies that showed no difference in neurocognitive outcomes, the patients received a single, brief exposure to anesthesia with mean case duration of 80 minutes or less.[97] A secondary analysis of one cohort suggested that having multiple exposures to general anesthesia in early childhood was associated with decreased processing speed and motor coordination, with parents reporting an increased incidence of behavior and reading problems.[100] A number of attempts have been made to investigate the utility of perioperative processed EEG monitoring to guide care in these younger patients. Some evidence supports the application of the adult BIS algorithm in children age above 12 months, but infant BIS values do not closely correlate with end-tidal sevoflurane concentrations. A recent study of healthy pediatric ambulatory surgery patients did not demonstrate the benefits of routine processed EEG monitoring when measured by total exposure to volatile anesthetic agents, recovery profile or readiness for PACU discharge.[101] By contrast, BIS monitoring may have advantages in guiding general anesthesia in developmentally delayed children, facilitating shorter times to spontaneous ventilation, opening eyes, and extubation, while decreasing mean PACU length of stay,[102] though further research is needed to determine whether this is indicated. As with adults, processed EEG may be a useful adjunct in this patient demographic, but is not a substitute for provider vigilance and contextual clinical judgment.

Monitoring Neuromuscular Blockade

Principles of Operation

Neuromuscular blocking drugs (NMDBs) are commonly used as part of a balanced anesthesia technique, facilitating laryngoscopy for endotracheal intubation and optimizing conditions for invasive procedures. Care must be taken in their selection, titration, and reversal. The inclusion of NMDBs in anesthetic practice has been shown to be a dose dependent risk factor for postoperative morbidity and mortality.[103,104] As such, monitoring the depth of neuromuscular blockade is crucial to providing safe anesthetic care. Monitoring the degree of neuromuscular blockade is a two-step process: first directly stimulating the nerve with an electrical impulse, and second, evaluating the evoked muscle response, or "twitch." Stand-alone nerve stimulators are designed to deliver a current at amplitudes ranging from 0 to 80 mA, most commonly as a series, or "train," of four (TOF). The clinician subjectively assesses the downstream effect of the evoked muscle response, noting the number of subsequent movements of the distal extremity as well as any perceived difference in strength of the movements. A decrease in the strength of subsequent twitches is often referred to as "fade." Neuromuscular monitors, by contrast, both stimulate the motor neuron upstream of the neuromuscular junction then measure the downstream response and, in some cases, measure the difference between the intensity of subsequent evoked responses in sequence, generating a TOF ratio.[105]

Neuromuscular monitors fall into three distinct categories: mechanomyography, acceleromyography, and electromyography. Mechanomyography machines directly measure the force generated by a distal extremity immediately following stimulation of the motor nerve. Though utilized in laboratory measurement of depth of neuromuscular blockade, these are not commercially available for use in clinical settings. With acceleromyography, a motor nerve is stimulated and subsequent acceleration of the innervated extremity is measured. Most often this involves stimulating the ulnar nerve and measuring the acceleration of the adductor policis. Newer electromyography-based monitors also function by stimulating an upstream motor nerve, and directly measure the resultant compound action potentials.

Electromyography may have advantages in cases where positioning of the downstream extremity limits its ability to move (e.g., when arms are tucked) as electromyographic monitoring does not require actual motion of the extremity.[106] Instead, adhesive monitors affixed to the innervated extremity measure the generated action potentials at the target muscle.[107]

Proper Use and Interpretation

A common method for monitoring neuromuscular blockade involves stimulating the ulnar nerve at the wrist, and observing the response of the adductor policis muscle. With proper placement of the stimulating electrodes on the wrist overlying the ulnar nerve, adduction of the thumb should only occur as a result of conducted nerve impulses, rather than direct muscle stimulation. For accurate measurement, the hand must be positioned in such a way that the thumb is free to move. Prior to the administration of NMDB, the patient's baseline TOF ratio should be measured. This value can later be referenced to the poststimulus response after the drug has been administered.[106]

Indications

Given that the use of NMDBs is associated with a dose-dependent increase in postoperative respiratory complications, the International Anesthesia Research Society released a 2018 consensus statement stating: "whenever a neuromuscular blocker is administered, neuromuscular function must be monitored by observing the evoked muscular response to peripheral nerve stimulation. Ideally, this should be done at the hand muscles (not the facial muscles) with a quantitative (objective) monitor."[103,108] Of note, despite this recommendation, monitoring of neuromuscular blockade continues to be underutilized, particularly in pediatric anesthesia cases.[109]

Contraindications

The authors note no contraindications to neuromuscular monitoring.

Common Problems and Limitations

Use of a nerve stimulator alone and having the clinician observer measure the downstream response may lead to imprecision, both in quantifying the relative strength of the evoked twitch, as well as in differentiating movement stimulated by action potentials at the neuromuscular junction from movement caused by direct muscle stimulation. When access to the extremities is limited, anesthesia personnel often place stimulating electrodes on the face with the aim of monitoring the response of the orbicularis oculi or the corrugator supercilii muscles. Improper placement may lead to direct stimulation (and contraction) of these muscles, causing the clinician to underestimate the degree of residual neuromuscular blockade. Acting on this erroneous measurement, the clinician may elect to give more neuromuscular blocker than necessary, or, of greater concern, lead them to underdose reversal agents when preparing their patient for emergence from anesthesia.

For optimal performance, the accelerometer of a neuromuscular monitor must be placed on a digit that can move freely. When the extremities are in a tucked position, this may limit their accuracy and utility. Even properly placed acceleromyography monitors can frequently report a baseline TOF ratio that is greater than 1 (as high as 1.6 with some models). This anomaly may cause acceleromyography to underestimate residual neuromuscular blockade.[107,110] Newer electromyography devices do not rely on actual muscle movement, enabling them to be applied to extremities that will be tucked. However, their accuracy may be hindered by the multiple sources of electromagnetic interference in the OR, including electrocautery. Further research is needed to justify electromyography as a replacement for acceleromyography in clinical practice.[106]

Future Trends in Monitoring

Anesthesiologists have been at the forefront of the incorporation of innovative biomedical devices and technologies into their practice. We will continue to adapt our practice to make use of new technologies to enhance patient safety. There are three trends in device design that appear most likely to lead to further improvements in our practice: greater automated marshaling of monitoring and clinical data, the dissemination of our current devices into wider hospital use, and the development of devices with greater algorithmic sophistication to obtain clinical data less invasively.

The Anesthesia Information Management Systems (AIMS) will continue to become more interconnected with patient monitoring devices, as well as with drug delivery systems such as infusion pumps and vaporizers. The AIMS will also begin to interface more deeply with hospital-wide Computerized Provider Order Entry (CPOE) systems, allowing patient clinical data and documentation to be available immediately to the anesthesiologist. The safety of the administration of intravenous medications will be enhanced by the routine use of machine-readable labels, whether by barcoding or radiofrequency identification (RFID), so that the intended administration of a medication will be known to the AIMS prior to the actual administration. The AIMS will make use of this information to alert to the potential for drug interactions and allergies during the case itself immediately prior to administration. The automatic availability of this data will allow the AIMS to provide decision support to the anesthesiologist, tracking the administration of intravenous medications and providing predictions of plasma and effect site concentrations to improve dose titration. Overall, improvements in the automated marshaling and display of patient data will assist the anesthesiologist with situational awareness. Further, using more intelligent alarm systems to decrease false-positive alerts will more accurately guide the anesthesiologist to aspects of the patient's management that require attention. The sophistication of AIMS user interfaces will continue to improve so that the interaction between the anesthesiologist and the tasks of computer-based monitoring and charting will become smooth, fast, natural, and efficient.

In the recent revision of the ASA Standards for Basic Monitoring, the indications for capnography have been broadened to include the evaluation of ventilation during moderate or deep sedation. Moderate sedation may be performed by clinicians untrained in the practice of anesthesia; the effect of this standard will be the dissemination of capnographic equipment previously used only by anesthesiologists to the wider care environment. Anesthesiologists should be at the forefront of educational efforts to ensure that our medical colleagues use these devices appropriately, enhancing patient safety.

11 A trend in the development of biomedical devices is toward devices that use complex algorithmic models to infer clinical data in a less invasive or more rapid manner. Examples are arterial waveform CO monitors that produce an estimate of CO from the arterial pressure tracing alone, noninvasive hemoglobin monitors that estimate serum hemoglobin from infrared pulse oximetry, target-controlled infusion pumps that make use of population pharmacokinetic and pharmacodynamics data to estimate the redistribution and effect of a medication, and processed EEG monitors that attempt to reduce an ensemble of EEG data to a quantitated end point of consciousness. These devices are examples of incredible biomedical sophistication, usually the product of decades of scientific research and subsequent engineering refinement. However, the algorithms that these devices use are generally derived from the responses of healthy volunteers. The protocols used for the development of the algorithms are often seemingly simplistic or artificial when compared to the complexity of actual anesthetic practice. The result is that, during their initial introduction to practice, the functionality of the devices in the sickest of patients is not necessarily well characterized or understood. To put it more briefly: it may work, but does it *really* work? It is our sickest patients who have the most to gain from devices that allow us to assess their clinical condition more rapidly and less invasively, but it is our sickest patients who are the most vulnerable should the devices tend to become inaccurate under just those clinical conditions. The limits of the reliability and clinical applicability of these devices must be a matter of concern for the practicing anesthesiologist. Though devices are becoming "smarter," that knowledge does not excuse us of the knowledge to know how to employ them wisely.

For additional information please see 18 Video 26-18 in the eBook bundled with this text.

For further review and interactivities, please see the videos and narrative interactive clinical vignettes (NICVs) accessible in the complimentary eBook bundled with this text. Access instructions are located on the inside front cover.

REFERENCES

1. American Society of Anesthesiologists. *Standards for Basic Anesthetic Monitoring*. 2020.
2. Merilainen PT. A differential paramagnetic sensor for breath-by-breath oximetry. *J Clin Monit*. 1990;6:65–73.
3. Roe PG, Tyler CK, Tennant R, Barnes PK. Oxygen analysers. An evaluation of five fuel cell models. *Anaesthesia*. 1987;42:175–181.
4. Barker L, Webb RK, Runciman WB, Van der Walt JH. The Australian Incident Monitoring Study. The oxygen analyser: applications and limitations – an analysis of 200 incident reports. *Anaesth Intensive Care*. 1993;21:570–574.
5. Kaddoum RN, Chidiac EJ, Zestos MM, Ahmed Z. Electrocautery-induced fire during adenotonsillectomy: report of two cases. *J Clin Anesth*. 2006;18:129–131.
6. Roy S, Smith LP. What does it take to start an oropharyngeal fire? Oxygen requirements to start fires in the operating room. *Int J Pediatr Otorhinolaryngol*. 2011;75:227–230.
7. Ortega R, Hansen CJ, Elterman K, Woo A. Videos in clinical medicine. Pulse oximetry. *N Engl J Med*. 2011;364:e33.
8. Barker SJ, Curry J, Redford D, Morgan S. Measurement of carboxyhemoglobin and methemoglobin by pulse oximetry: a human volunteer study. *Anesthesiology*. 2006;105:892–897.
9. Barker SJ. "Motion-resistant" pulse oximetry: a comparison of new and old models. *Anesth Analg*. 2002;95:967–972.
10. Nishiyama T. Pulse oximeters demonstrate different responses during hypothermia and changes in perfusion. *Can J Anaesth*. 2006;53:136–138.
11. Rolf N, Cote C. Diagnosis of clinically unrecognized endobronchial intubation in paediatric anaesthesia: which is more sensitive, pulse oximetry or capnography? *Paediatr Anaesth*. 1992;2:31–35.
12. Murat I, Constant I, Maud'huy H. Perioperative anaesthetic morbidity in children: a database of 24,165 anaesthetics over a 30-month period. *Paediatr Anaesth*. 2004;14:158–166.
13. Walder B, Lauber R, Zbinden AM. Accuracy and cross-sensitivity of 10 different anesthetic gas monitors. *J Clin Monit*. 1993;9:364–373.
14. Colman Y, Krauss B. Microstream capnograpy technology: a new approach to an old problem. *J Clin Monit Comput*. 1999;15:403–409.
15. Edmonds A, Stambaugh H, Pettey S, Daratha KB. Evidence-based project: cost savings and reduction in environmental release with low-flow anesthesia. *AANA J*. 2021;89:27–33.
16. Eger EI, 2nd, Saidman LJ, Brandstater B. Minimum alveolar anesthetic concentration: a standard of anesthetic potency. *Anesthesiology*. 1965;26:756–763.
17. Hendrickx JFA, De Wolf AM. End-tidal anesthetic concentration: monitoring, interpretation, and clinical application. *Anesthesiology*. 2022;136:985–996.
18. Avidan MS, Jacobsohn E, Glick D, et al. Prevention of intraoperative awareness in a high-risk surgical population. *N Engl J Med*. 2011;365:591–600.
19. Patel R, Lenczyk M, Hannallah RS, McGill WA. Age and the onset of desaturation in apnoeic children. *Can J Anaesth*. 1994;41:771–774.
20. Weiss M, Dullenkopf A, Fischer JE, Keller C, Gerber AC; European Paediatric Endotracheal Intubation Study G. Prospective randomized controlled multi-centre trial of cuffed or uncuffed endotracheal tubes in small children. *Br J Anaesth*. 2009;103:867–873.
21. Kugelman A, Zeiger-Aginsky D, Bader D, Shoris I, Riskin A. A novel method of distal end-tidal CO_2 capnography in intubated infants: comparison with arterial CO2 and with proximal mainstream end-tidal CO_2. *Pediatrics*. 2008;122:e1219–e1224.
22. Hagerty JJ, Kleinman ME, Zurakowski D, Lyons AC, Krauss B. Accuracy of a new low-flow sidestream capnography technology in newborns: a pilot study. *J Perinatol*. 2002;22:219–225.
23. Kleinman B, Powell S, Kumar P, Gardner RM. The fast flush test measures the dynamic response of the entire blood pressure monitoring system. *Anesthesiology*. 1992;77:1215–1220.
24. Golamari R, Gilchrist IC. Collateral circulation testing of the hand—is it relevant now? A narrative review. *Am J Med Sci*. 2021;361:702–710.
25. Tegtmeyer K, Brady G, Lai S, Hodo R, Braner D. Videos in clinical medicine. Placement of an arterial line. *N Engl J Med*. 2006;354:e13.
26. Levin PD, Sheinin O, Gozal Y. Use of ultrasound guidance in the insertion of radial artery catheters. *Crit Care Med*. 2003;31:481–484.
27. Vender JS, Watts DR. Differential diagnosis of hand ischemia in the presence of an arterial cannula. *Anesth Analg*. 1982;61:465–468.
28. Adelman RD, Morrell RE. Coarctation of the abdominal aorta and renal artery stenosis related to an umbilical artery catheter placement in a neonate. *Pediatrics*. 2000;106:e36.
29. Ishii S, Shime N, Shibasaki M, Sawa T. Ultrasound-guided radial artery catheterization in infants and small children. *Pediatr Crit Care Med*. 2013;14:471–473.
30. Venkataraman ST, Thompson AE, Orr RA. Femoral vascular catheterization in critically ill infants and children. *Clin Pediatr (Phila)*. 1997;36:311–319.

31. Iwashima S, Ishikawa T, Ohzeki T. Ultrasound-guided versus landmark-guided femoral vein access in pediatric cardiac catheterization. *Pediatr Cardiol*. 2008;29:339–342.
32. Weiss M, Balmer C, Cornelius A, Frey B, Bauersfeld U, Baenziger O. Arterial fast bolus flush systems used routinely in neonates and infants cause retrograde embolization of flush solution into the central arterial and cerebral circulation. *Can J Anaesth*. 2003;50:386–391.
33. Ng KG, Small CF. Survey of automated noninvasive blood pressure monitors. *J Clin Eng*. 1994;19:452–475.
34. Swei SC, Liou CC, Liu HH, Hung PC. Acute radial nerve injury associated with an automatic blood pressure monitor. *Acta Anaesthesiol Taiwan*. 2009;47:147–149.
35. Jones DW, Appel LJ, Sheps SG, Roccella EJ, Lenfant C. Measuring blood pressure accurately: new and persistent challenges. *JAMA*. 2003;289:1027–1030.
36. Bowen RES, Graetz TJ, Emmert DA, Avidan MS. Statistics of heart failure and mechanical circulatory support in 2020. *Ann Transl Med*. 2020;8:827.
37. van Egmond J, Hasenbos M, Crul JF. Invasive v. non-invasive measurement of arterial pressure. Comparison of two automatic methods and simultaneously measured direct intra-arterial pressure. *Br J Anaesth*. 1985;57:434–444.
38. Harrison MJ, Connor CW. Statistics-based alarms from sequential physiological measurements. *Anaesthesia*. 2007;62:1015–1023.
39. Block FE, Schulte GT. Ankle blood pressure measurement, an acceptable alternative to arm measurements. *Int J Clin Monit Comput*. 1996;13:167–171.
40. Emerick DR. An evaluation of non-invasive blood pressure (NIBP) monitoring on the wrist: comparison with upper arm NIBP measurement. *Anaesth Intensive Care*. 2002;30:43–47.
41. Singer AJ, Kahn SR, Thode HC, Jr., Hollander JE. Comparison of forearm and upper arm blood pressures. *Prehosp Emerg Care*. 1999;3:123–126.
42. Zahn J, Bernstein H, Hossain S, Bodian C, Beilin Y. Comparison of non-invasive blood pressure measurements on the arm and calf during cesarean delivery. *J Clin Monit Comput*. 2000;16:557–562.
43. König K, Casalaz DM, Burke EJ, Watkins A. Accuracy of non-invasive blood pressure monitoring in very preterm infants. *Intensive Care Med*. 2012;38:670–676.
44. West JB, Dollery CT, Naimark A. Distribution of blood flow in isolated lung; relation to vascular and alveolar pressures. *J Appl Physiol*. 1964;19:713–724.
45. Shah MR, Hasselblad V, Stevenson LW, et al. Impact of the pulmonary artery catheter in critically ill patients: meta-analysis of randomized clinical trials. *JAMA*. 2005;294:1664–1670.
46. Ortega R, Song M, Hansen CJ, Barash P. Videos in clinical medicine. Ultrasound-guided internal jugular vein cannulation. *N Engl J Med*. 2010;362:e57.
47. Saugel B, Scheeren TWL, Teboul JL. Ultrasound-guided central venous catheter placement: a structured review and recommendations for clinical practice. *Crit Care*. 2017;21:225.
48. Pronovost P, Needham D, Berenholtz S, et al. An intervention to decrease catheter-related bloodstream infections in the ICU. *N Engl J Med*. 2006;355:2725–2732.
49. Costello JM, Clapper TC, Wypij D. Minimizing complications associated with percutaneous central venous catheter placement in children: recent advances. *Pediatr Crit Care Med*. 2013;14:273–283.
50. Casado-Flores J, Barja J, Martino R, Serrano A, Valdivielso A. Complications of central venous catheterization in critically ill children. *Pediatr Crit Care Med*. 2001;2:57–62.
51. Branthwaite MA, Bradley RD. Measurement of cardiac output by thermal dilution in man. *J Appl Physiol*. 1968;24:434–438.
52. Mihm FG, Gettinger A, Hanson CW 3rd, et al. A multicenter evaluation of a new continuous cardiac output pulmonary artery catheter system. *Crit Care Med*. 1998;26:1346–1350.
53. Koo KK, Sun JC, Zhou Q, et al. Pulmonary artery catheters: evolving rates and reasons for use. *Crit Care Med*. 2011;39:1613–1618.
54. Kelly CR, Rabbani LE. Videos in clinical medicine. Pulmonary-artery catheterization. *N Engl J Med*. 2013;369:e35.
55. Pearl RG, Rosenthal MH, Nielson L, Ashton JP, Brown BW Jr. Effect of injectate volume and temperature on thermodilution cardiac output determination. *Anesthesiology*. 1986;64:798–801.
56. Egan JR, Festa M, Cole AD, Nunn GR, Gillis J, Winlaw DS. Clinical assessment of cardiac performance in infants and children following cardiac surgery. *Intensive Care Med*. 2005;31:568–573.
57. McLuckie A, Murdoch IA, Marsh MJ, Anderson D. A comparison of pulmonary and femoral artery thermodilution cardiac indices in paediatric intensive care patients. *Acta Paediatr*. 1996;85:336–338.
58. Harvey S, Harrison DA, Singer M, et al. Assessment of the clinical effectiveness of pulmonary artery catheters in management of patients in intensive care (PAC-Man): a randomised controlled trial. *Lancet*. 2005;366:472–477.
59. American Society of Anesthesiologists Task Force on Pulmonary Artery Catheterization. Practice guidelines for pulmonary artery catheterization: an updated report by the American Society of Anesthesiologists Task Force on Pulmonary Artery Catheterization. *Anesthesiology*. 2003;99:988–1014.
60. Thiele RH, Durieux ME. Arterial waveform analysis for the anesthesiologist: past, present, and future concepts. *Anesth Analg*. 2011;113:766–776.
61. Penaz J. Photoelectric measurement of blood pressure, volume and flow in the finger. Digest of the 10th International Conference on Medical and Biological Engineering. *Dresden*. 1973:102–104.
62. Martina JR, Westerhof BE, van Goudoever J, et al. Noninvasive continuous arterial blood pressure monitoring with Nexfin(R). *Anesthesiology*. 2012;116:1092–1103.
63. Langewouters GJ, Wesseling KH, Goedhard WJ. The static elastic properties of 45 human thoracic and 20 abdominal aortas in vitro and the parameters of a new model. *J Biomech*. 1984;17:425–435.
64. Maus TM, Lee DE. Arterial pressure-based cardiac output assessment. *J Cardiothorac Vasc Anesth*. 2008;22:468–473.
65. Biais M, Nouette-Gaulain K, Cottenceau V, et al. Cardiac output measurement in patients undergoing liver transplantation: pulmonary artery catheter versus uncalibrated arterial pressure waveform analysis. *Anesth Analg*. 2008;106:1480–1486.
66. Monnet X, Letierce A, Hamzaoui O, et al. Arterial pressure allows monitoring the changes in cardiac output induced by volume expansion but not by norepinephrine. *Crit Care Med*. 2011;39:1394–1399.
67. Meng L, Tran NP, Alexander BS, et al. The impact of phenylephrine, ephedrine, and increased preload on third-generation Vigileo-FloTrac and esophageal Doppler cardiac output measurements. *Anesth Analg*. 2011;113:751–757.
68. Monnet X, Anguel N, Naudin B, Jabot J, Richard C, Teboul JL. Arterial pressure-based cardiac output in septic patients: different accuracy of pulse contour and uncalibrated pressure waveform devices. *Crit Care*. 2010;14:R109.
69. Lorsomradee S, Cromheecke S, De Hert SG. Uncalibrated arterial pulse contour analysis versus continuous thermodilution technique: effects of alterations in arterial waveform. *J Cardiothorac Vasc Anesth*. 2007;21:636–643.
70. Slagt C, Beute J, Hoeksema M, Malagon I, Mulder JW, Groeneveld JA. Cardiac output derived from arterial pressure waveform analysis without calibration vs. thermodilution in septic shock: evolving accuracy of software versions. *Eur J Anaesthesiol*. 2010;27:550–554.
71. Shih BF, Huang PH, Yu HP, et al. Cardiac output assessed by the fourth-generation arterial waveform analysis system Is unreliable in liver transplant recipients. *Transplant Proc*. 2016;48:1170–1175.
72. Calamandrei M, Mirabile L, Muschetta S, Gensini GF, De Simone L, Romano SM. Assessment of cardiac output in children: a comparison between the pressure recording analytical method and Doppler echocardiography. *Pediatr Crit Care Med*. 2008;9:310–312.
73. Urbano J, Lopez J, Gonzalez R, et al. Measurement of cardiac output in children by pressure-recording analytical method. *Pediatr Cardiol*. 2015;36:358–364.
74. Frank SM, Fleisher LA, Breslow MJ, et al. Perioperative maintenance of normothermia reduces the incidence of morbid cardiac events. A randomized clinical trial. *JAMA*. 1997;277:1127–1134.
75. Kurz A, Sessler DI, Lenhardt R. Perioperative normothermia to reduce the incidence of surgical-wound infection and shorten hospitalization. Study of Wound Infection and Temperature Group. *N Engl J Med*. 1996;334:1209–1215.
76. Vaughan MS, Cork RC, Vaughan RW. Inaccuracy of liquid crystal thermometry to identify core temperature trends in postoperative adults. *Anesth Analg*. 1982;61:284–287.
77. Rampil IJ. A primer for EEG signal processing in anesthesia. *Anesthesiology*. 1998;89:980–1002.
78. Connor CW. A forensic disassembly of the BIS monitor. *Anesth Analg*. 2020;131:1923–1933.
79. Connor CW. Open reimplementation of the BIS algorithms for depth of anesthesia. *Anesth Analg*. 2022;135:855–864.
80. Mashour GA, Alkire MT. Consciousness, anesthesia, and the thalamocortical system. *Anesthesiology*. 2013;118:13–15.
81. Purdon PL, Pierce ET, Mukamel EA, et al. Electroencephalogram signatures of loss and recovery of consciousness from propofol. *Proc Natl Acad Sci USA*. 2013;110:e1142–e1151.
82. Kim D, Ahn JH, Jung H, Choi KY, Jeong JS. Effects of neuromuscular blockade reversal on bispectral index and frontal electromyogram during steady-state desflurane anesthesia: a randomized trial. *Sci Rep*. 2019;9:10486.
83. Messner M, Beese U, Romstock J, Dinkel M, Tschaikowsky K. The bispectral index declines during neuromuscular block in fully awake persons. *Anesth Analg*. 2003;97:488–491.
84. Doyle PW, Matta BF. Burst suppression or isoelectric encephalogram for cerebral protection: evidence from metabolic suppression studies. *Br J Anaesth*. 1999;83:580–584.
85. Brenner RP, Schwartzman RJ, Richey ET. Prognostic significance of episodic low amplitude or relatively isoelectric EEG patterns. *Dis Nerv Syst*. 1975;36:582–587.
86. Tirel O, Wodey E, Harris R, Bansard JY, Ecoffey C, Senhadji L. Variation of bispectral index under TIVA with propofol in a paediatric population. *Br J Anaesth*. 2008;100:82–87.
87. Whitlock EL, Villafranca AJ, Lin N, et al. Relationship between bispectral index values and volatile anesthetic concentrations during the maintenance phase of anesthesia in the B-unaware trial. *Anesthesiology*. 2011;115:1209–1218.
88. Hans P, Dewandre PY, Brichant JF, Bonhomme V. Comparative effects of ketamine on Bispectral Index and spectral entropy of the electroencephalogram under sevoflurane anaesthesia. *Br J Anaesth*. 2005;94:336–340.
89. Faraoni D, Salengros JC, Engelman E, Ickx B, Barvais L. Ketamine has no effect on bispectral index during stable propofol-remifentanil anaesthesia. *Br J Anaesth*. 2009;102:336–369.
90. Yufune S, Takamatsu I, Masui K, Kazama T. Effect of remifentanil on plasma propofol concentration and bispectral index during propofol anaesthesia. *Br J Anaesth*. 2011;106:208–214.
91. Crosby G. General anesthesia–minding the mind during surgery. *N Engl J Med*. 2011;365: 660–661.

92. Pousman RM, Eilers WA 3rd, Johns B, Jung H. Irritant contact dermatitis after use of bispectral index sensor in prone position. *Anesth Analg.* 2002;95:1337–1338.
93. Myles PS, Leslie K, McNeil J, Forbes A, Chan MT. Bispectral index monitoring to prevent awareness during anaesthesia: the B-Aware randomised controlled trial. *Lancet.* 2004;363:1757–1763.
94. Avidan MS, Zhang L, Burnside BA, et al. Anesthesia awareness and the bispectral index. *N Engl J Med.* 2008;358:1097–1108.
95. Davidson AJ, Smith KR, Blusse van Oud-Alblas HJ, et al. Awareness in children: a secondary analysis of five cohort studies. *Anaesthesia.* 2011;66:446–454.
96. Malviya S, Galinkin JL, Bannister CF, et al. The incidence of intraoperative awareness in children: childhood awareness and recall evaluation. *Anesth Analg.* 2009;109:1421–1427.
97. Liu X, Ji J, Zhao GQ. General anesthesia affecting on developing brain: evidence from animal to clinical research. *J Anesth.* 2020;34:765–772.
98. Sinner B, Becke K, Engelhard K. General anaesthetics and the developing brain: an overview. *Anaesthesia.* 2014;69:1009–1022.
99. Davidson AJ, Disma N, de Graaff JC, et al. Neurodevelopmental outcome at 2 years of age after general anaesthesia and awake-regional anaesthesia in infancy (GAS): an international multicentre, randomised controlled trial. *Lancet.* 2016;387:239–250.
100. Warner DO, Zaccariello MJ, Katusic SK, et al. Neuropsychological and behavioral outcomes after exposure of young children to procedures requiring general anesthesia: the Mayo Anesthesia Safety in Kids (MASK) Study. *Anesthesiology.* 2018;129:89–105.
101. Sullivan CA, Egbuta C, Park RS, Lukovits K, Cavanaugh D, Mason KP. The use of bispectral index monitoring does not change intraoperative exposure to volatile anesthetics in children. *J Clin Med.* 2020;9:2437.
102. Sargin M, Uluer MS, Ozmen S. The effects of bispectral index monitoring on hemodynamics and recovery profile in developmentally delayed pediatric patients undergoing dental surgery. *Paediatr Anaesth.* 2015;25:950–955.
103. McLean DJ, Diaz-Gil D, Farhan HN, Ladha KS, Kurth T, Eikermann M. Dose-dependent association between intermediate-acting neuromuscular-blocking agents and postoperative respiratory complications. *Anesthesiology.* 2015;122:1201–1213.
104. Thesleff S. An investigation of the muscle-relaxing action of succinyl-choline-iodide in man. *Acta Physiol Scand.* 1952;25:348–367.
105. Ortega R, Brull SJ, Prielipp R, Gutierrez A, De La Cruz R, Conley CM. Monitoring neuromuscular function. *N Engl J Med.* 2018;378:e6.
106. Bowdle A, Michaelsen K. Quantitative twitch monitoring: what works best and how do we know? *Anesthesiology.* 2021;135:558–561.
107. Kopman AF, Chin W, Cyriac J. Acceleromyography vs. electromyography: an ipsilateral comparison of the indirectly evoked neuromuscular response to train-of-four stimulation. *Acta Anaesthesiol Scand.* 2005;49:316–322.
108. Naguib M, Brull SJ, Kopman AF, et al. Consensus statement on perioperative use of neuromuscular monitoring. *Anesth Analg.* 2018;127:71–80.
109. Faulk DJ, Austin TM, Thomas JJ, Strupp K, Macrae AW, Yaster M. A survey of the society for pediatric anesthesia on the use, monitoring, and antagonism of neuromuscular blockade. *Anesth Analg.* 2021;132:1518–1526.
110. Bowdle A, Jelacic S. Progress towards a standard of quantitative twitch monitoring. *Anaesthesia.* 2020;75:1133–1135.

27 Echocardiography and Point-of-Care Ultrasound

MICHAEL HUA-GEN LI • SUNDAR KRISHNAN • BENJAMIN O'BRIEN • MADHAV SWAMINATHAN • SUSAN WRIGHT

KEY POINTS

1. Understanding the basic principles, utility, and pitfalls of ultrasound is required to optimize image quality and patient benefit, and to minimize patient harm.
2. Comprehensive standard-of-care echocardiographic examination involves a combination of two-dimensional (2D) and three-dimensional (3D) imaging, and Doppler techniques.
3. While global left and right ventricular *systolic* function can be visually estimated or quantitatively measured, several quantitative measurements are required for the diagnosis and grading of *diastolic* function.
4. Regional wall abnormalities are not always straightforward to evaluate, even among expert echocardiographers.
5. Speckle tracking and artificial intelligence are newer modalities that are evolving and will be more widely applied in the future.
6. The assessment of valve pathology should include consideration of the mechanism, etiology, severity, and the associated sequelae.
7. Peak velocity, mean gradient, and aortic valve area are commonly used to grade the severity of aortic stenosis.
8. Echocardiographic features differentiating cardiac tamponade from pericardial effusion include atrial collapse during ventricular systole and right ventricular collapse during diastole.
9. Point-of-care ultrasound (POCUS) for the anesthesiologist goes beyond assessment of cardiac function and hemodynamic status and includes assessment of lung pathology and gastric contents.
10. Certification and training for anesthesiologists in echocardiography and POCUS are available and evolving worldwide.

Introduction

Echocardiography and point-of-care ultrasound (POCUS) have become essential parts of perioperative and peri-interventional anesthesia practice.[1] After early adoption in the perioperative care of patients undergoing cardiac surgery–focused on preoperative diagnosis, perioperative hemodynamic assessment and monitoring, guidance of intervention, and evaluation of surgical results[2]—the last four decades have seen the use of POCUS spread to perioperative assessment and monitoring in noncardiac surgery[3,4] and beyond the operating room to critical care.[5] POCUS furthermore allows evaluation of other organs, such as the lung or stomach. Ultrasound is an established adjunct to interventional procedures, such as intravascular catheter placement and regional anesthesia. Echocardiography and ultrasound in general have therefore become ubiquitous tools for the anesthesiologist, and the application of ultrasound to patient management is now an integral part of modern anesthesia practice. This chapter describes the principles of ultrasound and practical applications of perioperative echocardiography and POCUS, as relevant to the general anesthesiologist.

Physics of Sound

Characteristics of Sound Waves

Knowledge of the characteristics of sound waves is important to an understanding of how ultrasound images are created. Ultrasound transducers use piezoelectric elements (PZEs), which are crystals or crystalline ceramics that expand and contract when an alternating current is applied to them, generating a sound wave that propagates through the adjacent medium, thereby undergoing compression and rarefaction.

The velocity of propagation of the sound wave (V) is equal to the product of the wavelength (λ) and the frequency (f) of the wave:

$$V = f \times \lambda$$

The frequency and the wavelength of the sound wave are therefore inextricably linked and inversely related (Fig. 27-1). With the velocity assumed to be constant, the frequency increases as the wavelength decreases, and *vice versa*. Ultrasound is sound comprising any frequencies higher than those in the audible range (i.e., greater than 20 kHz). In practice, diagnostic ultrasound utilizes high frequencies in the range of 2 to 10 MHz.

The creation of an ultrasound image depends on sound waves being reflected back to the transducer from structures in their path. When activated, each PZE in a transducer emits brief pulses of ultrasound (lasting a few microseconds) that are separated by longer periods of "listening" to receive the reflected signal. When the reflected ultrasound returns to the PZE, it generates an electrical signal that is interpreted by the ultrasound machine.

The ultrasound software measures the time that was taken for this signal to be reflected back to the transducer, from which it then calculates the distance, or depth, of the reflecting object along the scan line. Conveniently, the velocity of sound traveling through blood, muscle, and fat is broadly similar (Table 27-1), and for the purposes of generation of a two-dimensional (2D) ultrasound image, an averaged velocity of 1,540 ms^{-1} is used by the software to calculate the depth of a reflecting object. Sound reflected from deeper structures takes longer to return to the transducer and so these signals are drawn deeper in the constructed image displayed on the screen.

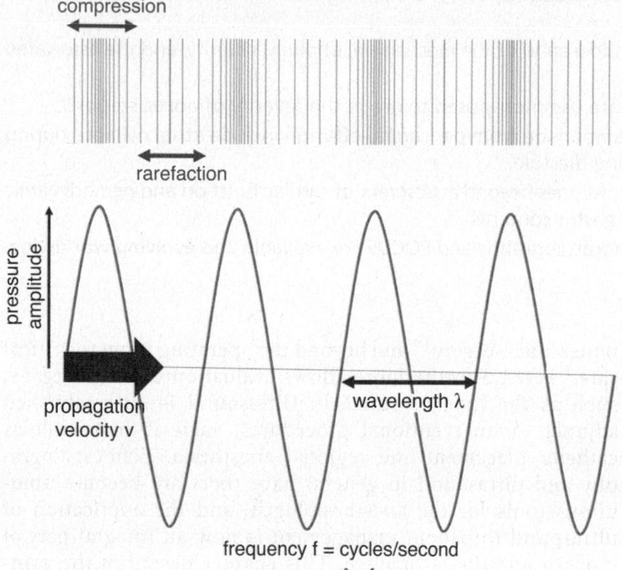

Figure 27-1 Characteristics of a sound wave.

Table 27-1 Velocity of Sound in Different Tissues

Average velocity of sound in soft tissue = 1,540 m/s	
Medium	**Velocity (m/s)**
Air	330
Lung	600
Bone	4,080
Muscle	1,580
Fat	1,450
Blood	1,560

Reflection

Reflection occurs when the ultrasound beam meets an interface between media of differing *acoustic impedance* (which is related to the density of the medium). The greater the difference in acoustic impedance at the interface, the greater the proportion of ultrasound that is reflected. The stronger the reflected signal, the brighter the object appears on the display. Therefore, most of the ultrasound that meets the surface of a structure that has high acoustic impedance, such as bone, is reflected back to the transducer, leaving an "acoustic shadow" in the image beyond the reflecting surface. This phenomenon also applies to metallic or calcified structures, such as prosthetic heart valves or plaques, which have a similarly high acoustic impedance (Fig. 27-2).

Conversely, homogeneous media such as blood do not reflect the ultrasound signal traveling through them because there is no change in acoustic impedance; blood-filled spaces such as blood vessels and cardiac chambers are therefore *echolucent* and typically appear black on screen.

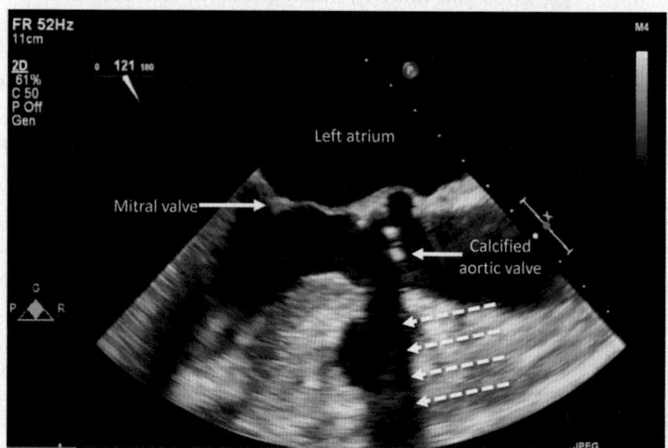

Figure 27-2 Acoustic shadow artifact. Acoustic shadow (*dashed lines*) formed in the far field by echodense calcification of the aortic valve obscuring any signals along the path of the ultrasound beam.

Resolution and Image Optimization

Temporal Resolution

Clinical 2D echocardiography is performed using *phased array* transducers, in which PZEs are fired in a phasic manner to direct the ultrasound beam in a specific direction. This allows a large area of scanning while maintaining a relatively small transducer footprint. A *sector* scan is typically compiled from 96 to 256 ultrasound scan lines. The rate at which this 2D scan image is refreshed (the *frame rate*) depends on how many scan lines are activated (sector width) and how far the ultrasound needs to travel into the tissues (sector depth). The sector width and depth can be set by the operator. The aim is to minimize the size of the sector such that it contains only the structures being studied, so that the frame rate, and therefore the *temporal resolution,* is maximized. A frame rate of approximately 25 fps is seen as smooth motion by the human eye. At frame rates below this, which may, for example, be seen in three-dimensional (3D) ultrasound imaging, the image appears jerky.

In *M-mode ("motion-mode") imaging,* the reflected signal from a single line of ultrasound is plotted against time (Fig. 27-3). As there is only one scan line, the temporal resolution is maximal since it is not hampered by the time taken for the signal to "sweep" across the field. M-mode imaging is therefore useful to examine the motion of rapidly moving structures, such as valve leaflets. It is also commonly used to measure distances along the scan line, though this may not be accurate due to incorrect angulation, and measurements should be taken in 2D images.

Spatial Resolution

For two reflectors in the path of the scan line to be distinguishable as separate structures, the duration of the emitted pulse of ultrasound needs to be short so that the signals reflected at successive interfaces do not merge. The shorter the wavelength, the shorter the achievable pulse duration. In practice the shortest pulse that can be emitted is 2 wavelengths, so two structures along the path of a line of ultrasound need to be more than one wavelength apart to generate distinct reflected signals. It follows that high-frequency transducers provide better resolution along the path of the scan line ("axial resolution") than low-frequency transducers.

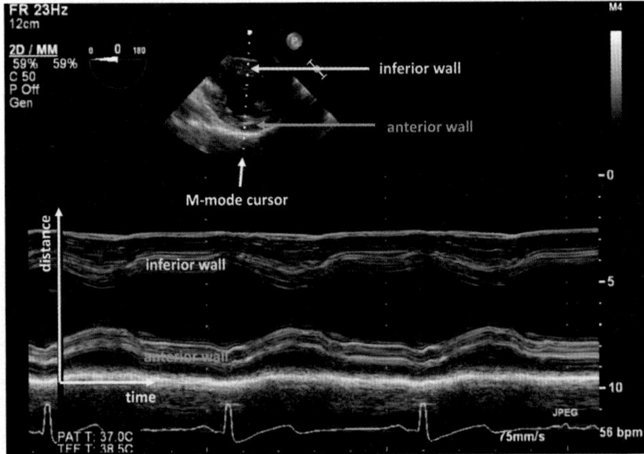

Figure 27-3 M-mode imaging. M-mode display of the left ventricle in a transgastric midpapillary short-axis view. The operator places the M-mode cursor in the required position on the 2D image. The position of structures on the *single line* is plotted against time.

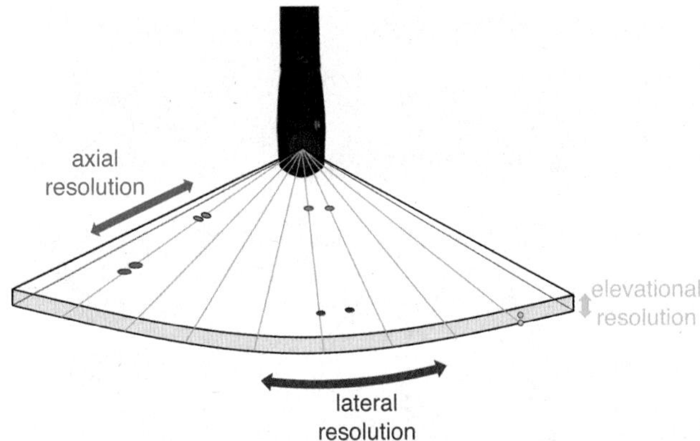

Figure 27-4 Spatial resolution. Spatial resolution of the ultrasound image. Lateral resolution (*red and orange dots*), axial resolution (*blue and purple dots*), and elevational resolution (*green dots*).

In practice, a 5-MHz transducer emits an ultrasound signal with a wavelength of just over 0.3 mm, which approximates to the axial resolution of the image. In order to be identified as separate structures, two reflectors lying along the scan line would therefore need to be more than 0.3 mm apart. Ultrasound signals emitted by a 10-MHz probe have half that wavelength and would therefore be able to achieve a greater axial resolution of 0.15 mm.

However, while high-frequency waves provide better axial resolution in an ultrasound image, they are absorbed by tissue to a greater degree than lower-frequency waves. This is relevant to diagnostic imaging, limiting the depth of a high-resolution image, as the strength of the high-frequency signal diminishes rapidly as the sound travels into tissue. A pediatric sonographer, for example, may select a higher-frequency echocardiographic probe to generate a high-resolution image over the smaller depth of field required. In contrast, the greater depth of field required to image an adult heart requires the use of a lower-frequency probe, albeit at the cost of image quality from lower axial resolution.

Since an ultrasound beam spreads out and is not parallel sided, scan lines diverge moving away from the transducer. The distance between the scan lines increases as they move toward the far end of the sector. Structures that lie between the scan lines are not registered and the echocardiography system averages the signals from adjacent lines to fill in the space between them in the ultrasound image (Fig. 27-4). The result of this in practical terms is that the ability of the machine to distinguish two structures side by side deeper in the scanned sector is lower than its ability to do so in the narrower part of the beam nearer the probe where the scan lines are closer together. In other words, the *lateral resolution* decreases with distance from the probe. The lateral resolution in a 2D ultrasound image is equal to approximately depth/50. At a depth of 5 cm, therefore, the lateral resolution is approximately 1 mm, while at a depth of 10 cm, it drops to approximately 2 mm. The shape of the beam may be manipulated by the operator by setting a focal point just deep to a structure of interest to ensure that it lies within a region where the beam is narrowest and therefore resolution is greatest.

Structures close to the probe are imaged best and the clinician should select imaging planes that place a structure of interest as close to the probe as possible. For example, there are no transesophageal echocardiography (TEE) imaging planes in which the pulmonic valve, one of the most anterior structures in the heart, is close to the probe, and structural assessment of the pulmonic valve is therefore frequently better performed using transthoracic echocardiography (TTE), where the surface probe is closer to the valve.

Elevational resolution is analogous to lateral resolution but applies to distinguishing structures that are positioned perpendicular

Figure 27-5 Reverberation and Mirror-Image artifact. Mirror-image artifact and reverberation generated by the strongly echogenic wall of the aortic arch. The aortic wall generates both reverberation artifact and a mirror-image artifact, resulting in an apparent second aorta.

to the sector scan. A 2D sector scan produces a tomographic image that is not completely flat but has a certain slice thickness, as the beam spreads. All objects existing in that slice are displayed as if they existed in one plane. Elevational resolution is approximately equal to the depth/30; so at a depth of 10 cm, it is approximately 3.3 mm.

Common Artifacts

1 Artifacts often occur when reflected ultrasound meets a second strong reflector in its path back to the transducer, leading the software to interpret the signal as returning from a deeper structure. Two mechanisms are particularly common:

1. "Back-and-forth" bouncing of the signal between parallel reflectors causes the complex returning signal to be displayed as a streak-like shape, called a "reverberation" or "comet tail" artifact.
2. When the returning ultrasound is deflected by an angled reflecting surface, the software might produce two images of one anatomical structure, both with the same distance to the angled reflection surface. This is called "mirror-image" artifact.

Both "reverberation artifact" and "mirror-image artifact" can occur in the same image. In the clinical application of TEE, this is most commonly seen during imaging of the descending thoracic aorta (Fig. 27-5). The aortic wall is a strong reflector. Ultrasound reflected by the wall further away from the probe may, on its return, bounce off the nearer wall before again being reflected back to the probe by the deeper wall. Some of the emitted signal, therefore, travels an extended distance before being received by the transducer, which the machine erroneously interprets as if the ultrasound had been reflected in a simple round trip by a second structure behind the aorta. The resulting mirror-image appearance of a "double" aorta can sometimes be mistaken for an aortic dissection.

Doppler Echocardiography

The Doppler Principle

When a sound wave is reflected by a moving object, the frequency 2
of the reflected signal is different from that of the emitted wave (Fig. 27-6):

- Sound reflected by an object moving away from the transducer has a lower frequency.
- Sound reflected by an object moving toward the transducer has a higher frequency.

The magnitude of the change in frequency, or *frequency shift*, depends on the velocity of the reflecting object moving toward or away from the transducer. The frequency shift of ultrasound reflected by moving red cells can be analyzed by the ultrasound machine to determine the velocity of blood flow.

The ultrasound machine can only register the component vector of the velocity that is directly toward or away from the transducer. If the Doppler signal is not well aligned with the direction of blood flow, then the calculated velocity will underestimate the true velocity of flow. Malalignment of 20 degrees corresponds to an underestimation of the true velocity by 6%. During an echocardiographic examination, the Doppler signal should therefore be placed within 20 degrees of the direction of blood flow to ensure a measurement error of less than 6%.

Doppler Imaging Modes

Pulsed Wave Doppler

The velocity of blood flow at a specific point in the heart can be measured by analyzing the Doppler shift of an ultrasound signal reflected by red blood cells at the chosen site. A cursor, or *sample volume*, can be positioned in a 2D image to determine the site of measurement. The ultrasound machine determines the

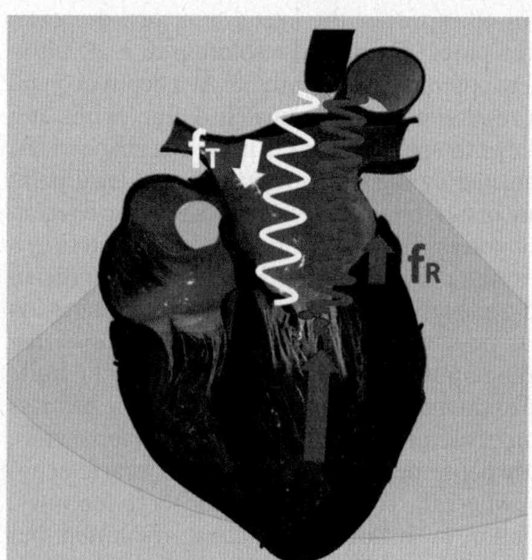

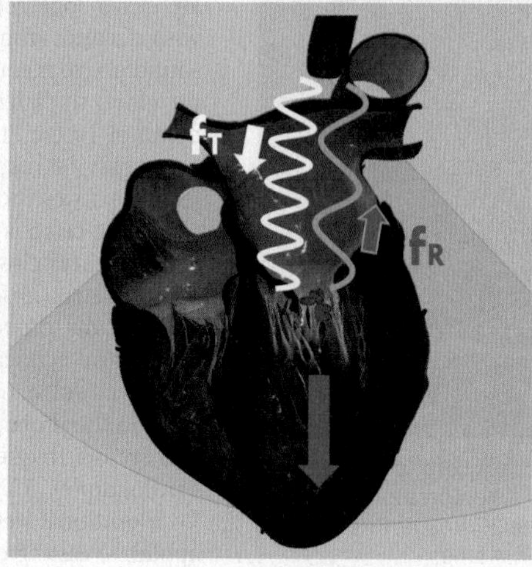

Figure 27-6 The Doppler principle. Sound reflected from an object moving toward the transducer (**left**) has a higher frequency (f_R) than the frequency (f_T) of the transmitted signal. Conversely, the frequency of the ultrasound reflected by an object moving away from the transducer is lower (**right**).

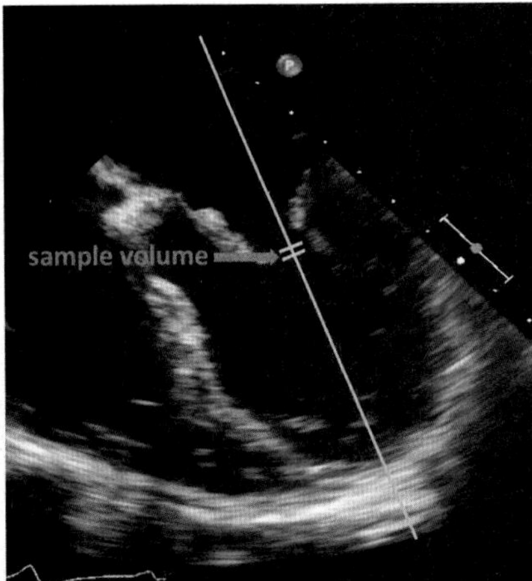

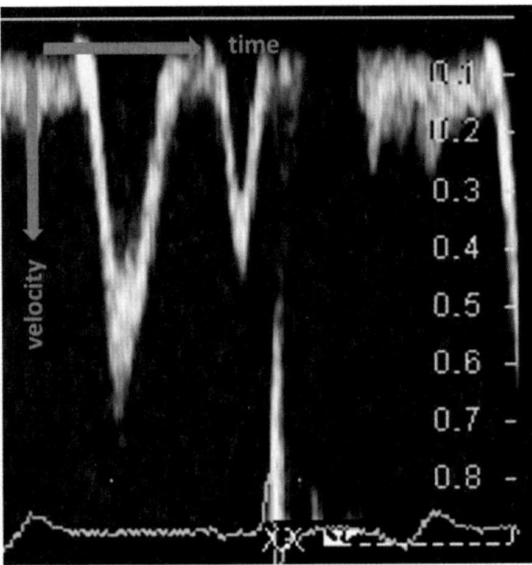

Figure 27-7 Pulsed wave Doppler spectral display. Pulsed wave Doppler spectral display of velocity of blood flow through the mitral valve in the midesophageal four-chamber view. The sample volume has been positioned by the operator at the level of the leaflet tips. Flow is away from the probe and therefore plotted below the baseline.

distance of the sample volume from the transducer, and calculates the time taken for a reflected ultrasound signal to return to the transducer from that point. One or several PZEs in the transducer will emit a pulse of ultrasound of known frequency and, after the calculated time for return of the signal from the site of the sample volume, will switch mode to receive the reflected signal. A subsequent ultrasound pulse is transmitted as soon as the reflection from the previous pulse is received. Analysis of the frequency shift of this reflected wave allows calculation of velocity of the reflecting red cells, equating to velocity of blood flow. The velocity of flow is plotted against time in a *spectral display* (Fig. 27-7).

A reflected wave needs to be sampled at least twice during one cycle for its wavelength and frequency to be measured. This can become difficult if the velocity is high and the sample volume is far from the transducer. The further the sample volume from the transducer, the lower the sample rate of the reflected signal, because the time taken for the signal to return to the transducer is longer. If the blood flow velocity is high, the frequency shift will also be high. The sample rate may be insufficient to sample this reflected signal twice in each cycle. This phenomenon is called *aliasing*, and it causes the machine to produce an ambiguous result in terms of the perceived direction of flow. In practice, this means that when the velocity increases above a certain limit (the *Nyquist limit*), the calculated velocity is displayed as being in the opposite direction to the true direction of flow. Aliasing limits the maximum velocity that can be measured at any particular point in the image. The advantage of PWD is that velocity can be measured at a precise location; the price of this specificity is the inability to measure high velocities.

Color Doppler Imaging

Color Doppler imaging is a form of PWD imaging. A region of interest (ROI) is positioned in a 2D ultrasound image by the sonographer. The ultrasound machine analyzes data received from multiple sample volumes within the ROI to determine the velocities of flow within the chosen area. These velocities are represented as colors within the ROI according to a color map: a key by which colors are assigned to specific velocities. Ultrasound machines have a range of color maps that the clinician can choose as appropriate for the study (Fig. 27-8).

The Nyquist limit is displayed by the color map on the ultrasound screen. As the velocity of flow exceeds the Nyquist limit it is represented by colors that lie at the opposite extreme of the color map, thereby visualizing the phenomenon of aliasing (Fig. 27-9).

Tissue Doppler Imaging

Tissue velocities can be measured in the same way that blood flow velocities are measured using PWD imaging, by placing a Doppler cursor at a point of interest in a 2D image (Fig. 27-10). Tissue

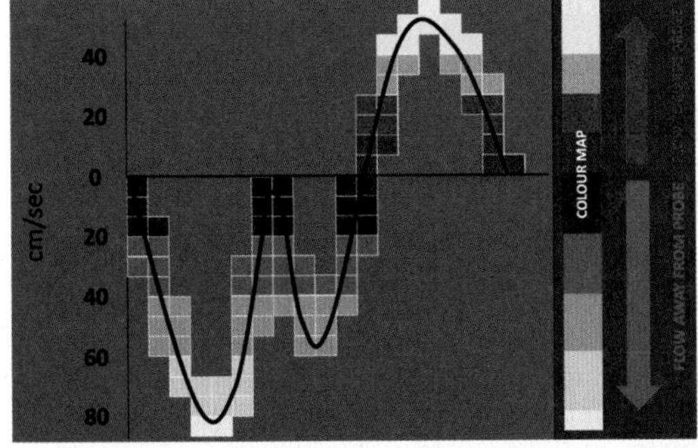

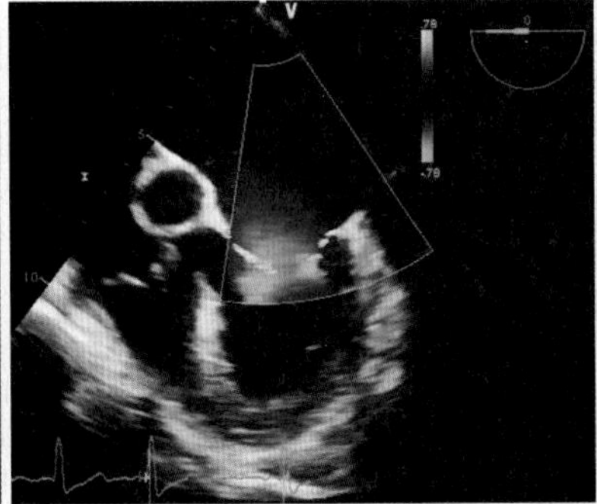

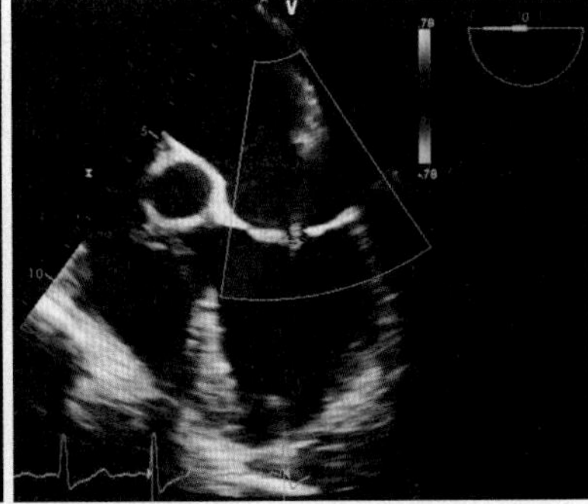

Figure 27-8 Color Doppler imaging. Each velocity is ascribed a color according to a color map selected by the operator (**left panel**). The most frequently used convention for color mapping is for flow away from the probe to be represented by blue shades, and flow toward the probe to be represented by red ("blue away, red toward" or "BART"). In this example, the region of interest has been positioned over the mitral valve and left atrium (LA) to interrogate transmitral flow. Normal forward flow from the LA to the left ventricle (away from the probe) is seen as blue in the central panel, higher velocities being seen as paler blue. A mitral regurgitant jet of blood entering the LA is flow toward the probe and is therefore predominantly red. Higher velocities are orange and yellow, according to the color map.

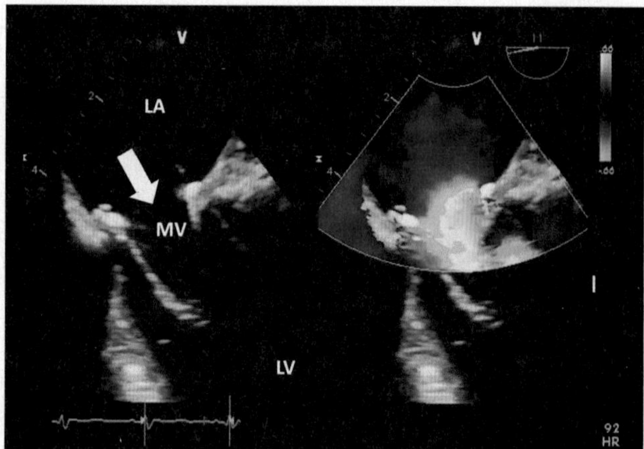

Figure 27-9 Aliasing. Color Doppler display of flow across a repaired mitral valve in an ME4C view. Flow approaching the mitral valve (MV) from the left atrium (LA) accelerates toward the orifice and is represented by increasingly pale blue colors (flow away from the probe). Once the velocity of flow exceeds the Nyquist limit of 66 cm/s, the color display aliases, and faster velocities are represented by yellow and then orange. Note that the fastest velocities in each direction on the color map are plotted next to each other in the image. This distinguishes aliasing from flow in opposite directions, where the slowest velocities are adjacent to each other in the image. LV, left ventricle; ME4C, midesophageal four chamber.

velocities are much lower than blood flow velocities, although they have higher amplitudes (and thus appear brighter).

Continuous Wave Doppler Imaging

CWD imaging (Fig. 27-11) can overcome this limitation on the maximum measurable velocity of flow that affects PWD. In CWD mode, a Doppler signal is continuously emitted by PZE, while the reflected signal from all points along the chosen path of ultrasound through the tissue is continuously received by an adjacent PZE. The receiving PZE continuously registers the velocity of blood flow at all points along the scan line. However, this means that the precise position of the highest velocity of flow along the interrogated scan line cannot be determined. Whereas PWD can suffer from the problem of *aliasing*, CWD suffers from so-called *range ambiguity*.

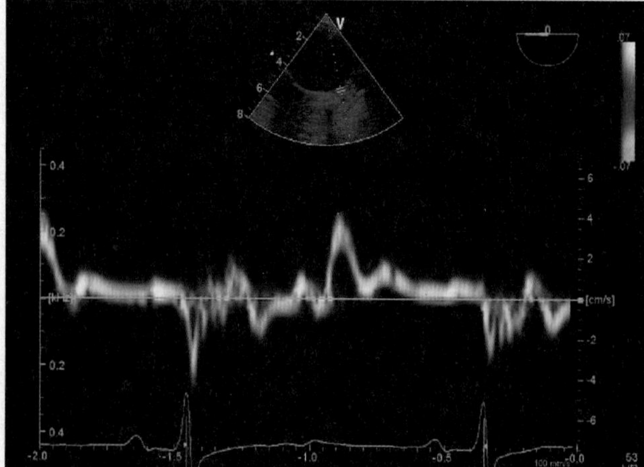

Figure 27-10 Tissue Doppler imaging. Tissue Doppler imaging spectral display of lateral mitral annular movement in an midesophageal four-chamber view.

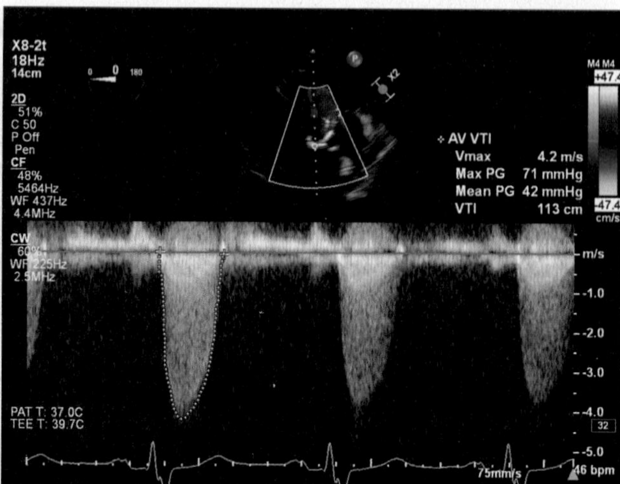

Figure 27-11 Continuous wave Doppler (CWD) imaging. Continuous wave Doppler display of an aortic stenosis jet in the deep transgastric five-chamber view. The high-velocity flow is directed from the left ventricular outflow tract through a stenotic aortic valve away from the probe. The spectral representation of this flow is therefore below the baseline.

Hemodynamic Assessment

Velocity

The velocity of flow can be measured using Doppler imaging. Velocities may be represented in a spectral display of velocity plotted against time or as a color Doppler image, as described above. Accurate measurement of velocity is dependent on careful positioning of the sample volume or continuous wave cursor in the ultrasound image, with particular attention to alignment of the Doppler signal with the direction of blood flow.

Gradient

The velocity of flow of fluid through an orifice is determined by the pressure gradient across the orifice and the area through which the fluid travels. This relationship is expressed in the Bernoulli equation, which also takes other variables such as fluid density and viscous friction into account. For the purposes of clinical echocardiography, the equation is used in a simplified form to allow calculation of the gradient across an orifice from the measured velocity of flow:

$$\text{Gradient} = 4 \times \text{Velocity}^2$$

Inputting a measured peak velocity (V_{max}) into the equation will provide the peak gradient. The peak gradient is used in the calculation of stenotic and regurgitant valvular lesions, which can then be used to either grade their severity or derive adjacent chamber or vessel pressures during the same point in the cardiac cycle (Table 27-2). When the outline of a velocity curve in a Doppler spectral display is traced, the machine can calculate a mean gradient by calculating the mean of the calculated instantaneous gradients throughout the period of flow (Fig. 27-12).

Stroke Distance, Stroke Volume, and Cardiac Output

Similarly, the area under a velocity curve (AUC) in a Doppler spectral display can be calculated if the waveform is traced by the

Table 27-2 Derivations of Cardiac Chamber Pressures

Pressure	Equation
RSVP or PASP	$= 4(V_{TR})^2 + RAP$
MPAP	$= 4(V_{early}\ PI)^2 + RAP$
PADP	$= 4(V_{end}\ PI)^2 + RAP$
LAP	$= SBP - 4(V_{MR})^2$
LVEDP	$= DBP - 4(V_{end\ AI})^2$

AI, aortic insufficiency; DBP, diastolic blood pressure; LAP, left atrial pressure; LVEDP, left ventricular end-diastolic pressure; MPAP, mean pulmonary artery pressure; MR, mitral regurgitation; PADP, pulmonary artery diastolic pressure; PASP, pulmonary artery systolic pressure; PI, pulmonic valve insufficiency; RAP, right atrial pressure; RVSP, right systolic ventricular pressure; SBP, systolic blood pressure; TR, tricuspid regurgitation; V, velocity.

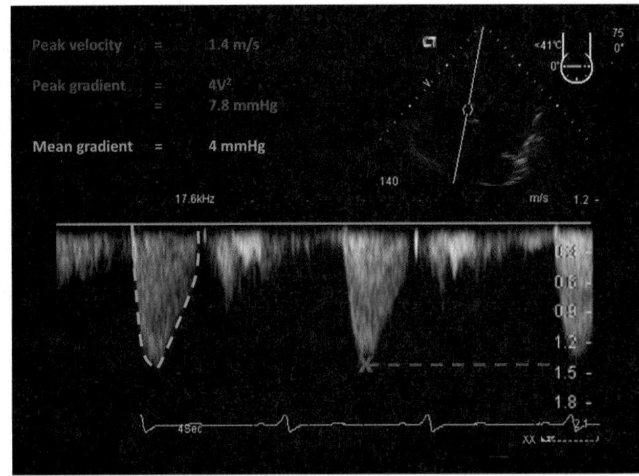

Figure 27-12 Calculation of gradients. Measurement of peak and mean gradients from the continuous Doppler display of flow through the aortic valve in a deep transgastric five-chamber view.

operator. This AUC is the integral of velocity (cm/s) over time (s) and has the units of distance (cm). Conceptually, this velocity time integral (VTI) of flow across an orifice during the cardiac cycle can be thought of as being the distance that a red cell would travel along the path of flow during that cardiac cycle, so the VTI can also be termed *"stroke distance."* If the VTI is multiplied by the cross-sectional area of the orifice, the resulting cylinder of volume is equal to the stroke volume through that orifice (Fig. 27-13).

By performing these measurements of flow across an orifice with a known cross-sectional area, such as the left ventricular outflow tract (LVOT), the stroke volume and therefore cardiac output can be calculated. Sequential VTI measurements can be used to track changes in stroke volume as a measure of response to changes in therapy, as the orifice area is assumed to remain constant in the patient being monitored.

The Continuity Equation

When the cross-sectional area of an orifice is unknown (e.g., the aortic valve [AV] area in aortic stenosis [AS]), the measurement of stroke volume allows calculation of this unknown orifice area by using the *continuity equation*. Based on the conservation of mass in fluid mechanics, the principle is that if two orifices are in sequence, the forward stroke volume across them is equal. However, valvular regurgitation and intracardiac shunts may render this assumption invalid.

Using the principle of continuity:

$$\text{stroke volume through orifice A} = \text{stroke volume through orifice B}$$
$$VTI_A \times \text{orifice area}_A = VTI_B \times \text{orifice area}_B$$

In clinical practice, the continuity equation is frequently used to calculate AV area as orifice A. The LVOT is commonly used as orifice B. The AV area can then be calculated from the VTIs at the LVOT and the AV, and the LVOT area.

Perioperative Echocardiography Imaging

Indications

The indications for ultrasound and particularly echocardiogra- 1
phy in clinical anesthesia practice have broadened rapidly with increasing appreciation of their benefits in many clinical settings.

When delivering perioperative care to patients undergoing cardiac surgery, specialist expertise is required to provide

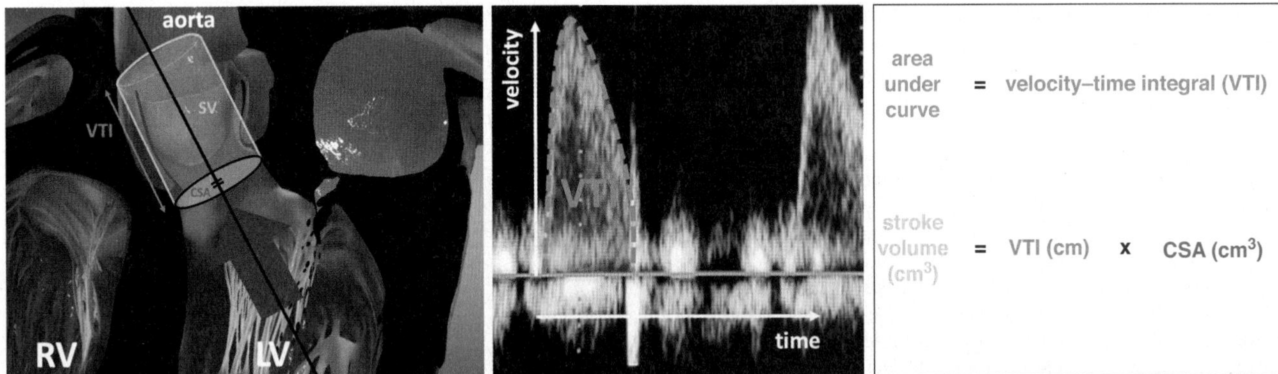

Figure 27-13 Calculation of stroke volume. The velocity time integral (VTI) of flow through an orifice such as the left ventricular tract (LVOT) is traced on a spectral Doppler display (in this case, pulsed wave Doppler) of flow velocity in the LVOT. The VTI, when multiplied by the cross-sectional area (CSA) of the orifice (in this example, calculated from the measured diameter of the LVOT on 2D imaging) gives the stroke volume. LV, left ventricle; RV, right ventricle.

Table 27-3 Indications for Perioperative Echocardiography in Anesthesia Practice

Modality	Setting		Uses
TEE	Intraoperative	Cardiovascular surgery	Hemodynamic monitor Confirmation of pathology Exclusion of additional pathology that will alter surgical plan Assessment of deairing of left heart Evaluation of surgical repair
		Noncardiovascular surgery	Hemodynamic monitor
	Critical care		Diagnosis in acute hemodynamic compromise Hemodynamic monitor Evaluation of response to therapy
	Resuscitation		Evaluation of adequacy of CPR Hemodynamic monitor Evaluation of response to therapy
TTE	Preoperative assessment		Evaluation of cardiac function and volume status
	Critical care		Diagnosis in acute hemodynamic compromise Hemodynamic monitor Evaluation of response to therapy
	Resuscitation		Identification of cause of cardiac arrest Hemodynamic monitor Evaluation of response to therapy

TEE, transesophageal echocardiography; TTE, transthoracic echocardiography.

comprehensive examination of both cardiac structure and function, reflected in the higher levels of training and accreditation recommended for cardiac anesthesiologists. Outside of the cardiac operating room, however, echocardiography can be applied in a more focused manner, with the emphasis on its application as an adjunct for hemodynamic management.[5,6] TEE is usually the main mode of imaging during intraoperative use because it does not interfere with the surgical field. Outside of the operating room, TTE is the preferred modality because it is less invasive. However, TEE may be required in patients with unfavorable body habitus, when drains or dressings limit access to the chest wall, or when certain structures such as the left atrial appendage need to be assessed. Indications for echocardiography in anesthesia practice are summarized in Table 27-3.[7,8]

Transesophageal Echocardiography

Complications and Contraindications

TEE is a semi-invasive procedure that carries a risk of patient injury. Evidence of esophageal injury following TEE has been seen at endoscopy in over 80% of patients who have undergone TEE for procedural guidance.[6] The vast majority of these injuries, which include mucosal lacerations, intramural hematomas, and evidence of thermal injury, resolve with conservative management and are of no clinical significance. Life-threatening complications such as major hemorrhage or perforation of the stomach or esophagus by the TEE probe are rare, but often fatal.[7] They are more likely in patients with pre-existing gastroesophageal pathology,[8] although many affected patients have no identifiable risk factors. Several large studies of patients undergoing TEE imaging during cardiac surgery report a mortality related to complications of up to 1 in 3,000.[7,9] Minor complications are more frequent and are usually transient in nature. The most common is postoperative odynophagia, which can be of significance in the development of postoperative respiratory complications. Others include minor oral bruising or laceration, sore throat, and chipped teeth. Accepted contraindications to the use of TEE are largely based on consensus opinion.[7,8] Commonly agreed contraindications are described in Table 27-4.

Probe Insertion and Manipulation

A disinfected TEE probe may be inserted with or without a sheath, depending on institutional practice. Acoustic gel should be applied to a TEE sheath before the probe is placed into it to displace any air that may hamper the transmission of

Table 27-4 Common Contraindications to Transesophageal Echocardiography

Absolute Contraindications

- Perforated viscus
- Gastroesophageal strictures
- Gastroesophageal masses
- Gastroesophageal diverticula
- Tracheoesophageal fistula
- Recent upper GI surgery
- Active oral, hypopharyngeal, or gastroesophageal hemorrhage

Relative Contraindications

- Previous radiation therapy to the neck or mediastinum
- Previous esophageal or gastric surgery
- History of upper GI hemorrhage
- Esophageal varices
- Active esophagitis
- Active gastric ulceration
- Coagulopathy

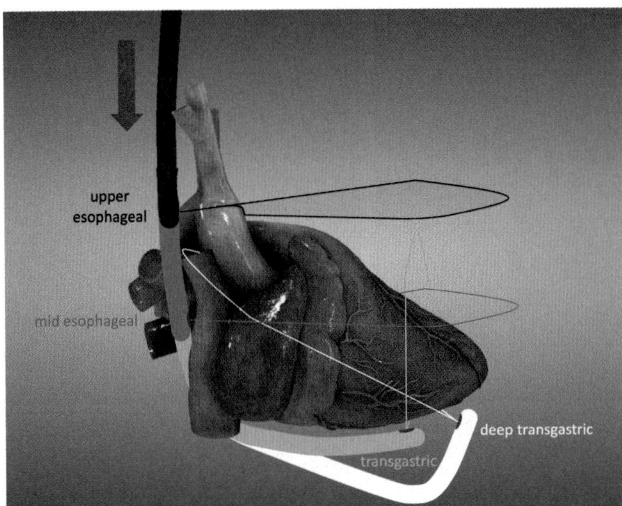

Figure 27-14 Tranesophageal echocardiography (TEE) probe positions. TEE probe tip positions relative to the heart for acquisition of standard imaging planes.

ultrasound. The sheath tip should be examined prior to insertion of the probe to ensure that there are no bubbles of air present. In an anesthetized patient, the lubricated probe may be inserted blindly, or a laryngoscope may be used to "straighten" the path of the probe through the oropharynx and into the upper esophagus to avoid trauma to the posterior pharyngeal wall. Insertion is aided by lifting the mandible forward, either by placing a thumb inside the patient's mouth behind the incisors, or by jaw thrust applied by an assistant. Neck flexion may also be of help. The lubricated probe should be inserted with constant gentle pressure and efforts should be abandoned if significant resistance is encountered. Images from the upper esophagus will appear when the probe has been inserted to a depth of 25 to 30 cm in adult patients.

A comprehensive knowledge of cardiac and mediastinal anatomy is central to achieving an understanding of probe manipulation and the orientation of images on the display screen. The esophagus passes directly behind the heart as it descends through the thorax to cross the diaphragm and open into the stomach. Although ultrasound images can be acquired at any point in this path, the standard imaging planes that make up a basic TEE study are most commonly acquired from the upper esophagus, midesophagus, and stomach (Fig. 27-14). The names of the imaging planes reflect the level from which they are acquired.

To achieve an imaging plane, the operator can apply the following movements to the TEE probe (Figs. 27-15 to 27-18):

- Advance/withdraw
- Turn left and right
- Anteflex/retroflex
- Left and right lateral flex
- Ultrasound plane rotation

The probe tip movements and ultrasound plane rotation are achieved using the control wheels and buttons on the probe handle. A typical arrangement of probe controls is shown in Figure 27-19.

The ultrasound plane—the fan of scan lines leaving the probe—can also be rotated smoothly through 180 degrees using the buttons or rocker switch on the probe handle. The degree of rotation is displayed on the ultrasound screen; 0-degree rotation is considered to be a horizontal plane (Fig. 27-20). The ultrasound plane always rotates in the same direction; the image edge that is positioned on the patient's right side when the imaging plane is horizontal (0 degrees) rotates inferiorly toward a vertical plane (90 degrees) and beyond to 180 degrees, which then produces a mirror image of the 0-degree plane.

Image Orientation

The narrower apex of the ultrasound image is most commonly positioned so it displays at the top of the ultrasound machine screen. By convention, when the transducer is in the esophagus and the imaging plane is horizontal (0 degrees), right-sided structures are displayed on the left side of the screen and left-sided structures on the right of the screen. As the esophagus lies posterior to the heart, the narrow apex of the image is posterior, and the wider far end, at the bottom of the screen, displays anterior structures.

As the ultrasound plane is rotated from 0 to 90 degrees, the image border on the left of the screen increasingly displays inferior structures and the right border of the image superior structures.

When the probe is advanced through the diaphragm, it curves anteriorly through almost 90 degrees to enter the patient's

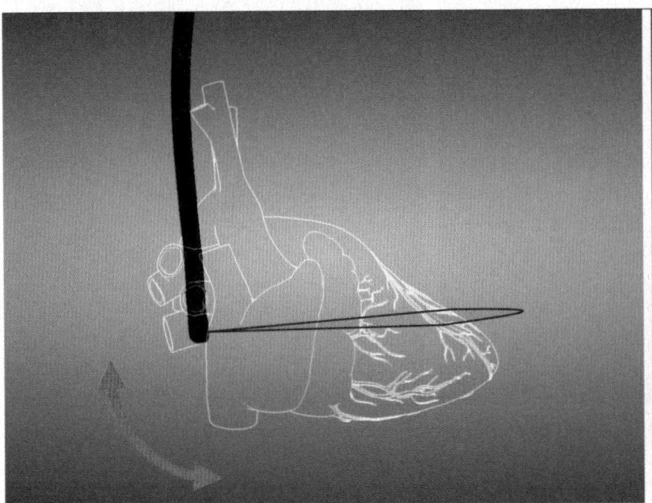

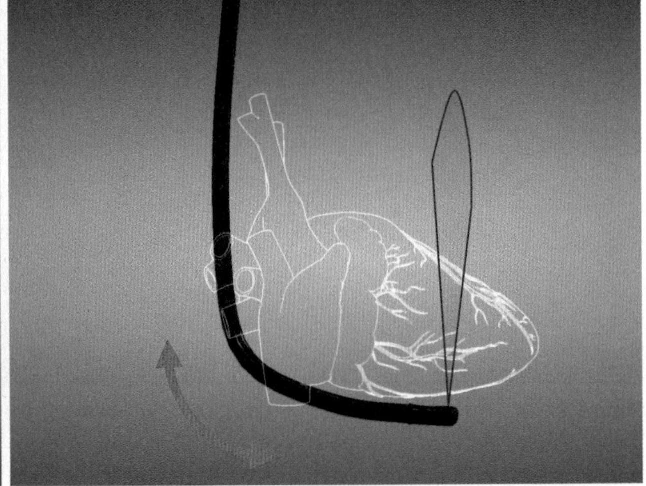

Figure 27-15 Advancing and withdrawing probe. Note that the probe passively curves anteriorly as it is advanced through the diaphragm and into the stomach.

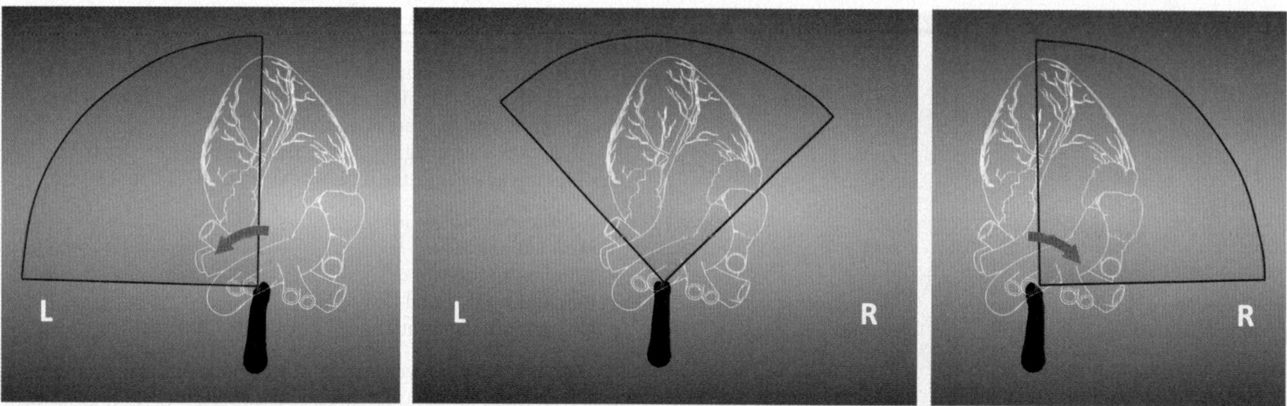

Figure 27-16 Turning the probe. Turning left ("counterclockwise") and right ("clockwise"). The direction of turn is named in relation to the patient's left and right sides.

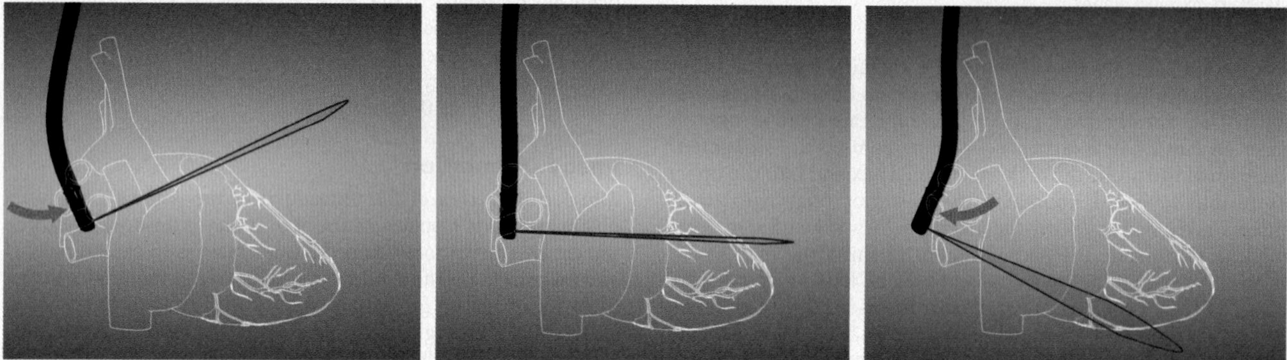

Figure 27-17 Probe anteflexion and retroflexion. Rotating the wheels on the probe handle anteflexes (*left image*) and retroflexes (*right image*) the probe tip from a neutral position (*center image*). The position of the ultrasound plane is significantly altered by these probe tip movements.

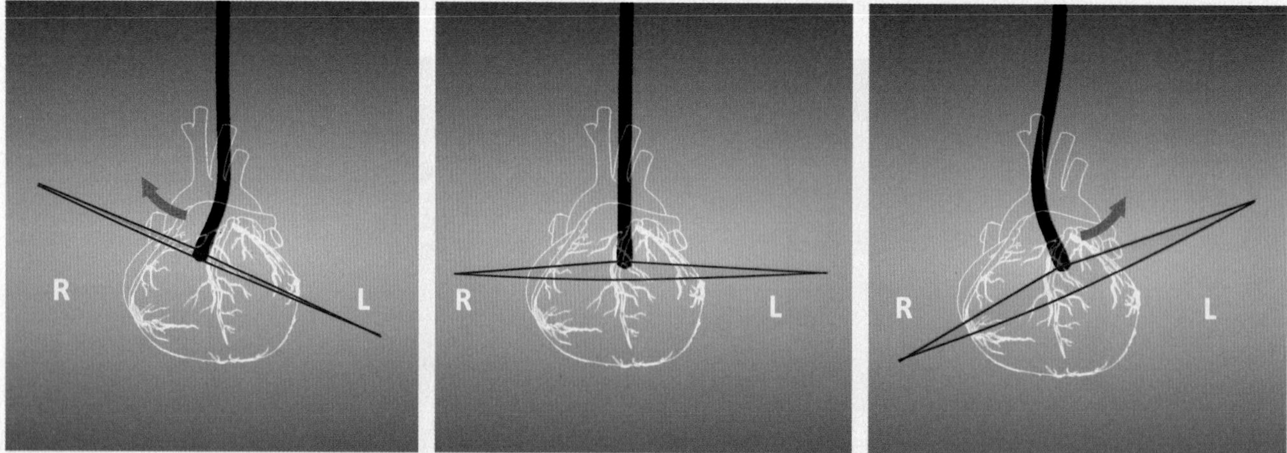

Figure 27-18 Probe lateral flexion. The probe tip can be flexed to the patient's right (*right image*) and left (*left image*) from a neutral position (*center*).

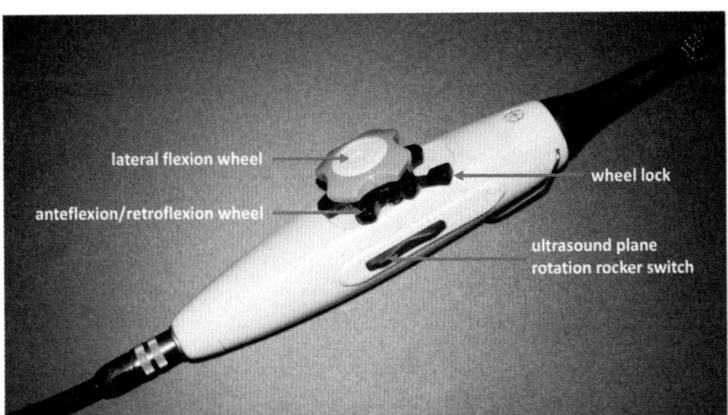

Figure 27-19 The typical tranesophageal echocardiography (TEE) probe handle. Typical configuration of controls on a TEE probe handle. The ability to lock the flexion wheels introduces potential for patient injury if the probe tip is locked in a flexed position and then advanced or withdrawn within the esophagus.

stomach and comes to lie below the heart. Structures closest to the probe (at the top of the screen) are therefore now inferior; those at the bottom of the screen are now superior. At 0 degrees of rotation, the left side of the image still displays right-sided structures and the right side of the image displays left-sided structures.

When the ultrasound plane is rotated through 90 degrees with the probe in the stomach, the image border on the left side of the screen moves to slice through anterior (apical) structures.

Principal TEE Imaging Planes

Most commonly, a system of 28 standard TEE imaging planes is used,[7] all of which form part of a comprehensive study and are part of the core knowledge base for cardiac anesthesiologists.

A smaller subset of these imaging planes commonly forms a "focused" or "basic" study sequence[10] that would be appropriate for intraoperative hemodynamic monitoring during noncardiac surgery or in a critical care setting.

Preferred terminology for imaging plane names varies between countries, institutions, and specialties. In general, imaging planes are named according to the transducer position, the principal structure imaged, and whether that structure is displayed in the short axis ("SAX," i.e., displaying the shorter dimension of the structure) or long axis ("LAX," i.e., displaying its longer dimension). The nomenclature used in this chapter is aligned with guidelines published by the American Society of Echocardiography (ASE) in 2013.[7]

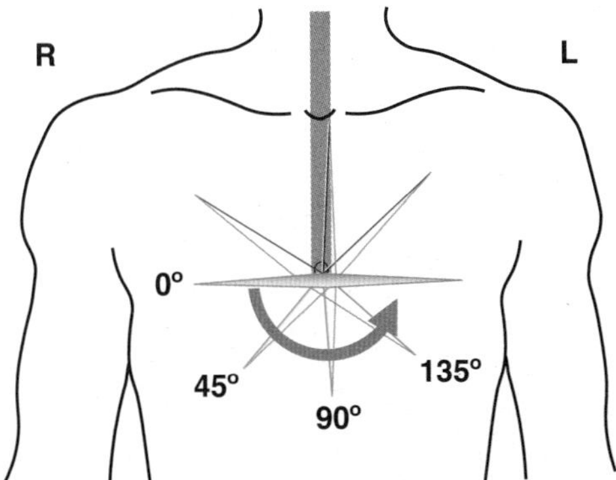

Figure 27-20 Tranesophageal echocardiography probe plane rotation. The ultrasound plane can be rotated electronically through 180 degrees. This is usually performed by pressing buttons or a rocker switch on the probe handle.

The order of the imaging sequence can vary according to clinical need, as planes that yield the most information relevant to the clinical setting may be prioritized for acquisition earlier in the sequence. Some clinicians prefer to perform a structure-based sequence, in which each cardiac structure in turn is comprehensively studied using several imaging planes. Others may prefer to order their study sequence based on the depth of the TEE probe tip, acquiring all midesophageal images before advancing the probe tip into the stomach to acquire the transgastric imaging planes. Twelve imaging planes that may make up a focused TEE study are described in Figure 27-21; they broadly follow the basic perioperative transesophageal echocardiography (PTE) sequence recommended by the ASE and the Society of Cardiovascular Anesthesiologists (SCA).[10] These views are described in further detail below.

Midesophageal Four Chamber View (ME 4C)

Advancing the probe 35 to 40 cm into the esophagus with the angle of plane rotation at 0 degrees will position the probe tip about half-way down the esophagus, posterior to the left atrium (LA), and the four cardiac chambers come into view (Fig. 27-22). In this "horizontal" position, the ultrasound plane usually cuts through the anterior wall of the left ventricle (LV), resulting in "foreshortening" of the LV. In order to remove foreshortening and "open up" the LV apex to achieve the correct ME4C view, the ultrasound plane should be aligned with the long axis of the heart. This invariably requires retroflexion of the probe tip to tilt the ultrasound plane inferiorly in the far end of the scanned area so that the plane slices through the apex rather than the anterior LV wall. A small amount of ultrasound plane rotation (0 to 20 degrees) may be needed to exclude the LV outflow tract from the image. This may bring the anterolateral papillary muscle into view.

The midesophageal four-chamber (ME4C) view is useful for assessment of

- cardiac dimensions
- biventricular function, both systolic and diastolic
- LV septal and lateral wall function
- mitral and tricuspid valve function
- atrial septum and ventricular septum

Turning the probe slightly to the left and right will center left heart or right heart structures in the image for closer examination.

Midesophageal Two Chamber View (ME 2C)

Keeping the left heart in the center of the image and rotating the ultrasound plane through approximately 90 degrees will display the LA and LV in a vertical plane (Fig. 27-23). Small adjustments by turning the probe to the left or right will ensure that the plane slices through the apex, rather than the lateral or septal wall of the LV. The inferior and anterior LV walls are seen. The anatomy of the left atrial appendage is variable, but it may be seen arising from the anterior left atrial wall in this view. The coronary sinus (CS) is seen in the inferior atrioventricular groove and the posteromedial papillary muscle group can frequently be visualized on the inferior LV wall.

The midesophageal two-chamber (ME2C) view is useful for assessment of:

- LV inferior and anterior wall function
- left atrial appendage for thrombus
- mitral valve (MV) function

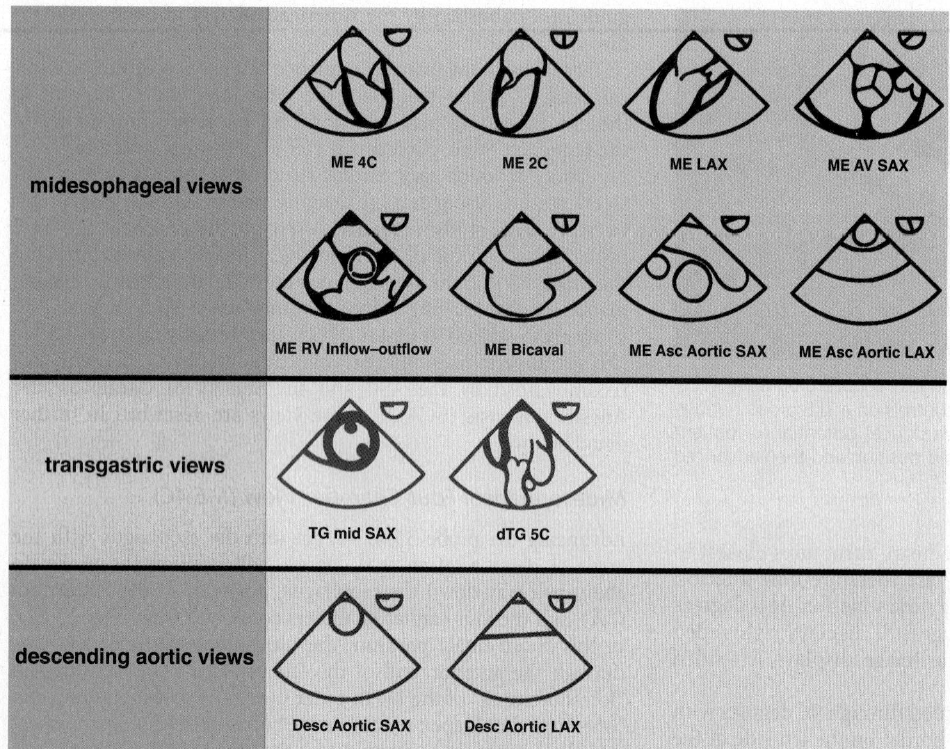

Figure 27-21 Basic transesophageal echocardiography imaging planes.

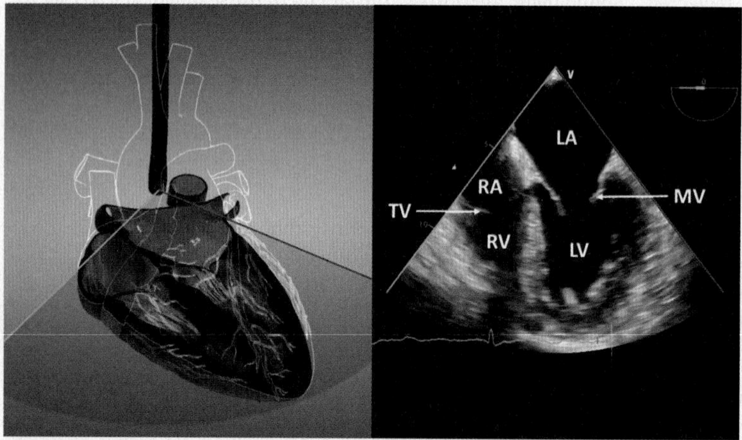

Figure 27-22 Midesophageal four-chamber view. RA, right atrium; RV, right ventricle; LA, left atrium; LV, left ventricle; TV, tricuspid valve; MV, mitral valve.

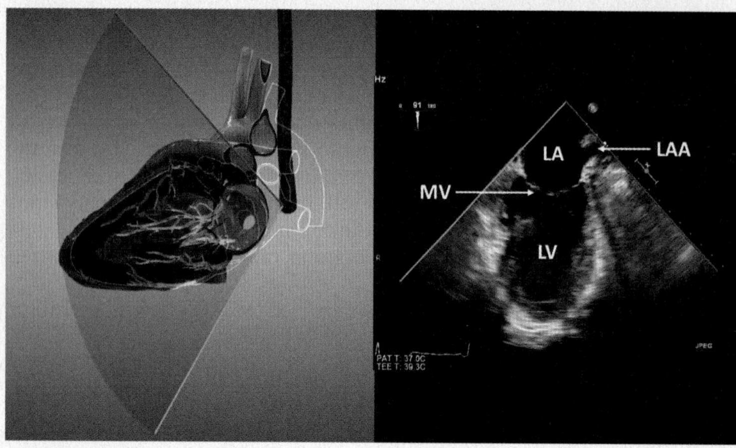

Figure 27-23 Midesophageal two-chamber view. LA, left atrium; LV, left ventricle; MV, mitral valve; LAA, left atrial appendage.

Midesophageal Long Axis View (ME LAX)

Further forward rotation of the ultrasound plane from the ME2C view to 120 to 150 degrees will bring the LV outflow tract and AV into view, along with a small portion of the RV outflow tract (Fig. 27-24). The MV is displayed on one of its natural axes, with the plane slicing through the A2 and P2 regions of the mitral leaflets perpendicular to the line of coaptation. Turning the probe from this position to the left and right will display A1/P1 and A3/P3 regions of the valve, respectively. This allows accurate localization of mitral leaflet pathology.

The midesophageal long-axis (MELAX) view is useful for assessment of:

- LV inferolateral and anteroseptal wall function
- MV pathology
- AV pathology
- the aortic root and region of aortomitral continuity
- the LV outflow tract for obstructive lesions, both structural and dynamic

Midesophageal Aortic Valve Short Axis View (ME AV SAX)

From the MELAX view, if the probe is withdrawn slightly and turned to the right to center the AV, rotating the ultrasound plane back to 30 to 40 degrees will produce a short-axis view of the valve (Fig. 27-25). The plane should slice through the leaflet tips of the AV so that in diastole, when the valve closes, there is no gap between the three leaflets, or "cusps." If a gap is visible in an otherwise normal valve, the probe is too low in the esophagus and the ultrasound plane is slicing through the body of the leaflets; withdrawing the probe slightly will elevate the plane to the level of the leaflet tips. The noncoronary cusp is adjacent to the atrial septum and septal pathology may be evident in this view. The coronary arteries arise from the sinuses of Valsalva at variable heights above the AV annulus; slightly withdrawing the probe may help to identify the coronary ostia.

The midesophageal aortic valve short-axis (ME AV SAX) view is useful for assessing:

- AV pathology
- aortic root pathology

Midesophageal Right Ventricular Inflow–Outflow View (ME RV Inflow-Outflow)

From the ME AV SAX view, the right heart can be "developed" by increasing the multiplane angle of rotation to 50 to 70 degrees (Fig. 27-26). To fully open the chamber of the RV, the probe may need to be advanced by 1 to 2 cm; from this point, small adjustments to the angle of plane rotation should result in both the tricuspid and pulmonic valves being visible.

The midesophageal right ventricular inflow–outflow (ME RV inflow–outflow) view is useful for assessment of:

- right heart pathology, particularly in the setting of congenital heart disease where intracardiac shunts may result in right heart volume or pressure overload
- RV free wall systolic function
- tricuspid and pulmonic valve pathology
- atrial septal pathology
- pericardial collections

Midesophageal Bicaval View (ME BC)

Further forward rotation of the ultrasound plane to 90 to 120 degrees and turning the probe slightly to the right will produce an midesophageal bicaval (ME bicaval) view (Fig. 27-27). Adjustment to bring both the inferior vena cava (IVC) and superior vena cava (SVC) into view usually involves small changes to the angle of rotation. The CS enters the right atrium adjacent to the IVC and care should be taken not to mistake it for the IVC when the angle of rotation is increased too much. The presence of the IVC in the image can be confirmed by advancing the probe to confirm that it extends below the diaphragm immediately adjacent to the liver.

The ME bicaval view is useful for

- assessment of the atrial septum for defects
- guidance for placement of cardiopulmonary bypass (CPB) and extracorporeal membranous oxygenation (ECMO) cannulae, CS cannulae, pulmonary artery (PA) catheters
- procedural guidance for transseptal puncture (e.g., in electrophysiologic intervention, such as ablation of atrial fibrillation)
- measurement of respiratory variation in caval diameter to evaluate the patient's volume status

Midesophageal Ascending Aorta Short Axis View (ME Asc Ao SAX)

In this view, the ascending aorta is imaged in a horizontal plane. From an ME bicaval view, therefore, the ultrasound plane is returned to 0-degree rotation and the probe is turned to the left to center the heart in the image before the probe is withdrawn past the AV to reveal the circular proximal ascending aorta above it (Fig. 27-28). The main pulmonary artery lies to the right of the aorta on the screen; the PA bifurcation and branch PAs can be seen, although the left pulmonary artery is often not seen beyond its most proximal portion due to the air-filled left main bronchus obstructing the image. In practice, the airways often extend between the esophagus and the aorta at this level and can make the view difficult to achieve at all. This anatomical relationship is also responsible for a TEE "blind spot" that includes the distal ascending aorta at levels above the midesophageal ascending aorta short-axis (ME asc aorta SAX) plane.

The ME asc aorta SAX view is useful for assessing

- proximal ascending aortic pathology such as atheroma and dissection
- main and branch PA abnormalities in congenital heart disease
- main pulmonary artery flow in the quantification of shunt
- the presence of thrombus in the pulmonary artery
- PA catheter placement

Midesophageal Ascending Aorta Long Axis (ME Asc Aorta LAX)

The long and short axes of any structure are orthogonal. If the ascending aorta is centered in the ME asc aorta SAX image and the ultrasound plane rotated through 90 degrees to a vertical plane, the ascending aorta will be shown in long axis as it passes anterior to the right pulmonary artery (Fig. 27-29). Again, the intervening airway may obscure some of the view, and in practice, the site of aortic cannulation for cardiopulmonary bypass can often not be seen.

This view is useful for assessment of

- proximal ascending aortic pathology, such as atheroma and dissection

Transgastric Midpapillary Short Axis View (TG SAX)

If the multiplane angle of rotation is returned to 0 degrees and the TEE probe carefully advanced a further 10 to 15 cm beyond the midesophageal level, it will move beyond the four-chamber view and the CS in the left inferior atrioventricular groove to pass immediately afterward into the stomach. The natural anatomy of the esophagus and stomach will passively direct the probe tip anteriorly through almost a right angle as it enters the stomach so

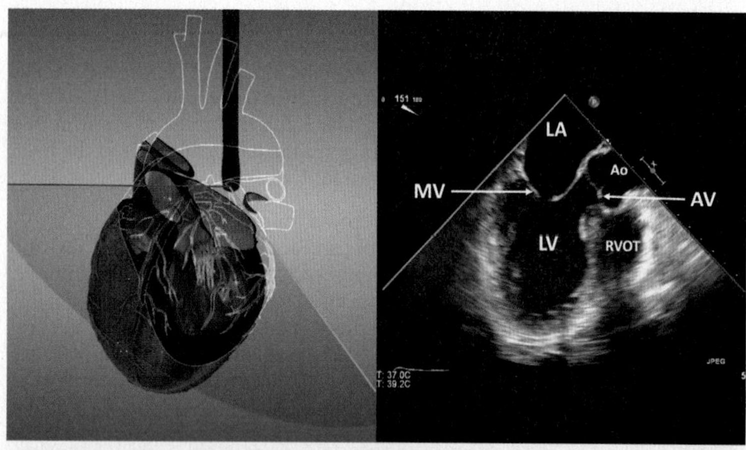

Figure 27-24 Midesophageal long-axis view. RVOT, right ventricular outflow tract; LA, left atrium; LV, left ventricle; MV, mitral valve; AV, aortic valve; Ao, proximal ascending aorta.

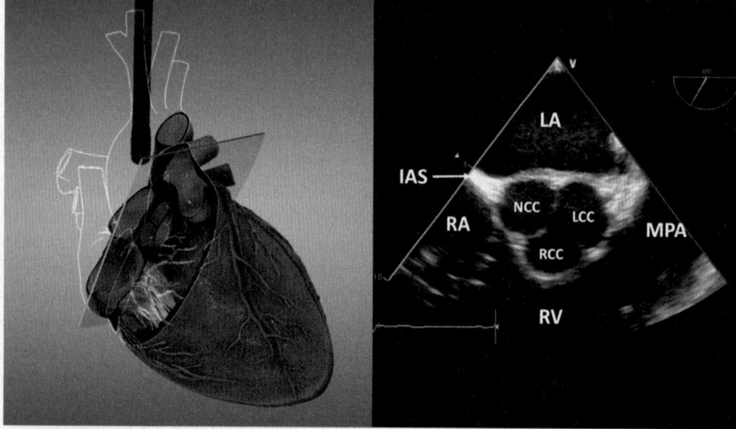

Figure 27-25 Midesophageal aortic valve short-axis view. NCC, aortic valve noncoronary cusp; LCC, aortic valve left coronary cusp; RCC, aortic valve right-coronary cusp; RA, right atrium; RV, right ventricle; MPA, main pulmonary artery; LA, left atrium; IAS, interatrial septum.

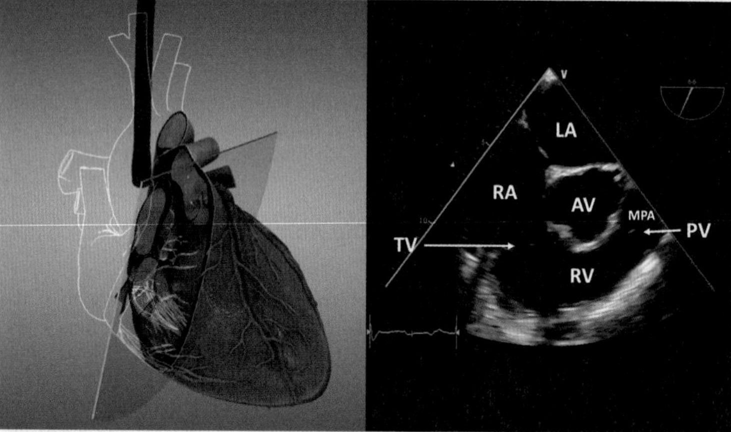

Figure 27-26 Midesophageal right ventricular inflow–outflow view. RA, right atrium; TV, tricuspid valve; RV, right ventricle; PV, pulmonic valve; MPA, main pulmonary artery; LA, left atrium; LV, left ventricle; MV, mitral valve; AV, aortic valve.

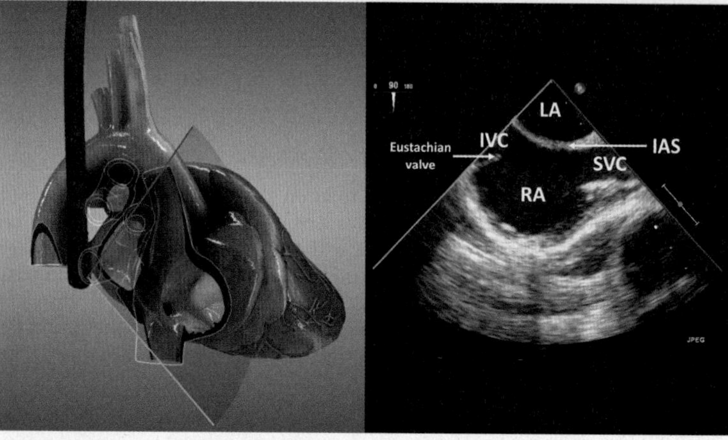

Figure 27-27 Midesophageal bicaval view. RA, right atrium; LA, left atrium; IAS, interatrial septum; IVC, inferior vena cava; SVC, superior vena cava.

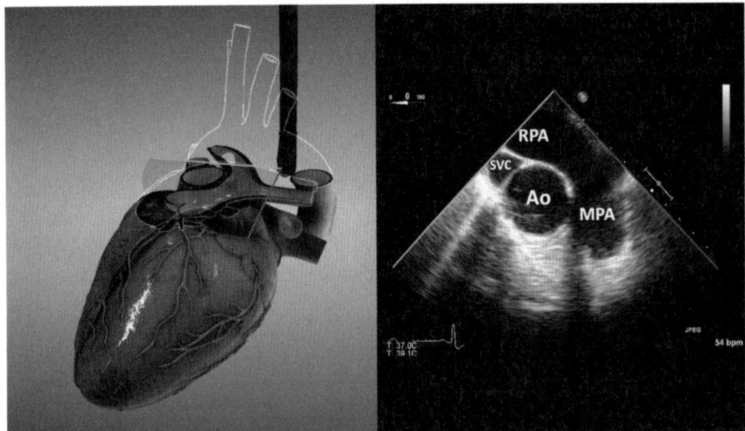

Figure 27-28 Midesophageal ascending aorta short-axis view. Ao, ascending aorta; MPA, main pulmonary artery; RPA, right pulmonary artery; SVC, superior vena cava.

that it comes to lie inferior to the heart. It is advanced until the LV is imaged in short axis at the level of attachment of the papillary muscles to the endocardium (Fig. 27-30). This view is important in the assessment of patient hemodynamics and is frequently the first view sought in the setting of acute hypotension. Withdrawing and advancing the probe from this view will produce images of the basal and apical levels of the LV, allowing comprehensive regional assessment.

Loss of contact with the esophageal mucosa when the probe enters the stomach can lead to loss of image quality; it can be restored by gentle anteflexion to establish contact with the gastric wall. In addition, gastric air can obscure the image; on rare occasions, it can be necessary to empty the stomach of air using an orogastric tube.

The transgastric midpapillary short-axis (TG mid SAX) view is useful for evaluation of

- LV dimensions
- biventricular systolic function, both global and regional
- ventricular septal position and motion in the scenario of right heart pressure and volume overload
- pericardial collections

Deep Transgastric Five Chamber

Advancing the probe deeper into the stomach and beyond the LV apex before applying extreme anteflexion and then slowly withdrawing allows the clinician to position the transducer close to the apex. This enables alignment of the Doppler cursor with flow across the LV outflow tract and aortic valve, which is not possible from the esophagus. In addition, pathology close to the LV apex may be imaged more clearly as it is positioned in the near field of the image (Fig. 27-31).

The deep transgastric five-chamber (dTG 5C) view is useful for assessment of

- AV gradient and area
- the LV outflow tract in the presence of AS or mechanical AV prosthesis that causes acoustic shadow across the LVOT in other imaging planes
- LV outflow tract VTI for estimation of stroke volume and cardiac output
- apical pathology, such as mural thrombus

Descending Aorta Short Axis

From the deep stomach, the probe is withdrawn to the lower esophagus. From a position where the heart is visible in the image, the probe is turned to the left until the heart is no longer visible and the circular descending aorta comes into view (Fig. 27-32). The sector depth should be reduced to approximately 6 cm. From this position, the entire thoracic descending aorta can be examined by slowly withdrawing the probe, making small turns to the left and right to keep the aorta centered in the image until it reaches the level of the distal aortic arch in the upper esophagus.

The descending aorta short-axis (desc aorta SAX) view is useful for

- assessment of descending aortic pathology, such as atheroma and dissection

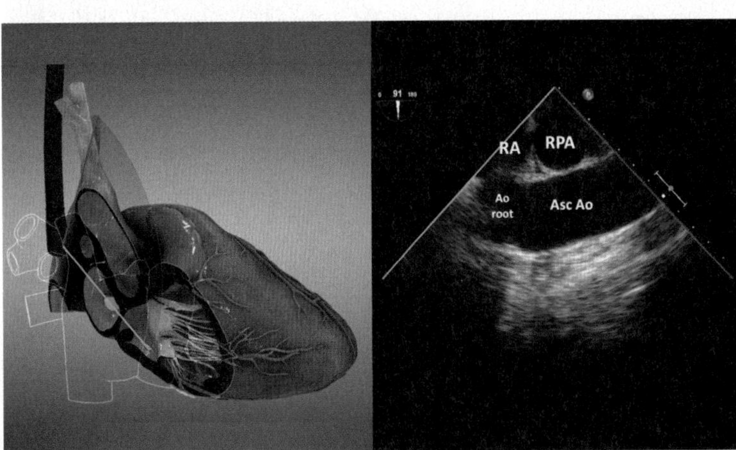

Figure 27-29 Midesophageal ascending aorta long-axis view. Ao root, aortic root; Asc Ao, ascending aorta; RPA, right pulmonary artery; RA, right atrium.

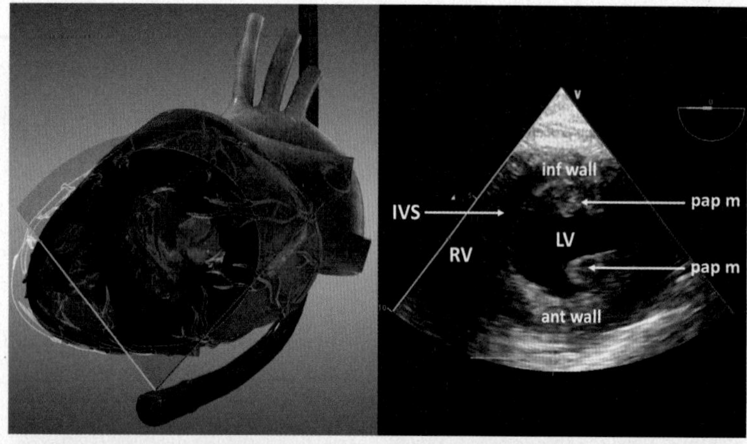

Figure 27-30 Transgastric mid short-axis view. LV, left ventricle; RV, right ventricle; IVS, interventricular septum; inf wall, inferior wall; ant wall, anterior wall; pap m, papillary muscle.

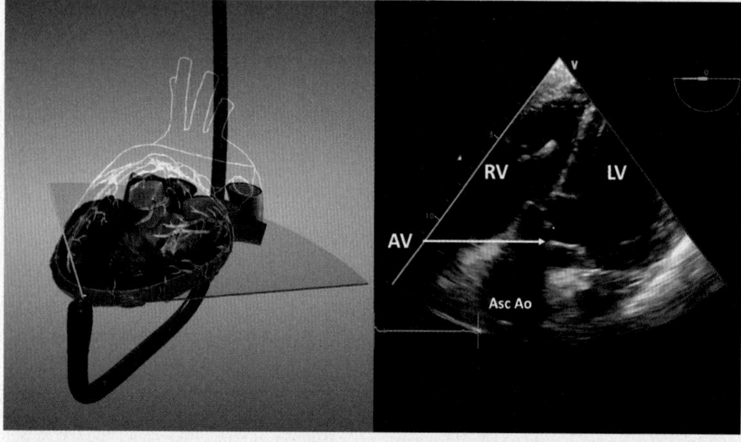

Figure 27-31 Deep transgastric five-chamber view. RV, right ventricle; LV, left ventricle; AV, aortic valve; Asc Ao, ascending aorta.

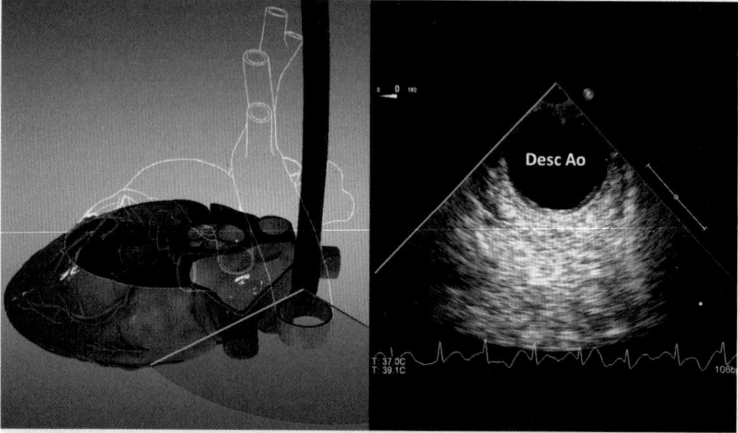

Figure 27-32 Descending aorta short-axis view. Desc Ao, descending aorta.

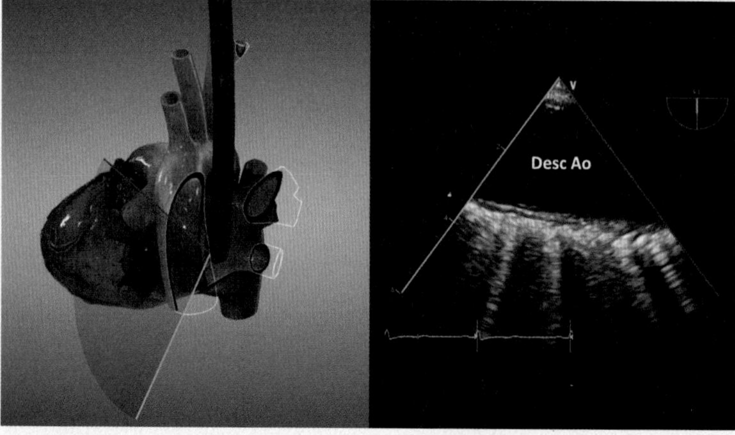

Figure 27-33 Descending aorta long-axis view. Desc Ao, descending aorta.

- procedural guidance for placement of guidewires, catheters, and mechanical support devices
- Imaging the left pleural space for pleural effusions

Descending Aorta Long-Axis View

From a desc aorta SAX view, the ultrasound plane is rotated through 90 degrees to image the descending aorta in the long axis (Fig. 27-33). As with the short-axis view, the probe can be advanced and withdrawn to examine the entire thoracic descending aorta.

The descending aorta long-axis (desc aorta LAX) view is useful for

- Assessment of descending aortic pathology, such as atheroma and dissection
- procedural guidance for placement of guidewires, catheters, and mechanical support

Focused Transthoracic Echocardiography: Basic and Advanced Views

Transthoracic imaging with focused cardiac ultrasound (FOCUS) provides adequate evaluation of cardiac anatomy and function in most patients and has been shown to be useful for rapid bedside identification of the cause of severe hemodynamic compromise.[11] More detailed cardiac evaluation using POCUS requires more advanced training.[5] Basic and advanced FOCUS views are listed in Table 27-5 and described in Figures 27-34 and 27-35.

By convention, the probe icon is on the top right of the ultrasound screen during TTE imaging. This icon edge on the screen corresponds to an index marker on one side of the TTE probe. To optimize transthoracic imaging, subtle probe manipulations from the standardized views are often necessary because of individual differences in patient anatomy. These probe movements include the following:

- Sliding: moving the probe toward or away from the marker
- Rocking: angling the probe along the axis of the imaging plane, lifting either the marker end or the nonmarker end very slightly off the patient's chest, such that structures can be seen to continue further
- Tilting: angling the probe orthogonal to the imaging plane, such that adjacent structures are visualized
- Rotation: moving the probe clockwise or anticlockwise, such that the structures can be imaged in various axes

Three-Dimensional Echocardiography

2

The structural and functional assessment offered by 3D TEE makes it an important tool in cardiac operating rooms.[12] 3D echocardiography requires a special 3D probe. By scanning multiple planes simultaneously, 3D ultrasound probes can generate a pyramidal dataset. Real-time 3D echocardiographic reconstruction then generates images that allow visualization of cardiac structures from any spatial point of view.[13] Further, the echocardiographer may virtually dissect the dataset, to focus on the structure of interest. Volume rendering of the display through a range of colors and opacities creates depth perception on the 2D screen. However, just like 2D imaging, optimal 3D echocardiography requires a balance between the size of the sector being scanned and the temporal resolution. Shorter depth and narrower pyramidal sectors increase temporal

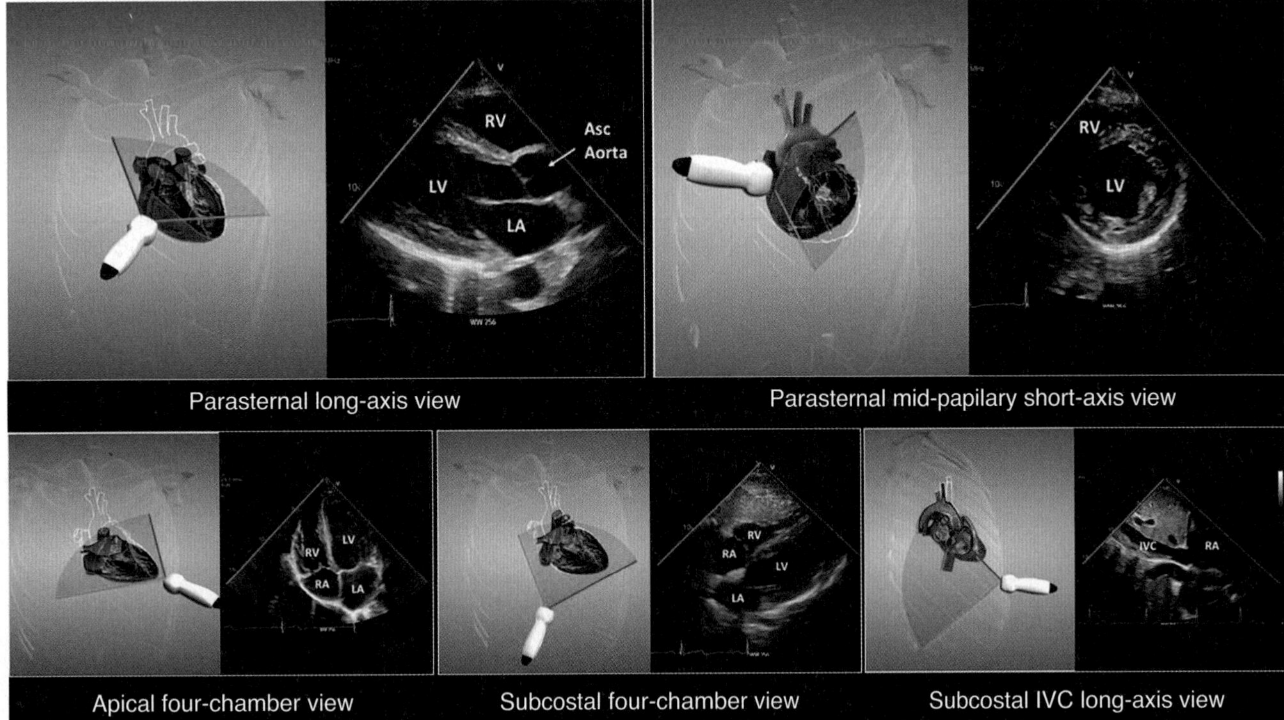

Figure 27-34 Basic focused cardiac ultrasound views.

Table 27-5 Basic and Advanced Focused Cardiac Ultrasound Views

	Probe Position	Marker Orientation	Remarks
Basic Focused Cardiac Ultrasound Views			
Parasternal long axis (PLAX)	Third or fourth intercostal space on the left edge of the sternum	Toward the right shoulder	Attempt to achieve a "horizontal" interventricular septum, with a clear view of aortic and mitral valves
Parasternal short axis (PSAX)	Third or fourth intercostal space on the left edge of the sternum	Toward the left shoulder	Mid-left ventricular view, with papillary muscles clearly seen
Apical four chamber (A4C)	At the cardiac apex	Toward the patient's left side	Attempt probe placement directly over left ventricular apex
Subcostal four chamber (SC4C)	Inferior to the xiphoid process	Toward the patient's left side	Hold the probe from above, to allow for a more horizontal imaging plane
Subcostal inferior vena cava (SC IVC)	Inferior to the xiphoid process	Cephalad direction	Distinguish inferior vena cava (IVC) from aorta by identifying hepatic veins or right atrium connected to IVC, or by noting transhepatic course of IVC. Rocking inferiorly and tilting slightly to the right allows clear visualization of the portal vein
Advanced Focused Cardiac Ultrasound Views			
Modified parasternal long axis: RV inflow (PS RV inflow)	Third or fourth intercostal space on the left edge of the sternum	Toward the right shoulder	From the parasternal long axis, tilt the probe toward the patient's right hip (tail toward left shoulder)
Modified parasternal long axis: RV outflow (PS RV outflow)	Third or fourth intercostal space on the left edge of the sternum	Toward the right shoulder	From the parasternal long axis, tilt the probe toward the patient's left shoulder (tail toward right hip)
Parasternal aortic valve short axis (PS AoV SAX)	Third or fourth intercostal space on the left edge of the sternum	Toward the patient's left side	From the parasternal short axis, tilt the probe medially
Apical five chamber (A5C)	At the cardiac apex	Toward the patient's left side	From the apical four-chamber, tilt the probe anteriorly
Apical two chamber (A2C)	At the cardiac apex	Toward the patient's left shoulder	From the apical four-chamber, rotate the probe counterclockwise 90 degrees
Apical three chamber (A3C)	At the cardiac apex	Toward the patient's left ear	From the apical two chamber, rotate the probe counterclockwise 30–45 degrees
Suprasternal (SS)	Suprasternal notch	Toward the patient's left scapula	Extend the neck as far as possible
Transhepatic	Anterior axillary line, seventh–ninth intercostal space	Cephalad	Achieve long-axis view of IVC when subcostal windows are not possible (e.g., because of subxiphoid drains and surgical dressings). Slight inferior rocking allows clear visualization of the portal vein

By convention, the probe icon is on the top right of the ultrasound screen during TTE imaging. This icon edge on the screen corresponds to an index marker on one side of the TTE probe.

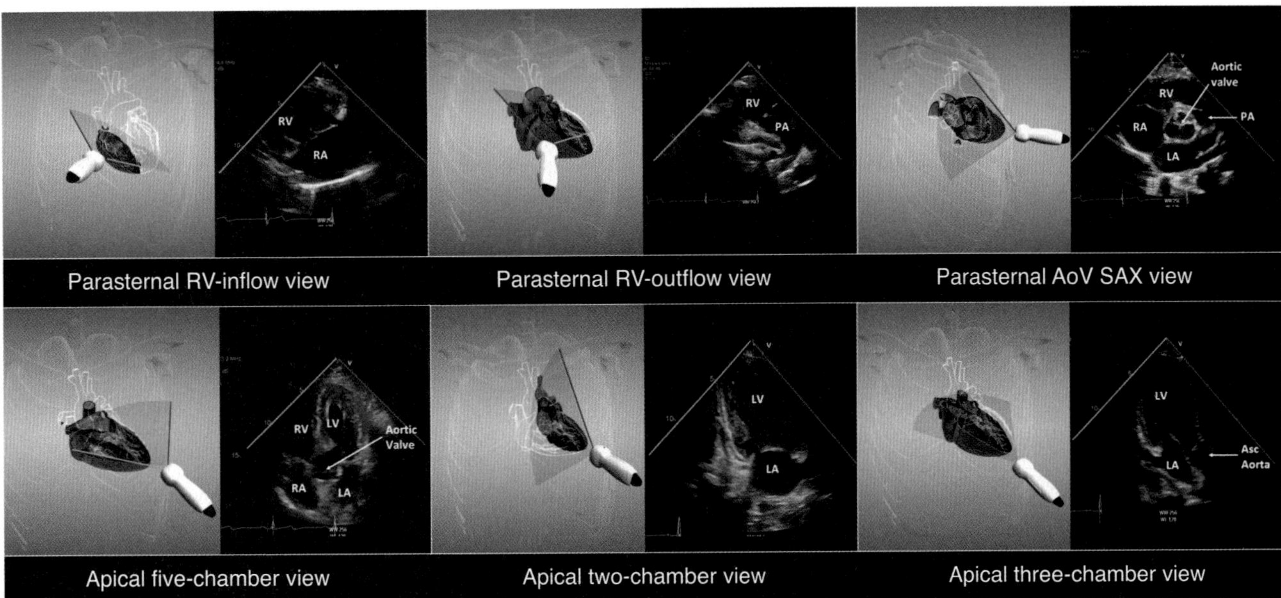

Figure 27-35 Advanced focused cardiac ultrasound views.

resolution. Multibeat, ECG-gated imaging offers improved frame rates on larger pyramidal datasets by stitching together narrower subvolumes.

Clinically, 3D TEE is used for evaluation of global and segmental ventricular wall motion, including evaluation of ventricular dyssynchrony. With software tools such as "semiautomated endocardial border detection" and "multiplanar reconstruction," a detailed view of left ventricular contraction can be presented. 3D imaging is also particularly useful for assessment of valvular structure and function, presented in realistic views akin to how they are seen in the surgical field. This is particularly true for the assessment of the MV, where an *en face* view can be easily obtained. Further, 3D TEE allows for better assessment of cardiac masses in relation to surrounding structures. A 3D-enabled TEE probe can also be used to evaluate structures in two planes simultaneously (e.g., short- and long-axis views

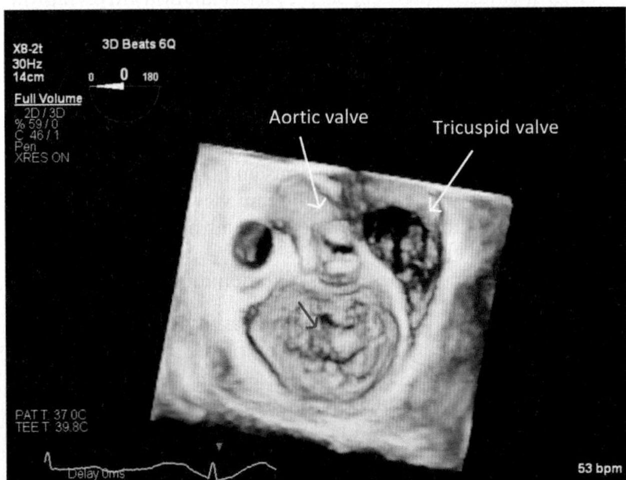

Figure 27-36 3D TEE imaging in the en face view. The surgeon's view, or the en face view, is used here to provide intraoperative localization of the lesion, in this case, a flail segment of the A2 segment of the anterior leaflet of the mitral valve, *highlighted by the red arrow*.

of a structure), allowing for a clearer understanding of the location of a pathology. For percutaneous procedures performed in hybrid operating rooms or cardiac catheterization labs (such as valve insertion, septal defect closure, and left atrial appendage closure), 3D TEE plays a vital role in guiding the proceduralist for the placement of wires, catheters, and devices. The realistic imaging offered by 3D TEE also enhances the communication of findings between the echocardiographer and the proceduralist (Fig. 27-36).

Clinical Echocardiography

Left Ventricle

Evaluation of the LV is one of the most studied, evidence-based components of the echocardiographic examination. It can be performed via qualitative measures alone in basic interrogation, but formal, comprehensive examinations will also use quantitative measures.

Normal Anatomy and Echocardiographic Appearance of the Left Ventricle

The LV appears as a longitudinal bullet-shaped cavity, with a rounded apex and cylindrical base, separated from the LA via the MV, and the right ventricle (RV) via the interventricular septum (Fig. 27-37). The cavity of the LV is echolucent, with endocardium and myocardium appearing comparatively textured and echodense. As the endocardium represents the interface between blood and tissue, it often appears brighter than surrounding tissue. A combination of longitudinal, circumferential, and radial forces causes the LV to contract and expel blood through the LVOT. On echocardiographic views, such as the ME4C in transesophageal and the A4C in transthoracic modalities, the LV base is seen to descend toward the apex.[14]

When interrogating the LV, "foreshortening" can lead to an apparent increase in wall thickness, inaccuracies in assessing wall motion, and the potential to overestimate systolic function. The walls of the LV can be divided into segments using the 17-segment model (also relevant for coronary supply), where the lateral wall

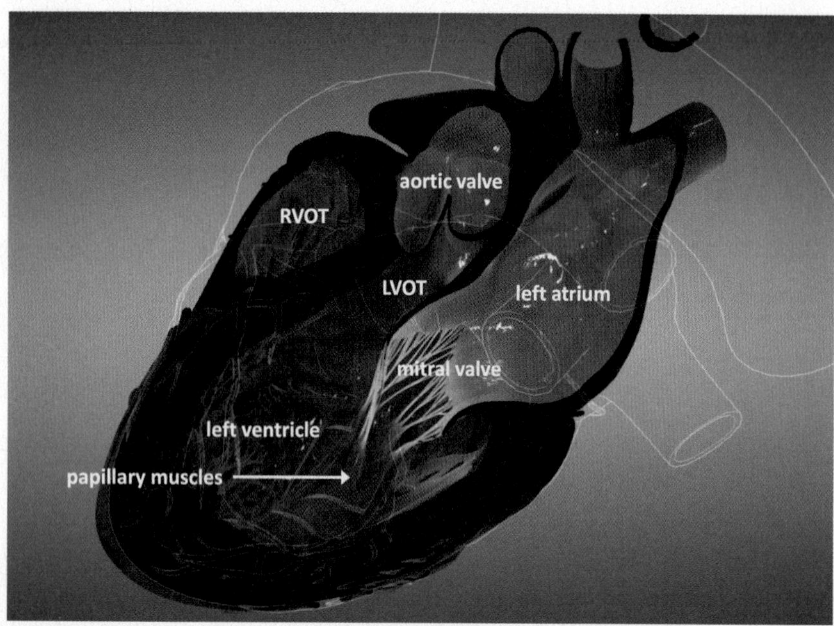

Figure 27-37 Anatomy of the left ventricle. The left ventricle is bordered by the mitral valve, aortic valve, ventricular septum, and the ventricular wall. Normally, the LV wall forms the apex of the heart. LVOT, left ventricular outflow tract; RVOT, right ventricular outflow tract.

is broadly supplied by the circumflex coronary artery, the anterior wall is supplied by the left anterior descending artery, and the inferior wall is supplied by the right coronary artery (Fig. 27-38).[15] These walls can be examined in their entirety either by progressively rotating the plane angle from the ME4C through to the ME2C and MELAX views in TEE, or rotating the transducer from the A4C to A2C and A3C in TTE. They can also be examined in the short axis via the TGSAX and the PSAX views, respectively, "sweeping" the ultrasound plane from base to apex to display the entire LV in short axis. Table 27-6 summarizes the views used to evaluate the LV.

Global Systolic Function

3 Measures of global systolic function can be performed qualitatively or quantitatively. Qualitative measures focus on visual estimation of the degree of wall thickening in systole, and the extent to which the LV cavity is reduced in size during systole. These are typically used in basic echocardiographic assessments in the absence of quantitative measures, but are also used by experienced

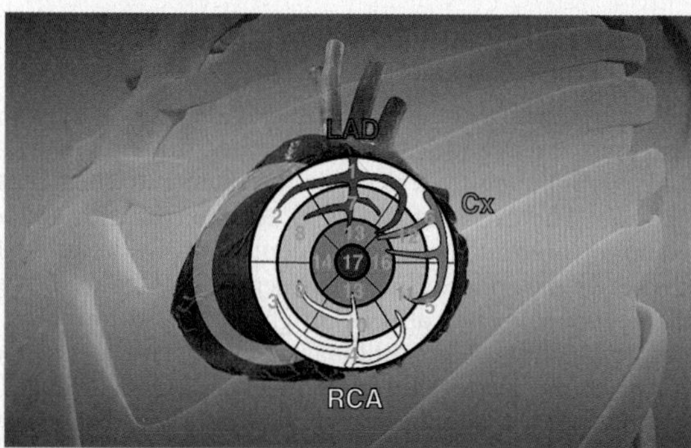

Figure 27-38 17-Segment model of the left ventricle. A 17-segment model of the LV with associated coronary distribution. 1—basal anterior, 2—basal anteroseptal, 3—basal inferoseptal, 4—basal inferior, 5—basal inferolateral, 6—basal anterolateral, 7—mid anterior, 8—mid anteroseptal, 9—mid inferoseptal, 10—mid inferior, 11—mid inferolateral, 12—mid anterolateral, 13—apical anterior, 14—apical septal, 15—apical inferior, 16—apical lateral, 17—apex.

echocardiographers to assess global systolic function in the setting of hemodynamic instability.

Fractional shortening (FS), fractional area change (FAC), and ejection fraction (EF) are commonly used quantitative measures (Table 27-7), and are best taken in their recommended views (Table 27-6).

- FS is the percentage change in LV basal diameter between end diastole and end systole.
- FAC is the percentage change in LV area at midpapillary level between end diastole and end systole (Fig. 27-39).
- EF is the percentage change in LV volume between end diastole and end systole. LV volumes are calculated using Simpson's method, the method of discs (MOD), which entails tracing the LV endocardial border in four- and two-chamber views at end diastole and end systole. Volumes for each measurement are calculated via thin slices of discs generated by tracing the endocardium. An alternative method is area–length (A–L) method, which consists of a calculation involving the long axis and the endocardial area of the LV (Fig. 27-40).

When tracing the endocardium, one should ensure that there is consistency of measurement. For example, if excluding the papillary muscles in the end-diastolic measurement, they should also be excluded in the end-systolic measurement. Accuracy is improved with more information, thus an EF obtained by measuring an average of two volumes in different views will provide more accurate information than a single diameter or area, as in the FS or FAC, respectively.

Several other modalities are used to quantify LV function.

- Evaluation of the descent of the mitral annulus toward the apex can be measured as mitral annular plane systolic excursion (MAPSE), which uses M-mode to assess the distance moved by the lateral mitral annulus (Fig. 27-41).[16]
- Tissue Doppler imaging (TDI) can also be used to measure the velocity of the lateral annular descent in systole (s prime, or s′).[17,18]
- Measuring the change in LV pressure over time (Dp/dt) requires a measurable mitral regurgitant velocity with CWD.[19] The time taken for the velocity to increase from 100 cm/s to 300 cm/s is measured by plotting the slope on the spectral tracing (Fig. 27-42). The

Table 27-6 Common Equivalent Two-Dimensional Transesophageal Echocardiography and Transthoracic Echocardiography Views for Important Cardiac Structures

Structure	Component	TEE View	TTE View
Left ventricle	Lateral and septal wall function	ME4C	A4C
	Anterior and inferior wall function	ME2C	A2C
	Anteroseptal and inferolateral wall function	MELAX	A3C and PLAX
	Mid-papillary short-axis LV function	TG mid SAX	PSAX
	Fractional shortening	TG mid SAX	PLAX
	Fractional area change	TG mid SAX	PSAX
	Ejection fraction	ME4C and ME2C	A4C and A2C
	Mitral annular motion	ME4C	A4C
	dP/dt	ME4C	A4C
	MPI	ME4C	A4C
	Transmitral diastolic inflow	ME4C	A4C
	LV dimensions	ME4C, TGmid SAX	PLAX
	LVOT VTI	Deep TG 5C	A5C and A3C
Right ventricle	Qualitative assessment of global systolic function	ME4C and RV inflow–outflow	A4C and PS AoV SAX
	Fractional area change	ME4C	A4C
	Wall thickness and dimensions	ME4C	A4C
	Tricuspid annular motion (TAPSE, S′)	ME4C[a]	A4C
	RIMP	ME4C[a]	A4C
Aortic valve	Structure	ME AV SAX and MELAX	PS AoV SAX and PLAX
	Systolic gradient	Deep TG	A5C and A3C
	LVOT diameter	MELAX	PLAX
	Vena contracta	MELAX	PLAX
	AR jet width	MELAX	PLAX
	Pressure half-time for regurgitation	Deep TG	A5C and A3C
Mitral valve	Structure	ME4C, ME2C, ME commissural view and MELAX	A4C, A2C, A3C and PLAX
	Diastolic gradient	ME4C and MELAX	A4C
	Vena contracta	ME4C and MELAX	A4C and PLAX
	Regurgitant jet area	ME4C, ME2C, and MELAX	A4C, A2C, A3C and PLAX
	Pulmonary venous flow	ME2C	A4C
Aorta		MELAX, ME Asc Aorta SAX, and ME Asc Aorta LAX Desc Aorta SAX Desc Aorta LAX	PLAX and SS

[a]Angle adjustment on the ultrasound machine is necessary to align the measurement along the direction of tissue movement.

Table 27-7 Assessment of Left Ventricular Systolic Function

Indices	Normal	Abnormal
FS	>26–45%	<25%
FAC	>41–60%	<40%
EF % (male, female)	>52%, >54%	Impairment Mild: 41–55%, 41–53% Moderate: 30–40%, 30–40% Severe: <30%, <30%
MAPSE	12–15 mm	EF <50%: <8 mm EF <30%: <7 mm
Lateral mitral valve annulus s'	>8 cm/s	<5 cm/s
dP/dt	>1,200 mmHg/s	<800 mmHg/s Severe: <500 mmHg/s
MPI	<0.4	>0.5

EF, ejection fraction; FAC, fractional area change; FS, fractional shortening; MAPSE, mitral annular plane systolic excursion; MPI, myocardial performance index.

software calculates the time and provides the Dp/dt value. Shorter times reflect rapidly increasing LV pressures in systole, while longer times are typically seen in the setting of poor LV function.

- The myocardial performance index (MPI) examines the ratio of time spent in isovolemic contraction (IVCT) and relaxation (IVRT) to ejection time (ET) and measures the efficiency of overall LV function.[20]

$$MPI = (IVCT + IVRT)/ET$$

As this value assesses the proportion of time the ventricle spends in isovolemic states over time spent in ejection, a higher proportion is indicative of worsening LV efficiency. Of the number of ways to obtain these values, an accepted method is via TDI of the lateral mitral annulus (Fig. 27-43). Since the goal is to ascertain the durations of AV opening (ET) and MV closure (IVCT+ET+IVRT), the sweep speed on the spectral Doppler should be increased to enable accurate measurement of time intervals.

Regional Systolic Function

Regional wall motion is assessed in each of the 17 segments, or 4
more broadly, by assessing the anterior, inferior, septal, and lateral walls of the LV. Wall motion is defined by wall thickening as either hyperkinetic, normal, hypokinetic, akinetic, or dyskinetic (Table 27-8).[21] Caution should be exercised as foreshortening or translocation of the ventricle can be misinterpreted as wall motion abnormality. In addition, conduction abnormalities and ventricular pacing may result in dyssynchronous contraction and the appearance of a regional wall abnormality where none exists. Assessment of regional wall motion can be challenging and, even among expert echocardiographers, there can be significant inter- and intraobserver variability in interpretation. The novice practitioner is hence cautioned against making all but the most obvious inferences.

Strain

Myocardial strain has been validated as an objective and reli- 5
able measure of systolic function. Strain captures local myocardial deformation, such as shortening or lengthening and thickening or thinning. It is measured using either speckle tracking, in which the relative positions of individual speckles in the myocardium are tracked through the cardiac cycle, or TDI. Longitudinal, radial, and circumferential strain can be measured to assess both regional and global systolic function. Strain values are normally negative for longitudinal and

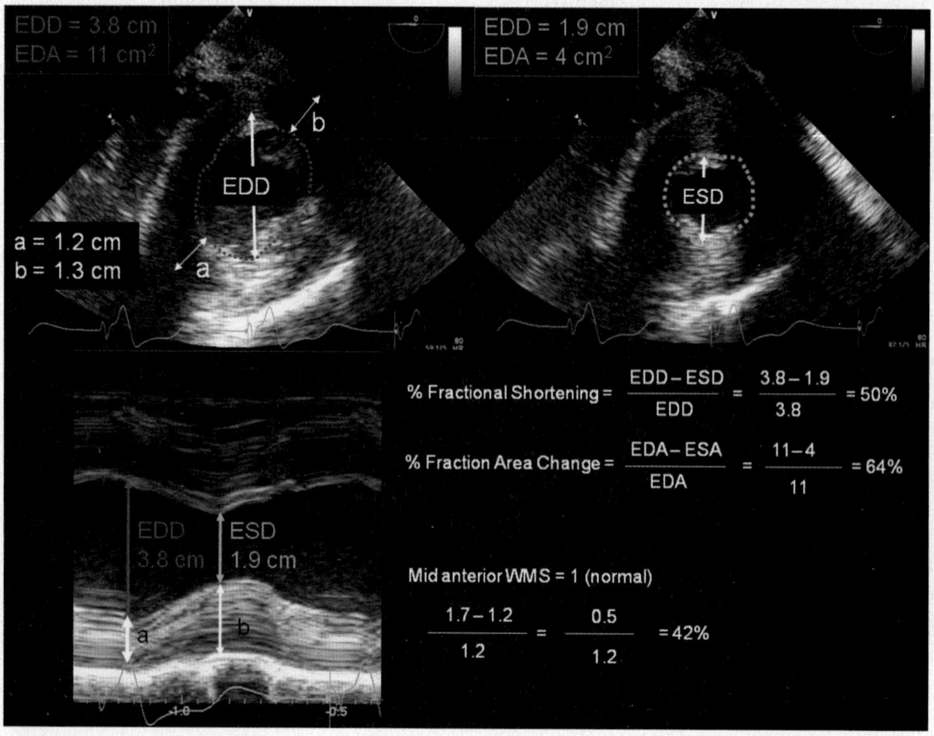

Figure 27-39 Fractional area change. Top panel: Evaluation of global LV function using diameter and area in end diastole (ED) and end systole (ES) in the transgastric short axis. Measurement of diameters (D), areas (A), and wall thickness. Wall thickness should be measured at ED in the anteroseptal and inferolateral wall segments. Bottom panel: Diameter and wall thickness measured using M-mode with the cursor crossing the middle of inferior (*top*) and anterior (*bottom*) segments. The percent change of wall thickness in each of these segments can be used to grade its regional function.

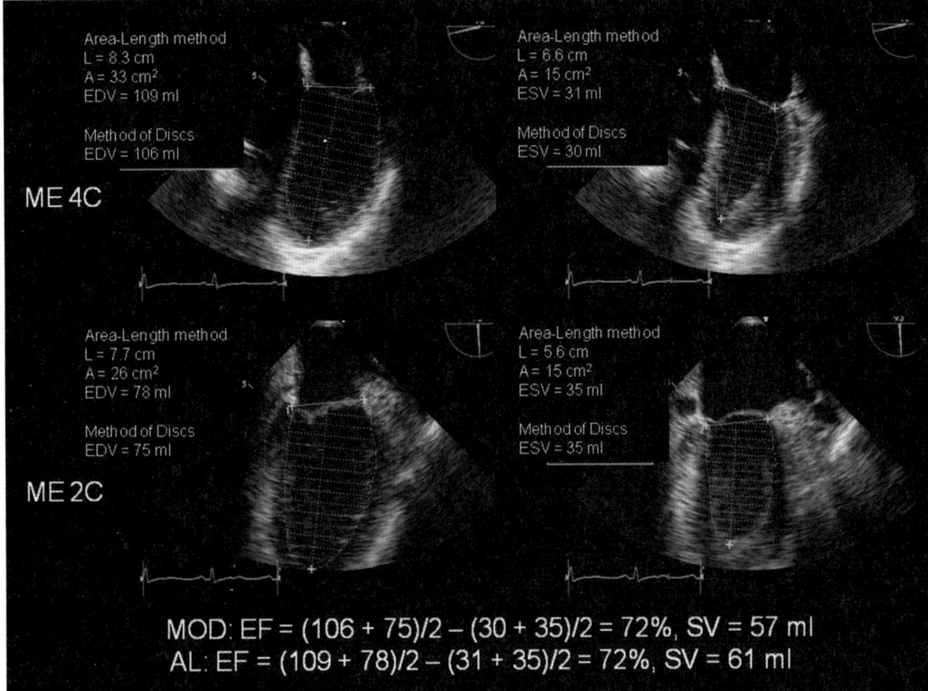

Figure 27-40 Volumetric quantification of left ventricular (LV) systolic function. Volumetric quantitation of LV systolic function, using traces of endocardium in the midesophageal four-chamber and midesophageal two-chamber end-diastolic and end-systolic frames. LV volumes are calculated by software using either the method of discs (MOD) or the area–length method (AL). EF, ejection fraction; EDV, end-diastolic volume; ESV, end-systolic volume; SV, stroke volume.

circumferential strain (myocardial shortening), and positive for radial strain (myocardial thickening). Strain rate describes the rate of change in myocardial length over time. Both strain and strain rate can be described in graphical format over the cardiac cycle, allowing for evaluation of regional function (Fig. 27-44).

Left Ventricular Diastolic Function

Active ventricular relaxation starts as LV pressure begins to fall in systole, when actin–myosin filaments in ventricular myocytes begin to decouple in an ATP-dependent process. Relaxation then continues throughout the ventricular filling phase, which starts when left atrial pressure exceeds left ventricular pressure, thereby opening the MV. The LV passively fills with blood until atrial and ventricular pressures equilibrate—diastasis—and further flow only occurs with atrial systole, which normally contributes 20% of LV end-diastolic volume (this proportion is higher when impaired relaxation reduces the amount of passive filling). A combination of impaired relaxation, increased ventricular stiffness, or pericardial constriction will result in diastolic dysfunction and subsequent rise in left atrial pressure. Ultimately, pulmonary hypertension (PHTN) and right ventricular failure can develop.[22]

Diastolic dysfunction is an independent predictor of perioperative and long-term morbidity and mortality.[23] Echocardiography plays a key role in the evaluation of its severity, and may help

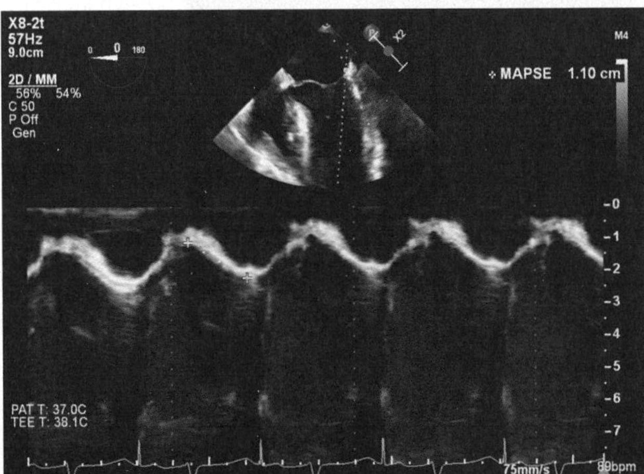

Figure 27-41 Mitral annular plane systolic excursion (MAPSE). A midesophageal four-chamber view in M-mode with the cut plane passing through the lateral mitral annulus, showing the mitral annular plane systolic excursion.

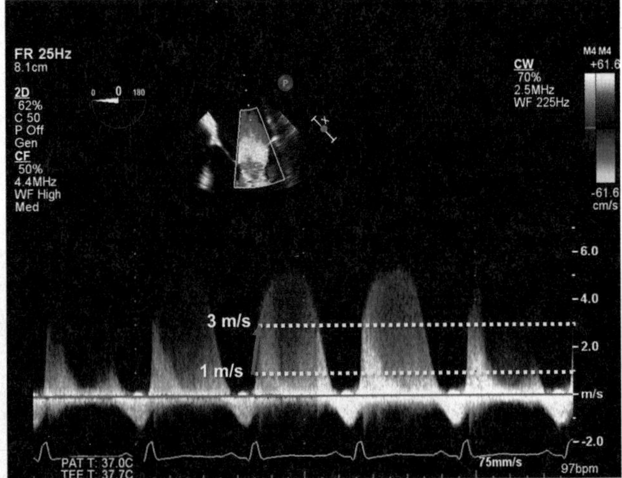

Figure 27-42 Assessment of systolic function by dP/dt. Continuous wave Doppler display of mitral regurgitant jet. The change in pressure over time is measured as the time taken (*slope of red arrow*) for the velocity to increase from 1 m/s to 3 m/s (*yellow dashed lines*).

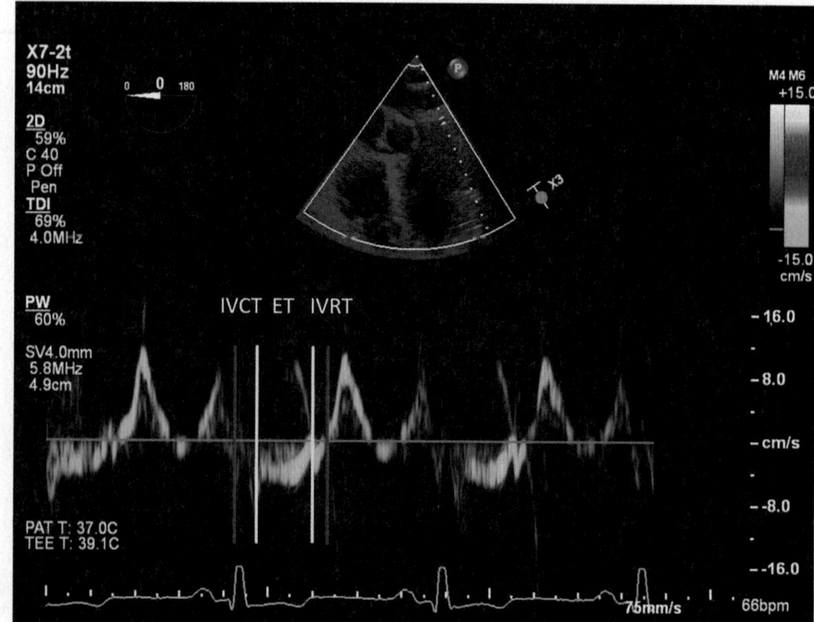

Figure 27-43 Myocardial performance index by tissue Doppler imaging. The isovolemic contraction time (IVCT) and isovolemic relaxation time (IVRT) is 0.16 seconds and the ejection time (ET), *bordered by the yellow line*, is 0.27 seconds. The myocardial performance index is therefore calculated at 0.59.

Table 27-8 Assessment of Regional Wall Motion

Systolic Wall Motion	Radial Shortening Toward Center of LV Chamber (%)	Wall Thickening (%)
Normal	>30%	>30%
Hypokinesis	10–30%	10–30%
Akinesis	None	None
Dyskinesis	Outward motion	None
Aneurysm	Outward motion	Thin-walled

with identification of the underlying etiology. Heart failure with preserved EF is a well-recognized clinical syndrome in which diastolic dysfunction plays a causal role. However, only a subset of patients with diastolic dysfunction will go on to develop clinically significant heart failure and therefore, echocardiographic findings must be correlated with a thorough history and physical examination.[24]

The progression of diastolic dysfunction is defined in a graded manner (see Table 27-9).[22] Evaluation of diastolic function is complex. The four formal components of assessment are as follows:

- Mitral inflow velocities
- TDI-derived mitral annular early velocity (e′)

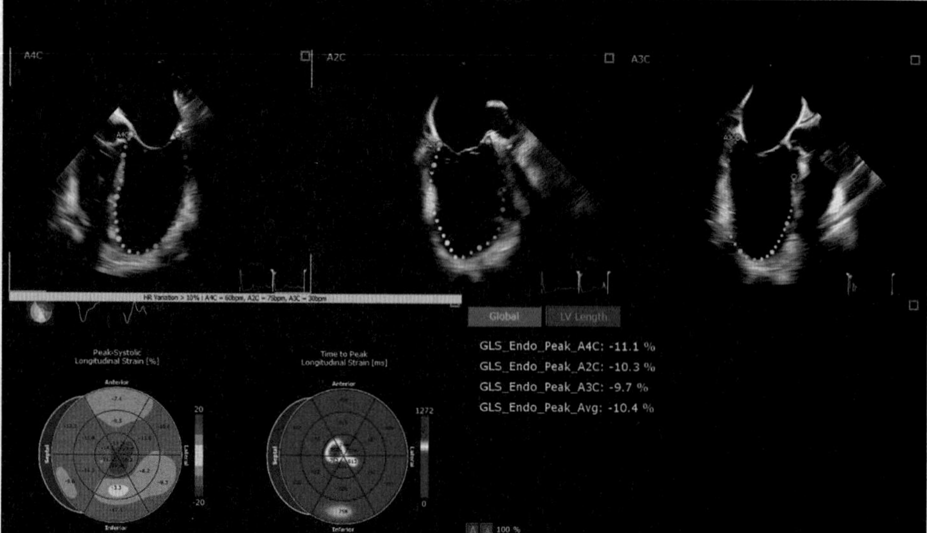

Figure 27-44 Strain. Left ventricular strain can be quantified using speckle tracking software. The example shown in this image reveals a global longitudinal strain of more than −15%, which is considered abnormal. The three imaging planes used in this image are the equivalent four-, two-, and three- chamber views in transthoracic and tranesophageal echocardiography.

Table 27-9 Differing Grades of Diastolic Dysfunction and Their Associated Features

	Normal	Grade 1	Grade 2	Grade 3
LV relaxation	Normal	Impaired	Impaired	Impaired
LAP	Normal	Normal or ↑	↑	↑
Mitral E/A ratio	≥0.8	<0.8	≥0.8–<2	≥2
Peak TR velocity >2.8 m/s	No	No	Yes	Yes
LAVI >34 mL/m^2	No	—	Yes	Yes

- Tricuspid regurgitant jet velocity (TR V_{max})
- Left atrial volume, indexed to body surface area (LAVI)

Early diastolic transmitral inflow velocity (E) and late mitral inflow velocity generated by atrial contraction (A) are measured by placing the pulse wave (PW) cursor at the tips of the MV leaflets in a four-chamber view. The mean of the lateral and septal e′ values, measured using PW TDI of the lateral and medial mitral annulus, is used for analysis of diastolic function. Left atrial volume is difficult to quantify with TEE due to its close proximity to the TEE probe, which makes it impossible to display the atrium fully. The left atrium is best viewed in TTE in the A4C and A2C views. A LAVI of greater than 34 mL/m^2 indicates diastolic dysfunction (Fig. 27-45). A TR V_{max} of greater than 280 cm/s reflects PHTN and is also suggestive of diastolic dysfunction (Fig. 27-46). Pulmonary venous flow velocity is also affected by diastolic function and can be used for supplementary evaluation, although this can be difficult to assess with TTE and therefore is best imaged with TEE. The ASE guideline remains the most widely used resource describing the assessment and interpretation of diastolic function (Fig. 27-47).[22]

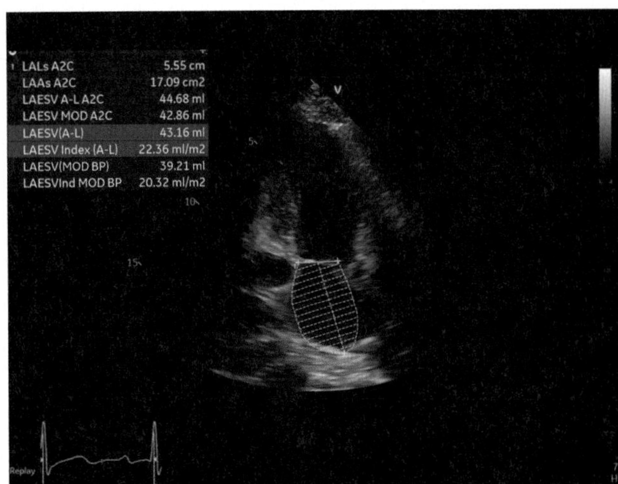

Figure 27-45 Left atrial volume index. Left atrial area is obtained during ventricular end systole (ES) in the transthoracic A4C and A2C view (seen below). Volume is calculated using the area–length method (A–L) or method of discs (MOD), and combined with body surface index, can be calculated left atrial volume index, a marker of diastolic dysfunction. LALs, left atrial length in systole; LAAs, left atrial area in systole.

Left Ventricular Pathology

Dilation

At end diastole, the normal LV end-diastolic diameter is <5.5 cm. Larger values may suggest chronic volume overload, for example, caused by mitral or AV regurgitation, or an associated cardiomyopathy.

Ventricular Aneurysms and Pseudoaneurysms

LV wall aneurysms are areas of thinned myocardium, which have wide bases or necks (Fig. 27-48) and are often due to ischemia. Pseudoaneurysms, in contrast, are areas of large outpouching through a rupture in the myocardium via a narrow base,

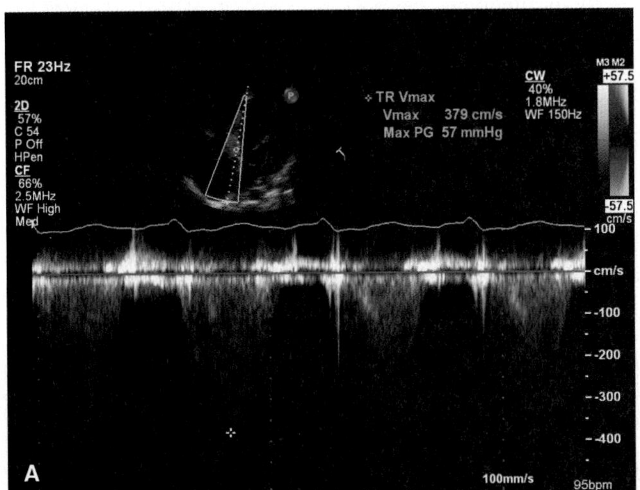

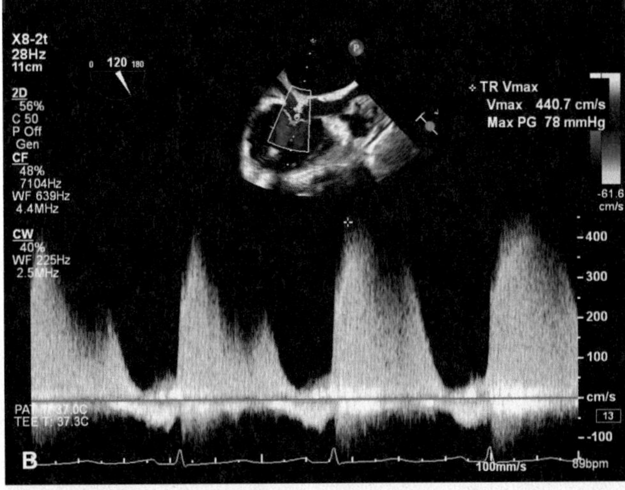

Figure 27-46 Tricuspid regurgitant peak jet velocity. Tricuspid regurgitant peak jet velocity (TR V_{max}) obtained in the transthoracic parasternal short-axis view (**Panel A**) and a modified bicaval view (**Panel B**). The maximum pressure gradient (max PG) is determined using the simplified Bernoulli equation. The right ventricular systolic pressure (RSVP)—a surrogate for pulmonary systolic artery pressure—can be estimated by adding the max PG to the right atrial pressure (RAP), a hemodynamic parameter that can be assumed from the central venous pressure obtained from a central venous catheter. Panel A shows an elevated TR V_{max} (>2.8 m/s) that would suggest an elevated RVSP (>36 mmHg)[90] and pulmonary hypertension (PHTN). (Reprinted from Bossone E, D'Andrea A, D'Alto M, et al. Echocardiography in pulmonary arterial hypertension: from diagnosis to prognosis. *J Am Soc Echocardiogr*. 2013;26(1):1–14. Copyright © 2013 Elseiver. With permission.)

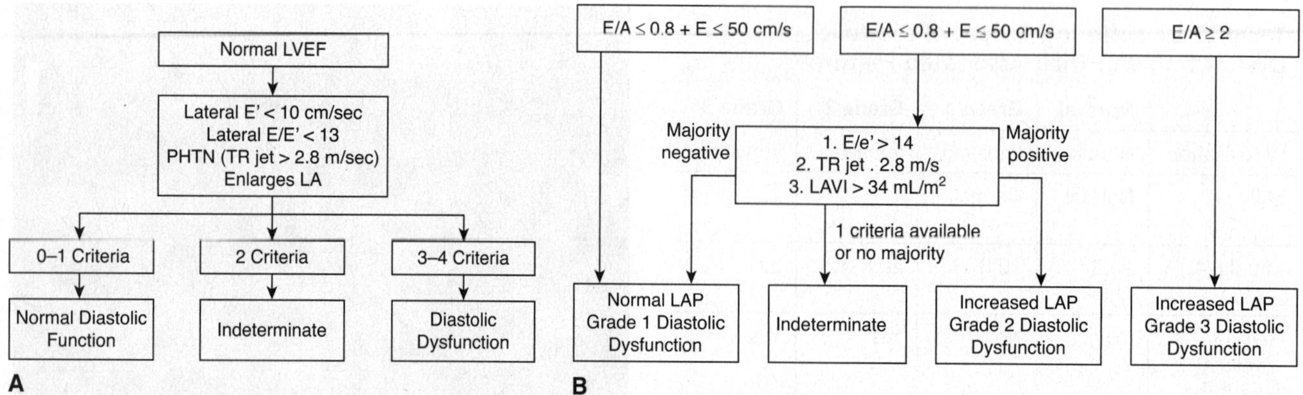

Figure 27-47 ASE Guideline Algorithm for the diagnosis of left ventricular diastolic dysfunction. Panel A describes grading of diastolic dysfunction. Panel B describes grading of diastolic dysfunction specifically in patients with depressed left ventricular ejection fraction (LVEF) and patients with myocardial disease and normal LVEF. Grading of dysfunction is based on identification of raised left atrial pressure. PHTN, pulmonary hypertension; TR, tricuspid regurgitation; LA, left atrium; LAP, left atrial pressure; LAVI, left atrial volume index. (Adapted from the 2016 American Society of Echocardiography recommendations for evaluation of left ventricular diastolic dysfunction.)

contained by the surrounding pericardium; these can be at high risk of uncontrolled rupture and tamponade. Both aneurysms and pseudoaneurysms are a potential source of thrombi and emboli due to their low-flow state and should be interrogated closely by the echocardiographer.[25]

Hypertrophy

Left ventricular wall hypertrophy generally occurs over months to years due to remodeling. Wall hypertrophy may be concentric or asymmetric. Diastolic LV wall septal or posterior thickness greater than 1.0 cm in women and 1.1 cm in men is considered to be abnormal, and greater than 1.5 cm and 1.7 cm, respectively, is considered severe. In hypertrophic obstructive cardiomyopathy (HOCM), LV hypertrophy causes obstruction. Turbulent flow can be seen in the LVOT on color Doppler imaging. This condition can also be associated with systolic anterior motion (SAM) of the anterior MV leaflet (Fig. 27-49). This is an important cause of low cardiac output often seen in the perioperative setting in patients with LV hypertrophy and hypovolemia from excessive blood loss, combined with hypercontractility from endogenous or administered catecholamines.

Right Ventricle

Assessment of the RV is more challenging than assessing the LV, owing to its asymmetric, crescentic shape (Fig. 27-50). The RV comprises a free wall, interventricular septum, and apex, with the tricuspid valve as its inflow, and the pulmonic valve as its outflow. The right coronary artery supplies most of the RV, although in a left dominant circulation, the posterior descending artery will supply the inferior RV wall. As it is part of a lower-pressure system, the RV wall tends to be thinner and more compliant than the LV, but more sensitive to changes in afterload.[14] It plays an important role in outcomes for patients with cardiorespiratory disease, mandating a greater awareness among anesthesiologists for early detection and management of RV dysfunction.

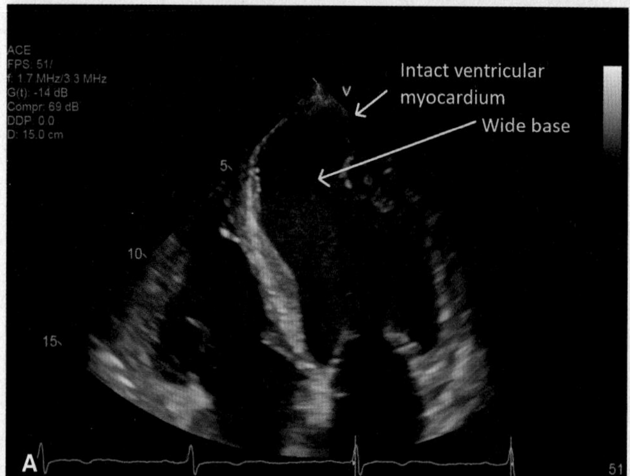

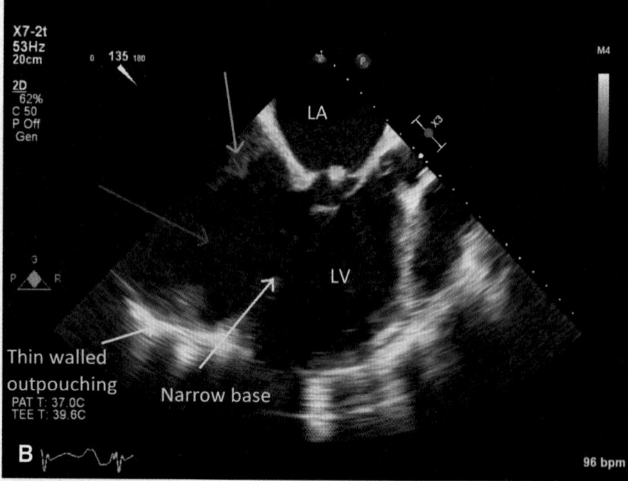

Figure 27-48 Ventricular aneurysms and pseudoaneurysms. The apical ventricular aneurysm (**Panel A**) shows an intact, but thinned, ventricular myocardium in the apical four chamber. Conversely, in a midesophageal long-axis view, the inferolateral left ventricular pseudoaneurysm (**Panel B**) has an outpouching through a narrow ventricular myocardial defect. This image is also significant for the echodense thrombus (*green arrow*), contrasted against the more echolucent blood (*red arrow*).

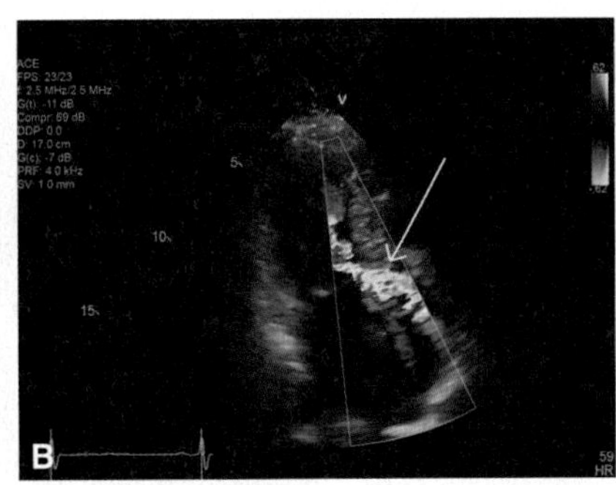

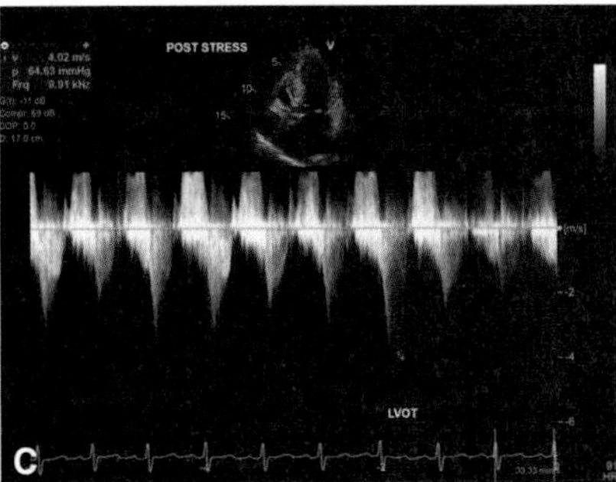

Figure 27-49 Hypertrophic obstructive cardiomyopathy. Septal hypertrophy in a patient with hypertrophic obstructive cardiomyopathy, visualized in a zoomed-in midesophageal long-axis view, with associated Systolic Anterior Motion (**Panel A**). Flow acceleration is seen as turbulent flow in the left ventricular outflow tract (LVOT) in the same patient with a prior apical three-chamber view, suggesting a narrowing in or proximal to the LVOT (**Panel B**). Following pharmacologic stress test, a peak LVOT gradient of greater than 50 mmHg is observed in CWD obtained from the A5C view (**Panel C**), consistent with dynamic LVOT obstruction.

Diameters and Wall Thickness

Quantitative echocardiographic assessment of the diameter and wall thickness of the right ventricle is more challenging than for the LV, in part due to a shape that makes standardized measurement difficult. A wall thickness >5 mm suggests of hypertrophy, and a basal diameter of >42 mm, mid-diameter >35 mm, or length >86 mm is suggestive of dilation.[26] Visual estimation of RV dilation can also be made relative to a normal LV: an RV more than two-thirds toward the LV apex suggests mild dilation, equivalent RV and LV length suggests moderate dilation, and a larger RV that extends beyond the LV apex suggests severe dilation (Fig. 27-51).

RV Systolic Function

3 The irregular shape of the RV precludes geometric assumptions like those used to calculate the function of the LV in 2D imaging. Since quantification of RV volumes and RV-EF is not possible in 2D imaging, the evaluation of RV systolic function is limited to measurements of distances, time, and areas:

- Tricuspid annular plane systolic excursion (TAPSE) is a commonly used measurement. It is measured in a four-chamber view using M-mode. The cursor is placed on the lateral tricuspid annulus; and its orientation adjusted such that it aligns with the direction of annular movement toward the apex of the RV. The distance that the tricuspid annulus travels toward the apex during systole is then quantified (Fig. 27-52). A value of less than 17 mm suggests at least mild dysfunction. A limitation of TAPSE is that it is a regional, rather than global, assessment of RV function. FAC is measured in the ME4C or A4C view, where the percentage change from end-diastolic to end-systolic area is calculated (Fig. 27-53). A value of less than 35% is indicative of RV dysfunction.
- TDI-derived measurements using lateral annular systolic velocity and right ventricular index of myocardial performance (RIMP)—similar in concept to the LV MPI—are best measured in the TTE A4C view, as alignment of the structures can be difficult to obtain by TEE.[14] TDI-derived lateral annular systolic velocity of less than 10 cm/s (Fig. 27-54) and a TDI-derived RIMP of greater than >0.55 indicate RV dysfunction.

Valvular Heart Disease

Echocardiography remains one of the principal methods for evaluating cardiac valvular pathology. The pulmonic valve is easier to image with TTE, while the MV is easier to image with TEE. The principles of echocardiographic imaging of pathologic valves are based on their anatomy, impact of lesions on surrounding structures, and quantification of severity of lesions. Regarding more detailed valvular anatomy, please refer to Chapter 12. 6

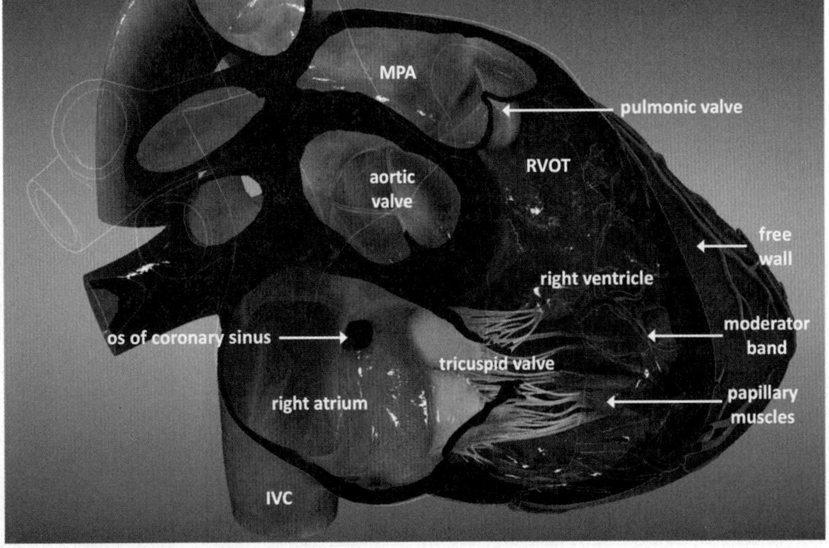

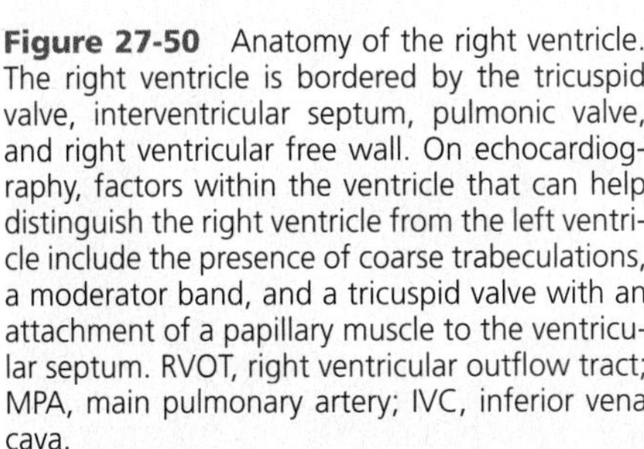

Figure 27-50 Anatomy of the right ventricle. The right ventricle is bordered by the tricuspid valve, interventricular septum, pulmonic valve, and right ventricular free wall. On echocardiography, factors within the ventricle that can help distinguish the right ventricle from the left ventricle include the presence of coarse trabeculations, a moderator band, and a tricuspid valve with an attachment of a papillary muscle to the ventricular septum. RVOT, right ventricular outflow tract; MPA, main pulmonary artery; IVC, inferior vena cava.

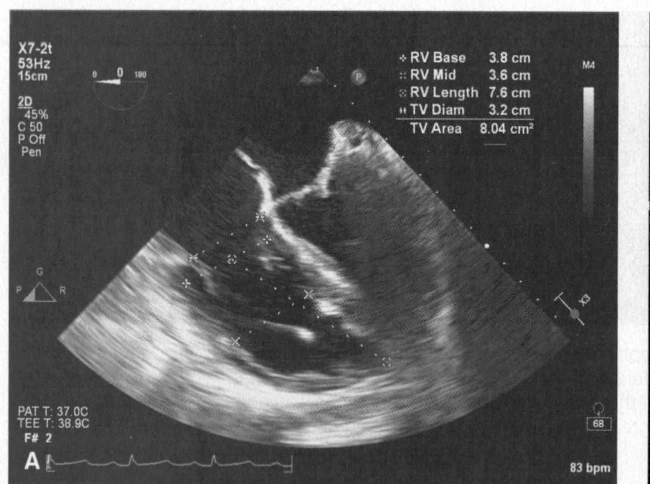

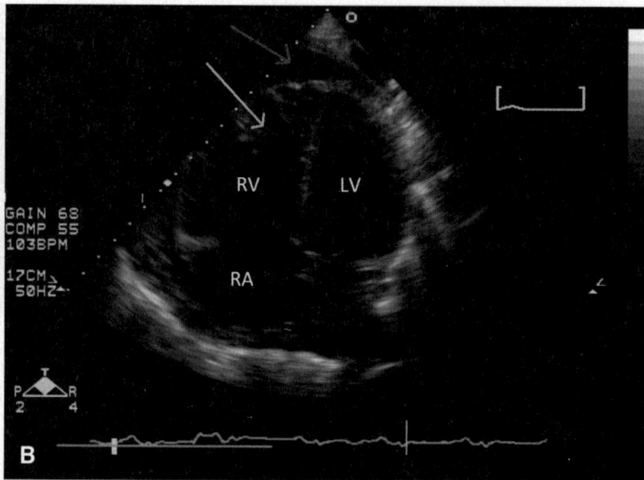

Figure 27-51 Right ventricular dimensions. Normal right ventricular dimensions as measured on the midesophageal four chamber (**Panel A**) is compared to a severely dilated right ventricle on the apical four chamber (**Panel B**). The right ventricle is identified by the moderator band seen with the *green arrow*. A small pericardial effusion is indicated by the *red arrow*. RA, right atrium; RV, right ventricle; LV, left ventricle; TV, tricuspid valve.

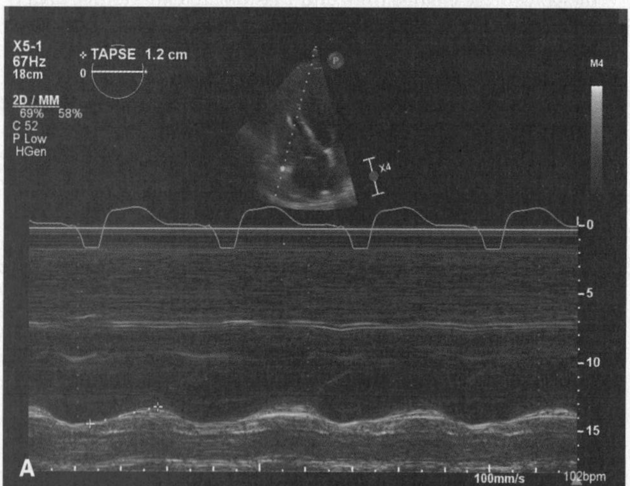

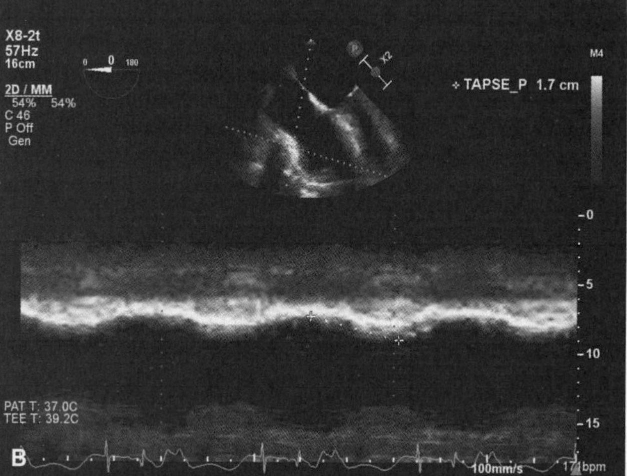

Figure 27-52 Tricuspid annular plane systolic excursion. Tricuspid Annular Plane Systolic Excursion (TAPSE) by M-mode echocardiography with an abnormal result shown in Panel A, performed in the apical four-chamber view. While TAPSE can be performed in tranesophageal views, as shown in Panel B, it commonly requires anatomical M-mode, a feature available only to certain ultrasound machines, allowing alignment of the M-mode plane between the lateral tricuspid annulus and the right ventricular apex.

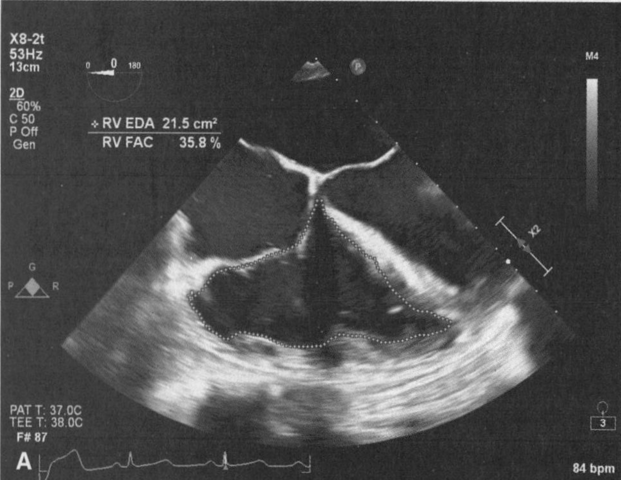

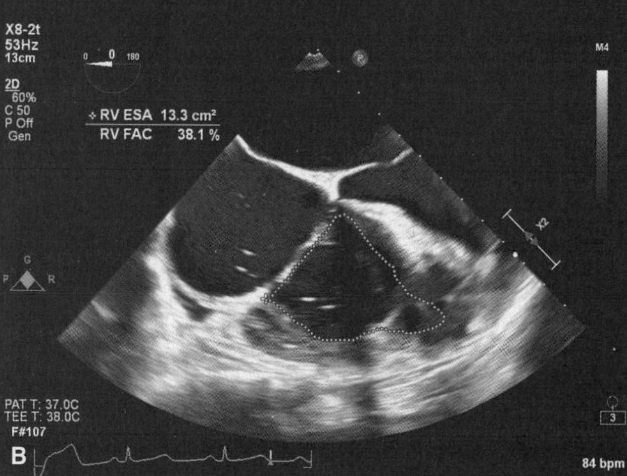

Figure 27-53 Right ventricular fractional area change. Normal right ventricular fractional area change (FAC), measuring the area of the RV in the midesophageal four-chamber view during end diastole (EDA), measured in Panel A, and end systole (ESA), measured in Panel B.

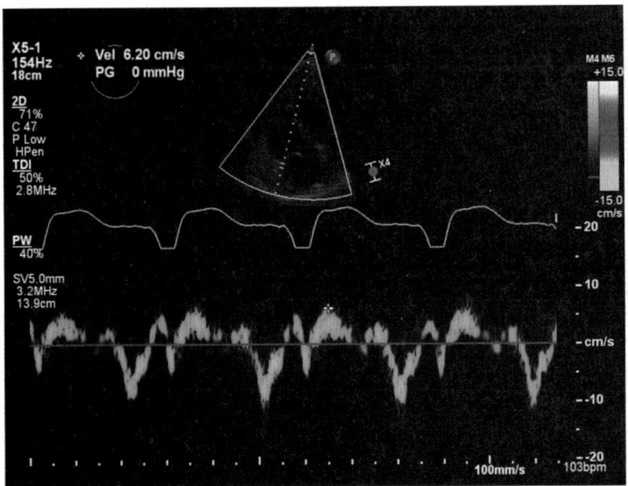

Figure 27-54 Right ventricular S′. An abnormal tricuspid valve annular S′ velocity measured in a patient with cardiomyopathy, taken in the apical four-chamber view.

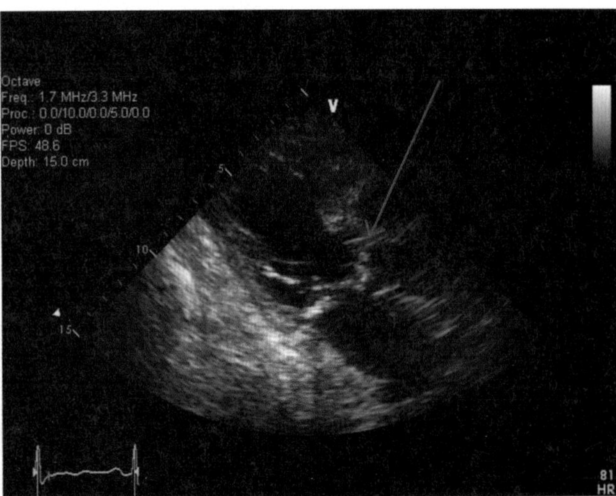

Figure 27-56 Significant aortic stenosis. In this parasternal long-axis view, minimal opening on the aortic valve (*red arrow*) is seen in systole, suggestive of significant aortic stenosis.

Table 27-6 describes the typical echocardiographic views for each valve. When estimating the severity of valvular lesions, there are some visual cues that may predict severe disease. For regurgitant or stenotic lesions, flow converges close to the pathologic valve, followed by turbulence after the valve lesion is crossed (Fig. 27-55). In significant stenotic lesions, minimal leaflet motion is seen throughout the cardiac cycle (Fig. 27-56).

Aortic Valve

It is important to appreciate the AV as a 3D structure that extends between the ventriculoaortic junction and the sinotubular junction. The normal AV has three leaflets, or cusps. Congenital abnormalities can range from unicuspid to quadricuspid valves. Each leaflet is bordered by a free margin, two commissures, the highest attachment point on either side of each leaflet, and a

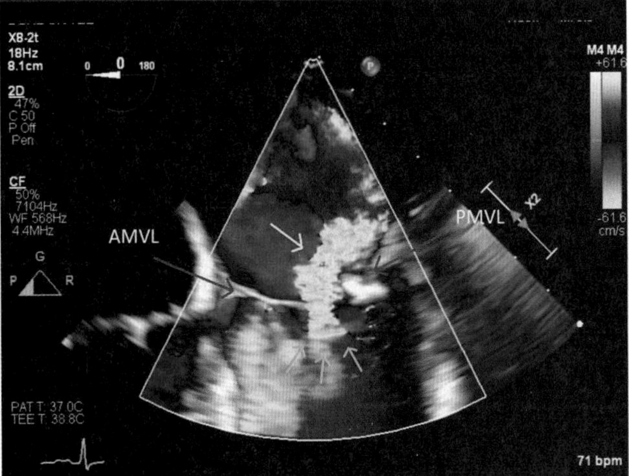

Figure 27-55 Flow convergence and turbulent flow seen in mitral regurgitation. A zoomed-in midesophageal four-chamber view of a Carpentier type 3 mitral regurgitation, with a restricted posterior leaflet and a posteriorly directed eccentric jet. The *green arrows* indicate the significant flow convergence upstream of the lesion and the *yellow arrow* indicates downstream turbulent flow, suggestive of severe mitral regurgitation. AMVL, Anterior mitral valve leaflet; PMVL, posterior mitral valve leaflet.

hinge which anchors the leaflet to the wall of the aorta. AV function is closely linked to its surrounding structures and *vice versa*. These structures include the sinuses of Valsalva, the sinotubular junction, coronary ostia, the anterior MV leaflet, and the LVOT (Fig. 27-57).

Aortic Stenosis

The most common causes for AS in the developed world are calcification and bicuspid valves. Globally, there is a high prevalence of rheumatic disease (Fig. 27-58).[27] In the ME AV SAX and the PSAX AV, it is important to assess the degree of opening of each leaflet and characterize its appearance and associated features. In calcific disease, the leaflet body will appear thick and stiff with significant echodense calcification, causing acoustic shadowing. In rheumatic disease, there is fusion between the edges of the leaflets along the commissures, while the leaflet body might be spared. Associated features seen with AS include aortic regurgitation (AR), diastolic dysfunction from LV hypertrophy, and poststenotic aortic root dilatation.

The severity of AS can be graded in several ways. Measurements of flow through the AV, such as peak velocity, peak and mean gradients are usually easy to obtain (Fig. 27-11), but these do not provide a quantitative assessment of AV area. The area of the AV orifice can be estimated in two ways:

1. Measurement via planimetry is best done in 3D but can be performed in 2D by tracing out the area of AV opening during systole. However, planimetry is often inaccurate because calcification may cause acoustic shadowing and it may not be possible to obtain the correct imaging plane exactly at the leaflet tips.
2. The recommended method of AV opening area estimation is derived from the continuity equation as described earlier, which requires the LVOT cross-sectional area, LVOT VTI using PWD of systolic flow, and the AV VTI from the CWD trace in systole:

$$\text{AV Area} = \text{VTI}_{\text{LVOT}} \times \text{CSA}_{\text{LVOT}} \div \text{VTI}_{\text{AV}}$$

The dimensionless index is also commonly used, which requires only the VTI at the AV and at the LVOT:

$$\text{Dimensionless Index} = \text{VTI}_{\text{LVOT}} \div \text{VTI}_{\text{AV}}$$

Table 27-10 provides a summary of parameters used to grade the severity of AS.

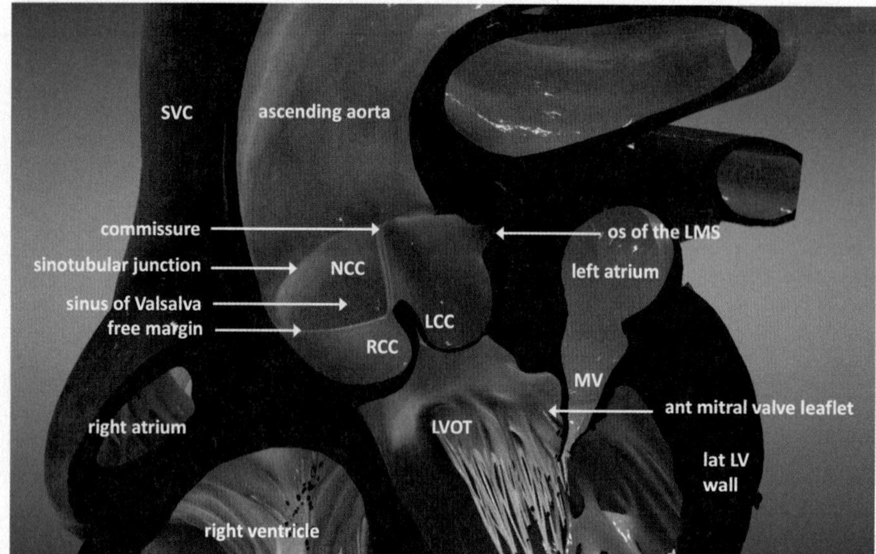

Figure 27-57 Aortic valve model. A model of the aortic valve showing the three cusps, or leaflets, with each leaflet bordered by a free margin and a curved line of attachment to the wall of the left ventricle outlet and aortic root. The aortic valve is closely related to the aorta, coronary os, left ventricular outflow tract (LVOT), and anterior mitral valve leaflet. NCC, noncoronary cusp; RCC, right coronary cusp; LCC, left coronary cusp; SVC, superior vena cava; LMS, left main stem coronary artery; ant, anterior; lat, lateral.

Aortic Regurgitation

AR may be due to primary AV disease or aortic root disease.[28] Primary valve disease commonly occurs due to congenital abnormalities, infective endocarditis, rheumatic heart disease, or as accompanying regurgitation in patients with AS. Common causes for aortic root dilatation include degenerative disease, or connective tissue disorders, such as Marfan syndrome. Further, patients with ascending aortic dissection can develop AR due to extension of the dissection to the aortic root, or because of prolapse of the dissection flap onto the valve leaflets, preventing complete closure.

Chronic AR may cause eccentric LV hypertrophy, and over time may result in a reduced EF. AR can be quantified by measuring the diameter of the regurgitant jet at its narrowest point, called the *vena contracta*. Other assessments include calculating the regurgitant jet to LVOT diameter ratio, or the AR pressure half-time by applying CWD across the AR jet. The trace on CWD may also appear denser in severe disease (see Tables 27-6 and 27-11 and Fig. 27-59).

Table 27-10 Grading the Severity of Aortic Stenosis

	Sclerosis	Mild	Moderate	Severe
Peak velocity	≤2.5	2.6–2.9	3.0–4.0	>4.0
Peak gradient (mmHg)	<20	20–40	41–70	>70
Mean gradient (mmHg)		<20	20–40	>40
Aortic valve area (cm^2)	>2	1.5–1.9	1.0–1.4	<1
Dimensionless index		>0.5	0.25–0.5	<0.25

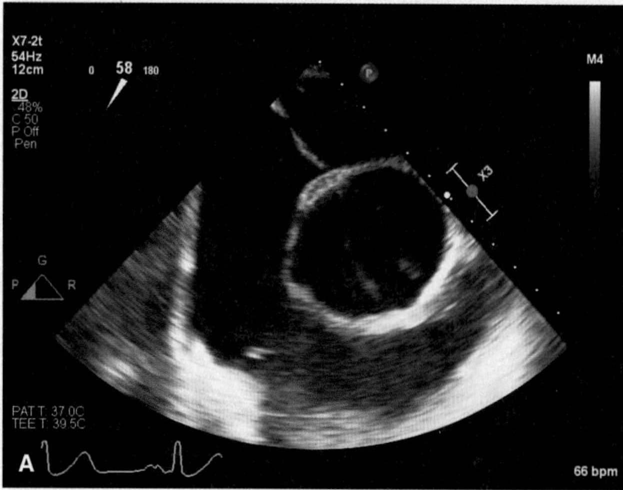

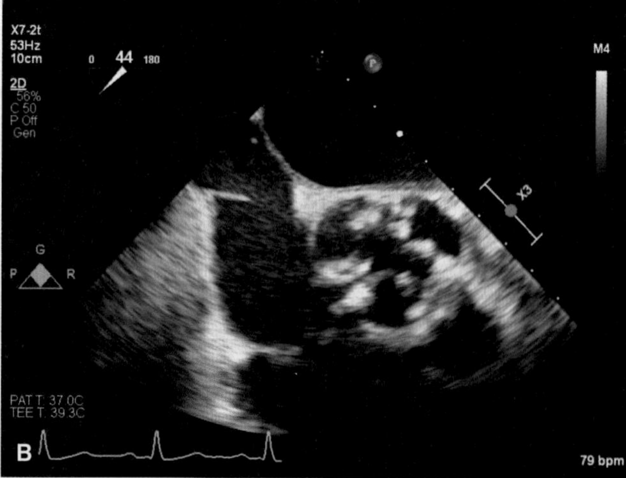

Figure 27-58 Common aortic valve pathologies. Bicuspid valve (**Panel A**) and calcific disease (**Panel B**) are the most common reasons for aortic stenosis in the developed world.

Table 27-11 Grading the Severity of Aortic Regurgitation

	Mild	Moderate	Severe
Vena contracta (mm)	<3	3–6	>6
Pressure half-time (ms)	>500	200–500	<200
Jet width to jet LVOT diameter (%)	<25	25–64	>64
Descending aorta diastolic flow reversal	Early	Intermediate	Holodiastolic
Density CWD jet	Faint	Faint	Dense

Mitral Valve

As described in Chapter 12: Cardiac Anatomy and Physiology, and illustrated in Figure 27-60, the MV consists of an anterior leaflet and posterior leaflet; the latter is usually divided into three scallops—P1, P2, and P3—opposed by three segments of the anterior leaflet—A1, A2, and A3. The structure of the MV is maintained by the saddle-shaped mitral annular ring, chordae tendineae, and associated anterolateral and posteromedial papillary muscles. In particular, the anterior leaflet of the MV is closely related to the AV, and forms part of the structure of the LVOT. This relationship can become relevant when there is SAM of the anterior mitral leaflet, whereby, the leaflet may be drawn into the LVOT during systole, causing LVOT obstruction. This condition may be seen in patients with hypovolemia, HOCM, or those who have undergone MV repair. In addition to standard 2D views to examine the MV (Table 27-6), 3D echocardiography is routinely used in the evaluation of MV pathology during cardiac surgery. MELAX usually provides the most effective view to interrogate

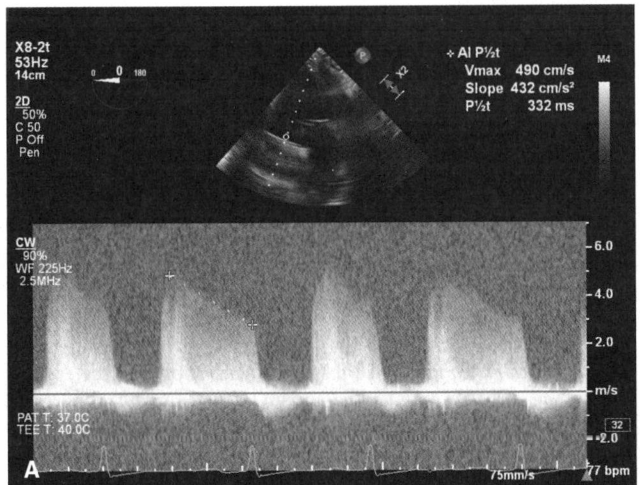

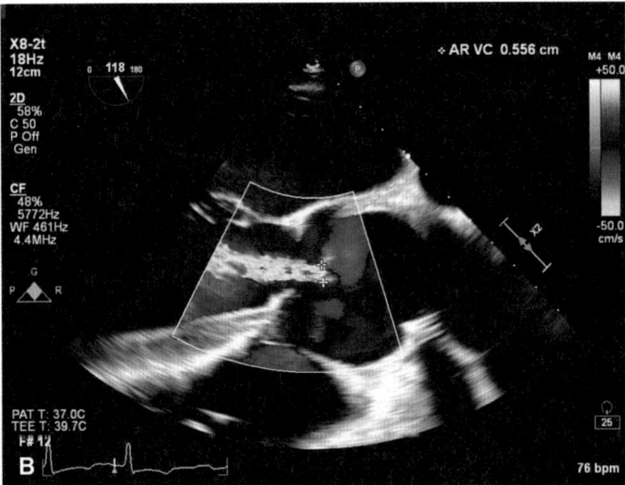

Figure 27-59 Aortic regurgitation. Aortic valve regurgitation/insufficiency (AR/AI) as measured by pressure half-time (P½t) seen in Panel A and vena contracta (VC) seen in Panel B. In arrhythmias such as atrial fibrillation as seen here, multiple measurements may need to be taken and averaged out.

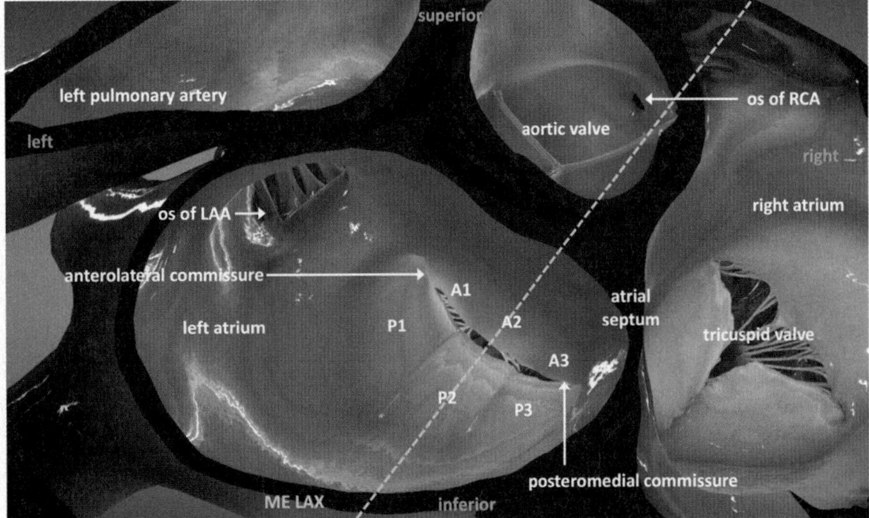

Figure 27-60 Mitral valve anatomy. Mitral valve anatomy as seen in the en face view, viewed from the left atrium, with the aortic valve seen above the mitral valve. The intersecting dotted plane of the midesophageal long axis (MELAX) view shows how the transesophageal echocardiographic probe can be manipulated left to view the A1/P1 segments, and right to view the A3/P3 segments. RCA, right coronary artery; LAA, left atrial appendage.

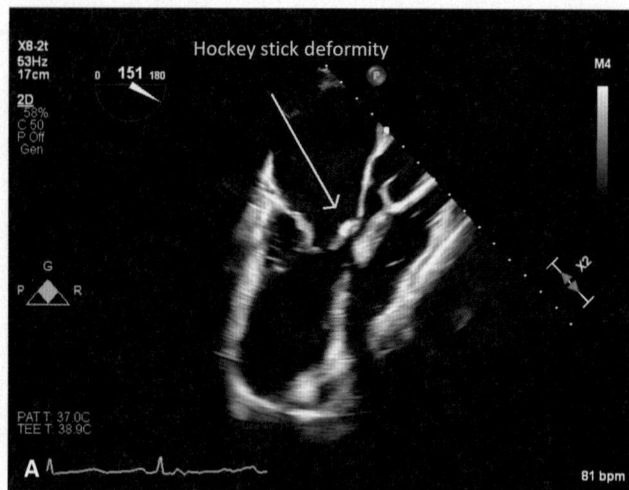

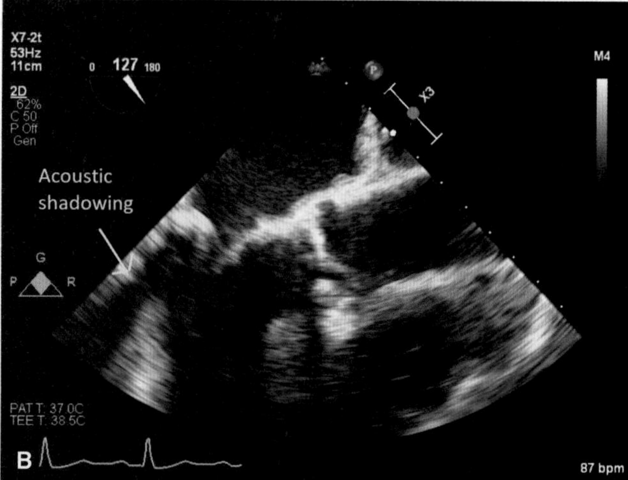

Figure 27-61 Rheumatic (**Panel A**) and calcific (**Panel B**) disease. In rheumatic mitral stenosis, there is typically bowing of the anterior mitral valve, or hockey stick deformity, as is seen on this midesophageal long-axis view. In calcified valvular disease, as is seen in Panel B with both calcified mitral and aortic valve disease, the valve appears hyperechoic, with acoustic shadowing beyond.

the individual leaflet as it cuts the MV in the anterior–posterior axis. Turning the probe from left to right allows examination of the entire valve so that masses and regurgitant lesions can be identified in relation to their position on the mitral leaflets.

Mitral Stenosis

The predominant causes of mitral stenosis (MS) are calcific disease of the mitral annulus, and rheumatic heart disease. As with rheumatic disease of the AV, the commissures fuse, causing the free leaflet bodies to form a dome shape in diastole, resulting in the characteristic "hockey stick" deformity (Fig. 27-61). Due to the restrictions to flow from the LA to the LV, MS is associated with an enlarged LA. The resulting blood stasis is seen as an echogenic swirling of blood flow in the LA, known as spontaneous echo contrast, or "smoke." Consequently, the chronically underfilled LV typically appears small by comparison (Fig. 27-62).

The severity of MS can be measured via planimetry or by the diastolic pressure gradient across the valve. Planimetry is more difficult to accurately perform in 2D, particularly due to the asymmetric nature of the MV, so measuring the orifice using planimetry in the appropriate plane in a 3D image may be a useful option. On spectral Doppler of transmitral inflow, the mean diastolic gradient can be measured by placing the CWD between the mitral leaflets in the appropriate view. The pressure half-time of the decelerating

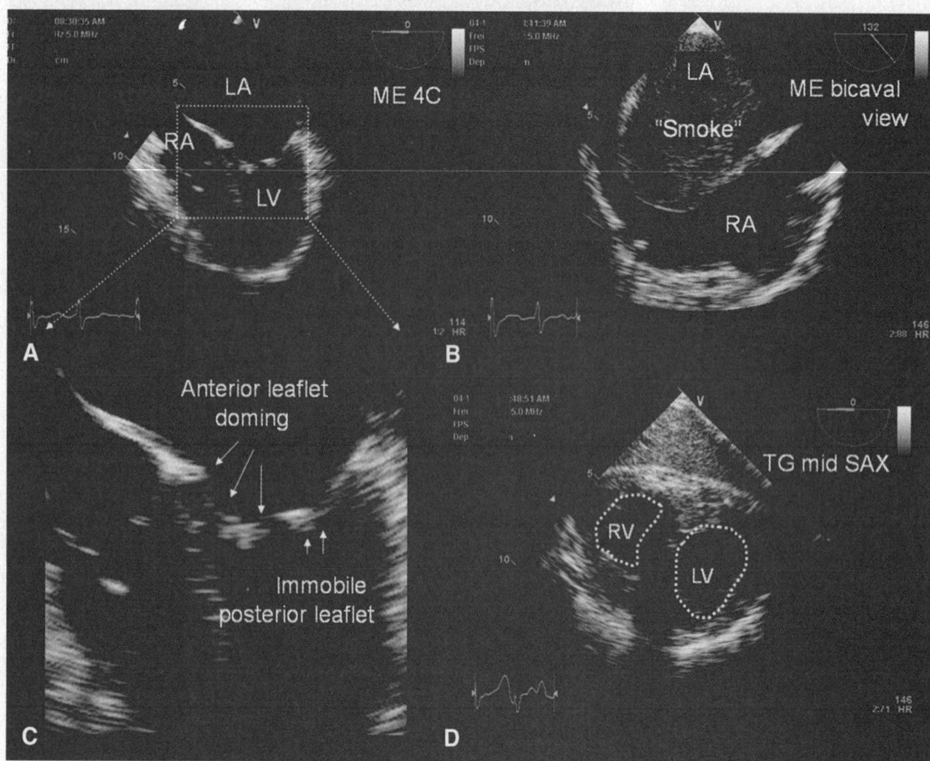

Figure 27-62 Associated features of mitral stenosis. **Panel A:** Left atrial dilation with bowing of the interatrial septum toward the right atrium, indicating a higher left atrial pressure, and a small left ventricle (LV), in the midesophageal four-chamber view. **Panel B:** Spontaneous echocardiography contrast, or "smoke," seen in the left atrium on midesophageal bicaval view, is suggestive of a low-flow state. Bowing of the interatrial septum toward the right atrium suggests a higher left atrial pressure. **Panel C:** An enlarged view of Panel A, the anterior mitral leaflet exhibits diastolic doming whereas the posterior mitral leaflet is immobile. **Panel D:** A comparatively small LV, as compared to the right ventricle, seen in a transgastric short-axis view.

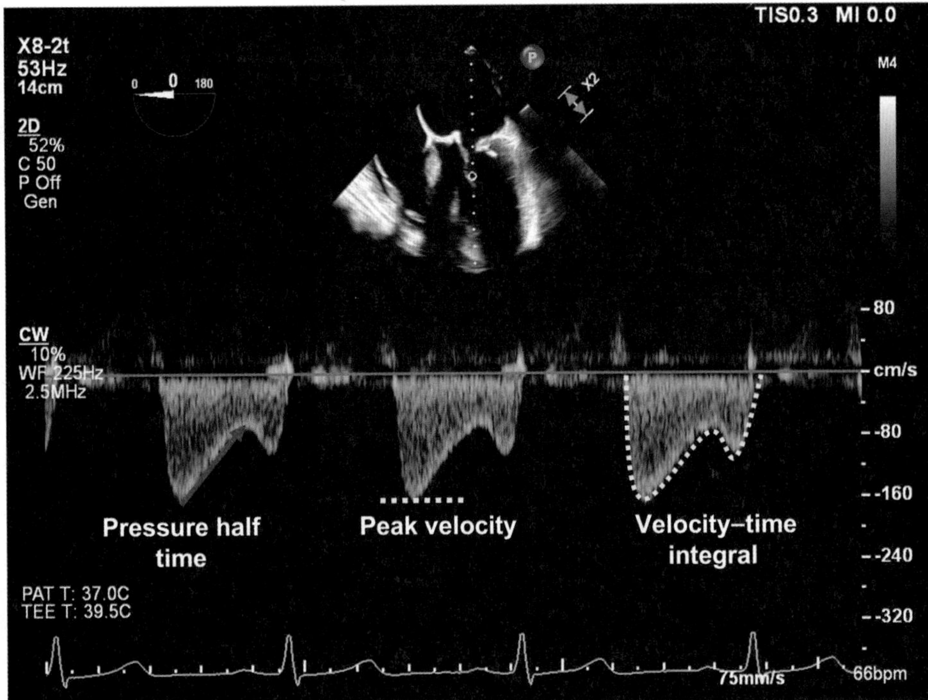

Figure 27-63 Assessment of mitral stenosis. Continuous wave Doppler across a stenotic mitral valve. Three tracings show measurement of pressure half-time (peak velocity and slope); peak velocity (peak gradient calculated using simplified Bernoulli equation); and velocity time integral (mean gradient calculated from area under the curve).

E-wave slope, starting at the peak and following the descent of the E wave, can also be used to quantify lesion severity (Fig. 27-63). Parameters used to grade the severity of MS are shown in Table 27-12.

Mitral Regurgitation

Mitral regurgitation (MR) can be primary (structural), or secondary (functional). Primary MR is most commonly caused by MV prolapse, leaflet perforation, or ruptured chordae tendineae, whereas in secondary MR, the MV is typically normal in morphology and the MR is related to LV dilation, or abnormal wall motion. The motion of the leaflets can be described according to the Carpentier classification (Fig. 27-64). Especially if leaflet motion is normal, one must then interrogate the MV annulus to assess for dilation, use color Doppler to look for regurgitation through a perforation in the MV and look for endocarditic vegetation. The presence of prolapsing or flail leaflets may suggest degenerative connective tissue disease, papillary muscle rupture, or chordal dysfunction. Restricted leaflets may be due to the causes of MS, for example, rheumatic disease, or may occur because of increased tension on the subvalvular structures due to ischemic cardiomyopathy.[29] Severe MR is initially associated with a dilated, hyperdynamic LV, along with LA enlargement and a bulging interatrial septum reflecting a relatively higher LAP. With progression of severe MR, LV systolic function decreases, and yet, LV function might still appear deceptively normal on echocardiography because of partial regurgitant emptying of the LV back into the LA.

The grading of MR severity is summarized in Table 27-13. The diameter of the *vena contracta* can be measured in both TEE and TTE. As with AR, the ratio of the regurgitation jet area to LA size is another measure of MR severity. TTE can capture the entirety of the LA area due to an increased distance from the probe, and is therefore the better technique for defining the jet area in the LA. The severity of eccentric jets might be underestimated. In severe MR, the pulmonary venous S wave is reversed.

Table 27-12 Grading Severity of Mitral Stenosis

	Mild	Moderate	Severe
Mean gradient (mmHg)	<5	5–10	>10
Pressure half-time (ms)	≤100	100–220	>220
Mitral valve area (cm^2)	>1.5	1–1.5	<1.0
Pulmonary artery systolic pressure (mmHg)	<30	30–50	>50

Tricuspid Regurgitation

Similar principles apply to determine the etiology, grading, and severity of tricuspid regurgitation (TR). Trivial or mild TR is commonly seen in around 90% of patients. The grading of severity of TR is summarized in Table 27-14.

Other Pathology

Diseases of the Aorta

Aortic dissection, aneurysms, and atheromatous disease can be detected by echocardiography. Pathology of the ascending aorta can sometimes be seen in the PLAX and SS views on TTE. TEE offers much clearer visualization of the ascending aorta in the ME asc aorta SAX and LAX views. As described earlier in this chapter, the presence of the tracheobronchial tree can make it difficult to assess the distal ascending aorta and proximal portion of the aortic arch by TEE, but this portion might be viewed in TTE via the SS view. The distal arch and thoracic aorta are best viewed by TEE the desc aorta SAX view. Distal to the diaphragm, surface ultrasound might again allow visualization of the abdominal aorta.

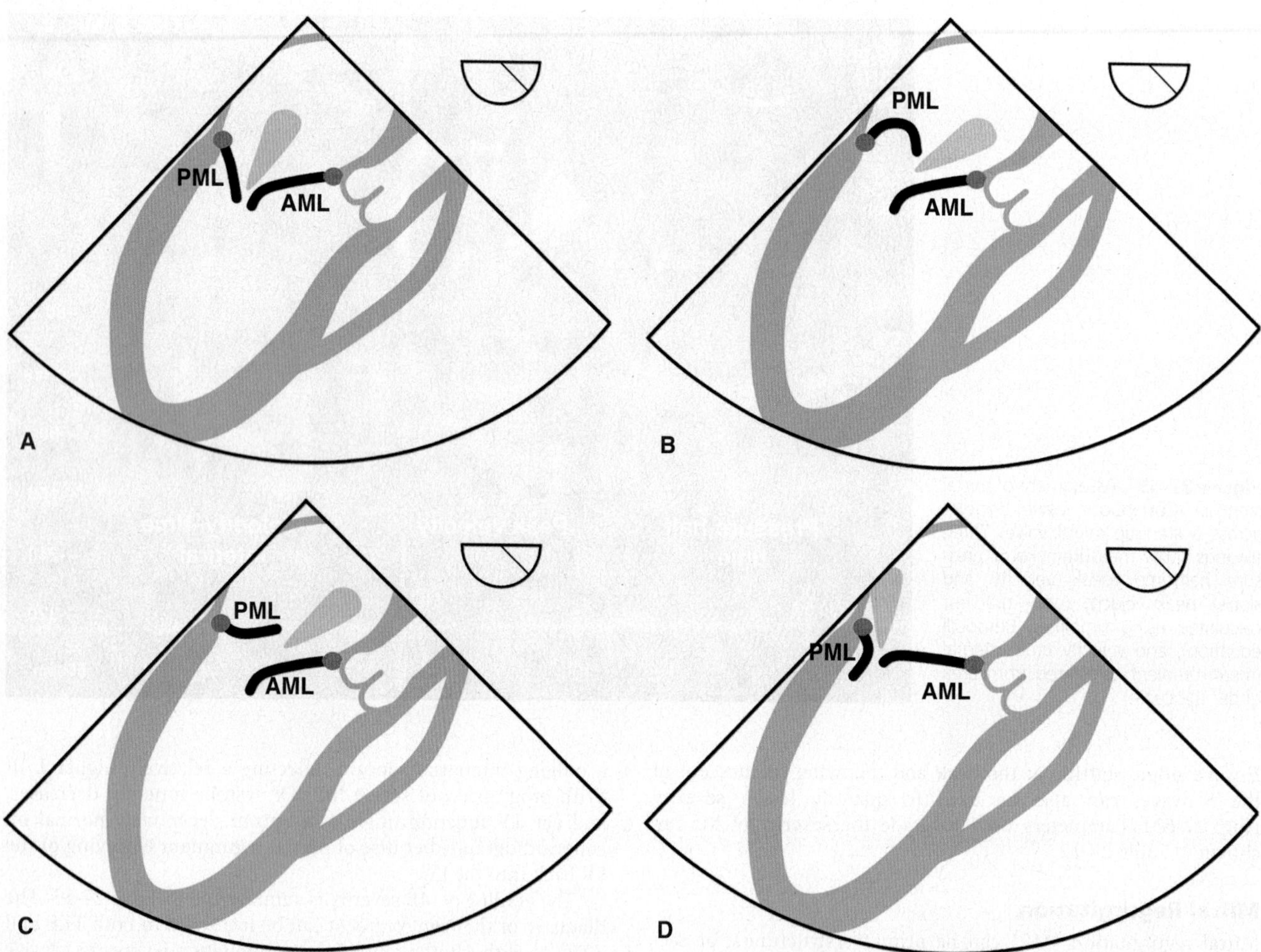

Figure 27-64 Carpentier classification of mitral regurgitation. Panels A to D are midesophageal long-axis views showing the Carpentier classification of mitral regurgitation, by type: Panel A: Type 1—normal leaflet motion, with central jet. Panel B (prolapse) and C (flail): Type 2—excessive leaflet motion, with jet away from lesion. Panel D: Type 3—restricted leaflet motion, with jet toward the lesion. AML, anterior mitral leaflet; PML, posterior mitral leaflet.

An aortic diameter of greater than 4 cm is indicative of an aneurysm, and a diameter of greater than 5.5 cm significantly increases the likelihood of rupture. In aortic dissection, the intimal layer becomes separated from the media layer, and a resulting flap can be visualized in affected portions of the aorta. It is important, for prognostic and interventional purposes, to detail the portions of aorta involved, the origin of the dissecting flap, and to be able to differentiate between the true and false lumen (Figs. 27-65 and 27-66). A Stanford type A aortic dissection necessitates urgent surgical intervention (Fig. 27-67). This may be associated with aortic regurgitation, pericardial effusion and tamponade, pleural effusions, or regional wall abnormalities, depending on the degree of dissection into the aortic root. The true lumen tends to be smaller and expands during systole. Thrombus, hematoma, and reduced or retrograde flow may be visualized in the false lumen.[30]

Table 27-13 Grading the Severity of Mitral Regurgitation

	Mild	Moderate	Severe
Vena contracta (mm)	<3	3–7	>7
Jet area (%LA)	<20	20–40	>40
Pulmonary venous S:D ratio	≥1	<1	S Reversal
Density of CWD jet	Faint	Faint	Dense

Table 27-14 Grading the Severity of Tricuspid Regurgitation

	Not Severe	Severe
Vena contracta (mm)	≤7	>7
Peak velocity (m/s)	≤2.4	>2.4
IVC diameter (cm)	≤2	>2
Hepatic vein diameter (cm)	≤1	>1
Hepatic vein S:D ratio	S>D	S reversal
Density of CWD jet	Faint	Dense

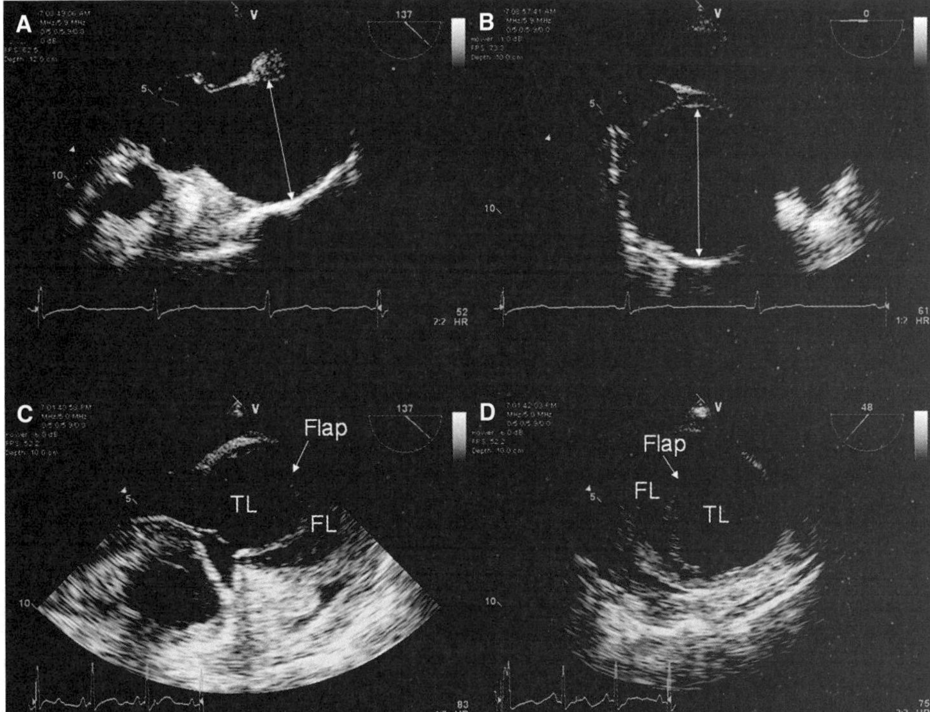

Figure 27-65 Aortic aneurysm. Aneurysm of the ascending aorta distal to the sinotubular junction seen in the midesophageal long-axis (**A**) and midesophageal aortic valve short-axis (**B**) views, with a measured diameter of 5 cm. In a separate case, a Stanford type A dissection is seen to originate from the sinotubular junction. The true lumen (TL) expands in systole and the flap bows toward the false lumen (FL). **D:** Dissection of the descending aorta as seen in the descending aorta short-axis view.

Intramural hematoma, a precursor of dissection, should still be treated similarly.

Aortic atheromas will appear brighter, due to calcium deposits, and tend to have a rougher surface (Fig. 27-68). Detailing atheromatous disease is important for open and percutaneous procedures requiring aortic manipulation to avoid potential distal embolization.

Pericardial Disease

The pericardium consists of an outer fibrosal and an inner serosal component. The pericardial cavity normally contains less than 50 mL of serous fluid, which can be seen in the transverse and oblique sinuses on TEE ME asc ao and ME2C views, respectively. As a fluid-filled space, this appears echolucent (Fig. 27-69), distinguishing it from a hematoma or a benign fat pad, which will

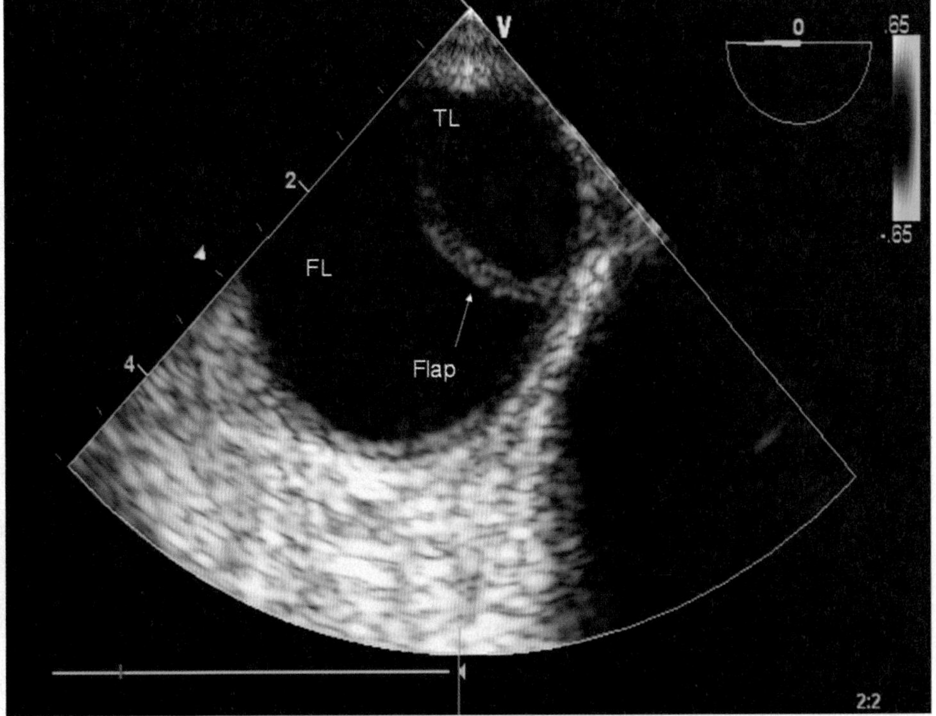

Figure 27-66 True and false lumens in aortic dissection. This descending aorta short-axis view shows a dissection of the descending aorta. The true lumen of the aorta contains endothelium, and therefore has a smooth endoluminal surface. The intimal flap usually bows toward the false lumen, particularly in systole. A relatively higher flow compared to the false lumen is demonstrated on color flow Doppler.

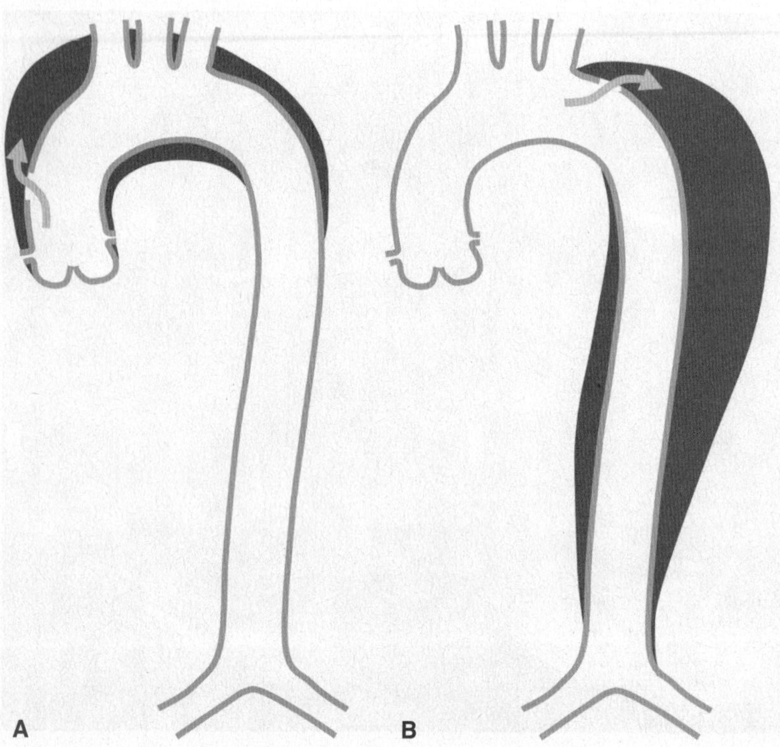

Figure 27-67 Classification of aortic dissections. Stanford criteria for aortic dissection: Stanford A indicates involvement of the ascending aorta and aortic arch—the aorta proximal to the left subclavian artery. Stanford B indicates involvement of the descending aorta—the aorta distal to the left subclavian artery.

appear more echodense. While multiple views must be taken to assess a pericardial effusion, initial views in the ME4C or the SC4C are appropriate to begin with.

Diseases of the pericardium (e.g., constrictive pericarditis or pericardial tamponade) can mimic ventricular diastolic dysfunction. Moreover, pericardial disease has to be differentiated from myocardial disease with similar initial appearance, such as restrictive cardiomyopathy. Several echocardiographic features can be useful in making this distinction. Ventricular systolic function in tamponade and constrictive pericarditis is typically not impaired, whereas it can be impaired in late restrictive cardiomyopathy. The constrictive effect of pericardium is likely to reduce movement of the lateral myocardial walls, but not the septal wall. Hence, the lateral e′ velocity may be reduced, but comparatively, the septal e′ velocity will be increased. Intravascular volume changes also tend to have a more dramatic effect in patients with constrictive pericarditis and pericardial tamponade, compared to patients suffering from restrictive cardiomyopathy. In spontaneously breathing patients, this is seen as a reduced mitral E velocity on inspiration and an increased mitral E velocity on expiration. The reverse is true in positive pressure ventilation. Finally, constrictive pericarditis is typically associated with an echogenic and thickened pericardial lining.

In patients with pericardial effusion, determination of the size, nature, and hemodynamic significance of the effusion is paramount to determining treatment, as well as anesthesia management. The appearance of pericardial effusions can be characterized

Figure 27-68 Aortic atheroma. Descending aortic short-axis view showing extensive atheromatous disease (*red arrow*).

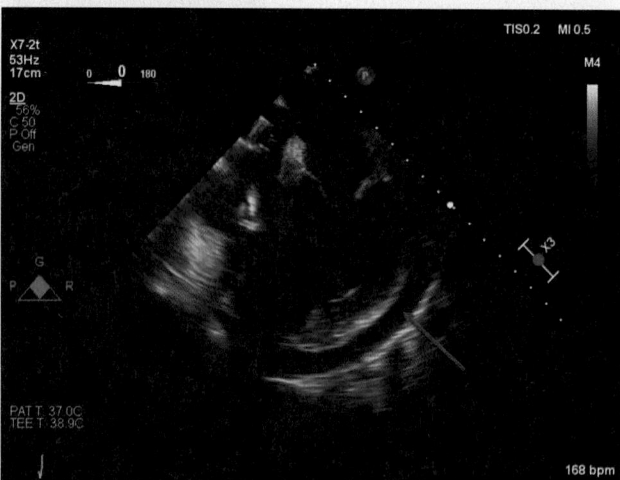

Figure 27-69 Pericardial effusion. Midesophageal four-chamber view showing a pericardial effusion (*arrow*). Any fluid in the pericardial space generally appears as an echolucent space.

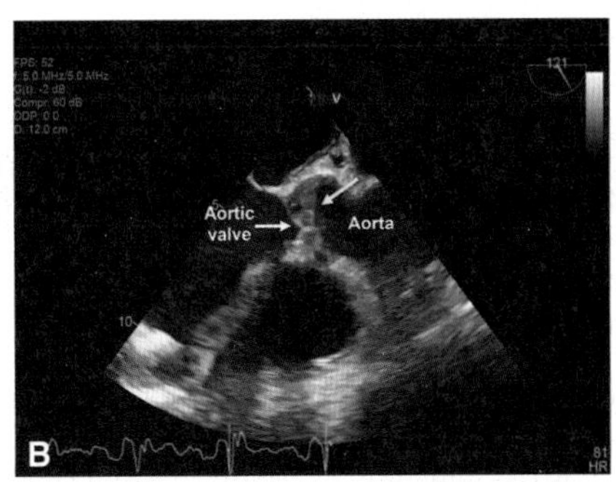

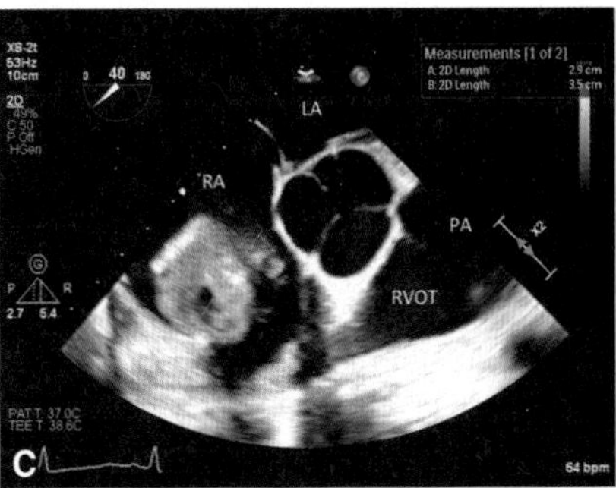

Figure 27-70 Cardiac masses. **Panel A:** Midesophageal four-chamber view showing a myxoma in the LA (*yellow arrow*). **Panel B:** Midesophageal aortic valve long-axis view showing a thrombus (*yellow arrow*) obstructing aortic valve opening. **Panel C:** Midesophageal aortic valve short-axis view showing a large vegetation on the tricuspid valve.

as transudative (echolucent) or exudative (echodense). Nonclotted blood will appear as a slow swirl of spontaneous contrast, while clotted blood will appear more echodense. Effusions may also appear loculated, with fibrin stranding. The degree of pericardial effusion can be described by its size and whether it is circumferential or localized. An important echocardiographic feature for distinguishing tamponade from effusion is the collapse of the cardiac chambers during their respective periods of relaxation. Low-pressure chambers are the first to show collapse. Early tamponade is suggested by early right atrial collapse during ventricular systole, with increasing severity indicated by early right ventricular collapse during diastole.[31] Presence of these findings will highlight the importance in maintaining chronotropy and preload during induction of anesthesia.

Cardiac Masses

Common cardiac masses include tumors, thrombi, and vegetations (Fig. 27-70). It is important to interrogate a cardiac mass from multiple views and angles, to establish its point of origin, extent, and size. The contour, echogenicity, consistency, and mobility of a mass also provide clues to its etiology. The most common cardiac tumor is a myxoma, which is benign and most commonly appears as a pedunculated or sessile mass in the atria. Thrombi typically appear homogenous, tend to aggregate in low-flow areas, such as the left atrial appendage, and may be heralded by spontaneous echo contrast. Vegetations tend to appear on valves and foreign bodies, such as catheters and wires, and appear irregular and hypermobile. TEE is typically the gold standard for assessing for cardiac thrombi and vegetations.[32]

Congenital Heart Disease

Improved survival rates due to advancements in pediatric cardiac surgery have increased the prevalence of adults with surgically treated congenital heart disease. Adults with congenital heart disease might present with a range of findings, such as intracardiac shunts (e.g., patent foramen ovale, atrial septal defect, or ventricular septal defect), bicuspid AV, coarctation of the aorta, or repaired tetralogy of Fallot. A PFO and ASD are best interrogated in the ME bicaval view in TEE by activating color Doppler and reducing the Nyquist aliasing velocity to 15 to 30 cm/s, so as to detect a low flow jet (Fig. 27-71). It is important to note the direction of the jet (left to right or right to left).

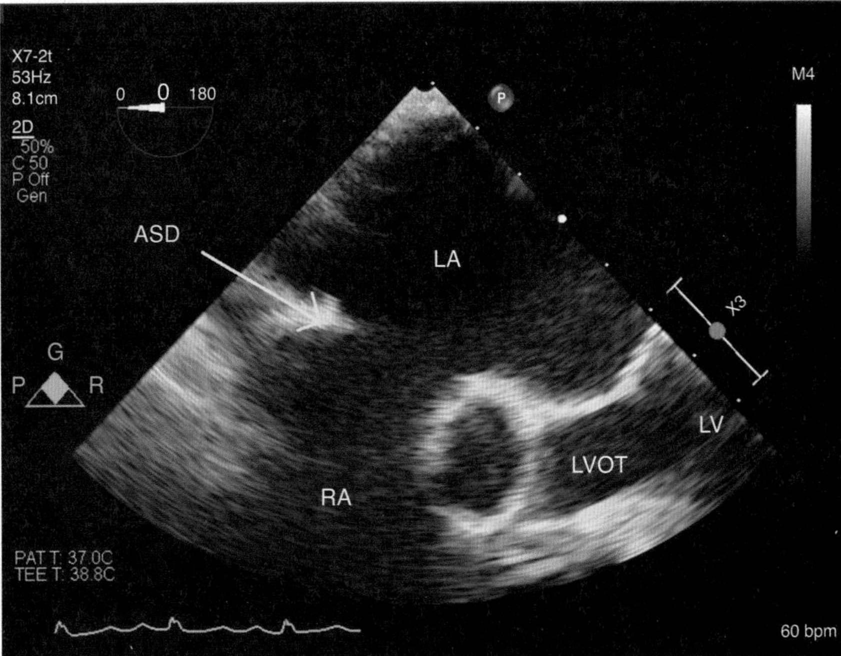

Figure 27-71 Intracardiac shunt. Secundum atrial septal defect visualized in the midesophageal five-chamber view.

Point-of-Care Ultrasound

Increased recognition of the utility of ultrasound imaging, and the proliferation of handheld and portable ultrasound devices, have contributed to the development of POCUS protocols and their application in routine clinical practice. POCUS allows anesthesiologists to use ultrasound at the bedside to perform rapid, goal-oriented assessments, and guide a variety of acute care procedures.[33,34] Further, the potential utility of POCUS spans the entire perioperative care spectrum.[34–36] While POCUS assessments can be used for almost all organ systems,[37] this chapter will focus on its use for cardiac, pulmonary, and gastric evaluation. Several acronyms involving the use of POCUS are in use. In the critical care environment, critical care echocardiography (CCE) and FOCUS are commonly used to describe the use of POCUS for bedside cardiac evaluation. The use of ultrasound for regional anesthesia is discussed separately in Chapters 35 and 36.

Consultative ultrasonography (performed by sonographers and interpreted by radiologists or cardiologists) requires comprehensive training in image acquisition and interpretation, uses advanced imaging techniques routinely, and is used to diagnose and grade the severity of a broad range of pathologies. In contrast, POCUS training is less extensive, and most evaluations are limited to the use of 2D ultrasound. Hence, POCUS is best used to answer specific clinical questions (Table 27-15). These evaluations can then be repeated over time to monitor the patient's response to therapy.

In essence, POCUS represents a disruptive innovation[38] that addresses immediate clinical needs in a cheaper, faster, and more accessible manner than consultative ultrasonography. However, it is important to remain aware that the utility of POCUS is limited by the provider's skill and knowledge, and that the visual information provided must be interpreted in conjunction with other clinical information.[39]

Table 27-15 Clinical Questions Generally Answered Using Point-of-Care Ultrasound (POCUS)

Clinicai Question	POCUS Features
Cardiovascular: basic questions	
Are there signs of severe LV systolic dysfunction?	1. LV walls thickening <30% during systole (best seen in PLAX and PSAX views) 2. LV chamber emptying <50% of its contents in two-dimensional (2D) views 3. MAPSE <8 mm on A4C view 4. Peripheral clues to low-flow state (minimal diastolic excursion of anterior mitral leaflet; minimal aortic valve systolic opening despite absence of calcification)
Are there signs of severe right ventricular (RV) dilation and systolic dysfunction?	1. Decreased RV free wall motion 2. Interventricular septum deviated toward left ventricle (best seen in PLAX, PSAX, or A4C views) 3. RV chamber emptying <35% of its contents in A4C view 4. RV/LV size >2/3 in A4C view 5. TAPSE <17 mm on A4C view
Is there significantly reduced venous return?	1. End-systolic LV cavity obliteration in the PSAX view combined with small LV end-diastolic dimension 2. Small IVC with significant respirophasic changes in subcostal views 3. Respiratory variation in IVC diameter (>15% in mechanically ventilated patients[a], >40% in spontaneously breathing patients[b]) 4. >10–15% respiratory variation in LVOT VTI, or in V_{max} for brachial or carotid arteries[c]
Is there a pericardial effusion?	Hypoechoic collection noticed between the heart and parietal pericardium in any views[d]
Are there significant valvular abnormalities?	Severe aortic stenosis: calcified aortic valve with minimal leaflet motion seen in parasternal long-axis (PLAX) view Severe mitral stenosis: calcified or thickened mitral valve leaflets with minimal diastolic opening seen in PSAX and apical views, along with a dilated left atrium Severe valvular regurgitation: coaptation defects clearly visible, with large regurgitant flow convergence zones on color Doppler in the chamber upstream to the regurgitation, along with large turbulent flow patterns in the downstream chamber Infective endocarditis: obvious echogenicities on the valvular surface[e]
Is there evidence of LVOT obstruction?	Hypertrophied basal ventricular septum, with systolic anterior motion of the anterior mitral leaflet, noticed on PLAX or A5C views

Table 27-15 Clinical Questions Generally Answered Using Point-of-Care Ultrasound (POCUS) (*Continued*)

Clinical Question	POCUS Features
Cardiovascular: advanced questions	
Is the stroke volume abnormal?	SV calculation based on LVOT VTI measured on A5C or A3C views, and LVOT diameter on PLAX view
Does the stroke volume respond to fluids, vasopressors, or inotropes?	LVOT VTI changes by >15–20% in response to therapeutic maneuver. LVOT is diameter is assumed to be unchanged between measurements
Is there an aortic dissection?	Dissection flap noticed in the ascending aorta on PLAX or SS views[e]
Is there a regional wall motion abnormality?	Segmental abnormality (<30%) in wall thickening, reproducible in multiple views[f]
Is the left atrial pressure elevated?	1. B-lines on lung ultrasound (see below) 2. Bowing of interatrial septum to the right throughout the cardiac cycle 3. E/A >2, or E/A 0.8–2 with (2 of 3) LA size (PLAX view) >5 cm, TR V_{max} >2.8 m/s, or E/e′ >14
Are there features of tamponade?	1. IVC plethora 2. Diastolic RV collapse (best identified on M-mode on the PLAX view) 3. RA collapse >1/3 of cardiac cycle 4. Exaggerated respiratory variation in valvular flow (Mitral >25%, tricuspid >40%)
Is the pulmonary pressure significantly elevated?	PASP calculation using TR V_{max} (modified PLAX view, AoV SAX view, or A4C view) and CVP demonstrates elevated pulmonary arterial pressure
Are there features of severe venous congestion?	IVC >2 cm on SC view, with (2 of 3) hepatic venous systolic reversal, portal venous pulsatility >50%, or interrupted systolic flow in interlobar renal vein
Pulmonary	
Is there a pneumothorax?	Ruled out by presence of lung sliding, B-lines, or lung pulse
Are there pleural effusions?	Hypoechoic areas, commonly seen in the posterior costophrenic angles
Is there pulmonary consolidation?	Deaerated lung, ultrasound appearance might be similar to the liver. For focal, subpleural disease, an irregular border with normal, aerated lung might be seen (shred sign)
Is there significant interstitial disease in the pulmonary parenchyma (cardiogenic pulmonary edema, acute respiratory distress syndrome (ARDS), pneumonia, or pulmonary fibrosis)?	Multiple B-lines in several intercostal spaces. Within the clinical context, different patterns might suggest specific differential diagnoses (e.g., unilateral interstitial syndrome is suggestive of a focal process whereas bilateral interstitial syndrome is suggestive of a diffuse process)
Is the diaphragm functioning appropriately?	>30% thickening of diaphragm with inspiration
Airway	
Is there an increased risk of difficulty with laryngoscopy and intubation?	Significant amount of anterior neck soft tissue on POCUS evaluation
Gastric	
Is there an increased risk of aspiration with induction of anesthesia?	Abnormally large volume of gastric content, or solid contents, on POCUS evaluation of the gastric antrum. Best seen by bringing the antrum into a dependent position by having the patient lay right lateral decubitus
Abdomen	
Is there free fluid in the abdomen?	Free fluid noticed in the left or right upper quadrant of the abdomen or on suprapubic views

[a]Controlled mechanical ventilation, tidal volumes 8 mL/kg.
[b]Specificity is much lower in spontaneously breathing patients.
[c]Respiratory variation parameters are valid only when all conditions are met: sinus rhythm, controlled mechanical ventilation with tidal volumes >8 mL/kg, normal intra-abdominal pressure, closed chest and normal right ventricle.
[d]Fat pad on the anterior RV surface is common and might be confused for a localized hematoma. Comparison with prior imaging could be useful. Left pleural effusions track posterior to the descending thoracic aorta on the initial (scout) PLAX view, which is acquired with increased depth.
[e]POCUS has poor sensitivity for ruling out infective endocarditis or aortic disease.
[f]Assessing regional wall motion abnormalities carries significant inter- and intra-observer variability, even among experts. The POCUS reader is advised to use significant caution confirming or ruling out segmental function abnormalities.

Focused Cardiac Ultrasound

Perioperative hypoperfusion can occur due to reduced venous return, left- or right-sided systolic dysfunction, PHTN, significant valvular abnormalities, LVOT obstruction, cardiac tamponade, or venous congestion. These can often be diagnosed, or ruled out, by POCUS evaluation with a low-frequency, phased-array probe. It is important, however, to avoid over-reliance on ultrasound data. Assessment of fluid status and volume responsiveness with ultrasound is particularly challenging.[40] Dynamic ultrasound parameters like respiratory variation in LVOT VTI are more predictive of volume responsiveness, but lose sensitivity in all but the most controlled circumstances.[41] Hence, hemodynamic assessment should always integrate ultrasound findings with other clinical data.

In small-scale studies, routine preoperative FOCUS has been shown to change perioperative management and positively impact clinical outcomes.[42,43] Common preoperative abnormalities identified included hypovolemia, or cardiovascular pathologies, such as heart failure, PHTN, and AS. For patients with severe hemodynamic instability or cardiac arrest, FOCUS is a valuable tool to rapidly diagnose the cause and guide therapy.[44] Similarly, FOCUS use in the PACU can lead to earlier identification of hypovolemia, distributive shock, and depressed systolic function, with the potential to reduce PACU length of stay.[36] Finally, the use of FOCUS is well established in the critical care setting.[45]

Evaluation of volume excess on ultrasound is being increasingly recognized as a method for estimating venous congestion and organ dysfunction. Importantly, the presence of multiple ultrasound signs of volume overload is significantly associated with an increase in risk of postoperative acute kidney injury.[46]

Lung Ultrasound

9

POCUS is used to evaluate various lung pathologies, including pleural effusion, pulmonary edema, consolidation, pneumothorax, and to confirm endobronchial intubation. POCUS has been repeatedly shown to perform better than chest radiographs in diagnosing these pathologies, and is often comparable to computed tomography.[47] Many different protocols have been described for systematic POCUS evaluation of the lungs. The bedside lung ultrasound in emergency (BLUE) protocol can be used for a standardized and systematic evaluation of pulmonary pathology in acute respiratory failure. Similarly, the fluid administration limited by lung sonography (FALLS) protocol has been developed for management of acute circulatory failure.[48]

Lung ultrasound can be performed with linear, phased array or curvilinear probes, depending on the patient's body habitus. At least three areas must be examined in each patient: anteriorly below the clavicle, anterolaterally in fourth to fifth intercostal space, and posterolaterally in the seventh to ninth intercostal space. The anterior and anterolateral evaluations should be done with depth reduced to 4 to 6 cm to evaluate the pleural surface well. The posterolateral examination should be done with an increased depth (typically 14 to 18 cm), such as to include the spine in the deeper sections of the image. In all views, the probe is oriented in a cephalad–caudad position, with ribs on either side of the image causing shadows and the hyperechoic pleural line about 1 to 2 cm deeper to the ribs. Figure 27-72 demonstrates the typical appearance of lung pathology on ultrasound.

The presence of B-lines, lung pulse, or lung sliding would rule out pneumothorax in the area of lung investigated.[49] B-lines, or comet-tails, are elongated, hyperechoic lines that project from subpleural pathology, with the artifacts extending all the way to

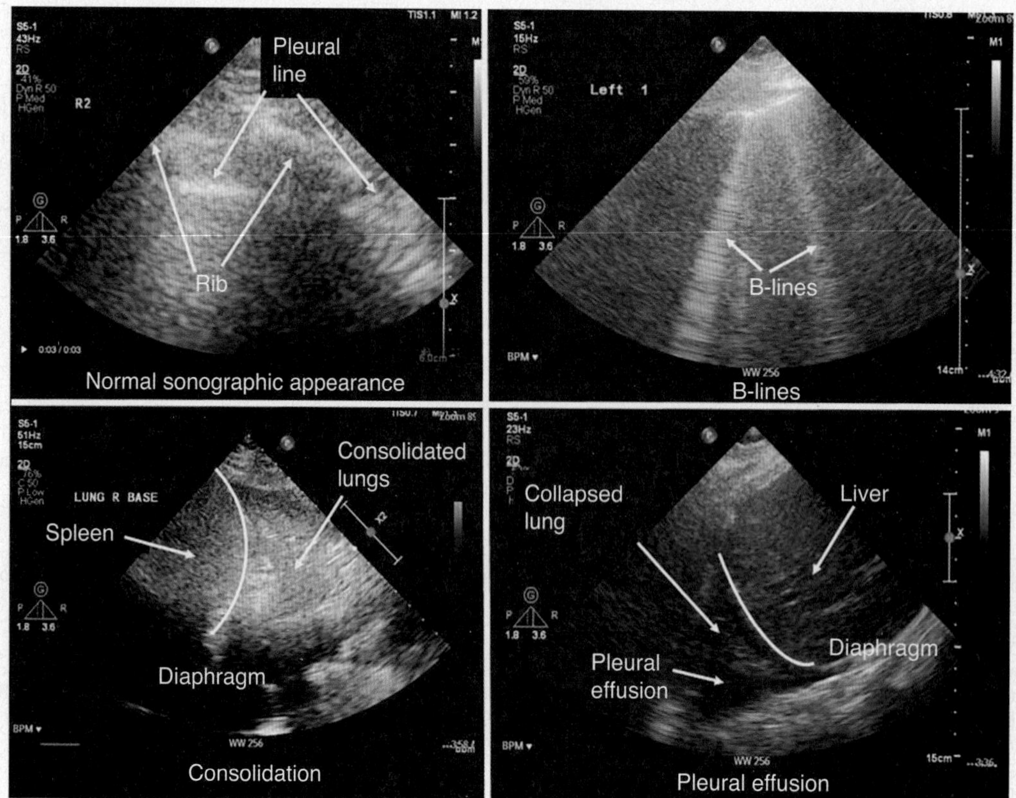

Figure 27-72 Common lung ultrasound findings.

the bottom of the screen, and move in concert with lung sliding. Lung pulse is the pulsation created at the pleural surface due to cardiac motion. Compared to lung sliding, lung pulse has a higher frequency and a smaller amplitude of motion. On M-mode ultrasound, lung sliding causes a "seashore sign" due to constant motion at the pleural surface, while the absence of lung sliding would appear as a "barcode sign." It is important to note that lung sliding is also absent with poorly ventilated lungs, contralateral endobronchial intubation, or pleural adhesions. The presence of a lung point (the visualization of a transition from presence to absence of lung sliding in the same screen) would be pathognomonic of pneumothorax, and suggests that the pneumothorax is partial, with some of the lung parenchyma remaining in contact with the parietal pleural surface.[50]

The presence of multiple B-lines (>2 in an interstitial space, or B-lines bunched together) signifies an interstitial syndrome, that is, cardiogenic pulmonary edema, ARDS, pneumonia, or interstitial fibrosis. Different patterns of B-lines have been shown to indicate specific pathologies.[51] Pleural effusions appear as hypoechoic areas in the costophrenic angles. Smaller effusions are only visible when the probe is angulated posteriorly. With larger effusions, the spine might be visible in the deeper sections of the image. Deaerated areas of the lung with compression atelectasis can often be seen within the pleural fluid. Simple effusions appear as uniformly hypoechoic collections, while complex effusions include scattered echogenic shadows. Septations can be seen within the fluid collection in loculated effusions, which might also appear primarily in nondependent areas.

Consolidation on lung ultrasound may be described as "sonographic hepatization" of the lung due to loss of aeration. Consolidation can be due to atelectasis or an infiltrative process, such as pneumonia. Atelectatic lung classically demonstrates volume loss and a homogenous lung parenchyma, whereas an infiltrative process like pneumonia typically shows preserved lung volume, heterogeneous lung tissue, and signs of internal airflow called "dynamic air bronchograms." Consolidation can be seen to impact the entire lobe of the lung, with visualization of the spine or viscera deeper to it. More commonly, a partial lobar consolidation pattern with a "shred sign" might be seen, causing a jagged border between consolidated and normal, aerated lung.

Finally, evaluation of diaphragmatic motion and thickening has been shown to correlate with respiratory mechanics, ability to wean from mechanical ventilation, and diaphragmatic dysfunction.[52]

Abdominal Ultrasound

POCUS evaluation of the volume and contents in the gastric antrum can be performed in the supine and right lateral decubitus (RLD) position. The gastric antrum is usually visualized with a curvilinear low-frequency probe in a cross-sectional plane under the left lobe of the liver in a parasagittal plane, with the abdominal aorta visible in the deeper planes. Based on the ultrasound dimensions of the antrum, gastric volume can then be estimated with a formula such as:

$$\text{Volume (mL)} = 27.0 + (14.6 \times \text{RLD CSA}) - (1.28 \times \text{Age})$$

where RLD is right lateral decubitus and CSA is cross-sectional area.[53]

In most studies, the presence of solid contents, or gastric fluid volume >1.5 mL/kg, is defined as "full stomach." Despite following fasting guidelines, up to 5% of patients presenting for elective surgery have been found to have full stomachs. The proportion of patients with full stomach could be up to 50% among those with diabetes, and in those presenting for emergency surgery. In test populations, gastric ultrasound carries a very high sensitivity and negative predictive value for diagnosing a full stomach.[54] However, there are no current professional guidelines replacing *nil per os* recommendations with gastric ultrasound evaluation. The ideal current use for gastric ultrasound is to diagnose a previously unrecognized full stomach.

The focused assessment with sonography for trauma (FAST) examination is widely used in emergency rooms as a bedside tool to evaluate for free fluid in the pericardium, abdomen, and pelvis. Similar applications for FAST have been described in the postanesthesia care unit.[36]

Other Uses of Ultrasound

Ultrasound-Guided Vascular Cannulation

Ultrasound guidance is now the standard of care for internal jugular venous cannulation.[55] It is also commonly used for subclavian and femoral venous cannulation, for radial and other arterial cannulation, and it can be helpful for peripheral venous access. Scanning the insertion site prior to prepping allows for identification of small or thrombosed vessels that are inappropriate for cannulation. During the cannulation attempt, real-time ultrasound guidance provides visualization of the needle tip and vascular structures, leading to avoidance of inadvertent vascular or lung injury, and a reduction in the total number of attempts. Moreover, in patients with mechanical cardiac support and absent arterial pulsatility, ultrasound guidance is invaluable for arterial cannulation. In patients undergoing minimally invasive cardiac surgery or placement of percutaneous mechanical cardiac support, ultrasound is again vital for visualization of wires and cannulae in appropriate chambers and vessels.

Standard precautions should be maintained regarding sterility of the ultrasound probe, ultrasound gel, operative area, and vascular catheter. Regarding ultrasound guidance of the needle, it is most important that after initial skin puncture, ultrasound imaging should be performed in a dynamic manner, staying ahead of, rather than following, the needle tip.[56] This technique allows guidance of the needle from subcutaneous tissue to blood vessel, and further tracking for a few millimeters into the blood vessel to continuously achieve the "bulls-eye" of the needle tip in the vessel lumen. During central venous cannulation, after initial needle or cannula entry, manometry should be performed to rule out arterial access.

Epicardial and Epiaortic Ultrasound

In cardiac surgical operating rooms, a probe covered in a sterile sheath can be used to perform ultrasound imaging within the surgical field, applied directly on the heart or the ascending aorta. In both cases, filling the mediastinal cavity with warm sterile saline enhances acoustic transmission, and hence improves image quality.

For patients with any contraindication to transesophageal imaging, the heart can be examined with epicardiac echocardiography using a high-frequency, phased-array transthoracic ultrasound probe. The described images are largely similar in orientation to TTE.[10] Epicardiac ultrasound has been described to be useful for evaluation of valvular and ventricular function during cardiac surgery.[57]

Ultrasound evaluation of the ascending aorta prior to cannulation and bypass grafting has been recommended as a strategy to reduce embolic neurologic events.[58] The use of epiaortic ultrasonography (EAU) is associated with a decreased risk of postoperative stroke. Imaging is performed with a high-frequency ultrasound probe. Creating a 1-cm gap ("standoff") between the probe and the aorta using saline or ultrasound gel in the sterile sheath helps to prevent an issue called near-field clutter. Despite current guidelines and evidence recommending routine use of EAU to reduce the risk of stroke in cardiac surgery, there is significant site-to-site variability in its use.[59] Anesthesiologists have a role in advocating for the use of EAU in cardiac surgical patients at high risk of stroke. In addition, EAU can be useful for examining parts of the ascending aorta and arch that are not clearly visualized on TEE.[60]

Out-of-OR Echocardiography

For patients undergoing transcatheter procedures under general anesthesia (e.g., AV implantation, MV repair, tricuspid valve repair, paravalvular leak repair, atrial septal defect closure, left atrial appendage closure) in the cardiac catheterization laboratory or hybrid operating rooms, TEE is used to perform preprocedure evaluation, guide wire access, device deployment, and for postdeployment evaluation.[61] The use of 3D TEE in these cases vastly improves the ability to accurately guide surgical intervention. TEE is similarly useful for evaluation of cardiac structure and function during extraction of pacemaker and defibrillator leads.

Training and Certification

10 The delivery of high-quality care is predicated on comprehensive training and assessment of competency. Structured training in echocardiography is part of most anesthesiology training programs around the world. The level of training is different in early training (residency) compared to advanced training (fellowship) programs. Certification, on the other hand, is provided by a regulatory body that attests to the completion of a knowledge assessment (a test), performance of a specific number of examinations (via a logbook) or demonstration of technical ability (in an observed practical examination) that imply acquisition of satisfactory skills.

Training in Perioperative Echocardiography

Structured training in perioperative echocardiography, in both TEE and TTE, is essential for providing high-quality care. Such training is usually part of subspecialty training and is based on national guidelines and recommendations.

Training programs are usually governed by accrediting organizations that define the specific components of training. For example, in the United States, the ASE, American College of Cardiology (ACC), and Society of Cardiovascular Anesthesiologists (SCA) provide recommendations for training in perioperative echocardiography within a fellowship program, both in cardiology and anesthesiology.[62,63] In the United States, these training recommendations are generally adopted by the Accreditation Council for Graduate Medical Education (ACGME), which accredits training programs.

Training in perioperative TEE has largely followed the recommendations made by the ASE and SCA in 2002, which detail the cognitive and technical skills required to perform a perioperative TEE examination.[63] Adult cardiothoracic anesthesiology fellowships are required to include advanced training in TEE, and these recommendations form the basis of any advanced training program in perioperative TEE around the world.

For basic perioperative TEE, specific training objectives are detailed in guidelines published by the ASE and SCA in 2013,[10] which form the basis for training in basic TEE during anesthesiology residency. The American Board of Anesthesiology expects that anesthesiology residency programs include echocardiographic recognition of normal cardiac anatomy using TEE,[64] while the ACGME includes the placement and use of TEE as a competency requirement for any accredited anesthesiology residency program.[65]

Trainees in cardiology are also required to undergo training in perioperative echocardiography, which has been included in the ACC core training requirements.[62,66]

Training in perioperative TTE is more challenging to describe, due to its remarkable versatility and consequent variability in its application across specialties. The use of ultrasound in medicine is vast, but its use as a point-of-care imaging tool to assist with bedside care in the perioperative area is narrower. The use of TTE for describing cardiovascular structure and function in the perioperative setting is also more limited and training requirements are not well defined. A guideline document from the ASE in 2020 describes the spectrum of ultrasound use for cardiovascular and hemodynamic assessment—from ultrasound-assisted physical examination (UAPE) to the traditional comprehensive TTE examination.[67]

Training in bedside TTE is well described in the critical care environment. In 2009, the Société de Réanimation de Langue Française and the American College of Chest Physicians published a consensus statement defining competency in critical care ultrasound, which included basic and advanced CCE.[68] Two years later, 11 critical care societies from all over the world jointly published training requirements in basic and advanced CCE.[69] The same group later published separate training standards in greater detail for advanced CCE.[70] This document describes the required views and number of examinations in both TTE and TEE that would assure a minimal degree of competence in the performance of advanced CCE. More recently, the ASE provided further guidance for echocardiography laboratories participating in training of physicians in cardiac POCUS and CCE.[67] While this document provides recommendations from a cardiology perspective for training noncardiology personnel, it also includes helpful terminology that distinguishes between UAPE, CCE, and TTE.

There are several guidelines focusing on training and competency requirements in critical care ultrasound that are broader in scope than those focused on echocardiography. For instance, in 2020, the European Society of Intensive Care Medicine published a framework for core critical care ultrasound competencies that recommends 15 echocardiographic competencies, but also includes thoracic, abdominal, and vascular ultrasound.[71] Similarly, training recommendations have been made by critical bodies around the world.[72,73]

Certification in Perioperative Echocardiography

In the United States certification in perioperative echocardiography, including basic and advanced TEE, and in critical care echocardiography, is provided by the National Board of Echocardiography (NBE). The NBE is an independent organization that was created from a partnership between the ASE and SCA to provide oversight of testing and certification for echocardiography in the United States. While testing evaluates cognitive skills, competence is certified with documentation of completion of a specific number of examinations under appropriate supervision. Those who pass an NBE examination are known as "testamurs" while certification provided upon appropriate documentation leads

Table 27-16 Certification Requirements in Perioperative Echocardiography and Critical Care

Domain	Testing	Number of Studies	Personally Performed	Supervised Learning	Certifying Agency	Country or Region
TEE	Basic TEE[a]	150	50	100	NBE	USA
	Advanced TEE[b]	300	150	150	NBE	USA
	TOE[c]	125	125	N/A	EACVI and EACTAIC	Europe
	TOE[d]	125	125	N/A	BSE	UK
	None[e]	180–200	130–150	50	ANZCA	Australia/NZ
	TEE[f]	N/A	N/A	N/A	JB-POT	Japan
	F-TEE[g]	100	100	N/A	IACTA	India
Critical Care	CCE[h]	150	150	N/A	NBE	USA
	ACCE[i]	250	250	N/A	BSE	UK
	EDEC[j]	135	135	N/A	ESICM	Europe

ACCE, Adult critical care echocardiography; ANZCA, Australia New Zealand College of Anaesthetists; BSE, British Society of Echocardiography; CCE, critical care echocardiography; EACTAIC, European Association of CardioThoracic Anesthesiology and Intensive Care; EACVI, European Association of Cardiovascular Imaging; EDEC, European Diploma in Advanced Critical Care Echocardiography; ESICM, European Society of Intensive Care Medicine; IACTA, Indian Association of Cardiovascular and Thoracic Anaesthesiologists; JB-POT, Japanese Board of PeriOperative TEE; NBE, National Board of Echocardiography (USA); TEE/TOE, transesophageal echocardiography.

[a]150 is the minimum number of studies of which at least 50 must be personally performed, interpreted, and reported.[74]

[b]Similar to Basic TEE requirements in terms of minimum number required.[75]

[c]Minimum of 75 required if candidate is also certified in transthoracic echocardiography by the EACVI.[76]

[d]Minimum of 75 required if candidate is also certified in transthoracic or TEE by the EACVI.[77]

[e]No formal examination/certification process outside of training requirements; minimum studies required are 50 comprehensive studies during initial training (or 30 each for transthoracic and TEE), 50 additional unsupervised with review, and another 100 comprehensive studies prior to completion of training.[78]

[f]JB-POT does not include number of exams required for certification.[79]

[g]Minimum of 100 studies required in logbook with validation of digital exams in 25 cases.[80]

[h]All exams must be clinically indicated and not part of limited, goal-directed exams.[81]

[i]Up to 50 of the minimum 250 required may be "second look" scans from previous comprehensive exams. Only 150 required if candidate is also certified in TEE/TOE by the BSE/EACVI.[82]

[j]Includes 100 transthoracic and 35 TEE cases.[83]

to a "diplomate" designation. Cognitive skills and competence are re-evaluated every 10 years for maintenance of certification. Although training in perioperative echocardiography is offered by various societies in the United States and around the world, testing and certification are either only offered by a few regulatory bodies (United States, United Kingdom, Europe, Japan) or included within general subspecialty training requirements (Australia and New Zealand). Several other countries have ongoing initiatives aimed at developing certification processes, while others recognize established certifications in the United States, United Kingdom, or Europe. A summary of testing and certification processes in various countries/regions is provided in Table 27-16.

While training goals are generally consistent across programs around the world, there is considerable variability in the certification process in different countries. The number of examinations required for certification in TEE or CCE differs among certifying bodies, which likely reflects uncertainty in how we define competency other than by testing. Training in perioperative echography, including CCE, will likely become more structured for residency now due to its value in clinical care, requirements of the curriculum, and widespread availability of echocardiographic simulators that allow training in a safe environment with tracking of learning metrics.[84–86]

For practitioners of perioperative medicine, echocardiography continues to be an invaluable tool in bedside care. Training programs and certification criteria will evolve alongside improvements in clinical care pathways and advances in technology.

Future Trends in Echocardiography

Artificial intelligence and machine learning have significant potential in standardizing subjective echocardiographic evaluation.[87] Pooling large datasets allows machine learning technologies to reduce interobserver variability. For novice users, artificial intelligence can provide guidance for image acquisition by displaying on-screen messages that suggest the most likely probe manipulations necessary to improve the desired view. The imaging on some devices can also overlay labels for various cardiac chambers, with a high recognition accuracy. There is evidence that novice users benefit from such imaging guidance in the outpatient clinic.[88] As of yet, the utility for similar imaging guidance in the postsurgical and ventilated patient population remains unproven.

The COVID pandemic has resulted in innovations that have improved the accessibility of POCUS expertise with tele-ultrasound.[89] Experts in non-COVID areas of the hospital, or even in another city or country, can provide live guidance and second opinions in the care of critically ill patients. Such a setup could also be modified for remote training in POCUS.

Another evolving area is intravascular ultrasound (IVUS) technology. Transducers are becoming ever more miniaturized, cheaper, and can be mounted at the tip of a catheter.

Conclusions

Ultrasound now has an established presence in every anesthesiologist's toolkit. From the limited and focused use of surface imaging for vascular cannulation to the relatively invasive comprehensive TEE examination that may potentially alter the surgical plan, ultrasound has enhanced our ability to manage patients throughout the perioperative period. Understanding of the technology that generates ultrasound images and correlation with patient anatomy and pathophysiology is key to successful clinical management. Training, certification, and ongoing acquisition of knowledge will be critical to ensuring that the highest quality of care is provided to our patients. Technology continues to evolve at a rapid pace, as do indications and uses of ultrasound. While artificial intelligence and machine learning may change the way we use ultrasound imaging, human intelligence will remain the cornerstone of any advance in patient care we may see in the future.

For additional information please see NICVs 27-1–27-3 and Videos 27-1–27-2 in the eBook bundled with this text.

Acknowledgment

The authors wish to acknowledge HeartWorks (Intelligent Ultrasound Ltd.) for providing the software to reconstruct anatomical and ultrasonographic images.

For further review and interactivities, please see the videos and narrative interactive clinical vignettes (NICVs) accessible in the complimentary eBook bundled with this text. Access instructions are located on the inside front cover.

REFERENCES

1. Eltzschig HK, Rosenberger P, Löffler M, Fox JA, Aranki SF, Shernan SK. Impact of intraoperative transesophageal echocardiography on surgical decisions in 12,566 patients undergoing cardiac surgery. *Ann Thorac Surg.* 2008;85(3):845–852.
2. Nicoara A, Scubas N, Ad N, et al. Guidelines for the use of transesophageal echocardiography to assist with surgical decision-making in the operating room: a surgery-based approach: from the American Society of Echocardiography in collaboration with the Society of Cardiovascular Anesthesiologists and the Society of Thoracic Surgeons. *J Am Soc Echocardiogr.* 2020;33(6):692–734.
3. Denault A, Ferraro P, Couture P, et al. Transesophageal echocardiography monitoring in the intensive care department: the management of hemodynamic instability secondary to thoracic tamponade after single lung transplantation. *J Am Soc Echocardiogr.* 2003;16(6):688–692.
4. Schulmeyer MCC, Santelices E, Vega R, Schmied S. Impact of intraoperative transesophageal echocardiography during noncardiac surgery. *J Cardiothorac Vasc Anesth.* 2006;20(6):768–771.
5. Subramaniam K, Subramanian H, Knight J, Mandell D, McHugh SM. An approach to standard perioperative transthoracic echocardiography practice for anesthesiologists-perioperative transthoracic echocardiography protocols. *J Cardiothorac Vasc Anesth.* 2022;36(2):367–386.
6. Freitas-Ferraz AB, Bernier M, Vaillancourt R, et al. Safety of transesophageal echocardiography to guide structural cardiac interventions. *J Am Coll Cardiol.* 2020;75(25):3164–3173.
7. Hahn RT, Abraham T, Adams MS, et al; American Society of Echocardiography, Society of Cardiovascular Anesthesiologists. Guidelines for performing a comprehensive transesophageal echocardiographic examination: recommendations from the American Society of Echocardiography and the Society of Cardiovascular Anesthesiologists. *Anesth Analg.* 2014;118(1):21–68.
8. American Society of Anesthesiologists and Society of Cardiovascular Anesthesiologists Task Force on Transesophageal Echocardiography. Practice guidelines for perioperative transesophageal echocardiography. An updated report by the American Society of Anesthesiologists and the Society of Cardiovascular Anesthesiologists Task Force on Transesophageal Echocardiography. *Anesthesiology.* 2010;112(5):1084–1096.
9. Ramalingam G, Choi SW, Agarwal S, et al; Association of Cardiothoracic Anaesthesia and Critical Care. Complications related to peri-operative transoesophageal echocardiography–a one-year prospective national audit by the Association of Cardiothoracic Anaesthesia and Critical Care. *Anaesthesia.* 2020;75(1):21–26.
10. Reeves ST, Finley AC, Skubas NJ, et al; Council on Perioperative Echocardiography of the American Society of Echocardiography, Society of Cardiovascular Anesthesiologists. Basic perioperative transesophageal echocardiography examination: a consensus statement of the American Society of Echocardiography and the Society of Cardiovascular Anesthesiologists. *J Am Soc Echocardiogr.* 2013;26(5):443–456.
11. Cowie B. Three years' experience of focused cardiovascular ultrasound in the peri-operative period. *Anaesthesia.* 2011;66(4):268–273.
12. Rong LQ. An update on intraoperative three-dimensional transesophageal echocardiography. *J Thorac Dis.* 2017;9(Suppl 4):S271–S282.
13. Lang RM, Badano LP, Tsang W, et al; American Society of Echocardiography, European Association of Echocardiography. EAE/ASE recommendations for image acquisition and display using three-dimensional echocardiography. *Eur Heart J Cardiovasc Imaging.* 2012;13(1):1–46.
14. Lang RM, Badano LP, Mor-Avi V, et al. Recommendations for cardiac chamber quantification by echocardiography in adults: an update from the American Society of Echocardiography and the European Association of Cardiovascular Imaging. *J Am Soc Echocardiogr.* 2015;28(1):1–39.e14.
15. Cerqueira MD, Weissman NJ, Dilsizian V, et al; American Heart Association Writing Group on Myocardial Segmentation and Registration for Cardiac Imaging. Standardized myocardial segmentation and nomenclature for tomographic imaging of the heart. A statement for healthcare professionals from the Cardiac Imaging Committee of the Council on Clinical Cardiology of the American Heart Association. *Circulation.* 2002;105(4):539–542.
16. Hu K, Liu D, Herrmann S, et al. Clinical implication of mitral annular plane systolic excursion for patients with cardiovascular disease. *Eur Heart J Cardiovasc Imaging.* 2013;14(3):205–212.
17. Simonson JS, Schiller NB. Descent of the base of the left ventricle: an echocardiographic index of left ventricular function. *J Am Soc Echocardiogr.* 1989;2(1):25–35.
18. Gulati VK, Katz WE, Follansbee WP, Gorcsan J 3rd. Mitral annular descent velocity by tissue Doppler echocardiography as an index of global left ventricular function. *Am J Cardiol.* 1996;77(11):979–984.
19. Chen C, Rodriguez L, Guerrero JL, et al. Noninvasive estimation of the instantaneous first derivative of left ventricular pressure using continuous-wave Doppler echocardiography. *Circulation.* 1991;83(6):2101–2110.
20. Tei C, Ling LH, Hodge DO, et al. New index of combined systolic and diastolic myocardial performance: a simple and reproducible measure of cardiac function–a study in normals and dilated cardiomyopathy. *J Cardiol.* 1995;26(6):357–366.
21. Kjøller E, Køber L, Jørgensen S, Torp-Pedersen C; Trace Study G. Short and long term prognostic importance of regional dyskinesia versus akinesia in acute myocardial infarction. *Heart.* 2002;87(5):410–414.
22. Nagueh SF, Smiseth OA, Appleton CP, et al. Recommendations for the evaluation of left ventricular diastolic function by echocardiography: an update from the American Society of Echocardiography and the European Association of Cardiovascular Imaging. *J Am Soc Echocardiogr.* 2016;29(4):277–314.
23. Fayad A, Ansari MT, Yang H, Ruddy T, Wells GA. Perioperative diastolic dysfunction in patients undergoing noncardiac surgery is an independent risk factor for cardiovascular events: a systematic review and meta-analysis. *Anesthesiology.* 2016;125(1):72–91.
24. Obokata M, Reddy YNV, Borlaug BA. Diastolic dysfunction and heart failure with preserved ejection fraction: understanding mechanisms by using noninvasive methods. *JACC Cardiovasc Imaging.* 2020;13(1 Pt 2):245–257.
25. Restrepo CS, Lane MJ, Murillo H. Cardiac aneurysms, pseudoaneurysms, and diverticula. *Semin Roentgenol.* 2012;47(3):262–276.
26. Rudski LG, Lai WW, Afilalo J, et al. Guidelines for the echocardiographic assessment of the right heart in adults: a report from the American Society of Echocardiography endorsed by the European Association of Echocardiography, a registered branch of the European Society of Cardiology, and the Canadian Society of Echocardiography. *J Am Soc Echocardiogr.* 2010;23(7):685–713; quiz 786–788.
27. Baumgartner H, Hung J, Bermejo J, et al; American Society of Echocardiography, European Association of Echocardiography. Echocardiographic assessment of valve stenosis: EAE/ASE recommendations for clinical practice. *J Am Soc Echocardiogr.* 2009;22(1):1–23; quiz 101–2.
28. El Khoury G, Glineur D, Rubay J, et al. Functional classification of aortic root/valve abnormalities and their correlation with etiologies and surgical procedures. *Curr Opin Cardiol.* 2005;20(2):115–121.
29. Zoghbi WA, Adams D, Bonow RO, et al. Recommendations for noninvasive evaluation of native valvular regurgitation: a report from the American Society of Echocardiography Developed in Collaboration with the Society for Cardiovascular Magnetic Resonance. *J Am Soc Echocardiogr.* 2017;30(4):303–371.
30. Evangelista A, Flachskampf FA, Erbel R, et al; European Association of Echocardiography. Echocardiography in aortic diseases: EAE recommendations for clinical practice. *Eur J Echocardiogr.* 2010;11(8):645–658.
31. Klein AL, Abbara S, Agler DA, et al. American Society of Echocardiography Clinical Recommendations for Multimodality Cardiovascular Imaging of Patients with Pericardial Disease: Endorsed by the Society for Cardiovascular Magnetic Resonance and Society of Cardiovascular Computed Tomography. *J Am Soc Echocardiogr.* 2013;26(9):965–1012.e15.

32. Habib G, Badano L, Tribouilloy C, et al; European Association of Echocardiography. Recommendations for the practice of echocardiography in infective endocarditis. *Eur J Echocardiogr.* 2010;11(2):202–219.
33. Bronshteyn YS, Anderson TA, Badakhsh O, et al; American Society of Anesthesiologists Ad Hoc Committee on PoCUS. Diagnostic point-of-care ultrasound: recommendations from an expert panel. *J Cardiothorac Vasc Anesth.* 2022;36(1):22–29.
34. Kalagara H, Coker B, Gerstein NS, et al. Point-of-care ultrasound (POCUS) for the cardiothoracic anesthesiologist. *J Cardiothorac Vasc Anesth.* 2022;36(4):1132–1147.
35. Ramsingh D, Runyon A, Gatling J, et al. Improved diagnostic accuracy of pathology with the implementation of a perioperative point-of-care ultrasound service: quality improvement initiative. *Reg Anesth Pain Med.* 2020;45(2):95.
36. Ramsingh D, Singh S, Canales C, et al. The evaluation point-of-care ultrasound in the post-anesthesia unit–a multicenter prospective observational study. *J Clin Med.* 2021; 10(11):2389.
37. Blanco P, Abdo-Cuza A. Point-of-care ultrasound in the critically ill pregnant or postpartum patient: what every intensivist should know. *Intensive Care Med.* 2019;45(8):1123–1126.
38. Weile J, Brix J, Moellekaer AB. Is point-of-care ultrasound disruptive innovation? Formulating why POCUS is different from conventional comprehensive ultrasound. *Crit Ultrasound J.* 2018;10(1):25.
39. Feilchenfeld Z, Kuper A, Whitehead C. Stethoscope of the 21st century: dominant discourses of ultrasound in medical education. *Med Educ.* 2018;52(12):1271–1287.
40. Millington SJ, Koenig S. Ultrasound assessment of the inferior vena cava for fluid responsiveness: making the case for skepticism. *J Intensive Care Med.* 2021;36(10):1223–1227.
41. Broch O, Renner J, Gruenewald M, et al. Variation of left ventricular outflow tract velocity and global end-diastolic volume index reliably predict fluid responsiveness in cardiac surgery patients. *J Crit Care.* 2012;27(3):325.e7–e13.
42. Canty DJ, Royse CF, Kilpatrick D, Bowyer A, Royse AG. The impact on cardiac diagnosis and mortality of focused transthoracic echocardiography in hip fracture surgery patients with increased risk of cardiac disease: a retrospective cohort study. *Anaesthesia.* 2012;67(11): 1202–1209.
43. Canty DJ, Royse CF, Kilpatrick D, Williams DL, Royse AG. The impact of pre-operative focused transthoracic echocardiography in emergency non-cardiac surgery patients with known or risk of cardiac disease. *Anaesthesia.* 2012;67(7):714–720.
44. Price S, Uddin S, Quinn T. Echocardiography in cardiac arrest. *Curr Opin Crit Care.* 2010; 16(3):211–215.
45. Levitov A, Frankel HL, Blaivas M, et al. Guidelines for the appropriate use of bedside general and cardiac ultrasonography in the evaluation of critically ill patients-part II: cardiac ultrasonography. *Crit Care Med.* 2016;44(6):1206–1227.
46. Beaubien-Souligny W, Rola P, Haycock K, et al. Quantifying systemic congestion with point-of-care ultrasound: development of the venous excess ultrasound grading system. *Ultrasound J.* 2020;12(1):16.
47. Xirouchaki N, Magkanas E, Vaporidi K, et al. Lung ultrasound in critically ill patients: comparison with bedside chest radiography. *Intensive Care Med.* 2011;37(9):1488–1493.
48. Lichtenstein DA. BLUE-protocol and FALLS-protocol: two applications of lung ultrasound in the critically ill. *Chest.* 2015;147(6):1659–1670.
49. Volpicelli G. Sonographic diagnosis of pneumothorax. *Intensive Care Med.* 2011;37(2): 224–232.
50. Lichtenstein D, Mezière G, Biderman P, Gepner A. The "lung point": an ultrasound sign specific to pneumothorax. *Intensive Care Med.* 2000;26(10):1434–1440.
51. Mojoli F, Bouhemad B, Mongodi S, Lichtenstein D. Lung ultrasound for critically ill patients. *Am J Respir Crit Care Med.* 2019;199(6):701–714.
52. Zambon M, Greco M, Bocchino S, Cabrini L, Beccaria PF, Zangrillo A. Assessment of diaphragmatic dysfunction in the critically ill patient with ultrasound: a systematic review. *Intensive Care Med.* 2017;43(1):29–38.
53. Perlas A, Mitsakakis N, Liu L, et al. Validation of a mathematical model for ultrasound assessment of gastric volume by gastroscopic examination. *Anesth Analg.* 2013;116(2): 357–363.
54. Kruisselbrink R, Gharapetian A, Chaparro LE, et al. Diagnostic accuracy of point-of-care gastric ultrasound. *Anesth Analg.* 2019;128(1):89–95.
55. Troianos CA, Hartman GS, Glas KE, et al; Councils on Intraoperative Echocardiography and Vascular Ultrasound of the American Society of Echocardiography. Guidelines for performing ultrasound guided vascular cannulation: recommendations of the American Society of Echocardiography and the Society of Cardiovascular Anesthesiologists. *J Am Soc Echocardiogr.* 2011;24(12):1291–1318.
56. Ueda K, Hussey P. Dynamic ultrasound-guided short-axis needle tip navigation technique for facilitating cannulation of peripheral veins in obese patients. *Anesth Analg.* 2017;124(3): 831–833.
57. Munirathinam GK, Kajal K, Jayant A, Dogra N, Singh H. Epicardial echocardiography as rescue modality for detection of dynamic right ventricular outflow tract obstruction in post pulmonary valve stenosis repair. *A A Pract.* 2019;13(10):396–398.
58. Glas KE, Swaminathan M, Reeves ST, et al; Council for Intraoperative Echocardiography of the American Society of Echocardiography, Society of Cardiovascular Anesthesiologists, Society of Thoracic Surgeons. Guidelines for the performance of a comprehensive intraoperative epiaortic ultrasonographic examination: recommendations of the American Society of Echocardiography and the Society of Cardiovascular Anesthesiologists; endorsed by the Society of Thoracic Surgeons. *Anesth Analg.* 2008;106(5):1376–1384.
59. Shapeton AD, Leissner KB, Zorca SM, et al. Epiaortic ultrasound for assessment of intraluminal atheroma; insights from the REGROUP trial. *J Cardiothorac Vasc Anesth.* 2020;34(3):726–732.
60. Rhoades D, Subramani S. Diagnostic challenges with transesophageal echocardiography for intraoperative iatrogenic aortic dissection: role of epiaortic ultrasound. *Ann Card Anaesth.* 2021; 24(1):83–86.
61. Zamorano JL, Badano LP, Bruce C, et al. EAE/ASE recommendations for the use of echocardiography in new transcatheter interventions for valvular heart disease. *Eur Heart J.* 2011; 32(17):2189–2214.
62. Wiegers SE, Ryan T, Arrighi JA, et al. 2019 ACC/AHA/ASE advanced training statement on echocardiography (revision of the 2003 ACC/AHA clinical competence statement on echocardiography): a report of the ACC Competency Management Committee. *J Am Coll Cardiol.* 2019;74(3):377–402.
63. Cahalan MK, Stewart W, Pearlman A, et al; Society of Cardiovascular Anesthesiologists, American Society of Echocardiography Task Force. American Society of Echocardiography and Society of Cardiovascular Anesthesiologists Task Force guidelines for training in perioperative echocardiography. *J Am Soc Echocardiogr.* 2002;15(6):647–652.
64. American Board of Anesthesiology (ABA). Initial certification in anesthesiology 2019. https://theaba.org/pdfs/Initial_Certification_Content_Outline.pdf. Published 2019. Accessed 02/24/2023.
65. Accreditation Council for Graduate Medical Education (ACGME). ACGME program requirements for graduate medical education in anesthesiology. 2020. https://www.acgme.org/globalassets/pfassets/programrequirements/040_anesthesiology_2022.pdf Published 2022. Accessed 02/24/2023.
66. Ryan T, Berlacher K, Lindner JR, Mankad SV, Rose GA, Wang A. COCATS 4 Task Force 5: training in echocardiography: endorsed by the American Society of Echocardiography. *J Am Soc Echocardiogr.* 2015;28(6):615–627.
67. Kirkpatrick JN, Grimm R, Johri AM, et al. Recommendations for echocardiography laboratories participating in cardiac point of care cardiac ultrasound (POCUS) and critical care echocardiography training: report from the American Society of Echocardiography. *J Am Soc Echocardiogr.* 2020;33(4):409–422.e4.
68. Mayo PH, Beaulieu Y, Doelken P, et al. American College of Chest Physicians/La Societe de Reanimation de Langue Francaise statement on competence in critical care ultrasonography. *Chest.* 2009;135(4):1050–1060.
69. Expert Round Table on Ultrasound in ICU. International expert statement on training standards for critical care ultrasonography. *Intensive Care Med.* 2011;37(7):1077–1083.
70. Expert Round Table on Echocardiography in ICU. International consensus statement on training standards for advanced critical care echocardiography. *Intensive Care Med.* 2014;40(5):654–666.
71. Wong A, Galarza L, Forni L, et al; ESICM Critical Care Ultrasound Group. Recommendations for core critical care ultrasound competencies as a part of specialist training in multidisciplinary intensive care: a framework proposed by the European Society of Intensive Care Medicine (ESICM). *Crit Care.* 2020;24(1):393.
72. Fagley RE, Haney MF, Beraud AS, et al. Critical care basic ultrasound learning goals for American anesthesiology critical care trainees: recommendations from an expert group. *Anesth Analg.* 2015;120(5):1041–1053.
73. Hu X, Xi X, Ma P, et al; China Critical Care Clinical Trials Group (CCCCTG) and the Task Force of Core Competencies in Intensive and Critical Care Medicine Training in China. Consensus development of core competencies in intensive and critical care medicine training in China. *Crit Care.* 2016;20(1):330.
74. National Board of Echocardiography. Application for certification in basic perioperative transesophageal echocardiography (basic PTEeXAM) Raleigh, NC: NBE; 2022. https://www.echoboards.org/wp-content/uploads/2022/11/BasicPTE_Cert_App-2022.pdf Published 2022. Accessed 02/2/2023.
75. National Board of Echocardiography. Application for certification in advanced perioperative transesophageal echocardiography (advanced PTEeXAM) Raleigh, NC: NBE; 2022. https://www.echoboards.org/wp-content/uploads/2022/11/AAdvPTE_Cert_App-2022.pdf. Accessed 02/24/2023.
76. European Society of Cardiology. EACVI adult transoesophageal echocardiography (TOE) certification: certification organised by the European Association of Cardiovascular Imaging (EACVI): EACVI; 2022. https://www.escardio.org/Education/Career-Development/Certification/Adult-Transoesophageal-Echo. Accessed 02/24/2023.
77. British Society of Echocardiography. Accreditation in adult transoesophageal (TOE) echocardiography information pack 2022. https://www.bsecho.org/common/Uploaded%20files/Accreditation/Accreditation%20Packs/TOE%20Accreditation%20Pack%20Apr%2022%20v6.pdf. Accessed 02/24/2023.
78. ANZCA. PG46(POM) guideline on training and practice of perioperative cardiac ultrasound in adults 2014. https://www.anzca.edu.au/getattachment/8181a47f-60e3-4d6b-9de8-fe42dac09079/PS46-Guideline-on-training-and-practice-of-perioperative-cardiac-ultrasound-in-adults. Accessed 02/24/2023.
79. Japanese Board of Perioperative Transesophageal Echocardiography. JB-POT certifying examination 2022. http://www.jb-pot.com/en/exam/18. Accessed 02/24/2023.
80. Indian Association of Cardiovascular and Thoracic Anaesthesiologists. Indian College of Cardiac Anaesthesia FTEE application form 2022. http://www.iacta.co.in/uploads/FTEE_Exam_Appl_form_revised.pdf. Accessed 02/24/2023.

81. National Board of Echocardiography. Application for certification in critical care echocardiography (CCEeXAM) 2022. https://www.echoboards.org/wp-content/uploads/2022/11/CCEeXAM-Cert_App-2022.pdf. Accessed 02/24/2023.
82. British Society of Echocardiography. Accreditation in adult critical care echocardiography information pack 2022. https://www.bsecho.org/common/Uploaded%20files/Accreditation/Accreditation%20Packs/ACCE%20Accreditation%20pack%20Apr%2022-v3.pdf. Accessed 02/24/2023.
83. European Society of Intensive Care Medicine. European diploma in advanced critical care echocardiography (EDEC) 2022. https://www.esicm.org/wp-content/uploads/2018/06/EDEC_Guidelines_2018.pdf. Accessed 02/24/2023.
84. Bose RR, Matyal R, Warraich HJ, et al. Utility of a transesophageal echocardiographic simulator as a teaching tool. *J Cardiothorac Vasc Anesth*. 2011;25(2):212–215.
85. Ferrero NA, Bortsov AV, Arora H, et al. Simulator training enhances resident performance in transesophageal echocardiography. *Anesthesiology*. 2014;120(1):149–159.
86. Neelankavil J, Howard-Quijano K, Hsieh TC, et al. Transthoracic echocardiography simulation is an efficient method to train anesthesiologists in basic transthoracic echocardiography skills. *Anesth Analg*. 2012;115(5):1042–1051.
87. Zamzmi G, Hsu LY, Li W, Sachdev V, Antani S. Harnessing machine intelligence in automatic echocardiogram analysis: current status, limitations, and future directions. *IEEE Rev Biomed Eng*. 2021;14:181–203.
88. Schneider M, Bartko P, Geller W, et al. A machine learning algorithm supports ultrasound-naïve novices in the acquisition of diagnostic echocardiography loops and provides accurate estimation of LVEF. *Int J Cardiovasc Imaging*. 2021;37(2):577–586.
89. Hussain A, Via G, Melniker L, et al. Multi-organ point-of-care ultrasound for COVID-19 (PoCUS4COVID): international expert consensus. *Crit Care*. 2020;24(1):702.
90. Bossone E, D'Andrea A, D'Alto M, et al. Echocardiography in pulmonary arterial hypertension: from diagnosis to prognosis. *J Am Soc Echocardiogr*. 2013;26(1):1–14.

Section 6

BASIC ANESTHETIC MANAGEMENT

28 Airway Management

ANTHONY TANELLA • JAIME B. HYMAN • WILLIAM H. ROSENBLATT

KEY POINTS

1. Management of the difficult airway, especially when unanticipated, requires flexibility and is paramount to safe perioperative care. Preoperative airway evaluation and planning favorably affects outcomes.
2. From infancy to childhood, the airway undergoes significant changes in its size, shape, and relation to the cervical spine.
3. The advent of the laryngeal mask airway, as well as other supraglottic airways, has revolutionized both routine and emergency airway management.
4. Airway management always begins with a thorough airway-relevant history and physical examination.
5. Preoxygenation (also termed *denitrogenation*) should be practiced in all cases when time allows.
6. Oxygenation should be optimized throughout the process of airway management.
7. The gold standard for verification of tracheal intubation is sustained detection of exhaled carbon dioxide.
8. The technique of rapid-sequence induction is performed to gain control of the airway in the shortest period of time after the ablation of protective airway reflexes with the induction of anesthesia.
9. In terms of airway management, the period of extubation may be far more treacherous than that of induction of anesthesia and tracheal intubation.
10. In most instances, awake intubation can be accomplished successfully if approached with care and patience. Awake airway management remains a mainstay of the American Society of Anesthesiologists' difficult airway guidelines.
11. Airway access via the extrathoracic trachea may be warranted when mask ventilation, supraglottic airway, and intubation all fail.

Perspectives on Airway Management

In the more than three decades since the publication of the first edition of this text, the field of airway management has undergone a vigorous revolution. The array of devices, algorithms, and pharmaceuticals in the modern airway armamentarium has increased exponentially. The final decade of the last century saw a significant increase in the application of supraglottic ventilation, followed by the introduction and widespread adoption of videolaryngoscopy (VL). More recently, pharmacologic and oxygenation tools have taken the spotlight.

Along with offering the provider better tools, technology has also aided in the creation of large databases of airway-related records with a wealth of information from which we can better understand the incidence of and contributing factors to adverse airway events.[1]

Techniques and practices in airway management have long been an important concern of anesthesia societies, as illustrated by the publication and revision of various difficult airway guidelines.[2,3] Despite advancements, analysis of the American Society of Anesthesiologists' (ASA) Closed Claims Database in the periods before and after year 2000 reveals disturbing trends.[4] There was a significant increase in the proportion of claims related to death and a greater proportion of claims from nonperioperative locations. Inadequate planning for airway management and judgment errors occurred in a majority of claims.[4] Although the closed claims data is useful, it has significant limitations, including its retrospective nature and the lack of denominator data.

Management of the difficult airway, especially when unantici- 1
pated, is paramount to safe perioperative care (1 Video 28-1).

Difficult and failed airway management accounts for 2.3% to 64.4% of anesthetic deaths.[5–7] The following steps are essential to safe airway management: (1) thorough airway history and physical examination; (2) consideration of the ease of rapid tracheal intubation by direct or indirect laryngoscopy; (3) preinduction formation of a management plan, which includes the use of non-tracheal tube ventilation (e.g., facemask and supraglottic airway [SGA]); (4) aspiration risk assessment; and (5) estimation of the risk that airway management procedures may fail.[8] This chapter will focus on routine and rescue airway management techniques that are the fundamentals upon which all airway management is based. Specialty-specific techniques (e.g., elective suspension laryngoscopy) will not be addressed.

Review of Airway Anatomy

2 The term *airway* refers to the nasal and oral cavities, pharynx, larynx, trachea, and principal bronchi. The airway in humans is primarily a conducting pathway. Because the oroesophageal and nasotracheal passages cross each other, anatomic and functional complexities have evolved for protection of the sublaryngeal airway against aspiration of food passing through the pharynx. Like other bodily systems, the airway is not immune from the influence of genetic, nutritional, and hormonal factors. From infancy to childhood, the airway undergoes significant changes in its size, shape, and relationship to the cervical spine.[9] Table 28-1 illustrates the anatomic differences in the larynx of infants and adults.

The laryngeal skeleton consists of nine cartilages (three paired and three unpaired); together, these house the vocal folds, which extend in an anterior–posterior plane from the thyroid cartilage to the arytenoid cartilages. The shield-shaped thyroid cartilage acts as the anterior "protective housing" of the vocal mechanism (Fig. 28-1). Movements of the laryngeal structures are controlled by two groups of muscles: the extrinsic muscles, which move the larynx as a whole; and the intrinsic muscles, which move the various cartilages in relation to one another. The larynx is innervated by the superior and recurrent laryngeal nerves, which are branches of the vagus nerve. Because the recurrent laryngeal nerves supply all the intrinsic muscles of the larynx (with the exception of the cricothyroid muscle), trauma to these nerves can result in vocal cord dysfunction. With unilateral recurrent laryngeal nerve injury, hoarseness is the primary symptom; the protective role of the larynx in preventing aspiration may also be compromised. Bilateral injury can result in complete airway obstruction due to unopposed vocal cord adduction as well as expose the patient to an increased risk of aspiration.

An important identifiable anatomic structure is the cricothyroid membrane (CTM), which joins the superior surface of the cricoid cartilage and the inferior edge of the thyroid cartilage. In

Table 28-1 Anatomic Differences between Infant and Adult Larynxes

Infant larynx proportionately smaller
Vertical location: C3–C5 in infant; C4–C6 in adult
Pliable laryngeal cartilage in the infant/child
Vocal folds: Anterior angle with respect to perpendicular axis of larynx in infant/child
Aryepiglottic folds closer to midline in infant/child
Epiglottis: Relatively longer, narrower, and stiffer in infant
Mucosa more vulnerable to trauma in infant

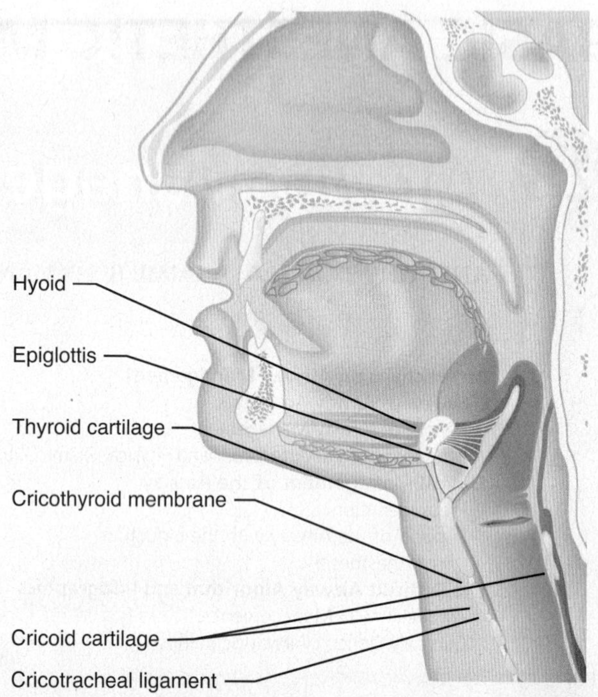

Figure 28-1 The major landmarks of the airway mechanism. Note that the cricoid cartilage is <1 cm in height in its anterior aspect but may be 2 cm in height posteriorly.

an adult, the membrane is typically 8 to 12 mm in width and 10.4 to 13.7 mm in height and is composed of a yellow elastic tissue that lies directly beneath the skin and a fascial layer. It can be identified 1 to 1.5 fingerbreadths below the laryngeal prominence (thyroid notch).[10] The membrane has a central portion known as the *conus elasticus* and two lateral thinner portions. Directly beneath the membrane is the laryngeal mucosa. Because of anatomic variability in the course of veins and arteries and the membrane's proximity to the vocal folds (which may be 0.9 cm above the ligaments' upper border), it is suggested that any incisions or needle punctures to the CTM be made in its inferior third and be directed posteriorly (a posterior probing needle will strike the back side of the signet ring-shaped cricoid cartilage). Identification of an appropriate incision or puncture site may be difficult. Alshareef et al.[11] found that only one-third of trainees were able to correctly identify the CTM. The use of ultrasound (US) facilitates identification, even in obese patients.[12] The ASA difficult airway guidelines suggest that every patient be evaluated for difficult surgical airway.[2] This should lead to routine examination of laryngeal structures, including the marking of surface anatomy and the use of US identification in at-risk patients (Fig. 28-2).[13]

At the base of the larynx, suspended by the underside of the CTM, is the signet ring–shaped cricoid cartilage. This cartilage is approximately 1 cm in height anteriorly, but almost 2 cm in height in its posterior aspect as it extends in a cephalad direction behind the CTM (Fig. 28-1). The tracheal cartilages are interconnected by fibroelastic tissue, which allows for expansion of the trachea in both length and diameter with inspiration/expiration and flexion/extension of the thoracocervical spine. Inferiorly, the trachea is suspended from the cricoid cartilage by the cricotracheal ligament.

The trachea measures approximately 15 cm in adults and is circumferentially supported by 17 to 18 C-shaped cartilages, with a membranous posterior surface overlying the esophagus. In adults, the first tracheal ring is anterior to the sixth cervical vertebra.

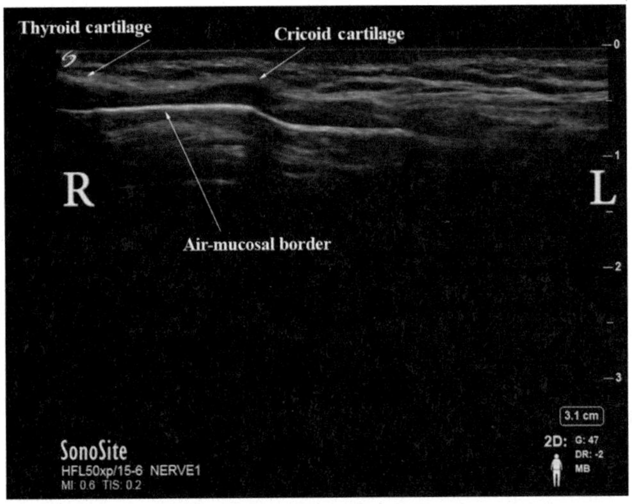

Figure 28-2 Ultrasound image of the cricothyroid membrane (CTM, midline sagittal).

The trachea ends at the carina (opposite the fifth thoracic vertebra), where it bifurcates into the principal bronchi. The right principal bronchus is larger in diameter than the left and deviates from the sagittal plane of the trachea at a less acute angle. For these reasons, aspirated materials, as well as a deeply inserted endotracheal tube (ETT), tend to gain entry into the right principal bronchus, although left-sided positioning cannot be excluded. Cartilaginous ring support continues through the first seven generations of bronchi.

History of Airway Management

Prior to 1874, mechanisms of airway obstruction were poorly understood. Opening the mouth with a wooden screw and drawing the tongue forward with a forceps or a steel-gloved finger was the extent of nonsurgical airway management.[14] Not until 1880 was it recognized that most airway obstruction resulted from the tongue falling against the posterior pharyngeal wall. Though it is possible that similar devices were employed toward the end of the first millennium, the first application of an SGA is credited to Joseph Thomas Clover (1825–1882), who used a nasopharyngeal tube for the delivery of chloroform anesthesia.[15] Over the next 50 years, several modifications of the basic oropharyngeal airway were described. In the 1930s, Ralph Waters introduced the now-familiar flattened tube oral airway. Arthur Guedel modified Waters' concept by fitting his airway within a stiff rubber envelope in an attempt to reduce mucosal trauma.

Tracheal intubation was first described in 1788 as a means of resuscitation of the "apparently dead,"[16] but was not used for the delivery of anesthesia until almost 100 years later. The forerunner of the modern oral ETT was designed by Joseph O'Dwyer in the 1880s. O'Dwyer cared for pediatric patients suffering airway obstruction secondary to diphtherial pseudomembrane formations. He was aware of the work of Emile Trousseau, a French physician who reported having performed over 200 tracheostomies in patients with diphtheria. Hoping to provide his patients nonsurgical relief from airway obstruction, O'Dwyer designed brass tracheal tubes that were placed in the larynx using blind digital intubation. Some 20 years later, German otolaryngologist Dr. Franz Kuhn (1866–1929) developed a flexometallic tube that resisted kinking and could be shaped to the patient's upper airway anatomy. Like O'Dwyer's tubes, it was inserted using a blind technique. The patients were intubated awake and the hypopharynx was sealed with oiled gauze packing.

Sir Ivan Magill and Stanley Rowbotham are credited with the initial development of modern tracheal intubation. Performing anesthesia for reconstructive facial surgery during World War I, they developed a two-tube nasal system. One narrow tube (gum elastic design) was passed through the nares and guided into the larynx using a surgical laryngoscope. The other tube was blindly passed into the pharynx to provide for the escape of gases. During use of this "Magill" tube, the exhaust lumen would occasionally pass blindly into the larynx, leading Sir Ivan to describe "blind nasal intubation."[17]

Cuffed SGAs were initially described in the early part of the 20th century. Three factors led to the development of these devices: (1) the introduction of cyclopropane (which was explosive and required an airtight circuit for appropriate gas containment); (2) appreciation that blind and laryngoscope-guided tracheal intubation remained a difficult task; and (3) a need for protection of the lower airway from blood and surgical debris in the upper airway.[15] The Primrose cuffed oropharyngeal tube, the Shipway airway (a Guedel oropharyngeal airway fitted with a cuff and a circuit connector designed by Sir Ivan Magill), and the Lessinger airway were predecessors of the modern supraglottic devices. In 1937, Leech introduced a "pharyngeal bulb gasway" with a noninflatable cuff that fit snugly into the hypopharynx.

The use of SGAs remained dominant until the introduction of curare in 1942 and the mass training of anesthesiologists in tracheal intubation in anticipation of casualties during World War II. The description by Mendelson[18] of gastric-content aspiration in parturients managed with a mask airway (66 of 44,016 patients, with 2 deaths) furthered the shift toward tracheal intubation in most surgical procedures. Within a few years, proficiency in direct laryngoscopy (DL) and tracheal intubation became a mark of professionalism. The advent of succinylcholine in 1951 furthered the dominance of tracheal intubation by providing rapid and profound muscle relaxation.

By 1981, two types of airway management prevailed—tracheal intubation and facemask ventilation with or without a Guedel airway. Although time-tested, both had faults. Tracheal intubation was associated with dental and soft tissue injury as well as cardiovascular stimulation. On the other hand mask ventilation, while less invasive, often required a prolonged hands-on-the-airway technique. These difficulties led to reconsideration of SGAs.

The advent of the laryngeal mask airway (LMA) and the subsequent introduction of other SGAs revolutionized both routine and emergency airway management. In 1981, Dr. Archie Brain conceived the idea of fitting a mask-like structure over the larynx. He believed that airway control could be achieved less traumatically than with tracheal intubation and more reliably than with facemask ventilation. The first prototypes of the LMA were built from the Goldman dental mask, fitted with a tracheal tube. The LMA Classic (Teleflex, Research Triangle Park, NC) was introduced into practice in the United Kingdom in 1989 and approved by the U.S. Food and Drug Administration in 1991. The variety of advanced models that followed (e.g., with intubation and gastric drainage capabilities) will be discussed later in this chapter. With the expiration of the early patents and the introduction of other design concepts (e.g., noninflatable masks), several additional devices applying the supraglottic concept were introduced.

Parallel to the development of SGAs, the concept of indirect laryngoscopy was gaining favor. Although fiberoptic devices were applied to the problem of difficult tracheal intubation as early as the 1960s, this technology was expensive and required a unique skill set. It was not until the late 1980s when the technology became readily available that skill in flexible fiberoptic airway management came to be considered critical to safe practice.[19] Bullard introduced the use of a fiberoptic bundle to the rigid laryngoscope. The Bullard laryngoscope (ACMI/Circon, Southborough, MA) incorporated optical and light-transmitting fiberoptic bundles into an anatomically shaped blade. A detachable stylet held the tracheal tube near the optic objective, which could be placed proximal to the larynx with minimal movement of the head and neck. The Bullard laryngoscope can be considered the vanguard of the modern videolaryngoscopes and optical and video stylets.[20] Fiberoptic elements were also incorporated into standard laryngoscope blades, such as the Storz Video-Macintosh blade (Karl Storz, Tuttlingen, Germany), which was developed by Dr. George Berci, a pioneer in endoscopic surgery.

The first years of the 21st century saw the era of VL begin, with the advent of inexpensive and miniaturized light-sensitive computer chip devices (e.g., complementary metal-oxide-semiconductors or CMOS). The Glidescope (Verathon, Bothell, WA) was the first of a generation of devices to use CMOS technology to visualize the larynx indirectly. The Glidescope's acutely angled blade placed the clinician's point of vision around the base of the tongue, obviating the need to establish a direct line of sight from the operator's eye to the larynx. Difficulty in placement of the ETT around the Glidescope's hyperangulated blade quickly led to the introduction of both specialized stylets and channeled-type laryngoscopes. Each of these advents will be discussed later in this chapter.

Limitations of Patient History and Physical Examination

4 Airway management always begins with a thorough airway-relevant history and physical examination, including a search for previously documented airway-related anesthetic events. When a patient requires more than routine care (anticipated or unanticipated), the patient should be made aware of diagnostic evaluations and therapeutic interventions that were employed. It is becoming common practice for a dedicated "difficult airway note" to be incorporated into electronic and paper medical records and for a "difficult airway letter" to be given to and reviewed with patients and their families, describing critical and unanticipated airway events. The patient may also be referred to difficult airway registries, such as MedicAlert (http://www.medicalert.org/everybody/difficult-airwayintubation-registry). In the absence of such documentation, the clinician should seek the records of past anesthetics, which may require contacting other institutions. When this information is not available and significant concern exists, there should be a low threshold for use of a more conservative approach to airway management (e.g., awake intubation). It is not unusual for a patient to be referred to a different facility or practitioner due to airway management concerns. Signs and symptoms related to potentially difficult airway management, including aspiration and risk of cardiovascular collapse, should be sought (Tables 28-2 and 28-3, 2 Video 28-2). Many congenital and acquired syndromes are associated with difficult airway management (Table 28-4).

The difficulty in developing the perfect airway evaluation tool lies in two interrelated areas: simplicity and interdependency.

Table 28-2 Physical Examination Features with Airway Management Implications

Physical Examination Feature	Significance
Mouth opening	Difficult blade insertion/tongue displacement if limited
Jaw protrusion	Difficult tongue displacement if limited
Dentition	Obstructed view (if large central incisors), increased risk of dental trauma (if poor or restored dentition), difficult mask ventilation (if edentulous)
Retrognathia	Difficult tongue displacement
Thyromental distance	Reflects neck mobility and degree of retrognathia
Mallampati grade	Describes the relationship between mouth opening, tongue size, and pharyngeal space
Presence of beard	Difficult mask seal
Airway pathology	Potential for difficult mask ventilation (obstructive masses/tissue, atypical facial contours) and laryngoscopy (friable tissue, atypical or absent landmarks, and limited mouth opening, jaw protrusion, tongue displacement, and neck mobility)

Table 28-3 Conditions with Airway Management Implications

Increased Risk of Difficult Laryngoscopy, Mask Ventilation, or SGA Ventilation

- History of failed or traumatic airway management
  - Dental damage or prolonged airway soreness after a previous anesthetic
- History of head/neck surgery or radiation therapy
- Various congenital and acquired syndromes (Table 28-4)
- Supraglottic pathology
  - Obstructive sleep apnea (BMI >35 kg/m^2, loud snoring, daytime somnolence, gasping or pauses in breathing during sleep)
  - Lingual tonsillar hyperplasia
- Acute airway pathology
  - Airway cyst or tumor
  - Airway bleeding
  - Stridor

Cervical spine disease or limited range of motion
Temporomandibular joint disease

Increased Aspiration Risk

Recent meal
Acute trauma
Acute gastrointestinal pathology
Acute narcotic therapy
Significant gastroesophageal reflux
Current intensive care unit admission
Pregnancy (gestational age ≥12 wk)
Postpartum (before second postpartum day)
Frequent pneumonia
History of voice change, vocal cord polyp, or coughing after eating/drinking
Systemic-disease associated with gastroparesis: diabetes mellitus, collagen vascular disease, advanced Parkinson disease, central nervous system tumors

Table 28-4 Syndromes Associated with Difficult Airway Management

Pathologic Condition	Features Affecting Airway Management
Congenital	
Pierre Robin sequence	Micrognathia, relative macroglossia, glossoptosis, cleft palate
Treacher Collins syndrome	Malar and mandibular hypoplasia, microstomia, choanal atresia
Down syndrome	Macroglossia, microcephaly, cervical spine abnormalities
Klippel–Feil syndrome	Congenital fusion of cervical vertebrae, decreased cervical range of motion
Cretinism	Macroglossia, compression or deviation of larynx/trachea by goiter
Cri du chat syndrome	Micrognathia, laryngomalacia, stridor
Alport syndrome	Maxillary hypoplasia, prognathism, cleft soft palate, tracheobronchial cartilaginous anomalies
Beckwith syndrome	Macroglossia
Cherubism	Mandibular and maxillary fibrous tissue overgrowth
Meckel syndrome	Microcephaly, micrognathia, cleft epiglottis
Neurofibromatosis type I (von Recklinghausen disease)	Tumors may occur in the larynx and right ventricle outflow tract. Increased incidence of pheochromocytoma
Hurler/Hunter syndrome	Stiff joints, upper airway obstruction due to infiltration of lymphoid tissue, abnormal tracheobronchial cartilages
Pompe disease	Muscle deposits, macroglossia
Acquired Infections	
Epiglottitis	Epiglottal edema
Croup	Laryngeal edema
Papillomatosis	Obstructive papillomas
Intraoral/retropharyngeal abscess	Airway distortion/stenosis, trismus
Ludwig angina	Airway distortion/stenosis, trismus
Arthritis	
Rheumatoid arthritis	Restricted cervical spine mobility, temporomandibular joint ankylosis, atlantoaxial instability
Ankylosing spondylitis	Ankylosis/immobility of cervical spine and temporomandibular joints
Tumors	
Cystic hygroma, lipoma, adenoma, goiter	Airway distortion or stenosis
Carcinoma of tongue/larynx/thyroid	Airway distortion or stenosis, fixation of larynx or adjacent tissues
Trauma	
Head/facial/cervical spine	Airway edema or hemorrhage, unstable facial or mandibular fractures, intralaryngeal damage
Miscellaneous Conditions	
History of head/neck radiation	Friable tissue, edema from impaired lymphatic drainage
Morbid obesity	Short, thick neck, large tongue, and obstructive sleep apnea are likely
Acromegaly	Macroglossia, prognathism
Acute burns	Airway edema, bronchospasm, decreased apnea tolerance

Several bedside physical evaluation measures have become widely used although their reproducibility and predictive value have been disputed (Table 28-5). Adequate evaluation may require endoscopic, radiologic, or other examinations that are impractical to perform universally in the perioperative setting.[21–23] Interdependency refers to the predictive value of one airway examination measure based on the findings of another. Details of the various examinations and their interdependency are discussed later in "Direct Laryngoscopy," under the topic of Functional Airway Assessment (FAA).

Historically, airway assessment has been synonymous with evaluation for the ease of DL, the end point being the anticipated ease of visualization of the larynx. The changing landscape of laryngoscopy (i.e., the rapid proliferation of indirect techniques, including VL) may make many of these evaluation indices irrelevant. Efforts to define attributes that identify patients who may be difficult to intubate by DL have been only modestly successful. In their meta-analysis of bedside screening tests used to predict difficult DL, Roth et al.[24] found these tests have only modest discriminative power (Table 28-6).

Table 28-5 Common Airway Assessment Elements

Examination	
Thyromental distance	Measured from tip of mentum to thyroid notch in neck-extended position
Mouth opening	Interincisor distance (or interalveolar distance when edentulous) with the mouth maximally opened
Mallampati score	See Figure 28-8
Head and neck mobility	Range of motion from full flexion to full extension
Ability to prognath	Capacity to bring lower incisors in front of upper incisors

Despite the disappointing performance of individual indexes, combinations of these tests or a combination of results from physical assessment and imaging studies offers improved predictability. Of course, some pathology will only present with the induction of anesthesia and/or attempts at laryngoscopy.[25–27] A simplified scoring system, studied on a multi-institution population of 3,763 patients,[28] found 5 attributes that could be used to predict difficult laryngoscopy (Table 28-7).[28]

Until recently, there was limited data on external airway findings that may indicate a risk of difficult *indirect* laryngoscopy.[29] The following preoperative findings contribute to failure of VL: scarring, radiation, masses or thickness of the neck, thyromental distance of less than 6 cm, limited cervical motion, and operator experience.[30] In 2016, based on a secondary analysis of 1,100 VL intubations, Aziz et al.[31] identified four distinct predictors of difficult acute-angle VL, including the attending anesthesiologist performing the intubation versus a supervised resident, otolaryngology or cardiac surgery patients, small mouth opening, and sniffing position (SP). Of note, the "supine sniffing" position was associated with more difficult VL compared to the "supine neutral" position, suggesting that this common position may be best avoided when initial plans include VL. Unexpectedly this study found an association between difficulty with VL and the attending anesthesiologist as compared with the supervised resident performing the intubation. The authors of that study make several suggestions to explain this:

1. The attending gravitating toward intubating the more difficult appearing patients themselves.
2. Residents benefiting from having the assistance of the attending.
3. Residents performing more frequent routine intubations.

In general, tracheal intubation should be considered nonroutine under the following conditions: (1) the presence of other equally important priorities to the management of the airway (such as a "full stomach" or emergency surgery); (2) abnormal airway anatomy; or (3) direct injury to the upper airway, larynx, spine, and/or trachea. Although the finding of abnormal anatomy is not synonymous with difficult airway management, it should kindle heightened suspicion.

Few studies have objectively determined findings that identify patients who will be difficult to mask ventilate as defined in Table 28-8(A). In a study of 1,502 patients, Langeron et al.[22] found 5% of patients to be difficult to mask ventilate, with only one patient in the series being impossible to mask ventilate. Table 28-8(B) describes the five independent clinical predictors found by Langeron, with the presence of two or more indicating a high likelihood of difficult mask ventilation. Using different criteria, Kheterpal et al.,[32] found 0.15% of patients to be impossible to mask ventilate. The same study showed that high Mallampati score, male sex, the presence of a beard, and a history of sleep apnea or neck radiation were independent predictors of impossible mask ventilation. More

Table 28-6 Summary of Pooled Sensitivity and Specificity of Difficult Laryngoscopy for Commonly Used Methods of Airway Evaluation[24]

Examination	Sensitivity (%)	Specificity (%)
Mouth opening	22	94
Mallampati classification	53	80
Thyromental distance	37	89
Sternomental distance	33	92
Upper lip bite	67	92

Table 28-7 Simplified Risk Score for Difficult Intubation[28]

Number of Risk Factors[a]	Incidence of Difficult Intubation
0	0
1	2%
2	4%
3	8%
4 or 5	17%

[a]Presence of upper front teeth, history of a difficult intubation, Mallampati >1, Mallampati of 4, mouth opening <4 cm.

Table 28-8 Assessment and Predictability of Difficult Mask Ventilation[22]

(A) Criteria for Difficult Mask Ventilation	
Inability for one anesthesiologist to maintain oxygen saturation >92%	
Significant gas leak around facemask	
Need for ≥4 L/min gas flow (or use of fresh gas flow button more than twice)	
No chest movement	
Two-handed mask ventilation needed	
Change of operator required	
(B) Independent Risk Factors for Difficult Mask Ventilation	
Risk Factors	**Odds Ratio**
Presence of a beard	3.18
Body mass index >26 ng/m^2	2.75
Lack of teeth	2.28
Age >55 yr	2.26
History of snoring	1.84

recently in a study of 46,804 patients, Lundstrøm et al.[33] found 1% of patients to be difficult to mask ventilate, with 0.05% being impossible to mask ventilate. Lundstrøm's difficult mask ventilation score added increasing age, shorter thyromental distance, and previous difficult tracheal intubation to the previously mentioned criteria to achieve a scoring algorithm with sensitivity and specificity of 85% and 59%, respectively.

US technology is widely used, portable, and provides rapid, real-time, dynamic images. Bedside US can confirm endotracheal intubation with both a sensitivity and specificity of 0.98.[34] It can also be used to identify the CTM, rule out esophageal intubation, predict postextubation stridor by measuring width of US acoustic shadow before and after cuff deflation,[35] and verify ventilation in the absence of CO_2 detection (assuring bilateral lung excursion).[36] Subglottic hemangiomas, papillomas, and laryngeal cysts and stenosis have also been identified by US. Another use for US imaging is the estimation of ETT (including double lumen) size. Although it may be possible to examine the upper airway for changes such as hypertrophic lingual tonsils, the clinical relevancy (e.g., impact on laryngoscopy and ventilation) of ultrasonography has not been studied[36] and the applications of US in preoperative airway evaluation are still limited. When using US for airway evaluation, the linear high-frequency transducer is the most useful probe.

Clinical Management of the Airway

Preoxygenation

5 Preoxygenation (3 Video 28-3) should be practiced in all cases when time allows. This procedure entails the replacement of the nitrogen volume of the lung (as much as 95% of the functional residual capacity) with oxygen in order to provide an apneic oxygen reservoir. Under ideal conditions, a healthy patient breathing room air ($FiO_2 = 0.21$) will experience oxyhemoglobin desaturation to a level of less than 90% after approximately 1 to 2 minutes of apnea. In the same patient, several minutes of preoxygenation with 100% O_2 via a tight-fitting facemask may support at least 8 minutes of apnea before desaturation occurs. Patients with pulmonary disease, obesity, or conditions affecting metabolism frequently evidence desaturation sooner, owing to decreased functional residual capacity, increased O_2 extraction, and/or right-to-left transpulmonary shunting. In one study, healthy nonobese patients breathing 100% O_2 preoperatively sustained an oxygen saturation of greater than 90% for 6 ± 0.5 minutes, as opposed to 2.7 ± 0.25 minutes for obese patients under the same conditions.[37]

Time-sparing methods of preoxygenation have also been described. Using a series of four vital capacity breaths of 100% O_2 over a 30-second period, a high arterial PaO_2 (339 mmHg) can be achieved, but the time to desaturation remains shorter than with traditional techniques.[38] A modified vital capacity technique, wherein the patient is asked to take eight deep breaths in a 60-second period, shows promise in terms of prolonging the time to desaturation.[38] The authors of the current chapter prefer the technique of applying a facemask, then allowing for tidal volume breathing of 100% oxygen at flows of 10 to 12 L/min. The mask is placed immediately after the patient has been made comfortable on the operating room table and remains in place during the application of monitors and preoperative time out.

Certain circumstances can limit the effectiveness of preoxygenation, as exemplified by the patient who experiences claustrophobia with the anesthesia facemask (which can almost always be overcome by having the patient hold the mask or by removing the mask and allowing the patient to breathe directly from the anesthesia machine circuit) or the use of self-inflating breathing bags (which do not deliver an FiO_2 of 100% during spontaneous breathing) or nasal-only masks (4 Video 28-4). Likewise, leaks around the facemask can allow entrainment of air, thereby reducing the FiO_2. Leaks as small as 4 mm (cross-sectional) can cause significant reductions in the inspired oxygen content.[39]

In the obese patient, bilevel positive airway pressure and reverse Trendelenburg position have been advocated to reach maximal preinduction arterial oxygenation and to delay oxyhemoglobin desaturation.[38,40] Apneic oxygenation can also delay the onset of oxyhemoglobin desaturation during apnea. In this technique, oxygen is insufflated at a rate of 3 to 60 L/min via a low-flow or high-flow nasal cannula upon induction of anesthesia.[38,41,42] This technique relies on the phenomenon of apneic oxygenation, a process by which gases are entrained into the alveolar space during apnea.

In addition, use of high-flow nasal cannula has been described to maintain oxygenation during awake intubation,[43] as well as during periods of prolonged apnea, such as during suspension laryngoscopy procedures. Its use in this context has been coined "Transnasal Humidified Rapid-Insufflation Ventilatory Exchange (THRIVE)."[44] Apneic durations of up to 55 minutes have been reported with this technique in select patients (i.e., nonobese and without pulmonary disease). Hypercapnia may occur to a more limited degree with this technique.[45] Carbon dioxide elimination with THRIVE is attributed to turbulent flow at the glottic opening, gas mixing in anatomical dead space, cardiobalismus, and other factors.[46,47] Conflicting results regarding carbon dioxide elimination were observed in studies using THRIVE in pediatric patients[48] and adult patients,[49] both of which found a time-dependent increase in hypercapnia consistent with minimal ventilatory effect.

Support of the Airway with the Induction of Anesthesia

Oxygenation should be optimized throughout the process of airway management. With the induction of anesthesia and the onset of apnea, ventilation and oxygenation must be supported. Traditional methods include the anesthesia facemask, SGA, and ETT. High-flow nasal oxygen has also been used. 6

The Anesthesia Facemask

With the induction of anesthesia, the patient's level of consciousness changes from the awake state, with a competent and protected airway, to the unconscious state, with an unprotected and potentially obstructed airway. This drug-induced central ventilatory depression, along with relaxation of the upper airway musculature, can lead rapidly to hypercarbia and hypoxia. The anesthesia facemask is the device most commonly used to and ventilate an apneic patient. Facemask ventilation is highly effective, minimally invasive, and requires the least sophisticated equipment, making it critical to initial management of the airway and delivery of anesthesia.

A facemask is gently held on the patient's face with the thumb and first finger of the operator's left hand, leaving the right hand free for other tasks (Fig. 28-3). Most modern masks can be distorted by the operator's fingers to form a seal around facial contours. Air leaks around the mask's edges can be prevented by gentle downward pressure in the awake patient or, if the patient is asleep, by pulling the mandible upward into the mask.[50] A two-handed jaw-thrust technique has been shown to be superior to the classic one-handed grip for this maneuver.[51] Elastic "mask straps" may also be used and can be particularly helpful for the clinician with short fingers or for "hands-off" preoxygenation while other tasks are being performed. Gas leaks should be avoided, and a common reason for suboptimal preoxygenation is a loose-fitting mask, which allows the entrainment of room air.[38]

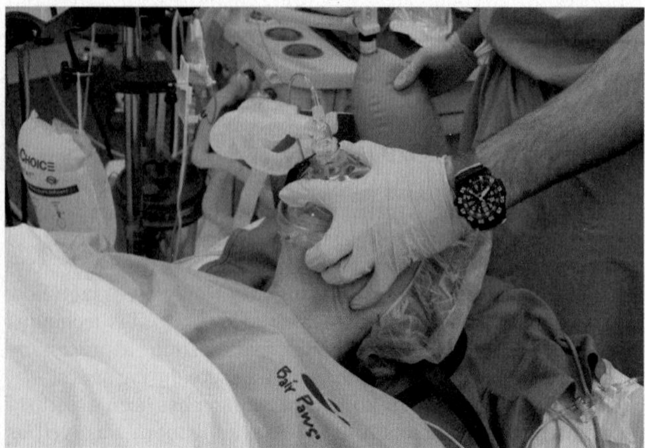

Figure 28-3 Holding the anesthesia mask on the face. The thumb and the first finger grip the mask in such a fashion that the anesthesia circuit (or self-inflating resuscitation bag) connection abuts the web between these digits. This allows the palm of the hand to apply pressure to the left side of the mask, while the tips of these two digits apply pressure over the right. The third finger helps to secure under the mentum, and the fourth finger is under the angle of the mandible or along the lower mandibular ridge. Mask straps (on pillow) may be used to complement the hand grip by securing the right side of the mask.

Appropriate positioning of the patient is paramount for delivery of positive-pressure ventilation via facemask. With the patient supine, "ramped," or in reverse Trendelenburg position, the head and neck are placed in the *sniffing* position, described later (see discussion of *tracheal intubation*). This position improves mask ventilation by anteriorizing the base of the tongue and the epiglottis.[52] In obese patients, mask ventilation may be improved through a 25-degree semi-Fowler position.[53]

After induction of anesthesia, a jaw thrust is achieved by upward displacement of the mandible into the mask. This maneuver raises the soft tissues of the anterior airway off the pharyngeal wall and allows for improved ventilation. In patients who are obese, edentulous, or bearded, two hands or a mask strap may be required to ensure an adequate mask seal. When two hands are required for holding the facemask, a second operator may be required to squeeze the reservoir bag. If necessary, the second operator can improve the mask's fit by providing additional jaw thrust and chin lift. The ventilator can also be used to deliver the breaths.

One useful, albeit poorly characterized, maneuver that aids in facemask ventilation is the *expiratory chin drop.* When positive-pressure inspiration is successful but is not followed by passive gas escape during expiration, allowing phasic head flexion and reducing chin/jaw lifting will often improve gas egress.

Well-secured dentures may improve the mask seal in an edentulous patient.[54] The advantage of this must be weighed against the risk of denture displacement or damage. Dentures may be removed when laryngoscopy is initiated.

A patient with normal lung compliance should require no more than 20 to 25 cm H_2O pressure for lung inflation, as measured on the anesthesia circle manometer. If more pressure is required, the adequacy of the mask technique should be reevaluated. This includes adjusting the mask fit, seeking aid with the mask hold, administering neuromuscular blockade, or considering adjuncts such as oral and nasal airways. Both oral and nasal airways can bypass upper airway obstruction by creating an artificial passage to the hypopharynx. Nasal airways are less likely to stimulate coughing, gagging, or vomiting in the lightly anesthetized patient but may cause epistaxis. For this reason, nasal airways are typically avoided in patients at high risk for bleeding (e.g., iatrogenic or pathologic coagulopathy, pregnancy, hereditary hemorrhagic telangiectasia, uncontrolled hypertension).

The nasal airway should be long enough to reach from the nostril to the thyroid notch when placed alongside the patient's face (NICV 28-1). It is inserted along the floor of the nose, in an anterior–posterior direction, and should always be prepared with water-soluble lubricant to reduce trauma to the highly vascular nasal mucosa. A vasoconstrictor agent (e.g., oxymetazoline or phenylephrine) may be applied before insertion of the nasal airway to decrease this risk. Resistance to insertion should prompt repositioning of the airway bevel, reassessment of the direction of insertion, or change to a smaller airway or the contralateral nostril.

The typical rounded oral airway is placed with its longitudinal concavity rotated in a rostrad direction. Once the distal end of the airway has been inserted to the level of the oropharynx, the device is rotated 180 degrees and insertion is continued to its ultimate position. This maneuver avoids displacement of the tongue into the hypopharynx and can be aided by caudad displacement of the tongue with a tongue depressor. A small oral aperture, intrapharyngeal mass or foreign body, intact gag reflex or otherwise light anesthesia may prevent oral airway placement. As will be discussed later, some intubating oral airways are large and have a rectangular cross-section. These devices tend to be too large for intraoral rotation and are inserted with the concavity facing caudally while the tongue is stabilized by a tongue depressor or held by the operator. Similar to nasal airway sizing, oral airways should reach from the teeth (or alveolar ridge) to the mandibular angle.

Obstruction to mask ventilation may be caused by laryngospasm, a local reflex closure of the vocal folds. Laryngospasm may be triggered by a foreign body (e.g., oral or nasal airway), saliva, blood, or vomitus touching the glottis. It may also result from pain or visceral stimulation. Hypoxia as well as noncardiogenic (negative pressure) pulmonary edema can result from continued spontaneous ventilation against closed vocal cords (or other obstruction). Management of laryngospasm consists of removing the offending stimulus (if identified), administering oxygen with continuous positive airway pressure (CPAP), deepening the plane of the anesthesia, and/or administering a rapid-acting neuromuscular blocker.[55]

The practice of withholding neuromuscular blocker prior to the establishment of adequate facemask ventilation, which has been a fixture of anesthetic teaching, has been called into question.[56,57] Objective evidence supports administration of depolarizing or nondepolarizing neuromuscular blocking agents simultaneously with anesthetic induction agents[56] to facilitate mask ventilation, SGA ventilation, and tracheal intubation. This is discussed in detail in the clinical cases later (Case 4).

If there are no contraindications (e.g., increased aspiration risk), mask ventilation can be the primary ventilatory technique for anesthetic maintenance. Otherwise, it is commonly used to administer anesthetic gases and/or oxygen and to facilitate ventilation until the anesthetic state is adequate for use of another means of airway support, such as an SGA or ETT. This decision should be made after careful consideration of the patient's coexisting diseases and surgical requirements.

Supraglottic Airways

Devices that isolate the airway above the vocal cords are referred to as SGAs. Although initially approved as a substitute for facemask ventilation and when tracheal intubation was not achievable, SGAs have now become widely used in many surgical cases traditionally managed with tracheal intubation.[58,59] SGAs are associated with a lower incidence of sore throat, coughing, and laryngospasm on emergence, as well with decreased reversible

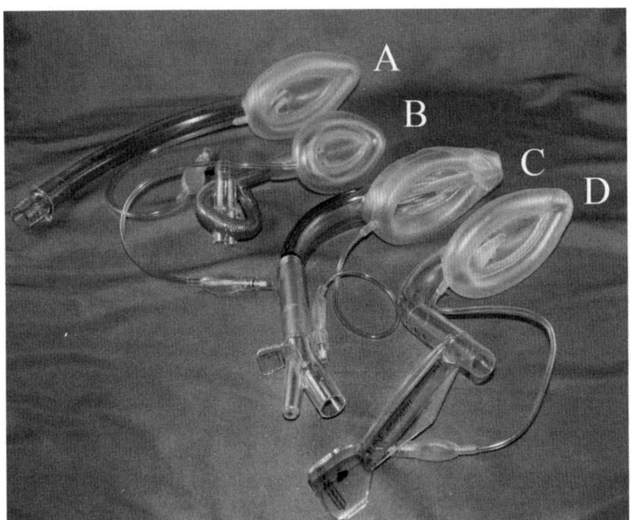

Figure 28-4 The family of laryngeal mask airways (from top): (**A**) Unique, (**B**) Flexible, (**C**) Supreme, (**D**) Fastrach.

bronchospasm compared to tracheal intubation.[60,61] Recent data suggests that more than 50% of anesthetics in the United States and United Kingdom are performed with SGAs.[58,62,63]

As the first device of its kind, a wealth of information exists on the LMA Classic and its subsequent iterations (Fig. 28-4). Much of this knowledge may be applied to newer SGAs as well. That this chapter devotes considerable text to the LMA family of devices is not meant to infer preference, but rather the availability of information.

The advent of the LMA as well as other SGAs has led some to question the relative safety of tracheal intubation.[64] This, along with the ASA Closed Claims Database information, lends support to the search for safe alternatives to tracheal intubation whenever possible.[65] Similarly, pharyngeal mucosa appears to be more resilient to trauma from SGAs relative to tracheal mucosa to damage from ETTs. In one animal study, mucosal injury from the LMA ProSeal (Teleflex, Research Triangle Park, NC) did not occur until more than 9 hours of continuous use.[66] The hemodynamic effects associated with airway management are also reduced with SGAs. Increases in heart rate, blood pressure, and intraocular pressure are all less during airway management with an SGA than with an ETT.[67,68]

First-Generation SGAs. The original SGA, the LMA Classic, is composed of a perilaryngeal mask and an airway barrel. The device is designed to sit in the hypopharynx with an anterior surface aperture overlying the laryngeal inlet. The mask has an inflatable cuff that fills the hypopharyngeal space, creating a seal that allows positive-pressure ventilation with up to 20 cm H_2O pressure. The adequacy of the seal depends on correct placement, appropriate size, and patient anatomy, and is less dependent on the cuff-filling pressure or volume. Attached to the posterior surface of the mask is a barrel (airway tube) which extends proximally from the mask's central aperture and can be connected to a self-inflating resuscitation bag or anesthesia circuit. While the LMA Classic is constructed of reusable silicone, several models constructed with silicone or polyvinyl chloride (PVC) became available from various manufacturers.

LMAs come in varying sizes, from neonatal to large adult, and appropriate size selection is critical to both successful use and complication avoidance. The manufacturer recommends that the clinician choose the largest size that will fit comfortably within the oral cavity. LMA insertion technique mimics the processes of swallowing. Just as a bolus of masticated food is pressed against the hard palate by the tongue, the operator applies the advancing tip of the LMA against the hard palate as it is introduced into the mouth. As with swallowing, head extension and neck flexion enlarge the space behind the tongue to allow passage into the hypopharynx. These functions allow a food bolus—and similarly an LMA—to reach its mark while avoiding contact with the anterior pharyngeal structures or stimulation of protective airway reflexes.

The insertion of the LMA (5 Video 28-5) as described by its inventor, Dr. Archie Brain, has been modified by a number of writers. Discussion of these various alternatives is beyond the scope of this text. The principles of LMA insertion can be applied to many other SGAs, though the individual manufacturer's recommendations should be consulted. The currently recommended insertion technique, illustrated in Figure 28-5, has a 94% success rate.[69] In this technique, the mask is completely deflated and the palatal surface is lubricated (with a nonlocal anesthetic containing lubricant). The operator's nondominant hand is placed under the occiput to flex the neck on the thorax and extend the head at the atlanto-occipital joint, creating a space behind the larynx (this action also tends to open the mouth).[70] The index finger of the dominant hand is placed in the cleft between the mask and barrel. The hard palate is visualized and the superior (nonaperture) surface of the mask is placed against it. Force is applied by the index finger in an upward direction toward the top of the patient's head. This causes the mask to flatten and follow the contour of the palate into the pharynx and hypopharynx. The index finger continues along this arc, continually applying an outward pressure until resistance from the upper esophageal sphincter is met. The most common error made by clinicians is the application of pressure with a posterior vector, causing the LMA's tip to impact the posterior pharyngeal wall, which may result in tip folding, device misplacement, and/or tissue trauma.

Prior to attachment of the anesthesia circuit, the LMA is inflated with the minimum amount of pressure that allows ventilation to 20 cm H_2O without an air leak (6 Video 28-6). The manufacturer recommends keeping the intracuff pressure under 60 cm H_2O; limited available evidence supports keeping the pressure under 44 mmHg.[71] When an adequate seal cannot be obtained with 60 cm H_2O cuff pressure, the LMA's positioning, sizing, or type should be re-evaluated. Light anesthesia and laryngospasm also may contribute to poor seal. With inflation, one should be able to observe a rising of the cricoid and thyroid cartilages and a lifting of the barrel out of the mouth by approximately 1 cm as the mask expands. If a midline position is not possible due to the patient's position or the surgical procedure, a flexible LMA (discussed later) should be considered. A bite block is recommended to prevent biting and occlusion of the LMA barrel. Cuff pressure should be measured after insertion and periodically monitored if nitrous oxide is being used.

Although the distal tip of the LMA mask sits in the esophageal inlet, it does not reliably seal it. The LMA was not designed to protect against the aspiration of gastric contents nor does it reliably do so. Despite this, when used in patients at low risk for regurgitation, the rate of aspiration during LMA use is similar to that in all non-LMA general anesthetics (approximately 2 in 10,000 cases).[72,73] The incidence of gastroesophageal reflux may be increased when compared with use of the facemask,[72] but when populations of patients considered to have a full stomach are studied, there is still a low incidence of aspiration noted with elective or emergency LMA use. Reports have included safe use in patients who are morbidly obese or have experienced frequent gastroesophageal reflux, those undergoing elective cesarean section or airway rescue during labor, and those presenting to emergency departments or paramedic crews.[74,75] During cardiopulmonary resuscitation, the incidence of gastroesophageal regurgitation is four times greater with a bag-valve mask than with an LMA.[76]

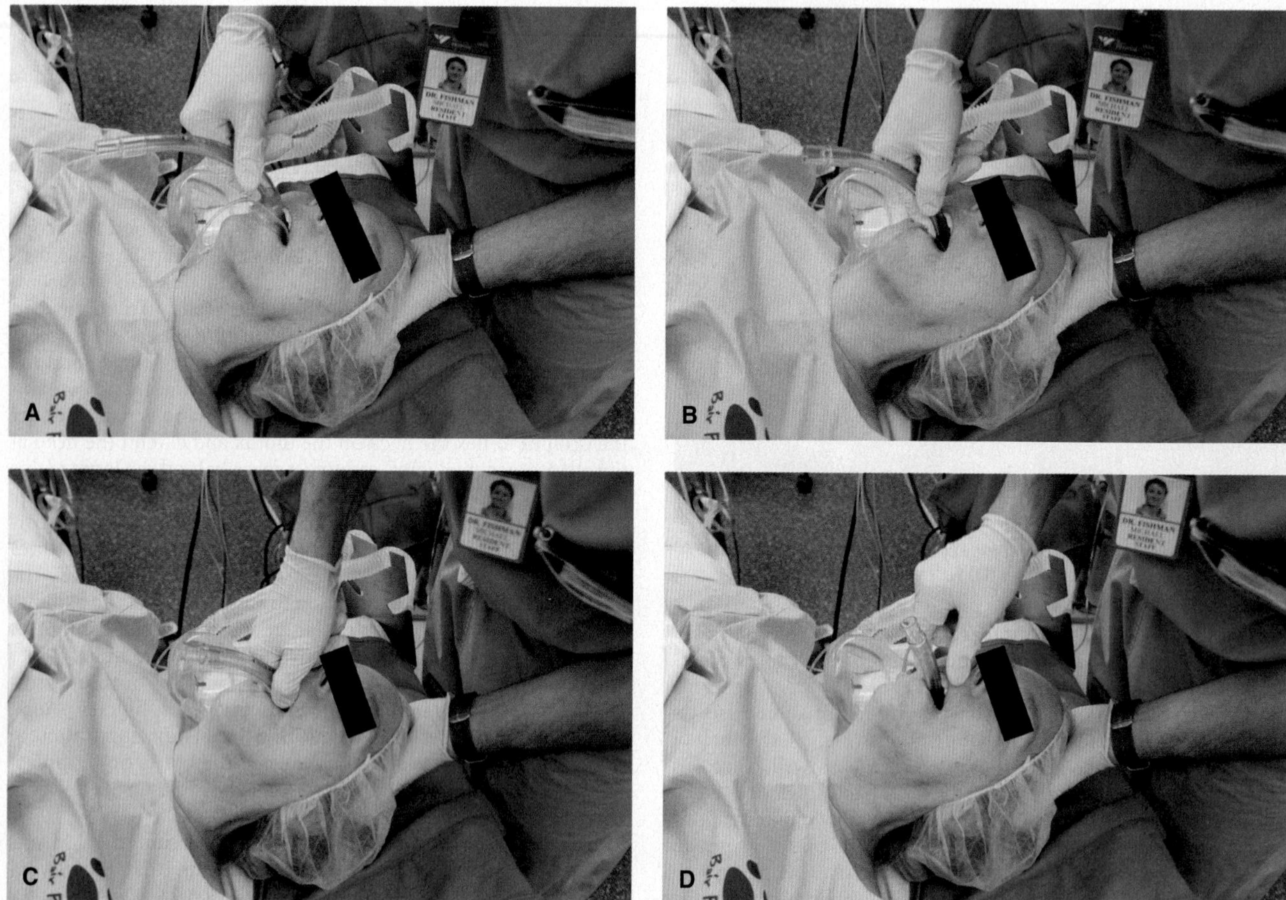

Figure 28-5 Insertion of the laryngeal mask airway (LMA). The LMA is inserted with the index finger of the dominant hand pressing with a force vector against the hard palate (**A** and **B**). The outward force vector is continued from the hard palate to the pharynx and hypopharynx (**C**) until the index finger meets resistance against the upper esophageal sphincter and is removed (**D**).

If at any time gastric contents are noted in an SGA barrel, maneuvers similar to those applied when using an ETT should be instituted. The SGA should be left in place, the barrel suctioned, the patient placed in Trendelenburg position, and 100% oxygen administered.

Although first introduced for use with spontaneous ventilation, the LMA has proved useful and safe for cases in which positive-pressure ventilation is either desired or preferred.[68,77] There is no difference in gastric inflation with positive-pressure ventilation (<17 cm H_2O) when comparing an LMA to an ETT.[78] With the LMA Classic, tidal volumes are limited to 8 mL/kg and airway pressure to 20 cm H_2O. These devices have been used successfully with supine, prone, lateral, oblique, Trendelenburg, and lithotomy positions. Although the manufacturer recommends use for a maximum of 2 to 3 hours, reports of use for more than 24 hours exist.[79] In a porcine model, Goldmann et al.[66] saw no evidence of mucosal changes with up to 9 hours of LMA ProSeal use, though mucosal damage was consistently evident after 12 hours.

The LMA Flexible. The introduction of flexible barrel SGAs (e.g., the LMA Flexible, Teleflex, Research Triangle Park, NC; Fig. 28-4) has permitted extension of SGA use to a variety of cases in which the airway is within the surgical field or shared with the surgical team (e.g., ophthalmologic or otolaryngologic procedures). These devices differ in design from traditional SGAs by the presence of a thin-walled, small-diameter, wire-reinforced (kink-resistant) barrel, which can be positioned out of the midline without affecting the hypopharyngeal position of the mask. This device was designed to be paired with a tonsillar mouth gag commonly used in oral and pharyngeal surgery.[80] In addition, the LMA Flexible has proved useful when heavy drapes are placed over the airway (e.g., ophthalmic procedures), when there is movement of the head during surgery (e.g., tympanostomy tubes), or when the LMA barrel cannot be secured in the midline (e.g., mid or lateral facial surgery). The use of this mask in surgery above the level of the hypopharynx, including tonsillectomy, affords a number of clinically important advantages over tracheal intubation (Table 28-9). When correctly placed, LMAs protect the airway from blood, secretions, and surgical debris from above the level of the mask better than tracheal tubes, which do not protect the trachea from liquids instilled into the pharynx.[81,82]

The SGA and Bronchospasm. SGAs produce significantly less reversible bronchospasm than ETTs. For this reason, they appear to be well suited to the patient with a history of or risk factors for bronchospasm who is not at risk for reflux or aspiration.[61] SGAs present a unique opportunity for the clinician to conveniently and effectively control the airway without introducing a foreign body into the trachea and stimulating the sensitive bronchial tree. When tracheal intubation is required for the surgical procedure and the patient is at high risk of bronchospasm, the Bailey maneuver can be employed. In this maneuver, the deflated LMA is placed behind the in situ ETT. The ETT is removed, the LMA is inflated, and emergence is conducted via the LMA.[83] Similarly, if an SGA

Table 28-9 Advantages of the Laryngeal Mask Airway in Supraglottic Surgery

Improved protection of the airway from blood and surgical debris
Reduced cardiovascular responses
Reduced coughing on emergence
Reduced intraoperative bronchospasm
Reduced laryngospasm after airway device removal
Improved oxygen saturation after airway device removal
Ability to administer oxygen until complete restoration of airway reflexes

was utilized as a conduit for tracheal intubation, the option exists to deflate the SGA cuff and leave the device in situ. When the ETT is no longer needed, it can be removed, leaving the SGA as the primary airway. This latter technique can be of great benefit in cases in which an ETT is needed intraoperatively but coughing or hypertension during emergence would be deleterious.

SGA Removal. An SGA should be removed either when the patient is deeply anesthetized or after protective airway reflexes have returned and the patient is able to open the mouth on command.[84] Removal during excitation stages of emergence can be accompanied by coughing and/or laryngospasm. Many clinicians remove the LMA fully inflated so that it acts as a "scoop" for secretions above the mask, allowing them to be carried out of the airway.[85]

Contraindications to SGA Use. SGAs do not reliably prevent the aspiration of regurgitated gastric contents. Thus, SGAs are contraindicated in clinical scenarios with an increased risk of regurgitation (e.g., full stomach, hiatal hernia with significant gastroesophageal reflux, intestinal obstruction, delayed gastric emptying, unclear history), though their use as an airway salvage technique in these populations is acceptable. Other contraindications include high airway resistance, glottic or subglottic obstruction, and limited mouth opening (<1.5 cm).[15]

Complications of SGA Use. Apart from aspiration, reported complications related to SGAs include laryngospasm, coughing, gagging, and other events characteristic of airway manipulation. The incidence of SGA-induced postoperative sore throat varies from 4% to 50% and is highly dependent on the study methods. No single device shows a consistently lower rate of dysphagia. All appear to be better than tracheal intubation in this regard, in which postoperative sore throat occurs in 30% to 60%.[86] Rare reports exist of nerve injury associated with SGA use, including damage to the hypoglossal, lingual, and/or recurrent laryngeal nerves. These injuries typically manifest within 48 hours postoperatively and resolve spontaneously in 1 hour to 18 months. Predisposing factors include the use of small masks, lidocaine lubrication, nitrous oxide, cuff overinflation, difficult or alternative insertion techniques, nonsupine positioning, and cervical bone or joint disease.[87] Pressure neuropraxia from the tube or cuff is the most common causal factor.

The Laryngeal Tube (King LT, Ambu, Ballerup, Denmark) consists of a single-lumen tube with distal and proximal low-pressure cuffs that are inflated via a common pilot valve (Fig. 28-6). When positioned correctly, the distal cuff obstructs the upper esophagus and the proximal cuff seals the oral and nasal pharynx. Apertures between the cuffs serve as orifices for spontaneous

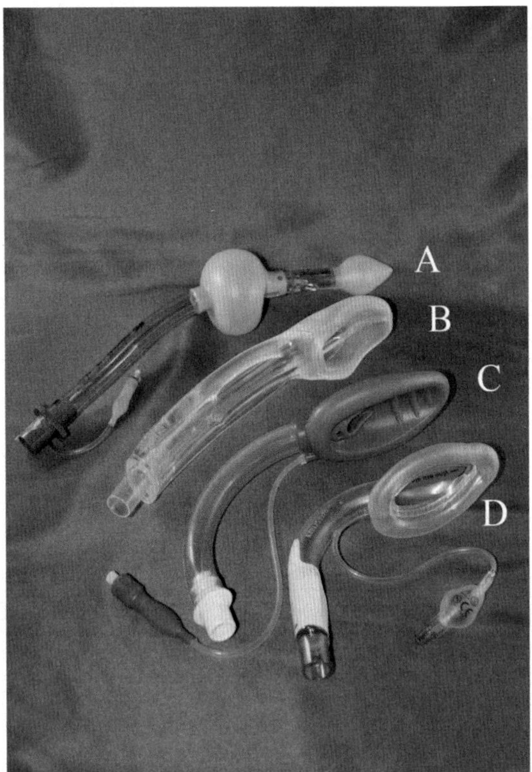

Figure 28-6 (**A**) The King LT, (**B**) I-Gel, (**C**) air-Q, and (**D**) Aura-I.

or positive-pressure ventilation. The King LT requires a mouth opening of at least 2.3 cm and is inserted either blindly or with the aid of a laryngoscope. The Laryngeal Tube Suction (King LTS-D, Ambu, Ballerup, Denmark) is a single-use device which adds a lumen terminating distal to the esophageal cuff, facilitating gastric drainage. One case report describes the successful use of the LTS-D as an emergency airway for a pregnant woman who underwent cesarean section but could not be intubated. The device improved oxygenation and facilitated drainage of gastric contents during the patient's emergence from a failed rapid-sequence intubation.[88]

The Laryngeal Tube is available in six sizes (0 to 5) suitable for children to large adults. In children under 10 years old, the Laryngeal Tube is less effective than the LMA during spontaneous or assisted ventilation and for fiberoptic evaluation of the airway.[89] The Laryngeal Tube is not recommended for children weighing less than 10 kg, as its use is associated with technical difficulties and inadequate ventilation.[90]

A cadaveric study demonstrated that mucosal pressures in the lateral pharynx, base of tongue, and posterior pharynx were similar between the Laryngeal Tube and LMA ProSeal. However, the pressure with the Laryngeal Tube was higher on the posterior hypopharynx, and the investigators expressed concern that this increased pressure might impede pharyngeal perfusion.[91] A case of acute tongue and uvula ulceration after use of the Laryngeal Tube has been reported.[92]

Cookgas air-Q. Developed by Dr. Daniel Cook, the air-Q perilaryngeal airway (Cookgas LLC, St. Louis, MO; Fig. 28-6) can function both as an elective SGA and a conduit for blind or flexible scope-aided intubation (described later in this chapter). A cuff grossly the shape of the LMA Classic cuff seals the perilaryngeal space and has airway seal pressures of 25 to 30 cm H_2O.[93] The device comes in sizes 0.5 to 4.5 and is inserted using a technique

Table 28-10 Features of the LMA ProSeal

Feature	Clinical Impact
Gastric drain	Confirmation of device positioning • Suprasternal notch test[a,85] • No gas leak via gastric port[b,84] Gastric tube placement • Active and passive gastric emptying Protection from gastric-content aspiration
Posterior cuff	Increased seal pressure
Bite block	Prevention of obstruction from biting Confers rotational stability Confirmation of device positioning—50% or more of the bite block should be within the oral cavity[85]
Placement	First insertion less successful than LMA Classic
Size choice	Size down from LMA Classic

[a]When a small amount of lubricant is used to occlude the gastric drain, gentle pressure on the suprasternal notch is reflected in movement of the lubricant meniscus.

[b]If the lubricant meniscus does not move with positive-pressure ventilation, there is no connection between the esophageal and laryngeal ports and ventilation is unlikely to cause gastric insufflation.

similar to that recommended for the LMA (see previous discussion). The inventor recommends filling the cuff with less than 10 mL of air, as a poor seal is often secondary to cuff *over*inflation. If, after insertion, the airway is obstructed, an up–down motion of the barrel often realigns the epiglottis. A recent innovation, the self-pressurizing air-Q, does not require cuff insufflation but rather varies intracuff pressure based on airway pressure. The self-pressurizing air-Q may improve flexible scope visualization for SGA-assisted intubation but does not appear to result in a higher cuff leak pressure.[94]

Second-Generation Supraglottic Airways. The LMA ProSeal was the first SGA with a gastric port and thus the first "second-generation" SGA (Table 28-10). The original intent of the ProSeal's gastric drain was to aid the clinician in the diagnosis of SGA malposition. The gastric drain also allows passive (regurgitation) and active (gastric tube insertion) emptying of the stomach.[95] The design of the ProSeal cuff improves airway seal during positive-pressure ventilation as compared with other first-generation LMA devices (≥40 cm H_2O). These advanced capabilities offer advantages in the care of obese patients, patients undergoing intra-abdominal procedures, and in airway resuscitation.[96–98] A single-use version of the ProSeal, the LMA Supreme (Teleflex, Research Triangle Park, NC), incorporates a fixed curvature and supports inspiratory pressures of greater than 35 cm H_2O[99,100] (Fig. 28-4).

The i-gel. This uniquely designed SGA has a solid elastomer gel body mounted on a plastic barrel without an inflatable cuff (Intersurgical Inc., East Syracuse, NY, Fig. 28-6). A drain tube runs from the distal tip, which sits over the esophageal inlet, to an outlet lateral to the airway circuit connector. A gastric tube may be placed via this drain (the largest size accommodating a 14-French tube), which also serves as a passage for passively regurgitated gastric contents. Airway leak pressures have been reported to range from 24 to 30 cm of water in adults. The incidence of sore throat appears to be less than with the LMA,[101] and some reports note a lower rate of visible blood on the device at the time of removal. The i-gel is reported to have modestly shorter insertion times, but slightly lower oropharyngeal leak pressures as compared to the LMA ProSeal.[102] Contrary to a widely held belief, the solid mask of the i-gel does not change shape as it is warmed by the pharyngeal mucosa (personal communication, Muhammed Nasir, MD).

Tracheal Intubation

The goal of DL is to produce a direct line of sight from the operator's eye to the larynx. This requires the creation of a new nonanatomic visual axis, achieved via maximal alignment of the axes of the oral and pharyngeal cavities, as well as displacement of the tongue. Unanticipated failure of DL is primarily a problem of tongue displacement, as inability to align the axes typically can be predicted by physical examination. As pointed out in the ASA Difficult Airway Practice Guidelines, multiple measures must be integrated in order to make sensible airway management decisions.[2] Roth et al.[24] published a meta-analysis of studies regarding airway physical examination scores and cautioned on the poor sensitivity and modest specificity of all routine tests.

In 1944, Bannister and MacBeth proposed a three-axis model to explain the anatomic relationships involved in airway axis alignment.[103] Based on this model, alignment of the laryngeal, pharyngeal, and oral axes would result in an adequate glottic view. This model explains the rationale of the intubation SP in which the neck is flexed by 35 degrees and the head extended by 15 degrees. This positioning is achieved by placing a support (around 7 cm in the adult) under the patient's occiput. The three-axis explanation has been challenged by Adnet et al.[97,104] who noted that, although extension at the atlanto-occipital joint maximally facilitated an oral cavity/pharyngeal alignment, no significant improvement was achieved with flexion of the cervical spine on the thorax.

Chou and Wu[105] proposed a two-axis/tongue-displacement model. This model does not depend on the alignment of all axes to create an in-line view of the larynx but rather maximizes the spaces between the alveolar ridge and laryngeal aperture through oropharyngeal alignment and tongue displacement. This concept may explain difficulties with DL as well as why common methods of airway assessment lack predictive power. This concept has been described as Functional Airway Assessment (FAA).[106]

FAA is a method of examining the functional nature of each of the anatomic correlates of the commonly used airway assessment indices. FAA places an emphasis on the interdependence of these anatomic characteristics rather than on their individual size or functional integrity. As explained by Chou and Wu,[105] when the head and neck are in the neutral position, the oral and pharyngeal axes are near perpendicular to each other. With maximal extension of a normal atlanto-occipital joint, 35 degrees or more of motion is attained (Fig. 28-7). This brings the angle between the oral and pharyngeal axes to 125 degrees. Although an improvement, it is certainly not the 180 degrees required for creating a line of sight to the glottis. Additional space must be created, which is accomplished by displacement of the tongue with the laryngoscope. Although atlanto-occipital extension cannot by itself allow direct laryngeal vision, it does provide anterior displacement of the mass of the tongue and bring the alveolar ridge into an improved position relative to the tongue and larynx. The extension of the atlanto-occipital joint also provides an advantage in mouth opening; Calder et al.[70] showed that maximal mouth opening is 26% greater in full atlanto-occipital extension as compared with the neutral head position. Mandibular mobility also facilitates displacement of the tongue away from the required visual axis—rotation and translation of the temporomandibular joint

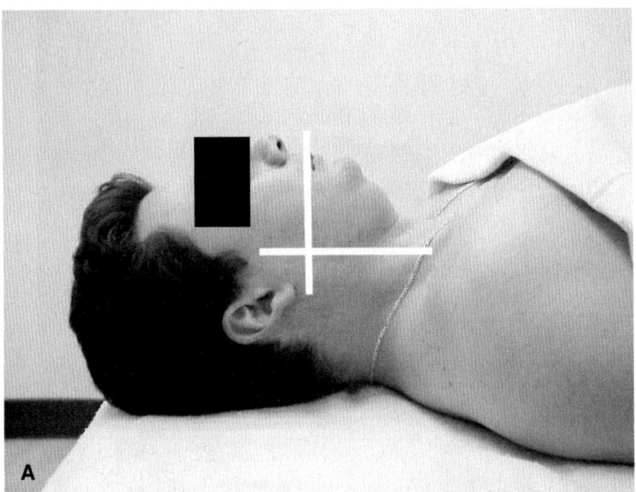

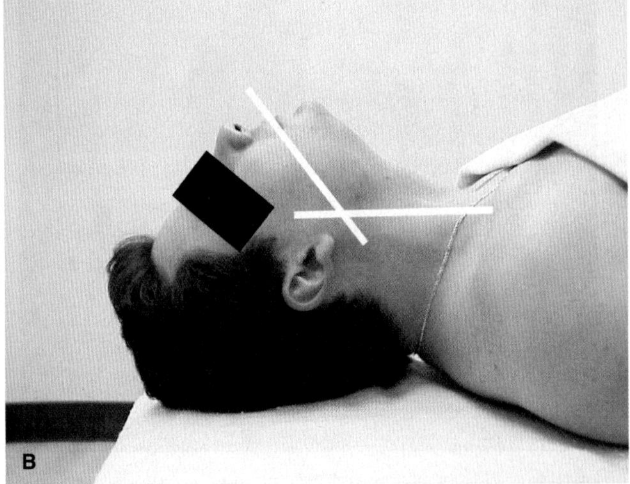

Figure 28-7 **A:** With the patient supine, the oral and pharyngeal axes do not overlap. **B:** Extension at the atlanto-occipital joint maximally overlaps the oral and pharyngeal axes.

results in relaxation of the tongue insertion as well as creation of the aperture width needed for instrumentation.

Using the FAA approach to airway evaluation also helps to explain the value of the popular, yet highly criticized, Mallampati and thyromental distance indices.[107] These two measures have historically been considered important because they approximate the relative mass of the tongue and the anterior–posterior borders of space into which it will be displaced by the laryngoscope, respectively (Fig. 28-8). As noted elsewhere, these indices have shown to have poor and/or variable predictive power. Two groups have studied the interrelated nature of these measures in a way that reveals why they perform poorly when considered individually. Ayoub et al.[108] found a high Mallampati score to be predictive of difficult DL when the thyromental distance was less than 4 cm. When the thyromental distance was more than 4 cm relative tongue size, as determined by the Mallampati classification, was not predictive. Iohom et al.[10] found similar results using a thyromental distance cut-off of 6 cm. The finding that the predictive power of the Mallampati improves when the mandible is short is consistent with the concept of FAA: when the mandibular space is restricted, tongue size is important. When the space is large, a tongue of any nonpathologic size should be accommodated easily. An exception to this may be a hypopharyngeal tongue, as described by Chou and Wu,[109] although, according to those authors, measurement of the mandibular hyoid distance should help in diagnosing this condition.

As noted earlier, a common cause of difficulty in DL is a pathologic increase in tongue size (7 Video 28-7). Ovassapian et al.[110] identified lingual tonsil hyperplasia as the most common cause of *unanticipated* difficult DL. In a review of all cases of unanticipated difficult DL in their institution from 1999 to 2000, 33 patients were identified. On fiberoptic examination, all patients were found to have lingual tonsil hyperplasia (Fig. 28-9).

Expanding on the SP, some have suggested positioning the patient with the external auditory meatus level with the patient's sternal notch (EAM-SN position). This is especially helpful in obese patients[111] to move the mass of the chest away from the airway and allow space for manipulation of the laryngoscope handle. This may require placing a wedge-shaped lift under the scapula, shoulders, and nape of neck. This raises the head and neck above the thorax, producing the EAM-SN position and allowing gravity to pull the pannus away from the airway.

After the head and neck have been positioned, the mouth is opened by one of two techniques. The first method encourages extension of the atlanto-occipital joint by the use of the right hand under the occiput. This maneuver is reserved for patients with stable cervical spines and leads to passive opening of the mouth, which can be accentuated by using the fourth finger of the left hand (holding the laryngoscope) to apply pressure over the chin in a caudad direction. In the second technique, which tends to be more effective but requires contact of the (gloved) hand with the teeth and/or gums, the right thumb applies caudad pressure to the mandibular canine/bicuspids on the patient's same side while the first or second finger, crossed below the thumb, applies cephalad pressure to the ipsilateral maxillary canine/bicuspid (Fig. 28-10). The goal of both techniques is rotation and translation of the temporomandibular joint to maximize the interincisor gap.

Direct Laryngoscope Blades. Two blades, each with a unique manner of application, are in common use (8 Video 28-8). Many other blades are described in the literature but will not be discussed here. There are some excellent reviews detailing these other devices.[112]

The Macintosh (curved) blade is used to displace the epiglottis out of the line of sight by placement of the distal tip in the vallecula and tensing of the glossoepiglottic ligament. The Miller (straight) blade reveals the glottis by compressing the epiglottis against the base of the tongue. Both blades include a flange along the left side of their length which is used to sweep the tongue to the left. Blades with a right-sided flange are available for the left-handed practitioner but are not found in common practice.

Blade size needs to be chosen appropriately and, on occasion, exchanged after a failed attempt at laryngoscopy. As a generalization, the Macintosh blade is regarded as advantageous whenever there is little room to pass an ETT (e.g., small mouth), whereas the Miller blade is considered better in the patient who has a small mandibular space, large incisors, or a large epiglottis.[55] Ultimately, the optimal blade tends to be the one with which the provider has the most experience.

During laryngoscopy, the laryngoscope handle is held in the left hand and the mouth opened as described earlier. The blade is inserted into the right side of the mouth, with care taken to avoid unnecessary contact with the lips or teeth. As the blade is advanced toward the epiglottis, the tongue is swept leftward and compressed into the mandibular space. Once reaching the base of the tongue (with the Macintosh blade in the vallecula or the Miller blade compressing the epiglottis against the base of the tongue), the operator's arm and shoulder lift in an anterior–caudad direction.

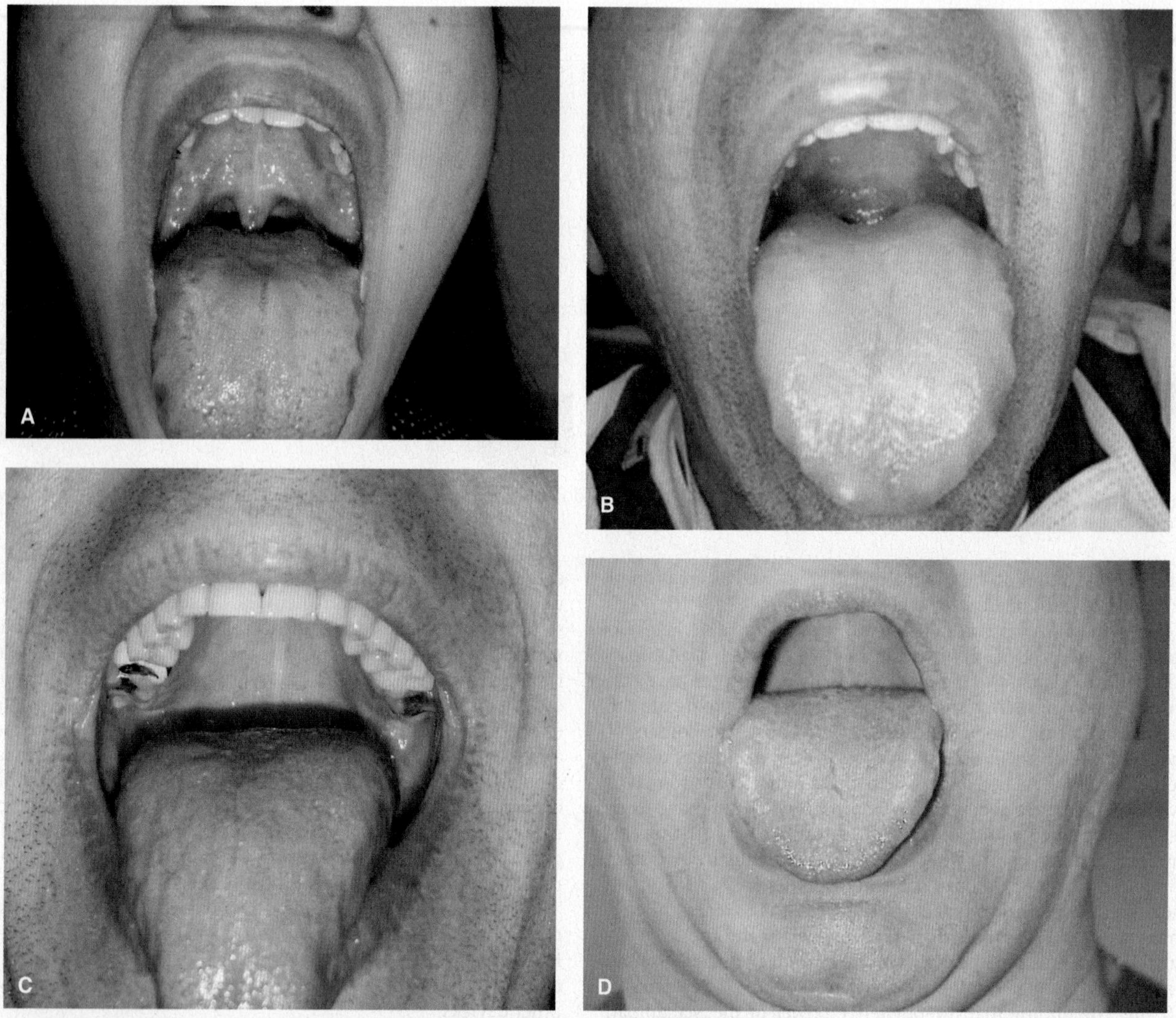

Figure 28-8 Mallampati/Samsoon–Young classification of the oropharyngeal view.[103] **A:** Class I: Uvula, faucial pillars, soft palate visible. **B:** Class II: Faucial pillars, soft palate visible. **C:** Class III: Soft and hard palate visible. **D:** Class IV: Only hard palate visible (added by Samsoon and Young).

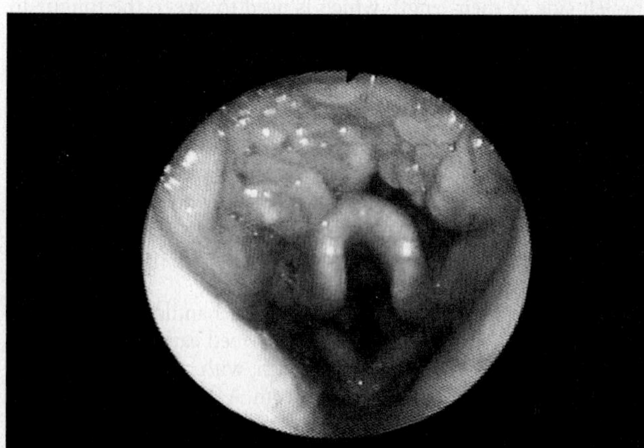

Figure 28-9 Lingual tonsil hyperplasia. The vallecula is filled with hyperplastic lymphoid tissue in a patient who had an unanticipated difficult direct laryngoscopy.

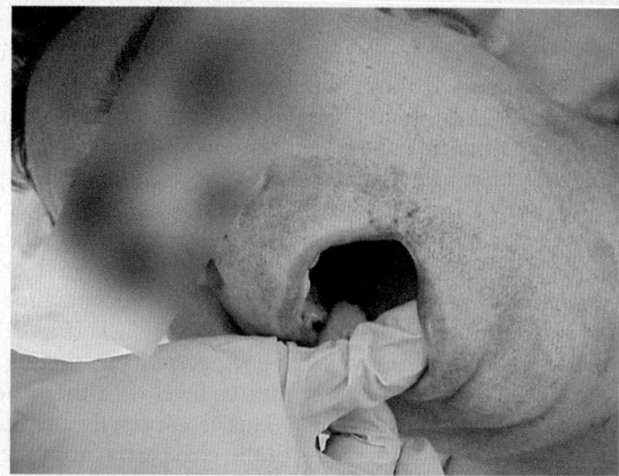

Figure 28-10 Picture of ipsilateral maxillary canine/bicuspid opening of oral cavity (aka scissoring open the mouth). The right thumb applies caudad pressure to the mandibular canine/bicuspids on the patient's same side while the first or second finger, crossed below the thumb, applies cephalad pressure to the ipsilateral maxillary canine/bicuspid. The goal is rotation and translation of the temporomandibular joint to maximize the interincisor gap.

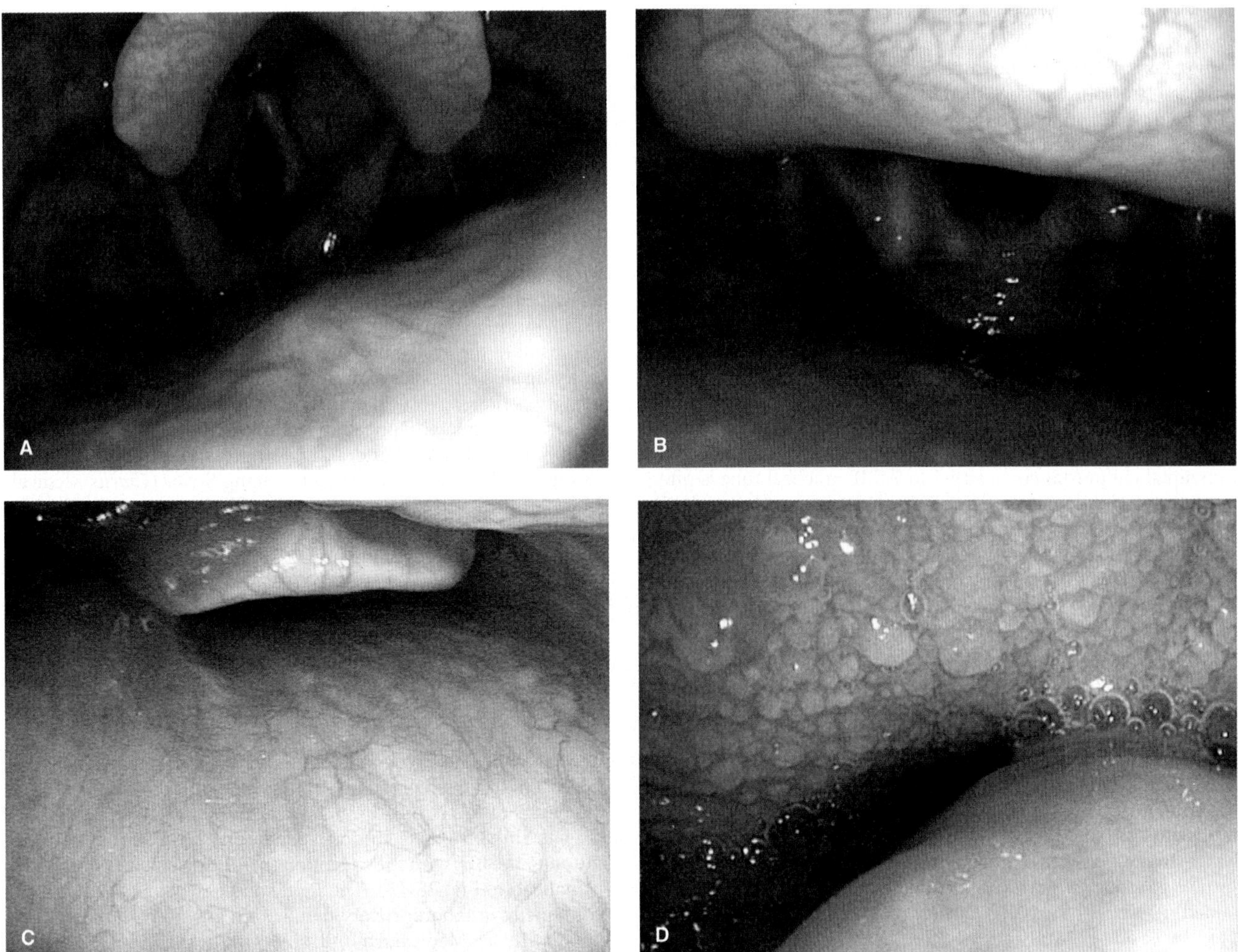

Figure 28-11 The Cormack–Lehane laryngeal view scoring system: grade 1 (**A**), grade 2 (**B**), grade 3 (**C**), and grade 4 (**D**).

With either blade, the laryngoscopist must avoid rotating the laryngoscope in a cephalad direction, bringing the proximal blade into contact with the upper incisors. Inserting either blade too deeply can result in the tip of the blade resting under the larynx itself such that forward pressure lifts the airway from view.

Special considerations apply to the technique of laryngoscopy and intubation in the infant and child. Because of the relatively larger size of the occiput in children, elevation of the head is not required to achieve an SP.[55] In fact, on occasion, the practitioner may need to elevate the thorax instead. Excessive hyperextension (>30%) at the atlanto-occipital joint may cause airway obstruction from the relative pliability of the trachea.[113] The comparatively short neck of a child gives the impression of an anterior position of the larynx and external laryngeal manipulation is often required to move the laryngeal inlet into view. A straight blade often is chosen, as it is helpful in displacing the stiff, omega-shaped epiglottis. Because the cricoid cartilage is the most rigid portion of the airway until 6 to 8 years of age, the anesthetist must be sensitive to resistance to advancement of an ETT that has easily passed the vocal folds. Due to the short length of the trachea, there is a higher risk of endobronchial intubation or accidental extubation with head movement (9 Video 28-9). Close attention should always be paid to the depth of the tube in pediatric patients.

A laryngeal view scoring system that has won general acceptance was developed by Cormack and Lehane,[114] who described four grades of laryngeal view. Grade 1 includes visualization of the entire glottic aperture, grade 2 includes visualization of only the posterior aspects of the glottic aperture, grade 3 is visualization of the tip of the epiglottis, and grade 4 is visualization of no more than the soft palate (Fig. 28-11). A Cormack–Lehane grade 3 or 4 is expected in 1.5% to 8.5% of adult laryngoscopies.[115] A modification of the Cormack and Lehane score was proposed by Yentis and Lee,[116] who noted that when a partial vocal cord view (2A) is achieved, tracheal intubation was significantly easier than when only the arytenoids and epiglottis were visualized (2B). A finer classification of a Cormack and Lehane grade 3 view has also been described. When the epiglottis can be manipulated with repositioning or an intubating bougie, it is referred to as a "3a" view and a nonmovable epiglottis constitutes a "3b" view.[117] The Cormack and Lehane grades are intended to describe the view at laryngoscopy, but they may also correlate with likelihood of successful tracheal intubation.[118]

Another view scoring system is based on the clinician's estimate of the percent of glottic opening (POGO) seen during laryngoscopy, for example, 0% to 100% of the span from anterior commissure to the interarytenoid notch. The POGO score has improved interexaminer reliability when compared to the Cormack and Lehane system and has been adopted by many researchers in the comparative evaluation of video laryngoscopy.[119]

If a satisfactory laryngeal view is not achieved, the backward–upward–rightward pressure (BURP) maneuver may be applied. In this maneuver, the larynx is displaced backward (B) against the cervical vertebrae, upward (U, superiorly) and to the patient's right (R), using pressure (P) over the thyroid cartilage. The BURP maneuver has been shown to improve the laryngeal view, decreasing the rate of difficult intubation in a study of 1,993 patients from 4.7% to 1.8%.[120] Similarly, Benumof and Cooper describe "optimal external laryngeal manipulation," which consists of pressing posteriorly and cephalad over the thyroid, hyoid, and cricoid cartilages.[121]

Once the larynx is visualized, the tracheal tube is inserted from the right-hand side, care being taken not to obstruct the view of the vocal cords. Whenever possible, the action of the ETT passing through the vocal cords should be witnessed by the laryngoscopist. This decreases the possibility of accidental esophageal placement or trauma to paraglottic structures. The tracheal tube cuff should be advanced at least 2 cm past the glottic opening to approximate a mid-tracheal placement. This should correlate to depths of 21 and 23 cm at the teeth for the typical adult female and male, respectively. Though allowances should be made for individual circumstances, a size 7 to 7.5 ID tracheal tube is often used in the adult female and size 7.5 to 8 ID in the adult male. To reduce the incidence of sore throat and hoarseness, smaller sizes may be appropriate for tracheal intubation when there is a low likelihood of need for postoperative mechanical ventilation.[122,123] In contrast, larger tracheal tubes may be desirable if pulmonary toilet or diagnostic or therapeutic bronchoscopy is to be part of the clinical course. Pediatric tracheal tube sizes are presented in detail in Table 28-11 (see also Chapter 42).

An alternative approach to DL has been described by Henderson.[124] In this "paraglossal" approach, a straight-bladed laryngoscope is introduced into the right side of the mouth and advanced between the tongue and palatine tonsil. The blade passes below the epiglottis, which is then elevated. This approach subjects the tongue to less compressive forces and may improve the view of the larynx in the presence of lingual tonsil hyperplasia.

7 The gold standard for verification of tracheal intubation is sustained detection of exhaled carbon dioxide (10 Videos 28-10, 11 28-11 and 12 28-12, NICV 28-2). In the absence of end-tidal carbon dioxide, the tracheal tube must be removed, and ventilation restored with face mask or SGA. Additional verification techniques include visualization of tube placement through the vocal folds, auscultation over the chest and abdomen, visualization of chest excursion, observation of humidity in the ETT, full return of tidal volume during expiration, use of a self-inflating bulb (TubeChek-B, Ambu, Ballerup, Denmark), flexible scope identification of tracheal anatomy, and US or chest x-ray.[125]

Table 28-11 Size and Length of Pediatric Tracheal Tubes Relative to Airway Anatomy

Age	Internal Diameter (mm)	Distance from Lips to Midtrachea[a] (cm)
Premature	2.5	8
Full term	3	10
1–6 mon	3.5	11
6–12 mo	4	12
2 yr	4.5	13
4 yr	5	14
6 yr	5.5	15
8 yr	6.5	16

[a]Add 2–3 cm for nasal tubes.

Although DL remains the most common method for tracheal intubation, it is far from successful in all cases and not always benign when successful. DL is reported to be difficult (Cormack and Lehane grade 3 or 4 view) or impossible in 4.4% and up to 0.43% of attempts, respectively.[126–128] Analysis of the ASA Closed Claims Database reveals that claims for laryngeal injury during intubation are declining.[4] Historically, 80% of laryngeal injury claims occurred during routine (nondifficult) tracheal intubation in which no injury was suspected.[65] This has led some to question whether routine tracheal intubation is as safe as assumed.[64]

Image-guided laryngoscopy is beginning to dominate modern airway management. The first decade of the 21st century saw a proliferation of optical and video-transmitting devices primarily as the result of the availability of inexpensive CMOS technology. The unifying characteristics of these laryngoscopes are that a direct line of sight is no longer needed from the provider's eye to the glottis.

Optical Stylets. Optical stylets incorporate both optical and light source elements into a single rigid stylet-like shaft. Some examples of these are the Shikani Seeing Stylet (*Clarus* Medical, LLC, Minneapolis, MN) and the Bonfils Intubation Fiberscope (BIF, Karl Storz, Tuttlingen, Germany; Fig. 28-12). Both require less cervical spine motion than DL.[129,130]

The BIF is a long rigid tubular device with conventional optical and light-transmitting fiberoptic elements.[131] The distal end has a 40-degree angulation, and the objective lens allows a 100-degree field of view. A proximal-end eyepiece can be used with the naked eye or fitted with a standard endoscopy camera. A cable (or battery-powered attachment) brings illumination from an external light source, and suction may be applied through a working channel. Laryngoscopy technique replicates the paraglossal approach discussed previously in this chapter. Sizes with external diameters of 2, 3.5, and 5 mm are available.

The Shikani Seeing Optical Stylet (SOS) has a similar configuration to the BIF, with the exception that the distal half of the stylet is malleable (Fig. 28-13). The light source may be cabled or self-contained with a proprietary handle or a green line laryngoscope handle (Rusch Medical, Duluth, GA). Unlike the BIF, the SOS uses a midline approach. Although the SOS can be used as an independent intubating device, it can also be employed as an adjunct to DL when a high Cormack and Lehane score is achieved. While the SOS is primarily an oral intubation device, it has been used also

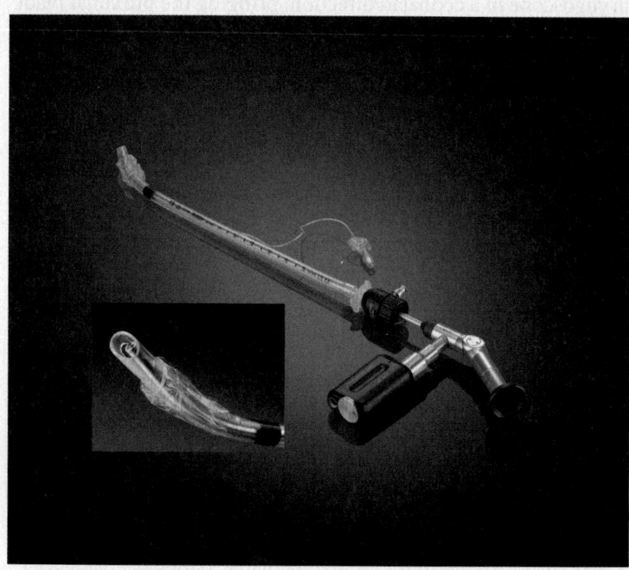

Figure 28-12 The Bonfils. (Copyright © KARL STORZ SE & Co. KG, Germany.) *Inset*: Objective end within tracheal tube.

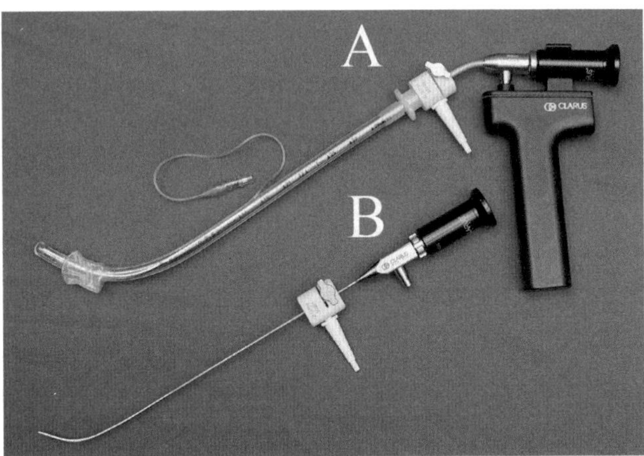

Figure 28-13 A: The Shikani Seeing Optical Stylet. (Used with permission from Clarus Medical, LLC, Minneapolis, MN.) B: The Levitan FPS.

for nasal intubation. The pediatric and adult SOSs can accommodate tracheal tubes as small as 2.5 and 5.5 mm ID, respectively.

The Levitan First Pass Success Scope (FPS, *Clarus* Medical, LLC, Minneapolis, MN) is a shorter (30-cm) version of the SOS designed to be used as an adjunct to DL when a poor laryngeal view is encountered (Fig. 28-13). The shorter length allows easier positioning by the laryngoscopist,[132] but standard tracheal tubes (6 mm ID or larger can be used) should be trimmed in length so that the objective lens is within the bevel.[133,134] The hypothetical benefits of using the device in this manner are reduced unanticipated difficult intubations and maintenance of alternative technique skills by incorporating this or similar devices into daily practice.[134]

The Clarus Video System (*Clarus* Medical, LLC, Minneapolis, MN; Fig. 28-14) marries the malleable stylet concept of the SOS with CMOS technology. A 4-in adjustable-angle LED screen is mounted on the handle and has a proprietary video-out port. The device also supports intubation via a transillumination technique by incorporating a distal, anteriorly positioned red diode that may be visible through the skin when the tip of the device is in the larynx.

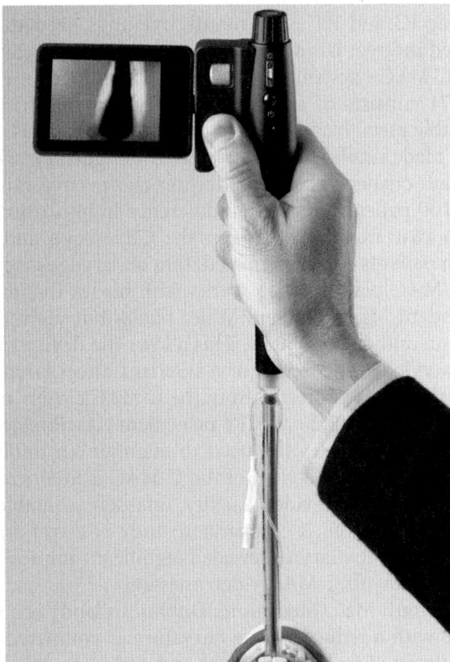

Figure 28-14 The Clarus Video System. (Used with permission from Clarus Medical, LLC, Minneapolis, MN.)

Videolaryngoscopy

VL mimics the operator actions of DL but places an imaging device toward the distal end of the laryngoscope blade. This moves the provider's point of view past the tongue, avoiding the need for a direct line of sight to the glottis. The ASA Difficult Airway Taskforce recommends that a videolaryngoscope be available as a first attempt or rescue device for all patients being intubated.[2] VL improves the ability to visualize the larynx, and intubation success approaches 97% to 98%. An added benefit is decreased cervical motion when compared with DL, which appears to be more pronounced with the channeled devices.

The first widely available videolaryngoscope was the Glidescope (Verathon, Bothell, WA; Fig. 28-15 and 13 Video 28-13). The Glidescope blade has both a light-emitting diode and a CMOS chip and is cabled to an LCD monitor.[135] The distal portion of the blade has a 60-degree angulation, making it a hyperangulated videolaryngoscope. The Glidescope design has several advantages[1]: It may be handled with a skill set similar to that used with conventional DL.[2] As the video apparatus is positioned close to the distal end of the blade, the operator "sees" from a position beyond the base of the tongue, and tongue displacement is not as critical as it is with DL. Similarly, with the optics positioned distal to the lingual tonsils, tonsillar hyperplasia should not affect the visual axis as it does with conventional DL.[3] The video apparatus eliminates fragile fiberoptic elements.[4] The airway image is displayed on a portable screen, allowing for observation by more

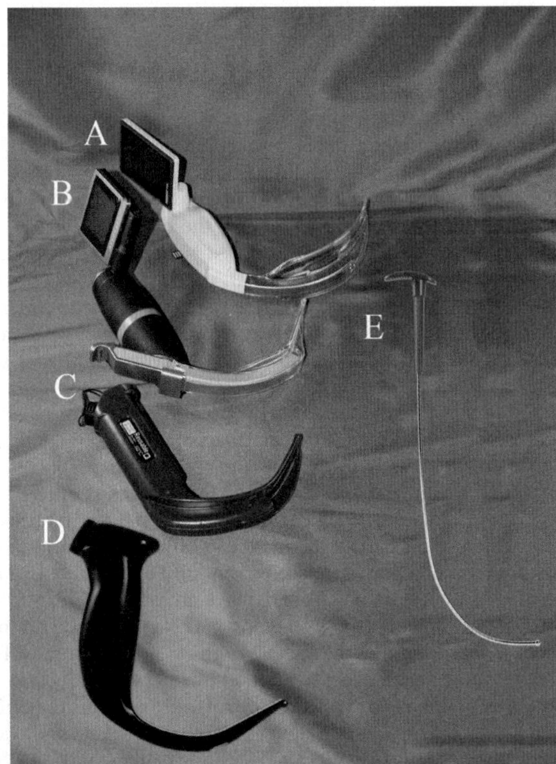

Figure 28-15 (A) McGRATH MAC and (B) McGRATH Series 5. ((A) McGRATH™ MAC and (B) McGRATH® Series 5 (Medtronic, Dublin, Ireland).) (C) Glidescope Multiuse blade, (D) GlideScope Spectrum LoPro S3 Single-use Video Laryngoscope. (Used with permission, © Verathon Inc.), and (E) GlideRite Reusable Rigid Stylet. (Used with permission, © Verathon Inc.)

than one individual (e.g., aid, mentor, student).[5] The 60-degree distal angulation reduces cervical spine motion by 50% at the C2–5 segments compared with Macintosh DL.[136]

When used by inexperienced operators, the Glidescope provides a better glottic view than DL (Cormack–Lehane grade 1 view in 85.7% vs. 48.9% of patients) and can obtain a Cormack–Lehane grade 1 or 2 view in 77% of patients in whom no glottic exposure was achieved by DL.[135] A large prospective, nonrandomized study of 1,755 patients showed a 98% intubation success rate with the Glidescope, including 96% success in patients predicted to be difficult by DL and 94% success in airway rescue after failed DL.[30] Although achieving an adequate laryngeal view with the VL appears relatively easy, ETT manipulation into the larynx appears to be more difficult. In one study, placement of the ETT required an additional 16 seconds (on average) when compared to DL.[135,137] This is likely due to difficulty in maneuvering the ETT around the hyperangulated blade. For this reason, the use of a stylet is advised.[138,139] A dedicated, nonmalleable stylet, the Gliderite Rigid Stylet (Verathon, Bothell, WA), has a 90-degree distal bend and may be used with various videolaryngoscopes. A study by Jones et al.[140] suggests that the angle of the ETT has greater impact on time to intubation than the Cormack and Lehane grade of the image. A 1 to 2 cm withdrawal of the stylet as the glottis is entered may facilitate advancement into the larynx as well as counterclockwise rotation of the tracheal tube as it is advanced off the stylet. Because the stylet is rigid, there is a concern that it may cause laryngeal or tracheal trauma. Insertion of the stylet into the larynx should be minimized.

Theoretically, the airway axes do not need to be aligned to achieve adequate glottic visualization with VL. Manipulation of the videolaryngoscope to the position needed for adequate image can cause cervical segment extension, though.[141] Care must be taken in that regard, especially if the cervical spine is unstable. The Glidescope has been successfully used to achieve tracheal intubation in patients with limited cervical spine movement because of ankylosing spondylitis and cervical spine trauma, but it may be difficult to use in patients with limited mouth opening.[142,143]

The classic Glidescope insertion technique follows the midline approach. After the uvula is visualized, the blade is advanced in the midline into the vallecula or is passed posterior to the epiglottis.[135] For patients with a limited mouth aperture, the blade can be inserted like a Guedel airway, with the Glidescope blade concavity facing rostrad and rotated 180 degrees counterclockwise once the distal tip is in the oropharynx. This maneuver displaces the tongue to the left and minimizes neck movements.

Practitioners must visualize to completion insertion of both the blade and the ETT into the oropharynx. Traumatic complications associated with the use of the videolaryngoscope have been related to blind manipulation of the ETT as it enters the airway but is not yet visualized on the video screen. Traumatic events, which appear to be more likely with the use of a rigid stylet, have been reported relating primarily to the soft palate, palatoglossal arch, right palatopharyngeal arch, and right anterior tonsillar pillar (Fig. 28-16).[144,145] Steps to avoid soft tissue trauma include: (1) assuring that the stylet is within the bevel of the ETT; (2) maintaining the ETT in a midline position and as close to the blade as possible; (3) focusing the operator's attention on the patient's oral cavity(as is done during DL, as the blade and then ETT are advanced into the mouth, occasionally glancing at the VL monitor. (Full attention is turned to the video image only when the distal ETT can be seen on the image monitor.); (4) avoiding levering of the blade inward, as this increases the "blind spot" inferiorly; (5) using the least force necessary to advance the ETT; and (6) practicing "reverse loading" of the ETT (as described later).[134] The potential for trauma to the oropharyngeal soft tissues due to

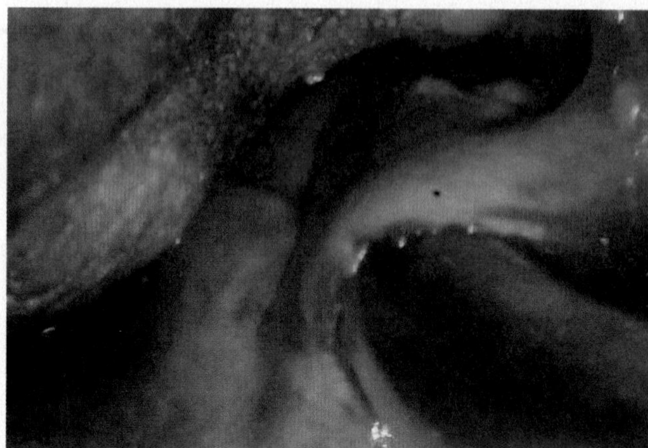

Figure 28-16 Passage of a tracheal tube through the right palatoglossal arch due to a blind spot created with videolaryngoscopy.

the above-described "blind spot" is similar for all videolaryngoscopes, unless true direct laryngoscopic technique is used.

Controlled studies have shown no significant advantage of the Glidescope in preventing hemodynamic responses to orotracheal intubation compared with the Macintosh direct laryngoscope.[146] The Glidescope has been used to facilitate nasotracheal intubation with a reduced time to intubation and higher first-time success rate when compared with DL. Reverse loading technique and use of a gum elastic bougie have also been described. Reverse loading entails bending the distal tip of the stylet in the opposite direction of the natural ETT curvature. This promotes a more posteriorly directed delivery of the ETT and decreases the chance of impingement on the anterior commissure or tracheal rings.[147]

A newer version of the Glidescope, the Glidescope Titanium (Verathon, Bothell, WA), has also been introduced. The new design is made of titanium and has two standard curved blades (MAC T3 and T4) as well as two low-profile acute-angle blades (LoPro T3 and T4). Plastic, single-use versions are also available (LoPro/Mac P3 and P4). The mouth openings needed for commonly used indirect laryngoscopes are listed in Table 28-12.

The C-MAC system (Karl Storz, Tuttlingen, Germany; Fig. 28-17) consists of an electronic laryngoscope handle with exchangeable metal blades. One of these, the D-Blade, is an hyperangulated blade similar to the Glidescope, designed for when difficult DL is anticipated. A large multicenter, prospective, randomized trial of 1,100 patients showed no difference in intubation success rate (with two attempts) between the Glidescope and C-MAC D-Blade in patients with anticipated difficult laryngoscopy.[148]

The C-MAC platform also works with blades that are identical to standard Macintosh and Miller blades but with integrated illumination and CMOS optics. This allows the device to be used as either a videolaryngoscope or a standard direct laryngoscope. Although the image projected from the C-MAC closely resembles that seen with the naked eye, ETT placement is facilitated because the video image obviates the need to maintain an unobstructed line of sight to the glottis. Use of the C-MAC is identical to standard DL, making the video facility uniquely valuable during supervised instruction. A comparison study of direct and video-assisted views of the larynx revealed significant improvement of the glottic view with C-MAC video assistance.[149]

The McGrath Mac (Medtronic, Dublin, Ireland) is a videolaryngoscope with a reduced blade curvature as compared to other hyperangulated videolaryngoscopes and a slimmer blade design (11.9 mm). The reduced curvature allows easier use as a direct laryngoscope and an improved screen allows shared viewing.

Table 28-12 Mouth Opening Needed for Commonly Used Indirect Laryngoscopes

Device	Mouth Opening Needed
Glidescope	17.4 mm
Glidescope Ranger[a]	
Glidescope Titanium[a]	
Glidescope LoPro	12.4 mm
Storz C-MAC (Mac 3)[a]	
Storz C-MAC (D-Blade)[a]	
Airtraq SP (size 0)	11 mm
Airtraq SP (size 1)	12 mm
Airtraq SP (size 2)	15 mm
Airtraq SP (size 3)	16 mm
Airtraq AVANT (sizes 2 and 3)	17 mm
McGrath Mac[a]	
McGrath Mac X[a]	
King Vision (size 1)	10 mm (nonchanneled)
King Vision (size 2)	10 mm (nonchanneled), 13 mm (channeled)
King Vision (size 3)	13 mm (nonchanneled), 18 mm (channeled)

[a]Company stated "No available data."

The "blind spot" noted with the Glidescope is reduced if a DL approach is used. Though there may be less concern for soft tissue trauma, the cautions mentioned earlier still apply. Another McGrath product, the McGrath X blade, has an acute angle tip for anticipated difficult airways, a slimmer design, and a portrait display to decrease blindspot size.

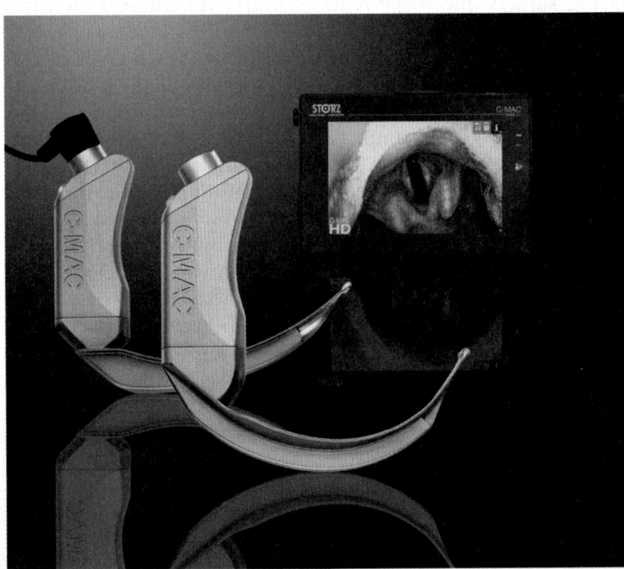

Figure 28-17 KARL STORZ C-MAC HD Video Laryngoscope. (Copyright © KARL STORZ SE & Co. KG, Germany.)

A configuration of videolaryngoscopes, termed "channeled scopes," employ a J-shaped channel that follows the course of the optical elements from the viewing element (optical or video imaging) to the distal objective lens or CMOS chip. DL accommodates for the right-angle nature of the airway by displacing the anterior structures; VL accommodates by placing the operator's point of view beyond the tongue. By contrast, the channeled devices replicate the near 90-degree relationship of the oral and pharyngeal axes, limiting the need for tissue displacement and cervical manipulation. A lubricated ETT is preloaded into the channel and guided in the same trajectory as the objective. When adequate visualization of the glottis is achieved, the ETT is advanced in the channel until observed approaching the larynx. In theory, as the tracheal tube is never in a blind spot, this technique should reduce the incidence of soft tissue trauma seen with the classic videolaryngoscope approach. The blades of channeled devices typically have an anatomic shape; therefore, neutral head and neck positions tend to result in improved glottic alignment. Minor manipulations of the videolaryngoscope may be needed to align the ETT and facilitate passage through the glottis.

The Airtraq optical laryngoscope (Prodol Meditec S.A., Vizcaya, Spain; Fig. 28-18 and 14 Video 28-14) is a single-use, anatomically shaped, channeled laryngoscope with periscopic optics. The device has a built-in antifog system and a low-temperature light that facilitates the laryngeal view. The Airtraq has been used successfully as a rescue device in patients after failed intubation with DL.[150] Anterior forces (e.g., those applied to the tongue) are reduced compared to that found with DL, but some cervical spine movement still occurs.[141] Reports of its use in awake patients, patients with cervical spine disease, and after failed DL have been published.[151] One study showed the need for fewer maneuvers to improve glottic exposure and fewer alterations in blood pressure and heart rate when compared with DL.[152] Reduced cervical spine movement in patients with midline axial stabilization also has been demonstrated. The Airtraq AVANT (Prodol Meditec S.A., Vizcaya, Spain) functions similarly, but with reusable prismatic optics sheathed in a disposable blade. A study of 100 patients showed better glottic visualization with the AVANT than with DL utilizing a Macintosh blade.[153]

The Airway Scope (Pentax AWS, AWS-S100; Hoya-Pentax, Tokyo, Japan) is a reusable, channeled device with a CMOS camera cord fitted into a single-use blade (Fig. 28-18). The handle incorporates a 2.4-in LCD monitor, the angle of which can be adjusted for easier viewing. The channel on the disposable blades accepts ETTs with internal diameters between 6.5 and 8.0 mm and incorporates a working channel that can be used for placement of a small suction

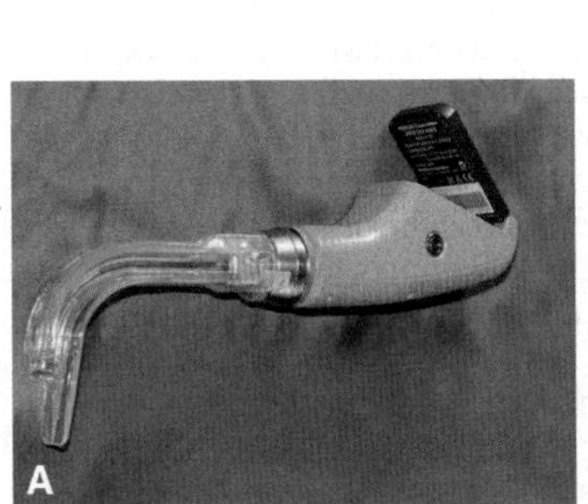

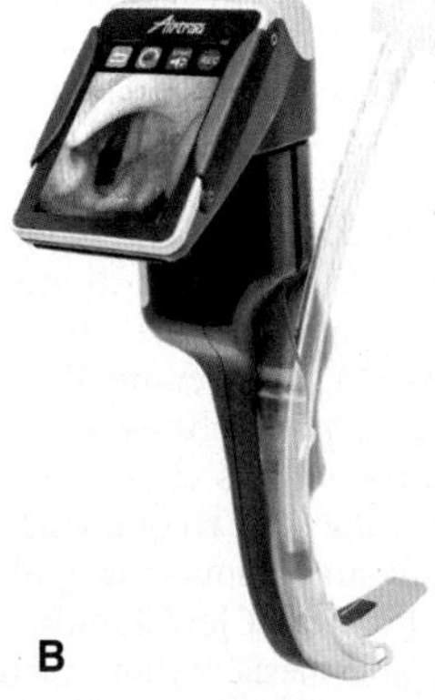

Figure 28-18 A: The Pentax Airway Scope. (Hoya-Pentax, Tokyo, Japan.) **B:** The Airtraq laryngoscope. (Used with permission from Prodol Meditec S.A., Vizcaya, Spain.)

catheter, injection of lidocaine, or insufflation of oxygen. Unlike the Airtraq, the manufacturer of the AWS recommends using the blade to lift the epiglottis (similar to using a Miller blade) prior to ETT insertion. The difference in technique appears to be related to the ETT being closer to the device tip during tube extrusion with the AWS than with the Airtraq.[154] In one small, nonblinded, non-crossover study, the AWS produced less of a hemodynamic response and had a higher intubation success rate than the Glidescope (100% vs. 96%) in patients predicted to be difficult by DL.[155] As with other channeled devices, the AWS has a higher success rate than the Glidescope in volunteers with restricted neck mobility.[30]

The KingVision Video Laryngoscope (Ambu, Ballerup, Denmark) includes a reusable, battery-operated OLED display and disposable channeled and nonchanneled blades. The device can therefore be used as a classic VL or as a channeled scope. The on-handle display gives a higher-quality image than most other VLs and includes a composite video-out port.

NPO Status and Rapid-Sequence Induction (15 Video 28-15)

Aspiration of gastric contents trails only failed intubation in frequency of reported adverse anesthesia-related events.[1] Induction of anesthesia profoundly depresses intrinsic reflexes that protect the airway from the entrance of foreign bodies, including regurgitated material (NICV 28-3, 16 Videos 28-16 and 17 28-17). In addition, manipulation of the upper esophageal inlet reduces the closing pressure of the lower esophageal sphincter. Many patients will present in situations in which aspiration is a significant risk (Table 28-13A) and rapid-sequence induction (RSI) is indicated. If, in addition, difficult airway management is anticipated, awake intubation is often chosen (see Airway Approach Algorithm below). When aspiration is of concern, pharmacologic therapy can help mitigate risk, with the goal of reducing both the volume and acidity of gastric contents. Obesity has long been considered a risk factor for gastric-content aspiration and preoperative treatment with gastric emptying and acid-reducing agents has been recommended,[156] though this remains controversial. Although initial studies touted the increased volume and decreased pH of gastric secretions in the obese fasting patient, others have refuted this claim.[157,158]

Control of Gastric Contents

Preventing pulmonary aspiration of gastric contents is a primary concern during airway management. Control of gastric contents involves (1) minimizing intake; (2) increasing gastric emptying; and (3) reducing gastric volume and acidity (Table 28-13B). Altered physiologic states (e.g., pregnant patients in labor and diabetes mellitus) and gastrointestinal pathology (e.g., bowel obstruction and peritonitis) adversely affect the rate of gastric emptying, thereby increasing aspiration risk. The extent of delayed gastric emptying with diabetes mellitus correlates well with the presence of autonomic neuropathy but not with age, duration of disease, HbA1c, or peripheral neuropathy. The difference in gastric emptying times between healthy patients and those with type I diabetes ranges from 30 minutes to 2 hours.[159] Human breast milk is cleared more rapidly than other milk products[160] and the ASA recommends a fasting period of 4 hours for breast milk and 6 hours for nonhuman milk, infant formula, and a light solid meal. Clear liquids can be administered up to 2 hours prior to anesthesia without increased risk for regurgitation and aspiration (Table 28-13C).[161]

Reduction of gastric acidity can be achieved with the aid of H_2-receptor antagonists and proton pump inhibitors (PPIs), which also reduce gastric volume. Famotidine given a few hours before surgery effectively reduces gastric volume and increases gastric pH better than ranitidine.[162] The PPIs rabeprazole, lansoprazole, and omeprazole are most effective when given in two successive doses: one the evening before and one the morning of anesthesia.[163,164] When given in a single dose, pantoprazole and ranitidine should be administered 1 hour before the induction of anesthesia.[165] This is in contrast to single-dose therapy with omeprazole, which is most effective when administered the night before surgery.[163,164,166] Sodium citrate oral solution increases gastric pH and is best administered within 1 hour preoperatively in a dose of 15 to 30 mL. When combined with metoclopramide (10 mg IV), sodium citrate (15 mL PO) reduces gastric volume by 33% and increases gastric pH by 38% versus unmedicated controls.[167] A nasogastric (NG) tube can also be used to reduce gastric volume prior to induction of anesthesia in patients at high risk of regurgitation. An NG tube in situ provides a passage for passive drainage of gastric contents and does not diminish the effectiveness of cricoid pressure.[168] NGs are best left in place and open to freely drain during induction of anesthesia. The presence of an NG tube does not guarantee an empty stomach, though, and may impair the function of the lower and upper esophageal sphincters.

Table 28-13 Pulmonary Aspiration: Patients at Risk for Aspiration, Methods to Reduce Aspiration Risk, and ASA Recommended Fasting Guidelines

(A) Patients at Risk of Aspiration
- Full stomach (recent ingestion)
- Diabetes mellitus (with peripheral neuropathy)
- Clinically significant gastroesophageal reflux/hiatal hernia
- Pregnancy
- Acute pain/acute opioid therapy, renal colic
- Bowel obstruction/intra-abdominal process
- Trauma/unknown timing of last meal

(B) Methods to Reduce Aspiration Risk
- Minimize intake: adequate preoperative fasting, clear liquids only if necessary
- Increase gastric emptying: prokinetics (e.g., metoclopramide)
- Reduce gastric volume and acidity: preinduction nasogastric tube, nonparticulate antacid (e.g., sodium citrate), H_2-receptor antagonists, proton pump inhibitors
- Airway protection: rapid placement of cuffed ETT after induction, cricoid pressure (controversial)

(C) Summary of Preoperative Fasting Recommendations[159]

Ingested Material:	Minimum Fasting Period:
• Clear liquids	2 hr
• Breast milk	4 hr
• Infant formula	6 hr
• Nonhuman milk	6 hr
• Light meal	6 hr
• Meal containing fatty foods or meat	≥8 hr

Rapid-Sequence Induction. RSI is indicated when there is increased risk of gastric content aspiration. The goal of RSI is to 8 gain control of the airway in the shortest amount of time after the ablation of protective airway reflexes with the induction of general anesthesia. In the RSI technique, an intravenous anesthetic induction agent is administered and immediately followed by a rapidly acting neuromuscular blocking drug. Laryngoscopy and intubation are performed as soon as neuromuscular blockade is confirmed. Historically, mask ventilation is omitted for concern of gastric insufflation. Classically, cricoid pressure is applied (Sellick maneuver), which entails the posterior displacement of the cricoid cartilage against the vertebral bodies, and cricoid pressure is maintained from the beginning of induction until confirmation of ETT placement. This maneuver is purported to ablate the esophageal lumen.

Early cadaveric studies showed that correctly applied cricoid pressure was effective in preventing gastric fluids from leaking into the pharynx. However, recently, MRI studies have suggested that the esophagus is laterally displaced in a majority of normal patients.[169] In addition, cricoid pressure may worsen the laryngoscopic view[170] and is contraindicated during active vomiting (risk of esophageal rupture), and with cervical spine or laryngeal fracture. There is also little evidence that omission of mask ventilation provides any clinical benefit, especially in patients with poor pulmonary reserve. In fact, if oxyhemoglobin desaturation occurs, gentle positive-pressure ventilation (<25 cm H_2O) is recommended as is, in the instance of poor laryngeal view, the release of cricoid pressure.[171] For these reasons, and the lack of randomized controlled trials evaluating outcomes related to the use of cricoid pressure,[172] some practitioners have abandoned classic RSI technique in favor of gentle mask ventilation, without cricoid pressure, while awaiting the effects of fast-acting paralytics.[173] If mask ventilation is omitted, high-flow oxygen via nasal cannula can be used to reduce the risk of oxygen desaturation via apneic oxygenation, as discussed earlier.

The Intubating Supraglottic Airways. Blind, flexible scope-aided, and stylet-guided intubation via SGAs has been widely reported, but many limitations have been described. In an effort to overcome these limitations, Brain et al. introduced a version of the LMA, the LMA Fastrach (Teleflex, Research Triangle Park, NC), designed specifically as a conduit to intubation (Fig. 28-4). Other manufacturers have introduced similar devices including the Aura-I (Ambu, Ballerup, Denmark) and the air-Q (Fig. 28-6). Most non-Fastrach devices require guided tracheal intubation (e.g., with a flexible intubation scope) during the intubation process. Expert groups, such as the Canadian Airway Focus Group Difficult Airway Society of the United Kingdom, recommend this visually guided approach.[174]

The mask of the LMA Fastrach differs from Dr. Brain's original LMA design with the incorporation of a vertically oriented, semirigid bar fixed at the proximal end of the bowl aperture. This "epiglottic elevating bar" sits beneath the epiglottis in the average-sized adult and guides the ETT toward the larynx. A handle at the proximal end of the barrel is used for insertion, repositioning, and removal of the device. Originally made of stainless steel and silicone, a plastic single-use version is available. The LMA Fastrach barrel can accommodate up to an 8 mm ID-cuffed ETT, which can be inserted blindly or over a flexible scope device. The Fastrach is designed to be used with a wire-reinforced tracheal tube, although the use of both standard and Parker Flex-Tip (Parker Medical, Englewood, CO) PVC tracheal tubes has been described.[175] The LMA Fastrach is available in sizes with cuffs equivalent to the size 3, 4, and 5 LMA Classics. Experience suggests that most adults between 40 and 70 kg are best managed with a size 4 Fastrach and heavier persons require a size 5.

In one study, blind intubation via the LMA Fastrach occurred in 97% of patients who were anticipated to have a difficult intubation; the remaining intubations were facilitated with adjunct use of a flexible intubation scope.[99]

Insertion technique for the LMA Fastrach is the same as for the LMA Classic. The position of the device can be optimized by lateral and anterior–posterior manipulation of the handle, known as the *Chandy maneuver* (after Dr. Chandy Verghese, Redding, UK).[176] A seemingly common cause of airway obstruction with the LMA Fastrach is down-folding of the epiglottis. This can be relieved with a smooth rotational movement of the inflated LMA Fastrach out of the airway (6 cm along the axis of insertion) and immediate replacement (the "up–down maneuver").

Blind tracheal intubation is undertaken only if the airway is clear, neuromuscular blockade established, and/or the patient is sufficiently anesthetized. After adequate ventilation and anesthesia are achieved, the ETT is advanced though the barrel. As the ETT exits the bowl aperture of the LMA Fastrach, the elevating bar is pushed anteriorly, carrying the epiglottis out of the way. If positioned correctly, the ETT can freely enter the glottis.

When blind intubation fails (esophageal insertion or inability to advance the ETT) and ventilation is adequate, the clinician can (1) continue with short surgical procedures using the Fastrach as a simple SGA (procedures longer than 15 minutes may be ill-advised because of the pressure exerted by the LMA Fastrach on pharyngeal tissues); (2) change to a different SGA; (3) intubate with the aid of a flexible intubation scope through the LMA; (4) remove the SGA and employ an alternative technique of tracheal intubation; or (5) perform a surgical airway while continuing ventilation via the SGA. This last procedure may be an underappreciated facility of all the SGAs, as these devices may serve as bridges while invasive airway procedures are performed.

Once successful intubation is confirmed by capnography, an intubating SGA may be removed. Though this is typically a requirement of the rigid devices (e.g., LMA Fastrach), some intubating SGAs (e.g., the Aura-I or air-Q) may be left in situ. For removal, the ETT circuit adapter is removed and the intubating SGA is withdrawn over the ETT. During the SGA removal, the ETT is stabilized either coaxially by a stabilizing rod (supplied by the manufacturer) or by Magill forceps holding the proximal tip of the ETT (as described by Rosenblatt and Murphy).[177] In the mid-removal position, a finger is placed in the mouth to stabilize the ETT while the SGA is fully retreated.

The pre-curved Aura-I intubating SGA lacks the rigid components as well as the epiglottic lifting bar concept of the LMA Fastrach. Because it does not apply as much pressure to pharyngeal mucosa, it can be left in situ after intubation or used for long periods as a simple SGA. When using an Aura-I for tracheal intubation, a flexible intubation scope should be used.

The air-Q SGA also forgoes the rigid components and epiglottic lifting bar. Unlike the devices discussed earlier, it lacks the 90-degree pre-curvature of the barrel. The air-Q barrel will accept a tracheal tube from 4.5 to 8.0 mm internal diameter (ID) and the keyhole-shaped airway outlet is designed to steer the ETT toward the larynx. For blind intubation, the ETT cuff is deflated, lubricated, and inserted into the device barrel. If the larynx is entered, advancement past 12 to 15 cm should occur with little resistance. If resistance is met, the air-Q can be repositioned and ETT advancement attempted again. Once tracheal intubation is confirmed, the device can be removed with the help of a specialized stylet provided by the manufacturer. In a study comparing like devices, the LMA Fastrach had a higher blind intubation success rate than the air-Q (99% vs. 77%, respectively, with two attempts), though greater than 95% of patients could be intubated with either device if flexible optical guidance was utilized.[178] Unlike the other intubating SGAs, a range of pediatric-sized air-Qs are available and intubation success rates of 95% have been achieved in infants.[179]

Extubation of the Trachea

9 Although a wealth of literature is focused on the field of tracheal intubation, more recent reviews have focused on the process of extubation after completion of surgery or prolonged ventilatory support.[180] Indeed, the period of extubation may be far more treacherous than that of intubation.[1]

Routine Extubation

Extubation of the trachea must not be considered a benign procedure, as it is fraught with its own set of potential complications (Table 28-14, 18 Video 28-18). Appropriately trained personnel and equipment should be immediately available at the time of extubation. This may range from a postanesthetic care unit nurse or respiratory therapist with a set of laryngoscopes to a surgeon prepared to perform an emergency invasive airway. An excellent reference exists in the Difficult Airway Society Extubation Guidelines that outline a strategic stepwise approach to decision-making before, during, and after both routine and "at-risk" extubations.[181]

Most adult patients are extubated after the return of spontaneous respiration, the resolution of neuromuscular block, and the demonstration of the ability to follow simple commands (Table 28-15). Prior to extubation, a suction catheter is typically used to remove supraglottic secretions or blood. If coughing or straining is contraindicated or hazardous (e.g., increased intracranial pressure), extubation may be performed while the patient is in a surgical plane of anesthesia and breathing spontaneously—the so-called deep extubation). Three considerations for deep extubation are (1) a history of easy mask ventilation following induction; (2) nonairway surgery; and (3) empty stomach. If deep extubation is desired and the patient is at risk of gastric content aspiration (e.g., full stomach) or upper airway obstruction (e.g., obstructive sleep apnea), the clinician needs to assess the relative risk of each potential morbidity (e.g., coughing vs. aspiration vs. obstruction).

Laryngospasm upon ETT removal accounts for 23% of all critical postoperative respiratory events in adults.[55] The mechanism of laryngospasm is the contraction of the lateral cricoarytenoids, the thyroarytenoid, and the cricothyroid muscles in response to stimulation of the vagus nerve. Potential stimuli include secretions, vomitus, blood, or foreign body in the airway, pelvic or abdominal visceral stimulation, and pain. Management of laryngospasm consists of the immediate removal of the offending stimulus (if identifiable), administration of oxygen with CPAP and, if other maneuvers are unsuccessful, the use of a small dose of short-acting induction or neuromuscular blocking agent.[55]

Table 28-14 Complications of Tracheal Extubation

Respiratory drive failure (e.g., residual anesthetic, decreased response to high CO_2/low O_2)
Hypoxia (e.g., atelectasis)
Upper airway obstruction (e.g., edema, residual anesthetic or paralytic, reduced upper airway tone)
Vocal fold–related obstruction (e.g., laryngospasm, vocal cord edema, or paralysis)
Tracheal obstruction (e.g., subglottic edema or tracheomalacia from prolonged intubation)
Bronchospasm (airway irritation from endotracheal tube)
Aspiration (from decreased gag and swallow reflexes)
Hypertension
Increased intracranial pressure
Increased ocular pressure
Increased pulmonary artery pressure
Increased bronchial stump pressure (e.g., after pulmonary resection)
Increased abdominal wall pressure (risk of wound dehiscence)

Table 28-15 Criteria for Routine "Awake" Postsurgical Extubation

Subjective clinical criteria:
- Breathing spontaneously
- Following commands
- Five-second sustained head lift
- Intact gag reflex
- Airway clear of debris
- Adequate pain control
- Minimal end-expiratory concentration of inhaled anesthetics

Objective criteria:
- Vital capacity ≥10 mL/kg
- Peak voluntary negative inspiratory pressure > −20 cmH_2O
- Tidal volume >6 mL/kg
- Sustained tetanic contraction (5 s)
- T1/T4 ratio >0.7–0.8
- Alveolar–arterial Pa_{O_2} gradient <350 mmHg (on Fi_{O_2} of 1)[a]
- Dead space to tidal volume ratio ≤0.6[a]

[a]Used during weaning from mechanical ventilation in the intensive care setting.

Patients who are not fully recovered from neuromuscular blockade are also at risk of airway obstruction and aspiration at the time of extubation.[182] This is in part due to incompetent pharyngeal function when the train-of-four (TOF) ratio remains less than 0.9.[183] Fortier et al.[184] found that 65% of patients who received nondepolarizing neuromuscular blocker and had been reversed with neostigmine still had residual neuromuscular blockade (TOF <0.9) at the time of extubation and 60% had residual neuromuscular blockade on arrival to the postanesthesia care unit (PACU). This data suggests that neostigmine alone cannot be relied on for adequate reversal, and vigilance is needed during intraoperative titration of neuromuscular blockade. In addition, peripheral nerve stimulation should be used to guide reversal. A new class of agents, cyclodextrins, are hollow-structure molecules capable of trapping other molecules within their core. The lipophilic core of the agent Sugammadex (Merck & Co., Whitehouse Station, NJ) so tightly encapsulates rocuronium or vecuronium molecules that it can remove blocking agents that are already bound to the neuromuscular junction. The trapped neuromuscular blocker is unavailable to bind elsewhere and excreted in the urine. This is discussed more thoroughly in Chapter 21.

Mechanical airway obstruction may also result in extubation failure; the risk is higher in patients with obstructive sleep apnea. Obstruction may result from trauma related to intubation (e.g., multiple failed attempts), surgical manipulation (e.g., lingual edema caused by mouth gags), and impaired lymphatic (e.g., after radiation therapy) or venous (e.g., with extreme neck flexion) drainage. Palatopharyngeal edema associated with anterior cervical spine procedures or hematomas (e.g., following endarterectomy) may also result in postextubation airway failure.

Unilateral vocal cord paralysis may result from trauma to the recurrent laryngeal nerve. If the contralateral nerve has been damaged previously, airway obstruction can occur due to unopposed vocal cord adduction. This may occur following neck or intrathoracic surgery or even after internal jugular line placement or endotracheal intubation. Transient vocal cord or swallowing dysfunction has been demonstrated in absence of injury, placing even healthy patients at risk of aspiration after general anesthesia. Many patients will undergo preoperative nasopharyngoscopy to assess the state of laryngeal function prior to one of these high-risk procedures.

Pharmacologic agents used during maintenance and emergence of anesthesia may also affect the success of extubation. Though low concentrations of potent inhalation anesthetics (e.g., 0.2 Minimal Alveolar Concentration [MAC]) do not alter the respiratory response to CO_2, they may blunt hypoxic drive. Opioids and, to a lesser extent, benzodiazepines affect both hypercarbic and hypoxic respiratory drives. Some nondepolarizing neuromuscular blocking agents also reduce the hypoxic ventilatory drive secondary to their effect on cholinergic receptors in the carotid body.[180,182]

A randomized controlled trial revealed that multiple-dose dexamethasone effectively reduced incidence of postextubation stridor in adult patients at high risk for postextubation laryngeal edema. In contrast, a single dose of dexamethasone given 1 hour before extubation did not reduce the number of patients requiring reintubation.[185]

Identification of Patients at Risk for Complications after Extubation

All patients should be evaluated for potentially difficult extubation just as they are evaluated for potentially difficult intubation. A number of clinical situations may place patients at increased risk for difficulty with oxygenation or ventilation at the time of extubation (Table 28-16).

A popular test used to predict postextubation airway competency is the detection of a leak on deflation of the ETT cuff (NICV 28-4). A meta-analysis showed that the absence of a cuff leak is associated with a higher risk of reintubation, but the presence of a detectable leak has low predictive value.[186]

When mask ventilation and intubation are without difficulty and there is no substantial reason to believe that an interim insult to the airway has occurred, extubation may be accomplished in a routine fashion. Even under these circumstances, one must always be prepared for emergent reintubation.

Approach to the Difficult Extubation

When there is a suspicion that a patient may have difficulty with oxygenation or ventilation after tracheal extubation, the clinician may opt for a number of management strategies. These range from continued ventilation, to the preparation of standby reintubation and/or surgical equipment and personnel, to the active establishment of a bridge or guide for reintubation or oxygenation.

Several types of obturators, which may be left in the airway for extended periods, are available for use in trial extubation (19 Video 28-19). These devices are generally referred to as airway exchange catheters (AECs). The success of first-pass reintubation is significantly higher, and the incidence of hypoxia is lower, in patients when an AEC is positioned in the airway.[187] One commercially available AEC is the Cook Airway Exchange Catheters (Cook Critical Care, Bloomington, IN) which is available in multiple sizes, has a central lumen, and rounded, atraumatic ends.

Despite their advantages, AECs have been associated with significant morbidity, and complication rates of up to 60% have been reported.[188] Complications have included loss of airway control, mucosal trauma, esophageal intubation, pneumothorax (even in the absence of gas insufflation), and death.[189] Specific cautions are often exercised to reduce complications with AECs, though little empiric literature is available.

Prior to placement of an AEC, the patient should meet extubation criteria and, in most cases, be fully preoxygenated. An AEC with an external diameter closest to the internal diameter of the ETT that would be used for reintubation should be chosen to prevent "hang-up" (see later under Use of the Flexible Intubation Scope).

When the patient is ready for extubation, the ventilator is disconnected and the distal end of the lubricated AEC is placed to the depth of the tracheal tube bevel. Most AECs have depth markings that may be matched with the markings on the ETT (Fig. 28-19). If care was taken with the initial tracheal tube positioning, this will result in a midtracheal positioning of the AEC and reduce the chance of endobronchial placement. As the ETT is removed, careful attention is paid to maintaining the AEC's position. If tracheal reintubation is required and the ETT will not pass through the glottis, lifting the tongue with a laryngoscope may

Table 28-16 Clinical Situations Presenting Increased Risk for Complications at Time of Extubation

Edema (local, generalized, or angioneurotic)	Airway narrowing
Thyroid surgery	Recurrent laryngeal nerve injury
Laryngoscopy (diagnostic)	Edema, laryngospasm (especially after biopsy)
Uvulopalatoplasty	Palatal and oropharyngeal edema
Obstructive sleep apnea	Upper airway obstruction
Carotid endarterectomy	Wound hematoma, glottic edema, nerve palsies
Maxillofacial trauma	Laryngeal fracture, mandibular/maxillary wires
Cervical vertebrae decompression/fixation	Supraglottic and hypopharyngeal edema
Anaphylaxis	Laryngotracheal narrowing
Upper cervical fracture	Prevertebral/retropharyngeal hematoma
Hypopharyngeal infections	Laryngotracheal narrowing
Hypoventilation syndromes	(e.g., residual anesthetic, central sleep apnea, myasthenia gravis, morbid obesity, severe chronic obstructive pulmonary disease)
Hypoxemic syndromes	(e.g., ventilation–perfusion mismatch, increased oxygen consumption, impaired alveolar oxygen diffusion, severe anemia)
Inadequate airway-protective reflexes	Increased aspiration risk

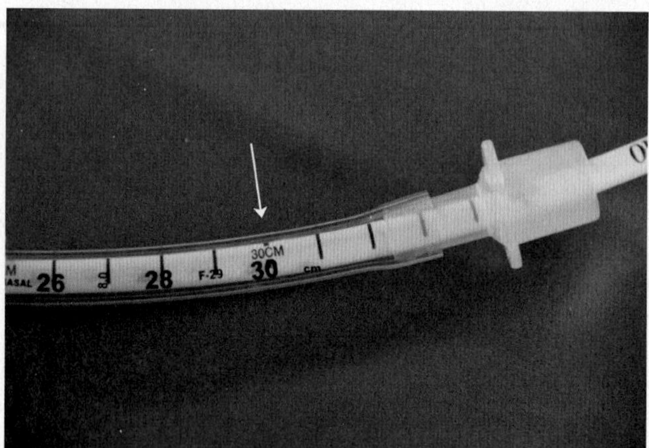

Figure 28-19 Markings of an airway exchange catheter (AEC) are aligned with the markings on the in situ tracheal tube. Aligning these marks as the AEC is inserted prevents bronchial trauma.

facilitate reintubation. A 2 or 3 cm withdrawal of the ETT, counterclockwise tracheal tube rotation (90 degrees), and reinsertion will often overcome "hang-up."

Similarly the Cook Staged Extubation Set (Cook Critical Care, Bloomington, IN) utilizes a flexible guidewire which is inserted into the ETT prior to extubation. This guidewire is left in place after extubation and is thought to be less irritating to the patient during the trial of extubation. If reintubation is indicated, the system includes a blunt tip catheter to slide over the guidewire, over which the ETT is advanced. Note that this system is multi-staged and while the guidewire may increase patient comfort during the extubation trial, it may require a longer period of time to execute tracheal re-inubtation compared to the AEC.

During removal of the ETT, a flexible intubation scope may be used to view tracheal structures. If extubation is tolerated, the bronchoscope can be slowly withdrawn into the subglottic region and the vocal folds and other structures visualized and evaluated.

The Difficult Airway Algorithm and Infographics

In 1992, the ASA Task Force on the Difficult Airway first published an algorithm that has become a staple of modern airway management. This algorithm has been revised and reissued in 2003, 2013 and 2022.[2] Up until recently, the most significant amendments to the ASA difficult Airway Algorithm (ASA-DAA) have been the repositioning of the SGA from the emergency to the non-emergency management pathway and the inclusion of VL as an option for both initial airway management and after failed tracheal intubation with DL (Fig. 28-20). In 2022, a decision tree tool for choosing between the Awake Intubation and Intubation after Induction of Anesthesia pathways was added. In addition, the 2022 guidelines include both adult and pediatric infographics that transform the historic Difficult Airway Algorithm in style and function.

The text of the ASA-DAA succinctly states the challenge of recommending practices for management of the difficult airway: "The difficult airway represents a complex interaction between patient factors, the clinical setting, and the skills of the practitioner" and this viewpoint is clearly reflected in the major update.

Entry into the pathways of the ASA-DAA, as well as the adult Infographic starts with the clinician's assessment of the risk of failure with core airway management modalities as well as other principle considerations. These factors are incorporated into a decision tree tool (Figs. 28-20 and 28-21 Part 1).[190] The clinician charged with management of the airway must consider the patient's physical examination and history, their own remote and recent experience, availability of tools (e.g., DL or VL) and capable aide, and the context in which care is being delivered (e.g., operating room versus inpatient ward). If, after this inductive assessment, the laryngoscopist concludes that laryngoscopy and intubation (of their choosing, for example, DL or VL) would be straightforward, they are directed to the Intubation after Induction of Anesthesia (ASA-DAA)/Airway Management with Induction of Anesthesia (Infographic) pathways. If, on the other hand, their assessment is that there may be difficulty with laryngoscopy and intubation, the question of ability to ventilate (by any means, for example, facemask or SGA) is considered. If, based on the factors elucidated above, there is any concern regarding ability to ventilate, the decision tree tool directs the clinician toward the Awake Intubation pathway. If facemask/SGA ventilation is assessed to be straightforward, the next step is to assess the risk of gastric content aspiration. The factors affecting the risk of gastric content regurgitation and aspiration are varied and discussed in detail elsewhere. This risk must be assessed by the clinician managing the patient's airway based on the patient's conditions (e.g., pregnant patient in labor), comorbidities (e.g., diabetes, trauma, gastroesophageal reflux disorder), *nil per os* status and other factors.[191] If the risk is significant and laryngoscopy and intubation may not be rapidly and efficiently achieved, again the Awake Intubation pathway is considered. Lastly, the question must be asked: should intubation fail and facemask and SGA ventilation prove unexpectedly inadequate, will the patient rapidly desaturate? Factors such as age, pregnancy, pulmonary physiology, reliability of preoxygenation, abnormal oxygen consumption (e.g., fever), and choice of induction agents will influence this assessment. In summary, concerns over the ability to rapidly correct loss of airway patency and ability to manage the airway drives the decision toward the Awake Intubation pathway in both the ASA-DAA and the Infographic.

An exception in the decision tree tool pathway is a patient who is unable to cooperate owing to cognitive disability, intoxication, depressed level of consciousness, or young age. Though the Awake Intubation pathway may be appropriate, it may need to be forgone in favor of techniques that maintain spontaneous ventilation (e.g., inhalational induction or titrated intravenous agents such as dexmedetomidine). Alternatively, the Airway Management after Induction of Anesthesia pathway may need to be entered with provisions for emergent invasive airway should it be needed.

Preparation of the patient for awake intubation is discussed later in this chapter. In most instances, awake intubation can be accomplished successfully if approached systematically with care and patience. When awake intubation fails, the clinician has a number of options that are integrated in the relevant pathways of the ASA-DAA and Infographic (Part 1) (Figs. 28-20 and 28-21): (1) postponing the surgical case and arranging specialized equipment or personnel for a return to the operating room; (2) electing an alternative technique of awake intubation; (3) choosing a regional anesthetic technique; or (4) if clinically indicated, persuing an invasive airway. The decision to proceed with regional anesthesia due to real or anticipated airway management difficulties must be considered in terms of risks and benefits (Table 28-17). Information from the ASA Closed Claims Database has identified failure of regional anesthesia as a source of serious complications when no airway strategy was preemptively considered.[190,192]

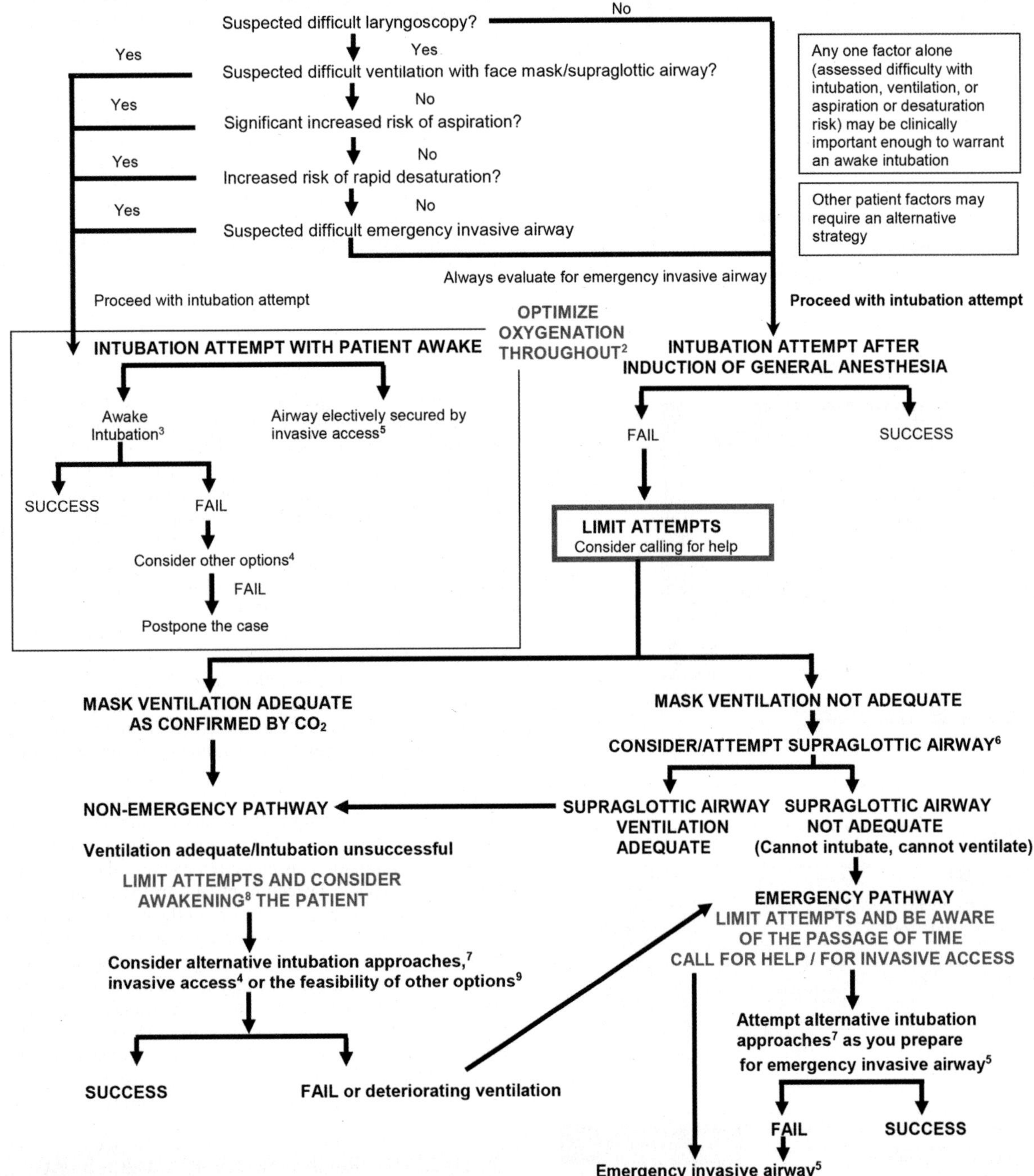

Figure 28-20 2022 American Society of Anesthesiologists Practice Guidelines for Management of the Difficult Airway.[193]

The ASA-DAA and the Infographic introduced in 2022 provide distinct guidance in the unanticipated difficult airway scenario (Box B in Figs. 28-20, 28-21 Infographic Part 3). When induction agents (with or without neuromuscular blockade) have been administered and the airway cannot be controlled as expected, vital management decisions must be made rapidly.

Key points of the unanticipated difficult intubation arm of the ASA-DAA have been discussed elsewhere. Apart from a few modifications, this algorithm has little changed since its last revision in 2013. However, one significant modification is the reduced emphasis on attempting to "wake the patient" when ventilation is deemed inadequate. Though a return to spontaneous ventilation

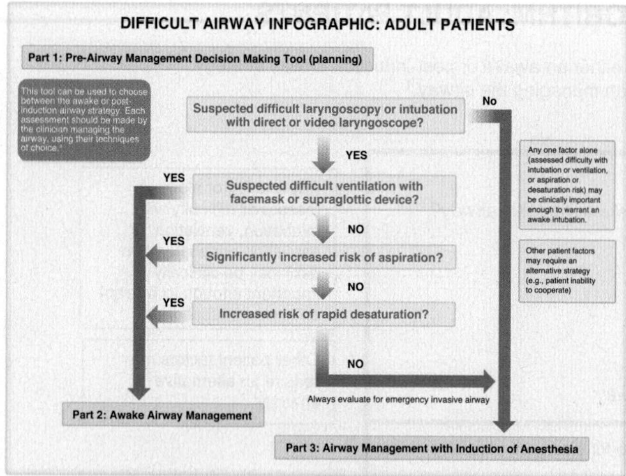

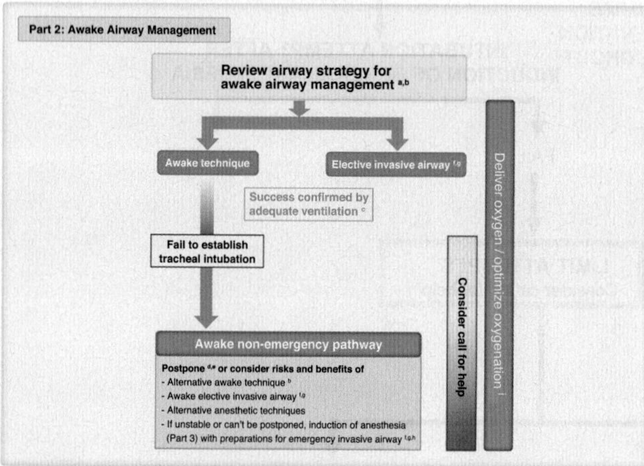

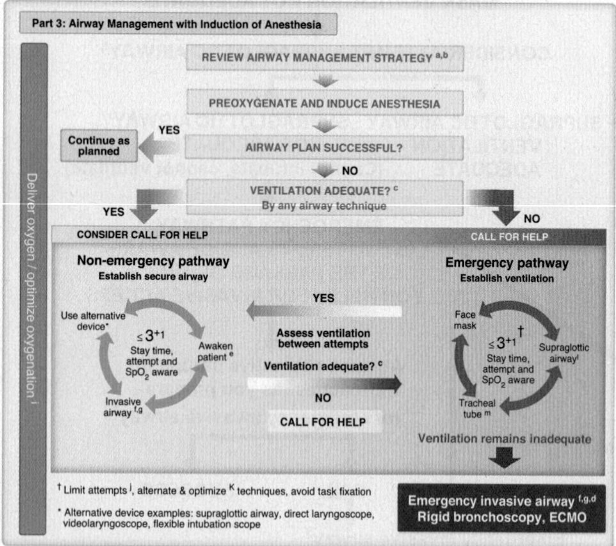

Figure 28-21 2022 American Society of Anesthesiologists Practice Guidelines for Management of the Difficult Airway.[193]

is encouraged, the Task Force on Management of the Difficult Airway wished to discourage the interruption of other rescue maneuvers in anticipation of the patient simply emerging from the crisis.

The series of Infographics are a significant addition to the ASA-DAA guidelines. Part 3 of the Infographic mirrors the difficulty with the airway management pathway of the traditional ASA-DAA. The Infographic Part 3 pathway begins with a review of the airway management strategy. Akin to the Surgical Sign-In procedure of the World Health Organization Surgical Safety Checklist, the airway managing team is encouraged to discuss concerning factors and plans prior to the induction of anesthesia[192] (Table 28-18).

Preoxygenation, as discussed elsewhere in this chapter, is encouraged in all cases, regardless of the anesthetic plan. The purpose of preoxygenation is to prolong the safe apneic period should the airway plan fail to maintain airway patency. In addition, Part 3 of the Infographic encourages continued oxygenation and optimization of oxygenation throughout the process of airway management (Table 28-19).

Within the context of the Airway Guidelines of the ASA, induction of anesthesia has historically referred to the induction of general anesthesia, as reflected in the ASA-DAA.[2] The Infographic, Part 3 includes a broader view of induction to include the induction of regional anesthesia, sedation anesthetic care, as well as general anesthesia. Once induction is complete, it is left to the clinician to evaluate the success of the airway plan, whether it be tracheal intubation, facemask or SGA ventilation, nasal cannula, or another technique. If the airway plan is successful, it is continued. If the airway plan is not successful, the question of adequacy of ventilation, as measured by end-tidal carbon dioxide (CO_2) is considered. Detection of CO_2 in the exhaled gas represents a near instantaneous indicator of the patency of the patient's airway. Historically, oxygen saturation was considered the critical indicator of gas exchange. This has been downgraded based on the appreciation of the delay in oxygen saturation that may occur after loss of airway patency due to the availably of pulmonary, arterial blood and tissue oxygen stores. Though end-tidal CO_2 offers an objective and qualitative assessment of airway patency, it may not reflect adequacy of gas exchange. Appropriate end-tidal CO_2 waveforms (clear upward and downward trace, separated by

Table 28-17 Regional Anesthesia (RA) for Patients with Likely Difficult Airways

May Consider RA	Should Not Consider RA
Superficial surgery	Cavity-invading surgery
Minimal sedation needed	Moderate or heavy sedation needed
Local infiltration adequate	Large-volume local anesthetic required or high risk of intravascular injection/absorption
Easy access to the airway	Poor access to the airway
Surgery can be halted at any time	Surgery cannot be stopped once started

Table 28-18 Review of Airway Management Strategy Prior to Anesthetic Induction[2]

Anatomic factors
Physiologic factors
Aspiration risk
Equipment and monitoring check
Primary airway management plan

Table 28-19 Optimization of Oxygenation Throughout Airway Management

Nasal cannula/High-flow humidified oxygen
Head elevated position
Noninvasive ventilation

a plateau) and quantitative minimums (e.g., 20 mm Hg) should be sought and are discussed elsewhere in this text. Adequacy of gas exchange is assessed using other factors: tidal volume, chest rise, sustained oxygen saturation. If ventilation is deemed adequate, the left-sided, nonemergency pathway is entered with the goal of establishing a secured airway. Three fundamental subpaths may be followed, each with a variety of options: (1) attempts at airway management with an alternative device; (2) awakening the patient; and (3) proceeding with an invasive airway.

Attempts at airway management, and in particular attempts at tracheal intubation and SGA placement should be limited. The authors of the 2022 ASA-DAA suggest that "A reasonable approach may be to limit attempts with any technique class (i.e., face mask, SGA, tracheal tube) to 3, with 1 additional attempt by a clinician with higher skills." This is based on evidence that more than 2 or 3 attempts with these modalities are unlikely to be successful, though the introduction of a new and more experienced operator may be fruitful.[194–197] However, each attempt introduces trauma to the airway that is likely to degrade the adequacy of ventilation that has been achieved. Each attempt should represent an effort to optimize conditions based on what the operator ascertains as the reasons for previous failures.

If at the time of initial attempts at airway management, or while working within the nonemergency pathway, ventilation is deemed inadequate, the emergency pathway is entered. Within this pathway the goal is the restoration of adequate ventilation. The operator is encouraged to cycle between the core techniques of airway management—tracheal intubation, facemask ventilation, or SGA ventilation. This may be influenced by operator experience, available devices, capable aid, and what information has been learned regarding the reason for failure at each juncture. Within the emergency pathway an additional consideration is the principle of constraint—additional attempts consume the safe apnea time. Progressing to more invasive options should be considered while the patient's oxygen saturation is maintained if evidence suggests the current path will likely be fruitless.

When the recommended number of attempts at each core modality have been exhausted, or oxygen saturation is failing or expected to fail imminently the Emergency Invasive Airway Pathway is entered (Fig. 28-21 Inforgraphic Part 3).

The Emergency Invasive Airway Pathway of the Infographic includes three modalities: surgical airway, extracorporeal membrane oxygenation (ECMO) and rigid bronchoscopy. Rigid bronchoscopy is most often used in the pediatric population where surgical manipulation of the larynx and trachea is highly discouraged; it has applications in the adult when surgical airway access is impossible (e.g., kyphosis). ECMO is included as an emerging resuscitation modality. Though time consuming to initiate, a reflection on the entry to the Infographic emergency pathway reveals ECMO's possible utility—patients whose physiology may be marginally supported by present, but inadequate airway patency and gas exchange.

Awake Airway Management

10 In most instances, awake intubation can be accomplished successfully if approached with care and patience. Awake airway management remains a mainstay of the ASA-DAA. The awake techniques provide maintenance of spontaneous ventilation in the event that the airway cannot be secured rapidly. Other benefits of the awake technique include increased size and patency of the pharynx; relative forward placement of the base of the tongue; posterior placement of the larynx; and the ability of the patient to cooperate (open the mouth, protrude the tongue, and take a deep breath to further open the airway for instrumentation) with the procedure.[194] In addition, the awake state confers some maintenance of upper and lower esophageal sphincter tone, thus reducing the risk of regurgitation. In the event of regurgitation, the patient can expel aspirated foreign bodies by cough to the extent that these reflexes have not been blunted by local anesthetics.[186] Finally, patients at risk for neurologic sequelae (e.g., patients with unstable cervical spine pathology) may undergo active sensory–motor testing after tracheal intubation and positioning. In an emergent situation, there may be cautions (e.g., cardiovascular stimulation in the presence of cardiac ischemia or ischemic risk, bronchospasm, increased intraocular or intracranial pressure) but no absolute contraindications to awake intubation. Contraindications to elective awake intubation include patient refusal (though with establishing trust and reassurance this can nearly always be overcome), inability to cooperate (e.g., child, profound mental disability, dementia, intoxication), or allergy to local anesthetics (though true IgE-mediated allergic reactions to local anesthetics is extremely rare).[195,196]

Once the clinician has decided to proceed with awake airway management, the patient must be prepared both physically and psychologically. Most adult patients will appreciate an explanation of the need for an awake intubation and will be more cooperative once they realize the importance of and rationale for any potentially uncomfortable procedures.

Along with an appropriate explanation, medication can be used to reduce anxiety. If sedatives are to be administered, the clinician must keep in mind that producing obstruction or apnea in the difficult airway patient can be devastating, and an overly sedated patient may not be able to cooperate with procedures or protect the airway from regurgitated gastric contents. Patients with sleep apnea may be particularly prone to airway obstruction, even with minimal sedation.

Although almost any sedative agent can be used, some general rules apply to all: dose judiciously, avoid polypharmacy (try to use no more than two agents), and have reversal agents on hand. Small doses of benzodiazepines (e.g., midazolam) are commonly used to alleviate anxiety without producing significant respiratory depression. These drugs may be given in intravenous or oral forms. Short-acting opioid receptor agonists (e.g., fentanyl or alfentanil boluses or low-dose remifentanil infusion) can also be used if judiciously titrated for their analgesic and antitussive effects. However, if adequately topicalized, little or no systemic analgesic should be needed.

Dexmedetomidine, a highly selective centrally acting α_2-adrenergic agonist, is also popular among clinicians for awake intubation because it causes relatively less respiratory depression. Dexmedetomidine has also been used for awake intubation in patients with local anesthetic allergy. The success of this technique is likely due to the combined anxiolytic, sedative, and analgesic properties of the drug.[197] A typical loading dose of dexmedetomidine is 1 mcg/kg intravenously over 10 minutes followed by a maintenance infusion of 0.2 to 0.7 mcg/kg/hr.[55] Dexmedetomidine, especially with boluses, may cause bradycardia and both hypo- and hypertension. Bradycardia is reliably treated with atropine or glycopyrrolate, which is often given as a pretreatment for bradycardia prophylaxis as well as for its antisialagogue effect. Hypotension can be corrected with phenylephrine or ephedrine, and hypertension is treated by decreasing the rate of or stopping the dexmedetomidine infusion. Deep sedation with any agent should not be confused with awake intubation, during which the patient remains responsive to verbal commands.

Administration of an antisialagogue is important to the success of awake intubation techniques, as even small amounts of saliva can obscure the objective lens of indirect optical instruments. Antisialagogues have the secondary benefit of increasing the effectiveness of topical anesthetics by limiting secretions that may act as a barrier to mucosal contact with the local anesthetic. In addition, copious salivary secretions may cause cough or laryngospasm. The commonly used antisialagogues are glycopyrrolate (0.2 to 0.4 mg intramuscularly or intravenously) or atropine (0.5 to 1 mg intramuscularly or intravenously). As the drying effects of these medications may take some time (approximately 15 to 30 minutes), they are best administered in the preoperative waiting area.

Vasoconstriction of the nasal passages is required if there is to be instrumentation of this part of the airway (20 Video 28-20). Oxymetazoline is a potent and long-lasting vasoconstrictor commonly used for this purpose. As with the antisialagogues, the effects of this medication are not immediate and should be administered in the preoperative waiting area.

If the patient is at increased risk for gastric regurgitation and aspiration, prophylactic measures should be undertaken as discussed above. Patients should also receive continuous supplemental oxygen until ETT placement is confirmed, either by low-flow or high-flow nasal cannula, depending on the patient's respiratory status and resources available.

Local anesthetics are a cornerstone of awake airway management (see Chapter 22). As an evolutionary necessity, the airway, from the base of the tongue to the bronchi, is exquisitely sensitive. Topical anesthesia and injected nerve block techniques have been developed to blunt the protective reflexes and provide airway analgesia.

Local anesthetics are both effective and potentially dangerous drugs. Because these agents are used within the tracheal–bronchial tree, there is potential for significant intravascular absorption. The clinician should have a thorough understanding of the mechanism of action, metabolism, toxicities, and acceptable cumulative doses of any drug they choose to employ. The toxic level of lidocaine, for example, is considered to be 4 μg/mL. In a human study, 400 or 800 mg of lidocaine gel was applied topically to the upper airway. Serial blood lidocaine levels were measured, peaking 60 to 70 minutes later at 0.57 and 1.39 μg/mL, respectively.[196] In another human study, using nebulized lidocaine of the same dose, serum levels of 2.8 and 6.5 μg/mL were measured within 10 minutes of dose completion, respectively.[199] This underscores the need for vigilance and forethought with local anesthetic dosing, especially when applied to the subglottic airways, as with nebulization.

Despite the myriad of local anesthetics available, only those most commonly used in airway preparation will be discussed here. In reality, the choice of local anesthetic has little to do with the success of the technique of awake intubation.[200]

Lidocaine, an amide local anesthetic, is available in a wide variety of preparations and doses. Topically applied, peak analgesia occurs within 15 minutes. This relatively rapid onset and breadth of preparations (e.g., liquid, gel, ointment) make it a common choice for airway topicalization.

Benzocaine, an ester local anesthetic, is popular among some clinicians because of its very rapid onset (<1 minute) and short duration (approximately 10 minutes) (NICV 28-5). It is available in 10%, 15%, and 20% solutions and has been combined with tetracaine in some preparations to prolong the duration of action.

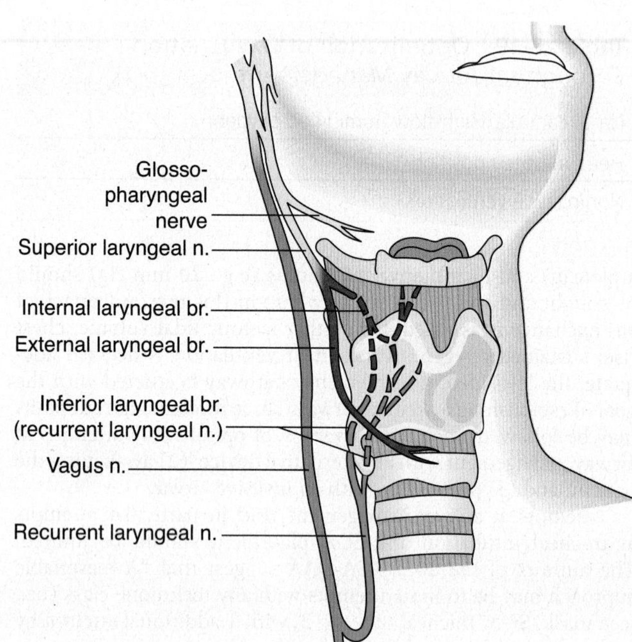

Figure 28-22 Airway innervation.

A 0.5-second aerosol administration of benzocaine can deliver as much as 30 mg of benzocaine. With the toxic dose being 100 mg, caution must be taken not to spray too liberally. Benzocaine may also produce methemoglobinemia (especially in children) which is treated with methylene blue (1 to 2 mg intravenously over several minutes).[201]

For awake airway management, local anesthetic therapy is directed to three anatomic areas: the nasal cavity/nasopharynx, the pharynx/base of the tongue, and the hypopharynx/larynx/trachea (Fig. 28-22).

In the authors' experience, consideration should be given to always include the nasal passages in the preparation for awake intubation for two reasons. First, if during the course of the awake intubation the plan is changed from the oral to the nasal route, preparation is complete. Second, much of the preparation of the nose with local anesthesia will also affect the pharyngeal airway. The nasal cavity is innervated by the greater and lesser palatine nerves (innervating the nasal turbinates and most of the nasal septum) and the anterior ethmoidal nerve (innervating the nares and anterior third of the nasal septum), which are distal branches of the trigeminal nerve (cranial nerve [CN] V). The palatine nerves arise from the sphenopalatine ganglion located posterior to the middle turbinate. Two techniques for palatine nerve block have been described. In the noninvasive nasal approach, cotton-tipped applicators soaked in local anesthetic are passed along the lower border of the middle turbinate until the posterior wall of the nasopharynx is reached and left there for 5 to 10 minutes. In the invasive oral approach, a needle is introduced into the greater palatine foramen, which can be palpated in the posterior-lateral aspect of the hard palate 1 cm medial to the second and third maxillary molars. A 25-gauge or 27-gauge needle is inserted in a superior/posterior direction to a depth of 2 to 3 cm, and 1 to 2 mL anesthetic solution is injected, taking care to avoid intravascular (sphenopalatine artery) injection. The anterior ethmoidal nerve can be blocked by cotton-tipped applicators soaked in local anesthetic and placed along the dorsal surface of the nose until the anterior cribriform plate is reached. The applicators are left in place for 5 to 10 minutes.

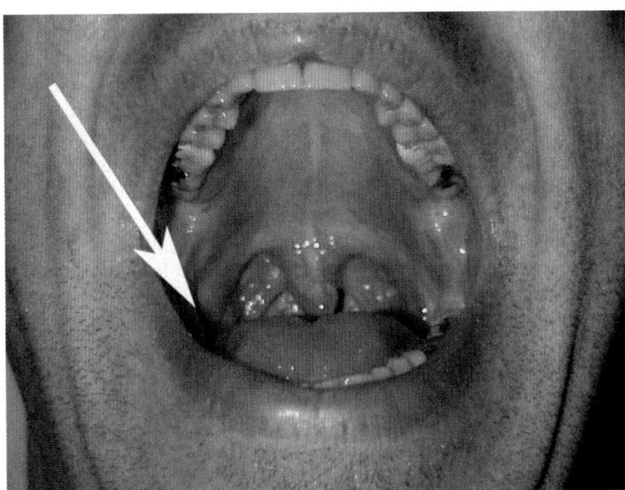

Figure 28-23 The palatoglossal arch (*arrow*) is a soft tissue fold that is a continuation of the posterior edge of the soft palate to the base of the tongue. A local anesthetic-soaked swab placed in the gutter along the base of the tongue is left in contact with the fold for 5 to 10 minutes to produce an ipsilateral glossopharyngeal nerve block.

The oropharynx is innervated by branches of the vagus, facial, and glossopharyngeal nerves. A wide variety of techniques may be used to anesthetize this part of the airway. The simplest techniques involve aerosolized local anesthetic solution, or a voluntary local anesthetic "swish and swallow."

The glossopharyngeal nerve (CN IX) travels anteriorly along the lateral surface of the pharynx and supplies sensory innervation to the posterior third of the tongue, walls of the pharynx (pharyngeal branch), tonsils (tonsillar branch), vallecula, and anterior surface of the epiglottis (lingual branch). As it also supplies the afferent limb for the pharyngeal (gag) reflex, anesthesia of the glossopharyngeal nerve is key to comfortable awake airway management.

The branches of the glossopharyngeal nerve are most easily accessed for local anesthetic block as they transverse the palatoglossal folds. These folds are seen as soft tissue ridges that extend from the posterior aspect of the soft palate to the base of the tongue bilaterally (Fig. 28-23). A noninvasive technique employs anesthetic-soaked cotton-tipped applicators held gently against the inferior most aspect of the bilateral folds for 5 to 10 minutes. When this noninvasive technique proves inadequate, local anesthetic can be injected in a similar manner. Standing on the contralateral side, the operator displaces the protruded tongue, a 25-gauge spinal needle is inserted into the fold near the floor of the mouth, and an aspiration test is performed. If air is aspirated, the needle has passed through-and-through the membrane and is withdrawn slightly prior to injection. If blood is aspirated, the needle tip is redirected more medially. The lingual branch is most readily blocked in this manner, but retrograde tracking of the injectate has also been demonstrated.[202] Even though it provides a reliable block, this more invasive technique is reported to be painful and may result in a bothersome and persistent hematoma.[203] A posterior approach to the glossopharyngeal nerve has also been described in the otolaryngologic literature. As the site of needle insertion is difficult to see behind the palatopharyngeal arch and in close proximity to the carotid artery, this advanced technique will not be described here, and the reader is referred to a more authoritative text.[55]

The superior laryngeal nerve is a branch of the vagus nerve (CN X). The internal branch of the superior laryngeal nerve provides sensory innervation to the base of the tongue, posterior surface of the epiglottis, aryepiglottic folds, and arytenoids. This branch originates lateral to the cornu of the hyoid bone, pierces the thyrohyoid membrane and travels under the mucosa in the pyriform recess. The external branch of the superior laryngeal nerve supplies motor innervation to the cricothyroid muscle and has no sensory component.

Several blocks of the internal branch have been described. In many instances, topical application of anesthetics in the pharyngeal/hypopharyngeal cavities will provide adequate analgesia. For a targeted noninvasive technique, the patient is asked to open their mouth widely and the tongue is grasped with a gauze pad. Right-angled forceps (e.g., Jackson–Krause forceps) with anesthetic-soaked cotton swabs are slid over the lateral tongue and into the pyriform sinuses bilaterally. The swabs are held in place for 5 minutes. An invasive block may be performed with the patient supine with the head extended. The clinician identifies the greater cornu of the hyoid bone beneath the angle of the mandible. Using one hand, medially directed pressure is applied to the contralateral hyoid cornu, displacing the hyoid toward the clinician. Caution must be taken to locate the carotid artery and displace it if necessary. The needle can then be inserted directly over the ipsilateral greater cornu and "walked" off the bone in an inferomedial direction until it can be passed through the thyrohyoid ligament to a depth of 1 to 2 cm. Before injecting local anesthetic, an aspiration test should be performed to ensure that either the pyriform sinus or a vessel has been entered. Local anesthetic (1.5 to 2 mL) is injected in the space between the thyrohyoid membrane and pharyngeal mucosa.

Sensory innervation of the vocal folds and the trachea is provided by the recurrent laryngeal nerve, another branch of the vagus nerve. Translaryngeal injection of local anesthetic is a simple technique that can produce adequate analgesia of these structures. A syringe with a fine needle or small-bore angiocatheter filled with a local anesthetic solution (e.g., 2 to 4 mL of 2% or 4% lidocaine) is inserted through the CTM perpendicular to the plane of the cervical spine. In this orientation, a needle advanced too far will likely impact the posterior aspect of the cricoid cartilage instead of puncturing the esophagus. In addition, this angle will help avoid trauma to the near-lying vocal folds. Constant retraction on the syringe plunger will result in air aspiration when the airway is entered, after which the anesthetic agent is injected. Coughing is likely to occur; thus, the needle should be stabilized to prevent mucosal abrasions. Alternatively, an angiocatheter can be advanced once air is aspirated, the needle removed, and the syringe reattached to administer the local anesthetic. Coughing can be advantageous for spread of local anesthesia; by having the patient exhale fully prior to injection, a breath will need to be taken prior to coughing, spreading the medication proximally before being spread distally by the cough.

Another effective technique of tracheal and vocal cord topicalization is to instill local anesthetic through the working channel of the flexible intubation scope. A disadvantage of this technique is that the local anesthetic can obscure the objective lens. This can be overcome by use of an epidural catheter, ideally multi-orificed inserted through the working channel, as described by Ovassapian.[204] Not only does this prevent obscuring of the view but it also allows "aiming" of the anesthetic stream.

Clinically Difficult Airway Scenarios

The clinician approaching the patient with a difficult airway has a vast armamentarium of instruments and techniques available.[205] Although this array can be confusing, textbook authors cannot dictate specific approaches in every situation; moreover, the variability of patient presentation makes specific recommendations difficult. Thus, in order to discuss management, the following section presents a number of brief clinical scenarios and the authors' preferred approach. Major alternative airway management techniques are discussed in this manner. All of the clinical cases described herein have been managed by the authors or a colleague. In these cases, as in actual practice, the first technique applied may not have been the best one. The principle of flexibility (and the willingness to change course quickly) will be emphasized repeatedly—the clinician must be prepared to alter their approach as the situation demands.

Case 1: Preoperative Endoscopy

A 52-year-old man presents for diagnostic DL, esophagoscopy, and biopsy of a base of the tongue tumor. The patient had sought otolaryngologic consultation after 6 months of progressive difficulty in swallowing and the sensation of fullness in his throat. Aside from sleep apnea requiring CPAP, he had no other medical issues and denied voice change or gastroesophageal reflux disease. In the preoperative holding area, oxymetazoline was applied to both nares, followed by 50 mg of 2% lidocaine viscous solution. A 3.2-mm diameter flexible intubation scope was then inserted via the more patent nostril. The scope's objective was positioned in the nasopharynx; on flexion, the epiglottis and glottis could be visualized. The patient was then taken to the operating room where general anesthesia was induced, mask ventilation performed and the trachea intubated using a videolaryngoscope.

Preoperative Endoscopic Airway Evaluation (PEAE)

Modeled on the airway examination employed by otolaryngologists in office consultations, PEAE can help guide airway management decisions.[23] In the case described, pathology of the hypopharyngeal airway complicated preoperative decision making—an airway mass might compromise tracheal intubation or facemask or SGA ventilation. As discussed earlier in the ASA Airway Guidelines Decision Tool, with only routine information available, an awake intubation might have been the best approach but was unnecessary in this case. By using PEAE to confirm the airway as nonthreatening, the decision could be made to proceed with routine induction of anesthesia. PEAE was studied in 148 patients presenting for intra-airway surgery. In 24% of patients, PEAE resulted in a modification of the initial clinically decided airway plan. Though clinical assessment dictated awake intubation in 44 patients, only 16 were judged to need awake intubation after PEAE. More importantly, 8 of 94 patients who were to have asleep airway management were switched to an awake technique after a concerning preoperative endoscopic examination.[23] PEAE typically requires less than 5 minutes to complete. During the examination, the clinician asks three key questions: (1) is there an obstruction to rapid intubation of the trachea; (2) is there a lesion that could interfere with the placement or function of an SGA; and (3) is there a lesion that routine laryngoscopy (direct or indirect) might dislodge or otherwise traumatize? An affirmative answer to any of these questions encourages awake intubation. As noted earlier, PEAE most often serves to reassure the clinician that lesions otherwise invisible on bedside physical examination will not be a hindrance to routine airway management. Likewise, PEAE can often reveal unexpectedly compromising lesions for which the clinician might have been otherwise unprepared. The use of PEAE has been expanded for evaluating at-risk airways after significant burn injuries[206] or predicting difficult intubation in any general anesthetic case.[207]

Case 2: Flexible Intubation Scope-aided Intubation

A 50-year-old man with symptomatic cervical vertebral disc herniation presents for disc resection and spinal fixation. His past medical history includes tobacco use, alcohol consumption, and gastroesophageal reflux. In the preoperative holding area, 0.4 mg of intravenous glycopyrrolate and bilateral nasal oxymetazoline are administered. Five percent lidocaine ointment (50 mg) is applied to the nares via long cotton-tipped applicators. Fifteen minutes later, in the operating room, when the patient reports a dry mouth, he receives 2 mg of intravenous midazolam, and topical anesthesia is administered to the remainder of the airway. An intubating oral airway is placed which does not elicit a gag reflex. A flexible intubation scope (FIS), preloaded with a 7.0-ID ETT, is advanced into the hypopharynx. The vocal ligaments are visualized and 4 mL of 4% lidocaine solution is injected toward the laryngeal and sublaryngeal structures through the accessory lumen of the FIS (Ovassapian catheter technique).[204] The distal end of the FIS is then advanced through the larynx and into the trachea until the carina is identified. The ETT is positioned above the carina and the FIS is removed. The anesthesia circuit is attached to the tracheal tube and a steady output of carbon dioxide is detected by capnography. A brief sensory and motor neurologic examination is performed by the attending surgeon, and general anesthesia is induced.

The Flexible Intubation Scope in Airway Management

In 1967, the technique of fiberoptic-aided intubation was first performed using a choledochoscope in a patient with Still disease (idiopathic, adult-onset arthritis) (21 Video 28-21).[208] By the late 1980s, it was recognized that the use of the flexible fiberoptic bronchoscope represented such a significant advancement in the management of the patient with a difficult airway that no anesthesiologist could afford not to be facile with the technique.[19] With advancements in imaging technology, the fragile optical strands of fiberoptic scopes have given way to video imaging via distally mounted cameras on the same flexible shafts. These flexible intubation scopes are the most versatile tools available for situations when it is difficult or dangerous to create a line of sight to the glottis.[205]

There is no firm indication for FIS intubation. There are, however, many clinical situations in which the FIS can be of unparalleled aid in securing the airway.[204] These include anticipated difficult intubation based on history or physical examination findings, unanticipated difficult intubation (in which other techniques have failed), upper or lower airway obstruction, unstable or fixed cervical spine disease, mass effect in the upper or lower airways, dental risk or damage, and awake intubation.[204] Unlike the other devices used to intubate the trachea, the FIS also allows visualization of structures below the level of the vocal folds. A FIS is also useful in verifying single- and double-lumen ETT placement, identifying subglottic pathology and facilitating pulmonary toilet (Fig. 28-24).

Unfortunately, clinicians rarely employ alternative techniques until a difficult situation arises. As with any critical competency, mastery of these techniques involves gaining and maintaining skills through use in *routine* airway management.[134] As an example, Heidegger et al. introduced a simple algorithm for incorporating flexible fiberoptic-aided tracheal intubation into daily practice as a routine alternative to DL. Their incidence of difficult intubation was 6 in 1,324 cases, or 0.049% – markedly lower than reported previously.[134]

Contraindications to FIS-aided intubation are relative (Table 28-20). Although FIS-aided intubation is a versatile and vital technique, there are several pitfalls, the most common of

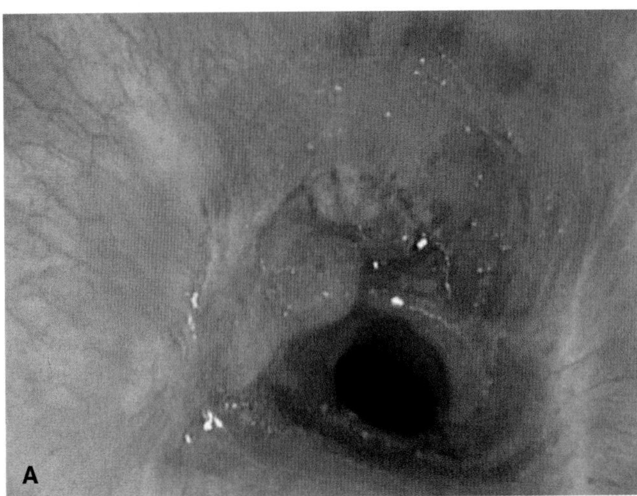

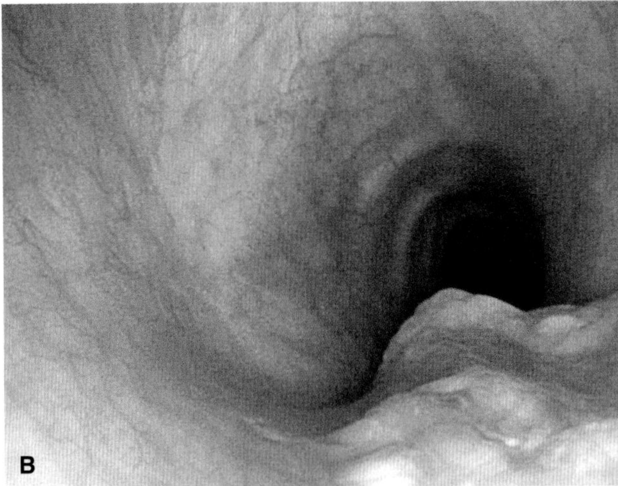

Figure 28-24 The flexible intubation scope may be useful for diagnosis and therapy below the level of the vocal ligaments, including examination of bronchial segments and pulmonary toilet. **A:** Laryngeal web found in an asymptomatic patient who had had one previous tracheal intubation. **B:** Tracheal mass in a patient with thyroid cancer.

which are listed in Table 28-21. Because the optical elements are small (the objective lens is typically 2 mm in diameter or smaller), minute amounts of airway secretions, blood, or traumatic debris can hinder visualization. Care must be taken to remove these obstacles from the airway beforehand. Administration of an antisialagogue (as discussed earlier) will produce a drying effect, but caution should be taken in patients who may not be able to tolerate an increase in heart rate. Vasoconstriction of the nose using topical oxymetazoline or phenylephrine reduces the chances of nasal bleeding if this route is chosen. If an awake FIS intubation is planned, the patient must be able to cooperate—a "quiet" airway, with little motion of the head, neck, tongue, and larynx, is vital to success. Finally, because FIS-aided intubation can require significant time (especially if the clinician is not facile with the device), hypoxia or impending airway loss is a contraindication and a more rapid method of securing the airway (e.g., SGA or emergency invasive airway) should be considered.

Any methods used for tracheal intubation in the asleep patient can also be employed for awake intubation. Awake intubation with video laryngoscopy,[209–213] combined video laryngoscopy and flexible intubation,[214,215] and SGA-guided flexible intubation[216,217] have been described.

Elements of the Flexible Intubation Scope

The early flexible intubation scopes were constructed with 10,000 to 30,000 glass fibers, 8 to 12 microns in diameter ("fiberscopes"). These devices tended to be fragile and difficult to repair. The new generation of video-based flexible scopes employs a light-sensitive CMOS chip in the distal insertion cord. This technology offers high-definition images at reduced production costs. A single-use version of this technology is available (aScope 3, Ambu, Ballerup, Denmark; Fig. 28-25).

Along with imaging elements, the insertion cord contains an *accessory lumen* or "working channel": a lumen, up to 2 mm in diameter, which travels from the distal tip to the handle. This can be used for applying suction, administering oxygen or medications (e.g., local anesthetics) or placing a wire for wire-guided airway exchange techniques (e.g., the Arndt Airway Exchange Catheter Kit, Cook Critical Care, Bloomington, IN). In general, flexible intubation scopes that are less than 2 mm in external diameter (e.g., pediatric) do not have a working channel.

The distal end of the insertion cord is hinged for movement. Two wires, traveling from the control lever in the handle down the length of the insertion cord control the movement of the distal tip in the sagittal plane. Coronal plane movement is accomplished by a combined use of the control lever and rotation of the *entire* FIS (from handle to distal end). It is key to keep the insertion cord completely straight as this maximizes rotational control by ensuring that rotation of the hand piece translates to identical rotation of the distal tip.

Table 28-20 Contraindications to Flexible Scope Intubation

Hypoxia
Significant airway secretions not relieved with antisialagogues and suction
Airway bleeding not relieved with suctioning
Local anesthetic allergy (for awake attempts)
Inability to cooperate (for awake attempts)

Table 28-21 Common Reasons for Failure of Flexible Scope Intubation

Lack of provider experience
Failure to adequately dry the airway: antisialagogue under-dose, rushed technique
Failure to adequately anesthetize the airway (awake patient)
Nasal cavity bleeding: inadequate vasoconstriction/lubrication, rushed technique
Obstructing base of tongue: insufficient tongue displacement (may require jaw thrust/tongue extrusion)
Hang-up: ETT/scope diameter ratio too large
Flexible scope fogging: suction or oxygen not attached to working channel, cold bronchoscope

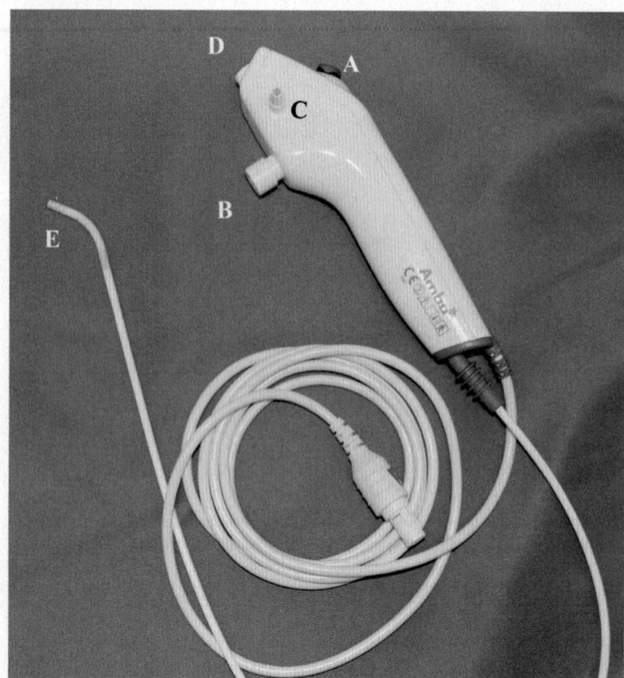

Figure 28-25 The Ambu aScope 3 single-use flexible intubation scope. (Ambu, Ballerup, Denmark). **A:** Directional control. **B:** Suction/oxygen activator valve. **C:** Suction/oxygen attachment port. **D:** Working channel access. **E:** Articulating objective end.

The final element of the flexible scope is the light source. In the fiberoptic devices, illumination of the objective is provided by one or two noncoherent bundles of glass fibers that transmit light from the handle to the distal tip. The light is provided either by a cord that emerges from the handle and is inserted into an endoscopic light source or a portable battery-operated light source on the handle. CMOS-based flexible scopes are fitted with an LED light source in the distal tip, obviating the need for glass bundles in the insertion cord.

Flexible bronchoscope-aided intubation is a technology-intense technique. Apart from the delicate optics, there are cameras, recorders, light sources, and a variety of disposable adjuncts that are typically required. Dedicated wheeled carts designed to carry equipment in a functional arrangement are often utilized.

Use of the Flexible Intubation Scope

The flexible intubation scope is held with the thumb over the control lever and the index finger poised over the working channel valve. The contralateral hand is used to steady and hold the insertion cord at the level of the patient. The art of endoscopy lies in the fine control required for steadying the bronchoscope while making minute directional adjustments and advancing the scope through the airway.

Traditionally, FISs are designed to be held in the left hand. The flexible scope insertion cord is lubricated with a medical-grade lubricant and threaded through the lumen of an ETT with the objective end emerging from the main ETT orifice. Once a clinically appropriate ETT is chosen, the FIS that best fits and fills the ETT lumen is employed. The greater the difference between the internal diameter of the ETT and the external diameter of the insertion cord, the greater the risk of "hang-up" on airway structures. There are limitations to this paradigm—smaller diameter scopes have less longitudinal strength and may be incapable of directing a tracheal tube.

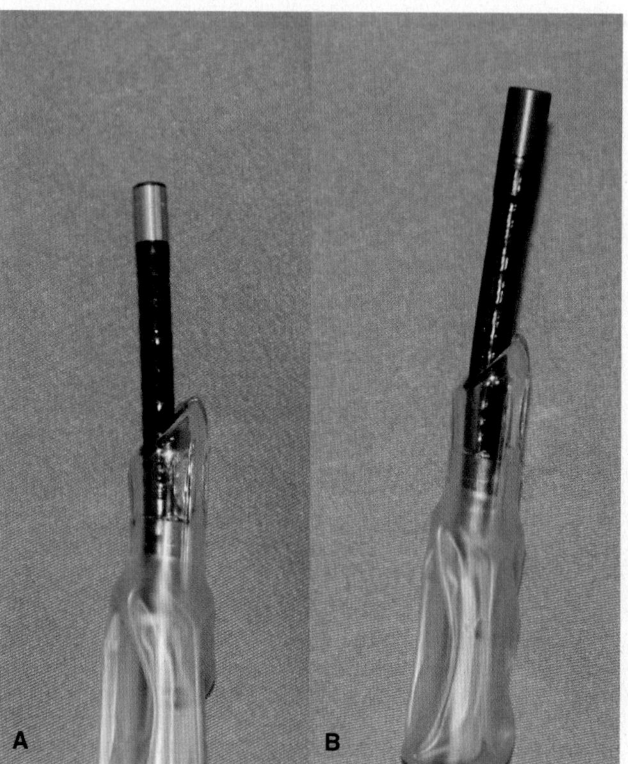

Figure 28-26 Size discrepancy between an airway exchange catheter or flexible intubation scope and a tracheal tube can create clefts that can trap tissues and hinder intubation. **A:** A 6.5-ID tracheal tube inserted over a 4.0-mm Storz Endovision F.I.V.E. scope with a notable cleft. (Copyright © KARL STORZ SE & Co. KG, Germany.) **B:** The same tracheal tube inserted over a 5.5-mm Storz Endovision F.I.V.E. scope with near-complete obliteration of the cleft.

"Hang-up" occurs when a cleft exists between the ETT and intubating guide (e.g., AEC, flexible scope insertion cord, gum-elastic bougie, retrograde wire, lighted stylet) because of a difference in their sizes (Fig. 28-26). This is most thoroughly described with flexible scope-aided intubation, for which it occurs in 20% to 30% of attempts.[204] Hang-up most commonly involves the right vocal cord, but may involve entrapment of the epiglottis, corniculate/arytenoid cartilages, or aryepiglottic folds. If hang-up occurs, rotation of the ETT 90 degrees counterclockwise places the bevel cleft anteriorly and improves passage.

Tracheal tube design may also affect hang-up. It has been suggested that the Parker Flex-Tip tracheal tube may pass the airway structures more easily than a standard ETT bevel.[218] The use of soft-tipped ETTs, asking the patient to inspire deeply during ETT advancement, and the "double setup," which uses a small ETT within a clinically adequate ETT (e.g., a 5.0 ID inside a 7.5 ID) to overcome the size differentials, all techniques that have been described to minimize the risk of hang-up.[219]

The route of intubation, either oral or nasal, is based on surgical needs, patient anatomy and clinical condition, and operator experience. The nasal route is considered anatomically easier by many clinicians, although cautions apply: the turbinates may obstruct ETT passage, bleed, be avulsed, or be painful when traumatized.[220] Nasal vasoconstrictors should be applied to reduce bleeding and promote nasal patency. The nasal tube should be softened in warm saline, water, or a blanket warmer[221] and well-lubricated prior to insertion. An ETT of the smallest size clinically acceptable should be chosen. However, a smaller diameter ETT may require a smaller diameter FIS which has less longitudinal

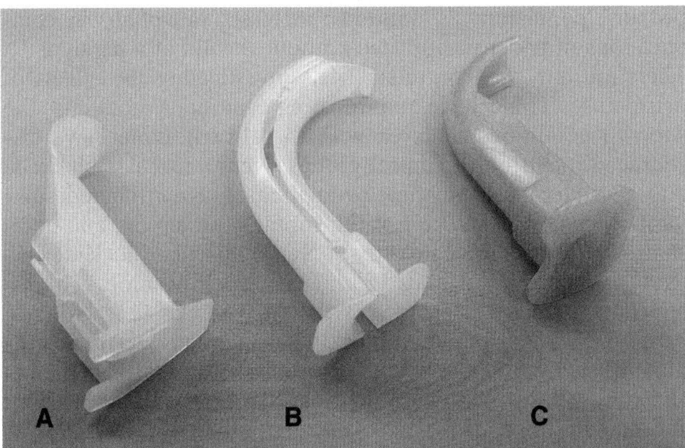

Figure 28-27 Intubating oral airways: (**A**) Ovassapian, (**B**) Berman and (**C**) Williams intubating oral airways.

strength and may be incapable of directing a tracheal tube. While mandibular advancement and/or tongue protrusion typically suffice, a variety of oral airways designed to facilitate flexible scope orotracheal intubation are commercially available. These devices function to provide a clear visual path from the oral aperture to the hypopharynx, keep the flexible scope and tracheal tube midline, prevent the patient from biting the insertion cord, and provide a clear airway for spontaneous or mask ventilation. The common characteristic of all intubating oral airways is a channel along the length of the airway that accommodates passage of an ETT.

The Ovassapian intubating oral airway (Fig. 28-27) provides two sets of semicircular, incomplete flexible flanges that stabilize the ETT (up to size 9 ID) in the midline and allow easy disengagement from the ETT after successful intubation. The flat lingual surface of the airway affords lateral and rotational stability. The Williams and the Berman airways both are molded plastic with circular internal lumens that guide the ETT toward the larynx. These airways have a smaller profile than the Ovassapian airway but tend to have less rotational stability. Because its internal lumen is a complete circle, the ETT circuit adapter must be removed prior to withdrawing a Williams airway. This may pose difficulty if the ETT has a fused circuit adapter. The Berman airway addresses this problem with a split along the length of one side. If the interincisor gap is adequate, malleable plastic seams on the contralateral side allow the airway to be removed laterally from around the ETT.

After successful navigation past the tongue (whether facilitated by tongue protrusion, mandibular advancement, or an intubating oral airway), the endoscopist visualizes the vocal folds. If glottic closure, gag, or coughing occurs, the operator may apply local anesthetic through the working channel, withdraw the scope and reinforce airway analgesia, or advance the scope into the larynx without further preparation. The action taken must be dictated by the individual clinical situation. In the elective scenario, there is likely to be time for additional airway preparation, whereas in the face of impending respiratory arrest, patient discomfort may need to be tolerated.

Once the larynx is entered, the flexible scope is advanced until the carina is visualized. The ETT is then advanced off the insertion cord and into the trachea. Simply having the flexible scope enter the trachea does not guarantee that the intubation will be successful; hang-up and accidental scope withdrawal (via coughing or inattention) may still occur. Therefore, in a patient with a critical airway, general anesthesia should not be induced until intratracheal tube placement is confirmed. The distance between the ETT and carina can be readily determined by advancing the scope to the carina and measuring how far it can be withdrawn before the objective re-enters the ETT bevel.

Table 28-22 Flexible Scope-Aided Intubation Techniques

Technique	Advantage
Endoscopy mask	Controlled (or assisted) ventilation maintained during or between attempts at flexible scope-aided intubation
Laryngeal mask	Excellent view of the larynx and ability to ventilate during or between attempts
Flexible scope-aided retrograde intubation	Guiding of the flexible intubating scope with a wire known to be in the trachea
Retrograde flexible intubation	Changing a tracheostomy to an oral or nasal tracheal tube when antegrade intubation is difficult or impossible
Flexible scope intubation with the aid of a rigid or video laryngoscope	Helpful with an obstructing mass or large epiglottis

The literature contains a number of variations and adjuncts to flexible scope-aided intubation. Table 28-22 lists several of these techniques.

Case 3: Failed Rapid-sequence Induction and the SGA

A 39-year-old man with obstructive sleep apnea (apnea-hypopnea index of 15) presents for elective uvulopharyngopalatoplasty. He has had no prior surgery. His maximal interincisor gap is 5 cm, thyromental distance is 7 cm, and his oropharyngeal view is a Samsoon–Young class 2.[222] *There is no limitation in neck flexion or extension. The patient has significant gastroesophageal reflux; thus, an RSI is planned. A hypnotic and neuromuscular blockade are administered. DL with a Macintosh 3 blade is made difficult by significant base-of-tongue hyperplasia, and all that can be visualized is a large epiglottis (Cormack–Lehane grade 3b view). The BURP maneuver does not improve glottic visualization. VL is utilized without improvement of the glottic view. Oxygen saturation has fallen from 100% to 92% and facemask ventilation is initiated with maintenance of cricoid pressure. Complete obstruction to ventilation is encountered. Placement of an oral airway, chin lift, jaw thrust, and two-person ventilation do not result in adequate mask ventilation. A size 5 LMA Classic (which had been prepared prior to induction) is inserted. A clear airway is immediately noted. A second dose of hypnotic is administered and the patient is intubated by the flexible scope aided passage of an Aintree Intubation Catheter (Cook Critical Care, Bloomington, IN). The LMA and flexible scope are removed and the Aintree catheter is used to guide a tracheal tube into position.*

The SGA in the Failed Airway

Kheterpal et al. found that 0.4% of patients presented difficulty in both mask ventilation and DL.[126] There have been many reports of cases in which the airway was rescued with an SGA.[223,224] A wealth of literature describes the use of the SGAs in both awake and unconscious patients in anticipated and unanticipated difficult airway situations, cervical spine injury, and pediatric dysmorphic syndromes.[96,97,187]

The characteristics of the SGAs that underlie their superiority as a tool in the management of the difficult airway are numerous: Their placement follows an intrinsic pathway (swallowing) which, unlike laryngoscopy, requires minimal tissue distortion; they can be utilized as part of a blind technique not hindered by blood, secretions, debris, and edema from previous attempts at laryngoscopy[225]; and, as the anatomic issues that result in difficult laryngoscopy do not necessarily result in difficult SGA placement, they are an excellent choice for airway rescue when laryngoscopy has failed. Because the success of SGA placement does not fully depend on anatomy that can be assessed on routine physical examination, many typical airway assessment measures do not apply.[226]

The major disadvantage of SGA use during cardiopulmonary resuscitation is the lack of mechanical protection from aspiration.[3,227,228] Despite these drawbacks, the rate of regurgitation during cardiopulmonary resuscitation with an LMA (3.5%) has been shown to be less than with bag-valve-mask ventilation (12.4%).[76] Even in cases of regurgitation, pulmonary aspiration is a rare event[72] and a secondary concern to life-threatening hypoxemia. Had one been available, an intubating SGA would have been an excellent choice in this case scenario.

Case 4: Flexibility and Back-up Planning in Difficult Airway Management

Thirteen hours after admission to the intensive care unit, a 76-year-old woman with head, neck, and facial trauma from a motor vehicle accident is noted to have progressive decline in her level of consciousness and respiratory effort. On examination, there appears to be an adequate interincisor gap and thyromental distance, but the oropharyngeal view and cervical range of motion cannot be evaluated. Because of the inability to evaluate her airway fully with respect to ease of intubation, an awake technique is chosen. Oropharyngeal blood from continued epistaxis suggests that adequate drying and analgesia of the airway may be difficult and that the use of a flexible intubation device may not be prudent. Techniques requiring significant patient preparation are not considered due to the rapid progression of the patient's respiratory failure. Blind nasal intubation is contraindicated based on the obvious facial trauma and the risk of cribriform plate disruption. Although the patient's altered mental status is believed to reflect an intracranial process, the risk of airway loss is felt to be the primary clinical hazard. Awake VL is attempted with manual in-line axial stabilization of the neck. After clearing fresh blood from the pharynx, a Cormack–Lehane grade 3 laryngeal view is obtained. Due to significant patient resistance (head and neck movement and biting of the laryngoscope), tracheal intubation is not achieved. The decision is made to proceed with RSI and intubation, with emergency cricothyrotomy as the back-up plan. After a head and neck surgeon is consulted and surgical preparation of the neck is completed, application of manual in-line stabilization, and preoxygenation, intravenous etomidate and succinylcholine are administered, DL is undertaken, the larynx is easily visualized, and the trachea is intubated.

Neuromuscular Blockade and Laryngoscopy

In the case described, the use of neuromuscular blockade significantly improved laryngeal visualization (22 Video 28-22). In one study, the use of neuromuscular blockade for DL increased intubation success rate and was associated with fewer intubation attempts, incidents of airway trauma, esophageal intubations, aspiration events, and even deaths.[229] A retrospective study in the pediatric population also found an increased rate of airway complications in patients intubated without the aid of a paralytic.[230] There are few well-controlled trials investigating the effects of neuromuscular blockade on intubating conditions though, as the superior conditions achieved with these medications have discouraged inclusion of control groups. Neuromuscular blockade improves laryngoscopic view by facilitating temporomandibular joint relaxation, relaxation of the supraglottic larynx, and anterior movement of the epiglottis.[231] Neuromuscular blockade also tends to fix the vocal folds in a neutral open position.[57] It also typically facilitates facemask ventilation. The classic teaching of withholding neuromuscular blocking agents until facemask ventilation has been demonstrated is rapidly being abandoned. Several studies show that neuromuscular blockade does not worsen and may improve mask ventilation.[56,232] When a neuromuscular blocker is administered with the induction agent there is less time between the beginning of apnea and ideal intubation conditions. Therefore, even if mask ventilation proves challenging, simultaneously administration of induction agent with neuromuscular blocker can increase the likelihood for tracheal intubation with ideal intubation conditions.

Changing Course

The scenario described in Case 4 is unusual in that the clinical situation necessitated abandoning the initial plan for awake intubation. The conditions described were more akin to the "crash" airway described by Walls.[233] In this case, the administration of a neuromuscular blocker, which might be considered contraindicated in the assessed difficult-to-intubate patient, allowed for full visualization of the larynx. Knowing that failure to intubate would likely result in loss of the airway, the clinical team was wisely prepared for an invasive emergency airway. Although the ASA decision tree is a valuable tool in the management of the difficult airway, the clinician must be prepared for cases that do not fit the mold. As stated earlier, adaptability in rapidly changing clinical scenarios is critical to the success of airway management.

Other Devices

An ever-increasing number of airway management devices are commercially available. Although encyclopedic coverage of these tools is beyond the scope of this chapter, a review of the more established equipment follows.

Esophageal Tubes with Laryngeal Openings

Esophageal tubes with laryngeal openings are SGAs with designs based on the propensity for blindly inserted oral tubes to enter the esophagus. They can be of single-lumen (King LT, Ambu, Ballerup, Denmark) and double-lumen (Combitube, Covidien, Mansfield, MA, and EasyTube, Teleflex, Research Triangle Park, NC) design with distal esophageal and proximal pharyngeal cuffs on either side of the laryngeal apertures, which act as ventilation ports (Fig. 28-28). When properly inflated, the cuffs prevent esophageal and oral leakage of gasses, making the larynx the route of least resistance for inspired gasses. These devices are quicker and easier for inexperienced providers to place than are ETTs.[234] This, combined with data showing the deleterious effects of repeat laryngoscopy,[235,236] has led to use of these devices by prehospital emergency providers who may have limited or infrequent experience with laryngoscopy.

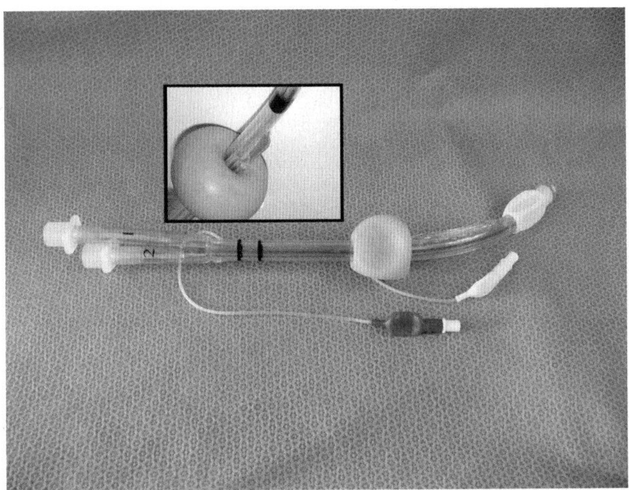

Figure 28-28 The Esophageal Tracheal Combitube. *Inset*: The fiberoptic port of the EasyTube.

Airway Introducers

Airway introducers are semimalleable stylets that may be blindly manipulated through the glottis when a poor laryngeal view is obtained (Cormack-Lehane grade 3 or 4) (23 Video 28-23). An ETT is then "threaded" over the introducer and into the trachea. These introducers, sometimes referred to as bougies, are generally low cost and highly portable. In the emergency department, first attempt emergency tracheal intubation success was higher using a bougie (98%) as compared with an ETT and stylet (87%).[237] The Eschmann introducer (Eschmann Health Care, Kent, England) is a 60-cm long, 15-French bougie with a 40-degree coudé tip 3.5 cm from its distal end. This introducer (also known as the *gum elastic bougie*) can be manipulated under the epiglottis, its angled segment directed anteriorly toward the larynx. Once it has entered the larynx and trachea, the operator often feels "clicks" as the bougie's tip passes over the cartilaginous structures of the anterior trachea. A similar device, the Frova Intubating Introducer (Cook Critical Care, Bloomington, IN) is a disposable device with a narrow internal lumen. Insufflation of oxygen via the lumen is discouraged due to reported cases of barotrauma. The lumen may also be used to detect carbon dioxide and to detect inadvertent esophageal placement. An optional "stiffening" stylet can be placed through the lumen to increase device rigidity.

Transcricothyroid Membrane Procedures

11 When intubation and mask and SGA ventilation fail, airway access via the extrathoracic trachea may be warranted (Table 28-23). Though the noninvasive tools of the modern airway armamentarium can manage most situations, the clinician must be familiar with these alternative techniques of intubation, oxygenation, and ventilation for both elective and emergency airway access.

Table 28-23 Criteria for Performing Emergent Invasive Airway Management

When all five criteria are met, an emergent invasive airway is indicated
Cannot intubate
Cannot ventilate
Cannot awaken patient
Supraglottic airway has failed
Clinically significant hypoxemia

Table 28-24 Equipment for Retrograde Wire Intubation

Angiocatheter (18 gauge or larger)
Luer-lock syringe (3 mL or larger)
Guide wire: • Type: J-type end preferable • Length: at least 2.5 times the length of a standard ETT (typically 110–120 cm) • Diameter: capable of passing via chosen angiocatheter
Other: scalpel blade, nerve hook, Magill forceps, silk suture

Retrograde Wire-Aided Tracheal Intubation

The technique involves the antegrade passage of an ETT into the airway using a wire that has been passed into the larynx via a percutaneous puncture through the cricothyroid or cricotracheal membrane. This wire is blindly passed in the cephalad direction into the hypopharynx, pharynx, and out of the mouth or nose and then used as an intubating conduit. The basic equipment used for retrograde intubation is listed in Table 28-24.

Retrograde wire-aired intubation (RWI) has been described in a number of clinical situations as a primary intubation technique (both elective and urgently) and for use after failed attempts at DL, fiberoptic-aided intubation, and LMA-guided intubation.[55] The most common indication for RWI is the inability to visualize the vocal folds owing to blood, secretions, unstable cervical spine or anatomic variations (e.g., upper airway malignancy, mandibular fracture, massive airway trauma). Contraindications include lack of access to the CTM or cricotracheal ligament (such as with severe neck deformity, obesity, or overlying mass), laryngotracheal disease (stenosis, malignancy, infection), coagulopathy, and overlying skin infection.

Common complications reported with RWI include bleeding, subcutaneous emphysema, pneumomediastinum, pneumothorax, breath-holding, a caudally traveling wire, and trigeminal nerve trauma.

Cricothyrotomy

Cricothyrotomy, cricothyroidotomy, coniotomy, and minitracheostomy are synonyms for establishing an air passage through the CTM. The CTM is a fibroelastic membrane that overlays the tracheal mucosa and is attached to the inferior border of the thyroid cartilage and superior edge of the cricoid cartilage. Although cricothyrotomy is the procedure of choice in an emergency situation, it may also be of use in elective situations when there is limited access to the trachea (e.g., severe cervical kyphoscoliosis). Cricothyrotomy is contraindicated in children younger than 6 years of age and in patients with laryngeal fractures.

Percutaneous Emergency Airway Access (PEAA), as a form of cricothyrotomy, is the most familiar to anesthesiologists (24 Video 28-24). The ASA Guidelines lists PEAA as an option in the "cannot mask ventilate/cannot intubate" (CNV/CNI) situation. PEAA is a simple and relatively safe means to sustain the patient's life in this critical situation.[55] Three techniques are commonly used for PEAA: narrow-bore catheter over a needle, large-bore cannula over a wire or trochar, and surgical incision with a blade[200] with or without a tube guide.[238] Success rates of these techniques vary greatly and are highly dependent on operator experience and the clinical scenario. As an example, the success rate of cannula cricothyrotomy performed by an anesthesia provider is roughly 50%,[1] while the success rate of an emergency surgical airway performed by a surgeon or trained prehospital provider is 90% to 100%.[1,239] This is not to suggest that PEAA be avoided by the anesthesia provider, but rather to advise that, if available, a surgeon experienced in cricothyrotomy may be the better choice for the initial attempt at surgical airway management.

A body of literature exists detailing the jerry-rigging of conveyance systems for PEAA and the use of intravenous catheters for transtracheal puncture. These systems have proven to be faulty, inadequate, and dangerous.[240] Catheters designed for intravenous infusion are known to kink in the airway.[241] Dedicated devices, such as the Cook transtracheal airway catheter (Cook Critical Care, Bloomington, IN), are made of kink-resistant materials and designed specifically for this task. The Ravussin translaryngeal catheter (VBM Medizintechnik, Sulz am Neckar Germany) is precurved to reduce kinking.

Before contemplating PEAA, the location of the CTM will need to be identified. With the aid of US, the CTM can be identified in 80% to 90% of adult patients.[12,242] The CTM should be identified in every patient as part of routine physical assessment; applying this examination to all patients should improve familiarity with the surface landmarks.[200] US can reveal the CTM as a lucent shadow between opaque cartilaginous structures and may be useful in emergency situations if immediately available.

When performing any emergency invasive airway, the patient is positioned supine with the head midline or extended on the neck and thorax (if not contraindicated by the clinical situation). After aseptic preparation, local anesthetic may be injected over the CTM (if the patient is awake and time permits). The clinician stands to the side of the patient with the dominant hand cephalad; the nondominant hand can be used to stabilize the larynx. A large-bore translaryngeal catheter (14 gauge or larger) attached to a 5- to 10-mL empty or fluid-filled (saline or local anesthetic) syringe is used. The catheter-needle is advanced at right angles to the plane of the cervical spine through the caudad third of the CTM. From the moment of skin puncture, there should be constant aspiration on the syringe plunger. Free aspiration of air confirms entrance into the airway (air-contrast technique) but does not indicate the direction that the catheter travels in the larynx; this is important, as cephalad advancement will not provide adequate oxygenation. Unless there is significant pulmonary fluid (e.g., blood or aspirated liquid), the aspiration of air should be incontrovertible. The needle–catheter assembly should be advanced slightly prior to threading of the catheter into the airway.

Once the catheter has been successfully placed, a high-pressure oxygen source should be attached. A 50-psi oxygen source with a metered and adjustable hand-controlled valve and a Luer-lock connector (Fig. 28-29) is down-regulated to 15 to 30 psi (central hospital supply or regulated cylinder) and delivered through the catheter. Insufflations should last 1 to 1.5 seconds at a rate of 12 insufflations per minute. Insufflation and expiration ratios, as well as driving pressure, are adjusted to provide visible chest excursion and recoil. If a 14-gauge catheter has been placed, this system will deliver a tidal volume of 400 to 700 mL. Low-pressure systems cannot provide enough flow to expand the chest adequately for oxygenation and ventilation (e.g., Ambu bag, 6 psi; anesthesia machine common gas outlet, 20 psi). It is important to remember that systems delivering pressurized oxygen require a path for gas egress.[243] Standard high-pressure regulating valves, as described earlier, are unidirectional and generally contraindicated when the upper airway is completely obstructed. Fortunately, this tends to be an uncommon situation. In any case, the clinician employing any type of translaryngeal oxygenation must strive to maintain upper airway patency with devices such as oral airways, nasal airways, or SGAs.

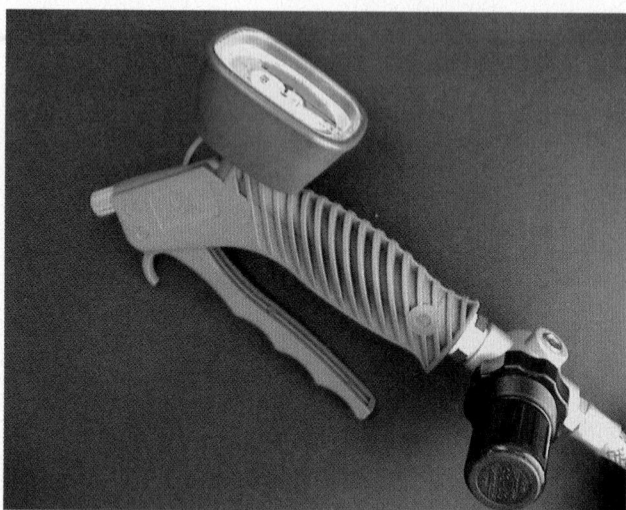

Figure 28-29 System for regulation of a high-pressure oxygen source for transtracheal jet ventilation.

PEAA can also be accomplished using low-flow oxygen delivery meters, which are common in the hospital environment. These systems can deliver a constant flow of 15 L/min and have been shown to be effective for resuscitation. In general, these devices utilize “flow interruption.” Flow is directed to the patient during the inspiratory phase, then diverted during expiration. As discussed earlier, jerry-rigged devices often fail to function as desired. For example, using a standard three-way stopcock as a flow diverter is potentially hazardous, as forward flow (inspiration) is never fully stopped.[244] The Enk flow modulator (Cook Critical Care, Bloomington, IN) is a hand-operated flow diverter that not only stops forward gas flow during the expiratory phase but also acts as a pathway for passive expiratory flow (Fig. 28-30). The Enk flow modulator has been used successfully in models of near and complete upper airway obstruction.[240]

A relatively newer concept in PEAA is expiratory ventilatory assistance.[245] Using the Bernoulli principle, the Ventrain (Ventinova Medical B.V., Eindhoven, The Netherlands; Fig. 28-30) is capable of *active* gas removal from a rescue catheter during the expiratory phase of PEAA. The benefit is the avoidance of air trapping in the

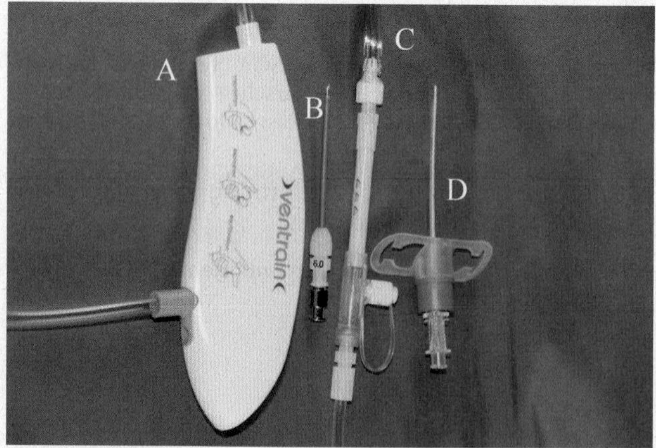

Figure 28-30 **A:** Ventrain. **B:** Cook Transtracheal Catheter. **C:** Enk flow modulator. **D:** Ravussin needle.

lungs, especially when the upper airway is completely obstructed. The device can achieve physiologic minute ventilation via a 2-mm ID transtracheal catheter[245] and has been effective in oxygenation and carbon dioxide removal in two large animal models.[246,247] In the first of these studies, the upper airways were critically or completely obstructed and the animals ventilated for 15 minutes via the Ventrain or a commercially available jet ventilation system. While both devices facilitated reoxygenation, the Ventrain was associated with superior minute ventilation (4.7 vs. 0.1 L/min), less acidosis (pH of 7.34 vs. 7.01), and decreased peak airway pressure on rescue (16 vs. 40 cm H_2O).[246] In the latter study, in a complete upper airway obstruction model, the peak airway pressure was significantly less with the Ventrain using an I:E of 1:1 (30 mbar) than with the jet ventilator at a ratio of 1:4 (50 mbar),[247] highlighting the benefit of expiratory ventilatory assistance. The Ventrain has also proven effective in both elective and emergent human airway management.[248,249]

Specialized percutaneous cricothyrotomy systems have been developed to improve the ease of transtracheal ventilation. These devices generally provide large-bore access adequate for oxygenation and ventilation with low-pressure systems. The Melker emergency cricothyrotomy catheter set (Cook Critical Care, Bloomington, IN) is placed using Seldinger technique and comes in a variety of cannula sizes (3.5-, 4-, and 6-mm ID, both cuffed and uncuffed). Preparation and positioning of the patient are the same as with needle cricothyrotomy. A 1- to 1.5-cm vertical incision, through the skin only, is made over the lower third of the CTM. Aiming 45-degrees caudally, a percutaneous puncture of the CTM is made with the provided 18-gauge needle–catheter assembly and syringe. After air is aspirated, the catheter is advanced into the trachea as described earlier. The provided guidewire is inserted through the catheter and into the trachea. The catheter is removed and the large-bore tracheal cannula, fitted internally with a curved dilator, is threaded onto the wire. The dilator is advanced through the CTM using firm pressure. Significant resistance on advancement typically indicates that the skin incision needs to be extended. Once the cannula–dilator assembly has been fully inserted, the dilator and wire are removed. The cannula's 15-mm circuit adapter is attached to a self-inflating resuscitation bag or anesthesia circuit and ventilation is initiated.

Other percutaneous needle systems include the Portex Cricothyroidotomy Kit (Smiths Medical, Minneapolis, MN) and the Quicktrach transtracheal catheter (VBM Medizintechnik, Sulz am Neckar, Germany). Nonneedle puncture techniques are beyond the scope of this text.

Severe complications of PEAA are typically related to barotrauma. Analysis of the ASA Close Claims Database reveals that 89% of patients who received transtracheal jet ventilation developed pneumothorax, pneumomediastinum, or subcutaneous emphysema[250]; bilateral tension pneumothorax has also been reported.[251] Causes of air insufflation into the paratracheal spaces include a misplaced cannula, multiple tracheal punctures, and cannula migration due to patient coughing.

The Scalpel-Bougie-Tube technique is perhaps the simplest PEAA method,. This technique requires three pieces of equipment: a scalpel, a bougie or tracheal tube introducer, and a small ETT (a 6.0 I.D. ETT is often recommended). Most importantly, it relies on the practitioner's ability to identify the CTM. Once identified, the scalpel, which is positioned axially, is used to cut down through the CTM and into the trachea. At this point, the blade can either be removed and a finger bluntly dissected into the trachea or the blade can be turned 90 degrees to dilate the opening. Once the cricothyrotomy is dilated, a bougie is inserted alongside the now sagitally positioned blade or finger and the ETT is advanced over the bougie. The ETT cuff should not be advanced more than a few centimeters into the trachea to avoid endobronchial intubation which can lead to bronchospasm or inadequate ventilation. A commonly used technique developed by the United States Veterans Administration and can be seen online at https://www.sharedfedtraining.org/external_content/DAARCweb/DAARC/index.html.

Conclusions

Apart from monitoring, management of the "routine" airway is the most common task of the anesthesia provider. Even during the administration of regional anesthesia, the airway must be monitored and possibly supported. The consequences of a lost airway are so devastating that the clinician can never afford a lackadaisical approach.

Although the ASA Task Force on Management of the Difficult Airway has given the medical community an immensely valuable tool in the approach to the patient with the difficult airway, judgment, experience, the clinical situation, and available resources all affect the appropriateness of airway plans.

If the last decade of the 20th century was the decade of the SGA, the first decades of the 21st century have witnessed the application of digital imaging to airway management. Although an increasingly vast array of devices exists, the clinician does not need to be expert in all the equipment and techniques, and no single device can be considered superior to another when viewed in isolation. Rather, a broad range of approaches should be mastered so that the failure of one does not preclude safe airway management and emergency rescue. The clinician's judgment and resources, both equipment and personnel, determine the effectiveness of any technique. When managing the difficult airway, flexibility prevails or rigidity.

For additional information please see 25 Videos 28.25 and 26 28.26 in the eBook bundled with this text.

For further review and interactivities, please see the videos and narrative interactive clinical vignettes (NICVs) accessible in the complimentary eBook bundled with this text. Access instructions are located on the inside front cover.

REFERENCES

1. Cook TM, Woodall N, Frerk C. Major complications of airway management in the UK: results of the Fourth National Audit Project of the Royal College of Anaesthetists and the Difficult Airway Society. Part 1: Anaesthesia †. *Br J Anaesth*. 2011;106(5):617–631.
2. Apfelbaum JL, Hagberg CA, Connis RT, et al. 2022 American society of anesthesiologists practice guidelines for management of the difficult airway*. *Anesthesiology*. 2022;136(1):31–81.
3. Frerk C, Mitchell VS, McNarry AF, et al. Difficult Airway Society 2015 guidelines for management of unanticipated difficult intubation in adults. *Br J Anaesth*. 2015;115(6):827–848.
4. Joffe AM, Aziz MF, Posner KL, Duggan LV, Mincer SL, Domino KB. Management of difficult tracheal intubation: a closed claims analysis. *Anesthesiology*. 2019;131(4):818–829.
5. Li G, Warner M, Lang BH, Huang L, Sun LS. Epidemiology of anesthesia-related mortality in the United States, 1999–2005. *Anesthesiology*. 2009;110(4):759–765.
6. Hove Lars D, Steinmetz J, Christoffersen JK, Møller A, Nielsen J, Schmidt H. Analysis of deaths related to anesthesia in the Period 1996–2004 from closed claims registered by the Danish patient insurance association. *Anesthesiology*. 2007;106(4):675–680.
7. Ellis SJ, Newland MC, Simonson JA, et al. Anesthesia-related cardiac arrest. *Anesthesiology*. 2014;120(4):829–838.
8. Rosenblatt WH. The airway approach algorithm: a decision tree for organizing preoperative airway information. *J Clin Anesth*. 2004;16(4):312–316.
9. Westhorpe RN. The position of the larynx in children and its relationship to the ease of intubation. *Anaesth Intensive Care*. 1987;15(4):384–388.
10. Iohom G, Ronayne M, Cunningham AJ. Prediction of difficult tracheal intubation. *Eur J Anaesthesiol*. 2005;20(1):31–36.

11. Alshareef H, Al Saawi A, Almazroua F, Alyami H, Reilly GO, Mitra B. Localisation of the cricothyroid membrane by digital palpation in the emergency department. *Postgrad Med J.* 2018;94(1114):442–445.
12. Kristensen MS, Teoh WH. Ultrasound identification of the cricothyroid membrane: the new standard in preparing for front-of-neck airway access. *Br J Anaesth.* 2021;126(1):22–27.
13. Kristensen MS, Teoh WH, Graumann O, Laursen CB. Ultrasonography for clinical decision-making and intervention in airway management: from the mouth to the lungs and pleurae. *Insights Imaging.* 2014;5(2):253–279.
14. Sykes WS. *Essays on the First Hundred Years of Anaesthesia*, vol. 3. Churchill Livingstone; 1982.
15. Brimacombe J. *Laryngeal Mask Anesthesia: Principles and Practice*, 2nd ed. Saunders Ltd.; 2004.
16. Brandt L. The first reported oral intubation of the human trachea. *Anesth Analg.* 1987; 66(11):1198–1199.
17. Magill IW. Endotracheal anaesthesia. *Proc R Soc Med.* 1928;22(2):83–88.
18. Mendelson CL. The aspiration of stomach contents into the lungs during obstetric anesthesia. *Am J Obstet Gynecol.* 1946;52(2):191–205.
19. Ovassapian A, Yelich SJ, Dykes MH, Golman ME. Learning fibreoptic intubation: use of simulators V. traditional teaching. *Br J Anaesth.* 1988;61(2):217–220.
20. Kaplan MB, Ward DS, Berci G. A new video laryngoscope—an aid to intubation and teaching. *J Clin Anesth.* 2002;14(8):620–626.
21. Breitmeier D, Wilke N, Schulz Y, et al. The lingual tonsillar hyperplasia in relation to unanticipated difficult intubation. *Am J Forensic Med Pathol.* 2005;26(2):131–135.
22. Langeron O, Masso E, Huraux C, et al. Prediction of difficult mask ventilation. *Anesthesiology.* 2000;92(5):1229–1236.
23. Rosenblatt W, Ianus AI, Sukhupragarn W, Fickenscher A, Sasaki C. Preoperative endoscopic airway examination (PEAE) provides superior airway information and may reduce the use of unnecessary awake intubation. *Anesth Analg.* 2011;112(3):602–607.
24. Roth D, Pace NL, Lee A, et al. Airway physical examination tests for detection of difficult airway management in apparently normal adult patients. *Cochrane Database Syst Rev.* 2018; 5(5):Cd008874.
25. Wilson ME, Spiegelhalter D, Robertson JA, Lesser P. Predicting difficult intubation. *Br J Anaesth.* 1988;61(2):211–216.
26. Patel SK, Whitten CW, Ivy R, et al. Failure of the laryngeal mask airway. *Anesth Analg.* 1998; 86(2):438–439.
27. Naguib M, Malabarey T, AlSatli RA, Al Damegh S, Samarkandi AH. Predictive models for difficult laryngoscopy and intubation. A clinical, radiologic and three-dimensional computer imaging study. *Can J Anaesth.* 1999;46(8):748–759.
28. Eberhart LHJ, Arndt C, Aust H-J, Kranke P, Zoremba M, Morin A. A simplified risk score to predict difficult intubation: development and prospective evaluation in 3763 patients. *Eur J Anaesthesiol.* 2010;27(11):935–940.
29. Cortellazzi P, Minati L, Falcone C, Lamperti M, Caldiroli D. Predictive value of the El-Ganzouri multivariate risk index for difficult tracheal intubation: a comparison of Glidescope ® videolaryngoscopy and conventional Macintosh laryngoscopy. *Br J Anaesth.* 2007;99(6): 906–911.
30. Aziz MF, Healy D, Kheterpal S, Fu RF, Dillman D, Brambrink AM. Routine clinical practice effectiveness of the Glidescope in difficult airway management: an analysis of 2,004 Glidescope intubations, complications, and failures from two institutions. *Anesthesiology.* 2011;114(1):34–41.
31. Aziz MF, Bayman EO, Van Tienderen MM, Todd MM, StAGE Investigator Group, Brambrink AM. Predictors of difficult videolaryngoscopy with GlideScope® or C-MAC® with D-blade: secondary analysis from a large comparative videolaryngoscopy trial. *Br J Anaesth.* 2016;117(1):118–123.
32. Kheterpal S, Martin L, Shanks AM, Tremper KK. Prediction and outcomes of impossible mask ventilation. *Anesthesiology.* 2009;110(4):891–897.
33. Lundstrøm LH, Rosenstock CV, Wetterslev J, Nørskov AK. The DIFFMASK score for predicting difficult facemask ventilation: a cohort study of 46,804 patients. *Anaesthesia.* 2019; 74(10):1267–1276.
34. Das SK, Choupoo NS, Haldar R, Lahkar A. Transtracheal ultrasound for verification of endotracheal tube placement: a systematic review and meta-analysis. *Can J Anaesth.* 2015; 62(4):413–423.
35. Sutherasan Y, Theerawit P, Hongphanut T, Kiatboonsri C, Kiatboonsri S. Predicting laryngeal edema in intubated patients by portable intensive care unit ultrasound. *J Crit Care.* 2013; 28(5):675–680.
36. Kristensen MS. Ultrasonography in the management of the airway. *Acta Anaesthesiol Scand.* 2011;55(10):1155–1173.
37. Jense HG, Dubin SA, Silverstein PI, O'Leary-Escolas U. Effect of obesity on safe duration of apnea in anesthetized humans. *Anesth Analg.* 1991;72(1):89–93.
38. Tanoubi I, Drolet P, Donati F. Optimizing preoxygenation in adults. *Can J Anaesth.* 2009; 56(6):449–466.
39. Kwei P, Matzelle S, Wallman D, Ong M, Weightman W. Inadequate preoxygenation during spontaneous ventilation with single patient use self-inflating resuscitation bags. *Anaesth Intensive Care.* 2006;34(5):685–686.
40. Boyce JR, Ness T, Castroman P, Gleysteen JJ. A preliminary study of the optimal anesthesia positioning for the morbidly obese patient. *Obes Surg.* 2003;13(1):4–9.
41. Ramachandran SK, Cosnowski A, Shanks A, Turner CR. Apneic oxygenation during prolonged laryngoscopy in obese patients: a randomized, controlled trial of nasal oxygen administration. *J Clin Anesth.* 2010;22(3):164–168.
42. Weingart SD, Levitan RM. Preoxygenation and prevention of desaturation during emergency airway management. *Ann Emerg Med.* 2012;59(3):165–175.e161.
43. Badiger S, John M, Fearnley RA, Ahmad I. Optimizing oxygenation and intubation conditions during awake fibre-optic intubation using a high-flow nasal oxygen-delivery system. *Br J Anaesth.* 2015;115(4):629–632.
44. Patel A, Nouraei SAR. Transnasal humidified rapid-insufflation ventilatory exchange (THRIVE): a physiological method of increasing apnoea time in patients with difficult airways. *Anaesthesia.* 2015;70(3):323–329.
45. Gustafsson IM, Lodenius Å, Tunelli J, Ullman J, Jonsson FM. Apnoeic oxygenation in adults under general anaesthesia using transnasal humidified rapid-insufflation ventilatory exchange (THRIVE) – a physiological study. *Br J Anaesth.* 2017;118(4):610–617.
46. Laviola M, Das A, Chikhani M, Bates DG, Hardman JG. Computer simulation clarifies mechanisms of carbon dioxide clearance during apnoea. *Br J Anaesth.* 2019;122(3): 395–401.
47. Hermez LA, Spence CJ, Payton MJ, Nouraei SAR, Patel A, Barnes TH. A physiological study to determine the mechanism of carbon dioxide clearance during apnoea when using transnasal humidified rapid insufflation ventilatory exchange (THRIVE). *Anaesthesia.* 2019;74(4): 441–449.
48. Riva T, Préel N, Theiler L, et al. Evaluating the ventilatory effect of transnasal humidified rapid insufflation ventilatory exchange in apnoeic small children with two different oxygen flow rates: a randomised controlled trial(). *Anaesthesia.* 2021;76(7):924–932.
49. Riva T, Greif R, Kaiser H, et al. Carbon dioxide changes during high-flow nasal oxygenation in apneic patients: a single-center randomized controlled noninferiority trial. *Anesthesiology.* 2022;136(1):82–92.
50. Bradley WPL, Lyons C. Facemask ventilation. *BJA Educ.* 2022;22(1):5–11.
51. Joffe AM, Hetzel S, Liew EC. A two-handed jaw-thrust technique is superior to the one-handed "EC-clamp" technique for mask ventilation in the apneic unconscious person. *Anesthesiology.* 2010;113(4):873–879.
52. Isono S, Tanaka A, Ishikawa T, Tagaito Y, Nishino T. Sniffing position improves pharyngeal airway patency in anesthetized patients with obstructive sleep apnea. *Anesthesiology.* 2005;103(3):489–494.
53. Chang JE, Seol T, Hwang JY. Body position and the effectiveness of mask ventilation in anaesthetised paralysed obese patients: a randomised cross-over study. *Eur J Anaesthesiol.* 2021; 38(8):825–830.
54. Conlon NP, Sullivan RP, Herbison PG, Zacharias M, Buggy DJ. The effect of leaving dentures in place on bag-mask ventilation at induction of general anesthesia. *Anesth Analg.* 2007; 105(2):370–373.
55. Hagberg CA. *Benumof's Airway Management (Second Edition)*, 4th ed. Mosby; 2017.
56. Joffe AM, Ramaiah R, Donahue E, et al. Ventilation by mask before and after the administration of neuromuscular blockade: a pragmatic non-inferiority trial. *BMC Anesthesiol.* 2015;15: 134–134.
57. Rizk MS, Zeineldine SM, El-Khatib MF, et al. [Nondepolarizing muscle relaxant improves direct laryngoscopy view with no effect on face mask ventilation]. *Rev Bras Anestesiol.* 2017; 67(4):383–387.
58. Rosenblatt W, Ovassapian A, Eige S. Use of the laryngeal mask airway in the United States. *Anesthesiology.* 1998;89(Supplement):575A.
59. Halaseh BK, Sukkar ZF, Hassan LH, Sia AT, Bushnaq WA, Adarbeh H. The use of ProSeal laryngeal mask airway in caesarean section – Experience in 3000 cases. *Anaesth Intensive Care.* 2010;38(6):1023–1028.
60. El-Boghdadly K, Bailey CR, Wiles MD. Postoperative sore throat: a systematic review. *Anaesthesia.* 2016;71(6):706–717.
61. Kim ES, Bishop MJ. Endotracheal Intubation, but not laryngeal mask airway insertion, produces reversible bronchoconstriction. *Anesthesiology.* 1999;90(2):391–394.
62. Ezri T, Szmuk P, Warters RD, Katz J, Hagberg CA. Difficult airway management practice patterns among anesthesiologists practicing in the United States: have we made any progress? *J Clin Anesth.* 2003;15(6):418–422.
63. Woodall NM, Cook TM. National census of airway management techniques used for anaesthesia in the UK: first phase of the fourth national audit project at the royal college of anaesthetists. *Br J Anaesth.* 2011;106(2):266–271.
64. Maktabi Mazen A, Smith Russell B, Todd Michael M. Is routine endotracheal intubation as safe as we think or wish? *Anesthesiology.* 2003;99(2):247–248.
65. Domino KB, Posner KL, Caplan RA, Cheney FW. Airway injury during anesthesia. *Anesthesiology.* 1999;91(6):1703-1703.
66. Goldmann K, Dieterich J, Rœssler M. Laryngopharyngeal mucosal injury after prolonged use of the ProSeal LMA in a porcine model: a pilot study. *Can J Anaesth.* 2007;54(10):822–828.
67. Lamb K, James MFM, Janicki PK. The laryngeal mask airway for intraocular surgery: effects on intraocular pressure and stress responses. *Br J Anaesth.* 1992;69(2):143–147.

68. Idrees A, Khan FA. A comparative study of positive pressure ventilation via laryngeal mask airway and endotracheal tube. *J Pak Med Assoc*. 2000;50(10):333–338.
69. McCrirrick A, Ramage DTO, Pracilio JA, Hickman JA. Experience with the laryngeal mask airway in two hundred patients. *Anaesth Intensive Care*. 1991;19(2):256–260.
70. Calder I, Picard J, Chapman M, O'Sullivan C, Crockard HA. Mouth opening. *Anesthesiology*. 2003;99(4):799–801.
71. Seet E, Yousaf F, Gupta S, Subramanyam R, Wong DT, Chung F. Use of manometry for laryngeal mask airway reduces postoperative pharyngolaryngeal adverse events. *Anesthesiology*. 2010;112(3):652–657.
72. Brimacombe JR, Berry A. The incidence of aspiration associated with the laryngeal mask airway: a meta-analysis of published literature. *J Clin Anesth*. 1995;7(4):297–305.
73. Warner MA, Warner ME, Weber JG. Clinical significance of pulmonary aspiration during the perioperative period. *Anesthesiology*. 1993;78(1):56–62.
74. Lee DH, Stang J, Reardon RF, Martel ML, Driver BE, Braude DA. Rapid sequence airway with the intubating laryngeal mask in the emergency department. *J Emerg Med*. 2021;61(5): 550–557.
75. Yao WY, Li SY, Sng BL, Lim Y, Sia AT. The LMA Supreme™ in 700 parturients undergoing cesarean delivery: an observational study. *Can J Anaesth*. 2012;59(7):648–654.
76. Stone BJ, Chantler PJ, Baskett PJF. The incidence of regurgitation during cardiopulmonary resuscitation: a comparison between the bag valve mask and laryngeal mask airway. *Resuscitation*. 1998;38(1):3–6.
77. Verghese C, Brimacombe JR. Survey of laryngeal mask airway usage in 11,910 patients. *Anesth Analg*. 1996;82(1):129–133.
78. Ahn JH, Jeong JS, Kang SH, et al. Comparison of intragastric pressure between endotracheal tube and supraglottic airway devices in laparoscopic hepatectomy: a randomized, controlled, non-inferiority study. *Medicine (Baltimore)* .2021:100(24):e26287.
79. Brimacombe J, Shorney N. The laryngeal mask airway and prolonged balanced regional anaesthesia. *Can J Anaesth*.1993;40(4):360–364.
80. Williams PJ, Bailey PM. Comparison of the reinforced laryngeal mask airway and tracheal intubation for adenotonsillectomy. *Br J Anaesth*. 1993;70(1):30–33.
81. Kaplan A, Crosby GJ, Bhattacharyya N. Airway protection and the laryngeal mask airway in sinus and nasal surgery. *Laryngoscope*. 2004;114(4):652–655.
82. Mao Z, Gao L, Wang G, et al. Subglottic secretion suction for preventing ventilator-associated pneumonia: an updated meta-analysis and trial sequential analysis. *Crit Care* .2016;20(1):353.
83. Nair I, Bailey PM. Use of the laryngeal mask for airway maintenance following tracheal extubation. *Anaesthesia*. 1995;50(2):174–175.
84. Goldmann K, Kuhlmann S, Gerlach M, Bornträger C. Geplante entfernung der kehlkopfmaske im aufwachraum. *Anaesthesist*. 2011;60(11):1002–1008.
85. Deakin CD, Diprose P, Majumdar R, Pulletz M. An investigation into the quantity of secretions removed by inflated and deflated laryngeal mask airways. *Anaesthesia*. 2000;55(5):478–480.
86. Aqil M, Khan MU, Mansoor S, Mansoor S, Khokhar RS, Narejo AS. Incidence and severity of postoperative sore throat: a randomized comparison of glidescope with macintosh laryngoscope. *BMC Anesthesiol*. 2017;17(1):127.
87. Brimacombe J, Clarke G, Keller C. Lingual nerve injury associated with the ProSeal laryngeal mask airway: a case report and review of the literature. *Br J Anaesth*. 2005;95(3):420–423.
88. Zand F, Amini A. Use of the Laryngeal Tube-S™ for airway management and prevention of aspiration after a failed tracheal intubation in a parturient. *Anesthesiology*. 2005;102(2): 481–483.
89. Bortone L, Ingelmo PM, Ninno GD, et al. Randomized controlled trial comparing the laryngeal tube and the laryngeal mask in pediatric patients. *Paediatr Anaesth*. 2006;16(3):251–257.
90. Keil J, Jung P, Schiele A, et al. [Interdisciplinary consensus statement on alternative airway management with supraglottic airway devices in pediatric emergency medicine: Laryngeal mask is state of the art]. *Anaesthesist*. 2016;65(1):57–66.
91. Keller C, Brimacombe J, Kleinsasser A, Loeckinger A. Pharyngeal mucosal pressures with the laryngeal tube airway versus ProSeal laryngeal mask airway. *Anasthesiol Intensivmed Notfallmed Schmerzther*. 2003;38(6):393–396.
92. Banchereau F, Delaunay F, Hervé Y, et al. Ulcérations oropharyngées suite à l'utilisation d'un tube laryngé S (Ann Fr Anesth Réanim 2006;25:884–7). *Annales Françaises d'Anesthésie et de Réanimation*. 2006;25(11–12):1134.
93. Galgon RE, Schroeder KM, Han S, Andrei A, Joffe AM. The air-Q(®) intubating laryngeal airway vs the LMA-ProSeal(TM): a prospective, randomised trial of airway seal pressure. *Anaesthesia*. 2011;66(12):1093–1100.
94. Lee JS, Kim DH, Choi SH, Ha SH, Kim S, Kim MS. Prospective, randomized comparison of the i-gel and the self-pressurized air-Q intubating laryngeal airway in elderly anesthetized patients. *Anesth Analg*. 2020;130(2):480–487.
95. Brain AIJ, Verghese C, Strube PJ. The LMA 'ProSeal'—a laryngeal mask with an oesophageal vent. *Br J Anaesth*. 2000;84(5):650–654.
96. Rosenblatt WH. The use of the LMA-ProSeal™ in airway resuscitation. *Anesth Analg*. 2003;97(6):1773–1775.
97. Awan R, Nolan JP, Cook TM. Use of a ProSeal TM laryngeal mask airway for airway maintenance during emergency caesarean section after failed tracheal intubation. *Br J Anaesth*. 2004;92(1):144–146.
98. Lu PP, Brimacombe J, Yang C, Shyr M. ProSeal versus the classic laryngeal mask airway for positive pressure ventilation during laparoscopic cholecystectomy†. *Br J Anaesth*. 2002;88(6):824–827.
99. Ferson DZ, Rosenblatt WH, Johansen MJ, Osborn I, Ovassapian A. Use of the intubating LMA-Fastrach™ in 254 patients with difficult-to-manage airways. *Anesthesiology*. 2001; 95(5):1175–1181.
100. Beleña JM, Gracia JL, Ayala JL, et al. The laryngeal mask airway supreme for positive pressure ventilation during laparoscopic cholecystectomy. *J Clin Anesth*. 2011;23(6):456–460.
101. de Montblanc J, Ruscio L, Mazoit JX, Benhamou D. A systematic review and meta-analysis of the i-gel®vs laryngeal mask airway in adults. *Anaesthesia*. 2014;69(10):1151–1162.
102. Shin HW, Yoo HN, Bae GE, et al. Comparison of oropharyngeal leak pressure and clinical performance of LMA ProSeal™ and i-gel® in adults: meta-analysis and systematic review. *J Int Med Res*. 2016;44(3):405–418.
103. Bannister F, Macbeth R. Direct laryngoscopy and tracheal intubation. *Lancet North Am Ed*. 1944;244(6325):651–654.
104. Adnet F, Borron SW, Lapostolle F, Lapandry C. The three axis alignment theory and the "Sniffing Position": perpetuation of an anatomic myth?. *Anesthesiology*. 1999;91(6):1964–1964.
105. Chou H-C, Wu T-L. Rethinking the three axes alignment theory for direct laryngoscopy. *Acta Anaesthesiol Scand*. 2001;45(2):261–262.
106. Rosenblatt WH. Preoperative planning of airway management in critical care patients. *Crit Care Med*. 2004;32(Supplement):S186–S192.
107. Mallampati SR, Gatt SP, Gugino LD, et al. A clinical sign to predict difficult tracheal intubation; a prospective study. *Can Anaesth Soc J*. 1985;32(4):429–434.
108. Ayoub C, Baraka A, el-Khatib M, Muallem M, Kawkabani N, Soueide A. A new cut-off point of thyromental distance for prediction of difficult airway. *Middle East J Anaesthesiol*. 2000;15(6):619–633.
109. Chou H-C, Wu T-L. Thyromental distance and anterior larynx: misconception and misnomer? *Anesth Analg*. 2003;1526–1527.
110. Ovassapian A, Glassenberg R, Randel GI, Klock A, Mesnick PS, Klafta JM. The unexpected difficult airway and lingual tonsil hyperplasia. *Anesthesiology*. 2002;97(1):124–132.
111. El-Orbany M, Woehlck H, Salem MR. Head and neck position for direct laryngoscopy. *Anesth Analg*. 2011;113(1):103–109.
112. Levitan RM. *The Airway Cam™ Guide to Intubation and Practical Emergency Airway Management*. Airway Cam Technologies, Inc.; 2004
113. Reiterer F, Abbasi S, Bhutani VK. Influence of head-neck posture on airflow and pulmonary mechanics in preterm neonates. *Pediatr Pulmonol*. 1994;17(3):149–154.
114. Cormack RS, Lehane J. Difficult tracheal intubation in obstetrics. *Anaesthesia*. 1984;39(11): 1105–1111.
115. Crosby ET, Cooper RM, Douglas MJ, et al. The unanticipated difficult airway with recommendations for management. *Can J Anaesth*. 1998;45(8):757–776.
116. Yentis SM, Lee DJH. Evaluation of an improved scoring system for the grading of direct laryngoscopy. *Anaesthesia*. 1998;53(11):1041–1044.
117. Cook TM. A new practical classification of laryngeal view. *Anaesthesia*. 2000;55(3):274–279.
118. Taboada M, Doldan P, Calvo A, et al. Comparison of tracheal intubation conditions in operating room and intensive care unit: a prospective, observational study. *Anesthesiology*. 2018;129(2):321–328.
119. Ochroch EA, Hollander JE, Kush S, Shofer FS, Levitan RM. Assessment of laryngeal view: percentage of glottic opening score vs Cormack and Lehane grading. *Can J Anaesth*. 1999;46(10):987–990.
120. Ulrich B, Listyo R, Gerig HJ, Gabi K, Kreienbühl G. Die schwierige intubation. *Anaesthesist*. 1998;47(1):45–50.
121. Benumof JL, Cooper SD. Quantitative improvement in laryngoscopic view by optimal external laryngeal manipulation. *J Clin Anesth*. 1996;8(2):136–140.
122. Cho HY, Yang SM, Jung CW, et al. A randomised controlled trial of 7.5-mm and 7.0-mm tracheal tubes vs. 6.5-mm and 6.0-mm tracheal tubes for men and women during laparoscopic surgery. *Anaesthesia*. 2022;77(1):54–58.
123. Karmali S, Rose P. Tracheal tube size in adults undergoing elective surgery – a narrative review. *Anaesthesia*. 2020;75(11):1529–1539.
124. Henderson JJ. The use of paraglossal straight blade laryngoscopy in difficult tracheal intubation. *Anaesthesia*. 1997;52(6):552–560.
125. Alerhand S. Ultrasound for identifying the cricothyroid membrane prior to the anticipated difficult airway. *Am J Emerg Med*. 2018;36(11):2078–2084.
126. Kheterpal S, Healy D, Aziz MF, et al. Incidence, predictors, and outcome of difficult mask ventilation combined with difficult laryngoscopy. *Anesthesiology*. 2013;119(6): 1360–1369.
127. Rose DK, Cohen MM. The airway: problems and predictions in 18,500 patients. *Can J Anaesth*. 1994;41(5):372–383.
128. Burkle CM, Walsh MT, Harrison BA, Curry TB, Rose SH. Airway management after failure to intubate by direct laryngoscopy: outcomes in a large teaching hospital. *Can J Anaesth*. 2005;52(6):634–640.
129. Turkstra TP, Pelz DM, Shaikh AA, Craen RA. Cervical spine motion: a fluoroscopic comparison of Shikani Optical Stylet vs Macintosh laryngoscope. *Can J Anaesth*. 2007;54(6): 441–447.

130. Rudolph C, Schneider JP, Wallenborn J, Schaffranietz L. Movement of the upper cervical spine during laryngoscopy: a comparison of the Bonfils intubation fibrescope and the Macintosh laryngoscope. *Anaesthesia*. 2005;60(7):668–672.
131. Halligan M, Charters P. A clinical evaluation of the Bonfils intubation fibrescope*. *Anaesthesia*. 2003;58(11):1087–1091.
132. Greenland KB, Liu G, Tan H, Edwards M, Irwin MG. Comparison of the Levitan FPS scope™ and the single-use bougie for simulated difficult intubation in anaesthetised patients. *Anaesthesia*. 2007;62(5):509–515.
133. Levitan RM. Design rationale and intended use of a short optical stylet for routine fiberoptic augmentation of emergency laryngoscopy. *Am J Emerg Med*. 2006;24(4):490–495.
134. Heidegger T, Gerig HJ, Ulrich B, Kreienbühl G. Validation of a simple algorithm for tracheal intubation: daily practice is the key to success in emergencies—an analysis of 13,248 intubations. *Anesth Analg*. 2001;92(2):517–522.
135. Cooper RM, Pacey JA, Bishop MJ, McCluskey SA. Early clinical experience with a new videolaryngoscope (GlideScope) in 728 patients. *Can J Anaesth*. 2005;52(2):191–198.
136. Turkstra TP, Craen RA, Pelz DM, Gelb AW. Cervical spine motion: a fluoroscopic comparison during intubation with lighted stylet, glidescope, and macintosh laryngoscope. *Anesth Analg*. 2005;101(3):910–915.
137. Sun DA, Warriner CB, Parsons DG, Klein R, Umedaly HS, Moult M. The GlideScope® Video Laryngoscope: randomized clinical trial in 200 patients. *Br J Anaesth*. 2005;94(3):381–384.
138. Kramer DC, Osborn IP. More maneuvers to facilitate tracheal intubation with the GlideScope. *Can J Anaesth*. 2006;53(7):737–737.
139. Kaplan MB, Berci G, Doyle DJ, et al. Videolaryngoscopy in the management of the difficult airway. *Can J Anaesth*. 2004;51(1):94–95.
140. Jones PM, Turkstra TP, Armstrong KP, et al. Effect of stylet angulation and endotracheal tube camber on time to intubation with the GlideScope®. *Can J Anaesth*. 2007;54(1):21–27.
141. Hindman BJ, Santoni BG, Puttlitz CM, From RP, Todd MM. Intubation biomechanics: laryngoscope force and cervical spine motion during intubation with Macintosh and Airtraq laryngoscopes. *Anesthesiology*. 2014;121(2):260–271.
142. Gunaydin B, Gungor I, Yigit N, Celebi H. The Glidescope ® for tracheal intubation in patients with ankylosing spondylitis. *Br J Anaesth*. 2007;98(3):408–409.
143. Easker DD, Policeni BA, Hindman BJ. Lateral cervical spine radiography to demonstrate absence of bony displacement after intubation in a patient with an acute type III odontoid fracture. *A A Case Rep*. 2015;5(2):25–28.
144. Raja J, Clyne S, Levine J, Tebbit C, Mair E. Otorhinolaryngology management of seven patients with iatrogenic penetrating injuries from GlideScope®: Our experience. *Clin Otolaryngol*. 2014;39(4):251–254.
145. Cooper RM. Complications associated with the use of the GlideScope® videolaryngoscope. *Can J Anaesth*. 2007;54(1):54–57.
146. Xue FS, Zhang GH, Li XY, et al. Comparison of hemodynamic responses to orotracheal intubation with the GlideScope® videolaryngoscope and the Macintosh direct laryngoscope. *J Clin Anesth*. 2007;19(4):245–250.
147. Allister DW, Parsons DG. 'Reverse loading' to facilitate Glidescope® intubation. *Can J Anaesth*. 2007;54(2):161–162.
148. Aziz MF, Abrons RO, Cattano D, et al. First-attempt intubation success of video laryngoscopy in patients with anticipated difficult direct laryngoscopy. *Anesth Analg*. 2016;122(3): 740–750.
149. Kaplan MB, Hagberg CA, Ward DS, et al. Comparison of direct and video-assisted views of the larynx during routine intubation. *J Clin Anesth*. 2006;18(5):357–362.
150. Maharaj CH, Costello JF, McDonnell JG, Harte BH, Laffey JG. The Airtraq®as a rescue airway device following failed direct laryngoscopy: a case series. *Anaesthesia*. 2007;62(6): 598–601.
151. Suzuki A, Toyama Y, Iwasaki H, Henderson J. Airtraq for awake tracheal intubation. *Anaesthesia*. 2007;62(7):746–747.
152. Maharaj CH, Buckley E, Harte BH, Laffey JG. Endotracheal intubation in patients with cervical spine immobilization. *Anesthesiology*. 2007;107(1):53–59.
153. Ueshima H, Kitamura A. Use of the new airtraq "Airtraq AVANT" in clinical settings. *J Clin Anesth*. 2015;27(5):441–442.
154. Suzuki A, Abe N, Sasakawa T, Kunisawa T, Takahata O, Iwasaki H. Pentax-AWS (airway scope) and Airtraq: big difference between two similar devices. *J Anesth*. 2008;22(2):191–192.
155. Malik MA, Subramaniam R, Maharaj CH, Harte BH, Laffey JG. Randomized controlled trial of the Pentax AWS®, Glidescope®, and Macintosh laryngoscopes in predicted difficult intubation. *Br J Anaesth*. 2009;103(5):761–768.
156. Mahajan V, Hashmi J, Singh R, Samra T, Aneja S. Comparative evaluation of gastric pH and volume in morbidly obese and lean patients undergoing elective surgery and effect of aspiration prophylaxis. *J Clin Anesth*. 2015;27(5):396–400.
157. Juvin P, Fèvre G, Merouche M, Vallot T, Desmonts JM. Gastric residue is not more copious in obese patients. *Anesth Analg*. 2001;93(6):1621–1622.
158. Harter RL, Kelly WB, Kramer MG, Perez CE, Dzwonczyk RR. A comparison of the volume and pH of gastric contents of obese and lean surgical patients. *Anesth Analg*. 1998;86(1):147–152.
159. Merio R, Festa A, Bergmann H, et al. Slow gastric emptying in type I diabetes: relation to autonomic and peripheral neuropathy, blood glucose, and glycemic control. *Diabetes Care*. 1997; 20(3):419–423.
160. Van Den Driessche M, Peeters K, Marien P, Ghoos Y, Devlieger H, Veereman-Wauters G. Gastric emptying in formula-fed and breast-fed infants measured with the 13C-octanoic acid breath test. *J Pediatr Gastroenterol Nutr*. 1999;29(1):46–51.
161. Practice guidelines for preoperative fasting and the use of pharmacologic agents to reduce the risk of pulmonary aspiration: application to healthy patients undergoing elective procedures: an updated report by the American society of anesthesiologists task force on preoperative fasting and the use of pharmacologic agents to reduce the risk of pulmonary aspiration. *Anesthesiology*. 2017;126(3):376–393.
162. Kulkarni PN, Batra YK, Wig J. Effects of different combinations of H_2 receptor antagonist with gastrokinetic drugs on gastric fluid pH and volume in children–a comparative study. *Int J Clin Pharmacol Ther*. 1997;35(12):561–564.
163. Nishina K, Mikawa K, Takao Y, Shiga M, Maekawa N, Obara H. A comparison of rabeprazole, lansoprazole, and ranitidine for improving preoperative gastric fluid property in adults undergoing elective surgery. *Anesth Analg*. 2000;90(3):717–721.
164. Nishina K, Mikawa K, Maekawa N, Takao Y, Shiga M, Obara H. A comparison of lansoprazole, omeprazole, and ranitidine for reducing preoperative gastric secretion in adult patients undergoing elective surgery. *Anesth Analg*. 1996;82(4):832–836.
165. Memiş D, Turan A, Karamanlioglu B, Saral P, Türe M, Pamukçu Z. The effect of intravenous pantoprazole and ranitidine for improving preoperative gastric fluid properties in adults undergoing elective surgery. *Anesth Analg*. 2003;97(5):1360–1363.
166. Escolano F, Castaño J, López R, Bisbe E, Alcón A. Effects of omeprazole, ranitidine, famotidine and placebo on gastric secretion in patients undergoing elective surgery. *Br J Anaesth*. 1992; 69(4):404–406.
167. Manchikanti L, Grow JB, Colliver JA, Hadley CH, Hohlbein LJ. Bicitra®(Sodium Citrate) and metoclopramide in outpatient anesthesia for prophylaxis against aspiration pneumonitis. *Anesthesiology*. 1985;63(4):378–384.
168. Vanner RG, Asai T. Safe use of cricoid pressure. *Anaesthesia*. 1999;54(1):1–3.
169. Smith KJ, Dobranowski J, Yip G, Dauphin A, Choi PT. Cricoid pressure displaces the esophagus: an observational study using magnetic resonance imaging. *Anesthesiology*. 2003;99(1): 60–64.
170. Levitan RM, Kinkle WC, Levin WJ, Everett WW. Laryngeal view during laryngoscopy: a randomized trial comparing cricoid pressure, backward-upward-rightward pressure, and bimanual laryngoscopy. *Ann Emerg Med*. 2006;47(6):548–555.
171. Alstrøm HB, Belhage B. [Cricoid pressure a.m. Sellick in rapid sequence intubation?]. *Ugeskr Laeger*. 2007;169(24):2305–2308.
172. Algie CM, Mahar RK, Tan HB, Wilson G, Mahar PD, Wasiak J. Effectiveness and risks of cricoid pressure during rapid sequence induction for endotracheal intubation. *Cochrane Database Syst Rev*. 2015;2015(11):CD011656
173. Brown JPR, Werrett G. Bag-mask ventilation in rapid sequence induction. *Anaesthesia*. 2009;64(7):784–785.
174. Law JA, Duggan LV, Asselin M, et al. Canadian airway focus group updated consensus-based recommendations for management of the difficult airway: part 2. Planning and implementing safe management of the patient with an anticipated difficult airway. *Can J Anaesth*. 2021; 68(9):1405–1436.
175. Kundra P, Sujata N, Ravishankar M. Conventional tracheal tubes for intubation through the intubating laryngeal mask airway. *Anesth Analg*. 2005;100(1):284–288.
176. Gerstein NS, Braude DA, Hung O, Sanders JC, Murphy MF. The FastrachTM Intubating Laryngeal mask airway®: an overview and update. *Can J Anaesth*. 2010;57(6):588–601.
177. Rosenblatt WH, Murphy M. The intubating laryngeal mask: use of a new ventilating-intubating device in the emergency department. *Ann Emerg Med*. 1999;33(2):234–238.
178. Karim YM, Swanson DE. Comparison of blind tracheal intubation through the intubating laryngeal mask airway (LMA FastrachTM) and the Air-QTM. *Anaesthesia*. 2011;66(3): 185–190.
179. Sinha R, Chandralekha, Ray BR. Evaluation of air-QTM intubating laryngeal airway as a conduit for tracheal intubation in infants – a pilot study. *Paediatr Anaesth*. 2011;22(2):156–160.
180. Miller KA, Harkin CP, Bailey PL. Postoperative tracheal extubation. *Anesth Analg*. 1995; 80(1):149–172.
181. Mitchell V, Dravid R, Patel A, et al. Difficult Airway Society Guidelines for the management of tracheal extubation. *Anaesthesia*. 2012;67(3):318–340.
182. Brull SJ, Murphy GS. Residual neuromuscular block. *Anesth Analg*. 2010;111(1):129–140.
183. Eriksson LI, Sundman E, Olsson R, et al. Functional assessment of the pharynx at rest and during swallowing in partially paralyzed humans. *Anesthesiology*. 1997;87(5):1035–1043.
184. Fortier L-P, McKeen D, Turner K, et al. The recite study. *Anesth Analg*. 2015;121(2):366–372.
185. Lee C-H, Peng M-J, Wu C-L. Dexamethasone to prevent postextubation airway obstruction in adults: a prospective, randomized, double-blind, placebo-controlled study. *Crit Care*. 2007;11(4):R72–R72.
186. Ochoa ME, del Carmen Marín M, Frutos-Vivar F, et al. Cuff-leak test for the diagnosis of upper airway obstruction in adults: a systematic review and meta-analysis. *Intensive Care Med*. 2009;35(7).
187. Mort TC. Continuous airway access for the difficult extubation: the efficacy of the airway exchange catheter. *Anesth Analg*. 2007;105(5):1357–1362.
188. Mort TC, Meisterling EM, Waberski W. A240 exchanging a tracheal tube in the ICU patient: a comparison of two exchangers with direct laryngoscopy. *Anesthesiology*. 1997;87.

189. Harris K, Chalhoub M, Maroun R, Elsayegh D. Endotracheal tube exchangers: should we look for safer alternatives? *Heart Lung*. 2012;41(1):67–69.
190. Rosenblatt WH, Yanez ND. A decision tree approach to airway management pathways in the 2022 difficult airway algorithm of the American society of anesthesiologists. *Anesth Analg*. 2022;134(5):910–915.
191. Warner MA, Meyerhoff KL, Warner ME, Posner KL, Stephens L, Domino KB. Pulmonary aspiration of gastric contents: a closed claims analysis. *Anesthesiology*. 2021;135(2):284–291.
192. Haynes AB, Weiser TG, Berry WR, et al. A surgical safety checklist to reduce morbidity and mortality in a global population. *N Engl J Med*. 2009;360(5):491–499.
193. Apfelbaum JL, Hagberg CA, Connis RT, et al. *Anesthesiology*. 2022;136(1):31–81.
194. Nandi PR, Charlesworth CH, Taylor SJ, Nunn JF, Doré CJ. Effect of general anaesthesia on the pharynx. *Br J Anaesth*. 1991;66(2):157–162.
195. Kvisselgaard AD, Krøigaard M, Mosbech HF, Garvey LH. No cases of perioperative allergy to local anaesthetics in the Danish anaesthesia allergy centre. *Acta Anaesthesiol Scand*. 2017; 61(2):149–155.
196. Trautmann A, Goebeler M, Stoevesandt J. Twenty years' experience with anaphylaxis-like reactions to local anesthetics: genuine allergy is rare. *J Allergy Clin Immunol Pract*. 2018;6(6): 2051–2058.e2051.
197. Madhere M, Vangura D, Saidov A. Dexmedetomidine as sole agent for awake fiberoptic intubation in a patient with local anesthetic allergy. *J Anesth*. 2011;25(4):592–594.
198. Nvdahl PA, Axelsson K. Venous blood concentration of lidocaine after nasopharyngeal application of 2% lidocaine gel. *Acta Anaesthesiol Scand*. 1988;32(2):135–139.
199. Wieczorek PM, Schricker T, Vinet B, Backman SB. Airway topicalisation in morbidly obese patients using atomised lidocaine: 2% compared with 4%. *Anaesthesia*. 2007;62(10):984–988.
200. Kristensen MS, Teoh WHL, Baker PA. Percutaneous emergency airway access; prevention, preparation, technique and training. *Br J Anaesth*. 2015;114(3):357–361.
201. McEvoy, GKASoH-SP. *AHFS Drug Information 2007*. American Society of Health-System Pharmacists; 2007.
202. Benumof JL. Management of the difficult adult airway. With special emphasis on awake tracheal intubation. *Anesthesiology*. 1991;75(6):1087–1110.
203. Sitzman TB, Rich GF, Rockwell JJ, Leisure GS, Durieux ME, DiFazio CA. Local anesthetic administration for awake direct laryngoscopy. *Anesthesiology*. 1997;86(1):34–40.
204. Ovassapian A. *Fiberoptic Endoscopy and the Difficult Airway*, 2nd ed. Lippincott-Raven.
205. Rosenblatt WH, Wagner PJ, Ovassapian A, Kain ZN. Practice patterns in managing the difficult airway by anesthesiologists in the United States. *Anesth Analg*. 1998;87(1):153–157.
206. Moshrefi S, Sheckter CC, Shepard K, et al. Preventing unnecessary intubations: a 5-year regional burn center experience using flexible fiberoptic laryngoscopy for airway evaluation in patients with suspected inhalation or airway injury. *J Burn Care Res*. 2019;40(3):341–346.
207. Gemma M, Buratti L, Di Santo D, et al. Pre-operative transnasal endoscopy as a predictor of difficult airway: a prospective cohort study. *Eur J Anaesthesiol*. 2020;37(2):98–104.
208. Murphy P. A fibre-optic endoscope used for nasal intubation. *Anaesthesia*. 1967;22(3):489–491.
209. Kramer A, Müller D, Pförtner R, Mohr C, Groeben H. Fibreoptic vs videolaryngoscopic (C-MAC(®) D-BLADE) nasal awake intubation under local anaesthesia. *Anaesthesia*. 2015; 70(4):400–406.
210. Mahran EA, Hassan ME. Comparative randomised study of GlideScope(®) video laryngoscope versus flexible fibre-optic bronchoscope for awake nasal intubation of oropharyngeal cancer patients with anticipated difficult intubation. *Indian J Anaesth*. 2016;60(12):936–938.
211. Abdellatif AA, Ali MA. GlideScope videolaryngoscope versus flexible fiberoptic bronchoscope for awake intubation of morbidly obese patient with predicted difficult intubation. *Middle East J Anaesthesiol*. 2014;22(4):385–392.
212. Rosenstock CV, Thøgersen B, Afshari A, Christensen AL, Eriksen C, Gätke MR. Awake fiberoptic or awake video laryngoscopic tracheal intubation in patients with anticipated difficult airway management: a randomized clinical trial. *Anesthesiology*. 2012;116(6):1210–1216.
213. Mendonca C, Mesbah A, Velayudhan A, Danha R. A randomised clinical trial comparing the flexible fibrescope and the Pentax Airway Scope (AWS)(®) for awake oral tracheal intubation. *Anaesthesia*. 2016;71(8):908–914.
214. Gómez-Ríos MA, Nieto Serradilla L. Combined use of an Airtraq® optical laryngoscope, Airtraq video camera, Airtraq wireless monitor, and a fibreoptic bronchoscope after failed tracheal intubation. *Can J Anaesth*. 2011;58(4):411–412.
215. Khan MF, Shamim F, Slote MU, Salim B, Abbas SA. Combined use of a videolaryngoscope and a flexible bronchoscope for awake tracheal intubation when front-of-neck airway is not an option. *Anaesth Rep*. 2021;9(1):12–15.
216. Shiraishi T. Awake insertion of the air-Q™ intubating laryngeal airway device that facilitates safer tracheal intubation in morbidly obese patients. *Br J Anaesth*. 2013;111(6):1024–1025.
217. Lim WY, Wong P. Awake supraglottic airway guided flexible bronchoscopic intubation in patients with anticipated difficult airways: a case series and narrative review. *Korean J Anesthesiol*. 2019;72(6):548–557.
218. Kristensen MS. The Parker Flex-Tip Tube versus a standard tube for fiberoptic orotracheal intubation. *Anesthesiology*. 2003;98(2):354–358.
219. Rosenblatt WH. Overcoming obstruction during bronchoscope-guided intubation of the trachea with the double setup endotracheal tube. *Anesth Analg*. 1996;83(1):175–177.
220. Ovassapian A, Yelich SJ, Dykes MM, Brunner EE. Fiberoptic nasotracheal intubation—incidence and causes of failure. *Anesth Analg*. 1983;62(7):692–695.
221. Lu PP, Liu HP, Shyr MH, et al. Softened endothracheal tube reduces the incidence and severity of epistaxis following nasotracheal intubation. *Acta Anaesthesiol Sin*. 1998;36(4):193–197.
222. Samsoon GLT, Young JRB. Difficult tracheal intubation: a retrospective study. *Anaesthesia*. 1987;42(5):487–490.
223. Martin SE, Ochsner MG, Jarman RH, Agudelo WE. Laryngeal mask airway in air transport when intubation fails. *J Trauma*. 1997;42(2):333–336.
224. Brimacombe JR, De Maio B. Emergency use of the laryngeal mask airway during helicopter transfer of a neonate. *J Clin Anesth*. 1995;7(8):689–690.
225. Gerstein NS, Braude DA, Hung O, Sanders JC, Murphy MF. The Fastrach intubating laryngeal mask airway: an overview and update. *Can J Anaesth*. 2010;57(6):588–601.
226. Brimacombe JR, Berry AM. Mallampati grade and laryngeal mask placement. *Anesth Analg*. 1996;82(5):1112.
227. Agro F, Frass M, Benumof JL, Krafft P. Current status of the Combitube™: a review of the literature. *J Clin Anesth*. 2002;14(4):307–314.
228. Keller C, Brimacombe J, Bittersohl J, Lirk P, von Goedecke A. Aspiration and the laryngeal mask airway: three cases and a review of the literature †. *Br J Anaesth*. 2004;93(4): 579–582.
229. Li J, Murphy-Lavoie H, Bugas C, Martinez J, Preston C. Complications of emergency intubation with and without paralysis. *Am J Emerg Med*. 1999;17(2):141–143.
230. Gnauck K, Lungo JB, Scalzo A, Peter J, Nakanishi A. Emergency intubation of the pediatric medical patient: use of anesthetic agents in the emergency department. *Ann Emerg Med*. 1994;23(6):1242–1247.
231. Sivarajan M, Joy JV. Effects of general anesthesia and paralysis on upper airway changes due to head position in humans. *Anesthesiology*. 1996;85(4):787–793.
232. Ikeda A, Isono S, Sato Y, et al. Effects of muscle relaxants on mask ventilation in anesthetized persons with normal upper airway anatomy. *Anesthesiology*. 2012;117(3):487–493.
233. Walls RM, Facep. Management of the difficult airway in the trauma patient. *Emerg Med Clin North Am*. 1998;16(1):45–61.
234. Ruetzler K, Roessler B, Potura L, et al. Performance and skill retention of intubation by paramedics using seven different airway devices—a manikin study. *Resuscitation*. 2011;82(5): 593–597.
235. Mort TC. Emergency tracheal intubation: complications associated with repeated laryngoscopic attempts. *Anesth Analg*. 2004;99(2):607–613.
236. Sakles JC, Chiu S, Mosier J, Walker C, Stolz U. The importance of first pass success when performing orotracheal intubation in the emergency department. *Acad Emerg Med*. 2013;20(1):71–78.
237. Driver BE, Prekker ME, Klein LR, et al. Effect of use of a bougie vs endotracheal tube and stylet on first-attempt intubation success among patients with difficult airways undergoing emergency intubation: a randomized clinical trial. *JAMA*. 2018;319(21):2179–2189.
238. Reardon R, Joing S, Hill C. Bougie-guided cricothyrotomy technique. *Acad Emerg Med*. 2010;17(2):225–225.
239. Hubble MW, Wilfong DA, Brown LH, Hertelendy A, Benner RW. A meta-analysis of prehospital airway control techniques part II: alternative airway devices and cricothyrotomy success rates. *Prehosp Emerg Care*. 2010;14(4):515–530.
240. Hamaekers AEW, Borg PAJ, Enk D. A bench study of ventilation via two self-assembled jet devices and the Oxygen Flow Modulator in simulated upper airway obstruction. *Anaesthesia*. 2009;64(12):1353–1358.
241. Sukhupragarn W, Rosenblatt WH. Kinking of catheters during translaryngeal jet ventilation: a bench model investigation of eight devices. *J Med Assoc Thai*. 2011;94(8):972–977.
242. Campbell M, Shanahan H, Ash S, Royds J, Husarova V, McCaul C. The accuracy of locating the cricothyroid membrane by palpation—an intergender study. *BMC Anesthesiol*. 2014; 14:108-108.
243. Hamaekers A, Borg P, Enk D. The importance of flow and pressure release in emergency jet ventilation devices. *Paediatr Anaesth*. 2008;19(5):452–457.
244. Lenfant F, Péan D, Brisard L, Freysz M, Lejus C. Oxygen delivery during transtracheal oxygenation. *Anesth Analg*. 2010;111(4):922–924.
245. Hamaekers AEW, Borg PAJ, Enk D. Ventrain: an ejector ventilator for emergency use. *Br J Anaesth*. 2012;108(6):1017–1021.
246. Berry M, Tzeng Y, Marsland C. Percutaneous transtracheal ventilation in an obstructed airway model in post-apnoeic sheep. *Br J Anaesth*. 2014;113(6):1039–1045.
247. Paxian M, Preussler NP, Reinz T, Schlueter A, Gottschall R. Transtracheal ventilation with a novel ejector-based device (Ventrain) in open, partly obstructed, or totally closed upper airways in pigs. *Br J Anaesth*. 2015;115(2):308–316.
248. Borg PAJ, Hamaekers AEW, Lacko M, Jansen J, Enk D. Ventrain ® for ventilation of the lungs. *Br J Anaesth*. 2012;109(5):833–834.
249. Willemsen MGA, Noppens R, Mulder ALM, Enk D. Ventilation with the Ventrain through a small lumen catheter in the failed paediatric airway: two case reports. *Br J Anaesth*. 2014; 112(5):946–947.
250. Peterson GN, Domino KB, Caplan RA, Posner KL, Lee LA, Cheney FW. Management of the difficult airway. *Anesthesiology*. 2005;103(1):33–39.
251. Bellemain A, Ghimouz A, Goater P, Lentschener C, Esteve M. Pneumothorax bilatéral au retrait du cathéter de jet ventilation à haute fréquence. *Ann Fr Anesth Reanim*. 2006;25(4): 401–403.

29 Patient Positioning and Potential Injuries

BRIDGET P. PULOS • REBECCA L. JOHNSON

KEY POINTS

1. The etiologies of postoperative peripheral neuropathies are often not clear. Although there are potential anatomic and neurophysiologic reasons, perioperative inflammation, resulting in microvasculitis, may be an important etiologic factor.
2. Stretching nerves 5% or more beyond their resting lengths may kink feeding arterioles and result in ischemia.
3. Padding provided by any number of different materials (e.g., gel or foam pads, blankets) should be used to widely disperse point pressure on body parts and soft tissues.
4. When possible, patients to be sedated or anesthetized should be placed in anticipated positions while they are awake to assure they are comfortable.
5. Permanent loss of vision can occur after nonocular surgical procedures, especially spine surgery performed in a prone position.

Positioning a patient for a surgical procedure is frequently a compromise between what the anesthetized patient can tolerate, both structurally and physiologically, and what the surgical team requires for access to its anatomic target. Establishment of the intended surgical posture may need to be modified to match the patient's tolerance. This chapter presents the significance of various positions in which a patient may be placed during an operation, briefly describes the techniques of establishing the positions, and discusses the potential complications of each posture. It also will present data that suggest perioperative inflammatory responses may play an important role in the development of peripheral, and potentially central, neuropathies.

It is very important for clinicians to understand the physiologic and potential pathologic consequences of patient positioning. A number of studies of large surgical populations have provided information on the frequency and natural history of rare perioperative events such as neuropathies and vision loss. However, these studies frequently have provided insufficient data to allow speculation as to potential mechanisms of injury. Based on the findings of these studies, investigators are continuing to seek and confirm mechanisms of injury and the efficacy of novel interventions to decrease the frequency of these perioperative events. Until these investigations are complete, the etiologic mechanisms for many potential positioning-related complications remain unknown.

The lack of solid scientific information on basic mechanisms of positioning-related complications often leads to medicolegal entanglements and notations on anesthesia and operating room records may be absent or uninformative. Careful descriptive notations about positions used during anesthesia and surgery, as well as brief comments about special protective measures such as eye care and pressure-point padding, are useful to include on the anesthesia record. In potentially complicated or contentious circumstances, a separate brief description of care documented in the patient's record is advisable. Only in this manner can subsequent inquiries be properly answered on behalf of either the patient or the anesthesiologist. When credible expanded knowledge that further delineates mechanisms of positioning-related complications is available, these issues and the care of patients will be improved.

General Principles

Without doubt, direct compression of neural and soft tissue may result in ischemia and tissue damage. Many efforts have been directed at provider education over the years to reduce direct tissue trauma from compression. Most anesthesia providers are taught from the start of their training that various maneuvers, pads, and positioning devices are useful to reduce point pressure on neural and soft tissues. Despite these efforts, neuropathies and soft tissue damage still occur. Is it a failure of education, the incorrect application of this information, or other issues that contribute to the continued presence of perioperative positioning injuries? Or perhaps, are there etiologic mechanisms at work that we do not yet understand?

Numerous studies and editorials suggest that we do not yet 1
fully understand the etiologic mechanisms of positioning issues.[1–4] These studies report inflammatory neuropathies in patients who developed severe postsurgical peripheral neuropathies. Surprisingly, the majority of these patients had widespread microvasculitic neuropathies, and many were responsive to immunologic modulation with high doses of corticosteroids. The inflammatory response may be dramatically altered in the perioperative period,

and microvasculitic neuropathy appears to be a previously unrecognized cause of peripheral neuropathy. For example, anesthetic drugs and transfusion of blood products are known to promote systemic inflammation.[5,6] Large epidemiologic studies will eventually help determine the role that this newly discovered etiology plays in the origin of perioperative neuropathies of all sorts. In the meantime, these reports serve as evidence that a number of perioperative neuropathies may, in fact, have no relationship to intraoperative positioning or management of physiologic factors.[4]

Viruses have been associated with central as well as peripheral neuropathies that develop in the perioperative period. As noted earlier, immunosuppression is present in a fairly significant proportion of patients undergoing major surgical procedures. This immunosuppression may provide opportunities for existing viruses or newly introduced viruses to activate, particularly in neural tissues. For example, the onset of shingles may be more frequent in surgical compared to general populations.[7]

2 Some positioning misadventures can, of course, cause tissue damage. Stretch of neural tissue may be an important factor in the development of peripheral and central neuropathies. Stretch of many mammalian nerves to 5% greater than their normal resting length has been shown repeatedly to lead to ischemia by reducing both arteriole and venule blood flow. The kinking of the arterioles and venules associated with neuronal stretch leads to ischemia.[8] If the ischemia is prolonged, it may result in permanent neural damage. The impact of stretch on other soft tissues is less well documented and would be highly dependent on the type of tissue and amount of stretch.

3 Point pressure on any soft tissue may reduce local blood flow and cause ischemia. There are many ways to reduce point pressure, but the most commonly used involve padding. Although there may be distinct differences in mechanical properties of various padding materials (e.g., gels, foam, textiles, and others), none have been proven to be significantly better than the others in reducing the frequency or severity of nerve or soft tissue damage perioperatively. The basic principle is to use any of these materials to protect nerves and soft tissues from point pressure, while avoiding creation of new pressure points by wrapping or securing padding too tightly.

Supine Positions

Variations of Supine Positions

Horizontal

In the traditional supine position, the patient lies on their back with a small pillow beneath the head (Fig. 29-1A). The arms are either comfortably padded and restrained alongside the trunk or abducted on well-padded arm boards. Either arm (or both) may be extended ventrally and the flexed forearm secured to an elevated frame in such a way that perfusion of the hand is not compromised, no skin-to-metal contact exists to cause electrical burns if cautery is used, and the brachial neurovascular bundle is neither stretched nor compressed at the axilla. The lumbar spine may need padded support to prevent a postoperative backache (see "Complications of Supine Positions"). Bony contact points at the occiput, elbows, and heels should be padded. Fortunately, most modern surgical tables have mattress pads that are sufficiently buoyant and thick to allow dispersion of point pressure.

Although the horizontal supine posture has a long history of widespread use, it does not place hip and knee joints in neutral positions and is poorly tolerated for prolonged periods by an immobilized, awake patient. When possible, contouring is recommended.

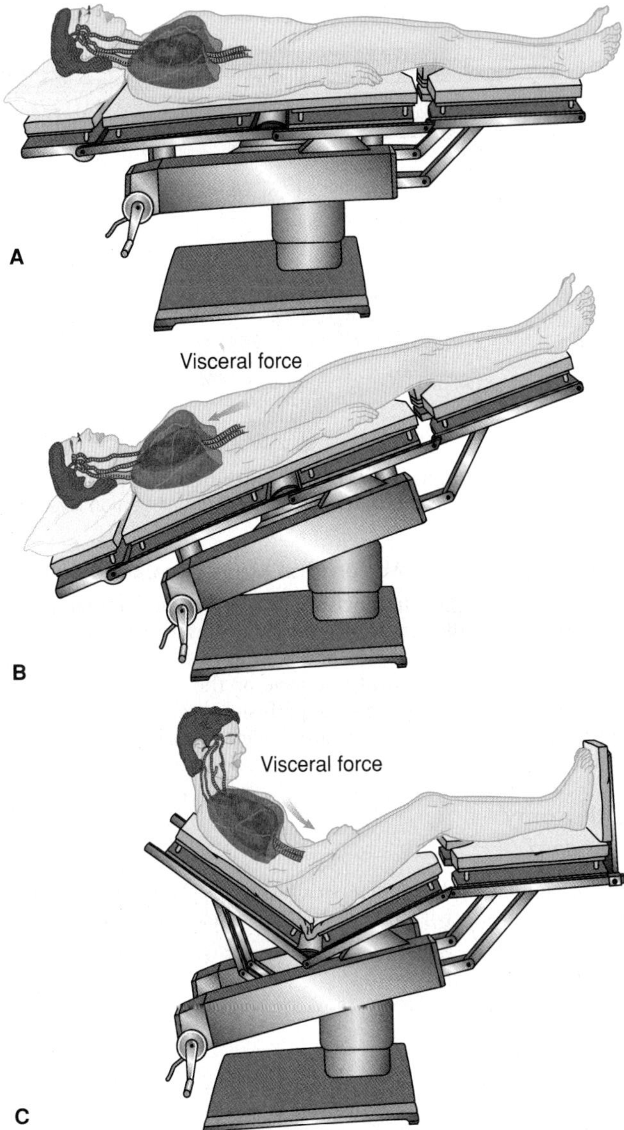

Figure 29-1 **A:** Supine adult with minimal gradients in the horizontal vascular axis. Pulmonary blood volume is greatest dorsally. Viscera displace the diaphragm cephalad. Cerebral circulation is slightly above heart level if the head is on a small pillow. **B:** Head-down tilt aids blood return from lower extremities but encourages reflex vasodilation, congests vessels in the poorly ventilated lung apices, and increases intracranial blood volume. **C:** Elevation of the head shifts abdominal viscera away from the diaphragm and improves ventilation of the lung bases. According to the gradient above the heart, pressure in arteries of the head and neck decreases; pressure in accompanying veins may become subatmospheric.

Contoured

A contoured supine posture (Fig. 29-2) has been termed the *lawn chair position*. It is established by arranging the surface of the operating table so that the trunk–thigh hinge is angulated approximately 15 degrees and the thigh–knee hinge is angulated a similar amount in the opposite direction. Alternatively, a rolled towel, pillow, or blanket can be placed beneath the patient's knees to keep them flexed. The patient of average height then lies comfortably with hips and knees flexed gently.

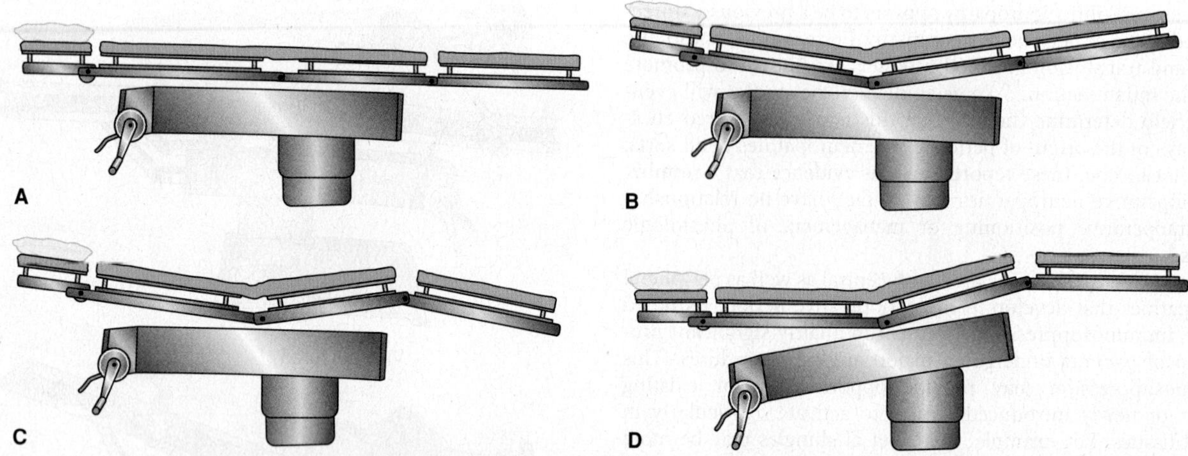

Figure 29-2 Establishment of the contoured supine (lawn chair) position. A: Traditional flat supine tabletop. **B:** Thighs flexed on trunk. **C:** Knees gently flexed in final body position. **D:** Trunk section leveled to stabilize floor-supported arm board.

Lateral Uterine or Abdominal Mass Displacement

With a patient in the supine position, a mobile abdominal mass, such as a very large tumor or a pregnant uterus, can rest on the great vessels of the abdomen and compromise circulation. This is known as the *aortocaval syndrome* or the *supine hypotensive syndrome*. A significant degree of perfusion can be restored if the compressive mass is rolled toward the left hemiabdomen by leftward tilt of the tabletop or by a wedge under the right hip.

Lithotomy

Standard

In the standard lithotomy position (Fig. 29-3), the patient lies supine, typically with one or both arms extended laterally to less than 90 degrees on arm boards. Each lower extremity is flexed at the hip and knee, and both limbs are simultaneously elevated and separated so that the perineum becomes accessible to the surgeon. For many gynecologic and urologic procedures, the patient's thighs are flexed approximately 90 degrees on the trunk and the knees are bent sufficiently to maintain the lower legs nearly parallel to the floor. More acute flexion of the knees or hips can threaten to angulate and compress major vessels at either joint. In addition, hip flexion to greater than 90 degrees on the trunk has been shown to increase stretch of the inguinal ligaments. Branches of the lateral femoral cutaneous nerves often pass directly through these ligaments and can be impinged and become ischemic within the stretched ligament.

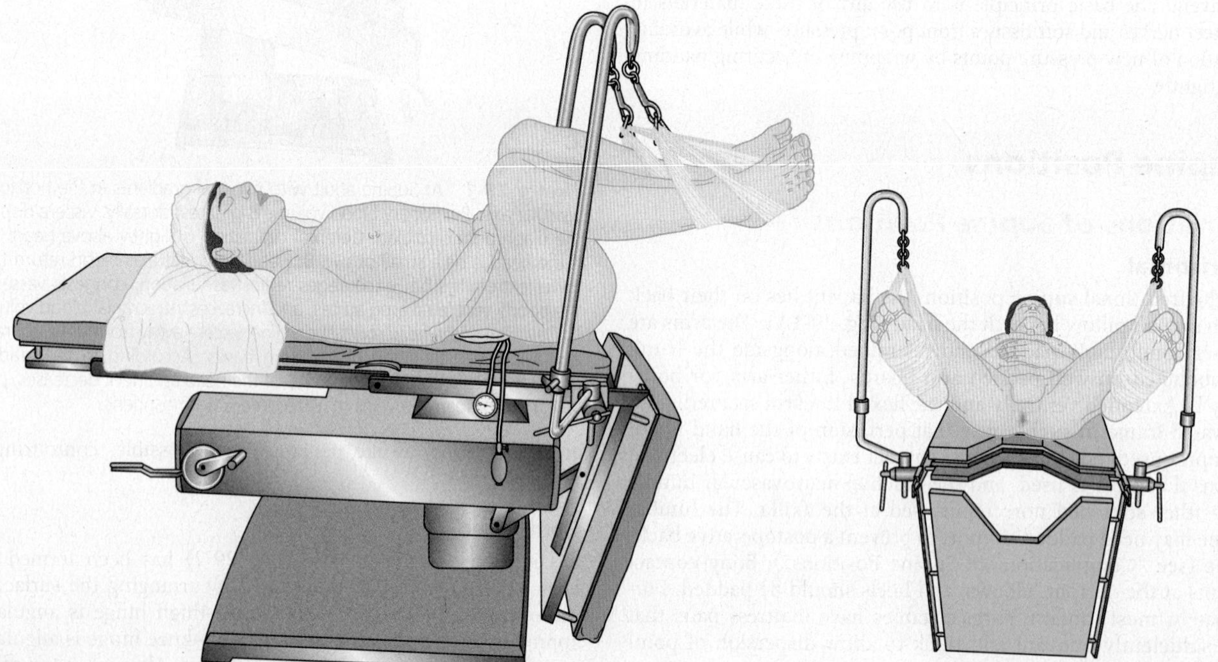

Figure 29-3 Standard lithotomy position with "candy cane" extremity support. Thighs are flexed approximately 90 degrees on the abdomen; knees are flexed enough to bring the lower legs grossly parallel to the torso section of the tabletop. Arms are retained on the boards, crossed on the abdomen, or snugged at the sides of patient.

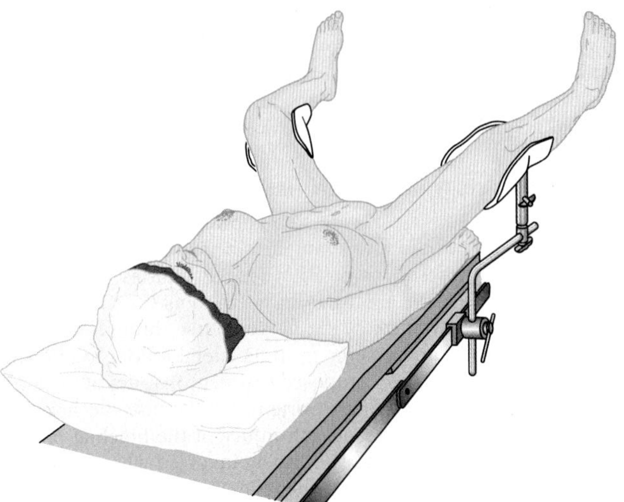

Figure 29-4 Low lithotomy position for perineal access, transurethral instrumentation, or combined abdominoperineal procedures.

Numerous devices are available to hold legs that are elevated during obstetric delivery or perineal operations (e.g., "candy canes" or stirrups). Each device should be fitted to the stature of the individual patient. Care should be taken to ensure that angulations or edges of the padded holder do not compress the popliteal space or the upper dorsal thigh. Compartment syndromes of one or both lower extremities have resulted from prolonged use of the lithotomy position with various types of support devices.[8]

Low

For most urologic procedures and for many procedures that require simultaneous access to the abdomen and perineum, the degree of thigh elevation in the lithotomy position is only approximately 30 to 45 degrees (Fig. 29-4). This reduces perfusion gradients to and from the lower extremities and improves access to a perineal surgical site for members of the operating team who may need to stand at the lateral aspect of either leg.

High

Some surgeons prefer to improve access to the perineum by suspending the patient's feet from high poles. The effect is to have the patient's legs almost fully extended on the thighs (Fig. 29-5) and the thighs flexed 90 degrees or more on the trunk. The posture produces a significant uphill gradient for arterial perfusion into the feet, requiring careful avoidance of systemic hypotension. There is considerable variation in lower extremity perfusion pressure in volunteers placed in high lithotomy positions; they all tend to have low perfusion pressures, however.[9,10] Less mobile patients may tolerate this posture poorly because of angulation and compression of the contents of the femoral canal by the inguinal ligament (Fig. 29-5A), or stretch of the sciatic nerve (Fig. 29-5B), or both.

Exaggerated

Transperineal access to the retropubic area requires that the patient's pelvis be flexed ventrally on the spine, the thighs almost forcibly flexed on the trunk, and the lower legs aimed skyward so that they are out of the way (Fig. 29-6). The result places the long axis of the symphysis pubis almost parallel to the floor. This exaggerated lithotomy position stresses the lumbar spine, produces a significant uphill gradient for perfusion of the feet, and may restrict ventilation because of abdominal compression by bulky thighs. If pre-existing painful lumbar spine disease is present, an

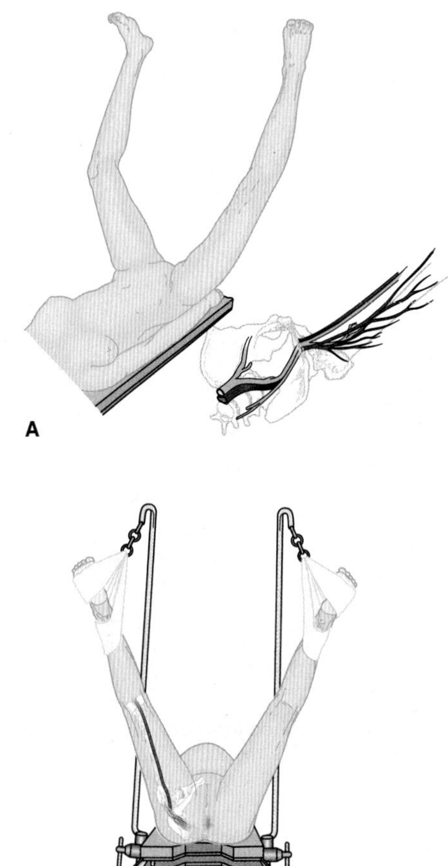

Figure 29-5 **High lithotomy position.** Note potential for angulation and compression/obstruction of contents of femoral canal (**A**, *inset*) or stretch of sciatic nerve (**B**). (Adapted and redrawn from McLeskey CH. *Geriatric Anesthesiology*. Williams & Wilkins; 1997:146.)

alternative surgical position may need to be chosen beforehand to avoid severely accentuating the lumbar distress after surgery. This position has been associated with a very high frequency of lower extremity compartment syndrome.[11] Maintenance of adequate perfusion pressure in the legs is important.

Complications of Supine Positions

Brachial Plexus Neuropathy

A 20-year review of malpractice closed claims cases involving positioning-related perioperative peripheral nerve injuries was published in 2019. Of these, 56% involved brachial plexus injuries, with the majority of those associated with supine and "arm out to the side" positioning.[12] The authors noted that although 92% of the claims involved "technical knowledge/performance" issues this may be an overestimation given the nature of closed claims analysis. A majority of claims involved a number of contributing factors and could be considered to be multifactorial.

Root Injuries

Shoulder braces placed tight against the base of the neck can compress and injure the roots of the brachial plexus when steep head-down positions are used (Video 29-1). Braces, if needed at all, are considered less harmful when placed more laterally over the acromioclavicular joint. In general, the use of shoulder braces should be discouraged. The same is true of straps or tape

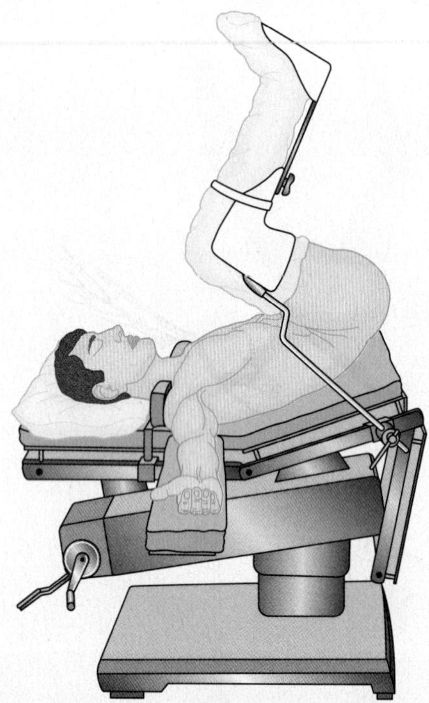

Figure 29-6 The exaggerated lithotomy position. Shoulder support may be needed to stabilize the torso. If used, it should be placed over the acromioclavicular area to minimize compression of the brachial plexus and adjacent vessels.

crisscrossed from above the shoulders to keep patients from sliding cephalad.

Supine positions do not usually threaten structures in the patient's neck unless considerable lateral displacement of the head occurs or if steep head-down tilt is added (2 Video 29-2). When lateral displacement of the head occurs, the roots of the brachial plexus on the side of the obtuse head–shoulder angle can be stretched and damaged. If the upper extremity is fixed to the operating table at the wrist (e.g., by wrist wrap or a sheet or towel used to tuck the arm), the stretch injury of the plexus can be accentuated as the head moves laterally away from the anchoring point of the wrist. Similarly, exaggerated rotation of the head away from an extended arm may be associated with a brachial plexus injury.

Sternal Retraction

Frequently, the patient undergoing a median sternotomy has both arms padded and secured alongside the torso. An alternative is to have both arms abducted.[13] Vander Salm et al.[14,15] described first-rib fractures and brachial plexus injuries associated with median sternotomies. They related the extent of the injury to the amount of retractor displacement of the rib, with the most severe injury being caused by displacement sufficient to produce a first-rib fracture. Roy et al.,[16] in a study of 200 consecutive adults scheduled for cardiac surgery via a median sternotomy, positioned the left arm either abducted and padded on an arm board with the palm supinated or secured by a draw sheet alongside the trunk; the right arm was always placed alongside the trunk. They found a 10% incidence of upper extremity nerve injury that was not influenced by internal mammary artery harvest, internal jugular vein catheterization, or left arm position. Surgical manipulation was more contributory than extremity positioning in producing trauma to the brachial plexus. Jellish et al.[13] reported that there is less slowing of somatosensory evoked potentials (SSEPs) of the ulnar nerve during sternotomy when both arms are abducted instead of tucked at the sides. However, they found no differences in perioperative symptoms between patients in the arm-abducted versus arm-at-side groups. Studies to ascertain the optimal arm positioning for patients undergoing median sternotomy are ongoing and definitive conclusions have not yet been reached.

Long Thoracic Nerve Dysfunction

A number of lawsuits have centered on postoperative serratus anterior muscle dysfunction and "winging" of the scapula (Fig. 29-7) alleged to be the result of position-related injuries to the long thoracic nerve, a nerve arising from nerve roots C5, C6, and C7. Because C5 and C6 fibers of the nerve course through the middle scalene muscle and emerge from its lateral border to join the fibers from C7, it has been proposed that neuropathies of the long thoracic nerve are traumatic in origin.[17,18] Because the nerve is not routinely involved in a stretch injury of the brachial plexus and because the plexus is not routinely involved when long thoracic nerve dysfunction occurs, the relationship between postoperative long thoracic neuropathy and patient positioning remains speculative. Based on evidence of Foo and Swann[19] plus data from various litigations, Martin[18] concluded that in the absence of demonstrable trauma, postoperative dysfunctions of the long thoracic nerve were quite likely the result of coincidental neuropathies, possibly of viral or inflammatory origin.

Axillary Trauma from the Humeral Head

Abduction of the arm on an arm board to greater than 90 degrees may thrust the head of the humerus into the axillary neurovascular bundle. This bundle typically lies on the flexion side of the shoulder joint. However, when the arm is abducted to greater than 90 degrees, the bundle is now on the extension side of the joint. The bundle is both compressed and stretched at that point, and its neural structures may be damaged. In the same manner, vessels can be compressed or occluded and perfusion of the extremity can be jeopardized.

Radial Nerve Compression

The radial nerve, arising from roots C6–8 and T1, passes dorsolaterally around the middle and lower portions of the humerus in the musculospiral groove. At a point on the lateral aspect of the arm, approximately three fingerbreadths proximal to the lateral epicondyle of the humerus, the nerve can be compressed against the underlying bone and injured. Pressure from the vertical bar of an anesthesia screen or a similar device against the lateral aspect of the arm, excessive cycling of an automatic blood pressure cuff, and compression at the midhumerus level by restrictive measures (sheets, towels, fabricated "toboggans") used to tuck the arms have been implicated in causing damage to the radial nerve. Other support devices, including arm boards and slings used when patients are positioned laterally, can directly compress the radial nerve as it wraps around the musculospiral groove.

Median Nerve Dysfunction

Isolated perioperative injuries to the median nerve are uncommon and the mechanism is usually obscure.[20,21] A potential source of injury is iatrogenic trauma to the nerve during access to vessels in the antecubital fossa, as might occur during venipuncture. Anecdotally, median nerve injury appears to occur primarily in men 20 to 40 years of age who cannot easily extend their elbows completely. Forced elbow extension after administration of muscle relaxants and while positioning the arms, with resultant stretch of the median nerve, has been suggested as one potential mechanism for this problem.

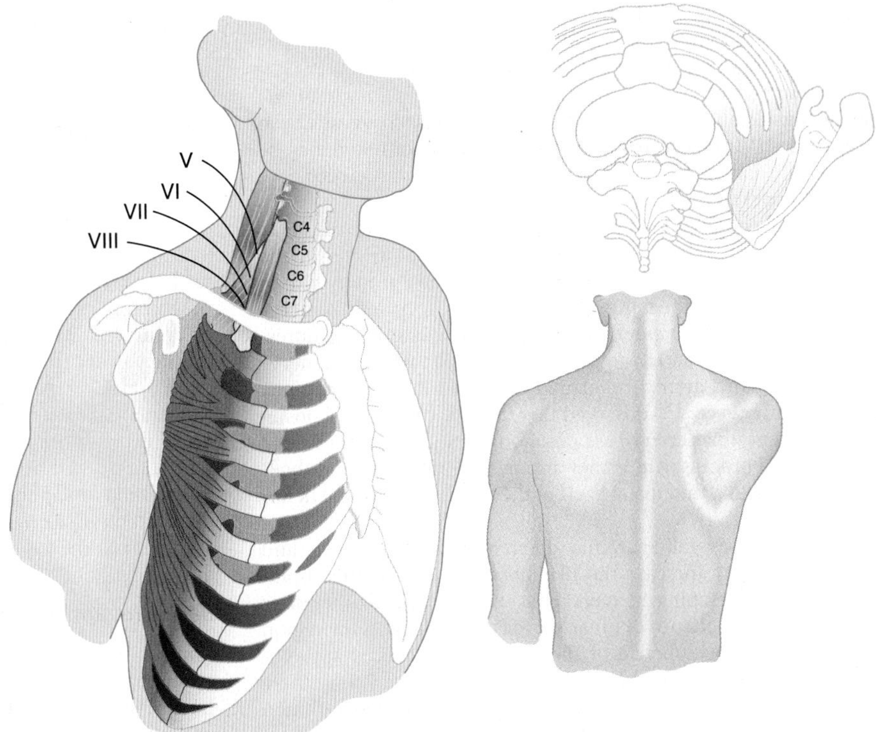

Figure 29-7 Scapular winging. The serratus anterior muscle (*upper right*) is supplied solely by the long thoracic nerve that branches immediately from C5, C6, C7, and sometimes C8 (*left figure*). Arising on the lateral ribs and inserting on the deep surface of the scapula, the muscle keeps the shoulder girdle approximated to the dorsal rib cage. Long thoracic nerve palsy allows dorsal protrusion of the scapula (*lower right*). See text for details.

Ulnar Neuropathy

The most common perioperative neuropathy involves the ulnar nerve (NICV 29-1 and Video 29-3). Improper anesthetic care and patient malpositioning were implicated as causative factors over a century ago[22,23] but a report in the 1970s suggested that external compression of the ulnar nerve during surgery was an uncommon causative factor.[24] A 2021 retrospective review of noncardiac surgical procedures in a large institution over a 4-year period found that the incidence of persistent perioperative ulnar neuropathy was 6.6 per 100,000 anesthetics and was increased with longer procedures.[25] Ulnar neuropathies can also develop in medical as well as surgical patients.[26] Thus, the mechanisms of perioperative ulnar neuropathy are unclear and may be multifactorial.

Typically, anesthesia-related ulnar nerve injury is thought to be associated with external nerve compression or stretch caused by malpositioning during the intraoperative period. Although this implication may be true for some patients, three findings suggest that other factors may contribute. First, patient characteristics (e.g., male gender, extremes of body mass index, history of cancer, and prolonged postoperative bed rest) are associated with these ulnar neuropathies.[24,27,28] Various reports suggest that 70% to 90% of patients who have this problem are men.[20,21,24–27] Second, many patients with perioperative ulnar neuropathies have a high frequency of contralateral ulnar nerve conduction dysfunction.[28] This finding suggests that many of these patients likely have asymptomatic but abnormal ulnar nerves before their anesthetics, and these abnormal nerves may become symptomatic during the perioperative period. Finally, many patients do not notice or complain of ulnar nerve symptoms until more than 48 hours after their surgical procedures.[26–28] A prospective study of ulnar neuropathy in 1,502 surgical patients found that none of the patients had symptoms of the neuropathy during the first 2 postoperative days.[29] Thus, it is not clear whether onset of symptoms indicates the time that an injury has occurred to the nerve.[30]

Elbow flexion can cause ulnar nerve damage by several mechanisms. In some patients, the ulnar nerve is compressed by the aponeurosis of the flexor carpi ulnaris muscle and cubital tunnel retinaculum when the elbow is flexed by greater than 110 degrees (Fig. 29-8).[31,32] In other patients, this fibrotendinous roof of the

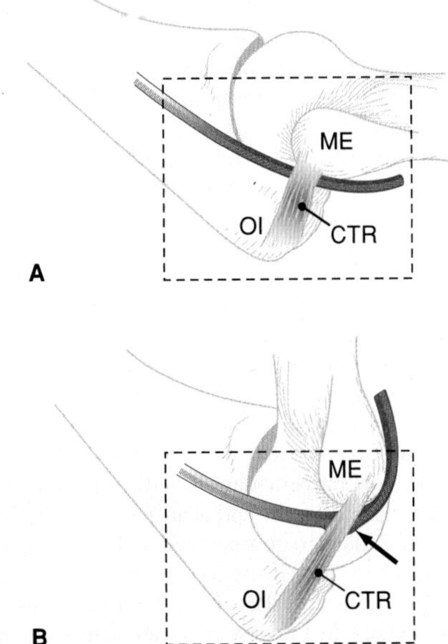

Figure 29-8 Medial-to-lateral view of right elbow. The cubital tunnel retinaculum (CTR) is lax in extension (**A**) as it stretches from the medial epicondyle (ME) to the olecranon (OI). The retinaculum tightens in flexion (**B**) and can compress the ulnar nerve (*arrow*). (Adapted and redrawn from O'Driscoll SW, Horii E, Carmichael SW, Morrey BF. The cubital tunnel and ulnar neuropathy. *J Bone Joint Surg Br*. 1991;73:615.)

cubital tunnel is poorly formed and can lead to anterior subluxation or dislocation of the ulnar nerve over the medial epicondyle of the humerus during elbow flexion. This displacement has been observed in approximately 16% of cadavers in whom the flexor muscle aponeurosis and supporting tissues have not been dissected.[33,34] It has been speculated that the ulnar nerve may be chronically damaged by recurrent mechanical trauma as the nerve is in subluxation over the medial epicondyle.[34]

External compression in the absence of elbow flexion also may damage the ulnar nerve.[35,36] Although compression within the medial epicondylar groove may be possible if the groove is shallower than normal, the bony groove usually is deep and the nerve is well protected from external compression.[37] External compression may occur distal to the medial epicondyle, where the nerve and its associated artery are relatively superficial. In an anatomic study, Contreras et al.[38] observed that the ulnar nerve and posterior recurrent ulnar artery pass posteromedially to the tubercle of the coronoid process, where they are covered only by skin, subcutaneous fat, and a thin distal band of the aponeurosis of the flexor carpi ulnaris.

There are several anatomic differences between men and women that may increase the likelihood of perioperative ulnar neuropathy developing in men. First, two anatomic differences may increase the chance of ulnar nerve compression in the region of the elbow. The tubercle of the coronoid process is approximately 1.5 times larger in men than women.[38] In addition, there is less adipose tissue over the medial aspect of the elbow of men compared with women of similar body fat composition.[38–40] Second, men may be more likely to have a well-developed cubital tunnel retinaculum than women, and the retinaculum, if present, is thicker. A thicker cubital tunnel retinaculum may increase the risk of ulnar nerve compression in the cubital tunnel when the elbow is flexed.

Clinical manifestations of ulnar nerve dysfunction vary with the location and extent of the lesion.[41] Nearly all patients have numbness, tingling, or pain in the sensory distribution of the ulnar nerves once they become symptomatic. However, there can be considerable ulnar nerve dysfunction before symptoms appear. Prielipp et al.[30] found that only 8 of 15 male volunteers with significant ulnar nerve conduction slowing noted any symptoms. More studies are needed to better understand the mechanism and natural history of ulnar neuropathy.

A significant proportion of patients have symptoms of bilateral ulnar nerve dysfunctions both before and after surgery.[29] Therefore, some have speculated that it might be helpful during the preanesthetic interview to inquire about a history of ulnar neuropathies ("crazy bone" problems) or previous surgery at the elbow. If such a history is indicated, the finding must be recorded and a discussion with the patient or family should present the possibility of a postoperative recurrence despite special precautions of padding and positioning.

The timing of recognition of neuropathy symptoms associated with ulnar nerve dysfunction may be quite important in establishing the origin of the postoperative syndrome. If ulnar hypesthesia or anesthesia is noted promptly after the end of anesthesia, as in the recovery area, the condition is likely to be associated with events that occurred during anesthesia or surgery. If the recognition is delayed for many hours, the likelihood of cause shifts from the intra-anesthetic period to postoperative events. In a review of closed claims, Cheney et al.[21] commented that postoperative ulnar dysfunction can occur as a result of events in the postanesthetic period and that nerve injury may develop in certain susceptible patients "despite conventionally accepted methods of positioning and padding."

Opioids may mask postoperative dysesthesias and pain, but even strong analgesics do not appear to mask a loss of sensation as a result of nerve dysfunction. It may be helpful to assess ulnar nerve function and record these observations before discharging the patient from the recovery room.

Other Supine Position Problems

Arm Complications

Arm boards should be securely attached to the operating table to prevent accidental release. An arm that is not properly secured can slip over the edge of the table or arm board, resulting in injury to the capsule of the shoulder joint by excessive dorsal extension of the humerus, fracture of the neck of an osteoporotic humerus, or injury to the ulnar nerve at the elbow. Conversely, in the unlikely event that the retaining strap or other holding device or cloth is excessively tight across the supinated forearm (Fig. 29-9), the potential exists for pressure to compress the anterior interosseous nerve, a branch of the median nerve in the upper forearm that courses with its artery along the volar surface of the tough interosseous membrane. The result is an ischemic injury to the distribution of the nerve and artery that resembles a compartment syndrome in the lower extremity and may require prompt surgical decompression.[42–44]

Backache and Paraplegia

4

Lumbar backache can be worsened by the ligamentous relaxation that occurs with general, spinal, or epidural anesthesia. Loss of normal lumbar curvature in the supine position is apparently the issue. As a general rule, when possible, patients should be placed in positions that are comfortable while they are awake prior to induction of anesthesia. Padding placed under the lumbar spine before the induction of anesthesia may help retain lordosis and make a patient with known lumbar distress more comfortable. Hyperlordosis should be avoided, however. Hyperextension of the lumbar spine, especially to an angulation of greater than 10 degrees at the L2–3 apex of the lumbar spine, may result in ischemia of the spinal nerves.[45] Multiple patients undergoing pelvic procedures have been reported to have developed paraplegia. In these patients, hyperlordosis was induced by retroflexing the operating room tables maximally, elevating kidney rests fully, and adding padding (e.g., towels, rolls, pillows, and even liter bags of crystalloid) under the lumbar spine to maximize hyperlordosis.

Compartment Syndrome

If, for whatever reason, perfusion to an extremity is inadequate, a compartment syndrome may develop. Characterized by ischemia,

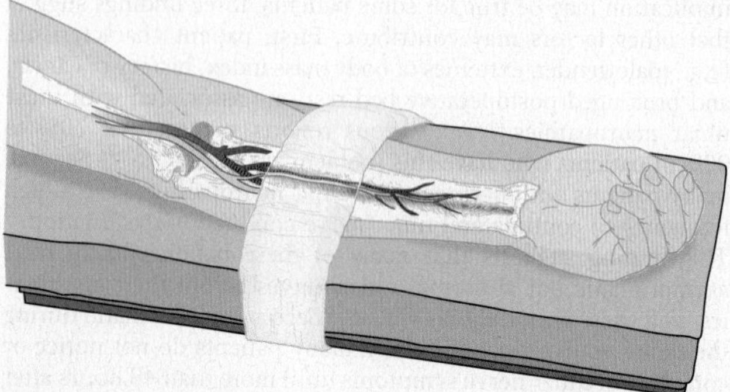

Figure 29-9 Arm restraint, if excessively tight, can compress the anterior interosseous nerve and vessel against the interosseous membrane in the volar forearm to produce an ischemic neuropathy. (Adapted and redrawn from McLeskey CH. *Geriatric Anesthesiology*. Williams & Wilkins; 1997:155.)

hypoxic edema, elevated tissue pressure within fascial compartments of the leg, and extensive rhabdomyolysis, the syndrome produces extensive and potentially lasting damage to the muscles and nerves in the compartment.

Causes of a compartment syndrome that may be associated with positioning factors while a patient is in any of the dorsal decubitus positions include (1) systemic hypotension and loss of perfusion pressure to the extremity (augmented by elevation of the extremity); (2) vascular obstruction of major leg vessels by intrapelvic retractors, by excessive flexion of knees or hips, or by undue popliteal pressure from a knee crutch; and (3) external compression of the elevated extremity by straps or leg wrappings that are too tight, by the inadvertent pressure of the arm of a surgical assistant, or by the weight of the extremity against a poorly supportive leg holder. A tight strap on an arm as well as tight "draw sheets" for maintaining arms at the patient's sides may compress the anterior interosseous neurovascular bundle and may be associated with an anterior interosseous neuropathy or a forearm or hand compartment syndrome.[43,44]

Several clinical characteristics seem to be associated with perioperative compartment syndrome. Prolonged lithotomy posture in excess of 5 hours has been a common factor in literature anecdotes of postlithotomy compartment syndromes. For lengthy procedures in the lithotomy position, well-padded holders that immobilize the limb by supporting the foot without compressing the calf or popliteal fossa seem to be the least threatening choice. Studies in healthy young volunteers have shown there is considerable variability in the perfusion pressure of the lower extremity in elevated legs.[9,10] Several volunteers had mean blood pressures when positioned in the high lithotomy position that were less than intracompartment pressures commonly measured in many lithotomy positions.

Perioperative compartment syndromes can occur in patients in positions other than lithotomy.[46] The frequency of this problem appears to occur as often (approximately 1 in 9,000 patients studied retrospectively) in anesthetized patients who are positioned laterally as in similar patients who are positioned in lithotomy. The difference between compartment syndromes in these two groups is that patients in a lateral decubitus position tend to have compartment syndromes of either arm, whereas those in a lithotomy position have compartment syndromes of the lower extremities.

Lateral Positions

There are several general positioning concepts to consider when placing a patient into a lateral decubitus position. Wrapping the legs and thighs in compressive bandages has been commonly used to combat venous pooling. Marked flexion of the lower extremities at knees and hips can partially or completely obstruct venous return to the inferior vena cava either by angulation of vessels at the popliteal space and inguinal ligament or by thigh compression against an obese abdomen. A small support placed just caudad of the downside axilla can be used to lift the thorax enough to relieve pressure on the axillary neurovascular bundle and prevent disturbed blood flow to the arm and hand. However, this chest support (improperly called an *axillary roll* by some) has not been proven to reduce the frequency of ischemia, nerve damage, or compartment syndrome to the downside upper extremity. It may, however, decrease shoulder discomfort postoperatively. Any padding should support only the chest wall and it should be periodically observed to ensure that it does not impinge on the neurovascular structures of the axilla.

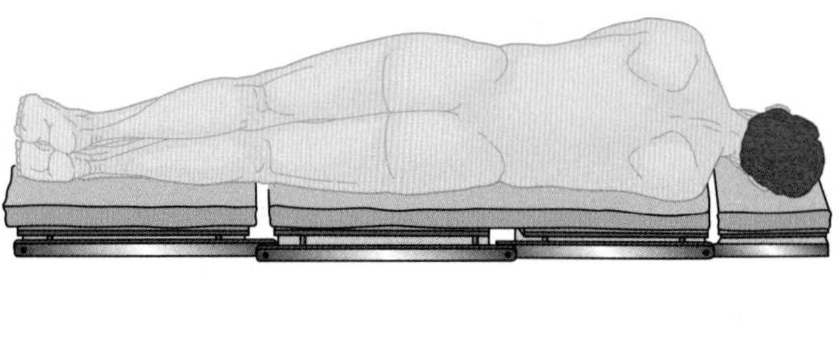

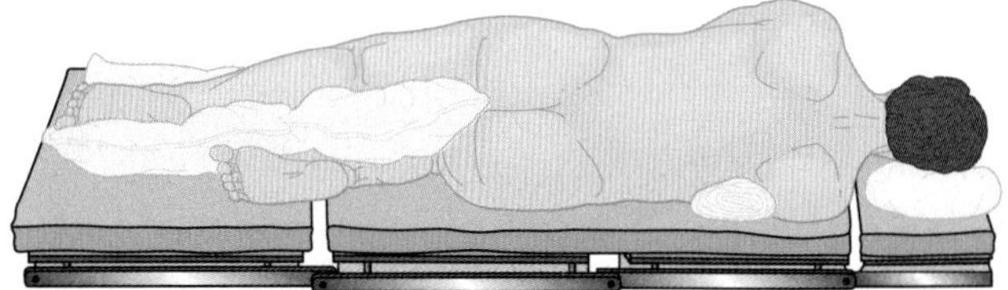

Figure 29-10 The standard lateral decubitus position. Proper head support, chest support, and leg pillow arrangements are shown in the *lower figure*. The downside leg is flexed at the hip and knee to stabilize the torso. Retaining straps and pad for the downside peroneal nerve are not shown.

Variations of Lateral Positions

Standard Lateral Position

In the standard lateral position (Fig. 29-10), the patient is rolled onto one side on a flat table surface and stabilized in that posture by flexing the downside thigh. The downside knee is bent to retain the leg on the table and improve stabilization of the trunk. The common peroneal nerve of that side is padded to minimize compression damage caused by the weight of the legs. The upside thigh and leg are extended comfortably, and pillows are placed between the lower extremities. The head is supported by pillows or a headrest so that the cervical and thoracic spines are properly aligned. A small pad, thick enough to raise the chest wall and prevent excessive compression of the shoulder or entrapment/compression of the neurovascular structures of the axilla, is placed just caudad to the downside axilla. This padding may support adequate perfusion of the downside hand and minimize circumduction of the dependent shoulder, which might stretch its suprascapular nerve.

Arms may be extended ventrally and retained on a single arm board with suitable padding between them, or they may be individually retained on a padded two-level arm support that can also help to stabilize the thorax. An alternate method of arm arrangement is to flex each elbow and place the arms on suitable padding on the table in front of the patient's face.

The patient is stabilized in the lateral position by the use of one or more retaining tapes or straps stretched across the hip and fixed to the underside of the tabletop. Care must be taken to see that the hip tapes or straps lie safely between the iliac crest and the head of the femur rather than over the head of the femur. An additional restraining tape or strap may be used across the thorax or shoulders if needed. Other methods, such as the use of "bean bag" or vacuum-supported retention devices, are commonly used. As with any such devices, it is essential to ensure that point pressure on bony prominences is minimized and body structures are appropriately supported.

Semisupine and Semiprone

Semilateral postures are designed to allow surgeons to reach anterolateral (semisupine) and posterolateral (semiprone) structures of the trunk. In the semisupine position, the upside arm must be carefully supported so that it is not hyperextended and

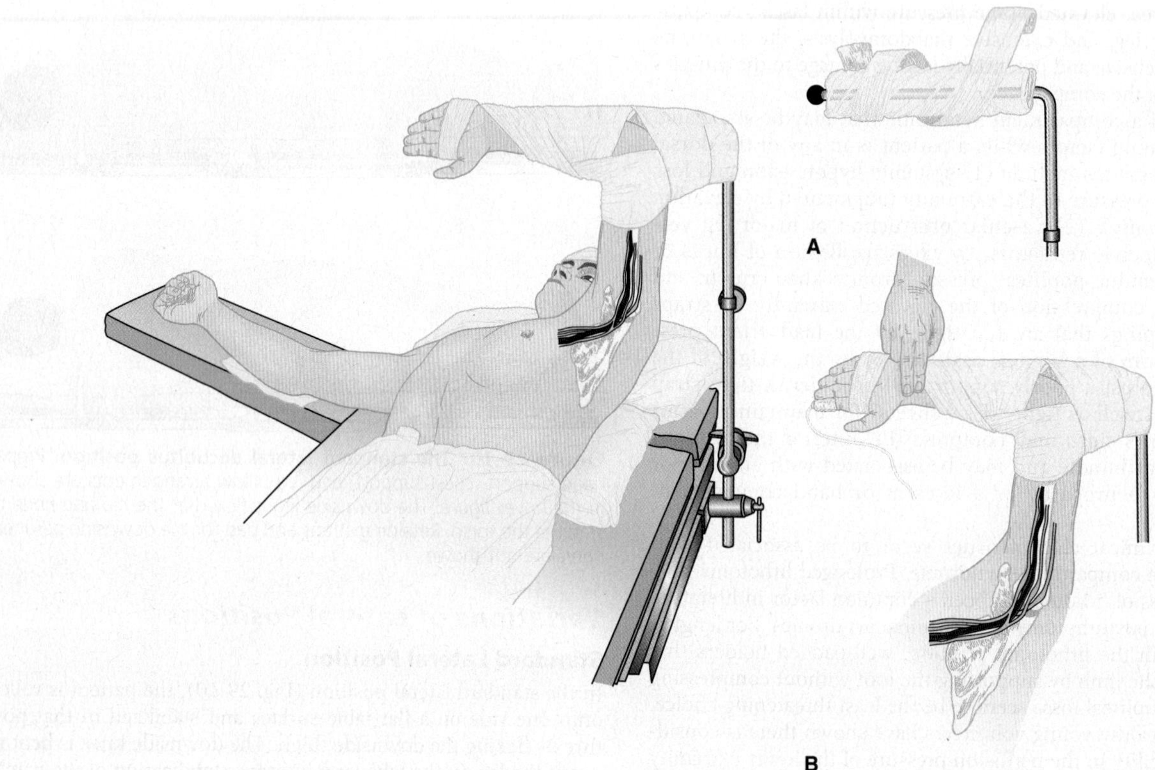

Figure 29-11 The semisupine position with dorsal pads supporting the torso, the extended arm padded at the elbow, and the elevated arm restrained on a well-cushioned, adjustable overhead bar (**A**). Axillary contents (**B**) are not under tension and are not compressed by the head of the humerus, and a pulse oximeter ensures that the digital circulation is not compromised. The position is safe only if the arm does not become a hanging mechanism to support the torso. (Adapted and redrawn from Collins VJ. *Principles of Anesthesiology*. 3rd ed. Lea & Febiger; 1993:176.)

no traction or compression is applied to the brachial and axillary neurovascular bundles (Fig. 29-11). The supporting bar should be well wrapped to prevent electrical grounding contact (Fig. 29-11A). Sufficient noncompressible padding should be placed under the torso and hip to prevent the patient from rolling supine and stretching the anchored extremity. The pulse of the restrained wrist should be checked to ensure adequate circulation in the elevated arm and hand (Fig. 29-11B).

Flexed Lateral Positions

Lateral Jackknife

The lateral jackknife position places the downside iliac crest over the hinge between the back and thigh sections of the table (Fig. 29-12). The tabletop is angulated at that point to flex the thighs on the trunk laterally. After the patient has been suitably positioned and restrained, the chassis of the table is tipped so that the uppermost surface of the patient's flank and thorax becomes essentially horizontal. As a result, the feet are below the level of the atria, and significant amounts of blood may pool in distensible vessels in each leg.

The lateral jackknife position is usually intended to stretch the upside flank and widen intercostal spaces as an asset to a thoracotomy incision. However, due to lumbar stress, restriction by the taut flank of upside costal margin motion, and pooling of blood in depressed lower extremities, the position has the potential to impose a significant physiologic insult. Once the rib-spreading retractor is placed in the incision, the position has reduced value for the rest of the operation and its use should be limited.

Kidney

The kidney position (Fig. 29-13) resembles the lateral jackknife position, but adds the use of an elevated rest (the *kidney rest*) under the downside iliac crest to increase the amount of lateral flexion and improve access to the upside kidney under the overhanging costal margin. Unlike the lateral jackknife position, the kidney position does not have a useful alternative for a flank approach to the kidney. Thus, the physiologic insults associated with the posture need to be limited by vigilant anesthesia and, hopefully, rapid surgery. Strict stabilizing precautions should be taken to prevent the patient from subsequently shifting caudad on the table in such a manner that the elevated rest relocates into the downside flank and becomes a severe impediment to ventilation of the dependent lung.

Complications of Lateral Positions

Eyes and Ears

Injuries to the dependent eye are unlikely if the head is properly supported during and after the turn from the supine to the lateral position. If the patient's face turns toward the mattress, however, and the lids are not closed or the eyes otherwise protected, abrasions of the ocular surface can occur. Direct pressure on the globe can displace the crystalline lens, increase intraocular pressure or, particularly if systemic hypotension is present, cause ischemia.

In the lateral position, the weight of the head can press the downside ear against a rough or wrinkled supporting surface. Careful padding with a pillow or a foam sponge is usually

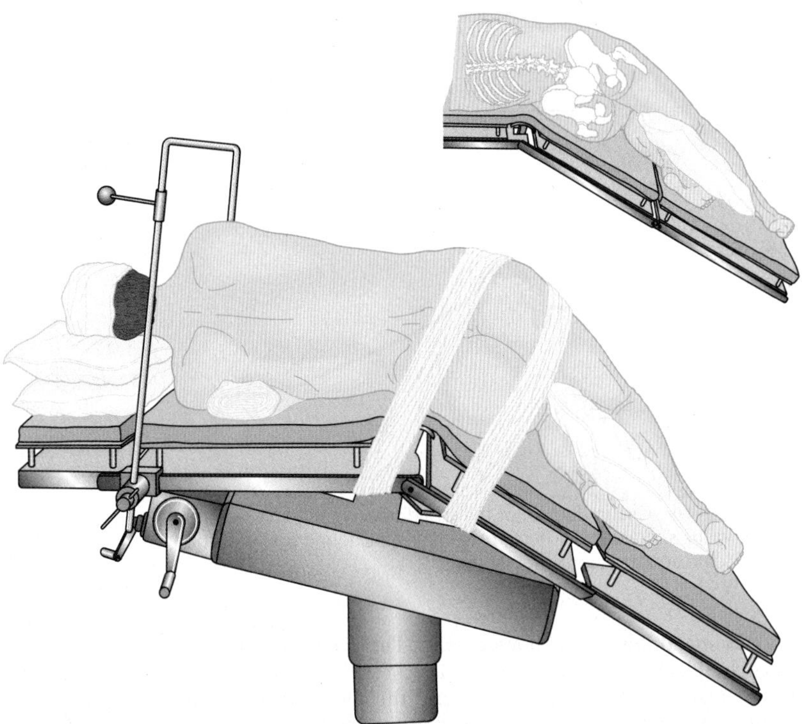

Figure 29-12 The lateral jackknife position, intended to open intercostal spaces. Note the properly placed restraining tapes (*large figure*) thrusting cephalad to retain the iliac crest at the flexion point of the table and prevent caudad slippage, which compresses the downside flank (*inset*).

sufficient protection against contusion of the ear. The external ear should also be palpated to ensure that it has not been folded over in the process of placing support beneath the head.

Neck

Lateral flexion of the neck is possible when the head of a patient in the lateral position is inadequately supported. If the cervical spine is arthritic, postoperative neck pain can be troublesome. Similarly, pain from a symptomatic protrusion of a cervical disk can be intensified.

Suprascapular Nerve

Ventral circumduction of the dependent shoulder can rotate the suprascapular notch away from the root of the neck (Fig. 29-14). Because the suprascapular nerve is fixed both paravertebrally and at the notch, circumduction can stretch the nerve and produce

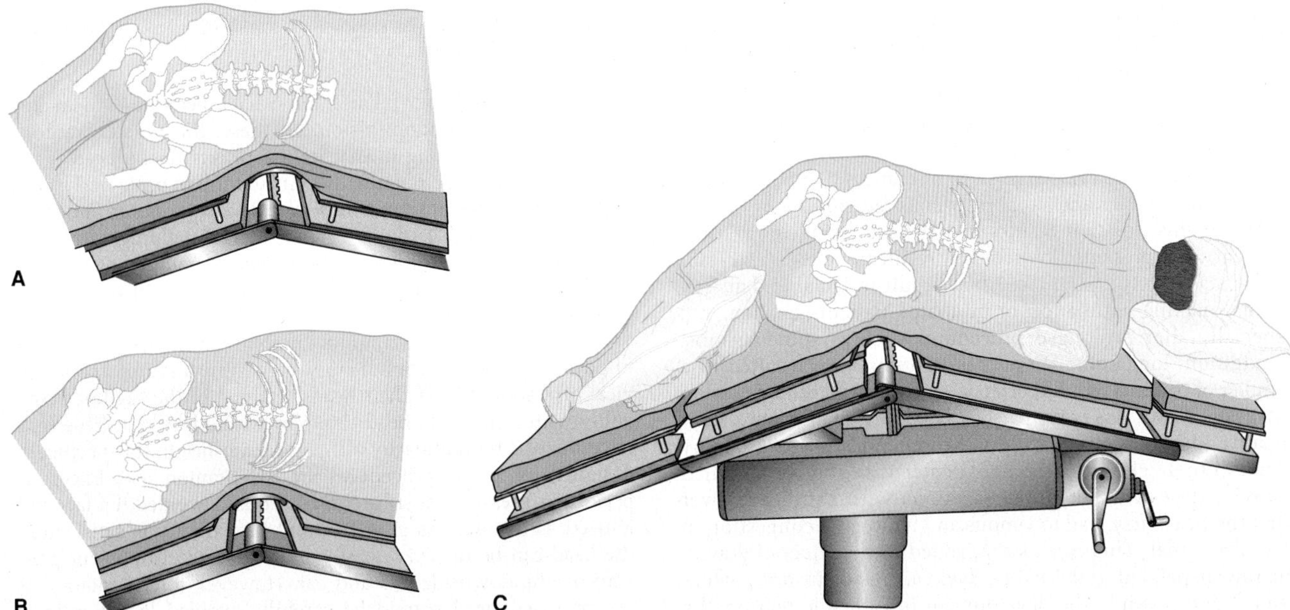

Figure 29-13 The flexed lateral (kidney) position. Upper panels show improper locations of the elevated transverse rest, the flexion point of the table, in the flank (**A**) or at the lower costal margin (**B**) to impede ventilation of the downside lung. The iliac crest at the proper flexion point (**C**), allowing the best possible expansion of the downside lung. Restraining tapes deleted for clarity.

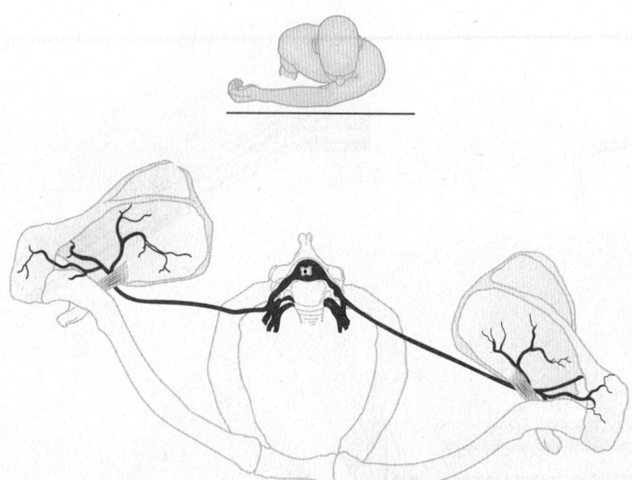

Figure 29-14 Circumduction of the arm displacing the scapula and stretching the suprascapular nerve between its anchoring points at the cervical spine and the suprascapular notch.

troublesome, diffuse, dull shoulder pain. The diagnosis is established by blocking the nerve at the notch and producing pain relief. Treatment may require resecting the ligament over the notch to decompress the nerve. A supporting pad placed under the thorax caudad of the axilla and thick enough to raise the chest off the shoulder may prevent a circumduction stretch injury to the nerve.

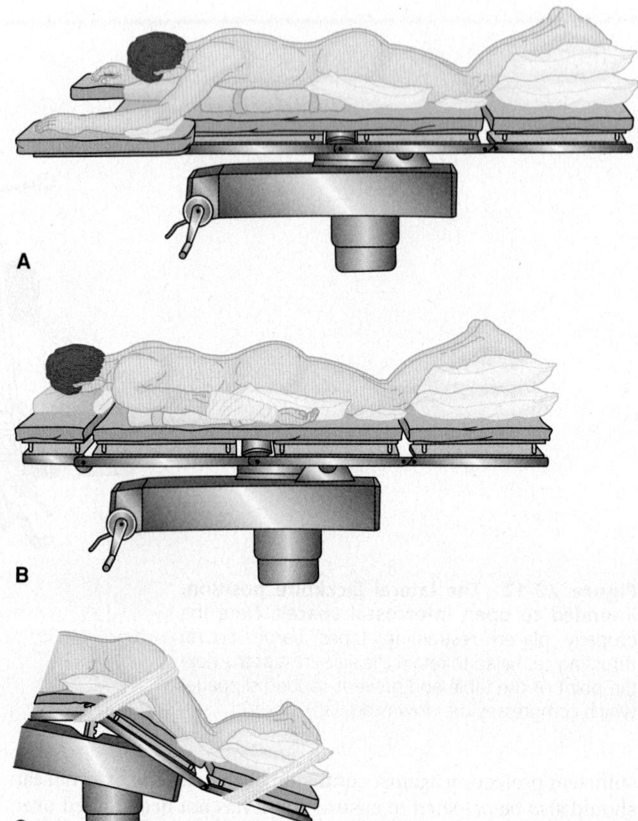

Figure 29-15 The classic prone position. A: Flat table with relaxed arms extended alongside the patient's head. Parallel chest rolls extended from just caudad of the clavicle to just beyond the inguinal area, with a pillow over the pelvic end. Elbows and knees are padded, and legs are bent at the knees. The head is turned onto a C-shaped pad, gel, or foam sponge that frees the downside eye and ear from compression. **B:** The same posture with arms snugly retained alongside the torso. **C:** Table flexed to reduce lumbar lordosis; subgluteal area straps placed after the legs are lowered to provide cephalad thrust and prevent caudad slippage.

Prone Positions

Full Prone

In the so-called *full prone position* (Fig. 29-15), the requirement to elevate the trunk off the supporting surface so that the ventral abdominal wall is freed of compression almost always results in the head and lower extremities being below the level of the spine. If the tabletop is angulated at the trunk–thigh hinge to remove the lumbar lordosis and separate the lumbar spinous processes, and if the chassis is then rotated head up sufficiently to level the patient's back, a significant perfusion gradient may develop between the legs and the heart. Wrapping the legs in compressive bandages, or the use of full-length elastic hosiery, minimizes pooling of blood in distensible vessels and supports venous return.

When this position results in the head being lower than the heart, the pressure gradient can result in venous and lymphatic stasis in the head. This may result in facial and airway edema, making extubation of intubated patients challenging, especially after prolonged procedures such as spine fusions. In addition, long spine surgical procedures have resulted in a number of patients who experience severe and permanent vision loss. This vision loss is primarily related to ischemic optic neuropathy. Although the etiology of the ischemic optic neuropathy is not entirely clear, a 2012 multicenter case-control designed study[47] suggested that prone positions with the head lower than the heart may lead to venous and lymphatic congestion in the optic canal. This congestion, added to the effect of gravity on the suspended globe of the eye, can result in optic nerve stretch and possibly the development of ischemic neuropathy (see later).[48]

Various pelvic, abdominal, and chest supports, including parallel rolls of tightly packed sheets, gels, padded and adjustable metal frames, and four-pillar frames, have been devised to free the abdomen from compression. Of these, the Wilson frame is particularly concerning in that its use results in the head being lower than the heart, potentially contributing to optic nerve congestion.[47] The use of frames may also produce opportunities for point pressure and if they are used, careful padding of contact points should be considered. The choice of equipment is based on the physique of the patient, the requirements of the surgical procedure, and availability.

Pronated patients with limited mobility of the neck, a history of postural neck pain, or a history suggesting a symptomatic cervical disk should have their heads retained in the sagittal plane, either with a skull-pin head clamp or with a face rest. Face rests have fluctuating popularity although foam headrests specifically designed for prone procedures are in common use. Excessive periocular pressure must be considered and avoided if a face rest is used. If the neck is pain free and its mobility is satisfactory, the head can be turned laterally and supported to prevent pressure on the downside eye and ear. However, forced rotation of the pronated head should be carefully avoided lest it induces postoperative neck pain or cervical nerve root or vascular compression. In addition, most patients described in the American Association of Anesthesiologists (ASA) Closed Claims database as having developed cervical neuropathies while positioned prone were found to have their heads rotated for greater than 3 hours. This information suggests that it may be reasonable to maintain the head in a neutral position when patients are anticipated to be positioned prone for greater than 3 hours.

When a patient is scheduled to be pronated after induction of anesthesia, it is worthwhile during the preanesthetic interview to obtain and record information about any limitations that may exist in their ability to raise the arms overhead during work or sleep. If the patient is symptomatic, it may be prudent to place the arms alongside the torso after pronation (see Thoracic Outlet Syndrome). If the arms are placed alongside the head (i.e., extended ventrally at the shoulder, flexed at the elbow, and abducted onto arm boards; the "surrender" position), the musculature about the shoulders should be under no tension, neither humeral head should stretch nor compress its axillary neurovascular bundle (i.e., shoulders should be abducted <90 degrees), ulnar nerves at the elbow should be padded, and the pulses at the wrists should remain full. Anterior (forward) flexion of the shoulders may reduce tension on the neurovascular structures of the axilla.

Complications of Prone Positions

Eyes and Ears

The eyes and ears may sustain injury in the prone position (4 Video 29-4). The eyelids should be closed, and each eye should be protected in some manner so that the lids cannot be accidentally separated and the cornea scratched. Instillation of lubrication in the eyes should be considered, although the value of this treatment is debated. The eyes should also be protected against the head turning after positioning and pressure being exerted on the globe. Monitoring wires and intravenous tubing should be checked after pronation to see that none has migrated beneath the head. If the head is retained in the sagittal plane, the eyes should be checked after positioning to ensure that they are safe from compression by any headrest.

Conjunctival edema usually occurs in the eyes of the pronated patient if the head is at or below the level of the heart. It is usually transient, inconsequential, and requires only reestablishment of the normal tissue perfusion gradients of the supine position, or of a slight amount of head-up tilt, to be redistributed. There does not appear to be any connection between this edema and the occurrence of posterior ischemic optic neuropathy.

Blindness

5 Permanent loss of vision can occur after nonocular surgical procedures, especially those performed in a prone position.[47,48] The occurrence of this devastating complication is associated particularly with extensive surgical procedures done in the prone position, such as reconstructive spine surgery, where there is associated blood loss, anemia, and hypotension.

Lee et al.[47] used data from the American Society of Anesthesiologists Visual Loss Registry to study ischemic optic neuropathy in spine fusion patients. Using a 1:4 case-control methodology, the authors found six risk factors, half of which strongly support their speculation that acute venous congestion of the optic canal is a potential etiology of ischemic optic neuropathy in this setting. The use of a Wilson surgical bed frame with its elevated curvature resulting in the head being lower than the heart, obesity with its potential elevation of intra-abdominal pressure in prone-positioned patients, and long anesthetic durations can all contribute to elevated venous congestion in the optic canal and potentially reduce optic nerve perfusion pressure. The authors also found that increased estimated blood loss, male gender, and lower colloid administration were independently associated with the development of ischemic optic neuropathy after spinal fusion surgery.

The ASA updated its Practice Advisory on this issue in 2019.[48] The recommendations for preoperative management are to review the patient's medical history for specific risk factors such as preexisting anemia, hypertension, diabetes, tobacco use, male sex, or obesity. Patients who are at high risk for perioperative visual loss in spine surgery should be informed of this potential devastating complication. The recommendations regarding intraoperative management involve maintenance of blood pressure as close to the patient's baseline as possible, ongoing communication with the surgeon, close attention to blood loss and fluid administration (monitor hemoglobin levels, use colloids in addition to crystalloids as indicated), and use of vasopressors to correct hypotension. The objectives of patient and head positioning should center on an attempt to reduce venous congestion in the optic canal. Consideration should be given to using positions that allow the patients' heads to be level with or higher than their hearts. Intraoperative positioning that helps reduce intra-abdominal pressure and, therefore, venous congestion, may be useful. The use of the Wilson frame and other positioning devices should be assessed carefully, with a goal to reduce pressure on the abdomen and to keep the head level with or higher than the heart. As with all procedural positioning, eyes should be checked regularly for compression. Since studies have found duration of anesthesia to be an independent risk factor for ischemic optic neuropathy in this population, it may be prudent to work with the spine surgeons to determine if there is merit to limiting the duration of surgeries that are anticipated to be prolonged, such as 6 hours or longer. Staging these procedures may be a judicious alternative.

Neck Problems

Anesthesia impairs reflex muscle spasm that protects the skeleton against motion that would be painful if the patient were alert. Lateral rotation of the head and neck of an anesthetized, pronated patient, particularly one with an arthritic cervical spine, can stretch relaxed skeletal muscles and ligaments and injure articulations of cervical vertebrae. Postoperative neck pain and limitation of motion can result. The arthritic neck is usually best managed by keeping the head in the sagittal plane when the patient is prone.

Extremes of head and neck rotation can also interfere with flow in either the ipsilateral or contralateral vessels to and from the head. Excessive head rotation can reduce flow in both the carotid[48] and vertebral systems.[49,50] Impaired cerebral perfusion is the obvious consequence.

Brachial Plexus Injuries

Stretch injuries to the roots of the brachial plexus (Fig. 29-16A) on the side contralateral to the turned face are possible if the contralateral shoulder is held firmly caudad by a wrist restraint. If an arm is placed on an arm board alongside the head, care must be taken to ensure that the head of the humerus is not stretching and compressing the axillary neurovascular bundle (Fig. 29-16B,C).

When an arm is placed on an arm board alongside the head, the forearm naturally pronates. As a result, the ulnar nerve, lying in the cubital tunnel (the groove between the olecranon process and the medial epicondyle of the humerus), is vulnerable to being compressed by the weight of the elbow (Fig. 29-16D). Consequently, the medial aspect of the elbow must be well padded and its weight borne across a large area to avoid point pressure.

Asking patients about their ability to work or sleep with arms elevated overhead may identify patients with *thoracic outlet obstruction*. A useful preoperative test if the history is in question is to have the patient clasp hands behind the occiput during the

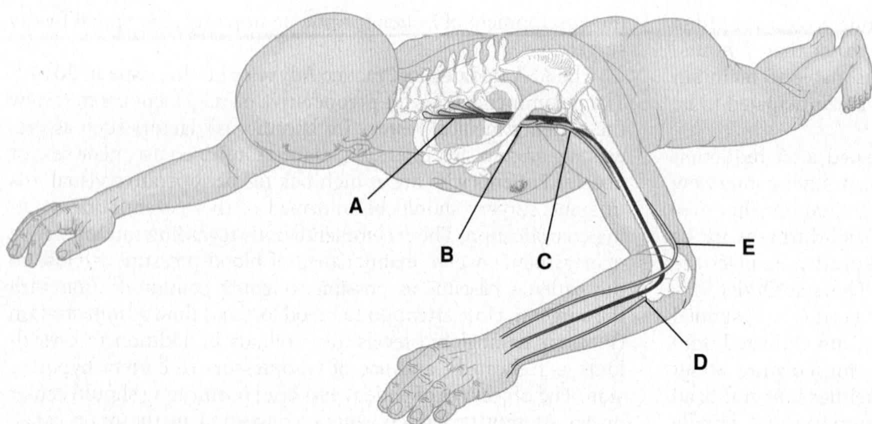

Figure 29-16 Sources of potential injury to the brachial plexus and its peripheral components when the patient is in the prone position. A: Neck rotation, stretching roots of the plexus. **B:** Compression of the plexus and vessels between the clavicle and first rib. **C:** Injury to the axillary neurovascular bundle from the head of the humerus. **D:** Compression of the ulnar nerve before, beyond, and within the cubital tunnel. **E:** Area of vulnerability of the radial nerve to lateral compression proximal to the elbow.

interview. If the patient describes dysesthesias, it may be prudent to keep the arms alongside the trunk in the prone position. Agonizing, debilitating, and unremitting postoperative pain has been known to follow overhead arm placement in pronated patients who have had prior discomfort in their arms in that position.

Breast Injuries

The breasts of a pronated woman can be stretched and injured along their sternal borders if forced laterally or medially by chest and abdominal wall supports. Direct pressure on breasts (particularly if breast prostheses are present) can cause ischemia to breast tissue and should be avoided. Multiple cases of breast tissue ischemia have been reported, often resulting in mastectomy and the need for reconstruction.

Abdominal Compression

Compression of the abdomen by the weight of the prone patient's trunk can cause viscera to force the diaphragm cephalad enough to impair ventilation. If intra-abdominal pressure approaches or exceeds venous pressure, return of blood from the pelvis and lower extremities is reduced or obstructed. Because the vertebral venous plexuses communicate directly with the abdominal veins, increased intra-abdominal pressure is transmitted to the perivertebral and intraspinal surgical field in the form of venous distention and increased difficulty with hemostasis. All of the various supportive pads and frames, when properly used, are designed to remove pressure from the abdomen and avoid these problems.

Stoma and Genitals

A stoma that drains visceral contents through the abdominal wall is at risk in the prone position if they lie against a part of any supporting frame or pad (5 Video 29-5). Compressive ischemia of the stomal orifice can cause it to slough. The same issue is present for genitals, especially the penis and scrotum of men turned prone.

Head-Elevated Positions

Variations of Head-Elevated Positions

Sitting

The classic *sitting position* for surgery places the patient in a semireclining posture on an operating table, with the legs elevated to approximately the level of the heart and the head flexed ventrally on the neck (NICV 29-2 and Fig. 29-17). Head flexion should not be sufficient to force the chin into the suprasternal notch (see "Midcervical Tetraplegia"). Elastic stockings or compressive wraps around the legs reduce pooling of blood in the lower extremities. The head often is held in place by some type of a face rest or by a three-pin skull fixation frame.

Supine—Tilted Head Up

A supine recumbent position with the head of the patient elevated is used for many operations involving the ventral and lateral aspects of the head (Fig. 29-18) and neck, and occasionally with the neck flexed, for transcranial access to the top of the brain. Its purpose is to improve access to the surgical target for the operating team as well as to drain blood and irrigation solutions away from the wound. The back section of the surgical table can be elevated as needed to produce a low sitting position (Fig. 29-18A) or the entire table can be rotated head high with the patient's extended legs supported by a footrest (Fig. 29-18B). Although the degree of tilt typically is not great, small pressure gradients are created along the vascular axis that can pool blood in the lower extremities or entrain air into patulous vessels that are incised above the level of the heart.

For operations around the shoulder joint, the patient may be placed in a head-elevated semisupine position (Fig. 29-19). The upper trunk typically is moved laterally until the raised surgical shoulder extends beyond the edge of the operating table. The torso is supported so that the hips are on the table, the surgical shoulder is off and above the table edge, and the head rests on either a pillow (Fig. 29-19A) or a headrest (Fig. 29-19B). Access is thereby provided to both the dorsal and ventral aspects of the shoulder girdle. The surgical arm remains on the front of the torso and is prepared and draped to be mobile in the surgical field.

Lateral—Tilted Head Up

The lateral position with the head somewhat elevated, a means of access to occipitocervical lesions, has also been referred to as the *park bench position*. All the stabilizing requirements needed for the usual lateral position apply. The head may be held firmly in a three-pin skull fixation holder, which can be readjusted as needed during surgery, or supported by pillows or padding. Although the degree of head elevation used typically is less than 15 degrees, the position does not completely remove the threat of air embolization. The anesthesiologist has good access to the patient's face and thorax for purposes of monitoring, manipulation, and resuscitation. Considerable attention should be directed to avoiding compression of neck veins, which can lead to an increase in intracranial pressure and to edema of the tongue.

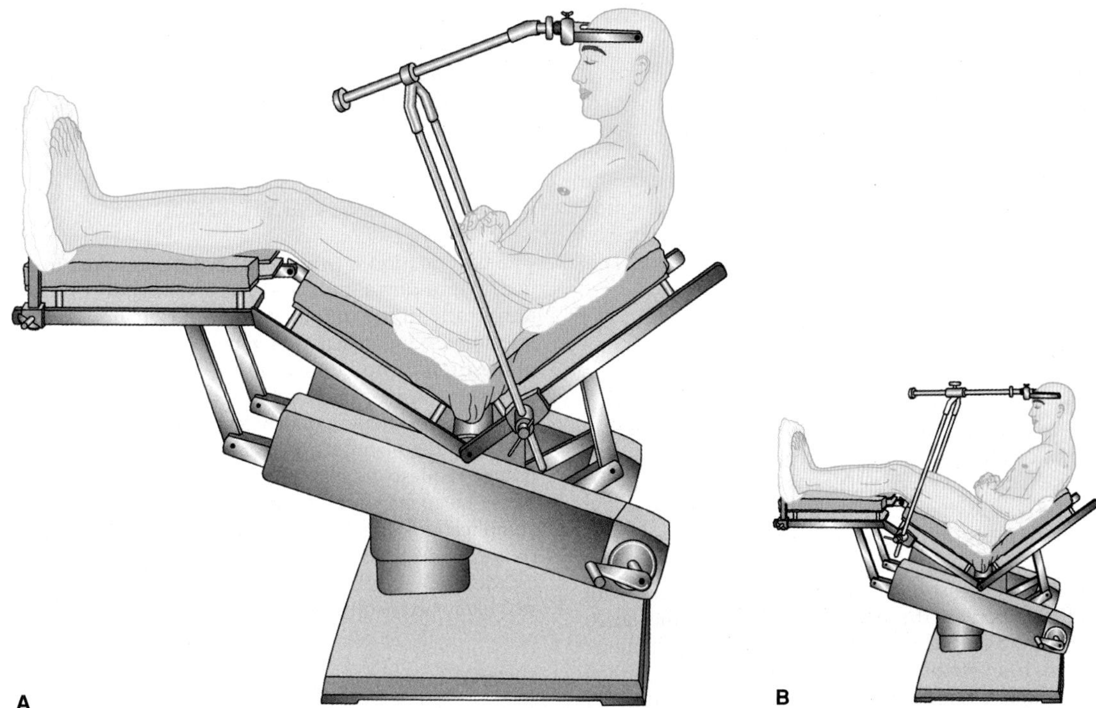

Figure 29-17 **A:** Conventional neurosurgical sitting position. The legs are at approximately the level of the heart and gently flexed on the thighs; the feet are supported at right angles to the legs; subgluteal padding protects the sciatic nerve. The frame of the head holder is *properly* clamped to the side rails of the back section in the event of hemodynamically significant air embolism. **B:** *Improper* attachment of the head frame to the table side rails at the thigh section. In this position, the patient's head could not be quickly lowered because it would require disengaging the skull clamp.

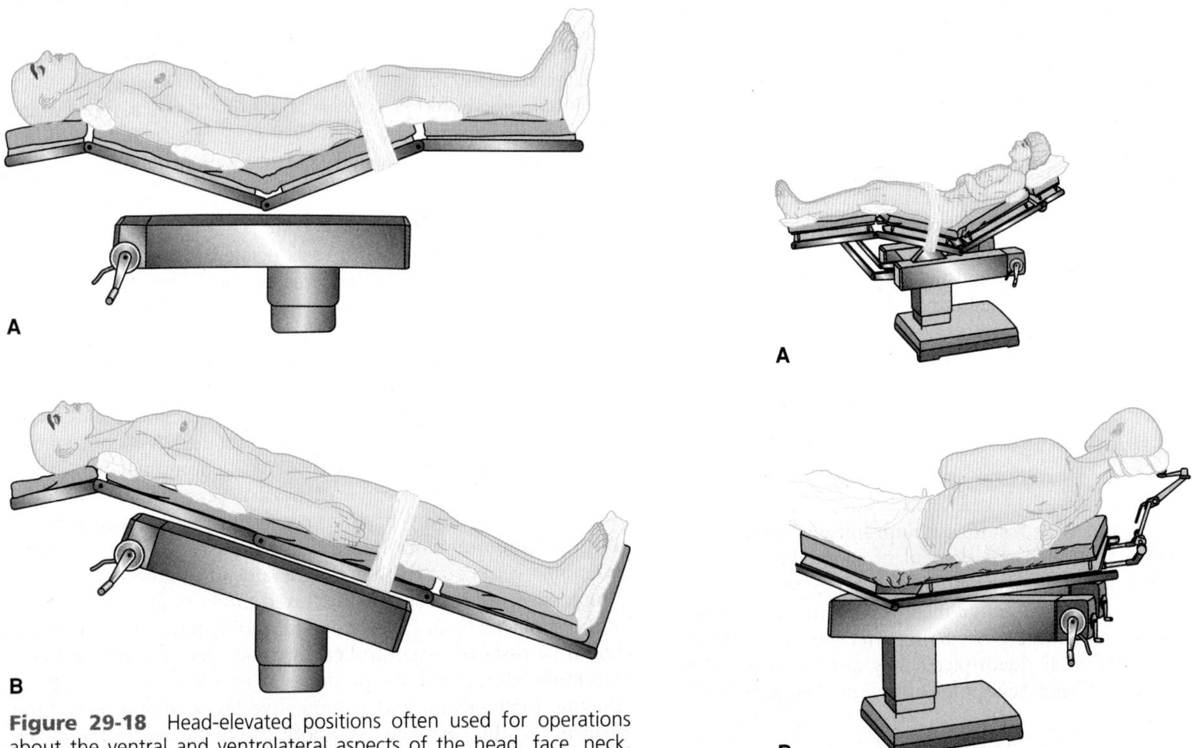

Figure 29-18 Head-elevated positions often used for operations about the ventral and ventrolateral aspects of the head, face, neck, and cervical spine. **A:** The legs are at approximately heart level and the gradient into the head is appreciable but slight. **B:** The flat table and footrest are useful when a thyroidectomy is planned under regional anesthesia.

Figure 29-19 **A:** The lawn chair position for surgery around the shoulder joint. **B:** The upper torso is rotated toward the nonsurgical shoulder and supported with a firm roll or pad.

Complications of Head-Elevated Positions

Postural Hypotension

In the anesthetized patient, establishing any of the head-elevated positions is frequently accompanied by some degree of reduction in systemic blood pressure. The normal protective reflexes are inhibited by drugs used during anesthesia. Measuring mean arterial pressures at the level of the circle of Willis is recommended by many to assess cerebral perfusion pressures more accurately. This recommendation, however, is controversial.[51–55]

Air Embolus

Air embolization is potentially lethal. In the bloodstream, air migrates to the heart, where it creates a compressible foam that destroys the propulsive efficiency of ventricular contraction and irritates the conduction system. Air can also move into the pulmonary vasculature, where bubbles obstruct small vessels and compromise gas exchange, or it can cross through a patent foramen ovale to the left side of the heart and the systemic circulation.

The potential for venous air embolization increases with the degree of elevation of the operative site above the heart. Although the occurrence of air emboli is a relatively frequent phenomenon in head-elevated positions, most of the emboli are small in volume, clinically silent, and recognizable only by sophisticated Doppler detection or echocardiographic (e.g., transesophageal) techniques. Nevertheless, the potential for dangerous accumulations of entrained air requires immediate detection of the embolization, a careful search for its portal of entry, and prompt treatment of its clinical effects.

Edema of the Face, Tongue, and Neck

Severe postoperative macroglossia, apparently because of venous and lymphatic obstruction, can be caused by prolonged, marked neck flexion. Postoperative need for a tracheostomy has been reported. Try to avoid placing the patient's chin firmly against the chest and use an oral airway to protect the endotracheal tube. Extremes of neck flexion, with or without head rotation, have been widely used to gain access to structures in the posterior fossa and cervical spine, but their potential for damage should be understood and excessive flexion–rotation avoided if possible. Moore et al.[56] have suggested that the primary mechanism may be neurologically determined rather than being the result of either vascular obstruction or local trauma. This problem also has been described with the use of transesophageal echocardiography probes.

Midcervical Quadriplegia

This devastating injury can occur after hyperflexion of the neck, with or without rotation of the head, and is attributed to stretching of the spinal cord with resulting compromise of its vasculature in the midcervical area. An element of spondylosis may be involved.[57,58] The result is paralysis below the general level of the fifth cervical vertebra. Although most reports in the literature have described the condition as occurring after the use of the sitting position, midcervical quadriplegia has also occurred after prolonged, nonforced head flexion for intracranial surgery in the supine position.

Sciatic Nerve Injury

Stretch injuries of the sciatic nerve can occur in some seated patients if the hips are markedly flexed without bending the knees. Prolonged compression of the sciatic nerve as it emerges from the pelvis is possible in a thin seated patient if the buttocks are not suitably padded. Foot drop may be the result of injuries to either the sciatic nerve or the common peroneal nerve and can be bilateral.

Head-Down Positions

The introduction of robotic procedures resulted in an increased use of head-down positions. The great majority of robotic procedures early in the introduction of the technology involved prostatectomies, colorectal, and gynecologic procedures. Thus, most of these initial procedures and the experience gained with robotic procedures were performed in the pelvis and lower abdomen. As with any introduction of new technology, there is a steep learning curve for the operators. Typically, early adopters of robotic technology requested steep head-down positions of supine patients. These steep head-down positions have resulted in a variety of complications that challenge anesthesia providers and patients. As the indications for and uses of robotic surgeries continue to increase new positioning challenges related to these procedures will likely be encountered.

Complications of Head-Down Positions

Head and Neck Injury

During the years coincident with the introduction of robotic surgery techniques, several patients suffered severe injury and even died from body shifts on operating room tables that were tilted severely head down. There are several anecdotes from medicolegal actions involving patients who slid off operating tables with resulting neck injuries. In one instance, a patient in a supine and very steep head-down position apparently somersaulted heels over head off of the operating room table and subsequently died from a massive intracranial bleed. Steep head-down tilt is not often warranted and should be actively discouraged when appropriate. Skilled operators often find that they need less steep head-down tilt as they gain experience and expertise with robotic procedures.

Brachial Plexopathy

There is a risk of brachial injuries associated with cephalad movement of the patient while the arms or shoulders are secured to the table. Cephalad movement when arms are fixated or when shoulder restraints with braces, tape, "bean bag" devices, or other torso restraints are used may result in stretch of the middle and lower divisions of the brachial plexus. If the cephalad movement results in a relative hyperabduction of the shoulder to greater than 90 degrees, the brachial plexus can be stretched as it courses distally around the hyperabducted head of the humerus.

Depending on the degree of head depression, the addition of tilt to the lithotomy position combines the worst features of both the lithotomy and the head-down postures. The weight of abdominal viscera on the diaphragm adds to whatever abdominal compression is produced by the flexed thighs of an obese patient or of one placed in an exaggerated lithotomy position. Ventilation should be assisted or controlled. Because elevation of the lower extremities above the heart produces an uphill perfusion gradient, systemic hypotension and compressive leg wrapping may limit perfusion to the periphery, and both can be factors in the development of compartment syndromes in the legs of patients in the lithotomy position. This perfusion gradient often is unpredictable and exaggerated, potentially increasing the risk of compartment syndrome.[9,10]

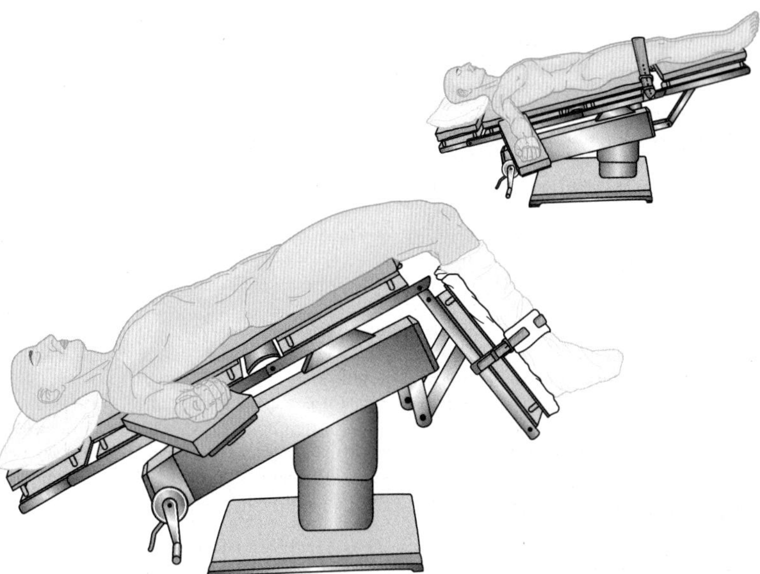

Figure 29-20 Head-down tilt. *Lower figure* shows traditional steep (30- to 45-degree) tilt. Leg restraints and knee flexion stabilize the patient, avoiding the need for wristlets or shoulder braces that threaten the brachial plexus. *Upper figure* shows 10 to 15 degrees of head-down tilt.

Cephalad displacement of the diaphragm and obstruction of its caudad inspiratory stroke accompany a head-down position because of gravity-shifted abdominal viscera. Consequently, the work of spontaneous ventilation is increased for an anesthetized patient in a posture that already worsens the ventilation–perfusion ratio by gravitational accumulation of blood in the poorly ventilated lung apices. During controlled ventilation, higher inspiratory pressures are needed to expand the lung.

Cranial vascular congestion and increased intracranial pressure can be expected to result from head-down tilt. For patients with known or suspected intracranial disease, the position should be used only in those rare instances in which a surgically useful alternate posture cannot be found. Maintenance of the position should then be as brief as possible.[59,60]

Steep head-down tilt positions (e.g., 30 to 45 degrees of head-down tilt) may require some means of preventing the patient from sliding cephalad out of position. The use of bent knees is occasionally used to retain the tilted patient in position (Fig. 29-20). Historically, shoulder braces, straps, or tape also have been used to prevent cephalad sliding in steep head-down tilt positions. These are best tolerated if placed over the acromioclavicular joints, but care must be taken to see that the shoulder is not forced sufficiently caudad to trap and compress the subclavian neurovascular bundle between the clavicle and the first rib. If they are placed medially against the root of the neck, they may easily compress neurovascular structures that emerge from the area of the scalene musculature. For these and other reasons, the use of shoulder braces and other retaining approaches has waned in popularity. In general, the use of steep head-down positions should be limited to only those portions of procedures in which their use is most important.[59,60]

Summary

There are many ways that patients can be injured during surgical procedures. Careful consideration of intraoperative and postoperative positioning may help reduce the frequency and severity of perioperative positioning–related adverse events. Although many complications that appear to be related to perioperative positioning may seem simple and preventable, the etiologic mechanisms of many of these problems are not readily apparent. Future investigations to determine the role of other potential etiologies, such as perioperative inflammatory responses, immunosuppression, and virus activation, for any position-related complications will be welcome.

For further review and interactivities, please see the videos and narrative interactive clinical vignettes (NICVs) accessible in the complimentary eBook bundled with this text. Access instructions are located on the inside front cover.

REFERENCES

1. Laughlin RS, Johnson RL, Burkle CM, Staff NP. Postsurgical neuropathy: a descriptive review. *Mayo Clin Proc.* 2020;95(2):355–369.
2. Staff NP, Dyck PJB, Warner MA. Postsurgical inflammatory neuropathy should be considered in the differential diagnosis of diaphragm paralysis after surgery. *Anesthesiology.* 2014;120:1057.
3. Laughlin RS, Dyck PJB, Watson JC, et al. Ipsilateral inflammatory neuropathy after hip surgery. *Mayo Clin Proc.* 2014;89:454–461.
4. Warner ME, Warner MA. Inflammatory neuropathy: a potentially treatable etiology of perioperative neuropathies. *Mayo Clin Proc.* 2014;89:434–436.
5. Ackerman RS, Luddy KA, Icard BE, Fernández JP, Gatenby RA, Muncey AR. The effects of anesthetics and perioperative medications on immune function: a narrative review. *Anesth Analg.* 2021;133:676–689.
6. Brand A. Immunological aspects of blood transfusions. *Transplant Immunol.* 2002;10:183–190.
7. Gilden DH, Katz RI. Surgical induction of zoster in a contralateral homologous dermatomal distribution. *Arch Neurol.* 2003;60:616–617.
8. Martin JT. Compartment syndromes: concepts and perspectives for the anesthesiologist. *Anesth Analg.* 1992;75:275–283.
9. Halliwill JR, Hewitt SA, Joyner MJ, Warner MA. Effects of various lithotomy positions on lower extremity blood pressures. *Anesthesiology.* 1999;89:1373–1376.
10. Pfeffer SD, Halliwill JR, Warner MA. Effects of lithotomy position and external compression on lower leg muscle compartment pressure. *Anesthesiology.* 2001;95:632–636.
11. Angermeier KW, Jordan GH. Complications of the exaggerated lithotomy position: a review of 177 cases. *J Urol.* 1994;151:866–868.
12. Grant I, Brovman EY, Kang D, Greenberg P, Saba R, Urman RD. A medicolegal analysis of positioning-related perioperative peripheral nerve injuries occurring between 1996 and 2015. *J Clin Anesth.* 2019;58:84–90.
13. Jellish WS, Blakeman B, Warf P, Slogoff S. Hands-up positioning during asymmetric sternal retraction for internal mammary artery harvest: a possible method to reduce brachial plexus injury. *Anesth Analg.* 1997;84:260–265.
14. Vander Salm TJ, Cereda JM, Cutler BS. Brachial plexus injury following median sternotomy. *J Thorac Cardiovasc Surg.* 1980;80:447–452.
15. Vander Salm TJ, Cutler BS, Okike ON. Brachial plexus injury following median sternotomy. Part II. *J Thorac Cardiovasc Surg.* 1982;83:914–917.

16. Roy RC, Stafford MA, Charlton JE. Nerve injury and musculoskeletal complaints after cardiac surgery: influence of internal mammary artery dissection and left arm position. *Anesth Analg*. 1988;67:277–279.
17. Gregg JR, Labosky D, Harty M, et al. Serratus anterior paralysis in the young athlete. *J Bone Joint Surg Am*. 1979;61:825–832.
18. Martin JT. Postoperative isolated dysfunction of the long thoracic nerve: a rare entity of uncertain etiology. *Anesth Analg*. 1989;69:614–619.
19. Foo CL, Swann M. Isolated paralysis of the serratus anterior: a report of 20 cases. *J Bone Joint Surg Br*. 1983;65:552–556.
20. Kroll DA, Caplan RA, Posner K, Ward RJ, Cheney FW. Nerve injury associated with anesthesia. *Anesthesiology*. 1990;73:202–207.
21. Cheney FW, Domino KB, Caplan RA, Posner KL. Nerve injury associated with anesthesia. *Anesthesiology*. 1999;90:1062–1069.
22. Büdinger K. Ueber Lähmungen nach Chloroform-Narkosen. *Archiv für Klinische Chiruque*. 1894;47:121.
23. Garriques HJ. Anaesthesia-paralysis. *Am J Med Sci*. 1897;113:81–89.
24. Wadsworth TG, Williams JR. Cubital tunnel external compression syndrome. *BMJ*. 1973;1: 662–666.
25. Pulos BP, Johnson RL, Laughlin RS, et al. Perioperative ulnar neuropathy: a contemporary estimate of incidence and risk factors. *Anesth Analg*. 2021;132:1429–1437.
26. Warner MA, Warner DO, Harper CM, Schroeder DR, Maxson PM. Ulnar neuropathy in medical patients. *Anesthesiology*. 2000;92:613–615.
27. Warner MA, Warner ME, Martin JT. Ulnar neuropathy. Incidence, outcome, and risk factors in sedated or anesthetized patients. *Anesthesiology*. 1994;81:1332–1340.
28. Alvine FG, Schurrer ME. Postoperative ulnar-nerve palsy. Are there predisposing factors? *J Bone Joint Surg Am*. 1987;69:255–259.
29. Warner MA, Warner DO, Matsumoto JY, Harper CM, Schroeder DR, Maxson PM. Ulnar neuropathy in surgical patients. *Anesthesiology*. 1999;90:54–59.
30. Prielipp RC, Morell RC, Walker FO, Santos CC, Bennett J, Butterworth J. Ulnar nerve pressure: influence of arm position and relationship to somatosensory evoked potentials. *Anesthesiology*. 1999;91:345–354.
31. Campbell WW, Pridgeon RM, Riaz G, Astruc J, Sahni KS. Variations in anatomy of the ulnar nerve at the cubital tunnel: pitfalls in the diagnosis of ulnar neuropathy at the elbow. *Muscle Nerve*. 1991;14:733–738.
32. O'Driscoll SW, Horii E, Carmichael SW, Morrey BF. The cubital tunnel and ulnar neuropathy. *J Bone Joint Surg Br*. 1991;73:613–617.
33. Childress HM. Recurrent ulnar nerve dislocation at the elbow. *J Bone Joint Surg*. 1956;38: 978–984.
34. Ashenhurst EM. Anatomical factors in the etiology of ulnar neuropathy. *Can Med Assoc J*. 1962;87:159–163.
35. Macnicol MF. Extraneural pressures affecting the ulnar nerve at the elbow. *Hand*. 1982;14:5–11.
36. Morell RC, Prielipp RC, Harwood TN, James RL, Butterworth JF. Men are more susceptible than women to direct pressure on unmyelinated ulnar nerve fibers. *Anesth Analg*. 2003;97:1183–1188.
37. Pechan J, Julis I. The pressure measurement in the ulnar nerve. A contribution to the pathophysiology of the cubital tunnel syndrome. *J Biomech*. 1975;8:75–79.
38. Contreras MG, Warner MA, Charboneau WJ, Cahill DR. The anatomy of the ulnar nerve at the elbow: potential relationship of acute ulnar neuropathy to gender differences. *Clin Anat*. 1998;11:372–378.
39. Shimokata H, Tobin JD, Muller DC, Elahi D, Coon PJ, Andres R. Studies in the distribution of body fat: I. Effects of age, sex, and obesity. *J Gerontol*. 1989;44:M66–M73.
40. Hattori K, Numata N, Ikoma M, Matsuzaka A, Danielson RR. Sex differences in the distribution of subcutaneous and internal fat. *Hum Biol*. 1991;63:53–63.
41. Chusid JG. *Correlative Neuroanatomy and Functional Neurology*. Lange Medical Publications; 1985:149.
42. Hill NA, Howard FM, Huffer BR. The incomplete anterior interosseous nerve syndrome. *J Hand Surg Am*. 1985;10:4–16.
43. Kies SJ, Danielson DR, Dennison DJ, Warner MA, Warner ME. Perioperative compartment syndrome of the hand. *Anesthesiology*. 2004;101:1232–1234.
44. Contreras MG, Warner MA, Carmichael SW, Spinner RJ. Perioperative anterior interosseous neuropathy. *Anesthesiology*. 2002;96:243–245.
45. Amoiridis G, Wöhrle JC, Langkafel M, Maiwurm D, Przuntek H. Spinal cord infarction after surgery in a patient in the hyperlordotic position. *Anesthesiology*. 1996;84:228–230.
46. Warner ME, LaMaster LM, Thoeming AK, Marienau ME, Warner MA. Compartment syndrome in surgical patients. *Anesthesiology*. 2001;94:705–708.
47. The Postoperative Visual Loss Study Group. Risk factors associated with ischemic optic neuropathy after spinal fusion surgery. *Anesthesiology*. 2012;116:15–24.
48. American Society of Anesthesiologists Task Force on Perioperative Visual Loss, North American Neuro-Ophthalmology Society, Society for Neuroscience in Anesthesiology and Critical Care. Practice advisory for perioperative visual loss associated with spine surgery 2019: an updated report by the American Society of Anesthesiologists Task Force on Perioperative Visual Loss, the North American Neuro-Ophthalmology Society, and the Society for Neuroscience in Anesthesiology and Critical Care. *Anesthesiology*. 2019;130: 12–30.
49. Sherman DG, Hart RG, Easton JD. Abrupt change in head position and cerebral infarction. *Stroke*. 1981;12:2–6.
50. Toole JF. Effects of change of head, limb and body position on cephalic circulation. *N Engl J Med*. 1968;279:307–311.
51. Cullen DJ, Kirby RR. Beach chair position may decrease cerebral perfusion. *APSF Newsletter*. 2007;22:25.
52. Cullen DJ, Kirby RR. Hazards of beach chair position explored. *APSF Newsletter*. 2008;22:8.
53. Munis J. The problems of posture, pressure, and perfusion. *APSF Newsletter*. 2007;22: 82–83.
54. Drummond JC, Hargens AP, Patel PM. Hydrostatic gradient is important – blood pressure should be corrected. *APSF Newsletter*. 2009;24:6.
55. Lanier WL. Cerebral perfusion: err on the side of caution. *APSF Newsletter*. 2009;24:1.
56. Moore JK, Chaudhri S, Moore AP, Easton J. Macroglossia and posterior fossa disease. *Anaesthesia*. 1988;43:382–385.
57. Hitselberger WE, House WF. A warning regarding the sitting position for acoustic tumor surgery. *Arch Otolaryng*. 1980;106:69.
58. Morandi X, Riffaud L, Amlashi SFA, Brassier G. Extensive spinal cord infarction after posterior fossa surgery in the sitting position: a case report. *Neurosurgery*. 2004;54:1512–1515.
59. Mills JT, Burris MB, Warburton DJ, Conaway MR, Schenkman NS, Krupski TL. Positioning injuries associated with robotic assisted urologic surgery. *J Urol*. 2013;190:580–584.
60. Pridgeon S, Bishop CV, Adshead J. Lower limb compartment syndrome as a complication of robot-assisted radical prostatetectomy: the UK experience. *BJU Int*. 2013;112:485–488.

30 Monitored Anesthesia Care

JESSICA R. BLACK • DANIEL L. WANG • SARA E. MEITZEN

KEY POINTS

1. Monitored anesthesia care (MAC) is a specific anesthesia service provided by a qualified anesthesiologist, thus can safely encompass the complete spectrum of sedation to general anesthesia if required.
2. The standards for preoperative evaluation, intraoperative monitoring, and the continuous presence of a member of the anesthesia care team are no different from those for general or regional anesthesia.
3. Indications for monitored anesthesia care include, but are not limited to, the nature of the procedure, the patient's clinical condition, and/or the need for deeper levels of analgesia and sedation than can be provided by moderate sedation (including potential conversion to a general or regional anesthetic).
4. The qualified anesthesiologist provider of monitored anesthesia care must be prepared to convert to general anesthesia and respond to the pathophysiology (airway and hemodynamic changes) of procedure and position in the management in induction of general anesthesia when necessary.
5. If the patient loses consciousness and the ability to respond purposefully, the anesthesia care is a general anesthetic, irrespective of whether airway instrumentation is required.
6. The important mechanisms whereby respiratory function may be compromised during monitored anesthesia care include the effects of sedatives and opioids on respiratory drive, upper airway patency, and protective airway reflexes.
7. The leading cause of death and severe nervous system injury during MAC is hypoxia due to suppression of spontaneous respiration by sedative–hypnotic drugs.
8. Burns, particularly around the head and neck, are an important cause of patient injury during MAC. The combination of electrocautery, supplemental oxygen, alcohol prep, and flammable drapes is particularly dangerous.
9. As a general principle, to avoid excessive levels of sedation, drugs should be titrated in small increments or by adjustable infusions rather than administered in larger doses according to predetermined notions of efficacy.
10. At the present time, no single drug can provide all the components of monitored anesthesia care (i.e., analgesia, anxiolysis, and hypnosis) with an acceptable margin of safety or ease of titratability.
11. If anesthesiologists are not willing or able to provide MAC or sedation/analgesia services, others, who are less qualified, are prepared to assume that role.

1 Monitored anesthesia care is a specific anesthesia service in which an anesthesiologist has been requested to participate in the care of a patient undergoing a diagnostic or therapeutic procedure and includes all the usual aspects of anesthetic care—a preprocedure evaluation, intraprocedure care, and postprocedure management. *Monitored anesthesia care does not describe the continuum of depth of sedation*. During monitored anesthesia care, the continuous attention of the anesthesiologist is directed at optimizing patient comfort and safety. Monitored anesthesia care usually (but not always) involves the administration of drugs with anxiolytic, hypnotic, analgesic, and amnestic properties, either alone or as a supplement to a local or regional technique. Monitored anesthesia care is provided by a qualified anesthesiologist, thus can safely encompass the complete spectrum of sedation from light sedation/analgesia to conversion to general anesthesia if required. The American Society of Anesthesiologists (ASA) has published several position statements, guidelines, and advisories on various topics that relate to monitored anesthesia care and moderate sedation. These are listed in Table 30-1 and are well worth reviewing.

Terminology

It is important to distinguish between the terms "monitored anesthesia care" and "moderate sedation/analgesia." In October 2018, the ASA House of Delegates reamended the statement titled "Distinguishing Monitored Anesthesia Care ("MAC") from Moderate Sedation/Analgesia (Conscious Sedation)."[1]

Moderate sedation/analgesia is the term used by the ASA in their published *Practice Guidelines for Moderate Procedural Sedation and Analgesia*.[2] During moderate sedation (conscious sedation), care needs to be provided by either a qualified anesthesia practitioner (defined as physician anesthesiologists, anesthesiology fellows, anesthesiology residents, certified anesthesiologist assistants [CAAs], and certified registered nurse anesthetists [CRNAs]) or a nonanesthesiologist sedation practitioner (defined as physicians, dentists, or podiatrists who have the training and licensure to administer moderate sedation). A proper preoperative history and physical, including airway examination, is required.

2 Sedation/analgesia provided by nonanesthesiologist providers should not intend to attain a level of sedation in which the patient is unresponsive. Monitored anesthesia care implies the potential for a deeper level of sedation than that provided by sedation/analgesia and is always administered or medically directed by a qualified anesthesiologist. The provider of MAC is prepared and qualified to convert to a general anesthetic if and when necessary. The standards for preoperative evaluation, intraoperative monitoring, and the continuous presence of a member of the anesthesia care team are no different from those for general or regional anesthesia.[3]

Conceptually, monitored anesthesia care utilizing sedation rather than general anesthesia is attractive because it should invoke less physiologic disturbance and allow a more rapid recovery than general anesthesia. It is instructive to review the ASA position statement that defines monitored anesthesia care[3]:

Monitored anesthesia care is a specific anesthesia service performed 3
by a qualified anesthesiologist for a diagnostic or therapeutic procedure. Indications for monitored anesthesia care include, but are not limited to, the nature of the procedure, the patient's clinical condition, and/or the need for deeper levels of analgesia and sedation than can be provided by moderate sedation (including potential conversion to a general or regional anesthetic).

Monitored anesthesia care includes all aspects of anesthesia care—a preprocedure assessment and optimization, intraprocedure care, and postprocedure management that is inherently provided by a qualified anesthesiologist as part of the bundled specific service. During monitored anesthesia care, the anesthesiologist provides or medically directs a number of specific services, including but not limited to:

- *Preprocedural assessment and management of patient comorbidity and periprocedural risk*
- *Diagnosis and treatment of clinical problems that occur during the procedure*
- *Support of vital functions inclusive of hemodynamic stability, airway management, and appropriate management of the procedure-induced pathologic changes as they affect the patient's coexisting morbidities*
- *Administration of sedatives, analgesics, hypnotics, anesthetic agents, or other medications as necessary for patient safety*
- *Psychological support and physical comfort*
- *Provision of other medical services as needed to complete the procedure safely.*

Monitored anesthesia care may include varying levels of sedation, 4
awareness, analgesia, and anxiolysis as necessary. The qualified 5
anesthesiologist provider of monitored anesthesia care must be prepared to convert to general anesthesia and respond to the pathophysiology (airway and hemodynamic changes) of procedure and

Table 30-1 American Society of Anesthesiologists Statements, Guidelines, and Practice Advisories Related to Monitored Anesthesia Care and Sedation/Analgesia.

Title of ASA Statement, Guideline, or Advisory	Date of Publication
Position on Monitored Anesthesia Care	October 2018
Statement on Respiratory Monitoring During Endoscopic Procedures	October 2019
Statement on Granting Privileges to Non-Anesthesiologist Physicians Supervising Deep Sedation	October 2017
Statement of Granting Privileges for Administration of Moderate Sedation to Practitioners	October 2021
Advisory on Granting Privileges for Deep Sedation to Non-Anesthesiologist Physicians	October 2017
Continuum of Depth of Sedation: Definition of General Anesthesia and Levels of Sedation/Analgesia	October 2019
Statement on Safe Use of Propofol	October 2019
Distinguishing Monitored Anesthesia Care (MAC) from Moderate Sedation/Analgesia (Conscious Sedation)	October 2018
Standards for Basic Anesthetic Monitoring	December 2020

position in the management in induction of general anesthesia when necessary. If the patient loses consciousness and the ability to respond purposefully, the anesthesia care is a general anesthetic, irrespective of whether airway instrumentation is required.

Monitored anesthesia care is a physician service provided to an individual patient. Whereas "moderate sedation/analgesia" is a service directed by the proceduralist who is preoccupied in focusing on successfully completing the scheduled procedure. The proceduralist may not be cognizant of ongoing pathophysiologic effects of sedatives given or procedure/position changes. Monitored anesthesia care should be subject to the same level of payment as general or regional anesthesia. Accordingly, the ASA Relative Value Guide provides for the use of proper base units, time, and any appropriate modifier units as the basis for determining payment.[*]

The ASA also states that monitored anesthesia care should be requested by the attending physician and be made known to the patient, in accordance with accepted procedures of the institution. In addition, the ASA states that the service must include the following:

- Performance of a preanesthetic examination and evaluation
- Prescription of anesthetic care
- Personal participation in, or medical direction of, the entire plan of care
- Continuous physical presence of the anesthesiologist or, in the case of medical direction, of the resident or CRNA being medically directed
- Proximate presence, or in the case of medical direction, availability of the anesthesiologist for diagnosis and treatment of emergencies

Furthermore, the ASA states that all institutional regulations pertaining to anesthesia services shall be observed, and all the usual services performed by the anesthesiologist shall be furnished, including but not limited to:

- Usual noninvasive cardiocirculatory and respiratory monitoring
- Oxygen administration, when indicated
- Administration of sedatives, tranquilizers, antiemetics, narcotics, other analgesics, β-blockers, vasopressors, bronchodilators, antihypertensives, or other pharmacologic therapy as may be required in the judgment of the anesthesiologist

Preoperative Assessment

The preoperative evaluation is an essential prerequisite to monitored anesthesia care and should be as comprehensive as that performed prior to any general or regional anesthetic (see Chapter 23). However, in addition to the usual evaluation for the patient who is scheduled to undergo general anesthesia, there are additional considerations unique to monitored anesthesia care that may ultimately determine the success or failure of the procedure.

Medical Status

The primary objective in the preoperative evaluation for patients undergoing monitored anesthesia care is to identify any physical and medical conditions that may increase the patient's risk of adverse events. Those conditions include severe cardiovascular disease (e.g., pulmonary hypertension), anxiety disorders, chronic pain (e.g., narcotic use), obstructive sleep apnea, morbid obesity, chronic renal failure, chronic hepatic disease, elderly patients (age >70), and ASA III to IV.[4] In a review of closed claims analyses in the United States, claims involving MAC tended to involve older and sicker (ASA III to V) patients, with respiratory depression representing the majority of claims.[5]

Airway

A proper evaluation of the patient's airway is essential as sedative agents can depress respiratory function. The anesthesiologist must be prepared for airway management at any point during the procedure should sedation become deeper than intended. Presence of beard, Mallampati score of III/IV, history of snoring, and limited mandibular protrusion can all be risk factors for difficult mask ventilation.[6] Knowledge of, and supplies for the difficult airway algorithm should be readily accessible if needed. In addition, routine preoperative fasting guidelines, as for general anesthesia, should be followed, and risk factors for aspiration should be identified and addressed, as patients with increased risk of aspiration may not be appropriate candidates for monitored anesthesia care.

Monitored Anesthesia Care Candidacy

There are several factors specific to the patient, the procedure, and the surgeon that must be considered when determining whether monitored anesthesia care is a safe and suitable option.

Patient Factors

Certain medical conditions may not be ideal for sedation. Aspiration risk (e.g., improper NPO status, morbid obesity, esophageal pathologies, symptomatic Gastroesophageal reflux disease [GERD]), anticipated difficult airway which may prolong rescue attempts (e.g., history of neck radiation, documented history of difficult intubation, limited mouth opening or neck extension, oropharyngeal pathologies), or inability to tolerate respiratory depression (e.g., severe pulmonary hypertension, intracranial pathology) may make general anesthesia a more appropriate option.

It is also important to evaluate the patient's ability to remain motionless and lie flat, as most, if not all, procedures require one or both conditions. Consequently, patients with severe anxiety, musculoskeletal pain, persistent cough, cognitive dysfunction, dementia, or tremors may require general anesthesia.

Finally, but perhaps the most important factor for a good MAC outcome is a motivated patient. Thus, it is essential to evaluate the patient's psychological preparedness for the planned procedure. It is also important to elicit the presence of coexisting sensorineural or cognitive deficits. Patient response and cooperation is sometimes required during procedures and hearing impairment or language barriers may make monitored anesthesia care more difficult. Verbal communication between physician and patient is vital for three reasons: as a monitor of the level of sedation and cardiorespiratory function, as a means of explanation and reassurance for the patient, and as a mechanism of communication when the patient is required to actively cooperate. As a wise attending once said, "Don't offer MAC to a patient you don't want to talk to."

Case Factors

When determining whether monitored anesthesia care is an appropriate choice for a procedure, the anesthesiologist must consider the depth of sedation needed (e.g., the need for paralysis), the length of case (e.g., tourniquet time), the level of fire risk, and most importantly, the ease of airway accessibility. Procedures

*Excerpted from American Society of Anesthesiologists. Position on Monitored Anesthesia Care (Amended October 17, 2018) © 2023 of the American Society of Anesthesiologists. A copy of the full text can be obtained from ASA, 1061 American Lane Schaumburg, IL 60173-4973 or online at www.asahq.org.

that prevent immediate access to the airway (e.g., head and neck procedures, prone procedures, procedures where patient is positioned with head away), may be more safely performed under minimal to no sedation, or general anesthesia.

Long procedure times can increase the opportunity for adverse events. Assuming the patient can tolerate lying in a certain position for a prolonged period (which is often unlikely), every moment that passes is another moment that the patient is sedated with an unsecured airway. As sedation is a continuum, the patient may reach deeper-than-intended levels, leading to disinhibition, respiratory, or hemodynamic compromise. In addition, some procedures combine regional anesthesia with sedation. Longer-than-anticipated procedures can lead to failure of regional anesthesia, or increased pneumatic tourniquet pain (should one be present), resulting in conversion to general anesthesia.[6]

It is important to be aware that supplemental oxygen administered during monitored anesthesia care can lead to a development of an oxygen-rich environment underneath drapes and increase the risk of fire. Due to fire risk, certain procedures near the mouth and nose may require intermittent or no supplemental oxygen, and intubation may be necessary if the patient is prone to developing hypoxemia without supplemental oxygen.

Last, the surgeon must also be amenable to monitored anesthesia care, with the expectation that the patient may move, become dissociated, and may require conversion to general anesthesia should the procedure be unable to be completed under MAC.

Conversion of Monitored Anesthesia Care to General Anesthesia

The anesthesiologist must always be prepared to convert from monitored anesthesia care to general anesthesia if factors prevent the procedure from continuing or patient safety is compromised (e.g., patient becomes combative, respiratory depression leading to hypoxia and hemodynamic compromise, aspiration, failure of regional anesthesia, complications of the procedure). In a retrospective study of 219,061 MAC cases, the most common reasons for conversion to general anesthesia were failed neuraxial or regional anesthesia, patient inability to tolerate monitored anesthesia care, and hypoxia or airway obstruction.[6] Factors that led to an inability to tolerate monitored anesthesia care included patient disinhibition, inability to stay still, and increasing sedation/analgesic requirements leading to deeper sedation. Experience of the anesthesia provider may also play a role as higher conversion rates were seen among residents and CRNAs versus attending anesthesiologists alone. Obese patients had a higher risk of conversion, likely due to the higher incidence of sleep apnea leading to airway obstruction and hypoxia. Other factors leading to conversion to general anesthesia included coughing, altered mental status, hemodynamic instability, aspiration, hypercarbia, loss of intravenous (IV) access, change of anticipated procedure type, prolonged surgical time, and surgeon request. Due to the myriad of issues that can arise during monitored anesthesia care, the anesthesia provider must be vigilant at all times and be prepared to readily convert to general anesthesia, if necessary.

Patient Expectations

Communicating and setting expectations with the patient is vital for successful monitored anesthesia care. To avoid potentially traumatizing experiences, there needs to be communication between the anesthesiologist and patient regarding what monitored anesthesia care entails; patients may be awake and have memories of their procedures; they may experience moments of discomfort or pain and may have to follow instructions periodically; and there is always the possibility for conversion to general anesthesia. Complaints of intraoperative awareness are due in part to discordance between the planned anesthetic and the patient's expectations of their experience. Some patients who expect to be unconscious throughout the procedure may receive moderate sedation and result in a higher incidence of reporting unintended awareness. Informed communication prior to the procedure can facilitate better patient experiences, and as a result, better experiences for the surgical team as well.

Monitoring during Monitored Anesthesia Care

American Society of Anesthesiologists Standards

The ASA standards for basic anesthesia monitoring are applicable to all levels of anesthesia care, including monitored anesthesia care. It is useful to review the components of the ASA standards that are pertinent to monitored anesthesia care as reaffirmed by the House of Delegates in October 2020.[7]

Communication and Observation

A conscientious and well-trained anesthesia provider is the single most vital monitor in the operating room (OR), and is expected to be present and in the room throughout the entirety of monitored anesthesia care. The provider's effectiveness will be markedly enhanced by the use of the basic quantitative and qualitative monitoring devices, which should be readily available in all ORs. It is important that the provider continually evaluates the patient's response to verbal stimulation to effectively titrate the level of sedation and to allow the earlier detection of neurologic or cardiorespiratory dysfunction. Continuous visual, tactile, and auditory assessment of physiologic function could include observation of the rate, depth, and pattern of respiration; palpation of the arterial pulse; and assessment of peripheral perfusion by extremity temperature and capillary refill. In addition, the patient should be continually observed for diaphoresis, pallor, shivering, cyanosis, and acute changes in neurologic status.

Pulse Oximetry

No monitor of oxygen transport has had a greater impact on the practice of anesthesiology than the pulse oximeter. Pulse oximetry is noninvasive, safe, and comfortable to the awake patient; it is also technically simple to apply and interpret, and allows continuous real-time monitoring of arterial oxygenation. The use of a quantitative measure of oxygenation is specifically mandated by the ASA standards for intraoperative monitoring. The important mechanisms whereby respiratory function may be compromised during monitored anesthesia care include the effects of sedatives and opioids on respiratory drive, upper airway patency, and protective airway reflexes. Additional important risk factors for arterial desaturation include obesity, pre-existing upper airway obstruction and respiratory disease, increased metabolic rate, general anesthesia, the extremes of age, surgical site, and patient positioning. The fundamental importance of monitoring oxygenation during monitored anesthesia care can be appreciated from the closed claim study of Caplan et al.[8] who examined 14 cases of sudden cardiac arrest in otherwise healthy patients who received spinal anesthesia. These major anesthetic mishaps occurred before the routine adoption of pulse oximetry. One of the major findings of this study was that cyanosis frequently heralded the onset of cardiac arrest, suggesting that unappreciated respiratory insufficiency may have played an important role. Further support for the use of pulse oximetry comes from the ASA Committee on Professional Liability analysis of closed anesthesia claims, which reveals that respiratory events constitute the single largest source of adverse outcomes. Furthermore, review of these cases suggests that pulse oximetry in combination with capnography would have prevented the adverse outcome in most cases.[5]

Capnography

Capnography can be used to monitor respiratory rate and—more importantly—aid in the early detection and management of airway obstruction, especially during the administration of supplemental oxygen where desaturation from hypoventilation may be delayed. There are numerous methods to monitor end-tidal carbon dioxide. Sidestream capnographs have been adapted for use with face masks, nasal airways, and nasal cannula and have been used successfully during monitored anesthesia care. Nasal cannula for oxygen delivery have been modified to provide an integrated port for respiratory gas sampling and are available commercially (Fig. 30-1). Alternatively, capnograph sampling lines can be attached to shortened IV catheters and inserted into simple face masks (Fig. 30-2). There is growing evidence that capnography may reduce risk associated with sedation/analgesia or monitored anesthesia care in both the pediatric and adult population. Waugh et al.[9] conducted a meta-analysis to determine if the addition of capnography identified more respiratory complications than standard monitoring alone. They reported that cases of respiratory depression were 17.6 times more likely to be detected if monitored with capnography. Soto et al.[10] observed patients undergoing MAC to determine if capnography would increase apnea detection rates over observation alone. All episodes of apnea greater than 20 seconds that occurred were not detected by the anesthesia provider but were detected by capnography. In a study of patients receiving upper endoscopy, pulse oximetry detected only about 50% of the episodes of apnea and disordered breathing (ADR) that were detected by capnography.[11] Hypoxemia, defined as a pulse oximeter arterial saturation (SpO_2) <90%, occurred an average of 45.6 seconds after the onset of ADR episodes. Respiratory depression was among one of the most common complications for patients receiving anesthesia in non-OR environments.[12] In closed claim analyses, inadequate oxygenation and ventilation were the most common damaging respiratory events in MAC cases and were commonly associated with oversedation and inadequate monitoring of ventilation.[5,12] Thus, with its low cost and enhanced patient safety, capnography should be utilized in every MAC case.

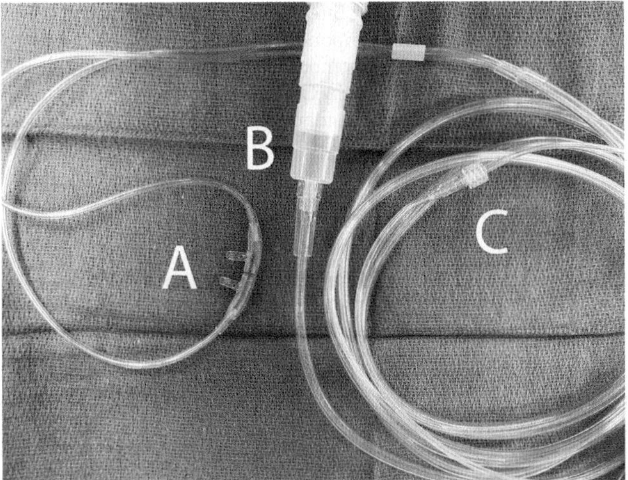

Figure 30-1 Nasal cannula with oxygen tubing and port for respiratory gas sampling. **A:** Nasal cannula. **B:** Oxygen tubing attached to 22- × 6-mm adapter attached to circuit*. **C:** Port for respiratory gas sampling (i.e., end-tidal CO_2 tubing) attached to machine end-tidal CO_2 tubing. *Oxygen tubing can be attached to circuit via 5.0 or 6.0 ETT connector as well (illustrated in Fig. 30-2). Circuit may be attached to machine breathing system or auxiliary common gas outlet (not available in all machines).

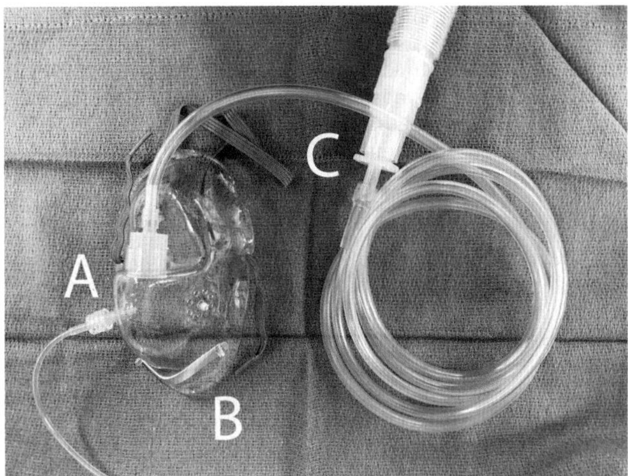

Figure 30-2 Modified IV catheter inserted into a simple face mask. **A:** End-tidal CO_2 tubing attached to 18-gauge IV catheter. **B:** Simple face mask. **C:** Oxygen tubing attached to 6.0 ETT connector (5.0 ETT works as well) attached to breathing circuit.

Cardiovascular System

At a minimum, the electrocardiogram (ECG) must be continuously displayed and the blood pressure measured and recorded at least every 5 minutes during monitored anesthesia care. The pulse should be monitored by palpation, oximetry, or auscultation. The selection of additional hemodynamic monitoring is usually determined more by the cardiovascular status of the patient than the magnitude of the procedure. Most procedures performed under monitored anesthesia care do not involve major hemorrhage, fluid shifts, or major physiologic trespass. Decisions concerning choice of monitoring for myocardial ischemia and other adverse hemodynamic events will need to be individualized on a case-by-case basis.

Temperature

It is an ASA standard for any patient receiving anesthesia to have temperature monitored when clinically significant changes in body temperature are intended, anticipated, or suspected.[7] Although sedation techniques used during monitored anesthesia care do not generally trigger malignant hyperthermia, there is potential for significant inadvertent hypothermia, particularly during neuraxial anesthesia. Even monitored anesthesia care techniques unaccompanied by regional anesthesia are associated with hypothermia at the extremes of age. At this time, there is no evidence suggesting that the morbidity associated with perioperative hypothermia is any less during monitored anesthesia care than during general anesthesia, and it is well described in high-risk patients—a group of patients very likely to undergo procedures under MAC. When hypothermia is significant, shivering may interfere with the planned procedure and markedly increase oxygen requirements, predisposing susceptible patients to myocardial ischemia or respiratory insufficiency. The major thermoregulatory defenses against hypothermia include vasoconstriction, shivering, and behavior (e.g., moving). Vasoconstriction and shivering can be impaired with administration of anesthesia. Behavioral thermoregulation is impaired even in the conscious patient. Regional anesthesia has major effects on thermoregulation. In the absence of reliable temperature monitoring, it is possible that the first indication of hypothermia may be the onset of shivering, by which time considerable central cooling may have already occurred.

Patients will frequently complain of feeling too warm when covered by heavy drapes. Although malignant hyperthermia is rare during monitored anesthesia care, hyperthermia is still possible as a result of thyroid storm or malignant neuroleptic syndrome. The subjective sensation of hyperthermia may also be the first indicator of important adverse events in evolution such as hypoxia, hypercarbia, cerebral ischemia, local anesthetic toxicity, and myocardial ischemia.

Monitoring Depth of Sedation

Multiple methods have been evaluated to assess the depth of sedation including clinical assessments and electroencephalogram. Aside from the ASA definitions,[13] most anesthesiologists do not use numeric scales to assess sedation levels. Nonetheless, they are included in this discussion, as many of the scales are used in intensive care settings, or for research purposes.

ASA Definitions of Sedation

The ASA outlines the spectrum of sedation based on patient responsiveness, airway intervention, and effects on spontaneous ventilation and cardiovascular function (Table 30-2).[13]

Minimal sedation maintains normal response to verbal stimuli. Airway, spontaneous ventilation, and cardiovascular function are unaffected. Moderate sedation (the depth of sedation often referred to as "conscious sedation") maintains purposeful response to verbal and light touch stimuli. Airway, spontaneous ventilation, and cardiovascular function are preserved. Deep sedation maintains purposeful response to repeated or painful stimuli but may lose responsiveness to verbal or light touch stimuli. Assistance may be required to maintain airway patency but cardiovascular function is usually maintained. General anesthesia defines a state where the patient is unarousable to painful stimuli. Airway support is often required and spontaneous ventilation is often inadequate, requiring positive pressure support. Furthermore, cardiovascular function may also be affected.

Ramsay Sedation Scale/Modified Ramsay Sedation Scale

The Ramsay Sedation Scale (RSS) was first described by Ramsay et al.[14] in 1974 observing ICU patients receiving alphaxalone–alphadolone for sedation. Six levels were formulated, three with the patient awake and three with the patient asleep. Awake levels depended on agitation and responsiveness: (1) anxious or agitated, (2) cooperative and oriented, and (3) responsive to commands only. Asleep levels depended on responses to tap or auditory stimuli: (4) brisk response, (5) sluggish response, and (6) no response. To adhere to The Joint Commission's (TJC's) sedation definitions (based on the ASA sedation definitions), a modified RSS was proposed in 2003 in a study involving patients receiving procedural sedation in the emergency department.[15] This scale added an additional level to both the awake and the asleep portions, increasing the total levels of sedation from six to eight.

Richmond Agitation Sedation Score

The Richmond Agitation Sedation Score (RASS) score was described in 2002 to assess level of consciousness and agitated behavior in Intensive Care Unit (ICU) patients.[16] The 10-level scale utilized three steps: observation, response to auditory stimuli, and response to physical stimuli. Since its introduction, the RASS score has been implemented to guide sedation levels in the ICU due to its high inter-rater reliability across physicians, nurses, and pharmacists. However, the use of the RASS score has not been widely explored with procedural sedation.

Modified Observer's Assessment of Alertness/Sedation Scale

The Observer's Assessment of Alertness/Sedation (OAA/S) Scale was described in 1990 to assess benzodiazepine antagonism with flumazenil in healthy adult patients.[17] Four areas of assessments are utilized (responsiveness, speech, facial expression, eyes) to generate a composite score from 1 (deep sleep) to 5 (alert). The scale demonstrated excellent inter-rater reliability and correlation with the responsiveness component most often correlating with the composite score. Various modifications have been published for the scale to better fit the ASA Continuum of Depth of Sedation. The scale has been utilized in many procedural sedation studies.

Table 30-2 Continuum of Depth of Sedation

	Minimal Sedation Anxiolysis	Moderate Sedation/Analgesia ("Conscious Sedation")	Deep Sedation/Analgesia	General Anesthesia
Responsiveness	Normal response to verbal stimulation	Purposeful[a] response to verbal or tactile stimulation	Purposeful response following repeated or painful stimulation	Unarousable, even with a painful stimulus
Airway	Unaffected	No intervention required	Intervention may be required	Intervention often required
Spontaneous ventilation	Unaffected	Adequate	May be inadequate	Frequently inadequate
Cardiovascular function	Unaffected	Usually maintained	Usually maintained	May be impaired

[a]Reflex withdrawal from a painful stimulus is not considered a purposeful response.

Adapted from ASA House of Delegates. Continuum of Depth of Sedation: Definition of General Anesthesia and Levels of Sedation/Analgesia, 2019. A copy of the full text can be obtained from ASA, 1061 American Lane, Schaumburg, IL 60173–4973 or online at www.asahq.org

Table 30-3 Assessments of Sedation

ASA Continuum of Depth of Sedation	Modified Ramsay Sedation Scale[15]	Richmond Agitation-Sedation Scale[16]	Modified Observer's Assessment of Alertness/Sedation Scale[17]
Minimal sedation (anxiolysis): normal response to verbal stimulation	1: Awake and alert, minimal or no cognitive impairment	+1 to +4: Scores indicate restlessness to combativeness and do not reflect anxiolysis 0: Alert and calm	5: Responds readily to name spoken in normal tone
Moderate sedation/analgesia ("conscious sedation"): purposeful response to verbal or tactile stimulation	2: Awake but tranquil, purposeful response to verbal commands at conversational level	−1: Not fully alert, but has sustained (more than 10 s) awakening, with eye contact, to voice	4: Lethargic response to name spoken in normal tone
	3: Appears asleep, purposeful responses to verbal commands at conversational level	−2: Briefly (less than 10 s) awakens with eye contact to voice	3: Responds after name called loudly or repeatedly or both
	4: Appears asleep, purposeful responses to verbal commands but at louder than usual conversational level, requiring light glabellar tap, or both	−3: Any movement (but no eye contact) to voice	2: Responds only after mild prodding or mild shaking
Deep sedation/analgesia: purposeful response following repeated or painful stimulation	5: Asleep, sluggish purposeful responses only to loud verbal commands, strong glabellar tap, or both	−4: No response to voice, but any movement to physical stimulation	1: Responds only to painful stimulation
	6: Asleep, sluggish purposeful responses only to painful stimuli		
	7: Asleep, reflex withdrawal to painful stimuli only (no purposeful responses)		
General anesthesia: unarousable even with painful stimulus	8: Unresponsive to external stimuli, including pain	−5: No response to voice or physical stimulation	0: No response to painful stimulation

A comparison of each sedation scale discussed in the text can be found in Table 30-3.

Processed Electroencephalography

The bispectral index (BIS) is a processed electroencephalography (EEG) parameter that was developed specifically to evaluate patient response during drug-induced anesthesia and sedation. Sedation monitoring is attractive because of the potential to titrate drugs more accurately, avoiding the adverse effects of both over- and underdosing. In addition, the aforementioned sedation scales are limited if the patient has neurologic deficits such as paralysis, aphasia, or deafness, and BIS monitoring may have potential advantages over conventional intermittent techniques of patient assessment.

The BIS has been shown to be a useful monitor of drug-induced sedation and recall in volunteers and has been shown to correlate with OAA/S scale scores during propofol-induced sedation in patients undergoing surgery with regional anesthesia. Liu et al.[18] found that an increasing depth of sedation was associated with a predictable decrease in BIS and absence of recall was associated with BIS values less than 80. These findings correspond with those of Kearse et al.[19] who found no intraoperative recall at BIS values below 79 during midazolam-, isoflurane-, and propofol-induced sedation. Despite studies supporting the use of BIS, other studies have shown significant variability and discrepancies between individual BIS scores and sedation levels.[20] BIS levels varied with the type of medication given and some patients who were wide awake had low BIS scores while other patients who were deeply sedated had high BIS scores. For BIS monitoring to become valuable, Drummond proposed that it needs to meet two conditions: *"First, not only must the average values yielded by the device in two distinct states* (e.g., *hemodynamically responsive* vs. *nonresponsive; aware* vs. *oblivious) be statistically different, but also the range of values seen in those two states should not overlap."*[21] Currently, the research is mixed and does not definitively meet the proposed criteria. Although the use of BIS to monitor sedation is appealing, conventional assessment of sedation is an important mechanism whereby continuous patient contact is maintained. Ideally, BIS monitoring will be employed in the future as an adjunct to clinical evaluation rather than as the primary monitor of consciousness. There is weak evidence supporting the use of other processed EEG monitoring systems for monitored anesthesia care (e.g., SedLine, Narcotrend, and spectral entropy).[4]

Supplemental Oxygen Administration

Hypoxia as a result of alveolar hypoventilation is a relatively common occurrence following the administration of sedatives, analgesics, and hypnotics. In the absence of significant lung disease, the administration of only modest concentrations of supplemental oxygen is frequently effective in restoring the patient's oxygen saturation to an acceptable level. This concept is well illustrated by reference to the familiar alveolar gas equation. An extreme example illustrates the point: An otherwise healthy adult male breathing room air receives a dose of an opioid that causes marked alveolar hypoventilation such that his alveolar PCO_2 is increased to 80 mmHg. The alveolar gas equation predicts that his arterial PO_2 will fall to approximately 40 mmHg as shown here:

$$P_AO_2 = PiO_2 - P_{ACO_2}/R$$

$$PiO_2 = FiO_2 \times (P_B - P_{H_2O})$$

$$PiO_2 = 0.21 \times (760 \text{ mmHg} - 47 \text{ mmHg}) = 150 \text{ mmHg}$$

$$P_AO_2 = 150 \text{ mmHg} - (80 \text{ mmHg}/0.8)$$

$$P_AO_2 = 50 \text{ mmHg}$$

where P_AO_2 is alveolar partial pressure of oxygen, PiO_2 is inspired partial pressure of oxygen, P_{ACO_2} is alveolar partial pressure of carbon dioxide, R is respiratory quotient, P_B is barometric pressure, and P_{H_2O} is water vapor pressure at body temperature.

Assuming a normal alveolar to arterial (A to a) gradient of 10 mmHg, his arterial partial pressure of oxygen (PaO_2) will be 40 mmHg, corresponding to an arterial oxygen saturation of 75%. If while initiating definitive therapy for hypoventilation this patient were to receive only a modest increase in inspired oxygen, a marked improvement in arterial saturation would be achieved:

$$FiO_2 \text{ increased to } 28\%$$

$$PiO_2 = 0.28 \times (760 \text{ mmHg} - 47 \text{ mmHg}) = 200 \text{ mmHg}$$

$$P_AO_2 = 200 \text{ mmHg} - (80 \text{ mmHg}/0.8)$$

$$P_AO_2 = 100 \text{ mmHg and } PaO_2 \sim 90 \text{ mmHg}$$

This theoretical example serves to highlight two important points. First, in isolated hypoventilation modest increases in inspired oxygen are remarkably effective at restoring oxygen saturation to acceptable levels. On the other hand, *a patient who is receiving minimal supplemental oxygen and has an acceptable oxygen saturation may have significant undetected alveolar hypoventilation*. The necessity to administer oxygen supplementation is controversial. Deitch et al.[22] reported that the use of supplemental oxygen (2 L/min) during sedation with midazolam and fentanyl did not reduce the occurrence of hypoxia compared to patients on room air. The investigators conducted a similar study evaluating the effect of 3 L/min of oxygen in patients receiving propofol. They reported no statistically significant difference in the incidence of hypoxemia when comparing those who received oxygen and those who did not (18% vs. 28%, respectively).[23] The authors claimed that physician recognition and correction of an obstructed airway was of greater significance than supplemental oxygen. Several studies have shown that capnography is more sensitive in detecting respiratory depression and apnea than pulse oximetry or by visual observation.[9–11] It should be noted that the data from the ASA closed claims analysis shows that respiratory depression associated with monitored anesthesia care accounted for over one-third of closed claim injuries in remote locations.[12] In order to improve prevention of hypoxic events, capnography should be utilized whether supplemental oxygen is used or not.

Head and Neck Fires with the Use of Supplemental Oxygen

7 From the ASA closed claims study of Bhananker et al.,[5] we learned
8 that the leading cause of death and severe nervous system injury
during MAC is hypoxia due to suppression of spontaneous respiration by sedative–hypnotic drugs. Although administration of supplemental oxygen is generally prudent, the authors of that study also note that the most common equipment-related problem was cautery fires, particularly around the head and neck. Thus, caution should be used when supplemental oxygen is administered to patients undergoing surgery in the head and neck. The combination of supplemental oxygen, electrocautery, alcoholic prep solution, and flammable drapes is particularly dangerous, especially when a tent of drapes around the patient's head creates a pocket of increased oxygen concentration. This pocket of enriched oxygen is due in part to the auxiliary ball-in-tube O_2 flowmeter delivering 100% O_2 via nasal cannula. The traditional heuristic rule of FiO_2 delivered to the patient is a 4% increase from a baseline of 20% for every liter-per-minute increase of 100% O_2 flow via nasal cannula.[24] However, the true effective FiO_2 may be slightly less. In a study measuring FiO_2 with mouth and tracheal gas sampling for oxygen delivered at various flow rates at 97% and 47% O_2, effective FiO_2 increased by 2.5% for every liter-per-minute increase of 97% O_2. For 47% O_2, FiO_2 only increased by about 1% for every liter-per-minute increase.[25] There was strong correlation between FiO_2 at the mouth and the trachea ($r = 0.96$, $P < .001$). However, these studies were not conducted with drapes present and a higher O_2 concentration may accumulate with drapes. There have been proposed strategies to deliver sub-100% O_2 mixtures via nasal cannula or simple face mask including connecting the oxygen tubing to the Y-piece of a circle breathing circuit with a 5- or 6-mm endotracheal tube (ETT) connector and adjusting the FiO_2 from the machine (Figs. 30-1 and 30-2), or by connecting the oxygen tubing to the auxiliary common gas outlet.[26] Venturi masks can deliver sub-100% FiO_2 mixtures by entraining room air, though its use should be avoided if drapes are present over the patient's face due to entrainment of oxygen-rich gas accumulated under the drapes. Venturi masks should also be avoided if cautery is used near the face. Recommendations to prevent fires during draping are listed in Table 30-4.

Table 30-4 Recommendations to Prevent Burn Injuries during MAC

Open face draping techniques; i.e., avoiding tent of drapes
Supplemental oxygen at lowest acceptable flows guided by SpO_2
Use of compressed air rather than oxygen to prevent CO_2 accumulation
Stopping oxygen flow 60 s prior to use of electrocautery
Avoidance of alcohol-based prep solutions
Awareness of the causes and prevention of surgical fires

Adapted with permission from Bhananker SM, Posner KL, Cheney FW, et al. Injury and liability associated with monitored anesthesia care—A closed claims analysis. *Anesthesiology*. 2006;104:228–234.

Techniques of Monitored Anesthesia Care

A variety of medications are commonly administered during monitored anesthesia care with the desired end points to provide patient comfort, maintain cardiorespiratory stability, improve operating conditions, and prevent recall of unpleasant perioperative events. It is helpful to delineate and individualize the goals for each patient in order to formulate an appropriate regimen, which frequently involves the administration of either individual or combinations of analgesic, amnestic, and hypnotic drugs. There should be a minimal incidence of side effects, such as cardiorespiratory depression, nausea and vomiting, delayed emergence, and dysphoria, and there should be a rapid and complete recovery. Ideally, the patient should be able to communicate during the procedure. Clinical experience suggests that a level of sedation that allows verbal communication is optimal for the patient's comfort and safety. If the level of sedation is deepened to the extent that verbal communication is lost, the risks of the technique approach those of general anesthesia with an unprotected and uncontrolled airway. However, because monitored anesthesia care is provided by anesthesiologists, the range of sedation may include deeper sedation techniques than those provided by nonanesthesiologists during sedation/analgesia.

The preanesthetic evaluation and plan should identify specific causes and provide specific therapy for pain, anxiety, and agitation. Pain may be treated by local or regional analgesia, systemic analgesics, or removal of the painful stimulus. Anxiety may be reduced by the use of an anxiolytic such as a benzodiazepine and reassurance by the anesthesiologist. Patient agitation may be a result of pain or anxiety or life-threatening factors such as hypoxia, hypercarbia, impending local anesthetic toxicity, and cerebral hypoperfusion. Other causes of pain and agitation include cycling of the blood pressure cuff, a distended bladder, hypothermia, hyperthermia, pruritus, nausea, positional discomfort, uncomfortable oxygen masks and nasal cannula, IV cannulation site infiltration, a member of the surgical team leaning on the patient, and prolonged pneumatic tourniquet inflation.

Pharmacologic Basis of Monitored Anesthesia Care Techniques

The ability to predict the effects of the drugs in our armamentarium demands an understanding of their pharmacokinetic and pharmacodynamic properties. This understanding is a fundamental prerequisite for the design of an effective sedation regimen and greatly increases the probability of producing the desired therapeutic effect. Context-sensitive half-time, effect-site equilibration time, and anesthetic/sedative drug interactions are fundamental concepts that are particularly useful in the context of monitored anesthesia care and are discussed in more detail in other chapters of this book.

9 The ultimate objective of any dosing regimen is to deliver a therapeutic concentration of drug to its site of action, which is determined by the unique pharmacokinetic properties of that drug in that particular patient (1 Video 30-1). The therapeutic response to a particular drug concentration is described by the pharmacodynamics of that particular patient–drug combination. There is a large degree of pharmacokinetic and pharmacodynamic variability, producing a significant variability in the dose–response relationship in clinical practice. Excessive sedation may result in cardiac or respiratory depression. Inadequate sedation may result in patient discomfort and potential morbidity from lack of cooperation. As a general principle, to avoid excessive levels of sedation, drugs should be titrated in small increments or by adjustable infusions rather than administered in larger doses according to predetermined notions of efficacy.[27] In an ideal dosing regimen, an effective concentration of drug is achieved and then adjusted according to the magnitude of the noxious stimulus. If the noxious stimulus is increased or decreased, the concentration is increased or decreased accordingly. By the end of the procedure, the drug concentration should have decreased to a level compatible with rapid recovery. This approach requires the easily titratable drugs such as propofol. When using drugs such as propofol, adjustable-rate continuous infusions are the most logical method of maintaining a desired therapeutic concentration. If intermittent bolus administration is used, significant fluctuations in drug concentration occur. Under these circumstances, the plasma concentrations are either above or below the desired therapeutic range for a significant proportion of the procedure (Fig. 30-3). Continuous infusions are generally superior to intermittent bolus dosing because they produce less fluctuation in drug concentration, thus reducing the number of episodes of inadequate or excessive sedation. Administration of drugs by continuous infusion rather than by intermittent dosing also reduces the total amount of drug administered and facilitates a more prompt recovery.[27]

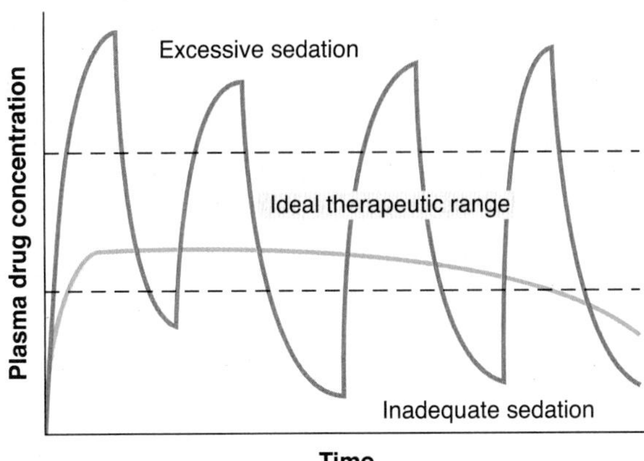

Figure 30-3 The changes in drug concentration during differing administration techniques. The *green line* represents a continuous infusion of a drug. In this situation, the drug is maintained within the therapeutic range for most of the procedure. The *orange line* represents the drug concentration resulting from intermittent bolus administration. The drug concentration is significantly above or below the desired therapeutic level for most of the procedure.

Distribution, Elimination, Accumulation, and Duration of Action

Following the administration of IV anesthetic drugs, the immediate distribution phase causes a brisk decrease in plasma levels as the drug is transported to the rapidly equilibrating vessel-rich group of tissues. There is a simultaneously occurring distribution of drug to the less well-perfused tissues such as muscle and skin. Over time, the drug is also distributed to the poorly perfused tissues such as bone and fat. Although the latter compartments are poorly perfused, they may accumulate significant amounts of lipophilic drugs during prolonged administration. This peripheral depot may contribute to a delayed recovery when the drug is eventually released back into the central compartment after its administration is discontinued. Redistributive factors are important determinants of drug effect and influence the plasma concentration of a drug in a time-dependent fashion.

Elimination Half-Life

Until recently, the elimination half-time was the predominant pharmacokinetic parameter used as the predictor of an anesthetic drug's duration of action. In everyday clinical practice, however, this parameter does not greatly enhance our ability to predict anesthetic drug disposition. Only in single-compartment models does the elimination half-time actually represent the time required for a drug to reach half of its initial concentration after administration. In a single-compartment model, elimination is the only process that can alter drug concentration. Intercompartmental distribution cannot occur because there are no other compartments for the drug to be distributed to and from. Most drugs in the anesthesiologist's armamentarium are lipophilic and are, therefore, more suited to multicompartmental modeling than single-compartment modeling. Similarly, other pharmacokinetic parameters, such as distribution half-time, distribution volume, intercompartmental rate constants, and so forth, do not provide us with a practical means of predicting drug disposition. In multicompartmental models, the metabolism and excretion of some IV anesthetic drugs may have only a minor contribution to the changes in plasma concentration when compared with the effects of intercompartmental distribution.

Context-Sensitive Half-Time

The concept of context-sensitive half-time was developed to improve the description and understanding of anesthetic drug disposition.[28] This concept has greatly improved our understanding of anesthetic drug disposition and is clinically applicable. The effect of distribution on plasma drug concentration varies in magnitude and direction over time and depends on the drug concentration gradients that exist between the various compartments. For example, during the early part of an infusion of a lipophilic drug, distributive factors will tend to decrease plasma concentrations as the drug is transported to the unsaturated peripheral tissues. Later, after the infusion is discontinued, drug will return from the peripheral tissues and re-enter the central circulation. The relative effect on plasma concentrations of distributive processes versus elimination varies over time and from drug to drug. The context-sensitive half-time describes the time required for the plasma drug concentration to decline by 50% after terminating an infusion of a particular duration.[28] This parameter is calculated by using computer simulation of multicompartmental models of drug disposition (Fig. 30-4). The context-sensitive

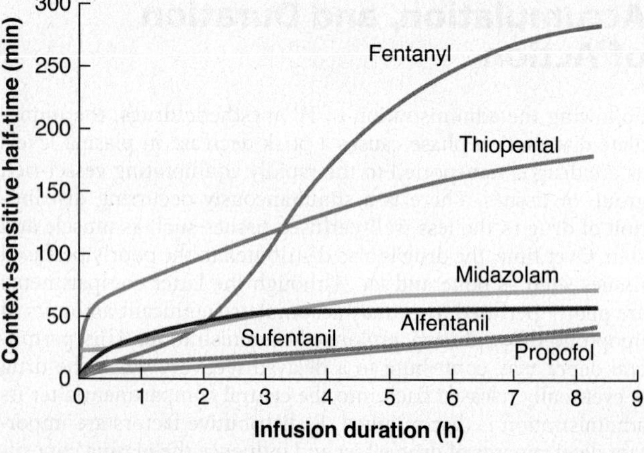

Figure 30-4 Context-sensitive half-time as a function of infusion duration. These data were generated from the computer model of Hughes et al. The context-sensitive half-time of propofol demonstrates a minimal increase as the duration of the infusion increases. Also note that for infusions of short duration, sufentanil has a shorter half-time than alfentanil. (Reproduced with permission from Hughes MA, Glass PSA, Jacobs JR. Context-sensitive half-time in multicompartment pharmacokinetic models for intravenous anesthetic drugs. *Anesthesiology*. 1992;76:334, with permission.)

half-time reflects the combined effects of distribution and metabolism on drug disposition. There are several interesting aspects of these data. First, the data confirm the clinical impression that as the infusion duration increases, the context-sensitive half-time of all the drugs increases; this phenomenon is not described in any way by the elimination half-life. The increase in context-sensitive half-time is particularly marked with fentanyl and thiopental. In the case of fentanyl, drug that is irreversibly eliminated from the plasma by hepatic clearance is immediately replaced by drug returning from the peripheral compartments. Thus, although fentanyl has a shorter *elimination* half-life than that of sufentanil (462 vs. 577 minutes), its *context-sensitive* half-time is much greater than that of sufentanil after an infusion of longer than 2 hours. The storage, and later release, of fentanyl from peripheral binding sites delay the decline in plasma concentration that would otherwise occur. *The context-sensitive half-times of all the drugs bear no constant relationship to their elimination half-times.* For example, compare also the context-sensitive half-times of propofol and thiopental (Fig. 30-4). Although the context-sensitive half-times of propofol and thiopental are comparable following a brief infusion, the context-sensitive half-time of thiopental increases rapidly following all but the shortest infusions. This finding confirms the clinical impression that thiopental is not an ideal drug for continuous infusion during ambulatory procedures. The context-sensitive half-time of propofol is prolonged to a minimal extent as the infusion duration increases. After an infusion of propofol, the drug that returns to the plasma from the peripheral compartments is rapidly cleared by metabolic processes and is, therefore, not available to slow the decay in plasma levels. This difference between thiopental and propofol is attributable to (1) the high metabolic clearance of propofol compared with thiopental, and (2) the relatively slow rate at which propofol returns to the plasma from peripheral compartments.

Alfentanil is the opioid that was, until the introduction of remifentanil, frequently studied, described, and promoted in the context of ambulatory techniques. Alfentanil has a very short elimination half-time, one-fifth that of sufentanil (111 vs. 577 minutes). However, despite the longer elimination half-time of sufentanil, its context-sensitive half-time is actually less than that of alfentanil for infusions up to 8 hours in duration. This phenomenon is explained in part by the huge distribution volume of sufentanil. After termination of a sufentanil infusion, the decay in plasma drug concentrations is accelerated not only by elimination but also by the continued redistribution of sufentanil into peripheral compartments. On the other hand, the small distribution volume of alfentanil equilibrates rapidly; therefore, peripheral distribution of drug away from the plasma is not a significant contributor to the decay in plasma concentration after an infusion. The data derived from computer simulation by Hughes et al.[28] show that the plasma decay of alfentanil is slower than that of sufentanil following infusions of similar duration to those used during conscious sedation. Thus, despite its short elimination half-time, alfentanil may not necessarily be superior to sufentanil.[29]

How Does the Context-Sensitive Half-Time Relate to the Time to Recovery?

Although the context-sensitive half-time represents a significant advance in our ability to describe drug disposition, this parameter does not directly describe how long it will take the patient to recover from monitored anesthesia care. The context-sensitive half-time merely describes how long it will take for the plasma concentration of the drug to decrease by 50%. The time to recovery depends on other additional factors. The difference between the plasma concentration at the end of the infusion and the

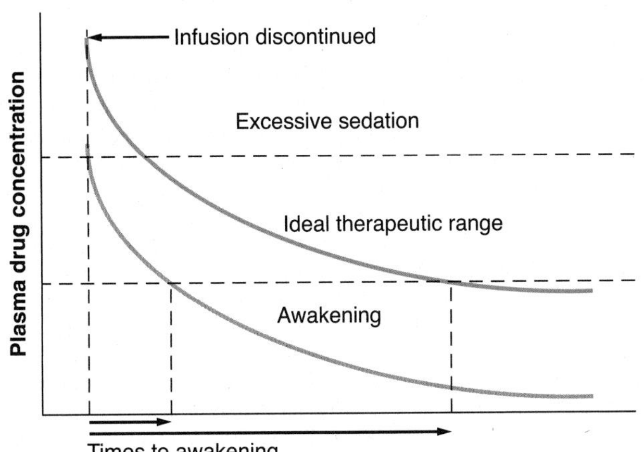

Figure 30-5 The context-sensitive half-time is not the sole determinant of the time it takes for the patient to awaken. This parameter merely reflects the time taken for the plasma concentration of a drug to decrease by 50%. The time to awakening is determined in addition by the difference in concentration at the end of the procedure and the concentration below which awakening will occur.

plasma concentration below which awakening can be expected is an obvious factor in determining time to recovery. For example, if the drug concentration is maintained at a level just above that required for awakening, the time to recovery will be more rapid than after an infusion during which the drug concentration is much greater than that required for awakening (Fig. 30-5). Furthermore, although context-sensitive half-time is a reflection of plasma drug decay, awakening from anesthesia is actually a function of effect-site (i.e., brain) concentration decay. Changes in effect-site concentration demonstrate a variable time lag behind changes in plasma drug concentration. Effect-site equilibration is a concept that is particularly relevant to IV sedation. When a drug is administered intravenously by bolus or infused rapidly, there is a delay before the onset of clinical effect. This delay occurs because the plasma is not usually the site of action but is merely the route by which the drug reaches its effect site. If some parameter of drug effect can be measured (e.g., power spectrum EEG analysis in the case of opioids), the half-time of equilibration between drug concentration in the blood and the drug effect can then be determined.[30] This parameter is abbreviated $t_{1/2}k_{e0}$. Drugs with a short $t_{1/2}k_{e0}$ will equilibrate rapidly with the brain and have a shorter delay in onset than drugs that have a longer $t_{1/2}k_{e0}$. Thiopental, propofol, and alfentanil have short $t_{1/2}k_{e0}$ values compared with midazolam, sufentanil, and fentanyl.

The $t_{1/2}k_{e0}$ allows predictions to be made of the time course of equilibration of the drug between the blood and the brain. A distinct time lag between the peak serum fentanyl concentration and the peak EEG slowing can be seen. In contrast, following alfentanil administration, the EEG changes closely parallel serum concentrations. The $t_{1/2}k_{e0}$ for fentanyl is 6.4 minutes compared with a $t_{1/2}k_{e0}$ of 1.1 minutes for alfentanil. Therefore, if an opioid is required to blunt the response to a single brief stimulus, alfentanil might represent a logical choice over fentanyl. The $t_{1/2}k_{e0}$ is an important determinant of bolus spacing when titrating drugs to clinical effect. In the case of drugs like midazolam and propofol, boluses of drug should be spaced far enough apart to allow the full peak effect to be clinically appreciated before further drug administration in order to avoid inadvertent overdosing.[31] For example, even if the shortest quoted equilibration half-time for midazolam (0.9 minutes) is used, it will take 2.7 (i.e., three half-times) minutes for effect-site concentrations to be 87.5% equilibrated. Other factors are also important determinants of bolus size and spacing. For example, a low cardiac output will markedly delay drug arrival at the site of action. If sufficient time is not given for the drug to take effect before giving additional drug increments, significant cardiorespiratory compromise may occur. Furthermore, the effects of initial doses of most drugs in anesthetic practice are terminated by redistribution, which depends on blood flow to redistribution sites. If there is reduced blood flow to redistribution sites because of pre-existing and iatrogenic decreases in cardiac output, the dangerous adverse effects of these drugs are likely to be both delayed and markedly prolonged. An example of this scenario is the patient with a hemodynamic compromise caused by a tachydysrhythmia who requires sedation for cardioversion. Careful, well-spaced, small boluses of drug should be given to induce the appropriate level of sedation, bearing in mind that it may take several minutes for the full effect of a small bolus dose to become apparent.

Drug Interactions

At the present time, no single drug can provide all the compo- 10
nents of monitored anesthesia care (i.e., analgesia, anxiolysis, and hypnosis) with an acceptable margin of safety or ease of titratability. Therefore, patient comfort is usually maintained with a combination of drugs. By acting synergistically, combinations of drugs enable reductions in the dose requirements of individual drugs. For example, the combination of propofol and fentanyl by infusion has been shown to produce a more rapid recovery and better stress response abolition than the use of propofol alone.[32] In addition, lower doses of each drug may reduce the untoward side effects associated with higher doses leading to increased patient satisfaction and decreased times to discharge. However, synergistic interaction may also extend to the undesirable interactions of the drugs such as cardiorespiratory depression.

Drug interactions may have both a pharmacodynamic and a pharmacokinetic basis and may vary depending on the combination of drugs being co-administered, the dose range over which these drugs are administered, and the specific clinical effect that is measured. For example, because fentanyl is primarily an analgesic rather than a hypnotic, it reduces propofol requirements for suppression of response to skin incision to a much greater degree than it reduces propofol requirements for induction of anesthesia.[32] On the other hand, because midazolam has significant hypnotic properties, it displays significant synergism with propofol when used to induce hypnosis and prevent movement in response to a painful stimulus.[33]

The plasma concentration of a drug at steady state that is required to abolish purposeful movement at skin incision in 50% of patients ($Cp_{ss}50$) is a measure of potency that is analogous to the familiar parameter of minimum alveolar concentration (MAC) of the volatile inhaled anesthetics. IV anesthetic interactions may be evaluated by their effect on the $Cp_{ss}50$ in a manner analogous to the expression of the effects of opioids on volatile anesthetic requirements in terms of MAC reduction.[33] For example, during general anesthesia, opioid requirements to suppress the responses to noxious stimuli are 10-fold higher when used as the sole agent compared with when they are used in conjunction with a nitrous oxide/potent inhaled vapor technique. This interaction persists at the lighter levels of anesthesia encountered during monitored anesthesia care. Therefore, it is likely that a rapid recovery would be facilitated by using opioids in combination with other agents (e.g., propofol/midazolam) rather than as the sole drug.

The interactions between propofol and opioids are important because these agents are frequently used during monitored anesthesia care. Interestingly, their drug interactions are dose dependent. For example, when analgesic concentrations of fentanyl (0.6 ng/mL) are used in combination with propofol for anesthesia, the $Cp_{ss}50$ of propofol is reduced by 50% compared with when propofol is used as the sole agent.[32] However, when the dose of fentanyl is increased, there is no significant further reduction of the $Cp_{ss}50$ for propofol beyond a fentanyl concentration of 3 ng/mL. Although the data presented here pertain to patients under general anesthesia, the findings have important implications for monitored anesthesia care.

These studies demonstrate that the potentiating effects of opioids on co-administered sedatives are pronounced within the dose range commonly used during monitored anesthesia care. Furthermore, the data suggest that the dose–response curve is likely to be steep within this dose range, thus supporting the clinical impression that significant increases in depth of sedation can occur with only modest increments in opioid or hypnotic/sedative dosage. The following clinical recommendations can be made: During monitored anesthesia care, the maximum benefit of opioid supplementation, in terms of potentiation of other administered sedatives, will accrue when the opioid is used in the analgesic dose range. Within this dose range, there is great potential for adverse cardiorespiratory interaction.

Opioid and benzodiazepine combinations are frequently used to achieve the components of hypnosis, amnesia, and analgesia. This drug combination displays marked synergism in producing hypnosis. Approximately 25% of the median effective dose for each individual drug is required in combination to induce hypnosis in 50% of patients.[34] If the combination were simply additive, hypnosis would be induced in only approximately 25% of patients. Even subanalgesic doses of alfentanil (3 μg/kg) produce a profound reduction in midazolam requirements for hypnosis.[34] This synergism also extends to the unwanted effects of these drugs, producing the life-threatening complications of respiratory and cardiac depression. Several fatalities have been reported after the use of midazolam, the majority of these being related to adverse respiratory events. In many of these cases, midazolam was used in combination with an opioid. The effects of midazolam and fentanyl on respiratory function in healthy volunteers have been examined by Bailey et al.[35] Whereas midazolam produced no significant respiratory effects alone, and fentanyl alone produced hypoxemia (oxyhemoglobin saturation ≤95%) in half of the subjects, the combination of midazolam 0.05 μg/kg and fentanyl 2 μg/kg resulted in hypoxemia in 11 of 12 subjects and apnea (no spontaneous respiratory effort for 15 seconds) in 6 of 12 subjects. The combination of midazolam and fentanyl places patients at high risk for developing hypoxemia and apnea. The respiratory depressant effects of this drug combination are likely to be even more significant in the patient with coexisting respiratory or central nervous system disease or at the extremes of age. In clinical practice, the clinical advantages of the synergy between opioids and benzodiazepines for the maintenance of patient comfort should be carefully weighed against the disadvantages of the potentially adverse effect of this drug combination on the cardiovascular and respiratory systems.

Specific Drugs Used for Monitored Anesthesia Care

Propofol

Propofol has become a popular choice for monitored anesthesia care due to its favorable side effect profile and ease of titratability. Propofol has many of the ideal properties of a sedative–hypnotic for use in monitored anesthesia care. Its pharmacokinetic profile, that is, a context-sensitive half-time that remains short even after infusions of prolonged duration and a short effect-site equilibration time, makes it an easily titratable drug with an excellent recovery profile. The quality of recovery and the low incidence of nausea and vomiting make propofol particularly well suited to ambulatory monitored anesthesia care procedures. Because of the aforementioned information, a significant body of experience with the use of propofol for monitored anesthesia care has emerged.

Propofol has significant advantages compared with benzodiazepines when used as the hypnotic component of a monitored anesthesia care technique. Although midazolam has a relatively short elimination half-time, its context-sensitive half-time is approximately twice that of propofol.[28] Whereas propofol is noted for the rapid return to clearheadedness, midazolam is often associated with prolonged postoperative sedation and psychomotor impairment, particularly in the elderly. Propofol in typical moderate sedation doses (25 to 75 μg/kg/min) has minimal analgesic properties. However, the unique advantages of propofol can be exploited to the maximum when propofol is used to provide sedation when the analgesic component is provided by a local or regional analgesic technique.[36,37]

The use of propofol (50 to 70 μg/kg/min) to provide sedation (defined as sleep with preservation of the eyelash reflex and purposeful reaction to verbal or mild physical stimulation) as an adjunct to spinal anesthesia for lower limb surgery has been examined.[36] After termination of infusions of approximately 100 minutes, patients regained consciousness in approximately 4 minutes. The authors also noted the ease with which general anesthesia could be induced if necessary by increasing the propofol infusion. Alternatively, if a deeper level of sedation was not intended, the propofol infusion could either be decreased or turned off.

The same group also compared propofol (60.5 μg/kg/min) with midazolam (4.3 μg/kg/min) as an adjunct to spinal anesthesia.[37] The propofol group had faster immediate recovery than the midazolam group (2.3 vs. 9.2 minutes to spontaneous eye opening). Furthermore, psychomotor function was comparable with baseline values following propofol sedation but did not return to baseline until 2 hours after midazolam administration. This study demonstrated that propofol produced less postoperative sedation, drowsiness, confusion, and clumsiness than midazolam.[36]

The beneficial effects of propofol on nausea and vomiting are a major feature of this drug. There is evidence that even subhypnotic doses (as little as 10 mg) of propofol possess direct antiemetic properties, particularly when combined with an antiemetic in patients at risk for nausea and vomiting.[38] On the other hand, even during low-dose infusions used for sedation, pain during injection of propofol may be troublesome in 33% to 50% of patients.[39]

Many strategies have been proposed to mitigate propofol injection pain including preadministration of lidocaine, lidocaine–propofol admixtures, cooled propofol, slower injection speeds, and more. A systematic review and meta-analysis including 177 randomized controlled trials (RCTs) and 25,260 adults examined multiple techniques to prevent propofol injection pain.[39] The most effective strategies were injection through the antecubital vein instead of a hand vein (RR 0.14, 95% CI 0.07–0.30) and pretreating with lidocaine and proximal venous occlusion (i.e., injecting IV lidocaine after application of proximal tourniquet) (RR 0.29, 95% CI 0.22–0.38). Although lidocaine–propofol admixture was deemed effective in reducing propofol injection pain (RR 0.40, 95% CI 0.33–0.48), the funnel plot for this intervention was asymmetrical, suggesting possible strong small study effect or reporting bias. Other interventions which showed efficacy included pretreatment with opioids (RR 0.49, 95% CI 0.41–0.59), ketamine (RR 0.52, 95% CI 0.46–0.57), and Nonsteroidal anti-inflammatory drug (NSAIDs) (RR 0.67,

Table 30-5 Published Strategies for Reducing the Pain on Intravenous Injection of Propofol

Using larger veins in antecubital fossa
Pretreating with lidocaine and proximal venous occlusion
Injection into a fast-running intravenous line
Diluting with 5% glucose or 10% intralipid
Adding lidocaine to propofol
Decreasing the speed of injection
Pretreatment with opioid
Cooling propofol to 4°C prior to injection
Injecting cooled saline (4°C) prior to injection
Discontinuing intravenous fluid administration during injection

95% CI 0.49–0.91). Strategies for reducing the pain of propofol administration are described in Table 30-5.

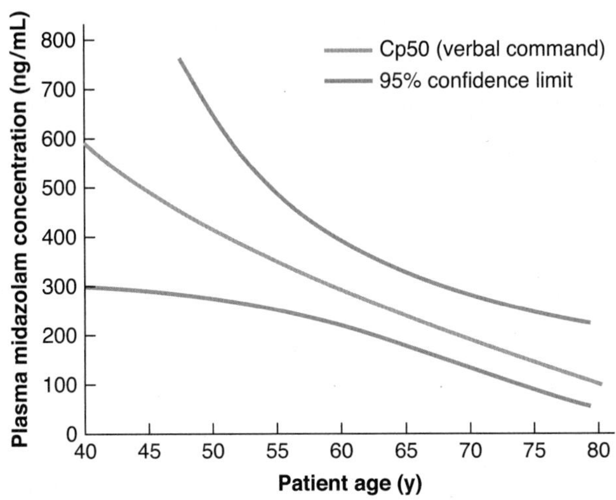

Figure 30-6 Midazolam Cp50 (the concentration at which 50% of subjects will fail to respond to a verbal command) as a function of age. There is a marked decrease in midazolam requirements as patient age increases. (Reproduced with permission from Jacobs JR, Reves JG, Marty J, et al. Aging increases pharmacodynamic sensitivity to the hypnotic effects of midazolam. *Anesth Analg.* 1995;80:143.)

Benzodiazepines

Benzodiazepines are commonly used during monitored anesthesia care for their anxiolytic, amnestic, and hypnotic properties. Patients presenting for diagnostic and surgical procedures frequently request some form of anxiolytic. Midazolam is usually administered prior to the start of the surgical or diagnostic procedures to facilitate amnesia and reduce the patient's level of anxiety. Midazolam's relatively short elimination half-life and decreased likelihood of concomitant drug interactions make it a superior choice to other benzodiazepines. However, when using midazolam as the sole anesthetic, there is often significant and prolonged psychomotor impairment.

With the availability of propofol, midazolam may be better used in a modified role by using lower doses prior to the start of a propofol infusion to provide the specific amnestic, and perhaps anxiolytic, component of a "balanced" sedation technique rather than as the major hypnotic component. A study in healthy volunteers demonstrated that propofol reduced the distribution and clearance of midazolam in a concentration-dependent manner.[40] The group reported increased plasma levels of midazolam ranging from 5% to 25% during increasing doses of propofol for monitored anesthesia care. This strategy allows the more evanescent and titratable propofol to provide the desired level of deep sedation in an adjustable manner according to the specific stimulus. The analgesic component, if required, of a balanced monitored anesthesia care technique may be provided by regional/local techniques or opioids. However, when using opioids with benzodiazepines, the potential for significant respiratory impairment should be considered.

The age of the patient should be taken into consideration when administering benzodiazepines. The dose of a particular benzodiazepine required to reach a desired clinical end point is reduced in elderly compared with younger patients. This difference in dosing requirements in elderly patients is mainly related to pharmacodynamic factors. As demonstrated by the threefold decrease in plasma concentration of midazolam, 50% of patients would be expected not to respond to verbal command (Cp50) in an 80-year-old patient compared with a 40-year-old patient (Fig. 30-6).[41]

Benzodiazepines are valuable components of monitored anesthesia care techniques because they enhance patient comfort, improve operating conditions, and provide amnesia. However, recovery of psychomotor and cognitive function may be significantly prolonged following benzodiazepine sedation, especially when compared with sedative–hypnotic techniques using propofol as the major component.[42] The specific benzodiazepine antagonist flumazenil provides the potential to improve the recovery profile of benzodiazepines by permitting the active termination of their sedative and amnestic effects without invoking adverse side effects. The availability of flumazenil to acutely reverse sedation with benzodiazepines can provide a margin of safety that is unavailable when using propofol. Consequently, midazolam may be the preferred sedative in the setting of a jeopardized airway, such as an awake tracheostomy, because it can be pharmacologically reversed. However, the potential for resedation remains an obstacle to the routine use of benzodiazepine reversal, particularly in patients undergoing ambulatory procedures. The effects of midazolam may recur up to 90 minutes following the administration of flumazenil.[42] Thus, it is possible that patients could be discharged prematurely to a less well-monitored area, or even out of the hospital in the case of ambulatory surgery, and later experience recurrence of benzodiazepine effects. Typical dose requirements for use of flumazenil are listed in Table 30-6.

Remimazolam

Remimazolam was approved by the food and drug administration (FDA) in 2020 as a new short-acting benzodiazepine for IV

Table 30-6 Recommended Regimen for the Use of Intravenous Flumazenil to Antagonize Benzodiazepine Effects

Initial recommended dose of 0.2 mg
If desired level of consciousness is not achieved in 45 s, repeat 0.2-mg dose
0.2-mg doses may need to be repeated every 60 s until a maximum of 1 mg is administered
Be aware of the potential for resedation

administration. Its structure allows agonism of γ-aminobutyric acid A ($GABA_A$) receptor activity while exhibiting metabolism to a nonpharmacologically active metabolite via nonspecific tissue esterases, similar to that seen with remifentanil.[43] It is mostly albumin bound and excreted in the urine. Clearance is not significantly different between normal renal function and end stage renal disease (ESRD). However, clearance is lower in patients with severe hepatic impairment (Child–Pugh score ≥10) and may need dose adjustments for these patients.[43] When compared with midazolam, remimazolam has a much shorter context-sensitive half-time (12 minutes vs. 122 minutes after 8-hour infusion), smaller mean volume of distribution (35 L vs. 82 L), higher mean clearance (70 L/h vs. 23 L/h), shorter mean terminal half-life (0.75 hours vs. 4.3 hours), and faster time to recovery (5.5 to 20 minutes vs. 40 minutes).[43] Like all benzodiazepines, it can be reversed with flumazenil. When administering remimazolam, the FDA recommends an initial IV dose of 5 mg over a 1-minute period followed by 2.5 mg IV doses over a 15-second time period with 2 minutes between administration of supplemental doses.[44]

In light of its unique metabolism, most would assume remimazolam would expedite recovery and facilitate a more rapid discharge from the postprocedure unit. However, large-scale RCTs utilizing remimazolam for monitored anesthesia care are lacking and some of the smaller studies that do exist utilize remimazolam as a continuous infusion, contrary to current FDA approvals. Thus, further studies are necessary before broad implementation of remimazolam for monitored anesthesia care can occur.

Opioids

Opioids are administered in the context of monitored anesthesia care to provide the specific analgesic component of a "balanced" technique. Opioids are indicated when regional or local anesthetic techniques are inappropriate or ineffective, and are typically administered immediately prior to the painful or invasive portion of the procedure. In addition, opioids may be indicated to blunt untoward hemodynamic and physiologic responses, a desirable effect in patients with significant cardiac disease. Pain relief may be required for factors other than the procedure itself, such as uncomfortable positioning, propofol injection, pneumatic tourniquet pain, or other pain not relieved by the local anesthetic technique. The choice of a particular opioid depends on several factors including cost, availability, time of onset, duration, and potential side effects. Opioids frequently administered during monitored anesthesia care include alfentanil, fentanyl, and remifentanil. Their adverse effects include respiratory depression, muscle rigidity, and nausea and vomiting, all of which are undesirable in the spontaneously breathing patient with an unprotected airway. A complicating issue is that the ability to predict the effect of a given dose of opioid in a particular patient is limited by significant interpatient pharmacokinetic and pharmacodynamic variability. Furthermore, the coadministration of sedative agents increases the risk of serious adverse events, particularly respiratory arrest. This problem is usually overcome in practice by the cautious incremental administration of small, carefully titrated boluses or by titrating infusions to the desired effect. A rule-of-thumb guide to time-to-peak effect after bolus administration of fentanyl, alfentanil, and sufentanil is 3.6 minutes, 1.4 minutes, and 5.6 minutes, respectively, as seen in a study by Shafer et al.[29]

The well-described phenomenon of patient awareness and subsequent recall of intraoperative events following high-dose opioid anesthesia is taken as evidence that opioids lack significant amnestic properties. However, when the effects of low-dose fentanyl on memory were specifically examined in volunteers, it was found that although the subjects appeared to be awake during the fentanyl infusion, there was significant memory impairment.[45] In this study, the degree of stimulation was probably less than that experienced by a patient undergoing a painful surgical procedure. Recall for a painful stimulus during an invasive procedure may not be impaired to the same degree as recall for the less noxious stimuli experienced by the subjects of this study. Aydin et al.[46] noted that the addition of fentanyl to local anesthesia during cataract surgery provided a significant difference in sedation levels; however, it was of brief duration. If amnesia is desired as part of a balanced technique, a sedative–hypnotic agent should be administered and the dose of both agents decreased to avoid any cardiorespiratory events.

Remifentanil

Remifentanil is a potent, ultrashort-acting opioid used during monitored anesthesia care to provide analgesia during brief, painful procedures. Remifentanil is typically administered as a bolus to achieve therapeutic analgesia followed by a continuous infusion. If the situation permits, the bolus should be avoided to decrease the incidence of adverse cardiorespiratory effects. It has been suggested that the administration of continuous infusions during monitored anesthesia care improves the operative conditions for the proceduralist.[47]

Remifentanil has pharmacodynamic properties similar to those of other potent μ-opioid receptor agonists such as fentanyl and alfentanil. However, remifentanil is predominantly metabolized by nonspecific esterases, generating an extremely rapid clearance and termination of effect and making it an attractive choice for patients with significant hepatic or renal disease.[48] Another major advantage is the intense analgesia of limited duration, which is advantageous to prevent respiratory depression after the stimulating portion of the procedure is completed. The context-sensitive half-time of remifentanil is consistently short, 3 to 5 minutes, increasing to a minimal degree with the duration of the infusion.[48] Furthermore, remifentanil has a short effect-site equilibration time ($t_{1/2}k_{e0}$) of 1 to 1.5 minutes. This $t_{1/2}k_{e0}$ is slightly longer than that of alfentanil (0.6 to 1.2 minutes) but much shorter than that of fentanyl (4 to 5 minutes) and morphine (approximately 20 minutes), and makes the onset of effect after drug administration very rapid, thus facilitating titration of effect during monitored anesthesia care.

In clinical practice, remifentanil has been used successfully as the analgesic component of sedation techniques for regional and local anesthesia. Its unique pharmacokinetic profile makes it well suited for monitored anesthesia care techniques. Published experience with the use of remifentanil suggests that it is possible to titrate remifentanil administration to provide effective analgesia with minimal respiratory depression. The published data can be used to generate some practical clinical guidelines,[49] which are discussed here:

1. The most desirable therapeutic end point for remifentanil administration is effective analgesia and patient comfort rather than sedation. Sedative drugs such as propofol or midazolam can be used in combination with remifentanil to provide the hypnotic–amnestic component of the sedation technique, remembering that the concomitant administration of midazolam decreases remifentanil dose requirements by up to 50%.[50]
2. Published data suggest that bolus administration of remifentanil is associated with an increased incidence of respiratory depression and chest wall rigidity. Because these side effects are likely to be related to high peak concentrations of drugs, it is recommended that remifentanil boluses be administered slowly (over 30 to 90 seconds) or avoided completely by using a pure infusion technique. If respiratory depression is promptly recognized and the remifentanil administration is reduced or discontinued, it should resolve within approximately 3 minutes.

Despite the pharmacokinetic advantages of remifentanil, the level of vigilance required for its administration should be no different from that for any other potent opioid. Although the offset time of remifentanil is rapid, it still requires the recognition of respiratory depression to trigger a downward adjustment in dosage. Similarly, the short $t_{1/2}k_{e0}$ of remifentanil suggests that sudden respiratory depression may occur in response to upward adjustments in dosage. Despite the potential for respiratory depression, the efficacy of remifentanil boluses during monitored anesthesia care has been investigated by several groups.[51]

3. The effects of coadministration of benzodiazepines and opioids are well documented. The addition of midazolam to provide the anxiolytic–sedative and amnestic components of a sedation technique has been shown to increase patient satisfaction and significantly reduce remifentanil dose requirements. Even relatively low-dose midazolam (2 mg IV) produces significant reductions in remifentanil requirements and patient anxiety. During breast or lymph node biopsy, remifentanil infusion requirements were 0.065 μg/kg/min when preceded by midazolam compared with 0.123 μg/kg/min when used alone.[50] The advantages of coadministration of small doses of midazolam include increased patient satisfaction, increased amnesia, decreased nausea and vomiting, and decreased anxiety. The disadvantages include a tendency toward increased respiratory depression, apnea, and excessive sedation.
4. Because most painful stimuli are of unpredictable duration and because the risk of adverse respiratory events is increased following bolus administration, the most logical method for the administration of remifentanil during monitored anesthesia care is by an adjustable infusion. This should ideally be preceded by a small bolus of midazolam. Most investigators have used infusion rates that start at 0.1 μg/kg/min approximately 5 minutes prior to the first painful stimulus. This initial "loading" infusion is then weaned to approximately 0.05 μg/kg/min to maintain patient comfort. The maintenance infusion is adjusted upward in response to pain or hemodynamic response or downward in response to excessive sedation, respiratory depression, or apnea. A typical incremental change in infusion rate is 0.025 μg/kg/min. The use of remifentanil infusions of 0.2 μg/kg/min is associated with an increased incidence of respiratory depression that is not necessarily associated with superior analgesia. As in the case of propofol administration, inadvertent interruption of remifentanil administration will result in abrupt offset of effect, which may result in patient discomfort, hemodynamic instability, and even morbidity due to patient movement. It is therefore very important to ensure that the drug delivery system is monitored carefully during the procedure. Remifentanil is supplied as a powder that must be reconstituted prior to use. It is particularly important when administering this drug to patients with an unsecured airway to ensure that there are no errors in drug dilution that would result in inadvertent dosing errors.

Typical adult dose recommendations for opioids and other drugs discussed in the text are listed in Table 30-7.

Ketamine

Ketamine, a phencyclidine derivative, is an intense analgesic frequently used as a component of pediatric sedation techniques and is rapidly gaining popularity in the adult population, particularly in the opioid-tolerant patient.[52] In addition to its analgesic

Table 30-7 Typical Dose Ranges of Sedative, Hypnotic, and Analgesic Drugs

Drug	Typical Adult Intravenous Dose Range (Titrated to Effect in Small Increments)
Benzodiazepines	
Midazolam	0.02–0.04 mg/kg (~1–2 mg) bolus prior to stimulus
Remimazolam	5 mg bolus over 1-min prior to stimulus, followed by 2.5-mg bolus with 2 min between administration of supplemental doses as necessary
Opioid Analgesics	
Alfentanil	5–20 μg/kg bolus 2 min prior to stimulus
Fentanyl	0.5–2 μg/kg bolus 2–4 min prior to stimulus
Remifentanil	Infusion 0.1 μg/kg/min 5 min prior to stimulus Wean to 0.05 μg/kg/min as tolerated Adjust up or down in increments of 0.025 μg/kg/min Reduce dose accordingly when co-administered with midazolam or propofol Avoid boluses
Hypnotics	
Propofol	0.25–0.5 mg/kg boluses
Ketamine "Ketofol"	25–75 μg/kg/min infusion 0.25–0.5 mg/kg boluses 0.25–0.5 mg/kg boluses 25–50 μg/kg/min infusion
Dexmedetomidine	Loading infusion: 0.5–1 μg/kg over 10–20 min
	Maintenance infusion: 0.2–0.7 μg/kg/h

properties, ketamine has a relatively high safety profile. When used in small doses, its use is associated with minimal respiratory and cardiovascular depression. Ketamine produces a dissociative state in which the eyes remain open with a nystagmic gaze. However, as the dose of ketamine increases, or when used in combination with other sedatives, a state of deep sedation and/or general anesthesia may be inadvertently achieved. It is often stated that increased oral secretions make laryngospasm more likely. The fear of laryngospasm is the underlying rationale for the frequent administration of an antisialagogue such as atropine or glycopyrrolate. Ketamine can elevate intracranial and intraocular pressure and is thus relatively contraindicated in patients with increased intracranial pressure and with glaucoma or open-globe injuries.[52] Patient movement may make ketamine less than ideal for procedures requiring a completely motionless patient. Although it has been suggested that airway reflexes are relatively preserved with ketamine, there is no convincing evidence to support this notion. Ketamine is frequently combined with a benzodiazepine to reduce the incidence of hallucinations associated with its use. However, this practice is controversial.[53]

When administered IV, ketamine should be given in small (0.25 to 0.5 mg/kg) increments, titrating to effect, with an onset of action of 1 to 2 minutes and an approximate duration of 20 to 60 minutes.

"Ketofol"

The combination of propofol and ketamine, nicknamed "ketofol," has been associated with a lower incidence of deleterious side effects than when each medication is given alone. Advantages of the administration of "ketofol" are predominately due to the ability of these drugs to balance the negative side effects of the other. For example, the analgesic effect of ketamine reduces the dosage of propofol required to complete an invasive or painful procedure. Some advantages include preserved hemodynamic stability, decreased nausea and vomiting, improved procedural conditions, and decreased airway complications.

While in theory, combining smaller doses of both medications may minimize their respective adverse effects, the literature is mixed. In a study of 100 females undergoing breast biopsy, propofol was administered with varying doses of ketamine.[54] No clinically significant respiratory depression occurred and there was a low incidence of psychomimetic effects. Moreover, several RCTs utilizing "ketofol" in the emergency department showed no significant differences in incidence of respiratory events compared with propofol alone.[55,56] Conversely, in a systematic review of six RCTs using a ketamine–propofol combination, there was a lower frequency of adverse respiratory events utilizing "ketofol" versus propofol alone in the emergency department.[57] However, adverse respiratory events were defined differently in each trial and many of the adverse events were not clinically significant (e.g., change in end-tidal CO_2, brief drop in oxygen saturation). Furthermore, another systematic review of 18 RCTs suggested that "ketofol" may result in less respiratory events requiring intervention, less hypotension, and less bradycardia than propofol alone.[58] Most recently, a systematic review in 2020 included 11 trials in pediatric patients examining "ketofol" versus single or combined agents.[59] Single agents included ketamine or propofol, and combinations included: ketamine–dexmedetomidine, propofol–dexmedetomidine, and propofol–fentanyl. Compared with single agents, the use of "ketofol" showed increased recovery time but had no significant effect on airway obstruction, apnea, desaturation, or nausea/vomiting. Compared with combined agents, the use of "ketofol" resulted in less hypotensive events but had no significant effect on recovery time, desaturation, or respiratory depression. Studies reporting on the use of "ketofol" should be interpreted and compared with caution, however, as each study may use different ratios of each drug.

While the data is mixed, meta-analyses have their limitations and patients may respond to "ketofol" differently. Ultimately, it is the anesthesiologist's responsibility to understand the pharmacology of the medications utilized and the appropriateness of clinical use based on the patient's comorbidities and surgical needs. There is no consensus on the exact mixture for "ketofol", and ratios as high as 1 mg of ketamine to 1 mg of propofol (i.e., 1:1), to as low as 1 mg of ketamine to 10 mg of propofol (i.e., 1:10) can be found in the literature with success. Regardless of ratio, dosing typically follows that of propofol: 0.25 mg/kg bolus followed by either a continuous infusion of 25 to 50 μg/kg/min or by incremental boluses of 0.25 to 0.5 mg/kg every 3 to 5 minutes. As ketamine is in the admixture, doses required to achieve the appropriate level of sedation should be less than when compared to propofol alone. However, problems may arise when repeated doses or prolonged administration of the drug combinations are required as the effects of ketamine may outlast that of propofol.

Dexmedetomidine

Dexmedetomidine is a selective α_2-receptor agonist that depresses central sympathetic function and produces sedation and analgesia. The α_2-agonists potentiate opioid-induced analgesia, benzodiazepine-induced hypnosis, and have potent MAC-sparing effects when administered with volatile agents. However, unlike propofol and benzodiazepines, dexmedetomidine does not appear to have amnestic properties.[60]

Dexmedetomidine induces a form of sedation resembling natural sleep from which the patient is easily and quickly aroused. It is most often delivered as an initial bolus of 0.5 to 1 μg/kg over 10 to 20 minutes, followed by a continuous infusion of 0.2 to 0.7 μg/kg/h. Compared with other sedative and analgesic drugs, dexmedetomidine appears to have relatively minor effects on respiratory function when used in the typical dose range.[60] However, dexmedetomidine should not be considered protective against respiratory depression because it can also decrease upper-airway patency,[61,62] though the ventilatory drive in response to obstruction may[61] or may not[62] be preserved. Occasional airway intervention to relieve obstruction and apnea may be required during dexmedetomidine administration, especially when used in combination with other respiratory depressants.[62]

Dexmedetomidine tends to decrease cerebral blood flow both directly via α_2-mediated constriction of cerebral blood vessels and indirectly via its effect on systemic pressure. However, there appears to be a concomitant decrease in cerebral metabolic rate.[63] To add further reassurance, the use of dexmedetomidine does not appear to be associated with an increase in the need for intracarotid shunting in patients undergoing awake carotid endarterectomy.[64] Dexmedetomidine has been used successfully in both adult and pediatric patients for monitored anesthesia care during the awake portions of craniotomies requiring patient cooperation for cortical speech mapping. Dexmedetomidine has been used as sedative supplementation to regional anesthesia during carotid endarterectomy. Under these circumstances, there were fewer fluctuations from the desired sedation level when compared with the combination of midazolam, fentanyl, and propofol.[64]

Dexmedetomidine can be used for sedation during instrumentation of the difficult airway. Patients undergoing fiberoptic intubation who are sedated using dexmedetomidine are generally comfortable yet cooperative (it even causes dry mouth!). Administration of α_2-agonist is associated with a reduction of sympathetic outflow and an increase in cardiac vagal activity; therefore,

Table 30-8 A Comparison of Some Important Properties of Propofol and Dexmedetomidine

	Propofol	Dexmedetomidine
Pain on injection	Yes	Minimal
Analgesic properties in subhypnotic doses	Minimal	Yes
Amnestic properties in subhypnotic doses	Significant	Insignificant
Time of onset with typical administration	Rapid	5–10 min
Restrictive regulations on use by non–anesthesia-trained providers	Yes	No
Potential for significant bradycardia	Minimal	Significant

hypotension and bradycardia may occur particularly during rapid IV infusion or bolus injection.[64] The α_2-agonists do have peripheral vasoconstrictive effects as well that can occasionally precipitate hypertension. Despite this phenomenon, the incidence of hypertensive episodes requiring intervention is lower when compared with an equivalent propofol-based technique.[64]

The lack of pain on injection and its analgesic and minimal adverse respiratory properties would seem to make dexmedetomidine a useful alternative to propofol in certain circumstances. However, when compared with propofol, the target sedation level takes longer to achieve with dexmedetomidine (25 vs. 10 minutes).[64] Furthermore, if loading boluses of dexmedetomidine are used to accelerate the onset of sedation, bradycardia and hypotension may occur. Although the use of dexmedetomidine may result in greater sedation, lower blood pressure, and improved analgesia in the recovery room when compared with propofol, the time to postanesthesia care unit (PACU) discharge is not significantly different.[64] On the contrary, secondary to its prolonged half-life of 2 hours, PACU times may be increased with the use of dexmedetomidine. Hypotension is the most frequently occurring adverse event and can linger for hours, delaying time to discharge.[65]

The analgesic properties of dexmedetomidine may make it a useful alternative to the use of propofol as a sole agent during painful procedures. However, the time taken to deliver the loading dose, the occasional need to rebolus, hypotension, bradycardia, and the relatively long recovery time may limit the utility of dexmedetomidine. On the other hand, the pain on injection of propofol and the legislative constraints on the administration of propofol by nonanesthesia-trained providers may make dexmedetomidine advantageous in certain circumstances. The properties of propofol and dexmedetomidine are compared in Table 30-8.

Complications during Monitored Anesthesia Care

The notion that monitored anesthesia care is safer or less harmful than general anesthesia (i.e., "it's just a MAC") is misleading and can create a false sense of security. In fact, the overall rate of complications surrounding MAC is similar to that for general anesthesia.[66] Monitored anesthesia care entails a fluctuating and dynamic range of sedation requiring frequent assessments and adjustments and has the potential for similar catastrophic cardiorespiratory complications as general anesthesia, but with the ever-present caveat: the patient has an unsecured airway!

Respiratory Depression

During monitored anesthesia care, there is significant potential for respiratory compromise, as highlighted by the ASA Closed Claims Database Study that examined claims related to MAC (NICV 30-1).[5] In that study, excessive sedation leading to respiratory compromise was the most common cause of death or central nervous system injury during MAC. An accompanying editorial noted that MAC is no less risky than general anesthesia in terms of occurrences of permanent brain injury and death for patients undergoing predominantly elective procedures in outpatient settings.[67] The adverse respiratory effects of sedation administration include adverse effects on respiratory drive, airway patency, and loss of airway protective reflexes. These effects result either directly as a result of sedative–hypnotic or opioid administration or indirectly as a consequence of brain stem hypoperfusion resulting from hypotension. There may also be a marked increase in the work of breathing because of increased upper airway resistance and adverse effects on respiratory system mechanics resulting from a decline in functional residual capacity.[68]

The upper airway is located outside the thorax. During inspiration, the pressure within the upper airway is subatmospheric; thus, there is a tendency for the upper airway to collapse under the influence of the surrounding atmospheric pressure. However, in the normal subject, this tendency for airway collapse is opposed by upper airway dilator muscle tone. These muscles increase the diameter and reduce the compliance of the upper airway. An increase in upper airway dilator muscle tone occurs during inspiration, commencing just prior to diaphragmatic contraction.[69] The coordinated activation of the diaphragmatic and upper airway respiratory muscles is critical in maintaining airway patency. However, upper airway dilator muscle control appears to be extremely sensitive to sedative–hypnotic drug administration. For example, sedative doses of benzodiazepines have been reported to increase inspiratory subglottic airway resistance by three- to four-fold[70] and to selectively suppress genioglossal muscle activity to a greater degree than diaphragmatic activity; furthermore, this effect is exaggerated in elderly patients. The response to this obstruction is a significant increase in intercostal and accessory muscle activity. However, this response is only partially effective because the increase in inspiratory force will further decrease intraluminal upper airway pressure, thus predisposing to further airway collapse. It is likely that these effects will be of greatest significance in patients with pre-existing respiratory compromise, such as elderly patients or those with chronic obstructive pulmonary disease. These patients often have limited respiratory reserve and are unable to increase their respiratory muscle activity in response to the increased work of breathing induced by sedation and may become hypercarbic, acidotic, and hypoxemic. Not surprisingly, the ASA Closed Claims Database Study showed that MAC-related adverse respiratory outcomes were overrepresented in the elderly and ASA physical status class III and IV populations.

Clinical experience would lead most anesthesiologists to predict that the administration of sedative–hypnotic drugs is associated with the depression of respiratory drive. However, the findings of scientific studies in this area are often conflicting and confusing. On occasion, they show minimal effects of sedative drugs, if any,[71] on ventilatory responsiveness. However, it is important to note that in many cases, the methods used to measure respiratory drive may affect the outcome of the study by stimulating the subject, thus attenuating the negative effect of the drug on respiratory drive. In clinical practice, it is likely that during regional anesthesia, there is a degree of deafferentation that will potentiate the respiratory depressant effects of sedative–hypnotic drugs.[72] Opioids have been demonstrated to depress the ventilatory response to hypercapnia and hypoxemia. Reports of the effects of sedative doses of benzodiazepines on carbon dioxide responsiveness have shown variable results, including no significant effect[73] and clinically significant depression.[74] However, when opioids and benzodiazepines are used in combination, there appears to be a consistent and marked negative effect on respiratory responsiveness. Although the addition of sedative doses of propofol to opioids showed little potentiation of the respiratory effects of opioids, caution is still warranted when combinations of sedative–hypnotics are used.

Aspiration

Competent laryngeal and upper airway reflexes are required to protect the lower airway from aspiration. However, protective laryngeal and pharyngeal reflexes are depressed by anesthesia and sedation. It is also well documented that protective airway reflexes are compromised by advanced age and debilitation. Therefore, it is likely that significant further impairment of airway reflexes occurs during sedation in the elderly or debilitated patient. Aspiration of gastric contents can potentially occur any time during the perioperative period, particularly if oral intake is allowed before the return of adequate upper airway protective reflexes. The time required for the return of protective reflexes varies considerably. For example, complete recovery of the swallowing reflex occurs approximately 15 minutes after the return of consciousness following propofol anesthesia.[75] However, the swallowing reflex is significantly depressed for up to 2 hours following the administration of midazolam, despite the return of normal consciousness.[76]

As protective airway reflexes alone cannot reliably prevent aspiration during monitored anesthesia care, patients who are deemed high risk of such complication should be maintained at the lightest level of sedation possible. Ideally, the patient should be awake enough to recognize the regurgitation of gastric contents and be able to protect their own airway. If the ability of the patient to protect their own airway cannot be reliably guaranteed and regurgitation/aspiration is thought to be a significant risk, placement of a cuffed ETT under general anesthesia should be seriously considered. Propofol has a particularly potent suppressive effect on upper airway protective reflexes.[77] This property of propofol is exploited by anesthesiologists in our daily clinical practice: it is used to facilitate LMA insertion, to prevent and treat laryngospasm, and to facilitate endotracheal intubation without the use of muscle relaxants. However, the obvious downside to propofol-induced protective reflex suppression is that propofol-based techniques with an unprotected airway might be associated with a greater likelihood of aspiration. There is some evidence to support this supposition. A large Medicare database–based study (>100,000 patients) retrospectively examined whether receiving anesthesia for screening colonoscopy was associated with an increase in complications, including aspiration pneumonia, requiring hospitalization within 30 days of colonoscopy.[78] Aspiration occurred more frequently in those patients receiving anesthesia services versus those who did not (0.14% vs. 0.1%).

Laryngospasm

Although protective laryngeal and pharyngeal reflexes are usually depressed by sedation, laryngospasm presents when the same reflexes become hyperstimulated. It typically occurs when stimulation of the laryngeal mucosa superior to the vocal cords (e.g., secretions), excites the vagus nerve via the internal branch of the superior laryngeal nerve (SLN). The motor response triggers contraction of the lateral cricoarytenoid (adduction and medial rotation of arytenoid cartilage) and thyroarytenoid muscles (shortening of vocal cords leading to glottic closure) via the recurrent laryngeal nerve, and the cricothyroid muscle (tensing of vocal cords) via the external branch of the SLN. Interestingly, splanchnic nerve stimulation has also been implicated in triggering vocal cord closure.[79] Repetitive suprathreshold stimulation of the SLN can result in heavy after-discharge activity which can result in the adductor motor output causing true laryngeal spasm, which in turn can result in vocal cord closure persisting beyond the cessation of the stimulus, potentially leading to hypoxemia, negative-pressure pulmonary edema, and subsequent cardiac arrest.[80] It is important to note that closure can occur at the true vocal cords, aryepiglottic folds, and vestibular folds.

Laryngospasm is a complication that can occur during any level of sedation. It can result in severe hypoxic injury or death in healthy patients if not recognized and dealt with promptly. Incidence of laryngospasm among 136,929 patients was 0.79% of all anesthetics performed.[81] Laryngospasm occurred more commonly in patients with pre-existing reactive airway disease or upper respiratory symptoms and was more common among younger patients than older patients.

Although the use of positive pressure ventilation (PPV) to "break" laryngospasm has been suggested in the past, its use should not be relied upon to treat laryngospasm in all cases. While PPV may be able to provide some ventilation if there is some patency of the true vocal cords, aryepiglottic folds, or vestibular folds, a complete closure of the true vocal cords can resist pressures of up to 140 mmHg.[82] Attempting to "break" a complete closure of the true vocal cords with PPV would be futile, though one would have successfully ventilated the stomach. The perceived success of PPV may rather be due to either coincidence that the laryngospasm self-resolved, or sufficient hypoxia or hypercarbia developed to depress the laryngospasm, or that the respiratory distress was not due to laryngospasm in the first place. Hypercarbia depresses adductor activity and severe hypoxemia (PaO_2 <50 mmHg) inhibits laryngospasm activity.[83] It is also possible that the true vocal cords may not be completely spasmed and instead there is a constriction of the false cords, in which case, the pressure to overcome has not been extensively studied. In either situation, aggressive PPV can increase the risk of aspiration, cranially displace the diaphragm due to gastric distention from PPV gases, and subsequently decrease the patient's functional residual capacity. The use of Larson's maneuver to terminate laryngospasm has been described in a 1998 correspondence.[84] A vigorous jaw thrust is applied by placing pressure to the area between the angle of the mandible, mastoid process, and the base of the skull, and can help relieve obstruction caused by collapse of upper airway tissues. However, this technique has only been described with anecdotal experience and the physiology supporting the termination of laryngospasm has not been definitively established. The thought behind the use of propofol or use of other agents to deepen sedation is that it depress laryngeal reflexes which will then hopefully "break" the laryngospasm. However, hope should not be relied upon as a definitive treatment. Rather, the use of succinylcholine or other nondepolarizing muscle relaxants to paralyze the muscles causing laryngospasm should be utilized early before permanent harm comes to the patient.

Cardiovascular Complications

The administration of different anesthetics can cause different hemodynamic changes and vasoactive medications should be readily at hand. Factors such as decreased effective arterial volume from NPO status, vagal cardiac reflexes (e.g., oculocardiac reflex, trigeminovagal reflex) seen in certain procedures, inadequate pain control or depth of sedation, anxiety, and fluid overload can all cause blood pressure derangements and arrhythmias. The control of certain factors such as pain and sedation are made more difficult due to potential respiratory depression in patients who do not have a protected airway during monitored anesthesia care. Risks of myocardial infarction are elevated during any procedure where hemodynamics can be altered, and vigilance is required to recognize changes in ECG pattern as well as a patient's report of angina. Cardiac arrest can always occur and one must be proficient with the Advanced Cardiac Life Support (ACLS) algorithm for resuscitation when needed. With all of the above-stated risks, vasoactive and emergency medications should be readily at hand for administration at a moment's notice.

Preparedness to Recognize and Treat Local Anesthetic Systemic Toxicity

Monitored anesthesia care is often provided in the context of regional or local anesthetic techniques. It is vitally important that the anesthesiologist responsible for the patient has a high index of suspicion and be fully prepared to recognize and treat local anesthetic systemic toxicity (LAST) immediately (see Chapter 22). This point deserves special emphasis, particularly in view of the fact that monitored anesthesia care is often provided to elderly or debilitated patients who have been deemed "unfit" for general anesthesia; these are the patients most likely to suffer adverse reactions to local anesthetic drugs. Even if the anesthesiologist caring for the patient in the OR does not perform the block personally, they are in a unique position to fulfill an important "preventive" role by advising the surgeon about the most appropriate volume, concentration, and type of local anesthetic drug or technique to be used.

LAST occurs when plasma concentrations of local anesthetic drug reach toxic levels. Plasma concentrations will increase when the rate of entry of drug into the circulation exceeds the rate of drug clearance from the circulation. The clinically recognizable effects of local anesthetics on the central nervous system are concentration dependent. At low concentrations, sedation and numbness of the tongue and circumoral tissues and a metallic taste are prominent features. As concentrations increase, restlessness, vertigo, tinnitus, and difficulty focusing may occur. Higher concentrations result in slurred speech and skeletal muscle twitching, which often herald the onset of tonic–clonic seizures.

The conduct of monitored anesthesia care may modify the individual's response to the potentially toxic effects of local anesthetic administration and adversely affect the margin of safety of a regional or local technique. For example, a patient with compromised cardiovascular function may experience a further decline in cardiac output during sedation. The resultant reduction in hepatic blood flow will reduce the clearance of local anesthetics that are metabolized by the liver and have a high hepatic extraction ratio, thereby increasing the likelihood of achieving toxic plasma concentrations. A patient receiving sedation may experience respiratory depression and a subsequent increase in $PaCO_2$. Hypercarbia adversely affects the margin of safety in several ways. By increasing cerebral blood flow, hypercarbia will increase the amount of local anesthetic that is delivered to the brain, thereby increasing the potential for neurotoxicity. By reducing neuronal axoplasmic pH, hypercarbia increases the intracellular concentration of the charged, active form of local anesthetic, thus also increasing its toxicity. In addition, hypercarbia, acidosis, and hypoxemia, all markedly potentiate the cardiovascular toxicity of local anesthetics. Furthermore, the administration of sedative–hypnotic drugs may interfere with the patient's ability to communicate the symptoms of impending neurotoxicity. However, the anticonvulsant properties of benzodiazepines may attenuate the seizures associated with neurotoxicity. In both of these circumstances, it is possible that the symptoms of cardiotoxicity will be the first evidence that an adverse reaction is occurring. Thus, appropriate treatment is delayed, or inadvertent intravascular injection is continued because of the absence of any clinical evidence of toxicity. Cardiovascular toxicity usually occurs at a higher plasma concentration than neurotoxicity, but when it does occur, it is usually much more difficult to manage than neurotoxicity. Although cardiotoxicity is usually preceded by neurotoxicity, it may on occasion be the initial presenting feature.

Closed Claims with Monitored Anesthesia Care

From the 1980s to the early 2020s, the proportion of closed claims associated with MAC has steadily increased.[85] In a 2006 study by Bhananker et al.,[5] the most common damaging respiratory event in MAC cases was inadequate oxygenation or ventilation. Death was the most common outcome associated with oversedation in MAC cases. Approximately half of the cases associated with sedation were judged to be preventable by better monitoring. A number of reasons can be attributed to adverse outcomes including distractions such as loud music, improperly functioning monitors, poor attention to monitor alarms, and delay in resuscitation due to patient positioning. MAC comprised the majority of non-OR anesthesia (NORA) claims.[86] Adverse respiratory events in NORA claims were twice that of OR claims.[86] Other adverse events included aspiration, burns, difficult or esophageal intubation, and medication errors.[85] NORA locations can present certain challenges such as unfamiliarity with room setup and equipment, inadequate lighting, lack of readily accessible resources or personnel, and room layouts which impede access to patients.[87] These are not excusable reasons for adverse events. Rather, the provider must optimize their working environment, have contingency plans, and provide constant vigilant monitoring to ensure patient safety. It is essential to remember that monitored anesthesia care is an anesthetic delivered to a patient with an unsecured airway experiencing dynamic changes in sedation and, subsequently, ventilation. Please see Chapter 33 for more detailed discussion of NORA.

Sedation and Analgesia by Nonanesthesiologists

Although anesthesiologists have specific training and expertise to provide sedation and analgesia, in clinical practice, minimal and moderate sedation services are frequently provided by nonanesthesiologists. Deep sedation is occasionally delivered by trained specialists, including emergency department physicians and intensivists. The specific reasons for nonanesthesiologist involvement differ from institution to institution and from case to case and include convenience, availability, and scheduling issues; perceived lack of anesthesiologist availability; perceived increased cost; and a perceived lack of benefit concerning patient satisfaction and safety when sedation and analgesia are provided by anesthesiologists. Despite our frequent noninvolvement in these cases, anesthesiologists are indirectly involved in the care of these patients by being required to participate in the development of institutional policies and procedures for sedation and analgesia, as mandated by TJC. To assist anesthesiologists in this process, an ASA task force developed practice guidelines for sedation and analgesia by nonanesthesiologists (see Table 30-1).[88,89]

As discussed previously, four levels of sedation are defined in the ASA practice guidelines on the continuum of depth of sedation and include minimal sedation, moderate sedation, deep sedation, and general anesthesia.[13] The guidelines emphasize that sedation and analgesia represent a continuum of sedation wherein patients can easily pass into a level of sedation deeper than intended. The statement contains a chart representing the clinical progression along this continuum (Table 30-2). When monitoring a sedated patient during a procedure, it is important to recognize when a patient becomes more deeply sedated than intended so that the care team can act appropriately to prevent cardiorespiratory compromise.

The sedation guidelines emphasize the importance of preprocedure patient evaluation, patient preparation, and appropriate fasting periods. The importance of continuous patient monitoring is discussed—in particular, the response of the patient to commands as a guide to the level of sedation. The appropriate monitoring of ventilation, oxygenation, and hemodynamics is also discussed, and recommendations are made for the contemporaneous recording of these parameters. The task force strongly recommends that an individual other than the person performing the therapeutic or diagnostic procedure be available to monitor the patient's comfort and physiologic status when administering moderate sedation. For deep sedation, the ASA requires an independent provider, different from the individual performing the procedure, dedicated to the administration of sedation and monitoring of the patient. Education and training of providers is recommended. Specific educational objectives include the potentiation of sedative-induced respiratory depression by concomitantly administered opioids, adequate time intervals between doses of sedative/analgesics to avoid cumulative overdosage, and familiarity with sedative/analgesic antagonists. At least one person with Basic Life Support training should be available during moderate sedation, with immediate availability (1 to 5 minutes) of personnel trained in ACLS. For procedures requiring deep sedation, the ASA recommends ACLS-trained personnel be present in the procedure room. This individual should have the ability to recognize airway obstruction, establish an airway, and maintain oxygenation and ventilation. The practice guidelines recommend that appropriate patient-sized emergency equipment be readily available, specifically including equipment for establishing an airway and delivering PPV with supplemental oxygen, emergency resuscitation drugs, and a working defibrillator. The presence of reliable IV access until the patient is no longer at risk for cardiorespiratory depression will improve safety. Adequate postprocedure recovery care with appropriate monitoring must be provided until discharge. Certain high-risk patient groups (e.g., uncooperative patients, extremes of age, severe cardiac, pulmonary, hepatic, renal, or central nervous system disease, morbid obesity, sleep apnea, pregnancy, and patients with alcohol or drug use disorders) will be encountered, and the guidelines recommend that preprocedure consultation with anesthesiologists, cardiologists, pulmonologists, and other specialists appropriate to the patient's comorbidities be performed *before* administration of sedation and analgesia by nonanesthesiologists.

The ASA released a statement in October 2005, amended in 2021, suggesting a framework for granting privileges that will help ensure competence of individuals who administer or supervise the administration of moderate sedation.[88] This statement suggests that the practitioner should complete formal training in (1) the safe administration of sedative and analgesic drugs used to establish a level of moderate sedation, and (2) rescue of patients who exhibit adverse physiologic consequences of a deeper-than-intended level of sedation. The ASA released an amended advisory in October 2017 on granting privileges for deep sedation to nonanesthesiologist sedation practitioners.[89] For procedures requiring deep sedation, the ASA statement limits administration to qualified nonanesthesiologist professionals trained to recognize and rescue patients from general anesthesia. The Centers for Medicare and Medicaid Services (CMS) define these professionals as physician anesthesiologists, nonanesthesiologist MD/DO, dentist, oral surgeon, CRNA, and CAA. Nonanesthesiologist physicians may not administer deep sedation without additional training and qualifications to recognize and rescue patients from general anesthesia. Requirements include, but are not limited to, the ability to perform a preoperative history and physical with airway assessment, understanding of the pharmacology of all potential medications (e.g., sedatives, analgesics, vasoactive drugs, antiarrhythmics) used, understanding of the risks and benefits of supplemental oxygen, recognition of ventilatory status, advanced airway management modalities including laryngoscopy and endotracheal intubation, ability to recognize depth of sedation and rescue patients if necessary, ACLS qualifications, and performance evaluation by the Director of Anesthesia Services prior to approval for administering deep sedation.

The CMS published revised hospital anesthesia services interpretive guidelines requiring hospitals to establish policies and procedures that address whether specific clinical situations involve "anesthesia" *versus* "analgesia" services. The CMS document places general anesthesia, monitored anesthesia care, deep sedation, and regional anesthesia under "anesthesia" services. These "anesthesia" services must be provided by a qualified anesthesiologist; a doctor of medicine or osteopathy, a dentist, oral surgeon, or podiatrist who is qualified to administer anesthesia under state law; an appropriately supervised CRNA or CAA, all who are separate from the practitioner performing the procedure. Moderate sedation and minimal sedation fall under "analgesia" services.[90] The statement released by the ASA on the safe use of propofol, most recently amended in 2019, is explicit that the drug should be administered only by "persons trained in the administration of general anesthesia, who are not simultaneously involved in these surgical or diagnostic procedures.... Failure to follow these recommendations could put patients at increased risk of significant injury or death."[91] In addition, even if moderate sedation is intended, the administration of propofol, ketamine, and etomidate is restricted to providers qualified to administer deep sedation and general anesthesia.[2]

Future Directions

Although the professional cost of anesthesia services is only a small fraction (3%) of the total physician services, the recent increase in spending on monitored anesthesia care is significant. Given the cost associated with anesthesiologist-administered sedation, and the increasing demand for large numbers of patients to receive sedation for procedures, it is not surprising that alternatives to anesthesiologist-administered sedation might be considered attractive.

Patient-Controlled Sedation and Analgesia

Techniques that allow the direct patient control of the level of sedation may positively affect patient satisfaction.[92] The degree of sedation desired by the patient varies significantly and the individual response to drugs is variable. Patient-controlled sedation appears to be an attractive solution to this problem. One approach to patient-controlled sedation has been to use a conventional patient-controlled analgesia (PCA) delivery system set to deliver 0.7-mg/kg boluses of propofol with a 3-minute lockout period.[92] Other approaches include fixed-dose combinations of 0.5-mg midazolam and 25-µg fentanyl with a 5-minute lockout interval between doses.[93] The pharmacokinetic profile of alfentanil is ideal for the treatment of short, discrete episodes of pain. These properties have been exploited during vaginal ovum retrieval procedures, when ultrasonically guided needles are passed through the vaginal wall under monitored anesthesia care. To this end, Zelcer et al.[94] used a PCA delivery system to allow self-administration of alfentanil during this procedure. After midazolam premedication and a loading dose of alfentanil, patients received 5-µg/kg boluses of alfentanil via the PCA pump with a mandatory 3-minute lockout period. Patient acceptability, alfentanil dosage, respiratory variables, and pain scores were similar to those obtained with physician-controlled analgesia. From the limited data that are available, intraoperative PCA during monitored anesthesia care appears to be an effective alternative to physician-administered analgesia.

Target-Controlled Infusions

Target-controlled infusions (TCI) are computers programmed with pharmacokinetic parameters with multicompartmental models and relevant patient characteristics (e.g., height, weight, age) to deliver a desired target concentration of a drug. One of the most widely approved TCI systems is the delivery of propofol with the Diprifusor TCI system.[95] This system has been approved in Europe and many other countries. However, since pharmacokinetics can vary depending on patient characteristics and comorbidities, the FDA did not approve this system for use in the United States without further developments. Since then, more open TCI systems have been developed utilizing generic propofol and different drugs, including models for remifentanil, sufentanil, and alfentanil.[95] To date, no TCI system has been approved for use in the United States.

Closed Loop Anesthesia Delivery Systems

Closed loop anesthesia delivery describes a technique in which an input variable (e.g., blood pressure, heart rate, BIS) is used to control the output (e.g., rate of drug administration).[96] Efforts have been made to develop different types of delivery systems including single-input single-output (SISO), multiple-input single-output (MISO), and multiple-input multiple-output (MIMO) closed loop systems. Systems tying propofol to BIS targets have been explored.[97] The use of closed-loop propofol delivery systems has also been demonstrated in conjunction with dexmedetomidine running at a static rate during maintenance.[98] Utilizing BIS as the controlled variable, the systems delivered less total propofol to the dexmedetomidine group as opposed to the nondexmedetomidine group. Though the use of closed-loop systems may be enticing to free the anesthesiologist to focus on acute changes in hemodynamic status or operative conditions, the application of these systems is still limited. Heart rate and blood pressure are influenced by much more than pain, and the system may be blind to measuring errors (e.g., electrocautery interaction with ECG, surgeon leaning on blood pressure cuff), or complex hemodynamic goals in certain pathologies (e.g., pulmonary hypertension, severe aortic stenosis, severe carotid stenosis). In addition, the assessment of hypnotic depth rests on the assumption that the BIS monitor is an accurate measure of sedation. As mentioned earlier, the literature supporting the BIS monitor as an accurate measure of sedation does not yet meet the criteria that Drummond[21] proposed. However, the potentials of the application of these delivery systems with the implementation of machine learning and artificial intelligence (AI) is vast. It is now possible for hypotensive events to be predicted by arterial waveform analysis based on machine learning.[99] With the immense data sets that can be gathered from electronic medical records and intraoperative data, machine learning may be able to eventually offer sophisticated analyses of multiple variables to modulate sedation, analgesia, paralytics, and hemodynamic control. The application of these systems can be used for all anesthetic management including regional, monitored anesthesia care, and general anesthesia. Oftentimes, the work of an anesthesiologist draws parallels with airline pilots. AI-controlled closed loop systems may eventually serve as an autopilot function with the anesthesiologist still at the helm.[100]

Conclusion

Through the use of monitored anesthesia care, an often terrifying and painful procedure can be made safe and comfortable for the patient. Monitored anesthesia care presents an opportunity for our patients to observe us at work. For the anesthesiologist, monitored anesthesia care presents an opportunity to provide a more prolonged and intimate level of care and reassurance to our patients that is in contrast to the more limited exposure that occurs during and after general anesthesia. Our airway management skills and our daily practice of applied pharmacology make us uniquely qualified to provide this service. Monitored anesthesia care presents us with an opportunity to display these skills and increase our recognition in areas outside the OR. The availability of drugs with a more favorable pharmacologic profile allows us to tailor our techniques to provide the specific components of analgesia, sedation, anxiolysis, and amnesia with minimal morbidity and to facilitate a prompt recovery. As the population ages, increasing numbers of patients will become candidates for monitored anesthesia care. Significant advances in nonsurgical fields (e.g., interventional radiology) will increase the number of procedures that are ideally performed under monitored anesthesia care. It is our responsibility to clearly demonstrate to our non-anesthesia colleagues that anesthesiologist-provided monitored anesthesia care contributes to the best outcome for our patients. If anesthesiologists are not willing or able to provide these services, others, who are less qualified, are prepared to assume that role.

Acknowledgments

We gratefully acknowledge the contributions of previous edition authors, Melissa M. Masaracchia, Kylene E. Halloran, Aaron J. Mancuso, and Simon C. Hillier, as portions of their chapter have been retained in this revision.

For further review and interactivities, please see the videos and narrative interactive clinical vignettes (NICVs) accessible in the complimentary eBook bundled with this text. Access instructions are located on the inside front cover.

REFERENCES

1. American Society of Anesthesiologists. Distinguishing Monitored Anesthesia Care ("MAC") from moderate sedation/analgesia. Updated October 2018. Accessed October 1, 2022. www.asahq.org
2. American Society of Anesthesiologists. Practice guidelines for moderate procedural sedation and analgesia. Updated March 2018. Accessed October 2, 2022. www.asahq.org

3. American Society of Anesthesiologists. Position on monitored anesthesia care. Updated October 2018. Accessed October 2, 2022. www.asahq.org
4. Hinkelbein J, Lamperti M, Akeson J, et al. European Society of Anaesthesiology and European Board of Anaesthesiology guidelines for procedural sedation and analgesia in adults. *Eur J Anaesthesiol*. 2018;35(1):6–24.
5. Bhananker SM, Posner KL, Cheney FW, Caplan RA, Lee LA, Domino KB. Injury and liability associated with monitored anesthesia care: a closed claims analysis. *Anesthesiology*. 2006;104(2):228–234.
6. Kim S, Chang BA, Rahman A, et al. Analysis of urgent/emergent conversions from monitored anesthesia care to general anesthesia with airway instrumentation. *BMC Anesthesiol*. 2021;21(1):183.
7. American Society of Anesthesiologists. Standards for basic anesthetic monitoring. Updated December 2020. Accessed October 2, 2022. www.asahq.org
8. Caplan RA, Ward RJ, Posner K, Cheney FW. Unexpected cardiac arrest during spinal anesthesia: a closed claims analysis of predisposing factors. *Anesthesiology*. 1988;68(1):5–11.
9. Waugh JB, Epps CA, Khodneva YA. Capnography enhances surveillance of respiratory events during procedural sedation: a meta-analysis. *J Clin Anesth*. 2011;23(3):189–196.
10. Soto RG, Fu ES, Vila H Jr, Miguel RV. Capnography accurately detects apnea during monitored anesthesia care. *Anesth Analg*. 2004;99(2):379–382.
11. Vargo JJ, Zuccaro G Jr, Dumot JA, Conwell DL, Morrow JB, Shay SS. Automated graphic assessment of respiratory activity is superior to pulse oximetry and visual assessment for the detection of early respiratory depression during therapeutic upper endoscopy. *Gastrointest Endosc*. 2002;55(7):826–831.
12. Metzner J, Posner KL, Domino KB. The risk and safety of anesthesia at remote locations: the US closed claims analysis. *Curr Opin Anaesthesiol*. 2009;22(4):502–508.
13. American Society of Anesthesiologists. Continuum of depth of sedation: definition of general anesthesia and levels of sedation/analgesia. Updated October 2019. Accessed October 2, 2022. www.asahq.org
14. Ramsay MA, Savege TM, Simpson BR, Goodwin R. Controlled sedation with alphaxalone-alphadolone. *Br Med J*. 1974;2(5920):656–659.
15. Gill M, Green SM, Krauss B. A study of the bispectral index monitor during procedural sedation and analgesia in the emergency department. *Ann Emerg Med*. 2003;41(2):234–241.
16. Sessler CN, Gosnell MS, Grap MJ, et al. The Richmond Agitation-Sedation Scale: validity and reliability in adult intensive care unit patients. *Am J Respir Crit Care Med*. 2002;166(10): 1338–1344.
17. Chernik DA, Gillings D, Laine H, et al. Validity and reliability of the observer's assessment of alertness/sedation scale: study with intravenous midazolam. *J Clin Psychopharmacol*. 1990;10(4):244–251.
18. Liu J, Singh H, White PF. Electroencephalographic bispectral index correlates with intraoperative recall and depth of propofol-induced sedation. *Anesth Analg*. 1997;84(1):185–189.
19. Kearse LA Jr, Manberg P, Chamoun N, deBros F, Zaslavsky A. Bispectral analysis of the electroencephalogram correlates with patient movement to skin incision during propofol/nitrous oxide anesthesia. *Anesthesiology*. 1994;81(6):1365–1370.
20. Ibrahim AE, Taraday JK, Kharasch ED. Bispectral index monitoring during sedation with sevoflurane, midazolam, and propofol. *Anesthesiology*. 2001;95(5):1151–1159.
21. Drummond JC. Monitoring depth of anesthesia: with emphasis on the application of the bispectral index and the middle latency auditory evoked response to the prevention of recall. *Anesthesiology*. 2000;93(3):876–882.
22. Deitch K, Chudnofsky CR, Dominici P. The utility of supplemental oxygen during emergency department procedural sedation and analgesia with midazolam and fentanyl: a randomized, controlled trial. *Ann Emerg Med*. 2007;49(1):1–8.
23. Deitch K, Chudnofsky CR, Dominici P. The utility of supplemental oxygen during emergency department procedural sedation with propofol: a randomized, controlled trial. *Ann Emerg Med*. 2008;52(1):1–8.
24. Shapiro BA, Peruzzi WT, Kozelowski-Templin R. *Clinical Application of Blood Gases*. 5th ed. Mosby-Year Book; 1994.
25. Markovitz GH, Colthurst J, Storer TW, Cooper CB. Effective inspired oxygen concentration measured via transtracheal and oral gas analysis. *Respir Care*. 2010;55(4):453–459.
26. Lampotang S, Gravenstein N, Paulus DA, Gravenstein D. Supplying sub-100% oxygen gas mixtures during monitored anesthesia care: respiratory monitoring and use of a venturi device. *Anesth Analg*. 2005;101(5):1407–1412.
27. Miner JR, Huber D, Nichols S, Biros M. The effect of the assignment of a pre-sedation target level on procedural sedation using propofol. *J Emerg Med*. 2007;32(3):249–255.
28. Hughes MA, Glass PS, Jacobs JR. Context-sensitive half-time in multicompartment pharmacokinetic models for intravenous anesthetic drugs. *Anesthesiology*. 1992;76(3):334–341.
29. Shafer Steven L, Varvel JR. Pharmacokinetics, pharmacodynamics, and rational opioid selection. *Anesthesiology*. 1991;74(1):53–63.
30. Scott JC, Ponganis KV, Stanski DR. EEG quantitation of narcotic effect: the comparative pharmacodynamics of fentanyl and alfentanil. *Anesthesiology*. 1985;62(3):234–241.
31. Mandema JW, Sansom LN, Dios-Vièitez MC, Hollander-Jansen M, Danhof M. Pharmacokinetic-pharmacodynamic modeling of the electroencephalographic effects of benzodiazepines. Correlation with receptor binding and anticonvulsant activity. *J Pharmacol Exp Ther*. 1991; 257(1):472–478.
32. Kazama T, Ikeda K, Morita K. The pharmacodynamic interaction between propofol and fentanyl with respect to the suppression of somatic or hemodynamic responses to skin incision, peritoneum incision, and abdominal wall retraction. *Anesthesiology*. 1998;89(4): 894–906.
33. Short TG, Plummer JL, Chui PT. Hypnotic and anaesthetic interactions between midazolam, propofol and alfentanil. *Br J Anaesth*. 1992;69(2):162–167.
34. Vinik HR, Bradley EL Jr, Kissin I. Midazolam-alfentanil synergism for anesthetic induction in patients. *Anesth Analg*. 1989;69(2):213–217.
35. Bailey PL, Pace NL, Ashburn MA, Moll JW, East KA, Stanley TH. Frequent hypoxemia and apnea after sedation with midazolam and fentanyl. *Anesthesiology*. 1990;73(5):826–830.
36. Smith I, Monk TG, White PF, Ding Y. Propofol infusion during regional anesthesia: sedative, amnestic, and anxiolytic properties. *Anesth Analg*. 1994;79(2):313–319.
37. White PF, Negus JB. Sedative infusions during local and regional anesthesia: a comparison of midazolam and propofol. *J Clin Anesth*. 1991;3(1):32–39.
38. Borgeat A, Wilder-Smith OH, Saiah M, Rifat K. Subhypnotic doses of propofol possess direct antiemetic properties. *Anesth Analg*. 1992;74(4):539–541.
39. Jalota L, Kalira V, George E, et al; Perioperative Clinical Research Core. Prevention of pain on injection of propofol: systematic review and meta-analysis. *BMJ*. 2011;342:d1110.
40. Pratila MG, Fischer ME, Alagesan R, Alagesan R, Reinsel RA, Pratilas D. Propofol versus midazolam for monitored sedation: a comparison of intraoperative and recovery parameters. *J Clin Anesth*. 1993;5(4):268–274.
41. Jacobs JR, Reves JG, Marty J, White WD, Bai SA, Smith LR. Aging increases pharmacodynamic sensitivity to the hypnotic effects of midazolam. *Anesth Analg*. 1995;80(1): 143–148.
42. Ghouri AF, Ruiz MA, White PF. Effect of flumazenil on recovery after midazolam and propofol sedation. *Anesthesiology*. 1994;81(2):333–339.
43. Antonik LJ, Goldwater DR, Kilpatrick GJ, Tilbrook GS, Borkett KM. A placebo- and midazolam-controlled phase I single ascending-dose study evaluating the safety, pharmacokinetics, and pharmacodynamics of remimazolam (CNS 7056): part I. Safety, efficacy, and basic pharmacokinetics. *Anesth Analg*. 2012;115(2):274–283.
44. Schüttler J, Eisenried A, Lerch M, Fechner J, Jeleazcov C, Ihmsen H. Pharmacokinetics and pharmacodynamics of remimazolam (CNS 7056) after continuous infusion in healthy male volunteers: part I. Pharmacokinetics and clinical pharmacodynamics. *Anesthesiology*. 2020;132(4):636–651.
45. Veselis RA, Reinsel RA, Feshchenko VA, et al. Impaired memory and behavioral performance with fentanyl at low plasma concentrations. *Anesth Analg*. 1994;79(5):952–960.
46. Aydin ON, Ugur B, Kir E, Ozkan SB. Effect of single-dose fentanyl on the cardiorespiratory system in elderly patients undergoing cataract surgery. *J Clin Anesth*. 2004;16(2):98–103.
47. Akcaboy ZN, Akcaboy EY, Albayrak D, Altinoren B, Dikmen B, Gogus N. Can remifentanil be a better choice than propofol for colonoscopy during monitored anesthesia care? *Acta Anaesthesiol Scand*. 2006;50(6):736–741.
48. Kapila A, Glass PS, Jacobs JR, et al. Measured context-sensitive half-times of remifentanil and alfentanil. *Anesthesiology*. 1995;83(5):968–975.
49. Servin F, Desmonts JM, Watkins WD. Remifentanil as an analgesic adjunct in local/regional anesthesia and in monitored anesthesia care. *Anesth Analg*. 1999;89(4S):28.
50. Avramov MN, Smith I, White PF. Interactions between midazolam and remifentanil during monitored anesthesia care. *Anesthesiology*. 1996;85(6):1283–1289.
51. Sá Rêgo MM, Inagaki Y, White PF. Remifentanil administration during monitored anesthesia care: are intermittent boluses an effective alternative to a continuous infusion? *Anesth Analg*. 1999;88(3):518–522.
52. Green SM. Research advances in procedural sedation and analgesia. *Ann Emerg Med*. 2007;49(1):31–36.
53. Sherwin TS, Green SM, Khan A, Chapman DS, Dannenberg B. Does adjunctive midazolam reduce recovery agitation after ketamine sedation for pediatric procedures? A randomized, double-blind, placebo-controlled trial. *Ann Emerg Med*. 2000;35(3):229–238.
54. Badrinath S, Avramov MN, Shadrick M, Witt TR, Ivankovich AD. The use of a ketamine-propofol combination during monitored anesthesia care. *Anesth Analg*. 2000;90(4):858–862.
55. Ferguson I, Bell A, Treston G, New L, Ding M, Holdgate A. Propofol or ketofol for procedural sedation and analgesia in emergency medicine-the POKER study: a randomized double-blind clinical trial. *Ann Emerg Med*. 2016;68(5):574–582.e1.
56. Andolfatto G, Abu-Laban RB, Zed PJ, et al. Ketamine-propofol combination (ketofol) versus propofol alone for emergency department procedural sedation and analgesia: a randomized double-blind trial. *Ann Emerg Med*. 2012;59(6):504–512.e1–2.
57. Yan JW, McLeod SL, Iansavitchene A. Ketamine-propofol versus propofol alone for procedural sedation in the emergency department: a systematic review and meta-analysis. *Acad Emerg Med*. 2015;22(9):1003–1013.
58. Jalili M, Bahreini M, Doosti-Irani A, Masoomi R, Arbab M, Mirfazaelian H. Ketamine-propofol combination (ketofol) vs propofol for procedural sedation and analgesia: systematic review and meta-analysis. *Am J Emerg Med*. 2016;34(3):558–569.

59. Foo TY, Mohd Noor N, Yazid MB, Fauzi MH, Abdull Wahab SF, Ahmad MZ. Ketamine-propofol (ketofol) for procedural sedation and analgesia in children: a systematic review and meta-analysis. *BMC Emerg Med*. 2020;20(1):81.
60. Ebert TJ, Hall JE, Barney JA, Uhrich TD, Colinco MD. The effects of increasing plasma concentrations of dexmedetomidine in humans. *Anesthesiology*. 2000;93(2):382–394.
61. Mishima G, Sanuki T, Sato S, Kobayashi M, Kurata S, Ayuse T. Upper-airway collapsibility and compensatory responses under moderate sedation with ketamine, dexmedetomidine, and propofol in healthy volunteers. *Physiol Rep*. 2020;8(10):e14439.
62. Lodenius Å, Maddison KJ, Lawther BK, et al. Upper airway collapsibility during dexmedetomidine and propofol sedation in healthy volunteers: a nonblinded randomized crossover study. *Anesthesiology*. 2019;131(5):962–973.
63. Drummond JC, Dao AV, Roth DM, et al. Effect of dexmedetomidine on cerebral blood flow velocity, cerebral metabolic rate, and carbon dioxide response in normal humans. *Anesthesiology*. 2008;108(2):225–232.
64. Arain SR, Ebert TJ. The efficacy, side effects, and recovery characteristics of dexmedetomidine versus propofol when used for intraoperative sedation. *Anesth Analg*. 2002;95(2):461–466.
65. Talke P, Richardson CA, Scheinin M, Fisher DM. Postoperative pharmacokinetics and sympatholytic effects of dexmedetomidine. *Anesth Analg*. 1997;85(5):1136–1142.
66. Domino K. Trends in anesthesia litigation in the 1990's: monitored anesthesia care claims. *ASA Newsl*. 1997;61:15–17.
67. Hug CC Jr. MAC should stand for maximum anesthesia caution, not minimal anesthesiology care. *Anesthesiology*. 2006;104(2):221–223.
68. Morel DR, Forster A, Bachmann M, Suter PM. Effect of intravenous midazolam on breathing pattern and chest wall mechanics in human. *J Appl Physiol Respir Environ Exerc Physiol*. 1984;57(4):1104–1110.
69. Gottfried SB, Strohl KP, Van de Graaff W, Fouke JM, DiMarco AF. Effects of phrenic stimulation on upper airway resistance in anesthetized dogs. *J Appl Physiol Respir Environ Exerc Physiol*. 1983;55(2):419–426.
70. Montravers P, Dureuil B, Desmonts JM. Effects of i.v. midazolam on upper airway resistance. *Br J Anaesth*. 1992;68(1):27–31.
71. Weil JV, McCullough RE, Kline JS, Sodal IE. Diminished ventilatory response to hypoxia and hypercapnia after morphine in normal man. N Engl J Med. 1975;292(21):1103–1106.
72. Pattinson KTS. Opioids and the control of respiration. *Br J Anaesth*. 2008;100(6):747–758.
73. Power SJ, Morgan M, Chakrabarti MK. Carbon dioxide response curves following midazolam and diazepam. *Br J Anaesth*. 1983;55(9):837–841.
74. Alexander CM, Gross JB. Sedative doses of midazolam depress hypoxic ventilatory responses in humans. *Anesth Analg*. 1988;67(4):377–382.
75. Rimaniol JM, D'Honneur G, Duvaldestin P. Recovery of the swallowing reflex after propofol anesthesia. *Anesth Analg*. 1994;79(5):856–859.
76. Lambert Y, D'Honneur G, Abhay K, Gall O, Duvaldestin P. Depression of swallowing reflex two hours after midazolam. *Anesthesiology*. 1991;75(3):A891–A891.
77. Sundman E, Witt H, Sandin R, et al. Pharyngeal function and airway protection during subhypnotic concentrations of propofol, isoflurane, and sevoflurane: volunteers examined by pharyngeal videoradiography and simultaneous manometry. *Anesthesiology*. 2001;95(5):1125–1132.
78. Cooper GS, Kou TD, Rex DK. Complications following colonoscopy with anesthesia assistance: a population-based analysis. *JAMA Intern Med*. 2013;173(7):551–556.
79. Brewer N, Bryant DS. The role of the splanchnics in the adductor spasm of the vocal cords following visceral traction. *Anesth Analg*. 1935;14(4):190.
80. Sasaki CT, Suzuki M. Laryngeal spasm: a neurophysiologic redefinition. *Ann Otol Rhinol Laryngol*. 1977;86(2 pt. 1):150–157.
81. Olsson GL, Hallen B. Laryngospasm during anaesthesia. A computer-aided incidence study in 136,929 patients. *Acta Anaesthesiol Scand*. 1984;28(5):567–575.
82. Brunton TL, Cash T. The valvular action of the larynx. *J Anat Physiol*. 1883;17(Pt 3):363–378.
83. Ikari T, Sasaki CT. Glottic closure reflex: control mechanisms. *Ann Otol Rhinol Laryngol*. 1980;89(3 Pt 1):220–224.
84. Larson CP Jr. Laryngospasm–the best treatment. *Anesthesiology*. 1998;89(5):1293–1294.
85. Metzner J, Posner KL, Lam MS, Domino KB. Closed claims' analysis. *Best Pract Res Clin Anaesthesiol*. 2011;25(2):263–276.
86. Woodward ZG, Urman RD, Domino KB. Safety of non-operating room anesthesia: a closed claims update. *Anesthesiol Clin*. 2017;35(4):569–581.
87. Melloni C. Anesthesia and sedation outside the operating room: how to prevent risk and maintain good quality. *Curr Opin Anaesthesiol*. 2007;20(6):513–519.
88. American Society of Anesthesiologists. Statement of granting privileges for administration of moderate sedation to practitioners. Updated October 2021. Accessed October 2, 2022. www.asahq.org
89. American Society of Anesthesiologists. Advisory on granting privileges for deep sedation to non-anesthesiologist physicians. Updated October 2017. Accessed October 2, 2022. www.asahq.org
90. Centers for Medicare and Medicaid Services. Revised hospital anesthesia interpretive guidelines. Published 2011. Accessed October 2022. www.asahq.org
91. American Society of Anesthesiologists. Statement on safe use of propofol. Updated October 2017. Accessed October 2, 2022. www.asahq.org
92. Rudkin GE, Osborne GA, Curtis NJ. Intra-operative patient-controlled sedation. *Anaesthesia*. 1991;46(2):90–92.
93. Park WY, Watkins PA. Patient-controlled sedation during epidural anesthesia. *Anesth Analg*. 1991;72(3):304–307.
94. Zelcer J, White PF, Chester S, Paull JD, Molnar R. Intraoperative patient-controlled analgesia: an alternative to physician administration during outpatient monitored anesthesia care. *Anesth Analg*. 1992;75(1):41–44.
95. Struys MMRF, De Smet T, Glen JIB, Vereecke HEM, Absalom AR, Schnider TW. The history of target-controlled infusion. *Anesth Analg*. 2016;122(1):56–69.
96. O'Hara DA, Bogen DK, Noordergraaf A. The use of computers for controlling the delivery of anesthesia. *Anesthesiology*. 1992;77(3):563–581.
97. Puri GD, Mathew PJ, Biswas I, et al. A multicenter evaluation of a closed-loop anesthesia delivery system: a randomized controlled trial. *Anesth Analg*. 2016;122(1):106–114.
98. Dutta A, Sethi N, Sood J, et al. The effect of dexmedetomidine on propofol requirements during anesthesia administered by bispectral index-guided closed-loop anesthesia delivery system: a randomized controlled study. *Anesth Analg*. 2019;129(1):84–91.
99. Hatib F, Jian Z, Buddi S, et al. Machine-learning algorithm to predict hypotension based on high-fidelity arterial pressure waveform analysis. *Anesthesiology*. 2018;129(4):663–674.
100. Cannesson M, Rinehart J. Closed-loop systems and automation in the era of patients safety and perioperative medicine. *J Clin Monit Comput*. 2014;28(1):1–3.

31 Ambulatory Anesthesia

PETER MANCINI

KEY POINTS

1. Procedures appropriate for ambulatory surgery are those associated with low rates of postoperative complications that do not require intensive physician or nursing management.
2. Society for Ambulatory Anesthesia issued a 2021 statement supporting cataract surgery in medically stable American Society of Anesthesiologists (ASA) IV patients at ambulatory surgery centers (ASCs), recognizing the procedure's low-risk profile, the enormous benefit of sight restoration, and ease of performing the procedure with topical anesthesia.
3. Medically stable ASA physical status III or IV patients may be appropriate candidates for ambulatory surgical procedures.
4. ASA, Society for Ambulatory Anesthesia, and American College of Chest Physicians agree that a procedure typically performed as an ambulatory procedure with local or regional anesthesia can also be performed as an ambulatory procedure in patients with obstructive sleep apnea (OSA).
5. The most recent ASA revised practice guidelines for preoperative fasting were published in 2017. The guidelines continue to allow a light meal up to 6 hours before an elective procedure and support a fasting period for clear liquids of 2 hours for all patients.
6. Regional and general anesthesia in the ambulatory setting are equally safe. However, even for experienced anesthesiologists, there is a failure rate associated with regional anesthesia.
7. Nerve blocks improve postoperative patient satisfaction and decrease postoperative nausea and vomiting (PONV) and postoperative pain.
8. Two primary concerns for ambulatory anesthesia are speed of wake-up and incidence of PONV.
9. It is important to distinguish between wake-up time and discharge time. Patients may emerge from anesthesia with desflurane and nitrous oxide significantly faster than after propofol or sevoflurane and nitrous oxide, though the ability to sit up, stand, and tolerate fluids and the time to fitness for discharge may be no different.
10. Nausea, with or without vomiting, is probably the most important factor contributing to a delay in discharge and an increase in unanticipated admissions after ambulatory surgery.
11. Widespread use of sugammadex in ambulatory anesthesia has not been shown to reduce postoperative pulmonary complications, and dosing neuromuscular blockade reversal should be guided by careful monitoring of neuromuscular block depth to ensure patient safety.

Ambulatory anesthesia is the delivery of anesthetic care to patients who will return home the same day they undergo a surgical procedure. It draws from the same skills, techniques, and science described in other chapters of this text. However, where ambulatory anesthesia is different is in its approach. The patient, the procedure, planning, and delivery of the anesthetic is chosen and tailored to avoid complications that will delay or prevent discharge home. This approach is not new. While no single individual invented ambulatory anesthesia, Drs John Ford and Wallace Reed (Fig. 31-1) opened a freestanding surgicenter in Arizona in accordance with the principles outlined in their classic 1971 paper.[1] Within several years, both the American Medical Association (AMA) and the ASA recognized the benefits and successes of surgicenters and formally endorsed the concept and practice of ambulatory anesthesia. Countless clinical questions would follow, and by the 1980s leaders in anesthesiology recognized the need for education and research. The Society for Ambulatory Anesthesia (SAMBA) in the United States and the British Association of Day Surgery were established, and by the 1990s, the International Association for Ambulatory Surgery (http://www.iaas-med.com) was formed, which now promotes worldwide development of ambulatory surgery and publishes a peer-reviewed journal, *Ambulatory Surgery*.[2]

The Place

Ambulatory surgery occurs in a variety of settings (NICV 31-1). Some centers are within a hospital while others are freestanding facilities that maintain affiliations with a hospital or health care

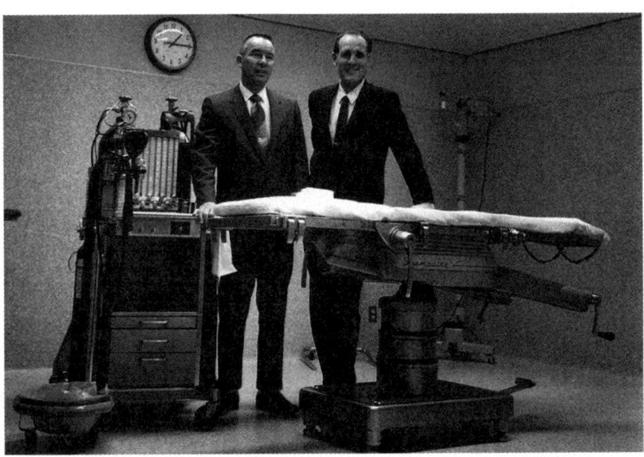

Figure 31-1 John Ford, M.D. (left) and Wallace Reed, M.D. (right) at the first surgicenter's opening day. February 12, 1970. *Acknowledgment: The Ambulatory Surgery Center Association.*

system. Others are entirely independent, and for-profit surgicenters market efficient service to surgeons and patients. In all these settings, predictable scheduling, brief operating room (OR) turnaround times, low risk of complications, and high reimbursement for procedures frequently make these facilities revenue sources. In the case of in-hospital or hospital-affiliated centers, they may subsidize less profitable departments and services. In the case of wholly private and independent ASCs, they are simply lucrative.[3] These economic forces do not always favor distribution of such centers based on clinical need, and evidence exists that they may worsen health care disparities along racial and socioeconomic lines.[4] In addition, private ASCs draw privately insured patients away from larger systems, creating concern that freestanding ambulatory surgery growth may force some hospitals out of business. This issue is particularly problematic in areas in which population density or median income is low. Surgeons may work exclusively in a freestanding facility and may not hold hospital staff privilege. Some hospitals have lost emergency department coverage for an entire surgical specialty because specialists in their geographic area work exclusively in independent ambulatory centers.

Procedures

What case is appropriate for an ambulatory surgical procedure? This question is fundamental in ambulatory anesthesia. Some centers set an arbitrary maximum duration of surgery time, for example, 4 hours. Others consider an ambulatory procedure as one that subjectively does not pose a significant safety risk or
1 require an overnight stay. In general, procedures appropriate for ambulatory surgery are those associated with postoperative care that is easily managed at home, have low rates of postoperative complications, and do not require intensive physician or nursing management. Establishing a low rate of postoperative complication depends on the relative aggressiveness of the facility, surgeon, patient, and payer. The list of procedures that match these goals is not static. Indeed, the relative complexity of outpatient surgeries has risen over time. Cervical spine surgery is now commonly performed in ASCs with an excellent safety record,[5] a practice unimaginable several decades ago. That does not mean that all ASCs are suitable places for all procedures performed on outpatients. Procedures of long duration, higher complexity, or those requiring specific resources (such as blood bank) are increasingly performed at some ASCs. Even complex oncologic surgeries are performed at more specialized ASCs affiliated with major cancer treatment centers.[6] Ultimately, enhanced recovery pathways and well-crafted administrative procedures are key to safety and success.

Patient Selection

Some have questioned the safety of ASCs. Deaths and adverse outcomes are reported both in medical literature and in news outlets. Anesthesia emergencies are rare but can occur even in healthy, carefully selected patients. An ambulatory surgery center must have the capability of managing such emergencies. A narrative review by Rajan in 2021[7] discusses the trend toward more complicated procedures and considers patient selection in the contemporary environment. Large retrospective data sets provide important outcome measures to insurers and Centers for Medicare & Medicaid Services (CMS) regarding unplanned complications in ambulatory surgery. Patient selection will depend on the regulatory environment which does vary between states. For instance, minimum age requirements for ASC eligibility will vary from state to state. Regardless of the regulatory environment, age is an important consideration in patient selection. For example, infants may not be appropriate for ambulatory surgery. Term infants whose postconceptual age (PCA) is less than 46 weeks, or preterm infants whose PCA is less than 60 weeks should be monitored for 12 hours after surgery because of risk of developing postoperative apnea (Fig. 31-2; Table 31-1).[8] Those requirements may prompt an ASC to refer patients to a hospital ambulatory center with the ability to monitor patients after normal working hours.

At the other extreme of life, advanced age alone is not a reason to disallow surgery in an ambulatory setting. However, advanced age can certainly complicate recovery. Some evidence identifies an association between postoperative morbidity and increased age following outpatient surgery. Large retrospective reviews do show an association between older age and hospital admission within 30 days of ambulatory surgery. This association remains even after adjusting for comorbidities that also increase the risk of admission during that 30-day recovery period (e.g., chronic renal failure, chronic obstructive pulmonary disease, current cancer treatment, and diabetes mellitus).[9]

The ASA physical status (PS) classification has a long history in anesthesia practice. While imperfect and heavily criticized for inconsistency between practitioners, recent recommendations do use this classification as a framework. The Rajan review summarizes several recommendations based on ASA-PS. ASA III patients should have their comorbidities optimized before having outpatient surgery. ASA IV patients who are medically stable should only undergo low-risk surgeries (e.g., cataract) at an ASC.
The example of cataracts warrants further discussion. In 2021, 2
SAMBA released a position statement on cataract surgery,[10] which is performed millions of times annually and has an enormous impact on sight preservation and quality of life improvement. The patient population is generally elderly, and significant comorbidities are common in this group. However, SAMBA is clear that cataract surgery is extremely low risk when performed with topical anesthesia. Failure to restore sight in these patients also leads to worse outcomes. This specific surgical problem illustrates how selection for ambulatory surgery is individualized and considers both the patient and procedure. Many patients who are candidates for outpatient cataract surgery would not be suitable candidates for procedures of even modestly greater risk.

Unplanned hospital admission is not necessarily a failure if it results in a better quality of care. With proper patient selection for typically elective ambulatory procedures, the incidence

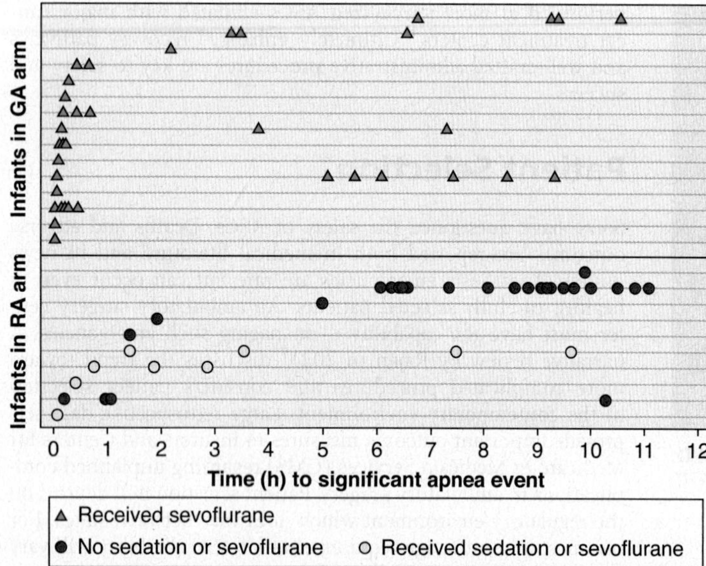

Figure 31-2 Apnea after regional and general anesthesia in infants. Regional anesthesia (RA) group further divided into those who received only regional anesthesia without sedation or general anesthesia (*closed circles*) and those who received spinal anesthesia and sedation or general anesthesia (*closed squares*). (Adapted from Davidson AJ, Morton NS, Arnup SJ, et al. General anesthesia compared to spinal anesthesia (GAS) consortium: apnea after awake regional and general anesthesia in infants: the general anesthesia compared to spinal anesthesia study-comparing apnea and neurodevelopmental outcomes, a randomized controlled trial. *Anesthesiology*. 2015;123(1):38–54.)

of hospital admission should be very low. Most medical problems that older individuals experience after ambulatory procedures are not related to patient age, but to specific organ dysfunction. For that reason, all individuals, whether young or old, should receive a careful preoperative history and physical examination.

3 Patients of ASA-PS III or IV are appropriate candidates for some ambulatory surgical procedures if their systemic diseases are medically stable. A large retrospective cohort study of ambulatory procedures at tertiary care centers in Massachusetts and New York between 2007 and 2017 examined unplanned hospital admission within 30 days of surgery.[11] Unplanned admissions were most often related to malignancy, nonsurgical site infections, and surgical complications, not patient age, procedure complexity, or ASA score.

Obese patients represent a special situation. In a meta-analysis of patients undergoing nonupper airway surgery, patients with or at high risk of obstructive sleep apnea (OSA) were more prone to adverse perioperative outcomes including respiratory, cardiac, and neurologic complications, and unplanned intensive care unit (ICU) transfer. Further, patients with sleep apnea had higher risk of hypoxemia postoperatively.[11] While not all obese patients have OSA, and not all OSA patients are obese, the overlap of both conditions is quite common, especially when BMI is over 50. The prior edition of this text recommended that these patients should probably be cared for as inpatients. However, a recent analysis of The American College of Surgeons National Surgical Quality Improvement Program (ACS-NSQIP) database from 2017 to 2018 revealed some surprising findings.[12] Super morbid obesity, defined as a BMI >50, was actually associated with lower rates of pulmonary complications after outpatient surgery than seen in obese patients with BMI between 40 and 50. These findings do not mean that BMI is unimportant in determining who should be excluded from ambulatory surgery. Rather, it supports careful screening of patients, which likely happened particularly well in these supermorbidly obese patients who were offered ambulatory surgery.

If electing to proceed as an outpatient, the anesthetic technique should be tailored to minimize narcotic usage, especially in the postoperative period. Patients with OSA who need more opioids may be at greater risk for apnea and should be observed for a longer period after their procedure. The ASA, SAMBA, and 4
American College of Chest Physicians published practice guidelines for the perioperative management of patients with OSA.[13–15] For patients with OSA, if a procedure is typically performed as an outpatient procedure and local or regional anesthesia is used, the procedure can also be performed as an ambulatory procedure. Conversely, those patients with OSA who are undergoing major surgery, or who are undergoing a procedure with an increased risk for perioperative complications, should not have their procedure performed as an ambulatory procedure.

Patients who undergo ambulatory surgery should have an adult take them home and stay with them afterward until the next morning to provide care. Before the procedure, the patient should receive information about the procedure, where it will be performed, laboratory studies that will be ordered, and dietary restrictions. The patient must understand before the procedure that an overnight stay is not intended. The patient, or some responsible adult, must ensure that all instructions are followed. Once at home, the patient must be able to tolerate the pain from the procedure, assuming adequate pain therapy is provided. The

Table 31-1 Guide to Determine Length of Stay for Infants after Surgery

Born (Weeks Postconception)	Age at Time of Surgery (Weeks Postconception)	Other Factors	Disposition
<37	<60		Admit overnight
>36	<46		Admit overnight
	<60	Still in PACU @ 9 PM	Admit overnight

PACU, postanesthesia care unit.

majority of patients are satisfied with early discharge, although a few prefer a longer stay in the facility. Patients for certain procedures such as laparoscopic cholecystectomy or transurethral resection of the prostate should live reasonably close to the ambulatory facility because postoperative complications may require their prompt return. However, "reasonably close" is not easily defined. This issue must be addressed by each facility for individual patients based on the planned procedure.

Preoperative Screening

Each outpatient facility should develop its own method of preoperative screening. The patient may visit the facility, or the staff members may telephone to obtain necessary information about the patient, including a complete medical history of the patient and family, the medications the patient is taking, and the problems the patient or the patient's family may have had with previous anesthetics. At some facilities, experienced nurses make those telephone calls. Screening may uncover logistical challenges that could lead to late cancelation, such as transportation or childcare needs. The process also provides the staff with an opportunity to remind patients of arrival time, suitable attire, and dietary restrictions (e.g., when to stop eating and drinking, no jewelry or makeup). Staff members can determine whether a responsible person is available to escort the patient to and from the facility and care for the patient at home after surgery. The screening is the ideal time for the anesthesiologist to talk to the patient, but if that is not possible, the anesthesiologist may review the screening record to determine whether additional evaluation by other consultants is necessary and whether laboratory tests are needed.

Table 31-2 A Guide to Medications Appropriate to Take Prior to Surgery

Medications that should be taken on the day of surgery:
β Blockers
Statins
Antiarrhythmics
Antihypertensives (except ACE I, ARB, diuretics)
Pulmonary inhalers
Pain medications (except NSAIDs)
Antiseizure medications
Hyperthyroid medications
Medications that should be avoided on the day of surgery:
ACE I/ARB (angiotensin-converting enzyme inhibitor/ angiotensin II receptor blockers)—risk of profound hypotension unresponsive to traditional treatments
Diuretics—hypokalemia and dehydration
Anticoagulants/antiplatelet—depending on surgery, surgeon, and underlying medical conditions—we leave these decisions up to surgeon and prescribing physician
Oral hypoglycemic agents
Vitamins which affect platelets (vitamin E)
Herbal supplements which may affect bleeding
Nonessential medications that can be continued on the day of surgery:
Hypothyroid medications
Antidepressants

Used with permission from Jill Zafar, Yale University Department of Anesthesiology.

Upper Respiratory Tract Infection

Following viral upper respiratory infections (URIs) in adults, airflow obstruction persists for up to 6 weeks (Fig. 31-3). For that reason, many agree that surgery should be delayed if an adult presents with a URI until 6 weeks have elapsed. In the case of children, whether surgery should be delayed for that length of time is questionable. In a year-long survey of almost 10,000 children who underwent surgery, URI was associated with an increased risk for perioperative respiratory adverse events only when symptoms were present or had occurred within the 2 weeks before the procedure.[16,17] The original Swiss study included children who were febrile or who had mucopurulent airway secretions and nevertheless had surgery. Of interest, children with these symptoms in the United States would have had their operations cancelled. Although a case may be cancelled because a child is symptomatic, the child may develop another URI when the procedure is rescheduled. Independent risk factors for adverse respiratory events in children with URIs include use of an endotracheal tube (vs. use of a laryngeal mask airway [LMA] or face mask), history of prematurity, history of reactive airway disease, history of parental smoking, surgery involving the airway, presence of copious secretions, and nasal congestion. In general, if a patient with a URI has a normal appetite, does not have a fever or an elevated respiratory rate, and does not appear toxic, it is probably safe to proceed with the planned procedure.

The COVID-19 pandemic presented additional questions and challenges for safety of anesthesia following infection. Although clinical recommendations have evolved rapidly, the most recent multidisciplinary guidelines published in the United Kingdom recommend avoiding surgery within 7 weeks of infection,[18] unless there is significant clinical risk of delaying surgery (e.g., a surgery aimed at diagnosing or removing a cancerous lesion). That risk-benefit decision should be individualized and include patient risk factors, severity of COVID symptoms, and risks of pulmonary complications associated with the procedure. These guidelines also recognize that patients with persistent symptoms may require a longer delay than 7 weeks.

Restriction of Food and Liquids Prior to Ambulatory Surgery

To decrease the risk of aspiration of gastric contents, we routinely ask patients not to eat or drink anything (*non per os* [NPO] or "nothing by mouth") for 8 hours before surgery. The most recent ASA revised practice guidelines for preoperative fasting were published in 2017 (Table 31-3).[19] A 2021 closed claims analysis of 115 cases of aspiration identified death in 57% of the claims and severe injury in 14%.[20] The anesthetic care was judged outside the standard of care in 59% of these claims. Pulmonary aspiration thus still presents a danger to even healthy, well patients undergoing relatively short outpatient surgeries under anesthesia. 5

Managing the Anesthetic: Premedication

Anxiety Reduction and Benzodiazepines

Most patients are anxious before scheduled surgery. Anxiety may begin as soon as the surgeon states that the patient needs an operation and may not end even after discharge from the outpatient facility. Reasons for anxiety include concerns about family, worry about pain after the procedure, fear of complications, and lack of social support. Preoperative reassurance from nonanesthesia staff,

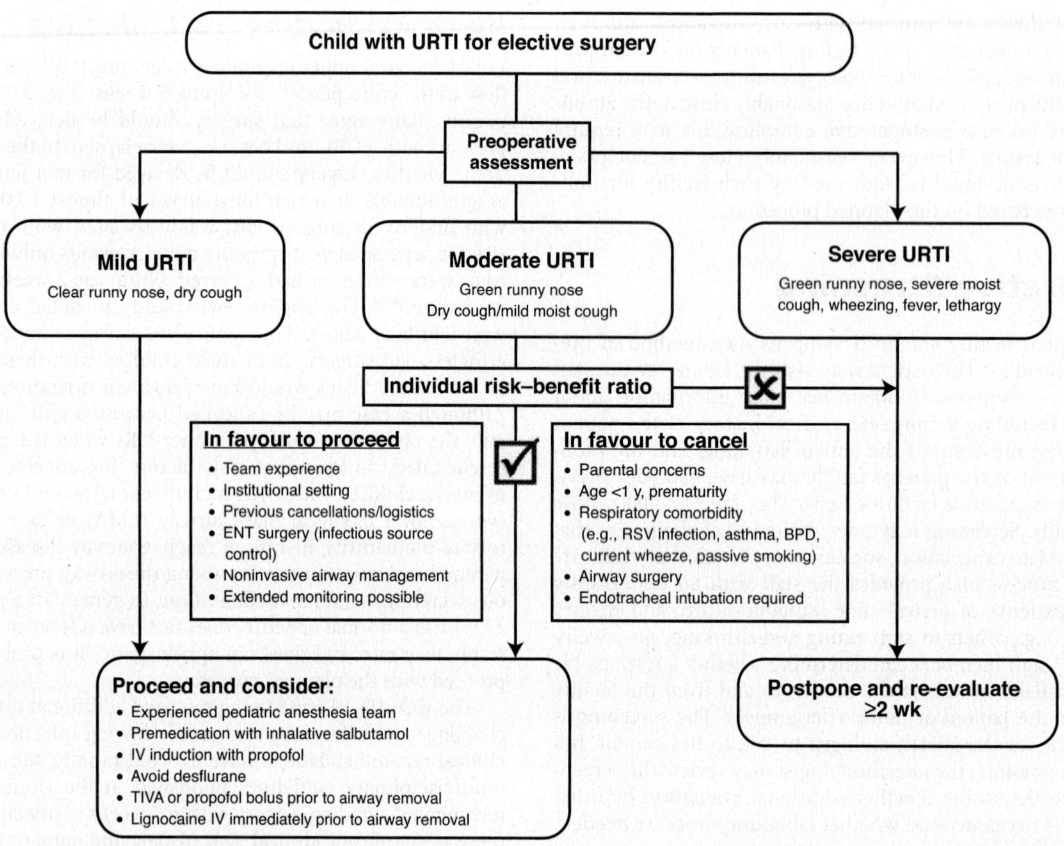

Figure 31-3 Children with upper respiratory tract infection. (Reprinted with permission from Regli A, Becke K, von Ungern-Sternberg BS. An update on the perioperative management of children with upper respiratory tract infections. *Curr Opin Anaesthesiol*. 2017;30(3):362–367.)

use of booklets or audiovisual instruction with information about the procedure, or a preoperative visit by the anesthesiologist can all help reduce preoperative anxiety. However, not all outpatients are anxious, and whether it is necessary to give every patient a preoperative drug to decrease anxiety is not clear. Further, even commonly used anxiolytics in modest doses do have side effects and should not be given if unnecessary. Midazolam, a benzodiazepine, is currently the drug most used to reduce preoperative anxiety and induce sedation. It can be administered intravenously and orally (Table 31-4). Large retrospective analysis does show an association between perioperative midazolam use and postoperative falls, delirium, and pulmonary complications.[21] Therefore, midazolam should not be used reflexively. If in doubt about patient anxiety, ask the patient; do not assume every patient needs a drug to reduce anxiety.

Table 31-3 Fasting Guidelines before Surgery

Food/Drink	Time to Fast Prior to Surgery (h)
Clear liquids (e.g., water, fruit juices without pulp, carbonated beverages, clear tea, and black coffee)	2
Breast milk	4
Infant formula	6
Nonhuman milk	6
Light meal (toast and clear liquids)	6
Meals that include fried or fatty foods or meat	8

Reprinted with permission from Practice Guidelines for Preoperative Fasting and the Use of Pharmacologic Agents to Reduce the Risk of Pulmonary Aspiration: Application to Healthy Patients Undergoing Elective Procedures: An Updated Report by the American Society of Anesthesiologists Task Force on Preoperative Fasting and the Use of Pharmacologic Agents to Reduce the Risk of Pulmonary Aspiration. *Anesthesiology*. 2017;126:376–393.

Opioids and Nonsteroidal Analgesics

Opioids can be administered preoperatively to sedate patients, control hypertension during tracheal intubation, and decrease

Table 31-4 A Guide to Premedication

A patient is seen at least 24 h before a scheduled procedure, expresses a desire for medication to relieve anxiety, or has anxiety that cannot be relieved with comforting: oral diazepam, 2–5 mg per 70 kg body weight the night before and at 6 AM on the day of surgery, even if surgery is scheduled for 1 PM or later.
A patient is seen for the first time in the preoperative holding area and seems to need medication: midazolam, 0.01 mg/kg intravenously, or in the OR, propofol, 0.7 mg/kg, intravenously.
For an anxious child, oral midazolam, 0.25 mg/kg, administered in the preoperative holding area.

OR, operating room.

pain before surgery. Opioid premedication prevents increases in systolic pressure in a dose-dependent fashion. After tracheal intubation, systolic, diastolic, and mean arterial blood pressures sometimes decrease below baseline values.

It would seem that preoperative administration of opioids or nonsteroidal anti-inflammatory drugs (NSAIDs) may be useful for controlling pain in the early postoperative period. The term "preventive analgesia" (as opposed to "preemptive analgesia") is used to mean treatment of postoperative pain for a longer duration than the effect of the target drug (e.g., at least 5.5 half-lives of the drug), so that the effect of the drug is more than its analgesic effect.[22,23] The drug then does not necessarily have to be administered before surgery.

Intraoperative Management: Choice of Anesthetic

6 There are several choices among anesthetic methods: general anesthesia, regional anesthesia, and local anesthesia. Regional and local anesthesia can be used with or without sedation. In ambulatory anesthesia, all three types are otherwise equally safe. This finding contrasts anesthesia for cesarean section where there are clear safety advantages to regional anesthesia. However, even for experienced anesthesiologists, there is a failure rate associated with regional anesthesia. Certainly, some procedures are possible only with a general anesthetic. For others, the preference of patients, surgeons, or anesthesiologists may determine selection.

The choice of anesthetic method may also influence time to recovery. In one retrospective study of patients undergoing ambulatory surgery at a large tertiary center, regional anesthesia use was associated with shorter PACU length of stay compared to general anesthesia; in addition, when regional anesthesia was used in conjunction with general anesthesia, PACU length of stay was shorter than when general anesthesia was used alone.[24] Patients who receive spinal anesthesia for ambulatory surgery may take longer to be discharged if micturition is required, though discharge instructions do not necessarily have to require a patient to micturate prior to discharge. In general, pain and postoperative nausea and vomiting (PONV) are greater after general anesthesia compared to regional anesthesia. When applying studies of regional anesthesia to everyday practice, one must recognize that the studies arise from centers where the authors are experienced in performing regional anesthesia and there are good systems to support the practice. Note also that anesthesiologists who are more experienced in performing regional anesthesia are more likely to provide regional anesthesia.

With regional anesthesia or sedation, some of the side effects of general anesthesia can be avoided. Performing a block may take longer than inducing general anesthesia, and the block may fail. However, performing the block beforehand in a preoperative holding area can obviate unnecessary delays that may prompt surgeons to discourage regional anesthetics for their cases despite the evidence that postoperative pain control is best with regional techniques. Surgeons might feel that regional anesthesia is beneficial, but the potential delay in establishing a block and perceived unpredictable success might detract from their enthusiasm for regional anesthesia.

Regional Techniques

Local anesthesia and regional anesthesia have long been used for ambulatory surgery. As early as 1963, for example, 56% of ambulatory procedures were performed with the use of these techniques.[25] Regional techniques commonly used for ambulatory surgery, in addition to spinal and epidural anesthesia, include local infiltration, brachial plexus and other peripheral nerve blocks, and intravenous regional anesthesia. General anesthesia can also be supplemented with regional nerve blocks.

An occasional patient may experience syncope when the needle for the regional block is inserted. This event is alarming to patients and providers. Needle phobia can be minimized by using oral premedication with benzodiazepines or intravenous sedation before starting the block, monitoring patients during the procedure, and having available atropine and vasopressors.[26] After a regional block, patients may still have a numb extremity (e.g., after a brachial plexus block) but otherwise meet all criteria for discharge. In such instances, the extremity must be well protected (e.g., with a sling for an upper extremity procedure) and patients must be cautioned to protect against injury because they are without normal sensations that would warn them of vulnerability. Reassurance that sensation will return should be provided.

Spinal Anesthesia

Children

Some centers use spinal anesthesia most commonly for ex-premature infants undergoing hernia repair because the risk of postoperative apnea is reduced and because neurodevelopmental outcome is likely less affected by spinal anesthesia compared to general. When planning spinal anesthesia, general anesthesia should be available as a backup because spinal anesthesia failure rates for this population are as high as 20%.[27] The same study found that although apnea in the immediate postoperative period may be lower with spinal anesthesia, it does not reduce the risk of apnea seen up to 12 hours after surgery. Furthermore, premature infants and those who have postoperative apnea within 30 minutes after surgery are more likely to have apnea up to 12 hours after surgery.

Adults

Spinal anesthesia is suitable for pelvic, lower abdominal, lower extremity, and even laparoscopic cholecystectomy surgery. Motor block of the legs may delay a patient's ability to walk. However, the use of a short-acting local anesthetic will minimize this problem. Different drugs and drug concentrations have been used for spinal anesthesia. Though any intrathecal local anesthetic can cause transient neurologic symptoms, lidocaine use is particularly problematic because of its high association with transient neurologic symptoms. Bupivacaine can be problematic for ambulatory surgical procedures because of its longer duration of action. In one study where spinal anesthesia was compared with either 0.75% hyperbaric bupivacaine 7.5 mg (n = 53) or 2% preservative-free 2-chloroprocaine 40 mg (n = 53), discharge readiness was 76 minutes faster with chloroprocaine.[28]

Although headache is a complication of lumbar puncture, smaller-gauge needles result in a lower incidence of postdural puncture headache. For those patients who do receive spinal anesthesia, it is incumbent on the anesthesiologist and the facility to have follow-up with telephone calls to ensure no disabling symptoms of headache have developed. If the headache does not respond to bed rest, analgesics, and oral hydration, the patient must return to hospital for a course of intravenous caffeine therapy or an epidural blood patch. Instructions regarding postdural puncture headache should be included in the preoperative consent process.

Epidural and Caudal Anesthesia

Epidural anesthesia typically takes longer to perform than spinal anesthesia. Onset with spinal anesthesia is more rapid, although recovery may be the same with either technique. When spinal anesthesia and epidural anesthesia are combined, the initial onset of block is faster than with epidural anesthesia alone. Epidural anesthesia is particularly advantageous for procedures where duration of surgery is unclear. Another advantage of the epidural block is that it can be performed outside the OR and avoids the problem of postdural puncture headache provided there is no "wet tap."

Peripheral Nerve Blocks

7 Nerve blocks are an important technique in ambulatory anesthesia. They improve patient satisfaction and reduce both PONV and postoperative pain. In a study of patients undergoing arthroscopic rotator cuff repair, most patients in the continuous interscalene brachial plexus block group had pain scores less than 4 compared to patients in the single-injection interscalene brachial plexus block group or the general anesthesia group whose pain scores were more than 4. These findings were observed on postoperative days 1, 2, and 7.[29] A designated room where regional anesthesia can be performed far enough in advance of the OR such that the block is effective by the time the patient enters the OR will reduce turnover time.[30] Counterintuitively, there was no difference in PACU times between with regional anesthesia and with or without general anesthesia; but PACU length of stay was shorter with regional anesthesia compared to general anesthesia alone.

Sedation and Analgesia

Many patients who undergo surgery with local or regional anesthesia prefer to be sedated and to have no recollection of the procedure. Sedation is important, in part, because injection with local anesthetics can be painful and lying on a hard OR table can be uncomfortable. Levels of sedation vary from light, during which a patient's consciousness is minimally depressed, to deep, in which protective reflexes are partially blocked and response to physical stimulation or verbal command may not be appropriate.

General Anesthesia

Induction

The drugs selected for general anesthesia determine how long patients stay in the PACU after surgery, and for some patients, whether they can be discharged to go home. Propofol is by far the most common induction agent in ambulatory anesthesia. Pentathol is no longer used clinically in the United States. Though the effect of drugs given for induction may appear transient, they can depress psychomotor performance for several hours. Propofol's half-life is 1 to 3 hours, and after an induction dose, impairment is apparent for only 1 hour. This compares very favorably to, for instance, methohexital which has a half-life of 6 to 8 hours. Propofol's dominance in ambulatory anesthesia is likely to be lasting.

However, pain on injection can be a problem with propofol, which is observed in approximately 60% of patients and is more likely when injected into dorsal hand veins.[31] Effective techniques to mitigate the discomfort include intravenous placement in larger antecubital veins and/or pretreatment with lidocaine. Typically, the latter is best done by occluding the vein with a tourniquet to provide venous stasis for 30 to 120 seconds, allowing lidocaine to topically anesthetize the vein before propofol administration. Most children and some adults prefer not to have an intravenous catheter inserted before the start of anesthesia. Sevoflurane has a relatively low blood–gas partition coefficient and the speed of induction is only slightly slower than propofol. In these cases, inhalational induction with sevoflurane can be hastened when the patient is told to breathe out to residual volume, take a vital capacity breath through a primed anesthesia circuit, and then hold the breath.

For short procedures, some patients may not require neuromuscular-blocking drugs; others may need brief paralysis (e.g., with succinylcholine) to facilitate tracheal intubation. Nondepolarizing drugs can be used to facilitate intubation and continue paralysis during the procedure. Large doses of rocuronium have rapid onset times that are similar to those with succinylcholine. Of course, paralysis is not needed to insert an endotracheal tube; drug combinations such as propofol, alfentanil, or remifentanil, with or without lidocaine, obviate the need for paralysis. Succinylcholine should be used with caution in children because of the possibility of cardiac arrest related to hyperkalemia, malignant hyperthermia, or unsuspected muscular dystrophy, particularly Duchenne disease. Many patients can experience painful postoperative myalgias after receiving succinylcholine.

Maintenance

Although many factors affect the choice of agents for maintenance of anesthesia, two primary concerns for ambulatory anesthesia are speed of wake-up and incidence of PONV. 8

Time to recovery may be measured by various criteria; however, for an ambulatory center, a patient may be considered "recovered" only when they are able to leave the center. Actual discharge from an ambulatory center, though, may depend on administrative issues such as a written order from a surgeon or anesthesiologist. The time necessary before a patient can be taken from the OR after completion of surgery, or a patient's ability to skip the PACU and go directly to phase II recovery, may be directly related to the anesthetic and may result in cost savings for an institution.

Does choice of maintenance agent affect recovery after anesthesia? Propofol, desflurane, and sevoflurane have characteristics that make them ideal for maintenance of anesthesia for ambulatory surgery. Propofol has a short half-life and, when used as a maintenance agent, results in rapid recovery and few side effects. Desflurane and sevoflurane, halogenated ether anesthetics with low blood–gas partition coefficients, seem to be ideal for general anesthesia for ambulatory surgery. Although total intravenous anesthetics are thought by many practitioners to have smoother wakeups and recoveries, no evidence favoring total intravenous maintenance in ambulatory anesthesia exists. In fact, a 2021 randomized trial showed that the selection of intravenous or inhalation maintenance anesthesia did not objectively affect postoperative recovery following total laparoscopic hysterectomy.[32]

Emergence and Recovery

It is important to distinguish between wake-up time and discharge time. Patients may emerge from anesthesia with desflurane and nitrous oxide significantly faster than after propofol or sevoflurane and nitrous oxide, although the ability to sit up, stand, and tolerate fluids and the time to fitness for discharge may be no different. Fast wake-up times may translate to bypass of phase I, which can result in cost savings. 9

Nausea, with or without vomiting, is probably the most important factor contributing to a delay in discharge of patients and an increase in unanticipated admissions of both children and adults after ambulatory surgery. Patients often fear PONV more than postoperative pain. Reducing risk factors can significantly decrease the incidence of PONV (Table 31-5). To decrease the risk of PONV: 10

- Use regional anesthesia.
- If general anesthesia is necessary, use a propofol infusion instead of an inhalation agent.

Table 31-5 Techniques to Decrease Postoperative Nausea and Vomiting Risk

Use regional anesthesia alone if possible
If general anesthesia is needed, use a propofol infusion instead of an inhalation agent
Avoid use of nitrous oxide for anesthesia maintenance, particularly for procedures longer than 1 h
Minimize use of perioperative opioids
Use sugammadex instead of neostigmine for reversal of neuromuscular blockade
Consider adequate hydration

- Avoid nitrous oxide.
- Minimize use of perioperative opioids.
- Use sugammadex instead of neostigmine to reverse neuromuscular blockade.
- Provide adequate hydration.

The incidence of emesis may be greater after nitrous oxide than after potent inhalation agents. Although many studies have shown that nitrous oxide can be used successfully for ambulatory anesthesia, there is evidence that when nitrous oxide is used for less than 1 hour, the risk of PONV is not increased.[33] Women have a higher incidence of PONV as do those with a previous history of PONV or motion sickness. Specific procedures, for example, laparoscopy, lithotripsy, major breast surgery, and ear, nose, or throat surgery, also have increased risk for PONV. The greater the number of risk factors, the greater the risk for nausea or vomiting after surgery.

Propensity to PONV is probably multifactorial and may include several genomic pathways; more study relating genetic makeup and possible treatment implications is needed. Treatment targets sites and pathways in the brain that are associated with PONV. Receptor antagonists, specifically selective serotonin antagonists (ondansetron, dolasetron, and granisetron), have been shown to have similar efficacy to help alleviate nausea and vomiting. Dopamine antagonists, antihistamines, and anticholinergic drugs are useful but are associated with extensive side effects. Combination of multiple drugs typically is more effective than one. For example, dexamethasone has an additive effect when included with ondansetron and droperidol. Other therapies useful in controlling PONV include acupuncture or acupressure,[34] supplemental fluid therapy, and clonidine (perhaps in part because it decreases anesthesia requirement).

Though much work has been focused on PONV, postdischarge nausea and vomiting (PDNV) is also an issue. In one study, the overall incidence of PDNV was almost 45%, and PDNV continued until day 7 for 6% of patients (Fig. 31-4).[35] Those who had a history of motion sickness, previous PONV, migraine headaches, and pain on activity postdischarge were more likely to have PDNV. Practitioners may use antiemetics to prevent PONV with merely the hope and assumption that they will prevent PDNV. However, evidence exists that more precise treatment is possible. A recent randomized trial showed that low-dose olanzapine (10 mg) preinduction is very effective in reducing postdischarge PDNV in ambulatory surgery.[36]

Paralysis

A nondepolarizing muscle relaxant given at induction lasts beyond the time that paralysis is needed or helpful for intubation. This is especially significant in ambulatory anesthesia where even cases that require intubation are often relatively short. The duration of action of rocuronium, vecuronium, and cisatracurium ranges from 25 to 40 minutes. Reversal agents must be used unless there is no doubt that muscle relaxation has fully worn off, which is highly unlikely in a short ambulatory case. Since publication of the prior edition, use of the reversal agent sugammadex has become widespread[37] and represents a significant practice change. Sugammadex is a gamma-cyclodextrin with a lipophilic core. It binds aminosteroid nondepolarizing muscle relaxants (rocuronium and vecuronium). While highly effective at reversing nondepolarized blockade, caution and careful pre- and postreversal motor assessment are still mandatory. A quality improvement (QI) review at a prominent academic center revealed that switching from neostigmine to sugammadex resulted in no reduction in the rates of pulmonary complications related to residual neuromuscular blockade.[38] Patient safety is still optimized when acceleromyography is used to monitor the extent of paralysis and the adequacy of reversal.[39] Furthermore, when quantitative monitoring of neuromuscular block depth guides reversal dosing, respiratory complications can be minimized (Fig. 31-5).[40] 11

The use of supraglottic airways, such as the LMA, provides several advantages for allowing a patient to return to baseline status quickly. Muscle relaxants are generally avoided. Coughing is less than with tracheal intubation. Anesthetic requirements, hoarseness, and sore throat are also reduced. Overall, cost savings result with the use of LMAs. Because of gastric insufflation, though, nausea and vomiting may be greater. After an LMA is inserted, there is a 1% failure rate requiring endotracheal tube insertion.[41] In the study of almost 16,000 patients, risk factors for failure included surgical table rotation, male gender, poor dentition, and increased body mass index.

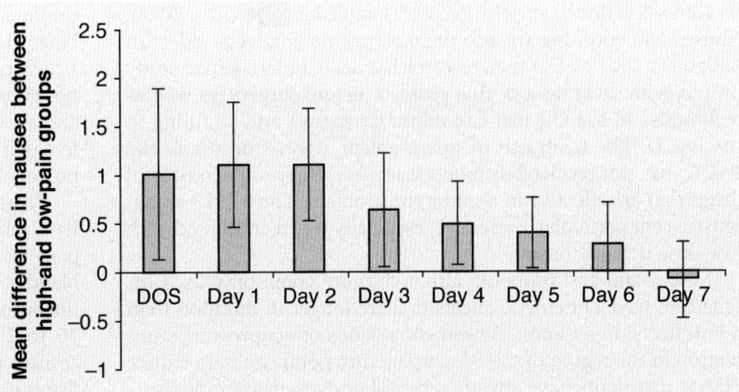

Figure 31-4 Mean differences in daily nausea scores between high- and low-pain groups, with 95% confidence intervals from day of surgery (DOS) to postoperative day 7. The largest difference was seen on the second day after surgery, followed by a gradual decrease. Differences on days 6 and 7 were not significant. (Adapted with permission from Odom-Forren J, Rayens MK, Gokun Y, et al. The relationship of pain and nausea in postoperative patients for 1 week after ambulatory surgery. *Clin J Pain*. 2015;31:845–851.)

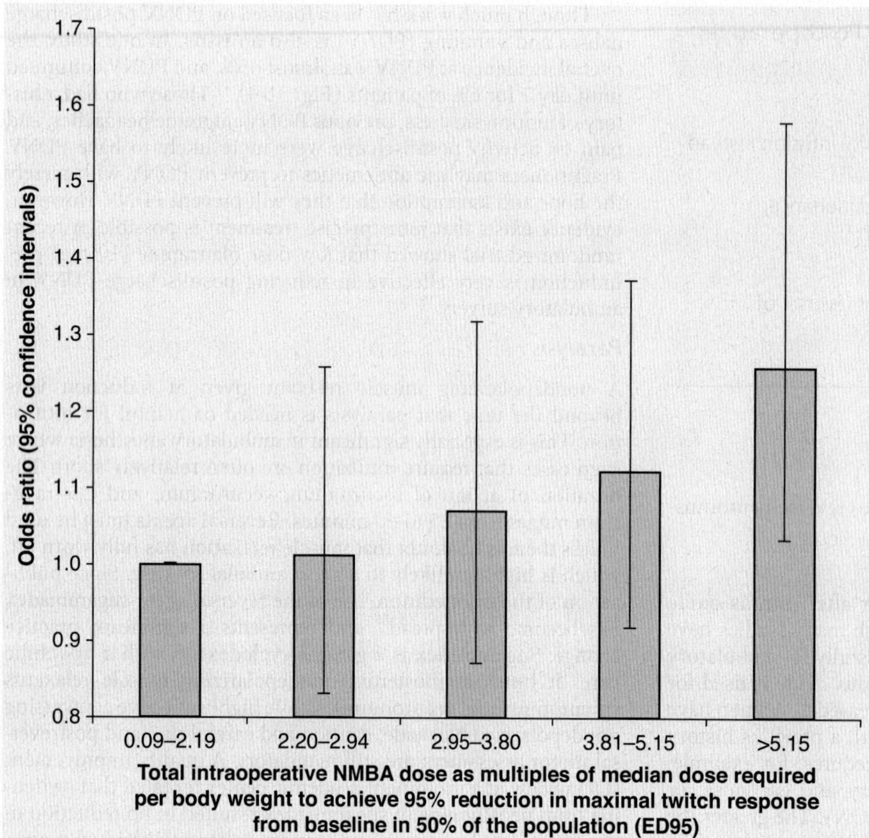

Figure 31-5 As the dose of neuromuscular blocking agent (intraoperative dose of atracurium, cisatracurium, rocuronium, or vecuronium) increases, the likelihood of respiratory complications increases. (Adapted with permission from McLean DJ, Diaz-Gil D, Farhan HN, Ladha KS, Kurth T, Eikermann M. Dose-dependent association between intermediate-acting neuromuscular-blocking agents and postoperative respiratory complications. *Anesthesiology*. 2015;122:1201–1213.)

Management of Postanesthesia Care

Managing common problems in the PACU quickly and effectively is as important as appropriate patient selection and choice of anesthetic technique if the patient is to return home on the day of surgery. The three most common reasons for delay in patient discharge from the PACU are drowsiness, nausea and vomiting, and pain. All three are a function of intraoperative management, but nausea, vomiting, and pain become most apparent in the PACU.

Nausea and Vomiting

Nausea and vomiting are the most common reasons both children and adults have protracted stays in the PACU or unexpected hospital admission due to anesthesia (see Chapter 12, Video 20-2). Nausea and vomiting are also the most common adverse effect in patients in the PACU. Much research has been undertaken to study prophylactic treatment of this problem before surgery, as well as techniques in the OR that can minimize nausea and vomiting in the PACU. The treatment of this problem, once it occurs in the PACU, has not received as much study. Yet, there are a variety of drugs that are effective in treating the problem. The 5-HT3 antagonists seem particularly effective, especially when combined with low-dose dexamethasone.

Midazolam and propofol, although more commonly used for sedation, have antiemetic effects that are longer in duration than their effects on sedation. Acupressure bands or acupressure stimulation in the region of the P6 acupuncture point can help reduce PONV. If patients have already received ondansetron prophylaxis in the OR, and then are nauseous in the PACU, another dose might not be effective. Based on a retrospective analysis of patients with nausea after receiving prophylactic ondansetron, established PONV was more effectively treated with promethazine than ondansetron; and promethazine, 6.25 mg intravenously, rather than higher doses was most effective.[42] More work is obviously needed to study effective therapies for treatment of PONV in the PACU. Finally, because pain may be associated with nausea, treatment of pain frequently decreases nausea. For a more complete discussion, consider the most recent 2020 consensus guidelines by Gan et al.[43]

Pain

Intraoperative opioid administration provides analgesia for both the intraoperative and postoperative course. Fentanyl is probably the most popular drug, although all other available opioids have been tried. All opioids can cause nausea, sedation, and dizziness, which can delay a patient's discharge. Nonsteroidal analgesics are not effective as supplements to blunt surgical stimuli during general anesthesia, although they are useful in controlling postoperative pain, particularly when given before skin incision. To control postoperative pain, combination therapy is most useful.

Postsurgical pain must be treated quickly and effectively. It is important for the practitioner to differentiate postsurgical pain from the discomfort of hypoxemia, hypercapnia, or a full bladder. Medications for pain control should be given in small intravenous doses (e.g., morphine 1 to 3 mg/70 kg or fentanyl 10 to 25 µg/70 kg). Intramuscular injection of opioid for pain control in the PACU is usually not necessary. Onset of action of drugs is faster after intravenous catheter administration than after oral administration. Control of postoperative pain may include administration of opioid analgesics or NSAIDs, the latter of which are not associated with respiratory depression, nausea, or vomiting. Fentanyl is the opioid frequently used to control postoperative pain for ambulatory surgery patients, although the analgesic effects of morphine and hydromorphone last longer. Patients who receive fentanyl for pain control may require additional injections and go home no sooner compared with patients who receive morphine. Oral tramadol/acetaminophen (T/A 37.5/325 mg) given after surgery and then as one tablet four times daily for 48 hours is an effective fixed drug combination for treating pain after discharge.[44] Nonsteroidal medications, such as ketorolac or ibuprofen, can also effectively control postoperative pain[45] and, compared with opioids, can give pain relief for a longer period, and are associated with less nausea and vomiting. Although NSAIDs can cause platelet dysfunction and increase bleeding, there is no evidence of increased postoperative bleeding due to NSAIDs for most ambulatory surgery procedures. When swelling and pain are problematic postoperatively, NSAIDs can be more effective than opioids in relieving both.

Although acetaminophen was used clinically late in the 19th century, it was not until early in the 21st century that the drug became available intravenously. Unlike opioids, acetaminophen is not associated with PONV or respiratory depression, and unlike NSAIDs, it is not associated with platelet dysfunction, gastritis, or renal toxicity. When given intravenously, first-pass hepatic exposure is limited, and the risk of hepatic injury is reduced. When given before surgical incision,[46] or postoperatively,[47] opioid requirement is reduced. Total daily dose of acetaminophen should not exceed 4 g/d and 2 g/d or less for patients with impaired liver or kidney function.

Preparation for Discharge

In addition to the PACU, most ASCs in the United States have phase II recovery. Patients remain in phase II recovery until they can tolerate liquids, walk, and/or (depending on the operation) void. Patients who undergo procedures under monitored anesthesia care can usually go straight to phase II recovery from the OR. Though it may seem that time and money are saved when a patient can bypass the PACU, nursing workload in phase II recovery might be greater and overall hospital costs may be no different than if a patient first recovers in the PACU.

Some criteria for discharge to home were created without scientific basis. One criterion is the ability to tolerate oral liquids before being discharged. Postoperative nausea may be greater if patients are required to drink liquids prior to discharge. Even though it is warranted after spinal or epidural anesthesia, the requirement that low-risk patients void before discharge may only lengthen their stay in the ASC facility, particularly if patients are willing to return to a medical facility if they are unable to void. Practical criteria for patient discharge from the OR, from the PACU, and from phase II recovery are needed such that there is no compromise in patient safety. However, the value of psychomotor tests to measure different phases of recovery, except for research purposes, is questionable.

Although scoring systems may be used to guide transfer from the PACU to the phase II recovery and from phase II recovery to home, they do little to test higher levels of function, such as the ability to use one's hands, to drive a car, or to remain alert long enough to drive. Patients may feel fine after they leave the hospital, but they should be advised against driving or other risky activities (e.g., operating power tools, swimming, climbing ladders, going back to work, or answering emails remotely) for at least 24 hours after a procedure. Once the patient leaves the medical facility, supervision may not be as good as it was in the hospital. Therefore, before a patient is discharged, dressings should be checked. It is wise to include the responsible person in all discharge instructions.

Patients should also be informed that they may experience pain, headache, nausea, vomiting, or dizziness and, if succinylcholine was used, generalized muscle aches and pains for at least 24 hours. A patient will be less stressed if the described symptoms are expected in the course of a normal recovery. Written instructions are important. The addition of written and oral education techniques at discharge has a significant impact on improving compliance.

For patients with a language barrier, consent forms, procedural explanation, and discharge information may have to be written in languages other than English and the services of an interpreter may be necessary. Nursing staff should assess the adult who will take the patient home to determine whether they are a responsible person. A responsible person is an adult who is physically and intellectually able to take care of the patient at home. Facilities should develop a method of follow-up after the patient has been discharged. At some facilities, staff members telephone the patient the next day to determine the progress of recovery; others use follow-up postcards.

Whenever we become innovative in the management of our outpatients, we must assess how a cost-effective, "no frills" approach to care affects patient safety. We must determine what we can do for the patient who lives alone, for the patient whose responsible person is unable to manage their needs, for the patient without means of transportation, and for the patient with limited insurance coverage. Hospital beds can be set aside for patients who require observation. Patients in these beds after an ambulatory surgical procedure are still considered outpatients. However, they are charged for the hours spent in the observation area. Some hospitals have joined with management firms to build a hospital hotel or medical motel close to the hospital itself. The hotel, usually a nonmedical facility, offers the outpatient a comfortable, inexpensive, and convenient place to recuperate while being cared for by family or nurses. Home health care nursing may be appropriate after surgical procedures such as reduction mammoplasty, abdominoplasty, vaginal hysterectomy, and major open ligament repairs of the knee. Prospective studies are needed to assess the quality of care and the effect that these innovative approaches have on patient safety.

Patient, procedure, availability and quality of aftercare, and anesthetic technique must be individually and collectively assessed to determine acceptability for ambulatory surgery. A delicate and balanced approach must be maintained between the patient's physical status, the proposed surgical procedure, and the appropriate anesthetic technique. The expertise of the anesthesiologist is necessary to provide that level of care safely and successfully.

Anesthesia for ambulatory surgery is a rapidly evolving specialty. Many patients who were once believed to be unsuitable for ambulatory surgery are now considered appropriate candidates. Operations once believed unsuitable for outpatients are now routinely performed in the morning, so patients can be discharged in the afternoon or evening. The availability of both shorter- and longer-acting analgesics as well as numerous antiemetics enables us to care for patients in ambulatory centers effectively. The appropriate anesthetic management begins before these patients come to the facility and continues not just during their operation but also through recovery. All are key to success.

Acknowledgments

Thanks to Yale University, Department of Anesthesiology.

For further review and interactivities, please see the videos and narrative interactive clinical vignettes (NICVs) accessible in the complimentary eBook bundled with this text. Access instructions are located on the inside front cover.

REFERENCES

1. Ford JL, Reed WA. The surgical center: concept, care, cost in freestanding facility. *Hospital Topics*. 1971;49(12):69–81.
2. Philip BK. A history of the Society for Ambulatory Anesthesia, *Amb Surg*. 1993;1(2):77–79.
3. Tanna N, Gibstein AR, Boll A, et al. Joint-venture ambulatory surgery centers: the perfect partnership. *Plast Reconstr Surg*. 2021;148(5):1149–1156.
4. Janeway MG, Sanchez SE, Chen Q, et al. Association of race, health insurance status, and household income with location and outcomes of ambulatory surgery among adult patients in 2 US states. *JAMA Surg*. 2020;155(12):1123–1131.
5. Gologorsky Y. Outpatient spine surgery: transition to the ambulatory surgery center. *World Neurosurg*. 2018;114:369–370.
6. Tokita H, Twersky R, Laudone V, et al. Complex cancer surgery in the outpatient setting: the Josie Robertson Surgery Center, *Anesth Analg*. 2020;131(3):699–707.
7. Rajan N, Rosero EB, Joshi GP. Patient selection for adult ambulatory surgery: a narrative review. *Anesth Analg*. 2021;133(6):1415–1430.
8. Davidson AJ, Morton NS, Arnup SJ, et al; General Anesthesia compared to Spinal anesthesia (GAS) Consortium. Apnea after awake regional and general anesthesia in infants: the General Anesthesia Compared to Spinal Anesthesia Study–comparing apnea and neurodevelopmental outcomes, a randomized controlled trial. *Anesthesiology*. 2015;123(1):38–54.
9. De Oliveira GS Jr, Holl JL, Lindquist LA, Hackett NJ, Kim JYS, McCarthy RJ. Older adults and unanticipated hospital admission within 30 days of ambulatory surgery: an analysis of 53,667 ambulatory surgical procedures. *J Am Geriatr Soc*. 2015;63(8):1679–1685.
10. Sweitzer B, Rajan N, Schell D, Gayer S, Eckert S, Joshi GP. Preoperative care for cataract surgery: the Society for Ambulatory Anesthesia position statement. *Anesth Analg*. 2021;133(6): 1431–1436.
11. Teja B, Raub D, Friedrich S, et al. Incidence, prediction, and causes of unplanned 30-day hospital admission after ambulatory procedures. *Anesth Analg*. 2020;131(2):497–507.
12. Hajmohamed S, Patel D, Apruzzese P, Kendall M, De Oliveira G. Early postoperative outcomes of super morbid obese compared to morbid obese patients after ambulatory surgery under general anesthesia: a propensity-matched analysis of a National Database. *Anesth Analg*. 2021;133(6):1366–1373.
13. American Society of Anesthesiologists Task Force on Perioperative Management of patients with obstructive sleep apnea. Practice guidelines for the perioperative management of patients with obstructive sleep apnea: an updated report by the American Society of Anesthesiologists Task Force on Perioperative Management of patients with obstructive sleep apnea. *Anesthesiology*. 2014;120:268–286.
14. Stierer TL, Collop NA. Perioperative assessment and management for sleep apnea in the ambulatory surgical patient. *Chest*. 2015;148:559–565.
15. Joshi GP, Ankichetty SP, Gan TJ, Chung F. Society for ambulatory anesthesia consensus statement on preoperative selection of adult patients with obstructive sleep apnea scheduled for ambulatory surgery. *Anesth Analg*. 2012;115:1060–1068.
16. von Ungern-Sternberg BS, Boda K, Chambers NA, et al. Risk assessment for respiratory complications in paediatric anaesthesia: a prospective cohort studay. *Lancet*. 2010;376:773–783.
17. Regli A, Becke K, von Ungern-Sternberg BS. An update on the perioperative management of children with upper respiratory tract infections. *Curr Opin Anaesthesiol*. 2017;30(3):362–367.
18. El-Boghdadly K, Cook TM, Goodacre T, et al. Timing of elective surgery and risk assessment after SARS-CoV-2 infection: an update: a multidisciplinary consensus statement on behalf of the Association of Anaesthetists, Centre for Perioperative Care, Federation of Surgical Specialty Associations, Royal College of Anaesthetists, Royal College of Surgeons of England. *Anaesthesia*. 2022;77(5):580–587.
19. Practice guidelines for preoperative fasting and the use of pharmacologic agents to reduce the risk of pulmonary aspiration: application to healthy patients undergoing elective procedures: an updated report by the American Society of Anesthesiologists Task Force on preoperative fasting and the use of pharmacologic agents to reduce the risk of pulmonary aspiration. *Anesthesiology*. 2017;126:376–393.
20. Warner MA, Meyerhoff KL, Warner ME, Posner KL, Stephens L, Domino KB. Pulmonary aspiration of gastric contents: a closed claims analysis. *Anesthesiology*. 2021;135:284–291.
21. Athanassoglou V, Cozowicz C, Zhong H, et al. Association of perioperative midazolam use and complications: a population-based analysis. *Reg Anesth Pain Med*. 2022;47(4):228–233.
22. Katz J, Clarke H, Seltzer Z. Review article: preventive analgesia: quo vadimus? *Anesth Analg*. 2011;113:1242–1253.
23. Kissin I. A call to reassess the clinical value of preventive (preemptive) analgesia. *Anesth Analg*. 2011;113:977–978.
24. Corey JM, Bulka CM, Ehrenfeld JM. Is regional anesthesia associated with reduced PACU length of stay? A retrospective analysis from a tertiary medical center. *Clin Orthop Relat Res*. 2014;472:1427–1433.
25. Cohen DD, Dillon JB. Anesthesia for outpatient surgery. *JAMA*. 1966;196:1114–1116.
26. Sokolowski CJ, Giovannitti JA Jr, Boynes SG. Needle phobia: etiology, adverse consequences, and patient management. *Dent Clin North Am*. 2010;54:731–744.
27. Frawley G, Bell G, Disma N, et al; General Anesthesia compared to Spinal anesthesia (GAS) Consortium. Predictors of failure of awake regional anesthesia for neonatal hernia repair: data from the general anesthesia compared to spinal anesthesia study-comparing apnea and neurodevelopmental outcomes. *Anesthesiology*. 2015;123:55–65.
28. Lacasse MA, Roy JD, Forget J, et al. Comparison of bupivacaine and 2-chloroprocaine for spinal anesthesia for outpatient surgery: a double blind randomized trial. *Can J Anaesth*. 2011;58:384–391.
29. Salviz EA, Xu D, Frulla A, et al. Continuous interscalene block in patients having outpatient rotator cuff repair surgery: a prospective randomized trial. *Anesth Analg*. 2013;117: 1485–1492.
30. Mercereau P, Lee B, Head SJ, Schwarz SKW. A regional anesthesia-based "swing" operating room model reduces non-operative time in a mixed orthopedic inpatient/outpatient population. *Can J Anaesth*. 2012;59:943–949.
31. Jalota L, Kalira V, George E, et al; Perioperative Clinical Research Core. Prevention of pain on injection of propofol: systematic review and meta-analysis. *BMJ*. 2011;342:d1110.
32. Niu Z, Gao X, Shi Z, et al. Effect of total intravenous anesthesia or inhalation anesthesia on postoperative quality of recovery in patients undergoing total laparoscopic hysterectomy: a randomized controlled trial. *J Clin Anesth*. 2021;73:110374.
33. Peyton PJ, Wu CY. Nitrous oxide-related postoperative nausea and vomiting depends on duration of exposure. *Anesthesiology*. 2014;120:1137–1145.
34. Lee A, Fan LT. Stimulation of the wrist acupuncture point P6 for preventing postoperative nausea and vomiting. *Cochrane Database Syst Rev*. 2009;(2):CD003281.
35. Odom-Forren J, Jalota L, Moser DK, et al. Incidence and predictors of postdischarge nausea and vomiting in a 7-day population. *J Clin Anesth*. 2013;25(7):551–559. doi: 10.1016/j.jclinane.2013.05.008
36. Hyman JB, Park C, Lin HM, et al. Olanzapine for the prevention of postdischarge nausea and vomiting after ambulatory surgery: a randomized controlled trial. *Anesthesiology*. 2020; 132(6):1419–1428.
37. Bash LD, Black W, Turzhitsky V, Urman RD. Neuromuscular blockade and reversal practice variability in the outpatient setting: insights from US utilization patterns. *Anesth Analg*. 2021;133(6):1437–1450.
38. Gen L, Freundlich RE, Gupta RK, et al. Postoperative Pulmonary Complications' Association with Sugammadex versus Neostigmine: a retrospective registry analysis. *Anesthesiology*. 2021;134:862–873.
39. Brull SJ, Prielipp RC. Reversal of neuromuscular blockade: "identification friend or foe." *Anesthesiology*. 2015;122:1183–1185.
40. McLean DJ, Diaz-Gil D, Farhan HN, Ladha KS, Kurth T, Eikermann M. Dose-dependent association between intermediate-acting neuromuscular-blocking agents and postoperative respiratory complications. *Anesthesiology*. 2015;122:1201–1213.
41. Ramachandran SK, Mathis MR, Tremper KK, Shanks AM, Kheterpal S. Predictors and clinical outcomes from failed Laryngeal Mask Airway Unique: a study of 15,795 patients. *Anesthesiology*. 2012;116:1217–1226.
42. Habib AS, Reuveni J, Taguchi A, White WD, Gan TJ. A comparison of ondansetron with promethazine for treating postoperative nausea and vomiting in patients who received prophylaxis with ondansetron: a retrospective database analysis. *Anesth Analg*. 2007;104: 548–551.
43. Gan TJ, Belani KG, Bergese S, et al. Fourth Consensus guidelines for the management of postoperative nausea and vomiting. *Anest Analg*. 2020;131(2):411–448.
44. Alfano G, Grieco M, Forino A, Meglio G, Pace MC, Iannotti M. Analgesia with paracetamol/tramadol vs. paracetamol/codeine in one day-surgery: a randomized open study. *Eur Rev Med Pharmacol Sci*. 2011;15:205–210.
45. White PF, Tang J, Wender RH, et al. The effects of oral ibuprofen and celecoxib in preventing pain, improving recovery outcomes and patient satisfaction after ambulatory surgery. *Anesth Analg*. 2011;112:323–329.
46. De Oliveira GS Jr, Castro-Alves LJ, McCarthy RJ. Single-dose systemic acetaminophen to prevent postoperative pain: a meta-analysis of randomized controlled trials. *Clin J Pain*. 2015;31:86–93.
47. Dahl JB, Nielsen RV, Wetterslev J, et al; Scandinavian Postoperative Pain Alliance (ScaPAlli). Post-operative analgesic effects of paracetamol, NSAIDs, glucocorticoids, gabapentinoids and their combinations: a topical review. *Acta Anaesthesiol Scand*. 2014;58:1165–1181.

32 Office-Based Anesthesia

LAURENCE M. HAUSMAN • DENNIS GRECH

KEY POINTS

1. An office-based anesthetic is one that is performed in an outpatient venue such as a freestanding medical or surgical office or procedure room that is not accredited as either an ambulatory surgery center (ASC) or a hospital.
2. Cost containment and patient convenience are the two major advantages of office-based procedures over traditional hospital-based procedures.
3. The disadvantages of office-based procedures are related to patient safety, reporting, quality improvement, and peer review. Thus, great care must be taken concerning these issues.
4. Office-based morbidity and mortality is usually the result of inadequate perioperative patient monitoring, oversedation, and thromboembolic events.
5. The injuries that occur in offices tend to be of greater severity than those that occur in ambulatory surgical centers. Twenty-one percent of the reported injuries sustained in offices were temporary and nondisabling in nature and 64% were permanent or led to death, whereas 62% of the injuries sustained in ambulatory surgical centers were temporary and nondisabling and only 21% were permanent or led to death.
6. The American Society of Plastic Surgeons acknowledged that the ideal patient for an office-based procedure has an American Society of Anesthesiology (ASA) physical status of 1 or 2. They recommended that ASA physical status 3 patients undergo an office-based procedure only after an anesthesia consultation and only have an office-based procedure performed under local anesthesia without sedation.
7. Pulmonary embolism arising from deep vein thrombosis remains an important risk of an office-based procedure.
8. When formulating a quality improvement program, there should be random chart reviews as well as key sentinel events that trigger a case review.
9. The anesthesiologist should function as a zealous patient advocate in assuring that an anesthetic only is performed in a safe anesthetizing location. Issues that must be sorted out and codified include equipment, monitoring in conformance with ASA standards, emergency drugs and equipment, controlled substance handling and storage, medical director and governance, plan for hospital admission if needed, fire prevention and preparedness, and accreditation.
10. Nonfatal injuries occurring during monitored anesthesia care were more likely to be permanent than the nonfatal injuries occurring during general anesthesia, which were more frequently temporary. Of all injuries occurring during monitored anesthesia care, 34% were fatalities.
11. In terms of smooth operation of an office-based anesthesia practice and patient satisfaction, prevention of postoperative nausea and vomiting and pain are paramount.

1 Office-based anesthesia (OBA) is a subset of both non-operating room anesthesia (NORA) and ambulatory anesthesia. NORA refers to any anesthetic that takes place outside of the traditional operating room (OR) or delivery room but often performed within a fully licensed hospital. NORA locations include endoscopy suites, invasive radiology suites, magnetic resonance imaging (MRI) machine, or an area in which electroconvulsive therapy (ECT) takes place. An ambulatory anesthetic is defined as one in which the patient arrives to the surgical venue on the day of the procedure, is anesthetized, and is discharged home later that same day.

An OBA is one that is performed in an outpatient venue such as a free-standing medical or surgical office or procedure room that is not accredited by a nationally accepted accrediting body as either an ambulatory surgery center (ASC) or as a hospital. The surgical/medical office often provides practitioners with the space for other activities such as consultation with new patients, the performance of routine history and physicals, and office administration. Office-based practices are generally confined to one specialty such as urology, gastroenterology, plastic surgery, or dentistry[1,2]; but, some surgical offices provide OR space for a number of surgical and procedural subspecialties under one roof.

Although an OBA practice may be an exciting alternative to the traditional hospital-based one, it requires the anesthesiologist to expand their role within the health care delivery system. The anesthesia provider must deliver safe anesthetics to patients that may be young or old, and although they usually are healthy, some are medically compromised. Many of the patients are scheduled to undergo complex procedures, thus the anesthesiologist must understand office safety and policy, legal and financial issues (such as antitrust laws, state laws and regulations), the need for possible accreditation, and billing and collection issues.[3,4] These are relatively new responsibilities for the anesthesiologist, who historically has worked as a member within a hospital department either in the private or academic setting, where these responsibilities are given to hospital administrators, lawyers, nurses, and other medical professionals. A further challenge to the office-based practitioner is that presently they have received little to no training in OBA within the anesthesia residency curriculum.[5]

Brief Historical Perspective of OBA

There have been reports of office-based surgery and anesthesia since the mid-19th century. In 1856, John Snow documented his experience in providing anesthesia with chloroform for 867 dental patients, and approximately 3,021 teeth were extracted in private dental offices under his care.[6] In addition to dental care, the family physician often performed house calls where numerous small surgical procedures such as the lancing of boils and repair of wounds were conducted within the comfort of the patient's home. The physician's private medical office was, likewise, utilized in the service of this type of surgical care.

As surgery became more invasive, the need for intensive perioperative physiologic monitoring became increasingly necessary. The capacity to administer blood products and the development of an extensive array of pharmaceutical agents began to play a role in health care, fostering the growth of larger health care delivery teams to assist in patient care. Over time, the inpatient hospital became the primary setting in which surgery would be performed.

Over the past several decades, as a result of both surgical and anesthetic advances, the surgical experience has again changed. Through innovations such as laparoscopic and endoscopic surgical capabilities, surgery has become increasingly less invasive and less painful. In addition, newer anesthetics have the benefit of a "fast-acting" profiles (associated with quick onsets and rapid termination of effect) and with fewer hemodynamic side effects, lending increasing numbers and types of procedures to be suitable for performance in outpatient and office-based venues.[7–9]

During the 1970s, fewer than 10% of all surgical and diagnostic procedures were performed on an ambulatory basis and, virtually all of these were performed in hospitals. Meaning that the patient still needed to register at a hospital, undergo surgery, and then be discharged home later that day. They did not go to a freestanding ASC.

By 1987, approximately 25 million, or 40% of all procedures, were performed on an ambulatory basis. In the United States, between 1984 and 1990, the number of office-based procedures increased from 400,000 to 1.2 million, and by 1994, 8.5% of all procedures were performed in offices.[10] In 1994, a landmark survey of the membership of the American Society of Plastic Surgeons (ASPS) revealed that 55% of the respondents performed the majority or all of their procedures in an office.[11] By the year 2000, approximately 75% of all procedures were performed on an outpatient basis; 17% in freestanding ASCs, and 14% to 25% (approximately 8 to 10 million) in physicians' offices.[12–16] By 2005, the American Hospital Association reported that while 82% of all procedures were performed on an ambulatory basis, 16% of all these ambulatory procedures were performed in private offices. By 2010, 17% to 24% of all surgical procedures (approximately 10,000,000 procedures) were performed in private surgical offices annually.[17] ASCs have continued to expand with centers with two or more ORs increasing, and those with one OR decreasing in number.[18] The most rapid growth of ASC has been in centers with nine or more ORs with pain procedures and orthopedic surgeries being the most common types of surgery in the ACS.[18] Endoscopies have increased threefold from 2014 to 2019 and are now the fourth most common procedure performed in an ASC. In addition, in a prospective cohort study that studied 129,007 patients (183,914 procedures), the American Society for Aesthetic Plastic Surgery (ASAPS) found that a 5% increase in office-based cosmetic procedures from 56.3% to 61.9% occurred from 2014 to 2015.[19] Currently, in a retrospective study that utilized multiple logistic regression analysis to analyze 2,089,830 cases, it was reported that over 65% of all surgical procedures are scheduled in an ambulatory setting,[20] with 10% to 12% being in an office-based facility.[19]

The Advantages and Disadvantages of Office-Based Surgery and Anesthesia

There are many advantages to an office-based procedure when 2
compared to a traditional hospital-based one, with one of the most obvious being cost containment (NICV 32-1).[21] Several components make up the actual cost of a given surgical procedure. In addition to the professional fees of both the proceduralist and the anesthesia provider (which are usually negotiated prior to an elective procedure), there is a facility fee charged by the hospital or ASC. This fee generally covers the associated costs to the specific site, and includes overhead such as maintenance, equipment, and staffing. It often constitutes a large component of the patient's overall charge. In an office, this amount can easily be predicted and is often significantly less. The reason for this discrepancy is that while the overhead costs in a small office are usually lower and managed, the comparable costs in a large tertiary care hospital can be both enormous and complicated to tease apart.[12,13,22,23]

To get a historical perspective of cost analysis, in 1994, Schultz determined the cost of an in-hospital laparoscopic inguinal hernia repair to be $5,494. When the same procedure was performed in an office, the price was decreased to $1,534. Similarly, the average cost of an in-hospital open inguinal hernia repair that same year was found to be $2,237, while only $894.79 when performed in a private office.[24] More recently, it has been reported that office-based ocular surgeries, performed under monitored anesthesia care (MAC), can cost 70% less than similar procedures performed in a hospital.[25] A recent study found that when dental rehabilitation is performed in an office, the cost is approximately 13 times less than when done in a hospital.[20] This resulted in an average savings of $6,800 per case.

Data from 1995 to 2019 demonstrated that ENT procedures performed in an outpatient clinic had considerably lower costs.[26] In addition, a comparison of 750 pediatric dental patients undergoing hospital-based general anesthesia (GA) *versus* OBA showed a decrease of 84.4% for anesthesia and facility fees if the treatment was provided in an office-based setting.[27] It is understandable why insurance companies now often offer incentives to surgeons who utilize an office location as their preferred surgical venue.[28]

Other clear advantages of office-based procedures include ease of scheduling (often with less "paperwork"), patient and surgeon convenience, decreased patient exposure to nosocomial infections, and both improved patient privacy and continuity of care, since an office is usually staffed by a small consistent group of personnel.[3,13,29,30]

There is evidence that, in addition to cost savings, office-based 3
procedures can be completed in less time than in a traditional

hospital-based setting. In a comparative study that looked at patients undergoing 135 dental procedures, 114 patients underwent an OBA and 23 underwent an anesthetic delivered in a hospital OR. The mean case duration in the office-based setting was 56.2 minutes (standard deviation 16.1) *versus* 130.9 minutes (standard deviation 20.3) in the hospital OR.[31]

In a retrospective analysis, Rashewsky et al. studied completed records of 98 cases of pediatric dental rehabilitation.[23] The total anesthesia time in the office-based setting was 157 minutes (standard deviation 97.2) *versus* 222 minutes (standard deviation 62.7) for the hospital OR setting.[27]

Safety is always a concern when considering an OBA. According to a systematic review of 10 studies, evidence supports the conclusion that similar levels of patient safety for procedures done in an ASC *versus* OBA exist.[32] Achieving a high degree of safety with OBA depends on a number of factors including proper patient selection, which will be discussed later in this chapter. Of note, a recent review confirmed that it is crucial that anesthesiologists and surgeons work together to identify patients that are appropriate for an office-based procedure.[33]

Along with advantages, there are, of course, potential disadvantages to an office-based procedure. As alluded to earlier, disadvantages often relate to issues regarding patient safety (both true and perceived), reporting issues, quality improvement, and the existence of peer review.[34] In some parts of the United States, no regulations governing office-based surgery and OBA exist. Therefore, there may be practicing surgical offices in some U.S. states where there is little to no oversight regarding the certification or qualification of either the surgeon or the anesthesiologist to perform the intended procedures. There would likewise be no oversight regarding the evaluation of the surgical office's policy regarding peer review, performance and quality improvement, documentation, general policies and procedures, and the reporting of adverse outcomes. The office could have no policies whatsoever. Fortunately, the number of such states without any regulations and/or oversight is rapidly decreasing (Table 32-1).[35] The number of states with existing regulations is ever-growing and the actual regulations are in a state of flux. It is imperative that the practicing anesthesiologist be familiar with all laws and regulations that exist in the location of their practice.[36] Failure to adhere to local regulations and standards could be considered professional misconduct or even result in a criminal prosecution.

Table 32-1 States Which Have Regulations Regarding Office-Based Surgery and Anesthesia[193]

Alabama	Indiana	North Carolina
Arkansas	Kansas	Ohio
Arizona	Kentucky	Oklahoma
Alaska	Louisiana	Oregon
California	Maine	Pennsylvania
Colorado	Maryland	Rhode Island
Connecticut	Massachusetts	South Carolina
Delaware	Michigan	Tennessee
Washington D.C	Mississippi	Texas
Florida	Nevada	Virginia
Georgia	New Jersey	Washington
Illinois	New York	

Office Safety

As mentioned earlier, safety in an office-based practice is always in question. Early media reports and newspaper articles raised the initial questions regarding the safety of office-based procedures.[37] These news pieces were usually a result of a bad surgical or anesthetic outcome in the area. The exposés in the lay press may be legitimate. In fact, the remote location of an office could conceivably confer an increased risk of injury during an OBA.[38]

Data reveal that injuries and deaths occurring in offices are often multifactorial in causation. Reasons include toxicity of local anesthetics, prolonged surgery with occult blood loss, pulmonary embolism, accumulation of multiple anesthetics resulting in oversedation, hypovolemia, hypoxemia, and the use of reversal drugs with short half-lives.[39–41] Both the Anesthesia Patient Safety Foundation and the American Society of Anesthesiologists (ASA) have emerged as leaders in the field of OBA safety and have advocated that the quality of care in office-based practice be no less than that of a hospital or freestanding ASC.[42] Thus, it is imperative to ensure that all safety precautions one may take for granted in a hospital be present in the surgical office.

In 1990, the mortality rate from anesthesia was approximately 1/100,000. By the year 2000, the rate had decreased to 1/250,000 in hospitals and 1/400,000 in freestanding ASCs.[43] Although the interpretation of these figures is open to debate, the decrease in mortality can be attributed, in part, to improvements in the training of the anesthesia providers, the safety profiles of the newer anesthetics, enhanced perioperative monitoring capabilities, and intrinsic safety mechanisms in place within the anesthetizing location. Since the majority of office-based patients are young and healthy, one would expect that anesthetics performed in offices would be at least as safe as those performed in hospitals, if not safer. However, reports of morbidity and mortality within office-based practices exist. In 1997, Morello et al. conducted a survey querying 418 accredited plastic surgeons' offices. They had a 57% response rate and found that over a 5-year period, 400,675 office procedures were performed; of these, 63.2% were cosmetic and 36.8% were reconstructive. Several outcomes were reviewed including hemorrhage, hypertension, hypotension, wound infection, need for hospital admission, and reoperation. There was an overall complication rate of 0.24%, and seven mortalities occurred, which were secondary to both surgery and anesthesia. These mortalities included two myocardial infarctions, (one following an augmentation mammoplasty, the other 4 hours after a rhinoplasty), one case of cerebral hypoxia during an abdominoplasty, one tension pneumothorax during a breast augmentation, one cardiac arrest during carpal tunnel surgery, one stroke 3 days following a rhytidectomy and brow lift, and one unexplained death.[44] These data represented an overall mortality rate of 1 in 57,000. A later report by Hoefflin et al., however, found no complications after 23,000 plastic surgical procedures that occurred in a single office under GA.[45] Similarly, Sullivan et al. retrospectively reviewed the results in an office performing over 5,000 surgical procedures by five independent plastic surgeons. The primary anesthetic technique during this period consisted of deep sedation in conjunction with local anesthesia or regional block, which was performed by an anesthesiologist supervising a certified registered nurse anesthetist (CRNA). No mortalities occurred over the 5-year period.[46] Bitar et al. retrospectively studied adverse outcomes in 3,615 consecutive patients undergoing

4,778 plastic surgery procedures in offices between 1995 and 2000. The anesthetics were MAC with midazolam, propofol, and an opioid, and again, no deaths were reported. Dyspnea occurred in 0.05% of patients, nausea and vomiting 0.2%, and there was a 0.05% rate of hospital admissions.[47] When analyzing these outcomes, it must be appreciated that, since the mortality rate from anesthesia is so low, an extremely large cohort group would be necessary to provide sufficient data to assess the relative risk of an OBA.

A more recent prospective cohort study of 183,914 cosmetic procedures (129,007 patients) demonstrated complication rates in OBA, ASCs, and hospitals of 1.3%, 1.9%, and 2.4%, respectively. The multivariate analysis showed a lower risk of developing complications in OBA compared to an ASC (relative risk [RR] 0.67, 95% confidence interval [CI] 0.59–0.77, $p < .01$) or a hospital (RR 0.59, 95% CI 0.52–0.68, $p < .01$).[20] The same study showed lower rates of hematomas, infections, and pulmonary dysfunction in office-based surgery (0.6%, 0.3%, and 0.1%) compared to ASCs (1.0%, 0.5%, and 0.1%) and hospitals (1.0%, 0.6%, and 0.2%, respectively, $p < .03$).[19]

A closer look at the more recent data supports the supposition that an office-based procedure is as safe as a procedure done in a more traditional setting. Keyes et al. looked at adverse events in offices accredited by the American Association for Accreditation of Ambulatory Surgical Facilities, Inc. (AAAASF) between 2001 and 2002. This group found no increase in morbidity and mortality in patients who had procedures with OBA, when compared to those having surgery in a freestanding ASC.[48,49] The group then analyzed the charts of 1,000,000 patients undergoing ambulatory procedures between 2001 and 2006. They found an overall mortality rate of 0.002% (with more than half the deaths being caused by a pulmonary embolism). They concluded that there is no increase in mortality for an ambulatory setting when compared to a freestanding hospital.[49] Similar results were reported by Soltani et al. when looking at 5,500,000 patients undergoing outpatient surgery.[50]

4 One important caveat when looking at safety records for office-based surgery is that there are no prospective randomized studies. All data presently available in the literature are from retrospective chart reviews.

When examining the relevant literature, it becomes clear that there have been a few studies that reported a poor outcome for patients undergoing office-based procedures. According to closed malpractice claims in Florida, Rao et al. reported 830 deaths and 4,000 injuries associated with OBA between 1990 and 1999. These claims accounted for 30% of all malpractice claims in that state. Other published data showed that office-based morbidity and mortality is usually the result of inadequate perioperative patient monitoring, oversedation, and thromboembolic events.[37,39,51] The challenge of acquiring accurate morbidity and mortality data for OBA is complicated by the fact that many offices are not required to report adverse events. In addition, although an anesthesiologist may not even be administering the anesthetic in an office, many complications may still be reported as "anesthetic related."

Why should the surgical venue affect the safety of a particular procedure? Again, the difference may be multifactorial. For example, traditional credentialing procedures, such as board certification and the granting or renewing of hospital privileges based on competency and proof of continuing medical education, may not be required or enforced in an office. Within and among offices, providers of anesthesia may also have varying degrees of both education and expertise. The provider may be an anesthesiologist, a nurse anesthetist, a dental anesthetist, or a surgeon with little or no training in anesthesia. Furthermore, safety within an anesthetizing location also depends on the perioperative patient monitoring capabilities within the space. Hospitals are mandated by the accrediting organizations to have defined standards of care for monitoring during the perioperative period. Since some U.S. states do not require accreditation of an office, monitoring standards may be lacking in nonaccredited surgical offices.[47]

There have been patient injuries reported during office-based procedures resulting from the use of obsolete and/or malfunctioning anesthesia machines, as well as from alarms that have not been serviced and/or are not functioning properly.[52] The ASA created guidelines for defining anesthesia machine obsolescence. The use of an obsolete anesthesia machine is prohibited if it lacks any essential safety features (e.g., oxygen ratio device, oxygen pressure failure alarm), if the machine has the presence of unacceptable features (e.g., copper kettles or vaporizers with rotary concentration dials that increase vapor concentration when the dial is turned clockwise), or if routine maintenance of the machine is no longer possible.[53]

Without prospective data regarding injuries occurring during 5
office-based surgery and anesthesia, closed claim databases offer the most reliable approximation. A review of ASA Closed Claims Project data, which incorporates information from the 35 liability insurers that indemnify approximately 50% of the practicing anesthesiologists in the United States, reveals that safety concerns in office-based practices are more than theoretical.[38,52] In 2001, there were 753 (13.7%) claims for ambulatory procedures and 14 (0.26%) for office-based ones. This small number of claims is most likely due to the 3- to 5-year time lag in reporting to the database.[43] ASA physical status 1 or 2 females who had undergone elective surgery under GA make up the majority of claims filed. This statistic parallels the profiles of trends seen in ORs and freestanding ASCs. The injuries that occur in offices tend to be of greater severity than those that occur in ASCs. Twenty-one percent of the reported injuries sustained in offices were temporary and nondisabling in nature and 64% were permanent or led to death, while 62% of the injuries sustained in ASCs were temporary and nondisabling and only 21% were permanent or led to death.[43] A study by Coté et al. concluded that the causes for injuries in offices ranged from human error to machine and equipment malfunction (Table 32-2).[54,55]

The Closed Claims Project database reveals that injuries during office-based procedures occur throughout the perioperative period and are multifactorial in etiology. The majority, 64%, occurred intra-operatively, while 14% occurred in the postanesthesia care unit (PACU) and 21% after discharge.[43] Half of these adverse events were respiratory and included airway obstruction, bronchospasm, inadequate oxygenation and ventilation, and unrecognized esophageal intubation. The second most common group of events was considered to be drug related, occurring 25% of the time. These included incorrect agents or doses, allergies, and malignant hyperthermia (MH). Cardiovascular and equipment-related injuries each occurred in 8% of incidents.[43]

Table 32-2 Causes of Injury in the Office-based Practice[46,47]

1. Inadequate resuscitation equipment
2. Inadequate monitoring (most commonly lack of pulse oximetry
3. Inadequate preoperative or postoperative evaluation
4. Human error
   a. Slow recognition of an event
   b. Slow response to an event
   c. Lack of experience
   d. Drug overdosage

The Closed Claims Project was a comparative study that contrasted 121 claims associated with MAC to claims associated with general (1,519) and regional anesthesia (312). The results demonstrated that office-based claims had a threefold increase in deaths when compared to ASCs. An editorial opinion concerning this article showed that 46% of these events may have been avoided by improved monitoring and better patient selection.[56]

An important point to consider when looking at adverse events is whether or not they were preventable. Again, according to the information in the Closed Claims Project database, only 13% of the events that occurred in ASCs were considered preventable, whereas 46% of the office-based ones were deemed so. Furthermore, all of the adverse respiratory events that occurred in the PACUs of offices could have been prevented had pulse oximetry and capnography been used. Care was deemed substandard in 50% of OBA claims and in 34% of ASC ones. In 2001, claims originating from an office-based procedure resulted in a monetary award 92% of the time, with a median payment of $200,000 (ranging between $10,000 and $2,000,000), whereas claims originating from ASC-based procedures were compensated only 59% of the time with a median payout of $85,000 (ranging between $34 and $14,700,000).[43]

Ensuring office-based practice safety is critical. In 2000, the Anesthesia Patient Safety foundation created a task force on patient safety for office-based surgical facilities. Its goal was to scrutinize OBA facilities and weigh the pros of efficiency and cost containment against the possible cons of decreased patient safety during OBA. As a result of this initiative, several studies on this topic were conducted. These studies, such as a multicenter prospective cohort study that looked at 31,010 liposuction procedures, showed less than 1% morbidity and mortality rates for OBA procedures.[57]

Three studies that included different treatment settings performed a subanalysis on mortality and serious adverse event (SAE) ratios. The first study focused on fatalities of patients undergoing liposuction. It showed that 23% of the fatalities occurred in the hospital ORs, 30% in an ASC, and 48% in an office-based setting.[58] Although alarming, this study included patients undergoing combined procedures, which could bias the data. A study by Hausman et al. reported different conclusions. This study found that SAE rate was highest in hospitals and ASCs and lowest in office-based surgical suites.[59] Kaoutzanis and colleagues' data reported serious adverse event SAE rates of 3.3% ($p < .01$), 2.3% ($p < .01$), and 1.6% ($p < .01$) in hospital, ASC, and OBA, respectively.[58] The last two studies eliminated patients undergoing combined procedures (*i.e.*, liposuction and rhinoplasty) in a systematic review study that looked at 24 studies.[60]

Historically, it should be mentioned that after several highly publicized office-based liposuction injuries and deaths in August 2000, the State of Florida placed a 90-day moratorium on all office-based procedures that utilized anesthetic depths greater than conscious sedation while an investigation could be undertaken. During that time, a safety panel comprised of surgeons, anesthesiologists, and other health care professionals was formed and charged with the task of developing recommendations to improve the safety record of office-based procedures. The panel's recommendations focused on factors including patient selection, preoperative evaluation and testing, procedures to be excluded, surgeon qualification, and facility standards.[30,61] Other major organizations that have played a leading role in developing standards for the office-based practitioner include the ASA, ASPS, the American Association of Nurse Anesthetists (AANA), and the American Medical Association (AMA).[42,61–63]

Patient Selection

Proper patient selection is important for a good outcome to an office-based procedure. Prior to presenting for an office-based procedure, the patient's medical condition should be optimally managed.[64] They should have a preoperative history and physical examination documented within 30 days prior to the procedure, and all pertinent laboratory tests as well as any medically indicated specialist consultation(s) must be readily available. Consent for the procedure and the anesthetic must also be in the chart. The anesthesiologist should have access to all of this information preoperatively and, when possible, contact the patient prior to the scheduled procedure.

If a patient's ASA physical status is 1 or 2, the surgeon's office should arrange the surgery as per office protocol. However, if a patient has significant comorbid conditions, a preoperative anesthesiology consultation should be obtained before scheduling the patient for office-based surgery. A protocol regarding the scheduling of patients with significant comorbidities has become increasingly important in OBA because, as OBA became more commonplace, the medical/surgical community began to include older and sicker patients in this venue. There are many office-based practices that perform procedures on ASA physical status 3 patients and several on ASA physical status 4 patients.[65]

Patient selection has always been a controversial topic among anesthesiologists practicing OBA because little morbidity and mortality data exist to support the inclusion or exclusion of specific populations. A similar problem happened during the development of hospital-based ambulatory surgery.

In 1982, Meridy reported that patients should not be excluded from undergoing ambulatory procedures based solely on their age, the type of procedure, or the duration of the planned procedure.[66] Conflicting recommendations do exist. One must always keep in mind the difference between an office-based practice and a freestanding ASC.

The ASPS has acknowledged that the ideal patient for an office-based procedure has an ASA physical status of 1 or 2. They recommended that ASA physical status 3 patients undergo an office-based procedure only after an anesthesia consultation and only have an office-based procedure performed under local anesthesia without sedation. The ASA also developed recommendations regarding patient selection.[67] It is important to realize that the office is often remote, and the anesthesiologist may be unable to get assistance should it be required. Thus, patient groups where development of anesthetic problems are anticipated or may develop should be avoided (Table 32-3). Individual anesthesiologists should therefore consider excluding certain patients with significant comorbid

Table 32-3 Unsuitable Candidates for an Office-Based Procedure

1. Poorly controlled diabetes
2. History of substance abuse
3. Seizure disorder
4. Malignant hyperthermia susceptibility
5. Potential difficult airway
   a. Morbid obesity
   b. Severe obstructive sleep apnea syndrome
6. NPO less than 8 h
7. No escort home
8. Previous adverse outcome from anesthesia
9. Significant drug allergies
10. Aspiration risk

conditions in order to avoid unanticipated problems. Again, these are recommendations that are not based on evidence-based medicine.

A recent retrospective study that utilized multiple logistic regression analysis to analyze 2,089,930 cases demonstrated that higher ASA physical status independently predicted increased medical complications, readmissions, and perioperative mortality for outpatient surgery across surgical subspecialties and anesthesia types. The authors also noted the ASA 4 patients had an 89-fold greater chance of mortality after ambulatory surgery when compared to ASA 1 patients. The authors suggest that patients with high ASA designation (3 and 4) receive their surgeries in a hospital-based setting.[20]

Morbidly obese patients and those with obstructive sleep apnea syndrome (OSAS) present unique and increasingly frequent challenges to the office-based practitioner.[68] Indeed, they are usually the same population, with estimates of 60% to 90% of all obstructive sleep apnea patients being obese (body mass index [BMI] ≥ 30 kg/m^2).[69,70] Confounding this problem is that the majority of the patients with OSAS have yet to be formally diagnosed.[71] In patients who have not been diagnosed with OSAS, the STOP-BANG (snoring, tiredness, observed apnea, high blood pressure, BMI, age, neck circumference, male gender) questionnaire is a helpful and highly sensitive tool.[72–74]

Looking sequentially at anesthesia events during the perioperative period, during the induction of GA, patients with OSAS are often difficult to ventilate and intubate. One of the first steps in the ASA algorithm for management of the difficult intubation is to call for help, which, in an office will only result is help from registered nurse (RNs) and surgeons. If the patients are intubated, patients with OSAS are likely to experience major anesthetic problems after extubation of the trachea.[75] These patients tend to be exquisitely sensitive to the respiratory depressant effects of even small dosages of sedation and/or opioids.[62] They are prone to respiratory distress after extubation or may suffer from respiratory arrest with postoperative sedation or analgesia.[55,76] Although perhaps clinically unimportant, transient hypoxia is often seen during the recovery phase of patients with OSAS.[77] Furthermore, respiratory depression may not be reversible with pharmacologic antagonism.[78] It has been recommended that a postoperative observational unit with close monitoring of oxygen saturation or an intensive care unit setting be used for monitoring the OSAS patient postoperatively.[79] It may thus be prudent to avoid performing GAs in which opioids are required during the perioperative period on any patient with severe OSAS, in an office-based venue.[80] A review of 13 trials of patients with OSA undergoing surgical procedures, including general, orthopedic, laparoscopic, and upper airway surgery, found no clinically significant adverse perioperative outcomes. The authors identified significant adverse outcomes as delayed discharge, readmission, need for a surgical airway, or incidence of anoxic brain injury. The OSAS patients did have a higher incidence of postoperative hypoxemia, but there was no increase in the requirement for postoperative ventilatory assistance or reintubation. An editorial opinion article that examined various studies, including a cohort study, looked at 2,139 patients. The authors note that these patients had an increase in laryngoscopy attempts, a less favorable grade of laryngoscopic view, and increased use of fiberoptic intubation.[56]

The authors of an editorial opinion article stressed the importance of having difficult airway apparatus such as a fiberoptic scope, video laryngoscopy, and supraglottic airway devices available as well as pharmacologic reversal agents sugammadex, neostigmine, naloxone, and flumazenil readily available. During recovery from anesthesia, OSAS patients should be fully monitored by a dedicated practitioner and always remain with the head of the bed elevated to prevent airway obstruction.[56] Patients should be placed on their own CPAP machines after sedation or GA if possible.[81] Monitoring for 60 minutes after patients have met the modified Aldrete PACU discharge criteria is also beneficial. In a prospective cohort study by Gali et al. that looked at 693 patients, the authors found that any patient experiencing adverse respiratory events, categorized as O_2 $<90\%$ on nasal cannula, RR <8 breaths per minute, apnea lasting more than 10 seconds, or pain–sedation mismatch, should be observed for an extended time and evaluated for possible hospital admission.[56] The ASA recommends that patients with OSAS undergoing ambulatory surgery receive at least 3 hours of postoperative observation before discharge to ensure adequate recovery and minimize airway compromise.

Preoperative evaluation of OSAS patients to determine the risk of gastric aspiration should be conducted, and when indicated, the use of proton-pump inhibitors, antacids, or histamine-2 blockers may be used. When dosing medications, use ideal body weight. In certain patients, the use of local anesthesia alone may be the safest option. If sedation is required, short-acting agents such as dexmedetomidine, nitrous oxide, or remifentanil should be used. Substituting nonopioid analgesics such as ketamine, acetaminophen, ketorolac, and corticosteroids will limit postoperative respiratory compromise. Limiting the use of medications that cause apnea such as propofol or methohexital and avoiding opioids with active metabolites such as hydromorphone or morphine are recommended. For postoperative pain, use of long-acting liposomal bupivacaine, ibuprofen, celecoxib, ketorolac, acetaminophen, gabapentin, or pregabalin can limit the need for postoperative opioids.[81]

Pulmonary embolism has long been known to be a significant cause of perioperative morbidity and mortality from office-based surgical procedures.[82,83] Recent studies have revealed that this risk has not dissipated with time.[49,50] Even in 1998, Reinisch et al. found that 0.39% (37/9,493) of patients who underwent rhytidectomy developed a deep vein thrombosis (DVT). Of these, 40.5% (15/37) went on to form a pulmonary embolism. Although GA had only accounted for only 43% of the anesthetic techniques used for the procedure, 83.7% of the embolic events were associated administration of GA.[84] Studies by Keys et al. and Soltani,[49,50] confirmed that PE, in 2014, remained an important risk of an office-based procedure. A multicenter survey study reported that there are 33,000 VTE events each year for patients undergoing plastic surgery.[85] Risk factors for the development of DVT appear in Table 32-4.[86] The ASPS recommends that patients be stratified according to risk and the prophylactic treatment be guided by risk (Table 32-5). A recent study on patients undergoing rhytidectomy

Table 32-4 Risk Factors for the Development of Deep Vein Thrombosis (DVT)

- Age greater than 40
- Antithrombin III deficiency
- Central nervous system disease
- Family history of DVT
- Heart failure
- History of a DVT
- Hypercoagulable states
- Lupus anticoagulant
- Malignancy
- Obesity
- Oral contraceptive use
- Polycythemia
- Previous miscarriage
- Radiation therapy for pelvic neoplasms
- Severe infection
- Trauma
- Venous insufficiency

Table 32-5 Recommended Treatment for Prevention of Deep Vein Thrombosis in Patients, Stratified by Risk[71]

Cohort	Treatment
Low Risk	
• No risk factors • Uncomplicated surgery • Short duration	• Comfortable position • Knees flexed at 5 degrees • Avoid constriction and external pressure
Moderate Risk	
• Age >40 with no other risks • Procedure >30 min • Oral contraceptive use	• Proper positioning • Intermittent pneumatic compression of calf or ankle (prior to sedation and continued until patient is awake and moving) • Frequent alterations of the OR table
High Risk	
• Age >40 with concomitant risk factors • Procedure >30 min	• Treatment as per patients with moderate risk • Preoperative hematology consultation with consideration of perioperative antithrombotic therapy

OR, operating room.

confirms that limiting total operative time is crucial in decreasing the risk of venous thromboembolism (VTE). Performing procedures under local anesthetic, limiting the number of procedures performed during an operative session, and a surgeon who performs a high number of these procedures, all tend to limit operative time and, therefore, lower the risk of VTE.[85] There is also evidence of increased risk of VTE when patients undergo abdominoplasty with another procedure such as liposuction or breast augmentation. Abdominoplasty was shown to have a VTE incidence of 1% to 3%. When performed in conjunction with a second procedure, risk of VTE increased. Likewise, Voss et al. compared intraoperative and postoperative morbidity in the following groups of patients: (1) abdominoplasty plus one of five common gynecologic procedures ($N = 76$); (2) one of the five gynecologic procedures alone, matched for age, weight, and time of operation ($N = 76$); and (3) abdominoplasty alone ($N = 70$) and reported a VTE incidence rate of 6.6% when abdominoplasty was performed along with gynecologic procedures.[85,87]

As more subspecialties begin to perform office-based procedures, and as the population ages, older and sicker patients will present for surgery and anesthesia.[88] The anesthesiologist must be the patient's advocate in the matter of safety. This advocacy can only result from a true understanding of how to adequately select appropriate patients for this unique surgical venue.

Surgeon Selection

The relationship between the surgeon and anesthesiologist must be one of mutual trust and understanding. Since the surgeon performing the procedure may also own the office, they must not put pressure on the anesthesiologist to perform an anesthetic if they believe that the patient or procedure is not appropriate.

The surgeon must have a valid medical license, registration, and Drug Enforcement Administration (DEA) certificate. They should be either board eligible or board certified by a recognized member of the American Board of Medical Specialties, and either have privileges to perform the proposed procedure in a local hospital, or have training and documented competency comparable to a practitioner who does have such privileges in a hospital. Although this requirement may sound intuitive, there have been cases reported of surgeons performing procedures for which they have little or no training.[13] In addition, the surgeon must have adequate liability insurance, at least equal to that carried by the anesthesiologist. If a lawsuit should arise and the surgeon is inadequately insured, the anesthesiologist may be held financially responsible, and become the "deep pocket." Similarly, the facility itself should have adequate liability insurance.

In addition, there should be a system in place for monitoring continuing medical education as well as peer review and ongoing quality improvement for the surgeon/proceduralist, anesthesiologist, and nursing staff. This is often not the case in a small, nonaccredited office-based practice.[13] If an anesthesia group provides care at more than one office, an overall peer review for the practice may be used; it need not be specific to each individual office site. Solo anesthesia practitioners are not exempt from this process. Anesthesiologist should only align themselves with the offices that have ongoing processes, or they should help to organize one. The peer review committee should include surgeons, anesthesiologists, and nursing staff. It should meet regularly and maintain a written record of minutes and recommendations. Similarly, continuing medical education must also be documented and at a minimum should be sufficient to meet relicensing requirements.

When formulating a quality improvement program, there should be random chart reviews as well as key sentinel events that trigger a case review (Table 32-6). It is imperative that this review be an open forum to ensure continued quality improvement of care, and not be biased or hindered by fear of litigation. Legal counsel should be sought to determine whether information disclosed at these meetings is discoverable in a court of law, should a malpractice claim arise. 8

Similar to the quality program, there should be dedicated committees for risk assessment, safety, and infection. All should have specific policies and procedures regarding the objectives and the

Table 32-6 Anesthetic-Related Sentinel Events that Should Trigger a Case Review and be Presented at a Performance Improvement/Quality Assurance Meeting

1. Death
2. Neurologic injury
3. Perioperative myocardial infarction (MI) or stroke
4. Aspiration
5. Reintubation
6. Return to the operating room
7. Peripheral nerve injury
8. Adverse drug reaction
9. Uncontrolled pain or nausea/vomiting
10. Unexpected hospital admission
11. Cardiac arrest
12. Dental injury
13. Incomplete charts
14. Controlled substance discrepancy
15. Patient complaints
16. Corneal Abrasion

MI, myocardial infarction.

everyday running of each committee. Each committee should be headed by a clearly delineated qualified health care worker. All findings of the committees should be reported throughout the organization, both upward to the governing body, laterally and downward as applicable.

Office Selection and Requirements

9 The anesthesiologist should function as a zealous patient advocate in assuring that an anesthetic only is performed in a safe anesthetizing location. The office needs to be appropriately equipped, stocked, and maintained to perform GA (Table 32-7). All supplies must be age and size appropriate for the patient population. If an anesthesia machine or ventilator is present, it must be regularly serviced and calibrated. If potent inhaled volatile agents or N_2O are used, there must be a functioning waste gas scavenging system. This system may be exhausted via a window or roof vent. However, the exhaust must not be situated such that there is a possibility that it will be vented back into the office or into any other inhabited space. Further, it must be in accordance with Occupational Safety and Health Administration (OSHA), as well as state and federal standards. Portable scavenging systems presently available can be safely used. Air testing for trace levels of anesthetic gases should be done on a regular basis. In an office without an exhaust system, only total intravenous anesthesia (TIVA) techniques should be employed if GA is desired.

All offices, even those without ventilators or anesthesia machines, require a means to deliver positive pressure ventilation to the patient's lungs. This can be achieved by using a self-inflating resuscitation device. An adequate supply of compressed oxygen must be present as well as a backup supply for use in an emergency. In offices that do not have a pipeline supply of oxygen, H cylinders are usually used and several E cylinders should be available in reserve. A policy must be in place describing the transport, storage, and disposal of medical gases, consistent with state and local laws. All equipment described in the ASA algorithm for management of the difficult airway should be present.[89] A readily available means to create an emergency surgical airway and jet ventilation capability may be lifesaving.

Table 32-7 Safe Delivery of OBA Requires the Availability of the Following Equipment

Monitors
Noninvasive blood pressure with an assortment of cuff sizes
Heart rate/ECG
Pulse oximeter
Temperature
Capnography
Airway supplies
Nasal cannulas
Oral airways
Facemasks
Laryngeal mask airways
Self-inflating bag-mask ventilation device
Laryngoscopes multiple sizes and styles (Mac and Miller)
Handles
Video laryngoscopes, various sizes
Various sizes of tracheal tubes
Stylettes
Emergency airway equipment (cricothyrotomy kit, transtracheal jet ventilation equipment)
Suction catheters, pharyngeal suction tips, and suction equipment
Cardiac defibrillator
Emergency drugs
ACLS drugs
Dantrolene and malignant hyperthermia supplies
Intravenous lipid infusion if nerve blocks are being performed
Anesthetic drugs
Vascular cannulation equipment

ACLS, advanced cardiac life support.

Recent advances in video laryngoscope technology have made their availability and use much more common. OBA delivery is well suited for the use of these handheld devices. Lewis et al. systematically reviewed 38 studies involving video laryngoscopy and found statistically significant decreases (odds ratio [OddsR] 0.35, 95% CI 0.19–0.65) in failed intubation rates.[90] In addition, they found statistically significant decreases in the incidences of laryngeal trauma (OR 0.68, 95% CI 0.48–0.96) and postoperative hoarseness (OR 0.57, 95% CI 0.36–0.88).[90]

Perioperative monitoring must adhere to the ASA standards for basic anesthetic monitoring.[91] These include continuous monitoring of heart rate and oxygen saturation, intermittent noninvasive blood pressure monitoring, end-tidal carbon dioxide ($EtCO_2$) monitoring and the capacity for both temperature monitoring, and continuous ECG. Monitors must be routinely serviced, calibrated, and repaired as per manufacturers' recommendations (preventative maintenance is usually performed annually). All monitors should have a backup battery supply and there should be an extra monitor available for an emergency. $EtCO_2$ monitoring should be utilized for all depths of sedation from moderation sedation through GA. Currently, the ASA only requires that sedation performed by anesthesiologists to utilize $EtCO_2$ monitoring. If sedation is performed by a nonanesthesiologist, the ASA does not require $EtCO_2$ monitoring. However, most accrediting bodies independently require $EtCO_2$ monitoring be performed for all depths of sedation. Monitoring policies must be entered into a policy manual and must be adhered to. Further, in 2014, the American Association of Oral and Maxillofacial Surgeons Board of Trustees mandated the use of capnography by all of its members for both deep sedation and GA, not just GA.[92]

All emergency drugs appearing on the American Heart Association Advanced Cardiac Life Support (ACLS) protocol should be immediately available in the office, in all patient areas. The expiration dates for these agents should be checked on a regular basis, and outdated drugs replaced. There should be a look-alike/sound-alike policy as well as a high-alert medication policy in the office.

A cardiac defibrillator with a battery backup must be immediately available and routinely checked and maintained, as should a source of suction including pharyngeal suction catheters. Having an "MH" cart containing at least 12 bottles of dantrolene (or its equivalent) is a requirement, if triggering agents are stocked in an office. A complete listing of MH supplies is available online at www.mhaus.org.[93] The office-based anesthesiologist should be familiar with the signs and symptoms of MH and be prepared to initiate treatment. It is recommended that the published MH algorithm be displayed in all areas where triggering agents are used. The office staff should undergo MH drills annually.

A protocol for the delivery and secure storage of controlled substances must be in place. A licensed anesthesiologist may supply these drugs in accordance with DEA regulations, as can any licensed physician with a current DEA registration certificate. Instead of transporting drugs, it is often more convenient to store them in the surgical office. In this situation, they must be stored in a double-locked storage cabinet installed in a secure location, in accordance with state and local regulations. The office in which the controlled substances will be dispensed must also be properly registered with the DEA. Drug accounting must be performed in accordance with state and federal regulations. Individual states have different provisions and regulations regarding the dispensing of controlled substances, and it is the responsibility of the dispensing physician to assure that the office-based practice is in compliance.

The office-based practice must be a legally recognized entity such as a corporation or solo/group practice. A medical director and a governing body, responsible for overall operations and ensuring high-quality patient care, must be identified for every office. There must be a chain of command within the organization, with clearly delineated responsibilities and qualifications. The governing body is ultimately responsible for the determining the mission statement of the practice and making sure that all local and state laws are followed. The governing body is also responsible for developing and reviewing all policies and procedures within the office-based practice. These notions even apply to solo practitioner offices. Policies and procedures will outline exactly how every aspect of the practice will run from administration and governance through clinical outcomes and infection tracing. The governing body should meet at least annually and among other duties, be responsible for the credentialing and privileging of all health care providers and review all aspects of the practice.

There must be a policy and procedures manual that outlines the responsibilities of the governing body, each staff member including nurses (circulating, scrub, and postop), physician assistants, surgical technicians, office staff, and administrators. The manual should include a description of the infection control policy, risk management, safety protocols, anesthesia policies, etc. All nurses should be licensed by the state and have training and education consistent with their responsibilities. Basic cardiac life support (BLS) certification should be mandatory and ACLS certification is preferable for nurses. In addition, either the anesthesiologist or the physician who supervises the anesthesia care provider must be ACLS or pediatric advanced life support (PALS) certified, depending on the patient population. There should always be at least one member of the health care team with current ACLS/PALS certification present in the office until the last patient has been physically discharged from the unit. This policy should be clearly stated in the written policy and procedure manual.

External and internal emergencies such as cardiac arrest, earthquakes, bomb scares, MH, hurricanes, fires, etc., can, and do, occur in office-based settings. (Table 32-8). Each office must have a plan in the procedural manual for delineating the responsibilities of each staff member, in the event of any of these occurrences.

Table 32-8 Emergencies Which Require Contingency Plans

1. Fire
2. Bomb/bomb threat
3. Power loss
4. Equipment malfunction
5. Loss of oxygen supply pressure
6. Cardiac or respiratory arrest in the waiting room, OR, or PACU
7. Earthquake
8. Hurricane
9. External disturbance such as a riot
10. Malignant hyperthermia
11. Massive blood loss
12. Emergency transfer of patient to a hospital

OR, operating room; PACU, postanesthesia care unit.

The physical structure of the office is an important consideration. There should be clear egress that would easily accommodate a stretcher carrying a mechanically ventilated patient. Adequate clearance and room for transport in an elevator must also be considered. The office should have mandatory quarterly drills dealing with both internal and external emergencies.

Destinations for a patient in need of an emergency unplanned hospital admission must be identified. Developing an office–hospital relationship is challenging, as hospitals may be reluctant to be involved in office mishaps. However, it is of utmost importance to have a formal written transfer agreement in place with a local hospital should an emergency requiring hospital admission occur. An alternative is to make sure the physicians in the office-based group have admitting privileges at a local hospital.

There should also be a plan in place regarding how the patient will be physically moved to a local hospital. Telephoning the emergency services number (911) is an acceptable plan for transportation, provided the response time is rapid. If 911 is unavailable in a specific city, or has a slow response time, the office should have a contractual agreement with a local ambulance company.

The office must be prepared to respond to an intraoperative fire. The ASA published an advisory on the prevention and management of a fire emergency.[94] Fire requires three components known as the "fire triad": an oxidizer (oxygen and nitrous oxide [N_2O]), an ignition source (electrocautery, laser, drill), and fuel (sponges, drapes, endotracheal tubes, solutions containing alcohol or other volatile compounds). The modern OR contains all three in great supply. The first step in fire prevention is education. All members of the surgical and anesthesia team must be educated on how fires are started, sustained, and prevented. There must be regularly scheduled fire drills that include all employees, even those with nonclinical duties. These drills should highlight the responsibilities of each staff member. A yearly meeting with the local fire marshal is often helpful.

Fire prevention is of the utmost importance. The ASA recommends that if flammable agents are used to prep the skin, they should be allowed to completely dry prior to draping the surgical field. The field should then be draped in a manner that does not allow for oxygen to accumulate. This is important because these accumulated pockets of oxygen may flow into the surgical field, where there is a source of ignition such as electrocautery. There must be communication between the surgeon and anesthesiologist when an oxygen-rich environment is created near a surgical site. This scenario is common during facial plastic surgery. Medical air insufflation or suctioning can be used to reduce oxygen accumulation and the use of N_2O should be avoided. When using an ignition source in an oxygen-rich environment, the ASA recommends reducing the oxygen flow as low as possible without creating hypoxia, and waiting several minutes to allow the oxygen to dissipate.[86]

The management of a fire will require recognizing the early signs, stopping the procedure and ignition source, extinguishing the fire, and delivering care to the patient. It may even be necessary to evacuate the building. In any case, it is imperative that all these steps be reviewed regularly and drills performed. The office should have at least a 1-hour firewall present to help prevent in the spread of the fire.

There must be contingency plans in the event of a power supply interruption or electrical failure. Each office should have an emergency generator capable of running necessary equipment and monitors; monitors should have battery backup power that is routinely checked. Battery reserve power will usually last for

1 1/2 hours, but should be verified for each piece of electrically powered equipment.

The office should keep patient records (including anesthesia records) in accordance with state statute of limitation laws, which is usually for a minimum of 5 to 7 years. Clinical paper records must be stored in a secure location consistent with health information protection and portability act (HIPPA) regulations, with access limited to medical professionals who are privileged to review these records. Similarly, the anesthesiologist should maintain their own records, which include the preanesthesia history and physical, informed consent, intraoperative documentation, and postoperative care record, as well as discharge orders. Electronic records should be stored consistent with HIPPA privacy regulations and recommendations.

Accreditation

One way to objectively evaluate an office is to have it be accredited by a nationally recognized accrediting agency. The ASA developed a classification of offices that stratifies them by the level of anesthetic depth that may be administered (Table 32-9).[67] Presently, many states require offices to be accredited and more are following suit. In states that do not require accreditation, there are benefits to an office voluntarily obtaining it. Accreditation often will allow the facility fee to be reimbursed by a third-party payer in medically necessary procedures.[95] It should be noted that presently Medicare and Medicaid will not pay a facility fee for an office-based procedure, accredited or nonaccredited. Another possible benefit of accreditation is that the patient may feel more comfortable undergoing a procedure in an office that has been accredited. As more states enact accreditation laws, facilities that are already accredited will ensure continuity of care at these locations.

Currently, there are three major accrediting bodies for office-based surgery offices, although several other agencies are also recognized. The Accreditation Association for Ambulatory Health Care (AAAHC) was the first major accrediting body, offering certification since 1998. The AAAASF, originally the Accreditation Association for Ambulatory Plastic Surgical Facilities (AAAAPSF), was the second, followed by The Joint Commission (TJC). To date, the most active organization in the accreditation of surgical offices is the AAAASF. Although its requirements are similar to those of AAAHC and TJC, the accreditation process is often less expensive. Changes are currently underway to allow AAAHC and TJC to be priced more competitively.[3] Each agency has different criteria for eligibility and different accreditation cycles pertaining to the time limit of a certificate.[96] The agencies deal with the entire perioperative spectrum of running a surgical office, ranging from the physical facility through patient care, governance, risk management, safety, infection, clinical record keeping, and administration (Table 32-10). Each agency has a workbook available to the practitioners to review all requirements of accreditation. Of note, the AAAHC can accredit not only the surgical office, but also anesthesia groups that provide OBA.

The accrediting agencies were developed, in part, to reduce some of the variability that exists among offices in regard to safety and administrative issues. Several professional societies are encouraging their members to perform procedures only in accredited facilities. The Society for Aesthetic Plastic Surgeons mandates that all of its members perform procedures only in offices that have been accredited by one of the nationally recognized accrediting agencies, or have been certified to participate in the Medicare program under title XVIII, or are licensed by the state. The actual improvement in safety conferred by performing surgery in an accredited office has yet to be determined, and there are those who suggest that it provides no advantage.[97] As long as there is no mandatory reporting system in place, it will be impossible to determine true incidence of morbidity associated with office-based practice. Presently, the only accrediting agency that requires reporting of all adverse outcomes in the AAAASF. In addition, several states have similar reporting mandates. Clearly, though safety in an office depends upon more than just accreditation, there must be constant vigilance by all members of the health care team.

Table 32-9 ASA Classification of Surgical Procedures[54]

Class A Minor surgical procedures Local, topical, or infiltration of local anesthetic No sedation preop or intraoperatively
Class B Minor or major surgical procedures Sedation via oral, rectal, or intravenous sedation Analgesic or dissociative drugs
Class C Minor or major surgical procedures General anesthesia Major conduction block anesthesia

Table 32-10 Factors Considered in Accrediting an Office for Surgical Procedures. A Complete Listing of Criteria Can Be Obtained from the Individual Agencies

1. Governance
2. Administration
3. Clinical records and electronic health records
4. Credentialing and privileging
5. Safety
6. Infection control
7. Physical layout of the office
8. Labs
9. Quality improvement
10. Personnel records
11. Surgeon qualification
    a. Training
    b. Local hospital privileges (surgical and admission)
12. Peer review
13. Anesthesiologist requirements and qualification
14. Staffing intra- and postoperatively
15. Monitoring capabilities both intra- and postoperatively
16. Ancillary care
17. Equipment
18. Drugs (emergency, controlled substances, routine medications)
19. BLS, ACLS/PALS certification
20. Temperature
21. Neuromuscular functioning
22. Patient positioning
23. Pre- and postanesthesia care/documentation
24. Quality assurance/peer review
25. Liability insurance
26. PACU evaluation
27. Discharge evaluation
28. Emergency preparedness (fire/admission/transfer, etc.)

ACLS, advanced cardiac life support; BCLS, basic cardiac life support; PACU, postanesthesia care unit; PALS, pediatric advanced life support.

Procedure Selection

Early in the development of office-based surgery, procedures were generally noninvasive and of short duration. However, as newer surgical and anesthetic techniques have evolved, longer and more invasive procedures have been successfully performed.[98–105] Suitable office-based procedures range the gamut from superficial incision and drainage of abscesses to more invasive microlaparoscopies.

Duration of procedure has long been correlated with the need for hospital admission, with procedures lasting more than 1 hour being associated with a higher incidence of unplanned admission.[106] Other data have shown that longer procedures are also often associated with an increased incidence of postoperative nausea and vomiting (PONV), postoperative pain, and bleeding[107,108] which may warrant hospital admission. For these reasons the ASPS recommended that procedures be limited to 6 hours and be completed by 3 PM, thus allowing for a full patient recovery during maximum office staffing.[61] In a systematic review and meta-analysis that examined 66 observational studies, Cheng et al. found that perioperative complications rise with prolonged procedure times.[109] As surgical time exceeds 2 hours, they found that complication rates increase by twofold (pooled OR = 1.99, 95% CI [1.41,2.83], $p < .001$).[109] The authors concluded that surgical care teams should prioritize operating efficiency and optimization of work flows to ensure intraoperative times are as brief as possible. In addition, when determining the suitability of a procedure one must consider the possibility of hypothermia, blood loss, or significant fluid shifts.[61]

Specific Procedures

Liposuction

Liposuction is the most common cosmetic procedure performed primarily by plastic surgeons and dermatologists.[110,111] It is accomplished by inserting hollow rods into small incisions in the skin, and suctioning subcutaneous fat into an aspiration canister. Superwet and tumescent techniques, introduced in the mid-1980s, utilize large volumes (1 to 4 cc) of infiltrate solution (0.9% saline or Ringer lactate with epinephrine 1:1,000,000 and lidocaine 0.025% to 0.1%) for each 1 cc of fat to be removed. Blood loss is generally 1% of the aspirate with these techniques.[112] The peak serum levels of lidocaine occur 12 to 14 hours after injection and decline over the subsequent 6 to 14 hours.[113,114] Although the maximum dose of lidocaine has been traditionally limited to 7 mg/kg, 35 to 55 mg/kg doses have been used safely because the tumescent technique results in a single compartment clearance similar to that of a sustained-release medication.[115]

Liposuction is not a benign procedure.[116] In 2000, a census survey of the 1,200 members of the ASAPS revealed an overall mortality rate of 19.1 per 100,000 liposuction procedures, with pulmonary embolism the diagnosis in 23.1% of deaths. Other etiologies of mortality included abdominal viscous perforation, anesthesia causes, fat embolism, infection, and hemorrhage; 28.5% of all deaths in this study were reported as of unknown or confidential etiology.[117] Risk factors identified included the use of multiliter wetting solution infiltration, megavolume aspiration causing massive third spacing, multiple concurrent procedures, anesthetic sedative effects yielding hypoventilation, and permissive discharge policies. The management of the postoperative period, with attention to fluid and electrolyte balance and pain control, is critical to an optimal outcome after liposuction. The patient's fluid deficit, maintenance, intraoperative loss, and third spacing should guide fluid management throughout the perioperative period. In general, an office liposuction should be limited to 5,000 mL of total aspirant which includes supernatant fat and fluid.[61]

Work performed by Halk et al. demonstrated that tumescent liposuction showed the lowest rate of SAEs, followed by the semi-tumescent, superwet, and wet techniques.[60] The authors found that use of GA and IV sedation also increased rate of SAE. Additional factors shown to increase the rate of SAE include adding abdominoplasty to the liposuction procedure, performing the liposuction in a hospital or ASC, and removing higher volumes of adipose tissue.[60] Kaoutzanis et al. found that type of facility where liposuction procedure is performed is an independent predictor of SAE.[57] Liposuction in hospitals was shown to have a higher risk of major complications compared to ASC or OBS locations with a relative risk of 1.36. The authors note that this may be because high-risk patients may be scheduled for their procedure in a hospital-based surgical facility.[57] Kaoutzanis found that although rare, hematoma, pulmonary dysfunction, surgical site infection, and VTE were the most common major complications.[57] Increased age, elevated BMI, combining other procedures with liposuction, and performing the procedure in a hospital setting were noted as risk factors for major SAEs. Halk et al. found that the most common SAEs for liposuction as an uncombined procedure were excessive blood loss requiring transfusion, infection, and VTE.[60]

Iverson et al. developed the following considerations and recommendations regarding office-based liposuction[30,61]:

1. Plastic surgeons should follow the current ASA Guidelines for Sedation and Analgesia.
2. GA can be used safely in the office setting.
3. GA has advantages for more complex liposuction procedures that include precise dosing of sedatives, controlled patient movement, and airway management.
4. Epidural and spinal anesthesia in the office setting are discouraged because of the possibility of vasodilatation, hypotension, and fluid overload.
5. Moderate sedation/analgesia augments the patient's comfort and is an effective adjunct to the anesthetic infiltrate solutions.

In 2002, 261 respondents to a survey sent to the membership of The American Society for Dermatologic Surgery reported no mortalities among 66,570 liposuction procedures performed in hospitals, ASCs, and offices. The authors reported adverse events, which mirrored those of the ASAPS. They found that SAEs occurred more frequently with procedures performed in hospital and ASCs than in offices. This observation may be due to the fact that in hospitals, liposuction is performed on sicker patients or that the procedures are associated with removal of a larger amount of fat. Interestingly, 71% of the offices surveyed were nonaccredited. Further, the authors reported that morbidity correlated better with the area of the body suctioned (abdomen and buttocks as compared to extremities, which has lower associated morbidity) than the facility in which the procedure took place.[118]

Aesthetics

Many facial aesthetic procedures such as blepharoplasty, rhinoplasty, and meloplasty are routinely performed in offices, usually under varying depths of MAC, but occasionally with GA. Facial plastic procedures that require use of a laser or even routine electrocautery, pose a problem for the anesthesiologist. Supplemental nasal oxygen in patients receiving sedation presents a fire hazard. Any supplemental oxygen must be turned off during periods of laser or electrocautery use about the face, and requires vigilance by the anesthesiologist who must be in constant communication with the surgeon. Methods for delivering supplemental oxygen to a patient having a facial procedure include nasal cannula, an oxygen hood, or placement of oxygen tubing in an oral/nasal airway. The latter usually requires a deeper level of sedation. The avoidance of supplemental oxygen when medically appropriate is ideal.

Breast

Procedures such as breast biopsy or augmentation, implant exchange, and transverse rectus abdominal muscle (TRAM) flap (*i.e.*, nipple construction or revisions) are routinely performed in office settings. Breast augmentation entails separating the pectoralis muscles from the chest wall, which is painful and usually requires GA, which can be accomplished by using either a laryngeal mask airway (LMA), or tracheal tube. The use of regional anesthesia with paravertebral nerve blocks has also been reported.[119] Breast surgery is associated with a high incidence of PONV, thus it is likely that patients undergoing breast surgery will require antiemetic medication in addition to postoperative analgesics.[120]

Gastrointestinal Endoscopy

Procedures performed by gastroenterologists include esophageal, gastric, and duodenal endoscopies (EGD) and colonoscopies. This patient population tends to be older, with significant comorbid conditions. Upper gastrointestinal (GI) procedures rarely require endotracheal intubation because, although many of these patients have gastroesophageal reflux, the stomach is emptied under direct visualization. The endoscopist may require patient participation such as swallowing. This can be achieved by administering small doses of propofol with or without midazolam.

Colonoscopy is uncomfortable secondary to the insertion and manipulation of the endoscope, and may be associated with cardiovascular effects, including dysrhythmias, bradycardia, hypotension, hypertension, myocardial infarction, and death. The mechanism of these cardiovascular effects is not known, but there is evidence that they may be mediated by the autonomic nervous system when stimulated by anxiety or discomfort.[121] Adding an opioid to midazolam during colonoscopy has been shown to improve patient tolerance of the procedure and decrease pain without increasing the frequency of respiratory events.[122] Interestingly, anesthetic techniques consisting of midazolam,[123] remifentanil/propofol, and fentanyl/propofol/midazolam[124] lower the number of episodes of heart rate variability which reflects sympathetic activation as seen on continuous electrocardiography and may contribute to the number of cardiovascular events that occur during colonoscopy.

Recently, the gastroenterology community has sought to be able to provide moderate or even deep sedation with propofol without the assistance of a trained anesthesiologist.[125] However, due to safety concerns, propofol may still only be given by an anesthesiologist as indicated in the product insert. In addition, the ASA "Statement on Safe Use of Propofol" states that "the practitioner administering propofol for sedation/anesthesia should, at a minimum, have the education and training to identify and manage the airway and cardiovascular changes which occur in a patient who enters a state of general anesthesia, as well as the ability to assist in the management of complications."[126] The AAAASF has, likewise, indicated that anesthesia professionals are best qualified to administer propofol sedation. Every office should clearly delineate who is privileged and credentialed to administer propofol.

Dentistry/Oral and Maxillofacial Surgery

N_2O has been used for most of the world's office-based dental anesthetics since 1884, when Horace Wells, himself a dentist, had N_2O administered for a wisdom tooth extraction by a colleague. It was Harry Langa, another dentist, who pioneered the concept of using lower concentrations of N_2O in combination with local anesthetics. This idea of "relative analgesia" was the forbearer of "conscious sedation."[127]

The American Association of Oral and Maxillofacial Surgeons studied a prospective cohort of patients who underwent oral and maxillofacial surgery (OMS) between January and December 2001 (NICV 32-2). Of the 34,191 patients included, 71.9% received deep sedation/GA, 15.5% conscious sedations, and 12.6% local anesthesia. The operating surgeon provided anesthesia services in 96% of cases, and anesthesia-specific hospitalization rate was 4 per 100,000, with no reported mortalities. The authors attributed this safety level to the use of pulse oximetry, blood pressure and ventilation monitoring, as well as administration of supplemental oxygen.[128] Newer studies have found that the majority of patients are satisfied with the use of office-based sedation and GA.[129] Patient's biggest concerns and reason for dissatisfaction continue to be pain, nausea and vomiting, or being "awake" during the procedure.[130] Because office-based OMS procedures are so common and patients are presenting with more comorbidities, it is likely that anesthesiologists will increase their presence in this arena. All American Association of OMS members agree to have their offices undergo a periodic anesthesia peer review process to assure that staff are trained and equipped to deliver safe anesthesia and deal with untoward events.[131] Delivery of anesthesia requires standard ASA monitoring including monitoring of blood pressure and temperature every 5 minutes, continuous ECG, pulse oximetry, and $EtCO_2$ monitoring. Ultra–short-acting anesthetic agents without active metabolites are ideal for use in the office-based dental anesthesia.[132]

Orthopedics/Podiatry

Orthopedic offices provide excellent locations for anesthesiologists who practice regional anesthesia. While knee arthroscopies can be performed with intraarticular local anesthesia and MAC, an adductor canal block with bupivacaine or ropivacaine, supplementing the intra-articular local anesthetic in an arthroscopically assisted anterior cruciate ligament (ACL) repair will provide long-acting postoperative analgesia. Interscalene, supraclavicular, infraclavicular, and axillary blocks avoid airway manipulations in patients undergoing upper extremity procedures, while ankle blocks or blocks of the sciatic nerve in the popliteal fossa provide anesthesia for operations on the lower extremity. All of these blocks can be supplemented with short-acting anxiolytic agents.

Spinal anesthetics in the office-based setting must be of short duration, secondary to limited PACU space. Lidocaine, which provides reliable short-acting analgesia, may be associated with an increased risk of transient neurologic symptoms (TNS) in the ambulatory patient population,[129] whereas using procaine–fentanyl spinals are associated with nausea and vomiting as well as pruritus.[133] When the neuraxial anesthetic wears off, postoperative pain may arise; therefore, the patient must be discharged with oral analgesics as well as contact information for both the surgeon and the anesthesiologist.

Gynecology/Genitourinary

Many procedures, such as dilation and curettage, vasectomy, and cystoscopy have been routinely performed in offices, often with local anesthesia and no sedation.[134] Recently, there has been an increase in more invasive procedures (on older patients) such as minilaparoscopies, ovum retrieval, prostate biopsies, and lithotripsy, necessitating an anesthesiologist's expertise.[135] A variety of anesthetic options are available for these procedures and the anesthetic choice depends on the surgeon, patient, and anesthesiologist's preferences.

Ophthalmology/Otolaryngology

Ophthalmologic procedures suitable for the office include cataract extractions, lacrimal duct probing, and ocular plastics. Topical anesthesia and periorbital or retrobulbar blocks are frequently used to provide analgesia. Supplemental sedation may be required. Otolaryngology procedures include endoscopic sinus surgery, turbinate resection, septoplasty, and myringotomy.[136] Again, combinations of topical and regional nerve blocks, with supplemental sedation are commonly employed, but occasionally GA is used.[137,138]

Pediatrics

Although no minimum age requirement for a child to undergo an OBA has been established, patients with postgestational age greater than 6 months and ASA physical status 1 or 2 may be reasonable candidates.[22] Appropriate OBA pediatric cases are usually dental, and chloral hydrate with N_2O has historically been the anesthetic choice of many dentists. The use of these agents is, however, associated with significant morbidity. Ross et al. found that in children between the ages of 1 and 9 years, 70 mg/kg of chloral hydrate with 30% N_2O resulted in hypoventilation in 94% of patients, which increased to 97% of patients when the chloral hydrate was combined with 50% N_2O.[22] This increase is significant in view of the findings of Coté et al. who reviewed 95 adverse sedation-related events in pediatric patients. In the 93% of these cases that resulted in permanent neurologic injury or death, the anesthetic was delivered by either an oral surgeon, periodontist, or CRNA supervised by a dentist.[54,55]

There are increasing numbers of ophthalmologic, (examination under anesthesia, lacrimal duct probing), otolaryngology (myringotomy), cast/dressing changes, and minor plastics procedures being performed on children in offices. The American Academy of Pediatrics, Section on Anesthesiology developed guidelines for the pediatric perioperative environment, which should be adhered to in the office setting (Table 32-11).[139]

Table 32-11 Guidelines for the Pediatric Perioperative Anesthesia Environment Include the Following Considerations:

Patient care facility and medical staff policies
Designation of operative procedures
Categorization of pediatric patients undergoing anesthesia
Annual minimal case volume to maintain clinical competence
Clinical privileges of anesthesiologists
Regular privileges
Special pediatric clinical privileges
Pain management
Patient care units
Preoperative evaluation and preparation units
Operating room
Anesthesiologists
Other health care providers involved in perioperative care
Clinical laboratory and radiologic services availability and capabilities
Pediatric anesthesia equipment and drugs including resuscitation cart
PACU
Nursing staff
Anesthesiologist/physician staff
Pediatric anesthesia equipment and drugs
Postoperative intensive care

PACU, postanesthesia care unit.

Anesthetic Techniques

The ASA recommends that anesthetics be provided or supervised by a fully licensed anesthesiologist.[67] If an anesthesiologist is directing anesthesia care, they must be immediately available throughout the entire perioperative period. Regulations in several states have questioned the need for this level of anesthesia training in the delivery of OBA. Some states allow for an anesthetic to be performed by a nonphysician anesthesia provider supervised by a licensed physician. In this situation, the supervising physician must be qualified to perform a preanesthetic focused history and physical examination as well as be immediately available throughout the perioperative period. They must know how to handle anesthetic-related emergencies and complications. The supervising physician must be ACLS certified.

OBA requires many levels of anesthesia, ranging from moderate sedation through regional and GA (1 Video 32-1).[140] Anesthesia is, however, a continuum and it is often impossible to predict how a patient will react. The ASA developed definitions regarding depths of anesthesia (Table 32-12). Patients will routinely drift between depths of sedation, thus it is imperative that the anesthesia provider or supervisor be able to rescue a patient from a deeper level of anesthetic than was anticipated.

When formulating an anesthetic plan, one must consider that all agents and techniques used should be short acting, and patients should be ready for discharge home soon after the completion of the procedure. Furthermore, any agents used should have a high safety profile, few side effects, and be cost-effective. One must not be under the false impression that sedation is inherently safer than GA. Cohen et al. reviewed data from 10,000 anesthetics and found monitored anesthesia care to have the highest rate of mortality of 208.85 per 10,000 anesthetics.[141] The complication rate related to MAC anesthetics is increasing, as its use expands.

10

The ASA Closed Claims Project database reveals that in the 1970s, sedation (often referred to as MAC) cases accounted for 1.6% of the claims, in the 1980s for 1.9%, and by the 1990s for 6% of the cases. The injuries sustained in patients receiving MAC ranged from emotional distress to death (Table 32-13). The percentage of claims resulting in mortality was identical for both MAC and GA cases. In the 1990s, when injuries other than death occurred during MAC anesthetics, they were more likely to be permanent, whereas injuries occurring during GA were more frequently temporary.[142] MAC anesthetics also tend to lead to litigation. Suits were filed in 90% of the MAC claims; 65% were settled, 20% went to judgment, and 15% were dismissed. The range of payout was $2,000 to $6,300,000 with a median of $75,000.[142]

Anesthetic Agents

Intravenous (IV) sedation (propofol, midazolam, fentanyl) is the most often used anesthetic technique in the OBA setting. When selecting an anesthetic for an office-based procedure, one must consider factors such as duration of action, presence of active metabolites, cost-effectiveness, and safety/side effects profile.

Table 32-12 Continuum of Depth of Sedation: Definition of General Anesthesia and Levels of Sedation/Analgesia

	Minimal Sedation Anxiolysis	Moderate Sedation/Analgesia ("Conscious Sedation")	Deep Sedation/Analgesia	General Anesthesia
Responsiveness	Normal response to verbal stimulation	Purposeful** response to verbal or tactile stimulation	Purposeful** response following repeated or painful stimulation	Unarousable even with painful stimulus
Airway	Unaffected	No intervention required	Intervention may be required	Intervention often required
Spontaneous Ventilation	Unaffected	Adequate	May be inadequate	Frequently inadequate
Cardiovascular Function	Unaffected	Usually maintained	Usually maintained	May be impaired

Developed By: Committee on Quality Management and Departmental Administration
Last Amended: October 23, 2019 (original approval: October 13, 1999).
https://www.asahq.org/standards-and-guidelines/continuum-of-depth-of-sedation-definition-of-general-anesthesia-and-levels-of-sedationanalgesia
Minimal sedation (anxiolysis) is a drug-induced state during which patients respond normally to verbal commands. Although cognitive function and physical coordination may be impaired, airway reflexes, and ventilatory and cardiovascular functions are unaffected.
Moderate sedation/analgesia ("conscious sedation") is a drug-induced depression of consciousness during which patients respond purposefully** to verbal commands, either alone or accompanied by light tactile stimulation. No interventions are required to maintain a patent airway, and spontaneous ventilation is adequate. Cardiovascular function is usually maintained.
**Reflex withdrawal from a painful stimulus is NOT considered a purposeful response.
Deep sedation/analgesia is a drug-induced depression of consciousness during which patients cannot be easily aroused but respond purposefully** following repeated or painful stimulation. The ability to independently maintain ventilatory function may be impaired. Patients may require assistance in maintaining a patent airway, and spontaneous ventilation may be inadequate. Cardiovascular function is usually maintained.
General anesthesia is a drug-induced loss of consciousness during which patients are not arousable, even by painful stimulation. The ability to independently maintain ventilatory function is often impaired. Patients often require assistance in maintaining a patent airway, and positive pressure ventilation may be required because of depressed spontaneous ventilation or drug-induced depression of neuromuscular function. Cardiovascular function may be impaired.

Ideal drugs should have a short half-life, be inexpensive, and not be associated with undesirable side effects such as nausea and vomiting.

Because of its desirable pharmacokinetics and pharmacodynamics, propofol, a di-isopropyl phenol molecule, has long been a mainstay of ambulatory anesthesia. It has a rapid onset (approximately 1 arm–brain circulation time), and because of rapid redistribution, has a short clinical duration of action (approximately 15 minutes). Its short context-sensitive half-time causes propofol's clinical effect to be terminated relatively quickly, even after relatively long infusion times (8 hours).[143] In addition to its hypnotic properties, it has an intrinsic antiemetic effect. Propofol may cause a burning sensation on injection or elicit an allergic reaction. It is also associated with bradycardia and respiratory depression, and it supports microbial growth. It can be used alone or in combination with other agents by intermittent boluses or continuous infusion.

Table 32-13 Patient Injuries During Sedation and MAC[142]

1. Death	34%
2. Brain damage	19%
3. Nerve damage	7%
4. Eye damage	12%
5. Myocardial infarction	4%
6. Stroke	4%
7. Burn	4%
8. Emotional distress	4%
9. Aspiration	4%

Fentanyl is the gold standard for "short-acting" narcotics It has an intermediate duration and does not cause histamine release. The use of remifentanil has also increased in popularity. Remifentanil, an ultra–short-acting opioid, when combined with propofol for conscious sedation, has been shown to provide discharge readiness within 15 minutes after colonoscopy. This time frame is a marked reduction from the 48 to 80 minutes reported after the traditional meperidine/midazolam technique.[144] Remifentanil is also an ideal drug for use during many office-based procedures such as facial cosmetic procedures, which can be quite painful while the local anesthetic is being injected after which is relatively painless. An important caveat to the use of remifentanil is that it may cause nausea and vomiting as well as apnea. Infusions of remifentanil are also associated with acute tolerance and hyperalgesia during the recovery phase, which may limit its utility.[145–148] In addition, it often requires the use of an infusion pump.

Ketamine, a phencyclidine derivative, has experienced a resurgence in popularity over the past several years in the OBA practice. The use of ketamine–propofol sedation has been described as an excellent way to provide a relaxed surgical field in a quiet, immobile patient, often eliminating the need for supplemental oxygen.[149] Ketamine functions as both an anesthetic and an analgesic. It does not depress respiration, and will increase laryngeal reflexes, thus decreasing the risk of aspiration. Furthermore, it is not associated with nausea and vomiting. Ketamine can, however, cause an increase in secretions as well as cause hallucinations. The latter can be decreased or eliminated by adding propofol or midazolam.[150–153] Glycopyrrolate can be used as an antisialagogue. Another advantage of ketamine is that it is relatively inexpensive.

Remimazolam is a new benzodiazepine that offers unique advantages over other IV benzodiazepines due to its pharmacokinetics and pharmacodynamics. The procedural advantages of remimazolam include a faster onset and offset of hypnotic effect and a low susceptibility for cardiovascular depression, respiratory depression, and injection pain. Standard dosages of remimazolam that are utilized include 0.075 mg/kg and 0.25 mg/kg. Early studies demonstrated that remimazolam had a short terminal half-life (70 ± 10 min), small volume of distribution, and very rapid clearance.[154] Remimazolam also has a short duration of action which, according to studies, ranges from 11 to 14 minutes after its last dose.[155] In the liver, remimazolam is hydrolyzed by carboxylesterase-1 (CES-1) into a carboxylic acid metabolite and methanol. Moreover, in case of any adverse events or to further lessen recovery times, flumazenil, a benzodiazepine antagonist, can reverse the effects of remimazolam.

Clonidine has been found to be useful in an office. Since it is an alpha-2 agonist, clonidine will help control blood pressure throughout the perioperative period, thus potentially minimizing blood loss.[156,157] In addition, it may decrease the total propofol usage.[128] Its use may, however, precipitate hypotension and oversedation.

Dexmedetomidine has also recently become a mainstay infusion drug for an office-based anesthetic.[158] It is a short-acting, alpha-2 adrenergic receptor agonist with sedative qualities. Dexmedetomidine permits patients to retain their respiratory drive and does not cause nausea and vomiting. An in-depth understanding of the pharmacologic, pharmacokinetic, and pharmacodynamic effects of dexmedetomidine are critical to not only maximize its safe and effective delivery in the ambulatory anesthesia setting, but also to broaden the scope of its usage.[159] Dexmedetomidine acts in the locus ceruleus and spinal cord resulting in sedation, analgesia, and a centrally mediated sympatholytic effect. It has been shown to reduce the anesthetic and opioid requirements both intraoperatively and postoperatively. The incidence of postoperative nausea, vomiting, delirium, and agitation is low with dexmedetomidine and it has minimal effect on respiratory drive. The main adverse event health care workers should be cautious of when administering dexmedetomidine is hemodynamic changes such as bradycardia, hypotension, and hypertension. In a randomized controlled trial (RCT) that studied 105 patients, Song et al. found that patients who received dexmedetomidine intraoperatively had almost a twofold increase in bradycardia compared with the control group.[160] In an RCT that studied 60 patients, Shariffudin et al. found a significant decrease in the systolic blood pressure, 104.3 (12.8) versus 114.2 (21.2) mmHg ($P < .05$) in patients without dexmedetomidine, at the 15-minute mark after infusion.[161] This phenomenon disappeared by the 20-minute mark and did not return for the remainder of the case. One way to mitigate this bradycardia and hypotension is to forgo a loading bolus and instead utilize a slower basal infusion rate. Health care providers should use caution when administering dexmedetomidine to patients who are less able to tolerate bradycardia. Further, dosing must be adjusted in patients with hepatic impairment, as dexmedetomidine is predominantly metabolized in the liver.[162]

TIVA is a common choice for non-OR anesthetics, and usually consists of propofol as the hypnotic component used in conjunction with fentanyl, remifentanil, or ketamine as the analgesic component. All of these drugs can be given by intermittent bolus or infusion. Mathews et al. found that remifentanil 0.085 μ/kg/min can substitute for 66% N_2O.[163] Advantages of TIVA over inhalation anesthesia include the avoidance of the need for gas scavenging and a reduced incidence of PONV. Since the availability of the newer less soluble inhalation agents (*e.g.*, desflurane and sevoflurane), many authors have compared recovery times from these agents with the recovery time after a total IV anesthetic using a propofol infusion.[164,165] Recently, Gupta conducted a meta-analysis of all such publications and reported an overall more rapid recovery from desflurane when compared to either isoflurane- or propofol-based anesthetics. Recovery was also found to be faster with sevoflurane when compared to isoflurane. However, there was more PONV as well as postdischarge nausea and vomiting in the isoflurane groups as compared to the propofol ones; for these considerations, isoflurane may not be the best choice of inhalation agent in non-OR locations. Overall, the inhalation agent groups required more antiemetic treatment than did the propofol groups.[166] Recent evidence has shown that TIVA with propofol and air/oxygen reduces the PONV risk by approximately 25%.[167]

Depth of anesthesia monitoring has been shown to decrease the time to extubation and discharge readiness.[168–170] A depth of anesthesia monitor has been described as useful in the office during MAC procedures, resulting in a possible decrease in total propofol usage.[171] Whether this type of monitoring will prove to be cost-effective or not, in office-based settings, remains to be seen.

Data regarding the perioperative use of dexmedetomidine in the ambulatory surgery setting are promising, albeit with some limitations related mostly to its half-life. Despite the synergistic properties of dexmedetomidine with respect to narcotics and volatile anesthetics, the lingering sedation may prolong discharge from the recovery room.

Dexmedetomidine has a rapid onset within 5 minutes and peak effect within 15 minutes. Dexmedetomidine is rapidly distributed, with a short redistribution half-life of 6 minutes, and undergoes hepatic metabolism, producing inactive metabolites mainly via glucuronidation and hydroxylation, with an elimination half-life of 2 hours. Despite being designed for IV use only, it is well absorbed through the nasal and buccal mucosa. Intranasal delivery lacks any burning sensation, so pediatric patients may tolerate intranasal dexmedetomidine to a higher degree than intranasal midazolam. Dexmedetomidine has a variety of clinical uses, including preoperative sedation, attenuation of hemodynamic responses to intraoperative stresses, controlled hypotension, and for procedural sedation. When used as the sole agent via continuous infusion, the loading dose is administered over 10 minutes, which facilitates a speedier onset, although can cause bradycardia and hypotension. It can also be used to decrease the incidence of emergence delirium in children without prolonging the time to discharge by use of subanesthetic doses. Clinical disadvantages of dexmedetomidine include a relatively slow induction time to avoid hemodynamic changes, and a variable quality of sedation among patients. The sedative profile produced by dexmedetomidine is similar to that associated with sleep.[172]

Any type of anesthesia from sedation through GA and regional anesthesia can be administered in an office setting safely but it is vital that the office be adequately equipped and staffed to rescue a patient from a deeper stage of anesthesia. Thus, if MAC is planned, GA must be anticipated.

Postanesthesia Care Unit

Following an office-based procedure, a patient should be able to sit in a chair or ambulate to an examination room to dress almost immediately postoperatively and be free of pain and PONV. All vital signs should be within 10% of baseline. A formal PACU may not be present, and the patient may be required to recover in the surgical suite. Regardless of where the patient recovers, it is important to adhere to all the ASA standards for monitoring and documentation throughout the postoperative period. Staffing in the recovery area must be adequate, and the use of a pulse oximeter is imperative.[173] It is recommended that there be at least one ACLS/PALS-certified member of the health care team present until the last patient has left the office.

11 Since PACU space in an office is often limited and the anesthesiologist may have multiple locations to attend in a single day, patient satisfaction and prevention of PONV and pain are paramount. The effect of these physiologic occurrences may also have a profound economic impact on an office surgical unit.[174] It is imperative that every anesthetic administered be designed to maximize postoperative patient alertness and mobility and minimize the risks of the need for a prolonged PACU stay. Twersky has recommended that the postanesthesia discharge scoring system and clinical discharge criteria used in ambulatory surgery also be used in the office-based setting.[175] Interestingly, there is a trend to discharge patients, particularly after colonoscopy, without escorts. This has been sanctioned in some states. In New York, regulations require that all patients undergoing a procedure with anesthesia be "discharged in the company of a responsible adult, unless exempted by a physician."[176] Specific data confirming the enhanced safety of this practice do not exist.

A timely discharge from the PACU also depends on adequate pain control. Opioids, nonopioid analgesic agents, supplementation by wound infiltration with local anesthetics, and peripheral nerve blocks often form the basis for a multimodal strategy for postoperative pain management. As detailed in a review paper, liposomal bupivacaine is a local anesthetic that uses multivesicular liposome technology to release its contents in a more consistent and prolonged manner, extending patient analgesia up to 72 to 96 hours.[177] Ilfed et al.'s review paper examined 76 RCTs and found that 11% of the trials reported a statistically significant improvement in postoperative pain control when utilizing liposomal bupivacaine.[178] As mentioned in a commentary, support for utilization of liposomal bupivacaine for postoperative pain control in OBA and other anesthesia settings continues to increase.[179] Additional literature states that the efficacy of liposomal bupivacaine correlates to larger dosage administration. Liposomal bupivacaine provides prolonged analgesia and opioid-sparing effects when compared to placebo and may even be used as a stand-alone medication.[177]

These effective pain relief techniques not only decrease the anesthetic and analgesic requirements during surgery but also reduce the need for opioid analgesics in the postoperative period, thus facilitating the recovery process.[180] Nonopioid analgesics (*e.g.*, acetaminophen) and nonsteroidal anti-inflammatory drugs (*e.g.*, ketorolac) are routinely used. Ketorolac decreases the incidence of PONV and patients tolerate oral fluids and meet discharge criteria sooner than those receiving opioids.[181] In an effort to minimize the potential for postoperative bleeding and risk of GI complications, more specific COX-2 inhibitors are being increasingly used as nonopioid adjuvants for minimizing postoperative pain.[182]

PONV is a major factor that impacts perioperative morbidity, patient satisfaction, and throughput times by prolonging PACU stays. In a review article that looked at eight RCTs, one prognostic study, and one post hoc analysis, it was found that PONV has been shown to impact up to 30% of all postop patients and up to 80% of patients with multiple risk factors for PONV.[183] In addition, nausea and vomiting has been implicated in increased costs due to prolonged postop recovery and unanticipated admissions.[185] PONV is also shown to increase perioperative morbidity from fluid and electrolyte imbalance, wound dehiscence, hemorrhage, and aspiration pneumonia.[183]

An optimal antiemetic regimen for OBA has yet to be established. However, since the etiology of PONV is multifactorial, combination prophylactic therapies may be beneficial in high-risk patients.[184] Many of the older first-line therapies are associated with sedation, drowsiness, and extrapyramidal side effects, and have been supplanted by 5-HT_3 antagonists such as ondansetron, dolasetron, and granisetron.[185] Dexamethasone has been shown to improve the efficacy of both 5-HT_3 antagonists[186] as well as dopamine antagonists when used for the prevention of PONV.[185] Dexamethasone has no utility as a rescue drug for PONV.

Recent literature recommends aprepitant as a mainstay for PONV prophylaxis in patients at high risk for PONV.[184] Based on a retrospective study that examined 338 patients, Therneau et al. recommend a single 40-mg dose of aprepitant in addition to a multimodal regimen, as the authors saw a reduction of PONV at 1 hour (OR [95% CI], 0.5 [0.30–0.80]; $p = .007$) and fewer emesis episodes at 48 hours (OR [95% CI], 0.45 [0.21–0.95]; $p = .04$).[187]

Routine PONV prophylaxis of all patients, though, has not been shown to offer any advantage over symptomatic treatment[188] and has associated costs. Prophylaxis should be considered for all patients with a high risk of PONV. Such patients include, young women having breast or gynecologic surgery, nonsmokers, or patients with a history of PONV. Ensuring adequate hydration (up to 20 mL/kg of crystalloid), to avoid orthostatic hypotension and, thus, prevent the release of emetogenic chemicals by decreasing blood flow to the midbrain emetic centers is an intervention that may be successful in the prevention of PONV.[185]

Regulations

Governmental oversight of office-based surgery varies among states; currently, regulations exist in the majority of states with others following. A complete list of regulations in each of the states is available online.[35] Whereas accreditation is often a voluntary certification of an office, in some states, regulations, which are governmental mandates imposed by the local or state government, exist. It is imperative that anesthesiologists embarking on an office-based practice familiarize themselves with any rules and regulations that govern practice in their particular state.

In 1994, California was the first state to adopt legislation regarding OBA and was soon followed by New Jersey. A closer look at these two states provides an example of the varied requirements being enforced by states throughout the country. California's regulations pertain to patients undergoing a GA, and do not address procedures performed under local, peripheral nerve block or sedation/anxiolytics administered in doses that do not affect a patient's life-preserving reflexes.[189] The regulations deal with issues ranging from office policy and mandatory reporting of adverse outcomes to surgeon and anesthesia provider qualifications.[189] California Health and Safety Code 1248-1248.85 mandates that surgical procedures occur only in offices that have been accredited or have been certified to participate in the Medicare Program under Title XVIII (42 U.S.C. Sec. 1395 et seq.), with very few exceptions.[190] In addition, offices must have a written plan in place that deals with issues regarding emergency admissions. Surgeons must have admitting privileges at a local licensed or accredited acute care hospital or have a written transfer agreement with a physician who does have such privileges. Offices must have an agreement with the hospital for the admission, in accordance with the hospital's system of quality assurance and peer review. California law also requires that offices have adequate patient monitoring throughout the perioperative period and have a system in place for the storage and maintenance of patient records. Any office that fails to comply with these regulations risks sanctions ranging from reprimand with or without monetary penalties to criminal prosecution.

New Jersey's administrative Code 13:35-4A.1-13:35-4A.18 develops criteria for patient selection. Only ASA physical status 1 and 2 patients may undergo general or regional anesthesia. ASA physical status 3 patients can undergo only conscious sedation. Providers of GA must be credentialed to do so by a hospital, and only appropriately credentialed physicians may supervise CRNAs. New Jersey law establishes guidelines regarding mandatory monitoring, emergency supplies that must be present, physician credentialing, and peer review. In contrast to California, New Jersey's regulations pertain to all patients undergoing surgical procedures regardless of the anesthetic depth. However, similar to California, violations may result in fines ranging from reprimand to license revocation and criminal prosecution.[191]

In states that have no regulations regarding office-based surgical procedures, any physician who holds a valid medical license may perform any procedure, they so choose, within their office without oversight. A surgeon may perform a procedure for which they may have had little to no training, and may sedate a patient without any training in anesthesia or airway management. In fact, there have been reported cases of patients undergoing procedures without any preoperative evaluation, pertinent labs, informed consent, intra- or postoperative monitoring or operative report, and without regard for sterile technique.[13] It is therefore imperative that the anesthesiologist continues to maintain the role of a zealous patient advocate, and help to educate the surgeon as to what constitutes a safe anesthetizing location.

Business and Legal Aspects

It is in the anesthesia provider's best interest to seek legal counsel and create a valid business model before embarking on a career in OBA. This model must consider the overhead costs associated with staffing and running a safe surgical office as well as the potential and probable case load and patient insurance mix. An OBA division within a department may provide benefits to an academic practice, in addition to the monetary ones. There may be an intangible benefit to the community it serves, as well enhancing the anesthesia training program.[5] It would however become necessary to involve the American Board of Anesthesiology (ABA) as well as the American College of Graduate Education (ACGME) to ensure that any resident rotation outside the ACGME approved hospital setting is acceptable.

Many OBA groups have formed either professional corporations or limited liability companies. Although not eliminating the need for liability insurance, both of these arrangements serve to protect the private assets of the anesthesiologists in the case of a malpractice claim.[3] Legal counsel may also prove to be beneficial in creating business plans that follow all state and federal laws regarding billing/collection and antitrust.[192]

It is imperative to have an aboveboard and legal relationship with every office in which anesthesia services are being delivered. Billing strategies must be legal and ethical. In this complex environment of third-party payers, it is quite easy to make legal errors. Ignorance of the law offers no protection or excuse, and one should seek the advice of expert billing agencies, even if one chooses not to outsource this responsibility. In calculating pricing, one must include all overhead charges such as drugs, equipment, time, and business expenses including malpractice insurance. A pricing structure with the surgeon must exist before embarking on a clinical relationship. One must outline specifically what will be provided by the office (e.g., IV equipment, antibiotics, monitors, etc.) and what the anesthesiologist will supply. These decisions take on further legal implications when the office is receiving a facility fee.

Conclusions

OBA continues to rapidly expand and pose unique challenges to anesthesiologists, who must not only provide medical care in remote environments, but also have a solid business sense and an extensive understanding of OR management. It is imperative that, although regulations have not kept pace with the growth of OBA, anesthesia providers make it their responsibility to help ensure that every possible safety measure is afforded to their patients. Decisions about appropriate patient/procedure selection and equipping anesthetizing locations must be made in conjunction with surgeons. All clinical decisions and anesthetic choices must take into consideration the need for rapid turnover and limited PACU availability. Any depth of anesthesia from minimal sedation through regional and GA may be delivered as long as the proper safeguards are in place.

The many advantages afforded by office-based surgery are fueling its evolution. As more complex procedures are performed on patients with advanced age, the anesthesiologist's role in providing safe and efficient care will become more challenging. The anesthesiologist's role in the providing of care and as serving as their patient's advocate is both complex and vital.

For further review and interactivities, please see the videos and narrative interactive clinical vignettes (NICVs) accessible in the complimentary eBook bundled with this text. Access instructions are located on the inside front cover.

REFERENCES

1. Twersky, Rebecca S. and Saad Mohammad. "Office-based Anesthesia: Successes and Challenges." *ASA Refresher Courses in Anesthesiology.* 41 (2013):125–134.
2. Levine, A. I., Govindaraj, S., & DeMaria, Jr., S. (2013). *Anesthesiology and Otolaryngology* (1st ed.). Springer New York.
3. Koch ME, Dayan S, Barinholtz D. Office-based anesthesia: an overview. *Anesthesiol Clin North Am.* 2003;21:417.
4. *Outpatient office-based surgery—federation of state medical boards.* (2002). Retrieved February 22, 2023, from https://www.fsmb.org/siteassets/advocacy/policies/outpatient-office-based-surgery.pdf
5. Hausman LM, Levine AI, Rosenblatt MA. A survey evaluating the training of anesthesiology residents in office-based anesthesia. *J Clin Anesth.* 2006;18:499.
6. Snow J. *On chloroform and other anesthetics.* John Churchill; 1858;314–315.
7. Tang J, White PF, Wender RH, et al. Fast-track office-based anesthesia: a comparison of propofol versus desflurane with antiemetic prophylaxis in spontaneously breathing patents. *Anesth Analg.* 2001;92(1):95–99.
8. White PF, Song D. New criteria for fast-tracking after outpatient anesthesia: a comparison with the modified Aldrete's scoring system. *Anesth Analg.* 1999;88(5):1069–1072.
9. Ambulatory surgery in the United States, 2006. Cullen, Karen A.;Hall, Margaret Jean; Golosinskiy, Aleksandr; National Center for Health Statistics (U.S.). January 28, 2009. URL: https://stacks.cdc.gov/view/cdc/5395
10. Lazarov SJ. Office-based surgery and anesthesia: where are we now? *World J Urol.* 1998; 16:384.
11. Courtiss EH, Goldwyn RM, Joffe JM, Hannenberg AA. Anesthetic practices in ambulatory surgery. *Plast Reconstr Surg.* 1994;93:792.
12. Wetchler BV. Online shopping for ambulatory surgery: let the buyer beware! *Ambul Surg.* 2000;8:111.
13. Quattrone MS. Is the physician office the wild, wild west of health care? *J Ambul Care Manage.* 2000;23:64.
14. Laurito CE. Report of educational meeting: the Society for Office-Based Anesthesia, Orlando, Florida, March 7, 1998. *J Clin Anesth.* 1998;10:445.
15. Russo, C.A. (Thomson Reuters), Elixhauser, A. (AHRQ), Steiner, C. (AHRQ), and Wier, L. (Thomson Reuters). *Hospital-Based Ambulatory Surgery, 2007.* HCUP Statistical Brief #86. February 2010. Agency for Healthcare Research and Quality, Rockville, MD. http://www.hcup-us.ahrq.gov/reports/statbriefs/sb86.pdf
16. Kurrekk MM, Twersky RS. Office-based anesthesia: how to start an office-based practice. *Anesthesiol Clin.* 2010;28:253–267.
17. Kurrek MM, Twersky RS. Office-based anesthesia, how to start an office-based practice. *Aneshtesiol Clin.* 2010:28(2):353–367.

18. 2021 Anesthesia Almanac. THE AMERICAN SOCIETY OF ANESTHESIOLOGISTS. September 8 2021. Accessed March 12 2022. https://www.asahq.org/-/media/sites/asahq/files/public/resources/analytics-research-services/2021-anesthesia-almanac.pdf?la=en&hash=404CEC03EBEE9D7BE5E0C3C24AA59EB835A25B54
19. Gupta V, Parikh R, Nguyen L, et al. Is office-based surgery safe? Comparing outcomes of 183,914 aesthetic surgical procedures across different types of accredited facilities. *Aesthet Surg J.* 2017;37(2):226–235. doi: 10.1093/asj/sjw138
20. Foley C, Kendall MC, Apruzzese P, De Oliveira GS. American Society of Anesthesiologists Physical Status Classification as a reliable predictor of postoperative medical complications and mortality following ambulatory surgery: an analysis of 2,089,830 ACS-NSQIP outpatient cases. *BMC Surg.* 2021;21:253.
21. Shapiro FE, Punwani N, Rosenberg NM, Valedon A, Twersky R, Urman RD. Office-based anesthesia: safety and outcomes. *Anesth Analg.* 2014;119(2):276–285.
22. Ross AK, Eck JB. Office-based anesthesia for children. *Anesthesiol Clin North Am.* 2002; 20:195.
23. Rashewsky S, Parameswaran A, Sloane C, Ferguson F, Epstein R. Time and cost analysis: pediatric dental rehabilitation with general anesthesia in the office and the hospital setting. *Anesth Prog.* 2012;59(4):147–153.
24. Schultz LS. Cost analysis of office surgery clinic with comparison to hospital outpatient facilities for laparoscopic procedures. *Int Surg.* 1994;79:273.
25. Bartamian M, Meyer DR. Site of service, anesthesia, and postoperative practice patterns for oculoplastic and orbital surgeries. *Ophthalmology.* 1996;103:1628.
26. Schimberg AS, Wellenstein DJ, van den Broek EM, et al. Office-based vs. operating room-performed laryngopharyngeal surgery: a review of cost differences. *Eur Arch Otorhinolaryngol.* 2019;276(11):2963–2973.
27. Saxen MA, Urman RD, Yepes JF, Gabriel RA, Jones JE. Comparison of anesthesia for dental/oral surgery by office-based dentist anesthesiologists versus operating room-based physician anesthesiologists. *Anesth Prog.* 2017;64(4):212–220.
28. Way JC, Culham BA. Establishment and cost analysis of an office surgical suite. *Can J Surg.* 1996;39:379.
29. Anello S. Office-based anesthesia: advantages, disadvantages and the nurse's role. *Plastic Surg Nurs.* 2002;22:107.
30. Iverson RE, Lynch DJ; ASPS Task Force on Patient Safety in Office-Based Surgery Facilities. Patient safety in office-based surgery facilities: II. Patient selection. *Plast Reconstr Surg.* 2002;110:1785.
31. Lalwani K, Kitchin J, Lax P. Office-based dental rehabilitation in children with special healthcare needs using a pediatric sedation service model. *J Oral Maxillofac Surg.* 2007;65:427–433.
32. Berglas NF, Battistelli MF, Nicholson WK, Sobota M, Urman RD, Roberts SCM. The effect of facility characteristics on patient safety, patient experience, and service availability for procedures in non-hospital-affiliated outpatient settings: a systematic review. *PLoS One.* 2018;13(1): e0190975.
33. Seligson E, Beutler SS, Urman RD. Office-based anesthesia: an update on safety and outcomes (2017-2019). *Curr Opin Anaesthesiol.* 2019;32(6):756–761.
34. Metzner J, Posner KL, Domino KB. The risk and safety of anesthesia at remote locations: the US closed claims analysis. *Curr Opin Anesthesiol.* 2009;22:502–508.
35. State requirements for accreditation. Accreditation Association for Ambulatory Health Care website. Accessed June 2, 2016. https://www.aaahc.org/news/enhanced-v42-standards/
36. Robert Singer, MD, FACS, Geoffrey R Keyes, MD, FACS, Foad Nahai, MD, FACS, FRCS (Hon), American Association for Accreditation of Ambulatory Surgical Facilities (AAAASF) History: Its Role in Plastic Surgery Safety, *Aesthetic Surgery Journal Open Forum*, Volume 1, Issue 2, June 2019, ojz008, https://doi.org/10.1093/asjof/ojz008
37. Arens JF. Anesthesia for office-based surgery: are we paying too high a price for access and convenience? *Mayo Clinic Proc.* 2000;75:225.
38. Missant C, Van de Velde M. Morbidity and mortality related to anesthesia outside the operating room. *Curr Opin Anesthesiol.* 2004;17:323–327.
39. Vila H Jr, Soto R, Cantor AB, Mackey D. Comparative outcomes analysis of procedures performed in physician offices and ambulatory surgery centers. *Arch Surg.* 2003;138;991.
40. Clayman MA, Caffee HH. Office surgery safety and the Florida moratoria. *Ann Plastic Surg.* 2006;56:78.
41. Melloni C. Morbidity and mortality related to anesthesia outside the operating room. *Minerva Anesthesiol.* 2005;325–334.
42. Stoelting RK. Office-based anesthesia growth provokes safety fears. *Anesthesia Patient Safety Foundation Newsletter.* 2000;15(1):1.
43. Domino KB. Office-based anesthesia: lessons learned from the closed-claims project. *ASA Newsletter.* 2001;65:9.
44. Morello DC, Colon GA, Fredricks S, Iverson RE, Singer R. Patient safety in accredited office surgical facilities. *Plast Reconstr Surg.* 1997;99:1496.
45. Hoefflin SM, Bornstein JB, Gordon M. General anesthesia in an office-based plastic surgical facility: a report on more than 23,000 consecutive office-based procedures under general anesthesia with no significant anesthetic complications. *Plast Reconstr Surg.* 2001;107:243.
46. Sullivan PK, Tattini CD. Office-based operatory experience: an overview of anesthetic technique, procedures and complications. *Med Health RI.* 2001;84:392.
47. Bitar G, Mullis W, Jacobs W, et al. Safety and efficacy of office-based surgery with monitored anesthesia care/sedation in 4778 consecutive plastic surgery procedures. *Plast Reconstr Surg.* 2003;111:150.
48. Keyes GR, Singer R, Iverson RE, et al. Analysis of outpatient surgery center safety using an internet based quality improvement and peer review program. *Plast Reconstr Surg.* 2004;113(6):1760–1770.
49. Keyes GR, Singer R, Iverson RE, et al. Mortality in outpatient surgery. *Plast Reconstr Surg.* 2008;122(1):245–250.
50. Soltani AM, Keyes GR, Singer R, Reed L, Fodor PB. Outpatient surgery and sequelae: an analysis of the AAAASF internet-based quality assurance and peer review database. *Clin Plast Surg.* 2013;40(3):465–473.
51. McDevitt NB. Deep vein thrombosis prophylaxis. *Plast Reconstr Surg.* 1999;104: 1923–1928.
52. Robbertze, R, Posner KL, Domino KB. Closed claims review of anesthesia for procedures outside the operating room. *Curr Opin Anesthesiol.* 2006;19:436–442.
53. American Society of Anesthesiologists Committee on Equipment and Facilities. Guidelines for determining anesthesia machine obsolescence. Accessed December 5, 2007. https://www.apsf.org/article/guidelines-published-for-determining-anesthesia-machine-obsolescence/
54. Coté CJ, Karl HW, Notteman DA, Weinberg JA, McCloskey C. Adverse sedation events in pediatrics: analysis of medications used for sedation. *Pediatrics.* 2000;106:663.
55. Coté CJ, Notteman DA, Karl HW, Weinberg JA, McCloskey C. Adverse sedation events in pediatrics: a critical incident analysis of contributing factors. *Pediatrics.* 2000;105:8–5.
56. Gupta R, Pyati S. Controversies in office-based anesthesia: obstructive sleep apnea considerations. *Minerva Anestesiol.* 2018;84(9):1102–1107.
57. Kaoutzanis C, Gupta V, Winocour J, et al. Cosmetic liposuction: preoperative risk factors, major complication rates, and safety of combined procedures. *Aesthet Surg J.* 2017;37(6): 680–694.
58. Grazer FM, de Jong RH. Fatal outcomes from liposuction: census survey of cosmetic surgeons. *Plast Reconstr Surg.* 2000;105(1):436–446; discussion 447–8.
59. Hausman LM, Levine AI, Rosenblatt MA. A survey evaluating the training of anesthesiology residents in office-based anesthesia. *J Clin Anesth.* 2006;18:499.
60. Halk AB, Habbema L, Genders RE, Hanke CW. Safety studies in the field of liposuction: a systematic review. *Dermatol Surg.* 2019;45(2):171–182.
61. Iverson R. ASPS Task Force on Patient Safety in Office-Based Surgery Facilities. Patient safety in office-based surgery facilities: I. Procedures in the office-based surgery setting. *Plast Reconstr Surg.* 2002;110:1337.
62. Tunajek SK. Office based procedure standards. *AANA J.* 1999;67:115.
63. American Medical Association House of Delegates at the I-01 Meeting. Office-based surgery core principles. *American Society of Anesthesiologists Newsletter.* 2004;68:14. https://www.aana.com/docs/default-source/sga-aana-com-web-documents-(all)/ama-actions-concerning-office-based-surgery-regulation.pdf?sfvrsn=938445b1_2
64. Haeck PC, Swanson JA, Iverson RE, et al; ASPS Patient Safety Committee. Evidence-based patient safety advisory: patient selection and procedures in ambulatory surgery. *Plast Reconstr Surg.* 2009;124:6S–38S.
65. Shapiro FE, Jani SR, Liu X, Dutton RP, Urman RD. Initial results from the national anesthesia clinical outcomes registry and overview of office-based anesthesia. *Anesthesiol Clin.* 2014;32:431–444.
66. Meridy HW. Criteria for selection of ambulatory surgical patients and guidelines for anesthetic management: a retrospective of 1553 cases. *Anesth Analg.* 1982;61:921.
67. American Society of Anesthesiologists Committee on Ambulatory Surgical Care and the American Society of Anesthesiologists Task Force on Office-Based Anesthesia. *Office-based anesthesia: considerations for anesthesiologists in setting up and maintaining a safe office anesthesia environment.* Park Ridge, Il. American Society of Anesthesiologists; 2000.
68. Haeck PC, Swanson JA, Iverson RE, Lynch DJ; ASPS Patient Safety Committee. Evidence-based patient safety advisory: patient assessment and prevention of pulmonary side effects in surgery. Part 1-obstructive sleep apnea and obstructive lung disease. *Plast Reconstr Surg.* 2009;124S:45S–56S.
69. Benumof JL. Obstructive sleep apnea in the adult obese patient: implications for arway management. *J Clin Anesth.* 2001;13:144.
70. Boushra NN. Anaesthetic management of patients with sleep apnea syndrome. *Can J Anaesth.* 1996;43:599.
71. Young T, Evans L, Finn L, Palta M. Estimation of the clinically diagnosed proportion of sleep apnea syndrome in middle-aged men and women. *Sleep.* 1997;20:705.
72. Chung F, Abdullah HR, Liao P. STOP-Bang Questionnaire: A Practical Approach to Screen for Obstructive Sleep Apnea. *Chest.* 2016 Mar;149(3):631-8. doi: 10.1378/chest.15-0903. Epub 2016 Jan 12. PMID: 26378880.
73. Chung F, Liao P, Farney R. Correlation between the stop-bang score and the severity of obstructive sleep apnea. *Anesthesiology.* 2015;122(6):1436–1437.
74. Chung F, Yang Y, Brown R, Liao P. Alternative scoring models of stop-bang questionnaire improve sensitivity to detect undiagnosed obstructive sleep apnea. *J Clin Sleep Med.* 2014;10(9):951–958.

75. Lofsky A. Sleep apnea and narcotic postoperative pain medication: a morbidity and mortality risk. *APSF Newsletter*. 2002;17:24e. https://www.apsf.org/article/special-article-sleep-apnea-and-narcotic-postoperative-pain-medication-a-morbidity-and-mortality-risk/
76. Xara D, Mendonça J, Pereira H, Santos A, Abelha FJ. Adverse respiratory eventsnafter general anesthesia in patients at high risk of obstructive sleep apnea. *Braz J Anesthesiol*. 2015;65(5)359–366.
77. Kurrek MM, Cobourn C, Wojtasik Z, Kiss A, Dain SL. Morbidity in patients with or at high risk for obstructive sleep apnea after ambulatory laparoscopic gastic banding. *Obes Surg*. 2011;21(10):1494–1498.
79. Samuels SI, Rabinov W. Difficulty reversing drug-induced coma in a patient with sleep apnea. *Anesth Analg*. 1986;65:1222.
79. Benumof JL. Creation of observational unit may decrease sleep apnea risk. *APSF Newsletter*. 2002;17:39.https://www.apsf.org/article/creation-of-observational-unit-may-decrease-sleep-apnea-risk/
80. Ankichetty S, Chung F. Considerations for patients with obstructive sleep apnea undergoingambulatory surgery. *Curr Opin Anesthesiol*. 2011;24(6):605–611.
81. Steed MB, Lyman A. Obstructive sleep apnea. In: Bouloux GF, ed. *Office Based Anesthesia Complications*. Springer, Cham; 2021. https://doi.org/10.1007/978-3-030-61427-0_9
82. Coldiron B, Shreve E, Balkrishnan R. Patient injuries from surgical procedures performed in medical offices: three years of Florida data. *Dermatol Surg*. 2004;30:1435.
83. Claymen MA, Seagle BM. Office surgery safety: The myths and truths behind the Florida moratoria–six years of Florida data. *Plast Reconstr Surg*. 2006;118:777.
84. Reinisch JF, Bresnick SD, Walker JW, Rosso RF. Deep venous thrombosis and pulmonary embolus after face lift: a study of incidence and prophylaxis. *Plast Reconstr Surg*. 2001 May;107(6): 1570-5; discussion 1576-7. doi: 10.1097/00006534-200105000-00044. PMID: 11335838.
85. Santos DQ, Tan M, Farias CL, Swerdloff JL, Paul MD. Venous thromboembolism after facelift surgery under local anesthesia: results of a multicenter survey. *Aesthetic Plast Surg*. 2014; 38(1):12–24.
86. Davison SP, Venturi ML, Attinger CE, Baker SB, Spear SL. Prevention of venous thromboembolism in the plastic surgery patient. *Plast Reconstr Surg*. 2004;114;43e.
87. Voss SC, Sharp HC, Scott JR. Abdominoplasty combined with gynecologic surgical procedures. *Obstet Gynecol*. 1986;67(2):181–185.
88. Galway U, Borkowski R. Office-based anesthesia for the urologist. *Urol Clin North Am*. 2013;40:497–515.
89. American Society of Anesthesiologists: Practice guidelines for management of the difficult airway: An updated report. *Anesthesiology* 2003;98:1269–1277.
90. Lewis SR, Butler AR, Parker J, Cook TM, Schofield-Robinson OJ, Smith AF. Videolaryngoscopy versus direct laryngoscopy for adult patients requiring tracheal intubation: a Cochrane Systematic Review. *Br J Anaesth*. 2017;119(3):369–383.
91. American Society of Anesthesiologists: Standards for basic anesthetic monitoring. ASA Directory of Members, 2001 (last amended October 21, 1998). American Society of Anesthesiologists; 2001:493
92. Matin MB, Gonzalez ML, Dodson TB. What factors influence community oral and maxillofacial surgeons' choice to use capnography in the office-based ambulatory anesthesia setting. *J Oral Maxillofac Surg*. 2015;73:1484.e1–1484.e10.
93. Gurunluoglu R, Swanson JA, Haeck PC, ASPS Patient Safety Committee. Evidence-based patient safety advisory: malignant hyperthermia. *Plast Reconstr Surg*. 2009;124:68S–81S.
94. American Society of Anesthesiologists Task Force on Operating Room Fires; Caplan RA, Barker SJ, Connis RT. Practice advisory for the prevention and management of operating room fires. *Anesthesiology*. 2008;108:786–801.
95. Moss E. MD office regs stalled in New Jersey. *APSF Newsletter*. 1997; Winter: 37. https://www.apsf.org/article/md-office-safety-regs-stalled-in-new-jersey/
96. Yates JA, American Society of Plastic Surgeons office-based surgery accreditation crosswalk. *Plastic Surg Nurs*. 2002;22:125.
97. Coldiron B. Office surgical incidents: 19 months of Florida data. *Dermatol Surg*. 2002;28:710.
98. Bing J, McAuliffe MS, Lupton JR. Regional anesthesia with monitored anesthesia care for dermatologic laser surgery. *Dermatol Clin*. 2002;20:123.
99. Morris KT, Pommier RF, Vetto JT. Office-based wire-guided open breast biopsy under local anesthesia is accurate and cost effective. *Am J Surg*. 2000;179:422.
100. Jones JS, Streem SB. Office-based cystoureteroscopy for assessment of the upper urinary tract. *J Endourol*. 2002;16:307.
101. Friedman O, Deutsch ES, Reilly JS, Cook SP. The feasibility of office-based laser-assisted tympanic membrane fenestration with tympanostomy tube insertion: the duPont Hospital experience. *Int J Pediatr Otorhinolaryngol*. 2002;62:31.
102. Jones JS, Oder M, Zippe CD. Saturation prostate biopsy with periprostatic block can be performed in the office. *J Urol*. 2002;168:2108.
103. Goldrath MH, Sherman AI. Office hysteroscopy and suction curettage: can we eliminate the hospital diagnostic dilitation and curettage? *Am J Obstet Gynecol*. 1985;152:220.
104. Armstrong M. Office-based procedures in rhinosinusitis. *Otolaryngol Clin North Am*. 2005; 38;1327–1338.
105. Siegel GJ, Seiberling KA, Haines KG, Aguado AS. Office CO2 laser turbinoplasty. *Ear Nose Throat J*. 2008;87;386–390.
106. Mingus ML, Bodian CA, Bradford CN, Eisenkraft JB. Prolonged surgery increases the likelihood of admission of scheduled ambulatory surgery patients. *J Clin Anesth*. 1997;9:446.
107. Fortier J, Chung F, Su J. Unanticipated admission after ambulatory surgery–a prospective study. *Can J Anaesth*. 1997;45;612.
108. Gold BS, Kitz DS, Lecky JH, Neuhaus JM. Unanticipated admission to the hospital following ambulatory surgery. *JAMA*. 1989;262:3008.
109. Cheng H, Clymer JW, Po-Han Chen B, et al. Prolonged operative duration is associated with complications: a systematic review and meta-analysis. *J Surg Res*. 2018;229:134–144.
110. American Society of Plastic Surgeons: 2007 quick facts: Cosmetic and reconstructive plastic surgery trends. https://www.plasticsurgery.org/documents/News/Statistics/2007/plastic-surgery-statistics-full-report-2007.pdf
111. American Society for Aesthetic and Plastic Surgery. Top 5 surgical and nonsurgical cosmetic procedures. http://www.surgery.org
112. Iverson RE, Lynch DJ; American Society of Plastic Surgeons Committee on Safety. Practice advisory on liposuction. *Plast Reconstr Surg*. 2004;113:1478.
113. Fodor PB, Watson JP. Wetting solutions in ultra-sound assisted lipoplasty: a review. *Clin Plast Surg*. 1999;26:289.
114. Klein JA. Tumescent technique for regional anesthesia permits lidocaine doses of 35 mg/kg. *J Dermatol Surg Oncol*. 1990;16:248.
115. Ostad A, Kageyama N, Moy RL. Tumescent anesthesia with lidocaine dose of 55 mg/kg is safe for liposuction. *Dermatol Surg*. 1996;22:921.
116. Martínez MA, Ballesteros S, Segura LJ, García M. Reporting a fatality during tumescent liposuction. *Forensic Sci Int*. 2008;178:e11–e16.
117. Grazer FM, de Jong RH. Fatal outcome from liposuction: census survey of cosmetic surgeons. *Plast Reconstr Surg*. 2000;105:436.
118. Housman TS, Lawrence N, Mellen BG, et al. The safety of liposuction: results of a national survey. *Dermatol Surg*. 2002;28:971.
119. Conveney E, Weltz CR, Greengrass R, et al. Use of paravertebral block anesthesia in the surgical management of breast cancer. Experience in 156 cases. *Ann Surg*. 1998;227:496.
120. Jaffe SM, Campbell P, Bellman M, Baildam A. Postoperative nausea and vomiting in women following breast surgery: an audit. *Eur J Anaesthesiol*. 2000;17:261.
121. Vawter M, Ruiz R, Alaama A, Aronow WS, Dagradi AE. Electrocardiographic monitoring during coloscopy. *Am J Gastroenterol*. 1975 Feb;63(2):155–7. PMID: 1130390.
122. Radaelli F, Meucci G, Terruzzi V, et al. Single bolus of midazolam versus bolus midazolam plus meperidine for colonoscopy: a prospective, randomized trial. *Gastrointest Endosc*. 2003; 57:329.
123. Ristikankare M, Julkunen R, Laitinen T, et al. Effect of conscious sedation on cardiac autonomic regulation during colonoscopy. *Scand J Gastroenterol*. 2000;9:990.
124. Petelenz M, Gonciarz M, Macfarlane P, et al. Sympathovagal balance fluctuates during colonoscopy. *Endoscopy*. 2004;36:508.
125. Training Committee. American Society for Gastrointestinal Endoscopy. Training guideline for use of propofol in gastrointestinal endoscopy. *Gastrointest Endosc*. 2004 Aug;60(2):167–72. doi: 10.1016/s0016-5107(04)01699-2. PMID: 15278039.
126. Institute for Safe Medication Practices. Propofol sedation: who should administer? Accessed November 5, 2011. https://www.asahq.org/standards-and-guidelines/statement-on-safe-use-of-propofol?&ct=91285098b4f8d051cd407fafc131371b1bafa2cf06f8dd8ed45d433d7e5a87451ab0fa353247aa7cfedd5ba8d9b73436d0f20624ef0dbb4ab1c078cf95be6e86
127. Finder RL. The art and science of office-based anesthesia in dentistry: a 150-year history. *Int Anesthesiol Clin*. 2003;41:1.
128. Perrott DH, Yuen JP, Andresen RV, Dodson TB. Office-based ambulatory anesthesia: outcomes of clinical practices of oral and maxillofacial surgeons. *J Oral Maxillofac Surg*. 2003;61:938.
129. Freedman JM, Li DK, Drasner K, Jaskela MC, Larsen B, Wi S. Transient neurologic symptoms after spinal anesthesia: an epidemiologic study of 1,873 patients. *Anesthesiology*. 1998; 89:633.
130. Coyle TT, Helfrick JF, Gonzalez ML, Andresen RV, Perrott DH. Office-based ambulatory anesthesia: factors that influence patient satisfaction with deep sedation/general anesthesia. *J Oral Maxillofac Surg*. 2005;63:163–172.
131. Verma P, Krishnan DG. Office-based anesthesia in oral and maxillofacial surgery-The American model and training. In: Bonanthaya K, Panneerselvam E, Manuel S, Kumar VV, Rai A, eds. *Oral and Maxillofacial Surgery for the Clinician*. Springer; 2021. https://doi.org/10.1007/978-981-15-1346-6_6
132. Kramer KJ, Brady JW. anesthetic agents commonly used by oral and maxillofacial surgeons. *Oral Maxillofac Surg Clin North Am*. 2018;30(2):155–164. doi: 10.1016/j.coms.2018.01.003
133. Mulroy MF, Larkin KL, Siddiqui A. Intrathecal fentanyl-induced pruritis is more severe in combination with procaine than with lidocaine or bupivicaine. *Reg Anesth Pain Med*. 2001;26:252.
134. Sardo ADS, Bettocchi S, Spinelli M, et al. Review of new office-based hysteroscopic procedures 2003–2009. *J Minim Invasive Gynecol*. 2010;17:436–448.
135. Wortman M. Instituting an office-based surgery program in the gynecologists office. *J Minim Invasive Gynecol*. 2010;17;673–683.
136. Jourdy DN, Kacker A. Regional anesthesia for office-based procedures in otorhinolaryngology. *Anesthesiology Clin*. 2010;28:457–468.
137. Woo P. Office-based laryngeal procedures. *Otolaryngol Clin North Am*. 2006;39:111–133.

138. Lan MC, Hsu YB, Chang SY, et al. Office-based treatment of vocal cord polyp with flexible laryngovideostroboscopic surgery. *J Otolaryngol Head Neck Surg*. 2010;39:90–95.
139. Hackel A, Badgwell JM, Binding RR, et al. Guidelines for the pediatric perioperative environment. American Academy of Pediatrics Section on Anesthesiology. *Pediatrics*. 1999; 103:512.
140. Tang J, Chen L, White PF, et al. Use of propofol for office-based anesthesia: effect of nitrous oxide on recovery profile. *J Clin Anesth*. 1999;11:226.
141. Cohen MM, Duncan PG, Tate RB. Does anesthesia contribute to operative mortality? *JAMA*. 1988;260:2859.
142. Karen B. Domino, Karen L. Posner, Robert A. Caplan, Frederick W. Cheney; *Awareness during Anesthesia*: A Closed Claims Analysis. *Anesthesiology* 1999;90:1053–1061 doi: https://doi.org/10.1097/00000542-199904000-00019
143. Hughes MA, Glass PS, Jacobs JR. Context-sensitive half-time in multicompartment pharmacokinetic models for intravenous anesthetic drugs. *Anesthesiology*. 1992;76:3340–3341.
144. Rudner R, Jalowiecki P, Kawecki P, Gonciarz M, Mularczyk A, Petelenz M. Conscious analgesia/sedation with remifentanil and propofol versus total intravenous anesthesia with fentanyl, midazolam, and propofol for outpatient colonoscopy. *Gastrointest Endosc*. 2003; 57:657.
145. Angst MS. Intraoperative use of remifentanil for tiva: postoperative pain, acute tolerance, and opioid-induced hyperalgesia. *J Cardiothorac Vasc Anesth*. 2015;29(1)S16–S22.
146. Thomas B. Remifentanil versus fentanyl in total intravenous anesthesia for lumbar spine surgery: a retrospective cohort study. *J Clin Anesth*. 2015;27:391–395.
147. Guignard B, Bossard AE, Coste C, et al. Acute opioid tolerance: intraoperative remifentanil increases postoperative pain and morphine requirement. *Anesthesiology*. 2000;93:409–417.
148. Liu Y, Zheng Y, Ga X, Ma Z. The efficacy of NMDA receptor antagonists for preventing remifentanil-induced increase in postoperative pain and analgesic requirement: a meta-analysis. *Minerva Anesthesiol*. 2012;78:653–667.
149. Friedberg BL. Facial laser resurfacing with the propofol-ketamine technique: room air, spontaneous ventilation (RASV) anesthesia. *Dermatol Surg*. 1999;25:569.
150. Friedberg BL. Propofol-ketamine technique: dissociative anesthesia for office surgery (a five year review of 1,264 cases). *Aesthetic Plast Surg*. 1999;23:70.
151. Friedberg BL. Propofol-ketamine technique. *Aesthetic Plast Surg*. 1993;17:297.
152. Friedberg BL. Hypnotic doses of propofol block ketamine-induced hallucinations. *Plast Reconstr Surg*. 1993;91:196.
153. Friedberg BL, Sigl JC. Clonidine premedication decreases propofol consumption during bispectral index (BIS) monitored propofol-ketamine technique for office-based surgery. *Dermatol Surg*. 2000;26:848.
154. Schüttler J, Eisenried A, Lerch M, Fechner J, Jeleazcov C, Ihmsen H. Pharmacokinetics and pharmacodynamics of remimazolam (CNS 7056) after continuous infusion in healthy male volunteers: Part I. Pharmacokinetics and clinical pharmacodynamics. *Anesthesiology*. 2020; 132(4):636–651.
155. Pantos MM, Kennedy DR, Nemec EC. Remimazolam: A novel option for procedural sedation in high risk patients. *J Pharm Pract*. 2021:8971900211027303.
156. Man D. Premedication with oral clonidine for facial rhytidectomy. *Plast Reconstr Surg*. 1994; 94:214.
157. Baker TM, Stuzin JM, Baker TJ, Gordon HL. What's new in aesthetic surgery? *Clin Plast Surg*. 1996;23:16.
158. Kumar P, Priya K, Kirti S, Johar S, Singh V. Dexmedetomidine supported office based genioplasty: a pilot study. *J Maxillofac Oral Surg*. 2015;14(3):750–753.
159. Mohamed M, Mason KP. Dexmedetomidine and ambulatory surgery. *ASA Newsletter*. 2015;79:24–26.
160. Song Y, Shim JK, Song JW, Kim EK, Kwak YL. Dexmedetomidine added to an opioid-based analgesic regimen for the prevention of postoperative nausea and vomiting in highly susceptible patients: a randomised controlled trial. *Eur J Anaesthesiol*. 2016;33(2):75–83.
161. Shariffuddin II, Teoh WH, Wahab S, Wang CY. Effect of single-dose dexmedetomidine on postoperative recovery after ambulatory ureteroscopy and ureteric stenting: a double blind randomized controlled study. *BMC Anesthesiol*. 2018;18:3.
162. Kaye AD, Chernobylsky DJ, Thakur P, et al. Dexmedetomidine in enhanced recovery after surgery (eras) protocols for postoperative pain. *Curr Pain Headache Rep*. 2020;24(5):21.
163. Mathews DM, Gaba V, Zaku B, Neuman GG. Can remifentanil replace nitrous oxide during anesthesia for ambulatory orthopedic surgery with desflurane and fentanyl? *Anesth Analg*. 2008;106:101–108.
164. Nathan N, Peyclit A, Lahrimi A, Feiss P. Comparison of sevoflurane and propofol for ambulatory anaesthesia in gynaecological surgery. *Can J Anaesth*. 1998;45:1148–1150.
165. Song D, Joshi GP, White PF. Fast-track eligibility after ambulatory anesthesia: a comparison of desflurane, sevoflurane and propofol. *Anesth Analg*. 1998;86:267–273.
166. Gupta A, Stierer T, Zuckerman R, Sakima N, Parker SD, Fleisher LA. Comparison of recovery profile after ambulatory anesthesia with propofol, isoflurane, sevoflurane and desflurane: a systematic review. *Anesth Analg*. 2004;98:632–641.
167. Gan TJ, Diemunsch P, Habib AS, et al; Society for Ambulatory Anesthesia. Consensus guidelines for the management of postoperative nausea and vomiting. *Anesth Analg*. 2014;118(1):85–113.
168. Drover DR, Lemmens JH, Pierce ET, et al. Patient state index: titration of delivery and recovery from propofol, alfentanil, and nitrous oxide anesthesia. *Anesthesiology*. 2002;97:82.
169. Gan TJ, Glass PS, Windsor A, et al. Bispectral index monitoring allows faster emergence and improved recovery from propofol, alfentanil, and nitrous oxide anesthesia. *Anesthesiology*. 1997;87:805.
170. Song D, Joshi GP, White PF. Titration of volatile anesthetics using bispectral analysis index facilitates recovery after ambulatory anesthesia. *Anesthesiology*. 1997;87:842.
171. Friedberg BL. The effect of a dissociative dose of ketamine on the bispectral index (BIS) during propofol hypnosis. *J Clin Anesth*. 1999 Feb;11(1):4–7. doi: 10.1016/s0952-8180(98)00117-2. PMID: 10396711.
172. Kramer KJ, Brady JW. Anesthetic agents commonly used by oral and maxillofacial surgeons. *Oral Maxillofac Surg Clin North Am*. 2018;30(2):155–164.
173. Singer R, Thomas PE. Pulse oximeter in the ambulatory aesthetic surgical facility. *Plast Reconstr Surg*. 1988;82:111.
174. Tang J, Chen X, White PF, et al. Antiemetic prophylaxis for office-based surgery-are the 5-HT3 receptor antagonists beneficial? *Anesthesiology*. 2003;98:293.
175. Chung F, Chan VW, Ong D. A postanesthetic discharge scoring system for home readiness after ambulatory surgery. *J Clin Anesth*. 1995;7:500.
176. Title: Part 755 - Free-Standing and Off-Site Hospital Based Ambulatory Surgery Services. New York Codes, Rules and Regulations. Section 755.6.f; Volume D. 2012.
177. Kaye AD, Armstead-Williams C, Hyatali F, et al. Exparel for postoperative pain management: a comprehensive review. *Curr Pain Headache Rep*. 2020;24:73. https://doi.org/10.1007/s11916-020-00905-4
178. Ilfeld BM, Eisenach JC, Gabriel RA. Clinical effectiveness of liposomal bupivacaine administered by infiltration or peripheral nerve block to treat postoperative pain. *Anesthesiology*. 2021;134(2):283–344.
179. Wells AV, Lippell R, Weinberg RY, Tedore TR, Akerman M. Liposomal bupivacaine to treat postoperative pain: comment. *Anesthesiology*. 2021;135:762–763.
180. White PF. The role of non-opioid analgesic techniques in the management of pain after ambulatory surgery. *Anesth Analg*. 2002;94:577.
181. Ding Y, White PF. Comparative effects of ketorolac, dezocine, and fentanyl as adjuvants during outpatient anesthesia. *Anesth Analg*. 1992;75:566.
182. Desjardins PJ, Shu VS, Recker DP, Verburg KM, Woolf CJ. A single preoperative oral dose of valdecoxib, a new cyclooxygenase-2 specific inhibitor, relieves post-oral surgery or bunionectomy pain. *Anesthesiology*. 2002;97:565.
183. Milnes V, Gonzalez A, Amos V. Aprepitant: a new modality for the prevention of postoperative nausea and vomiting: an evidence-based review. *J Perianesth Nurs*. 2015;30(5):406–417.
184. Gan TJ, Meyer TA, Apfel CC, et al. Society for ambulatory anesthesia guidelines for the management of postoperative nausea and vomiting. *Anesth Analg*. 2007;105:1615–1628.
185. Kovac AL. Prevention and treatment of postoperative nausea and vomiting. *Drugs*. 2000;59: 213.
186. Henzi I, Walder B, Tramèr MR. Dexamethasone for prophylaxis of postoperative nausea and vomiting: a quantitative systematic review. *Anesth Analg*. 2000;90:186.
187. Therneau IW, Martin EE, Sprung J, Kellogg TA, Schroeder DR, Weingarten TN. The role of aprepitant in prevention of postoperative nausea and vomiting after bariatric surgery. *Obes Surg*. 2018;28(1):37–43.
188. Scuderi PE, James RL, Harris L, Mims GR 3rd. Antiemetic prophylaxis does not improve outcomes after outpatient surgery when compared to symptomatic treatment. *Anesthesiology*. 1999;90:360.
189. Surgery in certain outpatient settings. California Codes Business & Professions Code, Division 2. Healing Arts. 2215–17, 2003.
190. California Health and Safety Code, Division 2. Licensing Provisions, Chapter 1.3. Outpatient setting. Cal. Health & Saf. Code. Section 1248.1 1995.
191. New Jersey Administrative Code: Title 13. Law and public safety: Chapter 35. Board of medical examiners: Subchapter 4A. Surgery, special procedures, and anesthesia services performed in an office setting. New Jersey Administrative Code: Title 13. 2003.
192. Manchikanti L, BcMahon EB. Physician refer thyself: Is stark II, Phase III the final voyage? *Pain Physician*. 2007;10:725–741.
193. Office-Based Surgery (OBS) Board-by-Board Status, Regulations, and Policies. Federation of State Medical Boards. Published May 2020. Accessed March 14, 2022. https://www.fsmb.org/siteassets/advocacy/key-issues/office-basedsurgery.pdf

33 Nonoperating Room Anesthesia

ADAM J. CLAESSENS • MICHAEL L. HALL

KEY POINTS

1 Nonoperating room (NOR) locations are remote from a hospital's main operating room sites.

2 A three-step approach that considers the patient, the procedure, and the environment is useful in considering any anesthetic in the NOR setting.

3 All significant patient comorbidities must be carefully assessed, and the appropriate level of sedation, general anesthesia, and level of monitoring determined by the anesthesiologist caring for the patient.

4 Procedural considerations are both general (e.g., duration, position, and level of discomfort) and specific to individual specialties.

5 Patients must receive the same standard of care at a NOR site as they do in the operating room, and the American Society of Anesthesiologists (ASA) has defined guidelines to be applied to the administration of anesthesia in NOR locations.[1]

6 The anesthetic and monitoring equipment used for nonoperating room anesthesia (NORA) must meet the same standards as equipment provided in the operating room.

7 Following NORA, the patient should be transported to an appropriate postanesthesia care unit (PACU), accompanied and monitored by anesthesia-trained personnel.

8 Environmental considerations in NOR locations include hazards such as radiation, magnetic resonance imaging, and the side effects of intravenous contrast agents.

General Principles

1 Nonoperating room anesthesia (NORA) refers to anesthesia that is provided at any location remote from the traditional operating room (OR) environment.[1] These locations include radiology departments, endoscopy suites, magnetic resonance imaging (MRI) scanners, and computed tomography (CT) scanners. This chapter will consider the care of the patient undergoing procedures in these locations. Discussion of anesthesia in stand-alone ambulatory centers, or offices, is addressed in Chapters 31 and 32. Anesthesia and analgesia provided for labor and delivery is discussed in Chapter 41.

Examination of recent data from the National Anesthesia Clinical Outcomes Registry (NACOR)[2] has estimated that NORA accounts for about 30% of anesthesia cases. While the number of OR anesthesia cases remains relatively static, NORA cases have steadily increased, particularly gastroenterologic procedures.[3]

Three-Step Approach to Nonoperating Room Anesthesia 2

Away from theOR, the anesthesiologist may lack familiar equipment and staff experienced in the care of the anesthetized patient. Backup anesthesia-trained personnel may be less immediately available in case of an emergency. NORA, therefore, presents unique challenges and a systematic approach using the simple three-step paradigm "the Patient, the Procedure, and the Environment" is recommended (Fig. 33-1).

The Patient

Patients presenting for NOR procedures tend to be older and of 3
higher ASA status than patients having surgery in the standard ORs. They are also more likely to receive monitored anesthesia care (MAC) or sedation than those undergoing OR procedures.[3] Patients may require sedation or anesthesia to tolerate

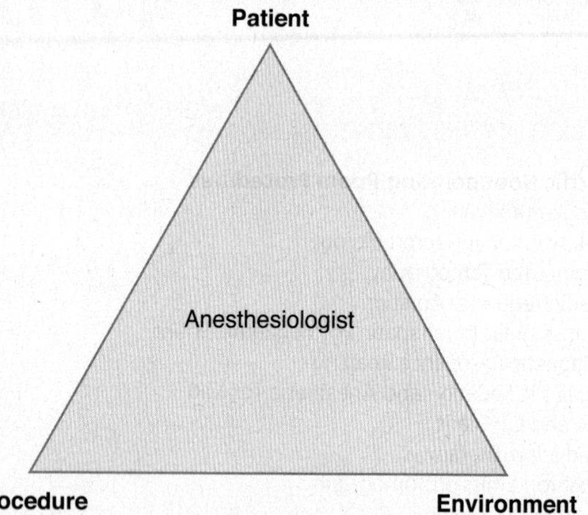

Figure 33-1 A three-step paradigm for nonoperating room anesthesia.

NOR procedures for several reasons (Table 33-1). Children commonly require sedation or anesthesia for diagnostic and therapeutic procedures.[4] Less invasive palliative procedures are increasingly being offered to patients too ill to tolerate a major surgical procedure, representing a continuing challenge for the NOR anesthesiologist. All patients presenting for NORA require a thorough preanesthetic assessment, standard preanesthesia care,[5] the development of a sound anesthetic plan with appropriate monitoring,[6] and the appropriate postanesthesia care.[7]

The Procedure

4 Common NOR procedures for which the patient may require anesthesia or sedation are listed in Table 33-2. The anesthesiologist must understand the nature of the procedure, including the position of the patient, how painful the procedure will be, and how long it will last. The optimum anesthesia plan provides safe patient care and facilitates the procedure. Discussions with the proceduralist must include contingencies for emergencies and adverse outcomes.

The Environment

5 The American Society of Anesthesiologists (ASA) has developed standards for NORA.[1] Prior to the anesthetic, the presence and

Table 33-1 Patient Factors Requiring Sedation or Anesthesia for Nonoperating Room Procedures

Claustrophobia, anxiety, and panic disorders
Cerebral palsy, developmental delay, and learning difficulties
Seizure disorders, movement disorders, and muscular contractures
Pain, both related to the procedure and other causes
Acute trauma with unstable cardiovascular, respiratory, or neurologic function
Raised intracranial pressure
Significant comorbidity and patient frailty (American Society of Anesthesiology physical status III, IV)
Children, especially those below 10 y

Table 33-2 Common Nonoperating Room Anesthesia Procedures

	Procedure
Radiologic imaging	Computed tomography Magnetic resonance imaging Positron emission tomography
Interventional radiology[a]	Vascular imaging, stenting, and embolization procedures Biopsy and/or drainage of lesions, tumors, cysts Radiofrequency ablation
	Transjugular intrahepatic portosystemic shunt
Interventional neuroradiology[a]	Occlusive ("closing") procedures • Embolization of cerebral aneurysm • Embolization of arteriovenous malformations • Embolization of vascular tumors "Opening" procedures in acute thromboembolic stroke, cerebral atherosclerosis, or cerebral vasospasm • Angioplasty • Stenting • Thrombolysis
Radiotherapy	Radiation therapy Intraoperative radiotherapy
Interventional cardiology[a]	
Cardiac catheterization laboratory	Diagnostic cardiac catheterization Percutaneous coronary interventions Percutaneous ventricular assist devices Percutaneous closure of septal defects Alcohol septal ablation Structural heart procedures • Transcatheter aortic valve replacement • Mitral valve repair for mitral regurgitation ("MitraClip") • Left atrial appendage occlusion
Electrophysiology laboratory (EPL)	Cardiac implantable electronic devices Electrophysiology studies with ablation Laser lead extraction
Other cardiac procedures	Cardioversion Diagnostic transesophageal echocardiography
Gastroenterology[a]	Upper gastroenterology endoscopy Esophageal dilatation or stenting Percutaneous endoscopic gastrostomy tube placement Endoscopic retrograde cholangiopancreatography Colonoscopy Liver biopsy
Psychiatry	Electroconvulsive therapy

[a]Diagnostic and therapeutic procedures.

Table 33-3 American Society of Anesthesiology Standards for Nonoperating Room Anesthetizing Locations[1]

1. Oxygen-reliable source—ideally piped and full backup E-cylinder
2. Suction-adequate and reliable
3. Scavenging system if inhalational agents are administered
4. Anesthetic equipment
   - Backup self-inflating bag capable of delivering at least 90% oxygen by positive pressure ventilation
   - Adequate anesthetic drugs, supplies, and equipment for intended anesthesia care
   - Adequate monitoring equipment to allow adherence to the ASA standards for basic monitoring[6]
   - Anesthesia machine with equivalent function to those in the operating rooms and maintained to the same standards
5. Electrical outlets
   - Sufficient for anesthesia machine and monitors
   - Isolated electrical power or ground fault circuit interrupters if "wet location"
6. Adequate illumination of patient, anesthesia machine, and monitoring equipment; battery-operated backup light source
7. Sufficient space for:
   - Personnel and equipment
   - Easy and expeditious access to patient, anesthesia machine, and monitoring equipment
8. Resuscitation equipment immediately available
   - Defibrillator/emergency drugs/cardiopulmonary resuscitation equipment
9. Adequately trained staff to support the anesthesiologist and a reliable means of two-way communication
10. All building and safety codes and facility standards should be observed
11. Postanesthesia care facilities[7]
    - Adequately trained staff to provide postanesthesia care
    - Appropriate equipment to allow safe transport to main postanesthesia care unit

proper functioning of all equipment needed for safe patient care must be established; this is described in Table 33-3. The location of immediately available resuscitation equipment should be noted and protocols developed with the local staff for dealing with emergencies, including cardiopulmonary resuscitation and the management of complications including anaphylaxis, malignant hyperthermia (MH), and local anesthetic systemic toxicity (LAST).

6 Anesthesia Equipment and Monitors

Anesthesia machines and monitors may or may not be provided in NOR locations. Small, portable anesthesia machines and monitors are available if a site does not offer a permanent anesthesia workstation. Anesthesia machines and monitors that remain in a NOR location need to undergo routine maintenance. Infrequent use may result in degradation of equipment and the use of preprocedural checks, preferably with a standardized checklist, cannot be overemphasized before embarking on NORA. If more advanced monitors (e.g., an arterial line, central venous pressure [CVP], or intracranial pressure [ICP] monitoring) are required, these devices should be readily available. A standardized anesthesia cart containing essential equipment that is checked and restocked after each case is recommended.

Patient Safety in Nonoperating Room Anesthesia

Patient safety is of utmost importance in all types of anesthesia, not least NORA.

Adverse Events

Significant adverse events occur infrequently in NOR locations, although the large multicenter studies needed to determine their true incidence are lacking. A recent study of the NACOR database[3] indicated that contrary to previous reports,[8] NORA procedures appear to have a lower incidence of both minor and major complications and mortality than OR procedures. However, the continued need for vigilance and attention to detail remains high in NORA. The ASA closed claims database has identified NORA as an area of liability for the anesthesiologist.[8] The gastroenterology suite, cardiac catheterization lab, and the emergency department are sites where adverse events are most likely to occur; and the elderly, medically complex patients there have been determined to be more at risk by both the closed claims and the NACOR analyses.[3,9] Respiratory depression secondary to oversedation was the most common type of adverse event in the closed claims study.[8,9] Capnography provides an early monitor of impending respiratory depression during sedation and is recommended.[6,10,11] Adverse events associated with NORA have been divided into minor and major and appear to be more frequent in patients undergoing radiology procedures and in cardiology locations (Table 33-4).[3]

Table 33-4 Complications of Nonoperating Room Anesthesia[3]

Minor Complications (in Order of Frequency)
Postoperative nausea and vomiting
Inadequate postoperative pain control
Hemodynamic instability
Minor neurologic complications such as postdural puncture headache (cardiology and radiologic locations)
Minor respiratory complications (cardiology and radiologic locations)
Complications related to central/intravenous lines (cardiology locations)
Need for opioid reversal (cardiology and radiologic locations)
Major Complications
Unintended patient awareness (gastroenterologic locations)
Anaphylaxis (radiology procedures and cardiology locations)
Need for upgrade of care
Serious hemodynamic instability
Respiratory complications
Need for resuscitation
Central and peripheral nervous system injury (radiology procedures and cardiology locations)
Vascular access–related complications (radiology procedures and cardiology locations)
Wrong patient/wrong site (radiology procedures and cardiology locations)
Fall or burn (radiology procedures and cardiology locations)

Reprinted with permission from Du AL, Robbins KS, Waterman RS, et al. National trends in nonoperating room anesthesia: procedures, facilities, and patient characteristics. *Curr Opin Anaesthesiol*. 2021;34(1):464–469.

Preprocedural Checklists

The use of checklists and pre- and postprocedural team briefings has been broadly embraced in OR practice and emerging evidence points toward improved patient outcomes when checklists are employed.[12,13] Similar systems should be adopted in NOR sites and recently a checklist has been proposed for use in interventional radiology suites.[14]

Standards of Care for Nonoperating Room Anesthesia

The ASA has published a number of guidelines and standards of care for preanesthesia[5] and postanesthesia[7] care, basic monitoring standards,[6] and MAC.[15] These standards apply to patients being cared for in all NOR sites in the same way as they do in the ORs. At the conclusion of the NOR procedure, the patient should be transported to a recovery area by a member of the anesthesia team who must provide a full verbal report to the recovery nursing staff. The recovery area should be equipped to the same standards as for postoperative patients.

7 Patient Transfer

Sick, unstable patients are often transferred back and forth between the intensive care unit, the ORs, and NOR locations for imaging, therapeutic, or diagnostic procedures. During transport, the patient should be accompanied by skilled personnel to evaluate, monitor, and support the patient's medical condition. A specialized transport team may contribute to reducing the number of critical incidents that occur during the transport of ventilated and critically ill patients.[16] Patients are often mechanically ventilated and receiving multiple drug infusions for both sedation and hemodynamic support. Portable ventilators are useful for transport; adequate supplies of oxygen must be available for the transfer. A manual self-inflating bag is essential in the event of ventilator failure. Infusion pumps and portable monitors should have adequate battery power for transit. The transport team should carry spare anesthetic and emergency drugs, equipment for intubation or reintubation, portable suction, and if the patient's condition requires, a portable defibrillator. It is vital to notify the destination area that the patient is in transit, so that appropriate preparations to receive the patient can be made in advance. It is also useful to send personnel ahead to secure the elevators to prevent delays during transfer.

Sedation and Anesthesia

Definition of Sedation and Anesthesia

Many NOR procedures are performed under sedation or MAC, for which the ASA has developed guidelines.[15] A consistent definition of these terms is essential for clear communication between the various stakeholders involved in provision of NORA. On January 14, 2011, the Centers for Medicare and Medicaid Services (CMS) issued a revision to Interpretive Guideline (IG) for Hospitals No. 482.52 concerning anesthesia services. This revised guideline places the responsibility and oversight for all anesthesia services under the direction of one suitably qualified physician, the "director of anesthesia services."[17] IG 482.52 defines "anesthesia," to mean general anesthesia, regional anesthesia, deep sedation/analgesia, or MAC. "Analgesia/sedation" is defined as local/topical anesthesia, minimal sedation, and moderate sedation/analgesia ("conscious sedation").

The Continuum of Anesthesia

Anesthesia exists along a continuum and the transition from minimal sedation to general anesthesia is not clear-cut (Table 33-5).[15,17–19] As sedation deepens, it is important to recognize the progressive blunting and loss of airway reflexes and patency, together with depression of spontaneous ventilation and cardiovascular function. The individual responsiveness of patients to different sedative agents varies, as do the levels of stimulation throughout a procedure. Medications given preprocedurally may interact or have a synergistic effect with sedative agents, contributing to respiratory depression. Consequently, during the course of a NOR procedure under sedation, the patient may drift to a deeper level than the one intended, including transitioning into general anesthesia with loss of airway reflexes and possibly airway obstruction. In any circumstances where a particular level of sedation is being provided, services must be immediately available to rescue a patient from a deeper-than-intended level of sedation or general anesthesia.[18]

Environmental Considerations for Nonoperating Room Anesthesia 8

X-Rays and Fluoroscopy

X-radiation (x-rays) are produced when electrons are accelerated through high voltage in a vacuum tube and collide with a metal

Table 33-5 Definition of General Anesthesia and Levels of Sedation/Analgesia[18]

	Minimal Sedation (Anxiolysis)	Moderate Sedation/Analgesia (Conscious Sedation)	Deep Sedation/Analgesia	General Anesthesia
Responsiveness	Normal response to verbal stimulation	Purposeful[a] response to verbal or tactile stimulation	Purposeful[a] response after repeated or painful stimulation	Unarousable, even with painful stimulus
Airway	Unaffected	No intervention required	Intervention may be required	Intervention often required
Spontaneous ventilation	Unaffected	Adequate	May be inadequate	Frequently inadequate
Cardiovascular function	Unaffected	Usually maintained	Usually maintained	May be impaired

[a]Reflex withdrawal from a painful stimulus is *not* considered a purposeful response.

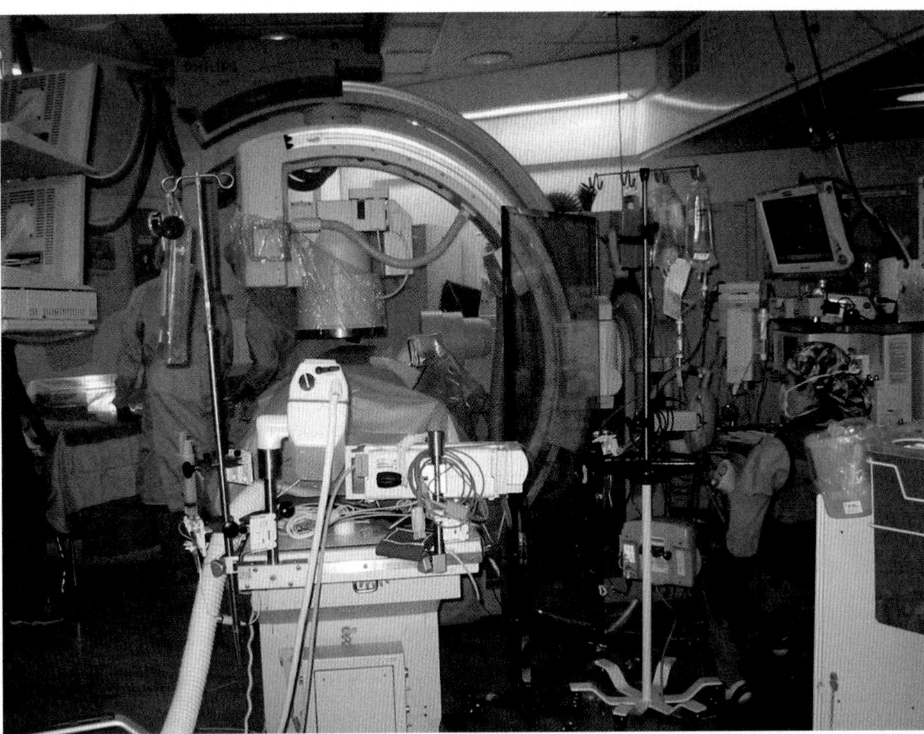

Figure 33-2 A radiology suite showing a C-arm and the high density of equipment that may separate the anesthesiologist from the patient.

target. In medical x-ray tubes, the target is usually tungsten or a more crack-resistant alloy of rhenium (5%) and tungsten (95%) (1 Video 33-1). X-ray production is determined by, and directly proportional to, the tube current and the voltage. Fluoroscopy is a technique used to obtain real-time moving images of the internal structures. The patient is positioned between the x-ray source and a fluorescent screen. By coupling the fluoroscope to an x-ray image intensifier and a video camera, the images can be recorded and played on a monitor. Fluoroscopy is widely and increasingly used in NOR locations including interventional radiology, cardiac catheterization, and electrophysiologic procedures and in the gastroenterology suite. Large, C-shaped, mobile fluoroscopy devices (C-arms) are used to provide images in multiple dimensions. The C-arm often impedes access to the patient by the anesthesiologist; and during C-arm movement (e.g., 3D rotational angiography, or "spins") risks dislodging intravascular lines and endotracheal tubes (Fig. 33-2).

Hazards of Ionizing Radiation

The effects of ionizing radiation on biologic tissues are classified as deterministic (dose related causing cell death and tissue damage) and stochastic (the development of cancer from direct DNA ionization or the creation of hydroxyl radicals from x-ray interactions with water molecules). Patient exposure to radiation during imaging and treatment varies depending on the type of procedure as well as patient- and operator-related factors.[20] For example, the radiation a patient receives from a simple chest x-ray is 0.02 millisieverts (mSv), and between 20 and 40 mSv for pulmonary angiography.[21] Exposure from fluoroscopy is 100 to 1,000 times greater than from simple x-rays. Standard procedures exist to minimize patient exposure to radiation and efforts to reduce occupational exposure for staff including anesthesiologists working in radiology suites are an important consideration. A number of terms are used to define exposure to radiation[22]; these are summarized in Table 33-6.

NOR staff, including anesthesiologists, must be aware of the hazards of occupational exposure to ionizing radiation and take appropriate measures to protect themselves.[23] Exposure to ionizing radiation may come from direct exposure and from scatter. Patients are subjected to direct exposure where the beam enters the skin, whereas staff members working in fluoroscopy suites are more at risk from scattered radiation. In general, the exposure to staff is 1/1,000th the entrance skin exposure at 1 m from the fluoroscopy tube. A recent study of radiation exposure to OR personnel during fluoroscopic-guided endovascular repair of thoracoabdominal aortic aneurysms using fenestrated endografts identified that anesthesiologists were likely to receive 15 times the dose of radiation compared to the scrub nurses even though both types of practitioners were at the same distance (7 feet) from the C-arm.[24] This finding was attributed to anesthesiologists being less likely to use the protective shielding during their patient care activities. Another recent study demonstrated that anesthesiologists working in the neurointerventional suite were at equal risk of developing cataracts as neuroradiologists, and that the radiation may even be directed away from the neuroradiologists and toward the anesthesiologist.[25] These studies highlight the need for anesthesiologists to be aware of the risks and the means to protect themselves from radiation, especially in areas where fluoroscopy is used.

Staff exposure to radiation can be minimized by taking certain precautions[22,23]:

1. *Limiting the time of exposure to radiation.*
2. *Increasing the distance from the source of radiation. (Dose rates are proportionate to the inverse square of the distance from the source.)*
3. *Using protective shielding* (lead-lined garments and fixed and/or movable shields).

Lead aprons, thyroid shields, and leaded eyeglasses are recommended despite being bulky and contributing to staff fatigue. Anesthesiology staff should consider using movable

Table 33-6 Common Terms Used in Radiation Exposure[22]

Term	Units	Definition	Notes
Exposure	Roentgen (R)—defined as 2.58 × 10^{-4} coulombs (C)/kg (SI units).	Quantity of x-radiation or gamma radiation required to produce an amount of ionization (electric charge) in air at standard temperature and pressure	Ionization measurements are often made in exposure rate, i.e., amount of exposure per unit time, e.g., fluoroscopy is measured in R/min
Absorbed dose	Rad (radiation absorbed dose) or Gray (Gy, the SI unit)	Amount of ionizing radiation absorbed by the body	Depends on exposure to x-ray beam and the tissue type A Gray represents 100 times more radiation than a Rad
Dose equivalent	Sievert (Sv) or roentgen equivalent in man (rem)	Absorbed dose multiplied by a radiation quality factor specific for the type of radiation	Measures the "harmfulness" of any radiation-absorbed dose
Effective dose	Sievert (Sv)	Dose equivalent to the entire body caused by irradiating only a localized area. Calculated by multiplying the dose equivalent by a weighting factor specific for the irradiated organ	Takes into account the differing radiosensitivity of different organs Used to estimate cancer risk for patients (stochastic effects) and to calculate equivalent whole-body exposure in staff wearing personal dosimeters for comparison with annual personnel dose limits

or fixed lead-lined glass shields so that they can gain easy access to their patients while protecting themselves from radiation.

4. *Measuring occupational exposure to radiation.*

The dose limits for occupational exposure to radiation established by the International Commission on Radiological Protection (IRCP) have been adopted in most countries.[26] In the United States, the National Council on Radiation Protection and Measurements (NCRP) recommends an occupational limit of 50 mSv in any single year and a lifetime limit of 10 mSv multiplied by the individual's age in years.[23,27] Health care workers including anesthesiologists should be issued individual dosimeter badges to monitor their cumulative exposure to radiation. These data should be regularly reviewed by the facility's radiation safety section or medical physics department.

Intravenous Contrast Agents

Intravenous contrast agents are commonly used in radiologic and MRI to enhance vascular imaging. Radiologic contrast media are iodinated compounds classified according to their osmolarity (high, low, or iso-osmolar), their ionicity (ionic or nonionic), and the number of benzene rings (monomer or dimer). Nonionic contrast agents cause less discomfort on injection and have a lower incidence of adverse reactions.[28] MRI contrast agents are also divided into ionic and nonionic compounds. They are chelated metal complexes containing gadolinium, iron, or manganese.

Adverse reactions to contrast agents may be divided into renal adverse reactions and hypersensitivity reactions.[29]

Renal Adverse Reaction

Contrast agents are eliminated via the kidneys, and contrast-induced nephropathy (CIN) associated with their use is estimated to account for nearly 10% of hospital-acquired acute renal failure.[30] CIN is defined as an increase in serum creatinine of 0.5 mg/dL or a 25% increase from the baseline within 48 to 72 hours after iodinated contrast medium administration. Chronic kidney disease is the most important predictor of CIN, increasing the risk by 20 times[30]; other risk factors for CIN include history of renal disease, prior renal surgery, proteinuria, diabetes mellitus, hypertension, gout, and use of nephrotoxic drugs. Preventative measures to avoid CIN include adequate hydration, maintaining a good urine output, and using sodium bicarbonate infusions to improve elimination of the contrast agent. Nephrotoxic medications such as nonsteroidal anti-inflammatory drugs, aminoglycosides, and diuretics should be avoided for 24 to 48 hours before and after the use of intravenous (IV) contrast agents. The efficacy of N-acetylcysteine and other agents such as fenoldopam, dopamine, calcium channel blockers, atrial natriuretic peptide, and L-arginine in mitigating CIN has not been proven.[31]

Hypersensitivity Reactions

Hypersensitivity reactions to contrast media are divided into immediate (<1 hour) and nonimmediate (>1 hour) reactions.[28,29] Mild immediate reactions occur in about 0.5% to 3% and severe reactions occur in 0.01% to 0.04%. Fatal hypersensitivity reactions may occur in about 1 per 100,000 contrast administrations. The frequency of nonimmediate reactions is much more variable (0.5% to 23%) related partly to difficulty in determining whether symptoms relate to contrast agents or not. The clinical manifestations of various hypersensitivity reactions to contrast media are outlined in Table 33-7.[32] Although widely used, the effectiveness of corticosteroids and antihistamines in preventing hypersensitivity reactions to contrast agents in unselected patients is doubtful.[33] Treatment of severe hypersensitivity reactions includes discontinuing the causative agent and supportive therapy, oxygen, intubating the trachea, cardiovascular support with fluids, vasopressors, and inotropes, and if required, bronchodilators.[29] Reactions to gadolinium-based contrast agents used for MRI are less frequent than to iodinated contrast agents. Hypersensitivity

Table 33-7 Clinical Manifestations of Immediate and Nonimmediate Hypersensitivity Reactions to Radiocontrast Agents[a,32]

Immediate Reactions
Pruritus
Urticaria
Angioedema/facial edema
Abdominal pain, nausea, diarrhea
Rhinitis (sneezing, rhinorrhea)
Hoarseness, cough
Dyspnea (bronchospasm, laryngeal edema)
Respiratory arrest
Hypotension, cardiovascular shock
Cardiac arrest
Nonimmediate Reactions
Pruritus
Exanthema (mostly macular or maculopapular drug eruption)
Urticaria, angioedema
Erythema multiforme minor
Fixed drug eruption
Stevens–Johnson syndrome
Toxic epidermal necrolysis
Graft-versus-host reaction
Drug-related eosinophilia with systemic symptoms (DRESS)
Symmetrical drug-related intertriginous and flexural exanthema (SDRIFE)
Vasculitis

[a]Most frequent are in italics.

Adapted with permission from Springer: Brockow K. Immediate drug hypersensitivity: epidemiology, clinical features, triggers and management. *Hautarzt*. 2014;65(5):409–414.

to gadolinium-containing agents occurs in 5.9 per 10,000 injections and the rate is higher (13 per 10,000) in patients undergoing abdominal MRI examinations. Severe reactions occur 1:10,000 to 1:40,000 and the mortality rate is 1 in a million injections.[34] Gadolinium-containing compounds have been associated with nephrogenic systemic fibrosis (NSF), a disease manifesting fibrosis of the skin and internal organs with some similarities to scleroderma in patients with renal insufficiency.[29,35]

Specific Nonoperating Room Procedures

Angiography

Angiography causes minimal discomfort and may be performed under local anesthesia with or without light sedation. Patients are required to remain completely motionless during these procedures, which may be lengthy, particularly spinal angiography. Neurologic disorders such as recent subarachnoid hemorrhage, stroke, and depressed level of consciousness or raised ICP may necessitate anesthesia with intubation for airway protection. Patients with chronic pain, morbid obesity, or pulmonary comorbidities may be unable to lay flat, requiring a deeper level of sedation or controlled ventilation with general anesthesia. Angiography is often performed via the femoral artery; the femoral vein may also be accessed when imaging arteriovenous malformations (AVMs) or dural venous abnormalities. Liberal use of local anesthetic at the puncture site precludes the need for IV analgesia. The injection of contrast media into the cerebral arteries may cause discomfort, burning, or pruritus around the face and eyes. Hypotension and bradycardia may also occur and discomfort from a full bladder as a result of fluid and IV contrast administration is a consideration in nonanesthetized patients. During angiography and other interventional radiologic procedures, the patient is placed on a moving gantry and the radiologist positions the patient to track catheters as they pass from the groin into the vessels of interest. It is vital to have extensions on all anesthesia breathing circuits, infusion lines, and monitors to prevent these implements from being accidentally dislodged as the radiologist swings the x-ray table back and forth. Care should be taken with positioning of radiopaque pieces of equipment. The electrocardiogram electrodes and metallic coils in the cuffs of endotracheal tubes may cause radiologic artifacts if they lie over the area being imaged.

Interventional Neuroradiology

A variety of neurosurgical conditions including neurovascular diseases are effectively managed by interventional neuroradiology.[36] These procedures may be subdivided as "occlusive" and "opening" procedures (Table 33-2).

Cerebral aneurysms and AVMs are particularly amenable to occlusive endovascular treatments.[37] A commonly employed technique is to insert detachable platinum coils into the abnormal vessel(s). Other occlusive agents include cyanoacrylates, biocompatible liquid embolic agents, and polyvinyl alcohol particles. These particles may also be used to produce temporary occlusion of blood vessels for preoperative embolization of vascular tumors, particularly meningiomas. In 2009, a large multicenter study, the International Subarachnoid Aneurysm Trial (ISAT) reported better outcomes in patients with ruptured anterior and posterior circulation aneurysms undergoing interventional neuroradiology compared to surgical clipping.[38] The benefits of coiling appear to be prolonged with the most recent follow-up of ISAT reporting the probability of disability-free survival to be significantly greater in the endovascular group compared to the neurosurgical group at 10 years.[39] The World Federation of Neurosurgical Societies' (WFNS's) poor grade for cerebral aneurysms in elderly patients did not clearly establish the superiority of one treatment or the other.[40,41] The management of an unruptured intracranial aneurysm depends on many factors including aneurysm size, shape, location, and patient comorbidity. In 2015, the American Heart Association and American Stroke Association jointly published guidelines for management of unruptured intracranial aneurysms.[42]

"Opening" procedures include the management of acute thromboembolic stroke and postsubarachnoid hemorrhage vasospasm. In the case of acute ischemic stroke, early (within 6 hours of symptoms) intervention to recanalize the occluded vessel by superselective intra-arterial thrombolytic therapy has been shown to improve outcome.[43,44] Specialized centers have developed various "stroke code protocols"[45] to manage these patients with the NOR anesthesiologist forming a key member of the team.

Procedural and Anesthetic Technique Considerations in Interventional Neuroradiology

For most interventional neuroradiologic procedures, arterial access is gained using a 6- or 7-French gauge sheath via the femoral or, rarely, the carotid or axillary artery. The umbilical vessels are an alternative route in neonates. Anticoagulation is required during and up to 24 hours after interventional radiologic procedures to prevent thromboembolism. Heparin, between 3,000 and 5,000 IU (50 to 70 IU/kg), followed by an infusion is used to keep the activated clotting time (ACT) between two and three times the patient's baseline.[43] At the end of the procedure, or in case of hemorrhage, heparin effect may be reversed with protamine. Protamine should always be given slowly and the patient monitored for anaphylaxis or hypotentsion. General anesthesia and conscious sedation are both suitable techniques for interventional neuroradiology, depending on the complexity of the procedure, the need for blood pressure manipulation, and the need for intraprocedural assessment of neurologic function.[36,43] The anesthetic management of patients undergoing endovascular treatment for acute ischemic stroke received much attention recently.[46,47]

Cases performed under general anesthesia and associated with hypotension have been related to poorer neurologic outcome compared to cases performed under local anesthesia and no hypotension. General anesthesia for interventional neuroradiology is usually conducted with endotracheal intubation and positive pressure ventilation, although the laryngeal mask airway (LMA) is a suitable alternative in selected cases.[48] Sedation techniques vary; propofol infusions are widely used, as are combinations of a benzodiazepine (usually midazolam) and opioid (usually fentanyl). The anesthesiologist may facilitate the procedure by manipulating systemic blood pressure and controlling end-tidal carbon dioxide tension. Controlled hypotension is often requested to facilitate embolization of AVMs and moderate hypertension may help reduce cerebral ischemia by maintaining cerebral perfusion. Certain procedures require patients to be awake for part of the procedure. The Wada test (injection of a small dose of a barbiturate or other anesthetic drug directly into one) is used to determine the dominant side for cognitive functions such as speech and memory. This procedure may be used prior to surgery for non–life-threatening conditions such as epilepsy. Permanent neurologic deficits follow embolization of AVMs in approximately 10% of cases.[49] The superselective anesthesia functional examination (SAFE), an extension of the Wada test, may be performed prior to permanent embolization by injecting anesthetic into the vessels to identify angiographically occult vessels that supply normal brain tissue.[50] The worldwide unavailability of amobarbital has led to the use of other agents in these tests including propofol[50,51] and etomidate.

Major complications of interventional neuroradiology are hemorrhagic, such as aneurysm rupture, intracranial vessel injury, or dissection; occlusive, such as displacement or fragmentation of embolic materials or vasospasm; or non–central nervous system (CNS) complications, such as contrast hypersensitivity, anaphylaxis, CIN, and hemorrhage at the peripheral vessel puncture site causing groin or retroperitoneal hematoma.[36,43]

Computed Tomography

CT scanners obtain a cross-sectional image in a few seconds, and spiral scanners can image a slice of the body in less than 1 second, minimizing problems with motion artifacts. The procedure is painless and most adults do not require sedation or anesthesia. There is an absolute requirement for the patient to remain motionless while the study is being performed and children or adults with psychologic or neurologic disorders preventing immobility may require sedation or anesthesia (Table 33-1). Contrast agents for CT imaging may be administered orally and the anesthesiologist needs to be aware of the possibility of a full stomach. CT scanning may be employed to facilitate invasive procedures such as abscess localization and drainage, ablation of bony metastases, and radiofrequency ablation (RFA) of malignancies. Patients with acute thoracic, abdominal, and cerebral trauma often require urgent imaging to facilitate diagnosis. These patients may develop hemorrhagic shock, raised ICP, depression of consciousness, and cardiac arrest in the CT scanner and must be adequately resuscitated and stabilized before transportation to the radiology department.

Radiofrequency Ablation

Percutaneous RFA is carried out in the radiology suite for treatment of primary and metastatic tumors in the liver, lung, adrenal gland, breast, thyroid, prostate, kidney, and spleen. A high-frequency alternating current is used to generate a localized heat source directly into the tumor causing coagulative necrosis and tumor cell death while avoiding injury to the surrounding tissues. The majority of these procedures are tolerated without sedation. If an anesthesiologist does become involved in the care of these patients, careful evaluation is required; patients may be in the later stages of their disease, have often failed surgical treatment, and may have undergone extensive radiation therapy and/or chemotherapy. Recently, high-frequency jet ventilation (HFJV) has been evaluated in patients undergoing anesthesia for RFA of liver tumors.[52] Positioning of the probe is critical and excursions of the diaphragm in ventilated or spontaneously ventilating patients may cause excessive movement; HFJV minimizes liver motion during these procedures. A variety of anesthesia techniques have been described for percutaneous RFA of hepatic tumors including general anesthesia, sedation, thoracic epidural, and thoracic paravertebral block.[53]

Transjugular Intrahepatic Portosystemic Shunt

Transjugular intrahepatic portosystemic shunt (TIPS) is a connection between the hepatic portal and systemic circulations created via a percutaneous catheter inserted in the internal jugular vein and directed into the liver. TIPS functions to decompress the portal circulation in patients with portal hypertension. Beneficial effects include reduction in bleeding from varices and control of refractory cirrhotic ascites. TIPS is often performed in patients who have failed to respond to medical therapy and may be used as a bridge to transplant in patients with poor liver function. The procedure causes minimal stimulation, lasts between 2 and 3 hours, and may be performed under sedation or general anesthesia.[54] Patients presenting for a TIPS procedure, in general, have significant hepatic dysfunction, and require careful preoperative assessment and intraoperative management. The considerations are outlined in Table 33-8 (see also Chapter 46).

Magnetic Resonance Imaging

Physical Principles

The physical principles of MRI are well described in detail elsewhere.[55] Briefly, when atoms with an odd number of protons in their nuclei, notably hydrogen, are subjected to a powerful static magnetic field, they align themselves with the magnetic field. If they are then intermittently exposed to a radiofrequency wave, the nuclei change their alignment. As the radiofrequency pulses are discontinued, the protons return to their original alignment ("relax") within the magnetic field and, as they do, they release energy. The release of energy over time (the relaxation time) is specific for given tissues and is used to generate the MRI signal. Magnetic field strengths are expressed in Gauss (G) and Tesla (T) (1 T = 10,000 G). The earth's magnetic field is approximately 0.3 to 0.7 G. MRI scanners used for clinical purposes generate a field of

Table 33-8 Considerations in Patients Presenting for the Transjugular Intrahepatic Portosystemic Shunt Procedure

Airway—risk of aspiration	Recent gastrointestinal bleeding Raised intragastric pressure due to ascites Decreased level of consciousness due to hepatic encephalopathy
CNS	Hepatic encephalopathy Altered mental status Variable response to anesthetic agents
Respiratory system	Decreased functional residual capacity due to ascites Pleural effusion Intrapulmonary shunts Pneumonia
Cardiovascular system	Associated alcoholic cardiomyopathy Altered volume status Acute hemorrhage from esophageal varices Intraperitoneal hemorrhage
Hematologic system	Coagulopathy Thrombocytopenia
Fluid balance	Ascites Risk of hepatorenal syndrome
Endocrine system	Tendency to hypoglycemia
Pharmacokinetics	Increased volume of distribution Decreased protein binding, drug metabolism, and elimination

CNS, central nervous system.

1.5 to 3 T, and machines generating magnetic fields from 4 to 9.4 T are used in research.

Hazards of MRI

MRI is devoid of the risks related to ionizing radiation; however, peripheral nerve stimulation (PNS) has been reported in biologic tissues exposed to radiofrequencies greater than 60 Hz (NICV 33-1). PNS results in sensory phenomena ranging from mild tingling to intolerable pain. MRI workers may experience transient vertigo-related symptoms and a metallic taste in the mouth when working in high (>3 T) magnetic fields.[56] Ferromagnetic implantable medical devices may move in the magnetic field with disastrous consequences. This issue is a particular concern in patients with cardiac pacemakers, which may also malfunction, and cerebral aneurysm clips.[57] Before entering the vicinity of the magnet, patients and staff need to complete a rigorous checklist to ensure that they have no ferrometallic objects in their bodies. The magnetic field takes several days to establish and is constantly present, decreasing in strength with distance from the center of the magnet. Ferromagnetic equipment such as IV poles, gas cylinders, laryngoscopes, and pens become potentially lethal projectiles if brought too close.

Considerable noise is generated by the rapidly alternating currents of the MRI scanner; this noise may exceed the occupational exposure limits, defined as a weekly average exposure of 99 dB and peak exposure of 140 dB.[58] Patients and staff should wear ear protection and staff should minimize time spent in the scanner. Cables and wires wound in loops may cause induction-heating effects and thermal injury may also occur in skin with large tattoos, especially those with ferromagnetic inks. Patient monitors, ventilator equipment, and electrical infusion pumps may all malfunction when they come too close to the magnetic field. The electrocardiogram is sensitive to the changing magnetic signals, and it is nearly impossible to eliminate all artifacts. The electrodes should be placed close together and toward the center of the magnetic field and the leads insulated from the patient's skin to avoid causing thermal injury. MRI-compatible devices have been developed; however, in the absence of MRI-compatible monitors, tube extensions can be used to keep standard infusion pumps and monitors at a distance.[55] An MRI sequence takes upward of 30 minutes and many patients find it difficult to stay still for long periods. It may become very warm within the coil of the magnet, often reaching 80 °F, adding to patient discomfort and is of particular concern in children whose temperatures should be monitored. Once a scan sequence is initiated, no one may enter or leave the scan room. In the case of an emergency, the MRI technicians should be notified, the scan sequence stopped, and the patient rapidly removed. Resuscitation attempts should take place outside the scanner because equipment such as laryngoscopes, oxygen cylinders, and cardiac defibrillators cannot be taken close to the magnet.

Anesthetic Technique

Claustrophobia is a real concern for up to 15% of all adult patients undergoing MRI necessitating sedation or even general anesthesia for them to complete the imaging studies.[59] Sedation may be provided by the oral route with benzodiazepines, as IV sedation or MAC. Interventions including the design of the MRI scanner, cognitive-behavioral strategies, prone positioning, and fragrance administration have also been reported to reduce anxiety during MRI scan.[60] Anesthesiologists often become involved with more complex patients such as those with obesity, obstructive sleep apnea (OSA), elevated ICP, movement disorders, developmental delay, and when there is potential for a difficult airway.

Pediatric Sedation and Anesthesia for MRI and CT Scans

In children, a combination of incomprehension, separation anxiety, and fear can result in noncooperation and intolerance of relatively brief periods of immobility. Most children younger than 5 years and some as old as 11 years, particularly those with developmental delay, require sedation or general anesthesia for successful acquisition of MRI or CT images.[61] There is ongoing debate about the optimal care and techniques for these cases.[62,63] The benefits of a "sedation-only" approach include ease of medication administration (oral, rectal, or sometimes IV), lower cost (a sedation-trained nurse rather than an anesthesiologist), and more rapid wakening and discharge home. Disadvantages include a higher failure rate than general anesthesia, airway complications arising from oversedation, unpredictable onset of enteral sedatives causing schedule delays, and inadequate analgesia during painful procedures. The choice of sedation or general anesthesia for a particular child is multifactorial and has been obfuscated in the past by the use of imprecise terms to describe the different clinical states.[64] As with all NORA, the standards of care for pediatric patients undergoing sedation and/or general anesthesia for MRI and CT imaging are the same as those in the OR. A checklist mnemonic, "SOAPME" (Suction, Oxygen, Airway equipment, appropriate Pharmaceuticals, Monitoring, and special

Equipment) can be used before embarking upon any pediatric sedation or anesthetic.[65]

Sedative Agents

Older sedation practices in pediatric patients included the use of oral chloral hydrate, "lytic cocktails," barbiturates, and the "feed, wrap, and scan" technique in otherwise healthy neonates avoiding sedation or anesthesia altogether. These techniques, however, are being superseded by the use of short-acting agents including propofol, remifentanil, and dexmedetomidine[4] which provide more reliable pharmacologic profiles and have preferable track records for adverse events.[66]

Radiation Therapy

External beam radiation is a common treatment for children with malignancies, making use of either highly tissue-targeted or total body irradiating (TBI) doses of x-rays. Proton beam therapy is a newer modality of this therapy, which has less potential for collateral injury to adjacent or beam-traversed tissues, a factor of utmost importance in pediatric patients at risk of long-term complications of radiation exposure.[67,68] Radiosensitive malignancies occurring in children are shown in Table 33-9. Tumors commonly involve vital structures such as the airway, thorax, mediastinum, heart, and CNS. Thorough preoperative assessment is essential, including assessment for elevated ICP in children with CNS tumors, and compressive symptoms of mediastinal masses. Many children receive concurrent cytotoxic or immunosuppressive chemotherapy and are at increased risk of sepsis, thrombocytopenia, and anemia. The challenges of anesthesia for children undergoing radiation therapy have recently been reviewed.[68–70] Patients are typically scheduled for a series of daily treatments, which can last upward of 45 minutes, over a 6-week period. Radiation doses in the range of 180 to 250 centiGray (cGy) are employed, so interfaced systems of closed-circuit television and telemetric microphones are used with standard monitoring to prevent staff from being exposed to high levels of radiation. In the event of a problem, shutdown of the radiation beam and immediate access to the patient (within 20 to 30 seconds) is crucial. Children older than 6 or 7 years can sometimes tolerate repeated treatment sessions without sedation or anesthesia using behavioral techniques,[70] although most require general anesthesia or deep sedation techniques with propofol.[71,72] Absence of movement is crucial to ensure treatment beam accuracy and immobilization devices, especially those applied to the face and head, are unpleasant for the child and may cause airway concerns for the anesthesiologist. Most children will have indwelling central venous access, avoiding the need for repeated IV puncture or inhalational induction. Radiation treatments are also used in adults who have a greater capacity than children to remain still without sedation or general anesthesia.

Table 33-9 Common Radiosensitive Tumors in Children

Primary CNS tumor—neuroblastoma, medulloblastoma
Acute leukemia—CNS leukemia
Radiosensitive ocular tumors—retinoblastoma
Intra-abdominal tumors—Wilms tumor
Rhabdomyosarcoma
Other tumors—Langerhans cell histiocytosis

CNS, central nervous system.

Positron Emission Tomography

Positron emission tomography (PET) scanning is a newer imaging modality using radiolabeled isotopes to measure tissue glucose uptake, thereby estimating tumor extent. Anesthesia concerns are similar to those for CT; studies typically take longer to complete which may affect choice of technique/agent. Patients are typically exposed to greater ionizing radiation from both isotope and CT sources.[55]

Gastroenterology

Procedures commonly performed in the gastrointestinal (GI) endoscopy suite are described in Table 33-2. Procedures may be performed under general anesthesia or sedation.[73] The American Gastroenterological Association reports that 98% of patients for upper and lower endoscopies receive sedation.[74] Of these, over one-third are performed in ambulatory surgery centers and only 29% of these procedures involve anesthesia care providers.[74,75] Controversy surrounds the administration of sedation for GI procedures both in the United States[74] and worldwide.[76] A wide variety of sedation techniques are practiced and gastroenterologists are increasingly advocating for the use of propofol sedation by nonanesthesiologists, citing the safety and efficacy of these techniques (nonanesthesiologist-administered propofol "NAAP" or nurse-administered propofol sedation "NAPS").[77,78] However, the use of propofol by those without expert airway skills remains controversial in the anesthesiology community.[79] It should, however, be noted that in recently published guidelines, gastroenterologists do universally agree that patients in ASA classes III or IV, for complex procedures, or with histories of adverse or inadequate responses to sedation require the involvement of an anesthesiologist.[76,80]

Upper Gastrointestinal Endoscopy

Upper GI endoscopy is performed for diagnostic procedures, such as biopsy, and for therapeutic procedures, such as retrieval of foreign bodies, treatment of esophageal varices with sclerotherapy or band ligation, dilation of esophageal strictures, and placement of a percutaneous endoscopic gastrostomy. Patients may have multiple comorbidities including gastroesophageal reflux, hepatic dysfunction, coagulopathy, and ascites. Sedation techniques or general anesthesia may be used after careful patient assessment and discussion with the endoscopist. Under general anesthesia, tracheal intubation is the gold standard to protect the airway and facilitate passage of the endoscope; however, an LMA may serve as an alternative device for airway management.[81] Local anesthetic (such as benzocaine) sprayed into the oropharynx to facilitate passage of the endoscope attenuates the gag reflex and may increase the risk of aspiration. A bite block is inserted to prevent the patient from biting down on the endoscope and damaging both the teeth and the endoscope. Procedures are performed in the prone or semiprone position with the patient's head rotated to the side, making the airway less accessible. Care and attention should also be paid to pressure areas, particularly the eyes, lips, and teeth, and extreme rotation of the neck should be avoided. Most procedures are brief, lasting 10 to 30 minutes, and are generally painless.

Endoscopic Retrograde Cholangiopancreatography

Endoscopic retrograde cholangiopancreatography (ERCP) is important in the diagnosis and treatment of both biliary and pancreatic diseases. During the procedure, the biliary and pancreatic duct systems are identified, instrumented, and therapeutic maneuvers such as the passage of stents or removal of stones carried out. The complication rate during ERCP is reported as between 5% and 10% with a mortality of 0.1% to 1%. Complications include acute pancreatitis, hemorrhage, and perforation.[82,83] Patients usually experience discomfort during ERCP and general anesthesia or deep sedation techniques are recommended for the procedure, which usually lasts between 20 and 80 minutes. The airway and patient positioning considerations are similar to those for GI endoscopy. Sphincter of Oddi manometry may be performed in which case drugs that affect sphincter pressure such as atropine, glycopyrrolate, glucagon, and various opioids should be avoided. Patients presenting for ERCP may have significant comorbidities including acute cholangitis with septicemia, abdominal ascites, jaundice with liver dysfunction and coagulopathy, bleeding from esophageal varices resulting in hypovolemia, or biliary stricture following major hepatobiliary surgery (including liver transplantation). Transient bacteremia may occur during endoscopy, and antibiotic prophylaxis is recommended for patients with cardiac valvular abnormalities. Gastroenterologists frequently use antispasmodics such as glucagon and IV hyoscyamine to reduce duodenal motility and improve operating conditions during endoscopy[84]; sinus tachycardia may occur.

Cardiology and Interventional Cardiology

The number of interventional cardiology and electrophysiology (EP) procedures has dramatically increased in most institutions over the last decade, with approximately 400,000 pacemakers and implantable cardiac defibrillators (ICDs) being placed each year in the United States.[85] As volumes and patient complexity increase anesthesiologists are playing a much more significant role in the EP and cardiac catheterization laboratories. Hybrid ORs with fluoroscopy capability are becoming more common in the design plans for new ORs and these are usually designed with the anesthesiologist in mind. Cardiac catheterization laboratories and EP laboratories are often simply modified to accommodate anesthesia providers. This retrofit can make for frequent territorial and ergonomic constraints.

Percutaneous Intervention

For patients with evidence of myocardial ischemia, cardiac catheterization and coronary angiography is an essential step in the diagnosis of coronary artery disease. Often, this step is followed by coronary angioplasty with stenting for intracoronary luminal obstructions that are more than 70% occluded.[86] The procedures are usually done with mild sedation administered by the catheterization laboratory team: blood pressure, ECG, and pulse oximetry are monitored and the patient breathes spontaneously with supplemental oxygen. However, the care of an anesthesiologist may be required for patients who are hemodynamically unstable, who are high risk for airway obstruction (e.g., high body mass index or OSA), or who are in cardiogenic shock either before or during the procedure. Early recognition of at-risk patients allows for coordination between the anesthesiologist and cardiologists to avoid hypoxia and hypercarbia, and potentially cardiac arrest. Certain percutaneous interventions (PCIs) have a higher level of complexity and can involve patients with significant comorbidities. Coronary atherectomy for chronic total occlusion can be time-consuming and technically difficult due to complex anatomy and general anesthesia may be required for cases with long duration or requiring immobility.[87] The anesthesiologist should prepare for potential hemodynamic instability with routine anesthetic monitors, possible arterial blood pressure monitoring, and good peripheral or central IV access. Cardiologists are often working through the femoral veins and in an emergency situation it is possible to link sterile IV tubing to the access sites for administration of inotropes and vasopressors.

Percutaneous Ventricular Assist Devices

Patients in cardiogenic shock or having high-risk PCI or EP procedures may benefit from the hemodynamic support provided by percutaneous ventricular assist devices. The TandemHeart (Cardiac Assist, Inc., Pittsburgh, PA) is a left atrial to femoral bypass system that offers flow rates up to 4.0 L/min through an external centrifugal pump. It is designed for short-duration support (14 to 162 hours for cardiogenic shock and 1 to 24 hours for high-risk PCIs).[88] The Impella (Abiomed Inc., Danvers, MA) is an axial flow device with different models that can support flow from 2.5 to 5.5 L/min. An Impella can be placed in the femoral or axillary arteries through the aortic valve and into the left ventricle. It is advantageous in high-risk coronary intervention procedures through improvement of coronary perfusion, LV offloading, and increasing cardiac output.[89] Percutaneous LV to aorta support devices such as Impella should be considered in high-risk PCI cases or cases with higher risk of hemodynamic collapse. Cardiac anesthesiologists often care for patients who are having these devices placed. Transesophageal echocardiography (TEE) guidance may be required for guiding the cannula's position and assuring it is not interfering with or damaging adjacent structures.

Percutaneous Closure of Septal Defects

A number of different devices have been introduced for the closure of patent foramen ovales (PFOs), atrial septal defects (ASDs), paravalvular leaks (PVLs), and ventricular septal defects (VSDs).[90,91] These devices are placed by the cardiologist under the guidance of fluoroscopy and ultrasound. The introduction of intracardiac echocardiography (ICE) has lessened the need for general anesthesia to facilitate TEE guidance.[92] PVL procedures often require general anesthesia and TEE guidance, while other cases (PFO, ASD, and VSD) may be done under sedation or general anesthesia, depending on patient and procedural factors. Special attention should be paid to avoiding air in any IV tubing as left-to-right shunts can be reversed with the drop in systemic vascular resistance that accompanies many anesthetic agents.

Alcohol Septal Ablation

Alcohol septal ablation offers an alternative to open heart myomectomy for patients with hypertrophic cardiomyopathy with equivalent mortality outcomes.[93] Specific septal perforator vessels are identified using coronary angiography and injection of approximately 3 mL of absolute ethanol into these vessels causes a controlled infarction of the hypertrophic septum.[94] This infarction can be visualized in real time on live echocardiography. Although most of the procedure requires only minimal sedation, the alcohol injection can be very painful and require a deeper level of sedation or analgesia.

Structural Heart Procedures

Transcatheter Aortic Valve Replacement

Calcific aortic stenosis affects almost 5% of adults over the age of 65.[95] Once symptoms of syncope and heart failure begin, median life expectancy is 3 years. However, surgical aortic valve replacement (SAVR) in elderly patients with multiple comorbidities can carry a mortality rate of up to 20%.[95] Transcatheter aortic valve replacements (TAVRs) use a sophisticated catheter delivery system to deploy a folded replacement valve through a sheath in the common femoral artery, subclavian artery, carotid artery, or via a minithoracotomy directly into the aorta or left ventricular apex.[95–98] Rapid ventricular pacing is used to minimize left ventricular ejection so that the new valve can be deployed into the correct position. Initially, TAVR was only offered to extremely high-risk surgical patients; however, ongoing studies have shown benefit in intermediate- and low-risk surgical risk patients.[99,100]

The CoreValve (Medtronic, Inc., Minneapolis, MN) is self-expanding and is made of bioprosthetic porcine pericardial tissue sutured into a malleable metal stent that is rigid at body temperature.[95] The compressed CoreValve is slowly deployed as its delivery system is pulled back and allows for some repositioning before the valve is fully released. The Edwards SAPIEN XT transcatheter heart valve (Edwards Lifesciences, Irvine, CA) is a bovine pericardial tissue valve in a cobalt–chromium alloy stent, which has a smaller diameter delivery system. This valve expands with a balloon within the native valve with the goal of displacing the native leaflets.[99]

Research and development in structural heart procedures is ongoing; with expected improved delivery systems, advancements in valve technology, as well as use in aortic insufficiency patients.[100] Initial experience with TAVR procedures required general anesthesia and TEE for all patients; however, many institutions are using sedation with transthoracic echo (TTE) standby.[101] These patients are at high risk for cardiac death during the procedure and experience frequent hemodynamic instability during the rapid ventricular pacing that is required for balloon valvuloplasty and for valve deployment.[101,102] Cardiopulmonary bypass standby is present for many patients. Given the physiologic sequelae of aortic stenosis, all patients undergoing TAVR procedures with a general anesthetic should have preinduction arterial line blood pressure monitoring. Central access in the neck or groin is essential for inotrope and vasopressor administration and large bore IV access is necessary for fluid resuscitation if blood loss is significant. The large cannulae that are exchanged in and out of the groin during the procedure can result in a surprising drop in hematocrit which should be checked frequently during the procedure. One-lung ventilation may be helpful in cases with a transapical approach or when directly cannulating the ascending aorta; this can be accomplished with either a double-lumen tube or a bronchial blocker. The goal for most of these procedures is to extubate the patient in the procedure room or shortly thereafter. Many of the patients are elderly and at high risk for delirium; thus, benzodiazepines and long-acting opioids should be avoided if possible.

Mitral Transcatheter Edge-to-Edge Repair

Mitral regurgitation (MR) is the most common valvular disorder in the aging population in the United States.[103] Cardiac surgical mitral valve repair should be offered to all surgical candidates with symptomatic MR.[104] In North America, the MitraClip (Evalve, San Francisco, CA) is intended to treat patients with moderately severe to severe symptomatic degenerative or functional MR who are considered too high risk for open heart surgery.[103,105,106] The MitraClip delivers a clip device percutaneously that mimics the Alfieri edge-to-edge repair to create a double-orifice mitral valve (Figs. 33-3 and 33-4).[107] The mitral transcatheter edge-to-edge repair (TEER) is a unique application that intervenes on a heart under echocardiographic guidance, allowing the clip grasp and effect on regurgitation to be evaluated in real time. In open heart surgery, the repair is done on a flaccid heart and the effect is evaluated after the heart is reperfused and beating. Recent evaluations have shown that the MitraClip is effective in reducing MR and improving LV remodeling. As well, mortality associated with the MitraClip is less than with surgery using the predicted outcomes surgical risk predictors.[103] Patients undergoing the MitraClip procedure receive a general anesthetic with invasive monitors and TEE.

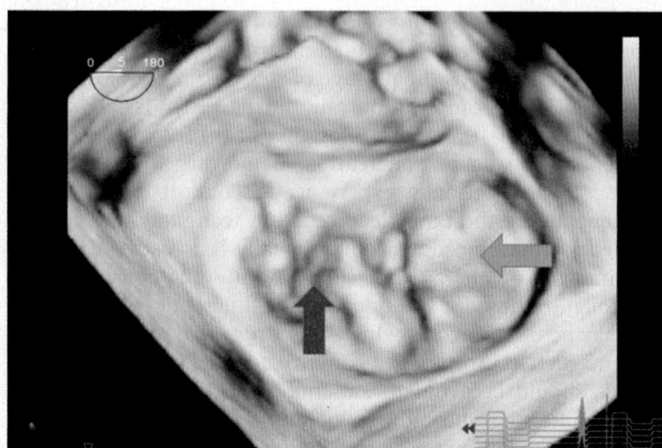

Figure 33-3 Three-dimensional en face view of mitral valve. *Blue arrow* points to A3 portion of anterior mitral leaflet. *Red arrow* points between P1 (**left**) and P2 prolapsing segments of the posterior leaflet with flail chordae visible. (Courtesy of Dr G.B. Mackensen MD, PhD, FASE.)

Left Atrial Appendage Occlusion

The left atrial appendage (LAA) is a source of clot formation in patients with atrial fibrillation and patients require lifelong anticoagulation to prevent this source of embolism. If the LAA can be removed, then anticoagulation is no longer necessary. Traditionally, LAA closures have been performed through median sternotomy; however, the Watchman (Boston Scientific, Minneapolis, MN) is a novel device that can be deployed directly into the LAA via a transfemoral catheter.[108] Presently, the Watchman is offered to patients with nonvalvular atrial fibrillation, a high risk of stroke, and intolerance or contraindication to oral anticoagulation.[109] The device has been shown to reduce hemorrhagic stroke and cardiovascular death when compared to warfarin, although

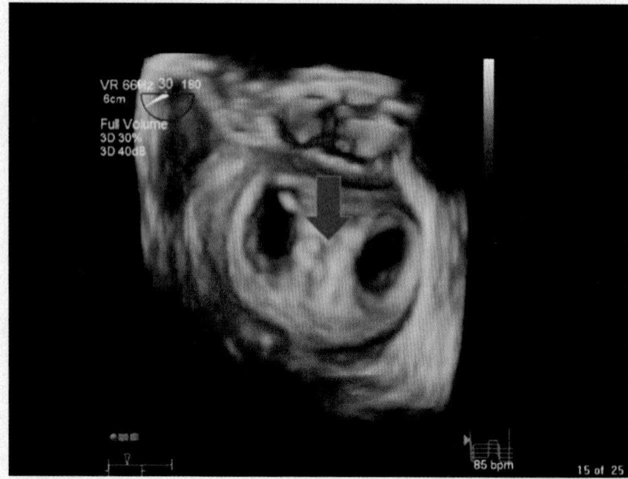

Figure 33-4 Three-dimensional en face view of mitral valve after two MitraClips deployed. *Purple arrow* shows where the two clips have been placed between A2 and P2 segments of the mitral valve. (Courtesy of Dr G.B. Mackensen MD, PhD, FASE.)

there is an increased incidence of ischemic stroke as a periprocedural event.[110] The procedure requires meticulous evaluation of the LAA by TEE to ensure the proper device is selected. Arterial catheters should be used to measure blood pressure for most of these procedures. ICE has been demonstrated to be a safe alternative to general anesthesia and TEE.

Electrophysiology

Like many catheterization laboratory procedures, sedation for EP procedures can sometimes be managed by cardiologists; however, both patient and procedure complexity often necessitate general anesthesia to facilitate a safe and comfortable experience for the patient. EP studies can be divided into cardiac implantable electronic devices (CIEDs) and EP studies with ablation.[111]

Cardiac Implantable Electronic Devices

CIEDs include pacemakers for symptomatic bradycardia and for chronic resynchronization therapy (CRT) and implantable cardioverter defibrillators (ICDs). These devices are usually implanted in the left pectoral area with one to three transvenous leads inserted into the axillary, subclavian, or cephalic veins.[112] Pacemakers can generally be placed under light sedation with local anesthetic to the skin for the pacemaker pocket; if significant patient comorbidities exist, it may be necessary to administer general anesthesia for this procedure. ICDs decrease the risk of sudden cardiac death by both primary and secondary prevention of ventricular tachycardia and ventricular fibrillation.[113] Primary prevention ICDs are indicated for those with an EF less than 35%, with NYHA class II to III symptoms who are on optimal heart failure medical therapy.[114] Secondary prevention ICDs are for patients who have had a documented ventricular fibrillation cardiac arrest or an episode of sustained ventricular tachycardia.[115] The implantation of the device is similar to the process for placing a pacemaker; however, the defibrillation threshold testing requires deeper sedation. CRT pacemakers are indicated for those with cardiomyopathy, an EF less than 35%, a left bundle branch block (LBBB), QRS duration less than 120 milliseconds, and NYHA class II to IV symptoms.[116] A lead is placed transvenously into the coronary sinus which allows for simultaneous pacing of the left and right ventricles: this reduces mortality (in NICM) and improves quality of life.[117,118] Many patients in heart failure are unable to lie flat for the duration of the procedure and placing a lead into the coronary sinus in someone with ventricular dilatation and valvular regurgitation can be challenging with sedation alone.[119]

EP Studies with Ablations

EP studies can be performed for risk stratification or to evaluate specific symptoms that suggest an arrhythmia[113]; however, it is uncommon to not pair these with concurrent ablation procedures, especially if the ablation is to treat tachyarrhythmias (Table 33-10).

The most common ablation procedures performed currently are for narrow complex tachycardias such as atrial fibrillation or atrial flutter and for wide complex tachycardias like polymorphic ventricular tachycardia. Patients with atrial fibrillation should be effectively anticoagulated or have a TEE assessment preablation to rule out an LAA thrombus. Ablation catheters are inserted via the femoral veins into the right heart to try to induce arrhythmias. Complex mapping techniques localize the source of the arrhythmia and an energy source is applied to ablate this source. Ablations can be performed with either radiofrequency or cryotherapy with the former being much more stimulating for the patient.[120] Saline irrigation is used to cool the energy delivery system and therefore can result in significant volume administration during long procedures.[121] The phrenic nerve lies close to the right upper pulmonary veins and is at risk during ablation. Avoidance of neuromuscular blockade will alert the electrophysiologist to phrenic irritation when this area is being ablated.[117] Although drugs that affect the sympathetic and parasympathetic systems can influence the sinus and atrioventricular nodes, there is little evidence to support the notion that general anesthesia affects inducibility of specific arrhythmias.[119,122] The duration of ablation procedures can be lengthy (4 to 8 hours) and mapping requires minute catheter adjustments that are sensitive to patient movement. The ablation process can also be painful and general anesthesia may be required. Invasive arterial blood pressure monitoring is helpful in these patients, especially for those with reduced ejection fractions in whom hemodynamically unstable arrhythmias might be induced.

Table 33-10 Arrhythmia Classification

Bradyarrhythmias
Sick sinus syndrome
Atrioventricular block
First-degree heart block
Second-degree heart block (Mobitz type I and II)
Third-degree heart block
Tachyarrhythmias
Regular rhythm, normal QRS complex
Sinus tachycardia
Atrioventricular nodal reentrant tachycardia
Atrioventricular reciprocating tachycardia—orthodromic
Junctional tachycardia
Atrial flutter
Irregular rhythm, narrow QRS
Atrial fibrillation
Multifocal atrial tachycardia
Frequent premature atrial contractions
Regular rhythm, wide QRS
Monomorphic ventricular tachycardia
Atrioventricular reciprocating tachycardia, antidromic
Regular supraventricular tachycardias with bundle branch block
Irregular rhythm, wide QRS
Polymorphic ventricular tachycardia
Ventricular fibrillation
Frequent premature ventricular contractions
Irregular supraventricular tachycardias with bundle branch block

Laser Lead Extractions

As pacemakers and ICDs become more widespread, so does the need for lead extractions. Device infections, lead endocarditis, thrombosis or venous stenosis, chronic pain due to leads/device, and nonfunctional leads are all reasons for lead removal.[123] Leads become well adhered to the subclavian vein and/or the endocardium which makes this particular procedure high risk for vascular or cardiac injury.[124,125] Vascular injury causing significant blood loss and cardiac tamponade is rare but the involved clinicians should be prepared for it. General anesthesia with large bore IV access and invasive blood pressure monitoring is essential; TEE is usually advisable for prompt evaluation of hemodynamic changes. A cardiac surgical team is often available or on standby for these procedures.[124] As expected, centers with higher lead extraction volume have a lower probability of complications and death.[126]

Cardioversions and Diagnostic TEEs

Cardioversion and TEE procedures are brief procedures but are exquisitely stimulating. Elective electrical cardioversions are ideally performed with a bolus of sedative/hypnotic anesthetic agent on fully monitored patients under the supervision of an anesthesiologist. Atrial fibrillation is the most common reason for an elective cardioversion, so it is necessary to rule out the presence of an LAA clot if the patient is not on therapeutic anticoagulation to avoid embolic complications.[127] TEE is the gold standard for evaluating the LAA.[128] Topical anesthesia in the pharynx with 4% lidocaine can facilitate TEE probe insertion and an infusion of low-dose propofol sedation provides patient comfort with spontaneous ventilation. Standard monitors should be applied, and although end-tidal CO_2 monitoring is not completely necessary, it can be very helpful. Many of the patients presenting for cardioversion and elective TEE have compromised cardiac function; thus, resuscitation drugs should be readily available.

The anesthesiologist may also be involved in elective TEEs for specific indications under the American Society of Echocardiography (ASE) guidelines including evaluation of suspected aortic dissection, determining suitability for valve repair, diagnosis of endocarditis, evaluation of persistent fever with an intracardiac device, and evaluation for LAA thrombus.[129] Anesthesiologists caring for these patients should ensure that there are no contraindications to TEE related to known esophageal pathology (strictures, varices, malignancy, recent ulcer or hemorrhage, Zenker diverticulum) or those with a history of unevaluated dysphagia.[129] Although topical anesthesia and sedation are usually sufficient, uncooperative patients and those with a potentially difficult airway should be prophylactically intubated and maintained on TIVA. In these situations, the anesthesiologist can help facilitate passage of the TEE probe using a laryngoscope.

Electroconvulsive Therapy

Electroconvulsive therapy (ECT) has had an important role in the management of depression, mania, and affective disorders since the 1930s (NICV 33-2).[130] Typically, it is performed three times a week for 6 to 12 treatments, followed by weekly or monthly maintenance therapy to prevent relapses.[131]

Physiologic Response to Electroconvulsive Therapy

The physiologic response to ECT includes generalized motor seizures and an acute cardiovascular response. The seizure usually lasts several minutes, and minimum seizure duration of 25 seconds is recommended to ensure adequate antidepressant efficacy.[132] The cardiovascular response includes transient bradycardia and occasional asystole giving way to more prominent hypertension and tachycardia. Increased cerebral blood flow, raised ICP and cardiac dysrhythmias, myocardial ischemia, infarction, or neurologic vascular events may be precipitated. Short-term memory loss is also common following ECT. Other sequelae include myalgias, bone fractures, joint dislocations, headache, emergence agitation, status epilepticus, and sudden death.

Anesthetic Considerations for ECT

Scalp electrodes are placed to monitor the electroencephalogram and a blood pressure cuff is applied to an extremity and inflated before muscle relaxant is administered to monitor the seizure. Patients presenting for ECT are often elderly, with multiple coexisting conditions.[133] Patients may be taking antidepressant medications which include tricyclic antidepressants, monoamine oxidase inhibitors, and selective serotonin reuptake inhibitors. Of these drugs, the monoamine oxidase inhibitors have the most significant interactions with anesthetic agents. The anesthetic requirements for ECT are described in Table 33-11.

Table 33-11 Anesthetic Consideration for Electroconvulsive Therapy

Anesthetic Requirements	Comments
Amnesia	With induction agent of choice
Airway management	Usually with bag–mask ventilation, although the laryngeal mask has been used with success[134]
Moderate hypocapnia	Improves the quality and duration of seizures[135]
Protection of the teeth and tongue during the seizure	Using a soft bite block
Prevention of seizure-related injuries (fractures and dislocations)	Small doses of muscle relaxant, e.g., succinic choline (0.75–1.5 mg/kg) are most commonly used unless there are contraindications
Control of hemodynamic responses	Labetalol; esmolol; and the calcium channel antagonists nifedipine, diltiazem, and nicardipine all attenuate the hemodynamic responses to ECT. Dexmedetomidine (1 μg/kg administered over 10 min just before induction of anesthesia) has been shown to be effective in controlling blood pressure without affecting seizure duration.[136]
Control or prevention of the parasympathetic effects of ECT (salivation, transient bradycardia, and asystole)	Can be prevented with glycopyrrolate or atropine
Analgesia to relieve postseizure myalgia	Ketorolac 15–30 mg is effective in younger patients Acetaminophen or aspirin may be used in older patients or where NSAIDs are contraindicated

ECT, electroconvulsive therapy; NSAID, nonsteroidal anti-inflammatory drug.

Most of the IV induction agents have been used for ECT,[133] despite their anticonvulsant effects. Methohexital (1 to 1.5 mg/kg), historically considered the "gold standard" agent, appears to have less anticonvulsant activity than the other agents. Etomidate (0.15 to 0.3 mg/kg) is generally associated with longer seizure duration and is the preferred agent of some psychiatrists, despite a slightly longer recovery and associated myoclonus. Propofol is more effective at attenuating the acute hemodynamic responses than etomidate and in small doses (0.75 mg/kg) seizure duration is usually acceptable.[137] Short-acting opioids, such as remifentanil, can be used to decrease the dose of induction agent and prolong seizure duration without reducing the depth of anesthesia.[138] Recently, ketamine, either alone or in combination, has been attributed intrinsic antidepressant effects when used as an anesthetic agent for ECT, although its effects are far from certain.[139]

Summary

The number and complexity of NOR procedures are steadily increasing. This increase has resulted in an expansion of anesthesia services in areas remote from the OR that may not be familiar to anesthesia providers. In preparing to administer anesthesia or sedation in a NOR site, a simple three-step approach can be followed. This approach involves giving careful consideration to the evaluation and the needs of the *patient*, the particular challenges posed by the *procedure*, and the hazards and limitations of the *environment*. In all cases, the standards of anesthesia care and monitoring should be no different than those provided in the conventional OR.

Acknowledgments

We gratefully acknowledge the contributions of previous edition authors, Karen J. Souter, Andrew J. Pittaway, and Carly Peterson, as portions of their chapter have been retained in this revision.

For further review and interactivities, please see the videos and narrative interactive clinical vignettes (NICVs) accessible in the complimentary eBook bundled with this text. Access instructions are located on the inside front cover.

REFERENCES

1. Committee on Standards and Practice Parameters. Statement on nonoperating room anesthetizing locations. Approved by the ASA House of Delegates on October 19, 1994, and last amended on October 17. 2018Accessed April 19, 2022. https://www.asahq.org/standards-and-guidelines
2. Nagrebetsky A, Gabriel RA, Dutton RP, Urman RD. Growth of nonoperating room anesthesia care in the United States: a contemporary trends analysis. *Anesth Analg.* 2017;124(4):1261–1267.
3. Du AL, Robbins K, Waterman RS, Urman RD, Gabriel RA. National trends in nonoperating room anesthesia: procedures, facilities, and patient characteristics. *Curr Opin Anaesthesiol.* 2021;34(1):464–469.
4. Tobias JD. Sedation of infants and children outside of the operating room. *Curr Opin Anaesthesiol.* 2015;28(4):478–485.
5. Committee on Standards and Practice Parameters. Basic standards for preanesthesia care. Approved by the ASA House of Delegates on October 14, 1987, and last affirmed on December 13, 2020. Accessed April 19, 2022. https://www.asahq.org/standards-and-guidelines
6. Committee on Standards and Practice Parameters. Standards for basic anesthetic monitoring. Approved by the ASA House of Delegates on October 21, 1986, and last amended on October 20, 2010, and last affirmed on December 13, 2020. Accessed April 19, 2022. http://www.asahq.org/standards-and-guidelines
7. Committee on Standards and Practice Parameters. Standards for postanesthesia care. Approved by the ASA House of Delegates on October 27, 2004, and last amended on October 23, 2019. Accessed April 19, 2022.http://www.asahq.org/standards-and-guidelines
8. Woodward ZG, Urman RD, Domino KB. Safety of non-operating room anesthesia. *Anesthesiol Clin.* 2017;35:569–581.
9. Metzner J, Domino KB. Risks of anesthesia or sedation outside the operating room: the role of the anesthesia care provider. *Curr Opin Anaesthesiol.* 2010;23(4):523–531.
10. Waugh JB, Epps CA, Khodneva YA. Capnography enhances surveillance of respiratory events during procedural sedation: a meta-analysis. *J Clin Anesth.* 2011;23(3):189–196.
11. Anwar A, Heller KO, Esper SA, Ferreira RG. Nonoperating room anesthesia: strategies to improve performance. *Int Anesthesiol Clin.* 2021;59(4):27–36.
12. Semel ME, Resch S, Haynes AB, et al. Adopting a surgical safety checklist could save money and improve the quality of care in U.S. hospitals. *Health Aff (Millwood).* 2010;29(9):1593–1599.
13. Hill MR, Roberts MJ, Alderson ML, Gale TC. Safety culture and the 5 steps to safer surgery: an intervention study. *Br J Anaesth.* 2015;114(6):958–962.
14. Lee MJ, Fanelli F, Haage P, Hausegger K, Van Lienden KP. Patient safety in interventional radiology: a CIRSE IR checklist. *Cardiovasc Intervent Radiol.* 2012;35(2):244–246.
15. Committee on Economics. Position on monitored anesthesia care. Approved by the House of Delegates on October 25, 2005, and last amended on October 17, 2018. Accessed April 19, 2022. https://www.asahq.org/standards-and-guidelines
16. Kue R, Brown P, Ness C, Scheulen J. Adverse clinical events during intrahospital transport by a specialized team: a preliminary report. *Am J Crit Care.* 2011;20(2):153–161.
17. ASA interpretive guidelines templates. Approved by the ASA Committee on Quality Management and Departmental Administration on May 19, 2011, and last amended on October 8, 2014. Accessed December 18, 2015. https://www.asahq.org/quality-and-practice-management/qmda-regulatory-toolkit/qmda-regulatory-toolkit-interpretive-guidelines-templates
18. Committee on Quality Management and Departmental Administration. Continuum of depth of sedation: definition of general anesthesia and levels of sedation/analgesia. Approved by the ASA House of Delegates on October 13, 1999, and last amended on October 23, 2019. Accessed April 19, 2022. https://www.asahq.org/standards-and-guidelines
19. Martel JP, Barnett SR. Sedation: definitions and regulations. *Int Anesthesiol Clin.* 2015;53(2):1–12.
20. Miller DL. Overview of contemporary interventional fluoroscopy procedures. *Health Phys.* 2008;95(5):638–644.
21. Semelka RC, Armao DM, Elias J Jr, Huda W. Imaging strategies to reduce the risk of radiation in CT studies, including selective substitution with MRI. *J Magn Reson Imaging.* 2007;25(5):900–909.
22. Mitchell EL, Furey P. Prevention of radiation injury from medical imaging. *J Vasc Surg.* 2011;53(1 Suppl):22S–27S.
23. Miller DL, Vañó E, Bartal G, et al; Cardiovascular and Interventional Radiology Society of Europe, Society of Interventional Radiology. Occupational radiation protection in interventional radiology: a joint guideline of the Cardiovascular and Interventional Radiology Society of Europe and the Society of Interventional Radiology. *J Vasc Interv Radiol.* 2010;21(5):607–615.
24. Mohapatra A, Greenberg RK, Mastracci TM, Eagleton MJ, Thornsberry B. Radiation exposure to operating room personnel and patients during endovascular procedures. *J Vasc Surg.* 2013;58(3):702–709.
25. Anastasian ZH, Strozyk D, Meyers PM, Wang S, Berman MF. Radiation exposure of the anesthesiologist in the neurointerventional suite. *Anesthesiology.* 2011;114(3):512–520.
26. Valentin J. ICRP, 2007. The 2007 Recommendations of the International Commission on Radiological Protection. ICRP publication 103. *Ann ICRP.* 2007,37;(2-4):1–332.
27. National Council on Radiation Protection and Measurements. *Recent applications of the NCRP public dose limit recommendations for ionizing radiation. NCRP Statement No 10.* National Council on Radiation Protection and Measurements; 2004.
28. Thomsen HS. Contrast media safety-an update. *Eur J Radiol.* 2011;80(1):77–82.
29. Beckett KR, Moriarity AK, Langer JM. Safe use of contrast media: what the radiologist needs to know. *Radiographics.* 2015;35(6):1738–1750.
30. Nicola R, Shaqdan KW, Aran K, Mansouri M, Singh A, Abujudeh HH. Contrast-induced nephropathy: identifying the risks, choosing the right agent, and reviewing effective prevention and management methods. *Curr Probl Diagn Radiol.* 2015;44(6):501–504.
31. McCullough PA. Radiocontrast-induced acute kidney injury. *Nephron Physiol.* 2008;109(4):p61–p72.
32. Brockow K. Immediate drug hypersensitivity: epidemiology, clinical features, triggers and management. *Hautarzt.* 2014;65(5):409–414.
33. Davenport MS, Cohan RH, Ellis JH. Contrast media controversies in 2015: imaging patients with renal impairment or risk of contrast reaction. *AJR Am J Roentgenol.* 2015;204(6):1174–1181.
34. Prince MR, Zhang H, Zou Z, Staron RB, Brill PW. Incidence of immediate gadolinium contrast media reactions. *AJR Am J Roentgenol.* 2011;196(2):W138–W143.
35. Zou Z, Zhang HL, Roditi GH, Leiner T, Kucharczyk W, Prince MR. Nephrogenic systemic fibrosis: review of 370 biopsy-confirmed cases. *JACC Cardiovasc Imaging.* 2011;4(11):1206–1216.
36. Guercio JR, Nimjee SM, James ML, McDonagh DL. Anesthesia for interventional neuroradiology. *Int Anesthesiol Clin.* 2015;53(1):87–106.

37. Fusco MR, Ogilvy CS. Surgical and endovascular management of cerebral aneurysms. *Int Anesthesiol Clin.* 2015;53(1):146–165.
38. Molyneux AJ, Kerr RSC, Birks J, et al; ISAT Collaborators. Risk of recurrent subarachnoid haemorrhage, death, or dependence and standardised mortality ratios after clipping or coiling of an intracranial aneurysm in the International Subarachnoid Aneurysm Trial (ISAT): long-term follow-up. *Lancet Neurol.* 2009;8(5):427–433.
39. Molyneux AJ, Birks J, Clarke A, Sneade M, Kerr RSC. The durability of endovascular coiling versus neurosurgical clipping of ruptured cerebral aneurysms: 18 year follow-up of the UK cohort of the International Subarachnoid Aneurysm Trial (ISAT). *Lancet.* 2015;385(9969):691–697.
40. Schulenburg E, Matta B. Anaesthesia for interventional neuroradiology. *Curr Opin Anaesthesiol.* 2011;24(4):426–432.
41. Ryttlefors M, Enblad P, Kerr RSC, Molyneux AJ. International subarachnoid aneurysm trial of neurosurgical clipping versus endovascular coiling: subgroup analysis of 278 elderly patients. *Stroke.* 2008;39(10):2720–2726.
42. Thompson BG, Brown RD Jr, Amin-Hanjani S, et al; American Heart Association Stroke Council, Council on Cardiovascular and Stroke Nursing, and Council on Epidemiology and Prevention; American Heart Association; American Stroke Association. Guidelines for the management of patients with unruptured intracranial aneurysms: a guideline for healthcare professionals from the American Heart Association/American Stroke Association. *Stroke.* 2015;46(8):2368–2400.
43. Lee CZ, Young WL. Anesthesia for endovascular neurosurgery and interventional neuroradiology. *Anesthesiol Clin.* 2012;30(2):127–147.
44. Furlan A, Higashida R, Wechsler L, et al. Intra-arterial prourokinase for acute ischemic stroke. The PROACT II study: a randomized controlled trial. Prolyse in Acute Cerebral Thromboembolism. *JAMA.* 1999;282(21):2003–2011.
45. Jauch EC, Saver JL, Adams HP, et al; American Heart Association Stroke Council; Council on Cardiovascular Nursing; Council on Peripheral Vascular Disease; Council on Clinical Cardiology. Guidelines for the early management of patients with acute ischemic stroke: a guideline for healthcare professionals from the American Heart Association/American Stroke Association. *Stroke.* 2013;44(3):870–947.
46. Davis MJ, Menon BK, Baghirzada LB, et al; Calgary Stroke Program. Anesthetic management and outcome in patients during endovascular therapy for acute stroke. *Anesthesiology.* 2012;116(2):396–405.
47. Abou-Chebl A, Yeatts SD, Yan B, et al. Impact of general anesthesia on safety and outcomes in the endovascular arm of Interventional Management of Stroke (IMS) III Trial. *Stroke.* 2015; 46(8):2142–2148.
48. See JJ, Manninen PH. Anesthesia for neuroradiology. *Curr Opin Anaesthesiol.* 2005;18(4): 437–441.
49. The Arteriovenous Malformation Study Group. Arteriovenous malformations of the brain in adults. *N Engl J Med.* 1999;340(23):1812–1818.
50. González JAJ, Llibre Guerra JC, Prince López JA, Vázquez Luna F, Rodríguez Ramos RM, Ugarte Suárez JC. Feasibility of the superselective test with propofol for determining eloquent brain regions in the endovascular treatment of arteriovenous malformations. *Interv Neuroradiol.* 2013;19(3):320–328.
51. Mikuni N, Takayama M, Satow T, et al. Evaluation of adverse effects in intracarotid propofol injection for Wada test. *Neurology.* 2005;65(11):1813–1816.
52. Raiten J, Elkassabany N, Gao W, Mandel JE. Medical intelligence article: novel uses of high frequency ventilation outside the operating room. *Anesth Analg.* 2011;112(5):1110–1113.
53. Piccioni F, Fumagalli L, Garbagnati F, Di Tolla G, Mazzaferro V, Langer M. Thoracic paravertebral anesthesia for percutaneous radiofrequency ablation of hepatic tumors. *J Clin Anesth.* 2014;26(4):271–275.
54. Scher C. Anesthesia for transjugular intrahepatic portosystemic shunt. *Int Anesthesiol Clin.* 2009;47(2):21–28.
55. Veenith T, Coles JP. Anaesthesia for magnetic resonance imaging and positron emission tomography. *Curr Opin Anaesthesiol.* 2011;24(4):451–458.
56. Institute of Physics. *MRI and the physical agents (EMF) directive.* Institute of Physics Report; 2008. Accessed November 3, 2015. https://studylib.net/doc/8116513/mri-and-the-physical-agents--emf--directive
57. Association of Anaesthetists of Great Britain and Ireland; Farling PA, Flynn PA, Darwent G, et al. Safety in magnetic resonance units: an update. *Anaesthesia.* 2010;65(7):766–770.
58. United States Department of Labor. Occupational Safety and Health Administration (OSHA) technical manual section III: Chapter 5. Noise. Accessed April 19, 2022. https://www.osha.gov/otm/section-3-health-hazards/chapter-5
59. Dewey M, Schink T, Dewey CF. Claustrophobia during magnetic resonance imaging: cohort study in over 55,000 patients. *J Magn Reson Imaging.* 2007;26(5):1322–1327.
60. Munn Z, Jordan Z. Interventions to reduce anxiety, distress and the need for sedation in adult patients undergoing magnetic resonance imaging: a systematic review. *Int J Evid Based Healthc.* 2013;11(4):265–274.
61. Kannikeswaran N, Mahajan PV, Sethuraman U, Groebe A, Chen X. Sedation medication received and adverse events related to sedation for brain MRI in children with and without developmental disabilities. *Paediatr Anaesth.* 2009;19(3):250–256.
62. Krauss B, Green SM. Training and credentialing in procedural sedation and analgesia in children: lessons from the United States model. *Paediatr Anaesth.* 2008;18(1):30–35.
63. Arthurs OJ, Sury M. Anaesthesia or sedation for paediatric MRI: advantages and disadvantages. *Curr Opin Anaesthesiol.* 2013;26(4):489–494.
64. American Academy of Pediatrics; American Academy of Pediatric Dentistry; Coté CJ, Wilson S; Work Group on Sedation. Guidelines for monitoring and management of pediatric patients during and after sedation for diagnostic and therapeutic procedures: an update. *Paediatr Anaesth.* 2008;18(1):9–10.
65. American Academy of Pediatrics; American Academy of Pediatric Dentistry, Coté CJ, Wilson S; Work Group on Sedation. Guidelines for monitoring and management of pediatric patients during and after sedation for diagnostic and therapeutic procedures: an update. *Pediatrics.* 2006;118(6):2587–2602.
66. Cravero JP. Risk and safety of pediatric sedation/anesthesia for procedures outside the operating room. *Curr Opin Anaesthesiol.* 2009;22(4):509–513.
67. Alonso-Basanta M, Lustig RA, Kennedy DW. Proton beam therapy in skull base pathology. *Otolaryngol Clin North Am.* 2011;44(5):1173–1183.
68. Chalabi J, Patel S. Radiation therapy in children. *Int Anesthesiol Clin.* 2009; 47(3):45–53.
69. McFadyen JG, Pelly N, Orr RJ. Sedation and anesthesia for the pediatric patient undergoing radiation therapy. *Curr Opin Anaesthesiol.* 2011;24(4):433–438.
70. Harris EA. Sedation and anesthesia options for pediatric patients in the radiation oncology suite. *Int J Pediatr.* 2010;2010:870921.
71. Buehrer S, Immoos S, Frei M, Timmermann B, Weiss M. Evaluation of propofol for repeated prolonged deep sedation in children undergoing proton radiation therapy. *Br J Anaesth.* 2007; 99(4):556–560.
72. Anghelescu DL, Burgoyne LL, Liu W, et al. Safe anesthesia for radiotherapy in pediatric oncology: St. Jude Children's Research Hospital Experience, 2004–2006. *Int J Radiat Oncol Biol Phys.* 2008;71(2):491–497.
73. Bryson EO, Sejpal D. Anesthesia in remote locations: radiology and beyond, international anesthesiology clinics: gastroenterology: endoscopy, colonoscopy, and ERCP. *Int Anesthesiol Clin.* 2009;47(2):69–80.
74. Cohen LB, Wecsler JS, Gaetano JN, et al. Endoscopic sedation in the United States: results from a nationwide survey. *Am J Gastroenterol.* 2006;101(5):967–974.
75. Goulson DT, Fragneto RY. Anesthesia for gastrointestinal endoscopic procedures. *Anesthesiol Clin.* 2009;27(1):71–85.
76. Dumonceau JM, Riphaus A, Schreiber F, et al. Non-anesthesiologist administration of propofol for gastrointestinal endoscopy: European Society of Gastrointestinal Endoscopy, European Society of Gastroenterology and Endoscopy Nurses and Associates Guideline. *Endoscopy.* 2015;47(12):1175–1189.
77. Rivera B. The current status of nurse-administered propofol sedation in endoscopy: an evidence-based practice nurse fellowship project. *Gastroenterol Nurs.* 2015;38(4):297–304.
78. Birk J, Bath RK. Is the anesthesiologist necessary in the endoscopy suite? A review of patients, payers and safety. *Expert Rev Gastroenterol Hepatol.* 2015;9(7):883–835.
79. Werner C, Smith A, Van Aken H. Guidelines on non-anaesthesiologist administration of propofol for gastrointestinal endoscopy: a double-edged sword. *Eur J Anaesthesiol.* 2011; 28(8):553–555.
80. Cohen LB, Ladas SD, Vargo JJ, et al. Sedation in digestive endoscopy: the Athens international position statements. *Aliment Pharmacol Ther.* 2010;32(3):425–442.
81. Osborn IP, Cohen J, Soper RJ, Roth LA. Laryngeal mask airway: a novel method of airway protection during ERCP: comparison with endotracheal intubation. *Gastrointest Endosc.* 2002; 56(1):122–128.
82. Garewal D, Powell S, Milan SJ, Nordmeyer J, Waikar P. Sedative techniques for endoscopic retrograde cholangiopancreatography. *Cochrane Database Syst Rev.* 2012;6:CD007274.
83. Garewal D, Vele L, Waikar P. Anaesthetic considerations for endoscopic retrograde cholangiopancreatography procedures. *Curr Opin Anaesthesiol.* 2013;26(4):475–480.
84. Lynch CR, Khandekar S, Lynch SM, Disario JA. Sublingual L-hyoscyamine for duodenal antimotility during ERCP: a prospective randomized double-blinded study. *Gastrointest Endosc.* 2007;66(4):748–752.
85. Ammannaya GKK. Implantable cardioverter defibrillators – the past, present and future. *Archives Medical Sci Atheroscler Dis.* 2020;5:e163–e170.
86. Faillace RT, Kaddaha R, Bikkina M, Yoganathan T, Parikh R, Casthley P. The role of the out-of-operating room anesthesiologist in the care of the cardiac patient. *Anesthesiol Clin.* 2009;27(1):29–46.
87. Vanneman MW. Anesthetic considerations for percutaneous coronary intervention for chronic total occlusions—a narrative review. *J Cardiothorac Vasc Anesth.* 2022;36(7): 2132–2142.
88. Kar B, Adkins LE, Civitello AB, et al. Clinical experience with the TandemHeart percutaneous ventricular assist device. *Tex Heart Inst J.* 2006;33(2):111–115.
89. Russo G, Burzotta F, Aurigemma C, Pedicino D, Romagnoli E, Trani C. Can we have a rationalized selection of intra-aortic balloon pump, Impella, and extracorporeal membrane oxygenation in the catheterization laboratory? *Cardiol J.* 2022;29:115–132.
90. Morray BH. Ventricular septal defect closure devices, techniques, and outcomes. *Interv Cardiol Clin.* 2019;8:1–10.
91. Kumar R, Jelnin V, Kliger C, Ruiz C E. Percutaneous paravalvular leak closure. *Cardiol Clin.* 2013;31:431–440.

92. Praz F, Wahl A, Schmutz M, et al. Safety, feasibility, and long-term results of percutaneous closure of atrial septal defects using the Amplatzer septal occluder without periprocedural echocardiography. *J Invasive Cardiol*. 2015;27(3):157–162.
93. Singh K, Qutub M, Carson K, Hibbert B, Glover C. A meta analysis of current status of alcohol septal ablation and surgical myectomy for obstructive hypertrophic cardiomyopathy. *Catheter Cardiovasc Interv*. 2016;88(1):107–115.
94. Alam M, Dokainish H, Lakkis NM. Hypertrophic obstructive cardiomyopathy-alcohol septal ablation vs. myectomy: a meta-analysis. *Eur Heart J*. 2009;30(9):1080–1087.
95. Horne A Jr, Reineck EA, Hasan RK, Resar JR, Chacko M. Transcatheter aortic valve replacement: historical perspectives, current evidence, and future directions. *Am Heart J*. 2014; 168(4):414–423.
96. Cormican D, Jayaraman A, Villablanca P, Ramakrishna H. TAVR procedural volumes and patient outcomes: analysis of recent data. *J Cardiothorac Vasc Anesth*. 2020;34:545–550.
97. Hamid A. Anesthesia for cardiac catheterization procedures. *Heart Lung Vessel*. 2014;6:225–231.
98. Morozowich ST, Sell-Dottin KA, Crestanello JA, Ramakrishna H. Transcarotid versus transaxillary/subclavian transcatheter aortic valve replacement (TAVR): analysis of outcomes. *J Cardiothor Vasc An*. 2021;36:1771–1776.
99. Stolker JM, Patel AY, Lim MJ, Hauptman PJ. Estimating the adoption of transcatheter aortic valve replacement by US interventional cardiologists and clinical trialists. *Clin Cardiol*. 2013;36(11):691–697.
100. Popma JJ, Deeb GM, Yakubov SJ, et al; Evolut Low Risk Trial Investigators. Transcatheter aortic-valve replacement with a self-expanding valve in low-risk patients. *N Engl J Med*. 2019; 380:1706–1715.
101. Mayr NP, Michel J, Bleiziffer S, Tassani P, Martin K. Sedation or general anesthesia for transcatheter aortic valve implantation (TAVI). *J Thorac Dis*. 2015;7(9):1518–1526.
102. Mahajan A, Chua J. Pro: a cardiovascular anesthesiologist should provide services in the catheterization and electrophysiology laboratory. *J Cardiothorac Vasc Anesth*. 2011;25(3): 553–556.
103. Velazquez EJ, Samad Z, Al-Khalidi HR, et al. The MitraClip and survival in patients with mitral regurgitation at high risk for surgery: a propensity-matched comparison. *Am Heart J*. 2015;170(5):1050–1059.e3.
104. Bonow RO, Carabello BA, Chatterjee K, et al; American College of Cardiology/American Heart Association Task Force on Practice Guidelines. 2008 Focused update incorporated into the ACC/AHA 2006 guidelines for the management of patients with valvular heart disease: a report of the American College of Cardiology/American Heart Association Task Force on Practice Guidelines (Writing Committee to revise the 1998 guidelines for the management of patients with valvular heart disease). Endorsed by the Society of Cardiovascular Anesthesiologists, Society for Cardiovascular Angiography and Interventions, and Society of Thoracic Surgeons. *J Am Coll Cardiol*. 2008;52(13):e1–e142.
105. Nyman CB, Mackensen GB, Jelacic S, Little SH, Smith TW, Mahmood F. Transcatheter mitral valve repair using the edge-to-edge clip. *J Am Soc Echocardiogr*. 2018;31:434–453.
106. Flint N, Price MJ, Little SH, et al. State of the art: transcatheter edge-to edge repair for complex mitral regurgitation. *J Am Soc Echocardiogr*. 2021;34:1025–1037.
107. Mauri L, Foster E, Glower DD, et al; EVEREST II Investigators. 4-Year results of a randomized controlled trial of percutaneous repair versus surgery for mitral regurgitation. *J Am Coll Cardiol*. 2013;62(4):317–328.
108. Holmes DR Jr, Kar S, Price MJ, et al. Prospective randomized evaluation of the Watchman left atrial appendage closure device in patients with atrial fibrillation versus long-term warfarin therapy: the PREVAIL trial. *J Am Coll Cardiol*. 2014;64(1):1–12.
109. Glikson M, Wolff R, Hindricks G. EHRA/EAPCI expert consensus statement on catheter-based left atrial appendage occlusion – an update. *Eurointervention* 2020;15:1133–1180.
110. Holmes DR Jr, Doshi SK, Kar S, et al. Left atrial appendage closure as an alternative to warfarin for stroke prevention in atrial fibrillation: a patient-level meta-analysis. *J Am Coll Cardiol*. 2015;65(24):2614–2623.
111. Peterson C, Prutkin JM, Robinson M, et al. Echocardiography for electrophysiology procedures. *Curr Anesthesiol Rep*. 2015;5(4):429–437.
112. Khazanie P, Hammill BG, Qualls LG, et al. Clinical effectiveness of cardiac resynchronization therapy versus medical therapy alone among patients with heart failure: analysis of the ICD Registry and ADHERE. *Circ Heart Fail*. 2014;7(6):926–934.
113. Epstein AE, DiMarco JP, Ellenbogen KA, et al; American College of Cardiology Foundation, American Heart Association Task Force on Practice Guidelines, Heart Rhythm Society. 2012 ACCF/AHA/HRS focused update incorporated into the ACCF/AHA/HRS 2008 guidelines for device-based therapy of cardiac rhythm abnormalities: a report of the American College of Cardiology Foundation/American Heart Association Task Force on Practice Guidelines and the Heart Rhythm Society. *J Am Coll Cardiol*. 2013;61(3):e6–e75.
114. Moss AJ, Zareba W, Hall WJ, et al; Multicenter Automatic Defibrillator Implantation Trial II Investigators. Prophylactic implantation of a defibrillator in patients with myocardial infarction and reduced ejection fraction. *N Engl J Med*. 2002;346(12):877–883.
115. Jiménez-Candil J, Hernández J, Martín A, et al. Differences in ventricular tachyarrythmias and antitachycardia pacing effectiveness according to the ICD indication (primary versus secondary prevention): an analysis based on the stored electrograms. *J Interv Card Electrophysiol*. 2015;44(2):187–195.
116. Chung ES, Leon AR, Tavazzi L, et al. Results of the predictors of response to CRT (PROSPECT) trial. *Circulation*. 2008;117(20):2608–2616.
117. Leyva F, Nisam S, Auricchio A. 20 Years of cardiac resynchronization therapy. *J Am Coll Cardiol*. 2014;64(10):1047–1058.
118. Doran B, Mei C, Varosy PD, et al. The addition of a defibrillator to resynchronization therapy decreases mortality in patients with nonischemic cardiomyopathy. *JACC Hear Fail*. 2021;9:439–449.
119. Buch E, Boyle NG, Belott PH. Pacemaker and defibrillator lead extraction. *Circulation*. 2011;123(11):e378–e380.
120. Lowe MD, Meara M, Mason J, Grace AA, Murgatroyd FD. Catheter cryoablation of supraventricular arrhythmias: a painless alternative to radiofrequency energy. *Pacing Clin Electrophysiol*. 2003;26:500–503.
121. Haddy S. Anesthesia for structural heart interventions. *Cardiol Clin*. 2013;31(3):455–465.
122. Mountantonakis SE, Elkassabany N, Kondapalli L, Marchlinski FE, Mandel JE, Hutchinson MD. Provocation of atrial fibrillation triggers during ablation: does the use of general anesthesia affect inducibility? *J Cardiovasc Electrophysiol*. 2015;26(1):16–20.
123. Tanawuttiwat T, Gallego D, Carrillo RG. Lead extraction experience with high frequency excimer laser. *Pacing Clin Electrophysiol*. 2014;37(9):1120–1128.
124. Bhatia M, Safavi-Naeini P, Razavi M, Collard CD, Tolpin DA, Anton JM. Anesthetic management of laser lead extraction for cardiovascular implantable electronic devices. *Semin Cardiothorac Vasc Anesth*. 2017;21:302–311.
125. Okamura H. Lead extraction using a laser system: techniques, efficacy, and limitations. *J Arrhythmia*. 2016;32:279–282.
126. Di Monaco A, Pelargonio G, Narducci ML, et al. Safety of transvenous lead extraction according to centre volume: a systematic review and meta-analysis. *Europace*. 2014;16(10): 1496–1507.
127. Priester R, Bunting T, Usher B, et al. Role of transesophageal echocardiography among patients with atrial fibrillation undergoing electrophysiology testing. *Am J Cardiol*. 2009; 104(9):1256–1258.
128. Wasmer K, Eckardt L. Management of atrial fibrillation around the world: a comparison of current ACCF/AHA/HRS, CCS, and ESC guidelines. *Europace*. 2011;13(10):1368–1374.
129. Flachskampf FA, Badano L, Daniel WG, et al; European Association of Echocardiography, Echo Committee of the European Association of Cardiothoracic Anaesthesiologists. Recommendations for transoesophageal echocardiography: update 2010. *Eur J Echocardiogr*. 2010;11(7):557–576.
130. UK ECT Review Group. Efficacy and safety of electroconvulsive therapy in depressive disorders: a systematic review and meta-analysis. *Lancet*. 2003;361(9360):799–808.
131. Ding Z, White PF. Anesthesia for electroconvulsive therapy. *Anesth Analg*. 2002;94(5): 1351–1364.
132. The Practice of Electroconvulsive Therapy: Recommendations for Treatment, Training, and Privileging: A Task Force Report of the American Psychiatric Association, 2nd ed. 2002.
133. MacPherson RD. Which anesthetic agents for ambulatory electro-convulsive therapy? *Curr Opin Anaesthesiol*. 2015;28(6):656–661.
134. Nishihara F, Ohkawa M, Hiraoka H, Yuki N, Saito S. Benefits of the laryngeal mask for airway management during electroconvulsive therapy. *J ECT*. 2003;19(4):211–216.
135. Sawayama E, Takahashi M, Inoue A, et al. Moderate hyperventilation prolongs electroencephalogram seizure duration of the first electroconvulsive therapy. *J ECT*. 2008;24(3): 195–198.
136. Begec Z, Toprak HI, Demirbilek S, Erdil F, Onal D, Ersoy MO. Dexmedetomidine blunts acute hyperdynamic responses to electroconvulsive therapy without altering seizure duration. *Acta Anaesthesiol Scand*. 2008;52(2):302–306.
137. Patel AS, Gorst-Unsworth C, Venn RM, Kelley K, Jacob Y. Anesthesia and electroconvulsive therapy: a retrospective study comparing etomidate and propofol. *J ECT*. 2006;22(3):179–183.
138. Chen ST. Remifentanil: a review of its use in electroconvulsive therapy. *J ECT*. 2011;27(4): 323–327.
139. McGirr A, Berlim MT, Bond DJ, et al. A systematic review and meta-analysis of randomized controlled trials of adjunctive ketamine in electroconvulsive therapy: efficacy and tolerability. *J Psychiatr Res*. 2015;62:23–30.

34 Anesthesia for the Older Patient

MICHELLE L. HUMEIDAN • ITAY BENTOV

KEY POINTS

1. The aging of America presents a medical and economic challenge to the entire healthcare system as older patients present for surgery in ever-increasing numbers.
2. Aging involves a gradual, cumulative process of damage and deterioration. The aging process affects connective tissue and cellular function, including the mitochondria, and inevitably leads to decreased function and, ultimately, frailty.
3. Determining the preoperative frailty status of a patient is essential to understanding perioperative risk. Frailty is associated with poorer postoperative outcomes and preoperative identification of a frail patient should prompt a tailored, risk-mitigation perioperative care plan.
4. Decreased organ reserve and increased sensitivity to anesthetic agents result from generalized body composition changes such as connective tissue stiffening and decreased muscle mass, plus impaired autonomic reflexes, and increased sensitivity to drugs.
5. Preoperative patient-centered care and multi-system evaluation focused on goals and risk-mitigation are critical for enhancing recovery of function after surgery. Planning for geriatric surgery has unique ethical considerations and should include discussions about informed consent, living wills, and advance directives. Risk modification should target education, prehabilitation, medication scrutiny, and discharge planning.
6. Intraoperative management must consider the increased sensitivity to drugs in the elderly patient, as well as an increased likelihood of hemodynamic, pulmonary, and thermoregulatory instability.
7. As older patients progress through the days following surgery, vigilance for neurologic and physiologic perturbations that can derail recovery is critical.
8. Analgesia is an important component of postoperative care but is made more difficult by the increased likelihood of adverse consequences from the analgesic regimen.
9. Perioperative complications, most notably pulmonary, cardiac, and central nervous system complications such as delirium or cognitive decline, occur more commonly in the elderly patient because of an interaction between comorbid disease and the decreased physiologic reserve of aging.

Age is not a particularly interesting subject. Anyone can get old. All you have to do is live long enough.

—*Don Marquis*

This quote suggests that aging is dull. To many medical practitioners, it is far worse than "dull." It is high risk due to the complexity of care and discouraging in its monetary reimbursement. To those concerned with the federal budget and personal expenses, medical care for the aged threatens to bankrupt the nation. Nevertheless, the impact of aging on the practice of medicine is far-reaching and profound, and therefore cannot be ignored. Just as children are not "little adults," the older patient is truly different from the younger adult counterpart. Information to guide care of the older surgical patient is more available than ever before from the American Society of Anesthesiologists (www.asahq.org), the Society for the Advancement of Geriatric Anesthesia (www.sagahq.org), the American College of Surgeons (ACS, www.facs.org/), and the American Geriatrics Society (www.americangeriatrics.org). All caregivers, including anesthesiologists, should be knowledgeable of the basics of aging to provide intelligent deviation from standard practices used with younger adults, especially when research evidence or expert guidance doesn't provide clear direction. In reality, caring for an older patient is rarely dull, if for no other reason than their diverse and fascinating lives. Anyone with a passing interest in physiology should enjoy the application of aging physiology to anesthetic management. Yes, their care is often time-consuming, stressful, and requires extra effort, but more often than not it provides the anesthesia caregiver the opportunity to truly practice medicine and make a positive impact on a vulnerable patient's life. Furthermore, the older patient is a prime candidate for the benefits provided by Enhanced Recovery After Surgery (ERAS) and perioperative surgical home (PSH) models of care.

Demographics and Economics of Aging

I advise you to go on living solely to enrage those who are paying your annuities. It is the only pleasure I have left.

—*Voltaire*

Every day in the United States, 10,000 people reach the milestone of their 65th birthday. When Social Security was initiated in 1935, only 6.1% of the U.S. population was older than 65 years. In 2019,

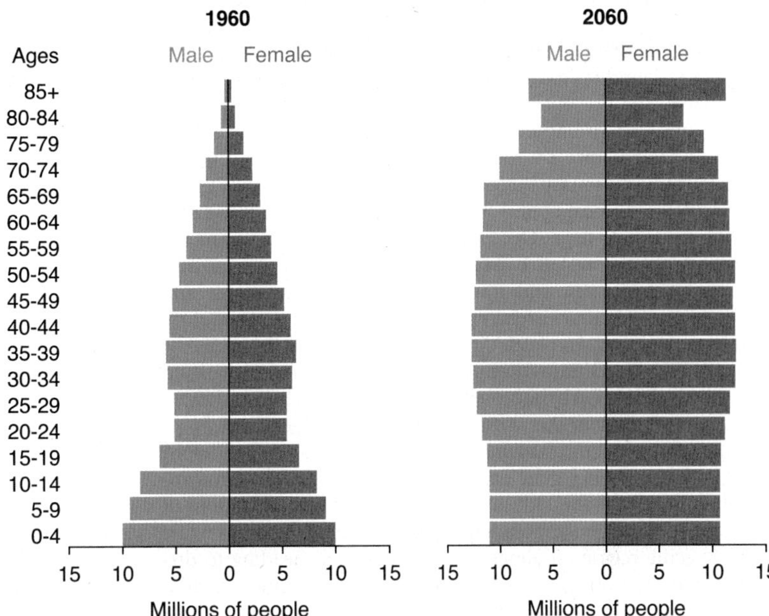

Figure 34-1 Past and Future Breakdown of Americans by age group. (Courtesy of the U.S. Census Bureau.)

this percentage had almost tripled to 16.5% representing 54 million people. We are about a quarter of the way into a timeline put forth by The U.S. Census Bureau projecting continued significant growth of this age bracket between 2010 and 2050. This equates to adults greater than age 65 years representing over 20% of the population (86 million people) in the near future. Currently, the average 65-year-old can expect to live another 19 years so the percentage of the U.S. population older than 85 is expected to nearly triple from 2010 to 2050 as well (from 1.8% to an estimated 4.8%). The growth of the U.S. population and its older subgroups is shown in Figure 34-1. The impact of these statistics is enormous with respect to medical care. In 2010, patients over 65 represented 13% of the population but accounted for 45% of the 167 million total U.S. inpatient days, a rate per capita more than five times greater than for those under 65. Based upon inpatient and ambulatory procedure data, an estimated 51 million inpatient procedures were performed in the United States in 2010. Of these, 37.3% were on patients older than 65 years. Likewise, older patients account for a third of annual outpatient procedures.

1 Federal spending for Medicare in 2021 was $696 billion ($875 gross) or just under 13% of the federal budget. This amount is approximately twice what was spent in 2000 after adjusting for inflation and represents an approximate 50% increase per enrollee. As impressive as Medicare expenditures may be, federal spending grossly underestimates the total cost of all healthcare spending for people over age 65. It is estimated that people over age 65 account for nearly half of the nation's healthcare costs, which totaled $4.1 trillion in 2020, or approximately 19.7% of the gross national product. In consequence, there is considerable pressure to contain healthcare costs, including physician reimbursement, by both private insurance companies and the federal government. Unfortunately, federal reimbursement to anesthesiologists is especially poor. In 2018, private insurance payments for anesthesia services were three and a half times more than Medicare payments. This percentage is in sharp contrast to all other specialties, for which Medicare reimbursement is approximately 83% of commercial rates. Although Medicare will reimburse at the 50% level for up to four concurrent medically directed procedures, academic programs had been at a disadvantage since faculty are not permitted to staff more than two procedures simultaneously if residents were involved. Fortunately, as of 2010, Medicare now reimburses academic institutions at 100% for two concurrent cases. In 2021, the No Surprises Act brought federal protections to consumers against surprise medical bills, bringing particular attention to the intricacy of understanding anesthesiology-associated costs due to the unique conversion-factor unit-of-payment for the specialty and complex provider structure, where settings with independent physicians, independent certified nurse anesthetists and dyad physician–nurse supervision models must be considered. Although significant variability exists in anesthesia services reimbursement across payers, this has not resulted in identification of access barriers to anesthesia providers for Medicare beneficiaries, even in traditionally underserved areas.

The Process of Aging

You can't help getting older, but you don't have to get old.
—*George Burns*

Aging involves a gradual, cumulative process of damage and deterioration. The aging process affects connective tissue and cellular function, including the mitochondria, and inevitably leads to decreased function and, ultimately, frailty. The question could be posed: Why is such a process allowed in nature? Classical evolutionary teleologic explanations would suggest that aging confers an advantage to the survival of the species. In the end of the 19th century, August Weismann theorized (and later abandoned his theory) that older members of a species need to remove themselves to sustain the turnover that is essential for evolution. Newer theories arose in the second part of the 20th century, such as mutation accumulation, which suggests that the random, detrimental mutations that do not cause mortality early in life will ultimately accumulate and lead to deterioration later in life. Another proposal 2 was antagonistic pleiotropy, meaning that a single gene has more than one phenotype (effect or trait). The phenotypes may prove beneficial in early life but detrimental in old age. Lastly, the disposable soma theory suggested that the organism must allocate energy to bodily functions and resources that are focused upon early survival, growth, and reproduction while compromising repair functions that would prevent deterioration with age. The existence of mechanisms that promote death (e.g., apoptosis, cellular senescence, and telomerase shortening) are used by some to support the classical evolutionary theories, and by others to criticize them.

A new, hierarchical approach to aging groups the mechanisms of aging into three tiers. The first tier is primary mechanisms, all of which are clearly negative. Examples of the first-tier mechanisms include: DNA damage and mitochondrial DNA mutations, and telomere loss. Telomeres are stretches of DNA at the ends of chromosomes, analogous to plastic tips on shoelaces. Without them the chromosome would unravel and stick to each other, which could scramble the DNA. Each time a cell divides, the telomeres get shorter, and when they become too short, the cell can no longer divide.

Another first tier mechanism is epigenetic drift: nongenetic DNA changes that influence gene expression. The most studied epigenetic phenomenon is the addition of methyl groups (methylation) of DNA. Most of the genome undergoes gradual demethylation while other, specific regions undergo hypermethylation, leading to disrupted transcription. Lastly, the production, folding, and degradation of proteins within the cell regulate their functionality. These pathways or homeostasis of proteins are referred to as proteostasis. Defective proteostasis has been implicated in several diseases such as diabetes and Alzheimer's, as well as the aging process.

The second tier includes antagonistic mechanisms that are primarily beneficial and protect the younger individual from damage or nutrient shortage. After prolonged use, however, these mechanisms themselves produce damage. Mechanisms in the second tier include senescence, a state in which the cell is alive and metabolically active but is not capable of dividing. Oxygen is important to providing large amounts of energy; however, reactive oxygen species such as peroxides and superoxides cause damage to DNA and proteins. Another second-tier mechanism is disrupted nutrient-sensing; for example, the mammalian target of rapamycin (mTOR) is a protein that senses cellular nutrient, oxygen, and energy levels. Activation of mTOR supports cell growth, proliferation, and survival. However, activation of mTOR is not without a price. Reduction in mTOR activity (e.g., due to a restrictive diet) has been found to increase life span in several animal models.[1] The last mechanism in the second tier is mitochondrial dysfunction; age is correlated not only with the accumulation of mitochondrial DNA mutations but also with a decline in respiratory chain function which may contribute to inefficient use of energy in the cell and reduced exercise capacity.

The third tier consists of integrative mechanisms which operate when the accumulated damage caused by the primary and antagonistic hallmarks cannot be compensated by tissue homeostatic mechanisms: stem cell numbers decline with age, suggesting that there has been a failure to replace damaged cells. Another mechanism is altered intercellular communication. Examples of intercellular communication are neurohormonal signaling processes such as renin–angiotensin, adrenergic, or insulin-IGF1 signaling pathways. Deregulated neurohormonal signaling in the aged is implicated in development of diseases such as hypertension, heart failure, diabetes, and malignancies.

The newly coined term "geroscience" refers to an interdisciplinary field which aims to understand the relationship between aging and age-related diseases.[2] A fundamental concept of geroscience is that numerous human diseases arise, at least in part, from aging itself. Aging is the major risk factor for diseases such as Alzheimer's, Parkinson's, and numerous malignancies. Studying aging mechanisms across a wide variety of pathologies raises an important question: are aging and disease different processes or are they, at least to some degree, inseparable? Elucidating each one of these processes could provide not just insight but potential solutions for the other. Though not specifically a disease of aging, the SARS-CoV-2 (COVID-19) pandemic clearly revealed an increased vulnerability in older patients with 75% of the individuals dying from the virus being 65 years of age or older. For younger people, 1 in 1,400 die from COVID-19, but that changes to 1 in 100 for older patients. Just 27 months after the first case was confirmed in the United States on January 20, 2020, over 1 million Americans have died from the novel coronavirus, and the global death toll is over 6 million, both likely significant underestimates. Postoperative surgical risks significantly increase in patients with a recent COVID-19 diagnosis. Major, elective surgery 0 to 4 weeks after SARS-CoV-2 infection is associated with an increased risk of postoperative complications including pneumonia, respiratory failure, pulmonary embolism and sepsis. Increased risk of postoperative pneumonia remains present until 8 weeks after SARS-CoV-2 infection based on our current understanding.[3]

Most of the gains in average human life span have been as the result of reducing those factors that cause premature death: predation, accidents, and disease. The inability to thwart aging entirely implies that the human life span is limited, and that if everyone died only of "old age," the age at death would end up being a bell-shaped curve centered at a certain value, probably around age 85. Nevertheless, it is possible that the bell-shaped curve could be shifted to a higher value, but how far it can be shifted is unclear. The focus of research has transitioned from just extending the number of years lived (life span) to extending the period during which one is generally healthy and free from serious comorbidities (healthspan). Several interventions (smoking cessation, weight loss, and exercise) have been shown to improve both life span and healthspan.[4]

Functional Reserve and the Concept of Frailty

Old age is no place for sissies.

—*Bette Davis*

Functional reserve represents the degree to which organ function can increase above the level necessary for basal activity. For healthy individuals, reserve peaks at approximately age 30, gradually declines over the next several decades, and then experiences more rapid decline beginning around the eighth decade. Assessment of reserve is something anesthesiologists perform all the time. For example, the ability to achieve a minimum of four metabolic equivalents appears to confer enough cardiovascular reserve to tolerate the stress of most surgical procedures.[5] As age advances, there emerges an extreme form of decreased reserve and limited resistance to stressors. This biologic syndrome is often referred to as frailty, and though significant overlap exists between frailty, disability, and comorbidity, they are not synonymous (Fig. 34-2). Determining the preoperative frailty status of a patient is essential to understanding perioperative risk. Frailty is associated with poorer postoperative outcomes and preoperative identification of a frail patient should prompt a tailored, risk-mitigation perioperative care plan. 3

Frailty can be conceptualized as a patient with a frail phenotype (weak, slowed down, low energy, fall-prone, and losing weight) or a patient with a critical burden of accumulating deficits (comorbidities, social stressors, mental and cognitive health dysfunction, physical decline, and poor nutrition). In community-dwelling older adults 65 years of age or more, 22.7% of the population is estimated to be frail, and this percentage nearly doubles in people

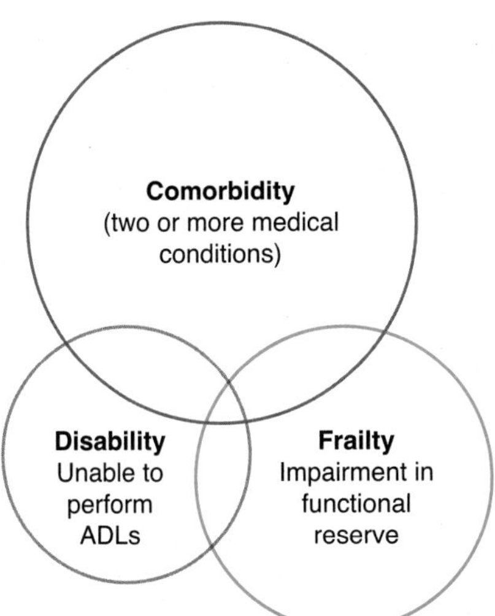

Figure 34-2 Comorbidity is defined as the presence of two or more chronic medical conditions. Disability is defined as the inability of a person to perform many of the activities of daily life (ADLs). Frailty occurs when there is impairment in physical and physiologic functional reserve. Comorbidity, disability, and frailty do not necessarily overlap.

aged 85 years or more.[6] Estimating the prevalence of frailty in the surgical population is complicated. One retrospective report based upon data from over 500,000 patients estimates that approximately 1 in 3 patients (29%) over age 65 presenting for major noncardiac surgery are frail. In this study, frail patients made up 41% of the emergency general surgery cohort in the same age group.[7] Though subject to variability dependent on the frailty assessment used, a similarly high percentage of patients aged 70 years and older (43%) presenting for cancer surgery are believed to be frail. Frail patients undergoing surgical procedures have a higher likelihood than nonfrail patients of experiencing mortality, morbidity, complications, prolonged hospital length of stay, and discharge to an institution.[8] Deploying process change to improve these poor outcomes is very challenging, when faced with the complex and pervasive barriers that currently limit resources available for effective healthcare delivery. Focusing on frail patients as an extremely vulnerable geriatric population is an opportunity for early gains when investing resources in perioperative care.

There are over 70 assessments for frailty. Although the diagnosis of frailty is often intuitive, there are two classical ways to define it. The first method is the frailty phenotype which is defined as a clinical syndrome in which three or more of the following criteria are present: unintentional weight loss (10 lb in past year), self-reported exhaustion, weakness (grip strength), slow walking speed, and low physical activity.[9] The Fried Phenotype assessment is highly validated, and several modifications exist. The second definition of frailty considers frailty in relation to deficit accumulation. The Frailty index is a list of symptoms, signs, diseases, and disabilities surveyed and scored in a binomial fashion (yes/no), from which the fraction of the positive deficits from the total number surveyed is calculated (e.g., 10 positive out of 40 surveyed equals a frailty index of 0.25).[10] Although the phenotype and index assessments do not necessarily identify the same patients, both predict mortality and institutionalization in community dwelling elderly.

In addition to the Fried Phenotype and related modifications and Frailty Index, the Clinical Frailty Scale and Edmonton Frail Scale are the most studied in surgical patients. The Clinical Frailty Scale is highly feasible in clinical settings (taking less than a minute or so) and can be useful for postoperative mortality and nonhome discharge risk stratification. The Edmonton Frail Scale is a better predictor of postoperative complications. The Fried Phenotype is strongly associated with postoperative delirium.[11] A summary of these and other commonly used frailty assessments is provided in Table 34-1. An area of intense investigation seeks to characterize objective radiographical markers of frailty and correlate these with clinical assessments.[12] This approach is exciting because imaging is often available for surgical patients that could be used opportunistically for frailty

Table 34-1 Frailty Screening Tools

Frailty Screening Tools (11,12)	Time to Administer	Type	Considerations
Clinical Frail Scale	<2 min	Observational	Associated with discharge to somewhere other than home and mortality. Does not require extra space or equipment
Edmonton Frailty Scale	<5 min	Observational/ patient-reported	Needs space, includes clock draw and timed getup and go tests. Software application available. Can predict postop complications
ACS NSQIP	5–10 min	Medical chart review	Limited to 30 days outcomes
Fatigue, Resistance, Ambulation, Illness, and Loss (FRAIL) Scale	5–10 min	Patient-reported	Simple administration. Not as widely studied as other assessments.
Risk Analysis Index	5–10 min	Patient-reported	Simple administration. Includes questions that are typically part of standard nursing interviews
Fried Phenotype	5–20 min	Observational	Most widely studied. Requires patient activity, special equipment. Associated with postoperative complications, including delirium
VESPA (short form)	10 min	Patient-reported	Modest sensitivity for postoperative complications
Frailty Index	10–13 min	Patient-reported	Does not require extra space or equipment. Associated with postoperative complications

For a more comprehensive list of frailty assessments, see Faller JW, Pereira DDN, de Souza S, Nampo FK, Orlandi FS, Matumoto S. Instruments for the detection of frailty syndrome in older adults: A systematic review. *PLoS One*. 2019 Apr 29;14(4):e0216166. doi: 10.1371/journal.pone.0216166. PMID: 31034516; PMCID: PMC6488093.

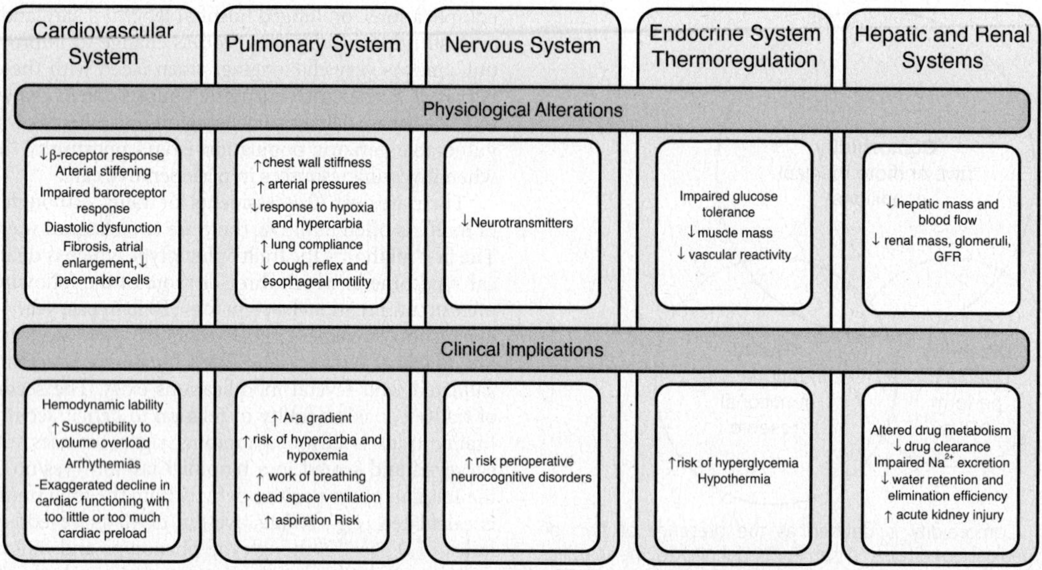

Figure 34-3 Common age-related changes in physiology.

assessment. Furthermore, there is promise in simple, noninvasive bedside procedures such as preoperative ultrasound measurements of quadriceps depth for identification of high-risk elderly patients.[13] Using objective radiologic methods for frailty identification could help tremendously with operationalization of frailty assessment. Raising awareness of positive frailty screening can improve outcomes.[14] Furthermore, when identified, frail patients can be further assessed to guide a targeted intervention plan.

The Physiology of Organ Aging

If I'd known I was going to live this long, I'd have taken better care of myself.

—James Hubert 'Eubie' Blake, age 100

Defining what constitutes "normal aging" is difficult. Is it what happens under the best of circumstances, or what happens to the "average" person? Comparisons of young and elderly subjects may not strictly reflect aging, as the elderly subjects may have experienced a much different diet, lifestyle, and environmental exposure than what the young group will have experienced by the time they become old. Following a group of healthy subjects over a long period is more likely to define the effects of aging, but not all available data come from such longitudinal studies. Studies that examine only the very old may underestimate the typical effects of aging because individuals generally do not achieve old age unless there is something intrinsically robust about them. The effects of aging vary considerably from one patient to another, and disease will interact with aging to further diminish functional organ reserve. A summary of the most consistently observed age-associated changes in physiology is provided in Figure 34-3.

Changes in Body Composition, and Liver and Kidney Aging

I have everything I had twenty years ago, only it's all a little bit lower.

—Gypsy Rose Lee

4 Changes in body composition are primarily characterized by a gradual loss of skeletal muscle and an increase in body fat, although the latter is more prominent in women (Fig. 34-4, Video 34-1, NICV 34-1). Basal metabolism declines with age, with most of the decline accounted for by the change in body composition. There is a reduction in total body water that reflects the reduction in cellular water that is associated with a loss of muscle and an increase in adipose tissue. Aging

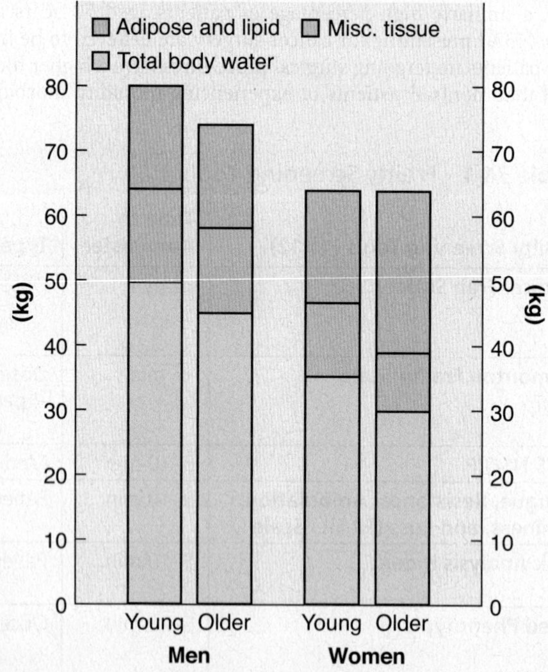

Figure 34-4 Age-related changes in body composition are gender-specific. In women, total body mass remains constant because increases in body fat (*upper shaded segment*) offset bone loss (*middle segment*) and intracellular dehydration (*lower shaded segment*). In men, body mass declines despite maintenance of body lipid and skeletal tissue elements because accelerating loss of skeletal muscle and other components of lean tissue mass produces marked contraction of intracellular water (*lower shaded segment*).

causes a small decrease in plasma albumin levels; however, there is a small increase in α_1-acid glycoprotein. The effect of these changes on drug protein binding and drug delivery appear to be minimal.

Liver mass decreases with age, and accounts for most, but not all, of the 20% to 40% decrease in liver blood flow.[15] There is also a modest reduction in phase I drug metabolism and bile secretion with age. Other than the effect of aging on drug metabolism, liver reserve should be more than adequate even in the very old in the absence of disease.

Renal cortical mass also decreases by 20% to 25% with age, but the most prominent effect of aging is the loss of up to half of the glomeruli by age 80. The decrease in the glomerular filtration rate of approximately 1 mL/min/yr after age 40 typically reduces renal excretion of drugs to a level where drug dosage adjustment becomes a progressively important consideration beginning at approximately age 60. Common comorbid conditions such as hypertension and diabetes can further decrease GFR (Fig. 34-5). Nevertheless, the degree of decline in glomerular filtration rate is highly variable and is likely to be much less than predicted in many individuals, especially those who avoid excessive dietary protein.

The aged kidney does not eliminate or retain sodium when necessary as effectively as that of a young adult. Part of the failure to conserve sodium when appropriate may be because of reduced aldosterone secretion. Similarly, the aged kidney does not retain or eliminate free water as rapidly as young kidneys when challenged by water deprivation or free water excess. Lastly, the sensation of thirst declines with age. In short, fluid and electrolyte homeostasis is more vulnerable in the older patient, particularly when an older patient suffers acute injury or disease and eating and drinking becomes more of a chore.

For the most part, functional endocrine decline does not interact with anesthetic management to any significant degree. However, aging is associated with decreased insulin secretion in response to glucose load, and also with increased insulin resistance, particularly in skeletal muscle. Thus, even healthy elderly patients may require perioperative insulin therapy more often than young adults, but the dose of insulin administered may need to be reduced.[16] Aging also results in decreases in testosterone, estrogen, and growth hormone production. The use of hormonal therapy to reduce sarcopenia, frailty in general, and cognitive decline and dementia is controversial, and does not have any current relevance to anesthetic management.

Central Nervous System Aging

By the time you're eighty years old you've learned everything. You only have to remember it.

—George Burns

Brain mass begins to decrease slowly beginning at approximately age 50 and declines more rapidly later, such that an 80-year-old brain has typically lost 10% of its weight. Neurotransmitter functions suffer more significantly, including dopamine, serotonin, γ-aminobutyric acid, and especially the acetylcholine system. The latter is especially important because of its connection to Alzheimer disease. Response times increase and learning is more difficult, but vocabulary, "wisdom," and past knowledge are better preserved. Nevertheless, of those individuals aged 85 and older, nearly half have significant cognitive impairment. In addition, some degree of atherosclerosis appears to be inevitable. Fortunately, and contrary to prior belief, the aged brain does make new neurons and is capable of forming new dendritic connections.

The major effect of brain aging on anesthetic management is the increased sensitivity to many anesthetic agents. Perhaps the best-known example is that after age 40 there is approximately a 6% decrease in minimum alveolar concentration (MAC) per decade (Fig. 34-6).[17] In addition, many intravenous agents produce an enhanced response in the older brain. These effects of aging are relatively simple to deal with in the clinical arena. More difficult to manage is the potential interaction of anesthesia, the stress of surgery, and a brain with minimal reserve. Age is a major risk factor for postoperative delirium and/or cognitive decline (see "Perioperative Complications").

Drug Pharmacology and Aging

I don't do alcohol anymore. I get the same effect just standing up fast.

—Unknown

Drugs typically have a more pronounced effect in an older patient. The cause can be either pharmacodynamic, in which case the target organ (often the brain) is more sensitive to a given drug tissue level, or pharmacokinetic, in which case a given dose of drug produces higher blood levels in older patients.

Most intravenous anesthetic drugs are highly lipid soluble and so begin to enter tissue even before fully mixed in the blood. The rate of transfer depends on the rate of delivery (i.e., the drug concentration in blood multiplied by the blood flow per gram of

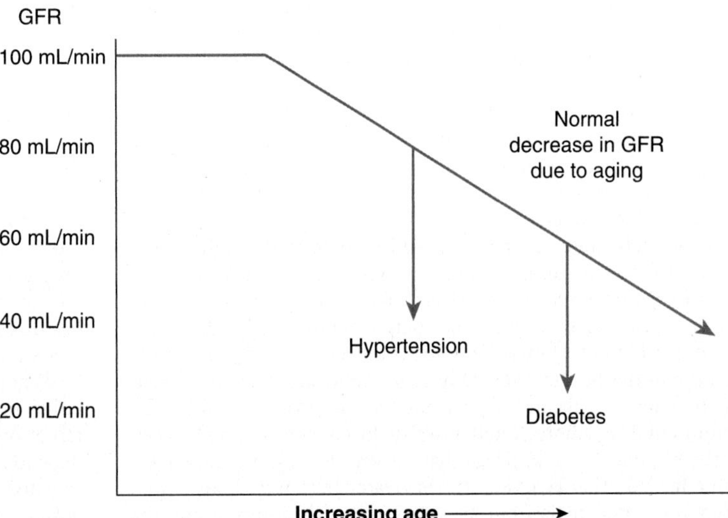

Figure 34-5 At around 40 years of age, glomerular filtration rate (GFR) decreases at a rate of 1 mL/min per year. In addition to this steady decrease, other common comorbid conditions such as hypertension and diabetes can further decrease GFR.

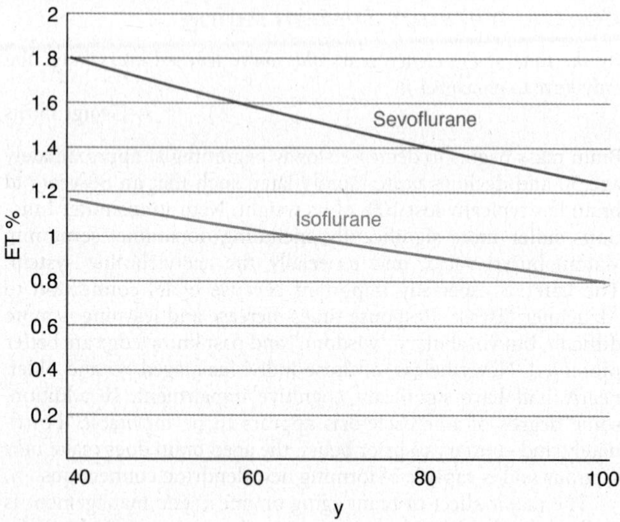

Figure 34-6 Minimum alveolar concentration (MAC) decreases with age for all volatile anesthetics. Illustrated above are the age-associated decreases in MAC for sevoflurane and isoflurane.

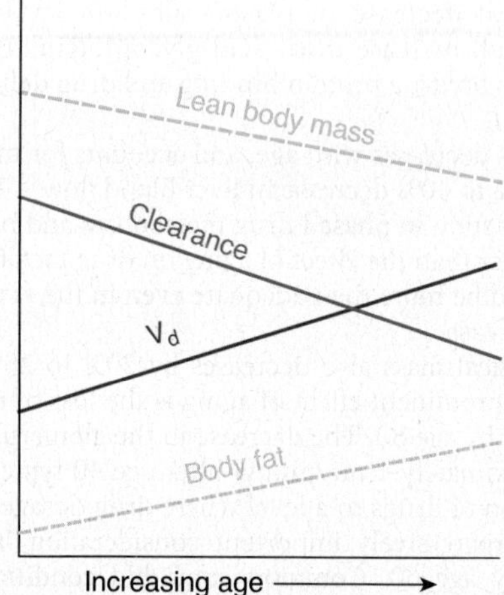

Figure 34-7 Changes in body composition with aging can lead to increased drug volume of distribution (V_d). Coupled with aging-associated decreases in clearance capability, the context-sensitive half-life of many drugs is increased in the elderly.

tissue), the concentration gradient of the drug between the blood and the tissue (i.e., a high gradient initially), the ease with which the drug crosses the blood and tissue membranes, and the solubility of the drug in the tissue. Thus, the vessel-rich group (brain, heart, kidney, muscle) will acquire drug much more rapidly than the vessel-poor group (fat, bone). Protein binding may affect transfer, with drugs that are highly protein-bound having a lower free concentration and a slower rate of transfer.

There are thus many ways for a drug bolus to have a more pronounced initial effect on older patients. The blood concentration is typically higher in older patients during the drug redistribution phase, partly because of a mildly contracted blood volume and partly because the reduction in muscle mass limits the rate and amount of drug removal by muscle. When drug blood levels remain higher for a longer time, more drug will be driven into highly perfused organs such as the brain (often the target organ) or the heart. A prime example of this phenomenon is sodium pentothal, and to a lesser degree, propofol.

Despite the fact that drugs typically have a greater effect on older patients, there is a general impression that bolus drugs take longer to achieve that greater effect. It is not entirely clear why this is so. Slower circulation is sometimes hypothesized, but total blood flow to any organ does not appear to decrease beyond that expected from the decrease in organ mass. Another possibility is a slower rate of transfer into the target organ. Drug effects are the result of tissue, not plasma concentrations. Brain–plasma equilibration is not instantaneous, and for at least some drugs (e.g., remifentanil), the equilibration half-life is prolonged in older brains. Why crossing the blood–brain barrier should take longer with age is not understood.

Ultimately though, the drug will distribute throughout the body based on tissue mass and solubility. Because most intravenous drugs used in anesthesia are highly lipid-soluble, most of the drug will end up in fat. How completely the drug is dispersed out of the blood and into the tissue is reflected by Vd_{ss}, the drug's volume of distribution at steady state. This variable is expressed as the liters of plasma that would be necessary to dilute the amount of drug administered down to the concentration observed in the plasma. As such, drugs that are very fat-soluble can have a value for Vd_{ss} that is several times greater than total body water. After the initial redistribution into vessel-rich group tissue, the drug will slowly diffuse back into the plasma as it continues to be absorbed into fat. In so doing, the target organ (e.g., brain) drug level will fall because the target organ is always in the vessel-rich group. Once a single therapeutic dose of a drug has fully distributed throughout the body, the blood and target organ drug levels are typically too low to have a meaningful clinical effect. However, very large doses, repeated doses, or infusions will eventually deliver enough drug to yield residual drug levels that produce therapeutic effects. At this point, the only way to decrease blood and target organ levels and eliminate the drug's effects is through metabolism. The elimination or metabolic half-life of a drug in the blood equals the volume of distribution at steady state (Vd_{ss}) divided by the clearance, where clearance represents the amount of blood from which drug is eliminated per minute.

The most prominent and consistent pharmacokinetic effect of aging is a decrease in drug metabolism, typically due to both a decrease in clearance and an increase in Vd_{ss} (Fig. 34-7). The increase in Vd_{ss} with age is likely due to the increase in body fat. Clearance decreases with age for any drug metabolized by the liver or kidney. When drug metabolism is via the liver, decreased liver mass and blood flow will decrease clearance for both high and low extraction drugs. In addition, elderly patients are often on a host of chronic medications, a setup for drug interactions as well as for inhibition of drug metabolism. Drugs with primarily renal elimination will experience decreased excretion because of reductions in glomerular filtration rate with aging. The net effect on drug metabolism is typically a doubling of the elimination half-life between old and young adults. However, with some drugs, the effect on half-life can be dramatic. In the case of diazepam, the half-life in hours is roughly equal to the patient's age (Fig. 34-8).[18] For a 72-year-old person, it would therefore require 3 days to metabolize half of a dose of diazepam. Such pharmacokinetics clearly illustrate why there is no place in modern medicine for the chronic use of diazepam and other drugs with similar half-lives when the desired effect is supposed to be transient (e.g., as a sleeping aid).

When dealing with infusions—or for that matter a series of bolus injections—the time it takes to decrease the blood and target organ drug levels to below the therapeutic threshold will depend on many factors. This is where the concept of the context-sensitive half-time proves useful; that is, the time necessary for a 50% decrease in plasma concentration following termination of

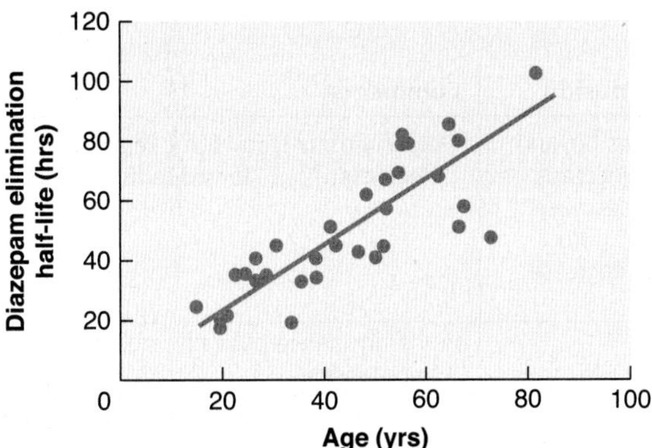

Figure 34-8 The effect of age on the elimination half-life of diazepam. The half-life in hours is equal to approximately the patient's age in years. (Reproduced with permission from Klotz U, Avant GR, Hoyumpa A, et al. The effects of age and liver disease on the disposition and elimination of diazepam in adult men. *J Clin Invest*. 1975;55:347; permission conveyed from Copyright Clearance Center, Inc.)

an infusion. At one extreme, if the residual level produced by the cumulative drug administration is still very low, then the drug effect will reverse quickly; the rapid redistribution of the most recently administered drug will lead to a rapid decrease in the blood level and termination of effect. At the other extreme, if there has been significant accumulation of drug in the body, and/or the maintenance blood level was high, then a long time may be required to decrease the drug levels enough to terminate the drug effect. As a general rule, the time to decrease the effect site drug concentration is increased most dramatically by aging when a large percentage decrease in plasma level is necessary to dip below the therapeutic threshold.

Review of the literature can yield a confusing picture when trying to ascertain which pharmacologic variable is most responsible for a given clinical effect. Table 34-2 summarizes some of this information for many of the common anesthetic drugs.[19] The effect of aging on sedative–hypnotic agents involves variations in both pharmacodynamic and pharmacokinetic properties. In contrast, the older brain appears to be more pharmacodynamically sensitive to opioids than in young adults, but the pharmacokinetics of opioids are largely unaffected by age.

Despite the loss of muscle and motor neurons with age, muscle relaxants do not appear to be more potent in the older patient when steady-state blood levels for a given level of paralysis are compared. Muscle relaxants often have a decreased initial volume of distribution, but this pharmacokinetic change does not seem to translate into smaller doses. The most commonly used relaxants, vecuronium and rocuronium, have modestly slowed metabolism with aging, so an increased duration of effect should be expected, especially with repetitive dosing. As such, the older patient is at greater risk for residual neuromuscular blockade (see section on Immediate Preoperative and Intraoperative Management).

Cardiovascular Aging

A man is as old as his arteries.

—*Thomas Sydenham*

Virtually all components of the cardiovascular system are affected by aging (NICV 34-2). The major changes include[1] decreased response to β-receptor stimulation;[2] stiffening of the myocardium, arteries, and veins;[3] changes in the autonomic nervous system with increased sympathetic activity and decreased parasympathetic activity;[4] conduction system changes; and[5] defective ischemic preconditioning. Although atherosclerosis appears to affect everyone by virtue of the fact that the mechanisms of aging contribute to the development of atherosclerosis, it is not clear that this inevitably leads to functional impairment or disease.

With age, there is increased sympathetic activity at rest and there is typically an exaggerated response to stimuli that increase sympathetic activity. Although there is decreased responsiveness of α-receptors with age, the swings in sympathetic activation during surgery can still produce significant changes in vascular resistance during anesthesia. These changes in vascular resistance contribute to the lability in blood pressure in the aged, as well as to a decrease in blood pressure when anesthesia removes the sympathetic tone.

The efficacy of baroreflex control of blood pressure decreases with age, caused primarily by a decrease in the heart rate response rather than a decrease in the baroreflex control of vascular tone itself. The decreased heart rate response to changes in blood pressure is in part due to lower vagal tone at rest, but the major mechanism is a decrease in the cardiac response to β-receptor stimulation. The mechanism does not appear to be a downregulation of β-receptors on the heart, but instead a defect in the intracellular coupling. Both heart rate and contractility increase less in response to endogenous release or exogenous administration of catecholamines. The increase in heart rate with exercise is therefore also diminished, as is maximal heart rate (often quoted as 220 minus age). This decrement contributes to decreased exertional capacity with age, even in trained individuals. The decrease in resting vagal tone may limit the increase in heart rate after administration of atropine or glycopyrrolate.

Conductance artery (aorta to arterioles) stiffening typically leads to systolic hypertension via two mechanisms. First, approximately half of the stroke volume remains in the thoracic aorta after ejection. Pressure must increase more to stretch out a stiffened aorta to accommodate that volume. Second, generalized arterial stiffening causes the pressure wave to transmit more rapidly. In vascular physiology, the pressure wave reflects off the arterial walls and branch points and returns to the thoracic aorta. In young people, the reflected waves do not return to the heart until after ejection is complete. These waves are responsible for the modest bump in pressure in the aortic root just after the dicrotic notch. These reflected waves return more rapidly in an older person because of the stiffer vessels, arriving by late ejection and increasing the pressure against which the left ventricle must pump to complete the stroke volume. This increased stress to the muscle stimulates hypertrophy.

Hypertrophy in and of itself stiffens the ventricle, but even worse, hypertrophy slows diastolic relaxation that, in turn, impairs ventricular filling in early diastole. The left ventricle now becomes more dependent on the atrial kick and requires an increase in left atrial pressure in order to preserve diastolic filling. The increase in atrial pressure is present at rest but can be quite dynamic with acute increases during stress such as tachycardia. This phenomenon, termed diastolic dysfunction, increases in severity with age. Most cases of congestive heart failure in very old persons are due to diastolic dysfunction and occur in the absence of clinically significant systolic dysfunction.

Adequate ventricular filling becomes more critical with age. The decreased response to β-receptor stimulation requires the ventricles to depend more on an adequate end-diastolic volume to generate enough contractile strength via the length–tension (Frank–Starling) relationship. Diastolic dysfunction requires an increase in central and pulmonary venous pressure to maintain that end-diastolic volume. The range in acceptable filling pressures ends up becoming narrower with age because too low a pressure results in inadequate filling. Since the normal pressure

Table 34-2 Effect of Age on Drug Dosing

Drug	Bolus Administration	Multiple Boluses or Infusion	Comments[a]
Propofol	20–60% reduction, dose on lean body mass, 1 mg/kg in very old	50% reduction, infusions beyond 50 min progressively increase the time required to decrease the blood level by 50% (but effect site levels may decrease faster in elderly)	↑ brain sensitivity (by some reports), decreased V_{cen}, slowed redistribution
Dexmedetomidine	Consider reduction	Consider reduction	Higher incidence of bradycardia and hypotension
Thiopental	20% reduction	20% reduction	= brain sensitivity, decreased V_{cen}, slowed redistribution
Etomidate	25–50% reduction	—	= brain sensitivity
Midazolam	Compared to age 20, modest reduction at age 60, 75% reduction at age 90	Similar to bolus (metabolic $t_{½}$ longer, but not meaningful unless very large doses are used)	↑↑ brain sensitivity
Morphine	Probably 50% reduction. Peak morphine effect is 90 min (though half of peak effect at 5 min)	Long effect site equilibration time translates into very slow reduction in effect on termination of infusion (4 hrs for 50% reduction)	Metabolite morphine-6-glucoronide build-up requires prolonged morphine use, but its renal excretion will make it very long acting
Fentanyl	50% reduction	50% reduction	↑ brain sensitivity, minimal changes in pharmacokinetics; delayed absorption from fentanyl patch
Alfentanil, sufentanil	50% reduction	50% reduction	Probably ↑ brain sensitivity, minimal changes in pharmacokinetics
Remifentanil	50% reduction	50% reduction	Slower blood–brain equilibration, suggesting slower onset and offset, modest decreased V_{cen}
Hydromorphone	No studies on aging exist, but assume increased potency in elderly	Assume 50% reduction	Compared with morphine, no active metabolite, faster onset
Methadone	No studies on aging exist, but assume increased potency in elderly	Assume 50% reduction	—
Meperidine	Use only for postoperative shivering	Do not use	Toxic metabolite normeperidine, whose renal excretion decreases with age
Vecuronium	Slower onset (≈33%)	Slower recovery times	Slightly greater liver metabolism than renal, age nearly doubles metabolic $t_{½}$
Mivacurium	Equally fast onset in young and old	Modest dose reduction for infusion, longer recovery time on repeated bolus	Elimination by plasma cholinesterase, modest prolongation of metabolic $t_{½}$ by age
Cisatracurium	Slower onset (≈33%)	No significant changes with age	Mostly Hoffmann elimination, modest prolongation of metabolic $t_{½}$ by age
Rocuronium	Minimally slower onset	—	Liver metabolism slightly greater than renal, modest increase in metabolic $t_{½}$ by age
Pancuronium	—	—	Primarily renal elimination, aging doubles metabolic $t_{½}$
Pipecuronium	Slower onset (≈50%), elderly may be *less* sensitive	—	Primarily renal elimination, no apparent change in metabolic $t_{½}$
Succinylcholine	Slower onset (≈40%)	—	
Edrophonium	Similar dosing and onset	—	↑ V_{cen}, primarily renal elimination, modest increase in metabolic $t_{½}$ by age
Neostigmine	Despite pharmacokinetic changes, some studies indicate need for increased dose with age	—	↑ V_{cen}, hepatic elimination, modest increase in metabolic $t_{½}$ by age

[a] V_{cen}, central volume of distribution or initial volume of distribution. Although V_{cen} does not have an anatomic correlate, a smaller V_{cen} will increase initial plasma levels and enhance transfer of the drug in the target organ (e.g., brain, muscle).

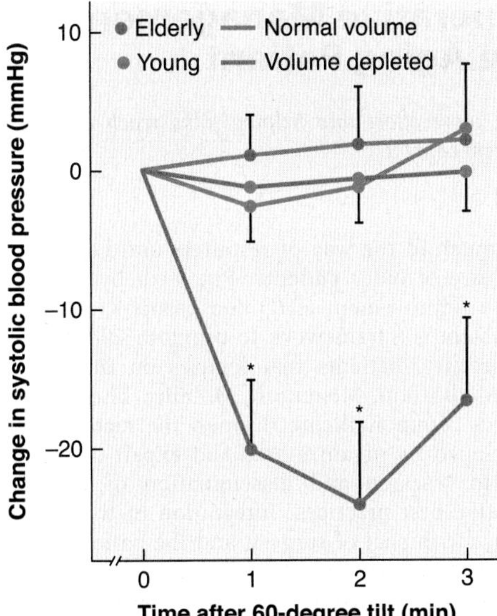

Figure 34-9 Young and elderly adults are subjected to a passive tilt test in their euvolemic state and after an approximate 2 kg of water and 100 mEq of sodium loss. With tilt, blood pools in the legs. Although young subjects tolerate tilt under both circumstances, the combination of hypovolemia and tilt exceeds the compensatory mechanisms of the older subjects. (Reproduced with permission from Shannon RP, Wei JY, Rosa RM, et al. The effect of age and sodium depletion on cardiovascular response to orthostasis. *Hypertension*. 1986;8:438.)

is already elevated, any further increase is that much closer to a pressure that results in fluid extravasation and adverse consequences such as pulmonary edema.

Unfortunately, aging also decreases the ability to maintain filling pressures in the acceptable range. The venous system serves as a reservoir for blood and buffers changes in blood volume in order to maintain ventricular filling at an appropriate level. However, veins stiffen with age. Venous stiffening impairs this buffering capacity and creates a situation where modest changes in venous blood volume may produce more dramatic changes in venous pressures and cardiac filling. In short, the system has become inherently more unstable as illustrated by the development of postural hypotension in elderly persons but not in young adults with mild hypovolemia (Fig. 34-9).

Rhythm disturbances may develop with age. Fibrosis of the conduction system may lead to conduction blocks, and loss of sinoatrial node cells may make the older patient more prone to sick sinus syndrome. The prevalence of atrial fibrillation climbs exponentially with age, perhaps in part because of atrial enlargement.

Aging appears to diminish or even eliminate any protective effect of ischemic preconditioning, a phenomenon whereby a brief period of myocardial ischemia will lessen the adverse effects of a subsequent, more prolonged ischemic event. "Warm-up angina" is the ability to achieve a higher level of exertion after first exercising to the point of angina. Starting around age 65, this increment in the level of exertion progressively diminishes with age. In younger adults, death or heart failure is a less frequent complication of a myocardial infarction if the patient had been experiencing angina within 2 weeks of the myocardial infarction. This protective effect of angina is not present in older adults.

This section began with a quote from Thomas Sydenham. Evidence is mounting that the quote is truly prophetic: arterial stiffening may indeed be a marker of physiologic age. One of the manifestations of arterial stiffening is a widened pulse pressure. Once the difference between systolic and diastolic pressure reaches 80 mmHg or more, there is a clear association with all-cause mortality; cardiovascular mortality; and a variety of morbidities including stroke, coronary disease, and renal failure.[20] Increased pulse pressure is also associated with increased morbidity and mortality after coronary artery bypass grafting.[20]

Pulmonary Aging

The most prominent effects of aging on the pulmonary system are increased stiffness of the chest wall and a decreased stiffness of the lung parenchyma. With aging, the thorax becomes more barrel-shaped which leads to flattening of the diaphragm. Less diaphragmatic curvature provides a mechanical disadvantage for the generation of negative pressure in the intrapleural space. The stiffened chest wall and flattened diaphragm increase the work of breathing. Combined with an age-related loss of muscle mass, it is easy to understand how the older patient will be more prone to fatigue when challenged by an increase in minute ventilation, and thus more likely to experience respiratory failure.

The decrease in lung tissue stiffness is due to a loss of elastin with age. Unlike elsewhere in the body, the elastin is not replaced with collagen and so older lungs become easier to inflate. There are several adverse effects of this increase in compliance. Small airways do not have enough inherent stiffness and so depend on tethering by the surrounding tissue to remain open. The degree of outward pull by the tissue depends on the stiffness of the tissue and the degree of stretch of the tissue. As the tissue loses its springiness, greater lung inflation is needed to produce the same amount of outward pull on the airways. The need for greater lung inflation to prevent small airway collapse is reflected by the increase in closing capacity with age (Fig. 34-10). Closing capacity typically exceeds functional residual capacity in the mid-60s, and will eventually exceed the tidal volume at some later age. Decreased lung tissue stiffness also increases ventilation–perfusion mismatch as each piece of

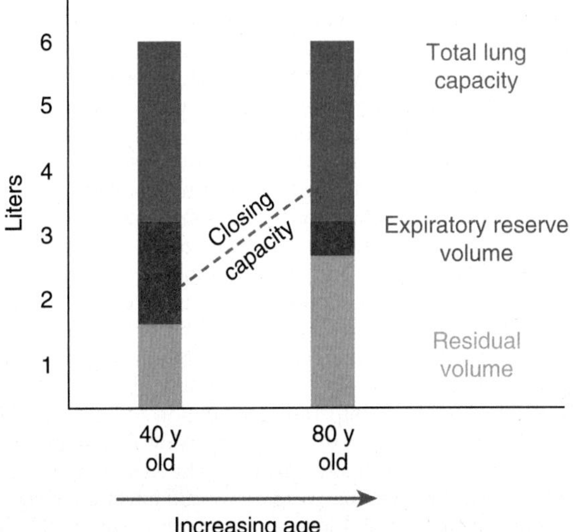

Figure 34-10 Changes in spirometry values with aging. There is virtually no change in total lung capacity. However, expiratory reserve volume decreases and residual volume increases. The sum of these—functional residual capacity—is largely unchanged. Note that closing capacity can exceed functional residual capacity leading to increased atelectasis.

lung tissue is less tethered to its neighbor, making ventilation less uniform. These changes, plus a modest reduction in alveolar surface area with age, contribute to a modest decline in resting PaO_2 with age.

Less-effective small airway tethering also leads to greater limitations during forced exhalation. At all ages, forced exhalation produces positive pressures in the intrapleural space that tends to compress intrathoracic airways. Only the airway connective tissue and lung tissue tethering oppose that compression. With less lung tissue tethering, airways compress at a larger lung volume in older subjects and produce a limitation in air flow during exhalation over a much larger percentage of the exhalation (e.g., the last 45% in a 70-year-old person) than in a younger subject (e.g., 20% in a 30-year-old person).[21]

Changes within the nervous system further influence the respiratory system. Aging leads to an approximate 50% decrease in the ventilatory response to hypercapnia, and an even greater decrease in the response to hypoxia, especially at night. Generalized loss of muscle tone with age applies to the hypopharyngeal and genioglossal muscles and predisposes elderly persons to upper airway obstruction. A high percentage, perhaps even 75%, of people over age 65 have sleep-disordered breathing, a phenomenon that may or may not be the same as sleep apnea, but which certainly places elderly patients at increased risk of hypoxia postoperatively.[22] Aging also results in less-effective coughing and impaired swallowing. Aspiration is a significant cause of community-acquired pneumonia and may well play a role in the development of postoperative pneumonia.[23]

Thermoregulation and Aging

In the past two decades there has been heightened awareness of the adverse consequences of perioperative hypothermia as well as improved methods to prevent hypothermia. Even outside the operating room, elderly individuals are prone to hypothermia when stressed by modestly cold environments that would not affect younger individuals. The initial response to a cold environment is vasoconstriction, and if that response is insufficient and the subject becomes colder, then shivering is the second response. Both mechanisms are triggered by decreases in core and/or skin temperature. The two temperatures interact such that a decrease in skin temperature of 1° is equivalent to a decrease in core temperature of approximately 0.2°.[24] Although there is great variability among the elderly over the degree to which vasoconstriction and shivering are impaired, one should anticipate that elderly patients will have not only impaired vasoconstriction but also decreased heat production due to a lower metabolism.

At all ages, both inhalational and some intravenous agents (e.g., propofol and alfentanil but not midazolam) alter the regulatory thresholds such that body temperature must fall by as much as 4°C (7°F) before initiation of vasoconstriction or shivering. Aging further impairs these thresholds by approximately 1°C (2°F), not only during general anesthesia but during spinal anesthesia as well.[24]

Given the impaired temperature regulation and decreased heat production of the elderly, it is not surprising that hypothermia occurs more frequently in older patients. The risks of hypothermia include myocardial ischemia, surgical wound infection, coagulopathy with increased blood loss, and impaired drug metabolism. Shivering places a significant metabolic stress on a patient and may not be well tolerated by a patient with borderline cardiac or pulmonary reserve. The prevention and treatment of hypothermia in an elderly patient does not appear to be any different than for younger adults.

Perioperative Management of the Aging Patient

We've put more effort into helping folks reach old age than into helping them enjoy it.

—Frank A. Clark

There is much in the way of resources and best-practice guidance for care of older patients. Put forth by the Institute for Healthcare Improvement (IHI) and partners, the Age-Friendly Health System is a framework to promote safe, evidence-based care of geriatric patients that focuses on the "4-M's": What Matters, Medication, Mentation, Mobility. These areas of focus repeat as a common theme through the materials and literature developed by organizations and expert consensus groups invested in research and dissemination of geriatric-focused perioperative best practices. Integration of the patient's medical status, the impact of surgery, and the patient's goals require a comprehensive approach that encompasses both preoperative optimization and potentially prolonged postoperative recovery. Healthcare organizations can now complete the Geriatric Surgical Verification (GSV) Program sponsored by the ACS. The program has over 30 components focused on preoperative screening to identify vulnerable patients, with creation, implementation, and interdisciplinary review of individualized management plans. Targeted vulnerabilities include, but are not limited to, malnutrition, impaired mobility or functional status, increased delirium risk and need for expert consultation.[25] Despite the growth of geriatric-focused clinical expertise, there is a lag in execution of recommended practices.[26] Leveraging other perioperative initiatives that have become popular could potentially help. Enhanced recovery protocols have been very effective in helping patients tolerate the stress of surgery and are becoming widespread.[27] The ASA supported PSH initiative is an even more comprehensive patient-centered, physician-led, interdisciplinary, and team-based care model, that strives to achieve better health, better healthcare, and reduced expenditures by implementing multidisciplinary interventions as soon as the need for surgery or a procedure is identified.[28,29] The identification of older patients who need specialized care and interventions to optimize perioperative management and improve the likelihood of maintained, if not improved, functional status after surgery is of paramount importance. Anesthesiologists have much more to offer to care of the surgical patients than simply providing optimal operating conditions. We have the most comprehensive knowledge of important perioperative physiology, pharmacology and intraoperative factors, and an established history of professional contributions to patient safety. It is worthwhile noting that since the 1990s, major innovations in anesthesiology have slowed, and this is potentially related to antagonism between innovation and the increasing demand for "compliance" of clinical behaviors in pursuit of efficiency and defect-free surgical care processes.[30] Evidence-based care should be rigorously implemented, but despite major improvements in anesthetic evaluation and care, significant problems continue to plague surgical patients, especially older ones. We must feel empowered to be curious about what can be done better and not allow compliance to yield complacency. It will serve our patients best if we use our unique understanding of care needs and broad medical knowledge to be effective coordinators of care programs and protocols to best optimize perioperative care, while also taking initiative to think about solutions to the most important perioperative challenges, unconstrained by conventional wisdom.

Evaluation and Care of the Older Surgical Patient in Preparation for Surgery

The American College of Surgeons National Surgical Quality Improvement Program (ACS NSQIP) and American Geriatrics Society (AGS) Best Practice Guidelines "Optimal Preoperative Assessment of the Geriatric Surgical Patient" provide a checklist of important components for comprehensive evaluation of older patients and suggest many feasible tools for assessment prior to surgery.[31] The Strong for Surgery Program is a condensed resource created by the ACS that highlights important components of preoperative risk stratification and offers basic patient optimization guidance. Fortunately, the majority of older surgical patients survive without major complication, but nonetheless an astounding one in four older surgical patients remain significantly compromised in some way postoperatively.[32]

5 Preoperative patient-centered care and multi-system evaluation focused on goals and risk-mitigation are critical for enhancing recovery of function after surgery. Planning for surgery should include discussions about informed consent, living wills, and ethical treatment of the older patient. Risk modification should include tailored interventions targeting education, prehabilitation, medication scrutiny, and discharge planning.

Although the goals of preoperative evaluation are no different than for any other patient, there are issues more common among the elderly population that should be raised. Older patients often recognize that the end of their life is no longer the theoretical consideration of youth, so they are more likely to have living wills, healthcare proxies, and healthcare directives in place at the time of surgery. Yet, they often have surgery near the end of life. A retrospective cohort survey of elderly Medicare beneficiaries found that almost a third undergo surgery in their last year of life and that over 18% undergo surgery in the last month of their lives.[33] The older patient's expectations for surgery may be much different than that of their younger counterparts, and medical practitioners must be careful not to judge a patient's decision making based on the practitioner's values or expectations. Such personal values are particularly important when questions of competence arise: the physician could be tempted to question competence if the patient's decision does not coincide with the opinion of the physician. A discussion of risks and benefits needs to include the probable degree of functional recovery and the speed with which that recovery is likely to occur. If healthcare directives prohibit various life-sustaining or resuscitative procedures, the patient/proxy and anesthesiologist must come to a mutual understanding of what will or will not be performed if an untoward event occurs in the perioperative period. Discussion of a patient's goals and values and consent to specific procedures can result in a "Limited Attempt at Resuscitation" agreement between the anesthesiologist and patient.[34]

The prospect of functional impairment of physical capabilities may be more worrisome to the older patient than even death. Elderly patients may require a long time to return to their preoperative level of function, assuming full recovery is even possible. For example, after major abdominal surgery, most older patients require at least 3 months for ADLs and independent ADLs to return to baseline.[35] Persistent disability at 6 months varies with the task. Although there is only a 9% incidence of persistent ADL deficits, there is a 19% incidence of deficit in independent ADLs, and a 52% incidence of diminished grip strength.

Functional impairment of neurocognition is common perioperatively. A significant change to nomenclature classifying cognitive dysfunction in surgical patients has occurred recently. To unify terminology in clinical and research settings, "perioperative neurocognitive disorders" (PNDs) is now used as the primary term for cognitive impairment identified in the pre *or* postoperative periods (see Perioperative Complications for more details).[36] Delirium remains a DSM-V diagnosis of acute onset change in mental functions with confusion and decreased awareness of surroundings, occurring within a week after surgery. This is an astoundingly common and costly complication in older surgical patients. Pre-existing cognitive dysfunction, also believed to be common (estimated in one study to be 25% of older patients presenting to preop clinic for orthopedic surgery[37]), is an important risk factor for postoperative complications, including delirium. Identification of patients with baseline cognitive deficits is prudent for risk stratification, but also has important implications for the informed consent process. Despite this, execution of preoperative cognitive evaluation occurs "rarely" or "never" for more than 80% of elderly patients.[26] Discussion of postoperative cognitive impairment is an important disclosure of risk when obtaining informed consent,[38] especially because of its high incidence, the gravity of which seems lost on patients, despite a high degree of awareness. A recent survey study of patients >70 years old preparing for surgery reported 83% of patients were aware of postoperative delirium, with several patients (16%) even reporting a previous personal experience with delirium, but concern about the effects of delirium was low (92% of respondents had no more than a "low-level" of concern).[39] Only one in four patients reported prior counseling on delirium, so there is a paucity of information being shared with patients, highlighting another missed opportunity for patient engagement in the preoperative period.

In conjunction with these important considerations, additional structured evaluation of the geriatric patient prior to surgery is warranted. A summary of best practices and resources for preoperative geriatric assessment from the ASA, AGS, and ACS is available (Table 34-3). Routine cognitive screening of older surgical patients is now recommended, and performance of the brief Mini-Cog assessment has been linked to speed of recovery, mortality risk and postoperative delirium risk. Additional core recommendations for promoting perioperative brain health include:

- Screening for depression (e.g., Patient Health Questionnaire–2 [PHQ-2])
- Use of a hospital-supported multidisciplinary team to manage delirium-mitigating processes including education about delirium (for care team and patients/family)
- Identification of patients at high risk
- Opiate-sparing pain management
- Minimization of pharmacologic agents associated with delirium such as those listed in the American Geriatrics Society Beers Criteria: a compendium of medications to avoid or consider with caution because they often present an unfavorable balance of benefits and harm for older people[40,41] (Table 34-4).

In the very old, dehydration, elder abuse, and malnutrition are all more common than generally appreciated. In the case of malnutrition, the deficit may be limited to isolated deficiencies such as vitamin D or B_{12}, or it may be more global and include inadequate caloric intake from poor oral hygiene or the "anorexia of aging" in which neuroendocrine changes lead to early satiety and diminished sense of taste.[42] Nutritional status is an underappreciated risk factor for surgery and should be evaluated preoperatively. The Veterans Affairs National Surgical Quality Improvement Program found albumin to be as sensitive an index for mortality or morbidity as any other single indicator, including the American Society of Anesthesiologists status.

Table 34-3 Preoperative Best Practice Guidelines for Older Adults and Implementation Strategies

Best Practice Guidelines	Implementation Strategies
Assess cognitive ability, capacity to understand the anticipated surgery	• Utilize a brief cognitive screening test such as the MoCA or Mini-Cog (MoCA-BLIND can be administered via telehealth) • Communicate results to PCP for longitudinal follow-up and to anesthesiologist/surgeon for risk stratification
Screen for depression	• Perform a brief depression screen with tools such as 2-question PHQ-2, longer instruments if initial screen is positive • Communicate results to PCP to consider management strategies with appropriate longitudinal follow-up • If patient has severe symptom burden, consider delaying surgery to optimize treatment
Identify patient's risk factors for developing postoperative delirium	• Use a standardized tool or template to quickly identify presence of risk factors, such as the table provided from the American College of Surgery[a] • Address modifiable risk factors • Provide standardized education to patients and family members directly or via prepared handouts
Screen for alcohol and other substance abuse/dependence	• Use a screening tool like the modified CAGE (cut down, annoyed, guilty, eye-opener) questionnaire[b] • For positive screens, consider perioperative prophylaxis for withdrawal syndromes, or potentially delaying surgery for preoperative abstinence or medical detoxification
Perform a preoperative cardiac evaluation according to the ACC/AHA[c] algorithm	• Estimate functional capacity in terms of metabolic equivalents (METs), with subsequent guideline-directed assessment
Identify the patient's risk factors for postoperative pulmonary complications and implement appropriate strategies for prevention	• Recognize that even without pulmonary disease, older adults are at higher risk for aspiration, atelectasis, and other complications
Document functional status, falls history	• Can collect this information at check-in or prior to appointment via telephone call • Document this information so it can be reviewed by inpatient providers
Measure frailty	• Tools such as the FiND-CFS[d] rapidly screen for frailty • Frail patients may need additional evaluation, optimization prior to surgery • Surgeons and anesthesiologists should be alerted of frailty status for risk stratification
Assess nutritional status, consider preoperative interventions	• Utilize short screening tools such as MNA-SF[e] • Provide standardized education encouraging protein intake • Consider referral to social work or nutritionist for at-risk patients
Take an accurate and detailed medication history, consider appropriate perioperative adjustments; monitor for polypharmacy	• Compare medications to the Beers list to identify high-risk medications[f] • Consider pharmacist referral • Discontinue high-risk, infrequently used medications (e.g., occasional benzodiazepines, sedatives) • Arrange PCP follow-up for more complex medication reviews • Leverage telehealth and E-consults to engage PCPs and other providers quickly
Determine the patient's treatment goals and expectations	• Tools such as the QPL[g] can be provided to patients and families prior to appointments to encourage thoughtful and efficient discussion • If patients' expectations for surgery do not align with their providers', consider referral back to surgeon to clarify goals of care
Determine patient's family and social support system	• Encourage presence of family member at preoperative appointment • Ask patients "Who will support you after surgery?" • Consider social work referral or delaying surgery if patients are unable to identify reliable support structure
Order appropriate preoperative diagnostic tests focused on elderly patients	• Hemoglobin, renal function, and albumin recommended for all older adults • Other testing should only be done with a clear indication

MoCA, Montreal Cognitive Assessment Test; PCP, primary care provider; PHQ-2, Patient Health Questionnaire-2.
[a]See section I-D of "Best Practice Guidelines" for a table of risk factors for postoperative delirium.[53]
[b]Modified CAGE Questionnaire.
[c]American College of Cardiology/American Heart Association.[5]
[d]FiND-CFS is the Frail Non-Disabled Survey and Clinical Frailty Scale.
[e]Mini Nutritional Assessment Short-Form.
[f]Beers Criteria for Potentially Inappropriate Medication Use in Older Adults.[41]
[g]Question-Prompt List.
Used with permission Zietlow KE, Wong S, Heflin MT, McDonald SR, Sickeler R, Devinney M, Blitz J, Lagoo-Deenadayalan S, Berger M. Geriatric Preoperative Optimization: A Review. *Am J Med*. 2022 Jan;135(1):39–48. doi: 10.1016/j.amjmed.2021.07.028. Epub 2021 Aug 18. PMID: 34416164; PMCID: PMC8688225.

Table 34-4 Common Perianesthesia Medications to Avoid

Drug	Rationale
Central Nervous System	
Antiemetics Examples: Metoclopramide, promethazine,[a,b] prochlorperazine[a]	Parkinsonian symptoms can be exacerbated by dopamine receptor antagonism [a]Additional anticholinergic properties [b]Additional antihistamine properties
Antidepressants Examples: Amitriptyline, clomipramine, nortriptyline, paroxetine, doxepin >6 mg/day	Highly anticholinergic, sedating, and can cause orthostatic hypotension; safety profile of low-dose doxepin (≤6 mg/day comparable to that of placebo)
Antihistamines (first generation) Examples: Diphenhydramine, hydroxyzine	Highly anticholinergic; sedating and clearance reduced with advanced age. ↑ risk of confusion, dry mouth, constipation Use diphenhydramine for severe allergic reaction as appropriate.
Antipsychotics, first (conventional) and second (atypical) generation	↑ risk of cerebrovascular accident (stroke), ↑ rate of cognitive decline and mortality in persons with dementia Antipsychotics for behavioral problems of dementia or delirium are not recommended unless nonpharmacologic options (e.g., behavioral interventions) have failed and the patient is a significant harm to self or others
Barbiturates	↑ risk of overdose at low dosages, tolerance and high rate of physical dependence
Benzodiazepines Examples: Short and intermediate acting: Alprazolam, lorazepam, midazolam Long acting: clonazepam, diazepam	↓ metabolism of long-acting agents in older adults All benzodiazepines increase risk of cognitive impairment, delirium, falls, fractures, and motor vehicle crashes in older adults May be appropriate for periprocedural anesthesia and other clinical scenarios (i.e., ethanol withdrawn, seizures, significant anxiety)
Nonbenzodiazepine, benzodiazepine receptor agonist hypnotics (i.e., "Z-drugs") Examples: Eszopiclone, zaleplon, zolpidem	Z drugs (Nonbenzodiazepine receptor agonist hypnotics) have minimal improvement in sleep latency and duration, and have benzodiazepine-like adverse effects
Pain Medications	
Meperidine	Safer alternatives available
Noncyclooxygenase-selective NSAIDs, oral. Examples: Aspirin >325 mg/day, ibuprofen, meloxicam, ketorolac (includes parenteral), indomethacin[a]	Significant gastrointestinal complications caused by NSAIDs occur in ~1% of patients treated for 3–6 mo and ~2–4% of patients treated for 1 yr. Risks are dose and duration related. Patients >75 years old are especially high risk. Can ↑ blood pressure and induce kidney injury. [a]Indomethacin is more likely than other NSAIDs to have adverse CNS effects. Of all the NSAIDs, indomethacin has the most adverse effects
Skeletal Muscle Relaxants	
Examples: Carisoprodol, chlorzoxazone, cyclobenzaprine, metaxalone, methocarbamol, orphenadrine	Anticholinergic adverse effects, sedation, increased risk of fractures; effectiveness at dosages tolerated by older adults questionable

All drugs listed above are strongly recommended to avoid by the 2019 American Geriatric Society Beers Criteria Update Expert Panel.[41]

Clearly there are many issues surrounding surgery in the elderly that are rarely present with younger patients. It is tempting to hypothesize that interventions before surgery targeting aging-specific care concerns, functional decline, and frailty could improve surgical outcomes. For patients scheduled for elective surgery, interventions provided before surgery (prehabilitation) do appear to be superior to similar interventions provided after surgery (rehabilitation), although a major obstacle is low patient adherence to the prehabilitation programs. Prehabilitation is a multifaceted approach for optimization before surgery to protect cognitive and physical functions and promote resiliency against perioperative stressors (Fig. 34-11).[43] The action of prehabilitating a patient can have varying degrees of intensity based upon baseline functionality, identified areas of risk and resources to support compliance. A significant challenge with evaluating the prehabilitation literature is that consistency is lacking in the prehabilitation programs studied. However, most studies do report an enhancement of cardiopulmonary functional status which is associated with a lower severity and rate of postoperative complications.[43] Further investigations specifically targeting older patients with prehabilitation are needed.[44]

Having traditionally focused on exercise-based interventions targeting aerobic, resistance, flexibility and balance training, surgery prehabilitation programs now also focus on lifestyle modifications (i.e., reduced alcohol consumption and smoking cessation), nutritional interventions (i.e., protein and multivitamin

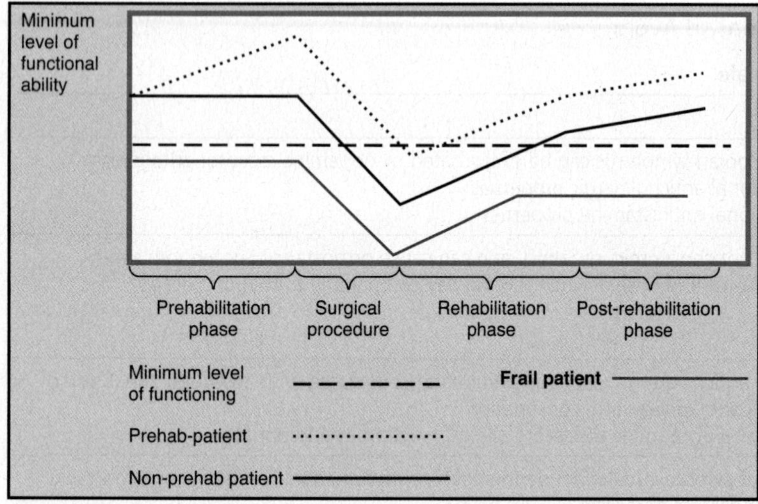

Figure 34-11 Through increasing reserve, prehabilitation can lower the amount of time patients experience impairment in functional abilities after surgery. Frail patients have reduced functional abilities at baseline and may experience a greater decline after surgery that remains persistent. The effects of prehabilitation in frail patients is an area of active investigation and may support allocation of healthcare resources for prehabilitation to this especially vulnerable population.

supplementation and immunonutrition) and behavioral health stress-coping mechanisms (i.e., relaxation and breathing exercises).[43] Recent publications have reported potential cost savings with prehabilitation for patients having major abdominal surgery.[45,46] "Cognitive exercises" for the protection or augmentation of preoperative cognitive reserve have potential for additional risk factor modification. Investigations into "brain gaming" for the prevention of PND have increased in light of evidence suggesting that only 12 hours of video-game training in older adults (60–85 years) over a 4-week period may produce lasting benefits in multi-tasking, working memory, and sustained attention.[47–49] Presurgical cognitive exercise deserves more study to further characterize the best cognitive protection strategies for elderly patients, in addition to multicomponent programs that include preoperative counseling, psychoeducation, and delirium risk reduction strategies (sensory orientation aids, nutrition, hydration, exercise, and stress management components).[50,51] A randomized pilot study in older surgical patients combining preoperative cognitive training and physical exercise demonstrated the feasibility of a comprehensive prehabilitation program for both cognitive and physical function.[52]

Immediate Preoperative and Intraoperative Management

Guidance on the optimal management of older surgical patients in the immediate perioperative phases of care has been summarized by the ACS and AGS (NICV 34-3). Prior to the OR, the patient's goals and treatment plan should be confirmed, especially if these have changed. Clarification of advance directives and determining who may act as the patient's legal decision makers are priorities. Implementation of a customized pain management plan with multimodal approaches and regional techniques as appropriate can lower mortality risk, reduce postoperative complications, and improve recovery after major surgery.[53]

6 Intraoperative management must take into account the increased sensitivity to drugs in the elderly patient, as well as an increased likelihood of hemodynamic, pulmonary, and thermoregulatory instability. Anesthetic care requires modification based upon the complex interaction of surgical stress, pharmacology and physiologic changes associated with both normal aging and age-linked disease states. During surgical positioning, special care should be taken to maintain skin integrity and limit pressure on peripheral nerves. Active patient warming strategies should be used to avoid hypothermia.

At this time, a single "best" anesthetic plan for older adults cannot be gleaned from the current evidence. For example, there are no magic bullets for the induction of general anesthesia in older patients. The effects of a bolus induction dose on a single patient are highly variable, so admittedly there is a certain amount of estimation and titration involved. In general, smaller doses are needed in comparison to young adults. It can be an effective strategy to use a lesser amount of a drug but to allow more time for the drug to achieve its peak target organ (brain) effect. A given blood level of propofol causes a greater decrease in brain activity in an older patient, but is likely to cause an even more dramatic decrease in blood pressure in comparison to the decrease observed in young adults. Many strategies can be used to minimize this decrease in blood pressure, usually by reducing the bolus amount of propofol via the use of adjuncts such as opioids or small doses of etomidate. Etomidate has been observed to produce less hypotension than propofol in older patients. An alternative approach is to induce with a propofol infusion of 400 μg/kg/min until the bispectral index (BIS) reaches 60.[54] Although swings in blood pressure may not be desirable, there is little evidence that even major, but brief, changes in blood pressure lead to adverse outcomes. The third PeriOperative ISchemic Evaluation (POISE-3) Trial will evaluate if a perioperative hypotension-avoidance strategy is superior to a hypertension-avoidance strategy in patients with or at risk of cardiovascular disease who are undergoing noncardiac surgery and chronically taking an antihypertensive drug.[55]

The influence of the anesthetic plan on postoperative outcomes is an area of active investigation. A recent important study in 1,600 older hip fracture patients randomized participants to either general anesthesia with a volatile agent or spinal anesthetic with sedation as needed for patient comfort. The primary outcome was a composite of postoperative death by day 60 and inability to walk independently at day 60. The primary composite outcome was not different between study groups (occurred in 18.5% of spinal anesthesia patients and 18% of GA patients). Other important indicators of postoperative recovery, delirium and hospital length of stay, were likewise similar between the groups. Thus, neither anesthetic approach is clearly superior in this patient population.[56] Delayed neurocognitive recovery occurred in 38 of 226 patients (16.8%) receiving total intravenous anesthesia (TIVA) and in 46 of 221 patients receiving sevoflurane anesthesia (20.8%) for laparoscopic abdominal surgery.[57] The THRIVE trial (Trajectories of Recovery after Intravenous Propofol vs. inhaled VolatilE anesthesia) is presently underway and is a large, pragmatic, comparative effectiveness, patient-level randomized controlled trial comparing postoperative quality of recovery and anesthetic safety among adult patients having either propofol based TIVA or volatile anesthesia for noncardiac surgery.[58] Although not specifically targeting elderly patients, the results are nonetheless anticipated, as little clear evidence exists for clinically important differences in postoperative outcomes between these anesthetic regimens. Growing evidence suggests that surgery-associated inflammation may be a more important cause of postoperative complications such as cognitive impairment, and may be of greater significance than the as-of-yet indistinguishable differences between anesthetic regimens.[57,59]

Whether general or neuraxial anesthesia is used, the maintenance phase of anesthesia will commonly result in a significant decrease in systemic blood pressure, more so than typically occurs in younger patients. Although decreases in both systemic vascular resistance and cardiac output likely occur, the decrease in vascular resistance is probably the largest contributor to the decrease in blood pressure. Figure 34-12 demonstrates this large decrease in vascular resistance and further shows that venous pooling is responsible for a decrease in preload that in turn decreases cardiac output. A large, multi-center retrospective cohort study of patients undergoing noncardiac surgery showed that a MAP <55 mm Hg was associated with increased odds of postoperative delirium, and this risk further grew with increasing duration of hypotension.[60] Because vascular resistance contributes significantly to the decrease in blood pressure during anesthesia, it has been argued that the use of α-agonists is an appropriate therapy and may be more effective than volume alone.[61] α-Agonists also promote venoconstriction, thereby shifting blood back to the central circulation and reducing the decrease in ventricular preload by venous pooling, and this presumably reduces the need for volume administration somewhat. Although vasoconstriction should not be used as a treatment for hypovolemia except as a stopgap measure, volume administration alone may not raise cardiac output enough to compensate for a large decrease in vascular resistance. Furthermore, this excess blood volume will shift from the periphery to the central circulation when sympathetic nervous system activity returns postoperatively. This excess central volume could push an elderly heart into diastolic heart failure immediately after surgery. In short, the appropriate balance between therapeutic vasoconstriction and volume administration in an older patient may be delicate, and dynamic with respect to the phase of perioperative care.

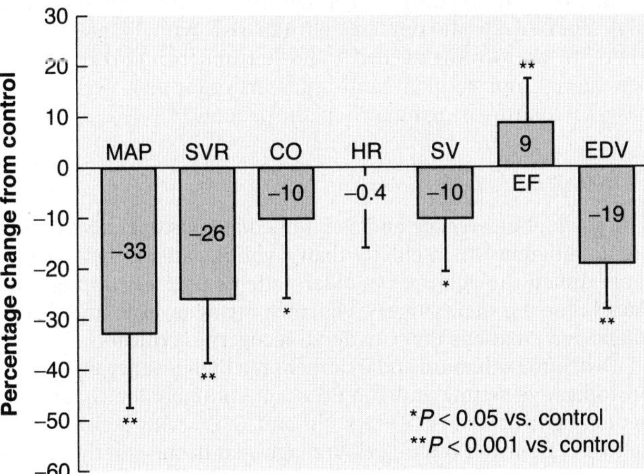

Figure 34-12 The response to total sympathectomy from spinal anesthesia as illustrated in older men with cardiac disease. Over 70% of the decrease in mean arterial blood pressure (MAP) was due to a decrease in systemic vascular resistance (SVR). Cardiac filling (end-diastolic volume [EDV]) was markedly diminished, but its effect on stroke volume (SV) and cardiac output (CO) was ameliorated by an increase in ejection fraction (EF). Although heart rate (HR) increased in some subjects and decreased in others, the overall effect was no change. (Reproduced with permission from Rooke GA, Freund PR, Jacobson AF. Hemodynamic response and change in organ blood volume during spinal anesthesia in elderly men with cardiac disease. *Anesth Analg*. 1997;85:99. Copyright © 1997 International Anesthesia Research Society.)

The choice between an endotracheal tube and a laryngeal mask airway involves many considerations, including body habitus, apparent frailty, surgical positioning, risk of regurgitation, and duration of surgery. The advantage of an endotracheal tube is the ability to guarantee control of ventilation and thereby prevent hypercarbia and intraoperative atelectasis, at the expense of adverse effects on mucociliary clearance and possibly on swallowing.

If positive-pressure ventilation is used, one important goal is to have the lung volume exceed closing capacity during the respiratory cycle in order to prevent atelectasis. This can be achieved either by using high tidal volumes or by using modest tidal volumes accompanied by positive end-expiratory pressure (PEEP). Initial studies have found that the lower tidal volume strategy tends to be associated with lower levels of inflammatory markers.[62] More recently, studies have appeared that also document a decreased incidence of perioperative pulmonary complications with the use of modest tidal volumes. Consequently, the modest tidal volume strategy plus PEEP as needed appears to be the preferred approach.

Another aspect of anesthetic management that is likely deleterious to the aging pulmonary system is the presence of residual neuromuscular blockade. This phenomenon is associated with adverse respiratory events such as hypoxia and airway obstruction.[63] Although initially observed with pancuronium, intermediate-acting neuromuscular blocking agents have also been implicated. Older patients are at almost double the risk of residual neuromuscular blockage and adverse respiratory events in comparison to middle-aged adults.[64] Although it is believed that reducing residual postoperative neuromuscular blockade may decrease pulmonary complications,[65] the best approach to achieving that goal is unclear. Complicating this picture is the observation that the use of neostigmine reversal may actually worsen residual blockade.[66] This observation argues for very careful use of nondepolarizing muscle relaxants in older patients. This adverse effect may be ameliorated by the use of neuromuscular transmission monitoring, presumably by permitting individualization of an appropriate dose of neostigmine,[67] but even this observation is controversial.[66] Perhaps the biggest change to pharmacologic options for anesthetic care in recent years has been the introduction of sugammadex for reversal of rocuronium and vecuronium. A sugammadex dose of 2 mg/kg effectively reverses deep neuromuscular blockade (only 2 TOF twitches present) in older adults, though the time to TOF ratio >0.9 was about 40 seconds longer in older compared to younger adults (2.9 minutes vs. 2.3 minutes, respectively).[68] If a faster reversal is desired in an emergency, administering an additional 1 mg/kg of sugammadex has been shown to shorten reversal time to less than 2 minutes in patients >70 years old.[69] A recent trial of approximately 200 patients showed that use of sugammadex (2 mg/kg) compared to neostigmine (0.07 mg/kg, max dose 5 mg) significantly reduced residual postoperative neuromuscular blockade. Larger studies are needed to determine if this translates to a decrease in postoperative pulmonary complications and ultimately better surgical outcomes.

Various anesthetic regimens have been studied to determine if particular amnestic agents, delivery approaches and pain management strategies change postoperative delirium risk in older patients. Unfortunately, these efforts have yielded no agreed-upon superior approach for neuroprotection.[38,40] Many postoperative nausea and vomiting prophylaxis strategies make use of Beers Criteria medications that may present an uneven balance of risks and benefits in older patients: prophylactic steroids, transdermal scopolamine, promethazine, and prochlorperazine all have cognitive impairment risks.

The utility of electroencephalography (EEG) for directed management of the anesthetic plan to lower postoperative complications remains an area of non-consensus. The ENGAGES randomized clinical trial involving 1,232 patients aged 60 years and older undergoing major surgery with volatile anesthetics, and compared postoperative outcomes and delirium rate between a BIS-guided anesthetic management group and a "usual care" group. The BIS-guided group had about a 0.1 MAC reduction. The 30-day mortality rate was lower in the BIS-guided group (0.65% vs. 3.07%) although no other postoperative comparisons showed relevant differences, including hypotension, PONV, delirium and serious complications.[70] The BALANCED trial was adequately powered to directly compare lighter (BIS target 50) to deeper (BIS target 35) anesthetic depths with more than 3,300 patients in each group, and more than double the reduction in volatile agent MAC was achieved between study groups compared to the ENGAGES trial. However, there was no benefit in either BIS group for postoperative mortality at 1 year, and no significant differences in serious adverse events after surgery such as infection and cardiac problems.[71] Through a subanalysis, which much be interpreted with caution, 515 patients from the BALANCED trial were evaluated for postoperative delirium and a significant reduction in delirium incidence was reported in the BIS 50 group (19%) compared to the BIS 35 group (28%, odds ratio 0.58 [95% confidence interval: 0.38–0.88, $P < .01$]). Likewise, cognitive function at 1-year postsurgery was significantly better in the lighter anesthesia group based upon the abbreviated mental test score (AMTS).[72] The SHARP randomized clinical trial of 217 elderly patients undergoing lumbar spinal fusion directly compared spinal anesthesia with targeted BIS-sedation[60–70] versus unguided general anesthesia. Researchers reported no difference in the primary outcome of postoperative delirium (25.2% in the spinal/BIS-sedation group vs. 18.9% in the unguided GA group). It is interesting that patients with pre-existing cognitive dysfunction, as determined by an MMSE score <27, had much lower delirium rates in the spinal/BIS-sedation group (17.7% vs. 43.5% for unguided GA group). Conversely, patients with normal preoperative cognition had lower delirium after unguided GA (12.1% vs. 26.6% in the spinal/BIS-sedation group).[73] However, the significance of this post-hoc analysis cannot be clearly determined.

The cumulative time of burst suppression has been correlated with the risk of postoperative delirium.[74] Nonetheless, current evidence does not support the routine use of processed EEG (e.g., BIS) specifically for the prevention of postoperative delirium. Nevertheless, two major practice guidance documents now recommend the use of intraoperative EEG monitoring to inform anesthetic management, although exactly how and what components of care to target is still controversial.[38,75] Avoidance of excessively deep levels of anesthesia is recommended in patients at high risk for postoperative delirium, though the evidence is limited and not consistent.[76] Coupling EEG guidance with cerebral oximetry is being investigated as a dual-monitoring approach to postoperative cognitive dysfunction risk-mitigation.[77] Potential consequences of lighter anesthesia must not be forgotten including undesired patient movement and recall.[70] One clear, unrefuted recommendation is that MAC dosages should be adjusted down with increasing age.[38]

Analgesia with meperidine should be avoided, except perhaps in small doses for shivering, as it is clearly a risk factor for delirium. There appears to be no superior choice among fentanyl, hydromorphone, and morphine.[78] Ketamine and dexmedetomidine have been investigated in clinical trials for their effect on postoperative cognitive recovery in older patients based upon their analgesic, antidepressant, and sedative properties. The Prevention of Delirium and Complications Associated with Surgical Treatments (PODCAST) trial determined that subanesthetic intraoperative doses of ketamine did not significantly decrease the risk of delirium, reporting similar incidence in study groups (19.45% and 19.82% in the intervention and placebo groups, respectively), and similar severity. Rather than preventing delirium, ketamine may increase negative psychoactive experiences.[79] Dexmedetomidine sedation decreases delirium risk in mechanically ventilated ICU patients and cardiac surgery patients, but its utility for perioperative cognitive protection in other surgical populations still needs to be established through clinical trials.[80,81] Gabapentin use has become common in multimodal opiate-sparing pain management strategies, but its risk–benefit analysis has been inconsistent. A recent large meta-analysis determined that although there were reductions in opiate use and pain with perioperative gabapentenoids and decreased postoperative nausea and vomiting, the increase in adverse events (visual disturbances and dizziness) did not support routine use in adults having surgery.[82] Gabapentinoids must be dose-adjusted for diminished renal function and there are serious concerns about overdose and adverse effects such as respiratory depression in older patients when opiates and gabapentinoids are used in combination. The newest Beer's Criteria recommendations highlight that use of gabapentinoids for opiate reduction is reasonable but must be done with extreme caution in older patients.[41] None of the volatile gases (desflurane, sevoflurane, isoflurane, and nitrous oxide) has superiority with regard to postoperative cognitive function.[83] Other pharmacologic agents of interest for postoperative cognitive protection include statins, melatonin, and clonidine.[84] The DEXACET randomized clinical trial reported a reduction in delirium risk with IV acetaminophen.[85] More work is needed to further understand the possible benefits of nonsteroidal anti-inflammatories and cycoloxegenase-2 inhibitors in aging orthopedic patients.[85,86]

Postoperative Care

The goals of emergence and the immediate postoperative period are no different for an elderly than a young patient; they are just more difficult to achieve. As older patients progress through the days following their surgery, vigilance for neurologic and physiologic perturbations that can derail recovery is critical.

Delirium evaluation and treatment is a high priority task in the postoperative setting and should occur routinely for all surgical patients greater than 65 years old and those with delirium risk factors.[31] Delirium often goes undiagnosed in the elderly patient as it is typically hypoactive (does not demonstrate behavior that draws attention). This characteristic is unfortunate because delirium is associated with an increased duration of hospitalization and its attendant costs, poorer long-term functional recovery, and increased mortality.[87] The Confusion Assessment Method is the gold standard for delirium diagnosis, however other instruments exist that are easier to administer like the 3-Minute Diagnostic Confusion Assessment Method (3D-CAM). It is important to consider precipitating conditions as prevention remains the best strategy for postoperative delirium. Nonpharmacologic risk-reduction strategies include daily physical activity and early mobility, cognitive reorientation with accessibility of assistive devices and aids, bedside presence of a family member whenever possible, sleep enhancement (e.g., sleep hygiene), pain management, nutrition and fluid repletion, appropriate medication usage (avoiding antipsychotics except for treatment of patients presenting a danger to themselves or others), prevention of constipation, and minimization of patient tethers (e.g., lines and drains).[31]

8 Analgesia is an important component of postoperative care but is made more difficult by the increased likelihood of adverse consequences from the analgesic regimen. Effective, multimodal opiate-sparing analgesia is of paramount importance. Narcotic administration represents a fine line between too much and too little, as both opiate use and inadequate pain control are associated with delirium. The standard approach to analgesia is to titrate to the desired effect, and the outcome should be good pain relief for patients of any age. There is no evidence that pain is any less severe or any less detrimental in an older patient than in young patients. However, there are impediments to achieving adequate analgesia in an older patient. Elderly patients sometimes underreport their pain level and may be more tolerant of their acute pain, perhaps partly because of the existence of chronic pain in their life. Older patients have more difficulty with visual analog scoring systems than verbal or numeric systems. If the patient is cognitively impaired, communication of pain is further complicated; indeed, demented patients often experience severe pain after hip surgery, but even mild cognitive impairment can lead to problems with pain assessment or with use of a patient-controlled analgesia machine. Failure to achieve adequate levels of analgesia is associated with numerous adverse outcomes, including sleep deprivation, respiratory impairment, ileus, suboptimal mobilization, insulin resistance, tachycardia, and hypertension. The apparent paradox of adequate analgesia is that opioids are the mainstay of postoperative analgesia, and opioids are capable of producing many of those same adverse outcomes. Therefore, as with all medical care of elderly patients, good judgment, caution, and frequent monitoring of analgesia and adverse effects are essential. Adjunctive medications such as nonsteroidal anti-inflammatory drugs have been shown to reduce opioid requirements and some of the opioid adverse effects, but often carry their own risks such as renal damage or gastrointestinal toxicity. Epidural analgesia is well known to provide analgesia that is superior to intravenous therapy, and this finding has been specifically replicated in the elderly.[88] Epidural analgesia led to a more rapid return of bowel function, earlier mobilization, and better nutritional status. Improvements in cardiopulmonary outcomes were equivocal.

Although many aspects of postoperative care are more likely to be the purview of the surgeon or the internist, there are some things that the anesthesiologist could and probably should be watchful for when performing a postoperative visit on an older patient. If a patient had a surgery with major fluid requirements, it is important to look for signs of fluid overload, including rales, dyspnea, tachypnea, and orthopnea, particularly around postoperative day 2 when third-space fluid tends to mobilize. A timely administration of a diuretic may prevent the development of overt pulmonary edema and the accompanying escalation of therapy and risk. Feel the pulse: atrial fibrillation is often paroxysmal and the more often someone looks for it, the more likely it will be detected. Additional important strategies for postoperative geriatric care are available in "Optimal Perioperative Management of the Geriatric Surgical Patient."[31] Aspiration precautions and aggressive pulmonary hygiene can lower the risk of pulmonary complications. Universal Fall Precautions and targeted fall prevention strategies are indicated in all older adult patients but should not introduce unnecessarily conservative management that interferes with mobilization. The ability to consume adequate nutrition should be evaluated daily, with expert consultation obtained as needed. Indwelling bladder catheters should be regularly evaluated for potential removal. Additional patient-centered components of geriatric postoperative care include family participation in care, early physical/occupational therapy consultation, geriatric consultation, and comprehensive discharge planning.

Integrated care of the postoperative surgical patient has been shown to positively impact postoperative recovery and outcomes.[89,90] The Hospital Elder Life Program (HELP)[91] care model can prevent delirium and other cognitive and functional decline in surgical patients.[53] The Acute Care for Elders (ACE) care model is linked to improved independent functioning, shorter length of stay and decreased costs. The Nurses Improving Care for Healthsystem Elderly (NICHE) care model is associated with improved institutional protocol compliance and clinical outcomes. Anesthesiologists should be prepared to support such programs as much as possible.

Perioperative Complications

My diseases are an asthma and a dropsy and, what is less curable, seventy-five.

—*Samuel Johnson*

The older patient is at increased risk for complications in the peri- 9
operative period, in part from comorbid disease and in part from the reduction in organ system reserve due to the aging process. Whether the aging process can be thought of as mere decreased reserve or subclinical disease is a matter of semantics. The result is the same: the elderly are at increased risk for almost every possible perioperative complication including cardiovascular, pulmonary, renal, central nervous system, wound infection, and death (Fig. 34-13).[92]

There is increasing evidence that anesthetic management may influence long-term outcomes. The elderly are particularly sensitive to the effect of anesthetics and thus may be more susceptible to the detrimental effects of anesthesia. Although specific sensitivity to anesthesia is difficult to define, several lines of evidence suggest that it can be attained by clinically available modalities. For example, an intraoperative state of "triple low" (a low concentration of volatile anesthetic that is accompanied by low blood pressure and a deep hypnotic level as defined by a BIS monitor) is associated with longer hospital stay and increased 1-month mortality.[93] Although association does not imply causation and

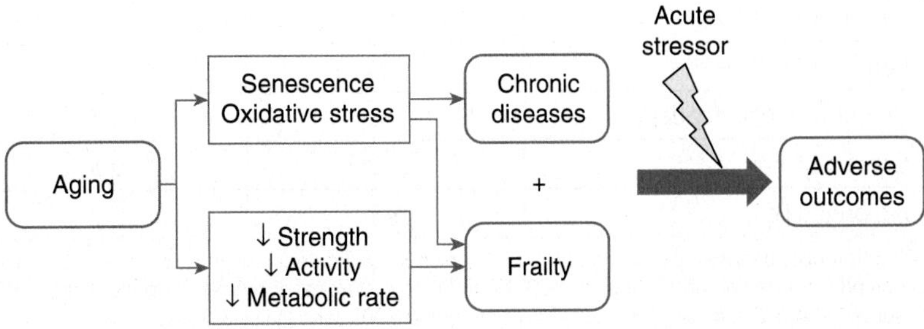

Figure 34-13 Schematic outlining some factors associated with normal aging that put patients at increased risk for adverse outcomes.

the "triple low" state may merely be a marker of low physiologic reserve, it is possible that identification of sensitivity may lead to improved outcomes. Additional studies show an association between intraoperative hypotension and other 1-month adverse outcomes including cardiac events, kidney dysfunction, and possibly stroke.[94,95] Age above 68 was an independent risk factor in one of these studies.[96] Another study that looked at 1-year mortality found no relation to intraoperative hypotension in the younger adult population, but found that the elderly subjects had a higher 1-year mortality that corresponded to the duration of the intraoperative hypotension.[97] Again, whether the hypotension is causal or just a marker is not clear, but these studies do suggest that permitting prolonged hypotension may not be a good idea.

Because the mechanisms of aging contribute not only to normal aging but also to the development and severity of disease, one might expect that age and disease would interact in their contribution to perioperative risk. Confirmation of such a hypothesis is provided by a prospective survey of nearly 200,000 anesthetics in France.[98] Both age and the number of chronic diseases are associated with an increased rate of complications, but what is particularly interesting is an apparent interaction between these two factors. Figure 34-14 demonstrates that, for any given age group, the number of complications increases with the number of comorbid diseases. To be young and sick likely represents a special case as suggested by the point representing the no more than 34-year-old group with three or more comorbid diseases. Ignoring that outlier, connecting the dots of equal number of comorbid diseases reveals a modest increase in risk with age for patients with zero comorbid disease, but examination of points for one, two, or three or more diseases reveals an effect with age that becomes increasingly larger. In other words, age appears to interact with comorbid disease to increase risk.

Complications of the cardiovascular and pulmonary systems are associated with the greatest perioperative mortality. The best database is provided by the Veterans Affairs National Surgical Quality Improvement Project, and much of the database involves examination of patients older than 80 (Table 34-5).[99] Although the perioperative complications of myocardial infarction or cardiac arrest carry higher associated mortality rates than pneumonia, prolonged intubation, or reintubation, the higher incidences of the pulmonary complications suggest that overall greater mortality results from pulmonary complications than from cardiac complications. That pulmonary complications are so significant

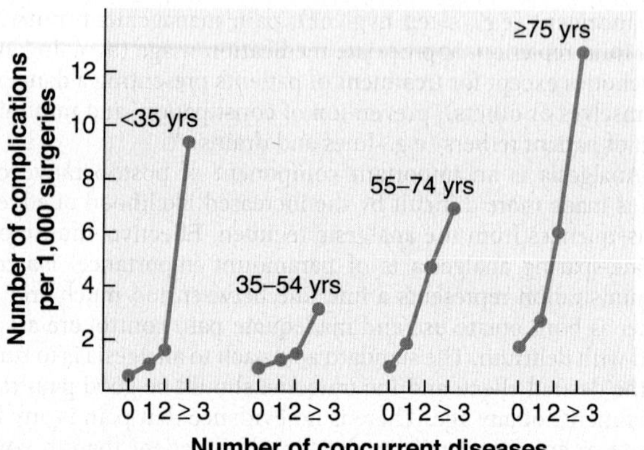

Figure 34-14 The interaction between age and comorbid disease. For each age bracket, as comorbid disease increases, so does the rate of complications. The effect of age on the complication rate is best visualized by examining points of equal comorbid disease. At zero disease, only a modest increase in complications is observed with increasing age. At ever-increasing degrees of comorbid disease, however, the increase in complications with age becomes more and more pronounced. (Reproduced with permission from Tiret L, Desmonts JM, Hatton F, Vourc'h G. Complications associated with anaesthesia–a prospective survey in France. *Can Anaesth Soc J*. 1986;33:336–344. With kind permission from Springer Science+Business Media.)

underscores the need for a better understanding of the mechanism of postoperative pneumonia, and particularly the likely contribution of silent aspiration.

Central nervous system complications are also a major source of morbidity and mortality. The most burdensome problems appear to be stroke, postoperative delirium, and postoperative cognitive decline. All have the potential to cause debilitating morbidity and an adverse impact on the patient's quality of life, their families, and the cost of medical care.

In a nonsurgical elderly population, there is an annual stroke incidence of approximately 1%. The incidence of perioperative stroke in the older general surgical population is approximately 0.5% (Table 34-5).[99–101] Risk factors include age, atrial fibrillation (odds ratio 2.0), history of a prior stroke or TIA (odds ratio at least 1.6), recent myocardial infarction, COPD or current smoking, acute renal dysfunction or chronic dialysis, the type of surgery, and a variety of

Table 34-5 Effect of Age on Selected Perioperative Complications and Associated Mortality[a]

	Complication Rate		Mortality Rate from the Complication	
Complication	***Age <80***	***Age ≥80***	***Age <80***	***Age ≥80***
Myocardial infarction	0.4	1.0	37.1	48.0
Cardiac arrest	0.9	2.1	80.0	88.2
Pneumonia	2.3	5.6	19.8	29.2
>48 hrs on ventilator	2.1	3.5	30.1	38.5
Required reintubation	1.6	2.8	32.3	44.0
Cerebrovascular accident	0.3	0.7	26.1	39.3
Coma >24 hrs	0.2	0.3	65.9	80.9
Prolonged ileus	1.2	1.7	9.2	16.0

[a]All differences between patients less than 80 versus 80 and older are significant at $P < .001$, except for coma mortality ($P = .004$).
Modified from Hamel MB, Henderson WG, Khuri SF, et al. Surgical outcomes for patients aged 80 and older: morbidity and mortality from major noncardiac surgery. *J Am Geriat Soc*. 2005;53:424. Copyright © 2005 John Wiley & Sons.

comorbid diseases including diabetes and renal or cardiovascular disease.[100–103] A particularly interesting risk factor, at least for cardiac surgery patients, is an elevated arterial pulse pressure.[104] This finding supports the concept that age-related changes can influence perioperative risk just as it appears to influence morbidity in the general population. The original PeriOperative ISchemic Evaluation study (POISE) raised the issue of perioperative β-blockade increasing the risk of stroke, but when chronic, less intense β-blockade is used that risk is not present.[105] Strokes typically occur well after surgery, on average 7 days later, although upward of half occur within 24 hours.[101,106] Most perioperative strokes are ischemic and presumably from thromboembolism originating in the heart or arteries. The contribution of hypotension to focal stroke is questionable, although the POISE study could be cited as evidence that hypotension increases stroke risk.[101] Mortality after a perioperative stroke is approximately twice that of a stroke in the general population, and overall mortality from perioperative stroke is at least 20%.[103,106]

As mentioned earlier, a recent significant change to nomenclature classifying cognitive dysfunction in surgical patients has occurred. *Perioperative neurocognitive disorders* (PND), which include delirium, are subclassified based upon DSM-V criteria and temporal association with the surgical procedure.[36] This shift in nomenclature and diagnostic criteria is an important step for clear identification, communication, and further study of very common and impactful perioperative cognitive conditions in older patients. The older term for persistent or late-onset cognitive impairment was *postoperative cognitive dysfunction* (POCD), a condition inherently more difficult to diagnose than delirium because outside of the obviously impaired patient, it requires sophisticated neuropsychologic testing, including baseline tests prior to surgery. Selection of tests, their timing, and what deficits are required to qualify as cognitive decline have proven problematic in the literature. Diagnosis of delirium remains consistent, with criteria for acute onset, waxing and waning alterations in attention and cognition occurring in the first 7 postoperative days. Not included in the diagnosis of POCD, DSM-V criteria for the category of general *neurocognitive disorders* (NCDs) include:

1. Presence of a subjective complaint by the patient, caregiver, or clinician
2. Objective decline (mild: 1–2 standard deviations below norms or controls; major: ≥2 standard deviations below norms or controls)
3. Evaluation of impact on activities of daily living (ADLs)

NCDs take the specifier "postoperative" if a new diagnosis is made after the expected surgical recovery time (30 days). Cognitive impairments based upon the same criteria but present between the window for postoperative delirium and NCDs are described as *delayed neurocognitive recovery* (dNCR, 7 to 30 days postsurgery).[36]

Animal studies provide the most evidence for anesthetic CNS toxicity. Many studies of animals (typically rodents) exposed to volatile anesthesia demonstrate impaired memory and diminished learning ability that persists for at least months after exposure.[107] Volatile anesthesia increases brain production of β-amyloid and abnormal τ-protein (leading to neurofibrillary tangles), both of which are associated with Alzheimer disease and also cell apoptosis.[107,108] However, other studies found that memory impairment and CNS chemical change only occurred in animals that had anesthesia plus surgery. Anesthesia without surgery was no different than control animals. Curiously, the anesthetics in these latter studies were fentanyl, droperidol, and chloral hydrate, thereby raising the possibility that not all anesthesia agents yield similar results. In addition to the potential neurodegenerative mechanism described above, cognitive decline could also result from a neuroinflammatory stress response to surgery and/or anesthesia.[109]

Postoperative delirium has received prioritized focus by perioperative clinicians and researchers because its incidence can exceed 50% for high-risk surgeries. Substantial physical, emotional, and financial costs occur to individuals, families, and healthcare systems (in excess of $150 billion per year in the United States). At least one in three cases is likely preventable.

The etiology of delirium is multifactorial. Risk factors include age, baseline low cognitive function (including mild cognitive impairment and dementia), depression, overall frailty, and general debility including dehydration or visual/auditory impairment.[110] The more risk factors present, the fewer perioperative stressors are required to push the patient over the edge to delirium.[87] Those additional stressors can include virtually any drug with central nervous system effects, including narcotics (especially meperidine), benzodiazepines (especially lorazepam), and drugs that possess anticholinergic properties (except perhaps glycopyrrolate). Other factors that likely contribute to delirium include sleep deprivation, being in an unfamiliar environment, and perioperative blood loss. Delirium is associated with hypotension (MAP < 55 mmHg)[60] and fluctuations in blood pressure.[111] Specific expert consensus statements exist for promoting perioperative brain health.[38,40] Once detected, management focuses on reversible risk factors such as optimizing current medications, pain management, and the sleep environment (Fig. 34-15).[112,113]

Much remains to be studied to better understand what is now referred to as *postoperative neurocognitive disorder* (NCD). Research using the newer "mild" and "major" subclassification

PREOPERATIVE FACTORS:

Age, baseline low cognitive function (including dementia), depression, frailty, and visual/auditory impairment

Surgical stress

DELIRIUM RISK

Deliriogenic medications

Foreign location

PRESENTATION:

Waxing and waning mental status often hypoactive

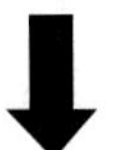

OUTCOMES:

Increased hospital length of stay, poor functional and cognitive recovery, and increased mortality

Figure 34-15 Delirium represents a condition of waxing and waning mental status. There are multiple factors that put patients at risk for delirium. Delirium is associated with poor outcomes for patients and increased cost to the healthcare system.

nomenclature is scarce, although the new utilization of DSM-V criteria of both objective and subjective criteria along with consideration for the impact on ADLs will most certainly result in more meaningful and impactful research than the POCD literature has produced to date. The question is whether anesthesia contributes to persistent cognitive impairment well after surgery, and if so, to what degree? At this time, understanding the POCD literature can still be valuable.

A seminal study not only examined surgical patients before and after surgery but included control subjects who were tested over time as well, but did not have surgery. At 3 months, a 10% incidence of POCD was observed in the patients who had surgery, in comparison to a 3% incidence of similar symptoms in those who did not.[114] Risk factors for POCD at 3 months after surgery include age, lower levels of education, prior history of stroke even in the absence of residual deficit, and POCD at hospital discharge.[115] Increased mortality at 1 year is associated with patients who demonstrate cognitive decline at both hospital discharge and at 3 months postoperatively.[115] A study that examined the association between exposure to surgery and anesthesia and cognitive function in 8,503 pairs of middle-aged and elderly twins identified 87 monozygotic and 124 dizygotic same-sexed twin pairs in whom one had major surgery and the other did not. A statistically significant but clinically negligible difference was found in neurocognitive testing. For example, when participants were asked to provide as many names of animals as possible in 1 minute, the mean number of animals named was 23.5 in those that were exposed to surgery versus 24.2 in those that were not.[116]

Regarding the first few days after surgery, a few observations have been made that are neither surprising nor particularly worrisome. First of all, there is a similar degree of cognitive deficit in all age groups, not just the elderly. Second, greater cognitive impairment can be observed with general anesthesia than with regional anesthesia.[117] Last, for the first few days, the choice of general anesthesia makes a difference with propofol $<$ desflurane $<$ sevoflurane in degree of cognitive decline. By 3 months, however, the presence of POCD is almost exclusively a problem in older patients.[118] Furthermore, no differences can be detected between general and regional anesthetic options.[119] By 1 year, even the best controlled studies suggest little or no demonstrable cognitive decline.[120] A longitudinal analysis of an Alzheimer disease database of patients who started with none to mild dementia showed the same overall rate of cognitive decline whether or not they had surgery or suffered a major illness.[121] Using before and after neuropsychologic testing, the incidence of POCD was compared for patients who underwent coronary angiography, total hip arthroplasty, or coronary artery bypass grafting.[122] At 1 week postoperatively, POCD was documented in 43% of the bypass graft patients and 17% for the hip replacement patients (angiography patients not tested at 1 week). At 3 months postprocedure, the incidence of POCD was 16% for both surgical groups and 21% for the angiography group (differences not significant). These two studies suggest there is no overall long-term adverse cognitive impact on patients, and that it is not the anesthetic which is to blame for whatever changes do occur. Effective treatment strategies for persistent postoperative cognitive impairment are still absent and therefore the best treatment seems to be prevention. Small, limited trials have assessed different strategies to reduce the incidence of POCD in animal models and in humans, but guidelines or recommendations that are supported by rigorous science are unavailable.

Delirium and postoperative NCD or POCD are often inappropriately perceived as a single entity along a time continuum. There may be an association between delirium and POCD, but if there is, the relationship has not been fully elucidated. Predictors of postoperative delirium such as hypoxemia were not found to be risk factors for POCD.[123] Furthermore, postoperative delirium has not been found to be a risk factor for cognitive dysfunction at 3 months.[124]

In the last 5 years, awareness of the significant risks posed by postoperative cognitive impairment has continued to grow. So what do we tell our patients about stroke, delirium, and postoperative NCD? This is not an easy question to answer, especially for cognitive decline. However, patients are usually satisfied to know the facts and are willing to accept the unknown, including the fact that there does not seem to be any clear evidence that basic anesthetic techniques differ in their impact on outcome. Furthermore, at least for POCD, some believe that the accumulated evidence does not support the concept of long-term POCD as a clinical problem and that patients can be reassured that surgery and anesthesia are unlikely to be implicated in causing persistent cognitive decline or dementia.[125] Hopefully, the concurrently growing interest in broader initiatives aimed at improving comprehensive geriatric surgical care, with multidisciplinary and multicomponent approaches to better preparing and managing older surgical patients, will ultimately result in focused and tailored function-preserving or even function-improving postoperative outcomes in our geriatric patients.

In summary, there are a few specific points about the conduct of anesthesia that can be made. Besides the obvious caveats ("avoid hypotension and hypoxia"), the basic approach to an anesthetic for an elderly patient can be described as cautious. Since stroke is likely a thromboembolic phenomenon, there may be little that can be done beyond standard, good anesthetic care. However, it is not clear that antiplatelet therapy needs to be discontinued for surgery as much as currently occurs. The efficacy of statins has also not been adequately assessed. As previously discussed, drug choices and dosage have a potentially major impact on delirium. Pain control with multimodal therapy to reduce opioid consumption is probably a good thing, but poor pain control may be as bad as too much opioid. Finally, it is not clear what the relationship is between anesthesia and cognitive decline, if there is one at all. Given that unsatisfactory statement, it seems reasonable to choose the anesthetic technique based on the other factors germane to the patient and surgery.

The Future

I will never be an old man. To me, old age is always 15 years older than I am.

—*Francis Bacon*

Improvements in surgical and anesthetic techniques that reduce the overall stress to the patient are permitting more surgeries to be performed on older and sicker patients than ever before. Nevertheless, the older patient will continue to experience the majority of perioperative adverse outcomes. Much remains to be accomplished in the quest to find ways to decrease the incidence and severity of those adverse outcomes. The most pressing issues are arguably the prevention of postoperative delirium, cognitive decline, pneumonia, respiratory failure, and cardiovascular complications. Improved pain-control techniques that also diminish side effects, especially to the brain and bowels, would be welcome. However, other realms of care are just in their infancy, most notably whether preoperative improvement in the functional status of frail patients is helpful. Targeted, coordinated comorbidity management, prehabilitation, rehabilitation, medication management, and delirium prevention strategies can improve postoperative outcomes for older surgical patients. To facilitate risk mitigation, implementation strategies for consideration have been published by several expert groups. Collectively, they require patient, family and surgical care team communication, education and goal-setting, in addition to engagement with primary care providers, utilization of expert consultation for the highest-risk patients, comprehensive medication management, and overall consideration of barriers to recovery. When caring for the elderly, especially the frail elderly, the overriding goal should be to produce as little stress to the patient as possible during both surgery and the subsequent hospitalization and recovery.

We must comment on the potentially crippling "human resource" gaps that are currently expanding in healthcare, particularly with regard to direct care workers for aging patients, who clearly require personal attention and physical assistance as major components of their care. Patient evaluation, and the development and execution of comprehensive care plans for complex elderly patients require focused time from a skilled geriatric clinician, an equally scare resource. Developments in artificial intelligence (AI) may revolutionize the way we care for geriatric surgical patients by addressing these problems and more. With approaches such as machine-learning and advanced health monitoring techniques, AI could facilitate any number of actions important to geriatric care, but high-quality research validation with standardized, healthcare-specific data metrics is needed. These innovations would need to be integrated into the existing clinical workflow, while prioritizing privacy and safety.

We must also acknowledge healthcare disparities as a significant problem for the delivery of high-quality care in the United States. Elderly Black patients are seen less often by specialists, receive less preventive care, lower-quality hospital care, and fewer expensive, technologic procedures. Older people in general may not be offered the most advanced surgical options, despite being a population that could benefit. Our understanding of the complex interplay between patient factors, healthcare disparities and the many elements that shape a surgical episode of care is woefully limited. Awareness of the inadequacies in both our practice and research efforts, and emphasis on addressing them is encouragingly a priority for the "big thinkers" in anesthesiology. Complete care of the geriatric surgical patients is multidisciplinary out of necessity. No single specialty possesses the total perspective, and the anesthesiologist's expertise is an important component of that care.

For further review and interactivities, please see the videos and narrative interactive clinical vignettes (NICVs) accessible in the complimentary eBook bundled with this text. Access instructions are located on the inside front cover.

REFERENCES

1. Bishop NA, Guarente L. Genetic links between diet and lifespan: shared mechanisms from yeast to humans. *Nat Rev Genet*. 2007;8:835–844.
2. Hayden EC. Age research: a new angle on 'old'. *Nature*. 2007;450:603–605.
3. Deng JZ, Chan JS, Potter AL, et al. The risk of postoperative complications after major elective surgery in active or resolved COVID-19 in the United States. *Ann Surg*. 2022;275:242–246.
4. Kennedy BK, Berger SL, Brunet A, e al. Geroscience: linking aging to chronic disease. *Cell*. 2014;159:709–713.
5. Fleisher LA, Fleischmann KE, Auerbach AD, et al. 2014 ACC/AHA guideline on perioperative cardiovascular evaluation and management of patients undergoing noncardiac surgery: a report of the American College of Cardiology/American Heart Association Task Force on practice guidelines. *J Am Coll Cardiol*. 2014;64:e77–137.
6. Song X, Mitnitski A, Rockwood K. Prevalence and 10-year outcomes of frailty in older adults in relation to deficit accumulation. *J Am Geriatr Soc*. 2010;58:681–687.
7. McIsaac DI, Wong CA, Huang A, Moloo H, van Walraven C. Derivation and validation of a generalizable preoperative frailty index using population-based health administrative data. *Ann Surg*. 2019;270:102–108.
8. McIsaac DI, Bryson GL, van Walraven C. Association of frailty and 1-year postoperative mortality following major elective noncardiac surgery: a population-based cohort study. *JAMA Surg*. 2016;151:538–545.
9. Fried LP, Tangen CM, Walston J, et al. Frailty in older adults: evidence for a phenotype. *J Gerontol A Biol Sci Med Sci*. 2001;56:M146–156.
10. Rockwood K, Mitnitski A. Frailty in relation to the accumulation of deficits. *J Gerontol A Biol Sci Med Sci*. 2007;62:722–727.
11. Aucoin SD, Hao M, Sohi R, et al. Accuracy and feasibility of clinically applied frailty instruments before surgery: a systematic review and meta-analysis. *Anesthesiology*. 2020;133:78–95.
12. Bentov I, Kaplan SJ, Pham TN, Reed MJ. Frailty assessment: from clinical to radiological tools. *Br J Anaesth*. 2019;123:37–50.
13. Canales C, Mazor E, Coy H, et al. Preoperative point-of-care ultrasound to identify frailty and predict postoperative outcomes: a diagnostic accuracy study. *Anesthesiology*. 2022;136:268–278.
14. Hall DE, Arya S, Schmid KK, et al. Association of a frailty screening initiative with postoperative survival at 30, 180, and 365 days. *JAMA Surg*. 2017;152:233–240.
15. Schmucker DL. Age-related changes in liver structure and function: Implications for disease ? *Exp Gerontol*. 2005;40:650–659.
16. Duggan EW, Carlson K, Umpierrez GE. Perioperative hyperglycemia management: an update. *Anesthesiology*. 2017;126:547–560.
17. Mapleson WW. Effect of age on MAC in humans: a meta-analysis. *Br J Anaesth*. 1996;76:179–185.
18. Klotz U, Avant GR, Hoyumpa A, Schenker S, Wilkinson GR. The effects of age and liver disease on the disposition and elimination of diazepam in adult man. *J Clin Invest*. 1975;55:347–359.
19. Lien CA, Suzuki T. Relaxants and their reversal agents. In: Silverstein JH, Rooke GA, Reves JG, McLeskey CH, eds. *Geriatric Anesthesiology*. 2nd ed. Springer; 2008:266–277.
20. Barodka VM, Joshi BL, Berkowitz DE, Hogue CW, Nyhan D. Review article: implications of vascular aging. *Anesth Analg*. 2011;112:1048–1060.
21. DeLorey DS, Babb TG. Progressive mechanical ventilatory constraints with aging. *Am J Respir Crit Care Med*. 1999;160:169–177.
22. Ancoli-Israel S, Coy T. Are breathing disturbances in elderly equivalent to sleep apnea syndrome? *Sleep*. 1994;17:77–83.
23. Marik PE, Kaplan D. Aspiration pneumonia and dysphagia in the elderly. *Chest*. 2003;124:328–336.
24. Sessler DI. Perioperative thermoregulation. In: Silverstein JH, Rooke GA, Reves JG, McLeskey CH, eds. *Geriatric Anesthesiology*. 2nd ed. Springer; 2008:107–122.
25. Optimal Resources for Geriatric Surgery: 2019 Standards: American College of Surgeons; 2018. https://www.facs.org/media/u4jf5j3k/geriatricsv_standards.pdf. Copyright © 2019 American College of Surgeons, 633 N. Saint Clair St., Chicago, IL 60611-3295. All rights reserved.
26. Deiner S, Fleisher LA, Leung JM, et al. Adherence to recommended practices for perioperative anesthesia care for older adults among US anesthesiologists: results from the ASA Committee on Geriatric Anesthesia-Perioperative Brain Health Initiative ASA member survey. *Perioperative Medicine*. 2020;9:6.
27. Gillis C, Ljungqvist O, Carli F. Prehabilitation, enhanced recovery after surgery, or both? A narrative review. *Br J Anaesth*. 2022;128:434–448.
28. Englesbe MJ, Lussiez AD, Friedman JF, Sullivan JA, Wang SC. Starting a surgical home. *Ann Surg*. 2015;262:901–903.
29. Mello MT, Azocar RJ, Lewis MC. Geriatrics and the perioperative surgical home. *Anesthesiol Clin*. 2015;33:439–445.
30. Hogan K. Malignant hypercompliance. *Anesthesiology*. 2017;126:759–762.
31. Chow WB, Rosenthal RA, Merkow RP, et al. Optimal preoperative assessment of the geriatric surgical patient: a best practices guideline from the American College of Surgeons National Surgical Quality Improvement Program and the American Geriatrics Society. *J Am Coll Surg*. 2012;215:453–466.
32. McIsaac DI, Wijeysundera DN, Huang A, Bryson GL, van Walraven C. Association of the hospital volume of frail surgical patients cared for with outcomes after elective, major noncardiac surgery: a retrospective population-based cohort study. *Anesthesiology*. 2017;126:602–613.
33. Kwok AC, Semel ME, Lipsitz SR, et al. The intensity and variation of surgical care at the end of life: a retrospective cohort study. *Lancet*. 2011;378:1408–1413.
34. Ethical Guidelines for the Anesthesia Care of Patients with Do-Not-Resuscitate Orders or Other Directives that Limit Treatment. American Society of Anesthesiologists; 2018.
35. Lawrence VA, Hazuda HP, Cornell JE, et al. Functional independence after major abdominal surgery in the elderly. *J Am Coll Surg*. 2004;199:762–772.
36. Evered L, Silbert B, Knopman DS, et al. Nomenclature Consensus Working G. Recommendations for the nomenclature of cognitive change associated with anaesthesia and surgery-2018. *British Journal of Anaesthesia*. 2018;121:1005–1012.
37. Culley DJ, Flaherty D, Fahey MC, et al. Poor performance on a preoperative cognitive screening test predicts postoperative complications in older orthopedic surgical patients. *Anesthesiology*. 2017;127:765–774.

38. Berger M, Schenning KJ, Brown CH, et al. Best practices for postoperative brain health: recommendations from the Fifth International Perioperative Neurotoxicity Working Group. *Anesthesia and Analgesia*. 2018;127:1406–1413.
39. Ragheb J, Khatibi N, McKinney A, et al. Patient perspectives on delirium and cognitive dysfunction after surgery: a cross-sectional survey. *Br J Anaesth*. 2022;128:e270–e273.
40. Hughes CG, Boncyk CS, Culley DJ, et al. American Society for Enhanced Recovery and Perioperative Quality Initiative Joint Consensus Statement on Postoperative Delirium Prevention. *Anesth Analg*. 2020;130:1572–1590.
41. Panel BtAGSBCUE. American Geriatrics Society 2019 Updated AGS Beers Criteria® for potentially inappropriate medication use in older adults. *J Am Geriatr Soc*. 2019;67: 674–694.
42. Rosenthal RA, Kavic SM. Assessment and management of the geriatric patient. *Crit Care Med*. 2004;32:S92–S105.
43. Carli F. Prehabilitation for the anesthesiologist. *Anesthesiology*. 2020;133:645–652.
44. Borrell-Vega J, Esparza Gutierrez AG, Humeidan ML. Multimodal prehabilitation programs for older surgical patients. *Anesthesiol Clin*. 2019;37:437–452.
45. Howard R, Yin YS, McCandless L, Wang S, Englesbe M, Machado-Aranda D. Taking control of your surgery: impact of a prehabilitation program on major abdominal surgery. *J Am Coll Surg*. 2019;228:72–80.
46. Barberan-Garcia A, Ubre M, Pascual-Argente N, et al. Post-discharge impact and cost-consequence analysis of prehabilitation in high-risk patients undergoing major abdominal surgery: secondary results from a randomised controlled trial. *Br J Anaesth*. 2019;123:450–456.
47. Anguera JA, Boccanfuso J, Rintoul JL, et al. Video game training enhances cognitive control in older adults. *Nature*. 2013;501:97–101.
48. Humeidan ML, Reyes JC, Mavarez-Martinez A, et al. Effect of cognitive prehabilitation on the incidence of postoperative delirium among older adults undergoing major noncardiac surgery: The Neurobics Randomized Clinical Trial. *JAMA Surg*. 2021;156:148–156.
49. O'Gara BP, Mueller A, Gasangwa DVI, et al. Prevention of early postoperative decline: a randomized, controlled feasibility trial of perioperative cognitive training. *Anesth Analg*. 2019.
50. Atkins KJ, Scott DA, Silbert B, Pike KE, Evered L. Preventing delirium and promoting long-term brain health: A Clinical Trial Design for the Perioperative Cognitive Enhancement (PROTECT) Trial. *J Alzheimers Dis*. 2021;83:1637–1649.
51. Olotu C, Lebherz L, Härter M, et al. Improvement of perioperative care of the elderly patient (PeriAge): protocol of a controlled interventional feasibility study. *BMJ Open*. 2019;9: e031837.
52. Rengel KF, Mehdiratta N, Vanston SW, et al. A randomised pilot trial of combined cognitive and physical exercise prehabilitation to improve outcomes in surgical patients. *Br J Anaesth*. 2021; 126:e55--e57.
53. Mohanty S, Rosenthal RA, Russell MM, Neuman MD, Ko CY, Esnaola NF. Optimal perioperative management of the geriatric patient: a best practices guideline from the American College of Surgeons NSQIP and the American Geriatrics Society. *J Am Coll Surg*. 2016;222: 930–947.
54. McEvoy MD, Reves J. Intravenous hypnotic anesthetics. In: Silverstein JH, Rooke GA, Reves JG, McLeskey CH, eds. *Geriatric Anesthesiology*. 2nd ed. Springer; 2008:229–245.
55. Marcucci M, Painter TW, Conen D, et al. Rationale and design of the PeriOperative ISchemic Evaluation-3 (POISE-3): a randomized controlled trial evaluating tranexamic acid and a strategy to minimize hypotension in noncardiac surgery. *Trials*. 2022;23:101.
56. Neuman MD, Feng R, Carson JL, et al. Spinal anesthesia or general anesthesia for hip surgery in older adults. *N Engl J Med*. 2021;385:2025–2035.
57. Li Y, Chen D, Wang H, et al. Intravenous versus volatile anesthetic effects on postoperative cognition in elderly patients undergoing laparoscopic abdominal surgery. *Anesthesiology*. 2021; 134:381–394.
58. THRIVE: Trajectories of Recovery after Intravenous Propofol vs Inhaled Volatile Anesthesia, ClinicalTrials.gov Identifier: NCT05346588. https://www.pcori.org/research-results/2021/thrive-trajectories-recovery-after-intravenous-propofol-vs-inhaled-volatile-anesthesia
59. Mahanna-Gabrielli E, Schenning KJ, Eriksson LI, et al. State of the clinical science of perioperative brain health: report from the American Society of Anesthesiologists Brain Health Initiative Summit 2018. *British Journal of Anaesthesia*. 2019;123:464–478.
60. Wachtendorf LJ, Azimaraghi O, Santer P, et al. Association between intraoperative arterial hypotension and postoperative delirium after noncardiac surgery: a retrospective multicenter cohort study. *Anesth Analg*. 2022;134:822–833.
61. Rooke GA. Cardiovascular aging and anesthetic implications. *J Cardiothorac Vasc Anesth*. 2003;17:512–523.
62. Güldner A, Kiss T, Serpa Neto A, et al. Intraoperative protective mechanical ventilation for prevention of postoperative pulmonary complications: a comprehensive review of the role of tidal volume, positive end-expiratory pressure, and lung recruitment maneuvers. *Anesthesiology*. 2015;123:692–713.
63. Grosse-Sundrup M, Henneman JP, Sandberg WS, et al. Intermediate acting non-depolarizing neuromuscular blocking agents and risk of postoperative respiratory complications: prospective propensity score matched cohort study. *BMJ*. 2012;345:e6329.
64. Murphy GS, Szokol JW, Avram MJ, et al. Residual neuromuscular block in the elderly: incidence and clinical implications. *Anesthesiology*. 2015;123:1322–1336.
65. Martinez-Ubieto J, Ortega-Lucea S, Pascual-Bellosta A, et al. Prospective study of residual neuromuscular block and postoperative respiratory complications in patients reversed with neostigmine versus sugammadex. *Minerva Anestesiol*. 2016;82:735–742.
66. Meyer MJ, Bateman BT, Kurth T, Eikermann M. Neostigmine reversal doesn't improve postoperative respiratory safety. *BMJ*. 2013;346:f1460.
67. Hunter JM. Antagonising neuromuscular block at the end of surgery. *BMJ*. 2012;345:e6666.
68. McDonagh DL, Benedict PE, Kovac AL, et al. Efficacy, safety, and pharmacokinetics of sugammadex for the reversal of rocuronium-induced neuromuscular blockade in elderly patients. *Anesthesiology*. 2011;114:318–329.
69. Shin S, Han DW, Lee HS, Song MK, Jun EK, Kim SY. Elderly patients require higher doses of sugammadex for rapid recovery from deep neuromuscular block. *Basic Clin Pharmacol Toxicol*. 2016;118:462–467.
70. Wildes TS, Mickle AM, Ben Abdallah A, et al. Effect of electroencephalography-guided anesthetic administration on postoperative delirium among older adults undergoing major surgery The ENGAGES Randomized Clinical Trial. *JAMA*. 2019;321:473–483.
71. Short TG, Campbell D, Frampton C, et al. Australian New Zealand C. Anaesthetic depth and complications after major surgery: an international, randomised controlled trial. *Lancet*. 2019;394:1907–1914.
72. Evered LA, Chan MTV, Han R, et al. Anaesthetic depth and delirium after major surgery: a randomised clinical trial. *Br J Anaesth*. 2021;127:704–712.
73. Brown CH, Edwards C, Lin C, et al. Spinal anesthesia with targeted sedation based on bispectral index values compared with general anesthesia with masked bispectral index values to reduce delirium: The SHARP Randomized Controlled Trial. *Anesthesiology*. 2021;135:992–1003.
74. Fritz BA, Kalarickal PL, Maybrier HR, et al. Intraoperative electroencephalogram suppression predicts postoperative delirium. *Anesth Analg*. 2016;122:234–242.
75. Evered LA, Goldstein PA. Reducing perioperative neurocognitive disorders (PND) through depth of anesthesia monitoring: a critical review. *Int J Gen Med*. 2021;14:153–162.
76. Chan MTV, Hedrick TL, Egan TD, et al. American Society for Enhanced Recovery and Perioperative Quality Initiative Joint Consensus Statement on the Role of Neuromonitoring in Perioperative Outcomes: Electroencephalography. *Anesth Analg*. 2020;130:1278–1291.
77. Ballard C, Jones E, Gauge N, et al. Optimised anaesthesia to reduce post operative cognitive decline (POCD) in older patients undergoing elective surgery, a randomised controlled trial. *PLoS One*. 2012;7:e37410.
78. Fong HK, Sands LP, Leung JM. The role of postoperative analgesia in delirium and cognitive decline in elderly patients: a systematic review. *Anesth Analg*. 2006;102:1255–1266.
79. Avidan MS, Maybrier HR, Ben Abdallah A, et al. Intraoperative ketamine for prevention of postoperative delirium or pain after major surgery in older adults: an international, multicentre, double-blind, randomised clinical trial. *Lancet*. 2017;390:267–275.
80. Pasin L, Landoni G, Nardelli P, et al. Dexmedetomidine reduces the risk of delirium, agitation and confusion in critically Ill patients: a meta-analysis of randomized controlled trials. *J Cardiothorac Vasc Anesth*. 2014;28:1459–1466.
81. Vlisides P, Avidan M. Recent advances in preventing and managing postoperative delirium. *F1000Res*. 2019;8.
82. Verret M, Lauzier F, Zarychanski R, et al. Perioperative use of gabapentinoids for the management of postoperative acute pain: a systematic review and meta-analysis. *Anesthesiology*. 2020;133:265–279.
83. Sprung J, Abcejo ASA, Knopman DS, et al. Anesthesia with and without nitrous oxide and long-term cognitive trajectories in older adults. *Anesth Analg*. 2020;131:594–604.
84. Mu JL, Lee A, Joynt GM. Pharmacologic agents for the prevention and treatment of delirium in patients undergoing cardiac surgery: systematic review and metaanalysis. *Crit Care Med*. 2015;43:194–204.
85. Subramaniam B, Shankar P, Shaefi S, et al. Effect of intravenous acetaminophen vs placebo combined with propofol or dexmedetomidine on postoperative delirium among older patients following cardiac surgery The DEXACET Randomized Clinical Trial. *JAMA*. 2019;321:686–696.
86. Memtsoudis S, Cozowicz C, Zubizarreta N, et al. Risk factors for postoperative delirium in patients undergoing lower extremity joint arthroplasty: a retrospective population-based cohort study. *Reg Anesth Pain Med*. 2019.
87. Sieber FE. Postoperative delirium in the elderly surgical patient. *Anesthesiol Clin*. 2009;27: 451–464, table of contents.
88. Carli F, Mayo N, Klubien K, Schricker T, Trudel J, Belliveau P. Epidural analgesia enhances functional exercise capacity and health-related quality of life after colonic surgery: results of a randomized trial. *Anesthesiology*. 2002;97:540–549.
89. McDonald SR, Heflin MT, Whitson HE, et al. Association of Integrated Care Coordination With Postsurgical Outcomes in High-Risk Older Adults: The Perioperative Optimization of Senior Health (POSH) Initiative. *JAMA Surg*. 2018;153:454–462.
90. Chen CCH, Li HC, Liang JT, et al. Effect of a modified hospital elder life program on delirium and length of hospital stay in patients undergoing abdominal surgery a cluster randomized clinical trial. *JAMA Surg*. 2017;152:827–834.
91. Inouye SK, Bogardus ST, Baker DI, Leo-Summers L, Cooney LM. The Hospital Elder Life Program: a model of care to prevent cognitive and functional decline in older hospitalized patients. Hospital Elder Life Program. *J Am Geriatr Soc*. 2000;48:1697–1706.

92. Bentov I, Reed MJ. Anesthesia, microcirculation, and wound repair in aging. *Anesthesiology*. 2014;120:760–772.
93. Sessler DI, Sigl JC, Kelley SD, et al. Hospital stay and mortality are increased in patients having a "triple low" of low blood pressure, low bispectral index, and low minimum alveolar concentration of volatile anesthesia. *Anesthesiology*. 2012;116:1195–1203.
94. Walsh M, Devereaux PJ, Garg AX, et al. Relationship between intraoperative mean arterial pressure and clinical outcomes after noncardiac surgery: toward an empirical definition of hypotension. *Anesthesiology*. 2013;119:507–515.
95. van Waes JA, van Klei WA, Wijeysundera DN, van Wolfswinkel L, Lindsay TF, Beattie WS. Association between intraoperative hypotension and myocardial injury after vascular surgery. *Anesthesiology*. 2016;124:35–44.
96. Kheterpal S, O'Reilly M, Englesbe MJ, et al. Preoperative and intraoperative predictors of cardiac adverse events after general, vascular, and urological surgery. *Anesthesiology*. 2009;110:58–66.
97. Bijker JB, van Klei WA, Vergouwe Y, et al. Intraoperative hypotension and 1-year mortality after noncardiac surgery. *Anesthesiology*. 2009;111:1217–1226.
98. Tiret L, Desmonts JM, Hatton F, Vourc'h G. Complications associated with anaesthesia–a prospective survey in France. *Can Anaesth Soc J*. 1986;33:336–344.
99. Hamel MB, Henderson WG, Khuri SF, Daley J. Surgical outcomes for patients aged 80 and older: morbidity and mortality from major noncardiac surgery. *J Am Geriatr Soc*. 2005;53:424–429.
100. Bateman BT, Schumacher HC, Wang S, Shaefi S, Berman MF. Perioperative acute ischemic stroke in noncardiac and nonvascular surgery: incidence, risk factors, and outcomes. *Anesthesiology*. 2009;110:231–238.
101. Ng JL, Chan MT, Gelb AW. Perioperative stroke in noncardiac, nonneurosurgical surgery. *Anesthesiology*. 2011;115:879–890.
102. Kaatz S, Douketis JD, Zhou H, Gage BF, White RH. Risk of stroke after surgery in patients with and without chronic atrial fibrillation. *J Thromb Haemost*. 2010;8:884–890.
103. Mashour GA, Shanks AM, Kheterpal S. Perioperative stroke and associated mortality after noncardiac, nonneurologic surgery. *Anesthesiology*. 2011;114:1289–1296.
104. Benjo A, Thompson RE, Fine D, et al. Pulse pressure is an age-independent predictor of stroke development after cardiac surgery. *Hypertension*. 2007;50:630–635.
105. Devereaux PJ, Yang H, Yusuf S, et al. Effects of extended-release metoprolol succinate in patients undergoing non-cardiac surgery (POISE trial): a randomised controlled trial. *Lancet*. 2008;371:1839–1847.
106. Kam PC, Calcroft RM. Peri-operative stroke in general surgical patients. *Anaesthesia*. 1997; 52:879–883.
107. Bittner EA, Yue Y, Xie Z. Brief review: anesthetic neurotoxicity in the elderly, cognitive dysfunction and Alzheimer's disease. *Can J Anaesth*. 2011;58:216–223.
108. Tang J, Eckenhoff MF, Eckenhoff RG. Anesthesia and the old brain. *Anesth Analg*. 2010; 110:421–426.
109. Hudson AE, Hemmings HC. Are anaesthetics toxic to the brain? *Br J Anaesth*. 2011;107:30–37.
110. Leung JM, Tsai TL, Sands LP. Brief report: preoperative frailty in older surgical patients is associated with early postoperative delirium. *Anesth Analg*. 2011;112:1199–1201.
111. Hirsch J, DePalma G, Tsai TT, Sands LP, Leung JM. Impact of intraoperative hypotension and blood pressure fluctuations on early postoperative delirium after non-cardiac surgery. *Br J Anaesth*. 2015;115:418–426.
112. Young J, Murthy L, Westby M, Akunne A, O'Mahony R, Group GD. Diagnosis, prevention, and management of delirium: summary of NICE guidance. *BMJ*. 2010;341:c3704.
113. Adults AGSEPoPDiO. American Geriatrics Society abstracted clinical practice guideline for postoperative delirium in older adults. *J Am Geriatr Soc*. 2015;63:142–150.
114. Moller JT, Cluitmans P, Rasmussen LS, et al. Long-term postoperative cognitive dysfunction in the elderly ISPOCD1 study. ISPOCD investigators. International Study of Post-Operative Cognitive Dysfunction. *Lancet*. 1998;351:857–861.
115. Monk TG, Weldon BC, Garvan CW, et al. Predictors of cognitive dysfunction after major noncardiac surgery. *Anesthesiology*. 2008;108:18–30.
116. Dokkedal U, Hansen TG, Rasmussen LS, Mengel-From J, Christensen K. Cognitive functioning after surgery in middle-aged and elderly Danish twins. *Anesthesiology*. 2016;124:312–321.
117. Wu CL, Hsu W, Richman JM, Raja SN. Postoperative cognitive function as an outcome of regional anesthesia and analgesia. *Reg Anesth Pain Med*. 2004;29:257–268.
118. Crosby G, Culley DJ. Surgery and anesthesia: healing the body but harming the brain? *Anesth Analg*. 2011;112:999–1001.
119. Rörtgen D, Kloos J, Fries M, et al. Comparison of early cognitive function and recovery after desflurane or sevoflurane anaesthesia in the elderly: a double-blinded randomized controlled trial. *Br J Anaesth*. 2010;104:167–174.
120. Silverstein JH, Timberger M, Reich DL, Uysal S. Central nervous system dysfunction after noncardiac surgery and anesthesia in the elderly. *Anesthesiology*. 2007;106:622–628.
121. Avidan MS, Searleman AC, Storandt M, et al. Long-term cognitive decline in older subjects was not attributable to noncardiac surgery or major illness. *Anesthesiology*. 2009;111:964–970.
122. Evered L, Scott DA, Silbert B, Maruff P. Postoperative cognitive dysfunction is independent of type of surgery and anesthetic. *Anesth Analg*. 2011;112:1179–1185.
123. Kazmierski J, Kowman M, Banach M, et al. Incidence and predictors of delirium after cardiac surgery: Results from The IPDACS Study. *J Psychosom Res*. 2010;69:179–185.
124. Jankowski CJ, Trenerry MR, Cook DJ, et al. Cognitive and functional predictors and sequelae of postoperative delirium in elderly patients undergoing elective joint arthroplasty. *Anesth Analg*. 2011;112:1186–1193.
125. Avidan MS, Evers AS. the fallacy of persistent postoperative cognitive decline. *Anesthesiology*. 2016;124:255–258.

35 Neuraxial Anesthesia

NICOLE Z. SPENCE • MARK C. NORRIS

KEY POINTS

1. A growing body of evidence suggests that spinal and epidural anesthesia are associated with less morbidity and mortality than general anesthesia. This association is strongest in patients undergoing major hip or knee surgery, and data continues to evolve.
2. The epidural space is not a homogeneous, continuous cylinder surrounding the subarachnoid space. Instead, discrete pockets of fat lie in the posterior and lateral epidural spaces. Epidural veins pass through the anterior and lateral space. Blood in an epidural needle or catheter suggests that you are not in the midline.
3. Develop a mental model of spinal anatomy that will allow you to systematically locate the subarachnoid or epidural space.
4. The hemodynamic effects of spinal and epidural anesthesia are proportional to the extent of local anesthetic block.
5. Patient variables (age, height, weight, etc.) minimally affect the spread of intrathecal and epidural medications.
6. Unrecognized *intrathecal (subarachnoid)* injection of local anesthetics is a common cause of morbidity during epidural block. Early signs of unintended intrathecal local anesthetic injection can be subtle and easily missed. Commonly used epidural doses, if injected intrathecally, can produce excessive levels of sensory and motor block.
7. *Intravenous* local anesthetics can produce seizures and cardiac arrest. Test doses and incremental injections are key safety steps to prevent this complication.
8. Patients receiving antithrombotic or thrombolytic medications are at increased risk of developing a spinal or epidural hematoma. Refer to the American Society of Regional Anesthesia and Pain Medicine Regional Guidelines for Antithrombotic and Thrombolytic Therapy for current recommendations.

Introduction

Subarachnoid spinal and epidural anesthesia are key techniques that every anesthesiologist should master. Subarachnoid or intrathecal anesthesia is commonly referred to as spinal anesthesia. Some use the term "peridural" instead of "epidural." Caudal block refers to injection into the caudal epidural space via the sacral hiatus. Neuraxial is a general term that includes both subarachnoid and epidural injection.

Subarachnoid injection of a small dose of local anesthetic can rapidly produce dense surgical anesthesia. Subarachnoid injection is almost always done in the lumbar region, below the termination of the spinal cord. Spinal anesthesia can provide excellent operating conditions for lower abdominal, pelvic, and lower extremity surgery. Most subarachnoid anesthetics are single injections and have a finite duration. Single-injection subarachnoid anesthesia will last 2 to 3 hours at most. Single-injection subarachnoid anesthesia is not a good choice for prolonged or unpredictable surgeries.

Continuous subarachnoid anesthesia with a catheter can provide extended duration block. However, continuous subarachnoid anesthesia requires a dural puncture with a larger gauge needle. Such needles can produce an unacceptably high incidence of headache, especially in younger patients (see "Complications"). Microsubarachnoid catheters, which could be inserted through a 25-gauge needle were associated with permanent neurologic injury and are no longer available. In addition, subarachnoid catheters can be mistaken for epidural catheters. Dangerous levels of block can occur if an epidural dose of medication is accidentally injected into a continuous subarachnoid catheter. Still, continuous subarachnoid anesthesia allows careful titration of medication, which provides better hemodynamic stability in fragile patients. In addition, subarachnoid catheters can be redosed as needed during prolonged surgeries.

Epidural anesthesia requires larger doses of local anesthetic and takes more time to establish. However, when a catheter is in the epidural space, local anesthetic can be injected repeatedly, and anesthesia can be prolonged to match the duration of the surgery. Epidural injection can safely be performed in the lumbar, thoracic, and even cervical regions. Lumbar epidural anesthesia and subarachnoid anesthesia can be used for many of the same procedures. Thoracic epidural anesthesia is a useful adjunct to general anesthesia for upper abdominal and thoracic surgeries and can be used to provide postoperative analgesia. Cervical epidural injection is rarely used for surgery; however, it is commonly used to treat pain associated with cervical disc disease. See Chronic Pain chapter for further discussion of cervical epidural injection.

The caudal canal is the lower extension of the epidural space. Caudal anesthesia and analgesia are uncommon in adults but can be useful for pediatric surgeries.

Epidural injection of medications also can provide analgesia. Dilute mixtures of local anesthetic and opioid can provide postoperative analgesia with minimal motor block. Epidural analgesia is a key element of many enhanced recovery after surgery (ERAS) protocols. The flexibility of continuous epidural block makes it an excellent choice for labor pain relief. Dilute local anesthetic and opioid solutions can provide labor *analgesia* with minimal maternal motor block and negligible effects on the progress and outcome of labor. Should surgical delivery be required, more concentrated local anesthetics can be administered via the epidural catheter to provide operative *anesthesia* (see OB Anesthesia chapter).

In some settings, the anesthesiologist may combine subarachnoid and epidural injections. This approach offers the rapid onset of dense anesthesia produced by subarachnoid injection of local anesthetic and the flexibility of an epidural catheter.

Indications and Contraindications

There are no absolute indications for subarachnoid or epidural anesthesia. Their use is determined by a combination of patient, surgeon, and anesthesiologist preferences. Contraindications to neuraxial anesthesia or analgesia include patient refusal, coagulopathy, hemodynamic instability, and infection at the site of injection.

Neuraxial Anesthesia and Outcome

1 Many investigators have compared patient outcomes associated with neuraxial and general anesthesia. Small randomized controlled trials examining major morbidity and mortality after high-risk and vascular surgeries yielded conflicting results.[1,2] By 2012, 40 studies including over 3,000 patients were available for meta-analysis.[3] Subarachnoid and epidural anesthesia were associated with a lower risk of death within 30 days of surgery (risk ratio [RR] 0.71). Neuraxial anesthesia also reduced the risk of postoperative pneumonia (RR 0.45), but not the risk of myocardial infarction (RR 1.17). Interestingly, adding neuraxial anesthesia to general anesthesia did not reduce the risk of death or myocardial infarction compared to general anesthesia alone. However, the combination of neuraxial and general anesthesia was associated with a reduced risk of postoperative pneumonia (RR 0.69).

Large, multi-institutional databases allow robust comparisons of neuraxial and general anesthesia. In more than 18,000 patients undergoing hip fracture surgery, neuraxial anesthesia was associated with a decreased risk of in-hospital death and pulmonary complications.[4] However, the same authors reported a follow-up study of more than 50,000 patients and did not find any decreased mortality after neuraxial anesthesia.[5] In contrast, neuraxial anesthesia was associated with lower 30-day mortality and fewer prolonged hospital stays in nearly 400,000 patients undergoing hip or knee replacement.[6] However, in a recent randomized controlled clinical trial, neuraxial anesthesia did not improve survival or ambulation 60 days after hip fracture surgery.[7] Interestingly, the incidence of postoperative delirium was similar between both anesthetics.[8]

Neuraxial anesthesia may improve outcomes in some subgroups of patients. A small retrospective review from a single institution found fewer postoperative pulmonary complications and arrhythmias, as well as shorter intensive care unit, stays among patients receiving regional instead of general anesthesia for lower extremity amputation.[9] A review of more than 5,000 patients with chronic obstructive pulmonary disease (COPD) found that regional anesthesia (subarachnoid, epidural, or peripheral nerve block) was associated with fewer adverse respiratory events (postoperative pneumonia, prolonged ventilator dependence, and unplanned postoperative intubation) than general anesthesia.[10] There were fewer wound infections, blood transfusions, pneumonias, and total infections associated with neuraxial versus general anesthesia among more than 14,000 patients undergoing total knee arthroplasty.[11] Hospital length of stay was also shorter in the patients who received neuraxial anesthesia.[12] Neuraxial anesthesia improves outcomes that predict readiness for hospital discharge, including pain and postoperative nausea and vomiting, in patients undergoing orthopedic joint surgeries and may subsequently decrease health care costs.[13,14] In contrast, a different review of more than 7,000 hip fracture patients found no anesthesia-related differences in mortality but an *increased* risk of superficial wound infection and urinary tract infection among patients receiving subarachnoid anesthesia.[15]

Some investigators have reported a lower risk of thromboembolism in patients receiving neuraxial anesthesia.[16] However, not all studies have confirmed this benefit.[6] There are insufficient data to determine if regional anesthesia improves outcomes for patients undergoing major vascular surgery.[17] One retrospective study of 822 patients found that regional anesthesia does *not* improve graft patency after lower extremity revascularization.[18]

An intriguing advantage of epidural anesthesia and analgesia might be improved survival after cancer surgery. Regional anesthesia and analgesia avoid the immunosuppression associated with general anesthesia and postoperative opioid analgesia. In a recent meta-analysis, epidural anesthesia and analgesia were associated with longer survival but no difference in cancer recurrence after surgery.[19] Recent data regarding the beneficial effect of epidural analgesia on cancer recurrence have been less promising.[20]

Anatomy

Subarachnoid and epidural anesthesia are exercises in applied anatomy. The anesthesiologist must have a thorough grasp of the relationships between surface landmarks and deeper structures. Text and two-dimensional images are a useful, but imperfect, way to learn vertebral anatomy. Careful examination of skeletal models can help. Recently, investigators have used high-resolution

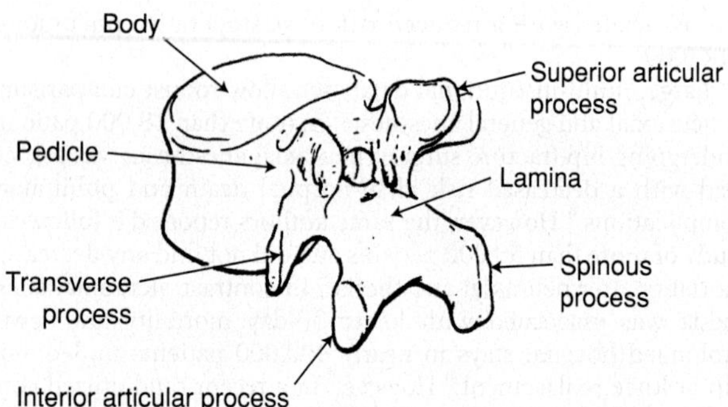

Figure 35-1 The vertebral body. (From Norris MC. *Obstetric Anesthesia*. 2nd ed. Lippincott Williams & Wilkins; 1999:286.)

magnetic resonance images to construct interactive virtual three-dimensional models of bony, ligamentous, and nervous structures of the spine (http://www.usra.ca/virtual-spine/vspine.php or http://pie.med.utoronto.ca/VSpine/index.htm).[21,22]

Vertebrae

The spine is comprised of 33 vertebrae: 7 cervical, 12 thoracic, 5 lumbar, 5 fused sacral, and 4 fused coccygeal. All vertebrae have the same structural components but with varying shapes and sizes. The vertebrae surround and protect the vertebral canal, which contains the spinal cord, cerebrospinal fluid (CSF), meninges, spinal nerves, and epidural space. Each vertebra has a body anteriorly, two pedicles that project posteriorly from the body, and laminae that connect the pedicles (Fig. 35-1). The transverse processes arise laterally from the junction of the pedicle and lamina, and the spinous process projects posteriorly from the union of the bilateral laminae. The paraspinous muscles and ligaments attach to these bony projections. The pedicles form the superior and inferior vertebral notches, through which the spinal nerves exit the vertebral canal. The lamina and pedicles meet at the superior and inferior articular processes, which form the joints that connect the adjacent vertebrae. The first and second cervical vertebrae, also referred to as the atlas and dens, have a unique appearance in that C1 lacks a vertebral body or spinous process and C2 has a large articulating process (dens).

Five fused vertebrae form the sacrum. In 0.9% to 6.4% of the population, sacralization (fusion of the L5 and S1 vertebrae) occurs.[23] Up to 60% of those with this variation have only unilateral fusion, known as hemisacralization.[23] The fifth sacral vertebra does not fuse posteriorly, forming the sacral hiatus, which provides access to the most caudal point of the epidural space. The sacral hiatus is usually open in children, but its patency varies in adults. The four coccygeal vertebrae fuse to form the coccyx, which represents a vestigial tail and serves as an anchor for the attachment of tendons, ligaments, and muscles.

In surgical and obstetric patients, neuraxial block is usually accomplished without the aid of imaging. Attaining the desired level for neuraxial block and avoiding complications requires familiarity with surface landmarks. Commonly identified landmarks include the C7 spinous process (vertebra prominens), the 12th rib, and the iliac crests. Many anesthesiologists use the line between the iliac crests (Tuffier line) to identify the L4–L5 interspace. However, this landmark commonly misleads even experienced anesthesiologists.[24] When possible, locating the L5–S1 interspace and counting cephalad may be a more reliable way to identify a specific lumbar interspace.[25] In obese patients, a midline skin crease and the gluteal cleft can help locate the midline.

Ligaments

Several ligaments stabilize the vertebral column. The anterior and posterior longitudinal ligaments link the vertebral bodies. Dorsally, the supraspinous and interspinous ligaments, as well as the ligamentum flavum, connect the vertebrae. The supraspinous ligament covers the tips of the spinous processes between C7 and the sacrum; from C7 to the external occipital protuberance, it continues as the ligamentum nuchae. The supraspinous ligament thins in the lower lumbar region, allowing greater flexion of the spine. The intraspinous ligament runs between spinous processes. It may contain slit-like, fat-filled cavities that can create a false loss of resistance during attempts to identify the epidural space. The intraspinous ligament merges with both supraspinous ligament and ligamentum flavum. The ligamentum flavum (yellow ligament) is a pair of dense trapezoid-shaped structures made mostly of elastin. The two ligaments fuse in the midline at an 80- to 90-degree angle. This fusion may be incomplete. Lumbar midline gaps occur in approximately 10% of patients (Fig. 35-2).[26] When attempting to locate the epidural space, aim to appreciate the "snap" of the supraspinous ligament, "mushy" intraspinous ligament, and "gritty" ligamentum flavum.

Epidural Space

The epidural space lies within the vertebral canal but outside the 2
dural sac. It extends from the foramen magnum to the end of the

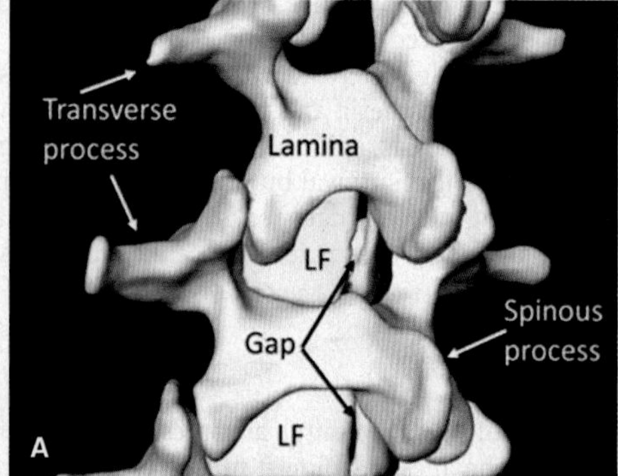

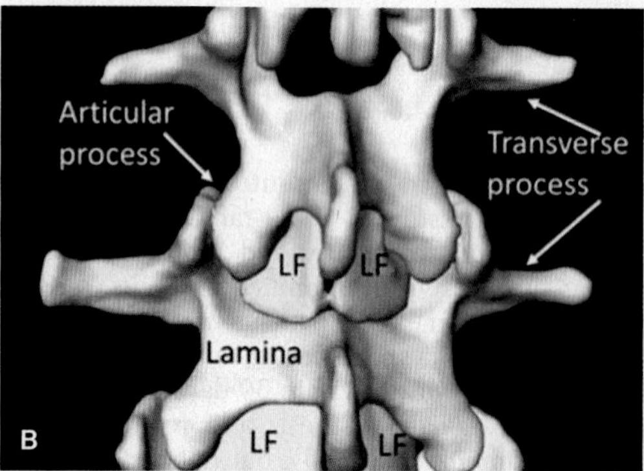

Figure 35-2 Three-dimensional reconstruction of human lumbar ligamentum flavum (LF). A: Posterior-lateral view. **B:** Posterior view. Note the gap (*arrow*) between the two halves of the ligamentum flavum. (Adapted with permission from Reina MA, Lirk P, Puigdellívol-Sánchez A, et al. Human lumbar ligamentum flavum anatomy for epidural anesthesia: reviewing a 3D MR-based interactive model and postmortem samples. *Anesth Analg*. 2016;122:903–907. Copyright © 2016 International Anesthesia Research Society.)

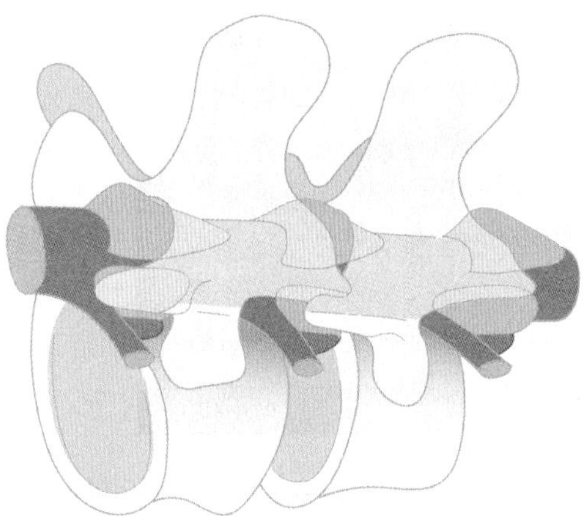

Figure 35-3 The compartments of the epidural space (*grey*) are discontinuous. Areas in between are potential spaces where the dural mater normally abuts the sides of the vertebral canal. (Adapted with permission from Hogan Q. Lumbar epidural anatomy: a new look by cryomicrotome section. *Anesthesiology*. 1991;75:767–775.)

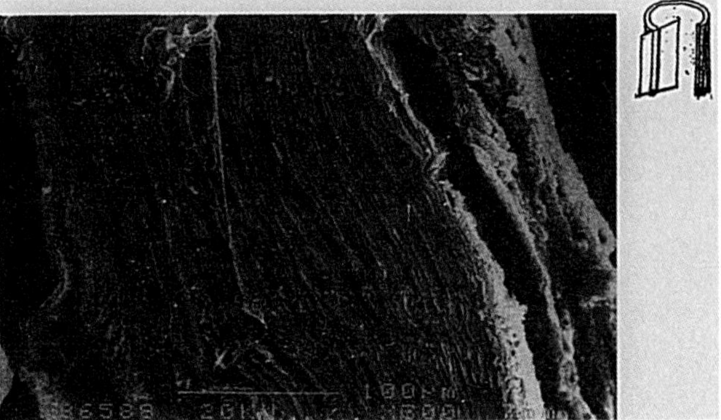

Figure 35-5 Scanning electron microscopic image of a radial longitudinal section of human dura mater. Total thickness is a composite of all concentric layers. (Adapted from Reina MA, Dittmann M, López Garcia A, van Zundert A. New perspectives in the microscopic structure of human dura mater in the dorsolumbar region. *Reg Anesth*. 1997;22:161–168.)

dural sac at S2. The epidural space is bound anteriorly by the posterior longitudinal ligament and posteriorly by the lamina and ligamentum flavum. Laterally, the epidural space extends to the pedicles where it communicates with the paravertebral space via the intervertebral foramina.[27] The epidural space is often absent because the dura intermittently abuts the bony and ligamentous structures of the spine. The remainder of the space consists of discontinuous, fat-filled pockets that open readily upon injection of air or liquid.[27] The cervical level contains no epidural fat. In the lumbar region, fat in the anterior and posterior aspects of the epidural space forms multiple, metameric, discrete collections (Fig. 35-3).[27,28] This fat may play an important role in the kinetics of epidural medications.[29]

Epidural veins are located mostly in the anterior epidural space. The intervertebral foramina allow transmission of intra-abdominal pressure into the epidural space. Conditions that increase intra-abdominal pressure (i.e., pregnancy) can cause engorgement of epidural veins, leading to more frequent venous cannulation or possibly enhancing the spread of injected medications.

Meninges

The meninges surround and protect the spinal cord, CSF, and nerve roots until they exit the foramina. The dura, arachnoid, and pia mater form three structurally distinct meningeal layers (Fig. 35-4).

Dura

The dura mater (hard mother) is the thickest, outermost meningeal layer. It is 270 to 280 μm thick and consists mostly of collagen fibers arranged in about 80 layers of very fine lamellae (Fig. 35-5). The external (epidural) surface contains bands of collagen fibers running in different directions. The dura also contains thick elastic fibers and fine granular material. The inner (subarachnoid) surface includes fine fibers that fuse with the arachnoid mater.[30] A potential subdural space exists between the dura and arachnoid mater. Drugs, needles, or catheters intended for the epidural or subarachnoid spaces rarely may end up in this subdural space (Fig. 35-6).

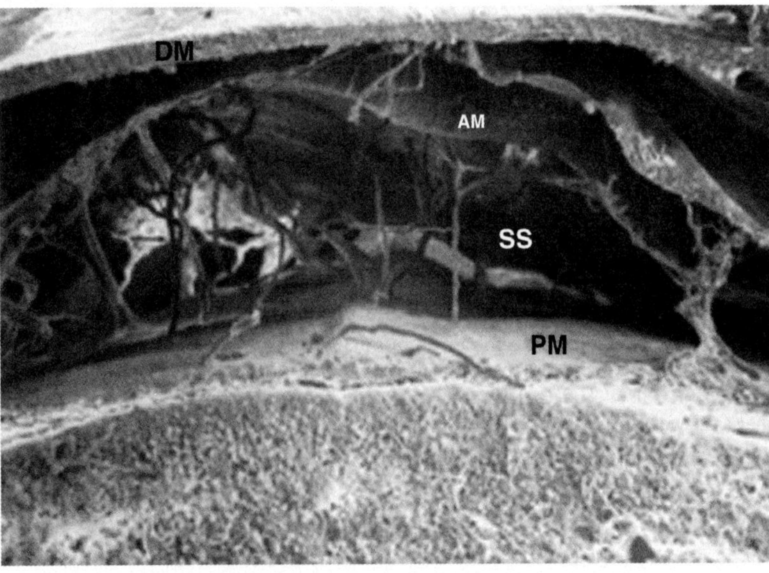

Figure 35-4 The spinal meninges of a dog, showing the pia mater (PM) in apposition to the spinal cord, the subarachnoid space (SS), the arachnoid mater (AM) with trabeculae stretching from the arachnoid mater to the pia mater, and the dura mater (DM). The separation between the arachnoid mater and the dural mater is the subdural space, which was created here as an artifact of preparation. (Adapted from Peters A, Palay SL, Webster H, eds. *The Fine Structure of the Nervous System: The Neurons and Supporting Cells*. WB Saunders; 1976. Copyright © 1976 Elsevier. With permission.)

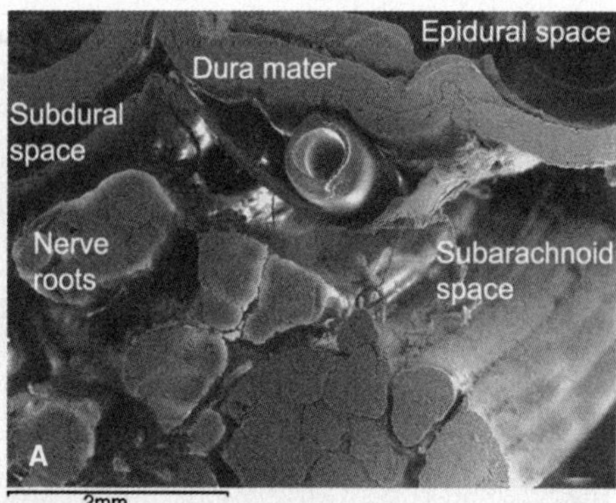

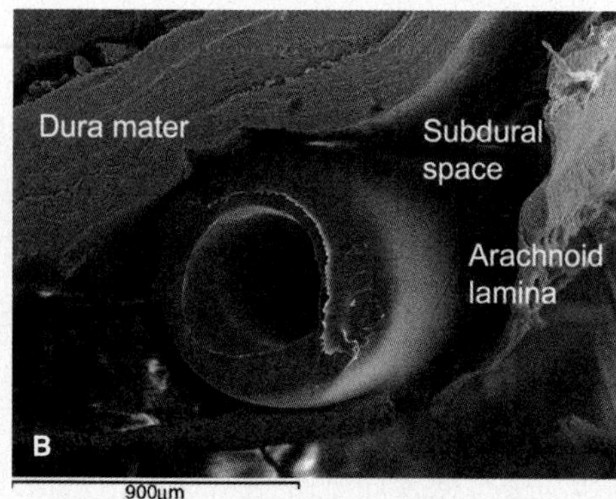

Figure 35-6 Human subdural space. A: Enhanced view (×20) of an epidural catheter inside a subdural space. **B:** Detail (×60) of **A.** Sample was obtained from a cadaver under scanning electron microscopy. (Adapted from Reina MA, Collier CB, Prats-Galino A, Puigdellívol-Sánchez A, Machés F, De Andrés JA. Unintentional subdural placement of epidural catheters during attempted epidural anesthesia: an anatomic study of spinal subdural compartment. *Reg Anesth Pain Med.* 2011;36:537–541.)

The dura mater is a continuation of the spinal meninges, extending from the foramen magnum to approximately S2 in adults, where it fuses with the filum terminale. It extends laterally with individual nerve roots and fuses with the epineurium near the intervertebral foramina.

Arachnoid

The arachnoid mater (spider mother) lies within the dura and has two portions. A compact laminar layer of flattened epithelial-like cells that are tightly connected to one another covers the inner surface of the dura mater. Then, a trabecular web-like portion extends to the pia mater (Fig. 35-7).[31] Because of this cellular architecture, the arachnoid, not the dura, hinders drug movement through meninges. The low permeability of the arachnoid mater keeps the CSF in the subarachnoid, not the subdural space.[32] Specialized intercellular junctions within the internal portion of the arachnoid mater explain its selective permeability.[33]

The spinal nerve roots traverse the dura and arachnoid membranes as they exit the vertebral foramina. Here, the arachnoid mater herniates through the dura and forms arachnoid granulations. These granulations provide an exit for material leaving the central nervous system.

Pia

The innermost layer of the spinal meninges is the pia mater (soft mother). The pia consists of flat overlapping cells that coat the spinal cord and nerve roots. The pial cells contain numerous fenestrations along the lumbar spinal cord and nerve roots (Fig. 35-8). Any role these fenestrations might play in the action of subarachnoid or epidural medications is speculative.[34]

Cerebrospinal Fluid

CSF is 99% water. Multiple minor components include protein, glucose, electrolytes, and neurotransmitters. In adult humans, the volume of CSF is 100 to 160 mL. For many years, we thought that CSF was primarily produced in the choroid plexus and then flowed from the ventricles to the subarachnoid space, where it was absorbed by arachnoid granulations. This hypothesis is incomplete and probably incorrect. The choroid plexus is not the sole site of CSF production, and the arachnoid granulations are not its primary absorption sites. CSF and interstitial fluid (IF) are

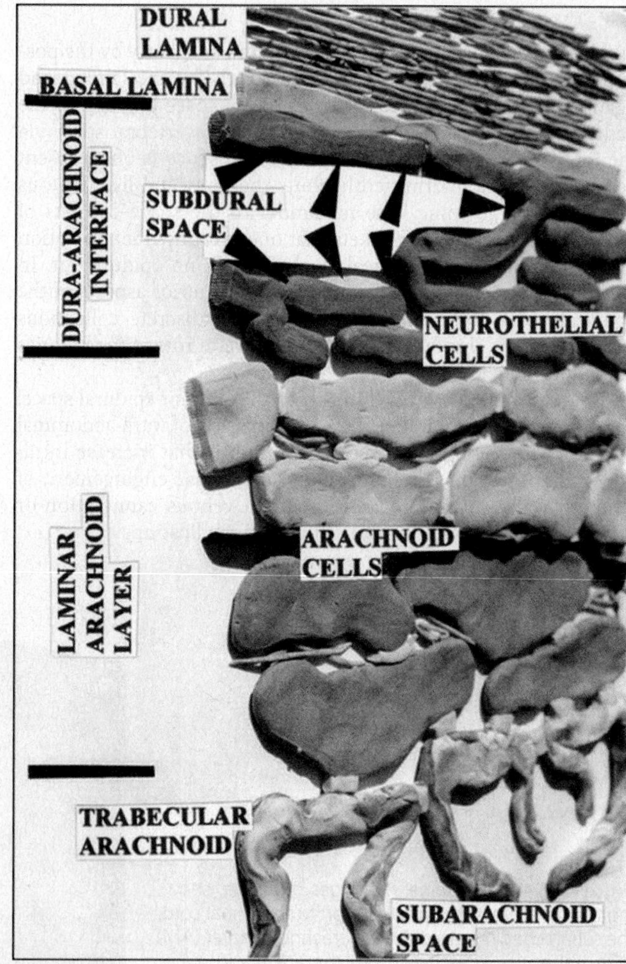

Figure 35-7 Dura–arachnoid interface model. From the **top:** the dural lamina (dura mater's most internal portion) is followed by the dura–arachnoid interface; the interface is filled with neurothelial cells, and forms the subdural space. **Below** are the laminar and trabecular portions of the arachnoid mater. (Adapted with permission from Reina MA, De Leon Casasola O, Lopez A, et al. The origin of the spinal subdural space: ultrastructure findings. *Anesth Analg.* 2002;94:991–995.)

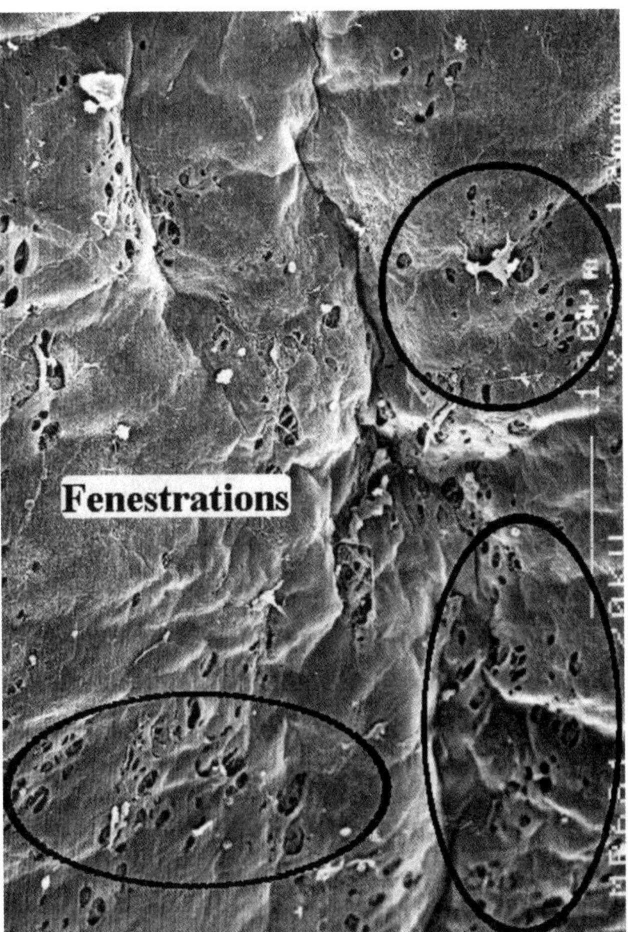

Figure 35-8 Fenestrations in the pial cellular layer at the level of the spinal cord. Numerous fenestrations appear in this scanning electron micrograph. (Adapted with permission from Reina MA, De Leon Casasola O, Villanueva MC, et al. Ultrastructural findings in human spinal pia mater in relation to subarachnoid anesthesia. *Anesth Analg*. 2004;98:1479–1485.)

closely related. They are both mainly produced and absorbed in the parenchymal capillaries of the brain and spinal cord. The lymphatic system also absorbs a considerable amount of CSF and IF.[35] CSF flow is not unidirectional. Instead, transmitted cardiac oscillations produce local mixing, whereas other drugs spread slowly by diffusion. Solutes are reabsorbed across capillary membranes into the bloodstream.[36]

Spinal Cord

In the first trimester fetus, the spinal cord extends to the end of the sacrum. The vertebral column grows faster than the spinal cord, and at birth, the cord usually ends at the level of the third lumbar vertebra. In adults, the cord most often ends at around L1. However, there is considerable interindividual variation. The cord ends at T12 in some adults but may extend to L3 in up to 10% of adults.

There are 31 pairs of spinal nerves, each with an anterior motor root and a posterior sensory root. These nerve roots arise from individual spinal cord segments. Each posterior sensory root innervates a specific dermatome (Fig. 35-9). The sympathetic nervous system arises from the intermediolateral grey matter of the T1 to L2 spinal cord segments. This grey matter contains the cell bodies of the preganglionic sympathetic neurons, whose axons travel with the corresponding spinal nerve through the intervertebral foramen. They then diverge and join the sympathetic chain ganglia.

The spinal nerves and their corresponding dermatomes are named for the foramina through which they exit the vertebral column (1 Video 35-1). In the cervical region, spinal nerves are named after the lower vertebrae (i.e., C5 exits between C4 and C5). Distal to the cervical portion of the column, the roots are named by the upper vertebrae (i.e., L2 emerges between L2 and L3). Since the vertebral column is longer than the spinal cord, the thoracic, lumbar, and sacral nerve roots traverse progressively greater distances from their originating spinal cord segment to their exiting foramina. The lumbar and sacral spinal nerves that extend beyond the tip of the cord are called the cauda equina. These nerve roots, covered only by pia mater, may be more susceptible to chemical injury than more proximal roots.

In one study examining magnetic resonance images of seven adults, the dural sac volume from S1 to T12 was 43 mL. The average CSF volume was 34 mL. The remaining 9 to 10 mL consisted of conus medullaris and nerve roots. The percentage of nerve volume to dural sac volume increased from 7% to 14% at L5, to 25% at L4, to 30% to 43% at T12. Upper lumbar punctures risk needle contact with the conus medullaris, and the cauda equina is vulnerable to contact with lower punctures.[37]

Ultrasound Anatomy of the Spine

Ultrasound can complement clinical examination when performing neuraxial blocks. Ultrasound examination of the lumbar spine can establish the depth of the epidural space, identify the precise intervertebral level, and locate the midline and interspinous/interlaminar spaces. This information can guide subsequent needle insertion. Systematic reviews suggest that ultrasound increases the success and reduces the technical difficulty of lumbar neuraxial blocks. Furthermore, ultrasound increases the first-pass success rate of combined spinal epidural (CSE) placement, even for experienced anesthesiologists.[38] Ultrasound may reduce the risk of traumatic procedures and may contribute to the safety of lumbar neuraxial blocks.[39]

Although real-time, ultrasound-guided approaches have been described,[40] most experts use ultrasound before attempting neuraxial block to locate landmarks. Once mastered, a preprocedure ultrasound examination can quickly identify the exact lumbar interspace, midline, skin puncture point, angle of needle insertion, and depth of the epidural space.[41]

The basic ultrasound examination of the lumbar spine consists of two scans: a paramedian longitudinal scan and a transverse or axial scan. The paramedian longitudinal view can identify specific interspace levels by scanning through interlaminar windows. Place a low-frequency curvilinear transducer longitudinally along the spine, parallel to it, 2 to 3 cm lateral to the midline. Tilt the probe slightly to aim the ultrasound beam toward the center of the spinal canal. Multiple vertebral levels can be seen in one scanned image. The structures seen in this view include sacrum, lamina, ligamentum flavum, and dorsal dura mater (Fig. 35-10).[41] The ligamentum flavum and dorsal dura mater appear as a single bright line in the interlaminar window. A deeper bright reflection emanates from the ventral dura/posterior longitudinal ligament/vertebral body complex. Once the desired level is identified in the paramedian longitudinal plane, turn the transducer perpendicular to the axis of the spine to view the entire interspace. The structures that can be seen in the axial plane include the ligamentum flavum and dorsal dura mater, ventral dura/posterior longitudinal ligament/vertebral body complex, articular processes, and transverse processes (Fig. 35-11).[41]

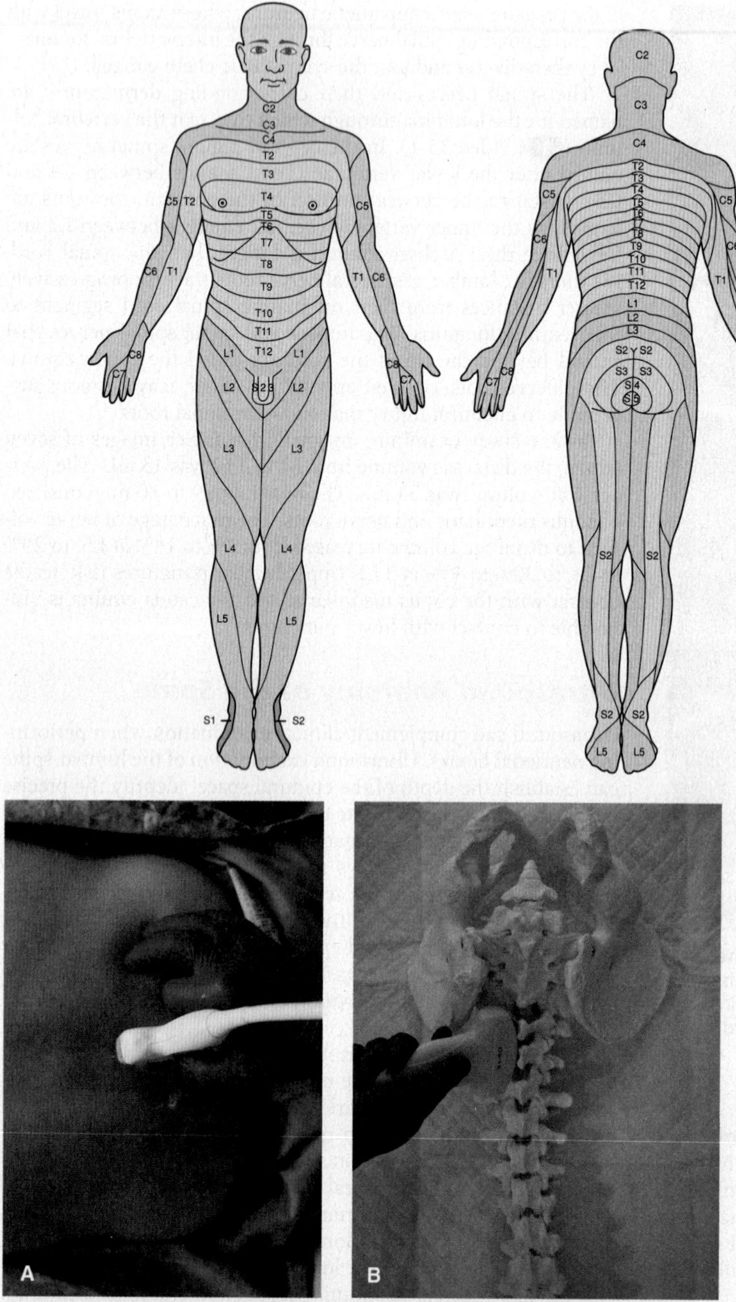

Figure 35-9 Human sensory dermatomes.

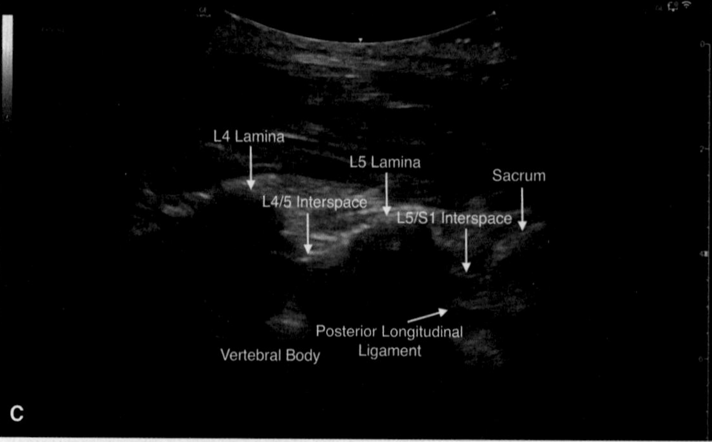

Figure 35-10 **A:** Scanning in the paramedian longitudinal plane. **B:** Probe oriented parallel to the axis of spine model. **C:** Ultrasound image with a typical saw-tooth sign: hyperechoic flat band on the right represents sacrum, saw-teeth indicate lamina, and the two parallel bands between saw-teeth correspond to the interspace containing the ligamentum flavum–dorsal dural unit (**upper**) and the ventral dura posterior longitudinal ligament–vertebral body complex (**lower**).

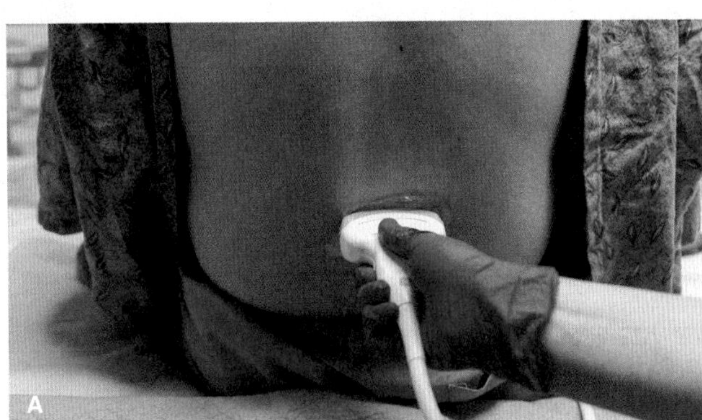

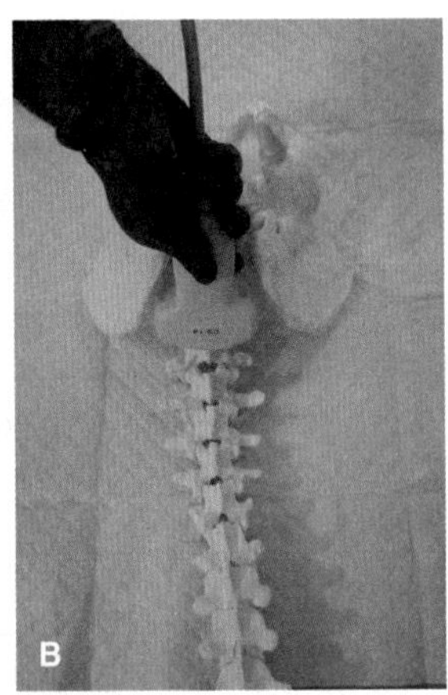

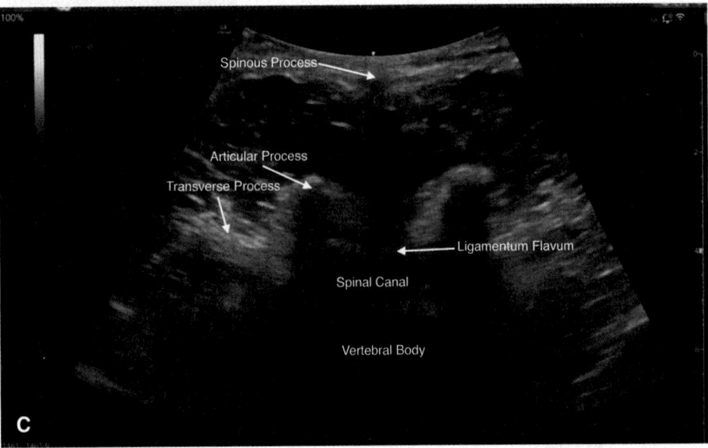

Figure 35-11 **A:** Scanning in the transverse plane. **B:** Probe oriented perpendicular to the axis of spine model. **C:** Typical ultrasound of a lumbar interspace: midline hyperechoic structures represent the ligamentum flavum–dorsal dura unit (**upper**) and the ventral dura posterior longitudinal ligament–vertebral body complex (**lower**); bilateral symmetrical hyperechoic lateral structures indicate articular and transverse processes with their acoustic shadows.

After acquiring the best image of the interspace structure and ligamentum flavum/dura, center the target interspace on the screen of the ultrasound machine. Then, holding the probe steady, mark the skin at the midline of both the vertical and horizontal edges of the probe. Remove the probe and connect the marks to make a cross. With a transverse probe, this cross will identify a midline puncture site (Fig. 35-12). With a longitudinal probe, the cross identifies a paramedian insertion site. By freezing the image on the ultrasound machine, one can also measure the depth of the ligamentum flavum/dura and estimate the best angle for needle insertion.[41]

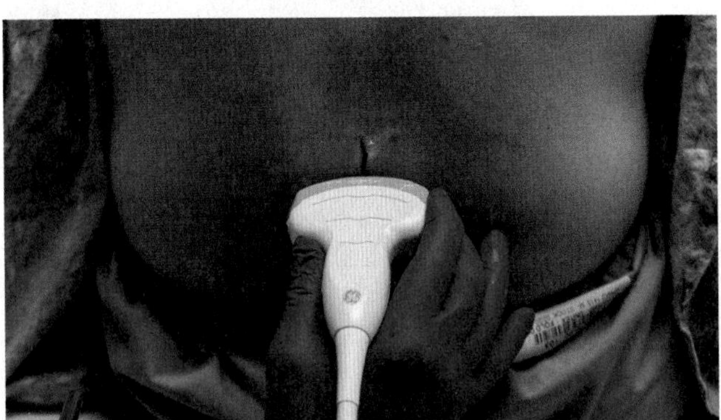

Figure 35-12 Vertical line marks midline; horizontal line marks the interspace. The intersection of these two lines indicates needle insertion location.

Technique

Patient Preparation

Equipment

Before inducing subarachnoid or epidural anesthesia, assemble all equipment you might need. This equipment should include the supplies needed to perform the block and emergency equipment required to treat rare, but potentially catastrophic complications. At a minimum, always monitor blood pressure and pulse oximetry. Subarachnoid anesthesia is usually induced in an operating room (OR) or nearby procedure room. Epidural anesthesia can be induced in a labor room, intensive care unit, or preoperative holding area. A dedicated cart can hold the needed supplies (Table 35-1).

Positioning

Most patients will either sit or lie on their side during induction of neuraxial anesthesia. Inserting a spinal needle with the patient in the prone jackknife position has been described but is rarely used in contemporary practice. One published report describes a real-time, ultrasound-guided approach to the L5–S1 interspace in prone patients.[40] The choice between sitting and lateral position depends on the proceduralist, the patient, and the procedure. Many physicians prefer the sitting position.[42] Thin patients (BMI [body mass index] <25) report being more comfortable in the lateral position. Obese patients (BMI >30) may prefer sitting.[43] Some clinical situations dictate the lateral position (i.e., hip fractures, labor analgesia in rapidly progressing patients, and certain emergency cesarean

Table 35-1 Suggested Contents for an Epidural Cart

Epidural Supplies
Epidural trays
Sterile gloves
Sterile prep applicators
Extra epidural needles/catheters
Extra loss-of-resistance syringes
Sterile dressings
Tape
Emergency Equipment
Self-inflating bag–valve mask
Oral airways
Working laryngoscope and blade
Endotracheal tubes/supraglottic airways
20% lipid emulsion, +/– syringes of phenylephrine and ephedrine

deliveries). Physicians should be comfortable inserting spinal and epidural needles with patients in either position to be able to use the approach most suitable for each patient and procedure.

When sitting, place the patient squarely on the operating table with back and buttocks at the near edge. Have the patient relax their shoulders and curve their back to flex the lumbar spine (Fig. 35-13). Tilting the operating table may help flex the patient's

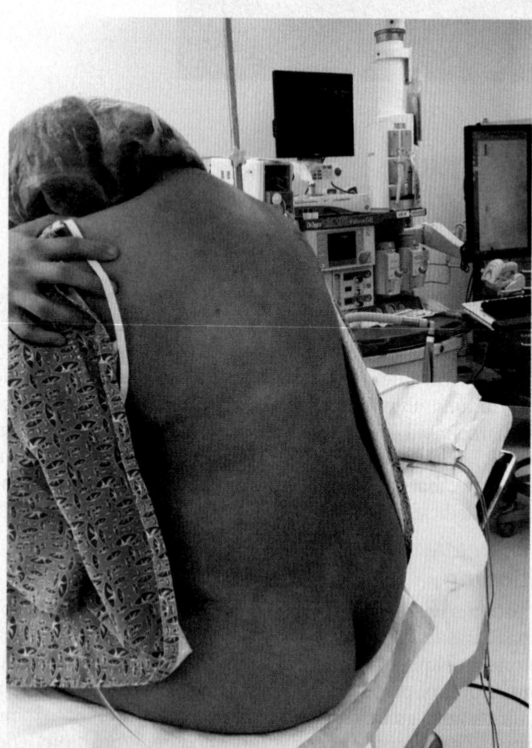

Figure 35-13 Sitting position for neuraxial block. Position the patient squarely on the bed or operating table with the buttocks at the edge near the operator. The patient's legs can be supported by the table, a stool, or (in Labor and Delivery) flexed on the bed. An assistant should provide support. Instruct the patient to relax their shoulders and flex their lumbar spine. ("Arch your back like a rainbow.")

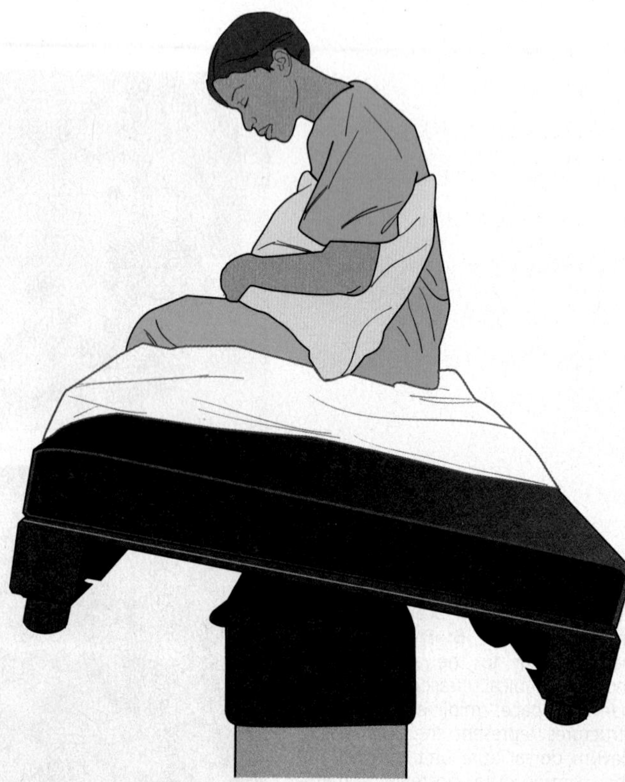

Figure 35-14 Tilting the operating table can encourage the patient to flex her hips and lumbar spine.

hips and lumbar spine, further opening the lumbar interspaces (Fig. 35-14).[44] Sitting obese patients, and those with poorly palpable landmarks, can make it easier to identify the midline and eventually subarachnoid or epidural space. When the patient is positioned properly, a line from the C7 vertebral prominence to the gluteal cleft identifies the midline.

When positioning laterally, bring the patient's back to the edge of the table. Position the hips and shoulders perpendicular to the bed (Fig. 35-15). Place a pillow under the patient's head. An assistant can help the patient bend their knees and hips and

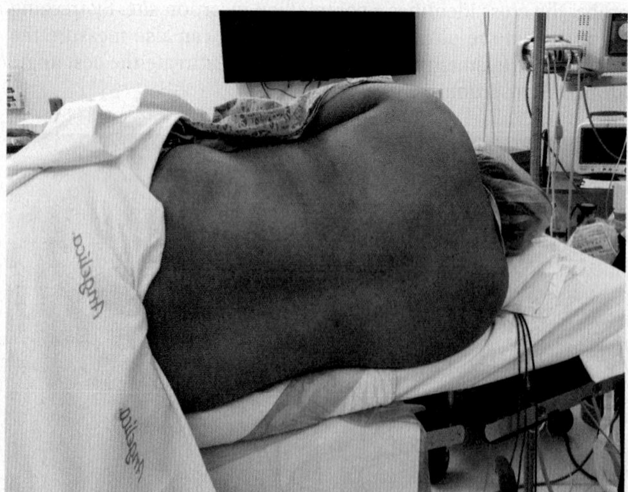

Figure 35-15 Lateral position for neuraxial block. The patient's hips and shoulders are even with the edge of the bed. The head and neck are supported to remain even with the spine.

flex their lumbar spine. The site of surgery and baricity of the local anesthetic will determine laterality of the subsequent block. When using hyperbaric drug, position the operative side down. With isobaric/hypobaric drug, put the operative side up. When inducing subarachnoid anesthesia for cesarean section with either hyperbaric or isobaric drug, place the patient on her *right* side, then turn supine after successful subarachnoid injection, and provide *left* uterine displacement.[45]

In either position, be mindful of patient comfort. Use blankets and pillows to keep them warm, comfortable, and appropriately covered. Light sedation with midazolam or fentanyl may sometimes be appropriate. Patients with painful fractures may need deeper sedation to allow appropriate positioning. In this case, small doses of ketamine or propofol may be useful. Although skilled pediatric anesthesiologists have a good record of safely inducing neuraxial anesthesia after induction of general anesthesia in children,[46] this approach is not prudent in adults.[47,48]

Skin Preparation

Aseptic technique is crucial. The American Society of Anesthesiologists (ASA) recommends removing jewelry (e.g., rings and watches), hand washing, sterile gloves, caps, and masks.[49] Use individual antiseptic packets to cleanse the skin. (Previously opened, multiple-use bottles of povidone–iodine can be contaminated.)[50] Both chlorhexidine with alcohol and povidone–iodine with alcohol provide effective skin decontamination.[51]

Needles

Spinal and epidural needles are categorized by the design of their tips (Fig. 35-16). Spinal needles may have a beveled cutting tip or a pencil-point noncutting tip. Pencil-point needles have a lower incidence of postdural puncture headaches (PDPHs) than cutting-tip needles. Most anesthesiologists use thin (smaller than 24-gauge) needles to limit the risk of PDPH. A shorter, but larger gauge, introducer needle helps puncture the skin and guide the flimsier spinal needle toward the subarachnoid space.

Epidural needles are usually larger than spinal needles (Fig. 35-16). This larger diameter improves the tactile feel as the needle advances through the ligamentum flavum and into the epidural space. In addition, an 18-gauge needle will allow passage of a 20-gauge catheter. Epidural needles usually have a curved tip to guide the catheter into the epidural space. Curved-tip epidural needles, as well as the straight-tipped Crawford needle, also can be used for caudal block.

Combined subarachnoid epidural block can be performed sequentially or as a needle-through-needle technique. The needle-through-needle technique can be done most simply with a long spinal needle and a regular epidural needle (Fig. 35-17). In this case, the spinal needle should protrude at least 1.5 cm beyond the tip of the epidural needle. Specialized needle-through-needle or needle-beside-needle combinations are also available (Fig. 35-16).

Spinal needles
Quincke
Sprotte
Whitacre
Greene
Epidural needles
Hustead
Tuohy
Crawford
Combined spinal/epidural needle

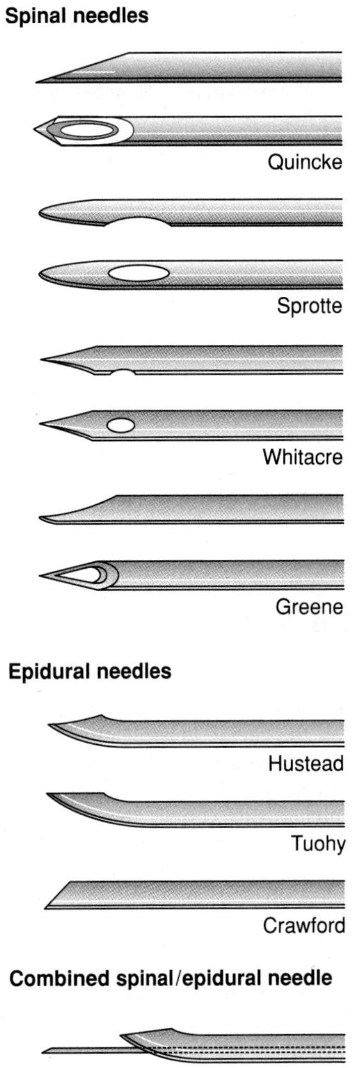

Figure 35-16 Some spinal and epidural needles. Needles are distinguished by their tip designs.

Approach

Lumbar neuraxial block can be performed with either a midline or paramedian approach (Fig. 35-18). The thoracic spinous processes slope steeply, and the thoracic spine does not flex as much as the lumbar spine. As a result, the thoracic epidural space is more easily entered using the paramedian approach.

Technique

3 Identifying the subarachnoid or epidural space is an exercise in applied anatomy. Understand the relationship between surface landmarks (i.e., the spinous process) and the target (the subarachnoid or epidural space). Sometimes, the needle will strike bone. Recognize which part of the vertebrae (spinous process, lamina) and where (midline, right, or left) the needle is touching and make an informed adjustment to redirect the needle toward the target (Fig. 35-19).

The midline approach is the most straightforward (2 Video 35-2). After positioning the patient, identify the midline by palpating the spinous processes. In obese patients, estimate the midline by imagining a line between the C7 prominence and the intergluteal cleft. Insert the needle in the middle to upper part of the desired interspace. In patients with poor landmarks, insert the needle in the presumed midline and explore. If the needle strikes bone, assess your location (spinous process: intermediate or shallow depth; lamina: deeper) and adjust your approach accordingly.

The paramedian approach requires some applied geometry. The insertion site is approximately 1 cm lateral to the superior edge of the inferior spinous process (Fig. 35-18). Angle the needle slightly cephalad and slightly medial, aiming for the midline at the estimated depth of the epidural or subarachnoid space. A bony obstruction at the estimated depth of the subarachnoid or

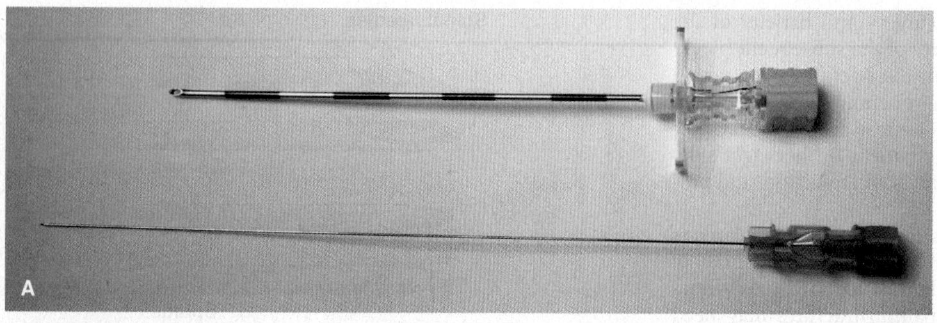

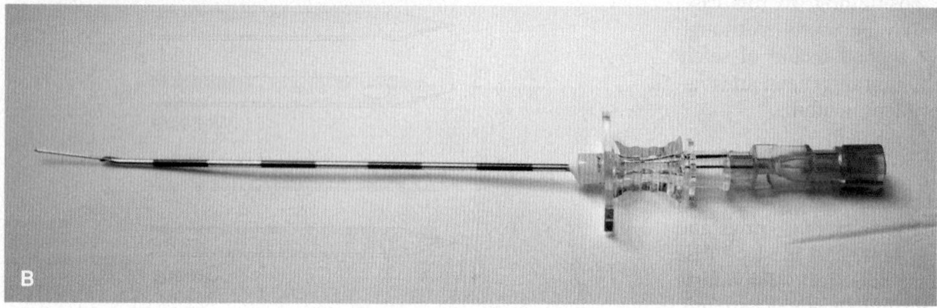

Figure 35-17 Combined spinal epidural using standard needles. **A:** An 18-gauge, 90-mm Tuohy needle and 27-gauge, 127-mm Whitacre needle side by side. **B:** Whitacre needle inserted through Tuohy needle.

epidural space is usually lamina. Most often, the needle strikes the upper edge of the lateral, lower lamina. Gradually, walk the needle cephalad until you enter the epidural or subarachnoid space. When attempting thoracic epidural needle placement, many experts intentionally contact the lamina of the vertebral body below the target interspace. This contact provides an estimation of the depth of the epidural space. The epidural needle can then be "walked up" the lamina and into the desired epidural space (Fig. 35-20).

Subarachnoid Spinal Anesthesia

After positioning the patient, preparing the skin, and applying a sterile drape, infiltrate the skin with a small amount of local anesthetic. A single pass with a finder needle may help identify the interspace. Injecting too much local anesthetic can obscure landmarks and make things more difficult. Using either a midline or paramedian approach, insert the introducer needle. Note that the introducer needle has a beveled tip. In the occasional thin or small patient, the introducer needle may accidentally enter the subarachnoid space. To limit the risk of PDPH in this situation, always insert the introducer needle as you would a cutting-tip spinal needle with the bevel oriented parallel to the longitudinal axis of the back. Next, pass the spinal needle through the shaft of the introducer needle and advance toward the subarachnoid space. Hold the hub of the spinal needle with your fingertips and appreciate the "clicks" and "pops" as the needle traverses the ligamentum flavum and the dura. Remove the stylet from the spinal needle after each pop to look for CSF. If the patient is sitting, CSF should appear promptly. If the patient is lying on their side (or prone), or if the spinal needle tip is angled downward, CSF may appear more slowly. If the spinal needle contacts bone, withdraw it into the shaft of the introducer needle and *pivot* the introducer slightly and reinsert the spinal needle (Fig. 35-21). If a midline introducer needle is inserted in the center of an interspace and the spinal needle contacts bone, it is

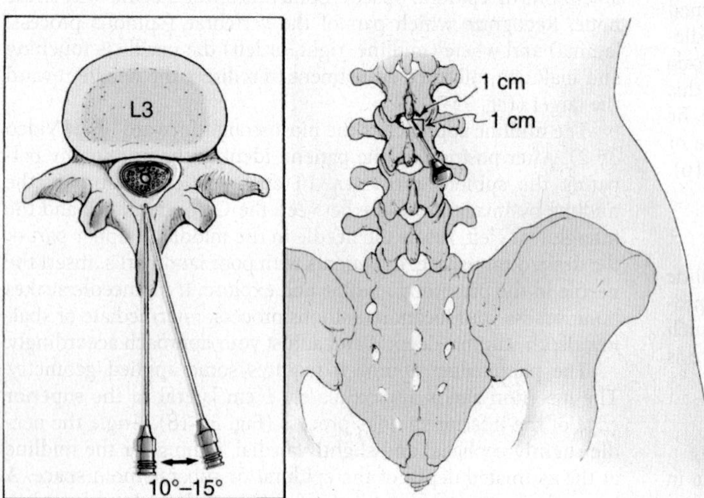

Figure 35-18 Vertebral anatomy of the lumbar midline and paramedian approaches. The midline approach requires anatomic projection in only two planes: sagittal and horizontal. The paramedian approach adds the oblique plane. The paramedian approach requires less lumbar flexion. The paramedian needle insertion site is 1 cm lateral and slightly below the cephalad edge of the more caudal spinous process. The needle is inserted 10 to 15 degrees off both sagittal and horizontal planes (*inset*). (Adapted from Chestnut DH, Wong CA, Tsen LC, et al., eds. *Chestnut's Obstetric Anesthesia: Principals and Practice*. 5th ed. WB Saunders; 2014:239. Copyright © 2014 Elsevier. With permission.)

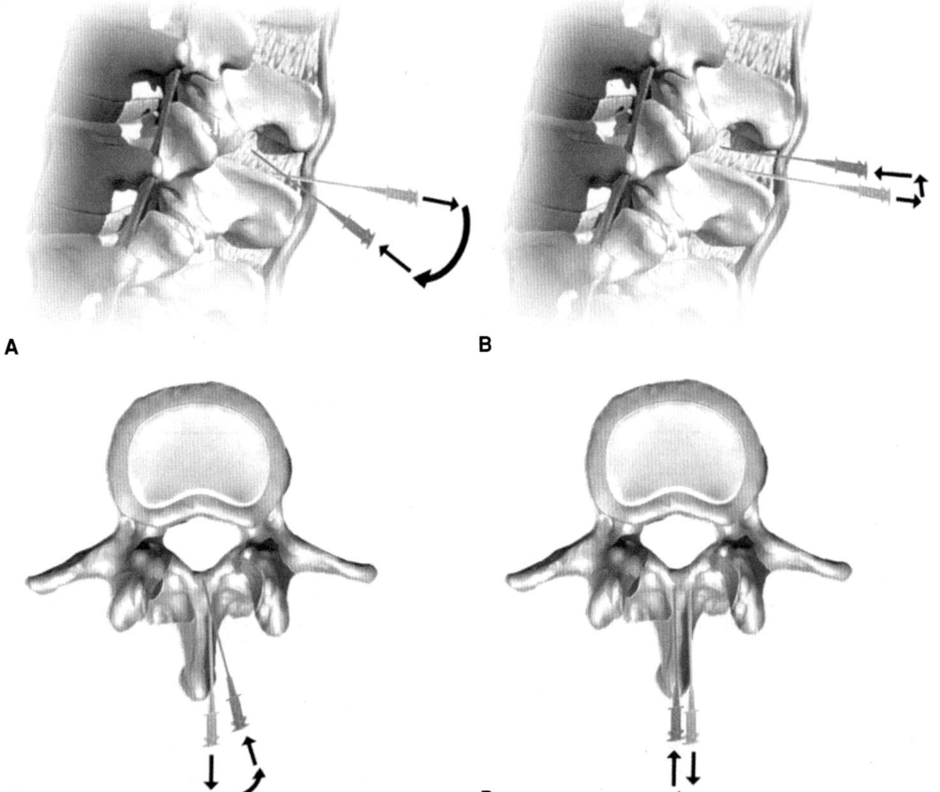

Figure 35-19 Troubleshooting contact with bones. The *gray* needle is the initial approach; the *blue* needle is the adjusted approach. **A:** If the needle is midline, redirect slightly more cephalad. **B:** Or, lift the needle after withdrawing it into the subcutaneous tissues. **C:** If the needle is off midline and contacting lamina, redirect as in **A. D:** Or, withdraw the needle into the subcutaneous tissue and shift as in **B.** (Adapted from Chestnut DH, Wong CA, Tsen LC, et al., eds. *Chestnut's Obstetric Anesthesia: Principals and Practice*. 5th ed. WB Saunders; 2014:239. Copyright © 2014 Elsevier. With permission.)

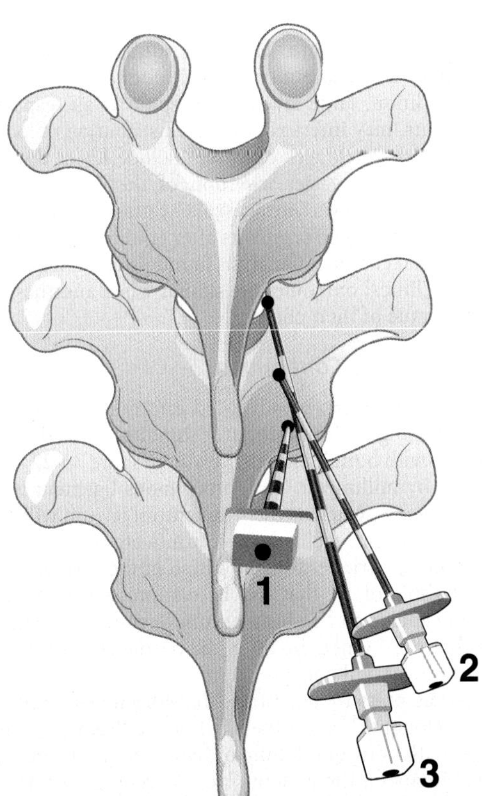

Figure 35-20 Thoracic epidural insertion: use the lamina as a depth marker and "walk" the needle into the epidural space.

most likely lamina of the lower vertebra (Fig. 35-19). By slowly redirecting the needle cephalad, you should be able to "walk off" the lamina and into the subarachnoid space. The spinal needle should advance a little deeper with each redirection. If you still do not enter the subarachnoid space, remove the spinal needle, palpate the back, and reassess the insertion site of your introducer needle.

Patients will occasionally report a transient paresthesia during spinal needle insertion. These paresthesias may be from needle to nerve root contact within the subarachnoid space[52] or they may emanate from the dura. Should a transient paresthesia occur, stop advancing the spinal needle, and withdraw the stylet. If you see CSF, inject the medication into the subarachnoid space. Do not inject if the paresthesia persists or recurs. Instead, remove and reposition the spinal needle.

Once clear CSF appears in the hub of the spinal needle, fix the needle in position with your nondominant hand and attach the syringe containing the medication. Aspirate gently. If using a hyperbaric solution, you will see birefringence (Schlieren lines), which indicates the mixing of solutions of differing baricities. Some experts recommend rotating the spinal needle 360 degrees to confirm free flow of CSF in four quadrants. This step is unnecessary.

Drug emerges directly from the tip of cutting-point needles, so needle bevel orientation has no effect on the subsequent level of subarachnoid block. Pencil-point needles have side holes, which produce directional flow of injected drug. Side-hole orientation, especially caudal versus cephalad, influences the distribution of both hyperbaric and isobaric local anesthetics.[53,54] In most cases, orient the side-hole toward the head to ensure adequate sensory block and to minimize the risks of local anesthetic pooling around the cauda equina (see Toxicity, below).

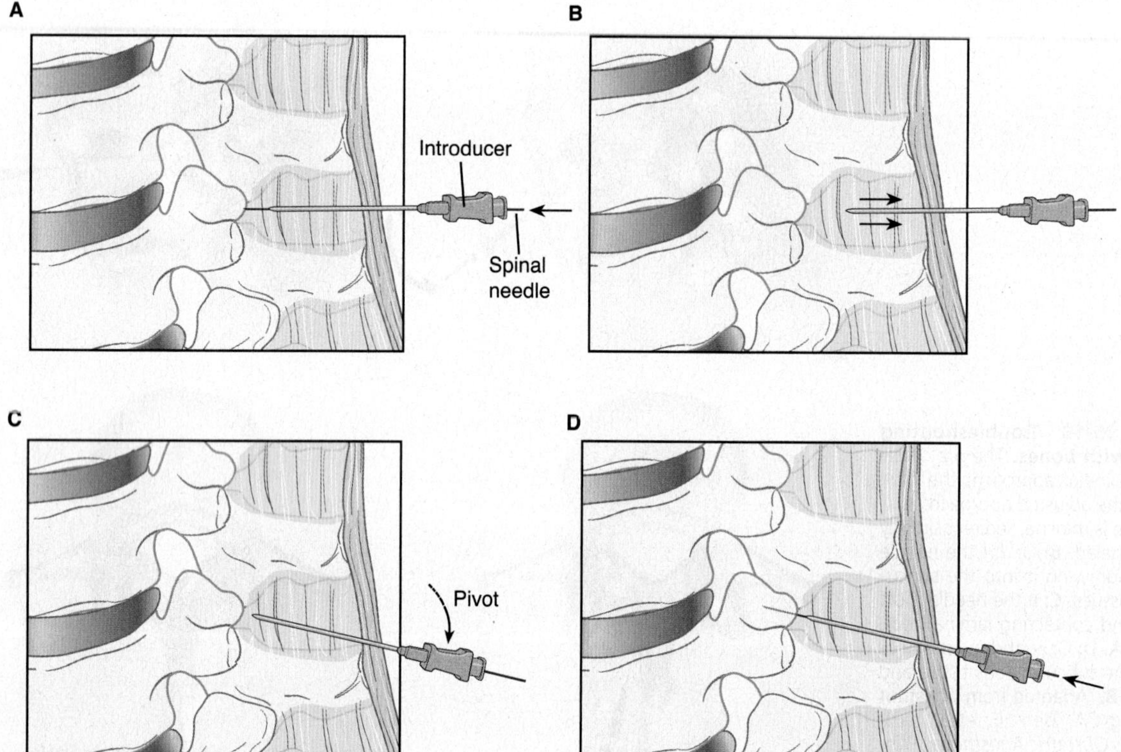

Figure 35-21 Using an introducer needle. If the spinal needle contacts bone (**A**), withdraw it into the shaft of the introducer needle (**B**). Otherwise, the spinal needle will merely bend, not change direction. After withdrawing the spinal needle, *pivot* the introducer (**C**) and reinsert the spinal needle (**D**).

Continuous Subarachnoid Spinal Anesthesia

After identifying the subarachnoid space with a large-gauge needle, insert an appropriately sized catheter 2 to 3 cm. The catheter will advance more easily and be more likely to lie cephalad to the insertion site if the bevel or orifice of the needle is directed toward the patient's head. Caudally directed catheters may cause pooling and maldistribution of local anesthetic, which has been associated with permanent neurologic injury (see Complications).

Epidural Anesthesia

The epidural space can be identified with either the hanging drop or loss-of-resistance technique. With the hanging drop technique, place a drop of saline at the hub of the epidural needle. As the needle enters the epidural space, the drop of liquid will be pulled into the needle. This technique relies on negative pressure within the epidural space. It is more reliable for thoracic than lumbar needle insertion.

Most anesthesiologists use a loss-of-resistance technique to identify the epidural space. When the tip of the epidural needle lies within the ligamentum flavum, there is resistance to injection. As the tip of the needle enters the epidural space, this resistance disappears. Common variations of the loss-of-resistance technique use air or saline in the loss-of-resistance syringe and intermittent or continuous pressure to advance the epidural needle.

Air versus Saline

Anesthesiologists often have a preference for air or saline in the loss-of-resistance syringe. Air has the advantage of simplicity. In addition, using air makes it easier to recognize an accidental or intentional dural puncture. However, intracranial air, injected after an accidental dural puncture, will produce an instant headache.[55] In addition, large amounts of epidural air, especially in smaller patients, may interfere with the distribution of local anesthetic. Proposed advantages of saline include fewer dural punctures, fewer PDPHs, easier insertion of the epidural catheter, fewer paresthesias, fewer intravascular catheters, better analgesia, and fewer unblocked segments after epidural local anesthetic injection. *But* a recent meta-analysis found **no** advantages of saline versus air.[56] Clinical outcomes are similar when anesthesiologists use the technique of their choice.[57]

Intermittent versus Continuous

The epidural needle can be advanced intermittently or continuously. When using an intermittent technique, grasp the epidural needle firmly with both hands as shown in Figure 35-22. Advance it millimeter by millimeter. The intraspinous ligament will present little resistance, whereas the ligamentum flavum will feel firm and gritty. In between each advance, firmly tap the plunger of the loss-of-resistance syringe. If using saline in the syringe, you may include a bubble of air that can be compressed with each tap. When the needle is in the ligamentum flavum, the plunger will recoil or "bounce." Once the tip of the needle enters the epidural space, the plunger will collapse.

Continuous pressure techniques have been described by Bromage[58] and Doughty[59] and others.[60] For the Bromage technique, make a fist with your nondominant hand and place your carpal–metacarpal joints on the patient's back. Firmly grasp the shaft of the epidural needle between your thumb and forefinger. Advance the needle slowly by rolling your fist into the patient's back. Meanwhile, use your dominant hand to apply continuous pressure to

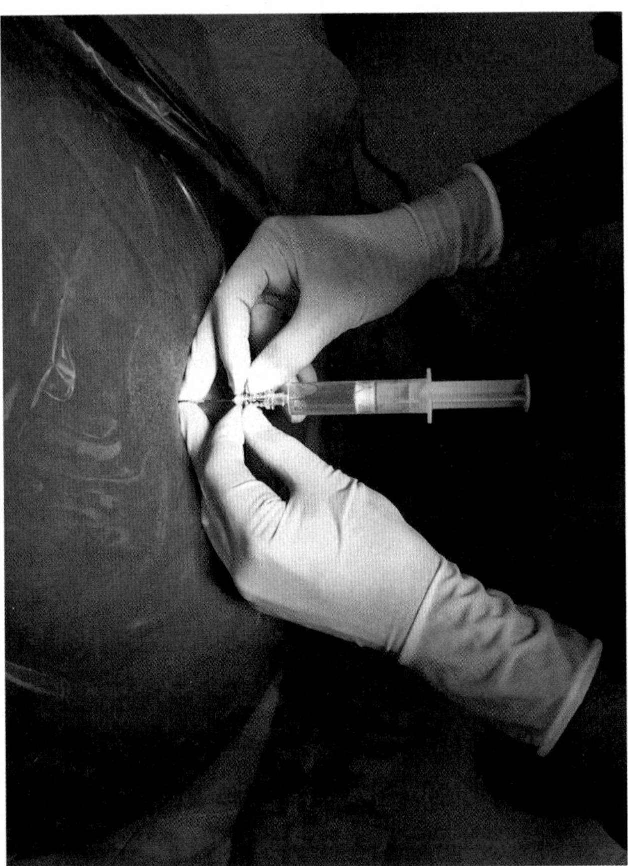

Figure 35-22 **Hand positions for intermittently advancing a needle toward the epidural space using a winged needle.** Grasping the wings with your index fingers and thumb, place your long fingers alongside the shaft at the site of insertion. Your thumb and index fingers advance the needle while the middle fingers control the needle's forward movement.

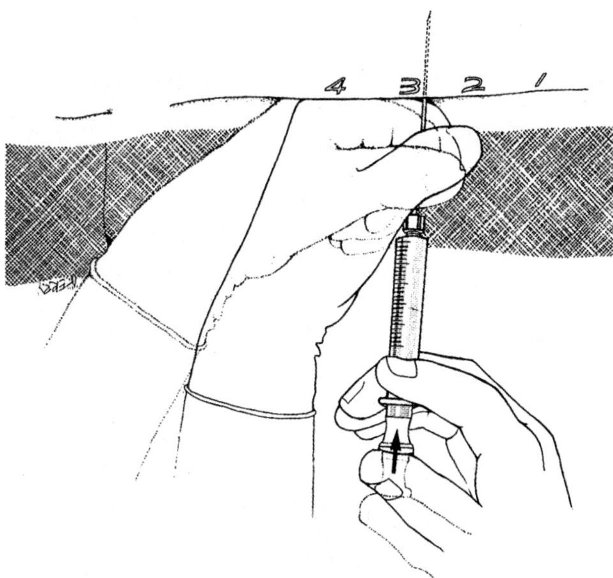

Figure 35-23 **The Bromage technique for identifying the epidural space.** Grip the needle shaft with the nondominant hand. Drive the needle forward by slowly extending the wrist and rocking forward on the knuckles. Use the thumb of the nondominant hand to apply constant pressure to the plunger of the syringe. The plunger will collapse when the tip of the needle enters the epidural space. (Reprinted with permission from Norris MC, ed. *Obstetric Anesthesia*. 2nd ed. Lippincott Williams & Wilkins; 1999:302; Original drawing from Bromage PR. *Epidural Analgesia*. WB Saunders, 1978:329, with permission.)

the plunger of the loss-of-resistance syringe, which can contain either air or saline. Stop advancing the needle when the plunger collapses (Fig. 35-23).

In the Doughty technique, the roles of the hands are reversed. Brace the epidural needle with your nondominant hand to control its advance. Grasp the barrel of the loss-of-resistance syringe with your dominant hand so the metacarpal head of your index finger is positioned on the end of the plunger (Fig. 35-24). Slowly advance the needle by balancing the driving pressure from your dominant hand with resistance from your bracing hand. Use the metacarpal head of the dominant index finger to exert pressure on the end of the plunger; you will perceive the loss of resistance immediately upon entering the epidural space.[59]

More common today are various "son-of-Doughty" techniques. Here, the driving pressure is applied directly to the plunger of a saline-filled loss-of-resistance syringe (Fig. 35-25).[60] When the tip of the needle enters the epidural space, the plunger collapses and the needle stops advancing.

As with the choice between air and saline, any technique done well is better than the best technique done poorly.

The Epidural Catheter

After identifying the epidural space, you can inject local anesthetic through either the needle or a catheter. Injecting through

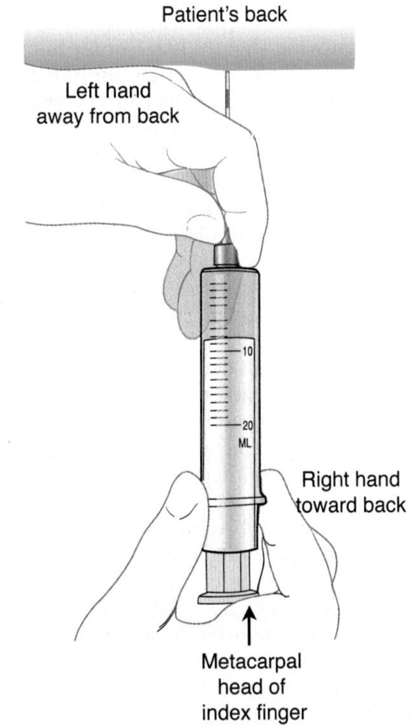

Figure 35-24 **The Doughty technique: the nondominant (left) hand braces the needle against the patient's back.** The dominant (**right**) hand advances the needle by grasping the hub while applying pressure to the plunger with the metacarpal head of the index finger. The right hand will feel the loss of resistance as soon as it occurs.

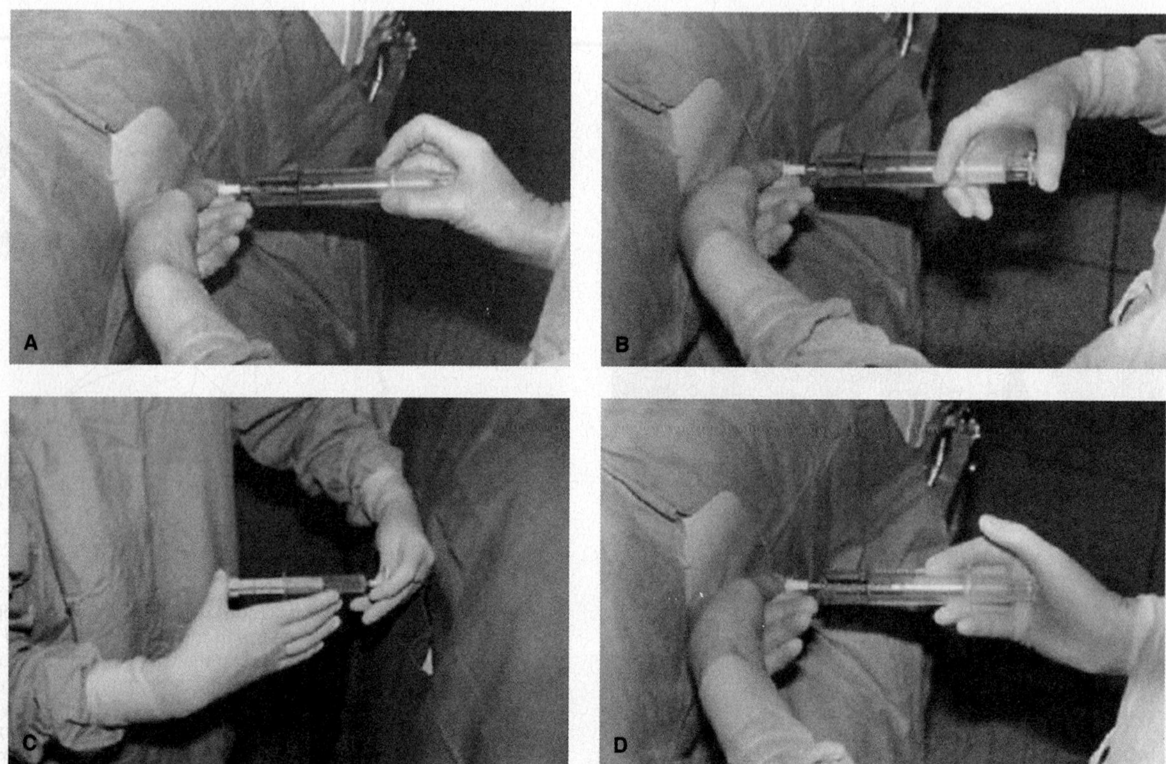

Figure 35-25 Hand positions for (A) the original Doughty technique and (B), (C), and (D) various "son-of-Doughty" techniques. (**A, B,** and **D** reprinted from Russell R, Porter J, Scrutton M. In: Reynolds F, ed. Pain Relief in Labour. London: BMJ Publishing; 1997. Copyright © 1997 John Wiley & Sons. **C** reprinted from Reynolds F. Hand positions and the 'son-of-Doughty' technique. *Anaesthesia*. 2005;60:717–718. Copyright © 2016 Association of Anaesthetists of Great Britain & Ireland.)

the needle will provide slightly faster onset but risks complications if drug is accidentally injected intrathecally or intravenously. Inserting a catheter into the epidural space encourages more careful injection of the initial dose of medication and allows the provision of epidural anesthesia or analgesia for as long as needed. Most epidural catheters are made of nylon or polyamide. Some are wire reinforced. Catheters can have a single orifice at the tip or multiple orifices along the distal end. Multiorifice catheters allow wider distribution of injected medication and, in laboring women, are associated with more extensive block and better analgesia. Nylon and polyamide catheters can be flimsy and kink at the hub of the epidural needle. Many come with "threading assist devices" that seat in the hub of the epidural needle and ease catheter insertion. Try to insert about 5 cm of catheter into the epidural space. Inserting less increases the chances that the catheter will become dislodged. Inserting more makes it more likely that the catheter will enter a blood vessel.[61] Although the orientation of the epidural needle bevel will determine the initial direction of the epidural catheter, it does not reliably aim the catheter in a cephalad or caudad direction. Most epidural catheters curl on themselves at the level of insertion. If you meet resistance while inserting the catheter, *do not* withdraw and try to reinsert. Some epidural needles have a sharp inner bevel that can shear the tip of a catheter. Instead, remove both needle and catheter together and reidentify the epidural space.

Once the epidural catheter is inserted, it is time to remove the needle. Hold the epidural catheter about 1 cm from the hub of the needle. Gently withdraw the needle, sliding it along the catheter until the hub meets your fingertips. Move your fingers back another centimeter and repeat the process. When the tip of the needle comes out of the skin, grasp the catheter between the needle and the skin and slide the needle off the catheter.

Combined Subarachnoid Spinal Epidural

Technique

The needle-through-needle technique is the most common method of combined spinal epidural (CSE) block. Because the conus medullaris sometimes extends to L2 or even L3, it is safest to perform a CSE block at the L3–L4 or L4–L5 interspaces (see Complications, below). First, identify the epidural space with your usual technique. Using air in the loss-of-resistance syringe will assure that any liquid flowing through the spinal needle is indeed CSF. After identifying the epidural space, insert a long, small-gauge spinal needle. You should feel some resistance as the tip of the spinal needle passes the tip of the epidural needle. Then, you will feel a subtle pop as the spinal needle pierces the dura. Stabilize the spinal needle by pinching the hubs of both needles between your thumb and finger (Fig. 35-26). Withdraw the stylet from the spinal needle and look for CSF. Once CSF is appreciated, carefully inject the subarachnoid medication, withdraw the spinal needle, and insert the epidural catheter.

Troubleshooting

The most common problem encountered with the needle-through-needle technique is failure to see CSF in the hub of the spinal needle (Fig. 35-27). Most often, the spinal needle has not entered the subarachnoid space. The epidural needle may not be in the epidural space or it may be directed laterally. Sometimes,

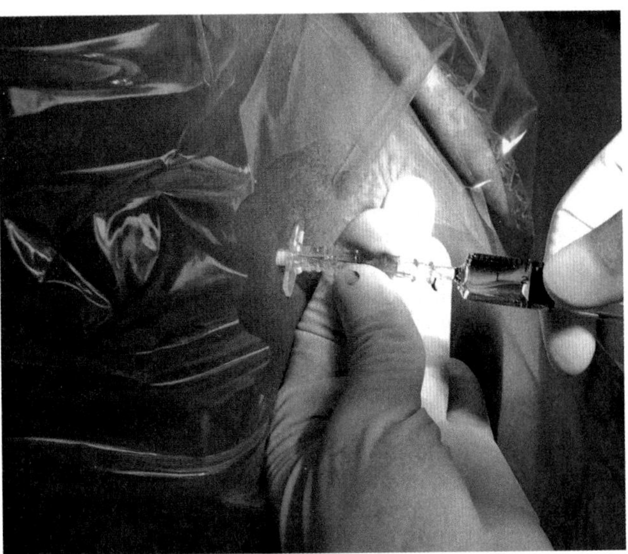

Figure 35-26 Hand position for stabilizing CSE needles. The thumb and index finger pinch the hubs of both spinal and epidural needles to fix the position of the spinal needle.

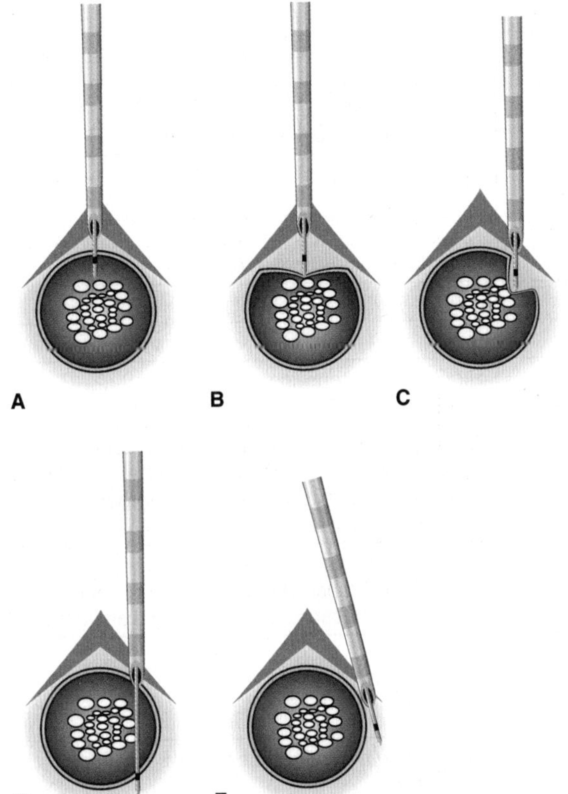

Figure 35-27 Different positions of epidural and spinal needles with the needle-through-needle CSE technique. A: The ideal position; a midline epidural needle guides the spinal needle into the subarachnoid space. **B:** Spinal needle too short; it indents but does not pierce the dura. **C:** Spinal needle too short and too lateral. **D:** Spinal needle too long; it has passed through the subarachnoid space. **E:** Spinal needle too lateral; the epidural needle is in the epidural space but it guides the spinal needle away from the dural sac. (Adapted with permission from Norris MC, ed. *Obstetric Anesthesia*. 2nd ed. Lippincott Williams & Wilkins; 1999:307.)

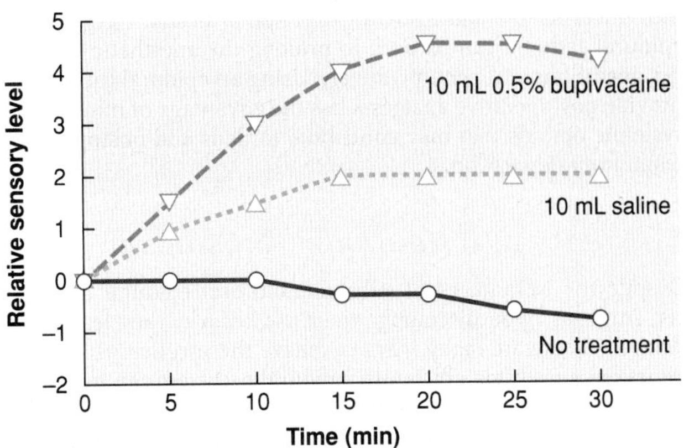

Figure 35-28 Spread of sensory block with CSE. Nonpregnant patients received 10 mg 0.5% bupivacaine intrathecally. After the maximum level of sensory block had been achieved, patients received nothing (O), 10 mL epidural saline (Δ), or 10 mL epidural bupivacaine (∇). (Adapted with permission from Norris MC, ed. *Obstetric Anesthesia*. 2nd ed. Lippincott Williams & Wilkins; 1999:309; Reprinted with permission from Stienstra R, Dahan A, Alhadi BZR, et al. Mechanism of action of an epidural top-up in combined spinal epidural anesthesia. *Anesth Analg*. 1996;83:382.)

the spinal needle does not extend far enough to penetrate the dura. This problem is more likely to occur if the patient is in the lateral position rather than sitting. Sometimes, rotating the spinal needle 360 degrees will be enough to enter the subarachnoid space. Otherwise, consider proceeding with an epidural technique or reidentifying the epidural space.

Drug Dosing

The CSE technique can alter the behavior of both intrathecal and epidural medications. Because the epidural catheter can be used to supplement the subarachnoid block, it is possible to use smaller doses of subarachnoid medication. Less intrathecal local anesthetic may limit the hemodynamic effects of subarachnoid anesthesia. Epidural injection of local anesthetic or saline can raise the level of sensory block even after the level of subarachnoid anesthesia has stabilized (Fig. 35-28). The presence of a small-gauge dural hole also may enhance the spread of subsequent epidural medications. This effect may be responsible for the improved labor epidural analgesia reported after previous 25-gauge needle dural puncture.[62] 4

Choice of Technique

Subarachnoid anesthesia, with its rapid onset of dense sensory block, is often the best choice for surgeries of known duration (usually <2 hours). Epidural anesthesia is slower in onset, which may be helpful when caring for hemodynamically fragile patients. In addition, the epidural catheter can be used for postoperative analgesia. Thoracic epidural analgesia is an important part of many ERAS protocols for patients undergoing major intra-abdominal and intrathoracic procedures. CSE anesthesia can offer the benefits of both techniques for lower abdominal and lower extremity surgeries. The intrathecal component can provide rapid anesthesia, whereas the epidural catheter can be used to extend anesthetic duration and provide postoperative analgesia. The CSE technique also is a good alternative to subarachnoid anesthesia in morbidly obese patients. It can be easier to find the subarachnoid space after identifying the epidural space with a 17- or 18-gauge needle than when using only a short introducer needle and a small-gauge spinal needle.[63] Again, the epidural catheter can be used to prolong the anesthetic for longer operations and postoperatively. Using an epidural catheter to provide postoperative analgesia has the advantage of minimizing systemic opioids that may contribute to ileus and postoperative respiratory depression.

Efficiency and Neuraxial Anesthesia

Despite the advantages of subarachnoid and epidural anesthesia, surgeons often discourage their use because they fear being delayed. There are many ways to relieve these concerns and use neuraxial anesthesia efficiently. Epidural catheters can be placed before the patient enters the OR. Some operating suites have designated procedure rooms or block rooms for this purpose. In other settings, epidural catheters can be placed in the preoperative holding area. Subarachnoid anesthesia kits can be opened in advance. Drugs can be drawn up into appropriately labeled sterile syringes. The kit can then be rewrapped and set aside, ready to use as soon as the patient enters the OR. Finally, performing subarachnoid and epidural blocks regularly will improve skills and build confidence, both yours and your surgeon's.

Pharmacology

Subarachnoid Anesthesia

Spread and Duration

Density and dose are the two most important factors that determine the spread and duration of subarachnoid anesthesia. Density is the ratio of the mass of a substance to its volume. Baricity is the ratio of two densities: here, the density of CSF and that of the local anesthetic. Currently used local anesthetics are made *hyperbaric* by mixing with dextrose. Most plain local anesthetic solutions are *isobaric* or slightly *hypobaric*. Table 35-2 offers suggestions for dose and baricity when performing subarachnoid anesthesia for various surgeries.

Hyperbaric local anesthetics are denser than CSF and will flow with gravity to the dependent areas of the spine, usually the

Table 35-2 Some Common Surgical Procedures that Can Be Done with Subarachnoid Spinal Anesthesia

Procedure	Level	Local Anesthetic	Comments
Obstetrics			
Cesarean section	≥T6	12–15 mg hyperbaric bupivacaine[a]	Lower doses may produce less hypotension but should be used as part of a combined subarachnoid epidural technique. Adding a lipophilic opioid may improve intraoperative analgesia.
Postpartum tubal ligation (minilaparotomy)	≥T8	10–12 mg hyperbaric bupivacaine	
Cervical cerclage	≥T10	5–7.5 mg hyperbaric bupivacaine	Faster discharge with smaller doses; 2-chloroprocaine can be used as an alternative
Orthopedics			
Hip fracture or replacement	≥T12	10–20 mg isobaric[b] bupivacaine	Sitting or lateral position with the operative side *up*
Knee replacement	≥T12	12–15 mg hyperbaric bupivacaine or 7–10 mg isobaric bupivacaine	Higher level if tourniquet used
Knee arthroscopy	≥T12	5–7.5 mg either isobaric or hyperbaric bupivacaine	Faster discharge with smaller dose. Lipophilic opioid may help with tourniquet pain. Alternatively, can use 40-mg preservative-free 2-chloroprocaine for outpatient procedures.
Ankle surgery	≥T12	At least 7.5 mg hyperbaric bupivacaine	Dose depends on expected duration of procedure. Combined subarachnoid epidural or peripheral nerve blocks can add postoperative analgesia.
Urology			
Cystoscopy	≥T10	2.5–5.0 mg isobaric or hyperbaric bupivacaine	Faster discharge with smaller dose
Transurethral resection of bladder tumor or prostate	≥T10	At least 7.5 mg isobaric or hyperbaric bupivacaine	Adjust dose according to expected duration of surgery.
Penile prosthesis	≥T10	12–15 mg hyperbaric bupivacaine	
General Surgery			
Inguinal hernia repair/open appendectomy	≥T8	12–15 mg hyperbaric bupivacaine	
Perianal/perirectal	Sacral	5–7.5 mg hyperbaric bupivacaine (lithotomy position)	Smaller doses of isobaric bupivacaine (2.5–5 mg) can be used if the patient will be prone.

[a]In the United States: 0.75% bupivacaine with 8.25% dextrose.
[b]Preservative-free 0.5% bupivacaine.

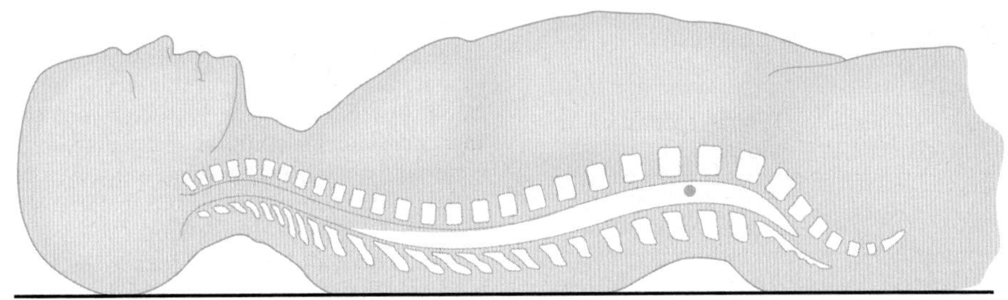

Figure 35-29 In the supine position, hyperbaric local anesthetics injected at the apex of the lumbar lordosis (*circle*) flow with gravity and pool in the sacrum and thoracic kyphosis. Thoracic pooling may be why hyperbaric solutions typically produce midthoracic levels of sensory block. (Reprinted with permission from Barash PG, Cullen BF, Stoelting RK, et al., eds. *Clinical Anesthesia*. 7th ed. Wolters Kluwer; 2015;917.)

upper thoracic region in supine patients (Fig. 35-29). Positioning patients upright or lateral can limit the initial spread of hyperbaric local anesthetic. But, when the patient returns to the supine position, even after 20 to 30 minutes, the sensory level reaches the usual midthoracic dermatomes.

Bulk displacement determines the initial spread of isobaric drug. Subsequently, movement of CSF by either transmission of cardiac pulsations[64] or gross patient movements (i.e., turning from lateral to supine position[65]) will determine the ultimate spread of block.

In nonpregnant patients, hyperbaric local anesthetics produce more consistent levels of sensory block than isobaric drug (Fig. 35-30).[66] Isobaric drugs produce longer blocks.[67] When used for subarachnoid anesthesia for cesarean section, there is little difference between equal doses of isobaric or hyperbaric bupivacaine.[68]

Patient Variables

5 Height, weight, BMI, and vertebral column length have no clinically significant effect on the spread of subarachnoid anesthesia. Increasing age is associated with slower onset and longer duration but no change in extent of subarachnoid block.[69] Both female gender and pregnancy increase motor blockade produced by intrathecal isobaric bupivacaine.[70] One small study reported that CSF volume correlated with the spread of subarachnoid anesthesia.[71] Pregnant patients will develop higher levels of sensory block than nonpregnant patients when given the same dose of intrathecal local anesthetic. This enhanced sensitivity disappears shortly after delivery.[72] In nonpregnant adults, increasing abdominal girth correlates with increasing extent of sensory block after intrathecal injection of isobaric bupivacaine.[73] Increases in intra-abdominal and consequently epidural space pressure associated with both pregnancy and obesity may enhance sensory spread by decreasing lumbar CSF volume.

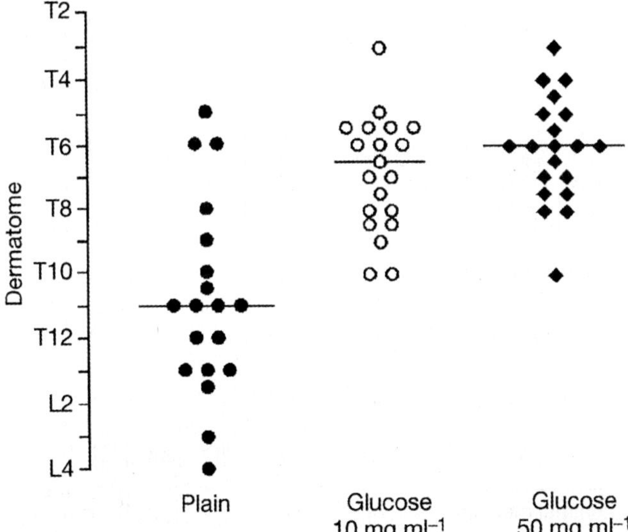

Figure 35-30 Range of sensory block after intrathecal injection of two different solutions of 0.5% tetracaine. Solutions containing dextrose, which are hyperbaric, produce more consistent levels of block than plain (isobaric) solutions. (Reprinted with permission from van Kleef JW, Veering BT, Burm AGL. Spinal anaesthesia with ropivacaine: a double-blind study on the efficacy and safety of 0.5% and 0.75% solutions in patients undergoing minor lower limb surgery. *Anesth Analg*. 1994;78(6):1125–1130.)

Local Anesthetic Dose

Within commonly used ranges (i.e., 7.5 to 12 mg hyperbaric bupivacaine), increasing the dose of local anesthetic does not significantly raise the level of block.[69] At some point (i.e., 15 mg hyperbaric bupivacaine), a higher sensory level will develop.[74] Larger doses of both hyperbaric and isobaric local anesthetics produce denser and longer-lasting anesthesia.

Adjuvants

Many drugs have been studied for their ability to prolong or improve subarachnoid anesthesia. Vasoconstrictors, such as epinephrine or phenylephrine, may prolong the intrathecal block by inhibiting absorption of intrathecal local anesthetics or by acting directly on spinal cord α-receptors. Vasoconstrictors prolong the duration of intrathecal tetracaine. They have no clinically significant effects on the duration of intrathecal lidocaine. Some studies report that epinephrine prolongs the duration of intrathecal bupivacaine.[75]

The α_2-agonists clonidine and dexmedetomidine prolong the duration of subarachnoid anesthesia and analgesia. Associated bradycardia may require atropine.[76] Larger doses of intrathecal clonidine also can cause hypotension and sedation.[77]

Lipid-soluble opioids (fentanyl or sufentanil) can enhance intraoperative anesthesia and provide a few hours of postoperative analgesia. Small doses of fentanyl (5 to 10 μg) are as effective as larger doses and produce less pruritus. Intrathecal preservative-free morphine, which is hydrophilic, can provide prolonged (12 to 24 hours) postoperative analgesia as it remains in the CSF but side effects, including pruritus, nausea, and vomiting, are common and challenging to treat. Rarely, intrathecal morphine can produce delayed respiratory depression.

Epidural Anesthesia

Lumbar epidural anesthesia can be used interchangeably with subarachnoid anesthesia in most cases. One exception is procedures involving the S1 dermatome (i.e., ankle surgery). S1 is the

Table 35-3 Recommendations for Epidural Anesthesia

Type of Surgery	Insertion Site	Typical spread of Block
Thoracic	T2–T6	T2–T6 (5–10 mL local anesthetic)
Abdominal	T6–L1	T1–L4 (10–20 mL local anesthetic)
Lower extremity or pelvic, peripheral vascular, obstetric	Lumbar L2–L5	T8–S5 (20 mL local anesthetic)
C8–T8 (upper level of sensory block)		

Modified with permission from Visser WA, Lee RA, Gielen MJM. Factors affecting the distribution of neural blockade by local anesthetics in epidural anesthesia and a comparison of lumbar versus thoracic epidural anesthesia. *Anesth Analg*. 2008;107:708–721.

largest nerve root in the body, and the onset of epidural block can be slow and incomplete. Thoracic epidural injection can provide segmental block, which can supplement general anesthesia for upper abdominal and intrathoracic surgeries (Table 35-3).

Spread of Block

Patient variables, drug dose, and site of injection are the main determinants of the spread of epidural block.[78] A given dose of local anesthetic will spread farther in older compared to younger patients. As a result, the risk of hypotension associated with epidural local anesthetics may be greater in older patients. Height, weight, and BMI have no clinically significant effects on the extent of epidural block. However, increases in intra-abdominal and consequently epidural space pressure associated with pregnancy and obesity may enhance sensory spread. Pregnant patients will develop more extensive block after a fixed dose of local anesthetic than nonpregnant patients.[79]

The extent of epidural block is proportional to the dose of local anesthetic injected. Mass of drug, not the volume injected, mostly determines the extent of sensory block. However, the relationship is not linear. A smaller dose produces a relatively greater spread (dermatomes/dose) than a larger dose.[78]

Site of injection has a major impact on the spread of epidural block. Small doses of local anesthetic (5 to 10 mL) will produce a band of anesthesia around the injection site. Lumbar injection spreads more cephalad than caudad, whereas upper thoracic injection blocks more dermatomes below than above the injection site (Fig. 35-31).[80]

Onset and Duration

Onset and duration of epidural anesthesia depend largely on the choice of anesthetic (Table 35-4). Some sign of sensory block should be detectable at the dermatomal level of injection within 5 to 10 minutes. The full extent of block usually develops within 20 to 30 minutes. Differences in onset time between local anesthetics are small and rarely clinically significant.[81] 2-Chloroprocaine has fastest onset but shortest duration followed by lidocaine and mepivacaine. The more potent drugs, bupivacaine and ropivacaine, have slower onset but the longer duration. Lidocaine produces relatively more motor block than

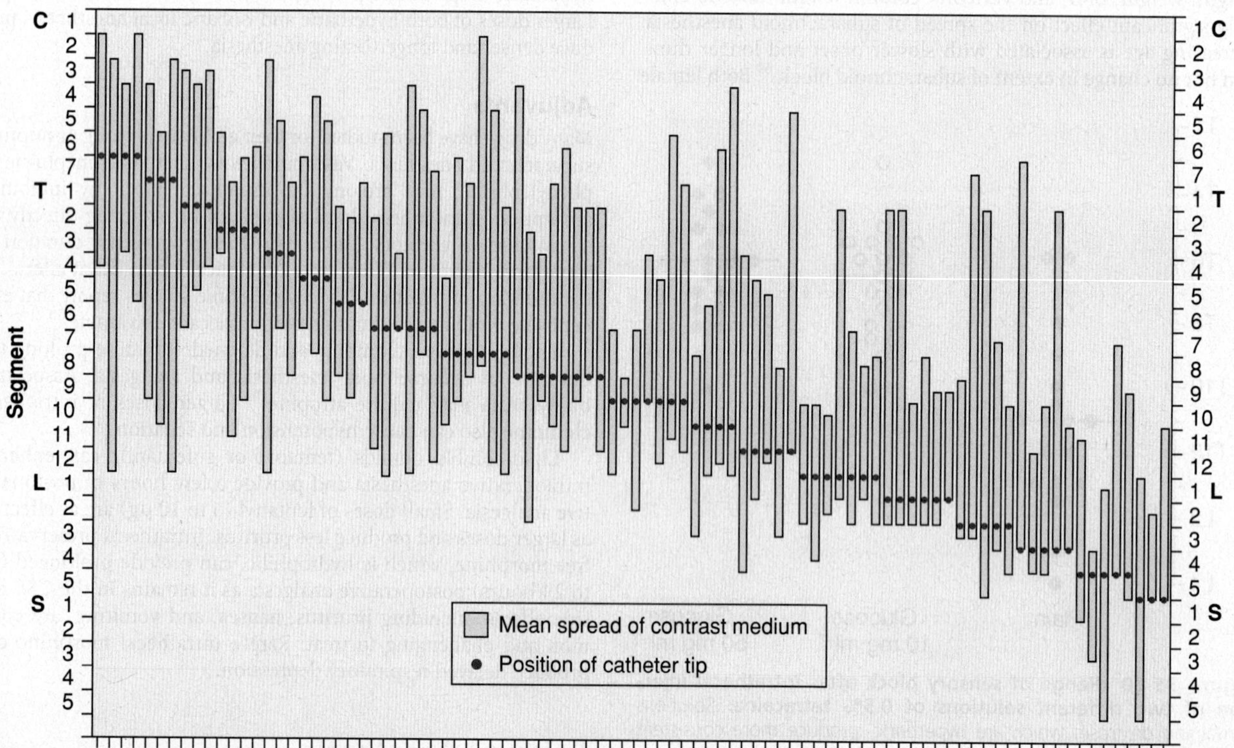

Figure 35-31 Mean radiographic spread after epidural injection of 5 mL iotrolan, 240 mg I/mL, in 90 patients. C, cervical segment; L, lumbar segment; S, sacral segment; T, thoracic segment. Cervical injection spreads more caudally, whereas lumbar injection spreads more cranially. (Adapted with permission from Yokoyama M, Hanazaki M, Fujii H, et al. Correlation between the distribution of contrast medium and the extent of blockade during epidural anesthesia. *Anesthesiology*. 2004;100:1504–1510.)

Table 35-4 Local Anesthetics Used for Surgical Epidural Block

Drug	Duration: Two-Dermatome Regression (min)	Duration: Complete Resolution (min)	Prolongation by Epinephrine (%)
2-Chloroprocaine 3%	45–60	100–160	40–60
Lidocaine 2%	60–100	160–200[a]	40–80[b]
Mepivacaine 2%	60–100	160–200	40–80
Ropivacaine 0.5–1.0%	90–180	240–420	None
Bupivacaine 0.5–0.75%[c]	120–240	300–460	None

[a]Motor block can outlast sensory block.
[b]Epinephrine also improves quality of sensory block.
[c]Use only 0.5% bupivacaine in obstetric patients.

sensory block. Postoperative patients may have pain before the motor block has completely regressed. Sensory block usually outlasts motor block with mepivacaine, ropivacaine, and bupivacaine.

Surgery often outlasts the duration of the initial epidural injection. Injecting half the initial dose once the block has regressed by two dermatomes should maintain an adequate level of block. Another way to maintain surgical anesthesia is to inject a fixed dose of drug at regular intervals. For lumbar epidural catheters, inject 5 mL 0.5% ropivacaine or bupivacaine every 60 minutes. Use the same approach with thoracic epidural catheters but inject a smaller volume (2.5 mL).

Adjuvants

Adjuvants can speed the onset, improve the quality, and prolong the duration of epidural block.[78]

Sodium Bicarbonate

Sodium bicarbonate raises the pH of commercially prepared local anesthetics, increasing the amount of nonionized, active drug. Adding sodium bicarbonate speeds the onset and increases the density of epidural local anesthetic block. These effects are most pronounced with lidocaine. Bupivacaine readily precipitates in the presence of sodium bicarbonate.

Epinephrine and α_2-Agonists

Epinephrine-induced vasoconstriction decreases systemic absorption of local anesthetics. In addition, stimulation of spinal cord α_2-receptors produces analgesia. Adding α_2-agonists (epinephrine, clonidine, or dexmedetomidine) to local anesthetic speeds the onset and improves the quality of epidural anesthesia. Clinically, adding epinephrine 5 μg/mL to lidocaine markedly improves the quality of epidural anesthesia for cesarean section. Patients who receive lidocaine with epinephrine are about half as likely to experience intraoperative pain or need conversion to general anesthesia compared with patients who receive plain lidocaine.[82] Epidural clonidine or dexmedetomidine intensifies and prolongs the effects of epidural local anesthetics.[83] These drugs also provide postoperative analgesia.[84] Sedation, however, is common.

Opioids

Epidural opioids also speed the onset and improve the quality of block produced by local anesthetics. Fentanyl, sufentanil, hydromorphone, and morphine are the most commonly used opioids. These drugs also can provide postoperative analgesia. Pruritus, nausea, and vomiting are common side effects, especially with epidural morphine.[85] Opioid-only epidural infusions are not as common. Although they do not cause motor block or hypotension, epidural opioid-only infusions can produce nausea and pruritus.

Test Doses

Currently, most clinicians use a blind technique to identify the epidural space and insert a catheter. Intended epidural catheters may be subarachnoid, subdural, intravascular, or elsewhere. Misplaced injection of drugs intended for the epidural space can have serious adverse consequences. To minimize these risks, all epidural catheters should be tested *throughout* their use. The purpose of these tests is twofold: to prove that the catheter is not in an unintended place (i.e., intrathecal or intravenous) *and* to prove that the catheter is indeed in the epidural space.

The most common cause of significant anesthetic-related morbidity and mortality in laboring women is unrecognized *intrathecal* injection of local anesthetics.[86,87] When inducing epidural anesthesia or analgesia, first inject a small dose of local anesthetic (i.e., 30 to 45 mg lidocaine or 5 to 10 mg bupivacaine) through the catheter and look for signs of subarachnoid anesthesia. Within 2 to 3 minutes of intrathecal local anesthetic injection, patients will note warmth and tingling in their legs or feet. Sensory block to cold and pinprick can be detected.[88] In parturients, intrathecal lidocaine will also produce some (but not complete) motor block by 3 minutes. In laboring women, rapid onset of analgesia should also alert to intrathecal injection. Pay close attention to the intrathecal test dose. Positive findings can be subtle and easily overlooked on a busy labor and delivery floor. 6

Be aware of two limitations of lidocaine as an intrathecal test dose in pregnant women. First, some women will report warmth in their legs and motor weakness after *epidural* injection of 30 to 45 mg lidocaine. As a result, a positive intrathecal test dose should be evaluated carefully to avoid removing an appropriately placed epidural catheter. Second, when injected into the subarachnoid space, even these small doses of lidocaine can produce extensive sensory and sympathetic block (Fig. 35-32). Dangerously high subarachnoid anesthesia can occur.[89] In one report, unplanned intrathecal injection of 45 mg lidocaine

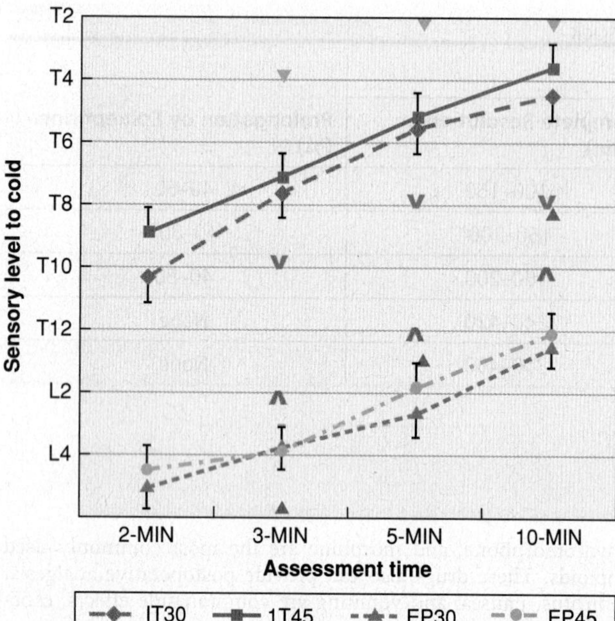

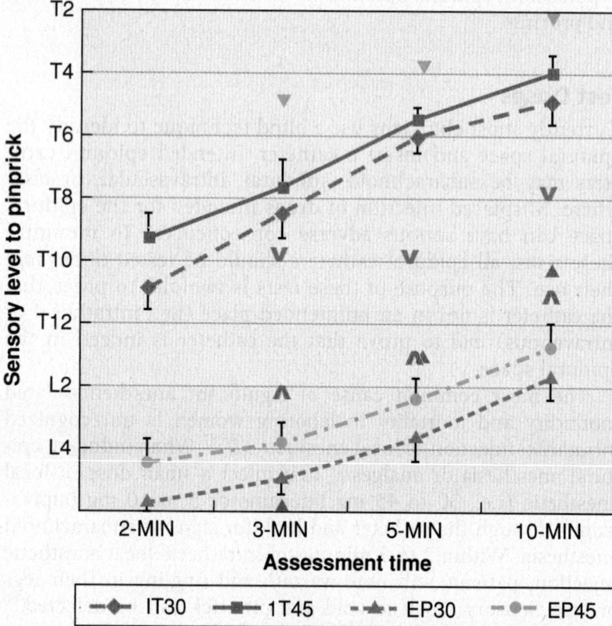

Figure 35-32 Spread of sensory block after intrathecal (IT) or epidural (EP) injection of 30 or 45 mg lidocaine. Both intrathecal doses produced significantly higher block than both epidural doses ($P < .01$ for each). IT30, intrathecal injection of 30 mg lidocaine; IT45, intrathecal injection of 45 mg lidocaine; EP30, epidural injection of 30 mg lidocaine; EP45, epidural injection of 45 mg lidocaine. The maximum and minimum outliers for each dose are added to demonstrate the overlap in sensory levels between epidural and intrathecal dosing. Maximum epidural outliers are represented by the *blue open triangle* for 30-mg dose, and *green solid triangle* for 45-mg dose. Minimum intrathecal outliers are represented by *black open triangle* for the 30-mg dose, and *red solid triangle* for the 45-mg dose. (Adapted with permission from Pratt S, Hess P, Vasudevan A. A prospective randomized trial of lidocaine 30 mg versus 45 mg for epidural test dose for intrathecal injection in the obstetric population. *Anesth Analg.* 2013;116:125–132.)

Table 35-5 Complications of Unintended Intrathecal Injection of 45 mg of Lidocaine in Parturients

Number of Patients (%)	Complication
8 (32%)	Hypotension prompting vasopressors (only)
3 (12%)	Cesarean delivery for nonreassuring fetal status (also received vasopressors)
4 (16%)	High spinal (shortness of breath, sensory level above T4, vasopressors)
10 (40%)	No complication

Data from Bolden N, Gebre E. Accidental dural puncture management: 10-year experience at an academic tertiary care center. *Reg Anesth Pain Med.* 2016;41:169–174.

produced clinically significant complications in 60% of patients (Table 35-5).[90]

7

Intravascular local anesthetic injection can produce seizures and even cardiac arrest. The most widely used intravenous test dose is lidocaine with epinephrine. Intravenous injection of epinephrine 15 μg will increase heart rate by at least 10 beats per minute and systolic blood pressure by at least 15 mmHg.[91] Unfortunately, sedation, general anesthesia, β-blockade, advancing age, and pre-existing neuraxial block can blunt this response. In laboring women, pain-induced tachycardia can be confused with a positive epinephrine response. In one study, the epinephrine test dose produced more false-positive than true-positive responses.[92]

In pregnant women, observation and aspiration will detect almost all intravascular catheters. Although it is tempting to withdraw an intravascular catheter until blood can no longer be aspirated, these catheters are often still in a blood vessel.[92]

Rarely, a catheter may be subdural (inside the dura mater but outside of the arachnoid mater) (Fig. 35-6).[93] Subdural catheters can present with varying degrees of sensory, motor, and sympathetic block. The subdural space extends cephalad to the floor of the third ventricle. Unrecognized subdural injection may be the cause of excessive epidural block. (The epidural space ends at the base of the skull and the cervical epidural space is very narrow. Lumbar *epidural* injection of local anesthetics should not produce cervical or higher levels of sensory block.)

The best test of an epidural catheter is to obtain level and density of blockade that are consistent with the local anesthetic injected. Thus, a laboring woman should develop bilateral sensory change and effective analgesia 20 to 30 minutes after receiving 10 to 15 mL of dilute local anesthetic or dilute local anesthetic with opioid solution. A surgical patient should notice warmth and numbness 5 to 10 minutes after receiving 2-chloroprocaine or lidocaine and 15 to 30 minutes after bupivacaine or ropivacaine. However, even a properly sited epidural catheter can migrate into a blood vessel or penetrate the dura.

Because no test dose is foolproof and even working epidural catheters can migrate, inject *all* drugs in increments small enough that they will not cause harm if misplaced (i.e., every dose is a "test" dose). Incremental injection may not detect intravascular catheters but should prevent systemic toxicity. If an epidural catheter does not behave as expected, do not inject more drug. Instead, remove and replace it.

Physiology

Central Nervous System

Site of Action

The exact site of action of subarachnoid and epidural anesthesia remains unknown. Local anesthetic can be detected throughout the spinal nerve rootlets and spinal cord after intrathecal injection. Local anesthetic injected into the epidural space diffuses through the dura and arachnoid and can be identified in the nerve rootlets and spinal cord as well.

Intrathecal local anesthetics reduce, but do not routinely eliminate, somatosensory evoked potentials (SSEPs). Cortical evoked potentials from direct spinal cord stimulation diminish but persist. These results suggest that some block of spinal cord conduction occurs, but that subarachnoid anesthesia occurs mostly within the spinal nerve roots.[94]

In monkeys, epidural local anesthetics alter evoked potentials in the nerve roots, dorsal root entry zone, and the long tracts of the spinal cord white matter.[95] In humans, epidural local anesthetics decrease SSEPs in areas of sensory block but not in dermatomes above or below,[96] suggesting a peripheral rather than spinal cord site of action.

Although intrathecal and epidural local anesthetics do not reach the brain, extensive neuraxial anesthesia does produce sedation. Neuraxial block also potentiates the effects of sedatives and decreases the minimum alveolar concentration of potent volatile anesthetic agents.[97,98]

Differential Nerve Block

Neuraxial local anesthetics have different potencies on motor, sensory, and sympathetic nerves. This differential block is largely related to the size of different nerves. Large motor nerves (and larger lumbar and sacral nerve roots) are most resistant to local anesthetic block. Sensory nerves have intermediate sensitivity. Preganglionic sympathetic fibers are the smallest and most sensitive to local anesthetics. These differences occur with both subarachnoid and epidural anesthesia. Analgesia (loss of sensation of sharpness to pinprick) extends two or more segments cephalad than anesthesia (loss of sensation to touch).[99] Sympathetic block (as measured by increase in skin temperature) may extend as many as six spinal segments higher than the upper limit of sensory block.[100]

Cardiovascular System

Subarachnoid

Intrathecal injection of local anesthetics produces extensive sympathetic block. Earlier investigators believed that venodilation and the subsequent fall in venous return led to lower cardiac output and hypotension. Intravenous fluids should help prevent or treat hypotension by this mechanism. Unfortunately, multiple studies have shown that increasing intravascular volume with infusions of crystalloid or colloid has little effect on the incidence of subarachnoid anesthesia-related hypotension. Recent studies monitoring cardiac output have clearly and consistently shown that cardiac output **increases** after induction of subarachnoid anesthesia and that a fall in systemic vascular resistance leads to lower blood pressures (Fig. 35-33).[101,102] The degree of hypotension varies widely among patients. Risk factors include pregnancy, hypovolemia, advanced age, obesity, concurrent general anesthesia, and sensory level above T6.[103]

Heart rate may increase, decrease, or remain unchanged. Thoracic levels of anesthesia can produce cardiac sympathetic block as the cardiac accelerator fibers exist from T1–T4. The resultant vagal predominance can decrease heart rate. A decrease in cardiac filling pressures may also stimulate vagally mediated bradycardia via the Bezold–Jarisch reflex. This bradycardia is usually benign but can occasionally be profound. Cardiac arrest has been reported.[104] A review of 14 closed anesthesia malpractice claims from the 1970s found that prompt treatment with ephedrine, atropine, and chest compressions, but delayed administration of epinephrine produced uniformly poor neurologic outcomes after subarachnoid anesthesia-associated cardiac arrest.[105] Unrecognized hypoxemia may have contributed to the earlier adverse outcomes. Recent cases with pulse oximetry monitoring had better outcomes.[104,106]

Epidural

Hypotension and bradycardia can also occur during epidural anesthesia. The major risk factors for hypotension are the extent and onset of sensory block: faster onset and more extensive block increase the frequency of hypotension.[107] Bradycardia (heart rate ≤45 beats per minute) is more common in males. Genetics also may alter the risk of hypotension after epidural anesthesia. One study, using phenylephrine requirement as a marker, found that β_2-adrenoreceptor gene variants altered vasopressor requirements during thoracic epidural anesthesia. These authors also reported that women required more vasopressors than men.[108]

Prevention and Treatment

Volume

Intravenous fluids have long been used to prevent or treat hypotension associated with neuraxial anesthesia. However, even large volumes of crystalloid (2 liters) do not reliably prevent maternal hypotension with neuraxial anesthesia for cesarean section.[109] Colloid infusion is more effective, but hypotension is still common.[110] Fluids infused after the induction of epidural anesthesia increase both blood pressure and plasma volume. However, they are no more effective than vasopressors and, when given in excess, cause complications of their own.[111] In parturients, rapid infusion of 750 mL crystalloid slightly increased cardiac output and decreased systemic vascular resistance. It also significantly increased markers of endothelial glycocalyx destruction.[112] (The endothelial glycocalyx is an intricate meshwork of proteoglycans and glycoproteins that line the vascular endothelium. An intact glycocalyx prevents extravasation of intravascular fluid by maintaining an oncotic gradient.)

Vasopressors

Ephedrine and phenylephrine are the most used vasopressors for prevention and treatment of hypotension associated with neuraxial anesthesia. In parturients during cesarean section, ephedrine raises blood pressure primarily by increasing stroke volume and cardiac output. Phenylephrine increases systemic vascular resistance and decreases cardiac output (Fig. 35-34).[113] However, since cardiac output increases with induction of subarachnoid anesthesia, it usually remains above baseline even after phenylephrine administration.[113] Changes in heart rate parallel the changes in cardiac output. Ephedrine usually increases heart rate, whereas phenylephrine causes a reflex slowing.[113]

Norepinephrine also can be used to prevent or treat maternal hypotension associated with subarachnoid anesthesia. Unlike phenylephrine, norepinephrine maintains heart rate and cardiac output.[114] The clinical implications of these findings remain to be seen. Vasopressin may be a treatment of last resort in severe

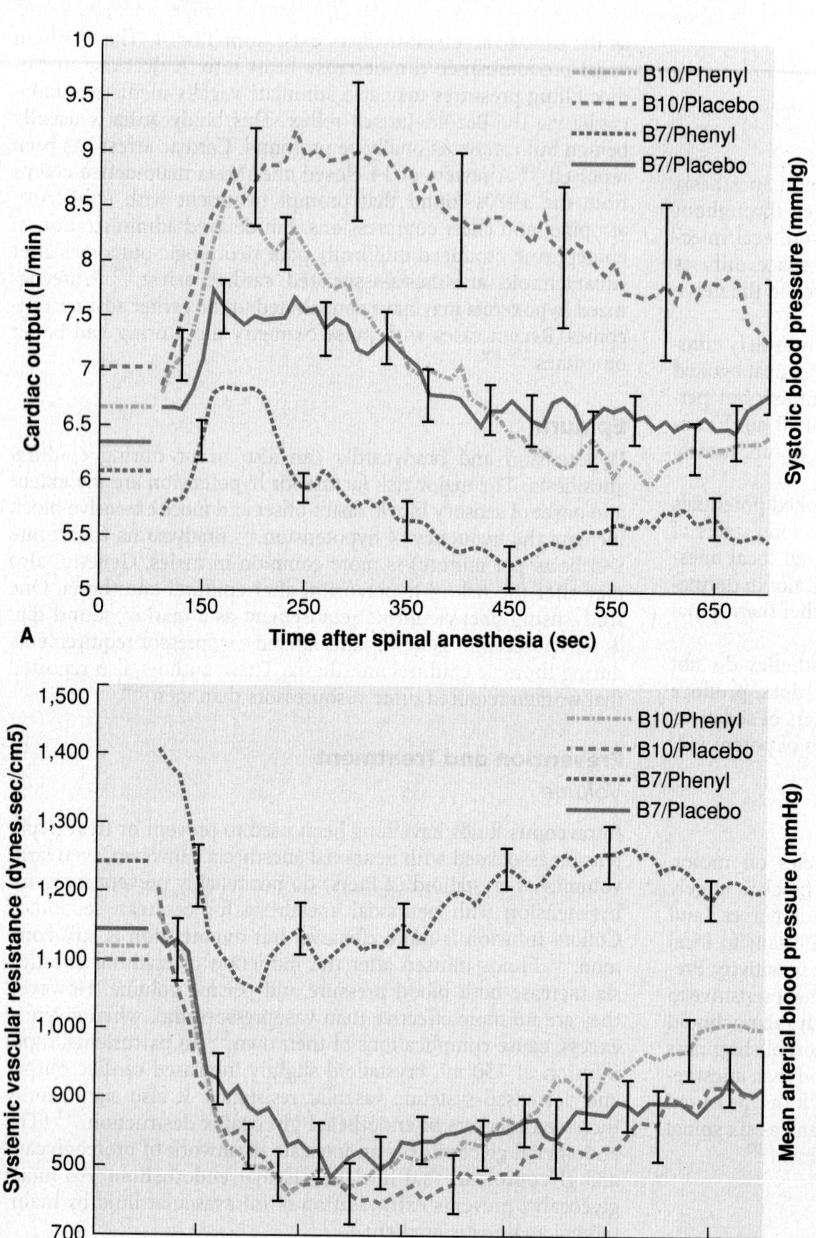

Figure 35-33 Mean differences in cardiac output (**A**) and systemic vascular resistance (**B**) in term parturients after intrathecal injection of 7 (B7) or 10 (B10) mg isobaric bupivacaine. Placebo patients received a normal saline intravenous infusion after injection. Phenyl patients received an intravenous infusion of phenylephrine after injection. (Adapted with permission from Langesaeter E, Rosseland LA, Shubhaug A. Continuous invasive blood pressure and cardiac output monitoring during cesarean delivery. *Anesthesiology*. 2008;109:856–863.)

hypovolemic hypotension or for patients taking medications that impair the renin–angiotensin system.

The Bezold–Jarisch reflex is an alternate explanation for the bradycardia that often accompanies hypotension after neuraxial anesthesia (NICV 35-1). This reflex is mediated by 5-hydroxytryptamine (5HT-3) serotonin receptors located in the vagus nerve and in ventricular myocardium. Activation of these receptors in response to systemic hypotension increases efferent vagal signaling, producing bradycardia, reduced cardiac output, and worsened hypotension.[115] Several groups have studied the effects of HT-3 receptor antagonists like ondansetron on the hemodynamic effects of neuraxial anesthesia. Meta-analysis of these results suggests that ondansetron may halve the risk of subarachnoid anesthesia-induced hypotension.[116] Ondansetron also limited the risk of bradycardia, nausea, and vomiting. Unfortunately, the small number of patients studied to date and the high likelihood of publication bias limits the strength of these conclusions.[117]

Respiratory System

Subarachnoid and epidural anesthesia have little effect on pulmonary function. Although patients often note chest tightness and dyspnea with thoracic levels of sensory block, respiratory function is usually unchanged. Subarachnoid block above T6 decreases forced vital capacity (FVC) and 1-second forced expiratory volume (FEV1) only in patients greater than 60 years of age.[118] While neuraxial anesthesia does not significantly interfere with respiration, it does prevent the patient from coughing effectively, particularly if the abdominal muscles

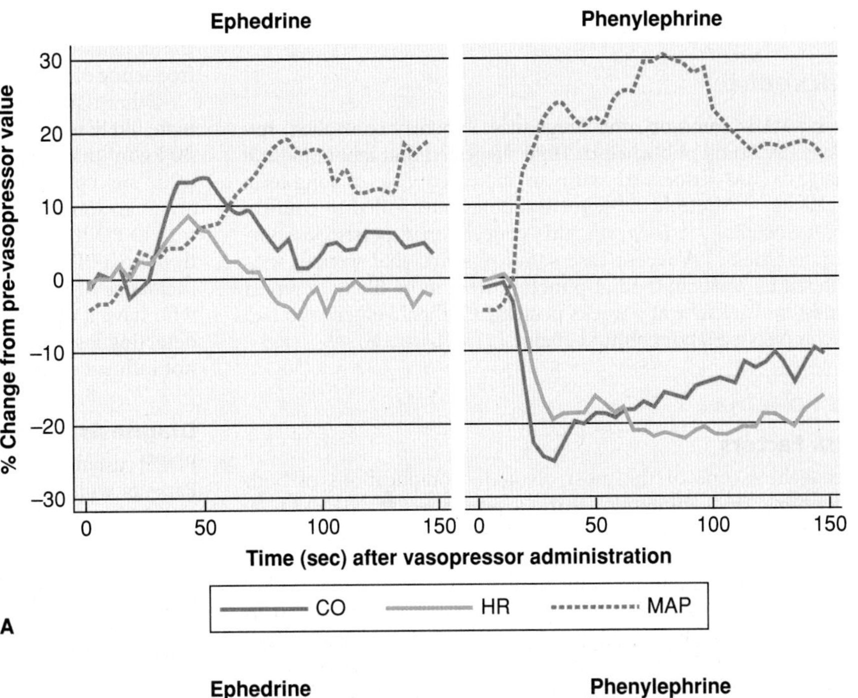

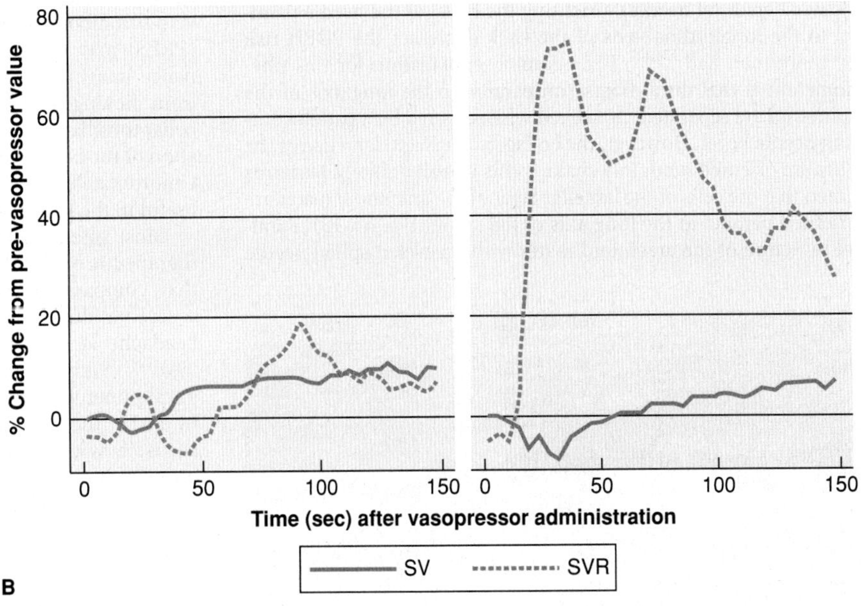

Figure 35-34 **A:** Percentage changes from prevasopressor values in cardiac output (CO), heart rate (HR), and mean arterial pressure (MAP) after the administration of phenylephrine or ephedrine. **B:** Percentage changes from prevasopressor values, in stroke volume (SV), and systemic vascular resistance (SVR) after the administration of phenylephrine or ephedrine. (Adapted with permission from Dyer RA, Reed AR, van Dyk D, et al. Hemodyamic effects of ephedrine, phenylephrine, and the coadministration of phenylephrine with oxytocin during spinal anesthesia for elective cesarean delivery. *Anesthesiology*. 2009;111:753–765.)

are affected. Neuraxial block of cervical levels can impair diaphragmatic function and produce significant respiratory compromise.

Gastrointestinal System

Neuraxial anesthesia-induced sympathetic blockade leads to unopposed vagal stimulation of the gastrointestinal system. Secretions increase, sphincters relax, and the bowel constricts. Many patients experience nausea and vomiting. Risk factors for nausea and vomiting include female gender, opioid premedication, and high level of block.[103] At cesarean section, nausea and vomiting are strongly associated with maternal hypotension.

Temperature Homeostasis

Hypothermia occurs routinely. Neuraxial anesthesia inhibits central thermoregulatory control. More importantly, blockade of peripheral sympathetic and motor nerves prevents vasoconstriction and shivering. As with general anesthesia, body temperature initially falls because heat redistributes from the core to the periphery. Heat loss continues through convection, radiation, and evaporation. Eventually, shivering may arise in the upper extremities, but this response does little to maintain body temperature.[119] Forced air warming, fluid warming, or both may limit the fall in maternal temperature after induction of subarachnoid anesthesia for cesarean section.[120]

Complications

Backache

Back pain is common after pregnancy. A poorly controlled, retrospective study published in 1990 suggested that labor epidural analgesia was associated with an increased risk of long-term backache.[121] Multiple subsequent studies have failed to confirm this association.[122] However, this concern may persist in some communities.[123] A recent case series reported that women who suffered an accidental dural puncture were more likely to report persistent backache at 6 weeks postpartum than women who had uncomplicated labor epidural analgesia (58% vs. 4%).[124]

Headache

Risk Factors

Headache is one of the most common complications of both intentional and unintentional dural puncture (NICV 35-2). The risk of PDPH correlates with the needle size, tip design, and bevel orientation. Pencil-point needles produce fewer headaches than similar-sized cutting-point needles. The smaller the needle, the lower the risk of PDPH. This relationship persists down to very fine (27-gauge) cutting-tip needles.[125] Twenty-four–gauge and smaller pencil-point needles carry similar PDPH risks. When using a cutting-tip needle (i.e., Quincke spinal needle or Tuohy or Hustead epidural needle), orienting the bevel of the needle parallel to the longitudinal axis of the back decreases the PDPH risk by more than half.[126,127] The common explanation for this phenomenon is that dural fibers run parallel to the long axis of the spine and are separated, not sliced when entered by a parallel cutting needle bevel. However, the collagen fibers and lamellae of the dura are oriented randomly, making this reason unlikely. Bernards noted that the cells of the lamellar layer of the arachnoid mater are oriented parallel to the long axis of the spine (Fig. 35-35). Parallel puncture of the arachnoid mater with a beveled spinal needle results in a narrow slit-like hole. Perhaps minimizing damage to the arachnoid, not the dura mater, is the key to decreasing the frequency of PDPH.[32]

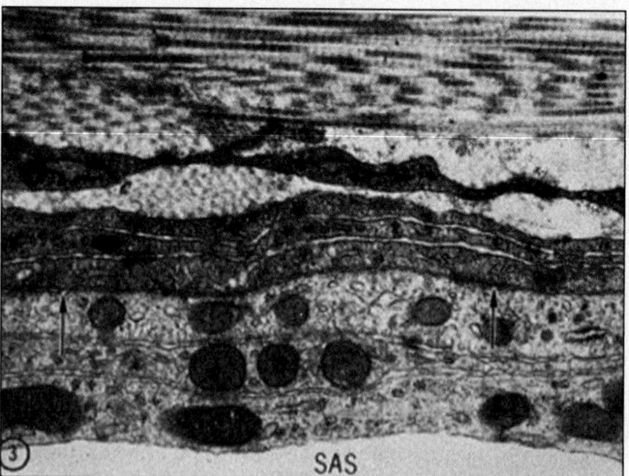

Figure 35-35 Transmission electron micrograph of the acellular dura mater (collagen bundles in the **top** one-third of the micrograph) and the cellular arachnoid mater (**bottom** two-thirds of the micrograph). *Arrows* indicate tight junctions, SAS indicates subarachnoid space, and *circled 3* identifies a mitochondrion. Note that the collagen bundles of the dura mater course in multiple planes (parallel, perpendicular, and oblique to the plane of section), whereas the arachnoid cells lie in a single plane oriented cephalocaudad. (Adapted from Bernards CM. Sophistry in medicine: lessons from the epidural space. *Reg Anesth Pain Med.* 2005;30:56–66.)

Other risk factors for PDPH include age; younger patients are *more* likely to develop PDPH and BMI; patients with a BMI above 30 kg/m^2 may be *less* likely to develop PDPH.[128] Females may be more susceptible to PDPH.[129] It is unknown if pregnant women are at greater risk than nonpregnant women. Patients with a history of PDPH or those with chronic headaches are more likely to develop a PDPH.[130] Observational studies have reported a higher incidence of PDPH in women who deliver vaginally versus those who have a cesarean section.[90,128] The choice of air or saline for detecting loss of resistance while locating the epidural space does not influence the incidence of PDPH.[56]

Diagnosis

PDPH usually develops 24 to 72 hours after dural puncture. Patients will complain of frontal and occipital pain that is made worse by standing and relieved by lying flat. Severe PDPH can also cause neck, shoulder, or back pain, which may not be relieved by lying down. Visual disturbances, vertigo, and cranial nerve palsies can occur.[131,132] Rarely, cortical vein thrombosis or subdural hematoma occur.[133,134] Death has been reported.[135] Differential diagnosis includes caffeine withdrawal, tension, migraine, or cluster headache. In parturients, preeclampsia, magnesium therapy, or nifedipine can cause headaches. Rarely, intracranial masses, cortical vein thrombosis, or posterior reversible encephalopathy syndrome (PRES) may be the cause. Gadolinium-enhanced magnetic resonance imaging (MRI) may show diffuse meningeal enhancement from meningeal vessel dilation. Other MRI findings include cerebellar tonsillar descent with crowding of the posterior fossa, obliteration of the basilar cisterns, and enlargement of the pituitary gland. Unfortunately, these findings are nonspecific.[130] Still, MRI may be useful in the patient with atypical, severe, or intractable headache.

Most often, PDPH will resolve within 5 to 7 days or after therapeutic epidural blood patch. However, two case series report that, compared to matched controls, parturients who suffered an accidental dural puncture had an increased incidence of chronic headache at 6 weeks (35% vs. 2%) and 24 months (28% vs. 5%).[124,136] Recent data support the association of unintentional dural puncture with an epidural needle and chronic headaches.[137] In 2021, the ASA issued a statement on PDPH management: https://www.asahq.org/standards-and-guidelines/statement-on-post-dural-puncture-headache-management.

The exact mechanism of PDPH is unknown. Loss of CSF through the iatrogenic dural tear seems to be the inciting factor. When the patient is upright, intracerebral CSF volume decreases. This change may cause the brain to sag toward the foramen magnum, stretching the pain-sensitive meningeal vascular covering. Alternatively, the diminished CSF volume may incite a compensatory increase in cerebral blood volume and produce a vascular headache.

Prevention

Anesthesiologists have tried many interventions to prevent PDPH. The three most widely studied approaches are prophylactic epidural blood patch, intrathecal catheter placement, and epidural morphine injection. Despite multiple studies of varying quality, prophylactic epidural blood patch has not been shown to consistently reduce the incidence of PDPH or the need for therapeutic blood patch.[138,139] Intrathecal catheters do not consistently prevent PDPH but may lower the need for epidural blood patch.[140–142] Epidural morphine may decrease the frequency and severity of PDPH. However, pruritus, nausea, and vomiting are common with epidural morphine.[143] Two small case series have reported that intrathecal injection of 10 mL saline, either immediately after accidental dural puncture or just before removing an intrathecal catheter, is associated with a decreased need for epidural blood patch.[90,144]

Treatment/Epidural Blood Patch

Once PDPH develops, most therapy is symptomatic. Bed rest will often relieve PDPH pain but does not shorten its duration.[145] Neither oral nor intravenous hydration has any effect on PDPH.[145] Patients with PDPH should have access to adequate analgesics. Acetaminophen, nonsteroidal anti-inflammatory drugs (NSAIDs), and opioids can be effective. Caffeine may relieve the symptoms of PDPH but the data supporting its use are weak.

Epidural blood patch is the definitive therapy for PDPH. The efficacy of epidural blood patch has clearly been established in small, but well-conducted, randomized prospective trials.[146] Most authors report that a single epidural blood patch cures 75% to 90% of PDPHs.[130,147] A second blood patch is usually effective for patients with incomplete relief or recurrent symptoms. However, a recent study reported a significantly lower success rate of epidural blood patch.[148] Only 67% of women reported headache relief after a single epidural blood patch. Fewer than 20% reported permanent relief. PDPH often recurred 4 to 5 days after the original blood patch. Twenty-one percent of the women received a second epidural blood patch.[146] Eleven percent of women in a series of 917 epidural blood patches collected from 30 hospitals in the United States received a second blood patch.[86]

Unresolved questions about epidural blood patch include the timing of the procedure in relation to the original dural puncture and the volume of blood that should be injected. Several retrospective chart reviews have suggested that epidural blood patch is more likely to provide headache relief if it is performed at least 72 hours after dural puncture compared with less than 24 hours after puncture.[147,148] However, these types of studies cannot control for headache severity. A more severe PDPH may have both a more rapid onset and be more difficult to cure with an epidural blood patch.

The initial reports of epidural blood patch used very small volumes (2 to 3 mL) of blood. Since then, the volume of blood injected has steadily increased. Most authors now recommend around 20 mL.[148] Patients often report back pain as blood is being injected into the epidural space. This pain usually recedes if the injection is halted. More blood can be injected after a moment or two. Stop adding more blood if the back pain returns immediately after resuming injection. Mild back pain is common after epidural blood patch. Serious complications are rare. However, epidural hematoma requiring surgical decompression has been reported.[149] One patient with idiopathic intracranial hypertension developed acute vision loss after rapid epidural injection of 25 mL autologous blood.[150]

Hearing Loss

Transient, low-frequency hearing loss can occur after subarachnoid anesthesia.[151] This complication may be more common in the elderly.[152] Hearing loss is presumably because of the effect of decreased CSF pressure on inner ear function. The risk of hearing loss is lower with smaller-gauge versus larger-gauge spinal needles.[151] Although hearing usually returns to normal in about 1 month, permanent loss has been reported.[153]

High Block/Total Subarachnoid Spinal Block

Subarachnoid and epidural anesthesia have enviable safety records. However, high levels of sensory block can occur (NICV 35-3). If unrecognized or not managed properly, high levels of block can produce respiratory compromise and cardiac arrest.[154] The exact frequency of these events is unknown. High neuraxial block (otherwise undefined) complicated approximately 1 in 4,000 obstetric neuraxial anesthetics.[86] Suggested, but unproven, risk factors for high block included obesity, short stature, subarachnoid block after failed epidural, repeat epidural after unintended dural puncture, and spinal deformity. A disturbingly common cause of high block in laboring women is unrecognized intrathecal injection during attempted labor epidural analgesia.[86,87,90]

High neuraxial block can produce both cardiac and respiratory instability. Extensive sympathetic block can lead to hypotension and bradycardia. Extensive sympathetic block combined with moderate to deep sedation (and presumed hypoxemia) can lead to sudden cardiac arrest, even in otherwise healthy young patients. In a series of 14 such arrests, prompt treatment with ephedrine, atropine, and chest compressions, but delayed administration of epinephrine produced uniformly poor neurologic outcomes. More rapid treatment with epinephrine might help counter the subarachnoid anesthesia-induced sympathetic block and lead to better results.[105] High neuraxial block can also produce significant respiratory compromise. Although patients often note chest tightness and dyspnea with thoracic levels of sensory block, respiratory function is usually unchanged. As the block ascends into the cervical regions, handgrip will weaken. Finally, blocks to C3–C5 will impair diaphragmatic function. These patients will only be able to whisper. They should be ventilated promptly and intubated if needed. When faced with a high level of sensory block after intrathecal injection of hyperbaric local anesthetic, you may be tempted to limit the rising block by placing the patient in reverse Trendelenburg position. Don't! This position may decrease the cephalad spread of sensory block, but Trendelenburg positioning will cause the patient's blood to pool in the legs, exacerbating the hypotensive effects of subarachnoid anesthesia. Reverse Trendelenburg position will also decrease blood flow to the brain, further hampering respiration. Instead, flex the patient's head at the neck. This may help prevent further cervical spread of hyperbaric local anesthetic. Continue to monitor the patient's respiratory and cardiovascular status and intervene as needed.

Systemic Toxicity

Local anesthetic systemic toxicity (LAST) can follow absorption from the epidural space or unrecognized intravascular injection. Signs and symptoms range from tinnitus and metallic taste to seizures and cardiac arrest. Important safety steps to prevent local anesthetic toxicity include incremental injection, limiting the total dose of local anesthetic, and using a test dose that contains a marker for intravascular injection.[91] Incremental injection of 3 to 5 mL of local anesthetic every 90 to 120 seconds is probably the most effective of these steps. Treatment of local anesthetic toxicity is discussed in Chapter 22.

Neurologic Injury

Neurologic injury is a rare, but potentially catastrophic complication of neuraxial block. Serious or permanent neurologic harm may occur after 1:20,000 to 35,000 neuraxial blocks.[86,155] Direct trauma, mass effect, and physiologic damage can cause neurologic injury.[156]

Needle Trauma

Spinal and epidural needles can damage both the spinal cord and nerve roots (Fig. 35-36). Although the spinal cord typically ends at

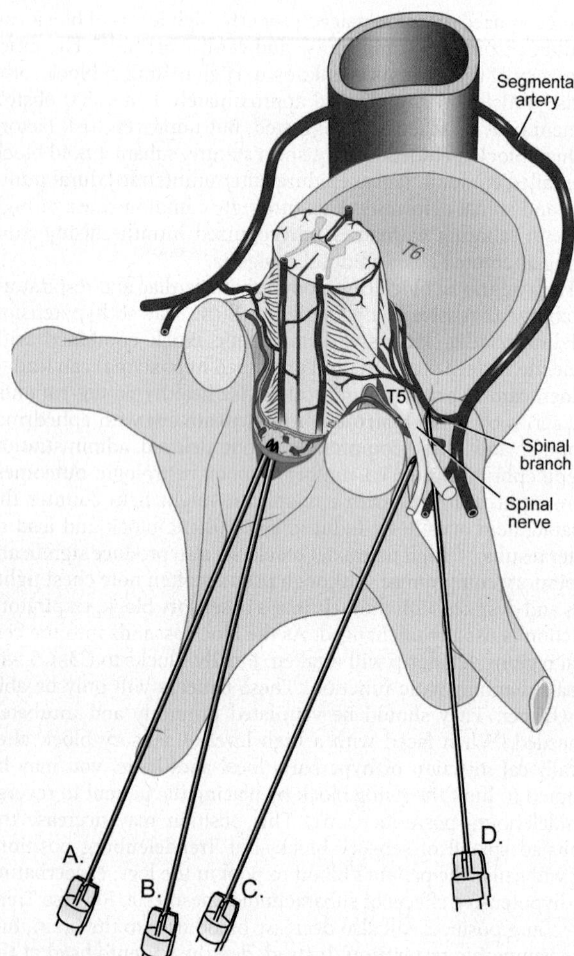

Figure 35-36 Midline or paramedian approaches (needles *A* and *B*) may directly traumatize the spinal cord, whereas unintentional lateral deviation of the needle (*C*) may contact the spinal nerve or the anterior or posterior primary ramus outside the foramen. Intentional lateral approaches, for example, transforaminal approach (needle *D*), have the potential to come near the spinal nerve or a spinal artery. Note that transforaminal approaches are typically at the cervical or lumbar levels, not the T6 level as illustrated. (Illustration by Gary J. Nelson. Reproduced from Neal JM, Kopp SL, Pasternak JJ, et al. Anatomy and pathophysiology of spinal cord injury associated with regional anesthesia and pain medicine: 2015 update. *Reg Anesth Pain Med.* 2015;40:506–525, with permission from BMJ Publishing Group Ltd.)

L1–L2 in adults, the exact termination varies, and the cord extends farther caudad in children. In addition, anesthesiologists using palpation often misidentify the lumbar interspaces and insert needles at a higher level than intended.[24] Permanent damage to the conus medullaris has been reported after attempted subarachnoid or CSE anesthesia at the presumed L2–L3 vertebral interspace.[157] In parturients, using the space just below, instead of above, the palpated intercristal line can decrease the frequency of inserting the spinal or epidural needle at or above L2–L3.[158] Lateral deviation of the needle may injure the spinal nerve or the anterior or posterior primary ramus outside the foramen (Fig. 35-36).[156]

The risk of direct spinal cord injury is highest with cervical epidural injection. The cervical epidural space is narrow, and the underlying spinal cord is vulnerable to needle trauma. Injury associated with cervical epidural injection was the most common damaging event in a recent review of pain medicine malpractice claims. Cervical epidural injections represent fewer than one-quarter of epidural injections but generate two-thirds of epidural injection–related claims.[159]

Mass Lesions

Mass lesions also can injure the spinal cord (Fig. 35-37). These 8
lesions can compress the spinal cord and decrease perfusion. Spinal cord ischemia or infarction can follow. Abscess and hematoma are the most widely studied compressive complications of neuraxial block. Significant hematoma may occur as often as 1:3,600 blocks or as rarely as 1:260,000.[155] Patients undergoing orthopedic procedures and those taking medications that interfere with coagulation are at greatest risk.[154,155,160,161] Hematoma is more common after epidural than subarachnoid block.[162] Hematoma also can occur after removing an epidural catheter. The American Society of Regional Anesthesia has a regularly updated guideline (https://www.asra.com/guidelines-articles/guidelines) that provides recommendations for the safe use of neuraxial block in patients taking antithrombotic or thrombolytic medications. The Society for

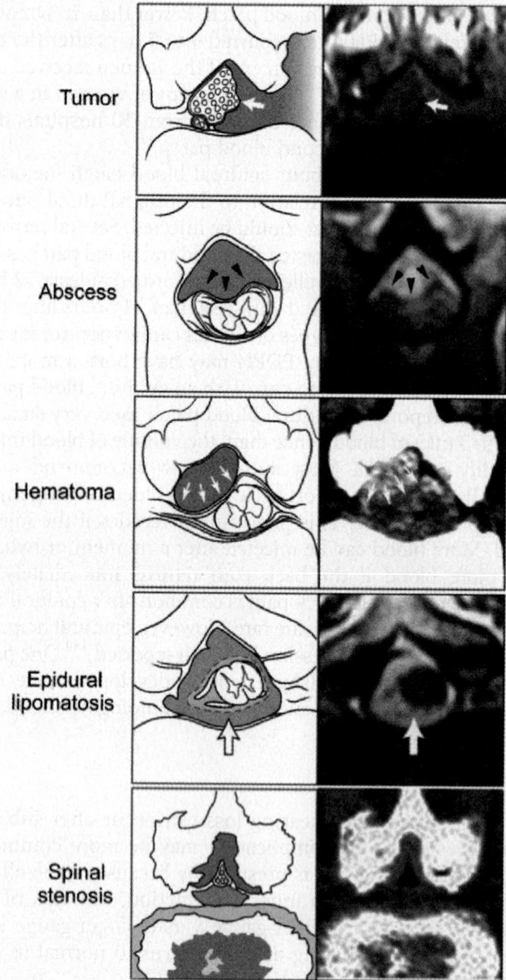

Figure 35-37 Extradural mass lesions. Note how various conditions can reduce spinal canal cross-sectional area and either directly compress the spinal cord or the cauda equina (*arrows*) or increase epidural space or CSF pressures through their mass effect (From Neal JM, Kopp SL, Pasternak JJ, Lanier WL, Rathmell JP. Anatomy and pathophysiology of spinal cord injury associated with regional anesthesia and pain medicine. 2015 update. *Reg Anesth Pain Med.* 2015;40:506–525.)

Obstetric Anesthesia and Perinatology recently published a consensus statement on neuraxial procedures for obstetric patients with thrombocytopenia.[163]

Epidural abscess is less common, complicating approximately 1:100,000 neuraxial blocks. Rarely, the combination of neuraxial local anesthetics and other mass lesions (tumors, lipomas, cysts, or granulomas) can produce compressive symptoms (Fig. 35-37).[156]

Patients with mass lesions may present with severe back pain. Other worrisome signs are persistent or recurrent sensory or motor block and bowel or bladder dysfunction. MRI provides more useful information about soft tissues and spinal canal pathology than computed tomography (CT). However, if MRI is not immediately available, CT can detect space-occupying lesions that may require immediate surgical intervention. Complete or partial neurologic recovery seems most likely if surgical decompression occurs within 8 to 12 hours of symptom onset.[156] However, complete recovery may occur even after a longer delay.[161] Figure 35-38 shows a systematic approach to the evaluation and treatment of a patient with suspected perioperative nerve injury.[164]

Hypoperfusion

Other potential causes of spinal cord ischemia include direct needle trauma to the spinal cord vasculature, prolonged hypoperfusion related to systemic hypotension, and spinal stenosis. Direct needle trauma to spinal vessels is extremely rare. Spinal cord ischemia or infarction related to systemic hypotension also is unusual. However, there are cases of ischemic spinal cord injury attributed to prolonged hypotension.[156] Risk factors may include spinal stenosis, anemia (reduced oxygen-carrying capacity), hypocapnia, raised intrathoracic pressure (e.g., during mechanical ventilation in lung-injured patients), extremes of patient position, chronic hypertension, unrecognized vascular abnormalities, and variation in the lower level of autoregulation of cerebral blood flow. Current guidelines, based only on expert opinion, suggest keeping blood pressure within 20% to 30% of

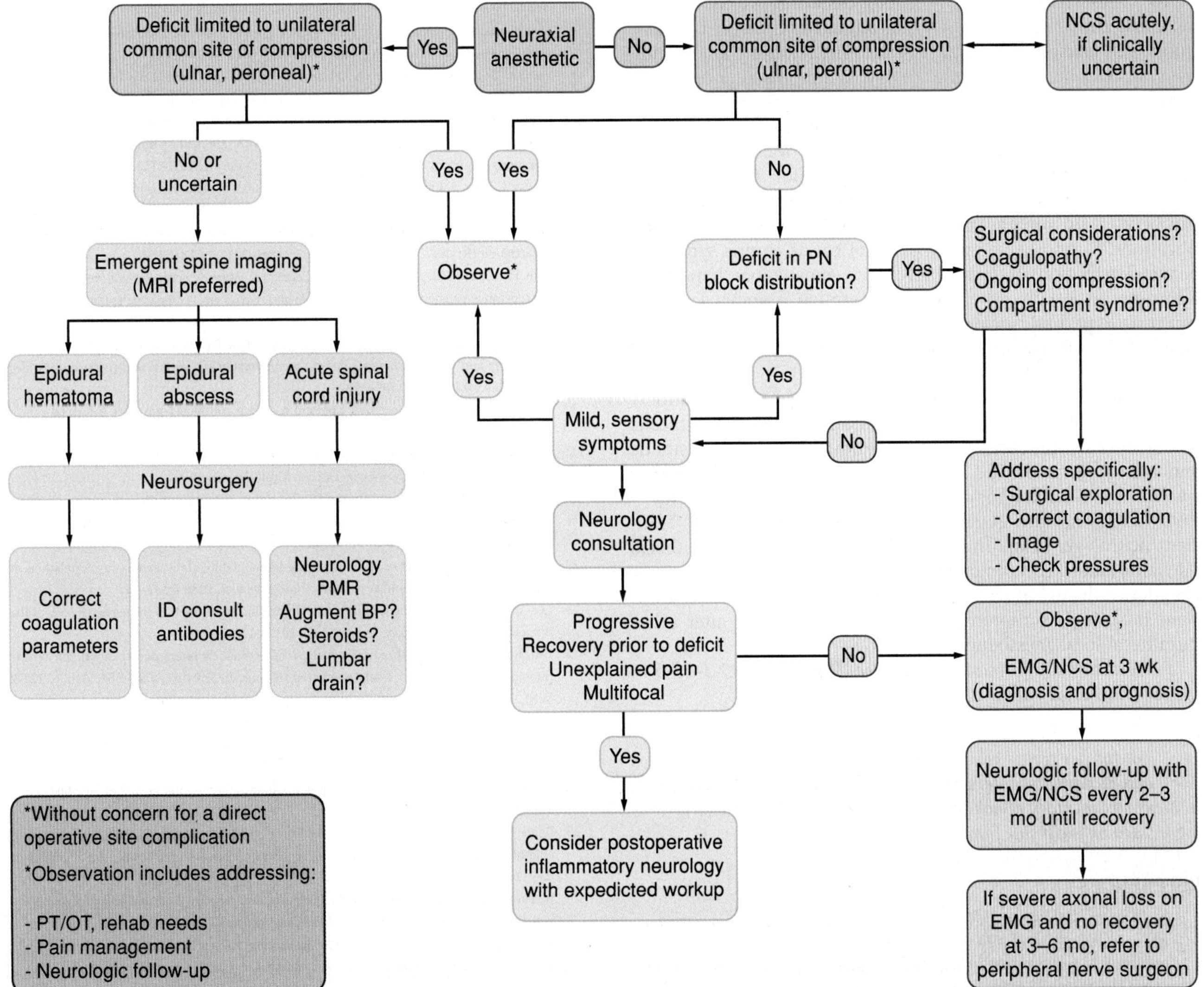

Figure 35-38 Approach to perioperative nerve injury. BP, blood pressure; EMG, electromyography; NCS, nerve conduction studies; PMR, physical medicine rehabilitation specialty consultation; PN, peripheral nerve. (Adapted from Watson JC, Huntoon MA. Neurologic evaluation and management of perioperative nerve injury. *Reg Anesth Pain Med*. 2015;40:491–501.)

baseline.[156] However, rare, uniquely susceptible patients may suffer spinal cord ischemia during an otherwise routine subarachnoid anesthetic.[165]

Spinal Stenosis

Pre-existing spinal stenosis may increase the risk of neurologic injury after neuraxial block. Osteoporosis can cause degenerative spinal stenosis. Also, hypertrophy of the ligamentum flavum and bony elements of the spinal canal can reduce spinal canal cross-sectional area, limiting space for the spinal cord and nerve roots. Spinal stenosis, combined with degenerative narrowing of the intervertebral foramina, may lead to increased vertebral canal pressure, and decreased spinal cord blood flow after neuraxial injection of local anesthetics. Currently, it is unclear if worsening neurologic symptoms after neuraxial block in patients with spinal stenosis represents an effect of the anesthetic or progression of the underlying disease.[162,166]

Chemical Injury

The cauda equina may be especially susceptible to chemical injury. These nerve roots travel long distances within the spinal canal and are not extensively myelinated.[156] Direct chemical injury can cause cauda equina syndrome, adhesive arachnoiditis, and, possibly, transient neurologic symptoms after neuraxial anesthesia. In the 1980s, a series of cases implicated unrecognized intrathecal injection of 2-chloroprocaine as a cause of cauda equina syndrome or adhesive arachnoiditis. Most, but not all, laboratory studies attributed this complication to the sodium bisulfate preservative. Today, preservative-free 2-chloroprocaine can be used for subarachnoid anesthesia without reported complications.[167] Another possible cause of cauda equina syndrome is maldistribution of local anesthetics, most often hyperbaric lidocaine, especially when injected through a spinal catheter. Injecting hyperbaric local anesthetic through a caudally directed, side-holed, pencil-point needle also can cause sacral pooling of drug.[53]

Transient neurologic symptoms (persistent low back, buttock, and leg pain) have been reported after subarachnoid anesthesia. The symptoms often present within 24 hours of a spinal anesthetic and are self-limited. The exact etiology of this complication is unclear. Some think it may represent subtle neurologic toxicity.[156] But, there is no firm evidence of neurologic pathology.[168] Transient neurologic symptoms are most associated with intrathecal lidocaine and the lithotomy position. Most anesthesiologists have abandoned the use of lidocaine for subarachnoid anesthesia. Transient neurologic symptoms are much less common after other intrathecal local anesthetics.[156,168]

For additional information please see *Videos 35-3–35-5 in the eBook bundled with this text.*

For further review and interactivities, please see the videos and narrative interactive clinical vignettes (NICVs) accessible in the complimentary eBook bundled with this text. Access instructions are located on the inside front cover.

REFERENCES

1. Yeager MP, Glass DD, Neff RK, Brinck-Johnsen T. Epidural anesthesia and analgesia in high-risk surgical patients. *Anesthesiology*. 1987;66:729–736.
2. Bode RH Jr, Lewis KP, Zarach SW, et al. Cardiac outcome after peripheral vascular surgery. Comparison of general and regional anesthesia. *Anesthesiology*. 1996;84:3–13.
3. Guay J, Choi PT, Suresh S, Albert N, Kopp S, Pace NL. Neuraxial anesthesia for the prevention of postoperative mortality and major morbidity: an overview of Cochrane Systematic Reviews. *Anesth Analg*. 2014;119:716–725.
4. Neuman MD, Silber JH, Elkassabany NM, Ludwig JM, Fleisher LA. Comparative effectiveness of regional versus general anesthesia for hip fracture surgery in adults. *Anesthesiology*. 2012; 117:72–92.
5. Neuman MD, Rosenbaum PR, Ludwig JM, Zubizarreta JR, Silber JH. Anesthesia technique, mortality, and length of stay after hip fracture surgery. *JAMA*. 2014;311:2508–2517.
6. Memtsoudis SG, Sun X, Chiu YL, et al. Perioperative comparative effectiveness of anesthetic technique in orthopedic patients. *Anesthesiology*. 2013;118:1046–1058.
7. Neuman MD, Feng R, Carson JL, et al; REGAIN Investigators. Spinal anesthesia or general anesthesia for hip surgery in older adults. *N Engl J Med*. 2021;385(22):2025–2035.
8. Li T, Li J, Yuan L, et al; RAGA Study Investigators. Effect of regional vs general anesthesia on incidence of postoeprative delirium in older patients undergoing hip fracture surgery: the RAGA randomized trial. *JAMA*. 2022;327(1):50–58.
9. Chery J, Semaan E, Darji S, Briggs WT, Yarmush J, D'Ayala M. Impact of regional versus general anesthesia on the clinical outcomes of patients undergoing major lower extremity amputation. *Ann Vasc Surg*. 2014;28:1149–1156.
10. Hausman MS Jr, Jewell ES, Engoren M. Regional versus general anesthesia in surgical patients with chronic obstructive pulmonary disease: does avoiding general anesthesia reduce the risk of postoperative complications? *Anesth Analg*. 2015;120:1405 1412.
11. Liu J, Ma C, Elkassabany N, Fleisher LA, Neuman MD. Neuraxial anesthesia decreases postoperative systemic infections risk compared with general anesthesia in knee arthroplasty. *Anesth Analg*. 2013;117:1010–1016.
12. Pugely AJ, Martin CT, Gao Y, Mendoza-Lattes S, Callaghan JJ. Differences in short-term complications between spinal and general anesthesia for primary total knee arthroplasty. *J Bone Joint Surg Am*. 2013;95(3):193–199.
13. Yap E, Wei J, Webb C, Ng K, Behrends M. Neuraxial and general anesthesia for outpatient total joint arthroplasty result in similarly low rates of major perioperative complications: a multicentered cohort study. *Reg Anesth Pain Med*. 2022;47:294–300.
14. Paziuk TM, Luzzi AJ, Fleischman AN, et al. General vs spinal anesthesia for total joint arthoplasty: a single institution observational review. *J Arthroplasty*. 2020;35(4):955–959.
15. Whiting PS, Molina CS, Greenberg SE, Thakore RV, Obremskey WT, Sethi MK. Regional anaesthesia for hip fracture surgery is associated with significantly more peri-operative complications compared with general anaesthesia. *Int Orthop*. 2015;39:1321–1327.
16. Modig J, Borg T, Karlstrom G, Maripuu E, Sahlstedt B. Thromboembolism after total hip replacement: role of epidural and general anesthesia. *Anesth Analg*. 1983;62:174–180.
17. Barbosa FT, Jucá MJ, Castro AA, Cavalcante JC. Neuraxial anaesthesia for lower-limb revascularization (Review). *Cochrane Database Syst Rev*. 2013;7:CD007083.
18. Wiis JT, Jensen-Gadegaard P, Altintas Ü, Seidelin C, Martusevicius R, Mantoni T. One-week postoperative patency of lower extremity in situ bypass graft comparing epidural and generalanesthesia: retrospective study of 822 patients. *Ann Vasc Surg*. 2014;28:295–300.
19. Sun Y, Li T, Gan TJ. The effects of perioperative regional anesthesia and analgesia on cancer recurrence and survival after oncology surgery: asystematic review and meta-analysis. *Reg Anesth Pain Med*. 2015;40:589–598.
20. Hasselager RP, Hallas J, Gögenurl. Epidural analgesia and recurrence after colorectal cancer surgery: a Danish retrospective registry-based cohort study. *Anesthesiology*. 2022;136:459–471.
21. Virtual Spine Model. Ultrasound for Regional Anesthesia (USRA). Published 2020. Accessed February 12, 2023. http://www.usra.ca/virtual-spine/vspine.php
22. Virtual Spine. Toronto General Hospital. Department of Anesthesia. Perioperative Interactive Education. Published 2012. Accessed February 12, 2023. http://pie.med.utoronto.ca/VSpine/index.htm
23. Avrahami E, Cohn DF, Yaron M. Computerized tomography, clinical and x-ray correlations in the hemisacralized fifth lumbar vertebra. *Clin Rheumatol*. 1986;5:332–337.
24. Lee AJ, Ranasinghe JS, Chehade JM, et al. Ultrasound assessment of the vertebral level of the intercristal line in pregnancy. *Anesth Analg*. 2011;113:559–564.
25. Pancaro C, Rajala B, Vahabzadeh C, et al. Sacral anatomical interspace landmark for lumbar puncture in pregnancy: a randomized trial. *Neurol*. 2020;94(6):e626–e634. doi: 10.1212/WNL.0000000000008749
26. Reina MA, Lirk P, Puigdellívol-Sánchez A, Mavar M, Prats-Galino A. Human lumbar ligamentum flavum anatomy for epidural anesthesia: reviewing a 3D MR-based interactive model and postmortem samples. *Anesth Analg*. 2016;122:903–907.
27. Hogan QH. Lumbar epidural anatomy. A new look by cryomicrotome section. *Anesthesiology*. 1999;75:767–775.
28. Reina MA, Franco CD, López A, Dé Andrés JA, van Zundert A. Clinical implications of epidural fat in the spinal canal. A scanning electron microscopic study. *Acta Anaesthesiol Belg*. 2009;60:7–17.
29. Bernards CM, Shen DD, Sterling ES, et al. Epidural, cerebrospinal fluid, and plasma pharmacokinetics of epidural opioids (Part 1): differences among opioids. *Anesthesiology*. 2003;99:455–465.
30. Reina MA, Dittmann M, López Garcia A, van Zundert A. New perspectives in the microscopic structure of human dura mater in the dorsolumbar region. *Reg Anesth*. 1997;22:161–166.
31. Reina MA, de Leon Casasola O, Lopez A, De Andrés JA, Mora M, Fernández A. The origin of the spinal subdural space: ultrastructure findings. *Anesth Analg*. 2002;94:991–995.
32. Bernards CM. Sophistry in medicine: lessons from the epidural space. *Reg Anesth Pain Med*. 2005;30:56–66.

33. Reina MA, Prats-Galino A, Sola RG, Puigdellívol-Sánchez A, Arriazu Navarro R, De Andrés JA. Structure of the arachnoid layer of the human spinal meninges: a barrier that regulates dural sac permeability. [Spanish]. *Rev Esp Anestesiol Reanim*. 2010;57:486–492. Spanish. doi: 10.1016/s0034-9356(10)70709-x.
34. Reina MA, De León Casasola Ode L, Villanueva MC, López A, Machés F, De Andrés JA. Ultrastructural findings in human spinal pia mater in relation to subarachnoid anesthesia. *Anesth Analg*. 2004;98:1479–1485.
35. Miyajima M, Arai H. Evaluation of the production and absorption of cerebrospinal fluid. *Neurol Med Chir (Tokyo)*. 2015;55:647–656.
36. Bulat M, Lupret V, Orehković D, Klarica M. Transventricular and transpial absorption of cerebrospinal fluid into cerebral microvessels. *Coll Antropol*. 2008;32:43–50.
37. Prats-Galino A, Reina MA, Puigdellívol-Sánchez A, Juanes Méndez JA, De Andrés JA, Collier CB. Cerebrospinal fluid volume and nerve root vulnerability during lumbar puncture or spinal anaesthesia at different vertebral levels. *Anaesth Intensive Care*. 2012;40:643–647.
38. Tao B, Liu K, Ding M, Xue H, Li X, Zhao P. Ultrasound increases the success rate of spinal needle placement through the epidural needle during combined spinal-epidural anaesthesia: a randomised controlled study. *Eur J Anaesthesiol*. 2021;38(3):251–258.
39. Perlas A, Chaparro LE, Chin KJ. Lumbar neuraxial ultrasound for spinal and epidural anesthesia: a systematic review and meta-analysis. *Reg Anesth Pain Med*. 2016;41:251–260.
40. Lee PJ, Tang R, Sawka A, Krebs C, Vaghadia H. Real-time ultrasound-guided spinal anesthesia using Taylor's approach. *Anesth Analg*. 2011;112:1236–1238.
41. Balki M. Locating the epidural space in obstetric patients—ultrasound a useful tool: continuing professional development. *Can J Anesth*. 2010;57:1111–1126.
42. Polley LS. Neuraxial techniques for labor analgesia should be placed in the lateral position. *Int J Obstet Anesth*. 2008;17:149–152.
43. Vincent RD, Chestnut DH. Which position is more comfortable for the parturient during induction of epidural anesthesia? *Int J Obstet Anesth*. 1991;1:9–11.
44. Jones AR, Carle C, Columb M. Effect of table tilt on ligamentum flavum length measured using ultrasonography in pregnant women. *Anaesthesia*. 2013;68:27–30.
45. Kapur D, Grimsehl K. A comparison of cerebrospinal fluid pressure and block height after spinal anaesthesia in the right and left lateral position in pregnant women undergoing cesarean section. *Eur J Anaesth*. 2001;18:668–672.
46. Taenzer AH, Walker BJ, Bosenberg AT, et al. Asleep versus awake: does it matter? Pediatric regional block complications by patient state: a report from the Pediatric Regional Anesthesia Network. *Reg Anesth Pain Med*. 2014;39:279–283.
47. Bromage PR, Benumof JL. Paraplegia following intracord injection during attempted epidural anesthesia under general anesthesia. *Reg Anesth Pain Med*. 1998;23:104–107.
48. Bernards CM, Hadzic A, Suresh S, Neal JM. Regional anesthesia in anesthetized or heavily sedated patients. *Reg Anesth Pain Med*. 2008;33:449–460.
49. American Society of Anesthesiologists Task Force on infectious complications associated with neuraxial techniques. Practice Advisory for the prevention, diagnosis, and management of infectious complications associated with neuraxial techniques. *Anesthesiology*. 2010;112:530–545.
50. Birnbach DJ, Stein DJ, Murray O, Thys DM, Sordillo EM. Providone iodine and skin disinfection before initiation of epidural anesthesia. *Anesthesiology*. 1998;88:668–672.
51. Birnbach DJ, Meadows W, Stein DJ, Murray O, Thys DM, Sordillo EM. Comparison of povidone iodine and DuraPrep, an iodophor-in-isopropyl alcohol solution, for skin disinfection prior to epidural catheter insertion in parturients. *Anesthesiology*. 2003;98:164–169.
52. Pong, RP, Gmelch BS, Bernards CM. Does a paresthesia during spinal needle insertion indicate intrathecal needle placement? *Reg Anesth Pain Med*. 2009;34:29–32.
53. Holman SJ, Robinson RA, Beardsley D, Stewart SF, Klein L, Stevens RA. Hyperbaric dye solution distribution characteristics after pencil-point needle injection in a spinal cord model. *Anesthesiology*. 1997;86:966–973.
54. Stroumpoulis K, Stamatakis E, Koutroumanis P, Loukeri A, Valsamidis D. Pencil-point needle bevel direction influences ED50 of isobaric ropivacaine with fentanyl in spinal anesthesia for cesarean delivery: a prospective, double-blind sequential allocation study. *Int J Obstet Anesth*. 2015;24:225–229.
55. Aida S, Taga K, Yamakura T, Endoh H, Shimoji K. Headache after attempted epidural block: the role of intrathecal air. *Anesthesiology*. 1998;88:76–81.
56. Antibas PL, do Nascimento Junior P, Braz LG, Vitor Pereira Doles J, Módolo NS, El Dib R. Air versus saline in the loss of resistance technique for identification of the epidural space. *Cochrane Database Syst Rev*. 2014;18;2014(7):CD008938. doi: 10.1002/14651858.CD008938.pub2.
57. Segal S, Arendt KW. A retrospective effectiveness study of loss of resistance to air or saline for identification of the epidural space. *Anesth Analg*. 2010;110:558–563.
58. Bromage PR. *Epidural Analgesia*. WB Saunders; 1978.
59. Doughty A. Paternity of the Doughty technique. *Anaesthesia*. 2005;60:1242–1243.
60. Reynolds F. Hand positions and the "son-of-Doughty" technique. *Anaesthesia*. 2005;60:717–718.
61. Beilin Y, Bernstein HH, Zucker-Pinchoff B. The optimal distance that a multiorifice epidural catheter should be threaded into the epidural space. *Anesth Analg*. 1995;81:301–304.
62. Capiello E, O'Rourke N, Segal S, Tsen LC. A randomized trial of dural puncture epidural technique compared with the standard epidural technique for labor analgesia. *Anesth Analg*. 2008; 107:1646–1651.
63. Ross VH, Dean LS, Thomas JA, Harris LC, Pan PH. Techniques in morbidly obese parturients undergoing cesarean delivery: time for initiation of anesthesia. *Anesth Analg*. 2014;118:168–172.
64. Hsu Y, Hettiarachchi HDM, Zhu DC, Linninger AA. The frequency and magnitude of cerebrospinal fluid pulsations influence intrathecal drug distribution: key factors for interpatient variability. *Anesth Analg*. 2012;115:386–394.
65. Xu F, Qian M, Wei Y, et al. Postural change from lateral to supine is an important mechanism enhancing cephalic spread after injection of interthecal 0.5% plain bupivacaine for cesarean section. *Int J Obstet Anesth*. 2015;24:308–312.
66. Whiteside JB, Burke D, Wildsmith JA. Spinal anesthesia with ropivacaine 5 mg/mL in glucose 10 mg/mL or 50 mg/mL. *Br J Anaesth*. 2001;86:241–244.
67. Malinovsky JM, Renaud G, Le Corre P, et al. Intrathecal bupivacaine in humans: influence of volume and baricity of solutions. *Anesthesiology*. 1999;91:1260–1266.
68. Sia AT, Tan KH, Sng BL, Lim Y, Chan ES, Siddiqui FJ. Use of hyperbaric versus isobaric bupivacaine for spinal anaesthesia for caesarean section. *Cochrane Database Syst Rev*. 2013; 31;(5):CD005143. doi: 10.1002/14651858.CD005143.pub2.
69. Hocking G, Wildsmith JAW. Intrathecal drug spread. *Br J Anaesth*. 2004;93:568–578.
70. Camorcia M, Capogna G, Columb MO. Effect of sex and pregnancy on the potency of intrathecal bupivacaine: determination of ED50 for motor block with the up-down sequential allocation method. *Eur J Anaesthesiol*. 2011;28:240–244.
71. Carpenter RL, Hogan QH, Liu SS, Crane B, Moore J. Lumbosacral cerebrospinal fluid volume is the primary determinant of sensory block extent and duration during spinal anesthesia. *Anesthesiology*. 1998;89:24–29.
72. Teoh WHL, Ithnin F, Sia ATH. Comparison of an equal-dose spinal anesthetic for cesarean section and for post partum tubal ligation. *Int J Obstet Anesth*. 2008;17:228–232.
73. Zhou QH, Xiao WP, Shen YY. Abdominal girth, vertebral column length, and spread of spinal anesthesia in 30 minutes after plain bupivacaine 5 mg/mL. *Anesth Analg*. 2014;119: 203–206.
74. De Simone CA, Leighton BL, Norris MC. Spinal anesthesia for cesarean section. A comparison of two doses of hyperbaric bupivacaine. *Reg Anesth*. 1995;20:90–94.
75. Katz D, Hamburger J, Gutman D, et al. The effect of adding subarachnoid epinephrine to hyperbaric bupivacaine and morphine for repeat cesarean delivery: a double-blind prospective randomized control trial. *Anesth Analg*. 2018;127(1):171–178.
76. Abdallah FW, Abrishami A, Brull R. The facilitatory effects of intravenous dexmedetomidine on the duration of spinal anesthesia: a systematic review and meta-analysis. *Anesth Analg*. 2013;117(1):271–278. doi: 10.1213/ANE.0b013e318290c566. Epub 2013 Apr 30.
77. De Kock M, Gautier P, Fanard L, Hody JL, Lavand'homme P. Intrathecal ropivacaine and clonidine for ambulatory knee arthroscopy. *Anesthesiology*. 2001;94:574–578.
78. Visser WA, Lee RA, Gielen MJM. Factors affecting the distribution of neural blockade by local anesthetics in epidural anesthesia and a comparison of lumbar versus thoracic epidural anesthesia. *Anesth Analg*. 2008;107:708–721.
79. Arakawa M. Does pregnancy increase the efficacy of lumbar epidural anesthesia? *Int J Obstet Anesth*. 2004;13:86–90.
80. Yokoyama M, Hanazaki M, Fujii H, et al. Correlation between the distribution of contrast medium and the extent of blockade during epidural anesthesia. *Anesthesiology*. 2004;100: 1504–1510.
81. Hillyard SG, Bate TE, Corcoran TB, Paech MJ, O'Sullivan G. Extending epidural analgesia for emergency caesarean section: a meta-analysis. *Br J Anaesth*. 2011;107:668–678.
82. Kinsella SM. A prospective audit of regional anaesthesia failure in 5080 caesarean sections. *Anaesthesia*. 2008;63:822–832.
83. Eisenach JC, De Kock M, Klimscha W. Alpha2-adrenergic agonists for regional anesthesia. A clinical review of clonidine (1984–1995). *Anesthesiology*. 1996;85:655–674.
84. Tong Y, Ren H, Ding X, Jin S, Chen Z, Li Q. Analgesic effect and adverse events of dexmedetomidine as additive for pediatric caudal anesthesia: a meta-analysis. *Paediatr Anaesth*. 2014;24(12):1224–1230. doi: 10.1111/pan.12519. Epub 2014 Sep 9.
85. Youssef N, Orlov D, Alie T, et al. What epidural opioid results in the best analgesia outcomes and fewest side effects after surgery? A meta-analysis of randomized controlled trials. *Anesth Analg*. 2014;119:965–977.
86. D'Angelo R, Smiley RM, Riley ET, Segal S. Serious complications related to obstetric anesthesia; the serious complication repository project of the Society for Obstetric Anesthesia and Perinatology. *Anesthesiology*. 2014;120:1505–1512.
87. Davies JM, Posner KL, Lee LA, Cheney FW, Domino KB. Liability associated with obstetric anesthesia: a closed claims analysis. *Anesthesiology*. 2009;110:131–139.
88. Pratt S, Vasudevan A, Hess P. A prospective randomized trial of lidocaine 30 mg versus 45 mg for epidural test dose for intrathecal injection in the obstetric population. *Anesth Analg*. 2013; 116:125–132.
89. Richardson MG, Lee AC, Wissler RN. High spinal anesthesia after epidural test dose administration in five obstetric patients. *Reg Anesth*. 1996;21:119–123.
90. Bolden N, Gebre E. Accidental dural puncture management: 10-year experience at an academic tertiary care center. *Reg Anesth Pain Med*. 2016;41:169–174.
91. Guay J. The epidural test dose: a review. *Anesth Analg*. 2006;102:921–929.
92. Norris MC, Ferrenbach D, Dalman H, et al. Does epinephrine improve the diagnostic accuracy of aspiration during labor epidural analgesia? *Anesth Analg*. 1999;88:1073–1076.

93. Reina MA, Collier CB, Prats-Galino A, Puigdellívol-Sánchez A, Machés F, De Andrés JA. Unintentional subdural placement of epidural catheters during attempted epidural anesthesia: an anatomic study of spinal subdural compartment. *Reg Anesth Pain Med.* 2011;36:537–541.
94. Boswell MV, Iacono RP, Guthkelch AN. Sites of action of subarachnoid lidocaine and tetracaine: observations with evoked potential monitoring during spinal cord stimulator implantation. *Reg Anesth.* 1992;17:37–42.
95. Cusick JF, Myklebust JB, Abrams SE. Differential neural effects of epidural anesthetics. *Anesthesiology.* 1980;53:299–306.
96. Dahl JB, Rosenberg J, Lund C, Kehlet H. Effect of thoracic epidural bupivacaine 0.75% on somatosensory evoked potentials after dermatomal stimulation. *Reg Anesth.* 1990;15:73–75.
97. Hodgson P, Liu SS, Gras TW. Does epidural anesthesia have general anesthetic effects: a prospective, randomized, double-blind, placebo-controlled trial. *Anesthesiology.* 1999;91:1687–1692.
98. Reinoso-Barbero F, Martínez-García E, Hernández-Gancedo, Simon AM. The effect of epidural bupivacaine on maintenance requirements of sevoflurane evaluated by bispectral index in children. *Eur J Anaesthesiol.* 2006;23:460–464.
99. Brull SJ, Greene NM. Zones of differential sensory block during extradural anaesthesia. *Br J Anaesth.* 1991;66:651–655.
100. Chamberlain DP, Chamberlain BD. Changes in the skin temperature of the trunk and their relationship to sympathetic blockade during spinal anesthesia. *Anesthesiology.* 1986;65:139–143.
101. Langesaeter E, Rosseland LA, Shubhaug A. Continuous invasive blood pressure and cardiac output monitoring during cesarean delivery: a randomized, double-blind comparison of low-dose versus high-dose spinal anesthesia with intravenous phenylephrine or placebo infusion. *Anesthesiology.* 2008;109:856–863.
102. Langesaeter E, Dyer RA. Maternal haemodynamic changes during spinal anaesthesia for caesarean section. *Curr Opin Anesthesiol.* 2011;24:242–248.
103. Tarkkila P, Isola J. A regression model for identifying patients at high risk of hypotension, bradycardia and nausea during spinal anesthesia. *Acta Anaesthesiol Scand.* 1992;36:554–558.
104. Kumari A, Gupta R, Bajwa SJS, Singh A. Unanticipated cardiac arrest under spinal anesthesia: an unavoidable mystery with review of current literature. *Anesth Essays Res.* 2014;8:99–102.
105. Caplan RA, Ward RJ, Posner K, Cheney FW. Unexpected cardiac arrest during spinal anesthesia: a closed claims analysis of predisposing factors. *Anesthesiology.* 1988;68:5–11.
106. Dyamanna DN, Bs SK, Zacharia BT. Unexpected bradycardia and cardiac arrest under spinal anesthesia: case reports and review of literature. *Middle East J Anaesthesiol.* 2013;22:121–125.
107. Curatolo M, Scaramozzin P, Venuti FS, Orlando A, Zbinden AM. Factors associated with hypotension after epidural blockade. *Anesth Analg.* 1996;83:1033–1040.
108. Frey UH, Karlik J, Herbstreit F, Peters J. β2-adrenoreceptor gene variants vasopressor requirements in patients after thoracic epidural anaesthesia. *Br J Anaesth.* 2011;112:477–484.
109. Norris MC. Hypotension during spinal anesthesia for cesarean section: does it affect neonatal outcome? *Reg Anesth.* 1987;12:191–194.
110. Mercier FJ, Diemunsch P, Ducloy-Bouthors A-S, et al; CAESAR Working Group. 6% Hydroxyethyl starch (130/0.4) vs. Ringer's lactate preloading before spinal anaesthesia for Caesarean delivery: the randomized, double-blind, multicentre CAESAR trial. *Br J Anaesth.* 2014;113:459–467.
111. Holte K, Foss NB, Svensén C, Lund C, Madsen JL, Kehlet H. Epidural anesthesia, hypotension and changes in intravascular volume. *Anesthesiology.* 2004;100:281–286.
112. Powell MF, Mathru M, Brandon A, Patel R, Frölich MA. Assessment of endothelial glycocalyx disruption in term parturients receiving a fluid bolus before spinal anesthesia: a prospective observational study. *Int J Obstet Anesth.* 2014;23:330–334.
113. Dyer RA, Reed AR, van Dyk D, et al. Hemodynamic effects of ephedrine, phenylephrine, and the coadministration of phenylephrine with oxytocin during spinal anesthesia for elective cesarean delivery. *Anesthesiology.* 2009;111:753–765.
114. Ngan Kee WD, Lee SWY, Ng FF, Tan PE, Khaw KS. Randomized double-blinded comparison of norepinephrine and phenylephrine for maintenance for blood pressure during spinal anesthesia for cesarean delivery. *Anesthesiology.* 2015;122:736–745.
115. Watts SW, Morrison SF, Davis RP, Barman SM. Serotonin and blood pressure regulation. *Pharmacol Rev.* 2012;64:359–388.
116. Gao L, Zheng L, Han J, Wang Y, Zheng J. Effects of prophylactic ondansetron on spinal anesthesia-induced hypotension: a meta-analysis. *Int J Obstet Anesth.* 2015;24:335–343.
117. Terkawi AS, Mavridis D, Flood P, et al. Does ondansetron modify sympathectomy due to subarachnoid anesthesia? Meta-analysis, meta-regression, and trial sequential analysis. *Anesthesiology.* 2016;124:846–869.
118. Oğurlu M, Sen S, Polatli M, Sirthan E, Gürsoy F, Cildağ O. The effect of spinal anesthesia on pulmonary function tests in old patients. *Tuberk Toraks.* 2007;55:64–70.
119. Sessler DI. Perioperative heat balance. *Anesthesiology.* 2000;92:578–596.
120. Sultan P, Habib AS, Cho Y, Carvalho B. The effect of patient warming during caesarean delivery on maternal and neonatal outcomes: a meta-analysis. *Br J Anaesth.* 2015;115:500–510.
121. MacArthur C, Lewis M, Knox EG, Crawford JS. Epidural anaesthesia and long term backache after childbirth. *BMJ.* 1990;301:9–12.
122. Reynolds F. Obstetric problems? Blame the epidural! *Reg Anest Pain Med.* 2008;33:472–476.
123. Orejuela FJ, Garcia T, Green C, Kilpatrick C, Guzman S, Blackwell S. Exploring factors influencing patient request for epidural analgesia on admission to labor and delivery in a predominantly Latino population. *J Immigr Minor Health.* 2012;14:287–291.
124. Ranganathan P, Golfeiz C, Phelps AL, et al. Chronic headache and backache are long-term sequelae of unintentional dural puncture in the obstetric population. *J Clin Anesth.* 2015;27:201–206.
125. Lambert DH, Hurley RJ, Hertwig L, Datta S. Role of needle gauge and tip configuration in the production of lumbar puncture headache. *Reg Anesth.* 1997;22:66–72.
126. Norris MC, Leighton BL, DeSimone CA. Needle bevel direction and headache after inadvertent dural puncture. *Anesthesiology.* 1989;70:729–731.
127. Richman JM, Joe EM, Cohen SR, et al. Bevel direction and postdural puncture headache: a meta-analysis. *Neurologist.* 2006;12:224–228.
128. Peralta F, Higgins N, Lange E, Wong CA, McCarthy RJ. The relationship of body mass index with the incidence of postdural puncture headache in parturients. *Anesth Analg.* 2015;121:451–456.
129. Wu CL, Rowlingson AJ, Cohen SR, et al. Gender and post-dural puncture headache. *Anesthesiology.* 2006;105:613–618.
130. Baysinger CL. Accidental dural puncture and postdural puncture headache management. *Int Anesthesiol Clin.* 2014;52:18–39.
131. Loures V, Savoldelli G, Kern K, Haller G. Atypical headache following dural puncture in obstetrics. *Int J Obstet Anesth.* 2014;23:246–252.
132. Hofer JE, Scavone BM. Cranial Nerve VI palsy after dural-arachnoid puncture. *Anesth Analg.* 2015;120:644–646.
133. Nepomuceno R, Herd A. Bilateral subdural hematoma after inadvertent dural puncture during epidural analgesia. *J Emerg Med.* 2013;44:e227–e230.
134. Cuypers V, Van de Velde M, Devroe S. Intracranial subdural haematoma following neuraxial anaesthesia in the obstetric population: a literature review with analysis of 56 reported cases. *Int J Obstet Anesth.* 2016;25:58–65.
135. Freedman RL, Lucas DN. MBRACE-UK: saving lives, improving mothers' care – implications for anesthetists. *Int J Obstet Anesth.* 2015;24:161–173.
136. Webb CAJ, Weyker PD, Zhang L, et al. Unintentional dural puncture with a Tuohy needle increases risk of chronic headache. *Anesth Analg.* 2012;115:124–132.
137. Ansari JR, Barad M, Shafer S, Flood P. Chronic disabling postpartum headache after unintentional dural puncture during epidural anaesthesia: a prospective cohort study. *Br J Anaesth.* 2021;127(4):600–607.
138. Bradbury CL, Singh SI, Badder SR, Wakely LJ, Jones PM. Prevention of post-dural puncture headache in the parturients: a systematic review and meta-analysis. *Acta Anaesthsiol Scand.* 2013;57:417–430.
139. Kaddoum R, Motlani F, Kaddoum RN, Srirajakalidindi A, Gupta D, Soskin V. Accidental dural puncture, postdural puncture headache, intrathecal catheters, and epidural blood patch: revisiting the old nemesis. *J Anesth.* 2014;28:628–630.
140. Verstraete S, Walters MA, Devroe S, Roofthooft E, Van de Velde M. Lower incidence of post-dural puncture headache with spinal catheterization after accidental dural puncture in obstetric patients. *Acta Anaesthiol Scand.* 2014;58:1233–1239.
141. Heesen M, Klöhr S, Rossaint R, Walters M, Straube S, van de Velde M. Insertion of an intrathecal catheter following accidental dural puncture: a meta-analysis. *Int J Obstet Anesth.* 2013;22:26–30.
142. Jagannathan DK, Arrianga AF, Elterman KG, et al. Effect of neuraxial technique after dural puncture on obstetric outcomes and anesthetic complications. *Int J Obstet Anesth.* 2015;25:23–29.
143. Al-metwalli RR. Epidural morphine injections for prevention of post dural puncture headache. *Anaesthesia.* 2008;63:847–850.
144. Charsley MM, Abram SE. The injection of intrathecal normal saline reduces the severity of post dural puncture headache. *Reg Anesth Pain Med.* 2001;26:301–305.
145. Arevalo-Rodriguez I, Ciapponi A, Munoz L, Roqué i Figuls M, Bonfill Cosp X. Posture and fluids for preventing post-dural puncture headache (Review). *Cochrane Database Syst Rev.* 2013;7:CD009199.
146. van Kooten F, Oedit R, Bakker SLM, Dippel DWJ. Epidural blood patch in post dural puncture headache: a randomised, observer-blind, controlled clinical trial. *J Neurol Neurosurg Psychiatry.* 2008;79:553–558.
147. Kokki M, Sjövall S, Keinänen M, Kokki H. The influence of timing on the effectiveness of epidural blood patches in parturients. *Int J Obstet Anesth.* 2013;22:303–309.
148. Paech MJ, Doherty DA, Christmas T, Wong CA; Epidural Blood Patch Trial Group. The volume of blood for epidural blood patch in obstetrics: a randomized, blinded clinical trial. *Anesth Analg.* 2011;113:126–133.
149. Mehta SP, Keogh BP, Lam AM. An epidural blood patch causing acute neurologic dysfunction necessitating a decompressive laminectomy. *Reg Anesth Pain Med.* 2014;39:78–80.
150. Pagani-Estévez GI, Chen JJ, Watson JC, Leavitt JA. Acute vision loss secondary to epidural blood patch. *Reg Anesth Pain Med.* 2016;41:164–168.
151. Cosar A, Yetiser S, Sizlan A, Yanarates O, Yildirim A. Hearing impairment associated with spinal anesthesia. *Acta Otolaryngol.* 2004;124:1159–1164.
152. Ok G, Tok D, Erbuyun K, Aslan A, Tekin I. Hearing loss does not occur in young patients undergoing spinal anesthesia. *Reg Anesth Pain Med.* 2004;29:430–433.

153. Kilickan L, Gürkan Y, Ozkarakas H. Permanent sensorineural hearing loss following spinal anesthesia. *Acta Anaesthesiol Scand.* 2002;46:1155–1157.
154. Lee LA, Posner KL, Domino KB, Caplan RA, Cheney FW. Injuries associated with regional anesthesia in the 1980s and 1990s: a closed claims analysis. *Anesthesiology.* 2004;101: 143–152.
155. Moen V, Dahlgren N, Irestedt L. Severe neurological complications after central neuraxial blockades in Sweden 1990–1999. *Anesthesiology.* 2004;101:950–959.
156. Neal JM, Kopp SL, Pasternak JJ, Lanier WL, Rathmell JP. Anatomy and pathophysiology of spinal cord injury associated with regional anesthesia and pain medicine. 2015 update. *Reg Anesth Pain Med.* 2015;40:506–525.
157. Reynolds F. Damage to the conus medullaris following spinal anaesthesia. *Anaesthesia.* 2001;56:238–247.
158. Srinivasan KK, Deighan M, Crowley L, McKeating K. Spinal anaesthesia for caesarean section: an ultrasound comparison of two different landmark techniques. *Int J Obstet Anesth.* 2014;23:206–212.
159. Pollak KA, Stephens LS, Posner KL, et al. Trends in pain medicine liability. *Anesthesiology.* 2015;123:1133–1141.
160. Pumberger M, Memtsoudis SG, Stundner O, et al. An analysis of the safety of epidural and spinal neuraxial anesthesia in more than 100,000 consecutive major lower extremity joint replacements. *Reg Anesth Pain Med.* 2013;38:515–519.
161. Bateman BT, Mhyre JM, Ehrenfeld J, et al. The risk and outcomes of epidural hematomas after perioperative and obstetric epidural catheterization: a report from the multicenter perioperative outcomes group research consortium. *Anesth Analg.* 2013;116:1380–1385.
162. Neal JM, Barrington MJ, Brull R, et al. The second ASRA practice advisory on neurologic complications associated with regional anesthesia and pain medicine: executive summary 2015. *Reg Anesth Pain Med.* 2015;40:401–430.
163. Bauer ME, Arendt K, Beilin Y, et al. The Society for Obstetric Anesthesia and Perinatology Interdisciplinary Consensus statement on neuraxial procedures in obstetric patients with thrombocytopenia. *Anesth Analg.* 2021;132(6):1531–1544.
164. Watson JC, Huntoon MA. Neurologic evaluation and management of perioperative nerve injury. *Reg Anesth Pain Med.* 2015;40:491–501.
165. Zaphiratos V, McKeen DM, Macaulay B, George RB. Persistent paralysis after spinal anesthesia for cesarean delivery. *J Clin Anesth.* 2015;27:68–72.
166. Kopp SL, Peters SM, Rose PS, Hebl JR, Horlocker TT. Worsening of neurologic symptoms after spinal anesthesia in two patients with spinal stenosis. *Reg Anesth Pain Med.* 2015;40: 502–505.
167. Goldblum E, Atchabahian A. The use of 2-chloroprocaine for spinal anaesthesia. *Acta Anaesthesiol Scand.* 2013;57:545–552.
168. Zaric D, Pace NL. Transient neurologic symptoms (TNS) following spinal anaesthesia with lidocaine versus other local anaesthetics. *Cochrane Database Syst Rev.* 2009:CD003006.

36 Peripheral Nerve Blockade

CHI-HO BAN TSUI • RICHARD W. ROSENQUIST

KEY POINTS

1. Peripheral nerve blocks (PNBs) deliver effective anesthesia and analgesia in a site-specific manner, with the potential for long-term benefits.
2. PNB safety and success require precise nerve identification and local anesthetic delivery. Improved ultrasound image resolution has recently shifted regional anesthesia from targeting particular nerves to the expanded use of interfascial plane blocks.
3. Ultrasound imaging provides real-time visualization of needle movement when approaching nerve structures, minimizing the risk of inadvertent needle contact with critical anatomy and potentially reducing complications. Although ultrasound technology is highly desirable as a tool for providing regional anesthesia, it requires extensive training and a complete understanding of both the equipment and the cross-sectional anatomy relevant to regional nerve blocks.
4. Peripheral nerve stimulators are excellent ultrasonography adjuncts for deep blocks, but they do not eliminate the risk of nerve injury. An awake and responsive adult patient may improve safety by reporting nerve contact or discomfort during injection.
5. Pediatric nerve block techniques are broadly comparable to those performed on adults, with the notable exception that they are routinely performed with the child under general anesthesia or sedation.
6. Nerve blocks that are anatomically related to bone or vascular features are more reliably and more accessibly performed using ultrasound guidance.
7. Larger quantities of local anesthetic may boost PNB success, but the dosage must be restricted to minimize systemic toxicity. Increased local anesthetic concentrations produce more reliable motor blocks. Ultrasound imaging may permit successful blocks with lower volumes of local anesthetics, but this has not been completely validated.
8. This chapter uses the most recent standardized nomenclature for regional anesthetic procedures, as recommended by the American Society of Regional Anesthesia and Pain Medicine (ASRA) and the European Society of Regional Anaesthesia and Pain Therapy (ESRA).

Introduction

1 Regional anesthesia allows for location-specific, long-lasting, and effective anesthesia and analgesia. It is appropriate for many surgical patients and has been shown to improve analgesia and reduce morbidity, mortality, and the need for reoperation after major surgical procedures. Peripheral nerve blocks (PNBs) can be used as the sole "surgical" anesthetic, as a supplement to general anesthesia to provide analgesia and muscle relaxation, or as the first step in providing prolonged postoperative analgesia, as with brachial plexus blocks or continuous peripheral nerve catheters. Compared to parenteral analgesics, a single-injection or continuous PNB can provide better analgesia while lowering the risk of side effects. Optimal pain relief with minimal side effects (e.g., nausea and vomiting) significantly improves patient outcomes, including patient satisfaction and earlier mobilization, meeting the need
2 for streamlined surgical services at a lower cost. Nonetheless, the safety and success of PNB techniques are highly dependent on the accurate delivery of the correct dose of local anesthetic. Even in experienced hands, there is an inherent failure rate associated with regional anesthesia, and the risk—albeit rare—of systemic toxicity, infection, bleeding, permanent nerve injury, or other physical injury. Nevertheless, many anesthesiologists and surgeons have benefited from using PNBs more frequently, guided by advances in knowledge (e.g., the properties of solutions during electrical nerve stimulation [NS]) and in technology (e.g., the introduction of anatomically based ultrasound [US] imaging).

Medical knowledge and procedures are continually evolving. While new developments provide the potential for enhanced patient care, they must be evaluated and compared to accepted techniques to assess their safety and efficacy. On the other hand, anatomic structures are static, and a solid understanding of human anatomy and its common variations will always be essential for performing regional anesthesia. This chapter discusses regional anatomy in depth while reviewing two current, common techniques for nerve localization and block performance: NS and

US imaging. Block approaches are presented in sections organized by body location. Special considerations for nerve blocks in pediatric patients will be addressed where appropriate. This chapter uses the latest standardized nomenclature for regional anesthetic procedures as proposed by the American Society of Regional Anesthesia and Pain Medicine (ASRA) and the European Society of Regional Anaesthesia and Pain Therapy (ESRA).

General Principles and Equipment

Regional anesthesia has long been regarded as an "art."[1] Until recently, real success with these techniques was confined to a few gifted individuals. The introduction of NS, which relies on physiologic responses of neural structures to electrical impulses, was the first step toward transforming regional anesthesia into a "science." There is considerable interindividual variation in the physiologic response to NS, further influenced by other factors such as injectates, physiologic solutions (e.g., blood), and comorbid disease.

3 Anatomically based US imaging is an exciting advance in regional anesthesia. This is a quantum leap in technology for those in the field, and realizing its potential benefits may encourage those anesthesiologists who had previously abandoned regional anesthesia techniques to resume or increase their use. Despite initial enthusiasm, US-guided regional anesthesia has a steep learning curve. NS and US imaging can be combined to increase block success. Used alone, US may allow good visualization of the needle and nerve and a reasonable estimate of the spread of the total dose of the local anesthetic. However, the identity of the nerve
4 may be unknown, especially for novice ultrasonographers. By stimulating the nerve, its identity may be determined objectively by observing the motor response to NS or, in some cases, the anatomic distribution of a paresthesia-like sensation in response to NS for a sensory nerve.

A successful PNB requires careful patient selection and the correct type, dose, and site of local anesthetic. The patient must be monitored during the procedure and before discharge, and ambulatory patients with home-going catheters should be monitored remotely with phone follow-up or home health care team visits until the catheter is removed and the block resolves.

Preblock Stage

Setup

For adults, it is preferable to perform regional blocks with the patient awake, prior to the operating room to allow sufficient "soak time." This is the time it takes local anesthetics to cross the cell membrane, block action potentials, and produce analgesia or surgical anesthesia. This specialized presurgical area, often referred to as a "block room," must have monitoring and resuscitation equipment and it must have supplies and equipment for common and advanced regional block techniques. Some important "block room" considerations:

- All supplies in this area must be readily identifiable and accessible to the anesthesiologist.
- The area should be sufficiently large to allow block performance, patient monitoring, and resuscitation.
- There should be equipment for monitoring, oxygen delivery, emergency airway management, suction, and the area should have sufficient lighting. In addition, cardiovascular resuscitation equipment (e.g., a crash cart) and local anesthetic systemic toxicity (LAST) treatment supplies should be readily available.
- A practically organized equipment storage cart is desirable. It should contain all the necessary equipment (including those required for emergency procedures), supplies, local anesthetics, needles, nerve stimulators, block trays, dressings, and resuscitation drugs. A US machine with a variety of probes should also be present.
- It is ideal to have a prepared specialty tray with sterile skin preparation and draping items, a marking pen and ruler for landmark identification, needles and syringes for skin infiltration, and specific block needles and catheters.
- A selection of sedatives, hypnotics, and intravenous anesthetics should be immediately available to prepare patients for regional anesthesia. These drugs should be titrated to maximize benefits and minimize adverse effects (high therapeutic index); short-acting medications with a high safety margin are desirable.
- Emergency drugs should include atropine, epinephrine, phenylephrine, ephedrine, propofol, midazolam, succinylcholine, and Intralipid. In addition, guidelines for resuscitation in the event of LAST should be laminated and kept with the Intralipid.

Monitoring

Skilled staff should monitor the patient while performing regional anesthesia. Standard monitoring includes electrocardiogram (ECG), noninvasive blood pressure (NIBP), and pulse oximetry. Sedated patients also need end-tidal CO_2 monitoring. Since vasovagal episodes are common during many regional procedures, the patient's level of consciousness should be checked often. There are no reliable techniques to detect real-time blood levels of local anesthetic, but adding pharmacologic markers like epinephrine can indirectly suggest an increasing systemic dose. Systemic toxicity can occur by rapid intravenous injection (within 2 minutes) or by delayed absorption (20 minutes). Patients who have received a PNB should be closely monitored for systemic toxicity for 30 minutes.

Stable vital signs following regional anesthesia must be present to fulfill discharge criteria from the recovery area. If the block has not begun to regress, appropriate protection for the anesthetized limb and complete instructions should be provided to the patient and their family before discharge. For inpatients, proper orders should be written to assure limb protection. Postoperatively, patients receiving perineural local anesthetic infusions should be followed by a skilled physician or a member of the Acute Pain Service.

Pediatric nerve blocks are often administered under general 5
anesthetic or deep sedation as children cannot be expected to articulate discomfort appropriately nor cooperate reliably with the procedure. As such, monitoring to reduce the risk of nerve damage (e.g., US, NS, and injection pressure) is critical in pediatric practice.[2]

Premedication and Sedation

Careful patient selection and education are the essential preparations for successful regional anesthesia, although appropriate sedation and analgesia can greatly assist with minimal adverse effects. Propofol, midazolam, fentanyl, ketamine, remifentanil, alfentanil, or a combination of these medication can induce sedation and analgesia. The drugs should be titrated to the patient, nerve block treatment, and length of surgery.

Documentation

Preblock checklists ensure correct block placement on the patient's body. Preoperative conditions should be documented, risks and benefits discussed, and consent obtained. For quality assurance, research, and medicolegal reasons, PNB procedures should be carefully documented.

Block Performance Stage

Common Techniques: Nerve Stimulation

Basics of Technique and Equipment

Electrical NS for regional anesthesia was first introduced in the 1960s. Low-current electrical impulses delivered through the needle can stimulate the motor fibers in peripheral nerves, thus indicating nerve proximity without needle contact and patient pain from paresthesia. Theoretically, NS methods should reduce nerve injury risk, but this has never been proven. NS can also be used to guide catheter placement: stimulating catheters were introduced to increase accuracy. However, NS relies on the physiologic responses of neural structures to the stimulating current, which varies widely.

Practical Guidelines

When using NS, depolarization of the nerve can be improved by using the positive (red) pole of the stimulator as the ground electrode and the negative (black) lead as the needle connection (known as cathodal preference). The ground electrode location is unimportant when using a constant-current nerve stimulator.[1] In general, the needle is in proximity to the nerve when the threshold for motor response is between 0.3 and 0.5 mA. Placing the needle to a point where the motor response only requires 0.1 to 0.2 mA may increase the chance of intraneural injection and should be avoided.[3] Once a satisfactory threshold response is obtained, 2 to 3 mL of local anesthetic is injected, and the operator watches for the disappearance of the motor twitch. This so-called "Raj test" was originally thought to result from the injected solution's physical displacement of the targeted nerve, although this response has also been attributed to a change in the electrical field at the needle–tissue interface. Electrically conducting solutions (e.g., local anesthetic or saline) reduce the current density at the needle tip, thereby increasing the current threshold for motor response, whereas nonconducting solutions (e.g., D5W) increase the current density and maintain or augment the twitch response (Fig. 36-1).[4] After a successful test, the remainder of the intended dose is injected in divided aliquots.

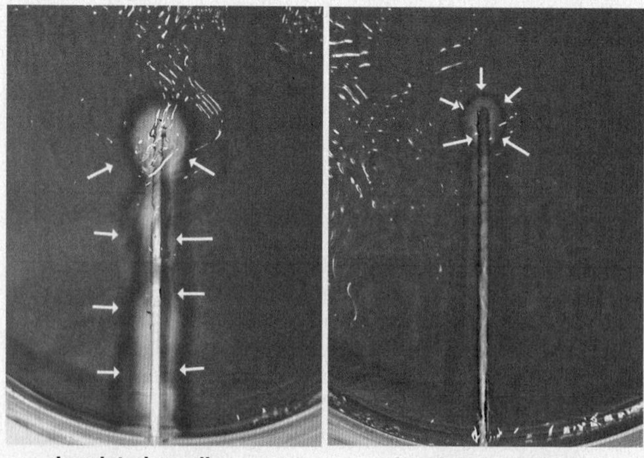

Figure 36-1 Current density is localized to the needle tip when using nonconducting solutions (e.g., D5W), thereby maintaining the motor response to the threshold current level during nerve stimulation.

Common Techniques: Ultrasound Imaging

Basics of Technique and Equipment

US imaging is a valuable regional anesthesia tool because it can determine the size, depth, and location of many nerves in their surroundings. Visualizing the moving needle, once inserted at an appropriate angle and within the US probe's plane, helps the anesthesiologist perform regional anesthesia. With US-guided PNB, the clinician can adjust needle or catheter placement under direct vision, leading to fewer needle attempts and the ability to use less local anesthetic. The ability to visualize critical adjacent structures (e.g., blood vessels, pleura) helps avoid complications. US images reflect anatomic structure contours based on tissue or fluid acoustic impedances. Sound waves reflect at interfaces between substances of different acoustic impedance, defining tissue contours. High US beam reflection from high-impedance/dense structures (e.g., bone, connective tissue) results in a bright (hyperechoic) image, often with acoustic shadowing underneath. Low-impedance structures reflect beams less and appear gray (hypoechoic). Minimal impedance structures/spaces (e.g., fluid in vessels) appear black (anechoic). Higher frequencies offer better surface spatial resolution (e.g., as for the brachial plexus at the supraclavicular fossa), but deep structure delineation requires lower frequencies (e.g., as for the sciatic nerve in the subgluteal region). Block location and depth determine the most suitable imaging transducer. It is important to master the field, gain, and Doppler effect functions on the US imaging system. Many nerves are near blood vessels: Doppler imaging helps distinguish them during US localization.

Practical Guidelines

Probe sterility is paramount if performing real-time or dynamic US guidance during block performance. This can be maintained by standard sleeve covers (Fig. 36-2A). For single-injection blocks, it is practical to use a sterile transparent dressing (e.g., Tegaderm; 3M Health Care, St Paul, MN) without the full cover of a sterile sleeve (Fig. 36-2B).[1]

One of the most common reasons for poor visualization is the lack of sufficient gel for skin-probe contact. It is helpful to first identify one or more reliable anatomic landmarks (bone or vessel) with a known relationship to the nerve structure. The clinician can localize the nerve at a location near this landmark and then proceed to follow, or "trace," the nerve to the optimal block location (Table 36-1).[1] To get the best possible view of the shaft and tip of the needle, it is imperative to align the needle shaft to the longitudinal axis ("in-plane" [IP]) of the US transducer (probe) (Fig. 36-2C). The nerve structure is often placed at the edge of the US screen to ensure adequate viewing distance for the needle shaft. An alternative approach uses a transverse or tangential ("out-of-plane" [OOP]) alignment, which only allows appreciation of the needle in cross-section (Fig. 36-2D).

After the needle is seen close to the nerve(s), a 1- to 2-mL injectate can be injected to visualize appropriate spread. If NS is being used to confirm nerve identity, D5W should be used to maintain accurate motor responses.[5] Some experts recommend combining US and NS techniques, where the nerve is sought primarily using visualization under US guidance. The nerve stimulator is set at 0.3 to 0.5 mA, and serves as an alert when the insulated needle tip is too close to the nerve (i.e., contacting or inside the nerve).

Other Related Equipment

Needles

The "short bevel" (i.e., 30 to 45 degrees) or "B bevel" is used and is claimed to reduce the potential for injury to nerves.[6] Other

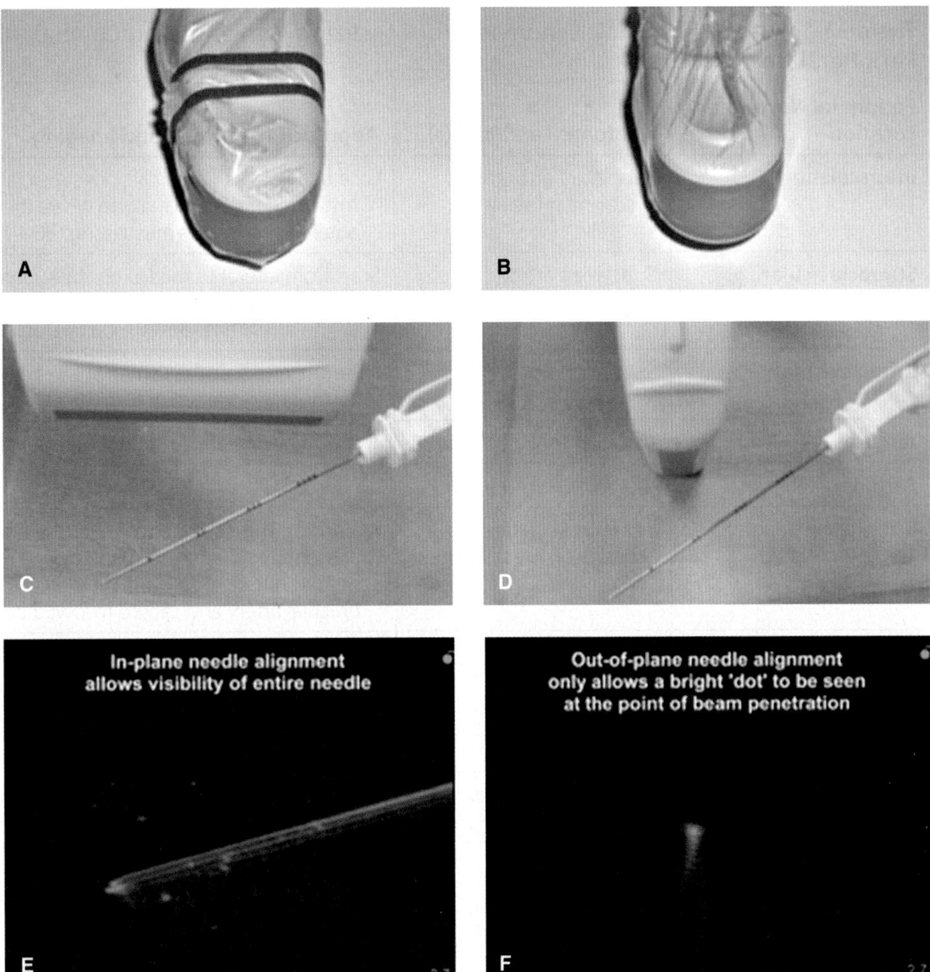

Figure 36-2 Probe sterility using the full cover of a sterile sleeve (**A**) and a sterile transparent dressing (e.g., Tegaderm; 3M Health Care, St Paul, MN) (**B**). In-plane (**C, E**) and out-of-plane (**D, F**) needle alignment and needle visibility on ultrasound.

modifications, such as the "pencil-point" needle, have been introduced to minimize nerve injury. Single-injection PNB techniques generally employ 22- to 24-gauge insulated needles with short bevels. Various echogenic needles are available for use; these needles possess special coatings, grooves, or "cornerstone" reflectors that enhance their acoustic reflectivity, allowing easier visualization when performing US-guided blocks.

Practical Tips

High-pressure injections into the nerve (especially intrafascicular injections) are associated with damage in animals.[7,8] Many techniques and devices have been proposed to limit peak injection pressure since considerable variation exists among anesthesiologists with regard to the amount of pressure they apply during injections. Disposable, in-line injection pressure monitors are available, although their ability to prevent long-term injury is not well documented. Alternatively, a compressed air injection technique (CAIT) has been described to limit the generation of excessive pressure during injection. With this method, some excess air is drawn into the syringe and compressed by 50% during the entire injection. This, in principle, maintains an injection pressure of approximately 760 mmHg (by Boyle's law, pressure × volume = constant) (Fig. 36-3), which is well below the 1,300 mmHg threshold considered to be an associated risk factor for clinically significant nerve injury.[1]

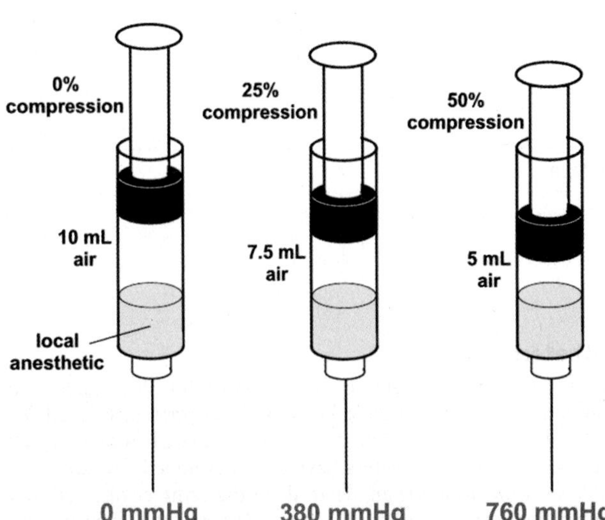

Figure 36-3 The compressed air injection technique (CAIT) avoids high pressure; 50% compression of air volume within the syringe corresponds to an injection pressure of 760 mmHg.

Table 36-1 Useful Anatomic Landmarks for Localizing Nerves during Common Ultrasound-Guided Peripheral Nerve Blocks

Peripheral Nerve Block Location	Anatomic Landmark(s)	Approach for Ultrasound Imaging
Interscalene	Subclavian artery and scalene muscles	Locate the plexus trunks/divisions superolateral to the artery at the supraclavicular fossa, and trace proximally to where the roots/trunks lie between the scalenus anterior and medius muscles (Fig. 36-19).
Supraclavicular	Subclavian artery	Scan from lateral to medial on the superior aspect of the clavicle to locate the pulsatile artery; the plexus trunks/divisions lie lateral and often superior to the artery (Fig. 36-20). Color Doppler is useful.
Infraclavicular	Subclavian/axillary artery and vein	Place the artery at the center of the field and locate the brachial plexus cords surrounding the artery (Fig. 36-21).
Axillary	Axillary artery	The terminal nerves surround the artery (Fig. 36-22).
Peripheral Nerves		
Radial nerve at anterior elbow	Humerus at spiral groove and deep brachial artery	To confirm the nerve's identity at the elbow, trace the nerve proximally and posteriorly toward the spiral groove of the humerus, just inferior to the deltoid muscle insertion. The nerve is located here adjacent to the deep brachial artery and can be followed back to the anterior elbow (Fig. 36-23).
Median nerve at forearm	Brachial artery	The large anechoic artery lies immediately lateral to the nerve (Fig. 36-25).
Ulnar nerve at forearm	Ulnar artery	Scan at the anteromedial surface of the forearm approximately at the junction of its distal third and proximal two-thirds, to capture the ulnar nerve as it approaches the ulnar artery on its medial aspect (Fig. 36-25).
Lumbar Plexus	Transverse processes	The plexus lies between and just deep to the lateral aspect (tips) of the processes (Fig. 36-34).
Femoral	Femoral artery	The nerve lies lateral to the artery (vein most medial) (Fig. 36-35). Insert the needle above the branching of the deep femoral artery.
Sciatic		
Classical/Labat	Ischial bone and inferior gluteal or pudendal vessels	The nerve lies lateral to the thinnest aspect of the ischial bone. The inferior gluteal artery generally lies medial to and at the same depth as the nerve (Fig. 36-39).
Subgluteal	Greater trochanter and ischial tuberosity	The nerve lies between the two bone structures (Fig. 36-40).
Popliteal	Popliteal artery	Trace the tibial and common peroneal nerves from the popliteal crease to where they form the sciatic nerve. At the crease, the tibial nerve lies adjacent to the popliteal artery. Scanning proximally to the sciatic bifurcation, the artery becomes deeper its distance from the nerve becomes greater (Fig. 36-41).
Ankle		
Tibial (posterior tibial)	Posterior tibial artery	The nerve lies posterior to the artery (Fig. 36-43).
Deep peroneal	Anterior tibial artery	The nerve lies lateral to the artery (Fig. 36-44).

Catheters

Continuous-infusion catheter kits suitable for PNB include a standard polyamide catheter, such as those previously used for epidural analgesia, combined with an insulated Tuohy needle with NS capability. Catheters have been developed that are amenable to stimulation via an electrode in the catheter tip, enabling confirmation of the catheter location. The recent reintroduction of catheter-over-needle assemblies allows the needle and catheter to be inserted as a single unit, avoiding the potential problems associated with threading the catheter through the needle. A catheter introduced over the needle is theoretically more stable and leakproof. These assemblies are discussed in more detail later. Precautions are required to maintain the sterility of the catheter and the insertion site.

Postblock Stage

Block Assessment and Monitoring

Following performance of a PNB, progression of the block should be monitored, and the patient's sensory and motor response in the blocked region should be assessed closely. Traditional block monitoring tools, which rely on applying cold stimuli (ice, alcohol swab) or touch (pinprick, pinch, monofilament), are generally subjective. Sensory assessment relies primarily on collecting feedback directly from the patient using validated pain rating scales. The most popular of these are variations on the 0 to 10 scale, with 0 indicating "no pain" and 10 indicating "worst pain imaginable." Other pain scales consist of or incorporate cartoons representing a series of faces in progressing severity of the pain; these scales are helpful for children and individuals who cannot communicate their pain verbally. Pain rating scales for individuals with dementia or other cognitive impairments are available and rely on the assessor's judgment of pain based on various physical and verbal cues.

Assessment of motor block is commonly performed by collecting a Bromage score[9] or equivalent based on a graded scale where the lowest score indicates the full range of movement and the highest score indicates complete block/no movement. As with sensory assessment, this method is subjective and relies on the assessor's ability to differentiate differing degrees of motor ability.

Discharge Criteria

Patients should have well-controlled pain upon discharge. Incorporating a standard level of pain relief (e.g., on a verbal rating scale) before discharge home or to the ward is prudent. Specific common risks for certain blocks should be discussed before discharge. It is necessary to provide in-depth instruction related to potential risks and their prevention if a patient is to be discharged home while an extremity is still anesthetized (i.e., if the block was performed to provide extended analgesia). Clear understanding of this information is essential for the patient and their caregivers (e.g., avoiding cooking with open heat to avoid a risk of burns to anesthetized areas, careful positioning to avoid the potential for developing pressure neuropathies). Written instructions, including the expected course, typical side effects, and 24-hour contact information, should be provided.

Avoiding Complications

Complication rates are as low as 8 per 10,000 for seizures resulting from LAST[10] and lower than 0.1% to 1% for nerve injury.[11,12] Only rare cases of severe chronic pain syndromes following regional anesthesia have been reported.[13] Careful attention to any unusual responses or reports of pain during block performance is important, as well as follow-up before and after discharge. Regrettably, these are often overlooked.

Patient Selection

Not all patients are suitable candidates for PNB. Patients scheduled for extremity, thoracic, abdominal, or perineal surgery should be considered potential candidates for peripheral regional anesthetic techniques. Adamant refusal of regional anesthesia by a patient or, in the case of children, by a parent/guardian is an absolute contraindication to the procedure. Other contraindications include local infection, systemic anticoagulation, and severe systemic coagulopathy. The presence of pre-existing neurologic disease is controversial, and although limited data are available in the case of spinal anesthesia, the safety concerning PNB is unclear. One must be cognizant of the potential to compound existing neurologic deficits; therefore, clearly documenting any deficiencies before the procedure and carefully discussing the potential risks and benefits is critical. It is imperative to follow applicable national and international guidelines, such as those set by the American Society of Anesthesiologists (ASA) for patient monitoring and those in place for anticoagulated patients, as provided by the ASRA.

Local Anesthetic Drug Selection, Toxicity, and Doses

This section will provide an overview of drug selection and toxicity during PNB. For a more detailed discussion of the pharmacology and toxicity of local anesthetics, the reader is referred to Chapter 22.

Rates of systemic and local toxicity and nerve injury with PNB 7
are generally low. Still, using available methods to reduce inadvertent intravascular and intraneural injection is warranted. It is important to note that lower concentrations of local anesthetic (e.g., 1% to 1.5% lidocaine, 0.125% to 0.5% bupivacaine) compared to those used for epidural anesthesia are appropriate for peripheral nerves. The neural toxicity of these anesthetics appears to be concentration dependent.[14] Lower concentrations are usually indicated to limit the total drug dose when larger volumes are required to anesthetize poorly localized peripheral nerves or block a series of nerves. Nevertheless, no clinical evidence suggests that prolonged nerve exposure (as with continuous PNB) to local anesthetic solutions of appropriate concentration predisposes to neurotoxic injury.[15]

Systemic toxicity is often related to accidental intravascular injection and rarely to administering an excessive quantity of local anesthetic to an appropriate site. The degree of systemic drug absorption and duration of anesthesia can also vary depending on the site of injection (i.e., the level of local vascularity) and the addition of vasoconstrictors. The highest blood levels of local anesthetic occur after intercostal blocks, followed by caudal, epidural, brachial plexus, intravenous regional, and lower extremity blocks. Equivalent doses of local anesthetic may produce only 3 to 4 hours of anesthesia when placed in the epidural space but 12 to 14 hours in the arm and 24 to 36 hours when injected along the sciatic nerve. Many believe that adding epinephrine (1:200,000 to 1:400,000) is advantageous in prolonging the block's duration and reducing local anesthetic systemic blood levels. However, this has more relevance to local anesthetics like lidocaine and less to ones like bupivacaine. Epinephrine is inappropriate in the vicinity of "terminal" blood vessels, such as in the digits, penis, or ear, or when using an intravenous regional technique. Oxygen, suction, monitoring, and appropriate resuscitation equipment must be immediately available if significant quantities of local anesthetic are to be used. Even small doses of local anesthetic may produce significant side effects when injected into susceptible regions such as the neck.

Animal studies[16] and case reports[17,18] have shown successful resuscitation from LAST by intravenous administration of Intralipid 20% (not the 10% lipid of propofol), using one or more boluses (each of 1 to 2 mL/kg or 100 mL) followed by a 30-minute infusion (0.5 mL/kg/min). However, the goal must be to prevent local anesthetic system toxicity from occurring in the first place. Intralipid should be used only as an acute resuscitation strategy when standard precautionary measures have failed.

Nerve Damage and Other Complications

Peripheral nerve injury may result from intraneural injection[19,20] or direct needle trauma.[21] Animal studies indicate that nerve injury most occurs when high injection pressures are applied intrafascicularly, particularly when highly concentrated local anesthetic solutions or their preservatives are used.[7,8,22] Thus, needle-related trauma without injection may result in injury of lesser magnitude than that from injection injury.[23] One major sequela from intrafascicular injection is endoneurial ischemia.[24] Although in some cases these syndromes resolve uneventfully, full recovery of some peripheral injuries may never occur or may require several months, a result of slow regeneration of injured peripheral nerves.[19] There is generally room around a peripheral nerve to accommodate modest low-pressure swelling, and so a hematoma around a peripheral nerve is not of the same significance or risk as in the enclosed epidural or subarachnoid space.

Complications may also result from other causes primary to the surgical procedure itself, such as patient positioning, proximity of the nerve to the surgical site, and tourniquet application.[25] These injuries cannot be said to result from the nerve block, but they may not be appreciated until the nerve block has regressed. It is essential to address patients' concerns and to try to relieve any pain or discomfort resulting from procedural complications.

Clinical Anatomy

Anatomical descriptions of major nerve structures, including plexuses and terminal/peripheral nerves, are discussed in this section. The section is divided based on regions of the body: head and neck, spine, upper extremity, trunk, and lower extremity.

Head and Neck

Trigeminal Nerve (Video 36-1)

The branches of the fifth cranial (trigeminal) nerve provide sensory and motor innervation of the face. The roots of this nerve arise from the base of the pons and send sensory branches to the large semilunar (trigeminal or Gasserian) ganglion, which lies on the dorsal surface of the petrous bone. Its anterior margin gives rise to three main branches: the ophthalmic, maxillary, and mandibular nerves (Fig. 36-4). A smaller motor fiber nucleus lies behind the main trigeminal ganglion and sends motor branches to the terminal mandibular nerve. The three major branches of the trigeminal nerve each have a separate exit from the skull:

- The uppermost ophthalmic branch passes through the sphenoidal fissure into the orbit. The main terminal fibers of this sensory nerve, the *frontal nerve*, run behind the center of the orbital cavity and bifurcate into the supratrochlear and supraorbital nerves. The *supraorbital* branch traverses the orbit along the superior border and exits on the front of the face in the easily palpated supraorbital notch; the *supratrochlear nerve* runs in a medial direction toward the trochlea.
- The *maxillary* nerve contains only sensory fibers. It exits the skull through the round foramen (foramen rotundum), passes beneath the skull anteriorly, and enters the sphenopalatine fossa. At this point, it lies medial to the lateral pterygoid plate on each side. At the anterior end of this channel, it moves superiorly to re-enter the skull in the infraorbital canal on the orbit floor and branches to form the zygomatic nerve, extending to the orbit, the short sphenopalatine (pterygopalatine) nerves, and the posterior dental branches. The anterior dental nerves arise from the main trunk as it passes through the infraorbital canal. The terminal infraorbital nerve penetrates through the inferior orbital fissure to the base of the orbit, to the infraorbital groove and canal (just below the eye and lateral to the nose), and reaches the facial surface of the maxilla. It then divides into the palpebral (lower eyelid), nasal (wing of the nose), and labial nerves (upper lip).
- The *mandibular* nerve is the third and largest branch of the trigeminal nerve and the only one to receive motor fibers. It exits the skull posterior to the maxillary nerve through the foramen ovale, forms a short thick trunk, and then divides into anterior and posterior trunks, mainly motor and sensory. The main branch (posterior trunk) continues as the inferior alveolar nerve medial to the ramus of the mandible and innervates the molar and premolar teeth. This nerve curves anteriorly to follow the mandible and exits as a terminal branch (mental nerve) through the mental foramen. The *mental* nerve provides sensation to the lower lip and chin. Other terminal nerves include the lingual nerve (floor of mouth and anterior two-thirds of tongue) and the auriculotemporal nerve (ear and temple).

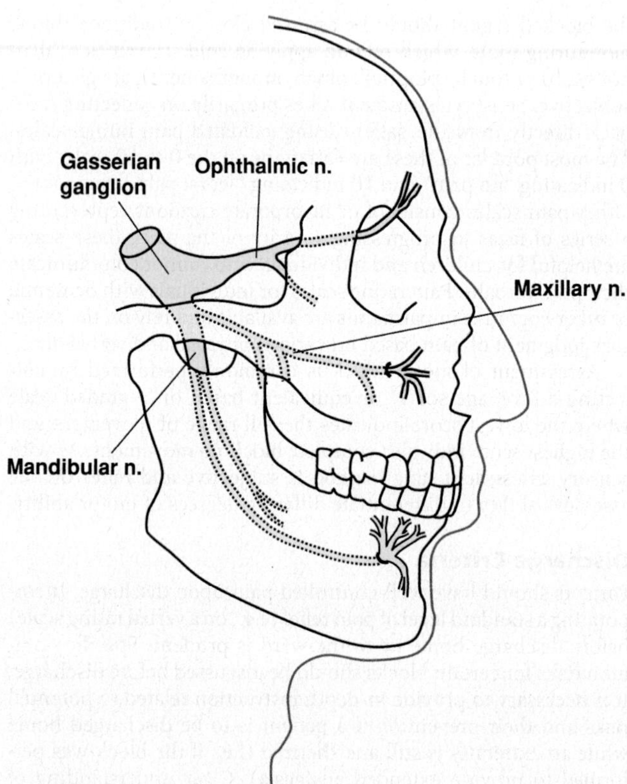

Figure 36-4 Major branches of the trigeminal nerve. The trigeminal nerve roots arise from the pons and form the large Gasserian (or semilunar) ganglion. The three major branches have separate exits from the skull. The main terminal fibers of the ophthalmic nerve—the frontal nerve—terminate as the supraorbital and supratrochlear nerves and exit their respective foramina. The maxillary and mandibular branches emerge from the skull medial to the lateral pterygoid plate. The maxillary nerve terminates as the infraorbital nerve (through the infraorbital foramen), and the mandibular nerve provides the inferior alveolar nerve (as well as motor branches), which exits at the mental foramen as the mental nerve.

Cervical Plexus

Sensory and motor fibers of the neck and posterior scalp arise from the anterior rami (branches) of the first four cervical (C1–C4) spinal nerves (Fig. 36-5). The cervical plexus is unique in that it divides early into cutaneous branches (penetrating the cervical fascia) and muscular branches (deeper branches that innervate the muscles and joints), which can be blocked separately (see Specific Techniques section). The dermatomes of the cervical nerves C2–C4 are illustrated in Figure 36-6.

Classic cervical plexus anesthesia along the tubercles of the vertebral body produces both motor and sensory blockade. The transverse processes of the cervical vertebrae form elongated troughs for the emergence of their nerve roots (Fig. 36-7). These troughs lie immediately lateral to a medial opening for the cephalad passage of the vertebral artery. The trough at the terminal end of the transverse process divides into an anterior and a posterior

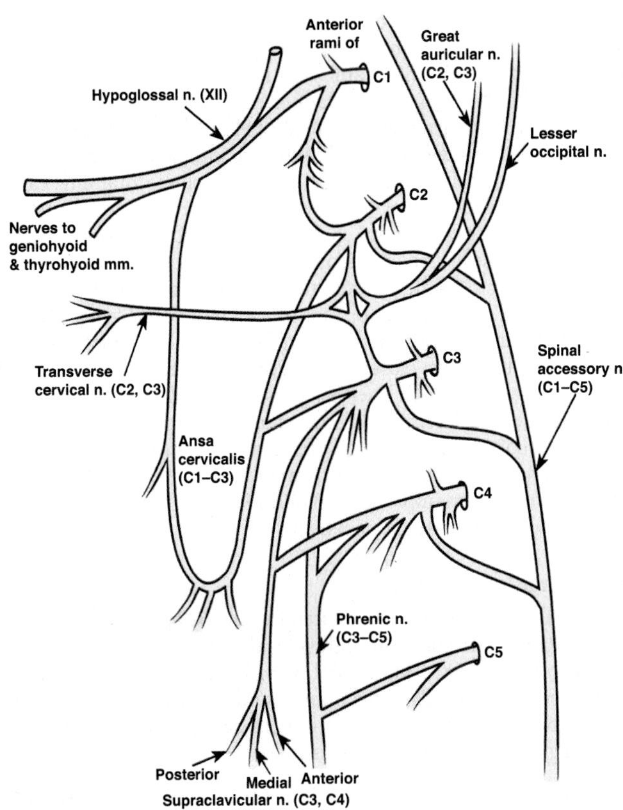

Figure 36-5 Schematic diagram of the cervical plexus, which arises from the anterior primary rami of C2–C4. The motor branches (including the phrenic nerve) curl anteriorly around the anterior scalene muscle and travel caudally and medially to supply the deep muscles of the neck. The sensory branches exit at the lateral border of the sternocleidomastoid muscle to supply the skin of the neck and the shoulder.

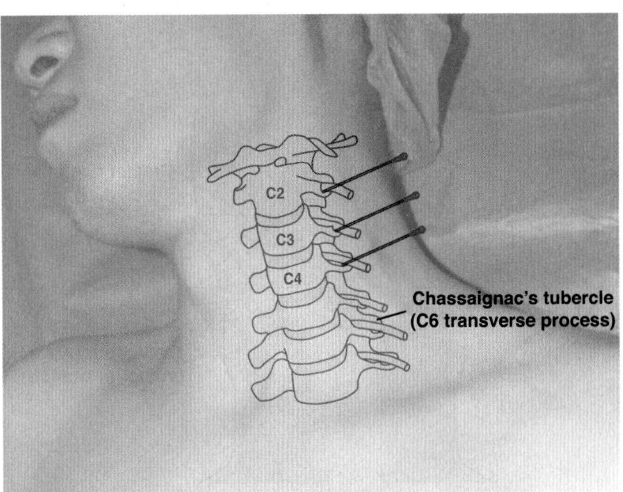

Figure 36-7 Needle insertion points and angles for deep cervical plexus block. The nerve roots exit the vertebral column via troughs formed by the transverse processes. Using caudad and posterior angulation, the needle is inserted to contact the articular pillars of C2–C4.

tubercle, which can often be easily palpated. These tubercles also serve as the attachments for the anterior and middle scalene muscles, which form a compartment for the cervical plexus and the brachial plexus immediately below. The compartment at this level is less developed than the one formed around the brachial plexus. The deep muscular branches curl anteriorly around the lateral border of the anterior scalene and then proceed caudally and medially. Many branches serve the deep anterior neck muscles. Still other branches include the inferior descending cervical nerve, the trapezius branch of the plexus, and the phrenic nerve, which give anterior branches to the sternocleidomastoid muscle as they pass behind it. The sensory fibers emerge behind

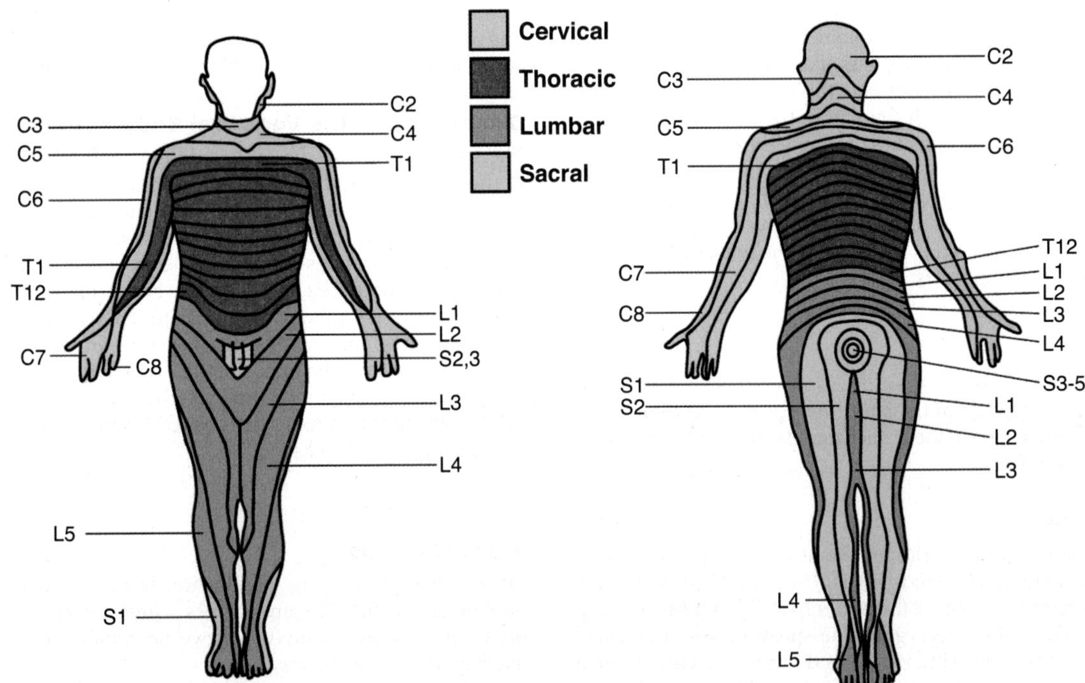

Figure 36-6 The cervical, thoracic, lumbar, and sacral dermatomes of the body.

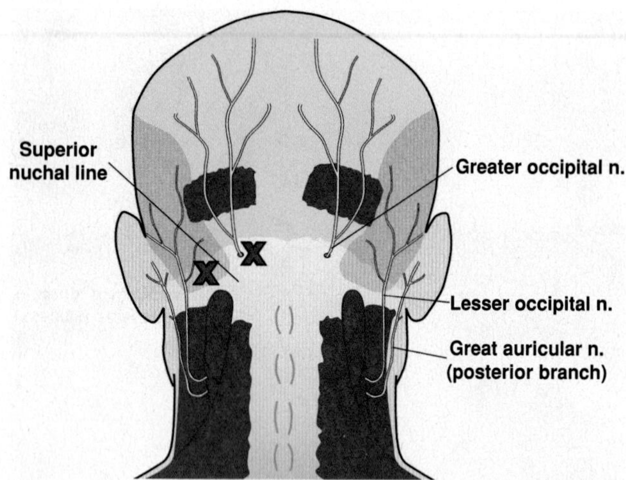

Figure 36-8 Greater and lesser occipital nerve anatomy, supply (*green*, greater occipital n.; *pink*, lesser occipital n.), and block needle insertion sites (X).

the anterior scalene muscle but separate from the motor branches and continue laterally to emerge superficially under the posterior border of the sternocleidomastoid muscle. The branches, including the lesser occipital nerve, great auricular nerve, transverse cervical nerve, and the supraclavicular nerves (anterior, medial, and posterior branches), innervate the anterior and posterior skin of the neck and shoulder.

Occipital Nerve

The ophthalmic branch of the trigeminal nerve provides sensory innervation to the forehead and anterior scalp. The remainder of the scalp is innervated by the greater and lesser occipital nerve fibers (Fig. 36-8).

The *lesser occipital nerve* arises from the superficial (cutaneous) cervical plexus (Fig. 36-5), traversing cephalad from the sternocleidomastoid muscle's posterior edge toward the top of the head, and divides into several branches. The *greater occipital nerve* arises from the posterior ramus of the second cervical spinal nerve (the cervical plexus arises from the anterior rami). It travels in a cranial direction to reach the skin in the area of the superior nuchal line while giving branches to supply the head and laterally toward the ear. These nerves can be blocked by superficial injection at the point on the posterior skull where they emerge from below the neck muscles. Alternatively, the greater occipital nerve may be blocked at the level of C2 between the semispinalis capitis and obliquus capitis muscles.

Spine

Spinal/epidural anesthesia is not discussed in this chapter. However, a basic description of the spinal nerves and vertebral structures is provided, given their relevance to the performance of other regional blocks.

Spinal Nerves

The spinal nerves are part of the peripheral nervous system, the cranial and autonomic nerves, and ganglia. There are 31 pairs of spinal nerves—8 cervical (C1–C8), 12 thoracic (T1–T12), 5 lumbar (L1–L5), 5 sacral (S1–S5), and 1 coccygeal. The spinal nerves are formed by the union of the ventral (anterior) and dorsal (posterior) spinal roots and consist of both motor and sensory fibers. In addition, all spinal nerves contain sympathetic fibers for supplying blood vessels, smooth muscle, and glands in the skin. The nerves give off sympathetic branches immediately after leaving the intervertebral foramen. Gray and white rami communicantes connect the spinal nerves to the sympathetic chain ganglia to allow preganglionic sympathetic fibers leaving the spinal cord (T1–L2/L3) to enter the chain and leave it again to be distributed with spinal nerves at all levels. Soon after exiting the intervertebral (spinal) foramina, each spinal nerve divides into a larger ventral and a smaller dorsal ramus (branches). The ventral rami course laterally and anteriorly of supplying the muscles, subcutaneous tissues (superficial fascia), and skin of the neck, trunk, and the upper and lower extremities (see the layout of dermatomes in Fig. 36-6). The dorsal rami course posteriorly and supply the paravertebral muscles, subcutaneous tissues, and back skin close to the midline. It is essential to realize that the first cervical (C1) nerve leaves the spinal cord and courses above the atlas (C1 vertebra). Consequently, the cervical nerves are numbered corresponding to the vertebra **inferior** to them. All other spinal nerves are numbered corresponding to the vertebral level **above** them. For example, the T3 and L4 spinal nerves exit below the T3 and L4 vertebrae, respectively.

Paravertebral Space

The paravertebral space is a bilateral wedge-shaped area between the individual vertebrae on both sides that extends the entire vertebral column length. The spinal nerves pass through this space, giving off their sympathetic branch and a small dorsal sensory branch before exiting from the intervertebral foramina. In the thoracic region, its boundaries are as follows:

- Medially: The vertebral body, intervertebral disc and foramen, and spinous processes (angulation decreases from T1 to L4/L5).
- Anterolaterally: The parietal pleura.
- Posteriorly: The costotransverse process, approximately 2.5 cm from the tip of the spinous process, is often in a slightly caudad orientation.

The intervertebral foramina at each level lie between the transverse processes and approximately 1 to 2 cm anterior to the plane formed by the transverse processes in their associated fasciae. At this point, the sympathetic ganglia lie close to the somatic nerves, and coincidental sympathetic block is usually attained.

Orientation of the Vertebral Body Processes

The spinous processes lie in the midline, with T7 at the distal tip of the scapulae and L4 at the level of the iliac crests. The transverse processes lie approximately 2.5 cm lateral to the spinous processes: At T1, the transverse process is directly lateral to its corresponding spinous process, but subsequent transverse processes in the midthoracic region are increasingly cephalad (i.e., the T7 transverse process is lateral to T6 spinous process). In the lumbar region, the spinous processes are straight, and the transverse processes lie opposite their respective spinous process. Variations in the anatomy of the vertebral column should be considered when determining the desired location for needle insertion during trunk blocks.

Upper Extremity

Brachial Plexus

The brachial plexus (Fig. 36-9) arises from the anterior primary rami of C5–C8 and T1 spinal nerves. The network consists of five *roots*, three *trunks*, six *divisions* (two per trunk), three *cords*, and five major terminal nerves.

The C5–T1 nerve roots emerge from their corresponding intervertebral foramina and then travel along the grooves between the

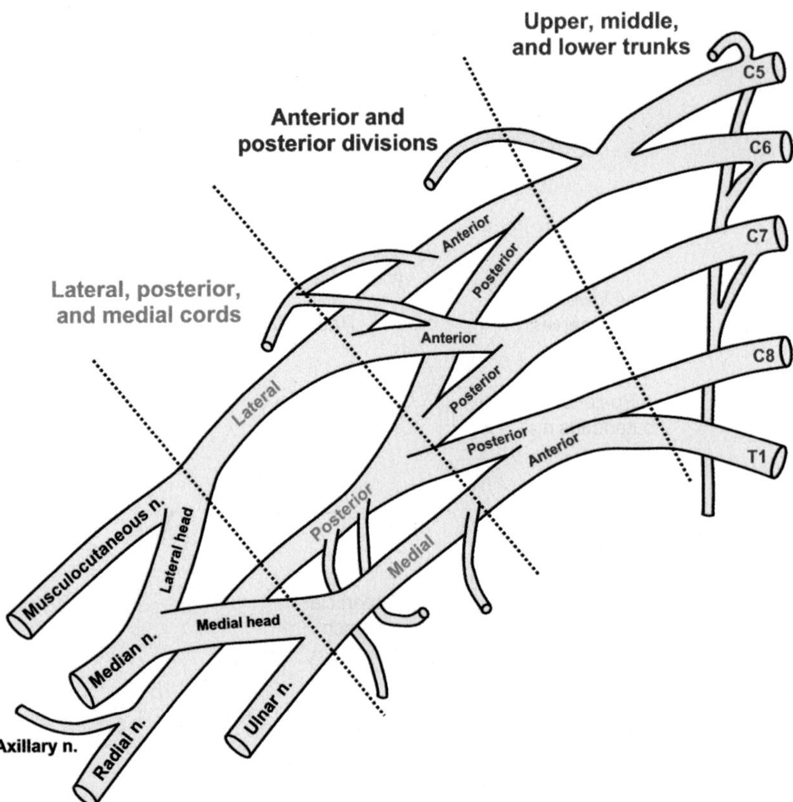

Figure 36-9 Schematic diagram of the brachial plexus. Not shown are the many branches, including the medial cutaneous nerves of the forearm and arm, which arise from the medial cord.

anterior and posterior tubercles of the corresponding transverse process. They finally emerge between the anterior and medius scalene muscles, above the second part of the subclavian artery and posterior to the vertebral artery. The C5 and C6 nerve roots unite to form the *upper (superior) trunk*, C7 continues as the *middle trunk*, and C8 and T1 converge into the *lower (inferior) trunk*. Fibrous sheaths (as part of the prevertebral fascia) surround the anterior and posterior aspects of the plexus and continue to envelop the plexus between the scalene muscles more distally (called the *interscalene fascial sheath* proximally and the *axillary sheath* distally). The three trunks travel inferolateral and cross the base of the posterior triangle of the neck (superficial) and the first rib (upper and middle trunks above the subclavian artery and lower trunk behind or below the artery). At the lateral border of the first rib, each trunk bifurcates into *anterior* and *posterior* divisions. Approximately at the level where the nerves course under the pectoralis minor muscle, the divisions converge to form three *cords: lateral cord*—anterior divisions of upper and middle trunks (C5–C7); *medial cord*—an anterior division of lower trunk (C8, T1); *posterior cord*—posterior divisions of all three trunks (C5–T1). The cords are grouped around the second part of the axillary artery (within 2.5 cm from its center). There are three parts of the axillary artery named for their positions above (medial to), behind, and below (lateral to) the pectoralis minor muscle. Typically, with a US probe placed to view the transverse axis of the cords, the medial cord lies inferior, the lateral cord superior, and the posterior cord posterior to the first part of the axillary artery. Immediately beyond the pectoralis minor muscle, the three cords diverge into the terminal branches, including the median, ulnar, radial, axillary, and musculocutaneous nerves. The phrenic nerve descends typically anterior to the scalenus anterior muscle. It crosses the muscle from lateral to medial as it descends and passes under the clavicle and through the superior thoracic aperture into the superior mediastinum, just medial to the external jugular vein. However, there is anatomic variation in the course of the phrenic nerve and it is not always anterior to the anterior scalene muscle.

Terminal Nerves of the Brachial Plexus

The anatomy of the peripheral nerves is outlined here, although the clinically related innervation patterns are included in each block's technique discussion. Figure 36-10 illustrates the courses of these nerves within the upper extremity. Figure 36-11 shows the cutaneous innervation of the terminal nerves of the upper extremity. The axillary nerve is an additional terminal nerve of the upper extremity, but the anatomy and block of this nerve will not be discussed here.

Radial Nerve (Originates from C5–C8 and T1 Roots, Upper and Middle Trunks, Posterior Divisions, and Posterior Cord)

This nerve originates deep (often posteromedial) to the axillary artery, descends within the axilla (giving off branches to the long head of the triceps brachii), passes between the medial and lateral heads of the triceps, and then descends obliquely across the posterior aspect of the humerus along the spiral (radial) groove at the level of the deltoid insertion. The nerve travels posterior and medial to the deep brachial artery of the arm. It reaches the lateral margin of the humerus 5 to 7 cm above the elbow before crossing over the lateral epicondyle and entering the anterior compartment of the arm. In front of the elbow, the nerve divides and continues as the superficial radial (sensory) and the deep posterior interosseous (motor) nerves.

Median Nerve (Originates from C5–C8, T1, All Trunks, and Lateral and Medial Cords)

In the axilla, this nerve often lies anterolateral to the axillary artery. The nerve descends along the medial aspect of the arm

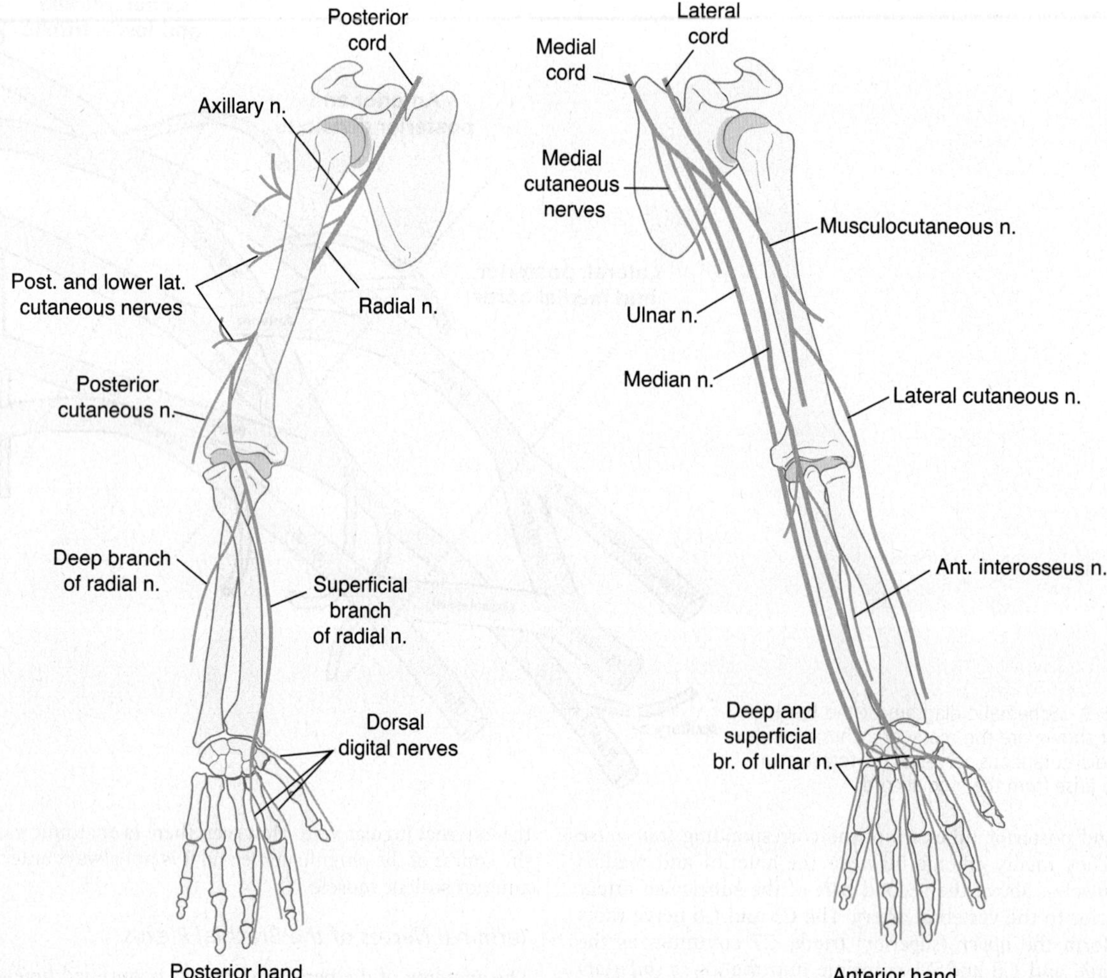

Figure 36-10 Courses of the terminal nerves of the upper extremity. The anterior view (**A**) shows branches from the lateral (musculocutaneous and median nerves) and medial (median and ulnar nerves) cords, while the posterior view (**B**) shows branches from the posterior cord (axillary and radial nerves).

lateral to the brachial artery. It crosses the artery, usually anteriorly, at the midpoint of the arm at the insertion of the coracobrachialis muscle. The nerve crosses the elbow lying medially on the brachialis muscle and just medial to the brachial artery and vein (all of these are medial to the biceps brachii tendon). Distal to the antecubital fossa, the nerve gives off the anterior interosseous nerve and cutaneous sensory branches.

Axillary n.

Medial cutaneous nerve of the arm

Medial cutaneous nerve of the forearm

Radial n.

Musculocutaneous n.

Ulnar n.

Median n.

Figure 36-11 Cutaneous innervation of the upper extremity.

Musculocutaneous Nerve (Originates from C5–C7 Roots, Upper and Middle Trunks, Anterior Divisions, and Lateral Cord)

This nerve leaves the fascial sheath of the plexus approximately at the level of the coracoid process; thus, the infraclavicular location is the most distal brachial plexus block for this nerve. Just distal (2 to 3 cm) to the pectoralis major muscle attachment, the nerve usually pierces the coracobrachialis muscle, after which it exits and comes to lie between the coracobrachialis muscle and the short and long heads of the biceps brachii muscle. Although it is difficult to observe using US, the nerve continues as the lateral cutaneous nerve of the forearm at the antecubital fossa and courses along the lateral aspect of the forearm, providing subsequent anterior and posterior branches.

Ulnar Nerve (Originates from C7–C8, T1 Roots, Lower Trunk, Anterior Division, and Medial Cord)

Initially, the nerve often courses between the axillary artery and vein (it may lie anteromedial to the artery and vein) and then along the medial aspect of the brachial artery to the midpoint of the humerus before passing posteriorly and following the anterior surface of the medial head of the triceps. The nerve then passes behind the medial epicondyle of the humerus (in the condylar groove), divides between the humeral and ulnar heads of the flexor carpi ulnaris, and lies on the medial aspect of the elbow joint. During its descent through the forearm, the nerve courses anteriorly to approach the ulnar artery directly anterior to the ulna at the junction of the lower third and upper two-thirds of the forearm. At the wrist, it crosses superficial to the flexor retinaculum and divides into superficial and deep branches. The ulnar artery lies anterolateral to the nerve at the wrist.

Anatomic Variation

There are many variations in the anatomy of the brachial plexus and the course of the terminal nerves and vascular elements. Some of these variations may contribute to difficulty performing PNB since there may be unexpected NS responses (e.g., if two nerves are conjoined) or poor localization by NS or by US imaging (e.g., if the nerve follows a substantially different path). Some examples are described here:

- The plexus may include anterior rami from C4 to C8 ("prefixed") or, less commonly, from C5 to T2 ("postfixed").
- The existence and characteristics of the connective tissue sheath that invests the plexus at various regions are controversial. A continuous, tubular sheath has been shown unlikely, especially in the axillary region. A more complex and septated structure may cause a nonuniform distribution of local anesthetic, supporting the finding that a multiple injection technique may be superior.[26] US guidance can be valuable in this location to ensure circumferential spread of local anesthetic around the nerves.
- The interscalene groove may vary in the relationship between the plexus roots, trunks, and muscles. For example, the C5 and C6 nerve roots may traverse either through or anterior to the anterior scalene muscle.
- In many cadaver specimens, no inferior trunk exists. A single cord or a pair of cords may develop. In some cases, no discrete posterior cord forms, with the posterior divisions diverging to form terminal nerves.
- The terminal nerves may lie in various relations to the axillary vessels. Combining NS- and US-guided techniques to confirm the nerve localization (NS) and obtain a circumferential spread of local anesthetic around each nerve (US) may improve block success.[27] The musculocutaneous nerve may fuse to or communicate with the median nerve, resulting in the former's absence from within the coracobrachialis muscle. Communication between the median and ulnar nerves in the forearm is common, with the median nerve replacing the innervation to various muscles normally supplied by the ulnar nerve.
- There may also be variations concerning the vessels within the arm, with aberrant formations including double axillary veins, a high origin of the radial artery, and double brachial arteries.

Trunk

Intercostal Nerves and Articulations

Intercostal Nerves

At the thoracic level, each anterior primary ramus enters a neurovascular bundle with its respective artery and vein and travels along the intercostal groove on the ventral caudal surface of each rib. The fasciae of the internal and external intercostal muscles provide the borders of the intercostal groove. As the intercostal nerves travel beyond the midaxillary line, they give off a lateral sensory branch. The main trunk continues to the anterior abdominal wall to provide sensory and motor innervation for the trunk and abdomen down to the pubis level. The intercostal groove becomes less well-defined anterior to the midaxillary line, and the nerves begin to move away from their protected position. The lowermost intercostal nerve (subcostal; 12th) is less proximal to its accompanying rib and is not as easy to identify and anesthetize using a classic intercostal blockade technique.

Costovertebral Articulations

The ribs articulate through two synovial joints with the vertebral column, each enclosed in fibrous capsules that are reinforced by ligaments. The *costovertebral joint* is a synovial articulation of the head of the rib with the demi-facets on the adjacent thoracic vertebral bodies and the corresponding intervertebral disc of the upper vertebral joint (except for the 1st, 10th, 11th, and 12th ribs, which articulate with a single vertebral facet). The *costotransverse joint* is a synovial joint between the articular facets on the ribs' tubercles and the thoracic vertebrae's transverse processes (except for the 11th and 12th ribs which lack this articulation as they do not possess tubercles). Penetration of the costotransverse ligament may occur during a paravertebral block.

Lumbar Spinal Nerves and Plexus

The spinal nerves at the lumbar level follow the same course as those of the thoracic level when leaving the intervertebral foramen, but the anterior (ventral) rami then form the lumbar plexus instead of continuing as intercostal nerves. The lumbar plexus (Fig. 36-12) is formed by the union of the anterior primary rami of L1–L3 and part of L4.

The upper nerve roots emerge from their foramina into a compartment lined by the fasciae of muscles anterior and posterior to it. The quadratus lumborum (QL) provides the posterior border of the compartment. The anterior border of the compartment is the rear fascia of the psoas muscle, through which the nerves pass. In anatomic relation to the psoas major muscle, the obturator (L2–L4) and accessory obturator nerves emerge from its medial border, the genitofemoral (L1, L2) pierces the muscle to lie on its anterior surface, and all others emerge from its lateral border.

The lumbar plexus supplies the skin and muscles of the lower part of the anterior abdominal wall (including the external genitalia) and the skin and muscles of the anterior and medial compartments of the thigh. L1 bifurcates into an *upper* part (iliohypogastric and ilioinguinal nerves) and *a lower* part, which joins with a branch from L2 to form the genitofemoral nerve. L3, with portions of L2 and L4, divides into *anterior* and *posterior divisions*. The anterior division forms the obturator (L2–L4) and accessory obturator (L3, L4, when present) nerves, whereas the posterior division forms the lateral (femoral) cutaneous nerve of the thigh (L2–L3) and the femoral nerve (L2–L4). The terminal nerves of the lumbar plexus are discussed in the Lower Extremity section.

Inguinal Nerves

The iliohypogastric nerve penetrates the transverse abdominal muscle just above the iliac crest, supplies the muscle, and divides into anterior and lateral cutaneous branches:

- The anterior branch pierces and supplies the internal oblique muscle just 2 cm medial to the anterior superior iliac spine. It then courses deep to the external oblique muscle and superior to the inguinal canal. It pierces the external oblique aponeurosis about 2 to 3 cm above the superficial inguinal ring, terminating subcutaneously in the skin of the suprapubic region.
- The lateral cutaneous branch supplies the anterolateral portion of the gluteal skin after piercing both the oblique muscles.

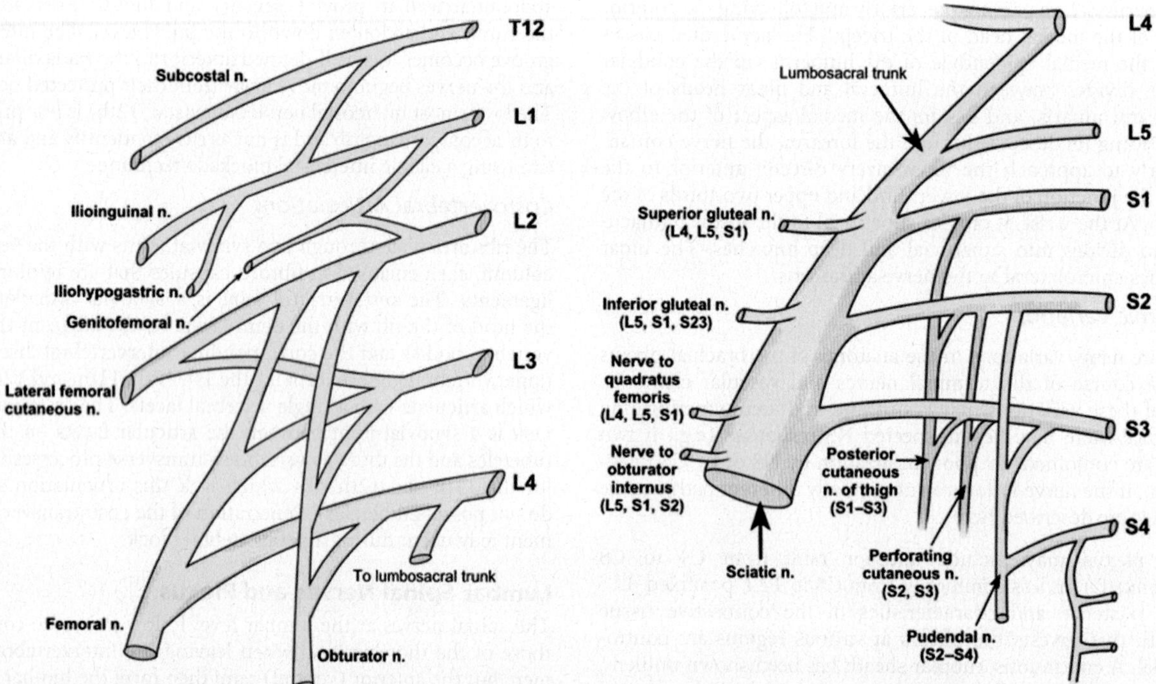

Figure 36-12 Schematic diagrams of the lumbar (**left**; L1–L4) and sacral (**right**; L4–S4) plexuses.

The ilioinguinal nerve pierces and supplies the internal oblique muscle and then enters the inguinal canal, where it traverses outside the spermatic cord to emerge through the superficial (external) inguinal ring (the external oblique aponeurosis), providing cutaneous innervation to the skin of the scrotum (or labium majus) and adjacent thigh.

Lumbosacral Plexus: Formation and Branches

At the medial border of the psoas major muscle, the lumbosacral trunk is formed by the union of a branch of L4 and the anterior ramus of L5. After exiting through the anterior sacral foramina, the anterior primary rami of S1–S4 join the lumbosacral trunk to form the sacral plexus (Fig. 36-12). The sacral plexus nerves converge toward the greater sciatic foramen anterior to the piriformis muscle on the posterior pelvic wall. The main terminal nerves are the sciatic nerve (continuation of the plexus) and the pudendal nerves ("terminal branches"). Several other small branches are given off, including muscular branches (e.g., inferior and superior gluteal nerves and nerves to the quadratus femoris, piriformis, obturator internus, and external sphincter muscles), cutaneous branches (e.g., posterior cutaneous nerve of the thigh), and visceral branches (pelvic splanchnic nerves). The gluteal vessels (superior and inferior) generally follow the course of the sacral nerves in the anterior plane. They can be used to help identify the sciatic nerve at its proximal course. Additional vascular structures that may be identified under US imaging are the pudendal vessels, which pass from the greater to lesser sciatic foramen between the sciatic and pudendal nerves.

Lower Extremity

Together, the lumbar and sacral plexuses supply the lower limb (Fig. 36-12). Cutaneous innervation in the lower extremity is shown in Figure 36-13. The lower extremity dermatomes are shown in Figure 36-6.

Terminal Nerves of the Lumbar Plexus

Genitofemoral Nerve (L1, L2)

This nerve leaves the lumbar plexus at the lower border of the L3 vertebra. It pierces and then lies anterior to the psoas major muscle before descending subperitoneal and behind the ureter. It divides into two branches (genital and femoral) at a variable distance above the inguinal ligament. The genital branch crosses the external iliac artery and traverses the inguinal canal. It supplies

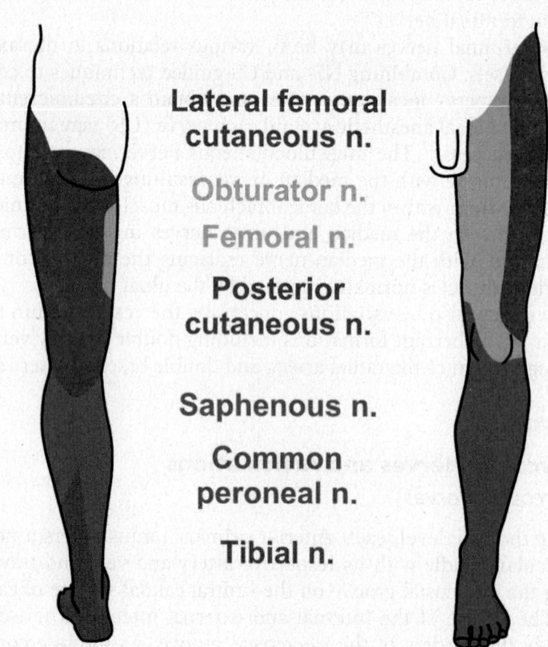

Figure 36-13 Cutaneous innervation of the lower extremity by terminal nerves.

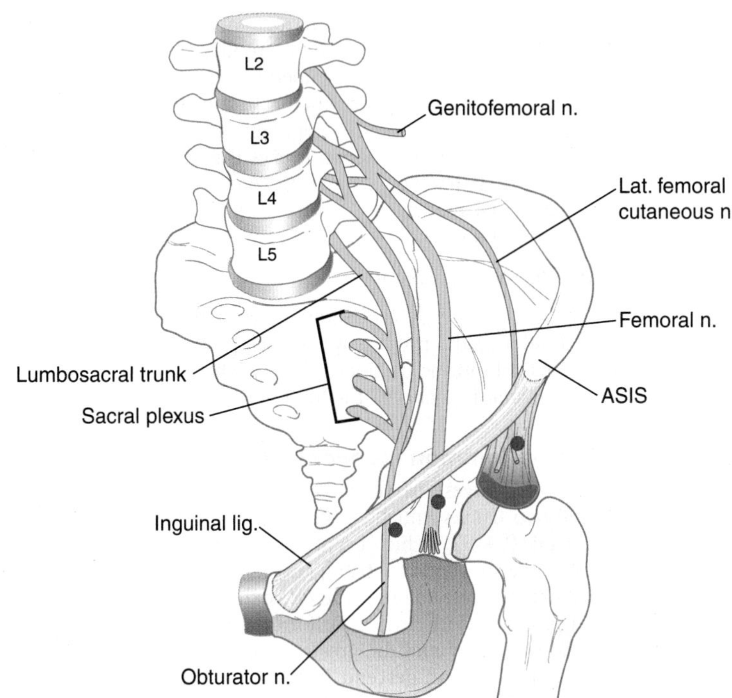

Figure 36-14 An illustration of the anterior pelvic area shows courses of major lumbar plexus branches. Needle insertion sites (*red dot*) for blocking the lateral femoral cutaneous, femoral, and obturator nerves are shown. ASIS, anterior superior iliac spine.

the cremaster muscle and skin over the scrotum and adjacent thigh (males) or the skin over the anterior part of labium majus and mons pubis (females). The femoral branch descends lateral to the external iliac artery, passes under the inguinal ligament, enters the femoral sheath lateral to the femoral artery, and pierces the anterior layer of the femoral sheath and fascia lata. It innervates the skin immediately below the crease of the groin anterior to the upper part of the femoral triangle.

Lateral Cutaneous Nerve of Thigh (aka, Lateral Femoral Cutaneous Nerve) (L2, L3)

This nerve passes obliquely from the lateral border of the psoas major muscle over the iliacus to enter the thigh below or through the inguinal ligament, variably medial to the anterior superior iliac spine (Fig. 36-14). On the right side of the body, the nerve passes posterolateral to the cecum, and on the left, it traverses behind the lower part of the descending colon. The nerve lies on top of the sartorius muscle before dividing into anterior (supplies skin over the anterolateral aspect of the thigh) and posterior (supplies skin on the lateral aspect of the thigh from the greater trochanter to the midthigh) branches. Occasionally, this nerve is a branch of the femoral nerve rather than its own nerve.

Femoral Nerve (L2–L4)

The femoral nerve is the largest nerve of the lumbar plexus, supplying muscles and skin on the anterior aspect of the thigh. It descends through the psoas major muscle and emerges low at its lateral border, coursing inferiorly between the iliacus and psoas major muscles to enter the thigh under the inguinal ligament (Fig. 36-14). At the inguinal ligament (the line running between the anterior superior iliac spine and the medial pubic tubercle) and just distal to it (in the femoral triangle), the nerve lies slightly deeper (0.5 to 1 cm) and lateral (approximately 1.5 cm) to the femoral artery; the vein is medial to the artery ("VAN" is the mnemonic for the anatomic relationship, starting medially). At the femoral (inguinal) crease (a few centimeters caudad to the inguinal ligament), the nerve lies underneath the fascia iliaca (iliopectineal fascia), deep to the fascia lata. Beyond the femoral triangle, the nerve branches into anterior (quite proximally) and posterior divisions. The anterior division gives muscular branches to the pectineus and sartorius muscles and cutaneous branches (intermediate and medial cutaneous nerves of the thigh) to the skin on the anterior aspect of the thigh. The posterior division sends muscular branches to the quadriceps femoris muscle and gives rise to the *saphenous nerve*, its largest cutaneous branch. The saphenous nerve follows the femoral artery, lying lateral to it within the adductor (Hunter's, subsartorial) canal and crossing it anteriorly to lie medial to the artery. Distal to the canal, the saphenous nerve leaves the artery to lie superficial at the medial aspect of the knee; the nerve then continues inferiorly (subcutaneously) with the lengthy (great) saphenous vein along the medial aspect of the leg down to the tibial aspect of the ankle. The saphenous branch supplies the skin on the medial aspect of the leg below the knee and the medial aspect of the foot; it provides articular branches to the hip, knee, and ankle joints.

Obturator Nerve (L2–L4)

The obturator nerve emerges from the medial border of the psoas major muscle at the pelvic brim to pass behind the common iliac vessels and lateral to the internal iliac vessels. It then courses inferiorly and anteriorly along the lateral wall of the pelvic cavity on the obturator internus muscle toward the obturator canal, through which it enters the upper part of the medial aspect of the thigh above and anterior to the obturator vessels. The nerve divides into its anterior and posterior branches near the obturator foramen (Fig. 36-14); the anterior branch passes into the thigh anterior to the obturator externus, descends in front of the adductor brevis, and behind the pectineus and adductor longus muscle, with its terminal cutaneous branches emerging as it courses alongside the femoral artery. It supplies the adductor longus, gracilis, adductor brevis (usually), and pectineus (often) muscles. Cutaneous branches supply the skin on the medial aspect of the thigh and perhaps to the medial knee. The nerve's posterior branch pierces the obturator externus muscle anteriorly and supplies it, then passes behind the adductor brevis muscle (sometimes supplies it) to descend on the anterior aspect of the adductor magnus muscle (medial to the anterior branch), which it supplies. There is no apparent cutaneous supply from this nerve. It uses the adductor canal with the femoral artery and vein to enter the popliteal fossa. It terminates as an articular branch to the back of the knee joint capsule (oblique popliteal ligament).

Accessory Obturator Nerve (L3, L4)

This nerve is present in about 30% of individuals. It descends along the medial border of the psoas major muscle, crosses the superior pubic ramus behind the pectineus muscle, supplies the muscle, and gives articular branches to the hip joint.

Sciatic, Tibial, and Common Peroneal Nerves

The sciatic nerve—the largest nerve of the body—is usually the conjunction of two trunks initially enveloped in a common sheath: a lateral trunk (L4–S2), which eventually emerges as the common peroneal nerve, and a medial trunk (L4–S3), which later becomes the tibial nerve. These combined nerves exit through the sciatic notch and pass anteriorly to the piriformis muscle to lie between the ischial tuberosity and the greater trochanter of the femur. They curve caudally and descend in the posterior thigh adjacent to the femur. The sciatic nerve bifurcates into the tibial and common peroneal nerves at a variable distance within the posterior thigh (often high in the popliteal fossa). The common peroneal nerve descends along the medial border of the biceps femoris muscle and then on the lateral border of the gastrocnemius muscle. At the fossa, it gives off the lateral sural nerve, which forms the lateral sural cutaneous nerve by joining the medial sural nerve supplied by the tibial nerve. It winds around the neck of the fibula and terminates as the deep and superficial peroneal nerves. In the posterior thigh, the tibial nerve is covered medially by the semitendinosus and semimembranosus muscles and laterally by the biceps femoris muscle. Beyond the knee joint, it is covered by both heads of the gastrocnemius muscle and then deep to the soleus muscle before coming to an end on the tibialis posterior muscle and finally on the posterior surface of the tibial shaft medial to the medial malleolus. Within the fossa, it gives off muscular branches (gastrocnemius, soleus, popliteus, and plantaris muscles) and the medial sural nerve (to join its lateral counterpart from the common peroneal nerve). In the lower leg and foot, it gives off muscular, articular (ankle), and cutaneous branches and terminates as the medial and lateral plantar nerves. The nerve is often called the posterior tibial nerve in the lower leg.

Nerves at the Ankle

By the time the femoral, tibial, and common peroneal nerves reach the ankle, five branches cross this joint to provide innervation for the skin and muscles of the foot.

Saphenous Nerve

The saphenous nerve is the superficial terminus of the femoral nerve and supplies the skin over the medial lower leg (Fig. 36-13). It leaves the femoral nerve proximally in the femoral triangle (Scarpa triangle), descends within the adductor canal, and courses beneath the sartorius muscle with the femoral artery (beginning lateral of the vessel at first and then crossing to the medial side superior to the artery just proximal of the lower end of the adductor magnus muscle). Further distally, the femoral artery departs from the sartorius muscle, traveling deep to continue as the popliteal artery at the adductor hiatus. At this location, the saphenous nerve continues its course under the sartorius muscle, traveling adjacent to the saphenous branch of the descending genicular artery. It runs superficially at the medial surface of the lower leg and in front of the heel.

Deep Peroneal Nerve (L5, S1)

This nerve lies anterior to the tibia and interosseus membrane and lateral to the anterior tibial artery and vein at the ankle. It travels deep to and between the tendons of the extensor hallucis longus and extensor digitorum longus muscles. Beyond the extensor retinaculum, it branches into medial and lateral terminal branches; the medial branch passes over the dorsum of the foot and supplies the first web space through two digital terminal branches, and the lateral branch traverses laterally and terminates as the second, third, and fourth dorsal interosseous nerves.

Tibial Nerve (aka, Posterior Tibial Nerve; S1–S3)

The tibial nerve joins the posterior tibial artery on the posterior aspect of the knee joint. It then runs deep through the lower third of the leg, where it emerges at the medial border of the calcaneal tendon (Achilles tendon). Behind the medial malleolus, it lies beneath several layers of fascia and is separated from the Achilles tendon only by the tendon of the flexor hallucis longus muscle. The nerve is posteromedial to the posterior tibial artery and vein, which are, in turn, posteromedial to the tendons of the flexor digitorum longus and tibialis posterior muscles. The nerve divides into the lateral and medial plantar nerves below the medial malleolus. The nerve innervates the ankle joint through its articular branches and the skin over the medial malleolus, the inner aspect of the heel (including the Achilles tendon), and the dorsum of the foot (through the medial and lateral plantar nerves) with its cutaneous branches.

Superficial Peroneal Nerve

The superficial peroneal nerve lies lateral to the deep peroneal nerve in the upper leg. The anterolateral aspect of the lower leg becomes superficial about 7 to 8 cm above the lateral malleolus. It divides into medial and lateral dorsal cutaneous nerves to supply the dorsum of the foot.

Sural Nerve

This nerve arises from the tibial (medial sural nerve) and common peroneal (lateral sural nerve) nerves. It emerges in the superficial compartment at a similar but posterior level to the superficial peroneal nerve, 7 to 8 cm above the lateral malleolus. It then curves around the malleolus at some distance (1 to 1.5 cm) to enter and innervate the lateral aspect of the dorsal surface of the foot.

Specific Techniques

The remainder of this chapter is devoted to the procedural details of specific blocks, arranged by body regions. Head and neck blocks are primarily performed using anatomic landmarks. Upper extremity, trunk, and lower extremity blocks are described using both NS and US imaging techniques. Unless otherwise stated, NS is performed with variable currents with a frequency of 2 Hz and pulse width of 0.1 ms. The suggested volumes of local anesthetic to use are for blocks performed with NS; US guidance may reduce the required volume in some instances. The figures in these sections will focus on combining the US- and the NS-guided techniques, although procedures for blind techniques using NS alone are also described. The figures include cadaveric sections obtained from the Visible Human Visualization Software, which show the anatomic arrangement of structures relevant to each block. Note that the figures are representative of the clinical scenario and technique, but sterile preparation has been omitted in order to show proper probe and needle handling more clearly.

Head and Neck

Regional anesthesia for the head and neck is diverse, and many head and neck surgical procedures are amenable to some form of regional block. Techniques range from local infiltration to field block to specific nerve blocks. Blocks can be used for ophthalmic, neurologic, ENT, plastic, and endocrine surgeries. Regional anesthesia techniques, such as trigeminal or occipital nerve block, may also be used for diagnostic and therapeutic purposes in acute and chronic pain syndromes. A regional technique may be the sole mode of anesthesia or may be incorporated into a balanced general anesthetic offering optimal postsurgical analgesia. The absence of definitive airway control is a frequent concern with regional techniques, since obtaining airway control intraoperatively can be challenging. Regional anesthesia of the head and neck depends primarily on local infiltration and specific nerve blocks placed with reliable anatomic landmarks, and elicitation of paresthesia is the primary method for nerve localization. NS and US imaging are not usually employed.

Trigeminal Nerve Blocks

Prepare the needle insertion site and other applicable skin areas with an antiseptic solution for every procedure, and use sterile equipment. All blocks described here use the extraoral route, although alternative intraoral routes may be suitable in many cases.

Semilunar (Gasserian) Ganglion Block

The most comprehensive block of the trigeminal nerve targets the central ganglion (Fig. 36-4, NICV 36-1). This block is usually performed under fluoroscopic guidance to treat disabling trigeminal neuralgia. Few operating room anesthesiologists perform this technically challenging block, which is used more often in chronic pain and will not be described in detail here.

Superficial Trigeminal Nerve Branch Block

Trigeminal block can be performed easily by injecting the three individual terminal superficial branches (supraorbital, infraorbital, and mental nerves). Each nerve is associated closely with its respective foramina, and all foramina lie in the same sagittal plane on each side of the face (approximately 2.5 cm lateral to the midfacial line passing through the pupil) (Fig. 36-15) and are easily located by US.[28] These foramina are readily palpable, and the nerves can be blocked with superficial injections of small quantities of local anesthetic. The bony landmarks are usually sufficient for routine anesthetic purposes. However, paresthesias are desirable when performing neurolytic blocks with alcohol. An additional block of the supratrochlear nerve is required if the field of anesthesia is to cross the midline. In general, fine, short needles (e.g., 24 to 26 gauge, 25 to 40 mm) and small syringes (1 to 5 mL) will be suitable for these blocks. The block is usually performed with the patient in the supine position.

Procedure

- *Supraorbital nerve (terminal nerve of the ophthalmic branch).* The supraorbital notch can be easily palpated at the upper medial angle of the orbit or located by the US, as shown in Figure 36-15. The needle is inserted, and local anesthetic (see Clinical Pearls) is injected slowly after aspiration, slightly outside the notch, producing anesthesia of the ipsilateral forehead.
- *Supratrochlear nerve (terminal nerve of the ophthalmic branch).* Anesthesia of the supratrochlear nerve is obtained with superficial infiltration of the upper internal angle of the orbital rim. This is needed if the field of anesthesia is to cross the midline.
- *Infraorbital nerve (terminal branch of the maxillary nerve).* The infraorbital foramen lies about 1 cm below the middle of the

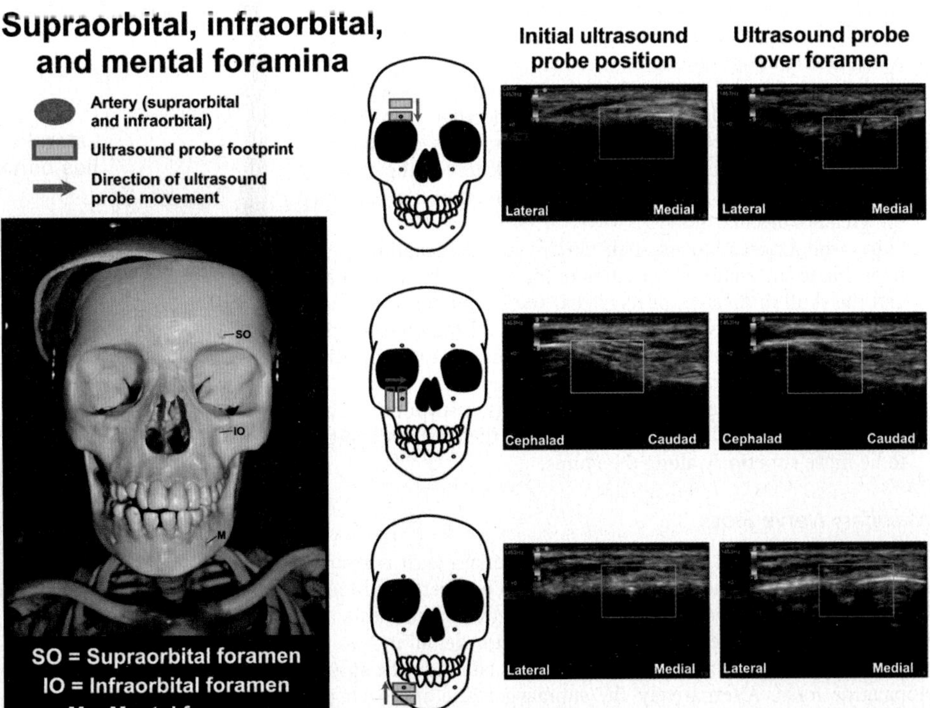

Figure 36-15 Ultrasound scanning of the supraorbital, infraorbital, and mental foramina. Discontinuation of the hyperechoic bony line indicates the position of the foramen.

lower orbital margin. If the foramen cannot be palpated directly, it can be identified by locating the discontinuity of the hyperechoic line on the US (Fig. 36-15).[28] The needle should be introduced in a cranial direction through a skin wheal approximately 0.5 cm below the expected opening. After making contact with the bone and withdrawing slightly, a small quantity of local anesthetic is injected. This block produces anesthesia of the middle third of the ipsilateral face.

- *Mental nerve (sensory terminal branch of the mandibular nerve).* The mental nerve emerges from its foramen, which lies inferior to the outer lip at the level of the second premolar, midway between the upper and lower borders of the mandible. The mental canal angles medially and inferiorly; therefore, needle insertion should start approximately 0.5 cm above and 0.5 cm lateral to the anticipated location of the orifice if it cannot be palpated directly. Again, using US can aid in identification of the foramen (Fig. 36-15). Slow injection after aspiration at the canal's opening produces anesthesia of the mandibular area. Injection directly into the canal should be avoided to reduce the risk of neural injury.

Clinical Pearls

- The choice of local anesthetic for all blocks will depend on the purpose of the block and the duration of anesthesia required (e.g., 1% mepivacaine for shorter procedures and 0.75% ropivacaine for more prolonged procedures). For surgical anesthesia, 2 to 5 mL of local anesthetic may be used, whereas diagnostic or therapeutic volumes or volumes for infants will be much smaller (0.5 to 1 mL).
- Blocks should be followed by local compression to prevent hematoma formation.
- PNB of the terminal branches of the trigeminal nerve offers a safe and effective alternative to local infiltration for soft tissue injury of the face. Despite this, local infiltration is often required to rectify incomplete anesthesia, especially of the supra- and infraorbital nerves.[29]
- Infraorbital nerve block may be performed for postoperative analgesia after cleft lip repair. Palpating anatomic landmarks for this block can be problematic in the neonate due to the developing facial configuration.
- Skull nerve blocks can be used for craniotomy procedures and are recommended to attenuate postoperative pain.[30] The nerves blocked to achieve successful anesthesia for craniotomy include the supraorbital and supratrochlear nerves, the greater and lesser occipital nerves, the auriculotemporal nerves, and the greater auricular nerve.
- Supraorbital nerve blocks often require supplementation, perhaps due to the anatomic variation of the nerve. The nerve may exit the skull undivided, or its medial and lateral branches may exit separately. For frame pin placement during stereotactic neurosurgery, failure to block the lateral branch may account for inadequate coverage.[31]
- During mental nerve block in older patients, resorption of the superior margin of the mandible will make the foramen appear to lie more superiorly along the ramus.

Maxillary Nerve Block

This block should be performed by practitioners with relevant and adequate experience. It is required when a superficial block of the infraorbital nerve does not produce adequate anesthesia or when anesthesia of the more proximal superior dental nerves is required. This can be performed with a block lateral to the sphenopalatine fossa. Alternatively, the suprazygomatic approach to the maxillary nerve (SZMN) block is well described.[32]

Lateral Approach to the Sphenopalatine Fossa

Procedure

- The patient either sits with the mouth slightly open or lies supine with a small towel under the occiput and the head turned slightly away from the side to be blocked.
- Above the zygomatic arch: The center of the upper zygomatic arch is marked. A 60- to 90-mm needle is introduced at 45 degrees caudally and medially toward the contralateral molar teeth. After paresthesia is elicited at the nostril, upper lip, and cheek, the needle is withdrawn slightly, and local anesthetic is injected slowly and incrementally and with frequent aspiration.
- Below the zygomatic arch (Fig. 36-16): The zygomatic arch is marked along its course, and the patient is asked to open and close the mouth slowly so that the curved upper border of the mandible can be identified. The mandibular fossa is palpated between the condylar and coronoid processes. The lowest point of the mandibular notch is palpated, and an "X" is marked at this spot, usually at the zygoma's midpoint. A local anesthetic skin wheal is raised at the "X" after appropriate skin preparation.
- With the patient's jaw in the open position, a 60- to 90-mm needle is introduced through the "X" at a 45-degree angle toward the dorsal part of the eyeball (cephalad and slightly anterior).
- The needle should contact the lateral portion of the pterygoid process (pterygoid plate) at a depth of 4 to 5 cm. The needle is then withdrawn and redirected slightly cephalad and anteriorly until it passes beyond the pterygoid plate and enters the pterygopalatine fossa at an additional depth of no more than 1 cm. Paresthesia in the nose or the upper teeth confirms nerve localization. The pterygopalatine fossa is highly vascular, so care must be exercised to avoid intravascular injection.
- Anesthesia can be achieved by injecting 5 mL into the pterygopalatine fossa, either upon obtaining the paresthesia or blindly advancing 1 cm beyond the pterygoid plate.

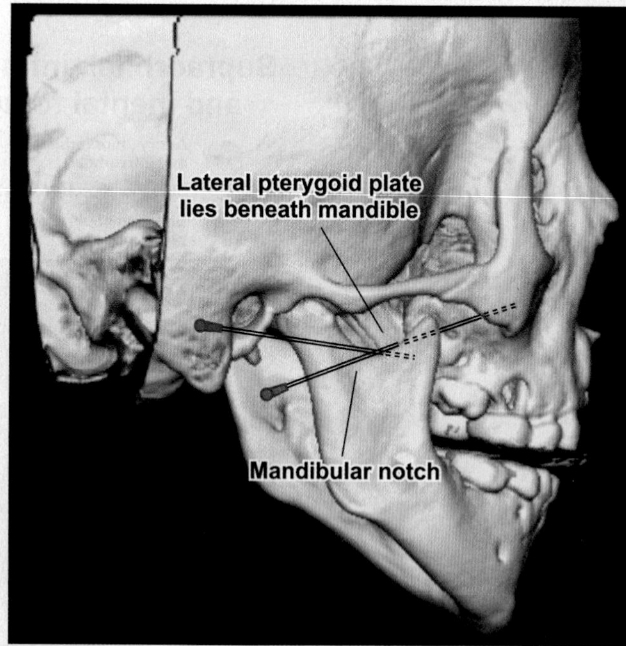

Figure 36-16 The lateral view of a computed tomography–scanned skull shows the bony landmarks and final needle insertion angles for the maxillary (*red needle*) and mandibular (*blue needle*) nerves. Each block procedure involves first reaching the lateral pterygoid plate (see text for details).

Clinical Pearls

- One concern during this block is the spread of local anesthetic to adjacent structures, especially to nerves in orbit. If pain occurs in the orbit region during the procedure, the injection should be stopped, and the needle should be withdrawn.
- Although the mainstay of treatment for trigeminal neuralgia continues to be pharmacologic or neuroablative, maxillary nerve block with extraoral mandibular nerve block has been reported to provide relief in some settings.[33]

Suprazygomatic Maxillary Nerve/Suprazygomatic Infratemporal–Pterygopalatine Fossa Injections

The SZMN blocking is a well-established, safe, and effective regional pain management approach after cleft palate surgery.[34,35] Recently, researchers used bilateral SZMN blocks, or more precisely suprazygomatic infratemporal–pterygopalatine fossa injections (Fig. 36-17), to provide opioid-sparing perioperative analgesia in pediatric adenotonsillectomy patients.[36]

Procedure Using Landmark Technique

SZMN block targets the maxillary division of the trigeminal nerve as it travels through the pterygopalatine fossa. It is traditionally described and administered as a landmark-based approach for the pediatric patient.

Needling: Following aseptic preparation, a 22-gauge, 5-cm nerve block needle is inserted perpendicular to the skin in the frontozygomatic angle formed by the posterior orbital rim and zygomatic arch in children of any age or weight (Fig. 36-17). When the needle makes contact with the larger wing of the sphenoid (approximately 10 to 15 mm deep), it is redirected caudally and anteriorly medially into the infratemporal fossa and advanced toward the pterygopalatine fossa until it finds osseous resistance (around 35 to 45 mm deep).

Local anesthetic spread: The amount of local anesthetic used per side is determined by weight and can range from 0.2 mL/kg to up to a maximum of 5 mL of 0.5% ropivacaine. If a total volume by weight is less than 5 mL of 0.5% ropivacaine, the calculated volume is diluted with normal saline to achieve a total volume of 5 mL.

Procedure Using Ultrasound Guidance

Scanning: US visualization of local anesthetic injection has been recently demonstrated utilizing a high-frequency linear US transducer (13 to 6 MHz) positioned in the infrazygomatic area and pointed cephalad at a 45-degree angle. The maxillary artery and vein can be seen deep in the infratemporal and pterygopalatine fossae. The needle tip can be difficult to view with this OOP scanning, and the nerve itself is rarely seen by ultrasonic imaging. Following local anesthetic injection, US imaging often shows the lifting of the soft tissues in the infratemporal and pterygopalatine fossas deep to the lateral pterygoid muscle between the maxilla (medial) and the coronoid process of the jaw (lateral).

Clinical Pearls

- The SZMN block is an injection that starts from a suprazygomatic approach that traverses a space, specifically the infratemporal fossa, to ultimately target a narrower deeper space, the pterygopalatine fossa.
- The maxillary nerve is not visualized when using US confirmation or guidance.
- Some experts believe that 5 mL of local anesthetic gives a more constant dispersion than a lower volume. However, a recent study found that 5 mL considerably surpasses the capacity of the pterygopalatine fossa, causing the drug to spread outside of the fossa.[37]
- The suprazygomatic infratemporal–pterygopalatine fossa injection is the injection of local anesthetic into a fossa rather than a perineural injection.[36]
- Numbness in the distribution of the maxillary nerve including the cheeks, nasal septum, philtrum, and soft palate can be used to confirm that the injectate has reached its intended target.
- The suprazygomatic infratemporal–pterygopalatine fossa injection alone does not provide complete analgesia of the palatine tonsils and adenoids. Sparing of the glossopharyngeal nerve is essential to maintain protective airway reflexes after surgery.[38]

Mandibular Nerve Block

This nerve can be blocked for dental and maxillary surgery, inferior dental pain, trigeminal neuralgia in the third branch, or temporomandibular joint dysfunction. It is the only branch of the

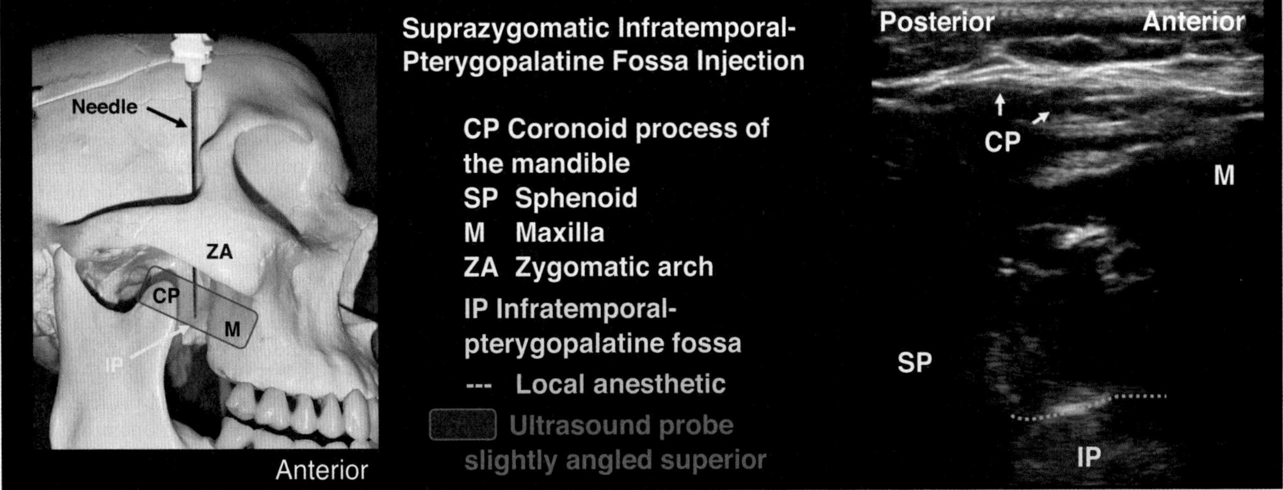

Figure 36-17 Injection of the suprazygomatic infratemporal–pterygopalatine fossa (commonly known as suprazygomatic maxillary nerve block). **Left:** A depiction of ultrasound probe placement on a model skeleton. **Right:** Ultrasound real-time image of a right suprazygomatic infratemporal–pterygopalatine fossa injection with local anesthetic deposition within the Infratemporal fossa.

trigeminal nerve where anesthesia carries the risk of losing motor (mastication) function.

Procedure

- The patient lies supine with the face in profile. Landmarks for the location of the mandibular fossa are the same as those described for maxillary nerve blockade.
- A 60- to 90-mm needle is introduced through the skin wheal and directed perpendicularly to the skin, without the cephalad angulation required for maxillary nerve anesthesia.
- When the pterygoid plate is contacted, the depth should be noted. The needle is then redirected posteriorly until it passes beyond the pterygoid plate. It should contact the nerve 0.5 to 1 cm deep from the point where the pterygoid plate was contacted (Fig. 36-17).
- Paresthesias of the lower jaw, lower lip, and lower incisors at a depth of approximately 4 to 4.5 cm confirm proximity to the nerve. Gentle exploration may be required in a cephalad and caudad direction, from the initial point where the needle passes posterior to the plate. After slight needle withdrawal, 5 to 10 mL of solution is injected incrementally with repeated aspiration to avoid intravascular injection. As with maxillary blockade, paresthesias can be painful to the patient.

Clinical Pearls

- Anesthesia of the auriculotemporal nerve is often delayed.
- Facial nerve anesthesia can occasionally be seen when large volumes are injected to block the mandibular nerve. This is of little consequence unless neurolytic agents are used.
- A more severe complication is the possibility of intravascular injection in this highly vascular area. Injection of local anesthetic should be performed incrementally with small quantities, and there should be constant observation for signs of toxicity.
- For patients with abnormal anatomy or accessory innervation to the mandible, alternatives to the standard mandibular block include the Gow-Gates and Akinosi–Vazirani blocks.[39]

Cervical Plexus Blocks

Anesthesia of the deep or superficial cervical plexus can be used for lateral or anterior neck procedures such as parathyroidectomy and carotid endarterectomy. During carotid surgery, local infiltration of the carotid bifurcation may be necessary to block reflex hemodynamic changes associated with glossopharyngeal stimulation.

Deep Cervical Plexus Block

Procedure

- The patient is supine with a small towel under the head, which is turned 45 degrees to the opposite side with a slight neck extension.
- Landmarks include the posterior edge of the sternocleidomastoid muscle, the caudal portion of the mastoid process, the angle of the jaw, and the transverse processes of cervical vertebrae C2–C5 (about 1.5 cm apart). If all transverse processes cannot be palpated, the most prominent tubercle of C6 (Chassaignac's) is marked. A line is drawn from the mastoid process along the sternocleidomastoid muscle to reach the transverse process of C6. Each transverse process of C2–C5 is marked approximately 0.5 to 1 cm behind the line; the transverse process of C2 lies about 1.5 cm inferior to the mastoid process.
- Skin infiltration is carried out at the "X" marks of C2–C4 and three needles (22 gauge, 3.5 to 5 cm) are introduced perpendicular to the skin and advanced about 30 degrees caudally with a slight posterior orientation (Fig. 36-7).
- After confirming contact with the transverse process, the needle is withdrawn slightly, and a syringe is connected to the needle. Two to three milliliters of local anesthetic solution are injected per segment for therapeutic or diagnostic purposes or blocks in children, whereas 5 to 10 mL per segment may be sufficient for surgical block (limiting the total to approximately 20 mL if superficial blocks are also performed).

Clinical Pearls

- The deep block may be performed by single injection at C3 or C4 as initially described by Winnie et al.[40] or by a standard three-injection technique.
- A recent anatomic study demonstrated that the longus capitis muscle is a suitable landmark for US-guided deep cervical plexus block.[41] With this approach, the deep cervical plexus and sympathetic trunk can be blocked.
- Paresthesia occurring during these blocks has been associated with more effective anesthesia.[42]
- Anesthesia for carotid endarterectomy may involve performing combined superficial and deep cervical plexus blocks, yet the benefit of combined over superficial block alone has been questioned.[43,44] There appears to be no difference between these two approaches in the amount of supplemental local anesthesia required.
- Several life-threatening complications may arise from deep cervical plexus block and this block is rarely administered. Injection may occur into the vertebral artery. Subarachnoid or epidural injections are possible if the needle is advanced too far medially into the vertebral foramen. This is more likely in the cervical region because of the longer dural sleeves accompanying these nerve roots. Careful patient monitoring should continue for 60 minutes after the block has been performed.
- Phrenic nerve palsy leading to hemidiaphragmatic paresis is common with deep cervical plexus block.[45] This block is not indicated in any patient who depends on the diaphragm for tidal ventilation and bilateral blocks are never recommended.
- Other well-described side effects include Horner syndrome (if the superior cervical or cervicothoracic ganglion is blocked),[46] stellate ganglion block,[47] and hoarseness due to recurrent laryngeal nerve block.

Superficial Cervical Plexus Block

This block is performed similarly to a deep cervical plexus block. It results in anesthesia only of the sensory fibers of the plexus.

Procedure

- An "X" is made at the midpoint of the posterior border of the sternocleidomastoid muscle.
- Local skin infiltration is performed with a fan-like injection using 10 to 20 mL of local anesthetic (0.1 to 0.2 mL/kg for children) along the posterior border of the sternocleidomastoid muscle 4 cm above and below the level of the midpoint (Fig. 36-18).

Clinical Pearls

- The most common approach for minimally invasive parathyroidectomy (involving a small unilateral incision rather than bilateral neck exploration) includes a combination of C2–C4 superficial cervical plexus block, infiltration along the incision line, and infiltration of the upper thyroid pedicle.[48] This approach can result in shorter anesthetic and operative times, leading to earlier hospital discharge and significantly better postoperative pain relief.[48,49]
- Initial studies of US-guided superficial cervical plexus block showed no added benefit over the blind technique,[50] although US guidance may be helpful in emergencies.[51]

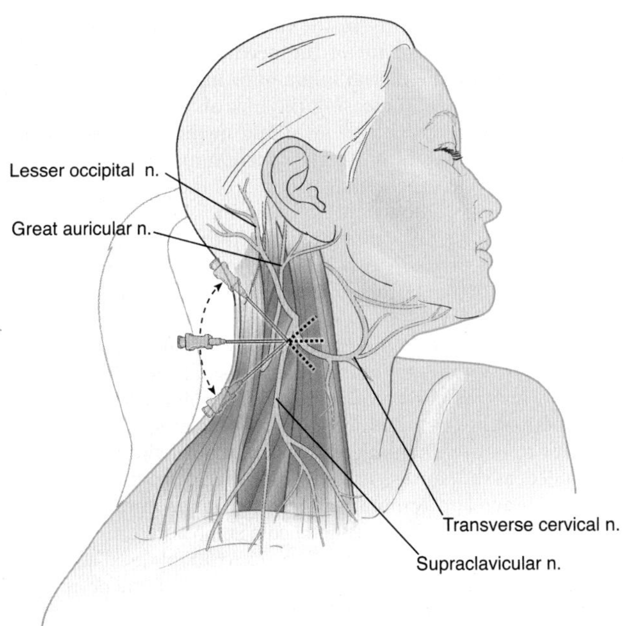

Figure 36-18 The lateral view of the head and neck shows the block needle insertion angles needed to perform superficial cervical plexus block. Initially, the needle is inserted perpendicular to the skin at the midpoint of the lateral border of the sternocleidomastoid muscle (where the external jugular vein crosses it). The needle can then be repositioned to superior and inferior angulations to reach the entire cervical plexus.

- Using a modified surgical approach, thyroid surgery has been performed under superficial cervical plexus block in combination with anterior field block.[52]
- Minimally invasive surgery may require conversion to general anesthesia when there is difficulty ensuring adequate protection of the recurrent laryngeal nerve or when the intraoperative diagnosis of parathyroid carcinoma or multiglandular parathyroid hyperplasia occurs.
- Phrenic nerve paralysis leading to diaphragmatic dysfunction,[42] vagus nerve block with resultant recurrent nerve paralysis,[53] and inadvertent intravascular injection field[54] have all been reported.

Occipital Nerve Blocks

The greater and lesser occipital nerves can be blocked by superficial injection at the points on the posterior skull, where they emerge from below the neck muscles. This block is rarely used for surgical procedures and is often applied as a diagnostic step in evaluating head and neck pain complaints.

Procedure

- The patient sits with their head tilted forward slightly to expose the prominent nuchal ridge of bone at the posterior base of the skull.
- The inferior nuchal line is palpated at one-third of the distance between the external occipital protuberance and the foramen magnum. A mark is placed on the nuchal line at the lateral border of the insertion of the erector muscles of the neck, usually 2.5 cm from the midline. At this point, the branches of the greater occipital nerve usually pass laterally from behind the muscle to cross the nuchal line. The nerve is located directly lateral to the easily palpated occipital artery. During its ascent along with the posterior skull, the lesser occipital nerve can be located an additional 2.5 cm away from the greater occipital nerve along the inferior nuchal line; a mark should also be placed here (Fig. 36-8).
- A short, fine needle (e.g., 25 mm 25 gauge) is introduced with a slight cranial angulation at each mark to the depth of the skull itself. After small withdrawal, local anesthetic is injected (e.g., 0.5 to 1 mL of 1% lidocaine for diagnostic procedures or 1 to 3 mL of 0.75% ropivacaine for therapeutic procedures). Paresthesias are occasionally encountered but are not essential for obtaining simple skin anesthesia.
- If more anterior scalp anesthesia is required, the lesser occipital nerve branches can also be blocked by advancing the needle subcutaneously from this point in an anterior direction toward the mastoid process. A band of anesthetic solution is deposited along the line between skin entry and the mastoid process using 2 to 3 mL of local anesthetic.

Clinical Pearls

- Block of the lesser occipital and greater auricular nerves (both blocked by subcutaneous injection from the angle of the mandible to the mastoid process) has successfully provided postoperative analgesia after otoplasty.[55] Reducing the requirement for opioid analgesia (with its associated nausea and vomiting) is essential due to the high incidence of pain and vomiting on the first postoperative day related to the surgical procedure alone.
- Greater occipital nerve block is commonly used for primary headache syndromes. The anterior region involving the trigeminal nerve is also blocked for chronic syndromes.[56] It has been reported for use with cervicogenic headaches, occipital neuralgia, migraines, and cluster headaches.[57]
- Complications with this technique are rare. Care must be taken not to advance the needle anteriorly under the skull, as the foramen magnum might be entered unintentionally with a long needle. Suboccipital approaches may be performed safely with US guidance. Local hematoma may be produced with superficial injection, but this is only a temporary problem.

Upper Extremity

Although many approaches to the brachial plexus have been described, there are traditionally four anatomic locations where local anesthetics are placed: (1) the interscalene groove near the cervical transverse processes, (2) the subclavian sheath at the first rib, (3) near the coracoid process in the infraclavicular fossa, and (4) surrounding the axillary artery in the axilla. The introduction of US imaging has increased the use of blocks at the supraclavicular fossa, as visualization of the subclavian artery and lung makes these critical structures easier to avoid. It is important to stress that clear visibility of the needle is essential for this block (and generally for all brachial plexus blocks). The appropriate choice of approach depends not only on the patient's anatomy but also on the site of surgery and the method used to locate nerve structures.

The terminal branches of the brachial plexus can also be anesthetized by local anesthetic injection along their peripheral course as they cross joint spaces, where they lie proximal to easily identifiable structures (Table 36-1), or by injection of a dilute local anesthetic solution intravenously below a pneumatic tourniquet on the upper arm ("intravenous regional" or Bier block). Using US may increase the locations where the terminal nerves can be successfully blocked. For example, the ulnar nerve can be blocked effectively at the medial surface of the midforearm, which may reduce the risk of ulnar nerve palsy posed by a block at the elbow near the cubital tunnel. As stated in the introduction to Specific Techniques, the use of combined US- and NS-guided techniques is stressed in the figures, and, for simplicity of viewing, the necessary sterile precautions are not shown.

Brachial Plexus Block

Interscalene Block

This block, as described by Winnie[58] in 1970, is indicated mostly for surgical anesthesia of the shoulder and upper arm, and forearm but is often insufficient for the hand (2 Video 36-2, 3 Video 36-3, NICV 36-2). It frequently spares the plexus's lowest branches, the C8 and T1 fibers, which innervate the forearm's caudad (ulnar) border. Nevertheless, recent reports provide evidence that a low interscalene block (below C6, just superior to the clavicle) may provide sufficient anesthesia and analgesia for procedures on the lower arm.[59,60] The patient is positioned supine, with their head faced slightly to the contralateral side. The main surface landmark used for this block—the sternocleidomastoid muscle—can be accentuated by asking the patient to reach for the ipsilateral knee and rotating the head approximately 45 degrees to the nonoperative side. The head should also be elevated slightly, and the patient should be instructed to take a deep breath since contraction of the scalenus muscles accentuates the interscalene groove. This groove lies immediately behind the lateral border of the clavicular head of the sternocleidomastoid muscle at the level of the cricoid cartilage (C6). As for all upper extremity procedures, prepare the needle insertion site and other applicable skin areas with an antiseptic solution and, if using US imaging, ensure sterility of the US probe with a standard sleeve cover or transparent dressing.

Procedure Using Nerve Stimulation Technique

- Landmarks: Using the maneuvers described earlier, the interscalene groove is palpated by rolling the fingers posteriorly off the lateral border of the sternocleidomastoid muscle; mark the groove as high as possible. After the patient relaxes, the prominent transverse process of C6 can often be felt directly in the groove and should be marked.
- Needling: A skin wheal is raised in the interscalene groove at the level of the cricoid. A 22-gauge, 36- to 50-mm insulated needle (shorter for pediatric patients) is introduced through the wheal. The needle is directed medially, caudally, and slightly posteriorly in the direction of the C6 transverse process. The caudad tilt of the needle is important to avoid either entering the neural foramen or injection into the dural nerve root sheath, increasing the risk of high-spinal anesthesia or spinal cord injury.[61] Avoiding medial placement using a mostly caudad and posterior direction may reduce the risks even more. The superficial structures of the plexus are located at an average, shallow depth of 5.5 mm.[62] Due to the compact arrangement of neck anatomy in children, an angled insertion may be needed (as opposed to perpendicular in adults) to avoid puncture of the vertebral artery or epidural/subarachnoid space.
- Nerve localization: Applying an initial current of 0.8 mA is sufficient for stimulation of the plexus (usually at a depth of 1 to 3 cm), and the current is reduced to aim for a threshold current of 0.4 mA before injection after obtaining an appropriate motor response. Diaphragmatic or trapezius twitches should be avoided, as they are associated with cervical plexus stimulation. A diaphragmatic response indicates that the phrenic nerve is being stimulated and that the needle is too anterior.
- Injection: After careful aspiration, 25 to 30 mL local anesthetic is injected in small increments to detect intraneural or intravascular placement of the needle.

Procedure Using Ultrasound Guidance (Fig. 36-19)

- Scanning: Two scanning techniques are recommended for viewing the brachial plexus at the interscalene level: (1) beginning anteriorly at the cricoid cartilage level (C6) with movement from anterior and medial to posterior and lateral toward the interscalene groove, and (2) scanning proximally from the supraclavicular fossa to the interscalene location.
- Appearance: At the supraclavicular fossa, the brachial plexus (trunks/divisions) can be seen in the short axis as a tightly enclosed cluster (i.e., honeycomb like), superior and lateral to the subclavian artery (Fig. 36-20). After proximally tracing the nerves toward the interscalene groove, the nerve structures (roots/trunks) are visualized in a sagittal oblique section as three (usually) or up to five round- or oval-shaped hypoechoic (see Common Techniques: Nerve Stimulation and Ultrasound Imaging section) structures, sometimes with a few internal punctate echoes, lying between the scalenus anterior and

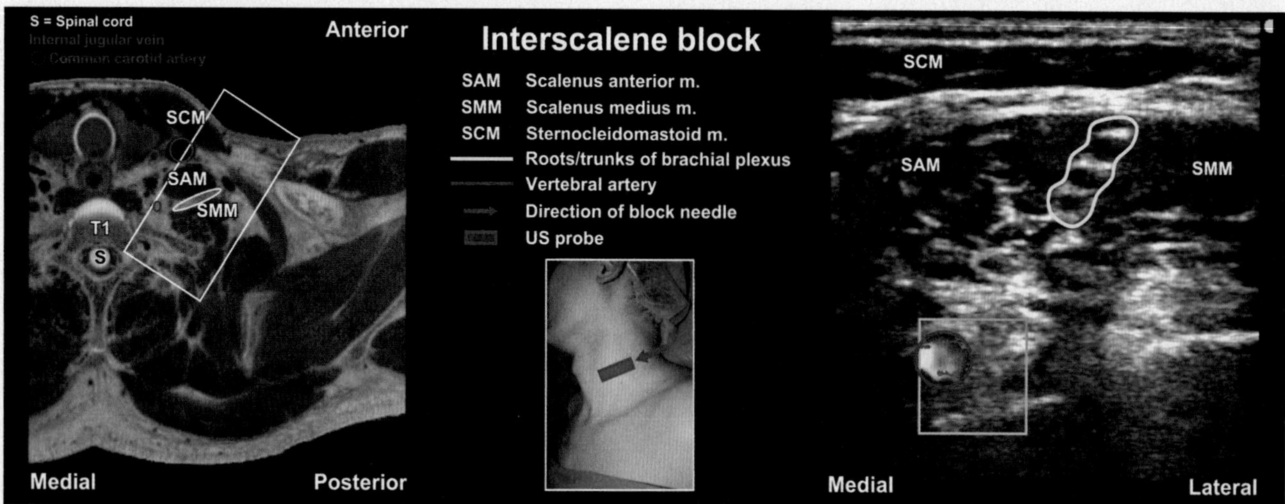

Figure 36-19 Anatomy arrangement for ultrasound-guided interscalene brachial plexus block. The block is performed by aligning an in-plane needle to a linear, high-frequency probe. To avoid the intervertebral foramen, the needle is directed laterally to medially with a slight caudal angulation. The plexus roots/trunks are typically seen as three or more round or oval-shaped hypoechoic structures sandwiched in the interscalene groove between the scalenus anterior and medius muscles. The vertebral artery is located medial and deep to the brachial plexus.

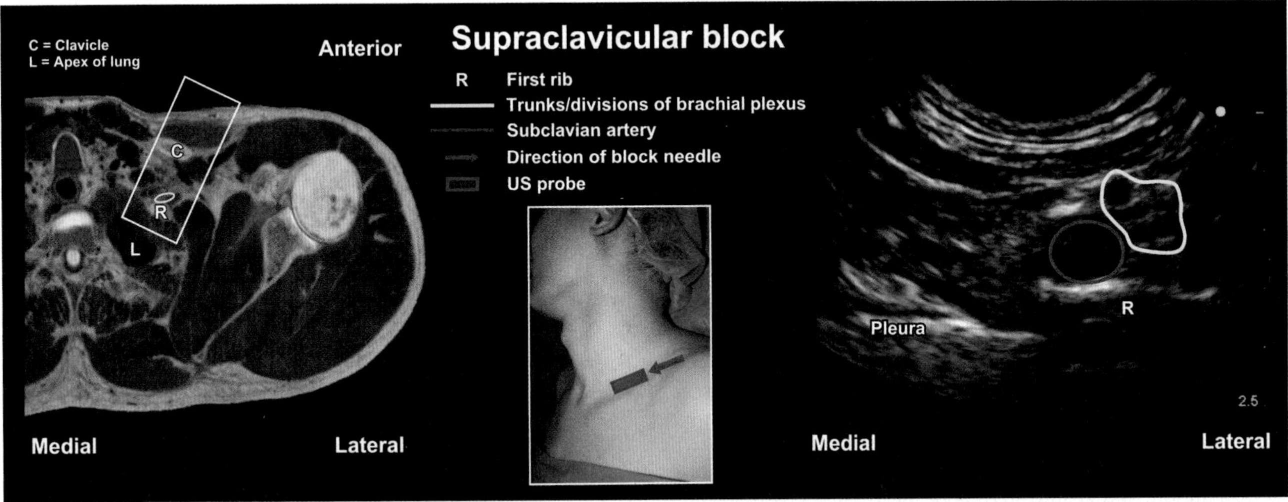

Figure 36-20 Arrangement of relevant anatomy for ultrasound-guided supraclavicular brachial plexus block. The block is performed using IP needle alignment to a small footprint curved probe with the needle inserted lateral to medial in a slightly sagittal plane. Color Doppler can be valuable to quickly locate the subclavian artery inferomedial to the plexus trunks/divisions.

medius muscles. The C8 and T1 roots may be difficult to identify because of their depth.[63,64]

- Needling: After infiltration of local anesthetics to the skin at the anticipated needle puncture site, a 22-gauge, 50-mm needle (insulated is recommended) is introduced either OOP (see Common Techniques section) or IP to the probe (Fig. 36-20) and advanced to a maximum of 3 cm for most patients. For the OOP needle insertion technique, the clinician stands beside or cephalad to the probe and places the initial needle puncture site cranial to the probe. The needle is typically angled somewhat caudally toward the US beam plane. For the IP needle insertion technique, the needle is moved from lateral to medial (still slightly caudad) and will first penetrate the scalenus medius muscle before entering the interscalene groove. It is recommended to use NS to enable further nerve localization. In children, the brachial plexus roots are relatively superficial at the interscalene level compared to adults. In infants, the roots may be only millimeters below the skin surface.
- Local anesthetic spread: A test injection of D5W is recommended and will help further confirm nerve localization with NS and estimate the pattern of local anesthetic spread. Local anesthetic should be deposited in the midst of the neural structures so that it spreads to surround the nerves circumferentially. Local anesthetic distention in this compartment can be seen by the US as a hypoechoic (fluid) expansion.

Clinical Pearls

- The use of long-acting local anesthetics may provide analgesia for 10 to 12 hours. For more extended analgesia, a continuous catheter is effective for procedures such as total shoulder replacement, although securing the catheters in the mobile neck tissues is challenging.
- Equal success has been achieved when any of the appropriate muscle responses are elicited as a positive stimulating test. Palpation of the muscle may confirm the motor response.
- Even though subarachnoid or intraneural injection can occur even when the threshold current is more than 0.4 mA, it is advisable to avoid injecting when the current responses are less than 0.4 mA.
- If a continuous block is indicated, the needle entry point may be moved a centimeter cephalad for the OOP approach, making the corresponding insertion angle a little steeper and more tangential to the course of the plexus. The bevel of the introducing needle should be directed laterally. Placement of a stimulating catheter may be aided by dilating the perineural space with D5W, which will allow the user to monitor the catheter's advancement to a location where the motor response is maintained at less than 0.5 mA.
- Securing catheters in the freely mobile neck is a challenge. Some prefer to secure the catheter by tunneling 3 to 4 cm below the skin by passing it back through an intravenous catheter that has been introduced subcutaneously near the entry site.
- During OOP US-guided technique, more than 45-degree needle angulation should be avoided, as the needle may be inserted too deep and directed toward the spinal cord.
- Complications from this approach are related to the structures in the tubercle's vicinity. The cupola of the lung is close, particularly on the right side, and can be contacted if the needle is directed too far caudally. Pneumothorax should be considered if cough or chest pain is produced while exploring for the nerve. If the needle is allowed to pass directly medially, it may enter the intervertebral foramen, and injection of local anesthetic may produce spinal or epidural anesthesia. The vertebral artery passes posteriorly at the level of the sixth vertebra to lie in its canal in the transverse process that can be seen as a pulsatile structure deep to the plexus; direct injection into this vessel can rapidly produce central nervous system toxicity and convulsions. Careful aspiration and incremental injections are essential to help avoid both of these potential problems.
- Even with appropriate injection, the local anesthetic solution can spread to adjacent nerves. It may produce cervical plexus block, including motor fibers to the diaphragm, which may be a problem in patients with respiratory insufficiency. A case report described an optimal spread of local anesthetic, and the possibility of using saline dilution should phrenic nerve block occur.[65]
- Horner syndrome is common because of the spread to the sympathetic chain on the anterior vertebral body.
- Neuropathy of the C6 root is a potential problem because the needle may unintentionally pin the nerve root against the tubercle and predispose it to intraneural injection. The needle should be withdrawn slightly if the first injection produces the characteristic "crampy" pain sensation.

- An alternative technique for blocking the roots of the brachial plexus is to perform a cervical paravertebral block,[66] which can utilize the bony landmarks of the vertebral column. This is high quality but advanced block and should be performed using US guidance. A lateral US view of the brachial plexus at the level of C6 allows visualization of the needle as it passes lateral to the C6 transverse process and into the interscalene space. This view avoids the challenges of viewing the brachial plexus from a posterior approach, where the bony structures may obscure the view of the needle and plexus.

Supraclavicular Block

The supraclavicular block targets the trunks and divisions of the brachial plexus, depending on the location of the injection site and the patient's anatomy (4 Video 36-4). Like the interscalene block, the patient is positioned supine with the head turned approximately 45 degrees to the contralateral side. Prepare the needle insertion site and other applicable skin areas with an antiseptic solution, and ensure sterility of the US probe with a standard sleeve cover or transparent dressing.

Procedure Using Nerve Stimulation Technique (Note that Most Clinicians Prefer to Perform this Block under US Guidance to Minimize Potential Complications; Some May Use Ns as an Adjunct Method with the US)

- Landmarks: The outline of the clavicle is drawn on the skin, and the midpoint of the clavicle is marked. An "X" is placed posterior to this midpoint in the interscalene groove, usually 1 cm behind the clavicle. Since the plexus lays immediately cephaloposterior to the subclavian artery, its pulse is a reliable landmark in thinner individuals.
- Needling: Local infiltration is performed at the site of the nerve, and a 2.5- to 5-cm, 22-gauge needle is introduced in the parasagittal plane at the superior border of the clavicle at the lateral edge of the sternocleidomastoid muscle insertion. An initial insertion angle of 45 degrees cephalad is recommended, with subsequent reductions in angle as necessary.[67] However, an angle of less than 20 degrees may lead to the needle contacting the pleura and subclavian vein before the plexus. The rib may be contacted with subsequent anteroposterior needle adjustment to contact the plexus but avoiding rib contact may be prudent. Careful lateral or medial exploration may be needed, but medially probing increases the risk of contacting the pleura. For children, a weight-dependent guide can help in determining needle insertion depth. In general, for a 10-kg child, the needle is inserted 10 mm; the depth of insertion increases by 3 mm for every 10 kg increase in weight until 50 kg. For children above this weight, insertion advances 1 mm for every 10 kg increase in weight (maximum depth should not be >35 mm). However, it would be preferable to use US as a guide.
- Nerve localization: Responses to NS can be helpful for confirmation of needle proximity to the separate trunks. Twitches of pectoralis, deltoid, biceps (upper trunk), triceps (upper/middle trunk), forearm (upper/middle trunk), and hand (lower trunk) muscles with a current intensity of 0.4 mA (0.1 to 0.3 ms) are acceptable. Distal responses (hand or wrist flexion or extension) best confirm placement within the fascia. Multiple nerve responses are not required.
- Injection: If a nerve response is produced during exploration, the anesthetic solution can be injected while the needle is fixed in position. 25 to 40 mL of local anesthetic will produce adequate analgesia. In children, the fascia surrounding the nerve trunks is less adherent than in adults, which may lead to a greater spread of local anesthetic.

Procedure Using Ultrasound Guidance (Fig. 36-20)

- Scanning: The probe is first placed in a coronal oblique plane at the lateral end and just above the upper border of the clavicle. It is then moved medially until an image of the subclavian artery appears on the screen. Some dorsal and ventral rotations of the probe may be necessary. With the subclavian artery in the middle of the screen, the plexus is located superolateral to the artery, and the neurovascular structures lie above the first rib. Small-footprint probes are generally used for scanning children since they offer better needle movement around the probe.
- Appearance: The subclavian artery is anechoic, hypodense, pulsatile, and round; color Doppler can further confirm its identity. Trunks/divisions of the brachial plexus appear as a cluster of hypoechoic "grape-like" structures consisting of usually three (more as one moves distally) hypoechoic nodules, all surrounded by a hyperechoic lining (presumably the connective tissues). With the probe in a coronal oblique plane, the plexus depth has been shown with MRI to be around 1.65 cm in males and 1.45 cm in females.[67,68] Medial and deep to the artery, the rib may be seen as a hyperechoic line with dorsal shadowing. The anechoic subclavian vein may be seen inferomedial to the artery.
- Needling: The selected needle insertion site is often more lateral with the US-guided technique than with NS techniques. The skin is infiltrated with local anesthetic, and a 22-gauge, 50-mm (or less) needle (insulated is recommended) is introduced with IP needle alignment to a curved, small footprint (Fig. 36-20) or linear probe. The needle is inserted immediately above the clavicle in a lateral-to-medial direction with a slight cephalad angle. It is recommended to have the concurrent use of NS for additional confirmation of nerve localization and as an additional monitor to prevent intraneural injection by having the threshold stimulation of more than 0.2 mA. See earlier for acceptable motor responses to NS.
- Local anesthetic spread: It is best to deposit local anesthetic next to the nerve structures immediately lateral to the subclavian artery on top of the first rib. Injection in this location will often lift the nerve structures superiorly away from the first rib and subclavian artery. The hypoechoic spread of local anesthetic surrounding the nerves may be seen on the US screen.

Clinical Pearls

- It is recommended to use US imaging combined with NS technique during this block to help avoid puncturing the pleura. When using US, it is critical to visualize both the first rib and the pleura and optimize the image such that the first rib covers the pleura, especially just lateral to the subclavian artery where the target of the needle tip is. Before needle insertion, measuring and being aware of the skin–pleura distance with US is critical. The responses to NS can be helpful in confirming needle proximity to the separate trunks.
- The primary challenge with US imaging in this region is the presence of a bony prominence (clavicle) and curved soft tissue contour that can interfere with imaging of the brachial plexus in the short axis. A curved array probe with a small footprint is extremely useful in this compact area.
- The lateral-to-medial IP needle approach will ensure that the needle approaches the nerve structures before reaching the subclavian artery (i.e., less chance of inadvertent vascular puncture). However, using a slightly sagittal plane (Fig. 36-20) may reduce the risk of pleural puncture. The needle should be viewed at all times when using a lateral-to-medial approach.
- The most significant risk when using this technique is pneumothorax, as the cupola of the lung lies just medial to the first rib, not far from the plexus. The risk of pneumothorax is greater on

the right side as the cupola of the lung is higher on that side. The risk is also greater in tall, thin patients. In children, the brachial plexus at this level is relatively superficial and close to the pleura; careful needle insertion must be exercised to avoid the risk of pneumothorax.

- This method does not introduce more complications than other methods of brachial plexus block.
- When using a catheter-over-needle method, a medial-to-lateral approach is indicated to reduce the risk of dislodgment.[69] This approach will place the needle tip in the corner immediately lateral to the subclavian artery and above the first rib.

Infraclavicular Block

Infraclavicular block targets the cords of the brachial plexus, and the nerves can be blocked next to the axillary artery's second part at the coracoid process level. Brachial plexus block in the infraclavicular area offers excellent analgesia for the entire arm and allows the introduction of continuous catheters to provide prolonged postoperative pain relief. The musculocutaneous and axillary nerves often branch off high in the axilla and can be missed with an axillary block approach; the infraclavicular approach blocks them more consistently. Multiple injections may be required for a successful infraclavicular block.

Infraclavicular blocks are indicated for the forearm, elbow, and hand surgeries. The patient is supine with the head turned approximately 45 degrees to the nonoperative side, and their arm may be either at their side with a hand on the abdomen or abducted with their palm placed behind their head. When preparing for this block, it is common to have the patient's elbow flexed and the hand resting on the abdomen to facilitate observation of motor responses generated with NS. Alternatively, externally rotating the arm and placing the hand behind the head stretches the cords and brings the nerves closer to the axillary artery, which may facilitate local anesthetic spread around the nerves. As always, prepare the needle insertion site and other applicable skin areas with an antiseptic solution and ensure sterility of the US probe with a standard sleeve cover or transparent dressing.

Procedure Using Nerve Stimulation Technique

Several approaches have been described for infraclavicular blocks, all with various needle puncture sites and angles of insertion. A lateral approach may improve plexus cord localization and reduce the risk of puncture to the pleura and axillary artery.[70]

- Landmarks: With the patient's arm adducted and their hand resting on their abdomen, the medial aspect of the coracoid process is palpated as one slips their finger off the clavicle.
- Needling: After skin preparation and skin wheal, a 50- to 90-mm, 18- to 22-gauge needle is inserted where the clavicle meets the medial aspect of the coracoid process, generally directed 0 to 15 degrees posterior to the horizontal plane (Fig. 36-21 illustrates this needle insertion when using US guidance). The 15-degree trajectory will likely increase the chances of contacting the more posteriorly located posterior or medial cords, which may improve analgesia. A greater angle may be required to achieve adequate responses to NS since local anesthetic injection at more than one cord may be beneficial. The cords should be approximately 4 to 6 cm deep (more than 7.5 cm insertion may risk pleural puncture).[70] The needle puncture site may be adjusted slightly caudad to this location. If the needle is placed 2.5 cm caudad to the coracoid process, a laterally projected needle directed toward the axillary artery may be effective.
- Nerve localization: The first response (elbow flexion) obtained is usually the musculocutaneous nerve arising from the lateral cord. A separate distal response must be obtained from the medial (distal flexors) and posterior (distal and proximal extensors) cords for complete hand anesthesia. A close examination of the movements of the fifth digit (pinkie) can be helpful to differentiate the cords, with lateral movement (i.e., pronation) representing the lateral cord, medial movement (i.e., flexion) representing the medial cord, and dorsal movement (i.e., extension) representing the posterior cord.[1] Some practitioners also advocate that eliciting a forearm response (pronation via the lateral cord) is essential for a complete block. The artery may be punctured easily at this point, and careful aspiration is required to prevent intravascular injection.
- Injection: If a musculocutaneous nerve response is obtained, the nerve or lateral cord can be blocked by injecting 5 to 10 mL of local anesthetic. Once responses in the hand are obtained, 25 mL of local anesthetic can be injected around the posterior and medial cords.

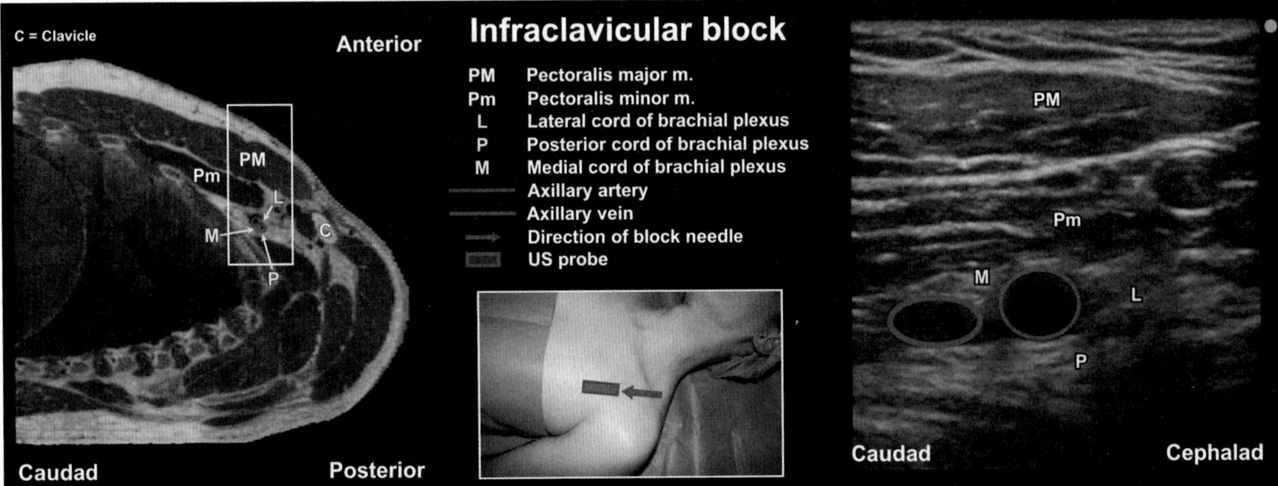

Figure 36-21 Arrangement of relevant anatomy for ultrasound-guided infraclavicular brachial plexus block. The block is performed using IP needle alignment to a linear probe and directing the needle 15 degrees posteriorly in a cephalad-to-caudad direction. In contrast to the more proximal blocks, the nerves (cords) appear hyperechoic due to higher fascial content and the relatively hyperechoic surrounding tissue (muscle).

Procedure Using Ultrasound Guidance (Fig. 36-21)

- Scanning: Immediately medial and inferior to the coracoid process, position a linear or curved lower frequency transducer (4 to 7 MHz), depending on body habitus, in a parasagittal plane, and capture the best possible short-axis view of the brachial plexus cords and axillary vessels. A higher frequency probe may be used if the patient is relatively thin or if the block is performed at a more medial location (not described here) where the nerves are more superficial.
- Appearance: The pectoralis major and minor muscles are separated by a hyperechoic lining (perimysium); the pectoralis major lies superficial and lateral to the pectoralis minor. Approximately 4 to 5 cm deeper lies the axillary neurovascular bundle. The large axillary vein lies medial and caudad to the artery. The lateral cord of the plexus is often readily visualized as a hyperechoic oval structure. However, the medial and posterior cords may not be easily identified since the medial cord lies between the axillary artery and vein. In contrast, the posterior cord can be hidden deep in an axillary artery acoustic shadow. In addition, the medial cord can be posterior or even slightly cephalad to the axillary artery. It is essential to realize that there is a great deal of individual anatomic variation in cord location around the artery. The nerve structures now appear hyperechoic rather than hypoechoic as seen more proximally, presumably due to an increase in the number of fascicles and amount of hyperechoic-appearing connective tissue.
- Needling: The skin is infiltrated with local anesthetic. For the single-injection technique, a 50- to 90-mm, 18- to 22-gauge insulated needle is suitable if using NS, whereas a 90-mm, 17- to 20-gauge needle can be used for catheter placement. An IP needle alignment will usually be most suitable; however, this may be difficult in young children due to the limited space between the clavicle and the US probe. The block needle is inserted cephalad to the probe and is then advanced caudally and posteriorly at approximately 30 degrees to the skin (IP insertion caudad to the probe is acceptable for young children in whom there is limited space cephalad to the probe). The cords should be found at a depth of 4 to 6 cm. It is recommended to combine US with NS for accurate nerve localization (e.g., musculocutaneous nerve or a specific cord) due to the high variability of cord location.
- Local anesthetic spread: Aim to place the needle and local anesthetic posterior to the axillary artery next to the posterior cord (spread from this location is optimal for complete block success). Before local anesthetic injection, performing a test dose with D5W is recommended to visualize spread and confirm nerve localization.[1] Inject 20 to 25 mL of local anesthetic around the posterior cord. If the local anesthetic spread is deemed inadequate to surround all cords, reposition the needle before injecting any additional local anesthetic.

Clinical Pearls

- In the past, numerous techniques were developed with modifications to localize nerves and avoid vessel and pleural punctures. Real-time guidance with US addresses some of these issues, although US-guided block techniques are continually being refined to determine the safest and most successful approaches.
- Techniques incorporating multiple injections may be easier and potentially safer under combined US and NS guidance, which provides direct visualization of the anatomic structures.
- If a catheter is to be threaded, the aim should be to elicit motor responses in the hand itself. The tip of the Tuohy needle (90 mm, 17 to 20 gauge) should be directed laterally to allow the catheter to run in the direction of the nerves.
- Compared to blocks at more proximal locations, the infraclavicular block has the advantage of lower risk of blocking the phrenic nerve or stellate ganglion. However, in some cases, continuous catheters may lie along one cord and fail to provide complete anesthesia and analgesia of the entire brachial plexus with small volume infusions. This may be overcome by intermittent boluses of larger volumes of local anesthetic.
- Vessel puncture is a potential complication; therefore, frequent aspiration should be performed. Lateral needle insertion will help avoid the risk of pneumothorax.

Axillary Block

The nerves targeted for axillary block course distally with the axillary artery and vein along the humerus from the apex of the axilla (Fig. 36-10). This block is helpful for elbow, forearm, and hand surgery. The ulnar, median, and radial nerves are the primary targets. The musculocutaneous nerve often leaves the plexus (via the lateral cord) proximal to this point. It may be blocked separately during the axillary block within the coracobrachialis muscle or at a midhumeral location beyond the coracobrachialis. Relative to the third part of the axillary artery, the usual course of the terminal nerves is as follows: the median nerve lies anterior and medial, the ulnar nerve lies posterior and medial, the musculocutaneous nerve lies anterior and lateral, and the radial nerve lies posterior and lateral. Because the single sheath may be broken up into separate compartments by fascial septa surrounding individual nerves in the axilla, some practitioners advocate that local anesthetic should be injected at multiple sites, in contrast to the single injections possible with proximal approaches. The patient is positioned supine with the arm abducted at 70 to 80 degrees and externally rotated with the elbow flexed at 90 degrees.

Procedure Using Nerve Stimulation Technique

- Landmarks: The axillary artery is marked as high in its course through the axilla as is practical. It is usually felt in the intramuscular groove between the coracobrachialis and the triceps muscles. It also passes between the insertions of the pectoralis major and the latissimus dorsi muscles on the humerus.
- Needling: A 30- to 50-mm, 22-gauge insulated needle is suitable for this block. After aseptic preparation, a skin wheal is raised over the proximal portion of the artery. The index and middle fingers of the nondominant hand straddle the artery just below this point, locating the pulsation and compressing the neurovascular bundle below the intended injection site. The needle is inserted in a slight cephalad direction, followed by a two-step, four-injection process with a puncture at locations just superior and inferior to the artery.
- Nerve localization: Ideally, the nerves serving the proposed surgery area are sought first with the NS technique. The median and the musculocutaneous nerves lie on the superior aspect of the artery (as viewed by the operator). In contrast, the ulnar and radial nerves lie below and behind the vessel. Obtaining a direct musculocutaneous nerve response (elbow flexion) indicates the localization of this particular nerve but not all nerves.
- Injection: Experience has shown that the most reliable approach is to perform injections around each individual nerve, 10 to 15 mL at each nerve location. Less volume may be required, but the minimum required dose/volume per nerve is currently unknown.

Procedure Using Ultrasound Guidance (Fig. 36-22)

- Scanning: High-frequency, linear probes are generally recommended (10 to 15 MHz) for imaging since the nerves are

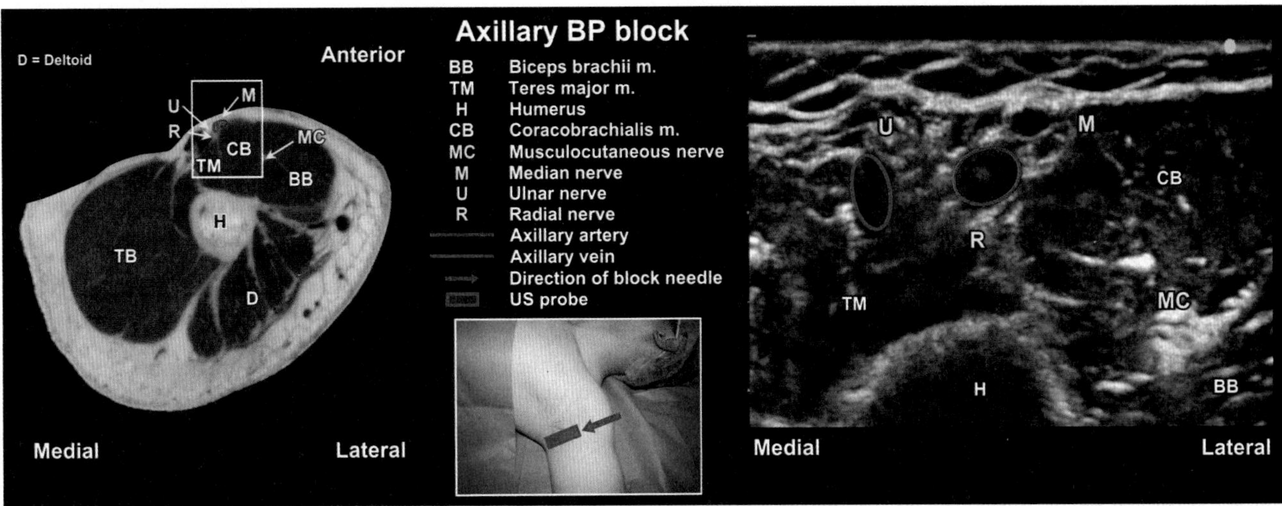

Figure 36-22 Arrangement of relevant anatomy for ultrasound-guided axillary brachial plexus block. The block is performed using IP needle alignment to a linear, high-frequency probe. Typically, the block needle is advanced in sequence to reach the median, ulnar, and radial nerves.

superficial (1 to 2 cm) below the skin. Small footprint probes are recommended for young children. The most proximal location at the apex of the axilla may be the best for viewing all of the terminal branches of the brachial plexus. The probe is perpendicular to the anterior axillary fold and cross-section to the humerus at the bicipital sulcus (and at the level of the axillary pulse) to capture the transverse or short-axis view of the neurovascular bundle.

- Appearance: In cross-section: The coracobrachialis and the biceps brachii muscles are seen laterally; the teres major and the triceps brachii muscles lay medially, the latter being deeper than the biceps brachii muscle. The anechoic and circular axillary artery lies centrally, adjacent to the biceps brachii and coracobrachialis muscles, and is surrounded by the nerves. The nerves appear round to oval in a short axis, generally appearing as hyperechoic masses due to a large amount of connective tissue (epi- and perineurium) interspersed within the hypoechoic nerve fascicles.

The *median* nerve is often located superficial and between the artery and the biceps brachii muscle; the *ulnar* nerve is usually located medial and superficial to the artery; the *radial* nerve lies deep to the artery at the midline (clockwise: median, ulnar, radial—but there are many variations). The *musculocutaneous* nerve is commonly located in the hyperechoic plane between the biceps brachii and coracobrachialis muscles.

- Needling: A 50-mm, 22-gauge insulated needle is suitable for the recommended combined US and NS technique. Both IP and OOP needle approaches can be used for axillary blocks. An OOP approach, with the needle distal to the probe and on the transverse axis to the nerve, is similar to the traditional blind procedure, except that the needle will be aligned at an angle rather than perpendicularly to optimize its visibility. An angle of 30 to 45 degrees from the skin, with the needle, placed approximately 1 to 2 cm caudad to the probe, may allow optimal needle visibility (see description of the walk-down technique in the section on Common Techniques: Nerve Stimulation and Ultrasound Imaging). The IP approach involves inserting the needle at an acute angle (20 to 30 degrees) into the skin in a lateral-to-medial direction (Fig. 36-22). Typically, the block needle is advanced to contact the median nerve. It is then crossed over the axillary artery to reach the ulnar nerve superficially and then finally behind the artery to the deeper radial nerve. Follow NS procedure if using this technique.
- Local anesthetic spread: Performing a test dose with D5W is recommended before local anesthetic application to visualize spread and confirm nerve localization. A proper injection is indicated by fluid space entirely around the nerve structure, with nerve movement away from the needle tip. Improper injection (e.g., injection outside the sheath) appears as partial asymmetrical fluid expansion not immediately adjacent to the nerve structure.

Clinical Pearls

- Although a multiple-injection NS technique has been used extensively for this and other blocks, it is important to consider that some spread of the local anesthetic solution will occur, and hypesthesia can occur unpredictably, limiting the identification of subsequent nerves. A recent evaluation of a two-injection technique—with one injection posterior to the axillary artery and the other to the musculocutaneous nerve—demonstrated that this approach might be as effective as blocking each of the ulnar, median, radial, and musculoskeletal nerves separately,[71] potentially minimizing unwanted spread to adjacent nerves.
- If forearm anesthesia is required and the musculocutaneous nerve was not localized previously, supplementary anesthesia of the musculocutaneous nerve should be attained using some reliable means of nerve localization (i.e., NS and US guidance) rather than blind injection into the coracobrachialis muscle. US imaging 1 to 2 cm distal to the axillary block location can identify the muscle and usually the nerve.
- Intercostobrachial and medial brachial cutaneous nerve blocks can be achieved by subcutaneous injections (5 mL in total) on the medial surface of the upper arm all the way from the biceps to triceps muscles. Both nerves are relatively small and difficult to visualize under US; however, local anesthetics can be infiltrated superficially above the median nerve toward the triceps.
- Perivascular infiltration and transarterial approaches are also traditionally performed for axillary block, although these techniques have been largely replaced by advanced technologies such as NS and US.
- For continuous nerve blocks, a 17- to 18-gauge Tuohy needle is required to facilitate catheter placement. Securing the catheter in the axilla may be challenging and require a short tunnel to stabilize the catheter.

- Axillary approaches to the brachial plexus are associated with minimal complications compared to proximal brachial plexus blocks. Neuropathy from needle puncture or intraneural injection of local anesthetic is the foremost consideration. However, this may be reduced with US imaging and careful attention to injection pressures during the block. Hematoma can occur if the axillary artery is punctured, but this is a self-limiting complication.

Terminal Upper Extremity Nerve Blocks

Upper extremity PNBs are of particular value as rescue blocks to supplement incomplete surgical anesthesia and to provide long-lasting selective analgesia in the postoperative period (5 Video 36-5). The peripheral nerves may be individually blocked at upper midhumeral, elbow, or wrist locations, depending on the specific nerve. If using US guidance, the elbow and forearm regions appear to be the most suitable block regions, and blocks at these sites may improve the accuracy of nerve localization and local anesthetic spread. The wrist is highly populated with tendons and fascial tissues (e.g., flexor and extensor retinacula), which, on US, can be challenging to distinguish from nerves and may also obscure visualization of nerves. With the help of color Doppler, US can be used to identify the nerves at many desirable locations, as they are often situated near blood vessels (Table 36-1). This chapter will focus on blocks for which NS and US imaging are most amenable but will also comment on nerve blocks at the wrist. Musculocutaneous nerve block at the upper midhumeral level is discussed in the section on Axillary Block. Figures 36-10 and 36-11 illustrate the courses and cutaneous innervation of the terminal nerves of the upper extremity.

Radial Nerve

The radial nerve can be blocked at the anterosuperior aspect of the lateral epicondyle of the humerus. The radial nerve supplies the posterior compartments of the arm and forearm, including the skin and subcutaneous tissues. It also innervates skin on the posterior aspect of the hand laterally near the base of the thumb, the index's dorsal aspect, and the ring finger's lateral half up to the distal interphalangeal crease. For radial nerve blocks, the patient is positioned supine with their arm slightly abducted, laterally rotated, and extended elbow.

Procedure Using Nerve Stimulation Technique

- Landmarks: A line is drawn on the anterior elbow between the medial and lateral epicondyles of the humerus. The radial nerve is located beneath this intercondylar line, approximately 1 to 2 cm lateral to the biceps tendon. This position should be marked with an "X."
- Needling: A 30- to 50-mm, 22- to 24-gauge insulated needle is used, and a skin wheal is raised at the "X." The needle is then inserted perpendicular to the plane passing through the humeral epicondyles.
- Nerve localization: The correct response to radial NS at this location is an extension (dorsiflexion) of the wrist and digits on the operative side. Elbow extension should not be elicited since the branch to the long head of the triceps has diverged proximally.
- Injection: Approximately 5 mL of local anesthetic are injected under low pressure.

Procedure Using Ultrasound Guidance (Fig. 36-23)

- Scanning: A linear probe in the frequency range of 5 to 10 MHz is suitable for scanning in most cases, although high-frequency (10- to 15-MHz) probes are recommended for children due to the short distance between the skin and the nerve. The radial nerve can first be located proximally at the level of the spiral (radial) groove of the humerus, where it lies immediately adjacent to the humerus and posteromedial to the deep brachial (profunda brachii) artery of the arm. The patient's arm should be internally rotated and placed with the hand over the abdomen on the opposite side of the body. The spiral groove lies immediately distal and posterior to the deltoid tubercle. Subsequent tracing of the nerve from this humeral location to the anterolateral elbow may facilitate its precise localization. To confirm its location, the probe can be rotated slowly to scan the nerve in the longitudinal and transverse planes at the elbow.
- Appearance: At the spiral groove of the humerus, the bone is relatively superficial and appears deep to the hypoechoic triceps brachii muscle as a demarcated hyperechoic oval shape with dark shadowing in its interior (not shown). The nerve appears oval and predominantly hyperechoic and is located in the posterior aspect of the humerus and immediately adjacent

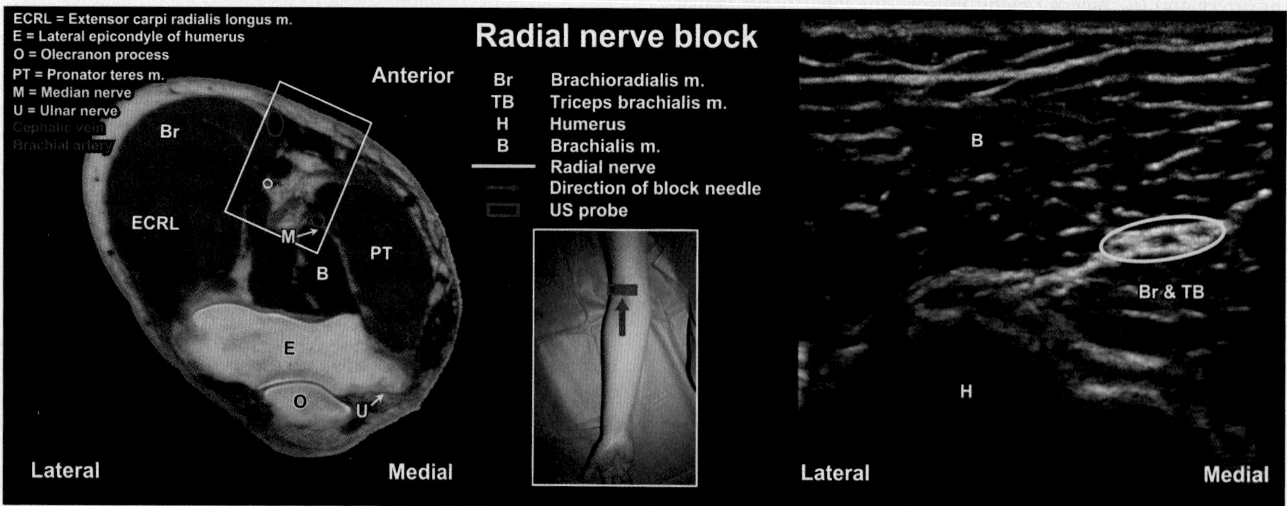

Figure 36-23 Arrangement of relevant anatomy for ultrasound-guided radial nerve block. The block is performed using an OOP needle alignment to a linear probe at the anterolateral elbow. The ideal placement will be a few centimeters above the elbow, where the nerve has not yet been divided into superficial and deep branches.

to the small, pulsatile deep brachial (profunda brachii) artery (as verified with Doppler). At a point just proximal to the anterior compartment of the elbow, the humerus appears to have changed shape and appears smaller and almost rectangular in cross-section. The hyperechoic radial nerve now lies at some distance from the humerus, is sandwiched between the brachialis and brachioradialis muscles, and appears oval shaped.

- Needling: A 30- to 50-mm, 22-gauge insulated needle is suitable if using NS. The needle can be aligned using IP and OOP (Fig. 36-23) approaches to block the nerve at the anterosuperior aspect of the lateral epicondyle of the humerus. The nerve should be blocked slightly above the elbow since it divides into deep and superficial branches approximately 2 cm above the elbow. The block needle is advanced to approach the target nerve on its side, preferably avoiding direct needle contact with the nerve.
- Local anesthetic spread: Performing a test dose with D5W is recommended before local anesthetic application to visualize spread and confirm nerve localization. The aim is to inject approximately 5 mL of local anesthetic and observe the spread around the nerve circumferentially.

Clinical Pearls

- Needle contact with the humerus indicates that the needle is too deep. In contrast, deep needle penetration without bone contact indicates that the needle is lateral to the humerus (beyond the bone).
- The radial nerve can be blocked at the wrist or lateral distal forearm adjacent to the radial artery. At the wrist, 3 mL of solution is injected into the "anatomic snuffbox" formed by the tendons of the extensor pollicis longus and extensor pollicis brevis tendons. A subcutaneous wheal is then raised from this point, extending over the dorsum of the wrist 3 to 4 cm onto the back of the hand. This approach is suboptimal for most procedures since the nerve divides immediately beyond the elbow and continues as the superficial radial (sensory) and deep posterior interosseous (motor) nerves.

Median Nerve

The median nerve can be blocked at the anterior elbow's midline or the anterior forearm's mid-to-distal aspect (Fig. 36-24).

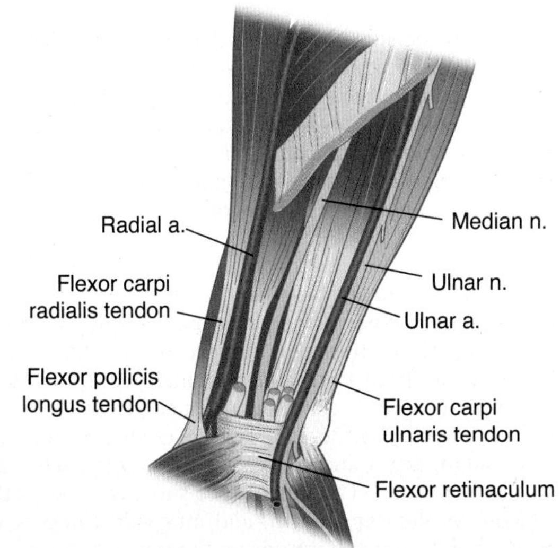

Figure 36-24 Illustration of the anterior forearm showing the courses of the median and ulnar nerves. The ulnar artery is a reliable landmark for localizing the ulnar nerve using ultrasound imaging.

The nerve is located adjacent (medial) to the brachial artery at the elbow, facilitating its localization here. In the forearm, the nerve can be located at its position lateral to the ulnar nerve. The median nerve supplies the skin anteriorly on the medial surface of the thumb, palm, and digits two to four, and posteriorly on the distal third of the second to fourth digits. It causes flexion at the metacarpophalangeal joints and extension at the interphalangeal joints of digits two and three. The nerve innervates muscles that produce flexion and opposition of the thumb, middle, and index fingers and pronation and flexion of the wrist. For blocks at the anterior wrist or anterior distal forearm, the patient's arm should be positioned next to the torso, with the elbow flexed slightly and the hand free to allow a wrist or thumb flexion response elicited by NS.

Procedure Using Nerve Stimulation Technique

At the elbow:

- Landmarks: As with radial nerve block, an intercondylar line is drawn, and the nerve is located where this line crosses the pulsation of the brachial artery, usually 1 cm to the ulnar side of the biceps brachii tendon.
- Needling: Using a 30- to 50-mm insulated needle, a skin wheal is raised at the point identified with landmarks (see earlier), and the needle is introduced perpendicularly.
- Nerve localization: Nerve responses to electrical stimulation are sought immediately adjacent to the artery. The optimal NS response for median nerve block at the elbow location is any one of the following or a combination thereof: flexion and opposition of the thumb, middle, and index fingers; flexion of the wrist; and pronation of the forearm.
- Injection: 5 mL of local anesthetic should be sufficient to block this nerve. Care should be taken to avoid intravascular and intraneural injection.

In the forearm:

- It may be challenging to locate this nerve blindly in the forearm using NS. However, transcutaneous electrical stimulation[72] or percutaneous electrode guidance[73,71] can be used to locate the nerve with a probe placed on or indenting the skin's surface. Once the nerve has been localized, an insulated needle is inserted perpendicular to the plane of the forearm, and NS responses are sought. A similar volume of local anesthetic should suffice.

Procedure Using Ultrasound Imaging (Fig. 36-25)

- Scanning: A high-frequency (10- to 15-MHz) linear probe can capture a transverse view of the nerve and localize the brachial artery at the elbow, where the nerve lies medial to both the artery and then the tendon of the biceps brachii muscle. At the anterolateral forearm, the nerve lies lateral to the ulnar nerve and artery (localizing the ulnar nerve first will help identify the median nerve). Color Doppler may be used to confirm the arteries' location.
- Appearance: At the elbow, the median nerve can be identified at approximately 1 to 2 cm in depth as a hyperechoic yet distinctly honeycomb-like structure, lying medial to the anechoic pulsatile brachial artery. Deep to the neurovascular structures lies the musculature of the superior aspect of the elbow (pronator teres and brachialis muscles) as a hypoechoic homogeneous mass. The nerve appears oval shaped and lateral to the ulnar artery at the forearm.
- Needling: OOP and IP techniques can be used for either block location. For OOP needling at the elbow (not shown), after adjusting the US image to place the nerve in the middle of the screen, insert a 30- to 50-mm insulated needle perpendicular to

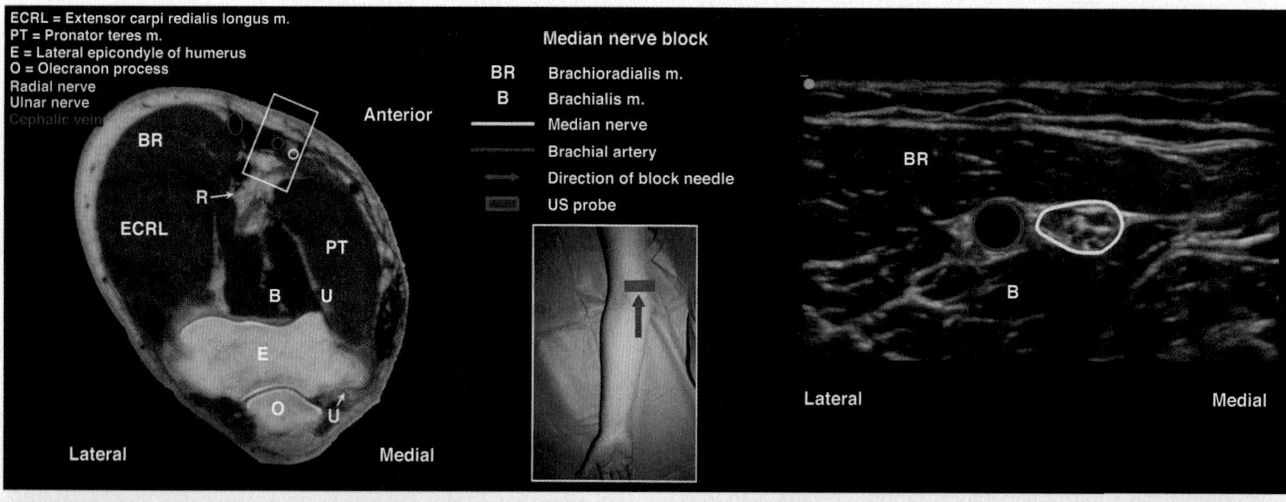

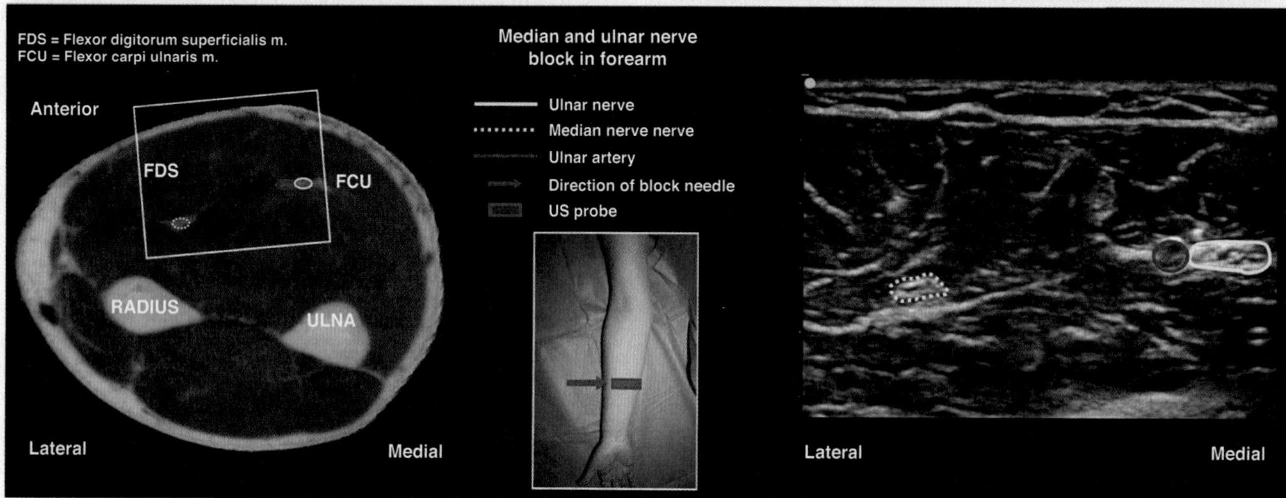

Figure 36-25 Arrangement of relevant anatomy for ultrasound-guided median and ulnar nerve block. **Top:** Ultrasound-guided median nerve block at the medial aspect of the elbow using an OOP approach. **Bottom:** Ultrasound-guided ulnar nerve block in the middistal forearm using an IP needle aligned to a small footprint, linear ("hockey stick") probe. For ulnar nerve block, the ideal location to avoid arterial puncture is where the nerve has yet to approach the ulnar artery fully.

the transversely placed probe at a 45- to 60-degree angle. If using the combined technique, the NS procedure should be followed. An IP technique with the needle in a medial-to-lateral direction may be advantageous at the elbow to allow easy tracking of the needle to ensure it avoids puncturing the brachial artery.

- Local anesthetic spread: After performing a test dose with D5W, the aim is to spread approximately 5 mL of local anesthetic around the nerve in a circular fashion, avoiding nerve contact and obtaining complete block.

Clinical Pearls

- The median nerve lies deep to the flexor retinaculum at the wrist, and there is always the potential risk of causing carpal tunnel syndrome due to elevated pressure within the tunnel following injection. For this reason, the elbow or forearm locations for blocking the median nerve are more logic choices.
- At the wrist, the median nerve lies between the tendons of the palmaris longus and the flexor carpi radialis muscles. If only the palmaris longus muscle can be felt, the nerve lies next to the radial side of its tendon. A skin wheal is raised, and a needle is inserted until it pierces the deep fascia. An injection of 3 to 5 mL of local anesthetic is sufficient to produce anesthesia.
- Aspiration of blood into the tubing during elbow block indicates brachial artery puncture. In this case, the needle should be reinserted after applying pressure to the puncture site until hemostasis is achieved. Contact with the humerus indicates that the needle is too deep. Localized contraction of the arm muscles (e.g., elbow flexion and forearm pronation) indicates the local muscles' stimulation and that the needle is likely too deep.

Ulnar Nerve

In the periphery, the ulnar nerve can be blocked at the elbow, forearm, or wrist. An ulnar nerve block may be used for rescue analgesia or surgical anesthesia for surgery on the fifth digit. At the junction of the distal third and proximal two-thirds of the medial forearm, the nerve is commonly located just medial to the pulsatile ulnar artery (Fig. 36-25). The US-guided technique is advised to avoid the artery and localize the nerve accurately when using this block location. The ulnar nerve supplies muscles that produce flexion of the ring (fourth) and little (fifth) fingers and ulnar deviation of the wrist. It innervates the skin over the medial surface (anterior and posterior) of the hand and digits four and five. Before performing the block, the patient's arm should be flexed at the elbow by 30 degrees and the forearm supinated. The forearm can rest on an arm board with an additional pillow under the wrist.

Procedure Using Nerve Stimulation Technique

At the elbow:

- Anesthetizing the ulnar nerve at the elbow may be uncomfortable for the patient. NS is not routinely used for localizing the ulnar nerve at the elbow since the nerve is easily located and palpated in the cubital tunnel (ulnar groove) between the medial epicondyle of the humerus and the olecranon process of the ulna. Only a small volume (1 to 4 mL) of local anesthetic should be injected if performing the block at this location.

In the forearm:

- Similar to the median nerve, it may be challenging to locate this nerve in the forearm using NS blindly. Transcutaneous electrical stimulation or percutaneous electrode guidance can be used to locate the nerve. Once the nerve has been localized, an insulated needle attached to a nerve stimulator is inserted perpendicular to the plane of the forearm, and appropriate motor responses are sought. The appropriate responses for ulnar nerve block at this location are flexion of the ring (fourth) and little (fifth) fingers and ulnar deviation of the wrist. Injection of 5 mL of local anesthetic is sufficient to block the nerve at the forearm. Combined US- and NS-guided technique provides good localization and accuracy with local anesthetic spread.

Procedure Using Ultrasound Guidance (Forearm, Fig. 36-25)

- Scanning: This block often uses a high-frequency (10- to 15-MHz) linear probe. The probe is placed transversely just above the midforearm level to view the ulnar nerve in a short axis as it approaches the ulnar artery. The nerve is positioned above the ulna and the belly of the flexor carpi ulnaris, on the arm's anterior surface, rather than medially to contact the bone. The operator should scan downward slowly until the nerve and pulsatile artery are viewed adjacent to each other (Doppler may be valuable here) and then retract the scan head slightly, so the artery and nerve appear clearly as separate structures (Fig. 36-25).
- Appearance: The nerve in the short axis is seen as a honeycomb-like, oval-shaped structure, including hypoechoic fascicular structures surrounded by hyperechoic tissue. The adjacent ulnar artery appears anechoic and roughly similar in size to the nerve and lateral to it. The median nerve may be seen at the lateral edge of the image and seems similar to the ulnar nerve in size and shape.
- Needling: During IP needling, the image should be adjusted so that the nerve is toward the most lateral edge of the screen for good visibility of the needle shaft (not shown in Fig. 36-25). A short (20- to 30-mm) needle can be used in a medial-to-lateral direction to reduce the risk of vascular puncture.
- Local anesthetic spread: The aim is to spread approximately 5 mL of local anesthetic around the nerve in a circular fashion to obtain a complete block while avoiding nerve contact. The local anesthetic injection will appear as an expansion of hypoechogenicity surrounding the nerve, which may separate the nerve from the artery.

Clinical Pearls

- When performing regional anesthesia at the elbow, direct injection after eliciting paresthesia or direct injection into the groove under pressure is not advised because of the nerve damage risk. Small volumes (1 to 4 mL) of local anesthetic should be used.
- During nerve block in the forearm, blood withdrawal into the tubing suggests ulnar artery puncture, and the needle should be reinserted after holding pressure. Contact with the ulna indicates that the needle is too deep.
- US imaging facilitates the unique approach of blocking the ulnar nerve in the forearm. This technique may reduce complications such as ulnar nerve neuritis or neurapraxia compared to blocks at the cubital tunnel behind the medial epicondyle.
- A linear or curved array US probe with a small footprint (26 mm; e.g., a "hockey stick" probe) may be used. This probe size is helpful for easy manipulation on the forearm and good needle alignment using the IP technique.
- At the wrist, the ulnar nerve lies between the ulnar artery and the flexor carpi ulnaris muscle tendon. A skin wheal is raised at the level of the styloid process on the palmar side of the forearm between these two landmarks, a small-gauge needle is inserted, and 3 mL of solution is injected into the area, with or without paresthesias.

Intravenous Regional Anesthesia (Bier Block)

Without NS or US, arm anesthesia can be provided by injecting local anesthetic into the venous system distal to an occluding tourniquet (NICV 36-3).

Procedure

- A small-gauge (20 or 22) intravenous catheter is inserted and taped on the dorsum of the hand in the arm to be blocked. A heparin lock or small syringe is attached, and saline is injected to maintain patency. A pneumatic tourniquet is applied over the upper arm. The tourniquet pressure should be set to 2.5 times the systolic blood pressure. The tourniquet should be inflated as a test to confirm that the pressure is sufficient to occlude distal arterial blood flow and should then be deflated again.
- The arm is elevated to promote venous drainage. An Esmarch bandage is then wrapped tightly around the limb from distal to proximal to produce further exsanguination. After exsanguination, the tourniquet is inflated to 300 mmHg or 2.5 times the patient's systolic blood pressure and is again tested for adequate occlusion of the distal radial pulse.
- The arm is returned to the horizontal position, a 50-mL syringe with 0.5% lidocaine (without preservative) is attached to the previously inserted cannula, and the contents are injected slowly. The forearm discolors, and the patient perceives a transient "pins and needles" sensation and warmth as anesthesia ensues over the following 5 minutes. Epinephrine should not be added to the local anesthetic solution.
- For short procedures, the cannula can be removed at this point. If surgery extends beyond 1 hour, the cannula can be left in place and used for reinjection after 90 minutes.
- Beyond 45 minutes of surgery, many patients experience discomfort at the level of the tourniquet. Special "double-cuff" tourniquets are available for this block to alleviate this problem. The distal cuff is inflated first, followed by the proximal cuff. The distal cuff is deflated, allowing anesthesia to be induced in the area under the distal cuff. If discomfort ensues, the distal cuff is inflated over the anesthetized area of skin, and the uncomfortable proximal cuff is released. This step is critical because the significant risk of this procedure is the premature release of the local anesthetic solution into the circulation. If a double cuff is used, both cuffs should be tested before starting, and the proper sequence for inflation and deflation should be followed meticulously. The potential for leakage of anesthetic into the circulation is greater with the narrower cuffs used in this double setup. Because the shifting process also increases the potential for unintentional anesthetic release, using a single, wider cuff may be better for short procedures.
- If surgery is completed in less than 20 minutes, the tourniquet is left inflated for at least that total period. If 40 minutes have elapsed, the tourniquet can be deflated as a single maneuver.

Between 20 and 40 minutes, the cuff can be deflated, reinflated immediately, and finally deflated after 1 minute to blunt the initial absorption of anesthetic into the systemic circulation. However, this may not truly lower the eventual peak plasma local anesthetic levels achieved.

- The duration of anesthesia is minimal after tourniquet release.
- Bupivacaine is contraindicated for Bier block due to its systemic cardiotoxicity.

Clinical Pearls

- The simplicity of this technique is offset by the potentially significant risk of systemic local anesthetic toxicity if the tourniquet fails or is released prematurely. Complications related to systemic toxicity include seizures, cardiac arrest, and death; other noted complications include nerve damage, compartment syndrome, and thrombophlebitis. Careful testing of the tourniquet and slow injection of a solution into a peripheral (not antecubital) vein will reduce the chance of leakage under the tourniquet. Systemic blood levels are time dependent, and careful attention should be paid to the sequence of tourniquet release and patient monitoring during this period. A separate intravenous site for injection of resuscitation drugs is needed and all appropriate resuscitative equipment must be available. However, with careful attention to these details, the Bier block is one of the most effective and reliable techniques available to the anesthesiologist.

Trunk: Interfascial Plane and Nerve Blocks

Anesthesia of the abdomen and chest is often obtained most simply with spinal and epidural injections of local anesthetics. However, epidural anesthesia carries concerns of systemic hypotension and epidural hematoma, limiting its use for some patients, and may be hazardous because of infection or coagulopathy. Thus, peripheral block of the spinal nerves in the paravertebral space or the intercostal or inguinal nerves can be suitable for many indications, particularly when a narrow band of anesthesia (intercostal or paravertebral) or reduced motor block is preferable. The sympathetic nerves separate from their somatic counterparts early in their course, making independent somatic and sympathetic blockade a practical consideration. In many clinical situations, it may be desirable to use intercostal blocks to avoid the combined anesthesia of the somatic and sympathetic fibers that occurs with neuraxial blocks. Likewise, although paravertebral blocks may result in somatic and sympathetic blocks, hemodynamic responses are often less than those encountered with epidural block. Sympathetic blocks are performed commonly at the major ganglia, particularly the stellate, celiac, and lumbar plexus. These blocks may require multiple injections and are technically more difficult than neuraxial anesthesia, but they offer advantages in specific clinical situations. The reader is referred to Chapter 56 for a discussion of these blocks.

Ilioinguinal and iliohypogastric nerve blocks are used for procedures in the inguinal area, including hernia repair and orchidopexy. A lumbar plexus block is not optimal in these cases since these nerves exit the plexus more cranially (L1–L2) than those targeted by the lumbar plexus block (L3–L5). Transversus abdominis plane (TAP) block[75,76] and rectus sheath blocks[77,78] can be performed for abdominal, umbilical, or other midline surgical procedures and are often performed bilaterally. Approaches to the rectus sheath block target the terminal branches of the 9th, 10th, and 11th intercostal nerves within the rectus sheath; ideally, injection is between the posterior rectus sheath and the rectus abdominis muscle. The TAP block aims to impede innervation of the abdominal wall up to the level of T8 by injecting local anesthetic between the transversus abdominis and internal oblique muscles. The initial technique of multiple injections of local anesthetic in the abdominal wall was modified to a single injection using the landmark technique of locating the "lumbar triangle of Petit."[79] US-guided regional techniques allow the layers of musculature to be identified, and needle insertion and local anesthetic deposition between the fascial layers can be visualized in real time. The TAP block has become more common in clinical practice as the approach has evolved.

A New Era of Interfascial Plane Blocks

Interfascial trunk blocks have gained in popularity due to their 8
accessibility and potential opioid-sparing characteristics. Even though they appear to have an effect on reducing somatic pain, they cannot be relied upon to provide a solid surgical or sympathetic block. Nevertheless, TAP blocks are a classic example of how US technology and image quality have led to a shift in regional anesthesia away from precision techniques that target specific nerves or plexuses to the idea of depositing local anesthesia in an interfascial plane which the nerves travel through. Interfascial plane blocks (Figs. 36-26 and 36-27) have become increasingly popular in both the chest and abdominal walls

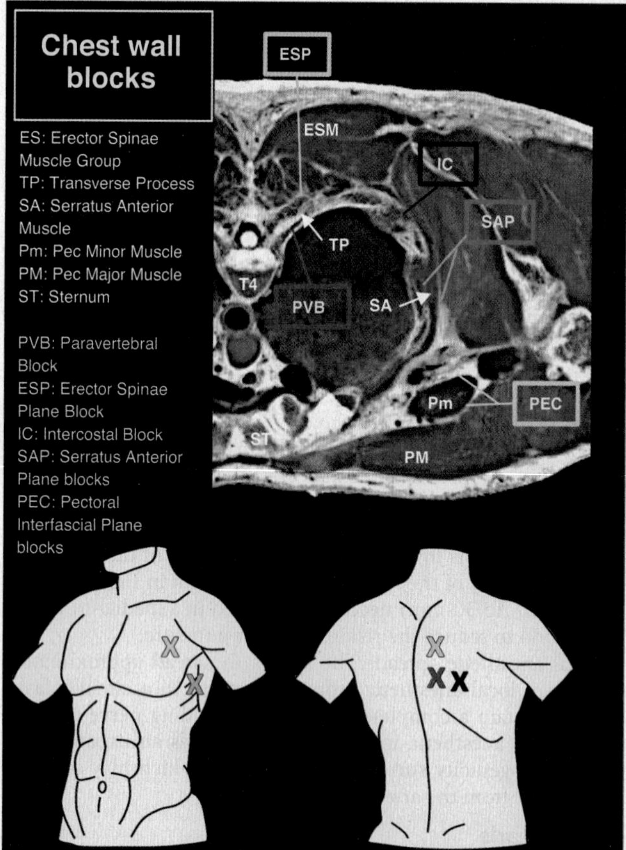

Figure 36-26 Variations of chest wall blocks. The erector spinae plane block is performed at the transverse process; moving the block site laterally allows the performance of an intercostal block, while moving the block site further laterally at the axillary line allows the performance of a serratus anterior plane block. Moving the insertion site anteriorly and superiorly allows the performance of pectoral interfascial plane blocks. **Bottom:** Needle insertion sites (X) for chest wall interfascial blocks, color-coded according to the **top** figure.

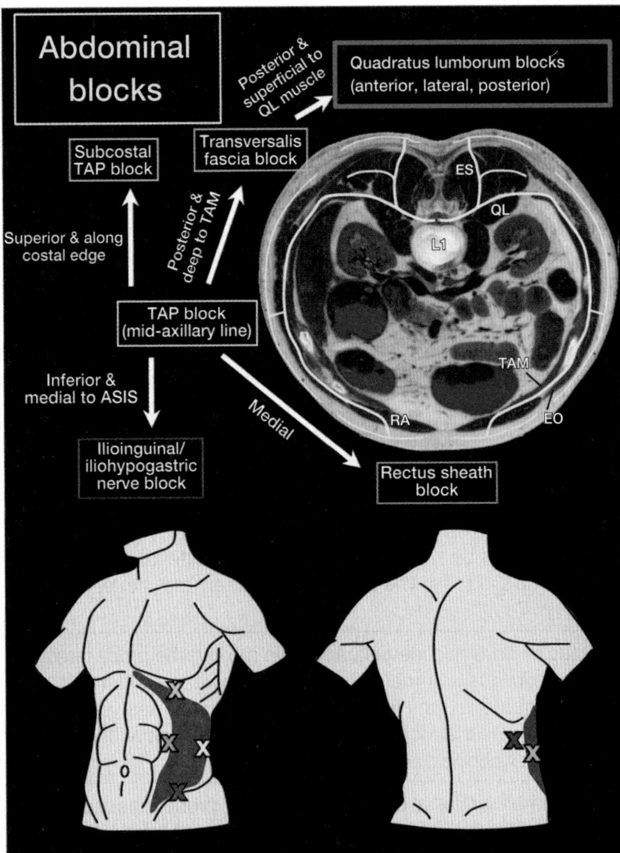

Figure 36-27 Variations of abdominal interfascial blocks. **Top:** The TAP block is performed at the midaxillary line; moving the block site medially allows the performance of a rectus sheath block while moving the block site posteriorly allows the performance of transversalis fascia and quadratus lumborum blocks. Moving the insertion site superiorly or inferiorly from the TAP insertion site allows the performance of subcostal TAP and ilioinguinal/iliohypogastric blocks, respectively. **Bottom:** Needle insertion sites (X) for abdominal field blocks, color-coded according to the **top** figure. The approximate location of the transversus abdominis muscle is indicated in *red*.

(e.g., erector spinae plane [ESP] block, pectoralis plane block [PEC], serratus anterior plane block [SAPB] and transversus abdominis, QL plane blocks). These new interfascial plane blocks aim to increase the overall efficiency and safety of regional anesthesia, usually with more superficial and more readily identifiable landmarks (Table 36-2). Nevertheless, a comparison of their analgesic efficacy with that of their older precision counterparts is needed.

Erector Spinae Plane Block

The ESP is a new interfascial plane block described as an alternative to neuraxial and paravertebral nerve blocks.[80] Located between the transverse process and the anterior aspect of the erector spinae muscle group, this forms the ESP. This fascial plane runs from T1 and the cervical vertebrae to the medial sacral crest on both sides of the spine. It is believed that its analgesic mechanism involves blocking the dorsal and ventral rami of the spinal nerves and sympathetic fibers, with diffusion and spreading both cranially and caudally to encompass numerous vertebral levels. Its appeal stems from the ease of single injection and catheter placement.[81]

Procedure Using Landmark technique

Using a landmark method similar to that used for the paravertebral block, one can mark the transverse processes 1 to 2.5 cm lateral to the spinous processes. A perpendicularly inserted needle contacts the transverse process. Once the needle contacts the transverse process, a single injection of local anesthetic is administrated after aspiration. If the initial injection encounters resistance, withdraw the needle slightly. However, US is strongly recommended to provide safe guidance for both single shot and catheter placement for ESP procedures.

Procedure Using Nerve Stimulation Technique

NS for the ESP block has not been established. A single-case report describes the advancement of an electrical NS-guided catheter from thoracic to cervical level within the ESP.[82]

Procedure Using Ultrasound Guidance (Fig. 36-28)

- Scanning: A linear probe with a high frequency (13 to 6 MHz) is typically used on an average adult. However, a curvilinear transducer with a lower frequency (8 to 3 MHz) may be required for a larger individual. The probe is positioned over the paraspinal skin in the cephalocaudal orientation at the thoracic or lumbar level. Slide the probe laterally until the transverse process is visualized. In the thoracic area, the transverse processes appear as shallow rectangular structures with hyperechoic outlines and acoustic shadowing, in contrast to the overlapping lines of the lamina and the deeper, smooth arcs of the ribs. The pleura appears as a hyperechoic line between the osseous ribs' acoustic shadowing.
- Needling: Using an IP method, the needle can be inserted superior or inferior to the probe, cephalad to caudal or caudal to cephalad, respectively. Once the needle tip reaches beneath the erector spine muscle and contacts the transverse process, a saline bolus should be administered through the needle to open and expand the collapsible ESP plane. If resistance is encountered, the needle should be withdrawn gently from the transverse process while remaining beneath the erector spinae muscle. In response to the injection pressure, the erector spinae muscle should be visible detaching from the transverse process. Following confirmation of the correct interfascial plane, the local anesthetic is injected after aspiration. The US probe can be scanned in a cephalad or caudad direction from the needle insertion site to ensure proper fascial plane distribution and spreading along the ESP.
- Local anesthetic spread: Ropivacaine 0.2% to 0.5% in 15 to 20 mL volumes has been suggested.

Clinical Pearls

- The ESP block is considered to have a lower risk of complications because of its utilization of the transverse process as an osseous backstop and its location away from neuraxial structures, major arteries, and pleura.[83]
- Early evidence shows considerable opioid-sparing effects in multiple operations, highlighting the ESP block's adaptability.[84]
- ESP, in particular, is more easily compressible, presumably reducing the risk of hematomas caused by cardiopulmonary bypass. With the ESP's anticipated improved safety profile and potential for opioid-sparing effects, this block has attracted much attention for its use in cardiac surgery patients.[85]

Paravertebral Block

Techniques

The paravertebral block is useful for segmental anesthesia, particularly in the upper thoracic segments. It is also useful if a more

Table 36-2 Useful Anatomic Landmarks for Localizing Interfascial Planes during Common Ultrasound-Guided Interfascial Plane Blocks

Interfascial Plane Location	Anatomic Landmark(s)	Approach for Ultrasound Imaging
Erector spinae plane (ESP)	Transverse process	A linear probe (13–6 MHz) is typically used on an average adult; however, a curvilinear transducer (8–3 MHz) may be required for a larger individual. At the thoracic or lumbar level, the probe is positioned over the paraspinal skin with cephalocaudal orientation. Slide the probe laterally until one can observe the transverse processes (rectangular shadow) without pleural in between (Fig. 36-28).
Interpectoral and pectoserratus	T3 and T4 anterior ribs; pectoralis and serratus muscles	After identifying the subclavian arteries, identify the second rib in this view. Slide the probe inferiorly to the third and fourth ribs. Pectoralis major is located above pectoralis minor. A very thin band of serratus anterior muscle overlies the ribs, with the pectoralis minor muscle sitting on top and tapering caudally. The thoracoacromial artery branches between the interpectoral planes.
Serratus anterior plane	T4 and T4 ribs	Slide the probe caudally and laterally to find the fourth and fifth midaxillary ribs. In this area, latissimus dorsi is superficial to serratus anterior (Fig. 36-32). Pleura are between rib shadows. The thoracodorsal artery may be seen above serratus anterior.
Transversus abdominis (TAP) plane block	The three layers of the abdominal muscles	To identify the rectus muscles midline first, and then moving the probe laterally reveals the external oblique, internal oblique, and transversus abdominis (Fig. 36-35) to the anterior axillary line above the iliac crest. The hyperechoic line beneath the transversus abdominis is the peritoneum. Below this is the peritoneal cavity, which shows bowel peristalsis.
Quadratus lumborum (QL)	TAP muscles; shamrock	Between the costal margin and iliac crest, the curvilinear probe is positioned in a transverse plane on the midaxillary line. Slide the probe posteriorly above the iliac crest to identify the transversus abdominis tapers and quadratus lumborum beneath it. At the level of the transverse process to detect the quadratus lumborum block structures (Fig. 36-36) yields an ultrasonic pattern like three shamrock leaves (i.e., the stem-transverse process and the three leaves-Psoas, Quadratus lumborum, and Erector Spinae).

proximal (central) block than that of the intercostal nerves is needed, such as to relieve the pain of herpes zoster or a proximal rib fracture. The thoracic paravertebral block is used for breast surgery and perioperatively for thoracic surgery. Thoracolumbar paravertebral anesthesia is used commonly for inguinal herniorrhaphy and postoperative analgesia following hip surgery. The lumbar paravertebral blockade has been used successfully for outpatient hernia operations, providing significant postoperative analgesia.

A single-injection paravertebral block used for surgical anesthesia has been shown to surpass general anesthesia concerning

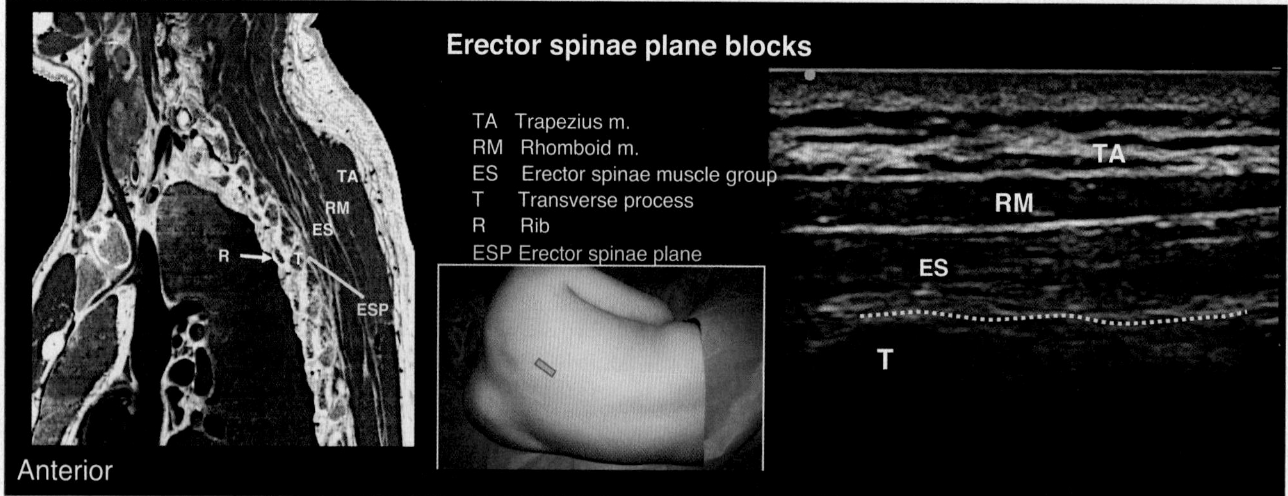

Figure 36-28 Erector Spinae plane block. A high-frequency linear probe is placed sagittal at the transverse process on the back, revealing the erector spinae muscle group. The needle is at an IP alignment to the probe and inserted in a caudad-to-cephalad or cephalad-to-caudad direction.

postoperative pain relief, the incidence of vomiting, and pain upon mobilization.[86] Paravertebral blocks are considered "unilateral epidurals" since they block spinal nerves selectively on the side of the anesthetic application. However, they also have the potential for epidural spread (i.e., they can be bilateral if desired). The anesthesia includes both somatic and sympathetic effects, with a reduced hemodynamic response (e.g., hypotension) compared to epidural anesthesia. This nerve block requires excellent knowledge of paravertebral anatomy but can be performed easily with experience.

The upper five ribs are more challenging to palpate laterally, and blocking their associated intercostal nerves is best performed with a paravertebral injection. This approach is technically more complex and has a slightly greater potential for complications because of the proximity of the lung and intervertebral foramina. The paravertebral block can be used at any level. At the lumbar spine, some prefer to perform a lumbar plexus block to reduce the number of injections and avoid sympathetic block. The injection is made into the triangular paravertebral space, just after the spinal nerve has left the intervertebral foramen. The nerve may be challenging to localize blindly using bony landmarks, and larger volumes of local anesthetic are often required. NS has been used to locate the nerve. US imaging can be performed before the block to improve bony landmark identification, particularly for obese patients or those with a spinal deformity. However, real-time US guidance can be challenging. It may offer limited additional value from preprocedural landmark identification since the overriding bone tissue reflects the US beam and causes dorsal shadowing, which obscures imaging (especially of the needle) to the depth of the paravertebral space. The paravertebral block is performed with the patient in the lateral, sitting, or prone position. If prone, a pillow is placed under the patient's abdomen to produce flexion of the thoracic and lumbar spine.

Procedure Using Nerve Stimulation or Loss-of-Resistance Technique

- Landmarks: The paravertebral approach varies depending on the spinal level and the respective orientation of the vertebral spinous and transverse processes (see Clinical Anatomy section). Thus, paravertebral blocks in the upper thoracic region are performed at each level by identifying the spinous process of the vertebra above the level to be blocked; in the lumbar region, the spinous process of the level to be blocked is used to locate the transverse process. The appropriate spinous processes for the region to be blocked are marked. Transverse lines are drawn across the cephalad border and extended laterally to overlie the transverse process (approximately 2.5 cm) (Fig. 36-29). Finally, the transverse processes are marked individually or by drawing a vertical line parallel to the spine joining the ends of the transverse lines. For a diagnostic block, a single nerve may need to be anesthetized. For pain control, several levels must be identified. Because of sensory overlap from multiple nerves, the injection of at least three segments (as in intercostal block) is required to produce a reliable segmental block.
- Needling: After aseptic skin preparation and patient sedation, skin wheals are raised at the marked transverse processes. A 22-gauge, 70-mm insulated needle is introduced through the skin wheal in the sagittal plane and directed slightly cephalad to contact the transverse process (usually at a depth of 2 to 4 cm in the thoracic region and 5 to 8 cm in the lumbar region) or—often likely—the costotransverse ligament. Gentle cephalad or caudad exploration may be required to identify the bone. The depth of the transverse process should be noted on the needle shaft. The needle is then withdrawn from the transverse process to the skin level and reinserted 10 degrees superiorly (to target the spinal nerve corresponding to the spinous process) or inferiorly (corresponding to the vertebral level below the spinous process) and 1 cm deeper than the point of bone contact. The needle should be angled slightly medially to avoid causing pneumothorax. There will be a subtle "give" at the midpoint between these landmarks (spinous and transverse processes), indicating entry into the paravertebral space.
- Nerve localization: For NS, an initial current of 2.5 to 5 mA is used, and the needle is advanced until contractions of the appropriate muscles (e.g., abdominal muscles with lumbar paravertebral block) are observed, after which the current intensity is reduced to localize the nerves at 0.5 to 0.6 mA. A test dose of local anesthetic will confirm nerve localization upon elimination of the nerve response, resulting from the current dissipation at the needle tip from the conducting solution.[4] For loss of resistance, a 22-gauge Tuohy needle is used. After walking off the transverse processes, a "pop" or loss of resistance may be felt when entering the paravertebral space.
- Injection: When the needle has entered the paravertebral space, 3 to 7 mL of local anesthetic, depending on the number of sites and patient size, is injected at each site following careful aspiration. Attention must be paid to the total milligram dose injected; the volume required to block each level limits the concentration that can be used and the total number of levels that can be blocked. If lumbar paravertebral injections are combined with intercostal blocks, both blocks' concentration and total volume may have to be reduced.

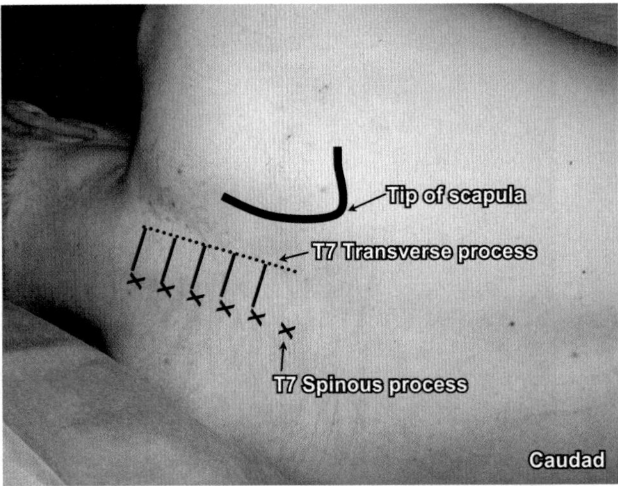

Figure 36-29 Landmarks for a paravertebral block at the thoracic spine. The spinous process of the level below the block (e.g., spinous process of T7 for a block at T6) is identified, and a line is drawn horizontally from the cranial aspect of the spinous process to mark the transverse process. The needle is inserted at appropriate spinal levels at the lateral line marking the transverse processes.

Procedure Using Ultrasound Imaging

Imaging for these blocks is often used before block performance (i.e., "preprocedural," "supported," or "off-line" imaging) rather than during (i.e., "real-time" or "on-line" imaging) to identify the deep bony landmarks, including the articular and transverse processes. A real-time US-guided paravertebral block is an advanced block and should only be performed by experienced personnel.

- Scanning: Placing the probe transversely at the midline will provide an overview of the vertebral lamina and processes and costal structures if viewing the thoracic spine (Fig. 36-30, *top*). A medial-to-lateral scan using a longitudinally placed probe

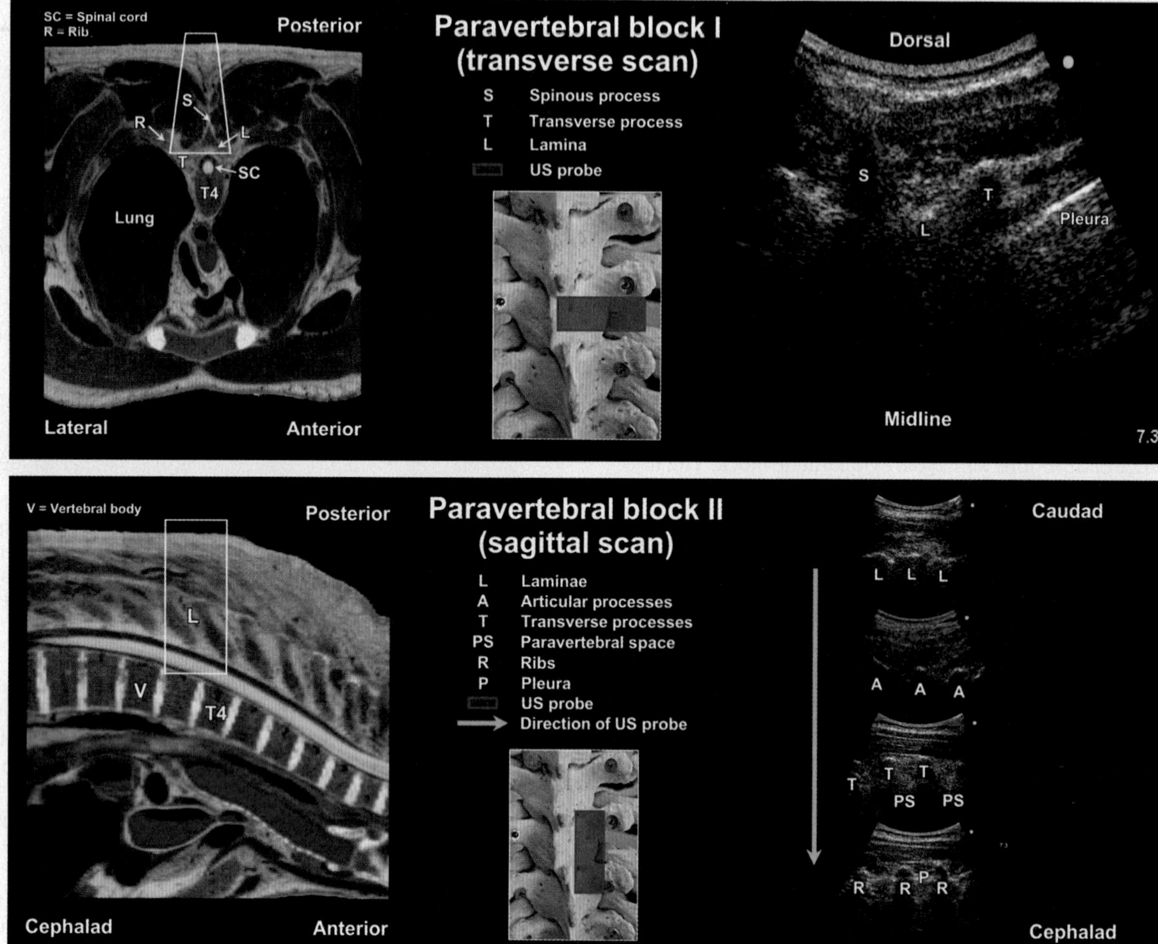

Figure 36-30 Arrangement of relevant anatomy and transverse probe placement for the thoracic paravertebral block. **Top:** The probe is first placed in the midline of the spine to capture a transverse view of the elements of the vertebral and costal (if thoracic spine). **Bottom:** The probe is then rotated longitudinally and moved laterally to view the laminae, articular processes, and transverse processes; the paravertebral space can be found deep to and between the latter.

can locate and mark important bony landmarks (Fig. 36-30, *bottom*). For this, a 5- to 7-MHz curved-array US probe (lower frequency for obese patients and higher frequency linear probes for thin adult or pediatric patients) is positioned in the sagittal plane on top of the spinous processes of the target thoracic or lumbar region. Subsequent lateral scanning will allow consecutive identification of the lamina, articular, transverse processes, and the ribs in the thoracic spine.

- Appearance: The initial transverse scan will show a hyperechoic outline of the vertebral spinous and transverse processes, the lamina, and (in the thoracic spine) the associated rib. The laminae will appear first as largely overlapping linear structures during the lateral scan with the probe placed longitudinally to the spine. The articular processes in the long axis appear as "multiple lumps," just lateral to the spinous processes, and are short rectangular structures with hyperechoic lines and underlying hypoechoic bony shadowing. Moving laterally, the transverse processes appear and will look similar to the articular processes; they will disappear from view when the probe is moved beyond their tips, which can help distinguish them from the articular processes and mark the lateral block location. Beyond the transverse processes, the rib heads appear as long shadows within hyperechoic borders, deep to the linear hyperechoic muscle fibers of the paravertebral muscles. The paravertebral space lies deep to the transverse processes, and the pleura can often be identified between and deep to the transverse process and the ribs.
- Needling: Since multiple injections are generally needed to completely cover all the dermatomes of the surgical area in clinical practice, US imaging is more suitable for a preblock assessment ("supported" US) to visualize and measure the depth of needle penetration required for the needle to contact the transverse processes. Needling will be identical to that for the blind technique, except that the depth of the transverse process will be known more accurately. It is possible to perform real-time US guidance using IP or OOP needle alignment. The reader is referred to Clinical Pearls for advice on important precautions when using US guidance.
- Local Anesthetic Spread: In adults, visualization of local anesthetic spread will be difficult if using real-time US guidance. The overlying bones largely reflect the US beam and obstruct visibility beyond the paravertebral space. However, the local anesthetic spread may be seen with US in young children (<2 to 3 years old) since the fusion of the neural arches, and vertebral bodies has not yet occurred, allowing good visibility into the paravertebral space.

Clinical Pearls

- Since the paravertebral space is well vascularized, an inadvertent vascular puncture will often occur, highlighting the need for frequent aspiration and injection in small aliquots.[87]
- Pneumothorax is more likely with a paravertebral technique than with intercostal block. The needle should be directed medially as it passes below the transverse process and never more than 2 cm beyond the transverse process. If cough or chest pain occurs, a chest radiograph should be performed to rule out pneumothorax.
- Subarachnoid injection is also more likely in the thoracic area because of the dural sleeves' extension to the intervertebral foramina level. Careful aspiration is important but may not prevent unintentional injection of local anesthetic into the intrathecal space. Total spinal anesthesia can result from a 5- to 10-mL injection. Systemic toxicity is also possible because of the need for large local anesthetic volumes.
- If attempting real-time US guidance of paravertebral block, it is important to observe the angulation of the needle, and the use of IP needle alignment may be most prudent. The needle should not be inserted in a significant medial direction as there is a risk of spinal cord injury from intraforaminal insertion and injection. Likewise, a lateral direction increases the risk of pneumothorax. If choosing to use real-time US guidance during block procedure, note that: (1) with the probe placed in the sagittal/longitudinal plane, OOP needling may be riskier, as it often requires the medial or lateral angulations described earlier, and (2) an IP needling approach can be riskier when the probe is placed in the coronal/transverse plane.
- Traditionally, paravertebral blocks and other trunk blocks are performed blindly, with either sole use of landmarks, including a loss of resistance to needle penetration of the costotransverse ligament for paravertebral block, or combined landmark and NS technique. US imaging may be beneficial for these blocks, particularly paravertebral blocks, to facilitate landmark localization. For example, preprocedural scanning can identify the tips of the transverse processes, which will help determine the correct needle insertion site. US may be beneficial for performing blocks in obese patients (where the depth of needle insertion will be modified) or those with anatomic variation (e.g., scoliosis).

Intercostal Nerve Block

Anesthesia of the intercostal nerves provides both motor and sensory anesthesia of the abdominal wall from the xiphoid to the pubis. Intercostal nerve block is used for acute and chronic pain conditions affecting the thorax and upper abdomen (e.g., postoperative analgesia after thoracotomies, various cardiac surgeries, and both open and laparoscopic cholecystectomies). It can be performed through several means, including continuous infusions into the subpleural space, interpleural catheters, and direct intercostal nerve block. The surgical site (i.e., intraoperative anatomic access) determines the available options.

These nerve blocks involve injections along the easily palpated sharp posterior angulation of the ribs, which occurs between 5 and 7 cm from the midline in the back. The blocks may be performed laterally (8 to 10 cm from the midline)[88] or more medially (immediately beyond the transverse processes). The upper levels T1–T5 may be most amenable to paravertebral block due to this region's overlying scapula and bulky paraspinal musculature. Intercostal nerve block of five or six levels is a viable procedure for providing analgesia and motor relaxation for upper abdominal procedures such as cholecystectomy and gastric surgery. Unilateral intracostal block is helpful in the management of pain from rib fractures and also reduces postoperative analgesic requirements in patients with subcostal incisions. This technique is also helpful in reducing the pain associated with the insertion of chest tubes or percutaneous biliary drainage procedures. Several adjacent segments must be blocked because of the overlap in the supply of the intercostal nerves.

The patient may be in the lateral, sitting, or prone position for intercostal blocks. For operative anesthesia, the prone position is most practical. A pillow is placed under the abdomen to provide slight flexion of the thoracic spine. The arms are draped over the edge of the stretcher or operating table so that the scapula falls away laterally from the midline. The anesthesiologist stands at the patient's side. Most anesthesiologists prefer to stand on the side that allows their dominant hand to hold the syringe at the caudad end of the patient.

Procedure Using Landmark-Based Technique

- Landmarks: The reader is referred to the Clinical Anatomy section (see earlier) for descriptions of the locations of the relevant landmarks. The spinous processes in the midline from T6 to T12 are marked. The ribs are then identified along the line of their most extreme posterior angulation. The 6th and 12th ribs are marked first at their inferior borders, and a line is drawn between these two points. The rest of the ribs between them are identified, and a mark is placed on the inferior border of each rib along the angled parasagittal plane identified by the first line between the 6th and 12th ribs.
- Needling: After aseptic preparation, light sedation is provided for the patient, and a skin wheal is raised at each mark on the inferior border of each respective rib. Starting with the lowest rib, the index finger of the cephalad hand retracts the skin above the identifying mark in a cephalad direction. Using the other hand, the anesthesiologist inserts a needle (22 gauge, 3.75 cm) directly onto the rib, maintaining a constant 10-degree cephalad angulation. After contact with the rib, the cephalad traction is slowly released, the cephalad hand takes over the needle and syringe, and the needle is allowed to "walk" down to below the rib at the same angle. The needle is then advanced approximately 4 mm under the rib.

Age influences the point of needle insertion in children. The needle is inserted at the intersection of the lower border of the rib with the midaxillary line in children below 10 years old or with the posterior axillary line in children above 10 years old, respectively. Anterior approaches are rarely used and will not be described here.

- Injection: Once in the intercostal groove, aspiration is performed, and 3 to 5 mL of local anesthetic solution (lower volumes for children <3 years old) is injected. The needling and injection procedure is repeated for each segmental level and for both sides. Since the intercostal space is highly vascularized, local anesthetics are absorbed rapidly. Toxic levels of local anesthetic may be encountered when using large volumes, which can quickly lead to neurologic or cardiovascular sequelae. Maximum doses should be calculated and followed carefully for these blocks.

Procedure Using Ultrasound Guidance

The ribs can be visualized easily using US. A high-frequency (5- to 15-MHz) probe is placed on a longitudinal axis. The rib will appear as a hyperechoic line casting a hypoechoic bony shadow underneath (Fig. 36-31). The pleurae can also be seen to "glitter" as they slide with respiration. The remainder of the procedure will be similar to the blind technique. If a more medial (proximal) intercostal nerve block is desired, such as to

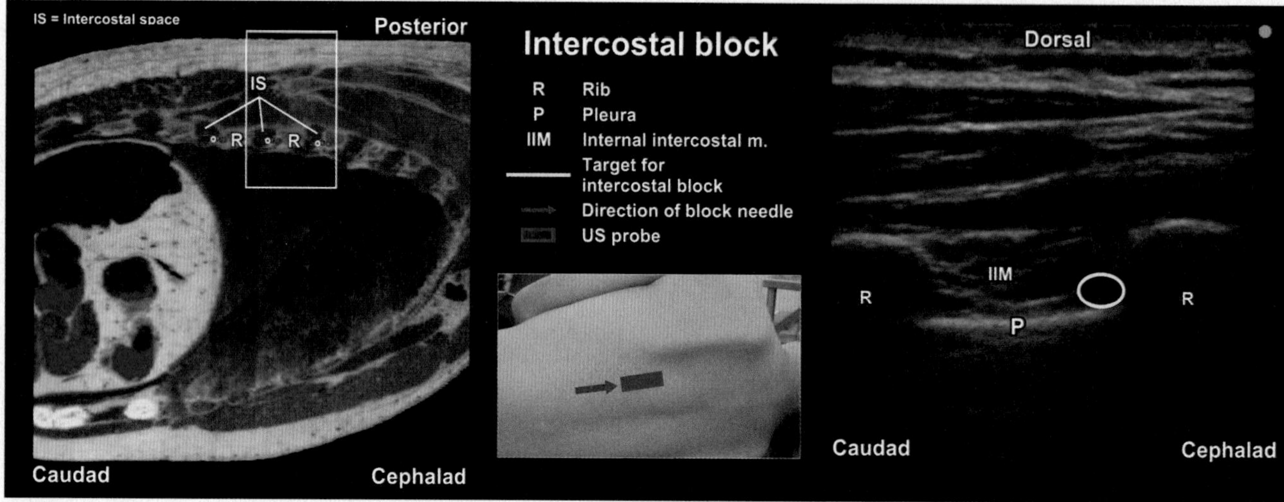

Figure 36-31 Arrangement of relevant anatomy for ultrasound-guided intercostal nerve block. The ultrasound image shows the hyperechoic lines of the ribs casting a hypoechoic bony shadow. The pleura is the hyperechoic line deep to that of the ribs and has a glittery appearance, especially on respiration.

relieve the pain of herpes zoster or proximal rib fractures, US imaging of the costotransverse joint and ribs may be helpful. The section on the paravertebral block describes and illustrates this imaging.

Clinical Pearls

- Intercostal nerve blocks can be supplemented by several somatic paravertebral nerve blocks or sympathetic blocks of the celiac plexus for abdominal procedures. Care should be taken to adjust the total dose of the drug in these combined techniques so that the maximal recommended amounts are not exceeded.
- The advantages of intercostal blocks over sole intravenous opioid use include superior analgesia, opioid-sparing, improved pulmonary mechanics (including earlier extubation), and reduced central nervous system depression. Intercostal blocks are often used in addition to systemic analgesia (e.g., intravenous, patient-controlled analgesia).
- Despite frequent concern about the incidence of pneumothorax with intercostal blocks, this complication is rare, mainly when US is used in inexperienced hands. This depends primarily on maintaining strict safety features of the described technique. Emphasis should be placed on absolute control of the syringe and needle at all times, particularly during the injection.
- A common complication is related to the sedation required to perform this block in the prone position. Overdose can lead to airway obstruction and respiratory depression in the prone position. Attention must be paid to the patient's mental status because this block produces the highest blood levels of local anesthetics compared to any other regional anesthetic technique. When the block is performed for postoperative pain relief, the dose should be reduced to 0.25% bupivacaine or ropivacaine to minimize the risk of toxicity.
- It is possible to produce partial spinal or epidural anesthesia if the injection is made close to the midline and the local anesthetic tracks along a dural sleeve to the epidural or subarachnoid space. Respiratory insufficiency can also be seen if the intercostal muscles are blocked in patients who depend on them for ventilation. Patients with chronic obstructive disease with ineffective diaphragm motion are not good candidates for this technique.

Serratus Anterior Plane Block

SAPB is a relatively new ultrasound-guided interfascial block performed in the axillary and lateral chest wall regions.[89,90] This block is lateral and posterior compared to the PEC blocks. Local anesthetic injections are given in the plane between the serratus anterior and latissimus dorsi muscles (superficial SAPB). The intercostobrachial nerve is located here, as are the lateral cutaneous branches of the intercostal nerves (T3–T9), the long thoracic, and the thoracodorsal nerve. Alternatively, local anesthetic injections have been administered between the serratus anterior muscle and the corresponding rib (deep SAPB). SAPBs, like other interfascial plane blocks, are characterized by a lack of sympathetic block.

Procedure Using Landmark Technique

On the anterior chest, the fifth rib can be palpated along the midaxillary line, to the left of the rib cage. While the clinician holds the fifth rib in place with the index and middle fingers along the rib with one hand, the needle is then inserted perpendicular to the skin and contacts the rib between the index and middle fingers with the other hand. Aspiration is performed before injecting the local anesthetic. The needle should be withdrawn slightly if resistance is encountered during the injection. Most clinicians use US guidance for this procedure.

Procedure Using Nerve Stimulation Technique

SAPB cannot be performed with NS because there are no major nerves to activate or stimulate.

Procedure Using Ultrasound Guidance (Fig. 36-32)

- Scanning: Start at the midclavicular line with a linear (13- to 6-MHz) probe. Slide the probe caudally and laterally until the fourth and fifth ribs in the midaxillary line are identified. In this region, the latissimus dorsi muscle is superficial to the serratus anterior muscle. Between each rib shadow is pleura. The thoracodorsal artery can be observed above the serratus anterior.
- Needling: The needle is typically advanced from the cephalad to the caudal direction in an IP approach. Depending on the desired block approach, the local anesthetic can be placed between the latissimus dorsi and serratus anterior muscles (superficial SAP) or more deeply (deep SAP) into this muscle between the serratus anterior muscle and the rib). Inject local anesthetic after negative aspiration.

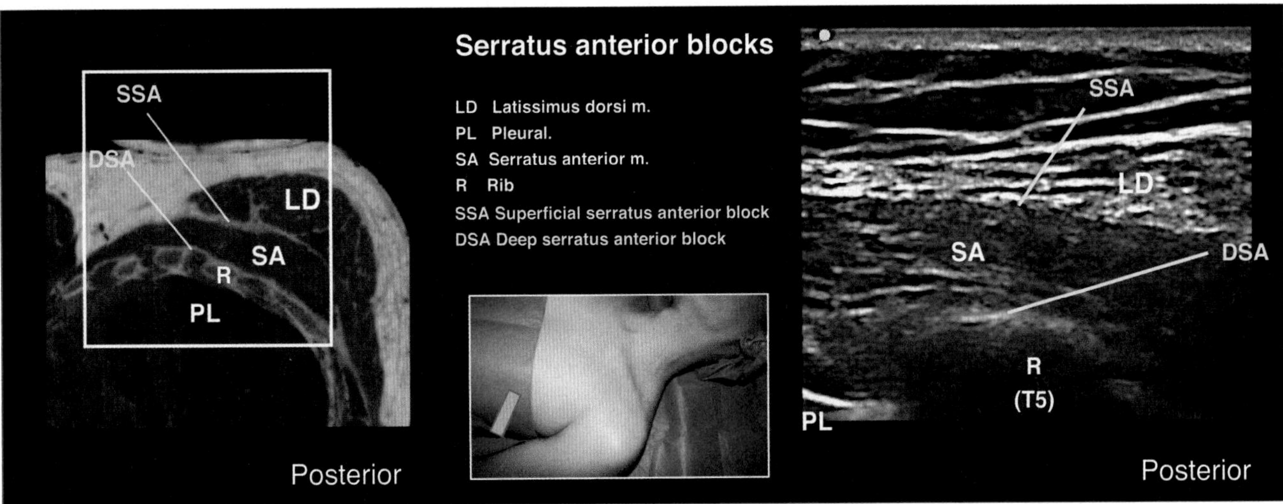

Figure 36-32 Arrangement of relevant anatomy for ultrasound-guided serratus anterior plane block.

- Local anesthetic spread: Ropivacaine 0.375% in 40 mL volumes has been suggested to produce better spread than 20 mL.[91]

Clinical Pearls

- An inadvertent injection of air into the superficial plane will block the visibility of the deep plane. Thus, if both the superficial and deep injection procedures are to be performed, the deeper injection should always be carried out first.
- Analgesic efficacy appears to be similar for both superficial and deep SAP injection.
- Compared to just systemic analgesia, the SAP block has been found to minimize postoperative pain and opioid intake in the first 24 hours after thoracic surgery.[92]
- Using an ultrasound-guided IP technique with the rib as a backstop, this block offers a minimal theoretical risk of pleural and neural tissue complications.
- Dislodgment can be a problem with preoperatively placed SAP catheters, which are challenging to keep in place intraoperatively unless there is careful planning.[93] It may be easier to place continuous SAP catheters after surgery to avoid interference with the surgical procedure.

Interpectoral [Pectoralis (PECS) 1] and Pectoserratus [Pectoralis (PECS) 2] Plane Blocks

The interpectoral[94] (PECS 1) and pectoserratus[95] (PECS 2) planes are newer interfascial anterior chest wall blocks[96] that have gained popularity because of their ease of use, safety, and ability to be performed with single needle insertion. The interpectoral plane block was initially proposed for use in breast surgery to alleviate surgical pain in the pectoralis major and minor muscles. The pectoserratus plane block was developed to block of the long thoracic, intercostobrachial nerves, and T3 to T6 intercostal nerves between the pectoralis minor and serratus anterior muscles for the insertion of breast expanders and subpectoral prostheses. The favorable safety profile of the interpectoral and pectoserratus plane blocks relies on the anatomical delineation of its superficial targets and the position of the ribs, which serve as a barrier against pleural penetration. Despite the presence of small branches of the thoracoacromial artery, the superficial location of the interpectoral and pectoserratus plane block allows hematoma complications to be managed by simple compression.[97] The interpectoral plane and pectoserratus plane blocks are often performed under US guidance to target the two interfascial planes between the pectoralis major, pectoralis minor, and serratus anterior muscle layers.

Procedure Using Nerve Stimulation Technique

The NS technique is not commonly used for interpectoral plane blocks.

Procedure Using Ultrasound Guidance

- Scanning: The patient is positioned supine with the arm slightly abducted for scanning. Figure 36-33 depicts the placement of a linear (13- to 6-MHz) probe in the deltopectoral groove below the clavicle (a similar location for performing an infraclavicular nerve block). After identifying the subclavian arteries, identify the second rib in this view. Inferiorly slide the probe to the level of the third and fourth ribs.
- Appearance: The serratus anterior muscle has the appearance of a very thin band of muscle overlying the ribs, with the pectoralis minor muscle sitting on top of it and tapering caudally. Pectoralis major is situated over pectoralis minor. The thoracoacromial artery has branches between the major and minor pectoral muscles. Care must be made to avoid these branches in the trajectory of the needle.
- Needling: The needle is usually inserted in a cephalad-to-caudad direction using the IP method. The deeper pectoserratus plane block is performed first as inadvertent injection of air will reduce the visibility of deeper structures. The needle tip is inserted between the serratus anterior and pectoralis minor muscles. Be certain that the anesthetic does not spread intramuscularly. Once the pectoserratus plane block has been completed, slowly withdraw the needle to inject local anesthetic between the pectoralis major and minor muscles to complete the shallower interpectoral plane block.
- Local anesthetic spread: Local anesthetic should spread in the two interfascial planes between the pectoralis major, pectoralis minor, and serratus anterior muscles. Typically, 10 mL of local anesthetic is administered into the deeper interfascial plane between the pectoralis minor and serratus anterior, after which the needle is slowly withdrawn, and another 10 mL of local anesthetic is delivered into the shallower plane between the pectoralis major and minor. Commonly, a total volume of 15 to 20 mL of ropivacaine 0.2% or 0.25% is preferred. The optimal dose, concentration, and volume of local anesthetic for the PECS blocks have not been definitively established.

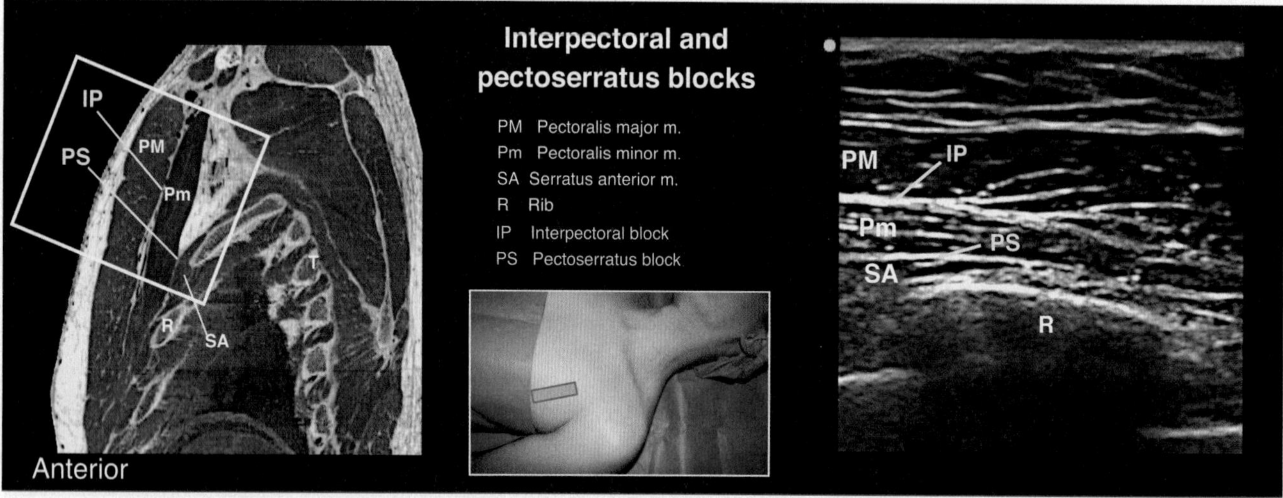

Figure 36-33 Arrangement of relevant anatomy for ultrasound-guided interpectoral and pectoserratus plane blocks.

Clinical Pearls

- Possible risks include infection, pneumothorax, hematoma, winging of the scapula from block of the long thoracic nerve, and local anesthetic toxicity.
- These blocks reduce postoperative pain intensity and opioid intake in the first 24 hours following breast surgery compared to systemic analgesia alone.[98] The interpectoral and pectoserratus plane PECS block has not been directly compared to neuraxial techniques or other chest wall blocks in large-scale randomized controlled trials.
- In addition to breast surgery, PECS blocks may be indicated for placement of pacemakers or implantable cardioverter defibrillators (ICDs), transapical transcatheter aortic valve implantation, minimally invasive mitral valve repair, port placement and removal, postherpetic neuralgia in the thoracic region, midshaft and distal collarbone surgery, and proximal anterior humeral surgery.
- Branches of the thoracoacromial artery are located between the major and minor pectoralis muscles and are frequently utilized as a landmark for the interfascial interpectoral plane.

Rectus Sheath Block

Procedure Using Landmark Technique

- The patient is positioned supine, and the umbilicus and linea semilunaris are identified. The external layer of the rectus sheath is marked on both sides, and a short-beveled needle is inserted at a point where the border of the rectus sheath intersects an imaginary horizontal line at the level of the umbilicus.
- The needle is advanced 60 degrees to the skin toward the umbilicus until a "pop" is felt as the needle penetrates the anterior rectus sheath. Local anesthetic is injected, and the exact steps are repeated for the other side.

Procedure Using Ultrasound Guidance

- Scanning: A linear probe (6 to 15 MHz) is placed transversely on the anterior abdominal wall lateral to the intended site of the incision. Penetration depth varies with the thickness of the subcutaneous layer.
- Appearance: At the midline, the linea alba can be seen between the bellies of the rectus muscle, whereas the peritoneum can be visualized behind the posterior rectus sheath (Fig. 36-34). The

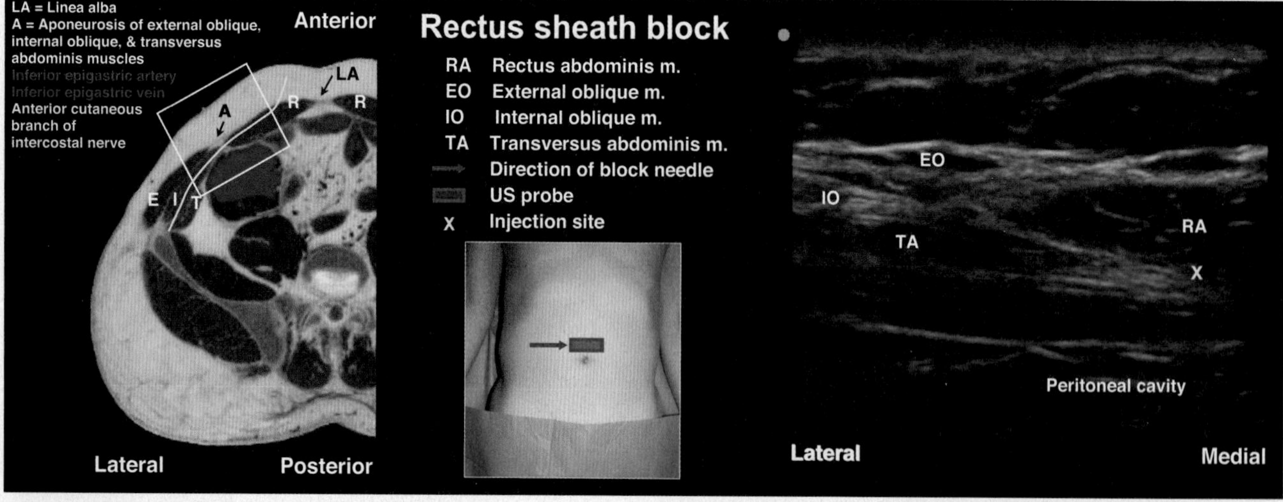

Figure 36-34 Arrangement of relevant anatomy for ultrasound-guided rectus sheath block. Placement of a transverse probe over the midline reveals the rectus abdominis and layers of the abdominal wall. Below these can be seen the peritoneum and peritoneal cavity. The needle is advanced in an IP alignment to the probe.

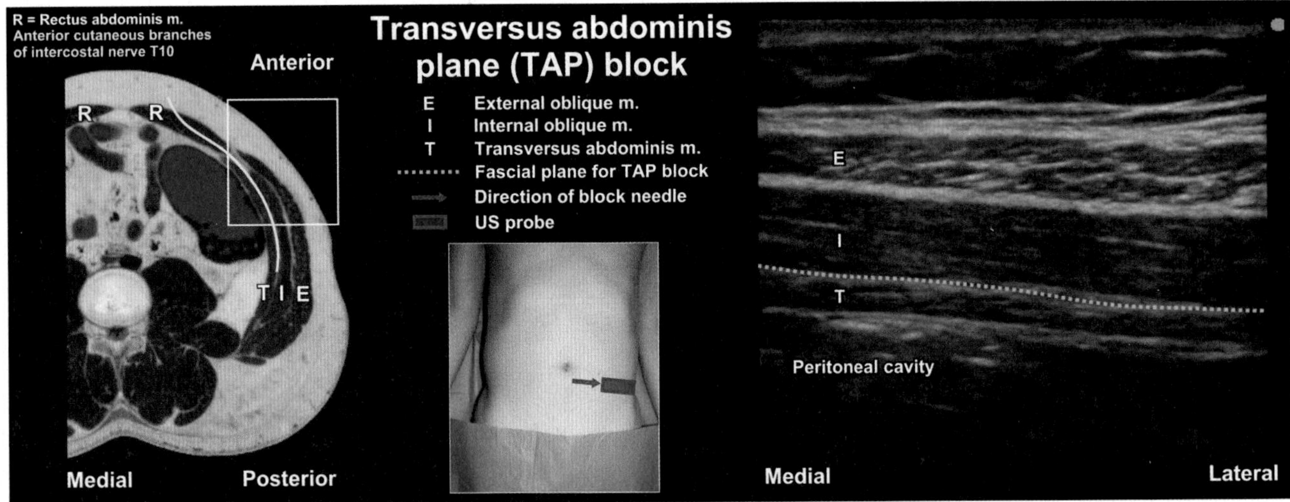

Figure 36-35 Arrangement of relevant anatomy for ultrasound-guided TAP block. A high-frequency linear probe is placed transversely above the iliac crest on the anterior axillary line, revealing the three layers of abdominal muscles, the peritoneum, and the peritoneal cavity. The needle is at an IP alignment to the probe, inserted in a medial-to-lateral direction.

external oblique, internal oblique, and transversus abdominis muscles can be seen lateral to the rectus muscle; the internal oblique muscle is on the same plane as the rectus muscle. Target nerves, which are not visible with US, are located between the internal oblique and transversus abdominis muscles before piercing the posterior rectus sheath and traversing the belly of the rectus muscle. The intended location of the injection is the lateral space between the posterior rectus sheath and the rectus muscle. Color Doppler may be used to identify and avoid the inferior epigastric vessels that run through the rectus muscle.

- Needling: A 22-gauge, 50- to 100-mm needle (depending on subcutaneous fat depth) is inserted IP in a lateral-to-medial direction. A lateral insertion point will help to avoid inferior epigastric vessels. The needle is aimed through the external and internal oblique muscles toward the lateral gutter of the rectus muscle directly superior to the posterior rectus sheath. With this approach, the needle does not penetrate the belly of the rectus muscle and avoids the inferior epigastric vessels.
- Local anesthetic spread: Injection of 1 to 2 mL D5W can confirm needle tip position. A volume of 10 mL (0.2 mL/kg for children) local anesthetic (e.g., 0.5% ropivacaine) is injected on each side. The hypoechoic spread between the posterior rectus sheath and the rectus muscle will be seen.

Transversus Abdominis Plane Block

Procedure Using Landmark Technique

- The patient is positioned supine, and the "triangle of Petit" is identified with the inferior margin, the iliac crest, the posterior margin, the latissimus dorsi muscle, and the external oblique muscle lying anterior.
- A blunted 22-gauge, 50- to 100-mm needle (depending on body habitus) is inserted perpendicularly, immediately posterior to the midaxillary line and above the iliac crest.
- The first and second "pops" will be felt as the needle traverses through the external and internal oblique muscles' fascial layer. The needle tip should be within the plane between the internal oblique and the transversus abdominis.

Procedure Using Ultrasound Guidance

- Scanning: This block often uses a high-frequency (10- to 15-MHz) linear probe. With the patient lying supine, the probe is placed transversely in the midline to identify the rectus muscles. The probe is moved laterally, and the three layers of muscles—the external oblique, the internal oblique, and the transversus abdominis—can be identified (Fig. 36-35). The probe should be positioned above the iliac crest in the anterior axillary line.
- Appearance: The intercostal nerves can be too small and scattered to be identified under US imaging; therefore, the TAP block is predominantly a muscular plane block. The three layers of the abdominal muscles can be identified clearly since the hyperechoic fascia separates them. Beneath the abdominal muscles is the peritoneum, which is the hyperechoic line seen on the US underneath the transversus abdominis. Below this lies the peritoneal cavity, where bowel peristalsis can be seen in real time.
- Needling: During IP needling, the image should be adjusted so that the three layers of the abdominal muscles and a small portion of the peritoneal cavity are in view. A 22-gauge, 100-mm needle can be used in a medial-to-lateral direction to reduce the risk of peritoneal puncture. It should aim toward the muscle plane between the internal oblique and transversus abdominis muscles.
- Local anesthetic spread: The aim is to spread 20 to 30 mL of local anesthetic without exceeding the toxic dose (e.g., 2 mg/kg of bupivacaine or 3 mg/kg of ropivacaine; one-tenth of these volumes for children), on either side of the abdomen for transverse incision across the midline (6 Video 36-6). The local anesthetic injection will appear as an expansion of hypoechogenicity deep to the fascial plane of the internal oblique and above that of the transversus abdominis muscle.

Clinical Pearls

- It is important to ensure local anesthetic spread in the correct fascial plane rather than injecting local anesthetic intramuscularly.
- Color Doppler should be employed to ensure the needle trajectory is clear of blood vessels within the abdominal muscles.
- For midline incisions of the abdomen, rectus sheath block (described above) can be performed by targeting the local anesthetic injection between the rectus abdominis muscle and the posterior rectus sheath, which is formed by the aponeurosis of the three layers of abdominal muscles.

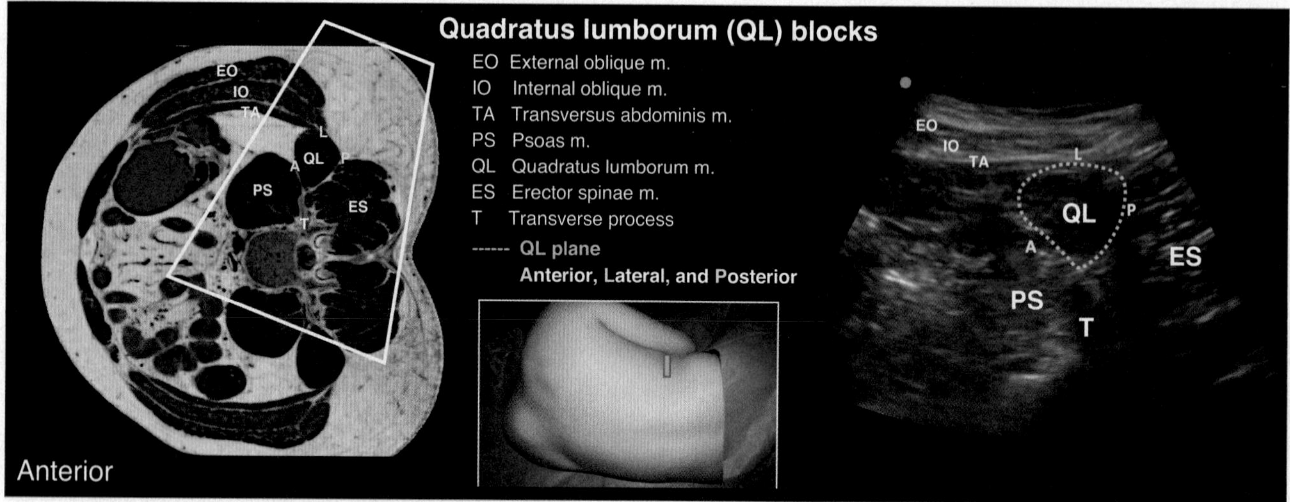

Figure 36-36 Quadratus lumborum (QL) plane blocks. Arrangement of relevant anatomy for ultrasound-guided QL plane block. A low-frequency curved probe is placed transversely above the iliac crest along the flank, revealing the three layers of abdominal muscles, the QL muscle, the psoas muscle, and the erector spinae muscle group. The needle is at an IP alignment to the probe, inserted anterior-to-posterior or posterior-to-anterior direction.

- TAP blocks have been demonstrated to provide adequate analgesia in the obstetric and general surgery populations.
- TAP catheters can be placed under direct vision by the surgeon to provide adequate continuous postoperative analgesia. Following the closure of the abdominal muscle layers, a catheter is inserted percutaneously above the incision, with the tip located at the most lateral point of the incision.
- TAP blocks can be modified into transversalis fascial plane (TFP) blocks by targeting the local anesthetic injection into the layer between the transversus abdominis muscle aponeurosis and the transversalis fascia. Local anesthetic will spread proximally over the inner surface of the QL muscle to anesthetize the proximal portions of the T12 and L1 nerves. The TFP block has been demonstrated to provide analgesia for anterior iliac bone graft harvesting.[99]

Other variations of abdominal field blocks have been described. Each block differs in the location where the injection is made (Fig. 36-35), but all use the transversus abdominis muscle as the primary landmark. The most well studied of these blocks are the rectus sheath block and ilioinguinal/iliohypogastric nerve block.

Quadratus Lumborum Block

The QL block is an abdominal wall interfascial plane block in which the local anesthetic is injected around the thoracolumbar fascia (TLF) on the anterior (QL3 or transmuscular), lateral (QL1), and posterior (QL2) aspects of the QL muscle.[100] The TLF is an extension of the muscular fascia of the abdominal wall. The QL block may offer analgesia to the paravertebral region through the TLF, which contains mechanoreceptors, nociceptors, and sympathetic fibers. It is believed that the diffusion of local anesthetic from the TLF into the paravertebral region and the involvement of sympathetic fibers in the TLF generate visceral analgesia that is absent in the TAP block. Cadaver and in vivo studies have demonstrated that dermatomal spread extends from T8 to L1 and consistently involves the iliohypogastric and ilioinguinal nerves.

Procedure Using Nerve Stimulation Technique

QL cannot be performed using NS because there are no major nerves to activate or stimulate.

Procedure Using Ultrasound Guidance (Fig. 36-36)

- Scanning: A curvilinear (C5-1 MHz) probe is used for most adult patients. To observe the three muscle layers for the TAP block, the probe is positioned in a transverse plane on the midaxillary line, between the costal margin and iliac crest. Slide the probe posteriorly above the iliac crest until the transversus abdominis tapers, and the QL is visible.
- Appearance: The anatomical structures of the adjacent muscles and bone are recognized by a US pattern resembling a shamrock with three leaves at the level of the transverse process. The anatomical structures are the shamrock's three leaves (psoas, QL, and erector spinae muscles) and stem (transverse process).
- Needling: The lateral QL (QL1) block targets the QL and transversus abdominis muscles. Tilting the probe caudally can increase transversus aponeurosis visibility. The needle is usually inserted IP to avoid damaging the ipsilateral kidney. Avoid intramuscular local anesthetic distribution.

The posterior QL (QL2) block targets the middle thoracolumbar fascial plane between the QL and erector spinae muscles. The best injection place is the lumbar interfascial triangle (LIFT) near the lateral margin of the erector spinae muscles. From anterior to posterior or posterior to anterior, the needle is inserted IP. Local anesthetic should reach the paravertebral space posteriorly.

The anterior QL (QL3 or transmuscular) block targets the QL and psoas muscles. To reduce needle travel, it is usually inserted posterior to anterior.

- Local anesthetic spread: Typically, 15 to 20 mL of ropivacaine 0.2% or 0.25% is administered into the interfascial planes.

Clinical Pearls

- A simple acronym mnemonic "PQRST" (Psoas, Quadratus lumborum, eRector Spinae, and Transverse process) describes the first or second letters of the names of these key structures.[101] With this acronym and the shamrock image, the names and relative positions of the anatomical structures can be easily remembered.
- Compared to systemic analgesia alone, the QL block reduces pain intensity and opioid intake in the early postoperative period following cesarean delivery and renal surgery.[102]

- The shamrock method not only describes the critical structures involved in QL blocks, but also lumbar plexus blocks.
- QL is considered a deep block. Careful needle visualization under US guidance should prevent peritoneal, bowel, or kidney puncture. The fourth lumbar artery in the TLF can develop significant hematomas if punctured in the setting of anticoagulation.
- Quadriceps weakness is evident after an anterior QL block because local anesthetic can spread to the fascia iliaca.

Ilioinguinal and Iliohypogastric Nerve Blocks

These blocks are performed quickly with a blind technique. However, US imaging may help improve the success rate of nerve localization and deposition of local anesthetic in the correct fascial plane proximal to the nerves.

Procedure Using Blind Technique (Single-Injection Fascial Click)

- Landmarks: The injection site is located at about 1 to 2 cm medial and 1 to 2 cm inferior to the anterior superior iliac spine.
- Needling and Injection: A 25-gauge, 36- to 50-mm blunted hypodermic needle can be used. The needle is inserted from the anterior abdomen (vertically) until a fascial click is detected, presumably at the junction of the internal oblique and transverse abdominis muscles. About 10 to 15 mL (0.3 to 0.5 mL/kg for children) of local anesthetic can be injected. An additional 0.5 to 1 mL local anesthetic can be injected subcutaneously to block the iliohypogastric nerve.

Procedure Using Ultrasound Guidance

- Scanning: Using a small footprint ("hockey stick") 5- to 10-MHz probe, placed in transverse axis, just medial and superior to the anterior superior iliac spine, the cross-sectional view of the ilioinguinal nerve can be captured lying between the internal oblique and transverse abdominis muscles.[103]
- Appearance: The nerves appear hypoechoic with many hyperechoic dots and a distinct hyperechoic rim (Fig. 36-37). They have an oval, somewhat "boomerang" shape and appear embedded between the fascicular hypoechoic-appearing muscles. In the more cranial position, the iliac bone, with its hyperechoic border and dorsal shadowing, may be captured on the medial aspect of the screen. The thin external oblique muscle lies superficial at the cranial position, but it may not be visible more inferiorly.
- Needling: An IP alignment, with the needle placed medial to lateral toward the probe, is preferred, although an OOP approach is also feasible.
- Local Anesthetic Spread: Depending on the number of distinct nerves localized, one or two injections can be made. The volume of local anesthetic may be lower when using US imaging if the nerves are well localized. In children, 0.075 mL/kg is effective for a single injection. An area of hypoechoic solution should be visualized adjacent to the nerve(s).

Clinical Pearls

- The ilioinguinal and iliohypogastric nerves may exist as a common trunk at the anterior superior iliac spine level, supporting US guidance for localizing the individual nerve.
- Since there is high variability in skin innervation from these nerves, it is impossible to confirm with clinical tests which nerve is blocked. Injecting lateral to the most laterally positioned ilioinguinal nerve or medial to the iliohypogastric nerve has been reported as one method to block these nerves individually.
- Complications of this block are generally volume related and include systemic toxicity and transient femoral nerve palsy. A recent assessment of the accuracy of the blind technique using US demonstrated that even in experienced hands, needles were inserted deep to the transversus abdominis muscle over 40% of the time.[104] This result reinforces the value of US in helping to prevent inaccurate needle placement or inappropriate anesthetic spread.

Penile Block

Penile block is used in children and adults for surgical procedures of the glans and shaft of the penis (7 Video 36-7). The dorsal nerves (terminal branches of the pudendal nerve; S2–S4) lie bilaterally on the outer aspect of the dorsal arteries of the penis. From the base of the penis, the nerves divide several times and encircle the shaft of the penis before reaching the glans. This

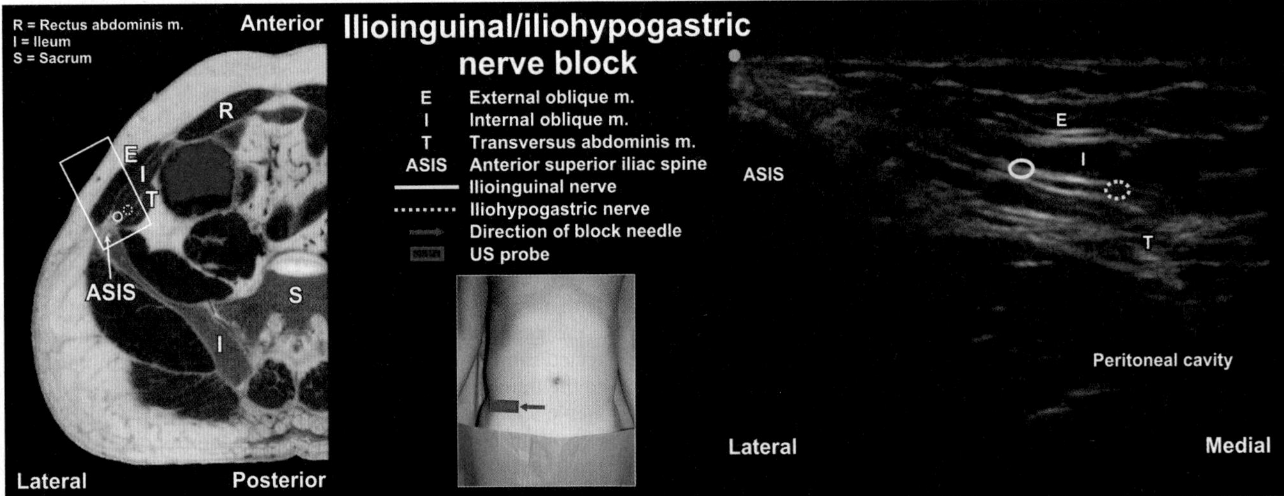

Figure 36-37 Arrangement of relevant anatomy for ultrasound-guided ilioinguinal/iliohypogastric nerve block. Transverse scanning on the abdomen just medial to the anterior superior iliac spine (ASIS) shows the nerves lying between the internal oblique and transversus abdominis muscles, just medial to the ASIS. These nerves can be blocked using an IP alignment and medial-to-lateral needle insertion to avoid puncturing the peritoneum.

block is often performed as a circumferential infiltration of the root of the penis (ring block). Two skin wheals are raised at the dorsal base of the penis, one on each side just below and medial to the pubic spine. A 25-gauge, 37.5-mm needle is introduced on each side, and 5 mL of anesthetic (0.5 to 1 mL for infants) is injected superficially and deep along the lower border of the pubic ramus to anesthetize the dorsal nerve. For a complete ring of infiltration, an additional 5 mL (adults) is infiltrated in the subcutaneous tissue around the underside of the shaft. A larger needle or a second injection site may be needed to complete the ring. 20 to 25 mL of 0.75% lidocaine or 0.25% bupivacaine usually suffices in adults. Epinephrine-containing solutions are contraindicated to avoid compromising penile circulation. US can be used to improve the efficacy of penile blocks and, in one study, was found to decrease postoperative pain and delay the administration of postoperative analgesics.[105] However, procedures using US were, on average, 10 minutes longer in duration compared to those performed blindly.

Lower Extremity

Combined blocks of the lumbar and sacral plexuses provide adequate surgical anesthesia to the entire lower extremity. An "anterior lumbar block" approach (also referred to as the "femoral three-in-one" approach) was first described by Winnie et al. in 1973[106]; this block was based on the assumption that a large volume of local anesthetic injected into the femoral nerve sheath would spread proximally to anesthetize the obturator and lateral femoral cutaneous nerves as well. However, reports of failures to obtain obturator nerve block with this approach led to the femoral block being considered an individual nerve block and indicated that the posterior lumbar block approach would be necessary to anesthetize the whole lumbar plexus reliably.

PNB is indicated when spinal or epidural techniques are contraindicated or when selective anesthesia of one leg or foot is needed. Because the anatomic landmarks identifying the fascial sheaths or compartments of the plexuses are not as clearly defined as those in the upper extremity, lower extremity blocks are often performed more distally, where the nerves have already separated into terminal branches. Thus, in addition to the fascial compartment approach (psoas block), peripheral approaches are described at the anterior and posterior hip, knee, and ankle.

Techniques

Lumbar Plexus Block (Psoas Compartment Block)

Several techniques for blocking the lumbar plexus using a posterior approach have been described. This block is often performed with a single injection at a point some distance lateral to the spinous process of L4 since the nerves of the lumbar plexus are in proximity between the transverse processes of L4 and L5. A more cephalad approach, near L3, may be used although there have been reports of renal subcapsular hematomas with blocks performed at this level. The psoas compartment block has the advantage of anesthetizing the entire lumbar plexus and provides anesthesia/analgesia of the anterolateral and medial thigh, the knee, and the cutaneous distribution of the saphenous nerve below the knee. Although the sacral nerve roots may be anesthetized, this block will likely not provide complete anesthesia/analgesia for the entire upper leg and a sciatic nerve block will usually also need to be performed. Continuous psoas compartment blocks with accompanying sciatic nerve block have been shown to be effective for anesthesia and perioperative analgesia in patients with hip fractures and after hip arthroplasty. The patient is placed in the lateral position, with the operative side up. Adequate sedation should be provided since the plexus lies deep, and the needle must penetrate several muscles.

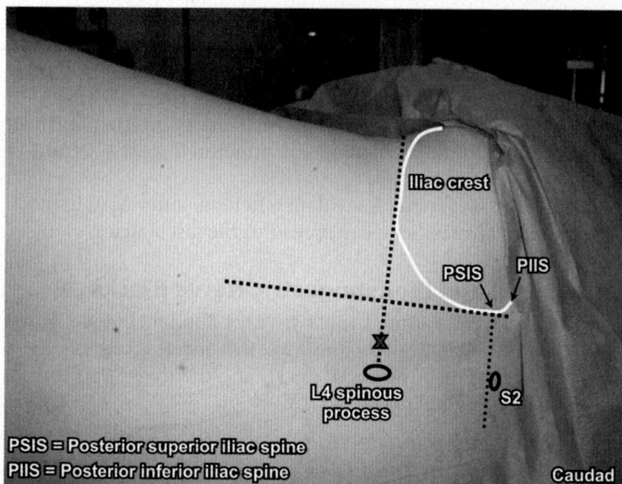

Figure 36-38 Surface landmarking for the lumbar plexus (psoas compartment) block. The needle insertion site (X) is one-third the distance along a horizontal line extending from the L4 transverse process to where it crosses a vertical line dissecting the posterior superior iliac spine.

Procedure Using Nerve Stimulation Technique

- Landmarks: The landmarks developed by Capdevila et al.[107] using computed tomography are illustrated in Figure 36-38. Compared to the depth of the lumbar plexus or transverse processes, the distance between the L4 spinous process and the lumbar plexus is not affected by body mass index. The spinous process of L4 is estimated to lie approximately 1 cm cephalad to a line between the tops of the iliac crests (the intercristal line); a horizontal line is drawn laterally from the L4 spinous processes to the far side of the body. A vertical line running parallel to the spine is then drawn at the point of the posterior superior iliac spine to intersect the horizontal line. The lumbar plexus is then located with an "X" below a point on the horizontal line and at the junction between the lateral third and medial two-thirds between the spine and posterior superior iliac spine. Based on computed tomography assessment, the mean skin-to-lumbar plexus depth at the level of L4 is 8.4 cm in adult men and 7.1 cm in adult women. The distance between the posterior edges of the transverse processes of the lumbar vertebrae and the lumbar plexus is about 1.8 cm. A strong correlation exists between weight and plexus depth in children; in one study, plexus depth ranged from 1.24 to 1.74 mm/kg in children aged 3 to 12 years.[108]
- Needling: A skin wheal is raised at the marked block site. An insulated needle (17 to 20 gauge for adults, 22 to 25 gauge for children, 110 to 150 mm long depending on body habitus) is inserted perpendicular to all planes at the "X" until contact with the L4 transverse process is made (approximately 5 to 6 cm deep). After contact, the needle is withdrawn and redirected caudad below the process to a maximum depth of 2 cm to the transverse process.
- Nerve localization: With the nerve stimulator set to deliver an output current of 1 to 1.5 mA, contraction of the quadriceps muscle (patellar twitch) is sought. The plexus is localized when a motor response is maintained at 0.3 to 0.5 mA. If a motor response is not obtained at first, moving the needle cautiously in a slight medial direction, without aiming toward the spinal cord, or in a direction 15 degrees caudad or cephalad may help.

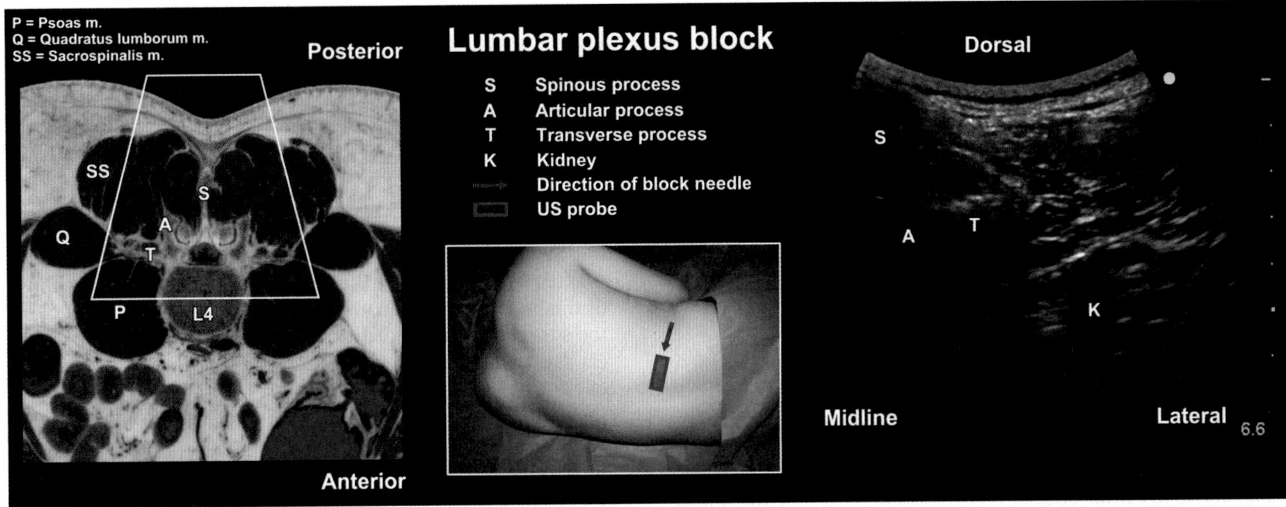

Figure 36-39 Arrangement of relevant anatomy for ultrasound-assisted lumbar plexus block. A curved array probe can be placed transversely to capture an overview of the spinous, articular, and transverse processes, with the psoas muscle just deep and lateral to the latter. Puncture of the kidney can be a potential complication of lumbar plexus block; if attempting real-time needle insertion, the safest needle alignment will be IP to a longitudinally placed probe over the L3–L5 transverse processes since the kidney may come to view at a more cephalad position.

- Injection: Once the plexus is localized, 30 to 40 mL of local anesthetic is injected, using careful aspiration and after administering a test dose to rule out intravascular, epidural, or subarachnoid placement. Fifteen to twenty minutes may be required for local anesthetic to spread to all the roots of the lumbar plexus. It will take longer to produce anesthesia of the caudad branches (the lower sacral fibers that form the tibial nerve), and they may not become anesthetized.

Procedure Using Ultrasound Guidance

The lumbar plexus is challenging to view adequately since the target structures are deep. Similar to paravertebral block, US imaging may be best for identifying the location and depth of the transverse processes before the block procedure. If there is a desire to perform the block at L3–L4, viewing the kidneys before and during the block may help prevent renal injury and hematoma. This is especially important in young children since the lower pole of the kidney can reach as low as L4–L5. Combining the NS technique with US is recommended to confirm the correct needle placement.

- Scanning: A curved array probe (5 to 8 MHz) is placed in the transverse plane in the midline at the level of the L4 spinous process to provide an overview of the L4 vertebra. The probe should be rotated with the longitudinal axis parallel to the spine, allowing a lateral scan to identify the tips of the transverse processes. The absence of associated ribs means that the tips of the transverse processes are fairly easily delineated. A 6- to 13-MHz "hockey stick" transducer may be used for young children and infants.
- Appearance: For adults and older children, the deep location of this block precludes clear visibility of the lumbar plexus. Indeed, the transverse processes (which are the primary landmarks) are often only vaguely delineated. Therefore, to survey the area, it is important to switch between transverse and longitudinal scanning between the spinous processes and the tip of the transverse processes. In the transverse scan, the spinous processes appear hypoechoic (likely due to the dorsal shadowing effect) and extend superficially. In contrast, the transverse processes are hyperechoic masses/lines at the lateral edge of the vertebra. The fascicular-appearing musculature is evident surrounding the vertebra yet poorly delineated by most compact US machines. In the longitudinal scan, the lateral tips of the transverse processes will be identified at the most lateral point where a hyperechoic nodule is viewed.
- Needling: Needling will be identical to that for the blind technique, except that the depth to the transverse process will be more accurately known. If choosing to perform a more cephalad approach above L4, real-time imaging may be helpful to view the kidneys (especially during inspiration when they fall toward L3–L4) (Fig. 36-39). An IP needle alignment to a longitudinal probe may be most suitable to avoid excessive medial or lateral needle angulation (see Paravertebral Blockade Clinical Pearls).
- Local anesthetic spread: When using US guidance, it will be challenging to view local anesthetic spread in all patients except young children. If seen, a hypoechoic mass will spread within the muscle mass lateral and deep to the transverse process.

Clinical Pearls

The psoas compartment block can be beneficial for placing a catheter to provide long-lasting analgesia; the catheter is held securely by the psoas muscles and kept away from any active joint region. After obtaining good localization with the stimulating needle (bevel facing caudad and lateral), a stimulating catheter is advanced 3 to 5 cm. In some cases, injecting a nonconducting solution such as D5W to expand the perineural space is helpful. Quadriceps muscle contraction should be maintained during catheter advancement with a stimulating catheter.

- Prepuncture US may be beneficial before needle insertion and catheter placement. Using a higher frequency (6- to 13-MHz) linear array transducer allows more accurate estimation of the depth and location of each transverse process, which may minimize the risks associated with needle/catheter insertion into the lumbar plexus.
- This block is contraindicated in patients with coagulopathy or bleeding diathesis. Complications include hematoma in the muscle sheath, retroperitoneal space, or kidney; infection; and catheter placement within the peritoneum. Neuropathy is possible, and unintended spread to the epidural or subarachnoid space has also been reported.

Separate Blocks of the Terminal Nerves of the Lumbar Plexus

Four terminal nerves of the lumbar plexus can be anesthetized in the lower extremity: the lateral femoral cutaneous, femoral, obturator, and saphenous. The block sites for the femoral, lateral femoral cutaneous, and obturator nerves are illustrated in Figure 36-14. The lateral femoral cutaneous nerve is occasionally blocked to provide sensory anesthesia for obtaining a skin graft from the lateral thigh. It can also be blocked as a diagnostic/therapeutic tool to identify cases of meralgia paresthetica (a neurologic disorder of the lateral femoral cutaneous nerve). The obturator nerve provides variable sensory supply to the medial aspect of the thigh and knee joint and gives off branches to the hip joint. Obturator nerve block can effectively prevent obturator reflex during transurethral bladder tumor resections, treat pain in the hip area, relieve adductor spasm (as seen in multiple sclerosis patients), or serve as a diagnostic tool when studying hip mobility. Saphenous nerve block often complements sciatic nerve block when anesthesia of the medial aspect of the ankle and foot is required. Procedures on the knee require anesthesia of the femoral and the obturator nerves, although postoperative analgesia of the knee can usually be provided by femoral nerve block alone. A continuous femoral nerve block can reduce side effects compared to continuous epidurals and facilitate rehabilitation. A US-guided infrapatellar nerve block has been described for use for postoperative analgesia after outpatient arthroscopic surgery.[109]

Femoral Nerve/Fascia Iliaca Block

Procedure Using Nerve Stimulation

- Landmarks: The patient is placed in the supine position, with slight external rotation of the femur. A pillow can be placed under the patient's hip to facilitate palpation of the femoral pulse and accentuate other pertinent landmarks for ease of palpation. The femoral artery descends at the "midinguinal point," at the junction between the medial third and lateral two-thirds of the inguinal ligament. However, it is most superficial at the femoral crease. It lies approximately 1 to 1.5 cm medial to the nerve. The inguinal crease is the skin fold located about 2.5 cm caudad and parallels the inguinal ligament (Clinical Anatomy of lower extremity).
- Needling: A skin wheal is raised lateral to the area where the femoral artery pulsation is felt, and a 50-mm, 22-gauge insulated needle is inserted perpendicular to the skin or using a cephalad angle of approximately 30 degrees. Aspiration is performed frequently since the femoral artery is situated close to the nerve.
- Nerve localization: Using NS, a quadriceps muscle response (patellar twitch preferably) is sought, with an endpoint of 0.5 mA used for accurate localization. Branches to the sartorius muscle arise inferior to the inguinal ligament and leave the femoral nerve proximal to the main block location site; a response of this muscle to stimulation often indicates that the needle is too superficial and medial to the main femoral nerve. For a fascia iliaca block, the loss-of-resistance technique is used instead of NS. The needle is placed vertically 5 cm lateral to the artery at the inguinal crease. Two pops are felt when the needle traverses the fascia lata and fascia iliaca and enters the iliopsoas muscle.
- Injection: Injection of 20 mL (or less) of local anesthetic should suffice for sole femoral nerve anesthesia. 20 to 30 mL of local anesthetic may be required for the fascia iliaca block. Intermittent injection with interval aspiration should be performed.

Procedure Using Ultrasound Guidance (Fig. 36-40)

- Scanning: A 10-MHz or higher transducer can be used for both blocks if the neurovascular structures are not located too deep (i.e., in thin individuals), as this will show a good distinction between the nerve and the surrounding vessels and muscles. A midrange 5- to 8-MHz linear transducer is recommended if the nerve and artery are deep (>4 cm). Position the probe transverse to the nerve axis at the level of the inguinal crease. The nerve should appear approximately 1 cm deep and 1.5 cm lateral to the femoral artery, depending on body habitus (color Doppler may be used to identify the femoral artery and vein). A 5- to 10-MHz "hockey stick" transducer can be used for most children.
- Appearance: The nerve lies about 1 cm lateral and deep to the large, circular, anechoic, and pulsatile femoral artery. The nerve often appears triangular in shape and of variable size due to its irregular course; early branching above the inguinal ligament can increase the transverse diameter of the nerve. The fascia lata (most superficial) and fascia iliaca (immediately adjacent

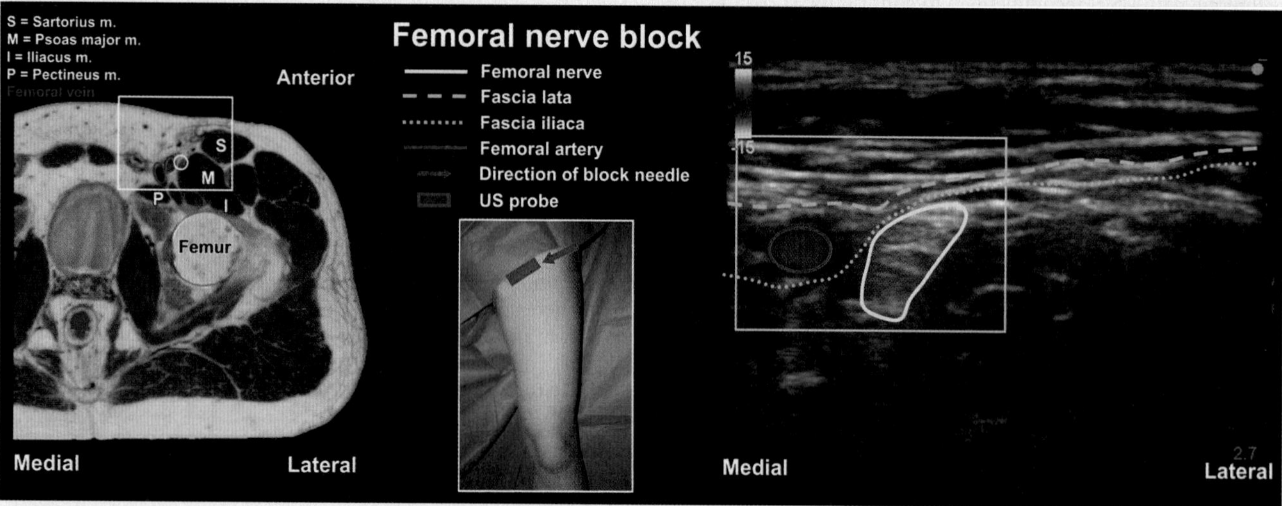

Figure 36-40 Arrangement of relevant anatomy for ultrasound-guided femoral nerve block. The probe is placed in a slightly oblique plane (at the level of and parallel to the inguinal crease) to capture the nerve in the short axis lateral to the femoral artery. The needle (not shown) can be visualized as it transects the fascia lata and iliaca. If IP needling is used, it should occur in a lateral-to-medial direction.

to the nerve and separating the nerve from the artery) may be seen as superficial to the femoral nerve and often appear bright and longitudinally angled.

- Needling: Place the nerve at the medial edge of the screen, with the probe capturing a transverse view of the neurovascular structures (8 Video 36-8). A 50-mm, 22-gauge needle (for single injection) can be inserted using IP needle alignment (Fig. 36-40). To maximize viewing, the needle should be inserted using an acute (30- to 45-degree) angle. IP blocks may be made more accessible by angling the needle tip slightly away from the nerve. In contrast, accuracy of catheter placement may be improved by tilting the needle hub in a caudad direction once the needle tip is positioned appropriately. Inserting the catheter perpendicular or parallel to the nerve does not affect the quality of analgesia, although the former technique may facilitate faster catheter insertion. Needle insertion for fascia iliaca block occurs 1 to 2 cm laterally to femoral nerve block and in a caudal–cephalad direction.
- Local anesthetic spread: Performing a test dose with D5W is recommended before local anesthetic application to visualize the spread and confirm nerve localization. The local anesthetic spread should occur within the fascial space surrounding the nerve. The solution may displace the nerve medially toward or laterally away from the artery.

Clinical Pearls

- When inserting a catheter, it is debatable whether a stimulating catheter improves placement, but using a solution to expand the perineural space is beneficial in some cases. If a stimulating catheter is used, injection of D5W for tissue expansion will maintain motor responses to NS.[4,5]
- With an IP needle alignment, lateral-to-medial needle insertion will ensure that the nerve is reached before encountering the femoral vessels.
- It is important to ensure that the US beam is perpendicular to the nerve's transverse axis to minimize the chance of anisotropic effects changing the echogenic properties of the structure. It has been shown that an approximate 10-degree cephalad or caudad tilt of the transducer can make the nerve isoechoic (similar appearing) to the underlying iliopsoas muscle.

Lateral Femoral Cutaneous Nerve

Using the NS technique, the lateral femoral cutaneous nerve can be localized at the inguinal crease, approximately 0 to 1 cm medial to the anterior superior iliac spine (Fig. 36-14). However, this mark may be highly variable and should be confirmed with NS. An insulated needle (22 gauge, 50 mm; 35 mm for children) is inserted using a perpendicular approach if the puncture is close to the anterior superior iliac spine or in a lateral direction at a distance. A "pop" may be felt as the needle penetrates the fascia lata. The primary endpoint for NS with this nerve is paresthesia over the lateral thigh (Fig. 36-14), with a current of approximately 0.5 to 0.6 mA. The sensory distribution may not extend proximal to the greater trochanter. 5 to 10 mL of local anesthetic is usually sufficient to obtain a block. A recent study demonstrated that nerve targeting might not be necessary in some cases; in patients undergoing knee surgery, injection of local anesthetic immediately under the inguinal ligament provided sufficient blockade without injecting directly around the nerve.[110]

Obturator Nerve

The obturator nerve branches early after its descent from the obturator foramen, and blocking the nerve within the foramen near the superior pubic ramus (i.e., before it branches) is often described using a blind technique. The patient is placed supine with their hip slightly externally rotated; the hip may be slightly flexed and abducted. The public tubercle is located, and a mark is placed 1.5 cm both inferior and lateral to it (this mark should resemble that in Fig. 36-14). An inguinal approach is another option and may result in higher block success rates and fewer needle attempts.

Procedure Using Nerve Stimulation Technique

- Nerve localization: An insulated needle (18 to 22 gauge, 90 to 100 mm for adults; 22 to 25 gauge, 35 to 50 mm for children) is inserted perpendicularly until contact with the inferior pubic ramus is obtained. The needle is then redirected laterally and caudally to enter the obturator foramen and is advanced 2 to 3 cm. Nerve localization can be greatly improved using NS with adductor muscle contraction at 0.5 mA as an endpoint.

Procedure Using Ultrasound Guidance (Fig. 36-41)

- Scanning: US-guided obturator block at the proximal thigh is based predominantly on the identification of three muscle layers: the adductor longus, adductor brevis, and adductor magnus muscles (from superficial to deep). The anterior branch of the obturator nerve usually lies on the lateral edge between the adductor longus and brevis muscles, whereas the posterior branch of the obturator nerve lies between the adductor brevis and magnus muscles; however, the obturator nerve shows a considerable degree of variability at this level. The anterior and posterior branches may be most easily visualized with the probe placed 2 cm laterally and distally to the pubic tubercle.[111] The depths of the anterior and posterior branches were 15.5 and 29.3 mm respectively, though tissue compression by the probe may influence this depth. The branches may be localized on either side of the adductor brevis muscle if the fascial planes of the muscles are highly visible (hyperechoic). The main (common) obturator nerve may be hard to view with US imaging. An IP needling technique and color Doppler can be used to help avoid adjacent blood vessels.
- Appearance: Using a high-frequency probe, US visualization of the three layers of muscle—adductor longus, adductor brevis, and adductor magnus—should be obtained. The anterior branches of the nerve usually appear as hypoechoic circles in between a hyperechoic layer formed by the adductor longus and brevis, whereas the posterior branches are located between the layers of the adductor brevis and magnus muscles at this level. The nerve can also be blocked more distally at the knee.
- Needling: To anesthetize the anterior branch of the obturator nerve, a 22-gauge needle is inserted in an IP fashion deep to the adductor longus muscle to deposit local anesthetic immediately beneath the muscle. Similarly, the needle can be inserted deeper to the adductor brevis to reach the posterior branch. 5 to 10 mL of local anesthetic should suffice.
- Local anesthetic spread: A homogeneous, hypoechoic spread pattern between the muscle layers should appear during the injection. It is important to avoid intramuscular injection.

Clinical Pearls

- Using cadavers and live subjects, Akkaya et al.[112] demonstrated that a hyperechoic triangle bordered by the superior pubic ramus, posterior edge of the pectineus muscle, and anterior aspect of the external obturator muscle is an ideal landmark to locate the obturator nerve, which lies just medial to the obturator vein.
- A report using US guidance suggested that a single injection of local anesthetic into the interfascial space between the adductor longus and adductor brevis muscles containing the anterior branch of the obturator nerve results in upward (cranial) spreading of anesthetic to block the posterior branch also.

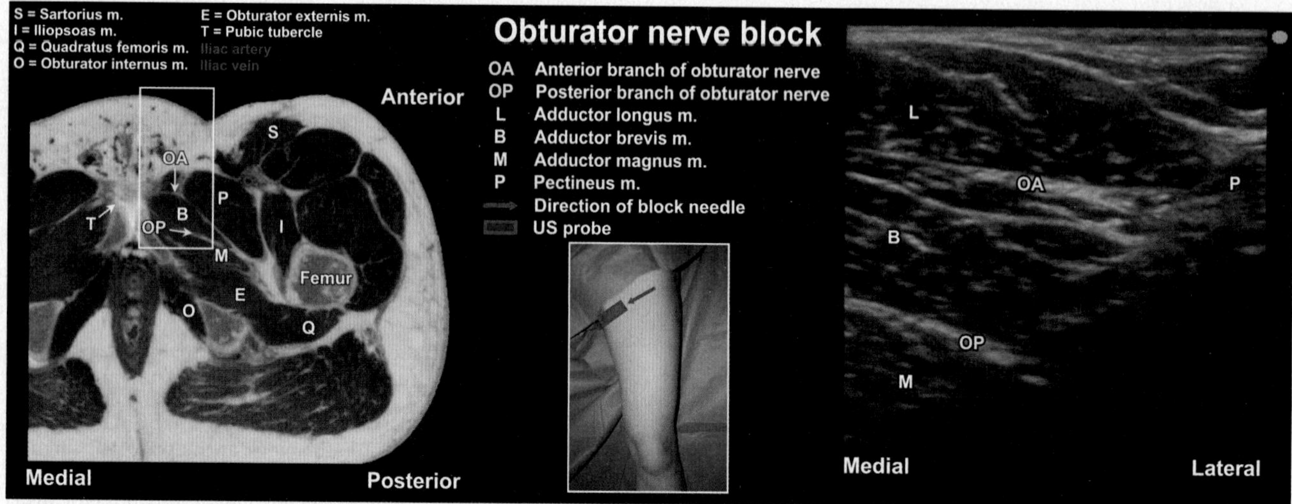

Figure 36-41 Arrangement of relevant anatomy for ultrasound-guided obturator nerve block (anterior and posterior branches) in the proximal thigh using an IP approach. It is important to identify the three adductor muscles—the adductor longus, adductor brevis, and adductor magnus (from superficial to deep). The pectineus muscle should also be in view on the lateral side since the anterior branch of the obturator nerve is sandwiched between the adductor longus and adductor brevis deep to the pectineus muscle.

Further spreading was encouraged by applying pressure distal to the needle insertion site.

- Aspiration is essential when injecting near the unbranched obturator nerve since the obturator artery lies adjacent to the nerve, and hemorrhage involving this artery can be life-threatening.

Saphenous Nerve

Many approaches to saphenous nerve blockade have been described, with needle placement at locations including the midthigh, surrounding the knee, or the ankle (as discussed in Ankle Block, below). US guidance has been commonly used with a transsartorius perifemoral approach.[113] Using the more proximally located and larger femoral artery (rather than the more distal saphenous branch of the descending genicular artery) as a landmark seems to help identify the sartorius muscle and nerve.

Procedure Using Nerve Stimulation Technique (Transsartorial)

- Landmarks: The sartorius muscle is palpated at the medial aspect of the knee joint by asking the patient to raise their extended leg 5 to 10 cm off the table. The block location is marked by the end of a 4-cm vertical line drawn from this point in a proximal direction.
- Needling: An insulated 22-gauge needle is inserted caudally at 45 degrees with a slight posterior angulation and advanced from the medial aspect of the knee in a slightly posterior and caudad direction to penetrate the sartorius muscle at a depth of approximately 2 to 3 cm.
- Nerve localization: Since the saphenous nerve is purely sensory, paresthesia at the medial malleolus should be felt with the nerve stimulator at 0.6 mA or less at a depth of 3 to 5 cm. Elicitation of paresthesia is not usually performed in children, as it can be uncomfortable or painful.
- Injection: Following careful aspiration, 10 mL of local anesthetic (e.g., 1.5% to 2% lidocaine) is injected.

Procedure Using Ultrasound Guidance (Fig. 36-42)

- Scanning: The sartorius muscle can be identified easily as being a superficial roof to the relatively prominent landmark of the femoral artery before the artery travels deep and becomes the popliteal artery via the adductor hiatus.[113] The nerve is located between the sartorius muscle and the artery in the thigh.
- Scanning: A high-frequency linear US transducer is placed transversely to the longitudinal axis of the extremity at the midthigh, approximately 10 to 12 cm proximal and 3 to 4 cm medial to the midpoint of the patella (9 Video 36-9). The femoral artery can be identified here with certainty by Doppler, which confirms the identity of the overlying sartorius muscle. The probe is scanned distally until it captures the point just before the femoral artery becomes the popliteal artery.
- Appearance: Using color Doppler is essential to visualize the femoral artery as a large hypoechoic structure at approximately 2 to 3 cm depth in average-sized individuals. The sartorius muscle can then be identified as a highly delineated, lip-shaped muscle with hyperechoic borders immediately superficial to the artery. The nerve can be blocked as it lies sandwiched between the artery and the muscle at this level, or it can be blocked more distally at the knee.
- Needling: A 22-gauge needle is inserted in an IP fashion to penetrate the sartorius muscle to deposit local anesthetic immediately beneath the muscle and medial to the artery. 5 to 10 mL of local anesthetic should suffice.
- Local anesthetic spread: A small hypoechoic mass on the medial surface of the femoral artery should appear during the injection.

Sciatic Nerve Block Using Gluteal, Subgluteal, Posterior Popliteal, and Anterior Approaches

A sciatic nerve block can be used with a lumbar plexus block for anesthesia of the lower extremity. Together with a saphenous nerve block, a sciatic block produces adequate anesthesia of the sole and the lower leg. The large sciatic nerve is deep within the gluteal region and may be difficult to locate blindly or with US. The numerous bony and vascular landmarks used to ease identification are beneficial during US-guided blockade of the sciatic nerve and its terminal branches (tibial and common peroneal nerves). Knowledge of anatomy is paramount with these blocks, and the block location and approach will ultimately depend on the surgical requirement.

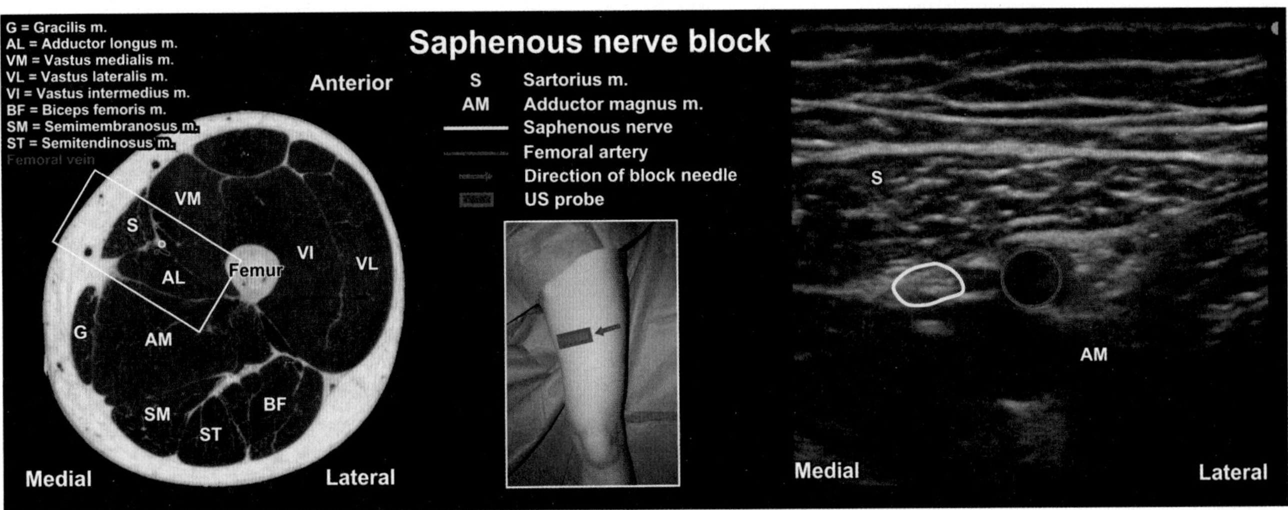

Figure 36-42 Arrangement of relevant anatomy for ultrasound-guided saphenous nerve block using a transsartorius perifemoral approach. The probe is placed in the transverse view where the femoral artery has yet to become the popliteal artery, approximately 10 to 12 cm proximal to and 3 to 4 cm medial to the midpoint of the patella. Using the large femoral artery as a landmark may benefit more distal approaches where the nerve lies adjacent to the smaller saphenous branch of the descending genicular artery (see text).

Posterior Sciatic Nerve Block: Classical Gluteal (Labat) Approach

Position the patient semiprone (Sims position) with the hip and knee flexed and the operative side uppermost.

Procedure Using Nerve Stimulation

- Landmarks (Fig. 36-43): An oblique line is drawn joining the posterior superior iliac spine to the midpoint of the greater trochanter (on its medial aspect). Next, a horizontal line is drawn joining the greater trochanter (at the above location) to the sacral hiatus. A perpendicular line drawn at the midpoint of the oblique line and reaching the parahorizontal line is the traditional puncture site. This intersection should be approximately 5 cm caudad along the perpendicular line.
- Needling: Raise a local anesthetic skin wheal after aseptic preparation. An insulated 100-mm (shorter for pediatric patients), 22-gauge needle is inserted perpendicular to the skin. For children, the depth to the nerve can be approximated as ~1 mm/kg weight, with less and more depth for younger and older individuals, respectively.
- Nerve localization: Nerve responses of the lower leg and foot are sought. If they are not obtained at the full depth of the needle, the needle is withdrawn to the skin and reintroduced at a location perpendicular to the course of the nerve. Bone contact typically requires lateral needle adjustment.
- Injection: Injection of 20 to 30 mL of local anesthetic (e.g., 0.75% ropivacaine, 1% mepivacaine, 0.5% bupivacaine) is performed. If several blocks are required (i.e., lumbar plexus and saphenous nerve), a reduced concentration of local anesthetic may be necessary to prevent exceeding the toxic dose.

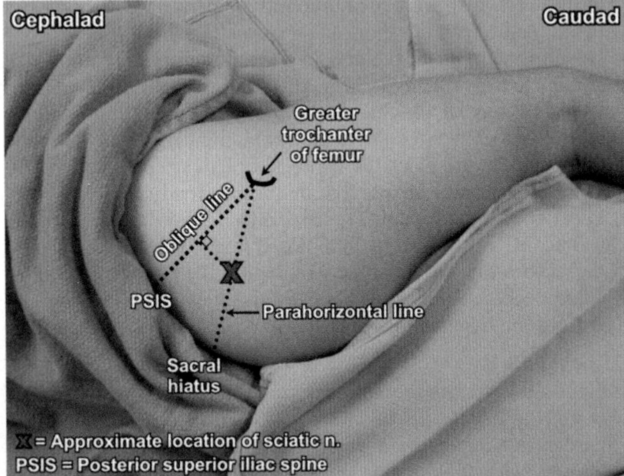

Figure 36-43 Landmarks for sciatic nerve block using a posterior gluteal (Labat) approach. This location will also serve as a reference point when applying ultrasound imaging.

Procedure Using Ultrasound Guidance (Fig. 36-44)

- Scanning: A curved, lower frequency 2- to 5-MHz probe (higher frequency for young children) is generally used for scanning the gluteal region. Moving the probe cephalad and caudad in the gluteal region will help examine the ischial bone (a hyperechoic line with bony shadowing underneath). The widest portion of this bone, with the ischial spine medial, should be located. The bulky gluteus maximus muscle will be seen superficial and posterior to the sciatic nerve. The internal pudendal vessels (artery and vein), which may be identified using color Doppler, are adjacent to the ischial spine, medial to the sciatic nerve and inferior gluteal artery. Alternatively, the nerve can be first located at the subgluteal region, at about the midpoint between the greater trochanter and the ischial tuberosity, and traced proximally. Bony landmarks (e.g., medial aspect of the greater trochanter, femoral condyles) are less visible in children, especially those under 7 years old.
- Appearance: The sciatic nerve in the gluteal region is found lateral to the ischial spine and superficial to the ischial bone. The nerve appears predominantly hyperechoic (bright) and is often broad and flat in the short axis of the US. Overlying the sciatic nerve is the large gluteus maximus, which is quite distinct from the usual "starry night" appearance. The inner muscle layers (superior and inferior gemellus muscles, obturator internus muscle, and quadratus femoris muscle) are often indistinct.

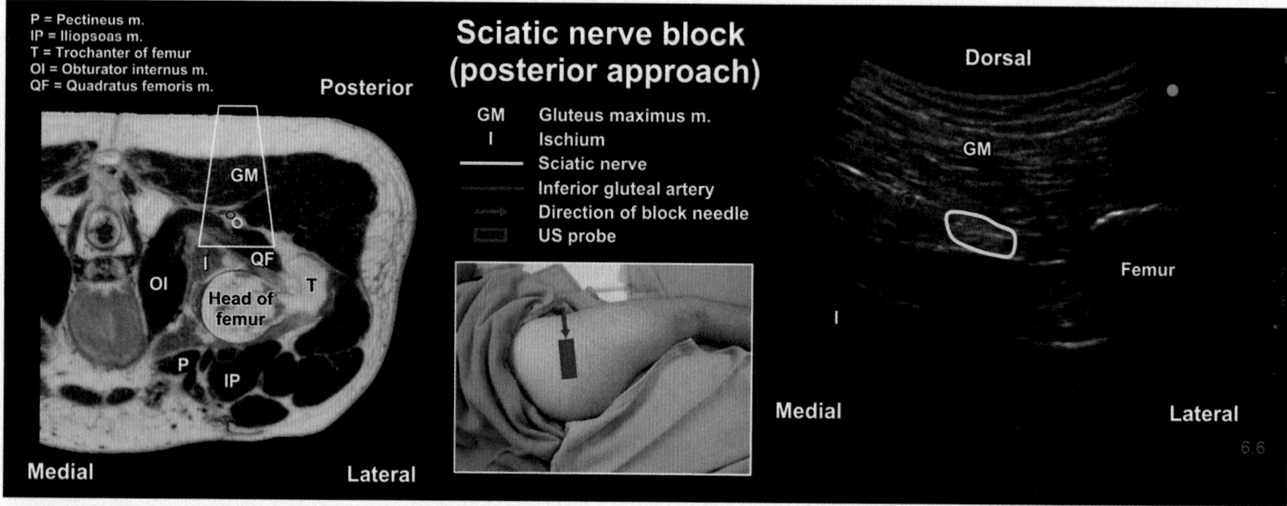

Figure 36-44 Arrangement of relevant anatomy for ultrasound-guided sciatic nerve block using a posterior gluteal (Labat) approach. An IP needle alignment to a curved low-frequency probe is used. A lateral-to-medial needle direction may help avoid puncture of the inferior gluteal or internal pudendal vessels.

- Needling: IP and OOP approaches are appropriate for US-guided sciatic nerve blocks in the gluteal region. The needle is inserted inferior to the probe in a cephaloanterior direction for an OOP approach. A fairly steep insertion angle will be required, but placing the needle slightly low to the probe will somewhat reduce the angle for better visibility of the needle. With the IP approach, the needle may be moved in a lateral-to-medial direction to penetrate the gluteus maximus muscle before reaching the sciatic nerve above the ischial bone (Fig. 36-44).
- Local anesthetic spread: Performing a test dose with D5W is recommended before local anesthetic application to visualize the spread and confirm nerve localization. Depositing the local anesthetic solution to spread entirely around the sciatic nerve is generally recommended.

Clinical Pearls

- For both IP and OOP needling approaches, scanning before needling will determine the angle, distance, and depth of needle penetration.
- The IP approach is often used for catheter insertion, and it is important to line up the site of needle insertion with the target nerve.

Posterior Sciatic Nerve Block: Subgluteal Approach

The patient is positioned semiprone (Sims position) with the hip and knee flexed and the foot resting on the dependent knee. In some patients, the supine position with the hip flexed, and knee bent is most comfortable or necessitated due to fracture or pain at the hip. The latter position requires an assistant to support the bent leg.

Procedure Using Nerve Stimulation Technique

- Landmarks: A horizontal line joins the medial aspect of the greater trochanter to the ischial tuberosity. The traditional puncture site is located on this line just medial to its midpoint.
- Needling: An insulated needle, 100 to 150 mm, depending on patient habitus, is used. The needle is inserted perpendicular to the skin. Shorter needles are recommended for use in children.
- Nerve localization: Similar responses for the classic gluteal approach are sought, with ankle responses preferable. It is essential to distinguish the nerve's tibial (inversion or plantar flexion) and common peroneal (eversion or dorsiflexion) components and obtain both responses or, at minimum, the tibial reaction.
- Injection: Injection of 20 to 30 mL of local anesthetic is sufficient. If additional blocks of the lower extremity are performed, a solution with a lower concentration should be considered to prevent exceeding the toxic dose of local anesthetic.

Procedure Using Ultrasound Guidance (Fig. 36-45)

- Scanning: A curved, lower frequency 2- to 5-MHz probe or a linear 4- to 7-MHz probe are suitable for scanning the subgluteal region; high-frequency probes are recommended for scanning young children. The center of the probe should be aligned with the midpoint of a line between the ischial tuberosity and the greater trochanter. If the sciatic nerve is hard to localize in the subgluteal region, it can be traced proximally from the bifurcation point at or near the apex of the popliteal fossa.
- Appearance: On the screen's lateral side, the greater trochanter's medial aspect appears almost pear shaped and hypoechoic when using a curved array probe. The sciatic nerve in the subgluteal region appears predominantly hyperechoic (bright) and is often elliptical in a short-axis view using US.
- Needling: Similar to the classic gluteal approach, IP and OOP plane needling can be performed, with the needle directed from lateral to medial for the IP technique. An insertion angle of approximately 45 degrees to the skin will provide the best view of the needle and reach the nerve, although steeper angles of 60 to 70 degrees may be required in obese individuals.
- Local anesthetic spread: The goal is to deposit local anesthetic (20 to 30 mL) next to, but not directly within, the sciatic nerve structure in the subgluteal region. During the injection, a hypoechoic local anesthetic fluid collection is often seen around the hyperechoic nerve within the sheath compartment.

Clinical Pearls

- Since a low-frequency curved array probe is necessary in many cases, the needle tip, as viewed with an IP approach, will be harder to identify than when using higher resolution linear probes. Nevertheless, this approach is used often since indwelling catheters are commonly placed in the subgluteal area. Using NS in addition to US guidance can confirm correct needle placement.

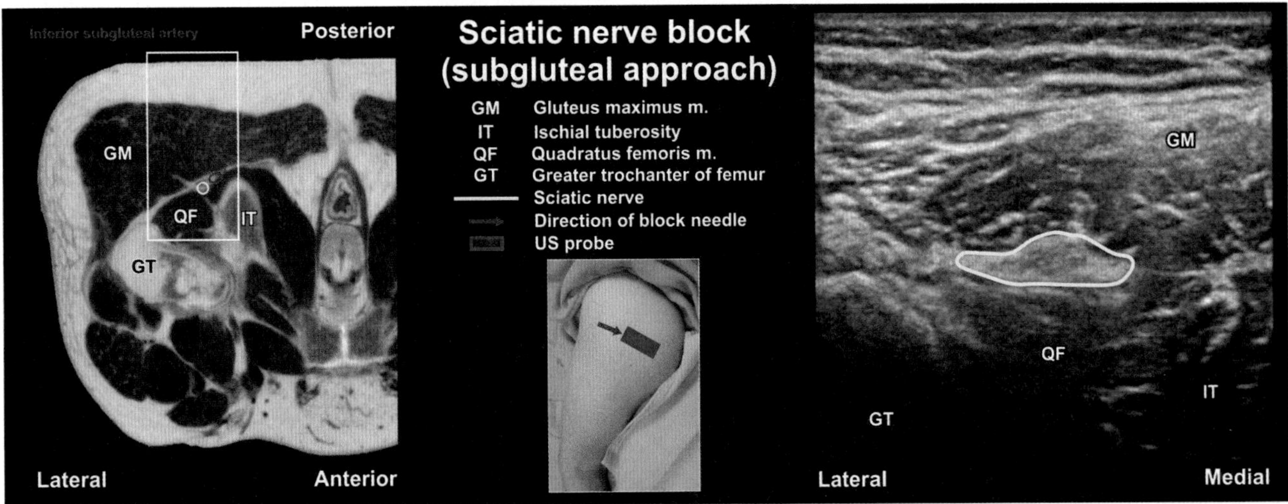

Figure 36-45 Arrangement of relevant anatomy for ultrasound-guided sciatic nerve block with a subgluteal approach. IP approaches are preferred since this approach is used often for indwelling catheter placement, especially in children. The medially positioned ischial tuberosity is not captured in this image but will serve as an excellent bony landmark in most circumstances.

Posterior Popliteal Sciatic Block

The sciatic nerve can be blocked below the hip at the lateral midfemoral or lateral popliteal locations in addition to the posterior popliteal location (10 Video 36-10).[114] When using US guidance, the posterior approach is preferred as it allows the needle to be placed close to the probe and thus may improve needle tracking and visibility. Furthermore, the posterior popliteal approach is most amenable to inserting indwelling catheters. The patient is positioned laterally or prone with the operative leg slightly flexed. Ideally, the ankles should be positioned beyond the end of the table so that motor responses to NS can be readily observed in the prone position. The landmarks become more visible when the knee is flexed against resistance.

Procedure Using Nerve Stimulation Technique

- Landmarks: The puncture site is often located at the tip of a triangle formed by the popliteal crease at the base, the biceps femoris tendon laterally, and the semimembranosus tendon medially (which generally lies medial to the tendon of the semitendinosus at this location). Alternatively, drawing lines 8 cm long in a cephalad direction from the insertion site of the medial and lateral tendons (above), the puncture point is at the midpoint of a line attaching the two (almost parallel) lines. It may be best to insert the needle at approximately 10 cm above the popliteal fossa to ensure that the sciatic nerve is blocked before bifurcation. For children, the distance between the popliteal fold and the needle insertion point can be calculated based on patient weight: less than 10 kg = 1 cm, 10 to 20 kg = 2 cm, 20 to 30 kg = 3 cm, and so forth.
- Needling: Depending on the patient, an insulated 50-mm, 22-gauge needle can be inserted at an angle of 45 degrees cephalad to the skin. A fan-wise search is conducted perpendicular to this line until the nerve is contacted. If the needle contacts the femur, the depth is noted; the nerve should lie midway between the skin and the femur.
- Nerve localization: NS elicits motor responses at the ankle or foot. The aim should be to localize the sciatic nerve before bifurcation into its tibial and common peroneal nerve components. If only ankle inversion and plantar flexion (tibial nerve) or eversion and dorsiflexion (common peroneal) are seen, adjust the needle insertion site a few centimeters cephalad to obtain complete ankle and foot movements. Otherwise, injecting after obtaining a sole tibial nerve response has been shown to provide similar success to that after both tibial and common peroneal responses (with two injections). Maintaining a motor response with currents less than 0.5 mA will help ensure the nerve–needle distance is appropriate for a successful block.
- Injection: 20 to 30 mL of local anesthetic should be deposited at the final needle location.

Procedure Using Ultrasound Guidance (Fig. 36-46)

- Scanning: A linear, higher frequency 10- to 15-MHz probe is commonly used for scanning the sciatic nerve transversely in the popliteal fossa. A "hockey stick" probe is suitable for most children. A distal-to-proximal scan can effectively locate the sciatic nerve in the posterior popliteal fossa before bifurcation (Fig. 36-46). At the popliteal crease, the transverse probe captures the tibial and common peroneal nerves, with the former being adjacent and lateral to the popliteal vessels (Doppler is valuable here). During a proximal scan, the tibial and common peroneal nerves approach each other and join to form the sciatic nerve.
- Appearance: At the level of the popliteal crease, the tibial and common peroneal nerves lie superficial and lateral to the popliteal vessels (the common peroneal nerve is the most lateral). Both nerves appear round to oval and hyperechoic compared to the surrounding musculature. The hyperechoic border of the femur (condyles) may be apparent. During the proximal scan, the tibial nerve moves away from the vessels and approaches the common peroneal nerve. More cephalad in the posterior thigh, the biceps femoris muscle lies superficial to the joining nerves and appears as a larger, oval-shaped structure with fewer internal punctate areas (hypoechoic spots) than the nerves. The sciatic nerve appears as a large, oval hyperechoic structure. The high fat and muscle content of the area may impair the visualization of the nerve itself. Furthermore, the probe often needs to be tilted for optimal imaging since the nerve becomes more superficial as it descends distally.
- Needling: An IP approach is performed commonly, especially if placing indwelling catheters. The probe is positioned directly above the sciatic nerve at or slightly cephalad to its bifurcation point so that the nerve is in the center of the image. The needle

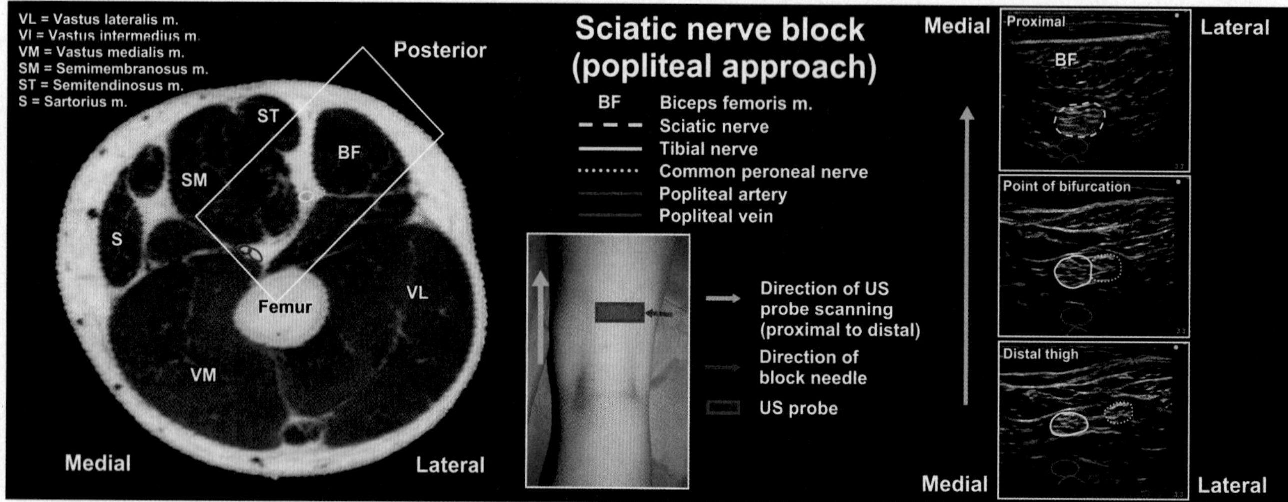

Figure 36-46 Arrangement of relevant anatomy for ultrasound-guided sciatic nerve block with a popliteal approach. The probe is placed initially at the popliteal crease. It is used to scan proximally to capture the sciatic nerve proximal to its bifurcation (i.e., the ideal block site), approximately 6 to 10 cm above the crease.

should be inserted at the caudal surface of the probe (especially if a catheter is to be inserted), with the needle tip contacting the skin approximately 3 to 4 cm caudal to the probe surface.

- Local anesthetic spread: For local anesthetic injection at the bifurcation, hypoechoic injectate will be seen to expand within the common epineural sheath. A circumferential spread producing a "donut" shape surrounding the hyperechoic nerve structure is preferable for injections above or below the bifurcation. Multiple injections (medial and lateral) may be required for complete circumferential spread.

Clinical Pearls

- The ideal needle insertion point for sciatic nerve block using the popliteal approach remains debatable. The tibial and common peroneal branches may be blocked separately or injection may occur between these nerves at the bifurcation.
- Several groups have provided evidence that injection distal (caudad), rather than proximal, to the bifurcation point results in faster block onset and improved sensory block. Recently, randomized comparison between a single subepineural injection at the neural bifurcation and separate injections around the tibial and peroneal divisions demonstrated a higher success rate and shorter performance, onset, and total anesthesia-related times with the former approach.[115]
- Compared to NS guidance alone, US guidance, either alone or in conjunction with NS, was shown to improve the success of both single-injection and catheter-delivered local anesthetic and patient outcomes concerning postoperative pain.
- The US probe may be rotated 90 degrees to show the sciatic nerve in the long axis. This helps differentiate the sciatic nerve from other nonneural structures.
- During needle insertion using an OOP approach, it may be helpful to use incremental needle angulations. The needle may be best tracked within the tissue if an initial shallow angle is used to identify the needle tip clearly as a hyperechoic dot, which can then be followed with subsequent steeper needle angulations (see the description of the "walk-down" technique under Practical Approaches for US guidance).

Anterior Sciatic Nerve Block

This block is most suitable for patients who cannot be positioned laterally. The block is indicated for surgery below the knee, with the only sensory deficiency being the medial strip of skin supplied by the saphenous nerve. The anterior block is performed on a short portion of the sciatic nerve close to the lesser trochanter of the femur. This block may cause more discomfort as the needle traverses through more muscle layers than other approaches to the sciatic nerve. The patient is positioned supine, with the leg blocked externally rotated slightly.

Procedure Using Nerve Stimulation Technique

- Landmarks: A line connecting the anterior superior iliac spine with the pubic tubercle (inguinal ligament) is drawn. A second line, parallel to the first, is drawn across the thigh from the greater trochanter. A line is drawn downward from a point at the medial third of the upper line; the nerve is usually located at the intersection of the perpendicular line and the lower of the two parallel lines. Alternatively, the nerve is located lateral to the femoral artery pulse at the level of the inguinal crease.
- Needling: This deep block will require a 22-gauge, 100- to 150-mm insulated needle.
- The needle is inserted perpendicular to the skin and advanced until contact with the femur occurs. The needle is then withdrawn slightly, angulated slightly medial and cephalad, and introduced 5 cm further.
- Nerve localization: Motor responses of the ankle joint or foot are sought.
- Injection: 20 to 30 mL of local anesthetic are injected after careful aspiration and a test dose.

Procedure Using Ultrasound Guidance (Fig. 36-47)

- Scanning: It is most common to use curved, lower frequency 2- to 5-MHz probes to scan the sciatic nerve in the proximal thigh. Place the probe over the proximal thigh approximately 8 cm distal to the femoral crease. A transversely placed probe is commonly used, although the nerve may be best visualized by placing the probe axis longitudinally along the course of the nerve. A longitudinal axis view of the nerve may improve its identification since it has a distinctive cable-like appearance. Moving in a medial-to-lateral direction may help capture an image of the nerve.
- Appearance: In the transverse axis, the sciatic nerve often appears oval or round, predominantly hyperechoic, medial, and posterior to the lesser trochanter, and deep to the adductor magnus muscle. If using Doppler, the femoral neurovascular

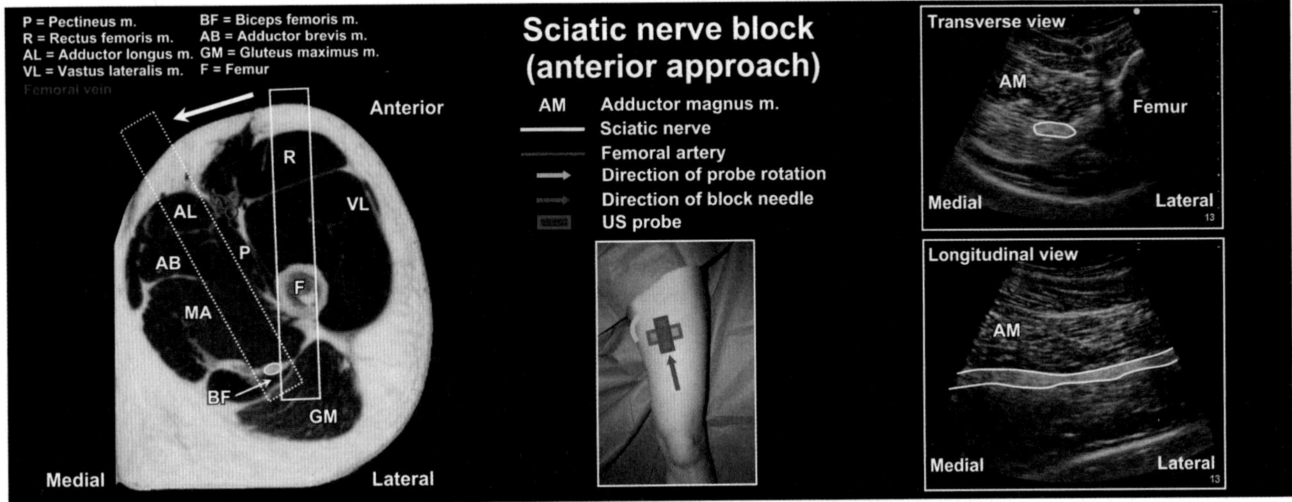

Figure 36-47 Arrangement of relevant anatomy for the ultrasound-guided sciatic block using an anterior approach. Transverse probe positioning allows a short-axis view of the nerve (upper US image). A longitudinally placed probe captures the long axis of the nerve (lower US image), which may be beneficial if the transverse view is difficult to capture due to bony shadowing from the lesser trochanter.

structures are seen superficial below the hyperechoic fascial tissue and lateral to the sciatic nerve when the leg is externally rotated. A longitudinal view captures a broad, linear, and hyperechoic cable of fibers and may allow easier nerve identification.[116]

- Needling: When using a probe positioned in the transverse axis to the nerve, an IP approach involves advancing the needle in a medial-to-lateral and anterior-to-posterior direction. An OOP approach involves inserting the needle along the midline of the probe at a location 2 to 3 cm inferior and perpendicular to the probe. If the probe is placed longitudinally, the needle direction for OOP alignment will be similar to that for the IP approach described earlier. Using an IP approach with the probe placed longitudinally, the needle will be placed in a cephalad-to-caudad direction, allowing it to be aimed easily toward a larger target (i.e., the cable-like sciatic nerve). Combining US and NS guidance is highly recommended for this procedure.
- Local anesthetic spread: After careful aspiration and injection of a small amount of D5W to visualize the anesthetic spread, inject the local anesthetic while ensuring it spreads circumferentially around the nerve.

Clinical Pearls

- Although depositing the local anesthetic around the nerve is desirable, it is technically challenging to reposition the needle on both sides of the nerve because of the nerve's depth within the muscle layers.
- As with other sciatic nerve blocks, if this block is combined with others, the local anesthetic may need to be diluted to reduce the risk of toxicity.
- Complications are rare but can include intravascular injection (e.g., femoral artery), infection in the injection area, hematoma formation, nerve injury, and potential CNS toxicity.

IPACK

Infiltration under US guidance between the popliteal artery and the capsule of the knee constitutes the IPACK block.[117] This block supposedly blocks the tibial, common peroneal, and obturator nerve articular branches in the popliteal region to provide analgesia for the knee.

Under US guidance, the technical benefit of IPACK versus deep surgical injection into the capsule is that the needle path may be monitored while avoiding the popliteal artery and sciatic nerve. While most experts expect this block to offer analgesic effects similar to the surgeon's local infiltration technique, there is no evidence to support IPACK being superior to local surgical infiltration.

Procedure Using Nerve Stimulation Technique

Because there is no major nerve to activate or stimulate, IPACK can only be defined and performed using ultrasonography.

Procedure Using Ultrasound Guidance (Fig. 36-48)

- Scanning: A linear, higher frequency (10- to 15-MHz) probe is typically used to scan the anatomical link between the popliteal artery and the femur. A "hockey stick" probe is suitable for the majority of children. In contrast to the popliteal sciatic block, the transverse probe is positioned on the medial thigh a few centimeters above the patella to capture the popliteal vessels illuminated with Doppler with the anterior border of the vastus medialis muscle and femur and the posterior wall of the sartorius and semimembranous muscles. Despite the probe being positioned on the medial thigh, a distal-to-proximal scan can still efficiently localize the sciatic nerve in the popliteal fossa before its bifurcation.
- Appearance: Visualize the vastus medialis muscle superficial to the outline of the curving hyperechoic line of the femoral shaft. Distally, the hyperechoic border of the femur (condyles) may be evident. Using Doppler, the pulsatile popliteal vessel can typically be located deep to the femoral shaft outline at a short distance posterior to the femur.
- Needling: A 22-gauge needle is inserted in IP fashion in between the popliteal vessels and femur, as shown in Figure 36-48.
- Local anesthetic spread: The aim is to inject local anesthetic into the area between the knee's posterior capsule and the popliteal artery. Insert the needle between the popliteal vessels and femur, then slowly withdraw the needle while injecting 10 to 15 mL of local anesthetic. While a total volume of 10 to 15 mL of ropivacaine 0.25% is the anesthetic of choice in many institutions, the ideal dose, concentration, and volume of local anesthetic for IPACK block have not been well established. The ideal injection level (i.e., above the

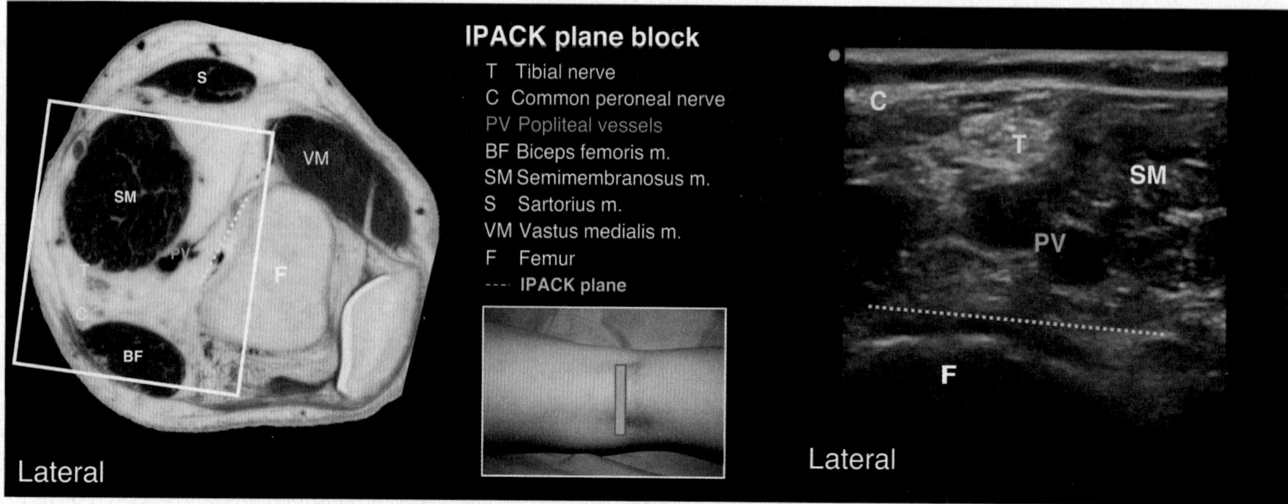

Figure 36-48 IPACK. Infiltration under ultrasound guidance between the popliteal artery and the knee capsule.

patella vs. at the level of the femoral condyle) also remains an open question.

Clinical Pearls

- Be aware that anesthetic spillage from an injection deeper and beyond the popliteal vessels is likely to produce an unintentional block of the sciatic nerve branches and the common peroneal nerve.
- In the absence of local infiltration analgesia, the IPACK block can be a motor-saving alternative to the tibial nerve block for knee surgery that might complement an adductor canal block.

Ankle Block

All five nerves of the foot can be blocked at the ankle level (See Chapter 22, Video 22-2). The superficial nerves—sural, superficial peroneal, and saphenous nerves—can be blocked by simple infiltration techniques. US guidance can be helpful in blocking the posterior tibial and deep peroneal (fibular) nerves, as their locations can be easily identified next to reliable landmarks (i.e., bones and vessels) visible to US.

Posterior Tibial Nerve

Procedure Using Landmark Technique

- Landmarks: The posterior tibial nerve is the major nerve to the sole of the foot. It can be approached with the patient either in the prone position or lying supine with the hip and knee flexed so that the foot rests on the bed. The medial malleolus is identified, along with the pulsation of the posterior tibial artery behind it. The nerve is located posterior to the artery.
- Needling: A needle is introduced through the skin just behind the posterior tibial artery and directed 45 degrees anteriorly, seeking paresthesia in the sole of the foot. Motor responses that may be seen with NS include twitches of the first (medial plantar branch) and fifth (lateral plantar branch) toes.
- Injection: 5 mL of local anesthetic produces anesthesia if paresthesia is identified. If not, a fan-shaped injection of 10 mL can be performed in the triangle formed by the artery, the Achilles tendon, and the tibia itself.

Procedure Using Ultrasound Guidance (Fig. 36-49)

- Scanning: A linear ("hockey stick") 10-MHz probe with a small footprint is positioned in transverse (short) axis to the nerve just posterior and inferior to the medial malleolus. Alternatively, the nerve can be identified 3 to 5 cm above the malleolus. Color Doppler may be helpful since the nerve lies posterior and deep to the posterior tibial artery at both locations. The nerve should be localized before it branches into the medial and lateral plantar nerves.
- Appearance: Immediately anterior to the artery lies the hypoechoic circular posterior tibial vein, although it may be compressed and not appear on the screen. Posterior to the artery, the nerve appears slightly more hyperechoic than the surrounding tissues and has a condensed, honeycomb-like structure.
- Needling: A 36- to 50-mm needle is inserted using an OOP approach with the needle caudal or an IP approach with the needle anterior to the transversely positioned probe.

Sural Nerve

The patient is placed either in the prone position or supine with the hip and knee flexed so that the foot rests on the bed. The posteriorly located sural nerve can be blocked by injection on the lateral side. Subcutaneous injection of 5 mL of local anesthetic behind the lateral malleolus, filling the groove between it and the calcaneus, produces anesthesia of the sural nerve. The effectiveness of a sural nerve block is improved using a perivascular approach (i.e., identifying the lesser saphenous vein 1 cm proximal to the lateral malleolus) rather than a traditional, surface landmark–based approach under US guidance.

Deep Peroneal Nerve

Procedure Using Landmark Technique

- Landmarks: The deep peroneal nerve is the major nerve to the dorsum of the foot and lies in the deep plane of the anterior tibial artery. The patient is positioned supine, generally with the leg extended. Pulsation of the artery is sought at the skin crease level on the ankle's anterior midline surface. If the artery is not palpable, the tendon of the extensor hallucis longus can be identified (the nerve lies immediately lateral to this) by asking the patient to extend the big toe.
- Needling and Injection: If the arterial pulse can be felt, 5 mL of local anesthetic is injected just lateral to it. If the artery is not palpable, the tendon of the extensor hallucis longus can be identified (see earlier). If using NS, toe extension is sought for this nerve. The injection can be made into the deep planes below the fascia using either one of these landmarks.

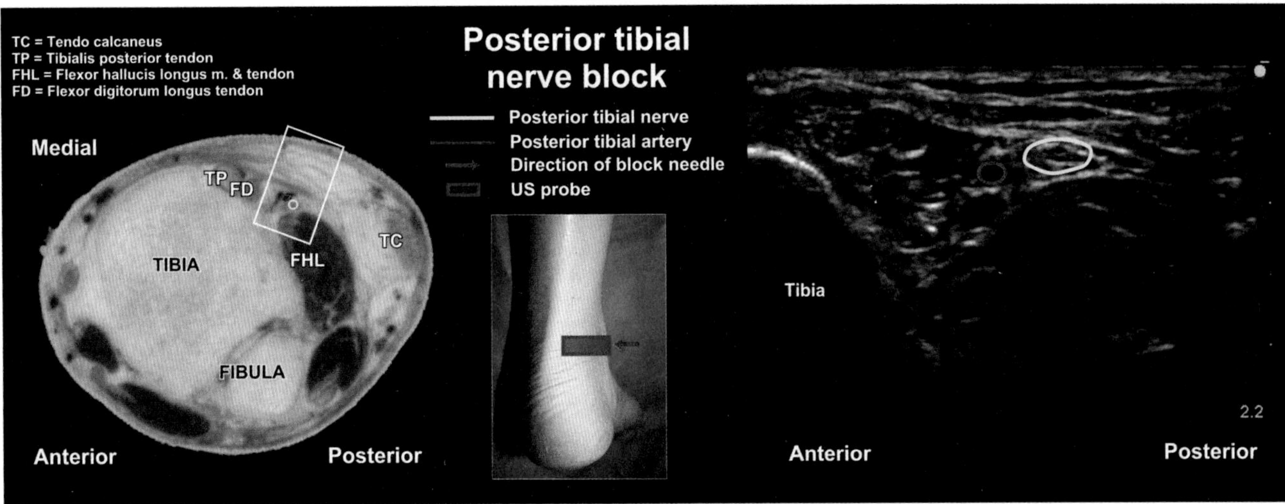

Figure 36-49 Arrangement of relevant anatomy for ultrasound-guided posterior tibial nerve block at the ankle using an IP approach. The nerve is imaged adjacent to the posterior tibial artery before the nerve divides into the medial and lateral plantar nerves.

Procedure Using Ultrasound Guidance (Fig. 36-50)

- Scanning: A small footprint linear ("hockey stick") 10-MHz probe is placed in transverse (short) axis to the nerve at the anterior surface of the ankle joint. Alternatively, the nerve can also be found 3 to 5 cm above the ankle joint. However, the nerve can be difficult to see, and only the artery can be located consistently. Color Doppler can be used at both locations to identify the anterior tibial artery lying medial to the nerve.
- Appearance: If seen, the nerve appears as a small cluster of hyperechoic, fascicular-appearing fibers immediately lateral to the artery, adjacent to the well-demarcated distal end of the tibia.
- Needling: An OOP approach is preferred here since tendons lie on either side of the nerve. A 36- to 50-mm needle is inserted OOP and caudal to the transversely positioned small footprint probe.
- Local anesthetic spread: Injecting 4 to 5 mL of local anesthetic lateral to the nerve will help avoid the anterior tibial artery, which lies medial. It is important to perform aspiration before injection.

Saphenous Nerve

The patient is placed supine with the leg extended. The saphenous nerve is anesthetized by infiltrating 5 mL of local anesthetic around the saphenous vein at the level where it passes anterior to the medial malleolus. A wall of anesthesia between the skin and the bone itself suffices to block the nerve. Alternatively, this nerve can be blocked at a more proximal site in the thigh. See the section on Separate Blocks of the Terminal Nerves of the Lumbar Plexus for more proximal approaches.

Superficial Peroneal Branches

A subcutaneous ridge of local anesthetic solution is injected along the skin crease between the anterior tibial artery and the lateral malleolus. This subcutaneous ridge overlies the subfascial injection used for the deep peroneal nerve. Another 5 to 10 mL of local anesthetic may be required to cover this area. The superficial peroneal nerve may be visualized using US, which may aid in a more accurate injection of local anesthetic.

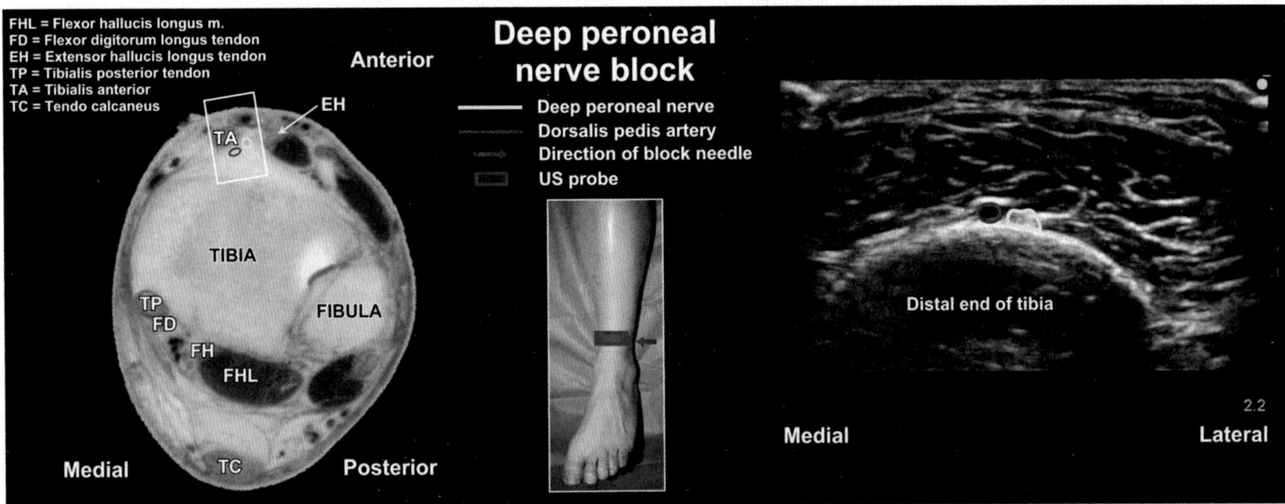

Figure 36-50 Arrangement of relevant anatomy for ultrasound-guided deep peroneal nerve block at the anterior ankle. If possible, the medially located anterior tibial artery should be localized with Doppler to differentiate between the nerve and surrounding tendons.

Clinical Pearls

- Anesthesia of the foot usually ensues within 15 minutes of these five injections.
- Complications of ankle block are rare, although neuropathy can be produced. Care should be taken not to pin any deep nerves against the bone at the time of injection. Epinephrine should not be added to local anesthetics to avoid compromising the distal circulation.
- US imaging for the deep nerves may help avoid bone contact and multiple injections with the infiltration technique.

Continuous Catheter Technique

Catheter insertion for continuous regional anesthesia, whether guided by NS or US, suffers from several fundamental problems owing to the design of current needle-catheter assemblies, including dislodgment or movement of the catheter, leakage at the insertion site, and imprecise catheter placement. The increasing popularity of US technology in regional anesthesia has facilitated the increased use of catheter-over-needle approaches to continuous catheter placement. Several commercially available catheter-over-needle kits are marketed throughout the world. The primary benefit of this approach is that the catheter is held tightly by the surrounding skin since the needle—which enables initial skin puncture—is housed within the catheter and is removed once the needle tip is located appropriately. This overcomes the typical problems described earlier in the traditional catheter-through-needle approach.[118]

Peripheral neuromodulation by electrical stimulation has recently emerged as a plausible analgesic approach in the management of acute pain, as an alternative to a reliance on local anesthetics to produce analgesia. Specifically, a dedicated neuromodulation electrode is implanted a short distance from or on the nerve.[119] An off-label use of a stimulating catheter for combining neuromodulation with pharmacologic local anesthetic blockade has been reported.[120] While evidence from a handful of researchers demonstrating the analgesic benefit of neuromodulation continues to accumulate, the safety and cost-effectiveness of its role in acute pain management has not been established.

Acknowledgments

The authors acknowledge the Ecole Polytechnique Federale de Lausanne, Switzerland, Visible Human Web Server (http://visiblehuman.epfl.ch) as the data source for the anatomic sections used in some of the figures. Most of the material was adapted from one of the author's (B.T.) textbooks, Atlas of Ultrasound and Nerve Stimulation-Guided Regional Anesthesia, 1st edition[1] and Pediatric Atlas of Ultrasound and Nerve Stimulation-Guided Regional Anesthesia.[2] B.T. also has contributed in part to the design of a continuous catheter over the needle.

For further review and interactivities, please see the videos and narrative interactive clinical vignettes (NICVs) accessible in the complimentary eBook bundled with this text. Access instructions are located on the inside front cover.

REFERENCES

1. Tsui BC. *Atlas of Ultrasound and Nerve Stimulation-Guided Regional Anesthesia*. 1st edition. Springer New York; 2007.
2. Tsui BCH, Suresh S. *Pediatric Atlas of Ultrasound- and Nerve Stimulation-Guided Regional Anesthesia*. Springer; 2015.
3. Borgeat A. Regional anesthesia, intraneural injection, and nerve injury: beyond the epineurium. *Anesthesiology*. 2006;105(4):647–648. doi:10.1097/00000542-200610000-00005
4. Tsui BCH, Wagner A, Finucane B. Electrophysiologic effects of injectates on peripheral nerve stimulation. *Reg Anesth Pain Med*. 2004;29(3):189–193. doi:10.1016/j.rapm.2004.02.002
5. Tsui BCH, Kropelin B, Ganapathy S, Finucane B. Dextrose 5% in water: fluid medium for maintaining electrical stimulation of peripheral nerves during stimulating catheter placement. *Acta Anaesthesiol Scand*. 2005;49(10):1562–1565. doi:10.1111/j.1399-6576.2005.00736.x
6. Selander D, Dhunér KG, Lundborg G. Peripheral nerve injury due to injection needles used for regional anesthesia: an experimental study of the acute effects of needle point trauma. *Acta Anaesthesiol Scand*. 1977;21(3):182–188. doi:10.1111/j.1399-6576.1977.tb01208.x
7. Hadzic A, Dilberovic F, Shah S, et al. Combination of intraneural injection and high injection pressure leads to fascicular injury and neurologic deficits in dogs. *Reg Anesth Pain Med*. 2004;29(5):417–423. doi:10.1097/00115550-200409000-00005
8. Selander D, Sjöstrand J. Longitudinal spread of intraneurally injected local anesthetics: an experimental study of the initial neural distribution following intraneural injections. *Acta Anaesthesiol Scand*. 1978;22(6):622–634. doi:10.1111/j.1399-6576.1978.tb01346.x
9. Bromage PR. *Epidural Analgesia*. WB Saunders; 1978:301–320.
10. Brown DL, Ransom DM, Hall JA, Leicht CH, Schroeder DR, Offord KP. Regional anesthesia and local anesthetic-induced systemic toxicity: seizure frequency and accompanying cardiovascular changes. *Anesth Analg*. 1995;81(2):321–328. doi:10.1097/00000539-199508000-00020
11. Borgeat A, Blumenthal S. Nerve injury and regional anaesthesia. *Curr Opin Anaesthesiol*. 2004;17(5):417–421. doi:10.1097/00001503-200410000-00011
12. Auroy Y, Narchi P, Messiah A, Litt L, Rouvier B, Samii K. Serious complications related to regional anesthesia: results of a prospective survey in France. *Anesthesiology*. 1997;87(3):479–486. doi:10.1097/00000542-199709000-00005
13. Kaufman BR, Nystrom E, Nath S, Foucher G, Nystrom A. Debilitating chronic pain syndromes after presumed intraneural injections. *Pain*. 2000;85(1-2):283–286. doi:10.1016/S0304-3959(99)00243-2
14. Selander D. Neurotoxicity of local anesthetics: animal data. *Reg Anesth*. 1993;18(6):461–468.
15. Ben-David B. Complications of peripheral blockade. *Anesthesiol Clin North America*. 2002;20(3):695–707. doi:10.1016/s0889-8537(02)00012-3
16. Weinberg GL, VadeBoncouer T, Ramaraju GA, Garcia-Amaro MF, Cwik MJ. Pretreatment or resuscitation with a lipid infusion shifts the dose—Response to bupivacaine-induced asystole in rats. *Anesthesiology*. 1998;88(4):1071–1075. doi:10.1097/00000542-199804000-00028
17. Litz RJ, Popp M, Stehr SN, Koch T. Successful resuscitation of a patient with ropivacaine-induced asystole after axillary plexus block using lipid infusion. *Anaesthesia*. 2006;61(8):800–801. doi:10.1111/j.1365-2044.2006.04740.x
18. Rosenblatt MA, Abel M, Fischer GW, Itzkovich CJ, Eisenkraft JB. Successful use of a 20% lipid emulsion to resuscitate a patient after a presumed bupivacaine-related cardiac arrest. *Anesthesiology*. 2006;105(1):217–218. doi:10.1097/00000542-200607000-00033
19. Fremling MA, Mackinnon SE. Injection injury to the median nerve. *Ann Plast Surg*. 1996;37(5):561–567. doi:10.1097/00000637-199611000-00019
20. Shah S, Hadzic A, Vloka JD, Cafferty MS, Moucha CS, Santos AC. Neurologic complication after anterior sciatic nerve block. *Anesth Analg*. 2005;100(5):1515–1517. doi:10.1213/01.ANE.0000150613.23987.92
21. Selander D, Edshage S, Wolff T. Paresthesiae or no paresthesiae? Nerve lesions after axillary blocks. *Acta Anaesthesiol Scand*. 1979;23(1):27–33. doi:10.1111/j.1399-6576.1979.tb01417.x
22. Gentili F, Hudson AR, Hunter D, Kline DG. Nerve injection injury with local anesthetic agents: a light and electron microscopic, fluorescent microscopic, and horseradish peroxidase study. *Neurosurgery*. 1980;6(3):263–272. doi:10.1227/00006123-198003000-00007
23. Enneking FK, Chan V, Greger J, Hadžić A, Lang SA, Horlocker TT. Lower-extremity peripheral nerve blockade: essentials of our current understanding. *Reg Anesth Pain Med*. 2005;30(1):4–35. doi:10.1016/j.rapm.2004.10.002
24. Selander D. Peripheral nerve injury after regional anesthesia. In: Finucane BT, ed. *Complications of Regional Anesthesia*. Churchhill Livingstone; 1999:105–115.
25. Winchell S, Wolfe R. The incidence of neuropathy following upper extremity nerve blocks. *Reg Anesth*. 1985;10(1):24–31.
26. Klaastad Ø, Smedby Ö, Thompson GE, et al. Distribution of local anesthetic in axillary brachial plexus block: a clinical and magnetic resonance imaging study. *Anesthesiology*. 2002;96(6):1315–1324. doi:10.1097/00000542-200206000-00009
27. Tsui B. Ultrasound-guidance and nerve stimulation: implications for the future practice of regional anesthesia. *Can J Anaesth*. 2007;54(3):165–170. doi:10.1007/bf03022635
28. Tsui BCH. Ultrasound imaging to localize foramina for superficial trigeminal nerve block. *Can J Anesth*. 2009;56(9):704–706. doi:10.1007/s12630-009-9129-3
29. Molliex S, Pascal J, Charier D, Perret D, Navez M, Auboyer C. Peripheral blocks of trigeminal nerve for facial soft-tissue surgery: learning from failures. *Eur J Anaesthesiol*. 2005;22(6):480–482. doi:10.1017/S0265021505260817
30. Nguyen A, Girard F, Boudreault D, et al. Scalp nerve blocks decrease the severity of pain after craniotomy. *Anesth Analg*. 2001;93(5):1272–1276. doi:10.1097/00000539-200111000-00048
31. Knize DM. A study of the supraorbital nerve. *Plast Reconstr Surg*. 1995;96(3):564–569. doi:10.1097/00006534-199509000-00007
32. Tsui BCH, Pan S, Smith L, Lin C, Balakrishnan K. Opioid-free tonsillectomy with and without adenoidectomy: the role of regional anesthesia in the "New Era." *Anesth Analg*. 2021;133(1):e7–e9. doi:10.1213/ANE.0000000000005567

33. Naja MZ, Al-Tannir M, Naja H, Ziade MF, Zeidan A. Repeated nerve blocks with clonidine, fentanyl and bupivacaine for trigeminal neuralgia. *Anaesthesia.* 2006;61(1):70–71. doi:10.1111/j.1365-2044.2005.04486.x
34. Mireault D, Cawthorn TR, Todd AR, Spencer AO. Suprazygomatic maxillary nerve block: an ultrasound and cadaveric study to identify correct sonoanatomical landmarks. *J Anesth.* 2021;35(1):150–153. doi:10.1007/s00540-020-02877-6
35. Echaniz G, De Miguel M, Merritt G, et al. Bilateral suprazygomatic maxillary nerve blocks vs. infraorbital and palatine nerve blocks in cleft lip and palate repair: a double-blind, randomised study. *Eur J Anaesthesiol.* 2019;36(1):40-47. doi:10.1097/EJA.0000000000000900
36. Lin C, Pan S, Barros VR, Meister K, Tsui BCH. Opioid-free postoperative pain management after adenotonsillectomy with nasal turbinate reduction using bilateral suprazygomatic infratemporal-pterygopalatine fossa injections: a case report. *A A Pract.* 2021;15(8):e01502. doi:10.1213/XAA.0000000000001502
37. Echaniz G, Chan V, Maynes JT, Jozaghi Y, Agur A. Ultrasound-guided maxillary nerve block: an anatomical study using the suprazygomatic approach. *Can J Anaesth.* 2020;67(2):186–193. doi:10.1007/S12630-019-01481-X
38. Smith L, Balakrishnan K, Pan S, Tsui BCH. Suprazygomatic maxillary (SZM) nerve blocks for perioperative pain control in pediatric tonsillectomy and adenoidectomy. *J Clin Anesth.* 2021;71:110240. doi:10.1016/j.jclinane.2021.110240
39. Haas DA. Alternative mandibular nerve block techniques: a review of the Gow-Gates and Akinosi-Vazirani closed-mouth mandibular nerve block techniques. *J Am Dent Assoc.* 2011:142. doi:10.14219/jada.archive.2011.0341
40. Winnie AP, Ramamurthy S, Durrani Z, Radonjic R. Interscalene cervical plexus block: a single injection technic. *Anesth Analg.* 1975;54(3):370–375.
41. Usui Y, Kobayashi T, Kakinuma H, Watanabe K, Kitajima T, Matsuno K. An anatomical basis for blocking of the deep cervical plexus and cervical sympathetic tract using an ultrasound-guided technique. *Anesth Analg.* 2010;110(3):964–968. doi:10.1213/ANE.0b013e3181c91ea0
42. Stoneham MD, Doyle AR, Knighton JD, Dorje P, Stanley JC. Prospective, randomized comparison of deep or superficial cervical plexus block for carotid endarterectomy surgery. *Anesthesiology.* 1998;89(4):907–912. doi:10.1097/00000542-199810000-00015
43. de Sousa AA, Filho MAD, Faglione W Jr, Carvalho GTC. Superficial vs combined cervical plexus block for carotid endarterectomy: a prospective, randomized study. *Surg Neurol.* 2005;63:S22–S25. doi:10.1016/j.surneu.2004.09.011
44. Pandit JJ, Bree S, Dillon P, Elcock D, McLaren ID, Crider B. A comparison of superficial versus combined (superficial and deep) cervical plexus block for carotid endarterectomy: a prospective, randomized study. *Anesth Analg.* 2000;91(4):781–786. doi:10.1097/00000539-200010000-00004
45. Castresana MR, Masters RD, Castresana EJ, Stefansson S, Shaker IJ, Newman WH. Incidence and clinical significance of hemidiaphragmatic paresis in patients undergoing carotid endarterectomy during cervical plexus block anesthesia. *J Neurosurg Anesthesiol.* 1994;6(1):21–23. doi:10.1097/00008506-199401000-00003
46. Masters RD, Castresana EJ, Castresana MR. Superficial and deep cervical plexus block: technical considerations. *AANA J.* 1995;63(3):235–243.
47. Stoneham MD, Knighton JD. Regional anaesthesia for carotid endarterectomy. *Br J Anaesth.* 1999;82(6):910–919. doi:10.1093/bja/82.6.910
48. Chen H, Sokoll LJ, Udelsman R. Outpatient minimally invasive parathyroidectomy: a combination of sestamibi-SPECT localization, cervical block anesthesia, and intraoperative parathyroid hormone assay. *Surgery.* 1999;126(6):1016–1021. doi:10.1067/msy.2099.101433
49. Miccoli P, Barellini L, Monchik JM, Rago R, Berti PF. Randomized clinical trial comparing regional and general anaesthesia in minimally invasive video-assisted parathyroidectomy. *Br J Surg.* 2005;92(7):814–818. doi:10.1002/bjs.5048
50. Tran DQH, Dugani S, Finlayson RJ. A randomized comparison between ultrasound-guided and landmark-based superficial cervical plexus block. *Reg Anesth Pain Med.* 2010;35(6):539–543. doi:10.1097/AAP.0b013e3181faa11c
51. Herring AA, Stone MB, Frenkel O, Chipman A, Nagdev AD. The ultrasound-guided superficial cervical plexus block for anesthesia and analgesia in emergency care settings. *Am J Emerg Med.* 2012;30(7):1263–1267. doi:10.1016/j.ajem.2011.06.023
52. Spanknebel K, Chabot JA, DiGiorgi M, et al. Thyroidectomy using local anesthesia: a report of 1,025 cases over 16 years. *J Am Coll Surg.* 2005;201(3):375–385. doi:10.1016/j.jamcollsurg.2005.04.034
53. Specht MC, Romero M, Barden CB, Esposito C, Fahey TJ 3rd. Characteristics of patients having thyroid surgery under regional anesthesia. *J Am Coll Surg.* 2001;193(4):367–372. doi:10.1016/S1072-7515(01)01048-1
54. Tobias JD. Cervical plexus block in adolescents. *J Clin Anesth.* 1999;11(7):606–608. doi:10.1016/S0952-8180(99)00104-X
55. Burtles R. Analgesia for "bat ear" surgery. *Ann R Coll Surg Engl.* 1989;71(5):332. doi:10.1016/s0022-3468(05)80045-4
56. Afridi SK, Shields KG, Bhola R, Goadsby PJ. Greater occipital nerve injection in primary headache syndromes—prolonged effects from a single injection. *Pain.* 2006;122(1–2):126–129. doi:10.1016/j.pain.2006.01.016
57. Anthony M. Cervicogenic headache: prevalence and response to local steroid therapy. *Clin Exp Rheumatol.* 2000;18(2 Suppl 19):S59–S64.
58. Winnie AP. Interscalene brachial plexus block. *Anesth Analg.* 1970;49(3):455–466.
59. Gadsden JC, Tsai T, Iwata T, Somasundarum L, Robards C, Hadzic A. Low interscalene block provides reliable anesthesia for surgery at or about the elbow. *J Clin Anesth.* 2009;21(2):98–102. doi:10.1016/j.jclinane.2008.06.031
60. Kim JH, Chen J, Bennett H, et al. A low approach to interscalene brachial plexus block results in more distal spread of sensory-motor coverage compared to the conventional approach. *Anesth Analg.* 2011;112(4):987–989. doi:10.1213/ANE.0b013e31820b5e8e
61. Benumof JL. Permanent loss of cervical spinal cord function associated with interscalene block performed under general anesthesia. *Anesthesiology.* 2000;93(6):1541–1544.
62. Yang WT, Chui PT, Metreweli C. Anatomy of the normal brachial plexus revealed by sonography and the role of sonographic guidance in anesthesia of the brachial plexus. AJR *Am J Roentgenol.* 1998;171(6):1631–1636. doi:10.2214/ajr.171.6.9843302
63. Demondion X, Herbinet P, Boutry N, Fontaine C, Francke JP, Cotten A. Sonographic mapping of the normal brachial plexus. *AJNR Am J Neuroradiol.* 2003;24(7):1303–1309.
64. Sheppard DC, Iyer RB, Fenstermacher MJ. Brachial plexus: demonstration at US. *Radiology.* 1998;208(2):402–406. doi:10.1148/radiology.208.2.9680567
65. Ip VHY, Tsui BCH. Continuous interscalene block: the good, the bad and the refined spread. *Acta Anaesthesiol Scand.* 2012;56(4):526–530. doi:10.1111/j.1399-6576.2012.02650.x
66. Boezaart AP, Koorn R, Rosenquist RW. Paravertebral approach to the brachial plexus: an anatomic improvement in technique. *Reg Anesth Pain Med.* 2003;28(3):241–244. doi:10.1053/rapm.2003.50049
67. Wedel DJ, Klaastad Ø, VadeBoncouer TR, Tillung T, Smedby Ö. An evaluation of the supraclavicular plumb-bob technique for brachial plexus block by magnetic resonance imaging. *Anesth Analg.* 2003;96(3):862–867. doi:10.1213/01.ane.0000048707.91577.83
68. Apan A, Baydar P, Yýlmaz S, et al. Surface landmarks of brachial plexus: Ultrasound and magnetic resonance imaging for supraclavicular approach with anatomical correlation. *Eur J Ultrasound.* 2001;13(3):191–196. doi:10.1016/S0929-8266(01)00131-8
69. Ip VHY, Tsui BCH. The catheter-over-needle assembly facilitates delivery of a second local anesthetic bolus to prolong supraclavicular brachial plexus block without time-consuming catheterization steps: a randomized controlled study. *Can J Anesth.* 2013;60(7):692–699. doi:10.1007/s12630-013-9951-5
70. Klaastad Ø, Smith HJ, Smedby Ö, et al. A novel infraclavicular brachial plexus block: the lateral and sagittal technique, developed by magnetic resonance imaging studies. *Anesth Analg.* 2004;98(1):252–256. doi:10.1213/01.ANE.0000094337.75996.AE
71. Imasogie N, Ganapathy S, Singh S, Armstrong K, Armstrong P. A prospective, randomized, double-blind comparison of ultrasound-guided axillary brachial plexus blocks using 2 versus 4 injections. *Anesth Analg.* 2010;110(4):1222–1226. doi:10.1213/ANE.0b013e3181cb6791
72. Ganta R, Cajee RA, Henthorn RW. Use of transcutaneous nerve stimulation to assist interscalene block. *Anesth Analg.* 1993;76(4):914–915. doi:10.1213/00000539-199304000-00063
73. Urmey WF, Grossi P. Percutaneous electrode guidance and subcutaneous stimulating electrode guidance: modifications of the original technique. *Reg Anesth Pain Med.* 2003;28(3):253–255. doi:10.1053/rapm.2003.50128
74. Urmey WF, Grossi P. Percutaneous electrode guidance: a noninvasive technique for prelocation of peripheral nerves to facilitate peripheral plexus or nerve block. *Reg Anesth Pain Med.* 2002;27(3):261–267. http://www.ncbi.nlm.nih.gov/pubmed/12016599
75. McDonnell JG, O'Donnell B, Curley G, Heffernan A, Power C, Laffey JG. The analgesic efficacy of transversus abdominis plane block after abdominal surgery: a prospective randomized controlled trial. *Anesth Analg.* 2007;104(1):193–197. http://ovidsp.ovid.com/ovidweb.cgi?T=JS&PAGE=reference&D=med5&NEWS=N&AN=17179269
76. O'Donnell BD, McDonnell JG, McShane AJ. The transversus abdominis plane (TAP) block in open retropubic prostatectomy. *Reg Anesth Pain Med.* 2006;31(1):91. doi:10.1016/j.rapm.2005.10.006
77. Courreges P, Poddevin F, Lecoutre D. Para-umbilical block: a new concept for regional anaesthesia in children. *Paediatr Anaesth.* 1997;7(3):211–214. doi:10.1046/j.1460-9592.1997.d01-79.x
78. Ferguson S, Thomas V, Lewis I. The rectus sheath block in paediatric anaesthesia: new indications for an old technique? *Paediatr Anaesth.* 1996;6(6):463–466. doi:10.1046/j.1460-9592.1996.d01-24.x
79. Rafi AN. Abdominal field block: a new approach via the lumbar triangle. *Anaesthesia.* 2001;56(10):1024–1026. doi:10.1046/j.1365-2044.2001.02279-40.x
80. Forero M, Adhikary SD, Lopez H, Tsui C, Chin KJ. The erector spinae plane block a novel analgesic technique in thoracic neuropathic pain. *Reg Anesth Pain Med.* 2016;41(5):621–627. doi:10.1097/AAP.0000000000000451
81. Chin KJ, El-Boghdadly K. Mechanisms of action of the erector spinae plane (ESP) block: a narrative review. *Can J Anaesth.* 2021;68(3):387–408. doi:10.1007/s12630-020-01875-2
82. Tsui BCH, Ip VHY. Can electrical nerve stimulation guidance assist in cervical erector spinae plane block catheter placement for total shoulder arthroplasty? *Can J Anaesth.* 2019;66(11):1417–1418. doi:10.1007/s12630-019-01457-x
83. Tsui BCH, Kirkham K, Kwofie MK, et al. Practice advisory on the bleeding risks for peripheral nerve and interfascial blockade: rooted in evidence. *Can J Anaesth.* 2020;67(3):379–380. doi:10.1007/s12630-019-01520-7
84. Tsui BCH, Fonseca A, Munshey F, McFadyen G, Caruso TJ. The erector spinae plane (ESP) block: a pooled review of 242 cases. *J Clin Anesth.* 2019;53:29–34. doi:10.1016/j.jclinane.2018.09.036

85. Saadawi M, Layera S, Aliste J, Bravo D, Leurcharusmee P, Tran DQ. Erector spinae plane block: a narrative review with systematic analysis of the evidence pertaining to clinical indications and alternative truncal blocks. *J Clin Anesth.* 2021;68:110063. doi:10.1016/j.jclinane.2020.110063
86. Pusch F, Freitag H, Weinstabl C, Obwegeser R, Huber E, Wildling E. Single-injection paravertebral block compared to general anaesthesia in breast surgery. *Acta Anaesthesiol Scand.* 1999;43(7):770–774. doi:10.1034/j.1399-6576.1999.430714.x
87. Naja Z, Lönnqvist PA. Somatic paravertebral nerve blockade: incidence of failed block and complications. *Anaesthesia.* 2001;56(12):1184–1188. doi:10.1046/j.1365-2044.2001.02084-2.x
88. Pourseidi B, Khorram-Manesh A. Effect of intercostals neural blockade with Marcaine (bupivacaine) on postoperative pain after laparoscopic cholecystectomy. *Surg Endosc.* 2007;21(9):1557–1559. doi:10.1007/s00464-006-9181-9
89. Biswas A, Castanov V, Li Z, et al. Serratus plane block: a cadaveric study to evaluate optimal injectate spread. *Reg Anesth Pain Med.* 2018;43(8):854–858. doi:10.1097/AAP.0000000000000848
90. Xie C, Ran G, Chen D, Lu Y. A narrative review of ultrasound-guided serratus anterior plane block. *Ann Palliat Med.* 2021;10(1):700–706. doi:10.21037/apm-20-1542
91. Kunigo T, Murouchi T, Yamamoto S, Yamakage M. Injection volume and anesthetic effect in serratus plane block. *Reg Anesth Pain Med.* 2017;42(6):737–740. doi:10.1097/AAP.0000000000000649
92. Marshall K, McLaughlin K. Pain management in thoracic surgery. *Thorac Surg Clin.* 2020;30(3):339–346. doi:10.1016/j.thorsurg.2020.03.001
93. Kim RK, Brodt J, MacArthur JW, Tsui BCH. Continuous serratus anterior plane block: a team approach. *J Cardiothorac Vasc Anesth.* 2022;36(4):1217–1218. doi:10.1053/j.jvca.2021.10.036
94. Blanco R. The "pecs block": a novel technique for providing analgesia after breast surgery. *Anaesthesia.* 2011;66(9):847–848. doi:10.1111/J.1365-2044.2011.06838.X
95. Blanco R, Fajardo M, Parras Maldonado T. Ultrasound description of Pecs II (modified Pecs I): a novel approach to breast surgery. *Rev Esp Anestesiol Reanim.* 2012;59(9):470–475. doi:10.1016/J.REDAR.2012.07.003
96. El-Boghdadly K, Wolmarans M, Stengel AD, et al. Standardizing nomenclature in regional anesthesia: an ASRA-ESRA Delphi consensus study of abdominal wall, paraspinal, and chest wall blocks. *Reg Anesth Pain Med.* 2021;46(7):571–580. doi:10.1136/rapm-2020-102451
97. Tsui BCH, Kirkham K, Kwofie MK, et al. Practice advisory on the bleeding risks for peripheral nerve and interfascial plane blockade: evidence review and expert consensus. *Can J Anaesth.* 2019;66(11):1356–1384. doi:10.1007/s12630-019-01466-w
98. Hussain N, Brull R, McCartney CJL, et al. Pectoralis-II myofascial block and analgesia in breast cancer surgery: a systematic review and meta-analysis. *Anesthesiology.* 2019;131(3):630–648. doi:10.1097/ALN.0000000000002822
99. Hebbard PD. Transversalis fascia plane block, a novel ultrasound-guided abdominal wall nerve block. *Can J Anaesth.* 2009;56(8):618–620. doi:10.1007/s12630-009-9110-1
100. Elsharkawy H, El-Boghdadly K, Barrington M. Quadratus lumborum block: anatomical concepts, mechanisms, and techniques. *Anesthesiology.* 2019;130(2):322–335. doi:10.1097/ALN.0000000000002524
101. Tsui BC. "PQRST": the shamrock method for lumbar plexus blocks. *J Clin Monit Comput.* 2017;31(6):1333–1334. doi:10.1007/s10877-016-9964-z
102. Jin Z, Liu J, Li R, Gan TJ, He Y, Lin J. Single injection auadratus lumborum block for postoperative analgesia in adult surgical population: a systematic review and meta-analysis. *J Clin Anesth.* 2020;62:109715. doi:10.1016/j.jclinane.2020.109715
103. Willschke H, Marhofer P, Bösenberg A, et al. Ultrasonography for ilioinguinal/iliohypogastric nerve blocks in children. *Br J Anaesth.* 2005;95(2):226–230. doi:10.1093/bja/aei157
104. Randhawa K, Soumian S, Kyi M, Khaira H. Sonographic assessment of the conventional "blind" ilioinguinal block. *Can J Anesth.* 2010;57(1):94–95. doi:10.1007/s12630-009-9211-x
105. Faraoni D, Gilbeau A, Lingier P, Barvais L, Engelman E, Hennart D. Does ultrasound guidance improve the efficacy of dorsal penile nerve block in children? *Paediatr Anaesth.* 2010;20(10):931–936. doi:10.1111/j.1460-9592.2010.03405.x
106. Capdevila X, Macaire P, Dadure C, et al. Continuous psoas compartment block for postoperative analgesia after total hip arthroplasty: new landmarks, technical guidelines, and clinical evaluation. *Anesth Analg.* 2002;94(6):1606–1613. doi:10.1097/00000539-200206000-00045
107. Kirchmair L, Enna B, Mitterschiffthaler G, et al. Lumbar plexus in children: a sonographic study and its relevance to pediatric regional anesthesia. *Anesthesiology.* 2004;101(2):445–450. doi:10.1097/00000542-200408000-00026
108. Lundblad M, Kapral S, Marhofer P, Lönnqvist PA. Ultrasound-guided infrapatellar nerve block in human volunteers: description of a novel technique. *Br J Anaesth.* 2006;97(5):710–714. doi:10.1093/bja/ael241
109. Hara K, Sakura S, Shido A. Ultrasound-guided lateral femoral cutaneous nerve block: comparison of two techniques. *Anaesth Intensive Care.* 2011;39(1):69–72. doi:10.1177/0310057x1103900111
110. Soong J, Schafhalter-Zoppoth I, Gray AT. Sonographic imaging of the obturator nerve for regional block. *Reg Anesth Pain Med.* 2007;32(2):146–151. doi:10.1016/j.rapm.2006.10.012
111. Akkaya T, Ozturk E, Comert A, et al. Ultrasound-guided obturator nerve block: a sonoanatomic study of a new methodologic approach. *Anesth Analg.* 2009;108(3):1037–1041. doi:10.1213/ane.0b013e3181966f03
112. Tsui BCH, Özelsel T. Ultrasound-guided transsartorial perifemoral artery approach for saphenous nerve block. *Reg Anesth Pain Med.* 2009;34(2):177–178. doi:10.1097/AAP.0b013e31819a273e
113. Dang CP. Midfemoral block: a new lateral approach to the sciatic nerve. *Anesth Analg.* 1999;88(6):1426. doi:10.1213/00000539-199906000-00052
114. Tran DQH, Dugani S, Pham K, Al-Shaafi A, Finlayson RJ. A randomized comparison between subepineural and conventional ultrasound-guided popliteal sciatic nerve block. *Reg Anesth Pain Med.* 2011;36(6):548–552. doi:10.1097/AAP.0b013e318235f566
115. Tsui BCH, Özelsel TJP. Ultrasound-guided anterior sciatic nerve block using a longitudinal approach: "expanding the view." *Reg Anesth Pain Med.* 2008;33(3):275–276. doi:10.1016/j.rapm.2007.11.008
116. Chan E, Howle R, Onwochei D, Desai N. Infiltration between the popliteal artery and the capsule of the knee (IPACK) block in knee surgery: a narrative review. *Reg Anesth Pain Med.* 2021;46(9):784–805. doi:10.1136/rapm-2021-102681
117. Tsui BCH, Tsui J. Less leakage and dislodgement with a catheter-over-needle versus a catheter-through-needle approach for peripheral nerve block: an ex vivo study. *Can J Anaesth.* 2012;59(7):655–661. doi:10.1007/s12630-012-9713-9
118. Ilfeld BM, Said ET, Finneran JJ, et al. Ultrasound-guided percutaneous peripheral nerve stimulation: neuromodulation of the femoral nerve for postoperative Analgesia following ambulatory anterior cruciate ligament reconstruction: a proof of concept study. *Neuromodulation.* 2019;22(5):621–629. doi:10.1111/ner.12851
119. Sondekoppam RV, Ip V, Tsui BCH. Feasibility of combining nerve stimulation and local anesthetic infusion to treat acute postamputation pain: a case report of a hybrid technique. *A A Pract.* 2021;15(6):e01487. doi:10.1213/XAA.0000000000001487
120. Winnie AP, Ramamurthy S, Durrani Z. The inguinal paravascular technic of lumbar plexus anesthesia: the "3-in-1 block." *Anesth Analg.* 1973;52(6):989–996.

Section 7

ANESTHESIA SUBSPECIALITY CARE

37 Anesthesia for Neurosurgery

JOHN PATRICK F. BEBAWY • LAURA B. HEMMER • JEFFREY J. PASTERNAK

KEY POINTS

1 The brain receives approximately 70% of its blood supply from two internal carotid arteries anteriorly and 30% from two vertebral arteries posteriorly forming the basilar artery, that subsequently converge to form the circle of Willis, an anastomotic ring at the base of the skull.

2 The spinal cord receives its blood supply from one anterior spinal artery and two posterior spinal arteries. The anterior spinal artery originates from 6 to 8 major radicular arteries derived from the aorta, with the largest one being the artery of Adamkiewicz (usually occurring at T11 or T12 and generally supplying T8 to the conus medullaris terminus).

3 Cerebral blood flow (CBF) is regulated by "flow-metabolism coupling," whereby increases in regional neuronal electrical activity require corresponding increases in regional blood flow. Such coupling occurs on the order of seconds, with very little variation in the amount of oxygen extraction by the brain tissue (i.e., CBF matches cerebral metabolic rate of oxygen consumption ($CMRO_2$) very quickly and efficiently in the healthy brain).

4 Moderate changes in mean arterial pressure (MAP) (or cerebral perfusion pressure) will yield a consistent CBF of 50 mL/100 g/min, due to the normal brain's ability to autoregulate its blood flow. Cerebral autoregulation of blood flow is thought to remain intact between a MAP of approximately 60 and 160 mmHg and functions by altering cerebrovascular resistance (CVR) on the order of 5 to 60 seconds. The alteration in CVR is accomplished in both a rapid phase ("dynamic autoregulation") and a slow phase ("static autoregulation").

5 CBF is linearly associated with arterial carbon dioxide tension ($PaCO_2$) between 20 and 80 mmHg. Hyper- and hypoventilation, both patient-determined and iatrogenic, play critical roles in decreasing or increasing CBF, respectively. A change in $PaCO_2$ of 1 mmHg roughly correlates to a similar change in CBF of 1 to 2 mL/100 g/min. Below the lower limit of this linear effect (i.e., with $PaCO_2$ below 20 mmHg), maximal cerebral vasoconstriction leads to tissue hypoxia and a reflex vasodilation.

6 Intravenous drugs, such as propofol, etomidate, benzodiazepines, and barbiturates, decrease CBF by virtue of a drug-induced decrease in $CMRO_2$ and subsequent flow-metabolism coupling. Autoregulation and $PaCO_2$ responsiveness remain intact with these agents.

7 Potent volatile anesthetics, such as isoflurane, sevoflurane, and desflurane, are direct cerebral vasodilators. However, this direct vasodilation is offset by a drug-induced decrease in $CMRO_2$, and via flow-metabolism coupling, an attenuation of the direct effect on CBF. This leads to minimal, if any, increase in CBF at lower doses. However, at high doses, where maximal suppression of $CMRO_2$ has occurred, are direct vasodilatory effects observed leading to a dose-dependent increase in CBF. Furthermore, autoregulation is inhibited with potent volatile anesthetic drugs in a dose-dependent fashion, although the cerebral vasculature remains responsive to changes in $PaCO_2$.

8 The Monro–Kellie doctrine states that "an increase in the volume of one intracranial compartment will lead to a rise in intracranial pressure (ICP) unless it is matched by an equal reduction in the volume of another compartment." Since the brain parenchyma is relatively incompressible, cerebrospinal fluid (CSF) and cerebral blood volume play an integral role in accommodating increases in ICP.

9 The most commonly used modalities of evoked potential monitoring are somatosensory evoked potentials, motor evoked potentials, and electromyography, with brainstem auditory evoked potentials and visual evoked potentials being less commonly used. Anesthetic drugs play a major role in facilitating the success of intraoperative evoked potential monitoring.

10 Reliable pharmacologic and nonpharmacologic therapies to prevent neuronal ischemic injury are currently not readily available for use in the perioperative period. At the present time, one can only hope to attenuate injury by preventing secondary insults to surrounding neuronal tissue (e.g., ensuring adequate oxygen and substrate delivery).

11 The preoperative evaluation of the neurosurgical patient is of paramount importance to ensure a safe and successful anesthetic. Specific problems must be identified so as to formulate appropriate plans for intraoperative and postoperative management. For patients with intracranial mass lesions, the most important fact to ascertain is the presence and extent of intracranial hypertension and this should be assumed until information proves otherwise. Choice of drugs for maintenance of general anesthesia depends to a great extent on the ICP and whether neuromonitoring is being employed.

Introduction

Neuroanesthesia is the practice of perioperative medicine related to the treatment of diseases or injury to the central nervous system (CNS) or peripheral nervous system (PNS). The CNS encompasses the brain and spinal cord, whereas the PNS includes all of the peripheral nerves of the body emanating from the brain and spinal cord. As such, neuroanesthesia is the provision of anesthesia and analgesia for a multitude of procedures, including invasive, minimally invasive, neurodiagnostic, and neurointerventional procedures, and involving the brain, spinal cord, and peripheral nerves.

Neuroanatomy

The CNS is composed of the brain and the spinal cord. The brain is enclosed by the cranium, a fixed bony cavity, and is physically and functionally divided into two compartments: the supratentorium and the infratentorium (Fig. 37-1). The supratentorium contains the paired cerebral hemispheres and the diencephalon that is composed of the thalamus and hypothalamus. Each cerebral hemisphere is divided into four lobes (frontal, temporal, parietal, and occipital). Eloquent cortical areas are generally considered to be regions responsible for gross motor function and language. The primary somatosensory and motor cortex strips lie adjacent to the central sulcus in the parietal and frontal lobes, respectively, and extend inferiorly to the Sylvian fissure. Cortical regions that are responsible for language are located in the left hemisphere in almost all right-handed people as well as in the majority of left-handed people. The two primary regions responsible for language are Broca area, located in the premotor frontal cortex and responsible for language formation, and Wernicke area, located in the posterior superior temporal cortex and responsible for language acquisition. Lesions in Broca area lead to expressive aphasia whereas those in Wernicke area cause receptive aphasia.

The extrapyramidal system consists of a group of brain structures that modify motor function but are not components of the corticospinal tract and primary motor cortex. These structures include the basal ganglia (comprised of the caudate nucleus, globus pallidus, putamen, substantia nigra, and red nucleus), cerebellum, and components of the auditory and vestibular pathways. Dysfunction of structures in the extrapyramidal system results in difficulty with motor control without frank weakness, which includes Parkinson disease, essential tremor, and ataxia.

The diencephalon lies cephalad to the midbrain and is composed of the thalamus and hypothalamus. The thalamus acts as a sensory and motor "relay station," functionally and physically connecting the cortex with the rest of the nervous system. The hypothalamus, lying below the thalamus, has autonomic and endocrine functions and is connected to the pituitary gland via the infundibulum.

The limbic system consists of a group of structures that play a role in cognitive function, memory consolidation, and emotional

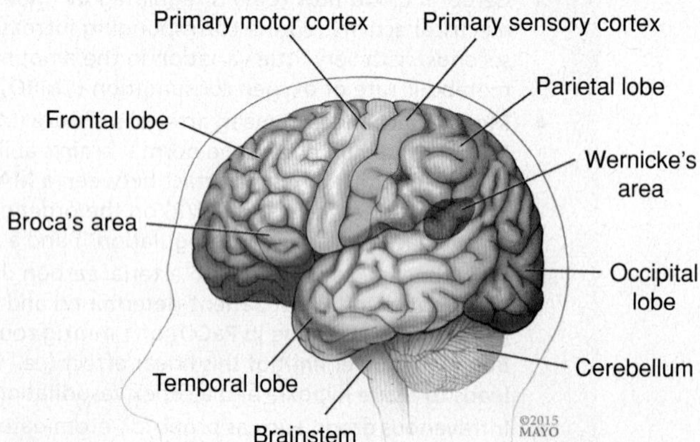

Figure 37-1 Gross anatomy of the brain. (Used with permission of Mayo Foundation for Medical Education and Research, all rights reserved.)

responses. Components of the limbic system include, but are not limited to, the hippocampus, amygdala, part of the hypothalamus, and some regions of the cortex (e.g., insular region). The hypothalamus, although generally considered a component of the diencephalon, also functions in the limbic system due to its role in the regulation of autonomic and endocrine function in addition to modulation of behavior and sexual function.

The infratentorium encompasses the brainstem and the cerebellum. The brainstem is comprised of the midbrain, pons, and medulla and is responsible for consciousness via the reticular activating system, a variety of autonomic functions including respiratory and cardiovascular control, and many reflexes (e.g., cough/gag, pupillary reflexes). The brainstem contains nuclei for cranial nerves III to XII. The cerebellum, among the most rudimentary parts of the brain, lies in the posterior fossa and is responsible for such actions as processing proprioceptive input and establishing axial posture and gait.

1 The brain receives approximately 70% of its blood supply from two internal carotid arteries anteriorly and 30% from two vertebral arteries posteriorly forming the basilar artery, that subsequently converge to form the circle of Willis, an anastomotic ring at the base of the skull (Fig. 37-2). The common carotid artery, originating from the aortic arch, divides at the level of the thyroid cartilage into the internal and external carotid arteries. The internal carotid artery traverses the skull base through the foramen lacerum and subsequently travels through the cavernous sinus and into the carotid groove. Thereafter, the artery divides into the posterior communicating artery (PCOM), the anterior cerebral artery (ACA), and the middle cerebral artery (MCA).

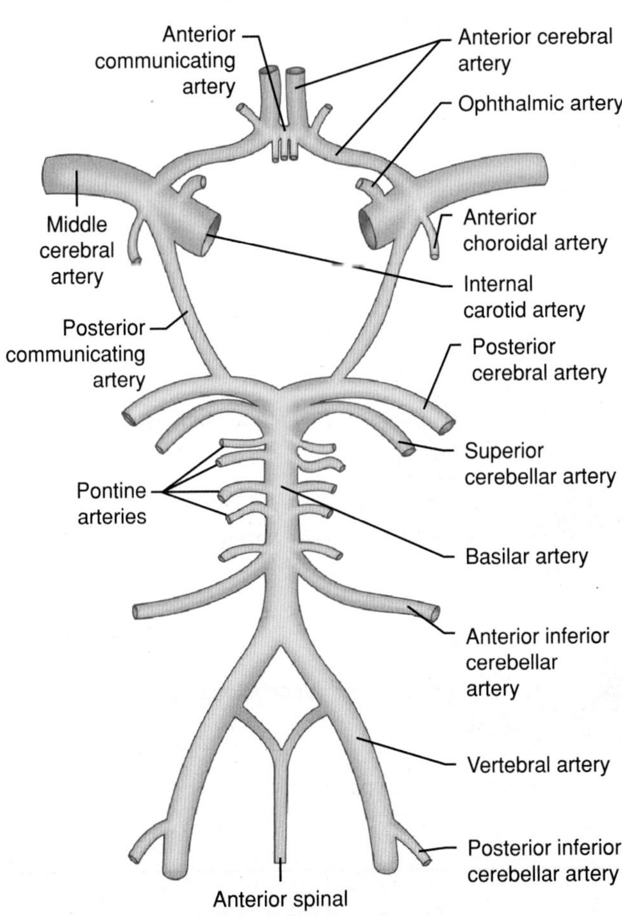

Figure 37-2 The circle of Willis, demonstrating the anterior and posterior blood supply to the brain.

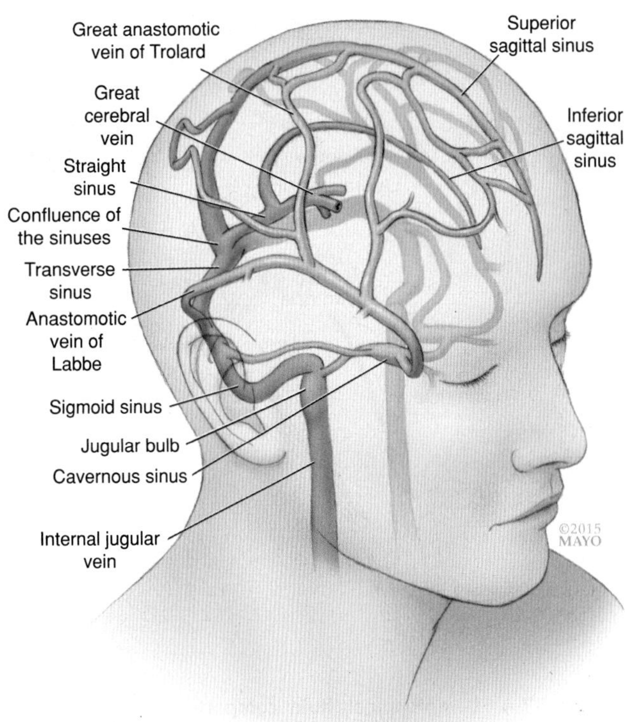

Figure 37-3 Gross anatomy of the venous drainage system of the brain, including the major venous sinuses. (Used with permission of Mayo Foundation for Medical Education and Research, all rights reserved.)

The bilateral vertebral arteries originate from the subclavian arteries and converge to form the basilar artery at the pontomedullary junction. When reaching the midbrain (along the ventral surface of the brainstem), the basilar artery divides into the posterior cerebral arteries (PCAs) and also anastomoses with the PCOMs, thus completing the circle of Willis. Interestingly, less than 50% of people demonstrate a "complete" circle of Willis.

The venous system of the brain consists of both deep and superficial veins that ultimately drain into the dural venous sinuses (Fig. 37-3). These sinuses are valveless endothelialized channels lying between the dura mater and skull periosteum. All of the sinuses eventually drain into the sigmoid sinus and thereafter into the internal jugular veins.

The entire CNS is insulated from its bony encasement by cerebrospinal fluid (CSF) that is produced mostly by the choroid plexus of the lateral and third ventricles (Fig. 37-4). The average volume of CSF in an adult is approximately 150 mL. CSF is created at a rate of 15 to 20 mL/h and moves from these ventricles via the aqueduct of Sylvius to the fourth ventricle. From there, CSF flows out of the fourth ventricle via the foramen of Magendie and the lateral foramina of Luschka to the subarachnoid space in the cranium. It does so via a series of interconnected cisterns at the base of the brain, to be subsequently reabsorbed into the dural venous sinuses, primarily the superior sagittal sinus, via arachnoid villi and granulations. Some CSF traverses the foramen magnum, entering the subarachnoid space within the spinal column.

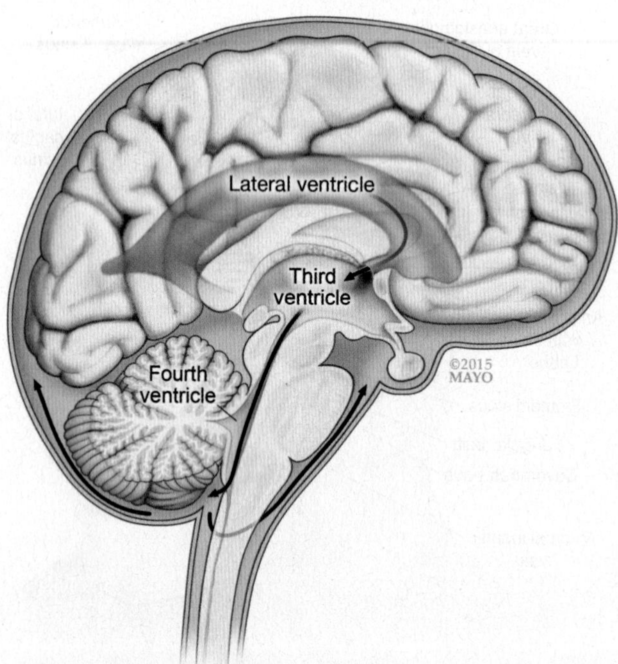

Figure 37-4 Cerebrospinal fluid compartments within and around the brain. This includes the ventricular system and gross cerebral spinal fluid flow patterns. (Used with permission of Mayo Foundation for Medical Education and Research, all rights reserved.)

This movement of CSF is important for acute and chronic compensation in elevated ICP states.

The spinal column is composed of 33 vertebrae (7 cervical, 12 thoracic, 5 lumbar, and 9 fused sacral and coccygeal), with nerve roots leaving the enclosed spinal cord and exiting through corresponding intervertebral foramina. The spinal cord itself is composed of central gray matter, the dorsal columns containing tracts responsible for proprioception and light touch, lateral spinothalamic tracts responsible for pain and temperature, and outer white matter containing the lateral corticospinal tracts (Fig. 37-5). The lateral gray columns contain the cell bodies of the preganglionic neurons that eventually enter the sympathetic chain (running on either side of the vertebral bodies), arising from T1 to L2 or L3. The spinal cord itself terminates at L1 or L2 in adults, ending in structures known as the conus medullaris terminus and filum terminale.

The spinal cord receives its blood supply from one anterior spinal artery and two posterior spinal arteries (Fig. 37-6). The anterior spinal artery originates from six to eight major radicular arteries derived from the aorta, with the largest one being the artery of Adamkiewicz (usually occurring at T11 or T12 and generally supplying T8 to the conus medullaris terminus). Thus, the artery of Adamkiewicz is responsible for supplying arterial blood to the anterior two-thirds of the spinal cord. The posterior spinal arteries originate from the posterior cerebral circulation and supply the dorsal horns and white matter (posterior third of the spinal cord).

Various regions of the brain and spinal cord responsible for distinct functions are shown in Table 37-1.

2

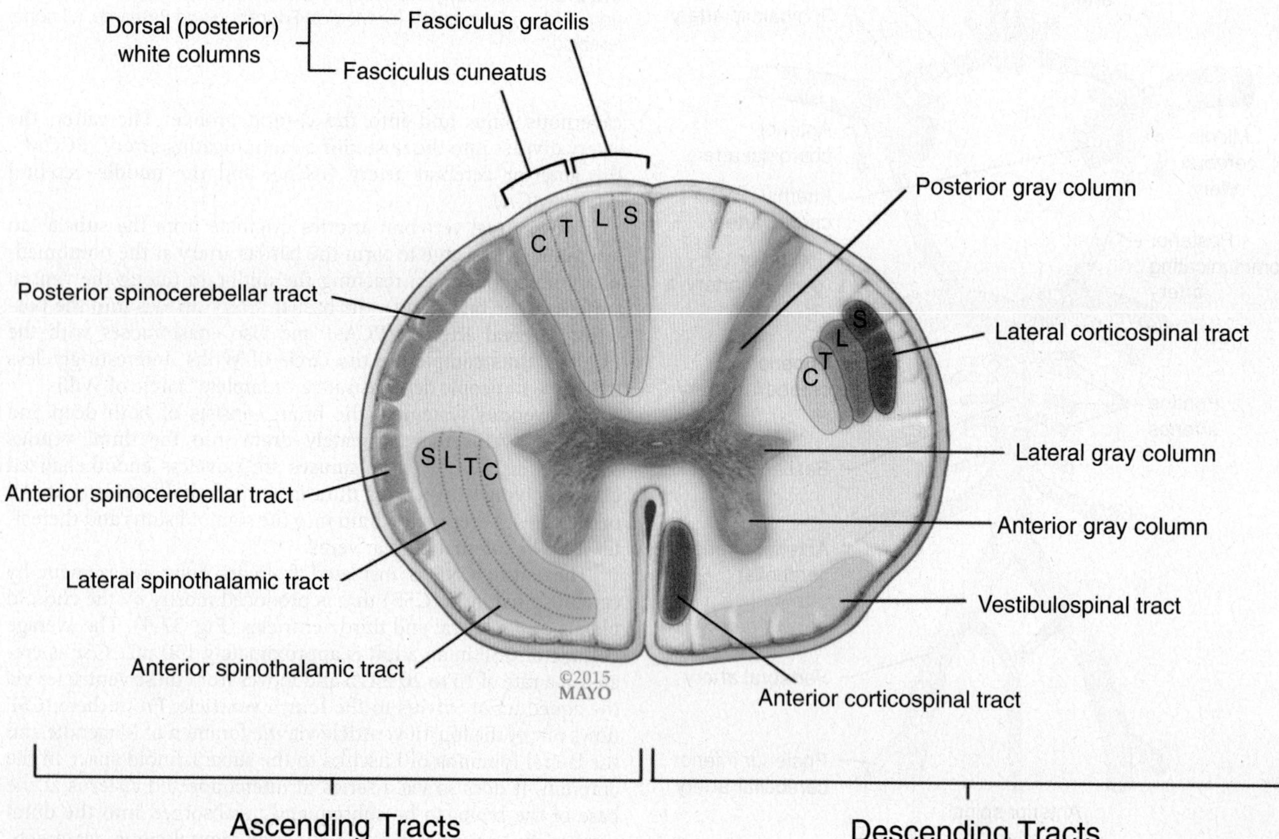

Figure 37-5 Major ascending and descending spinal cord tracts (cross-section). C, cervical; T, thoracic; L, lumbar; and S, sacral. (Used with permission of Mayo Foundation for Medical Education and Research, all rights reserved.)

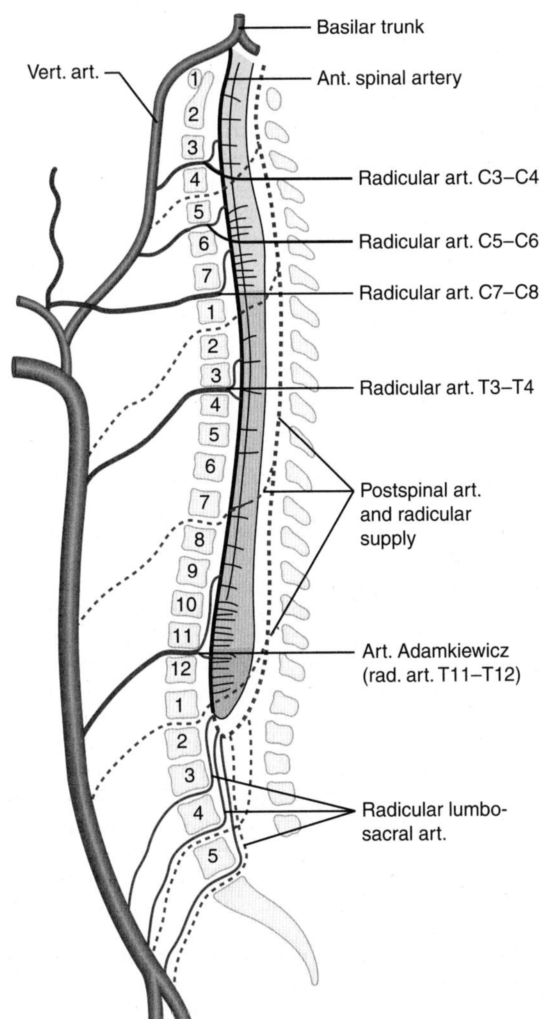

Figure 37-6 The spinal cord blood supply. Note that the cervical spine is served by the posterior circulation emanating from the circle of Willis.

Neurophysiology

Although the adult brain accounts for only 2% of total body weight, it is responsible for 20% of total body oxygen consumption and 25% of total body glucose consumption. The cerebral metabolic rate of oxygen consumption ($CMRO_2$) is normally 3 to 3.8 mL/100 g/min and brain glucose consumption is approximately 5 mg/100 g/min. Normal cerebral blood flow (CBF) is 50 mL/100 g/min or 750 mL/min. Therefore, the brain receives about 15% of the cardiac output to meet these high metabolic requirements. The brain depends on a continuous supply of oxygen and glucose, with irreversible injury potentially occurring after only 4 to 5 minutes of global ischemia.[1]

CBF is regulated by "flow-metabolism coupling," whereby 3
increases in regional neuronal electrical activity require corresponding increases in regional blood flow. Such coupling occurs on the order of seconds, with very little variation in the amount of oxygen extraction by the brain tissue (i.e., CBF matches $CMRO_2$ very quickly and efficiently in the healthy brain).

CPP is the difference between mean arterial pressure (MAP) 4
and either intracranial pressure (ICP) or central venous pressure (CVP), depending on which is higher. CBF itself is equal to CPP/cerebrovascular resistance (CVR). Fortunately, even moderate changes in MAP (or CPP) will yield a consistent CBF of 50 mL/100 g/min, due to the normal brain's ability to autoregulate its blood flow. Cerebral autoregulation of blood flow is thought to remain intact between a MAP of approximately 60 to 160 mmHg and functions by altering CVR on the order of 5 to 60 seconds (Fig. 37-7). However, the lower limit of autoregulation (LLA) is likely to be not only higher than a MAP of 60 mmHg but also dynamic throughout the day and differs among individuals. In those with otherwise healthy brains, the LLA may be as high as a MAP of 80 mmHg in some individuals.[2] The alteration in CVR is accomplished in both a rapid phase ("dynamic autoregulation") and a slow phase ("static autoregulation"). Dynamic autoregulation is thought to respond to pulsatility changes more closely linked to the systolic systemic blood pressure, whereas static autoregulation is a phenomenon that accommodates to changes in MAP over longer time intervals.[3] Above the upper limit of autoregulation and below the LLA, CBF is pressure dependent. Below the LLA maximal cerebral vasodilation occurs and cerebral

Table 37-1 Functionality of CNS Structures

Anatomic Location	Structure	Function
Postcentral gyrus	Primary somatosensory cortex	Sensation
Precentral gyrus	Primary motor cortex	Movement
Occipital lobe	Primary visual cortex	Vision
Temporal lobe	Primary auditory cortex	Hearing
Wernicke area (angular gyrus of dominant hemisphere)	Primary language association cortex	Language
Broca area (frontal lobe of dominant hemisphere)	Primary language expression cortex	Language
Frontal lobe	Primary personality cortex	Personality/Intellect
Temporal lobe	Limbic cortex	Emotion
Temporal lobe	Hippocampus	Memory
Diencephalon	Hypothalamus	Vegetative regulation
Brain stem	Reticular activating system	Consciousness
Brain stem	Vasomotor center	Circulatory/respiratory control
Spinal cord	Dorsal horn (sensory)/ventral horn (motor)	Movement/sensation/reflexes

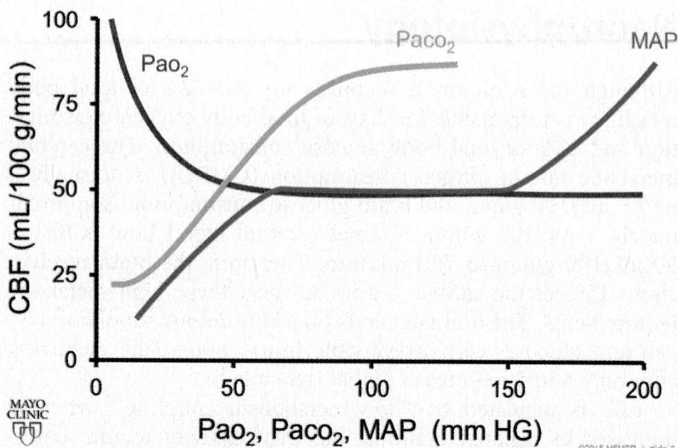

Figure 37-7 Autoregulation in the central nervous system: cerebral blood flow (CBF) remains constant between mean arterial pressures (MAP) of approximately 60 to 160 mmHg (*blue*). CBF varies linearly between arterial carbon dioxide partial pressures ($PaCO_2$) of 20 to 80 mmHg (*green*). Cerebral blood flow remains constant above an arterial oxygen partial pressure (PaO_2) of 50 mmHg (*red*). (Used with permission of Mayo Foundation for Medical Education and Research, all rights reserved.)

ischemia can result. Above the upper limit of autoregulation, cerebral vessels are maximally vasoconstricted and increases in perfusion pressure may lead to disruption of the blood–brain barrier (BBB), cerebral edema, or cerebral hemorrhage. CVR changes responsible for CBF autoregulation are the result of myogenic tone changes in response to transmural pressure changes in small arteries and arterioles, neurogenic forces where neuroglial cells secrete neurotransmitters with vasoactive properties that contribute to the diameter of moderate- and small-diameter vessels, metabolic responses in local microenvironments that alter vasomotor response in small vessels, and endothelial responses that impact cerebrovascular tone from endothelial paracrine signals.[3] The autoregulatory curve is shifted rightward in cases of chronic hypertension. Anesthetics, especially the potent volatile anesthetics, have a dose-dependent effect of decreasing the extent of autoregulation.

5 Besides MAP, other physiologic parameters play an important role in regulating CBF. Arterial carbon dioxide tension ($PaCO_2$) is the most important of these variables. CBF is linearly associated with $PaCO_2$ between 20 and 80 mmHg (Fig. 37-7). Hyper- and hypoventilation, both patient determined and iatrogenic, play critical roles in decreasing or increasing CBF, respectively. A change in $PaCO_2$ of 1 mmHg roughly correlates to a similar change in CBF of 1 to 2 mL/100 g/min. Below the lower limit of this linear effect (i.e., with $PaCO_2$ below 20 mmHg), maximal cerebral vasoconstriction leads to tissue hypoxia and a reflex vasodilation. This phenomenon is the basis for spontaneous hyperventilation that develops in response to acutely elevated ICP. This beneficial reflex, however, can be detrimental as low regional CBF and ischemia can occur.[4] Furthermore, the effect of hyperventilation on CBF and ICP is only sustainable for approximately 6 hours, as the pH of the CSF will renormalize.

Oxygen tension in the arterial blood (PaO_2) has minimal effect on CBF unless marked hypoxemia (PaO_2 <50 mmHg) occurs, below which CBF increases dramatically (Fig. 37-7). When PaO_2 is greater than 350 mmHg, slight cerebral vasoconstriction can occur. It is unclear why this reflex occurs, but it may be a method by which the brain protects itself from "oxygen toxicity" (i.e., oxygen-free radical formation). Temperature is also an important determinant of CBF, with a 6% to 7% decrease in CBF per 1°C decrease in core temperature.

Regional CBF is more complex than global CBF (as described earlier) and is governed by both humoral and neurogenic factors. Certain circulating catecholamines and other mediators such as α_1-adrenergic agonists, ionic calcium, endothelin, and thromboxane A_2 may have cerebral vasoconstrictive effects, whereas other factors such as β_2-adrenergic agonists, nitric oxide, adenosine, and prostaglandins play a role in regional cerebral vasodilation.[5,6] Neurogenic influences over local regulation of CBF include effects mediated by the release of acetylcholine, dopamine, serotonin, and substance P.

Anesthetics can have profound effects on CBF. Intravenous drugs, such as propofol, etomidate, benzodiazepines, and barbiturates, decrease CBF by virtue of a drug-induced decrease in $CMRO_2$ and subsequent flow-metabolism coupling. Autoregulation and $PaCO_2$ responsiveness remain intact with these agents. Opioids have very little effect on $CMRO_2$, CBF, autoregulation, or $PaCO_2$ responsiveness. Ketamine is unique in that it increases CBF and $CMRO_2$, with little effect on autoregulation or $PaCO_2$ responsiveness.[7] 6

Potent volatile anesthetics, such as isoflurane, sevoflurane, and desflurane are direct cerebral vasodilators. However, this direct vasodilation is offset by a drug-induced decrease in $CMRO_2$, and via flow-metabolism coupling, an attenuation of the direct effect on CBF. These effects lead to minimal, if any, increase in CBF at lower doses. However, at high doses where maximal suppression of $CMRO_2$ has occurred, direct vasodilatory effects are observed leading to a dose-dependent increase in CBF.[8] Furthermore, autoregulation is inhibited with potent volatile anesthetic drugs in a dose-dependent fashion, although the cerebral vasculature remains responsive to changes in $PaCO_2$. Nitrous oxide is a direct cerebral vasodilator and causes minimal effect on $CMRO_2$.[9] Nitrous oxide may have a variable effect on cerebral autoregulatory capacity leading to preserved autoregulation during propofol anesthesia but further impairment of autoregulation during sevoflurane anesthesia. 7

Spinal cord physiology is very similar to brain physiology in that autoregulation is maintained and spinal cord perfusion pressure (SCPP) = MAP − SSSP (spinal subarachnoid space pressure). The specific effects of different anesthetic drugs on spinal cord physiology are not as well characterized as the effects of these drugs on the brain.

Pathophysiology

ICP is the pressure within the intracranial cavity, which is a closed vault containing the brain parenchyma (1,400 mL), CSF (150 mL), and the cerebral blood volume (CBV) (150 mL). The Monro–Kellie doctrine states that "an increase in the volume of one intracranial compartment will lead to a rise in ICP unless it is matched by an equal reduction in the volume of another compartment."[10] Since the brain parenchyma is relatively incompressible, CSF and CBV play an integral role in accommodating increases in ICP. CSF will tend to egress out of the cranial cavity and into the spinal subarachnoid space, whereas CBV will be decreased by both a reflex arterial vasoconstriction and increased venous efflux from the brain and venous sinuses. Since these compartments are relatively low in volume, their ability to compensate for large increases in ICP is greatly limited. When these compensatory effects are exhausted, a small increase in volume can lead to a dramatic increase in the pressure within the cranium (Fig. 37-8). The results can be neurologically devastating with impaired perfusion and possible herniation of the brain. Herniation can cause irreversible brain injury or even death. Hence, meticulous care in those patients in whom elevated ICP is suspected is critical. 8

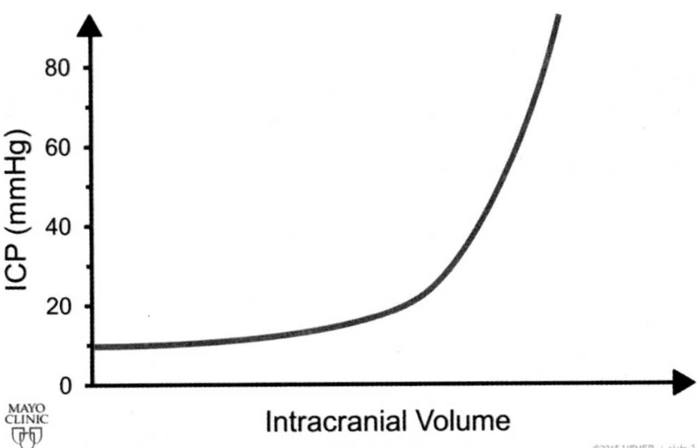

Figure 37-8 Intracranial elastance curve. The intracranial elastance curve is composed of three sections. Intracranial pressure (ICP) remains low and relatively constant at low volumes until the "elbow" of the curve is reached. At this point, small changes in volume lead to moderate changes in pressure. When a critical intracranial volume is reached, the pressure increases precipitously. (Used with permission of Mayo Foundation for Medical Education and Research, all rights reserved.)

Precautions include avoiding hypoventilation, maintaining adequate CPP, implementing techniques to reduce intracranial volume (i.e., mannitol, CSF diversion, cerebral vasoconstricting anesthetics), and considering decompressive craniectomy.

Normal ICP is 7 to 15 mmHg. Poor neurologic outcome is associated with prolonged ICP above 20 to 25 mmHg. Normal ICP is subject to fluctuation with such activities as the Valsalva maneuver or patient position. Kety and Schmidt demonstrated in 1948 that increases in ICP can lead to CBF reduction, which led many investigators to question the safe management of elevated ICP in terms of its effects on cerebral ischemia.[11]

The intracranial elastance curve is quite useful in visualizing the ICP–volume relationship (1 Video 37-1). The initial "flat part of the curve," where intracranial elastance is low, demonstrates that in nonpathologic brain states, changes in intracranial volume are compensated for quite easily by CSF and CBV buffering. When this compensation is exhausted ("elbow of the curve") and elastance increases, small increases in volume lead to rapid rises in ICP. Cerebral elastance ($E = dP/dV$) can be estimated with invasive cerebral and spinal monitoring devices (e.g., lumbar drain, extraventricular drain).

Elevated ICP may be caused by a variety of pathophysiologic mechanisms. The most common contributing factor to increased ICP is cerebral edema. Edema in the brain is generally classified into three major types: cytotoxic, vasogenic, and interstitial. Cytotoxic edema is characterized by increased *intracellular* water. This commonly occurs in the setting of cerebral ischemia, where failure of membrane ionic pumps leads to accumulation of ions, and thus water, within cells. Vasogenic edema occurs when there is loss of integrity of the BBB, leading to accumulation of extracellular water. Vasogenic edema commonly occurs in regions of brain surrounding tumors, abscesses, or contusions. Dexamethasone is effective at decreasing only vasogenic edema, due in part to its effect at upregulating expression of proteins responsible for the integrity of the tight junctions between endothelial cells in the brain.[12] Interstitial edema is characterized by increased extracellular fluid in the setting of an intact BBB. Interstitial edema occurs in patients with hydrocephalus due to permeation of CSF into the interstitial space and in those with a significant osmotic difference between the brain interstitial space and the intravascular space as occurs in acute hyponatremia. In many circumstances, cerebral edema may be due to a combination of cytotoxic, vasogenic, and interstitial edema.

In addition to edema, there are a variety of other causes that can contribute to intracranial hypertension. Increased CBV, because of either increased arterial inflow or decreased venous efflux, can lead to increases in ICP. Increased arterial inflow is due to cerebral arterial vasodilation from factors such as use of vasodilatory drugs, hypercapnia, severe hypoxemia, or acidosis and decreased venous efflux can be caused by jugular venous obstruction, or elevated pressures within the airways. Likewise, inadequate CSF absorption, due to diminished absorption at the arachnoid villi as may occur with subarachnoid hemorrhage (SAH) or obstructive hydrocephalus as may occur with tumor, can cause hydrocephalus and elevated ICP. Last, mass effect from tumors, hematomas, or abscesses can elevate ICP by a direct space-occupying effect.

Clinical symptoms of intracranial hypertension include headache, nausea, vomiting, and papilledema. As ICP continues to increase, Cushing triad, consisting of hypertension, bradycardia, irregular respiration, may appear. Patients risk brain herniation and death with very severe intracranial hypertension. The signs of herniation will depend on the structures that are herniating and may include pupillary dilation, oculomotor weakness, absent pupillary light reflex, and cardiorespiratory arrest. Radiologically, computed tomography (CT) is most commonly used, and ICP elevation may manifest itself as effacement of sulci, compression of the ventricles, midline shift, or even ventriculomegaly, depending on the etiology.

Acute spinal cord injury is distinctly different from chronic spinal cord injury. Although both may involve loss of sensory, motor, and possibly autonomic function below the level of injury, flaccid paralysis and hypotension are evident in the acute phase whereas spastic paralysis, pain, and possible risk for autonomic hyperreflexia are observed in the chronic phase. Acute spinal cord compression, due to trauma or tumor, is usually a surgical emergency, as time to decompression has been correlated with functional outcome in some populations.[13] The role of steroids in preventing secondary injury is much more controversial.[14] Cervical injuries necessitate extremely careful management of the airway, and these injuries are associated with more physiologic perturbations than lower injuries, including diaphragmatic paralysis, cardiac disturbances, and death.

Monitoring

Central Nervous System Function

The most important monitor of CNS function is the neurologic examination of an awake and responsive patient. Although some neurosurgical procedures are specifically performed with mild sedation, most are performed in patients who receive general anesthesia. In this latter circumstance, other modes to monitor the integrity of the nervous system may be necessary. Electrophysiologic monitoring techniques are commonly used in the operating room to assess the functional integrity of the nervous system during surgeries that might put neurologic structures at risk. There is some agreement that these monitoring techniques can detect reversible changes in neurologic function in the patient during general anesthesia, allowing a surgical or physiologic change of plan that may avert permanent neurologic injury. However, there is a paucity of definitive data in the form of randomized controlled trials to prove that such monitoring will prevent neurologic injury and improve outcomes.[15]

The most commonly used modalities of intraoperative neu- 9
rophysiologic monitoring are somatosensory evoked potentials

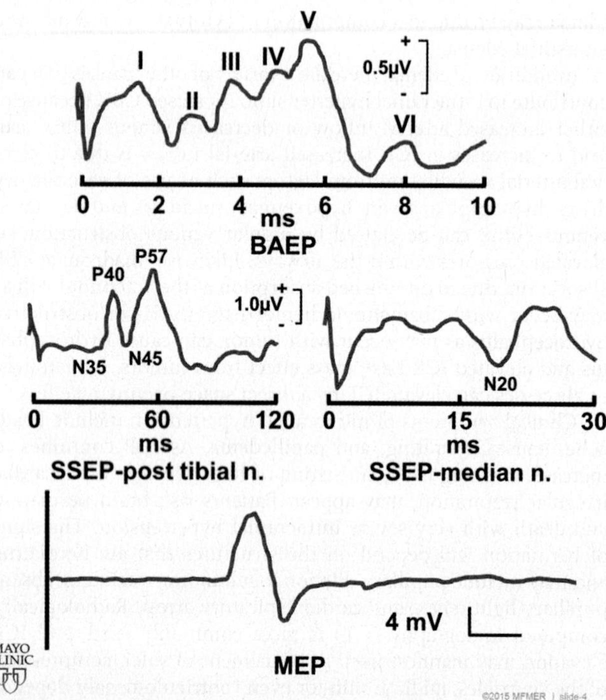

Figure 37-9 Representative brainstem auditory evoked potential (BAEP), somatosensory evoked potential (SSEP), and motor evoked potential (MEP) tracings. (Used with permission of Mayo Foundation for Medical Education and Research, all rights reserved.)

(SSEPs), motor evoked potentials (MEPs), and electromyography (EMG), with brainstem auditory evoked potentials (BAEPs) and visual evoked potentials (VEPs) being less commonly used (Fig. 37-9, NICV 37-1). The peaks and troughs of evoked potential waveforms can be characterized by two parameters: amplitude and latency. Amplitude, measured in microvolts (for SSEPs and BAEPs) or microvolts or millivolts (for MEPs), refers to the measured signal voltage of a peak relative to a baseline voltage or an adjacent peak. Latency, usually measured in milliseconds, refers to the delay in peak signal following stimulation and reflects transit time along the neural pathway.

SSEPs are elicited in a cyclical, repetitive manner from a peripheral nerve (e.g., median, ulnar, posterior tibial) and usually measured at the level of the subcortex (upper cervical spine, inion) and cortex (scalp). Stimuli predominantly travel via the posterior column/medial lemniscus pathway in the CNS. This modality is especially useful for monitoring the integrity of the peripheral nerves, dorsal columns of the spinal cord, the brainstem, the subcortex, and the sensory cortex of the brain. Any insult to this pathway may alter the SSEP response. Since sensory tracts decussate at the brainstem before proceeding through the thalamus and up to the sensory cortex, stimuli are recorded on the contralateral scalp. Notably, SSEPs are inherently small in amplitude, requiring a prolonged stimulation time, signal averaging, conversion from analog to digital format, and signal filtration to achieve a stable waveform. Therefore, it may take minutes to obtain a waveform. Muscle relaxants may be helpful as they tend to remove artifact caused by spontaneous EMG activity. SSEPs are commonly used during spine surgery, especially when posterolateral sensory elements are at risk of ischemia from surgical distraction. They may also be useful during neurovascular brain surgery to ensure sufficient perfusion to the somatosensory cortex during procedures that may put this cortex at risk, such as cerebral aneurysm clipping. Lower extremity SSEPs tend to correlate with the integrity of cortex supplied by the ACA whereas upper extremity SSEPs tend to correlate with the cortex supplied by the MCA distribution. The commonly used definitions of "significant changes" to the SSEP waveform include a decrease in the amplitude by 50% or an increase in the latency by 10% although experienced practitioners consider baseline drift and reproducibility and adapt warning criterion to account for these changes.[16]

MEPs are produced at the level of the cortex by direct stimulation of the cerebral cortex or by indirect stimulation of the scalp. MEP signals are usually measured as compound muscle action potentials (CMAPs) at the muscular level. MEPs are useful for assessing the motor cortex and the anterolateral spinal cord (containing the corticospinal tracts) during surgeries that may put these structures at risk. Stimulation may be performed magnetically or electrically, with the latter being the more common method. Indirect electrical stimulation of the motor cortex, via scalp electrodes, is performed, usually in a single pulse or train of pulses that travels caudad and depolarizes the upper motor neurons in the spinal cord, summating in the ventral horn. From here, the signal travels to the α-motor neurons via the internuncial pathways, descending to the motor endplates, where muscle movement related to an action potential can be measured. Unlike SSEPs, MEPs do not require signal averaging or filtration and are produced by a single pulse or train of a few pulses requiring only seconds. Measurement of a response in muscles is severely inhibited by muscle relaxants. MEPs are useful during spine surgery, especially when anterior elements are at risk, and during intracranial surgery during procedures where the motor cortex or descending motor pathway are at risk for injury or ischemia. Although there is no formal definition of "significant changes" that warrant concern for altered neural pathway function, a decrease in amplitude of 50% is considered "significant" as is a need to increase the stimulation intensity required to maintain a reproducible signal. Latency of MEPs has much less of a role in defining a worrisome change than with SSEPs.

EMG is a monitoring modality that is used to continually assess the integrity of distinct peripheral or cranial nerves or nerve roots. Spontaneous neural electrical activity can be monitored or, in stimulated EMG, electrical current can be induced in a nerve and then that signal can be detected as a means to monitor nerve integrity or identify a nerve. EMG is sensitive to both mechanical and thermal injury. EMG, unlike SSEPs and MEPs, is not a monitor of ischemia. Needle electrodes are placed in a muscle known to be innervated by a particular nerve root, and if that nerve root is disturbed, EMG activity is recorded from that muscle. For example, EMG can be monitored in muscles innervated by spinal nerves during spine surgery or in muscles innervated by cranial nerves during various intracranial procedures that may put cranial nerves at risk, such as during acoustic neuroma resection. In addition, a surgeon may use stimulated EMG to identify cranial nerves during surgery. "Triggered EMG," as is commonly performed with pedicle screw testing during spine surgery, relies on direct stimulation of the screws being placed within the bony pedicle. If there is disruption of the bony pedicle, and hence contact or near contact between the screw and neural elements, the amount of current necessary to stimulate the corresponding nerve root will be much less than if the pedicle were intact.[17] Like MEPs, EMG is particularly sensitive to the effects of muscle relaxants.

BAEPs are used to assess the integrity of the auditory canal, tympanic membrane, hair cells, spiral ganglion, vestibulocochlear nerve (cranial nerve VIII), cochlear nuclei, superior olivary complex, lateral lemniscus, inferior colliculus, and medial geniculate thalamic nuclei. A device that produces auditory stimuli (i.e., clicking sounds) is placed in the external auditory canal and responses are recorded from the scalp. Thousands of signals are averaged, yielding a typical waveform consisting of six waves. In general, any injury to cranial nerve VIII will affect all of the waves after wave I, decreasing their amplitude and prolonging their latency. Retraction on the cerebellum may prolong the latency of the tracing between waves I and V. BAEPs are often performed during surgery at or near the brainstem such as microvascular decompression of cranial nerves V or VII or for acoustic neuroma resection. Fortunately, BAEPs are extremely robust with little effect from any anesthetic regimen.

VEPs are used to assess the integrity of the visual pathway, including the eye, optic nerve, optic chiasm, and visual cortex in the occipital lobe. A bright stimulus is applied to the eyes using special goggles or contact lenses, and responses are recorded from scalp electrodes. VEPs may be useful during surgery at or near the optic chiasm or the occipital cortex. Unfortunately, VEPs are exquisitely sensitive to almost any anesthetic regimen and the difficulty in the ability to obtain and interpret the signals make them very infrequently used, although technologic advances have led to more reported successful intraoperative use.[18]

Influence of Anesthetic Technique on Evoked Potentials

Anesthetic drugs play a major role in facilitating the success of intraoperative evoked potential monitoring. With regard to cortical SSEPs, potent volatile anesthetics and nitrous oxide have the greatest inhibitory effect causing a decrease in amplitude and an increase in wave latency. These drugs may limit the acquisition of robust SSEP signals, doing so in a nearly linear dose-dependent fashion. Robust signals can, however, usually be obtained in neurologically intact patients with up to 0.5 minimum alveolar concentration (MAC) of inhaled agent.[19] In neurologically impaired patients, such as those with peripheral neuropathy, total intravenous anesthesia (TIVA) might be required and is commonly performed with a hypnotic (e.g., propofol) and an opioid infusion. Nitrous oxide has more of a depressant effect on signal amplitude rather than latency. Intravenous anesthetics such as propofol tend to have a very limited effect on SSEPs, unless administered in very high doses. Likewise, opioids tend to increase latency and decrease amplitude of SSEPs, especially with bolus administration, but they have minimal clinically significant impact on SSEPs.[20] Etomidate and ketamine are exceptions in that they actually can increase cortical amplitudes at clinical doses and have been used to enhance SSEP waveforms. Muscle relaxants are generally beneficial for SSEP monitoring as they eliminate myogenic interference. Last, it is important to note that these anesthetic effects are much less prominent with regard to subcortical, cervical, and peripheral signal acquisition, as these areas are much more resistant to the inhibitory effects of anesthesia.[21]

MEPs elicited from the scalp are exquisitely sensitive to the effects of anesthesia. Potent volatile anesthetics are greatly inhibitory to the acquisition of MEPs, though doses of 0.5 MAC can still be used in most cases. Above this concentration, a nonlinear and greatly accelerated suppression of MEP amplitudes occurs. As with SSEPs, nitrous oxide depresses MEP amplitudes. Intravenous anesthetics are generally conducive to MEP acquisition, except at very high doses. As such, TIVA is commonly employed when MEPs are being monitored, and TIVA should especially be used when difficulty in obtaining adequate baseline MEPS is anticipated, such as in patients with neuromuscular deficits.[21] Like SSEPs, ketamine and etomidate may improve MEP amplitudes and lower the electrical threshold required to obtain a response, although higher bolus doses have been reported to decrease MEP amplitudes.[22,23] Muscle relaxants must be given very judiciously or avoided completely so as not to abolish the MEP response or prohibitively increase its variability, rendering it difficult to follow over time.

Muscle relaxants can impair or, with deep neuromuscular blockade, abolish, EMG signals. Inhaled and intravenous anesthetics have very little effect on the acquisition of spontaneous or "triggered" EMG. Hence, it is wise to avoid muscle relaxation or reverse the effects of muscle relaxants prior to pedicle screw testing or cranial nerve identification.

BAEPs, as mentioned earlier, are quite robust regardless of the anesthetic regimen being used. Small increases in latency can be seen with deep inhalational or intravenous anesthesia. Notably, cold irrigation fluids at the brainstem will also cause some increases in interwave latencies.

VEPs are the most sensitive neuromonitoring modality with regard to anesthesia. Inhalational-based anesthetics, with and without nitrous oxide, are more inhibitory to VEPs than TIVA techniques in general. One proposed anesthetic technique for facilitating VEP monitoring might involve an opioid-based TIVA with muscle relaxants and BIS monitoring although other techniques may be used.[18,24]

Cerebral Perfusion

Transcranial Doppler Ultrasonography

Transcranial Doppler ultrasonography (TCD) is a tool used in neurology, neurosurgery, and neurocritical care. An ultrasound probe is placed over a "window" that is a thinner region of the cranium, such as the temporal bone above the zygomatic arch, to measure blood flow velocities in major cerebral vessels, including the MCA, PCA, and ACA and the basilar artery. The ultrasound probe emits a high-frequency sound wave that reflects off red blood cells and returns to the probe at a different frequency determined by the Doppler Effect. Specifically, the velocity of blood cells relative to the ultrasound probe will cause a change in the frequency of ultrasound waves that are reflected back to the probe. This "Doppler shift" is proportional to the velocity of blood and the sign (positive or negative) of the Doppler shift is determined by direction of blood flow. Positive (increase in frequency) occurs when blood is moving toward the probe and negative (decrease in frequency) occurs when blood is moving away from the probe. Flow velocity that is greater than expected can indicate stenosis, emboli, or vasospasm. It is important to note that TCD cannot determine actual CBF (reported as flow; which is unit volume per unit time). Rather, TCD measures blood flow velocity (in units of m/s). This distinction is significant as decreased arterial diameter will lead to an increased blood flow velocity but a decrease in blood flow volume. However, in other circumstances, such as cerebral autoregulatory failure, increases in CBF velocity occur with increases in CBF. Therefore, thoughtful interpretation of TCD data is required.[25] Also, other parameters that can influence CBF and blood flow velocity must be held constant to minimize their effect on the data. These variables include $PaCO_2$, systemic blood pressure, angle of insonation, and doses of drugs that can impact cerebral hemodynamics including anesthetics. Most TCD monitors are capable of deriving a variety of parameters in addition to mean flow velocity, including pulsatility of the waveform, which reflects distal CVR—commonly called the *pulsatility index*. TCD is also useful in quantifying the status of both static and dynamic autoregulation, using parameters known as the *index of autoregulation* and the *rate of restoration of flow velocity*, respectively.

Laser Doppler Flowmetry

Laser Doppler flowmetry (LDF) is a relatively new monitoring technology used to quantify blood flow in human tissue such as the brain. LDF employs a very small fiberoptic laser that is 0.5 to 1 mm in diameter and is implanted into the brain. LDF measures the Doppler shift caused by passing red blood cells in microscopic vessels in real time. Unlike ultrasound that uses sound waves, LDF is based on the Doppler shift in the frequency of light. This signal is then processed to yield the regional CBF. Such measurements are useful in detecting the effects of various physiologic changes, such as anemia and hyperventilation, on CBF. LDF yields measurements of CBF similar to the Xenon (^{133}Xe) washout technique, one of the established gold standard techniques used to determine CBF.[26]

Intracranial Pressure Monitoring

ICP monitoring is a useful tool for patients suffering from any cause of elevated ICP. ICP monitoring is probably most studied in patients with traumatic brain injury (TBI) at risk for intracranial hemorrhage, worsening cerebral edema, and diminished CPP. Normal ICP is 7 to 15 mmHg, and monitoring is generally initiated when ICP is thought to be above 20 mmHg or one is unable to assess for increased ICP by clinical means. ICP greater than 40 mmHg represents severe, life-threatening intracranial hypertension. Knowledge of the ICP alone can be useful but further information about cerebral well-being can be obtained from observing changes in ICP over time. Specifically, the presence of characteristic Lundberg waves can provide valuable information about the state of the brain. There are three, classically described Lundberg waves: A, B, and C (Fig. 37-10). "A waves," also called plateau waves, occur in the setting of severely exhausted compensatory mechanisms for elevated ICP. ICP increases to 50 to 100 mmHg and remains elevated for minutes. "A waves" occur due to intense vasodilation in response to decreased cerebral perfusion and are always pathologic. "B waves" are elevations in ICP of 20 to 30 mmHg above baseline, occurring once or twice per minute and reflecting changes in vascular tone when CPP is at the LLA. "C waves" are small oscillations occurring four to eight times per minute, where ICP is in the normal range, and reflect systemic changes in vasomotor tone, with little pathologic significance.

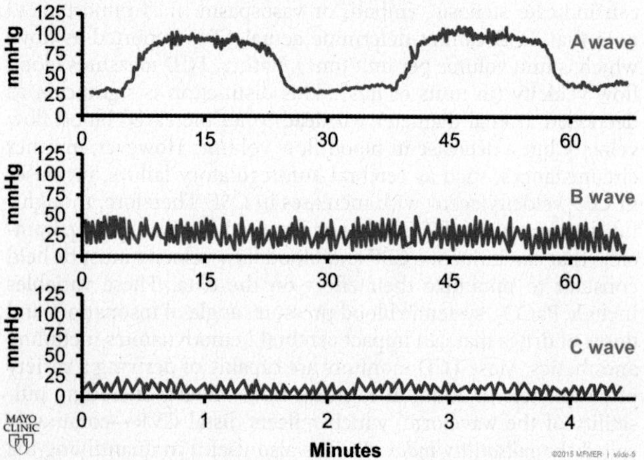

Figure 37-10 Lundberg A, B, and C wave morphologies. (Used with permission of Mayo Foundation for Medical Education and Research, all rights reserved.)

Monitoring can be accomplished using a variety of devices, most of which are invasive at this time, with a few notable exceptions (e.g., CT scan, optic nerve sheath diameter).[27] Although invasive modalities allow for actual pressure measurement, they have associated risks (described later). Noninvasive modalities, although associated with fewer risks, rely on surrogate variables to estimate ICP and therefore are prone to inaccuracy. The most commonly used device is a ventriculostomy or external ventricular drain (EVD) that measures ICP by way of a transducer (zeroed at the external auditory meatus) connected via tubing placed in the lateral ventricle.[28] Currently, the EVD is the gold standard of ICP monitoring. In addition to pressure transduction, a ventriculostomy also allows for drainage of CSF to attenuate elevated ICP and to provide CSF samples for laboratory diagnostic purposes. Also, a ventriculostomy can be used to deliver drugs, such as antibiotics and thrombolytic agents. There are certain disadvantages with EVD monitoring, including difficulty in placement, fluid leaks, clots, and air bubbles, all of which can lead to inaccurate recording. Most notably, infection is a great risk, since the intraventricular drain pierces the meninges and brain parenchyma. CSF sepsis can lead to increased morbidity and mortality in these patients, and aseptic technique in placement of EVDs is of prime importance. Vigilance is required when managing patients with an EVD (or its lumbar drain equivalent) due to the potential risks, and clinicians involved in the perioperative care of patients with these devices must be competent in their setup, assessment, and maintenance.

Intraparenchymal devices are also used to measure ICP, though much less frequently. Two such systems currently exist. The first is a microtransducer system attached to a flexible wire, and the second is a fiberoptic system with a pressure transducer at its tip. Both systems require a hollow screw to be inserted in the skull, whereby the wire or fiberoptic cables can traverse the brain parenchyma. These systems are highly accurate (second only to EVDs), are more easily placed than a ventriculostomy, and are associated with fewer infectious and hemorrhagic risks. Unfortunately, these devices are incapable of removing CSF or allowing drugs to be administered into the CSF.

Subarachnoid "bolts" are not commonly used anymore, but remain an alternative to EVDs. These systems rely on a small bolt that is threaded through a burr hole in the skull, with the tip placed 1 mm beneath the dura. The bolt is then attached to a stopcock assembly and transducer. Subarachnoid bolts are capable of diverting CSF, with lower infectious and hemorrhagic risks than EVDs, but are notoriously inaccurate in measuring ICP; therefore, they are rarely used. Epidural sensor/transducer systems have lower infectious and hemorrhagic risks than EVDs. They are unacceptably inaccurate, however, reflecting only the epidural space and not the entire intracranial compartment.

Cerebral Oxygenation and Metabolism Monitors

Other devices used to monitor the homeostasis of the brain, including its oxygenation and metabolism, are available but may not be commonly employed in the clinical setting. Jugular bulb venous oximetry is the most common of these techniques and involves a fiberoptic catheter placed in a retrograde fashion into the internal jugular vein. The catheter is advanced cephalad beyond the common facial vein and into the jugular bulb that lies at the skull base. Proper placement entails x-ray confirmation of the catheter tip at the level of the mastoid process. This catheter is capable of measuring the mixed cerebral/jugular bulb venous oxygen saturation ($SjVO_2$) that is indicative of the brain's global oxygen consumption/extraction. Other metabolites that can be measured from this source include lactate and glucose concentrations. Measurement can be accomplished by serial sampling, but this method only gives information about the status of the brain at single points in time. Furthermore, extracranial blood may contaminate the sample. More useful perhaps is the continuous fiberoptic measurement of $SjVO_2$. High $SjVO_2$ (80% to 85%) may reflect high oxygen delivery or low $CMRO_2$ whereas low $SjVO_2$ usually indicates low oxygen delivery (e.g., low CBF or hypoxemia) or high $CMRO_2$. $SjVO_2$ below 55%, commonly used to define critical jugular bulb desaturation, may be caused by cerebral ischemia in the setting of systemic hypotension or markedly elevated ICP. $SjVO_2$ may be useful in guiding hyperventilation that results in a reduction in $SjVO_2$ due to vasoconstriction, with the goal of maintaining the saturation above 55%.

Other monitors used to measure cerebral metabolism include brain tissue oxygen monitors and microdialysis catheters. Brain tissue oxygen monitors measure the partial pressure of oxygen ($PbtO_2$) in a portion of brain interstitium 15 to 20 mm wide, directly and invasively, via a Clark-type electrode.[29] $PbtO_2$ is normally 25 to 48 mmHg. $PbtO_2$ values reflect the balance between oxygen supply and demand in the region of brain surrounding the electrode. Factors that affect $PbtO_2$ include local oxygen delivery, predicted by the fraction of inspired oxygen, cardiac output, hemoglobin concentration, local oxygen extraction, PaO_2, and CBF. Generally, values below 20 mmHg in pathologic brain states are considered significant and may portend secondary injury to otherwise healthy brain tissue. Indications for brain tissue oxygen monitoring are most commonly TBI and SAH, and experience is growing with this type of monitoring.

Cerebral microdialysis is becoming more popular in neurocritical care units.[30] A filamentous catheter is placed into the brain parenchyma, consisting of outer and inner tubes and a semipermeable membrane at its tip. A pump is used to perfuse the inner catheter with a crystalloid solution that is iso-osmolar with CSF. At the tip of the catheter, metabolites in the extracellular fluid are driven by a concentration gradient into the outer tubing and are eventually collected into a microvial. This solution is then analyzed for its metabolite contents and their concentrations, including glucose, pyruvate, lactate, glutamate, and glycerol. Clinical correlation, with attention to the location of the catheter tip and comparison of values over time, is required. Although glucose, pyruvate, and lactate concentrations are measures of adequate aerobic metabolism, glutamate, and glycerol levels represent ischemic neuronal stress and cell membrane degradation, respectively. Indeed, one of the major limitations of cerebral microdialysis as well as brain tissue oxygen monitors is that findings will depend on the location of measurement. For example, measurement of values obtained from regions of brain remote from the site of brain injury might indicate minimal, if any, abnormality. Therefore, microdialysis and measurement of oxygen partial pressure is best obtained from locations where "at risk" brain exists.

Last, cerebral oximetry, which uses near-infrared spectroscopy technology, has become more prevalent in clinical use.[31] This technology involves a noninvasive, transcutaneous, measurement of regional cerebral blood oxygenation (rSO_2) over the frontal cortices bilaterally. Oxygenation is given as a percentage of maximum hemoglobin saturation. This reflects the contribution of both arterial and venous blood. A decrease of at least 20% from baseline values is considered significant hypoxia, though definitive data in this regard do not exist. Mechanistically, light from the probe placed on the forehead is transmitted through the skull. Hemoglobin oxygen saturation is determined by the ratio of the absorbances of two or more different wavelengths of light allowing for the determination of oxyhemoglobin and deoxyhemoglobin. This technology differs from pulse oximetry in that it uses two photodetectors, thereby allowing for subtraction of the absorbance from hemoglobin in the scalp and skull. Specifically, near-field photodetection is subtracted from far-field photodetection, yielding a value of brain tissue oxygenation. Cerebral oximetry also differs from pulse oximetry in that it does not rely on pulsatile blood flow. Regional estimates of cerebral oxygenation in the frontal cerebral cortices provide a sensitive method of detecting changes in oxygen delivery due to the very limited oxygen reserve of this highly metabolic area. Factors that may play a role in averting long-term injury based on low cerebral oximetry values include increasing systemic blood pressure, increasing cardiac output, increasing supplemental oxygen, increasing $PaCO_2$ to ameliorate cerebral vasoconstriction, or red blood cell transfusion to increase oxygen-carrying capacity and delivery.

Cerebral Protection

Ischemia and Reperfusion

Because of its high rate of oxygen and glucose consumption, inability to store substrate, and inability to dispose of toxic metabolites quickly, the brain is especially susceptible to rapid ischemic injury. With the accumulation of intracellular calcium (Ca^{2+}) under ischemic conditions, neuronal damage quickly occurs and is compounded by the accumulation of lactic acid. Global ischemia, as can occur during severe hypotension and severe anemia, may be responsive to interventions that restore total cerebral perfusion and oxygen-carrying capacity, such as cardiopulmonary resuscitation (CPR) or red blood cell transfusion. Focal ischemia occurs due to a regional insult such as an embolus or arterial disruption. Treatment of focal ischemia must be focused on restoring perfusion to the ischemic regions of brain. In cases of focal ischemia, a penumbra of salvageable tissue usually surrounds a necrotic core of dead parenchyma. Efforts must also be directed at restoring oxygen and substrate delivery to the ischemic penumbra that is being supplied by some collateral circulation. Much of the research being performed in cerebral protection today deals with this concept of "saving the penumbra," and practical methods include augmentation of CPP and reducing brain edema in the acute setting (see later). Another area under study is that of reperfusion and "reperfusion injury."[32] Specifically, reperfusion of previously ischemic brain tissue can actually worsen neurologic outcome largely due to the production of free radicals derived from oxygen and mediators of inflammation and exacerbation of injury of the microvasculature upon restoration of flow.

Hypothermia

Induced systemic hypothermia has been regarded as a potentially beneficial intervention in certain subgroups of the neurologically injured population, though definitive human studies regarding its consistent efficacy have been lacking. Theoretically, hypothermia should be extremely protective to the brain and spinal cord from a metabolic standpoint, as it lowers the $CMRO_2$ of the CNS to a much greater extent than anesthetics are capable of doing. Although anesthetics can cause an isoelectric EEG, reducing the brain's metabolic activity by up to 60%, hypothermia can do far more by reducing even the brain's homeostatic need for oxygen, required for basic neuronal survival. Animal models have shown that cerebral protection is possible with even a decrease of 1°C in core temperature, demonstrating that the possible protective effects of hypothermia on the CNS are not simply a result of decreased metabolism, but rather may involve other mechanisms as well.

The use of hypothermia in patients with global ischemia may be promising. Profound hypothermia in humans (27°C), as is currently used for cold-cardiopulmonary bypass, and deep hypothermia (12°C to 18°C) used during circulatory arrest, have been shown to provide cerebral protection. Earlier data showed that when adults who have sustained an out-of-hospital cardiac arrest and experience return of spontaneous circulation are cooled to 32°C to 34°C for 12 to 24 hours, neurologic outcome may be improved.[33] However, more recent data do not support a robust benefit from hypothermia in this cohort.[34] Clinical improvement has also been seen in neonates with hypoxic–ischemic encephalopathy treated with mild hypothermia within 6 hours of delivery.[35]

The use of hypothermia in those with focal ischemia is less promising. The Intraoperative Hypothermia for Aneurysm Surgery Trial (IHAST) demonstrated no improvement in neurologic outcome but higher rates of infectious complications in patients who had cerebral aneurysm clipping with mild total-body hypothermia compared to those that had normothermic management.[36] Data involving TBI patients and mild hypothermia have yielded mixed results.[37]

What is clearly known in both humans and animals is that cerebral hyperthermia is detrimental, with focal cerebral ischemic infarct size in animals tripling for each 1°C rise in core temperature.[38] Hyperthermia must be avoided in the setting of cerebral ischemia.

Pharmacologic Therapy for Cerebral Protection

As with induced hypothermia, there is promise for cerebral protection in the setting of neuronal ischemia by both anesthetic and nonanesthetic drugs. However, most of these data comes from animal stroke models and not definitive human studies. Anesthetics may mitigate the effects of CNS ischemia both by their reduction on $CMRO_2$ as well as by other molecular mechanisms. Volatile anesthetics may reduce ischemia-induced glutamate release, increase the availability of antiapoptotic mediators, activate adenosine triphosphate (ATP)-dependent potassium channels, reduce excitotoxic stressors, and augment CBF.[39] Likewise, barbiturates (of proven benefit in focal ischemia in animal studies), nitrous oxide, propofol, etomidate, ketamine, and lidocaine have been associated with beneficial effects on cerebral ischemia in animal and preclinical studies.[40] In clinical practice, ketamine has generally been avoided in neurosurgical patients over concern for its ability to elevate ICP. However, at least for mechanically ventilated patients, this concern appears unfounded and more recent focus has again been on its ability to provide neuroprotection. Clinical use remains rare for this purpose, however, as more randomized, controlled clinical data are needed.[41]

Nonanesthetic agents, too, have been the focus of many studies for their possible neuroprotective effects. Calcium-channel blockers, by inhibiting the effects of voltage-gated calcium channels, have been investigated, although they do not seem clinically useful for this indication. Likewise, magnesium has been investigated as a possible neuroprotective agent, by virtue of its antagonistic effect on various voltage-gated and transmitter-activated channels, though so far human clinical studies are disappointing although magnesium, when given antenatally, may decrease risk of cerebral palsy in children born prematurely.[42]

Other agents, such as free radical scavengers,[43] erythropoietin (activates antiapoptotic pathways and decreases inflammation),[44] and statins for their upregulation of nitric oxide synthase and both anti-inflammatory and antioxidative effects are currently under investigation.[45] Despite ongoing, and often promising, work in this field, it is important to note that a single and definitive neuroprotective agent in human clinical studies has never been identified.

Glucose and Cerebral Ischemia

As mentioned earlier, ischemia is rapidly detrimental to the nervous system not only because of oxygen starvation but also because glucose is the only substrate that can be aerobically metabolized by the brain under normal conditions. Glucose is not stored in the nervous system, so when glucose is reduced or absent due to limited cerebral circulation, ATP is no longer produced at a rate that supplies the energy requirement of neurons and cellular injury quickly ensues. Cerebral glucose consumption (5 mg/100 g/min) parallels $CMRO_2$, so hypoxemia and hypoglycemia are roughly equally detrimental to the brain. With cerebral ischemia and hypoglycemia, lactate is metabolized to some extent in the brain, but with much less efficacy than glucose. Hyperglycemia (serum blood glucose over 180 mg/dL) in the setting of cerebral ischemia has also been shown to worsen neurologic outcomes, presumably by worsening cerebral acidosis in an anaerobic setting, in which glucose is converted to lactic acid.[46]

A Practical Approach

Reliable pharmacologic and nonpharmacologic therapies to prevent neuronal ischemic injury are currently not readily available for use in the perioperative period. One can only hope to attenuate injury. With some exceptions, inhaled and intravenous anesthetics may protect the brain from ischemic injury. For surgeries in which there is planned regional ischemia, such as temporary clipping of cerebral vessels during aneurysm surgery, propofol given in a large bolus (1 to 2 mg/kg) followed by a high-dose infusion (150 μg/kg/min) is often used and titrated to induce burst suppression *prior* to the planned ischemia. In cardiac or neurologic surgeries in which circulatory and pulmonary arrest is planned, such as aortic arch repair or giant basilar aneurysm clipping, deep hypothermia (12°C to 18°C) can be instituted to protect the nervous system. Another example of practical neurologic protection involves the placement of a lumbar CSF drain prior to thoracoabdominal aortic aneurysm repair. This technique is used to lower CSF pressure and ostensibly maintain spinal cord perfusion when radicular arteries originating from the aorta are at surgical risk. 10

Anesthetic Management

Preoperative Evaluation

The preoperative evaluation of the neurosurgical patient is of paramount importance to ensure a safe and successful anesthetic. Specific problems must be identified so as to formulate appropriate plans for intraoperative and postoperative management. For patients with intracranial mass lesions, the most important fact to ascertain is the presence and extent of intracranial hypertension and this should be assumed until information proves otherwise. This information can be obtained most readily from the history and physical examination, CT and magnetic resonance imaging (MRI) scans, and ICP measurements, if available. Patients with elevated ICP may complain of headaches, dizziness, visual or gait disturbances, nausea or vomiting, and seizures. On physical examination, such patients may exhibit abnormalities such as altered level of consciousness, confusion, papilledema, loss of strength or sensation, and cranial nerve dysfunction. 11

Radiologic studies are generally most helpful in quantifying the degree of ICP derangement with "slit ventricles," or a shift of midline brain structure of more than 5 mm indicating advanced pathology. As part of a preoperative evaluation of the neurosurgical patient, findings on routine blood tests can also prove useful. A careful evaluation of laboratory values may demonstrate electrolyte disturbances, which can be due to pituitary pathology (e.g., syndrome of inappropriate antidiuretic hormone secretion [SIADH]), diuretics, steroids, or anticonvulsants being taken by the patient.

In patients with elevated ICP, premedication must be carefully titrated, or avoided completely. Benzodiazepines and opioids, even in small doses, can depress respiration, leading to elevated $PaCO_2$ and subsequent exacerbation of intracranial hypertension. Also, in patients with preexisting or resolved motor deficits, even sedative doses of common anesthetic drugs, especially those with significant GABA-ergic activity, have been shown to exacerbate or "unmask" these deficits.[47] Corticosteroids, such as dexamethasone, and anticonvulsants should be continued preoperatively.

Preoperative evaluation of patients presenting for spine surgery, especially in the acute setting, should focus on the airway examination, current hemodynamic conditions, the level of injury, the degree of injury (complete vs. incomplete), the timing of injury, and the complete neurologic examination. Carefully planning for endotracheal intubation and subsequent hemodynamic management of these patients is vital, as advanced airway techniques and careful fluid management with concomitant vasopressor use may be required.

Induction of Anesthesia and Airway Management

Induction of general anesthesia and airway management are critically important periods, especially in those patients who have elevated ICP, an unsecured aneurysm, or cervical spinal cord injury. Constant attention to hemodynamics is critical in patients with elevated ICP in order to maintain CPP. To that end, the induction of general anesthesia in patients with elevated ICP should be "slow and controlled," with constant attention to the blood pressure throughout the process. In many cases, preinduction arterial catheterization, osmotic diuresis, or CSF drainage may be helpful. Hypotension must be avoided. Patients with elevated ICP may receive a short-acting opioid and lidocaine (1.5 mg/kg) intravenously to blunt the sympathetic response to laryngoscopy. Also, hypoventilation and hypercapnia should be avoided. Following induction of anesthesia, a muscle relaxant should be administered. Succinylcholine should be used with caution in patients with preexisting motor deficits as upregulation of nicotinic receptors at the neuromuscular junction can lead to increased risk of hyperkalemia. Also, succinylcholine can increase ICP but this effect is of short duration.[48] During intubation, strict control of blood pressure is important, as a rapid increase in arterial blood pressure will worsen ICP, especially in patients with autoregulatory failure, or put an unsecured aneurysm at risk of rupture. Hypotension and decreased CPP can also be detrimental. In the case of a cervical spinal cord injury, maintenance of MAP is very important during induction of anesthesia, whereas the actual performance of intubation may require more complex techniques (e.g., awake fiberoptic intubation, midline and sagittal stabilization) to ensure that the spinal cord is not further compromised.

Maintenance of Anesthesia

The maintenance of general anesthesia in neurosurgical patients requires regimens that vary depending on the hemodynamic and monitoring goals for that procedure (2 Video 37-2). For intracranial surgeries, ICP control is paramount until the dura mater is opened. To this end, once Mayfield fixation of the head and positioning are safely completed, mannitol (0.5 to 1.5 g/kg) may be administered if ICP control is needed, as are steroids (e.g., dexamethasone 10 mg) and, in some cases, a prophylactic anticonvulsant. Choice of drugs for maintenance of general anesthesia depends to a great extent on the ICP and whether neuromonitoring is being employed. For patients with elevated ICP, volatile anesthetics are often limited to 0.5 MAC, if used at all, to minimize the degree of cerebral vasodilation and inhibition of autoregulation that can result. Anesthesia is either maintained or supplemented with intravenous drug infusions such as propofol with or without a short-acting opioid such as remifentanil or sufentanil. This regimen works well in neuromonitoring cases as well, where more than 0.5 MAC of volatile agent may interfere with SSEP and MEP monitoring. Muscle relaxants are generally used, unless limited by MEP or EMG monitoring, and nitrous oxide may be considered in select neurosurgical cases. Because of its mild vasodilating effects, potential for expanding pneumocephalus, and unfavorable effects on neuromonitoring, N_2O should be avoided in cases where the patient has significantly increased ICP, the potential for intradural air, or where it will interfere with monitoring modalities. In the absence of muscle relaxant, immobility can be achieved with remifentanil infusions. Throughout the procedure, CPP must be maintained, possibly requiring a vasopressor. Although it is possible that vasopressor choice may affect intracranial capillary flow and hence brain oxygenation beyond its impact on arterial tone, especially in the setting of a disrupted BBB, there is currently insufficient evidence to recommend certain vasopressors over others for most neurosurgical patients.[49] If autoregulation is greatly inhibited due to the disease process or the anesthetic drugs, CBF will be directly dependent on MAP, thus hypertension should be avoided. In cases of acute spinal cord injury, many of the same principles apply to maintenance of anesthesia, as spinal cord perfusion (especially in cervical spine surgery) and the ability to perform neuromonitoring are of great concern.

Ventilation Management

Ventilatory management of patients undergoing neurosurgery is also a key consideration. For patients undergoing an intracranial procedure, tidal volume should be maintained at 6 to 8 mL/kg to minimize potential inflammatory injury to the lungs, with peak pressures kept at less than 40 cmH_2O. These principles hold especially true for patients with SAH or TBI, who may already exhibit acute lung injury (ALI) or adult respiratory distress syndrome (ARDS). Positive end-expiratory pressure (PEEP) should be minimized unless needed to improve oxygenation, as it increases intrathoracic pressure and may impede cerebral venous drainage, although low PEEP levels appear to be well tolerated for most patients.[49] Positive pressure ventilation (PPV) is generally used for neurosurgical procedures, as it allows direct control of $PaCO_2$, and is especially beneficial during sitting craniotomies, where negative intrathoracic pressure may contribute to the development of venous air embolism (VAE).

Fluids and Electrolytes

For many years, the teaching of fluid maintenance during craniotomy was to keep the patient "dry" to minimize the amount of reactive cerebral edema both during the surgery and postoperatively. This strategy is generally not considered optimal, as the primary goal of fluid management in neurosurgical cases should be to maintain cerebral perfusion, which is a more important consideration and will actually lessen the amount of cerebral edema produced.[50] Hence, the goal of fluid management should be to keep the patient euvolemic. Isotonic or slightly hypertonic solutions (e.g., 0.9% sodium chloride) should be used if large amounts of fluid are to be administered. Hypotonic solutions, such as Ringer lactate, when administered in large amounts, can contribute to cerebral edema. Glucose-containing solutions are avoided, as hyperglycemia is detrimental to cerebral metabolism (see section Glucose and Cerebral Ischemia), and because glucose is quickly metabolized and not osmotically active, leaving free water that can worsen brain edema.

Depending on patient comorbidities and length of the surgery, electrolyte derangements may be common and require close monitoring (NICV 37-2). Certainly, patients with SIADH, diabetes insipidus (DI), or cerebral salt wasting syndrome, will require careful monitoring of electrolytes. Hypertonic saline (3%) supplementation (given slowly at a rate of 50 to 100 mL/h, and with the serum sodium level checked hourly) may be required in moderate to severe hyponatremic states. Rapid rises in serum sodium (more than 3 to 4 mEq/L/h) must be avoided as this poses a risk for central pontine myelinolysis. In patients with DI, hypotonic solutions such as Ringer lactate or 0.45% sodium chloride might be required, and their administration should be carefully titrated based on volume status and serum electrolyte concentrations. Mannitol, especially at large doses, can cause mild electrolyte derangements which are generally short lived (e.g., hyponatremia, hyperkalemia), and these should be monitored and possibly corrected.[51] Also, diuresis from mannitol can result in dehydration that can impair cerebral perfusion. Sodium chloride solution (0.9%), given in large amounts, can cause hyperchloremic metabolic acidosis and subsequent acute kidney injury due to renal tubular acidosis.

Transfusion Therapy

The transfusion of blood products may be required perioperatively in patients having neurosurgical procedures. Preoperatively, coagulation studies, if available, should be carefully noted and are required in patients receiving anticoagulants. Preoperative coagulopathies should be corrected as intraoperative or postoperative bleeding can have a significantly adverse impact on outcome. Neurosurgical patients having nonurgent surgery should have a platelet count over 100,000/mm^3. For patients having craniotomy for indications that would generally carry a low risk for intraoperative bleeding, a "type and screen" with a negative antibody screen may be adequate. Red blood cells that are "typed and crossed" should be available for procedures with high risk for bleeding such as neurovascular procedures (e.g., aneurysm clipping, arteriovenous malformation [AVM] resection) or tumor craniotomies that invade the cranial sinuses. For coagulopathies that may develop with the release of brain tissue thromboplastin, fresh frozen plasma, platelets, and cryoprecipitate may be needed. Complex spine surgery (especially with planned osteotomies or due to tumor) is usually associated with more profound blood loss, volume shifts, and the need for transfusion therapy. In these cases, multiple units of blood products should be immediately available and frequent monitoring of the complete blood count (CBC) and coagulation studies should be performed.

Glucose Management

As discussed earlier, glucose management is very important in neurosurgical cases for the prevention of both hypo- and hyperglycemia. In 2001, van den Berghe et al.[52] showed that strict glycemic control (i.e., target serum glucose concentration of 80 to 110 mg/dL) in critically ill surgical patients was associated with improved outcome. Strict glycemic control has been associated with increased risk for hypoglycemia that can be detrimental to the brain.[53] To reduce the risk of both hypoglycemia and excessive hyperglycemia, most authors agree that serum glucose during neurosurgical procedures should be maintained in the 90 to 180 mg/dL range. Intraoperative hyperglycemia >180 mg/dL has also been associated with an increase in postoperative infections after craniotomy.[54] For hyperglycemia exceeding this range, short-acting insulin should be readily available and can be given intravenously as a bolus with or without an infusion. In these cases, monitoring of serum glucose must be frequent enough to capture episodes of hypoglycemia.[55] In cases of hypoglycemia, 50% dextrose should be available, and 20 to 50 mL of this solution is administered with further titration based on continued close monitoring of serum glucose concentration.

Emergence

Emergence from general anesthesia following neurosurgical procedures requires meticulous attention to hemodynamic and ventilatory parameters, while also ensuring a prompt neurologic examination. Postcraniotomy hypertension is a well-described, albeit poorly understood, phenomenon, but can certainly be detrimental as it may increase bleeding from the surgical site and worsen cerebral edema.[56] Careful analgesia (so as not to obtund the patient postoperatively) is helpful to minimize risk for hypertension, but usually antihypertensive medications are required. These can include labetalol, esmolol, nicardipine, or clevidipine. Control of hypertension is especially important for patients emerging from cerebral AVM resection, as bleeding from the resection bed may be significant. In patients having undergone posterior fossa surgery, and those in whom a preexisting ventilatory disturbance was present due to brainstem compromise, emergence may be much slower and the time to safe extubation more prolonged. Coughing on emergence for all patients should be avoided due to the risk of bleeding and elevation in ICP. A low-dose remifentanil infusion and/or either intravenous or intratracheal lidocaine may be helpful in this regard. Likewise, postoperative nausea and vomiting should be prophylactically treated in these cases for the same reasons. Dexamethasone used for this indication should be avoided in patients in whom the diagnosis of lymphoma is being considered (or at least delayed until an adequate pathology specimen is obtained), as steroids can causes tumor lysis of lymphoma and potentially interfere with diagnosis. Also, dexamethasone should also be avoided following pituitary surgery as it can suppress the hypothalamic–pituitary–adrenal axis and significantly increase the false positive rate for diagnosis of postoperative hypopituitarism.[57]

Common Surgical Procedures

Surgery for Tumors

One of the most common indications for neurosurgery is the removal of both benign and malignant tumors that emanate from or spread to the CNS or PNS. In adults, supratentorial lesions are more common and include tumors derived from support cells in the CNS (e.g., gliomas, astrocytomas, oligodendrogliomas), meningiomas, or metastases. The most common metastatic tumors to the brain include melanoma or those that originate in the lung, breast, or kidney. Infratentorial tumors in the posterior fossa are more common in children and include medulloblastoma, pilocytic astrocytoma, ependymoma, and brainstem glioma.

Independent of their histology, the morbidity of brain tumors is associated with their size, rate of growth, and proximity to and invasion of nearby structures. Furthermore, glial disruption of the BBB may cause significant vasogenic edema, which may persist even after tumor resection, and autoregulation is usually impaired in parenchyma surrounding tumors.[58] Fortunately, most brain tumors grow slowly, allowing adaptive and compensatory mechanisms to accommodate increases in ICP due to edema or mass effect. Unfortunately, this same fact often leads to delayed diagnosis.

The anesthetic management of these patients must take all of these factors into account, as patients with dangerously elevated ICP preoperatively must be treated with great caution, sometimes requiring preoperative CSF diversion and dexamethasone. Surgery for intracranial tumors can be safely accomplished with a careful preoperative evaluation and a smooth induction, maintenance, and emergence regimen. Preoperative assessment should include an understanding of the lesion site and dimensions, plan for surgical approach, neurologic symptomatology, ICP concerns, and medical comorbidities. Anxiolysis with benzodiazepines must be carefully considered, as even small increases in $PaCO_2$ in otherwise asymptomatic patients can quickly lead to dangerously elevated ICP due to increased intracranial elastance. Steroids and anticonvulsants should be continued, and in many cases supplemented, prior to and during craniotomy. Hemodynamic instability during any part of the anesthetic should be minimized due to the possibility of impaired autoregulation in peritumoral brain parenchyma. Hypertension can increase the risk of bleeding and exacerbate brain edema. Generally, propofol is administered for induction of general anesthesia. Lidocaine (1 to 1.5 mg/kg) and fentanyl (1 to 2 μg/kg) may be given intravenously to blunt the hemodynamic and ICP response to laryngoscopy. Adequate vascular access (usually two large-bore peripheral intravenous catheters, and arterial catheter, and possibly a central venous catheter) is mandatory for brain tumor resection. ICP and CPP are of great concern throughout these procedures, and an arterial catheter is very helpful to monitor CPP closely while also allowing the titration of $PaCO_2$ by revealing its gradient with end-expired CO_2 via arterial blood gas measurement. After vascular access is established and any neuromonitoring modalities are applied, the head fixation device is usually applied to the skull. The hemodynamic response is similar to laryngoscopy, and optimal control of blood pressure must again be sought, often by using propofol, opioids, or short-acting β-adrenergic antagonists such as esmolol.

Excessive flexion, extension, or rotation of the neck may impair cerebral venous drainage via compression of the internal jugular veins. A head-up position is also favorable to promote venous drainage. PEEP should be used cautiously, as this may also impair venous drainage, although if oxygenation is impaired, PEEP up to 10 cmH_2O can be considered. In patients with large tumors or known significant intracranial hypertension, efforts should be made to decrease brain volume for optimal surgical exposure and to minimize retractor-related edema. This can include mild hyperventilation and use of mannitol (0.5 to 1.5 g/kg) or hypertonic saline (3% starting at 50 to 100 mL/h with hourly sodium surveillance). The osmolarity of similar volumes of 20% mannitol and 3% hypertonic saline are nearly equivalent, and clinical trials indicate that hypertonic saline is at least as effective, if not more effective, than mannitol in treating elevated ICP.[59] Furthermore, hypertonic saline may be more effective than mannitol for brain relaxation in elective craniotomy surgery.[51] Mannitol should be given as a bolus to achieve its full effect, although great care should be taken in patients with congestive heart failure, pulmonary edema, or renal failure as the initial elevation in central circulatory volume may be detrimental in these patients prior to the diuretic phase. Mannitol doses near the higher end of the dose range mentioned above may also be associated with an increased risk of rebound intracranial edema.[60] For maintenance of general anesthesia, the choice of anesthetics is heavily dictated by avoiding increases in ICP (at least until the dura is open), maintaining CPP, neuromonitoring requirements, and ensuring a rapid emergence. Short-acting and easily titratable drugs are generally preferred. These include propofol, remifentanil, sevoflurane, desflurane, and possibly nitrous oxide unless otherwise contraindicated. Muscle relaxants are beneficial if not precluded by neuromonitoring. Fluid maintenance should be accomplished with dextrose-free iso-osmolar crystalloids or colloids, with the goal of euvolemia (see earlier).

Patients who demonstrated a normal level of consciousness (Glasgow Coma Score [GCS] of 13 to 15) preoperatively are generally extubated at the conclusion of the case, and, as with induction, hemodynamic stability is paramount during this period. Aberrations in blood pressure, usually systemic hypertension, can lead to worsening cerebral edema or tumor resection bed bleeding postoperatively, and short-acting and easily titratable drugs, such as labetalol, nicardipine, or esmolol should be immediately available. Coughing or vomiting after extubation, which may both worsen ICP, can be minimized with careful opioid titration (such as a remifentanil intravenous infusion of 0.05 mcg/kg/min)[61] and a prophylactic antiemetic. Adequate analgesia must be ensured as well, as craniotomy can be associated with a significant amount of pain.[62] At the same time, avoiding analgesic doses which may obtund the patient and preclude a careful neurologic assessment postoperatively is vitally important. In this regard, the use of short-acting opioids (i.e., remifentanil, fentanyl), local anesthetic infiltration, intravenous acetaminophen, or dexmedetomidine can be considered.[63,64]

Due to their proximity to the brainstem, infratentorial tumors and tumors of the posterior fossa may be associated with more hemodynamic perturbations intraoperatively and postoperatively, as well as changes in respiratory control and arousal levels postoperatively. These patients may more frequently require postoperative intubation and mechanical ventilation due to altered levels of consciousness or delayed emergence. After elective craniotomy, there is wide variation among institutions for ICU admission postoperatively. In general, patients with new neurologic deficits (particularly reduced consciousness or deficits of lower cranial nerves), or who have other indication for delayed extubation, should be considered for ICU admission.[65]

In adults, tumors of the posterior fossa include acoustic neuromas, metastases, meningiomas, and hemangioblastomas. Because of their proximity to the brainstem and cranial nerves, these tumors can cause altered respiratory patterns, cardiac dysrhythmias, or cranial nerve dysfunction. Surgery for these tumors can be performed in the prone, lateral, or sitting positions, and may require specific cranial nerve monitoring, such as EMG or BAERs of cranial nerves. The sitting position requires special attention, as the risk of VAE is increased.

VAE occurs when the operative site is above the level of the right atrium in the presence of open, noncollapsible venous channels. VAE occurs in 30% to 75% of all sitting posterior fossa surgery, but is usually hemodynamically insignificant. It is estimated that 8% to 15% of VAE episodes cause significant hemodynamic change.[66,67] When air is entrained into the heart and pulmonary circulation, it can lead to impaired gas exchange, intrapulmonary shunting, hypoxemia, and a concomitant decrease in end-expired CO_2. If air entrainment becomes severe, arrhythmias, decreased cardiac output, severe pulmonary hypertension, and hemodynamic collapse can result. Monitoring for VAE in the sitting position may include precordial Doppler ultrasonography, which can detect 0.25 mL of air in the heart. A more sensitive monitor is transesophageal echocardiography, which is much more cumbersome, invasive, and requires an observer familiar with this technique. Also, transesophageal echocardiography may not allow for continuous monitoring for air as the device will cease working when probe temperature rises. However, transesophageal echocardiography allows for a quantitative assessment of intracardiac air whereas precordial Doppler sonography is a qualitative monitor for VAE (i.e., indicates only if air is present in the heart).

Prevention of VAE entails decreasing the height difference between the operative site and the heart as much as possible, maintaining euvolemia, and the use of bone wax by the surgeon to occlude visibly open dural venous sinuses or larger veins. Treatment of VAE includes notifying the surgeon to flood the surgical field, administering 100% oxygen, aspirating air through a multiorifice central venous catheter positioned at the junction of the superior vena cava and right atrium, and supportive hemodynamic care. Depending on the degree of hemodynamic perturbation, treatment may include vasopressors, fluids, inotropes, and adjusting the OR table position so that the head is at the level of the heart. This final maneuver is saved for severe or unremitting manifestations of VAE as it likely will disrupt the surgical field. A retrospective case series found position change to be effective in treating the hemodynamic and respiratory changes resulting from VAE.[68] If nitrous oxide was being used, it should be stopped because nitrous oxide may increase air bubble volume, potentially exacerbating the clinical effects of VAE. The application of PEEP, although theoretically favorable, can exacerbate systemic hypotension.

Pituitary Surgery

Pituitary surgery is usually performed endoscopically and transnasally. Anesthetic concerns for pituitary surgery include systemic manifestations of any associated endocrinopathy, electrolyte and fluid disturbances caused by endocrine disease, SIADH, or DI, and inadvertent surgical trespass into the cavernous sinus or internal carotid artery. Patients with a sellar mass may exhibit visual field defects, and a careful history and physical examination preoperatively is important to differentiate between organic and anesthetic causes of visual problems after surgery.

Growth hormone (GH)-secreting tumors cause acromegaly. A large mandible and hypertrophy of tissue leads to decreased airway aperture and predisposes to obstructive sleep apnea and difficulty with mask ventilation and intubation. Also, a smaller sized endotracheal tube and additional tools and strategies to secure the airway, such as awake fiberoptic intubation or a video laryngoscope–based intubation may be considered. Furthermore, longstanding acromegalics are prone to cardiac rhythm disturbances and hypertrophic cardiomyopathy, and caution with cardiac depressant medications is warranted.

Adrenocorticotropic hormone (ACTH)-secreting tumors cause Cushing syndrome by causing hypercortisolism. Cushing syndrome is associated with glucose intolerance or diabetes mellitus, increased skin fragility (potentially making peripheral intravenous access difficult), impaired wound healing, and secondary hypertension. There are data to suggest, however, that Cushing syndrome is not significantly associated with airway difficulty.[69]

Patients with thyroid-stimulating hormone (TSH)-secreting pituitary adenomas should be rendered euthyroid before surgery unless vision is threatened. Such patients may have inadvertently been treated for Graves disease preoperatively, thereby decreasing the production of free T4 and T3 hormones and reducing the amount of negative feedback to the pituitary adenoma, which may predispose to rapid tumor growth.

SIADH is common in patients with sellar tumors due to compression of the posterior pituitary and an excess of circulating antidiuretic hormone (ADH). SIADH may lead to intravascular volume overload and hyponatremia. Extracellular body water is usually normal, and edema or hypertension is usually not characteristic. Treatment of perioperative SIADH involves water restriction (to the extent that it is safe to do so), treating the underlying cause, demeclocycline (a tetracycline antibiotic that inhibits ADH action in the renal tubules), and desmopressin for persistent or severe cases.[70] The hallmark of DI is polyuria with dilute urine. Fluid replacement is required.[70]

Because accidental surgical entry into the cavernous sinus or internal carotid artery is an infrequent complication of pituitary surgery, adequate vascular access and an arterial catheter are recommended. A lumbar subarachnoid catheter is sometimes placed before or after pituitary surgery. Intraoperatively, injection of air or sterile saline or withdrawal of CSF can facilitate exposure of the tumor as increases or decreases in intracranial volume can serve to move the sellar structures inferiorly or superiorly, respectively. Postoperatively, a lumbar CSF drainage catheter can be used to drain CSF when a dural sealant or fat graft has been used and reduce the risk for chronic CSF leakage.

Cerebral Aneurysm Surgery and Endovascular Treatment

The development of cerebral aneurysms and their likeliness to rupture is associated with age over 40 years, female sex, cigarette smoking, systemic hypertension, and connective tissue disorders. Ruptured aneurysms are the most common cause of spontaneous SAH, accounting for 80% of nontraumatic SAH. Aneurysms are thought to arise from turbulent blood flow at arterial branching points, causing "sac-like" or "fusiform" dilatations. Cerebral aneurysms most commonly occur at the anterior communicating arteries (40%), PCOMs (25%), and MCA (25%), with only 10% arising from the vertebrobasilar system.

Following SAH, an acute increase in ICP is accompanied by a decrease in CPP. These changes result in an increase in systemic blood pressure to maintain CBF. Patients may present with severe headache (classically, the "worst headache of my life"), nausea and vomiting, photophobia, seizures, focal neurologic deficits, and altered consciousness. A noncontrast head CT scan is usually sufficient to diagnose SAH, but more sophisticated imaging, such as digital-subtraction angiography, CT angiography, or MRI angiography, is required to identify the location and morphology of the aneurysm.

Cerebral aneurysms and their neurologic sequelae are categorized in a variety of ways for both treatment and prognostication. The Hunt and Hess Grading Scale (based on clinical symptoms) (Table 37-2), the World Federation of Neurological Surgeons

Table 37-2 Hunt and Hess Grading System

Hunt and Hess Grade	Clinical Symptoms
0	Unruptured aneurysm/asymptomatic
1	Minimal headache, slight nuchal rigidity
2	Moderate to severe headache, nuchal rigidity, cranial nerve palsy
3	Mildly obtunded, confused, focal deficits
4	Severely obtunded, hemiparesis, early decerebrate posturing
5	Coma, decerebrate posturing

Table 37-3 World Federation of Neurological Surgeons (WFNS) Grading Scale

WFNS Grade	Glasgow Coma Scale Score	Motor Deficit
1	15	No
2	14–13	No
3	14–13	Yes
4	12–7	Yes or no
5	6–3	Yes or no

Grading Scale (based on GCS and motor deficits) (Table 37-3), and the Fisher Grade System (based on radiologic bleeding) (Table 37-4) are commonly used. Aneurysm size is an important factor when considering management. "Small" aneurysms are less than 10 mm in diameter, "large" aneurysms are 10 to 24 mm in diameter, and "giant" aneurysms are more than 24 mm in diameter. Rupture risk increases with aneurysm diameter, with those larger than 6 mm generally requiring treatment.

Preoperative assessment must include knowledge of the aneurysm size and location and whether it is intact or ruptured. Caring for patients with ruptured aneurysms must take into account the presence and possibility of rebleeding, vasospasm of cerebral arteries, hydrocephalus, cardiac dysfunction, neurogenic pulmonary edema, and seizures. Cerebral vasospasm rarely occurs within 72 hours of rupture. Surgical or endovascular treatment of ruptured aneurysms is generally undertaken within the first 48 hours after presentation of SAH, to minimize the risk of rebleeding but prior to increased risk for cerebral vasospasm. Cardiac and pulmonary conditions should be optimized to the greatest extent possible, which may require inotropes, antiarrhythmics, hypertonic saline supplementation if SIADH or cerebral salt wasting syndrome are present, maintenance of euvolemia, and maintenance of tissue oxygenation, all without delay of surgical treatment. Furthermore, enteral nimodipine and a statin drug should be administered. Nimodipine is the only intervention that decreases risk for cerebral vasospasm. Statins, via their pleotropic effects, may also decrease risk of vasospasm.

Aneurysms amenable to surgical clipping are usually saccular as opposed to fusiform in morphology. Great caution must be taken to minimize risk for rupture by avoiding hypertension during intubation, head fixation, and during the surgical procedure. Also, in patients with prior rupture, adequate CPP must be maintained as ICP may be elevated. Anesthetic induction is controlled with the above-mentioned ICP considerations in mind. In those with prior rupture, CPP is maintained, sometimes requiring careful vasopressor use to also prevent hypertension that can increase risk for rerupture.

Table 37-4 Fisher Grade System

Fisher Grade	Blood on Computed Tomography Scan
1	No subarachnoid blood seen
2	Diffuse vertical layers of blood <1 mm thick
3	Localized clot and/or vertical layer of blood ≥1 mm thick
4	Intracerebral or intraventricular clot with diffuse or absent subarachnoid hemorrhage

In patients without prior rupture and a normal ICP, excessive hypertension should be avoided. A maintenance anesthetic technique similar to the one described earlier for brain tumors is used because neuromonitoring may be employed to detect regional ischemia. No optimal maintenance anesthetic regimen for improved neurologic outcome has been identified, so a balanced anesthetic technique that takes into account the above considerations is appropriate. During exposure of the aneurysm, although not fully supported by human clinical data, burst suppression on the EEG may be desired to decrease the impending ischemic burden on the brain from temporary occlusion of large cerebral vessels.[71] Burst suppression can be accomplished with propofol administered as a 1- to 2-mg/kg bolus followed by infusion of 100 to 150 μg/kg/min. Additional vasopressor may be required during this time to maintain CPP.

Prior to direct clipping of the aneurysmal neck, the surgeon may place one or more temporary clips on parent or feeding arteries to "soften" the neck and make it more amenable to direct clipping while minimizing the chances of rupture. Alternatively, when temporary clips are anatomically difficult to place, adenosine 0.3 to 0.4 mg/kg may be safely given as a bolus to cause a transient (3- to 5-second) circulatory arrest allowing safe permanent clip application.[72,73] Other techniques, such as deep hypothermic circulatory arrest (DHCA), retrograde suction decompression, or rapid ventricular pacing achieve the same end point but are logistically more difficult to perform. During temporary and permanent clipping, SSEP and MEP monitoring may be performed more frequently as this is the time during which the brain is at greatest ischemic risk.

Inadvertent rupture is possible during dissection around the aneurysm. A plan must be in place to contend with this potentially devastating complication, including the availability of blood products and adenosine (0.3 to 0.4 mg/kg), or another rapidly acting antihypertensive medication (e.g., sodium nitroprusside), for rescue. In this regard, large-bore intravenous access is required, especially for large aneurysms over 10 mm and ruptured aneurysms, and central venous access is recommended.

Endovascular treatment of aneurysms involves groin arterial access and the deployment of coils into the aneurysmal sac to occlude blood flow into the sac. A Cochrane review (which included the International Subarachnoid Aneurysm Trial [ISAT]) concluded that outcome was better in patients in good clinical condition post aneurysmal rupture with coiling versus clipping.[74] However, both microsurgical and endovascular techniques have undergone technologic advances and appropriateness of one technique compared to the other for different patient populations is still being determined.[71] Also, certain aneurysms may not be amenable to coiling, due to their morphology. The major disadvantage of coiling is incomplete obliteration of the aneurysm, requiring recoiling that may be necessary in up to 30% of cases. General anesthesia with muscle relaxation is used, as movement should be prevented. An arterial catheter is needed to monitor the blood pressure closely and to obtain blood samples for coagulation measurements at repeated intervals, as heparin is administered periodically. The anesthesiologist should communicate closely with the interventionalist throughout the procedure, as any extravasation of dye into the brain parenchyma may be indicative of aneurysmal or feeding vessel rupture. In this circumstance, protamine must be immediately available to reverse the effects of heparin, and hyperventilation, mannitol, burst suppression, and placement of an EVD should be available on an emergency basis. Emergency craniotomy is a likely intervention. Embolism of coils to unintended locations in the brain is also possible throughout the procedure; thus, a prompt neurologic examination at the conclusion of the procedure is important.

Arteriovenous Malformations

Cerebral AVMs are congenital abnormalities in which a plexus of arteries and "arterialized" veins form a nidus that may lead to cerebral hemorrhage, headaches, seizures, or signs of cerebral ischemia due to a "steal" effect. AVMs are usually detected between the ages of 10 and 40 years, with approximately 70% being supratentorial. Morphologically, these structures have a nidus of dysplastic vessels of varying size and are drained by one or more superficial or deep veins. Characteristically, there is no capillary bed between arteries and veins within AVMs. These lesions can be diagnosed by MRI or cerebral angiography, and treatment modalities include stereotactic radiosurgery, embolization in the interventional radiology suite as stand-alone therapy, or embolization prior to a planned surgical resection to minimize intraoperative bleeding, burden, or improve curativity. The Spetzler–Martin Grading System is used to predict surgical outcome. It is based on size, eloquence of adjacent brain, and pattern of venous drainage (i.e., superficial vs. deep) of the AVM (Table 37-5). Notably, about 7% of cerebral AVMs include a flow-related cerebral aneurysm as well.

Vascular access, more than in any other intracranial neurosurgical procedure, is of great importance, and a central venous catheter is highly recommended. The greatest risk of AVM resection is bleeding, both intraoperatively and postoperatively. Surgical hemostasis can be challenging due to poor visualization of arterial and especially venous vessels and postoperatively. Strict control of blood pressure is required to maintain CPP without worsening blood loss from the resection bed due to ongoing systemic hypertension. At the same time, avoidance of hypotension is crucial as these patients often present with seizures or focal neurologic deficits due to an ischemic "steal" phenomenon. Because most AVMs are high-flow and low-resistance shunts, the incidence of sudden rupture with *acute* rises in systemic blood pressure (as with direct laryngoscopy) is low unless there is an accompanying aneurysm. Blood products should be immediately available, and antihypertensives are often needed, especially during emergence from anesthesia. The phenomenon of normal perfusion pressure breakthrough (NPPB), is controversial in terms of its mechanism, but clinically relevant to the anesthesiologist. NPPB is thought to be a type of autoregulatory inhibition caused by the AVM affecting the surrounding "normal" brain, in which previously normal cerebral vessels are maximally vasodilated due to longstanding "steal" caused by the AVM. After the AVM has been resected, these "vasoparalyzed" vessels are unable to vasoconstrict, leading to cerebral hyperemia, cerebral edema, headache, and possibly increased risk for postoperative bleeding. Another phenomenon that may lead to perioperative hyperemia and postoperative morbidity is "occlusive hyperemia." This phenomenon is primarily related to arterial and venous obstruction occurring in normal brain tissue that surrounded the AVM due to surgical disruption of these vessels. This obstruction can impact flow in brain parenchyma that surrounded the AVM leading to ischemia from poor arterial flow, edema, and increased risk for hemorrhage from impaired venous outflow. Postoperatively, up to 50% of patients may experience seizures, thus prophylactic anticonvulsants are typically administered. Neuromonitoring is increasingly used during cerebral AVM resections, and a maintenance anesthetic regimen that allows neuromonitoring may be required. Arterial catheterization and careful induction and intubation, as described with cerebral aneurysms, are standard.

Table 37-5 Spetzler–Martin Grading System

Feature of Arteriovenous Malformation	Score
Size	
Small (<3 cm)	1
Medium (3–6 cm)	2
Large (>6 cm)	3
Adjacent Brain	
Noneloquent	0
Eloquent	1
Venous Drainage Pattern	
Superficial	0
Deep	1

Carotid Surgery

Surgery to remove carotid plaque that may be causing symptomatic cerebral ischemia is generally indicated when the plaque burden is over 70% occlusive in the ICA. Up to 20% of strokes may be due to cerebral ischemia caused by intimal narrowing of the ICA, either unilaterally or bilaterally. Carotid revascularization has proven to be a useful procedure for reducing the risk of stroke in cases of severe occlusion of the ICA (i.e., 70% to 99% occlusion) in the presence of symptoms of ischemia. However, benefit in less severe occlusive states or in asymptomatic patients may not outweigh risks and medical management may be preferred.[75] Procedural treatments of carotid artery stenosis include carotid endarterectomy or carotid artery stenting. The most significant advantage of carotid endarterectomy over stenting is that it has an overall lower incidence of postoperative stroke (particularly in older patients) and restenosis, whereas potential disadvantages of this surgery include the need for a general or regional anesthetic technique, a possible increased risk for cardiac events, and a higher incidence of cranial nerve dysfunction.[76] However, carotid artery stenting may be accomplished with very minimal sedation and carries a lower incidence of cranial nerve injury, although it has been associated with a higher risk of restenosis and stroke in the postprocedural period.

Carotid endarterectomy is performed either "awake" with regional anesthesia or "asleep" with general anesthesia. Neither technique has been found to be superior at improving neurologic outcome.[77] "Awake" carotid surgery usually involves a superficial and sometimes deep cervical plexus block to provide anesthesia within the C2 to C4 dermatomes. Low-dose analgesia and sedation with remifentanil or propofol may be considered. It is important to ensure that the patient is responsive to commands and able to perform manual tasks on the contralateral side. This technique requires a cooperative patient who is able to tolerate lying flat for a prolonged period of time, and patients with chronic obstructive pulmonary disease or uncompensated congestive heart failure may be unsuitable candidates. Advantages of an "awake" technique include a direct monitor of the patient's neurologic status, better hemodynamic stability, shorter hospital length of stay, and decreased bleeding complications. If the patient becomes agitated, confused, or unresponsive following carotid occlusion, the anesthesiologist should assume that cerebral ischemia has ensued and assure adequate perfusion and oxygenation by increasing systemic blood pressure up to 20% greater than preoperative values.

"Asleep" carotid surgery employs general endotracheal anesthesia and frequently some form of monitoring for cerebral ischemia is used.[78] EEG is probably the most common and ischemia presents as ipsilateral slowing of oscillations. SSEPs and MEPs can also be used with ischemia appearing as a decrease in waveform amplitude or an increase in waveform latency. Carotid stump pressure is the pressure measured in the internal carotid artery distal to the cross-clamp and is thought to reflect adequate collateral blood flow via the circle of Willis. A stump pressure greater than 50 mmHg is desirable. Cerebral oximetry or TCD are other, less commonly employed techniques used to monitor for cerebral ischemia. To date, no modality of neuromonitoring has been shown to reliably ensure adequate collateral blood flow.

General anesthesia provides the advantages of a motionless patient, the ability to ensure eucapnia, and control of the airway at all times. Eucapnia is preferred, as hyperventilation will cause cerebral vasoconstriction and decreased CBF, whereas hypoventilation and hypercapnia may lead to a "steal" phenomenon from watershed areas of cerebral perfusion.

Regardless of the type of anesthesia performed, invasive arterial blood pressure monitoring is preferred as operative morbidity is generally due to neurologic complications whereas mortality is usually due to cardiac complications. Therefore, blood pressure control is critical. Patients are generally chronically hypertensive preoperatively and may have cardiovascular disease and other significant comorbidities. Blood pressure should be maintained at baseline levels prior to cross-clamping. Patients having regional anesthesia often maintain baseline blood pressure but those having general anesthesia may require pharmacologic manipulation of blood pressure. Cross-clamping occurs above and below the area of plaque, usually at the levels of the common carotid artery below and the ICA above and heparinization is commonly performed prior to cross-clamping. Upon cross-clamp occlusion of the common carotid artery, blood pressure should be augmented to improve collateral flow from the contralateral side, often requiring a vasopressor. During manipulation of the carotid baroreceptor, bradycardia and possibly hypotension are not uncommon, and the surgeon may infiltrate the carotid sinus with lidocaine to prevent this response. Following restoration of flow in the carotid artery, hypertension may persist, probably due to surgical denervation of the carotid baroreceptor. Since cerebral vessels distal to the stenotic carotid artery have been maximally vasodilated, autoregulation may not be intact. Hypertension with cerebral vasomotor paralysis can lead to cerebral edema and increased risk for cerebral hemorrhage. Any neurologic compromise postoperatively may also be indicative of cerebral emboli or ICA thrombosis, and patients must be monitored closely for these complications. Lastly, the anesthesiologist must be keenly aware of the potential for a postoperative neck hematoma, which may quickly compromise the airway. Immediate intubation, which may be more difficult, and surgical exploration of the wound is required. When airway management is complicated by an expanding neck hematoma, consideration should be given to immediate decompression of the airway by surgical incision opening.

Other modalities of treating ICA stenosis, including carotid angioplasty and transcarotid artery revascularization, have gained popularity in the last few years, with some evidence supporting their safety and efficacy over traditional endarterectomy.[79]

Epilepsy Surgery

Epilepsy affects about 1% of the general population and is characterized by recurrent seizure activity of both the generalized and partial varieties. Complex partial seizures, including temporal lobe epilepsy, are most common. They involve an initial focus of abnormal neuronal discharge that spreads with a subsequent loss of consciousness. Epilepsy may occur idiopathically, or as part of a constellation of symptoms related to head injury, tumors, neurovascular disease, metabolic derangement, or infection. Approximately 30% of patients with drug-resistant epilepsy undergo surgical treatment for their disease.[80] Perioperative management of patients having surgery for epilepsy requires a keen understanding of the pharmacologic effects of both anesthetics and antiepileptic drugs. Surgery for epilepsy is generally indicated when there is a discrete epileptic focus, most frequently identified in the temporal lobe. Thus, temporal lobectomy with amygdalohippocampectomy is a common surgical procedure performed for the treatment of epilepsy. Recently, stereoencephalography (SEEG) has been used as a less invasive technique to identify potentially resectable epileptogenic foci.[81] During the SEEG implantation procedure, electrodes are implanted into the brain via burr holes with stereotactic guidance and general anesthesia. Postoperatively, patients are admitted to an epilepsy monitoring unit to attempt to identify a resectable epileptogenic foci. If an epileptogenic focus is identified, the patient returns to the operating room for craniotomy for electrode removal and focus resection. If a focus could not be identified, the electrodes are removed with sedation. Patients in whom a focus can be identified may be candidates for laser interstitial thermal therapy (LITT).[82] During LITT, a fiberoptic probe is placed stereotactically via a burr hole into an epileptogenic focus and a laser beam is directed into the lesion to thermally ablate the focus with real-time MRI guidance. LITT avoids the need for a craniotomy. LITT has also been used to ablate brain tumors.

Preoperative evaluation is critical, with particular attention paid to the patient's preoperative antiepileptic regimen, their known side effects, and in some cases plasma concentrations of drugs with known therapeutic windows. Antiepileptic drugs are generally continued throughout the perioperative period unless seizure focus mapping is intended. Antiepileptics can induce liver enzymes and increase the metabolism of muscle relaxants, opioids, and dexmedetomidine, leading to a need for higher dosages.[83] Each anesthetic drug has its own profile of excitatory and inhibitory effects on seizure activity. Thus, if used improperly, anesthetic drugs can be detrimental to seizure focus mapping. Benzodiazepines should be avoided when electrocorticography (ECoG) is planned. Induction of anesthesia with propofol, a muscle relaxant, and an opioid is acceptable. During maintenance of anesthesia and prior to ECoG, any anesthetic regimen conducive for craniotomy can be used, but 30 minutes prior to ECoG initiation, propofol infusion should be stopped and potent volatile anesthetic decreased to 0.5 MAC or stopped. To prevent awareness, scopolamine, nitrous oxide, and high-dose opioid infusion can be used with very little adverse effect on ECoG. Dexmedetomidine may also be useful. The patient should be counseled about the possibility of intraoperative awareness. In some cases, methohexital, etomidate, or alfentanil (50 μg/kg) can be used to enhance epileptiform activity and assist in mapping.[84] Once ECoG is complete, the general anesthetic technique used prior to ECoG can be resumed during the focus resection. Postoperatively, patients should be monitored closely for seizure activity. Seizures may signify postoperative bleeding, metabolic derangements, hypercapnia, or hypoxemia and should be treated aggressively to avoid cerebral damage or status epilepticus.

Awake Craniotomy

Craniotomy performed with monitored anesthesia care, also known as "awake craniotomy," has gained popularity in some institutions and is used in cases in which a lesion lies adjacent to primary cortex that controls motor function, speech, or sensory function. Awake craniotomy allows for speech, motor, or sensory cortical mapping in real time, hence facilitating a more aggressive resection of the tumor and minimizing risk to function.

A motivated patient is critical to the success of the procedure. Preoperative assessment should include a detailed explanation of the anesthetic so as to ensure cooperation and allay anxiety. Awake craniotomy can be performed with the patient sedated for the duration of the procedure, or with an "asleep–awake–asleep" technique employing a supraglottic airway device general anesthesia prior to and following the awake mapping. During awake mapping, the airway device is removed so that the patient can communicate, and then replaced after the induction of anesthesia following mapping. Alternatively, most patients tolerate sedation for surgical closure.

An arterial catheter is placed and sedation prior to and following awake mapping may be facilitated with propofol, remifentanil, or dexmedetomidine infusions. Comparison of sedation for awake craniotomy with a propofol–remifentanil combination versus dexmedetomidine found similar sedation and intraoperative brain mapping efficacy between groups, but lower rates of respiratory depression in the dexmedetomidine group.[85] A selective scalp nerve block may be performed preoperatively, either unilaterally or bilaterally, blocking the six nerves which innervate the scalp and dura mater: the supratrochlear, supraorbital, zygomaticotemporal, auriculotemporal, lesser occipital, and great occipital nerves.[86] Otherwise, the surgeon may choose to perform a field block. Care must be taken to avoid local anesthetic toxicity, particularly as the surgeon infiltrates the dura mater with additional local anesthetic. During cortical mapping, surgeons use electrical stimulation with a probe stimulator in conjunction with neuropsychologic testing to map critical cortical regions. Thus the surgeon can determine safe resection margins, particularly if the tumor is located near major language areas in cortex (usually located in the left hemisphere).

Regardless of the anesthetic technique used, close attention to the airway is critical, as hypoventilation and hypercapnia are detrimental to surgical exposure and apnea requiring emergency intubation may be very difficult in a patient whose head is turned and fixed in a head holder. The surgical drape should be positioned in a manner allowing direct and constant access to the patient's face. Careful padding and positioning should be accomplished before any sedation is administered to ensure patient comfort for the duration of surgery. Last, is the importance of constant communication with the patient, not only to facilitate speech or motor testing but also to comfort the patient who may be anxious.

Complications of awake craniotomy intraoperatively include a disinhibited or uncooperative patient, oversedation prohibitive to neuropsychologic testing, respiratory depression, airway obstruction, intractable brain edema, seizures, or uncontrollable pain. Seizures should be treated with cold saline applied to the brain surface by the surgeon and a small bolus of propofol (20 mg) intravenously. Postoperatively, patients may be observed in the PACU or the ICU with similar considerations as any craniotomy, including adequate analgesia.

For patients who are poor awake craniotomy candidates, surrogate testing during general anesthesia can be performed with motor or sensory mapping, but language function cannot be monitored in this manner. Recently, advances in mapping and monitoring speech function have occurred, and may be available as a monitoring option in the future.[87,88]

Anesthesia and Traumatic Brain Injury

TBI is a significant public health problem in the developed and underdeveloped world, accounting for 15% to 20% of mortality in people 5 to 35 years old. TBI is often associated with other trauma such as thoracic, abdominal, and orthopedic injuries. It is important to note that the primary insult to the brain is often irreversible. Death following TBI is often associated with secondary insults from hypotension, hypoxemia, and malignantly increased ICP due to hematoma or edema. Emergency and anesthetic management of patients with TBI should focus on minimizing these secondary insults to optimize perfusion of the injured brain. Patients presenting with TBI are stratified according to the GCS on presentation (3 to 15). GCS 13 to 15 corresponds to mild head injury, GCS 9 to 12 corresponds to moderate head injury, and GCS below 9 represents severe head injury. Patients with TBI are often intubated when GCS is 8 or less owing to high risk for impaired airway protection. A GCS of 8 or less also corresponds to high mortality. ICP monitoring is frequently used in patients with acute TBI and can be instituted in the emergency department with an EVD, where mannitol, hyperventilation, and propofol or barbiturates can be used to control elevated ICP. Operative management, such as decompressive craniectomy, is normally indicated for depressed skull fractures, dural breech, midline shift more than 5 mm, basal cistern compression, refractory ICP elevation, and acutely expanding intracranial hemorrhage, including subdural and epidural hematomas.[89]

Anesthetic Management

Patients presenting with TBI are assumed to have concomitant cervical spine injury, and intubation, if not already performed, must take this into account. Furthermore, 40% of patients will have an associated life-threatening injury. A detailed but rapid primary survey, along with a focused neurologic examination is critical. Hypoxemia is common, treatment of which may be complicated by pulmonary injury. Anesthetic drug administration must be tailored to avoid systemic hypotension as patients may have hypovolemia from an associated injury. Succinylcholine is controversial following an acute closed head injury; it may raise ICP transiently but can be used if there is a need to rapidly secure an airway and no other contraindications to its use exist. Nasal intubation is contraindicated if a basilar skull fracture is present or presumed. Attention must be paid to hemodynamics, as systolic blood pressure should be maintained at ≥100 mmHg for patients aged 50 to 69 years old and at ≥110 mmHg for patients aged 15 to 49 years old or above 70 years old.[89] Fluid resuscitation and vasopressors are often needed to assure an adequate systemic and cerebral perfusion pressure. There is evidence that achieving euvolemia with hypertonic saline may be beneficial in TBI patients, especially pediatric patients, as intravascular volume is repleted and CPP is maintained with less cerebral edema.[90] Euglycemia should be maintained. Intravascular access should include an arterial catheter and large-bore intravenous cannulae, and possibly a central venous catheter. Cross-matched red blood cells and other blood products should be available, and results relating to hemoglobin concentration and clotting function should be reviewed.

Choice of an anesthetic maintenance technique depends on an understanding of ICP management (discussed earlier). Mannitol or hypertonic saline may be required to control edema. Hyperventilation should not continue beyond 2 to 6 hours, as its effect to decrease ICP may not be durable after this time. After this acute phase of hyperventilation, a $PaCO_2$ of 30 to 35 mmHg is desirable. Of particular importance for TBI management, CPP should always be kept above 60 mmHg, and perhaps above 70 mmHg, to maintain cerebral perfusion but excessive hypertension should be avoided to reduce risk of exacerbating edema or increasing risk for hemorrhage.[89] The release of brain tissue thromboplastin into the systemic circulation may lead to disseminated intravascular coagulation and coagulopathy must be aggressively sought and treated. Likewise, ARDS or neurogenic pulmonary edema may be present, and a lung-protective ventilation strategy using PEEP and low tidal volumes may be needed to maintain oxygenation.

Complications that may occur during and immediately following operative management of TBI include seizures, intracranial hemorrhage, sudden and profound hypotension following decompression of large hematomas, and cerebral edema. The latter can be treated with propofol, mannitol and/or hypertonic saline, temporary hyperventilation, CSF diversion, and possibly avoiding replacement of the bone flap at the conclusion of surgery.

Extubation at the conclusion of surgery depends on the degree of ICP elevation, the severity of injury, and concomitant injuries. Most patients are admitted to the neurointensive care unit after surgery and require continued intubation, mechanical ventilation, and sedation.

Anesthesia for Spine Trauma and Complex Spine Surgery

Spinal Cord Injury

Acute spinal cord injury often necessitates emergency surgery to stabilize the spinal column and prevent secondary injury. Cervical spine injuries are most common, as this is the most mobile part of the spine. Cervical injuries are also the most devastating injuries from a neurologic perspective. Cervical cord injuries cause more functional motor, sensory, and autonomic deficits than lower cord injuries. Also, higher cord injuries can impact respiratory muscle function to a greater extent with intercostal function being impacted by thoracic and cervical injuries and phrenic function being impaired by lesions at C5 or higher. Although voluntary respiratory effort remains with injury at the C4 level, vital capacity may be diminished by up to 25%. Sympathetic nervous system function is usually impaired following higher thoracic and cervical cord injuries and cardiac accelerator nerve function (derived from the T1 to T5 segments), may lead to profound hypotension and bradycardia. Likewise, temperature control is lost with SCI because of a loss of sweating function and cutaneous vasodilation due to loss of sympathetic function. The American Spinal Injury Association (ASIA) score is used to stratify spinal cord injury based on sensory, motor, and reflex function (Table 37-6).

Following acute spinal cord injury, spinal cord autoregulation is impaired and the phenomena of spinal shock may be present. Spinal shock is characterized by sensory–motor deficits below the level of the injury and flaccid paralysis, usually lasting up to 6 weeks. After this initial period, spasticity of the affected muscles tends to occur. Hypotension can result from autonomic impairment and hypovolemia associated with other injuries (e.g., long bone fractures, intra-abdominal bleeding). During this time, it is critical to prevent secondary injury by providing aggressive hemodynamic support. Although primary injury may be due to stretching, compression, or transection of the spinal cord or its blood supply due to hyperflexion, hyperextension, or impingement of the fractured spinal column, secondary injury is a more complicated biochemical phenomenon involving the release of inflammatory mediators, cytokines, and amino acids leading to cellular edema, apoptosis, and free radical formation. As with TBI, mitigating these secondary insults, by avoiding hypoxemia, hypotension, and worsening cord edema, is of paramount importance in ensuring the best outcome possible. Comorbid injuries are common in patients with acute SCI, including TBI, nonvertebral fractures, facial injuries, chest or abdominal injuries (including pneumothorax and pulmonary contusion), and traumatic amputations, and may cause or contribute to hypotension and hypoxemia. Life-threatening injuries must be addressed while ensuring that spinal alignment is maintained to avoid adding secondary injury to the spinal cord.

Table 37-6 American Spinal Injury Association (ASIA) Impairment Scale

ASIA Impairment Class	Deficit	Deficit Description
A	Complete	No motor or sensory function
B	Incomplete	Sensory but no motor function below neurologic level including S4–5
C	Incomplete	Motor function preserved below neurologic level + ≥50% key muscles have severe weakness
D	Incomplete	Motor function preserved below neurologic level + ≥50% key muscles have mild weakness
E	None/Intact	Normal motor and sensory function

Initial Management

Patients presenting with acute spinal cord injury, depending on the level and extent of injury, may be compromised from a ventilatory and hemodynamic standpoint, and immediate control of these parameters is crucial. A detailed neurologic examination is critical to establish the operative plan and subsequent prognostication. Airway management in cervical spinal injury focuses on maintaining in-line stabilization throughout, and may require the use of fiberoptic intubation or other adjuncts to secure the airway. In a stable patient, radiographic studies are helpful in assessing the degree of cervical injury and options for intubation. However, plain x-ray imaging of the cervical spine is not sensitive for ligamentous injury thus underestimating risk. In the setting of spinal cord compression, awake fiberoptic intubation may be preferred, as it allows for neurologic examination immediately postintubation.[91] Succinylcholine is safe in the initial 24 hours following spinal cord injury as new junctional and extrajunctional nicotinic receptors have not yet been fully expressed. In addition to intravenous fluids and blood products, vasopressors and inotropes are often required to support the blood pressure as hypotension and anemia can contribute to secondary injury of the spinal cord. Arterial blood pressure monitoring and large-bore intravenous access (preferably central venous access) are required. MAP should be maintained above 85 to 90 mmHg to ensure adequate spinal cord perfusion for at least 7 days from the date of injury.[92]

Other strategies to protect the spinal cord, such as corticosteroids, naloxone, or hypothermia, have received some attention, but convincing human data for these therapies is lacking. Corticosteroids have received particular attention in this regard, both in animal and human studies. The mechanism to account for their potential neuroprotective effect is thought to include reduction of vasogenic edema, improvement of spinal cord perfusion, anti-inflammatory effects, and free radical scavenging. The most comprehensive human trials were the National Acute Spinal Cord

Injury Studies (NASCIS) I to III, which demonstrated that early steroid intervention may improve neurologic outcome in SCI patients. These studies were highly suspect, however, in that their results were not reproducible, their populations were skewed, and survival or quality of life did not improve with the intervention (methylprednisolone). Furthermore, corticosteroids are known to have untoward effects, including the predisposition to infection and glucose dysregulation that must be weighed against their potential benefits. Guidelines published in 2013, and endorsed by the American Association of Neurological Surgeons and the Congress of Neurological Surgeons did not recommend the use of corticosteroids in patients with acute spinal cord injury. However, more recent guidelines published in 2017, recommend that high dose methylprednisolone for 24 hours be offered in acute spinal cord injury for patients presenting within 8 hours of injury.[93]

Intraoperative Management

The choice of technique for maintenance of anesthesia in patients with spinal cord injury should focus on two key considerations: maintaining blood pressure and allowing for intraoperative neuromonitoring. Complex spine surgery, which often involves multiple level fusions and osteotomies, should also take into account the real possibility of significant, and sometimes profound, surgical bleeding and the need for postoperative mechanical ventilation following massive transfusion. For these lengthy and extensive surgeries, great care must be paid to surgical prone positioning, and recognition of the potential for hypotension to occur with change to the prone position is necessary to proactively manage such an occurrence.[94] Allowing the abdomen to be free from compression during prone positioning is important to decrease abdominal pressure, thereby decreasing epidural venous plexus pressure, thereby decreasing blood loss during thoracolumbar surgery.[95] Depending on the spinal levels requiring intervention and the extent of the planned surgery, the patient may be placed in head-fixation device. Clearly, adequate intravascular access is important to establish before prone positioning. Measurements of arterial blood gas, coagulation parameters, hemoglobin concentration, and platelet counts should be undertaken frequently, as coagulopathy and anemia are quite common and need to be corrected rapidly as they can contribute to secondary injury. Close communication with the surgeon is important, as these large operations often may benefit from early closure and staging of the procedure. Use of antifibrinolytics, such as tranexamic acid, can decrease risk of bleeding with minimal, if any, increased risk for thrombotic complications.[96] In noninfectious, nontumor cases, intraoperative cell salvage can be quite helpful in reducing the total amount of allogeneic blood transfused. Other blood-sparing techniques, such as acute normovolemic hemodilution and deliberate hypotension, have largely fallen out of favor, due to the known harmful effects of anemia and hypotension on the neurologic and cardiovascular systems. Postoperative pain control can be particularly challenging in complex spine surgery patients.[97] A single bolus dose of methadone intraoperatively has been shown to reduce postoperative analgesic requirements, improve pain scores, and even provide analgesic benefit lasting months.[98] Emphasis has also been placed on multimodal management, including some less traditional methods of pain control after major spine surgery, such as regional blocks, which have shown promising results.[99]

Complications of Anesthesia for Spine Surgery

Fortunately, complications specifically related to anesthesia for spine surgery are rare, but they are often devastating when they occur (NICV 37-3). Postoperative visual loss (POVL) is one such complication, with an incidence of 0.088 to 1.2 per 1,000 after spine surgery. Most cases are due to posterior ischemic optic neuropathy, whereas central retinal artery occlusion and cortical blindness are less common. Risk factors include male sex, obesity, use of the Wilson frame, longer surgery duration, and high estimated blood loss, whereas use of colloid may be protective. An ASA Practice Advisory recommends informing high-risk patients preoperatively about the risk of POVL.[100] Ophthalmologic consultation should be immediately undertaken if this complication is suspected.

Another complication of spine surgery is anterior spinal artery syndrome. This syndrome is caused by sustained hypoperfusion of the anterior spinal artery, owing to either surgical distraction or hypotension, and leads to motor weakness. MEPs may be helpful in detecting and averting this devastating complication.

Deliberate hypotension, hypothermia, and hypovolemia may predispose spine surgery patients to the formation of deep venous thromboses (DVT) and subsequent pulmonary emboli (PE). Lumbar fusion is associated with an incidence of symptomatic DVT of up to 4%, with a 2% incidence of PE. Because prophylaxis with an anticoagulant is often impossible prior to spine surgery for fear of worsening blood loss and formation of epidural hematoma, an inferior vena cava filter should be considered for certain high-risk patients prior to surgery.

Autonomic dysreflexia (AD) is an important physiologic phenomenon that is not a complication of spine surgery, but rather a late complication of complete SCI. AD occurs weeks to months after such injury, in 60% to 80% of such SCI patients, and is characterized by a profound hypertensive response to any stimulus below the level of injury, such as distention of a hollow organ such as the bladder, pain, or surgery. The most common manifestation of AD is profound systemic hypertension, accompanied by headache, profuse sweating, and flushing above the level of injury and oftentimes bradycardia, cardiac dysrhythmias, or cardiac dysfunction. The pathophysiology of this phenomenon is thought to be due to a disruption of descending inhibitory tracts with intact sympathetic reflex arcs below the level of injury. The primary goal in patients at risk for AD is prevention. Triggers should be minimized (i.e., appropriate bowel and bladder care) and anesthesia should still be used for painful or stimulating procedures in insensate regions. Treatment of an acute episode of AD involves removing the inciting stimulus and deepening the level of anesthesia along with the administration of potent vasodilators. Recommended vasodilators include calcium-channel blockers, nitrates, or hydralazine. There is some controversy regarding the preferred anesthetic technique for these patients, although general and spinal anesthesia are usually preferred to epidural anesthesia or mild-to-moderate sedation. Spinal anesthesia has the advantage over epidural anesthesia as it is usually a denser block and does not risk sparing of sacral segments that may occur with epidural anesthesia. If general anesthesia is used, succinylcholine should be avoided as it may trigger a profound hyperkalemic response. As with all neurosurgical patients, careful monitoring for these patients in the postoperative period is critical, as AD may manifest itself at this time.

Conclusion

The perioperative care of neurosurgical patients requires a sound understanding of neurophysiologic and neuropharmacologic principles, the timely application of these principles, and vigilance to often rapidly changing clinical conditions. At the core of neuroanesthesia practice are the ideas of maintaining cerebral oxygen and substrate delivery, facilitating intraoperative neuromonitoring, and assuring for a rapid emergence to facilitate neurologic examination in appropriate patients. Expert application of the requisite knowledge to achieve these goals, along with efficient resource utilization, will provide the safest neurologic outcome possible for this vulnerable patient population.

For further review and interactivities, please see the videos and narrative interactive clinical vignettes (NICVs) accessible in the complimentary eBook bundled with this text. Access instructions are located on the inside front cover.

REFERENCES

1. Xu F, Liu P, Pascual JM, Xiao G, Lu H. Effect of hypoxia and hyperoxia on cerebral blood flow, blood oxygenation, and oxidative metabolism. *J Cereb Blood Flow Metab*. 2012;32(10):1909–1918.
2. Sanders RD, Degos V, Young WL. Cerebral perfusion under pressure: is the autoregulatory 'plateau' a level playing field for all? *Anaesthesia*. 2011;66(11):968–972.
3. Rivera-Lara L, Zorrilla-Vaca A, Geocadin RG, Healy RJ, Ziai W, Mirski MA. Cerebral autoregulation-oriented therapy at the bedside: a comprehensive review. *Anesthesiology*. 2017;126(6):1187–1199.
4. Meng L, Gelb AW. Regulation of cerebral autoregulation by carbon dioxide. *Anesthesiology*. 2015;122(1):196–205.
5. Claassen JAHR, Thijssen DHJ, Panerai RB, Faraci FM. Regulation of cerebral blood flow in humans: physiology and clinical implications of autoregulation. *Physiol Rev*. 2021;101(4):1487–1559.
6. Koch KU, Mikkelsen IK, Espelund US, et al. Cerebral macro- and microcirculation during ephedrine versus phenylephrine treatment in anesthetized brain tumor patients: a randomized clinical trial using magnetic resonance imaging. *Anesthesiology*. 2021;135(5):788–803.
7. Schmidt A, Ryding E, Akeson J. Racemic ketamine does not abolish cerebrovascular autoregulation in the pig. *Acta Anaesthesiol Scand*. 2003;47(5):569–575.
8. Kuroda Y, Murakami M, Tsuruta J, Murakawa T, Sakabe T. Preservation of the ration of cerebral blood flow/metabolic rate for oxygen during prolonged anesthesia with isoflurane, sevoflurane, and halothane in humans. *Anesthesiology*. 1996;84(3):555–561.
9. Dashdorj N, Corrie K, Napolitano A, Petersen E, Mahajan RP, Auer DP. Effects of subanesthetic dose of nitrous oxide on cerebral blood flow and metabolism: a multimodal magnetic resonance imaging study in healthy volunteers. *Anesthesiology*. 2013;118(3):577–586.
10. Macintyre I. A hotbed of medical innovation: George Kellie (1770-1829), his colleagues at Leith and the Monro-Kellie doctrine. *J Med Biogr*. 2014;22(2):93–100.
11. Kety SS, Skenkin HA, Schmidt CF. The effects of increased intracranial pressure on cerebral circulatory functions in man. *J Clin Invest*. 1948;27(4):493–499.
12. Dietrich J, Rao K, Pastorino S, Kesari S. Corticosteroids in brain cancer patients: benefits and pitfalls. *Expert Rev Clin Pharmacol*. 2011;4(2):233–242.
13. La Rosa G, Conti A, Cardali S, Cacciola F, Tomasello F. Does early decompression improve neurological outcome of spinal cord injured patients? Appraisal of the literature using a meta-analytical approach. *Spinal Cord*. 2004;42(9):503–512.
14. Bracken MB. Steroids for acute spinal cord injury. *Cochrane Database Syst Rev*. 2012;1:CD001046.
15. Holdefer RN, MacDonald DB, Skinner SA. Somatosensory and motor evoked potentials as biomarkers for post-operative neurological status. *Clin Neurophysiol*. 2015;126(5):857–865.
16. MacDonald DB, Dong C, Quatrale R, et al. Recommendations of the International Society of Intraoperative Neurophysiology for intraoperative somatosensory evoked potentials. *Clin Neurophysiol*. 2019;130(1):161–179.
17. Holdefer RN, Heffez DS, Cohen BA. Utility of evoked EMG monitoring to improve bone screw placements in the cervical spine. *J Spinal Disord Tech*. 2013;26(5):E163–E169.
18. Hayashi H, Kawaguchi M. Intraoperative monitoring of flash visual evoked potential under general anesthesia. *Korean J Anesthesiol*. 2017;70(2):127–135.
19. Sloan TB, Toleikis JR, Toleikis SC, Koht A. Intraoperative neurophysiological monitoring during spine surgery with total intravenous anesthesia or balanced anesthesia with 3% desflurane. *J Clin Monit Comput*. 2015;29(1):77–85.
20. Higgs M, Hackworth RJ, John K, Riffenburgh R, Tomlin J, Wamsley B. The intraoperative effect of methadone on somatosensory evoked potentials. *J Neurosurg Anesthesiol*. 2017;29(2):168–174.
21. Rabai F, Sessions R, Seubert CN. Neurophysiological monitoring and spinal cord integrity. *Best Pract Res Clin Anaesthesiol*. 2016;30(1):53–68.
22. Furutani K, Deguchi H, Matsuhashi M, Mitsuma Y, Kamiya Y, Baba H. A bolus dose of ketamine reduces the amplitude of the transcranial electrical motor-evoked potential: a randomized, double-blinded, placebo-controlled study. *J Neurosurg Anesthesiol*. 2021;33(3):230–238.
23. Yang LH, Lin SM, Lee WY, Liu CC. Intraoperative transcranial electrical motor evoked potential monitoring during spinal surgery under intravenous ketamine or etomidate anaesthesia. *Acta Neurochir (Wien)*. 1994;127(3–4):191–198.
24. Rozet I, Metzner J, Brown M, et al. Dexmedetomidine does not affect evoked potentials during spine surgery. *Anesth Analg*. 2015;121(2):492–501.
25. Czosnyka M, Brady K, Reinhard M, Smielewski P, Steiner LA. Monitoring of cerebrovascular autoregulation: facts, myths, and missing links. *Neurocrit Care*. 2009;10(3):373–386.
26. Rejmstad P, Akesson G, Hillman J, Wardell K. A laser Doppler system for monitoring of intracerebral microcirculation. *Annu Int Conf IEEE Eng Med Biol Soc*. 2012;2012:1988–1991.
27. Khan MN, Shallwani H, Khan MU, Shamim MS. Noninvasive monitoring intracranial pressure—A review of available modalities. *Surg Neurol Int*. 2017;8:51.
28. Lele AV, Hoefnagel AL, Schloemerkemper N, et al. Perioperative management of adult patients with external ventricular and lumbar drains: guidelines from the society for neuroscience in anesthesiology and critical care. *J Neurosurg Anesthesiol*. 2017;29(3):191–210.
29. Ngwenya LB, Burke JF, Manley GT. Brain tissue oxygen monitoring and the intersection of brain and lung: a comprehensive review. *Respir Care*. 2016;61(9):1232–1244.
30. Zeiler FA, Thelin EP, Helmy A, Czosnyka M, Hutchinson PJA, Menon DK. A systematic review of cerebral microdialysis and outcomes in TBI: relationships to patient functional outcome, neurophysiologic measures, and tissue outcome. *Acta Neurochir (Wien)*. 2017;159(12):2245–2273.
31. Wong ZZ, Chiong XH, Chaw SH, et al. The use of cerebral oximetry in surgery: a systematic review and meta-analysis of randomized controlled trials. *J Cardiothorac Vasc Anesth*. 2022;36:2002–2011.
32. Lin L, Wang X, Yu Z. Ischemia-reperfusion injury in the brain: mechanisms and potential therapeutic strategies. *Biochem Pharmacol (Los Angel)*. 2016;5(4):213.
33. Bernard SA, Smith K, Cameron P, et al. Induction of prehospital therapeutic hypothermia after resuscitation from nonventricular fibrillation cardiac arrest*. *Crit Care Med*. 2012;40(3):747–753.
34. Dankiewicz J, Cronberg T, Lilja G, et al. Hypothermia versus normothermia after out-of-hospital cardiac arrest. *N Engl J Med*. 2021;384(24):2283–2294.
35. Shankaran S. Therapeutic hypothermia for neonatal encephalopathy. *Curr Opin Pediatr*. 2015;27(2):152–157.
36. Todd MM, Hindman BJ, Clarke WR, Torner JC; Intraoperative Hypothermia for Aneurysm Surgery Trial I. Mild intraoperative hypothermia during surgery for intracranial aneurysm. *N Engl J Med*. 2005;352(2):135–145.
37. Shaefi S, Mittel AM, Hyam JA, Boone MD, Chen CC, Kasper EM. Hypothermia for severe traumatic brain injury in adults: recent lessons from randomized controlled trials. *Surg Neurol Int*. 2016;7:103.
38. Favero-Filho LA, Borges AA, Grassl C, Lopes AC, Sinigaglia-Coimbra R, Coimbra CG. Hyperthermia induced after recirculation triggers chronic neurodegeneration in the penumbra zone of focal ischemia in the rat brain. *Braz J Med Biol Res*. 2008;41(11):1029–1036.
39. Wang H, Li P, Xu N, et al. Paradigms and mechanisms of inhalational anesthetics mediated neuroprotection against cerebral ischemic stroke. *Med Gas Res*. 2016;6(4):194–205.
40. Bilotta F, Stazi E, Zlotnik A, Gruenbaum SE, Rosa G. Neuroprotective effects of intravenous anesthetics: a new critical perspective. *Curr Pharm Des*. 2014;20(34):5469–5475.
41. Gregers MCT, Mikkelsen S, Lindvig KP, Brochner AC. Ketamine as an anesthetic for patients with acute brain injury: a systematic review. *Neurocrit Care*. 2020;33(1):273–282.
42. Lingam I, Robertson NJ. Magnesium as a neuroprotective agent: a review of its use in the fetus, term infant with neonatal encephalopathy, and the adult stroke patient. *Dev Neurosci*. 2018;40(1):1–12.
43. Jelinek M, Jurajda M, Duris K. Oxidative stress in the brain: basic concepts and treatment strategies in stroke. *Antioxidants (Basel)*. 2021;10(12):1886.
44. Larpthaveesarp A, Ferriero DM, Gonzalez FF. Growth factors for the treatment of ischemic brain injury (growth factor treatment). *Brain Sci*. 2015;5(2):165–177.
45. O'Regan C, Wu P, Arora P, Perri D, Mills EJ. Statin therapy in stroke prevention: a meta-analysis involving 121,000 patients. *Am J Med*. 2008;121(1):24–33.
46. Wass CT, Lanier WL. Glucose modulation of ischemic brain injury: review and clinical recommendations. *Mayo Clin Proc*. 1996;71(8):801–812.
47. Rizk AA, Venkatraghavan L, Shankar JJS, Schaller B, Chowdhury T. Reappearance of neurological deficits in pathologic brain: are sedatives and opioids culprits? a systematic review. *J Neurosurg Anesthesiol*. 2022;34(1):14–20.
48. Cottrell JE. Succinylcholine and intracranial pressure. *Anesthesiology*. 2018;129(6):1159–1162.
49. Thorup L, Koch KU, Upton RN, Ostergaard L, Rasmussen M. Effects of vasopressors on cerebral circulation and oxygenation: a narrative review of pharmacodynamics in health and traumatic brain injury. *J Neurosurg Anesthesiol*. 2020;32(1):18–28.
50. Ryu T. Fluid management in patients undergoing neurosurgery. *Anesth Pain Med (Seoul)*. 2021;16(3):215–224.
51. Zhang W, Neal J, Lin L, et al. Mannitol in critical care and surgery over 50+ years: a systematic review of randomized controlled trials and complications with meta-analysis. *J Neurosurg Anesthesiol*. 2019;31(3):273–284.

52. van den Berghe G, Wouters P, Weekers F, et al. Intensive insulin therapy in critically ill patients. *N Engl J Med*. 2001;345(19):1359–1367.
53. Bilotta F, Caramia R, Paoloni FP, Delfini R, Rosa G. Safety and efficacy of intensive insulin therapy in critical neurosurgical patients. *Anesthesiology*. 2009;110(3):611–619.
54. Gruenbaum SE, Toscani L, Fomberstein KM, et al. Severe intraoperative hyperglycemia is independently associated with postoperative composite infection after craniotomy: an observational study. *Anesth Analg*. 2017;125(2):556–561.
55. Bebawy JF, Ramaiah VK, Hemmer LB, Gupta DK. Clinical pharmacology of insulin confounds stroke trials. *Ann Neurol*. 2012;71(1):148.
56. Bebawy JF, Houston CC, Kosky JL, et al. Nicardipine is superior to esmolol for the management of postcraniotomy emergence hypertension: a randomized open-label study. *Anesth Analg*. 2015;120(1):186–192.
57. Burkhardt T, Rotermund R, Schmidt NO, Kiefmann R, Flitsch J. Dexamethasone PONV prophylaxis alters the hypothalamic-pituitary-adrenal axis after transsphenoidal pituitary surgery. *J Neurosurg Anesthesiol*. 2014;26(3):216–219.
58. Bebawy JF. Perioperative steroids for peritumoral intracranial edema: a review of mechanisms, efficacy, and side effects. *J Neurosurg Anesthesiol*. 2012;24(3):173–177.
59. Ali A, Tetik A, Sabanci PA, et al. Comparison of 3% hypertonic saline and 20% mannitol for reducing intracranial pressure in patients undergoing supratentorial brain tumor surgery: a randomized, double-blind clinical trial. *J Neurosurg Anesthesiol*. 2018;30(2):171–178.
60. Li S, Sun H, Liu X, et al. Mannitol improves intraoperative brain relaxation in patients with a midline shift undergoing supratentorial tumor surgery: a randomized controlled trial. *J Neurosurg Anesthesiol*. 2020;32(4):307–314.
61. Ghodraty MR, Hasani V, Bagheri-Aghdam A, et al. Remifentanil infusion during emergence moderates hemodynamic and cough responses to the tracheal tube: a randomized controlled trial. *J Clin Anesth*. 2016;33:514–520.
62. Gottschalk A, Berkow LC, Stevens RD, et al. Prospective evaluation of pain and analgesic use following major elective intracranial surgery. *J Neurosurg*. 2007;106(2):210–216.
63. Rajan S, Hutcherson MT, Sessler DI, et al. The effects of dexmedetomidine and remifentanil on hemodynamic stability and analgesic requirement after craniotomy: a randomized controlled trial. *J Neurosurg Anesthesiol*. 2016;28(4):282–290.
64. Song J, Ji Q, Sun Q, Gao T, Liu K, Li L. The opioid-sparing effect of intraoperative dexmedetomidine infusion after craniotomy. *J Neurosurg Anesthesiol*. 2016;28(1):14–20.
65. Badenes R, Prisco L, Maruenda A, Taccone FS. Criteria for intensive care admission and monitoring after elective craniotomy. *Curr Opin Anaesthesiol*. 2017;30(5):540–545.
66. Mammoto T, Hayashi Y, Ohnishi Y, Kuro M. Incidence of venous and paradoxical air embolism in neurosurgical patients in the sitting position: detection by transesophageal echocardiography. *Acta Anaesthesiol Scand*. 1998;42(6):643–647.
67. Young ML, Smith DS, Murtagh F, Vasquez A, Levitt J. Comparison of surgical and anesthetic complications in neurosurgical patients experiencing venous air embolism in the sitting position. *Neurosurgery*. 1986;18(2):157–161.
68. Abcejo AS, Pasternak JJ, Perkins WJ. Urgent repositioning after venous air embolism during intracranial surgery in the seated position: a case series. *J Neurosurg Anesthesiol*. 2019;31(4):413–421.
69. Nemergut EC, Zuo Z. Airway management in patients with pituitary disease: a review of 746 patients. *J Neurosurg Anesthesiol*. 2006;18(1):73–77.
70. Dunn LK, Nemergut EC. Anesthesia for transsphenoidal pituitary surgery. *Curr Opin Anaesthesiol*. 2013;26(5):549–554.
71. Sharma D. Perioperative management of aneurysmal subarachnoid hemorrhage. *Anesthesiology*. 2020;133(6):1283–1305.
72. Bebawy JF, Gupta DK, Bendok BR, et al. Adenosine-induced flow arrest to facilitate intracranial aneurysm clip ligation: dose-response data and safety profile. *Anesth Analg*. 2010;110(5):1406–1411.
73. Bebawy JF, Zeeni C, Sharma S, et al. Adenosine-induced flow arrest to facilitate intracranial aneurysm clip ligation does not worsen neurologic outcome. *Anesth Analg*. 2013;117(5):1205–1210.
74. Lindgren A, Vergouwen MD, van der Schaaf I, et al. Endovascular coiling versus neurosurgical clipping for people with aneurysmal subarachnoid haemorrhage. *Cochrane Database Syst Rev*. 2018;8:CD003085.
75. Messas E, Goudot G, Halliday A, et al. Management of carotid stenosis for primary and secondary prevention of stroke: state-of-the-art 2020: a critical review. *Eur Heart J Suppl*. 2020;22(Suppl M):M35–M42.
76. Howard G, Roubin GS, Jansen O, et al. Association between age and risk of stroke or death from carotid endarterectomy and carotid stenting: a meta-analysis of pooled patient data from four randomised trials. *Lancet*. 2016;387(10025):1305–1311.
77. Lewis SC, Warlow CP, Bodenham AR, et al; GALA Trial Collaborative Group. General anaesthesia versus local anaesthesia for carotid surgery (GALA): a multicentre, randomised controlled trial. *Lancet*. 2008;372(9656):2132–2142.
78. Li J, Shalabi A, Ji F, Meng L. Monitoring cerebral ischemia during carotid endarterectomy and stenting. *J Biomed Res*. 2017;31(1):11–16.
79. Malas MB, Leal J, Kashyap V, Cambria RP, Kwolek CJ, Criado E. Technical aspects of transcarotid artery revascularization using the ENROUTE transcarotid neuroprotection and stent system. *J Vasc Surg*. 2017;65(3):916–920.
80. Cascino GD, Brinkmann BH. Advances in the surgical management of epilepsy: drug-resistant focal epilepsy in the adult patient. *Neurol Clin*. 2021;39(1):181–196.
81. Cardinale F, Rizzi M, Vignati E, et al. Stereoelectroencephalography: retrospective analysis of 742 procedures in a single centre. *Brain*. 2019;142(9):2688–2704.
82. Le S, Ho AL, Fisher RS, et al. Laser interstitial thermal therapy (LITT): seizure outcomes for refractory mesial temporal lobe epilepsy. *Epilepsy Behav*. 2018;89:37–41.
83. Flexman AM, Wong H, Riggs KW, et al. Enzyme-inducing anticonvulsants increase plasma clearance of dexmedetomidine: a pharmacokinetic and pharmacodynamic study. *Anesthesiology*. 2014;120(5):1118–1125.
84. Kacar Bayram A, Yan Q, Isitan C, Rao S, Spencer DD, Alkawadri R. Effect of anesthesia on electrocorticography for localization of epileptic focus: literature review and future directions. *Epilepsy Behav*. 2021;118:107902.
85. Goettel N, Bharadwaj S, Venkatraghavan L, Mehta J, Bernstein M, Manninen PH. Dexmedetomidine vs propofol-remifentanil conscious sedation for awake craniotomy: a prospective randomized controlled trial. *Br J Anaesth*. 2016;116(6):811–821.
86. Osborn I, Sebeo J. "Scalp block" during craniotomy: a classic technique revisited. *J Neurosurg Anesthesiol*. 2010;22(3):187–194.
87. Aydinlar EI, Dikmen PY, Kocak M, Sahillioglu E, Pamir MN. Intraoperative motor speech mapping under general anesthesia using long-latency response from laryngeal muscles. *Clin Neurol Neurosurg*. 2020;190:105672.
88. Martin J, Tyrand R, Lopez U, et al. Language monitoring in brain surgery under general anesthesia. *J Neurosurg Anesthesiol*. 2020;32(3):268–272.
89. Carney N, Totten AM, O'Reilly C, et al. Guidelines for the management of severe traumatic brain injury, Fourth Edition. *Neurosurgery*. 2017;80(1):6–15.
90. Piper BJ, Harrigan PW. Hypertonic saline in paediatric traumatic brain injury: a review of nine years' experience with 23.4% hypertonic saline as standard hyperosmolar therapy. *Anaesth Intensive Care*. 2015;43(2):204–210.
91. Farag E. Airway management for cervical spine surgery. *Best Pract Res Clin Anaesthesiol*. 2016;30(1):13–25.
92. Walters BC, Hadley MN, Hurlbert RJ, et al. Guidelines for the management of acute cervical spine and spinal cord injuries: 2013 update. *Neurosurgery*. 2013;60(CN_suppl_1):82–91.
93. Fehlings MG, Wilson JR, Tetreault LA, et al. A clinical practice guideline for the management of patients with acute spinal cord injury: recommendations on the use of methylprednisolone sodium succinate. *Global Spine J*. 2017;7(3 Suppl):203S–211S.
94. Yoon H-K, Lee H-C, Chung J, Park H-P. Predictive factors for hypotension associated with supine-to-prone positional change in patients undergoing spine surgery. *J Neurosurg Anesthesiol*. 2020;32(2):140–146.
95. Hoefnagel AL, Rajan S, Martin A, et al. Cognitive aids for the diagnosis and treatment of neuroanesthetic emergencies: consensus guidelines on behalf of the Society for Neuroscience in Anesthesiology and Critical Care (SNACC) education committee. *J Neurosurg Anesthesiol*. 2019;31(1):7–17.
96. Winter SF, Santaguida C, Wong J, Fehlings MG. Systemic and topical use of tranexamic acid in spinal surgery: a systematic review. *Global Spine J*. 2016;6(3):284–295.
97. Lamperti M, Tufegdzic B, Avitsian R. Management of complex spine surgery. *Curr Opin Anaesthesiol*. 2017;30(5):551–556.
98. Murphy GS, Avram MJ, Greenberg SB, et al. Postoperative pain and analgesic requirements in the first year after intraoperative methadone for complex spine and cardiac surgery. *Anesthesiology*. 2020;132(2):330–342.
99. Rajan S, Devarajan J, Krishnaney A, George A, Rasouli JJ, Avitsian R. Opioid alternatives in spine surgery: a narrative review. *J Neurosurg Anesthesiol*. 2022;34(1):3–13.
100. American Society of Anesthesiologists Task Force on Perioperative Visual Loss, North American Neuro-Ophthalmology Society, Society for Neuroscience in Anesthesiology and Critical Care. Practice advisory for perioperative visual loss associated with spine surgery 2019: an updated report by the American Society of Anesthesiologists Task Force on perioperative visual loss, the North American Neuro-Ophthalmology Society, and the Society for Neuroscience in Anesthesiology and Critical Care. *Anesthesiology*. 2019;130(1):12–30.

38 Anesthesia for Thoracic Surgery

EDMOND COHEN • JAMES B. EISENKRAFT

KEY POINTS

1. Determine prior to the commencement of anesthesia whether the patient will be able to tolerate the planned lung resection.
2. Preoperative assessment of vital capacity is critical because at least three times the tidal volume is needed for an effective cough.
3. Smoking increases airway irritability, decreases mucociliary transport, and increases secretions. It also decreases forced vital capacity and forced expiratory flow 25% to 75%, thereby increasing the incidence of postoperative pulmonary complications
4. The absolute indications for lung separation using a double-lumen tube are for protection against spillage of blood, infectious material, or lavage fluid from one lung to the other, or for ventilation in the case of a bronchopleural fistula or bullae. Pneumonectomy or lobectomy are relative indications.
5. The most important advance in checking the proper position of a double-lumen tube or a bronchial blocker is the pediatric flexible fiberoptic bronchoscope.
6. During one-lung ventilation (OLV), the dependent lung should be ventilated using a tidal volume that results in a plateau airway pressure <25 cmH_2O at a rate adjusted to maintain a $PaCO_2$ of 35 ± 3 mmHg.
7. The choice of anesthetic technique for OLV must take into consideration the effects on oxygenation and therefore on hypoxic pulmonary vasoconstriction.
8. The need for OLV is much greater with video-assisted thoracoscopic surgery than with open thoracotomy because it is not possible to retract the lung during VATS, unlike during open thoracotomy.
9. The potential advantages offered by high-frequency positive pressure ventilation are that lower tidal volume and inspiratory pressure result in a quiet lung field for the surgeon, with minimal movement of the airway, lung tissue, and mediastinum.
10. Myasthenia gravis is a disorder of the neuromuscular junction, characterized by weakness and fatigability of voluntary muscles with improvement following rest. Surgical thymectomy is a commonly performed therapy.
11. Adequate pain relief is essential to avoid atelectasis from limited inspiratory thoracic cage expansion. It also makes the patient more comfortable postoperatively.

Introduction

Thanks to more than 100 years of improvements in anesthesia and surgical techniques, complex thoracic procedures are now routinely performed in patients who would not have been considered candidates in the past. One-lung ventilation (OLV) is a critical part of thoracic anesthesia practice, and is essential for lung, esophageal, mediastinal, spinal, and cardiac procedures performed via thoracic approaches. Minimally invasive intrathoracic procedures rely heavily on OLV for adequate surgical exposure. The wide variety of double-lumen endotracheal tubes (DLTs) and endobronchial blockers that are currently available enables OLV to be provided safely and reliably for virtually all patients.

Lung Cancer

Lung cancer is currently estimated to be responsible for 1.59 million deaths annually worldwide.[1] It is by far the leading cause of cancer death, responsible for almost 25% of all cancer deaths. Each year, more people die from lung cancer than from colon, breast, and prostate cancers combined. The American Cancer Society estimates that in the United States in 2022, there will be 236,740 new cases of lung cancer (117,910 in men and 118,830 in women) resulting in about 130,180 deaths (68,820 in men and 61,360 in women) (Fig. 38-1). On a positive note, the number of new lung cancer cases continues to decrease due to people stopping smoking and advances in early detection and treatment.

The overall risk of developing lung cancer is greater in women than in men (1 in 13 vs. 1 in 16). Most lung cancers are found in the older population, the average age at time of diagnosis is about 70 years. Less than 2% of all cases occur in those aged 45 years or less.[2] The increased incidence of lung cancer has led to an increase in the amount of noncardiac thoracic surgery performed in the United States.

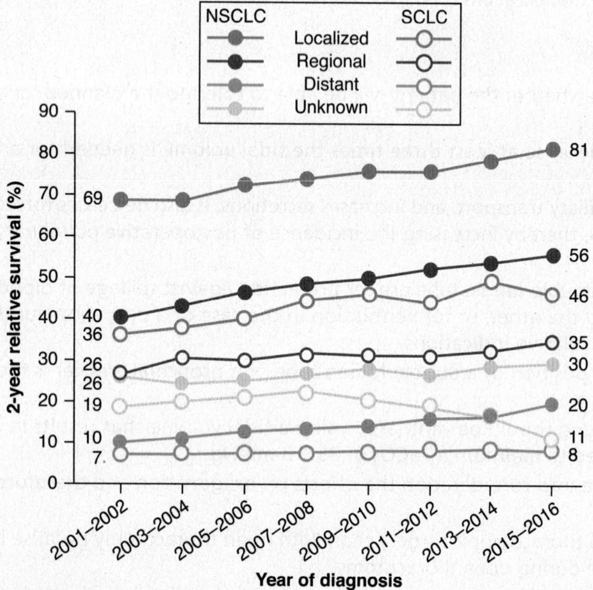

Figure 38-1 Cancer statistics 2021. Trends in 2-year relative survival for lung cancer by subtype and stage at diagnosis, 2001 to 2016. Survival is based on patients diagnosed during 2001 to 2016, all followed through 2017. NSCLC indicates non–small cell lung cancer; SCLC, small cell lung cancer. (Reprinted from Siegel RL, Miller KD, Fuchs HE, et al. Cancer Statistics, 2021. *CA A Cancer J Clinicians.* 2021;71(1):7–33. Copyright © 2021 American Cancer Society.)

In this chapter, the physiologic, pharmacologic, and clinical considerations for the patient undergoing pulmonary surgery are reviewed, followed by sections on anesthesia for diagnostic and therapeutic procedures, high-frequency ventilation, and special situations, including bronchopleural fistula (BPF) and tracheal reconstruction. A discussion of myasthenia gravis (MG) is included because of its relationship to the thymus gland and because thymectomy is one of the most commonly performed surgical procedures in these patients. The chapter concludes with a review of the postoperative management of the patient who has undergone noncardiac thoracic surgery.

Preoperative Evaluation

All patients undergoing thoracic surgery, regardless of age, type of 1
planned surgery, or extent of underlying disease, should be thoroughly evaluated for comorbid risk factors. These include but are not limited to the severity of their underlying pulmonary disease, the presence of cardiovascular disease, nutritional status, and any or all medical conditions whose modification could potentially improve outcome.

The main purposes of a comprehensive preoperative evaluation before thoracic surgery are to assess the risk associated with anesthesia and surgery throughout the perioperative period; to identify, modify, and optimize the treatment of comorbidities that may affect perioperative outcome; and to provide the basis for the design of an appropriate, individually tailored, anesthetic plan. It is important to determine whether the patient will be able to tolerate the planned lung resection. Additional benefits include patient education and informed consent, providing advanced knowledge to clinicians when preparation needs vary from the usual routine, and avoiding delay or cancellation on the day of surgery.

The most common complications following thoracic surgery are pulmonary in nature; the most frequent are pneumonia and atelectasis. It is more difficult to predict postoperative pulmonary complications following elective cardiothoracic surgery compared with noncardiothoracic surgery. Thoracic surgery is known to be high risk, and patient factors that have been associated with increased risk include advanced age, poor general health status, chronic obstructive pulmonary disease (COPD), body mass index greater than 30 kg/m^2, low forced expiratory volume in 1 second (FEV_1), and low predicted postoperative FEV_1.

History

Age has repeatedly been shown to be an independent predictor of operative risk and postoperative complications, resulting in increased morbidity and mortality.[3–5] In addition, age is one of the more prominent risk factors for the development of atrial fibrillation in the postoperative period. Pulmonary complications following surgery increase after the fifth decade of life. Although there is no upper age limit that precludes a patient from surgery, physiologic age is likely a better predictor of outcome than chronologic age. Elderly patients with adequate cardiopulmonary reserve and without additional significant risk factors may still have an acceptable level of risk for surgery.

Dyspnea

Dyspnea occurs when the requirement for ventilation is greater than the patient's ability to respond appropriately. Dyspnea is quantified by the degree of physical activity required to produce it, the level of activity possible (e.g., ability to walk on level ground or climb stairs), and management of daily activities. Severe exertional dyspnea usually implies a significantly diminished ventilatory reserve and an FEV_1 later 1,500 mL, with possible need for postoperative ventilatory support.

Cough

Recurrent productive cough for 3 months of the year for 2 consecutive years is necessary to make the diagnosis of chronic bronchitis. Cough indirectly increases airway irritability. If the cough is productive, the volume, consistency, and color of the sputum should be assessed. Sputum should be cultured to rule out infection and to establish whether there is a need for preoperative antibiotic therapy. Blood-stained sputum or episodes of gross hemoptysis should alert the anesthesiologist to the possibility of a tumor invading the respiratory tract (e.g., the main stem bronchus), which might interfere with endobronchial intubation.

Cigarette Smoking

Cigarette smoking is the main risk factor for developing lung cancer and, in the United States, is linked to about 90% of lung cancers. Using other tobacco products such as cigars or pipes also increases the risk for lung cancer. Tobacco smoke is a toxic mix of more than 7,000 chemicals. Cigarette smokers have a 15 to 30 times greater likelihood of developing and/or dying from lung cancer than nonsmokers. Former smokers have a lower risk of lung cancer than if they had continued to smoke, but their risk is still greater than the risk for people who never smoked. Stopping smoking at any age decreases the risk of lung cancer.[4]

Smoking is a well-established risk factor for COPD and heart disease and dramatically increases, up to 20-fold, the risk of lung and esophageal cancers. Smokers have increased postoperative morbidity with a positive correlation between the frequency of postoperative pulmonary complications and the increasing number of pack-years. In a large retrospective study, Matsuoka et al.[5] assessed the relationship between preoperative smoking habits and postoperative pulmonary complications in 1,248 thoracic surgical patients who underwent lobectomy. The incidence of postoperative complications was higher in smokers than in nonsmokers, and the frequency of respiratory-related complications increased along with the number of pack-years. However, they found no relationship between the length of the preoperative smoking cessation period and the frequency of postoperative complications. Therefore, while patients who have stopped smoking have a lower risk of postoperative respiratory-related complications when compared with patients who are actively smoking, the optimal duration of cessation is unclear. Some thoracic surgeons require that their patients stop smoking for a minimum of 2 weeks before surgery, but a majority of thoracic surgeons do not require smoking cessation at all if that would delay the procedure, as there are concerns about disease progression during the cessation period.

Chronic Obstructive Pulmonary Disease

COPD is the most common comorbid condition in the thoracic surgical population, and is the third leading cause of death in the United States. It is estimated that 3.8 million adults in the United States are currently diagnosed with COPD, and it is widespread in both the general and smoking population. COPD is associated with abnormal and permanent enlargement of the airspaces in the lung with destruction of the alveolar walls, which results in loss of gas exchange surface area, air-trapping, and hyperinflation of the airspaces distal to the terminal bronchioles. This leads to compromised lung mechanics, hypercapnia, dyspnea, and hypoxia that often require oxygen therapy. It is a progressive and debilitating disease which, in its final stages, greatly impacts the patient's quality of life and increases health care utilization.

In addition to patient history and physical examination findings, the severity of COPD can be categorized on the basis of the results of PFT-predicted values by using the criteria established in the Global Initiative for Obstructive Lung Disease.[6] COPD is a major patient-related risk factor that is predictive of postoperative pulmonary complications, including postoperative pneumonia, prolonged mechanical ventilation, and respiratory failure requiring reintubation. Severe COPD may also result in right ventricular dysfunction or cor pulmonale, complicating intraoperative management.

Exercise Tolerance

Patients who can walk up three or more flights of stairs are at reduced risk, and those unable to climb two flights are generally at increased risk. The best evaluation is actually the history of the patient's quality of life. An otherwise healthy patient, with good exercise tolerance, generally does not require additional screening tests. Quality of life measures alone have been shown to correlate poorly with such measures as FEV_1, diffusion capacity for carbon monoxide (DLCO), and exercise testing, and should not substitute for actual testing.

Risk Factors for Acute Lung Injury

In some cases, thoracic surgery may lead to acute lung injury (ALI) postoperatively. Perioperative risk factors that have been identified include preoperative alcohol abuse and patients undergoing pneumonectomy. Intraoperative risk factors include high ventilatory pressures and administration of excessive amounts of fluid. Poor preoperative pulmonary function and positive fluid balance on postoperative day 1 have been identified as independent risk factors for lung injury in patients undergoing open thoracotomy.[7]

Physical Examination

The physical examination of the patient should address the following aspects.

Respiratory Pattern

The presence of cyanosis and clubbing, the breathing pattern, and the type of breath sounds should be noted.

Cyanosis. The presence of peripheral cyanosis (in the fingers, toes, or ears) should be distinguished from causes of poor circulation (acrocyanosis). The presence of central cyanosis (in the buccal mucosa) is usually secondary to arterial hypoxemia. If cyanosis is present, the arterial hemoglobin saturation with oxygen is 80% or less (PaO_2 <50 to 52 mmHg), which indicates a limited margin of respiratory reserve.

Clubbing. Clubbing of fingers and toes is often seen in patients with chronic lung disease, malignancies, or congenital heart disease associated with right-to-left shunt.

Respiratory Rate and Pattern. A patient's inability to complete a normal sentence without pausing for breath is an indication of severe dyspnea. Inspiratory paradox, the abdomen moving in while the chest moves out, suggests diaphragmatic fatigue and respiratory dysfunction. The patient should be assessed for paroxysmal retraction (Hoover sign), limited diaphragmatic movement because of hyperinflation, asymmetry of chest movement secondary to phrenic nerve involvement, hemothorax, pleural effusion, and pneumothorax. The pattern and rate of breathing have important roles in distinguishing between obstructive and restrictive lung diseases. For constant minute ventilation, the work done against airflow resistance decreases when breathing is slow and deep. Work done against elastic resistance decreases when breathing is rapid and shallow (e.g., as in pulmonary infarct or pulmonary fibrosis).

Breath Sounds. Wet sounds (crackles) are usually caused by excessive fluid in the airways and indicate sputum retention or edema. Dry sounds (wheezes) are produced by high-velocity gas flow through bronchi and are a sign of airway obstruction. Distant sounds are an indication of emphysema and possibly bullae. The trachea should be in the midline. Displacement of the trachea may be secondary to a number of causes, including mediastinal mass, and should alert the anesthesiologist to a potentially difficult intubation of the trachea or airway obstruction on induction of anesthesia.

Evaluation of the Cardiovascular System

Cardiac complications are the second most common cause of perioperative morbidity and mortality after pulmonary morbidity in patients undergoing thoracic surgery. The reported incidence of an adverse cardiac event following major pulmonary surgery is approximately 10% to 15%. As smoking both increases the incidences of cardiac disease by over 60% and causes lung cancer, this is not surprising. As intrathoracic surgery itself is associated with increased risk of cardiac complications, an electrocardiogram before surgery is appropriate even in otherwise asymptomatic individuals, and is recommended in all patients above the age of 65 years. Anginal symptoms, suspected valvular disease, arrhythmias, shortness of breath, or a history of cardiac disease warrant an appropriate evaluation and noninvasive cardiac testing.

One of the most important factors in the evaluation of a patient scheduled for thoracic surgery is the presence of an increase in pulmonary vascular resistance (PVR) secondary to a fixed reduction in the cross-sectional area of the pulmonary vascular bed. The pulmonary circulation is normally a low-pressure, high-compliance system capable of handling an increase in blood flow by recruitment of normally underperfused vessels. This acts as a compensatory mechanism that normally prevents an increase in pulmonary arterial pressure. In COPD, there is distention of the pulmonary capillary bed with decreased ability to tolerate an increase in blood flow (decreased compliance). Such patients demonstrate an increase in PVR when cardiac output increases because of a decreased ability to compensate for an increase in pulmonary blood flow. This results in pulmonary hypertension, signs of which include a narrowly split second heart sound, increased intensity of the pulmonary component of the second heart sound, and right ventricular and atrial hypertrophy. An increase in PVR is of significance in the management of the patient during anesthesia because several factors, such as acidosis, sepsis, hypoxia, and application of positive end-expiratory pressure (PEEP), all further increase the PVR and increase the likelihood of right ventricular failure.

In patients with ischemic or valvular heart disease, the function of the left side of the heart should also be carefully evaluated.

Electrocardiogram

A patient with COPD may present with electrocardiographic features of right atrial and ventricular hypertrophy and strain. These include a low-voltage QRS complex due to lung hyperinflation and poor R-wave progression across the precordial leads. An enlarged P-wave ("P pulmonale") in standard lead II is diagnostic of right atrial hypertrophy. The electrocardiographic changes of right ventricular hypertrophy are an R/S ratio of greater than 1 in lead V_1 (i.e., R-wave voltage exceeds S-wave voltage).

Chest Radiography

Hyperinflation and increased vascular markings are usually present with COPD. Prominent lung markings often occur in bronchitis. Lung markings are decreased in emphysema, particularly at the bases, where actual bullae may be present in severe cases. Hyperinflation, with an increased anteroposterior chest diameter, may be present, together with an enlarged retrosternal air space of greater than 2 cm in diameter seen in a lateral chest radiograph.

The location of the lung lesion should be assessed by posteroanterior and lateral projections on chest radiography. In addition to tracheal or carinal shift, a mediastinal mass may indicate difficulty with ventilation, a difficult and bloody dissection, difficulty in placing a double-lumen tube (DLT; because of deviation of the main stem bronchus), or a collapsed lobe owing to bronchial obstruction with possible sepsis. Review of a computed tomography (CT) study is also useful, and often provides more information about tumor size and location than the chest radiograph.

Arterial Blood Gas Analysis

A common finding in arterial blood gas analysis of patients with COPD is hypoventilation and CO_2 retention. The "blue bloaters" (chronic bronchitis) are cyanotic, hypercarbic, hypoxemic, and usually overweight. They are in a state of chronic respiratory failure and have a decreased ventilatory response to CO_2. In these patients, the high $PaCO_2$ increases cerebrospinal fluid bicarbonate concentration, the medullary chemoreceptors become reset to a higher level of CO_2, and sensitivity to CO_2 is decreased. Such patients hypoventilate when given high concentrations of oxygen to breathe because of a decreased hypoxic drive.

The "pink puffers" (patients with emphysema) are typically thin, dyspneic, and pink, with essentially normal arterial blood gas values. They present with an increase in minute ventilation to maintain their normal $PaCO_2$, which explains the increase in work of breathing and dyspnea. The preoperative PaO_2 correlates with the intraoperative PaO_2 during OLV, but the intraoperative PaO_2 during two-lung ventilation correlates more closely.

Pulmonary Function Testing and Evaluation for Lung Resectability

There are three goals in performing pulmonary function tests in a patient scheduled for lung resection. The first goal is to identify the patient at risk of increased postoperative morbidity and mortality. In thoracic surgery for lung cancer, the specific question is: How much lung tissue may be safely removed without making the patient a pulmonary cripple? This should be weighed against the 1-year mean survival rate of the patient with surgically untreated lung carcinoma. The second goal is to identify the patient who will need short- or long-term postoperative ventilatory support. The third goal is to evaluate the beneficial effect and reversibility of airway obstruction with the use of bronchodilators.

Effects of Anesthesia and Surgery on Lung Volumes

Anesthesia and postoperative medications can cause changes in lung volumes and ventilatory pattern. Total lung capacity (TLC) decreases after abdominal surgery but not after surgery on an extremity. Vital capacity is decreased by 25% to 50% within 1 to 2 days after surgery and generally returns to normal after 1 to 2 weeks. Residual volume (RV) increases by 13%, whereas expiratory reserve volume decreases by 25% after lower abdominal surgery and 60% after upper abdominal and thoracic surgery. Tidal volume (V_T) decreases by 20% within 24 hours after surgery and gradually returns to normal after 2 weeks. Pulmonary compliance decreases by 33% with similar reductions in functional residual capacity (FRC) secondary to small airway closure.

Most of the patients who undergo lung resection are smokers with a certain degree of COPD. They are prone to postoperative complications in direct relation to the amount of lung to be resected (lobectomy or pneumonectomy) and to the severity of the preoperative lung disease.

Spirometry

2 Forced vital capacity (FVC), FEV_1, maximum voluntary ventilation (MVV), and RV/TLC correlate with outcome following thoracic surgery. An abnormal preoperative vital capacity can be identified in 30% to 40% of postoperative deaths. A patient with an abnormal vital capacity has a 33% likelihood of complications and a 10% risk of postoperative mortality.

FEV_1 is a more direct indication of airway obstruction. In the past, an FEV_1 of less than 800 mL in a 70-kg man had been considered an absolute contraindication to lung resection. However, with the advent of thoracoscopic surgery and improved postoperative pain management, patients with smaller lung volumes are now successfully undergoing surgery. It is preferable to indicate the FEV_1 as a percentage of predicted value, rather than just using the actual results in liters, as the implications of the absolute value may differ depending on the patient and the percentage of predicted value takes into account the patient's age and size. The ratio FEV_1/FVC is useful in differentiating between restrictive and obstructive pulmonary diseases. This ratio is normal in restrictive disease because both FEV_1 and FVC decrease, whereas in obstructive disease the ratio is usually low because the FEV_1 is markedly decreased compared to the FVC. MVV is a nonspecific test and is an indicator of both restriction and obstruction. Although MVV has not been systematically evaluated as a predictor of morbidity, it is generally accepted that an MVV less than 50% of predicted value is an indication of high risk. A ratio of RV to TLC (RV/TLC) of greater than 50% is generally indicative of a high-risk patient for pulmonary resection. By multiplying the preoperative FEV_1 by the percentage of lung tissue expected to remain following resection, a predicted postoperative FEV_1 can be calculated. Patients with a predicted postoperative FEV_1 value above 40% are at reduced risk and those with predicted postoperative FEV_1 below 30% are at increased risk. Those patients who fall into the latter category are more likely to need postoperative ventilation.

Flow–Volume Loops

The flow–volume loop displays essentially the same information as a spirometer but is more convenient for measurement of specific flow rates (Fig. 38-2). The shape and peak airflow rates during expiration at high lung volumes are effort dependent, but indicate the patency of the larger airways. Effort-independent expiration occurs at low lung volumes and usually reflects small airway resistance, best measured by forced expiratory flow (FEF) during the middle half of the FVC ($FEF_{25\% \text{ to } 75\%}$).

In general, patients with obstructive airway disease (Fig. 38-3), such as asthma, bronchitis, and emphysema, have grossly decreased FEV_1/FVC ratios because of increased airway resistance and a decrease in FEV_1. Peak expiratory flow rate and MVV are usually decreased, whereas TLC increases secondary to increases in RV. In these patients, the effort-independent portion of the flow–volume curve is markedly depressed inward, with reduction of the flow rate at 25% to 75% of FVC.

In patients with restrictive disease (Fig. 38-3), such as pulmonary fibrosis and scoliosis, there is a decrease in FVC with a relatively normal FEV_1. Because the airway resistance is normal, FEV_1/FVC is also normal. TLC is markedly decreased, whereas MVV and $FEF_{25\% \text{ to } 75\%}$ are usually normal. The flow–volume curves of these patients are normal in shape, but the lung volumes and peak flow rates are decreased.

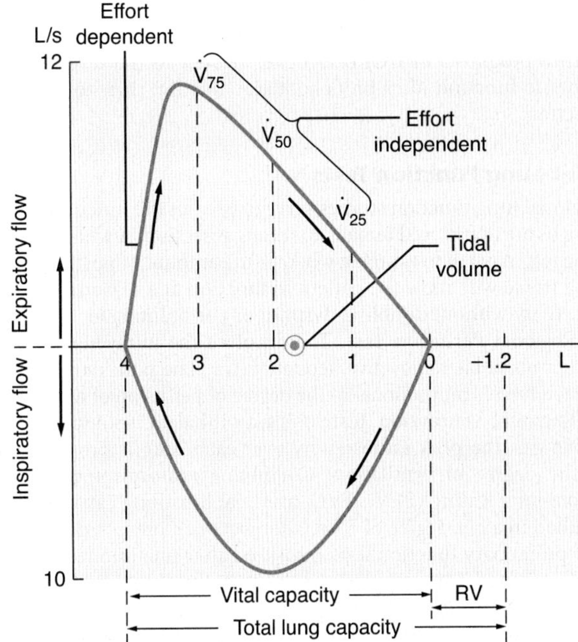

Figure 38-2 Flow–volume loop in a normal subject. $\dot{V}_{75}$, $\dot{V}_{50}$, and $\dot{V}_{25}$ represent flow at 75%, 50%, and 25% of vital capacity, respectively. RV, residual volume. (Adapted from Goudsouzian N, Karamanian A. *Physiology for the Anesthesiologist*. 2nd ed. Appleton-Century-Crofts; 1984.)

Significance of Bronchodilator Therapy. Pulmonary function tests are usually performed before and after bronchodilator therapy to assess the reversibility of the airway obstruction. This is useful in the assessment of the degree of airway obstruction and the patient's effort ability. After treatment with bronchodilators, increases in peak expiratory flow compared with baseline indicate reversibility of airway obstruction (often seen in asthmatic patients). A 15% improvement in pulmonary function tests may

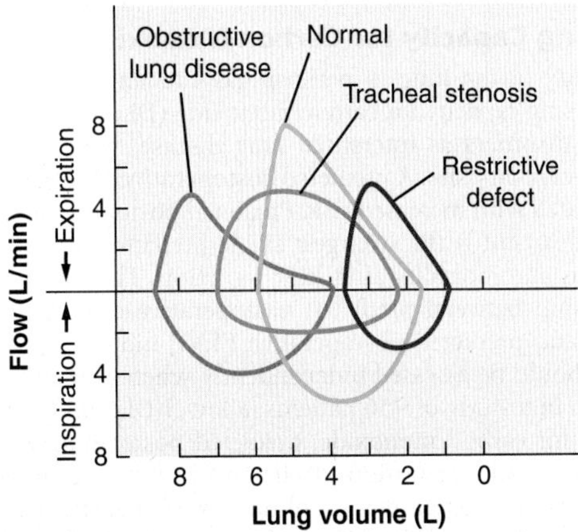

Figure 38-3 Flow–volume loops relative to lung volumes in a normal subject, in a patient with COPD, in a patient with fixed obstruction (tracheal stenosis), and in a patient with pulmonary fibrosis (restrictive defect). Note the concave expiratory form in the patient with COPD and the flat inspiratory curve in the patient with a fixed obstruction. (Adapted from Goudsouzian N, Karamanian A. *Physiology for the Anesthesiologist*. 2nd ed. Appleton-Century-Crofts; 1984.)

be considered a positive response to bronchodilator therapy and indicates that this therapy should be initiated before surgery. The overall prognosis of COPD is better related to the level of spirometric function after bronchodilator therapy than to baseline function.

Split-Lung Function Tests

Regional lung function studies serve to predict the function of the lung tissue that would remain after lung resection. A whole (two)-lung test may fail to estimate whether the amount of postresection lung tissue will allow the patient to function at a reasonable level of activity without disabling dyspnea or cor pulmonale.

Regional Perfusion Test. This involves the intravenous injection of insoluble radioactive xenon (^{133}Xe). The peak radioactivity of each lung is proportional to the degree of perfusion of each lung.

Regional Ventilation Test. Using an inhaled, insoluble radioactive gas, the peak radioactivity over each lung is proportional to the degree of ventilation. Combining radiospirometry with whole-lung testing (FEV_1, FVC, maximal breathing capacity) has resulted in a fair degree of correlation between predicted volumes and pulmonary function tests measured after pneumonectomy.

Computed Tomography and Positron Emission Tomography Scans. Patients normally undergo CT scanning. The CT scan provides anatomic sections through the chest and can delineate the size of a tumor. It can also reveal if there is airway or cardiovascular compression.

Positron emission tomography (PET) scans use a glucose analog that is labeled with a radionuclide positron emitter. This scan can detect tumor based on the metabolic activity. Because malignant tumors grow at such a fast rate compared with healthy tissue, the tumor cells will use up more of the sugar that has the radionuclide attached to it. There is greater uptake by malignant mediastinal lymph nodes than benign nodes. PET may be more accurate than CT for mediastinal staging. Currently, PET scans can be used to further evaluate lesions that are seen on a CT scan. The PET scan can also be used to follow the results of lung cancer treatments.

The CT and PET scans can be done at the same time to produce a PET–CT scan. A mass that is seen on the CT scan is more likely to be malignant if it also demonstrates enhanced glucose uptake on the PET scan.

Diffusing Capacity for Carbon Monoxide

The ability of the lung to perform gas exchange is reflected by the diffusing capacity for carbon monoxide (DLCO). It is impaired in such disorders as interstitial lung disease, which affects the alveolar-capillary site. A predicted postoperative DLCO below 40% is associated with increased risk. Predicted postoperative diffusing capacity percent is the strongest single predictor of risk of complications and mortality after lung resection. There is little interrelationship between predicted postoperative diffusing capacity percent and predicted postoperative FEV_1, indicating that these values should be assessed independently when estimating operative risk. In a study of 956 patients, a lower DLCOPPO (diffusing capacity for carbon monoxide, predicted postoperative) and the preoperative administration of chemotherapy were found to be predictive of postoperative complications. In that study, FEV_1 was not found to be predictive of complications.[8] In another study, the DLCOPPO was the most predictive factor for postoperative morbidity and mortality.[9] It has been demonstrated that PPO FEV_1 and DLCO are predictive for postoperative pulmonary complications in both minimally invasive and open lobectomies.[10] If the PPO FEV_1 and DLCO are greater than 60%, the patient is at low risk, and no further testing is needed.

Maximal Oxygen Consumption

Cardiopulmonary exercise testing (CPET) is a safe and reliable examination that objectively evaluates the function of both the heart and lungs under load. The inability to perform a preoperative CPET suggests that the patient has limited aerobic capacity and may not be suitable for thoracic surgery. Although there are numerous CPET indices, the most critical in assessing suitability for lung resection is the peak oxygen consumption (VO_2 max), which is defined as the maximum oxygen uptake by the body despite increasing workload. Thus, VO_2 max reflects the upper limit of the cardiovascular response and reflects overall cardiorespiratory fitness. In patients undergoing lung resection, perioperative complications have been associated with lower VO_2 max, and risk stratification is defined by the following:

- VO_2 max >20 mL/kg/min or >75% predicted can safely undergo planned lung resection, including pneumonectomy with good prognosis.
- VO_2 max between 10 and 15 mL/kg/min or between 35% and 75% predicted have increased risk of perioperative morbidity and mortality when compared with patients with VO_2 max >75%.
- VO_2 max <10 mL/kg/min or <35% predicted are extremely high risk for postoperative morbidity and mortality and is often regarded as a relative contraindication to major anatomic resections. In such cases, a reduction of the originally planned resection may be required or a nonoperative treatment modality may need to be pursued.[11]

A simpler test that can be performed is exercise oximetry—a decrease of 4% during exercise is associated with increased risk. A 6-minute walk test of less than 2,000 feet has been correlated both with a VO_2 max below 15 mL/kg/min and with a decrease in oximetry reading during exercise. It has been suggested that the percentage of predicted VO_2 max may be a better indicator for risk, and a threshold of 50% to 60% could be established without an increase in surgical mortality. Brunelli and Fianchini[12] had patients climb the maximum number of stairs possible: patients who were able to climb more than 14 m could safely undergo surgery, whereas those who were able to climb less than 12 m, with predicted postoperative function FEV_1 below 35%, were not considered suitable candidates for major lung resection. The inability to do maximal stair climbing has been correlated with an increased mortality following major lung resection.[13] In a recent study, climbing to 20 m with a speed of at least 15 m/min, correlated with meeting qualifying criteria for pneumonectomy. The results for stair climbing correlated with VO_2 consumption during treadmill exercise. Climbing 22 m has been correlated with VO_2 of at least 15 mL/kg/min, although stair climbing testing is not standardized.[14] Evaluating lung function with spirometry and DLCO and estimating peak oxygen consumption helps to predict the risk of postoperative complications. An 11-point scoring scale has been developed for predicting postoperative pulmonary complications: ASA physical status of 3 or higher, emergency or high-risk surgery, and history of CHF or chronic lung disease were independent predictors for reintubation following extubation.[15] The preoperative evaluation of the patient for lung resection is summarized in Figure 38-4.

Preoperative Preparation

Enhanced recovery after surgery protocols and postoperative pulmonary rehabilitation are now ingrained in perioperative pathways, but preoperative rehabilitation, or prehabilitation, is a relatively new concept. The aim of thoracic prehabilitation is to

Whole-lung function

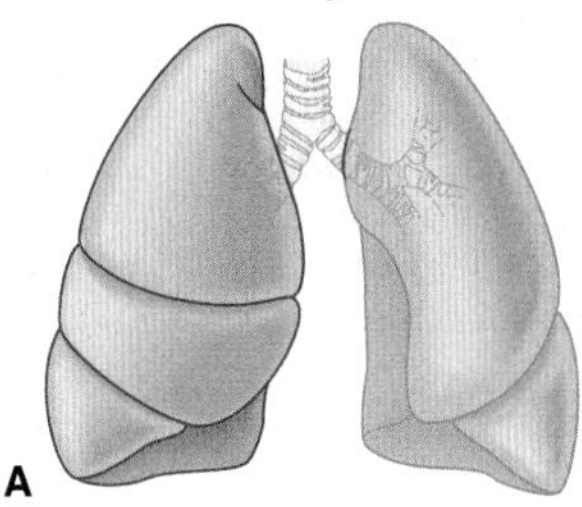

Split-lung function

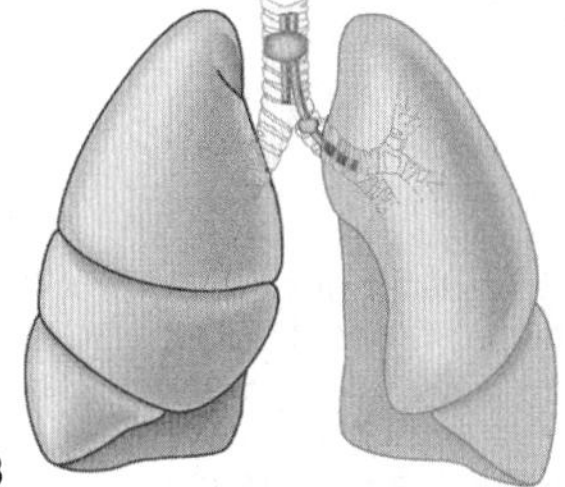

Figure 38-4 The order of tests to determine the cardiopulmonary status of the patient and the extent of lung resection that would be tolerated. **A:** The whole-lung function test is a basic screening test. **B:** The split-lung function tests are regional tests to determine the involvement of the diseased lung to be removed. ABG, arterial blood gas; FVC, forced vital capacity; FEV_1, forced expiratory volume in 1 second; VC, vital capacity; MVV, maximum voluntary ventilation; RV/TLC, residual volume/total lung capacity; DLT, double-lumen tube, DL_{CO}, diffusing capacity for carbon monoxide. (Adapted with permission from Neustein SM, Cohen E. Preoperative evaluation of thoracic surgical patients. In: Cohen E, ed. *The Practice of Thoracic Anesthesia*. JB Lippincott; 1995:187.)

reduce perioperative risk for patients who are suitable for surgery or, in some cases, to move a patient who was previously unfit for surgery into a group which is suitable for surgery. For both these cohorts, the chance of survival may be increased.[16]

The wide spectrum of physiologic changes that occur during thoracic surgery puts patients at great risk of developing postoperative complications. Morbidity and mortality increase when these changes are superimposed on an acutely or chronically compromised patient. Several conditions, including infection, dehydration, electrolyte imbalance, wheezing, obesity, cigarette smoking, cor pulmonale, and malnutrition show particular correlations with postoperative complications. Proper, vigorous preoperative preparation can improve the patient's ability to face surgery with a decreased risk of morbidity and mortality. It is important that conditions predisposing to postoperative complications be rigorously treated before surgery.

Smoking

3 There is a high prevalence of smoking among patients presenting for surgery, and there is extensive evidence that these patients are at increased risk for development of postoperative respiratory complications. Smoking increases airway irritability, decreases mucociliary transport, decreases FVC and $FEF_{25\% \text{ to } 75\%}$, and increases secretions, thereby increasing the incidence of postoperative pulmonary complications. In contrast, cessation of smoking for a period of longer than 4 to 6 weeks before surgery is associated with a decreased incidence of postoperative complications. Furthermore, cessation of smoking 48 hours before surgery has been shown to decrease the percentage of carboxyhemoglobin, to shift the oxyhemoglobin dissociation curve to the right, and to increase oxygen availability. It should be emphasized, however, that most of the beneficial effects of cessation of smoking, such as improvement in ciliary function, improvement in closing volume, increase in $FEF_{25\% \text{ to } 75\%}$, and reduction in sputum production usually occur 2 to 3 months after smoking has ceased. In one study, there was no evidence of a paradoxical increase in postoperative complications in patients who stopped smoking within 2 months before undergoing thoracic resection for lung tumor. Smoking is associated with increased mortality and pulmonary complications, but these can be decreased by preoperative cessation; the risk decreases with a longer cessation. A recent study indicated that the discontinuation of smoking for more than 8 weeks prior to surgery can help improve postoperative pulmonary function. One meta-analysis indicated that there was no improvement with cessation of smoking for less than 8 weeks,[17] but another meta-analysis indicated a progressive improvement with each week of abstinence from smoking.[18–20]

Nutrition

Low BMI is a known risk factor for patients undergoing lung resection surgery. This is a modifiable risk factor, and several scoring systems exist to detect malnutrition.[19,20] Every patient interaction is an opportunity to reinforce the importance of optimizing the nutritional state. There is no accepted definition for perioperative malnutrition, which should encompass both under- and overnourished states. Although overnourished patients are at risk of postoperative complications, undernourished patients with lung cancer may be sarcopenic and have limited reserve to cope with the insult of surgery. Avoiding malnutrition and supporting anabolism are basic perioperative goals, which can be met with screening, referral to dietetics, and nutritional prehabilitation.[21] Treatment can take the form of oral nutritional supplements, vitamins, immunonutrition, protein, and carbohydrate loading.

The American Society for Enhanced Recovery and Perioperative Quality Initiative published a Joint Consensus Statement on Nutrition Screening and Therapy Within a Surgical Enhanced Recovery Pathway. A proposed perioperative nutrition screen (PONS) determines the presence of nutrition risk based on a patient's BMI, recent changes in weight, reported recent decrease in dietary intake, and preoperative albumin level (Fig. 38-5). In

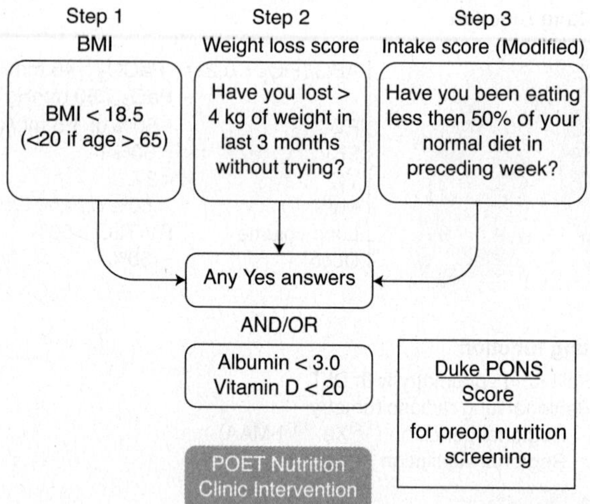

Figure 38-5 Perioperative nutrition screen (PONS). The PONS determines the presence of nutrition risk based on a patient's body mass index, recent changes in weight, reported decrease in dietary intake, and preoperative albumin level. In addition, the PONS includes evaluation of a preoperative albumin level, as this is a predictor of postoperative complications, including morbidity/mortality. BMI, Body Mass Index. (Reprinted with permission from Wischmeyer PE, Carli F, Evans DC, et al. American society for enhanced recovery and perioperative quality initiative joint consensus statement on nutrition screening and therapy within a surgical enhanced recovery pathway. *Anesthesia and Analgesia*. 2018;126:1883–1895.)

addition, the PONS includes evaluation of preoperative albumin level, as this is a predictor of postoperative complications, including morbidity/mortality.[22]

Infection

Although not all surgeons routinely administer antibiotics prophylactically to their patients, any infection present before surgery should be vigorously treated. Treatment of the acutely ill patient depends on the results of the Gram stain of the sputum and blood cultures, and broad-spectrum antibiotics are commonly used. Cefazolin is routinely administered perioperatively, unless the patient is already receiving antibiotics or has modifying circumstances such as an allergic history. To be most effective, antibiotics need to be given prior to skin incision. In one prospective study, the incidence of mortality was lower in the group treated with prophylactic antibiotics compared with the untreated group (9% vs. 17%), and a lower incidence of postoperative pulmonary infection was also found.[23]

Hydration and Removal of Bronchial Secretions

Correction of hypovolemia and electrolyte imbalance should be accomplished before surgery because adequate hydration decreases the viscosity of bronchial secretions and facilitates their removal from the bronchial tree. Humidification of inspired gas is extremely useful. The use of mucolytic drugs, such as acetylcysteine (Mucomyst), or oral expectorants (potassium iodide) can be beneficial to patients with viscous secretions. Commonly used methods for removing secretions from the bronchial tree include postural drainage, vigorous coughing, chest percussion, deep breathing, and the use of an incentive spirometer. These modalities often require patient cooperation and frequent verbal encouragement to maximize the benefit.

Wheezing and Bronchodilation

The presence of acute wheezing represents a medical emergency, and elective surgery should be postponed until effective treatment has been instituted. Chronic wheezing is often seen in patients with COPD and is attributable to the presence of gas flow obstruction secondary to smooth muscle contraction, accumulation of secretions, and mucosal edema. Smooth muscle contraction may occur in small airways only (detectable by changes in $FEF_{25\% \text{ to } 75\%}$) or may be widespread, with a large reduction of FEV_1 and FVC. The efficacy of bronchodilators in reversing the bronchospastic component is extremely important. A trial of bronchodilators and measurement of their effects on pulmonary function should be performed in any patient who shows evidence of airflow obstruction. Several classes of bronchodilators are available.

Sympathomimetic Drugs

Sympathomimetic drugs increase the formation of 3′, 5′-cyclic adenosine monophosphate (cAMP). The balance between cAMP, which produces bronchodilation, and cyclic guanosine monophosphate (cGMP), which produces bronchoconstriction, determines the state of contraction of the bronchial smooth muscle. Increasing cAMP production, therefore, causes relaxation of the bronchial tree. Sympathomimetic drugs, such as epinephrine, isoproterenol, isoetharine, and ephedrine, all have mixed β_1 and β_2 sympathetic agonist effects. The β_1 (cardiac effects) of these drugs are often undesirable in patients with COPD. Selective β_2 sympathomimetic drugs, such as albuterol, terbutaline, and metaproterenol, given as inhaled aerosols, are the preferred drugs for the treatment of bronchospasm, particularly in patients with cardiac disease.

Phosphodiesterase Inhibitors

Phosphodiesterase inhibitors inhibit the breakdown of cAMP by cytoplasmic phosphodiesterase. The methylxanthines, such as aminophylline, increase the level of cAMP, resulting in bronchodilation. In addition, aminophylline improves diaphragmatic contractility and increases the patient's resistance to fatigue. Therapeutic blood levels of aminophylline are 5 to 20 μg/mL and can be achieved by infusing a loading dose of 5 to 7 mg/kg over 20 minutes, followed by a continuous intravenous infusion of 0.5 to 0.7 mg/kg/h. Aminophylline may cause ventricular dysrhythmias, and this side effect should be borne in mind when treating patients who have myocardial ischemia. Because newer medications have fewer side effects, aminophylline is now rarely used.

Steroids

Although not true bronchodilators, steroids are traditionally considered to decrease mucosal edema and may prevent the release of bronchoconstricting substances. They are of questionable benefit in acute bronchospasm. Steroids may be administered orally, parenterally, or in aerosol form, such as beclomethasone by inhaler.

Cromolyn Sodium

Cromolyn sodium stabilizes mast cells and inhibits degranulation and histamine release. It is useful in the prevention of bronchospastic attacks but is of little value in the treatment of the acute situation.

Parasympatholytic Drugs

Parasympatholytics include atropine and ipratropium. In the past, atropine has been avoided in patients with COPD and bronchitis because of the concern regarding increases in the viscosity of mucus produced by this agent. However, atropine blocks the formation of cGMP and therefore has a bronchodilator effect.

Pulmonary Rehabilitation

Sekine et al. reported that pulmonary rehabilitation led to reduced hospital stay and improved postoperative FEV_1, compared with a historical control group.[23] The pulmonary rehabilitation included education in a variety of areas such as breathing, exercise, and nutrition. Preoperative physical therapy in patients undergoing surgery for lung cancer led to better oxygenation and shortened hospital stay in the treatment group. Prehabilitation must be multimodal. It is the sum of marginal gains from several interventions that are themselves complementary. It requires invested resources, infrastructure, organization, and an acceptance of the longer-term benefits for surgical outcomes, value for money, and public health.[24] Thoracic surgical patients awaiting resection of cancer have limited time available between diagnosis and surgery, and other related hospital appointments or treatments might place both a physical and psychological burden on the patient.

Intraoperative Monitoring

All patients undergoing anesthesia for thoracic surgical procedures require adherence to the Standards of Basic Anesthetic Monitoring of the American Society of Anesthesiologists (ASA) (see Chapter 26). In particular, these include an electrocardiogram (lead II and, if possible, V_5), chest or esophageal stethoscopes for heart and breath sound auscultation, and a temperature probe. A chest stethoscope may be placed over the dependent hemithorax to assess dependent lung ventilation. Pulse oximetry, which is a standard of care, is especially valuable during thoracic surgery because hypoxemia may occur during OLV.

Dysrhythmias occur commonly both during and after thoracic surgery, making the usual need for continuous electrocardiographic monitoring even more important. Intraoperative supraventricular tachyarrhythmias may be caused by cardiac manipulation. Dysrhythmias that occur during OLV may be a sign of inadequate oxygenation or ventilation. Postoperative dysrhythmias may be related to sympathetic nervous system stimulation from pain or to a decreased pulmonary vascular bed following lung resection. Patients who present for lung resection often have COPD due to cigarette smoking, have right-sided heart strain, and are prone to multifocal atrial tachyarrhythmias.

The axis of electrocardiogram lead II parallels that of the P-wave, making this lead useful for dysrhythmia detection. The simultaneous monitoring of lead V_5 also allows for monitoring of anterolateral wall myocardial ischemia. The use of multiple leads increases the sensitivity for ischemia detection. The following invasive monitors are also indicated and have led to marked improvements in patient care.

Direct Arterial Catheterization

Peripheral arterial catheterization has become an essential tool for the anesthesiologist in the management of patients undergoing major thoracic surgical procedures. It allows for continuous beat-to-beat measurement of blood pressure and frequent sampling of arterial blood gases. Continuous blood pressure readings are critical during thoracic surgery because surgical manipulations may result in cardiac compression and there may be sudden bleeding. Immediate recognition of these changes allows time for proper identification of the etiology and the institution of appropriate treatment.

Serial arterial blood gas analyses are performed as needed in the management of patients undergoing one-lung anesthesia or during cases in which a part of the lung may be "packed away" for a period. Arterial hypoxemia may occur because of an inadequate hypoxic pulmonary vasoconstriction (HPV) response and shunting of mixed venous blood through the collapsed lung. Significant changes in acid–base status and hyperventilation or hypoventilation can also be identified.

A radial artery catheter can be placed in either extremity during thoracic surgery. For a mediastinoscopic examination, one approach is to place the catheter in the right arm and to use it to monitor for possible compression of the innominate artery by the mediastinoscope. This can help avoid central nervous system complications that might result from inadequate cerebral blood flow via the right carotid artery (see "Mediastinoscopy"). The other approach would be to place the arterial catheter in the left radial artery, allowing for continuous blood pressure measurements, uninterrupted by innominate artery compression. If this is done, a pulse oximeter probe should be placed on the right upper extremity to monitor for innominate artery compression. During thoracotomy, placement of the arterial catheter in the dependent arm can be used to monitor for possible axillary artery compression, which may occur if the patient is not properly positioned. For a brief thoracoscopy case in a relatively healthy patient, it would be acceptable to proceed without an arterial catheter, as long as the pulse oximeter is functioning reliably. Such an example might be a healthy patient presenting for bilateral VATS sympathectomy for hyperhidrosis.

The patient undergoing a pulmonary resection, and especially a right pneumonectomy, is at risk for postoperative pulmonary edema. It is especially important to not fluid overload such a patient, as the likelihood of postoperative edema is greater with increased intraoperative fluid administration. It would be preferable to be able to identify whether the patient would be likely to respond favorably to a fluid bolus prior to its administration. The central venous pressure (CVP) may not accurately reflect intravascular volume status, and is no longer recommended as a guide for fluid responsiveness. Systolic pressure variation (SPV) and pulse pressure variation (PPV) have been reported as being able to predict fluid responsiveness. Cannesson et al. found a PPV greater than 13% predicted fluid responsiveness, less than 9% predicted that the patient would not be responsive, and 9% to 13% reflected a gray zone.[25] Stroke volume variation has been reported to predict fluid responsiveness, specifically in patients undergoing thoracic surgery, during OLV.

Central Venous Pressure Monitoring

The CVP may reflect the patient's blood volume, venous tone, and right ventricular performance; however, it is also affected by central venous obstructions and alterations of intrathoracic pressure such as PEEP. The CVP reflects right-sided heart function, not left ventricular performance. Catheters for measuring CVP may be placed for thoracotomies, and in particular, patients undergoing pneumonectomy. Uses of CVP catheters or large-bore introducers include (1) insertion of a transvenous pacemaker where necessary, (2) infusion of vasoactive drugs, and (3) insertion of a pulmonary artery (PA) catheter, which may subsequently be required during surgery or in the postoperative period.

The CVP catheter can be placed centrally from either the external or the internal jugular vein, from the subclavian veins, or from one of the arm veins. The success rate is highest using the right internal jugular vein, and a pacemaker or PA catheter can be inserted most easily from this vein. The major disadvantage of using the external jugular vein during thoracotomy is that the catheter often kinks when the patient is turned to the lateral decubitus position. The subclavian technique leads to a higher incidence of pneumothorax, which can be disastrous if it occurs in the dependent lung during OLV. If necessary and if possible, a subclavian catheter should be placed ipsilateral to the surgery. As discussed earlier, the CVP is no longer considered an accurate guide for fluid responsiveness. However, it is a common practice among thoracic anesthesiologists to place a CVP catheter for certain thoracic cases such as esophagectomy and pneumonectomy.

Pulmonary Artery Catheterization

The PA catheter is most reliably inserted through the right internal jugular vein using a modified Seldinger technique. Insertion of the PA catheter through either the external jugular vein or the subclavian vein often leads to obstruction of the catheter when the patient is placed in the lateral decubitus position. Misinterpretation of data from a PA catheter is a real risk in a patient with cardiac and pulmonary diseases undergoing thoracic surgery with OLV. These errors can be produced by altered ventilatory modes, the location of the PA catheter tip, ventricular compliance changes, or ventricular interdependence.[26] A major limitation of the PA catheter is the assumption that the pulmonary capillary wedge pressure (PCWP) provides a good approximation of left ventricular end-diastolic volume. The use of PCWP directly to assess preload assumes a linear relationship between ventricular end-diastolic volume and ventricular end-diastolic pressure. However, alterations in ventricular compliance affect this pressure–volume relationship during surgery. Decreases in ventricular compliance can occur with myocardial ischemia, shock, right ventricular overload, or pericardial effusion. Numerous investigators have demonstrated a poor correlation between PCWP and left ventricular end-diastolic volume in acutely ill patients. This correlation is further worsened by the application of PEEP. In addition, ventricular interdependence can cause misdiagnosis when the interventricular septum encroaches on the left ventricular cavity, leading to increased values of PCWP. A PCWP associated with a decreased cardiac output can be interpreted as left ventricular failure, when in fact, left ventricular end-diastolic volume may not be increased but decreased because of compression of the left ventricle by a distended right ventricle. This situation can occur with acute respiratory failure and high levels of PEEP. Techniques such as echocardiography, which directly measure ventricular dimensions, may facilitate resolution of this complex situation.

Because most of the pulmonary blood flow is to the right lower lobe, the tip of a flow-directed PA catheter is usually located in the right lower lobe. During a left thoracotomy with OLV, the catheter tip would then be in the dependent lung and should provide accurate hemodynamic measurements. However, during a right thoracotomy with OLV, the catheter tip would most likely be in the nondependent lung, and may not be accurate. The use of intraoperative mean PA pressure has been reported to be an indicator of safety for lung resection under thoracotomy.[26] The authors concluded that following occlusion of the main PA, upper safety limits of 33 mmHg for right, and 35 mmHg for left thoracotomy could be used. The authors noted that the difference between sides was minimal, and less than expected. The monitoring of mixed venous oxygen saturation has been evaluated in patients undergoing one-lung anesthesia; changes in mixed venous oxygen saturation were mainly dependent on changes in arterial oxygen saturation.[27] Currently, the use of the PA catheter for monitoring during thoracic surgery is generally unnecessary, and may be reserved for patients with pulmonary hypertension.

Transesophageal Echocardiography

Transesophageal echocardiography (TEE) is a useful intraoperative monitor for ventricular function, valvular function, and wall motion changes that might reflect ischemia. Its use in thoracic surgical patients has been limited, but it is widely used in patients undergoing lung transplant. The use of TEE requires special training, and may not be available at all centers. A recent review concluded that although the intraoperative use of TEE is not routinely indicated, it may be useful for diagnosing right ventricular dysfunction in the setting of hypotension or arrhythmias following lung resection. Right ventricular dysfunction may occur during OLV, clamping of the PA for pneumonectomy, or lung transplantation. TEE may be used to help determine if it is necessary to initiate cardiopulmonary bypass during lung transplantation.

TEE may be useful in visualizing hilar lung tumors, and evaluating possible extension into the heart. In one study, central lung tumors were able to be seen with TEE in nine of nine patients, peripheral lung tumors in one of three patients, and an anterior mediastinal mass in one of one patient.[28] TEE also revealed PA compression in five patients and PA infiltration in two patients. In another study investigating echocardiographic recognition of mediastinal tumors, TEE revealed that these tumors were often adjacent to the heart and identified those patients in whom there was compression of the innominate vein or PA, or infiltration of the heart.

Intraoperative TEE has also been used to reveal tumor invasion of the heart, which indicates that a resection by thoracotomy without cardiopulmonary bypass is not feasible.[29] In one case report, TEE monitoring during an attempted resection of a tumor invading the left atrium showed embolization of the tumor. Fragments of the tumor were seen to pass through the aortic valve. This patient subsequently died of disseminated metastases. In an exploratory thoracotomy for hemothorax, intraoperative TEE revealed the presence of a subacute aortic dissection, which was believed to be the cause of the hemothorax. TEE was used intraoperatively to evaluate a large anterior mediastinal mass, providing data on right ventricular outflow compression, and ventricular contractility and filling status. In another recent report, a mediastinal mass was diagnosed intraoperatively using TEE; in that case, the mass had been misdiagnosed preoperatively with transthoracic echocardiography as a pericardial effusion.

Additional Noninvasive Monitoring

Although data are presently limited, it has been reported that decreased cerebral oximetry values by absolute cerebral oximetry during OLV have been correlated with postoperative complications.[30] In a subsequent study, larger decreases in cerebral oxygen saturation occurred in patients with better preoperative lung function.[30] At this time, the data are still too limited to recommend cerebral oximetry as a routine monitor during thoracic surgery.

A meta-analysis of the use of noninvasive cardiac output measurements during surgery revealed poor agreement with thermodilution. Noninvasive cardiac output measurements are not commonly utilized during thoracic surgery and thus are recommended at this time.[31]

Monitoring of Oxygenation and Ventilation

Oxygenation

During the administration of all thoracic surgical anesthetics, the concentration of inspired oxygen in the breathing system must be measured using an oxygen analyzer with a low oxygen concentration limit alarm: this is a basic monitoring standard. Such analyzers vary in sophistication from fuel cells to rapidly responding paramagnetic analyzers that monitor oxygen breath by breath and display an oxygram (analogous to, and a mirror image of, the capnogram). Adequacy of blood oxygenation must be ensured, and adequate illumination and exposure of the patient are helpful to assess the color of shed blood or the presence of cyanosis of the lips, nail beds, or mucous membranes. Most patients undergoing thoracic surgical or diagnostic procedures have an arterial catheter in place for continuous monitoring of blood pressure and sampling of arterial blood for blood gas analyses.

Pulse oximetry is a standard of care for noninvasive assessment of blood oxygenation. The use of pulse oximetry is especially important during OLV, when rapid assessment of oxygenation is critical. A low SpO_2 reading provides the clinician with an indication for blood gas sampling and laboratory analysis of arterial blood. The traditional two-wavelength pulse oximeter may display spurious readings of SpO_2 in the presence of dyshemoglobins, methemoglobin, and carboxyhemoglobin. Multiwavelength (8 or 12 wavelengths) pulse oximeters are available that can measure carboxyhemoglobin, methemoglobin, deoxygenated hemoglobin, and oxygenated hemoglobin (HbO_2%).[32] Continuous noninvasive monitoring of total hemoglobin concentration is also available.

Ventilation

All patients must be continually monitored to ensure adequacy of ventilation. Monitoring includes qualitative signs such as chest excursion (visual observation of the lungs when the chest is open) and auscultation of breath sounds. In addition, during OLV, a stethoscope can be placed on the chest wall under the ventilated dependent lung. During controlled ventilation, circuit low- and high-pressure alarms with an audible signal must be used. The respiratory rate, V_T, minute volume, and inflation pressures should be monitored.

Adequacy of ventilation is confirmed by monitoring arterial blood gas analyses, and $PaCO_2$ in particular. This may be estimated continuously and noninvasively by capnography. The end-tidal CO_2 concentration represents alveolar CO_2 ($PaCO_2$), which approximates $PaCO_2$. There is normally a small arterial-to-alveolar CO_2 difference (4 to 6 mmHg), depending on alveolar dead space. The capnogram waveform is also helpful in diagnosing airway obstruction, incomplete relaxation, and even malposition of the DLT.[33] During OLV, systemic hypoxemia is usually a greater problem than hypercarbia. This is because CO_2 is approximately 20 times more diffusible than oxygen and $PaCO_2$ is more dependent on ventilation, compared with PaO_2, which is more dependent on perfusion.

Physiology of One-Lung Ventilation

Physiology of the Lateral Decubitus Position. Ventilation and blood flow under physiologically routine conditions are discussed in Chapter 15. These variables will now be considered as they pertain to the lateral decubitus position under six circumstances that are encountered during thoracic surgery.

Lateral Position, Awake, Breathing Spontaneously, Chest Closed. In the lateral decubitus position, the distribution of blood flow and ventilation is similar to that in the upright position, but turned by 90 degrees (Fig. 38-6). Blood flow and ventilation to the dependent lung are significantly greater than that to the nondependent lung. Good matching at the level of the dependent lung results in adequate oxygenation in the awake patient who is breathing spontaneously. There are two important concepts in this situation. First, because perfusion is gravity dependent, the vertical hydrostatic pressure gradient is smaller in the lateral than in the upright position; therefore, zone 1 is usually less extended. Second, in regard to ventilation, the dependent hemidiaphragm is pushed higher into the chest by the abdominal contents compared with the nondependent lung hemidiaphragm. During spontaneous ventilation, the conserved ability of the dependent diaphragm to contract results in an adequate distribution of V_T to the dependent lung. Because most of the perfusion is to the dependent lung, the matching in this position is maintained similar to that in the upright position.

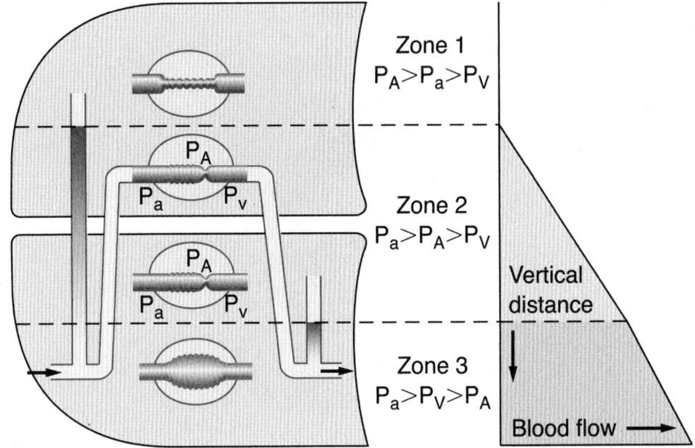

Figure 38-6 Schematic representation of the effects of gravity on the distribution of pulmonary blood flow in the lateral decubitus position. Vertical gradients in the lateral decubitus position are similar to those in the upright position and cause the creation of West zones 1, 2, and 3. Consequently, pulmonary blood flow increases with lung dependency, and is largest in the dependent lung and least in the nondependent lung. P_a, pulmonary artery pressure; P_A, alveolar pressure; P_V, pulmonary venous pressure. (Adapted from Benumof JL. Physiology of the open-chest and one lung ventilation. In: *Thoracic Anesthesia*. Churchill Livingstone; 1983:288. Copyright © 1983 Elsevier. With permission.)

Lateral Position, Awake, Breathing Spontaneously, Chest Open. Controlled PPV is the most common way to provide adequate ventilation and ensure gas exchange in an open-chest situation. Frequently, thoracoscopy is performed using intercostal blocks with the patient breathing spontaneously to allow proper lung examination. The thoracoscope provides an adequate seal of the open chest to prevent a "free" open-chest situation. Two complications can arise from the patient breathing spontaneously with an open chest. The first is mediastinal shift, usually occurring during inspiration (Fig. 38-7). The negative pressure in the intact hemithorax, compared with the less negative pressure of the open hemithorax, can cause the mediastinum to move vertically downward and push into the dependent hemithorax. The mediastinal shift can create circulatory and reflex changes that may result in a clinical picture similar to that of shock and respiratory distress. Sometimes, depending on the severity of the distress, it may be necessary to convert emergently to general anesthesia in order to intubate the patient and initiate PPV. The anesthesiologist must be prepared to intubate in lateral position without disturbing the surgical field.

The second phenomenon is paradoxical breathing (Fig. 38-8). During inspiration, the relatively negative pressure in the intact hemithorax compared with atmospheric pressure in the open hemithorax can cause movement of air from the nondependent lung into the dependent lung. The opposite occurs during expiration. This gas movement reversal from one lung to the other represents wasted ventilation and can compromise the adequacy of gas exchange. Paradoxical breathing is increased by a large thoracotomy or by an increase in airway resistance in the dependent lung.

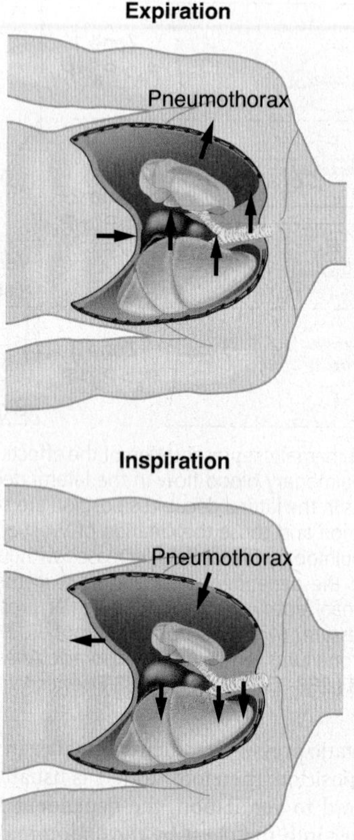

Figure 38-7 Schematic representation of mediastinal shift in the spontaneously breathing, open-chested patient in the lateral decubitus position. During inspiration, negative pressure in the intact hemithorax causes the mediastinum to move downward. During expiration, relative positive pressure in the intact hemithorax causes the mediastinum to move upward. (Adapted from Tarhan S, Moffitt EA. Principles of thoracic anesthesia. *Surg Clin North Am.* 1973;53:813. Copyright © 1973 Elsevier. With permission.)

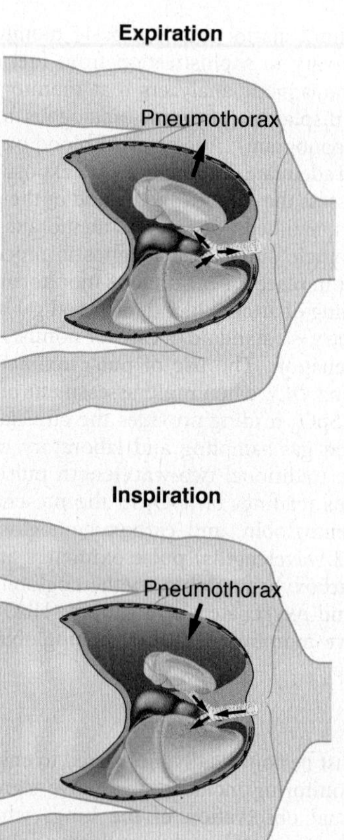

Figure 38-8 Schematic representation of paradoxical respiration in the spontaneously breathing, open-chested patient in the lateral decubitus position. During inspiration, movement of gas from the exposed lung into the intact lung and movement of air from the environment into the open hemithorax cause collapse of the exposed lung. During expiration, the reverse occurs, and the exposed lung expands. (Adapted from Tarhan S, Moffitt EA. Principles of thoracic anesthesia. *Surg Clin North Am.* 1973;53:813. Copyright © 1973 Elsevier. With permission.)

PPV or adequate sealing of the open chest eliminates paradoxical breathing.

Lateral Position, Anesthetized, Breathing Spontaneously, Chest Closed. The induction of general anesthesia does not cause significant change in the distribution of blood flow, but it has an important impact on the distribution of ventilation. Most of the V_T enters the nondependent lung, and this results in a significant mismatch. Induction of general anesthesia causes a reduction in the volumes of both lungs secondary to a reduction in FRC. For several reasons, any reduction in volume in the dependent lung is of a greater magnitude than that in the nondependent lung. First, the cephalad displacement of the dependent diaphragm by the abdominal contents is more pronounced and is increased by paralysis. Second, the mediastinal structures pressing on the dependent lung or poor positioning of the dependent side on the operating table prevents the lung from expanding properly. These factors will move the lungs to a lower volume on the S-shaped volume–pressure curve (Fig. 38-9). The nondependent lung moves to a steeper position on the compliance curve and receives most of the V_T, whereas the dependent lung is on the flat (noncompliant) part of the curve.

Lateral Position, Anesthetized, Breathing Spontaneously, Chest Open. Opening the chest has little impact on the distribution of perfusion. However, the upper lung is now no longer restricted by the chest wall and is free to expand, resulting in a

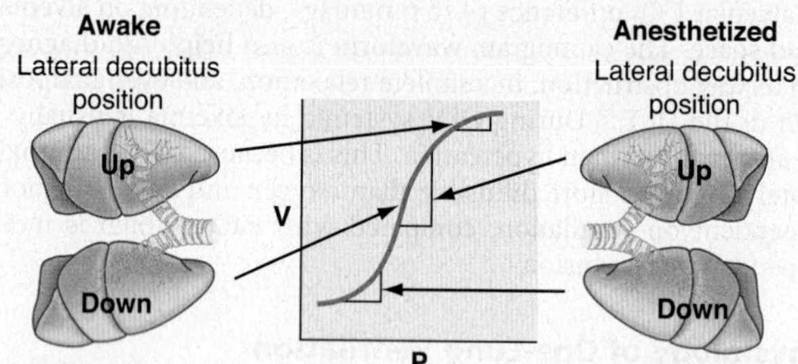

Figure 38-9 The left side of the schematic shows the distribution of ventilation in the awake patient (closed chest) in the lateral decubitus position, and the right side shows the distribution of ventilation in the anesthetized patient (closed chest) in the lateral decubitus position. The induction of anesthesia has caused a loss in lung volume in both lungs, with the nondependent (**up**) lung moving from a flat, noncompliant portion to a steep, compliant portion of the pressure–volume curve, and the dependent (**down**) lung moving from a steep, compliant part to a flat, noncompliant part of the pressure–volume curve. Thus, the anesthetized patient in the lateral decubitus position has most tidal ventilation in the nondependent lung (where there is the least perfusion) and less tidal ventilation in the dependent lung (where there is the most perfusion). V, volume; P, pressure. (Adapted from Benumof JL. *Anesthesia for Thoracic Surgery*. WB Saunders; 1987:112. Copyright © 1987 Elsevier. With permission.)

Figure 38-10 This schematic of a patient in the lateral decubitus position compares the closed-chested anesthetized condition with the open-chested anesthetized and paralyzed condition. Opening the chest increases nondependent lung compliance and reinforces or maintains the larger part of the tidal ventilation going to the nondependent lung. Paralysis also reinforces or maintains the larger part of tidal ventilation going to the nondependent lung because the pressure of the abdominal contents (P_{AB}) pressing against the upper diaphragm is minimal, and it is therefore easier for positive-pressure ventilation to displace this less resisting dome of the diaphragm. V, volume; P, pressure. (Adapted from Benumof JL. *Anesthesia for Thoracic Surgery*. WB Saunders; 1987:112. Copyright © 1987 Elsevier. With permission.)

further increase in mismatch as the nondependent lung is preferentially ventilated, owing to a now increased compliance.

Lateral Position, Anesthetized, Paralyzed, Chest Open. During paralysis and PPV, diaphragmatic displacement is maximal over the nondependent lung, where there is the least amount of resistance to diaphragmatic movement caused by the abdominal contents (Fig. 38-10). This further compromises the ventilation to the dependent lung and increases the mismatch.

OLV, Anesthetized, Paralyzed, Chest Open. During two-lung ventilation in the lateral position, the mean blood flow to the nondependent lung is assumed to be 40% of cardiac output, whereas 60% of cardiac output goes to the dependent lung (Fig. 38-11). Normally, venous admixture (shunt) in the lateral position is 10% of cardiac output and is equally divided as 5% in each lung. Therefore, the average percentage of cardiac output participating in gas exchange is 35% in the nondependent lung and 55% in the dependent lung.

OLV creates an obligatory right-to-left transpulmonary shunt through the nonventilated, nondependent lung because the percentage of cardiac output participating in gas exchange in that lung is zero by definition. In theory, an additional 35% should be added to the total shunt during OLV. However, assuming active HPV, blood flow to the nondependent hypoxic lung will be decreased by 50% and therefore becomes (35/2) = 17.5%. 5% must be added to this to account for the obligatory shunt through the nondependent lung, and, therefore, the shunt through the nondependent lung is 22.5% (Fig. 38-11). Together with the 5% shunt in the dependent lung, the total shunt fraction during OLV is 22.5% + 5% = 27.5%. This results in a PaO_2 of approximately 150 mmHg for an inspired oxygen fraction (FIO_2) of 1.0.[34]

Because 72.5% of the perfusion is directed to the dependent lung during OLV, the matching of ventilation in this lung is important for adequate gas exchange. The dependent lung is no longer on the steep (compliant) portion of the volume–pressure curve because of reduced lung volume and FRC. There are several reasons for this reduction in FRC, including general anesthesia, paralysis, pressure from abdominal contents, compression by the weight of mediastinal structures, and suboptimal positioning on the operating table. Other considerations that impair optimal ventilation to the dependent lung include absorption atelectasis, accumulation of secretions, and the formation of a transudate in the dependent lung. All these create a low $\dot{V}/\dot{Q}$ ratio and a large $P(A–a)O_2$ gradient.

One-Lung Ventilation

In any given case, the anesthesiologist must distinguish between 4
the need for lung separation versus lung isolation (Table 38-1). Most procedures use OLV for lung separation; only a few require isolation for lung protection. This distinction of lung isolation versus lung separation is important when selecting the method to provide OLV. When lung protection is necessary, DLTs are preferable to endobronchial blockers (BBs) because the low-pressure high-volume cuff of the BB would not provide an adequate protective seal to prevent contamination of the dependent lung. The use of blockers limits the ability to perform robust suctioning and removal of debris or thick pus before balloon deflation. Furthermore, once the balloon of the blocker is deflated, the nondiseased lung becomes subject to contamination from the diseased lung.

Lung Isolation

Whenever the nondiseased lung is threatened with contamination by blood or pus from the diseased lung, the nondiseased lung

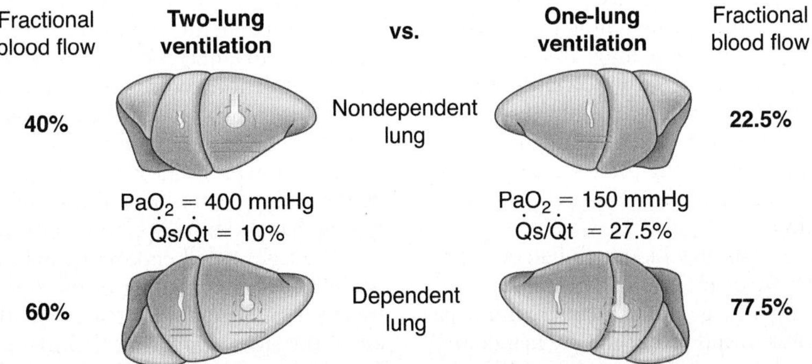

Figure 38-11 Schematic representation of two-lung ventilation versus one-lung ventilation (OLV). Typical values for fractional blood flow to the nondependent and dependent lungs, as well as PaO_2 and $\dot{Q}_s/\dot{Q}_t$ for the two conditions, are shown. The $\dot{Q}_s/\dot{Q}_t$ during two-lung ventilation is assumed to be distributed equally between the two lungs (5% to each lung). The essential difference between two-lung ventilation and OLV is that, during OLV, the nonventilated lung has some blood flow and therefore an obligatory shunt, which is not present during two-lung ventilation. The 35% of total flow perfusing the nondependent lung, which was not shunt flow, was assumed to be able to reduce its blood flow by 50% by hypoxic pulmonary vasoconstriction. The increase in $\dot{Q}_s/\dot{Q}_t$ from two-lung to OLV is assumed to be due solely to the increase in blood flow through the nonventilated, nondependent lung during OLV. (Adapted from Benumof JL. *Anesthesia for Thoracic Surgery*. WB Saunders; 1987:112. Copyright © 1987 Elsevier. With permission.)

Table 38-1 Indications for One-lung Ventilation

Absolute
1. Isolation of each lung to prevent contamination of a healthy lung
a. Infection (abscess, infected cyst)
b. Massive hemorrhage
2. Control of distribution of ventilation to only one lung
a. Bronchopleural fistula
b. Bronchopleural cutaneous fistula
c. Unilateral cyst or bullae
d. Major bronchial disruption or trauma
3. Unilateral lung lavage
4. Video-assisted thoracoscopic surgery
Relative
1. Surgical exposure—high priority
a. Thoracic aortic aneurysm
b. Pneumonectomy
c. Lung volume reduction
d. Minimally invasive cardiac surgery
e. Upper lobectomy
2. Surgical exposure—low priority
a. Esophageal surgery
b. Middle and lower lobectomies
c. Mediastinal mass resection, thymectomy
d. Bilateral sympathectomies

Modified from Benumof JL. Physiology of the open-chest and one lung ventilation. In: Kaplan JA, ed. *Thoracic Anesthesia*. Churchill Livingstone; 1983:299. Copyright © 1983 Elsevier. With permission.

must be isolated to prevent potentially life-threatening complications. Furthermore, the nondiseased lung must maintain adequate gas exchange. Lung isolation may be lifesaving by simply preventing drowning or severe contamination of the ventilated lung from the nondependent lung. Lung protection will prevent further deterioration of overall pulmonary function. Cases requiring lung isolation include hemoptysis, empyema, or where any contaminant in the noninvolved lung could lead to severe atelectasis, pneumonia, sepsis, and inadequate ventilation. A large bronchopleural or bronchocutaneous fistula can result in little or no ventilation. In this situation, the decreased resistance to flow in the affected lung results in most of the PPV being directed toward the diseased lung. This results in minimal ventilation of the normal lung, resulting in inadequate gas exchange. Conversely, a relatively noncompliant transplanted lung cannot compete with the better compliance of the native lung, and as a result, the healthy transplanted lung can be severely underventilated. Yet another scenario involves a lung with bullous or cystic disease, or a lung with tracheobronchial disruption. Tension pneumothorax or tension mediastinum could result during these scenarios from the increased airway pressures that are often observed with OLV in the lateral decubitus position.

Patients with alveolar proteinosis may require unilateral bronchopulmonary lavage, which involves multiple instillations of large fluid volumes into the target lung with subsequent drainage of the effluent fluid. Lung isolation and protection are mandatory to avoid lung cross-contamination and drowning caused by the large volume of fluid required to perform the lavage.

Lung Separation

Lung separation facilitates surgical exposure by providing a still operating field, avoiding lung trauma, and improving gas exchange. Operations such as repair of thoracic aneurysms, pneumonectomy, pulmonary lobectomies (especially of the upper lobe), video-assisted thoracoscopic surgery (VATS), esophageal surgery, and anterior spinal surgery, all benefit from the optimized surgical exposure afforded by lung separation and OLV. Lung protection further improves recovery by minimizing instrumentation and trauma to the operated, nonventilated, nondependent lung. In cases of unilateral lung trauma, oxygenation and recovery may be optimized with OLV by improving $\dot{V}/\dot{Q}$ matching.

Methods of Lung Separation

Double-Lumen Endobronchial Tubes[35]

Double-lumen endobronchial tubes are currently the most widely used means of achieving lung separation and OLV. There are several different types of DLT, but all are essentially similar in design in that two endotracheal tubes are "bonded" together. One lumen is long enough to reach a main stem bronchus, and the second lumen ends with an opening in the distal trachea. Lung separation is achieved by inflation of two cuffs: a proximal tracheal cuff and a distal bronchial cuff located in the main stem bronchus (see "Placement of Double-Lumen Tubes"). The endobronchial cuff of a right-sided tube is slotted or otherwise designed to allow ventilation of the right upper lobe because the right main stem bronchus is too short to accommodate both the right lumen tip and a right bronchial cuff.

Robertshaw Tube. The Carlens tube (which had a carinal hook) was the first clinically available DLT and was used by pulmonologists for split function spirometry testing (Fig. 38-12A). Subsequently, the Robertshaw-design DLT (which lacked a carinal hook) was developed to facilitate thoracic surgery (Fig. 38-12B). This DLT is available in left- and right-sided forms. The absence of a carinal hook facilitates insertion. The tube design has the advantages of having D-shaped, large-diameter lumens that allow easy passage of a suction catheter, offer low resistance to gas flow, and have a fixed curvature to facilitate proper positioning and reduce the possibility of kinking. The original red rubber Robertshaw tubes were available in three sizes: small, medium, and large. A single-use replica of the original red rubber Robertshaw design DLT is shown in Figure 38-13. Red rubber tubes are rarely used now and have been replaced by clear, polyvinyl chloride (PVC) disposable Robertshaw-design DLTs. These are available in both right-sided and left-sided versions for the 35 French (Fr), 37 Fr, 39 Fr, and 41 Fr sizes. A 32-Fr left-sided DLT is available for small adults, and a 28 Fr for use in pediatric cases. The advantages of the disposable tubes include the relative ease of insertion and proper positioning as well as easy recognition of the blue color of the endobronchial cuff when fiberoptic bronchoscopy is used. Other advantages are the confirmation of the position on a chest radiograph using the radiopaque lines in the wall of the tube and the continuous observation of tidal gas exchange and respiratory moisture through the clear plastic. The right-sided endobronchial tube is designed to minimize occlusion of the opening of the right upper lobe bronchus, featuring a right endobronchial cuff that is doughnut shaped to allow the right upper lobe ventilation slot to ride over the opening of the right upper lobe bronchus. The tube is also suitable for use in long-term ventilation in the intensive care unit (ICU) because it has a high-volume, low-pressure cuff. These disposable PVC tubes are generally considered the tubes of choice for achieving lung separation and OLV. In addition to the disposable PVC Robertshaw design DLT, there are novel DLTs that are less frequently used (Fig. 38-13).[35]

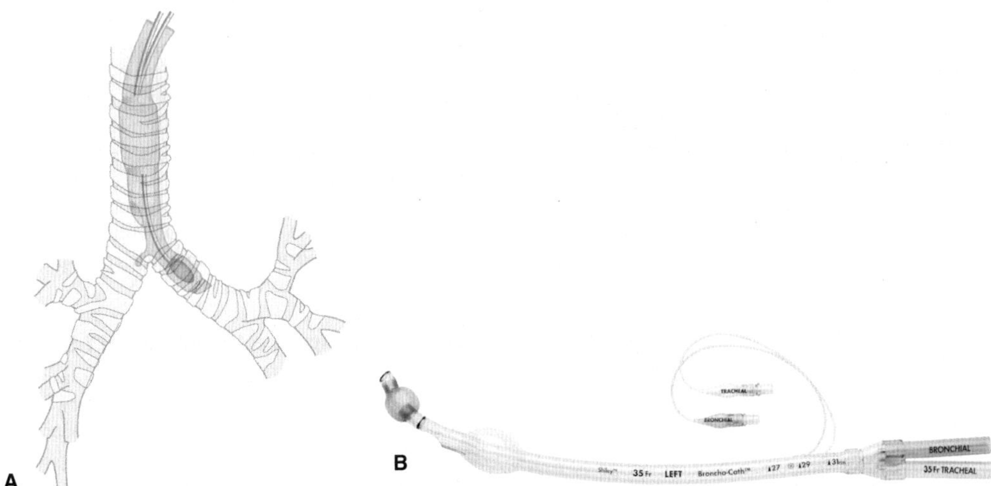

Figure 38-12 **A:** Left main stem endobronchial intubation using a Carlens tube. Note carinal "hook" used for correct positioning. (Derived from Hillard EK, Thompson PW. Instruments used in thoracic anaesthesia. In: Mushin WW, ed. *Thoracic Anaesthesia*. Blackwell Scientific; 1963:315.) **B:** A left-sided Robertshaw type double-lumen tube constructed from polyvinyl chloride. (© 2023 Medtronic. All rights reserved. Used with the permission of Medtronic)

The Silbroncho tube (Fuji Systems Corporation, Tokyo, Japan) is D shaped with a flexible wire-reinforced bronchial tip that allows the tube to be inserted at an angle of >50 degrees without kinking the bronchial lumen. It is useful in patients who require lung isolation after left upper lobectomy. In such patients, expansion of the left lower lobe causes the left main bronchus (LMB) to rotate upward and make a 90-degree angle from the trachea, which often prevents a conventional DLT from being placed in the LMB without kinking.[36] The tube is available only in a left-sided version.[37]

The Papworth BiVent tube (P3 Medical, Bristol, UK) is a divided single-lumen tube with a forked tip that rests on the carina. An integrated bronchial blocker can then be advanced into the operative lung. This tube eliminates the need for endobronchial intubation, and lung isolation can be achieved without the need for bronchoscope-guided blocker placement.

Silbroncho	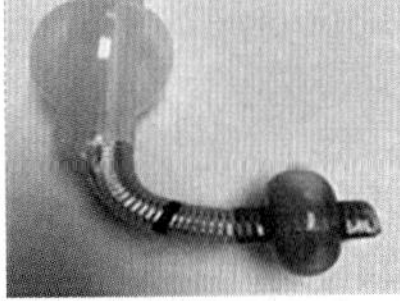	■ Can be inserted at > 50° angle without kinking of the bronchial lumen ■ Flexible wire-reinforced bronchial tip	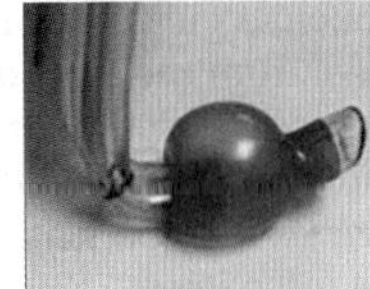	Conventional DTL stiffness prevents it passing through >50° angle into the left main bronchus without kinking the bronchial lumen
Papworth BiVent Tube	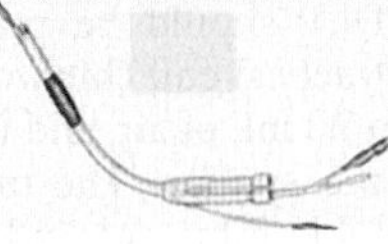	■ A divided single-lumen tube ■ Eliminates the need for endobronchial intubation ■ Can achieve lung isolation without the need for FB	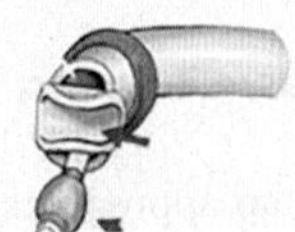	A forked tip that rests on the carina
ET View DLT	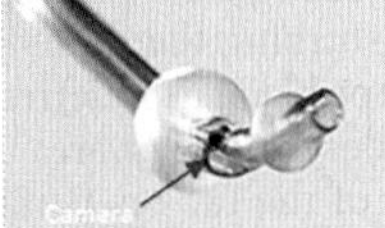	■ An integrated video camera ■ Provides a continuous real-time view of tube position	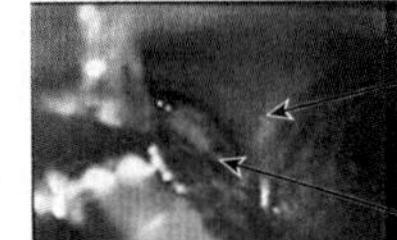	Carina L-DLT image throught the ET view Bronchial cuff
A single use Robertshaw DLT	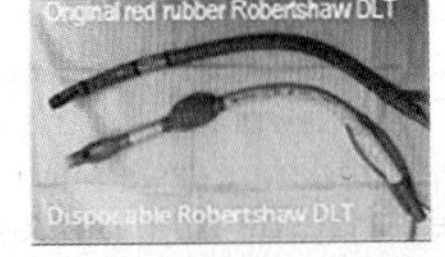	■ Single use replica of the original red rubber Robertshaw DLT ■ Less likely displaced intraoperatively	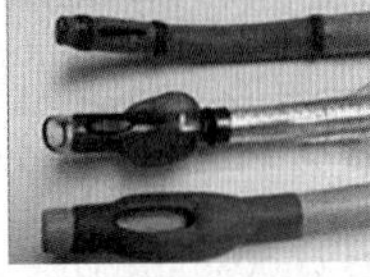	longer ventilating slot. Increases the chance of alignment with the right upper lobe orifice
ECOM DLT	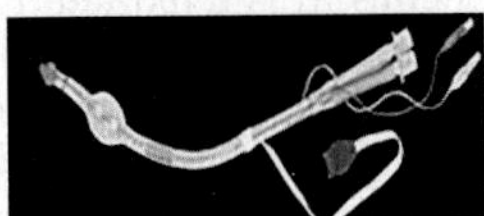	■ Continuous CO Monitoring ■ Potentially be useful during lung transplantation, off-pump cardiac surgery	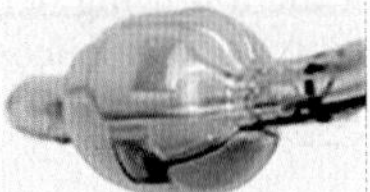	Electrodes on the Bronchial Cuff

Figure 38-13 Novel double-lumen tubes. CO indicates cardiac output; DLT, double-lumen tube; ET, endotracheal tube; FB, fiberoptic bronchoscope; L-DLT, left-sided double-lumen tube. See text for descriptions. (Reprinted with permission from Cohen E. Current practice issues in thoracic anesthesia. *Anesthesia & Analgesia*. 2021;133(6):1520–1531.)

The VivaSight-DL (Ambu Inc., Columbia, MO, USA / ET View Ltd., Misgav, Israel) has recently been introduced to clinical practice. It is a disposable DLT that incorporates a high-resolution camera embedded on the DLT between the tracheal cuff and the bronchial cuff.[38] This device allows continuous real-time viewing of the DLT position, which can be important in cases where the patient's head is away from the anesthesiologist, such as during robotic thoracic surgery. The VivaSight tube is also available as a single-lumen tube (VivaSight-SL), through which an independent blocker may be inserted without the need of a fiberoptic bronchoscope. A prospective study of 71 adult patients compared intubation times using either the VivaSight-DL or a conventional DLT. The duration of intubation with visual confirmation of tube position was significantly reduced using the VivaSight-DL compared with the conventional DLT (51 vs. 264 seconds). None of the patients allocated to the VivaSight-DL required fiberoptic bronchoscopy during intubation or surgery. One limitation of the VivaSight compared with a fiberoptic bronchoscope is that the position of the camera is set at the distal part of the tracheal lumen and therefore it cannot be used to inspect either the left or right main stem bronchus if this is deemed necessary. Thus, the VivaSight DLT will not completely eliminate the use of a fiberoptic bronchoscope in lung isolation procedures, but may instead lead to a significant reduction in use. Other studies of this tube have compared it favorably to conventional Robertshaw DLTs and found that it can be cost-effective when compared to routine Robertshaw/fiberoptic bronchoscope approaches.[39] In addition to decreasing the need for perioperative fiberoptic bronchoscopy, the VivaSight can also guide bronchial blocker placement by visualization of the bronchial blocker position at the carinal level. This real-time continuous monitoring of position can be useful during right-side isolation with a bronchial blocker, where the margin for malposition is smaller.

The ECOM DLT (ECOM Medical, CONMED Corporation, Utica, NY) has electrodes on the bronchial cuff that enable real-time monitoring of impedance changes from the ascending aorta and provides an estimate of cardiac output. This tube can potentially be useful during lung transplantation or off-pump cardiac surgery where lung collapse is required, or for patients with cardiac comorbidities who undergo lung resection.

Selection of DLT Size: Formulas, CT Scans, and Ultrasound

In order to provide lung separation, an appropriately sized DLT must be selected. Too large a tube may result in herniation of the bronchial cuff and/or cause tracheal or bronchial damage, while an undersized tube may dislocate intraoperatively with failure of lung separation.

The optimal size of DLT should allow the bronchial lumen to pass into the desired mainstem bronchus with minimal resistance and permit a bronchial seal when the bronchial cuff is inflated. A left-sided DLT is preferred for both left- and right-sided procedures. A left-sided DLT was selected for 1,166 of the 1,170 patients in one report, and was used successfully in over 98% of those patients. No consensus exists as to how to best determine DLT size and most anesthesiologists choose the DLT size based on their personal experience. Use of the following height/gender decision criteria resulted in a >90% incidence of successful positioning and a similar rate of effective lung separation:

- Women <1.6 m (63 in) → 35 Fr
- Women >1.6 m → 37 Fr
- Men <1.7 m (67 in) → 39 Fr
- Men >1.7 m → 41 Fr

Typically, most women will need a 37-Fr DLT and most men can be adequately managed with a 39-Fr DLT. The authors recommended selecting the largest DLT that will safely fit the bronchus. This will provide less resistance to ventilation, requires less air and pressure in the bronchial cuff to form a seal, and is less likely to dislocate or migrate distally. However, the common practice of fiberoptic bronchoscopy has decreased the risk of undetected distal placement or migration of the bronchial tip. One study showed that the routine use of a 35-Fr DLT in adults regardless of height was not associated with an increase in hypoxemia or any other adverse clinical outcomes.

Chest Imaging as a Guide for DLT Selection

Although patient height is often used as a basis for selecting a DLT, as above, the correlation between airway size and height is poor. Tracheal and bronchial dimensions can be directly measured from the chest radiograph or chest CT scan. The size of the LMB is a relevant factor when sizing a DLT but, unlike the trachea, it is not clearly visible on chest x-ray in >50% of cases. However, since tracheal width is closely correlated with LMB width, LMB width can be estimated as 0.68 × tracheal width. The average depth of insertion from the lips of left DLT placement in a 170-cm tall man or woman has been estimated at 28 to 29 cm with approximately ± 1.0 cm for each 10-cm change in height.

Two-dimensional ultrasound measurements of tracheal size have also been used to estimate correct DLT size.[40] When compared to measurements of LMB by CT scan, ultrasound estimates of tracheal size correlated with the CT scan measurements and placement of DLTs chosen based on ultrasound measurement were uniformly successful. Chest ultrasound has also been used to confirm correct DLT position and in comparative trials has demonstrated greater sensitivity to correct placement than auscultation.[41] The use of ultrasound to verify DLT placement may represent an alternative option if fiberoptic bronchoscopy is not available.

Placement of Double-Lumen Tubes

This section concentrates on the insertion of disposable Robertshaw-design DLTs because they are the most widely used. Before insertion, the DLT should be prepared and checked. (1 Video 38-1) The tracheal cuff (high volume, low pressure) can accommodate up to 20 mL of air, and the bronchial cuff can be checked using a 3-mL syringe. The tube should be coated liberally with water-soluble lubricant and the stylet should be withdrawn, lubricated, and gently placed back into the bronchial lumen without disturbing the tube's preformed curvature. A Macintosh laryngoscope blade is preferred for intubation of the trachea because it provides the largest area through which to pass the tube. The insertion of the tube is performed with the distal concave curvature facing anteriorly. After the tip of the tube is past the vocal cords, the stylet is removed and the tube is rotated through 90 degrees. A left-sided tube is rotated 90 degrees to the left, and a right-sided tube is rotated to the right. Advancement of the tube ceases when moderate resistance to further passage is encountered, indicating that the tube tip has been firmly seated in the main stem bronchus. It is important to remove the stylet before rotating and advancing the tube to avoid tracheal or bronchial laceration. Rotation and advancement of the tube should be performed gently and under continuous direct laryngoscopy to prevent hypopharyngeal structures from interfering with proper positioning. Once the tube is believed to be in the proper position, a sequence of steps should be performed to check its location.

First, the tracheal cuff should be inflated, and equal ventilation of both lungs established. If breath sounds are not equal, the tube is probably too far down, and the tracheal lumen opening is in a main stem bronchus or is lying at the carina. Withdrawal of the tube by 2 to 3 cm usually restores equal breath sounds. The second step is to clamp the right side (in the case of the left-sided tube) and remove the right cap from the connector. Then the bronchial cuff is slowly inflated to prevent an air leak from the bronchial lumen around the bronchial cuff into the tracheal lumen. This ensures that excessive pressure is not applied to the bronchus and helps avoid laceration. Inflation of the bronchial cuff rarely requires greater than 2 mL of air. The third step is to remove the clamp and check that both lungs are ventilated with both cuffs inflated. This ensures that the bronchial cuff is not obstructing the contralateral hemithorax, either totally or partially. The final step is to clamp each side selectively and watch for absence of movement and breath sounds on the ipsilateral (clamped) side; the ventilated side should have clear breath sounds, chest movement that feels compliant, respiratory gas moisture with each tidal ventilation, and no gas leak. If peak airway pressure during two-lung ventilation is 20 cmH_2O, it should not exceed 40 cmH_2O for the same V_T during OLV.

Other methods that have been used for ensuring the correct placement of a DLT include fluoroscopy, chest radiography, selective capnography, and use of an underwater seal. Determination of the presence of gas leaks when positive pressure is applied to one lumen of a DLT is easily done in the operating room (OR). If the bronchial cuff is not inflated and positive pressure is applied to the bronchial lumen of the DLT, gas will leak retrograde around the bronchial cuff and return through the tracheal lumen. If the tracheal lumen is connected to an underwater seal system, gas will be seen to bubble up through the water. The bronchial cuff can then be gradually inflated until no gas bubbles are seen and the desired cuff seal pressure is attained. This test is of extreme importance when absolute lung separation is needed, such as during bronchopulmonary lavage.

5 The introduction of the pediatric flexible fiberoptic bronchoscope has been the most important advance in checking for proper positioning of a DLT (Fig. 38-14). Smith et al.[42] showed that when the disposable DLT was believed to be in correct position by auscultation and physical examination, subsequent fiberoptic bronchoscopy showed that 48% of tubes were, in fact, malpositioned. Such malpositions, however, are usually of no clinical significance.[43] When using a left-sided DLT, the bronchoscope is usually first introduced through the tracheal lumen. The carina is visualized, but no bronchial cuff herniation should be seen. The bronchial cuff of the disposable DLT is easily visualized because of its blue color. The upper surface of the blue endobronchial cuff should be just below the tracheal carina. The bronchoscope should then be passed through the bronchial lumen, and the left upper lobe bronchial orifice should be identified. When a right-sided DLT is used, the carina should be visualized through the tracheal lumen but, more importantly, the orifice of the right upper lobe bronchus should be identified when the bronchoscope is passed through the right upper lobe ventilating slot of the DLT. Pediatric fiberoptic bronchoscopes are available in several sizes: 5.6 mm, 4.9 mm, and 3.6 mm in external diameter. The 3.6-mm diameter bronchoscope is easily passed through all sizes of DLT. The 4.9-mm diameter bronchoscope can be passed through DLTs of 37 Fr and larger. In general, it is recommended that the largest bronchoscope size that can pass through the lumen of the DLT be used because this provides better visualization and facilitates identification of the bronchial anatomy.

Problems of Malposition of the Double-Lumen Tube

The use of a DLT is associated with a number of potential problems, the most important of which is malposition. There are six main malposition possibilities to consider.

1. The DLT may be accidentally directed to the side opposite the desired main stem bronchus. In this case, the lung opposite the side of the connector clamp will collapse. Inadequate separation, increased airway pressures, and instability of the DLT usually occur. In addition, because of the morphology of the DLT curvatures, tracheal or bronchial lacerations may result. If a left-sided DLT is inserted into the right main stem bronchus, it obstructs ventilation to the right upper lobe. It is therefore essential to recognize and correct such a malposition as soon as possible.
2. The DLT may be passed too far down into either the right or the left main stem bronchus (Fig. 38-15). In this case, breath sounds are very diminished or not audible over the contralateral side. This situation is corrected when the tube is withdrawn and the opening of the tracheal lumen is above the carina.
3. The DLT may not be inserted far enough, leaving the bronchial lumen opening above the carina. In this position, good breath sounds are heard bilaterally when ventilating through the bronchial lumen. No breath sounds are audible when ventilating through the tracheal lumen because the inflated bronchial cuff obstructs gas flow arising from the tracheal lumen. The cuff should be deflated and the DLT rotated and advanced into the desired main stem bronchus.
4. A right-sided DLT may occlude the right upper lobe orifice. The mean distance from the carina to the right upper lobe orifice is 2.3 ± 0.7 cm in men and 2.1 ± 0.7 cm in women.[44] With right-sided DLTs, the ventilatory slot in the side of the bronchial catheter must overlie the right upper lobe orifice to permit ventilation of this lobe. However, the margin of safety is extremely small, and varies from 1 to 8 mm.[45] It is therefore difficult to ensure proper ventilation to the right upper lobe and avoid dislocation of the DLT during surgical manipulation. When right endobronchial intubation is required, a disposable right-sided DLT is perhaps the best choice because of the slanted doughnut shape of the bronchial cuff, which allows the ventilation slot to ride off the right upper lobe ventilation orifice and increases the margin of safety.
5. The left upper lobe orifice may be obstructed by a left-sided DLT. Traditionally, it was believed that the take-off of the left upper lobe bronchus was at a safe distance from the carina and that it would not be obstructed by a left-sided DLT. However, the mean distance between the left upper lobe orifice and the carina is 5.4 ± 0.7 cm in men and 5 ± 0.7 cm in women.[44] The average distance between the openings of the right and left lumens on the left-sided disposable tubes is 6.9 cm. Therefore, an obstruction of the left upper lobe bronchus is possible while the tracheal lumen is still above the carina. There is also a 20% variation in the location of the blue endobronchial cuff on the disposable tubes because this cuff is attached to the tube at the end of the manufacturing process.
6. Bronchial cuff herniation may occur and obstruct the bronchial lumen if excessive volumes are used to inflate the cuff. The bronchial cuff has also been known to herniate over the tracheal carina, and in the case of a left-sided DLT, to obstruct ventilation to the right main stem bronchus.

Tracheal laceration or rupture is a rare complication with DLTs (Fig. 38-16). Overinflation of the bronchial cuff, inappropriate

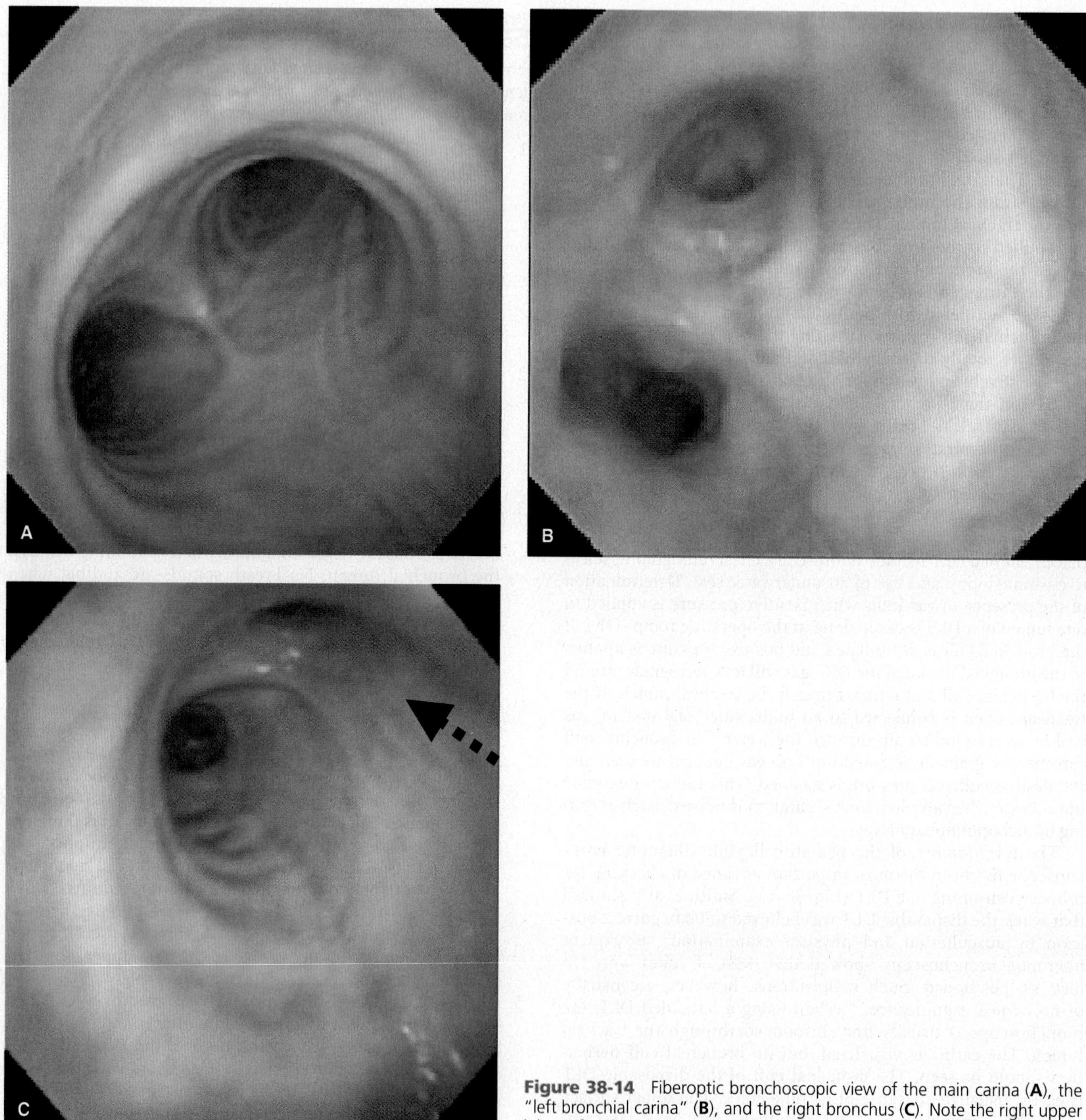

Figure 38-14 Fiberoptic bronchoscopic view of the main carina (**A**), the "left bronchial carina" (**B**), and the right bronchus (**C**). Note the right upper lobe orifice (*arrow*).

positioning, and trauma owing to intraoperative dislocation resulting in bronchial rupture have been described in association with the Robertshaw tube and the disposable DLT. Therefore, the pressure in the bronchial cuff should be assessed and decreased if the cuff is found to be overinflated. If absolute separation of the lungs is not needed, the bronchial cuff should be deflated and then reinflated slowly to avoid excessive pressure on the bronchial walls. The bronchial cuff should also be deflated during any repositioning of the patient unless lung separation is absolutely required during this time.

In a prospective trial, 60 patients were randomly assigned to two groups. OLV was achieved with either an endobronchial blocker (blocker group) or a DLT (double-lumen group). Postoperative hoarseness and sore throat were assessed at 24, 48, and 72 hours following surgery. Bronchial injuries and vocal cord lesions were examined by bronchoscopy immediately after surgery. Postoperative hoarseness occurred significantly more frequently in the double-lumen group compared with the blocker group (44% vs. 17%, respectively). Similar findings were observed for vocal cord lesions (44% vs. 17%).[46] The incidence of bronchial injuries was comparable between groups. Clayton-Smith et al.[47] performed a review and meta-analysis of 39 randomized controlled trials comparing bronchial blockers with DLTs. They concluded that while bronchial blockers are associated with a lower incidence of airway injury, DLTs can be placed more rapidly and reliably.

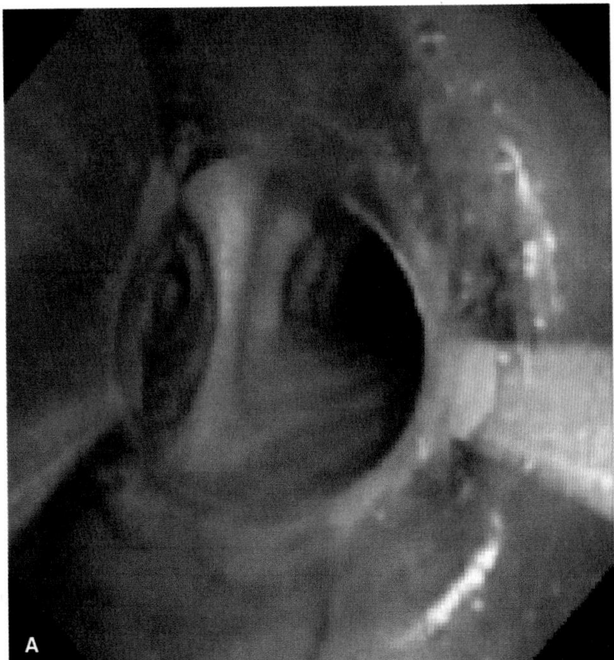

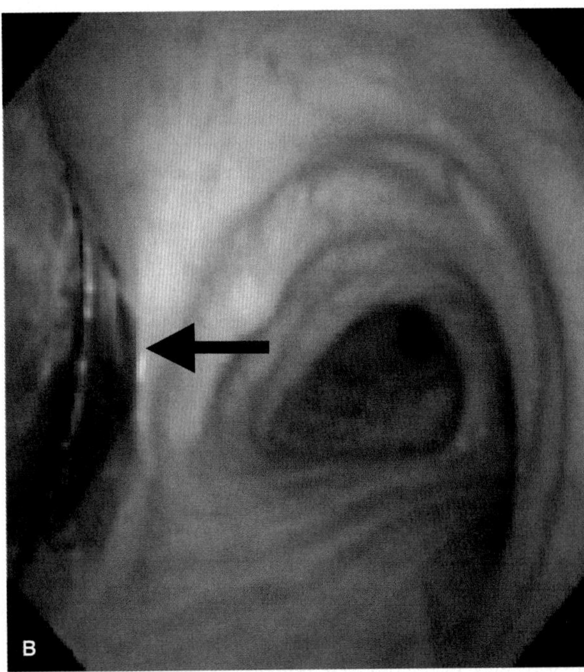

Figure 38-15 Malposition of the left bronchial limb of the double-lumen tube (DLT). **A:** The limb is too far into the left bronchus because the cuff is not evident. **B:** DLT is withdrawn and the balloon is now in view, indicating appropriate position of the DLT (*arrow*).

Lung Separation in the Patient with a Tracheostomy

Occasionally, a patient with a permanent tracheostomy is scheduled for surgery that requires lung isolation. Examples of such patients include those who have undergone resection of a tumor in the floor of the mouth or on the base of the tongue, followed by extensive reconstructive surgery with the creation of a permanent tracheal stoma. Routine follow-up may reveal a lung lesion that requires a diagnostic procedure. Conventional double-lumen endobronchial tubes are designed to be inserted through the mouth, not through a tracheal stoma. The standard DLTs are usually too stiff to negotiate the curve required for insertion through a tracheal stoma and are difficult to position. A separately inserted bronchial blocker may permit adequate lung separation.

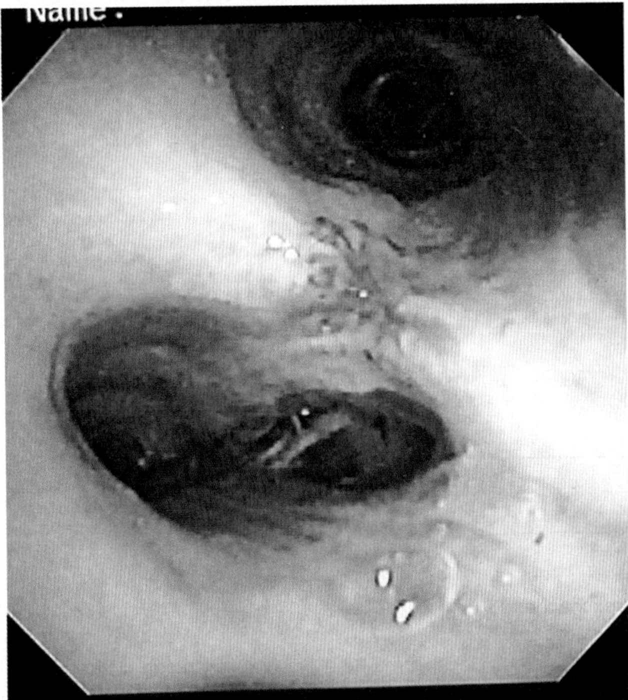

Figure 38-16 Bronchoscopic view showing laceration in left mainstem bronchus.

Saito et al.[48] described a spiral, wire-reinforced, double-lumen endobronchial tube made of silicone (Koken Medical, Tokyo, Japan) that is designed for placement through a tracheostomy. The middle section of the tube consists of two thin-walled silicone catheters with an internal diameter of 5 mm, glued together and reinforced with a stainless-steel spiral wire and covered with a silicone coating with two pilot balloons. The distal section, which contains the bronchial lumen and the bronchial cuff, is made of wire-reinforced silicone to avoid excessive flexibility. The dimensions are based on the Mallinckrodt DLT (Hazelwood, MD). The bronchial cuff is located 1.2 cm from the tip, and the distance between the tip orifice and the tracheal orifice is 4.9 cm. In a clinical trial in patients with permanent tracheal stomas, the tubes functioned well in achieving lung separation, with no sign of kinking or movement, and permitted easy passage of a suction catheter.

In a recent study, 70 cases were identified in patients who had a tracheostomy in situ.[49] These cases were divided into two groups: a fresh tracheostomy stoma <7 days ($n = 6$) or long-term stoma >7 days ($n = 64$). Information was collected regarding the devices used to manage the airway and lung isolation techniques. The devices used to manage the airway include the Shiley cuffed low-pressure tracheostomy tube, single-lumen endotracheal tube (SLT), or DLT. Devices used to manage OLV included SLTs, with or without bronchial blockers, or DLTs. Flexible fiberoptic bronchoscopy was used to assess the airway and confirm the position of the lung isolation device. Six cases had an early-stage fresh tracheostomy stoma where the Shiley tracheostomy tube was used for ventilation followed by the use of a bronchial blocker. In contrast, in patients who had a long-term stoma, the following devices were used:

- An SLT plus a bronchial blocker in 38 cases.
- A Shiley tracheostomy tube plus bronchial blocker in 15 cases.
- An SLT guided into a selective bronchus in seven cases.
- A DLT in four cases.

In all cases, flexible fiberoptic bronchoscopy was used and no complications occurred secondary to airway management or OLV. In patients undergoing thoracic surgery and OLV with a fresh tracheostomy stoma in situ, the authors recommended the use of the Shiley tracheostomy tube plus a bronchial blocker. In patients with a long-term tracheostomy stoma, an SLT can be used to intubate a single bronchus selectively.[49] In addition, an SLT or a Shiley tube can be used in conjunction with an independent bronchial blocker, such as the Arndt wire-guided bronchial blocker, Cohen tip-deflecting blocker, Fuji Uniblocker, or EZ-Blocker. DLTs are the least frequently used device for OLV in tracheostomized patients.[49]

Lung Separation in the Patient with a Difficult Airway

An airway may be recognized initially as difficult when conventional laryngoscopy reveals a grade III or IV view. When separation of the lungs is required and the patient has a clearly recognized difficult airway, then awake intubation using a flexible fiberoptic bronchoscope can be used to place a DLT, Univent tube, or single-lumen tube (SLT) (Fig. 38-17). The SLT may then be exchanged for a DLT or Univent tube using a tube exchanger. Furthermore, depending on the extent and duration of the surgical procedure, and the amount of fluid shift, an airway that was not initially classified as difficult may become difficult secondary to facial edema, secretions, and laryngeal trauma from the initial intubation.[50]

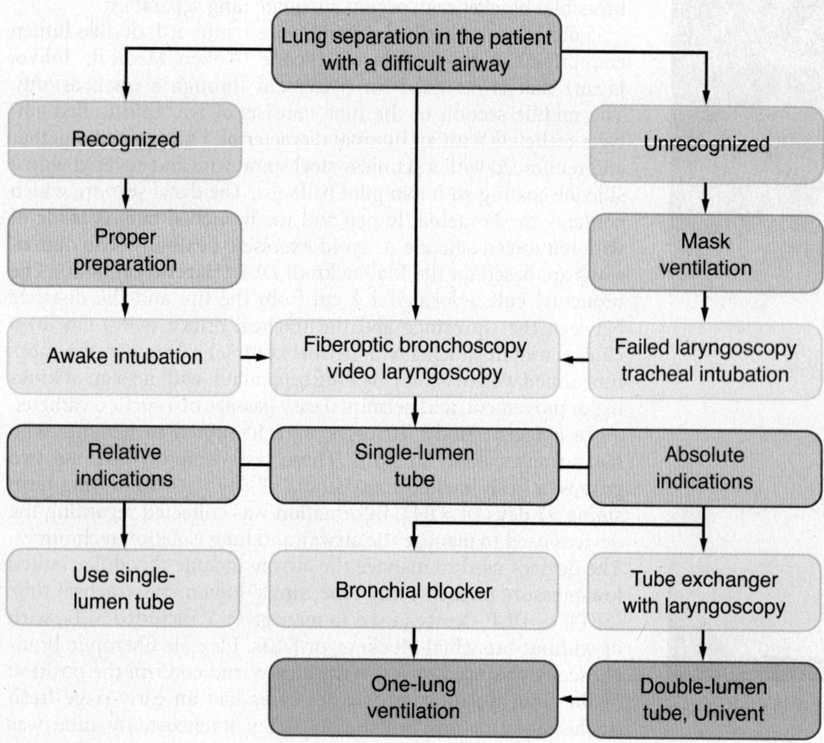

Figure 38-17 Lung separation in the patient with a difficult airway. (Adapted with permission from Cohen E, Benumof JL. Lung separation in the patient with a difficult airway. *Curr Opin Anesthesiol.* 1999;12:29.)

A logical approach to lung separation is shown in Figure 38-17. The same approach may be used for the patient with an unrecognized difficult airway and a failure to intubate with conventional laryngoscopy. When using a DLT over a fiberoptic bronchoscope, the anesthesiologist should keep in mind that the DLT is a bulky tube with a large external diameter whose length leaves only a limited part of the fiberoptic bronchoscope available for manipulation. In addition, the mismatch between the flexibility of the fiberoptic bronchoscope and the rigidity of the DLT makes it more difficult to advance the DLT over the bronchoscope. The Univent tube has the same bulky external diameter and is also often difficult to pass between the vocal cords, particularly in a patient who is awake.

If a Single-Lumen Tube Can Be Successfully Placed

If a failure to provide lung separation could result in a life-threatening situation, there are two possibilities to provide OLV when an SLT is already in place. First, depending on the indication for lung isolation, a tube exchanger can be used to switch to a DLT or a Univent tube. The second possibility is to direct a bronchial blocker through the SLT into the selected main stem bronchus. However, the DLT remains the definitive choice: the Univent or bronchial blocker may offer only limited protection or an inadequate seal in cases such as lung lavage, pulmonary abscess, or hemoptysis.

Use of a Tube Exchanger

Several tube exchangers are commercially available (Cook Critical Care, Bloomington, IN; Sheridan Catheter Corporation, Argyle, NY). These tube exchangers are available in a wide range of external diameters with depth markings in centimeters. They are easily adapted for either oxygen insufflation or jet ventilation. The size of the tube exchanger and the size of the tube to be inserted should be tested before use in a patient. The 11-Fr tube changer

Table 38-2 Indications for the Use of Endobronchial Blockers

The Difficult Airway
Avoids the need for tube exchange (DLT to SLT)
Following laryngeal surgery
Patient with a tracheostomy
Distorted bronchial anatomy due to compression by aneurysm or tumor
Patient who requires nasotracheal intubation

Management
Makes possible segmental blockade in a patient who cannot tolerate OLV
Morbid obesity
Small size and pediatric patients
Patients from the ICU who arrive to the OR tracheally intubated

Surgical Procedures not Involving the Lung
Esophageal surgery
Spine surgery that requires a transthoracic approach
Minimally invasive cardiac surgery

DLT, double-lumen tube; ICU, Intensive care unit; OLV, one-lung ventilation; OR, operating room SLT, single-lumen tube.

will pass through a 35-Fr to 41-Fr DLT, whereas the 14-Fr tube exchanger will not pass through a 35-Fr DLT. To prevent lung laceration, the tube exchanger should never be inserted against resistance. First generation of tube exchangers was very stiff, and posed a risk for tracheal or bronchial laceration. Tube exchangers are now available that have a soft flexible tip: these should be safer to use and less likely to cause airway laceration. Finally, when passing any tube over an airway guide, a laryngoscope should be used to facilitate passage of the tube over the airway guide past supraglottic tissues.

Use of Modern Bronchial Blockers

Lung separation can be achieved with a reusable bronchial blocker (2 Video 38-2, NICV 38-1). Magill described an endobronchial blocker that is placed using a bronchoscope and directed to the nonventilated lung. Inflation of the cuff at the distal end of the blocker serves to block ventilation to that lung. The lumen of the blocker permits suctioning of the airway distal to the catheter tip. Depending on the clinical circumstance, oxygen can be insufflated through the catheter lumen. A conventional tracheal tube is then placed in the trachea. This technique can be useful in achieving selective ventilation in children younger than 12 years of age. However, because the blocker balloon requires a high distending pressure, it may easily slip out of the bronchus into the trachea, obstructing ventilation and losing the seal between the two lungs. This displacement can be secondary to changes in position or to surgical manipulation. The loss of lung separation can be life-threatening if it was performed to prevent spillage of pus, blood, or fluid from bronchopulmonary lavage. For this reason, bronchial blockers are rarely used for these types of cases.

Indications for the use of a bronchial blocker are shown in Table 38-2. An independently passed bronchial blocker may be used with an SLT to obtain lung isolation, thereby avoiding the use of a DLT in a patient with a difficult airway. The use of a bronchial blocker also eliminates the potential risk of needing to change a DLT to an SLT at the conclusion of the procedure. Historically, Fogarty vascular embolectomy catheters were used for lung separation, but there is no indication for their use in the current practice of thoracic anesthesia. The balloon of the Fogarty is high pressure, low volume, and there is no lumen to allow egress of gas from the lung to facilitate deflation. Modern individual blockers are discussed in the chronologic order in which they were developed and introduced into practice. The characteristics of the various bronchial blockers are summarized in Table 38-3.

Univent Tube. The Univent (Fuji Systems Corp., Tokyo, Japan) is a single-lumen tracheal tube with a movable endobronchial blocker (Fig. 38-18, 3 Video 38-3). In the Univent tube, the bronchial blocker is housed in a small channel bored into the wall of the tube. The blocker contains a high-volume, low-pressure balloon, and is angled to permit external direction into the desired bronchus under direct fiberoptic bronchoscopic vision. After intubation of the trachea, the movable blocker is manipulated into the desired main stem bronchus with the aid of a fiberoptic bronchoscope. The Univent tube may be ideal for cases in which a tube change (e.g., from single to double lumen) may be difficult (e.g., mediastinoscopy followed by thoracotomy), or in cases of bilateral lung transplantation. The Univent tube has the advantage common to all bronchial blockers: it is an SLT, and there is no need to change the tube at the end of the procedure if postoperative ventilatory support is required. This is particularly important in cases of difficult intubation, altered anatomy of the airway, or prolonged surgery with airway edema, such as thoracic aortic aneurysm surgery or extensive neurosurgical procedures on the spine with massive fluid replacement. It is also possible to suction through the blocker lumen or to apply continuous positive airway pressure (CPAP) to improve oxygenation in cases of hypoxemia.

Table 38-3 Comparison of Bronchial Blockers (BBs)

	Arndt Blocker	Cohen Blocker	Uniblocker	EZ Blocker
Size	5 Fr, 7 Fr, 9 Fr	9 Fr	9 Fr	7 Fr
Guidance feature	Wire loop to snare FOB	Deflecting tip	Prefixed bend	Double-lumen bifurcated tip
Recommended Tracheal tube size	9 Fr 8 mm 7 Fr 7 mm 5 Fr 4.5 mm	8 mm	8 mm	8 mm
Central lumen	1.8 mm	1.8 mm	2 mm	
Murphy eye	Present in 9 Fr	Present	None	None
Disadvantages	BB not visualized during insertion	Expensive	No steering mechanism. Prefixed bend	Lumen too small. Impossible to suction

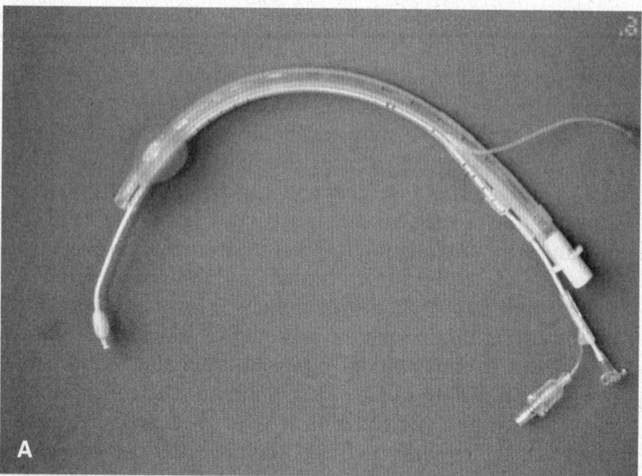

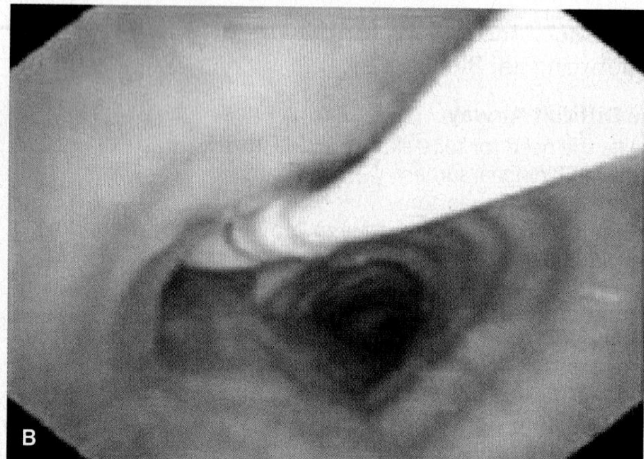

Figure 38-18 **A:** The Univent tube also allows lung separation using a single-lumen endotracheal tube. **B:** The Univent bronchial blocker positioned in left main stem bronchus.

The disadvantages of the Univent tubes are that correct positioning of the blocker may be difficult to achieve or maintain and that the external diameter of the tube is relatively large. The bulky external diameter can make it difficult to pass the tube between the vocal cords. Many anesthesiologists prefer to avoid postoperative ventilation with such a large-diameter tube, and may change it to a standard tube at the conclusion of the surgery. The blocker can dislocate during surgical manipulation, and satisfactory bronchial seal and lung separation are sometimes difficult to achieve.

The Univent bronchial blocker is somewhat stiff and sometimes cannot be easily directed into the main bronchus. This is particularly true for the left side. The bronchial blocker on first-generation Univent tubes was difficult to direct as the blocker would tend to spin (torque) on its long axis, which made it difficult to control. A second-generation Torque Control Blocker Univent was introduced more recently. It consists of a silicon endotracheal tube that has a high friction coefficient. The Torque Control Blocker provides better control and facilitates direction of the blocker into the target main stem bronchus.

Arndt Blocker. In an attempt to overcome these potential problems, the Arndt snare-guided bronchial blocker was introduced (Cook Critical Care) (Fig. 38-19A). It is a wire-guided catheter with a loop snare. A fiberscope is passed through the loop of the bronchial blocker and then guided into the desired bronchus. The blocker is then slid distally over the fiberscope and into the selected bronchus. Bronchoscopic visualization confirms blocker placement and bronchial occlusion. The balloon is available in spherical or elliptic shape. The set contains a multiport adapter, which allows uninterrupted ventilation during the positioning of the blocker. The wire may then be removed, freeing the 1.6-mm lumen for use as a suction port or for oxygen insufflation to the nondependent lung. With the first generation of this device, it was not possible to reinsert the wire once it had been pulled out, losing the ability to redirect the bronchial blocker if necessary. External reinforcement of the wire now allows for its reintroduction through the lumen. Finally, the external diameter necessitates a large size SLT (at least 8 mm) to be able to accommodate the bronchial blocker. The Arndt blocker is available in a 7 Fr and a 5 Fr pediatric size. One disadvantage of the Arndt blocker is that it is advanced blindly over the FB into the desired main bronchus; occasionally, the tip of the blocker may get caught at the carina or at the Murphy eye of the SLT.

Cohen Blocker. The Cohen Flexitip endobronchial blocker (Cook Critical Care) is designed for use as an independent bronchial blocker. It is inserted through an SLT with the aid of a small-diameter (4 mm) fiberoptic bronchoscope (Fig. 38-19B).[51] The blocker has a rotating wheel that deflects the soft tip by more than 90 degrees and easily directs it into the desired bronchus. The blocker cuff is a pear-shaped, high-volume, low-pressure balloon inflated via 0.4-mm lumen inside the wall of the blocker. In general, inflation of the cuff with between 6 mL and 8 mL of air provides an adequate seal of the bronchus. It is best to inflate the cuff under direct visualization via the fiberoptic bronchoscope. The cuff is a distinctive blue color that is easily recognizable by fiberoptic bronchoscopy. The blocker itself is 9 Fr, and has a central main lumen (1.6 mm) that allows limited suctioning of secretions and insufflation of oxygen to the collapsed lung in case of hypoxemia. The blocker and the fiberoptic bronchoscope do not have to pass through the tracheal tube at the same time for placement; the blocker can be passed ahead of the FB beyond the tracheal tube tip. This blocker can therefore be used even with a 7-mm endotracheal tube.

Uniblocker. Fuji Systems introduced a 9-Fr balloon-tipped, angled blocker with a multiple port adapter that is essentially the same design as the Univent tube blocker, but can be used as an independent blocker passed via a special connector through a standard tracheal tube (Fig. 38-19C).

EZ-Blocker. The most recent addition to the endobronchial blocker design is the EZ Blocker (Teleflex, Morrisville, NC). This is a 7-Fr, 4-lumen, 75-cm, disposable endobronchial blocker to facilitate selective lung ventilation (Fig. 38-19D). It has a symmetric Y-shaped bifurcation and both branches have an inflatable cuff and a central lumen. The bifurcation resembles the bifurcation of the trachea. During insertion via a standard tracheal tube, each of the two distal ends is placed into a main stem bronchus. The selected lung is isolated by inflating the blocker's balloon to the least volume necessary to occlude the main stem bronchus under bronchoscopic visualization. This blocker should offer an advantage during bilateral procedures because each lung can be deflated without the need for repositioning the blocker.[52]

The effectiveness of lung isolation among three devices—a left-sided DLT, a Torque Control Blocker Univent, and a wire-guided Arndt—has been compared in a prospective randomized trial. There was no significant difference in tube malpositions among the three groups: It took longer to position the Arndt blocker (3 minutes) compared with the left-sided DLT (2 minutes) and the Univent (2 minutes). Excluding the time for tube placement, the Arndt group also took longer for the lung to collapse (26 minutes), compared with the DLT group (17 minutes) or the Univent group (19 minutes). Furthermore, unlike the other two groups, the majority of the Arndt patients required suction to achieve lung

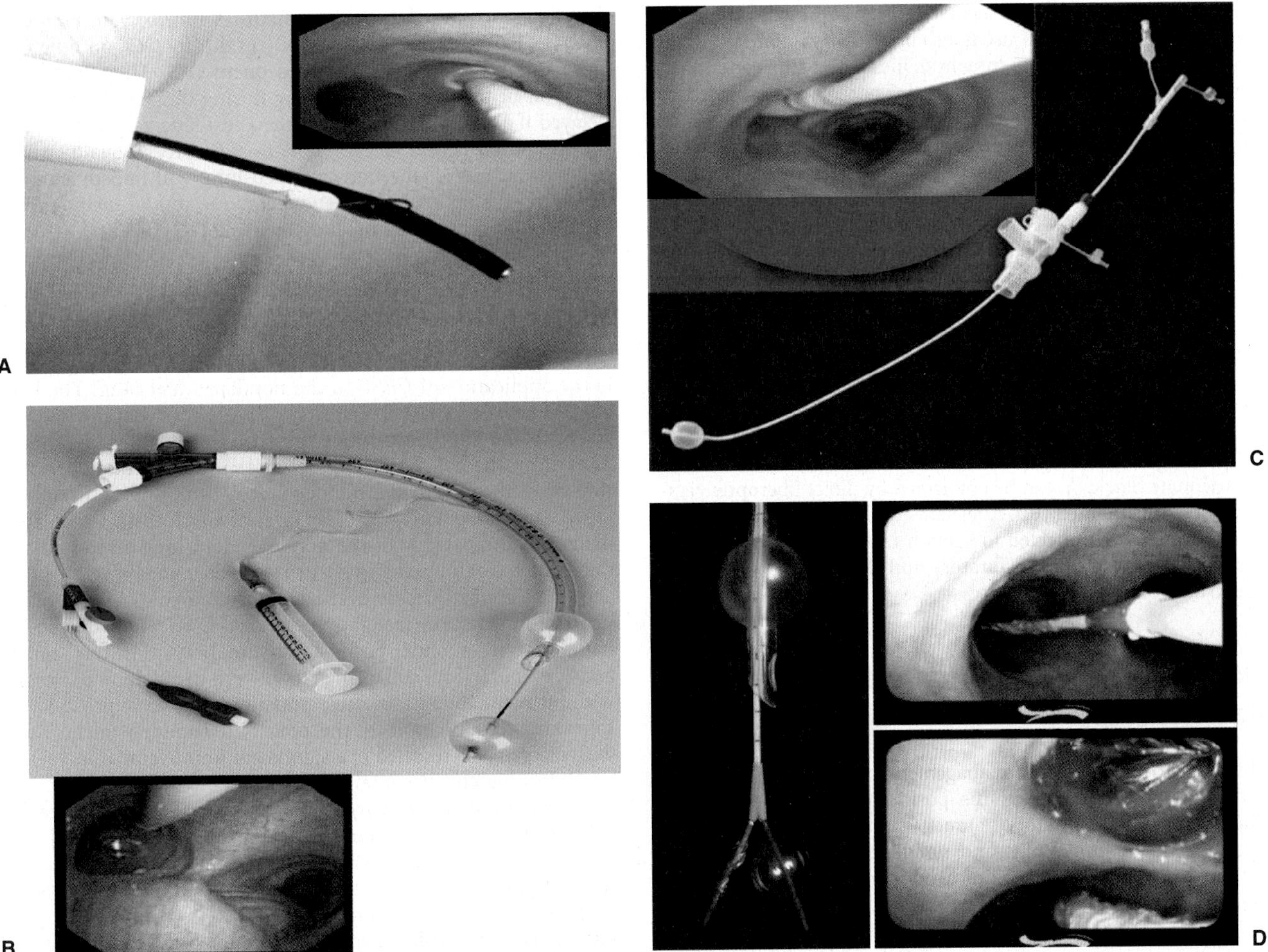

Figure 38-19 **A:** Arndt blocker. **B:** Cohen blocker. **C:** Uniblocker. **D:** EZ blocker.

collapse. Once lung isolation was achieved, overall surgical exposure was rated excellent for all three groups. One minute longer to position a bronchial blocker or 6 minutes longer to collapse the lung is insignificant when considering the overall duration of the thoracic procedure. Hence, patient safety and risk/benefit should be the controlling factors when choosing methods for lung isolation.

A further study evaluated the use of the Cohen blocker, the Arndt blocker, the Uniblocker, and DLT (four groups of 26 patients in each group). No difference was found between the groups in the time taken to insert these lung isolation devices or in the quality of the lung collapse.[53] The grading was done by the operating surgeons who were blinded as to which device was used. The number of cuff dislocations was higher among the three bronchial blocker (BB) groups compared to the DLT. Regardless of the type of BB or DLT selected to provide OLV, the decision as to which technique to use depends on the clinical circumstances and the physician's experience and comfort with a particular device. It is important, however, that the clinician should not limit their practice to the use of only one device but rather be versatile and comfortable in the use of several.

A recent comprehensive meta-analysis and randomized controlled trials analysis was performed for a comparison of the efficacy and adverse effects of DLTs and BBs in thoracic surgery.[47] The authors performed a systematic literature search for RCTs comparing BBs and DLTs using databases up to October 2013. The search produced 39 RCTs published between 1996 and 2013. The authors concluded that DLTs were quicker to place and less likely to be incorrectly positioned than BBs. BBs were associated with a lower incidence of postoperative sore throat, hoarseness, and fewer airway injuries than DLTs. Most importantly, no significant difference between the BBs and the DLT was shown for either the time taken for adequate lung collapse or the quality of the lung collapse.

DLTs have been used to achieve lung separation for more than 50 years and will remain the "gold standard" for lung separation. However, there are many clinical situations where the DLT may not be the method of choice or may be impossible to use. The anesthesiologist should become familiar with the various devices used to achieve lung separation. Bronchial blockers can be safely and effectively used either for simple procedures such as a brief wedge resection or for more complex extended procedures such as lobectomy or pneumonectomy. The fact that there are several BBs available for clinical use may be a reflection of the search for the ideal blocker. It is of benefit to the patient if the need to change tubes (DLT to SLT) during the case or at case end can be avoided because this change may expose the patient to a period during which the airway is unprotected.[54]

Double-Lumen Tube or Bronchial Blocker?

The decision whether to use a DLT or a BB is most commonly based on surgeon and anesthesiologist preference. When both lungs need to be ventilated separately, a DLT provides the most control of ventilation. DLT use is also particularly important when protection of the dependent lung from life-threatening contamination from the diseased lung is required. The isolation provided by the low-pressure, high-volume BB cuff is less reliable under such circumstances. If a tumor is occupying the main bronchus or an open sleeve resection is necessary, a contralateral DLT should be used. Sleeve resection is an open bronchial procedure and any isolation device placed in the surgical field will interfere with the bronchial anastomosis. Bilateral procedures, such as a double lung transplant, or bilateral sympathectomy are also best managed using a DLT because of the need to ventilate both lungs independently.[55]

Studies of BB use suggest that they are more likely to dislodge intraoperatively than a DLT. Proper locking of the BB inside the ET tube may decrease this likelihood, as may greater attention to securing the ET tube. Since BBs have low-pressure, high-volume cuffs, the peak airway pressure should be kept below 30 cmH_2O to prevent gas bypassing the cuff.

Adequate blockade can be confirmed by direct fiberoptic visualization of the inflated cuff. Alternatively, the lumen of the BB can be intermittently connected to suction to assure that no discrepancy exists between the inspiratory and the expiratory volumes due to suctioning of leaked gas.

Management of One-Lung Ventilation

This section discusses the management of OLV in a paralyzed patient in the lateral decubitus position with an open chest. The roles of the respiratory parameters of FIO_2, V_T, respiratory rate, dependent lung PEEP, and nondependent lung CPAP are reviewed. A comprehensive clinical approach to the management of OLV is presented.

Confirmation of Correct Position of the DLT or Bronchial Blocker

Following intubation with a DLT or placement of a bronchial blocker, the correct position should be checked by clinical assessment, visualization of chest movement, auscultation, and pressure/volume flow profile. In modern anesthesia practice, a standard 4.0-mm fiberscope should be passed down the tracheal lumen to check for correct depth, or alongside the bronchial blocker that was passed through the single-lumen tracheal tube. It is a common practice to visualize the tip of the blue bronchial cuff at the level of the carina to ensure that the left upper lobe orifice is not obstructed. Once the patient is turned into the lateral position, the position of the DLT should be rechecked to exclude dislocation of the tube during positioning.

Inspired Oxygen Fraction

An FIO_2 of 1 is generally recommended during OLV. A high oxygen concentration serves to protect against hypoxemia during the procedure and provides a higher margin of safety. A high FIO_2 may, however, cause absorption atelectasis and potentially further increase the amount of shunt because of collapsed alveoli. The use of an FIO_2 less than 1 during OLV has the potential benefits of decreasing the risk of absorption atelectasis and, if N_2O is used, may allow potent inhaled anesthetics to be used in lower concentrations. Some clinicians use an O_2 80%/N_2O 20% mixture as long that the SpO_2 is maintained in a safe range. The rate of the lung collapse during OLV was addressed by Ko et al.[56] They compared the effects of three different gas mixtures (air/oxygen, FIO_2 0.4; N_2O/O_2, FIO_2 0.4; and oxygen, FIO_2 1) during OLV on lung collapse and oxygenation during subsequent OLV: They found that deflation of the nonventilated lung during thoracic surgery was delayed if air was used as part of the anesthetic gas mixture during the initial period of OLV. For thoracic procedures in which delayed collapse of the nonventilated lung will impede surgical exposure, the optimal anesthetic technique should include thorough denitrogenation of the lung by using FIO_2 of 1.

Continuous Positive Airway Pressure to the Nondependent Lung

The single most effective maneuver to increase PaO_2 during OLV is the application of CPAP to the nondependent lung. The beneficial effects of CPAP 10 cmH_2O ($CPAP_{10}$) are not attributable solely to the effect of positive pressure in diverting blood flow away from the collapsed lung because (in dogs) the hyperinflation of nitrogen into the nondependent lung under 10 cmH_2O failed to improve PaO_2. A lower level of CPAP (5 to 10 cmH_2O) maintains the patency of the nondependent lung alveoli, allowing some oxygen uptake to occur in the distended alveoli. CPAP should be applied after delivering an inspiratory V_T to the nondependent lung to keep it slightly expanded. CPAP, applied by insufflation of oxygen under positive pressure, keeps this lung "quiet" and prevents it from collapsing completely. Insufflation of oxygen without maintaining a positive pressure failed to improve PaO_2. Intermittent reinflation of the collapsed (nondependent) lung with oxygen also resulted in a significant improvement in PaO_2.[57]

Unfortunately, in contemporary practice, most thoracic procedures are initiated thoracoscopically, such that the application of CPAP to the nondependent lung is generally not acceptable to most surgeons. During VATS, the lung should be well collapsed to allow the surgeon an optimal view of the surgical field and to palpate the lesion in the lung parenchyma. In addition, it is difficult to place the stapler on a lung that is not completely collapsed, resulting in an increased incidence of postoperative air leak.

Tidal Volume

Over the past two decades, the incidence of hypoxemia during OLV has decreased from 25% to 4% to 5%, most likely due to the routine use of fiberoptic bronchoscopy to confirm the correct position of the DLT/BB and the use of protective lung ventilation strategies which include the use of low V_T, PEEP, and recruitment maneuvers (RMs).[58] Of greater concern is the risk of ALI from stretching of the lung parenchyma from the delivery of large V_Ts. On the other hand, the use of a small V_T of 6 mL/kg without PEEP can lead to the formation of atelectasis in the dependent lung.[59]

The multicenter, prospective ARDS Network trial demonstrated that a smaller V_T of 6 mL/kg, rather than a traditional 12 mL/kg, significantly decreased in-hospital mortality in ICU patients.[60] Several subsequent clinical studies have confirmed the benefit of small V_T in ARDS patients.[61] These patients have a decreased lung capacity due to the presence of atelectatic areas that cannot be recruited despite the application of high levels of PEEP. They should be treated as having a "baby lung"[62] and ventilated with a small V_T to avoid overdistension of the rest of the ventilated lung. It is unclear, however, if this protective low V_T strategy in ARDS patients is applicable to the perioperative environment, specifically during OLV where, for the most part, patients do not have unrecruited atelectasis. In fact, in a retrospective analysis of over 30,000 patients (not thoracic or cardiac), the 30-day mortality rate was lower when a V_T of 8 to 9 mL/kg was used intraoperatively.

Blank et al.[63] analyzed the data from the Society of Thoracic Surgery that reported postthoracic procedure complications in 1,019 patients. They found that in a large proportion of the patients, the use of a large VT of 8 to 9 mL/kg during OLV was inversely proportional to the incidence of respiratory complications. The discrepancy between the ICU data and the thoracic surgical population can be explained by the fact that, to date, there is no evidence to confirm that the data derived from ARDS ICU patients are applicable to patients undergoing a thoracic procedure. Most thoracic surgery patients have a lung lesion accidentally discovered during a routine screening. In addition, thoracic patients are exposed to PPV only for the limited period of OR time compared to ICU patients who are prone to the risk of parenchymal damage from prolonged ventilatory support.[64]

The application of protective lung ventilation may be more complex in the lateral position. Unlike in the supine position where the relative blood flow to each lung is basically unchanged, in the lateral position, the ventilated lung is subjected to increased blood flow distribution due to the effect of gravity. During OLV, HPV in the nondependent lung further increases the proportion of blood that flows to the dependent lung. Consequently, the dependent lung may receive more than 70% of the total pulmonary blood flow, resulting in a hyperemia that is injurious to the pulmonary vasculature and may create additional shear stress, and possible damage to the endothelial glycocalyx.[65]

Positive End-Expiratory Pressure

The application of PEEP during thoracic surgery has an intraoperative effect on arterial oxygenation and on postoperative pulmonary complications. The beneficial effect of selective PEEP at 10 cmH_2O ($PEEP_{10}$) to the dependent lung is caused by an increased lung volume at end-expiration (FRC), which improves the ventilation/perfusion (V/Q) relationship in the dependent lung (Fig. 38-20). During OLV, PEEP also prevents alveolar closure at end expiration in the dependent lung and thus prevents repetitive intratidal opening and collapse of the airway.

Studies evaluating whether the application of PEEP to the dependent lung would improve arterial oxygenation were not encouraging and showed either no change, a decrease, or a slight increase in PaO_2. High levels of PEEP can reduce regional blood flow and protect the dependent lung from capillary overdistention. The negative effect of PEEP on PaO_2 during OLV is based on the increased compression of small interalveolar vessels, which increases the PVR accompanied by the diversion of blood flow to the nondependent lung, increasing the transpulmonary shunt. Nevertheless, PEEP does play an important role during OLV:

First, each time a patient is anesthetized and mechanically ventilated, atelectatic areas will form in the dependent part of the lung, particularly when low VT is used for protective lung ventilation. PEEP will prevent or at least decrease the extent of the atelectatic areas in the lung.

Second, studies that concluded that PEEP worsens the PaO_2 during OLV need to be carefully analyzed. Almost 40 years ago, the first report of the application of PEEP during OLV found that it decreased the PaO_2. However, in that study, the mean PaO_2 during OLV when PEEP was applied was 150 mmHg; clearly there was no clinical need to improve oxygenation. Whether the application of PEEP will improve or worsen the arterial oxygenation depends on the FRC. The application of PEEP to a patient with a low PaO_2 may increase the lung volume to normal FRC, which in turn results in a lower PVR and an improved V/Q ratio. With a higher PaO_2, the patient already has an adequate dependent lung FRC, so the applied PEEP may negatively affect the redistribution of blood flow away from the dependent lung. The same concept

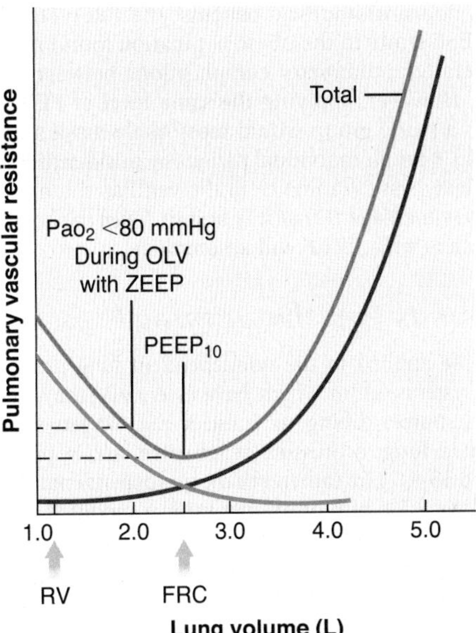

Figure 38-20 Effect of 10 cmH_2O positive end-expiratory pressure (PEEP) on functional residual capacity (FRC). It is postulated that, in patients having PaO_2 below 80 mmHg with zero end-expiratory pressure (ZEEP), FRC is low. $PEEP_{10}$ increases FRC and thereby increases PaO_2. OLV, one-lung ventilation; $PEEP_{10}$, positive end-expiratory pressure (10 cmH_2O); RV, residual volume.

was described by Slinger et al.[66] who showed that patients would selectively benefit from the application of PEEP during OLV when kept at an FRC volume in the dependent lung at which PVR was lowest.

Third, as previously mentioned, data on the effect of PEEP and protective lung ventilation strategy were derived from studies conducted in ICU patients. These findings may not always be applicable to the typical patient who presents for lung resection.

Finally, the same level of PEEP may not be universally applied to all patients. One size may not fit all, but rather PEEP should be individualized. Each patient has an individual level of PEEP that best fits their lung compliance at FRC lung volume. Analysis across the entire sample of patients, receiving the same level of PEEP, may not truly represent each patient's ideal ventilatory parameters. This concept was recently addressed using the driving pressure (DP) as the single best value for ideal ventilatory parameters. The optimum respiratory system compliance is when the PEEP is titrated to the lowest DP and *individualized for each patient.*[67] The concept of individualized PEEP is not new. A recent study evaluated PEEP guided by electrical impedance tomography (EIT) during OLV in elderly patients undergoing VATS. EIT is a noninvasive, medical imaging method that allows the reconstruction of dynamic pulmonary images in real time. The device forms a continuous tomographic map of the pulmonary ventilation resulting from the changes in chest conductivity caused by changes in lung-gas distributions from low-energy electrical signals. The authors studied 100 patients assigned to either the $PEEP_5$ or to EIT group ($PEEP_{EIT}$), and all were ventilated with a TV of 6 mL/kg. PEEP application was either fixed at 5 cmH_2O or individually titrated following EIT imaging for optimal oxygenation. At 1 hour into OLV, PaO_2/FiO_2 was 93 mmHg higher, lung compliance was 4.4 mL/cmH_2O higher, and the DP was 4.9 cmH_2O lower in the $PEEP_{EIT}$ group than in the $PEEP_5$ group.[68] The application of low PEEP (2 cmH_2O) versus high PEEP (12 cmH_2O) was evaluated in two prospective multicenter studies in noncardiothoracic patients: the PROVHILO trial and the PROBESE study in the obese population found no differences in postoperative pulmonary complications between these levels of PEEP.[67] However, applying the same level of PEEP across all patients in a study group would most likely mask any beneficial effect of PEEP for an individual patient by misidentifying the ideal DP to achieve best compliance in the ventilated lung. Ultimately, the takeaway message is that it is best to *"open the lung and keep it open"* which is what PEEP will accomplish.

Continuous Positive Airway Pressure

CPAP can be applied to the nondependent lung using a number of simple systems, all of which have essentially the same features: an oxygen source, tubing to connect the oxygen source to the nonventilated lung, a pressure relief valve, and a pressure gauge (4 Video 38-4). The catheter to the nondependent lung is usually insufflated with 5 L/min of oxygen using a modified Ayre's T-piece (pediatric) circuit, and the valve on the expiratory limb is adjusted to the desired pressure as read on the attached gauge. Instead of a pressure gauge or manometer inserted into the circuit, a spring-loaded adjustable PEEP valve can be used. The amount of CPAP applied should be titrated to the clinical circumstances. In most cases, even low levels of CPAP may be sufficient to increase the PaO_2 to an accepted safe level. CPAP greater than 10 cmH_2O is not beneficial because it creates an overdistention that interferes with surgical exposure and may have undesirable hemodynamic consequences.

High-frequency ventilation with oxygen to the nondependent lung and conventional ventilation (CV) to the dependent lung have also been used to improve PaO_2 during OLV (see "High-Frequency Ventilation").

Recruitment Maneuvers

RMs have the purpose of opening atelectatic areas of the lung which, once opened, should continue to remain patent with the application of PEEP. Many investigators believe that ventilator-induced lung injury (VILI) propagates from these atelectatic zones, rather than from continuously aerated alveoli that are repeatedly overstretched. Eliminating these atelectatic interfaces with RM is the primary objective of an "open lung" approach to safe ventilation. RM can be achieved by the application of 35 to 40 cmH_2O sustained airway pressure for 30 to 40 seconds or by 5 cmH_2O incremental increases in PEEP maintained for five breaths until reaching a final PEEP of 20 cmH_2O, plateauing at a pressure of 40 cmH_2O.[69]

RM is the most controversial part of protective ventilation (PV), with conflicting literature regarding its clinical value in both ARDS, anesthesia with two-lung ventilation, and OLV in particular. Performing an RM during lung resection carries significant challenges. Overpressure leaks past the bronchial cuff securing the operative lung may create unwanted stress on bronchial stumps and anastomoses. Impeded venous return during an RM can create cardiovascular depression and worsen hypoxia by reducing blood flow through the ventilated lung. Arnal et al.[70] reported that "during the recruiting effort, the incremental gain achieved by sustained inflation wanes progressively as the risk for adverse consequences builds." Although most of the hypotensive episodes caused by RM are rather transient, the efficacy of RM with sustained high pressure has been questioned. Marini stated that "although sustained inflation is commonly deployed and is still actively researched as a recruiting technique, there are good reasons to retire it from clinical practice. Stepwise approaches to the maximum applied pressure are perhaps more effective than abrupt applications of the same peak pressure, and the graded rise of mean pressure is generally better tolerated."[71]

Driving Pressure

DP is defined as the difference between plateau pressure and PEEP (Plat-PEEP), and can also be expressed as the ratio of V_T to respiratory system compliance. It depends on the V_T as well as on the relative balance between the amount of aerated lung at end expiration and end inspiration at different levels of PEEP. DP is derived from the interaction between the ventilatory parameters set by the anesthesiologist and the patient's total thoracic compliance.[72] In randomized controlled trials of mechanical ventilation in ARDS patients, DP is the variable that was most strongly associated with mortality. Amato et al.[73] conducted a multilevel analysis of data from 3,562 patients with ARDS which concluded that, among the ventilation parameters, DP was most strongly associated with survival even with "protective" lung ventilation. Individual changes in V_T or PEEP were not independently associated with survival unless the changes led to reductions in DP. The optimization of DP has thus been considered a tool to optimize mechanical ventilation during surgery and to improve outcome.

Park et al.[74] confirmed the significance of DP during OLV. In a double-blind, randomized study of 292 patients undergoing thoracic surgery, they compared DP-guided ventilation with conventional PV. The PV group (n = 147) received conventional PV during OLV: V_T 6 mL/kg, PEEP 5 cmH_2O, and RM. The DP group (n = 145) received the same V_T and recruitment, but with titrated individualized PEEP to produce the lowest DP during OLV. Ventilating the lungs using the lowest DP is equivalent to ventilating according to the patient's "functional lung size," which will avoid underdistention (atelectasis) or overdistension (barotrauma). Postoperatively, the number of patients who developed pneumonia or ARDS was smaller in the DP group.

Mechanical Power

Mechanical Power (MP) is the energy delivered from the ventilator to the respiratory system per unit of time. Briefly, the energy delivered to the respiratory system is composed of a static component, due to PEEP, and a dynamic cyclic component, due to DP and V_T above PEEP, plus the additional pressure required to generate gas flow. During each breath delivered by the ventilator, a certain amount of power is used to overcome the resistance of the airways and to expand the thorax wall. MP is expressed in Joules/minute (J/min). For volume-controlled ventilation, it is calculated as:

$$\text{Mechanical Power} = 0.098 \times RR \times V_T \times [P_{peak} - \tfrac{1}{2} \times (P_{Plat} - PEEP)]$$

MP is a single variable that combines volume, pressure, flow, and RR. Clinical changes in respiratory rate have the potential to affect the MP strongly.

The extent of lung injury depends on the total amount of mechanical energy delivered by the ventilator per unit of time. Serpa Neto et al.[75] analyzed multicenter data from 8,207 critically ill patients, with the primary outcome of in-hospital mortality. They concluded that high MP was independently associated with in-hospital mortality, ICU mortality, 30-day mortality, ventilator-free days, and ICU and hospital length of stay, regardless of V_T used.

The role of MP during thoracic surgery has been investigated. In the lateral decubitus position, the weight of the contralateral hemithorax adds to restriction of the dependent chest wall. The MP generated to ventilate the dependent lung is therefore expected to increase. This was confirmed in a prospective study by Chiumello et al.[76] who evaluated the MP, lung elastance, chest wall elastance, and esophageal pressure in the supine and lateral positions, with two and OLV, with both closed and open chest, before and after surgery. The authors found that the MP delivered to the dependent lung and the respiratory system elastance increased during OLV in the lateral position compared to the supine position. The chest wall elastance increased in the lateral position with two-lung ventilation as compared to supine, while opening the chest was associated with a decrease in the respiratory system and chest wall elastance. Interestingly, reducing the V_T did not result in a decrease in the MP. The authors concluded that, "Although we cannot suggest any clinical mechanical power threshold for possible injury, our data suggest that only the decrease of V_T from 8 to 5 mL/kg of ideal body weight did not reduce the mechanical power. Thus, the dependent lung might undergo an underappreciated amount of injury." The MP equation could be easily implemented and displayed by the ventilator's software. Rather than following intraoperative parameters such as V_T or the peak airway pressure, monitoring the MP may help estimate the contribution of ventilator-related causes of lung injury.

Therapeutic Hypercarbia

OLV is known to cause an inflammatory response and ALI.[77] Hypercapnia has been shown to have beneficial effects in patients with lung injuries such as ARDS. Gao et al.[78] studied the effect of deliberate hypercapnia on the inflammatory responses to OLV in patients undergoing lobectomy. Fifty patients having lobectomy under intravenous anesthesia were randomly assigned to ventilation with either an oxygen/air mixture (goal $PaCO_2$ of 35 to 45 mmHg) or an oxygen/air/CO_2 mixture (goal $PaCO_2$ of 60 to 70 mmHg). FIO_2 was maintained at greater than 0.8 during OLV. The duration of OLV was not significantly different between the two groups (means ~ 180 minutes). Alveolar lavage fluid was collected and assayed for inflammatory factors. The authors found that induced hypercapnia during the OLV period inhibited the local inflammatory response, decreased airway pressure, increased lung compliance, and improved PaO_2/FIO_2 following surgery. No severe adverse effects were reported in relation to the therapeutic hypercarbia. The potential beneficial effect of inhalation of CO_2 during OLV merits further investigation in patients receiving potent inhaled anesthetics, which have already been shown to inhibit the inflammatory response during lung surgery.

Clinical Approach to the Management of One-Lung Ventilation

6 Once the patient is in the lateral decubitus position, the placement of the DLT should be rechecked. Two-lung ventilation should be maintained for as long as possible. When OLV needs to be instituted, it is generally recommended that an FIO_2 of 1 be used (Table 38-4). The lung should be ventilated using a V_T that results in a plateau airway pressure less than 25 cmH_2O at a rate adjusted to maintain $PaCO_2$ at 35 ± 3 mmHg. This is usually monitored indirectly with the use of a capnometer or other multigas analyzer. The following measures are recommended during OLV: use of PV with low V_T 6 to 7 mL/kg, application of PEEP to the dependent lung, frequent RMs, and restriction of the volume of fluid administered.

After initiation of OLV, depending on the lung pathology and the intensity of HPV, PaO_2 can continue to decrease for up to 45 minutes. Frequent monitoring of arterial blood gases and use of a pulse oximeter continue throughout the operative period. It is also essential to work closely with the surgeon in case reinsufflation of the lung is necessary. If hypoxemia occurs during OLV, the position of the DLT should be rechecked using a fiberoptic bronchoscope. If the dependent lung is not severely diseased, a satisfactory PaO_2 on two-lung ventilation should not decrease to dangerously hypoxic levels on OLV. If a left thoracotomy is being performed using a right-sided DLT, ventilation to the right upper lobe should be ensured. After the tube position has been confirmed as correct, $CPAP_{10}$ should be applied to the nondependent lung after a V_T that expands the lung. In most cases, this is sufficient to increase the PaO_2 to a safe level. During thoracoscopy, application of CPAP is usually not possible because it impedes the surgeon. This is especially so during VATS procedures. In this case, PEEP to the ventilated lung may be tried. In the very rare case in which the PaO_2 remains low despite these maneuvers, intermittent two-lung ventilation can be reinstituted with the surgeon's cooperation. Also, if a pneumonectomy is being performed, depending on the stage of surgical dissection, ligation of the PA eliminates the shunt.

During OLV, the peak airway pressure, the actual V_T delivered (measured by a spirometer), the shape of the capnogram, and, if available, the pressure–volume loop, should be checked continuously. A sudden increase in peak airway pressure may be secondary to tube dislocation because of surgical manipulation, resulting in impaired ventilation. In addition, the ability to auscultate by a stethoscope over the dependent lung is extremely important. If there is any doubt about the stability of the patient, or if the patient becomes hypotensive, dusky, or tachycardic, two-lung ventilation should be resumed until the problem has been resolved. Because of pericardial manipulation (during left thoracotomy in particular) and pulling on the great vessels, cardiac dysrhythmias and hypotension are not uncommon. Cardiotonic drugs should be prepared and kept available for use during any thoracic surgical procedure. Most thoracic surgical procedures represent only relative indications for OLV, and the benefits of OLV should always be weighed against the risks to the patient.

Attention should be directed toward the protection of the ventilated lung. PV should be used with a low V_T and the lowest peak airway pressure (e.g., with an I:E ratio of 1:1), with a high respiratory rate or using pressure control ventilation. Patients with COPD are of particular concern because the application of PEEP may cause dynamic hyperinflation secondary to the increase in respiratory rate to maintain $PaCO_2$.

Frequent recruiting maneuvers should be applied to reduce the amount of atelectasis in the dependent lung. They should be applied with a sustained peak pressure of 40 cmH_2O to be effective. Fluid administration during the procedure must be limited to avoid fluid overload that could increase pulmonary capillary permeability. The risk of ALI and fluid overload increases in proportion to the amount of lung parenchyma resected.[79]

Table 38-4 Clinical Approach to One-lung Ventilation (OLV) Management

1. Use FIO_2 of 1
2. Ventilate with a V_T of 6–8 mL/kg with PEEP 5 cmH_2O
3. Respiratory rate to maintain $PaCO_2$ between 35 and 40 mmHg
4. Check the DLT/endobronchial blocker position subsequent to the lateral decubitus positioning
5. If peak airway pressure exceeds 40 cmH_2O during OLV, DLT/endobronchial blocker malposition should be excluded
6. For hypoxemia, apply CPAP 10 cmH_2O to the nondependent lung (not during VATS)
7. If additional correction of hypoxemia is necessary, add PEEP 5–10 cmH_2O to the ventilated lung
8. Frequent recruiting maneuvers
9. Avoid fluid overload
10. TIVA may be preferable to inhalation anesthetics
11. If necessary, intermittently inflate and deflate the operated lung

CPAP, continuous positive airway pressure; DLT, double-lumen tube; PEEP, positive end-expiratory pressure; TIVA, total intravenous anesthetic; VATS, video-assisted thoracoscopic surgery; V_T, tidal volume.

7 A balanced anesthetic technique using inhalational agents with low rates of propofol infusion alone or in combination with remifentanil is the technique of choice during OLV. It should have the least inhibitory effect on HPV and decrease the transpulmonary shunt through the nonventilated lung. Karzai et al.[58] published an excellent review on the prediction, prevention, and treatment of hypoxemia during OLV.

Yang et al.[80] compared the PV with CV strategies in two groups of 50 patients each undergoing OLV. The CV strategy consisted of FIO_2 1, V_T 10 mL/kg, zero end-expiratory pressure (ZEEP), and VCV; the PV strategy consisted of FIO_2 0.5, V_T 6 mL/kg, PEEP 5 cmH_2O, and PCV. During OLV, although 58% of the PV group needed an increased FIO_2 to maintain an SpO_2 greater than 95%, peak airway pressure was significantly lower than in the CV group, whereas the mean $PaCO_2$ values remained at 35 to 40 mmHg in both groups. Importantly, in the PV group, the incidence of the primary end point of pulmonary dysfunction was significantly lower than in the CV group (incidence of PaO_2/FIO_2 <300 mmHg, lung infiltration, or atelectasis: 4% vs. 22%). The mechanical ventilation strategies used during OLV are discussed in a recent comprehensive review by Sçentürk et al.[81] Walsh et al.[82] concluded that recent evidence from prospective randomized controlled trials of the ventilation of ICU patients without ARDS suggests that clinically important outcomes do not differ between patients who are ventilated with a low or a higher V_T, or with low versus higher PEEP. During OLV, while protective lung ventilation (via manipulation of V_T, PEEP, and DP) may be prudent, there is limited evidence that it reduces pulmonary complications.

Conclusion of the Surgical Procedure

Depending on the extent and the duration of the surgical procedure and the degree of fluid shift, an airway that was initially not classified as difficult may become difficult secondary to facial edema, secretions, and laryngeal trauma from the original intubation. In these cases, when planning to provide lung separation, consideration should be given to the postoperative period and the appropriate tube placed. Many procedures that are not considered to represent absolute indications for lung separation are lengthy and complex. Complex lung resection, with or without chest wall resection, thoracoabdominal esophagogastrectomy, thoracic aortic aneurysm resection with or without total circulatory arrest, or an extensive vertebral tumor resection, may result in facial edema, secretion, and hemoptysis, requiring postoperative ventilatory support. Other indications for postoperative ventilatory support are marginal respiratory reserve, unexpected blood loss or fluid shift, hypothermia, and inadequate reversal of residual neuromuscular blockade. One should always plan in advance for the postoperative period when selecting the method of lung separation. A close dialog with the surgical team is of vital importance.

If a Univent tube was used to provide OLV, the blocker may be fully retracted and the Univent tube can be used as an SLT. If an independent bronchial blocker was used, then the blocker is removed, leaving the SLT in place. The problem arises when a DLT was inserted for lung separation. In a patient with a difficult airway and subsequent facial edema, the DLT may be left in place after surgery.

If the decision to leave the DLT in place is made, it is important to keep in mind that the ICU staff is usually less experienced in managing such a tube, which may easily become dislocated. In addition, it is more difficult to suction through the lumens, and a longer, narrower suction catheter is needed to reach the tip of the endobronchial lumen. Another possibility is to withdraw the DLT to place the 19 to 20 cm mark at the teeth so that the endobronchial lumen is above the carina and both lungs can be ventilated via the bronchial lumen. Tracheal extubation from the DLT should be considered after diuresis and steroid therapy to allow reduction of the facial and airway edema.

If it is necessary to change the DLT to an SLT, a tube exchanger should be used to maintain access to the airway, as previously discussed. The tube exchanger can be passed through the bronchial limb of the DLT. Alternatively, the tube exchange may be performed under direct vision using one of several commercially available video laryngoscopes, such as the GlideScope (Verathon Medical), C-Mac (Karl Storz), or the McGrath (Aircraft Medical). With these video laryngoscopes, the tube exchanger can be placed under direct vision between the vocal cords alongside the existing tube to permit passage of an SLT (Fig. 38-21). The Airtraq DL

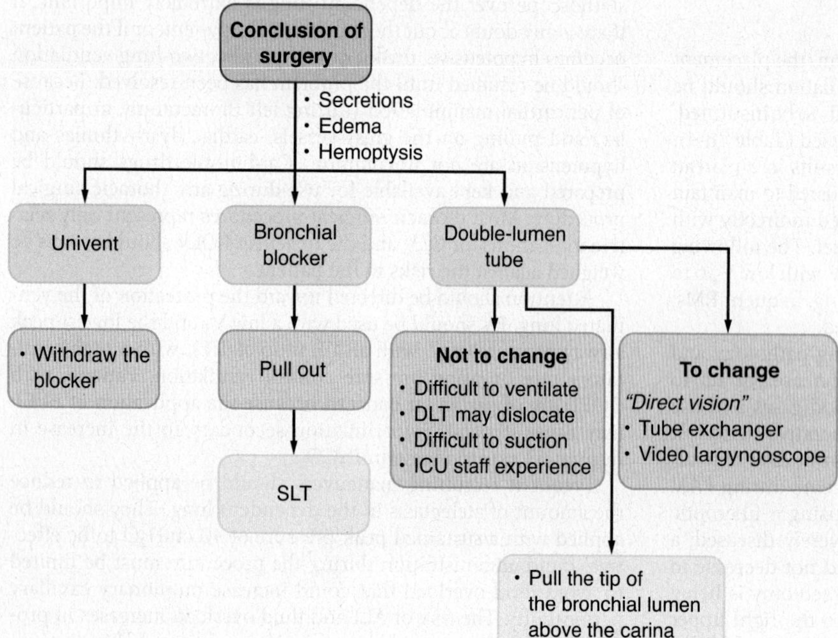

Figure 38-21 Conclusion of the surgical procedure. See text for discussion. SLT, single-lumen tube; DLT, double-lumen tube; ICU, intensive care unit.

(King Systems) is a disposable video blade that is manufactured with a large channel that is large enough to accommodate a DLT.

Choice of Anesthesia for Thoracic Surgery

Traditionally, potent inhaled anesthetics were the agents of choice for OLV since they decrease airway reactivity by direct action on the airway musculature of the bronchial tree. Of concern was their potential inhibitory effect on HPV with an increase in the transpulmonary shunt during OLV. This effect, however, was not supported by clinical trials that compared inhaled agents with TIVA.[83]

De Conno et al.[84] compared the effect of propofol and sevoflurane on the pulmonary inflammatory response before and after OLV. There was an attenuated inflammatory reaction with sevoflurane associated with significantly fewer pulmonary complications. A study by Schilling et al.[85] compared the effects of desflurane, sevoflurane, and propofol on pulmonary and systemic inflammation in patients undergoing open thoracic surgery. They found that the increase in alveolar concentrations of proinflammatory mediators in the ventilated lung was suppressed by desflurane and sevoflurane, while it was enhanced during propofol anesthesia. However, that increase was not associated with higher incidence of postoperative pulmonary complications. In a prospective study, Beck-Schimmeret et al.[86] compared desflurane with propofol in 240 patients undergoing OLV and found no difference in complications during hospital stay and within a 6-month postoperative period. To date, there is a lack of solid evidence that the use of TIVA overall necessarily benefits the patient.

Preconditioning with inhaled agents has a lung protective effect due to inhibition of proinflammatory mediators.[87] The proposed mechanism whereby inhaled anesthetics protect the lung is by maintaining the tight junctions between epithelial cells and preventing the leakage of inflammatory factors from the capillaries into the alveoli. Zona Occludens 1 (OZ-1) is a tight junction protein that acts as a scaffold which anchors the cells to prevent capillary leakage. Englert et al.[88] demonstrated in an animal lung model, with endotoxin-induced inflammation and injured epithelium, that the normally observed decrease in tight junction protein OZ-1 was prevented by preconditioning with isoflurane. Another mechanism by which inhaled anesthetics protect the lung is the preservation of glycocalyx in the epithelial cells. The glycocalyx is a carpet of microtubules that lines the inner surface of the capillary endothelial cells, and it regulates the normal patterns of fluid fluxes across semipermeable membranes. An intact glycocalyx layer tends to decrease leukocyte and platelet adhesion to the endothelium. Deterioration of the glycocalyx during ischemia–reperfusion injury and the presence of inflammatory mediators such as cytokines contribute to increased vascular permeability. It has been demonstrated that sevoflurane stabilizes and reduces glycocalyx shedding in postischemic vessels, which prevents the postischemic adhesion of leukocytes and platelets in a dose-dependent manner. This may explain the beneficial outcomes associated with the use of volatile anesthetics after ischemia–reperfusion.

Tubeless Thoracic Surgery

Tubeless thoracic procedures are procedures that are performed without an endotracheal tube while the patient is spontaneously breathing. Initially defined as an "awake" procedure, the term was updated to "tubeless" since these procedures are performed with sedation/regional block while maintaining spontaneous ventilation. Avoiding PPV fulfills the goal of performing a less traumatic, safe operation with decreased postoperative pain and an expeditious postoperative recovery. The initial concern was that an iatrogenic surgical pneumothorax can be detrimental and would not be tolerated by a spontaneously breathing patient.

In 2004, Pompeo et al.[46] reported the resection of pulmonary nodules by conventional VATS under intravenous anesthesia without endotracheal intubation. Under direct thoracoscopic vision, the vagus nerve was blocked using lidocaine sprayed to effectively abolish the cough reflex.[89] A report of 40 consecutive patients, who underwent uniportal tubeless VATS pulmonary resection using multilevel intercostal nerve blocks and intrathoracic vagal block with no in-hospital mortality, concluded that nonintubated uniportal VATS appears to be a feasible and valid surgical option for appropriately selected patients, depending on the surgeon's experience.

The Tor Vergata Hospital in Rome, Italy, has formed the "Awake Thoracic Surgery Research Group" dedicated to performing thoracic operations in nonintubated patients. They report more than 1,000 various tubeless procedures successfully performed with a low conversion rate. Some of these procedures were performed uniportal tubeless. In a large meta-analysis by Zhang et al.,[90] tubeless VATS was compared with conventional VATS. Tubeless VATS patients had a lower postoperative complication rate, shorter global in-OR time, hospital stay, anesthesia time, chest-tube placement time, reduced chest pain, and lower perioperative mortality rate.

The quality of life after tubeless versus intubated VATS pleurodesis for malignant pleural effusion was evaluated in a study of 198 tubeless and 193 intubated pleurodesis patients. The tubeless group had shorter total OR time, shorter duration of postoperative pleural fluid drainage, shorter postoperative hospital stay, lower mortality and morbidity, and lower costs. Quality of life was similar between groups, although dyspnea and early postoperative improvement in physical function were significantly better in the tubeless group.

Why choose a tubeless thoracic procedure? Exposure to positive pressure is not beneficial to the lung. There is a clear advantage for the lung when it is not subjected to positive pressure ventilation. The use of PPV is indicated when the patient has surgical, anesthetic, or pathologic reasons for inadequate ventilation and oxygenation, and the use of an artificial airway is indicated when the patient's own airway is likely to be compromised. However, mechanical ventilation has a number of potential side-effects such as pressure-induced injury, lung overdistension from volutrauma, release of a variety of proinflammatory mediators, atelectasis, and potential laryngeal or tracheal injuries. Avoidance of muscle relaxants will reduce the degree of atelectasis in the dependent zone of the lung from diaphragmatic dysfunction, and will maintain ventilation–perfusion matching. Eliminating the potential for residual neuromuscular blockade is particularly important in the thoracic surgical patient with compromised lung mechanics due to hyperinflation, or in MG. Avoidance of airway irritation, chest tube, or urinary catheter insertion ultimately will improve patient satisfaction. Finally, tubeless procedures offer the potential for surgery to patients who may otherwise be considered too high risk for general endotracheal anesthesia.

Several regional techniques have been used, including thoracic epidural, paravertebral block, intercostal block, serratus anterior plane block, and transversus thoracic plane block. A thoracic epidural can provide analgesia for the procedure and the postoperative period, but it would be hard to justify placing an epidural for procedures of short duration. Alternative regional blocks such as serratus anterior plane block, or transverse thoracic plane block depend on the patient, the procedure and the anesthesiologist's comfort and preference. The surgeon can supplement with vagal nerve blockade and local anesthetic spray of the pleura to block the cough reflex. Sedation can be managed with propofol infusion, fentanyl, remifentanil, dexmedetomidine, or ketamine. Oxygen saturation should be maintained with using a nonrebreather oxygen facemask, high-flow nasal cannula, positive-pressure nasal oxygen mask, or LMA.

A number of issues must be considered for tubeless procedures. The patient must be able to cooperate, have a BMI <40, and should not have a difficult airway in case an emergency intubation is needed. The procedures should be carefully selected and the surgeon should be comfortable and skilled in tubeless procedures. Close communication and collaboration between the surgeon and the anesthesiologist are crucial. Hypotension can result from mediastinal shift. Paradoxical breathing can occur, in which air from the nondependent lung moves into the dependent lung in inspiration, and in the opposite direction during exhalation. This wasted ventilation results in hypoxemia and hypercarbia that can be treated by applying a slight positive pressure with the face mask, which will usually stabilize the patient immediately.

At the present time, there are no clear guidelines for tubeless procedures and the extent of the procedures performed varies from country to country.

Robotic Thoracic Surgery

Robotic-assisted thoracoscopic surgery (RATS) offers the surgeon three-dimensional depth perception and allows fine motor movements and significant degrees of freedom at the tip of the robotic instruments.[91] Currently, the Da Vinci surgical robotic system (Intuitive Surgical, Sunnyvale, CA, USA) is the only available system with a cost of around $2 million.

A variety of thoracic procedures are performed using RATS, including wedge resection, lobectomy or pneumonectomy, thymectomy, resection of mediastinal masses, and esophageal procedures. The use of robotic procedures ignited controversies regarding the role and cost of this approach. A retrospective study compared 184 patients undergoing RATS versus VATS lung resection and found no improvement in any clinical outcomes, while RATS procedures took longer and cost significantly more. Another study found that a RATS lobectomy cost more than twice that of VATS lobectomy, but less than half of an open lobectomy.

Robotic thoracic procedures have implications for anesthetic management.

First, these procedures are relatively invasive and require the establishment of at least four ports, which is in contrast to the trend of performing minimally invasive surgery such as a uniportal approach. The increase in the number of ports will require diligent management of postprocedure pain and an epidural or paravertebral block should be considered. Potential intercostal nerve damage from the ports may lead to chronic postoperative pain. However, the combination of a smaller port size and a different angulation of the instruments in the incisions is believed to make RATS surgery less painful than VATS.

Second, in many RATS procedures, the surgeon insufflates the hemithorax with CO_2 to enhance lung collapse on the operative side. Pressure-controlled ventilation may provide superior PaO_2 and lower peak airway pressures during CO_2 insufflation. CO_2 insufflation often causes hypotension, so the anesthesiologist must remain in close communication with the surgeon to reduce the insufflation pressure, if necessary.[92] The anesthesiologist must be vigilant to the possibility of DLT/BB displacement from movement of the tracheobronchial tree and frequent variation in the delivered V_T.

Third, during RATS, the patient may be turned 90 degrees away from the anesthesia workstation. This orientation makes it difficult for the anesthesiologist to perform fiberoptic bronchoscopy during the procedure to monitor the correct positioning of the DLT. The use of a DLT with an embedded video camera provides continuous visualization of the carina and potentially earlier indication of impending displacement.

Whether RATS is superior to VATS for lobectomy remains the subject of debate. There are only a few reports comparing RATS lobectomy with conventional VATS lobectomy. One study compared in-hospital mortality, complications, length of stay, and cost for patients undergoing RATS lobectomy or VATS lobectomy; a total of 2,498 robotic-assisted and 37,595 thoracoscopic lobectomies were analyzed. RATS lobectomy was found to be associated with a higher rate of intraoperative injury and bleeding than VATS lobectomy, and at a significantly greater cost. Despite these issues with robotic surgery, the number of RATS procedures is increasing worldwide, possibly due to the perception that robotic surgery is cutting-edge technology that may improve the reputation of an institution. It is unclear at this time how much the availability of robotic surgery will attract patients. Hopefully, when additional devices become available, commercial competition will drive the cost down.

Anesthesia for Diagnostic Procedures

Bronchoscopy

Early bronchoscopes were rigid tubes, but in 1966, the Machida and Olympus Companies introduced the first practical fiberoptic bronchoscopes (Video 38-5). Since then, they have been improved dramatically and have simplified many otherwise complicated bronchoscopies. The indications for bronchoscopy are shown in Table 38-5 and the instruments of choice in Table 38-6. Operator preferences and experience may play a major role in the choice of instrument.

Before bronchoscopy is performed, the patient must be evaluated for chronic lung disease, respiratory obstruction, bronchospasm, coughing, hemoptysis, and infectivity of secretions. Medications should be reviewed, and the need for a more major procedure should always be anticipated: bronchoscopy may lead to thoracotomy or sternotomy. The planned technique for bronchoscopy should be discussed with the surgeon before the operation, and all equipment and connectors should be checked for compatibility. Monitoring during bronchoscopy should include an electrocardiogram, a blood pressure cuff, a precordial stethoscope, and a pulse oximeter. If thoracotomy is planned, an arterial cannula should also be placed, as well as other monitors (e.g., PA or CVP catheters) that may be indicated by the patient's condition. Many anesthetic techniques are useful for bronchoscopy.

Local Anesthesia

The patient should first be pretreated with a drying agent such as glycopyrrolate. The local anesthetics most commonly used are lidocaine and tetracaine. In all cases, the total dose of anesthetic must be considered and the potential for toxicity recognized. A nebulizer can be used to spray the oropharynx and base of the tongue, or the patient may gargle with viscous (2%) lidocaine. Alternatively, the tongue may be held forward, and pledgets soaked in local anesthetic held in each piriform fossa using Krause

Table 38-5 Indications for Bronchoscopy

Diagnostic
Cough
Hemoptysis
Wheeze
Atelectasis
Unresolved pneumonia
Diffuse lung disease
Preoperative evaluation
Rule out metastases
Abnormal chest radiograph
Assess local disease recurrence
Recurrent laryngeal nerve palsy
Diaphragm paralysis
Acute inhalation injury
Exclude tracheoesophageal fistula
During mechanical ventilation
Selective bronchography
Therapeutic
Foreign bodies
Accumulated secretions
Atelectasis
Aspiration
Lung abscess
Reposition endotracheal tubes
Placement of endobronchial tubes
Laser surgery of the airway

Adapted from Landa JF. Indications for bronchoscopy. *Chest*. 1978; 73(Suppl):686. Copyright © 1978 Elsevier. With permission.

forceps to achieve block of the internal branch of the superior laryngeal nerve. Tracheal anesthesia is achieved by a transtracheal injection of local anesthetic, or by spraying the vocal cords and trachea under direct vision using a laryngoscope or through the suction channel of the fiberoptic bronchoscope. Alternatively, a superior laryngeal nerve block can be performed by an external approach, and a glossopharyngeal block can be used to depress the gag reflex. These blocks cause depression of airway reflexes, so patients must be kept on nothing-by-mouth status for several hours after the examination. If fiberoptic bronchoscopy is to be performed transnasally, the nasal mucosa should be pretreated topically with 4% cocaine, or viscous lidocaine may be administered through the nares. Local anesthesia for bronchoscopy has the advantages of a patient who is awake, cooperative, and breathing spontaneously. Sedatives may be added to make the patient more comfortable. Disadvantages of local anesthesia include poor tolerance of any bleeding by the patient and the occasional lack of patient cooperation.

Table 38-6 Instruments of Choice for Bronchoscopy

Rigid
Foreign bodies
Massive hemoptysis
Vascular tumors
Small children
Endobronchial resections
Fiberoptic/Flexible
Mechanical problems of neck
Upper lobe and peripheral lesions
Limited hemoptysis
During mechanical ventilation
Pneumonia, for selective cultures
Positioning of double-lumen tubes
Difficult intubation
Checking position of endotracheal tube
Bronchial blockade

Adapted from Landa JF. Indications for bronchoscopy. *Chest*. 1978; 73(Suppl):686. Copyright © 1978 Elsevier. With permission.

General Anesthesia

General anesthesia for bronchoscopy is often combined with topical laryngeal anesthesia so less general anesthesia is needed. A balanced technique uses N_2O/O_2, incremental doses of an intravenous drug such as propofol, an opioid, and a neuromuscular blocking drug. A potent inhalational anesthesia technique is also satisfactory. Alternatively, an intravenous-based technique may be used to avoid contamination of the OR atmosphere by potent inhaled agents. If desired, limited scavenging of waste gases may be achieved by placing a suction catheter in the patient's oropharynx. Unless there is some contraindication, ventilation of the lungs is usually controlled. In any patient undergoing a thoracic diagnostic procedure for a suspected malignancy, the possibility of the myasthenic syndrome with sensitivity to nondepolarizing muscle relaxants must always be considered. The doses of neuromuscular blocking drugs should be titrated to effect using a neuromuscular monitoring system.

Rigid Bronchoscopy

A modern rigid ventilating bronchoscope is essentially a hollow tube with a blunted, beveled tip. Various sizes and designs are available; however, in all of them, a side arm is provided for connection to an anesthetic gas source. A number of techniques have been described for maintaining ventilation and oxygenation during rigid bronchoscopic examination.[93]

Apneic Oxygenation. After preoxygenation and induction of general anesthesia, skeletal muscle paralysis, and cessation of intermittent PPV, the $PaCO_2$ increases. During the first minute, the increase is approximately 6 mmHg. Subsequently, the average rate of increase is 3 mmHg/min.[94] Oxygen is insufflated at 10 to 15 L/min through a small catheter placed above the carina. The apneic period should be kept to the minimum necessary, particularly in high-risk patients, because the technique is limited by buildup of CO_2, respiratory acidosis, and cardiac dysrhythmias.

Apnea and Intermittent Ventilation. Oxygen and anesthesia gases are delivered to the bronchoscope via the anesthesia circuit (see Chapter 28, Video 28-24). Ventilation is possible only when the eyepiece is in place, which limits the period for instrumentation by the surgeon. Intermittent ventilation of the lungs is achieved by squeezing the reservoir bag. In this way, assuming a good bronchoscope fit in the airway, compliance is constantly monitored, the risk of barotrauma is reduced, and V_T may be estimated. The disadvantage of this technique is that there may be a leak around the bronchoscope, which could lead to hypoventilation and hypercarbia. Packing of the oropharynx can reduce the leak, and improve ventilation in the case of such a gas leak.

Sanders Injection System. Oxygen from a high-pressure source (50 psig) is delivered, using a controllable pressure-reducing valve and toggle switch, to a 2.5- to 3.5-cm 18- or 16-gauge needle inside and parallel to the long axis of the bronchoscope.[95] When the toggle switch is depressed, the jet of oxygen entering the bronchoscope entrains room air, and the air–oxygen mixture resulting at the distal tip of the bronchoscope emerges at a pressure to provide adequate ventilation and oxygenation. The intraluminal tracheal pressure depends on the DP from the reducing valve, the size of the needle jet, the length, internal diameter, and the design of the bronchoscope. Increasing the size of the needle jet increases the total gas flow for any given DP. For each combination of gas-driving pressure, jet orifice, and bronchoscope diameter, only one inflation pressure can be attained, regardless of the volume or compliance of the lung. As long as the proximal end of the bronchoscope is open, the system is strictly pressure limited, and the pressure does not increase because of obstruction at the distal end. Pressure varies inversely with the cross-sectional area of the bronchoscope, so insertion of a suction catheter or biopsy forceps into the lumen causes the intratracheal pressure to increase. Provided there is not a tight fit between the bronchoscope and the airway, the risk of barotrauma is low. If the fit is tight, DP should be decreased.

The advantages of the Sanders system are that because continuous ventilation is possible (because the presence of an eyepiece is not necessary for ventilation of the lungs), the duration of the bronchoscopy procedure is minimized, but the efficiency also permits extended bronchoscopy. A disadvantage is that entrainment of air by the oxygen jet results in a variable FIO_2 at the distal end of the bronchoscope, ventilation of the lungs may be inadequate if compliance is poor, and adequacy of ventilation may be difficult to assess.

Mechanical Ventilator. Ventilation of the lungs may be achieved by connecting a mechanical ventilator to an anesthesia circuit that is connected to the bronchoscope side arm. One disadvantage of this ventilation technique is the presence of a leak of anesthesia gases, and consequentially, light anesthesia.

High-Frequency Positive-Pressure Ventilation. High-frequency positive-pressure ventilation (HFPPV) has been used in conjunction with rigid bronchoscopy and has been compared with the Sanders injector in patients with tracheobronchial stenosis. With HFPPV of up to 150 breaths/min, blood gases were identical with both techniques. At a frequency of 500 breaths/min, oxygenation deteriorated and CO_2 was not removed effectively. HFPPV has the advantage that the tracheobronchial wall remains immobilized during ventilation.

Fiberoptic Bronchoscopy

New generations of fiberscopes, with their improved optics and smaller diameters, have revolutionized bronchoscopy (see Chapter 28, Video 28-21). The flexibility has also been applied in preoperative assessment of the airway, management of difficult tracheal intubations, endotracheal tube positioning and change, bronchial toilet, correct positioning of DLTs, bronchial blockade, and evaluation of the larynx and trachea. Nasal fiberoptic bronchoscopy under topical anesthesia is well tolerated by most awake patients. The administration of an antisialagogue such as glycopyrrolate is useful in reducing secretions. Oral insertion is also possible in both awake and asleep patients and should be performed with a bite block in place to prevent damage to the bronchoscope.

Physiologic Changes Associated with Fiberoptic Bronchoscopy. In all patients, insertion of the fiberoptic bronchoscope is associated with hypoxemia. The average decline in PaO_2 is 20 mmHg and lasts for 1 to 4 hours after the procedure. By 24 hours, the blood gas tensions are usually back to normal. It is therefore recommended that if the initial PaO_2 is 70 mmHg ($FIO_2 = 0.21$), bronchoscopy should be performed only with the administration of supplemental oxygen. This can be provided using mouth-held nasal prongs, a special face mask with a diaphragm through which the fiberscope can be passed, or an endotracheal tube with a T-piece diaphragm adapter.

During and after fiberoptic bronchoscopy, patients experience increased airway obstruction. In a study of 35 patients, insertion of the bronchoscope was associated with an increase in FRC (17% to 30%) and decreases in PaO_2, vital capacity, FEV_1, and forced inspiratory flow.[95] All returned to baseline by 24 hours. These changes are believed to be secondary to direct mechanical activation of irritative reflexes in the airway and, possibly, to mucosal edema. They may be avoided if atropine, either intramuscular or aerosolized into the airway, is administered before the procedure.

The standard adult fiberoptic bronchoscope has an external diameter of 5.7 mm and a 2-mm diameter suction channel. If suction at 1 atm is applied to the fiberscope, air is removed at a rate of 14 L/min. If the fiberscope is in the airway, this causes decreases in FIO_2, PaO_2, and FRC, leading to decreased PaO_2. Suctioning should therefore be kept brief. The adult fiberscope can be passed through endotracheal tubes of 7 mm or greater internal diameter. Clearly, passage through an endotracheal tube decreases the cross-sectional area available for ventilating the patient, so if fibroscopy is planned, an endotracheal tube of the largest possible diameter should be used.

Insertion of the bronchoscope also causes a significant PEEP effect that may result in barotrauma in ventilated patients. If PEEP is already being used, it should be discontinued before passage of the fiberscope. A postendoscopy chest radiograph is advisable to exclude the presence of mediastinal emphysema or pneumothorax. In patients whose tracheas are intubated with endotracheal tubes of less than 7 mm internal diameter, the use of pediatric fiberscopes, which have smaller diameters, would be more appropriate.

The suction channel of the adult fiberoptic bronchoscope has been used to oxygenate and ventilate the lungs of patients. By attaching a jet ventilation system (similar to that used to drive the Sanders injector for rigid bronchoscopy) to the suction connection at the head of a fiberoptic bronchoscope, successful ventilation of the lungs of patients undergoing gynecologic procedures was achieved.[96] A DP of 50 psig of oxygen was used with a ventilatory rate of 18 to 20 breaths/min. This technique permitted adequate ventilation of patients with normally compliant lungs and chest walls. Ventilation of the lungs should be performed only with the tip of the instrument in the trachea because a more peripheral location may produce barotrauma.

Neodymium-yttrium-aluminum garnet (Nd-YAG) lasers are used for the resection of obstructing and endobronchial lesions. This procedure is performed under general anesthesia. The lasers may be introduced into the bronchial tree through a fiberoptic bundle passed via the suction port of the fiberoptic bronchoscope. During laser resection, FIO_2 should be kept to a minimum and titrated to oxygen saturation (as continuously monitored by pulse oximeter) to make endotracheal fire less likely. Laser therapy of bronchial tumors is also possible using a rigid bronchoscope. HFPPV through a rigid bronchoscope provides satisfactory operating conditions for laser resection of tracheal tumors and has the advantage of producing airway immobility.

Complications of Bronchoscopy

Complications of rigid bronchoscopy include mechanical trauma to the teeth, hemorrhage, bronchospasm, loss of a surgical sponge into the bronchial tree, bronchial or tracheal perforation, subglottic edema, and barotrauma. The incidence of complications is much lower with fiberoptic bronchoscopy. Nevertheless, complications may arise owing to overdose with topical anesthetic, insertion trauma, local trauma, hemorrhage, upper airway obstruction related to passage of the instrument through an area of tracheal stenosis, hypoxemia, and bronchospasm. In most cases, it is best to intubate the trachea with an endotracheal tube after bronchoscopy under general anesthesia. This permits avoidance or treatment of some of these problems, particularly the increased airway irritability. Intubation also facilitates effective suctioning of the trachea and bronchi, and allows the patient to recover more gradually from general anesthesia.

Diagnostic Procedures for Mediastinal Mass

Patients with an anterior mediastinal mass may present a special problem for the anesthesiologist (6 Video 38-6, NICV 38-2). Although such masses may cause obvious superior vena cava obstruction, they may also cause obstruction of major airways and cardiac compression, which are less obvious and may become apparent only on induction of anesthesia. Many cases of anesthetic-related airway compression from anterior mediastinal mass have been reported. In one case, total occlusion of the trachea starting 2 to 3 cm above the carina and extending to both main stem bronchi was observed, and a bronchoscope was passed through the obstruction.[97] In the second case of this report, extrinsic compression of the left main stem bronchus occurred on inspiration during recovery from anesthesia. In the third case, flow–volume studies were performed with the patient in the upright and supine positions, with marked reductions in FEV_1 and peak expiratory flow in the latter position. These findings suggested potential obstruction with onset of anesthesia; radiation therapy to the mediastinum was commenced, after which the flow–volume studies showed improved function. The planned surgical procedure was then performed under local anesthesia. In a subsequent series of 105 patients with mediastinal masses, the incidence of intraoperative cardiorespiratory complications was 38%, and the incidence of postoperative respiratory complications was 11%.[98] No cases of airway collapse were reported during anesthesia. In this series, patients were at increased risk of complications if there were preoperative cardiorespiratory signs and symptoms, obstructive and restrictive dysfunction on pulmonary function tests, and greater than 50% tracheal compression on CT scan. In another series of patients with mediastinal mass, four patients had abnormal spirometry but underwent general anesthesia without sequelae.[99] In severe cases of airway compression, the femoral vessels should be cannulated prior to induction of anesthesia so that if the airway is lost completely, cardiopulmonary bypass can be instituted immediately.[100]

If the mass is sensitive to radiation therapy, this may shrink the tumor and make an induction of general anesthesia less hazardous. However, a serious potential disadvantage of preoperative radiation therapy is that it may affect tissue histologic appearance, thereby preventing an accurate diagnosis. If the patient is a child, it may be difficult to obtain tissue samples under local anesthesia alone, and there may be no adequate alternative to general anesthesia. No fatalities occurred in a series of 44 patients aged 18 years or younger with anterior mediastinal masses who underwent general anesthesia before radiation or chemotherapy. However, seven patients did have airway compromise.[101] In another report on a series of children, it was found to be safe to induce general anesthesia if the CT scan revealed that the tracheal cross-sectional area and peak expiratory flow rates were at least 50% of predicted. Airway obstruction caused by an anterior mediastinal mass has been attributed to changes in lung and chest wall mechanics associated with changes in position or with onset of paralysis in muscles that previously maintained airway patency. Preoperative evaluation of a patient with an anterior mediastinal mass to avoid life-threatening total airway obstruction is shown in Figure 38-22. It is important to determine in the history if the patient has dyspnea in the supine position and to examine the CT scan to determine the extent of the tumor and its effect on surrounding structures. If such obstruction occurs, it may be relieved by passage of a rigid bronchoscope or reinforced anode tube past the obstruction, by direct laryngoscopy, or by changing the position of the patient.

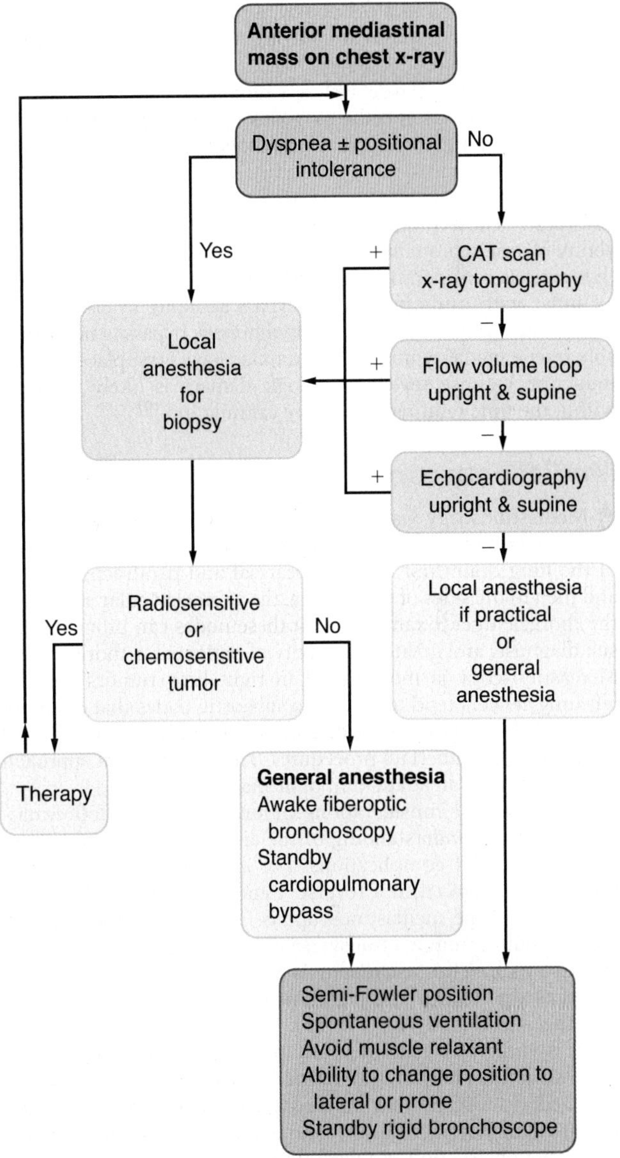

Figure 38-22 Flow chart describing the preoperative evaluation of the patient with an anterior mediastinal mass. + indicates positive finding; – indicates negative workup. (Reprinted with permission from Neuman GG, Weingarten AE, Abramowitz RM, Kushins LG, Abramson AL, Ladner W. The anesthetic management of the patient with an anterior mediastinal mass. *Anesthesiology*. 1984;60:144.)

In a situation in which the biopsy procedure cannot be performed under local anesthesia and there is concern that muscle paralysis may result in airway compression, fiberoptic intubation of the awake patient followed by general anesthesia with spontaneous ventilation has been described. During spontaneous inspiration, the normal transpulmonary pressure gradient distends the airways and helps maintain their patency, even in the presence of extrinsic compression. Airway collapse and inability to ventilate have been reported in a previously asymptomatic patient with a mediastinal mass despite spontaneous ventilation with an inhaled anesthetic and an endotracheal tube.[102] This resulted in sudden cardiopulmonary collapse. PPV was impossible, a rigid bronchoscopy was requested and the surgeons began to prepare femoral vessel access for emergent cardiopulmonary bypass. Fortunately, the airway patency was re-established when the patient's spontaneous respiratory efforts improved as he awoke from general anesthesia. The authors emphasize the need for immediate availability of a rigid bronchoscope and that if a patient is at high risk, then serious consideration should be given to insertion of femoral cannulae with cardiopulmonary bypass standing by before general anesthesia is induced. Cardiopulmonary bypass is not a suitable rescue modality unless the cannulae have been placed before induction because severe neurologic damage is likely to occur within the time required to achieve cannulation.[103]

Mediastinoscopy

Mediastinoscopy was introduced as a means of assessing the spread of bronchial carcinoma (7 Video 38-7). The lymphatics of the lung drain first to the subcarinal and paratracheal areas, and then to the sides of the trachea, the supraclavicular areas, and the thoracic duct. Examination of these nodes can provide a tissue diagnosis and greater selectivity of patients for thoracotomy. Mediastinoscopy is most useful in right lung tumors because left lung cancers tend to spread to subaortic nodes that are more accessible by an anterior mediastinoscopy in the second or third interspace (Chamberlain procedure). The transcervical approach to the thymus is an adaptation of mediastinoscopy.

The anesthetic considerations for mediastinoscopy follow naturally from an understanding of the anatomy of this procedure and its potential complications. For cervical mediastinoscopy, the patient is placed in a reverse Trendelenburg (i.e., head-up) position, and the mediastinoscope is inserted into the superior mediastinum through a transverse incision just above the suprasternal notch. The instrument is advanced along the anterior aspect of the trachea and passes behind the innominate vessels and the aortic arch (Fig. 38-23). The left recurrent laryngeal nerve is vulnerable as it loops around the aortic arch, and any of these structures may be traumatized. Because of scarring, previous mediastinoscopy may be considered a contraindication to a repeat examination. Relative contraindications include superior vena cava obstruction, tracheal deviation, and aneurysm of the thoracic aorta.

Preoperative evaluation should include a search for airway obstruction or distortion. Review of a CT scan is very helpful in this regard. Evidence of impaired cerebral circulation, history of stroke, or signs of the Eaton–Lambert syndrome resulting from oat cell carcinoma should be sought. Blood must be available for the procedure because hemorrhage from major vessels is a real risk and may be life-threatening.

Most surgeons and anesthesiologists prefer general anesthesia using an endotracheal tube and continuous ventilation because this offers a more controlled situation and greater flexibility in terms of surgical manipulation. The anesthetic technique should include a muscle relaxant to prevent the patient from coughing because this may produce venous engorgement in the chest or trauma by the mediastinoscope to surrounding structures.

The incidence of morbidity with mediastinoscopy has been reported as 1.5% to 3.0%, and that of mortality as 0.09%. The most common complication is hemorrhage (0.73%) because of the proximity of major vessels and the vascularity of certain tumors. Tamponade may be the only recourse, and thoracotomy or median sternotomy may be required to achieve hemostasis.

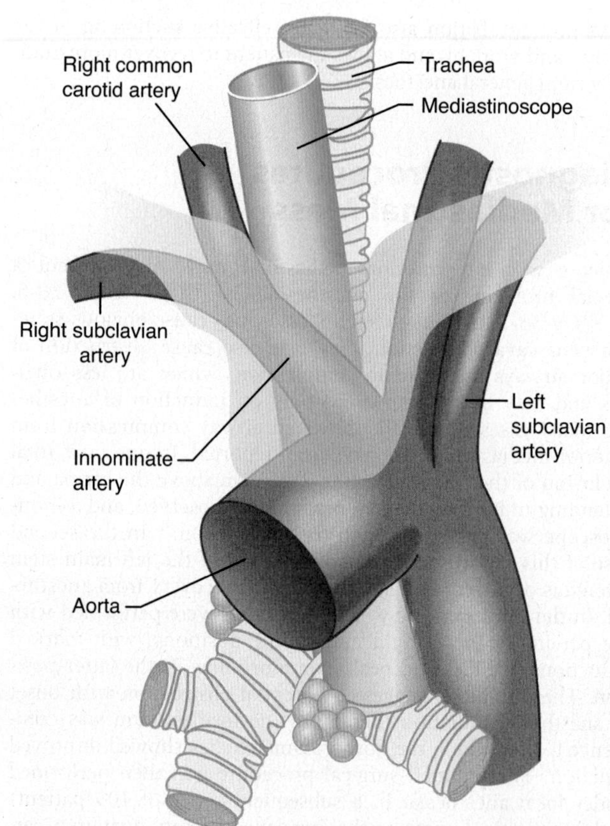

Figure 38-23 Anatomic relationships during mediastinoscopy. Note the position of the mediastinoscope behind the right innominate artery and aortic arch and anterior to the trachea. (Adapted from Carlens E. Mediastinoscopy: A method for inspection and tissue biopsy in the superior mediastinum. *Dis Chest*. 1959;36:343. Copyright © 1959 Elsevier. With permission.)

Needle aspiration of any structure is essential before any biopsy is taken. If severe bleeding occurs, induced arterial hypotension may be helpful in reducing the size of the tear in a vessel. If bleeding is venous, fluids given via an upper limb vein may enter the mediastinum, in which case a large-bore catheter should be placed in a lower limb vein. A venous laceration may also result in air embolism, particularly if the patient is breathing spontaneously. Some recommend the use of a precordial Doppler probe if the risk of air embolism is likely.

Pneumothorax is the second most common complication (0.66%). It is usually right sided, often recognized at the time of the occurrence, and is treated according to the size. A symptomatic pneumothorax should be treated by chest tube decompression.

Recurrent laryngeal nerve injury occurred in 0.34% of cases and was permanent in 50% of these cases. The nerve may be damaged by the mediastinoscope or be involved in tumor. Unilateral injury to the recurrent laryngeal nerve may result in hoarseness. If both recurrent laryngeal nerves are damaged, upper airway obstruction may result. Autonomic reflexes may be triggered by manipulation of the trachea or the aorta, the latter having pressor receptors located in the arch. Vagally mediated reflexes may be blocked by atropine.

The mediastinoscope can inadvertently compress the innominate artery, causing reduced blood flow in the right subclavian artery, right vertebral artery, and right common carotid artery. This can cause the appearance of a "factitious cardiac arrest" in which the right radial pulse disappears and no pulse oximetry reading can be obtained from the right hand, all in the presence of a normal electrocardiogram. A normal right radial pulse should return once the pressure on the innominate artery from the mediastinoscope is removed. Compression of the innominate can be of much greater clinical severity if it causes reduced blood flow to the right hemisphere of the brain. There is a greater risk of right-sided cerebral ischemia if there is a history of impaired cerebral circulation or transient ischemic attacks or if a carotid bruit is present. Transient left hemiparesis may occur after mediastinoscopy. It is therefore recommended that blood pressure be monitored in the left arm and that the right radial pulse be monitored continuously during mediastinoscopy. A decrease in the right radial pulse amplitude is an indication for repositioning the mediastinoscope, especially in a patient with a history of cerebrovascular disease.

Other reported complications include acute tracheal collapse, tension pneumomediastinum, mediastinitis, hemothorax, and chylothorax. A chest radiograph taken in the immediate postoperative period is a useful precaution in all patients after mediastinoscopy.

Thoracoscopy

Thoracoscopy (medical thoracoscopy) involves the insertion of an endoscope into the thoracic cavity and pleural space. It is used for the diagnosis of pleural disease, effusions, and infectious disease (especially in immunosuppressed patients and those with acquired immunodeficiency syndrome) and for staging procedures, chemical pleurodesis, and lung biopsy. It is usually performed by the pulmonary physician in the clinic, under local anesthesia. It is also used in therapeutic procedures such as CO_2 laser treatment of spontaneous pneumothorax or bullous emphysema and Nd-YAG laser vaporization of malignant pleural tumors. A small incision is made in the lateral chest wall, and with the insertion of the instrument, fluid and biopsy specimens are easily obtained.

This procedure may be performed using local, regional, or general anesthesia, the choice depending on the expected duration of the procedure and the physical status of the patient. Pneumothorax is a potential complication of an intercostal block, but it would not have clinical sequelae during a thoracoscopy because it is created as part of the surgical procedure. The collapse of the lung provides the surgeon with a working space, and a chest tube is placed at the conclusion of the surgery. The addition of a stellate ganglion block helps suppress the cough reflex that is sometimes provoked during manipulation of the hilum of the lung.

When air enters the pleural cavity under inspection, a partial pneumothorax occurs, permitting good surgical visualization. Changes in PaO_2, $PaCO_2$, and cardiac rhythm are usually minimal when the procedure is performed using local or regional anesthesia.

With local anesthesia, the spontaneous pneumothorax is usually well tolerated because the skin and chest wall form a seal around the thoracoscope and limit the degree of lung collapse. Occasionally, however, the procedure is poorly tolerated, and general anesthesia must be induced. The insertion of a DLT with the patient in the lateral position may be difficult, in which case the patient may be temporarily placed in the supine position for the intubation.

If general anesthesia is required, a DLT is preferable to an SLT because PPV via an SLT would interfere with endoscopic visualization. In addition, if pleurodesis is being performed, general anesthesia through a DLT allows for re-expansion of the lung and avoids the pain associated with instillation of talc for recurrent pneumothorax.

Video-Assisted (Minimally Invasive) Thoracoscopic Surgery

VATS entails making small incisions in the chest wall, which allows the introduction of a video camera and surgical instruments into the thoracic cavity. In general, it is performed by a thoracic surgeon in the OR under general anesthesia. Although the first thoracoscopy was performed by Jacobeus in 1910, using what was at that time a cystoscope, in more recent years, the surgical techniques, instruments, and video technology have been improved to permit a wide variety of procedures to be performed using VATS. These now include diagnostic procedures for evaluation of pleural disease and effusions, staging of lung cancer, and the identification of parenchymal disease, including nodules, mediastinal tumors, and pericardial disease. They also include therapeutic procedures such as operations for pleural disease, including pleurodesis, decortication and drainage of empyema, resection of lung tissue or bullae, pericardial window or stripping, and esophageal surgery. Lung lobectomies are now usually performed by VATS, and an increasing number are being performed robotically.

Anesthesia Considerations

8

As with a traditional thoracotomy, the patient needs to be in the lateral decubitus position, and lung collapse is needed for adequate surgical exposure. This generally mandates the use of a lung-separation technique. VATS is most commonly performed under general anesthesia with OLV. The need for OLV is much greater in VATS procedures than in open thoracotomy procedures. This is because during VATS, it is not possible to retract the lung, whereas during open thoracotomy lung retraction is possible. Deflation of the nondependent (operated) lung should begin as soon as possible following tracheal intubation and patient positioning because it can take more than 30 minutes to achieve complete collapse of the lung. Also, the surgeon enters the thoracic cavity much sooner during VATS than with open thoracotomy. Suction applied to the airway can help facilitate a more rapid deflation of the lung. In some cases, carbon dioxide is insufflated into the pleural cavity to facilitate visualization. Insufflation pressures should be maintained as low as possible and the CO_2 inflow rate kept less than 2 L/min. Higher pressures can cause mediastinal shift, hemodynamic compromise, increases in airway pressure, and increases in end-tidal CO_2. The clinical picture of hemodynamic compromise is similar to that seen with tension pneumothorax. Significant hemodynamic changes can be produced when pressures as little as 5 mmHg are used to insufflate CO_2 into the chest cavity.

CPAP is commonly used for the treatment of hypoxemia during OLV for thoracotomy and is usually very effective. However, during VATS, CPAP interferes with the surgical exposure and is therefore best avoided. It is preferable to use PEEP to the nonoperated (dependent lung). It may be necessary to tolerate a lower PaO_2 during VATS compared to an open thoracotomy.[104]

Postoperative Concerns

There is less pain after VATS than after open thoracotomy, and an epidural catheter is usually placed before surgery only if there is a likelihood that a thoracotomy may need to be performed. Although a lobectomy can be performed by VATS, sometimes, conversion to an open thoracotomy may be required. The patient's respiratory function is better preserved after VATS, and their recovery is faster. However, postoperative dysrhythmias, which commonly occur after thoracotomy, have also been reported after VATS. Other complications that may occur include bleeding, pulmonary edema, and pneumonia.

Anesthesia for Special Situations

Management of patients with BPF, empyema, cysts, and bullae, as well as those requiring tracheal reconstruction, is considered here. Many of these patients are appropriately managed using high-frequency ventilatory techniques; therefore, these techniques are described first.

High-Frequency Ventilation

With conventional PPV, V_T and respiratory rates usually exceed or approach those in the normal, spontaneously breathing patient. Gas transport to the alveoli occurs by convection in the larger airways, and then by convection and molecular diffusion in the more distal airways and alveoli. High-frequency ventilation differs from conventional PPV in that smaller V_T and more rapid rates are used. Gas transport may depend more on molecular diffusion, high-velocity flow, and coaxial gas flow in the airways, with gas in the center moving distally and that in the periphery moving proximally.

There are several different types of high-frequency ventilation.[105] HFPPV uses small V_T at rates of 60 to 120 breaths/min (1 to 2 Hz). The ventilator used has a negligible internal compliance so the V_T generated, which usually approximates the dead space volume, equals the volume set on the ventilator and represents all fresh gas. The high instantaneous gas flows that are generated facilitate gas exchange and movement in the conducting airways.

HFPPV may be delivered by an open or a closed system. An example of the former is the percutaneous placement of a transtracheal catheter or placement of a catheter through the nose or mouth with its distal end above the carina. Inflow is intraluminal and outflow is extraluminal. This technique has been used during bronchoscopy, tracheal resection, and reconstructive surgery. When open systems are used, the gas outflow pathway is not established mechanically and depends on natural airway patency. It is therefore subject to compromise. Also, aspiration is a potential complication with open systems.

The closed system is superior because it integrates both airway patency and outflow protection. A closed system is represented by a catheter placed in a short segment of an endotracheal tube for delivery of the HFPPV, whereas the remainder of the tube lumen represents the exit pathway for gas. A quadruple-lumen endotracheal tube (Hi-Lo Jet Tracheal Tube, Mallinckrodt, Inc.) has been designed specifically for delivery of HFPPV. One lumen is for the HFPPV delivery, one for gas outflow, one for cuff inflation, and one for measuring airway pressures at the distal end of the tube. The use of a closed system also permits application of PEEP, a situation not possible with an open arrangement.

High-frequency jet ventilation (HFJV) uses a pulse of a small jet of fresh gas introduced from a high-pressure source (50 psig) into the airway through a small catheter or additional lumen in an endotracheal tube. Rates used are usually 100 to 400 breaths/min. The fresh gas jet entrains gas from an injection cannula side-port reservoir. This system is somewhat analogous to the Sanders injector system described in the "Bronchoscopy" section, and FIO_2 is similarly variable. The jet and entrained gas flows cause forward motion of the mass of gas in the airways. HFJV can be used with an open system or with a closed arrangement, as described earlier. In the latter, PEEP may be added to enhance oxygenation. Also, with use of high fresh gas flows from an anesthesia circuit, inhaled anesthetics may be delivered as an entrained gas mixture.

High-frequency oscillation ventilation uses a mechanism that oscillates gas at rates of 400 to 2,400 breaths/min. It has not been described in association with thoracic surgical procedures. In this system, V_T is small (50 to 80 mL), and gas exchange occurs through enhanced molecular diffusion and coaxial airway flow.

The potential advantages offered by HFPPV during thoracic anesthesia are that lower V_T and inspiratory pressures result in a quiet lung field for the surgeon, with minimal movements of airway, lung tissue, and mediastinum. Thus, HFPPV has been used to ventilate both the nondependent and the dependent lung during thoracic surgical procedures, with adequate arterial blood gas measurements obtained throughout. At high frequencies (>6 Hz), however, CO_2 retention may become a problem.

HFJV has been used to ventilate the nondependent lung to improve PaO_2 during one-lung anesthesia, whereas the dependent lung is ventilated with conventional intermittent PPV. PaO_2 increased compared with that obtained during simple collapse of the nondependent lung. A study comparing HFJV with CPAP to the nondependent lung during conventional intermittent PPV to the dependent lung found that both improved PaO_2 significantly during closed and open stages of the surgery. When the chest was open, HFJV maintained satisfactory cardiac output, whereas CPAP usually decreased cardiac output; however, there were no significant differences in $PaCO_2$ between HFJV and CPAP. Because similar increases in PaO_2 may be obtained using selective CPAP to the nondependent lung and with much simpler equipment than that necessary to deliver high-frequency ventilation, the use of CPAP would seem preferable to high-frequency ventilation to increase PaO_2 during most one-lung anesthesia situations.

The lower pressures and V_T associated with high-frequency ventilation result in only a small leak through BPFs, and HFJV is now generally considered the conservative treatment of choice in this condition. Another advantage of high-frequency ventilation is that the rapid-rate small V_T can be delivered through small tubes or catheters so if an airway has to be divided, the passage of a small tube across the surgical field permits ventilation of the distal airway and lung tissue. This use has been applied during sleeve resection of the lung, tracheal reconstruction, and surgery for tracheal stenosis. In all three situations, the surgeon is able to work easily around the small catheter used to provide the high-frequency ventilation.

Bronchopleural Fistula and Empyema

A BPF is an abnormal communication between the bronchial tree and the pleural cavity. Occasionally, there is an additional communication to the surface of the chest, a cutaneous BPF. BPF occurs most commonly after pulmonary resection for carcinoma. Other causes include traumatic rupture of a bronchus or bulla (sometimes caused by barotrauma or PEEP), penetrating chest wound, or spontaneous drainage into the bronchial tree of an empyema cavity or lung cyst. The incidence of BPF is higher after pneumonectomy than following other types of lung resection. The problems associated with BPF and empyema are that PPV may result in contamination of healthy lung, loss of air, decreased alveolar ventilation leading to CO_2 retention, and the development of a tension pneumothorax.

If an empyema is present, it should be drained under local anesthesia before any surgery to close the BPF. Drainage is performed with the patient sitting up and leaning toward the affected side. Empyemas are often loculated, and complete drainage is not always possible. A drain to an underwater seal system is left in the cavity before administration of anesthesia for surgery of the BPF. After drainage of an empyema, a chest radiograph should be obtained to determine the efficacy of the procedure.

The priorities in the anesthetic management of BPF are the isolation of the affected side in terms of contamination and ventilation. The ideal approach is intubation of the trachea while the patient is awake using a DLT with the patient breathing spontaneously. Supplemental oxygen should be administered, and the patient should be constantly reassured. Neuroleptanalgesia is satisfactory in providing a suitably cooperative patient, and the airway is then pretreated with topical anesthesia. The endobronchial tube selected should be such that the bronchial lumen is on the side opposite the BPF. Selection of the largest possible tube provides a close fit in the trachea, which helps stabilize the tube. Once the tube is adequately positioned in the trachea, there may be a considerable outpouring of pus from the tracheal lumen if an empyema is present; therefore, this lumen should be immediately suctioned using a large-bore suction catheter. The healthy and possibly the affected lung may then be ventilated; adequacy of oxygenation and ventilation is assessed by pulse oximetry and arterial blood gas analysis.

An alternative technique is to insert the DLT under general anesthesia, with the patient breathing spontaneously to avoid a tension pneumothorax. With either technique, the chest drainage tube must be left unclamped to avoid any bouts of coughing and to prevent the buildup of a tension pneumothorax in the event that a predisposing valvular mechanism exists. In patients who do not have an empyema, use of an SLT has been described and may be satisfactory if the BPF and air leak are small. A rapid-sequence induction with ketamine or propofol followed by a relaxant has also been described, but is associated with considerable risk of contamination and tension pneumothorax.

BPF may also be treated conservatively using various ventilatory techniques. Thus, the bronchus of the normal lung may be intubated and ventilated, allowing the BPF the opportunity to rest and heal. This approach may result in an intolerable shunt, however, and PEEP may be necessary to maintain PaO_2. Differential lung ventilation using a DLT has also been described, the healthy lung being ventilated with normal V_T, while the affected lung is exposed to a smaller V_T or to CPAP with oxygen at pressures just below the critical opening pressure of the fistula. The critical opening pressure of the BPF can be assessed by determining the lowest level of CPAP that must be applied to the bronchus on the affected side to produce continuous bubbling through the underwater seal chest drain.

For a large BPF, HFJV may be the nonsurgical treatment of choice. The use of small V_T results in minimal gas loss through the fistula, which may heal more quickly. In addition, hemodynamic effects are usually minimal and spontaneous efforts at ventilation are usually abolished, thereby decreasing the work of breathing and eliminating the need for relaxants or excessive sedation.

Lung Cysts and Bullae

Air-filled cysts of the lung are usually bronchogenic, postinfective, infantile, or emphysematous. They may be associated with COPD or be an isolated finding. A bulla is a thin-walled space filled with air that results from the destruction of alveolar tissue. The walls are, therefore, composed of visceral pleura, connective tissue septa, or compressed lung tissue. In general, bullae represent an area of end-stage emphysematous destruction of the lung.

Patients may be considered for surgical bullectomy when dyspnea is incapacitating, when the bullae are expanding, when there are repeated pneumothoraces owing to rupture of bullae, or if the bullae compress a large area of normal lung. Most of these patients have severe COPD and CO_2 retention, and little functional respiratory reserve. The first consideration in management is maintenance of a high FIO_2. If the bulla or cyst communicates with the bronchial tree, PPV may cause it to expand or even to rupture, if it is compliant, producing a situation analogous to tension pneumothorax. If the bulla is very compliant, most of the applied V_T may be wasted in this additional dead space. Nitrous oxide should be avoided because it causes expansion of any air spaces in the body, including bullae. Once the chest is open, even more of the V_T may enter the compliant bulla, which is no longer limited by chest wall integrity, and an increase in ventilation is needed until the bulla is controlled.

The anesthetic management of these patients is challenging, particularly if the disease is bilateral. Ideally, a DLT is inserted with the patient awake or under general anesthesia but breathing spontaneously. The avoidance of PPV (when possible) helps decrease the likelihood of the potential problems described previously, although oxygenation may be precarious with spontaneous ventilation. Once the endotracheal tube is in place, each lung may be controlled separately, and adequate ventilation can be applied to the healthy lung if bilateral disease is not present. Gentle PPV with rapid, small V_T and pressures not to exceed 10 cmH_2O may be used during the induction and maintenance of anesthesia, especially if the bullae have been shown to have no or only poor bronchial communication by preoperative ventilation scanning. While the surgery is being performed, as each bulla is resected, the operated lung can be separately ventilated to check for air leaks and the presence of additional bullae.

If PPV is to be applied before the chest is opened, the possibility of a tension pneumothorax must be kept in mind, and treatment should be readily available. The diagnosis of pneumothorax may be made by a unilateral decrease in breath sounds (this may be difficult to distinguish in a patient with bullous disease), increase in ventilatory pressure, progressive tracheal deviation, wheezing, or cardiovascular changes. Treatment of a pneumothorax involves the rapid placement of a chest tube. An added risk of chest tube placement is the creation of a cutaneous BPF, which causes problems for ventilation. Alternatively, general anesthesia is induced only after the surgeon has prepared the operative field and draped the patient. In the event of sudden deterioration in the patient's condition during induction, the surgeon may perform an immediate median sternotomy. In any event, the time from induction of anesthesia to sternotomy must be kept to a minimum.

To avoid these problems in a patient with known bullae, HFJV has been used in a patient with a large bulla undergoing coronary artery bypass graft and in another patient undergoing bilateral bullectomy. If bilateral bullectomy is to be performed, a median sternotomy is usually used. Benumof[106] described the use of sequential OLV using a DLT in the management of a patient needing bilateral bullectomy. The side with the largest bulla and least lung function, as assessed before surgery by ventilation and perfusion scans, should be operated on first. In this way, the lung with the better function should support gas exchange first. If hypoxemia develops during this one-lung situation, application of CPAP to the nonventilated lung during the deflation phase of a tidal breath should increase PaO_2.

Unlike most cases of pulmonary resection, patients after bullectomy are left with a greater amount of functional lung tissue than was previously available to them, and the mechanics of respiration are improved. At the end of the procedure, the DLT is replaced by an SLT, and the patients generally require several days to be weaned from the ventilator. During this time, the positive airway pressure used should be minimized to avoid causing a pneumothorax owing to rupture of suture or staple lines or of residual bullae.

Anesthesia for Resection of the Trachea

Tracheal resection and reconstruction are technically difficult for the surgeon and challenging for the anesthesiologist. Indications for this type of procedure include congenital lesions (agenesis, stenosis), neoplasia (primary or secondary), injuries (direct or indirect), infections, and postintubation injuries (caused by an endotracheal tube or tracheotomy). For the surgical team, the major problems are maintenance of ventilation to the lungs while the airway is being operated on and postoperative integrity of the anastomoses. In this respect, the presence of lung disease sufficiently severe to require postoperative ventilatory support is a relative contraindication to tracheal resection or reconstruction.

Monitoring of these patients should include placement of an arterial cannula in the left radial artery to permit continuous measurement of blood pressure during periods of innominate artery compression. Steroids should be administered to help reduce any tracheal edema, and a high F_{IO_2} should be used throughout the procedure to ensure an adequate oxygen reserve at all times in the FRC so that temporary interruptions of ventilation are less likely to produce hypoxemia.

Numerous methods have been reported to provide oxygenation and ventilation of the lungs during these procedures. A small-bore reinforced anode tube may be placed through and distal to an upper tracheal lesion so resection may occur around the tube. This technique is useful only in mild stenoses. Alternatively, an endotracheal tube may be passed through the glottis to above the stenosis, and a sterile endotracheal or bronchial tube may later be inserted into the trachea opened distal to the site of stenosis, with the sterile anesthesia tubing being led across the surgical field. After resection of the lesion, the sterile and distally placed endotracheal tube is withdrawn, and the upper tube (originally passed through the glottis) is advanced across the anastomosis. With low tracheal or bronchial lesions, resection and reconstruction may be performed around an endobronchial or DLT. During these procedures, the patient is kept in a head-down position to minimize aspiration of blood and debris into the alveoli, and ventilation must be carefully monitored throughout the procedure.

Clearly, the presence of a large-bore tube in the airway may make these resections technically difficult, and the use of high-frequency ventilation techniques may improve surgical access. Thus, a small-diameter catheter or catheters may be placed across or through the stenotic lesion or transected airway(s) and ventilation to the distal airways and lungs maintained using HFPPV or HFJV. Potential disadvantages of these high-frequency ventilation techniques are that, by necessity, the system is "open" (see "High-Frequency Ventilation"), and egress of gas during exhalation may be compromised if the stenosis is tight. Also, the catheter may become occluded by blood and become displaced, and distal aspiration of debris or blood may occur. With complex resections, two anesthesia teams with two machines and anesthesia circuits or sets of ventilating equipment may be necessary to ensure adequate ventilation of the two distal airway segments. During carinal resections, HFPPV to the left lung alone usually provides adequate oxygenation and ventilation.

After tracheal resection or reconstructive surgery, patients should be positioned with the neck and head flexed to reduce tension on the anastomotic suture lines. In some cases, this is maintained by using sutures between the chin and the anterior chest wall. Extubation of the trachea is performed as early as possible to minimize tracheal trauma due to the endotracheal tube and cuff.

Bronchopulmonary Lavage

This procedure involves irrigation of the lung and bronchial tree, and is used as a treatment for alveolar proteinosis, radioactive dust inhalation, cystic fibrosis, bronchiectasis, and asthmatic bronchitis. Lung lavage is performed under general anesthesia using a DLT so one lung may be ventilated while the other is being treated with lavage fluid.[107]

The preoperative assessment of these patients should include ventilation–perfusion scans so lavage can be performed first on the more severely affected lung (i.e., the one with the least ventilation). If involvement is equal, the left lung is generally lavaged first because gas exchange should be better through the larger, right lung. Patients are premedicated and supplied with supplemental oxygen en route to the OR.

Anesthesia is induced with an intravenous drug and maintained with an inhaled agent in oxygen to maintain the highest possible F_{IO_2}. Muscle relaxation facilitates placement of the DLT, and the cuff seal should be checked to maintain perfect separation at a pressure of 50 cmH_2O to prevent leakage of lavage fluid around the cuff. A fiberoptic bronchoscope is useful to check the position of the bronchial cuff of the DLT. Monitoring should include an arterial catheter, and a stethoscope should be placed over the ventilated lung to check for rales, the presence of which may indicate leakage of lavage fluid into this lung.

The patient is maintained on an F_{IO_2} of 1 throughout the procedure. Before lavage, this serves to denitrogenate the lungs so only oxygen and carbon dioxide remain. Instillation of fluid then allows these gases to be absorbed, resulting in greater access by the fluid to the alveolar spaces than if the more insoluble nitrogen bubbles remained.

Once the trachea is intubated, the patient is turned so the side to be lavaged is lowermost, and the DLT position and seal are checked once again. With the patient in a head-up position, warmed heparinized isotonic saline is infused by gravity from a reservoir 30 cm above the midaxillary line into the catheter to the dependent lung, while the nondependent lung is ventilated. When fluid ceases to flow in (usually after 700 to 1,000 mL in an adult), the patient is placed in a head-down position and fluid is allowed to drain out. The lavage is continued until the effluent is clear (as opposed to the milky fluid that drains initially when lavage is being performed for alveolar proteinosis), at which point the lung is suctioned and ventilation is re-established with large V_T (and pressures) because compliance is decreased owing to loss of surfactant. With each lavage, inflow and outflow volumes are monitored so the patient is not "drowned" in fluid, and there is no excessive absorption or leakage to the ventilated side. At least 90% of the saline volume should be recovered with each lavage. Two-lung ventilation is re-established and, as compliance improves, an air–oxygen mixture (i.e., addition of nitrogen) may be introduced to help maintain alveolar patency. After a further period of ventilation, in most patients, the trachea can be extubated in the OR. In the posttreatment period, patients are encouraged to cough and engage in breathing exercises to fully re-expand the treated lung. From 3 days to 1 week after lavage of the first lung, the patient may return to the OR for lavage of the other lung.

Problems sometimes encountered with this procedure include spillage of lavage fluid from the treated to the ventilated lung. This must be managed by stopping the lavage and ensuring functional separation of the lungs before continuing. DLT positioning is critical. Spillage may cause profound decreases in oxygenation, which may necessitate terminating the procedure and maintaining two-lung ventilation with oxygen and PEEP.

During periods when lavage fluid is being instilled into the dependent lung, oxygenation usually improves because the increased intra-alveolar pressure caused by the fluid produces diversion of the pulmonary blood flow to the nondependent, ventilated lung. Conversely, when the fluid is drained out of the dependent lung, hypoxemia may occur. In some cases in which severe hypoxemia was anticipated during right lung lavage, the risk has been reduced by passing a balloon-tipped catheter into the right main PA (checked by radiography) and inflating the balloon during periods of right lung drainage. In this way, blood flow to the dependent, right, nonventilated lung is minimized during periods of drainage. This technique is not without risk (e.g., PA rupture) and is reserved for those patients considered to be at greatest risk for hypoxemia during lavage. If the patient has recently had a diagnostic open lung biopsy, a BPF may be present. If this is a possibility, a chest tube should be inserted on the side of the BPF, and this side should be lavaged first. The chest drain is removed several days later.

Limitations in the sizes of available DLTs preclude their use for lavage in patients weighing less than 40 kg. In such cases, cardiopulmonary bypass may be required to provide oxygenation during lavage.

Myasthenia Gravis

10 The thoracic anesthesiologist will most likely have to manage patients with MG for thymectomy, which is now considered the treatment of choice in most cases of MG. MG is a disorder of the neuromuscular junction, the function of which is altered routinely in the modern practice of anesthesia. The incidence of MG appears to be increasing. The most accurate estimate of incidence of MG was around 30/1,000,000 per year. The incidence in children and adolescents aged 0 to 19 years was found to be between 1 and 5/1,000,000 per year. These rates may well be an underestimate of the true incidence rates, as mild cases will have been missed and cases in the elderly will have been misdiagnosed.[107] People of any age may be affected, but peaks of incidence occur in the third decade for women and the fifth decade for men. MG is a chronic disorder characterized by a clinical course of fluctuating painless weakness and fatigability of voluntary muscles with improvement following rest. Onset is usually slow and insidious, any skeletal muscle or group of muscles may be affected, and the condition is associated with relapses and remissions. The most common onset is ocular; if the disease remains localized to the eyes for 2 years, the likelihood of progression to generalized MG is low. In some cases, the disease is generalized and may involve the bulbar musculature, causing problems with breathing and swallowing. Peripheral muscle involvement may cause weakness, clumsiness, and difficulty in holding up the head or in walking. A commonly used clinical classification of MG[109] is shown in Table 38-7.

In MG, there is a decrease in the number of postsynaptic acetylcholine receptors (AChRs) at the endplates of affected muscles. This causes a decrease in the margin of safety of neuromuscular transmission. MG is an autoimmune disorder, and about 80% of the affected patients have detectable circulating antibodies to the nicotinic AChR. These anti-AChR antibodies may cause complement-mediated lysis of the postsynaptic membrane or direct blockade of the receptors, or may modulate the receptor turnover such that the degradation rate exceeds the resynthesis rate. Studies of the endplate area show loss of synaptic folds and a widening of the synaptic cleft. A variable proportion of the patients who do not have anti-AChR antibodies have antibodies to muscle-specific tyrosine kinase (MuSK).[110]

The diagnosis of MG is suspected from the patient's history and confirmed by clinical, pharmacologic, electrophysiologic, or immunologic testing. Patients cannot sustain or repeat muscular contraction. The electrical counterpart of this is a decrement in the compound muscle action potentials evoked by repetitive stimulation of a motor nerve. This is the most specific of the nerve tests for MG but it can be performed only on certain muscles, which may not be the ones affected in an individual patient. Mechanical and electrical (electromyography) decrements improve with 2 to 10 mg of intravenous edrophonium (Tensilon test). MG patients characteristically are sensitive to nondepolarizing muscle relaxants. When the routine electromyographic results are equivocal, a regional nondepolarizing muscle relaxant test may be performed using a tourniquet to isolate the limb and limit the action of the drug. In the regional nondepolarizer muscle relaxant test, electromyograms are performed before and after the administration of 0.2 mg of curare. In equivocal cases, a positive result of a test for anti-AChR antibodies is considered diagnostic.

Table 38-7 Clinical Classification of Myasthenia Gravis (MG)

Class	Description
I	Ocular myasthenia—involvement of ocular muscles only. Mild with ptosis and diplopia. Electrophysiologic testing of other musculature is negative for MG.
IA	Ocular myasthenia with peripheral muscles showing no clinical symptoms but showing a positive electromyogram for MG.
II	Generalized myasthenia
IIA	Mild—slow onset, usually ocular, spreading to skeletal and bulbar muscles. No respiratory involvement. Good response to drug therapy. Low mortality rate.
IIB	Moderate—as IIA but progressing to more severe involvement of skeletal and bulbar muscles. Dysarthria, dysphagia, difficulty chewing. No respiratory involvement. Patient's activities limited. Fair response to drug therapy.
III	Acute fulminating myasthenia—rapid onset of severe bulbar and skeletal weakness with involvement of muscles of respiration. Progression usually within 6 mos. Poor response to therapy. Patient's activities limited. Low mortality rate.
IV	Late severe myasthenia—severe MG developing at least 2 yrs after onset of group I or group II symptoms. Progression of disease may be gradual or rapid. Poor response to therapy and poor prognosis.

Adapted from Osserman KE, Genkins G. Studies in myasthenia gravis: a review of a 20-year experience in over 1200 patients. *Mt Sinai J Med.* 1971;38:497. Copyright © 1971 John Wiley & Sons.

Medical Therapy

Anticholinesterases are used to prolong the action of acetylcholine at the postsynaptic membrane and may also exert their own agonist effect at the AChRs. Anticholinesterases are the most commonly used medical therapy in MG (Table 38-8). Interestingly, no randomized controlled trial has been conducted on the use of acetylcholinesterase inhibitors in patients with MG because the response in observational studies is so obvious that a placebo group could not be justified.[111] Myasthenic patients learn to regulate their medication and titrate the dose for optimum effect. Overdosage causes the muscarinic effects of acetylcholine and may cause a cholinergic crisis. Underdosage causes weakness or a myasthenic crisis. In a patient with weakness, distinction between the two types of crisis may be made by performing a Tensilon test or by examining pupillary size, which will be large (mydriatic) in a myasthenic crisis but small (miotic) in a cholinergic crisis. Muscarinic side effects are treatable with atropine.

Table 38-8 Anticholinesterase Drugs Used to Treat Myasthenia Gravis

	Dose (mg)			
Drug	***Oral***	***IV***	***IM***	***Efficacy***
Pyridostigmine (Mestinon)	60	2	2–4	1
Neostigmine (Prostigmine)	15	0.5	0.7–1	1

IM, intramuscular; IV, intravenous.

The immunologic basis of MG has led to the use of short- and long-term immunosuppressive drugs. Steroids are used for short-term immunosuppression, whereas for long-term effect azathioprine, cyclophosphamide, cyclosporine, methotrexate, mycophenolate mofetil, rituximab, and tacrolimus have been used. Steroids often produce initial deterioration before an improvement. The usual regimen is prednisone 1 mg/kg on alternate days. Rapid short-term immunomodulation has been achieved in acute exacerbations or to improve muscle strength prior to surgery. Plasma exchange or plasmapheresis may produce dramatic but transient improvements in muscle strength with decreases in anti-AChR and anti-MuSK titers, as well as other inflammatory mediators. Usually reserved for severe MG, plasma exchange has been shown to improve respiratory function in both operated and non-operated patients with MG. Plasmapheresis causes a decrease in plasma cholinesterase levels that may prolong the effect of drugs such as succinylcholine that are normally broken down by this enzyme system.

Long-term immunomodulation is achieved by surgical thymectomy.[112] Abnormalities are found in 75% of thymus glands removed from patients with MG (85% show hyperplasia, 15% show thymoma). After thymectomy, approximately 75% of patients either go into remission or show some improvement. Thymectomy is always indicated in those patients with thymoma, and is now considered the treatment of choice in most patients with MG, except for those in Osserman class I (Table 38-7). Response to thymectomy is best if it is performed within the first 3 years following diagnosis. Clinical outcome from thymectomy is equivalent whether performed via a transsternal or video-assisted thoracoscopic approach. A report describing anesthesia concerns in 17 patients who underwent robotic-assisted thoracoscopic thymectomy suggested that refinement of the surgical technique and positioning are required.[113]

Management of General Anesthesia

When possible, patients with MG should be admitted for elective surgery while in remission.[114] On admission, the patient's physical and emotional states should be optimized. Other diseases occasionally associated with MG should be excluded (Table 38-9).[115] The patient's current drug therapy should be reviewed and possible drug interactions considered. Because patients are less active while in the hospital, their anticholinesterase dosage may need to be decreased. If the patient has a history of respiratory disease or bulbar involvement, preoperative evaluation should include respiratory function studies. Breathing exercises and instruction in the use of incentive spirometers may be indicated. Patients should be told of the possible need for postoperative intubation of the trachea and ventilation of the lungs. Ideally, patients with MG should be scheduled to be the first case of the day in the OR. Patients receiving steroid therapy should receive perioperative coverage. Interactions with other immunosuppressant drugs must be considered and if the patient is in crisis, preoperative plasmaphereses may be necessary.

Because the trachea is to be intubated and the lungs ventilated for the planned procedure in the patient with MG, traditional practice is to withhold anticholinesterase therapy on the morning of surgery so that the patient is weak on arrival at the OR.[116] This avoids interactions with other drugs used in the OR. Anticholinesterase therapy may be continued if the patient is physically or psychologically dependent on it. Others recommend continuing pyridostigmine, including an oral dose just before induction. Premedication is satisfactorily achieved with a benzodiazepine or barbiturate. Opioids are usually avoided because of the risk of producing respiratory depression.

Monitoring should be dictated by the patient's state and planned surgical procedure, but should include an assessment of neuromuscular transmission (by means of a mechanomyogram/twitch monitor, an integrated electromyographic monitor, a kinemyograph, or an accelograph monitor) if agents affecting neuromuscular transmission are to be used.

Induction of anesthesia is readily achieved with a short-acting barbiturate (if available) or propofol. In elective cases, intubation of the trachea, maintenance, and relaxation are readily achieved using potent inhaled anesthetics. Anesthesia may be deepened using a potent inhaled agent and the trachea intubated under its effect. Myasthenic patients are more sensitive than normal patients to the neuromuscular depressant effects of the potent inhaled agents. In patients with MG, isoflurane at 1.9 MAC end-tidal concentration induced a neuromuscular block of 30% to 50%, whereas halothane at 1.8 MAC induced a block of 10% to 20%. Both agents produced fade in the train-of-four ratio of 41% and 28%, respectively.[117] The less-soluble inhaled agents, sevoflurane and desflurane, are even more easily administered and withdrawn; they are now the most commonly used anesthetic drugs for patients with MG. Nitahara et al.[118] studied the neuromuscular effects of sevoflurane in 16 myasthenic patients and 12 normal patients. As expected, they found a concentration-dependent decrease in T1 and T4/T1 values. The depressant effects of sevoflurane were more prominent in those myasthenic patients with baseline T4/T1 less than 0.90. Whichever agent is used, at the end of the procedure, the inhaled agent is discontinued and recovery of neuromuscular function begins. Experience with desflurane in MG patients undergoing video-assisted thoracoscopic thymectomy was similar.

Table 38-9 Disorders Associated with Myasthenia Gravis

Thymoma
Thyroid disease
Hyperthyroidism
Hypothyroidism
Thyroiditis
Idiopathic thrombocytopenic purpura
Rheumatoid arthritis
Systemic lupus erythematosus
Anemias
Pernicious
Hemolytic
Multiple sclerosis
Ulcerative colitis
Leukemia
Lymphoma
Convulsive disorders
Extrathymic neoplasia
Sjögren syndrome
Scleroderma

Nondepolarizing Relaxants. In some cases, patients with MG cannot tolerate the cardiovascular depressant effects of the potent inhaled anesthetics, in which case neuromuscular blocking drugs may be used, titrating dose against monitored effect. Patients with MG are sensitive (i.e., show a decrease in ED_{50} and ED_{95} when compared with non-MG patients) to nondepolarizing neuromuscular blocking drugs.[119] All nondepolarizing relaxants have been successfully and uneventfully used with careful monitoring in patients with MG. Since the sensitivity of any individual MG patient is unknown, these drugs should be titrated in 1/10 of the usual dose. Cisatracurium may be preferred because of its short elimination half-life, small volume of distribution, lack of cumulative effect, and high clearance. Sensitivity to nondepolarizing relaxants is increased during the coadministration of a potent inhaled anesthetic.

Other intermediate-duration nondepolarizing agents such as vecuronium and rocuronium may be used; long-acting relaxants are best avoided in patients with MG. If necessary, the residual relaxation produced by nondepolarizers may be reversed by increments of anticholinesterase drugs, where neuromuscular transmission is carefully monitored to obtain maximum antagonism yet avoid a cholinergic crisis. All anticholinesterases have been safely used. The sensitivity of patients with MG to nondepolarizing relaxants is very variable, depending on the individual patient, the severity of MG, and the treatment. MG patients who have a T4/T1 ratio less than 0.9 in the preanesthetic period show increased sensitivity to atracurium. Neuromuscular monitoring using train-of-four stimulation should begin in the preinduction period following administration of adequate analgesia (fentanyl, 2 μg/kg). Itoh et al.[120] found that patients with ocular MG were less sensitive to vecuronium than were those with generalized MG. They also found that in patients with clinical MG, sensitivity to vecuronium was unrelated to the presence or absence of antibodies to the AChR. Seronegative patients were as sensitive to vecuronium as seropositive patients. There are conflicting reports as to the sensitivity of patients with MG in remission. All such patients should be considered sensitive to nondepolarizers until proven otherwise.

Sugammadex is a novel cyclodextrin drug that is designed to bind rocuronium with a great affinity. Before the introduction of sugammadex, anticholinesterase drugs were the only options for antagonism of residual neuromuscular blockade, and in MG patients anticholinesterases must be administered with caution so as to avoid myasthenic or cholinergic crises. Sugammadex has been reported to provide very rapid, complete, and lasting recovery from deep levels of rocuronium-induced neuromuscular blockade in normal patients. Sugammadex has since been reported to safely reverse deep rocuronium-induced neuromuscular blockade within 210 seconds in a patient with MG. Sugammadex offers significant advantages in the management of the MG patient.[121]

Succinylcholine. Myasthenic patients are resistant to the neuromuscular blocking effects of succinylcholine. The ED_{95} is 2.6 times normal in these patients.[122] Clinically, however, the use of succinylcholine has been without incident, with the usual clinical doses producing adequate relaxation for endotracheal intubation and a normal recovery time, despite the occasionally reported early onset of phase II block. Doses of 0.2 to 1 mg/kg have been used in a number of patients with MG, and most did not show fasciculation before becoming paralyzed. Fade in response to train-of-four stimulation was observed in some patients during recovery, but recovery was not delayed. Prior administration of an anticholinesterase may complicate the response to succinylcholine by delaying its metabolism.

When a rapid-sequence intubation of the trachea is required, rapid onset of muscle relaxation may be achieved with succinylcholine or with moderate doses of a nondepolarizer in the latter case, with an associated prolongation of effect. A succinylcholine (1.5 mg/kg)–vecuronium (0.01 mg/kg) sequence has been safely used in three patients with MG for thymectomy. A combination technique of intubating dose rocuronium–sugammadex may replace succinylcholine for the MG patient who requires rapid-sequence induction.

Nonrelaxant Techniques. Because of concerns over the use of muscle relaxants in MG patients, there are many reports of successful use of nonrelaxant techniques. Della Rocca et al.[123] studied 68 consecutive MG patients undergoing transsternal thymectomy randomized to receive propofol/O_2/N_2O/fentanyl or sevoflurane/N_2O/O_2/fentanyl. All were tracheally extubated in the OR, and none required intubation for postoperative respiratory depression. Sevoflurane has been used as the sole anesthetic combined with intrathecal sufentanil–morphine for analgesia in an adult patient who underwent transsternal thymectomy. Propofol anesthesia combined with thoracic epidural anesthesia has been reported for thymectomy in MG. Another reported technique used propofol combined with epidural bupivacaine and sufentanil. The authors of those reports commented that the shift away from the use of muscle relaxants provided optimal operating condition and improved patient comfort.

Baraka et al.[124] described a 19-year-old myasthenic patient with a thymoma who received remifentanil and sevoflurane anesthesia for a 2-hour thymectomy. Although the trachea was extubated 10 minutes after discontinuation of remifentanil, the patient was unresponsive to verbal stimuli and remained somnolent for 12 hours. Because the patient had been receiving pyridostigmine for the months prior to surgery, they suggest that the delayed arousal may have been the result of possible inhibition by pyridostigmine of the nonspecific esterases that normally hydrolyze remifentanil.

Other Drug Interactions. Medications with neuromuscular blocking properties should be used with caution in patients with MG, particularly if relaxants are being used concurrently. Such drugs include antiarrhythmics (quinidine, procainamide, calcium channel blockers), diuretics (by causing hypokalemia), nitrogen mustards, quinine, and aminoglycoside antibiotics. Dantrolene has been used safely in a patient with MG.

Recovery from Anesthesia. Recovery from anesthesia must be carefully monitored in these patients. Extubation of the trachea should be performed when the patients are responsive and able to generate negative inspiratory pressures of greater than –20 cmH_2O. After extubation of the trachea, patients are carefully observed in the recovery area or the ICU. As soon as possible, patients should resume their usual pyridostigmine regimen. Cases of mild respiratory depression may be treatable with parenteral anticholinesterase; more severe cases may require reintubation of the trachea and mechanical ventilation of the lungs. In the immediate postoperative period, postthymectomy patients often show a marked improvement in their condition and a decreased need for anticholinesterase therapy.

Postoperative Respiratory Failure

Myasthenic patients are at increased risk for development of postoperative respiratory failure. There have been several attempts to predict before surgery which patients with MG will require prolonged postoperative ventilation of the lungs.[125] For patients who underwent transsternal thymectomy, positive predictors were a duration of MG more than 6 years, history of chronic respiratory disease other than that directly caused by MG, pyridostigmine dosage more than 750 mg/d, and a preoperative vital capacity less than 2.9 L. This predictive system was not found useful when applied in patients with MG undergoing transsternal thymectomy at other centers, and of no value in patients with MG undergoing other types of surgical procedures.[126] A study of 52 MG patients following thymectomy concluded that those patients who received more than 250 mg of pyridostigmine were at greater risk for respiratory failure requiring reintubation. A more recent scoring system to predict postoperative myasthenic crisis and need for ventilatory support has been proposed which cites as its chief risk factors advanced staging of the patient's MG (bulbar involvement and rapid progression conferring greater risk), BMI greater than 28, history of prior myasthenic crisis, duration of symptoms more than 2 years, and association with a pulmonary resection.[127] Each patient should therefore be treated on their own merits.

A study of patients undergoing transsternal thymectomy suggested that the need for postoperative mechanical ventilation correlated best with preoperative maximum static expiratory pressure. It was concluded that expiratory weakness, by reducing cough efficacy and ability to clear secretions, was the main predictive determinant. Adequate clearance of secretions is essential in these patients and may occasionally necessitate bronchoscopy.

In general, the postoperative morbidity in terms of respiratory failure is lower after transcervical rather than transsternal thymectomy. Techniques described that may be useful in reducing postoperative ventilatory failure include preoperative plasma exchange and high-dose perioperative steroid therapy. If the anticipated duration of the surgical procedure is 1 to 2 hours, preoperative oral anticholinesterase therapy may be of value because the peak effect of the drug coincides with the conclusion of the surgical procedure and attempts at tracheal extubation.

Postoperative Care

In the immediate postoperative period, pain relief for patients with MG is usually provided by opioid analgesics, such as meperidine, but in reduced doses. The analgesic effect of morphine and other opioid analgesics has been reported to be increased by anticholinesterases, which has led to the recommendation that the dose of opioid analgesics be reduced by one-third in patients receiving anticholinesterase therapy. Combined regional and general anesthesia techniques have also been used to provide good surgical conditions and improved postoperative analgesia in patients with MG undergoing thymectomy. Combined epidural–general anesthesia has been reported to provide excellent intraoperative and postoperative conditions for both surgeon and patient.

Myasthenic Syndrome (Eaton–Lambert Syndrome)

The myasthenic syndrome is a very rare immune-mediated disorder of neuromuscular transmission, associated with antibodies to the presynaptic voltage-gated calcium channel. The prevalence is estimated to be about 1/100,000. It is associated with small cell carcinoma of the lung in 50% to 60% of cases. Complaints of weakness may be mistaken for MG, but in Eaton–Lambert syndrome, symptoms do not respond to administration of anticholinesterases or steroids, and activity improves strength. The defect in this condition is prejunctional, is associated with diminished release of acetylcholine from nerve terminals, and improved by agents such as 4-aminopyridine,[128] guanidine, and germine that increase repetitive firing. Affected patients are particularly sensitive to the effects of all muscle relaxants, which should be used with great caution or avoided entirely. Other therapies have included immunosuppression, immune globulins, and plasmapheresis.

The possibility of Eaton–Lambert syndrome should be considered in all patients with known malignant disease and those patients undergoing diagnostic procedures for suspected carcinoma of the lung. Anesthesia considerations in these patients are essentially the same as in those with MG.[129]

Postoperative Management and Complications

Postoperative Pain Control

After extubation of the trachea, respiratory therapy and pain management become critical components of postoperative care. Adequate postoperative pain control is necessary to ensure a good respiratory effort. Administration of intravenous opioids has been the standard form of pain management for years. The administration of sufficient opioid to treat pain adequately may cause sedation and respiratory depression. Patient-controlled analgesia (PCA) has been reported to decrease the amount of postoperative pain, drug use, sedation, and pulmonary complications. PCA also eliminates the delays associated with personnel-administered medications and in general is very well accepted by patients. 11

There are other intravenous medications that can be used for pain management in addition to opioids. Low-dose ketamine infusion at 0.05 mg/kg/h was reported to be a useful adjunct to epidural analgesia for postthoracotomy pain management. Small doses of ketamine added to morphine for PCA administration have been shown to reduce the amount of morphine administered, improve respiratory parameters, and reduced the incidence of oxygen desaturation below 90% during the first three postoperative nights. Ketamine may provide an anti-inflammatory effect. Ketamine can also be administered via the epidural route to relieve postthoracotomy pain.

Gabapentin has been successful in reducing pain following thoracic surgery. Gabapentin may also reduce the incidence of postoperative delirium, and one approach could be to administer 900 mg 1 to 2 hours preoperatively. Gabapentin has been reported to be not effective in reducing the ipsilateral shoulder pain that may occur following thoracic surgery, but local injection of the periphrenic fat pad has been shown to reduce this pain.

Intercostal nerve blocks can decrease pain and improve postoperative respiratory function. The intercostal blocks can be performed internally or externally before or after surgery using a standard technique. However, the easiest method during thoracic surgery is to have the surgeon perform the blocks under direct vision from inside the thorax while the chest is open. Bupivacaine 0.25% to 0.5%, in doses of 2 to 5 mL, can be placed in the five intercostal spaces around the incision and in intercostal spaces where chest tubes will be placed. This provides 6 to 24 hours of moderate pain relief, but patients still complain of diaphragmatic and shoulder discomfort caused by the chest tubes. Larger volumes of local anesthetics should not be used in the intercostal space because of the high absorption rate and attendant systemic toxicity that can be produced, as well as the possibility of pushing the drug centrally and producing a paravertebral sympathetic or epidural block with central sympatholysis and severe hypotension. The intraoperative placement of catheters in intercostal grooves allows for a continuous postoperative intercostal nerve block. The technique reduces pain and improves pulmonary function. Placement of a catheter in the paravertebral space allows for blockade of multiple levels of intercostal nerves. This technique has been reported to provide good analgesia, and with fewer side effects than epidural analgesia. Paravertebral block may be as effective as epidural analgesia for pain relief following thoracic surgery, and is a good alternative. Another approach to postoperative pain control after thoracic surgery is the use of epidural or subarachnoid opioids. Epidural morphine produces profound analgesia lasting from 16 to 24 hours after thoracotomy and does not cause a sympathetic block or sensory or motor loss. These are significant advantages over systemic opioids or infiltration of local anesthetics. Epidural opioids are most effective at alleviating pain when administered at the thoracic level. Epidural morphine has been shown to decrease pain and improve respiratory function in postthoracotomy patients.

On the basis of a meta-analysis of 100 studies in the National Library of Medicine's PubMed database from 1966 to 2002, Block et al.[130] concluded that epidural analgesia was superior to parenteral medication; this was true regardless of agent used in the epidural catheter or the level of catheter placement. There may be a reduction in both morbidity and mortality with epidural or spinal analgesia. The technique most commonly employed in academic medical centers in the United States is an infusion of bupivacaine together with a narcotic such as fentanyl administered via a thoracic epidural catheter. Data in the pediatric population are limited; in one study of adolescent patients, the use of thoracic epidural analgesia provided better postoperative pain relief following minimally invasive pectus excavatum repair. Acetaminophen may be a useful adjunct to thoracic epidural analgesia for treatment of ipsilateral shoulder pain following thoracotomy. Ketorolac may be given postoperatively, but carries a risk of bleeding if given intraoperatively.

Subarachnoid (intrathecal) morphine, in a dose of 10 to 12 µg/kg, has been successfully used after thoracic surgery.[131] With this technique, the drug acts directly on the spinal cord, and analgesia can be produced with a smaller dose than by the epidural or intravenous routes. When morphine is given intrathecally before the induction of anesthesia, a decrease in the dose of anesthetic drugs required may occur. All patients who have received subarachnoid or epidural opioids must be closely observed for potential side effects, including delayed respiratory depression, urine retention, pruritus, nausea, and vomiting. These effects appear to be dose-related and may be reversed with naloxone. Despite over 30 years of usage, it is still not clear what dosage is optimal for this type of surgery.

Noxious stimuli, including surgical incision, may lead to changes in the central nervous system that exacerbate postoperative pain. The administration of analgesic agents before surgery is termed preemptive analgesia and may prevent these neuroplastic changes, thereby decreasing postoperative pain. This has more recently been termed preventive analgesia. In an early study of preemptive analgesia, the administration of lumbar epidural fentanyl before thoracotomy incision reduced postoperative pain scores and use of PCA morphine by a small but significant amount, compared with administration of lumbar epidural fentanyl after skin incision. On the basis of a meta-analysis of randomized controlled studies published between 1966 and 2004, Bong et al.[132] concluded that thoracic epidural preemptive analgesia did not provide a statistically significant reduction in postoperative pain, but was associated with a trend toward a reduction in the incidence of such pain. A subsequent study investigating the preemptive analgesic effect of infiltration of the surgical incisions with lidocaine prior to bilateral VATS incisions did help relieve pain for 24 hours, but not thereafter. In that study, since there was a bilateral incision, the infiltration was only done on one side, and each patient served as their own control.

Interpleural analgesia is another technique for postoperative pain treatment. The injection of local anesthetic between the pleural layers can block multiple intercostal nerves and/or pain fibers traveling with the thoracic sympathetic chain. The surgeon can place the catheter under direct vision while the chest is open. The chest tubes should not be suctioned for approximately 15 minutes after injection of local anesthetic to avoid loss of the anesthetic into the drainage. The surgeon can also place in the wound a soaker catheter, through which local anesthetics can be administered postoperatively. The On-Q PainBuster (I-Flow Corporation, Lake Forrest, CA) can be used for this purpose, and is an effective adjunct in alleviating pain following thoracic surgery. There may be chronic pain following thoracotomy, and also following VATS, even though the incisions are smaller with this approach.[133] In one report, women were more likely than men to suffer from both perioperative pain and chronic pain. If chronic postoperative pain occurs, it is important to treat it early and aggressively.

There is a high incidence of chronic pain following thoracotomy.[134] Approximately one-third of these have a neuropathic component. Chronic postthoracotomy pain has been reported to occur with an incidence of approximately 30% to 50%. Successful prevention and management of postthoracotomy chronic pain is hindered by an inadequate understanding of the pathophysiology. Thoracic epidural analgesia may reduce development of this chronic pain syndrome. Peripheral nerve stimulation may provide relief in some cases. Although ketamine reduces pain acutely, it does not have a long-term effect, either intravenously or by the epidural route. Although celecoxib has been shown to improve acute postoperative pain following thoracic surgery as an adjunct to epidural analgesia, there is no data on an impact on postthoracotomy pain syndrome. Once developed, postthoracotomy chronic pain is difficult to treat, as it is a form of neuropathic pain.

In recent years, the use of VATS has become more common, and is often the initial approach for thoracic surgery. Although there can be expected to be less pain and respiratory impairment following VATS compared with thoracotomy, it is still important to have a pain management strategy as there can be a significant amount of postoperative pain. Acute postoperative pain may be either myofascial or neuropathic in origin. These can cause neuroplastic changes, which may result in chronic pain. In one study, there was a 47% incidence of chronic pain reported following VATS. The incidence of chronic pain after VATS may be comparable with that following thoracotomy. The pain that occurs may be related to trauma to intercostal nerves by insertion of the surgical trocars or by compression during the surgery. In addition, an incision will be required to extract a lobe in the case of a lobectomy, which may exacerbate pain further.

If there is a relatively high likelihood of the surgeon converting the VATS to a thoracotomy, it may be preferable to place a thoracic epidural. If the preoperative lung function is poor, such that the patient may have difficulty breathing adequately postoperatively or may not tolerate systemic opioids, it also may be more prudent to place an epidural for that situation also. In contrast, for patients with good lung function who are scheduled to undergo a VATS in which a thoracotomy is unlikely, an epidural is probably unnecessary. The use of intercostal or paravertebral block combined with systemic opioids via PCA should be sufficient. In the United Kingdom, that approach has been reported to be more common for VATS lobectomy than the use of epidural analgesia.[135] In that survey, only 46% of patients undergoing VATS had a thoracic epidural placed. In contrast with an epidural, the paravertebral block is unilateral, and does not cause a sympathectomy. The administration of local anesthetic via the chest tubes is another approach which can successfully treat postoperative pain. In a recent update in which the literature was reviewed regarding pain management for VATS, it was concluded that an epidural is not necessary.[136] The use of a single shot, multilevel, paravertebral block has been recommended for VATS in a recent update on the use of paravertebral blocks for thoracic surgery. The placement of a paravertebral catheter for VATS was shown to be effective for postoperative pain management in a prospective randomized trial.

Complications Following Thoracic Surgery

Atelectasis

Patients who require thoracotomy often have pre-existing pulmonary disease that, when combined with the operative procedure, is likely to result in significant pulmonary dysfunction and possibly pneumonia. There is a reduction in respiratory complications with epidural analgesia including atelectasis and pneumonia. Atelectasis, the most significant cause of postoperative morbidity, has been reported to occur in up to 100% of patients undergoing thoracotomy for pulmonary resection. It occurs more commonly in the basal lobes than in the middle or upper lung regions. It may be secondary to reduction of normal respiratory effort due to splinting from pain, obesity, intrathoracic blood and fluid accumulation, and decreased compliance, all of which lead to rapid, shallow, constant V_T. Such a respiratory pattern produces small airway closure and obstruction with inspissated secretions, resulting ultimately in alveolar air resorption and terminal airway collapse. A poor cough and limited clearance of secretions add to the problem. Other sources of atelectasis include mucus plugging, which can obstruct a lobe or even an entire lung, and incomplete re-expansion of the remaining lung tissue after one-lung anesthesia.

The diagnosis of atelectasis can be made by clinical findings, chest radiography, or arterial blood gas analysis. This problem is best resolved by increasing resting lung volume or FRC. The latter can be increased by an increase in transpulmonary pressure (difference between airway pressure and interpleural pressure) or in lung compliance.

The tracheas of many patients can be extubated shortly after thoracic surgical procedures. These patients should be observed in the OR for at least 5 minutes following extubation, and many will require a high FiO_2 by face mask. Some patients with COPD undergoing extensive thoracic surgical procedures require postoperative ventilation to avoid atelectasis and other pulmonary complications. Mechanical ventilation increases airway pressure and, to a lesser extent, interpleural pressure; therefore, transpulmonary pressure increases.

The use of incentive spirometry and CPAP has been shown to reduce postoperative complications. Additional modalities that may be helpful in preventing atelectasis include bronchodilator treatment, coughing and clearance of secretions, chest physiotherapy, mobilizing the patient, and providing adequate analgesia. Atelectasis caused by collapse of lung tissue distal to a mucus plug can be treated by positioning the patient in the lateral decubitus position with the fully expanded lung in the dependent position. This improves matching and facilitates clearance of mucus from the nondependent obstructed lung. However, the patient should not be placed with the operative side in the dependent position after a pneumonectomy because of the risk of cardiac herniation.

The other major complications after thoracic surgery can be grouped into cardiovascular, pulmonary, and related problems.

Cardiovascular Complications

Cardiovascular complications are often the most difficult to manage in patients with associated respiratory insufficiency. The low cardiac output syndrome and postoperative cardiac dysrhythmias may be life-threatening. Invasive hemodynamic monitoring may be needed to assist in diagnosis and fluid management therapy. Other diagnostic modalities, such as echocardiography, may be required to rule out the presence of pericardial effusions or tamponade after opening the pericardium during certain types of thoracic surgical procedures. The low cardiac output syndrome must be differentiated from hypovolemia resulting from intrathoracic hemorrhage, tamponade, pulmonary emboli, or the effects of mechanical ventilation with PEEP. Postoperative fluid administration can lead to pulmonary edema resulting from the resection of lung tissue and the concomitant reduction of the pulmonary vascular bed. Re-expansion of a chronically collapsed lung may in some cases lead to re-expansion pulmonary edema (RPE); rapid re-expansion and drainage of large amounts of pleural fluid increase the risk for RPE.[137] A postoperative pulmonary embolism can originate from the remaining PA stump. Therapeutic interventions for postoperative myocardial dysfunction include inotropic drugs, vasodilators, and combinations of these drugs, as needed, to improve ventricular function. The goal is to shift the Starling function curve up and to the left by reducing preload of either the left or right side of the heart and increasing cardiac output. Vasodilators are very effective at decreasing right ventricular afterload and improving right ventricular function because this side of the heart is especially afterload-dependent. Combinations of inotropes and vasodilators, such as dopamine and nitroglycerin, or combined drugs, such as milrinone, can be especially useful in the treatment of right-sided heart failure.

Postoperative cardiac dysrhythmias are common after thoracic surgery. Patients following pulmonary resection have postoperative supraventricular tachycardias with a frequency and severity proportional to both their age and the magnitude of the surgical procedure. Many factors contribute to these dysrhythmias, including underlying cardiac disease, degree of surgical trauma, intraoperative cardiac manipulation, stimulation of the sympathetic nervous system by pain, a reduced pulmonary vascular bed, effects of anesthetics and cardioactive drugs, and metabolic abnormalities.

In a series of 300 thoracotomies for lung resection, atrial fibrillation occurred in 20% of patients with malignant disease but in only 3% with benign disease. A similar incidence of dysrhythmias is observed after pneumonectomies. Multifocal atrial tachycardia often occurs in patients with COPD and concomitant right-sided cardiac dysfunction. The right side of the heart may be further strained by the reduction in the size of the pulmonary vasculature from the lung resection, especially after right pneumonectomy.

The prophylactic use of digitalis in thoracic surgical patients is controversial, particularly in patients with signs of congestive heart failure. Arguments against its use include the potential toxic effects of the drug and the difficulty in assessing adequacy of digitalization in the absence of heart failure. A prospective, placebo-controlled, randomized study demonstrated no advantage to prophylactic digitalization of patients undergoing thoracic surgery. Part of the argument for its use is the drug's efficacy in reducing the incidence of potentially fatal complications in older patients. In some studies, it has been reported to reduce the incidence of perioperative dysrhythmias. If digitalis therapy is to be instituted, normokalemia should be ensured to reduce the likelihood of digitalis toxicity.

More recently, newer drugs have replaced digitalis for dysrhythmia control. Supraventricular tachycardias can be treated with other agents such as β-blockers or calcium channel–blocking drugs, after ruling out underlying reversible physiologic abnormalities, such as hypoxia.[138] Amiodarone has been reported to be effective in restoring and maintaining sinus rhythm. Verapamil has been the standard treatment for these problems until the introduction of the ultrashort-acting β-blocker, esmolol. Esmolol, in an intravenous loading dose of 500 μg/kg given over 1 minute followed by an infusion of 50 to 200 μg/kg/min, has been shown to be effective in the control of supraventricular tachycardias. Esmolol has been shown to be equally effective in controlling the ventricular rate in patients with postoperative atrial fibrillation or flutter and in increasing the conversion rate to regular sinus rhythm from 8% to 34%. Owing to its short duration of action (β elimination half-life of 9 minutes) and β_1-cardioselectivity, it is the drug of choice in the postoperative period to control these dysrhythmias.

Bleeding and Respiratory Complications

Hemorrhage and pneumothorax are always major concerns after intrathoracic surgery. Although there is less pain following VATS compared with thoracotomy, the risk of bleeding and intraoperative complications may be higher. Because of these problems, interpleural thoracostomy tubes with an underwater seal system are routinely used after thoracic surgery. Slippage of a suture on any major vessel or airway in the chest can lead to the slow or rapid development of hypovolemic shock or a tension pneumothorax. Drainage of more than 200 mL/h of blood is an indication for surgical re-exploration for hemorrhage. Management of the pleural drainage system is fraught with confusion. The chest bottles must be kept below the level of the chest, and the tubes should not be clamped during patient transport. These tubes can be lifesaving, but errors in technique can lead to serious complications. The creation of a pneumothorax in the nonoperative chest by central venous catheter placement is very hazardous because this lung is essential both intraoperatively during one-lung anesthesia and postoperatively after contralateral lung resection. Dehiscence of the bronchial stump may lead to the formation of a BPF, which carries a mortality rate of 20%. Surgical treatment may be needed, in which case ventilation of the patient's lungs may be difficult because of loss of V_T through the fistula. A double-lumen endobronchial tube positioned in the contralateral main stem bronchus or the use of HFJV may be required for safe management. HFJV allows ventilation with lowered peak airway pressures. However, there have been reports in which ventilation by HFJV was difficult. If a double-lumen endobronchial tube is placed, the lung with the fistula can be ventilated independently with either CPAP or HFJV.

Neurologic Complications

Central and peripheral neurologic injuries can occur during intrathoracic procedures. Such injuries often result in serious and disabling loss of function. Peripheral nerves can also be injured, either in the chest or in other parts of the body, by pressure or stretching. The nerve injury may be apparent immediately after surgery or may not become obvious until several days later. These patients often complain of a variety of unpleasant sensations, including paresthesias, cold, pain, or anesthesia in the area supplied by the affected nerves. The brachial plexus is especially vulnerable to trauma during thoracic surgery, owing to its long superficial course in the axilla between two points of fixation, the vertebrae above, and the axillary fascia below. Stretching may be the primary cause of damage to the brachial plexus, with compression playing only a secondary role. Branches of the brachial plexus may also be injured lower in the arm by compression against objects such as an ether screen or other parts of the operating table. Intrathoracic nerves can be directly injured during a surgical procedure by being transected, crushed, stretched, or cauterized. The recurrent laryngeal nerve can become involved in lymph node tissue and injured at the time of a node biopsy, especially when the biopsy is performed through a mediastinoscope. This nerve can also be injured during tracheostomy or radical pulmonary dissections. The phrenic nerve may be injured during pericardiectomy, radical pulmonary hilar dissections, division of the diaphragm during esophageal surgery, or dissection of mediastinal tumors.

Prevention is the treatment of choice for these intraoperative nerve injuries. Analgesics may be necessary to control postoperative pain in the distribution of the nerve injury and to aid in maintaining joint mobility during the healing phase.

For additional information please see NICVs 38-3 and 38-4 in the eBook bundled with this text.

For further review and interactivities, please see the videos and narrative interactive clinical vignettes (NICVs) accessible in the complimentary eBook bundled with this text. Access instructions are located on the inside front cover.

REFERENCES

1. Cancer: fact sheet no. 297. World Health Organization website. Updated February 2015; accessed January 10, 2016. http://www.who.int/mediacentre/factsheets/fs297/en/
2. American Cancer Society. What are the key statistics about lung cancer. Last accessed July 10, 2022. http://www.cancer.org/cancer/lungcancer-non-smallcell/detailedguide/non-small-cell-lung-cancer-key-statistics
3. Gupta S, Fernandes RJ, Rao JS, Dhanpal R. Perioperative risk factors for pulmonary complications after non-cardiac surgery. *J Anaesthesiol Clin Pharmacol*. 2020;36:88–93.
4. Centers for Disease Control and Prevention. What are the risk factors for lung cancer? Centers for Disease Control Website. Accessed January 10, 2016. http://www.cdc.gov/cancer/lung/basic_info/risk_factors.htm
5. Matsuoka K, Yamada T, Matsuoka T, Nagai S, Ueda M, Miyamoto Y. Preoperative smoking cessation period is not related to postoperative respiratory complications in patients undergoing lung cancer surgery. *Ann Thorac Cardiovasc Surg*. 2019;25:304–310.
6. Vogelmeier CF, Criner GJ, Martinez FJ, et al. Global strategy for the diagnosis, management, and prevention of chronic obstructive lung disease 2017 report. *Am J Respir Crit Care Med*. 2017;195:557–582.
7. Yao S, Mao T, Fang W, Xu M, Chen W. Incidence and risk factors for acute lung injury after open thoracotomy for thoracic diseases. *J Thorac Dis*. 2013;5:455–460.
8. Amar D, Munoz D, Shi W, Zhang H, Thaler HT. A clinical prediction rule for pulmonary complications after thoracic surgery for primary lung cancer. *Anesth Analg*. 2010;110:1343–1348.
9. Ferguson MK, Vigneswaran WT. Diffusing capacity predicts morbidity after lung resection in patients without chronic obstructive pulmonary disease. *Ann Thorac Surg*. 2008;85: 1158–1165.
10. Zhang R, Lee SM, Wigfield C, Vigneswaran WT, Ferguson MK. Lung function predicts pulmonary complication regardless of the surgical approach. *Ann Thorac Surg*. 2015;99:1761–1767.
11. Brunelli A, Kim AW, Berger KI, Addrizzo-Harris DJ. Physiologic evaluation of the patient with lung cancer being considered for resectional surgery: diagnosis and management of lung cancer 3rd edition. American College of Chest Physicians evidence-based clinical practice guidelines. *Chest*. 2013:143.
12. Brunelli A, Al Refai M, Monteverde M, Borri A, Salati M, Fianchini A. Stair climbing test predicts cardiopulmonary complications after lung resection. *Chest*. 2002;121:1106–1110.
13. Bernasconi M, Koegelenberg CFN, von Groote-Bidingmaier F, et al. Speed of ascent during stair climbing identifies operable lung resection candidates. *Respiration*. 2012;84:117–122.
14. Spyratos D, Zarogoulidis P, Porpodis K. Preoperative evaluation for lung cancer resection. *J Thorac Dis*. 2014;6:S162–S166.
15. Brueckmann B, Villa-Uribe JL, Bateman BT, et al. Development and validation of a score for prediction of postoperative respiratory complications. *Anesthesiology*. 2013;118:1276–1285.
16. Batchelor TJP, Rasburn NJ, Abdelnour-Berchtold E, et al. Guidelines for enhanced recovery after lung surgery: recommendations of the Enhanced Recovery After Surgery (ERAS®) Society and the European Society of Thoracic Surgeons (ESTS). *Eur J Cardiovasc Surg*. 2019; 55:91–115.
17. Myers K, Hajek P, Hinds C, McRobbie H. Stopping smoking shortly before surgery and postoperative complications: a systematic review and meta-analysis. *Arch Intern Med*. 2011;171: 983–989.
18. Lugg ST, Tikka T, Agostini PJ, et al. Smoking and timing of cessation on postoperative pulmonary complications after curativeintent lung cancer surgery. *J Cardiothorac Surg*. 2017;12:52.
19. Lumb AB. Pre-operative respiratory optimisation: an expert review. *Anaesthesia*. 2019;74: 43–48.
20. Vigano A, Kasvis P, Di Tomasso J, Gillis C, Kilgour R, Carli F. Pearls of optimizing nutrition and physical performance of older adults undergoing cancer therapy. *J Geriatr Oncol*. 2017;8: 428–436.
21. Gillis C, Wischmeyer PE. Pre-operative nutrition and the elective surgical patient: why, how and what? *Anaesthesia*. 2019;74:27–35.
22. Wischmeyer PE, Carli F, Evans DC, et al. American Society for Enhanced Recovery and Perioperative Quality Initiative joint consensus statement on nutrition screening and therapy within a surgical enhanced recovery pathway. *Anesth Analg*. 2018;126:1883–1895.

23. Sekine Y, Chiyo M, Iwata T, et al. Perioperative rehabilitation and physiotherapy for lung cancer patients with chronic obstructive pulmonary disease. *Jpn J Thorac Cardiovasc Surg.* 2005;53:237–243.
24. Levy N, Grocott MPW, Carli F. Patient optimisation before surgery: a clear and present challenge in peri-operative care. *Anaesthesia.* 2019;74:3–6.
25. Cannesson M, Le Manach YL, Hofer CK, et al. Assessing the diagnostic accuracy of pulse pressure variations for the prediction of fluid responsiveness. *Anesthesiology.* 2011;115:231–241.
26. Koji A. Mean pulmonary artery pressure under thoracotomy as an indicator of safety for lung resection. *J Jpn Assoc Chest Surg.* 2001;15:561.
27. Thys DM, Cohen E, Eisenkraft JB. Mixed venous oxygen saturation during thoracic anesthesia. *Anesthesiology.* 1988;69:1005–1009.
28. Pothoft G, Curtius JM, Wassermann K, et al. Transesophageal echography in staging of bronchial cancers. *Pneumologie.* 1992;446:111–117.
29. Neustein SM, Cohen E, Reich DL, Kirschner P. Transesophageal echocardiography and the intraoperative diagnosis of left atrial invasion by carcinoid tumor. *Can J Anaesth.* 1993;40: 664–666.
30. Kazan R, Bracco D, Hemmerling TM. Reduced cerebral oxygen saturation measured by absolute cerebral oximetry during thoracic surgery correlates with postoperative complications. *Br J Anaesth.* 2009;103:811–816.
31. Peyton PJ, Chong SW. Minimally invasive measurement of cardiac output during surgery and critical care: a meta-analysis of accuracy and precision. *Anesthesiology.* 2010;113:1220–1235.
32. Barker SJ. Pulse oximetry. Chapter 11. In: Ehrenwerth J, Eisenkraft JB, Berry JM, eds. *Anesthesia Equipment: Principles and Applications.* 3rd ed. Elsevier; 2021:253–270.
33. Gravenstein N, Jaffe MB. Capnography. Chapter 10. In: Ehrenwerth J, Eisenkraft JB, Berry JM, eds. *Anesthesia Equipment: Principles and Applications.* 3rd ed. Elsevier; 2021:239–252.
34. Benumof JL. Isoflurane anesthesia and arterial oxygenation during one-lung ventilation. *Anesthesiology.* 1986;64:419–422.
35. Cohen E. Current practice issues in thoracic anesthesia. *Anesth Analg.* 2021;133(6):1520–1531.
36. Langiano N, Fiorelli S, Deana C, et al. Airway management in anesthesia for thoracic surgery: a "real life" observational study. *J Thorac Dis.* 2019;11:3257–3269.
37. Lohser J, Brodsky JB. Silbronco double-lumen tube. *J Cardiothorac Vasc Anesth.* 2006;20: 129–131.
38. Koopman EM, Barak M, Weber E, et al. Evaluation of a new double-lumen endobronchial tube with an integrated camera (VivaSight-DL™): a prospective multicentre observational study. *Anaesthesia.* 2015;70:962–968.
39. Larsen S, Holm JH, Sauer TN, Andersen C. A cost effectiveness analysis comparing the VivaSight double lumen tube and a conventional double-lumen tube in adult patients undergoing thoracic surgery involving one-lung ventilation. *Pharmacoecon Open.* 2020;4:159–169.
40. Roldi E, Inghileri P, Dransart-Raye O, et al. Use of tracheal ultrasound combined with clinical parameters to select left double-lumen tube size: a prospective observational study. *Eur J Anaesthesiol.* 2019;36:215–220.
41. Parab SY, Kumar P, Divatia JV, Sharma K. A prospective randomised controlled double blind study comparing auscultation and lung ultrasonography in the assessment of double lumen tube position in elective thoracic surgeries involving one lung ventilation at a tertiary care cancer institute. *Korean J Anesthesiol.* 2019;72:24–31.
42. Smith G, Hirsch N, Ehrenwerth J. Sight and sound: Can double-lumen endotracheal tubes be placed accurately without fiberoptic bronchoscopy? *Br J Anaesth.* 1987;58:1317.
43. Cohen E, Neustein SM, Goldofsky S, Camunas JL. Incidence of malposition of PVC and red rubber left-sided double lumen tubes and clinical sequelae. *J Cardiothorac Vasc Anesth.* 1995; 9:122–127.
44. Benumof JL, Partridge BL, Salvatierra C, Keating J. Margin of safety in positioning modern double-lumen endotracheal tubes. *Anesthesiology.* 1987;67:729–738.
45. Pompeo E, Mineo D, Rogliani P, Sabato AF, Mineo TC. Feasibility and results of awake thoracoscopic resection of solitary pulmonary nodules. *Ann Thorac Surg.* 2004;78:1761–1768.
46. Knoll H, Ziegeler S, Schreiber JU, et al. Airway injuries after one-lung ventilation: a comparison between double-lumen tube and endobronchial blocker: a randomized, prospective, controlled trial. *Anesthesiology.* 2006;105:471–477.
47. Clayton-Smith A, Bennett K, Alston RP, et al. A comparison of the efficacy and adverse effects of double-lumen endobronchial tubes and bronchial blockers in thoracic surgery: a systematic review and meta-analysis of randomized controlled trials. *J Cardiothorac Vasc Anesth.* 2015; 29:955–966.
48. Saito T, Naruke T, Carney E, Yokokawa Y, Hiraga K, Carlsson C. New double-lumen intrabronchial tube (Naruke tube) for tracheostomized patients. *Anesthesiology.* 1998;89:1038–1039.
49. Campos JH, Musselman ED, Hanada S, Ueda K. Lung isolation techniques in patients with early-stage or long-term tracheostomy: a case series report of 70 cases and recommendations. *J Cardiothorac Vasc Anesth.* 2019;33(2):433–439.
50. Cohen E, Benumof JL. Lung separation in the patient with a difficult airway. *Curr Opin Anesthesiol.* 1999;12:29–35.
51. Cohen E. The Cohen flexitip endobronchial blocker: an alternative to a double lumen tube. *Anesth Analg.* 2005;101:1877–1879.
52. Mourisse J, Liesveld J, Verhagen A, et al. Efficiency, efficacy, and safety of EZ-blocker compared with left-sided double-lumen tube for one-lung ventilation. *Anesthesiology.* 2013;118:550–561.
53. Narayanaswamy M, McRae K, Slinger P, et al. Choosing a lung isolation device for thoracic surgery: a randomized trial of three bronchial blockers versus double-lumen tubes. *Anesth Analg.* 2009;108:1097–1101.
54. Cohen E. Strategies in lung isolation: to block or not to block? *Can J Anaesth.* 2016;63: 797–801.
55. Campos JH. Which device should be considered the best for lung isolation: double-lumen endotracheal tube versus bronchial blockers. *Curr Opin Anaesthesiol.* 2007;20:27–31.
56. Ko R, McRae K, Darling G, et al. The use of air in the inspired gas mixture during two-lung ventilation delays lung collapse during one-lung ventilation. *Anesth Analg.* 2009;108:1092–1096.
57. Malmkvist G. Maintenance of oxygenation during one-lung ventilation: effect of intermittent reinflation of the collapsed lung with oxygen. *Anesth Analg.* 1989;68:763–766.
58. Karzai W, Schwarzkopf K. Hypoxemia during OLV: prediction, prevention and treatment. *Anesthesiology.* 2009;110:1402–1411.
59. Güldner A, Kiss T, Serpa Neto A et al, Intraoperative protective mechanical ventilation for prevention of postoperative pulmonary complications: A comprehensive review of the role of tidal volume, positive end-expiratory pressure, and lung recruitment maneuvers. *Anesthesiology.* 2015;123:692–713.
60. Brower RG, Matthay MA, Morris A, Schoenfeld D, Thompson BT, Wheeler A; The Acute Respiratory Distress Syndrome Network. Ventilation with lower tidal volumes as compared with traditional tidal volumes for acute lung injury and the acute respiratory distress syndrome. *N Engl J Med.* 2000;342:1301–1308.
61. Ball L, Robba C, de Abreu MG, Pelosi P. Lung protection during one-lung ventilation: another piece in the puzzle. *Eur J Anaesthesiol.* 2018;35:724–726.
62. Gattinoni L, Pesenti A. The concept of "baby lung." *Intensive Care Med.* 2005;31:776–784.
63. Blank RS, Colquhoun DA, Durieux ME, et al. Management of one-lung ventilation: impact of tidal volume on complications after thoracic surgery. *Anesthesiology.* 2016;124:1286–1295.
64. Lohser J, Slinger P. Lung injury after one-lung ventilation: a review of the pathophysiologic mechanisms affecting the ventilated and the collapsed lung. *Anesth Analg.* 2015;121: 302–318.
65. Roth JV. Complications of one-lung ventilation: is it the blood flow or the ventilation? *Anesthesiology.* 2016;125:1246–1254.
66. Slinger PD, Kruger M, McRae K, Winton T. Relation of the static compliance curve and positive end-expiratory pressure to oxygenation during one-lung ventilation. *Anesthesiology.* 2001;95:1096–1102.
67. Pereira SM, Tucci MR, Tonelotto BFF, et al. Individual positive end expiratory pressure settings optimize intraoperative mechanical ventilation and reduce postoperative atelectasis. *Anesthesiology.* 2018;129:1070–1081.
68. Liu K, Huang C, Xu M, et al. PEEP guided by electrical impedance tomography during one-lung ventilation in elderly patients undergoing thoracoscopic surgery. *Ann Transl Med.* 2019;7:757.
69. Ferrando C, Mugarra A, Gutierrez A, et al. Setting individualized positive end-expiratory pressure level with a positive end-expiratory pressure decrement trial after a recruitment maneuver improves oxygenation and lung mechanics during one-lung ventilation. *Anesth Analg.* 2014;118:657–665.
70. Arnal J-M, Paquet J, Wysocki M, et al. Optimal duration of a sustained inflation recruitment maneuver in ARDS patients. *Intensive Care Med.* 2011;37:1588–1594.
71. Marini JJ. Recruitment by sustained inflation: time for a change. *Intensive Care Med.* 2011;37:1572–1574.
72. Bugedo G, Retamal J, Bruhn A. Driving pressure: a marker of severity, a safety limit, or a goal for mechanical ventilation?. *Crit Care.* 2017;21:199.
73. Amato MBP, Meade MO, Slutsky AS et al. Driving pressure and survival in the acute respiratory distress syndrome. *N Engl J Med.* 2015;372:747–755.
74. Park M, Ahn HJ, Kim JA, et al. Driving pressure during thoracic surgery: a randomized clinical trial. *Anesthesiology.* 2019;130:385–393.
75. Serpa Neto A, Deliberato RO, Johnson AEW, et al; PROVE Network Investigators. Mechanical power of ventilation is associated with mortality in critically ill patients: an analysis of patients in two observational cohorts. *Intensive Care Med.* 2018;44:1914–1922.
76. Chiumello D. Paolo Formenti P, Bolgiaghi L, et al. Body position alters mechanical power and respiratory mechanics during thoracic surgery. *Anesth Analg.* 2020;130:399–401.
77. Sugasawa Y, Yamaguchi K, Kumakura S, et al. The effect of one-lung ventilation upon pulmonary inflammatory responses during lung resection. *J Anesth.* 2011;25:170–177.
78. Gao W, Liu DD, Li D, Cui GX. Effect of therapeutic hypercapnia on inflammatory responses to one-lung ventilation in lobectomy patients. *Anesthesiology.* 2015;122:1235–1252.
79. Rivers EP. Fluid-management strategies in acute lung injury: liberal, conservative, or both? *N Engl J Med.* 2006;354(24):2598–2600.
80. Yang M, Ahn HJ, Kim K, et al. Does a protective ventilation strategy reduce the risk of pulmonary complications after lung cancer surgery? A randomized controlled trial. *Chest.* 2011;139:530–537.
81. Sçentürk M, Slinger P, Cohen E. Intraoperative mechanical ventilation strategies for one-lung ventilation. *Best Pract Res Clin Anaesthesiol.* 2015;29:357–369.
82. Walsh SP, Shaz D, Amar D. Ventilation during lung resection and critical care:comparative clinical outcomes. *Anesthesiology.* 2022;137:473–483.

83. Kozian A, Schilling T, Fredén F, et al. One-lung ventilation induces hyperperfusion and alveolar damage in the ventilated lung: an experimental study. *Br J Anaesth*. 2008;100:549–559.
84. De Conno E, Steurer MP, Wittlinger M, et al. Anesthetic-induced improvement of the inflammatory response to one-lung ventilation. *Anesthesiology*. 2009;110:1316–1326.
85. Schilling T, Kozian A, Senturk M, et al. Effects of volatile and intravenous anesthesia on the alveolar and systemic inflammatory response in thoracicsurgical patients. *Anesthesiology*. 2011;115:65–74.
86. Beck-Schimmer B, Bonvini JM, Braun J, et al. Which anesthesia regimen is best to reduce morbidity and mortality in lung surgery? A multicenter randomized controlled trial. *Anesthesiology*. 2016;125:313–321.
87. Collins SR, Blank RS, Deatherage LS, Dull RO. The endothelial glycocalyx: emerging concepts in pulmonary edema and acute lung injury. *Anesth Analg*. 2013;117:664–674.
88. Englert JA, Macias AA, Amador-Munoz D, et al. Isoflurane ameliorates acute lung injury by preserving epithelial tight junction integrity. *Anesthesiology*. 2015;123:377–388.
89. Pompeo E. Pathophysiology of surgical pneumothorax in the awake patient. In: Pompeo E. ed. *Awake Thoracic Surgery (Ebook)*. Bentham Science Publishers; 2012:9–18.
90. Zhang K, Chen HG, Wu WB, et al. Non-intubated video-assisted thoracoscopic surgery vs. intubated video-assisted thoracoscopic surgery for thoracic disease: a systematic review and meta-analysis of 1,684 cases. *J Thorac Dis*. 2019;11:3556–3568.
91. Zirafa CC, Romano G, Key TH, Davini F, Melfi F. The evolution of robotic thoracic surgery. *Ann Cardiothorac Surg*. 2019;8:210–217.
92. Heller JA, Bhora FY, Heller BJ, Cohen E. Robotic-assisted thoracoscopic lung surgery: anesthetic impact and perioperative experience. *Minerva Anestesiol*. 2018;84:108–114.
93. Pathak V, Welsby I, Mahmood K, Wahidi M, MacIntyre N, Shofer S. Ventilation and anesthetic approaches for rigid bronchoscopy. *Ann Am Thorac Soc*. 2014;11:628–634.
94. Frumin MJ, Epstein RM, Cohen G. Apneic oxygenation in man. *Anesthesiology*. 1959;20:789–798.
95. Matsushima Y, Jones RL, King EG, Moysa G, Alton JD. Alterations in pulmonary mechanics and gas exchange during routine fiberoptic bronchoscopy. *Chest*. 1984;86:184–188.
96. Satyanarayana T, Capan L, Ramanathan S, Chalon J, Turndorf H. Bronchofiberscopic jet ventilation. *Anesth Analg*. 1980;59:350–354.
97. Neuman GG, Weingarten AE, Abramowitz RM, Kushins LG, Abramson AL, Ladner W. The anesthetic management of the patient with an anterior mediastinal mass. *Anesthesiology*. 1984;60:144–147.
98. Béchard P, Létourneau L, Lacasse Y, Côté D, Bussières JS. Perioperative cardiorespiratory complications in adults with mediastinal mass: incidence and risk factors. *Anesthesiology*. 2004;100:826–834.
99. Hnatiuk OW, Corcoran PC, Sierra A. Spirometry in surgery for anterior mediastinal masses. *Chest*. 2001;120:1152–1156.
100. Tempe DK, Arya R, Dubey S, et al. Mediastinal mass resection: femorofemoral cardiopulmonary bypass before induction of anesthesia in the management of airway obstruction. *J Cardiothorac Vasc Anesth*. 2001;15:233–236.
101. Ferrari LR, Bedford RF. General anesthesia prior to treatment of anterior mediastinal masses in pediatric cancer patients. *Anesthesiology*. 1990;72:991–995.
102. Gardner JC, Royster RL. Airway collapse with an anterior mediastinal mass despite spontaneous ventilation in an adult. *Anesth Analg*. 2011;113:239–242.
103. Slinger PD, Karsli C. Management of a patient with a large anterior mediastinal mass: recurring myths. *Curr Opin Anaesthesiol*. 2007;20:1–3.
104. Lohser J. Managing hypoxemia during minimally invasive thoracic surgery. *Anesthesiol Clin*. 2012;30:683–697.
105. Courey AJ, Hyzy RC. High frequency ventilation in adults. UpToDate website. Updated May 2015. http://www.uptodate.com/contents/high-frequency-ventilation-in-adults
106. Benumof JL. Sequential one-lung ventilation for bilateral bullectomy. *Anesthesiology*. 1987;67:268–272.
107. Cohen E, Eisenkraft JB. Bronchopulmonary lavage: effects on oxygenation and hemodynamics. *J Cardiothorac Anesth*. 1990;4:609–615.
108. McGrogan A, Sneddon S, de Vries CS. The incidence of myasthenia gravis: a systematic literature review. *Neuroepidemiology*. 2010;34:171–183.
109. Osserman KE, Genkins G. Studies in myasthenia gravis: review of a twenty-year experience in over 1200 patients. *Mt Sinai J Med*. 1971;38:497–537.
110. McConville J, Farrugia ME, Beeson D, et al. Detection and characterization of MuSK antibodies in seronegative myasthenia gravis. *Ann Neurol*. 2004;55:580–584.
111. Mehndiratta MM, Pandey S, Kuntzer T. Acetylcholinesterase inhibitor treatment for myasthenia gravis. *Cochrane Database Syst Rev*. 2011;16:CD006986.
112. Cata JP, Lasala JD, WilliamsW, Mena GE. Myasthenia gravis and thymoma surgery: a clinical update for the cardiothoracic anaesthesiologist. *J Cardiovasc Thoracic Anesth*. 2019;33:2537–2545.
113. Maurizi G, D'Andrilli A, Sommella L, Venuta F, Rendina EA. Transsternal thymectomy. *Thorac Cardiovasc Surg*. 2015;63(3):178–186.
114. Blichfeldt-Lauridsen L, Hansen BD. Anesthesia and myasthenia gravis. *Acta Anaesthesiol Scand*. 2012;56:17–22.
115. Gilhus NE, Nacu A, Andersen JB, Owe JF. Myasthenia gravis and risks for comorbidity. *Eur J Neurol*. 2015;22:17–23.
116. Tripathi M, Kaushik S, Dubey P. The effect of use of pyridostigmine and requirement for vecuronium with myasthenia gravis. *J Postgrad Med*. 2003;49:311–314.
117. Nilsson E, Muller K. Neuromuscular effects of isoflurane in patients with myasthenia gravis. *Acta Anaesthesiol Scand*. 1990;34:126–131.
118. Nitahara K, Sugi Y, Higa K, Shono S, Hamada T. Neuromuscular effects of sevoflurane in myasthenia gravis patients. *Br J Anaesth*. 2007;98:337–341.
119. Eisenkraft JB, Book WJ, Papatestas AE. Sensitivity to vecuronium in myasthenia gravis: a dose-response study. *Can J Anaesth*. 1990;37:301–306.
120. Itoh H, Shibata K, Nitta S. Difference in sensitivity to vecuronium between patients with ocular and generalized myasthenia gravis. *Br J Anaesth*. 2001;87:885–889.
121. de Boer HD, Shields MO, Booij LHDJ. Reversal of neuromuscular blockade with sugammadex in patients with myasthenia gravis: A case series of 21 patients and review of the literature. *Eur J Anaesthesiol*. 2014;31:715–721.
122. Eisenkraft JB, Book WJ, Mann SM, Papatestas AE, Hubbard M. Resistance to succinylcholine in myasthenia gravis: a dose-response study. *Anesthesiology*. 1988;69:760–763.
123. Della Rocca G, Coccia C, Diana L, et al. Propofol or sevoflurane anesthesia without muscle relaxants allow the early extubation of myasthenic patients. *Can J Anaesth*. 2003;50:547–552.
124. Baraka AS, Haroun-Bizri ST, Georges FJ. Delayed postoperative arousal following remifentanil-based anesthesia in a myasthenic patient undergoing thymectomy. *Anesthesiology*. 2004;100:460–461.
125. Eisenkraft JB, Papatestas AE, Kahn CH, Mora CT, Fagerstrom R, Genkins G. Predicting the need for postoperative mechanical ventilation in myasthenia gravis. *Anesthesiology*. 1986;65:79–82.
126. Grant RP, Jenkins LC. Prediction of the need for postoperative mechanical ventilation in myasthenia gravis: thymectomy compared to other surgical procedures. *Can Anaesth Soc J*. 1982;29:112–116.
127. Leuzzi G, Meacci E, Cusumano G, et al. Thymectomy in myasthenia gravis: proposal for a predictive score of postoperative myasthenic crisis. *Eur J Cardiothorac Surg*. 2014;45:e76–e88.
128. Keogh M, Sedehizadeh S, Maddison P. Treatment for Lambert-Eaton myasthenic syndrome. *Cochrane Database Syst Rev*. 2011:CD003279.
129. Weingarten TN, Araka CN, Mogensen ME, et al. Lambert-Eaton myasthenic syndrome during anesthesia: a report of 37 patients. *J Clin Anesth*. 2014;28:648–653.
130. Block BM, Liu SS, Rowlingson BA, Cowan AR, Cowan JA Jr, Wu CL. Efficacy of postoperative epidural analgesia: a meta-analysis. *JAMA*. 2003;290:2455–2463.
131. Askar FZ, Kocabas S, Yucel S, Samancilar O, Cetin H, Uyar M. The efficacy of intrathecal morphine in post-thoracotomy pain management. *J Int Med Res*. 2007;35:314–322.
132. Bong CL, Samuel M, Ng JM, Ip-Yam C. Effects of preemptive epidural analgesia on post-thoracotomy pain. *J Cardiothorac Vasc Anesth*. 2005;19:786–793.
133. Gotoda Y, Kambara N, Sakai T, Kishi Y, Kodama K, Koyama T. The morbidity, time course and predictive factors for persistent post-thoracotomy pain. *Eur J Pain*. 2001;5:89–96.
134. Wildgaard K, Ravn J, Kehlet H. Chronic post-thoracotomy pain: a critical review of pathogenic mechanisms and strategies for prevention. *Eur J Cardiothorac Surg*. 2009;36:170–180.
135. Kotemane NC, Gapinath N, Vaja R. Analgesic techniques following thoracic surgery: a survey of United Kingdom practice. *Eur J Anaesthesiol*. 2010;27:897–899.
136. Kaplowitz J, Papadakos PJ. Acute pain management for video-assisted thoracoscopic surgery: an update. *J Cardiothorac Vasc Anesth*. 2012;26(2):312–321.
137. Neustein SM. Reexpansion pulmonary edema. *J Cardiothorac Vasc Anesth*. 2007;21:887–891.
138. Ciriaco P, Mazzone P, Canneto B, Zannini P. Supraventricular arrhythmia following lung resection for non-small-cell lung cancer and its treatment with amiodarone. *Eur J Cardiothorac Surg*. 2000;18:12–16.

39 Anesthesia for Cardiac Surgery

SANDEEP KHANNA • JENNIFER M. HARGRAVE • ABEY ABRAHAM, YASDET MALDONADO • SURENDRASINGH CHHABADA • NELSON BURBANO-VERA • NIKOLAOS J. SKUBAS

KEY POINTS

1. The hemodynamic goals for patients with coronary artery disease are to control heart rate, avoid hypo- and hypervolemia, and assure adequate perfusion pressure.
2. Volatile anesthetics precondition the myocardium against reperfusion injury and help reduce myocardial infarct size.
3. Manipulating preload, afterload and heart rate helps to promote forward flow in patients with regurgitant valvular disease.
4. In patients with aortic dissection, preventing hypertension and tachycardia are crucial to avoiding progression of dissection.
5. Mecanical Circulatory Support (MCS) reduces left ventricular stroke work and myocardial oxygen demand and provides adequate systemic and coronary perfusion in patients with cardiogenic shock.
6. Contemporary anesthetic regimens for elective cardiac surgical procedures provide a balanced anesthetic that is based on use of short-acting, fast-emergence drugs to facilitate early recovery.

Introduction

Anesthetizing patients who undergo cardiac surgery is a dynamic, intellectually challenging, and demanding hands-on experience. The cardiac anesthesiologist should have a thorough understanding of normal and altered cardiac physiology, cardiovascular and anesthetic pharmacology and be cognizant of the physiologic alterations associated with cardiopulmonary bypass (CPB) and attendant surgical procedures.

Coronary Artery Disease

The goal of perioperative care for the patient undergoing coronary artery bypass graft (CABG) surgery is the prevention or treatment of myocardial ischemia and to decrease the incidence of perioperative myocardial infarction. Hemodynamic management should avoid factors that increase myocardial oxygen demand ($M\dot{V}O_2$), particularly during the vulnerable pre-CPB period. Optimizing oxygen delivery to the myocardium is critical, since most

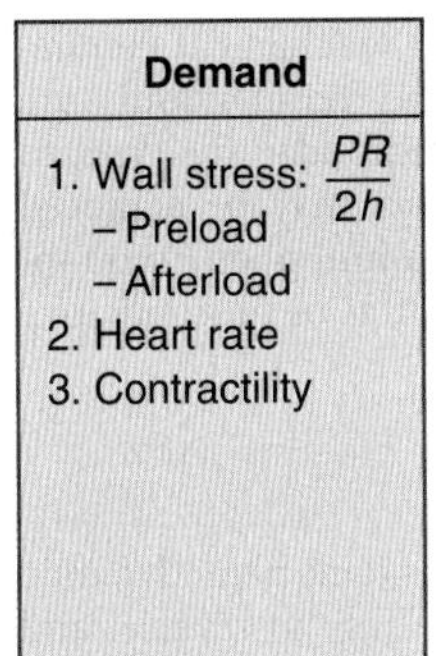

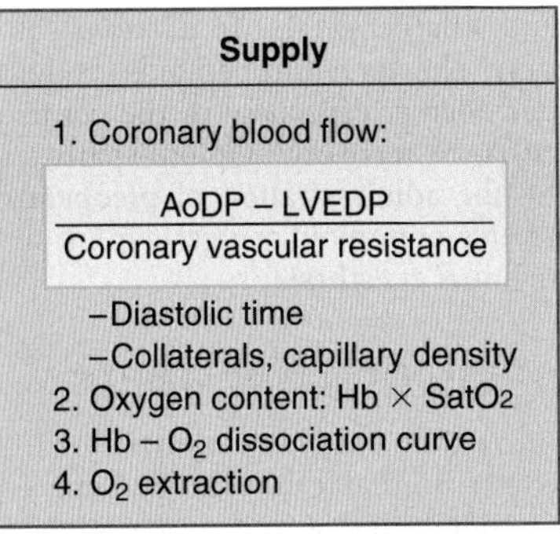

Figure 39-1 Determinants of myocardial oxygen balance. P, intracavitary pressure; R, ventricular radius; h, wall thickness; AoDP, diastolic arterial pressure; LVEDP, left ventricular end-diastolic pressure; Hb, hemoglobin; $SatO_2$, arterial oxygen saturation.

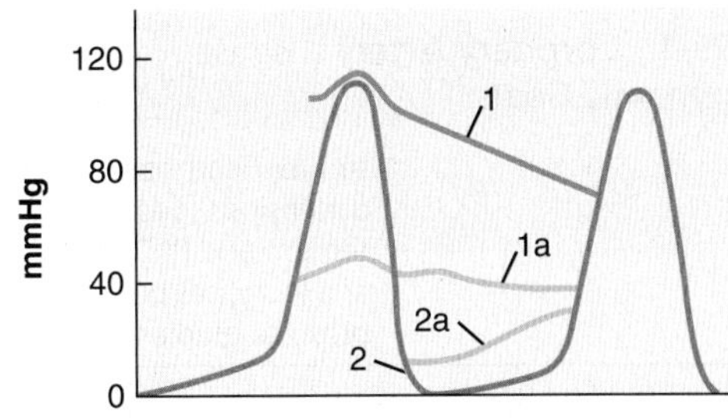

Figure 39-2 The pressure relationships between the aorta (*1*) and the left ventricle (*2*) determine coronary perfusion pressure. In coronary artery disease, myocardial perfusion may be compromised by decreased pressure distal to a significant stenosis (*1a*) (not quantifiable clinically) and/or by an increase in left ventricular end-diastolic pressure (*2a*). (Adapted from Gorlin R. *Coronary Artery Disease*. WB Saunders; 1976:75. Copyright © 1976 Elsevier. With permission.)

ischemic events occur with minimal or no change in $M\dot{V}O_2$.[1,2] The determinants of myocardial oxygen supply and demand are shown in Figure 39-1 and are also discussed in Chapter 12, Cardiac Anatomy and Physiology.

Myocardial Oxygen Demand

The principal determinants of $M\dot{V}O_2$ are wall stress, heart rate, and contractility.[3] According to Laplace's law, wall stress is directly proportional to intracavitary pressure and radius and inversely proportional to wall thickness. Thus, $M\dot{V}O_2$ is reduced by decreasing afterload (blood pressure) and preventing or promptly treating ventricular distention (hypervolemia).

Myocardial Oxygen Supply

Increases in $M\dot{V}O_2$ can be addressed by augmenting coronary blood flow. Arterial blood oxygen content and myocardial oxygen extraction are infrequent reasons for intraoperative myocardial ischemia because blood volume and oxygenation are usually well controlled during anesthesia. In addition, coronary sinus blood is desaturated (Po_2 of 15 to 20 mmHg) so that further oxygen extraction cannot counterbalance a significantly increased $M\dot{V}O_2$. Therefore, the principal interventions to favor the balance oxygen supply versus $M\dot{V}O_2$ are by regulation and facilitation of coronary blood flow.

Coronary Blood Flow

Coronary blood flow is regulated by several factors including heart rate, perfusion pressure, vascular tone of the coronary circulation, and metabolism and is affected by the severity of intraluminal obstructions. The LV has the greatest metabolic requirements due to its greater systolic shortening when compared to the right ventricle (RV),[3] and its subendocardium is most vulnerable to ischemia since it is directly exposed to intracavitary pressures and its perfusion takes place almost entirely during diastole. The RV subendocardium is perfused in both diastole and systole, assuming pulmonary hypertension is not present.

The LV coronary perfusion pressure is often defined as the gradient between aortic diastolic pressure (AoDP) and LV end diastolic pressure (LVEDP; usually approximated by the pulmonary artery wedge pressure). This pressure gradient is decreased in the presence of intraluminal obstruction or increased myocardial vascular tone (Fig. 39-2). A lower LVEDP is ideal for improving perfusion (higher-pressure gradient) and reducing $M\dot{V}O_2$ (decreased LV volume and wall stress). On the other hand, increasing perfusion pressure by raising the aortic pressure will increase $M\dot{V}O_2$, but this is not as important, since tachycardia is the main cause of intraoperative and perioperative increases in $M\dot{V}O_2$.

Alterations in the tone of the small intramyocardial arterioles regulate diastolic vascular resistance, allowing matching of oxygen supply with $M\dot{V}O_2$ over a wide range of perfusion pressures.[4] The difference between autoregulated (basal) flow and blood flow available under conditions of maximal vasodilation is termed *coronary vascular reserve* and is normally three to five times higher than basal flow. As epicardial coronary stenosis becomes more pronounced, progressive vasodilation of arterioles preserves basal flow, but at the cost of a reduced reserve. Autoregulation of subendocardial coronary flow is lost once perfusion pressure decreases to below 40 mmHg. Signs, symptoms, and metabolic evidence of ischemia develop whenever $M\dot{V}O_2$ increases above available coronary vascular reserve.

Reversible ischemia may be caused by an inadequate supply of oxygen to the myocardium and/or the inability to respond to an increased $M\dot{V}O_2$. Irreversible injury to the myocardium can occur if coronary blood flow is occluded for longer than 20 minutes, leading to myocardial cell death and necrosis. Supply-induced ischemia results from a transient coronary occlusion from vasospasm or thrombus, while demand-induced ischemia develops from the inability to increase coronary blood flow and oxygen delivery to the myocardium in response to increases in $M\dot{V}O_2$. In either situation, the consequence is subendocardial ischemia and decreased LV compliance.

Stunned myocardium refers to temporary myocardial dysfunction due to ischemia and normalizes once tissue perfusion is completely restored. No cell death occurs in stunning, but it may take several days or longer for the myocardium to recover, even after adequate blood flow has been restored. Hibernating myocardium refers to abnormal function from chronically reduced coronary blood flow, usually secondary to a fixed stenosis. Hibernating myocardial cells downregulate their metabolism and oxygen demand to maintain viability in response to decreased oxygen supply.[5]

Necrotic and viable myocardium (stunned or hibernating) are difficult to differentiate with echocardiography, as they both appear hypokinetic. Studies such as single-photon emission CT (SPECT) or low-dose dobutamine stress echocardiography can help to identify viable myocardium that may be amenable to revascularization. The current data for revascularization in patients with CAD and LV systolic dysfunction remains inconclusive with the most recent guidelines for CABG surgery published in 2021 recommending that the choice of revascularization in such patients should be based on clinical indications, regardless of sex, race, or ethnicity and made by a multidisciplinary Heart Team.[6]

Table 39-1 Coronary Artery Disease: Hemodynamic Goals

Preload	↓	A smaller heart size (TEE dimensions) decreases wall tension and PADP (LVEDP) and increases perfusion pressure gradient
Afterload	Maintain	Hypertension is better than hypotension
Contractility	↓	If LV function is normal
Rate	↓	
Rhythm	Sinus	Correct arrhythmias
$M\dot{V}O_2$		Monitor for and treat "supply"-related disturbances
Post-CPB		No need for increased PADP (LVEDP)

↑, increase; ↓, decrease; PADP, pulmonary artery diastolic pressure; LVEDP, left ventricular end-diastolic pressure; $M\dot{V}O_2$, myocardial oxygen consumption; CPB, cardiopulmonary bypass; TEE, transesophageal echocardiography.

Hemodynamic Goals

The primary goal of any successful cardiac anesthetic is prevention of myocardial ischemia and prompt identification and treatment of new ischemic episodes by reducing and controlling the factors (Table 39-1) affecting $M\dot{V}O_2$ (heart rate, contractility, and wall tension) and optimizing coronary blood flow (maintaining coronary perfusion pressure and increasing diastolic time). It is important to remember that peripheral arterial systolic pressure
1 is different (usually higher) than aortic root pressure. Thus, the hemodynamic goals for patients with coronary artery disease are a slower heart rate, avoidance of ventricular distention, and adequate blood pressure. Of the preoperative medications that benefit coronary patients, statins and β-blockers are essential. β-Blockers are associated with a decreased incidence of both atrial and ventricular dysrhythmias.[7]

Selection of Anesthetic

The choice of anesthetic should be based on known hemodynamic, pharmacologic, and pharmacokinetic effects of each drug as they apply to the patient and their comorbidities and the relative cost–benefit ratio of each agent. Hemodynamic changes are minimized in patients with severe myocardial depression if drugs are titrated to the desired effect, thus facilitating a safe anesthetic. In general, the use of low-dose opioid-based general anesthesia, addition of regional anesthetic techniques, and time-directed protocols for enhanced recovery have similar risks of mortality and major postoperative complications compared to conventional care, and appear to be safe in patients considered to be at low-to-moderate risk. Enhanced recovery protocols are associated with a reduced time to extubation, shortened ICU, and hospital length of stay.[7,8]

Opioids

The primary advantages of opioids are lack of myocardial depression, maintenance of a stable hemodynamic state, and reduction of heart rate. They are supplemented with benzodiazepines and volatile agents. To decrease the time of mechanical ventilation, shorter-acting opioids (sufentanil and remifentanil) are considered, especially in the context of mutimodal analgesia to enhance recovery.[9] Opioid-sparing anesthesia may be achieved by the administration of preoperative acetaminophen, intraoperative nonopioid analgesic infusions, and intra- or postoperative regional anesthesia.

Inhalation Anesthetics

All volatile anesthetic agents have dose-dependent hemodynamic effects, titratable myocardial depression, are easy to reverse, and provide amnesia and suppression of sympathetic responses to surgical stress. Volatile anesthetics precondition the myocardium 2
against reperfusion injury and help reduce myocardial infarct size. This beneficial effect has been shown when volatile anesthetics are administered before a period of prolonged ischemia ("anesthetic preconditioning") as well as during reperfusion ("anesthetic postconditioning").[10] When compared to total intravenous anesthesia, desflurane or sevoflurane is associated with decreased mortality and morbidity after cardiac surgery.[11] Multimodal anesthetic schemes based on combinations of opioids and any of the volatile anesthetics are advantageous with minimal untoward effects.

The three main volatile agents used in clinical practice today are desflurane, isoflurane, and sevoflurane. Isoflurane has the greatest degree of coronary vasodilation, however this effect is clinically insignificant in doses less than 1 MAC. Clinical studies titrating isoflurane to clinical rather than pharmacologic end points have not shown increased episodes of ischemia or a worsened outcome.[10] Desflurane and sevoflurane have the fastest recovery of all volatile anesthetics. Desflurane has a rapid uptake and distribution, allowing it to be useful in cases in which hemodynamic changes mandate rapid changes in anesthetic depth. When studying sympathetic nervous system activity, Helman et al.[12] found an increase in sympathetic activity and myocardial ischemia in patients anesthetized with desflurane as the sole anesthetic agent for coronary artery bypass surgery compared with patients anesthetized with sufentanil.

Intravenous Sedative Hypnotics

An alternative adjuvant anesthetic to a low-dose opioid technique is a titratable intravenous infusion of a short-acting sedative, such as midazolam, propofol, ketamine, or dexmedetomidine. These can be continued postoperatively in the ICU and afford a predictable and fairly rapid awakening after discontinuation. Compared to volatile anesthetics, propofol was associated with less favorable effects on cardiac function, higher need for inotropic support, and elevated plasma troponins after cardiac surgery in elderly patients.[13,14] Dexmedetomidine may provide for a faster emergence however it should not be used to reduce atrial fibrillation or delirium in cardiac surgery patients.[14]

Treatment of Ischemia

Anesthetics or vasoactive drugs affect heart size, heart rate, and myocardial perfusion pressure. The principal vasoactive drugs are nitrates, β-blockers, peripheral vasoconstrictors, and calcium entry blockers. Clinical scenarios for their use are given in Table 39-2. Volatile anesthetics can also be used to control blood pressure and reduce contractility.

Nitrates

Nitroglycerin is the drug of choice for the treatment of acute myocardial ischemia. It acts via systemic venodilation and coronary

Table 39-2 Treatment of Intraoperative Ischemia

Clinical Manifestation	Suggested Intervention
Increased Demand	
↑ Heart rate	Administer β-blocker, ↑ Anesthetic depth
↑ Blood pressure	↑ Anesthetic depth
↑ PCWP	Nitroglycerin
Decreased Supply	
↓ Heart rate	Atropine, pacing
↓ Blood pressure	↓ Anesthetic depth, administer vasoconstrictor
↑ PCWP	Nitroglycerin, inotrope
No Changes	
	Nitroglycerin, calcium channel blockers, consider heparin

↑, increase(d); ↓, decrease(d); PCWP, pulmonary capillary wedge pressure.

arterial dilation, which is effective in both stenosed coronaries and collateral beds. Prophylactic use of nitroglycerin does not prevent intraoperative ischemia or decrease postoperative cardiac complications.[15] At higher doses, nitroglycerin dilates systemic arteries and may cause systemic hypotension, which is counterproductive for the treatment of myocardial ischemia, as compensatory tachycardia may increase $M\dot{V}O_2$. Nitroglycerin may also cause methemoglobinemia at higher doses and with prolonged administration.

Sodium Nitroprusside

Sodium nitroprusside decreases peripheral vascular resistance via its metabolic or spontaneous reduction to nitric oxide. Similar to nitroglycerin, sodium nitroprusside improves ventricular compliance in the ischemic myocardium. Dosing should be reduced in the presence of hepatic and/or renal disease. It deteriorates in the presence of light and the solution container should be wrapped in a nontransparent material.

Adverse effects of sodium nitroprusside administration include cyanide and thiocyanate toxicity, rebound hypertension, intracranial hypertension, blood coagulation abnormalities, and pulmonary shunting. In vitro findings suggest that cardiac surgical patients may be at an increased risk of cyanide toxicity.[16] Cyanide is a metabolite of sodium nitroprusside. Toxic blood levels (>100 µg/dL) occur when more than 1.0 mg/kg sodium nitroprusside is administered within 2 hours or when more than 0.5 mg/kg/hr is administered within 24 hours. The presenting signs of cyanide toxicity include the triad of elevated mixed venous O_2 (SvO_2), tachyphylaxis and metabolic acidosis.[17] The patient may also appear flushed. A greater risk of cyanide toxicity exists in patients who are nutritionally deficient in cobalamin (vitamin B_{12} compounds) or receive dietary substances containing sulfur. Measurement of blood cyanide and pH will enable detection of abnormalities in high-risk patients for whom larger than recommended amounts of sodium nitroprusside have been used. Treatment should consist of discontinuing the infusion, administering 100% O_2, amyl nitrate (inhaled) or intravenous sodium nitrite and intravenous thiosulfate. Treatment with hydroxocobalamin is recommended in those patients with abnormal renal function.

Vasoconstrictors

Vasoconstrictors (phenylephrine, norepinephrine, vasopressin) are useful adjuncts in the prevention and treatment of ischemia: they increase systemic blood pressure, thereby improving coronary perfusion pressure, at the expense of increasing afterload and perhaps $M\dot{V}O_2$. Concomitant venoconstriction increases venous return and LV preload. In most situations, the increase in coronary perfusion pressure more than offsets any increase in wall tension. Peripheral vasoconstriction is needed during episodes of systemic hypotension, especially those caused by reduced surgical stimulation or drug-induced vasodilation. No single vasoconstrictor is superior. Occasionally, a combination of vasoconstrictors (e.g., norepinephrine and vasopressin) may be needed to achieve the desired blood pressure.[18]

β-Blockers

β-Adrenergic blockade improves myocardial oxygen balance by decreasing chronotropy and inotropy. Indications for β-blockers include treatment of sinus tachycardia unrelated to light anesthesia or hypovolemia, decreasing the ventricular response to supraventricular dysrhythmias and control of ventricular dysrhythmias.[19] The use of β-blockers should aim to reduce the heart rate and increase diastolic filling time without simultaneously decreasing perfusion pressure and cardiac output. These therapeutic targets are even more important, since the POISE study revealed that death and stroke were side effects of perioperative β-blockade.[19] Current intravenous preparations include metoprolol, labetalol, and esmolol. Metoprolol has the purported advantage of β_1-selectivity and is less likely to trigger bronchospasm in patients with reactive airway disease. Labetalol combines β- and α-blocking properties and is useful in treating hyperdynamic and hypertensive states. Esmolol is a short-acting β_1-blocker that is cardioselective, with a half-life of 9.5 minutes. It is particularly useful in treating transient increases in heart rate owing to episodic sympathetic stimulation.

The most recent guidelines for CABG surgery were published in 2021.[6] Notable summary statements related to anesthetic management include:

- The maintenance anesthetic agent likely does not play as large a role as previously thought, however volatile anesthesia may facilitate earlier extubation.
- Nonopioid analgesia should be offered as part of a multimodal strategy.
- The use of TEE in isolated CABG is less established but may aid in determining the cause of hemodynamic changes and for monitoring ventricular function and segmental wall motion abnormalities.
- Use of PACs should be reserved for patients who are older and/or with congestive heart failure, pulmonary hypertension, or concomitant valve disease.

The reader is encouraged to consult the full document at *https://www.jacc.org/doi/epdf/10.1016/j.jacc.2021.09.006*, (accessed April 29, 2023).

Valvular Heart Disease

The prevalence of valvular heart disease (VHD) continues to be a source of patient morbidity and mortality. In 2021 the American Heart Association reported that the incidence of VHD was 65 percent 100,000 people-years.[20] Aortic stenosis remains the most prevalent

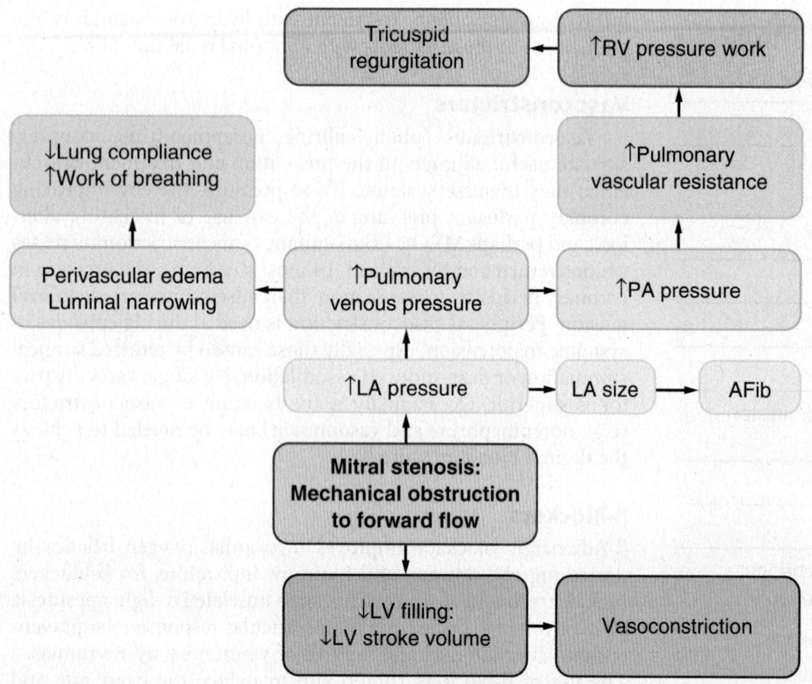

Figure 39-3 Pathophysiology of mitral stenosis. RV, right ventricle; PA, pulmonary artery; LA, left atrium; AFib, atrial fibrillation; LV, left ventricle.

diagnosis at 47.2% followed by mitral regurgitation at 24.2% and aortic regurgitation at 18%.

VHD management remains a challenge because the primary valvular disease impacts cardiac output and the secondary, compensatory mechanisms also contribute to morbidity and mortality. For example, mitral regurgitation or mitral stenosis may lead to increased pressures within the left atrium and subsequently increased pressure within the pulmonary vasculature, resulting in pulmonary hypertension, which can result in increased right ventricular afterload and failure.

The American Heart Association (AHA) and American College of Cardiology (ACC) has established extensive VHD management guidelines that focus on preventing the development of detrimental compensatory mechanisms and improving the quality of life.[21] Recent innovations increased the number of percutaneous or minimally invasive surgical approaches for treating VHD, facilitating either quicker recovery for patients or allowing to high risk, previously nonsurgical candidates an opportunity for interventional treatment. Finally, echocardiography remains the standard for diagnosis and monitoring of the progression of VHD. Because of the complexities associated with VHD physiology and the difficulty of perioperative care, preoperative imaging may be indicated along with intraoperative transesophageal echocardiography monitoring (refer to Chapter 27). The following sections provide a preview of the various VHDs, associated pathophysiology, and an understanding of optimal perioperative anesthetic management.

Mitral Stenosis

Mitral valve stenosis (MS) is due to leaflet thickening and commissural fusion, typically due to rheumatic heart disease or mitral annular calcification (NICV 39-1). Rheumatic disease remains the most common cause of MS worldwide. Other causes include radiation valvulitis, congenital causes (parachute mitral valve, cor triatriatum), and obstructive lesions such as an atrial myxoma[22] in native valves and degenerative changes in prosthetic valves.

Pathophysiology

The physiologic sequelae of MS are depicted in Figure 39-3. The normal MV area is 4 to 6 cm^2. With worsening stenosis, a transmitral gradient develops between the LA and LV (usually at an area <2 cm^2) (1 Video 39-1). The increasing left atrial pressures (LAPs) result in: (i) increased risk of pulmonary hypertension which will leads to compensatory RV hypertrophy, dilation, and then eventual RV failure with associated tricuspid regurgitation (TR), and (ii) increased LAP, LA dilation, and increased risk of atrial arrhythmias (atrial fibrillation is present in about 40% of patients with MS). Ultimately, there is decreased LV stroke volume due to poor LV filling in diastole.

The Gorlin formula can be used for calculation of the MVA[23]:

$$\text{Valve area} = \text{flow}/(K \cdot \sqrt{\text{Pressure gradient}})$$

where flow is cardiac output/diastolic filling time; pressure gradient is the difference between LAP and LVDP; and *K* is a hydraulic pressure constant (this calculation assumes no regurgitant flow). At a constant MVA, the formula can be rearranged to delineate which factors contribute to an elevated LAP.

$$\text{LAP} - \text{LVDP} = [(\text{cardiac output})/(\text{diastolic time})/(K \cdot \text{MVA})]^2$$
$$\text{or LAP} = \text{LVDP} + [\text{flow}/(K \cdot \text{MVA})]^2$$

Hence, anything that increases cardiac output or decreases diastolic filling time will result in increased LAP. This explains why high cardiac output conditions such as pregnancy or infection can increase LAP and result in pulmonary edema. Similar LAP increases will occur with atrial fibrillation, which decreases diastolic filling time.

The definitive treatment for MS is surgical management: MV replacement, repair or balloon mitral valvotomy. The medical therapy for MS should aim to slow the heart rate (with β- or calcium channel blockers) to promote diastolic LV filling. If patients with MS develop acute AF, immediate rate control is paramount

Table 39-3 Mitral Stenosis: Hemodynamic Goals

Parameter	Goal	Comment
Preload	Maintain	Maintain, avoid hypovolemia
Afterload		Prevent ↑ RV afterload (due to pulmonary vasoconstriction hypoxia, hypercarbia); treat systemic hypotension with vasopressors
Contractility	↑ RV	May be decreased in long-standing pulmonary hypertension (LV: usually intact)
Rate	Maintain	At low end of normal; avoid and treat tachycardia
Rhythm		Control ventricular response in atrial fibrillation
$M\dot{V}O_2$		Not a problem
Post-CPB		LV preload and filling pressures may be elevated; cardiac function does not improve immediately

↑, increase(d); RV, right ventricle; $M\dot{V}O_2$, myocardial oxygen consumption; CPB, cardiopulmonary bypass; MV, mitral valve; LV, left ventricle.

Table 39-4 Mechanisms of Mitral Regurgitation

Cause	Characteristics	Location
Degeneration	Excessive motion due to prolapse or flail	Leaflet
	Redundant tissue	
	Ruptured chordae	
Rheumatic	Thickened, calcified, restricted leaflets	Leaflet
	Commissural fusion	
Congenital	Cleft mitral valve, double orifice mitral valve	Leaflet
Miscellaneous	Drug-related (fenfluramine)	Leaflet
Endocarditis	Perforation(s)	Leaflet
	Vegetations	
Myocardial infarction	Papillary muscle rupture	Tensor apparatus
Dilated cardiomyopathy	Annular dilatation	Annulus
Ischemic heart disease	Papillary muscle dysfunction	Tensor apparatus

with pharmacologic measures, followed by synchronized cardioversion if needed.

Anesthetic Considerations

The hemodynamic goals for MS are listed in Table 39-3. Patients with MS are at risk for developing pulmonary edema and RV failure. Consequently, tachyarrhythmias, hypervolemia, and preventing further increases in right ventricular afterload should be avoided. Hypoxemia, hypercapnia, acidosis, and hypothermia increase pulmonary vascular resistance and can precipitate right ventricular failure in MS and should also be avoided. Many induction anesthetic agents may cause hypotension with reflex tachycardia. The mainstay of pharmacologic treatment is with β-blockers or rate selective calcium channel blockers. A fluid bolus may not be ideal to offset the hypotension given the fixed stenotic MVA and risk of pulmonary edema.

After TEE insertion, one should ensure there is no thrombus present in the LA or its appendage, given the risk of atrial fibrillation. The period of post-CPB is crucial as the chronically under-filled LV is at risk of distension post mitral valve repair or replacement. In addition, RV dysfunction is also of concern, especially in the presence of elevated pulmonary arterial pressures. One may need to consider inotropic agents to augment RV function and effect pulmonary arterial vasodilation. The echocardiographic evaluation of MS is described in Chapter 27.

Mitral Regurgitation

Primary mitral regurgitation (MR) is due to intrinsic pathology of the mitral valve apparatus (leaflets, chordae, or papillary muscles). Causes include MV prolapse, mitral annular calcification, rheumatic disease, and infective endocarditis. Secondary MR occurs in the presence of LV dysfunction. Causes include coronary artery disease and nonischemic (dilated) cardiomyopathy. The mitral valve leaflets are normal however the change in LV geometry can result in apical tethering of the mitral valve leaflets or mitral annular dilation. Classification of MR can be based on leaflet motion; (i) MR with normal leaflet mobility due to perforation secondary to endocarditis, (ii) MR with excessive leaflet motion due to prolapse or flail or degenerative conditions, such as Barlow disease or fibroelastic deficiency, or, finally (iii) MR with restrictive leaflet motion attributed to rheumatic heart disease or dilated cardiomyopathy. The various mechanisms of MR are highlighted in Table 39-4. Treatment options for MR include percutaneous MV repair (MitraClip), transcatheter MV replacement, or surgical repair or replacement with conventional sternotomy or a minimally invasive approach.[22,24]

Pathophysiology

The pathophysiology of mitral regurgitation varies based on an acute versus chronic presentation (Fig. 39-4, 2 Video 39-2). Normally, LV pressure exceeds LA pressure during isovolumetric contraction, thus forcing closure of MV. With MR, the incompetent MV allows retrograde systolic blood flow into the LA. Over time, the LA dilates and the LV hypertrophies, with the former increasing the risk of atrial fibrillation. Eccentric LV hypertrophy initially allows for a normal or increased stroke volume, however with time LV systolic dysfunction ensues. Overall, the degree of MR depends on the effective regurgitant orifice area of the MV, LA compliance, systolic ejection time, systemic vascular resistance, and the pressure gradient between the LV and LA.

With acute MR, the LA and LV have not had time to adapt, hence patients are prone to pulmonary edema given the acutely increased LA pressures. Furthermore, LVEDP increases, and LV stroke volume decreases. These patients may require pharmacologic support, along with use of circulatory assist devices, such as an intra-aortic balloon pump.

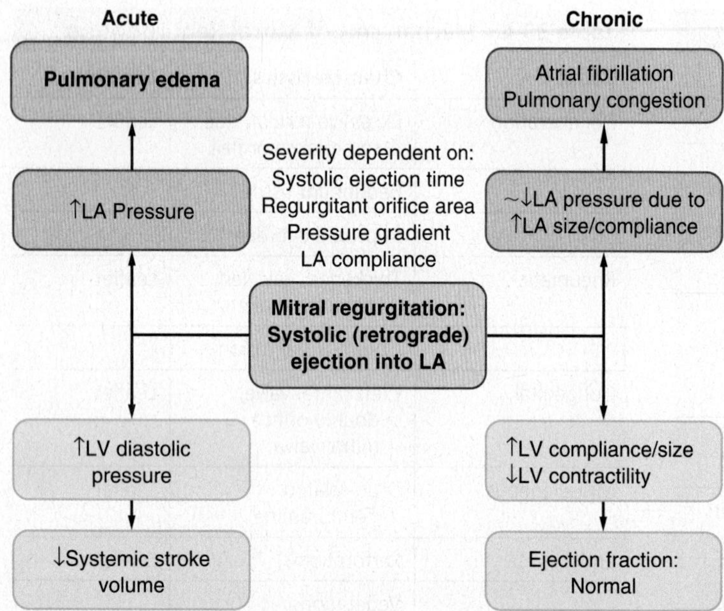

Figure 39-4 Pathophysiology of mitral regurgitation. LA, left atrial; LV, left ventricular.

MR presents unique loading conditions for the LV: there are two outflow tracts for LV blood flow, the aortic valve (AV) and mitral valve. Regurgitant flow through the mitral valve provides a low impedance pathway, hence a patient's LV ejection fraction (EF) may overestimate true systolic function. With MV repair or replacement, the LV can eject blood only through the LVOT, which provides a normal impedance pathway. Postbypass, this can unmask existing LV systolic dysfunction, as LV afterload has now increased. Use of inotropes and vasodilators can help support LV function, and thus help separate from bypass.

Anesthetic Considerations

3 Manipulating preload, afterload and heart rate helps to promote forward flow in patients with valve disease. The hemodynamic goals for MR are highlighted in Table 39-5. Minimizing afterload and achieving a faster heart rate helps promote forward (systemic) flow and decreased regurgitation (retrograde flow) in patients with chronic MR. Maintaining sinus rhythm ensures atrial contribution and thus maximizes LV diastolic filling. Adequate anesthetic depth and use of vasodilators are encouraged. Furthermore, a faster heart rate will decrease systolic duration, and thus time taken for MR. If mitral valve repair (MVr) is planned, the risk of systolic anterior motion (SAM) of the anterior MV leaflet should be assessed in the pre-bypass period. If the risk is high, it is likely the anterior MV leaflet will be dragged toward the interventricular septum in systole, thus causing LVOT obstruction. Some of the risk factors for SAM post-MVr include bileaflet prolapse, posterior leaflet height >15 mm, coaptation-septum (C-sept) distance <25 mm and an LV end-diastolic diameter <45 mm.[25]

The echocardiographic evaluation of MR and its surgical treatment are described in Chapter 27.

Tricuspid Stenosis

Tricuspid stenosis is relatively rare, with an incidence of around 3% worldwide. The most common cause of tricuspid stenosis is rheumatic heart disease. Other causes include congenital lesions, such as Ebstein anomaly, and infective endocarditis. Treatments include surgical valve replacement or repair.[26]

The hemodynamic goals are maintaining a higher preload, and contractility. Sinus rhythm is crucial, and aberrant arrhythmias must be promptly controlled with medications or cardioversion.

Tricuspid Regurgitation

TR can be classified into primary (10% to 15%) and functional. Primary TR is due to an abnormality with the tricuspid valve apparatus. Causes include Ebstein anomaly, rheumatic disease, and carcinoid disease. Functional TR occurs when there is annular dilation and leaflet tethering secondary to left heart disease causing pulmonary hypertension, right ventricular failure, or atrial fibrillation. As TR worsens, RV volume overload and dysfunction ensues, ultimately causing hepatic congestion, peripheral edema, and ascites. Treatment typically involves surgical replacement or

Table 39-5 Mitral Regurgitation: Hemodynamic Goals

Parameter	Goal	Comment
Preload	↑ Slightly	
Afterload	↓	With anesthetics, arterial vasodilators
Contractility		(May be ↑) titrate myocardial depressants carefully
Rate	↑ Slightly	↑ Avoid bradycardia
Rhythm		Control ventricular response if atrial fibrillation present
$M\dot{V}O_2$		Compromised if MR coexists with ischemic heart disease
Post-CPB		↑ Inotropy (afterload is increased with competent valve)

↑, increase(d); ↓, decrease(d); $M\dot{V}O_2$, myocardial oxygen consumption; MR, mitral regurgitation; CPB, cardiopulmonary bypass.

repair, however there has been recent advances in transcatheter tricuspid valve repair techniques. Hemodynamic goals include maintaining preload, sinus rhythm and a faster heart rate to minimize regurgitant flow. In the event of failure, inotropic agents are indicated. It is of paramount importance that factors that increase pulmonary vascular resistance, such as hypoxemia, hypercapnia, and acidosis, are avoided.[27]

Hypertrophic Cardiomyopathy

Hypertrophic cardiomyopathy is an autosomal dominant condition involving asymmetric left ventricular (LV) hypertrophy, typically involving the basal interventricular septum. Its prevalence is 0.16% to 0.29%. Histologically, there is evidence of myocyte hypertrophy and interstitial fibrosis. Hypertrophic cardiomyopathy is a known cardiac risk factor for sudden death, with associated complications such as atrial fibrillation.[28]

Pathophysiology

The physiologic consequences of LV hypertrophy are highlighted in Figure 39-5 (see also NICV 39-2). Around one-third of patients with hypertrophic cardiomyopathy have a degree of dynamic left ventricular outflow tract (LVOT) obstruction. This is due to bulging of the hypertrophied septum, along with SAM of the anterior mitral valve leaflet, which encroaches the LVOT. The LVOT gradient increases when LV cavity size decreases; this can result from decreased preload and afterload, or increased myocardial contractility. As the anterior mitral valve leaflet is dragged into the LVOT, a posteriorly directed mitral regurgitation jet can develop. In the presence of primary mitral valve disease, there may be additional MR jets.

In hypertrophic cardiomyopathy, there is an imbalance between myocardial oxygen supply (reduced as the coronary arteries demonstrate luminal narrowing) and demand (increased due to LV hypertrophy). Overall, patients may experience ischemic symptoms at rest or with exercise, in the absence of atherosclerotic coronary artery disease.

Anesthetic Considerations

Surgical treatment options include alcohol septal ablation or septal myectomy. The former involves injecting ethanol into one of the septal perforator branches, resulting in infarction of the proximal interventricular septum, thus decreasing the LVOT obstruction. The aim of surgical septal myectomy is to effect a resting peak gradient of <30 mmHg across the LVOT. The anesthetic management of patients with hypertrophic cardiomyopathy includes (a) maintaining preload, (b) maintaining afterload (using alpha-adrenergic agonists), (c) minimizing increases in contractility, (d) avoiding tachycardia, and (e) maintaining sinus rhythm (Table 39-6).

Table 39-6 Hypertrophic Cardiomyopathy: Hemodynamic Goals

Parameter	Goal	Comment
Preload	Maintain or ↑	Treat as in aortic stenosis
Afterload	↑	Treat hypotension aggressively with α-adrenergic agonists
Contractility	↓	
Rate	Maintain	β-Blockers
Rhythm	Sinus	Consider atrial pacing modalities (PAC, esophageal)
$M\dot{V}O_2$		Not a problem
Post-CPB		Start with volume and vasoconstrictors; avoid inotropes. Check carefully for residual LVOT gradient and SAM; rule out ventricular septal defect

↑, increase; ↓, decrease; LVOT, left ventricular outflow tract; LVEDP, left ventricular end-diastolic pressure; LV, left ventricle; PAC, pulmonary artery catheter; $M\dot{V}O_2$, myocardial oxygen consumption; CPB, cardiopulmonary bypass; SAM, systolic anterior motion.

Some patients may have aortic stenosis in combination with hypertrophic cardiomyopathy, hence it is important to distinguish between dynamic LVOT obstruction and valvular aortic stenosis. With echocardiography, the distinct appearances of systolic velocities can help distinguish the two entities.[29]

Aortic Valve Stenosis

A normal AV consists of three symmetrical semilunar cusps contained within the aortic annulus and suspended from the aortic root's sinuses of Valsalva. The cusps are named according to their relationship with the coronary ostia: right, left, and noncoronary (adjacent the interatrial septum) (Fig. 39-6). Aortic valve stenosis (AS) remains one of the most common VHDs typically caused by

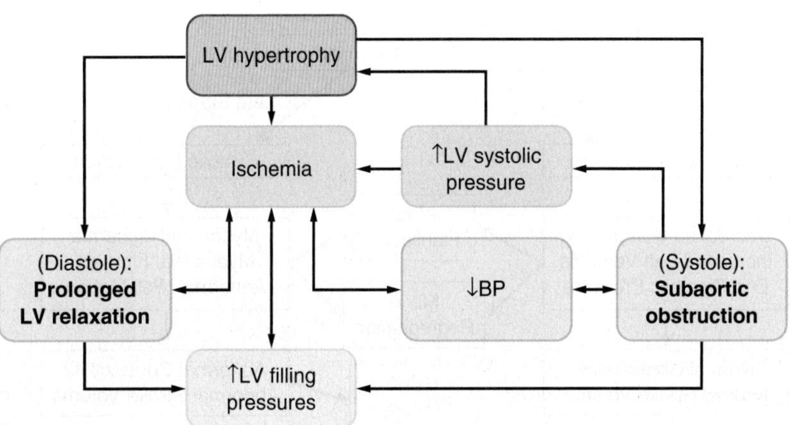

Figure 39-5 Pathophysiology of primary left ventricular (LV) hypertrophy in hypertrophic cardiomyopathy. BP, blood pressure.

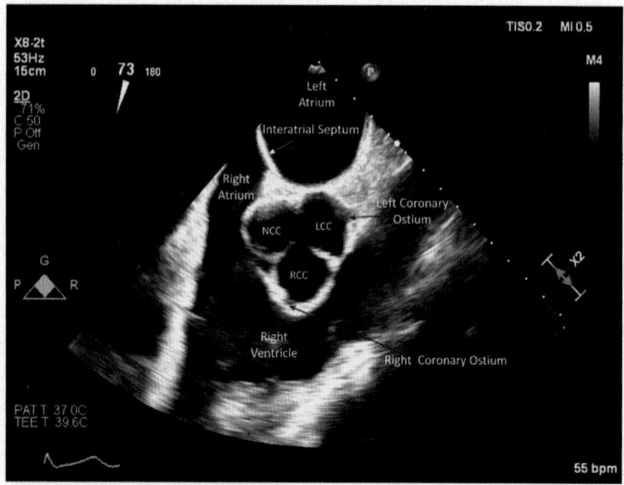

Figure 39-6 Transesophageal echocardiography mid-esophageal short axis of the aortic valve. NCC, aortic valve non-coronary cusp; RCC, aortic valve right coronary cusp; LCC, aortic valve left coronary cusp.

a degenerative process, although congenital anomalies, such as a bicuspid AV, account for the second most common cause of AS. Deposits of calcium are characteristic of the degenerative process as a response to constant mechanical stress throughout the cardiac cycle. The autoimmune process of rheumatic heart disease resulting in AS and aortic insufficiency (AI) is seen in underdeveloped countries. Similar to the mechanism of mitral stenosis, rheumatic heart disease may cause commissural fusion of the AV cusps. The diagnosis and severity of AS is based on the AV area and pressure gradients. A normal AV area is 2 to 4 cm^2. The AHA and the ACC provide guidelines for classifications of mild, moderate, and severe AS (Table 39-7).[21] Although with normal LV function, sufficient pressure is generated to cause elevated peak velocities and pressure gradients across the AV, a dysfunctional LV may produce "normal" AV pressure gradients. If LV dysfunction is present, additional investigation with dobutamine (to provide pharmacologic stress) should be used to appropriately diagnose "pseudo" (normal AV area at increased systolic pressure) or "low flow, low gradient" (small AV area regardless of systolic pressure) AS.

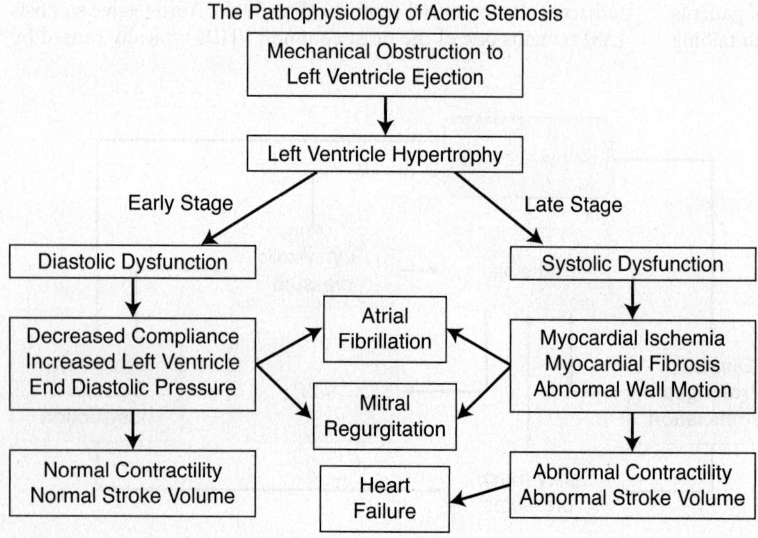

Figure 39-7 The early and late stages of aortic stenosis pathophysiology.

Table 39-7 Aortic Stenosis: Classifications

	Mild	Moderate	Severe
Peak Aortic Valve Velocity	2.6–3.0 (m/s)	3–4 (m/s)	>4 (m/s)
Transvalvular Pressure Gradient	<20 mmHg	20–40 (m/s)	>40 mmHg
Aortic Valve Area	>1.5 cm^2	1.0–1.5 cm^2	<1.0 cm^2

Pathophysiology

Recent guidelines recommend aggressive treatment of AS.[28] Life expectancy, following the development of specific symptoms, is 5 years for angina, 3 years for syncope, and 2 years for dyspnea. Minimally invasive treatments, such as transcatheter aortic valve replacement (TAVR), are options for patients considered at high risk for surgical AV replacement.[30]

As AV area decreases, LV workload increases. Over time, this results in LV hypertrophy. Hypertrophy of the LV decreases the LV wall stress, according to La Place's law:

Wall Stress = (Pressure × Volume) / Wall Thickness

The compensatory mechanism of concentric LV hypertrophy increases the risk of myocardial ischemia and LV diastolic dysfunction (Fig. 39-7). With LV hypertrophy, LV mass and basal myocardial requirement of oxygen increase. In addition, the increased LV mass may prevent the perfusion of endocardial coronary arteries increasing the possibility of ischemia.

With LV hypertrophy, ventricular relaxation decreases resulting in diastolic dysfunction and a higher LV end-diastolic pressure (LVEDP), that is, decreased compliance. Myocardial perfusion via the coronary arteries is directly dependent on the LVEDP:

Coronary perfusion pressure = Aortic diastolic pressure – LVEDP

As diastolic dysfunction and myocardial oxygen requirements increase secondary to LV hypertrophy, AS patients are at significant risk of myocardial ischemia, especially during periods of hypotension and/or with concurrent coronary artery disease (3 Video 39-3). In AS LV afterload is determined by the stenotic AV, and stroke volume depends upon preload; AS is considered a "preload dependent" state. Providing adequate volume to fill the left atrium is necessary to facilitate diastolic LV filling. With progressive diastolic dysfunction the probability of atrial fibrillation increases. The "atrial kick" of sinus rhythm remains critical to preserved LV diastolic filling and cardiac output.

Anesthetic Considerations of Aortic Stenosis

The ideal hemodynamic environment for the patient with AS is summarized in Table 39-8 (see also NICV 39-3 and 39-4). According to published reports, patients undergoing noncardiac surgery with both severe and moderate AS have increased risk of both 30-day mortality and postoperative myocardial infarction.[31] A minimally invasive treatment for AS is TAVR. The American Heart Association's Valvular Heart Disease Guidelines published in 2020 noted that low- or moderate-risk noncardiac surgical procedures in patients with asymptomatic severe AS are reasonable, with invasive hemodynamic monitoring along with advanced perioperative monitoring via a pulmonary artery catheter or transesophageal echocardiography.[21]

Considering the increased risk in the AS patient population, an anesthesiologist must maintain physiologic goals appropriate for AS patients: (i) immediate detection and treatment of systemic arterial hypotension to preserve coronary perfusion, (ii) avoidance of extremes in heart rates; tachycardia increases myocardial oxygen requirements, which is already increased in AS patients secondary to LV hypertrophy. Although bradycardia may increase LV diastolic filling time, the stroke volume is unable to increase proportionally due to the decreased compliance of the LV. With "fixed" afterload from the stenotic AV and the previously discussed limited ability to increase the LV stroke volume, heart rate contributes significantly to cardiac output.

Table 39-8 Aortic Stenosis: Hemodynamic Goals

Parameter	Goal	Comment
Preload	Maintain or ↑	Preload depended condition
Afterload	Maintain or ↑	Coronary perfusion gradient
Contractility	Normal	Normal in the early stage, but may have decreased function in late stages
Rate	Normal	Bradycardia decreased cardiac output Tachycardia increases O_2 requirement
Rhythm	Sinus	Consider cardioversion or rate control if in a nonsinus rhythms
$M\dot{V}O_2$	Normal	Increases with disease progression Avoid tachycardia and treat hypotension

$M\dot{V}O_2$, myocardial oxygen consumption.

Aortic Insufficiency

Aortic valve insufficiency (AI) is classified by normal AV leaflet motion, AV leaflet prolapse and AV leaflet restriction (4 Video 39-4).[32] Normal leaflet motion results in AI as a result of annular dilatation secondary to aortopathies or perforation of an AV cusp (as a result of bacterial endocarditis). Prolapse of a leaflet may be the result of a bicuspid AV, aortic dissection (AD), trauma or destruction by infectious process. Restriction of the AV cusp is seen during degeneration from calcification, thrombosis, vegetations, or rheumatic heart disease.

Pathophysiology

AI results in volume and pressure overload of the LV because of the retrograde, diastolic filling as a result of the incompetent AV.[33] Mild acute AI is often tolerated with minimal hemodynamic changes because LVEDP and volume are mildly increased (Fig. 39-8).

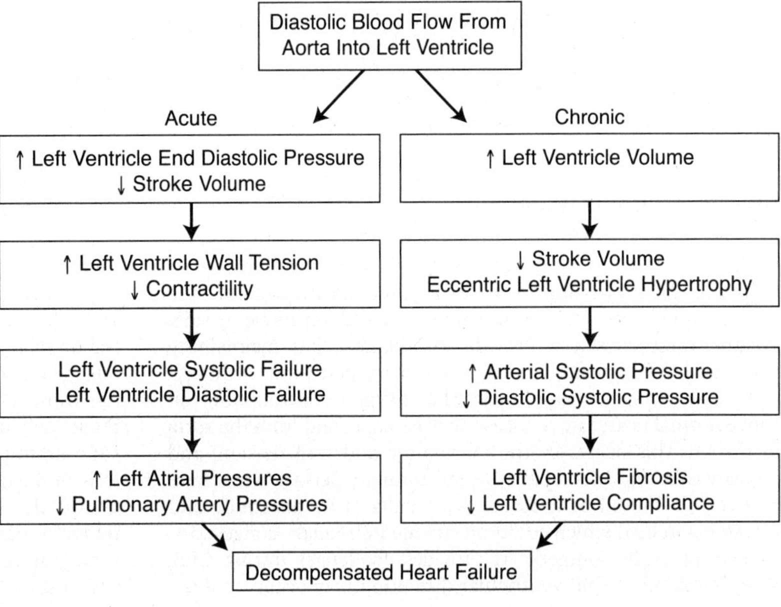

Figure 39-8 The acute and chronic pathophysiology of aortic insufficiency.

Table 39-9 Aortic Insufficiency: Hemodynamic Goals

Parameter	Goal	Comment
Preload	↑ Slightly	↑ Slightly
Afterload	↓	Vasodilation (to decrease regurgitant fraction)
Contractility		Usually adequate
Rate	↑	Reduces left ventricular volume and increases diastolic aortic pressure
Rhythm	Normal	
$M\dot{V}O_2$	Normal	Increases as aortic insufficiency progresses

$M\dot{V}O_2$, myocardial oxygen consumption.

Patients acutely developing significant AI will present with decompensated heart failure (HF), since the LV has not had the time to develop compensatory mechanisms. Coronary perfusion of the LV becomes compromised as the systemic diastolic pressure decreases with the retrograde flow into the LV and the LVEDP is increased. In addition, the increased LV volume and pressure may result in mitral regurgitation, increased LAPs and pulmonary hypertension, resulting in right ventricular dysfunction. As an attempt to preserve cardiac output, tachycardia and vasoconstriction to increase mean arterial pressure (MAP) will occur. These compensatory mechanisms increase myocardial oxygen requirements and subsequently may lead to HF. Patients presenting with acute mild AI typically respond to diuresis and vasodilatation, while patients with severe acute AI will often require emergent AV intervention.

The slower progression of chronic AI allows for the LV to remodel and compensate for increased pressures and volume. As the LV cavity size increases gradually and out of proportion to the LV wall thickness (eccentric LV hypertrophy), LV wall stress increases. Unlike in severe acute AI, the increase in compliance prevents significant changes in the LVEDP, so that although the LV may eject more than twice the normal stroke volume, the myocardial oxygen requirements do not increase. The diastolic runoff and the moderate vasodilation reduce LV afterload and increase the arterial pulse pressure. In chronic AI, patients are often asymptomatic until remodeling (fibrosis of the myocardium) decreases LV compliance resulting in decompensated HF. Intervention should occur prior to irreversible myocardial changes.[21]

Anesthetic Considerations

Anesthetic management in patients with AI focuses on promoting cardiac output and decreasing the regurgitant volume of AI (Table 39-9). Preventing increases in afterload may require the use of vasodilators such as nicardipine or sodium nitroprusside. Volatile anesthetics also provide vasodilation, but maintaining adequate MAPs remains crucial to coronary perfusion. Although tachycardia may increase myocardial oxygen consumption, an above normal heart rate reduces the diastolic runoff from the aorta to the LV. This decreases the LV volume and wall tension, and increases diastolic blood pressure and coronary perfusion gradient. Bradycardia should be avoided as it results in LV distention and elevations in LAP, which could precipitate pulmonary congestion.

During cardiac surgery, AI provides challenges during CPB. With initiation of CBP, ventricular distention may occur until the LV is separated from the systemic circulation with the aortic cross clamp or is emptied via an LV vent catheter. Arresting the heart via cardioplegia also remains a challenge. The incompetent AV prevents anterograde cardioplegia delivery in the aortic root from entering the coronary arteries. Cardioplegia administration during severe AI includes direct injection into the coronary ostia (after aortotomy) or retrograde administration via the coronary sinus.

Aortic Diseases

Pathology of the aorta originates from many different conditions: inflammation, trauma, genetic disorders, wall stress alterations from flow through a bicuspid AV, chronic hypertension, and others.[34] Aortopathies develop and progress due to stiffing of the aortic tissue secondary to alterations in aortic wall composition. The number of smooth muscle cells and elastin fibers decrease, and their arrangement becomes increasingly erratic. Aortic aneurysm (dilation of the aorta), AD (tearing of the aortic intima), or intramural hematoma (bleeding between the walls of the aorta) remains the three conditions that often require urgent intervention.

Aortic Dissection

Acute aortic syndromes consist of three categories of aortic pathology: AD, intramural hematoma, and penetrating ulcers.[35] Risk factors for AD include hypertension in elderly patients and connective tissue disorders, such as Marfan, Ehlers–Danlos, and Loeys–Dietz syndromes in younger patients. An AD results from an intimal tear that allows blood to escape from the true lumen and create a false lumen within layers of aortic media (Fig. 39-6). The accumulation of blood within the false lumen can extend proximally or distally and compromise branch vessels, freely rupture into the pericardium or thoracic cavity, or detach the AV leaflets to cause acute AI. Two classifications systems are used to describe the extent of ADs: the DeBakey system and the Stanford system.[36] DeBakey classifies dissections into three types: type I—intimal tear in the ascending aorta with extension of the dissection to the descending aorta; type II—tear in the ascending aorta with dissection confined to the ascending aorta; and type III—tear beginning in the descending aorta. The Stanford classification system is simpler: type A dissections involve the ascending aorta, and type B dissections do not involve the ascending aorta. Acute AD of the ascending aorta (type A) has a mortality rate of 1% to 2% per hour after onset of symptomatology and is a true surgical emergency. A type B AD distal to the left subclavian artery has a 30-day mortality of 10%. Type B AD may be managed medically unless indications of organ malperfusion develop or pain persists. Intramural hematomas originate from ruptured vasa vasorum in the media and may progress to an AD. Treatment for an intramural hematoma follows the guidelines for an AD.

Clinical presentations of AD include pain in the chest (type A) or back or abdomen (type B). Depending on the progression of the dissection, cerebral and coronary perfusion may be compromised. Cardiac tamponade remains a concern if the aortic wall has thinned or ruptured allowing blood to fill the pericardium. Pulse deficits in extremities and/or differences in blood pressure are important to detect and related to impaired blood flow to a limb. It is important to diagnose correctly the type of AD as this determines the proper treatment. A variety of diagnostic techniques are accurate. Contrast-enhanced spiral computed tomography or magnetic resonance imaging is more sensitive and specific than TEE.[34]

Surgery is the definitive treatment for patients with type A acute AD to decrease mortality by closing the intimal tear and preventing expansion of the false lumen. In addition, surgical intervention addresses potential cerebral and coronary malperfusion, cardiac tamponade, and AV disruption. Surgical repair consists of composite graft, with or without reimplantation of the coronaries, replacement of the AV, and cerebral vessel anastomosis. The addition of stent placement in the proximal descending aorta is becoming common. Type B ADs are managed medically in the absence of organ malperfusion. If intervention is required, endovascular aortic stents remain the most common approach.

Anesthetic Considerations

Acute AD is a surgical emergency. The anesthesiologist must anticipate hemodynamic compromise during the induction period. Prior to induction, LV function, presence of pericardial tamponade, and the competency of the AV should be assessed with transthoracic echocardiography. For induction and in the pre-CPB period, sympathetic surge suppression and maintenance of adequate perfusion are priorities. Patients will often present with antitachycardia therapy, such as β-blocker infusions, and vasodilators in preoperative care. As volatile anesthesia is initi-
4 ated, vasodilators may be weaned off. Prevention of hypertension and tachycardia during direct laryngoscopy and sternotomy remain crucial to avoid progression of AD. Adequate intravenous access and invasive hemodynamic monitoring, including TEE, are important. The hemodynamic goals are shown in Table 39-10.

If the AD involves the aortic arch, hypothermic circulatory arrest is utilized to facilitate replacement of the damaged aorta. Cerebral metabolic oxygen requirements decrease sufficiently at 18 °C to allow for cessation of systemic blood flow for approximately 30 minutes.[37] Adjuncts used to improve cerebral protection include retrograde (via a superior vena cava cannula) or selective antegrade (direct cannulation the axillary artery or cerebral vessels) cerebral perfusion. These techniques may prolong the cooling of cerebral tissue and flush out embolic matter and ischemic metabolites.

Table 39-10 Acute Aortic Dissection: Hemodynamic Goals

Parameter	Goal	Comment
Preload	Normal	If tamponade, ↑ preload
Afterload	↓	With anesthetics, analgesics, vasodilators (nitroprusside, nicardipine): keep systolic BP <100–120 mmHg
Contractility	↓	β-blockers unless ventricle dysfunction
Rate	↓ to <60–80 bpm	Use β-blocker; ensure contractility is adequate
Rhythm		Control ventricular response (If atrial fibrillation present)
$M\dot{V}O_2$	Normal	Compromised if aortic dissection involves coronary vessels

bpm, beats per minute; $M\dot{V}O_2$, myocardial oxygen consumption.

Aortic Aneurysm

The classification of aortic aneurysms is based on their morphology (saccular, fusiform, or diffuse) as well as their location within the thoracic aorta (aortic root, ascending aorta, arch, descending aorta). According to the most recent guidelines, in an average size patient, an aortic segment >4 cm in maximal diameter is aneurysmal.[34] Typically, aneurysms are asymptotic although if large enough, compression of the airway or the recurrent laryngeal nerve may be the presenting clinical symptom. As discussed previously, dilation of the ascending aorta may cause AI. The gold standard for detection and sizing is contrast-enhanced computed tomography scanning and magnetic resonance angiography. Since the risk for rupture increases abruptly as aortic aneurysms reach a diameter of 6 cm, surgery is indicated for ascending aortic aneurysms greater than 5.5 cm.

If the aneurysm is isolated to the ascending aorta, a simple supracoronary composite graft is required. If AI is present secondary to aortic dilatation, with an otherwise normal AV, a valve-sparing procedure (David procedure) is performed. If the aortic root is significantly dilated or the AV is pathologic, a composite aortic repair (Bentall procedure) is performed using a composite graft with either a mechanical or biologic prosthetic AV sewn into its proximal end. Aneurysms of the descending thoracic aorta are most commonly addressed with endovascular aortic stent grafts. Descending aorta stent grafts interrupt lumbar artery perfusion of the spinal cord and are associated with postoperative paraplegia (13% to 17%).

Anesthetic Considerations

The anesthetic management priorities complement management of ADs (Table 39-10). Decreasing strain on the aorta by decreasing contractility and MAP are a priority. If the aneurysm extends into the aortic arch, hypothermic circulatory arrest may be required. Endovascular repair of the descending thoracic aorta may require drainage of cerebrospinal fluid improving spinal cord perfusion pressure. Continuous drainage of cerebrospinal fluid during stent deployment and in the postoperative period to maintain a cerebrospinal fluid pressure below 10 mmHg is the current recommendation.

Heart Failure

By 2030, 1 in 33 Americans will suffer from HF, 9 million patients will seek care related to HF and the cost will increase to an estimated 70 billion dollars. The increasing prevalence of HF has been attributed to an aging population and prolonged survival in patients with cardiovascular disorders including coronary artery disease and cardiomyopathy. In 2013, ACC/AHA published guidelines for management of HF patients and these guidelines were revised in 2022.[38,39]

Definition, Classification, and Staging of Heart Failure

HF is a progressive clinical syndrome that is characterized by reduced cardiac performance, related to impaired ventricular filling and/or systolic blood ejection. Diastolic and systolic HF result in dyspnea, decreased exercise tolerance, and fatigue. Diagnosis is with clinical assessment complemented by imaging studies (echocardiography) and cardiac biomarkers (brain natriuretic peptide) (Table 39-11). Clinical suspicion of HF should prompt evaluation of LV EF and assessment of functional status.

Table 39-11 Diagnosis of Heart Failure

Assessment Modality	Comments
History and Physical Examination	Symptoms: Dyspnea on exertion, orthopnea or PND, abdominal swelling, fatigue and recent weight gain Signs: Audible S3, lung rales, presence of pedal edema and/or ascites, raised JVP, +ve hepatojugular reflex
Modified Framingham clinical criteria: Diagnosis requires 2 major or 1 major + 2 minor criteria	Major Criteria: PND, orthopnea, elevated JVP, presence of S3, Cardiomegaly on CXR, Pulmonary edema on CXR, weight loss ≥ 4.5 kg in 5 days in response to presumed HF treatment Minor Criteria: Bilateral leg edema, dyspnea on ordinary exertion, nocturnal cough, hepatomegaly, pleural effusion, tachycardia (HR >120 beats/min)
Laboratory evaluation	BNP, liver and renal function tests, serum electrolytes, TSH, CBC, Urinalysis, HbA1c, lipid profile
Other modalities	Echocardiography CXR Stress testing Left and Right heart catheterization

BNP, brain natriuretic peptide; CBC, complete blood count; CXR, chest x-ray; HF, heart failure; HR, heart rate; JVP, jugular venous pressure; PND, paroxysmal nocturnal dyspnea; S3, third heart sound; TSH, thyroid-stimulating hormone.

The New York Heart Association (NYHA) classification, first published in 1928 and last updated in 1994 is used to assess severity of functional impairment in HF. Its popularity stems from its simplicity, ability to predict peak oxygen consumption, and to prognosticate and evaluate efficacy of treatment. Interpretation challenges stem from subjectivity and nonspecificity. In addition, noncardiac conditions such as emphysema, obesity, anemia, and neuromuscular diseases lead to fatigue and dyspnea with exercise. Efforts to lend objectivity to functional assessment led to the development of other classification schemes.[40]

Based on LV EF, HF can be classified as:

- HF with reduced EF (HFrEF, EF ≤ 40%)
- HF with preserved EF (HFpEF, EF ≥ 50%)
- HF with improved EF (HFimEF, previously documented EF of ≤ 40% improves to >40% on follow-up)
- HF with mildly reduced EF (HFmrEF, EF between 41% and 49%)

Staging of HF (Table 39-12), allows visualization of chronic HF as a progressive process that commences as asymptomatic systolic or diastolic impairment (Stages A and B), progresses to a symptomatic state (Stage C) and culminates as advanced or end stage HF (Stage D).[39] Unlike the NYHA classification, patients cannot revert back to a previous state in the staging schema. For example, a patient with Stage C HF designation is at risk of progressing to Stage D but cannot revert back to either Stage A or B HF. In contrast, a patient presenting in NYHA class IV, can revert to a NYHA functional class II, with appropriate guideline-directed medical therapy (GDMT).

Temporal categorization of HF is arbitrary but clinically important. Consequently, patients who have had HF for some time (months to years) are labeled as having "*chronic HF*." Patients with HF symptoms and signs that have remained unchanged on optimal guideline-directed management therapy, for at least 1 month have "*stable HF*." New-onset or "de novo" HF presents in patients who previously did not exhibit clinical manifestations of HF. This can occur acutely; for example, during infective endocarditis or subacutely as in a patient with dilated cardiomyopathy who is asymptomatic until they develop dyspnea and present for evaluation. Acute HF syndrome or decompensated HF, often necessitates urgent therapy and/or hospital admission and generally occurs when chronic stable HF deteriorates. Patients often present with

Table 39-12 Staging of Heart Failure

Stage of HF	Definition	Examples
A	At high risk for HF. No evidence of structural heart disease or symptoms of HF.	Patients with hypertension or diabetes mellitus.
B	Signs or symptoms of HF are absent (pre-HF, asymptomatic). Evidence of structural heart disease is present.	Patients with, asymptomatic valvular disease such as aortic valve stenosis with left ventricular hypertrophy.
C	Patient reports prior or current symptoms of HF. (Symptomatic) Evidence of structural heart disease is present.	Symptomatic valvular disease. Patient with degenerative mitral regurgitation with dyspnea, fatigue or chest pain during exercise.
D	Refractory, advanced or end-stage HF necessitating specialized interventions.	NYHA Class IV patient with recurrent hospitalizations for HF decompensation

HF, heart failure; NYHA, New York Heart Association.

Table 39-13 Definition of Cardiogenic Shock

Name of Trial/Guidelines	Definition of Cardiogenic Shock
2022 AHA/ACC/HFSA Guideline for the management of heart failure	• I. SBP <90 mmHg or MAP < 60 mmHg for ≥30 min or catecholamines to maintain SBP >90 mmHg or MAP >60 mmHg. • II. Other hemodynamic parameters: CI <2.2 L/min/m^2, PCWP >15 mmHg, CPO <0.6 watts, Shock index (HR/SBP) >1, RV shock (PAPI <1, CVP/PCWP >0.6) • III. Presence of hypoperfusion (at least one of the following criteria): a. Altered mental status b. Cold/clammy skin and extremities c. Urine output <30 mL/h d. Lactate >2.0 mmol/L

AHA/ACC/HFSA, American Heart Association/American College of cardiology/Heart Failure Society of America; CI, Cardiac Index; CPO, cardiac power output; HR, heart rate; MAP, mean arterial pressure; PCWP, pulmonary capillary wedge pressure; RV, right ventricle; SBP, systolic blood pressure.

worsening dyspnea secondary to severe pulmonary congestion, with or without a low cardiac output and/or systemic hypoperfusion. Patients suffering from advanced or refractory HF remain in NYHA III–IV functional status despite optimal GDMT and suffer from recurrent episodes of pulmonary or systemic congestion, low output or malignant arrhythmias causing >1 unplanned visit or hospitalization in the last 6 months.[39]

Pathophysiology of Chronic Heart Failure

In HFrEF, a dysregulated neurohormonal response, including activation of the renin–angiotensin–aldosterone and sympathetic nervous systems leads to sodium and fluid retention, ventricular remodeling, and vasoconstriction.[41] In HFpEF, emerging evidence suggests that microvascular endothelial inflammation and dysfunction promote fibrosis and ventricular hypertrophy leading to increased LVEDP, pulmonary hypertension, and atrial fibrillation.[42] GDMT for treating HF patients includes lifestyle modifications, pharmacotherapy, electrophysiology procedures, and surgical interventions.

Cardiogenic Shock

Clinically, cardiogenic shock (CS) is characterized by persistent hypotension, hypoperfusion, and low cardiac index.[39] Acute coronary syndromes and progressive HF remain the leading causes and typically affect the elderly. The SHOCK trial in 1999 suggested a hemodynamic definition, modifications of which have been subsequently incorporated in other guidelines and landmark trials (Table 39-13).[43,44]

CS is a continuum that extends from a pre-shock to a refractory shock state and frequently necessitates institution of pharmacotherapy and mechanical circulatory support (MCS) to address hypoperfusion (Table 39-14).[44]

Table 39-14 Stages of Progression of Cardiogenic shock

Risk Category	Defining Features	Biochemical Markers and Hemodynamic Parameters
A: At risk	Patients are "at risk" for developing cardiogenic shock but are not currently experiencing signs/symptoms of cardiogenic shock.	• Normal lactate • Normotensive (SBP ≥100) • CI ≥ 2.5, CVP < 10, $M\dot{V}O_2$ sat ≥ 65%
B: Beginning	Evidence of relative hypotension or tachycardia without hypoperfusion. These patients are considered to be experiencing "beginning" of cardiogenic shock	• Normal lactate, elevated BNP • SBP < 90 OR MAP < 60, PR ≥ 100 • CI ≥ 2.2, $M\dot{V}O_2$ sat ≥ 65%
C: Classical	Patients demonstrate "Classic" cardiogenic shock: Hypotension and hypoperfusion are manifest. In addition to inotropes and vasopressors, mechanical circulatory support excluding extracorporeal membrane oxygenation may be required.	• Lactate ≥2, doubling of serum Cr • Increased LFTs, elevated BNP • SBP < 90 OR MAP <60 with need for drugs to maintain BP above cut off levels for hypotension • CI < 2.2, PCWP > 15, RAP/PCWP ratio ≥ 0.8
D: Doom or Deteriorating	Cardiogenic shock is refractory to therapies and patient is deteriorating rapidly. Consider initiating or mobilizing extracorporeal membrane oxygenation support.	• Stage C and deteriorating. • Multiple vasopressor/inotropes OR addition of MCS device needed to maintain adequate tissue perfusion
E: Extremis or "Trying to die"	Patients in "Extremis" include those who are experiencing cardiac arrest with ongoing cardiopulmonary resuscitation and/or extracorporeal membrane oxygenation cardiopulmonary resuscitation.	• No SBP/MAP in the absence of ongoing resuscitation • PEA or refractory ventricular tachycardia/ fibrillation • Persistent hypotension despite maximal support

BNP, brain natriuretic peptide; CI, cardiac index (L/min/m^2); CVP, central venous pressure (mmHg); Cr, creatinine; MCS, mechanical circulatory support; $M\dot{V}O_2$ sat, mixed venous oxygen saturation; MAP, mean arterial pressure (mmHg); PCWP, pulmonary capillary wedge pressure (mmHg); PEA, pulseless electrical activity; PR, pulse rate (beats/min); RAP, right atrial pressure (mmHg); SBP, systolic blood pressure.

Mechanical Circulatory Support (MCS) in Cardiogenic Shock: When and Why?

Vasoactive medications such as norepinephrine, epinephrine, and vasopressin are often initiated to maintain perfusion in CS. However, they increase $M\dot{V}O_2$, worsen ischemia, increase myocardial work, and exacerbate the risk of developing malignant arrhythmias.
5 Unlike vasoactive medications, MCS reduces LV stroke work and $M\dot{V}O_2$, in conjunction with providing adequate systemic and coronary perfusion in CS patients. An ideal MCS device leads to restoration of MAP and cardiac index, and a decrease in pulmonary capillary wedge pressure, LVEDP, and LV end-diastolic volume. These hasten recovery of the failing ventricle. Biochemically, resolution of hypoperfusion is demonstrated by a decreasing serum lactate level and rising mixed venous oxygen saturation.

MCS devices can be categorized by:

1. Method of implantation: Percutaneous versus Surgical
2. Intended duration of deployment: Short term (days to weeks) versus Durable (months to years)
3. Ventricle supported: Left, right versus biventricular support

The purpose of short-term MCS devices is to provide "bridge to recovery," that is, support the myocardium until recovery. Short-term MCS devices are most often used in *acute* CS, as in postcardiotomy shock, inability to wean from CPB, acute myocardial infarction, high-risk percutaneous coronary intervention, ablation of refractory ventricular fibrillation/tachycardia, fulminant myocarditis, and postcardiac arrest.

In contrast, durable MCS devices such as the Heartmate II and III LV assist devices (LVADs) are used to provide "bridge to transplantation" in patients with end-stage or advanced HF who are awaiting heart transplantation (bridge to transplantation) and "destination therapy" in those patients who do not qualify for heart transplantation but need long-term MCS.

Nondurable or short-term MCS devices help stabilize patients with acute CS allowing for decision making regarding need for long-term, durable MCS or heart transplantation. Short-term MCS are categorized by the ventricle assisted:

1. LV assistance: IABP (Intra-aortic balloon pump), Impella (2.5, CP, 5 and 5.5), Tandem Heart (TH)
2. RV assistance: Impella RP, TH Right Atrium-Pulmonary Artery and percutaneous right ventricular assist device (pRVAD)
3. Biventricular assistance: VA ECMO (venous-arterial extracorporeal membrane oxygenation), combinations of LV-RV Impella devices, LV Impella and TH RA-PA or pRVAD devices

Below is a brief summary on commonly used MCS devices: IABP, LV Impella, and VA ECMO and durable LVADs.[45,46]

IABP: It consists of a 25-cm long, sausage-shaped balloon composed of nonthrombogenic polyurethane mounted on a 90-cm vascular catheter; helium gas is used for inflating and deflating the balloon. It uses the principle of synchronized counter-pulsation: blood volume is moved in a direction "counter" to normal flow to assist the beating heart (Fig. 39-9). Electrocardiographic signals trigger inflation and deflation. The balloon is inflated during diastole (T wave–P wave interval) and deflated during systole (R wave–T wave interval). Balloon inflation elevates aortic diastolic blood pressure (diastolic augmentation) increasing the coronary perfusion gradient and pushes blood distally; presystolic balloon deflation lowers systemic diastolic pressure facilitating LV ejection. Imprecise timing of balloon deflation reduces effectiveness of the device. As other devices provide more robust cardiac output augmentation and decreases in LVEDP, the use of IABP is declining.[47,48]

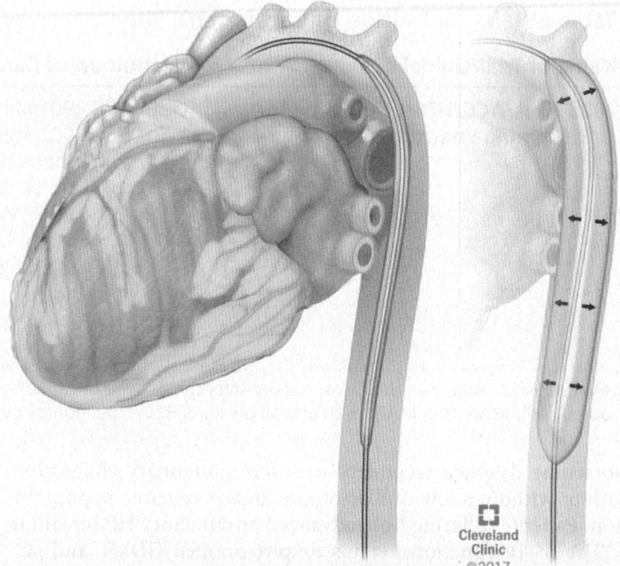

Figure 39-9 IABP deflates at commencement of systole (left) and inflates at beginning of diastole (right). (Reprinted with permission, Cleveland Clinic Foundation © 2022. All Rights Reserved.)

LV Impella: The basic design incorporates a continuous, nonpulsatile, axial flow: an Archimedes screw pump aspirates LV blood and expels it into the aorta, allowing for immediate unloading, as well as, near ideal conditions for recovery of the failing LV (Fig. 39-10). In addition, decreases in LVEDP and LV wall tension minimize $M\dot{V}O_2$ and increases in MAP, cardiac output, and coronary perfusion improve systemic perfusion. Effective LV unloading

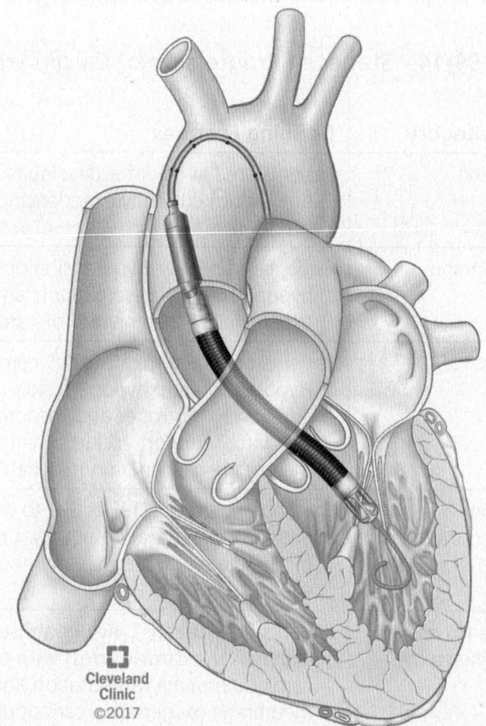

Figure 39-10 Impella device decompresses the left ventricle by withdrawing blood from the cavity and ejecting it into the ascending aorta. (Reprinted with permission, Cleveland Clinic Foundation © 2022. All Rights Reserved.)

also decreases pulmonary venous pressures and pulmonary vascular resistance, boosting RV function and potentially biventricular synchrony. In contrast to IABP support, Impella assistance is independent of cardiac rhythm and augments cardiac output regardless of the severity of tachyarrhythmias. Extent of cardiac flow augmentation is also much greater compared to IABP support.[49]

VA ECMO: VA ECMO provides biventricular support and can be employed centrally or peripherally. In peripheral VA ECMO, the femoral or internal jugular vein is accessed with a cannula (venous inflow) to aspirate blood from the venous system which is then circulated via a nonpulsatile centrifugal pump through a membrane oxygenator-heater and returned to the systemic arterial vasculature via cannulas in a femoral or axillary artery (Fig. 39-11). Unlike the Impella devices that augment cardiac flow and output in a physiologic anterograde manner, circulatory support with VA ECMO is a nonphysiologic retrograde perfusion technique. Consequently, institution of VA ECMO often raises total peripheral resistance, increases LV wall tension and can lead to paradoxical elevation of LVEDP. Such changes can potentially worsen subendocardial myocardial ischemia, hinder recovery of the failing LV, reduce LV contractility, and precipitate cardiogenic pulmonary edema. Pooling of blood in the compromised LV can lead to formation of an intracavitary thrombus. To prevent these complications, LV venting is utilized via surgical or percutaneous vent placement or use of IABP and Impella devices in conjunction with VA ECMO.[50]

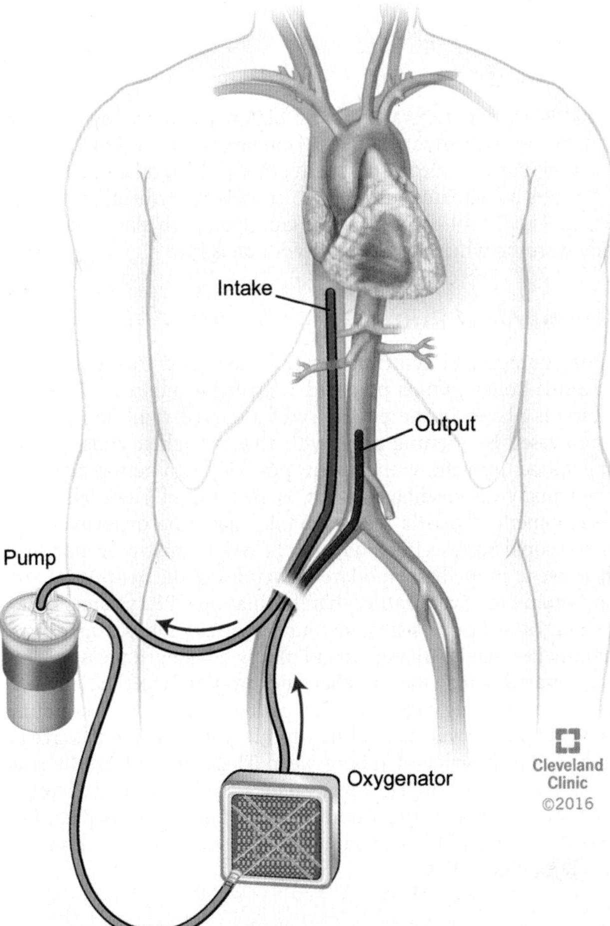

Figure 39-11 In VA ECMO, deoxygenated blood is removed from the inferior vena cava, oxygenated and then propelled into the aorta with the help of a centrifugal pump. (Reprinted with permission, Cleveland Clinic Foundation © 2022. All Rights Reserved.)

For extracorporeal cardiopulmonary resuscitation (ECPR) VA ECMO is established within 20 minutes of cardiac arrest. Other MCS devices are not suitable for use in cardiac arrest patients with inability to achieve return of spontaneous circulation (ROSC).[51]

Complications associated with use of MCS devices include hemolysis, bleeding, infection, thrombocytopenia, and distal limb ischemia when femoral or axillary arterial access is established.

Long-Term or Durable Left Ventricular Assist Devices

Durable LVADs provide long-term MCS for "bridge to transplantation" and "destination therapy." The current devices provide nonpulsatile continuous systemic flow via a centrifugal pump (third-generation devices: Heart Ware, Heartmate III) or an axial pump (second-generation device: Heartmate II). Unlike axial pumps, centrifugal pumps minimize the use of mechanical pivot bearings. This decreases pump mechanical damage, hemolysis, and potential for thrombus formation in the device. CPB is used for device insertion to minimize hemodynamic instability and optimize the surgical field. An inflow connection allows blood from the LV to be pumped by the centrifugal or axial LVAD pump into the ascending aorta via an outflow connection. The pump contains an impeller or rotatory blade that is magnetically assisted; rotations of this blade create flow from LV into the ascending aorta.

Nonpulsatile flow attenuates systolic and diastolic components of arterial pressure; consequently, MAP is monitored to determine adequacy of end-organ perfusion. Overall flow is governed by interplay between preload (LV pressure) and afterload (MAP). Low MAP leads to hypoperfusion while high MAP decreases flow and is associated with adverse neurologic events. Suggested optimal MAP in these patients ranges from 70 to 90 mmHg. Importantly, adequacy of LV preload depends upon RV function. Deterioration of RV function from increased pulmonary vascular resistance, ischemia, arrhythmias or tamponade will impede LV filling. As the LV cavity is continuously emptied by the LVAD pump, poor LV filling leads to suctioning of the interventricular septum at the inflow connection ("suction event"). In addition to causing ventricular irritability, suction events compromise effective RV ejection due to mechanical distortion of the interventricular septum. Thus, effective LVAD functioning depends upon optimization of RV function, LV preload and afterload. Inotropic agents such as epinephrine, dobutamine, and milrinone as well as inhaled agents such as nitric oxide and iloprost are often used to support the RV and help maintain low PVR. Warfarin and aspirin are often commenced in LVAD patients to prevent pump thrombosis and stroke. Major noncardiac surgery necessitates discontinuation of anticoagulation and perioperative heparin bridging in these patients. Other pertinent anesthetic considerations are described in Table 39-15.[52–54]

Cardiopulmonary Bypass

CPB circuitry replaces heart and lung function during cardiac surgery to:

1. Provide a bloodless and motionless surgical field
2. Oxygenate and ventilate
3. Maintain organ perfusion and oxygen delivery
4. Manage temperature including hypothermia for organ protection during surgery and rewarming prior to weaning from CPB
5. Provide inhalational or intravenous anesthesia

Table 39-15 Patients with Durable Left Ventricular Assist Device presenting for Noncardiac Surgery: Anesthetic Considerations

- Communicate with Heart Failure/LVAD team to ascertain type of LVAD, baseline parameters, anticoagulation status and presence of device-related complications.
- Consider invasive arterial blood pressure monitoring, central venous access if duration of procedure is long, involves laparoscopic or thoracoscopic insufflation and/or major bleeding or fluid shifts.
- A PAC and/or TEE monitoring should be considered in patients with poor RV function
- Use warming devices to maintain normothermia.
- Hemodynamic goals: MAP in the 70–90 mmHg range, optimal RV and LV filling.
- Adequacy of perfusion can be assessed by cerebral oximetry monitoring or measuring serial serum lactate levels and/or mixed venous oxygen saturation.
- Minimize PVR: Avoid hypoxemia, hypercarbia and high intrathoracic pressures during mechanical ventilation.
- Support RV function: Inotropic agents such as epinephrine, dobutamine, and milrinone as well as inhaled agents such as nitric oxide, epoprostenol, and iloprost are helpful.
- Anesthesia induction and maintenance often requires judicious and reduced doses of anesthetic drugs; intravenous drugs may take longer to act.
- Bleeding related to anticoagulation with heparin and MCS induced hemolysis and/or thrombocytopenia may necessitate packed red blood cell transfusions.
- Thromboelastography/metry guides need for transfusion of platelets, cryoprecipitate, and fresh frozen.
- Acute hemodynamic instability may be due to inadequate volume resuscitation, suction events, acute RV failure, malfunctioning of MCS device, cardiac tamponade, superimposed sepsis, severe ARDS, pneumothorax, and/or ongoing bleeding.
- Consider anticoagulation status prior to instituting central neuraxial or regional blockade.

ARDS, acute respiratory distress syndrome; LV, left ventricle; LVAD, left ventricular assist device; MAP, mean arterial pressure; MCS, mechanical circulatory support; PAC, pulmonary artery catheter; PVR, pulmonary vascular resistance; RV, right ventricle; TEE, transesophageal echocardiography.

Basic components of CPB circuitry include venous drainage cannulae, a reservoir for collecting venous blood, a mechanical pump to propel the blood, an oxygenator, heat exchanger, arterial filter (to trap debris), and arterial return cannula. Additional components such as delivery set to administer cardioplegia, cannulae for venting, external cardiotomy reservoir to collect shed blood and a hemoconcentrator are often added. CPB circuitry also includes inline blood gas monitoring capability, volatile agent vaporizers, and warning monitors (Fig. 39-12, 5 Video 39-5, 6 Video 39-6).[36,55–57]

Venous Cannulae and Cannulation Strategies

Venous cannulas drain blood from the SVC, IVC, RA, and coronary sinus into the venous reservoir. Cavae are cannulated with "dual or multistage" cannula or individual "single-stage" cannulae. Dual- or multistage cannulae have multiple apertures embedded into a single cannula and are employed when surgery (CABG, AV, and/or aortic surgery) does not necessitate opening of the RA and consequently, risk of air entrainment is minimal. Cannula kinking may occur during surgery when the surgeon rotates the heart, and this impedes drainage. Bicaval cannulation is necessary whenever surgery necessitates incising the RA (mitral and tricuspid valve). Smaller cannulae with shorter lengths help to decrease the need for using large volumes of prime solution and minimized hemodilution. Alternative approaches for venous drainage include cannulation of the (typically right) femoral vein and advancing a multi-stage cannula into the SVC (under TEE guidance). This is often employed during minimally invasive cardiac surgery (MICS) where the heart is approached through a thoracotomy rather than a sternotomy or when there is a high risk of accidentally entering the heart during sternotomy as may occur during re-do cardiac surgery. Complications associated with venous cannulation include bleeding, arrhythmias, and malposition that may result in venous congestion and inadequate venous drainage.

Venous Reservoir

Blood is drained via gravity into a high-capacitance low-pressure venous reservoir situated 40 to 70 cm below the level of the heart. Vacuum may be added to augment gravity-aided drainage. Venous reservoirs are situated just before the CPB mechanical pump, can accept 4 to 5 L of blood, and are equipped with alarms that provide warning when the reservoir volume is low.

Mechanical Pumps

Roller pumps and centrifugal pumps are used to propel blood forward. Roller pumps predated centrifugal pumps; a length of tubing is placed in the periphery of a curved rigid housing and compressed by rotating arms with rollers at their ends, propelling blood forward without the possibility of retrograde flow. Their many disadvantages, such as shearing of blood elements, development of plastic micro emboli, cavitation or formation of microscopic bubbles in blood, and the risk for disconnection limit their use to propelling blood from suctioning and venting into the cardiotomy reservoir, rather than facilitating CPB systemic flow.

Centrifugal pumps are constrained vortex pumps consisting of an impeller that is situated a rigid plastic housing; a pressure drop is generated across the impeller and propels blood radially outward in a centrifugal fashion. They are associated with less trauma to blood cells, lower risk of line rupture, lower risk of massive air emboli, and absence of tubing wear. These are universally used for CPB systemic flow. However, an increase in afterload decreases flow output of centrifugal pumps and a flow meter is placed on the arterial side of the CPB circuit to assess adequacy of flow (see also 7 Video 39-7).

Oxygenators

Oxygenators are the "lungs" of the CPB circuitry: they transfer oxygen to and remove carbon dioxide from venous blood. In the 1980s, bubble oxygenators were predominantly used; gas exchange was

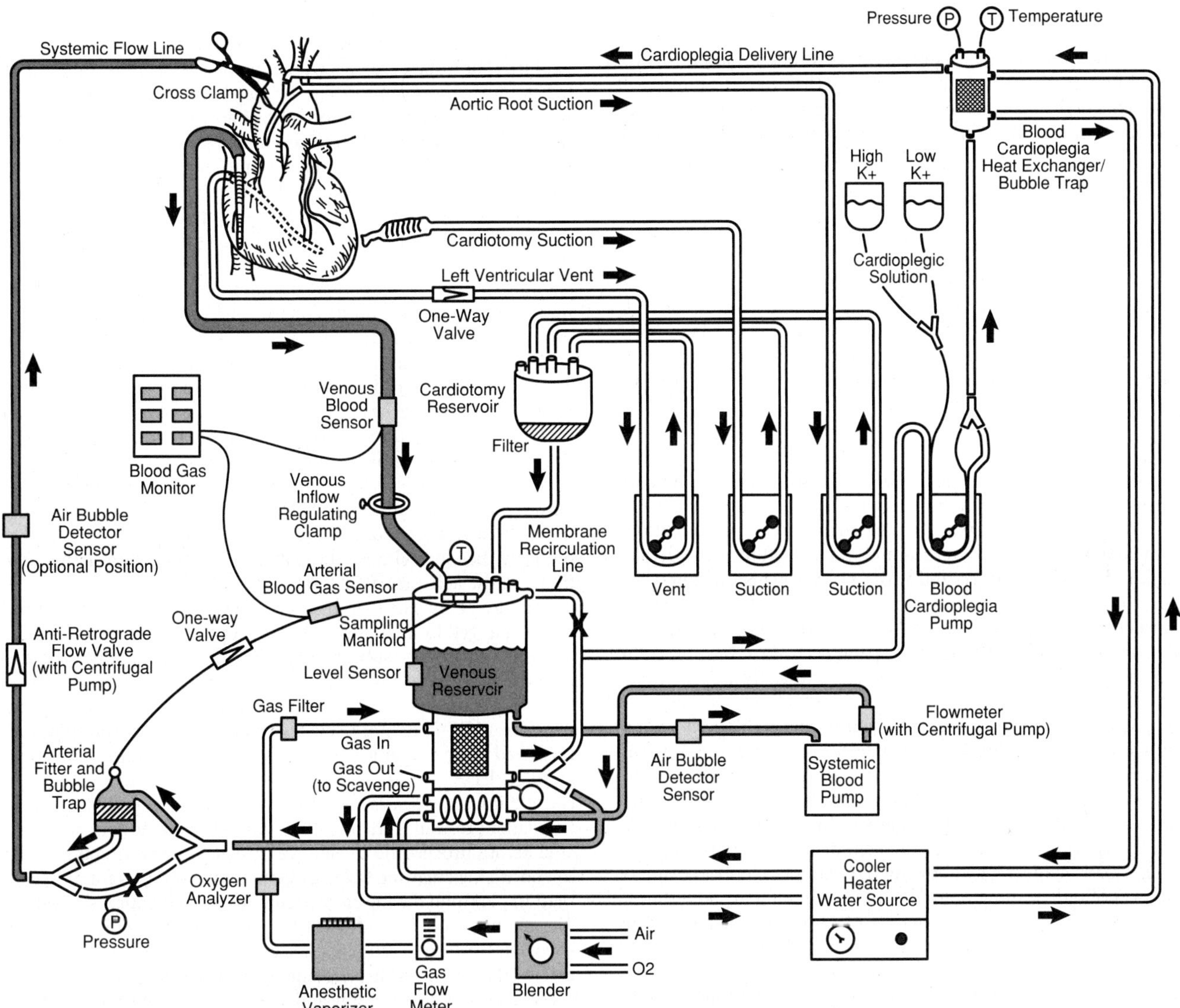

Figure 39-12 Cardiopulmonary bypass circuitry. (Reproduced with permission from Barry AE, Chaney MA, London MJ. Anesthetic management during cardiopulmonary bypass: a systematic review. *Anesth Analg*. 2015;120(4):749–769.)

effected by bubbling oxygen through blood. However, this resulted in increased destruction of blood elements and risked formation of microbubbles and air emboli. Membrane oxygenators have replaced bubble oxygenators in contemporary clinical practice. They consist of bundles of hollow-fiber capillaries of microporous polypropylene contained within a plastic housing. The blood flows externally around the bundles while the fresh gas flow is blown through the hollow bundles. As the blood and gas phases are separated by a thin membrane, gas exchange occurs via simple diffusion similar to native lungs. The partial pressure of arterial oxygen can be changed by varying the FiO_2 while the rate of carbon dioxide removal can be altered by varying the total gas flow or "sweep rate." Volatile anesthetics move freely into blood across these oxygenators and can be used to maintain anesthesia during CPB.

Heat Exchangers

Heater–cooler units or exchangers are counter-current devices to circulate heated or cooled water around the fibers of the oxygenator to maintain a precise temperature.

Arterial Cannulae and Cannulation Strategies

Arterial cannulation returns oxygenated, temperature-controlled blood from the CPB machine to the systemic circulation. The ascending aorta is typically cannulated (central approach). Alternative sites are used if the ascending aorta has palpable plaques or significant atheroma burden is identified with epiaortic ultrasound or if the RV or aorta are abutting the sternum in redo surgeries. Such sites are femoral, subclavian, axillary, or innominate arteries (peripheral approach). Common femoral artery is often cannulated during MICS, AD surgery, and when there is a need for emergent establishment of CPB.

Mechanical complications associated with aortic cannulation include plaque dislodgement with embolization, dissection, and malpositioning. AD after institution of CPB is diagnosed from low systemic arterial pressure, high arterial line pressure (>300 mmHg) in the CPB circuitry, loss of venous drainage, and bluish discoloration of the aorta. TEE can help corroborate the diagnosis.

Arterial Line Filter and Pressure Monitor

Before the oxygenated, temperature-controlled blood is propelled into the systemic circulation (via the arterial cannula), it passes through an arterial line filter to help trap gaseous and nongaseous (tissue debris, thrombi, and fat particles) emboli. Arterial line pressure is monitored proximal to this filter to detect occlusion of the filter.

Ancillary Components

Ancillary components include roller pumps to deliver temperature-controlled cardioplegia, vent and decompress the LV, provide ultrafiltration/hemoconcentration to remove excess water (thus increasing the patient's hematocrit), as well as suction the shed mediastinal blood into the main venous reservoir after filtering it.

Pump Prime

Priming solutions fill and de-air the CPB circuit. There is no consensus on an optimal priming solution; local tradition often dictates its composition. Crystalloid based solutions with additions such as albumin (to decrease fluid extravasation and edema), mannitol (diuretic effect), and various electrolytes including calcium (to prevent hypocalcemia) and magnesium (antiarrhythmic effect) are used. Heparin is added for anticoagulation. The volume of priming solution is based on the patient's body surface area; the average prime volume for adults is approximately 1.5 L. Hemodilution from priming solutions decreases blood viscosity and may help counteract the effect of hypothermia on blood flow during CPB. However, dilutional anemia decreases oxygen-carrying capacity and blood may be added to maintain a sufficient hematocrit on CPB especially in children, small adults, and anemic patients. In adults, the target hematocrit for CPB ranges from 21% to 24%. Autologous priming may help decrease the priming volume. This is achieved by allowing the patient's blood to displace the crystalloid priming solution in the circuit into an external reservoir in a retrograde manner ("RAP or retrograde autologous priming"). The external reservoir is then excluded from the CPB circuitry. Priming volume can be substantially decreased with use of mini extracorporeal CPB circuits with shorter tubing lengths (80 to 150 cm), allowing for reduction of priming volume to around 0.5 to 0.8 L. The reduction in surface area and priming volume helps decrease blood usage during CPB.[57]

Anticoagulation

Systemic anticoagulation is required prior to cannulation and initiation of CPB as contact between the patient's blood and CPB components activates the coagulation cascade. In the absence of anticoagulation, wide spread thrombosis would ensue. Unfractionated heparin is the anticoagulant of choice for CPB given its reliable action and ease of reversal with protamine. It is an indirect anticoagulant, which inhibits the coagulation cascade by binding to antithrombin III (AT) via a specific pentasaccharide sequence. Heparin binding results in a 1,000-fold stronger AT inhibition on thrombin (IIa) and factor Xa, thereby fibrin clot is unable to form.[58]

Prior to CPB initiation, heparin is typically injected intravenously in doses ranging from 300 to 500 units/kg (heparinization). Its peak onset of action is <5 minutes and systemic anticoagulation is achieved rapidly. Its half-life is approximately 90 minutes under normothermic conditions and progressively increases during hypothermic states.

The anticoagulant effect of heparin is monitored via point-of-care tests, such as activated clotting time (ACT) and/or blood-heparin concentrations. ACT requires addition of whole blood to tubes containing contact phase activators (celite or kaolin). The tubes are subsequently rotated and the time taken for clot formation is measured. In the absence of heparin, normal ACT values range from 80 to 160 seconds. In general, ACTs >400 to 480 seconds are considered acceptable for the initiation of CPB. In addition to heparin, ACT is often prolonged by factors such as hypothermia, hemodilution, severe thrombocytopenia, and hypo- or dysfibrinogenemia. In contrast, acquired or congenital deficiency of AT may result in failure of achieving target ACT values despite administration of large doses of heparin (>600 units/kg).[59] Administration of commercially available plasma-derived or recombinant AT concentrate (up to 1,000 units) may be necessary in such circumstances to achieve target ACT values.

Heparin concentrations that are safe for CPB vary from 3 to 3.5 IU/mL. This can be determined with an automated method, by adding known doses of protamine to a heparinized sample of blood sequentially, until the optimum dose of protamine that produces a clot in the shortest amount of time is determined.

Partial thromboplastin time (PTT) cannot differentiate between a safe and unsafe level of heparin anticoagulation during CPB; heparin blood concentration >1 IU/mL causes the sampled blood to become almost incapable of clotting within the time frame of the activated PTT test.

Allergy to heparin or history of heparin-induced thrombocytopenia (HIT) may necessitate using alternative anticoagulants. There are two subtypes of HIT. HIT-I is generally mild and characterized by a transient decrease in platelet count following heparin administration, typically within first few days of heparin exposure. HIT-II is more severe, characterized by autoimmune-mediated platelet count decrease due to the formation of platelet factor (PF) 4/heparin antibodies that activate platelets and can cause clinically devastating thrombosis. In these patients, it may be prudent to wait until anti-PF4 antibodies are no longer detectable before proceeding to elective cardiac surgery. It is important to consult vascular medicine or hematology services for anticoagulation planning during cardiac surgery in such patients. Bivalirudin and argatroban are direct thrombin inhibitors and have been successfully used to establish safe anticoagulation in patients with active HIT who need urgent/emergent cardiac surgery. The use of these agents is uncommon and the reader is advised to consult one of the several reviews on this subject.[60]

Blood Conservation in Cardiac Surgery

Although transfusion of blood and its components is often necessary and life-saving during cardiac surgery, it is critical to emphasize that these resources are finite, expensive, and not risk-free (infection, incompatibility reactions, transfusion error, TRALI, TACO). Patient blood management is focused on managing anemia, optimizing coagulation status and includes blood conservation strategies to facilitate rational transfusion practices. Preoperative identification of patients at high risk (advanced age, presence of preoperative anemia and abnormal coagulation status) who may need perioperative transfusions is encouraged. Iron deficiency should prompt therapy with supplemental iron days to weeks prior to elective cardiac surgery. Patients who refuse blood transfusions or suffer from non–iron deficiency anemia may benefit from preoperative therapy with erythropoietin-stimulating agents with or without iron supplementation. Patients on dual antiplatelet therapy, warfarin or novel anticoagulants need clear instructions on timing of stopping these medications to minimize the risk of intraoperative bleeding from medication-related coagulation dysfunction. Laboratory or point-of-care testing may help determine residual effect of such anticlotting medications prior to surgery. Activation of fibrinolytic pathways during cardiac surgery with or without CPB, increases perioperative bleeding. Synthetic antifibrinolytic agents such as epsilon-aminocaproic acid (EACA) and tranexamic acid inhibit fibrinolysis by binding to plasminogen and blocking its ability to bind lysine residues of fibrinogen. Intraoperative use of EACA and tranexamic acid is associated with decreased post-CPB bleeding and transfusion needs.

Negative effects of CPB include activation of the coagulation cascade, consumption of clotting factors, and platelet dysfunction. Acute normovolemic hemodilution (ANH) entails removing 1 to 2 units of whole blood from a patient prior to systemic heparinization and CPB, and is a reasonable method to decrease bleeding and transfusion risk by excluding a portion of the patient's blood from the effects of CPB. Returning this blood post-CPB helps mitigate coagulopathy by providing active platelets and functional coagulation factors. However, this technique may not be suitable in all patients as withdrawal of patient's blood and replacement with crystalloid solution can itself precipitate anemia and a potential supply/demand mismatch. Consequently, caution is advised in patients with preoperative anemia, high-grade left main coronary artery disease, severe aortic stenosis, and hemodynamically unstable patients.

Preservation of adequate hematocrit during CPB, may necessitate combining ANH with retrograde autologous priming (RAP). RAP is achieved by allowing the patient's blood to displace the crystalloid priming solution in the CPB circuit into an external reservoir in a retrograde manner. Hypotension during this maneuver may necessitate treatment with vasoconstrictors or application of Trendelenburg positioning. Although the practice of RAP is not associated with improvements in mortality, it helps decrease CPB-related hemodilution and reduces extravascular lung water in cardiac surgical patients. Similar to RAP, reductions in priming volume can be achieved with using minimally invasive extracorporeal circulation (MiECC) systems that incorporate shorter tubing and closed CPB circuits to reduce blood transfusions. Pursuing a restrictive threshold for RBC transfusion (≤7.5 g/dL) and using viscoelastic tests such as thromboelastography or rotational thromboelastometry to guide blood component therapy helps conserve blood without jeopardizing patient safety.

Transfusion of cell-salvaged blood is another key method of intraoperative blood conservation in cardiac surgery. Following processing, units of shed mediastinal blood may have hematocrits of as high as 70%. However, platelets and coagulation factors are removed in the washing process during cell salvage. Thus, while reinfusion of cell-salvaged blood may decrease need for RBC transfusions, it does not mitigate coagulopathy. Absolute contraindications to the use of intraoperative cell salvage include admixture of blood with topical hemostatic agents, sterile water or toxic solutions such as alcohol, hydrogen peroxide or povidone-iodine. Its use in infection and malignancy is decided on a case-to-case basis.

Removing excess fluid via modified ultrafiltration is another technique used in conjunction with CPB to reduce postoperative bleeding and transfusion needs. It employs a semipermeable membrane, and the hydrostatic pressure differential across it separates plasma water from low–molecular-weight solutes, intravascular cell components, and plasma proteins, leading to hemoconcentration. In addition, this technique may also help decrease levels of circulating inflammatory mediators.[61,62]

Myocardial Protection

Myocardial protection of the heart from ischemic damage during CPB is achieved via: institution of hypothermia, induction of cardioplegia to facilitate arrest, and decompression of the LV; the goal is to minimize myocardial metabolic function.

For each degree centigrade reduction in temperature below 37°C, cellular metabolism decreases by approximately 8%; at 28°C the metabolic rate falls to 50%. While most cardiac surgeries are performed with mild (>28°C) or moderate (20° to 28°C) systemic hypothermia, some surgeries such as aortic arch replacement or pulmonary endarterectomy require deep (<20°C) hypothermia. Systemic hypothermia provides myocardial and neurologic protection during cardiac surgery by reducing oxygen consumption, preserving high-energy phosphate substrates, and inhibiting excitatory neurotransmitter release.

In addition to systemic hypothermia, topical myocardial cooling is achieved by bathing the heart with cold (ice) solution and infusing cold (10° to 15°C), hyperkalemic (8 to 20 mEq/L) cardioplegia solution. Cardioplegia solutions are either crystalloid or blood-crystalloid solutions with a supranormal concentration of potassium that precipitate diastolic cardiac arrest when injected into the coronary vasculature. These solutions can be infused into the coronary vessels antegrade, retrograde, or a combination of both. In antegrade application, cardioplegia is delivered proximal to the aortic cross-clamp, into the aortic root at a pressure of 60 to 100 mmHg or directly into the coronary ostia if significant AI or coronary artery disease is present. In the retrograde application, a catheter is placed inside the coronary sinus and cardioplegia is delivered (200 to 400 mL/min) to a venous pressure of 30 to 50 mmHg. Retrograde cardioplegia is often used in combination with antegrade to maximize myocardial protection especially in patients with severe coronary artery disease, when the presence of obstructive plaques can limit antegrade spread of cardioplegia. In addition, during coronary artery bypass surgery, use of individual grafts to deliver cardioplegia after completion of the distal anastomoses may help maximize myocardial protection. Cold cardioplegia is typically administered every 20 to 30 minutes but single shot administration, especially of the del Nido solution (1 part of blood + 4 parts of crystalloid + additives including lidocaine, magnesium sulfate, sodium bicarbonate, mannitol, and potassium chloride) in cases of anticipated short aortic cross clamp times is also reasonable. Warm/tepid (normothermic) cardioplegia can also be employed, and has been associated with better postoperative cardiac indices. Unlike cold cardioplegia, normothermic cardioplegia needs to be delivered continuously. Arrest of cardiac activity typically occurs within minutes (30 to 60 seconds with antegrade application, 2 to 4 minutes with retrograde delivery) of cardioplegia delivery. Washout of cardioplegia over time, leads to resumption of electrical activity.

Lastly, it is important to make sure that the LV is being appropriately vented during CPB. This can be easily monitored with TEE. LV distension increases wall tension and oxygen consumption, leading to poor myocardial protection. Vigilance is recommended, especially in patients with severe AI in whom the leaky valve may allow the antegrade cardioplegia to seep into the LV cavity instead of the coronary ostia. LV distension and lack of rapid electrical arrest ensue under such conditions.[36,55–57]

Preoperative and Intraoperative Management

Preoperative Considerations

Preoperative visits are important for decision making. A multidisciplinary approach is important and the following steps need to be executed:

1. Performance of a thorough history and physical examination.
2. Assessment of current comorbidities, need for further optimization, and confirmation of primary cardiac diagnosis.

The time frame between the visit and proposed surgical date and whether further optimization will affect outcomes are important to consider.
3. Detailed review of prior testing and assessment for additional investigations.
4. Detailed review of and clear instructions to patients regarding perioperative medication management. Most cardiovascular medications are continued until the day of surgery including aspirin and β-blockers for CABG surgery. Certain guidelines advocate for discontinuing RAAS blockers (ACEIs, ARBs, ARNIs) prior to cardiac surgery. As institutional practices vary, the reader is encouraged to consult authoritative published resources.[63,64] Without appropriate perioperative management of ongoing anticoagulant therapy, unnecessary delay of surgical care may occur. Consequently, discontinuation of oral anticoagulants (such as apixaban, dabigatran, fondaparinux, and warfarin) and perioperative bridging in patients on warfarin therapy, should be clearly communicated to patients, as well as surgical teams.[65,66]
5. Assessment of current electrophysiologic therapies such as CIEDs or MCS devices such as LVADs.
6. Evaluation of perioperative risk for complications, morbidity and mortality. EuroScore and Society of Thoracic Surgeons risk calculators, two popular validated tools, help assess these parameters.
7. Initiation of conversations regarding goals of care, advanced directives, and end of life decisions.
8. Identification of factors that may affect perioperative care such as heparin or protamine allergy, difficulty in obtaining blood for transfusion purposes due to antibodies, history of or anticipated difficult airway management, contraindications to performing TEE, presence of central venous stenosis that may complicate placement of central access devices and presence of severe peripheral arterial disease that may influence the choice of MCS if needed.
9. Elicitation of patient and family concerns with regard to their anesthetic and perioperative management. The anesthetic plan should be explained and informed consent obtained.
10. Discussion of expectations regarding postoperative pain with exploration of multimodal analgesia and regional blocks as components of pain management.

Premedication and Anxiolysis

Premedication alleviates patient anxiety and helps improve patient experience. Selection of drug and dosage depends on the patient's age, hemodynamic state, level of distress, and location. We would also like to emphasize the important role of empathy-based communication for allaying patients' fears and worries. In contemporary practice settings, patients typically receive minimal or no sedation until completion of regulatory paperwork and performance of a multidisciplinary huddle that utilizes a surgical safety checklist to ensure patient safety. Thereafter, sedation is employed prior to placing preinduction invasive lines. Optimal levels of sedation (mild to moderate) help alleviate hypertension, tachycardia, and/or coronary vasospasm. However, deep levels of sedation are best avoided, especially in hemodynamically tenuous patients who may be keenly susceptible to myocardial depressant effects of anxiolytic drugs.

Monitoring

Various monitoring modalities used during anesthetic care have been described extensively in Chapter 26. Standard ASA monitoring (pulse oximetry, electrocardiography, and noninvasive arterial blood pressure monitoring) should be established when patients arrive in the operating room.

Electrocardiogram

A 5 electrode configuration (left-arm, left-leg, precordial, right-arm, and right-leg) is employed intraoperatively to provide electrocardiographic information including heart rate, rhythm, and presence of ischemia. Leads V5 and II are selected for display as monitoring these leads allows for detection of arrhythmias, as well as approximately 90% of all ischemic episodes.

ECG changes in specific leads can broadly help localize the region of the heart experiencing ischemia and/or the affected arterial territory as follows:

Leads I, aVL, V5, and V6 (lateral LV wall); left circumflex and/or left anterior descending territory (LAD).

Leads II, III, and aVF (inferior LV wall); right coronary artery territory.

Leads V1 to V4 (anteroseptal and anterior LV wall); LAD territory.

Temperature

During CPB patients are often allowed to drift to mild–moderate hypothermia and then rewarmed after completion of surgical repair. Temperature is monitored at various sites to characterize the patient's thermal condition. Common temperature monitoring sites include core sites, such as bladder, nasopharynx, tympanum and pulmonary artery, and peripheral sites, such as skin and rectum; the latter often lag behind core temperature and are rarely useful.[67,68]

Arterial Blood Pressure

Invasive arterial monitoring during cardiac surgery is from the radial, femoral, brachial, and axillary arteries. Criteria for determining the site of arterial catheterization include accessibility, convenience, lack of proximal stenosis, rate of complications, and avoidance of the dominant hand. Equally important is to accommodate surgical needs. For example, if in a right-hand dominant patient undergoing CABG the surgical plan includes using the left radial artery as an arterial conduit, the right brachial or radial artery should be catheterized. Similarly, right brachial or radial artery is preferentially catheterized in patients undergoing procedures involving the descending thoracic aorta because the left subclavian artery may be included in the proximal aortic clamp.

Brachial arterial catheterization is rarely associated with complications.[69] Post-CPB, radial artery pressure may under-represent central aortic pressure substantially; the pressure discrepancy may be as much as 30 mmHg. The mechanism remains unclear and may be related to decreased radial artery diameter due to fall in arterial elasticity, marked vasoconstriction, or vasospasm.[70] Consequently, when the radial artery is catheterized during cardiac surgery, it is important to consider that post-CPB hypotension may be spurious and related to pressure discrepancy. Although the central aortic pressure can be estimated by direct palpation by the surgeon, direct measurement by either femoral artery catheterization or with a needle placed directly into the aorta are suggested to ensure accurate assessment.

Central Venous Pressure and Pulmonary Artery Catheter

Central venous catheterization in cardiac surgical patients facilitates:

1. Safe infusion of cardioactive drugs
2. Measurement of right atrial (RAP) or central venous pressure (CVP)

3. Analysis of CVP waveform morphology
4. Large volume resuscitation

However, CVP is not an accurate representation of cardiac preload and LV filling pressure, especially in the presence of severe LV failure, pulmonary hypertension, or reduced LV compliance. Pulmonary artery catheterization, overcomes these shortcomings, provides a trove of hemodynamic data (stroke volume, cardiac output, PVR and SVR), allows for mixed venous blood sampling and facilitates hemodynamic management. In addition, PACs with pacing capabilities are useful for providing a reliable rate and rhythm in patients with bradyarrhythmias. Routine PAC use in cardiac surgery varies greatly among institutions and is likely influenced by patient risk factors (low EF, presence of CS or MCS device, and increased risk for vasoplegia), practice type, geographic location, and surgeon preference. Pulmonary artery perforation and infarction are rare, but major complications associated with PAC use and may be related to catheter migration to a distal position in the pulmonary artery, over inflation of the catheter tip balloon or accidentally leaving the balloon inflated at or after insertion. As these complications are associated with significant morbidity and mortality, close attention should be devoted to using the optimal volume of air for balloon inflation and making sure that the balloon is deflated after suitable positioning of the PAC is achieved. Distal migration of the PAC often occurs with cardiac manipulation, and acute preload changes. Consequently, retracting the PAC a few centimeters prior to CPB initiation may help prevent "overwedging" and possible pulmonary artery rupture.[71]

Echocardiography

Currently, perioperative TEE is recommended for all patients undergoing open heart and thoracic aortic surgery. Use of TEE during conventional CABG surgery, is not mandatory but encouraged to refine the preoperative diagnosis, detect new or unsuspected abnormalities and assess the results of the surgical intervention. In elective cardiac surgery, pre-CPB TEE is used to:

1. Confirm the preoperative diagnosis.
2. Evaluate presence of severe aortic atherosclerotic disease that may alter aortic cannulation or aortic cross clamp site.
3. Rule out new findings that may alter surgical plan, such as the presence of a persistent left SVC that may alter the plan for delivery of retrograde cardioplegia.
4. Guide volume resuscitation, especially in circumstances when the ventricles are noncompliant or failing.

Post-CPB, TEE helps assess adequacy of de-airing (open heart surgery), the appropriateness of the surgical intervention, and inadvertent consequences of CPB or surgery (new regional wall motion abnormalities, RV failure from embolism, worsening valvular regurgitation or AD). In addition, as LV compliance worsens after CPB, TEE helps assess ventricular filling. Please see Chapter 27 for a review of TEE applications.[72]

Neurologic Monitoring

Neurologic complications such as stroke, postoperative cognitive dysfunction, and delirium are the second leading cause of morbidity and mortality after cardiac surgery. Along with increased likelihood of long-term care and decreased quality of life, these complications substantially increase cost of care. The goal of neurologic monitoring in cardiac surgery is to assess adequacy of cerebral oxygen delivery, especially during the unique physiologic circumstances created by CPB. Current monitoring techniques include bispectral index monitoring, electroencephalography and assessment of evoked potentials, near-infrared spectroscopy (cerebral oximetry) and less frequently, transcranial Doppler blood flow measurement in the middle cerebral artery. It is unclear whether application of such monitoring decreases the incidence of perioperative neurologic complications.

The etiology of perioperative neurologic complications is believed to be ischemic injury, either related to emboli (air, atheroma, other particulate matter) or cerebral hypoperfusion in susceptible patients (e.g., pre-existing cerebrovascular disease). Ischemic strokes vastly outnumber hemorrhagic strokes in the perioperative setting, tend to be focal and most likely are a consequence of macroembolization. Cognitive dysfunction probably results from microembolization, hypoperfusion, inflammation, and/or silent infarctions. Risk factors for neurologic complications include advanced age (>70 years), pre-existing cerebrovascular disease (e.g., carotid artery stenosis >80%), history of prior stroke, peripheral vascular disease, ascending aortic atheroma, and diabetes. Surgical risk factors that influence neurologic outcomes include the duration of CPB, intracardiac procedure (e.g., valve replacement), aortic pressure, excessive warming during and following CPB, and perioperative hypotension.[73] Intraoperative hyperglycemia, hypoglycemia, and postoperative glycemic variability have been associated with neurocognitive injury.[74–76]

Embolization during cardiac surgery is related to aortic atheroma burden; patients with mobile atheromas are most susceptible. Suggested surgical strategies for patients with severely diseased aortas who are at increased risk of stroke, include performing surgery under hypothermic fibrillatory arrest with LV venting and avoidance of aortic cross-clamping, applying a single cross-clamp (i.e., distal and proximal grafts performed during same cross-clamp), relocation of proximal grafts to an area of nondiseased aorta, no proximal grafts (internal mammary arteries only), using off-pump coronary artery bypass, or hypothermic circulatory arrest with resection and graft replacement of the diseased aortic segment.

Cerebral oximetry, which is based on the Beer-Lambert law and principles of optical spectrometry, has gained widespread clinical acceptance due to ease of application, interpretation of monitoring data, and validated protocols to treat desaturations. Numerical values of regional cerebral saturation ($rScCO_2$) range from 60% to 80%. It is important to get bilateral baseline values, prior to administration of sedative medications and oxygen. An absolute decrease of $rScCO_2$ value to ≤50% or a decrement from the baseline value ≥20% should prompt treatment. Interventions include repositioning of malpositioned CPB cannulae, increasing pump flow, augmenting MAP, altering sweep or ventilation to ensure normocarbia, increasing inspiratory oxygen concentrations to treat hypoxemia, deepening anesthesia level, and transfusing blood to maintain a hemoglobin level ≥8 g/dL. Standardized protocols-based treatment of cerebral oximetry-related desaturations may help decrease the incidence of postoperative cognitive dysfunction after cardiac surgery.[77]

Selection of Anesthetic Drugs

The term *fast-track* in cardiac anesthesia was first introduced by Engelman and associates in 1994, in their article "Fast-Track Recovery of the Coronary Bypass Patient."[78] Improvements in technology and surgical techniques led to a surge in cardiac procedures in the 1990s creating logistical challenges for perioperative teams. Limited availability of operating rooms and ICU space, in conjunction with increased costs associated with cardiac surgical perioperative care prompted a change in anesthesia practice to achieve early extubation and minimize ICU length of stay. This led to abandonment of the high-dose opioid technique that had gained popularity in the 1980s. Although the high-dose opioid technique provided cardiovascular stability, its use was

associated with prolonged mechanical ventilation and increased
6 perioperative resource utilization.[79] Contemporary anesthetic regimens for elective cardiac surgical procedures are comprised of short-acting, fast-emergence drugs to facilitate early tracheal extubation. Induction is with etomidate or propofol and amnesia with volatile anesthetics or propofol-based TIVA. Short-acting benzodiazepines are often used to supplement these anesthetics, especially on CPB. Adequate depth of anesthesia is ensured by an MAC of ≥0.8 pre-CPB; the concentration of the volatile anesthetic can be measured in the exhaust line of the oxygenator during CPB. The depth of anesthesia can be monitored (bispectral index) intraoperatively. Volatile anesthetics are preferred during cardiac surgery and CPB since they have been associated with favorable postoperative morbidity and mortality outcomes. It is important to note that hemodilution during CPB decreases the blood/gas partition coefficient of volatile anesthetics while hypothermia increases it. Consequently, these opposing effects often counterbalance each other during CPB.

Analgesia is typically multimodal and includes: low-dose opioids, regional anesthetic blocks and/or ketamine and lidocaine infusions. Although hemodilution during CPB reduces the total concentration of propofol and opioids, concomitant reduction in protein concentration, often leads to increase in the unbound fraction of these drugs. In addition, hypothermia during CPB decreases drug metabolism via hepatic and renal pathways, leading to prolonged elimination half-lives of these drugs. Interestingly, remifentanil infusions can be decreased by 30% per 5°C drop in temperature during CPB, as its organ-independent elimination is temperature-dependent and decreases with hypothermia. Intermediate-acting muscle relaxants such as rocuronium, vecuronium, atracurium, and cis-atracurium are preferred, with neuromuscular monitoring-guided re-dosing. A rapidly adjustable anesthetic depth should be used to match the varying intensity of surgical stress. Tracheal intubation, skin incision, sternotomy, pericardiotomy, and manipulation of the aorta are events associated with intense stimulation and sympathetic response.[76]

Intraoperative Management

It is important for the anesthesiology team to be familiar with the surgical steps of the intended surgery as this helps anticipate surgical needs and expectations, and to prepare accordingly.

In conventional on-pump CABG, saphenous vein grafts and the internal mammary artery are used as conduits to "bypass" a stenosed epicardial coronary artery. Postinduction, the patient's chest and legs are prepped. The approach to the heart and IMA is via a median sternotomy. The IMA can be mobilized in a pedicled manner (proximal origin from the subclavian artery is kept intact) or it can be transected and used as a "free graft." Low tidal volume ventilation as well as frequent ventilation "holds" may be needed to optimize exposure during harvesting. The saphenous vein grafts are harvested by another surgical team/member simultaneously. Subsequently, heparin is administered centrally and a sample of blood (arterial or venous) is drawn 3 minutes later. Adequacy of anticoagulation (ACT > 400 to 480 seconds) is confirmed and the aorta and atria are cannulated. Prior to aortic cannulation, the surgical team will palpate the aorta to assess calcification. Absence of atheroma may be confirmed with precannulation epiaortic ultrasound scanning as it is important to cannulate the aorta in a nonatheromatous segment to decrease perioperative stroke. The perfusionist and surgeon assess appropriateness of cannulation prior to commencing CPB, followed by the surgeon placing an aortic cross clamp (typically in the distal ascending aorta) and delivery of antegrade cardioplegia, with or without retrograde cardioplegia to arrest the heart and provide cardiac standstill in a bloodless field. CABG entails performing distal and proximal anastomoses; distal anastomoses involve suturing the IMA or saphenous vein graft to the target diseased vessel. After completion of the proximal anastomoses (attaching the graft to the ascending aorta), the aortic cross clamp is removed, and the heart is allowed to beat. Alternatively, a partially occluding aortic cross clamp is applied to facilitate construction of the proximal anastomoses. The patient is subsequently weaned off CPB, decannulated and heparin anticoagulation is reversed with protamine. Successful grafting is proven by measuring conduit flow via a transit-time flowmeter. Indices such as mean graft flow (>20 mL/min) and pulsatility index (ideally <3, acceptable <5) indicate patency and quality of grafting.[80,81]

Preparation

A checklist-based approach to prepare the operating room prior to arrival of the patient should be utilized (Table 39-16) to standardize organization and resources across different teams. Heparin

Table 39-16 Anesthetic Preparation for Cardiac Surgery
Anesthesia Machine
Routine check
Airway
Nasal cannula for O_2
Ventilation/intubation equipment, including difficult airway devices
Suction
Inspired gas humidifier
Circulatory Access
Catheters (peripheral and central venous and arterial access)
Intravenous fluids and infusion tubing and pumps
Fluids warmer
Monitors
Standard ASA: ECG leads, blood pressure cuff, pulse oximeter, neuromuscular blockade monitor
Temperature probes (nasal, tympanic, bladder, rectal)
Transducers (arterial, pulmonary, and central venous pressure) zeroed and functioning
Cardiac output computer: Proper constant inserted
Awareness monitor (BIS)
Anticoagulation (ACT) monitor(s)
Recorder/printer
Medications
General anesthetic: hypnotic/induction, amnestic/benzodiazepine, volatile, opioid, muscle relaxant
Heparin (predrawn)
Cardioactive
• Predrawn: nitroglycerin/nicardipine, $CaCl_2$, phenylephrine/ephedrine, epinephrine
• Infusions: nitroglycerin, inotrope
Antibiotics
Miscellaneous
Pacemaker with battery
Defibrillator/cardioverter with external paddles and ECG cables
Ultrasound system for central venous line insertion
Compatible blood in operating room

ASA, American Society of Anesthesiologists; ECG, electrocardiogram; BIS, bispectral index; ACT, activated clotting time.

may be drawn up prior to induction of anesthesia in the unlikely event of the need to "crash" onto CPB. Typed and cross-matched blood should be readily available for rare blood types or if antibodies are present, prior to anesthesia induction.

Preinduction Period

The preoperative encounter in the holding area is a great opportunity to demonstrate empathy and cement trust between the patient and the anesthesiology team. Patients may have varied levels of anxiety and treatment with sedatives, with or without oxygen supplementation may be needed. Once standard ASA monitors are connected (peripheral oxygen saturation monitor, ECG leads, and noninvasive blood pressure cuff) and baseline vital signs are recorded, teams conduct a multidisciplinary huddle, which involves identifying the correct patient, type of surgery, site of surgery (if applicable), surgical equipment needs, availability of blood for transfusion, patient allergies, and antibiotic prophylaxis. Vascular access prior to induction is individualized for each patient. Peripheral intravenous cannulae are inserted after site infiltration with local anesthetic. An invasive arterial catheter is inserted prior to induction of anesthesia and central venous cannulation is performed following tracheal intubation. However, it is reasonable to establish invasive monitoring after induction in stable patients at minimal risk of decompensation during induction. Once hemodynamic monitoring is established, baseline values for all hemodynamic parameters should be recorded, along with baseline values of arterial blood gases, hematocrit, blood glucose, and ACT.

Induction and Intubation

Induction goal is a smooth transition from consciousness to appropriate anesthetic depth with minimal hemodynamic perturbations. Use of short-acting and hemodynamically stable drugs is emphasized. Patients with hemodynamic instability may require vasopressors/inotropes preinduction. Awake intubation should be prioritized in patients with known or suspected difficult airway. The response to tracheal intubation can be mitigated with opioids, β-blockers or deepening the level of anesthesia. Following successful tracheal intubation, central venous cannulation and TEE probe placement are accomplished. The need for pulmonary artery catheterization should be clarified in the "huddle." Monitoring for assessing depth of anesthesia is initiated either preinduction or immediately after induction.

Preincision Period

There is minimal stimulation during the period from tracheal intubation until skin incision. The surgical team attends to insertion of a urinary bladder catheter, temperature probe, positioning, preparing, and draping. During this period, completion of a comprehensive TEE examination as well as ANH (if planned and feasible) is done. In the event of hypotension, decreasing the anesthetic depth and/or use of vasoconstrictors are used to support the systemic and coronary perfusion pressure.

Incision to Bypass

Skin incision, sternotomy, and pericardiotomy are periods of intense surgical stimulation that may cause hypertension and tachycardia, and may even induce ischemia. Deepening the anesthetic, vasodilators and short acting β-blockers help to rebalance myocardial oxygen demand and supply. Hypotension, related to decrease venous return, can occur during manipulation of the heart to facilitate atrial cannulation; appropriate treatment may range from observation to vasoconstrictors. Hemodynamically significant supraventricular dysrhythmias may occur during atrial cannulation and should be treated with synchronized cardioversion. Refractory hypotension or surgical bleeding may warrant rapid cannulation and institution of CPB. Adequate intravascular volume may attenuate the extent of hypotension. This is a critical period and continuous observation of the surgical field is essential.

New or worsening of pre-existing ischemia can also precipitate refractory hypotension. Presence of new RWMAs, mitral regurgitation (TEE), ST segment alterations (ECG), and increased LV filling pressure (PAC) are indicators of ischemia. If it occurs, it should be treated appropriately and the surgeon notified.

Cardiopulmonary Bypass

Heparin 400 IU/kg is administered and satisfactory levels of anticoagulation (ACT > 400 to 480 seconds) are confirmed. Subsequently, cavoatrial and aortic cannulation are achieved. Once CPB is initiation it is important to confirm adequacy of venous drainage (no pulsatility on CVP or PA waveforms), unobstructed arterial flow (appropriate systemic arterial pressure and line pressure), sufficient gas exchange (ABG: arterial oxygen saturation, PaO_2, $PaCO_2$) and depth of anesthesia (Bispectral index monitoring). With establishment of full CPB (flow 2.2 to 2.4 L/min/m^2 or 50 to 60 mL/kg/min), lung ventilation is withheld. Although MAP may decrease to 30 to 40 mmHg initially due to the hemodilution effect of the CPB prime and cessation of pulsatile flow, the perfusionist quickly adjusts flow rates and alters vascular resistance with use of vasoconstrictors to restore a MAP between 50 and 80 mmHg. Currently, the optimal MAP during CPB is unknown.

Monitoring and Management during Bypass

During CPB, it is important to continue monitoring hemodynamic parameters (MAP, CVP, PA pressure, LA pressure, heart rate and rhythm), temperature, depth of anesthesia, adequacy of neuromuscular blockade, arterial and venous blood gases, adequacy of anticoagulation (ACT), and urine output. With commencement of CPB, CVP should trend toward zero. High CVP values may reflect incomplete venous decompression and presence of venous congestion. This should be addressed promptly as high venous pressures compromise tissue perfusion pressure. Difficulty in maintaining perfusion pressure targets should prompt the examination of cannulae to exclude mechanical obstruction to flow (NICV 39-5).

The common causes of blood pressure perturbations during CPB are highlighted in Table 39-17. After adequate flow is achieved on CPB, cooling is initiated (gradient between arterial outflow and venous inflow is kept <10°C). Most cardiac surgeries including CABG are performed under mild hypothermia (>28°C). Depth of anesthesia monitors such as bispectral index monitor and assessment of volatile anesthetic concentration in the oxygenator's exhaust line may help ensure adequacy of anesthetic plane during CPB. Clinical signs that suggest inadequate anesthetic depth are unreliable during CPB. Special attention should be directed to interpretation of arterial and venous blood gases. Increasing serum lactate, low mixed venous oxygen saturation and presence of acidosis suggest inadequate perfusion. Increases in serum glucose (>180 mg/dL) and serum potassium levels (due to cardioplegia) may necessitate insulin therapy (to maintain blood glucose between 140 and 180 mg/dL) and modified ultrafiltration (for K^+ >6.5 mEq/L). A low urine output (<0.5 mL/kg/hr) should prompt examination of catheter and collection tubing for obstruction. However, urine output during CPB is not associated with postoperative renal dysfunction. Postoperative renal failure is most likely related to aggravation of pre-existing renal dysfunction or persistent low cardiac output following CPB.

Table 39-17 Checklist during Cardiopulmonary Bypass

Laboratory Values	Heparinization Adequate	ACT or Other Method
	ABGs Hematocrit, Na^+, K^+, ionized Ca^{2+}, glucose	Is there acidosis?
Anesthetic	Discontinue ventilation	
Monitors		
Arterial hypotension	Inadequate venous return Pump Arterial cannula Decreased vascular tone Transducer/monitor malfunction	Venous cannula malposition, clamp, kink, air lock Bleeding, hypovolemia, IVC obstruction, table too low Poor occlusion, low flow Misdirected, kinked, partially clamped, aortic dissection Anesthetics, hemodilution, idiopathic Radial artery cannula malpositioned, dampened waveform
Arterial hypertension	Pump Arterial cannula Vasoconstriction Transducer/monitor malfunction:	High flow Misdirected Light anesthetic plane, response to hypothermia Radial artery cannula malpositioned/kinked
Venous pressure	Decreased Increased	Transducer higher than atrial level? True obstruction of chamber drainage (CVP: right, PCWP/LA: left heart)
Adequate body perfusion Temperature Urine output	Flow and pressure? Acidosis Mixed venous blood oxygen saturation	
Patient/field	Heart Cyanosis, venous engorgement, skin temperature Movement Signs of light anesthesia/hypercapnia	Distention, fibrillation Breathing/diaphragmatic movement
Support	Assist/adequacy of pump flow	Anesthetics/vasodilators for hypertension Constrictors for hypotension

ACT, activated clotting time; ABGs, arterial blood gases; IVC, inferior vena cava; CVP, central venous pressure; PCWP, pulmonary capillary wedge pressure; LA, left atrium; EEG, electroencephalogram.

Rewarming, De-Airing, and Removal of Aortic Cross Clamp

When surgical repair is near completion, the surgeon will requests the perfusionist to gradually rewarm the patient. During rewarming it is important to ensure the following:

1. The temperature gradient between the perfusate and patient's blood temperature should not exceed 4° to 6°C to prevent formation of gas bubbles in the patient's blood.
2. The patient's blood temperature should not exceed 37°C to minimize temperature-related blood damage and neurologic injury.
3. The rate of rewarming should not exceed 0.5°C/min. A slower rate of rewarming has been associated with better cognitive function 6 weeks post-CABG surgery.
4. Maintenance of adequate depth of anesthesia (MAC ≥0.8 for volatile anesthetics or BIS of 40 to 60) is important to prevent patient awareness as hypothermia dissipates.

Once surgical repair is completed, residual intracardiac air is removed via de-airing. The anesthesiologist recruits and ventilates the lungs to remove air from the pulmonary veins, the perfusionist fills up the heart by clamping the venous line and the patient is placed in Trendelenburg position before removing the aortic cross clamp (to direct bubbles away from carotid arteries). Surgeons often mechanically shake or massage the heart to dislodge bubbles that are adherent to the chamber walls. TEE helps confirm the effectiveness of the de-airing process. Intravenous lidocaine (100 mg) is often administered for ventricular fibrillation prophylaxis prior to aortic cross clamp removal. However, it is not uncommon for the ventricles to fibrillate and in such a circumstance, defibrillation with internal paddles should be done. Subsequently, the heart is allowed to beat (if native rhythm is present) or externally paced at 80 to 90 beats/min via epicardially placed ventricular (and /or atrial) pacing wires in preparation to separate from CPB.

Table 39-18 Checklist before Separation from Cardiopulmonary Bypass

Laboratory Values
Hematocrit, ABGs
K^+: possibly elevated (cardioplegia)
Ionized Ca^{2+}
Anesthetic/machine
Lung compliance: Evaluate (hand ventilation)
Lungs are expanded, no atelectasis, both are ventilated (manual or mechanical)
Vaporizers: Off
Alarms: On
Monitors
Normothermia (37°C nasopharyngeal, 35.5°C bladder, 35°C rectal)
ECG: Rate, rhythm, ST
Transducers re-zeroed and leveled
Arterial and filling pressures
Recorder (if available)
Patient/field
Look at the heart!
De-aired: Check lead II, TEE
Eyeball contractility, size, rhythm
LV vent clamped/removed, caval snares released
Bleeding: No major sites (grafts, suture lines, LV vent site)
Vascular resistance: CPB flow $\propto$ MAP ÷ resistance
Support
As needed

ABGs, arterial blood gases; ECG, electrocardiogram; TEE, transesophageal echocardiography; LV, left ventricle; CPB, cardiopulmonary bypass; MAP, mean arterial pressure.

Discontinuation of Cardiopulmonary Bypass

To minimize errors during discontinuation of CPB, we encourage using a checklist-based approach (Table 39-18). At our institution, we use an "A to H" mnemonic to prepare for this crucial event.

A: Ensure adequacy of **anesthesia** (MAC or BIS) and functioning of **audio-visual** monitors. All invasive hemodynamic monitors should be re-zeroed and clearly visible to the whole team. The volume of pulse oximeter should be restored to audible range.

B: " **Breathe**": recruitment maneuvers followed by lung protective mechanical ventilation.

C: Optimize **circulatory** parameters (heart rate/rhythm, systemic and pulmonary pressures) and initiate inotropes/vasopressors as needed (see below). Revisit pharmacologic therapy and need to escalate to MCS in case of failure to wean. Pacing may be initiated to achieve optimal heart rate (70 to 100 bpm) especially if the intrinsic HR is inadequate and rhythm is nonsinus. Although asynchronous modes can be employed, a DDD mode is preferred as this minimizes the chances of a "R on T" phenomenon when the patient's intrinsic heart rate recovers to an adequate level (>70 bpm).

D: Ensure complete **de-airing** is achieved.

E: Optimize **electrolytes and acid–base status** (calcium [1.09 to 1.3 mmol/L], potassium [4 to 5.5 mEq/L], pH >7.3).

F: **Foster warmth**; ensure adequate rewarming and consider increasing operating room temperature and/or using a heated breathing circuit to prevent post-CPB decrease in patient's core temperature.

G: **Go over issues collaboratively.** It is important to communicate issues that may influence successful weaning from CPB with the surgical and perfusion team. Issues may include, but are not limited to, ongoing bleeding, assessment of coagulation parameters, transfusion requirements, initiation/adjustment of vasoactive medications including inhaled pulmonary vasodilators, need for MCS, and post-repair TEE findings.

H: Ensure adequate **hemoglobin levels** (≥7 g/dL).

During discontinuation of CPB, incremental occlusion of venous cannulae in conjunction with measured decreases in CPB flow allows the heart to gradually fill and eject. Hemodynamic parameters (MAP, CO, PA pressure, CVP), TEE data and direct inspection of the heart (contractility, rhythm, and ventricular filling), help guide the need for vasoactive pharmacologic support during this period. Possible causes that may impede weaning from CPB are summarized in Table 39-19. Occasionally, despite best efforts at de-airing, coronary air embolism occurs during weaning, leading to diffuse ST segment elevation, arrhythmias, and right ventricular dysfunction. In such circumstances, it is best to revert back to CPB, unload the LV and ensure a higher perfusion pressure. These maneuvers help expel the air bubbles from the coronary circulation and improve cardiac performance. Separation from CPB can be straightforward (need of no or one vasoactive medication), difficult (need for multiple vasoactive medications) or very difficult (need for MCS). Common intravenous vasoactive drugs and infusion doses used during this period include:

A. Vasopressors: Norepinephrine (0.1 to 1µ/kg/min), vasopressin (0.01 to 0.05 units/min), phenylephrine (1 to 3 µ/kg/min)
B. Inotropes: Epinephrine (0.1 to 1 µ/kg/min), milrinone (0.3 to 0.7 µ/kg/min after a bolus of 25 to 50 µ/kg over minutes)
C. Vasodilators: nitroglycerin and sodium nitroprusside (0.5 to 5 µ/kg/min). For pulmonary hypertension, inhaled epoprostenol (0.01 to 0.05 µ/kg/min) can be delivered via a dedicated ICU ventilator.

If systemic perfusion remains inadequate despite pharmacologic escalation, MCS is required. Various MCS devices and anesthetic management of patients in CS have been discussed previously in this chapter (NICV 39-6 and 8 Video 39-8).

A persistently low MAP after weaning from CPB can be attributed to multiple factors (Table 39-20) and requires targeted

Table 39-19 Etiology of Right or Left Ventricular Dysfunction after Cardiopulmonary Bypass

Ischemia
Inadequate myocardial protection
Intraoperative infarction
Reperfusion injury
Coronary spasm
Coronary embolism (air, thrombus, calcium)
Technical difficulties (kinked or clotted grafts)
Uncorrected Structural Defects
Nongraftable vessels, diffuse coronary artery disease
Residual or new valve pathology
Hypertrophic cardiomyopathy
Shunts
Preexisting cardiac dysfunction
CPB-Related Factors
Excessive cardioplegia
Unrecognized cardiac distention

Table 39-20 Low Mean Arterial Pressure during and after Weaning from Cardiopulmonary Bypass: Causes and Treatment

Diagnoses	Data Derived from PAC					Data Derived from TEE		Suggested Intervention
	CVP	PAP	PCWP	CI	SVR	LV Function	RV Function	
LV dysfunction	Normal to high	Normal to high	High	Low	Variable	Dilated LV, poor contractility	Normal	Escalate inotropes, consider VAD
RV dysfunction	High	Normal or low	Normal to high	Low	Variable	Normal	Dilated RV, poor contractility, possible TR	Escalate inotropes, initiate pulmonary vasodilators, consider VAD
Bi-ventricular dysfunction	High	Variable	Normal to high	Low	Variable	Dilated LV, poor contractility	Dilated RV, poor contractility, possible TR	Escalate inotropes, initiate pulmonary vasodilators, consider VAD or VA-ECMO
LVOTO	Low	Low	Low	Low	Low	Hyper-dynamic, SAM of MV leaflet and LVOTO seen.	Normal to hyper-dynamic	Administer Volume, initiate vasopressor, decrease HR
Hypo-volemia	Low	Low	Low	Low	Normal to high	Hyperdynamic	Hyperdynamic	Administer volume
Vasoplegia	Normal to low	Normal to low	Normal to low	High	Low	Hyperdynamic	Hyperdynamic	Administer volume, initiate vasopressor

CI, Cardiac Index; CVP, central venous pressure; PAP, pulmonary artery pressure; PCWP, pulmonary capillary wedge pressure; LV, left ventricle; LVAD, left ventricular assist device; LVOTO, left ventricular tract obstruction; MV, mitral valve; PAC, pulmonary artery catheter; RV, right ventricle; SAM, systolic anterior motion; SVR, systemic vascular resistance; TEE, transesophageal echocardiography; TR, tricuspid regurgitation; VAD, ventricular assist device; VA-ECMO, venoarterial extracorporeal membrane oxygenation.

treatment. Continuous reassessment of the situation is necessary to document the efficacy of treatment.

Retrospective studies of patients undergoing CABG with or without concomitant valve surgery showed that wall motion score index, combined CABG and mitral valve surgery, LV EF <35%, reoperation, moderate-to-severe MR, and aortic cross-clamp time were independent predictors for use of inotropes (39% of patients).[82] Low cardiac output syndrome is defined as hemodynamic instability necessitating the use of >2 vasoactive drugs to maintain systemic perfusion on the first postoperative day or need for MCS during or within 5 days of surgery; it independently predicts hospital mortality, resource utilization, and costs.[83] Lastly, elevated MAP after weaning from CPB should prompt reassessment of depth of anesthesia, need for analgesia, status of preload and administration of vasodilatory medications if the SVR is increased.

Postcardiopulmonary Bypass

After successful weaning from bypass, important steps include venous decannulation, reversal of heparin anticoagulation with protamine, aortic decannulation, return of residual pump blood, achievement of hemostasis, chest closure, and transport to the ICU. Venous decannulation entails removal of venous cannulae by the surgical team and closure of atrial/caval sites. Heparin anticoagulation is neutralized with protamine, a polycationic protein derived from salmon sperm. Protamine dose can be determined using a fixed ratio (1-mg protamine to 100 U heparin) or automated heparin-protamine titration assays. Protamine is given before the aorta is decannulated as its administration can be accompanied with significant adverse reactions (anaphylaxis, anaphylactoid reaction, severe pulmonary hypertension with concomitant RV failure) that may necessitate reverting to CPB. In addition, slow administration of protamine is important as rapid infusion leads to profound systemic hypotension. While true anaphylaxis to protamine is rare, catastrophic acute pulmonary hypertension may occur in about 1% of patients. Thromboxane and C5a anaphylatoxin have been implicated in mediating this reaction (NICV 39-7).

We typically administer a "test dose" (10 mg) of protamine prior to slowly administering (over 5 to 10 minutes) the complete dose. If there are no adverse reactions noted after protamine test-dose administration, aortic decannulation is accomplished. Pump suckers are discontinued at this stage to avoid introducing protamine into the pump circuit.

Residual pump blood in the venous reservoir can then be transfused directly to the patient or processed via a "cell saver" device before returning it to the patient. With direct infusion, patients benefit from functional platelets and clotting factors present in the residual pump blood. However, this may necessitate administration of additional protamine as residual pump blood is heparinized. Processing the residual pump blood via a cell-saver device, removes heparin, obviating the need for additional protamine administration. However, platelets and clotting factors are also removed during the "washing" process employed by the cell-saver device.

Persistent residual bleeding in the field after protamine administration may result from inadequate surgical hemostasis, thrombocytopenia, insufficient heparin neutralization, dilution of coagulation factors, hypothermia, platelet dysfunction, and rarely "heparin rebound." Blood product transfusion guided by point of care testing may be effective. Chest closure should occur after adequate hemostasis. A transient decrease in blood pressure after chest closure is rectified with volume resuscitation. However, persistent or refractory hypotension may necessitate chest reopening to rule out cardiac tamponade, a kinked coronary bypass graft, or other causes of shock. Consequently, it may be best to remove the TEE probe *after* chest closure has been safely completed. The anesthesiology team is responsible for ensuring an orderly and safe transfer of the patient from the operating room to the ICU.[76]

Minimally Invasive Cardiac Surgery (MICS) for Myocardial Revascularization

Minimally Invasive Cardiac Surgery prioritizes avoidance of a complete median sternotomy. Instead, surgical repair is accomplished via one or more, smaller chest incisions (thoracotomy, mini-sternotomy, and transverse sternotomy) with or without the aid of CPB. In addition, MICS can be performed with or without robotic assistance. Suggested benefits include less pain, decreased scarring, and shorter recovery times. Currently, myocardial revascularization, aortic, mitral or tricuspid valve surgery, closure of atrial septal defects, and surgical ablation of atrial fibrillation can be achieved with MICS. Percutaneous valve replacement/repair procedures are also becoming popular approaches in selected patients who have prohibitive surgical risk. Anesthetic considerations for each procedure are unique and the reader may benefit from perusing previously published literature.[84–86] We would like to focus our discussion on two nontraditional myocardial revascularization approaches:

- Minimally direct coronary artery bypass (MIDCAB) surgery
- Off-pump coronary artery bypass (OPCAB) grafting.

In the classic MIDCAB, LIMA harvesting and anastomosis to LAD is approached via a limited left chest thoracotomy. This necessitates left lung isolation (double lumen endotracheal tube or a single-lumen endotracheal tube with a bronchial blocker). Patients are placed supine with 30-degree elevation of the left hemithorax and the left arm is tucked. The chest and groins are prepared in the event that sternotomy and emergent conversion to femoral–femoral bypass is needed. The pericardium is opened to visualize the LAD through an anterolateral thoracotomy incision (4th or 5th left intercostal space). The LIMA is dissected, heparin administered (target ACT >300 seconds), and LIMA to LAD anastomosis is performed on the beating heart. Pure pressure or vacuum-assisted myocardial stabilizer devices help stabilize the heart during this process. Subsequently, protamine is administered, hemostasis achieved, and a left pleural chest tube/drain is placed before thoracotomy closure. Typically, MIDCAB is employed when one or two vessel CABG is needed (LIMA to LAD or composite graft off LIMA to another coronary artery).

OPCAB avoids use of CPB and aortic cross clamping; the intention with this approach is to achieve revascularization while minimizing deleterious effects of CPB such as stroke and renal injury. Approach to the pericardial cavity is via a median sternotomy. LIMA and other conduits are harvested for multiarterial grafting. Heparin is administered to achieve an acceptable ACT (300 seconds or institutional preference). A generous pericardiotomy is necessary to facilitate cardiac mobilization. This is turn, improves target vessel access. Although the anteriorly situated LAD is relatively easy to access, grafting the inferior and/or lateral wall target vessels requires the heart to be lifted out of the pericardial cradle (*verticalization*). In a *verticalized* heart, its apex is at the zenith and in this position forward systemic ejection and stroke volume are compromised. Suction devices help achieve this position while stabilization devices (Octopus/Medtronic, Ultima II/Guidant, and Acrobat-i/Macquet) are needed to compress the ventricles to achieve local immobility to facilitate grafting. Epicardial pacing wires may be placed prior to cardiac manipulation to enable pacing to a target heart rate of 80 bpm to increase stroke volume. Institutional preferences govern order of revascularization. More often than not, vessels are grafted as follows: anterior, then inferior and finally lateral wall vessels. Mechanical distortion of the heart and coronary occlusion during the procedure may prompt the surgical team to use intracoronary shunts to mitigate ongoing myocardial ischemia and accompanying hemodynamic compromise. Technical difficulties or refractory hemodynamic instability may necessitate abandoning the OPCAB approach and employing conventional CPB to achieve adequate revascularization. Anesthetic considerations for OPCAB surgery are listed in Table 39-21.

While the OPCAB approach may lead to decreased rates of transfusion, renal injury and resource utilization, it is associated with higher rates of incomplete revascularization and is technically challenging. Interestingly, stroke rates between OPCAB and on-pump CABG are similar despite the absence of CPB associated emboli, lack of aortic manipulation and use of a "no touch" technique in OPCAB.[87]

Minimally Invasive and Robotic Valvular Surgery

Over the past few decades, MICS has been a quickly developing field in the arena of mitral valve repair and AV replacement. Initially, MICS for the mitral valve was approached through a right-sided anterior lateral minithoracotomy, yet as endoscopic and robotic technology has increased, robotic approaches have become highly utilized. While the minithoracotomy incision remains small, the robotic approach allows mitral valve repairs to be completed with five, small port incisions. Anesthetic management essential to these MICS techniques requires isolation of the right lung. Since the access to cardiac structures is only available

Table 39-21 Anesthetic Considerations for OPCAB Surgery

1. Monitoring and vascular access: invasive arterial blood pressure monitoring, central venous access, consider PAC when LV function is poor or severe mitral regurgitation is present, TEE is essential unless contraindicated. ECG and TEE may not be able to detect ischemia during cardiac mobilization especially verticalization of the heart.
2. Prioritize normothermia: Use warming devices, heated breathing circuits and optimize operating room temperature
3. Hemodynamic compromise may be related to positioning of the heart, stabilizer application, worsening of myocardial ischemia, atrial compression, and compromised preload.
4. Utilize Trendelenburg positioning, volume administration, and vasoactive medications to counteract hemodynamic instability during surgery.
5. Be wary of RV dysfunction and compromised graft patency: These will lead to persistent or refractory hemodynamic instability
6. Ensure immediate availability and expertise to institute CPB and MCS.

CPB, cardiopulmonary bypass; MCS, mechanical circulatory support; OPCAB, Off-pump coronary artery bypass; PAC, pulmonary artery catheter; RV, right ventricle; TEE, transesophageal echocardiography.

through small incisions, CPB must be initiated through a peripheral approach. The femoral artery and femoral vein are most commonly accessed, and optimal draining of the right side of the heart is done via a superior vena cava venous cannula inserted via the right internal jugular vein.[88]

MICS for surgical AV replacement utilizes a right sided mini anterior thoracotomy, just lateral to the sternum in the 4th intercostal space. The anterior position of the AV in the thorax, allows access through a 3-cm incision. Similarly to mitral valve surgery, right lung isolation is required along with peripheral cannulation for CPB. Since the AV is positioned anteriorly, complete draining of the right side of the heart is not required for visualization; therefore, a peripheral superior vena cava cannula is not required.[89]

Percutaneous Approaches to Valvular Disease

Over the past 20 years, TAVR or transcatheter aortic valve insertion (TAVI) has been shown to be noninferior to surgical AV replacement in the PARTNER trials.[90,91] Traditionally, an expandable AV is delivered through the femoral artery across the AV and then the deployed with balloon inflation, although certain AV models self-expand without a balloon. Stroke remains a risk with the potential showering of calcium from the degenerative native AV, although devices inserted in the carotid arteries to "strain" for debris remain an option. Anesthetic management is usually monitored anesthesia care, although institutional preferences for general anesthesia exist. Vascular and structural injury remains the greatest risk during the procedure: AV annular disruption, AD, ventricle tear, femoral artery injury, etc. These rare but catastrophic events require that the anesthesiologist plan with the team for pre-determined rescue strategies.

Percutaneous options for MV regurgitation include the MitraClip for patients considered to be high risk for surgery. The MitraClip provides an edge-to edge grasping and pulling together of the pathologic regions of the mitral valve. Randomized control trials report successful outcomes both in degenerative and functional MR.[91] These procedures are performed under general anesthesia with transesophageal echocardiography guiding the interventional cardiologist through the proper location placement of the MitraClip. The femoral vein is accessed and the delivery device is guided across the interatrial septum. Under echocardiographic and fluoroscopic guidance the clip is positioned and the MR impact assessed prior to deployment.

Postoperative Considerations

The acuity and complexity of cardiac surgical procedures and patients present challenges within the postoperative period. Surgical anastomosis involving high-pressured cardiac structures have the possibility of continued bleeding in the postoperative period. Coagulopathy, surgical bleeding, cardiac tamponade, organ failure, atrial fibrillation, respiratory failure, and pain management are issues that must be addressed in the cardiac intensive care unit. In addition, enhanced recovery after cardiac surgery (ERACS) guidelines are encouraging expedient discharge for an appropriate patient population.[7]

Indications for Re-Exploration

Reported reexploration of postoperative cardiac surgical patients occurs in approximately 4.2% of patients with 3.9 percent of patients returning to the operating room specifically for bleeding.[92] A trigger to return to the operative room for reexploration includes hemodynamic instability, anemia, and persistent chest tube output exceeding 200 mL/hr, despite correction of coagulopathy. Delaying re-exploration may lead to cardiac tamponade, which will further decrease cardiac output, organ perfusion and impact long-term prognosis. During postoperative cardiac tamponade, the elevated pericardial pressure compresses the cardiac chambers and falsely elevates the measured intracardiac pressures. Collapse of the cardiac chambers, seen with echocardiography, remains the diagnostic gold standard. Chambers with the lowest intracardiac pressure are most commonly compressed, such as the right and left atria along with the RV. Since the stroke volume is limited, tachycardia remains the primary component of cardiac output. Systemic vascular resistance significantly increases to increase venous return and fill the right side of the heart. Diastolic filling of the ventricles is closely dependent on respiration-induced ventricular interdependence. During mechanical inspiration the increased intrathoracic pressure will impede the RV and augment the LV filling. As a result, the diastolic tricuspid flow will decrease while the diastolic mitral flow will increase. This increased MV flow is a result of increased intrathoracic pressure "compressing" the intrathoracic pulmonary veins driving blood into the LV. During spontaneous respiration, the reciprocal scenario of chamber filling occurs (see also NICV 39-8).

Cardiac tamponade requires emergency surgical exploration. If the patient is extubated, systemic vascular resistance should not be compromised by induction of anesthesia. Ketamine is often the induction agent of choice. The surgical team must be ready for immediate sternotomy, which often includes prepping the chest and a fully gowned and gloved surgical team prior to induction. The anesthesiologist must also be aware that upon reopening the sternum, systemic blood pressures will significant increase. If surgical anastomosis was a challenge secondary to diseased tissues, this acute elevation in blood pressure may induce additional bleeding.

Children with Congenital Heart Disease

Introduction

The incidence of congenital disease (CHD) remains stable worldwide (17.9 per 1,000 live births) and its prevalence continues to increase.[93] Pediatric cardiac anesthesiologists are challenged during the perioperative management of children with CHD due to the high complexity and heterogeneity of cardiac lesions. The pathophysiology of a wide variety of cardiac lesions can be best understood by envisioning the pathway that blood must follow to maintain systemic and pulmonary blood flow ("anatomy dictates the physiology"). Table 39-22 classifies various types of lesions by their physiologic impact. A combination of more than one defect is quite common (see also NICV 39-9).

Preoperative Evaluation

History

In infants, HF manifests through feeding difficulties, easy fatigability, lethargy, labored breathing, and ultimately a failure to thrive. In the older child, it causes easy fatigability, shortness of breath, and dyspnea on exertion. The child's age and weight, baseline oxygen saturation, medications, supplemental oxygen requirement, associated comorbidities, and anticipated duration of surgery and CPB must be considered. Previous surgical history and cardiac catheterization data provide a thorough understanding of anatomy, residual lesions, and vessel patency (occlusion or thrombus).

Physical Examination

The physical examination of a child should seek to evaluate baseline status and clinical features of congenital cardiac lesions. Children with uncompensated lesions usually presents with failure to thrive, diaphoresis, tachycardia, rales and/ or jugular venous distension, which could be secondary to pulmonary hypertension and/ or poor peripheral oxygenation and perfusion. Extremities should be examined for cyanosis, clubbing, edema, and pulse volume. It is important to measure blood pressures in the arms and legs in all patient with suspected CHD and children with hypertension to rule out coarctation of aorta. In children with history of classic subclavian to pulmonary artery (Blalock–Taussig shunt) or subclavian artery flap used for coarctation of aorta repair, upper extremity pulses may be reduced or absent on the side of the shunt. The overall incidence of extracardiac anomalies in children with CHD may be as high as 20%.[94]

Laboratory Evaluations

Children with cyanotic lesions present with polycythemia. Polycythemia results as a consequence of bone marrow stimulation (via release of erythropoietin from the kidneys) from arterial desaturation. Polycythemia can lead to hyperviscosity, peripheral sludging, and reduced oxygen delivery. Sludging is augmented by dehydration from preoperative fasting and by hypothermia. In patients with hematocrit >70%, consideration should be given to preoperative electrophoresis if symptomatic hyperviscosity is present. Polycythemia can induce a low-grade disseminated intravascular coagulation with activation of fibrinolysis, degranulation of platelets, and consumption of coagulation factors. Newborns often have inadequate coagulation factors because of immaturity of hepatic function. Moreover, significant coagulation factor dilution and platelet dysfunction occurs on CPB. Platelet count, prothrombin time, and PTT should be evaluated. Children on diuretic therapy are at risk for hypokalemia, particularly if they are receiving digitalis. Infants, particularly those with congestive HF, are also at risk for both hypoglycemia and hypocalcemia. Children who have undergone major cardiac procedures earlier in their lives may have been exposed to blood or blood products and are at increased risk of having abnormal serum antibodies to various blood antigens. Hence, samples of a child's blood should be sent to the blood bank for possible cross-matching.

Table 39-22 Physiologic Effects of Congenital Cardiac Lesions

Volume overload (ventricle or atrium) resulting in increased pulmonary blood flow • Atrial septal defect: ↑ flow, ↓ pressure • Ventricular septal defect: ↑ flow, ↑ pressure • Patent ductus arteriosus: ↑ flow, ↑ pressure • Endocardial cushion defect: ↑ flow, ↑ pressure
Cyanosis resulting from obstruction to pulmonary blood flow • Tetralogy of Fallot • Tricuspid atresia • Pulmonary atresia
Pressure overload to the ventricle • Aortic stenosis • Coarctation of the aorta • Pulmonary stenosis
Cyanosis due to a common mixing chamber • Total anomalous venous return • Truncus arteriosus • Double outlet right ventricle • Single ventricle
Cyanosis due to separation of the systemic and pulmonary circulation • Transposition of the great vessels

↑, increase; ↓, decrease.

Cardiac Evaluations

Echocardiography delineates most of the cardiac anatomy and permits noninvasive measurement of ventricular size and function, cardiac output, and severity of valve dysfunction. Cardiac catheterization is reserved for patients with poor echocardiographic windows or unclear findings. Cardiac MRI and three-dimensional printed heart models are used to demonstrate complex anatomy in order to delineate the surgical plan. The chest radiograph of a child with CHD should be evaluated for cardiac position, size, shape, abnormal vessels, right aortic arch, scimitar syndrome (hypoplasia/aplasia of one or more lobes of right lung and hypoplasia of right pulmonary artery), aberrant pulmonary vessels, abnormal position of bronchi, vascular rings, or associated pulmonary abnormalities (e.g., pneumonia, atelectasis, or emphysema). The ECG should be reviewed for rate and rhythm abnormalities.

Premedication

The purpose of the premedication is to have a calm child without loss of protective airway reflexes or hemodynamic compromise. This will facilitate separation of the child from parents and ease the fear and anxiety associated with the perioperative period.

Monitoring

In addition to standard monitors, additional monitors used during open heart procedures include peripheral and central temperature monitoring, invasive blood pressure, and CVP monitoring, LAP monitoring via a catheter placed by the surgeon intraoperatively (in selected cases) and transesophageal echocardiography (TEE). Of note, airway or aortic arch compression can occur after TEE probe placement in smaller patients (<4 kg).

Intraoperative Management

Inhalational agents are predominately used as induction and maintenance agents in pediatric cardiac patients. However, patients with poor ventricular function, pulmonary hypertension and those with critical dependence on SVR and/or PVR will need intravenous access preinduction and avoidance or limitation of anesthetic agents that can further compromise hemodynamic function. Anesthetic aims are to balance total pulmonary blood flow (Qp) to total systemic blood flow (Qs), contractility and heart rate, and maintain systemic perfusion. For example, vigilance is required during induction while oxygenating and ventilating children with left to right shunt lesions (e.g., VSD, AV canal). On the other hand, inhalation induction is slow in patient with right to left shunt lesion (e.g., TOF). It is prudent to de-air the intravenous catheters and lines to avoid paradoxical air embolism. The choice of anesthetic agents following induction is governed by ventricular function, anticipated use of CPB, and the possibility of mechanical ventilation or tracheal extubation at the end of the case. Opioids are used routinely to limit the stress response in the pre-CPB phase.

Neonatal myocardial morphology and performance is distinct: limited preload reserve, afterload mismatch, reduced ventricular compliance and contractile mass, increased interventricular dependence and incomplete autonomic sympathetic system with dominant parasympathetic innervation are some of the characteristics of the neonatal myocardium.

Neonates and infants undergoing cardiac surgery and deep hypothermic CPB can generate a significant hormonal stress response. No specific relationship between opioid dose and stress response has been established. Of special note is the marked reduction in neuromuscular blocking requirements during hypothermic bypass.

Advances in CPB, surgical, and anesthetic techniques have significantly improved the survival of children with CHD. However, CPB produces marked hemostatic derangements including: dilution of red blood cells and blood clotting factors, activation of the clotting cascade and consumption of clotting factors and platelets, and activation of the fibrinolytic pathway.

Aminocaproic acid or tranexamic acid are used to attenuate coagulopathy during pediatric cardiac surgery associated with CPB.

Separation from CPB will require pharmacologic and/or pacing support in some patients.

In lesions in which the presence of increased PVR is known or suspected, addition of inhaled pulmonary vasodilators may be beneficial.

Tracheal Extubation and Postoperative Ventilation

Children with simple lesions who have undergone procedures that do not involve ventricular incisions (atrial septal defect, ventricular septal defect) can often be extubated at the conclusion of surgery or shortly thereafter in the ICU.[95]

Children most at risk for ventilatory failure following cardiac surgery include those younger than 6 months, with complex surgeries requiring long CPB time and circulatory arrest time,

Down syndrome, pulmonary hypertension requiring preoperative ventilatory support, postoperative cardiovascular and pulmonary complications, or those requiring high inotropic support.

In infants, nasal continuous positive airway pressure can be employed instead of mechanical ventilation. In patients with Fontan physiology (passive pulmonary circulation), decreasing PVR is paramount and is very much dependent on adequate ventilation. The potentially detrimental effects of endotracheal intubation and positive pressure ventilation offset this advantage. Positive pressure ventilation is known to have a deleterious effect on pulmonary blood flow in patients with Fontan physiology. Resumption of pain-free spontaneous respiration does enhance hemodynamic performance in these patients.[3]

As a part of multimodal analgesia, regional anesthetic techniques are commonly used to supplement intraoperative anesthesia and provide postoperative analgesia, and to facilitate early tracheal extubation. For example, caudal (epidural) opioids or intercostal nerve blocks can be used in aortic coarctation repair in or ligation of a patent ductus arteriosus. Ultrasound guided bilateral paravertebral blocks, or interfacial plane block such as erector spine plane block, transverse thoracic muscle plane block are used to enhance postoperative recovery and opioid reduction.[5] Reported benefits of regional techniques include decreased stress response, improved pulmonary and gastrointestinal function, and potential for cost reduction.[96,97]

Postoperative Monitoring

Low Cardiac Output Syndrome (LCOS)

The incidence of LCOS is high after congenital heart surgery. Approximately 25% of children experience a decreased cardiac index (<2 L/min/m^2) within 6 to 18 hours postoperatively.[98,99] Ventricular dysfunction, change in the loading condition, SVR and PVR, ventriculotomy, myocardial edema, refractory arrhythmias and residual lesions are some of the common factors leading to hemodynamic and physiologic abnormalities causing LCOS. Close monitoring including assessment of tissue oxygenation (mixed venous oxygen saturation and lactate trends) and cardiovascular function, ventricular preload optimization, judicious use of inotropic agents and mechanical ventilation to decrease oxygen demand and afterload, and in rare instance MCS are used.

Pulmonary Hypertension Crisis

The RV is extremely sensitive to increases in afterload. Hence, acute pulmonary hypertension may lead to severe circulatory compromise and cardiac arrest. Pulmonary hypertension crisis is characterized by a rapid increase in pulmonary artery pressure (exceeding systemic arterial pressure), evidenced by an abrupt decrease in $EtCO_2$, hypoxemia, hypotension, and increased CVP and bronchospasm. Close monitoring, early recognition in high-risk patients, and timely intervention are vital in the prevention of cardiac dysfunction, LCOS and hemodynamic collapse. Patients should be managed with 100% oxygen, moderate hyperventilation, epinephrine and calcium and inotropes, inhaled pulmonary vasodilators, and correction of metabolic and respiratory acidosis.

Adults with Congenital Heart Disease

The survival of patients with CHD has increased significantly in the last four decades.[100] As a result, it is estimated that the number of adults with CHD (ACHD) is greater than the number of children with CHD in the United States. In addition, the current distribution of age at death in ACHD approximates that of the general population. Adults with repaired or palliated CHD now present to the operating room in greater numbers requiring different types of cardiac and noncardiac procedures. Despite overall survival benefits, the perioperative death rates in this group are higher than for their peers. Some of the most common CHD found in adults after repair or palliation include atrial septal defects, ventricular septal defects, tetralogy of Fallot (after transannular patch), common atrioventricular canal defects (atrioventricular septal defects), coarctation of the aorta, transposition of the great arteries (after atrial switch or arterial switch operations), and congenitally corrected transposition of the great arteries (after double switch operation). The appropriate perioperative care of ACHD depends on the amount of residual lesion after repair, functional status and complexity of the surgical procedure. Anesthesiologists with expertise in congenital heart disease are better suited to care for patients with moderate or severe residual lesions, significant pulmonary hypertension and single ventricle patients.

For further review and interactivities, please see the videos and narrative interactive clinical vignettes (NICVs) accessible in the complimentary eBook bundled with this text. Access instructions are located on the inside front cover.

REFERENCES

1. Thygesen K, Alpert JS, Jaffe AS, et al. Fourth universal definition of myocardial infarction (2018). *J Am Coll Cardiol*. 2018;72(18):2231–2264.
2. Smit M, Coetzee AR, Lochner A. The pathophysiology of myocardial ischemia and perioperative myocardial infarction. *J Cardiothorac Vasc Anesth*. 2020;34(9):2501–2512.
3. Spinale FG. Assessment of cardiac function–basic principles and approaches. *Compr Physiol*. 2015;5(4):1911–1946.
4. Johnson NP, Gould KL, De Bruyne B. Autoregulation of coronary blood supply in response to demand: JACC review topic of the week. *J Am Coll Cardiol*. 2021;77(18):2335–2345.
5. Kloner RA, Jennings RB. Consequences of brief ischemia: stunning, preconditioning, and their clinical implications: part 2. *Circulation*. 2001;104(25):3158–3167.
6. Lawton JS, Tamis-Holland JE, Bangalore S, et al. 2021 ACC/AHA/SCAI Guideline for Coronary Artery Revascularization: Executive Summary: A Report of the American College of Cardiology/American Heart Association Joint Committee on Clinical Practice Guidelines. *Circulation*. 2022;145(3):e4–e17.
7. Engelman DT, Ben Ali W, Williams JB, et al. Guidelines for perioperative care in cardiac surgery: enhanced recovery after surgery society recommendations. *JAMA Surg*. 2019;154(8):755–766.
8. Grant MC, Isada T, Ruzankin P, et al. Results from an enhanced recovery program for cardiac surgery. *J Thorac Cardiovasc Surg*. 2020;159(4):1393–1402.
9. Grant MC, Isada T, Ruzankin P, et al. Opioid-sparing cardiac anesthesia: secondary analysis of an enhanced recovery program for cardiac surgery. *Anesth Analg*. 2020;131(6):1852–1861.
10. Pagel PS, Crystal GJ. The discovery of myocardial preconditioning using volatile anesthetics: a history and contemporary clinical perspective. *J Cardiothorac Vasc Anesth*. 2018;32(3): 1112–1134.
11. Landoni G, Lomivorotov VV, Nigro Neto C, et al. Volatile anesthetics versus total intravenous anesthesia for cardiac surgery. *N Engl J Med*. 2019;380(13):1214–1225.
12. Helman JD, Leung JM, Bellows WH, et al. The risk of myocardial ischemia in patients receiving desflurane versus sufentanil anesthesia for coronary artery bypass graft surgery. The S.P.I. Research Group. *Anesthesiology*. 1992;77(1):47–62.
13. Cromheecke S, Pepermans V, Hendrickx E, et al. Cardioprotective properties of sevoflurane in patients undergoing aortic valve replacement with cardiopulmonary bypass. *Anesth Analg*. 2006;103(2):289–296.
14. Turan A, Duncan A, Leung S, et al. Dexmedetomidine for reduction of atrial fibrillation and delirium after cardiac surgery (DECADE): a randomised placebo-controlled trial. *Lancet*. 2020; 396(10245):177–1785.
15. Ali IS, Buth KJ, Maitland A. Impact of preoperative intravenous nitroglycerin on in-hospital outcomes after coronary artery bypass grafting for unstable angina. *Am Heart J*. 2004;148(4): 727–732.
16. Cheung AT, Cruz-Shiavone GE, Meng QC, et al. Cardiopulmonary bypass, hemolysis, and nitroprusside-induced cyanide production. *Anesth Analg*. 2007;105(1):29–33.
17. Hottinger DG, Beebe DS, Kozhimannil T, Prielipp RC, Belani KG. Sodium nitroprusside in 2014: a clinical concepts review. *J Anaesthesiol Clin Pharmacol*. 2014;30(4):462–471.
18. Egi M, Bellomo R, Langenberg C, et al. Selecting a vasopressor drug for vasoplegic shock after adult cardiac surgery: a systematic literature review. *Ann Thorac Surg*. 2007;83(2):715–723.
19. Oprea AD, Lombard FW, Kertai MD. Perioperative β-adrenergic blockade in noncardiac and cardiac surgery: a clinical update. *J Cardiothorac Vasc Anesth*. 2019;33(3):817–832.
20. Virani SS, Alonso A, Aparicio HJ, et al. Heart Disease and Stroke Statistics-2021 Update: A Report From the American Heart Association. *Circulation*. 2021;143(8):e254–e743.
21. Otto CM, Nishimura RA, Bonow RO, et al. 2020 ACC/AHA Guideline for the Management of Patients With Valvular Heart Disease: Executive Summary: A Report of the American College of Cardiology/American Heart Association Joint Committee on Clinical Practice Guidelines. *Circulation*. 2021;143(5):e35–e71.
22. Harb SC, Griffin BP. Mitral valve disease: a comprehensive review. *Curr Cardiol Rep*. 2017; 19(8):73.
23. Gorlin R, Gorlin SG. Hydraulic formula for calculation of the area of the stenotic mitral valve, other cardiac valves, and central circulatory shunts. I. *Am Heart J*. 1951;41(1):1–29.
24. Harky A, Botezatu B, Kakar S, Ren M, Shirke MM, Pullan M. Mitral valve diseases: pathophysiology and interventions. *Prog Cardiovasc Dis*. 2021;67:98–104.
25. Varghese R, Itagaki S, Anyanwu AC, Trigo P, Fischer G, Adams DH. Predicting systolic anterior motion after mitral valve reconstruction: using intraoperative transoesophageal echocardiography to identify those at greatest risk. *Eur J Cardiothorac Surg*. 2014;45(1):132–137.
26. Cevasco M, Shekar PS. Surgical management of tricuspid stenosis. *Ann Cardiothorac Surg*. 2017;6(3):275–282.
27. Zoller JK, Gregory SH. Anesthetic considerations for transcatheter tricuspid valve repair. *J Cardiothorac Vasc Anesth*. 2020;34(7):1942–1951.
28. Marian AJ, Braunwald E. Hypertrophic cardiomyopathy: genetics, pathogenesis, clinical manifestations, diagnosis, and therapy. *Circ Res*. 2017;121(7):749–770.
29. Nagueh SF, Phelan D, Abraham T, et al. Recommendations for Multimodality Cardiovascular Imaging of Patients with Hypertrophic Cardiomyopathy: An Update from the American Society of Echocardiography, in Collaboration with the American Society of Nuclear Cardiology, the Society for Cardiovascular Magnetic Resonance, and the Society of Cardiovascular Computed Tomography. *J Am Soc Echocardiogr*. 2022;35(6):533–569.
30. Makkar RR, Thourani VH, Mack MJ, et al. Five-year outcomes of transcatheter or surgical aortic-valve replacement. *N Engl J Med*. 2020;382(9):799–809.
31. Samarendra P, Mangione MP. Aortic stenosis and perioperative risk with noncardiac surgery. *J Am Coll Cardiol*. 2015;65(3):295–302.
32. Boodhwani M, de Kerchove L, Glineur D, et al. Repair-oriented classification of aortic insufficiency: impact on surgical techniques and clinical outcomes. *J Thorac Cardiovasc Surg*. 2009; 137(2):286–294.
33. Bekeredjian R, Grayburn PA. Valvular heart disease: aortic regurgitation. *Circulation*. 2005; 112(1):125–134.
34. Hiratzka LF, Bakris GL, Beckman JA, et al. 2010 ACCF/AHA/AATS/ACR/ASA/SCA/SCAI/SIR/STS/SVM guidelines for the diagnosis and management of patients with Thoracic Aortic Disease: a report of the American College of Cardiology Foundation/American Heart Association Task Force on Practice Guidelines, American Association for Thoracic Surgery, American College of Radiology, American Stroke Association, Society of Cardiovascular Anesthesiologists, Society for Cardiovascular Angiography and Interventions, Society of Interventional Radiology, Society of Thoracic Surgeons, and Society for Vascular Medicine. *Circulation*. 2010; 121(13):e266–e369.
35. Vilacosta I, San Román JA, di Bartolomeo R, et al. Acute aortic syndrome revisited: JACC state-of-the-art review. *J Am Coll Cardiol*. 2021;78(21):2106–2125.
36. Bechtel A, Huffmyer J. Anesthetic management for cardiopulmonary bypass: update for 2014. *Semin Cardiothorac Vasc Anesth*. 2014;18(2):101–116.
37. Yan TD, Bannon PG, Bavaria J, et al. Consensus on hypothermia in aortic arch surgery. *Ann Cardiothorac Surg*. 2013;2(2):163–168.
38. Heidenreich PA, Albert NM, Allen LA, et al. Forecasting the impact of heart failure in the United States: a policy statement from the American Heart Association. *Circ Heart Fail*. 2013;6(3):606–619.
39. Heidenreich PA, Bozkurt B, Aguilar D, et al. 2022 AHA/ACC/HFSA Guideline for the Management of Heart Failure: A Report of the American College of Cardiology/American Heart Association Joint Committee on Clinical Practice Guidelines. *Circulation*. 2022;145(18):e89 5–e1032.
40. Goldman L, Hashimoto B, Cook EF, Loscalzo A. Comparative reproducibility and validity of systems for assessing cardiovascular functional class: advantages of a new specific activity scale. *Circulation*. 1981;64(6):1227–1234.
41. Murphy SP, Ibrahim NE, Januzzi JL Jr. Heart failure with reduced ejection fraction: a review. *JAMA*. 2020;324(5):488–504.
42. Redfield MM. Heart failure with preserved ejection fraction. *N Engl J Med*. 2016; 375(19):1868–1877.
43. Hochman JS, Sleeper LA, Webb JG, et al. Early revascularization in acute myocardial infarction complicated by cardiogenic shock. SHOCK Investigators. Should we emergently revascularize occluded coronaries for cardiogenic shock. *N Engl J Med*. 1999;341(9):625–634.
44. Baran DA, Grines CL, Bailey S, et al. SCAI clinical expert consensus statement on the classification of cardiogenic shock: This document was endorsed by the American College of Cardiology (ACC), the American Heart Association (AHA), the Society of Critical Care Medicine (SCCM), and the Society of Thoracic Surgeons (STS) in April 2019. *Catheter Cardiovasc Interv*. 2019;94(1):29–37.
45. Peura JL, Colvin-Adams M, Francis GS, et al. Recommendations for the use of mechanical circulatory support: device strategies and patient selection: a scientific statement from the American Heart Association. *Circulation*. 2012;126(22):2648–2667.
46. Balthazar T, Vandenbriele C, Verbrugge FH, et al. Managing patients with short-term mechanical circulatory support: JACC review topic of the week. *J Am Coll Cardiol*. 2021;77(9):1243–1256.
47. González LS, Chaney MA. Intraaortic balloon pump counterpulsation, Part I: history, technical aspects, physiologic effects, contraindications, medical applications/outcomes. *Anesth Analg*. 2020;131(3):776–791.
48. González LS, Chaney MA. Balloon pump counterpulsation part ii: perioperative hemodynamic support and new directions. *Anesth Analg*. 2020;131(3):792–807.
49. Subramaniam K, Boisen M, Shah PR, Ramesh V, Pete A. Mechanical circulatory support for cardiogenic shock. *Best Pract Res Clin Anaesthesiol*. 2012;26(2):131–146.
50. Keebler ME, Haddad EV, Choi CW, et al. Venoarterial extracorporeal membrane oxygenation in cardiogenic shock. *JACC Heart Fail*. 2018;6(6):503–516.
51. Peberdy MA, Gluck JA, Ornato JP, et al. Cardiopulmonary resuscitation in adults and children with mechanical circulatory support: A Scientific Statement From the American Heart Association. *Circulation*. 2017;135(24):e1115–e1134.
52. Dalia AA, Cronin B, Stone ME, et al. Anesthetic management of patients with continuous-flow left ventricular assist devices undergoing noncardiac surgery: an update for anesthesiologists. *J Cardiothorac Vasc Anesth*. 2018;32(2):1001–1012.
53. Chung M. Perioperative management of the patient with a left ventricular assist device for noncardiac surgery. *Anesth Analg*. 2018;126(6):1839–1850.
54. Han JJ, Acker MA, Atluri P. Left ventricular assist devices. *Circulation*. 2018;138(24): 2841–2851.

55. Wahba A, Milojevic M, Boer C, et al. 2019 EACTS/EACTA/EBCP guidelines on cardiopulmonary bypass in adult cardiac surgery. *Eur J Cardiothorac Surg*. 2020;57(2):210–251.
56. Barry AE, Chaney MA, London MJ. Anesthetic management during cardiopulmonary bypass: a systematic review. *Anesth Analg*. 2015;120(4):749–769.
57. Hessel EA, 2nd. What's new in cardiopulmonary bypass. *J Cardiothorac Vasc Anesth*. 2019;33(8):2296–2326.
58. Shore-Lesserson L, Baker RA, Ferraris VA, et al. The Society of Thoracic Surgeons, The Society of Cardiovascular Anesthesiologists, and The American Society of ExtraCorporeal Technology: Clinical Practice Guidelines-Anticoagulation During Cardiopulmonary Bypass. *Anesth Analg*. 2018;126(2):413–424.
59. Chen Y, Phoon PHY, Hwang NC. Heparin resistance during cardiopulmonary bypass in adult cardiac surgery. *J Cardiothorac Vasc Anesth*. 2022;36(11):4150–4160.
60. Rehfeldt KH, Barbara DW. Cardiopulmonary bypass without heparin. *Semin Cardiothorac Vasc Anesth*. 2016;20(1):40–51.
61. Tibi P, McClure RS, Huang J, et al. STS/SCA/AmSECT/SABM update to the clinical practice guidelines on patient blood management. *Ann Thorac Surg*. 2021;112(3):981–1004.
62. Raphael J, Mazer CD, Subramani S, et al. Society of Cardiovascular Anesthesiologists Clinical Practice Improvement Advisory for Management of Perioperative Bleeding and Hemostasis in Cardiac Surgery Patients. *Anesth Analg*. 2019;129(5):1209–1221.
63. Lomivorotov VV, Efremov SM, Abubakirov MN, Belletti A, Karaskov AM. Perioperative management of cardiovascular medications. *J Cardiothorac Vasc Anesth*. 2018;32(5):2289–2302.
64. Sousa-Uva M, Head SJ, Milojevic M, et al. 2017 EACTS Guidelines on perioperative medication in adult cardiac surgery. *Eur J Cardiothorac Surg*. 2018;53(1):5–33.
65. Tafur A, Douketis J. Perioperative management of anticoagulant and antiplatelet therapy. *Heart*. 2018;104(17):1461–1467.
66. Baumann Kreuziger L, Karkouti K, Tweddell J, Massicotte MP. Antithrombotic therapy management of adult and pediatric cardiac surgery patients. *J Thromb Haemost*. 2018;16(11):2133–2146.
67. Sessler DI. Perioperative temperature monitoring. *Anesthesiology*. 2021;134(1):111–118.
68. Grocott HP. Perioperative temperature and cardiac surgery. *J Extra Corpor Technol*. 2006; 38(1):77–80.
69. Singh A, Bahadorani B, Wakefield BJ, et al. Brachial arterial pressure monitoring during cardiac surgery rarely causes complications. *Anesthesiology*. 2017;126(6):1065–1076.
70. Kanazawa M, Fukuyama H, Kinefuchi Y, Takiguchi M, Suzuki T. Relationship between aortic-to-radial arterial pressure gradient after cardiopulmonary bypass and changes in arterial elasticity. *Anesthesiology*. 2003;99(1):48–53.
71. Rozental O, Thalappillil R, White RS, Tam CW. To swan or not to swan: indications, alternatives, and future directions. *J Cardiothorac Vasc Anesth*. 2021;35(2):600–615.
72. Nicoara A, Skubas N, Ad N, et al. Guidelines for the Use of Transesophageal Echocardiography to Assist with Surgical Decision-Making in the Operating Room: A Surgery-Based Approach: From the American Society of Echocardiography in Collaboration with the Society of Cardiovascular Anesthesiologists and the Society of Thoracic Surgeons. *J Am Soc Echocardiogr*. 2020;33(6):692–734.
73. Hogue CW Jr, Palin CA, Arrowsmith JE. Cardiopulmonary bypass management and neurologic outcomes: an evidence-based appraisal of current practices. *Anesth Analg*. 2006;103(1):21–37.
74. Lazar HL, McDonnell M, Chipkin SR, et al. The Society of Thoracic Surgeons Practice Guideline Series: Blood Glucose Management During Adult Cardiac Surgery. *Annals of Thoracic Surgery*. 2009;87(2):663–639.
75. Liu Y, Chen K, Mei W. Neurological complications after cardiac surgery: anesthetic considerations based on outcome evidence. *Curr Opin Anaesthesiol*. 2019;32(5):563–567.
76. Kunst G, Milojevic M, Boer C, et al. 2019 EACTS/EACTA/EBCP guidelines on cardiopulmonary bypass in adult cardiac surgery. *Br J Anaesth*. 2019;123(6):713–757.
77. Ali J, Cody J, Maldonado Y, Ramakrishna H. Near-infrared spectroscopy (NIRS) for cerebral and tissue oximetry: analysis of evolving applications. *J Cardiothorac Vasc Anesth*. 2022;36(8 Pt A):2758–2766.
78. Engelman RM, Rousou JA, Flack JE 3rd, et al. Fast-track recovery of the coronary bypass patient. *Ann Thorac Surg*. 1994;58(6):1742–1746.
79. Bainbridge D, Cheng DC. Early extubation and fast-track management of off-pump cardiac patients in the intensive care unit. *Semin Cardiothorac Vasc Anesth*. 2015;19(2):163–168.
80. Niclauss L. Techniques and standards in intraoperative graft verification by transit time flow measurement after coronary artery bypass graft surgery: a critical review. *Eur J Cardiothorac Surg*. 2017;51(1):26–33.
81. Sousa-Uva M, Neumann FJ, Ahlsson A, et al. 2018 ESC/EACTS Guidelines on myocardial revascularization. *Eur J Cardiothorac Surg*. 2019;55(1):4–90.
82. McKinlay KH, Schinderle DB, Swaminathan M, et al. Predictors of inotrope use during separation from cardiopulmonary bypass. *J Cardiothorac Vasc Anesth*. 2004;18(4):404–408.
83. Duncan AE, Kartashov A, Robinson SB, et al. Risk factors, resource use, and cost of postoperative low cardiac output syndrome. *J Thorac Cardiovasc Surg*. 2022;163(5):1890–8.e10.
84. White A, Patvardhan C, Falter F. Anesthesia for minimally invasive cardiac surgery. *J Thorac Dis*. 2021;13(3):1886–1898.
85. Parnell A, Prince M. Anaesthesia for minimally invasive cardiac surgery. *BJA Educ*. 2018; 18(10):323–330.
86. Vernick W, Atluri P. Robotic and minimally invasive cardiac surgery. *Anesthesiol Clin*. 2013; 31(2):299–320.
87. Lazar HL. Should off-pump coronary artery bypass grafting be abandoned? *Circulation*. 2013; 128(4):406–413.
88. Burns DJP, Wierup P, Gillinov M. Minimally Invasive Mitral Surgery: Patient Selection and Technique. *Cardiol Clin*. 2021;39(2):211–220.
89. Glauber M, Miceli A, Gilmanov D, et al. Right anterior minithoracotomy versus conventional aortic valve replacement: a propensity score matched study. *J Thorac Cardiovasc Surg*. 2013;145(5):1222–1226.
90. Leon MB, Smith CR, Mack MJ, et al. Transcatheter or surgical aortic-valve replacement in intermediate-risk patients. *N Engl J Med*. 2016;374(17):1609–1620.
91. Davidson LJ, Davidson CJ. Transcatheter treatment of valvular heart disease: a review. *Jama*. 2021;325(24):2480–2494.
92. Ruel M, Chan V, Boodhwani M, et al. How detrimental is reexploration for bleeding after cardiac surgery? *J Thorac Cardiovasc Surg*. 2017;154(3):927–935.
93. Wu W, He J, Shao X. Incidence and mortality trend of congenital heart disease at the global, regional, and national level, 1990-2017. *Medicine (Baltimore)*. 2020;99(23):e20593.
94. Ko JM. Genetic syndromes associated with congenital heart disease. *Korean Circ J*. 2015;45(5): 357–361.
95. Mittnacht AJ, Hollinger I. Fast-tracking in pediatric cardiac surgery-the current standing. *Ann Card Anaesth*. 2010;13:92–101.
96. Raj N. Regional anesthesia for sternotomy and bypass—Beyond the epidural. *Pediatr Anesth*. 2019;29:519–529.
97. Lofland GK. The enhancement of hemodynamic performance in Fontan circulation using pain free spontaneous ventilation. *Eur J Cardiothorac Surg*. 2001;20:114–119.
98. Chandler HK, Kirsch R. Management of the Low Cardiac Output Syndrome Following Surgery for Congenital Heart Disease. *Curr Cardiol Rev*. 2016;12(2):107–111.
99. Naito Y, Aoki M, Watanabe M, et al. Factors affecting systemic oxygen delivery after Norwood procedure with Sano modification. *Ann Thorac Surg*. 2010;89(1):168–173.
100. Verheugt CL, et al. Mortality in adult congenital heart disease. *European Heart Journal*. 2010;31(10):1220–1229.

40 Anesthesia for Vascular and Endovascular Surgery

ELIZABETH A. VALENTINE • E. ANDREW OCHROCH

KEY POINTS

1. Atherosclerosis is the most common underlying pathophysiologic mechanism for the development of cardiovascular disease.
2. The same risk factors that lead to coronary artery disease also lead to vascular disease in other major vascular beds, including the cerebral, aortic, and peripheral circulation.
3. Improvements in the medical management of patients with atherosclerotic risk factors with antiplatelet agents, β-blockers, angiotensin-converting enzyme inhibitors, statins, and strict glucose control have revolutionized the management of vascular surgery patients. Meticulous optimization of comorbid conditions plays a critical role in the reduction of perioperative morbidity and mortality in this patient population.
4. Most vascular surgery patients are at elevated perioperative risk of major adverse cardiac events, which remain the single most important cause of both short- and long-term morbidity and mortality following vascular surgery.
5. The pathophysiology of aneurysmal aortic disease is a clinically distinct degenerative process, although many of the risk factors are shared between degenerative and atherosclerotic vascular disease.
6. Endovascular procedures have transformed the field of vascular surgery with an increasing number of procedures being performed via a minimally invasive approach. Perioperative improvements in morbidity and mortality must be weighed against the long-term risks of decreased durability and increased need for repeat intervention.

Introduction

Atherosclerotic cardiovascular disease (ASCVD) is the most important cause of morbidity and mortality in both the United States and throughout the world. More than 80 million adults in the United States carry a diagnosis related to ASCVD. Globally, ASCVD has overtaken communicable diseases as the leading cause of death worldwide. ASCVD currently accounts for more than 17.3 million deaths worldwide per year, and this number is expected to increase to greater than 23.6 million deaths by 2030 due to an aging population.[1,2] Advances in medical management have led to an overall decrease in the total number of deaths attributable to ASCVD over recent years, although nearly one out of every three deaths in the United States is related to ASCVD.[3]

Emphasis on increased screening and the increasing age of the population in Western societies will likely increase the number of vascular procedures performed on a yearly basis. It has been estimated that 1 to 2 million vascular procedures will be performed annually in the United States by the year 2030.[4] Improvements in optimal medical management may delay the need for surgical interventions until severe systemic ASCVD disease is present. As a result of recent advances in endovascular techniques, many patients who previously would be deemed too high risk for the operating room are increasingly considered surgical candidates. This combination of a high-risk patient population and complex, high-risk surgical procedures makes vascular anesthesia challenging even for the experienced clinician. Despite both the medical and surgical issues that this patient population presents, surgical mortality has fallen from greater than 25% for major aortic reconstruction in the 1960s to as low as 3% today. This is largely due to improved perioperative optimization and management. The anesthesiologist may have greater influence in reducing morbidity and mortality in vascular surgery than in any other area of anesthesia.

This chapter begins with a discussion of the pathophysiology of ASCVD and a suggested approach to the preoperative evaluation and perioperative optimization of vascular surgery patients. Coronary artery disease (CAD) will be discussed in particular detail, given the high incidence of concomitant CAD in vascular surgery patients and the increased morbidity and mortality in this patient population. The specific surgical goals, anatomic considerations, and perioperative concerns for cerebrovascular, aortic, and lower extremity revascularization will be discussed in the context of optimal anesthetic management and accounting for surgical technique (open vs. endovascular repair).

Vascular Disease

Pathophysiology of Atherosclerosis

Atherosclerosis is the most common pathophysiologic mechanism underlying cardiovascular disease. At its simplest definition, atherosclerosis is a generalized inflammatory disorder of the arterial tree. Putative mechanisms include endothelial damage, hemodynamic shear stress, inflammation from chronic infections, hypercoagulability with resultant thrombosis, and 1

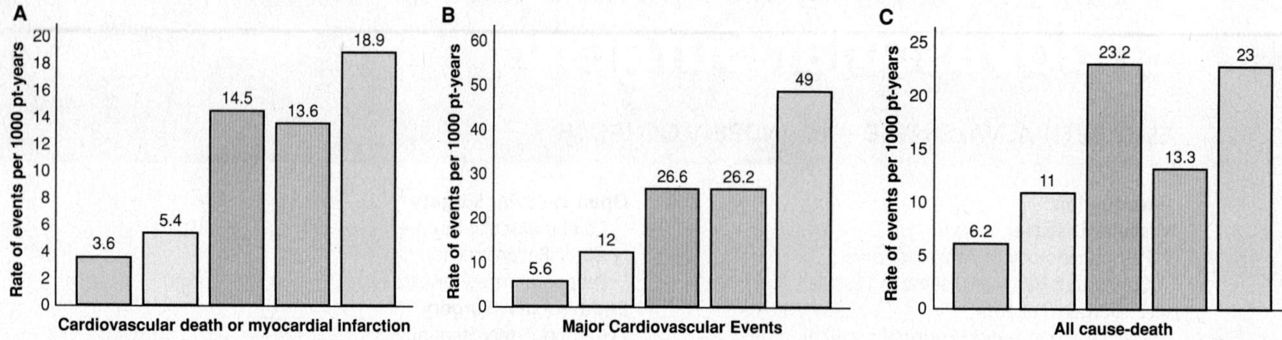

Figure 40-1 Rate of cardiovascular death, myocardial infarction, or major adverse cardiac event by presence, severity, and extent of coronary artery disease (CAD). Both obstructive and nonobstructive atherosclerotic plaque may result in significant cardiovascular morbidity and mortality. Overall disease burden may be as important a contributor as individual plaque characteristics to adverse events. (Reprinted with permission from Bittencourt MS, Hulten E, Ghoshhajra B, et al. Prognostic value of nonobstructive and obstructive coronary artery disease detected by coronary computed tomography angiography to identify cardiovascular events. CAD is coronary artery score, SIS is coronary segment involvement score. *Circ Cardiovasc Imaging*. 2014;7:282–291.)

the destructive effect of low-density lipoproteins (LDLs). Atherosclerotic plaque formation is a complex process involving endothelial dysfunction, lipid deposition, smooth muscle proliferation, and the proliferation of inflammatory and immunogenic mediators.[5]

The development of atherosclerosis occurs in two stages: injury and response to injury. An intact vascular endothelium serves as a barrier between the blood and the more thrombogenic subendothelial tissues. Injured epithelial cells express leukocyte adhesion molecules that increase the adherence of macrophages and other leukocytes. Increased permeability of the damaged endothelium permits entry of leukocytes and LDL particles into the subendothelial space, and modified LDL particles induce leukocyte adhesion. The earliest recognizable lesion of atherosclerosis is this "fatty steak" which is comprised of lipid-rich macrophages and T lymphocytes that accumulate within the intima of the vessel wall. Monocyte-derived macrophages act as scavenging and antigen-presenting cells and produce further proinflammatory mediators. A variety of cytokines and growth factors (including monocyte chemotactic protein-1, macrophage and granulocyte-macrophage colony stimulating factors, intercellular adhesion molecule-1, tumor necrosis factor α, and interleukins 1, 3, 6, 8, and 18) further recruit activated immune and smooth muscle cells. In this enriched environment, macrophages transform into foam cells. Foam cells and extracellular lipid form the core of the plaque, which is surrounded by smooth-muscle cells and a collagen-rich matrix. The progression of atherosclerotic plaque ultimately narrows the intravascular lumen and contributes to an imbalance between oxygen supply and demand. Depending on location of the atherosclerotic plaque, the end result is ischemia of the coronary, cerebral, mesenteric, or peripheral circulation.

The traditional teaching is that of the "vulnerable plaque" model. That is, over time, inflammatory mediators and proteolytic enzymes may weaken the thin fibrous cap overlying the atheromatous plaque, making it particularly prone to ulceration, rupture, and acute thrombosis. Historically, treatment of presumed high-risk lesions was the focus of great effort. However, more recent evidence suggests that although such high-risk features may be valuable as a surrogate for overall disease burden, no conclusive evidence exists to support that high-risk plaque characteristics are an independent risk factor for a clinical event.[5] Focus on overall atherosclerotic disease burden rather than individual plaque features may be as, if not more, important (Fig. 40-1). When plaque rupture is the culprit event, platelets play a pivotal role. Platelet polymorphisms have been found to be an independent risk factor following vascular surgery.[6]

Concurrent Vascular Disease in Vascular Surgery Patients

The underlying risk factors for atherosclerotic disease are simi- 2
lar regardless of plaque location, though individual risk factors may be more strongly associated with disease in one vascular bed than another. Some risk factors, such as a strong family history, nonwhite ethnicity, male sex, and increasing age, are outside a patient's control. Modifiable risk factors include smoking, atherogenic dyslipidemia (hypertriglyceridemia, elevated LDL, and decreased high-density lipoprotein [HDL]), abdominal obesity, hypertension, insulin resistance, renal insufficiency, and proinflammatory states.[7,8] With aggressive lifestyle and pharmacologic interventions, atherosclerotic disease progression can be significantly slowed.

ASCVD in one vascular bed often predicts significant disease in other areas of the body (Fig. 40-2).[7] The presence of cerebrovascular disease (CVD) has long been used as a surrogate marker for

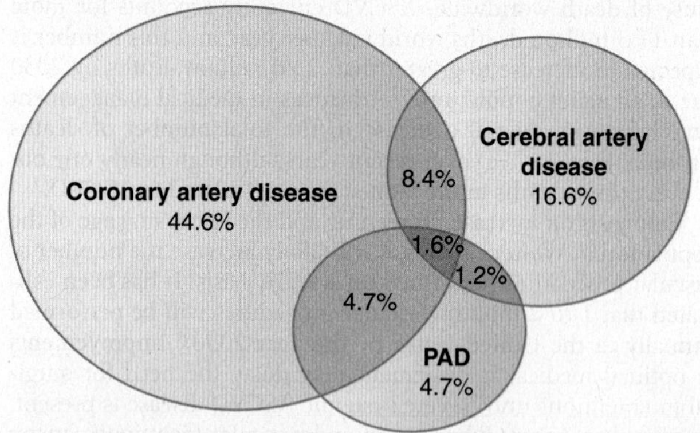

Figure 40-2 Typical overlap of atherosclerotic cardiovascular disease by vascular bed. Atherosclerotic disease in one vascular bed often predicts disease in other areas. (Reprinted from Norgren L, Hiatt WR, Dormandy JA, et al. Inter-Society Consensus for the Management of Peripheral Arterial Disease [TASC II]. *J Vasc Surg*. 2007;45[Suppl S]: S5–S67. Copyright © 2007 The Society for Vascular Surgery. Published by Mosby, Inc. With permission.)

Table 40-1 Coronary Artery Disease (CAD) Severity for Vascular Surgery Patients Who Underwent Routine or Selective Coronary Angiography[a]

	Patients With Coronary Artery Disease	
	Routine Surveillance (%)	***Suspected Disease (%)***
Normal coronaries	14	4
Mild to moderate CAD	49	18
Advanced but compensated CAD	22	34
Severe, correctable CAD	14	34
Severe, inoperable CAD	1	10

[a]A significant portion of patients who underwent coronary artery angiography prior to vascular surgery were found to have advanced disease. This held true even for patients without a high clinical suspicion for significant coronary artery disease.

Adapted with permission from Hertzer NR, Beven EG, Young JR, et al. Coronary artery disease in peripheral vascular patients: a classification of 1000 coronary angiograms and results of surgical management. *Ann Surg*. 1984;199:223–233.

CAD. Multiple studies have demonstrated an association between carotid intima-media thickness (CIMT) and CAD and cardiovascular death. A meta-analysis of the literature demonstrated that for each 0.1-mm increase in CIMT, the future risk of myocardial infarction (MI) was increased by 10% to 15%.[9] Conversely, every 0.01 mm/yr decrease in the progression of CIMT has been associated with a nearly 20% reduction of the risk of nonfatal MI.[9] The overall presence of carotid atherosclerotic plaque, independent of CIMT, also predicts an increase in incidence of MI and cardiovascular death.[10]

Hertzer et al.[11] performed coronary angiography on 1,000 consecutive patients presenting for elective vascular surgery and identified an overall prevalence of CAD of approximately 50% in this patient population. Severe, correctable CAD was noted in 25% of the entire series (Table 40-1). Surgically correctable disease was more frequent in patients with known risk factors for coronary disease than those without (34% vs. 14%). Subsequent analysis demonstrated that the severity of CAD could be accurately predicted by clinical risk factors.[12] The absence of (1) diabetes mellitus, (2) prior angina, (3) previous MI, or (4) history of congestive heart failure (CHF) predicted the absence of severe CAD with a positive predictive value of 96%. The absence of critical CAD (greater than or equal to 70% stenosis of left main or triple vessel disease) could be predicted with a positive predictive value of 94% in patients without (1) prior angina, (2) previous MI, or (3) history of CHF.

The clinical prevalence of CAD or CVD in patients with diagnosed peripheral artery disease (PAD) ranges from 40% to 60%. The extent of CAD, measured by either computed tomography (CT) detection of coronary artery calcium or coronary angiography, correlates with the ankle–brachial index.[7] Approximately 10% to 30% of patients with documented CAD have concurrent PAD. Concurrent carotid and peripheral arterial disease occurs in approximately 25% to 50% of patients. Autopsy studies have demonstrated that patients with fatal MI are twice as likely to have a significant disease in the cerebral and peripheral arterial beds.

Medical Optimization Prior to Vascular Surgery

Cardiovascular complications are a major source of morbidity and 3
mortality following vascular surgery. Nearly 10% of patients demonstrate evidence of significant myocardial injury in the perioperative period, and 2% of patients suffer a major adverse cardiac event (MACE).[13–15] Patient who experience an MI following noncardiac surgery have an elevated in-hospital mortality rate of 15% to 25%, and nonfatal perioperative MI is an independent predictor for cardiovascular death in the 6 months following surgery.[14] Thus, medical optimization of ASCVD in the perioperative period has been a focus of significant study.

Lifestyle modifications such as regular exercise, weight loss, diet modification, and smoking cessation may forestall the progression of atherosclerotic disease and improve fitness for surgery. Patients undergoing vascular surgery should also be aggressively treated for underlying medical conditions that predispose to ASCVD such as hypertension, dyslipidemia, and diabetes. Improvements in pharmacologic therapy have revolutionized the care of patients with atherosclerotic disease. It is worth noting that many of the landmark trials that currently dictate recommendations for surgical intervention were performed at a time when best medical therapy for atherosclerotic disease was significantly limited as compared to today. In the modern era of multimodal treatment with β-blockade, statins, intensive glucose control, antiplatelet therapies, and pharmacologic aids for smoking cessation, it is conceivable that a larger number of patients may be appropriately managed with medical, rather than surgical, therapy. That is, with improved medical management, the number needed to operate on to prevent an untoward cardiovascular event may be even higher than the current literature suggests. Trials comparing modern-day intensive medical therapy versus intervention, either open or endovascular, are actively underway.[16]

Perhaps the most widely studied medical intervention in the perioperative period is the use of β-blockade. A significant proportion of postoperative ischemic events are thought to be secondary to a persistently exaggerated sympathetic response. Substantial elevations in heart rate increase myocardial oxygen demand while simultaneously decreasing oxygen supply, with resultant demand ischemia. It has been proposed that modulating this heart rate response may decrease both the incidence and severity of the ischemia (Fig. 40-3).[17,18] Several randomized controlled studies demonstrated a significant benefit to β-blockade as a means to reduce the risk of MACE,[18,19] although other studies have failed to validate these findings.[20,21] The PeriOperative ISchemic Evaluation (POISE-1) trial, a large randomized controlled trial of more than 8,000 patients, found that perioperative β-blockade was associated with a decrease in perioperative MI, at the expense of an even greater increased risk of death or stroke.[22] Current recommendations for the role of perioperative β-blockade in noncardiac surgery released by the American College of Cardiology (ACC) and American Heart Association (AHA) reviewed 17 large (>100 patients) randomized controlled or cohort studies comparing perioperative β-blockade against placebo in adult patients undergoing noncardiac surgery.[13] For patients started on β-blockade 1 day or less before surgery, this review demonstrated an overall moderate reduction in nonfatal MI, even with the exclusion of the DECREASE studies. There was, however, an overall increased risk of all-cause death and trend toward increased risk of cardiovascular death. There was also a significant increase in the risk of nonfatal stroke and for significant hypotension and bradycardia in the group receiving β-blockade. For patients in whom β-blockade was initiated 2 or more days prior to surgery, current data were deemed insufficient to recommend for or against β-blockade

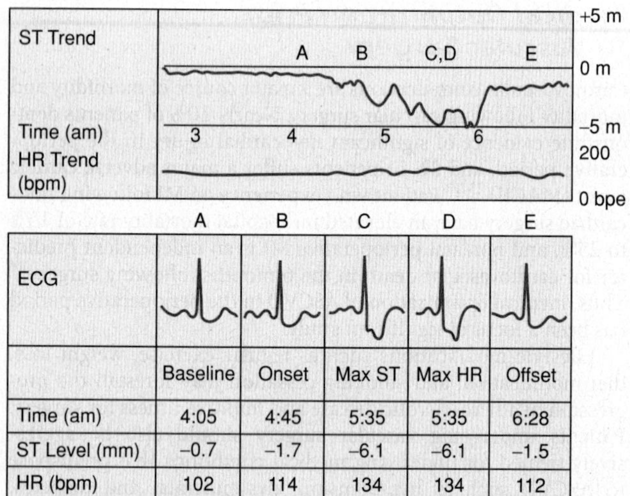

	Baseline	Onset	Max ST	Max HR	Offset
Time (am)	4:05	4:45	5:35	5:35	6:28
ST Level (mm)	−0.7	−1.7	−6.1	−6.1	−1.5
HR (bpm)	102	114	134	134	112

Figure 40-3 ST segment changes with heart rate (HR) during an ischemic episode. Tachycardia can increase the myocardial oxygen demand (due to increased work) while decreasing supply (due to decreased diastolic filling time), culminating in demand ischemia. (Reprinted from Mangano DT, Hollenberg M, Fegert G, et al. Perioperative myocardial ischemia in patients undergoing noncardiac surgery–I: Incidence and severity during the 4 day perioperative period. The Study of Perioperative Ischemia [SPI] Research Group. *J Am Coll Cardiol.* 1991;17:843–850. Copyright © 1991 Elsevier. With permission.)

therapy in the perioperative period. Further multicenter, randomized controlled trials are needed to address this gap in knowledge.

The 2014 update to the ACC/AHA clinical practice guideline for perioperative cardiovascular evaluation and management of patients undergoing noncardiac surgery also made specific recommendations regarding the management of perioperative β-blockade.[23] This task force recommended that β-blockers should be continued in the perioperative period in patients who are chronically on β-blocker therapy (Class I, Level of Evidence B) and that it may be reasonable to begin β-blockers in the perioperative period on those patients with intermediate- to high-risk myocardial ischemia noted on preoperative testing (Class IIb, LOE C) or in patients with three or more cardiac risk factors (Class IIb, LOE B). It is reasonable to start such therapy in advance of surgery to establish safety and tolerability (Class IIb, Level of Evidence: B). They further recommend that β-blockers should not be started on the day of surgery (Class III, LOE B).

Studies of perioperative β-blockade specific to the vascular surgery population have found similar conclusions to those in the general surgical population. A retrospective cohort analysis of the Society for Vascular Surgery Vascular Quality Initiative (SVS-VQI) found that, exclusive of high-risk open abdominal aortic aneurysm repair (OAR), preoperative institution of β-blockade did not decrease mortality or rate of MACE, but did increase the rates of other adverse events following major vascular surgery.[24] The Perioperative Beta Blockade (POBBLE)[21] trial evaluated more than 100 patients undergoing infrarenal vascular surgery and the Metoprolol after Vascular Surgery (MaVS)[20] included nearly 500 patients undergoing abdominal aortic surgery, axillofemoral revascularization, or infrainguinal revascularization. Both studies failed to find a significant difference in MACE between patients who received β-blockers in the perioperative period and placebo. A recent Cochrane Review concluded that there is no evidence that perioperative β-blockade reduces all-cause mortality, cardiovascular mortality, nonfatal MI, arrhythmia, heart failure, stroke, or composite cardiovascular events in patients undergoing vascular surgery.[25] It further concluded that strong evidence suggests that β-blockade increases the risk of perioperative bradycardia and hypotension.

As a result of a shift in both the strength and direction of evidence, the practice of β-blocker initiation in the immediate perioperative period has precipitously declined over recent years (Fig. 40-4), although the practice remains relatively common in patients with higher cardiac risk and those undergoing vascular surgery.[26] The choice of β-blocker in the perioperative

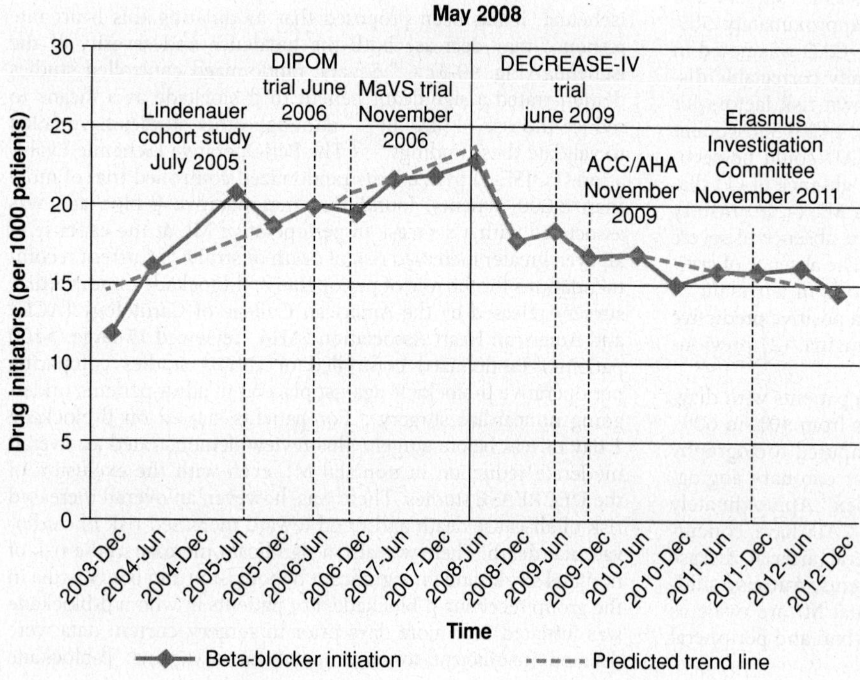

Figure 40-4 Temporal trends in β-blockade initiation within 30 days of surgery from 2003 to 2012. Following the influential POISE trial, the practice of perioperative β-blockade initiation within 30 days of surgery decreased significantly. ACC/AHA, American College of Cardiology/American Heart Association. (Reprinted from Patorno E, Wang SV, Schneeweiss S, et al. Patterns of beta-blocker initiation in patients undergoing intermediate- to high-risk noncardiac surgery. *Am Heart J.* 2015;170:812–820.e6. Copyright © 2015 Elsevier. With permission.)

period has also been studied. An epidemiologic analysis of nearly 40,000 high-risk patients found a decreased mortality at both 30 days and 1 year in patients who received atenolol as compared to metoprolol.[27] A retrospective analysis of nearly 60,000 patients found that both preoperative metoprolol (compared to atenolol) and intraoperative metoprolol (compared to esmolol or labetalol) was associated with an increased risk of stroke after noncardiac surgery.[28]

The marked sympathetic stimulation that occurs in the perioperative period has led to significant interest in α_2-adrenergic agonists to blunt the surgical stress response and reduce cardiovascular morbidity and mortality. Evidence for the utility of α_2-agonists in the perioperative period is conflicting. Though early studies suggested that the perioperative use of α_2-agonists reduces intraoperative myocardial ischemia, postoperative catecholamine levels, and mortality in high-risk noncardiac surgery,[29,30] more recent evidence calls the perioperative benefit of α_2-agonists into question. The PeriOperative ISchemic Evaluation-2 (POISE-2) trial was a multicenter, international, randomized, blinded trial that evaluated over 10,000 patients with, or at risk for, ASCVD undergoing noncardiac surgery.[31] In this study, α_2-agonists did not reduce the incidence of perioperative MI or the composite outcome of death or nonfatal MI. Patients receiving α_2-agonists had more clinically significant hypotension and an increased incidence of nonfatal cardiac arrest. In light of these recent findings, the most recent ACC/AHA guidelines state that α_2-agonists are not recommended for prevention of MACE in patients undergoing noncardiac surgery (Class III; LOE B).[23] Although evidence to support the initiation of α_2-agonists is lacking, it is important to recognize that the abrupt discontinuation of this class of medication in patients who are chronic users can result in a rebound sympathetic surge including profound hypertension and tachycardia, diaphoresis, and pulmonary edema. Thus, the relative risks and benefits of continuing versus withdrawing this class of medication must be considered in patients who chronically receive α_2-agonists.

Renin–angiotensin system (RAS) blockers (including angiotensin-converting enzyme inhibitors and angiotensin-receptor blockers) are a commonly used class of antihypertensive agents that have several benefits in regard to prevention of acute cardiovascular events independent of their antihypertensive effects. The RAS has been shown to influence the progression of ASCVD via effects on inflammation, endothelial function, and overall plaque stability.[32] RAS blocking agents have demonstrated beneficial effects on ventricular remodeling following acute MI,[33] ischemia–reperfusion injury,[34] and perioperative acute kidney injury.[35] Despite beneficial long-term effects, a recent large, retrospective study in the cardiac surgery population found an increased risk of perioperative morbidity (including significant vasoplegia, need for inotropic support, dysrhythmia, and renal dysfunction) and mortality when ACE inhibitors were continued in the perioperative period.[36] A similar association was found between perioperative RAS blockade and 30-day mortality following major vascular surgery.[37] To date, no studies provide definitive evidence for the independent ability of RAS blockers to reduce perioperative cardiovascular risk, and further randomized controlled trials are warranted. The most recent ACC/AHA guidelines suggest that continuation of RAS blocking agents is reasonable in the perioperative period (Class IIa; LOE B), and that if they stopped preoperatively, it is reasonable to restart as soon as clinically feasible (Class IIa; LOE C).[23] However, many choose to hold this class of medication in the preoperative period due to a well-recognized association between RAS blocking medications and refractory vasoplegia.

Statins are widely utilized for both primary and secondary prevention of ASCVD for their beneficial effects on lipid profile. More recent evidence also suggests more pleiotropic effects on events critical to the surgical stress response. Statins have been shown to inhibit the inflammatory response, reduce ischemia–reperfusion injury, reduce thrombosis, enhance fibrinolysis, decrease platelet reactivity, and restore endothelial function.[38] Use of preoperative statins has been associated with reduced cardiac morbidity and mortality following both cardiac and vascular surgery.[39–41] The abrupt discontinuation of statins interferes with endothelial functioning and increases markers of inflammation and oxidative stress in acute coronary syndromes,[42] and the discontinuation of statins in the postoperative period is similarly associated with increased in-hospital death and myonecrosis.[40] Meta-analyses specific to the vascular surgery population have had conflicting results on perioperative outcomes. One analysis found no difference in 30-day mortality or MACE in patients not already receiving a statin medication following noncardiac vascular surgery,[43] whereas another found no significant difference in cardiovascular mortality but a lower risk of all-cause mortality, MI, stroke, and the composite outcome of MI, stroke, and death.[44] The ACC/AHA recommendations propose that patients who take a statin should be continued on this medication during the perioperative period (Class I; LOE B). They further suggest that it is reasonable to initiate treatment in patients undergoing vascular surgery if statin naïve (Class IIa; LOE B).[23]

Antiplatelet agents are commonly employed for secondary prevention of MACE. Multiple studies have found that antiplatelet agents, and particularly dual antiplatelet therapy (DAPT), can reduce the rate of ischemic events; furthermore, aspirin withdrawal syndrome has been associated with acute perioperative cardiovascular events.[45] Patients who have suffered previous ischemic stroke should be continued on mono or dual antiplatelet therapy,[46] and evidence suggests that patients undergoing carotid endarterectomy (CEA) have a lower rate of perioperative stroke when antiplatelet agents are continued in the perioperative period.[47] Similarly, DAPT is essential following coronary stent implantation.[23] Despite the purported benefits of antiplatelet agents, however, a review from the Vascular Quality Initiative found no difference in the rate of in hospital MI or death in patients who did and did not receive antiplatelet agents before major vascular surgery.[48] There was, however, an increased rate of blood loss for all procedures and increased transfusion rate for infrainguinal bypass. Similarly, the POISE-2 trial found no difference in the primary outcome of composite of death or nonfatal MI at 30 days between those who did and did not receive aspirin, or in the secondary outcome which also included nonfatal stroke.[49] A greater risk of major bleeding was observed in the aspirin group. In contrast to these two trials, a recent prospective review from the Vascular Study Group of New England evaluated the use of clopidogrel, aspirin, or DAPT for more than 10,000 patients at 15 centers undergoing nonemergent CEA, lower extremity bypass, endovascular aortic repair (EVAR), and OAR and found no difference in major bleeding complications between the three groups.[50] Thus, although the use of antiplatelet agents is important for long-term management of ASCVD, the purported risks and benefits of antiplatelet therapy in the perioperative period must be carefully weighed in noncardiac, noncarotid vascular surgery.

The lack of perceived benefit of aspirin on perioperative MI observed in the Vascular Quality Initiative and POISE-2 studies may be related to a difference in the causative mechanism of MI in the perioperative period compared to the nonoperative setting. Specifically, type I MI (characterized by morphologically complex coronary plaque prone to rupture and thrombus) may not be the dominant mechanism in the perioperative setting but rather a demand ischemia (Type II MI) caused by a mismatch in arterial supply and demand, which may be exacerbated by major bleeding on the resultant anemia, hypotension, and tachycardia.[51] The most recent ACC/AHA guidelines suggest that the management of perioperative antiplatelet therapy should be determined by consensus of the treating clinicians (Class I; LOE C). It may be reasonable to continue aspirin in patients undergoing nonemergent/nonurgent noncardiac surgery who have not had previous coronary stenting when the perceived risk of MACE outweighs the risk of increased bleeding (Class IIb; LOE B). These guidelines recommend against the initiation or continuation of aspirin in patients undergoing elective noncardiac, noncarotid surgery who have not had previous coronary stenting (Class III; LOE B), unless the risk of ischemic event is greater than the risk of surgical bleeding (Class III; LOE C).[23]

Hyperglycemia has been associated with increased morbidity and mortality in critically ill patients. Of the oral hypoglycemic agents, it is reasonable to hold sulfonylureas due to the risk of hypoglycemia in the settling of preoperative fasting. Metformin is associated with lactic acidosis and should also be held preoperatively due the increased risk of lactic acidosis with hypovolemia and renal dysfunction (which may be comorbid or provoked by iodinated contrast agents used during endovascular procedures). Sodium-glucose co-transport type 2 inhibitors (SGLT-2i) are a newer class of drugs that are increasingly used to treat type 2 diabetes mellitus that have been associated with perioperative euglycemic ketoacidosis and should be temporarily discontinued for at least 3 days prior to surgery according to the Food and Drug Administration safety labeling.[52] When other antihyperglycemics are suspended, patients can be managed with insulin, which is the treatment modality most intensively studied in the perioperative period. Initial work suggested that tight glucose control (glucose 80 to 110 mg/dL) in critically ill patients led to significant decrease in mortality and multiorgan system failure, resulting in a call for stringent control of hyperglycemia in hospitalized patients.[53] Subsequent studies, however, have failed to replicate these results and instead have found an increase in unrecognized hypoglycemia and an increased risk of death in patients in the intensive glucose control group.[54,55] Hyperglycemia may exacerbate neurologic injury and thus may be especially important for carotid and thoracic aortic procedures with elevated risk of perioperative stroke. In the intraoperative period, both hyperglycemia and tight glucose control have been associated with an increased risk of adverse outcomes.[56] Thus, although severe hyperglycemia should be avoided, it is likely prudent to maintain glucose levels in the 140 to 180 mg/dL range rather than attempt normoglycemia.

It has been suggested that anemia (hematocrit <28%) may increase the incidence of postoperative myocardial ischemia and MACE in high-risk patients undergoing noncardiac surgery,[57] and a traditional practice is to transfuse patients deemed high risk for adverse cardiac events to a hematocrit of 30%. More recently, two studies have suggested no benefit to liberal (hemoglobin goal 10 to 12 mg/dL) rather than restrictive (hemoglobin goal 7 to 8 mg/dL) transfusion practices.[58,59] The Functional Outcomes in Cardiovascular Patients Undergoing Surgical Hip Fracture Repair (FOCUS) trial,[59] in specific, found no outcomes differences between patients transfused intraoperatively with a restrictive versus liberal strategy, even in a perceived high-risk population. Studies on perioperative transfusion in vascular surgery have produced mixed results; both transfusion and perioperative anemia have been independently associated with increased 30-day morbidity and mortality.[60,61] Perioperative transfusion should be based on evidence of compromised end-organ perfusion, rate and cause of blood loss, and likelihood of obtaining control of ongoing hemorrhage.

Cardiac morbidity and mortality is higher following vascular surgery than after other types of noncardiac surgery, and the presence of uncorrected CAD appears to double the 5-year mortality following vascular surgery. Given the high likelihood of concurrent CAD in patients presenting for vascular surgery, and given that myocardial revascularization may have long-term benefits in patients with triple vessel CAD, left main disease, or poor left ventricular (LV) function, the question of preoperative coronary revascularization prior to elective vascular surgery has been a subject of study. Initial observational studies suggested that preoperative cardiac revascularization improves patient outcomes prior to high-risk noncardiac surgery.[62,63] Whether preoperative coronary revascularization actually protects against perioperative MACE is controversial in prospective studies. Monaco and colleagues[64] randomized more than 200 patients undergoing vascular surgery to routine preoperative coronary angiography versus selective angiography based on the results of noninvasive testing and risk stratification. Myocardial revascularization was more common in the routine surveillance group, although there was no significant different in in-hospital MACE rate between groups. Notably, however, long-term survival and freedom from death/cardiovascular events was improved in the group who underwent routine preoperative coronary angiography (Fig. 40-5). The multicenter Coronary Artery Revascularization Prophylaxis (CARP) trial evaluated more than 500 patients who underwent prophylactic cardiac revascularization prior to major vascular surgery based on the presence of ischemia on a noninvasive stress imaging study.[65] Patients were randomized to either percutaneous coronary intervention (PCI) or coronary artery bypass (CABG). With aggressive medical therapy (>80% of patients on β-blockers, >70% on aspirin, and >50% on statins in both groups), no long-term benefit was noted with preoperative revascularization. A subsequent subgroup analysis examined the value of CABG versus PCI and found that patients who underwent CABG had fewer MIs and shorter hospital stays than their counterparts in the PCI group.[66] This difference may be due to more complete revascularization in the CABG group. It is worth noting that the CARP study randomized patients on the basis of abnormal stress testing, whereas the Monaco study performed coronary angiography on all patients in the routine group. Thus, in the CARP study, patients with CAD but limited or no ischemia at stress testing may have missed on a benefit to revascularization prior to the procedure. Furthermore, most patients in the CARP trial had single-vessel or two-vessel disease with normal LV ejection fraction. Exclusion criteria in this study included left main disease or ejection fraction less than 20%, thus limiting patients with more severe disease. A subsequent analysis of the CARP data found that patients with unprotected left main disease may be the only subset of patients who benefits from prophylactic revascularization.[67] In large part due to the CARP trial, preoperative coronary revascularization (either surgical or interventional) is not recommended prior to even high-risk surgery, unless revascularization is independently indicated according to current practice guidelines.[68]

For patients who have suffered recent MI who need noncardiac surgery, evidence suggests that the risk of postoperative MI decreases significantly with time. Furthermore, the risk of postoperative MI may be modified by the occurrence and type of revascularization performed (CABG vs. PCI) prior to elective surgery.[69] Current guidelines recommend waiting at least 60 days following MI before elective noncardiac surgery in the absence of intervention.[23] For patients for whom preoperative coronary revascularization is deemed necessary prior to elective surgery, the timing of originally proposed procedure depends on the type of coronary intervention performed. The most recent ACC/AHA guidelines make no specific recommendation on appropriate timing on noncardiac surgery following CABG. In this case, the clinical urgency of the procedure, medical optimization, and overall

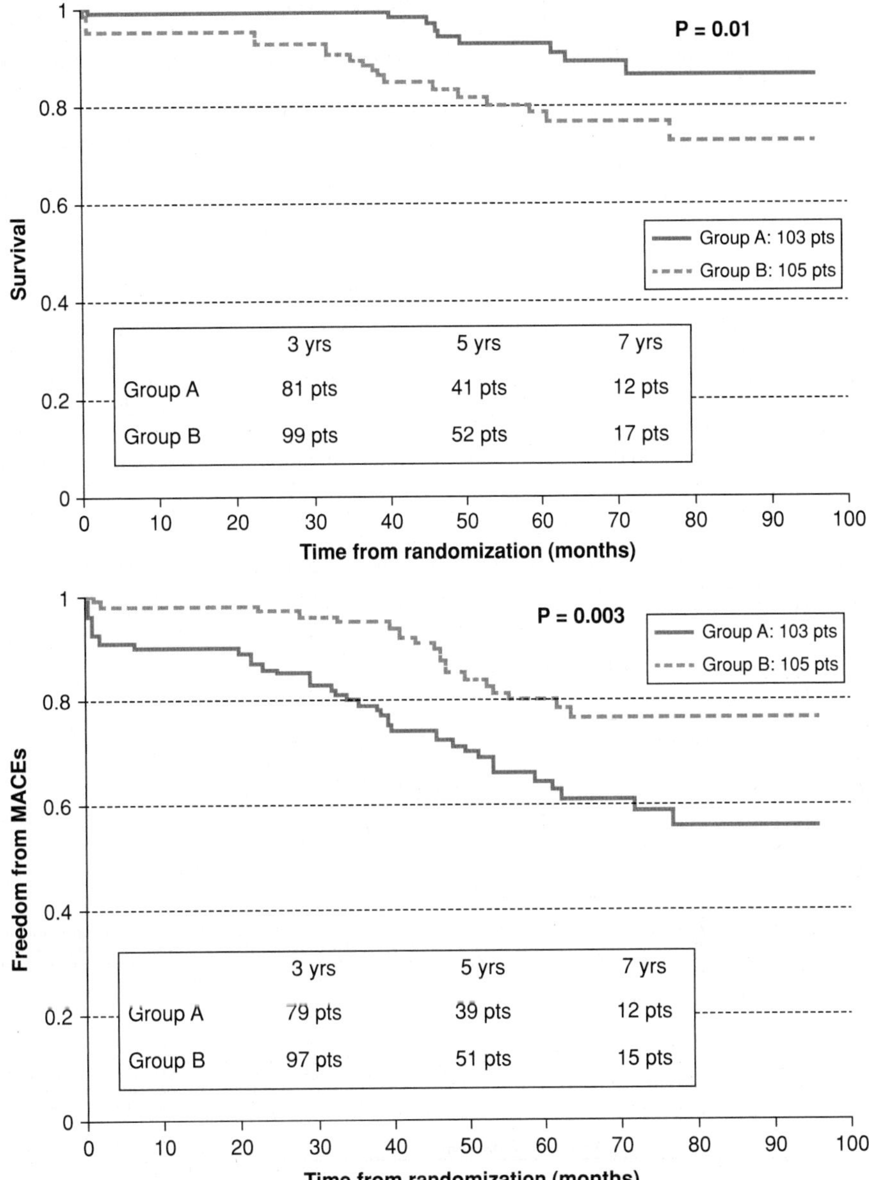

Figure 40-5 Cumulative survival and freedom from major adverse cardiac event for routine versus selective coronary angiography prior to major vascular surgery in intermediate- to high-risk patients. Long-term survival, and survival free from MACE, were greater in the group who underwent routine preoperative coronary angiography. (Reprinted from Monaco M, Stassano P, Di Tommaso L, et al. Systematic strategy of prophylactic coronary angiography improves long-term outcome after major vascular surgery in medium- to high-risk patients: a prospective, randomized study. *J Am Col Cardio.* 2009;54:989–996. Copyright © 2009 Elsevier. With permission.)

fitness of surgery must all be taken into consideration. Specific recommendations are made following PCI, and the ACC/AHA released a focused update on duration of dual antiplatelet therapy (DAPT) for patients with CAD in 2016.[70] The updated guidelines suggest delaying elective noncardiac surgery 30 days following bare metal stent (BMS) placement and ideally 6 months following drug-eluting stent (DES) placement (Class I; LOE B-NR). For patients treated with DAPT following coronary stent placement who must undergo surgical procedures that mandate discontinuation of their platelet receptor inhibitor (P2Y12) therapy, it is recommended that aspirin be continued when possible and the P2Y12 inhibitor be restarted as soon as possible following surgery (Class 1; LOE C-EO). A consensus decision among treating clinicians as to the relative risk of surgery and the discontinuation or continuation of antiplatelet agents can be useful (Class IIa; LOE C-EO). Elective noncardiac surgery after DES placement for whom P2Y12 inhibitor must be discontinued may be considered after 3 months if the risk of further delaying surgery outweighs the expected risk of stent thrombosis (Class IIb; LOE C-EO). Elective noncardiac surgery should not be performed within 30 days following BMS placement or within 3 months for DES implantation in patients in whom DAPT will need to be discontinued perioperatively (Class III; LOE B-NR).

Preoperative Anesthesia Evaluation for Vascular Surgery

The purpose of the preoperative anesthesia evaluation is to delineate the extent of any underlying comorbid pathology and medically optimize the patient for surgery. In vascular surgery, the preoperative assessment predominantly focuses on the presence of, or risk factors for, coronary or noncoronary ASCVD. A careful history must be taken to define the extent of any diagnosed ASCVD and to screen for any undiagnosed concurrent disease (e.g., angina or equivalent, symptoms of transient ischemic attack

(TIA), or mesenteric or peripheral ischemia). Physical examination should evaluate for any evidence of end-organ involvement (e.g., diminished pulses, S_4 gallop, or residual deficit from previous stroke) or cardiovascular decompensation (e.g., new or worsened murmur, jugular venous distention, third heart sound on cardiac auscultation, rales, shortness of breath, or peripheral edema). It is important to evaluate the control of any comorbid conditions such as diabetes or hypertension. The strong association between smoking and vascular disease mandates a thorough assessment of any underlying pulmonary disease. Medications should be optimized as discussed earlier.

For any major vascular surgery, it is prudent to obtain baseline laboratory studies. A complete blood count should be obtained due to the risk of major blood loss and possibility of concurrent medical diseases that may predispose to anemia. Coagulation studies should be considered if the patient is on anticoagulant medications or if regional anesthesia is anticipated. A metabolic panel should be obtained due to an increased likelihood of underlying renal insufficiency with resultant electrolyte abnormalities. It is also useful to have a baseline given an elevated risk of postoperative renal dysfunction. Cardiac biomarkers (e.g., troponin I, N-terminal pro-brain natriuretic peptide, cystatin C, and C-reactive protein) and risk factors identified on advanced imaging modalities (coronary artery calcium scores or CIMT) have long been studied for their ability to predict long-term cardiovascular outcomes; their utility in the perioperative setting to predict high-risk patients, however, is a relatively new area of interest.[71] A preoperative 12-lead electrocardiogram (ECG) is reasonable as a baseline because of the increased risk of perioperative MACE. A preoperative echocardiogram to assess LV function is reasonable for patients with previously documented LV dysfunction, worsening clinical status or if not assessed within the previous year, or for patients with dyspnea of unknown origin.[23] Routine echocardiography in asymptomatic patients cannot be recommended.

Determining which patients require additional preoperative 4
cardiac testing is a source of frequent debate. Vascular surgery patients are known to be at elevated risk of perioperative MACE. It has been predicted that postoperative troponin elevation and MI predict a 26% and 55% lower survival rate, respectively, in the 5 years following vascular surgery compared with patients who do not experience an event (Fig. 40-6).[72] Thus, significant effort has focused on identifying patients at elevated cardiac risk. Conversely, over utilization of advanced testing modalities can put undue stress on the health-care system, result in false positive tests, delay necessary surgery, and ultimately cause patient harm in further invasive workup and treatment. The most

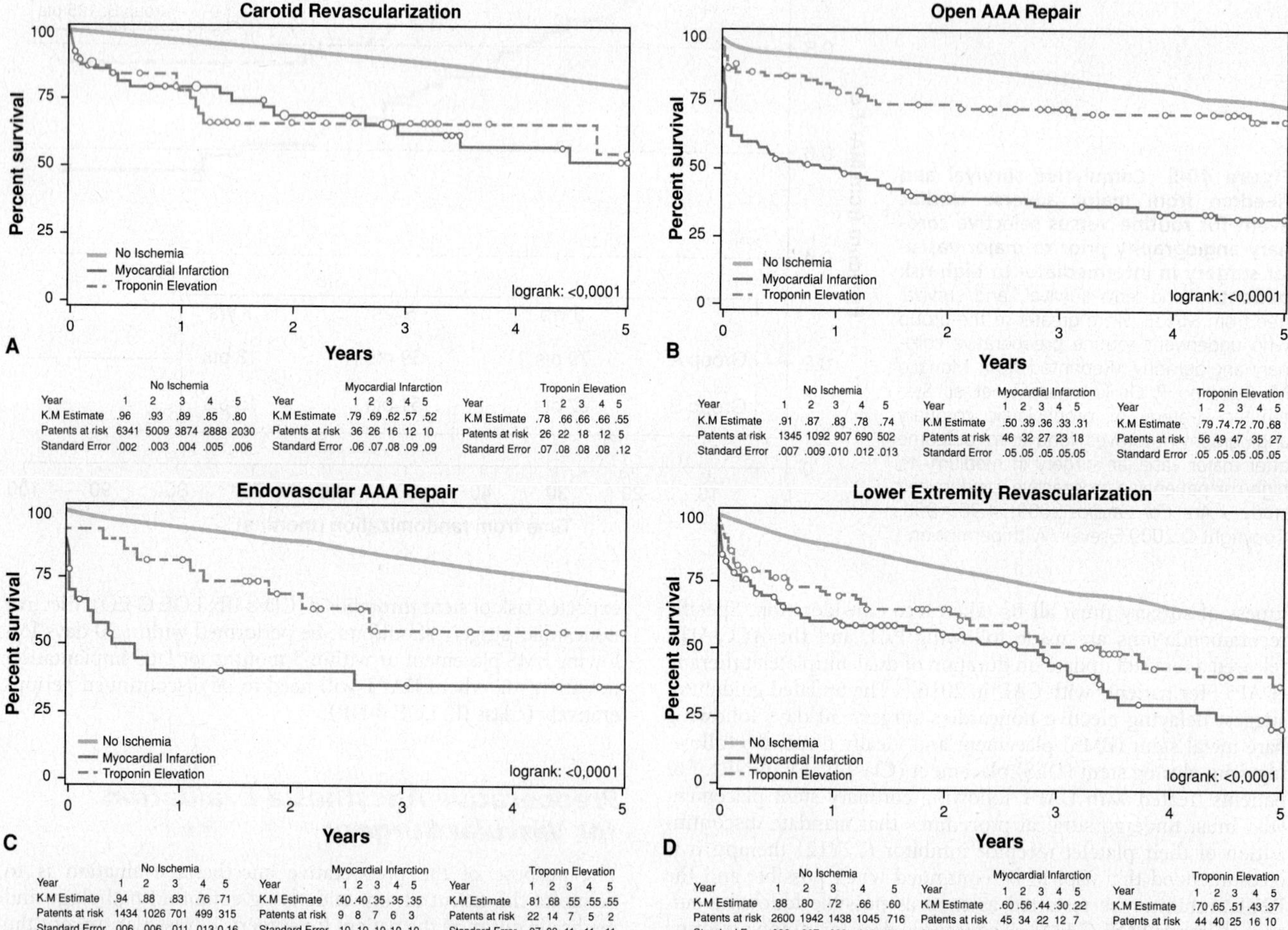

Figure 40-6 Univariate Kaplan–Meier (*K-M*) survival curves, stratified according to postoperative myocardial ischemia, for different major vascular surgical procedures. Vascular surgery patients who suffer from perioperative myocardial ischemia have significantly worse outcomes with decreased survival at 5 years for (A) carotid, (B) open aortic, (C) endovascular aortic, and (D) peripheral interventions. AAA, abdominal aortic aneurysm. (Reprinted from Simons JP, Baril DT, Goodney PP, et al. The effect of postoperative myocardial ischemia on long-term survival after vascular surgery. *J Vasc Surg*. 2013;58:1600–1608. Copyright © 2013 Elsevier. With permission.)

well-recognized clinical practice guidelines for perioperative cardiovascular evaluation for patients undergoing noncardiac surgery are jointly developed by the ACC/AHA and were most recently revised in 2014 (Fig. 40-7).[23] The first step in evaluation for fitness for surgery is to determine the urgency of surgery. Clinical emergencies (e.g., ruptured abdominal aortic aneurysm [AAA]) should proceed to the operating room without delay and with best medical optimization in the time available, recognizing that the risk of perioperative MACE is elevated in this situation. Situations that are urgent, but not emergent (e.g., critical limb

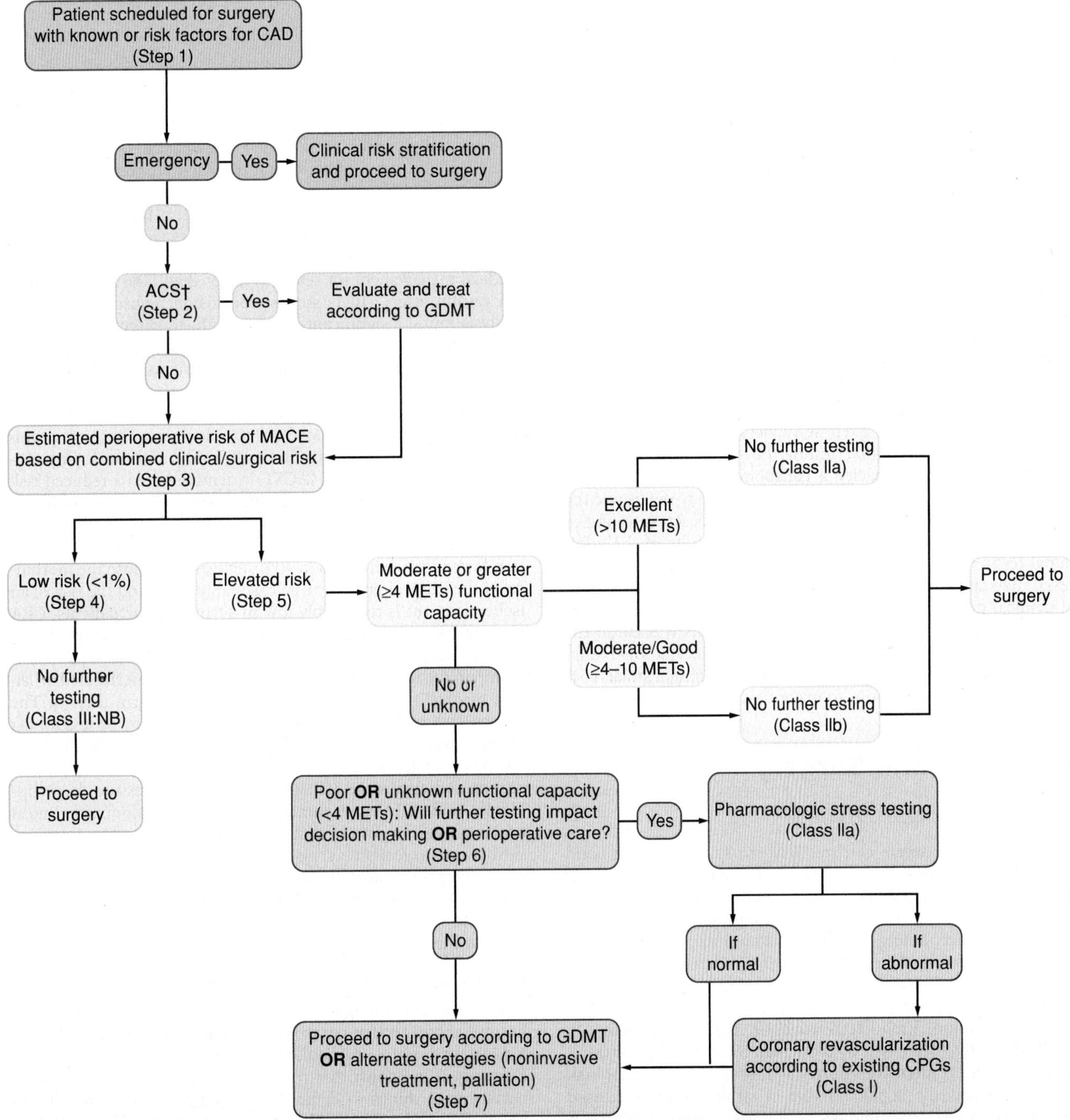

Figure 40-7 Proposed algorithm for cardiovascular evaluation and management of patients undergoing noncardiac surgery. In this most recent iteration of the ACC/AHA clinical practice guidelines, individual consideration of patient medical versus surgical risk has been combined into overall perioperative risk. A combination of clinical urgency, patient risk of major adverse cardiac event, and patient functional status helps to guide the necessity of further preoperative cardiac work up. CAD, coronary artery disease; ACS, acute coronary syndrome; GDMT, guideline directed medical therapy; MACE, major adverse cardiac event; MET, metabolic equivalent; NB, no benefit; CPG, clinical practice guideline. (Reprinted with permission from 2014 ACC/AHA Guideline on Perioperative Cardiovascular Evaluation and Management of Patients Undergoing Noncardiac Surgery: Executive Summary. *Circulation*. 2014;130:2215–2245. © 2014 American Heart Association, Inc.)

ischemia [CLI]) may allow for an abbreviated cardiac workup, if such workup will impact clinical management. The second step is to evaluate whether the patient has an acute coronary syndrome (new, crescendo, or unstable angina; MI within the last 60 days) or other major cardiac pathophysiology (symptomatic heart failure; new or worsening valvular heart disease; or unstable arrhythmia or conduction disease). If present, these conditions should be evaluated and optimized per clinical practice guidelines prior to elective surgery. The third step involves estimation of perioperative risk of MACE based on combined clinical and surgical risk factors. Commonly used risk estimations include the American College of Surgeons National Surgical Quality Improvement Program risk calculator[73] or the revised cardiac risk index (RCRI).[74] The Vascular Study Group of New England has developed a vascular surgery-specific model for the prediction of cardiac events that more accurately predicted the risk of cardiac complications in vascular surgery patients than the RCRI, which was found to underestimate the risk of MACE by 1.7- to 7.4-fold in vascular surgery patients.[75] Independent predictors of MACE in this study included increasing age, smoking, insulin-dependent diabetes, CAD, CHF, abnormal cardiac stress test, long-term β-blocker therapy, chronic obstructive pulmonary disease, and elevated creatinine. Regardless of the risk calculator used, functional status dictates the necessity for further cardiac workup prior to surgery for any patient deemed at elevated (>1%) risk of perioperative MACE. Patients with moderate (4 metabolic equivalents [METs]) to excellent (>10 METs) exercise capacity may proceed to surgery with no further cardiac testing. For patients with poor or unknown functional capacity, a collaborative decision must be made between the patient and treating clinicians to determine the next step. Further cardiac testing (in the form of stress testing or cardiac catheterization) is reasonable if the results of the additional testing will change management decisions (e.g., coronary revascularization prior to planned surgery, further optimization of medical management, or adopting an alternative plan for palliative care). Since most vascular surgery patients will fall in the elevated risk category and many will have poor to unknown functional status due to comorbid conditions, additional cardiac testing is not unreasonable prior to major vascular procedures.

Open Vascular Surgery

Cerebrovascular Disease

An imbalance between cerebral oxygen supply and demand leads to cerebral ischemia, which can be temporary or permanent. Approximately 800,000 patients per year suffer a stroke in the United States. Stroke is the fifth leading cause of death in the United States, accounting for approximately 1 in every 19 deaths.[3] Equally importantly, the combination of significant psychological consequences and new disability may lead to a profound impact on quality of life. Stroke has been called the most burdensome chronic condition. From 2009 to 2019, the age-adjusted U.S. stroke death rate decreased by more than 5% (37.0 per 100,000), primarily due to intensive efforts to control cardiovascular risk factors, whereas the actual number of stroke deaths increased 16.4% during the same time period. Efforts to control hypertension appear to have had the greatest influence on the decline in stroke mortality, although improved management of diabetes mellitus and hyperlipidemia, as well as aggressive smoking cessation campaigns, have also contributed.

Most strokes are ischemic, rather than hemorrhagic, in origin. Carotid atherosclerotic disease accounts for approximately 20% of all ischemic strokes, although the mechanism of pathophysiology is typically embolic rather than occlusive. Stroke symptomatology depends on the distribution of ischemia. Carotid disease may manifest as transient attacks of monocular blindness (amaurosis fugax), paresthesia, weakness or clumsiness, facial drooping, or speech problems. These symptoms may resolve spontaneously after a short period. Any focalized neurologic deficit lasting less than 24 hours' duration with no evidence of permanent infarction is known as a TIA. It has been estimated that up to 15% of strokes are heralded by TIA,[76] and the most important risk factor for future stroke is the presence of recent TIA symptoms. The risk of stroke following TIA is elevated in the initial days to weeks following the initial event.[76] Thus, TIA symptoms should prompt an immediate workup and referral for definitive intervention.

Several high profile randomized controlled trials have demonstrated clinical benefit for CEA for both symptomatic and asymptomatic carotid atherosclerosis. The North American Symptomatic Carotid Endarterectomy (NASCET) trial,[77] European Carotid Surgery Trial (ECST),[78] and Veterans Affairs Cooperative Studies (VACS) Program,[79] all demonstrated a benefit for CEA over best medical management for severe (greater than 70% to 80%) internal carotid artery (ICA) stenosis occlusion. Subsequent pooled analysis found a significant 5-year benefit to surgery for patients with greater than 70% stenosis, a marginal benefit for patients with 50% to 70% stenosis, no benefit in patients with 30% to 49% stenosis, and an increased risk of ipsilateral ischemic stroke in patients with less than 30% stenosis.[80] There was no benefit to treatment of lesions of less than 50% stenosis. The Asymptomatic Carotid Atherosclerosis Study (ACAS)[81] and the Asymptomatic Carotid Surgery Trial (ACST)[82] demonstrated a reduced risk of stroke for asymptomatic carotid disease, albeit less robust. A meta-analysis of trials of asymptomatic patients found a small absolute risk reduction of about 1% per year for surgical intervention for patients with 50% to 70% stenosis.[83] Because the morbidity of the surgical procedure is reasonably high, and the risk of an ischemic event is reasonably low in asymptomatic patients, CEA is justifiable only if the operative morbidity and mortality is lower than the natural risk of ischemic events in an untreated patient. It is important to recognize that these trials were performed when best medical therapy consisted primarily of aspirin therapy. The relative risk reduction of surgical intervention may be less robust in the current era of multimodal medical treatment with diet and lifestyle changes; smoking cessation campaigns; dual antiplatelet agents; and aggressive management of blood pressure, hyperlipidemia, and diabetes. A parallel multicenter randomized clinical trial is actively underway that seeks to compare modern intensive medical management versus CEA plus intensive management, while the parallel arm will assess intensive medical management versus CAS plus intensive medical management.[16] The goal of this trial is to inform clinical decision making in the modern era of medical therapy.

Preoperative Evaluation and Preparation

The appropriate timing for CEA has been subject to debate. There has been concern that operative risk may be increased early after a neurologic event, particularly for large or evolving strokes.[84] However, it is known that transient neurologic symptoms are a harbinger of things to come. In one study of more than 1,700 patients who presented with index TIA, more than 10% returned with an acute stroke within 90 days, and nearly half of these strokes occurred within 2 days.[85] Analysis of pooled data from the NASCET and ECST trials demonstrated that for patients with greater than or equal to 70% stenosis, the attributable risk reduction for any ipsilateral stroke or any stroke or death within 30 days decreased from 30% when surgery occurred within 2 weeks to 18% at 2 to 4 weeks and 11% at 4 to 12 weeks.[84,86] Thus, for symptomatic patients in whom surgical intervention is warranted, most recent recommendations favor definitive intervention within 2 weeks of the index event (COR 2a, LOE C-LD).[86]

It is reasonable to obtain a cardiac evaluation due to the known association between carotid and CAD; however, definitive intervention should not be delayed for extensive cardiac evaluation even in those patients with known cardiac disease because of the urgent nature of the surgery. It is prudent to treat all patients undergoing CEA as if they have underlying CAD with strict hemodynamic control. Fifty percent of patients with TIA or stroke due to CVD will have an abnormal stress test despite no report of angina; in 60% of these patients, the CAD will be severe by coronary angiography.[87] The approach to patients with both severe CAD and CVD is controversial, with proponents for both staged and synchronous repair. Because these operations are relatively rare (especially in symptomatic patients), current evidence comes primarily from poor-quality case series performed over many years, making generalizability to current practice difficult. Current guidelines provide no clear consensus on how this situation should be managed.

Neurophysiologic Monitoring and Preserving Neurologic Integrity During Carotid Endarterectomy

Most strokes in the perioperative period are embolic in origin. Hypoperfusion related to temporary occlusion ("cross-clamping") of the carotid artery during surgery can also lead to cerebral ischemia. Cross-clamping acutely disrupts blood flow to the ipsilateral hemisphere, even if flow was markedly diminished by severe stenosis. In this case, blood supply to the brain will depend entirely on collateral flow from an intact circle of Willis. Autopsy studies have found that the majority of specimens demonstrated anatomic anomalies in the circle of Willis.[88] Hypoplasia was the most frequently noted anomaly (24%) (Fig. 40-8), and an incomplete circle due to complete absence of a vessel was noted in an additional 6%. Furthermore, even an anatomically intact circle of Willis may not provide adequate cerebral blood if collateral perfusion is compromised by occlusive disease of the contralateral carotid or vertebral arteries, or if the patient becomes relatively hypotensive compared to baseline.

A temporary carotid shunt can be employed to bypass the cross-clamp and restore cerebral blood flow. Significant practice variation exists among surgeons regarding the use of carotid shunts in CEA. Some surgeons never use shunts and rely on expedient surgery and meticulous hemodynamic control (including permissive hypertension) to maintain adequate collateral cerebral perfusion pressures. Others may shunt selectively based on changes in neurophysiologic monitoring, and still others shunt routinely. Shunt placement is not an entirely benign undertaking, with morbidity including atheromatous or air emboli, arterial dissection, nerve injury, hematoma, infection, and long-term restenosis. Perhaps most compellingly, shunting has been demonstrated to be unnecessary in approximately 85% of patients.[89] Furthermore, a shunt is only beneficial if the cause of neurologic dysfunction is inadequate blood flow. However, the majority of studies suggest that as many as 65% to 95% of all neurologic deficits during CEA are caused by thromboembolic events. A review of the literature found no difference in outcomes including rate of all stroke, ipsilateral stroke, or death up to 30 days after surgery between selective and routine shunting.[90]

Neurophysiologic monitoring is commonly employed to assess overall cerebral perfusion and to help determine which patients may benefit from carotid shunting. Some monitoring techniques, such as electroencephalography (EEG), somatosensory-evoked potentials (SSEP), and motor-evoked potentials (MEP), assess the overall integrity of cerebral function. Others, including transcranial Doppler (TCD) or carotid stump pressure, assess the blood flow in the large cerebral vessels. A third group, including near-infrared spectroscopy (NIRS) and jugular venous bulb saturation, estimate cerebral metabolism. The gold standard for cerebral monitoring remains serial neurologic examination on an awake patient. No matter the modality employed, the goal of neurophysiologic monitoring is to identify patients who may benefit from selective shunting and to avoid shunting in patients where it is unnecessary.

EEG monitoring is perhaps the most commonly employed neurophysiologic monitor for carotid surgery. EEG records the electrical activity of the brain, and changes in cerebral blood flow can be reflected in the EEG waveform. Normal cerebral blood flow is approximately 50 mL/min/100 g brain tissue. In the perioperative period, decreases in cerebral blood flow as low as approximately 22 mL/min/100 g brain tissue may be well tolerated with no EEG changes.[91] EEG deterioration usually begins below a threshold of approximately 15 to 18 mL/min/100 g brain tissue, and frank cellular failure appears to occur below 10 to 12 mL/min/100 g brain tissue (Fig. 40-9). The most common manifestations of cerebral ischemia on EEG are ipsilateral slowing and/or attenuation. Deterioration in EEG can be noted within seconds of carotid cross-clamping, and these changes are typically reversible with appropriate augmentation of hemodynamics and/or temporary shunt placement.

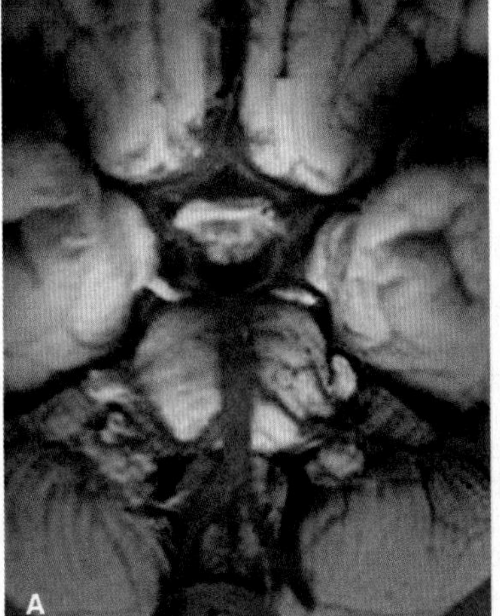

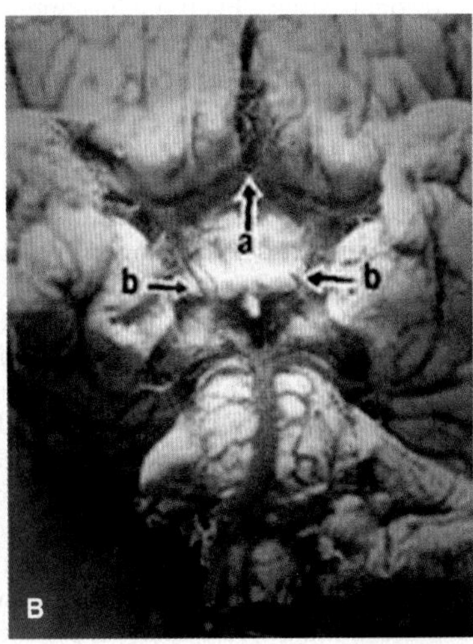

Figure 40-8 Intact and hypoplastic circle of Willis. (**A**) demonstrates an anatomically normal circle of Willis. (**B**) demonstrates hypoplastic (*a*) anterior and (*b*) posterior communicating arteries. (Reprinted with permission from Iqbal S. A comprehensive study of the anatomical variations of the circle of Willis in adult human brains. *J Clin Diagn Res*. 2013;7(11):2423–2427.)

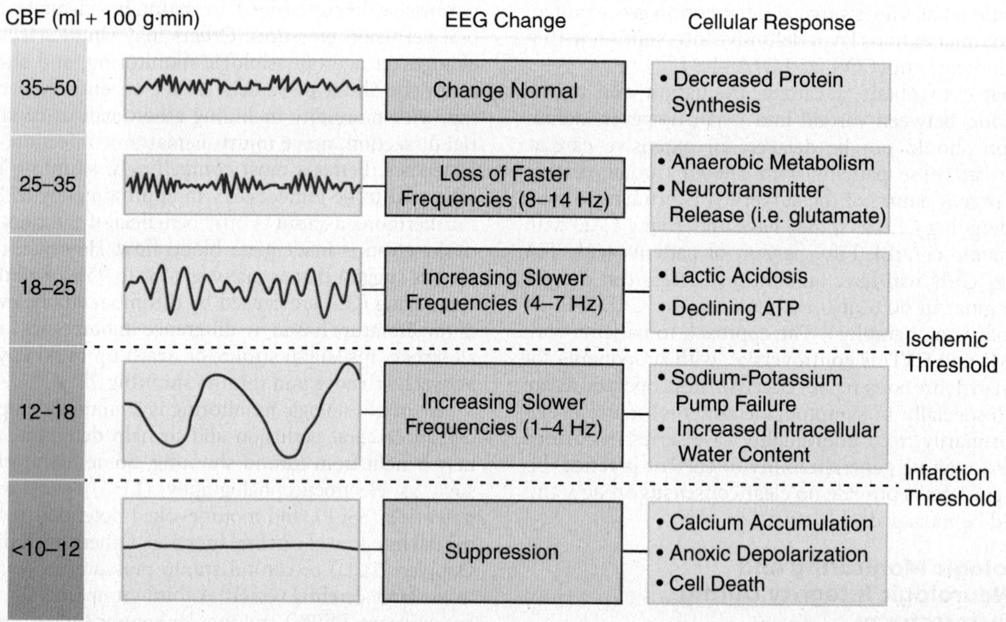

Figure 40-9 Characteristic electroencephalogram (EEG) changes with reduction in cerebral blood flow. Decreases in cerebral blood flow are associated with characteristic changes in the EEG and predictable cellular response. CBF, coronary blood flow; EEG, electroencephalogram; ATP, adenosine triphosphate. (Reprinted with permission from Foreman B, Claassen J. Quantitative EEG for the detection of brain ischemia. *Crit Care.* 2012;16[2]:216.)

EEG monitoring is not without limitations. The sensitivity of EEG for predicting cerebral ischemia is poor; in one series of more than 300 patients, EEG identified cerebral ischemia in fewer than 60% of patients with a false-positive rate of 1%.[92] In patients with pre-existing or fluctuating neurologic deficits, the EEG may be falsely negative. In these patients, there may be areas of brain parenchyma that are electrically silent or immediately adjacent to regions of infarction, and therefore not reliably monitored by EEG. These still-viable regions may progress to irreversible injury over the length of the procedure. EEG monitors cortical structures and not deep brain structures, and strokes in this distribution will be missed. Interpretation of EEG may be complicated by other intraoperative parameters such as hypothermia or rapid or sudden changes in anesthetic depth, although in general EEG changes secondary to anesthetic agents are more likely to be bilateral, whereas changes due to cross-clamping or hypoperfusion tend to involve the ipsilateral hemisphere. Finally, it is important to recognize that EEG is a global monitor of cerebral activity. It is unable to reliably detect strokes related to smaller thromboembolic phenomena, which is the most likely etiology of perioperative stroke.

SSEP monitoring employs electrical stimuli to peripheral nerves and evaluates the amplitude and latency of the signal over the cerebral cortex. In contrast to EEG, which only evaluates cortical functioning, SSEP monitoring also reflects the deep brain structures. Most commonly, the median and/or tibial nerves are assessed. A decrease in signaling for the median nerve suggests hypoperfusion in the watershed of the middle cerebral artery, whereas deterioration of tibial nerve signaling may reflect ischemia of the parenchyma supplied by the anterior cerebral artery. A decrease in signal amplitude of greater than 50% is typically accepted as indicative of ischemia, which may occur when cerebral blood flow is critically low (i.e., at 15 mL/min/100 g brain tissue). SSEP monitoring may be particularly useful in patients with baseline cerebral ischemia in whom EEG interpretation is more difficult. However, SSEPs are sensitive to virtually all commonly used anesthetic agents which may complicate intraoperative interpretation and lead to a high false-positive rate. A light plane of anesthesia must be maintained if increased latencies and decreased amplitude of SSEP are to be ascribed to inadequate cerebral perfusion. False negatives with intraoperative SSEP monitoring have also been described; focal ischemia of the internal capsule has been suggested as a potential mechanism in this circumstance. Although some studies have been optimistic about the value of SSEP monitoring, others have questioned both the sensitivity and specificity of SSEP for the detection of cerebral ischemia. A comparison of different neurophysiologic monitoring techniques demonstrated a sensitivity of approximately 80% and a specificity of 57% for the detection of cerebral ischemia.[93] Monitoring motor, rather than sensory, evoked potentials is one mechanism to overcome this problem. To monitor MEP, transcranial electrodes are utilized to stimulate the cerebral cortex, and motor response in the contralateral extremity is recorded. In one recent study, the use of MEP in addition to SSEP was more sensitive for detection of cerebral ischemia.[94] In this study, there were no false-negative results with MEP as compared to a 1.5% false-negative rate when SSEPs were used alone. MEPs, however, can be exquisitely sensitive to anesthetic interference (neuromuscular blockade, in particular, is avoided) and may be more prone to false positives and unnecessary intervention (such as blood pressure augmentation or temporary shunt placement).

TCD measures the maximum velocity of blood flow through the middle cerebral artery as a surrogate for cerebral blood flow. TCD may be particularly useful in the detection of microembolic phenomena that may be missed by more global measures of cerebral functioning. In a small case series, TCD predicted neurologic events despite a normal intraoperative EEG.[95] Detection of microembolic showers, particularly during surgical manipulation, may allow for the operative team to alter the surgical plan to prevent further neurologic insult. TCD is also useful in confirming that cerebral blood flow remains at an acceptable level after carotid cross-clamping or, if a shunt is used, to confirm that flow through the shunt is adequate. TCD may be particularly useful in postoperative surveillance because most strokes occur after, rather than during, CEA. In addition to microembolic showers, TCD can also identify patients with acute postoperative thrombosis or those at risk for cerebral hyperperfusion syndrome. TCD has the benefits of being quick, easy to apply, more easily interpretable without expertise (as compared to EEG or evoked potentials), and allows for serial evaluation. Disadvantages to TCD include operator dependence and technical limitation. In approximately 10% to 20% of patients, adequate temporal windows (a prerequisite for accurate monitoring) cannot be obtained.

Carotid stump pressure estimates ipsilateral hemispheric blood flow by directly measuring the pressure in the carotid stump distal to the clamp. Purported advantages of this technique are that it is a direct gauge of collateral cerebral perfusion, quick to obtain, cost effective, and does not require sophisticated equipment or expert interpretation. Stump pressures greater than 40 to 50 mmHg are generally considered adequate to avoid temporary shunt placement, although a critical value for stump pressure is not known. Some patients may have adequate perfusion below values of 40 to 50 mmHg, whereas others may not have sufficient collateral flow despite maintaining stump pressure above this range. A retrospective series of more than 400 patients performed under regional anesthesia found that a stump pressure cutoff of 40 mmHg was as reliable as EEG monitoring in predicting cerebral ischemia on cross-clamp application during CEA.[96] The generalizability to patients undergoing CEA under general anesthesia is unclear.

NIRS uses the relative absorption of specific wavelengths of light by oxyhemoglobin and deoxyhemoglobin to estimate frontal lobe cerebral perfusion (rSO_2) and estimate cerebral oxygen balance. A decrease in rSO_2, theoretically, reflects a decrease in cerebral blood flow below a critical level. NIRS is easily portable, inexpensive, and simple to interpret without special training. Limitations include potential inaccuracy over areas of previous infarction, as well as in the fact that NIRS is a global assessment of cerebral oxygenation only in the frontal grey matter. Thus, ischemia in other areas of the brain may be missed. Data on the sensitivity and specificity of NIRS for predicting cerebral ischemia during CEA are conflicting. One study performed under regional anesthesia demonstrated that a drop in rSO_2 more than 19% following carotid cross-clamping has sensitivity of 100% and specificity of 98% (yielding PPV of 82% and NPV of 100%) for predicting need for temporary shunt placement,[97] whereas another using the same device and ischemic threshold demonstrated a sensitivity of 60% and a specificity of 25%.[98] Whether these results are applicable to CEA performed under general anesthesia is unclear.

Anesthetic Considerations for Carotid Endarterectomy

In general, premedication with sedatives is avoided to facilitate rapid emergence and immediate assessment of a neurologic examination (NICV 40-1). If deemed necessary, the smallest effective dose of midazolam should be titrated to effect. Once in the operating room, standard monitors should be applied. Invasive blood pressure monitoring is recommended due to the potential for hemodynamic lability as a result of surgical or anesthetic manipulation. Care should be taken to maintain hemodynamics within 20% of the patient's baseline range due to potential shifts in cerebral autoregulation. Rarely is invasive central monitoring with a central venous or pulmonary artery catheter necessary, unless dictated by specific patient risk factors. At least one medium- to large-bore intravenous access should be obtained, although the risk of major blood loss or fluid shifting in this procedure is low.

CEA can be performed under either general or regional anesthesia. A regional anesthetic allows for continuous monitoring of a patient's neurologic status, which is the ultimate monitor for cerebral ischemia. An abrupt change in mental status will alert the operative team sooner and more definitely than indirect neuromonitoring methods and will also avoid morbidity associated with unnecessary interventions. Regional anesthesia avoids hemodynamically labile periods such as induction and emergence of general anesthesia as well as the need to administer negative inotropic anesthetic agents to patients with underlying cardiovascular disease. Superficial cervical plexus blockade has been found to be as efficacious as deep or combined block while avoiding the known complications of a deep cervical plexus block.[99] Complications associated with deep cervical plexus block include accidental subarachnoid injection with resultant brainstem anesthesia; intravascular injection with potential seizure; or accidental blockade of the phrenic, vagus, or recurrent laryngeal nerves with respiratory complications. Patient cooperation is vital as the patient will have to lie still for the duration of the operation (inability to communicate, orthopnea, and painful arthritis are relative contraindications) and patients cannot be claustrophobic as the surgical drapes will be in close proximity to the patient's face.

General anesthesia affords improved patient comfort, particularly for highly anxious patients, and may allow for more frank intraoperative communication among the operative team. Perhaps most compellingly, it avoids an urgent conversion to general anesthesia should complications arise such as deterioration of neurologic status or oversedation. It is not uncommon for the operating room table to be positioned with the head away from the anesthesia provider to allow the surgical team adequate room to work. Thus, emergent conversion to general anesthesia, with an ongoing operation in the neck, is not a trivial task. Overall conversion rates to general anesthesia are generally less than 5%;[100] nevertheless, the ability to rapidly convert to general anesthesia in case of surgical or anesthetic misadventure must be ensured.

Whether one anesthetic technique is superior to the other has been the subject of extensive debate. The most well-known study in this patient population is the General Anesthesia versus Local Anesthesia for carotid surgery (GALA) trial,[100] an international, multicenter, randomized controlled trial of more than 3,500 patients. There was no difference in the primary end point of proportion of patients with stroke, MI, or death between randomization and 30 days after surgery between the two groups. A meta-analysis of 14 randomized trials involving more than 4,500 operations (the largest trial included being the GALA trial) similarly demonstrated no difference in death, stroke, or MI rates between the general and local anesthesia groups (Fig. 40-10).[101] There were also no differences in major morbidity, postoperative cardiovascular or pulmonary complications, hospital length of stay, or patient satisfaction between the two groups. Currently available literature does not suggest a benefit of one anesthetic approach over another. Rather, a mutually agreeable decision should be made between the surgeon and anesthesiologist, bearing in mind patient preference and potential limitations. Regardless of technique chosen, the anesthetic goals are the same: mitigate perioperative cerebral insult, ensure hemodynamic stability, and allow for a smooth and rapid emergence for anesthesia to allow for early neurologic assessment.

General anesthesia for CEA is typically performed with an endotracheal tube (ETT), although the use of laryngeal mask airway (LMA) has been described. An ETT offers a more secure airway, potentially better control of gas exchange, and may distort the anatomy of the neck less than an LMA. An LMA may cause less hemodynamic lability during periods of induction and emergence since direct laryngoscopy is avoided. General anesthesia is

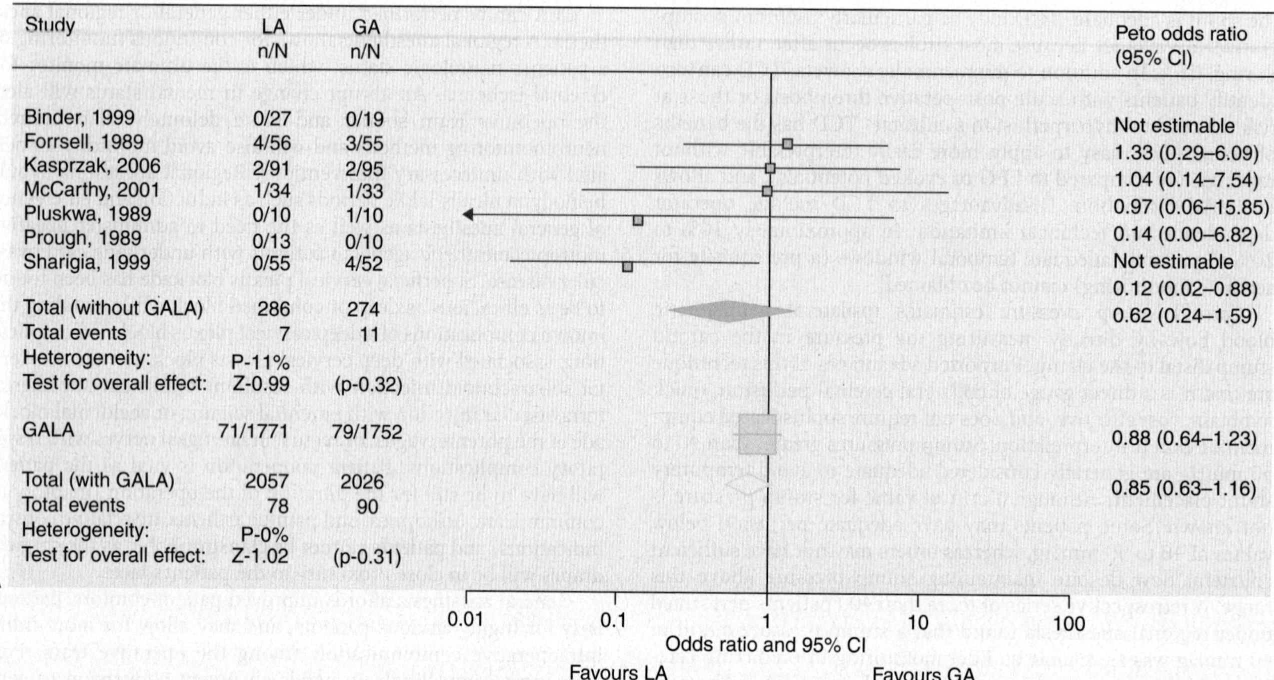

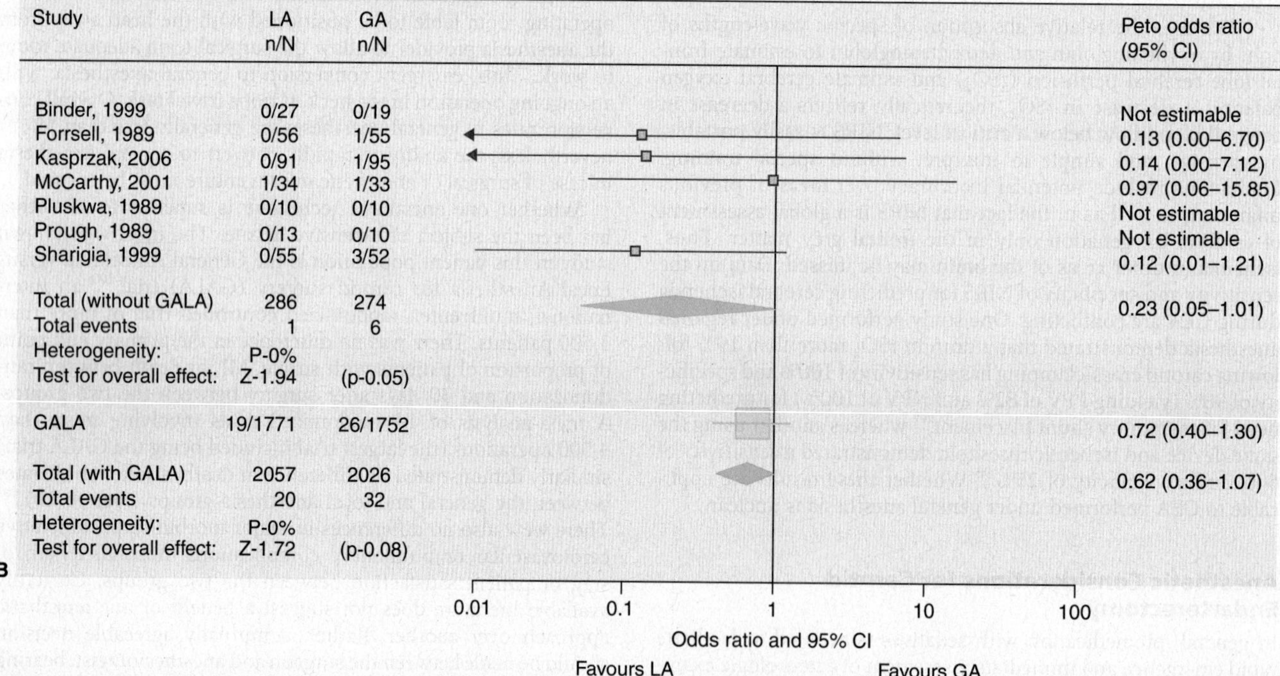

Figure 40-10 Odds ratio for outcome of (A) stroke or death, or (B) death for carotid endarterectomy performed under general versus local anesthesia. Plots show odds ratios and 95% confidence interval for the specified outcomes. No difference in any of the primary outcomes was noted in either the GALA trial or a meta-analysis of the literature. GA, general anesthesia; LA, local anesthesia. (Reprinted from Lewis SC, Warlow CP, Bodenham AR, et al. General anaesthesia versus local anaesthesia for carotid surgery [GALA]: a multicentre, randomised controlled trial. *Lancet*. 2008;372:2132–2142. Copyright © 2008 Elsevier. With permission.)

maintained at a "light" level that ensures amnesia but minimally interferes with neurophysiologic monitoring. Typically, a balanced technique is favored and a variety of agents have been successfully employed. General anesthesia is typically induced with a short-acting hypnotic agent, titrated to effect. Both etomidate and propofol decrease cerebral metabolic rate and thus cerebral oxygen requirements. Etomidate may preserve cardiovascular stability and thus be beneficial for patients in whom cardiac reserve is limited. The addition of a short-acting opioid such as fentanyl or remifentanil is frequently employed to blunt the hemodynamic stimulation of intubation. The trachea may be sprayed with atomized lidocaine prior to intubation in an attempt to minimize stimulation by the ETT during surgery and to prevent coughing upon emergence. Small amounts of short-acting opioid can be titrated intraoperatively as needed; however, large doses or long-acting opioids are typically avoided so as to not confound the neurologic examination at the end of surgery. The combined use of a cervical plexus block and/or surgeon-administered local anesthetic can significantly reduce or eliminate the need for perioperative opioids. Muscle relaxation is not mandated for this surgery, but often allows for a "lighter" plane of anesthesia and reduces muscular interference with the EEG.

General anesthesia can be maintained with either volatile or intravenous agents. No evidence has reliably demonstrated a benefit for one technique over another.[102,103] No differences in intraoperative hemodynamics have been described between inhalational and intravenous anesthetic techniques. Patients undergoing a propofol-based anesthetic have been noted to have fewer intraoperative regional wall motion abnormalities suggestive of ischemia than those undergoing isoflurane-based anesthetics; however, no postoperative differences in troponin levels, EKG changes, or clinical outcomes were noted in study.[102] The transient intraoperative regional wall motion abnormalities were attributed to isoflurane-induced ventricular loading changes as a result of arterial and venous dilation, unrelated to myocardial oxygen balance. Intravenous anesthesia with propofol and remifentanil may be associated with less hemodynamic lability upon emergence of anesthesia,[103] at the expense of longer recovery room stays and medical intervention for hypertension.[102] The authors attribute this difference not to the ultrashort duration of action of analgesia, but rather the more rapid awakening from propofol/remifentanil than isoflurane/fentanyl-based regimens. This assertion is supported by comparable pain scores and analgesic requirements. The more rapid recovery from intravenous-based anesthetic techniques and ability to obtain a postoperative neurologic examination makes intravenous-based anesthetics attractive to many providers. Intravenous regimens had the added benefit of lower rates of postoperative nausea and vomiting, which prevents retching on a fresh neck incision and may decrease the risk of postoperative hematoma, a feared complication. Intravenous techniques, at approximately nine times the cost of inhalational based anesthetics, were less cost effective in comparison. Regardless of whether an inhalation or intravenous based technique is chosen, short-acting agents are preferable to allow for rapid awakening. Desflurane or sevoflurane may be preferable to isoflurane due to their rapid offset and salutary effects on cognitive recovery and cerebral ischemia.[104]

Normocapnia should be maintained during CEA. Hyperventilation may lead to cerebral vasoconstriction and decreased cerebral blood flow during critical periods of carotid cross-clamping. Hypercapnia may be equally detrimental if it leads to dilation of the cerebral vasculature in normal areas of the brain, whereas vessels in ischemic areas are already maximally dilated and are unable to further respond. The net effect is a "steal" phenomenon with diversion of blood flow from hypoperfused to normal areas of the brain. Hypothermia can depress cerebral activity and decrease cellular oxygen requirements below the minimum levels normally required to maintain cellular viability. In theory, hypothermia represents the most effective method of cerebral protection; even a mild decrease in temperature may reduce ischemic damage to the brain. However, even mild hypothermia can induce shivering that significantly increases myocardial oxygen consumption and work. Currently, the literature provides no definitive evidence to support the hypothesis that hypothermia protects that brain sufficiently to justify the myocardial risks imposed by hypothermia and shivering.

Patients are nearly always extubated at the end of the surgical procedure. A deep extubation may be considered in those patients who were easy to ventilate, intubate, and are at minimal risk for aspiration. The rationale for deep extubation is to mitigate the hemodynamic lability that may accompany emergence and to prevent coughing or straining against an ETT with a fresh vascular anastomosis in the neck. Tight blood pressure control must continue through extubation and into the postoperative period. Whether performed before or after extubation, neurologic integrity must be confirmed prior to leaving the operating room. New neurologic deficits may lead to noninvasive imaging, cerebral angiography, or surgical re-exploration. It is rare to require postoperative intensive care unit (ICU) monitoring, and this is typically limited to particularly high-risk patients.

Postoperative Considerations

The paradox of carotid surgery is that, though the goal is to reduce the long-term patient risk of stroke, the patient incurs a small but real risk of perioperative stroke. The historical incidence of postoperative stroke following CEA has been estimated to be approximately 6%.[77,78] Three interventions in the modern era, however, have decreased the incidence of perioperative stroke to approximately 1%: improved perioperative medication management, perioperative neurophysiologic monitoring, and perioperative hemodynamic control.[105] Cerebral hyperperfusion syndrome (CHS) is a rare but devastating complication of CEA, reported in up to 3% of cases.[106] CHS occurs as a consequence of impaired cerebral autoregulation following relief of high-grade stenosis, which may result in ipsilateral cerebral edema, headache, seizures, focal neurologic deficit, or intracerebral hemorrhage. Management of CHS consists of pharmacologic control of hypertension and limitation of rises in cerebral perfusion. Early recognition and treatment are paramount, and complete recovery is possible.

Hemodynamic lability is common in the perioperative period; hypertension is more common than hypotension. Both acute tachycardia and hypertension may precipitate acute myocardial ischemia and failure, and hypertension is associated with CHS as discussed earlier. Post-CEA hypertension is significantly associated with adverse events such as stroke, death, and a trend toward cardiac complications, whereas postoperative hypotension and bradycardia do not appear to correlate with adverse primary or secondary outcomes. A large review of more than 60,000 patients suggests the risk of perioperative MI is below 1%.[107] Despite the low incidence, MI remains a leading cause of death following CEA. Appropriate perioperative medication management as discussed earlier is critical to decrease the risk of MACE. Uncontrolled pain may contribute to hemodynamic lability, although it is important to balance pain control with the need to follow neurologic status. Total perioperative fluid should be limited in this case due to relatively small intraoperative losses (either blood or evaporative), a short surgical time with limited exposure, and frequent diastolic dysfunction. Fluid overload is relatively common cause of demand ischemia, congestion, and respiratory or cardiovascular morbidity following CEA. Other common causes of hypertension should also be ruled out such as full bladder, hypoxemia, or hypercarbia. Once secondary causes of hypertension are ruled out, pharmacologic treatment should be initiated with goal hemodynamics typically within 20% of the patient's baseline values. In some centers, a postoperative ECG is obtained in the recovery room to evaluate for new ischemia.

Postoperative respiratory insufficiency following CEA may result from underlying pulmonary pathophysiology, recurrent laryngeal nerve or hypoglossal nerve injury, neck hematoma, or altered carotid body chemoreceptor response to hypercapnia or hypoxia. Surgical manipulation may damage the nerve supply to the carotid body, resulting in impaired chemo- and baroreceptor responses. Although unilateral loss of carotid body chemoreceptor function is unlikely to be significant, a bilateral loss may prevent the patient from appropriately increasing ventilation in response to hypercapnia or hypoxemia. This may be particularly important for a patient undergoing CEA who has had previous contralateral surgery. Supplemental oxygen should be supplied in the postoperative period. Similarly, drugs that depress respiratory drive (e.g., narcotics) should be limited and avoided whenever possible. Cranial nerve injury is usually temporary.

Wound hematomas develop in up to 2% of patients following CEA. Small hematomas which are likely caused by venous oozing may be managed conservatively with reversal of residual heparin or with compression. A rapidly expanding hematoma is a clinical emergency and must be evaluated immediately due to the risk of tracheal compression and impending loss of airway. Impaired lymphatic drainage can produce sudden and severe pharyngolaryngeal edema; it is prudent to have difficult airway equipment (including videolaryngoscopy, small ETT, and surgical airway equipment) available prior to reinstrumentation of the airway. A high index of suspicion for arterial bleeding may preclude the ability to open and evacuate the hematoma at bedside. Management of a rapid enlarging or symptomatic hematoma is best undertaken in the operating room, both for airway management and surgical re-exploration.

Aortic Reconstruction

Surgical manipulation of the aorta can result in significant and potentially catastrophic effects on patient hemodynamics (NICV 40-2). The anesthetic management of aortic reconstruction is perhaps the most technically challenging for the vascular anesthesiologist. Aortic surgery typically comes in two flavors: reconstruction for aneurysmal disease or reconstruction for aortic dissection.

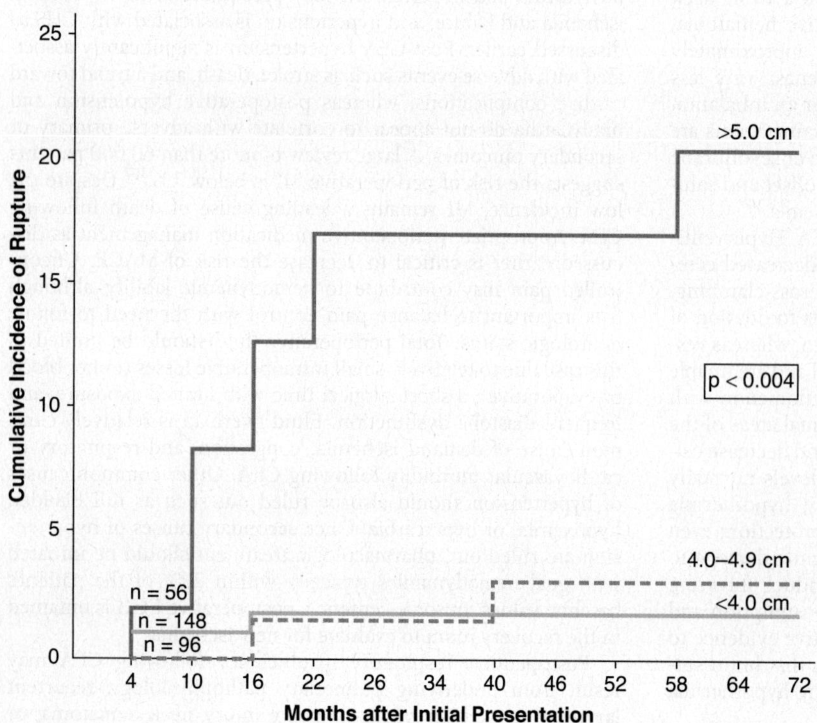

An aneurysm is defined as a greater than 50% dilation of normal expected arterial diameter; for most patients, this corresponds to an abdominal aortic diameter greater than 3.0 cm. The abdominal aorta is the most frequent location of arterial aneurysm, occurring approximately nine times more frequently than a thoracic aortic aneurysm. Approximately 15% of aortic aneurysms involve both the thoracic and abdominal aorta. Thoracic aortic aneurysms are discussed in more detail in the chapter on Anesthesia for Cardiac Surgery. AAAs are classified as infrarenal, juxtarenal, or suprarenal. Approximately 85% of AAAs are infrarenal, with a minority involving the suprarenal aorta.[108] It is vital to understand the location of the aneurysm because it will dictate the level of aortic cross-clamp applied, which has significant implications for the anesthetic management.

Though many of the risk factors are shared between the two processes, the pathophysiology of aortic aneurysm formation is distinct from atherosclerotic disease. Aortic aneurysm formation is a degenerative process involving the degradation of aortic wall connective tissue (primarily, the medial and adventitial layers), inflammation and immune responses, and biomechanical wall stress. The size of the aortic aneurysm is the single most important predictor of subsequent rupture and mortality. A prospective study followed 300 consecutive patients who were initially managed nonoperatively.[109] The median increase in aneurysm diameter was 0.3 cm per year. The 6-year cumulative incidence of rupture was 1% in patients among patients with aneurysms less than 4.0 cm, 2% for patients with aneurysms 4.0 to 4.9 cm, but 20% among patients with aneurysms more than 5.0 cm in diameter (Fig. 40-11). Current recommendations are for serial monitoring of known aneurysms and surgical repair when AAAs exceed 5.5 cm for men or 5.0 cm to 5.4 cm for women.[108] Other risk factors for rupture include rapid growth, symptomatology (e.g., abdominal or back pain), aneurysm shape (saccular vs. fusiform), sex, family history, and degree of control of other comorbidities. Aneurysm rupture is nearly always lethal with mortality rates of 85% to 90%.[110] Thus, close clinical following of known aneurysms is essential, particularly as they enlarge.

Figure 40-11 Cumulative incidence of abdominal aortic aneurysm rupture, according to aneurysm diameter at diagnosis. The incidence of rupture is significantly higher for aneurysms greater than 5.0 cm in diameter. (Reprinted from Guirguis EM, Barber GG. The natural history of abdominal aortic aneurysms. *Am J Surg.* 1991;162:481–483. Copyright © 1991 Elsevier. With permission.)

Acute aortic dissection is a life-threatening medical catastrophe that is associated with very high rates of morbidity and mortality. The hallmark lesion of aortic dissection is a tear in the intimal layer of the arterial wall that creates a false lumen, which is then propagated by pulsatile blood flow. Aortic dissections are classified anatomically and temporally. Acute dissections are those in which clinical symptomatology has lasted fewer than 14 days. Dissections with symptoms exceeding 2 weeks' duration are deemed chronic. Approximately half of aortic dissections originate from the ascending aorta; ascending aortic aneurysms are a surgical emergency. Death from an ascending aortic aneurysm is usually due to acute aortic regurgitation, pericardial tamponade, or myocardial ischemia secondary to coronary ostial compromise. The next most common site of origin is just distal to the left subclavian artery, in the vicinity of the ligamentum arteriosum. Isolated abdominal aortic dissections are rare, with a reported incidence of 1.3%.[111] Death from acute descending aortic dissection is typically secondary to end-organ compromise due to malperfusion of the visceral vessels. Uncomplicated descending aneurysms may be managed medically, whereas complicated (i.e., visceral or limb compromise) require surgical intervention.

Pathophysiology of Aortic Occlusion and Reperfusion

The pathophysiologic response to aortic cross-clamping depends on the level of the occlusion, the overall volume status of the patient, and overall cardiac function (Fig. 40-12).[112] Aortic cross-clamping has little to no effect on heart rate. The most dramatic and consistent effect of aortic cross-clamping is an increase in systemic vascular resistance and mean arterial pressure as a result of the sudden impedance to aortic flow. The extent to which afterload increases depends upon the level at which the cross-clamp is applied. Infrarenal cross-clamping may increase arterial blood pressure 2% to 10%, where as a supraceliac clamp has a significantly greater effect and may increase the mean arterial pressure up to 50% (Table 40-2).

A complex interaction between splanchnic venous tone, blood volume redistribution, coronary blood flow, and myocardial contractility may result in an increase or decrease in cardiac preload, central filling pressures, and cardiac output (Fig. 40-13). Placement of the aortic cross-clamp results in blood volume redistribution proximal to the clamp placement. Infraceliac cross-clamping is relatively well tolerated compared with supraceliac cross-clamping. With lower clamping, blood volume can shift into the compliant splanchnic vasculature, thus limiting preload changes. With the placement of a supraceliac cross-clamp, the splanchnic circulation is unable to absorb this shift in blood volume. Instead, the decrease in splanchnic arterial flow is associated with a decrease in venous capacitance as a result of elastic recoil. The net result is an increase in venous return, central filling pressures, and cardiac output. The increase in preload and afterload increases myocardial work, which in turn leads to coronary

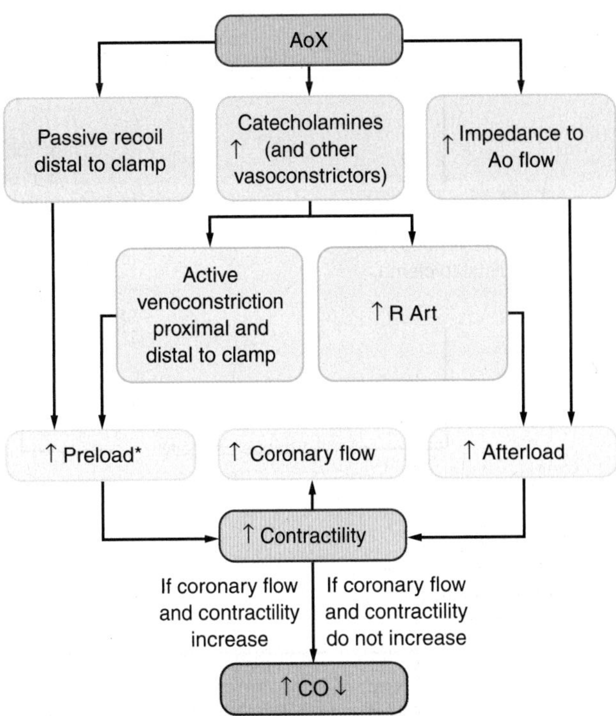

Figure 40-12 Systemic hemodynamic response to aortic cross-clamping (AoX). Preload does not necessarily increase. The most dramatic and consistent effect of aortic cross-clamping is an increase in systemic vascular resistance and mean arterial pressure as a result of the sudden impedance to aortic flow. Ao, aorta. (Adapted with permission from Gelman S. The pathophysiology of aortic cross-clamping and unclamping. *Anesthesiology*. 1995;82(4):1026–1060.)

Table 40-2 Effect of Level of Aortic Occlusion on Changes in Cardiovascular Variables[a]

	% Change in Variable, by Level of Aortic Occlusion		
Cardiovascular Variable	***Supraceliac***	***Suprarenal***	***Infrarenal***
Mean arterial blood pressure	54	5	2
Pulmonary capillary wedge pressure	38	10	0
End diastolic area	28	2	9
End systolic area	69	10	11
Ejection fraction	−38	−10	−3
Abnormal motion of wall, % of patients	92	33	0
New myocardial infarction, % of patients	8	0	0

[a]The degree of hemodynamic derangements with aortic cross clamping is dictated in large part by the level of aortic occlusion.
Adapted from Roizen MF, Beaupre PN, Alpert RA, et al. Monitoring with two-dimensional transesophageal echocardiography. Comparison of myocardial function in patients undergoing supraceliac, suprarenal-infraceliac, or infrarenal aortic occlusion. *J Vasc Surg*. 1984;1(2):300–305.

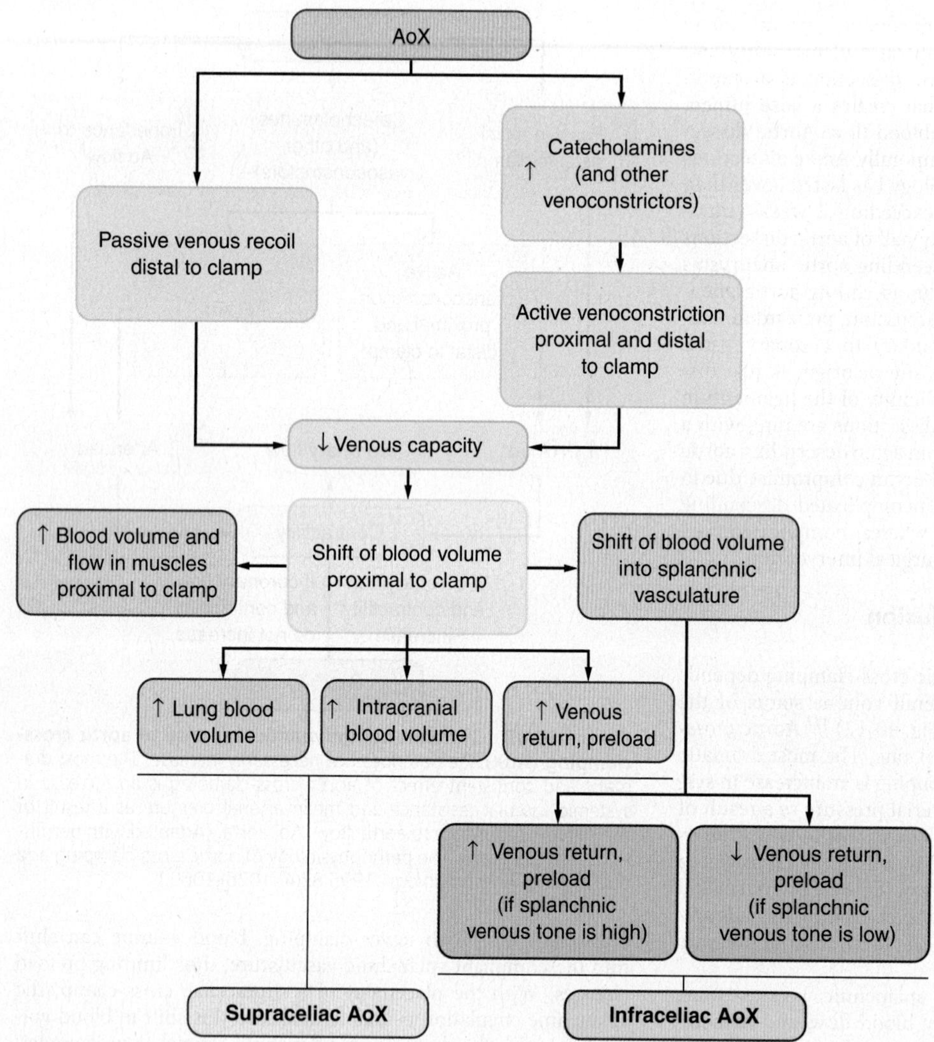

Figure 40-13 Blood volume redistribution following aortic cross-clamp (AoX) placement. Passive venous recoil distal the aortic cross-clamp results in a shift in blood volume from distal to the aortic occlusion to proximal to the occlusion. If the aorta is occluded above the level of the celiac axis, the splanchnic reserve is redistributed to the organs and tissues proximal to the clamp. If an infraceliac cross-clamp is placed, the blood volume may shift into the splanchnic system in addition to other organs proximal to the clamp. The ability to shift into or out of the splanchnic vasculature accounts for variability in preload augmentation. (Adapted with permission from Gelman S. The pathophysiology of aortic cross-clamping and unclamping. *Anesthesiology*. 1995; 82(4):1026–1060.)

vasodilation to maximize coronary blood flow and oxygen delivery. Patients with limited cardiac reserve, such as those with a decreased ejection fraction or significant CAD (in whom the coronary vasculature is already maximally dilated), may not tolerate this increase in myocardial work. In such cases, myocardial ischemia or failure may develop. New LV wall abnormalities have been demonstrated in up to one-third of patients with a suprarenal aortic cross-clamp placement, and more than 90% of patients with a supraceliac aortic cross-clamp.[113] Patients with an infrarenal cross-clamp, by comparison, did not have evidence of regional wall motion abnormalities during cross-clamp placement. Despite a decrease in ejection fraction, cardiac output and stroke volume increased by expanding the cavity size of the left ventricle.

Anticipation of aortic cross-clamp placement should prompt hemodynamic manipulation. A pragmatic approach is to initially use esmolol to decrease heart rate to a target of around 60 to 65 beats per minute. This decreases the risk of myocardial oxygen imbalance. Direct vasodilators are then employed to control arterial pressure. This can be accomplished via bolus (+/– continuous infusion) of intravenous vasodilating agents (e.g., sodium nitroprusside, nitroglycerin, or nicardipine), local anesthetic administration via thoracic epidural, or deepening of anesthetic depth. The goal is to offset the increase in afterload and myocardial work with systemic vasodilation. It is important to recognize that attempts to normalize systemic vascular resistance above the level of the clamp can even further compromise blood flow distal to the clamp. It is critical to maintain a perfusion pressure below the level of the cross-clamp that will not potentiate visceral or spinal cord ischemia.

There are two distinct aortic unclamping events. Even if the initial aortic clamp was supraceliac, the anastomosis is most commonly infrarenal. Once the proximal anastomosis is made, the clamp is moved from native aorta to graft in order to allow reperfusion of the celiac and renal beds. This is usually hemodynamically insignificant due to the relatively short duration of ischemia and rapid reapplication of the cross-clamp distal to the visceral vessels until the distal anastomosis (or, in the case of bifurcated graft, anastomoses) are completed. The subsequent release of the distal clamp(s) results in the release of inflammatory mediators, decreased cardiac output, hypoxemia-mediated vasodilation, and a reactive hyperemia that ultimately culminates in profound vasodilation and arterial hypotension (Fig. 40-14). Systemic vascular resistance may decrease up to 80%, with similarly profound decrease in LV pressure. A relative central hypovolemia develops as blood pools in tissue distal to the cross-clamp. Various therapies have been employed to counteract this response, with no evidence to suggest superiority of one method over another. Most anesthesiologists employ some degree of volume loading during the period of cross-clamp application. Vasoconstrictors such as phenylephrine or norepinephrine, or inotropic agents such as

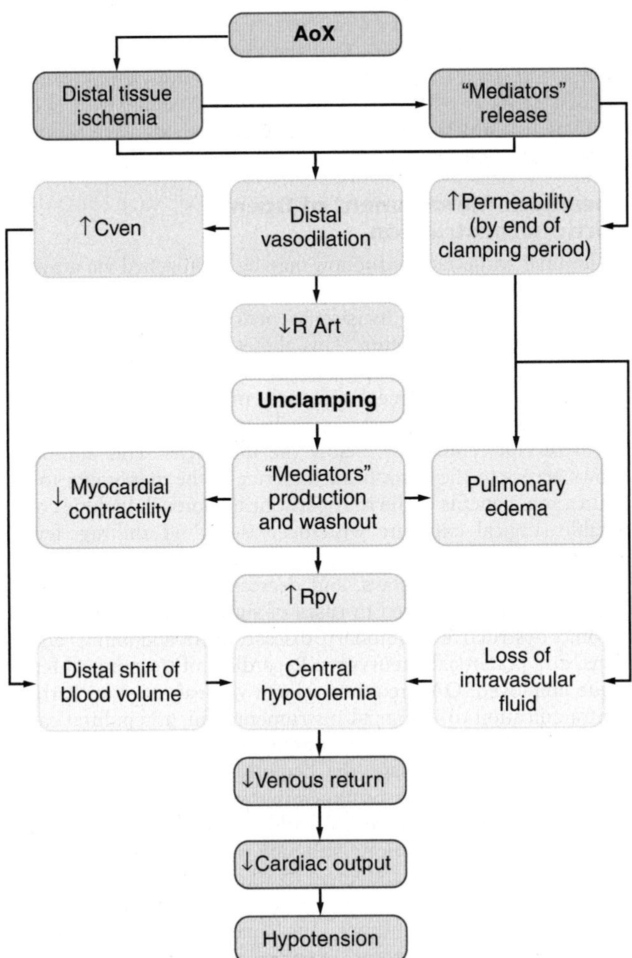

Figure 40-14 Hemodynamic response to aortic cross-clamp (AoX) release. A complex cascade of events, including release of inflammatory mediators, distal vasodilation, increased vascular permeability, and decreased myocardial contractility results in a relative central hypovolemia, decreased cardiac output, and systemic hypotension. (Adapted with permission from Gelman S. The pathophysiology of aortic cross-clamping and unclamping. *Anesthesiology*. 1995;82(4):1026–1060.)

epinephrine or calcium chloride are frequently employed in conjunction with volume loading. It may also be prudent to decrease anesthetic depth and/or discontinue epidural infusions in anticipation of these predictable changes. Preferable to pharmacologic manipulation is a gradual release of the cross-clamp to allow for a slow, controlled release of vasoactive and cardiodepressant mediators. If bilateral iliac clamps are employed, the lower extremities can be reperfused sequentially to allow for a more controlled release and appropriate resuscitation. Clear communication with the vascular surgeon is vital to coordinate appropriate management. For example, bleeding at the anastomosis requires immediate reclamping; if vasopressors and inotropes are administered as boluses and then the clamp is reapplied, profound proximal hypertension can ensue.

Renal Hemodynamics and Renal Protection

Postoperative mortality is four- to fivefold higher in those who develop acute renal failure when compared with those who do not. Preoperative renal dysfunction is the most powerful predictor of postoperative renal dysfunction. There is no proven renal protective strategy other than minimizing the length of ischemia and avoidance of profound or prolonged hypotension.[114] Though the level of the cross-clamp can markedly impact renal blood flow, renal failure is a commonly encountered source of perioperative morbidity even with infrarenal cross-clamp placement. The incidence of acute renal failure is approximately 5% following infrarenal cross-clamping and approaches 13% after suprarenal cross-clamping. With suprarenal occlusion, renal blood flow decreases by up to 80%. Blood flow is not only reduced but also redistributed, favoring flow to the cortical and juxtamedullary layers over the hypoxia-prone renal medulla.[115] Even with an infrarenal occlusion, renal blood flow is decreased by nearly 50% compared to baseline, whereas renal vascular resistance increases by almost 70%. These alterations are predominantly a result of neurohumoral activation rather due to changes in hemodynamics or cardiac output. Physiologic fluctuations do not immediately revert after the release of cross-clamping and may persist for at least 30 minutes beyond systemic cardiovascular return to baseline. Thus, the best initial management of decreased urine output in the immediate post–cross-clamping period may be to wait and observe for recovery.

Many different pharmacologic methods of renal protection have been advocated, most centering on improving renal blood flow or glomerular flow. Mannitol increases diuresis and functions as a free radical scavenger. No clinical trials to date have demonstrated any reduction in the incidence of postoperative renal failure in patients undergoing repair of an AAA who have been given mannitol. Diuretics, and particularly loop diuretics, are often considered in the case of low urine output, despite the fact that no significant correlation has been demonstrated between intraoperative mean urinary output or lowest hourly urinary output and the development of acute renal insufficiency. The use of diuretic medications for the sole purpose of increasing urine output only converts an oliguric to polyuric renal failure while significant fluid shifting may result in depletion of intravascular volume, adding further renal insult. Diuretics should be reserved only for patients who are demonstrably volume overloaded and then used judiciously to effect. Dopamine does not appear to improve postoperative renal dysfunction. Fenoldopam, a selective dopamine agonist, has shown promise in some clinical trials but results have been conflicting in cardiovascular surgery.[114,116] Ali and colleagues[117] investigated the role of ischemic preconditioning on renal and myocardial injury with aortic cross-clamping and found a beneficial effect on both. In this study, ischemic preconditioning was found to decrease the incidence of postoperative renal insufficiency by 23%.

Spinal Cord Ischemia and Protection

The spinal cord is supplied primarily by the single anterior and paired posterior spinal arteries, arising from the posterior circulation (Fig. 40-15). The posterior spinal arteries supply approximately 25% of spinal cord blood flow and supply the sensory tracts of the posterior columns. The anterior spinal artery supplies the anterolateral cord, including motor tracts, and supplies 75% of the spinal cord blood flow. The anterior spinal artery is fed by a series of radicular arteries arising from the aorta, although collateralization is variable. This leaves areas of the spinal cord vulnerable to watershed ischemia, particularly with aortic occlusion or prolonged hypotension. The single most important radicular artery supplying the thoracolumbar cord is derived from the artery of Adamkiewicz. The artery of Adamkiewicz originates between T8 and T12 in 75% of cases and at the level of L1 or L2 in an additional 10% of cases.

Spinal cord ischemia is a feared complication of aortic reconstruction and occurs in up to 10% of patients involving a distal

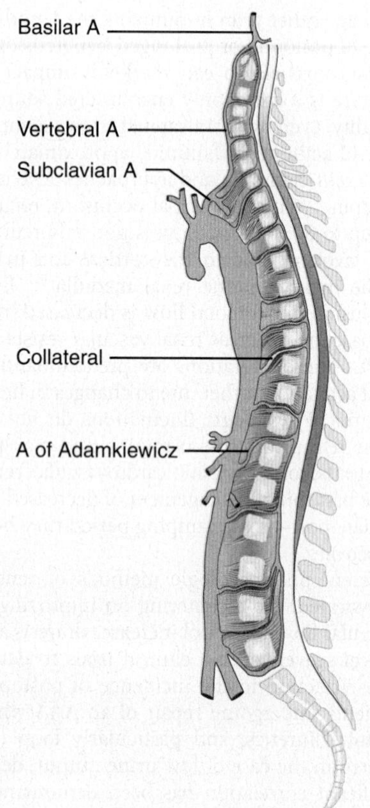

Figure 40-15 Vascular supply to the spinal cord. The singular anterior spinal artery and paired posterior spinal arteries arise from the posterior circulation and provide blood supply to the spinal cord. Radicular arteries arising from the aorta supplement this blood supply. The artery of Adamkiewicz is the most clinically significant contributor. Variability in collateral flow helps to explain, in part, the unpredictability of paraplegia following aortic surgery. (Adapted from Piccone W, DeLaria GA, Najafi H. Descending thoracic aneurysms. In: Bergan JJ, Yao JST, eds. *Aortic Surgery*. WB Saunders; 1989:249. Copyright © 1989 Elsevier. With permission.)

aortic repair. Pertinent risks for spinal cord ischemia include previous aortic surgery (particularly with vascular exclusion of major thoracic radicular collaterals), open surgical repair, aortic cross-clamp location and duration, length of aortic replacement, and intraoperative hypotension/hypoperfusion. The definitive measures to prevent spinal cord ischemia are a short cross-clamp time, maintenance of normal cardiac function, and higher perfusion pressures. Segmental sequential surgical repair may minimize the duration of ischemia to any given vascular bed. A markedly reduced incidence of neurologic deficits has been reported in thoracoabdominal aortic repairs when distal aortic perfusion is used in combination with cerebral spinal fluid (CSF) drainage, placed either prophylactically or for rescue.[118] The rationale behind CSF drainage is that spinal cord perfusion pressure can be augmented either by increasing the forward driving pressure (MAP) or by relieving any obstructing pressure (CSF pressure). In the setting of aneurysmal disease and major vascular reconstruction, it may be practically problematic to augment MAP to the degree necessary to ensure adequate perfusion. Autoregulatory mechanisms that occur with aortic cross-clamping results in a reflexive increase in CSF pressure, effectively lowering spinal cord perfusion pressure. CSF drainage, then, favors improved spinal cord perfusion. When employed, CSF monitoring is usually continuous, and CSF is slowly removed to maintain a CSF pressure less than 12 mmHg. Although commonly used in thoracic or thoracoabdominal aortic repairs (see the chapter on Anesthesia for Cardiac Surgery), this technique is less commonly employed for isolated AAAs as perfusion of the artery of Adamkiewicz is less likely at risk unless there has been previous extensive thoracic aortic artery replacement.

Anesthetic Management of Open Aortic Reconstruction

Abdominal aortic reconstruction may be approached via a transabdominal or retroperitoneal approach. In the first case, a thoracoabdominal midline incision is performed and the aorta is accessed via the peritoneum. This allows generous exposure and is usually favored for complex aortic reconstruction or replacement. In the retroperitoneal approach, incision is made over the lateral border of the left rectus muscle, from the level of the 12th rib to several centimeters below the umbilicus. This approach allows access to the aorta from the crux of the diaphragm to its bifurcation. Benefits of the retroperitoneal approach include comparable surgical exposure with decreased fluid shifting, fewer postoperative pulmonary complications, faster return of bowel function, shorter ICU stays, and decreased hospital costs. This technique may be favored in cases of significant truncal obesity, chronic obstructive pulmonary disease, intra-abdominal adhesions, and juxtarenal aneurysms. Regardless of the surgical technique employed, OAR requires a large vertical incision. Barring contraindication to neuraxial instrumentation, an epidural catheter should be considered. A functional epidural may be used intraoperatively to manage the hemodynamic lability of aortic cross-clamping, decrease postoperative sympathetic stimulation, aid in postoperative pain control, and potentially aid in weaning from mechanical ventilation. Although most ischemic complications are the result of dislodgment of atheromatous material from the diseased aorta and not de novo clot formation, most surgeons nevertheless administer intravenous heparin to reduce the risk of thromboembolic events before aortic cross-clamping. If neuraxial instrumentation is attempted, heparin dosing should be delayed per current guidelines.[119] In the case of traumatic placement or intravascular catheter, a frank consideration of the risks and benefits of proceeding to surgery versus delaying the case must be undertaken by the operative team due to the small but catastrophic risk of epidural hematoma.

General anesthesia is typically employed for open repair of AAA. Induction of general anesthesia and intubation can be associated with dramatic hemodynamic lability and sympathetic stimulation, which may put the aneurysm at risk of rupture. It is prudent to ensure adequate blood product availability in the operating room and large-bore peripheral intravenous access prior to the induction of general anesthesia. There is no single "best" induction technique; regardless of agents chosen, the goal is a smooth induction with stable hemodynamics and avoidance of tachycardia or hypertension. Preinduction placement of an arterial line may aid in appropriate titration of induction agents. Central venous catheterization is generally employed for monitoring volume trends and for the reliable delivery of vasoactive medication. Cardiac function is commonly assessed with either a pulmonary artery catheter or transesophageal echocardiography. Either technique can provide valuable information about cardiac functioning and volume status. Echocardiography is the most sensitive marker for new regional wall motion abnormalities and direct visualization of appropriate ventricular filling. Pulmonary artery catheterization can be useful both intraoperatively and postoperatively to guide resuscitation. The use of pulmonary artery catheters has been the subject of debate, with conflicting evidence as to their benefit in high-risk surgical patients.[120,121]

Virtually all anesthetic drugs and techniques have been described for aortic reconstructive surgery. The ability to maintain hemodynamic equilibrium and attend to detail is far more important than the choice of drug. Volatile agents may improve preconditioning mechanisms should myocardial ischemia occur.[122] These effects have been demonstrated in animal models and in cardiac, although not vascular, surgery. The maintenance anesthetic is designed to maintain hemodynamics within 20% of the baseline range. An array of short-acting vasoactive agents (including vasodilators, vasopressors, and inotropes) should be on hand to immediately treat hemodynamic lability.

For the period prior to cross-clamp placement, the patient is kept slightly hypovolemic (typically, as assessed by CVP, pulmonary catheter wedge pressure or echocardiography) to limit hypertensive extremes with aortic occlusion. At the time of cross-clamp placement, vasodilating infusions may be required. Alternatively, deepening the anesthetic or injection of the epidural catheter with local anesthetic will increase vasodilation, although both of these approaches require careful attention to avoid unintended hypotension. When there is concern about spinal cord perfusion, it may be prudent to allow permissive hypertension, to the extent possible, above the level of the clamp to provide higher distal perfusion pressure and avoid distal ischemia. This choice may come at the expense of myocardial well-being.

After the vascular clamps are placed and the aneurysm sac is incised, blood loss is swift from any vessels arising from the aorta between the two clamps. Adequate peripheral and central venous access is imperative. Blood loss can be considerable without the onset of hypotension or tachycardia because a significant portion of the vascular tree is excluded from circulation during aortic occlusion. An autotransfusion device should be employed to reduce the amount of autologous blood needed. It is prudent to volume load during the period of aortic cross-clamping in anticipation for the vasoplegic washout and reactive hyperemia that will occur with the removal of aortic cross-clamp. This augmentation of central volume will then fill the increased capacitance distal to the aortic clamp when it is subsequently released.

Immediately prior to the removal of the aortic clamp, vasodilating agents are discontinued. The surgeon opens the aortic clamp gradually to ensure that severe hypotension or bleeding does not develop. Ongoing fluid resuscitation and vasopressor and inotropic support is frequently necessary. Severe refractory hypotension can be temporarily abated with reapplication of the aortic cross-clamp until appropriate measures can be instituted. Over the course of the reconstruction, there may be frequent instances of cross-clamp application and release to limit the ischemic time to vital organs and to "test" the anastomoses. It is imperative for the anesthesiologist to be flexible and adaptable, and to have a variety of short-acting vasoactive agents available for hemodynamic manipulation. Each time the cross-clamp is removed, a "washout" of vasoactive agents occurs with the potential for hemodynamic instability. Central and pulmonary filling pressures may be elevated despite systemic hypotension because of the washout of lactic acid and other inflammatory mediators, which results in pulmonary vasoconstriction and cardiac stunning.

At the end of the procedure, the decision regarding emergence and extubation must take into account any ongoing hemodynamic instability, metabolic derangements, and ongoing need for resuscitation. β-Blocking agents are continued in the perioperative period, as tolerated. Redosing of the epidural catheter allows for adequate pain control and may help with weaning from mechanical ventilation, particularly in patients with concomitant chronic obstructive pulmonary disease. For those patients who remain intubated, the use of the epidural catheter for pain control permits a reasonably light intravenous sedation, which allows for continued monitoring of neurologic status.

Peripheral Artery Disease

It has been estimated that up to 20% of the population is affected by PAD. Though the majority of patients are asymptomatic, PAD is a risk factor for adverse cardiovascular events, with an annual rate of 5% to 7%.[7,123] Risk factors include nonwhite race, male gender, age, smoking, diabetes, hypertension, dyslipidemia, chronic renal insufficiency, hyperviscous/hypercoagulable states, hyperhomocysteinemia, and patients with elevated inflammatory markers. There are three clinical indications for elective surgery for PAD: intermittent claudication (IC), ischemic rest pain or ulceration, or gangrene.

Most patients with PAD have either asymptomatic disease or IC, defined as reproducible discomfort in a defined muscle group that is induced by activity and relieved with rest. Approximately 10% to 35% of patients with PAD will present with symptoms of IC. The clinical manifestations of IC depend on the location of the occlusion, its severity, and the presence (or absence) of collateral blood flow. Aortoiliac occlusive disease (AIOD), or "inflow" disease, tends to result in claudication in the buttock or hip. AIOD usually originates in the distal aorta or proximal common iliac arteries. "Outflow" disease, defined as femoropopliteal or infrapopliteal lesions, results in claudication of the thigh or leg.

IC is the first and most common symptom associated with PAD. The natural history of PAD is typically indolent with a slow, progressive decline in function. Aggressive management of risk factors with pharmacologic, exercise, and lifestyle modification prevents disease progression in the vast majority of cases. Because of the relatively slow and benign progression of symptoms, the decision for surgical intervention for IC must be individualized. Decision making should consider response to therapy, loss of function, and effect on quality of life. A very active person may be debilitated by relatively mild symptoms, whereas more severe symptoms may be well tolerated by a sedentary individual.

Chronic limb ischemia (CLI) occurs when the existing arterial blood flow is unable to meet even basal metabolic demands, resulting in rest pain, ulceration, and gangrene. CLI is an especially aggressive manifestation of PAD associated with more severe, multisegmental occlusion. Risk factors for accelerated disease progression include age, diabetes, smoking, and hyperlipidemia. PAD progresses to CLI in approximately 1% to 2% of the population. Patients with CLI may have progressive ischemia and are at variable risk for imminent limb loss; thus, urgent surgical intervention is warranted. It is estimated that within 1 year, 25% of patients will progress to amputation, and an additional 25% will die from cardiovascular causes.[7,123] Not surprisingly, these patients also have more severe ASCVD in other vascular beds. Approximately 50% of patients with CLI will have concomitant CAD, with a higher mortality from MI or stroke among patients with CLI compared to less aggressive forms of PAD. These patients, then, are at elevated perioperative risk due to both medical and surgical factors related to disease severity.

AIOD may be repaired via direct reconstruction (aortoiliac or aortofemoral bypass), or with extra-anatomic reconstruction (axillary-femoral +/– femoral-femoral bypass). Direct reconstruction has better long-term patency rates (greater than 80%), at the expense of greater perioperative morbidity and mortality. Extra-anatomic bypass, although less morbid, has also proven less durable, with 5-year patency rates are reported between 55% and 80%.[123] As such, extra-anatomic bypass is typically reserved for patients deemed particularly high risk for direct surgical reconstruction due to previous graft or stent complications, infection, or previous intra-abdominal surgery with resultant abdominal adhesions. Open revascularization of infrainguinal disease depends on the level of the lesion(s), and may involve the femoral, popliteal, or infrapopliteal vessels.

Anesthetic Management of Lower Extremity Revascularization

The anesthetic management of AIOD depends on whether anatomic or extra-anatomic bypass is performed. Anesthetic considerations for aortofemoral bypass are similar to OAR. Barring contraindication, a preinduction epidural catheter should be considered for postoperative pain control. General anesthesia with an ETT is typically employed due to the length of the case as well as the potential for hemodynamic lability. Large-bore peripheral IV access and an arterial line should be placed to help guide resuscitation and to allow instantaneous assessment of hemodynamic changes. Although aortic cross-clamping and uncross-clamping is required for aortofemoral bypass, it is typically better tolerated than for aneurysmal disease because the patient is already accustomed to high aortic resistance. Hemodynamics tend to be more stable both as a result of clamp location (typically, distal aortic) as well as the likelihood of extensive collateralization related to chronic atherosclerotic obstruction. This stands in stark contrast to aneurysmal disease, which features limited pre-existing collateral flow. Central venous access is reasonable to ensure reliable delivery of necessary vasoactive medications. Additional cardiac monitoring, such as pulmonary artery catheter placement or transesophageal echocardiography, may be considered depending on patient and surgical factors.

By definition, extra-anatomic bypass does not involve aortic manipulation and thus avoids the need for aortic cross-clamping and uncross-clamping (1 Video 40-1). Typically, extra-anatomic bypass is undertaken from the axillary artery to the ipsilateral femoral artery, +/– subsequent femoral to femoral artery bypass. Less hemodynamic lability is noted with axillary and femoral artery cross-clamping than with aortic cross-clamping. Thus, although large-bore peripheral IV and arterial line placement is still prudent, the need for extensive central or cardiac monitoring is less critical unless independently indicated due to medical comorbidities. Arterial line placement should be contralateral to the surgical bypass, as arterial cross-clamp placement will render an ipsilateral arterial line nonfunctional. The extra-anatomic bypass must be tunneled subcutaneously in the mid-axillary line to prevent kinking of the graft, which may be more sympathetically stimulating than cross-clamp placement. Close attention must be paid to prevent untoward hemodynamic swings or patient movement during this period.

The choice of anesthetic technique for infrainguinal revascularization is individualized for each patient. Lower extremity revascularization can be performed under general, neuraxial, or regional anesthesia. Purported benefits of regional anesthesia include avoidance of hyperdynamic responses to tracheal intubation and extubation, blunted perioperative catecholamine response, improved vascular blood flow, higher graft patency rates, and lower pulmonary complications. A review of the NSQIP database compared nearly 15,000 patients receiving neuraxial (spinal or epidural) versus general anesthesia for lower extremity revascularization.[124] In this study, neuraxial anesthesia was associated with a decreased likelihood of reintervention, decreased rates of graft failure, and decreased rates of postoperative respiratory and cardiovascular complications. In an analysis of patients in the NSQIP database with CLI, however, no differences in perioperative morbidity were noted between patients who underwent general versus neuraxial anesthesia.[125] A Cochrane review of general versus regional anesthesia for lower extremity revascularization concluded that there was insufficient evidence to rule out clinically important differences for most clinical outcomes (mortality, MI, or rate of lower-limb amputation).[126] Thus, anesthetic technique should be governed by clinical expertise, patient, and surgeon preferences.

Morbidity and mortality following lower extremity revascularization is typically cardiac in origin. A review of the NSQIP database suggests an overall cardiac mortality rate of 2.7% with 30-day combined mortality/major morbidity rate of nearly 20%.[127] Patients who undergo surgery for CLI as compared to IC are at increased risk, likely due to greater disease burden and more technically challenging repairs due to multilevel, extensive disease.

Endovascular Surgery

The advent of the endovascular era has revolutionized the field of vascular surgery. Endovascular procedures are minimally invasive and are generally associated with decreased perioperative mortality and major morbidity, shorter hospital and intensive care stays, and quicker return to baseline function, particularly for the elderly or frail. In addition to a lower level of surgical stress, endovascular techniques may obviate the need for general anesthesia. Despite overall improvements in short- and intermediate-term outcomes, long-term benefits to endovascular repairs have not been sustained. In addition, endovascular repairs have proven less durable and more prone to reintervention than traditional open repairs. In this section, we will consider the anesthetic implications for endovascular approaches to vascular disease. 6

Carotid Artery Stenting

Carotid artery angioplasty and stenting was first described in the late 1970s and early 1980s, but early complications related to distal plaque embolization during stent deployment limited initial enthusiasm for an endovascular approach to cerebral vascular disease. The development of embolic protection devices in the 1990s led to a renewed interest in an endovascular approach to carotid disease, especially in patients deemed high risk for open surgery. Five landmark randomized controlled trials have compared traditional open CEA to carotid artery stenting.[128–132] A 2020 meta-analysis of the current data concluded that, for symptomatic patients, carotid artery stenting was associated with a higher risk of periprocedural stroke or death than endarterectomy, mostly attributable to minor, nondisabling strokes occurring in the elderly population. Beyond the periprocedural period, carotid stenting was as effective in preventing recurrent stroke as endarterectomy.[133]

These findings stand in contrast to head-to-head trials of endovascular versus open repairs in other vascular beds (such as treatment of aortic and peripheral disease, discussed later), where short-term perioperative morbidity and mortality tend to be improved with endovascular treatment. Most of the differences in perioperative morbidity were limited to the elderly. Long-term outcomes beyond the perioperative period, including functional outcomes, are comparable between patients who undergo open versus endovascular intervention for carotid disease. At present, the contemporary literature fails to reach a consensus on the superiority of either open or endovascular technique for the treatment of carotid disease. Individual medical, surgical, and operator considerations must be weighed in the decision for open versus endovascular repair (OVER). Though CEA remains the gold standard for repair, continuous advances in endovascular techniques are changing the trends in the management of carotid disease. Advances in technology, cerebral protection devices, and operator skill have impacted outcomes for endovascular carotid artery stenting since the initial landmark studies were done. Studies evaluating outcomes for carotid artery stenting in the modern era are currently ongoing.[16,134]

Transcarotid artery revascularization (TCAR) is a novel hybrid approach to carotid artery revascularization that involves a small cutdown on the common carotid artery and deployment of a carotid stent. TCAR creates a temporary reversal of cerebral blood flow via a novel cerebral protection device. Perioperative outcomes reported from the Safety and Efficacy Study for Reverse Flow Used During Carotid Artery Stenting Procedure (ROADSTER) and ROADSTER-2 trials report the lowest perioperative stroke rates (1.4%) for endovascular techniques, which are equivalent to open CEA,[135,136] and a lower risk of stroke and death than traditional transfemoral carotid artery stenting.[137] Carotid stenting is strongly preferred over open repair for reoperation, for very high lesions, and in patients who have had neck radiation.

A major benefit of carotid artery stenting lies in the ability to continuously monitor neurologic integrity during the procedure. The minimally invasive vascular approach requires little, if any, sedation beyond local anesthetic to the access site. It is vital that the patient remains alert and cooperative with the proceduralist for serial neurologic examinations. A candid preoperative discussion to set appropriate patient expectations is perhaps the most critical anesthetic intervention. The lowest necessary doses of short-acting sedatives should be titrated to effect; patient disinhibition must be avoided. Standard intraoperative monitoring and a single medium- to large-bore peripheral intravenous line is typically sufficient for the procedure; invasive arterial access may be considered but is rarely warranted. In an emergency, arterial pressure may be monitored from the surgical access site. It is important to recognize that carotid angioplasty and stent deployment may trigger the carotid baroreceptor reflex, with resultant bradycardia and hypotension, similar to external carotid manipulation. If this occurs, cessation of manipulation should extinguish the response; prophylaxis with an anticholinergic agent may be considered. Altered postoperative carotid baroreceptor function is possible as with open repair; hemodynamic instability should be treated as for CEA.

Endovascular Aortic Repair

Prior to the endovascular era, options for AAA management were limited to OAR or medical management. The morbidity and mortality associated with OAR are significant. At the same time, the risk of rupture increases significantly as aneurysms enlarge, with a near 100% mortality rate for out-of-hospital rupture. The advent of the endovascular era has revolutionized the management of AAAs. Initially, this technique was reserved for high-risk patients with straightforward anatomy deemed unfit for open surgical repair. Recent advances in stent technology and surgical skill, including customized fenestrated and branched modular stents and chimney techniques, have made endovascular repair an option for patients who previously would have been considered unfit due to anatomic considerations. In fact, the broad application of EVAR technology has rapidly overtaken the use of OAR as the primarily modality for AAA treatment.[138] In 2000, EVAR accounted for 5.2% of AAA repairs. In 2004, EVAR surpassed OAR as the more commonly employed technique. By 2010, this percentage had risen dramatically to 74%. Endovascular repair has also become the treatment modality of choice for complicated acute type B dissections.[108]

Several rigorous, large, multicenter, randomized controlled trials have addressed the issue of open versus endovascular aneurysm repair.[139–142] The Dutch Randomized Endovascular Aneurysm Management (DREAM), EndoVascular Aneurysm Repair (EVAR), and OVER trials all demonstrated significantly lower perioperative mortality with EVAR than with OAR, although this benefit was lost in intermediate- to long-term follow-up. The Aneurysme de l'aorte abdominale: Chirurgie versus Endoprothese (ACE) trial, in contrast, found no significant difference in perioperative or longer-term mortality between the EVAR and OAR groups, although it is worth noting that these patients were considered low- to intermediate-risk for surgery. Taken together, a pooled analysis of these results suggests a decrease in short-term mortality, but no significant difference in either intermediate- (up to 4 years) or long-term outcomes.[143] Major operative morbidity, including myocardial, neurologic, and renal complications, were similar in pooled analysis. Pulmonary complications were found to be significantly higher in the OAR compared to EVAR group, and a similar trend was noted in pulmonary-related deaths. The long-term reintervention rate was significantly higher in the EVAR than OAR group; the unique complication profile of endovascular repair necessitates a lifetime of surveillance. In general, the majority of reinterventions are also endovascular with low associated morbidity and mortality. Even so, repeated exposure to radiation and contrast exposure, and potentially surgery and anesthesia, should be considered when deciding between open- versus endovascular-based interventions. An otherwise young, fit patient with a lower perioperative risk profile may be a reasonable candidate for OAR to avoid the associated risks of lifetime surveillance and potential for reintervention; however, a review of the NSQIP database suggests that the perioperative reduction in mortality and major morbidity persists even in patients deemed low risk for infrarenal OAR.[144]

The EVAR-2 trial was designed to compare maximum medical therapy versus EVAR in patients deemed unfit for OAR.[145] Patient factors that were associated with ineligibility for OAR included major cardiac, pulmonary, or renal comorbidities. This trial concluded that EVAR reduces aneurysm-related, but not overall, mortality as compared to medical therapy. Presumably, the same factors that made patients too high risk for OAR likely contributed to a high subsequent rate of all cause mortality. Thus, the authors suggest that patients with a poor life expectancy due to coexisting disease do not benefit from EVAR.

A question that persists after the EVAR-2 trial is which patients, in particular, should be considered high risk for endovascular repair. Table 40-3 lists the baseline risk factors that significantly predicted mortality with a corresponding score, derived from 67,000 patients who underwent EVAR in the inpatient Medicare database.[146] The vast majority of patients (96.6%) had additive scores below 10, which correlated with a 30-day mortality of less than 5%, whereas less than 1% had a mortality rate greater than 10%. Thus, although a high-risk cohort exists that should not be treated with EVAR due to prohibitively high 30-day mortality, that cohort is quite small. The EVAR Risk Assessment model has been shown to predict not only perioperative mortality but also morbidity, mid-term survival, and reintervention rates.[147] The 10 variables included in this model were self-reported fitness, American Society of Anesthesiologists physical status score, history of stroke/transient ischemic attack, age, aneurysm angle, infrarenal neck length, white cell count, respiratory assessment, diabetes and statin therapy. Fitness alone predicted perioperative mortality better than any other factor.

Evolution of Endovascular Repair for Complex Aneurysms

The field of endovascular surgery has rapidly expanded since Parodi[148] first described the use of a custom-made Dacron tube

Table 40-3 Risk Scores for 30-day Mortality for EVAR Patients[a]

Risk Factor	Score
Renal failure with dialysis	7
Lower extremity ischemia	5
Age ≥85 yrs	4
Liver disease	3
Congestive heart failure	3
Age 80–84 yrs	2
Female	2
Neurologic comorbidity	2
Chronic pulmonary disease	1
Surgeon case experience <3	1
Hospital annual volume <7	1
Age 57–59 yrs	1

[a]A total score between 10 and 12 predicts a 5% mortality rate. A total score greater than 13 predicts a 10% operative rate.
EVAR, EndoVascular Aneurysm Repair.
Adapted from Egorova N, Giacovelli JK, Gelijns A, et al. Defining high-risk patients for endovascular aneurysm repair. *J Vasc Surg*. 2009;50(6):1271–1279.e1. Copyright © 2009 Elsevier. With permission.

endograft, which limited its use to infrarenal aortic segments only. The development of bifurcated and modular grafts soon followed, allowing for extension beyond the aortic bifurcation. Until recently, however, device design constraints excluded patients with more complicated anatomy from endovascular repair. Patients with juxta- or suprarenal aneurysms, for example, were not candidates for endovascular repair because the visceral vasculature may arise from the aneurysmal aorta: blood flow to these critical organs would have been interrupted by the graft. Similarly, up to 15% of infrarenal aneurysms have an inadequate length of normal infrarenal aorta to allow for an adequate proximal seal without compromising visceral blood flow. Recent advances in stent technology have revolutionized management of these more complicated repairs. The development of fenestrated or branched grafts (f/b-EVAR) allows for continued blood flow to visceral organs while still permitting proximal graft extension. These devices are custom made based on three-dimensional reconstructions (typically, CT angiography) so that the fenestrations or branches are appropriately positioned for the corresponding arterial orifices. Because these devices are custom designed, they are costly and take significant time to manufacture. Thus, they are typically not an option for emergent repair. An alternative technique is that of a chimney graft (Ch-EVAR). With this approach, a distinct endograft is positioned in parallel to the body of the main aortic stent graft (between the aortic wall and the main stent) to allow for preserved flow to the visceral branch (Fig. 40-16). The "snorkel" technique allows for blood flow from above the level of the main stent while the "periscope" technique allows blood flow from below. The end result is preservation of visceral blood flow to vessels that otherwise would have been excluded by the main body of the graft. A "sandwich" technique has even been described, in which the visceral snorkels are sandwiched between two segments of aortic grafts. Chimney grafts are available "off the shelf" and thus remain an option

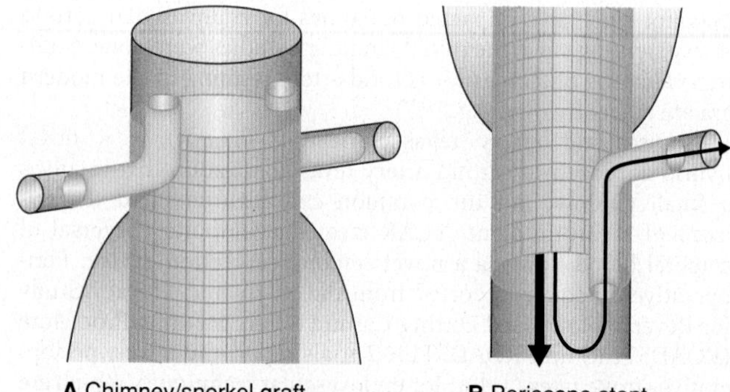

Figure 40-16 Snorkel and periscope stents. Coaxial placement of stents into vital mesenteric vessels allow for both adequate blood flow to visceral organs and exclusion of the aneurysm sac for supra- or juxtarenal aneurysms or aneurysms with insufficient proximal (**A**) or distal (**B**) landing zones. In the case of a periscope, blood exiting the body of the main stent flows back up into the coaxial periscope, providing blood flow to the visceral branch that would otherwise be excluded from the circulation. (Reprinted with permission from Wilson A, Zhou S, Bachoo P, Tambyraja AL. Systematic review of chimney and periscope grafts for endovascular aneurysm repair. *Br J Surg*. 2013; 100(12):1557–1564.)

in urgent situations in which no time exists to manufacture a custom-made fenestrated stent. They are also less prohibitively expensive than their custom-made counterparts.

No randomized controlled trials exist to compare the use of open, fenestrated, or chimney techniques for complex aneurysm repairs. It is important to recognize the inherent bias in the published literature. Patient cohorts are likely not comparable based on pre-existing morbidity, complexity of anatomy, and urgency of procedure. A recent systematic review demonstrated a trend toward decreased perioperative mortality with f/b-EVAR compared to OAR, but this was accompanied by a trend toward higher mortality in longer-term follow-up. Neither difference reached statistical significance.[149] As with any technique, an early steep learning curve must be considered in the interpretation of these data. In addition, this technique was primarily reserved for high-risk patients who were not suitable candidates for open repair in the early years. Further study to evaluate outcomes is ongoing now that f/b-EVAR has become a standard practice in major aortic centers.

The perioperative mortality rate for Ch-EVAR has been demonstrated to be comparable to OAR (4% to 5%) but higher than for standard EVAR.[150] Both the medical complexity of the patient and surgical complexity of the aneurysm are likely to account for this difference. One concern for the Ch-EVAR approach is an increased risk of a type I endoleak (discussed below) due the coaxial deployment of the main and chimney stents. A review of the literature concluded that Ch-EVAR clearly produced more endoleaks than f/b-EVAR, although many of these were successfully treated intraoperatively with additional balloon dilation or disappeared during subsequent follow-up.[151] Ch-EVAR was also associated with an increased risk of ischemic stroke compared to either OAR or f/b-EVAR. The chimney technique requires vascular access from the brachial or axillary artery in order to appropriately align and deploy the chimney graft. This upper extremity approach, particularly in patients with atherosclerotic or difficult arch anatomy, increases the risk for iatrogenic stroke.[151] Ch-EVAR remains a valuable technique, particularly for complex patients with urgent need for surgical repair who cannot wait for the design of a customized fenestrated stent. The technical success and patency rates in the short- and intermediate-term are promising for both f/b-EVAR and Ch-EVAR, although long-term results have yet to be determined.

Anesthetic Management of Endovascular Aneurysm Repair

EVAR can be successfully performed under almost any type of anesthesia including local, regional, neuraxial, and general techniques. Concurrent use of antiplatelet agents or therapeutic anticoagulation may preclude the use of neuraxial or regional anesthetics. Patient factors, such as inability to lie flat for an extended period or an inability to effectively communicate, may sway the provider toward general anesthesia. Finally, surgical considerations such as the anticipated duration or difficulty of surgery must be considered. Many nonrandomized analyses address the question of local or regional versus general anesthesia for EVAR. A review of more than 5,500 patients in the NSQIP database demonstrated a decrease in pulmonary morbidity and a 10% to 20% decrease in hospital length of stay when local or regional anesthesia was used as compared to general anesthesia.[152] A review of the Vascular Quality Initiative suggested that patients undergoing EVAR for ruptured AAA may benefit from local anesthesia over general anesthesia with lower perioperative mortality rates, transfusion rates, pulmonary complications, and ICU length of stay.[153] A meta-analysis of the current literature suggests a decrease in operative time, hospital stay, and postoperative complications with local compared to general anesthesia, in spite of the fact that patients receiving local anesthesia tended to be older with an increased burden of cardiovascular or respiratory disease.[154] However, there are no randomized controlled trials to suggest the superiority of one technique over another.

The minimally invasive nature of EVAR means that hemodynamic changes should be relatively insignificant during the case; however, the possible need for urgent conversion to general anesthesia must always be considered if another anesthetic technique is primarily employed. The perioperative conversion rate from EVAR to OAR is less than 1% and may occur in the setting of difficult arterial access, vessel dissection, poor anatomic parameters, stent malposition or migration, or aneurysm rupture. Adequate resuscitative equipment such as cell saver and rapid infusion devices should be readily available. Two large-bore peripheral intravenous lines should be placed and adequate blood product availability should be ensured.

Most stents self-deploy without ballooning. If aortic ballooning is needed for stent deployment, which produces transient hemodynamic changes analogous to external cross-clamping, short periods of hypertension and increased afterload should be anticipated. These episodes typically do not require intervention due to their brevity. Blood loss should be minimal in experienced hands but complex endovascular repairs (i.e., f/b-EVAR or Ch-EVAR) can involve significant and insidious blood loss. In case of rupture, emergent proximal control is first obtained via endoscopic balloon occlusion which may then require open conversion. In this setting, proximal arterial access is indispensable due to the hemodynamic changes anticipated during OAR. Central venous access is not typically warranted for EVAR because hemodynamic changes are rare during routine surgery, vasoactive infusions are rarely warranted, and postoperative ICU stay is rare. Exceptions to this rule may include thoracic endovascular aneurysm repair (TEVAR) cases or complex abdominal repairs. Central venous access may be considered for TEVAR for the ability to rapidly place a pulmonary artery catheter should that case convert to an open TAAA, which would require cardiopulmonary bypass, or in case vasoactive infusions are required perioperatively to maintain spinal cord perfusion (as discussed in the chapter on Anesthesia for Cardiac Surgery). Central venous access may be considered for snorkel/chimney cases because each additional stent placed requires separate arterial sheaths. These cases can be longer, more complicated, and associated with greater blood loss. Thus, more aggressive resuscitation and/or vasoactive infusions may be necessary. Before device insertion, systemic anticoagulation with intravenous heparin will be requested with a goal activated clotting time (ACT) of 200 seconds or longer. At the time of device deployment, the patient will be asked to hold their breath (or, for anesthetized patients, a request will be made to hold ventilation) to allow for accurate stent deployment. At the same time, a request for temporary lowering of the mean arterial pressure may be made to minimize distal migration of the stent. After device deployment, a completion angiogram is performed to evaluate for technical success and any complications related to the procedure. Anticoagulation is then reversed, and the patient is typically extubated in the operating room.

Complications of Endovascular Aneurysm Repair

The unique complication profile related to endovascular repair mandates a lifetime of surveillance and a higher rate for reintervention as compared to OAR (29.6% vs. 18.1%).[139] Most reinterventions are graft-related complications including endoleaks, stent graft occlusion, migration, kinking, or infection. The majority of reinterventions tend to be catheter-based with limited morbidity and mortality. Nevertheless, each iterative intervention exposes the patient to the risks of radiation, iodinated contrast dye, and potentially the risks of anesthesia.

The most common indication for reintervention following EVAR is for endoleak. An endoleak is characterized by persistent blood flow into the aneurysm sac outside of the stent graft. The failure to exclude the aneurysm from the circulation may cause an increase in sac pressure over time, expansion, and potential rupture. Endoleaks complicate approximately 10% to 25% of EVAR cases[155,156] and require reintervention in upward of 12%.[156] Five types of endoleaks exist (Fig. 40-17). Types I and III involve direct communication with the systemic arterial circulation and thus mandate reintervention. Type I endoleaks are typically treated with repeat balloon molding or proximal or distal stent extension, whereas stent relining is the treatment for Type III endoleaks. The treatment of Type II endoleaks, caused by retrograde filling of the aneurysm sac by branch vessels, is controversial. Though retrograde flow can lead to aneurysm enlargement and increase in sac pressure, the majority of these aneurysms remain stable or decrease in size due to low flow and spontaneous thrombosis. If treatment is warranted, endovascular embolization of the feeding vessel is typically employed. Type IV endoleaks are related to graft porosity and are typically self-limited once the patient's coagulation status returns to baseline. Type V endoleak, also called "endotension," refers to an enlarging aneurysm sac without demonstrable endoleak. The etiology of endotension has not been completely elucidated. Although there may be a role for conservative management or endovascular reintervention, open conversion is the mainstay of management for endotension. Endoleak remains the single leading cause of late (more than 30-day) conversion to open repair, accounting for more than 60% of late reinterventions.[157] The incidence of late conversions has been reported to be as low as 2% but more recent evidence suggests a rate as high as 4%. This may be related to the increased number of endovascular repairs, and particularly complex endovascular repairs, performed. Late conversion to open repair is a technically challenging procedure with a relatively high mortality rate, particularly if performed emergently. Mortality rates for nonelective repair have been reported to be as high as 30%.[157]

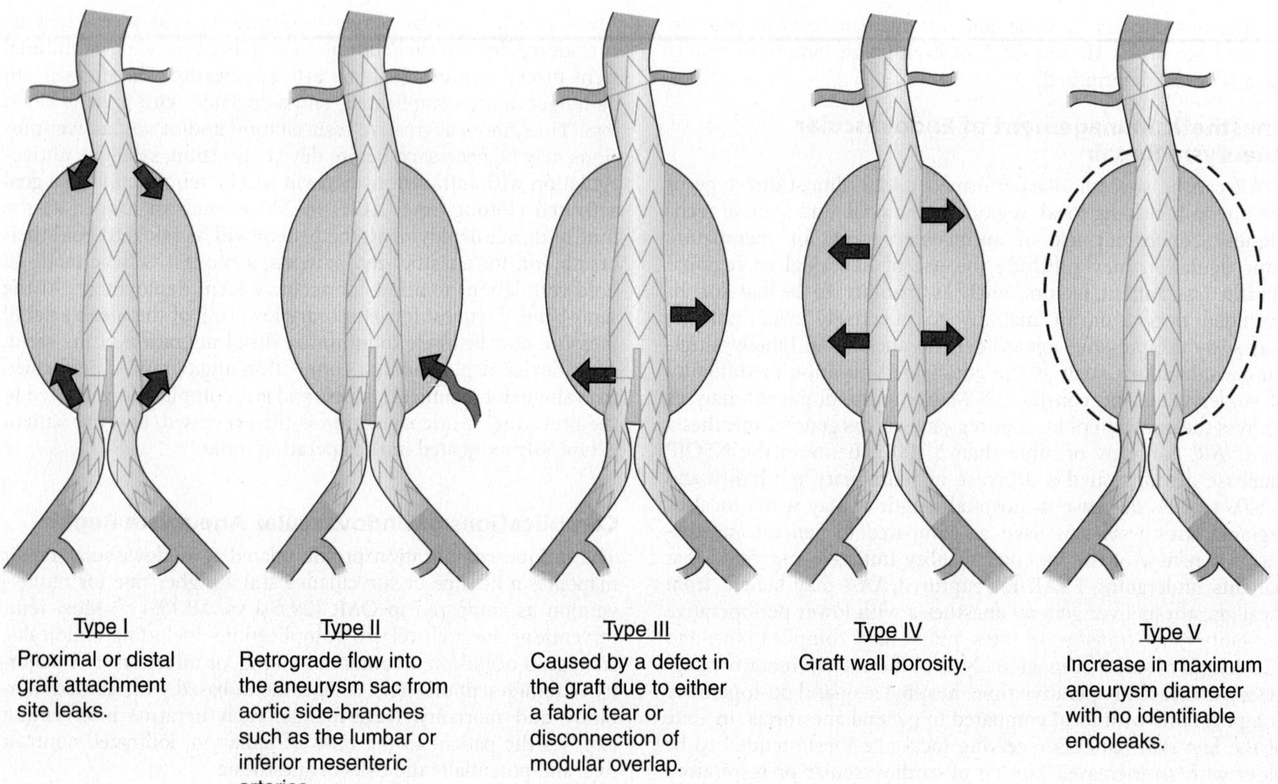

Figure 40-17 Types of endoleaks. Five types of endoleaks exist depending on the mechanism of persistent blood flow. Subsequent management depends on the type of endoleak present. The possibility of endoleak requires lifelong surveillance following EVAR, and endoleak remains the primary indication for late reintervention. (Reprinted with permission from England A, McWilliams R. Endovascular aortic aneurysm repair [EVAR]. *Ulster Med J.* 2013;82[1]:3–10.)

The pulsatile nature of blood flow results in an ongoing downward pressure on the stent graft and may result in stent migration. Over time, this may re-expose the aneurysm to systemic pressurization. Risk factors include aneurysm anatomy (e.g., hostile angulation of the aortic neck or short proximal landing zone) and graft properties (e.g., inadequate fixation and short overlaps). Aortic stent graft infection occurs in up to 1% of cases and may be a result of direct primary contamination or occur later from a secondary source. Clinical findings may be nonspecific such as fever, back pain, or leukocytosis. Initial treatment involves broad-spectrum antibiotics but may require explantation of the stent graft and open bypass. Stent graft kinking or infolding occurs in less than 5% of cases but may result in flow-restricting stenosis, graft thrombosis, and occlusion. Acute occlusion is frequently treated with catheter-directed thrombolysis or may be treated with mechanical thrombectomy if pharmacologic treatment is contraindicated.

Renal damage after EVAR is multifactorial. Preoperative renal insufficiency best predicts perioperative renal failure/dialysis need. Serial creatinine or GFR should be followed to ensure that the patient has sufficiently recovered from diagnostic angiography prior to surgery. The best way to limit renal damage is to limit contrast use. Gadolinium and CO_2 have been used. Better x-ray equipment and operator experience allows for lower contrast dosing. Preoperative fluid loading with 1 mL/kg/hr over 12 hours prior to surgery seems to be optimum management, but most patients present as outpatients. Thus, an initial fluid loading by the anesthesiologist seems prudent. Sodium bicarbonate infusions and *N*-acetyl cysteine infusions may play a small role in preventing renal damage.

Endovascular Management of Peripheral Artery Disease

The Inter-Society Consensus for the Management of PAD (TASC II) recommends endovascular revascularization for focal, discrete lesions and open surgical revascularization for severe disease.[7] Evidence suggests, however, that national trends in revascularization approach skew heavily toward endovascular repair even for more diffuse, complex disease. Endovascular interventions have increased more than threefold while open peripheral bypass surgery has decreased by more than 40% in recent years.[158] This trend is likely due, in large part, to continued improvement in the technology available for endovascular repair (e.g., stents, imaging techniques, and drug–device combinations). This paradigm shift is reflected in the most recent recommendations from the Society for Vascular Surgery practice guidelines, which endorse endovascular treatment as a reasonable first-line approach in most circumstances, even for complex disease.[123] In some cases, a hybrid approach to PAD may be employed. The development of hybrid operating rooms, with a full array of imaging equipment, allows for real-time decision making and completion of multiple procedures (both endovascular and open) under one anesthetic. Ultimately, the decision making must take into account disease severity and location, patient risk factors, and proceduralist skill.

Few randomized controlled trials exist to guide management decisions for the surgical management of PAD; the majority of the evidence is based on observational data. No large randomized controlled trials have compared OVER for complex AIOD. A systematic review of more than 5,300 patients undergoing OVER demonstrated greater perioperative morbidity and mortality but better long-term durability with open repair.[159] The Bypass versus Angioplasty in Severe Ischaemia of the Leg (BASIL) trial was a multicenter, randomized controlled trial that demonstrated that endovascular therapy resulted in less short-term morbidity and similar amputation-free survival for femoropopliteal disease.[160] For patients who survived at least 2 years, however, open revascularization was associated with increased overall survival and a trend toward amputation-free survival. The Best Endovascular versus Best Surgical Therapy in Patients with Critical Limb Ischemia (BEST-CLI) trial is a prospective, multicenter, randomized controlled trial designed to compare treatment efficacy, functional outcomes, cost-effectiveness, and quality of life for patients suffering from CLI that is currently ongoing.[161] Endovascular repair of infrapopliteal disease has traditionally been reserved for patients with CLI due to limited success and unacceptable rates of restenosis, dissection, and thrombosis early after the intervention. However, the advent of new technologies, particularly DESs, is changing the treatment paradigm for infrapopliteal disease. Several recent randomized controlled trials and meta-analyses support the use of DESs for symptomatic infrapopliteal disease that is anatomically suitable for intervention.[162]

Endovascular repair of PAD is typically performed under local anesthesia or monitored anesthesia care. Small doses of short-acting agents should be used to allow for patient cooperation throughout the procedure. The patient must be able to tolerate lying flat on the procedure table for several hours. Patients who are particularly anxious or who are unable to cooperate may require general anesthesia. Because the risk of blood loss is minimal and significant hemodynamic alterations are not anticipated intraoperatively, invasive hemodynamic monitoring is rarely indicated for these procedures. A single medium- to large-bore intravenous line is sufficient for vascular access.

Conclusion

Vascular surgery patients are generally elderly patients with significant cardiovascular disease in multiple vascular beds. They frequently have complex comorbid medical problems including CAD, COPD, diabetes mellitus, and renal insufficiency. A thorough preoperative evaluation for concurrent disease and pharmacologic optimization is paramount. The use of preoperative cardiac testing is controversial but current recommendations suggest it is reasonable to obtain preoperative cardiac testing for patients with poor or unknown exercise capacity if it will change perioperative management. Major morbidity in the perioperative setting is related to cardiovascular events; therefore, the heart should be the major focus of the anesthesiologist's attention. The skill of the anesthesiologist can greatly influence perioperative outcome. The field of vascular surgery is increasingly moving toward an endovascular focus, and open repair is increasingly reserved for more severe or surgically complex disease. Improvements in imaging technique, equipment, and proceduralist skill are pushing the frontiers of what can be accomplished via minimally invasive techniques, although the long-term outcomes of many recent advances remain to be seen. Endovascular surgery has its own unique complication profile that mandates a lifetime of postprocedural surveillance.

For further review and interactivities, please see the videos and narrative interactive clinical vignettes (NICVs) accessible in the complimentary eBook bundled with this text. Access instructions are located on the inside front cover.

REFERENCES

1. Laslett LJ, Alagona P, Clark BA, et al. The worldwide environment of cardiovascular disease: prevalence, diagnosis, therapy, and policy issues: a report from the American College of Cardiology. *J Am Coll Cardiol*. 2012;60(25 Suppl):S1–S49.
2. Smith SC, Collins A, Ferrari R, et al. Our time: a call to save preventable death from cardiovascular disease (heart disease and stroke). *Circulation*. 2012;126(23):2769–2775.
3. Tsao CW, Aday AW, Almarzooq ZI, et al. Heart Disease and Stroke Statistics-2022 Update: A Report From the American Heart Association. *Circulation*. 2022;145(8):e153–e639.
4. Anderson PL, Gelijns A, Moskowitz A, et al. Understanding trends in inpatient surgical volume: vascular interventions, 1980-2000. *J Vasc Surg*. 2004;39(6):1200–1208.
5. Libby P, Theroux P. Pathophysiology of coronary artery disease. *Circulation*. 2005;111(25):3481–3488.
6. Faraday N, Martinez EA, Scharpf RB, et al. Platelet gene polymorphisms and cardiac risk assessment in vascular surgical patients. *Anesthesiology*. 2004;101(6):1291–1297.
7. Norgren L, Hiatt WR, Dormandy JA, et al. Inter-Society Consensus for the Management of Peripheral Arterial Disease (TASC II). *J Vasc Surg*. 2007;45(Suppl S):S5–S67.
8. Grundy SM. Metabolic syndrome update. *Trends Cardiovasc Med*. 2016;26(4):364–373.
9. Goldberger ZD, Valle JA, Dandekar VK, Chan PS, Ko DT, Nallamothu BK. Are changes in carotid intima-media thickness related to risk of nonfatal myocardial infarction? A critical review and meta-regression analysis. *Am Heart J*. 2010;160(4):701–714.
10. Wyman RA, Mays ME, McBride PE, Stein JH. Ultrasound-detected carotid plaque as a predictor of cardiovascular events. *Vasc Med*. 2006;11(2):123–130.
11. Hertzer NR, Beven EG, Young JR, et al. Coronary artery disease in peripheral vascular patients. A classification of 1000 coronary angiograms and results of surgical management. *Ann Surg*. 1984;199(2):223–233.
12. Paul SD, Eagle KA, Kuntz KM, Young JR, Hertzer NR. Concordance of preoperative clinical risk with angiographic severity of coronary artery disease in patients undergoing vascular surgery. *Circulation*. 1996;94(7):1561–1566.
13. Wijeysundera DN, Duncan D, Nkonde-Price C, et al. Perioperative beta blockade in noncardiac surgery: a systematic review for the 2014 ACC/AHA guideline on perioperative cardiovascular evaluation and management of patients undergoing noncardiac surgery: a report of the American College of Cardiology/American Heart Association Task Force on Practice Guidelines. *Circulation*. 2014;130(24):2246–2264.
14. Devereaux PJ, Goldman L, Cook DJ, Gilbert K, Leslie K, Guyatt GH. Perioperative cardiac events in patients undergoing noncardiac surgery: a review of the magnitude of the problem, the pathophysiology of the events and methods to estimate and communicate risk. *CMAJ*. 2005;173(6):627–634.
15. Vascular Events In Noncardiac Surgery Patients Cohort Evaluation (VISION) Study Investigators, Devereaux PJ, Chan MTV, et al. Association between postoperative troponin levels and 30-day mortality among patients undergoing noncardiac surgery. *JAMA*. 2012;307(21):2295–2304.
16. Howard VJ, Meschia JF, Lal BK, et al. Carotid revascularization and medical management for asymptomatic carotid stenosis: Protocol of the CREST-2 clinical trials. *Int J Stroke*. 2017;12(7):770–778.
17. Mangano DT, Hollenberg M, Fegert G, et al. Perioperative myocardial ischemia in patients undergoing noncardiac surgery–I: Incidence and severity during the 4 day perioperative period. The Study of Perioperative Ischemia (SPI) Research Group. *J Am Coll Cardiol*. 1991;17(4):843–850.
18. Mangano DT, Layug EL, Wallace A, Tateo I. Effect of atenolol on mortality and cardiovascular morbidity after noncardiac surgery. Multicenter Study of Perioperative Ischemia Research Group. *N Engl J Med*. 1996;335(23):1713–1720.
19. Beattie WS, Wijeysundera DN, Karkouti K, McCluskey S, Tait G. Does tight heart rate control improve beta-blocker efficacy? An updated analysis of the noncardiac surgical randomized trials. *Anesth Analg*. 2008;106(4):1039–1048.
20. Yang H, Raymer K, Butler R, Parlow J, Roberts R. The effects of perioperative beta-blockade: results of the Metoprolol after Vascular Surgery (MaVS) study, a randomized controlled trial. *Am Heart J*. 2006;152(5):983–990.
21. Brady AR, Gibbs JSR, Greenhalgh RM, Powell JT, Sydes MR, POBBLE trial investigators. Perioperative beta-blockade (POBBLE) for patients undergoing infrarenal vascular surgery: results of a randomized double-blind controlled trial. *J Vasc Surg*. 2005;41(4):602–609.
22. POISE Study Group, Devereaux PJ, Yang H, et al. Effects of extended-release metoprolol succinate in patients undergoing non-cardiac surgery (POISE trial): a randomised controlled trial. *Lancet*. 2008;371(9627):1839–1847.
23. Fleisher LA, Fleischmann KE, Auerbach AD, et al. 2014 ACC/AHA guideline on perioperative cardiovascular evaluation and management of patients undergoing noncardiac surgery: executive summary: a report of the American College of Cardiology/American Heart Association Task Force on Practice Guidelines. *Circulation*. 2014;130(24):2215–2245.
24. Scali S, Patel V, Neal D, et al. Preoperative β-blockers do not improve cardiac outcomes after major elective vascular surgery and may be harmful. *J Vasc Surg*. 2015;62(1):166–176.e2.
25. Mostafaie K, Bedenis R, Harrington D. Beta-adrenergic blockers for perioperative cardiac risk reduction in people undergoing vascular surgery. *Cochrane Database Syst Rev*. 2015;1:CD006342.

26. Patorno E, Wang SV, Schneeweiss S, Liu J, Bateman BT. Patterns of β-blocker initiation in patients undergoing intermediate to high-risk noncardiac surgery. *Am Heart J*. 2015;170(4): 812–820.e6.
27. Wallace AW, Au S, Cason BA. Perioperative β-blockade: atenolol is associated with reduced mortality when compared to metoprolol. *Anesthesiology*. 2011;114(4):824–836.
28. Mashour GA, Sharifpour M, Freundlich RE, et al. Perioperative metoprolol and risk of stroke after noncardiac surgery. *Anesthesiology*. 2013;119(6):1340–1346.
29. Ellis JE, Drijvers G, Pedlow S, et al. Premedication with oral and transdermal clonidine provides safe and efficacious postoperative sympatholysis. *Anesth Analg*. 1994;79(6):1133–1140.
30. Wallace AW, Galindez D, Salahieh A, et al. Effect of clonidine on cardiovascular morbidity and mortality after noncardiac surgery. *Anesthesiology*. 2004;101(2):284–293.
31. Devereaux PJ, Sessler DI, Leslie K, et al. Clonidine in patients undergoing noncardiac surgery. *N Engl J Med*. 2014;370(16):1504–1513.
32. Husain K, Hernandez W, Ansari RA, Ferder L. Inflammation, oxidative stress and renin angiotensin system in atherosclerosis. *World J Biol Chem*. 2015;6(3):209–217.
33. Sayer G, Bhat G. The renin-angiotensin-aldosterone system and heart failure. *Cardiol Clin*. 2014;32(1):21–32.
34. Lazar HL. The use of angiotensin-converting enzyme inhibitors in patients undergoing coronary artery bypass graft surgery. *Vascul Pharmacol*. 2005;42(3):119–123.
35. Benedetto U, Sciarretta S, Roscitano A, et al. Preoperative angiotensin-converting enzyme inhibitors and acute kidney injury after coronary artery bypass grafting. *Ann Thorac Surg*. 2008;86(4):1160–1165.
36. Miceli A, Capoun R, Fino C, et al. Effects of angiotensin-converting enzyme inhibitor therapy on clinical outcome in patients undergoing coronary artery bypass grafting. *J Am Coll Cardiol*. 2009;54(19):1778–1784.
37. Railton CJ, Wolpin J, Lam-McCulloch J, Belo SE. Renin-angiotensin blockade is associated with increased mortality after vascular surgery. *Can J Anaesth*. 2010;57(8):736–744.
38. Le Manach Y, Coriat P, Collard CD, Riedel B. Statin therapy within the perioperative period. *Anesthesiology*. 2008;108(6):1141–1146.
39. Schouten O, Boersma E, Hoeks SE, et al. Fluvastatin and perioperative events in patients undergoing vascular surgery. *N Engl J Med*. 2009;361(10):980–989.
40. Le Manach Y, Godet G, Coriat P, et al. The impact of postoperative discontinuation or continuation of chronic statin therapy on cardiac outcome after major vascular surgery. *Anesth Analg*. 2007;104(6):1326–1333.
41. Berwanger O, Le Manach Y, Suzumura EA, et al. Association between pre-operative statin use and major cardiovascular complications among patients undergoing non-cardiac surgery: the VISION study. *Eur Heart J*. 2016;37(2):177–185.
42. Heeschen C, Hamm CW, Laufs U, et al. Withdrawal of statins increases event rates in patients with acute coronary syndromes. *Circulation*. 2002;105(12):1446–1452.
43. Sanders RD, Nicholson A, Lewis SR, Smith AF, Alderson P. Perioperative statin therapy for improving outcomes during and after noncardiac vascular surgery. *Cochrane Database Syst Rev*. 2013;(7):CD009971.
44. Antoniou GA, Hajibandeh S, Hajibandeh S, Vallabhaneni SR, Brennan JA, Torella F. Meta-analysis of the effects of statins on perioperative outcomes in vascular and endovascular surgery. *J Vasc Surg*. 2015;61(2):519–532.e1.
45. Gerstein NS, Schulman PM, Gerstein WH, Petersen TR, Tawil I. Should more patients continue aspirin therapy perioperatively?: clinical impact of aspirin withdrawal syndrome. *Ann Surg*. 2012;255(5):811–819.
46. Smith SC, Benjamin EJ, Bonow RO, et al. AHA/ACCF Secondary Prevention and Risk Reduction Therapy for Patients with Coronary and other Atherosclerotic Vascular Disease: 2011 update: a guideline from the American Heart Association and American College of Cardiology Foundation. *Circulation*. 2011;124(22):2458–2473.
47. Batchelder A, Hunter J, Cairns V, Sandford R, Munshi A, Naylor AR. Dual antiplatelet therapy prior to expedited carotid surgery reduces recurrent events prior to surgery without significantly increasing peri-operative bleeding complications. *Eur J Vasc Endovasc Surg*. 2015;50(4):412–419.
48. De Martino RR, Beck AW, Hoel AW, et al. Preoperative antiplatelet and statin treatment was not associated with reduced myocardial infarction after high-risk vascular operations in the Vascular Quality Initiative. *J Vasc Surg*. 2016;63(1):182–189.e2.
49. Devereaux PJ, Mrkobrada M, Sessler DI, et al. Aspirin in patients undergoing noncardiac surgery. *N Engl J Med*. 2014;370(16):1494–1503.
50. Stone DH, Goodney PP, Schanzer A, et al. Clopidogrel is not associated with major bleeding complications during peripheral arterial surgery. *J Vasc Surg*. 2011;54(3):779–784.
51. Smit M, Coetzee AR, Lochner A. The pathophysiology of myocardial ischemia and perioperative myocardial infarction. *J Cardiothorac Vasc Anesth*. 2020;34(9):2501–2512.
52. Thiruvenkatarajan V, Meyer EJ, Nanjappa N, Van Wijk RM, Jesudason D. Perioperative diabetic ketoacidosis associated with sodium-glucose co-transporter-2 inhibitors: a systematic review. *Br J Anaesth*. 2019;123(1):27–36.
53. van den Berghe G, Wouters P, Weekers F, et al. Intensive insulin therapy in critically ill patients. *N Engl J Med*. 2001;345(19):1359–1367.
54. NICE-SUGAR Study Investigators, Finfer S, Chittock DR, et al. Intensive versus conventional glucose control in critically ill patients. *N Engl J Med*. 2009;360(13):1283–1297.
55. Griesdale DEG, de Souza RJ, van Dam RM, et al. Intensive insulin therapy and mortality among critically ill patients: a meta-analysis including NICE-SUGAR study data. *CMAJ*. 2009;180(8):821–827.
56. Jiang J, Li S, Zhao Y, et al. Intensive glucose control during the perioperative period for diabetic patients undergoing surgery: An updated systematic review and meta-analysis. *J Clin Anesth*. 2021;75:110504.
57. Nelson AH, Fleisher LA, Rosenbaum SH. Relationship between postoperative anemia and cardiac morbidity in high-risk vascular patients in the intensive care unit. *Crit Care Med*. 1993; 21(6):860–866.
58. Hébert PC, Wells G, Blajchman MA, et al. A multicenter, randomized, controlled clinical trial of transfusion requirements in critical care. Transfusion Requirements in Critical Care Investigators, Canadian Critical Care Trials Group. *N Engl J Med*. 1999;340(6):409–417.
59. Carson JL, Terrin ML, Noveck H, et al. Liberal or restrictive transfusion in high-risk patients after hip surgery. *N Engl J Med*. 2011;365(26):2453–2462.
60. Obi AT, Park YJ, Bove P, et al. The association of perioperative transfusion with 30-day morbidity and mortality in patients undergoing major vascular surgery. *J Vasc Surg*. 2015;61(4): 1000–1009.e1.
61. Kougias P, Sharath S, Mi Z, Biswas K, Mills JL. Effect of postoperative permissive anemia and cardiovascular risk status on outcomes after major general and vascular surgery operative interventions. *Ann Surg*. 2019;270(4):602–611.
62. Foster ED, Davis KB, Carpenter JA, Abele S, Fray D. Risk of noncardiac operation in patients with defined coronary disease: The Coronary Artery Surgery Study (CASS) registry experience. *Ann Thorac Surg*. 1986;41(1):42–50.
63. Eagle KA, Rihal CS, Mickel MC, Holmes DR, Foster ED, Gersh BJ. Cardiac risk of noncardiac surgery: influence of coronary disease and type of surgery in 3368 operations. CASS Investigators and University of Michigan Heart Care Program. Coronary Artery Surgery Study. *Circulation*. 1997;96(6):1882–1887.
64. Monaco M, Stassano P, Di Tommaso L, et al. Systematic strategy of prophylactic coronary angiography improves long-term outcome after major vascular surgery in medium- to high-risk patients: a prospective, randomized study. *J Am Coll Cardiol*. 2009;54(11):989–996.
65. McFalls EO, Ward HB, Moritz TE, et al. Coronary-artery revascularization before elective major vascular surgery. *N Engl J Med*. 2004;351(27):2795–2804.
66. Ward HB, Kelly RF, Thottapurathu L, et al. Coronary artery bypass grafting is superior to percutaneous coronary intervention in prevention of perioperative myocardial infarctions during subsequent vascular surgery. *Ann Thorac Surg*. 2006;82(3):795–800; discussion 800–801.
67. Garcia S, Moritz TE, Goldman S, et al. Perioperative complications after vascular surgery are predicted by the revised cardiac risk index but are not reduced in high-risk subsets with preoperative revascularization. *Circ Cardiovasc Qual Outcomes*. 2009;2(2):73–77.
68. Lawton JS, Tamis-Holland JE, Bangalore S, et al. 2021 ACC/AHA/SCAI Guideline for Coronary Artery Revascularization: A Report of the American College of Cardiology/American Heart Association Joint Committee on Clinical Practice Guidelines. *Circulation*. 2022;145(3):e18–e114.
69. Livhits M, Gibbons MM, de Virgilio C, et al. Coronary revascularization after myocardial infarction can reduce risks of noncardiac surgery. *J Am Coll Surg*. 2011;212(6):1018–1026.
70. Levine GN, Bates ER, Bittl JA, et al. 2016 ACC/AHA Guideline Focused Update on Duration of Dual Antiplatelet Therapy in Patients With Coronary Artery Disease: A Report of the American College of Cardiology/American Heart Association Task Force on Clinical Practice Guidelines: An Update of the 2011 ACCF/AHA/SCAI Guideline for Percutaneous Coronary Intervention, 2011 ACCF/AHA Guideline for Coronary Artery Bypass Graft Surgery, 2012 ACC/AHA/ACP/AATS/PCNA/SCAI/STS Guideline for the Diagnosis and Management of Patients With Stable Ischemic Heart Disease, 2013 ACCF/AHA Guideline for the Management of ST-Elevation Myocardial Infarction, 2014 AHA/ACC Guideline for the Management of Patients With Non-ST-Elevation Acute Coronary Syndromes, and 2014 ACC/AHA Guideline on Perioperative Cardiovascular Evaluation and Management of Patients Undergoing Noncardiac Surgery. *Circulation*. 2016;134(10):e123–e155.
71. Zarinsefat A, Henke P. Update in preoperative risk assessment in vascular surgery patients. *J Vasc Surg*. 2015;62(2):499–509.
72. Simons JP, Baril DT, Goodney PP, et al. The effect of postoperative myocardial ischemia on long-term survival after vascular surgery. *J Vasc Surg*. 2013;58(6):1600–1608.
73. Bilimoria KY, Liu Y, Paruch JL, et al. Development and evaluation of the universal ACS NSQIP surgical risk calculator: a decision aid and informed consent tool for patients and surgeons. *J Am Coll Surg*. 2013;217(5):833–842.e1-3.
74. Ford MK, Beattie WS, Wijeysundera DN. Systematic review: prediction of perioperative cardiac complications and mortality by the revised cardiac risk index. *Ann Intern Med*. 2010; 152(1): 26–35.
75. Bertges DJ, Goodney PP, Zhao Y, et al. The Vascular Study Group of New England Cardiac Risk Index (VSG-CRI) predicts cardiac complications more accurately than the Revised Cardiac Risk Index in vascular surgery patients. *J Vasc Surg*. 2010;52(3):674–683, 683.e1–683.e3.
76. Easton JD, Saver JL, Albers GW, et al. Definition and evaluation of transient ischemic attack: a scientific statement for healthcare professionals from the American Heart Association/American Stroke Association Stroke Council; Council on Cardiovascular Surgery and Anesthesia; Council on Cardiovascular Radiology and Intervention; Council on Cardiovascular Nursing; and the Interdisciplinary Council on Peripheral Vascular Disease. The American

Academy of Neurology affirms the value of this statement as an educational tool for neurologists. *Stroke*. 2009;40(6):2276–2293.

77. Barnett HJ, Taylor DW, Eliasziw M, et al. Benefit of carotid endarterectomy in patients with symptomatic moderate or severe stenosis. North American Symptomatic Carotid Endarterectomy Trial Collaborators. *N Engl J Med*. 1998;339(20):1415–1425.
78. Randomised trial of endarterectomy for recently symptomatic carotid stenosis: final results of the MRC European Carotid Surgery Trial (ECST). *Lancet*. 1998;351(9113):1379–1387.
79. Hobson RW, Weiss DG, Fields WS, et al. Efficacy of carotid endarterectomy for asymptomatic carotid stenosis. The Veterans Affairs Cooperative Study Group. *N Engl J Med*. 1993;328(4):221–227.
80. Rerkasem A, Orrapin S, Howard DP, Rerkasem K. Carotid endarterectomy for symptomatic carotid stenosis. *Cochrane Database Syst Rev*. 2020;9:CD001081.
81. Endarterectomy for asymptomatic carotid artery stenosis. Executive Committee for the Asymptomatic Carotid Atherosclerosis Study. *JAMA*. 1995;273(18):1421–1428.
82. Halliday A, Mansfield A, Marro J, et al. Prevention of disabling and fatal strokes by successful carotid endarterectomy in patients without recent neurological symptoms: randomised controlled trial. *Lancet*. 2004;363(9420):1491–1502.
83. Chambers BR, Donnan GA. Carotid endarterectomy for asymptomatic carotid stenosis. *Cochrane Database Syst Rev*. 2005;(4):CD001923.
84. Rothwell PM, Eliasziw M, Gutnikov SA, Warlow CP, Barnett HJ, Carotid Endarterectomy Trialists Collaboration. Endarterectomy for symptomatic carotid stenosis in relation to clinical subgroups and timing of surgery. *Lancet*. 2004;363(9413):915–924.
85. Johnston SC, Gress DR, Browner WS, Sidney S. Short-term prognosis after emergency department diagnosis of TIA. *JAMA*. 2000;284(22):2901–2906.
86. Kleindorfer DO, Towfighi A, Chaturvedi S, et al. 2021 Guideline for the Prevention of Stroke in Patients With Stroke and Transient Ischemic Attack: A Guideline From the American Heart Association/American Stroke Association. *Stroke*. 2021;52(7):e364–e467.
87. Chimowitz MI, Poole RM, Starling MR, Schwaiger M, Gross MD. Frequency and severity of asymptomatic coronary disease in patients with different causes of stroke. *Stroke*. 1997;28(5):941–945.
88. Iqbal S. A comprehensive study of the anatomical variations of the circle of Willis in adult human brains. *J Clin Diagn Res*. 2013;7(11):2423–2427.
89. Aburahma AF, Mousa AY, Stone PA. Shunting during carotid endarterectomy. *J Vasc Surg*. 2011;54(5):1502–1510.
90. Chongruksut W, Vaniyapong T, Rerkasem K. Routine or selective carotid artery shunting for carotid endarterectomy (and different methods of monitoring in selective shunting). *Cochrane Database Syst Rev*. 2014;(6):CD000190.
91. Guarracino F. Cerebral monitoring during cardiovascular surgery. *Curr Opin Anaesthesiol*. 2008;21(1):50–54.
92. Hans SS, Jareunpoon O. Prospective evaluation of electroencephalography, carotid artery stump pressure, and neurologic changes during 314 consecutive carotid endarterectomies performed in awake patients. *J Vasc Surg*. 2007;45(3):511–515.
93. Moritz S, Kasprzak P, Arlt M, Taeger K, Metz C. Accuracy of cerebral monitoring in detecting cerebral ischemia during carotid endarterectomy: a comparison of transcranial Doppler sonography, near-infrared spectroscopy, stump pressure, and somatosensory evoked potentials. *Anesthesiology*. 2007;107(4):563–569.
94. Malcharek MJ, Ulkatan S, Marinò V, et al. Intraoperative monitoring of carotid endarterectomy by transcranial motor evoked potential: a multicenter study of 600 patients. *Clin Neurophysiol*. 2013;124(5):1025–1030.
95. Costin M, Rampersad A, Solomon RA, Connolly ES, Heyer EJ. Cerebral injury predicted by transcranial Doppler ultrasonography but not electroencephalography during carotid endarterectomy. *J Neurosurg Anesthesiol*. 2002;14(4):287–292.
96. Calligaro KD, Dougherty MJ. Correlation of carotid artery stump pressure and neurologic changes during 474 carotid endarterectomies performed in awake patients. *J Vasc Surg*. 2005;42(4):684–689.
97. Ritter JC, Green D, Slim H, Tiwari A, Brown J, Rashid H. The role of cerebral oximetry in combination with awake testing in patients undergoing carotid endarterectomy under local anaesthesia. *Eur J Vasc Endovasc Surg*. 2011;41(5):599–605.
98. Stilo F, Spinelli F, Martelli E, et al. The sensibility and specificity of cerebral oximetry, measured by INVOS - 4100, in patients undergoing carotid endarterectomy compared with awake testing. *Minerva Anestesiol*. 2012;78(10):1126–1135.
99. Pandit JJ, Satya-Krishna R, Gration P. Superficial or deep cervical plexus block for carotid endarterectomy: a systematic review of complications. *Br J Anaesth*. 2007;99(2):159–169.
100. GALA Trial Collaborative Group, Lewis SC, Warlow CP, et al. General anaesthesia versus local anaesthesia for carotid surgery (GALA): a multicentre, randomised controlled trial. *Lancet*. 2008;372(9656):2132–2142.
101. Rerkasem A, Orrapin S, Howard DP, Nantakool S, Rerkasem K. Local versus general anaesthesia for carotid endarterectomy. *Cochrane Database Syst Rev*. 2021;10:CD000126.
102. Jellish WS, Sheikh T, Baker WH, Louie EK, Slogoff S. Hemodynamic stability, myocardial ischemia, and perioperative outcome after carotid surgery with remifentanil/propofol or isoflurane/fentanyl anesthesia. *J Neurosurg Anesthesiol*. 2003;15(3):176–184.
103. Mutch WA, White IW, Donen N, et al. Haemodynamic instability and myocardial ischaemia during carotid endarterectomy: a comparison of propofol and isoflurane. *Can J Anaesth*. 1995;42(7):577–587.
104. Umbrain V, Keeris J, D'Haese J, et al. Isoflurane, desflurane and sevoflurane for carotid endarterectomy. *Anaesthesia*. 2000;55(11):1052–1057.
105. Naylor AR, Sayers RD, McCarthy MJ, et al. Closing the loop: a 21-year audit of strategies for preventing stroke and death following carotid endarterectomy. *Eur J Vasc Endovasc Surg*. 2013;46(2):161–170.
106. van Mook WNKA, Rennenberg RJMW, Schurink GW, et al. Cerebral hyperperfusion syndrome. *Lancet Neurol*. 2005;4(12):877–888.
107. Boulanger M, Cameliere L, Felgueiras R, et al. Periprocedural myocardial infarction after carotid endarterectomy and stenting: systematic review and meta-analysis. *Stroke*. 2015;46(10):2843–2848.
108. Chaikof EL, Dalman RL, Eskandari MK, et al. The Society for Vascular Surgery practice guidelines on the care of patients with an abdominal aortic aneurysm. *J Vasc Surg*. 2018;67(1):2–77.e2.
109. Guirguis EM, Barber GG. The natural history of abdominal aortic aneurysms. *Am J Surg*. 1991;162(5):481–483.
110. Kent KC. Clinical practice. Abdominal aortic aneurysms. *N Engl J Med*. 2014;371(22):2101–2108.
111. Trimarchi S, Tsai T, Eagle KA, et al. Acute abdominal aortic dissection: insight from the International Registry of Acute Aortic Dissection (IRAD). *J Vasc Surg*. 2007;46(5):913–919.
112. Gelman S. The pathophysiology of aortic cross-clamping and unclamping. *Anesthesiology*. 1995;82(4):1026–1060.
113. Roizen MF, Beaupre PN, Alpert RA, et al. Monitoring with two-dimensional transesophageal echocardiography. Comparison of myocardial function in patients undergoing supraceliac, suprarenal-infraceliac, or infrarenal aortic occlusion. *J Vasc Surg*. 1984;1(2):300–305.
114. Sheinbaum R, Ignacio C, Safi HJ, Estrera A. Contemporary strategies to preserve renal function during cardiac and vascular surgery. *Rev Cardiovasc Med*. 2003;4(Suppl 1):S21–S28.
115. Wahlberg E, Dimuzio PJ, Stoney RJ. Aortic clamping during elective operations for infrarenal disease: the influence of clamping time on renal function. *J Vasc Surg*. 2002;36(1):13–18.
116. Bove T, Zangrillo A, Guarracino F, et al. Effect of fenoldopam on use of renal replacement therapy among patients with acute kidney injury after cardiac surgery: a randomized clinical trial. *JAMA*. 2014;312(21):2244–2253.
117. Ali ZA, Callaghan CJ, Lim E, et al. Remote ischemic preconditioning reduces myocardial and renal injury after elective abdominal aortic aneurysm repair: a randomized controlled trial. *Circulation*. 2007;116(11 Suppl):I98–105.
118. Haunschild J, VON Aspern K, Misfeld M, Davierwala P, Borger MA, Etz CD. Spinal cord protection in thoracoabdominal aortic aneurysm surgery: a multimodal approach. *J Cardiovasc Surg (Torino)*. 2021;62(4):316–325.
119. Horlocker TT, Vandermeulen E, Kopp SL, Gogarten W, Leffert LR, Benzon HT. Regional anesthesia in the patient receiving antithrombotic or thrombolytic therapy: American Society of Regional Anesthesia and Pain Medicine Evidence-Based Guidelines (Fourth Edition). *Reg Anesth Pain Med*. 2018;43(3):263–309.
120. Sandham JD, Hull RD, Brant RF, et al. A randomized, controlled trial of the use of pulmonary-artery catheters in high-risk surgical patients. *N Engl J Med*. 2003;348(1):5–14.
121. Heringlake M, Sedemund-Adib B, Grossherr M, Heinze H, Klaus S. The use of a pulmonary artery catheter does not increase mortality in critical cancer care and can reduce the mortality of high-risk surgical patients. *Anaesthesist*. 2007;56(3):275–276; author reply 276, 278–280.
122. Tanaka K, Ludwig LM, Kersten JR, Pagel PS, Warltier DC. Mechanisms of cardioprotection by volatile anesthetics. *Anesthesiology*. 2004;100(3):707–721.
123. Society for Vascular Surgery Lower Extremity Guidelines Writing Group, Conte MS, Pomposelli FB, et al. Society for Vascular Surgery practice guidelines for atherosclerotic occlusive disease of the lower extremities: management of asymptomatic disease and claudication. *J Vasc Surg*. 2015;61(3 Suppl):2S–41S.
124. Singh N, Sidawy AN, Dezee K, et al. The effects of the type of anesthesia on outcomes of lower extremity infrainguinal bypass. *J Vasc Surg*. 2006;44(5):964–968; discussion 968–970.
125. Ghanami RJ, Hurie J, Andrews JS, et al. Anesthesia-based evaluation of outcomes of lower-extremity vascular bypass procedures. *Ann Vasc Surg*. 2013;27(2):199–207.
126. Barbosa FT, Jucá MJ, Castro AA, Cavalcante JC. Neuraxial anaesthesia for lower-limb revascularization. *Cochrane Database Syst Rev*. 2013;(7):CD007083.
127. LaMuraglia GM, Conrad MF, Chung T, Hutter M, Watkins MT, Cambria RP. Significant perioperative morbidity accompanies contemporary infrainguinal bypass surgery: an NSQIP report. *J Vasc Surg*. 2009;50(2):299–304, 304.e1–4.
128. Mas JL, Trinquart L, Leys D, et al. Endarterectomy versus angioplasty in patients with symptomatic severe carotid stenosis (EVA-3S) trial: results up to 4 years from a randomised, multicentre trial. *Lancet Neurol*. 2008;7(10):885–892.
129. Gurm HS, Yadav JS, Fayad P, et al. Long-term results of carotid stenting versus endarterectomy in high-risk patients. *N Engl J Med*. 2008;358(15):1572–1579.
130. Eckstein HH, Ringleb P, Allenberg JR, et al. Results of the Stent-Protected Angioplasty versus Carotid Endarterectomy (SPACE) study to treat symptomatic stenoses at 2 years: a multinational, prospective, randomised trial. *Lancet Neurol*. 2008;7(10):893–902.

131. Bonati LH, Dobson J, Featherstone RL, et al. Long-term outcomes after stenting versus endarterectomy for treatment of symptomatic carotid stenosis: the International Carotid Stenting Study (ICSS) randomised trial. *Lancet*. 2015;385(9967):529–538.
132. Brott TG, Hobson RW, Howard G, et al. Stenting versus endarterectomy for treatment of carotid-artery stenosis. *J Engl J Med*. 2010;363(1):11–23.
133. Müller MD, Lyrer P, Brown MM, Bonati LH. Carotid artery stenting versus endarterectomy for treatment of carotid artery stenosis. *Cochrane Database Syst Rev*. 2020;2:CD000515.
134. Halliday A, Bulbulia R, Bonati LH, et al. Second asymptomatic carotid surgery trial (ACST-2): a randomised comparison of carotid artery stenting versus carotid endarterectomy. *Lancet*. 2021;398(10305):1065–1073.
135. Kwolek CJ, Jaff MR, Leal JI, et al. Results of the ROADSTER multicenter trial of transcarotid stenting with dynamic flow reversal. *J Vasc Surg*. 2015;62(5):1227–1234.
136. Kashyap VS, Schneider PA, Foteh M, et al. Early outcomes in the ROADSTER 2 study of transcarotid srtery revascularization in patients with significant carotid artery disease. *Stroke*. 2020;51(9):2620–2629.
137. Schermerhorn ML, Liang P, Eldrup-Jorgensen J, et al. Association of transcarotid artery revascularization vs transfemoral carotid artery stenting with stroke or death among patients with carotid artery stenosis. *JAMA*. 2019;322(23):2313–2322.
138. Dua A, Kuy S, Lee CJ, Upchurch GR Jr, Desai SS. Epidemiology of aortic aneurysm repair in the United States from 2000 to 2010. *J Vasc Surg*. 2014;59(6):1512–1517.
139. De Bruin JL, Baas AF, Buth J, et al. Long-term outcome of open or endovascular repair of abdominal aortic aneurysm. *N Engl J Med*. 2010;362(20):1881–1889.
140. United Kingdom EVAR Trial Investigators, Greenhalgh RM, Brown LC, et al. Endovascular versus open repair of abdominal aortic aneurysm. *N Engl J Med*. 2010;362(20):1863–1871.
141. Becquemin JP, Pillet JC, Lescalie F, et al. A randomized controlled trial of endovascular aneurysm repair versus open surgery for abdominal aortic aneurysms in low- to moderate-risk patients. *J Vasc Surg*. 2011;53(5):1167–1173.e1.
142. Lederle FA, Freischlag JA, Kyriakides TC, et al. Long-term comparison of endovascular and open repair of abdominal aortic aneurysm. *N Engl J Med*. 2012;367(21):1988–1997.
143. Paravastu SCV, Jayarajasingam R, Cottam R, Palfreyman SJ, Michaels JA, Thomas SM. Endovascular repair of abdominal aortic aneurysm. *Cochrane Database Syst Rev*. 2014;(1): CD004178.
144. Siracuse JJ, Gill HL, Graham AR, et al. Comparative safety of endovascular and open surgical repair of abdominal aortic aneurysms in low-risk male patients. *J Vasc Surg*. 2014;60(5): 1154–1158.
145. Sweeting MJ, Patel R, Powell JT, Greenhalgh RM, EVAR Trial Investigators. Endovascular repair of abdominal aortic aneurysm in patients physically ineligible for open repair: very long-term follow-up in the EVAR-2 randomized controlled trial. *Ann Surg*. 2017;266(5):713–719.
146. Egorova N, Giacovelli JK, Gelijns A, et al. Defining high-risk patients for endovascular aneurysm repair. *J Vasc Surg*. 2009;50(6):1271–1279.e1.
147. Cowled P, Boult M, Barnes M, Fitridge RA. Update of a model to predict outcomes after endovascular aneurysm repair. *Ann Vasc Surg*. 2021;75:430–444.
148. Parodi JC, Palmaz JC, Barone HD. Transfemoral intraluminal graft implantation for abdominal aortic aneurysms. *Ann Vasc Surg*. 1991;5(6):491–499.
149. Antoniou GA, Juszczak MT, Antoniou SA, Katsargyris A, Haulon S. Editor's choice—Fenestrated or branched endovascular versus open repair for complex aortic aneurysms: meta-analysis of time to event propensity score matched data. *Eur J Vasc Endovasc Surg*. 2021;61(2): 228–237.
150. Wilson A, Zhou S, Bachoo P, Tambyraja AL. Systematic review of chimney and periscope grafts for endovascular aneurysm repair. *Br J Surg*. 2013;100(12):1557–1564.
151. Katsargyris A, Oikonomou K, Klonaris C, Töpel I, Verhoeven EL. Comparison of outcomes with open, fenestrated, and chimney graft repair of juxtarenal aneurysms: are we ready for a paradigm shift? *J Endovasc Ther*. 2013;20(2):159–169.
152. Edwards MS, Andrews JS, Edwards AF, et al. Results of endovascular aortic aneurysm repair with general, regional, and local/monitored anesthesia care in the American College of Surgeons National Surgical Quality Improvement Program database. *J Vasc Surg*. 2011;54(5): 1273–1282.
153. Faizer R, Weinhandl E, El Hag S, et al. Decreased mortality with local versus general anesthesia in endovascular aneurysm repair for ruptured abdominal aortic aneurysm in the Vascular Quality Initiative database. *J Vasc Surg*. 2019;70(1):92–101.e1.
154. Deng J, Liu J, Rong D, et al. A meta-analysis of locoregional anesthesia versus general anesthesia in endovascular repair of ruptured abdominal aortic aneurysm. *J Vasc Surg*. 2021;73(2): 700–710.
155. Chen J, Stavropolous SW. Management of Endoleaks. *Semin Intervent Radiol*. 2015;32(3): 259–264.
156. Ilyas S, Shaida N, Thakor AS, Winterbottom A, Cousins C. Endovascular aneurysm repair (EVAR) follow-up imaging: the assessment and treatment of common postoperative complications. *Clin Radiol*. 2015;70(2):183–196.
157. Kouvelos G, Koutsoumpelis A, Lazaris A, et al. Late open conversion after endovascular abdominal aortic aneurysm repair. *J Vasc Surg*. 2015;61(5):1350–1356.
158. Goodney PP, Beck AW, Nagle J, Welch HG, Zwolak RM. National trends in lower extremity bypass surgery, endovascular interventions, and major amputations. *J Vasc Surg*. 2009;50(1): 54–60.
159. Indes JE, Pfaff MJ, Farrokhyar F, et al. Clinical outcomes of 5358 patients undergoing direct open bypass or endovascular treatment for aortoiliac occlusive disease: a systematic review and meta-analysis. *J Endovasc Ther*. 2013;20(4):443–455.
160. Adam DJ, Beard JD, Cleveland T, et al. Bypass versus angioplasty in severe ischaemia of the leg (BASIL): multicentre, randomised controlled trial. *Lancet*. 2005;366(9501): 1925–1934.
161. Farber A, Rosenfield K, Siami FS, Strong M, Menard M. The BEST-CLI trial is nearing the finish line and promises to be worth the wait. *J Vasc Surg*. 2019;69(2):470–481.e2.
162. Antoniou GA, Chalmers N, Kanesalingham K, et al. Meta-analysis of outcomes of endovascular treatment of infrapopliteal occlusive disease with drug-eluting stents. *J Endovasc Ther*. 2013;20(2):131–144.

41 Obstetric Anesthesia

HOLLY B. ENDE • FEYCE M. PERALTA • CYNTHIA A. WONG

KEY POINTS

1. Airway edema may be particularly severe in women with preeclampsia, in those who have pushed during the second stage of labor, or with concurrent use of tocolytic agents.
2. As oxygen consumption increases during pregnancy, the maternal cardiovascular system adapts to meet the metabolic demands of a growing fetus.
3. The driving force for placental drug transfer is the concentration gradient of free drug between maternal and fetal blood.
4. Labor analgesia may benefit mother and fetus and should not be withheld if requested.
5. Benefits of neuraxial anesthesia for cesarean delivery include avoiding airway manipulation, decreasing aspiration risk, minimizing fetal anesthetic exposure, and allowing the mother to remain awake during childbirth.
6. A rapid-sequence induction of anesthesia, application of cricoid pressure, and intubation with a cuffed tracheal tube are usually performed for pregnant women receiving general anesthesia after 20 weeks of gestation.
7. Pregnant women are at a higher risk for developing postdural puncture headache due to their age and sex.
8. Pregnancy and parturition are considered "high risk" when accompanied by conditions unfavorable to the well-being of the mother, fetus, or both.
9. Preeclampsia includes a spectrum of end-organ manifestations of the disease—severe hypertension or other end-organ disease is termed preeclampsia with severe features.
10. Hemorrhage is the leading cause of maternal mortality worldwide.
11. Cardiovascular conditions are now responsible for over a quarter of all pregnancy-related deaths in the United States.
12. Obese parturients are more likely to have antenatal comorbidities, which may adversely affect outcomes.
13. In the setting of nonobstetric surgery during pregnancy, no data suggest that any one anesthetic technique is preferred over another, provided oxygenation and blood pressure are maintained and hyperventilation is avoided.

Anatomic and Physiologic Changes of Pregnancy

Pregnancy is characterized by significant anatomical and physiologic changes in several maternal organ systems. These changes are primarily attributed to shifts in hormone production (e.g., progesterone) and the mechanical compression inflicted by the gravid uterus and are necessary to meet the new demands of the growing fetus and uterus. The changes vary by gestational age and return to normal within the first several months after birth (Table 41-1).

Airway and Pulmonary Changes

1 Capillary engorgement of nasal, oropharyngeal, and laryngeal mucosa occurs throughout pregnancy and can be more prominent at birth due to increased extracellular fluid and hormonal changes. Airway edema can also worsen in parturients with preeclampsia, those who have pushed during the second stage of labor, and for those receiving tocolytic therapy. Therefore, insertion of devices via the nasal route (e.g., nasopharyngeal airways, endotracheal tubes, nasogastric tubes) should be done carefully to minimize the risk of bleeding. Mallampati scores tend to increase throughout pregnancy and labor. These airway changes are compounded by breast engorgement, which may make tracheal intubation attempts more difficult. Hence, the use of a short-handled laryngoscope is recommended for parturients when tracheal intubation is needed.

An increase in progesterone causes bronchodilation. There is a small increase in the respiratory rate along with a 45% increase in tidal volume (TV), resulting in a 50% increase in minute ventilation at term.[1] The functional residual capacity (FRC) decreases by up to 30% at term due to decreases in residual volume (RV) by approximately 25% and expiratory reserve volume (ERV) by approximately to 20%. Closing volume and closing capacity do not change during pregnancy, but the decrease in FRC, exacerbated by conditions such as obesity, supine position, or the induction of anesthesia, contributes to airway closure during normal tidal volume breathing and increase the risk of hypoxemia. The increase in alveolar ventilation coupled with a decrease in FRC enhances the maternal uptake and elimination of inhalational anesthetics. There is minimal decrease in the total lung capacity; the decrease in the vertical lung diameter due to cephalad displacement of the diaphragm is compensated by an increase in chest anteroposterior and transverse diameters. The forced expiratory volume in 1 second (FEV1), forced vital capacity (FVC), FEV1/FVC ratio, and dead space remain relatively unchanged during pregnancy. Specifically, anatomic dead space increases from the dilation of large airways but alveolar dead space decreases due to an increase in cardiac output (CO). These changes do not differ between singleton and twin pregnancies.

Basal oxygen consumption increases by up to 21% during pregnancy accompanied by an increase in CO_2 production. Oxygen consumption increases most dramatically during labor (45% in the first stage, 75% in the second stage of labor), especially for parturients not receiving neuraxial analgesia.[2] Pregnancy is a state of incompletely compensated respiratory alkalosis with maternal pH ranging between 7.42 and 7.46 and $PaCO_2$ decreasing to approximately 30 mmHg at term. The PaO_2 increases from approximately 93 mmHg to 106 mmHg.[1] Apnea is poorly tolerated due to the increase in oxygen consumption coupled with decreases in RV, ERV, and FRC, resulting in early desaturation during rapid sequence induction of general anesthesia.

Table 41-1 Summary of Physiologic Changes of Pregnancy at Term

Variable	Change	Amount
Plasma volume	↑	40–50%
Total blood volume	↑	40%
Hemoglobin	↓	11–12 g/dL
Fibrinogen	↑	100%
Serum cholinesterase activity	↓	20–30%
Systemic vascular resistance	↓	20–50%
Cardiac output	↑	30–50%
Systemic blood pressure	↓	Slight
Functional residual capacity	↓	20–30%
Minute ventilation	↑	50%
Alveolar ventilation	↑	70%
Oxygen consumption	↑	20%
Carbon dioxide production	↑	35%
Arterial carbon dioxide tension	↓	10 mmHg
Arterial oxygen tension	↑	10 mmHg
Minimum alveolar concentration	↓	32–40%

↑, increase; ↓, decrease.

Cardiovascular Changes

As oxygen consumption increases during pregnancy, the maternal cardiovascular system adapts to the metabolic demands of the growing fetus, resulting in an overall state of hyperdynamic circulation. The early increase in progesterone, relaxin, and other hormones results in peripheral vasodilation, leading to a decrease in systemic vascular resistance by 20% to 50% starting as early as 8 weeks of gestation.[3] CO increases by 30% to 50% during pregnancy, beginning in the first trimester.[4] This increase is the result of increases in stroke volume by 20% to 50% and heart rate by 15%. CO is highest during the second stage labor (due to increases in uterine contractions and the sympathetic nervous system response to pain and anxiety) and immediately following delivery (due to relief of the inferior vena cava obstruction and contraction of the uterus, which facilitates autotransfusion from the uterus to the central circulation). These values decline rapidly, returning to prelabor levels within several hours after delivery and to prepregnancy values within 2 weeks after delivery. 2

Increased estrogen, volume overload, as well as increased stretch and force demand, all contribute to the reversible left ventricular hypertrophy (50% increase in mass at term) and diastolic dysfunction observed during pregnancy.[5]

Beginning early in pregnancy, systolic blood pressure (BP), mean arterial pressure (MAP), and diastolic BP decrease; the decrease in peripheral vascular resistance outweighs the increase in CO.[6] Arterial BP begins to increase during the third trimester and returns to prepregnancy levels postpartum. Both central venous pressure and pulmonary capillary wedge pressure remain relatively unchanged during pregnancy.

In the supine position, there is near complete occlusion of the vena cava at term by the gravid uterus, resulting in a decrease in preload and a consequent fall in stroke volume and CO by approximately 25%.[7] These changes are usually observed after the second trimester of pregnancy and can lead to significant maternal hypotension, compensatory tachycardia, nausea, altered mental status, and decreased uterine perfusion (which can compromise fetal well-being). The uterine blood flow increases dramatically during pregnancy from 50 to 100 mL/min in a nonpregnant woman to 700 to 900 mL/min at term. Renal blood flow increases by 60%. Pregnancy decreases the overall response to endogenous and exogenous vasoconstrictors (e.g., angiotensin II, epinephrine, norepinephrine, phenylephrine, arginine vasopressin).[8]

Hematology and Coagulation

During pregnancy, the total blood volume is increased by 40%, creating a state of relative volume overload. The increase in plasma volume has been attributed to a substantial activation of the renin–angiotensin–aldosterone system, which increases mineralocorticoid activity and leads to sodium and water retention.[9] Red blood cell mass is also increased by approximately 20%. However, its increase lags in comparison to the increase in plasma volume, causing a state of relative anemia; normal pregnancy hemoglobin levels may be as low as 11 g/dL. This relative anemia peaks at 32 to 34 weeks of gestation.

Pregnancy is associated with decreased anticoagulant activity (decreases Protein S concentration, resistance to protein C, decreased fibrinolysis). The concentration of all procoagulant factor levels, except factors XI and XIII, increase. Fibrinogen concentration is markedly increased compared to the nonpregnant state, ranging from 400 to 500 mg/dL or higher.[10] Acute decreases in fibrinogen concentration are an early predictor of the severity of postpartum hemorrhage.[11,12] Activated partial thromboplastin time (APTT), prothrombin time (PT), thrombin time (TT), and international normalized ratio (INR) remain normal in the absence of anticoagulants or coagulopathy. Although the platelet count decreases due to increased consumption and hemodilution occurring in the third trimester, most platelet counts remain within the normal limit. Lower platelet values ($100 - 150 \times 10^9$/L) are seen in 5% to 10% of healthy pregnancies at term.[13] During normal pregnancy, leukocyte count ranges from 8,000 to 10,000/mm.

Gastrointestinal System

Pregnancy increases the risk for gastric content aspiration due to anatomic and physiologic changes in the gastrointestinal system. There is an upward displacement of the stomach by the gravid uterus, altering its axis and increasing intragastric pressure. Lower esophageal sphincter (LES) tone decreases because of progesterone-induced muscle relaxation. LES relaxation allows displacement of the intra-abdominal segment of the esophagus into the thorax. Gastric emptying is not significantly delayed in nonlaboring patients, but is delayed during labor.[14,15] Systemic opioids administered to parturients for labor analgesia can lead to a delay in gastric emptying. In contrast, epidural analgesia may facilitate gastric emptying due to better pain relief compared to labor without epidural analgesia.[16] The gastrointestinal changes of pregnancy return to the prepregnancy state by 24 to 48 hours postpartum.

Renal System

Pregnancy causes renal vasculature vasodilation, resulting in a 60% increase in renal plasma flow and glomerular filtration rate (GFR) by the end of the first trimester. The increase in GFR leads to decreases in serum creatinine, urea, and uric acid values and increased clearance of drugs. The normal serum creatinine value in pregnancy is 0.5 to 0.6 mg/dL. Values greater than 1.0 mg/dL warrant further investigation.

Hepatic System

Pseudocholinesterase activity is lower during early pregnancy and reaches a maximal decrease on the third postpartum day when levels may be 20% to 33% lower than the nonpregnant state. This is due to both hemodilution and reduced synthesis by the liver. Despite this decrease, a dose adjustment for succinylcholine is not indicated as pseudocholinesterase activity can by reduced by as much as 50% before increased sensitivity to succinylcholine occurs.[17] An exception is in patients with HELLP (hemolysis, elevated liver enzymes, low platelets) syndrome, when pseudocholinesterase activity can be significantly reduced.[18]

Endocrine System

Increasing levels of human chorionic gonadotropin (hCG) activate the thyroid stimulating hormone receptors in the thyroid gland, leading to transient hyperthyroidism.[19] In late pregnancy, there is a relative resistance to insulin and a compensatory increase in insulin synthesis and secretion. Fetal insulin levels are independent of maternal insulin production but dependent on maternal glucose which crosses the placenta. Poor maternal glucose control can increase the risk of neonatal hypoglycemia after delivery. Chronic maternal hyperglycemia increases the risk of macrosomia and shoulder dystocia.

Placental Transfer and Fetal Exposure to Anesthetic Drugs

The human placenta acts as the interface between the mother and fetus and holds important functions, including gas exchange, transfer of nutrients and waste products between maternal and fetal plasma, transfer of immunity by transfer of immunoglobulins from the mother to the fetus, and secretion of hormones that are important for fetal growth and development.

Placental Drug Transfer

Most drugs, including many anesthetic agents, readily cross the placenta. The driving force for placental drug transfer is the concentration gradient of free drug between the maternal and fetal plasma. Other factors include the physicochemical characteristics of the drug (e.g., molecular size, lipid solubility, pH difference between maternal–fetal blood, degree of ionization, protein binding), placental thickness, placental surface area, and uteroplacental blood flow. Placental transfer of drugs occurs by one of the following mechanisms: simple diffusion, facilitated diffusion using a carrier, active transport using adenosine triphosphate (ATP), and pinocytosis. 3

Simple diffusion is the most common mechanism for the transfer of drugs across the placenta. It follows Fick's law of diffusion, which states that the rate of diffusion per unit time is directly proportional to the surface area of the membrane (placenta) and the concentration gradient across it, and inversely proportional to the thickness of the membrane:

$$Q/t = KA(C_m - C_f)/D$$

where Q/t is the rate of diffusion, K is the diffusion constant, A is the surface area available for exchange, C_m is the concentration of free drug in maternal blood, C_f is the concentration of free drug in fetal blood, and *D* is the thickness of the diffusion barrier. The diffusion constant (*K*) depends on the physicochemical characteristics of the drug. Compounds with a molecular weight of less than 500 Da readily diffuse across the placenta, whereas those with molecular weights between 500 and 1,000 Da are more restricted. Of note, most drugs used in anesthesia practice have molecular weights less than 500 Da.

Highly lipophilic drugs readily diffuse across biologic membranes, including the placenta. The degree of ionization is also important because only the nonionized form of the drug crosses the placental membrane. The degree of ionization depends on the pKa of the drug and the pH of maternal blood. The relative concentrations of drug existing in the nonionized and ionized forms can be predicted from the Henderson–Hasselbalch equation:

$$\text{pH} = \text{pKa} + \log(\text{conjugate base acid}).$$

The pKa is the pH at which the concentrations of free base and acid are equal. Ion trapping occurs when the lower pH in the fetus results in an increased proportion of ionized drug. The ionized molecules are unable to diffuse back across the placenta into maternal circulation, leading to fetal drug accumulation.

Anesthetic medications vary in their ionization and lipophilicity. Local anesthetics and opioids are weak bases with pKa values above physiologic pH (7.7 to 8.1) with variable lipid solubility. Propofol is very lipid soluble and able to cross the placenta easily. Volatile anesthetic agents also readily cross the placenta as they are highly lipophilic and have low molecular weights. In contrast, muscle relaxants are highly ionized and less lipophilic, and their rate of placental transfer is limited. While placental transfer of local anesthetics and lipid-soluble opioids occurs after epidural administration, fetal plasma concentrations are in the nano- to micromolar range.

The rate of drug passage across the placenta is inversely proportional to protein binding. However, if enough time is allowed for fetal–maternal equilibrium to be approached, a substantial accumulation of highly protein-bound drugs, such as bupivacaine, can occur in the fetus.[20]

The driving force for placental drug transfer, via simple diffusion, is the concentration gradient of free drug between the maternal and fetal blood. On the maternal side, the administered dose, the mode and site of administration, and, in the case of local anesthetics, the use of vasoconstrictors, influence the maternal plasma concentration. The rates of distribution, metabolism, and excretion of the drug, which may vary at different stages of pregnancy, are also important. In general, higher doses result in higher maternal blood concentrations.

The absorption rate of the drug into maternal plasma varies with the site of drug injection. Compared with other forms of administration, an intravenous bolus results in the highest blood concentrations. Increased maternal blood concentrations after repeated drug administration depend on the dose and frequency of reinjection in addition to the pharmacokinetic characteristics of the drug. The elimination half-life of amide local anesthetic agents is relatively long, so repeated injections may lead to accumulation in the maternal plasma. In contrast, 2-chloroprocaine, an ester local anesthetic, undergoes rapid enzymatic hydrolysis in the presence of pseudocholinesterase and does not accumulate.

Uteroplacental Blood Flow

Factors that decrease placental blood flow (e.g., aortocaval compression, hypotension, or hemorrhage) can decrease drug delivery to the fetus. During labor, uterine contractions intermittently reduce perfusion of the placenta. If a uterine contraction coincides with a rapid decline in plasma drug concentration after an intravenous bolus injection, less drug may be delivered to the fetus.

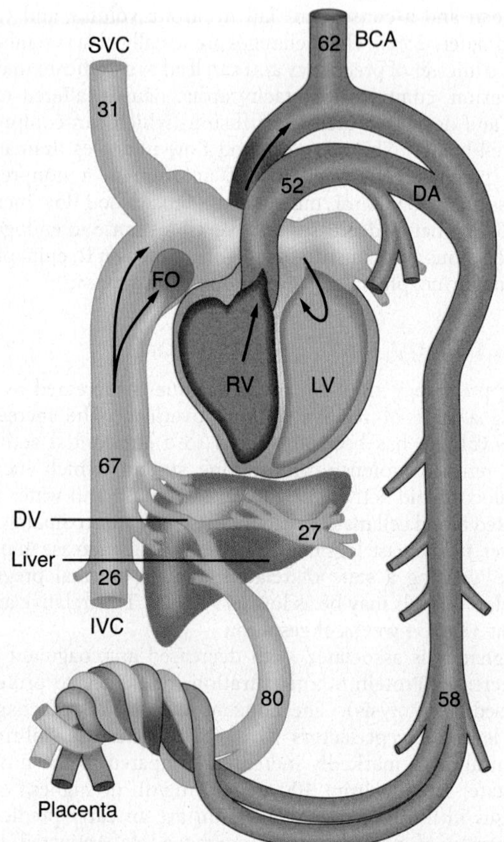

Figure 41-1 Diagram of the circulation in the mature fetal lamb. The numerals indicate the mean oxygen saturation (%) in the great vessels of six lambs: Right ventricle (RV), left ventricle (LV), superior vena cava (SVC), inferior vena cava (IVC), brachiocephalic artery (BCA), foramen ovale (FO), ductus arteriosus (DA), ductus venosus (DV). (Used with permission from Cold Spring Harbor Laboratory Press, from Born GVR, Dawes GS, Mott JC, et al. Changes in the heart and lungs at birth. *Cold Spring Harb Symp Quant Biol.* 1954;19:103.)

Several characteristics of the fetal circulation delay equilibration between the umbilical arterial and venous blood, and thus mitigate the depressant effects of anesthetic drugs (Fig. 41-1). Blood in the umbilical vein carries drugs to the fetus. The liver is the first fetal organ perfused by the umbilical venous blood. Substantial uptake by the fetal liver has been demonstrated for a variety of drugs, including thiopental, lidocaine, and halothane. During its transit to the arterial side of the fetal circulation, the drug is progressively diluted as blood in the umbilical vein becomes admixed with fetal venous blood draining from the gastrointestinal tract, the lower extremities, the head and upper extremities, and finally, the lungs. Because of the unique pattern of fetal circulation, continuous administration of anesthetic concentrations of nitrous oxide during elective cesarean delivery causes newborn depression only if the induction-to-delivery interval exceeds 5 to 10 minutes. Rapid placental transfer of volatile inhalation agents results in detectable umbilical vein and artery concentrations after 1 minute.[21] Fetal regional blood flow changes can also affect the uptake of drugs by individual fetal organs. For example, during asphyxia and acidosis, a greater proportion of the fetal CO perfuses the fetal brain, heart, and placenta. In asphyxiated baboon fetuses, infusion of lidocaine resulted in increased drug uptake in the heart, brain, and liver compared with control fetuses that were not asphyxiated.[22]

Fetus and Newborn

Because the movement of drug molecules is bidirectional between maternal and fetal circulation, the placenta is the main portal of exit from, as well as entry to, the fetus. Drugs that reach the fetus undergo metabolism and excretion depending on the existing concentration gradient of the free drug across the placenta.

The fetus can excrete the drug back to the mother once the concentration gradient of the free drug across the placenta has been reversed. With local anesthetics, this may occur even though the total plasma drug concentration in the mother exceeds that in the fetus because protein binding is lower in the fetus.[23] Only 2-chloroprocaine, which is rapidly metabolized in fetal blood, avoids accumulation in the fetus during periods of acidosis.[24] In both term and preterm newborns, the liver contains enzymes essential for the biotransformation of amide local anesthetics. The metabolic clearance in the newborn is similar to the adult, and renal clearance greater than the adult. Elimination half-life is prolonged in the newborn due to a greater volume of distribution of the drug. It is not completely understood whether the fetus and the newborn are more sensitive than the adult to the depressant and toxic effects of local anesthetics. The relative central nervous system (CNS) and cardiorespiratory toxicity of lidocaine have been studied in adult ewes and lambs (fetal and neonatal).[25] The doses required to produce toxicity in the fetal and neonatal lambs were greater than those required in the adult, although serum concentrations at which toxicity occurred were not different. In the fetus, this was attributed to placental clearance of drug into the mother and maintenance of blood gas tensions during convulsions. In the newborn, a larger volume of distribution was thought to be responsible for the higher doses needed to induce toxic effects.

Finally, multiple studies have evaluated the effect of anesthetic agents on the developing brain. Both volatile anesthetic and N-methyl-D-aspartate (NMDA) receptor antagonist administration have been associated with neuroapoptosis and related neurohistologic and neuropathologic disturbances in rodent and nonhuman primate models,[26] raising concerns that anesthetic exposure to the fetus or during the neonatal period may lead to clinically significant neurologic adverse effects.[27] Reassuringly, however, children exposed to regional or general anesthesia for cesarean birth do not have an increased incidence of learning disabilities compared to children born vaginally, suggesting that brief antenatal exposure to anesthetic medications does not negatively impact early neurodevelopment.[28] Postnatally, a single exposure to general anesthesia during early childhood also does not appear to cause long-term neurocognitive dysfunction in retrospective cohort and sibling-matched human studies.[29] While a link between labor epidural analgesia and autism in offspring was recently proposed, a preponderance of evidence now refutes that association.[30]

Analgesia for Labor and Vaginal Delivery

4 Labor analgesia may benefit the mother and fetus and should not be withheld if requested. Most women experience moderate-to-severe pain during parturition. In the first stage of labor, pain is caused by uterine contractions, associated with dilation of the cervix and stretching of the lower uterine segment. Pain impulses are carried in visceral afferent type C fibers which accompany the sympathetic nerves. During the first stage of labor, pain is referred to the T10 to L1 spinal cord segments. In the late first and second stages of labor, additional pain impulses from distention of the vaginal vault and perineum are carried by the pudendal nerves, composed of sacral fibers (S2 to S4).

In addition to relieving pain and anxiety, well-conducted obstetric analgesia may confer additional benefits to mother and fetus. During the first and second stages of labor, epidural analgesia blunts the sympathetic surges that occur with painful uterine contractions and nonvoluntary "bearing down," thus avoiding increases in maternal heart rate and BP and decreases in uterine blood flow. In reducing maternal secretion of catecholamines, epidural analgesia may convert a previously dysfunctional labor pattern to normal. Maternal analgesia may also benefit the fetus by preventing maternal hyperventilation, which can reduce fetal arterial oxygen tension by causing a leftward shift of the maternal oxygen–hemoglobin dissociation curve.

The most frequently chosen methods for relieving the pain of parturition are psychoprophylaxis, systemic medication, and neuraxial analgesia. Inhalation analgesia, spinal analgesia, and paracervical blockade are less commonly used. General anesthesia is rarely necessary but may be indicated for uterine relaxation in complicated deliveries. Labor varies in length and intensity, as does individual tolerance to pain and desire for pain relief. Women should be educated about the options for labor analgesia and supported in their choice for method of pain control. Neonatal outcomes appear to be similar for healthy women who deliver without pharmacologic analgesia and for women who receive analgesia.

Nonpharmacologic Methods of Labor Analgesia

Nonpharmacologic methods to relieve the pain of childbirth include childbirth education, emotional support, massage, aromatherapy, audiotherapy, and therapeutic use of heat and cooling. More advanced techniques that require specialized training or equipment include hydrotherapy, intradermal water injections, biofeedback, transcutaneous electrical nerve stimulation (TENS), acupuncture or acupressure, and hypnosis. There are varying levels of evidence to support each of these analgesic methods.[31]

Prepared Childbirth and Psychoprophylaxis

The philosophy of prepared childbirth maintains that lack of knowledge, misinformation, fear, and anxiety can heighten a patient's response to pain and consequently increase the need for analgesics. The most popular method of prepared childbirth was introduced by Lamaze. It provides an educational program on the physiology of parturition and attempts to diminish cortical pain perception by encouraging responses such as specific patterns of breathing and focused attention on a fixed object.[32] Scientific data as to whether childbirth education and psychoprophylaxis are effective in reducing childbirth pain are inconsistent and lack scientific rigor. Education, intense motivation, and cultural beliefs can influence the affective and behavioral responses to pain, although their true effect on pain sensation is less clear.

Other Nonpharmacologic Methods

Continuous labor support refers to the presence during labor of nonmedical support by a trained person. Prospective, controlled trials and several systematic analyses have concluded that women who receive continuous labor support have shorter labors, fewer operative deliveries, fewer analgesic interventions, and better overall satisfaction.[33] Systematic reviews of randomized controlled trials of hydrotherapy (water baths) have concluded that women experience less pain and use less analgesia, without change in the duration of labor, rate of operative delivery, or neonatal outcome.[34] Intradermal water injection consists of the injection of 0.05 to 0.1 mL of sterile water at four sites on the lower back to treat back pain during labor. Although some randomized controlled trials have found that the technique is effective in reducing severe back pain during labor, a 2012 meta-analysis of seven studies concluded that there is little robust evidence that sterile water injections are effective for low back pain or other labor pain.[35] Hypnosis requires prenatal training of the mother by a trained hypnotherapist. A meta-analysis concluded that the small number of available trials precludes drawing conclusions about the usefulness of hypnotherapy for pain management during labor, although the technique shows some promise.[36] The results of studies using TENS are inconsistent, but in general, labor pain does not appear to be lessened by TENS, nor does TENS lower the use of other analgesic modalities.[37] In a meta-analysis including 13 trials, women who were randomized to receive acupuncture or acupressure versus control (no or "false" acupuncture) had modestly lower pain scores.[38] Similarly, relaxation techniques may also reduce pain intensity and improve satisfaction with pain relief compared to standard care.[39]

Systemic Medication

The advantages of systemic analgesics include ease of administration and patient acceptability. However, the drug, dose, time, and method of administration must be chosen carefully to avoid maternal or neonatal side effects. Opioids are used most commonly, while sedative–hypnotic and ketamine use is rare.

Opioids

Systemic opioids are commonly administered for labor analgesia, although existing data suggest that they provide little significant analgesia.[40] Meperidine was historically the most commonly used systemic analgesic for the treatment of labor pain. Meperidine can be administered by intravenous (effective analgesia in 5 to 10 minutes) or intramuscular (peak effect in 40 to 50 minutes) injection. Use has declined in recent decades due to concerns of lack of efficacy and its side effects. The major side effects of opioids are nausea and vomiting, maternal sedation, depression of ventilation, orthostatic hypotension, and neonatal depression. Meperidine may cause transient alterations of the fetal heart rate (FHR), such as decreased beat-to-beat variability and mild bradycardia. The risk of neonatal depression is related to the interval from the last drug injection to delivery. Placental transfer of an active metabolite, normeperidine, which has a long elimination half-life in the neonate (62 hours), has also been implicated in contributing to neonatal depression and subtle neonatal neurobehavioral dysfunction.

Synthetic opioids such as fentanyl, alfentanil, and remifentanil are more potent than meperidine; however, their use during labor is limited by their short duration of action. These drugs offer an advantage when analgesia of rapid onset but short duration is necessary (e.g., with forceps application). For more prolonged analgesia, fentanyl or remifentanil can be administered with patient-controlled delivery devices.[41] However, patient-controlled analgesia (PCA) administration of opioids carries the potential for drug accumulation and the risk of neonatal depression. Remifentanil has the theoretical advantage of rapid onset and offset compared with other opioids. Bolus doses ranging from 0.2 to 1 µg/kg with lockout intervals from 1 to 5 minutes and background infusion rates from 0 to 0.1 µg/kg/min have been described. Background infusions with PCA should be used with caution due to potential for drug accumulation in an obtunded mother. As with other systemic opioid techniques, it is unclear whether remifentanil PCA can provide satisfactory analgesia without an unacceptably high incidence of maternal, fetal, and neonatal side effects.[42]

Opioid agonists–antagonists, such as butorphanol (1 to 2 mg) and nalbuphine (10 mg), administered via intravenous or intramuscular injection, have also been used for obstetric analgesia (NICV 41-1). These drugs have the proposed benefits of a lower incidence of nausea, vomiting, and dysphoria. Unlike meperidine, these drugs are biotransformed into inactive metabolites and have a "ceiling effect" on depression of ventilation.

If naloxone is necessary to correct opioid-induced respiratory depression in the newborn, the drug should be given directly to the newborn intramuscularly (0.1 mg/kg). Preemptive administration to the mother just before birth is discouraged, as it reverses maternal analgesia at a time when it is most needed. In addition, in some instances, it has caused maternal pulmonary edema and even cardiac arrest.

Ketamine

Ketamine is a potent analgesic; however, it may also induce unacceptable amnesia, preventing maternal recall of the birth. Nonetheless, ketamine is a useful adjuvant to inadequate regional analgesia during vaginal delivery or for obstetric manipulations. In low doses (0.2 to 0.4 mg/kg), ketamine provides adequate analgesia without causing neonatal depression. Constant communication is required with the patient to ensure that awareness and appropriate airway reflexes are preserved.

Neuraxial Analgesia

Regional techniques provide excellent analgesia with minimal depressant effects on the mother and the fetus. The most common regional techniques in obstetric anesthesia include neuraxial blocks (epidural, combined spinal–epidural [CSE], dural-puncture epidural [DPE], spinal). Paracervical, pudendal, and lumbar sympathetic blocks are rarely performed. Hypotension resulting from sympathectomy is the most frequent complication of neuraxial blockade. Therefore, maternal BP should be monitored at regular intervals, typically every 2 to 5 minutes, for approximately 15 to 20 minutes after the initiation of the block and at routine intervals thereafter. The use of neuraxial analgesia may be contraindicated in the presence of coagulopathy, acute hypovolemia, or infection at the site of needle insertion. Chorioamnionitis without frank sepsis is not a contraindication to neuraxial blockade in obstetrics, provided antibiotics have been administered.

Epidural Analgesia

Epidural analgesia may be used for pain relief during labor and vaginal delivery, and if necessary, converted to surgical anesthesia for cesarean delivery. For labor, low concentrations of local anesthetic are usually combined with lipid-soluble opioids. Combining drugs allows the use of lower doses of both drugs, thus minimizing side effects and complications of each. Long-acting amides such as bupivacaine or ropivacaine are most frequently used because they produce excellent sensory analgesia while sparing motor function at low concentrations (<0.1%). Although some studies have found that ropivacaine is associated with less motor blockade than equipotent doses of bupivacaine, there was no difference in the rate of operative vaginal delivery among women randomized to receive epidural levobupivacaine, bupivacaine, or ropivacaine for maintenance of labor analgesia.[43]

Analgesia for the first stage of labor may be achieved with approximately 10 mL of bupivacaine or ropivacaine (0.125%)

combined with fentanyl (50 to 100 μg) or sufentanil (5 to 10 μg) injected into the mid- or low-lumbar epidural space. Because catheter aspiration is not always diagnostic, particularly when using single-orifice epidural catheters, some experts believe that a test dose should be administered to improve detection of an intrathecally or intravascularly placed catheter. Alternatively, the analgesic dose should be injected incrementally.

Epidural labor analgesia is maintained by the intermittent or continuous administration of the local anesthetic–opioid solution until delivery. Typical solutions include bupivacaine (0.0625% to 0.1%) or ropivacaine (0.08% to 0.15%). The addition of fentanyl (1 to 2 μg/mL) or sufentanil (0.3 to 0.5 μg/mL) allows for more dilute local anesthetic solutions to be administered. Continuous infusions are administered at 10 to 12 mL/h. Alternatively, analgesia may be maintained with patient-controlled epidural analgesia (PCEA) with similar solutions of local anesthetic and opioid. PCEA results in greater patient satisfaction, lower average hourly bupivacaine dose, less motor block, and need for fewer physician interventions[44] compared with a continuous epidural infusion. Common PCEA parameters include a parturient-administered bolus dose of 5 to 10 mL, a lockout interval of 10 to 20 minutes, and a background infusion of 0 to 10 mL/h. Thirty percent to 50% of the hourly dose is often administered as a background infusion.

The timed, or programmed, intermittent epidural bolus (PIEB) technique is a newer method for maintaining epidural analgesia. The epidural infusion pump is programmed to deliver a bolus dose at regular intervals. Bolus administration of drugs results in better distribution of the solution in the epidural space compared to continuous infusion. Randomized controlled trials comparing this technique with continuous epidural infusion or with PCEA have shown lower anesthetic dose, greater patient satisfaction, and a lower incidence of motor block and instrumental vaginal delivery.[45] Typical pump settings are a programmed bolus dose of 5 to 10 mL and a programmed bolus interval of 30 to 60 minutes. PIEB is often combined with PCEA.

If operative vaginal delivery (forceps or vacuum) is required, the sacral dermatomes may be blocked with 10 mL of bupivacaine (0.25% to 0.5%), lidocaine (1%), or 2-chloroprocaine (2% to 3%) to produce dense sacral analgesia.

Combined Spinal–Epidural Analgesia

CSE analgesia combines the rapid, reliable onset of profound analgesia resulting from spinal injection with the flexibility and longer duration associated with a continuous epidural technique. After identification of the epidural space using a 9-cm epidural needle, a longer (127 mm), pencil-point spinal needle is advanced into the subarachnoid space through the epidural needle. After intrathecal injection, the spinal needle is removed and an epidural catheter is inserted. Intrathecal injection of fentanyl (10 to 25 μg) or sufentanil (2 to 5 μg) alone or more commonly in combination with bupivacaine (1.25 to 2.5 mg) produces profound analgesia lasting for 90 to 120 minutes with minimal motor block. Spinal opioid alone can provide complete analgesia for the latent phase of labor. However, the addition of local anesthetic is necessary for satisfactory analgesia during the active phase of labor. Continuous epidural analgesia, PCEA, or PIEB may be initiated following the spinal injection to maintain analgesia.

The most common side effects of intrathecal opioids are pruritus, nausea, vomiting, and urinary retention. The incidence of pruritus is lower if opioid is co-administered with local anesthetic.[46] Rostral spread resulting in delayed respiratory depression may occur; the risk is highest in the first 30 minutes after injection. It is rare with the use of fentanyl or sufentanil. Transient nonreassuring FHR patterns may occur after initiation of either epidural or spinal analgesia, with or without opioids; however, the incidence is higher after CSE compared to epidural analgesia.[47] Presumably, uterine tachysystole and decreased uteroplacental perfusion occur as a result of rapid decrease in circulating maternal epinephrine levels after initiation of analgesia or as a result of hypotension after sympatholysis. The incidence of emergency cesarean delivery, however, is no greater after CSE than after conventional epidural analgesia.[47]

Parturients in early labor, or with preload-dependent medical conditions (e.g., aortic stenosis), may particularly benefit from opioid-only CSE analgesia. Spinal opioid provides complete analgesia without the need for local anesthetic in early labor, thus avoiding an acute decrease in preload associated with neuraxial local anesthetic administration, and almost always allows motivated women to ambulate without motor block. Multiparous women with advanced cervical dilation also benefit from CSE analgesia in which both intrathecal opioid and local anesthetic are injected. The onset of sacral analgesia is accomplished significantly faster and with less drug compared to epidural analgesia. Some experts advocate the cautious use of CSE analgesia in women who may require urgent cesarean delivery or are at increased risk from general anesthesia (e.g., morbidly obese or anticipated difficult airway) because the spinal component of a CSE may initially mask the functional assessment of the epidural catheter. However, epidural catheters placed as part of a CSE technique fail less frequently during labor and intrapartum cesarean delivery compared to catheters sited with a traditional epidural technique. In addition, placement of an epidural catheter as part of a CSE does not delay recognition of catheter failure.[48]

Dural-Puncture Epidural Analgesia

A combined spinal–epidural procedure without subarachnoid medication injection is known as DPE analgesia. The advantage of DPE compared with CSE is avoidance of potential fetal bradycardia which is associated with that technique. Potential advantages of DPE over traditional epidural analgesia include confirmation of midline placement via presence of CSF return as well as greater transfer of epidurally administered medications into the intrathecal space. Purported benefits of the DPE include faster analgesia onset, faster sacral spread, fewer asymmetric blocks, and decreased need for catheter replacement compared to traditional epidural analgesia. Studies comparing epidural to DPE analgesia have shown conflicting results. Current evidence does not provide strong support for the DPE compared to epidural technique.[49] After the initial DPE procedure, analgesic initiation and maintenance mirror that of traditional epidural analgesia.

Spinal Analgesia

A single subarachnoid injection for labor analgesia has the advantage of fast and reliable onset of neural blockade, and it is technically easier to initiate compared with epidural analgesia. However, repeated intrathecal injections may be required for a long labor, thus increasing the risk of postdural puncture headache (PDPH). Spinal analgesia with fentanyl (15 to 25 μg) or sufentanil (2 to 5 μg) in combination with plain bupivacaine (1.25 to 2.5 mg) may be appropriate in the multiparous patient with anticipated imminent delivery. A potential disadvantage of single-shot spinal analgesia is that the duration of labor, even in a rapidly progressing multiparous woman, may be longer than anticipated. Furthermore, if the woman requires urgent cesarean delivery, a new anesthetic will need to be initiated. However, spinal anesthesia is a safe and effective alternative to general anesthesia or pudendal nerve block for operative delivery in parturients without pre-existing epidural analgesia.

Impact of Neuraxial Analgesia on Labor

Because of ethical considerations and methodologic difficulties, it is difficult to design clinical trials to examine the effects of neuraxial analgesia on the progress of labor and mode of delivery. Randomized controlled trials have found no difference in the rate of cesarean birth in women who received neuraxial compared with systemic opioid labor analgesia.[50] Meta-analyses suggest that neuraxial analgesia does not prolong the first stage of labor, although the data are heterogeneous.[50] There has been concern that early initiation of epidural analgesia during the latent phase of labor (<4 cm cervical dilation) in nulliparous women may result in a higher incidence of dystocia and cesarean birth. However, a meta-analysis of randomized trials found no difference in the rate of cesarean birth in women randomized to early neuraxial compared with systemic opioid analgesia.[51] Neuraxial analgesia is, however, associated with prolongation of the second stage of labor in nulliparous women, possibly owing to a decrease in expulsive forces or malposition of the vertex.[50] Although the American College of Obstetricians and Gynecologists (ACOG) traditionally defined abnormally prolonged second stage of labor as more than 3 hours in nulliparous women with epidural analgesia and more than 2 hours in women without epidural analgesia, a 2014 consensus document developed jointly by the ACOG and the Society for Maternal-Fetal Medicine (SMFM) stated that "a specific absolute maximum length of the time spent in second stage labor beyond which all women should undergo operative delivery has not been identified."[52] In addition, they suggested that longer durations (beyond the traditional 3 hours) may be appropriate on an individual basis. Prolongation of the second stage in women with epidural analgesia may be minimized by the use of dilute local anesthetic solutions in combination with opioid.[53]

Alternative Regional Anesthetic Techniques

Alternative regional anesthetic techniques to block sensory afferent input from the uterus and cervix during labor exist but are used rarely in modern obstetric practice. Bilateral paracervical block interrupts transmission of nerve impulses from the uterus and cervix during the first stage of labor. Five to ten milliliters of dilute local anesthetic solution are injected submucosally via the vagina into the left and right lateral vaginal fornices. This technique has fallen out of favor due to association with poor fetal outcomes. Paravertebral lumbar sympathetic block is an alternative if contraindications to neuraxial analgesia are present. Unfamiliarity and technical difficulties associated with the performance of the block and risks of intravascular injection have decreased its use in standard practice.

The pudendal nerves, which derive from the sacral nerve roots (S2 to S4) and supply the vaginal vault, perineum, rectum, and parts of the bladder, can be anesthetized transvaginally where they loop around the ischial spines (1 Video 41-1). Ten milliliters of dilute local anesthetic solution deposited behind each sacrospinous ligament can provide adequate anesthesia for outlet forceps delivery and episiotomy repair.

Inhalation Analgesia and General Anesthesia

Nitrous oxide (50% by volume in oxygen) is the most frequently used inhalation agent for labor analgesia. Parturients are trained to intermittently self-administer the admixture at the onset of a contraction. Studies are conflicting as to whether nitrous oxide provides benefit to the parturient; its safety for the fetus and the neonate has also not been well studied.[54] A major disadvantage of inhalation labor analgesia is the need for a waste gas scavenging system—nitrous oxide is a greenhouse gas.

General anesthesia is rarely used for vaginal delivery, and precautions against gastric aspiration must always be observed (see General Anesthesia in the section Anesthesia for Cesarean Delivery). General anesthesia may be required when time constraints prevent induction of regional anesthesia. Potent inhalation drugs (1.5 to 2 MAC for short periods) can provide uterine relaxation for obstetric maneuvers such as second twin delivery, breech presentation, or postpartum manual removal of a retained placenta. However, in current practice, intravenous nitroglycerin (50 to 250 μg) has largely replaced the need for general anesthesia for uterine relaxation.

Anesthesia for Cesarean Delivery

The most common indications for cesarean delivery include arrest of dilation, nonreassuring fetal status, cephalopelvic disproportion, malpresentation, prior cesarean delivery, and prior uterine surgery (2 Video 41-2). The choice of anesthesia depends on the urgency of the procedure, the condition of the mother and fetus, and the mother's wishes. Most patients undergoing cesarean delivery receive spinal or epidural anesthesia. Neuraxial techniques have several advantages, such as avoidance of airway manipulation and decreased risk of pulmonary aspiration, avoidance of depressant anesthetic drugs (which cross the placenta and cause neonatal depression), facilitation of awake birth (allowing the mother to experience childbirth), and lower operative blood loss.

5

Preoperative Preparation, Monitoring, and Positioning

Aspiration prophylaxis is commonly administered prior to cesarean delivery due to the increased risk of gastroesophageal reflux and aspiration in pregnancy. Specific medications may include any combination of nonparticulate antacid, H_2-receptor antagonist, and dopamine-receptor antagonist. Sedative premedication is usually not necessary. Standard monitors are sufficient for uncomplicated cesarean deliveries, although BP should be measured frequently (every 1 to 3 minutes) for the first 20 minutes after initiation of anesthesia. Patients should be positioned with left uterine displacement to avoid aortocaval compression in the supine position. There is no evidence that intraoperative supplemental oxygen offers any benefit to the mother or fetus in the absence of maternal hypoxemia.[55]

Neuraxial Anesthesia

Surgical anesthesia up to the T4 dermatome is necessary to perform cesarean delivery without maternal discomfort. The most common complication of neuraxial anesthesia is hypotension and the attendant risk of decreased uteroplacental perfusion (see Hypotension in the section Anesthetic Complications). Measures to decrease the incidence and severity of hypotension include left uterine displacement, intravenous fluid administration, and the continuous infusion of prophylactic vasopressors.

Spinal Anesthesia

Subarachnoid block is the most commonly administered neuraxial anesthetic for cesarean delivery because of its simplicity, speed of onset, and reliability. Hyperbaric 0.75% bupivacaine (12.0 to 13.5 mg [1.6 to 1.8 mL]) is used most frequently for cesarean delivery in the United States, as it reliably provides 90 to 120 minutes of surgical anesthesia.

Despite an adequate dermatomal level for surgery, women may experience varying degrees of visceral discomfort, nausea, or vomiting intraoperatively, particularly during exteriorization of the uterus and traction on abdominal viscera. Improved perioperative anesthesia can be provided with the addition of fentanyl (10 to 20 μg), sufentanil (2.5 to 5 μg), or morphine (0.1 to 0.15 mg) to the local anesthetic solution. Fentanyl has a rapid onset but is short acting and provides little additional postoperative analgesia. In contrast, morphine has a longer latency than fentanyl but will also provide analgesia for 12 to 18 hours after delivery.

Epidural Anesthesia

In contrast to spinal anesthesia, epidural anesthesia is associated with a slower onset of action and a larger drug requirement to establish adequate sensory block. The major advantages of epidural compared with single-shot spinal anesthesia are the ability to titrate the extent and duration of anesthesia. To avoid unintentional intrathecal or intravascular injection, correct placement of the epidural needle and catheter is essential. Aspiration of the epidural catheter for blood or cerebrospinal fluid is not reliable for detection of catheter misplacement, particularly with single-orifice catheters. Thus, most anesthesiologists administer a test dose before the initiation of surgical anesthesia. A small dose of local anesthetic (e.g., lidocaine, 45 mg, or bupivacaine, 5 mg) readily produces identifiable sensory and motor blocks if injected intrathecally. Addition of epinephrine (15 μg) with careful hemodynamic monitoring may signal intravascular injection if followed by a transient increase in heart rate and BP. A negative test, although reassuring, does not eliminate the need for incremental administration of local anesthetic.

The most commonly used agents for obstetric epidural anesthesia in the United States are 2% lidocaine with epinephrine, 5 μg/mL (1:200,000) and 3% 2-chloroprocaine. Adequate anesthesia is usually achieved with 15 to 25 mL of either local anesthetic solution, administered in divided doses over 5 to 10 minutes. 2-Chloroprocaine provides rapid onset of a reliable block with minimal risk of systemic toxicity because of its extremely high rate of metabolism in maternal and fetal plasma. However, 2% lidocaine with epinephrine and sodium bicarbonate (1 mEq/10 mL lidocaine) and fentanyl may also be used when the rapid conversion of pre-existing epidural labor analgesia to surgical anesthesia is required for urgent cesarean delivery.[56] Lidocaine should be administered with epinephrine, as lidocaine without epinephrine does not consistently provide satisfactory surgical anesthesia. Bupivacaine is no longer commonly used for obstetric epidural anesthesia, as it is associated with a greater risk of local anesthetic systemic toxicity (LAST) compared with other amide local anesthetics. Unintentional intravascular injection of bupivacaine is associated with a high incidence of maternal mortality.[57] Ropivacaine 0.5% combined with fentanyl may be used for surgical anesthesia, as the risk of toxicity is less than that of bupivacaine. A meta-analysis of studies comparing different anesthetic solutions for extension of labor epidural analgesia for cesarean delivery concluded that ropivacaine provided denser anesthesia compared with bupivacaine or levobupivacaine.[56]

Combined Spinal–Epidural Anesthesia

Advantages of CSE anesthesia for cesarean delivery include the rapid onset of a dense block with a low anesthetic dose and the ability to extend the duration of anesthesia. In addition, the epidural catheter can be used to provide continuous postoperative analgesia when needed. There is a lower incidence of breakthrough pain and intraoperative shivering and higher maternal satisfaction with CSE compared to epidural anesthesia for cesarean delivery.[58] Several variations of the CSE technique have been described. A common technique uses the same spinal dose of local anesthetic as is used for conventional spinal anesthesia. In sequential CSE anesthesia, a smaller spinal dose is expected to result in inadequate anesthesia for some patients. After 15 minutes, if anesthesia is inadequate, the block is extended by injecting supplemental local anesthetic via the epidural catheter. Although the incidence of hypotension is lower with this technique compared with full-dose spinal anesthesia, the induction to incision time is prolonged.

General Anesthesia

General anesthesia may be necessary when absolute or relative contraindications exist to neuraxial anesthesia (e.g., coagulopathy, hemorrhage with unstable maternal vital signs, severe aortic stenosis) or when the need for emergency delivery precludes neuraxial blockade (NICV 41-2). Preoperative airway evaluation is particularly important in pregnant women because the inability to intubate the trachea and provide effective ventilation is the leading cause of maternal death related to anesthesia.[59] Equipment to manage the difficult airway should be immediately available.[60] Mallampati classification scores worsen during labor in some parturients. If airway difficulties are anticipated, a neuraxial anesthetic technique should be considered or an awake tracheal intubation performed.

To minimize the risk of hypoxemia during induction of anesthesia, denitrogenation for 3 to 5 minutes with a tight-fitting mask is essential. In an emergency, four deep breaths with 100% oxygen may suffice. Although somewhat controversial,[61] a rapid-sequence induction of anesthesia, application of cricoid pressure, and intubation with a cuffed tracheal tube are usually performed for all pregnant women undergoing general anesthesia after 20 weeks of gestation. Airway management guidelines from the Obstetric Anaesthetists' Association and the Difficult Airway Society suggest that the head-up position and gentle mask ventilation with cricoid pressure may be used to prolong the safe apnea period.[62] Low- or high-flow nasal cannula oxygen, administered during the apneic period, including during laryngoscopy, may also prolong the safe apneic period.[63]

Induction with a sedative–hypnotic (e.g., propofol [2 mg/kg], ketamine [1 mg/kg], or etomidate [0.2 to 0.3 mg/kg]) is followed by succinylcholine (1 to 1.5 mg/kg) or rocuronium (1.0 mg/kg) to facilitate tracheal intubation. Historically, succinylcholine has been the preferred muscle relaxant. However, with the availability of sugammadex, high-dose rocuronium is a safe alternative to achieve deep neuromuscular blockade rapidly. A trained assistant applies cricoid pressure until the airway is properly secured with a cuffed endotracheal tube. Once correct placement of the endotracheal tube is confirmed with capnography and auscultation, the obstetrician may proceed with incision.

If there is difficulty in securing the airway, the mother should be ventilated with 100% oxygen before a subsequent attempt at tracheal intubation is made. Although some experts advise attempting to maintain cricoid pressure throughout, this practice may actually make visualization of the glottis and mask ventilation more difficult in some patients. The American Society of Anesthesiologists' Difficult Airway Algorithm should be modified to include assessment of fetal status and the need for immediate delivery (Fig. 41-2).[62,64] It may be safer to awaken the patient and reassess the method of induction and intubation, rather than to persist with traumatic efforts at tracheal intubation. However, if the fetus is in extremis, airway management with a mask or supraglottic airway device may be an acceptable alternative.[62]

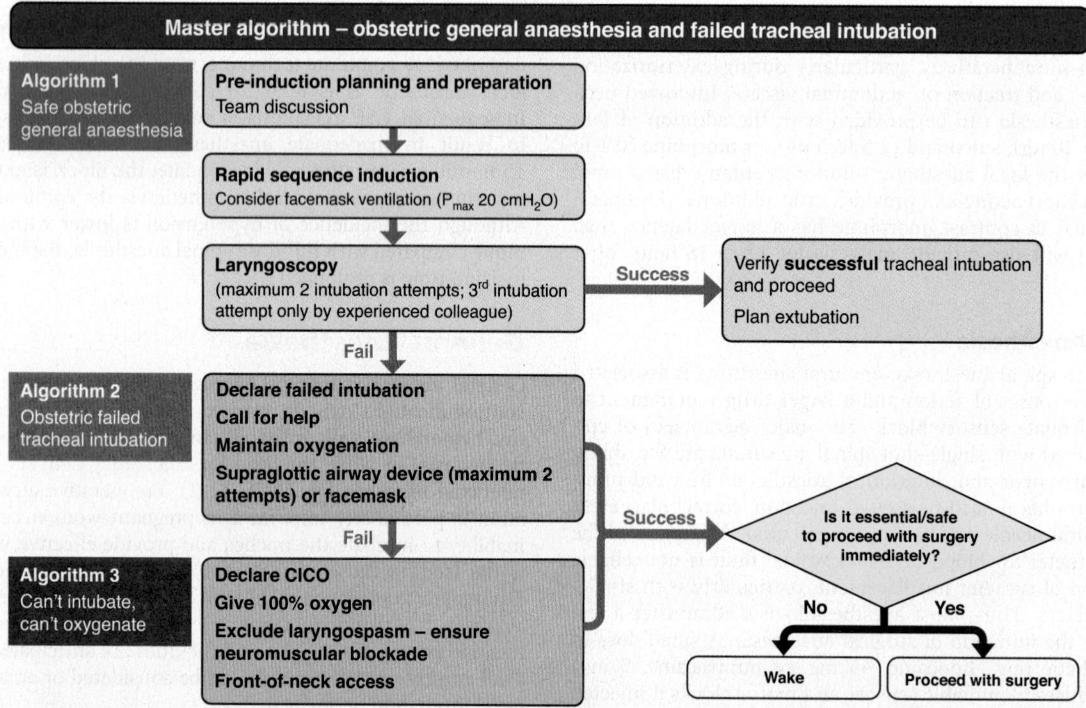

Figure 41-2 Obstetric Anaesthetists' Association and Difficult Airway Society master algorithm for management of obstetric general anesthesia and failed tracheal intubation. CICO, cannot intubate, cannot oxygenate. P_{max}, maximal inflation pressure. (Reproduced from Mushambi MC, Kinsella SM, Popat M, et al. Obstetric Anaesthetists' Association and Difficult Airway Society guidelines for the management of difficult and failed tracheal intubation in obstetrics. *Anaesthesia*. 2015;70:1286–1306, with permission from Obstetric Anaesthetists' Association/Difficult Airway Society.)

In the interval between tracheal intubation and delivery, anesthesia is usually maintained with a 50:50 mixture of nitrous oxide in oxygen and a volatile anesthetic agent. In the past, it was common to limit the volatile agent concentration to 0.5 MAC to limit fetal exposure before delivery and to limit uterine relaxation after delivery. However, the incidence of intraoperative awareness appears to be unacceptably high with this technique.[65] Indeed, a significant number of women had bispectral index values greater than 60 during general anesthesia with sevoflurane 1% in nitrous oxide 50%.[66] Therefore, higher concentrations of volatile agent should be used before delivery. After delivery, the nitrous oxide concentration can be increased and intravenous amnestics (e.g., midazolam) and opioids can be administered to supplement the low concentration of volatile anesthetic.

General anesthesia for cesarean delivery is associated with lower neonatal Apgar scores at 1 minute compared with neuraxial anesthesia; however, the Apgar scores at 5 minutes are comparable. Therefore, an individual trained in neonatal resuscitation should be present at delivery of the infant when general anesthesia is used. After delivery, prophylactic intravenous oxytocin is administered to decrease the risk of uterine atony. At the end of the procedure, the trachea is extubated once all extubation criteria have been met.

Postoperative Analgesia

Multimodal analgesia, including systemic nonsteroidal anti-inflammatory drugs, acetaminophen, and long-acting neuraxial opioids, is optimal for postoperative pain management. Prolonged (12 to 24 hours) postoperative pain relief can be provided by intrathecal morphine (50 to 150 μg) or epidural morphine (1 to 3 mg).[67,68] Side effects of neuraxial morphine include nausea, vomiting, and pruritus. Delayed respiratory depression is a rare but potentially devastating complication; therefore, patients who receive neuraxial opioids must be monitored carefully in the postoperative period.[68] Morbidly obese women may be at higher risk for respiratory depression. PCEA with a dilute solution of local anesthetic and lipid-soluble opioid can be considered for postoperative analgesia in patients with risk factors for uncontrolled pain. Abdominal wall nerve block techniques (transversus abdominis plane [TAP] block or quadratus lumborum [QL] block) have also been described after cesarean delivery. While these blocks do not provide additional benefit when added to intrathecal morphine,[69] TAP or QL block, or wound infiltration with local anesthetic should be considered for patients who did not receive neuraxial morphine or in whom neuraxial morphine has less effect (e.g., those on buprenorphine).

Very small amounts of maternally administered medications cross into breast milk, and even smaller amounts are absorbed from the neonatal gut; therefore, most analgesics administered in standard doses are considered safe with breastfeeding. Notable exceptions include codeine, tramadol, and meperidine.

Anesthetic Complications

Pulmonary Aspiration

The risk of inhalation of gastric contents is increased in pregnant women compared to nonpregnant controls. Pregnancy reduces the competency of the LES and changes the anatomic relationship between the esophagus and stomach, increasing the occurrence of gastroesophageal reflux. While gastric emptying is not delayed during pregnancy or early labor, data suggest that gastric transit times increase as labor progresses.[14,70] Women who have recently eaten, are laboring, have received systemic opioids, or have frequent heartburn are of greatest concern for pulmonary aspiration. Comprehensive airway evaluation, prophylactic administration of nonparticulate antacids, and use of regional anesthesia decrease the risk of aspiration. Rapid sequence induction is recommended if general anesthesia is required for cesarean delivery, unless an anticipated difficult airway warrants awake intubation.

Hypotension

Neuraxial anesthesia is frequently associated with hypotension. BP should be monitored frequently (every 2 to 3 minutes) after the induction of neuraxial anesthesia. Techniques to reduce the incidence of hypotension during neuraxial anesthesia include left uterine displacement, intravenous fluid, and vasopressor administration. Maintaining the maternal BP close to baseline reduces the incidence of maternal nausea and vomiting and is associated with higher umbilical artery pH values.[71] The administration of an intravenous bolus of crystalloid solution at the time of induction of neuraxial analgesia (co-load) is as effective as administration of the same volume of solution prior to the initiation of anesthesia (preload).[72]

Phenylephrine is equally efficacious to ephedrine for treating maternal hypotension and results in less fetal acidosis; thus, phenylephrine is preferred for the prevention and treatment of neuraxial anesthesia-induced hypotension in pregnancy.[73] Phenylephrine may be administered as a bolus dose (100 to 150 μg) to treat hypotension[74] or as a continuous prophylactic infusion (starting rate, 25 to 50 μg/min).[75] Managing spinal anesthesia-induced hypotension using a prophylactic phenylephrine infusion results in fewer physician interventions and less patient nausea than treating hypotension with bolus-dose phenylephrine after it occurs.[76] Because phenylephrine may result in reflex bradycardia and decreased CO, some experts have proposed using norepinephrine to prevent and treat hypotension due to its β-adrenergic agonist effects. The relative potency of norepinephrine to phenylephrine is approximately 11:1, and thus the suggested dose of IV bolus norepinephrine for this indication is 6 μg.[77,78]

Total Spinal Anesthesia

High or total spinal anesthesia is a rare complication of neuraxial local anesthetic injection that occurs after excessive cephalad spread of local anesthetic in the subarachnoid or epidural space. Unintentional intrathecal administration of epidural medication as a result of dural puncture or catheter migration may also result in this complication. The clinical presentation includes rapid ascent of sensory–motor blockade, dyspnea, inability to phonate, and difficulty swallowing. Profound hypotension may lead to brainstem and cerebral hypoperfusion and cause loss of consciousness. Immediate vasopressor administration, rapid fluid administration, left uterine displacement, and leg elevation might be necessary to achieve hemodynamic stability. Rapid control of the airway is essential, and tracheal intubation may be necessary to ensure oxygenation without aspiration.

Local Anesthetic Systemic Toxicity

LAST is a potential complication of local anesthetic administration by any route and most commonly manifests clinically as neurologic or cardiovascular sequelae (see Chapter 22). Resuscitation equipment (intravenous access, airway equipment, emergency medications, and suction) should be readily available when administering local anesthetics. To avoid LAST, strict adherence to recommended local anesthetic doses, methods to detect misplaced needles and catheters (e.g., use of ultrasound), needle and catheter aspiration before injection, and fractional administration of local anesthetic dose are essential.

Despite these precautions, life-threatening convulsions and, rarely, cardiovascular collapse may occur. Seizure activity should be treated with an intravenous benzodiazepine, such as midazolam (1 to 5 mg), or other sedative–hypnotic. Circulation, ventilation, and oxygenation must be maintained. Lipid emulsion (20%, 1.5 mL/kg over 1 minute, followed by 0.25 mL/kg/min for at least 10 minutes after attainment of hemodynamic stability) should be administered concurrently with basic and advanced cardiac life support protocols.[79] Vasopressin, calcium channel blockers, and β-adrenergic blockers should be avoided. Amiodarone may be used to treat ventricular dysrhythmias, particularly those due to bupivacaine. Failure to respond to lipid emulsion and vasopressor therapy should prompt consideration of cardiopulmonary bypass.

Postdural Puncture Headache

By virtue of age and sex, pregnant patients are at higher risk for developing PDPH (see Chapter 35). In addition, after delivery, reduced pressure in the epidural space may increase the risk of cerebrospinal fluid leakage through a dural puncture, and estrogen withdrawal after delivery of the placenta may exacerbate vascular headaches.

The incidence of PDPH is related to the size of the dural puncture, ranging from greater than 70% with a 16-gauge needle to less than 1% with 25-gauge needles. The incidence of headache is reduced with the use of pencil-point needles (Whitacre or Sprotte), compared with cutting bevel (Quincke) spinal needles. Conservative treatment is indicated in the presence of mild-to-moderate discomfort, and includes bed rest, hydration, and simple analgesics. Caffeine (500 mg intravenously or 300 mg orally) has also been used in the treatment of PDPH, but the therapeutic effect is transient. Severe headache that does not respond to conservative measures is best treated with an autologous epidural blood patch. Using aseptic technique, approximately 20 mL of the patient's blood is injected into the lumbar epidural space.[80] Prophylactic administration of autologous blood (after delivery, before removal of the epidural catheter) does not influence the incidence and severity of PDPH, although the duration of headache is shorter compared with expectant management.[81] Data supporting the use of intrathecal catheter placement for prevention of PDPH are inconsistent.[82] PDPH is a self-limited condition; however, recent data suggest that unintentional dural puncture and PDPH are associated with long-term neurologic and psychologic sequelae, including chronic headache, chronic back pain, auditory impairment, and postpartum depression.[83]

Neurologic Injury

Neurologic sequelae of neuraxial blockade, although rare, have been reported. Direct trauma to nerve roots or the spinal cord by a needle or catheter produce immediate pain. Needle or catheter advancement should stop immediately on patient complaint of paresthesia or pain, and if the symptom does not resolve within seconds, the needle or catheter should be withdrawn and repositioned. Anesthetic agents should *not* be injected in the presence of paresthesias. Infections are rare; epidural abscess is usually caused by skin contaminants and meningitis by contamination of drugs or needles with clinicians' nasopharyngeal flora (streptococcus viridans).[84] Epidural hematoma usually occurs in association with coagulation defects. Nerve root irritation recovery may be protracted, lasting weeks or months. Postpartum peripheral nerve injuries, termed obstetric palsies, are more common than anesthesia-related nerve injury and may result from obstetric instrumentation, lithotomy position, or compression of nerves by the fetal head.[85]

Maternal Mortality

While maternal mortality has increased in the United States in recent decades, anesthesia-related deaths have declined to record lows, with only 0.2% of maternal deaths in 2011 to 2013 attributable to anesthesia complications.[86] Historically, general anesthesia has been associated with a higher rate of anesthesia-related deaths compared to neuraxial anesthesia. However, that safety margin has narrowed, with the risk ratio for general to neuraxial anesthesia now only 1.7 (95% confidence interval 0.6 to 4.6).[59] In a review of anesthesia-related maternal mortality 1979 to 2002, mortality was most often associated with cesarean delivery (86%), and the leading causes of death were intubation failure or induction problems (23%), respiratory failure (20%), and high spinal or epidural block (16%).[59]

In the event of maternal cardiac arrest, cardiopulmonary resuscitation should be initiated immediately with two important modifications to American Heart Association (AHA) algorithms: (1) manual left uterine displacement should be performed to decrease aortocaval compression whenever the uterus is at the level of the umbilicus or higher; (2) preparations should be taken to evacuate the uterus (resuscitative hysterotomy) during the initial resuscitation. If return of spontaneous circulation is not achieved with the usual resuscitation measures, perimortem cesarean delivery should be performed, ideally within 5 minutes of the cardiac arrest.[87] The patient should not be moved to an operating room to perform the hysterotomy, as this wastes valuable time. Rather, the delivery should be performed at the site of the arrest. In addition, if magnesium is infusing, it should be discontinued, and calcium should be administered if magnesium toxicity is suspected.

Management of High-Risk Parturients

8 Pregnancy and parturition are considered "high risk" when accompanied by conditions unfavorable to the well-being of the mother, the fetus, or both. Maternal conditions may be related or unrelated to the pregnancy. Specific pregnancy-related conditions include hypertensive disorders of pregnancy, gestational diabetes mellitus, placenta previa, or placental abruption. Chronic medical conditions unrelated to pregnancy include cardiac, renal, neurologic, or hematologic disease as well as asthma, obesity, and substance use disorder. These conditions may or may not affect the pregnancy or be affected by it. Advanced maternal age (AMA)—usually defined as age greater than 35 years at the time of delivery—is associated with increased risk of maternal and fetal complications. Prematurity (gestation <37 weeks), postmaturity (gestation ≥42 weeks), intrauterine growth restriction (IUGR), and multiple gestation constitute high-risk fetal conditions. During labor and delivery, fetal malpresentation (breech, transverse lie), umbilical cord compression (prolapse, nuchal cord), precipitous labor, or intrauterine infection may increase the risk to the mother or the fetus.

In general, the anesthetic management of the high-risk parturient is based on the same maternal and fetal considerations as the management of healthy mothers and fetuses. These include optimization of maternal cardiovascular function and oxygenation, maintenance of adequate uteroplacental blood flow, facilitation of a painless and atraumatic delivery, and avoidance of significant fetal medication exposures. However, many high-risk conditions are associated with diminished physiologic reserve, and thus many of these functions may be compromised prior to the induction of anesthesia. For example, even brief episodes of maternal hypotension following initiation of spinal anesthesia for cesarean birth can lead to significant fetal acidosis in the setting of pre-existing uteroplacental insufficiency (e.g., preeclampsia, diabetes). In addition, high-risk parturients may be prescribed multiple medications for treatment of their comorbidities. Thus, anesthesiologists must be familiar with potential interactions between these drugs and the anesthetic medications they plan to administer.

Women with high-risk pregnancies may require advanced levels of care and the participation of specialists (e.g., maternal–fetal medicine specialists, cardiologists, neonatologists, obstetric anesthesiologists, intensivists) in their care. In order to reduce maternal morbidity and mortality and minimize disparities in obstetric care, the ACOG has defined a classification system for levels of maternal care (Table 41-2).[88] This classification scheme should be used to determine the risk-appropriate level of care for all mothers, especially those with high-risk conditions.

Hypertensive Disorders of Pregnancy

Hypertensive disorders of pregnancy, which complicate up to 10% of pregnancies, are a major cause of maternal morbidity and mortality (NICV 41-3).[89] The ACOG defines four categories of hypertensive disorders—chronic hypertension, gestational hypertension, preeclampsia, and chronic hypertension with superimposed preeclampsia.[90] Chronic hypertension refers to pre-existing hypertension or hypertension that develops during pregnancy prior to 20 weeks of gestation. Gestational hypertension describes the condition of elevated BP after 20 weeks of gestation without proteinuria or signs of end-organ damage. Preeclampsia is defined by hypertension accompanied by proteinuria or other signs or
symptoms of end-organ involvement. Preeclampsia includes a 9
spectrum of end-organ manifestations of the disease—severe hypertension or other end-organ disease is termed preeclampsia with severe features (Table 41-3). Chronic hypertension with superimposed preeclampsia describes the development of preeclampsia in a patient previously diagnosed with chronic hypertension. Eclampsia is defined by new-onset convulsions in a patient with hypertensive disease and no other cause for seizures. HELLP syndrome is a particular form of preeclampsia with severe features characterized by *h*emolysis, *e*levated *l*iver enzymes, and *l*ow *p*latelet count (thrombocytopenia).

Pathophysiology

The pathophysiology of preeclampsia is incompletely understood.[91] Placental ischemia plays a primary role. Multiple etiologic factors may converge to cause the syndrome of preeclampsia. These include endothelial cell dysfunction, intravascular inflammation, and syncytiotrophoblast stress. Maternal, fetal, and placental causes have been identified.[92] In women with preeclampsia, there appears to be an imbalance between proangiogenic factors (vascular endothelial growth factor [VEGF]) and antiangiogenic factors (tyrosine kinase 1 [sFlt-1]).[91]

Systemic Effects

Neurologic

While global cerebral blood flow is not diminished in preeclampsia, focal hypoperfusion may occur due to intense vasoconstriction. Cerebral edema and small foci of degeneration have been attributed to hypoxia. Petechial hemorrhage is common after the onset of convulsions. Related symptoms include headache,

Table 41-2 Maternal Levels of Care

	Birth Center	Level I	Level II	Level III	Level IV
Definition	Care for low-risk women expected to have an uncomplicated birth	Care of low- to moderate-risk pregnancies; ability to detect and stabilize unanticipated maternal or fetal issues until transfer to higher level of care	Level I capabilities plus care of appropriate high-risk antepartum, intrapartum, and postpartum conditions	Level II capabilities plus care of more complex maternal medical conditions, obstetric complications, and fetal conditions	Level III capabilities plus onsite medical and surgical care of the most complex maternal conditions and critically ill parturients and fetuses
Examples of appropriate patients	Term singleton vertex fetus with anticipated uncomplicated delivery	Uncomplicated twin gestation, preeclampsia, labor after cesarean	Placenta previa with no prior uterine surgery, anticipated complicated cesarean delivery	Moderate maternal cardiac disease, suspected invasive placentation	Severe maternal cardiac disease, severe pulmonary hypertension, need for organ transplant
Anesthesia requirement		Anesthesia services readily available at all times	Anesthesiologist readily available at all times	Board-certified anesthesiologist physically present at all times, director of obstetric anesthesia services with obstetric anesthesiology fellowship training or experience in obstetric anesthesiology	Board-certified anesthesiologist with obstetric anesthesiology fellowship or obstetric anesthesiology experience physically present at all times
Delivery provider minimum requirement	Midwife	Qualified birthing professional, physician with privileges to perform emergency cesarean delivery	Obstetrician readily available at all times, obstetric leadership is board-certified in obstetrics-gynecology	Board-certified obstetrician-gynecologist physically present at all times	Board-certified obstetrician-gynecologist physically present at all times
Maternal–fetal medicine specialist requirement			Available for consultation onsite, by phone, or by telemedicine, as needed	Available at all times onsite, by phone, or by telemedicine with inpatient privileges	Available at all times for consultation and management

The American College of Obstetricians and Gynecologists and the Society for Maternal-Fetal levels of maternal care. Adapted from American College of Obstetricians and Gynecologists. Levels of maternal care. *Am J Obstet Gynecol.* 2015 Mar;212(3):259–271. Copyright © 2015 Elsevier. With permission.

Table 41-3 Severe Features of Preeclampsia

Systolic blood pressure ≥160 mmHg OR diastolic blood pressure ≥110 mmHg
- On two occasions, ideally separated by 4 h but can be expedited to facilitate antihypertensive treatment

Neurologic disturbances
- New-onset headache not accounted for by alternative diagnosis and unresponsive to analgesic medication
- Visual disturbances

Pulmonary edema

Thrombocytopenia
- Platelet count <100 × 10^9/L

Liver dysfunction
- Elevation of liver enzyme values to more than twice upper limit of normal
- Severe persistent right upper quadrant pain unresponsive to analgesic medication

Renal insufficiency
- Serum creatinine >1.1 mg/dL
- Serum creatinine doubling from baseline

Adapted with permission from Gestational Hypertension and Preeclampsia: ACOG Practice Bulletin, Number 222. *Obstet Gynecol.* 2020;135:e237–e260.

vertigo, cortical blindness, hyperreflexia, and convulsions. BP elevation correlates poorly with the incidence of seizures. Cerebral hemorrhage and pulmonary edema are leading causes of death in women with eclampsia or preeclampsia with severe features.

Hepatic

Decreased blood supply to the liver may lead to periportal necrosis. Subcapsular hemorrhage can result in right upper quadrant or epigastric pain. Rarely, the overstretched liver capsule may rupture causing massive hemorrhage into the abdominal cavity. Aspartate aminotransferase, lactate dehydrogenase, and alkaline phosphatase may be elevated, whereas bilirubin is unaltered.

Renal

In the kidneys, swelling of glomerular endothelial cells and deposition of fibrin lead to a constriction of the capillary lumina. Renal blood flow and GFR decrease, resulting in reduced uric acid clearance and, in severe cases, reduced clearance of urea and creatinine. Oliguria and proteinuria are characteristic symptoms of severe preeclampsia. The severity of renal involvement is reflected in the degree of proteinuria, which may reach nephrotic levels of 10 to 15 g/24 h.

Pulmonary

Pulmonary edema occurs in approximately 2% of patients with preeclampsia with severe features as a result of magnesium infusion, circulatory overload, heart failure, or aspiration of gastric contents during convulsions. Pulmonary ventilation–perfusion mismatch has also been reported in severe cases; however, arterial oxygen tension typically remains within normal limits. Airway edema, which may also occur, is of great concern because it may lead to difficulty in tracheal intubation.

Vascular

Although preeclampsia is accompanied by exaggerated retention of water and sodium, a shift of fluid and proteins from the intravascular into the extravascular compartment may result in hypovolemia, hypoproteinemia, and hemoconcentration. This phenomenon may be further exacerbated by proteinuria. The risk of uteroplacental hypoperfusion and poor fetal outcome correlates with the degree of maternal plasma and protein depletion. The mean plasma volume in women with severe preeclampsia can be up to 30% to 40% below normal.[93] Volume expansion may improve maternal tissue perfusion in patients with severe disease, but must be balanced against the risk of pulmonary edema.

Hematologic

Adherence of platelets at sites of endothelial damage may result in consumptive coagulopathy and thrombocytopenia, with platelet counts typically ranging from 100×10^9/L to 150×10^9/L. Elevated levels of fibrin degradation products are found less frequently, and plasma fibrinogen concentrations remain normal unless there is placental abruption. Prolongation of prothrombin and partial thromboplastin times indicates consumption of procoagulant factors.

Fetal

Reduction in placental intervillous blood flow may occur, despite elevated maternal BP, due to vasoconstriction or the development of occlusive lesions in decidual arteries. Reduced placental blood flow leads to chronic fetal hypoxia and malnutrition. The risks of IUGR, premature birth, and perinatal death are substantially higher than in normal pregnancies and correlate with the severity of preeclampsia.

General Management

The ACOG recommends that women at high risk of developing preeclampsia initiate prophylactic low-dose aspirin therapy (81 mg/d) between 12 and 28 weeks of gestation (ideally prior to 16 weeks) and continue this therapy until delivery.[90] If preeclampsia develops, the definitive treatment is delivery of the fetus and placenta; however, the decision to pursue delivery or expectant management depends on the severity of maternal disease and the gestational age of the fetus. Expectant management can occur until term (37 weeks' gestational age) for patients with gestational hypertension or preeclampsia without severe features. In the presence of severe features, expectant management can be considered prior to 34 weeks' gestational age; however, delivery is indicated at or beyond this time when the fetal benefits of continued gestation are thought to be outweighed by the risk of maternal complications of continuing the pregnancy. During periods of expectant management, goals are to improve maternal organ and fetal perfusion, normalize BP, correct clotting abnormalities, and prevent or control convulsions. Concerning results of fetal surveillance (e.g., low fetal biophysical profile, absent or reversed diastolic flow on umbilical artery Doppler examination) may necessitate delivery at earlier gestational ages.

Antihypertensive Therapy

Antihypertensive therapy in preeclampsia is used to lower the risk of cerebral hemorrhage, myocardial ischemia, and renal injury in the mother while maintaining tissue and fetal perfusion. The ACOG recommends rapid treatment of hypertension within 30 to 60 minutes when the systolic BP is above 160 mmHg or the diastolic BP is above 110 mmHg.[90] Labetalol and hydralazine are the most commonly used intravenous antihypertensives; however, oral nifedipine may also be used to treat acute hypertension. Invasive arterial BP monitoring may be useful for patients with severely elevated BPs, but central venous pressure monitoring is infrequently used. Transthoracic echocardiography may be used to assess heart function, intravascular volume, and the presence of pulmonary edema. Close hemodynamic monitoring should be extended at least 24 hours into the postpartum period. Preeclampsia may present in the postpartum period.

Magnesium

The mainstay of seizure prevention and therapy for women with preeclampsia with severe features or eclampsia is magnesium sulfate (see Chapter 16). Magnesium sulfate is administered as an intravenous loading dose of 4 to 6 g over 20 to 30 minutes, with therapeutic blood levels (4 to 8 mEq/L) subsequently maintained by continuous infusion of 1 to 2 g/h. Magnesium ions cross the placenta readily and may lead to fetal and neonatal hypermagnesemia; however, magnesium concentrations in the umbilical cord blood are not associated with low Apgar scores or ventilatory depression at birth. Indeed, magnesium therapy has been shown to provide neuroprotective benefits for the fetus and to reduce the risk of cerebral palsy.[94]

Anesthetic Management

Epidural, spinal, or CSE analgesia for labor and delivery may be used in women with preeclampsia. In volume-repleted patients positioned with left uterine displacement, neuraxial analgesia does not cause an unacceptable reduction in BP and may significantly improve placental perfusion. An older study using radioactive xenon found that placental intervillous blood flow increases by up to 75% after the induction of epidural analgesia (10 mL of bupivacaine 0.25%).[95]

Women with preeclampsia are at increased risk for cesarean birth. Historically, spinal anesthesia was avoided in women with severe preeclampsia due to concern for catastrophic hypotension caused by sudden onset of extensive sympathectomy in the setting of intravascular volume depletion. Subsequent studies have shown that women with severe preeclampsia, in fact, demonstrate lower risk of hypotension than normotensive women during spinal anesthesia for cesarean birth.[96] The incidence and severity of hypotension is similar with spinal and epidural anesthesia.[97] It is important to note that women with severe preeclampsia need to be adequately prepared prior to neuraxial anesthesia with judicious hydration and control of BP. Relative hypotension should be avoided with the judicious intraoperative use of vasopressors—an acute decrease in BP is poorly tolerated by both the mother and fetus.

General anesthesia is occasionally required in women with preeclampsia due to contraindication to neuraxial anesthesia or emergency status; several potential hazards should be considered in these circumstances. Rapid-sequence induction of anesthesia and tracheal intubation may be difficult because of edema of the tongue, epiglottis, or pharynx (see Chapter 28). In patients with impaired coagulation, laryngoscopy and tracheal intubation may provoke profuse bleeding. Marked systemic and pulmonary hypertension occurring at intubation and extubation increases the risk of cerebral hemorrhage and pulmonary edema; these hemodynamic changes should be minimized with appropriate antihypertensive therapy. The use of ketamine and ergot alkaloids should be avoided in the setting of uncontrolled hypertension. Magnesium may prolong the effects of neuromuscular blockers through its actions on the myoneural junction. Therefore, nondepolarizing muscle relaxants should be administered with caution and accompanied by neuromuscular blockade monitoring to avoid overdose. Consumptive coagulopathy, if present, predisposes patients to postpartum hemorrhage and need for transfusion (see Chapter 17).

Obstetric Hemorrhage

10 Worldwide, obstetric hemorrhage remains the leading cause of maternal mortality, causing approximately 25% of maternal deaths. The vast majority of these deaths occur in low-resource settings; however, there is evidence that the rate and severity of hemorrhage are increasing in developed nations, including the United States.[98]

Antepartum Hemorrhage

Antepartum hemorrhage complicates 3% to 5% of pregnancies and is a leading contributor to both maternal and perinatal mortality worldwide.[99] It occurs most commonly in association with placenta previa and placental abruption. Placenta previa refers to abnormal placental implantation on the lower uterine segment with partial-to-total occlusion of the internal cervical os. Risk factors for placenta previa include a uterine scar from prior cesarean birth or other surgery, tobacco use, AMA, multiparity, and multiple gestation. The risk for placenta previa and placenta accreta spectrum increases in a "dose-dependent" manner with the number of previous cesarean deliveries and greater parity. The diagnosis should be suspected whenever a patient presents with painless, bright red vaginal bleeding, usually after the seventh month of pregnancy. The diagnosis is confirmed by ultrasonography. If bleeding is not profuse and the fetus is immature, expectant management is warranted to prolong pregnancy. Admission to a high-risk unit is advisable if contractions or acute bleeding are present. Intravenous access and typed and cross-matched blood should be available. In severe cases, or if the fetus is mature at the onset of symptoms, prompt cesarean birth is indicated. Vaginal birth is contraindicated in the setting of placenta previa.

Neuraxial anesthesia is the preferred technique for delivery in patients with placenta previa, provided the mother is hemodynamically stable and no contraindications exist. General anesthesia is associated with greater blood loss and greater need for transfusion. Placenta previa is associated with both uterine atony and placenta accreta, both of which may lead to postpartum hemorrhage. The risk of placenta accreta in women with previa increases from 3% in primary cesarean deliveries to 61% in patients with three prior cesareans.[100]

Placental abruption complicates approximately 1% of deliveries, usually in the final 10 weeks of gestation (NICV 41-4). Risk factors include tobacco use, trauma, cocaine use, multiple gestation, hypertension, preeclampsia, AMA, and preterm premature rupture of membranes. While maternal mortality is rare (<1%), the perinatal mortality rate ranges from 9% to 12% in developed countries.[101] The diagnosis of placental abruption is based on the presence of uterine tenderness and hypertonus as well as vaginal bleeding of dark, clotted blood. Bleeding may be concealed if the placental margins have remained attached to the uterine wall. If the blood loss is severe, changes in the maternal BP and pulse rate, indicative of hypovolemia may be present.

When placental separation is more than 50%, stillbirth is the likeliest outcome. Management of abruption depends on presentation, gestational age, and the degree of compromise. Management of milder cases of abruption includes artificial rupture of amniotic membranes and oxytocin augmentation of labor, if required. Distant from term, expectant management with close observation is reasonable. In the presence of nonreassuring fetal status, an emergency cesarean birth may be indicated. If fetal death has occurred in the setting of severe abruption, attempted vaginal birth is reasonable if the mother is stable. Placental abruption can lead to coagulation abnormalities, including disseminated intravascular coagulation. Coagulation studies should be followed closely and preparation for massive blood loss and resuscitation is indicated. Neuraxial analgesia and anesthesia are appropriate if the mother is hemodynamically stable and coagulation parameters are normal.

Postpartum Hemorrhage

Postpartum hemorrhage has historically been defined as blood loss greater than 500 mL after vaginal birth or greater than 1,000 mL after cesarean birth (NICV 41-5). Recent guidance published by the ACOG, however, defines postpartum hemorrhage as blood loss ≥1,000 mL after any type of delivery or any volume of blood loss accompanied by signs or symptoms of hypovolemia within 24 hours after birth.[102] Postpartum hemorrhage may occur in the setting of uterine atony, abnormal placentation, and genital tract trauma (Table 41-4). The incidence of postpartum hemorrhage is increasing in the United States, mainly due to an increase in uterine atony, which accounts for >70% of cases.[98] Predisposing factors for atony include multiple gestation, labor induction or augmentation, cesarean birth, polyhydramnios, chorioamnionitis, hypertensive disorders of pregnancy, and antepartum hemorrhage, among others.[103]

Abnormal placentation, a spectrum of diseases including placenta accreta, placenta increta, and placenta percreta (termed placenta accreta spectrum), is a serious and life-threatening cause of postpartum hemorrhage. As the incidence continues to increase, placenta accreta is becoming the leading cause of cesarean hysterectomy.[104] The average blood loss during delivery of patients with placenta accreta is 3 to 5 L. When abnormal placentation is suspected or known, delivery is usually scheduled at 34 to 36 weeks of gestation via planned cesarean hysterectomy.[105] Under controlled, elective conditions, complications can be minimized. The use of vascular occlusive balloon catheters (placed in the internal iliac arteries or aorta prior to surgical delivery) is controversial and is currently not recommended by the ACOG

Table 41-4 Etiologies of Postpartum Hemorrhage

Uterine atony
Genital tract trauma Episiotomy Perineal laceration Vaginal laceration Cervical laceration
Retained products of conception
Abnormally invasive placenta Placenta accreta Placenta increta Placenta percreta
Coagulation defects Inherited Acquired
Uterine inversion

Table 41-5 Uterotonic Therapy

Drug	Dose	Side Effects
Oxytocin[a]	Bolus 1–3 IU IV, start infusion 2.5–15 IU/h[b] or Infusion 18–36 IU/h IV[b]	Hypotension, tachycardia
Methylergonovine[c]	0.2 mg IM q2–4h	Hypertension, vasoconstriction Coronary vasospasm
15-Methylprostaglandin F_2 alpha[c]	0.25 mg IM q15–60 min	Bronchospasm ↑ pulmonary vascular resistance Nausea
Misoprostol[c]	800–1,000 µg PR/PO q2h	Fever Nausea

IM, intramuscularly; IV, intravenous; PO, orally (or sublingual or buccal); PR, rectally; ↑, increase.
[a]Oxytocin is administered prophylactically.
[b]Lower doses are used for elective caesarean delivery, higher doses are used for intrapartum caesarean delivery.
[c]Additional therapeutic uterotonic usually administered in the setting of uterine atony.

although the technique is used in some institutions. Ureteral stents may be considered on a case-by-case basis.

Anesthetic Management

The anesthesiologist's role in management of obstetric hemorrhage includes both maternal resuscitation and provision of anesthesia for cesarean birth, cesarean hysterectomy, or dilation and curettage. The choice of anesthetic technique depends on the anticipated duration and urgency of the surgery as well as maternal hemodynamic, volume, and coagulation status. General anesthesia is indicated in the presence of uncontrolled hemorrhage and/or severe coagulation abnormalities. Neuraxial anesthesia, usually CSE or epidural anesthesia, has been successfully used for hysterectomy in planned, controlled situations.

Treatment of postpartum hemorrhage may require aggressive uterotonic therapy for atony (Table 41-5), intrauterine balloon tamponade, or evacuation of the uterus for retained products of conception. If there is a need for dilation and curettage, the anesthesiologist may be asked to provide uterine relaxation. This can be accomplished in the awake patient with sublingual or intravenous nitroglycerin or with volatile agents if the patient is receiving general anesthesia.

Maternal resuscitation in the setting of hemorrhage may require rapid tracheal intubation if significant hemodynamic instability occurs, in addition to obtaining large-bore intravenous, arterial, and possibly central venous access. All of these tasks may be challenging in the parturient and consideration should be given to performing them in advance of an anticipated hemorrhage or early during the course of bleeding. Prompt transfusion of blood component therapy is crucial for replacement of blood loss, maintenance of tissue oxygenation, and correction of coagulopathy.

Transfusion practices for postpartum hemorrhage have been adapted from published studies of trauma patients, given that hypothermia, metabolic acidosis, and coagulopathy commonly occur in both traumatic and obstetric hemorrhage. Transfusion of packed red blood cells and plasma in a 1:1 ratio decreases mortality from hemorrhage in trauma patients, and early administration of platelets and cryoprecipitate has also become common in hemostatic resuscitation protocols for major traumatic hemorrhage (see Chapter 53). Transfusion of cryoprecipitate or fibrinogen concentrate should be considered early in obstetric hemorrhage because decreased fibrinogen levels strongly correlate with severity of postpartum hemorrhage.[12,106] Obstetric hemorrhage is associated with the rapid development of consumptive and dilutional coagulopathy which can be quickly assessed using viscoelastic assessment (i.e., thromboelastography [TEG] or rotational thromboelastometry [ROTEM] [see Chapter 17]) of coagulation.

Other treatment options are available to decrease transfusion requirements and reduce blood loss. The antifibrinolytic drug tranexamic acid has been shown to decrease bleeding in both elective cesarean birth as well as postpartum hemorrhage. The use of tranexamic acid was associated with decreased death due to bleeding in a large, international, randomized trial, and its early use is now recommended in resuscitation for postpartum hemorrhage.[107] Intraoperative cell salvage, historically avoided because of concerns about the risk of amniotic fluid contamination, has been implemented safely during cesarean birth in many centers.[108]

All obstetric units should have protocols in place for the management of obstetric hemorrhage, which include antepartum risk assessment, diagnosis, and management of high-risk patients and intraoperative management of hemorrhage (e.g., obstetric rapid-response team, massive transfusion protocols).[109]

Heart Disease

The incidence of heart disease during pregnancy is steadily increasing due to AMA and associated cardiovascular risk factors. In addition, advancement in care of women with congenital heart disease has led to improved survival into adulthood and childbearing years.[110] Cardiovascular conditions are now responsible for over a quarter of all pregnancy-related deaths in the United States.[86] Many forms of maternal cardiovascular disease are exacerbated by physiologic changes of pregnancy related to stroke volume, heart rate, CO, blood volume, and systemic vascular resistance. For this reason, cardiac decompensation occurs most commonly during the third trimester, during labor and delivery, and during the immediate postpartum period, when physiologic changes are most pronounced.

Evaluation of pre-existing heart disease is crucial, and a multidisciplinary approach is necessary when managing patients with complicated cardiac disease during pregnancy. Diagnosing a new cardiac condition during pregnancy can be challenging due to typical pregnancy symptoms mimicking those of cardiac disease. For example, shortness of breath and venous stasis from aortocaval compression can be difficult to distinguish from pulmonary and peripheral edema associated with congestive heart failure. Flow murmurs may be difficult to distinguish from those due to pathologic valvular lesions. For the anesthesiologist, it is particularly important to understand how the hemodynamic consequences of different anesthetic techniques might adversely affect mothers with specific cardiac lesions. Invasive monitoring during labor and delivery is rarely indicated with the possible exceptions of women with pulmonary hypertension, right-to-left shunts, and coarctation of the aorta. Because hemodynamic changes observed during labor and delivery persist into the postpartum period, invasive monitoring, if used, should continue for 24 to 48 hours postpartum.

Importantly, anesthesiologists should have knowledge of risk stratification for pregnant patients with cardiac disease. The modified World Health Organization (mWHO) risk classification defines four risk classes, with specific examples of cardiac lesions belonging to each class.[111] Patients with mWHO risk class III or IV should be referred to facilities with higher maternal levels of care.

Congenital Heart Disease

The risks of pregnancy in patients with congenital heart disease vary depending on the severity of the underlying structural defect and whether surgical correction has occurred.

Many patients with successful surgical repair will go on to have asymptomatic, uncomplicated pregnancies. In contrast, patients with uncorrected or partially corrected lesions may experience cardiac decompensation due to physiologic changes associated with pregnancy and delivery.

Patients in mWHO risk class I or II can generally be cared for in local hospitals, without the need for transfer to a higher level of maternal care. Specific cardiac lesions in these classes include repaired patent ductus arteriosus, repaired tetrology of Fallot, and repaired aortic coarctation. Patients with corrected or small uncorrected ventricular septal defects or atrial septal defects require no special care. With larger or symptomatic defects, neuraxial analgesia will minimize the increase in SVR associated with elevated catecholamines, thus minimizing left-to-right shunting. In severe, untreated left-to-right shunts, Eisenmenger syndrome can occur, resulting in pulmonary hypertension and reversal of flow to a right-to-left shunt. Pregnancy is not well tolerated in this setting and mortality can be as high as 20% to 50%.[112] Management is challenging, and these patients should be referred to Level IV maternal care centers. Consideration should also be given to refer patients with Fontan circulation, unrepaired cyanotic heart disease, and atrioventricular septal defects to high-risk centers.

Valvular Heart Disease

Anesthetic management of patients with valvular heart disease includes tailoring hemodynamic goals to the specific valvular lesion (Table 41-6) as well as managing anticoagulation in patients with mechanical heart valves. Maternal morbidity and mortality are greatest with left-sided stenotic valvular lesions and those accompanied by ventricular dysfunction or pulmonary hypertension. Symptoms of left-sided stenotic lesions are exacerbated by the physiologic changes of pregnancy. Pregnancy-induced increases in blood volume, heart rate, and CO contribute to pulmonary edema, heart failure, arrhythmias, and even death in these patients, with the greatest risk during labor and immediately following delivery. In contrast, valvular regurgitant lesions are generally well tolerated during pregnancy—decreased afterload associated with pregnancy and neuraxial procedures can improve maternal hemodynamics.

In patients requiring therapeutic anticoagulation due to mechanical valves, warfarin is often discontinued during the first trimester due to teratogenic effects but is usually restarted during the second trimester and continued to near term. Warfarin is typically transitioned to unfractionated heparin prior to delivery.[113] The Society for Obstetric Anesthesia and Perinatology recommends holding intravenous unfractionated heparin for 4 to 6 hours, and low-molecular-weight heparin for 24 hours, prior to performing a neuraxial procedure for labor analgesia or cesarean anesthesia.[114] Resuming anticoagulation after delivery requires coordination with the obstetric and cardiology teams.

Table 41-6 Hemodynamic Goals with Valvular Heart Lesions

Lesion	Goal
Aortic stenosis	Sinus rhythm Maintain HR Avoid ↓ SVR Maintain venous return
Aortic insufficiency	Mild ↑ HR Avoid ↑ SVR
Mitral stenosis	Sinus rhythm ↓ HR Maintain SVR Maintain venous return
Mitral insufficiency	Sinus rhythm Mild ↑ HR Avoid ↑ SVR Avoid ↑ venous return

HR, heart rate; ↑, increase; ↓, decrease; SVR, systemic vascular resistance.

Pulmonary Hypertension

Pulmonary hypertension is defined as mean pulmonary artery pressure ≥25 mmHg, and pulmonary *arterial* hypertension (PAH) describes a subset of pulmonary hypertension with elevated pulmonary vascular resistance and normal left ventricular filling pressures. Although uncommon in pregnancy, PAH is associated with very high maternal mortality. Pregnancy is discouraged in these patients, and termination is advised should pregnancy occur. Antepartum and peripartum care in a regional prenatal health center (Maternal Level of Care IV) is recommended.

The mode of delivery for patients with PAH is controversial. Vaginal delivery is associated with smaller hemodynamic shifts and decreased risk of bleeding. However, emergency cesarean delivery for maternal or fetal deterioration may be required. Planned cesarean delivery offers the advantage of ensuring optimal conditions and availability of experienced staff.

Pain during labor and vaginal delivery is especially detrimental because it may further increase pulmonary vascular resistance and decrease CO. Neuraxial analgesia is useful in attenuating these hemodynamic changes. General and epidural anesthesia have been used successfully for cesarean delivery; however, single-shot spinal anesthesia is not recommended due to the abrupt decrease in SVR associated with this technique. Maternal mortality from PAH is estimated between 16% and 30%, with most deaths due to right heart failure during labor or the early postpartum period.[112]

Cardiomyopathy

Peripartum cardiomyopathy is left ventricular systolic dysfunction occurring late in pregnancy or in the first 6 weeks postpartum. Most cases are diagnosed after delivery. It occurs in approximately 1 in 3,000 births and is associated with a maternal mortality of 10% to 25%.[112] Peripartum cardiomyopathy is a diagnosis of exclusion; the cause is thought to be related to myocarditis or an abnormal immune response. Risk factors include AMA, multiparity, multiple gestation, smoking, diabetes, obesity, and preeclampsia.[112] Good long-term prognosis is related to recovery of left ventricular function within 6 months of delivery. Left ventricular ejection fraction of less than 30% at diagnosis, significant left ventricular dilation, and involvement of the right ventricle are associated with adverse outcomes, and these patients should be counseled against future pregnancies. Medical management includes preload optimization, afterload reduction, and therapy to improve myocardial contractility. Some patients require thromboprophylaxis or automatic implantable cardioverter defibrillator placement. Intrapartum anesthetic management goals include avoiding bradycardia, maintaining afterload and contractility, ensuring normovolemia, and preventing development of pulmonary edema.

Ischemic Heart Disease

Acute myocardial infarction during pregnancy is rare, occurring in 1 in 20,000 women; however, it is associated with high maternal (7%) and fetal (7%) mortality.[112] Approximately one in five maternal cardiac deaths is the result of coronary artery disease. As more women with risk factors become pregnant, this complication will continue to increase in frequency. The left anterior descending artery is most commonly affected, with 18% of infarcts associated with coronary spasm (i.e., normal angiogram) and 43% associated with spontaneous coronary artery dissection. Risk factors include smoking, obesity, AMA, diabetes, hypertension, and hyperlipidemia. Women older than 35 years are at greatest risk, and the risk is 30-fold higher in women older than 40 years, compared to those younger than 20 years. Ergot alkaloids should be avoided in women with ischemic heart disease because they can lead to coronary vasospasm. Cocaine use has also been implicated in coronary spasm.

Diagnosis of myocardial ischemia may be difficult, as symptoms of ischemia may mimic common nonspecific complaints during pregnancy. Thus, the greatest obstacle to diagnosis is a low index of suspicion. Cardiac troponin I levels are increased if cardiac muscle injury occurs; however, preeclampsia and gestational hypertension are also accompanied by an increase in troponin levels. Therefore, ECG is an important diagnostic tool.

Delivery within 2 weeks of the infarct is associated with a high rate of reinfarction and death. Thus, delaying delivery, if possible, should be considered. Vaginal delivery is associated with lower morbidity and mortality than cesarean delivery. Intrapartum monitoring should mimic intraoperative monitoring of the nonobstetric patient with a recent myocardial infarction.

Arrhythmias

Tachyarrythmias, including atrial fibrillation and paroxysmal supraventricular tachycardia, are the most common arrhythmias in pregnant patients and occur in approximately 1 in 2,000 pregnancies. These arrhythmias may present for the first time or increase in frequency during pregnancy due to atrial stretching which is exacerbated by pregnancy-associated physiologic changes in the cardiovascular system. Adenosine or electrical cardioversion is recommended in the setting of hemodynamic instability, while pharmacologic rhythm control is the preferred treatment for stable atrial fibrillation. Ventricular tachycardia, ventricular fibrillation, bradyarrhythmias, and atrioventricular block are rare during pregnancy.[112]

Aortic Disease

Heritable or acquired aortic disease is rare but may cause fatal complications in pregnancy. Many syndromes are known to be associated with both aneurysm and dissection of the thoracic aorta, including Marfan syndrome, Loeys–Dietz syndrome, and Ehlers-Danlos type IV. Marfan syndrome affects approximately 1 in 5,000 patients and is associated with an overall 3% risk of aortic dissection during pregnancy.[112] Risk is increased to 10% in patients with aortic root diameter >40 mm, history of prior dissection, or recent rapid aortic root dilation.[110] Any patient with aortic root diameter >45 mm should be counseled to avoid pregnancy. β-Adrenergic blockers are recommended in women with aortopathy during pregnancy, as they have been shown to reduce the risk of aortic dissection.

Diabetes Mellitus

Diabetes mellitus complicates approximately 7% of pregnancies, with gestational diabetes constituting the majority of cases (nearly 90%).[115] Pregestational diabetes includes type 1 cases, caused by autoimmune destruction of pancreatic β cells, and type 2 cases, caused by insulin resistance and relative insulin deficiency. Gestational diabetes mellitus is defined as diabetes or glucose intolerance that is first diagnosed during pregnancy. The incidence of gestational diabetes is increasing across all ethnic and racial groups corresponding with rising rates of obesity.[116] Gestational diabetes mellitus is associated with adverse pregnancy outcomes, including macrosomia, neonatal hypoglycemia, hyperbilirubinemia, and intrauterine fetal demise, as well as an increased risk of obesity and diabetes in offspring. Women with gestational diabetes mellitus are at increased risk for development of type 2 diabetes later in life.[117]

Pre-existing type 1 or 2 diabetes is also associated with adverse pregnancy outcomes, including congenital malformations. Diabetes-associated vasculopathy, nephropathy, and retinopathy may be exacerbated by pregnancy. Tight glycemic control before and during pregnancy may decrease the risk of these adverse outcomes. Normal physiologic changes of pregnancy can trigger diabetic ketoacidosis, especially in patients with type 1 diabetes. Diabetic ketoacidosis occurs at lower glucose levels in pregnancy due to enhanced lipogenesis and ketogenesis. β-Adrenergic agonist therapy and glucocorticoid administration (e.g., administered to enhance fetal lung maturity in the setting of preterm delivery) may also increase the likelihood of developing this complication. Although maternal mortality from diabetic ketoacidosis is unusual, fetal mortality is high.

Guidelines for the management of diabetes during pregnancy focus on glycemic control. Glucose levels should be maintained near physiologic levels throughout pregnancy, and insulin therapy is preferred if glucose levels are not well controlled with diet and exercise.[115,118] Maternal insulin requirements increase progressively during the second and third trimesters. Fetal surveillance is more intense in women with diabetes. Antenatal surveillance with twice-weekly nonstress tests often begins at 28 weeks of gestation. Current evidence does not support the superiority of vaginal or planned cesarean delivery in women with estimated fetal weight >4,500 g; therefore, the ACOG recommends counseling individual women on the risks and benefits of both modes of delivery.[115]

There is no compelling evidence that one analgesic or anesthetic technique is superior to another when caring for parturients with diabetes. Patients with pregestational diabetes should be assessed for comorbidities such as hypertension and renal disease. Neuraxial labor analgesia does not appear to alter peripartum insulin and glucose requirements. Intrapartum blood glucose levels should be monitored frequently, and glucose administration and insulin therapy should be titrated to maintain maternal glucose concentration between 60 and 120 mg/dL in the peripartum period. Insulin requirements typically begin to decrease shortly after delivery.

Obesity

In the United States, obesity complicates more than half of all pregnancies, with significant implications for anesthetic and obstetric management. Women with obesity are more likely to have antenatal comorbidities, such as hypertension, diabetes mellitus, and obstructive sleep apnea.[119] Obstetric outcomes may also be affected by maternal obesity, as there is a greater risk of macrosomia, prolonged labor, failed induction, and cesarean delivery.[120] Antepartum anesthetic consultation of parturients with morbid obesity should be considered to evaluate comorbidities, anticipate potential complications, and generate a multidisciplinary care plan. The use of general anesthesia for cesarean delivery is higher in parturients with obesity, and difficult tracheal intubation is more likely than in nonobese peers. Thus, anesthetic evaluation should include a thorough airway examination and alternative airway equipment must be readily available during delivery. Continuous neuraxial analgesia is the preferred option for pain relief during labor because it avoids potential sedation or obtundation from systemic medication administration. Most importantly, a well-functioning neuraxial anesthetic for labor may be used for anesthesia for operative vaginal or cesarean delivery, thus avoiding general anesthesia and airway manipulation. For cesarean delivery, the choice of anesthetic depends on maternal and fetal conditions. Of note, difficult epidural catheter placement, number of attempts, and likelihood of epidural failure are all associated with increasing body mass index. Obesity is further associated with an increased risk for maternal mortality related to increased incidence of infection, diabetes, preeclampsia, uterine atony and hemorrhage, and thromboembolism. Anesthesia-related morbidity and mortality are also increased, primarily related to airway difficulties.[119] For these reasons, women with obesity require more intensive monitoring in the postpartum period.

Advanced Maternal Age

As reproductive technologies improve and more women are delaying childbearing, pregnancies in women of AMA are becoming more prevalent. In the United States in 2020, the mean age of mothers at the time of first delivery was over 27 years.[121,122] Comorbidities and obstetric complications, such as gestational diabetes, hypertensive diseases, placenta previa, and placental abruption, are more common in parturients with AMA. Pregestational hypertension occurs more frequently in patients over 30 years of age, and patients with chronic hypertension are more likely to develop superimposed preeclampsia, deliver preterm, and deliver via cesarean than normotensive patients.[123] Further, older parturients are more likely to require prolonged hospitalization and to be admitted to the intensive care unit than those who are younger.

Perinatal complications are also significantly increased in patients with AMA. Multiple gestations, both naturally occurring and via assisted reproduction, are more common in older gravidae. The incidence of miscarriage, congenital anomalies, preterm delivery, fetal growth restriction, low birth weight, and intrauterine and neonatal death increase with advancing age.[121]

Anticoagulation

Several physiologic changes of pregnancy predispose patients to thrombosis including increased platelet aggregation, increased coagulation factor levels (II, VII, VIII, IX, X, XII, XIII, von Willebrand Factor), and decreased endogenous anticoagulants (protein C, protein S). As a result, venous thromboembolism is now a leading cause of maternal death in the United States. Expanding use of thromboprophylaxis to decrease morbidity and mortality from thromboembolism has significant impacts on antepartum and intrapartum anesthetic management. The Society for Obstetric Anesthesia and Perinatology has published obstetric-specific guidance for use of neuraxial anesthesia following varying doses of prophylactic and therapeutic anticoagulation medications.[114]

Maternal Cardiac Arrest

Cardiac arrest during hospitalization for delivery occurs in approximately 1 in 12,000 delivery admissions.[124] In the event of cardiac arrest after approximately 20 weeks of gestation, continuous manual left uterine displacement should be maintained during cardiopulmonary resuscitation. Considerations specific to pregnancy include intravenous access placement above the diaphragm to ensure proper circulation of medications, anticipation of difficult airway, and discontinuation of magnesium sulfate if applicable. Preparations should be made to evacuate the uterus (termed perimortem cesarean delivery or resuscitative hysterotomy) while resuscitative measures are ongoing. If return of spontaneous circulation is not achieved, the uterus should be evacuated, ideally within 5 minutes of the cardiac arrest.[87] This improves both maternal and infant survival.

Preterm Delivery

Preterm delivery, or delivery prior to 37 completed weeks of gestation, occurs in approximately 11% of all births and accounts for up to 35% of neonatal deaths.[125] In general, the mortality and morbidity rates are higher among preterm infants than among small-for-gestational-age infants of comparable weight. Severe problems that may develop in preterm infants are respiratory distress syndrome, intracranial hemorrhage, hypoglycemia, hypocalcemia, and hyperbilirubinemia. With improved neonatal intensive care, preterm infants who weigh over 1,500 g often survive without severe long-term impairment. The very low birth weight infant (<1,500 g) is still at greater risk for significant long-term impairment.

In the absence of contraindications, obstetricians may administer uterine relaxants (tocolytics) in an effort to stop preterm contractions. Contraindications include uterine infection, severe hemorrhage, nonreassuring fetal status, and fetal death or anomalies incompatible with life. When appropriate, tocolysis may delay delivery long enough for maternal glucocorticoid administration which improves fetal lung maturity. Calcium channel blockers, prostaglandin inhibitors, and β-adrenergic agonists are medication classes used for tocolysis. While magnesium does attenuate uterine contractions, its use solely as a tocolytic is not recommended. Magnesium may, however, be used in the setting of preterm labor prior to 34 weeks' gestation to reduce the risk of cerebral palsy.[94]

The premature infant is more vulnerable than the term newborn to the effects of drugs used in obstetric analgesia and anesthesia. However, there have been few systematic studies to determine the maternal and fetal pharmacokinetics and dynamics of drugs throughout gestation. There are several postulated causes of enhanced drug sensitivity in the preterm newborn, including the following:

- Less plasma protein available for drug binding
- Higher bilirubin levels (competes for protein binding sites)
- Poorly developed blood–brain barrier allowing greater drug access to the fetal CNS
- Decreased drug metabolism and excretion.

In selection of the anesthetic drugs and techniques for delivery of a preterm infant, concerns regarding drug effects on the newborn are far less important than prevention of asphyxia and trauma to the fetus. Preterm infants with breech presentation are usually delivered by cesarean as are very low birth weight infants (<1,500 g) due to concern for head entrapment during vaginal delivery. If unanticipated vaginal delivery occurs with a breech infant, general anesthesia with volatile anesthetic agents or nitroglycerin may be needed for uterine relaxation if head entrapment occurs.

The administration of tocolytic medications also has several implications for anesthetic management. Calcium channel blockers can cause vasodilation and myocardial depression, leading to systemic hypotension, as well as cardiac conduction defects. β-Adrenergic agonists produce significant maternal tachycardia and can cause pulmonary edema in rare cases. Magnesium sulfate, if used for fetal and neonatal neuroprotection, can exacerbate hypotension and potentiate neuromuscular blockade of both depolarizing and nondepolarizing muscle relaxants.

Substance Use Disorder

The most commonly used substances during pregnancy are alcohol, tobacco, cocaine, marijuana, opioids, and amphetamines. Substance use disorder may result in obstetric crises that require the intervention or assistance of an anesthesiologist and may significantly impact intrapartum anesthetic management. Diagnosis of the patient who is not under the acute effect of a substance at admission may be made when she, or her infant, develops withdrawal symptoms or the newborn is diagnosed with a syndrome related to in utero exposure. Women often use more than one drug; therefore, the newborn's presentation may reflect the impact of multiple drug exposures, acute, chronic, or both.

Tobacco

Tobacco is the most commonly used substance during pregnancy. Smoking during pregnancy has been associated with spontaneous abortion, IUGR, premature rupture of membranes, placental previa, placenta abruption, preterm delivery, impaired respiratory function in newborns, and sudden infant death syndrome. The pregnant patient who smokes is at greater risk for bronchitis, pneumonia, and asthma. Nicotine causes vasoconstriction and thus may decrease placental blood flow and oxygen delivery to the fetus. Paradoxically, however, smoking appears to be protective for the development of preeclampsia.

Alcohol

Heavy alcohol consumption may be associated with liver disease, coagulopathy, cardiomyopathy, esophageal varies, and altered drug metabolism in pregnant women. In the fetus, maternal alcohol use is linked to fetal alcohol syndrome. The prevalence of fetal alcohol syndrome is approximately one-third of infants of heavy drinkers (>28 g absolute alcohol or two drinks per day). Neurobehavioral deficits and IUGR have been demonstrated in infants of moderate drinkers (>14 g absolute alcohol or one drink per day). The parturient who uses alcohol is at further increased risk for pulmonary aspiration compared with the average pregnant woman. Acute alcohol withdrawal may present within 6 to 48 hours of abstinence; thus, it may occur intrapartum or postpartum. The signs and symptoms of alcohol withdrawal include nausea and vomiting, hypertension, tachycardia, dysrhythmias, seizures, and cardiac failure.

Opioids

The prevalence of opioid use and abuse during pregnancy is rapidly increasing, with nearly one in five women in the United States filling an opioid prescription while pregnant. For women seeking treatment for opioid use disorder during pregnancy, opioid agonist pharmacotherapy with buprenorphine or methadone is recommended due to worse outcomes with medically supervised withdrawal.[126]

The anesthetic management of a woman with opioid use disorder should include continuation of opioids throughout labor and into the postpartum period to prevent acute opioid withdrawal. Thus, methadone or buprenorphine for opioid maintenance should also be continued. Neuraxial labor analgesia and cesarean delivery anesthesia are safe in these patients; the efficacy of local anesthetics is not affected by chronic opioid use. In contrast, neuraxially administered opioids are likely to have diminished effect due to opioid receptor downregulation and occupation of opioid binding sites by methadone or buprenorphine.

Women who chronically use opioids are likely to have increased opioid requirements perioperatively if cesarean delivery is required. Due to difficulties with postoperative pain control, patients on chronic opioids should be offered multimodal cesarean analgesia, including regular administration of nonsteroidal anti-inflammatory drugs and acetaminophen, truncal nerve blocks, and postoperative neuraxial analgesia. Mixed opioid agonists–antagonists such as nalbuphine are contraindicated in the setting of chronic opioid use due to the risk of precipitating withdrawal. Neonates of mothers with opioid use disorder should be monitored for neonatal abstinence syndrome, which is characterized by gastrointestinal, autonomic, and CNS dysfunction.[126]

Marijuana

Marijuana is frequently used by women of childbearing age. Δ-9-Tetrahydrocannabinol (THC) readily crosses the placenta and may directly affect the fetus. It has been associated with IUGR.[127] Pregnant women who chronically smoke marijuana have an increased incidence of respiratory problems, including bronchitis and emphysema, and thus may be at risk for respiratory complications related to general anesthesia. Acute marijuana use may be associated with cardiovascular stimulation at moderate doses and myocardial depression at higher doses.

Cocaine

Women acutely ingesting cocaine generally display euphoria, tachycardia, and hypertension (Table 41-7). More serious manifestations may include seizure and coma, myocardial infarction, pulmonary edema, and subarachnoid hemorrhage. Cerebrovascular accidents associated with cocaine use may result from severe hypertension leading to cerebral hemorrhage or vasospasm causing cerebral infarction. Sudden death may occur from a lethal ventricular dysrhythmia. Therapy is supportive, primarily aimed at controlling cardiovascular and CNS consequences. Cocaine use in the first trimester may cause congenital anomalies. Later in

Table 41-7 Anesthetic Considerations Associated with Cocaine and/or Amphetamine Use

- Uncontrolled hypertension
- Cardiac dysrhythmias (ventricular tachycardia/fibrillation)
- Myocardial ischemia
- Ephedrine-resistant hypotension with neuraxial blockade (use direct-acting agent)
- Acute intake may increase MAC of volatile agents
- Chronic use may decrease MAC of anesthetic agents
- May have increased sensitivity to arrhythmogenic effects of volatile agents

MAC, minimum alveolar concentration.

pregnancy, cocaine use may be associated with premature labor, IUGR, uteroplacental insufficiency, or placental abruption.

The choice of anesthetic depends on maternal and fetal conditions, the planned procedure (vaginal or cesarean delivery), and urgency. Sympathetic stimulation associated with general anesthesia and laryngoscopy may cause uncontrolled hypertension, tachycardia, and life-threatening dysrhythmias in women using cocaine. Pure β-adrenergic antagonist medications should be avoided because of the potential for worsening hypertension related to unopposed α-adrenergic receptor stimulation by cocaine. The minimum alveolar concentration of anesthetics may be increased with acute ingestion and decreased with chronic exposure to cocaine.

Cocaine use may also complicate neuraxial anesthesia. Cocaine is a local anesthetic, and systemic toxicity may be additive when using amide local anesthetics for epidural anesthesia. Ester local anesthetics compete with cocaine for metabolism, resulting in decreased metabolism of both drugs. Chronic cocaine use may be associated with thrombocytopenia. The incidence and severity of hypotension related to neuraxial anesthesia may be greater in parturients who chronically use cocaine compared with controls, and hypotension may be more difficult to treat. Direct-acting vasoactive agents are more effective and predictable for treating hypotension than indirect-acting agents (e.g., ephedrine).

Amphetamines

Amphetamines are noncatecholamine sympathomimetic drugs. They are often abused in conjunction with other CNS stimulants such as cocaine. They can be taken orally, intravenously (methamphetamine), or smoked (crystal methamphetamine). Ecstasy is an analog of methamphetamine. Amphetamine use leads to an increased release of norepinephrine, causing hypertension, tachycardia, dysrhythmias, dilated pupils, hyperpyrexia, proteinuria, agitation, confusion, and seizures. These signs and symptoms closely resemble those of cocaine use. Methamphetamine use has been associated with stroke in pregnant women as well as fetal and infant deaths. Amphetamines taken early in pregnancy can result in fetal anomalies and low birth weight infants. Later in pregnancy, placental abruption may lead to fetal death. The anesthetic management of patients who use amphetamines is similar to that of patients who use cocaine.

Fetal Monitoring

Intrapartum fetal monitoring is routinely performed and it is important that the anesthesiologist understand the basic principles of the technology as well as the interpretation of results.

Electronic Fetal Monitoring

Intrapartum electronic monitoring includes assessment of the FHR as well as tocodynamometry to monitor for uterine contractions (NICV 41-6).[128] External fetal monitoring is performed most commonly and uses data obtained indirectly from transducers secured to the mother's abdomen with adjustable straps. Doppler ultrasound (which detects fetal heart motion) is the most used method of obtaining FHR signals; however, newer technologies allow monitoring of fetal heart electrical activity. Both methods estimate R wave-to-R wave intervals to calculate the FHR. Uterine activity is concurrently monitored with a tocodynamometer triggered by the changing shape of the uterus during contractions. External tocodynamometry is mostly qualitative, displaying the frequency and duration of contractions but not their intensity. The advantage of external monitors is that they can be applied without rupture of membranes, even before the onset of labor.

While external monitors are reliable in most cases, internal FHR and contraction monitoring are occasionally required when certain conditions (e.g., maternal obesity, polyhydramnios) make external monitoring technically challenging. Internal monitoring requires rupture of membranes and a cervical dilation of at least 1.5 cm. An electrocardiogram (ECG) electrode is attached to the presenting part to assess the fetal ECG. A transcervical, saline-filled catheter is connected to a transducer to quantitatively monitor uterine contraction frequency and strength.

Fetal Heart Rate Interpretation

The process of labor involves repetitive uterine contractions which transiently decrease blood flow and oxygen delivery to the fetus. While most fetuses tolerate these normal physiologic changes, characteristic FHR patterns may indicate inadequate fetal reserve, reduced oxygenation, or acidosis. The following FHR variables are considered when fetal well-being is being assessed: baseline heart rate, variability, presence of accelerations, and presence and type of decelerations.

The baseline FHR is the average heart rate during a 10-minute segment and normally ranges between 110 and 160 beats per minute.[128] Persistently elevated rates may be associated with chronic fetal distress, maternal fever, or administration of drugs such as ephedrine and atropine. Abnormally low rates may be encountered in fetuses with congenital heart block or as a late occurrence in the setting of fetal hypoxia and acidosis.

FHR variability refers to fluctuations in the FHR baseline over time. Variability is quantified by the amplitude of the peak to the trough heart rate and normally ranges between 6 and 25 beats per minute.[128] FHR variability reflects the beat-to-beat adjustments of the parasympathetic and sympathetic nervous systems to a variety of internal and external stimuli and is mediated by the CNS, the peripheral nervous system, and the cardiac conduction system. Presence of normal variability is a reassuring sign of normal fetal acid–base status. Asphyxia leading to fetal CNS depression may cause decreased variability; therefore, a smooth FHR tracing without variability may be an ominous finding. However, drugs that depress the CNS (sedatives, opioids, barbiturates, anesthetics) can also decrease FHR variability. Atropine may decrease variability by blocking the transmission of control impulses to the cardiac pacemaker. An acceleration of FHR is an abrupt increase over baseline and is a reassuring sign that the fetus is not acidemic.[128]

A deceleration is a decrease in FHR below baseline, and the type of deceleration is determined by the timing of the deceleration in relation to uterine contractions (Fig. 41-3, Video 41-3). Early decelerations are characterized by a symmetrical, gradual decrease in FHR, beginning with the onset of the contraction, nadiring with the peak of the contraction, and returning to baseline as the uterus relaxes. Early decelerations reach a nadir 30 seconds or more after the onset of the deceleration.[128] This type of deceleration has been attributed to fetal head compression leading to increased vagal tone, and is not associated with systemic hypoxemia or acidosis.

Late decelerations are also symmetric and gradual in onset. However, they begin after the onset of a uterine contraction and the nadir of the deceleration occurs well after the contraction peak, at least 30 seconds after deceleration onset.[128] Late decelerations are most worrisome, as they are commonly caused by CNS or myocardial ischemia resulting from uteroplacental insufficiency and fetal hypoxemia.

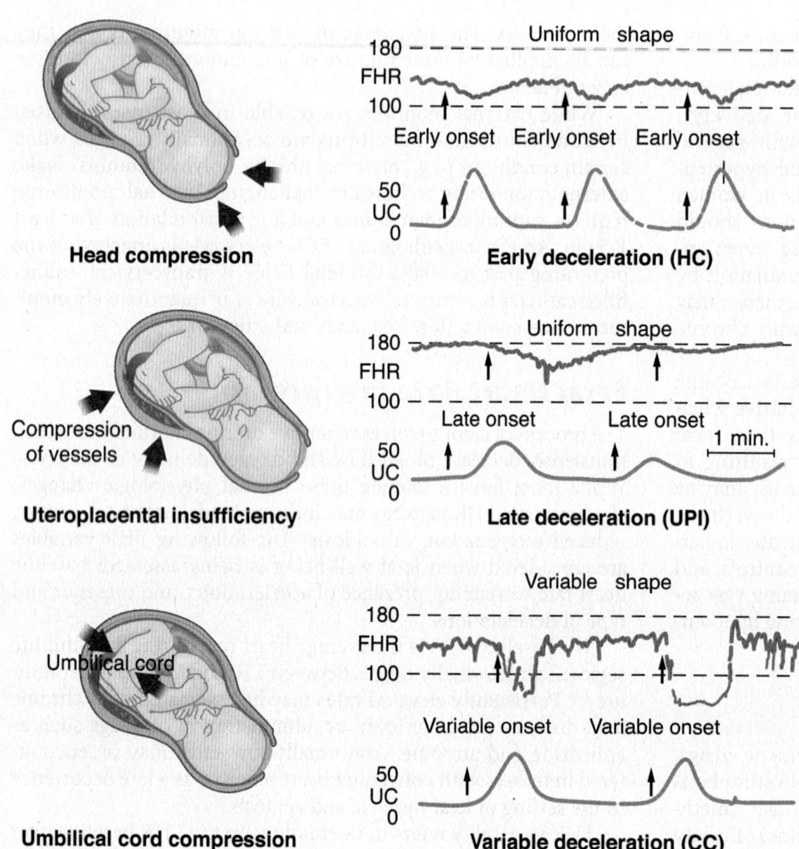

Figure 41-3 Classification and mechanism of fetal heart rate patterns. HC, head compression; UPI, uteroplacental insufficiency; CC, cord compression. (Adapted from Hon EH. *An Introduction to Fetal Heart Rate Monitoring*. Harty Press; 1969:29.)

Variable decelerations are the most common periodic pattern observed in the intrapartum period. They are variable in shape and abrupt in onset, with the heart rate nadir occurring within 30 seconds of the onset.[128] Variable decelerations occur due to umbilical cord compression that results in activation of the carotid baroreceptor reflex. Although the initial FHR changes are of reflex origin, fetal asphyxia may result in fetal hypoxemia, CNS insult, or direct myocardial depression if the cord compressions are frequent or prolonged. Recurrent (occur with at least one-half of contractions) or prolonged (≥15 beats per minute below baseline lasting between 2 and 10 minutes) decelerations are correlated with fetal acidosis; urgent delivery should be considered.[129]

The ACOG currently recommends a three-tiered system for the evaluation of FHR tracings (Table 41-8).[128] Category I tracings are those with normal baseline and variability, and no late or variable decelerations. They correlate strongly with normal fetus acid–base status at the time of observation. Category III tracings are abnormal. They are characterized by absent variability with any one of the following: recurrent late decelerations, recurrent variable decelerations, or bradycardia (FHR <100 beats per minute). Sinusoidal patterns (a sine wave–like pattern) also fall into category III. Category III tracings may be corrected by improving fetal oxygenation, correction of maternal hypotension or aortocaval compression, or by taking measures that reduce uterine activity. If the heart rate pattern does not respond to these conservative measures (i.e., in utero resuscitation), imminent delivery may be required. Finally, Category II tracings include all those that are not classified as either category I or III. They are predictive of neither normal nor abnormal acid–base status and require continued observation and assessment.

Currently, experts agree that a normal category I FHR tracing is reassuring for fetal well-being. Consensus also exists regarding the potentially ominous nature of category III tracings. However, FHR patterns between these extremes present a clinical dilemma. Category II tracings demonstrate a high false-positive rate for adverse neonatal outcomes and may lead to unnecessary cesarean deliveries. Recent recommendations regarding the approach to a category II tracing emphasize that clinicians should consider time spent with a category II tracing and progress of labor when determining delivery plans.[129]

The ACOG recognizes that FHR monitoring suffers from excessive inter- and intraobserver variability in interpretation. Continuous monitoring is associated with an increase in both operative vaginal and cesarean deliveries, but it is not associated with a decreased incidence of cerebral palsy.[128] Thus, while the ACOG recommends continuous FHR analysis for parturients with high-risk conditions, it allows intermittent FHR monitoring in uncomplicated mothers and fetuses.

Newborn Resuscitation in the Delivery Room

Of the approximately 3.5 million infants born in the United States each year, 10% require resuscitation in the delivery room.[130] The following factors may contribute to depression of the newborn: medications used during labor and delivery (including anesthetic agents), birth trauma, and birth asphyxia (i.e., hypoxia and hypercapnia with metabolic acidosis).

Fetal Asphyxia

Fetal asphyxia, the best-studied cause of neonatal depression, usually develops because of diminished placental perfusion. The

Table 41-8 Three-Tier Fetal Heart Rate Interpretation System

Category I

Category I fetal heart rate (FHR) tracings include all of the following:

- Baseline rate: 110–160 beats per minute (bpm)
- Baseline FHR variability: moderate
- Late or variable decelerations: absent
- Early decelerations: present or absent
- Accelerations: present or absent

Category II

Category II FHR tracings include all FHR tracings not categorized as Category I or Category III.

Category II tracings may represent an appreciable fraction of those encountered in clinical care.

Examples of Category II FHR tracings include any of the following:

Baseline rate

- Bradycardia not accompanied by absent baseline variability
- Tachycardia

Baseline FHR variability

- Minimal baseline variability
- Absent baseline variability not accompanied by recurrent decelerations
- Marked baseline variability

Accelerations

- Absence of induced accelerations after fetal stimulation

Periodic or episodic decelerations

- Recurrent variable decelerations accompanied by minimal or moderate baseline variability
- Prolonged deceleration >2 min but <10 min
- Recurrent late decelerations with moderate baseline variability
- Variable decelerations with other characteristics, such as slow return to baseline, "overshoots," or "shoulders"

Category III

Category III FHR tracings include either:

- Absent baseline FHR variability and any of the following:
  - Recurrent late decelerations
  - Recurrent variable decelerations
  - Bradycardia
- Sinusoidal pattern

Reprinted with permission from Macones GA, Hankins GDV, Spong CY, et al. The 2008 National Institute of Child Health and Human Development Workshop on Electronic Fetal Monitoring: Updates on Definitions, Interpretations, and Research Guidelines. *Obstet Gynecol.* 2008;112(3):661–666.

normal fetus is neither hypoxic nor acidotic before labor. Experimental data have revealed that transplacental gradients for pH and $PaCO_2$ are approximately 0.05 pH units and 5 mmHg, respectively. Although fetal oxygen tension is low, oxygen saturation is 80% to 85% by virtue of the leftward shift of the fetal oxyhemoglobin dissociation curve.

During labor, uterine contractions decrease or even eliminate blood flow through the intervillous space of the placenta. Umbilical cord compression occurs during the final stages of approximately one-third of vaginal deliveries. Thus, mild degrees of hypoxia and acidosis occur even during normal labor and delivery and play an important role in initiation of ventilation immediately after birth. On average, healthy, vigorous infants have a pH of 7.24, and a $PaCO_2$ of 56 mmHg at birth.

Severe fetal asphyxia occasionally develops because of maternal or fetal complications, such as uterine tachysystole, premature separation of the placenta, maternal hypotension, tight nuchal umbilical cord, or prolapsed cord. During asphyxia, changes in acid–base status are rapid. The decrease in pH results from accumulation of carbon dioxide (respiratory acidosis) and end products of anaerobic metabolism (metabolic acidosis). After oxygen stores are exhausted, the ability of fetal brain and myocardium to derive energy from anaerobic metabolism is essential for survival. However, anaerobic glycolysis is pH dependent, and its rate is greatly diminished when the pH decreases below 7.0. Other untoward effects of severe hypoxia and acidosis include myocardial depression, resulting from a decrease in responsiveness to catecholamines; a right shift of the fetal oxyhemoglobin dissociation curve, resulting in reduced oxygen delivery; and an increase in pulmonary vascular resistance, which plays an important role during circulatory changes at birth.

Neonatal Adaptations at Birth

During birth and through the early hours and days of life, many morphologic and functional changes take place, with the cardiovascular and ventilatory systems undergoing the most dramatic alterations. In the normal newborn, two events occur almost simultaneously within seconds of delivery: cessation of umbilical circulation through the placenta and expansion of the lungs. These events change the fetal circulation toward the adult type.

Survival of the neonate depends primarily on prompt establishment of effective ventilation and expansion of the lungs, which dilates the pulmonary vascular bed, resulting in decreased resistance and a significant increase in pulmonary blood flow. Pulmonary vascular resistance further decreases as oxygen tension increases and carbon dioxide levels decrease. As soon as pulmonary resistance decreases, the foramen ovale undergoes functional closure because of relative pressure changes across the valve of the foramen (Fig. 41-1). Cessation of the umbilical circulation reduces pressure in the inferior vena cava and right atrium, whereas the increase in pulmonary blood flow increases venous return and pressure in the left atrium. The smooth muscle of the ductus arteriosus constricts in response to increased oxygen tension in the newborn's blood. Catecholamines, which exist in increased concentrations in the newborn, particularly during the first 3 hours of life, also constrict the ductus arteriosus. In contrast, prostaglandins I_2 and E_2, produced by the wall of the ductus arteriosus, relax the ductal smooth muscle. Functional closure of the ductus arteriosus may take hours, even days. Thus, shunting may still occur in the neonatal period, its direction depending on relative resistances in the pulmonary and systemic vascular beds.

CO and its distribution also increase. These changes closely parallel the increase in oxygen consumption. The redistribution of CO also leads to increases in myocardial, renal, and gastrointestinal blood flow, and decreases in cerebral, adrenal, and carotid flow.

During fetal life, respiratory gas exchange takes place through the placenta. Delivery of the infant's trunk relieves the thoracic compression that occurs as the infant passes through the birth canal, and the thorax and lungs expand. Most infants initiate respiratory efforts within a few seconds of birth. Negative pressures in excess of 40 cm H_2O bring about the initial entry of air into fluid-filled alveoli. In the mature, normal neonate, the lungs expand almost completely after the first few breaths, and the pressure–volume changes achieved with each respiration resemble those of the adult. After lung expansion, the FRC approximates 70 mL in the term newborn and changes little over the first 6 days of life. The TV varies between 10 and 30 mL, and the breathing frequency ranges from 30 to 60 breaths per minute. Minute ventilation thus exceeds 500 mL. After delivery and prompt lung expansion, reoxygenation is rapid, but it takes 2 to 3 hours to achieve a relatively normal acid–base balance, primarily by pulmonary excretion of carbon dioxide. By 24 hours, the healthy neonate has reached the same acid–base state as that of the mother before labor.

Resuscitation

The delivery room must be prepared for prompt and adequate treatment of severe neonatal depression at birth. Members of the delivery room team should be trained in resuscitation methods because both mother and infant may encounter difficulty simultaneously. One person should be designated specifically to care for the newborn during every delivery. When continued resuscitation is anticipated, a team of skilled personnel should be present. Equipment necessary for emergency resuscitation should be checked carefully before delivery. The algorithm for neonatal resuscitation in the delivery room is provided in Figure 41-4.

Evaluation and Treatment

The AHA has released guidelines to advise the practitioner providing neonatal resuscitation (NICV 41-7).[130] The initial appraisal of the newborn should start from the moment of birth, with particular attention to the following three questions:

- Is the newborn the result of a term gestation?
- Is the newborn crying or breathing vigorously?
- Does the newborn have good muscle tone?

If the answer to all three questions is "yes," then the baby does not require further resuscitation and should be placed skin to skin with its mother, if practical. In this scenario, umbilical cord clamping should also be delayed at least 30 seconds to improve fetal outcomes. If the answer to any of the above questions is "no," then further resuscitation should be provided, with the following steps taken in the order listed.

Initial Stabilization

The infant should be placed supine under a radiant heat source, with the head maintained low in the sniffing position. Breathing should be stimulated by slapping the infant's soles lightly or rubbing the back. Suctioning is only needed in the presence of obvious secretions, as it may provoke vagally induced bradycardia.

Assessment of Respirations and Heart Rate

Presence of respiration versus apnea is assessed, and respiratory efforts are judged as unlabored versus gasping or labored. An assistant should listen to the heartbeat immediately, indicating the rate by finger movement, or the rate can be detected from pulsation of the umbilical cord. Normally, the newborn's heart rate is above 100 beats per minute.

Ventilation

If the newborn is apneic or gasping, or if the heart rate is below 100 beats per minute after initial stabilization, positive pressure ventilation (PPV) should be initiated via bag and mask at a rate of 40 to 60 breaths per minute. The initial breath may require pressures of 30 to 40 cm H_2O. Subsequent inflation pressures should be reduced to 15 to 20 cm H_2O in an infant with normal lungs. A small plastic oropharyngeal airway may help maintain patency of the upper airway. Tracheal intubation may be required if bag–mask ventilation is ineffective or prolonged. The administration of oxygen is controversial because studies demonstrate that both hypoxemia and excessive oxygen administration may be harmful to neonates; meta-analyses suggest that room air resuscitation is associated with lower mortality than that with 100% oxygen.[131] Therefore, it is recommended that preductal pulse oximetry guide oxygen therapy with attention to target saturations listed in the box in Figure 41-4, and that oxygen therapy be titrated to heart rate response.

Chest Compressions

If the heart rate remains below 60 beats per minute after adequate ventilation with oxygen for 30 seconds, chest compressions should be initiated. The operator should encircle the chest with both hands, supporting the back and compressing the chest with the opposing thumbs; alternatively, one may compress the chest with two fingers. Compressions should take place on the lower third of the sternum to a depth that is one-third of the anterior–posterior diameter of the chest. Care must be taken not to interfere with ventilation. Recommendations call for a 3:1 compression-to-ventilation ratio, with 90 compressions and 30 breaths delivered per minute. Cardiac compressions should be maintained until the heart rate exceeds 60 beats per minute.

Medications and Volume Expansion

Persistent neonatal bradycardia is most often a result of hypoxemia, and usually responds to ventilatory efforts. If the heart rate continues to be less than 60 beats per minute despite adequate ventilation with 100% oxygen, the newborn may require epinephrine, intravascular volume expansion, or both. Epinephrine 0.01 to 0.03 mg/kg should be administered intravenously as soon as vascular access is established. In the absence of intravenous access, one may consider endotracheal administration of 0.05 to 0.1 mg/kg. The use of naloxone or other medications in the delivery room is no longer recommended.

Hypovolemia frequently follows severe birth asphyxia because a greater-than-normal portion of fetal blood remains in the placenta. The infant may appear pale and have low arterial pressure, tachycardia, and tachypnea. If the heart rate does not respond to other measures, acute blood volume expansion may be accomplished with the intravenous administration of normal saline or lactated Ringer solution 10 mL/kg over 5 to 10 minutes, or, when blood loss is suspected, a similar volume of O-negative blood. Albumin is not recommended (Table 41-9).

The Apgar Score

The scoring system introduced by Apgar is a useful method of clinically evaluating the infant; the standard of care is to perform this assessment at 1 and 5 minutes after delivery (Table 41-10).

Exit Procedure

The EXIT (ex utero intrapartum treatment) procedure, which maintains uteroplacental support for a period of time after partial delivery of the fetus, is employed for certain fetal conditions that pose an immediate threat to neonatal life on separation from the placental circulation. The most common indications are large fetal neck masses and reversal of tracheal occlusion from clips placed for congenital diaphragmatic hernia. The usual procedure involves partial delivery of the fetus, surgical treatment of fetal pathology (e.g., attainment of a patent fetal airway), and, finally, delivery of the fetus and clamping of the umbilical cord.

Anesthetic considerations include maintenance of uterine relaxation during the phase of fetal manipulation, administration

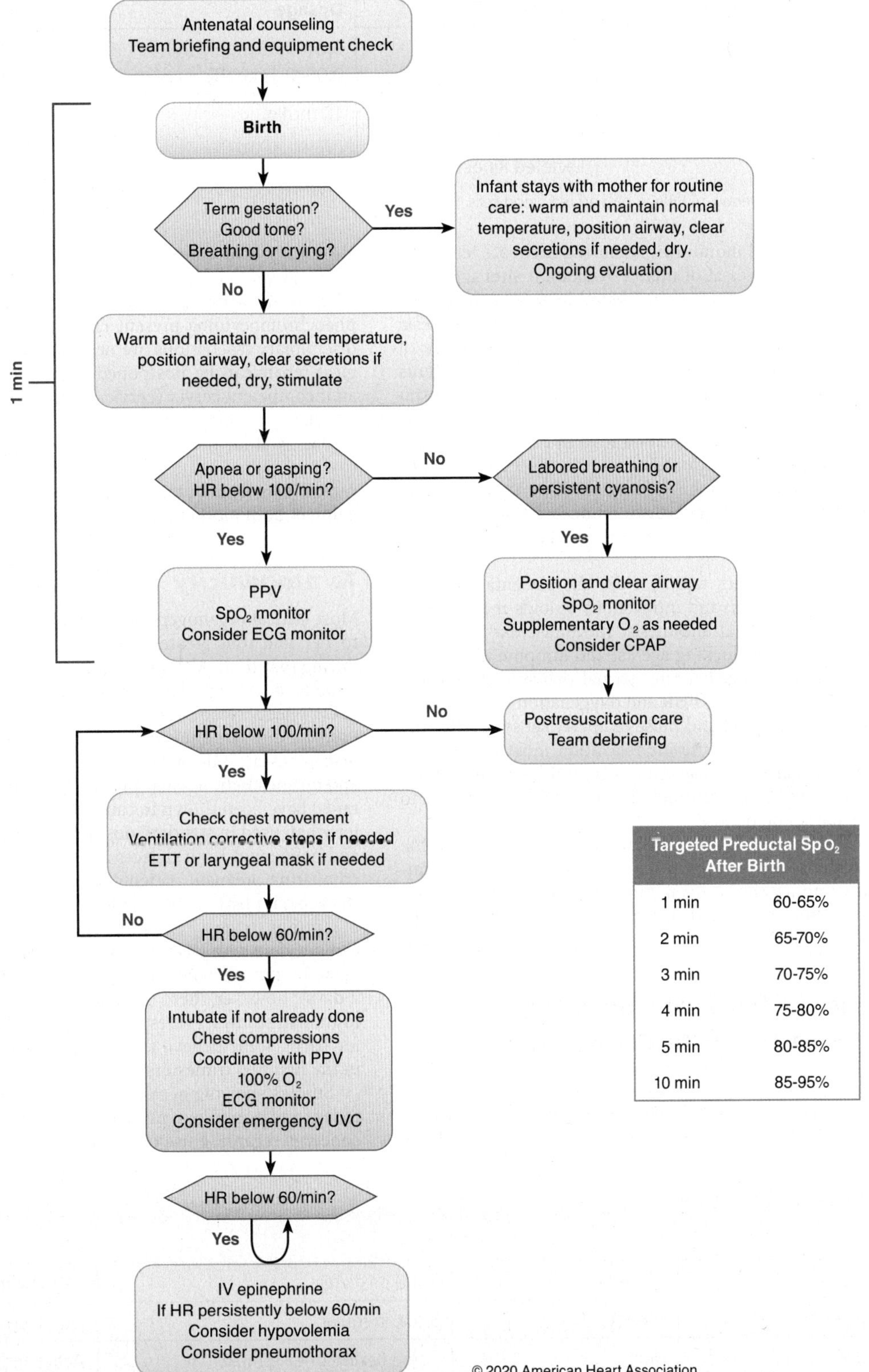

Targeted Preductal SpO2 After Birth	
1 min	60-65%
2 min	65-70%
3 min	70-75%
4 min	75-80%
5 min	80-85%
10 min	85-95%

Figure 41-4 American Heart Association neonatal resuscitation algorithm. HR, heart rate; PPV, positive pressure ventilation; SpO_2, pulse oximeter; ECG, electrocardiogram; ETT, endotracheal tube; UVC, umbilical vein catheter; IV, intravenous; CPAP, continuous positive airway pressure. (Reprinted with permission from 2020 American Heart Association Guidelines for CPR & ECC—Part 5: Neonatal Resuscitation. *Circulation*. 2020;142:S524–S550. © 2020 American Heart Association, Inc.)

Table 41-9 Therapeutic Guidelines for Neonatal Resuscitation

Drug or Volume Expander	Concentration	Dosage	Route/Rate
Epinephrine	1:10,000	0.01–0.03 mg/kg (IV) 0.05–0.1 mg (IT)	IV or IT Give rapidly
Volume expanders	PRBCs Normal saline Lactated Ringer	10 mL/kg	Give over 5–10 min

IT, intratracheally; IV, intravenously; PRBCs, packed red blood cells.

of fetal anesthesia, fetal monitoring, ensuring adequate fetal oxygenation, and rapid reversal of uterine relaxation after umbilical cord clamping to minimize maternal blood loss. Most often, the mother is anesthetized with deep inhalation general anesthesia following a standard rapid-sequence induction. Maintenance of anesthesia with high concentrations of volatile anesthetic agents provides uterine relaxation during the procedure; however, intravenous nitroglycerin may also be used for this purpose.[132] The use of high inspired inhalational anesthesia or nitroglycerin may be associated with maternal hypotension. Therefore, intravenous vasopressors may be required to ensure adequate uteroplacental blood flow. Use of volatile anesthetic concentrations less than 2 MAC is recommended to minimize untoward effects on uterine blood flow.

Inhalational anesthetics rapidly cross the placenta and contribute to fetal anesthesia, and intravenous opioids may be used to provide additional fetal anesthesia. Intramuscular anesthetic agents, neuromuscular blocking agents, and atropine are administered to the fetus as needed after partial delivery. During the period of fetal manipulation, FHR and oxygenation can be monitored by sterile ultrasound and pulse oximetry sensors. After the umbilical cord is clamped, uterine relaxation must be reversed rapidly by decreasing the inspired concentration of inhalation agent and administering uterotonic agents such as oxytocin to minimize maternal blood loss.

Usually, two anesthetic teams are employed: one to tend to the mother and the other to care for the fetus/newborn. Communication and coordination between surgical (obstetric and pediatric), pediatric, anesthesia, and nursing teams are mandatory for successful outcomes.

Anesthesia for Nonobstetric Surgery in the Pregnant Woman

In the United States, approximately 1% of pregnant women require nonobstetric surgical interventions during pregnancy (NICV 41-8).[133] The most frequent nonobstetric procedures are excision of ovarian cysts, appendectomy, cholecystectomy, breast biopsy, and surgery related to trauma. Serious conditions such as intracranial aneurysms, cardiac valvular disease, and pheochromocytoma present rarely during pregnancy and multidisciplinary discussions are necessary to determine whether surgical repair can be postponed until after delivery. Treatment of an incompetent cervix (cervical cerclage) typically occurs in early pregnancy or midpregnancy.

The goal for treating patients undergoing nonobstetric operative procedures is the same as for any patient: safe perioperative care. This goal is complicated by the need to consider the well-being of both mother and fetus.

Teratogenicity

Most critical organogenesis occurs in the first trimester (days 31 to 71), and thus greatest concern for structural teratogenicity is during that time. Although many commonly used anesthetics are teratogenic at high doses in animals, few studies support teratogenic effects of anesthetic or sedative medications in the doses used for human anesthesia care. Conventional doses of benzodiazepines are safe when needed to treat perioperative anxiety, and no anesthetic agents (propofol, etomidate, ketamine, barbiturates) have been shown to cause teratogenicity during any trimester when used in standard doses. Importantly, rates of miscarriage and congenital birth defects are not significantly different when comparing pregnant patients undergoing nonobstetric surgery to the general obstetric population.

Nitrous oxide causes inhibition of methionine synthetase and can interfere with DNA synthesis. It has been shown to be teratogenic in animals when administered for prolonged periods (1 to 2 days); however, there is no definitive evidence of teratogenicity in human studies.[134] Despite this, given the potential mechanism for harm, some believe that nitrous oxide use is contraindicated in the first two trimesters.

Studies showing accelerated neuronal cell death in immature rodent and nonhuman primate brains exposed to anesthetics raise concerns regarding use of general anesthesia during pregnancy.[26]

Table 41-10 Apgar Scores

Sign	0	1	2
Heart rate	Absent	<100 beats/min	>100 beats/min
Respiratory effort	Absent	Slow, irregular	Good, crying
Muscle tone	Limp	Some flexion of extremities	Active motion
Reflex irritability	No response	Grimace	Cough, sneeze, or cry
Color	Pale, blue	Body pink, extremities blue	Completely pink

The score for each of 5 domains is summed. A score of 8–10 is normal, 4–7 indicates moderate impairment, 0–3 indicates need for immediate resuscitation.

It is premature to suggest that impairment seen in the developing brain with general anesthesia in animal models can be extrapolated to humans. Studies in humans are inconclusive regarding whether short anesthesia exposure in utero or in early childhood is associated with adverse childhood outcomes.[29,135]

Anesthetic Implications of Pregnancy Physiology

Induction and emergence from general anesthesia are more rapid than in the nonpregnant state because of increased minute ventilation, decreased FRC, and decreased MAC of volatile agents; these changes are observed as early as 8 to 10 weeks of gestation. Supine hypotensive syndrome can occur as early as the second trimester. Although gastric emptying is essentially normal in pregnancy, it may be markedly slower in women with the need for emergency surgery. Gastroesophageal sphincter tone is decreased after 20 weeks of gestation, thus precautions should be taken to limit risk for aspiration and to avoid morbidity if it occurs. The effects of altered physiology during pregnancy are not limited to general anesthesia. Pharmacodynamic and anatomic changes during pregnancy lead to increased sensitivity to local anesthetics; thus, the amount of local anesthetic administered should be reduced by 25% to 30% during any trimester. Increased volume of distribution for both hydrophilic and lipophilic drugs as well as decreased protein binding influence drug pharmacokinetic properties. Hepatic metabolic enzymes are variably affected by pregnancy.

Intrauterine fetal asphyxia is avoided by maintaining maternal PaO_2, $PaCO_2$, and uterine blood flow. $PaCO_2$ can affect uterine blood flow as maternal alkalosis may cause direct vasoconstriction. Alkalosis also shifts the oxyhemoglobin dissociation curve, resulting in the release of less oxygen to the fetus at the placenta. Maternal hypotension leads to a reduction in uterine blood flow and thus fetal hypoxia. Increases in uterine tone, as occurs with increased uterine irritability, will also decrease uterine blood flow.

Anesthetic Management for Nonobstetric Surgery

Elective surgery should be delayed until the patient is no longer pregnant and has returned to her nonpregnant physiologic state (approximately 2 to 6 weeks postpartum). Procedures that can be scheduled with some flexibility but cannot be delayed until postpartum are best scheduled in the second trimester. This lessens the risk for teratogenicity (greatest concern in first trimester) or preterm labor (greatest concern in third trimester) (Fig. 41-5). In general, appropriate care for the mother results in the best outcomes for the fetus. Thus, diagnostic imaging, anesthesia, and surgery should proceed, if indicated.

In the setting of emergency surgery, no data suggest that any well-conducted anesthetic technique is preferred over another, provided oxygenation and BP are maintained and hyperventilation is avoided. Regional anesthesia confers the advantage of limited fetal medication exposure, while general anesthesia offers the uterine relaxation associated with volatile agents. Left uterine displacement should be used, if possible, during the second and third trimesters, and aspiration prophylaxis should be administered to all pregnant patients after approximately 20 weeks of gestation. At a minimum, pre- and postoperative FHR and uterine activity should be assessed.[136]

Practical Suggestions

The following approach to anesthesia during pregnancy is suggested (Fig. 41-5, 4 Video 41-4):

1. Anesthesiologists and surgeons should obtain consultation from an obstetrician before performing nonobstetric surgery in pregnancy.
2. The patient's apprehension should be allayed as much as possible by personal reassurance during the preanesthetic visit and by adequate sedation and premedication, if indicated.
3. Pain should be relieved whenever present.

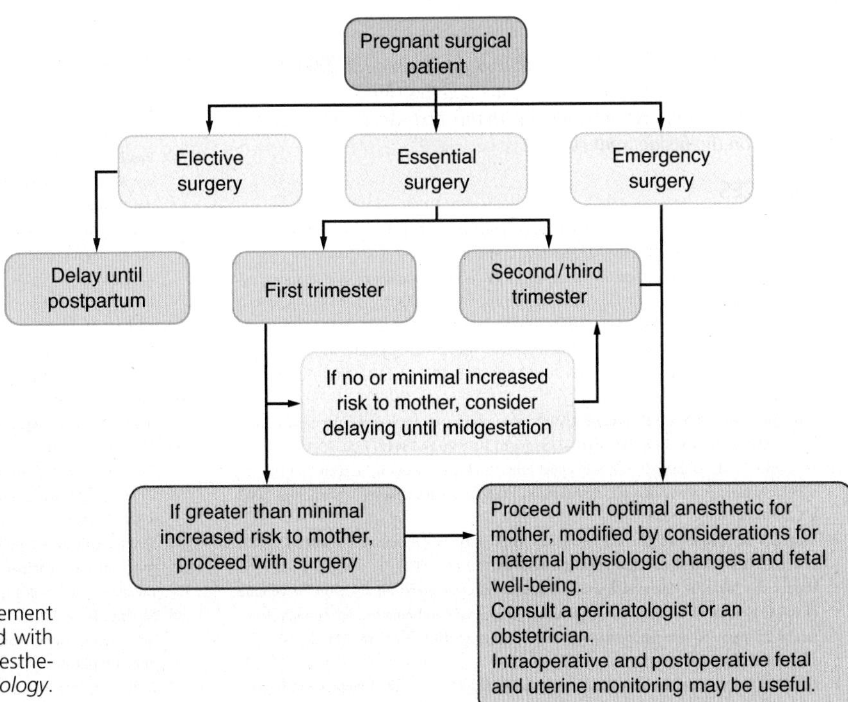

Figure 41-5 Recommendations for management of parturients and surgical procedures. (Adapted with permission from Rosen MA. Management of anesthesia for the pregnant surgical patient. *Anesthesiology.* 1999;91(4):1159–1163.)

4. A nonparticulate antacid should be administered within half an hour before induction of anesthesia. Ranitidine and metoclopramide may be useful.
5. Beginning in the second trimester, uterine displacement should be maintained.
6. Hypotension related to spinal or epidural anesthesia should be prevented as much as possible by rapid intravenous infusion of crystalloid solution during induction of anesthesia and prophylactic vasopressor use.
7. General anesthesia should be preceded by careful denitrogenation.
8. The risk of aspiration should be minimized by application of cricoid pressure and rapid tracheal intubation with a cuffed tube.
9. Choice of anesthetic agents is at the discretion of the anesthesia provider in consultation with the surgeon and patient; no currently used medications have demonstrated teratogenic effects in human studies at any gestational age when used in standard doses.
10. Avoid maternal hyperventilation and monitor end-expiratory $PaCO_2$ or arterial blood gases. Pregnancy is associated with chronic respiratory alkalosis, and $PaCO_2$ should be maintained within that adjusted baseline.
11. At a minimum, FHR should be assessed in the immediate preoperative and postoperative period. FHR may be monitored continuously or intermittently throughout surgery and anesthesia, provided that placement of the transducer does not encroach on the surgical field. The decision to monitor the fetus should be made in conjunction with the obstetrician based on the severity of maternal disease, the potential for fetal jeopardy, viability of the fetus, and immediate availability of a physician able to perform an emergency cesarean delivery.
12. Uterine tone may also be monitored with an external tocodynamometer if the uterus reaches the umbilicus or above. Monitoring uterine activity should be continued after the operation, and tocolytic agents may be required.

For additional information please see Chapter 15, Video 15-3 in the eBook bundled with this text.

For further review and interactivities, please see the videos and narrative interactive clinical vignettes (NICVs) accessible in the complimentary eBook bundled with this text. Access instructions are located on the inside front cover.

REFERENCES

1. LoMauro A, Aliverti A. Respiratory physiology of pregnancy: physiology masterclass. *Breathe (Sheff)*. 2015;11(4):297–301. doi:10.1183/20734735.008615
2. Hagerdal M, Morgan CW, Sumner AE, Gutsche BB. Minute ventilation and oxygen consumption during labor with epidural analgesia. *Anesthesiology*. 1983;59(5):425–427. doi:10.1097/00000542-198311000-00011
3. Ngene NC, Moodley J. Physiology of blood pressure relevant to managing hypertension in pregnancy. *J Matern Fetal Neonatal Med*. 2019;32(8):1368–1377. doi:10.1080/14767058.2017.1404569
4. van Oppen AC, Stigter RH, Bruinse HW. Cardiac output in normal pregnancy: a critical review. *Obstet Gynecol*. 1996;87(2):310–318. doi:10.1016/0029-7844(95)00348-7
5. Schannwell CM, Zimmermann T, Schneppenheim M, Plehn G, Marx R, Strauer BE. Left ventricular hypertrophy and diastolic dysfunction in healthy pregnant women. *Cardiology*. 2002 97(2):73–78.
6. Sanghavi M, Rutherford JD. Cardiovascular physiology of pregnancy. *Circulation*. 2014; 130(12):1003–1008. doi:10.1161/CIRCULATIONAHA.114.009029
7. Higuchi H, Takagi S, Zhang K, Furui I, Ozaki M. Effect of lateral tilt angle on the volume of the abdominal aorta and inferior vena cava in pregnant and nonpregnant women determined by magnetic resonance imaging. *Anesthesiology*. 2015;122(2):286–293. doi:10.1097/aln.0000000000000553
8. Gant NF, Daley GL, Chand S, Whalley PJ, MacDonald PC. A study of angiotensin II pressor response throughout primigravid pregnancy. *J Clin Invest*. 1973;52(11):2682–2689. doi:10.1172/JCI107462
9. Lumbers ER, Pringle KG. Roles of the circulating renin-angiotensin-aldosterone system in human pregnancy. *Am J Physiol Regul Integr Comp Physiol*. 2014;306(2):R91–R101. doi:10.1152/ajpregu.00034.2013
10. Thornton P, Douglas J. Coagulation in pregnancy. *Best Pract Res Clin Obstet Gynaecol*. 2010;24(3):339–352. doi:10.1016/j.bpobgyn.2009.11.010
11. Tang J, Lin Y, Mai H, et al. Meta-analysis of reference values of haemostatic markers during pregnancy and childbirth. *Taiwan J Obstet Gynecol*. 2019;58(1):29–35. doi:10.1016/j.tjog.2018.11.004
12. Charbit B, Mandelbrot L, Samain E, et al; PPH Study Group. The decrease of fibrinogen is an early predictor of the severity of postpartum hemorrhage. *J Thromb Haemost*. 2007;5(2):266–273. doi:10.1111/j.1538-7836.2007.02297.x
13. Valera MC, Parant O, Vayssiere C, Arnal JF, Payrastre B. Physiologic and pathologic changes of platelets in pregnancy. *Platelets*. 2010 21(8):587–595. doi:10.3109/09537104.2010.509828
14. Macfie AG, Magides AD, Richmond MN, Reilly CS. Gastric emptying in pregnancy. *Br J Anaesth*. 1991;67(1):54–57. doi:10.1093/bja/67.1.54
15. Wong CA, Loffredi M, Ganchiff JN, Zhao J, Wang Z, Avram MJ. Gastric emptying of water in term pregnancy. *Anesthesiology*. 2002;96(6):1395–1400.
16. Bouvet L, Schulz T, Piana F, Desgranges FP, Chassard D. Pregnancy and labor epidural effects on gastric emptying: a prospective comparative study. *Anesthesiology*. 2022;136(4):542–550. doi:10.1097/ALN.0000000000004133
17. Blitt CD, Petty WC, Alberternst EE, Wright BJ. Correlation of plasma cholinesterase activity and duration of action of succinylcholine during pregnancy. *Anesth Analg*. 1977;56(1):78–83. doi:10.1213/00000539-197701000-00019
18. Lurie S, Sadan O, Oron G, et al. Reduced pseudocholinesterase activity in patients with HELLP syndrome. *Reprod Sci*. 2007;14(2):192–196. doi:10.1177/1933719107299871
19. Cooper DS, Laurberg L. Hyperthyroidism in pregnancy. *Lancet Diabetes Endocrinol*. 2013; 1(3):238–249. doi: 10.1016/S2213-8587(13)70086-X
20. Kuhnert PM, Kuhnert BR, Stitts JM, Gross TL. The use of a selected ion monitoring technique to study the disposition of bupivacaine in mother, fetus, and neonate following epidural anesthesia for cesarean section. *Anesthesiology*. 1981;55(6):611–617.
21. Dwyer R, Fee JP, Moore J. Uptake of halothane and isoflurane by mother and baby during caesarean section. *Br J Anaesth*. 1995;74(4):379–383.
22. Morishima HO, Covino BG. Toxicity and distribution of lidocaine in nonasphyxiated and asphyxiated baboon fetuses. *Anesthesiology*. 1981 54(3):182–186.
23. Kennedy RL, Miller RP, Bell JU, et al. Uptake and distribution of bupivacaine in fetal lambs. *Anesthesiology*. 1986;65(3):247–253.
24. Kuhnert BR, Kuhnert PM, Prochaska AL, Gross TL. Plasma levels of 2-chloroprocaine in obstetric patients and their neonates after epidural anesthesia. *Anesthesiology*. 1980;53(1): 21–25.
25. Morishima HO, Pedersen H, Finster M, et al. Toxicity of lidocaine in adult, newborn, and fetal sheep. *Anesthesiology*. 1981;55(1):57–61.
26. Jevtovic-Todorovic V, Brambrick A. General anesthesia and young brain: what is new? *J Neurosurg Anesthesiol*. 2018;30(3):217–222. doi:10.1097/ana.0000000000000432
27. Andropoulos DB. Effect of anesthesia on the developing brain: infant and fetus. *Fetal Diagn Ther*. 2018 43(1):1–11. doi:10.1159/000475928
28. Sprung J, Flick RP, Wilder RT, et al. Anesthesia for cesarean delivery and learning disabilities in a population-based birth cohort. *Anesthesiology*. 2009;111(2):302–310. doi:10.1097/ALN.0b013e3181adf481
29. Sun LS, Li G, Miller TL, et al. Association between a single general anesthesia exposure before age 36 months and neurocognitive outcomes in later cildhood. *JAMA*. 2016;315(21):2312–2320. doi:10.1001/jama.2016.6967
30. Butwick AJ, Abrams DA, Wong CA. Epidural labour analgesia and autism spectrum disorder: is the current evidence sufficient to dismiss an association? *Br J Anaesth*. 2022;128(3):393–398. doi:10.1016/j.bja.2021.12.017
31. Melillo A, Maiorano P, Rachedi S, et al. Labor analgesia: a systematic review and meta-analysis of non-pharmacological complementary and alternative approaches to pain during first stage of labor. *Crit Rev Eukaryot Gene Expr*. 2022 32(2):61–89. doi:10.1615/CritRevEukaryotGeneExpr.2021039986
32. Scott JR, Rose NB. Effect of psychoprophylaxis (Lamaze preparation) on labor and delivery in primiparas. *N Engl J Med*. 1976;294(22):1205–1207.
33. Hodnett ED, Gates S, Hofmeyr GJ, Sakala C. Continuous support for women during childbirth. *Cochrane Database Syst Rev*. 2013;7:CD003766. doi:10.1002/14651858.CD003766.pub5
34. Cluett ER, Burns E. Immersion in water in labour and birth. *Cochrane Database Syst Rev*. 2009;2:CD000111. doi:10.1002/14651858.CD000111.pub3
35. Derry S, Straube S, Moore RA, Hancock H, Collins SL. Intracutaneous or subcutaneous sterile water injection compared with blinded controls for pain management in labour. *Cochrane Database Syst Rev*. 2012;1:CD009107. doi:10.1002/14651858.CD009107.pub2
36. Madden K, Middleton P, Cyna AM, Matthewson M, Jones L. Hypnosis for pain management during labour and childbirth. *Cochrane Database Syst Rev*. 2016;2016(5):CD009356. doi:10.1002/14651858.CD009356.pub3
37. Bedwell C, Dowswell T, Neilson JP, Lavender T. The use of transcutaneous electrical nerve stimulation (TENS) for pain relief in labour: a review of the evidence. *Midwifery*. 2011;27(5):e141–e148. doi:10.1016/j.midw.2009.12.004.

38. Smith CA, Collins CT, Crowther CA, Levett KM. Acupuncture or acupressure for pain management in labour. *Cochrane Database Syst Rev*. 2011;7:CD009232. doi:10.1002/14651858.CD009232
39. Smith CA, Levett KM, Collins CT, Crowther CA. Relaxation techniques for pain management in labour. *Cochrane Database Syst Rev*. 2011;12:CD009514. doi:10.1002/14651858.CD009514
40. Ullman R, Smith LA, Burns E, Mori R, Dowswell T. Parenteral opioids for maternal pain relief in labour. *Cochrane Database Syst Rev*. 2010;9:CD007396. doi:10.1002/14651858.CD007396.pub2
41. Ronel I, Weiniger CF. Non-regional analgesia for labour: remifentanil in obstetrics. *BJA Educ*. 2019;19(11):357–361. doi:10.1016/j.bjae.2019.07.002
42. Jelting Y, Weibel S, Afshari A, et al. Patient-controlled analgesia with remifentanil vs. alternative parenteral methods for pain management in labour: a Cochrane systematic review. *Anaesthesia*. 2017;72(8):1016–1028. doi:10.1111/anae.13971
43. Beilin Y, Guinn NR, Bernstein HH, Zahn J, Hossain S, Bodian CA. Local anesthetics and mode of delivery: bupivacaine versus ropivacaine versus levobupivacaine. *Anesth Analg*. 2007;105(3):756–763.
44. van der Vyver M, Halpern S, Joseph G. Patient-controlled epidural analgesia versus continuous infusion for labour analgesia: a meta-analysis. *Br J Anaesth*. 2002;89(3):459–465.
45. Xu J, Zhou J, Xiao H, et al. A systematic review and meta-analysis comparing programmed intermittent bolus and continuous infusion as the background infusion for parturient-controlled epidural analgesia. Sci Rep. 2019;9(1):2583. doi:10.1038/s41598-019-39248-5
46. Asokumar B, Newman LM, McCarthy RJ, Ivankovich AD, Tuman KJ. Intrathecal bupivacaine reduces pruritus and prolongs duration of fentanyl analgesia during labor: a prospective, randomized controlled trial. *Anesth Analg*. 1998; 87(6):1309–1315.
47. Abrão KC, Francisco RPV, Miyadahira S, Cicarelli DD, Zugaib M. Elevation of uterine basal tone and fetal heart rate abnormalities after labor analgesia: a randomized controlled trial. *Obstet Gynecol*. 2009;113(1):41–47. doi:10.1097/AOG.0b013e31818f5eb6
48. Booth JM, Pan JC, Ross VH, Russell GB, Harris LC, Pan PH. Combined spinal epidural technique for labor analgesia does not delay recognition of epidural catheter failures: A single-center retrospective cohort aurvival analysis. *Anesthesiology*. 2016;125(3):516–524. doi:10.1097/aln.0000000000001222
49. Segal S, Pan PH. Dural puncture epidural for labor analgesia: is it really an improvement over conventional labor epidural analgesia? *Anesthesiology*. 2022;136(5):667–669. doi:10.1097/aln.0000000000004187
50. Anim-Somuah M, Smyth RM, Cyna AM, Cuthbert A. Epidural versus non-epidural or no analgesia for pain management in labour. *Cochrane Database Syst Rev*. 2018;5(5):Cd000331. doi:10.1002/14651858.CD000331.pub4
51. Sng BL, Leong WL, Zeng Y, et al. Early versus late initiation of epidural analgesia for labour. *Cochrane Database Syst Rev*. 2014;10:CD007238. doi:10.1002/14651858.CD007238.pub2
52. American College of Obstetricians and Gynecologists (College), Society for Maternal-Fetal Medicine; Caughey AB, Cahill AG, Guise JM, Rouse DJ. Safe prevention of the primary cesarean delivery. *Am J Obstet Gynecol*. 2014;210(3):179–193. doi:10.1016/j.ajog.2014.01.026
53. Sultan P, Murphy C, Halpern S, Carvalho B. The effect of low concentrations versus high concentrations of local anesthetics for labour analgesia on obstetric and anesthetic outcomes: a meta-analysis. *Can J Anaesth*. 2013;60(9):840–854. doi:10.1007/s12630-013-9981-z
54. Likis FE, Andrews JC, Collins MR, et al. Nitrous oxide for the management of labor pain: a systematic review. *Anesth Analg*. 2014;118(1):153–167. doi:10.1213/ANE.0b013e3182a7f73c
55. Chatmongkolchart S, Prathep S. Supplemental oxygen for caesarean section during regional anaesthesia. *Cochrane Database Syst Rev*. 2016;3(3):Cd006161. doi:10.1002/14651858.CD006161.pub3
56. Hillyard SG, Bate TE, Corcoran TB, Paech MJ, O'Sullivan G. Extending epidural analgesia for emergency Caesarean section: a meta-analysis. *Br J Anaesth*. 2011;107(5):668–678. doi:10.1093/bja/aer300
57. Albright GA. Cardiac arrest following regional anesthesia with etidocaine or bupivacaine. *Anesthesiology*. 1979;51(4):285–287. doi:10.1097/00000542-197910000-00001
58. Choi DH, Ahn HJ, Kim JA. Combined low-dose spinal-epidural anesthesia versus single-shot spinal anesthesia for elective cesarean delivery. *Int J Obstet Anesth*. 2006;15(1):13–17. doi:10.1016/j.ijoa.2005.05.009
59. Hawkins JL, Chang J, Palmer SK, Gibbs CP, Callaghan WM. Anesthesia-related maternal mortality in the United States: 1979-2002. *Obstet Gynecol*. 2011;117(1):69–74. doi:10.1097/AOG.0b013e31820093a9
60. American Society of Anesthesiologists. Practice guidelines for obstetric anesthesia: an updated report by the American Society of Anesthesiologists Task Force on Obstetric Anesthesia and the Society for Obstetric Anesthesia and Perinatology. *Anesthesiology*. 2016;124(2):270–300. doi:10.1097/aln.0000000000000935
61. de Souza DG, Doar LH, Mehta SH, Tiouririne M. Aspiration prophylaxis and rapid sequence induction for elective cesarean delivery: time to reassess old dogma? *Anesth Analg*. 2010;110(5):1503–1505. doi:10.1213/ANE.0b013e3181d7e33c
62. Mushambi MC, Kinsella SM. Obstetric Anaesthetists' Association/Difficult Airway Society difficult and failed tracheal intubation guidelines–the way forward for the obstetric airway. *Br J Anaesth*. 2015;115(6):815–818. doi:10.1093/bja/aev296.
63. Ellis R, Laviola M, Stolady D, Valentine RL, Pillai A, Hardman JG. Comparison of apnoeic oxygen techniques in term pregnant subjects: a computational modelling study. *Br J Anaesth*. 2022;129(4):581–587. doi:10.1016/j.bja.2022.06.021
64. Apfelbaum JL, Hagberg CA, Connis RT, et al. 2022 American Society of Anesthesiologists practice guidelines for management of the difficult airway. *Anesthesiology*. 2022;136(1):31–81. doi:10.1097/aln.0000000000004002
65. Pandit JJ, Andrade J, Bogod DG, et al; Royal College of Anaesthetists; Association of Anaesthetists of Great Britain and Ireland. 5th National Audit Project (NAP5) on accidental awareness during general anaesthesia: summary of main findings and risk factors. *Br J Anaesth*. 2014;113(4):549–559. doi:10.1093/bja/aeu313
66. Chin KJ, Yeo SW. Bispectral index values at sevoflurane concentrations of 1% and 1.5% in lower segment cesarean delivery. *Anesth Analg*. 2004;98(4):1140–1144. doi:10.1213/01.Ane.0000103186.64302.38
67. Sultan P, Halpern SH, Pushpanathan E, Patel S, Carvalho B. The effect of intrathecal morphine dose on outcomes after elective cesarean delivery: a meta-analysis. *Anesth Analg*. 2016;123(1):154–164. doi:10.1213/ane.0000000000001255
68. Bauchat JR, Weiniger CF, Sultan P, et al. Society for Obstetric Anesthesia and Perinatology consensus statement: monitoring recommendations for prevention and detection of respiratory depression associated with administration of neuraxial morphine for cesarean delivery analgesia. *Anesth Analg*. 2019;129(2):458–474. doi:10.1213/ane.0000000000004195
69. Tan HS, Taylor C, Weikel D, Barton K, Habib AS. Quadratus lumborum block for postoperative analgesia after cesarean delivery: a systematic review with meta-analysis and trial-sequential analysis. *J Clin Anesth*. 2020;67:110003. doi:10.1016/j.jclinane.2020.110003
70. Nimmo WS, Wilson J, Prescott LF. Narcotic analgesics and delayed gastric emptying during labour. *Lancet*. 1975;1(7912):890–893. doi:10.1016/s0140-6736(75)91687-6
71. Ngan Kee WD, Khaw KS, Ng FF. Comparison of phenylephrine infusion regimens for maintaining maternal blood pressure during spinal anaesthesia for Caesarean section. *Br J Anaesth*. 2004;92(4):469–474. doi:10.1093/bja/aeh088
72. Banerjee A, Stocche RM, Angle P, Halpern SH. Preload or coload for spinal anesthesia for elective Cesarean delivery: a meta-analysis. *Can J Anaesth*. 2010;57(1):24–31. doi:10.1007/s12630-009-9206-7
73. Lee A, Ngan Kee WD, Gin T. A quantitative, systematic review of randomized controlled trials of ephedrine versus phenylephrine for the management of hypotension during spinal anesthesia for cesarean delivery. *Anesth Analg*. 2002;94(4):920–926. doi:10.1097/00000539-200204000-00028
74. George RB, McKeen D, Columb MO, Habib AS. Up-down determination of the 90% effective dose of phenylephrine for the treatment of spinal anesthesia-induced hypotension in parturients undergoing cesarean delivery. *Anesth Analg*. 2010;110(1):154–158. doi:10.1213/ANE.0b013e3181c30b72
75. Allen TK, George RB, White WD, Muir HA, Habib AS. A double-blind, placebo-controlled trial of four fixed rate infusion regimens of phenylephrine for hemodynamic support during spinal anesthesia for cesarean delivery. *Anesth Analg*. 2010;111(5):1221–1229. doi:10.1213/ANE.0b013e3181e1db21
76. Siddik-Sayyid SM, Taha SK, Kanazi GE, Aouad MT. A randomized controlled trial of variable rate phenylephrine infusion with rescue phenylephrine boluses versus rescue boluses alone on physician interventions during spinal anesthesia for elective cesarean delivery. *Anesth Analg*. 2014;118(3):611–618. doi:10.1213/01.ane.0000437731.60260.ce
77. Mohta M, Dubey M, Malhotra RK, Tyagi A. Comparison of the potency of phenylephrine and norepinephrine bolus doses used to treat post-spinal hypotension during elective caesarean section. *Int J Obstet Anesth*. 2019;38:25–31. doi:10.1016/j.ijoa.2018.12.002
78. Onwochei DN, Ngan Kee WD, Fung L, Downey K, Ye XY, Carvalho JCA. Norepinephrine intermittent intravenous boluses to prevent hypotension during spinal anesthesia for cesarean delivery: a sequential allocation dose-finding study. *Anesth Analg*. 2017;125(1):212–218. doi:10.1213/ANE.0000000000001846
79. Neal JM, Neal EJ, Weinberg GL. American Society of Regional Anesthesia and Pain Medicine local anesthetic systemic toxicity checklist: 2020 version. *Reg Anesth Pain Med*. 2021; 46(1):81–82. doi:10.1136/rapm-2020-101986
80. Paech MJ, Doherty DA, Christmas T, Wong CA; Epidural Blood Patch Trial Group. The volume of blood for epidural blood patch in obstetrics: a randomized, blinded clinical trial. *Anesth Analg*. 2011;113(1):126–133. doi:10.1213/ANE.0b013e318218204d
81. Scavone BM, Wong CA, Sullivan JT, Yaghmour E, Sherwani SS, McCarthy RJ. Efficacy of a prophylactic epidural blood patch in preventing post dural puncture headache in parturients after inadvertent dural puncture. *Anesthesiology*. 2004;101(6):1422–1427. doi:10.1097/00000542-200412000-00024
82. Apfel CC, Saxena A, Cakmakkaya OS, Gaiser R, George E, Radke O. Prevention of post-dural puncture headache after accidental dural puncture: a quantitative systematic review. *Br J Anaesth*. 2010;105(3):255–263. doi:10.1093/bja/aeq191
83. Mims SC, Tan HS, Sun K, et al. Long-term morbidities following unintentional dural puncture in obstetric patients: a systematic review and meta-analysis. *J Clin Anesth*. 2022;79:110787. doi:10.1016/j.jclinane.2022.110787
84. Centers for Disease Control and Prevention (CDC). Bacterial meningitis after intrapartum spinal anesthesia - New York and Ohio, 2008-2009. *MMWR Morb Mortal Wkly Rep*. 2010;59(3): 65–69.

85. Wong CA, Scavone BM, Dugan S, et al. Incidence of postpartum lumbosacral spine and lower extremity nerve injuries. *Obstet Gynecol.* 2003;101(2):279–288. doi:10.1016/s0029-7844(02)02727-8
86. Creanga AA. Maternal mortality in the United States: a review of contemporary data and their limitations. *Clin Obstet Gynecol.* 2018;61(2):296–306. doi:10.1097/GRF.0000000000000362
87. Merchant RM, Topjian AA, Panchal AR, et al; Adult Basic and Advanced Life Support, Pediatric Basic and Advanced Life Support, Neonatal Life Support, Resuscitation Education Science, and Systems of Care Writing Groups. Part 1: executive summary: 2020 American Heart Association guidelines for cardiopulmonary resuscitation and emergency cardiovascular care. *Circulation.* 2020;142(16_suppl_2):S337–s357. doi:10.1161/cir.0000000000000918
88. American College of Obstetricians and Gynecologists and Society for Maternal–Fetal Medicine Obstetric care consensus no. 9: Levels of maternal care. *Obstet Gynecol.* 2019;134(2):e41–55. doi: 10.1097/AOG.0000000000003383
89. Ananth CV, Keyes KM, Wapner RJ. Pre-eclampsia rates in the United States, 1980-2010: age-period-cohort analysis. *BMJ.* 2013;347:f6564. doi:10.1136/bmj.f6564
90. American College of Obstetricians and Gynecologists. Gestational hypertension and preeclampsia: ACOG Practice Bulletin, Number 222. *Obstet Gynecol.* 2020;135(6):e237–e260. doi:10.1097/AOG.0000000000003891
91. Jung E, Romero R, Yeo L, et al. The etiology of preeclampsia. *Am J Obstet Gynecol.* 2022; 226(2S):S844–S866. doi:10.1016/j.ajog.2021.11.1356
92. Erez O, Romero R, Jung E, et al. Preeclampsia and eclampsia: the conceptual evolution of a syndrome. *Am J Obstet Gynecol.* 2022;226(2S):S786–S803. doi:10.1016/j.ajog.2021.12.001
93. Chesley LC. Plasma and red cell volumes during pregnancy. *Am J Obstet Gynecol.* 1972; 112(3):440–450.
94. American College of Obstetricians and Gynecologists. Committee Opinion No. 455: magnesium sulfate before anticipated preterm birth for neuroprotection. *Obstet Gynecol.* 2010; 115(3):669–671. doi:10.1097/AOG.0b013e3181d4ffa5
95. Jouppila P, Jouppila R, Hollmén A, Koivula A. Lumbar epidural analgesia to improve intervillous blood flow during labor in severe preeclampsia. *Obstet Gynecol.* 1982;59(2): 158–161.
96. Aya AGM, Mangin R, Vialles N, et al. Patients with severe preeclampsia experience less hypotension during spinal anesthesia for elective cesarean delivery than healthy parturients: a prospective cohort comparison. *Anesth Analg.* 2003;97(3):867–872. doi:10.1213/01.ANE.0000073610.23885.F2
97. Wallace DH, Leveno KJ, Cunningham FG, Giesecke AH, Shearer VE, Sidawi JE. Randomized comparison of general and regional anesthesia for cesarean delivery in pregnancies complicated by severe preeclampsia. *Obstet Gynecol.* 1995;86(2):193–199. doi:10.1016/0029-7844(95)00139-i
98. Bateman BT, Berman MF, Riley LE, Leffert LR. The epidemiology of hemorrhage in a large, nationwide sample of deliveries. *Anesth Analg.* 2010;110(5):1368–1373. doi:10.1213/ANE.0b013e3181d74898
99. Royal College of Obstetricians & Gynaecologists. *Antepartum hemorrhage (Green-top Guideline No. 63).* 2011. Accessed 23 May, 2022. https://www.rcog.org.uk/guidance/browse-all-guidance/green-top-guidelines/antepartum-haemorrhage-green-top-guideline-no-63/
100. Silver RM, Landon MB, Rouse DJ, et al. Maternal morbidity associated with multiple repeat cesarean deliveries. *Obstet Gynecol.* 2006;107(6):1226–1232. doi:10.1097/01.AOG.0000219750.79480.84
101. Tikkanen M. Placental abruption: epidemiology, risk factors and consequences. *Acta Obstet Gynecol Scand.* 2011;90(2):140–149. doi:10.1111/j.1600-0412.2010.01030.x
102. Sharp HT, Johnson JV, Lemieux LA, Currigan SM. Executive summary of the reVITALize initiative: standardizing gynecologic data definitions. *Obstet Gynecol.* 2017;129(4):603–607. doi:10.1097/AOG.0000000000001939
103. Ende HB, Lozada MJ, Chestnut DH, et al. Risk factors for atonic postpartum hemorrhage: a systematic review and meta-analysis. *Obstet Gynecol.* 2021;137(2):305–323. doi:10.1097/AOG.0000000000004228
104. Bateman BT, Mhyre JM, Callaghan WM, Kuklina EV. Peripartum hysterectomy in the United States: nationwide 14 year experience. *Am J Obstet Gynecol.* 2012;206(1):63.e1–63.e8. doi:10.1016/j.ajog.2011.07.030
105. American College of Obstetricians and Gynecologists; Society for Maternal-Fetal Medicine. Obstetric care consensus No. 7: placenta accreta spectrum. *Obstet Gynecol.* 2018;132(6):e259–e275. doi:10.1097/AOG.0000000000002983
106. Girard T, Mörtl M, Schlembach D. New approaches to obstetric hemorrhage: the postpartum hemorrhage consensus algorithm. *Curr Opin Anaesthesiol.* 2014;27(3):267–274. doi:10.1097/ACO.0000000000000081
107. WOMAN Trial Collaborators. Effect of early tranexamic acid administration on mortality, hysterectomy, and other morbidities in women with post-partum haemorrhage (WOMAN): an international, randomised, double-blind, placebo-controlled trial. *Lancet.* 2017;389(10084): 2105–2116. doi:10.1016/S0140-6736(17)30638-4
108. Liumbruno GM, Liumbruno C, Rafanelli D. Intraoperative cell salvage in obstetrics: is it a real therapeutic option? *Transfusion.* 2011;51(10):2244–2256. doi:10.1111/j.1537-2995.2011.03116.x
109. Main EK, Goffman D, Scavone BM, et al. National Partnership for Maternal Safety: consensus bundle on obstetric hemorrhage. *Anesth Analg.* 2015;121(1):142–148. doi:10.1097/AOG.0000000000000869
110. Arendt KW, Lindley KJ. Obstetric anesthesia management of the patient with cardiac disease. *Int J Obstet Anesth.* 2019;37:73–85. doi:10.1016/j.ijoa.2018.09.011.
111. American College of Obstetricians and Gynecologists. ACOG Practice Bulletin No. 212 Summary: pregnancy and heart disease. *Obstet Gynecol.* 2019;133(5):1067–1072. doi:10.1097/AOG.0000000000003244
112. Regitz-Zagrosek V, Roos-Hesselink JW, Bauersachs J, et al; ESC Scientific Document Group. 2018 ESC Guidelines for the management of cardiovascular diseases during pregnancy. *Eur Heart J.* 2018;39(34):3165–3241. doi:10.1093/eurheartj/ehy340
113. Mehta LS, Warnes CA, Bradley E, et al; American Heart Association Council on Clinical Cardiology, Council on Arteriosclerosis, Thrombosis and Vascular Biology, Council on Cardiovascular and Stroke Nursing, Stroke Council. Cardiovascular considerations in caring for pregnant patients: a scientific statement from the American Heart Association. *Circulation.* 2020;141(23):e884–e903. doi:10.1161/CIR.0000000000000772
114. Leffert L, Butwick A, Carvalho B, et al. The Society for Obstetric Anesthesia and Perinatology consensus statement on the anesthetic management of pregnant and postpartum women receiving thromboprophylaxis or higher dose anticoagulants. *Anesth Analg.* 2018; 126(3):928–944. doi:10.1213/ANE.0000000000002530
115. American College of Obstetricians and Gynecologists. ACOG Practice Bulletin No. 190: gestational diabetes mellitus. *Obstet Gynecol.* 2018;131(2):e49–e64. doi:10.1097/AOG.0000000000002501
116. Shah NS, Wang MC, Freaney PM, et al. Trends in gestational diabetes at first live birth by race and ethnicity in the US, 2011-2019. *JAMA.* 2021;326(7):660–669. doi:10.1001/jama.2021.7217
117. Mulholland C, Njoroge T, Mersereau P, Williams J. Comparison of guidelines available in the United States for diagnosis and management of diabetes before, during, and after pregnancy. *J Womens Health (Larchmt).* 2007;16(6):790–801. doi:10.1089/jwh.2007.CDC7
118. American College of Obstetricians and Gynecologists' Committee on Practice Bulletins—Obstetrics. ACOG Practice Bulletin No. 201: pregestational diabetes mellitus. *Obstet Gynecol.* 2018;132(6):e228–e248. doi:10.1097/AOG.0000000000002960
119. Taylor CR, Dominguez JE, Habib AS. Obesity and obstetric anesthesia: Current Insights. *Local Reg Anesth.* 2019;12:111–124. doi:10.2147/LRA.S186530
120. Tonidandel A, Booth J, D'Angelo R, Harris L, Tonidandel S. Anesthetic and obstetric outcomes in morbidly obese parturients: a 20-year follow-up retrospective cohort study. *Int J Obstet Anesth.* 2014;23(4):357–364. doi:10.1016/j.ijoa.2014.05.004
121. Attali E, Yogev Y. The impact of advanced maternal age on pregnancy outcome. *Best Pract Res Clin Obstet Gynaecol.* 2021;70:2–9. doi:10.1016/j.bpobgyn.2020.06.006
122. Osterman M, Hamilton B, Martin JA, Driscoll AK, Valenzuela CP. Births: final data for 2020. *Natl Vital Stat Rep.* 2021;70(17):1–50.
123. Vigil-De Gracia P, Montufar-Rueda C, Smith A. Pregnancy and severe chronic hypertension: maternal outcome. *Hypertens Pregnancy.* 2004 23(3):285–293. doi:10.1081/PRG-200030315
124. Mhyre JM, Tsen LC, Einav S, Kuklina EV, Leffert LR, Bateman BT. Cardiac arrest during hospitalization for delivery in the United States, 1998-2011. *Anesthesiology.* 2014;120(4):810–818. doi:10.1097/ALN.0000000000000159
125. Walani SR. Global burden of preterm birth. *Int J Gynaecol Obstet.* 2020;150(1):31–33. doi:10.1002/ijgo.13195
126. American College of Obstetricians and Gynecologists. Committee Opinion No. 711: opioid use and opioid use disorder in pregnancy. *Obstet Gynecol.* 2017;130(2):e81–e94. doi:10.1097/AOG.0000000000002235
127. American College of Obstetricians and Gynecologists. Committee Opinion No. 722: marijuana use during pregnancy and lactation. *Obstet Gynecol.* 2017;130(4):e205–e209. doi:10.1097/aog.0000000000002354
128. American College of Obstetricians and Gynecologists. ACOG Practice Bulletin No. 106: intrapartum fetal heart rate monitoring: nomenclature, interpretation, and general management principles. *Obstet Gynecol.* 2009;114(1):192–202. doi:10.1097/AOG.0b013e3181aef106
129. Timmins AE, Clark SL. How to approach intrapartum category II tracings. *Obstet Gynecol Clin North Am.* 2015;42(2):363–375. doi:10.1016/j.ogc.2015.01.013
130. Aziz K, Lee CHC, Escobedo MB, et al. Part 5: neonatal resuscitation 2020 American Heart Association guidelines for cardiopulmonary resuscitation and emergency cardiovascular care. *Pediatrics.* 2021;147(Suppl 1). doi:10.1542/peds.2020-038505E
131. Davis PG, Tan A, O'Donnell CPF, Schulze A. Resuscitation of newborn infants with 100% oxygen or air: a systematic review and meta-analysis. *Lancet.* 2004;364(9442):1329–1333. doi:10.1016/S0140-6736(04)17189-4
132. Dick JR, Wimalasundera R, Nandi R. Maternal and fetal anaesthesia for fetal surgery. *Anaesthesia.* 2021;76(Suppl 4):63–68. doi:10.1111/anae.15423
133. Stewart MK, Terhune KP. Management of pregnant patients undergoing general surgical procedures. *Surg Clin North Am.* 2015;95(2):429–442. doi:10.1016/j.suc.2014.10.007
134. Smith BE, Gaub ML, Moya F. Teratogenic effects of anesthetic agents: nitrous oxide. *Anesth Analg.* 1965;44(6):726–732.
135. Bleeser T, Van Der Veeken L, Fieuws S, et al. Effects of general anaesthesia during pregnancy on neurocognitive development of the fetus: a systematic review and meta-analysis. *Br J Anaesth.* 2021;126(6):1128–1140. doi:10.1016/j.bja.2021.02.026
136. American College of Obstetricians and Gynecologists. ACOG Committee Opinion No. 775: nonobstetric surgery during pregnancy. *Obstet Gynecol.* 2019;133(4):e285–e286. doi:10.1097/AOG.0000000000003174

42 Neonatal Anesthesia

SHIVANI G. MUKKAMALA • JUSTIN B. LONG

KEY POINTS

1. Understanding the physiologic changes that occur during the transition from fetal to neonatal life is crucial to the anesthetic management of the neonate. The circulatory, pulmonary, hepatic, and renal systems are all affected in this process.
2. Important physiologic and anatomic factors account for the rapid rate of desaturation observed in neonates. These include an increase in oxygen consumption, a higher closing volume, a high ratio of minute ventilation to functional residual capacity, and a pliable rib cage.
3. Persistent pulmonary hypertension of the newborn is a pathologic condition that can be primary but often is secondary to other conditions, including meconium aspiration, sepsis, congenital diaphragmatic hernia, or pneumonia. Understanding the pathophysiologic characteristics of this condition helps guide therapy.
4. Knowledge of the major anatomic differences between the infant and the adult airway helps one understand why the infant's airway is often described as "anterior" and why airway management may be challenging. These differences include a relatively large tongue, a cephalad glottis with anterior slanting vocal folds, a larger occiput, and a narrowing at the cricoid ring.
5. Careful attention must be given to the choice of anesthetic agents and dosing of such agents in the neonatal population. Ongoing maturational changes in the renal and hepatobiliary systems, which occur during the first 30 days of life, will affect the metabolism and elimination of many anesthetic agents.
6. Although a host of anesthetic techniques are available, including regional anesthesia, multiple factors are considered when choosing an anesthetic plan for the neonate. These include the surgical requirements, the need for postoperative ventilation, the cardiovascular stability of the neonate, and the anticipated method of postoperative pain control.
7. Special considerations must be addressed when planning an anesthetic for a neonate. Some of the controversial issues include the risk of postoperative apnea, the role of oxygen concentration in the development of retinopathy of prematurity, and the neurocognitive effects of anesthetic agents on the fetal and neonatal brain.
8. True surgical emergencies are uncommon in the neonatal period. Knowledge of conditions with comorbidities, such as tracheoesophageal fistula, omphalocele, and congenital diaphragmatic hernia, and a thorough preoperative evaluation and stabilization of such neonates cannot be overemphasized.

Physiology of the Infant and the Transition Period

An infant's first year of life is characterized by a miraculous growth in size and maturity. The body weight alone changes by a factor of three, and there is no other period in extrauterine life when changes occur so rapidly. Before birth, fetal growth and development depend on the genetic composition of the fetus, the mother's placental function, and potential exposure to chemicals or infectious agents that can affect the mother, fetus, or both. After birth, the newborn must rapidly adjust to the extrauterine environment to survive. The dramatic changes in functions of several systems will determine the viability of the neonate, as well as its ability to grow and develop properly.

The newborn period has been defined as the first 24 hours of life, and the neonatal period as the first 28 days of life. There is significant change in many physiologic systems during both of the periods. The first 72 hours are especially significant for the cardiovascular, pulmonary, and renal systems. The changes in these systems are interrelated; inadequate progression of change or a disease state altering one of these systems can quickly alter the maturation of one or more of the other systems. Understanding the differences in these systems from the older child, as well 1 as the changes that occur in the neonatal period, is important in developing a comprehensive anesthetic approach.

The Cardiovascular System

Fetal Circulation

The fetal circulation is characterized by a parallel system in which both ventricles pump most of their output into the systemic circulation. Less than 10% of the combined cardiac output goes through the fetal circulation as a result of the ductus arteriosus (Fig. 42-1A). The placenta provides oxygenated blood into the ductus venosus, the inferior vena cava, and then into the right atrium. In the right atrium, the majority of the oxygenated blood primarily flows through the foramen ovale into the left atrium, bypassing the right ventricle and the pulmonary vascular bed. This preferential flow across the foramen occurs because of the relatively low pressure in the left atrium compared with that of the right atrium. Some blood from the right atrium does flow through the right ventricle and into the main pulmonary artery. The pulmonary vascular resistance is quite high in utero because of alveolar collapse and compression of blood vessels, inhibiting flow through the pulmonary circulation. The pulmonary vascular resistance is also high at this point because of the relatively low arterial partial pressure of oxygen (PaO_2) and pH of the blood that does flow through the vessels. Some blood in the pulmonary artery does flow through the pulmonary circulation and then into the left atrium, but the majority of flow goes through the ductus arteriosus into the descending aorta.

Changes at Birth

After birth, all shunts are eliminated or start to close quickly.[1] The placental shunt is eliminated and the ductus venosus is closed. The newborn's left ventricle now pumps blood into the higher-pressure systemic circulation exclusively. Expansion of the lungs and initiation of breathing lead to dramatic changes in both the circulatory and pulmonary systems (Fig. 42-1B). As alveoli fill with air, the compression of the pulmonary alveolar capillaries is relieved, reducing pulmonary vascular resistance and promoting flow through the pulmonary circulation. This blood is now oxygenated, raising the PaO_2, and further reducing pulmonary vascular resistance. Although the change in the first minutes to hours is dramatic, it usually takes 3 to 4 days for the pulmonary vascular resistance to decrease to normal levels. The foramen ovale will usually functionally close in the first hour of life as the increase in left atrial pressure from increased pulmonary circulation after the initiation of breathing exceeds right atrial pressure. The foramen is closed by a flap of tissue. This foramen can reopen if there is a relative increase in right atrial pressure such as is seen with elevated pulmonary vascular resistance or fluid overload. Anatomic closure usually occurs in the first year of life but may remain

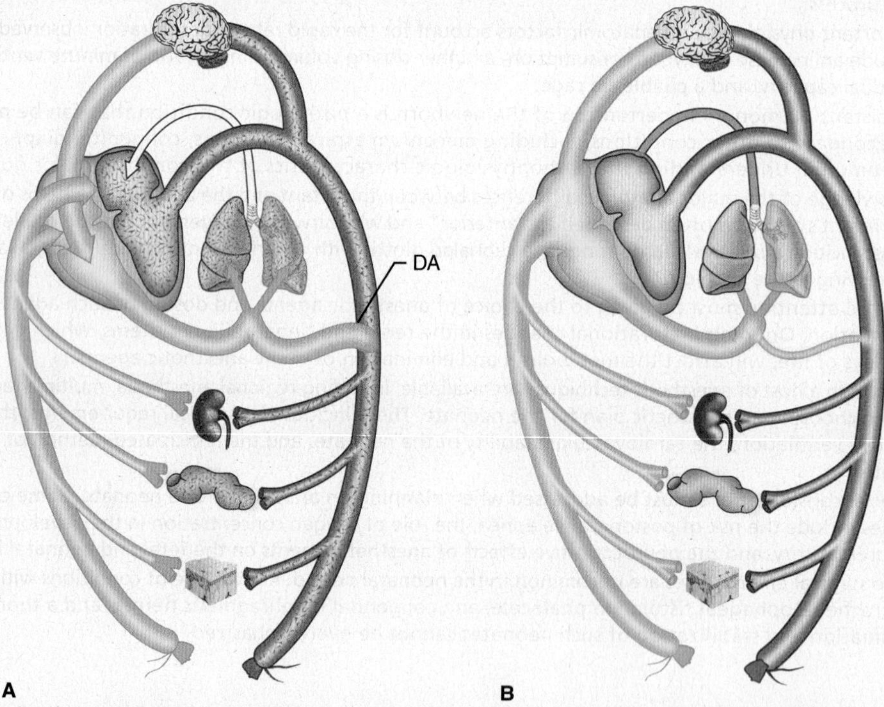

Figure 42-1 **A:** Schematic representation of the fetal circulation. Oxygenated blood leaves the placenta in the umbilical vein (*vessel without stippling*). Umbilical vein blood joins blood from the viscera (represented here by the kidney, gut, and skin) in the inferior vena cava. Approximately half of the inferior vena cava flow passes through the foramen ovale to the left atrium, where it mixes with a small amount of pulmonary venous blood, and this relatively well-oxygenated blood (*denoted by stippling*) supplies the heart and brain by way of the ascending aorta. The other half of the inferior vena cava stream mixes with superior vena cava blood and enters the right ventricle (blood in the right atrium and ventricle has little oxygen). Because the pulmonary arterioles are constricted, most of the blood in the main pulmonary artery flows through the ductus arteriosus (DA) so the descending aorta's blood has less oxygen (*heavy stippling*) than does blood in the ascending aorta (*light stippling*). **B:** Schematic representation of the circulation in the normal newborn. After expansion of the lungs and ligation of the umbilical cord, pulmonary blood flow and left atrial and systemic arterial pressures increase. When left atrial pressure exceeds right atrial pressure, the foramen ovale closes so all inferior and superior vena cava blood leaves the right atrium, enters the right ventricle, and is pumped through the pulmonary artery toward the lung. With the increase in systemic arterial pressure and decrease in pulmonary artery pressure, flow through the ductus arteriosus becomes left to right, and the ductus constricts and closes. The course of circulation is the same as in the adult. (Reprinted with permission from Phibbs R. Delivery room management of the newborn. In: Avery GB, ed. *Neonatology, Pathophysiology and Management of the Newborn*. 2nd ed. JB Lippincott; 1981:184.)

probe-patent into adulthood in 10% to 20% of patients. The ductus arteriosus starts to close in the first day of life and is usually functionally closed in the second day of life. *In utero*, patency of the ductus was maintained by the combined relaxant effects of low oxygen tension and endogenously produced prostaglandins, especially prostaglandin E_2. In a full-term neonate, oxygen is the most important factor controlling ductal closure. When the PaO_2 of blood in the ductus rises to about 50 mmHg, the muscle in the vessel constricts. It should be noted that the ductus of a preterm infant is less responsive to increased oxygen, even though its musculature is developed.

Myocardial function is different in the neonate. The neonatal cardiac myocyte has less organized contractile elements than the child or adult.[2] Not only are there fewer myofibril elements, but they are not organized in parallel roles, as seen in the child and adult heart, making them less efficient. The neonate myocyte also has a less mature sarcoplasmic reticulum system. The underdeveloped sarcoplasmic reticulum is associated with a decrease in Ca^{2+}-adenosine triphosphatase activity, an important component of contractility. As the sarcoplasmic reticulum matures, the efficiency of calcium transport and subsequent contractility increase.[3] The neonatal myocardium cannot generate as much force as that of the older child and is relatively noncompliant. Consequently, there is limited functional reserve in the neonatal period, with afterload increases particularly poorly tolerated. After birth, there are dramatic changes in the myocardium. As the work of the ventricles increases secondary to high stroke volume and increased vascular resistance, these myocytes grow quickly in number and size. This growth is more dramatic in the left ventricle than the right ventricle because of the rise in systemic vascular resistance and fall in pulmonary vascular resistance. Cardiac output is markedly different in the neonate, up to 400 mL/kg/min, falls in infancy to around 200 mL/kg/min, and is 100 mL/kg/min by adolescence approaching adult values of 70 to 80 mL/kg/min.

Especially in the first 3 months of life, the parasympathetic nervous system influence on the heart is more mature than the sympathetic system and the myocardium does not respond to inotropic support as well as the older child or adult. There is animal evidence that there are maturational changes in β-adrenergic receptor function that explain the decreased responsiveness to inotropes in the neonate.[4] The neonatal myocardium has increased glycogen stores and higher rates of anaerobic glycolysis, which may explain its relative resistance to hypoxia and better performance in the presence of an ischemic insult. Because the myocardium is relatively noncompliant in the newborn, preload changes can increase stroke volume and cardiac output, but not as effectively as in the older child.[5] In other words, the Frank–Starling relationship is present in the neonatal heart but is not as effective as in the adult. Therefore, the clinical implication of a noncompliant ventricle is that, in the absence of significant increases in stroke volume, cardiac output is not well maintained in the presence of bradycardia. Finally, neonates have immature baroreceptors. The baroreceptor is responsible for reflex tachycardia that occurs in response to hypotension. Therefore, the immaturity of this reflex would limit the neonate's ability to compensate for hypotension by increasing heart rate. In addition, the baroresponse of the neonate is more depressed than that of the adult at the same level of anesthesia.

In summary, the neonatal heart has some significant differences when compared to the mature heart. Resting cardiac output is much higher relative to body weight than in the adult because of the higher O_2 consumption per kilogram of body weight. Stimulation of the myocardium produces a limited increase in contractility and cardiac output. The sympathetic nervous system, which usually provides the important chronotropic and inotropic

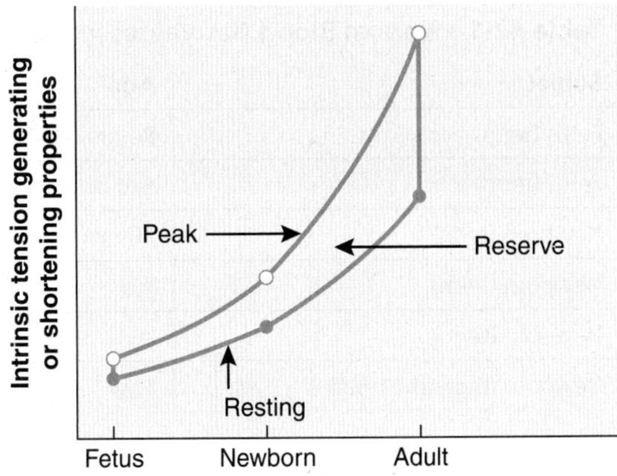

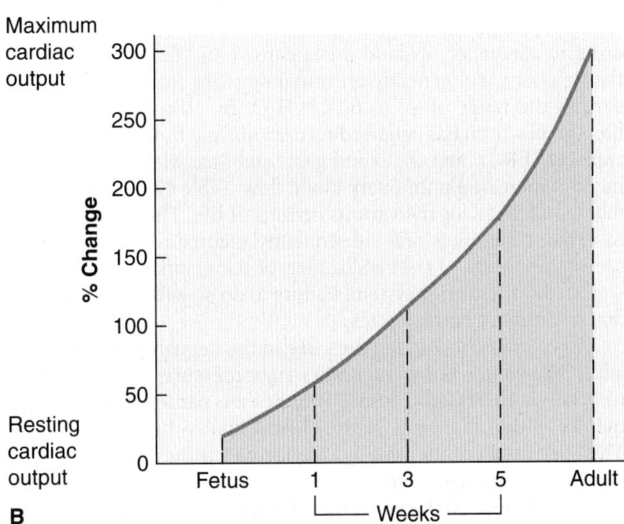

Figure 42-2 Schema of reduced cardiac reserve in fetal and newborn animal hearts compared with adult hearts. **A:** In the newborn infant, resting cardiac muscle performance is close to a peak of ventricular function because of limitations in diastolic, systolic, and heart rate reserve. **B:** Similarly, pump reserve early in life is limited by these factors and by much higher resting cardiac output relative to body weight, compared with that in adults. (Reprinted from Friedman WF, George BL. Treatment of congestive heart failure by altering loading conditions of the heart. *J Pediatr*. 1985;106:700. Copyright © 1985 Elsevier. With permission.)

support to the mature circulation during stress, is severely limited in the neonate because of relative lack of development when compared with the parasympathetic nervous system. Even in the absence of stress, the neonatal heart has limited ability to increase cardiac output compared with the mature heart (Fig. 42-2). The resting cardiac output of the immature heart is close to the maximal cardiac output, so there is limited reserve. The mature heart can increase cardiac output by 300%, whereas the immature heart can only increase cardiac output by 30% to 40%.

The Pulmonary System

The pulmonary system develops rapidly during the last trimester, with important changes in both the number of alveoli and the maturity of the pulmonary vascular system.[6] These systems have not matured enough to provide adequate gas exchange until about 24 to 26 weeks' gestation. The airways and alveoli continue to grow after birth, with alveoli increasing in number until about 8 years of age.[7] With the initiation of ventilation, the pulmonary

Table 42-1 Normal Blood Gas Values in the Neonate

Subject	Age	PaO_2 (mmHg)	$PaCO_2$ (mmHg)	pH
Fetus (term)	Before labor	25	40	7.37
Fetus (term)	End of labor	10–20	55	7.25
Newborn (term)	10 min	50	48	7.20
Newborn (term)	1 h	70	35	7.35
Newborn (term)	1 wk	75	35	7.40
Newborn (preterm, 1,500 g)	1 wk	60	38	7.37

system changes dramatically. The alveoli transition from a fluid-filled to an air-filled state and a normal ventilatory pattern with normal volumes develops in the first 5 to 10 minutes of life. In order to adequately expand the collapsed and fluid-filled alveoli, the newborn will generate an initial negative intrathoracic pressure in the range of 40 to 60 cm H_2O. By 10 to 20 minutes of life, the newborn has achieved its near-normal functional residual capacity (FRC), and the blood gases stabilize with the establishment of increased pulmonary blood flow. Table 42-1 lists the normal blood gases for the various periods of life. The initial breaths to expand the lungs and subsequently maintain FRC are necessary components of the stabilization of the ventilatory system, as well as the circulatory system. Failure to do so will quickly lead to deterioration of both systems.

2 Tidal volume is roughly the same in the neonate as the child or adult on a volume/kilogram body weight measure, but the respiratory rate is increased. Closing volumes are particularly high and may be within the range of the normal tidal volume (Fig. 42-3). This increased minute ventilation mirrors the higher oxygen consumption in neonates, which is about double that seen in an adult. Because the FRC in the newborn is comparable to that of the older child or adult, but the minute ventilation is much higher, the ratio of minute ventilation to FRC is two to three times higher in the newborn. The clinical significance of this ratio is twofold. First, anesthetic induction with a volatile anesthetic agent should be faster, as should emergence. Second, the decrease in FRC relative to minute ventilation and oxygen consumption means that there is less "oxygen reserve" in the FRC compared to that of older children and adults. There will be a more rapid drop in arterial oxygen levels in the newborn in the presence of apnea or hypoventilation. Table 42-2 compares normal respiratory parameters in the normal newborn and adult.

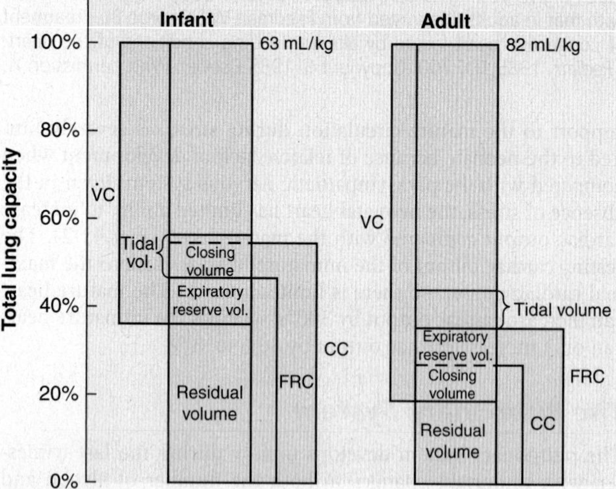

Figure 42-3 Static lung volumes of infants and adults. CC, closing capacity; FRC, functional residual capacity; VC, vital capacity. (Used with permission of Thomas, from Smith CA, Nelson NM. *Physiology of the Newborn Infant*. 4th ed. Springfield, IL: Charles C Thomas; 1976:207, permission conveyed from Copyright Clearance Center, Inc.)

Lung compliance is relatively low, but chest wall compliance is relatively high, compared to that of older children. The pliable rib cage gives less mechanical support than in the older child, leading to significant retractions with less efficient gas exchange and functional airway closure, thus increasing the work of breathing. The intercostal muscles are poorly developed at birth, with the diaphragm providing most of the gas exchange. The diaphragm in the neonate has two types of fibers, the type 1, slow twitch, high-oxidative fibers that give sustained contraction with very little fatigue, and the type 2, fast twitch, low-oxidative fibers that give quick contractions but fatigue easily. The distribution of these fibers in the newborn shows only about 25% type 1 fibers, whereas 55% of the fibers are type 1 in the mature diaphragm at about 2 years of age. The preterm newborn has even fewer type 1 fibers at birth, in the 10% range. This relative lack of type 1 fibers means that the newborn, especially the preterm, is at risk for diaphragmatic fatigue in the presence of significant resistance to ventilation or periods of hyperventilation.

Finally, the continued presence of surfactant is necessary to maintain both the distensibility of the alveoli and the maintenance of an FRC at exhalation. Decreased surfactant production, due to prematurity or other conditions such as maternal diabetes, can cause respiratory distress syndrome (RDS). The decreased surfactant can cause alveolar collapse, decrease in lung compliance, hypoxia, increased work of breathing, and respiratory failure. Commercially available surfactant is extraordinarily useful to both treat and prevent RDS in susceptible patients. In addition, surfactant

Table 42-2 Comparison of Normal Respiratory Values in Infants and Adults

Parameter	Infant	Adult
Respiratory frequency (breaths/min)	30–50	12–16
Tidal volume (mL/kg)	7	7
Dead space (mL/kg)	2–2.5	2.2
Alveolar ventilation (mL/kg/min)	100–150	60
Functional residual capacity (mL/kg)	27–30	30
Oxygen consumption (mL/kg/min)	7–9	3

can improve gas exchange in preterm neonates who may not have RDS, but are stressed by sepsis, heart failure, or other systemic problems.[8] Delivered through an endotracheal tube, it can be used prophylactically in the very preterm newborn to prevent RDS, as well as treat neonates who have developed RDS.

In addition to the mechanical aspects of the pulmonary system, control of breathing has unique aspects in the neonatal period, especially in the preterm neonate. Neonates respond less to hypercapnia than the older child. In addition, neonates respond to hypoxia with a brief period of hyperventilation, followed by hypoventilation. The initial hyperventilatory response is prevented by hypothermia, further increasing risk of hypoventilatory response to hypoxia. Finally, a periodic breathing pattern is common in neonates, especially in preterm newborns, and can persist up to a year of age.

Persistent Pulmonary Hypertension of the Newborn

3 The pulmonary circulation is extremely sensitive to oxygen, pH, and nitric oxide, a variety of mediators such as adenosine and prostaglandins, and mechanical factors such as lung inflation. Figure 42-4 illustrates the correlation of the mean pulmonary artery pressure with age during the first 3 days of life. Hypoxia and acidosis, along with inflammatory mediators, may cause pulmonary artery pressure either to persist at a high level or, after initially decreasing, to increase to pathologic levels. The result is termed *persistent pulmonary hypertension of the newborn* (PPHN), sometimes referred to as *persistent fetal circulation*. PPHN occurs in term and preterm infants, usually caused by precipitating conditions such as severe birth asphyxia, meconium aspiration, sepsis, congenital diaphragmatic hernia (CDH), and maternal use of nonsteroidal anti-inflammatory drugs with *in utero* constriction of the ductus arteriosus, although it is often idiopathic. Other risk factors include maternal diabetes, maternal asthma, and cesarean delivery.[9]

Elevated pulmonary vascular resistance causes both the ductus arteriosus and foramen ovale to remain open, with subsequent right-to-left shunting bypassing the pulmonary circulation. These changes result in profound hypoxia from right-to-left shunting and a normal or elevated $PaCO_2$. The hypoxemia is often noted to be out of proportion to the other presenting signs of respiratory and cardiovascular compromise. Treatment starts with correcting any predisposing disease (hypoglycemia, polycythemia) and improving poor tissue oxygenation. The response to therapy is often unpredictable. However, the goals are to achieve a PaO_2 of 60 to 100 mmHg and maintain normocapnia.[10]

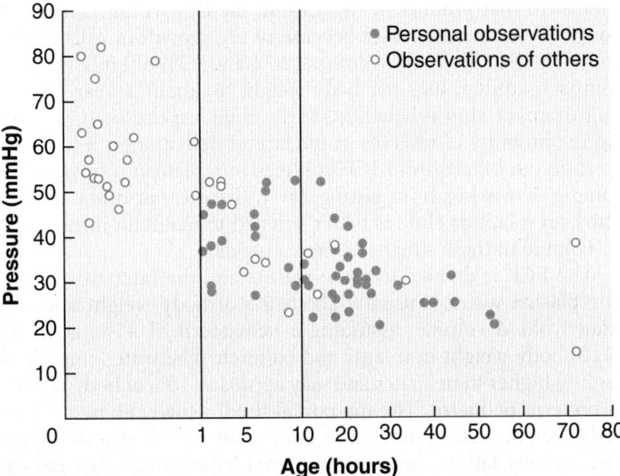

Figure 42-4 Correlation of mean pulmonary arterial pressure with age in 85 normal-term infants studied during the first 3 days of life. (Adapted from Emmanouilides GC, Moss AJ, Duffie ER, et al. Pulmonary arterial pressure changes in human newborn infants from birth to 3 days of age. *J Pediatr*. 1964;65:327. Copyright © 1964 Elsevier. With permission.)

In addition to standard mechanical ventilation, high-frequency ventilation, exogenous surfactant, inhaled nitric oxide (iNO), alkalinization, and extracorporeal membrane oxygenation (ECMO) have been used with varying degrees of success. In particular, the use of iNO is becoming more common and is indicated when the newborn expresses an oxygen index (OI) ≥15 ($OI = [Paw_{MEAN} \times FiO_2 \times 100]/PaO_2$ where Paw_{MEAN} = mean airway pressure, FiO_2 = fraction of inspired O_2). However, iNO has not been shown to reduce the need for ECMO in neonates with CDH.[11,12] iNO remains the only U.S. Food and Drug Administration (FDA) approved medication for treatment of PPHN. Additional vasodilator therapy with prostacyclin (epoprostenol), phosphodiesterase inhibitors (sildenafil), and endothelin receptor antagonists (bosentan) have varying levels of success beyond the neonatal period, into infancy. Success in treatment, and in survival, varies directly with correcting the underlying cause. Significant prognostic factors for PPHN are the ability of therapy to reduce pulmonary vascular resistance and the occurrence of associated complications, such as ischemic encephalopathy.

Maintenance of right ventricular function is paramount to survival in PPHN. Use of dobutamine in a normotensive patient may provide inotropy and decreased systemic vascular resistance, which could increase right-to-left shunting and offload the right ventricle.[13] Therapy is now often guided with the use of point-of-care echocardiography as its availability continues to grow and technology improves.[14] Preoperative assessment of the echocardiogram by the pediatric anesthesiologist may help predict what problems may be encountered in the operative environment. Also, the availability of very small transesophageal echocardiogram (TEE) probes make the possibility of real-time monitoring of cardiac function in the operating room a reality. However, insertion of even the smallest TEE probes requires close attention to ventilator parameters in very small (<3 kg) neonates.[15]

Meconium Aspiration

One of the most important pulmonary challenges in the newborn period is *meconium aspiration*. Interference with the normal maternal placental circulation in the third trimester may cause fetal hypoxia. Fetal hypoxia can result in an increase in the amount of muscle in the blood vessels of the distal respiratory units. Figure 42-5 illustrates the muscle increase found in blood vessels of a series of 11 infants who died of PPHN.[16] Chronic fetal hypoxia leads to the passage of meconium *in utero*. The fetus breathes *in utero* so the meconium mixed with amniotic fluid enters the lung. Meconium aspiration can be a marker of chronic fetal hypoxia in the third trimester. This condition is different from the meconium aspiration that occurs during delivery. Meconium at birth is thick and tenacious, and mechanically obstructs the tracheobronchial system. Meconium aspiration syndrome leads to varying degrees of respiratory failure, which can be fatal despite all current treatment modalities.

Current recommendations for intubation and suctioning for newborns at delivery with frank meconium aspiration or meconium staining (approximately 10% of newborns) emphasize a conservative approach.[17] Routine oropharyngeal suctioning of meconium is recommended immediately at the time of delivery, but tracheal intubation and suctioning should be performed selectively. If the newborn is vigorous and crying, no further suctioning

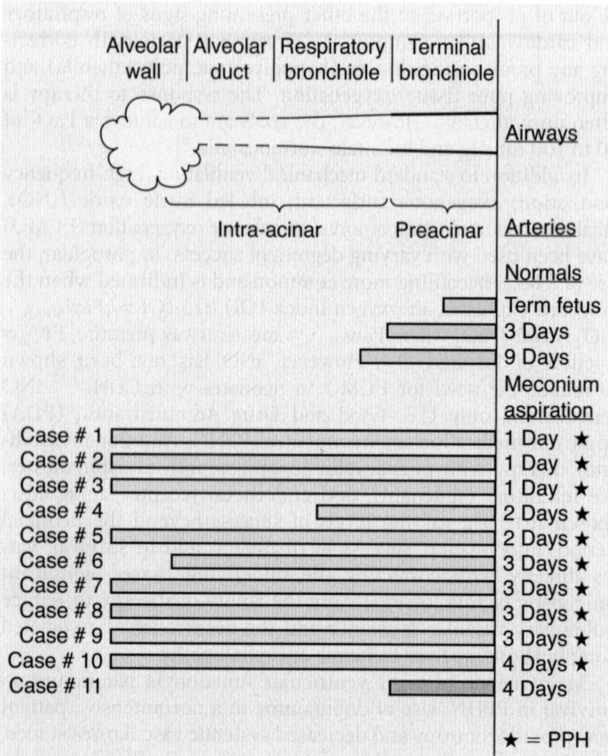

Figure 42-5 Diagram of muscle extension along pulmonary arterial branches (*shaded bars*). In the normal newborn, virtually no intra-acinar artery is muscular. In 9 of 10 infants with meconium aspiration and persistent pulmonary hypertension of the newborn (PPHN), muscle extended into the most peripheral arteries; the infant with meconium aspiration without PPHN (case 11) had normal intra-acinar arteries. (Reprinted from Murphy JD, Vawter GF, Reid LM. Pulmonary vascular disease in fetal meconium aspiration. *J Pediatr*. 1984;104:758. Copyright © 1984 Elsevier. With permission.)

is needed. If meconium is present and the newborn is depressed, the trachea should be intubated and meconium and other aspirated material suctioned from beneath the glottis. If meconium is retrieved and no bradycardia is present, reintubate and suction. If there is bradycardia, administer positive pressure ventilation and consider suctioning again later once the neonate is stabilized.

The Renal System

In utero, most of the fetal waste material is removed by the maternal placenta. In effect, the fetal kidneys are passive, receiving relatively little renal blood flow and having a low glomerular filtration rate (GFR).[18] There are four major reasons for the low renal blood flow and GFR: low systemic arterial pressure, high renal vascular resistance, low permeability of the glomerular capillaries, and the small size and number of glomeruli. *In utero*, the kidneys receive only about 3% of the cardiac output, whereas they will receive about 25% of cardiac output in adulthood. At birth, this changes dramatically. The systemic arterial pressure increases, the renal vascular resistance decreases, and the kidneys now receive a progressively increased part of the cardiac output. At birth, the GFR is low, but increases significantly in the first few days of life, doubles in the first 2 weeks, and reaches adult levels by about 2 years of age. The limited ability of the newborn's kidney to concentrate or dilute urine results from this low GFR and decreased tubular function. However, during the first 3 to 4 days, the circulatory changes increase renal blood flow and GFR, improving the neonate's ability to concentrate and dilute the urine. Part of the improvement in renal function is the establishment of gradients in the medullary interstitium that promotes resorption of sodium. This maturation continues in the normal, full-term neonate and the kidneys are approximately 60% mature by 1 month of age. Urine output is low in the first 24 hours but increases to an expected level of at least 1 to 2 mL/kg/hr. Urine output, after the first day of life, of less than 1 mL/kg/hr should be considered indicative of either hypovolemia or decreased renal function from another cause.

Despite rapid maturation of renal function and increased capacity of the neonatal kidneys, they still have limitations. From an anesthetic standpoint, the half-life of medications excreted by means of glomerular filtration will be prolonged.[19] The relative inability to conserve water means that neonates, especially in the first week of life, tolerate fluid restriction poorly. In addition, the inability to excrete large amounts of water means the newborn tolerates fluid overload poorly. The newborn kidney is better able to conserve sodium than excrete sodium, making hypernatremia a risk if excess sodium is administered. However, because of the lack of tonicity in the medullary interstitium shortly after birth, there will be some obligate sodium loss in the first days of life. Sodium loss improves as the countercurrent multiplier is developed in the interstitium.

Fluid and Electrolyte Therapy in the Neonate

Total body water (TBW), which is usually described in terms of percent of body weight, varies by both age and gestational status. The highest TBW is found in the fetus but decreases to about 80% of body weight for a term neonate at birth. Preterm neonates have a higher TBW than term infants, 85% of body weight, up to 90% of body weight in very low–birth-weight (VLBW) preterm neonates. TBW decreases during the first 6 months of life to about 60% of body weight, remaining this level through childhood.

TBW is distributed between two compartments, intracellular fluid (ICF) and extracellular fluid (ECF). The ECF volume is larger than the ICF volume in the fetus and newborn, usually in the 40% (ECF) and 20% (ICF) of body weight ranges. This ratio is the inverse of the ECF and ICF relationship observed in infants and children. There is a significant diuresis and natriuresis after birth that produces a decrease in the ECF volume. In addition, ICF volume increases because of the growth of cells in the body. The ECF and ICF volumes (20% and 40% of body weight) approach adult values per body weight by about 1 year of age. This dramatic shift is beneficial to the child, especially in increasing the mobility of reserves in the face of dehydration. Fluid can be easily mobilized from ICF volumes to replenish intravascular volume that is lost from fasting, fever, diarrhea, or other causes. Thus, an infant or child is better situated to maintain intravascular volume in these situations than a neonate.

The ECF is divided into the plasma and the interstitial fluid. The plasma water is usually about 5% of body weight and the related blood volume, assuming a hematocrit of 45%, is about 8% of body weight in infants and children. The water content is slightly higher in neonates and may approach 10% of body weight in preterm neonates. The interstitial fluid, usually about 15% of body weight, can demonstrate large increases in disease states such as liver failure, heart failure, renal failure, and other causes fluid retention, such as pleural effusions or ascites. Any condition that decreases oncotic pressure, such as loss of albumin in liver failure, promotes the loss of fluid into the interstitial fluid. On the other hand, raised hydrostatic pressures, such as seen in heart failure, can result in fluid leaving the plasma and accumulating in the interstitial space. Conditions that result in translocation of fluid from the plasma to the interstitial spaces, whether because of decreased oncotic pressure or increased hydrostatic pressure, are of significant consequence to the neonate. Loss of fluid from the plasma volume compromises the intravascular volume, potentially decreasing the perfusion of vital organs and systems.

The blood volume in the normal full-term newborn is approximately 90 mL/kg and approximately 100 mL/kg in preterm, VLBW, or critically ill newborns. However, these estimates of intravascular volumes are variable between studies. Approximately half of the intravascular volume in a newborn is plasma volume. For all practical purposes, electrolyte values in the neonatal period are the same as in the child and adult except for potassium, which can be about 1 to 2 mmol/L higher than average for the first 2 days of life.[20]

Maintenance fluid requirements increase during the first days of life. They have been estimated to be 60, 75, 90, 105, 120, 135, and 150 mL/kg/24 hr for the first 7 days of life, respectively. For the rest of the neonatal period, a maintenance rate of 150 mL/kg/24 hr is appropriate.[21]

The appropriate type of maintenance fluid depends on several issues. Because of ongoing sodium loss secondary to the inability of the neonatal distal tubule to respond fully to aldosterone, intravenous fluids in the neonate must contain some sodium. Most operations on neonates involve loss of blood and ECF, which must be replaced with a fluid of similar electrolyte content (i.e., a near-isotonic solution such as lactated Ringer or PlasmaLyte). Hypotonic solutions should not be used to replace these losses because they can cause significant hyponatremia. Thus, if the neonate is already stable on a maintenance solution, it is reasonable to continue this maintenance at a constant rate, adding balanced salt solution, colloid, or blood products as needed to offset ongoing surgical or insensible losses.

The other issues for fluid choice in the neonate center on appropriate glucose administration. In most cases, maintenance fluids containing 10% glucose and 0.2% saline with 20 mmol/L of potassium are reasonable in the first 48 hours of life. Beyond that time period, full-term infants may do well with 5% glucose instead of 10%, although preterm infants will often require the higher glucose load longer. Newborns of diabetic mothers, those who are small for gestational age, and those who have had continuous glucose infusions stopped have particular problems with hypoglycemia. These infants need to have their blood glucose values monitored. Neonates who are scheduled for surgery and have been receiving intravenous (parenteral) nutrition or supplementary glucose must continue to receive that fluid during surgery or must have their glucose levels monitored because of concerns of hypoglycemia. There is little consensus on the issue of what constitutes hypoglycemia.[22]

The concern about hypoglycemia must be balanced against the potential augmentation of ischemic injury from iatrogenic hyperglycemia. Interestingly, there are observational reports examining neonates undergoing cardiac surgery in which high glucose concentrations during or after the surgery were not associated with worse neurodevelopmental outcomes.[23] This finding supports the contention that avoiding hypoglycemia may be preferable to restricting glucose in newborns and risking hypoglycemia, at least in those having cardiac surgery.

Blood Component Therapy in the Neonate

Most of the basic principles of blood component therapy are the same in newborns and older children and adults. The first principle is to ensure adequate circulating intravascular volume and add components, as needed. However, there are a few important differences. These differences are related to the interconnection of maternal and fetal blood circulations and the flow of some, but not all elements, across the placenta, the incompletely developed immune system of the neonate, and the small intravascular volume of the neonate. The indications in the perioperative period for red blood cells are similar to those for adults, but the target values in available guidelines are higher. Recent neonatal literature supports more restrictive thresholds for transfusion including VLBW neonates. Newer restrictive thresholds in the first week of life may be as low as 9 g/dL and decrease to 7 g/dL after 2 weeks of life. Periprocedural transfusion planning should include the overall risk of bleeding during the perioperative period and concomitant cardiopulmonary disease.[24] Platelets should be kept above 50,000/μL for invasive procedures and above 100,000/μL for bleeding neonates. Platelet recommendations are based on expert consensus and older pediatric data, not prospective studies in neonates specifically.

The hemoglobin in transfused blood is hemoglobin A, as opposed to the hemoglobin F, which is present in the neonatal circulation at birth. An advantage of the transfused blood is better release of oxygen at the tissue level from hemoglobin A. Fresh blood cells have the advantage of lower potassium levels than older blood, although washed or frozen cells prevent this problem. This difference becomes especially important during rapid, massive transfusion. Transfusion-associated graft-versus-host disease is a rare but potentially deadly complication of red blood cell transfusion. Transfused lymphocytes in the donor blood attack the recipient bone marrow and other tissues, causing fever, pancytopenia, diarrhea, and hepatitis. To prevent this, gamma irradiation of cellular blood components is used to destroy lymphocytes and prevent transfusion-associated graft-versus-host disease. Therefore, irradiated blood is routinely used for transfusion of preterm infants and, in many centers, for all neonates and infants under 6 months of age. Leukocyte reduction by filtration is also used to reduce cytomegalic virus transmission, decrease risk of alloimmunization, and decrease febrile hemolytic transfusion reactions. There is decrease in retinopathy of prematurity (ROP), bronchopulmonary dyplasia, and length of hospital stay when leukocyte reduction is used for transfusions in premature neonates.[25] Finally, because there is very weak expression of the ABO antigens at birth, ABO typing, Rh typing, and an initial antibody screen are commonly done prior to transfusion, although crossmatching is not always needed.

The Hepatic System

The functional capacity of the liver is immature in the newborn, especially synthetic and metabolic functions. Although most enzyme systems for both normal function and drug metabolism are present at birth, the systems have not yet been induced.[26] *In utero*, the maternal circulation and metabolism were responsible for the majority of drug elimination. As the newborn develops, the different hepatic metabolic pathways mature at different rates. Conjugation by sulfation and acetylation are relatively well developed in the newborn, with conjugation with glutathione and glucuronidation less well developed.[27] Some of these pathways do not achieve adult levels of activity until after 1 year of age.[28] Because of this immaturity, some drugs that undergo hepatic biotransformation, such as morphine, have prolonged elimination half-lives in newborns. Other drugs, such as lidocaine, do not undergo prolonged elimination in the newborn. In some drugs, such as caffeine, the lack of hepatic metabolism of the drug is balanced by excretion of an increased amount of unchanged drug through the kidney. Up to 85% of unmetabolized caffeine may be found in the urine in the newborn, compared with 1% in the adult.[29]

Finally, decreased metabolism of a drug may actually increase its safety profile. Acetaminophen undergoes less biotransformation by the cytochrome P450 system in the newborn, producing less reactive metabolites that are toxic. Paradoxically, neonates can tolerate dosages of acetaminophen that would be hepatotoxic in adults.[30] Synthetic function of the liver is also altered in the neonatal period. Levels of albumin and other proteins necessary for binding of drugs are low in term newborns (and are even lower in preterm infants) and impacts the ability to bind drugs, producing greater levels of free drug. This phenomenon is especially true for the binding of alkaline drugs that bind to α-1–acid glycoprotein, such as synthetic opioids and local anesthetics. The ability to bind to existing albumin may also be altered by hyperbilirubinemia for some medications. The need for exogenous vitamin K in the newborn is a consequence of this decreased ability. Because of decreased synthetic function, neonatal hepatic glycogen stores are low, especially in the preterm infant, increasing the risk of hypoglycemia in response to stress.

Anatomy of the Neonatal Airway

4 The anatomic and maturational factors unique to the neonatal airway are important to understand in order to effectively manage the airway (Fig. 42-6). Although traditional teaching is that all neonates, especially preterm infants, are *obligate* nasal breathers, the majority of neonates are actually *preferential* nose breathers.[31] Anything that obstructs the nares can compromise the neonate's ability to breathe.[32] For this reason, bilateral choanal atresia of the nasopharynx can be a life-threatening surgical condition for the neonate. The airway needs to be secured or the atresia opened to ensure adequate ventilation. The large tongue occupies relatively more space in the infant's oropharynx, promoting both soft tissue obstruction of the upper airway and increasing the difficulty of direct laryngoscopic examination and intubation of the infant's trachea. In the normal adult, the glottis is at the level of C5–C6. In the full-term infant, the glottis is at the level of C4, and in the premature infant, it is at the level of C3. The combination of a large tongue and a relatively cephalad glottis means that on laryngoscopic examination it is more difficult to establish a direct line of vision between the mouth and the larynx; there is relatively more tissue in a smaller distance. Therefore, the infant's larynx appears to be *anterior*, although the more anatomically accurate description is *cephalad*. The epiglottis is omega- or tubular-shaped, with a stubby base and thick, bulky aryepiglottic folds, making it difficult to elevate with a laryngoscope blade. Because the tip of the epiglottis lies at C1, its close apposition with the soft palate allows the newborn to simultaneously suckle and breathe, which contributes to the *preferential* nasal breathing found in the neonate. The vocal cords are anterior-slanting, making visualization more challenging. The slanting also occasionally provides some obstruction to the passage of the endotracheal tube, which is especially true with either nasal or "blind" intubation attempts because the bevel of the tube may hang up in the anterior commissure of the angulated vocal cords instead of easily passing into the subglottic larynx.

Complicating anatomic factors in infants

Narrow nares
Large tongue
High glottis
C4
Slanting vocal cords
Large occiput
Narrow cricoid ring

Figure 42-6 Complicating anatomic factors in infants. (Adapted from Smith RM. *Smith's Anesthesia for Infants and Children*. 4th ed. Mosby; 1980:16. Copyright © 1980 Elsevier. With permission.)

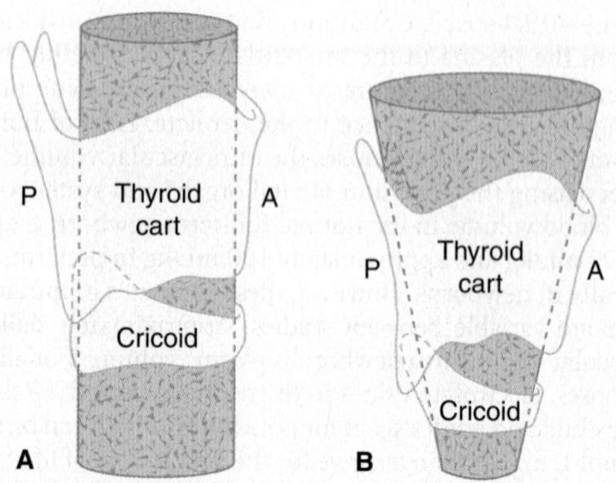

Figure 42-7 Configuration of the adult (**A**) versus the infant (**B**) larynx. The adult larynx has a cylindrical shape. The infant larynx is funnel-shaped because of the narrow, undeveloped cricoid cartilage. A, Anterior; P, Posterior. (Adapted from The pediatric airway, In: Ryan JF, Coté CJ, Todres ID, eds. *A Practice of Anesthesia for Infants and Children*. 2nd ed. Orlando, FL: Grune & Stratton; 1992:61. Copyright © 1992 Elsevier. With permission.)

The neonatal subglottic area is funnel-shaped, unlike the infant, child, or adult airway (Fig. 42-7). In adults, the narrowest aspect of the upper airway is at the vocal cords, but in the neonate there is further narrowing ending at the level of the cricoid ring, the first complete cartilaginous ring. Although studies have challenged the funnel shape in infants and children, there has been no study further clarifying this relationship in neonates.[33,34] Because this narrowing is susceptible to trauma from intubation or too large an endotracheal tube, uncuffed tubes have traditionally been used in the neonatal period, although cuffed tubes are increasingly popular. The use of newer, cuffed, small volume, high resistance endotracheal tubes have been demonstrated to provide an adequate airway with marginal changes to the diameter of the airway leading most anesthesiology practitioners to now use a cuffed tube, in even neonates and young infants.[35] Though cuffed endotracheal tubes may be gaining ground in use, it does not appear that they have supplanted the use of uncuffed endotracheal tubes in neonates.[36] Although the glottic opening may actually be the smallest measured point in the pediatric airway, it is more distensible than the cricoid ring, the first complete cartilaginous ring in the airway, thus, the cricoid ring is functionally the smallest cross-sectional area in the airway. An endotracheal tube that passes easily through the glottic opening may not advance beyond the less distensible cricoid ring.

Finally, the infant has a large occiput so the head flexes forward onto the chest when the infant is lying supine with their head in the midline. Further flexion of the neck can cause obstruction.

Extreme extension can also obstruct the airway, so a midposition of the head with slight extension is preferred for airway maintenance. Rarely, this may require placing a small roll at the base of the neck and shoulders.

Anesthetic Drugs in Neonates

5 The pharmacokinetics of drugs in neonates are different than in older children and adults. Factors affecting the metabolism of drugs in neonates include a larger volume of distribution, decreased protein binding, decreased body fat percentage, and immature renal and hepatic function. The following physiologic changes alter pharmacokinetics and pharmacodynamics in neonates:

- Volume of distribution. TBW represents a greater proportion of body weight in premature and full-term neonates, which increases the necessary dose for medications that are water soluble.
- Protein binding. Neonates have decreased protein and hence have a decrease in protein binding of most drugs. This leads to increased free drug levels, which leads to increased activity and toxicity of drugs that are predominantly protein bound.
- Fat content. Neonates have a decreased amount of fat and muscle mass, which leads to greater levels of drugs that are primarily redistributed to muscle and fat. Decreased renal and hepatic function predisposes neonates to increased blood levels from normal doses that are used for induction and maintenance of anesthesia.

Neurotoxicity of anesthetic agents is a topic that has received much attention in the literature as well as in popular media. However, most surgical procedures in the neonatal period are not elective. There is a detailed discussion of neurotoxicity of anesthetic agents presented in Chapter 43.

Intravenous Agents

Anticholinergics

Anticholinergics, such as atropine and glycopyrrolate, are used frequently in neonates. They may be helpful in decreasing secretions and the response to vagal stimulation on intubation. The dose of atropine is 10 μg/kg if given intravenously and 20 μg/kg if given intramuscularly. Intramuscular administration may be desirable in certain situations, prior to induction of anesthesia, especially in emergency surgeries. Caution should be exercised if neonates have other associated congenital abnormalities, particularly narrow-angle glaucoma in which case anticholinergics could increase intraocular pressure. Glycopyrrolate, a synthetic quaternary ammonium compound, has a longer duration of action than atropine and may potentially have fewer central effects because of decreased penetration of the blood–brain barrier.

Midazolam

Midazolam is a water-soluble benzodiazepine that can be used for premedication in infants prior to surgery. Clearance of midazolam is lower in neonates and premature infants, and hence caution must be exercised with the amount of midazolam used. If combined with opioids, intravenous midazolam can cause severe hypotension. A common modality for midazolam administration in neonatal intensive care units (NICUs) is by continuous infusion. If a patient is receiving midazolam infusion, care should be taken to avoid large doses of opioids to prevent hypotension.

Sedative/Hypnotics

The common sedative/hypnotics used in neonates include propofol, thiopental, and ketamine.

Thiopental

Because of an ongoing shortage of thiopental in North America, it is now rarely used there. Because of the large volume of distribution in neonates, it may be necessary to use large doses of thiopental for induction of anesthesia. However, because of its reduced clearance, the effect may last longer than anticipated. Thiopental can cause hypotension in neonates who are volume depleted, especially in infants presenting for emergency surgery. It should be avoided in neonates with congenital heart disease because of its effect on myocardial function, leading to hypotension. A dose of 2 to 4 mg/kg is usually well tolerated by most neonates for induction of anesthesia. When compared with intubation without any hypnotic, the use of intravenous thiopental demonstrated adequate maintenance of heart rate and blood pressure.[37]

Propofol

Propofol, a phenol derivative sedative/hypnotic, is a commonly used induction agent in infants and children. In a randomized trial comparing intravenous propofol with atropine, succinylcholine, and morphine, it was noted that propofol maintained adequate hemodynamics in neonates.[38] There is variability in elimination of propofol in neonates and preterm infants with longer elimination times.[39] Hence, while using propofol, it is important to reduce the dose to ensure early wake up and extubation. Propofol is the most commonly used intravenous induction agent in the United States.

Ketamine

Ketamine, an *N*-methyl-D-aspartic acid (NMDA) antagonist, is used for induction of anesthesia in neonates who may have cardiovascular instability. An induction dose of 2 mg/kg intravenously with a higher dose of 4 to 7 mg/kg is used intramuscularly. Although it produces hemodynamic stability, it can cause an increase in oral secretions. There have been significant alterations in excitotoxic cells in the animal model when exposed to NMDA receptor antagonists such as ketamine with resultant concern about potential neurodegenerative changes with their exposure.[40] All of these experimental models were using very high doses of ketamine, unlike what is routinely recommended for induction of anesthesia in neonates. In addition, there are also other sets of experimental data in animal studies that demonstrate a beneficial effect of ketamine in an experimental pain model.[41] Ketamine is still used frequently in neonates with congenital heart disease for induction of anesthesia.

Dexmedetomidine

Dexmedetomidine is an α-2 receptor agonist that can be used for sedation in neonates. Although it, as many drugs, has not been FDA-approved for use in the neonatal population, some centers have begun to employ this drug in the intensive care unit or as an adjunct to general anesthesia. FDA phase 2 and 3 trials indicate that dexmedetomidine is effective for sedation of term and preterm neonates receiving mechanical ventilation, but preterm neonates exhibited decreased plasma clearance and increased elimination half-life of the drug. A study of 127 infants and neonates revealed that dexmedetomidine is likely to be safe in this patient population at doses similar to those used in adult intensive care for sedation, 0.2 to 0.6 μg/kg/hr.[42] Blood pressure and heart rate should be monitored as drop in systolic blood pressure and episodes of bradycardia may be noted. Dexmedetomidine may reduce required doses of midazolam and fentanyl needed to achieve the same level of sedation. Animal studies suggest that dexmedetomidine may be less neurotoxic than other traditionally used agents, such as midazolam.[43]

Opioids

Opioids are used extensively in the management of anesthesia in neonates. The advantage of using opioids is their ability to maintain cardiovascular stability during major surgery. The common opioids used in neonates include fentanyl, morphine, and remifentanil. Infants who are on long-term doses of opioids may develop dependence and require further treatment with methadone, a longer-acting opioid.[44]

Fentanyl

This synthetic opioid is commonly used for sedation in the neonate in the intensive care unit as well as in the operating room. A dose of 2 to 4 μg/kg/hr can maintain hemodynamic stability in these infants during surgery. The use of fentanyl in association with benzodiazepines may lead to hypotension and hemodynamic instability. Sedation with a combination of opioids and benzodiazepines for more than a week in neonates has been associated with worse neurodevelopmental outcomes than when either agent is used alone.[45] Fentanyl may result in respiratory depression even with small doses. Continuous infusions may predispose to respiratory depression more frequently than bolus doses.[46] Chest wall rigidity and glottic rigidity have been described with fentanyl. Small doses, as little as 1 to 2 μg/kg, can result in significant chest wall rigidity, leading to desaturation and need for mechanical ventilation. There is no significant maturational change in the brain associated with fentanyl, compared with morphine. Hence, the sensitivity to fentanyl will not significantly change as the infant matures. Fentanyl continues to be the mainstay in newborns for sedation and analgesia.

Morphine

The kinetics of morphine have been studied in newborns, and premature babies have been shown to have decreased clearance. Morphine clearance (range, 0.8 to 6.5 mL/min/kg) directly correlates with gestational age ($r = 0.60$; $P < .01$) and birth weight ($r = 0.55$; $P < .01$).[47] Because of decreased clearance, dosing in neonates, especially premature infants, should occur on a 4- to 6-hour basis to allow for more predictable clearance of the drug.[48] Morphine is used frequently in the intensive care unit for postoperative pain control. Morphine infusions in the perioperative period have resulted in minor prolongation of postoperative ventilation. However, increased incidence of apnea or hypotension was not observed in neonates despite prolonged morphine infusions after successful extubation.[49]

Morphine is metabolized to morphine-3-glucoronide and morphine-6-glucoronide. Morphine-6-glucoronide predisposes to respiratory depression. The sensitivity to morphine-6-glucoronide increases with age because of increased maturation of the neuronal receptors.[50]

Remifentanil

Remifentanil is an ultra short–acting opioid that is metabolized by nonspecific esterases in plasma and tissues and has a half-life of less than 10 minutes. The pharmacokinetics of remifentanil in neonates are similar to that of older children.[51] Remifentanil can be used for maintenance of anesthesia with avoidance of volatile anesthetic agents. The use of remifentanil infusion facilitated tracheal extubation in infants in a randomized trial when compared with volatile agents.[52]

Methadone

Methadone is a long-acting opioid that is used in neonates and infants in NICUs, particularly when withdrawal from opioids is suspected. The FDA "black box" warning against the use of methadone in patients with prolonged QT intervals on their electrocardiogram is a valid concern and infants on long-term methadone use should be carefully monitored with serial ECGs. However, it is used frequently in managing opioid tolerance without significant complication.[44]

Neuromuscular Blocking Agents

Neuromuscular blocking agents (NMBAs) are frequently used during neonatal anesthesia to facilitate tracheal intubation, assist with controlled ventilation, relax abdominal musculature, and ensure immobility. Factors that influence the choice of agent include the time of onset, duration of action, cardiovascular effects, drug availability, and mechanism of clearance/elimination.

Succinylcholine

Succinylcholine, the only depolarizing muscle relaxant available, has the most rapid onset time of all the NMBAs. Neonates and infants have a larger ECF volume, leading to a larger volume of distribution and an increased dose requirement compared with children and adults. Thus, the recommended intravenous dose of succinylcholine for neonates and infants is 3 mg/kg, compared with 2 mg/kg in children, with an onset time of 30 to 45 seconds and duration of 5 to 10 minutes. The recommended intramuscular dose of succinylcholine is 4 mg/kg, with an onset time of 3 to 4 minutes and duration of approximately 20 minutes. Caution should be exercised when administering a second dose of succinylcholine because this can lead to vagally mediated bradycardia or sinus arrest. Pretreatment with atropine is recommended.[53]

Use of succinylcholine in boys younger than 8 years is controversial. Reports of hyperkalemia with cardiac arrest in such children with unrecognized muscular dystrophy has led some clinicians to take the position that succinylcholine should not be used routinely for this group of patients. The occurrence of this problem is approximately 1 in 250,000 anesthetics, with a mortality rate of 50%. Although a concern in young children, it is not a problem in the neonatal period. Succinylcholine is still recommended in rapid-sequence situations, potential difficult airway, or if there are airway emergencies with progressive desaturation. When it is evident that a neonatal airway is obstructed by laryngospasm or other reason and no progress is made in ventilation, intramuscular or intravenous succinylcholine should be administered. Hyperkalemia can be recognized by peaked T waves. However, the clinician may not see this particular electrocardiographic change because it occurs 2 to 3 minutes after drug administration, when the anesthesiologist is tending to the airway. The hyperkalemia interferes with cardiac conduction, leading to a bradycardia and, if severe enough, cardiac arrest.

Nondepolarizing Agents

The neonate's neuromuscular junction is more sensitive to nondepolarizing muscle relaxants, and the neonate has a larger volume of distribution because of a large ECF volume. These two effects tend to balance each other; therefore, the dose of a nondepolarizing muscle relaxant for an infant is similar to that for a child on an mg/kg basis. Ongoing organ maturation has a tremendous impact on the metabolism and clearance of the nondepolarizing agents. As a result, there is considerable variability and unpredictability in the duration of action of these agents in the neonatal period. Dosing should be titrated to effect and, when possible, guided by monitoring neuromuscular function with a nerve stimulator. However, reliable twitch monitoring may be challenging in this age group.

Intermediate Nondepolarizing Agents

Rocuronium

Rocuronium appears to be the drug of choice among the intermediate-acting, nondepolarizing muscle relaxants for neonates. The intubating dose of rocuronium is 0.6 mg/kg. The length of action of rocuronium in the neonate is similar to that in the older infant or child following an equipotent dose.[54] Smaller doses (0.45 mg/kg) have been demonstrated to provide adequate relaxation and predictable recovery in newborn infants. However, if a larger dose of rocuronium, 1 to 1.2 mg/kg, is administered to avoid using succinylcholine during a rapid-sequence induction, then rocuronium will be a relatively long-acting muscle relaxant. Rocuronium is metabolized by the liver; however, there are no active metabolites of rocuronium which is unlike vecuronium. Rocuronium has mild vagolytic properties and may slightly increase heart rate.

Vecuronium

Although vecuronium is considered an intermediate-acting muscle relaxant in children and adults, in infants younger than 1 year it is considered to be a long-acting muscle relaxant. The duration of action of vecuronium is approximately twice that observed in children because of liver immaturity. Vecuronium undergoes primarily hepatic metabolism with production of active metabolites that are dependent on renal excretion. The recommended dose of vecuronium is 0.1 to 0.15 mg/kg, with an onset time of 90 seconds and duration of action of 60 to 90 minutes in the neonate. Even with increased doses, vecuronium has no effect on the cardiovascular system.

Pancuronium

Pancuronium is a long-acting NMBA with a pharmacokinetic profile similar to vecuronium. The recommended dose of 0.1 to 0.15 mg/kg has an onset time of 120 seconds and duration of 60 to 75 minutes. Unlike vecuronium, however, pancuronium primarily undergoes renal excretion. Pancuronium has vagolytic and sympathomimetic actions that cause tachycardia and an increase in blood pressure.[55] In a relatively normal neonate with a normal blood pressure and normal blood volume, the use of pancuronium may result in hypertension, which has the potential to increase blood loss and increase the risk of hemorrhage in the extremely premature neonate. The risk for prolonged neuromuscular blockade in neonates, especially with altered renal function, makes pancuronium less desirable in neonates and infants undergoing minor outpatient surgical procedures. Prolonged use has been associated with sensorineural hearing loss in infants.[56]

Cis-atracurium

Cis-atracurium is an intermediate-acting NMBA of the bisbenzyltetrahydroisoquinolinium class. The unique aspect of this agent within its class is a lack of histamine release. The most important fact about this drug is its degradation through Hoffman elimination, which is an organ-independent chemodegradative mechanism. Because its elimination is not kidney or liver dependent, it offers a reliable recovery time even in neonates. In fact, when used for prolonged infusion in infants and neonates in intensive care, it offers a more reliable recovery time than vecuronium.[57] One theoretical concern with administration of *cis*-atracurium is the accumulation of one metabolite, laudanosine, which can decrease the seizure threshold. However, this does not seem to be relevant at clinical doses of *cis*-atracurium.[58] The typical dose is 0.15 to 0.2 mg/kg, has an onset time of 150 seconds, and a half-life of approximately 25 minutes.

Reversal Agents

The unpredictable nature of the NMBAs in the neonatal population, as well as the inability to accurately assess neuromuscular function in many situations, necessitates reversal of all nondepolarizing NMBA in neonates. Neostigmine is the most common agent used for reversal of nondepolarizing muscle relaxants in neonates. Neostigmine in a dose of 0.07 mg/kg requires 10 minutes for a 90% reversal of neuromuscular block. Anticholinergic drugs such as atropine or glycopyrrolate must be coadministered to decrease the incidence of bradycardia. Neostigmine administered without an anticholinergic is the most common drug error leading to perioperative cardiac arrest in the pediatric population.[59] Though restricted to off-label indications for children by the FDA, sugammadex has been successfully used to reverse neuromuscular blockade. The drug works by encapsulation and noncompetitive binding of aminosteroid neuromuscular-blocking agents, rocuronium and vecuronium. A retrospective study of 1,946 pediatric patients including neonates who received sugammadex compared with 4,136 pediatric patients who received neostigmine, demonstrated a shorter time from administration of reversal agent to time out of operating room in the neonatal group receiving sugammadex. No adverse effects differences were noted between the two groups.[60] Future studies in the neonatal population may help demonstrate the safety and efficacy of sugammadex as a reversal agent.

Volatile Agents

Volatile agents are used for maintenance of anesthesia in the neonatal period. Although halothane was the most commonly used volatile agent for many years and had a reasonable safety profile, the introduction of sevoflurane has clearly made a difference to the use of volatile agents in neonates. Isoflurane is used for maintenance of anesthesia for longer surgical procedures and desflurane may be desirable for rapid awakening in certain cases. Each of these agents will be discussed here.

Halothane

Halothane is still commonly used in developing countries but is not currently used in the United States nor other developed countries. Its long history for induction of anesthesia and its ease of use still make it a desirable agent in children. Halothane has a weak muscle relaxant property, facilitating induction and intubation without the use of a muscle relaxant. Halothane is a potent bronchodilator and may reduce the airway reflexes associated with intubation. The use of high doses of halothane for procedures including bronchoscopic evaluation of the airway may lead to significant myocardial depression. Infants less than 8 weeks old and with a history of RDS with longer period of preoperative fasting are prone to hypotension. Halothane also sensitizes the myocardium to cardiac dysrhythmias.

Isoflurane

Isoflurane is a common maintenance volatile agent in neonates and infants. Its pungent odor does not allow its use for mask induction. Isoflurane has a greater effect in potentiation of muscle relaxation and hence plays an important role as a maintenance anesthetic. It is important to remember that the dose of muscle relaxants should be reduced when isoflurane anesthesia is used because of potentiation. Isoflurane has less myocardial depression when compared with halothane in neonates.[61]

Sevoflurane

This volatile agent offers an advantage for rapid induction and rapid awakening. It has a less pungent smell than isoflurane, making it ideal for mask induction. Its pharmacodynamics have been studied in neonates and children with a reasonable safety profile.[62] In children with congenital cardiac disease, it has been shown to produce fewer hemodynamic changes when compared with isoflurane.[63] Although it produces less myocardial depression, it has a greater effect on respiratory depression compared with halothane. Minute ventilation and respiratory frequency are significantly lower during sevoflurane anesthesia compared with halothane anesthesia. There is also significantly less thoracoabdominal asynchrony during sevoflurane anesthesia.[64]

Desflurane

Desflurane was touted to be the best volatile agent in children because of its partition coefficient being close to that of nitrous oxide, thereby allowing a rapid uptake. However, the pungent nature of the drug makes it impossible to use for inhalation induction of anesthesia. When compared with sevoflurane, infants who were preterm were noted to wake up sooner with desflurane, but there were no reductions in postoperative respiratory events.[65] One MAC of desflurane in a neonate is estimated to be 9.2% end-tidal concentration.[66] Pungency increasing the risk of laryngospasm and bronchospasm make this volatile agent less attractive in neonates. In an animal model using neonatal mice, mice exposed to desflurane had greater neuroapoptosis than mice exposed to equipotent doses of isoflurane or sevoflurane.[67]

Local Anesthetics

Local anesthetic solutions are represented by two main classes, the amino-amides (amides) and the amino-esters (esters). The main difference between the two classes is that the amides undergo enzymatic degradation by the liver and the esters are hydrolyzed by plasma cholinesterases.

Amides

These are commonly used local anesthetic solutions in neonates and infants. Local anesthetics used in common clinical practice belonging to this class include lidocaine, bupivacaine, ropivacaine, and *levo*-bupivacaine. The main characteristics differentiating these drugs are their speed of onset, duration of action, and potential for cardiac toxicity. The ability of neonatal liver enzymes to metabolize and their ability to oxidize and reduce these drugs are decreased when compared with adults.[68] At approximately 3 months of age, the conjugation of these drugs in the liver reaches adult levels.

Local anesthetic solution levels have been shown to be higher in children undergoing intercostal nerve blocks compared with adults.[69] After caudal administration of local anesthetics, peak plasma level is obtained in children and adults in approximately 30 minutes.[70] The steady-state volume of distribution (Vd_{SS}) for amides is increased in children compared with adults, although clearance (CL) is similar.[70] Elimination half-life ($t_{1/2}$) is related to the volume of distribution and clearance as follows: $t_{1/2} = (0.693 \times Vd_{SS})/CL$. This results in a larger Vd_{SS} and prolongation of the elimination half-life, especially if a continuous infusion is used. Also, due to decreased circulating α-1–acid glycoprotein levels in neonates, more free (active) local anesthetic circulates in the bloodstream.

The systemic absorption of local anesthetics is often based on the site of injection. On a decreasing scale, the incidence of complications with local anesthetic solution injections decreases, with the highest concentrations seen in the intercostal area followed by the caudal space, the epidural space, and peripheral nerve blocks. With newer techniques in regional anesthesia, including ultrasound guidance, the volume and dose of local anesthetic solution can be significantly reduced.[71]

Bupivacaine. Bupivacaine is one of the most used local anesthetic solutions in infants and children. The pharmacokinetics and the pharmacodynamics have been well studied in infants and children. The concentration of the local anesthetic solution used depends on the site of injection, the desired density of blockade (motor and sensory), and the potential for cardiovascular and neurotoxicity. The concomitant use of other local anesthetics including infiltration anesthesia must be considered before a total volume of local anesthetic solution is determined. This is especially true in neonatal surgery in which large quantities of local anesthetic solution can be injected for skin infiltration. If upper safe limits are likely to be approached, it is reasonable to avoid local anesthetic solution for infiltration and use a dilute epinephrine solution instead for vasoconstriction. The preferred concentration for peripheral nerve blockade is 0.25% bupivacaine or 0.2% ropivacaine, and the preferred concentration for single dose caudal is 0.25% or 0.125% solution of bupivacaine or 0.2% ropivacaine. When a continuous infusion is desired, a 0.1% or 0.125% solution of bupivacaine is preferred. In premature infants and in infants weighing under 1 kg, we prefer using 0.0625% bupivacaine, or intermittent bolus dosing every 12 hours. Although clear guidelines do not exist for local anesthetic solutions, a rough rule of thumb is to use 0.2 mg/kg/hr for continuous infusions of bupivacaine and 2 mg/kg for bolus doses.[72]

Metabolism and Toxicity. Bupivacaine in the circulation is heavily bound to α-1–acid glycoprotein. Levels of this circulating protein are lower in the neonatal period.[73] Bupivacaine is a racemic mixture of the *levo* and *dextro* enantiomers. Although the *levo* enantiomer is the active form that provides the clinical effect of the local anesthetic solution, the *dextro* enantiomer is responsible for the adverse effects related to local anesthesia, including cardiac toxicity and neurotoxicity.

The major adverse effect of bupivacaine is toxicity related to the cardiovascular and the CNS systems. Local anesthetics cross the blood–brain barrier and can cause alterations in the CNS functions. Continuous infusions in neonates can predispose them to CNS toxicity sooner than older infants.[74] In pediatric patients, the incidence of cardiac toxicity occurs sooner than neurotoxicity,[74] which may be partly because children may be anesthetized, and devastating neurotoxicity may not be noticed until significant cardiac toxicity is seen. Manifestation of bupivacaine toxicity may also be affected by the concomitant use of volatile agents for general anesthesia.

Dosage. Bupivacaine can be used for most peripheral nerve blocks as well as for epidural and caudal infusions in infants and children. The maximum dosage suggested for bolus injections in the caudal space or epidural space for older children is 4 mg/kg and 2 mg/kg for neonates and infants.[73] Dosage recommendations for continuous infusions are 0.4 mg/kg/hr in older children and 0.2 mg/kg/hr in neonates and infants.[26] The concentration of the solution used for peripheral nerve blocks is usually 0.25%, bearing in mind the ceiling limit for maximum dosage. Higher concentration such as 0.375% may be necessary for surgical blockade without sedation. An example of a continuous infusion in a 4-kg neonate will be 0.2 mg/kg/hr; this will be equivalent to 0.8 mL/hr of a 0.1% solution of bupivacaine (1 mg/mL of bupivacaine).

Ropivacaine. Ropivacaine is an amide local anesthetic. It is a *levo* enantiomer with relatively less cardiovascular and CNS side effects compared with bupivacaine.[75] The pharmacokinetics of ropivacaine are such that caudal blocks with ropivacaine (2 mg/kg) in children (aged 1 to 8 years) result in plasma concentrations of ropivacaine well below toxic levels in adults.[75] This dose was also noted to produce less motor block but provide adequate analgesia. Mean maximum plasma concentration of total ropivacaine at 2 mg/kg was 0.47 mg/L. A threshold of CNS toxicity was noted at a plasma concentration of 0.6 mg/L. Body weight–adjusted clearance was the same as in adults (5 mL/min/kg). Ropivacaine clearance depends on the unbound fraction of ropivacaine rather than the liver blood flow.

Toxicity. Although the safety of ropivacaine has been demonstrated in animal experiments, there have been reports of CNS toxicity and cardiac toxicity associated with the use of epidural ropivacaine. It is important to understand that an overdose of ropivacaine can cause toxicity, making close attention to dosage as important with ropivacaine as with other local anesthetics. Our recommended dose is bolus dose of 2 mg/kg and an infusion rate of 0.2 mg/kg/hr in neonates.

Levobupivacaine. *Levo*-bupivacaine is a newer *levo* enantiomer that has fewer adverse effects than bupivacaine.[76] There are fewer pediatric trials available in literature. Because of the common use of bupivacaine in children and its low incidence of complications, *levo*-bupivacaine is not used abundantly in general pediatric anesthesiology practice. It is currently not available for use in the United States, although it is widely used in other parts of the world.

Toxicity. *Levo*-bupivacaine, in the animal model, has been shown to have less cardiac toxicity with lower degree of myocardial depression than bupivacaine. Although it is less toxic, the recommended doses remain the same for *levo*-bupivacaine as bupivacaine.

Lidocaine. Lidocaine is a frequently utilized amide local anesthetic with an intermediate duration of action. It is used for postoperative catheter infusions because its level can be measured in most hospital laboratories in a time-efficient manner. A variety of concentrations are readily available on the market. A concentration of 1.5% in the epidural space is generally considered to be adequate for surgical blockade, whereas peripheral nerve blocks are typically done with 2% for surgical block. Lidocaine has a high hepatic extraction ratio, so its clearance is based on hepatic blood flow. Lidocaine has a longer half-life and volume of distribution in the neonate. Furthermore, the relatively low level of α-1–acid glycoprotein in neonates increases the proportion that is not protein-bound in the serum. When utilized for spinal blockade, the possibility of transient neurologic symptoms is significant, so other local anesthetics have supplanted much of its use in spinal anesthesia.

Toxicity. Lidocaine has been an attractive local anesthetic for postoperative continuous infusion in the neonatal population. Because lidocaine has other uses in the intensive care setting, most hospital laboratories can measure its level reasonably quickly. Thus, serum levels of lidocaine may be monitored in the setting of continuous infusions for safety. Furthermore, convulsions are typically noted before the onset of cardiac toxicity, which may confer a greater safety level over bupivacaine.

Esters

Ester local anesthetics are metabolized by plasma cholinesterases. As a result, in populations with lower circulating pseudocholinesterase levels, there is a modestly increased serum half-life of these drugs. This includes infants and neonates particularly. The duration of action of the drug is short; hence, a continuous infusion of chloroprocaine is recommended versus frequent bolus dosing.

2-Chloroprocaine. This drug is experiencing a resurgence within the neonatal population as interest in its safety profile has reinvigorated its use. Even though neonates have a lower level of circulating pseudocholinesterase, the plasma half-life of chloroprocaine remains short. The plasma half-life of chloroprocaine in adults is 23 seconds, whereas in neonates it is 43 seconds. The plasma half-life of lidocaine, an intermediate-acting amide local anesthetic, is 90 to 120 minutes. Thus, the toxicity profile of chloroprocaine is expected to be much better across a range of doses, though studies in neonates have not been specifically designed to answer this clinical question.

Dosing. After a bolus dose of 1.5 mL/kg, a continuous infusion of chloroprocaine at 1.5 mL/kg/hr of 3% 2-chloroprocaine has been used to achieve a level of T4 to T2 through an intravenous catheter placed in the sacral canal.[77] This level will be effective in producing complete surgical anesthesia for neonates' major abdominal surgery. Lower doses such as 1 mL/kg bolus and an infusion of 1 mL/kg/hr have been used successfully for inguinal and penoscrotal surgery.[78] Given the high concentrations of local that can be used, motor block is easy to achieve with this local anesthetic. Postoperative infusion of chloroprocaine through an epidural catheter is a relatively common practice in neonates as observed in the Pediatric Regional Anesthesia Network (PRAN) database.

Management of Local Anesthetic Systemic Toxicity

Lipid emulsion therapy reverses the effects of LAST. Lipid should be readily available if local anesthetics are being used in neonates. There is a report where an infant received a caudal block which resulted in cardiac toxicity which was treated successfully with lipid rescue.[79] Although guidelines specific to neonatal administration of lipid rescue do not exist, lipid administration across a wide range of doses appears to be safe in neonates.[80] The present recommended dose of lipid rescue for LAST is 1.5 mL/kg bolus, which may be repeated for continued instability, followed by continuous infusion of 0.25 mL/kg/min, which may be increased for continued hypotension.[81]

Topical Anesthesia

Several local anesthetic preparations are now available for topical use. The most common local anesthetic preparations for topical use include lidocaine, tetracaine, benzocaine, and prilocaine. When these are applied to skin, they produce an effective but relatively short duration of analgesia. One topical anesthetic formulation, eutectic mixture of local anesthetic (EMLA), is a mixture of lidocaine 2.5% and prilocaine 2.5% and is used extensively for topical anesthesia in neonates, particularly for circumcision and venipunctures. The preparation should be applied under an occlusive bandage for 45 to 60 minutes to obtain effective cutaneous analgesia. Although the incidence of methemoglobinemia from prilocaine is not very common in neonates, caution should be exercised when applying large doses of EMLA for procedures.[82]

Newer topical anesthetic solutions are now available that may offer a faster rate of onset. LMX-4, a 4% liposomal lidocaine solution can be used as topical anesthesia. There is no need for an occlusive dressing when LMX-4 is used, and it has the same efficacy as EMLA.[83] Liposome-encapsulated lidocaine or tetracaine has been shown to remain in the epidermis after topical application, affording a fast and lasting anesthetic effect.

Anesthetic Management of the Neonate

Effective evaluation, preparation, and anesthetic management of the neonate depend on appropriate knowledge, clinical skills, and vigilance on the part of the anesthesiologist. For safe and effective care, the anesthesiologist must take extraordinary caution to understand the status of the patient, the nature of the planned surgery, and the potential need for stabilization and preparation before surgery. After ensuring that the patient has been adequately prepared, the anesthesiologist needs to develop a detailed plan that encompasses the issues of anesthetic equipment and monitoring, airway management, drug choice, fluid management, temperature control, anticipated surgical needs, pain management, and postoperative care.

Studies have shown that morbidity and mortality related to anesthesia is higher in infants, especially neonates, compared with infants, older children, and adults.[59,84,85] The rate of major complications may be as high as 23% in neonates undergoing surgical procedures and are more frequent in reoperations, surgery for CDH, gestational age less than 32 weeks at birth, and abdominal surgery.[86] There are probably several causes for the higher complication rate observed with neonatal surgery, including the emergency nature of most surgical procedures that are performed at this age, the physiologic instability of the neonate, the relative lack of experience most clinicians have with patients in this age range, and the technical challenges of monitoring and treating a very small patient. Because of the specialized nature of neonatal surgery and care, it is important that each institution that provides care to these patients has the resources of equipment, critical care facilities, nursing, laboratory, blood bank, and social work necessary to meet the needs of these patients and their families, as well as systems in place to guarantee a robust quality assurance emphasis on the provision of care. Both the American Academy of Pediatrics and the American Society of Anesthesiologists have provided guidance to many of the systems issues that should be addressed in institutions caring for these patients.[87] Physicians who agree to participate in this care need to have the preparation and ongoing experience needed to provide a consistent, expert level of care.

In the distant past, concerns about physiologic instability and other challenges of caring for neonates led some practitioners to use minimal or no anesthesia for both minor and major procedures. It is now widely recognized that neonates have stress responses similar to those of older patients, and the lack of adequate anesthetic care is as inhumane in the neonate as it is in the older child or adult.[88] The neurologic system in neonates is sufficiently developed to transmit painful stimuli and lack of pain control may result in a higher morbidity rate, increased pain to subsequent events, and increased neuroendocrine response to painful stimuli.[89] Consequently, the same attention to adequate analgesia and anesthesia needs to be paid to the neonate as to other patients.

Preoperative Considerations

Preanesthetic Evaluation—History

The preanesthetic planning process starts with an evaluation of the course of intrauterine growth, events of labor and delivery, and the immediate postpartum course of the patient. The amount of history available to the anesthesiologist may vary widely. If the mother had received prepartum and postpartum care in the same institution where the neonate is admitted, a significant amount of detail may be available. If the neonate is transferred from another institution, there may be limited information available. Best efforts should be made to get as much relevant information as possible, with an emphasis on maternal factors that may have affected fetal growth as well as the status of the neonate. Additional history of the child's course since birth is important, with a particular focus on the signs that identifies the surgical condition that is to be treated. Important factors include the history of feeding and hydration, need for oxygenation or ventilatory support, cardiovascular abnormalities, and any evidence of CNS problems such as seizures or intraventricular hemorrhage. Finally, an estimation of the gestational status is made, with an emphasis on the issues of prematurity and intrauterine growth retardation with subsequent small-for-gestational age status and VLBW neonates.

The World Health Organization's definition of prematurity is less than 37 weeks' gestation at birth. The determination of gestational age is based on the estimated date of full-term delivery, as well as physical examination of the newborn. Although these indicators are generally widely agreed on, they are subject to some degree of variation in interpretation. The greater the degree of prematurity, the more physiologic abnormalities will be expected. The implications for anesthesiologist are that the more preterm a newborn is, the greater the variability of responsiveness to anesthetic agents, fluids, vasoactive medications, and the stress of the surgical procedure.

In addition to prematurity, there is a second, related classification system. Low birth weight, defined as a birth weight of less than 2,500 g, can be due to prematurity, poor intrauterine growth, or both. Prematurity and intrauterine growth retardation are associated with increased neonatal morbidity and mortality, and it is difficult to completely separate factors associated with prematurity from those associated with intrauterine growth retardation. For discussion purposes, preterm infants are often divided into subgroups. Newborns born at 35 to 37 weeks' gestation are considered near term. These newborns have a lower incidence of major physiologic abnormalities typical of the more preterm newborn. Although they usually do not have significant pulmonary abnormalities, they may have some feeding problems or hyperbilirubinemia. This degree of prematurity does not usually have a significant impact on anesthetic management. However, infants born between 30 and 34 weeks' gestation are much more likely to show some abnormalities related to prematurity that can complicate anesthetic management.[90]

Although RDS had previously been a significant source of morbidity in this population, the widespread use of exogenous surfactant has decreased the incidence dramatically, as well as the later complications of chronic lung disease. This group does have more problems with inadequate feeding, persistent patency of the ductus arteriosus, apnea in response to stress, and temperature instability. However, infants born more prematurely than 30 to 34 weeks' gestation begin to demonstrate significant physiologic abnormalities related to prematurity.

For infants with VLBW, defined as less than 1,500 g, the presence of complicating problems and morbidity and mortality are inversely related to birth weight. Major surgery in VLBW infants is associated with a 50% greater risk of mortality or neurodevelopmental impairment at 18 to 22 months of age versus normal birth weight. RDS is found in approximately 80% of infants weighing 501 to 750 g, in 65% of those 751 to 1,000 g, in 45% between 1,001 and 1,250 g, and in 25% between 1,251 and 1,500 g. In addition, symptomatic intraventricular hemorrhage is found in about 25% of infants weighing 501 to 750 g, in 12% between 751 and 1,000 g, in 8% between 1,001 and 1,250 g, and in 3% between 1,251 and 1,500 g. Other complications, such as sepsis, necrotizing enterocolitis (NEC), and bronchopulmonary dysplasia (BPD) are very high in infants with VLBW. Table 42-3 lists some of the most common abnormalities found in the preterm population that have implications for anesthetic evaluation, preparation, and management.

Preanesthetic Evaluation—Physical Examination

Physical examination of the newborn is focused by the condition requiring surgical intervention. Hydration is often an important issue because of both fasting and losses related to the surgical lesion. Clinical signs of dehydration include a sunken fontanel, poor skin turgor, dry mucous membranes, sunken eyes, poor skin perfusion, delayed capillary refill, hypothermia, tachycardia, or absent urine output. If there are clinical signs of dehydration,

Table 42-3 Abnormalities Associated With the Preterm Infant: Common Anesthetic Concerns

Respiratory	Respiratory Distress Syndrome Apnea Pneumothorax, pneumomediastinum Pneumonia Pulmonary hemorrhage Bronchopulmonary dysplasia
Cardiovascular	Patent ductus arteriosus Hypotension Bradycardia Pulmonary hypertension Persistent transitional circulation Congenital heart disease
Central nervous system	Intraventricular hemorrhage Hypoxic–ischemic encephalopathy Seizures Kernicterus Drug withdrawal
Metabolic	Hypoglycemia Hyperglycemia Hypocalcemia Hypothermia Metabolic acidosis
Renal	Hyponatremia Hypernatremia Hyperkalemia Poor urine output
Gastrointestinal	Poor feeding Necrotizing enterocolitis Intestinal obstruction
Hematologic	Anemia Hyperbilirubinemia Vitamin K deficiency
Other	Retinopathy of prematurity Sepsis and infections

efforts should be made to correct the deficits before surgery, except in extreme, life-threatening situations. Physical examination also focuses on the respiratory and cardiovascular systems. The presence of any cardiovascular abnormalities should be noted, including poor perfusion or pulses, abnormal rhythm or rate, a murmur or gallop, hepatomegaly, or other signs of either heart failure or poor perfusion. The presence of a murmur is of concern in the neonatal period and warrants further evaluation, which is best done by a pediatric cardiologist. An electrocardiogram and echocardiogram will help define whether there is significant cardiovascular disease present that will affect the anesthetic management. Although this evaluation may take some effort and time, it is worthwhile to ensure that the anesthesiologist can plan the child's care with full knowledge of the limitations cardiovascular disease can impose.

The respiratory system also must be examined in some detail. The presence of stridor or other evidence of airway obstruction, such as sternal or chest wall retractions, should be identified and investigated. Although upper airway obstruction is relatively rare in the newborn, laryngeal webs, cysts of the tongue or supraglottic region, vocal cord paralysis after a traumatic delivery, and hemangiomas of the airway can cause obstruction and need to be identified. In addition, newborns that have been previously intubated may have some degree of subglottic edema related to previous intubation. More likely are signs of lower airway disease such as tachypnea, grunting, rhonchi, retractions, and cyanosis. This may be related to the early development of RDS, but may also represent meconium aspiration, pneumonia, pneumothorax, or heart failure. The cause of any respiratory distress needs to be evaluated expeditiously prior to anesthesia to identify treatable causes and begin therapy.

Preanesthetic Evaluation—Laboratory

Most laboratory investigations are related to the underlying surgical condition such as radiography, computed tomography, magnetic resonance imaging, and echocardiography. However, most newborns will have, at a minimum, a blood count and glucose level drawn. The hemoglobin in a newborn is primarily fetal hemoglobin, which has a higher affinity for oxygen than adult hemoglobin. Because of this higher affinity, the hemoglobin dissociation curve is shifted to the left, releasing less oxygen to the tissues than adult hemoglobin. Newborns have a higher hemoglobin than the infant or child, often in the 15 to 18 g/dL range.[91] Rarely, a newborn will have significant polycythemia, with hemoglobin levels above 20 g/dL. If symptomatic, these patients may benefit from therapeutic phlebotomy and volume replacement.

Glucose levels obtained close to the time of the proposed surgery are important. The stressed newborn, especially the stressed preterm or small-for-gestational age newborn, are at particular risk for hypoglycemia.[92] A glucose level between 60 and 80 mg/dL is expected in a full-term newborn, with a preterm often 10 mg/dL below that. Although there is some controversy about what constitutes hypoglycemia in these populations, most agree that levels less than 45 mg/dL warrant therapy with additional dextrose. Patients with diabetic mothers, those who have not been receiving either enteral or parenteral feeds, those who are VLBW, and those who have been septic are especially susceptible to hypoglycemia and require frequent monitoring and modification of parenteral fluids.

Other laboratory studies, such as electrolyte determinations and coagulation profiles, are indicated in specific patients. Hypocalcemia is especially troubling because signs of hypocalcemia are nonspecific. Unexplained hypotension, irritability, or even seizures can be presenting signs. Hypocalcemia is a problem with preterm newborns but can also be seen in full-term newborns who have a delay in starting enteral feedings. Hyponatremia is not uncommon in newborns who have been receiving solutions with little or no salt in the first days of life, although hypernatremia may occur if there is inadequate resuscitation of the dehydrated patient when water loss is greater than salt loss. The longer a newborn has received parenteral fluids, the greater the chance of electrolyte abnormalities because of the difficulty in matching ongoing losses with replacement in the presence of an immature kidney.

Coagulation parameters are different in newborns compared with adults.[93] Although platelet counts in term newborns are usually similar to adult values, lower values are frequently seen in the preterm. Unexplained thrombocytopenia can be an early sign of sepsis, and a falling count should be an impetus to look for other signs of sepsis. Other coagulation tests are different in both the full-term and preterm newborn. The prothrombin time and partial thromboplastin time levels are about 10% longer in the newborn, but prothrombin time values approach adult levels in the first week of life and partial thromboplastin time levels within the first month of life. Prevention of early vitamin K deficiency bleeding (VKDB) of the newborn is the purpose of intramuscular vitamin K administration after birth and is standard of care in the United States.[94]

Preanesthetic Plan

The anesthesiologist has a host of anesthetic techniques from which to choose and can tailor the anesthetic to the requirements of the surgery and the condition of the neonate. Major factors that should be considered in planning the anesthetic include (1) anticipated blood loss and necessity for blood products to be available before beginning the case, (2) monitoring requirements, including invasive monitoring techniques, (3) additional equipment needs for airway and vascular access, (4) transport requirements, (5) postoperative recovery location risk of postoperative ventilation requirements, and (6) plan for postoperative pain relief. Both the medical status of the patient and the planned surgical procedure will impact this planning. The anesthesiologist has the responsibility of clarifying any medical issues with the neonatologist before finalizing the plan, as well as clarifying any issues related to the planned procedure with the surgeon. Occasionally, as planning progresses, it becomes obvious that the patient needs further medical resuscitation or evaluation before it is prudent to proceed with the procedure.

Once the anesthetic plan is clear, it should be discussed with the available parent or caregiver who has legal custody of the child. Informed consent is a process by which the anesthesiologist explains their understanding of the patient's status, the planned procedure, the plan for anesthetic management, alternatives to the plan, and some discussion of risks and benefits. Although there may be rare circumstances in which the legal guardian is not available to provide consent, efforts should be made in all except the most emergent of situations to have this discussion. It should be stressed that informed consent is a process, not a document. The goal of informed consent is to help the parent understand what care is being proposed, the risks and benefits involved, and reasonable alternatives. It is the discussion, in terms understandable to the parent, that is the basis of true informed consent.

Premedication

Premedication is not commonly used for neonatal anesthetics (1 Video 42-1). Sedation is not usually necessary, and analgesics are rarely indicated before taking the patient to the operating room. Atropine or glycopyrrolate may be used for vagolytic effect before induction. Because of the dominance of the parasympathetic nervous system, bradycardia on induction or in response to inhalation agents is of concern. Manipulation of the airway or administration of succinylcholine may cause bradycardia in neonates without administration of atropine or glycopyrrolate. Although it is not requisite to administer a vagolytic, it should be among the drugs immediately available and additional vigilance from the anesthesiologist is necessary to quickly respond to bradycardia. Although a dose of 20 μg/kg of atropine is most frequently used to prevent bradycardia, the question of a minimum dose of 100 to 200 μg has been a source of controversy. However, it appears that prior concerns over paradoxical bradycardia with small doses of atropine have not been evident in clinical trials, leading to a practice reversal where the minimum dose of atropine is no longer commonly used.[95]

Intraoperative Considerations

Monitoring

Neonatal patients are at a disadvantage when it comes to perioperative monitoring because of their small size. Many of the monitoring modalities that are easily employed in older children and adults are very difficult in the neonate. Other monitors that are used may occasionally not provide reliable information for technical reasons. Examples of this include neuromuscular blockade monitoring and automated blood pressure monitoring. Invasive monitoring such as arterial line and central venous line catheters may be technically difficult to insert, especially in the preterm. However, improvements in ultrasound guidance have made line placement much more efficient and the development of small TEE probes has extended this useful monitoring technique into the neonatal population, including premature newborns.[15] The overarching goal of monitoring should be to establish American Society of Anesthesiologists standard monitors at the beginning of the case and add invasive monitoring, as appropriate.

Although physical observation of the patient is important in preanesthetic evaluation, it is difficult to use this monitor effectively during a surgical procedure. Observation of the patient's color, capillary refill, warmth of skin, muscle tone, fullness of fontanelle, and chest expansion are useful monitors, but they are difficult to reliably observe once the patient is covered with surgical drapes. There is a large dependence on electronic monitors during most of the procedure. However, it should be remembered that heart and breath sounds heard through a precordial or esophageal stethoscope, the compliance determined during hand ventilation, the appearance of bleeding in the surgical field, and trends noted in the anesthetic record are all important observations that the anesthesiologist can use as part of the overall assessment of the patient.

Pulse oximetry is one of the most important monitors in neonatal anesthesia. Flexible probes designed for pediatric patients should be used. Placement is sometimes difficult because of the small fingers of the neonate. It may be necessary to place the probe across the web space between the thumb and the first finger, around the lateral aspect of the hand, or on the foot. Many anesthesiologists will place and check two pulse oximeter probes at the beginning of the case because of the clinical experience of having one probe malfunctioning secondary to changes in perfusion during the case. Because there may be differences in preductal and postductal saturations, probes on the left hand or either leg may give lower values than a probe on the right hand in the setting of high pulmonary pressures or low systemic pressures. Especially in the first 2 weeks of life, there is a preponderance of fetal hemoglobin. The pulse oximeter does not compensate for the left shift of the hemoglobin desaturation curve, and pulse oximeter values read about 2% higher than arterial blood saturations.[96]

The hallmark of the pediatric anesthesiologist had been the precordial stethoscope. Precordial stethoscopes have the advantage of being simple and effective in allowing continuous monitoring of heart rate, heart rhythm, strength of heart sounds, and breath sounds. A softening of heart sounds often is indicative of a drop in blood pressure. The esophageal stethoscope is more secure and less susceptible to external noise compared to the precordial stethoscope, while also providing the ability to measure core temperature. However, there has been recent skepticism about the usefulness of the stethoscope,[97] and a survey of pediatric anesthesiologists in the United Kingdom and Ireland revealed relatively little use of the precordial or esophageal stethoscope.[98]

The electrocardiograph is useful primarily to assess heart rate and rhythm. It is sometimes difficult to get the leads to adhere properly but wiping the skin with alcohol before placement is often helpful. These leads, once applied, can bind tightly to skin, and care must be taken when removing them to avoid removal of skin, especially in the preterm newborn. ST–T wave abnormalities may be an indicator of significant electrolyte disturbances, but abnormalities related to myocardial ischemia are not common in the perioperative period unless coronary perfusion pressures are compromised.

Blood pressure measurements are important in the management of all newborns. Noninvasive automated machines are commonly used, but it is important that a proper-sized cuff—one-half to two-thirds of the length of the upper arm—be used, and that the arterial indicator, adjacent to the exit of the hoses, be placed over the artery. The cuff should not be routinely cycled excessively, more than every 3 minutes, because of the danger of venous stasis, especially in preterm neonates. In some cases, it is not possible to get reliable readings from an automated machine. An effective alternative is to use a manual cuff and place a Doppler probe over the brachial or radial artery. This system gives reliable systolic blood pressures over a very wide range; the Doppler probe can detect flow, even at very low blood pressures when the automated cuff may fail.

Direct arterial blood pressure monitoring offers the double advantage of accurate blood pressure readings and the ability to withdraw blood samples. A 22-gauge catheter is often used in full-term neonates and a 24-gauge catheter in preterm neonates. A variety of sites can be used, including the radial, dorsalis pedis, and posterior tibial arteries. Less commonly, the brachial, axillary, or femoral arteries are used. Ultrasound guidance is a valuable tool in the placement of arterial access, especially in neonates. Some patients may come to the operating room with an umbilical arterial line in place. Although these can be used for monitoring, umbilical lines have both infectious and embolic risks, and may be in the way of the surgical field. All arterial lines should be flushed, either continuously or intermittently, with small amounts of heparinized saline, but caution should be used because even small amounts of flush can transmit significant pressure retrograde and cause embolic damage to the brain.

Central venous monitoring is occasionally used in neonatal surgery. Access to blood samples and central venous pressures can be especially useful in procedures, such as gastroschisis repair, in which there are anticipated large changes in both blood loss and third-space losses. Central catheters can also be used for the administration of blood, total parenteral nutrition, and vasoactive drug infusion. Insertion of these lines can be in a variety of sites, including the subclavian, internal jugular, femoral, or external jugular veins using special precautions to maintain sterile technique.

Percutaneous insertion may be assisted by ultrasound guidance. Central lines can be both challenging to insert, but also associated with significant complications related to infection, thrombosis, and emboli. Meticulous technique with insertion and maintenance of the line will help minimize these complications. The use of ultrasound guidance is now routine in U.S. children's hospitals to provide a presumably safe and consistent method for gaining central venous access; however, a meta-analysis did not demonstrate any significant decrease in complications when ultrasound was used to place internal jugular access versus placement by landmark techniques.[99] The rate of complications with central line placement is lowest when the right internal jugular vein is used for central access in infants.[100] Peripherally inserted central catheter (PICC), are now common in neonatal practice and associated with a relatively low rate of complications, especially when the axillary vein site is used for access.[101]

Although there may be some differential between capnography and arterial pCO_2 readings, the trend data are accurate and the shape of the waveform can give significant information about changes in ventilation, obstruction, and rebreathing. Airway pressure measurements are particularly useful in assessing changes in resistance or compliance. Although it has been traditional that hand ventilation was important in determining changes in airway and chest compliance, there is controversy about the reliability of the "feel of the hand on the bag."[102,103] Airway pressure measurements are also useful in adapting adult anesthesia ventilators for use in neonatal and pediatric patients, using peak airway pressures as a guide for setting tidal volume.[104]

Anesthetic Systems

There is a long tradition in pediatric anesthesia of using semi-open, nonrebreathing systems for general anesthesia in newborns. Circuits such as the Jackson-Rees adaptation of the Ayre's T-piece and the Bain circuit have been the most commonly used. These, and related circuits, have the advantages of light weight, easy-to-open valves or lack of valves, rapid response to changes in anesthetic concentration, minimal work of breathing, and high circuit compliance. On the other hand, they require relatively high gas flows and require some modification for mechanical ventilation. These circuits were especially popular when spontaneous ventilation was more commonly used than it is now in neonatal patients. As the use of these circuits has diminished, familiarity with their use and application has dropped in favor of the semi-closed, rebreathing circle systems used in adult patients. There will be slower change in anesthetic concentration, less circuit compliance, and larger compression volume with these circuits, but they give the advantage of using the same circuit on patients of all ages, less environmental pollution with anesthetic gases, and allow accurate tidal volume delivery with modern anesthesia machines.

Because the loss of both heat and humidity through the endotracheal tube is of concern in the neonate, the anesthetic circuit should incorporate features to minimize water and heat loss. In the past, heated vaporizers were added to the circuit for this purpose. However, there is a danger of patient absorption of water and fluid overload with their use, as well as concerns about overheating the patient or an airway burn. It is now common to use a combination of low gas flows[105] and a disposable, neonatal humidity and heat exchanger in the circuit.[106]

Finally, the anesthesia machine used for anesthetizing neonates should have the capacity to administer medical air. There are two reasons for this. First, if nitrous oxide is contraindicated, such as in the newborn with bowel obstruction, air is mixed with oxygen to prevent the administration of only 100% oxygen. This is also used to minimize the risk of ROP by avoiding prolonged administration of 100% oxygen in preterm neonates. Second, some patients, such as those with hypoplastic left heart syndrome, may benefit from the administration of air with additional oxygen. Without an air flowmeter in the system, this will not be possible.

Induction of Anesthesia

There is no one method of induction and maintenance of anesthesia that is best for all patients. The current medical status of the patient, the surgical condition, the presence of ongoing fluid or blood losses, the gestational age of the patient, recent fasting, and the experience of the anesthesiologist are all important considerations. Most neonates who come to the operating room will have vascular access already established; if not, the first task before induction is to establish adequate vascular access after applying monitors. Although it may rarely be appropriate to use an inhalational induction if vascular access is difficult in the older newborn, near a month of age, it is mandatory to establish access first in the newborn who is preterm, medically unstable, has a full stomach, has a potentially difficult airway, or has ongoing fluid losses.

Airway Management

Establishing the airway in the neonate requires an appreciation of the differences between the newborn and the adult airway, as discussed earlier. It is rare to administer anesthesia in the newborn period without establishing an artificial airway. Although, with meticulous technique, a mask airway can successfully be used for short periods of time, the tolerances of mask fit, adequate airway pressure, and avoidance of gastric distention are small, making this a poor choice for any but the briefest of operations. In addition, controlled ventilation is used more commonly today than spontaneous ventilation for surgical procedures, making an artificial airway necessary.

Awake intubation has been used to secure the airway without the danger of loss of airway during the procedure, but it can be a traumatic experience for both the patient and the anesthesiologist, accompanied by pain, bradycardia, breath holding, desaturation, and tissue trauma.[107] The desaturation associated with this technique can be ameliorated by using an oxyscope, a Miller laryngoscope blade that has a side channel to allow insufflation of oxygen during the procedure. However, this technique is usually reserved for patients with severe hemodynamic compromise, an extraordinarily distended and tense abdomen, or a presumed difficult airway, especially the newborn with micrognathia. In the latter situation, the addition of sedation with an opioid or topical application of local anesthetic can help decrease some of the trauma of the procedure. It has also been suggested that an awake intubation may be best for the anesthesiologist who is not very experienced in intubating newborns. It may be better to have a more experienced clinician, if available, attend to the airway in that situation.

Most newborns are intubated after a rapid-sequence induction. Preoxygenation is useful in adding additional safety to the procedure. Although there may be a minor concern about a period of hyperoxia in the preterm, there is no evidence that a short exposure such as preoxygenation will increase the risk of ROP. Agents for induction and muscle relaxation are discussed elsewhere. If there is concern about the difficulty of intubation, it may be prudent to induce anesthesia, ensure adequacy of mask ventilation, and then give the muscle relaxant.

Positioning for intubation is based on the known differences in the neonatal airway. Because of the large occiput, the newborn already has a flexed neck. No changes in position are usually needed, although additional extension of the head may be accomplished by a shoulder roll. A Miller no. 1 blade is commonly used for the full-term newborn and a Miller no. 0 in the preterm, although there are other available blades that individual practitioners may prefer. Sliding the blade down the right side of the mouth allows the blade to be seated with minimal overlap by the tongue (Fig. 42-8). The tip of the blade is advanced to lift the epiglottis directly instead of placing it in the vallecula, as is commonly done with older patients. Every patient's anatomy is different, but if the laryngoscope is advanced in the direction parallel to the handle, one will get the best visualization. If the glottis is not easily seen, cricoid pressure can be applied with the little finger of the hand holding the handle or by an assistant, often improving the view (Fig. 42-9).

Uncuffed tubes have traditionally been used in newborns to minimize cuff pressure on the subglottic larynx, especially at the level of the cricoid cartilage. Although there has been interest in the use of cuffed tubes in newborns and infants,[108] many clinicians continue to use uncuffed tubes in newborns to maximize the internal diameter (ID) and gas flow characteristics for a given external diameter of tube. Modern cuffed endotracheal tubes make minimal sacrifice in tube diameter to allow for the presence of a cuff, which has renewed interest in cuffed endotracheal tubes, especially among anesthesiologists. Although various formulas have been proposed for how far to advance an uncuffed tube, it is prudent to use the depth markers at the end of the tube to ensure under direct vision that the tip is advanced 2 or 3 cm past the vocal cords. A 3- or 3.5-mm ID uncuffed tube is usually appropriate for a full-term newborn and a 2.5-mm ID tube is used in preterms, especially those under 1,500 g body weight. Once inserted, the presence of a positive capnograph tracing, bilateral expansion of the thorax, and bilateral breath sounds are used to ensure proper placement. Although some anesthesiologists prefer to advance the endotracheal tube past the carina and then withdraw until bilateral breath sounds are heard, there are two major disadvantages to the technique: trauma to the airway and lack of a guarantee that the tip of the tube is not sitting right at the carina, increasing the chance of migration into a bronchus with head movement. Finally, listen for an air leak at an airway pressure of about 20 cm H_2O to ensure that the tube is not too large for the airway, increasing the chances of subglottic edema and damage.

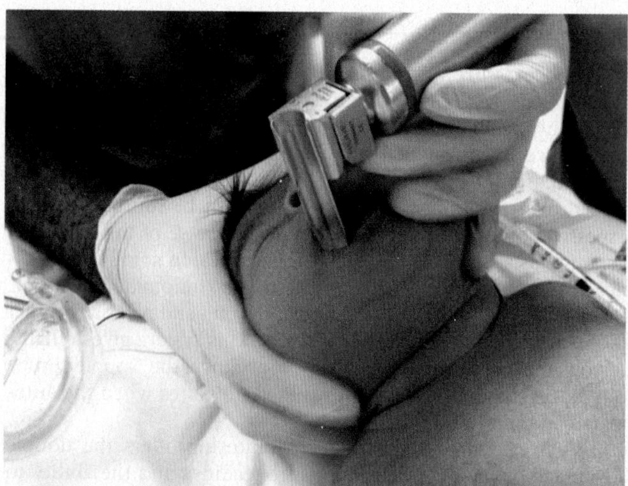

Figure 42-8 Insertion of Miller blade down the right side of the tongue. The blade is then turned and pressure is applied in the direction of the handle.

If intubation proves difficult, there are a variety of options. A supraglottic airway (SGA) can be used to provide ventilation in newborns as small as 1-kg body weight as preparations are made to use other intubating techniques.[109] The SGA has also successfully been used as the primary airway device in very small patients, but has not been extensively studied.[110] It is possible to use the SGA as a guide for blind intubations in newborns with the use of a styletted tube.[111] The light wand can also be used in newborns, and

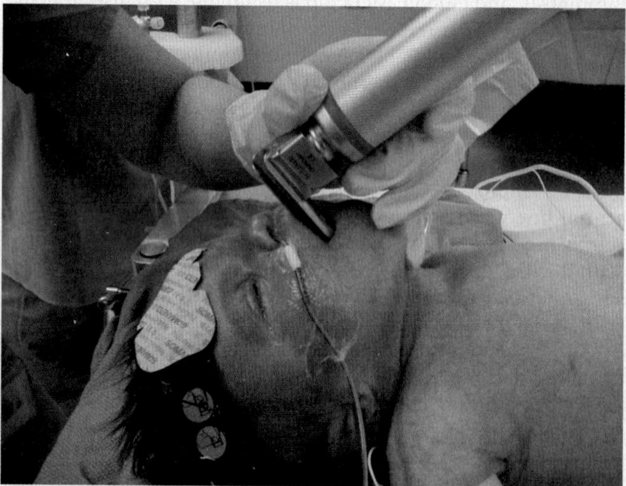

Figure 42-9 Cricoid pressure applied with little finger.

can be particularly useful in the newborn with micrognathia or retrognathia because of the ability to mold the wand to a "hockey stick" configuration with a sharp angle.[112] Fiberoptic laryngoscopy, the most flexible of intubating tools routinely used in older children and adults, can also be used in the newborn. Fiberscopes are currently available that accept endotracheal tubes as small as 2.5-mm ID. Insertion of the fiberscope can be done directly or through an SGA. An SGA as a conduit has been particularly useful in directly intubating newborns that could not be visualized by routine approaches.[113]

Finally, an old technique that is used infrequently is digital intubation in which two fingers are advanced along the midline of the tongue and onto the epiglottis, with a styletted tube then advanced between the two fingers.[114] Once the airway is secured, ventilation is usually controlled during neonatal surgical procedures with hand ventilation or, more commonly, mechanical ventilation. After establishing a baseline of acceptable ventilation, it is important to continuously monitor the peak airway pressures, chest expansion, return volume, pulse oximetry, and capnograph tracings for changes. Initial tidal volumes of 6 to 7 mL/kg and rates of 20 to 25 breaths per minute are a reasonable starting point for most patients. With this rate and volume setting, it would be expected that peak airway pressures be approximately 20 cm H_2O. A level of positive end-expiratory pressure (PEEP) of 3 to 5 cm H_2O can be useful in preventing atelectasis. Lung protective strategies applied in the NICU may be appropriate to continue in the operating room,[115] which is facilitated by the modern anesthesia ventilator. Of course, this strategy must be modified for some patients with severe coexisting disease.

Mechanical ventilation of the neonate can be challenging for the anesthesiologist. Many of the patients presenting for surgery during the neonatal period will have complicating factors such as BPD or frequent mucous plugging that make ventilation continuously challenging during the case. Modern anesthetic systems make ventilation much easier than in the past, even in the smallest patients. Although the standard has been to use pressure control ventilation in this population, all modes of ventilation are now readily available on modern anesthesia machines. In the NICU, volume control ventilation has started to replace pressure control ventilation due to its more predictable and consistent delivery of a set minute ventilation. Table 42-4 shows the modes of ventilation and breath synchronization most commonly used in neonates. Use of high-frequency ventilation in the operative setting will require use of a specialized ventilator and close consultation with a critical care physician and respiratory therapist. Table 42-5 lists some of the advantages and disadvantages to use of pressure control, volume targeted, and high-frequency ventilation.

Table 42-4 Common Ventilator Strategies in Neonates

- Conventional ventilation
  - Breath initiation
    - Intermittent mandatory ventilation
    - Synchronized intermittent mandatory ventilation
    - Pressure support ventilation
    - Neurally adjusted ventilatory assist
  - Pressure-limited ventilation
    - Pressure-control
  - Volume-targeted ventilation
    - Volume-control
    - Volume-guarantee
    - Pressure-regulated volume control
- High-frequency ventilation
  - High-frequency oscillator ventilation
  - High-frequency jet ventilation
  - High-frequency flow interrupter

Table 42-5 Advantages of Particular Ventilator Strategies in Neonates

Mode	Advantages	Disadvantages
Pressure control ventilation	• Easy to use due to long-standing widespread use worldwide • Supported by almost all ventilators • Less affected by large leaks around endotracheal tube	• Constant variation in tidal volume and minute ventilation • Rapid changes in lung compliance may lead to volutrauma, hyperventilation, desaturation, or hypoventilation • Increased work of breathing during spontaneous breaths
Volume-targeted ventilation	• Standard, targeted tidal volume, resulting in a predictable minute ventilation • Associated with lower rate of death or bronchopulmonary dysplasia in NICU management of acute respiratory failure[116] • Reduces rates of pneumothorax, hypocarbia, days of ventilation, and significant neurologic injury over pressure control ventilation[117]	• Requires ventilators with capability of measuring very small tidal volumes • Relies on pressure limits set in ventilator (risk of single point of failure) • More difficult to implement than PCV due to complexity of the ventilators • Large leaks around endotracheal tube may significantly affect reliability of ventilation
High-frequency ventilation	• May provide better ventilation and oxygenation in neonates with severe respiratory disease • Allows for small tidal volumes that are less than total dead space but allow for oxygenation and ventilation • Minimizes barotrauma and volutrauma	• No significant morbidity or mortality advantage over conventional ventilation • Additional cost and difficulty of operation over conventional ventilation • Anesthesia providers are not very familiar with optimization of these devices • Difficult for use during transport or non-ICU locations

Impact of Surgical Requirements on Anesthetic Technique

6 Every procedure has its own unique challenges. With any surgery, issues related to presurgical resuscitation, perioperative fluid and blood loss, heat loss from the surgical field, likely perioperative complications, and the likely need for postoperative intubation and ventilation should be anticipated, both on the basis of experience and communication about the unique needs of the upcoming procedure. There is a dramatic increase in the use of laparoscopic and thoracoscopic approaches to lesions, even in the smallest neonates. The considerations for these approaches are different from open procedures. There may be less blood, fluid, and heat loss, but there are additional issues related to positioning, insufflation pressures in the chest and abdomen, and prolonged surgical time. As new techniques evolve, close communication between the anesthesiologist and the surgeon is necessary to ensure adequate preparation, monitoring, and resolution of problems or complications.

Uptake and Distribution of Anesthetics in Neonates

Various reasons for the faster uptake of anesthetics in infants have been proposed: (1) the ratio of alveolar ventilation to FRC is 5:1 in the infant and 1.5:1 in the adult; (2) in the neonate, more of the cardiac output goes to the vessel-rich group of organs, which includes the heart and the brain; (3) the neonate has a greater cardiac output per kilogram of body mass; and (4) the infant has a lower blood gas partition coefficient for volatile anesthetics. One not well-recognized factor that may result in higher concentrations of volatile anesthetics being administered to infants has to do with the use of nonrebreathing systems such as the Bain or a Mapleson "D" circuit. When an adult circle system is used with infant tubes and bag, the clinician experienced with this equipment is used to reading the inspired, end-tidal, and dialed concentrations of the volatile anesthetic. In the circle system, the inspired concentration is a result of the combination of the end-tidal concentration that is rebreathed through the soda lime absorber and the dialed concentration. The inspired concentration is always lower than the dialed concentration unless the flow rates are so high that a nonrebreathing system has been created. In the nonrebreathing system, the dialed concentration is the inspired concentration. Clinicians who use both systems are accustomed to these subtle differences. However, if the clinician switches back and forth between the circle system and a nonrebreathing circuit, but does so infrequently, there is a danger of not recognizing the possibility of excessive overpressure of volatile anesthetics with the nonrebreathing systems.

Anesthetic Dose Requirements of Neonates

Neonates and premature infants have lower anesthetic requirements than older infants and children.[68] The easiest way to remember the minimum alveolar concentration (MAC) values is that the MAC value in the mature state (i.e., late teenager or adult) is the same as for a full-term infant. By 6 months of age, the MAC value has increased by 50%. In the premature infant, the MAC value decreases by 20% to 30%. However, for sevoflurane anesthesia the highest MAC requirement may be the full-term neonate, decreasing throughout life to adult values (Fig. 42-10).

The reasons for the lower MAC requirements are believed to be an immature nervous system, progesterone from the mother, and elevated blood levels of endorphins, coupled with an immature

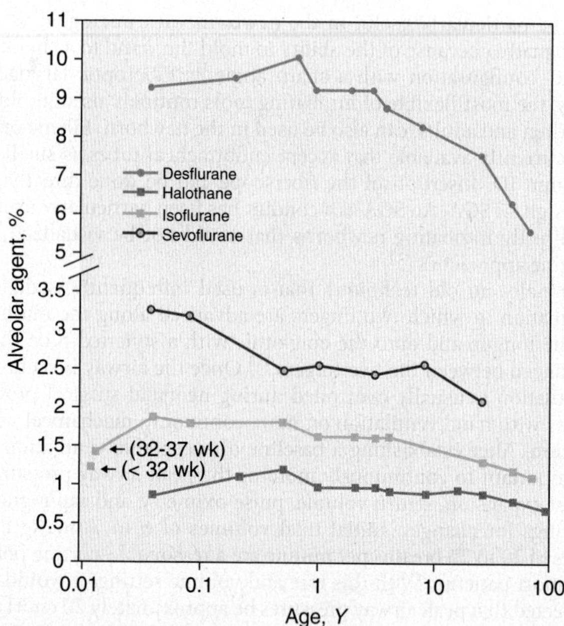

Figure 42-10 Effect of age on minimum alveolar concentration (MAC) of anesthetic gases. (Reprinted with permission from Miller RD, Greeley WJ. *Atlas of Anesthesia: Pediatric Anesthesia*, Vol. 7. 1st ed. Churchill Livingstone; 1999.)

blood–brain barrier. Progesterone has been shown to reduce the MAC of the pregnant mother. The newborn infant has elevated progesterone levels, similar to those of the mother. Elevated levels of β-endorphin and β-lipotropin have been demonstrated in infants in the first few days of postnatal life. Endorphins do not cross the blood–brain barrier in adults; however, it is believed that the neonate's blood–brain barrier is more permeable and that endorphins may pass into the CNS, thus elevating the pain threshold and reducing the MAC requirement.

Regional Anesthesia

There has been a tremendous increase in the use of regional anesthesia in infants and children. In general, regional techniques are combined with general anesthesia to permit early extubation and provide postoperative pain relief. Useful regional anesthesia techniques include spinal anesthesia, caudal anesthesia, epidural analgesia, penile block, and other peripheral nerve blocks (Table 42-6). Regional anesthesia may even have other

Table 42-6 Regional Anesthesia Techniques Useful in Neonates

Central neuraxial
Epidural (lumbar, thoracic, caudal)
Spinal
Peripheral nerve blocks
Infraorbital block
Brachial plexus block (supraclavicular, infraclavicular, axillary)
Lateral femoral cutaneous block
Penile block
Ilioinguinal block
TAP block (transversus abdominis plane block)
Scalp blocks

applications outside surgery, including management of neonatal limb ischemia.[118] Combined regional and general anesthesia is commonly provided for neonates for multiple procedures. The use of ultrasonography has revolutionized the use of regional anesthesia as vascular structures can be easily avoided while still providing a regional blockade.[119] It is important to remember that the dosage of local anesthetic solution used is limited and lipid emulsion is available to potentially treat any intravascular injections.[120]

Spinal Anesthesia

Regional anesthesia can be provided as a sole anesthetic or in combination with general anesthesia. The use of sole regional anesthesia in neonates and infants is for avoidance of general anesthetics, for either theoretical decreased risk of apnea or decreased risk of neurotoxicity. Although neurotoxicity trials are still ongoing, it has been shown that spinal anesthesia decreases early apnea following surgery in premature neonates, but does not decrease the risk of overall apnea following surgery in premature neonates.[121] For patients receiving combined general and regional anesthesia, early extubation is possible because the addition of regional anesthetic techniques eliminates the need for intraoperative narcotics in neonates, reduces or eliminates the need for muscle relaxants, and reduces the concentration of volatile agents needed for relaxation.[122] Spinal anesthesia has been reported to be effective when used as the sole anesthetic technique in premature and high-risk infants, but this technique requires excellent cooperation between the anesthesiologist and an experienced surgeon.[123] Although this is technically feasible, because of increasing advancements in general anesthesia techniques, we may be able to provide safer anesthesia with fewer complications by using general anesthesia.[124] Even high doses of spinal anesthetic provide a relatively short time of surgical anesthesia.

Some patients may benefit from providing a caudal block in addition to the spinal anesthetic. This technique seems to provide a longer duration of surgical anesthesia. Total spinal anesthesia, produced either with a primary spinal technique or secondary to an attempted epidural puncture, will present as apnea, rather than as hypotension, because of the lack of sympathetic tone in infants. The exact mechanism for the lack of cardiovascular change with spinal anesthesia in infants and young children is not clear. Consequently, the first indication of a high spinal is falling oxygen saturation rather than a falling blood pressure. Sedation can be added to regional anesthesia but may cause problems with apnea in ex-premature infants.[125]

Caudal Block

Caudal epidural block is frequently used for abdominal surgery in neonates and is the most commonly used regional anesthetic technique in neonates and infants (NICV 42-1). There are several different techniques described for performing a caudal block. The landmarks are the coccyx, the two sacral cornua, and the posterior superior iliac spines (Fig. 42-11). Several needle types may be used, but the "pop" through the sacrococcygeal ligament is best observed with a blunt-tipped needle, whereas an intravenous catheter advanced over a needle may provide additional confirmation of sacral canal entry. The caudal space is identified by "pop" through the sacrococcygeal ligament, ease of local anesthetic injection, and absence of subcutaneous swelling upon dose delivery. Once the sacrococcygeal ligament is penetrated and there is a loss of resistance, gentle aspiration is applied to the needle to assure there is no blood or cerebrospinal fluid. Injection of the anesthetic is then attempted. If there is difficulty in injecting the solution, then the tip of the needle is not in the caudal space and must be repositioned. The needle is not advanced up the sacral canal after proper placement in the caudal epidural space has been accomplished, this avoids dural puncture and accidental intrathecal injection. Other methods to identify the caudal space have been described, including a stimulation technique[126] and ultrasound guidance.[127] Epinephrine is added to local anesthetic solutions for the purposes of determining if there is an intravascular injection of the anesthetic. Evidence of an intravascular injection include (1) peaked T waves (which may be of relatively short duration), (2) increase in heart rate, and (3) increase in blood pressure. Another technique to minimize the potential difficulties of an intravascular injection is to fractionate the dose by dividing the total dose into three aliquots and waiting approximately 20 to 30 seconds between each aliquot before continuing the injection. Caudal blocks are safe procedures as demonstrated in a large prospective database (PRAN) with very minimal risk overall so long as appropriate precautions are taken during performance.[128]

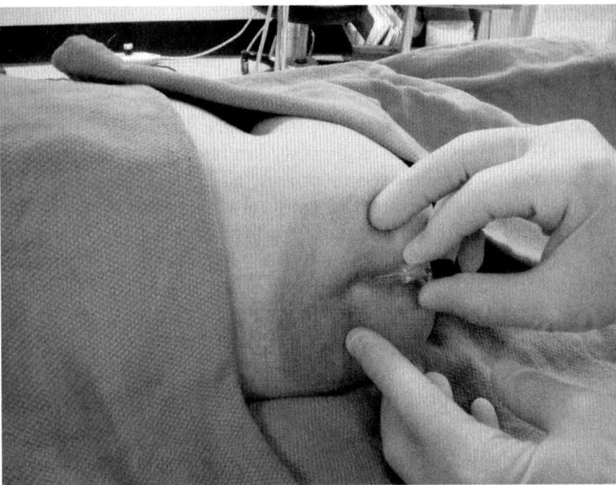

Figure 42-11 Caudal block. The sacral cornua are identified. A styletted needle is introduced into the caudal space through the sacral hiatus. A "pop" is felt as the sacrococcygeal ligament is accessed. After aspiration, 0.8 to 1 mL/kg of local anesthetic solution is injected. This provides analgesia for hernia repair, circumcisions, and lower abdominal surgeries.

Caudal anesthesia is particularly effective at reducing the concentrations of volatile anesthetics needed, as well as relaxants and opioids. In addition, a single-injection caudal anesthetic can provide analgesia for 6 to 8 hours. The most common local anesthetics currently in use are 0.125% bupivacaine, 0.25% bupivacaine, or 0.2% ropivacaine. Epinephrine, 1:200,000, is added to local anesthetics to assist in determining if there has been an intravenous injection. Ropivacaine has been reported to be less cardiodepressant than equipotent doses of bupivacaine. If a caudal catheter is placed, an infusion of ropivacaine, bupivacaine, lidocaine, or chloroprocaine can be administered and provide analgesia for several days postoperatively. Current recommendations for infusions in neonates and young infants are for an initial loading dose of 0.2 to 0.25 mg/kg of bupivacaine; after 1 to 2 hours, an infusion can be begun in a dose of 0.2 mg/kg/hr.[72] The addition of clonidine, 1 to 2 μg/kg, to local anesthetic for caudal block has been used, but may not enhance analgesia.[129] Opioids can also be used for epidural infusions. However, caution must be exercised in neonates and infants who may be prone to apnea with even moderate doses of opioids in the epidural space. Ultrasonography can be used for localization of the caudal space in infants whose anatomy may not be apparent.[127]

Epidural Analgesia

With the introduction of newer and smaller needles and epidural catheters, we are able to provide epidural analgesia in neonates and infants. Although some practitioners prefer using a caudal route to place catheters in the epidural space, lumbar and thoracic epidural catheters can be easily placed in neonates.[130] Ultrasound or fluoroscopy can be used to provide additional reassurance of successful placement into the epidural space. Use of neuraxial catheters for postoperative analgesia in neonates has a low serious complication rate (0.3%) while adverse events such as catheter malfunction, contamination, and vascular puncture are more common.[131] It is imperative to limit the dose of local anesthetic solution in neonates and children to avoid toxicity.

Peripheral Nerve Blocks

Common peripheral nerve blocks in neonates include penile blocks, ilioinguinal nerve blocks, lateral femoral cutaneous blocks, transversus abdominis plane (TAP) blocks, brachial plexus blocks, and head and neck blocks for neurosurgical procedures.

Penile Block

This is a relatively simple block that can be performed easily. The dorsal nerves of the penis are located on either side of the shaft of the penis. A ring block using local anesthetic without epinephrine can be used to provide analgesia following circumcision.[132] The dorsal penile nerves may also be approached more proximally, using the pubic symphysis as the primary landmark and injecting the nerves at approximately the 2 o'clock position and 10 o'clock position if the pubic symphysis is at the 12 o'clock position. Because the penis is innervated by the two dorsal penile nerves which are branches of the bilateral pudendal nerves and also innervated by the perineal nerves which are also branches of the pudendal nerves, the ventral surface of the penis may need a ring block with care to avoid the urethra for complete block of the penis. All of these techniques have also been described with ultrasound.[133]

Ilioinguinal Nerve Block

The ilioinguinal and iliohypogastric nerves supply sensory innervation to the inguinal area. These nerves can be easily visualized while operating. However, we find that blockade of these nerves can provide adequate postoperative analgesia (Fig. 42-12). The anterior superior iliac spine is identified. Immediately medial to the anterior superior iliac spine, a needle is inserted toward the umbilicus and local anesthesia is fanned into the area. The advantage with the use of ultrasonography is the ability to significantly reduce the dose of local anesthesia.[71] In fact, that study found the volume for ilioinguinal nerve block can be effectively reduced to 0.075 mL/kg of local anesthetic solution.

TAP Block

The TAP is a virtual space that exists between the internal oblique and the transversus abdominis muscle (NICV 42-2). This plane carries the thoracolumbar fibers from T8 to L1 (Fig. 42-13). This block has successfully been used to provide analgesia for infants and neonates undergoing major abdominal surgery, including colostomy placement.[134] This block provides cutaneous pain relief following abdominal procedures but does not provide visceral pain relief. It is a safe block in neonates with no evidence of toxicity.[135]

Lateral Femoral Cutaneous Nerve Block

The lateral femoral cutaneous nerve is a sensory branch of the lumbar plexus that supplies cutaneous innervation over the lateral aspect of the thigh. This block is particularly useful in neonates who undergo muscle biopsies of the lateral thigh.[122]

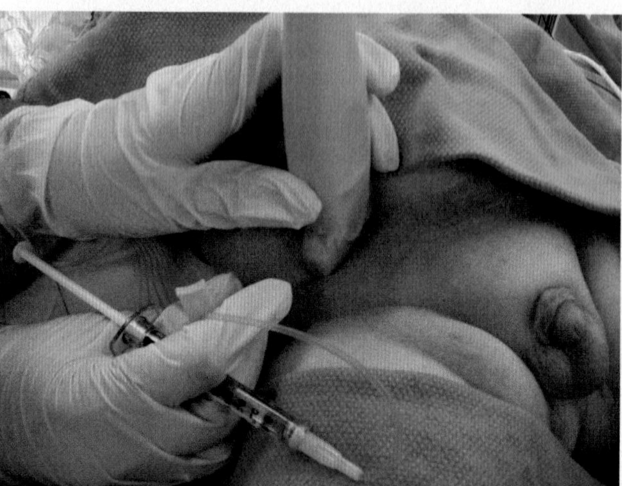

Figure 42-12 Ilioinguinal nerve block. Using a linear ultrasound probe, the anterior superior iliac spine is identified. The layers of the abdomen including the external oblique, transversus abdominis, and iliacus muscles are identified. The ilioinguinal and iliohypogastric nerves are located under the internal oblique muscle and in the plane between the internal oblique and the transversus abdominis muscle. A 27-gauge needle is inserted under ultrasound guidance in this plane. After aspiration, 0.075 to 0.1 mL/kg of local anesthetic solution is injected. This block can be used for pain relief following hernia surgery.

Brachial Plexus Block

This is performed for major limb surgery including major hand and arm surgical procedures. Using ultrasonography during the axillary approach to identify each branch of the brachial plexus allows selective block of each nerve,[136] thus reducing the total dose of local anesthetic. A single shot supraclavicular approach to the brachial plexus can also be used for providing analgesia for upper extremity surgery. It is important to visualize using

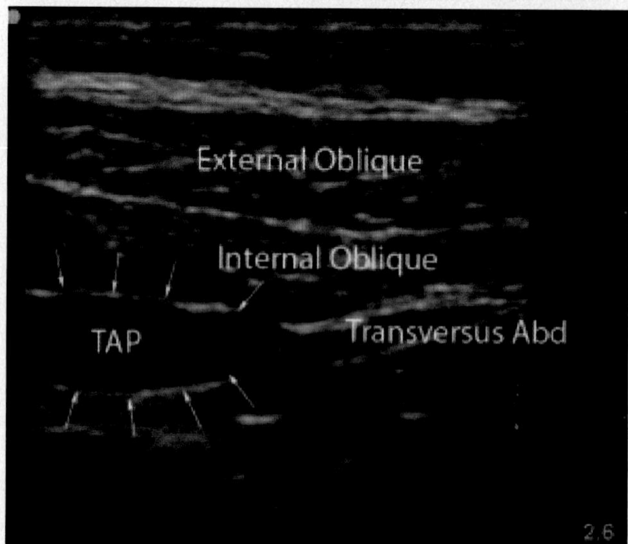

Figure 42-13 TAP (transversus abdominis plane) block using a linear ultrasound probe with a small footprint (25 mm), the abdominal wall is scanned from medial to lateral, the three layers of the abdominal muscles are recognized, a needle is inserted into the space between the internal oblique and the transversus abdominis muscle while hydro-dissecting to find the plane, 0.5 mL/kg of 0.125% bupivacaine is injected into each side to provide analgesia for the abdominal wall.

ultrasonography because the pleura is relatively close to the area of interest and injection. For sustained pain relief, an infraclavicular catheter may be used and is easily held in place by additional muscle and fascial layers which make this a preferable approach to catheter placement for upper extremity surgery.[137]

Neurosurgical Blocks

Peripheral nerve blocks of the head and neck are useful for many surgical procedures. These may be useful in the sick neonate who requires a neurosurgical procedure. Peripheral nerve blocks of the trigeminal nerve and occipital nerve branches may be used to provide analgesia while avoiding general anesthesia.[138]

Postoperative Pain Management

The concepts of postoperative pain management are well known to most anesthesiologists. The use of intraoperative epidural anesthesia followed by postoperative epidural local anesthetics or opioids has been popular in older children and adults, and these techniques are being applied to neonates. In addition, most neonatologists are experienced with the intravenous administration of opioids for patient comfort. Each technique has its own risks and benefits. Commonly used systemic treatments for postoperative pain are listed in Table 42-7.

Oral Routes

Oral routes of medications have been used for decades in neonates and children for managing pain. The commonly used oral analgesics include nonsteroidal analgesics including acetaminophen (10 to 15 mg/kg) and ibuprofen (5 to 10 mg/kg), as well as opioids, including hydrocodone (0.1 mg/kg) and oxycodone (0.05 mg/kg). There may be some pharmacogenetic changes associated with the use of codeine in infants; thus, it is falling out of favor in use across all ages.[139]

Rectal Routes

Rectal suppositories are used frequently in neonates and infants for managing pyrexia. Rectal acetaminophen is commonly used for postoperative analgesia. A larger dose than is usually given orally is needed in infants to achieve adequate blood levels, because of unreliable absorption. A dose of 20 to 30 mg/kg of rectal acetaminophen is generally recommended for postoperative pain control. Diclofenac, a commonly available rectal suppository in Europe, is frequently used in infants for postoperative pain control.

Table 42-7 Postoperative Pain Control for Neonates and Infants

Intravenous Opioids: morphine, fentanyl, methadone NSAIDs: ketorolac, ibuprofen Acetaminophen
Oral Acetaminophen Ibuprofen Hydrocodone Oxycodone Codeine
Rectal Acetaminophen Diclofenac
Regional and local anesthesia

NSAIDs, nonsteroidal anti-inflammatory drugs.

Intravenous Analgesia

Opioids are the mainstay of analgesia in neonates and infants in the postoperative period. Morphine and fentanyl are frequently used in the NICU for analgesia. However, the potential for opioid tolerance after prolonged infusion of opioids is somewhat common. To decrease the likelihood of opioid tolerance,[44] one can rotate opioids or add other medications including continuous intravenous naloxone[140] and intravenous methadone. Other intravenous nonsteroidal anti-inflammatory medications and intravenous acetaminophen have been introduced. Although not FDA approved for use in neonates, IV acetaminophen use has been gaining great interest in children for analgesia.[141] It is common to use decreased doses in neonates, 10 mg/kg, whereas the usual dose in older children is 15 mg/kg. Intravenous ketorolac, a nonsteroidal anti-inflammatory drug, has been used successfully in neonates and infants for pain control at a dose of 0.5 mg/kg.[142] Use of ketorolac in postsurgical neonates <21 days of age or <37 weeks corrected gestational age has been associated with increased risk of bleeding.[143]

Postoperative Ventilation

The choice of an anesthetic drug should be guided by the need for postoperative management of ventilation, as well as the drug's effects on the circulation and other organs. If the surgical procedure or the neonate's condition is such that postoperative ventilation is likely, the prolonged respiratory effects of opioids or any other drug are of little concern. However, if the surgical procedure is relatively short and by itself does not require postoperative ventilation, the clinician should carefully select drugs, as well as doses of anesthetic drugs and relaxants, that will not necessitate prolonged postoperative ventilation or intubation. Postoperative ventilation places the neonate at added risk because of the problems associated with mechanical ventilation, the trauma to the subglottic area, and the potential development of postoperative subglottic stenosis or edema. However, if there is any question about the neonate's ability to maintain protective airway reflexes or normal ventilation after anesthesia, the neonate should be returned to the recovery room or NICU with the trachea intubated, with controlled mechanical ventilation.

Special Considerations

Maternal Drug Use during Pregnancy

Many drugs taken during pregnancy can affect the fetus and neonate. One area of special concern is substance abuse. During pregnancy, maternal drug use of cocaine, marijuana, and others leads to a host of problems for the neonate. Cocaine use, for instance, results in a reduced catecholamine reuptake, which may result in the accumulation of catecholamines. This accumulation has circulatory effects on the uterus, the umbilical blood vessels, and the fetal cardiovascular system. Three major problems affecting the infant are premature birth, intrauterine growth retardation, and cardiovascular abnormalities, including low cardiac output.[144] The cardiac output and stroke volume are reduced on the first day of life but return to normal by the second day. The clinical implication of this finding is that these neonates may be unstable enough in the first day of life that it may be advantageous to postpone surgery, if possible, until the second or third day of life. There is also an increase in structural cardiovascular malformations and electrocardiographic abnormalities. The most frequent lesions are peripheral pulmonary stenosis, right ventricular conduction delay, right ventricular hypertrophy, and ST segment and T-wave changes.[145] Preanesthetic history should elicit the use of drugs, including illicit use, if possible, to evaluate potential alteration of the anesthetic approach.

Temperature Control and Thermogenesis

The newborn is at risk for significant metabolic derangements caused by hypothermia. Newborns, and especially preterms, do not have the normal compensatory mechanisms that infants and children have when exposed to a cold environment. The newborn does not shiver, increase activity, or effectively vasoconstrict like older children or adults do in response to cold. In addition, the newborn has a larger body surface area-to-weight ratio that promotes heat loss, as well as low levels of subcutaneous fat for insulation. The newborn's primary mechanism by which to compensate for heat loss is nonshivering thermogenesis.[146] When there is a 2° centigrade gradient between core and skin, there is a release of norepinephrine into the bloodstream. Norepinephrine stimulates increased metabolism in a specialized tissue, brown fat, which contains a high concentration of mitochondria and has abundant vascular supply. Stimulated lipolysis results in heat production, with side effects of increased oxygen consumption and production of ketone bodies and water. Ketone production causes both a metabolic acidosis and osmotic diuresis. The aerobic activity results in diversion of cardiac output to the deposits of brown fat around the kidneys, under the sternum, and between the scapulae. Because the diuresis, diversion of cardiac output away from the core circulation, and metabolic acidosis are maladaptive, every effort should be made to prevent nonshivering thermogenesis in the newborn.

Efforts to minimize nonshivering thermogenesis in the newborn are based on minimizing heat loss, both during transport to and from the NICU and in the operating room. Transport should be done with the newborn in an incubator or in an open bed with overhead heaters. This will prevent heat loss from conduction and radiation. In the operating room, the room temperature is raised to its maximal level to minimize loss by conduction. Placing the patient on a forced-air warming blanket can reduce conductive heat loss. Using plastic wrap or commercially available covers and hats to minimize heat loss from the head and all other areas not in the surgical field is also beneficial. The goal of all these activities is to maintain a neutral thermal environment, minimizing the stress that hypothermia can induce in the perioperative period. A complicating factor is that anesthetic agents can reduce or eliminate thermogenesis, removing any ability to compensate for cold stress.[147]

Respiratory Distress Syndrome

Because of the enormous technical ability of the neonatologist and the resources of NICUs, many small infants survive, and some will require surgery. One of the frequent problems of preterm infants is the occurrence of the RDS secondary to a deficiency of surfactant. As discussed earlier, the use of exogenous surfactant has been widely used in premature infants of low birth weight either to prevent or to treat RDS. As a result, fewer infants now die of this entity, and the incidence of complications related to RDS has dropped. One of the long-term consequences of RDS is BPD (NICV 42-3). BPD refers to a continuum of chronic disease of the lung parenchyma and airways, as well as neurodevelopment that occurs in preterm infants, especially those born under 32 weeks' gestation, who have survived RDS.[148] The theories of the cause of this condition include toxicity from oxygen administration, infection, inflammation, and barotrauma. Characteristics include airway smooth muscle hyperplasia, peribronchiolar fibrosis, enlarged alveoli, and disorganized pulmonary vasculature. Many patients improve as they age, but reactive airways, recurrent pulmonary infections, and a prolonged oxygen requirement are seen in some patients. Anesthetic concerns in these patients include evaluation of baseline oxygenation and potential presence of active bronchoconstriction. These patients often benefit from prophylactic bronchodilator therapy before induction. The baseline measure of oxygenation is important because these patients have less pulmonary oxygen reserve and may desaturate quickly with induction of anesthesia and hypoventilation. In patients with severe BPD, ventilatory management may be complicated by poor lung compliance and hyperinflation, as well as reactive airway disease. Although postanesthetic ventilation is not usually required, a high index of suspicion should be used if there is significant clinical evidence of poor lung function preoperatively.

Postoperative Apnea

Apnea and bradycardia are well-recognized, major complications during and after surgery in neonates.[149] The infants at highest risk are those born prematurely, those with multiple congenital anomalies, those with a history of apnea and bradycardia, and those with chronic lung disease. The etiology of neonatal apnea is multifactorial. Decreased ventilatory control and decreased responsiveness to hypoxia and hypercarbia may be potentiated by anesthetic agents. Respiratory muscle fatigue may also play a role because neonates have a smaller percentage of type I fibers in their diaphragm and intercostal muscles. In addition, hypothermia and anemia also contribute to the development of postoperative apnea.[150] The treatment of postoperative apnea or bradycardia may be as simple as tactile stimulation. However, some infants require mask ventilation or even prolonged intubation and ventilatory support. Infants with life-threatening apnea and bradycardia before surgery may be receiving CNS stimulants. Caffeine and theophylline (metabolized to caffeine) act by increasing central respiratory drive and lowering the threshold of response to hypercarbia, as well as stimulating contractility in the diaphragm. Caffeine is favored because of its wider therapeutic margin and decreased propensity for toxicity. Administering caffeine prophylactically to infants at risk of postoperative apnea to ensure adequate serum levels may prevent the need for prolonged periods of postoperative ventilatory support. The recommended loading dose is 10 mg/kg caffeine. Spinal anesthesia may reduce the risk of early postoperative apnea but does not reliably decrease the overall risk of postoperative apnea in premature infants.

The question remains as to which infant should be admitted and monitored after outpatient surgery and for how long. The most conservative approach is to monitor all infants younger than 60 weeks' postconceptual age overnight after surgery. Although the incidence of significant apnea and bradycardia is highest in the first 4 to 6 hours after surgery, it can occur up to 12 hours after surgery. In addition, the incidence of apnea directly correlates to postconceptual age. The risk of apnea goes up the younger the gestational age at birth. An insightful approach to interpreting the various small studies is to stratify the risk of apnea, as done by Cote et al.[150] Using a meta-analysis, the study determined that the risk of apnea could be correlated with a combination of gestational age and postconceptual age. Using 95% confidence limits, the authors found that the probability of apnea in nonanemic infants free of recovery room apnea was not less than 5% until postconceptual age was 48 weeks with gestational age of 35 weeks. This risk was not less than 1%, until a postconceptual age of 56 weeks with a gestational age of 32 weeks or a postconceptual age of 54 weeks and gestational age of 35 weeks. This type of analysis allows the clinician to determine which patients should be admitted on not only the criteria of gestational and postconceptual ages but also the amount of risk they are willing to assume.

Retinopathy of Prematurity

7 As the survival rate of increasingly preterm infants has grown, there is increasing concern about the development of ROP (NICV 42-4). The very preterm infant, especially those under 1,200 g of weight, are at highest risk, with an incidence of significant disease about 2%. Acute retinal changes are seen in about 45% of susceptible preterm neonates, but there is spontaneous regression in most, permitting development of normal vision. Other infants will progress to a severe form of ROP and potentially permanent blindness. Several complex factors may be responsible for the development of ROP. In the fetus, developing blood vessels grow gradually from the macula toward the edges of the developing retina. In full-term newborns, this process is complete at birth or in the first few weeks but continues for a longer period in the preterm infant. These growing vessels are at risk for vasoconstriction and subsequent hemorrhage, followed by disorganized neovascularization or scarring. This scarring and lack of normal growth can eventually cause the retinal network to peel away resulting in retinal detachment. The spectrum or stages of disease is classified as follows:

Stage I. Mildly abnormal blood vessel growth. Many children who develop stage I improve with no treatment and eventually develop normal vision.

Stage II. Moderately abnormal blood vessel growth. Many children who develop stage II improve with no treatment and eventually develop normal vision. The disease resolves on its own without further progression.

Stage III. Severely abnormal blood vessel growth. The abnormal blood vessels grow toward the center of the eye instead of following their normal growth pattern along the surface of the retina. Some infants who develop stage III disease improve with no treatment and eventually develop normal vision. However, when infants have a certain degree of stage III and "plus disease" develops, treatment is considered. Plus disease means that the blood vessels of the retina have become enlarged and twisted, indicating a worsening of the disease. Treatment at this point provides a good chance of preventing retinal detachment.

Stage IV. Partially detached retina.

Stage V. Completely detached retina.

The most common cited cause of ROP is hyperoxia from administered oxygen, but hypoxemia, hypotension, sepsis, intraventricular hemorrhage, and other stresses have been implicated. At one time, there was concern that exposure to bright ambient light could cause ROP, but this has been disproven.[151] Although there may be spontaneous regression in early stages, there may also be progression to advanced stages and retinal detachment. The most common therapies involve using cryotherapy or laser therapy to destroy peripheral areas of the retina, slowing or reversing the abnormal growth of blood vessels. This is done to preserve the central vision from continuing distortion of the abnormal vessels in the periphery, although there is some loss of peripheral vision with this therapy.[152] In advanced stages, partial retinal detachment can be treated with a scleral buckle or vitrectomy.

Cryotherapy and laser therapies, as well as advanced procedures, are usually performed under general anesthesia in the operating room, although it is occasionally done at bedside with sedation in ventilated patients. These surgical procedures do not involve blood loss or significant surgical stress, but they do depend on a still surgical field for periods ranging from 30 to 90 minutes. The primary anesthetic challenge in these patients is related to the extreme prematurity and small size of the patients. Adequate monitoring, vascular access, and thermal stability are common challenges to management.

The risks of the development of ROP from hyperoxia have been of concern to anesthesiologists who anesthetize preterm infants for any type of surgery. Whether supplemental oxygen during anesthesia contributes to development of ROP has been a long-standing question in neonatal anesthesia. There is no direct answer to this question, but some evidence from a large, collaborative study helps provide some guidance. Premature infants with confirmed early stages of ROP and a median pulse oximetry below 94% saturation were randomized to a conventional oxygen arm with pulse oximetry targeted at 89% to 94% saturation or a supplemental arm with pulse oximetry targeted at 96% to 99% saturation for at least 2 weeks.[153] The patients were then re-examined for progression of disease. Use of supplemental oxygen at pulse oximetry saturations of 96% to 99% did not cause additional progression of pre-threshold ROP. This study demonstrates that the use of supplemental oxygen for a prolonged period of time, not just for the short duration of a general anesthetic, was not deleterious as long as the pulse oximetry readings were kept in the 96% to 99% range. Consequently, keeping pulse oximetry readings in this range during an anesthetic should not be responsible for causing a progression of ROP in susceptible patients.

Neurodevelopmental Effects of Anesthetic Agents

There has been recent concern about the potential deleterious impact of anesthetic drugs on the developing brain. A variety of studies have shown that prolonged exposure of animal models to anesthetic agents can lead to neurodegenerative changes in the developing brain of neonatal rats.[154] However, these exposures to volatile agents and ketamine were for prolonged periods, the equivalent of several weeks of continuous exposure in the human. Nonetheless, this is an area of great concern for anesthesiologists.[155] Animal experiments have demonstrated neurocognitive changes in animals exposed to NMDA receptor antagonists such as ketamine, volatile agents such as isoflurane, as well as other agents including midazolam. The collective data that are currently available in literature do not support the withdrawal of these drugs from the practice of neonatal anesthesia. There has been a general recommendation to delay nonurgent surgery in children under 3 years of age made by the FDA/IARS public/private partnership, SmartTots[156]; however, neonatal surgical problems cannot usually be delayed safely for years.

The neurotoxicity data seem to be reproducible in rodents but not in other species. Future prospective trials with prospective neurocognitive testing of infants exposed to anesthesia are needed. There currently exists no conclusive evidence to demonstrate the deleterious effect of inhaled or intravenous anesthetics on neurocognitive function in neonates and infants. Results from a prospective randomized general anesthesia and spinal study (GAS) has demonstrated no significant differences in neurocognitive outcomes in infants undergoing short procedures such as hernia repair.[157] Several retrospective studies including data about children from a particular county in Minnesota has some data to lead to believe that there may be an association with the development of learning disability especially when exposed to multiple anesthetics before 2 years of age.[158] Although the data generated a lot of interest, it is important to understand that we need more concrete data and prospective studies to demonstrate that there are indeed clinically apparent neurocognitive changes associated with exposure to anesthesia in neonates and infants. A meta-analysis published regarding neurodevelopmental outcomes after noncardiac neonatal surgery revealed a number of risk factors for worse neurodevelopmental outcomes and the primary surgical lesion was among the most important factors.[159] Certainly, anesthesic exposure alone cannot account for the wide range of neurodevelopmental outcomes observed in neonates with major congenital anomalies.

Surgical Procedures in Neonates

Surgical procedures in neonates are functionally divided into two periods: those performed in the first week and those performed in the first month. There has been a strong trend in recent years to put an emphasis of presurgical stabilization before taking the newborn to the operating room. This stabilization has reduced the emergency nature of newborn surgeries. Many procedures that used to be done on an emergency basis, even in the middle of the night, such as repair of CDH or omphalocele, are now done days later, after initial therapy has been instituted. Exceptions to this include gastroschisis, which is usually corrected within 12 to 24 hours, airway lesions such as webs that are causing significant airway obstruction, and acute subdural/epidural hematomas from traumatic delivery. In most cases, however, a period of 1 to 3 days can be allowed for stabilization of the newborn or transport to an appropriate pediatric center for treatment. There is more to neonatal emergency surgery than just the immediate anesthetic and surgical procedures. Many of these infants require the support services of specialized nursing units, pediatric radiologists, pediatric intensive care physicians, specialized laboratory facilities, and they must have their complete care be the main consideration of where their surgery should be done. Many procedures are now performed using minimally invasive techniques which decreases postoperative morbidity and pain and facilitates early extubation.

Surgical Procedures in the First Week of Life

The most frequent major surgical procedures performed in the first week of life are for CDH, omphalocele and gastroschisis, tracheoesophageal fistula (TEF), intestinal obstruction, and myelomeningocele. Some of these conditions, such as CDH, omphalocele, gastroschisis, and myelomeningocele, are obvious at birth. It may take hours or days for a TEF or intestinal obstruction to manifest. Because of the lack of expertise many hospitals have in the care of these patients, the transfer of these neonates to hospitals with greater expertise is often prudent after initial stabilization of the patient. Most hospitals that have expertise in these patients have a transport team that is well qualified to help with stabilization and transport. Those centers that do not have transport teams often have extensive protocols and procedures to work with the sending institution to help ensure the safe transfer of the patient.

Two confounding factors in neonatal surgery are prematurity and associated congenital anomalies. The presence of one congenital anomaly increases the likelihood of another one. In conditions such as TEF, the mortality rate from an associated congenital heart defect is higher than that from the surgical correction of the TEF. Prematurity, particularly when associated with RDS, may adversely affect surgical outcome. The use of surfactant in the treatment of the RDS has greatly increased the number of survivors and has decreased the complexity of the issues of the infant with a combination of TEF and RDS. A neonatologist should be consulted in the case of any neonate with a congenital defect who is considered for surgery. The most serious associated congenital lesion is that of the cardiovascular system. More than 10% of infants with CDH have a cardiac anomaly,[160] with a higher incidence in newborns with associated syndromes, and approximately 15% to 25% of infants with TEF have an associated congenital cardiac anomaly.[161]

Congenital Diaphragmatic Hernia

CDH occurs with an incidence of approximately 1 in 4,000 live births. Traditionally, the mortality rate from CDH was in the range of 40% to 50%. The new strategy of permissive hypercapnia and delayed surgical repair has resulted in survival rates of more than 75% in some centers.[162] However, the morbidity remains high in survivors. A brief discussion of the embryologic characteristics of CDH will help the clinician understand the potentially enormous postoperative problems that may be encountered.

Embryology

Early in fetal development, the pleuroperitoneal cavity is a single compartment. The gut is herniated or extruded to the extraembryonic coelom during the ninth to tenth weeks of fetal life. During this period, the diaphragm develops to separate the thoracic and abdominal cavities (Fig. 42-14). The development of the

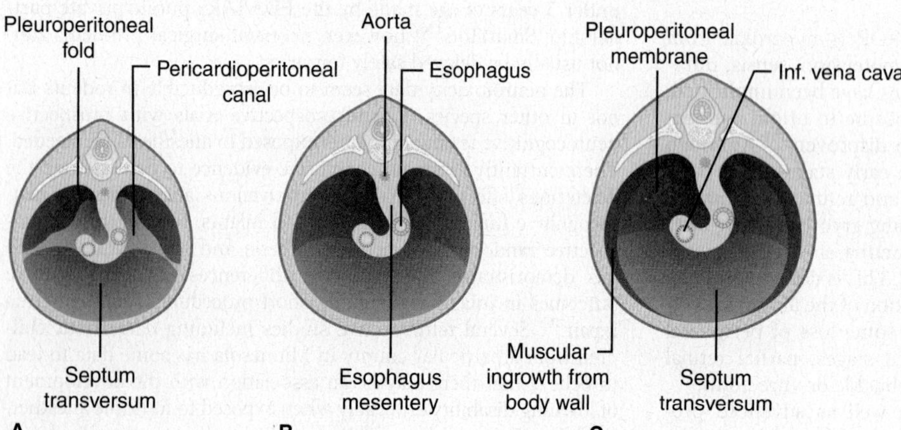

Figure 42-14 Schematic drawings illustrating the development of the diaphragm. **A:** The pleuroperitoneal folds appear at the beginning of the sixth week. **B:** The pleuroperitoneal folds have fused with the septum transversum and the mesentery of the esophagus in the seventh week, thus separating the thoracic cavity from the abdominal cavity. **C:** In a transverse section at the fourth month of development, an additional rim derived from the body wall forms the most peripheral part of the diaphragm. (Adapted with permission from Langman J. Body cavities and serous membranes. In: Sadler TW, ed. *Langman's Medical Embryology*. 5th ed. Williams & Wilkins; 1985:147.)

diaphragm is usually completed by the seventh fetal week. In the ninth to tenth weeks, the developing gut returns to the peritoneal cavity. If there is delay or incomplete closure of the diaphragm, or if the gut returns early and prevents normal closure of the diaphragm, a diaphragmatic hernia will develop, producing varying degrees of herniation of the abdominal contents into the chest. The left side of the diaphragm closes later than the right side, which results in the higher incidence of left-sided diaphragmatic hernias (foramen of Bochdalek). Approximately, 90% of hernias detected in the first week of life are on the left side.

Clinical Presentation

The clinical presentation and the outcome from a diaphragmatic hernia are varied. The bowel contents may compress the lung buds and prevent development, leading to bilateral hypoplastic lungs with very little chance for survival. In most instances, however, a moderately small diaphragmatic hernia may develop later in fetal life, so the lung is normal but compressed by the abdominal viscera. At the mild end of the scale, the infant might have a relatively normal pulmonary vascular bed with varying degrees of persistent pulmonary hypertension that may rapidly revert to normal. In more severe defects, significant pulmonary hypoplasia and abnormal pulmonary vasculature lead to greater mortality, largely a result of ongoing pulmonary hypertension.

After closure of the pleuroperitoneal membrane, muscular development of the diaphragm occurs. Incomplete muscularization of the diaphragm results in the development of a hernia sac because of intra-abdominal pressure. The condition is known as eventration of the diaphragm, and the diaphragm may extend well up into the thoracic cavity. The other possibility is that the innervation of the diaphragm is incomplete and the muscle is atonic. Eventration of the diaphragm is usually not symptomatic in the first week of life.

Antenatal Diagnosis

The diagnosis of CDH can be made prenatally by fetal ultrasonography or fetal magnetic resonance imaging. Antenatal diagnosis has led to the identification of a "hidden mortality" in CDH, fetuses who did not survive gestation and neonates who died before diagnosis. Various factors have been proposed to identify predictability of survival, including early gestation diagnosis, severe mediastinal shift, polyhydramnios, a small lung-to-thorax transverse area ratio, and the herniation of liver or stomach. New techniques in fetal surgery, such as temporary endoscopic fetal tracheal occlusion, may prove beneficial to fetuses with CDH who are identified to be at risk for not surviving to term.[163] The other obvious advantage of prenatal diagnosis is that plans can be made for maternal or neonatal transport to a center with advanced neonatal critical care with availability of ECMO. Early repair, on ECMO, or delayed repair with treatment of pulmonary hypertension on ECMO prior to repair remains an area of controversy, with literature in support of both approaches.[164,165] However, it is clear that introduction of ECMO has improved survival compared to historical data.[166]

Clinical Presentation

The occurrence of symptoms depends on the degree of herniation and interference with pulmonary function. At times, the degree of interference is so great that the neonate's clinical condition begins to deteriorate immediately and, in other situations, it may be several hours before the infant's condition is fully appreciated. In the severely affected newborn, the initial clinical findings are usually classic and readily discerned. The infant has a scaphoid abdomen secondary to the absence of intra-abdominal contents, which have herniated into the chest. Breath sounds on the affected side are reduced or absent. The diagnosis can be confirmed with a radiograph (Fig. 42-15). Immediate supportive care entails tracheal intubation and control of the airway along with decompression of the stomach. Excessive airway pressure carries a high risk for pneumothorax before and after the repair.

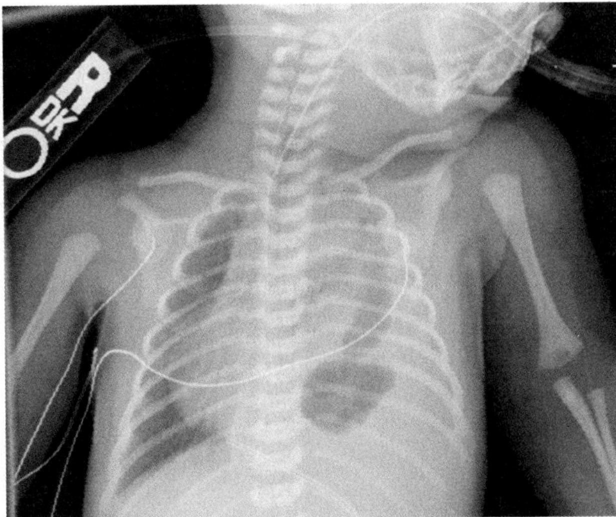

Figure 42-15 Infant with left-sided congenital diaphragmatic hernia. Note the loop of bowel gas in left hemithorax.

Preoperative Care

CDH was traditionally treated as a surgical emergency. The infants were taken immediately to surgery for decompression and repair. The thought was that removing the abdominal viscera from the thorax would allow for re-expansion of the atelectatic lung and improved oxygenation. However, as the pathophysiology of CDH was more clearly defined—pulmonary hypoplasia associated with a hyperreactive and hypoplastic pulmonary vasculature—a strategy of preoperative stabilization with delayed surgical repair was adopted.

The stabilization of an infant with CDH may require multiple treatment modalities. The use of aggressive ventilation strategies to induce respiratory alkalosis has been abandoned secondary to the high incidence of iatrogenic lung injury. Conventional ventilation with permissive hypercapnia is now favored. The goal is to maintain preductal arterial saturation above 85% using peak inspiratory pressures below 25 cm H_2O and allowing the $PaCO_2$ to rise to 45 to 55 mmHg.[162] High-frequency oscillatory ventilation, in addition to nitric oxide, has been used in place of conventional ventilation in an attempt to reduce barotrauma and has been demonstrated to be beneficial.[167] Neonates born with CDH may also have a component of surfactant deficiency, and studies have shown improvement in oxygenation in those infants given surfactant prophylactically. These have been well demonstrated in animal experiments when compared with tracheal ligation.[168]

The use of ECMO in infants with CDH was initiated in the mid-1980s. Despite extensive literature on the subject, there remains an ongoing debate as to whether ECMO improves survival in neonates with CDH. The Congenital Diaphragmatic Hernia Study Group analyzed data from the multicenter CDH Registry and determined that ECMO improves the survival rate in CDH neonates with a predicted high risk of mortality (≥80%) based on birth weight and 5-minute Apgar score. Right-sided CDH is associated with a higher risk of mortality than a left-sided defect, despite the use of ECMO.[169] Repair of a right-sided CDH can be seen in Figure 42-16.

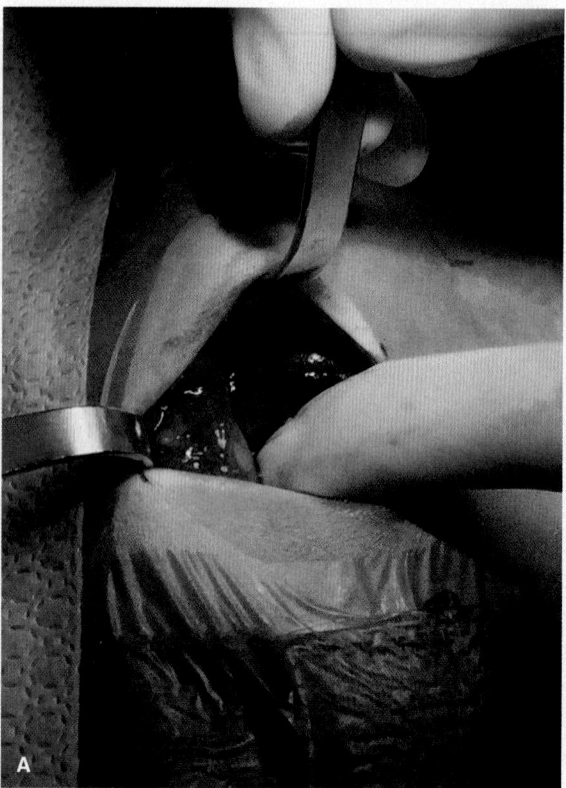

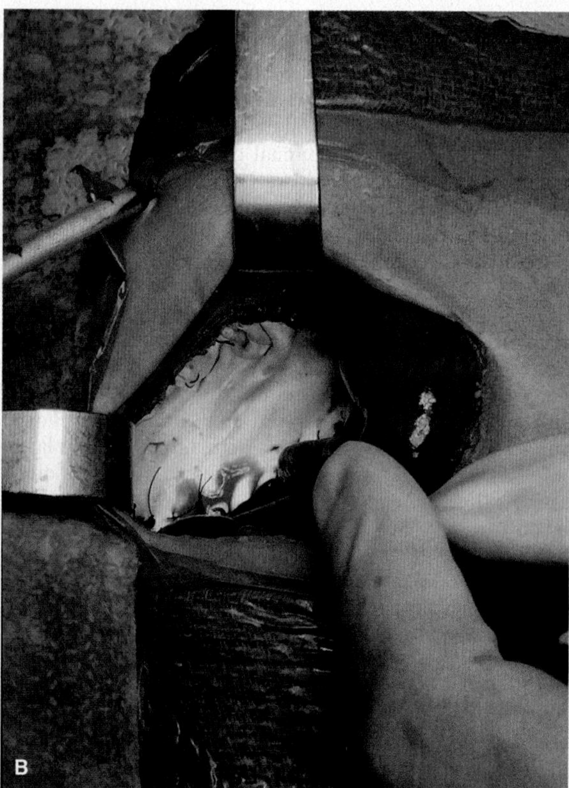

Figure 42-16 Another infant with congenital diaphragmatic hernia. In this patient, the defect is in the right diaphragm. **A:** The liver herniated into the right chest cavity. **B:** The complete repair with Gore-Tex graft material and the liver appropriately located in the abdominal cavity. (Photographs courtesy of Rashmi Kabre, MD.)

Perioperative Care

Because delayed surgical repair of CDH is now the norm, neonates with CDH frequently present to the operating room already intubated and on some form of ventilatory support. Despite a period of preoperative stabilization, some infants still have a component of reactive pulmonary hypertension. The goals of ventilatory management are to ensure adequate oxygenation and avoid barotrauma. Any sudden deterioration in oxygen saturation with or without associated hypotension should raise suspicion of pneumothorax. It is important to avoid hypothermia because this increases the oxygen requirement and could precipitate pulmonary hypertension. Blood loss and fluid shifts are usually not a problem, although maintenance of intravascular volume is essential to avoid acidosis, which could also precipitate pulmonary hypertension. Preoperative preparation may include multimodal treatment of pulmonary hypertension with nitric oxide, sildenafil (PDE-5 inhibitor), milrinone (PDE-3 inhibitor), epoprostenol or iloprost (PGI_2 inhibitor), bosentan (endothelin inhibitor), and imatinib (platelet-derived growth factor inhibitor) which have all been attempted with varying degrees of success.[170]

Anesthetic Technique

The anesthetic technique chosen depends on the size of the defect and the anticipated postoperative respiratory status. In those infants who will remain intubated after surgery, inhalation agents and opioids may be used as tolerated. In those infants with a small defect, who present to the operating room with little or no respiratory distress, it may be beneficial to avoid intraoperative opioids and provide regional or neuraxial analgesia in anticipation of extubation. The use of nitrous oxide should be avoided, particularly in those situations in which abdominal closure could be difficult. Muscle relaxation is often needed to facilitate abdominal closure.

Postoperative Care

Infants with CDH require intensive postoperative care. Recovery depends on the degree of pulmonary hypertension and pulmonary hypoplasia. It was previously believed that pulmonary hypoplasia was responsible for most deaths; however, it is now believed that potentially reversible pulmonary hypertension may be responsible for as much as 25% of reported deaths.

There is evidence to suggest that cardiac development is impaired in infants with CDH. Relative left ventricular hypoplasia with an attenuated muscle mass and cavity size have been described.

Omphalocele and Gastroschisis

Although omphalocele and gastroschisis sometimes appear similar and may be confused, they have entirely different origins and associated congenital anomalies.[171] During the fifth to tenth weeks of fetal life, the abdominal contents are extruded into the extraembryonic coelom, and the gut returns to the abdominal cavity at approximately the tenth week. Failure of part of or all the intestinal contents to return to the abdominal cavity results in an omphalocele that is covered with a membrane called the amnion (Fig. 42-17). The amnion protects the abdominal contents from infection and the loss of ECF. The umbilical cord is found at approximately the apex of the sac. Gastroschisis, in contrast, develops later in fetal life, after the intestinal contents have returned to the abdominal cavity. It results from interruption of

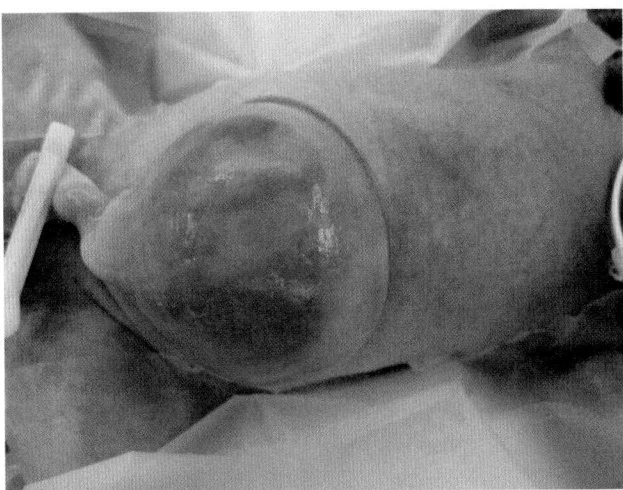

Figure 42-17 Omphalocele on day 1 of life. Note the abdominal contents covered in amnion and umbilical cord protruding from the apex of the sac. (Photograph courtesy of Matthew S. Clifton, MD, FACS, FAAP.)

the omphalomesenteric artery, which results in ischemia and atrophy of the various layers of the abdominal wall at the base of the umbilical cord. The gut then herniates through this tissue defect. The degree of herniation may be slight, or major amounts of the abdominal viscera may be found outside the peritoneal cavity. The umbilical cord is found to one side of the intestinal contents (Fig. 42-18).

The intestines and viscera are not covered by any membrane and therefore are highly susceptible to infection and loss of ECF. There is a very high incidence of associated congenital anomalies with omphalocele, but much lower with gastroschisis.[172] Neurodevelopmental outcomes are generally worse in omphalocele than with gastroschisis.[159] The Beckwith–Wiedemann syndrome consists of mental retardation, hypoglycemia, congenital heart disease, a large tongue, and an omphalocele. Congenital heart lesions are found in approximately 20% of infants with omphalocele. Other associated congenital defects are found with gastroschisis and omphalocele; most involve the gastrointestinal tract and consist primarily of intestinal atresia, stenosis, or malrotation. Because of the uncovered gut irritating the uterine lining, premature delivery is more common in gastroschisis patients.

Antenatal Diagnosis

The overall incidence of these defects is about 1:5,000 live births. Screening for abdominal wall defects is accomplished through the use of maternal serum α-fetoprotein (AFP). AFP is a normal protein present in fetal tissues during fetal development. Closure of the abdominal wall and the neural tube (see "Myelomeningocele") prevents release of large quantities of this protein into the amniotic fluid. High levels of AFP in the amniotic fluid can cross the placenta and be detected in maternal blood. Thus, abnormal levels of maternal serum AFP in the mother raise concerns over the possibility of either an abdominal wall defect or a neural tube defect in the fetus, as do high levels of AFP in fluid obtained during amniocentesis. Levels tend to be higher when the defect is gastroschisis instead of omphalocele. The primary method of definitive fetal diagnosis of gastroschisis and omphalocele is ultrasonography. Eighty-eight percent of patients with gastroschisis and 69% with omphalocele were diagnosed prenatally with ultrasound.[173] An advantage of ultrasound is the ability to diagnose other complicating abnormalities, such as cardiac defects.

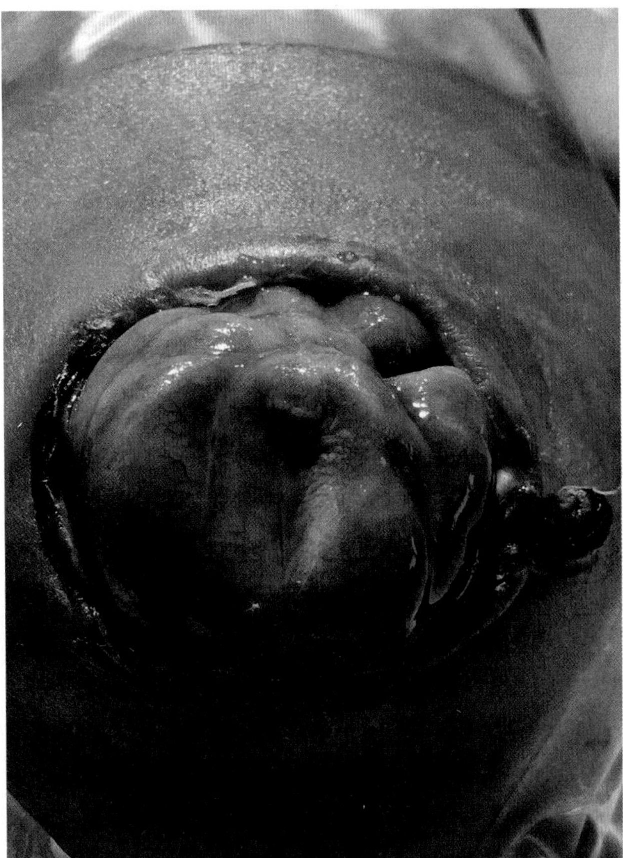

Figure 42-18 Gastroschisis. Note the umbilical cord is found to the side of the abdominal contents which are not covered in a sac. (Photograph courtesy of Linda Zekas, MSN, APN.)

Preoperative Care

Most neonates with gastroschisis or omphalocele diagnosed prenatally are delivered by cesarean section. The advantages of this are the ability to prevent trauma to the exposed bowel and to allow better coordination of the various medical specialties needed for immediate surgical management of the defect. Priorities in the delivery room care unique to an infant with gastroschisis are the need to protect the exposed bowel and minimize fluid and temperature loss. An effective way to achieve these goals involves placing the defect and lower body in a sterile, clear plastic bag to protect the defect and minimize heat and fluid loss. The bag can be filled with warm saline and a drawstring can be used to tighten the bag against the infant's body.

Preoperative stabilization of the neonate with an abdominal wall defect includes management of respiratory insufficiency, establishment of adequate intravenous access, and an assessment for associated congenital anomalies. It is expected that a significantly higher incidence of congenital anomalies will be found in omphalocele patients. Respiratory failure at birth in infants with omphalocele is a significant predictor of mortality. Lung hypoplasia and abnormal thoracic development may be significant in infants with large omphaloceles. A difficult airway can be present in the patient with Beckwith–Wiedemann syndrome because of the large tongue.

Surgery is not urgent in the neonate with an omphalocele and can be delayed for several days until the infant is assessed and stabilized. In those infants with severe respiratory distress or congenital heart disease who are too unstable for surgery, nonsurgical treatment with topical antiseptics and delayed closure is an option.[174] Although there has been some interest in nonoperative, bedside-staged closure of gastroschisis defects, primary operative closure continues to be the most common approach.[175]

Perioperative Care

The two major perioperative concerns are fluid loss and ventilation. The fluid volume management of the infant often entails administration of large amounts of full-strength, balanced salt solution. The adequacy of the peripheral circulation and urine output is an indicator of the adequacy of the intravascular volume resuscitation. Both conditions may present an intraoperative challenge to the anesthesiologist because with an omphalocele, after the amniotic membrane is removed, large volumes of fluid may transude or exude from the exposed abdominal viscera. The fluid that is lost is ECF, which should be replaced with a balanced salt solution even in neonates. An arterial line is often used for blood pressure monitoring and frequent blood gas monitoring to assess acid–base status.

If the defect in the abdominal wall is small, a primary repair of the deficit can be accomplished. However, with a large defect, it may be difficult to return the abdominal viscera to the peritoneal cavity because the muscle and peritoneum are underdeveloped. Because of concern for the increase in the volume of gas in the intestine, nitrous oxide should not be used. Muscle relaxation is necessary to allow closure of the abdomen. With moderate-sized abdominal wall defects, it may not be possible to close the peritoneum, but there may be sufficient skin to close the defect. With large defects, the peritoneal cavity may be too small to contain the viscera, and attempted closure can impair circulation to the bowel, kidneys, and lower extremities, as well as compromise respiration. A pulse oximeter probe on the foot can be helpful in monitoring circulation to the lower extremities during abdominal wall closure.

Attempts have been made to find objective criteria by which to determine whether the infant will tolerate primary closure of the defect, and to avoid or minimize the circulatory and ventilatory problems. One method has been to measure intragastric pressure in infants who undergo primary closure. Intragastric pressure is measured by placing a nasogastric tube in the stomach and using a column of saline to measure the pressure.[176] Studies have used the criteria that if the intragastric pressure was less than 20 mmHg, primary closure can proceed. Above 20 mmHg pressures during closure, delayed closure and placement of a Dacron silo were used. With this approach, primary closure has been successful when used, with faster return to full feeds and shorter hospital length of stay compared with patients treated by delayed closure. Complications have been less with primary closure using this approach. Another method to predict successful closure of abdominal wall defects is to use central venous pressure, an increase with closure of the fascia of greater than 4 mmHg is predictive of unsuccessful primary closure.[177]

If primary closure is impossible, a silo (Fig. 42-19) is incorporated into the abdominal wall to contain and cover the abdominal viscera. The repair is then staged from this point onward. Every 2 or 3 days, the size of the silo is reduced, in much the same fashion that a tube of toothpaste is squeezed. The infant may feel some degree of discomfort as the peritoneum and skin are stretched. Institutions vary in how they accomplish the delay closure, with some surgeons bringing the patient to the operating room for each stage and others doing this at bedside, often with the assistance of small doses of ketamine or other analgesics. Some of these patients remain on mechanical ventilation during this period, and others are extubated. In either case, both blood pressure and oxygen saturation should be closely monitored during and immediately after

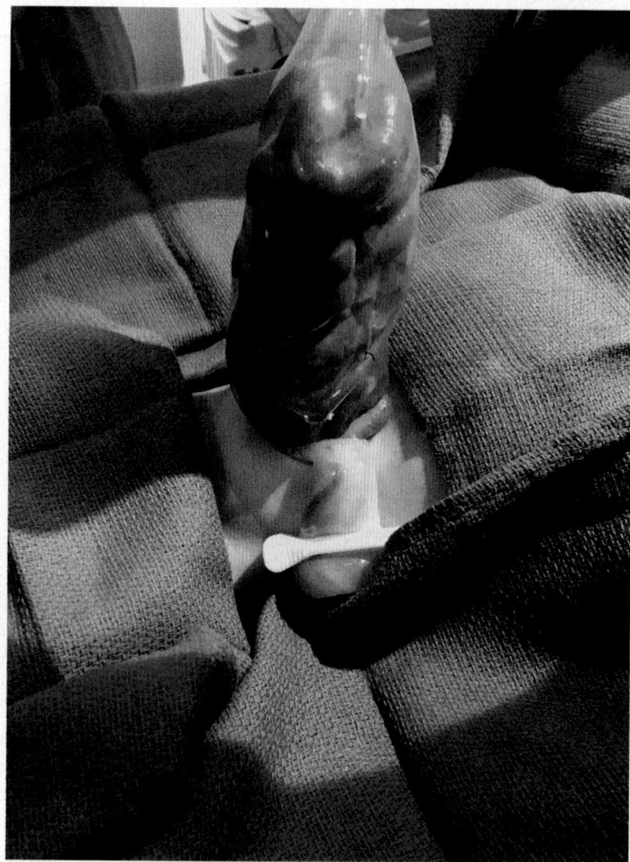

Figure 42-19 Silo placement on neonate with gastroschisis. The abdominal contents are now within a large silo, suspended above the neonate, with the umbilical cord observed protruding from one side of the defect. (Photograph courtesy of Linda Zekas, MSN, APN.)

each stage of closure to ensure that the increase in abdominal and intrathoracic pressure does not significantly impede ventilation, oxygenation, and venous return. In some cases, further reduction must be delayed until there is more abdominal growth. This situation requires clinical judgment. After several stages of silo reduction, the final operation is complete closure of the abdominal wall defect under full anesthesia with complete muscle relaxation.

Postoperative Care

The postoperative care of infants with omphalocele or gastroschisis is critical. Some need tracheal intubation and assisted ventilation of the lungs for days to weeks. The ventilatory status of the patient is especially critical in omphalocele patients because up to half of these patients are born with pulmonary hypoplasia, making the balance of increased abdominal pressures and adequate ventilation and oxygenation especially challenging. Additional complications include postoperative hypertension and edema of the extremities. The increased abdominal pressure can reduce the circulation to the kidneys, which results in a release of renin. Renin activates the renin–angiotensin–aldosterone system, which is believed to cause the hypertension.

Tracheoesophageal Fistula

The treatment of esophageal atresia and TEF can be both challenging and satisfying for the anesthesiologist (NICV 42-5). Death in the perioperative period typically results from prematurity or from an associated congenital heart defect. TEF occurs

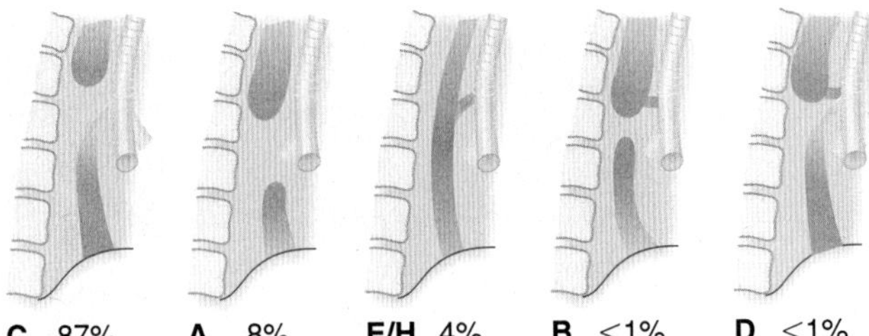

Figure 42-20 Diagrams of the five most commonly encountered forms of esophageal atresia and tracheoesophageal fistula, shown in order of frequency. (Adapted from Herbst JJ. Gastrointestinal tract. In: Behrman RE, Kleigman RM, Nelson WE, et al., eds. *Nelson's Textbook of Pediatrics*. 14th ed. WB Saunders; 1992:942. Copyright © 1992 Elsevier. With permission.)

in approximately 1 in 3,000 live births. Approximately 85% consist of a fistula from the distal trachea to the esophagus and a blind proximal esophageal pouch. In 10% of cases, there is a blind proximal esophageal pouch with no TEF (Fig. 42-20). The embryologic defect results from imperfect division of the foregut into the anteriorly positioned larynx and trachea and the posteriorly positioned esophagus; the division should occur between the fourth and fifth weeks of intrauterine life. Fifty percent of affected infants have associated congenital anomalies, of which approximately 15% to 25% involve the cardiovascular system.

Clinical Presentation

Atresia of the esophagus leads to inability of the fetus to swallow amniotic fluid and the subsequent development of polyhydramnios (NICV 42-6). Ultrasound may well raise the possibility of a congenital anomaly. For that reason, if polyhydramnios is present, attempts should be made to pass a nasogastric tube shortly after delivery. Passing a nasogastric tube is not routine in the delivery room; therefore, the diagnosis may not become apparent until the infant is fed. Cyanosis and choking with oral feedings should raise suspicion.

There are two major complications of esophageal atresia with a distal tracheal fistula: aspiration pneumonia and dehydration. The presence of a distal TEF increases the likelihood of reflux of gastric juice up the esophagus and into the pulmonary system. Dehydration results from the fact that the proximal esophagus does not communicate with the stomach. Therefore, preoperative preparation of these infants is aimed at evaluation and treatment of the pulmonary system, as well as at ensuring adequate hydration and electrolyte balance. Rarely, the degree of reflux and pneumonia is so great that a gastrostomy must be performed to protect the pulmonary system, and a period of several days is needed to improve the general condition of the infant. However, if the infant is in good condition, primary repair can be performed at 24 to 48 hours. This consists of ligation of the fistula and a primary repair with approximation of the two ends of the esophagus.

Anesthetic Considerations

The repair of TEF can be done in the conventional method or by using video-assisted thoracoscopic surgery (VATS) method. Both methods and the anesthetic implications for each technique will be described here. The presence of a gastrostomy reduces the potential for reflux of gastric juice during the surgical procedure. If a gastrostomy is present, the gastrostomy tube should be open to air and left at the head of the table under the anesthesiologist's observation to avoid kinking and obstruction.

Conventional Open TEF Closure. There are three approaches to tracheal intubation after induction of anesthesia. One is to use an inhalation induction, followed by topical spray of lidocaine and intubation while the infant is breathing spontaneously. Another technique is to use an intravenous or inhalation induction and intubate the trachea after muscle paralysis. This technique may lead to distention of the fistula and stomach with excessive positive-pressure ventilation. When controlled ventilation of the lungs is used, attempts must be made to minimize the distention of the stomach and the potential for reflux. If a gastrostomy tube is in place, the point is moot. A third technique is to intubate the neonates awake with mild sedation. This technique can protect the airway while reducing the chances of aspiration. Alternatively, because the fistula is usually located just above the carina on the posterior wall of the membranous trachea, the endotracheal tube can be placed just distal to the TEF. To do this, the endotracheal tube is inserted until it enters a main-stem bronchus, judged by unilateral expansion of the chest and unilateral breath sounds. The endotracheal tube is then slowly withdrawn until bilateral chest movement and breath sounds are confirmed.

The endotracheal tube might inadvertently enter the fistula when the infant is turned or during surgical manipulation. Intubation of the fistula should be suspected if there is increased difficulty in ventilation of the lungs, as well as decreased oxygen saturation and end-tidal CO_2. Because these findings may also be present when the lung is packed away to perform the surgery and because there are other explanations for these findings, intubation of the fistula should always be included in the differential diagnosis. If, at any time, ventilation is difficult and desaturation is occurring, the surgeon must stop the procedure while the situation is clarified. The surgeon will be able to palpate the tip of the tube in the fistula if this is the problem.

The localization and isolation of H-type fistulas can be difficult. In this situation, direct laryngoscopy and bronchoscopy is performed by the surgeon, the fistula is identified, and a guidewire is fed through the fistula tract into the esophagus. The infant is then intubated, with care taken not to dislodge the guidewire. Once intubated, esophagoscopy is performed, the guidewire is visualized and brought out through the mouth. In this way, the surgeon can use fluoroscopy to determine the level of the fistula and decide whether a cervical or thoracic approach is necessary. During surgery, the anesthesiologist can apply traction to the wire loop to facilitate the localization of the fistula by the surgeon.

Endoscopic TEF Repair. The use of endoscopic methods for repair of TEF is popular in pediatric surgery.[178] The infant should be kept spontaneously breathing until the fistula is ligated. Maintenance of spontaneous ventilation can be challenging considering that these infants may not tolerate the use of potent inhalation agents while spontaneous ventilation is established. The anesthetic management is challenging, particularly due to airway management, hypercapnia, and hypothermia.[179]

Postoperative Care

Although there have been great advances in the treatment of TEF and esophageal atresia, postoperative care can be complicated by associated congenital heart disease, RDS, and a need for continued postoperative ventilation. The compression of the lung for several hours, along with pre-existing aspiration pneumonia in some of these infants, suggest the need, in the more difficult cases, for a short period of postoperative ventilation, or at least intubation with PEEP, as the most conservative technique for postoperative airway management. Some infants are in excellent condition at the time of surgery with no complicating factors and, therefore, could be considered for extubation immediately at the end of surgery or shortly thereafter. If extubation of the trachea is planned for the end of surgery, the anesthetic technique must be tailored accordingly. Neuraxial anesthesia as part of the technique is useful in these situations, reducing the concentration of maintenance volatile anesthetics, the amount of muscle relaxants, and the need for intraoperative narcotics. These catheters may remain in place after the procedure to allow for postoperative pain control with local anesthetic by continuous infusion or intermittent bolus. Another option is to place a unilateral, ultrasound-guided paravertebral block which can again provide analgesia for the hemithorax that is the operative site.[180]

A high percentage of infants with esophageal atresia have residual defects of the tracheobronchial tree and esophagus for many years. These defects include tracheomalacia, gastroesophageal reflux, esophageal stricture, and recurrent fistulas.

Intestinal Obstruction

A useful way of classifying gastrointestinal obstruction is to group lesions proximal and distal to the pylorus. Obstruction of the upper gastrointestinal tract is manifested by vomiting, especially after feeds, whereas obstruction of the lower gastrointestinal tract may present with abdominal distention, little or no stool passed, hematochezia, signs of pain, and vomiting.

Upper Gastrointestinal Tract Obstruction

The most common cause of upper gastrointestinal obstruction in the newborn is pyloric stenosis, but pyloric stenosis does not usually present in the first week of life (NICV 42-7). Other rare causes of obstruction, such as congenital webs, may occur. If there has been persistent vomiting, this usually means that a deficit of fluids or electrolytes will develop in the infant. Persistent vomiting results in the greatest deficit of sodium. Another major concern in the infant with upper gastrointestinal tract obstruction is aspiration of gastric contents.

The anesthetic management of these patients is directed toward ensuring adequate relaxation for abdominal exploration, repair of the congenital defect, and closure of the abdomen. Nitrous oxide can be used in high intestinal obstruction because there is essentially no gas in the upper gastrointestinal tract. The next concern is whether the infant's trachea should be extubated at the end of surgery. If the infant is robust, extubation of the trachea at the end of surgery can be anticipated. The preferred technique is for general anesthesia combined with neuraxial anesthesia. This allows light levels of volatile agent and minimal muscle relaxant use, and results in early extubation. Opioids may be administered, although the impact on the ability to ventilate at the end of the procedure should be considered. If the infant is moderately debilitated or if the surgical incision is extensive, a period of postoperative ventilation may well be indicated, particularly if moderate doses of opioids have been used.

Lower Gastrointestinal Tract Obstruction

Intestinal obstruction in the newborn can result from a variety of lesions. These include imperforate anus, duodenal atresia, jejunoileal atresia (Fig. 42-21), intussusception, malrotation, volvulus, choledochal cyst, or meconium ileus. Although these are all different in etiology, their presentation is similar. The problems associated with lower gastrointestinal tract obstruction usually develop within 1 to 7 days after birth. It may take this long for the lesion to become evident because it is low in the gastrointestinal tract. An imperforate anus should be recognizable shortly after birth. However, once intestinal obstruction is diagnosed in the newborn, it becomes a surgical emergency as these patients may deteriorate rapidly. Some of these infants may have vomiting secondary to the obstruction, which poses a problem for fluid and electrolyte management. An enormous amount of fluid can be sequestered within the intestinal tract. This fluid is essentially ECF and has high sodium content. Therefore, these infants should be prepared expeditiously for surgery and have a serum sodium level of at least 130 mEq/L as well as a urine output of 1 to 2 mL/kg/hr. In addition to fluid and electrolyte disturbances, delayed diagnosis or treatment of these patients can result in increased abdominal pressure, leading to respiratory failure from pressure on the diaphragm and aspiration pneumonitis, as well as sepsis. Finally, some of these conditions are associated with other congenital anomalies that complicate preanesthetic evaluation and anesthetic management.[181] Duodenal atresia, for instance, can be associated with trisomy 21, cystic fibrosis, imperforate anus, or renal abnormalities.

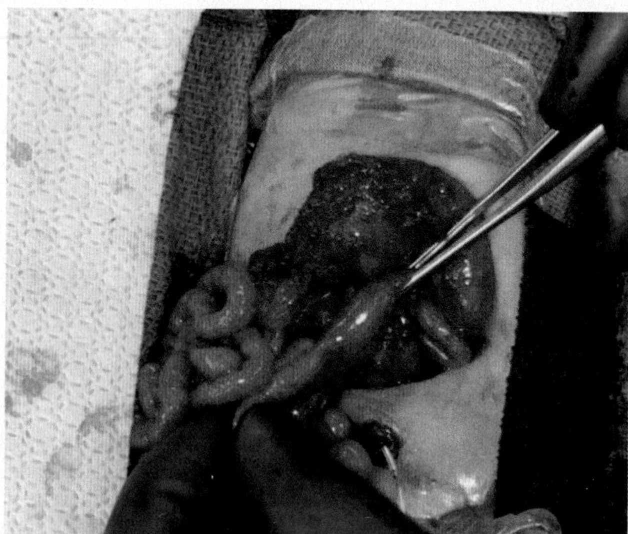

Figure 42-21 Jejunal atresia. (Photograph courtesy of Kurt Heiss, MD.)

The preanesthetic evaluation and perioperative management is similar for all these lesions. Preanesthetic evaluation is focused on the stabilization of fluid and electrolyte status, ensuring adequate oxygenation and ventilation, hemodynamic support if the patient is septic, and identification of complicating issues such as other congenital abnormalities.

In the operating room, the need for invasive arterial and central venous monitoring is determined by the status of the patient and the urgency of the procedure. The primary anesthetic considerations are the same as those in the preoperative period, including ongoing fluid and electrolyte resuscitation. Because these cases are usually emergent and there may be associated vomiting and abdominal distention, either an awake intubation or rapid-sequence induction and intubation is indicated. Although awake intubation may be the best approach if the patient has a probable difficult airway or has hemodynamic decompensation, a rapid-sequence induction and intubation after preoxygenation is the approach normally taken. Any induction agent can be used if judicious doses are chosen, but ketamine or etomidate are often chosen because of a concern about cardiovascular instability.

Anesthetic agents for maintenance during these cases are chosen based on the patient's status and the likely surgical course. Nitrous oxide should not be used in any infant who has gaseous distention of the intestine, which is easily determined from the preoperative radiograph. Providing adequate muscle relaxation for surgery can be accomplished with various anesthetic techniques such as volatile anesthesia, muscle relaxants, and caudal or epidural block.[182] Remifentanil is sometimes used in newborns and infants because of its titratability and short duration of action, potentially increasing the options for extubation at the end of the case for some patients.[183]

The criteria for tracheal extubation at the end of surgery are the same as those described for upper gastrointestinal tract obstruction. When in doubt, it is prudent to leave the tracheal tube in place and provide a period of postoperative ventilation during which the patient's status can be re-evaluated before deciding that extubation is safe.

Myelomeningocele

Clinical Presentation

Myelomeningocele is the most common congenital primary neural tube defect. Despite the known ability of folic acid supplementation during pregnancy to largely prevent this defect, the lesion still occurs in approximately 0.5 to 1 of every 1,000 live births.[184] It results from failure of neural tube closure during the fourth week of gestation. Neural tube defects can be identified on prenatal ultrasound. Elevated maternal serum AFP detects 50% to 90% of open neural tube defects but has a false-positive rate of 5%. Amniotic fluid AFP is more reliable and typically used for confirmation after elevated serum levels.

By definition, the lesion involves both the meninges and neural components, as compared with a meningocele, which does not contain neural elements. The infant is born with a cystic mass on the back comprising a neural placode, arachnoid, dura, nerve tissue and roots, and cerebrospinal fluid. The lesion most commonly occurs in the lumbosacral or sacral region, although it can extend to the thoracic region. The bony canal is also malformed, leading to multiple orthopedic problems as the child matures. Urologic complications correlate with the level of the spinal lesion.

Newborns born with myelomeningocele have an associated anomaly of the brainstem known as the Arnold–Chiari II (Chiari II) malformation. The Chiari II malformation is characterized by caudal displacement of the cerebellar vermis through the foramen magnum, caudal displacement of the medulla oblongata and the cervical spine, kinking of the medulla, and obliteration of the cisterna magna.[185] The cause of Chiari II malformation rests in the small size of the skull housing the posterior fossa, forcing CNS contents out during development. Hydrocephalus requiring shunting develops in approximately 80% to 90% of infants with myelomeningocele. In contrast, only 20% of patients have symptoms of brainstem dysfunction as a result of the Chiari II malformation, but the mortality rate among those symptomatic patients is high. Complications of brainstem dysfunction include stridor, apnea and bradycardia, aspiration pneumonia, sleep-disordered breathing patterns, vocal cord paralysis, lack of coordination, and spasticity. If the symptoms are not improved by shunting, posterior fossa decompression is necessary.[186]

The infant with a myelomeningocele is usually operated on within the first 24 to 48 hours of life, thus reducing the risk for development of ventriculitis or progressive neurologic deficits. Most centers close the defect and place a shunt at the same time. However, some centers may delay placement of a shunt until the infant develops symptoms of hydrocephalus. There is ongoing work to determine the benefits of intrauterine repair of myelomeningocele, hopefully with the benefits of decreased development of a Chiari II malformation, decreased hydrocephalus, and increased lower limb function. As these studies continue, the role of intrauterine repair will become clearer.[187]

Preoperative Care

The preoperative stabilization period focuses on the prevention of infection, maintenance of ECF volume, avoidance of hypothermia, and assessment for other congenital anomalies. The exposed neural placode is susceptible to trauma, leakage, and infection. The infant is usually placed in the prone position, and the placode is covered with warm saline-soaked gauze to prevent desiccation. Because of the high risk of infection, antibiotic therapy is initiated in the preoperative period. Rupture of the cyst on the back can lead to ongoing cerebrospinal fluid leakage. This fluid is replaced with a full-strength, balanced salt solution. The infant is also assessed for any potentially life-threatening congenital anomalies.

Perioperative Care

The high prevalence of clinical latex allergy and latex sensitization in children with myelomeningocele has drawn much attention and led many individuals to believe that these patients have an impaired immune system that makes them more susceptible to latex allergy. The likely cause of the increased incidence of latex sensitization is repeated exposure to latex products through frequent hospitalizations and surgical procedures, as well as a program of daily bladder catheterization for those with neurogenic bladders.[188]

Positioning is critical in the infant with myelomeningocele. For induction of anesthesia, the infant may be placed supine with the defect resting in a "doughnut" to minimize trauma. Alternatively, the induction can be performed with the infant in the lateral position, although this makes intubation more challenging. The infant is turned prone for surgery. Rolls are positioned to ensure the abdomen and chest are free, avoiding pressure on the epidural venous plexus to minimize bleeding and allow adequate ventilation.

In most instances, the infant has an intravenous line placed before surgery and an intravenous induction is performed. Succinylcholine may be used to facilitate intubation without risking hyperkalemia.[189] Because increased intracranial pressure is rarely present before closure of the defect, inhalational induction is an alternative in the infant with difficult intravenous access. The anesthetic management of these newborns is rarely complicated unless there are other congenital anomalies that warrant special attention. There is no advantage of one technique over another because of the surgical lesion. Because these patients are usually extubated at the end of the case, a technique that allows this is usually chosen. Regional anesthesia has been reported as a safe adjunct or alternative to general anesthesia in the neonate with myelomeningocele.

Postoperative Care

These infants must be monitored closely in the postoperative period. Respiratory complications, including stridor, apnea and bradycardia, cyanosis, and respiratory arrest, may develop after surgery in these infants with known brainstem abnormalities and potential disorders of central respiratory control. In addition, infants who were not shunted during repair may show signs of hydrocephalus, including lethargy, vomiting, seizures, apnea and bradycardia, or cardiovascular instability. These infants need to return to the operating room for insertion of a shunt. Although most of these patients will eventually require a shunt, only about one-third of the patients receive one during the initial hospitalization.[190]

Hydrocephalus

Hydrocephalus in the first month of life may have several causes. It may occur after closure of a meningomyelocele because of the Chiari II malformation, it may be congenital in origin, or it may be related to intraventricular hemorrhage, especially in the very preterm newborn. The cranial sutures in the neonate are open, so intracranial pressure increases are blunted or minimized. However, infants with hydrocephalus eventually have an increase in head size and sometimes in intracranial pressure, resulting in lethargy, vomiting, and cardiorespiratory problems.

The anesthetic approach and the technique for tracheal intubation depend on the infant's condition. The major concern is protection of the airway and control of intracranial pressure. Awake tracheal intubation, crying, struggling, and straining can increase intracranial pressure. A rapid-sequence induction of anesthesia to control the airway and intracranial pressure is preferred. Volatile drugs, nitrous oxide, and opioids are all reasonable choices for maintenance of anesthesia, with no evidence that one technique is superior. Noninvasive intracranial pressure measurements in neurologically normal preterm infants have shown a decrease in intracranial pressure with all drugs, including ketamine, fentanyl, and isoflurane. The failure of volatile anesthetics and ketamine to increase intracranial pressure as in adults is attributed to the compliance of the neonate's open-sutured cranium. After surgery, the trachea of these infants may remain intubated if they were experiencing periods of apnea or bradycardia before surgery because of the intracranial abnormalities. If not, the trachea can be extubated as soon as the protective reflexes of the airway have recovered.

Surgical Procedures in the First Month of Life

Surgical procedures in the first month also are considered an emergency, or at least urgent surgery. The most frequent surgical procedures in the first month are exploratory laparotomy for NEC, inguinal hernia repair, correction of pyloric stenosis, patent ductus arteriosus (PDA) ligation, a shunt procedure for hydrocephalus, and placement of a central venous catheter.

Necrotizing Enterocolitis

NEC is a disease that primarily affects premature infants who have survived the first days of life, although it can be seen in full-term newborns. One of the theories about NEC is that earlier, more rapid feeding places infants at greater risk for development of NEC. The incidence of NEC among VLBW infants varies between 5% and 15%.[191] The exact pathophysiology of NEC has been the source of much study and some controversy, although it is likely multifactorial.[192] The condition is characterized by a cascade of pathologic events, beginning with an immature distal small and sometimes large intestine that has a decreased ability to absorb substrate, leading to stasis. The most common site is the ileocolic region, but it can be seen in other areas and can be discontinuous, giving a patchy appearance. Stasis encourages bacterial proliferation, which leads to local infection. The picture is complicated by further pooling of fluid. The ischemia and infection may lead to necrosis of the intestinal mucosa, followed by perforation. The perforation leads to gangrene of the gut wall, fluid loss, peritonitis, septicemia, and disseminated intravascular coagulation. The first signs that NEC may be abdominal distention, irritability, and the development of metabolic acidosis, followed by radiologic evidence of pneumatosis intestinalis, portal venous air, or free abdominal air. NEC is primarily a medical disease and is treated by cessation of oral intake, administration of antibiotics, fluid and electrolyte therapy, insertion of an orogastric tube, hemodynamic support, and in some cases, the insertion of a peritoneal drain. In nonresponsive cases, the infant becomes more septic with severe peritonitis, and the only solution is to perform an exploratory laparotomy to remove the gangrenous bowel and create an ileostomy.

The preoperative problems are an acute abdomen with severe peritonitis, necrosis, and gangrene of the intestine, septicemia, metabolic acidosis, and hypovolemia. These neonates may also have disseminated intravascular coagulation. Preparation of the patient is directed toward stabilization of these problems. By the time the newborn becomes a surgical candidate, the septicemia, coupled with the distended abdomen and the overall clinical deterioration of the infant, often has necessitated the use of intubation and ventilation in the NICU. Appropriate laboratory investigations include an arterial blood gas, hemoglobin, glucose, electrolytes, and coagulation profile. The deteriorating status of the patient may compromise both resuscitation efforts and the desire to establish adequate vascular access and monitoring, but focused efforts should be made to provide multiple vascular access lines, an arterial line, and central venous access.

The anesthetic requirements are continuation of resuscitation, provision of abdominal relaxation for the surgery, and careful titration of anesthetic drugs. These infants are often so critically ill that they are very sensitive to the depressant effects of anesthesia. If the patient is not already intubated and ventilated, a rapid-sequence induction with ketamine and succinylcholine is often used. The only caution with this technique is that some patients with NEC have significant hyperkalemia secondary to dead bowel, making the use of succinylcholine problematic. High dose rocuronium is a reasonable alternative in that situation. Maintenance of anesthesia is usually based on an opioid technique, supplemented with additional doses of ketamine or, if the patient's condition improves, low-dose inhalation agent. The use of nitrous oxide should be avoided because of the gas pockets in the abdomen.

These infants are among the most challenging cases in pediatric anesthesia. The fluid loss can be enormous, both because of surgical losses and third-space losses. Fluid management starts with full-strength, balanced salt solution for maintenance of blood pressure and urine output. Blood products are often needed during these cases. If the hematocrit is below 30% to 35%, red blood cells should be administered. Based on both preoperative and intraoperative laboratory work, fresh-frozen plasma, platelets, and cryoprecipitate may be needed. Due to bleeding, activated factor 7 or other prothrombotic agents may be needed. Inotropic support may also be needed. The surgical technique and length of surgery is variable, depending on the findings at laparotomy. A combination of bowel resection, primary anastomoses, and enterostomies may be used. At the end of the procedure, these infants are returned intubated and ventilated to the intensive care unit, where resuscitation is continued. Long-term survival is based on several factors, including the degree of prematurity, associated congenital abnormalities, the degree of surviving bowel, the total length of affected bowel, and subsequent complications. Mortality rates, especially in newborns weighing less than 1,500 g, are poor with recent studies demonstrating 25% to 50% mortality before discharge.[193,194]

Inguinal Hernia Repair in the Neonate

The development of a hernia in the premature infant or neonate is a different clinical problem from the development of a hernia in an infant older than 1 year. In infants younger than 2 months who need inguinal hernia repair, there is a higher incidence of prematurity, history of RDS, history of incarceration, and congenital heart disease.[195] In preterms, the incidence of hernia may approach 20% to 30%. There is a concern about new or recurring incarceration in these patients, making hernia repair less an elective procedure than in older infants. Consequently, once identified, these patients usually are repaired within a relatively short time. If the patient is currently hospitalized, it is common to repair the hernia before discharge. Otherwise, the surgery should be scheduled within days to weeks of diagnosis.

Anesthetic Techniques for Hernia Repair

Surgical procedures below the umbilicus can be performed with either general or regional anesthesia. The choice of whether to use general or regional anesthesia depends on the preference of the surgeon and/or the anesthesiologist and expected length of procedure. However, the choice is influenced by the underlying status of the patient, previous complications, and the known risk of preterm patients to develop apnea and bradycardia during and after these procedures. There is a risk in any preterm for apnea and bradycardia after stressful procedures, but this has been most widely studied in association with inguinal hernia repair. Apneic events are inversely related to both gestational age and postconceptual age. The incidence of apnea is less in small-for-gestational age infants. Anemia increases the incidence of apneic events. Apneic events at home are associated with a higher incidence in the perioperative period. There have been multiple studies that were recently analyzed to determine if the choice of regional or general anesthetic techniques decreased the incidence of apnea and bradycardia.[196] Use of spinal anesthesia without sedatives does not decrease the risk of late apnea in preterm neonates in the best evidence to date. Consequently, the choice of anesthetic should not be based solely on the risk of preventing apneic spells. An adjunct that has some evidence in support of its use to minimize apneic spells is caffeine. The use of preservative-free caffeine in a single dose of 10 mg/kg has been suggested to decrease the incidence of apneic spells.

Regional anesthesia can be used entirely for the surgery or as an adjunct to reduce general anesthetic requirements and provide postoperative analgesia. Other methods of providing intraoperative anesthesia and postoperative analgesia include the ilioinguinal–iliohypogastric nerve block or local infiltration. Ilioinguinal–iliohypogastric nerve block with 0.25% bupivacaine or 0.2% ropivacaine, with epinephrine, can be administered shortly after the induction of general anesthesia and affords excellent postoperative analgesia.

Discharge after inguinal hernia repair to home is an area of some controversy. There is significant institutional variation on the issue of monitoring for postoperative apnea, with the decision to admit overnight usually based on the postconceptual age in preterm neonates. Some centers use 46 weeks postconceptual age as the lower limit for admission, but other centers will use up to 60 weeks postconceptual age as the limit. No matter what limits are used, if the infant has apneic or bradycardic spells during the perioperative period, he or she should be monitored in-house until the infant has been apnea-free for at least 12 hours.

Pyloric Stenosis

Pyloric stenosis is a relatively frequent surgical disease of the neonate and infant. It most commonly appears between weeks 2 and 6 of life. The pathologic characteristics include hypertrophy of the pyloric smooth muscle with edema of the pyloric mucosa and submucosa. This process, which develops over a period of days to weeks, leads to progressive obstruction of the pyloric valve, causing persistent vomiting. The vomiting leads to varying losses of fluids and electrolytes. The diagnosis is usually made at an early stage in the development of symptoms, especially with the help of ultrasound, so it is rare to find an infant with severe fluid and electrolyte derangements. However, an infant is occasionally seen whose problem has developed slowly over a period of weeks, resulting in severe fluid and electrolyte derangements. The stomach contents contain sodium, potassium, chloride, hydrogen ions, and water. The classic electrolyte pattern in infants with severe vomiting is hyponatremic, hypokalemic, and hypochloremic metabolic alkalosis with a compensatory respiratory acidosis. The anesthesiologist, pediatrician, and surgeon are all responsible for preparing these infants for surgery. Pyloric stenosis is a medical emergency, not a surgical emergency. The patient should not be operated on until there has been adequate fluid and electrolyte resuscitation. The infant should have normal skin turgor, and the correction of the electrolyte imbalance should produce a sodium level that is greater than 130 mEq/L, a potassium level that is at least 3 mEq/L, a chloride level that is greater than 85 mEq/L (trending upward), and a urine output of at least 1 to 2 mL/kg/hr. These patients need a resuscitation fluid of balanced salt solution and, after the infant begins to urinate, the addition of potassium.

Anesthetic Management

It is prudent to pass a large orogastric tube and aspirate the stomach contents because of the significant volume that may be present.[197] This procedure greatly reduces the quantity of gastric fluid. A rapid-sequence induction is advisable because of the potential for additional volume in the stomach. Although awake intubation had been popular with some clinicians in the past, it is associated with a higher incidence of complications and is traumatic to the child.[107] These patients should have been fully resuscitated before coming to surgery, so there is little reason for an awake intubation. Anesthesia can be maintained by almost any technique the clinician prefers. There has been a need for muscle relaxation only for a short period during pyloromyotomy. Some surgeons may require muscle relaxation because most of these are now performed using minimally invasive laparoscopic procedures (Fig. 42-22). Careful attention must be paid to ventilation and blood pressure as the abdominal pressure is increased during insufflation for laparoscopy. Controlled ventilation reduces or eliminates the need for muscle relaxants for this surgery. At the end of the case, the patient should be wide awake before extubation. A TAP block can be provided using ultrasound guidance for postoperative pain relief with good analgesia or local infiltration at laparoscopic port sites. Intravenous or rectal acetaminophen is commonly administered for pain relief as well.

Ligation of a Patent Ductus Arteriosus

As the number of small premature infants who survive has increased, so also has the number of infants who have a PDA with heart failure and respiratory failure (NICV 42-8). Prostaglandins relax the smooth muscle of the ductus so it cannot constrict. Indomethacin, a prostaglandin synthetase inhibitor,

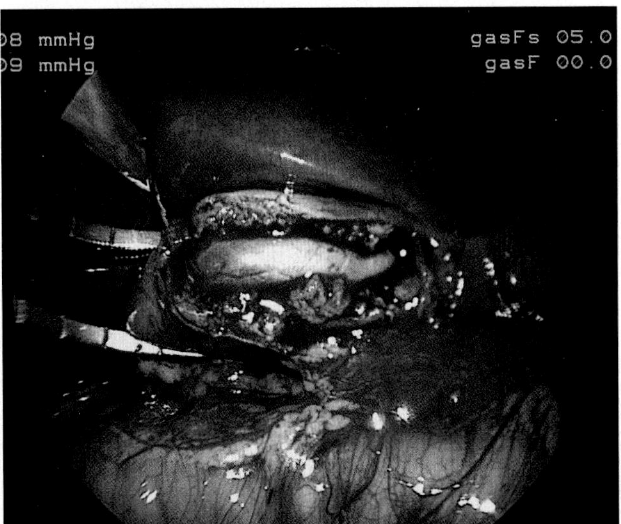

Figure 42-22 Laparoscopic repair of pyloric stenosis. In this image, the surgical cleft created in the hypertrophic muscles of the pylorus can be seen. This surgical intervention is curative of pyloric stenosis. (Photograph courtesy of Timothy Lautz, MD.)

can be administered to encourage closure of the ductus. However, indomethacin is often unsuccessful in the small premature infant because of the lack of muscle within the ductus. Infants with a PDA and heart failure need maximal medical management with fluid restriction, diuretics, and inotropes. These infants are at special risk because of the reduced blood volume and precarious cardiopulmonary system. If the surgery is performed in the operating room, special attention is taken to maintain normothermia, ventilation, and oxygenation during transport. If the surgery is performed at bedside in the NICU, the anesthesiologist must take time before the procedure to establish where he or she will be situated, the location of all venous access, and that all drugs and fluids are already prepared. An opioid-based technique with muscle relaxant is a frequent choice for anesthesia. Probably the biggest challenge during these cases is the diagnosis and management of hypotension. There can be sudden, catastrophic blood loss if the ductus arteriosus ruptures during the procedure. Consequently, syringes of a balanced salt solution, albumin, and blood should be immediately available. The other common cause of hypotension is compression of the lungs, heart, and great vessels by the surgeon as they are gaining exposure. There must be a balance between stopping the procedure to allow the heart and blood pressure to recover versus the need to proceed with the operation. The answer comes in close communication between the anesthesiologist and the surgeon. These patients usually remain intubated after procedure, without a need to reverse the muscle relaxant. Residual opioid will provide good analgesia for the immediate postoperative period. Hypotension is frequently encountered in the postoperative period due to postligation syndrome in which cardiac function becomes transiently diminished due to increased afterload from the PDA ligation.

There are two newer techniques for closing the PDA in infants that are increasing in popularity.[198] Video-assisted thoracoscopic surgery (VATS) uses small endoscopes inserted through a series of small thoracotomy incisions to guide instruments to ligate the ductus. VATS can be done either in the operating room or, rarely, at bedside. The other approach is used by cardiologists in the cardiac catheterization to occlude the ductus arteriosus with a coil. Transcatheter PDA occlusion devices are now being placed in neonates weighing <1 kg.[199] A test clamp is often used to demonstrate continued aortic flow to the lower extremities and an improvement in diastolic blood pressure from decrease of diastolic run-off to the ductus arteriosus.

Placement of a Central Venous Catheter

The use of a central venous catheter for monitoring serum electrolytes, for parenteral nutrition, and for administering medications is a well-established part of modern perioperative care. It can be placed either as part of the surgical procedure or at some other time as a separate procedure. The three major concerns in central venous catheter placement are airway management, pneumothorax, and bleeding. The anesthetic technique depends on the infant's condition. If general anesthesia is selected, then intubation or laryngeal mask airway have each been successfully used. A pneumothorax may occur with attempts at subclavian vein puncture. The first indication of pneumothorax may be a decreasing oxygen saturation, hypotension, or difficulty with ventilation of the lungs. Because fluoroscopic imaging is often used for central venous catheter placement, it can also be used rapidly to diagnose a pneumothorax. If not, the chest should be rapidly aspirated for both diagnostic and therapeutic reasons. Bleeding is an unusual but serious complication of central venous catheter placement. It usually manifests in the perioperative period as hemothorax or as hypovolemia with a decreasing hematocrit and/or blood pressure. Establishing intravenous access before proceeding with a central line is problematic for some patients. The reason for the central line may very well be the inability to obtain peripheral access, and the clinician is left with a trade-off between prolonged attempts at starting an intravenous catheter versus proceeding directly to obtain central venous line placement.

PICCs, placed in either the upper extremity or the femoral vein, are now in common practice. Often, these lines may be placed with local anesthetic only or with mild sedation, with ketamine for example. Strict attention to skin preparation, sterile glove and drape use, and minimizing access to the central line are components important to diminish catheter-related sepsis. Subclavian approach has a higher incidence of problems during line placement than internal jugular or femoral approaches but may have fewer associated infections and fewer overall problems with the line once it is in use. PICCs have not been well-studied in the neonatal population but continue to grow in their popularity.

Summary

The anesthetic management of the newborn is among the most challenging to anesthesiologists. A strong knowledge of neonatal anatomy, physiology, and pharmacology is needed, as well as an appreciation of the disease states and surgical procedures that are unique to this population. A thorough preanesthetic evaluation and preparation, a concise plan, and meticulous technique are the basis of an effective approach. The patient's neonatologist or pediatrician and the surgeon are strong allies in providing the best care, and close communication with them is necessary. Finally, the clinical status of a newborn can change remarkably quickly. Strict attention to detail and prospective management are the hallmarks of the anesthesiologist skilled in providing care in these difficult cases. Use of current technology including ultrasound guidance is suggested for facilitating vascular access as well as regional anesthesia for pain management in these fragile infants. 8

Acknowledgment

The authors of this edition would like to thank Dr. Santhanam Suresh and Dr. Steve Hall for their contributions to previous versions of this chapter as well as their career-long dedication to the field of pediatric anesthesiology.

For further review and interactivities, please see the videos and narrative interactive clinical vignettes (NICVs) accessible in the complimentary eBook bundled with this text. Access instructions are located on the inside front cover.

REFERENCES

1. Friedman AH, Fahey JT. The transition from fetal to neonatal circulation: normal responses and implications for infants with heart disease. *Semin Perinatol*. 1993;17(2):106–121.
2. Baum VC, Palmisano BW. The immature heart and anesthesia. *Anesthesiology*. 1997;87(6): 1529–1548.
3. Fu JD, Li J, Tweedie D, et al. Crucial role of the sarcoplasmic reticulum in the developmental regulation of Ca2+ transients and contraction in cardiomyocytes derived from embryonic stem cells. *FASEB J*. 2006;20(1):181–183.
4. Auman JT, Seidler FJ, Tate CA, Slotkin TA. Are developing beta-adrenoceptors able to desensitize? Acute and chronic effects of beta-agonists in neonatal heart and liver. *Am J Physiol Regul Integr Comp Physiol*. 2002;283(1):R205–R217.
5. Kishkurno S, Takahashi Y, Harada K, Ishida A, Tamura M, Takada G. Postnatal changes in left ventricular volume and contractility in healthy term infants. *Pediatr Cardiol*. 1997;18(2): 91–95.

6. Hislop A. Developmental biology of the pulmonary circulation. *Paediatr Respir Rev.* 2005;6(1):35–43.
7. Mansell AL, Collins MH, Johnson E Jr, et al. Postnatal growth of lung parenchyma in the piglet: morphometry correlated with mechanics. *Anat Rec.* 1995;241(1):99–104.
8. Engle WA. American Academy of Pediatrics Committee on Fetus and Newborn. Surfactant-replacement therapy for respiratory distress in the preterm and term neonate. *Pediatrics.* 2008;121(2):419–432.
9. Hernandez-Diaz S, Van Marter LJ, Werler MM, Werler MM, Louik C, Mitchell AA. Risk factors for persistent pulmonary hypertension of the newborn. *Pediatrics.* 2007;120(2):e272–e282.
10. Jain A, McNamara PJ. Persistent pulmonary hypertension of the newborn: advances in diagnosis and treatment. *Semin Fetal Neonatal Med.* 2015;20(4):262–271.
11. Konduri GG, Solimano A, Sokol GM, et al. A randomized trial of early versus standard inhaled nitric oxide therapy in term and near-term newborn infants with hypoxic respiratory failure. *Pediatrics.* 2004;113(3 Pt 1):559–564.
12. Steinhorn RH. Nitric oxide and beyond: new insights and therapies for pulmonary hypertension. *J Perinatol.* 2008;28(Suppl 3):S67–S71.
13. Noori S, Seri I. Neonatal blood pressure support: the use of inotropes, lusitropes, and other vasopressor agents. *Clin Perinatol.* 2012;39(1):221–238.
14. El-Khuffash A, Herbozo C, Jain A, Lapointe A, McNamara PJ. Targeted neonatal echocardiography (TnECHO) service in a Canadian neonatal intensive care unit: a 4-year experience. *J Perinatol.* 2013;33(9):687–690.
15. Scohy TV, Gommers D, Jan ten Harkel AD, Deryck Y, McGhie J, Bogers AJ. Intraoperative evaluation of micromultiplane transesophageal echocardiographic probe in surgery for congenital heart disease. *Eur J Echocardiogr.* 2007;8(4):241–246.
16. Murphy JD, Vawter GF, Reid LM. Pulmonary vascular disease in fatal meconium aspiration. *J Pediatr.* 1984;104(5):758–762.
17. Velaphi S, Vidyasagar D. Intrapartum and postdelivery management of infants born to mothers with meconium-stained amniotic fluid: evidence-based recommendations. *Clin Perinatol.* 2006;33(1):29–42, v-vi.
18. Drukker A, Guignard JP. Renal aspects of the term and preterm infant: a selective update. *Curr Opin Pediatr.* 2002;14(2):175–182.
19. Alcorn J, McNamara PJ. Ontogeny of hepatic and renal systemic clearance pathways in infants: part I. *Clin Pharmacokinet.* 2002;41(12):959–998.
20. Nash PL. Potassium and sodium homeostasis in the neonate. *Neonatal Netw.* 2007;26(2):125–128.
21. Chawla D, Agarwal R, Deorari AK, Paul VK. Fluid and electrolyte management in term and preterm neonates. *Indian J Pediatr.* 2008;75(3):255–259.
22. Cornblath M, Ichord R. Hypoglycemia in the neonate. *Semin Perinatol.* 2000;24(2):136–149.
23. Ballweg JA, Wernovsky G, Ittenbach RF, et al. Hyperglycemia after infant cardiac surgery does not adversely impact neurodevelopmental outcome. *Ann Thorac Surg.* 2007;84(6):2052–2058.
24. Girelli G, Antoncecchi S, Casadei AM, et al. Recommendations for transfusion therapy in neonatology. *Blood Transfus.* 2015;13(3):484–497.
25. Fergusson D, Hebert PC, Lee SK, et al. Clinical outcomes following institution of universal leukoreduction of blood transfusions for premature infants. *JAMA.* 2003;289(15):1950–1956.
26. Alcorn J, McNamara PJ. Pharmacokinetics in the newborn. *Adv Drug Deliv Rev.* 2003;55(5):667–686.
27. Strassburg CP, Strassburg A, Kneip S, et al. Developmental aspects of human hepatic drug glucuronidation in young children and adults. *Gut.* 2002;50(2):259–265.
28. Leeder JS, Kearns GL. Pharmacogenetics in pediatrics. Implications for practice. *Pediatr Clin North Am.* 1997;44(1):55–77.
29. Bory C, Baltassat P, Porthault M, Bethenod M, Frederich A, Aranda JV. Metabolism of theophylline to caffeine in premature newborn infants. *J Pediatr.* 1979;94(6):988–993.
30. Green MD, Shires TK, Fischer LJ. Hepatotoxicity of acetaminophen in neonatal and young rats. I. Age-related changes in susceptibility. *Toxicol Appl Pharmacol.* 1984;74(1):116–124.
31. deAlmeida VL, Alvaro RA, Haider Z, et al. The effect of nasal occlusion on the initiation of oral breathing in preterm infants. *Pediatr Pulmonol.* 1994;18(6):374–378.
32. Miller MJ, Carlo WA, Strohl KP, Fanaroff AA, Martin RJ. Effect of maturation on oral breathing in sleeping premature infants. *J Pediatr.* 1986;109(3):515–519.
33. Dalal PG, Murray D, Messner AH, Feng A, McAllister J, Molter D. Pediatric laryngeal dimensions: an age-based analysis. *Anesth Analg.* 2009:108(5):1475–1479.
34. Litman RS, Weissend EE, Shibata D, Westesson P. Developmental changes of laryngeal dimensions in unparalyzed, sedated children. *Anesthesiology.* 2003;98(1):41–45.
35. Weiss M, Dullenkopf A, Fischer JE, Keller C, Gerber AC, European Paediatric Endotracheal Intubation Study Group. Prospective randomized controlled multi-centre trial of cuffed or uncuffed endotracheal tubes in small children. *Br J Anaesth.* 2009;103(6):867–873.
36. Flynn PE, Black AE, Mitchell V. The use of cuffed tracheal tubes for paediatric tracheal intubation, a survey of specialist practice in the United Kingdom. *Eur J Anaesthesiol.* 2008;25(8):685–688.
37. Bhutada A, Sahni R, Rastogi S, Wung JT. Randomised controlled trial of thiopental for intubation in neonates. *Arch Dis Child Fetal Neonatal Ed.* 2000;82(1):F34–F37.
38. Ghanta S, Abdel-Latif ME, Lui K, Ravindranathan H, Awad J, Oei J. Propofol compared with the morphine, atropine, and suxamethonium regimen as induction agents for neonatal endotracheal intubation: a randomized, controlled trial. *Pediatrics.* 2007; 119(6):e1248–e1255.
39. Allegaert K, Peeters MY, Verbesselt R, et al. Inter-individual variability in propofol pharmacokinetics in preterm and term neonates. *Br J Anaesth.* 2007;99(6):864–870.
40. Bhutta AT. Ketamine: a controversial drug for neonates. *Semin Perinatol.* 2007;31(5):303–308.
41. Anand KJ, Garg S, Rovnaghi CR, Narsinghani U, Bhutta AT, Hall RW. Ketamine reduces the cell death following inflammatory pain in newborn rat brain. *Pediatr Res.* 2007;62(3):283–290.
42. Estkowski LM, Morris JL, Sinclair EA. Characterization of dexmedetomidine dosing and safety in neonates and infants. *J Pediatr Pharmacol Ther.* 2015;20(2):112–118.
43. Luo J, Guo J, Han D, Li H. [Comparison of dexmedetomidine and midazolam on neurotoxicity in neonatal mice]. *Sheng Wu Yi Xue Gong Cheng Xue Za Zhi.* 2013;30(3):607–610.
44. Suresh S, Anand KJ. Opioid tolerance in neonates: a state-of-the-art review. *Paediatr Anaesth.* 2001;11(5):511–521.
45. Puia-Dumitrescu M, Comstock BA, Li S, et al. Assessment of 2-year neurodevelopmental outcomes in extremely preterm infants receiving opioids and benzodiazepines. *JAMA Netw Open.* 2021;4(7):e2115998.
46. Vaughn PR, Townsend SF, Thilo EH, McKenzie S, Moreland S, Denver KK. Comparison of continuous infusion of fentanyl to bolus dosing in neonates after surgery. *J Pediatr Surg.* 1996;31(12):1616–1623.
47. Saarenmaa E, Neuvonen PJ, Rosenberg P, Fellman V. Morphine clearance and effects in newborn infants in relation to gestational age. *Clin Pharmacol Ther.* 2000;68(2):160–166.
48. Bhat R, Chari G, Gulati A, Aldana O, Velamati R, Bhargava H. Pharmacokinetics of a single dose of morphine in preterm infants during the first week of life. *J Pediatr.* 1990;117(3):477–481.
49. El Sayed MF, Taddio A, Fallah S, De Silva N, Moore AM. Safety profile of morphine following surgery in neonates. *J Perinatol.* 2007;27(7):444–447.
50. Murphey LJ, Olsen GD. Morphine-6-beta-D-glucuronide respiratory pharmacodynamics in the neonatal guinea pig. *J Pharmacol Exp Ther.* 1994;268(1):110–116.
51. Davis PJ, Cladis FP. The use of ultra-short-acting opioids in paediatric anaesthesia: the role of remifentanil. *Clin Pharmacokinet.* 2005;44(8):787–796.
52. Davis PJ, Galinkin J, McGowan FX, et al. A randomized multicenter study of remifentanil compared with halothane in neonates and infants undergoing pyloromyotomy. I. Emergence and recovery profiles. *Anesth Analg.* 2001;93(6):1380–1386.
53. Hannallah RS, Oh TH, McGill WA, Epstein BS. Changes in heart rate and rhythm after intramuscular succinylcholine with or without atropine in anesthetized children. *Anesth Analg.* 1986;65(12):1329–1332.
54. Rapp HJ, Altenmueller CA, Waschke C. Neuromuscular recovery following rocuronium bromide single dose in infants. *Paediatr Anaesth.* 2004;14(4):329–335.
55. Gronert BJ, Brandom BW. Neuromuscular blocking drugs in infants and children. *Pediatr Clin North Am.* 1994;41(1):73–91.
56. Cheung PY, Tyebkhan JM, Peliowski A, Ainsworth W, Robertson CM. Prolonged use of pancuronium bromide and sensorineural hearing loss in childhood survivors of congenital diaphragmatic hernia. *J Pediatr.* 1999;135(2 Pt 1):233–239.
57. Reich DL, Hollinger I, Harrington DJ, Seiden HS, Chakravorti S, Cook DR. Comparison of cisatracurium and vecuronium by infusion in neonates and small infants after congenital heart surgery. *Anesthesiology.* 2004;101(5):1122–1127.
58. Fodale V, Santamaria LB. Laudanosine, an atracurium and cisatracurium metabolite. *Eur J Anaesthesiol.* 2002;19(7):466–473.
59. Bhananker SM, Ramamoorthy C, Geiduschek JM, et al. Anesthesia-related cardiac arrest in children: update from the Pediatric Perioperative Cardiac Arrest Registry. *Anesth Analg.* 2007;105(2):344–350.
60. Gaver RS, Brenn BR, Gartley A, Donahue BS. Retrospective analysis of the safety and efficacy of sugammadex versus neostigmine for the reversal of neuromuscular blockade in children. *Anesth Analg.* 2019;129(4):1124–1129.
61. Murray DJ, Forbes RB, Mahoney LT. Comparative hemodynamic depression of halothane versus isoflurane in neonates and infants: an echocardiographic study. *Anesth Analg.* 1992;74(3):329–337.
62. Lerman J, Sikich N, Kleinman S, Yentis S. The pharmacology of sevoflurane in infants and children. *Anesthesiology.* 1994;80(4):814–824.
63. Russell IA, Miller Hance WC, Gregory G, et al. The safety and efficacy of sevoflurane anesthesia in infants and children with congenital heart disease. *Anesth Analg.* 2001;92(5):1152–1158.
64. Brown K, Aun C, Stocks J, Jackson E, Mackersie A, Hatch D. A comparison of the respiratory effects of sevoflurane and halothane in infants and young children. *Anesthesiology.* 1998;89(1):86–92.
65. Sale SM, Read JA, Stoddart PA, Wolf AR. Prospective comparison of sevoflurane and desflurane in formerly premature infants undergoing inguinal herniotomy. *Br J Anaesth.* 2006;96(6):774–778.
66. Taylor RH, Lerman J. Minimum alveolar concentration of desflurane and hemodynamic responses in neonates, infants, and children. *Anesthesiology.* 1991;75(6):975–979.
67. Kodama M, Satoh Y, Otsubo Y, et al. Neonatal desflurane exposure induces more robust neuroapoptosis than do isoflurane and sevoflurane and impairs working memory. *Anesthesiology.* 2011;115(5):979–991.

68. Mazoit JX. Pharmacokinetic/pharmacodynamic modeling of anesthetics in children. therapeutic implications. *Paediatr Drugs*. 2006;8(3):139–150.
69. Rothstein P, Arthur GR, Feldman HS, Kopf GS, Covino BG. Bupivacaine for intercostal nerve blocks in children: blood concentrations and pharmacokinetics. *Anesth Analg*. 1986;65(6): 625–632.
70. Ecoffey C, Desparmet J, Maury M, Berdeaux A, Giudicelli JF, Saint-Maurice C. Bupivacaine in children: pharmacokinetics following caudal anesthesia. *Anesthesiology*. 1985;63(4): 447–448.
71. Willschke H, Bosenberg A, Marhofer P, et al. Ultrasonographic-guided ilioinguinal /iliohypogastric nerve block in pediatric anesthesia: what is the optimal volume? *Anesth Analg*. 2006;102(6):1680–1684.
72. Berde CB. Convulsions associated with pediatric regional anesthesia. *Anesth Analg*. 1992;75(2):164–166.
73. Rapp HJ, Molnar V, Austin S, et al. Ropivacaine in neonates and infants: a population pharmacokinetic evaluation following single caudal block. *Paediatr Anaesth*. 2004;14(9):724–732.
74. McCloskey JJ, Haun SE, Deshpande JK. Bupivacaine toxicity secondary to continuous caudal epidural infusion in children. *Anesth Analg*. 1992; 75(2):287–290.
75. Hansen TG, Ilett KF, Reid C, Lim SI, Hackett LP, Bergesio R. Caudal ropivacaine in infants: population pharmacokinetics and plasma concentrations. *Anesthesiology*. 2001;94(4):579–584.
76. Chalkiadis GA, Eyres RL, Cranswick N, Taylor RH, Austin S. Pharmacokinetics of levobupivacaine 0.25% following caudal administration in children under 2 years of age. *Br J Anaesth*. 2004;92(2):218–222.
77. Tobias JD, O'Dell N. Chloroprocaine for epidural anesthesia in infants and children. *AANA J*. 1995;63(2):131–135.
78. Henderson K, Sethna NF, Berde CB. Continuous caudal anesthesia for inguinal hernia repair in former preterm infants. *J Clin Anesth*. 1993;5(2):129–133.
79. Shah S, Gopalakrishnan S, Apuya J, Shah S, Martin T. Use of Intralipid in an infant with impending cardiovascular collapse due to local anesthetic toxicity. *J Anesth*. 2009;23(3): 439–441.
80. Mirtallo JM, Dasta JF, Kleinschmidt KC, Varon J. State of the art review: Intravenous fat emulsions: Current applications, safety profile, and clinical implications. *Ann Pharmacother*. 2010;44(4):688–700.
81. Neal JM, Mulroy MF, Weinberg GL. American Society of Regional Anesthesia and Pain Medicine. American Society of Regional Anesthesia and Pain Medicine checklist for managing local anesthetic systemic toxicity: 2012 version. *Reg Anesth Pain Med*. 2012;37(1): 16–18.
82. Couper RT. Methaemoglobinaemia secondary to topical lignocaine/prilocaine in a circumcised neonate. *J Paediatr Child Health*. 2000;36(4):406–407.
83. Lehr VT, Taddio A. Topical anesthesia in neonates: clinical practices and practical considerations. *Semin Perinatol*. 2007;31(5):323–329.
84. Braz LG, Modolo NS, do Nascimento P Jr, et al. Perioperative cardiac arrest: a study of 53,718 anaesthetics over 9 yr from a Brazilian teaching hospital. *Br J Anaesth*. 2006;96(5):569–575.
85. Murat I, Constant I, Maud'huy H. Perioperative anaesthetic morbidity in children: a database of 24,165 anaesthetics over a 30-month period. *Paediatr Anaesth*. 2004;14(2):158–166.
86. Catre D, Lopes MF, Madrigal A, et al. Predictors of major postoperative complications in neonatal surgery. *Rev Col Bras Cir*. 2013;40(5):363–369.
87. Section on Anesthesiology and Pain Medicine, Polaner DM, Houck CS, American Academy of Pediatrics. Critical elements for the pediatric perioperative anesthesia environment. *Pediatrics*. 2015;136(6):1200–1205.
88. Anand KJ, Carr DB. The neuroanatomy, neurophysiology, and neurochemistry of pain, stress, and analgesia in newborns and children. *Pediatr Clin North Am*. 1989;36(4):795–822.
89. Prevention and management of pain and stress in the neonate. American Academy of Pediatrics. Committee on Fetus and Newborn. Committee on Drugs. Section on Anesthesiology. Section on Surgery. Canadian Paediatric Society. Fetus and Newborn Committee. *Pediatrics*. 2000;105(2):454–461.
90. Tomashek KM, Shapiro-Mendoza CK, Davidoff MJ, Petrini JR. Differences in mortality between late-preterm and term singleton infants in the United States, 1995–2002. *J Pediatr*. 2007;151(5):450–456, 456 e451.
91. Ozyurek E, Cetintas S, Ceylan T, et al. Complete blood count parameters for healthy, small-for-gestational-age, full-term newborns. *Clin Lab Haematol*. 2006;28(2):97–104.
92. Deshpande S, Ward PlattM. The investigation and management of neonatal hypoglycaemia. *Semin Fetal Neonatal Med*. 2005;10(4):351–361.
93. Lippi G, Salvagno GL, Rugolotto S, et al. Routine coagulation tests in newborn and young infants. *J Thromb Thrombolysis*. 2007;24(2):153–155.
94. American Academy of Pediatrics Committee on Fetus and Newborn. Controversies concerning vitamin K and the newborn. American Academy of Pediatrics Committee on Fetus and Newborn. *Pediatrics*. 2003;112(1 Pt 1):191–192.
95. Barrington KJ. The myth of a minimum dose for atropine. *Pediatrics*. 2011; 127(4):783–784.
96. Shiao SY. Effects of fetal hemoglobin on accurate measurements of oxygen saturation in neonates. *J Perinat Neonatal Nurs*. 2005;19(4):348–361.
97. Hubmayr RD. The times are a-changin': should we hang up the stethoscope? *Anesthesiology*. 2004;100(1):1–2.
98. Watson A, Visram A. Survey of the use of oesophageal and precordial stethoscopes in current paediatric anaesthetic practice. *Paediatr Anaesth*. 2001; 11(4):437–442.
99. Sigaut S, Skhiri A, Stany I, et al. Ultrasound guided internal jugular vein access in children and infant: a meta-analysis of published studies. *Paediatr Anaesth*. 2009;19(12): 1199–1206.
100. Han SH, Kim SD, Kim CS, et al. Comparison of central venous catheterization sites in infants. *J Int Med Res*. 2004;32(6):563–569.
101. Panagiotounakou P, Antonogeorgos G, Gounari E, Papadakis S, Labadaridis J, Gounaris AK. Peripherally inserted central venous catheters: frequency of complications in premature newborn depends on the insertion site. *J Perinatol*. 2014;34(6):461–463.
102. Schily M, Koumoukelis H, Lerman J, Creighton RE. Can pediatric anesthesiologists detect an occluded tracheal tube in neonates? *Anesth Analg*. 2001;93(1):66–70.
103. Spears RS Jr, Yeh A, Fisher DM, Zwass MS. The "educated hand." Can anesthesiologists assess changes in neonatal pulmonary compliance manually? *Anesthesiology*. 1991;75(4):693–696.
104. Tobin MJ, Stevenson GW, Horn BJ, Chen EH, Hall SC, Coté CJ. A comparison of three modes of ventilation with the use of an adult circle system in an infant lung model. *Anesth Analg*. 1998;87(4):766–771.
105. Hunter T, Lerman J, Bissonnette B. The temperature and humidity of inspired gases in infants using a pediatric circle system: effects of high and low-flow anesthesia. *Paediatr Anaesth*. 2005;15(9):750–754.
106. Luchetti M, Pigna A, Gentili A, Marraro G. Evaluation of the efficiency of heat and moisture exchangers during paediatric anaesthesia. *Paediatr Anaesth*. 1999;9(1):39–45.
107. Cook-Sather SD, Tulloch HV, Cnaan A, et al. A comparison of awake versus paralyzed tracheal intubation for infants with pyloric stenosis. *Anesth Analg*. 1998;86(5):945–951.
108. Salgo B, Schmitz A, Henze G, et al. Evaluation of a new recommendation for improved cuffed tracheal tube size selection in infants and small children. *Acta Anaesthesiol Scand*. 2006;50(5):557–561.
109. Lonnqvist PA. Successful use of laryngeal mask airway in low-weight expremature infants with bronchopulmonary dysplasia undergoing cryotherapy for retinopathy of the premature. *Anesthesiology*. 1995;83(2):422–424.
110. Jagannathan N, Ramsey MA, White MC, Sohn L. An update on newer pediatric supraglottic airways with recommendations for clinical use. *Paediatr Anaesth*. 2015;25(4):334–345.
111. Hansen TG, Joensen H, Henneberg SW, Hole P. Laryngeal mask airway guided tracheal intubation in a neonate with the Pierre Robin syndrome. *Acta Anaesthesiol Scand*. 1995;39(1):129–131.
112. Fisher QA, Tunkel DE. Lightwand intubation of infants and children. *J Clin Anesth*. 1997; 9(4):275–279.
113. Cain JM, Mason LJ, Martin RD. Airway management in two of newborns with Pierre Robin Sequence: the use of disposable vs multiple use LMA for fiberoptic intubation. *Paediatr Anaesth*. 2006;16(12):1274–1276.
114. Moura JH, da Silva GA. Neonatal laryngoscope intubation and the digital method: a randomized controlled trial. *J Pediatr*. 2006;148(6):840–841.
115. Feldman JM. Optimal ventilation of the anesthetized pediatric patient. *Anesth Analg*. 2015; 120(1):165–175.
116. Wheeler K, Klingenberg C, McCallion N, Morley CJ, Davis PG. Volume-targeted versus pressure-limited ventilation in the neonate. *Cochrane Database Syst Rev*. 2010(11):CD003666.
117. Wheeler KI, Klingenberg C, Morley CJ, Davis PG. Volume-targeted versus pressure-limited ventilation for preterm infants: a systematic review and meta-analysis. *Neonatology*. 2011;100(3):219–227.
118. Piersigilli F, Bersani I, Giliberti P, et al. Neonatal limb ischemia: caudal blockade and NIRS monitoring. *Eur J Pediatr*. 2014;173(12):1599–1601.
119. Marhofer P, Willschke H, Kettner S. Imaging techniques for regional nerve blockade and vascular cannulation in children. *Curr Opin Anaesthesiol*. 2006;19(3):293–300.
120. Weinberg GL, Ripper R, Murphy P, et al. Lipid infusion accelerates removal of bupivacaine and recovery from bupivacaine toxicity in the isolated rat heart. *Reg Anesth Pain Med*. 2006;31(4):296–303.
121. Davidson AJ, Morton NS, Arnup SJ, et al. Apnea after awake regional and general anesthesia in infants: The General anesthesia compared to spinal anesthesia study–Comparing apnea and neurodevelopmental outcomes, a randomized controlled trial. *Anesthesiology*. 2015; 123(1):38–54.
122. Suresh S, Wheeler M. Practical pediatric regional anesthesia. *Anesthesiol Clin North America*. 2002;20(1):83–113.
123. Williams RK, Adams DC, Aladjem EV, et al. The safety and efficacy of spinal anesthesia for surgery in infants: the Vermont Infant Spinal Registry. *Anesth Analg*. 2006;102(1): 67–71.
124. Suresh S, Hall SC. Spinal anesthesia in infants: is the impractical practical? *Anesth Analg*. 2006;102(1):65–66.
125. Welborn LG, Rice LJ, Hannallah RS, Broadman LM, Ruttimann UE, Fink R. Postoperative apnea in former preterm infants: prospective comparison of spinal and general anesthesia. *Anesthesiology*. 1990;72(5):838–842.
126. Tsui BC, Tarkkila P, Gupta S, Kearney R. Confirmation of caudal needle placement using nerve stimulation. *Anesthesiology*. 1999;91(2):374–378.

127. Marhofer P, Bosenberg A, Sitzwohl C, Willschke H, Wanzel O, Kapral S. Pilot study of neuraxial imaging by ultrasound in infants and children. *Paediatr Anaesth*. 2005;15(8): 671–676.
128. Suresh S, Long J, Birmingham PK, De Oliveira GS Jr. Are caudal blocks for pain control safe in children? An analysis of 18,650 caudal blocks from the Pediatric Regional Anesthesia Network (PRAN) database. *Anesth Analg*. 2015;120(1):151–156.
129. Wheeler M, Patel A, Suresh S, et al. The addition of clonidine 2 microg.kg-1 does not enhance the postoperative analgesia of a caudal block using 0.125% bupivacaine and epinephrine 1:200,000 in children: a prospective, double-blind, randomized study. *Paediatr Anaesth*. 2005;15(6):476–483.
130. Willschke H, Bosenberg A, Marhofer P, et al. Epidural catheter placement in neonates: sonoanatomy and feasibility of ultrasonographic guidance in term and preterm neonates. *Reg Anesth Pain Med*. 2007;32(1):34–40.
131. Long JB, Joselyn AS, Bhalla T, et al. The use of neuraxial catheters for postoperative analgesia in neonates: A Multicenter Safety Analysis from the Pediatric Regional Anesthesia Network. *Anesth Analg*. 2016;122(6):1965–1970.
132. Brady-Fryer B, Wiebe N, Lander JA. Pain relief for neonatal circumcision. *Cochrane Database Syst Rev*. 2004(4):CD004217.
133. Sandeman DJ, Dilley AV. Ultrasound guided dorsal penile nerve block in children. *Anaesth Intensive Care*. 2007;35(2):266–269.
134. Bielsky A, Efrat R, Suresh S. Postoperative analgesia in neonates after major abdominal surgery: 'TAP' our way to success! *Paediatr Anaesth*. 2009;19(5):541–542.
135. Suresh S, De Oliveira GS Jr. Blood bupivacaine concentrations after transversus abdominis plane block in neonates: a prospective observational study. *Anesth Analg*. 2016;122(3): 814–817.
136. Marhofer P, Greher M, Kapral S. Ultrasound guidance in regional anaesthesia. *Br J Anaesth*. 2005;94(1):7–17.
137. Marhofer P, Sitzwohl C, Greher M, Kapral S. Ultrasound guidance for infraclavicular brachial plexus anaesthesia in children. *Anaesthesia*. 2004;59(7):642–646.
138. Suresh S, Voronov P. Head and neck blocks in children: an anatomical and procedural review. *Paediatr Anaesth*. 2006;16(9):910–918.
139. Williams DG, Patel A, Howard RF. Pharmacogenetics of codeine metabolism in an urban population of children and its implications for analgesic reliability. *Br J Anaesth*. 2002; 89(6):839–845.
140. Cheung CL, van Dijk M, Green JW, Tibboel D, Anand KJ. Effects of low-dose naloxone on opioid therapy in pediatric patients: a retrospective case-control study. *Int Care Med*. 2007;33(1):190–194.
141. Pacifici GM, Allegaert K. Clinical pharmacology of paracetamol in neonates: a review. *Curr Ther Res Clin Exp*. 2015;77:24–30.
142. Papacci P, De Francisci G, Iacobucci T, et al. Use of intravenous ketorolac in the neonate and premature babies. *Paediatr Anaesth*. 2004;14(6):487–492.
143. Aldrink JH, Ma M, Wang W, Caniano DA, Wispe J, Puthoff T. Safety of ketorolac in surgical neonates and infants 0 to 3 months old. *J Pediatr Surg*. 2011;46(6):1081–1085.
144. Rayburn WF. Maternal and fetal effects from substance use. *Clin Perinatol*. 2007;34(4): 559–571, vi.
145. Lipshultz SE, Frassica JJ, Orav EJ. Cardiovascular abnormalities in infants prenatally exposed to cocaine. *J Pediatr*. 1991;118(1):44–51.
146. Hackman PS. Recognizing and understanding the cold-stressed term infant. *Neonatal Netw*. 2001;20(8):35–41.
147. Plattner O, Semsroth M, Sessler DI, Papousek A, Klasen C, Wagner O. Lack of nonshivering thermogenesis in infants anesthetized with fentanyl and propofol. *Anesthesiology*. 1997;86(4):772–777.
148. Ehrenkranz RA, Walsh MC, Vohr BR, et al. National Institutes of Child Health and Human Development Neonatal Research Network. Validation of the National Institutes of Health consensus definition of bronchopulmonary dysplasia. *Pediatrics*. 2005;116(6):1353–1360.
149. Long JB, Fiedorek MC, Oraedu O, Austin TM. Neonatal intensive care unit patients recovering in the post anesthesia care unit: An observational analysis of postextubation complications. *Paediatr Anaesth*. 2019;29(12):1186–1193.
150. Cote CJ, Zaslavsky A, Downes JJ, et al. Postoperative apnea in former preterm infants after inguinal herniorrhaphy. A combined analysis. *Anesthesiology*. 1995;82(4):809–822.
151. Kennedy KA, Fielder AR, Hardy RJ, et al. Reduced lighting does not improve medical outcomes in very low birth weight infants. *J Pediatr*. 2001;139(4):527–531.
152. Reynolds JD, Dobson V, Quinn GE, et al. Evidence-based screening criteria for retinopathy of prematurity: natural history data from the CRYO-ROP and LIGHT-ROP studies. *Arch Ophthalmol*. 2002;120(11):1470–1476.
153. Lloyd J, Askie L, Smith J, et al. Supplemental oxygen for the treatment of prethreshold retinopathy of prematurity. *Cochrane Database Syst Rev*. 2003;2003(2):CD003482.
154. Fredriksson A, Ponten E, Gordh T, Eriksson P. Neonatal exposure to a combination of N-methyl-D-aspartate and gamma-aminobutyric acid type A receptor anesthetic agents potentiates apoptotic neurodegeneration and persistent behavioral deficits. *Anesthesiology*. 2007;107(3):427–436.
155. Soriano SG, Anand KJ. Anesthetics and brain toxicity. *Curr Opin Anaesthesiol*. 2005;18(3): 293–297.
156. Rappaport BA, Suresh S, Hertz S, Evers AS, Orser BA. Anesthetic neurotoxicity–clinical implications of animal models. *N Engl J Med*. 2015;372(9):796–797.
157. McCann ME, de Graaff JC, Dorris L, et al. Neurodevelopmental outcome at 5 years of age after general anaesthesia or awake-regional anaesthesia in infancy (GAS): an international, multicentre, randomised, controlled equivalence trial. *Lancet*. 2019;393(10172):664–677.
158. Flick RP, Katusic SK, Colligan RC, et al. Cognitive and behavioral outcomes after early exposure to anesthesia and surgery. *Pediatrics*. 2011;128(5):e1053–e1061.
159. Stolwijk LJ, Lemmers PM, Harmsen M, et al. Neurodevelopmental outcomes after neonatal surgery for major noncardiac anomalies. *Pediatrics*. 2016;137(2):e20151728.
160. Lin AE, Pober BR, Adatia I. Congenital diaphragmatic hernia and associated cardiovascular malformations: type, frequency, and impact on management. *Am J Med Genet C Semin Med Genet*. 2007;145C(2):201–216.
161. Greenwood RD, Rosenthal A. Cardiovascular malformations associated with tracheoesophageal fistula and esophageal atresia. *Pediatrics*. 1976;57(1):87–91.
162. Harting MT, Lally KP. Surgical management of neonates with congenital diaphragmatic hernia. *Semin Pediatr Surg*. 2007;16(2):109–114.
163. Peralta CF, Jani JC, Van Schoubroeck D, Nicolaides KH, Deprest JA. Fetal lung volume after endoscopic tracheal occlusion in the prediction of postnatal outcome. *Am J Obstetr Gynecol*. 2008;198(1):60:e61–60:e65.
164. Fallon SC, Cass DL, Olutoye OO, et al. Repair of congenital diaphragmatic hernias on Extracorporeal Membrane Oxygenation (ECMO): does early repair improve patient survival? *J Pediatr Surg*. 2013;48(6):1172–1176.
165. West KW, Bengston K, Rescorla FJ, Engle WA, Grosfeld JL. Delayed surgical repair and ECMO improves survival in congenital diaphragmatic hernia. *Ann Surg*. 1992;216(4):454–460; discussion 460–452.
166. Ssemakula N, Stewart DL, Goldsmith LJ, Cook LN, Bond SJ. Survival of patients with congenital diaphragmatic hernia during the ECMO era: an 11-year experience. *J Pediatr Surg*. 1997;32(12):1683–1689.
167. Ng GY, Derry C, Marston L, Choudhury M, Holmes K, Calvert SA. Reduction in ventilator-induced lung injury improves outcome in congenital diaphragmatic hernia? *Pediatr Surg Int*. 2008;24(2):145–150.
168. Rodrigues CJ, Tannuri U, Tannuri AC, Maksoud-Filho J, Rodrigues AJ Jr. Prenatal tracheal ligation or intra-amniotic administration of surfactant or dexamethasone prevents some structural changes in the pulmonary arteries of surgically created diaphragmatic hernia in rabbits. *Rev Hosp Clin Fac Med Sao Paulo*. 2002;57(1):1–8.
169. Fisher JC, Jefferson RA, Arkovitz MS, Stolar CJ. Redefining outcomes in right congenital diaphragmatic hernia. *J Pediatr Surg*. 2008;43(2):373–379.
170. van den Hout L, Sluiter I, Gischler S, et al. Can we improve outcome of congenital diaphragmatic hernia? *Pediatr Surg Int*. 2009;25(9):733–743.
171. Hwang PJ, Kousseff BG. Omphalocele and gastroschisis: an 18-year review study. *Genet Med*. 2004;6(4):232–236.
172. Ledbetter DJ. Gastroschisis and omphalocele. *Surg Clin North Am*. 2006;86(2):249–260, vii.
173. Henrich K, Huemmer HP, Reingruber B, Weber PG. Gastroschisis and omphalocele: treatments and long-term outcomes. *Pediatr Surg Int*. 2008;24(2):167–173.
174. Lee SL, Beyer TD, Kim SS, et al. Initial nonoperative management and delayed closure for treatment of giant omphaloceles. *J Pediatr Surg*. 2006; 41(11):1846–1849.
175. Owen A, Marven S, Jackson L, et al. Experience of bedside preformed silo staged reduction and closure for gastroschisis. *J Pediatr Surg*. 2006; 41(11):1830–1835.
176. Olesevich M, Alexander F, Khan M, Cotman K. Gastroschisis revisited: role of intraoperative measurement of abdominal pressure. *J Pediatr Surg*. 2005; 40(5):789–792.
177. Yaster M, Buck JR, Dudgeon DL, et al. Hemodynamic effects of primary closure of omphalocele/ gastroschisis in human newborns. *Anesthesiology*. 1988;69(1):84–88.
178. Nguyen T, Zainabadi K, Bui T, Emil S, Gelfand D, Nguyen N. Thoracoscopic repair of esophageal atresia and tracheoesophageal fistula: lessons learned. *J Laparoendosc Adv Surg Tech A*. 2006;16(2):174–179.
179. Zani A, Lamas-Pinheiro R, Paraboschi I, et al. Intraoperative acidosis and hypercapnia during thoracoscopic repair of congenital diaphragmatic hernia and esophageal atresia/ tracheoesophageal fistula. *Paediatr Anaesth*. 2017;27(8):841–848.
180. Thompson ME, Haynes B. Ultrasound-guided thoracic paravertebral block catheter experience in 2 neonates. *J Clin Anesth*. 2015;27(6):514–516.
181. Dalla Vecchia LK, Grosfeld JL, West KW, Rescorla FJ, Scherer LR, Engum SA. Intestinal atresia and stenosis: a 25-year experience with 277 cases. *Arch Surg*. 1998;133(5):490–496; discussion 496–497.
182. Cucchiaro G, De Lagausie P, El-Ghonemi A, Nivoche Y. Single-dose caudal anesthesia for major intraabdominal operations in high-risk infants. *Anesth Analg*. 2001;92(6):1439–1441.
183. Welzing L, Roth B. Experience with remifentanil in neonates and infants. *Drugs*. 2006;66(10): 1339–1350.
184. Shaer CM, Chescheir N, Schulkin J. Myelomeningocele: a review of the epidemiology, genetics, risk factors for conception, prenatal diagnosis, and prognosis for affected individuals. *Obstetr Gynecol sur*. 2007;62(7):471–479.
185. McLone DG, Dias MS. The Chiari II malformation: cause and impact. *Child's Nerv Syst*. 2003;19(7–8):540–550.

186. McLone DG. Care of the neonate with a myelomeningocele. *Neurosurg Clin N Am*. 1998;9(1):111–120.

187. Sutton LN. Fetal surgery for neural tube defects. *Best Pract Res Clin Obstet Gynaecol*. 2008;22(1):175–188.

188. Shah S, Cawley M, Gleeson R, O'Connor J, McGeady S. Latex allergy and latex sensitization in children and adolescents with meningomyelocele. *J Allergy Clin Immunol*. 1998;101(6 Pt 1):741–746.

189. Dierdorf SF, McNiece WL, Rao CC, Wolfe TM, Means LJ. Failure of succinylcholine to alter plasma potassium in children with myelomeningocoele. *Anesthesiology*. 1986;64(2):272–273.

190. Sin AH, Rashidi M, Caldito G, Nanda A. Surgical treatment of myelomeningocele: year 2000 hospitalization, outcome, and cost analysis in the US. *Child's Nerv Syst*. 2007;23(10):1125–1127.

191. Lee JS, Polin RA. Treatment and prevention of necrotizing enterocolitis. *Semin Neonatol*. 2003;8(6):449–459.

192. Srinivasan PS, Brandler MD, D'Souza A. Necrotizing enterocolitis. *Clin Perinatol*. 2008;35(1):251–272, x.

193. Catre D, Lopes MF, Madrigal A, Oliveiros B, Viana JS, Cabrita AS. Early mortality after neonatal surgery: analysis of risk factors in an optimized health care system for the surgical newborn. *Rev Bras Epidemiol*. 2013;16(4):943–952.

194. Blakely ML, Lally KP, McDonald S, et al. Postoperative outcomes of extremely low birth-weight infants with necrotizing enterocolitis or isolated intestinal perforation: a prospective cohort study by the NICHD Neonatal Research Network. *Ann Surg*. 2005;241(6):984–989; discussion 989–994.

195. Lau ST, Lee YH, Caty MG. Current management of hernias and hydroceles. *Sem Pediatr Surg*. 2007;16(1):50–57.

196. Craven PD, Badawi N, Henderson-Smart DJ, O'Brien M. Regional (spinal, epidural, caudal) versus general anaesthesia in preterm infants undergoing inguinal herniorrhaphy in early infancy. *Cochrane Database Syst Rev*. 2003;(3):CD003669.

197. Cook-Sather SD, Tulloch HV, Liacouras CA, Schreiner MS. Gastric fluid volume in infants for pyloromyotomy. *Can J Anaesth*. 1997;44(3):278–283.

198. Jacobs JP, Giroud JM, Quintessenza JA, et al. The modern approach to patent ductus arteriosus treatment: complementary roles of video-assisted thoracoscopic surgery and interventional cardiology coil occlusion. *Ann Thorac Surg*. 2003;76(5):1421–1427; discussion 1427–1428.

199. Sathanandam SK, Gutfinger D, O'Brien L, et al. Amplatzer Piccolo Occluder clinical trial for percutaneous closure of the patent ductus arteriosus in patients ≥700 grams. *Catheter Cardiovasc Interv*. 2020;96(6):1 266–1276.

43 Pediatric Anesthesia

SALLY E. RAMPERSAD • BUKOLA OJO • ELIZABETH E. HANSEN • ERICA L. HOLLAND • RACHEL M. FELDMAN • KATHERINE R. GENTRY

KEY POINTS

1. Children with certain syndromes have facial features that can make tracheal intubation and/or mask ventilation difficult. Pediatric anesthesiologists should be familiar with these syndromes.
2. The process of "informed consent" entails obtaining permission from parents/legal guardians and may involve seeking *assent* from the child depending on their capacity to understand and make medical decisions.
3. Perioperative critical events including pulmonary aspiration, respiratory adverse events, cardiovascular instability, malignant hyperthermia, and anaphylaxis can be mitigated with adequate preoperative planning, multidisciplinary care, and use of standardized protocols.
4. The preoperative assessment is critical in optimizing patients and guiding the perioperative plan, including considerations for decreasing airway hyperreactivity, management of upper airway obstruction, anxiolysis, and glycemic control.
5. Management of the difficult airway in children should be approached differently than adults, as awake tracheal intubation is unlikely to be tolerated. Use of video laryngoscopy should be considered for the first attempt.

6 Induction of anesthesia can be achieved by inhalation of anesthetic gasses or IV medications, and care should be taken to make this experience pleasant and atraumatic for pediatric patients, with use of premedication and distraction.

7 We recommend avoidance of nitrous oxide and desflurane due to environmental concerns, as they are potent greenhouse gasses, and safe alternatives exist. Total intravenous anesthesia plus regional anesthesia where appropriate, can provide a superior experience for the patient and are less harmful to the environment.

8 Regional anesthesia (both neuraxial and peripheral nerve techniques) are safe in pediatrics and should be an integral component of multimodal analgesia.

9 Pediatric patients are at increased risk for respiratory complications during induction, emergence, and recovery from anesthesia. Perioperative respiratory adverse events (PRAEs) include bronchospasm, laryngospasm, severe persistent coughing, airway obstruction, apnea, oxygen desaturations, and stridor. The patients at highest risk include neonates, those with a current or recent upper respiratory infection, and those with chronic lung disease.

10 Emergence delirium is more common in the pediatric population. Emergence delirium typically manifests as a period of restlessness, inconsolability, lack of eye contact with caregivers, lack of purposeful activity, and lack of awareness of surroundings. A variety of prevention techniques have been trialed in the pre- and intraoperative phases of care. Dexmedetomidine is often the first-line agent chosen for treatment due to demonstrated efficacy.

Anatomy and Physiology

The anatomy and physiology of the neonate is discussed in Chapter 42, Neonatal Anesthesia. Pharmacology of anesthesia agents in neonates is also discussed in Chapter 42. Many of the attributes of the neonate are still present in the infant and young child and some of the considerations are pertinent to older children too.

Airway

The airway of infants and children is anatomically and physiologically different from the adult airway, and understanding these differences is key to managing the airway safely. Table 43-1 summarizes these differences. Infants and young children, have large heads and the occiput is prominent, such that the child's head will naturally rest in a flexed position and the head may easily fall from side to side. Flexion or overextension of the head can result in an obstructed airway, so care must be taken to maintain a neutral position. Pediatric patients tend to have a relatively large tongue as compared to adults. The jaw thrust maneuver can be very effective at opening the pediatric airway, with care taken to avoid pressure on the soft tissues in the submental triangle. Young infants, like neonates, are obligate nose breathers, or prefer nose breathing, so anything that obstructs the nose, such as secretions or a nasogastric tube, can increase difficulty with ventilation. A common airway problem in infants and young children is upper airway obstruction due to laryngomalacia. In this condition, the supraglottic structures converge on the glottic opening during inspiration blocking or partially blocking air entry through the glottis. The child may have suprasternal and supraclavicular retractions, paradoxical collapse of the chest wall and/or sternum with exaggerated diaphragmatic excursions. Upper airway obstruction in laryngomalacia is often relieved by constant positive airway pressure (CPAP). Laryngomalacia usually resolves with age and without treatment.[1]

1 There are several congenital syndromes that are associated with difficulties with mask ventilation and/or with intubation in pediatric patients. Some, such as Pierre Robin sequence (defined as micrognathia, airway distress in the first 24 to 48 hours after birth, and glossoptosis), improve with age, although in severe cases a surgical airway may be needed. In contrast, other airway anomalies, such as Treacher Collins syndrome (hypoplasia of the zygomatic complex, cheekbones, jaw, palate and mouth, with downward slanting palpebral fissures) become progressively more difficult to manage with age, with both difficulties in mask ventilation and tracheal intubation. The large tongue in Down syndrome and in Beckwith–Wiedemann syndrome can make mask ventilation difficult, as can the facial anomalies that are seen in Crouzon syndrome and Apert syndrome. A full description of all syndromes that affect pediatric patients is beyond the scope of this chapter, but readers are referred to the excellent text by Baum and O'Flaherty[2] which lists all of the important syndromes and their anesthetic considerations.

The infant airway differs from the adult airway in that it is a funnel shape rather than cylindrical (see Fig. 43-1). The cricoid

Table 43-1 Anatomic Features of the Upper Airway in Infants Compared with Adults

Head	Larger occiput in the infant naturally positions the head in the "sniffing" position Stabilize the head against lateral rotation Obligate nose breathers for the first few months
Mouth	Relative large tongue volume in the mouth in the infant reduces the available space for instrumentation Edentulous
Neck	Larynx is more cephalad in the neck (C3–C4) in the infant Epiglottis is omega shaped and longer Vocal cords slant caudally at their insertion in the arytenoids Narrowest part of the upper airway is the cricoid ring (a solid circumferential, cartilaginous structure) covered by pseudostratified columnar epithelium Trachea is short (4–5 cm)
Tracheobronchial tree	Acute angle of the right mainstem bronchus at the carina Turbulent gas flow until the fifth bronchial division (resistance is inversely related to the radius to the fifth power)

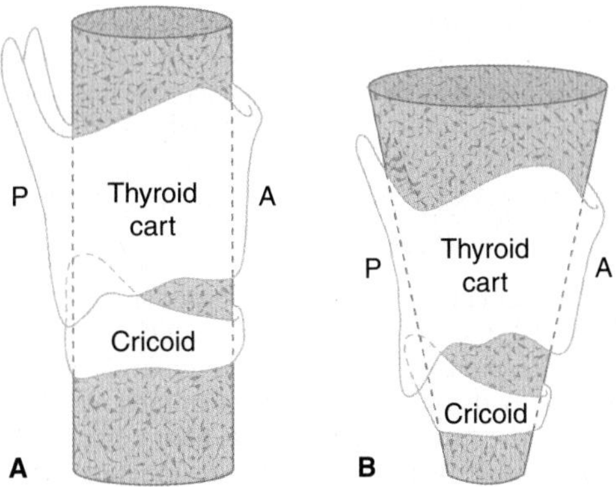

Figure 43-1 Configuration of the adult (**A**) versus the infant (**B**) larynx. The adult larynx has a cylindrical shape. The infant larynx is funnel-shaped because of the narrow, undeveloped cricoid cartilage. A, Anterior; P, Posterior. (Adapted from The pediatric airway, In: Ryan JF, Coté CJ, Todres ID, eds. *A Practice of Anesthesia for Infants and Children*. 2nd ed. Grune & Stratton; 1992:61. Copyright © 1992 Elsevier. With permission.)

ring is the only complete ring of cartilage in the airway and functionally forms the narrowest point. It is covered with pseudostratified, columnar epithelium that is loosely adherent and swells easily with infection or trauma, such as pressure from an endotracheal tube. Using Poiseuille's law, with laminar flow, the resistance to flow through a tube is proportional to the inverse of the 4th power of the radius. With turbulent flow, which may occur in the upper airway, particularly if the child is crying, resistance is even greater, proportional to the inverse of the 5th power of the radius.[3] Therefore, a 50% reduction in the radius of the cricoid ring increases the pressure drop by 32-fold, greatly increasing the work of breathing, which can result in respiratory failure if sustained. Care must therefore be taken to correctly size the endotracheal tube (described later in the chapter), so as not to cause swelling that might manifest as stridor upon removal of the airway device.

Another anatomic feature is the short length of the trachea in the infant and child. Persistent oxygen desaturation may be an indicator of unintentional endobronchial intubation. The physiology and pathophysiology of the respiratory system, described for neonates in Chapter 42, persists in infants and young children. They are prone to oxygen desaturation and to respiratory failure due to the greater alveolar ventilation to functional residual capacity (FRC) ratio in the child (5:1) compared with the adult (1.5:1), as well as increased oxygen consumption in infants and children as compared to adolescents and adults. There is increased compliance of the rib cage (due to both anatomic and physiologic features), reduced compliance of the lungs (due to the relative lack of elastin in the infant), and reduced percent of type 1 fibers (slow-twitch, high oxidative muscle fibers) in the diaphragm predisposing the basal segments of the lungs to atelectasis under the weight of the abdomen.

Cardiovascular

In infants and children, important cardiovascular congenital anomalies can still be a significant factor in anesthesia. For example, right-to-left shunts can slow the speed of mask induction.[4] In the early years, cardiac output is more dependent on heart rate than in the adult due to a limited ability of the pediatric heart to increase stroke volume, due to the ratio of contractile to noncontractile fibers in the heart muscle. Hypotension in the child with a normal or increased heart rate is most often due to hypovolemia

Table 43-2 Normal Range of Resting Heart Rates and Blood Pressure in Children

Age	Heart Rate (beats/min)	Blood Pressure (mmHg)
0–3 mos	100–150	65–85/45–55
3–6 mos	90–120	70–90/50–65
6–12 mos	80–120	80–100/55–65
1–3 yrs	70–110	90–105/55–70
3–6 yrs	65–110	95–110/60–75
6–12 yrs	60–95	100–120/60–75
>12 yrs	55–85	110–135/65–85

Adapted from Bernstein D. History and physical examination. In: Kliegman RM, Stanton BF, Geme JW, et al, eds. *Nelson Textbook of Pediatrics*. 19th ed. Saunders Elsevier; 2011:1529–1536.

and is ideally managed with fluids rather than vasopressors (except in those with congenital heart disease [CHD] and in some forms of shock). Typical heart rates and blood pressures increase with age and are shown in Table 43-2. A useful formula taught in the Pediatric Advanced Life Support (PALS) course, from the American Heart Association, is that for children aged 1 to 10 years of age, the 5th percentile for systolic blood pressures is 70 + 2× age in years and the 50th percentile is 90 + 2× age in years. The 5th percentile is taken as the cutoff for hypotensive shock in the PALS algorithms.[5] Children compensate well for loss of volume and will often keep a normal blood pressure until about 20% of blood volume is lost.

Central Nervous System

Physiology

Oxygen consumption in the brain of children (5.5 mL/100 g/min) is 50% greater than that in adults (3.5 mL/100 g/min)[6] and overall cerebral blood flow (CBF) is 50% to 70% greater than in adults (70 to 110 mL/min/100 g vs. 50 mL/min/100 g) in order to meet that oxygen consumption. Autoregulation is intact in full-term and nonstressed infants.

Neuroapoptosis

Animal studies, suggest that most general anesthetics and sedatives that act on *N*-methyl-D-aspartate (NMDA) or gamma-aminobutyric acid (GABA) receptors, cause apoptosis in newborn rodents and nonhuman primates. Only α-2 agonists, opioids, muscle relaxants, and possibly xenon appear to lack this effect. In animal studies of anesthetic effects on cognitive development, the more agents that were administered and the longer the duration of anesthesia, the worse the cognitive effects. This led to concern that anesthesia could cause apoptosis in humans, and in December 2016, the Federal Drug Administration (FDA) released a statement recommending that anesthesia should be limited for children aged 3 years or younger.[7] Their specific statement was "repeated or lengthy use of general anesthetic and sedation drugs during surgeries or procedures in children younger than 3 yr old or in pregnant women during their third trimester may affect the development of children's brains." Several studies have subsequently sought to replicate and to confirm these findings. A multinational randomized, controlled trial, the GAS study,[8] compared infants of less than

60 weeks' postmenstrual age who were born at more than 26 weeks' gestation and were undergoing inguinal herniorrhaphy, without previous exposure to general anesthesia or risk factors for neurologic injury. Patients were assigned to receive either a general anesthetic or a spinal anesthetic. Neurocognitive tests done at 2 and 5 years did not show any difference in IQ or in learning outcomes between the two groups. In a separate study, siblings who were discordant for anesthesia exposure at age <36 months were also compared and likewise did not show a difference in neurocognitive deficits.[9] In practical terms the FDA's recommendation has meant that some elective surgeries may be delayed until children are aged 3 years or older. However, for the most part the reported human studies are reassuring that brief anesthesia exposure is not harmful to children. More studies are needed to look at patients who have multiple or very prolonged exposures.

Pharmacology

Developmental Pharmacology

Basic pharmacology is covered in chapter 11. There are some important differences in pediatrics. Two major proteins that bind drugs are synthesized in the liver: albumin and α1-acid glycoprotein. The concentration of albumin, which binds acidic drugs, is reduced at birth and in children with liver disease, cancer, nephropathy, and malnutrition. The concentration of α1-acid glycoprotein, which binds basic drugs, such as lidocaine, is also reduced at birth but increases with increasing age, as well as during periods of stress and inflammation.[10] Reduced plasma concentrations of both albumin and α1-acid glycoprotein in neonates and infants leads to an increase in the free fraction of drugs, leading to a greater dose reaching the effect site and exerting physiologic as well as possible toxic effects. For example, the free fraction of lidocaine in young infants is greater than in older children.[10]

Termination of the action of most intravenous (IV) drugs depends on their metabolism through phase 1 reactions (e.g., hydroxylation and oxidation) and/or phase 2 reactions (e.g., glucuronidation) in the liver. The rates at which these enzyme systems mature vary widely among and within individuals. Genetic polymorphisms of several families of enzymes may dramatically affect the activity of each enzyme, resulting in a wide range of activity from zero to rapid and/or excessive. An important example of this is the opioid codeine, which may be very rapidly metabolized to its active metabolite, morphine, in "rapid metabolizers," resulting in excessive sedation and possibly death. Conversely, it may be very slowly metabolized in "slow metabolizers" resulting in lack of effectiveness. For this reason, it is no longer recommended as an analgesic for children and has been removed from the formularies at many institutions. The FDA issued a black box warning for codeine in 2017, stating that codeine and tramadol are no longer recommended for children less than 12 years for age.[11] This warning was an extension of the caution that the FDA had previously released about not using codeine after adenotonsillectomy. Phase 1 reactions are responsible for the majority of drug metabolism in the liver acting via the cytochrome P450 enzyme system. Isozyme systems responsible for phase 1 reactions mature from birth, reaching adult activity levels by 1 to 5 years of age. Phase 2 enzymes, which conjugate drugs and metabolites for excretion, are also immature at birth, which is why bilirubin can reach toxic levels in neonates; however, these systems also mature quickly with age. Termination of the action of many anesthetic drugs depends on either redistribution of the active compound away from the effect site to other vessel-rich organs or muscle, or metabolism in the liver and/orexcretion by the kidneys. Final elimination of the metabolic byproducts and residual active parent compounds depends on renal perfusion and elimination. The glomerular filtration rate is markedly reduced in the neonate and young infant but matures throughout childhood reaching adult rates by 5 to 15 years of age.

Inhalational Anesthetics

Inhalational anesthetics provide rapid onset and offset of action. Correctly dosed, there are limited adverse effects on the cardiovascular and respiratory systems, although children with CHD and also those with certain subtypes of mitochondrial disorders may require more cautious dosing. Halothane has largely disappeared from North American anesthetic practice, having been replaced by sevoflurane as the induction agent of choice for pediatric patients. For further discussion of inhalational agents, the reader is referred to Chapter 18. Although desflurane has favorable pharmacokinetic and in vivo metabolic characteristics (e.g., minimal blood and tissue solubilities and resistance to metabolism), it is not a good induction agent for children due to its propensity to cause airway irritability. Furthermore, desflurane is a potent greenhouse gas due to its persistence in the atmosphere.[12] Pediatric anesthesiologists have a duty to attend to all aspects of children's health and, in the opinion of the authors of this chapter, that means making the best choices to combat climate change. We therefore have chosen to discontinue the use of desflurane completely at our institution.

Pharmacokinetics

The rate at which inhaled anesthetics are washed into the body and become clinically effective is determined by three factors that reflect drug delivery to the lungs: inspired concentration, alveolar ventilation, and FRC. In addition, there are three factors which determine the rate of removal of anesthetic from the lungs: cardiac output, solubility, and the alveolar-to-venous anesthetic partial pressure gradient. The drug fraction in the alveolus (F_A) divided by the fraction in the inspired gas (F_I) is known as the "wash-in ratio" (F_A/F_I). The wash-in ratio increases from 0 toward 1 in the shape of an exponential curve for all inhalational anesthetics. The relative wash-in of the volatile anesthetics is inversely related to their solubility in blood; that is, the lower the solubility in blood, the more rapid the wash-in. For more details on inhaled anesthetics the reader is referred to Chapter 18. The wash-in curve for inhalational anesthetics is characterized by the simple exponential equation

$$F_A/F_I = 1 - e^{-kt}$$

where k is a constant (k = 1/time constant [τ]) and t is time in minutes. τ is the ratio of the volume of the organ to the blood flow to that organ. The smaller the time constant, the more rapidly F_A/F_I equilibrates. The time constants for most organs in children are less than those in adults, explaining in part the rapid equilibration of halothane in children compared with adults (Fig. 43-2).

In the case of infants and children, four factors explain the more rapid wash-in of halothane compared with adults. These factors are (1) greater alveolar ventilation in infants as compared to adults; (2) greater distribution of cardiac output to the vessel rich group in infants as compared to adults; and (3) reduced tissue and (4) reduced blood solubility of inhaled anesthesia agents in infants.

Infants and children have both a greater alveolar ventilation-to-FRC ratio and oxygen demand compared to adults. Increases in alveolar ventilation speed the equilibration of inspired to alveolar

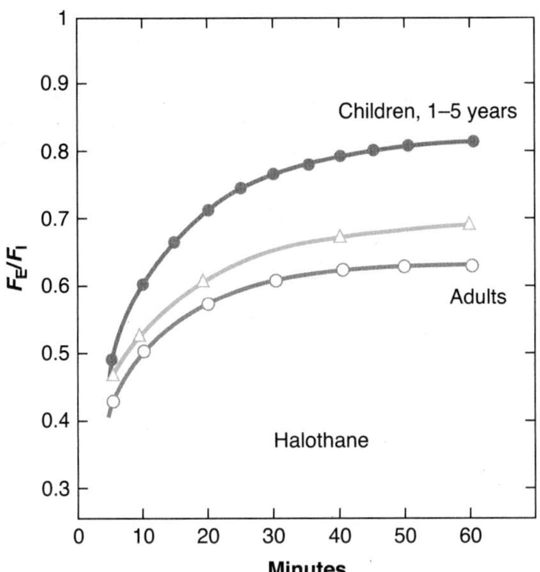

Figure 43-2 The more rapid wash-in of halothane in children compared with adults. The fractional end-tidal to inspired ratio (F_E/F_I) of halothane (*Y*-axis) over time (*X*-axis). The two *lower curves* (with *open symbols*) are from adults. (Adapted with permission from Salanitre E, Rackow H. The pulmonary exchange of nitrous oxide and halothane in infants and children. *Anesthesiology.* 1969;30:391.)

anesthetic partial pressures.[13] Although a greater cardiac output should slow the rate of increase in FA/FI, it actually speeds the equilibration in neonates and infants due to high perfusion of the vessel-rich group (VRG) (comprised of the heart, brain, gastrointestinal (GI) organs, kidneys, and endocrine glands) which comprises 18% of the body's weight in infants compared with only 8% in adults. Hence, the greater cardiac output in infants speeds the equilibration of FA/FI in the VRG, which takes up most of the anesthetic during the first couple of hours of anesthesia. The third factor is the reduced tissue solubility (including brain, muscle, and heart) of all inhalational agents in infants compared with that in adults.[14] The solubility of all inhalational anesthetics is reduced in tissues in infants compared with adults including the brain, muscle, and heart. The fourth factor is the reduced solubility of anesthetic in blood in infants, which speeds the wash-in of inhalational anesthetics.[15]

In contrast to the more soluble anesthetics of the past, the current inhalational anesthetics are much less soluble in both blood and tissues. Because changes in alveolar ventilation and cardiac output affect the wash-in of less soluble anesthetics to a lesser extent than more soluble anesthetics, the wash-in of more modern anesthetics such as sevoflurane and desflurane anesthetics is only marginally more rapid in infants than in adults.

There is safety in maintaining spontaneous ventilation during an inhalational induction of anesthesia. As depth of anesthesia increases, ventilation decreases and slows further uptake of anesthetic. If ventilation is controlled at this time, with the vaporizer setting still high (e.g., 8% for sevoflurane, 5% for halothane), the depth of anesthesia increases quickly, with depressant effects on the heart. This was a noted cause of cardiac arrest in the Pediatric Perioperative Cardiac Arrest (POCA) registry, especially with halothane.[16] Awareness of this issue and a change to the sevoflurane use have reduced its occurrence. Of note, the highest vaporizer setting for sevoflurane (8%) is approximately 4× MAC, whereas the highest setting for halothane (5%) is approximately 7× MAC.

Left-to-right shunts have limited effects on the uptake and distribution of inhalational anesthetics provided the cardiac output is maintained. However, right-to-left shunts present a more complex clinical situation. It is much more difficult to maintain an adequate depth of anesthesia with sevoflurane in infants with significant right-to left shunts—either an intrapulmonary or intracardiac shunt—and supplemental IV anesthesia is often required.

Pharmacodynamics

In children, the minimal alveolar concentration (MAC) of inhalational agents is known to vary substantively with age. As the fetus matures and reaches term, the MAC increases, peaking in infants 1 to 6 months of age, and then decreases steadily thereafter with increasing age (Fig. 43-3). The MAC of halothane is 25% less in children with cognitive dysfunction, especially those taking antiseizure drugs.[17]

Respiration

Airway responses to inhalational anesthetics depend on both the concentration and the particular anesthetic administered. Halothane and sevoflurane infrequently trigger reflex responses, while isoflurane and desflurane are quite irritating to the airway and are not recommended for inhalational induction of anesthesia in infants and children. Hence, in children with asthma, sevoflurane is preferable. In both children and adults with refractory status asthmaticus, inhalational anesthetics have been effective in treating bronchospasm in the intensive care unit.

Cardiovascular

Inhaled anesthetics depress cardiac function in a dose-dependent manner in adults and in children. Halothane is particularly prone to causing brady-dysrhythmias and was often given with an anticholinergic such as atropine. Halothane is also associated with

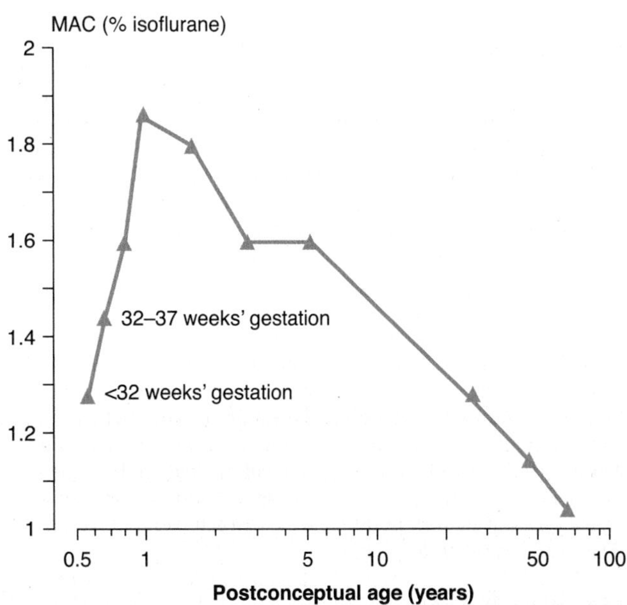

Figure 43-3 Age and the MAC of isoflurane from premature infants to adults. (Adapted with permission from LeDez KM, Lerman J. The minimum alveolar concentration [MAC] of isoflurane in preterm neonates. *Anesthesiology.* 1987;67:301–307.)

ventricular dysrhythmias, particularly in the presence of circulating epinephrine.

Central Nervous System

Autoregulation of CBF in children of all ages is similar to that in adults, although it occurs at greater blood flow rates.[6] The lower limit of autoregulation in children of all ages appears to be similar (mean arterial pressure [MAP] of ~60 mmHg).

Renal

Inhalational anesthetics do not exert substantive effects on the kidneys in children except through their metabolism: the kidney is a site of degradation of inhalational anesthetics. Nephrotoxicity due to inorganic fluoride was a concern with some earlier anesthetics, such as methoxyflurane, but is not a concern with more modern agents.

Hepatic

There are few data regarding the effects of inhalational anesthetics on hepatic function in children. However, isolated cases of hepatic dysfunction in children have been reported after uses of every inhalational anesthetic. Most children who develop hepatic dysfunction recover without further treatment. In the case of halothane hepatitis, serologic markers in the form of antibodies to hepatic cell membrane antigens have been detected. Use of sevoflurane, isoflurane, and desflurane has not generally been associated with hepatic dysfunction and there is no concern about repeated exposures.

In Vitro Metabolism

Degradation of inhalational anesthetics in the presence of carbon dioxide absorbents has been the subject of intense research and concern in both adults and children. Sevoflurane may be degraded via the Cannizzaro reaction in carbon dioxide absorbents. The reaction is accelerated in the presence of increased temperature and barium hydroxide, strong bases (potassium hydroxide), very low fresh gas flow, large sevoflurane concentrations, and desiccated absorbent. The reaction releases five compounds, of which compound A is the most common. Nephrotoxic concentrations of compound A are more than 100 ppm; in children 1 MAC sevoflurane produces 16 ppm after 5.6 MAC hours in a circle circuit with a 2 L/min fresh gas flow.[18] To date, there have been no instances of compound A–induced nephrotoxicity in children.

Intravenous

Like inhalational anesthetics, IV anesthetic drugs are distributed first to the VRG and then to the muscle, vessel-poor, and fat groups. The primary anesthetic effect occurs when an adequate brain concentration is achieved; thereafter, the anesthetic is redistributed to other tissues and metabolized to terminate its action. These anesthetics are described in detail in Chapter 19. This section will focus on agents of particular importance in pediatric anesthesia and important differences between pediatric and adult dosing and indications.

Induction Agents

Propofol

Propofol (diisopropylphenol) is the most commonly used IV induction agent in children. This highly lipophilic drug distributes rapidly to the VRG to effect its anesthetic action. Its action is terminated by redistribution, followed by hepatic and extrahepatic metabolism. To achieve the ~3 mcg/mL blood concentration required for general anesthesia, a 50% greater induction and infusion dosing schedule is required in young children compared to adults.[19] The ED50 and ED90 of propofol necessary to insert a laryngeal mask airway (LMA) in children is 3.5 and 5.4 mg/kg, respectively. The dose of propofol necessary to facilitate tracheal intubation in children during sevoflurane anesthesia is 1 to 2 mg/kg. Propofol is an integral part of total IV anesthesia (TIVA) for maintenance of anesthesia in children undergoing medical/radiologic evaluations and surgery. For painless medical or radiologic (e.g., MRI, radiation therapy) procedures in young children, an initial infusion rate of 15 mg/kg/hr (250 mcg/kg/min) of propofol is recommended after either an inhalational or an IV induction. This dose may have to be increased to stop spontaneous movement, particularly in those with neurocognitive impairment or who are younger. Conversely, the infusion rate may be reduced in older children. Based on pharmacokinetic modeling to maintain a blood concentration of ~3 mcg/mL, the infusion rate is decreased in a stepwise manner during prolonged surgery to facilitate rapid emergence. Target-controlled infusions (TCIs) that use pre-set algorithms are used in Europe, but not in the United States.

Propofol causes pain in 70% or more of patients during IV induction of anesthesia; the pain is greater when it is injected into a small vein. The pain can be lessened by the simultaneous administration of an inhalational agent or by administering IV lidocaine 0.5 to 1 mg/kg prior to the propofol (some advocate using the lidocaine to perform a mini-Bier block). Propofol has profound effects on the airway and respiration. After an induction dose, there is often transient apnea followed by a rapid return of spontaneous respiration. Airway obstruction may occur and is effectively managed with a jaw thrust in most children. Propofol relaxes the upper pharyngeal muscles and facilitates acceptance of an LMA. Propofol is the only anesthetic with effective antiemetic properties and may be used for children with a history of postoperative nausea and vomiting (PONV) and in emetogenic surgeries such as strabismus surgery.

In 1992, Parke et al. reported the potential concern for metabolic acidosis and fatal myocardial failure after propofol infusion in children, now known as propofol infusion syndrome (PRIS).[20] They described five patients admitted for respiratory illness who required tracheal intubation and sedation. In all cases the patients developed a worsening metabolic acidosis, bradycardia and myocardial dysfunction within 5 days that was refractory to resuscitative measures and resulted in death. For this reason, propofol is not recommended as a long-term sedative in pediatric patients. At our institution, propofol infusions are limited to 24 hours in duration. Patients with mitochondrial disorders are particularly sensitive to PRIS at much lower propofol doses and infusion durations; thus, it is recommended that patients with mitochondrial disorders should receive only a single bolus of propofol and that alternative agents should be used to induce and to maintain anesthesia/sedation.[21]

Ketamine

Ketamine is a phencyclidine derivative that offers enormous flexibility in the clinical care of children. This anesthetic can be used as a premedication (oral, nasal, rectal, or intramuscular [IM]), a general anesthetic induction agent (IV or IM), a maintenance agent as an infusion (IV), or as a neuraxial analgesic (caudal/epidural). Clearance of ketamine is reduced in neonates, but reaches adult levels by 6 months of age. Oral ketamine may be used for premedication in a dose of 5 to 6 mg/kg. It may cause nausea and vomiting postoperatively; nightmares are not common by this route. The dose of intranasal ketamine is 3 to 6 mg/kg. Rectal ketamine can result in prolonged duration of recovery due to the larger larger dose requirement (6 to 10 mg/kg) compared to other routes. For IM use, 2 to 5 mg/kg ketamine sedates an uncooperative child in 3 to 5 minutes with a duration of action of 30 to 40 minutes. General anesthesia may be induced with 1 to 2 mg/kg IV, a technique that is useful in children with cyanotic heart disease, septic shock, and conditions in which spontaneous respiration should be preserved, such as the child with an anterior mediastinal mass. Ketamine may also be given as a continuous infusion. It is used occasionally for perioperative analgesia and may be useful as an opioid avoidance strategy in children with obstructive sleep apnea. Preservative-free ketamine has been used for neuraxial analgesia. Side effects associated with ketamine include increased secretions, nystagmus, and nausea/ vomiting. The last effect may occur in up to 33% of children. Nightmares and hallucinations have been reported after ketamine but appear to be very infrequent. Coadministration of midazolam and awakening in a dark, quiet environment may reduce the risk of postoperative nightmares. Ketamine has historically been contraindicated in children with increased intracranial pressure and in those at risk for seizures, although the evidence for both is weak. Ketamine is useful for brief painful procedures where there is a need to preserve airway reflexes, such as sedation for reduction of a fracture in the Emergency Department.

Etomidate

An induction dose of 0.3 mg/kg etomidate IV is recommended in children. Use is typically limited to situations where there is hemodynamic instability due to concerns that it may cause transient adrenal suppression—of particular concern in patients with sepsis or who are critically ill. Like propofol it can also cause pain on injection.

Neuromuscular Blocking Agents

Succinylcholine

The depolarizing muscle relaxant succinylcholine is no longer used routinely to secure the airway of children requiring tracheal intubation. Succinylcholine is comprised of two joined acetylcholine molecules and acts by depolarizing the the neuromuscular endplate. It creates good intubation conditions with rapid onset (30 to 60 seconds) and rapid offset (within 5 minutes) without the need for reversal. The IV dose of succinylcholine is 3 to 4 mg/kg in neonates and infants, 2 mg/kg in children, and 1 mg/kg in adolescents. In contrast, an IM dose of 4 mg/kg paralyzes 100% of children within 1 to 2 minutes, although the duration may be as great as 20 minutes. Sublingual succinylcholine may be given if there is a need for rapid paralysis prior to gaining IV access: the onset is faster than IM, but slower than IV. Side effects associated with succinylcholine include dysrhythmias (particularly bradycardia), rhabdomyolysis with hyperkalemia and myoglobinuria, raised intraocular pressure, fasciculations, and malignant hyperthermia (MH). Succinylcholine causes bradycardia via acetylcholine-associated activation of the vagus nerve. Many anesthesia providers routinely give a dose of 20 mcg/kg of atropine just prior to succinylcholine in order to offset the bradycardia or asystole that can occur with a single dose, particularly in the very young. Rhabdomyolysis is most likely to occur in patients who have MH or who have myopathies. It may also occur in children with, upper and lower motor neuron disorders, burns greater than 24 to 48 old, severe sepsis, and chronic immobilization. It is possible for a myopathy that has not yet been diagnosed to present as an episode of hyperkalemia when succinylcholine is used. MH is described in detail below and in Chapter 24. It can present for the first time in children, who are receiving their first general anesthetic.

Succinylcholine metabolism can be variable, as its action is terminated by pseudocholinesterase (or plasma cholinesterase). There is genetic variation in this enzyme that can result in the duration of paralysis being as short as 5 minutes or as long as several hours. See Chapter 21 for a detailed description of the genetics and testing for this condition. Prolonged paralysis due to genetic variation may present in pediatric patients who are receiving their first general anesthetic. If prolonged paralysis occurs, management involves maintaining sedation and respiratory support until the paralysis resolves, as well as subsequent pseudocholinesterase testing.

Rocuronium

Rocuronium is a steroidal muscle relaxant that is an analog of vecuronium. The IV dose should be adjusted according to the child's age: the ED95 in infants is 0.25 mg/kg and in children is 0.4 mg/kg. In healthy children during sevoflurane anesthesia, 0.3 to 0.4 mg/kg rocuronium provides suitable intubating conditions in 2 to 3 minutes and permits antagonism within 20 minutes. Twice the ED95 (~0.6 mg/kg) provides relaxation in 1 to 1.5 minutes. At 3 to 4 × ED95 (0.9 to 1.2 mg/kg) IV rocuronium yields similar intubating conditions to succinylcholine within 60 seconds and may be used for rapid sequence induction (RSI). The concern that a high dose of rocuronium will lead to paralysis that is not reversible at the end of shorter cases has now been resolved due to the availability of sugammadex (described below). Recovery after rocuronium in infants is prolonged compared with that in children as a result of the reduced clearance and increased volume of distribution.

Cisatracurium

Cisatracurium is one of the 10 isomers of atracurium and has largely supplanted atracurium because it is more potent than atracurium, has more specificity for the receptor and has fewer side effects such as histamine release. It is degraded by Hofmann elimination with a typical duration of action of 30 to 50 minutes. Neither renal nor hepatic dysfunction affects the duration of action of cisatracurium. Side effects associated with the administration of cisatracurium are minimal.

Neostigmine

Neostigmine is an anticholinesterase that prevents the breakdown of acetylcholine at the neuromuscular junction and is the most widely used agent for antagonism of nondepolarizing neuromuscular blockade. It is given with an anticholinergic, usually glycopyrrolate, to balance the bradycardia that occurs (due to the effect of acetylcholine at the nicotinic receptors) if it is given alone. The typical dose in pediatrics is 0.05 mg/kg neostigmine and 0.01 mg/kg glycopyrrolate (or 0.02 mg/kg atropine). It is not effective if given to a patient who still has a high degree of neuromuscular blockade (see Chapter 21). Doses can be repeated if full reversal is not achieved, but care must be taken to avoid exceeding 0.1 mg/kg neostigmine, as acetylcholine-associated weakness may occur.

Sugammadex

This γ-cyclodextrin compound is a cylindrical oligosaccharide that uniquely binds rocuronium (and to a lesser extent vecuronium) to eliminate its neuromuscular blocking activity. It can be administered in the presence of moderate to profound rocuronium-induced neuromuscular blockade and can provide a direct intervention for a "cannot ventilate, cannot intubate" situation. A dose of 16 mg/kg can be used for successful reversal 3 minutes after administration of an intubating dose of rocuronium.

The rocuronium/sugammadex complex is excreted unchanged in the kidney. In children and adolescents, a single dose of 2 mg/kg or more given after partial recovery (two twitches of the train-of-four) from rocuronium yielded a train-of-four ratio of 0.9 in approximately 2 minutes. Experience with sugammadex in pediatrics has greatly increased over the past few years[22] and it is now the default reversal agent at many pediatric institutions in the United States. Because sugammadex is so effective at reversing neuromuscular blockade due to rocuronium, some providers have become less vigilant about monitoring for residual weakness with a twitch monitor, although many would argue that there is still strong evidence that monitoring is necessary.[23,24] It is still the case that a child who is partially reversed will have an increased likelihood of postoperative respiratory events, thus, it is our opinion that monitoring of neuromuscular blockade remains essential. In adolescents, sugammadex reduces the effectiveness of birth control medications for up to a week after its use. It is usual practice to disclose this possibility to patients who are taking, or who could be taking birth control medications.

Opioids and Analgesics

Opioids are discussed in detail in Chapter 20.

Morphine

Perioperative analgesia can usually be accomplished with an intraoperative IV dose of 50 to 100 mcg/kg and postoperative doses of 50 mcg/kg morphine. Perioperative infusions of morphine may also be administered. Morphine may be administered orally and has also been used in the epidural space.

Fentanyl

This semisynthetic opioid is a widely used intraoperative analgesic in children. This very lipid-soluble opioid is bound primarily to α1-acid glycoprotein in blood and has a very rapid onset of action, hemodynamic stability, and brief duration of action after a single dose. It may be used via the IV, IM, oral, intranasal, and caudal/epidural routes. Doses of 1 to 3 mcg/kg IV are often used to attenuate responses to surgery in conjunction with other agents. Much higher doses are used for cardiac surgery, or as a primary agent for surgery in very sick neonates, as it provides very stable hemodynamics. Intranasal dosing can be useful in situations where a child is in pain, but there is difficulty with obtaining IV access.

Meperidine

Doses of 0.25 to 0.5 mg/kg of meperidine are sometimes used for attenuation of shivering; however, it is rarely used in other perioperative settings.

Remifentanil

Remifentanil is a unique μ-receptor opioid that undergoes spontaneous degradation in blood by tissue esterases, with an elimination half-life of approximately 5 minutes that is independent of the duration of infusion. With this brief half-life, remifentanil is usually administered as a continuous infusion. Infusion rates typically range from 0.05 to 0.25 mcg/kg/min, with the dose adjusted according to the presence of concomitant drugs such as inhalational anesthetics. It is often used as one of the agents in a balanced TIVA (e.g., spine fusion). When administered in large doses, remifentanil may cause hypotension, bradycardia, and chest wall rigidity. Prolonged administration has resulted in tachyphylaxis.

Hydromorphone

Hydromorphone is a long-acting opioid analgesic. This μ-opioid receptor agonist is 5- to 10-fold more potent than morphine. Bolus dosing is 10 to 20 mcg/kg IV. It can also be used in IV infusions and in the epidural space. Unlike morphine, hydromorphone does not have metabolites that are sedating or that can accumulate in renal failure, so it is the preferred long-acting opioid for children with renal impairment.

Codeine

Codeine was the mainstay of postoperative analgesia in children for decades, but has fallen out of favor for the reasons discussed above, namely highly variable metabolism that results in unpredictable clinical effects, with the risk of overdose and death.

Alfentanil

Alfentanil is a short-acting, water-soluble opioid related to fentanyl. Its short duration of action makes it suitable for brief, stimulating or painful procedures, such as airway instrumentation or bone marrow aspiration. Boluses of 50 to 100 mcg/kg are often used to attenuate the response to procedural pain or stimulation. Alfentanil can also be given as a continuous infusion.

Acetaminophen

Acetaminophen is a nonsteroidal analgesic and antipyretic. It is an effective analgesic for mild-to-moderate pain in children. Acetaminophen has no anti-inflammatory properties and is also free of platelet inhibiting properties. Oral doses of 10 to 15 mg/kg or rectal doses of 30 to 40 mg/kg yield adequate blood concentrations. Absorption after oral administration is rapid (~10 to 15 minutes) whereas after rectal administration it is slow and variable (1 to 2 hours). With an elimination half-life of 2 to 4 hours after any route, repeat doses may be administered every 4 to 6 hours, while maintaining the maximum 24-hour dose at less than 90 mg/kg.

An IV dose of 10 to 15 mg/kg may be administered every 4 to 6 hours. It is essential that warnings and cross-referencing to all areas of the medication administration record are utilized, because it is easy for a dose of acetaminophen given during a different phase of care, or even at home, to be missed and for a subsequent dose to be given too soon.[25] For example, an oral dose of acetaminophen is given as a premedication before surgery, followed by an IV dose given during the procedure, with a cumulative dose that is excessive and could potentially cause liver damage.

Ketorolac

Ketorolac is a parenteral nonsteroidal anti-inflammatory drug (NSAID) available for use in children. It possesses anti-inflammatory and analgesic properties for mild-to-moderate perioperative pain and, like other NSAIDs, also inhibits platelet adhesion by reducing the synthesis of thromboxane. Ketorolac may be administered in doses of 0.5 to 1 mg/kg, with 0.5 mg/kg (maximum 30 mg) being the most common dose administered to children. The elimination half-life in infants and children is quite variable at 2 to 6 hours.

The side effects of ketorolac have raised concerns limiting its use in the perioperative period. Some surgeons avoid ketorolac during tonsillectomy and adenoidectomy because of the risk of bleeding from COX-2 inhibition of platelet aggregation. Current evidence indicates that ketorolac increases the incidence of bleeding after adenotonsillectomy in adults, but not in children. There is evidence that ketorolac inhibits bone healing in animals, but not in humans; therefore, the anesthesia team and surgeon should reach consensus regarding its use during orthopedic surgery. All NSAIDs may trigger severe bronchoconstriction in asthmatics, thus ketorolac is relatively contraindicated in this population. Rarely, idiosyncratic renal failure has been reported after a single dose, which in most instances resolves spontaneously. Many institutions have protocols where ketorolac is withheld if urine output is low.

Ibuprofen and Other Oral NSAIDs

Ibuprofen is a widely used analgesic, antipyretic, and anti-inflammatory agent in the perioperative period in children. A dose of 10 to 15 mg/kg oral (maximum 2,400 mg/24 hours) is widely prescribed for mild-to-moderate postoperative pain, although some limit its use when postoperative bleeding is anticipated or in patients with renal impairment. Diclofenac, naproxen, and meloxicam have also been used as oral NSAIDs in the perioperative period, with the same precautions and relative contraindications as ketorolac and ibuprofen.

Sedatives

Midazolam

The benzodiazepine midazolam is the most widely used anxiolytic in children in North America. It is water soluble, with a rapid onset of action when administered orally and a brief elimination half-life, making it useful as an oral premedication. Midazolam may be administered by the oral, sublingual, intranasal, IV, IM, and rectal routes. Midazolam is metabolized by CYP450 3A4 enzyme system; this enzyme reaches 30% to 40% of adult levels by 1 month and adult levels by 1 year. The effects of midazolam may be antagonized by IV flumazenil in a dose of 0.01 mg/kg, which may be repeated to a maximum dose of 0.2 mg.

Dexmedetomidine

Dexmedetomidine is an α2-agonist sedative whose relative affinity for α2:α1 receptors is eightfold greater than clonidine. It may be administered via the oral, nasal, IV, IM, and rectal routes. The oral dose, which requires 30 to 60 minutes to provide sedation, is 2 to 4 mcg/kg, with increasing doses being more effective, but with delayed recovery. The intranasal dose is 1 to 2 mcg/kg with 1 mcg/kg sedating ~60% of children within 1 hour. The dose of IV dexmedetomidine may include a loading dose of 1 mcg/kg infused over 10 minutes, followed by an IV infusion of 0.3 to 0.7 mcg/kg/hr. This infusion rate must be carefully transcribed because, unlike other drugs, the infusion rate is in mcg/kg/hr, not mcg/kg/min. When a loading dose is administered before the infusion, the risk of hypotension in the peri-induction period increases, but may be attenuated with fluid loading. The pharmacokinetics of dexmedetomidine in children show a rapid early redistribution phase (half-life of 7 minutes) and a slow terminal elimination (half-life of ~2 hours). Unlike other sedative and anxiolytics, dexmedetomidine exerts its clinical effects via α2 receptors with sedation in the locus coeruleus, and its hemodynamic manifestations via both direct and indirect actions on the sympathetic nervous system. The unique feature of this sedative/anxiolytic is the absence of substantial respiratory depression. It decreases the MAC of inhalational anesthetics approximately 30%, provides suitable sedation for radiologic investigations, facilitates awake fiberoptic intubation and awake craniotomy, provides sedation that is closest to natural sleep, provides analgesia, reduces emergence delirium, and facilitates motor- and sensory-evoked potential monitoring during spine surgery. Side effects of dexmedetomidine relate primarily to its hemodynamic effects. Bradycardia has been reported after larger infusion rates (up to 2 to 3 mcg/kg/hr) and in younger infants, with an incidence as great as 16%. Care should be taken not to treat the bradycardia with glycopyrrolate as profound hypertension may occur. At our institution dexmedetomidine has been used widely in opioid-free protocols as part of a multimodal approach that may include acetaminophen, ketorolac, and/or regional techniques to eliminate opioids for several surgeries, including adenotonsillectomy and some urologic surgeries.[26]

Resuscitation Medications

Epinephrine

Pediatric anesthesiologists often have epinephrine available for emergency use in cardiac arrests or symptomatic unstable bradycardia in a dose of 0.1 mL/kg of 1:10,000 (100 mcg/mL). The drug can also be diluted to 1:100,000 (10 mcg/mL) for incremental use for bronchospasm, hypotension, or in the early phases of an anaphylactic reaction.

Atropine

Atropine is used in doses of 20 mcg/kg to treat or to prevent bradycardia due to vagal stimulation, such as during strabismus surgery with traction on the extraocular muscles. It is given to prevent succinylcholine-associated bradycardia due to its action at the acetylcholine receptor. It may also be used to treat hypoxia-induced bradycardia in conjunction with improving oxygenation.

Preoperative Assessment and Preparation

Informed Consent, Assent, and Parental Permission

Obtaining informed consent for medical or surgical care is fundamental to the ethical practice of medicine. This practice is grounded in the ethical principle of respect for autonomy—that is, a person's right to hold views, to make their own decisions, and to act based upon personal values and beliefs.[27] Legally, however, individuals are not considered to be autonomous agents until they have reached the age of majority—18 years in most U.S. states. In the care of children, therefore, the process of 2
"informed consent" actually entails obtaining permission from parents/legal guardians and may involve seeking *assent* from the child depending on their capacity to understand and make medical decisions. Children vary in their ability to synthesize information and make decisions; in general, children 14 years and older have demonstrated adult-level competence.[27,28] It is generally thought that children 7 to 13 years old are developing decision-making capacity, and that adolescents 14 and older have that capacity. Healthcare providers therefore have an obligation to help children understand their condition and the proposed treatment in a developmentally appropriate manner, and increasingly involve them in decision-making as they mature. There may be times, however, when a child does not assent to treatment that healthcare providers and parents believe to be in the child's best interests. In such cases, the parents' permission generally overrides the child's dissent.[29]

In the pediatric setting, the preanesthesia evaluation and "consent" conversation can be challenging. Consent must be obtained in a short time frame, often upon the first meeting between the anesthesiology provider and the patient and their guardian. Pediatric anesthesiologists aim to achieve a delicate balance of adequately informing parents of risks while simultaneously assuaging anxiety and building rapport with the child, given that in a matter of minutes they will be escorting the child into the operating room.

Generally accepted components of informed consent include a description of the proposed plan; discussion of alternatives, risks, and benefits; assessment of comprehension; and solicitation of a decision.[30] Gentry et al. analyzed preanesthesia conversations for elements of informed consent and found that while the majority of conversations included discussion of the plan and anesthetic risks and benefits, anesthesiologists rarely solicited a parent's decision to proceed.[31] In a recent systematic review, Feinstein et al. identified 22 studies on the topic of informed consent in pediatric anesthesia, noting that most studies focus on parental understanding utilizing self-administered questionnaires, while very few studies focus on the pediatric patient themselves—their preferences, understanding, or refusal to assent.[32]

On rare occasions, parents refuse recommended medical or surgical interventions. While parents are granted wide latitude to make decisions on behalf of their children, their authority is not absolute. When parental refusals of care place a child at significant risk of serious harm, the Harm Principle can help clinicians consider whether state intervention is warranted to override parental authority.[33] In this author's anesthetic practice, the issue that most frequently prompts invoking the Harm Principle is that of parents who are Jehovah's Witnesses who refuse blood products on behalf of their children. While partnering with families to formulate a plan that avoids blood transfusion is ideal, in an emergency situation in which a child would die if they did not receive a blood transfusion, the Harm Principle generally supports providing the transfusion despite parental refusal in order to save the child's life. In so doing, the child can survive in order to reach the age of majority and decide whether or not to adhere to the tenets of the Jehovah's Witness faith.

Fasting Guidelines

Preoperative fasting is a period before a procedure when patients are not to orally ingest liquids or solids. The purpose of this is to reduce the risk of perioperative pulmonary aspiration of gastric contents.[34] Pulmonary aspiration is associated with a spectrum of severe adverse outcomes including acid-associated aspiration pneumonitis, infection, obstruction, respiratory failure, acute respiratory distress syndrome, and death. Ascertaining a patient's fasting status is a crucial part of the preoperative evaluation of a patient's predisposing risk factors for aspiration. Some predisposing risk factors for pulmonary aspiration include, emergency surgery, postinfectious and inflammatory etiologies including norovirus or other viral illnesses, motility disorders (including gastroesophageal reflux, small bowel failure, GI obstruction, achalasia, and diabetes mellitus), trauma, connective tissue disorders like muscular dystrophy and dysautonomia.

Current pediatric fasting guidelines mirror adult guidelines (Table 43-3).

Recent studies in children have shown no significant difference in the incidence of aspiration,[35–37] as well as decreased risk of low blood pressure during anesthesia,[5] when clear fluid fasting is decreased from 2 hours to 1 hour. Using point-of-care ultrasound, gastric emptying times have also been shown to be less than 1 hour for clear fluids.[38] The body of literature supporting decreasing pediatric clear liquid fasting guidelines to 1 hour has resulted in foreign consensus on a 1-hour pediatric clears guideline,[39–41] as well as, change in some U.S. institutional guidelines.[42] U.S. pediatric society guidelines remain as in Table 43-1 as of this writing. The risks and benefits of proceeding with general anesthesia should be weighed in patients who do not meet fasting guidelines. For instance, in emergent cases, mitigating measures may be taken prior to anesthesia. This includes premedication (e.g., nonparticulate antacids or, if there is time, prophylactic proton pump inhibitors) and RSI (described below in induction methods section).

Occasionally, patients may present with gum-chewing. A meta-analysis in adult patients showed statistical but likely nonclinically significant increase in gastric fluid volume and no change in gastric pH in healthy patients who chewed gum preoperatively.[43] Although no studies have been done in children, the decision to proceed with surgery may be made on a case-by-case basis considering a patient's other risk factors and nature of the procedure.

Table 43-3 American Society of Anesthesiologists Preoperative Fasting Guidelines

Fasting Recommendations

Ingested Material	Minimum Fasting Period
• Clear liquids	2 hrs
• Breast milk	4 hrs
• Infant formula	6 hrs
• Nonhuman milk	6 hrs
• Light meal	6 hrs
• Fried foods, fatty foods, or meat	Additional fasting time (e.g., 8 or more hours) may be needed

Practice Guidelines for Preoperative Fasting and the Use of Pharmacologic Agents to Reduce the Risk of Pulmonary Aspiration: Application to Healthy Patients Undergoing Elective Procedures: An Updated Report by the American Society of Anesthesiologists Task Force on Preoperative Fasting and the Use of Pharmacologic Agents to Reduce the Risk of Pulmonary Aspiration. *Anesthesiology*. 2017 Mar;126(3):376–393. Table 1.

Laboratory Testing

Routine preoperative laboratory tests are not recommended. Laboratory and imaging tests should only be performed to optimize specific medical comorbidities and surgery. For example, some tests may help with risk assessment of pediatric neurosurgical patients, complete blood count in patients with malignancies, bleeding disorders, or expected high blood loss surgeries.[44] Similarly, in patients with CHD presenting for elective cases, laboratory tests should be based on clinical presentation and history. Preoperative electrolyte panels and hemoglobin (Hb) A1c levels may modify management in patients with renal failure or diabetes mellitus, respectively. Hematologic tests may be required in infants with certain underlying history, including prematurity, CHD, and previous transfusion. When labs are drawn in infants, efforts should be made to use lab tubes requiring the smallest allowable aliquots. Preoperative hematologic tests should be reviewed in patients with a history of sickle cell disease. Recent recommendations suggest that routine preoperative pregnancy testing may pose more ethical and medicolegal concerns than otherwise. Preoperative pregnancy tests should be offered to patients of child-bearing age with a uterus, for whom the result would change the perioperative management. This test should not be mandatory, and patients should be allowed to make an informed decision.[45] In cases involving adolescent patients, providers should have a conversation with patients separate from their guardians.

Upper Respiratory Tract Infection (URI)

Children with a URI prior to anesthesia have increased airway reactivity and are at high risk of perioperative respiratory adverse events (PRAEs), which include hypoxia, laryngospasm, bronchospasm, increased respiratory secretions, and potentially respiratory failure. In a large multicenter European study of severe perioperative critical events, 6.3% of children presented with a URI within 2 weeks of the procedure and the overall incidence of severe respiratory critical events was 3.1%. These events were most common in infants and preschool children. Inhalational induction and airway management with either a supraglottic airway or endotracheal tube were associated with higher risk of PRAEs.[46] Use of a supraglottic airway instead of an endotracheal tube in patients with a URI decreases the incidence of cough, but does not appear to impact the incidence of major PRAEs.[47] However, in pediatric patients in general, regardless of the presence of URI, supraglottic airways appear to lower the incidence of major PRAEs.[48] Albuterol premedication decreases the incidence of PRAEs in children scheduled for tonsillectomies and should be considered in this population.[49] One risk assessment tool for decision-making on proceeding with anesthesia in patients with URI is the COLDS score which stands for: Current signs and symptoms, Onset of symptoms, Lung disease, Device to be used for airway management, and Surgery type (major or minor, airway vs. non-airway).[50] A large cohort study in Australia found that risks of PRAEs were highest in patients who had symptoms of a URI within the previous 2 weeks, whereas the risks of PRAEs were significantly decreased in patients whose symptoms were present 2 to 4 weeks prior.[51]

Asthma

Asthma is also associated with increased airway reactivity and risk of PRAEs. Preoperative evaluation should include the age of onset, most recent exacerbation, most recent use of bronchodilators or steroids, hospital admissions, emergency department or urgent care visits, recent pulmonary function tests, and physical examination for wheezes. A preoperative pulmonary consultation prior to anesthesia is recommended in patients with severe asthma and may help with postoperative disposition planning. This is especially important in patients scheduled for procedures impacting the respiratory system (e.g., scoliosis surgery) or those with a history of underlying restrictive lung disease. Patients at risk for PRAEs may benefit from an IV propofol induction technique instead of an inhalational induction.[52]

Obstructive Sleep Apnea (OSA)

OSA is the occurrence of prolonged partial upper airway obstruction (hypopnea) and/or intermittent complete obstruction (apnea) during sleep. Symptoms include snoring, breathing pauses, daytime somnolence, night-time enuresis, cognitive deficits, pulmonary hypertension, and cardiac dysfunction. The gold standard for diagnosis is a polysomnography, although many children may not have access to this study. First-line treatment for OSA in patients with adenotonsillar hypertrophy is adenotonsillectomy. This procedure is associated with some morbidity including PRAEs, bleeding, dehydration, PONV, and pain. Postoperative hemorrhage after adenotonsillectomy may be early or late, and is an emergency that may be complicated by difficult airway in a previously straightforward airway, hypotension, aspiration, and need for blood administration. OSA patients should be monitored postoperatively until they can maintain an adequate oxygen saturation on room air and while sleeping. Risk factors for PRAEs that should factor into the decision to admit adenotonsillectomy patients overnight include, age younger than 3 years, severe OSA (defined as an apnea/hypopnea index of >10 on polysomnogram [PSG]),[53] current URI, and comorbidities such as pulmonary hypertension, cardiac abnormalities, obesity, craniofacial anomalies, and neuromuscular disorders.[54] Caution should be taken with sedation and pain management in children with OSA, as chronic intermittent hypoxia increases opioid receptor activation and lowers the requirement for pain medication in OSA patients. OSA patients will therefore benefit from an opioid-sparing anesthetic. Multimodal analgesia may include NSAIDs, which have been shown to be safe perioperatively,[55] acetaminophen, ketamine, and dexmedetomidine. As discussed in the pharmacology section, codeine should not be administered postoperatively in adenotonsillectomy patients.

Prematurity

Prematurity and gestational age <60 weeks are strong risk factors for postoperative apnea in infants. Other factors that increase the risk of apnea include anemia (<12 g/dL Hb) and certain comorbidities (e.g., intraventricular hemorrhage). Low birth weight is also a risk factor for bradycardia and desaturation. Spinal anesthesia, without pre- or intraoperative sedative use, is associated with decreased incidence of early postoperative apnea in preterm neonates scheduled for inguinal hernia repair, but does not affect the incidence of late apnea.[56–58] Given the unclear evidence of the neurodevelopmental impact of certain general anesthetics on neonates and infants, a spinal or regional anesthetic technique should be considered and opioids avoided, to limit the risk of apnea and bradycardia in this population. Caffeine is the first-choice treatment for apnea of prematurity and can be considered during perioperative planning in high-risk patients. Optimal maintenance dosing varies, as different regimens have been reported with no clear optimal dosing.[59] Tachycardia has been reported at higher doses. Given the risk of apnea in former preterm infants receiving a general anesthetic, our institution admits former preterm infants <50 weeks postconceptional age (PCA), although many institutions having a policy of admitting infants <60 weeks PCA.[60]

Malignant Hyperthermia (MH)

MH is a potentially fatal inherited skeletal muscle disorder that results in a hypermetabolic crisis in affected patients exposed to halogenated inhalational agents or succinylcholine. Most MH patients have inherited mutations in the RYR1, STAC3, or CACNA1S genes (Fig. 43-4).[61] A defect in the ryanodine receptor causes excess myoplasmic calcium release when patients are exposed to triggering agents.

Obtaining and verifying a family history of MH is important, as there are few diagnostic centers that perform the gold standard, diagnostic, halothane contracture test. When there is a possible direct family history, MH precautions should be taken per the Malignant Hyperthermia Association of the United States (MHAUS). However, verifying the credibility of the history is key. In some situations, a family member died under anesthesia, but this may have been an older patient undergoing major surgery with a non-anesthesia cause of death. MH cases do not necessarily need to be first case starts, as activated charcoal filters now have a short washout time, achieving a volatile agent concentration of <5 ppm almost instantaneously.[62,63] Consensus (MHAUS) guidelines state that a lack of formal MH susceptibility testing should not limit administration of a general anesthesic. Rather, non–MH triggering agents should be administered and all anesthetic sites should be prepared to recognize and treat an MH crisis. All anesthetic sites should have MH interventions immediately available and accessible including generic dantrolene or Ryanodex (a preparation containing dantrolene that is easier to reconstitute than generic dantrolene). Ryanodex consists of 250 mg of dantrolene/vial, 125 mg of mannitol, and only requires 5 mL of sterile water for dissolution. Trigger-free techniques for patients with suspected MH risk include TIVA agents (e.g., propofol, opioids, dexmedetomidine), nitrous oxide, and local or regional anesthetics. Sensitive

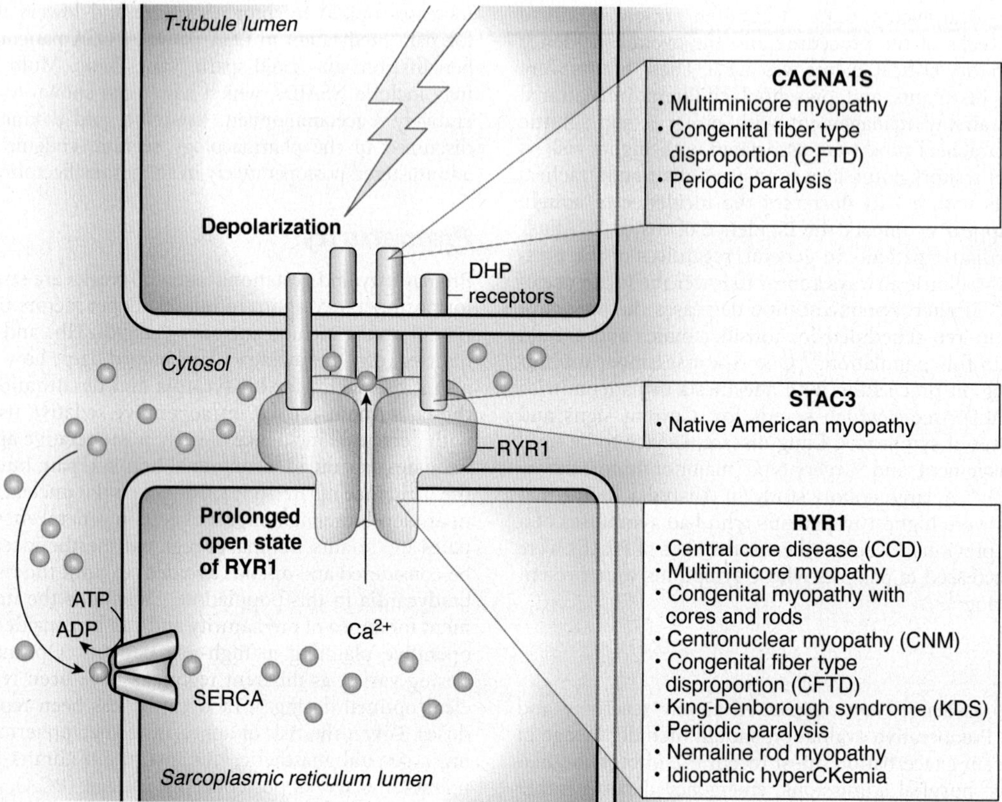

Figure 43-4 Image illustrating the location of mutations in malignant hyperthermia-susceptible patients. (Reprinted with permission from Litman RS, Griggs SM, Dowling JJ, et al. Malignant hyperthermia susceptibility and related diseases. *Anesthesiology*. 2018;128(1):159–167. (Figure 1))

monitors for MH signs include end-tidal CO_2, temperature, and heart rate monitors. MH management priorities are dantrolene administration, hyperventilation, and cooling, the latter of which is secondary to the first two. A Foley catheter should be placed for urine monitoring and serial arterial blood gases obtained to monitor for and manage the associated metabolic acidosis.

Myopathies

Some patients with muscular dystrophies or other myopathies may be predisposed to rhabdomyolysis, requiring careful anesthetic planning. Duchenne's muscular dystrophy is a result of an X-linked recessive mutation in the gene for dystrophin, with typical onset in early childhood and rapid progression of muscular weakness involving the cardiorespiratory system. Patients with Duchenne's may have an MH-like presentation with rhabdomyolysis, hyperthermia, and hyperkalemia, when exposed to MH-triggering agents. The exact mechanism is unclear.[64] The adverse reaction to triggering anesthetics in Duchenne's is mostly acute rhabdomyolysis, while MH is characterized by a hypermetabolic state. Management should therefore involve cessation and avoidance of halogenated agents and succinylcholine, maintaining cardiac output, and hyperkalemia management.[65] A trigger-agent free anesthetic is recommended in these patients.

Mitochondrial Disease

Patients with mitochondrial disease have a genetic disorder that impairs mitochondrial function and manifests as disorders of organs and systems with high-energy requirements, including the neurologic, hepatic, skeletal muscle, and cardiorespiratory systems. Mutations can involve both mitochondrial DNA and nuclear DNA genes. These patients can have significant myopathy and may develop adverse reactions to various medications and anesthetic agents. Metabolic stressors such as fasting, hypo- and hyperglycemia, hypotension, hypothermia, prolonged tourniquet use, and sepsis should be avoided but urgently managed if present, as they can lead to lactic acidosis. Mitochondrial disease patients should undergo careful assessment and planning prior to the procedure that includes a thorough history of baseline exercise capacity, cardiorespiratory, and metabolic status. Anesthetic care should limit fasting times, include IV fluids and maintenance dextrose on patients with a history of lactic acidosis, and avoid Ringers lactate solution. The patient's mitochondrial therapies should be continued in the perioperative period.[66]

Propofol and other drugs with lipid carriers should be avoided or limited as they can impair mitochondrial function. Some patients may tolerate propofol for limited induction and bolus doses, but infusions should be avoided as they can cause PRIS (see above), which is associated with metabolic acidosis and rhabdomyolysis. Patients with PRIS can have elevated levels of creatine kinase, troponin I, myoglobinuria, and respiratory chain (RC) complex IV, as well as a reduced RC cytochrome oxidase ratio. With regard to anesthetic agents, adverse RC complex reactions depend on the specific gene mutation and include the following.[66,67]

- Inhibitors of RC complex I: barbiturates, etomidate, propofol, halothane, isoflurane, bupivacaine, articaine, benzodiazepines
- Inhibitors of RC complex II: propofol, benzodiazepines
- Inhibitors of RC complex III: etomidate (mild), propofol, benzodiazepines
- Inhibitor of RC electron transport: sevoflurane

Slow incremental titration of anesthetics while monitoring anesthetic depth with a processed electroencephalography (EEG) system can be helpful.[66]

Sickle Cell Disease

Sickle cell disease (SCD) is a highly morbid blood disorder caused by a single nucleotide mutation in the gene that codes for the *Beta* globin chain of Hb, resulting in the substitution of the amino acid glutamate by valine. The resulting protein is called hemoglobin S (HbS). SCD is an autosomal recessive disease, thus affected patients typically are homozygous for HbS and are designated as HbSS. In some cases, patients have one HbS gene and another hemoglobinopathy, such as thalassemia. Normal adult Hb is designated HbA and fetal Hb is HbF.

SCD is commonly detected in newborn screening, affecting over 90,000 Americans regardless of ethnicity.[68] Genomic studies indicate that the HbS mutation arose ~7,000 years ago in a region of Africa where malaria was endemic.[69] The mutation has persisted in sub-Saharan Africa and other tropical regions because the carrier state is protective against malaria. Due to the transatlantic slave trade, most patients with SCD in the United States are Black. However, SCD also occurs in non-Black patients. Anesthesiologists should be aware of how racism and bias harm patients with SCD. Disbelieving a patient's reports of pain,[70] prescribing less pain medication,[71] and describing patients negatively[72] are some examples of how racial biases may manifest in the care of SCD patients of color. Approaches reduce the impact of racism in patients with SCD include[73]:

- Universal screening for social determinants of health
- Developing partnerships with patients and staying open to education on the impact of racism on patients' experience
- Avoiding use of stigmatizing language such as the word "sickler"

The anesthetic history for patients with SCD should assess for previous stroke, acute chest syndrome, OSA, hematologic and coagulopathy abnormalities, response to analgesic and sedative medications, functional capacity, and other specific cardiovascular symptoms. Interdisciplinary perioperative planning should include the patient's hematologist, surgeon, and anesthesiologist. The anesthetic plan should include risk mitigation strategies for bleeding, dehydration, infection, respiratory complications, thrombosis, pain, extremes of temperature, acid–base imbalances, hypotension, and atelectasis. Patients with HbSS SCD scheduled for high-risk surgery should undergo red cell exchange (RCE) regardless of Hb level. For low- or moderate-risk surgery, a partial exchange or RCE is recommended if the Hb is >9 g/dL and a simple transfusion, partial exchange, or RCE, if the Hb is <9 g/dL. For such patients receiving hydroxyurea and with an Hb >9 g/dL, no transfusion is recommended for low-risk surgeries.[74]

Other Hematologic Disorders

Patients with personal or family history of bleeding disorders should also undergo interdisciplinary preoperative assessment and planning, including those with factor V Leiden mutation, Von Willebrand disease (phenotype varies by type), or thalassemia.

Anterior Mediastinal Mass

Interdisciplinary care of children with an anterior mediastinal mass allows for prompt diagnosis and a tailored anesthetic approach that considers the patient's symptoms, cardiac, and respiratory anatomy. In patients with concerning findings such as, tracheobronchial compression of >50% or an echocardiogram showing a tamponade or compression of major vessels, or symptoms like orthopnea, general anesthesia should be avoided for biopsy procedures.[75] Sedative agents that are less likely to compromise respiratory drive (e.g., ketamine, dexmedetomidine) or that have reversal agents are prudent choices in these patients.

Subacute Bacterial Endocarditis Prophylaxis

Updated guidelines from the American College of Cardiology and the American Heart Association recommend antibiotic prophylaxis against the development of rheumatic fever in patients scheduled for dental procedures involving gingival tissue manipulation, oral mucosa perforation, or manipulation of the periapical region of the teeth. Patients at highest risk of developing and experiencing adverse outcomes from infective endocarditis, include those with prosthetic cardiac valves or repair materials, patients with previous infective endocarditis, unrepaired cyanotic CHD, repaired CHD with residual leaks, and cardiac transplant patients with an abnormal valve.[76] There is no evidence to support prophylaxis in nondental procedures, including GI or genitourinary procedures, or in previously uninfected patients.

Obesity

Obesity in children is often associated with other medical comorbidities such as upper airway obstruction, OSA, insulin resistance, and gastroesophageal reflux. Children with severe obesity scheduled for tonsillectomy are more likely to have perioperative complications.[77] Obese children may be anesthetized with either IV or inhalational anesthesia, preferably with an opioid-free or -sparing technique using analgesic adjuncts to decrease the risk of apnea or hypopnea in the perioperative period. As with other medical conditions associated with social stigma, anesthesiologists should ensure that children with obesity are not exposed to language or behaviors that incite shame and worsen mental health.

Diabetes Mellitus

Patients with type 1 and type 2 diabetes mellitus should undergo careful perioperative assessment and planning. Perioperative management recommendations of the Diabetes Workgroup of the Society for Pediatric Anesthesia for patients with type 1 diabetes mellitus (DM1) include recommendations for preoperative evaluation, planning, laboratory testing, and insulin/fluid regimens for elective and emergency surgery.[78] DM1 patients ideally should be scheduled for first case starts and their insulin regimen, dosage, and timing, insulin to carbohydrate ratio, correction factor, and glucose targets verified preoperatively. Elective surgeries should be delayed in patients with poor glycemic control until optimization or a sustainable plan is in place. PONV prophylaxis is important in DM1 patients to promote rapid resumption of oral intake and baseline insulin regimen postoperatively.

Patients with type 2 diabetes (DM2) should also have their glycemic control optimized prior to elective procedures and have a perioperative glycemic control protocol in place during procedures. Patients with uncontrolled DM2 are at risk for aspiration due to ileus from neuropathy.

Autism

The preoperative preparation for children with autism deserves special mention. The group Autism Speaks defines autism as "a broad range of conditions characterized by challenges with social skills, repetitive behaviors, speech and nonverbal communication." According to the Centers for Disease Control, autism affects an estimated 1 in 44 children in the United States.[79] Preoperative experiences (e.g., fasting overnight, coming to a hospital, changing into a hospital gown, meeting many new people, and waiting) as well as the clinical environment (e.g., brightly lit, cold rooms, ambient noise of the preoperative area, and a lack of familiar, comforting objects) can be disruptive and stressful to patients with autism. Recent publications have addressed this issue and recommended approaches to facilitate the perioperative care of children with autism including: involve parents early to identify the individual's needs and to establish a plan; adapt the environment to facilitate distraction and self-soothing and encourage families to bring comforting items; minimize unnecessary waiting; customize communication strategies recognizing that children with autism may do better communicating with pictures rather than verbal language; and shift away from a sole focus on sedation or restraint of the combative or uncooperative patient, and instead focus on the factors that lead a child to act in those ways.[80–82] Child-Life specialists can be an invaluable resource for supporting children with autism and anxiety through the entire perioperative experience.

Preoperative History

3 Preoperative evaluation of children should entail a focused and systems-based history because perioperative critical events can be mitigated with adequate preoperative planning, multidisciplinary care, and use of standardized protocols. Selected conditions that warrant additional considerations include.

- Seizure disorder: antiepileptic medication regimen, nature and frequency of seizures, timing of last seizure, rescue dosing, recent liver function tests, disorders involving other organ systems
- Trisomy 21: cervical spine films in patients >3 years old (instability suggested if the atlanto-dens interval is >4 to 5 mm),[83] echocardiograms and previous cardiac surgeries, history of cardiovascular abnormalities, previous airway management, OSA or upper airway obstruction, pulmonary hypertension, hematologic abnormalities, prematurity, cognitive and functional status, and medications.[84]
- CHD: anatomy and physiology of the defect, electrocardiogram (ECG), echocardiograms, recent cardiac catheterization reports, baseline room air oxygen saturation, oxygen needs at baseline, blood pressure in both arms (if not contraindicated), and recent cardiology notes.
- Malignancies: therapeutic history including complications, chemotherapy medications (and associated adverse reactions), history of radiation, blood counts and need for transfusion prior to procedures, electrolytes, medication regimen (including for nausea, pain or mucositis).

Allergies

Perioperative anaphylaxis has been reported to occur in 0.003% of procedural cases, with 11% requiring cardiopulmonary resuscitation, and a 1.6% fatality rate.[85] Severe allergic reactions may require cancellation of the planned procedure. Most common causes of these reactions include antibiotics, neuromuscular blocking agents and reversal agents,[86] and opioids. Other triggers for anaphylactic reactions include latex, protamine, antifibrinolytic agents, dyes, blood products, or products made from animal extracts, such as rabbit thymoglobulin. Although studies have shown low cross-reactivity to cephalosporins in penicillin-allergic patients, the risk of cross-reactivity varies depending on the R1 (C6/C7) side chain similarity. Aminocephalosporins (amoxicillin, ampicillin, cephalexin, cefadroxil, cefprozil, and cefaclor) have the highest risk of cross-reactivity. Cephalosporins with low R1 side chain similarity scores—hence low cross-reactivity—include cefazolin, cefotaxime, ceftriaxone, cefpodoxime, and cefepime.[87] Propofol use in patients allergic to egg or soy is a potential issue because propofol formulations contain egg lecithin (found in egg yolk) and soybean oil. However, there is no current evidence connecting allergies to egg or soy with an allergy to propofol.[88]

Another related reaction is drug hypersensitivity in patients with systemic mastocytosis, a clonal mast cell disorder resulting in proliferation of mast cells in tissues, in particular the skin and bone marrow. Triggers that cause mast cell activation and mediator release may result in pruritus, angioedema, abdominal pain, and anaphylaxis. Exposure to some perioperative drugs such as morphine and NSAIDs may result in anaphylaxis.[89] Like other suspected anaphylactic triggers, a serum tryptase level may be obtained when a drug hypersensitivity reaction is suspected in patients with mastocytosis.

Preoperative Physical Examination

A focused physical examination that includes the airway, cardiac, 4
respiratory, and neurologic examination is necessary before anesthetizing children and can help guide the perioperative plan. For example, abnormal vital signs may suggest potential issues (e.g., bradycardia in a ventriculoperitoneal shunt patient may indicate shunt obstruction, hypertension in a patient with autonomic dysreflexia). A lower-than-expected oxygen saturation may suggest cardiac anomalies, anemia, hypotension, methemoglobinemia, motion, skin dyes, or blue or green fingernail polish. Drug-induced methemoglobinemia may be caused by dapsone, local anesthetics like benzocaine, phenacetin, antimalarial drugs like chloroquine, and smoke. Organ-specific assessments may include:

- Airway: Mallampati score (school-aged children or cooperative younger children), tongue examination, craniofacial anomalies, chin—anterior and profile views, neck range-of-motion.
- Respiratory: abnormal lung sounds may be due to bronchospasm, URI or pneumonia and may require further imaging or pulmonary consultation.
- Cardiovascular: murmurs require a thorough history for cardiac symptoms (e.g., syncope, arrhythmias, tachycardia, or heart failure symptoms such as shortness of breath); new diastolic murmurs warrant a cardiology consultation.
- Piercings, dental hardware, loose teeth.
- Neurologic: Understanding the patient's baseline neurologic status may impact case urgency and postoperative management.

Preoperative Preparation

Anxiolysis

Nonpharmacologic: There is currently no evidence that parental presence at induction reduces children's anxiety; however, parental presence may be helpful to enhance the child's perspective of safety. When parents are less anxious, children are more cooperative. A quiet environment, video games, and related devices have been shown to facilitate anesthetic induction. Music therapy has not been shown to be beneficial.[90]

Pharmacologic: Midazolam is commonly used in oral, IV, or nasal form as a preoperative anxiolytic. Dexmedetomidine has been shown to be a comparable to midazolam[91] and is safe in children with CHD.[92] Some combinations of sedatives can also be effective, including nasal dexmedetomidine and oral ketamine.[93]

Other preoperative considerations include aspiration prophylaxis, bronchodilators for prevention of PRAEs in children with asthma or URI, and airway local anesthetics for anticipated difficult airway in older children needing awake intubation. When blood loss is anticipated, preparations should be made for antifibrinolytic agents, autologous transfusion, and use of intraoperative blood salvage. Perioperative antibiotic choice should be discussed as a team and follow institutional antibiotic stewardship guidelines.

Induction of Anesthesia

Equipment

Checklists can help to ensure that the anesthetizing location is properly and completely prepared. Appropriately sized equipment should be available for each child, including self-inflating Ambu-bag, working anesthesia machine, airway supplies, monitors, suction, IV supplies, fluids, and medications.

Airway Management Supplies

Appropriately sized face masks, oral and nasal airways, laryngoscope blades, tracheal tubes, and supraglottic devices (e.g., LMAs) should be present in all anesthetizing locations. Cushioned face masks that fit the contour of the child's face should be used. Clear masks allow identification of either fluid or solid material in the event of emesis or oral and nasal secretions. Oral airways are often used once the patient is deeply anesthetized to maintain a patent airway in conjunction with a jaw thrust maneuver to sufficiently open the airway during mask ventilation.

Straight, direct laryngoscope blades (Miller, Philips, or Wisconsin) are sometimes preferred for exposing the glottis of infants and small children, although the curved Macintosh blade is most often used in children and can provide a similar view to that of the Miller blade in children 1 month to 2 years of age.[94] Video laryngoscopes have become commonplace in pediatric airway management as both a primary and backup method of visualizing the airway, a teaching tool, as the initial method of exposing the airway in neonates[95] and in COVID-positive patients to reduce exposure of staff to aerosols.[96] Both standard-geometry (similar to the Macintosh blade) and hyperangulated geometry video laryngoscopes are available.

For laryngoscopy, the child is often positioned flat on the table with the head stabilized with a gel ring to prevent lateral movement. A shoulder roll may also be helpful, especially in neonates, to facilitate glottic visualization. In infants and children with limited oxygen reserve or difficult airway, supplying oxygen during laryngoscopy with nasal cannula may delay oxygen desaturation.[97]

Laryngeal Mask Airways

Use of LMAs is common in pediatric anesthesia for surgeries that do not require tracheal intubation and in patients with a low risk of aspiration. In selected pediatric patients, complications with LMAs are infrequent, but can include sore throat, gastric insufflation, aspiration, airway obstruction, large airway leak, laryngospasm, and bronchospasm, many of which can also occur with tracheal intubation.[98]

Several types of LMA exist, each with their own properties and advantages. Sizing for LMAs is typically weight-based, although an LMA will occasionally not seat well in the glottis even (with adjustments in cuff pressure) and need to be replaced with a size larger or smaller. Very small-sized LMAs can be used in neonates.[99] Some LMAs have modifications that allow gastric or esophageal venting, and some can even be used to facilitate intubation with a fiberoptic bronchoscope in a difficult airway.[100]

Endotracheal Tubes

The appropriate size and type of endotracheal tube should be selected based on the child's age and size (Table 43-4). In most pediatric patients, cuffed endotracheal tubes are used, as they allow delivery of more consistent tidal volumes and positive end-expiratory pressure (PEEP), with less leak and ambient contamination of anesthetic gasses. Modern cuffed tubes have high-volume, low-pressure cuffs that exert less pressure on the trachea compared to older versions. Cuff pressure can also be monitored and many modern anesthesia machines can report leak volumes by measuring the difference between delivered and exhaled volumes.

Ensuring the appropriate depth of the endotracheal tube is critical for pediatric patients. In a neonate, the distance between the glottis and the carina is very small, and the ETT may become dislodged or endobronchial with movement of as little as 1 cm. Nasal endotracheal tubes may be used for patients in whom an oral tube is contraindicated due to anatomy or surgical requirements (e.g., dental restoration, oral and craniofacial surgery). Depth of nasal tubes is typically 20% to 30% more than an oral tube. Nasal RAE tubes are curved at a set depth for each size, so must be selected carefully to ensure the tube is long enough to pass into the trachea.

Oral RAE tubes can be used for oral surgery and are commonly used for tonsillectomy and adenoidectomy. Similar to nasal RAE tubes, care must be taken to ensure the bend of the tube is at the appropriate depth to reduce the risk of accidental extubation.

Pediatric anesthesiologists occasionally care for patients with tracheostomy tubes. Cuffed tracheostomy tubes can be left in place for anesthesia if appropriate for the patient and surgery type. Uncuffed tracheostomy tubes are often replaced with a cuffed

Table 43-4 Guidelines for Endotracheal Tube Sizing in Infants and Children.

Age	Uncuffed Size (ID in mm)	Cuffed Size (ID in mm)	Depth (at gums in cm)
Preterm (<1,500 g)	2.5		6–7
Preterm (>1,500 g)	3		7–9
Term	3.5	3	9–10
Neonate–6 months	4	3.5	
0.5–1.5 years		Age (years)/4 + 3	
>2 years	Age (years)/4 + 4	Age (years)/4 + 3.5	Height (cm)/10 + 5

ETT through a mature stoma for the duration of surgery. Some tracheostomy tubes are MRI compatible, but some are not and will need to be replaced for MRI. Consultation with the patient's otolaryngologist may be necessary.

Ventilation Strategies

Historically, pressure-control ventilation was preferred in pediatric anesthesia, both to reduce the risk of high peak pressures causing barotrauma and to avoid issues with the compliance of the breathing circuit when using volume-control settings. However, modern anesthesia machines address these concerns with customizable settings and pressure limits that can maintain a fixed tidal volume down to 15 to 20 mL, and thus can be used for neonates. However, premature infants are often maintained on the neonatal intensive care unit (ICU) ventilators during anesthesia. For more details on neonatal ventilation, please refer to Chapter 42.

Monitors

The American Society of Anesthesiologists (ASA) standards of care for patient monitoring during anesthesia include ECG, blood pressure, pulse oximetry, capnography, and temperature. Additional monitors may be used depending on the patient's medical or anesthetic condition (e.g., depth of anesthesia monitor). Many infants and preschool-aged children do not tolerate the application of monitors while awake, however. Although induction of anesthesia is usually well tolerated and safe in expert hands, effort should be made to apply at least a pulse oximeter before inducing anesthesia. The remaining monitors should be applied as soon as the child loses consciousness. Certain monitors are impractical or unsafe in some settings. For example, conventional ECG monitoring in MRI may pose a risk of burns and is often omitted in children without a history of cardiac disease.

Capnography

Capnography measures the expired carbon dioxide tension and can be used to assess respiratory rate/apnea and anesthetic effects on respiratory drive. Sidestream capnography requires aspiration of gas obtained from the elbow of the circle breathing circuit into a separate analyzer, whereas the mainstream monitoring detects carbon dioxide with an integrated detector in the breathing circuit. Sidestream capnography provides accurate data, even in neonates who have small tidal volumes. Specialized adapters to minimize dead space can be used in neonates and may further improve the accuracy of capnography. In many modern anesthesia machines, the volume used for gas sampling is returned to the circle system, which reduces leak and allows for lower fresh gas flows. Mainstream capnography is rarely used in pediatric anesthesia, particularly in infants and neonates, because it increases dead space, must be fitted at the endotracheal tube/elbow, and is heavy—which can lead to kinking or obstructing of the endotracheal tube. Capnography is also used in sedated patients who are breathing spontaneously through a face mask or through baffled nasal prongs. This noninvasive but accurate technique allows continuous assessment of ventilation in remote sites such as the MRI/CT scanners and radiation oncology.

Temperature

Monitoring of core body temperature can be achieved in a variety of ways, depending on patient factors and the site of surgery. In larger children, a temperature Foley catheter may be placed. Monitoring at the mid-esophagus is ideal, though rectal or nasopharyngeal temperature probes may also be used. If monitoring core temperature is not feasible due to patient anatomy or competition with the surgical site, alternative monitors may be used. Axillary or skin temperature monitoring is more likely to be affected by ambient temperature, is less accurate, and is associated with increased risk of death in MH-susceptible patients.[101] Accurate monitoring of temperature is critical for early detection of MH, fever, and hypothermia. Hypothermia delays emergence from inhalational anesthesia, decreases the rate of metabolism of many medications, and increases risk of surgical site infections.

Heat loss is common during anesthesia, and the large surface area-to-body weight ratio for small pediatric patients makes this process more rapid than in adults. Heat loss occurs through radiation, convection, evaporation, and conduction. The effects of anesthesia promote redistribution of blood from the central core to the periphery, further exacerbating heat loss to the environment. For cases that are expected to last longer than 1 hour or in vulnerable patients, active warming is recommended.

Strategies for active warming include increasing the ambient temperature of the operating room, radiant overhead warming devices, forced-air warmers, and heated mattresses. In neonates and infants, use of radiant warmers and a preheated operating room are especially important. The heater must be placed an appropriate distance from the patient to reduce the risk of burns. Heat loss can be reduced by wrapping exposed areas of the anesthetized child with plastic sheets or blankets, IV fluid warmers, use of low fresh gas flows, and a humidity trap in the breathing circuit. Use of preoperative and intraoperative forced air warmers remains the most important and effective modality. These warmers may predispose to airborne contamination and possible surgical infection, although evidence is conflicting. Many surgeons request the forced air warmer be turned off when the skin is cleaned and resume heating after the surgical drapes are in place.

Active warming in the MRI scanner is challenging, however most patients remain normothermic due to warming effects of the magnet and use of warmed blankets. In infants, active warming may be necessary and can be achieved with MRI compatible portable chemical heaters.

Depth of Anesthetic Monitoring

Awareness under anesthesia has been reported at a rate of 0.0025% to 0.1% in children receiving general anesthesia for elective surgery.[102] The incidence is higher in cardiac and open abdomen procedures. Maintaining adequate depth of anesthesia can be achieved using a minimum, end-tidal, age-adjusted, anesthetic MAC of 0.7, and/or the use of processed EEG monitoring. Various processed EEG monitoring has been widely used in adult anesthesia care, but is unreliable for certain medications and at some stages of development. One such monitor (SedLine, Masimo, Irvine, CA) provides EEG waveforms converted into spectrograms that may be more useful in pediatric patients.[103] Use of these monitors in pediatric anesthesia remains an area of active investigation.

Other Monitors

Invasive blood pressure monitoring is routinely used in pediatric cardiac and transplant surgery, as well as neurosurgical, craniofacial, general, or orthopedic surgery where significant blood loss is expected or there is a need for continuous blood pressure monitoring or frequent blood sampling. Placement of arterial lines in pediatric patients can be challenging, and use of ultrasound has become routine. Catheters must be appropriately sized for the target vessel.

Neuromuscular blockade monitoring is recommended whenever muscle blocking agents are used.[104] Quantitative monitors

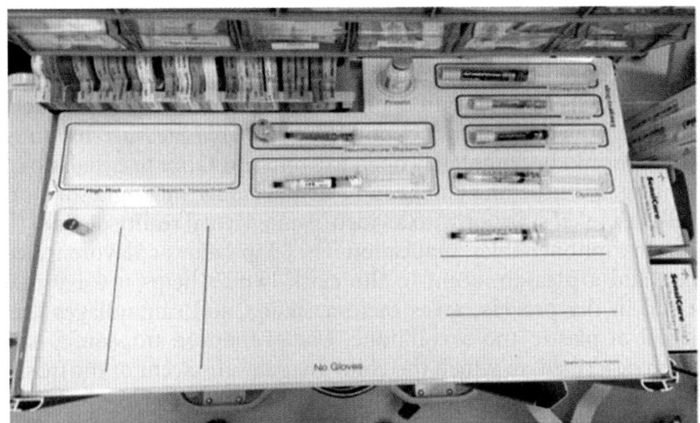

Figure 43-5 Anesthesia medication template showing the overall design. Syringes fit into designated cells in the top half of the template and the lower half is flexible space for other medications and to use as workspace.

have quickly become the gold standard, as qualitative monitoring has been shown to be insensitive and unreliable.[105] Quantitative twitch monitors can be used in children including neonates.[106] Use of sugammadex (see above) is associated with decreased use of monitoring among pediatric anesthesiologists.[24] Residual paralysis contributes to airway obstruction, atelectasis, and increased risk of other postoperative airway complications that may require reintubation.

Emergency Drugs

Emergency drugs should always be available before inducing anesthesia, including propofol, epinephrine, atropine, and succinylcholine. Prefilled syringes are preferred due to their longer duration of stability. Drawing up rarely used medications that are discarded after each case leads to increased cost and waste. However, medications that must be immediately available in an emergency should be well organized and easy to find. Use of a systematic cart top is associated with a reduced error rate in simulated emergencies[107] (Fig. 43-5). Syringes with a small gauge (23G or 25G) needle should be prepared to facilitate intramuscular or sublingual injection, and doses should be precalculated to reduce cognitive load during an emergency. "Code sheets" with prepopulated weight-based doses are invaluable and should accompany the patient in their chart to any anesthetizing location.[108] The Society for Pediatric Anesthesia publishes critical events cards and a smartphone application that can be used as cognitive aids during an emergency.[109] A syringe of propofol (1 to 2 mg/kg) can be used to rapidly increase depth of anesthesia, treat bronchospasm, laryngospasm, or emergence delirium. Vasoactive medications such as epinephrine, ephedrine, and phenylephrine should be available if the patient is critically ill, has CHD, or is undergoing high-risk surgery.

Airway Management—Special Considerations

Full Stomach and Rapid Sequence Induction

The term "full stomach" refers to the presence of residual solid or liquid foods in the stomach at induction of anesthesia, a condition that places the child at risk for regurgitation and aspiration. A full stomach is assumed to be present in children who require emergency surgery and have not waited the appropriate recommended fasting time (see preoperative section above), infants with pyloric stenosis, those with gastric dysmotility syndromes including short gut, and those who display evidence of gastroparesis. A full stomach may also accompany trauma, pain, and stress of the injury, as well as by the administration of opioids that delay gastric emptying.

In patients who have a full stomach, rapid sequence or modified RSI should be considered to reduce the risk of aspiration by securing the airway quickly after consciousness is lost. Preoxygenation is a key component of RSI, although this may be challenging in uncooperative pediatric patients who do not tolerate a mask. Premedication with midazolam or dexmedetomidine can help facilitate mask acceptance. Preoxygenation should begin as soon as possible while monitors are placed and patient positioning occurs, and continue until exhaled oxygen concentration increases to above 90% or oxygen saturation is greater than 97%.[110] Neonates and infants have shorter apneic oxygenation times than older children and adults due to their lower FRC and higher oxygen consumption. Therefore, in the former population the risks and benefits of modified RSI—which involves gentle positive pressure ventilation—should be weighed against the risk of rapid desaturation and multiple attempts at securing the airway when attempting a conventional RSI. One method of modified RSI technique involves gentle low-pressure (10 to 20 cm H_2O) mask ventilation as the muscle relaxant takes effect.[111] In the ultra-modified RSI technique, transnasal humidified rapid insufflation ventilatory exchange can be used.[112]

Cricoid pressure may be applied at the start of induction of anesthesia, although debate remains regarding its usefulness. In infants and children, too much pressure on the anterior neck can obstruct the trachea, as the cricoid ring is softer and more compressible.[113]

Medication choice in pediatric RSI may differ from adult practice; however, the principles of achieving adequate tracheal intubation conditions as quickly as possible are the same. A rapid onset hypnotic medication is given, followed by either rocuronium 1.2 mg/kg or succinylcholine 2 mg/kg for rapid muscle relaxation. As noted above, succinylcholine should be avoided in patients with known or suspected myopathies and MH susceptibility, as rhabdomyolysis and subsequent hyperkalemic cardiac arrest have been noted in such patients. If the risk of aspiration is determined to be greater than the risk of undiagnosed myopathy and the faster onset of succinylcholine is desired, emergency medications must be immediately available: atropine to counteract bradycardic effects, and IV calcium to treat hyperkalemia and cardiac arrhythmias.

Difficult Airway

Updated guidelines for management of the difficult airway were recently published by the ASA.[114] Key points for pediatric practice include: ask for help before you start, use supplemental oxygen during and between attempts, use advanced airway techniques (e.g., video laryngoscopy) for your first attempt, do not persist with failing techniques, do not persist with failing providers, and do not delay emergency front of neck access if you cannot oxygenate.[114]

Complications in patients with a difficult airway are highest among patients under 10 kg, patients who have a short thyromental distance, and when there are more than two attempts at tracheal intubation.[115]

Use of newer technology is common in management of children with a difficult airway.[95] Video laryngoscopes are widely 5 available and should be utilized as an initial method, either alone or in combination with a fiberoptic bronchoscope.[3] The Airtraq device is useful in the pediatric difficult airway patients including those with cervical spine immobility,[116] and has the additional advantage of being portable and battery operated. Tracheal intubation through supraglottic devices has also been achieved with and without the assistance of fiberoptic bronchoscopy.[117]

Lung Isolation

Single-lung ventilation, or lung isolation, may be necessary for certain surgical procedures or patient conditions. Using appropriately sized devices is critical. The smallest-sized double-lumen tube (26Fr) is not small enough for patients under age 8 years. Bronchial blockers can be used intraluminal to the endotracheal tube in larger pediatric patients or extraluminal to the tube in smaller patients.[118–120] Depending on which lung requires isolation, intentional right mainstem intubation can be used for infants, although care should be taken to choose the correct size tube.[121]

Anesthesia for Airway Surgery

Children undergoing airway surgery can be anesthetized with TIVA techniques that include propofol, dexmedetomidine, ketamine, and/or short-acting opioids such as remifentanil or alfentanil. This can provide general anesthesia while preserving native airway and spontaneous ventilation, with supplemental oxygen by nasal cannula or laryngoscope side port. Alternatively, positive pressure by endotracheal tube, jet ventilation, apneic oxygenation are used. The airway should be topicalized with atomized lidocaine, and steroids are often administered to reduce airway swelling. Clear and ongoing communication between the anesthesia and surgical teams will help ensure that appropriate depth of anesthesia is provided, along with adequate ventilation and oxygenation.[122]

Airway surgery occasionally requires the use of cautery or laser. Understanding the fire triad (oxidizer—oxygen or nitrous oxide; fuel—plastic endotracheal tube, instruments, and other commonly used items; and ignition source—laser, cautery, static electricity) and the institutional fire safety plan can reduce the risk of airway fire.

Induction Techniques

In North America, the most common technique for inducing anesthesia in children undergoing elective surgery is an inhala-
6 tional induction with sevoflurane. Many children tolerate this extremely well with preparation by the anesthesia team and child life specialists, distraction methods, parental presence, and/or premedication. Although multiple studies demonstrate that parental presence is not more effective at alleviating parents' or children's anxiety than midazolam or distraction, presence at induction is something many parents desire.[123] Inviting a parent to be present for induction (when deemed to be safe) honors the parent–child relationship and may contribute to family satisfaction with their perioperative experience.[124] If the child had a poor previous experience with anesthesia, it is important to understand the details of that experience and tailor the anesthetic to minimize their anxiety.

The child can be positioned sitting or lying on the operating room table or on the lap of a caregiver for induction of anesthesia. The child or caregiver may have a preference, and it is best to accommodate that whenever feasible and safe.

For a cooperative patient, a pulse oximeter (with more monitors as tolerated) is placed, then a flavored face mask is applied over the mouth and nose with oxygen. The sevoflurane can then be gradually introduced while preparing the child for the new smell. Fresh gas flow should not exceed the patient's minute ventilation, as flows higher than minute ventilation do not speed the onset of anesthesia and contribute to waste of agent.[125] If fresh gas flow exceeds minute ventilation, an open circuit is created, which may be preferred for induction. The adjustable pressure-limiting valve should be completely open to avoid resistance to exhalation. During this time, the child can be distracted by singing a song or telling a joke/ story, or with a video, game, virtual reality device,[126] or smartphone/tablet application.[127,128] Lip balm or flavored oils can add a pleasant scent to the mask, which helps involve the child in the process, gives them a choice, and camouflages the smell of plastic and sevoflurane. Use of induced troposmia has been described, in which the child imagines the scent of the mask will change to their favorite smell.[129]

Sevoflurane can be increased gradually or in one step from 0% to 8%. With low flows, the amount of sevoflurane in the circuit will steadily increase and the smell will be less noticeable. Nitrous oxide had previously been used routinely for inhalation induction due to its ability to speed induction through the second gas effect;[130] whether this translates to a clinically significant difference is unclear.[131] In addition, concerns about its negative environmental impact are leading to a decline in its use. As the child loses consciousness, they are placed supine. If apnea or hypopnea occurs, assisted mask ventilation may be required. Maintaining 8% sevoflurane until IV access has been established may reduce the risk of inadequate anesthetic depth; however, Trisomy 21 patients and cardiac patients may not tolerate this, especially if IV access is not rapidly obtained.

Use of the J-tip (subcutaneous needleless injection device) for local anesthetic infiltration may facilitate more rapid IV placement in a patient undergoing stage 2 of anesthesia, by preventing involuntary withdrawal of the limb. Prioritizing prompt IV access allows additional IV anesthetic medications to be administered to deepen the patient and to facilitate airway management.

If an LMA or endotracheal tube is inserted, confirmation of placement should then occur. Bilateral breath sounds, the presence of a sustained waveform on capnography, and no audible air entry over the upper epigastrium confirm proper placement of the airway device. After inflation of the cuff of the LMA, absence of excessive air leak at 20 cm H_2O confirms proper LMA placement. The inspired concentration of sevoflurane may be reduced to 2% to 3% inspired or maintenance of anesthesia can be transitioned to TIVA (see below).

For older children (usually >6 years of age) who understand how to hold their breath, a single vital capacity breath induction of anesthesia can be considered.[132] With this technique, rapid loss of eyelash reflex occurs. The patient is coached to inhale fully through the mouth, hold their breath, and then exhale to residual volume. This is practiced with the mask prior to induction. The anesthesia breathing circuit should be primed with 8% sevoflurane and oxygen, as use of nitrous oxide is unnecessary and will not increase the speed of induction.

The role of nitrous oxide has been reexamined in recent years. Concerns over safety as well as environmental impact have risen. Waste anesthesia gas exposure is a workplace hazard for operating room personnel as a tight mask seal is impossible to maintain at all times. Operating room workers or patient caregivers may be pregnant and wish to reduce their exposure to nitrous oxide. Nitrous oxide is known to expand in gas-filled spaces such as the inner ear, the cuff of an airway device, bowel gasses, and others. It is a risk factor for PONV, especially if used as part of maintenance of anesthesia. There is concern for adverse outcomes in patients (or staff) with MTHFR or other gene mutations, which may not be immediately apparent. Nitrous oxide may also have
neurotoxic effects in vulnerable patients.[133] Given the worsening 7

climate crisis, many have called for elimination of nitrous oxide use given its high global warming potential and ozone depleting properties.[134] Using nitrous oxide as part of the delivered gas mixture reduces the fraction of inspired oxygen. During the higher risk time of induction of anesthesia, use of 100% oxygen provides additional safety if laryngospasm or bronchospasm occurs.

Intravenous Induction

Establishing IV Access

Some patients may benefit from premedication with oral midazolam, intranasal or oral dexmedetomidine, intramuscular or oral ketamine, or other premedication to help facilitate IV placement. These approaches may be particularly useful for children with MH-susceptibility and myopathies in whom an inhalational anesthetic must be avoided, and in patients with aspiration risk in whom an RSI is to be performed. IV inductions have been shown to have lower incidence of respiratory complications in high-risk patients.[52]

Topical local anesthetic should be applied to the skin to reduce the pain of the IV needle puncture in awake patients. Many formulations exist, including creams, such as eutectic mixture of local anesthetics (EMLA), topical lidocaine cream (LMX), and 4% tetracaine (Ametop), that require 30 to 60 minutes to take effect, and J-tip injections of lidocaine that work rapidly, but are loud and can cause pain or skin trauma in a minority of patients.

Obtaining vascular access is difficult in a subset of pediatric patients. Risk factors for difficult IV placement access include younger age, female sex, darker skin color, obesity, prematurity, end-stage renal disease, CHD, higher ASA physical status, and emergency surgery.[135] Use of ultrasound for vascular access is becoming routine and can decrease the number of attempts.

Once IV access has been established, there are many medications available for induction of anesthesia, including propofol, ketamine, dexmedetomidine, and etomidate (see above).

Propofol is the most widely used IV induction agent. It can cause discomfort when injected into the small peripheral veins of children, and several strategies have been utilized to reduce this. Pretreatment with dexmedetomidine, ketamine, or opioid analgesic 2 to 3 minutes prior to propofol injection can be effective. Some inject lidocaine just prior to propofol or mix lidocaine with propofol. To adequately anesthetize the vein, a modified Bier block is most effective, especially when the IV is in a hand vein.[136]

Propofol is a very safe induction agent for pediatric patients. A bolus injection of propofol causes transient hypopnea or apnea with a minor decrease in heart rate and blood pressure, although this is generally well tolerated in pediatric patients. Teenagers may require a higher dose of propofol on induction, occasionally up to 5 mg/kg. Use of cannabis can increase propofol requirements further.[137] Premedication with dexmedetomidine 2 to 3 minutes prior to administration of propofol has been used to decrease propofol requirements[138] and can be given prior to preoxygenation.

Ketamine is also used for induction of anesthesia, although there are concerns for infrequent postoperative dysphoria or nightmares. It is useful in patients with cardiovascular instability or cyanotic heart disease. Lower doses can be used as part of a balanced anesthetic and for postoperative pain. Dexmedetomidine can be used as a premedication (see above) or in combination with other induction agents. Doses of 0.5 to 1 mcg/kg are well tolerated. Transient bradycardia can be observed. Etomidate is effective for induction of anesthesia and is used in a subset of pediatric patients, including those with cardiovascular instability. Care must be taken regarding the common side effect of adrenal suppression for up to 24 hours after both a single dose and a brief infusion of etomidate (see Chapter 19 for more details).

Problems during Induction of Anesthesia

Hemoglobin Oxygen Desaturation

During induction of anesthesia, airway obstruction, hypoventilation, and apnea can occur. Pulse oximetry should be monitored as soon as possible, as well as clinical observation of breathing and signs of cyanosis. Oxygen desaturation can be due to apnea, atelectasis, or intrapulmonary shunting, in addition to upper airway obstruction, bronchospasm, or laryngospasm. Maintaining a patent airway and delivering 100% oxygen with continuous positive airway pressure (CPAP) typically of 5 to 10 cm H_2O with care to not exceed pressures of 20 cm H_2O. If higher pressures are used, oxygen may insufflate the stomach, which could decrease the ability to ventilate due to increased intra-abdominal pressure.

Laryngospasm

Laryngospasm is a potentially life-threatening complication that occurs in 0.4% to 10% of children during induction and emergence from anesthesia.[139,140] Laryngospasm is the reflex closure of false and true vocal cords resulting in complete airway obstruction. Incomplete laryngospasm is the incomplete closure of the vocal cords through which some air movement can take place, although it is with significant patient effort and inspiratory stridor. Both must be recognized and treated quickly to prevent oxygen desaturation and bradycardia. Clinical signs of laryngospasm include stridor, suprasternal and supraclavicular retractions, and paradoxical chest movements known as "rocking." Loss of capnography and absence of movement of the reservoir bag can also signal laryngospasm.

Risk of laryngospasm is higher in patients with recent URI, who receive inhalational compared to IV anesthesia, and who have inadequate depth of anesthesia during airway management. The risk is lower in patients who are cared for by pediatric anesthesiologists and those with more experience.[140]

Treatment of laryngospasm requires a rapid response that includes applying a well fitted mask with 100% oxygen and continuous positive pressure of 15 to 20 cm H_2O, increasing the depth of anesthesia, typically with IV propofol, and instructing an assistant to call for help. If airway irritation from blood or secretions is suspected, the glottis should be suctioned and the mask quickly repositioned. An assertive jaw thrust should be applied by lifting the mandible anteriorly into the mask, which has the benefit of reducing airway obstruction and providing a painful stimulus to induce crying. Laryngospasm cannot persist when the patient begins to vocalize or cry.

If positive pressure, 100% oxygen, jaw thrust maneuver, and/or deepening the patient with propofol all fail to break the laryngospasm, desaturation and bradycardia may begin to develop. At this point, ensure that help has been called and consider repeating the dose of propofol, administering succinylcholine (1 to 2 mg/kg IV or 4 to 5 mg/kg IM if no IV access), and assessing other etiologies including airway obstruction and bronchospasm.

Bradycardia

Bradycardia is a heart rate below the normal range for age (see physiology section above). Younger pediatric patients do not tolerate bradycardia due to their dependence on rate for cardiac output, and thus it should be promptly evaluated and treated, including initiating CPR per PALS protocols if indicated. The most common causes of bradycardia in children are hypoxia and medications including succinylcholine, dexmedetomidine, sevoflurane (especially in trisomy 21 patients and those with CHD),[141] and halothane.

Treatment depends on the cause and hemodynamic consequences of bradycardia. Removing or decreasing offending agents or improving oxygenation can restore adequate heart rate without pharmacologic treatment. If pharmacologic treatment is needed, atropine, epinephrine, or in certain situations isoproterenol can be given.

Maintenance of Anesthesia

Techniques

Inhalational anesthetics, supplemented with IV analgesics and antiemetics, have been the mainstay of anesthesia for many years. TIVA has emerged as an appealing alternative. Using inhalational anesthetics allows one to continuously measure the end-tidal anesthetic concentrations of inhaled agents. Currently, isoflurane, sevoflurane, and desflurane are used to maintain anesthesia in children; however, many anesthesiologists and hospitals have abandoned use of desflurane given its negative environmental profile and airway irritant properties. The global warming potential of desflurane is 2,540 times that of carbon dioxide over a 100-year period (GWP100).[142,143]

TIVA has become the primary anesthetic technique for children at risk for MH,[144] muscular disorders,[145] those undergoing airway surgery,[122,146] those undergoing spine surgery with motor-evoked potential monitoring, those with a history of severe perioperative nausea and vomiting, and, in some institutions, for all children. Propofol, dexmedetomidine, and ketamine are used in combination as general anesthetics as part of a TIVA. Use of dosing tables or TCI can help guide dosing, but is not approved in the United States.[103] Propofol anesthetics are associated with lower emergence agitation and lower environmental footprint.[142,147–149] Dosing for bolus and infusions of propofol is described above. Use of a dose calculator for propofol can enable an estimate to be made of the total amount that will be needed for the case, thus minimizing medication waste.

Supplemental nonopioid analgesics such as ketamine, dexmedetomidine, acetaminophen, and ketorolac are used during both inhalational and IV anesthesia to prevent physiologic responses and movement to pain. Remifentanil is often administered as an infusion, whereas other opioids (alfentanil, fentanyl, morphine, hydromorphone, and methadone) are commonly administered by IV boluses. Muscle relaxants are necessary in specific surgical or patient situations, although most pediatric anesthetics do not require their use.

Regional anesthesia is safe in children, can be used as part of a balanced anesthetic, and provides excellent postoperative analgesia for many types of surgeries. It is discussed at length below.

Fluid Management

IV fluids are administered for most general anesthetics in pediatrics to maintain normovolemia. However, for short cases, such as tympanostomy tubes, in which an IV is not generally placed, IV fluids are omitted. An appropriately sized bag of fluids is prepared with a graduated buretrol and microdrip tubing for patients under 1 year of age, to minimize the risk of administering more fluids than intended. Care must be taken in premature infants and neonates, in whom use of 10-mL saline flushes after medications can contribute to significant volume administration. Tubing should have a manual controller, a valve to prevent retrograde flow of medications, and a port for IV medication administration. Following strict hand hygiene and using of a separate clean injection port manifold reduces the risk of contamination from "dirty" sections of the anesthesia workspace and has been shown to reduce central line–associated infections.[150]

Crystalloid isotonic balanced salt solutions that do not contain glucose are the standard for IV fluids for most children. These include Ringers lactate, Normosol, Plasmalyte, and Isolyte. For healthy children undergoing ambulatory surgery and in whom fasting time is not prolonged, the goal of replacing a calculated fluid deficit using the traditional "4-2-1 rule" has been largely replaced with providing smaller volumes or maintenance rate of 10 mL/kg/hr or a total of 20 mL/kg for day surgery. With the adoption of Enhanced Recovery After Surgery (ERAS) principles, fluid restricted approaches have become more common. Excess fluid administration is associated with increased complications, impaired recovery, and increased hospital length of stay in children undergoing abdominal surgery.[151] For patients undergoing major surgery with large fluid shifts, insensible losses, or significant bleeding, fluids management is goal-directed to vital signs, urine output, etc.

In patients under age 6 months, those receiving total parenteral nutrition (TPN), continuous feeds, or who have metabolic conditions that predispose them to hypoglycemia, a dextrose containing fluid should be administered as a continuous infusion, with blood glucose checks performed to ensure normoglycemia. Healthy children who have not had prolonged fasting times may become hyperglycemic with administration of glucose containing fluids. Bolus dosing of glucose containing hypotonic fluids is avoided, as it has been associated with adverse events including seizures, cerebral edema, and death. TPN can be continued, although lipids are typically discontinued due to concern for medication incompatibilities.

Monitoring of electrolytes may be necessary for specific patients or surgery types such as craniofacial surgery, which can be associated with hyponatremia. Normal saline contributes to hyperchloremic metabolic acidosis and is no longer routinely used except in specific circumstances. Ringers lactate is avoided for most neurosurgical cases, in patients with renal failure (as it contains potassium), and patients with mitochondrial myopathies who do not process lactate normally.[21]

Albumin is used as a plasma expander in pediatric patients, especially neonates, although evidence that it is superior to crystalloid is lacking.

Blood Transfusion Therapy

Transfusion of blood products in pediatric anesthesia requires careful attention to volume of administration, especially in smaller patients. Blood volume should be estimated (85–90 mL/kg in neonates, 75–80 mL/kg in infants, 70–75 mL/kg in children), and maximum allowable blood loss (MABL) can be calculated using the following formula:

$$\text{MABL} = \text{Estimated Blood Volume} \times (\text{starting hematocrit} - \text{target hematocrit})/\text{starting hematocrit}$$

Target hematocrit is generally chosen between 20% and 25%, though specific patient populations may require a higher target (e.g., preterm infants, term newborns, patients with cyanotic CHD, critically ill patients, patients with SCD). Discussion with the intensivists, cardiac team, and hematologist may be very useful for these special populations. Blood loss up to the MABL may be replaced with crystalloid at a ratio of 3:1 crystalloid to volume of blood loss. If estimated blood loss approaches the MABL, and further bleeding is expected, blood transfusion should be considered. Discussion with the surgical team prior to and during surgery is key to planning for IV access, availability of a blood warmer and blood. If blood loss is anticipated, a cell saver may be employed by the surgical team. Cross-matched blood should be ordered early, to give the blood bank time to obtain the appropriate products, especially in patients who have antibodies that make cross-matching difficult.

Blood volume lost should not be replaced 1:1, but rather to achieve the patient's target hematocrit. It has been estimated that 4 to 5 mL/kg of packed RBCs will increase Hb concentration by 1 g%. If large volumes of blood transfusion are required, a massive transfusion protocol can be used to ensure availability of resources and provision of a balanced transfusion strategy of providing erythrocytes and fresh frozen plasma, platelets and cryoprecipitate.[152] Frequent laboratory evaluations of blood chemistry, hematocrit, and coagulation factors can help guide therapy and detect electrolyte derangements such as hyperkalemia and hypocalcemia. Use of antifibrinolytics to reduce risk of bleeding and laboratory monitoring of coagulation are discussed in Chapter 17.

Prophylaxis for Postoperative Vomiting

Most pediatric patients are at risk for PONV and benefit from routine antiemetic administration and strategies to reduce the use of emetogenic medications. PONV risk is increased in patients with a history of motion sickness, prior PONV, and those undergoing higher-risk surgery (inguinal/orchidopexy, abdominal surgery, tonsillectomy and adenoidectomy, strabismus, and middle ear surgery). Choice of anesthetics can impact PONV risk—volatile anesthetics, nitrous oxide, and opioids all contribute and should be minimized whenever possible. Pain should be controlled primarily without opioids and instead use regional anesthesia when possible. A multimodal approach includes NSAIDs, acetaminophen, dexmedetomidine, and ketamine (see pharmacology section).

Routine use of antiemetic therapy can reduce the rate of PONV significantly. Dexamethasone and ondansetron are considered standard first-line antiemetics for patients over age 2 and without a contraindication to either medication. Dexamethasone should be avoided in most oncology patients, however, especially those at risk of tumor lysis syndrome. Scopolamine patches can be safely used in children over age 10, but must be applied early as the onset of action is 2 to 3 hours. Other antiemetics include diphenhydramine, metoclopramide and aprepitant.

Regional Anesthesia

8 Regional anesthesia is an integral component of multimodal analgesia for postoperative pain management. Regional anesthesia not only improves postoperative pain scores and decreases opioid consumption, but it decreases the surgical stress response, contributes to better wound healing, facilitates earlier return of bowel function, decreases length of stay, and increases patient and family satisfaction. Regional anesthesia can prevent the long-term pathologic responses to pain.[153]

For many years, the caudal block was the mainstay of pediatric regional anesthesia. However, with the increasing availability and efficiency of ultrasound, neuraxial blocks have been progressively replaced by peripheral nerve blocks. The Pediatric Regional Anesthesia Network (PRAN), a multicenter collaborative registry, conducted a review of over 100,000 neuraxial and peripheral blocks in children from 2007 to 2015.[154] The relative proportion of peripheral blocks to neuraxial blocks increased from approximately 25% in 2007 to around 50% in 2015. Similarly, the technology used for peripheral nerve blocks is predominantly ultrasound-guided, compared to nerve stimulator or anatomical landmarks.

Medical Decision Making

Unique to children, in addition to weighing the risks, benefits and the type of surgery, the size of the patient plays a large role when choosing a regional technique. To avoid toxicity, blocks more proximal to nerve origins (epidural or erector spine plane) are sometimes necessary to cover a large number of dermatomes with a small volume of anesthetic.

The pediatric population has a lower risk of perioperative deep vein thrombosis; therefore, lumbar epidurals and bilateral lower extremity peripheral nerve catheters are more common, as early ambulation is not as critical in the immediate postsurgery days. In addition, fewer pediatric patients are on systemic anticoagulation, as compared to adults.

When preparing pediatric patients for regional anesthesia, expectation management is limited or sometimes impossible depending on patient development. Nonetheless, setting realistic expectations with the parents/caregivers is critical to success. Some children, after an initial regional anesthesia experience, decide that they absolutely do not like the feeling of having their body part "asleep" and refuse regional anesthesia for subsequent surgeries. Pediatric patients cannot always express what they are feeling, nor be helpful in evaluation of a block coverage; therefore, the post-operative evaluation and management of regional anesthesia includes using a variety of pain evaluation scales and objective data. It is sometimes possible to test for dermatomal level, even in a neonate, using a glove filled with ice cubes. In areas with a good sensory block the baby will not respond to the coldness of the ice, but they flinch when the ice is touched in areas where sensation is intact.

Pharmacology and Dosing

Age-related changes in hepatic and renal maturity, plasma protein levels, volume of distribution, and cardiac output explain alterations in pharmacokinetics and pharmacodynamics of local anesthetics in children. Neonates and infants are at higher risk than older children for local anesthetic systemic toxicity due to these differences.

Amide local anesthetics (bupivacaine, ropivacaine, levobupivacaine) are metabolized by cytokine P450 enzymes that are immature in infants and children. Intrinsic clearance of amide local anesthetics is one-third that of adults at 1 month of age, and two-thirds at 6 months.[155] Clearance is significantly improved by 2 to 3 years of age, but not reaching full capacity until approximately 8 years of age. Ester local anesthetics, specifically chloroprocaine, are metabolized by plasma pseudocholinesterase and therefore useful as the agent for continuous infusions in neonates.

The primary binding protein of amide local anesthetics is α1-acid glycoprotein. Its plasma levels are exceedingly low at birth, but increase over the first year of life. This results in a higher plasma-free fraction of amide local anesthetics. However, α1-acid glycoprotein is also an acute phase protein, which increases with stress (surgery, infection) negating this effect to a variable degree.

Due to their larger volumes of distribution, peak plasma concentration after a single injection of local anesthetics is decreased in neonates and infants. Repeated injections or continuous infusions, however, will result in drug accumulation.

Children have relatively high baseline heart rates and cardiac output. This results in accelerated vascular absorption of drugs from tissues leading to higher initial plasma concentrations, as well as shorter drug duration.

Overall, ropivacaine and levobupivacaine are less cardiotoxic than bupivacaine, but with similar effect and duration, and are therefore used more commonly in children.[155]

High-level evidence is not yet available to guide dosage of local anesthetics in children, but there are current consensus guidelines according the European and American Societies of Regional Anesthesia.[155] Single injection caudal analgesia is dosed based on the desired dermatomal level of coverage, meaning 0.5 mL/kg for sacral dermatomes, 1 mL/kg to reach lumbar dermatomes, and 1.25 mL/kg to attempt to reach lower thoracic dermatomes. Similarly, loading doses for continuous epidural analgesia are approximately 0.4 to 0.6 mL/kg depending on catheter tip level. For continuous epidural infusions, maximum recommended rates of amide local anesthetics are 0.2 mg/kg/hr in infants less than 3 months of age, 0.3 mg/kg/hr for less than 1 year, and 0.4 mg/kg/hr if greater or equal to 1 year of age. For ester local anesthetics, the respective rates are 0.2 mg/kg/hr, 0.3 mg/kg/hr, and 0.5 mg/kg/hr.

Data for peripheral nerve block dosing are lacking. The location of the block affects systemic absorption and should be considered. Common anesthetics include bupivacaine, levobupivacaine, and ropivacaine. For single injections, suggested doses for upper and lower extremity blocks are 0.5 to 1.5 mg/kg and 0.25 to 0.75 mg/kg for fascial plane blocks.[155] For continuous catheters, using 0.2% ropivacaine or 0.125% bupivacaine, suggested rates are 0.1 to 0.3 mg/kg/hr.[156]

Safety and Complications

In general, blocks peripheral to the neuraxial space pose less risk, supporting the use of peripheral nerve blocks. However, PRAN has demonstrated excellent overall safety for all blocks. In their 2018 review of 100,000 cases of neuraxial and peripheral nerve blocks, there were no cases of permanent neurologic deficit. The rate of transient neurologic deficit was low at 2.4 per 10,000, and the incidence of local anesthesia toxicity was also low at 0.76 per 10,000. There is less risk when performed by specialized pediatric anesthesiologist, especially with patients less than 6 months of age.[154]

The current standard of care for pediatric regional anesthesia is to perform blocks under general anesthesia. This has been shown to be safe without any increased risk.

Regional Techniques—Neuraxial

Spinal Block

Spinal block is infrequently used in pediatrics, with indications primarily in preterm infants and neonates. (See Neonatal Anesthesia, Chapter 42, Spinal anesthesia.) A spinal anesthetic should be considered in infants with difficult airways, those in respiratory distress, or for short, superficial lower abdominal surgeries (commonly the neonatal inguinal hernia repair). Spinals are significantly shorter acting in infants as compared to adults. Bradycardia and hypotension are less common. Babies can be soothed with sucrose and a pacifier, and due to the lack of afferent peripheral input they tend to fall asleep. Unintentional high spinal blockade presents with apnea.

Epidurals (Caudal, Lumbar, and Thoracic)

Epidural analgesia for postoperative pain management is applicable for a broad range of surgeries, from lower extremities to abdominal and thoracic indications. Relative or absolute contraindications include systemic or localized (at the site) infection, concurrent anticoagulation or coagulopathy, central nervous system pathology or neurologic deficits, and previous spinal surgery.

Caudal epidurals remain a useful technique in children less than 2 to 3 years of age but can be successfully performed in children up to 6 to 8 years of age. The sacral hiatus lies between the sacral cornua at the apex of an equilateral triangle with the line between the posterior superior iliac spines forming the base.

A number of needles are available. Caudal, angiocath, or butterfly needles have been described. The needle can be advanced into the sacral hiatus at a 30- to 45-degree angle through the skin and the sacrococcygeal ligament until a "loss" is felt. The needle should be carefully advanced only a few millimeters without resistance. When using an angiocath, the cannula should be threaded into the caudal space. Advancing the needle too far can result in dural puncture. After negative aspiration, incremental injection of local anesthetic (0.1 to 0.2 mL/kg) is administered.

Careful observation of the ECG tracing during injection is critical to detect intravascular injection. Classic signs of toxicity are masked by general anesthesia. ECG changes are an early sign of a positive test dose and include tachycardia and ST segment/T-wave changes.

Ultrasound is increasingly used as a teaching tool to aid caudal placement and may result in higher success rate with fewer complications.[157] Ultrasound can also be used to confirm catheter placement to the lumbar or thoracic level, or to confirm epidural spread of local anesthetic in infants.

Leakage around epidural catheters in infants is a challenge. This is multifactorial—including a shallow epidural space, multiorifice catheters, and the difference between the needle and catheter size.

Regional Techniques—Peripheral

With the advent of ultrasound, peripheral nerve block use has increased.[154] The use of ultrasound has been shown to have faster onset times, decreasing doses requirements, and lower block failure rates.[158] In addition, ultrasound use reduces the risk of vascular puncture and local anesthetic toxicity in peripheral nerve blocks.[159] Peripheral nerve blocks, such as pudendal nerve block, have a longer duration of action than single shot neuraxial (caudal) blocks. In children, peripheral nerve and muscle plane targets tend to be shallow allowing for better definition with high-frequency ultrasound probes.

Various approaches to the brachial plexus have been described for upper limb procedures such as syndactyly or polydactyly, tumor excisions, and upper extremity fractures. For lower extremity procedures, such as hip and pelvic osteotomies for hip dysplasia, tendon lengthening for spasticity, club foot repair, and knee arthroscopic procedures, peripheral nerve block options include lumbar plexus, femoral and lateral femoral cutaneous, adductor canal and sciatic nerve blocks. Sympathetic blockade can be used for vasodilation for arterial spasm or chronic pain syndromes in both the upper and lower limbs.

Truncal nerve blocks are essentially fascial plane blocks, and these nerves can be blocked anywhere from their origins to their terminal branches. Truncal nerve blocks include paraspinal blocks (paravertebral, erector spinae), lateral blocks (serratus anterior, quadratus lumborum, intercostal, transversus abdominal plane) and blocks to the anterior terminal branches (rectus sheath, ilio-inguinal-iliohypogastric). These are indicated for minimally invasive thoracic and abdominal surgeries or for those patients with contraindications to neuraxial blocks.

Common peripheral nerve blocks for cleft lip and palate surgery include suprazygomatic maxillary and infraorbital blocks.

Maxillary blocks are technically difficult and should only be performed by experienced practitioners.

Placing continuous catheters in ambulatory patients is possible and provides safe, high-quality, outpatient pain management when appropriately set up with patient support and education. Typical ambulatory peripheral nerve catheters are kept in place for approximately three days with a predetermined infusion rate of local anesthetic, based on the patient's weight, delivered through a commercial device (such as an elastomeric pump). The patient and family are instructed on how to properly remove the nerve catheter. Since postoperative pain is significantly improved by postoperative day three, the transition off the peripheral nerve catheter is not commonly difficult. It is important to have contact information for the patient and family, in order to communicate with them daily to troubleshoot issues and provided support until catheter removal and expected sensation has returned. It is also necessary to have a qualified person available by pager or phone if a patient with a home catheter needs urgent assistance, most often this is the anesthesiologist or resident on-call.

Emergence and Recovery from Anesthesia

Tracheal Extubation

Tracheal extubation may be performed with the patient deeply anesthetized or awake with return of protective airway reflexes. Each technique has notable risks and benefits. The decision to perform an awake versus deep extubation is based on provider comfort and experience, patient-specific factors such as aspiration risk, and procedure-specific factors as explained below. Nursing experience level and staffing in the postanesthesia care unit (PACU) may also be a factor.

An awake extubation is performed when the patient has return of protective airway reflexes. Various criteria are used to determine readiness for awake extubation. Depending on age and developmental status, following commands may not be attainable in the pediatric population. For patients under 7 years old without a difficult airway who have undergone a volatile-based anesthetic, the following five features have been significantly associated with tracheal extubation success:

1. conjugate gaze
2. facial grimace
3. eye opening
4. purposeful movement, and
5. tidal volume greater than 5 mL/kg[160]

Importantly, there is a direct correlation between tracheal extubation success and number of predictors present, such that extubation success increases from 88.3% with one predictor present to 100% with five predictors present.[160] Conversely, factors associated with an unsuccessful extubation include:

1. URI within 7 days of the procedure
2. premedication with midazolam in patients over one year old, and
3. end-tidal carbon dioxide ($ETCO_2$) greater than 55 mmHg.[160]

Successful tracheal extubation does not have a universal definition but may be defined as

1. lack of oxygen desaturation below 92% or desaturation below 92% for <30 seconds and
2. patient requiring CPAP with 100% oxygen for <30 seconds.

Extensive literature exists on predictors of successful tracheal extubation in ICU patients, in whom other cardiopulmonary data (such as level of ventilatory support) are more likely to impact longer-term extubation success.

MAC values are also an important consideration for determining readiness for tracheal extubation, but caution must be taken because end-tidal volatile anesthetic concentration does not necessarily equate to the concentration of volatile anesthetic in the brain.[161] Like other age-dependent MAC values (see above), MAC-awake values change with age, generally increasing until 6 months of age and then decreasing with older age. Some providers employ the "no touch" technique, in which the patient is not stimulated during emergence until the end-tidal concentration of volatile anesthetic reaches a certain threshold (i.e., 0.2% sevoflurane) whereas others will directly stimulate the patient at slightly higher MAC values to assess for specific signs of extubation readiness.

A deep tracheal extubation is performed with the patient deeply anesthetized, often with the intention of facilitating a smoother emergence. Since coughing is less likely to occur in patients who are extubated deep, patients are less likely to experience hypertension, tachycardia, and increased intracranial pressure.[162] This may result in a decreased risk of postoperative bleeding, particularly for intracranial surgery. Intraocular pressure is less likely to rise during a deep extubation, which may be desirable for patients who have undergone intraocular procedures. Decreased coughing may also lead to less airway irritation, which can decrease the risk for postoperative hoarseness and secretions.

For a deep extubation, the patient should be in deep plane of anesthesia and should have adequate oxygenation and ventilation on minimal ventilator settings. Contraindications include inadequate training of PACU staff to manage deeply anesthetized patients, presence of copious oral secretions or bleeding, high risk for pulmonary aspiration, difficult airway, OSA, or significant airway obstruction during induction.

To perform a deep tracheal extubation, the oropharynx is cleared with suctioning. Various tests such as deep suctioning or jaw thrust are performed to ensure the patient is under an adequate depth of anesthesia. The patient should not demonstrate any response to stimulation, such as movement or sustained apnea. After adequate spontaneous ventilation is confirmed, the patient is preoxygenated with 100% FIO_2 before endotracheal tube removal. Due to the risk for airway obstruction, some providers will choose to insert an oral airway or nasal trumpet, assuming no contraindications, for every patient that is extubated deep. Others will elect to insert an adjunctive airway only if there is evidence of obstruction and inadequate ventilation with a natural airway, since airway placement has the potential to precipitate laryngospasm, coughing, and breath holding with emergence.[163] The anesthetic is turned off as soon as adequate ventilation has been demonstrated.

In general, pediatric patients are at increased risk for postextubation respiratory complications including hypoxia due to increased oxygen consumption from increased metabolic rate, immature alveolar development, and increased dead space (see above).[162] An important consideration with either technique is that the patient should not be in stage 2 of anesthesia, the excitatory phase of emergence, when the endotracheal tube is removed. Extubation during stage 2 places the patient at risk for breath holding, laryngospasm, upper airway obstruction, and aspiration. Deep extubation has been associated with a decreased incidence of cough and desaturation as compared to awake extubation, but an increased risk of airway obstruction.[162]

Tracheal extubation may occur in either the operating room or PACU, depending on institutional practices and provider

Table 43-5 Causes of Delayed Emergence from Anesthesia in Children

Cause	Investigation/Intervention
Anesthetic-related	
Residual anesthetic effects: Inhalational anesthetics, opioids, propofol	• End-tidal concentration • Evaluate total drug dose
Nonanesthesia medications: Recreational drug use (cocaine, crack), herbal medicines (valerian, St. John wort)	• History; drug toxicology screen
Depressed neuromuscular junction, residual neuromuscular blockade, or pseudocholinesterase deficiency	• Assess train-of-four
Hypothermia	• Measure the child's temperature. • Introduce heating modalities as indicated (e.g., forced air warmer, heat operating room)
Severe hypercapnia (minimum alveolar concentration CO_2 ~200–245 mmHg)	• Blood gas and end-tidal CO_2
Metabolic/other	
Hypo or hyperglycemia; diabetic ketoacidosis	• Measure blood glucose, urinary glucose, and ketones • Arterial blood gas and electrolytes for pH and anion gap
Electrolyte and metabolic disorder	• Serum electrolytes (e.g., hyponatremia, hypomagnesemia)
Acid–base disturbance	• Blood gas analysis (anion gap or non-anion gap acidosis)
Encephalopathy	• Hepatic, renal, endocrinopathy (e.g., hypothyroidism, Addison disease), or sepsis • Blood gas analysis, electrolytes, and blood cultures if indicated
Cerebrovascular accident/hypoxic-insult	• Check bilateral pupil size • Check responsiveness to light and pain stimulus bilaterally • Assess the presence of a gag reflex, symmetrical limb reflexes • Assess the fontanelle pressure in infants

judgment. If the patient has been demonstrated to have a difficult airway, extubation is likely to be safer in the operating room with appropriate personnel and difficult airway equipment immediately available. Similarly, for a patient who remains at risk for pulmonary aspiration, it may be most prudent to remain in the operating room so that the airway can quickly and safely be resecured if necessary. Extubation in the PACU, particularly deep extubation, requires that appropriate rescue supplies are available and PACU staff are comfortable with airway management.

LMA Removal

LMA removal may also be performed with the patient deeply anesthetized or awake. The incidence of respiratory complications with deep versus awake LMA removal mirrors that associated with deep versus awake endotracheal tube removal. In the absence of contraindications, deep LMA removal may decrease the risk of certain airway complications including cough and desaturation, but may increase the risk of airway obstruction.[162]

Delayed Emergence

Causes of delayed emergence are similar in pediatric and adult patients, although unique considerations exist in the pediatric population. Due to the wide distribution of body weights in the pediatric population, there is risk for drug dosing errors. Teenage patients may be hesitant to disclose recreational drug use in the presence of parents or guardians. Neonates, particularly premature neonates, are prone to hypothermia and hypoglycemia.

With delayed emergence, a comprehensive assessment of potential anesthetic, metabolic, and neurologic causes should include those listed in Table 43-5.

Evaluation typically includes:

1. assessment of vital signs and end-tidal volatile concentration,
2. review and verification of medications given,
3. train-of-four assessment,
4. blood gas, glucose, and electrolyte measurement, and
5. neurologic examination.

Tests for liver or kidney function may be indicated based on the clinical scenario. Imaging such as head CT may be indicated if these investigations fail to provide a suspected cause for the delayed emergence.

Transport to PACU

Transport from the operating room to PACU represents a particularly high-risk portion of the anesthetic. Providers may fail to recognize apnea or airway obstruction due to distraction caused by competing tasks and lack of monitoring equipment. Wake Up Safe (a Pediatric Anesthesia Quality Improvement Initiative in the United States) has described inadequate monitoring during transport to the PACU as a recurrent factor contributing to pediatric cardiac arrest in the PACU.[164] The absence of rescue airway equipment may lead to delays in treatment even when respiratory complications are detected during transport.

Prior to exiting the operating room, adequate hemodynamics, airway patency, oxygenation, ventilation, and pain control should be established. Patients should be accompanied by a provider who is comfortable managing the pediatric airway. Clinical signs

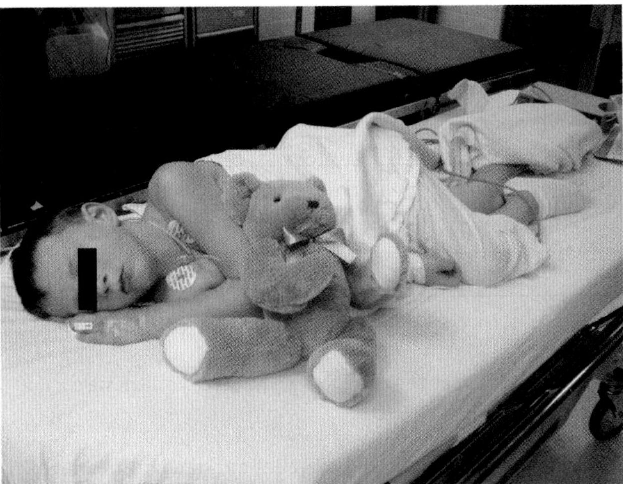

Figure 43-6 Position of the child after tracheal extubation in preparation for transfer to PACU and the pediatric ICU. This is known as the "recovery position" with the child lying in the lateral decubitus position, neck extended, and mouth opened. In this position, oropharyngeal secretions, blood, or vomitus will drain onto the mattress rather than collect in the parapharyngeal region and trigger upper airway reflex responses.

and symptoms may not be apparent in patients with borderline oxygenation until severe hypoxia is present.[165] Routine use of monitors including pulse oximetry is not the standard at all institutions but should be considered for high-risk patients or longer transport routes from other anesthetizing locations. Patients are often transported with supplemental oxygen in the form of nasal cannula or blowby with a Mapleson circuit, although this is not necessarily required for low-risk patients who have already demonstrated adequate spontaneous ventilation and oxygenation on room air.

Patient positioning should be optimized for airway patency during transport. A shoulder roll may be effective at preventing or relieving airway obstruction, but supporting the airway with a jaw thrust, chin lift, and/or CPAP may continue to be necessary to maintain airway patency. Alternatively, lateral positioning has been shown to improve the success of jaw thrust and chin lift maneuvers to relieve airway obstruction in post tonsillectomy pediatric patients.[163] The lateral position also facilitates drainage of secretions and can decrease the chance of pulmonary aspiration if the patient has an episode of emesis. The recovery position is pictured and described in Figure 43-6.

PACU Complications

Respiratory Complications

Perioperative Respiratory Adverse Events (PRAEs)

9 PRAEs are a common cause of morbidity and mortality in pediatric anesthesia. PRAEs include:

1. bronchospasm
2. laryngospasm
3. severe persistent coughing
4. airway obstruction
5. apnea
6. oxygen desaturations, and
7. stridor.[166]

PRAEs are most common during induction, emergence, and recovery.[166] They are responsible for approximately half of the cardiac arrests that occur during emergence and recovery from anesthesia.[5] Up to 10% of pediatric patients in the PACU may experience a PRAE.[166]

A multitude of risk factors exist for PRAEs. Patient-related risk factors include:

1. younger age (neonates are at particularly high risk)
2. recent or active URI, and
3. chronic lung disease (including asthma, bronchopulmonary dysplasia, cystic fibrosis).

Procedure-related risk factors are:

1. airway procedures, and
2. procedures that increase the risk of blood or secretions in the airway.

Anesthetic-related risk factors include;

1. tracheal intubation
2. multiple attempts at airway instrumentation,
3. use of neuromuscular blockers, and
4. opioid administration.[166]

Treatment for PRAEs depends on prompt recognition and availability of rescue airway equipment and medications in PACU. The PACU may or may not be staffed by an attending anesthesiologist, but one should always be available for an immediate response when needed. In addition, PACU nurses should be regularly trained in recognition and early management of PRAEs.[166] Treatment begins with administration of supplemental oxygen and airway support maneuvers (including CPAP, jaw thrust, and chin lift) as the provider makes a diagnosis and prepares for tailored treatment. This may include oral/nasal airway placement for airway obstruction, albuterol and/or epinephrine for bronchospasm, or racemic epinephrine and/or systemic steroids for stridor. Intubation equipment should always be available in PACU for severe PRAEs.

Postoperative Apnea

Risk factors for postoperative apnea include low gestational age, observed apnea at home, and anemia. Small-for-gestational age infants have a decreased risk.[167] The exact age at which infants are no longer susceptible to postoperative apnea has yet to be determined. Thus, institutional guidelines vary with regard to required postoperative monitoring guidelines for infants. At the authors' institution, term infants <4 weeks old and preterm infants <50 weeks postmenstrual age are admitted for overnight monitoring. Infants with other risk factors may also be appropriate for extended monitoring. Infants at highest risk are generally admitted to a monitored bed for up to 12 hours or overnight.[168]

Postoperative Stridor

Due to a smaller upper airway, pediatric patients are more susceptible to stridor from airway narrowing. Edema, blood, or secretions that lead to even small degrees of airway narrowing can markedly increase airway resistance.[169] Recall that Poiseuille's equation defines resistance as inversely related to the fourth power of radius. In a crying infant with turbulent airflow, airway resistance is inversely related to the fifth power of radius. The differential diagnosis for stridor in the pediatric patient includes foreign body aspiration, viral croup, epiglottitis, bacterial tracheitis, and

Table 43-6 Scoring System for the Pediatric Anesthesia Emergence Delirium (PAED) Scale[a]

	Not At All	Just a Little	Quite a Bit	Very Much	Extremely
The child makes eye contact with the caregiver	4	3	2	1	0
The child's actions are purposeful	4	3	2	1	0
Child is aware of their surroundings	4	3	2	1	0
The child is restless	0	1	2	3	4
The child is consolable	0	1	2	3	4

[a]Higher scores are directly related with emergence delirium.
Reprinted with permission from Sikich N, Lerman J. Development and psychometric evaluation of the pediatric anesthesia emergence delirium scale. *Anesthesiology*. 2004;100(5):1138–1145.

retropharyngeal abscess.[10] Postextubation stridor is commonly due to laryngeal edema.[170]

Postextubation stridor typically manifests within 30 minutes after tracheal extubation. Risk factors include (1) use of a larger endotracheal tube compared to that recommended for the patient's size, (2) prolonged tracheal intubation, and (3) history of multiple intubations or multiple intubation attempts.[169,170] Evidence continues to be inconclusive on whether cuffed versus uncuffed endotracheal tubes are protective against airway complications including postextubation stridor.[171]

Treatment for postextubation stridor in PACU includes administration of humidified oxygen, nebulized racemic epinephrine, and IV corticosteroids. Racemic epinephrine is presumed to cause local vasoconstriction, leading to decreased edema. IV corticosteroids will decrease the inflammatory response and blood vessel permeability over a more prolonged period.[169] For patients who have received racemic epinephrine, it is essential to monitor for recurrence of symptoms once the effect of the nebulized solution has worn off. The duration of monitoring varies by institution. If stridor is severe and leading to respiratory insufficiency or failure at any point, reintubation with a smaller endotracheal tube will be necessary.

Negative Pressure Pulmonary Edema

Negative pressure pulmonary edema (NPPE) is noncardiogenic pulmonary edema that develops following severe acute upper airway obstruction. The incidence is reported as 0.05% to 0.1% for all anesthetics. Risk factors include male gender, younger age, prolonged procedure time, active smoking, and endotracheal intubation.[172] Muscular teenagers—who are able to generate large intrathoracic negative pressure—should be considered high risk. NPPE may develop immediately and concurrently with acute airway obstruction (such as during complete endotracheal tube obstruction or postextubation laryngospasm) or following relief of chronic upper airway obstruction (such as post-tonsillectomy).[173] The large negative intrathoracic pressure that is generated to overcome airway obstruction leads to changes in the pressure gradient between the alveoli/interstitial lung space and the pulmonary capillaries. The result is transudation of fluid into the interstitial and alveolar space.[173]

Patients typically present with hypoxia, course breath sounds, and pink, frothy sputum within an hour of an event causing acute airway obstruction. Alternative diagnoses such as cardiogenic pulmonary edema, fluid overload, and anaphylaxis should be considered. The airway should be managed as necessary depending on the degree of respiratory insufficiency. This will often include tracheal intubation, but noninvasive positive pressure ventilation may also be used. CPAP and diuretics are standard treatment.[173] Fortunately, most patients respond well to treatment without long-term sequelae.

Emergence Delirium

Emergence delirium (ED) is more common in the pediatric population, with a reported incidence of up to 80%.[148] ED typically manifests as a period of agitation, or rarely, a period of hypoactivity, in the first 30 minutes after emergence from general anesthesia. The Pediatric Anesthesia Emergence Delirium (PAED) scale is a validated scoring system for ED.[174] It can be helpful in differentiating ED from pain, since there may be overlapping manifestations of the two. The PAED relies on assessment of five criteria:

1. eye contact with caregiver,
2. purposeful activity,
3. awareness of surroundings,
4. restlessness, and
5. inconsolability (see Table 43-6).

Lack of eye contact, lack of purposeful activity, lack of awareness of surroundings, restlessness, and inconsolability are associated with higher scores, which are directly correlated with ED.[174]

ED can lead to patient morbidity, delayed discharge, and increased PACU staffing requirements. Complications may include bleeding from or injury to surgical sites, dislodgement of lines and monitoring devices, and persistent negative behavioral patterns in the postoperative period.[175] Risk factors for ED may include volatile anesthetic exposure (particularly sevoflurane), certain types of surgery including ophthalmology and otorhinolaryngology procedures, patient age around 3 to 7 years old, patient anxiety, pre-existing maladaptive behavior, and negative behaviors during induction.[176]

Strategies to decrease the incidence of ED ideally begin in the preoperative period, with attempts to treat anxiety, provide distraction, and prepare the patient for what to expect with developmentally appropriate education. Intraoperative prevention techniques may focus on minimizing exposure to sevoflurane by using a propofol-based TIVA for maintenance, and pre- or intraoperative administration of dexmedetomidine. In a randomized clinical trial, dexmedetomidine at 0.5 mcg/mL following induction of anesthesia was associated with a decreased incidence of ED compared to placebo (31.1% vs. 53.3%) in 2- to 7-year-old patients undergoing tonsillectomy with sevoflurane for maintenance of anesthesia.[175] Depth of anesthesia as measured by processed EEG has not been shown to correlate with ED incidence in the pediatric population. Benzodiazepine premedication has not been shown to decrease ED, whereas ketamine or melatonin premedication has been shown to have some benefit.[176]

A large variety of treatment strategies have been trialed for treatment of ED, including use of propofol, opioids, or dexmedetomidine. In the absence of contraindications, dexmedetomidine is often the first-line agent chosen due to demonstrated efficacy and the additional analgesic and antiemetic effects.

Vomiting

As observed in the adult population, PONV is one of the most common adverse events in PACU in the pediatric population. It continues to be a leading cause for unplanned hospital admission. Estimates for the incidence of PONV range from 8% to 42%, a value higher than that seen in adults.[177] The rate of postdischarge nausea and vomiting in children has been reported to be 14%, lower than the estimated 30% to 50% incidence in adults having outpatient surgery.[177] Importantly, the risk factors for PONV in the pediatric population differ from those observed in adults. Preoperative risk factors include:

1. age greater than or equal to 3 years old
2. history of PONV or motion sickness
3. family history of PONV, and
4. postpubertal female sex.[178]

Intraoperative risk factors include:

1. strabismus surgery
2. adenotonsillectomy
3. otoplasty
4. surgery greater than or equal to 30 minutes
5. volatile anesthetic use, and
6. anticholinesterase administration.[178]

In the postoperative period, administration of long-acting opioids[178] and aggressive oral fluid hydration before patients elect to drink are risk factors.[179]

As in adults, PONV prevention strategies include use of propofol-based TIVA rather than volatile anesthetic for maintenance of anesthesia, opioid sparing techniques, and liberal IV fluid therapy.

Opioid-sparing techniques include regional and neuraxial blocks, as well as administration of non-narcotic analgesics such as dexmedetomidine, ketamine, and acetaminophen.[177,178] Antiemetic prophylaxis should be based on risk factors. If no risk factors are present, it may be reasonable to avoid prophylaxis. Those with one or two risk factors should receive dual prophylaxis, and those with three or more risk factors (high risk) should receive triple antiemetic prophylaxis. The combination of ondansetron (50 to 100 mcg/kg) and dexamethasone (0.15 mg/kg) as dual prophylaxis is most strongly supported in the literature. Propofol TIVA is often added as the third agent for triple prophylaxis.[177,178]

Other antiemetics that have demonstrated safety in the pediatric population (although not necessarily FDA approved for prevention of nausea in children) include aprepitant (NK1 receptor antagonist), promethazine (antihistamine), dimenhydrinate (antihistamine), droperidol (antidopaminergic, used in doses less than 10 to 15 mcg/kg with a maximum dose of 1.25 mg due to the risk of QT prolongation), and other 5HT3 antagonists including granisetron and palonosetron.[178] Scopolamine patches have also been used in the perioperative period, particularly for patients who will receive opioids. For patients who develop PONV despite prophylaxis, treatment should include a different pharmacologic class of medication than was previously given. A medication within the same class is unlikely to provide benefit if given within 6 hours of the original dose. Acupuncture or acupressure may also be beneficial as rescue or preventative treatment.[178]

Many other nonpharmacologic treatment strategies have been studied for PONV prophylaxis and treatment. Data are inconclusive on the beneficial impact of preoperative carbohydrate drinks, aromatherapy with peppermint or isopropyl alcohol, ginger, supplemental oxygen, and chewing gum in recovery.[178]

Pain

The experience of pain in PACU is associated with increased agitation and anxiety, as well as increased risk for development of persistent postsurgical pain.[180] Ongoing assessment and treatment of pain are critical components of PACU care. Unique challenges exist for pain assessment in the pediatric population, particularly for young or developmentally delayed patients. For patients able to self-report, commonly used pain scales include the Visual Analog Scale (VAS), Numeric Rating Scale (NRS), and Wong–Baker Faces Pain rating scale. For patients unable to self-report, the FLACC scale may be used. This involves observer assessment of Facial expression, Leg position and movement, Activity level, presence of Crying, and degree of Consolability.[181] Unfortunately, there is no gold-standard measurement tool that works across all ages and developmental stages. Although not currently a part of standard practice, research is ongoing to develop more objective pain assessment tools that rely on assessment of autonomic responses (such as cardiovascular sympathetic response or pupillary dilation) to nociceptive stimulation.

Treatment of pain in PACU should focus on multimodal analgesia with:

1. nonopioid analgesics such as acetaminophen and NSAIDs,
2. neuraxial and regional techniques, and
3. opioids analgesics titrated to effect.

Patient-controlled epidural or intravenous analgesia (PCEA or IV PCA) may be particularly beneficial for patients with the developmental capability to use these devices.[182] Based on cohort studies in the pediatric population and randomized controlled trials in adults, the Society for Pediatric Anesthesia supports PCA as a safe and efficacious option for opioid delivery in the pediatric population.[182] In addition, PCA use may be associated with higher patient satisfaction scores when compared to intermittent IV opioid administration.[182] For patients who do not have the physical or developmental capability to use a standard PCA, nurse-controlled analgesia is an alternative that has also been shown to be safe and efficacious. Importantly, this is only recommended in settings where nurses have extensive training and are supported by institutional guidelines.[182] Data comparing intermittent PCA bolus dosing with intermittent PCA bolus dosing plus a background continuous infusion have been mixed in regard to overall analgesia, impact on sleep quality, and adverse events such as respiratory depression.[182] Thus, use of a background continuous infusion is often based on patient- and situation-specific risk factors such as preoperative use of opioids. Patients receiving any form of opioid therapy should have regular, developmentally appropriate pain assessments to guide therapy.

For additional information please see NICVs 43-1–43-3 and Video 43-1 in the eBook bundled with this text.

For further review and interactivities, please see the videos and narrative interactive clinical vignettes (NICVs) accessible in the complimentary eBook bundled with this text. Access instructions are located on the inside front cover.

REFERENCES

1. MacLean JE. Laryngomalacia in infancy improves with increasing age irrespective of treatment. *J Clin Sleep Med.* 2021;17(4):619–620.
2. Baum V, O'Flaherty J. *Anesthesia for Genetic, Metabolic and Dysmorphic Syndromes of Childhood*, 3rd ed. Lippincott Williams & Wilkins (LWW); 2015.
3. Campbell M, Sapra A. Physiology, airflow resistance. *StatPearls [Internet]*. 2022. https://www.ncbi.nlm.nih.gov/books/NBK554401/. Accessed August 9, 2022. Published April 28, 2022.
4. Tanner GE, Angers DG, Barash PG, et al. Effect of left-to-right, mixed left-to-right, and right-to-left shunts on inhalational anesthetic induction in children: a computer model. *Anesthesia and analgesia*. 1985;64(2):101–107.
5. AHA. *Pediatric Advanced Life Support Provider Manual (International English)*. 9 American Heart Association, Incorporated; 2020.
6. Szabó EZ, Luginbuehl I, Bissonnette B. Impact of anesthetic agents on cerebrovascular physiology in children. *Paediatr Anaesth.* 2009;19(2):108–118.
7. US Federal Drug Administration. Food and Drug Administration Drug Safety Communication: FDA approves label changes for use of general anesthetic and sedation drugs in young children. https://www.fda.gov/Drugs/DrugSafety/ucm554634.htm. Published 2017. Accessed August 2, 2022.
8. McCann ME, de Graaff JC, Dorris L, et al. Neurodevelopmental outcome at 5 years of age after general anaesthesia or awake-regional anaesthesia in infancy (GAS): an international, multicentre, randomised, controlled equivalence trial. *Lancet.* 2019;393(10172):664–677.
9. Sun LS, Li G, DiMaggio CJ, et al. Feasibility and pilot study of the Pediatric Anesthesia NeuroDevelopment Assessment (PANDA) project. *J Neurosurg Anesthesiol.* 2012;24(4):382–388.
10. Lerman J, Strong HA, LeDez KM, et al. Effects of age on the serum concentration of alpha 1-acid glycoprotein and the binding of lidocaine in pediatric patients. *Clin Pharmacol Ther.* 1989;46(2):219–225. /bib>
11. US Federal Drug Administration. FDA Drug Safety Communication: FDA restricts use of prescription codeine pain and cough medicines and tramadol pain medicines in children; recommends against use in breastfeeding women. https://www.fda.gov/drugs/drug-safety-and-availability/fda-drug-safety-communication-fda-restricts-use-prescription-codeine-pain-and-cough-medicines-and#:~:text=carry%20this%20Contraindication.-,A%20new%20Warning%20to%20the%20drug%20labels%20of%20codeine%20and,risk%20of%20serious%20breathing%20problems. Published 2018. Accessed August 2, 2022.
12. Silva G, Waberski A, Bryant J. Eliminating Desflurane. Society for Pediatric Anesthesia. https://pedsanesthesia.org/wp-content/uploads/2021/08/Eliminiating-Desflurane.pdf. Published 2021. Accessed August 17, 2022.
13. Eger EI. *Anesthetic Uptake and Action*. Williams & Wilkins; 1974.
14. Lerman J, Schmitt-Bantel BI, Gregory GA, Willis MM, Eger EI 2nd. Effect of age on the solubility of volatile anesthetics in human tissues. *Anesthesiology*. 1986;65(3):307–311.
15. Lerman J, Gregory GA, Willis MM, Eger EI 2nd. Age and solubility of volatile anesthetics in blood. *Anesthesiology*. 1984;61(2):139–143.
16. Morray Jeffrey P, Geiduschek Jeremy M, Ramamoorthy C, et al. Anesthesia-related cardiac arrest in children: Initial Findings of the Pediatric Perioperative Cardiac Arrest (POCA) Registry. *Anesthesiology*. 2000;93(1):6–14.
17. Frei FJ, Haemmerle MH, Brunner R, Kern C. Minimum alveolar concentration for halothane in children with cerebral palsy and severe mental retardation. *Anaesthesia.* 1997;52(11):1056–1060.
18. Frink EJ, Jr., Green WB, Jr., Brown EA, et al. Compound A concentrations during sevoflurane anesthesia in children. *Anesthesiology*. 1996;84(3):566–571.
19. McFarlan CS, Anderson BJ, Short TG. The use of propofol infusions in paediatric anaesthesia: a practical guide. *Paediatr Anaesth.* 1999;9(3):209–216.
20. Parke TJ, Stevens JE, Rice AS, et al. Metabolic acidosis and fatal myocardial failure after propofol infusion in children: five case reports. *BMJ.* 1992;305(6854):613–616.
21. Niezgoda J, Morgan PG. Anesthetic considerations in patients with mitochondrial defects. *Paediatr Anaesth.* 2013;23(9):785–793.
22. Franz AM, Chiem J, Martin LD, et al. Case series of 331 cases of sugammadex compared to neostigmine in patients under 2 years of age. *Pediatric Anesthesia.* 2019;29(6):591–596.
23. Blobner M, Hollmann MW, Luedi MM, Johnson KB. Pro-Con debate: Do we need quantitative neuromuscular monitoring in the era of sugammadex? *Anesth Analg.* 2022;135(1):39–48.
24. Faulk DJ, Austin TM, Thomas JJ, et al. A Survey of the Society for Pediatric Anesthesia on the Use, Monitoring, and Antagonism of Neuromuscular Blockade. *Anesthesia and analgesia.* 2021;132(6):1518–1526.
25. SPA. PCA. WAKE UP SAFE: The Pediatric Anesthesia Quality Improvement Initiative Warning: Risk of acetaminophen overdose. Society for Pediatric Anesthesia. https://wakeupsafe.org/wp-content/uploads/2018/10/acetaminophen_warning.pdf. Published 2018. Accessed August 17, 2022.
26. Franz AM, Martin LD, Liston DE, et al. In Pursuit of an Opioid-Free Pediatric Ambulatory Surgery Center: A Quality Improvement Initiative. *Anesth Analg.* 2021;132(3):788–797.
27. Beauchamp TLCJ. *Principles of Biomedical Ethics*. 7th ed. Oxford University Press; 2009.
28. Unguru Y. *Pediatric decision-making: informed consent, parental permission, child assent, in Clinical Ethics in Pediatrics: A Case-Based Textbook*. Cambridge University Press; 2011.
29. Weithorn LA, Campbell SB. The competency of children and adolescents to make informed treatment decisions. *Child Dev.* 1982;53(6):1589–1598.
30. Braddock CH, 3rd, Fihn SD, Levinson W, Jonsen AR, Pearlman RA. How doctors and patients discuss routine clinical decisions. Informed decision making in the outpatient setting. *J Gen Intern Med.* 1997;12(6):339–345.
31. Gentry KR, Lepere K, Opel DJ. Informed consent in pediatric anesthesiology. *Paediatr Anaesth.* 2017;27(12):1253–1260.
32. Feinstein MM, Pannunzio AE, Lobell S, Kodish E. Informed consent in pediatric anesthesia: a narrative review. *Anesthesia & Analgesia.* 2018;127(6):1398–1405.
33. Diekema DS. Parental refusals of medical treatment: the harm principle as threshold for state intervention. *Theor Med Bioeth.* 2004;25(4):243–264.
34. Practice Guidelines for Preoperative Fasting and the Use of Pharmacologic Agents to Reduce the Risk of Pulmonary Aspiration: Application to Healthy Patients Undergoing Elective Procedures: An Updated Report by the American Society of Anesthesiologists Task Force on Preoperative Fasting and the Use of Pharmacologic Agents to Reduce the Risk of Pulmonary Aspiration*. *Anesthesiology*. 2017;126(3):376–393.
35. Beck CE, Rudolph D, Mahn C, et al. Impact of clear fluid fasting on pulmonary aspiration in children undergoing general anesthesia: Results of the German prospective multicenter observational (NiKs) study. *Paediatr Anaesth.* 2020;30(8):892–899.
36. Beach ML, Cohen DM, Gallagher SM, Cravero JP. Major adverse events and relationship to nil per os status in pediatric sedation/anesthesia outside the operating room: A Report of the Pediatric Sedation Research Consortium. *Anesthesiology*. 2016;124(1):80–88.
37. Andersson H, Hellström PM, Frykholm P. Introducing the 6-4-0 fasting regimen and the incidence of prolonged preoperative fasting in children. *Paediatr Anaesth.* 2018;28(1):46–52.
38. Beck CE, Witt L, Albrecht L, et al. Ultrasound assessment of gastric emptying time after a standardised light breakfast in healthy children: A prospective observational study. *Eur J Anaesthesiol.* 2018;35(12):937–941.
39. Rosen D, Gamble J, Matava C. Canadian Pediatric Anesthesia Society statement on clear fluid fasting for elective pediatric anesthesia. *Can J Anaesth.* 2019;66(8):991–992.
40. Linscott D. SPANZA endorses 1-hour clear fluid fasting consensus statement. *Pediatric Anesthesia.* 2019;29(3):292–292.
41. Thomas M, Morrison C, Newton R, Schindler E. Consensus statement on clear fluids fasting for elective pediatric general anesthesia. *Pediatric Anesthesia.* 2018;28(5):411–414.
42. Isserman R, Elliott E, Subramanyam R, et al. Quality improvement project to reduce pediatric clear liquid fasting times prior to anesthesia. *Pediatric Anesthesia.* 2019;29(7):698–704.
43. Ouanes JP, Bicket MC, Togioka B, et al. The role of perioperative chewing gum on gastric fluid volume and gastric pH: a meta-analysis. *J Clin Anesth.* 2015;27(2):146–152.
44. Dasenbrock HH, Smith TR, Robinson S. Preoperative laboratory testing before pediatric neurosurgery: an NSQIP-Pediatrics analysis. *J Neurosurg Pediatr.* 2019;24(1):92–103.
45. ASA Committee on Quality Management and Departmental Administration: Pregnancy Testing Prior to Anesthesia and Surgery [press release]. October 13, 2021. Accessed August 3, 2022. https://www.asahq.org/standards-and-guidelines/pregnancy-testing-prior-to-anesthesia-and-surgery#:~:text=The%20ASA%20Practice%20Advisory%20for,alter%20the%20patient's%20medical%20management
46. Habre W, Disma N, Virag K, et al. Incidence of severe critical events in paediatric anaesthesia (APRICOT): a prospective multicentre observational study in 261 hospitals in Europe. *Lancet Respir Med.* 2017;5(5):412–425.
47. de Carvalho ALR, Vital RB, de Lira CCS, et al. Laryngeal mask airway versus other airway devices for anesthesia in children with an upper respiratory tract infection: a systematic review and meta-analysis of respiratory complications. *Anesth Analg.* 2018;127(4):941–950.
48. Li L, Zhang Z, Yao Z, et al. The impact of laryngeal mask versus other airways on perioperative respiratory adverse events in children: A systematic review and meta-analysis of randomized controlled trials. *Int J Surg.* 2019;64:40–48.
49. von Ungern-Sternberg BS, Sommerfield D, Slevin L, et al. Effect of albuterol premedication vs placebo on the occurrence of respiratory adverse events in children undergoing tonsillectomies: The REACT Randomized Clinical Trial. *JAMA Pediatr.* 2019;173(6):527–533.
50. Lee LK, Bernardo MKL, Grogan TR, et al. Perioperative respiratory adverse event risk assessment in children with upper respiratory tract infection: Validation of the COLDS score. *Paediatr Anaesth.* 2018;28(11):1007–1014.
51. von Ungern-Sternberg BS, Boda K, Chambers NA, et al. Risk assessment for respiratory complications in paediatric anaesthesia: a prospective cohort study. *Lancet.* 2010;376(9743):773–783.
52. Ramgolam A, Hall GL, Zhang G, Hegarty M, von Ungern-Sternberg BS. Inhalational versus intravenous induction of anesthesia in children with a high risk of perioperative respiratory adverse events: a randomized controlled trial. *Anesthesiology*. 2018;128(6):1065–1074.

53. Schwengel DA, Dalesio NM, Stierer TL. Pediatric obstructive sleep apnea. *Anesthesiol Clin.* 2014;32(1):237–261.
54. Marcus CL, Brooks LJ, Draper KA, et al. Diagnosis and management of childhood obstructive sleep apnea syndrome. *Pediatrics.* 2012;130(3):576–584.
55. Bongiovanni T, Lancaster E, Ledesma Y, et al. Systematic review and meta-analysis of the association between non-steroidal anti-inflammatory drugs and operative bleeding in the perioperative period. *J Am Coll Surg.* 2021;232(5):765–790.e761.
56. Dohms K, Hein M, Rossaint R, et al. Inguinal hernia repair in preterm neonates: is there evidence that spinal or general anaesthesia is the better option regarding intraoperative and postoperative complications? A systematic review and meta-analysis. *BMJ Open.* 2019;9(10):e028728.
57. Jones LJ, Craven PD, Lakkundi A, Foster JP, Badawi N. Regional (spinal, epidural, caudal) versus general anaesthesia in preterm infants undergoing inguinal herniorrhaphy in early infancy. *Cochrane Database Syst Rev.* 2015;2015(6):Cd003669.
58. Davidson AJ, Morton NS, Arnup SJ, et al. Apnea after Awake Regional and General Anesthesia in Infants: The General Anesthesia Compared to Spinal Anesthesia Study–Comparing Apnea and Neurodevelopmental Outcomes, a Randomized Controlled Trial. *Anesthesiology.* 2015;123(1):38–54.
59. Chen J, Jin L, Chen X. Efficacy and safety of different maintenance doses of caffeine citrate for treatment of apnea in premature infants: a systematic review and meta-analysis. *Biomed Res Int.* 2018;2018:9061234.
60. Thompson DR, Orr R, Haberkern CM. A survey of pediatric hospitals: admission criteria for ex-prematurely born infants and term newborns following anesthesia. *Paediatr Anaesth.* 2012;22(11):1141–1143.
61. Litman RS, Griggs SM, Dowling JJ, Riazi S. Malignant hyperthermia susceptibility and related diseases. *Anesthesiology.* 2018;128(1):159–167.
62. Heiderich S, Thoben C, Dennhardt N, et al. Preparation of Dräger Atlan A350 and General Electric Healthcare Carestation 650 anesthesia workstations for malignant hyperthermia susceptible patients. *BMC Anesthesiol.* 2021;21(1):315.
63. Neira VM, Al Madhoun W, Ghaffari K, et al. Efficacy of malignant hyperthermia association of the united states-recommended methods of preparation for malignant hyperthermia-susceptible patients using Dräger Zeus anesthesia workstations and associated costs. *Anesth Analg.* 2019;129(1):74–83.
64. Rohde D, Schmitt HJ, Winterpacht A, Münster T. Duchenne muscular dystrophy and malignant hyperthermia: a genetic study of the ryanodine receptor in 47 patients. *Eur J Anaesthesiol.* 2014;31(6):341–342.
65. Gray RM. Anesthesia-induced rhabdomyolysis or malignant hyperthermia: is defining the crisis important? *Paediatr Anaesth.* 2017;27(5):490–493.
66. Hsieh VC, Krane EJ, Morgan PG. Mitochondrial Disease and Anesthesia. *Journal of Inborn Errors of Metabolism and Screening.* 2017;5:2326409817707770.
67. Finsterer J, Segall L. Drugs interfering with mitochondrial disorders. *Drug Chem Toxicol.* 2010;33(2):138–151.
68. Farooq F, Mogayzel PJ, Lanzkron S, Haywood C, Strouse JJ. Comparison of US Federal and Foundation Funding of Research for Sickle Cell Disease and Cystic Fibrosis and Factors Associated With Research Productivity. *JAMA Netw Open.* 2020;3(3):e201737.
69. Steinberg M. Pathophysiology of sickle cell disease. *UpToDate.* 2022. Accessed August 12, 2022.
70. Labbé E, Herbert D, Haynes J. Physicians' attitude and practices in sickle cell disease pain management. *J Palliat Care.* 2005;21(4):246–251.
71. Sabin JA, Greenwald AG. The influence of implicit bias on treatment recommendations for 4 common pediatric conditions: pain, urinary tract infection, attention deficit hyperactivity disorder, and asthma. *Am J Public Health.* 2012;102(5):988–995.
72. Sun M, Oliwa T, Peek ME, Tung EL. Negative patient descriptors: documenting racial bias in the electronic health record. *Health Aff (Millwood).* 2022;41(2):203–211.
73. Power-Hays A, McGann PT. When actions speak louder than words - racism and sickle cell disease. *N Engl J Med.* 2020;383(20):1902–1903.
74. Oyedeji CI, Welsby IJ. Optimizing management of sickle cell disease in patients undergoing surgery. *Hematology Am Soc Hematol Educ Program.* 2021;2021(1):405–410.
75. Fleming JM, Ross S, Hoffman LM, et al. Pediatric mediastinal mass algorithm: A quality improvement initiative to reduce time from presentation to biopsy. *Paediatr Anaesth.* 2021;31(8):885–893.
76. Otto CM, Nishimura RA, Bonow RO, et al. 2020 ACC/AHA Guideline for the Management of Patients With Valvular Heart Disease: A Report of the American College of Cardiology/American Heart Association Joint Committee on Clinical Practice Guidelines. *Circulation.* 2021;143(5):e72–e227.
77. Gleich SJ, Olson MD, Sprung J, et al. Perioperative outcomes of severely obese children undergoing tonsillectomy. *Paediatr Anaesth.* 2012;22(12):1171–1178.
78. Martin LD, Hoagland MA, Rhodes ET, et al. Perioperative management of pediatric patients with type 1 diabetes mellitus, updated recommendations for anesthesiologists. *Anesth Analg.* 2020;130(4):821–827.
79. What is Autism. Autism speaks. https://www.autismspeaks.org/what-autism. Accessed August 18, 2022.
80. Berglund IG, Björkman B, Enskär K, Faresjö M, Huus K. Management of children with autism spectrum disorder in the anesthesia and radiographic context. *J Dev Behav Pediatr.* 2017;38(3):187–196.
81. Thompson DG, Tielsch-Goddard A. Improving management of patients with autism spectrum disorder having scheduled surgery: optimizing practice. *J Pediatr Health Care.* 2014;28(5):394–403.
82. Koski S, Gabriels RL, Beresford C. Interventions for paediatric surgery patients with comorbid autism spectrum disorder: a systematic literature review. *Arch Dis Child.* 2016;101(12):1090–1094.
83. Bertolizio G, Saint-Martin C, Ingelmo P. Cervical instability in patients with Trisomy 21: The eternal gamble. *Paediatr Anaesth.* 2018;28(10):830–833.
84. Lewanda AF, Matisoff A, Revenis M, et al. Preoperative evaluation and comprehensive risk assessment for children with Down syndrome. *Paediatr Anaesth.* 2016;26(4):356–362.
85. Wakimoto M, Miller R, Kim SS, et al. Perioperative anaphylaxis in children: A report from the Wake-Up Safe collaborative. *Paediatr Anaesth.* 2021;31(2):205–212.
86. Yamada Y, Yamamoto T, Tanabe K, et al. A case of anaphylaxis apparently induced by sugammadex and rocuronium in successive surgeries. *J Clin Anesth.* 2016;32:30–32.
87. Picard M, Robitaille G, Karam F, et al. Cross-reactivity to cephalosporins and carbapenems in penicillin-allergic patients: two systematic reviews and meta-analyses. *J Allergy Clin Immunol Pract.* 2019;7(8):2722–2738.e2725.
88. Asserhøj LL, Mosbech H, Krøigaard M, et al. No evidence for contraindications to the use of propofol in adults allergic to egg, soy or peanut†. *Br J Anaesth.* 2016;116(1):77–82.
89. Bonadonna P, Pagani M, Aberer W, et al. Drug hypersensitivity in clonal mast cell disorders: ENDA/EAACI position paper. *Allergy.* 2015;70(7):755–763.
90. Manyande A, Cyna AM, Yip P, Chooi C, Middleton P. Non-pharmacological interventions for assisting the induction of anaesthesia in children. *Cochrane Database Syst Rev.* 2015;2015(7):Cd006447.
91. Pasin L, Febres D, Testa V, et al. Dexmedetomidine vs midazolam as preanesthetic medication in children: a meta-analysis of randomized controlled trials. *Paediatr Anaesth.* 2015;25(5):468–476.
92. Qiu L, Cao L, Lang Z, et al. Preoperative sedation in children with congenital heart disease: 50% and 95% effective doses, hemodynamic effects, and safety of intranasal dexmedetomidine. *J Clin Anesth.* 2022;81:110908.
93. Qiao H, Xie Z, Jia J. Pediatric premedication: a double-blind randomized trial of dexmedetomidine or ketamine alone versus a combination of dexmedetomidine and ketamine. *BMC Anesthesiol.* 2017;17(1):158.
94. Passi Y, Sathyamoorthy M, Lerman J, Heard C, Marino M. Comparison of the laryngoscopy views with the size 1 Miller and Macintosh laryngoscope blades lifting the epiglottis or the base of the tongue in infants and children <2 yr of age. *Br J Anaesth.* 2014;113(5):869–874.
95. Garcia-Marcinkiewicz AG, Kovatsis PG, Hunyady AI, et al. First-attempt success rate of video laryngoscopy in small infants (VISI): a multicentre, randomised controlled trial. *Lancet.* 2020;396(10266):1905–1913.
96. Matava CT, Kovatsis PG, Lee JK, et al. Pediatric Airway Management in COVID-19 Patients: Consensus Guidelines From the Society for Pediatric Anesthesia's Pediatric Difficult Intubation Collaborative and the Canadian Pediatric Anesthesia Society. *Anesth Analg.* 2020;131(1):61–73.
97. Kleine-Brueggeney M, Grosshauser M, Greif R. Apneic oxygenation in pediatric anesthesia. *Curr Opin Anaesthesiol.* 2022;35(3):361–366.
98. Luce V, Harkouk H, Brasher C, et al. Supraglottic airway devices vs tracheal intubation in children: a quantitative meta-analysis of respiratory complications. *Paediatr Anaesth.* 2014;24(10):1088–1098.
99. Stein ML, Park RS, Kovatsis PG. Emerging trends, techniques, and equipment for airway management in pediatric patients. *Paediatr Anaesth.* 2020;30(3):269–279.
100. Metterlein T, Dintenfelder A, Plank C, Graf B, Roth G. A comparison of various supraglottic airway devices for fiberoptical guided tracheal intubation. *Braz J Anesthesiol.* 2017;67(2):166–171.
101. Larach MG, Brandom BW, Allen GC, et al. Malignant hyperthermia deaths related to inadequate temperature monitoring, 2007-2012: a report from the North American malignant hyperthermia registry of the malignant hyperthermia association of the United States. *Anesth Analg.* 2014;119(6):1359–1366.
102. Lee AC, Redding AT, Tjia I, Rana MS, Heitmiller E. Self-reported awareness during general anesthesia in pediatric patients: a study from wake up safe. *Paediatr Anaesth.* 2021;31(6):676–685.
103. Yuan I, Xu T, Kurth CD. Using electroencephalography (EEG) to guide propofol and sevoflurane dosing in pediatric anesthesia. *Anesthesiol Clin.* 2020;38(3):709–725.
104. Fülesdi B, Brull SJ. Quantitative neuromuscular monitoring: "Love All, Trust a Few, Do Wrong to None". *Anesth Analg.* 2022;135(1):35–38.
105. Naguib M, Brull SJ, Kopman AF, et al. Consensus statement on perioperative use of neuromuscular monitoring. *Anesth Analg.* 2018;127(1):71–80.
106. Driessen JJ, Robertson EN, Booij LH. Acceleromyography in neonates and small infants: baseline calibration and recovery of the responses after neuromuscular blockade with rocuronium. *Eur J Anaesthesiol.* 2005;22(1):11–15.

107. Grigg EB, Martin LD, Ross FJ, et al. Assessing the impact of the anesthesia medication template on medication errors during anesthesia: a prospective study. *Anesth Analg.* 2017;124(5):1617–1625.
108. Ernst KD. Resources recommended for the care of pediatric patients in hospitals. *Pediatrics.* 2020;145(4).
109. SPA. PEDI CRISIS APP®. In: Society for Pediatric Anesthesia; 2017. Accessed July 31, 2022. https://pedsanesthesia.org/pedi-crisis-app/
110. Noce J, Olvera D, Davis D. The optimal preoxygenation target to avoid desaturation during pediatric rapid sequence intubation. *Air Medical Journal.* 2022;41(1):26.
111. Abdallah C, Hannallah R. Use of modified rapid sequence tracheal intubation in pediatric patients. *Saudi J Anaesth.* 2014;8(2):249–255.
112. Ayanmanesh F, Abdat R, Jurine A, et al. Transnasal humidified rapid-insufflation ventilatory exchange during rapid sequence induction in children. *Anaesth Crit Care Pain Med.* 2021;40(2):100817.
113. Walker RW, Ravi R, Haylett K. Effect of cricoid force on airway calibre in children: a bronchoscopic assessment. *Br J Anaesth.* 2010;104(1):71–74.
114. Peyton MBPMaJ. ASA difficult airway NEW guidelines. https://ronlitman.substack.com/p/asa-difficult-airway-new-guidelines. Published 2021. Accessed July 26, 2022.
115. Fiadjoe JE, Nishisaki A, Jagannathan N, et al. Airway management complications in children with difficult tracheal intubation from the Pediatric Difficult Intubation (PeDI) registry: a prospective cohort analysis. *Lancet Respir Med.* 2016;4(1):37–48.
116. White MC, Marsh CJ, Beringer RM, et al. A randomised, controlled trial comparing the Airtraq™ optical laryngoscope with conventional laryngoscopy in infants and children. *Anaesthesia.* 2012;67(3):226–231.
117. Wong DT, Yang JJ, Mak HY, Jagannathan N. Use of intubation introducers through a supraglottic airway to facilitate tracheal intubation: a brief review. *Can J Anaesth.* 2012;59(7):704–715.
118. Kapoor R, Singh Heir J. Pediatric one-lung ventilation: additional considerations when using bronchial blockers for lung isolation. *Anesth Analg.* 2021;132(6):e112–e113.
119. Templeton TW, Piccioni F, Chatterjee D. An update on one-lung ventilation in children. *Anesth Analg.* 2021;132(5):1389–1399.
120. Hammer GB. Single-lung ventilation in infants and children. *Paediatr Anaesth.* 2004;14(1):98–102.
121. Lazar A, Chatterjee D, Templeton TW. Error traps in pediatric one-lung ventilation. *Paediatr Anaesth.* 2022;32(2):346–353.
122. Bradley J, Lee GS, Peyton J. Anesthesia for shared airway surgery in children. *Paediatr Anaesth.* 2020;30(3):288–295.
123. Shih MC, Elvis PR, Nguyen SA, Brennan E, Clemmens CS. Parental presence at induction of anesthesia to reduce anxiety-a systematic research and meta-analysis. *J Perianesth Nurs.* 2022;38(1):12–20.
124. Shafer JS, Jenkins BN, Fortier MA, et al. Parental satisfaction of child's perioperative care. *Paediatric anaesthesia.* 2018;28(11):955–962.
125. Feldman JM. Managing fresh gas flow to reduce environmental contamination. *Anesth Analg.* 2012;114(5):1093–1101.
126. Jung MJ, Libaw JS, Ma K, et al. Pediatric distraction on induction of anesthesia with virtual reality and perioperative anxiolysis: a randomized controlled trial. *Anesth Analg.* 2021;132(3):798–806.
127. Low DK, Pittaway AP. The 'iPhone' induction - a novel use for the Apple iPhone. *Paediatr Anaesth.* 2008;18(6):573–574.
128. Seiden SC, McMullan S, Sequera-Ramos L, et al. Tablet-based Interactive Distraction (TBID) vs oral midazolam to minimize perioperative anxiety in pediatric patients: a noninferiority randomized trial. *Paediatric anaesthesia.* 2014;24(12):1217–1223.
129. Fukumoto M, Arima H, Ito S, et al. Distorted perception of smell by volatile agents facilitated inhalational induction of anesthesia. *Paediatric anaesthesia.* 2005;15(2):98–101.
130. Peyton PJ, Horriat M, Robinson GJB, et al. Magnitude of the second gas effect on arterial sevoflurane partial pressure. *Anesthesiology.* 2008;108:381–387.
131. O'Shea H, Moultrie S, Drummond GB. Influence of nitrous oxide on induction of anaesthesia with sevoflurane. *Br J Anaesth.* 2001;87(2):286–288.
132. Lee SY, Cheng SL, Ng SB, et al. Single-breath vital capacity high concentration sevoflurane induction in children: with or without nitrous oxide? *Br J Anaesth.* 2013;110(1):81–86.
133. Schmitt EL, Baum VC. Nitrous oxide in pediatric anesthesia: friend or foe? *Curr Opin Anaesthesiol.* 2008;21(3):356–359.
134. Devlin-Hegedus JA, McGain F, Harris RD, et al. Action guidance for addressing pollution from inhalational anaesthetics. *Anaesthesia.* 2022;77(9):1023–1029.
135. Ballard HA, Hajduk J, Cheon EC, et al. Clinical and demographic factors associated with pediatric difficult intravenous access in the operating room. *Paediatr Anaesth.* 2022;32(7):792–800.
136. Jalota L, Kalira V, George E, et al. Prevention of pain on injection of propofol: systematic review and meta-analysis. *BMJ.* 2011;342:d1110.
137. Flisberg P, Paech MJ, Shah T, et al. Induction dose of propofol in patients using cannabis. *Eur J Anaesthesiol.* 2009;26(3):192–195.
138. Nagoshi M, Reddy S, Bell M, et al. Low-dose dexmedetomidine as an adjuvant to propofol infusion for children in MRI: a double-cohort study. *Paediatr Anaesth.* 2018;28(7):639–646.
139. Hampson-Evans D, Morgan P, Farrar M. Pediatric laryngospasm. *Paediatric anaesthesia.* 2008;18(4):303–307.
140. Al-alami AA, Zestos MM, Baraka AS. Pediatric laryngospasm: prevention and treatment. *Curr Opin Anaesthesiol.* 2009;22(3):388–395.
141. Kraemer FW, Stricker PA, Gurnaney HG, et al. Bradycardia during induction of anesthesia with sevoflurane in children with Down syndrome. *Anesth Analg.* 2010;111(5):1259–1263.
142. Sherman J, Le C, Lamers V, et al. Life cycle greenhouse gas emissions of anesthetic drugs. *Anesth Analg.* 2012;114(5):1086–1090.
143. Sherman J. Yale Gassing Greener App. Accessed June 4, 2022. https://jscalc.io/calc/H7gGXIL4tmDJHOxh
144. Rosenberg H, Pollock N, Schiemann A, et al. Malignant hyperthermia: a review. *Orphanet J Rare Dis.* 2015;10:93.
145. Kynes JM, Blakely M, Furman K, Burnette WB, Modes KB. Multidisciplinary perioperative care for children with neuromuscular disorders. *Children (Basel).* 2018;5(9).
146. Wang JT, Peyton J, Hernandez MR. Anesthesia for pediatric rigid bronchoscopy and related airway surgery: tips and tricks. *Paediatr Anaesth.* 2022;32(2):302–311.
147. Kanaya A, Kuratani N, Satoh D, et al. Lower incidence of emergence agitation in children after propofol anesthesia compared with sevoflurane: a meta-analysis of randomized controlled trials. *J Anesth.* 2014;28(1):4–11.
148. Moore AD, Anghelescu DL. emergence delirium in pediatric anesthesia. *Paediatr Drugs.* 2017;19(1):11–20.
149. Chandler JR, Myers D, Mehta D, et al. Emergence delirium in children: a randomized trial to compare total intravenous anesthesia with propofol and remifentanil to inhalational sevoflurane anesthesia. *Paediatr Anaesth.* 2013;23(4):309–315.
150. Martin LD, Rampersad SE, Geiduschek JM, et al. Modification of anesthesia practice reduces catheter-associated bloodstream infections: a quality improvement initiative. *Paediatr Anaesth.* 2013;23(7):588–596.
151. Sanford EL, Zurakowski D, Litvinova A, Zalieckas JM, Cravero JP. The association between high-volume intraoperative fluid administration and outcomes among pediatric patients undergoing large bowel resection. *Paediatr Anaesth.* 2019;29(4):315–321.
152. Diab YA, Wong EC, Luban NL. Massive transfusion in children and neonates. *Br J Haematol.* 2013;161(1):15–26.
153. Bosenberg A. Benefits of regional anesthesia in children. *Paediatr Anaesth.* 2012;22(1):10–18.
154. Walker BJ, Long JB, Sathyamoorthy M, et al. Complications in pediatric regional anesthesia: an analysis of more than 100,000 blocks from the pediatric regional anesthesia network. *Anesthesiology.* 2018;129(4):721–732.
155. Suresh S, Ecoffey C, Bosenberg A, et al. The European Society of Regional Anaesthesia and Pain Therapy/American Society of Regional Anesthesia and Pain Medicine Recommendations on Local Anesthetics and Adjuvants Dosage in Pediatric Regional Anesthesia. *Reg Anesth Pain Med.* 2018;43(2):211–216.
156. Lönnqvist PA, Ecoffey C, Bosenberg A, Suresh S, Ivani G. The European society of regional anesthesia and pain therapy and the American society of regional anesthesia and pain medicine joint committee practice advisory on controversial topics in pediatric regional anesthesia I and II: what do they tell us? *Curr Opin Anaesthesiol.* 2017;30(5):613–620.
157. Jain D, Hussain SY, Ayub A. Comparative evaluation of landmark technique and ultrasound-guided caudal epidural injection in pediatric population: A systematic review and meta-analysis. *Paediatr Anaesth.* 2022;32(1):35–42.
158. Tsui BC, Pillay JJ. Evidence-based medicine: Assessment of ultrasound imaging for regional anesthesia in infants, children, and adolescents. *Reg Anesth Pain Med.* 2010;35(2 Suppl):S47–54.
159. Ecoffey C, Bosenberg A, Lonnqvist PA, et al. Practice advisory on the prevention and management of complications of pediatric regional anesthesia. *J Clin Anesth.* 2022;79:110725.
160. Templeton TW, Goenaga-Díaz EJ, Downard MG, et al. Assessment of common criteria for awake extubation in infants and young children. *Anesthesiology.* 2019;131(4):801–808.
161. Davidson AJ, Wong A, Knottenbelt G, et al. MAC-awake of sevoflurane in children. *Paediatr Anaesth.* 2008;18(8):702–707.
162. Koo CH, Lee SY, Chung SH, Ryu JH. Deep vs. awake extubation and LMA removal in terms of airway complications in pediatric patients undergoing anesthesia: a systemic review and meta-analysis. *J Clin Med.* 2018;7(10).
163. Arai YP, Fukunaga K, Hirota S, Fujimoto S. The effects of chin lift and jaw thrust while in the lateral position on stridor score in anesthetized children with adenotonsillar hypertrophy. *Anesth Analg.* 2004;99(6):1638–1641.
164. Christensen RE, Haydar B, Voepel-Lewis TD. Pediatric cardiopulmonary arrest in the postanesthesia care unit, rare but preventable: Analysis of Data From Wake Up Safe, The Pediatric Anesthesia Quality Improvement Initiative. *Anesth Analg.* 2017;124(4):1231–1236.
165. Coté CJ, Goldstein EA, Coté MA, Hoaglin DC, Ryan JF. A single-blind study of pulse oximetry in children. *Anesthesiology.* 1988;68(2):184–188.
166. von Ungern-Sternberg BS. Respiratory complications in the pediatric postanesthesia care unit. *Anesthesiol Clin.* 2014;32(1):45–61.
167. Coté CJ, Zaslavsky A, Downes JJ, et al. Postoperative apnea in former preterm infants after inguinal herniorrhaphy. A combined analysis. *Anesthesiology.* 1995;82(4):809–822.
168. Kuan CC, Shaw SJ. Anesthesia for major surgery in the neonate. *Anesthesiol Clin.* 2020;38(1):1–18.

169. Maloney E, Meakin GH. Acute stridor in children. *Continuing Education in Anaesthesia Critical Care & Pain*. 2007;7(6):183–186.
170. Pluijms WA, van Mook WN, Wittekamp BH, Bergmans DC. Postextubation laryngeal edema and stridor resulting in respiratory failure in critically ill adult patients: updated review. *Crit Care*. 2015;19(1):295.
171. Dariya V, Moresco L, Bruschettini M, Brion LP. Cuffed versus uncuffed endotracheal tubes for neonates. *Cochrane Database Syst Rev*. 2022;1(1):Cd013736.
172. Tsai PH, Wang JH, Huang SC, Lin YK, Lam CF. Characterizing post-extubation negative pressure pulmonary edema in the operating room-a retrospective matched case-control study. *Perioper Med (Lond)*. 2018;7:28.
173. Bhaskar B, Fraser JF. Negative pressure pulmonary edema revisited: Pathophysiology and review of management. *Saudi J Anaesth*. 2011;5(3):308–313.
174. Sikich N, Lerman J. Development and psychometric evaluation of the pediatric anesthesia emergence delirium scale. *Anesthesiology*. 2004;100(5):1138–1145.
175. Shi M, Miao S, Gu T, et al. Dexmedetomidine for the prevention of emergence delirium and postoperative behavioral changes in pediatric patients with sevoflurane anesthesia: a double-blind, randomized trial. *Drug Des Devel Ther*. 2019;13:897–905.
176. Mason KP. Paediatric emergence delirium: a comprehensive review and interpretation of the literature. *Br J Anaesth*. 2017;118(3):335–343.
177. Kovac AL. Postoperative nausea and vomiting in pediatric patients. *Paediatr Drugs*. 2021;23(1):11–37.
178. Gan TJ, Belani KG, Bergese S, et al. Fourth Consensus Guidelines for the Management of Postoperative Nausea and Vomiting. *Anesth Analg*. 2020;131(2):411–448.
179. Goodarzi M, Matar MM, Shafa M, Townsend JE, Gonzalez I. A prospective randomized blinded study of the effect of intravenous fluid therapy on postoperative nausea and vomiting in children undergoing strabismus surgery. *Paediatr Anaesth*. 2006;16(1):49–53.
180. Luo J, Min S. Postoperative pain management in the postanesthesia care unit: an update. *J Pain Res*. 2017;10:2687–2698.
181. Wong C, Lau E, Palozzi L, Campbell F. Pain management in children: Part 1—Pain assessment tools and a brief review of nonpharmacological and pharmacological treatment options. *Can Pharm J (Ott)*. 2012;145(5):222–225.
182. Cravero JP, Agarwal R, Berde C, et al. The Society for Pediatric Anesthesia recommendations for the use of opioids in children during the perioperative period. *Paediatr Anaesth*. 2019;29(6):547–571.

Section 8

ANESTHESIA FOR SELECTED SURGICAL SERVICES

44 Anesthesia for Laparoscopic and Robotic Surgeries

GERARDO RODRIGUEZ • SHARMA E. JOSEPH

KEY POINTS

1 Small incisions, decreased postoperative pain, and lower surgical complication rates are some of the benefits of laparoscopy over laparotomy.

2 Pneumoperitoneum and positioning cause physiologic changes that are important for the anesthesiologist to understand.

3 Patients with a body mass index (BMI) >40 kg/m^2 and obesity-related comorbidities tend to have more perioperative complications when undergoing laparoscopic surgery compared to those without such conditions.

4 Advances in robotic-assisted laparoscopy have expanded its application to multiple subspecialties.

5 Access to the patient during robotic-assisted surgery may be limited, which is especially significant in the event of an intraoperative cardiopulmonary or airway emergency.

6 Severe hypercarbia and acidosis from absorbed carbon dioxide (CO_2) can lead to reduced inotropy, dysrhythmias, and arterial vasodilation.

7 High intra-abdominal pressures (IAP), combined with hypovolemia, can severely impair venous return and cardiac filling.

8 Migration of the endotracheal tube into a bronchus is a risk during laparoscopic surgery. This is due to displacement of the diaphragm into the thorax caused by abdominal insufflation, as well as Trenelenburg positioning.

9 Renal blood flow, glomerular filtration, and urine output are reduced during pneumoperitoneum.

10 The assessment of neuromuscular blockade during laparoscopic surgery can be highly subjective.

11 Major vascular injuries occur rarely during abdominal entry but are associated with significant morbidity and mortality.

12 Severe hypotension during pneumoperitoneum should be treated with desufflation and may require conversion to an open procedure.

13 Risk factors for complications related to subcutaneous emphysema include operative time more than 200 minutes, elevated BMI, high IAP, and Nissen fundoplication surgery.

14 Tension capnothorax is a life-threatening condition that requires a high index of suspicion and immediate action from the operating room team.

15 Preemptive multimodal pain management strategies and postoperative nausea and vomiting prophylaxis facilitate rapid patient recovery after laparoscopic surgery.

Introduction

1 Over a century ago, laparoscopy was first introduced as a therapeutic alternative to laparotomy. Since then, the field of laparoscopic surgery has evolved, to the extent that it has now become a conventional approach for many surgical diseases traditionally treated with open procedures. In fact, laparoscopy is now the gold-standard technique for cholecystectomy and bariatric surgery. The growth of the specialty has been fueled by the many benefits of "minimally invasive" surgery (Table 44-1). Improved surgical cosmesis, reduced postoperative pain, faster return to work, and lower surgical complications are among the benefits.[1–4] Advances in anesthesia have further accelerated the expansion of laparoscopy beyond inpatient facilities. Today, many surgeries that once required prolonged hospital stays are now performed in outpatient and short-stay facilities.[5–9] The creation of protocolized, fast-track programs that maximize the benefits of minimally invasive surgery have improved surgical outcomes and reduced healthcare costs.[10]

Despite its advantages, the practice of laparoscopic surgery imposes technical challenges for the surgeon, derived from the act of operating through small access ports, using long, rigid surgical instruments—all while having a limited sense of pressure and depth. The application of robotics to laparoscopic surgery has helped overcome many of these challenges. Robotic-assisted laparoscopic surgery provides surgeons with a close approximation of the fine motor skills and depth of vision used in open surgery, while allowing the surgeon to be positioned comfortably away from the operating room table.

2 Despite its many benefits, laparoscopy also poses some disadvantages for both patients and medical providers (Table 44-2). Physiologic derangements—particularly affecting the cardiopulmonary system—are common during pneumoperitoneum and are further aggravated by nonsupine positioning frequently used in laparoscopy. A patient's age and comorbidities can greatly affect the severity of pneumoperitoneum-related changes. In robotic surgery, long operative time and limited access to the patient due to prominent robotic equipment can further complicate management of urgent conditions.

This chapter provides an overview of the anesthetic management of adult patients undergoing laparoscopic and robotic-assisted abdominal or pelvic surgery.

Laparoscopic Surgery

Surgical Approach and Positioning

Laparoscopic surgery is a minimally invasive surgical technique where specialized tubes are inserted for surgical access. Skin incisions approximately 1 cm in length facilitate insertion of rigid tubes called *trocars*. Trocars are sharp, multiport, one-way conduits used to insufflate gas and insert various specialized surgical instruments. Intraperitoneal viewing is conducted using a video-capable telescopic camera (laparoscope).

Exposure of the intraperitoneal space can be achieved either by intraperitoneal pressurization (pneumoperitoneum) or by gasless abdominal wall retraction.

Conventional laparoscopy uses carbon dioxide (CO_2) for intraperitoneal (e.g., bariatric and cholecystectomy surgery) and extraperitoneal (e.g., adrenal and inguinal hernia repair surgery) insufflation (NICV 44-1). In contrast to other insufflation gases such as helium and nitrous oxide, CO_2 has a desirable safety profile. CO_2 is highly soluble in blood, facilitating rapid pulmonary removal and minimizing the consequences of inadvertent extraperitoneal or intravascular insufflation. CO_2 is nonflammable, nonoxidizing, and safe to use with electrocautery. Despite its favorable safety profile, CO_2 insufflation has known side effects.

Intraperitoneal insufflation is generally established by creating a small subumbilical incision through which a stainless steel, spring-loaded, blunt needle called a *Veress needle* is inserted. An automated, self-regulating insufflator with adjustable preset parameters is connected to the Veress stopcock to deliver low-flow rates of CO_2 until adequate abdominal distention is achieved. Maximal preset intra-abdominal pressures (IAP) above 15 mmHg should be avoided to minimize CO_2-related complications and cardiopulmonary instability. The Veress needle is replaced with a trocar for laparoscope insertion. Several other incisions are then made, through which trocars are sequentially inserted under direct visualization and transillumination to avoid inadvertent intra-abdominal injury. The surgery is conducted using a laparoscope for video monitoring and various long, handheld surgical instruments. If the surgeon's hand is needed for intra-abdominal tissue manipulation or large specimen extraction, a larger surgical access can be provided for a laparoscopic hand-assisted approach. A single 5- to 7.5-cm abdominal wall opening is made for insertion of a flexible, self-retaining, circular sleeve used for intra-abdominal hand insertion.

As an alternative to CO_2 pneumoperitoneum, exposure of the intraperitoneal space can be achieved by external abdominal wall retraction, called abdominal wall lift. This infrequent technique requires a specialized horizontal lifting apparatus inserted into the abdominal wall which suspends the anterior abdominal wall away from the abdominal viscera. Despite the benefits of avoiding gas insufflation and its side effects, abdominal wall lift is generally believed to be inferior to pneumoperitoneum due to longer operative times and an unclear safety profile.[11]

Nonsupine patient positioning is often required during laparoscopic surgery. Bed tilting is usually needed to passively optimize surgical exposure with minimal surgical retraction. Steep, reverse Trendelenburg position (i.e., "head up") exposes upper abdominal structures, as needed in gastric bypass surgery. Steep Trendelenburg position (i.e., "head down") is used to expose lower

Table 44-1 Benefits of Laparoscopic Surgery

Patient Specific	Surgeon Specific	Anesthesiologist Specific
Improved cosmetic results	↓ Medical risk	↓ Neurohormonal stress response
Shorter recovery time	↓ Postoperative complications	↓ Opioid requirements
Earlier return to work	Earlier return of bowel function	↓ Postoperative pain
Faster return to normal activities		↓ Fluid shifts
↓ Costs		↓ Postoperative respiratory dysfunction

Table 44-2 Disadvantages of Laparoscopy Surgery

Patient Specific	Surgeon Specific	Anesthesiologist Specific
↑Risk of PONV	Highly specialized training	Pneumoperitoneum-induced stress response
Referred pain from CO_2 insufflation	Ergonomics Limited tactile sense Longer operating times Complex equipment and setup Use in reoperation or scar tissue more challenging	Positioning risks Mechanical ventilatory challenges Extraperitoneal CO_2-related complications Limited access to patient (robotic surgery)

PONV, postoperative nausea and vomiting.

abdominal structures, such as in uterine or prostate surgery. The lateral jackknife position is used to expose the retroperitoneal space during radical nephrectomy. Leftward tilting exposes the appendix, whereas rightward tilting exposes the left colon. The addition of lithotomy is dependent on the need for genital, urologic access. An in-depth discussion on patient positioning and potential injuries is available elsewhere in this textbook.

Ambulatory Laparoscopic Surgery

The earliest reports of outpatient laparoscopy date back to the 1970s, when it was first used in gynecologic surgeries such as tubal ligation and were found to be associated with minimal complications and low readmission rates.[12–14] Since then, general surgical procedures have surpassed all other outpatient laparoscopic surgeries performed worldwide. Laparoscopic cholecystectomy for symptomatic cholelithiasis is now the most commonly performed outpatient laparoscopic surgery. Its safety and dependability has been well established.[5,6,15]

Ambulatory laparoscopic surgery is also being performed in the bariatric population with increasing frequency. Common laparoscopic weight-loss procedures include gastric bypass, sleeve gastrectomy, and adjustable gastric band. Gastric banding is the most performed outpatient bariatric laparoscopic surgery.[8,16]

The expansion of sleeve gastrectomy and gastric bypass into the ambulatory setting is due to advancements in minimally invasive surgery, patient screening, and anesthetic management. Nonetheless, postoperative complications, unanticipated admissions, and relatively high readmission rates raise concerns for the suitability and safety of these procedure being performed in the outpatient setting. Causes for unanticipated readmission in both gastric bypass and sleeve gastrectomy surgery include dysphagia, nausea, and uncontrolled pain. More serious complications include unexpected gastric leaks, gastrointestinal bleeding, and pulmonary embolism (PE).[9,16,17]

3 Appropriate patient presurgical screening is necessary for optimizing surgical results and avoiding unexpected complications. Assessing the body mass index (BMI) and severity of obesity-related comorbidities is important for preoperative risk stratification. Patients with a BMI of less than 40 kg/m^2 and well-optimized comorbid conditions, such as type II diabetes, heart disease, and obstructive sleep apnea, may have an acceptable risk for ambulatory surgery. Patients with a BMI greater than 40 kg/m^2 and poorly managed obesity-related comorbidities have a greater risk of morbidity.[18]

In-depth reviews of the practice of ambulatory anesthesia (see Chapter 31) and anesthesia in obesity are presented elsewhere (see Chapter 45).

Robotic Laparoscopic Surgery

4 Robotic laparoscopic surgery is a highly sophisticated technologic variation on conventional laparoscopic surgery, requiring modification of both surgical and anesthetic management.[1–4] The approach was developed to address several limitations of conventional laparoscopy, including reduced range of motion and instrument dexterity, and a two-dimensional (2D) view of the operative field. The advanced technology has greatly expanded the application of laparoscopic surgery. Although it was first popularized in urology for radical prostatectomies, robotic-assisted surgery has since gained ground in other fields, in part due to improved surgical outcomes, lower complication rates, shortened lengths of hospital stay, and better ergonomics for the surgeon. It currently has applications and Food and Drug Administration (FDA) approval in other types of urologic surgeries, general laparoscopic surgeries, general noncardiovascular thoracoscopic surgeries, thoracoscopically-assisted cardiotomy procedures, and may be used with adjunctive mediastinotomy to perform coronary anastomosis during cardiac revascularization (Table 44-3).

Robotic surgery is most commonly performed employing the Da Vinci surgical system (Intuitive Surgical Inc., Sunnyvale, CA) that uses a surgeon control console, a robot cart with interactive surgical arms, and a high-definition (HD) three-dimentional (3D) video tower (Fig. 44-1). Similar to conventional laparoscopy, robotic laparoscopic surgery entails the creation of a pneumoperitoneum, insertion of a video laparoscope, and insertion of trocars for surgical access. Next, a surgical robot is positioned near the patient, with robotic arms inserted into the insufflated abdominal cavity. The robotic arms are controlled remotely by a surgeon seated at an ergonomically designed control console. Remote handling of instruments via a specialized control allows for movements that mimic natural maneuvers, improved degrees of freedom, and optimal surgical instrument rotation and pivoting. Surgical visualization is achieved via a goggle viewfinder with an HD, magnified, 3D video display. An assistant near the surgical

Table 44-3 Examples of Robotic-Assisted Laparoscopic Surgery

Cardiac Coronary artery bypass, valvuloplasty
Thoracic Lung resection, esophagectomy
Gastrointestinal Fundoplication, colectomy, gastrectomy, hepatectomy
Urologic Radical cystectomy, pyeloplasty, prostatectomy
Gynecologic, Oncologic Hysterectomy, lymph-node dissection, oophorectomy

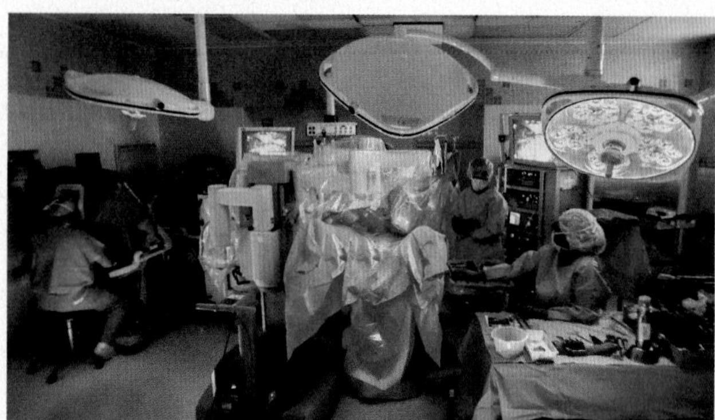

Figure 44-1 Robotic surgery room setup. Surgeon at the console (**left**), robot and patient (**center**), and video tower (**right**).

field provides surgical support, such as robotic arm adjustments, tissue retraction, and suctioning. Other clinicians in the operating room suite visualize the laparoscopic surgical field using 2D HD video screens.

5 Anesthetic management during laparoscopic robotic surgery requires preparing for patient accessibility limitations and adjusting for patient positioning challenges. Prominent robotic equipment near the patient can greatly limit anesthesia provider access to the patient. Though newer surgical robotic systems are becoming more compact, with thinner robotic arms and improved motorized maneuverability functions for steering and engaging, the robotic systems in use today have a large footprint near and above the operating room bed. In the rare event of an airway or cardiopulmonary emergency, the robotic surgical arms must first be carefully disengaged from the trocars before the robot can be removed safely and the patient positioned in a manner consistent with that needed for airway management or cardiopulmonary resuscitation.

Steep Trendelenburg positioning used in many robotic surgeries requires vigilance on the part of the whole intraoperative team. The risk of ocular injury in steep Trendelenburg during robotic surgery may be greater than in conventional laparoscopic surgery (see Complications Related to Surgery). Robotic arms often extend above the patient's face in this position, increasing the risk of both accidental endotracheal tube dislodgement and facial injury. Careful endotracheal tube taping and protective foam padding can be placed on the patient's face for extra security.

Physiologic Impact of Laparoscopy

Laparoscopic surgery induces complex physiologic changes that impact multiple organ systems. Direct mechanical stress as well as neuroendocrine stimulation are the primary forces responsible for most of the physiologic derangements observed during these procedures. The magnitude of these effects is modified by a patient's preexisting comorbidities, surgical factors, and anesthetic technique.[19]

Cardiovascular System

The cardiovascular system is exquisitely challenged during laparoscopy by multiple stressors on preload, inotropy, rhythm, and afterload (Table 44-4). The cumulative effect is an increase in mean arterial pressure (MAP), myocardial oxygen demand, pulmonary vascular resistance (PVR), and systemic vascular resistance (SVR). Modifiable factors that affect hemodynamics during

Table 44-4 Causes of Hemodynamic Changes During Laparoscopy

Determinants of Blood Pressure in Laparoscopy[a]	Effect on Blood Pressure
Preload (Venous Return)	
IVC compression	↑ or no change
Intra-abdominal organ compression	↑ or no change
Trendelenburg position	↑
Cardiac Output or Inotropya	
Venous return	↑ or no change
Peripheral vasoconstriction	↑ or no change
Rhythm (Brady- or Tachyarrhythmia[a])	
Hypercapnia/acidosis	↑ or no change
Hypoxia	↓ or no change
Peritoneal irritation	↑,↓ or no change
Afterload and MAP[a]	
Hypercapnia/acidosis	↑,↓ or no change

[a]Autonomic nervous system stimulation and neurohumoral factors, such as catecholamines, vasopressin, and cortisol released during laparoscopy contribute to these physiologic changes.
IVC, inferior vena cava; MAP, mean arterial pressure.

laparoscopy include the intravascular volume status of the patient, positioning, baseline comorbidities, and surgical technique.

CO_2 gas is highly soluble and during insufflation, it rapidly moves from the peritoneal cavity into the circulation. Prolonged surgeries and high insufflation pressures can lead to increased CO_2 absorption. Systemic CO_2 then exerts both direct and indirect effects on the cardiovascular system via adrenergic pathways. Mild hypercarbia ($PaCO_2$ of 45 to 50 mmHg) alters hemodynamics very little, whereas severe hypercarbia ($PaCO_2$ 55 to 70 mmHg) and acidosis can lead to myocardial depression, dysrhythmias from catecholamine-induced myocardial sensitization, and systemic vasodilation. Further complicating the response of the myocardium to transient hypercarbia is the potential for acute elevations in right ventricular afterload from hypercarbia-induced pulmonary vasoconstriction. The potential hemodynamic effects of severe hypercarbia are counteracted by sympathetic nervous system stimulation that concurrently produces tachycardia, an increase in MAP, and vasoconstriction from an increase in SVR.[20] 6

The peritoneum and abdominal viscera are highly innervated by autonomic nerve fibers. Stimulation of these autonomic pathways during pneumoperitoneum typically results in sympathetic nervous system activation, catecholamine release, activation of the renin–angiotensin system, and release of the neurohypophysial hormone vasopressin (antidiuretic hormone).[21] This potent endogenous hormone can cause intense vasoconstriction, an increase in MAP, and an increase in left ventricular afterload. Left ventricular wall tension and myocardial work needed to maintain intraventricular pressure and cardiac index (CI), respectively, are increased when there is a significant increase in SVR. Mechanical stretch on the peritoneum and abdominal viscera can result in parasympathetic stimulation through the vagus nerve, but sympathetic tone usually predominates.

Intravascular volume status is an important modifier of the mechanical effects of pneumoperitoneum.[20] In instances where low right atrial pressures reflect low cardiac filling volumes, an increase in IAP can result in compression of the inferior vena cava (IVC),

Table 44-5 Causes of Pulmonary Changes During Laparoscopy

Anatomic Displacement	V/Q Mismatch	Altered Lung Mechanics
Cranial cephalad displacement	Lung-volume reduction/uneven gas distribution	↓ Lung compliance
Diaphragm elevation	↑ Alveolar–arterial oxygen gradient	↑ Lung resistance
Endobronchial intubation	↑ Airway pressure	↑ Pleural pressure

causing a decrease in venous return and cardiac filling. In contrast, where high right atrial pressures reflect high cardiac filling volumes, the IVC can resist collapse, resulting in a rapid but transient increase in venous return from splanchnic compression.

7 Patient positioning can further modify the effects of IAP. Steep Trendelenburg positioning during pneumoperitoneum may augment venous return and cardiac filling.[22] In contrast, reverse Trendelenburg positioning during pneumoperitoneum can result in an increase in SVR and minor reductions in CI that are soon reversed. Initiating insufflation while supine and maintaining IAP within the recommended range (12 to 15 mmHg) can minimize any reduction in preload.[19] Nonetheless, extremely high IAP, especially in the setting of hypovolemia, can result in severe compression of the venous system as well as a perilous reduction in venous return and cardiac filling.

Preoperative comorbidities have varying effects on hemodynamics. Morbidly obese patients undergoing laparoscopic gastric bypass surgery show similar hemodynamic changes as nonbariatric patients. It is hypothesized that the morbidly obese better tolerate insufflation because of an intrinsically elevated IAP (9 to 10 mmHg) compared with nonobese patients.[23] Geriatric patients can generally tolerate laparoscopic surgery. However, complex hemodynamic changes in elderly patients with cardiovascular disease may be significant during pneumoperitoneum, despite a lack of observable myocardial ischemia by electrocardiogram.[24] In geriatric patients with at least one cardiac risk factor (i.e., history of hypertension, coronary artery disease, heart failure, or myocardial ischemia), the initiation of pneumoperitoneum in the supine position results in an increase in SVR and a reduction in ejection fraction (EF) and CI. Preload and left ventricular stroke work index (LVSWI) remain unchanged. Trendelenburg positioning increases preload, EF, and CI. Return to supine positioning with desufflation decreases SVR below baseline and increases EF, CI, and LVSWI—all to above baseline. In patients with significant pulmonary hypertension or right ventricular failure, ventricular function may be strained in the setting of changing preload and PVR. Acute increases in preload can strain an already stressed right ventricle. Hypercarbia and acidosis can lead to increased pulmonary vasoconstriction and right ventricular afterload, in addition to impaired inotropy. Significant volume loading of a dilated right ventricle can in turn compress the left ventricle through the mechanism of ventricular interdependence, leading to reduced global ventricular function.

The type of surgical procedure may also influence the degree of hemodynamic derangement. Surgical disruption of the esophageal hiatus during laparoscopic fundoplication may increase mediastinal and pleural pressures, resulting in a significant reduction in CI. Laparoscopic robotic prostatectomy results in hemodynamics similar to conventional laparoscopic surgery.[25,26] In a healthy patient placed in steep Trendelenburg position during robotic prostatectomy, ventricular filling pressure is increased, whereas cardiac markers of ventricular performance remain unchanged.

Respiratory System

Laparoscopic abdominal surgery exerts changes to the pulmonary 8
system by mechanically displacing thoracic structures, altering lung mechanics (i.e., volumes, compliance, resistance) and disrupting gas exchange through ventilation–perfusion mismatch (Table 44-5). An early effect of insufflation is displacement of the diaphragm into the thorax, which can be further aggravated by Trendelenburg positioning.[19] This shifts the carina cephalad, increasing the risk of endobronchial intubation. Elevated IAP and diaphragmatic displacement also lead to compression of the lung bases, atelectasis, intrapulmonary shunting, and hypoxemia. However, abnormally low levels of oxygen are rarely observed in patients with normal preoperative pulmonary function. The change in pulmonary compliance are observed as an increase in airway pressure during positive pressure ventilation. Furthermore, steep Trendelenburg positioning with pneumoperitoneum can produce close to a 50% reduction in lung compliance.[26] Ventilator adjustments may be needed to minimize peak airway pressure while maintaining acceptable minute ventilation. Hypercarbia from CO_2 pneumoperitoneum frequently requires adjustments in mechanical ventilation.

Hypercarbia routinely develops in all patients undergoing laparoscopic surgery from the absorption of intraperitoneal CO_2 into the circulatory system (Table 44-6). The concentration

Table 44-6 Causes of Severe Hypercarbia During Laparoscopy

Excessive CO_2 Absorption	Excessive CO_2 Production	Inadequate CO_2 Removal
CO_2 venous embolism	Hypermetabolic conditions (e.g., fever, malignant hyperthermia)	Hypoventilation
Subcutaneous emphysema	Morbid obesity	Endobronchial intubation
Capnothorax (CO_2 pneumothorax)		Atelectasis
Capnomediastinum		Cardiogenic shock
Capnopericardium		Exhausted CO_2 absorber

Table 44-7 Causes of Hypoxia During Laparoscopy

Preexisting Comorbidities	Inadequate O_2 Supply or Gas Exchange	Low Cardiac Output
Morbid obesity	Hypoventilation	Vena cava compression
Cardiopulmonary disease (e.g., congestive heart failure, chronic obstructive pulmonary disease)	Atelectasis	CO_2 venous embolism
	Endobronchial intubation Low inspired oxygen concentration	Capnothorax (CO_2 pneumothorax) Capnomediastinum Capnopericardium Acute dysrhythmias Severe hemorrhage

gradient that develops preferentially drives CO_2 from the pulmonary capillaries into the alveolar network, where it is removed during exhalation and measured by capnography as end-tidal CO_2 ($ETCO_2$). Exhaled CO_2 and the degree of gas absorption vary based on the route of insufflation, preoperative comorbidities, and intraoperative pathology. Extraperitoneal insufflation results in accumulation of CO_2 gas in an amount that is influenced by injection site, degree of tissue gas dissection, and perfusion differences of gas-dissected tissue. This is distinctly different from intraperitoneal insufflation, where gas in injected into the peritoneal cavity via a gas circulating circuit, resulting in a more predictable amount of CO_2 gas accumulation and elimination. Though extraperitoneal insufflation compared to intraperitoneal insufflation might result in more CO_2 absorption, a steady state of elimination can be reached within about 30 minutes.[27] In severe emphysema, the normal elimination of insufflated CO_2 may be prolonged due to pathologic disruption of alveolar network architecture.

In healthy patients undergoing intraperitoneal laparoscopy, hypercarbia and changes in pulmonary mechanics may have limited clinical significance. Compensatory hyperventilation can readily normalize hypercapnia. Despite speculation that ventilation–perfusion mismatch contributes to hypercapnia, minimal changes occur in alveolar dead space and pulmonary shunting during prolonged and steep Trendelenburg positioning with pneumoperitoneum used in robotic-assisted hysterectomy and prostatectomy.[28] Elevated $ETCO_2$ levels with a stable $PaCO_2$ in these types of surgeries is likely due to insufflated CO_2 absorption and not impaired alveolar ventilation.

Hypoxia during laparoscopy is usually due to a transient ventilation–perfusion mismatch that is commonly attributed to intrapulmonary shunting (Table 44-7). Physiologic and anatomical changes induced during pneumoperitoneum and extreme positioning can reduce the number of ventilated alveolar units being perfused. A reduction in functional residual capacity (FRC) in the supine position, or a preprocedural reduction in functional alveolar units might increase the risk of hypoxia during laparoscopy. Nonetheless, in a porcine animal model, there is evidence of improved arterial oxygenation during insufflation, mediated by hypoxic pulmonary vasoconstriction.[29,30]

Morbid obesity and chronic obstructive pulmonary disease (COPD) are common preexisting conditions that may complicate ventilation and gas exchange during laparoscopy. Compensating for hypercarbia, managing inspiratory resistance, and maintaining normoxia in morbidly obese patients are common intraoperative dilemmas. While extreme hypercarbia is detrimental, mild hypercarbia can improve tissue oxygenation, cause vasodilatation, and induce a rightward shift of the oxyhemoglobin dissociation curve.[31,32] Even before the induction of pneumoperitoneum, morbidly obese patients can have an inspiratory resistance about 70% higher than nonobese patients. After Trendelenburg positioning, inspiratory resistance increases significantly. A sizable reduction in FRC from pneumoperitoneum and Trendelenburg positioning may greatly impair PaO_2.[33] High BMI alone may also be a predictor of impaired PaO_2, despite compensatory ventilatory maneuvers.[34] Compared to healthy adults, morbidly obese patients are more likely to experience a prolonged return to baseline exhaled CO_2 after cessation of pneumoperitoneum, which may extend the need for ventilatory support.[35]

In patients with advanced COPD, severe hypercarbia and limited correlation with standard capnography is expected. A reduced number of intact pulmonary units and decreased effective alveolar ventilation can lead to a rapid and severe rise in $PaCO_2$ during pneumoperitoneum that may be refractory to hyperventilation maneuvers. Increased alveolar physiologic space in these patients leads to a wide $PaCO_2$–$ETCO_2$ difference. As a result, $ETCO_2$ monitoring in COPD may underestimate the actual $PaCO_2$.

Regional Perfusion Effects

In healthy patients undergoing laparoscopy, the splanchnic, renal, cerebral, and ocular organ systems undergo physiologic changes that are transient and of limited clinical significance; however, under certain circumstances, these changes have the potential to induce deleterious end-organ effects (Table 44-8). The magnitude of physiologic derangement and likelihood of iatrogenic injury from laparoscopy are modified by the patient's underlying pathophysiology.

Splanchnic blood flow may decrease both from external compression during pneumoperitoneum and systemic vasoconstriction from released neuroendogenous hormones. Increased IAP produced during pneumoperitoneum is known to reduce hepatic vein flow.[36] This may be advantageous during laparoscopic hepatic transection surgery; CO_2 peritoneum between 10 and 14 mmHg is sometimes used to minimize bleeding.[37] Diminished mesenteric blood flow during pneumoperitoneum has been implicated in unusual cases of intraoperative mesenteric ischemia in patients with underlying cardiovascular compromise.[38] Although splanchnic vasodilatation from absorbed CO_2 may offset any potential reductions in mesenteric blood flow in healthy patients, caution should be used in patients with known impairments in intestinal arterial flow, such as chronic mesenteric ischemia.

Renal function is reduced during pneumoperitoneum. 9
Increased IAP and the neurohumoral effects of pneumoperitoneum

Table 44-8 Causes of Regional Perfusion Changes During Laparoscopy

Cerebral	Splanchnic	Systemic Vasculature
↑ Cerebral blood flow	↓ or no change in intestinal flow Hypercapnic mesenteric vasodilatation Pneumoperitoneum-induced bowel compression	↓ Femoral vein flow IVC compression
↑ Intracranial pressure	↓ Hepatic flow Pneumoperitoneum-induced hepatic compression ↓ Renal flow Pneumoperitoneum-induced renal compression	

IVC, inferior vena cava

may account for reductions in renal blood flow, glomerular filtration, and urine output. Prolonged exposure to high insufflation pressure has been shown to correlate with reduced urine output; however, permanent renal sequelae are rare.[39] A reduction in renal perfusion induces vasopressin release, which results in reduced free water excretion and is associated with an increase in abdominal cavity pressure.[40] The use of surrogate renal injury biomarkers may facilitate the creation of a risk stratification tool that might better predict the likelihood of pneumoperitoneum related-acute kidney injury (AKI) based on preoperative variables.[41] Preoperative risk factors for renal dysfunction, such as hypertension and chronic kidney disease, may increase the risk of AKI postoperatively.[41] In bariatric surgery, increasing BMI and both insulin- and noninsulin-dependent diabetes mellitus have been associated with an increased risk of AKI within 72 hours of surgery.[42]

Both intracranial pressure and cerebral perfusion increase during Trendelenburg positioning and pneumoperitoneum, likely due to diminished cerebral venous outflow and hypercarbia-induced cerebral hyperperfusion.[43] Although the cerebral venous blood fraction is increased due to a reduction in cerebral venous drainage, regional cerebral tissue oxygen saturation is also increased, possibly due to an increase in cerebral oxygen delivery resulting from elevated cerebral perfusion pressure and cerebral hyperperfusion.[44] Though these physiologic changes are usually well-tolerated in healthy patients, prolonged steep Trendelenburg positioning with pneumoperitoneum has been associated with acute postoperative cerebral edema.[45] Patients with known or occult cerebral vascular disease or intracranial tumor are at increased risk of complications.

Intraocular pressure (IOP) increases during robotic prostatectomy in steep Trendelenburg positioning.[46] The determinants of elevated IOP in this setting are theorized to be elevations in central venous pressure (CVP) from Trendelenburg positioning and increased choroidal blood volume from hypercarbia. Rare cases of postoperative blindness after prolonged steep Trendelenburg positioning in laparoscopic prostatectomy[47] and colorectal surgery[48] have been reported. However, the role of increased IOP in the development of postoperative ischemic optic neuropathy remains controversial. Preexisting diseases, such as atherosclerotic disease, diabetes, and glaucoma, may lower the threshold of tolerance to acute intraocular derangements during laparoscopic surgery.

Intraoperative Management

General endotracheal anesthesia (GETA), muscle relaxation, and controlled mechanical ventilation remains the preferred anesthetic technique for laparoscopic surgery. Some factors that make laparoscopic surgery best suited for GETA versus other anesthetic techniques include extreme patient positioning, discomfort from pneumoperitoneum, prolonged operative times, and induced cardiopulmonary derangements. However, regional anesthesia might be suitable for brief laparoscopic procedures with minimal positioning changes.[20]

Monitoring

Electrocardiography, noninvasive blood pressure, capnography, pulse oximetry, and body temperature monitoring are mandatory. Neuromuscular and brain function monitoring are implemented at clinician discretion. Invasive or advanced noninvasive monitoring, such as arterial catheter, pulse contour analysis, pulmonary artery catheter, or echocardiography may be considered if significant preexisting cardiopulmonary disease is present. Reliability of CVP monitoring may be compromised, especially during steep Trendelenburg positioning.

Anesthesia Maintenance

Inhaled Anesthetics and Propofol

Desflurane and sevoflurane are inhaled anesthetics with short-acting and easily titratable properties, ideally suited for laparoscopic and robotic surgeries.[38] Propofol-based total intravenous anesthesia (propofol-TIVA) is an alternative that may be especially beneficial in patients with a history of postoperative nausea and vomiting (PONV).[49] Propofol's antiemetic properties may be mediated by its effect on gamma-aminobutyric acid receptor activity and olfactory cortex synaptic transmission.[50] However, there is no convincing evidence that propofol-TIVA is superior to volatile anesthetics.[51]

Nitrous Oxide

The use of nitrous oxide (N_2O) during laparoscopic surgery is controversial. During anesthesia, N_2O is believed to diffuse into air spaces such as intestinal lumina, leading to adverse pressurization. However, detectable intestinal distension and disruption of laparoscopic surgical conditions do not appear to occur during N_2O-based anesthesia.[52] N_2O is avoided by some practitioners due to a potentially greater risk of PONV. Although the risk of PONV with N_2O-based anesthetics seems to be greater than non-N_2O based anesthetics (particularly in young female patients) the overall risk in laparoscopy appears to be equivocal.[53] Additionally, the PONV risk associated with N_2O appears to be overcome using antiemetic prophylaxis or the addition of propofol to the anesthetic. N_2O is known to support combustion during a spark ignition. During an N_2O-based anesthetic, N_2O has been shown to accumulate to a combustible level in the peritoneal cavity within as little as 30 minutes.[54] Nonetheless, the incidence of spontaneous intra-abdominal laparoscopic surgical fire with N_2O is exceedingly rare. This may be explained by the mechanical circulation of peritoneal gases during pneumoperitoneum.

Pharmacologic Adjuncts

A number of pharmacologic adjuncts are available to minimize intraoperative sympathetic stimulation and optimize postoperative recovery following laparoscopic procedures. Remifentanil significantly suppresses sympathetic stimulation and the neuroendocrine stress response during pneumoperitoneum[55] without the prolonged respiratory effects of longer-acting opioids. Dexmedetomidine infusion during bariatric surgery reduces fentanyl use, PONV, and recovery room length of stay.[56] Lidocaine infusion administered during laparoscopic abdominal surgery has been associated with significant early postoperative pain reduction, as well as faster return of gastrointestinal motility.[57–60] Wound infiltration or intraperitoneal instillation with a local anesthetic is routinely performed as part of a preemptive analgesia strategy.[61,62] Improvements in early postoperative pain scores have been shown with both wound infiltration[63,64] and intraperitoneal installation[65,66] of a long-acting local anesthetic. Continuous local anesthetic wound infiltration may have a role in laparoscopic-assisted surgical procedures with longer incisions.[62] Paracetamol and nonsteroidal anti-inflammatory drugs (NSAIDs) are also commonly used adjuncts that reduce opioid requirements.[67]

Neuromuscular Blockade

10 Neuromuscular blocking agents are routinely used to improve surgical exposure during pneumoperitoneum. Still, controversy remains about how to best define the role of neuromuscular blockade (NMB) in laparoscopic surgery,[68] while minimizing the potential respiratory complications associated with residual paralysis. Subjective assessments of surgical working conditions during laparoscopy continue to vary among surgeons and anesthesia providers, as well as between surgeons. Satisfaction scores regarding surgical conditions during laparoscopy are consistently higher during deep versus conventional NMB.[69–71] Small trials show a correlation between deep NMB and improved surgical exposure during laparoscopy at IAPs less than 15 mmHg,[72,73] which supports the notion that more muscle relaxation provides better surgical exposure. Nonetheless, undetected residual paralysis and impaired hypoxic-ventilatory response remain significant patient safety risks associated with deep NMB.[74,75] Suffice it to say, monitoring of neuromuscular function and the use of reversal agents are imperative, especially when deep NMB is maintained. However, monitoring of neuromuscular function can be challenging since a patient's arms are often tucked during laparoscopic and robotic procedures and monitoring of the facial nerve is notoriously flawed. The widespread availability of sugammadex has facilitated the ability to quickly reverse the effects of nondepolarizing muscle relaxants with minimal side effects.[76,77]

Mechanical Ventilation

Volume control (VCV) and pressure control (PCV) ventilation with positive end-expiratory pressure (PEEP) are the conventional modes of ventilation used during general endotracheal anesthesia (GETA). Both modes of ventilation are suitable to handle the transient effects of laparoscopy on lung mechanics and to control minute ventilation during pneumoperitoneum.[78] Extreme positioning during pneumoperitoneum creates unique challenges relevant to each mode. During VCV in steep Trendelenburg, tidal volume remains constant while peak airway pressure increases and lung compliance decreases. In PCV, peak airway pressure remains constant while tidal volume typically decreases. Reverse Trendelenburg usually induces the opposite ventilatory effects—that is, lower peak airway pressure and increased compliance during VCV, and increased tidal volume during PCV. Though switching from VCV to PCV during Trendelenburg may result in dynamic lung mechanic improvements, the effects do not appear to result in significant static lung changes, better oxygenation, or any other measurable benefits.[79]

Compensatory hyperventilation and PEEP may be employed if either hypercarbia or hypoxia occur. Hypercapnia during laparoscopic cholecystectomy in a healthy patient may be corrected by increasing minute ventilation to about 25% above baseline.[80] Ventilation strategies that utilize PEEP can significantly improve ventilation–perfusion matching.[81] The use of PEEP during pneumoperitoneum for extended laparoscopy may improve oxygenation.[82] Furthermore, alveolar recruitment maneuvers (ARM) with the application of PEEP may help prevent the development of ventilator-induced lung injury by keeping alveoli open; this is especially true in obese patients.

PEEP in the presence of insufflation can increase intrathoracic pressure and contribute to a decrease in preload and a subsequent decrease in CI. This is especially true in the context of hypovolemia. However, the expected physiologic consequences of intrathoracic pressure on preload may vary based on habitus and patient position. The combination of ARM and PEEP in obese patients to improve oxygenation and lung compliance does not appear to harm MAP.[78] A position where the head is elevated above the level of the heart can promote venous pooling to the lower extremities, thereby transiently reducing preload. Additional factors that may alter the degree of preload reduction and subsequent hemodynamic variability include upper torso angle above 0 degrees, PEEP level, preoperative comorbidities, ventilator mechanics, and magnitude of insufflation pressure. Still, in a healthy patient positioned in a semifowler position, judicious PEEP can be hemodynamically safe, while improving ventilatory mechanics and oxygenation during pneumoperitoneum.[83,84] The physiologic mechanisms that determine these variable observations continue to be explored.

Low tidal volumes (6 to 8 mL/kg ideal body weight) and optimized PEEP (5 to 10 cm H_2O, or greater) continue to be the key components to minimizing the risk of ventilator-induced lung injury.[85,86] The rationale for lung-protective ventilation strategies in the operating room borrows from experience managing acute respiratory distress syndrome in the intensive care unit. The ideal inspired oxygen fraction (FiO_2) continues to be debated.[87] Intraoperative oxygen delivery at high concentration is speculated to have secondary benefits for PONV reduction, improved wound healing, and optimal ventilation–perfusion matching. The mechanisms by which oxygen reduces risks in the aforementioned categories remain mostly unknown. Nevertheless, prolonged exposure to 100% oxygen can result in alveolar nitrogen wash out and subsequent absorption atelectasis. States of hyperoxia can induce reactive oxygen species that may cause molecular and cellular injury and ultimately pulmonary oxygen toxicity and injury.

Body Temperature

Temperature control and monitoring during laparoscopic surgery should follow standard American Society of Anesthesiologists (ASA) guidelines. Active forced-air warming is effective in preventing hypothermia and is an important strategy to avoid postoperative surgical site infections.[88] The effects of CO_2 gas insufflation on heat loss during laparoscopic surgery is controversial. CO_2 gas used in laparoscopy is stored as a cold, liquid in pressurized cylinders. Phase transition from liquid to gas results in rapid heat extraction from the environment and release of cold, desiccated gas. Convective heat losses during insufflation have been theorized to be worse when intraperitoneal contents are exposed to cold, dry CO_2 gas.[89] This has led to the practice of actively warming and humidifying insufflated gas with an inline heating device.[90] However, insufflation with heated and humidified versus cold and dry CO_2 gas has not been shown to be superior in terms of preventing hyperthermia.[91]

Fluid Management

Pneumoperitoneum may create volume shifts that can alter expected perioperative fluid therapy goals. In patients undergoing ambulatory laparoscopic cholecystectomy, intraoperative fluid loading with 40 mL/kg compared with 15 mL/kg of Ringer's lactate resulted in unexpected improvements in postoperative pulmonary function, exercise capacity, and overall well-being. Surgical stress markers were also reduced.[92] These findings suggest a benefit to volume loading in the healthy patient undergoing elective ambulatory laparoscopy. However, in patients with comorbidities undergoing major abdominal laparoscopic surgery, fluid loading may be deleterious.

Classic hemodynamic and physiologic indicators used to guide intraoperative fluid administration may not be reliable during laparoscopic surgery. Pneumoperitoneum and steep Trendelenburg positioning alter the predictive value of heart rate, blood pressure, and CVP. Pneumoperitoneum also limits the value of urine output as a surrogate for intravascular volume status. Intraoperative monitors for goal-directed fluid therapy, such as esophageal Doppler, pulse contour analysis, and bioreactance, are available for use at a clinician's discretion. Though restricted fluid therapy approaches have gained momentum recently, insufficient evidence exists regarding the optimal total volume delivery, fluid timing, and role of intraoperative hemodynamic monitoring. In laparoscopic bariatric surgery, high-volume loading (10 mL/kg/h) compared to low-volume loading (4 mL/kg/h) of Ringer's lactate resulted in similar rates of oliguria with no difference in the risk of renal dysfunction.[93,94]

Complications Related to Surgery

Despite having an excellent safety profile, perioperative complications during laparoscopic surgery still occur and are most attributable to abdominal entry technique, pneumoperitoneum, or patient positioning.[95,96] Risk factors for complications include upper abdominal procedures, robotic surgery, and significant preexisting diseases.[97–101] Some complications encountered intraoperatively require emergent conversion to open laparotomy.

Intraoperative

Intra-abdominal Injuries

11 Over 50% of complications related to laparoscopy occur as a result of Veress needle and/or primary trocar insertion during abdominal entry.[95] Major vessels at risk for injury during midline abdominal entry include the abdominal aorta, iliac vessels, and IVC. Abdominal entry away from the midline puts other vessels at risk, such as the superior and inferior mesenteric arteries, epigastric artery, and other small vessels of the abdominal wall. Vessels proximal to the site of surgical dissection are at increased risk of injury; this includes the cystic and hepatic artery during laparoscopic cholecystectomy, and the dorsal vein complex during robotic prostatectomy. Though frank bleeding from a major vascular injury may be visible, it often remains occult, requiring clinicians to have a high level of suspicion throughout the procedure. The anesthesiologist should be prepared for immediate surgical conversion to an open laparotomy to control severe bleeding, while managing possible hemodynamic instability due to hemorrhagic shock. Intraoperative testing and interpretation of hematocrit as an assessment of acute blood loss should be performed cautiously, given the confounding effects of preoperative hematocrit collection, active bleeding, and intravascular dilution from crystalloid infusion. Transfusion triggers should be made on an individualized basis, taking into account estimated blood loss as well as the patient's hemodynamics and coexisting diseases. Despite these considerations, in general, the risk of bleeding complications during laparoscopic procedures is rare and routine preoperative type and screen testing is not necessary.[102,103]

Gastrointestinal structures can be injured during both abdominal entry and the intra-abdominal portion of the procedure.[95] Bowel injuries are infrequent but are a major cause of morbidity and mortality. Because many intestinal injuries go unrecognized, when they do occur, the risk of postoperative intra-abdominal sepsis is high, making it a common cause of death related to laparoscopy. Deflation of the stomach with an orogastric tube should be routinely performed prior to the start of surgery to minimize the risk of gastric injury during left upper quadrant trocar insertion. Bladder perforation and ureter ligation or transection are also possible during secondary trocar placement or in the context of dissection during laparoscopic hysterectomy. Low urine output, hematuria, and more rarely, pneumaturia may be signs of urologic injury during surgery. If suspected, the presence of an injury can be confirmed and possibly repaired via cystoscopy. Postoperative lower abdominal discomfort, unexpected gross hematuria, or rapidly rising serum creatinine should trigger immediate suspicion of occult injury.

Cardiopulmonary

Acute cardiovascular complications associated with laparoscopy 12
include hypertension, hypotension, dysrhythmias, and rarely, cardiac arrest. Hemodynamic and pulmonary changes are mediated by CO_2 insufflation, increased IAP, and hypercarbia. Initial insufflation at an IAP of 5 mmHg in normovolemic patients leads to an increase in venous return due to displacement of blood from the splanchnic vasculature, a rise in cardiac output, and hypertension. Catecholamine release further aggravates hypertension by increasing afterload. Catecholamine release and hypercarbia can also lead to tachyarrhythmias. As IAP increases to 15 mmHg, the IVC is compressed and venous return to the heart decreases, leading to a decrease in cardiac output and hypotension. Impaired venous return is also mediated by a sustained elevation in right atrial pressure. Peritoneal distention during abdominal insufflation can trigger vagally mediated bradyarrhythmias and even asystole.[104] Slower insufflation, lower IAP, and premedication with glycopyrrolate can diminish the vagal response and prevent cardiovascular collapse. If bradycardia occurs, the surgeon should be asked to open the laparoscopic port and deflate the abdomen to reduce IAP. Slow reinsufflation with lower IAP should be attempted. Conversion to open laparotomy or termination of surgery may be indicated if there is recurrent hypotension. Transient hypotension usually responds to a decrease in volatile anesthetics, volume loading, or decrease in IAP. Refractory hypotension may require immediate abdominal decompression, return to neutral patient position, and exploration for occult life-threatening conditions such as severe bleeding or capnothorax. Acute hypertension may be ameliorated by adjusting the depth of anesthesia. More severe cases may require short-acting vasoactive agents.

Pulmonary complications that develop during laparoscopy can present as acute hypercarbic (Table 44-6) or hypoxemic

(Table 44-7) events. Hypercarbia can lead to systemic vasodilatation, arrhythmias, and myocardial depression. Hypercarbia can also increase PVR and impact preload in patients with pulmonary hypertension or right ventricular failure. An increase in minute ventilation is usually effective to maintain partial pressure of CO_2 in or near the normal range. Refractory hypercarbia may require cessation of insufflation. If severe hypercarbia persists during emergence, particularly in the setting of significant pulmonary disease and obstructive sleep apnea, persistent ventilatory support should be considered. Treatment of hypoxemia should be swift, focusing on confirming O_2 delivery and endotracheal tube positioning. Immediate pneumoperitoneum release, 100% O_2 ventilation, and neutral positioning should be instituted for refractory hypoxia.

CO_2 Extravasation

Subcutaneous Emphysema

13 The inadvertent introduction of CO_2 gas into subcutaneous, preperitoneal, or retroperitoneal tissue leads to trapped gas pockets called subcutaneous emphysema.[105] Extension of extraperitoneal CO_2 gas along fascial planes can lead to distant anatomic areas being affected, such as the upper and lower extremities, neck, and face, as well as large cavities, such as the thorax, mediastinum, and pericardium. Risk factors for the development of subcutaneous emphysema include operative times greater than 3.5 hours, IAP >15 mmHg, higher insufflation flow rates, greater number of surgical ports, placement of cannulas outside the peritoneal cavity, $ETCO_2$ >50 mmHg, lower BMI, older patient age, and Nissen fundoplication surgery (NICV 44-2).[105,106] Subcutaneous emphysema may present as crepitus on physical exam but often remains undetected unless a computed tomography or X-ray is performed postoperatively. Unexplained sudden or persistent hypercarbia may be an early sign of subcutaneous emphysema.[107] The treatment of subcutaneous emphysema includes hyperventilation, and if inadequate, peritoneal desufflation. Reinsufflation at a lower IAP is recommended if pneumoperitoneum must be resumed. Postoperative treatment is supportive. Extravasated CO_2 resolves within 24 hours due to its high rate of diffusion. If concerns for persistent or recurrent hypercarbia from subcutaneous emphysema exist during the postoperative recovery, clinicians should maintain oxygen therapy and monitor for somnolence and acute respiratory acidosis by arterial blood gas. Cervical emphysema should be evaluated with a chest X-ray, and the airway should be evaluated for signs of obstruction.

Capnothorax

Carbon dioxide gas accumulation within the pleural space is called capnothorax. It is an unintentional complication of CO_2 insufflation that occurs when CO_2 travels outside the peritoneum, enters the mediastinum, and subsequently dissects along the parietal pleura. Tension capnothorax may occur from uncontrolled pressurization of the thoracic cavity, leading to an increase in intrathoracic pressure, mediastinal shift, decreased venous return, and subsequent right ventricular compression—a potentially life-threatening condition.[96,105]

Insufflated CO_2 can pass from the abdomen into the thorax and pleural space through various routes.[108,109] These include trauma to the diaphragm or falciform ligament. There are also several anatomic and congenital diaphragmatic defects in the diaphragm that connect the abdominal and thoracic cavities, most notably the aortic hiatus, esophageal hiatus, and caval opening. Risk factors for capnothorax are similar to those for subcutaneous emphysema; however, greater risk exists during procedures near the diaphragm (e.g., Nissen fundoplication).[100,107]

Early signs of capnothorax include palpable subcutaneous 14
emphysema in the upper torso, severe hypercarbia; on electrocardiogram, changes in the electrical axis and amplitude reduction may be observed. Physical exam findings include reduced breath sounds bilaterally or unilaterally as well as reduced chest excursion.[110] Tension capnothorax may present more acutely with high peak airway pressure, hypoxia, and severe hypotension.[109] Tension capnothorax can be life-threatening and may be difficult to diagnose intraoperatively; a high index of suspicion and quick communication with the surgical team is necessary. Transthoracic echocardiography is increasingly being used to assess intraoperative lung pathology, including pneumothorax.[111] However, its role in diagnosing capnothorax has not been well defined.

Primary treatment of capnothorax is immediate peritoneal desufflation. Hyperventilation can be used to expedite CO_2 reabsorption. Also, the addition of PEEP can reduce the pressure gradient between the abdomen and the thorax during both inspiration and expiration. Close observation is usually adequate for healthy patients with minimal physiologic derangements.[108,109,111] Patients with baseline cardiac dysfunction are more likely to require supportive therapy. Hemodynamically unstable patients should be supported with fluids or vasoactive agents while the capnothorax resolves. In severe cases, emergent needle decompression or chest tube insertion may be necessary intraoperatively. If tension capnothorax and hemodynamic instability recur after reinsufflation, termination of laparoscopy and conversion to an open surgical procedure is indicated.

Other thoracic structures rarely at risk for CO_2 dissection and compression include the mediastinum and pericardium. Capnomediastinum and capnopericardium may be associated with severe hemodynamic instability due to excessive pressure on the large mediastinal vascular structures and cardiac chambers. Treatment and postoperative management are similar to tension capnothorax.

Venous Gas Embolism

Venous CO_2 gas embolism is a potentially fatal complication of laparoscopy that occurs when a large volume of CO_2 gas enters a vein, artery, or solid organ, circulates to the heart, and results in increased pulmonary arterial pressure and resistance to right ventricular outflow. Decreased pulmonary venous return leads to decreased left ventricular preload and cardiac output which may result in cardiovascular collapse.[112] Although the consequence of CO_2 embolism is catastrophic, clinically significant emboli are rare. The availability of ultrasound for intraoperative monitoring has allowed clinicians to identify previously undetected gas emboli during laparoscopic surgery. Clinicians using intraoperative transesophageal echocardiography (TEE) have reported subclinical CO_2 gas emboli in approximately 20% of patients undergoing laparoscopic radical prostatectomies and nearly 100% of patients undergoing laparoscopic total hysterectomies.[113,114]

The etiology of a venous CO_2 gas embolism during laparoscopic surgery is multifactorial. Direct Veress needle insertion into a vein or solid organ during insufflation could potentially result in CO_2 entry into the venous system. Injured or transected vessels during laparoscopic surgical dissection may also provide a portal for gas ingress into the venous system. Round ligament transection and broad ligament dissection during laparoscopic hysterectomy have resulted in gas emboli.[114] The deep dorsal venous complex may be an entry point for CO_2 gas during radical prostatectomies.[115] Patient positioning may play a role in the degree of CO_2 gas entrainment into the right heart chambers. Trendelenburg position likely results in elevated CVPs, potentially minimizing susceptibility to significant gas emboli during pneumoperitoneum. Steep

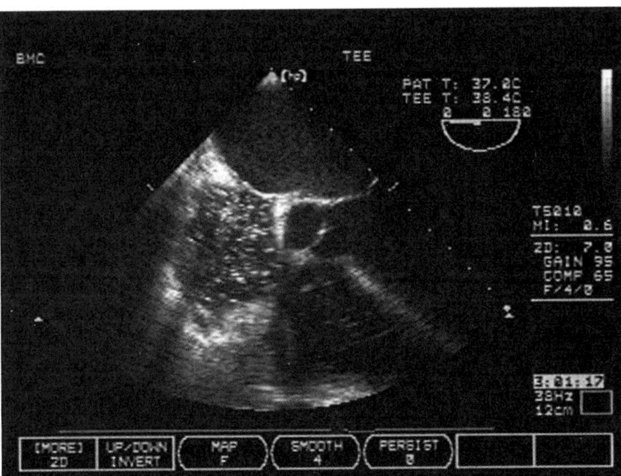

Figure 44-2 Venous air embolism of the right atrium visible with transesophageal echocardiographic monitoring.

Trendelenburg positioning during robotic radical prostatectomies appears to protect against venous gas embolism compared to open radical retropubic prostatectomies.[115,116]

The diagnosis of venous CO_2 gas embolism is usually dependent on recognition of the constellation of clinical signs. Acute tachycardia, cardiac arrhythmias, QRS complex widening, hypotension, hypoxemia, and low $ETCO_2$ may be observed. Physical exam findings may include cyanosis and a "mill wheel" murmur by auscultation. TEE is considered the most sensitive method for detecting gas emboli in the heart.[117] A large bolus of CO_2 gas would appear as a near white-out of the right heart chambers, potentially leading to a right ventricular air lock (Fig. 44-2). Because tiny air bubbles are present in most peripherally injected solutions, clinicians using TEE must be ready to distinguish CO_2 gas bubbles from peripherally injected bubbles. This can be facilitated by viewing the IVC during TEE monitoring.

Treatment of CO_2 gas embolism includes immediate termination of pneumoperitoneum and abdominal decompression. Advanced cardiac life support should be initiated for cardiac arrest. Rapid intravenous fluid should be used to treat hypotension. CO_2 gas removal may be accelerated with hyperventilation and administration of 100% O_2. The patient may be placed in Trendelenburg with a left lateral decubitus position to help minimize the severity of right ventricular air lock.

Patient Shifting and Falls

Potential injury related to patient positioning is fairly common in laparoscopic procedures, particularly in robot-assisted laparoscopy. Patients undergoing laparoscopy in steep reverse Trendelenburg and steep Trendelenburg are at risk of unexpectedly shifting downward or upward, respectively, on the operating room table. Operating rooms table falls are rare but potentially devastating.[118] The anesthesiologist should actively take part in safely positioning and securing the anesthetized patient. A patient in steep Trendelenburg may be secured from moving by using an operating table belt strap. Additional accessories include underbody skid prevention pads or a surgical "beanbag." During steep reverse Trendelenburg positioning, a padded footrest can be attached to the operating room table to keep a patient from shifting down and off the table. Careful attention should be paid to pressure points that may be created by securing devices.

Peripheral Nerve and Brachial Plexus Injuries

Patient positioning is responsible for a large proportion of nerve injuries acquired intraoperatively.[119] The mechanism of injury may involve excessive compression, stretch, and/or ischemia. Risk factors include prolonged operative times, high BMI, inadequate padding, arm tucking, steep Trendelenburg positioning, and improper use of positioning equipment (e.g., "beanbag" or stirrups). Brachial plexopathy is associated with steep Trendelenburg positioning and longer operative time in laparoscopic colorectal surgery.[120] In robotic prostatectomy, caudad shoulder displacement during steep Trendelenburg is another known causative factor.[121] Recommendations for risk reduction continue to evolve. In the meantime, careful attention to positioning throughout the operative course is imperative.

Ocular Injuries

The most frequent adverse ocular events during laparoscopic surgery are corneal abrasions and perioperative visual loss.[122] Corneal abrasions most commonly occur due to external factors, such as direct ocular trauma or corneal exposure; reduced production and distribution of lacrimal film may also be a factor. During robotic surgery, the camera system may come into contact with the patient's face. The use of protective devices like face masks and foam padding in addition to eye taping minimize this risk. Steep Trendelenburg positioning during laparoscopic robotic surgery is associated with increased IOP which may increase the risk of perioperative visual loss.[123] Additional risk factors for perioperative blindness may include external ocular pressure and excess fluid replacement.[124]

Airway Edema

Prolonged steep Trendelenburg position during robotic prostatectomy and some gynecologic surgeries together with large volume fluid resuscitation may induce facial and pharyngolaryngeal edema, which can lead to airway compromise postoperatively. Placing the patient in a recumbent sitting position often helps expedite reversal of orofacial edema during emergence and postoperative recovery. Performing an endotracheal tube cuff leak test prior to extubation may be helpful; however, how well this test rules out significant laryngeal edema in the intraoperative, noncritically ill patient is not well defined. If concerns for severe airway edema exist, continued postoperative intubation and ventilatory support is prudent.

Postoperative Complications

Respiratory Dysfunction

A significant benefit of laparoscopy over laparotomy is reduced postoperative respiratory complications. Albeit rare, the potential for postoperative respiratory dysfunction after laparoscopy surgery still exists and may be related to coexisting diseases, surgery-specific factors, and intraoperative challenges during mechanical ventilation. In bariatric surgery, patients with active reflux disease may be at risk for postoperative aspiration events and exacerbation of reactive airway disease.[125] Significant subcutaneous emphysema in the setting of coexisting lung disease may overwhelm a patient's ability to compensate for severe hypercarbia. Diaphragmatic dysfunction after laparoscopy has been reported[126] and can infrequently lead to respiratory dysfunction.[127]

Venous Thrombosis

The prevalence of deep venous thrombosis (DVT) and PE associated with laparoscopic surgery is low. Activation of the coagulation cascade and venous outflow obstruction during CO_2 pneumoperitoneum are the mechanisms associated with acute venous thromboembolism (VTE) in the context of laparoscopic surgery.[128] Surgical disease, associated comorbidities, and age are the most likely factors associated with VTE risk.[129] The prevalence of in-hospital VTE after laparoscopic cholecystectomy increases with age, but overall remains low.[129,130] Obesity is known to be associated with increased hypercoagulability, especially in women.[131] Lymph-node dissection during radical prostatectomy carries an increased risk of DVT and PE postoperatively, albeit lower if the surgery is performed robotically.[132]

Postoperative Management

Acute Pain Management

15 Postoperative pain has a significant impact on patient recovery, early mobilization, length of hospital stay, and return to normal activity. Compared to open abdominal surgery, laparoscopic surgery results in less and shorter duration of pain and reduced opioid consumption.[133] A number of surgical techniques during laparoscopy can reduce the severity of postoperative pain. These include the use of lower IAP, shorter duration of pneumoperitoneum, and evacuation of subdiaphragmatic CO_2 prior to wound closure.[134] Preemptive multimodal analgesia that relies on nonopioids, such as NSAIDS, cyclooxygenase-2 (COX-2) inhibitors, and acetaminophen is ideal. Although the role of transversus abdominis plane block remains unclear, this procedure remains a viable option for postoperative pain management after laparoscopic surgery.[135] Neuraxial analgesia is not routinely used unless the risk of conversion to laparotomy is high.[136]

Postoperative Nausea and Vomiting

Patients undergoing laparoscopic surgery are at greater risk of PONV than patients undergoing nonlaparoscopic surgery. PONV risk is particularly high in laparoscopic cholecystectomy.[137] In laparoscopic bariatric surgery, PONV is a common cause of prolonged anesthesia recovery.[138] Preoperative PONV risk stratification is useful in identifying those patients most likely to require antiemetic prophylaxis.[139]

Conclusion

Laparoscopic surgery has become a revolutionary alternative to many open surgical procedures. Its ability to provide surgeons the means to operate with minimal surgical trauma while providing patients a shorter postoperative recovery has made it critical to the growth of ambulatory surgery. The introduction of robotics has further expanded the applications of laparoscopy. For the anesthesia provider, "minimally invasive" surgery requires maximally attentive anesthesia. Pneumoperitoneum in conjunction with extreme patient positioning induces transient, but significant, multiorgan derangements that require short-term manipulation to minimize complications. Preemptive multimodal analgesia and PONV prophylaxis are also important to optimizing patient recovery.

For further review and interactivities, please see the videos and narrative interactive clinical vignettes (NICVs) accessible in the complimentary eBook bundled with this text. Access instructions are located on the inside front cover.

REFERENCES

1. Weinberg L, Rao S, Escobar PF. Robotic surgery in gynecology: an updated systematic review. *Obstet Gynecol Int*. 2011;2011:852061.
2. Finkelstein J, Eckersberger E, Sadri H, Taneja SS, Lepor H, Djavan B. Open versus laparoscopic versus robot-assisted laparoscopic prostatectomy: the European and US Experience. *Rev Urol*. 2010;12(1):35–43.
3. Hanly EJ, Talamini MA. Robotic abdominal surgery. *Am J Surg*. 2004;188(4A Suppl):19S–26S.
4. Mack MJ. Minimally invasive and robotic surgery. *JAMA*. 2001;285(5):568–572.
5. Gurusamy K, Junnarkar S, Farouk M, Davidson BR. Meta-analysis of randomized controlled trials on the safety and effectiveness of day-case laparoscopic cholecystectomy. *Br J Surg*. 2008;95(2):161–168.
6. Gurusamy KS, Junnarkar S, Farouk M, Davidson BR. Day-case versus overnight stay in laparoscopic cholecystectomy. *Cochrane Database Syst Rev*. 2008;(1):CD006798.
7. Thomas H, Agrawal S. Systematic review of day-case laparoscopic fundoplication. *J Laparoendosc Adv Surg Tech A*. 2011;21(9):781–788.
8. Thomas H, Agrawal S. Systematic review of same-day laparoscopic adjustable gastric band surgery. *Obes Surg*. 2011;21(6):805–810.
9. Thomas H, Agrawal S. Systematic review of 23-hour (outpatient) stay laparoscopic gastric bypass surgery. *J Laparoendosc Adv Surg Tech A*. 2011;21(8):677–681.
10. Walter CJ, Collin J, Dumville JC, Drew PJ, Monson JR. Enhanced recovery in colorectal resections: a systematic review and meta-analysis. *Colorectal Dis*. 2009;11(4):344–353.
11. Gurusamy KS, Koti R, Davidson BR. Abdominal lift for laparoscopic cholecystectomy. *Cochrane Database Syst Rev*. 2013;8:CD006574.
12. Gunning JE RB. Evolution of endoscopic surgery. In: White RA, ed. Endoscopic Surgery. Mosby Year Book; 1991:1–9.
13. Brash JH. Outpatient laparoscopic sterilization. *Br Med J*. 1976;1(6022):1376–1377.
14. Thompson B, Wheeless RC. Outpatient sterilization by laparoscopy: a report of 666 patients. *Obstet Gynecol*. 1971;38(6):912–915.
15. Vaughan J, Gurusamy KS, Davidson BR. Day-surgery versus overnight stay surgery for laparoscopic cholecystectomy. *Cochrane Database Syst Rev*. 2013;7:CD006798.
16. Hinojosa MW, Varela JE, Parikh D, Smith BR, Nguyen X-M, Nguyen NT. National trends in use and outcome of laparoscopic adjustable gastric banding. *Surg Obes Relat Dis*. 2009;5(2):150–155.
17. Abou Rached A, Basile M, El Masri H. Gastric leaks post sleeve gastrectomy: review of its prevention and management. *World J Gastroenterol*. 2014;20(38):13904–13910.
18. Joshi GP, Ahmad S, Riad W, Eckert S, Chung F. Selection of obese patients undergoing ambulatory surgery: a systematic review of the literature. *Anesth Analg*. 2013;117(5):1082–1091.
19. O'Malley C, Cunningham AJ. Physiologic changes during laparoscopy. *Anesthesiol Clin North Am*. 2001;19(1):1–19.
20. Collins LM, Vaghadia H. Regional anesthesia for laparoscopy. *Anesthesiol Clin North Am*. 2001;19(1):43–55.
21. Sammour T, Mittal A, Loveday BPT, et al. Systematic review of oxidative stress associated with pneumoperitoneum. *Br J Surg*. 2009;96(8):836–850.
22. Gannedahl P, Odeberg S, Brodin LA, Sollevi A. Effects of posture and pneumoperitoneum during anaesthesia on the indices of left ventricular filling. *Acta Anaesthesiol Scand*. 1996;40(2):160–166.
23. Nguyen NT, Wolfe BM. The physiologic effects of pneumoperitoneum in the morbidly obese. *Ann Surg*. 2005;241(2):219–226.
24. Harris SN, Ballantyne GH, Luther MA, Perrino AC Jr. Alterations of cardiovascular performance during laparoscopic colectomy: a combined hemodynamic and echocardiographic analysis. *Anesth Analg*. 1996;83(3):482–487.
25. Falabella A, Moore-Jeffries E, Sullivan MJ, Nelson R, Lew M. Cardiac function during steep Trendelenburg position and CO_2 pneumoperitoneum for robotic-assisted prostatectomy: a trans-oesophageal Doppler probe study. *Int J Med Robot*. 2007;3(4):312–315.
26. Lestar M, Gunnarsson L, Lagerstrand L, Wiklund P, Odeberg-Wernerman S. Hemodynamic perturbations during robot-assisted laparoscopic radical prostatectomy in 45° Trendelenburg position. *Anesth Analg*. 2011;113(5):1069–1075.
27. Kadam PG, Marda M, Shah VR. Carbon dioxide absorption during laparoscopic donor nephrectomy: a comparison between retroperitoneal and transperitoneal approaches. *Transplant Proc*. 2008;40(4):1119–1121.
28. Schrijvers D, Mottrie A, Traen K, et al. Pulmonary gas exchange is well preserved during robot assisted surgery in steep Trendelenburg position. *Acta Anaesthesiol Belg*. 2009;60(4):229–233.
29. Strang CM, Fredén F, Maripuu E, Hachenberg T, Hedenstierna G. Ventilation-perfusion distributions and gas exchange during carbon dioxide pneumoperitoneum in a porcine model. *Br J Anaesth*. 2010;105(5):691–697.

30. Strang CM, Ebmeyer U, Maripuu E, Hachenberg T, Hedenstierna G. Improved ventilation-perfusion matching by abdominal insufflation (pneumoperitoneum) with CO_2 but not with air. *Minerva Anestesiol*. 2013;79(6):617–625.
31. Hager H, Reddy D, Mandadi G, et al. Hypercapnia improves tissue oxygenation in morbidly obese surgical patients. *Anesth Analg*. 2006;103(3):677–681.
32. Fleischmann E, Herbst F, Kugener A, et al. Mild hypercapnia increases subcutaneous and colonic oxygen tension in patients given 80% inspired oxygen during abdominal surgery. *Anesthesiology*. 2006;104(5):944–949.
33. Pelosi P, Croci M, Ravagnan I, et al. The effects of body mass on lung volumes, respiratory mechanics, and gas exchange during general anesthesia. *Anesth Analg*. 1998;87(3):654–660.
34. Sprung J, Whalley DG, Falcone T, Wilks W, Navratil JE, Bourke DL. The effects of tidal volume and respiratory rate on oxygenation and respiratory mechanics during laparoscopy in morbidly obese patients. *Anesth Analg*. 2003;97(1):268–274.
35. Perilli V, Vitale F, Modesti C, Ciocchetti P, Sacco T, Sollazzi L. Carbon dioxide elimination pattern in morbidly obese patients undergoing laparoscopic surgery. *Surg Obes Relat Dis*. 2012;8(5):590–594.
36. Takagi S. Hepatic and portal vein blood flow during carbon dioxide pneumoperitoneum for laparoscopic hepatectomy. *Surg Endosc*. 1998;12(5):427–431.
37. Tranchart H, O'Rourke N, Van Dam R, et al. Bleeding control during laparoscopic liver resection: a review of literature. *J Hepatobiliary Pancreat Sci*. 2015;22(5):371–378.
38. Leduc LJ, Mitchell A. Intestinal ischemia after laparoscopic cholecystectomy. *JSLS*. 2006;10(2):236–238.
39. Nguyen NT, Perez RV, Fleming N, Rivers R, Wolfe BM. Effect of prolonged pneumoperitoneum on intraoperative urine output during laparoscopic gastric bypass. *J Am Coll Surg*. 2002;195(4):476–483.
40. Joris JL, Chiche JD, Canivet JLM, Jacquet NJ, Legros JJ, Lamy ML. Hemodynamic changes induced by laparoscopy and their endocrine correlates: effects of clonidine. *J Am Coll Cardiol*. 1998;32(5):1389–1396.
41. Calvert S, Shaw A. Perioperative acute kidney injury. *Perioper Med*. 2012;1(1):1–11.
42. Weingarten TN, Gurrieri C, McCaffrey JM, et al. Acute kidney injury following bariatric surgery. *Obes Surg*. 2013;23(1):64–70.
43. Halverson A, Buchanan R, Jacobs L, et al. Evaluation of mechanism of increased intracranial pressure with insufflation. *Surg Endosc*. 1998;12(3):266–269.
44. Kalmar AF, Foubert L, Hendrickx JFA, et al. Influence of steep Trendelenburg position and CO_2 pneumoperitoneum on cardiovascular, cerebrovascular, and respiratory homeostasis during robotic prostatectomy. *Br J Anaesth*. 2010;104(4):433–439.
45. Pandey R, Garg R, Darlong V, Punj J, Chandralekha, Kumar A. Unpredicted neurological complications after robotic laparoscopic radical cystectomy and ileal conduit formation in steep Trendelenburg position: two case reports. *Acta Anaesthesiol Belg*. 2010;61(3):163–166.
46. Hoshikawa Y, Tsutsumi N, Ohkoshi K, et al. The effect of steep Trendelenburg positioning on intraocular pressure and visual function during robotic-assisted radical prostatectomy. *Br J Ophthalmol*. 2014;98(3):305–308.
47. Weber ED, Colyer MH, Lesser RL, Subramanian PS. Posterior ischemic optic neuropathy after minimally invasive prostatectomy. *J Neuroophthalmol*. 2007;27(4):285–287.
48. Kumar G, Vyakarnam P. Postoperative vision loss after colorectal laparoscopic surgery. *Surg Laparosc Endosc Percutan Tech*. 2013;23(2):e87–e88.
49. Kumar G, Stendall C, Mistry R, Gurusamy K, Walker D. A comparison of total intravenous anaesthesia using propofol with sevoflurane or desflurane in ambulatory surgery: systematic review and meta-analysis. *Anaesthesia*. 2014;69(10):1138–1150.
50. Collins GG. Effects of the anaesthetic 2,6-diisopropylphenol on synaptic transmission in the rat olfactory cortex slice. *Br J Pharmacol*.1988;95(3):939–949.
51. Herling SF, Dreijer B, Wrist LG, Thomsen T, Møller AM. Total intravenous anaesthesia versus inhalational anaesthesia for adults undergoing transabdominal robotic assisted laparoscopic surgery. *Cochrane Database Syst Reviews*. 2017;4(4):CD011387.
52. Taylor E, Feinstein R, White PF, Soper N. Anesthesia for laparoscopic cholecystectomy. Is nitrous oxide contraindicated? *Anesthesiology*. 1992;76(4):541–543.
53. Fernández-Guisasola J, Gómez-Arnau JI, Cabrera Y, del Valle SG. Association between nitrous oxide and the incidence of postoperative nausea and vomiting in adults: a systematic review and meta-analysis. *Anaesthesia*. 2010;65(4):379–387.
54. Neuman GG, Sidebotham G, Negoianu E, et al. Laparoscopy explosion hazards with nitrous oxide. *Anesthesiology*. 1993;78(5):875–879.
55. Watanabe K, Kashiwagi K, Kamiyama T, et al. High-dose remifentanil suppresses stress response associated with pneumoperitoneum during laparoscopic colectomy. *J Anesth*. 2014;28(3):334–340.
56. Tufanogullari B, White PF, Peixoto MP, et al. Dexmedetomidine infusion during laparoscopic bariatric surgery: the effect on recovery outcome variables. *Anesth Analg*. 2008;106(6):1741–1748.
57. Kranke P, Jokinen J, Pace NL, et al. Continuous intravenous perioperative lidocaine infusion for postoperative pain and recovery. *Cochrane Database Syst Rev*. 2015;7:CD009642.
58. Marret E, Rolin M, Beaussier M, Bonnet F. Meta-analysis of intravenous lidocaine and postoperative recovery after abdominal surgery. *Br J Surg*. 2008;95(11):1331–1338.
59. McCarthy GC, Megalla SA, Habib AS. Impact of intravenous lidocaine infusion on postoperative analgesia and recovery from surgery: a systematic review of randomized controlled trials. *Drugs*. 2010;70(9):1149–1163.
60. Vigneault L, Turgeon AF, Côté D, et al. Perioperative intravenous lidocaine infusion for postoperative pain control: a meta-analysis of randomized controlled trials. *Can J Anaesth*. 2011;58(1):22–37.
61. Kehlet H, Gray AW, Bonnet F, et al. A procedure-specific systematic review and consensus recommendations for postoperative analgesia following laparoscopic cholecystectomy. *Surg Endosc*. 2005;19(10):1396–1415.
62. Thornton PC, Buggy DJ. Local anaesthetic wound infusion for acute postoperative pain: a viable option? *Br J Anaesth*. 2011;107(5):656–658.
63. Loizides S, Gurusamy KS, Nagendran M, Rossi M, Guerrini GP, Davidson BR. Wound infiltration with local anaesthetic agents for laparoscopic cholecystectomy. *Cochrane Database Syst Rev*. 2014;3:CD007049.
64. Gurusamy KS, Nagendran M, Guerrini GP, Wilson MS. Intraperitoneal local anaesthetic instillation versus no intraperitoneal local anaesthetic instillation for laparoscopic cholecystectomy. *Cochrane Database Syst Rev*. 2014;3:CD007337.
65. Kahokehr A, Sammour T, Soop M, Hill AG. Intraperitoneal use of local anesthetic in laparoscopic cholecystectomy: systematic review and meta-analysis of randomized controlled trials. *J Hepatobiliary Pancreat Sci*. 2010;17(5):637–656.
66. Kahokehr A, Sammour T, Srinivasa S, Hill AG. Systematic review and meta-analysis of intraperitoneal local anaesthetic for pain reduction after laparoscopic gastric procedures. *Br J Surg*. 2011;98(1):29–36.
67. Barazanchi AWH, MacFater WS, Rahiri JL, et al. Evidence-based management of pain after laparoscopic cholecystectomy: a PROSPECT review update. *Br J Anaesth*. 2018;121(4):787–803.
68. Kopman AF, Naguib M. Laparoscopic surgery and muscle relaxants: is deep block helpful? *Anesth Analg*. 2015;120(1):51–58.
69. Martini CH, Boon M, Bevers RF, Aarts LP, Dahan A. Evaluation of surgical conditions during laparoscopic surgery in patients with moderate vs deep neuromuscular block. *Br J Anaesth*. 2014;112(3):498–505.
70. Blobner M, Frick CG, Stäuble RB, et al. Neuromuscular blockade improves surgical conditions (NISCO). *Surg Endosc*. 2015;29(3):627–636.
71. Dubois PE, Putz L, Jamart J, Marotta M-L, Gourdin M, Donnez O. Deep neuromuscular block improves surgical conditions during laparoscopic hysterectomy: a randomised controlled trial. *Eur J Anaesthesiol*. 2014;31(8):430–436.
72. Staehr-Rye AK, Rasmussen LS, Rosenberg J, et al. Surgical space conditions during low-pressure laparoscopic cholecystectomy with deep versus moderate neuromuscular blockade: a randomized clinical study. *Anesth Analg*. 2014;119(5):1084–1092.
73. Van Wijk RM, Watts RW, Ledowski T, Trochsler M, Moran JL, Arenas GW. Deep neuromuscular block reduces intra-abdominal pressure requirements during laparoscopic cholecystectomy: a prospective observational study. *Acta Anaesthesiol Scand*. 2015;59(4):434–440.
74. Plaud B, Debaene B, Donati F, Marty J. Residual paralysis after emergence from anesthesia. *Anesthesiology*. 2010;112(4):1013–1022.
75. Broens SJL, Boon M, Martini CH, et al. Reversal of partial neuromuscular block and the ventilatory response to hypoxia: a randomized controlled trial in healthy volunteers. *Anesthesiology*. 2019;131(3): 467–476.
76. Murphy GS, Brull SJ. Residual neuromuscular block: lessons unlearned. Part I: definitions, incidence, and adverse physiologic effects of residual neuromuscular block. *Anesth Analg*. 2010;111(1):120–128.
77. Brull SJ, Murphy GS. Residual neuromuscular block: lessons unlearned. Part II: methods to reduce the risk of residual weakness. *Anesth Analg*. 2010;111(1):129–140.
78. Aldenkortt M, Lysakowski C, Elia N, Brochard L, Tramèr MR. Ventilation strategies in obese patients undergoing surgery: a quantitative systematic review and meta-analysis. *Br J Anaesth*. 2012;109(4):493–502.
79. Balick-Weber C-C, Nicolas P, Hedreville-Montout M, Blanchet P, Stéphan F. Respiratory and haemodynamic effects of volume-controlled vs pressure-controlled ventilation during laparoscopy: a cross-over study with echocardiographic assessment. *Br J Anaesth*. 2007;99(3):429–435.
80. Baraka A, Jabbour S, Hammoud R, et al. End-tidal carbon dioxide tension during laparoscopic cholecystectomy: correlation with the baseline value prior to carbon dioxide insufflation. *Anaesthesia*. 1994;49(4):304–306.
81. Hazebroek EJ, Haitsma JJ, Lachmann B, Bonjer HJ. Mechanical ventilation with positive end-expiratory pressure preserves arterial oxygenation during prolonged pneumoperitoneum. *Surg Endosc*. 2002;16(4):685–689.
82. Meininger D, Byhahn C, Mierdl S, Westphal K, Zwissler B. Positive end-expiratory pressure improves arterial oxygenation during prolonged pneumoperitoneum. *Acta Anaesthesiol Scand*. 2005;49(6):778–783.
83. Futier E, Constantin J-M, Pelosi P, et al. Intraoperative recruitment maneuver reverses detrimental pneumoperitoneum-induced respiratory effects in healthy weight and obese patients undergoing laparoscopy. *Anesthesiology*. 2010;113(6):1310–1319.

84. Valenza F, Vagginelli F, Tiby A, et al. Effects of the beach chair position, positive end-expiratory pressure, and pneumoperitoneum on respiratory function in morbidly obese patients during anesthesia and paralysis. *Anesthesiology*. 2007;107(5):725–732.
85. Fernandez-Bustamante A, Hashimoto S, Serpa Neto A, Moine P, Vidal Melo MF, Repine JE. Perioperative lung protective ventilation in obese patients. *BMC Anesthesiol*. 2015;15:56.
86. Coppola S, Froio S, Chiumello D. Protective lung ventilation during general anesthesia: is there any evidence? *Crit Care*. 2014;18(2):210.
87. Hovaguimian F, Lysakowski C, Elia N, Tramèr MR. Effect of intraoperative high inspired oxygen fraction on surgical site infection, postoperative nausea and vomiting, and pulmonary function: systematic review and meta-analysis of randomized controlled trials. *Anesthesiology*. 2013;119(2):303–316.
88. Madrid E, Urrútia G, Roqué i Figuls M. Active body surface warming systems for preventing complications caused by inadvertent perioperative hypothermia in adults. *Cochrane Database Syst Rev*. 2016;4(4):CD009016.
89. Gray RI, Ott DE, Henderson AC, Cochran SA, Roth EA. Severe local hypothermia from laparoscopic gas evaporative jet cooling: a mechanism to explain clinical observations. *JSLS*. 1999;3(3):171–177.
90. Davis SS, Mikami DJ, Newlin M, et al. Heating and humidifying of carbon dioxide during pneumoperitoneum is not indicated: a prospective randomized trial. *Surg Endosc*. 2006;20(1):153–158.
91. Birch DW, Manouchehri N, Shi X, Hadi G, Karmali S. Heated CO_2 with or without humidification for minimally invasive abdominal surgery. *Cochrane Database Syst Rev*. 2011;(1):CD007821.
92. Holte K, Klarskov B, Christensen DS, et al. Liberal versus restrictive fluid administration to improve recovery after laparoscopic cholecystectomy: a randomized, double-blind study. *Ann Surg*. 2004;240(5):892–899.
93. Matot I, Paskaleva R, Eid L, et al. Effect of the volume of fluids administered on intraoperative oliguria in laparoscopic bariatric surgery: a randomized controlled trial. *Arch Surg*. 2012; 147(3):228–234.
94. Chakravartty S, Sarma DR, Patel AG. Rhabdomyolysis in bariatric surgery: a systematic review. *Obes Surg*. 2013;23(8):1333–1340.
95. Magrina JF. Complications of laparoscopic surgery. *Clin Obstet Gynecol*. 2002;45(2):469–480.
96. Joshi GP. Complications of laparoscopy. *Anesthesiol Clin North Am*. 2001;19(1):89–105.
97. Coelho JCU, Campos AC, Costa MAR, Soares RV, Faucz RA. Complications of laparoscopic fundoplication in the elderly. *Surg Laparosc Endosc Percutan Tech*. 2003;13(1):6–10.
98. Pareek G, Hedican SP, Gee JR, Bruskewitz RC, Nakada SY. Meta-analysis of the complications of laparoscopic renal surgery: comparison of procedures and techniques. *J Urol*. 2006; 175(4):1208–1213.
99. Fischer B, Engel N, Fehr J-L, John H. Complications of robotic assisted radical prostatectomy. *World J Urol*. 2008;26(6):595–602.
100. Coelho RF, Palmer KJ, Rocco B, et al. Early complication rates in a single-surgeon series of 2500 robotic-assisted radical prostatectomies: report applying a standardized grading system. *Eur Urol*. 2010;57(6):945–952.
101. Lasser MS, Renzulli J 2nd, Turini GA 3rd, Haleblian G, Sax HC, Pareek G. An unbiased prospective report of perioperative complications of robot-assisted laparoscopic radical prostatectomy. *Urology*. 2010;75(5):1083–1089.
102. Dexter F, Ledolter J, Davis E, Witkowski TA, Herman JH, Epstein RH. Systematic criteria for type and screen based on procedure's probability of erythrocyte transfusion. *Anesthesiology*. 2012;116(4):768–778.
103. Usal H, Nabagiez J, Sayad P, Ferzli GS. Cost effectiveness of routine type and screen testing before laparoscopic cholecystectomy. *Surg Endosc*. 1999;13(2):146–147.
104. Yong J, Hibbert P, Runciman WB, Coventry BJ. Bradycardia as an early warning sign for cardiac arrest during routine laparoscopic surgery. *Int J Qual Health Care*. 2015;27(6): 472–477.
105. Ott DE. Subcutaneous emphysema—beyond the pneumoperitoneum. *JSLS*. 2014;18(1):1–7.
106. Murdock CM, Wolff AJ, Van Geem T. Risk factors for hypercarbia, subcutaneous emphysema, pneumothorax, and pneumomediastinum during laparoscopy. *Obstet Gynecol*. 2000;95(5): 704–709.
107. Phillips S, Falk GL. Surgical tension pneumothorax during laparoscopic repair of massive hiatus hernia: a different situation requiring different management. *Anaesth Intensive Care*. 2011; 39(6):1120–1123.
108. Joris JL, Chiche JD, Lamy ML. Pneumothorax during laparoscopic fundoplication: diagnosis and treatment with positive end-expiratory pressure. *Anesth Analg*. 1995;81(5):993–1000.
109. Yee R, Hyde PR, Currie JS. Pneumothorax during laparoscopic Nissen fundoplication. *Anaesth Intensive Care*. 1996;24(1):93–96.
110. Hawasli A. Spontaneous resolution of massive laparoscopy-associated pneumothorax: the case of the bulging diaphragm and review of the literature. *J Laparoendosc Adv Surg Tech A*. 2002;12(1):77–82.
111. Ueda K, Ahmed W, Ross AF. Intraoperative pneumothorax identified with transthoracic ultrasound. *Anesthesiology*. 2011;115(3):653–655.
112. Cottin V, Delafosse B, Viale JP. Gas embolism during laparoscopy: a report of seven cases in patients with previous abdominal surgical history. *Surg Endosc*. 1996;10(2):166–169.
113. Hong J-Y, Kim WO, Kil HK. Detection of subclinical CO_2 embolism by transesophageal echocardiography during laparoscopic radical prostatectomy. *Urology*. 2010;75(3):581–584.
114. Kim CS, Kim JY, Kwon J-Y, et al. Venous air embolism during total laparoscopic hysterectomy: comparison to total abdominal hysterectomy. *Anesthesiology*. 2009;111(1):50–54.
115. Hong JY, Kim JY, Choi YD, Rha KH, Yoon SJ, Kil HK. Incidence of venous gas embolism during robotic-assisted laparoscopic radical prostatectomy is lower than that during radical retropubic prostatectomy. *Br J Anaesth*. 2010;105(6):777–781.
116. Fors D, Eiriksson K, Arvidsson D, Rubertsson S. Gas embolism during laparoscopic liver resection in a pig model: frequency and severity. *Br J Anaesth*. 2010;105(3):282–288.
117. Couture P, Boudreault D, Derouin M, et al. Venous carbon dioxide embolism in pigs: an evaluation of end-tidal carbon dioxide, transesophageal echocardiography, pulmonary artery pressure, and precordial auscultation as monitoring modalities. *Anesth Analg*. 1994;79(5): 867–873.
118. Dauber MH, Roth S. Operating table failure: another hazard of spine surgery. *Anesth Analg*. 2009;108(3):904–905.
119. Sukhu T, Krupski TL. Patient positioning and prevention of injuries in patients undergoing laparoscopic and robot-assisted urologic procedures. *Curr Urol Rep*. 2014;15(4):398.
120. Eteuati J, Hiscock R, Hastie I, Hayes I, Jones I. Brachial plexopathy in laparoscopic-assisted rectal surgery: a case series. *Tech Coloproctol*. 2013;17(3):293–297.
121. Phong SV, Koh LKD. Anaesthesia for robotic-assisted radical prostatectomy: considerations for laparoscopy in the Trendelenburg position. *Anaesth Intensive Care*. 2007;35(2): 281–285.
122. Roth S, Thisted RA, Erickson JP, Black S, Schreider BD. Eye injuries after nonocular surgery: a study of 60,965 anesthetics from 1988 to 1992. *Anesthesiology*. 1996;85(5):1020–1027.
123. Newman NJ. Perioperative visual loss after nonocular surgeries. *Am J Ophthalmol*. 2008; 145(4):604–610.
124. American Society of Anesthesiologists Task Force on Perioperative Visual Loss; North American Neuro-Ophthalmology Society; Society for Neuroscience in Anesthesiology and Critical Care. Practice Advisory for Perioperative Visual Loss Associated with Spine Surgery 2019: An Updated Report by the American Society of Anesthesiologists Task Force on Perioperative Visual Loss, the North American Neuro-Ophthalmology Society, and the Society for Neuroscience in Anesthesiology and Critical Care. *Anesthesiology*. 2019;130:12–30
125. Avriel A, Warner E, Avinoach E, et al. Major respiratory adverse events after laproscopic gastric banding surgery for morbid obesity. *Respir Med*. 2012;106(8):1192–1198.
126. Sharma RR, Axelsson H, Oberg A, et al. Diaphragmatic activity after laparoscopic cholecystectomy. *Anesthesiology*. 1999;91(2):406–413.
127. Sadovnikoff N, Maxwell LG. Respiratory failure after laparoscopic cholecystectomy in a patient with chronic hemidiaphragm paralysis. *Anesthesiology*. 1997;87(4):996–998.
128. Milic DJ, Pejcic VD, Zivic SS, et al. Coagulation status and the presence of postoperative deep vein thrombosis in patients undergoing laparoscopic cholecystectomy. *Surg Endosc*. 2007;21(9):1588–1592.
129. Stein PD, Matta F, Sabra MJ. Pulmonary embolism and deep venous thrombosis following laparoscopic cholecystectomy. *Clin Appl Thromb Hemost*. 2014;20(3):233–237.
130. Stein PD, Matta F. Pulmonary embolism and deep venous thrombosis following bariatric surgery. *Obes Surg*. 2013;23(5):663–668.
131. Stein PD, Beemath A, Olson RE. Obesity as a risk factor in venous thromboembolism. *Am J Med*. 2005;118(9):978–980.
132. Tyritzis SI, Wallerstedt A, Steineck G, et al. Thromboembolic complications in 3,544 patients undergoing radical prostatectomy with or without lymph node dissection. *J Urol*. 2015;193(1):117–125.
133. Veldkamp R, Gholghesaei M, Bonjer HJ, et al. Laparoscopic resection of colon cancer: consensus of the European Association of Endoscopic Surgery (EAES). *Surg Endosc*. 2004;18(8): 1163–1185.
134. Atak I, Ozbagriacik M, Akinci OF, et al. Active gas aspiration to reduce pain after laparoscopic cholecystectomy. *Surg Laparosc Endosc Percutan Tech*. 2011;21(2):98–100.
135. Baeriswyl M, Kirkham KR, Kern C, Albrecht E. The analgesic efficacy of ultrasound-guided transversus abdominis plane block in adult patients: a meta-analysis. *Anesth Analg*. 2015 121(6):1640–1654.
136. Levy BF, Tilney HS, Dowson HMP, Rockall TA. A systematic review of postoperative analgesia following laparoscopic colorectal surgery. *Colorectal Dis*. 2010;12(1):5–15.
137. Apfel CC, Heidrich FM, Jukar-Rao S, et al. Evidence-based analysis of risk factors for postoperative nausea and vomiting. *Br J Anaesth*. 2012;109(5):742–753.
138. Weingarten TN, Hawkins NM, Beam WB, et al. Factors associated with prolonged anesthesia recovery following laparoscopic bariatric surgery: a retrospective analysis. *Obes Surg*. 2015;25(6):1024–1030.
139. Gan TJ, Belani KG, Bergese S, et al. Fourth consensus guidelines for the management of postoperative nausea and vomiting. *Anesth Analg*. 2020;131(2):411–448.

45 Anesthesia and Obesity

ANA FERNANDEZ-BUSTAMANTE • BRENDA A. BUCKLIN

KEY POINTS

1. Obese patients may have significant cardiovascular disease and appear asymptomatic because they often have limited exercise tolerance.
2. Elevated liver function tests (mostly elevated alanine aminotransferase) are seen in many obese patients, but no clear correlation exists between abnormalities of routine liver function tests and the capacity of the liver to metabolize drugs.
3. A neck circumference of ≥40 cm is the biggest predictor of difficult mask ventilation, difficult laryngoscopy, and difficult endotracheal intubation.
4. Evidence of obstructive sleep apnea (OSA) and obstructive hypoventilation syndrome (OHS) should be obtained preoperatively because they are frequently associated with difficult airway management and increased perioperative pulmonary complications.
5. Blood pressure measurements can be falsely elevated if a cuff is too small. In the supine position, forearm measurements with a standard cuff can be used when upper arm measurements are challenging.
6. The "ramped" position elevates the obese patient's upper body above the chest and improves laryngoscopic view compared with the standard "sniffing" position.
7. Larger doses of induction agents may be required by obese patients because blood volume, muscle mass, and cardiac output increase linearly with the degree of obesity. An increased dose of succinylcholine is necessary because of an increase in pseudocholinesterase activity.
8. Positive end-expiratory pressure is the only ventilatory parameter that has consistently been shown to improve respiratory function in obese patients but it decreases venous return, cardiac output, and subsequent oxygen delivery.
9. Prompt but safe extubation reduces the likelihood that the morbidly obese patient will become ventilator dependent, especially in patients with cardiopulmonary disease.
10. Because of the risk of perioperative hypoxemia and apnea in obese patients, postoperative pain management should include opioid-sparing multimodal analgesic techniques. Regional anesthetic techniques reduce the risk of opioid-related complications.
11. Obese patients who have received either neuraxial or parenteral opioids require careful postoperative monitoring. Delayed respiratory depression with centrally administered neuraxial opioids, when coupled with a potentially difficult airway in the obese patient, suggests that close monitoring is prudent.
12. Morbid obesity is a major independent risk factor for deep venous thrombosis and sudden death from acute postoperative pulmonary embolism. Mobilization in the morbidly obese is often difficult but critically important in the prevention of postoperative complications.

Definition and Epidemiology

Introduction

The World Health Organization defines obesity as a condition with excess body fat to the extent that health and well-being are adversely affected.[1] Rates of obesity worldwide have nearly tripled since 1975.[2] Estimates suggest that the age-adjusted prevalence of obesity has increased from 30.5% to 42.4% during the time period from 1999 to 2000 to 2017 to 2018 in the United States.[3] The prevalence of severe obesity also increased from 4.7% to 9.2% during the same time period. Prevalence of obesity in the United States is unevenly distributed geographically, by race and ethnicity, and by socioeconomic status. The Centers for Disease Control and Prevention (CDC) monitor the epidemiology of obesity and publish periodically updated data at http://www.cdc.gov/obesity/.

Obesity-related conditions including diabetes, cardiovascular disease, sleep apnea, nonalcoholic fatty liver disease (NAFLD), osteoarthritis, and some types of cancer are leading causes of preventable, premature death in this population.[4] Although there has been an exponential increase in the number of bariatric procedures performed, obese and morbidly obese patients undergo all types of surgical procedures. Surgery in this patient population is considered high risk but careful planning, preoperative risk assessment, adequate anesthetic management, strict venothrombotic event prevention, and effective postoperative pain control will all help to reduce the risk. With appropriate perioperative management, obese surgical patients can achieve safe and effective surgical outcomes.

The definition of obesity includes the presence of excessive body weight for the patient's age, gender, and height, and is based or estimated on the calculation of the following concepts:

- Ideal body weight (IBW) is a concept derived by life insurance companies by referencing height–weight tables. It is the weight associated with the lowest mortality rate for a given height and gender and can be estimated using Broca index:
  IBW (kg) = height (cm) – x, where x is 100 for adult males and 105 for adult females.
- Predicted body weight (PBW) is a similar concept as the IBW, more commonly used in the medical literature. PBW is usually calculated with the following formulas in adults[5]:
  Males: PBW (kg) = $50 + 0.91 \times$ (height [cm] – 152.4);
  Females: PBW (kg) = $45.5 + 0.91 \times$ (height [cm] – 152.4)
- Lean body weight (LBW) is the total body weight (TBW) minus the adipose tissue. It is a combination of body cell mass, extracellular water, and nonfat connective tissue. It approximates 80% and 75% of TBW for males and females, respectively, although more accurate formulas like the following have been proposed[6]:
  Males: $1.10 \times \text{TBW} - 0.0128 \times \text{BMI} \times \text{TBW}$;
  Females: $1.07 \times \text{TBW} - 0.0148 \times \text{BMI} \times \text{TBW}$
  In morbidly obese patients, increasing the IBW by 20% to 30% gives an estimate of LBW. In nonobese and nonmuscular individuals, TBW approximates IBW.[6]
- Body mass (Quetelet) index (BMI) is used in clinical practice to estimate the degree of obesity:

$$\text{BMI} = \frac{\text{body weight (kg)}}{\text{height}^2\text{ (m)}}$$

Obesity is defined as having a BMI ≥30 kg/m^2. Obesity is further classified according to systemic disease risk (Table 45-1). Morbid obesity, defined as a BMI ≥40 kg/m^2, can also be further classified into super obesity (BMI 50 kg/m^2) and super–super obesity (BMI 60 kg/m^2). BMI differentiates obese from nonobese adults and it estimates body fat because it adjusts for height while strongly correlating with body weight; however, it cannot distinguish between overweight and overfat, as heavily muscled individuals can be easily classified as overweight using BMI. Therefore, other factors such as age and fat content and distribution (i.e., waist circumference and waist-to-hip ratio) should be taken into consideration, along with other health risk predictors that use the concept of BMI.

The anatomic distribution of body fat has associated pathophysiologic implications.[7] In android (central) obesity, adipose tissue is located predominantly in the upper body (truncal distribution) and is associated with increased oxygen consumption and increased incidence of cardiovascular disease. Visceral fat is particularly associated with cardiovascular disease and left ventricular dysfunction. In gynecoid (peripheral) obesity, adipose tissue is located predominantly in the hips, buttocks, and thighs. This fat is less metabolically active, so it is less closely associated with cardiovascular disease. Body circumference indices such as waist circumference, waist-to-height ratio, and waist-to-hip ratio help to classify these patterns of obesity (e.g., android vs. gynecoid obesity) and correlate with mortality and the risk for developing obesity-related diseases. Waist circumference correlates with abdominal fat and is an independent risk predictor of disease.

Management of Obesity

Medical Therapy

Indications for drug treatment include a BMI ≥30 kg/m^2 or a BMI between 27 and 29.9 kg/m^2 in conjunction with an obesity-related medical complication. Although conventional treatments of obesity including lifestyle changes and medications have demonstrated little success in long-term weight loss,[8,9] medications are often used to treat obesity because of their ability to reduce energy intake, increase energy utilization, or decrease absorption of nutrients. Phentermine, phentermine–topiramate, lorcaserin, bupropion–naltrexone, liraglutide, and orlistat are FDA-approved antiobesity medications.[10] Most pharmacologic therapies target appetite mechanisms with the exception of orlistat. Phentermine (Adipex-P) is primarily a noradrenergic and possibly dopaminergic sympathomimetic amine that decreases appetite. Although it

Table 45-1 Classification of Obesity and Systemic Disease Risk According to Waist Circumference

		Waist Circumference/Risk	
BMI (kg/m^2)	**Description**	***Male: <102 cm Female: <88 cm***	***Male: ≥102 cm Female: ≥88 cm***
<18.5	Underweight		
18.5–24.9	Normal		
25.0–29.9	Overweight		
30.0–34.9	Obesity (class I)	Average	Average
35.0–39.9	Obesity (class II)	Increased	High
≥40	Morbid obesity (class III)	High	Very high
≥50	Super obesity	Very high	Very high
≥60	Super–super obesity	Extremely high	Extremely high

BMI, body mass index.

is only approved for 3 months' use, it can induce tachycardia, palpitations, and hypertension, as well as dependence, abuse, and withdrawal symptoms. It is no longer combined with fenfluramine (Phen-Fen) due to concerns of pulmonary hypertension and valvular heart disease. It is now being combined with topiramate (Topamax), although this combination often causes dry mouth, paresthesias, constipation, insomnia, and dizziness.[11] Lorcaserin is a serotonin receptor antagonist and stimulates the serotonin type 2c receptor. Bupropion is a dopamine and norepinephrine reuptake inhibitor,[12] which stimulates pro-opiomelanocortin neurons. In combination with naltrexone, the efficacy of bupropion is enhanced due to the release of feedback inhibition of pro-opiomelanocortin neurons that naltrexone potentiates. Liraglutide is associated with weight loss without an effect on appetite. It promotes weight loss by preventing resorption of glucose and water in the renal tubules.[13] Orlistat (OTC Alli, prescribed Xenical), or tetrahydrolipstatin, blocks the absorption of dietary fat by inhibiting lipases in the gastrointestinal tract. It leads to weight loss and to improved blood pressure, fasting blood glucose levels, and lipid profile. Fat malabsorption causes common complaints of oily spotting, liquid stools, fecal urgency, flatulence, and abdominal cramping. Chronic use of orlistat may result in fat-soluble vitamin deficiency. A prolonged prothrombin time with a normal partial thromboplastin time during orlistat treatment may reflect vitamin K deficiency and this coagulopathy should be corrected 6 to 24 hours before elective surgery.

Although over-the-counter preparations are widely used as a weight loss strategy, evidence to support their efficacy and safety is limited. Plant extracts or herbs are often used to combat obesity and include substances with alleged properties: pancreatic lipase inhibitors (e.g., caffeine, green or black tea), appetite suppressants (e.g., hoodia, Korean ginseng, ephedra, sunflower oil), stimulants of energy expenditure (e.g., acai berry, caffeine), regulators of lipid metabolism (e.g., soybean, fish oil, oolong tea, caffeine).[14] The American Society of Anesthesiologists warns patients to tell their anesthesiologists about medications they are taking, including vitamins, herbs, and other supplements. Since these products can interfere with anesthesia, they can cause complications during surgery.[15]

Bariatric Surgery

Bariatric surgery is currently the most effective treatment for morbid (class III) obesity. Although current guidelines recommend bariatric surgery for patients with BMI >40 kg/m^2 or BMI >35 kg/m^2 with obesity-related comorbidities not controlled with medical therapy,[16] there are recent calls to alter the threshold for bariatric surgery to BMI 35 kg/m^2 or BMI 30 kg/m^2 with comorbidities in order to reduce the lifetime cost associated with diabetes, hypertension, high cholesterol, colon cancer, and cardiovascular disease.[17] Procedures are classified into malabsorptive (e.g., jejunoileal bypass and biliopancreatic diversion, biliopancreatic diversion with duodenal switch), restrictive (vertical-banded gastroplasty, adjustable gastric banding, sleeve gastrectomy), or combined (Roux-en-Y gastric bypass [RYGB]). The RYGB combines gastric restriction with a minimal degree of malabsorption. RYGB, adjustable gastric banding, sleeve gastrectomy, and vertical-banded gastroplasty can all be performed laparoscopically. Laparoscopic bariatric surgery is associated with less postoperative pain, lower morbidity, faster recovery, and less "third-spacing." Several procedures (e.g., jejunoileal bypass) are no longer performed as bariatric operations due to the risk for revisions and adverse health effects. RYGB is the most commonly performed bariatric procedure and produces safe short- and long-term weight loss in severely obese patients. With RYGB, patients lose an average of 50% to 60% excess body weight and show a BMI decrease of approximately 10 kg/m^2 during the first 12 to 24 postoperative months. Type II diabetes resolves in a majority of patients. Sleeve or partial gastrectomy is the second most commonly performed restrictive bariatric procedure. Laparoscopic adjustable gastric banding (LAGB) is a restrictive gastric operation that utilizes an adjustable inflatable band to alter stomach capacity for individual weight loss needs. Vertical-banded gastroplasty also restricts food intake.

Less invasive bariatric techniques are being developed. An implantable abdominal vagal nerve stimulator is placed laparoscopically and emits electrical impulses to control gastric emptying and signal the satiety center in the brain.[18] This device can be adversely affected by defibrillation, electrocautery, lithotripsy, magnetic resonance imaging, and therapeutic radiation. Intragastric balloons and prostheses, at different stages of development, are placed endoscopically as a temporary measure to increase satiety. They are often considered to be a bridge to more definitive bariatric procedures. Adequate control of postoperative nausea and vomiting is critical to avoid possible lead and balloon dislodgement.

Pathophysiology

Obesity comes with adverse health implications for multiple organ systems (Video 45-1, NICV 45-1). Table 45-2 provides a list of the most relevant organ systems with implications for clinical management. These systems will be discussed separately in this section.

Respiratory System

Fat accumulation on the thorax and abdomen decreases chest wall and lung compliance. Decreased lung compliance is partially explained by increased pulmonary blood volume because of an overall increase in blood volume. Increased elastic resistance and decreased compliance of the chest wall are further reduced while supine, leading to shallow and rapid breathing, increased work of breathing, and limited maximum ventilatory capacity. Respiratory muscle efficiency is below normal in obese individuals. Decreased pulmonary compliance leads to decreased functional residual capacity (FRC), vital capacity, and total lung capacity. Reduction in FRC is primarily a result of reduced expiratory reserve volume (ERV), but the relationship between FRC and closing capacity, the volume at which small airways begin to close, is adversely affected (Fig. 45-1). Decreases in FRC and ERV are the most commonly reported abnormalities of pulmonary function in obese patients.[19] Residual volume and closing capacity are unchanged. Reduced FRC (due to decreased ERV) can result in lung volumes below closing capacity in the course of normal tidal ventilation, leading to small airway closure, ventilation–perfusion mismatch, right-to-left shunting, and arterial hypoxemia. Anesthesia and supine positioning worsen this situation such that up to a 50% reduction in FRC occurs in the obese anesthetized patient compared with 20% in the nonobese individual. Forced expiratory volume in 1 second and forced vital capacity are usually within normal limits. ERV is the most sensitive indicator of the effect of obesity on pulmonary function.

Obesity increases oxygen consumption and carbon dioxide production even at rest. This is because of the metabolic activity of excess fat and the increased workload on supportive tissues. The body attempts to meet these metabolic demands by increasing both cardiac output and alveolar ventilation. Basal metabolic activity is usually within normal limits in relationship to body

Table 45-2 Implications of Medical Consequences of Obesity

System	Practical Anesthesia Key Points
Respiratory	Increased risk of perioperative hypoxemia Careful monitoring needed Use of supplemental oxygen CPAP (when indicated) Nonsupine positioning (if possible) Extreme caution when administering respiratory depressants
Cardiovascular	Increased blood volume, cardiac output, left ventricular thickness Increased proinflammatory and prothrombotic mediators Higher perioperative complications related to hypertension, thromboembolic events, and left ventricular diastolic dysfunction
Gastrointestinal	Risk of regurgitation Higher gastric volume and lower pH increase risk of severe pneumonitis should aspiration occur Current fasting preoperative guidelines (6 h for solids, 2 h for clear liquids) are acceptable Careful assessment of preoperative liver function is recommended
Endocrine/metabolic	High prevalence of hyperglycemia, insulin resistance, and diabetes Careful perioperative glucose monitoring Metabolic syndrome (combination of central obesity, hypertension, dyslipidemia, and impaired glucose metabolism) is frequent and doubles the cardiovascular risk
Genitourinary	Increased risk of renal disease Higher incidence of preeclampsia and eclampsia
Neurologic	Careful positioning with extra padding needed
Hematology	Increased hypercoagulability and risk of perioperative thromboembolic events Preoperative polycythemia suggests prolonged sleep apnea
Musculoskeletal	Increased prevalence of osteoarthritis
Psychology/psychiatry	Depression, reduced self-esteem, social stigma

CPAP, continuous positive airway pressure.

surface area and normocapnia is usually maintained by an increase in minute ventilation. This requires increased oxygen consumption because most obese patients retain their normal response to hypoxemia and hypercapnia. Arterial oxygen tension in morbidly obese patients' breathing room air is lower than that predicted for similarly aged nonobese subjects in both sitting and supine positions. Chronic hypoxemia may lead to polycythemia, pulmonary hypertension, and cor pulmonale.

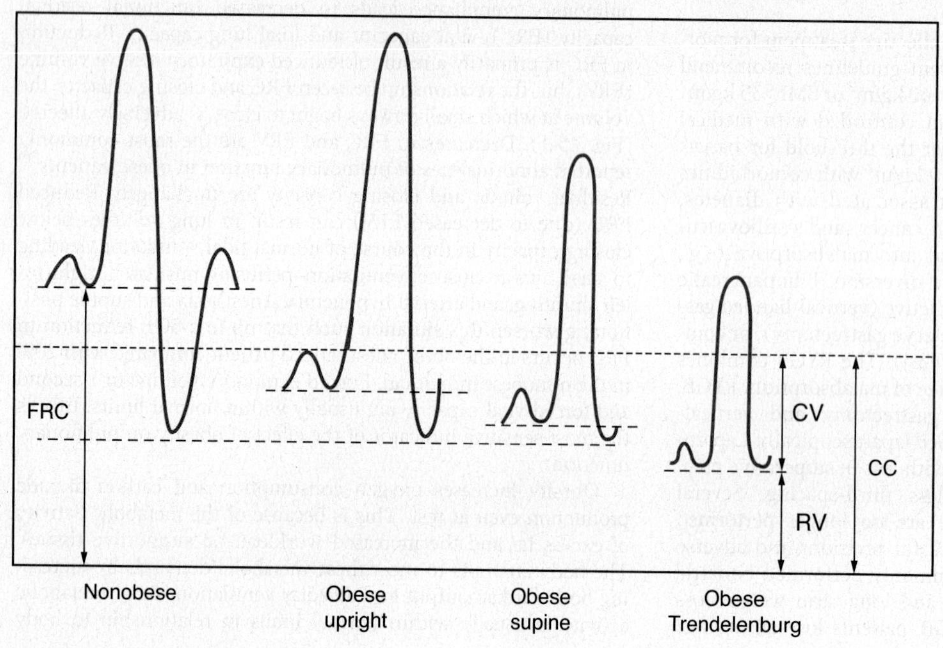

Figure 45-1 Effects of obesity, positioning, and anesthesia on lung volumes. FRC, functional residual capacity; CC, closing capacity; CV, closing volume; RV, residual volume.

Obese patients often suffer from obstructive sleep apnea (OSA) characterized by periodic, partial, or complete obstruction of the upper airway during sleep (2 Video 45-2). In obese patients, sleep apnea is more likely to result from airway obstruction produced by excess soft tissue. However, centrally mediated forms of sleep apnea can also occur. Physiologic abnormalities resulting from OSA include hypoxemia, hypercapnia, pulmonary hypertension, systemic vasoconstriction, hypertension, and secondary polycythemia (from recurrent hypoxemia). These result in an increased risk of ischemic heart disease and cerebrovascular disease. Right ventricular failure can occur from hypoxic pulmonary vasoconstriction. Respiratory acidosis is usually limited only to periods of sleep.

The gold standard diagnostic technique is overnight polysomnography (OPS). The inconvenience, time, and expense of polysomnography lead to a significant fraction of obese patients with suspicious but no formal diagnosis of OSA presenting for surgery.[20] Screening questionnaires such as the STOP-BANG and others[21] are increasingly used for identifying patients at high risk for OSA. Suggestive signs of OSA include witnessed episodes of apnea during sleep, BMI 35, neck circumference 16 inches (40 cm), hyperinsulinemia, and elevated glycosylated hemoglobin. Symptoms of snoring, frequent arousals during sleep and daytime sleepiness, impaired concentration, memory problems, and morning headaches are common but not predictive.[22] Ideally, a thorough preoperative evaluation for OSA should occur long enough before elective surgery to allow preparation of a perioperative management plan. Preoperative initiation of continuous positive airway pressure (CPAP), especially in severe OSA cases, should be considered.[23] A recent study found improvements in blood pressure and glucose and lipid metabolism in obese OSA patients treated with CPAP in addition to a weight loss intervention.[24] The frequent lack of compliance or intolerance to CPAP has spearheaded the development of alternative therapies; the implantable hypoglossal stimulator has shown promising results in a selected group of OSA patients. In general, patients with either confirmed or suspected OSA should be considered at high risk of presenting with a difficult airway and postoperative pulmonary complications and should be managed accordingly.[25] For the prevention of postoperative pulmonary complications in these patients with or at high risk for OSA, experts recommend a semiupright position, continuous pulse-oximetry monitoring, a focus to avoid opioid-based analgesia, and therapy with titrated oxygen and/or CPAP as needed to avoid hypoxemia and hypoventilation.[26]

Obesity hypoventilation (Pickwickian) syndrome (OHS) may result from long-term OSA and is seen in 5% to 10% of morbidly obese patients. OHS is a combination of obesity and chronic hypoventilation that is frequently misdiagnosed and untreated,[27] resulting in pulmonary hypertension and cor pulmonale, increased risk of postoperative complications, and death.[28] The presence of both obesity (BMI >30 kg/m^2) and awake arterial hypercapnia ($PaCO_2$ >45 mmHg) in the absence of known causes of hypoventilation supports the diagnosis. Prolonged OSA also alters the control of breathing, leading to CNS-mediated apneic events with an increased reliance on hypoxic drive for ventilation. The main ventilatory impairment of OHS is alveolar hypoventilation independent of intrinsic lung disease in a patient with obesity, daytime hypersomnolence, hypercapnia, hypoxemia, and polycythemia. Right ventricular failure eventually ensues. These patients also have an increased sensitivity to the respiratory depressant effects of general anesthetics.

Cardiovascular and Hematologic Systems

Total blood volume is increased in the obese individual, but on a volume-to-weight basis, it is less than in nonobese individuals (50 mL/kg compared with 70 mL/kg). Most of this extra volume is distributed in adipose tissue. Renal and splanchnic blood flows are increased. Cardiac output increases with increasing weight by as much as 20 to 30 mL/kg of excess body fat because of ventricular dilation and increases in stroke volume. The resulting increased left ventricular wall stress leads to hypertrophy, reduced compliance, and impairment of left ventricular filling (diastolic dysfunction) with elevated left ventricular, diastolic pressure, and pulmonary edema. When left ventricular wall thickening fails to keep pace with dilation, systolic dysfunction ("obesity cardiomyopathy") and eventual biventricular failure results (Fig. 45-2).

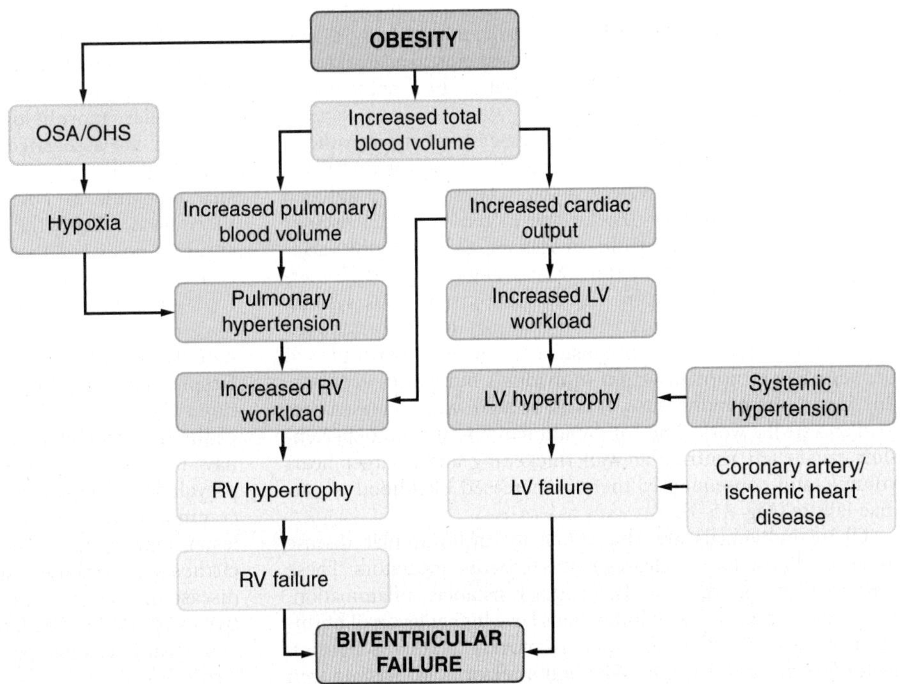

Figure 45-2 Interrelationship of cardiovascular and pulmonary sequelae of obesity. OSA, obstructive sleep apnea; OHS, obesity hypoventilation syndrome; LV, left ventricular; RV, right ventricular.

1 Obesity accelerates atherosclerosis. Symptoms such as angina or exertional dyspnea occur only occasionally because morbidly obese patients often have very limited mobility and may appear asymptomatic even when they have significant cardiovascular disease.

Blood flow to fat is 2 to 3 mL/100 g of tissue. Excess fat requires an increase in cardiac output, to parallel an increase in oxygen consumption. This leads to a systemic arteriovenous oxygen difference that remains normal or slightly above normal. Intraoperative ventricular failure may occur from rapid intravenous fluid administration (indicating left ventricular diastolic dysfunction), the negative inotropism of anesthetic agents, or pulmonary hypertension precipitated by hypoxia or hypercapnia. Cardiac dysrhythmias may be precipitated by fatty infiltration of the conduction system, hypoxia, hypercapnia, electrolyte imbalance, coronary artery disease, increased circulating catecholamines, OSA, and myocardial hypertrophy. Frequent electrocardiogram (ECG) findings seen in morbidly obese patients include low QRS voltage, multiple criteria for left ventricular hypertrophy (LVH) and left atrial enlargement, and T-wave flattening in the inferior and lateral leads. In addition, there is a leftward shift of the P-wave, QRS complex, and T-wave axes, lengthening of the corrected QT interval, and prolongation of the QT interval. Substantial weight reduction reverses many of these ECG abnormalities.

Cardiac output rises faster in response to exercise in the morbidly obese and is often associated with a rise in left ventricular end-diastolic pressure and pulmonary capillary wedge pressure. Similar changes occur during the perioperative period, which should prompt a low threshold for performing detailed cardiac investigations. Many obese patients have mild-to-moderate hypertension, with a 3- to 4-mmHg increase in systolic and a 2-mmHg increase in diastolic arterial pressure for every 10 kg of weight gained. Normotensive obese patients have reduced systemic vascular resistance, which rises with the onset of hypertension. Their expanded blood volume causes increased cardiac output, but a lower calculated systemic vascular resistance leads to the same level of arterial blood pressure. The renin–angiotensin system plays a major role in the hypertension of obesity by increasing circulating levels of angiotensinogen, aldosterone, and angiotensin-converting enzyme. As little as 5% reduction in body weight leads to a significant reduction in renin-angiotensin activity in both plasma and adipose tissue, contributing to a reduction in blood pressure.[29]

Obese patients have normal-to-increased level of sympathetic nervous system activity, which predisposes to insulin resistance, dyslipidemia, and hypertension.[30] These obesity-induced comorbidities are responsible for the increased cardiovascular risk in obese patients. Insulin resistance enhances the vasopressor activity of norepinephrine and angiotensin II. Hyperinsulinemia further activates the sympathetic nervous system, causing sodium retention and contributing to obesity-induced hypertension. Hypertension causes concentric hypertrophy of the ventricle in normal-weight individuals but causes eccentric dilation in obese individuals. It is associated with increased preload and stroke work. The combination of obesity and hypertension causes left ventricular wall thickening and a larger heart volume, and consequently, there is increased likelihood of cardiac failure (Fig. 45-3).

Obese individuals are also prone to cardiovascular disease because adipose tissue releases many bioactive mediators. These can result in abnormal lipids, insulin resistance, inflammation, and coagulopathies. Obese individuals have higher levels of fibrinogen (a marker for the inflammatory process of atherosclerosis), factor VII, factor VIII, von Willebrand factor, and plasminogen activator inhibitor-1 (PAI-1). Increased levels of fibrinogen, factor VII, factor VIII, and hypofibrinolysis are associated with hypercoagulability. High factor VIII levels are associated with increased cardiovascular mortality. Increased fasting triglyceride levels correlate with increased factor VII concentrations, and postprandial lipemia causes activation of factor VII. Endothelial dysfunction induced by insulin increases von Willebrand factor and factor VIII levels, predisposing to fibrin formation. Increased secretion of PAI-1 inhibits the fibrinolytic system and is associated with visceral obesity.[31]

Gastrointestinal System

Gastric volume and acidity are increased, hepatic function is altered, and drug metabolism is adversely affected by obesity. Many fasting morbidly obese patients who present for elective surgery have gastric volumes in excess of 25 mL and gastric fluid pH <2.5 (the generally accepted volume and pH indicative of high risk for pneumonitis should regurgitation and aspiration occur). Delayed gastric emptying occurs because of increased abdominal mass that causes antral distention, gastrin release, and a decrease in pH with parietal cell secretion.[32] Abdominal obesity increases intragastric pressure, increasing the frequency of transient lower esophageal sphincter relaxation, and/or hiatal hernia formation. An increase of >3.5 kg/m^2 in BMI is associated with a 2.7-fold increase in risk for developing new reflux symptoms.[32] An increased incidence of hiatal hernia and gastroesophageal reflux further increase aspiration risk.

Gastric emptying is faster with high-energy content intake such as fat emulsions, but because of larger gastric volume (up to 75% larger), the residual volume is increased. The combination of hiatal hernia, gastroesophageal reflux, and delayed gastric emptying, coupled with increased intra-abdominal pressure and high-volume/low-pH gastric content, puts the obese patient at risk for increased incidence of severe pneumonitis should aspiration occur. However, unpremedicated nondiabetic fasting obese surgical patients who are free from significant gastroesophageal pathology are unlikely to have high-volume, low-pH gastric contents after routine preoperative fasting. They should follow the same fasting guidelines as nonobese patients and be allowed to drink clear liquids up until 2 hours before elective surgery.[33] Weight loss significantly improves gastroesophageal reflux symptoms.

Peculiar morphologic and biochemical abnormalities of the liver are associated with obesity and include fatty infiltration (high prevalence of NAFLD), inflammation (nonalcoholic steatohepatitis or NASH), focal necrosis, and cirrhosis. Fatty infiltration reflects the duration rather than the degree of obesity. Histologic and liver function test abnormalities are relatively common, but clearance usually is not reduced. Abnormal liver function tests are seen in up to one-third of obese patients who have no evidence of concomitant liver disease. The most common abnormality is an increased alanine aminotransferase (ALT). Despite these histologic and enzymatic changes, no clear correla- 2
tion exists between liver function abnormalities and the capacity of the liver to metabolize drugs.[34] Morbidly obese patients who have undergone intestinal bypass surgery have a particularly high prevalence of hepatic dysfunction and cholelithiasis. This is also common in the general obese population due to abnormal cholesterol metabolism. The high prevalence of NAFLD, NASH, and cirrhosis necessitates careful assessment for pre-existing liver disease in obese patients scheduled for surgery. Features suggestive of NASH include hepatomegaly, elevated liver enzymes, and abnormal liver histology (steatosis, steatohepatitis, fibrosis, and cirrhosis).

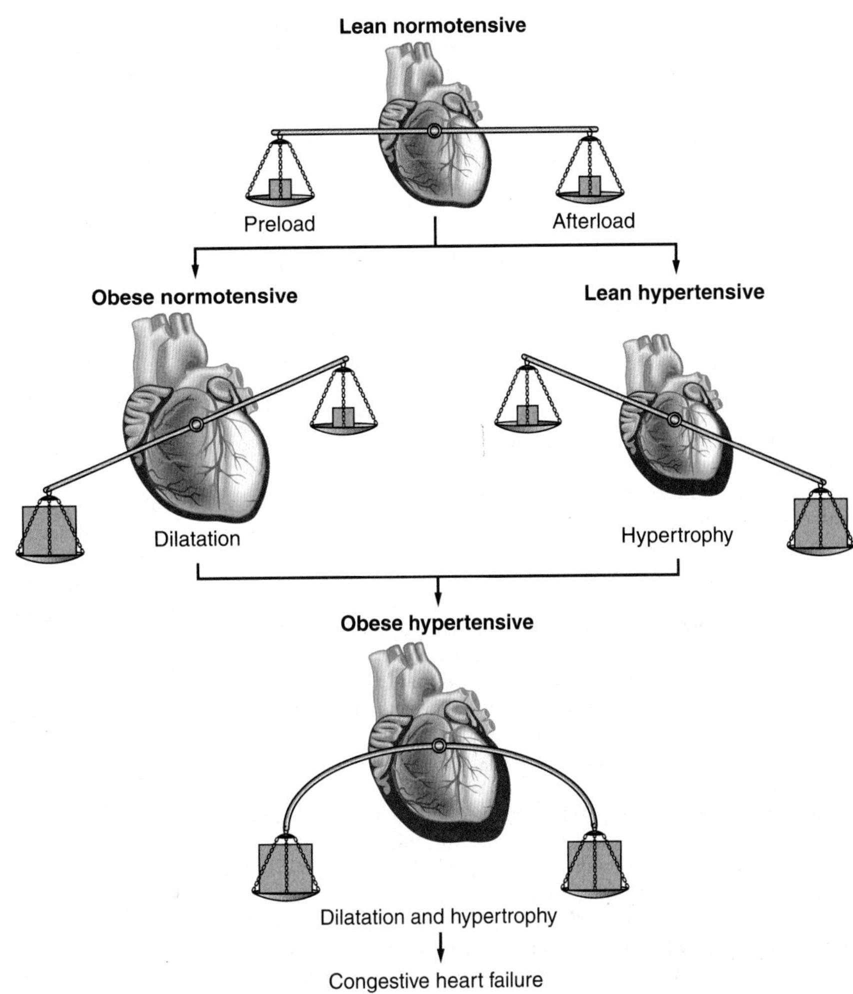

Figure 45-3 Adaptation of the heart to obesity and hypertension. (Reprinted from Messerli FH: Cardiovascular effects of obesity and hypertension. *Lancet.* 1982;1:1165. Copyright © 1982 Elsevier. With permission.)

Renal and Endocrine Systems

Impaired glucose tolerance in the morbidly obese is reflected by a high prevalence of type II diabetes mellitus as a result of resistance of peripheral adipose tissue to insulin.[30] Many obese patients have an abnormal glucose tolerance test, and the relative risk of developing diabetes increases by 25% for every 1 kg/m^2 increase in BMI above 22 kg/m^2.[30] Hyperglycemia, insulin resistance, and diabetes predispose obese patients to wound infections and an increased risk of myocardial infarction. Exogenous insulin may be required perioperatively even in obese patients with type II diabetes mellitus to oppose the catabolic response to surgery. In addition to these concerns, subclinical hypothyroidism occurs in about 25% of all morbidly obese patients. Thyroid-stimulating hormone levels are frequently elevated, suggesting the possibility that obesity leads to a state of thyroid hormone resistance in peripheral tissues. Hypothyroidism may be associated with hypoglycemia, hyponatremia, and impaired hepatic drug metabolism.

Obesity is associated with glomerular hyperfiltration as evidenced by increased renal blood flow and increased glomerular filtration rate. Excessive weight gain increases renal tubular resorption and impairs natriuresis through activation of the sympathetic and renin-angiotensin system as well as physical compression of the kidney. With prolonged obesity, there may be a loss of nephron function, with further impairment of natriuresis and further increases in arterial pressure. However, the increased risk of acute kidney injury by obesity *per se* is unclear.[35] Obesity-related glomerular hyperfiltration decreases after weight loss, which decreases the incidence of overt glomerulopathy.

Metabolic Syndrome. Metabolic syndrome, sometimes referred to as syndrome X and insulin resistance syndrome, is a cluster of metabolic abnormalities associated with an increased risk of diabetes and cardiovascular events. Individuals with this syndrome have up to a fivefold greater risk of developing type 2 diabetes mellitus (if not already present) and are also twice as likely to die from a myocardial infarction or stroke compared with those without the syndrome.[36] Furthermore, patients with metabolic syndrome are more likely to have perioperative adverse events including cardiovascular, pulmonary, and renal complications and wound infections.[37] Although there are several different definitions of metabolic syndrome, the National Cholesterol Education Program (NCEP) Adult Treatment Panel III (ATP III) definition is the most widely used.[38] It defines metabolic syndrome when three out of the following five conditions exist: (1) central obesity: waist circumference 102 cm (40 in) in males, 88 cm (35 in) in females; (2) dyslipidemia: triglycerides 150 mg/dL; (3) dyslipidemia: HDL 40 mg/dL in males, 50 mg/dL in females; (4) hypertension: 130/85 mmHg or use of antihypertensives; and (5) elevated fasting glucose: 100 mg/dL (5.6 mmol/L) or use of medication for hyperglycemia. Weight loss and lifestyle changes can improve metabolic syndrome features.[36] Bariatric surgery resolves metabolic syndrome in more than 95% of patients who achieve expected weight loss.[39]

Pharmacology

Pharmacologic Principles

General pharmacokinetic principles dictate, with certain exceptions, that drug dosing should take into consideration the volume of distribution (VD) for administration of the loading dose, and the clearance for the maintenance dose. A drug that is mainly distributed to lean tissues should have the loading dose calculated based on LBW. If the drug is equally distributed between adipose and lean tissues, dosing should be calculated based on TBW. For maintenance, a drug with similar clearance values in both obese and nonobese individuals should have the maintenance dose calculated based on LBW. However, a drug whose clearance increases with obesity should have the maintenance dose calculated according to TBW. Use of LBW and TBW in drug dosing for obese individuals is still under discussion.[40]

The relative volume of the central compartment in which drugs are first distributed remains unchanged in obese patients, but absolute body water content is decreased. Lean body and adipose tissue mass are increased, affecting lipophilic and polar drug distribution (Fig. 45-4). The VD in obese patients is affected by multiple factors including reduced total body water, increased total body fat, increased lean body mass, altered protein binding, increased blood volume, increased cardiac output, increased blood concentrations of free fatty acids, triglycerides, cholesterol, and α1-acid glycoprotein, lipophilicity of the drug, and organomegaly.[6] Increased redistribution of a drug prolongs its elimination half-life even when clearance is unchanged or increased. Hyperlipidemia and an increased concentration of α1-acid glycoprotein may affect protein binding, leading to a reduction in free drug concentration. Plasma albumin and total plasma protein concentrations and binding are not significantly changed by obesity, but when compared with normal-weight individuals, a relative increase in plasma protein binding may be evident. Splanchnic blood flow, blood volume, and cardiac output are all increased in obese patients. In contrast to the expected decrease in bioavailability of orally administered medications because of increased splanchnic blood flow, there is no significant difference in absorption and bioavailability when comparing obese and normal-weight subjects. Drugs that undergo phase I metabolism (oxidation, reduction, hydrolysis) are generally unaffected by changes induced by obesity, whereas phase II reactions (glucuronidation, sulfation) are enhanced.[6]

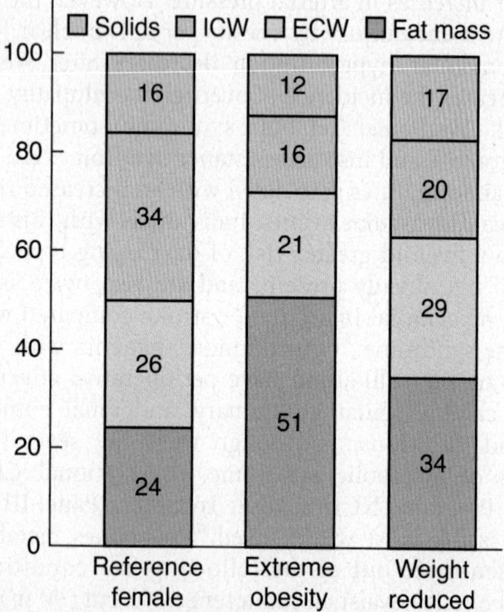

Figure 45-4 Body composition in extremely obese and weight-reduced states compared with reference female values. ICW, intracellular water; ECW, extracellular water. (Reprinted from Das SK, Roberts SB, Kehayias JJ, et al: Body composition methods in extreme obesity. *Am J Physiol Endocrinol Metab* 2003;284:E1080.)

Histologic abnormalities of the liver are common in the obese, with concomitant deranged liver function tests, but drug clearance is not usually affected. Renal clearance of drugs is increased in obesity because of increased renal blood flow and glomerular filtration rate.[41] As a result of the increases in glomerular filtration rate and tubular secretion, drugs such as cimetidine and aminoglycoside antibiotics that depend on renal excretion may require increased dosing. Highly lipophilic substances such as barbiturates and benzodiazepines show significant increases in VD for obese individuals.[6] These drugs have a more selective distribution to fat stores and therefore a longer elimination half-life but with comparable clearance values to normal individuals. Less lipophilic compounds have little or no change in VD with obesity. Exceptions to this rule include the highly lipophilic drugs digoxin, procainamide, and remifentanil. Drugs with weak or moderate lipophilicity may be dosed on the basis of LBW. Adding 20% to the estimated IBW dose of hydrophilic medications is sufficient to include the obese patient's extra lean mass. Nondepolarizing muscle relaxants can be dosed in this manner. A recent study evaluated recovery times after reversal of neuromuscular blockade with sugammadex in obese (BMI >30 kg/m) and nonobese (BMI <30 kg/m) patients, and found that recovery time did not correlate with BMI.[42] Sugammadex dosing can therefore be based on actual body weight in both obese and nonobese patients.

Increased blood volume in the obese patient decreases plasma concentrations of rapidly injected intravenous drugs. Fat, however, has poor blood flow, and doses calculated on actual body weight could lead to excessive plasma concentrations. Calculating initial doses based on LBW with subsequent doses determined by pharmacologic response to the initial dose is a reasonable approach. Repeated injections may accumulate fat, leading to a prolonged response because of subsequent release from this large depot. Table 45-3 presents dosing guidelines for intravenous agents when used in obese patients.[43]

Other Perioperative Agents

Patients' usual medications should be continued until the time of surgery, with the possible exception of certain antihypertensives, insulin, and oral hypoglycemics. Antibiotic prophylaxis is usually indicated because of an increased incidence of wound infections in the obese. A recent prospective, cross-sectional study of 896 patients undergoing RYGBs determined that the rate of surgical site infection was less in patients receiving a continuous infusion of cefazolin (1.55%) throughout the procedure compared to patients receiving either bolus dose ampicillin/sulbactam (4.16%) versus Ertapenem (1.98%).[44] Anxiolysis and prophylaxis against both aspiration pneumonitis and deep vein thrombosis (DVT) should be addressed preoperatively. Oral benzodiazepines are reliable for anxiolysis and sedation, and intravenous midazolam can be titrated in small doses for anxiolysis during the immediate preoperative period. Dexmedetomidine can be advantageous in this patient population because of its minimal respiratory depressant effects. Pharmacologic

Table 45-3 Intravenous Drug Dosing in Obesity[42,43]

Drug	Dosing	Practical Anesthesia Key Points
Thiopental	Induction: LBW (somewhat increased)	Increased initial dose due to increased blood volume, CO, muscle mass. Rapid distribution from plasma to periphery. Increased absolute dose. Prolonged duration of action due to high lipophilicity and increased V_D. Longer elimination half-life.
Propofol.	Induction: LBW (somewhat increased) Maintenance infusion: TBW	Short duration of action due to rapid redistribution. Highly lipophilic. Cardiac output is major determinant of peak plasma concentration. Increased V_D at steady state and increased clearance prevent increases in elimination half-life Total clearance and V_D at steady state correlate with body weight during maintenance infusion. Negative cardiovascular effects. High affinity for fat and well-perfused organs. High hepatic extraction and conjugation relate to TBW.
Succinylcholine	TBW	Pseudocholinesterase activity increases linearly with increasing weight and large extracellular fluid compartment. Dose of succinylcholine should be increased.
Rocuronium	LBW	Dosing according to LBW to prevent delayed recovery due to increased V_D. Faster onset and longer duration when dosed according to TBW. Pharmacokinetics and pharmacodynamics not altered in obese female patients.
Vecuronium	LBW	Prolonged action when dosed according to TBW. Dosing according to LBW to prevent delayed recovery due to increased V_D and impaired hepatic clearance. Obesity does not alter distribution or elimination of the drug.
Atracurium	LBW	V_D, absolute clearance, and elimination half-life unchanged by obesity. Unchanged dose per unit body weight without prolongation of recovery because of organ function-independent elimination.
Cis-atracurium	LBW	Pharmacokinetics similar to atracurium but prolonged duration of action when dosed according to TBW.
Benzodiazepines		Highly lipophilic drugs with larger V_D in obese patients result in longer duration of action. Midazolam has potential for prolonged sedation because larger initial doses are required to achieve adequate serum concentrations.
Fentanyl	LBW	Measured total body clearance has a nonlinear relationship to TBW and overestimates plasma concentration. Fentanyl dosing based on a derived LBW or "pharmacokinetic mass" model correlates better with clearance than TBW dosing. Dosing based on TBW overestimates dose requirements in the obese patient.
Sufentanil.	LBW	Highly lipid soluble Increased V_D and prolonged elimination half-life, which correlates with degree of obesity. Distributes extensively in excess body fat. Similar pharmacokinetic parameters in obese and nonobese predict similar plasma concentrations. Overestimation of plasma concentration occurs in the morbidly obese range (BMI >40 kg/m^2).
Remifentanil	LBW	Pharmacokinetics similar in obese and nonobese patients (i.e., more closely related to lean body mass than LBW. Systemic clearance and V_D corrected per kilogram of TBW is significantly smaller in the obese patient. Consider age and lean body mass for dosing.
Dexmedetomi-dine	TBW	Highly selective α_2-adrenergic agonist. Sedative-hypnotic, anesthetic-sparing analgesic, sympatholytic properties. Lacks significant effects on respiration. Ideal analgesic adjuvant in the morbidly obese patient. As part of a balanced anesthetic, infusion rates of 0.2 to 0.7 μg/kg/h produce clinically effective sedation with decreased analgesic and anesthetic requirements.
Neostigmine	TBW	Prompt early reversal but delayed full recovery during neostigmine-induced reversal of vecuronium dosed according to TBW.
Sugammadex		A modified γ-cyclodextrin compound that encapsulates rocuronium, (and other steroid-based neuromuscular blockers to a lesser extent). May prove invaluable for more rapid and complete neuromuscular blockade reversal in obese patients.

BMI, body mass index; LBW, lean body weight; TBW, total body weight; V_D, volume of distribution.
Adapted with permission from Ogunnaike BO, Jones SB, Jones DB, et al. Anesthetic considerations for bariatric surgery. *Anesth Analg*. 2002;95(6):1793–1805.
Adapted from Monk TG, Rietbergen H, Woo T, Fennema H. Use of sugammadex in patients with obesity: a pooled analysis. *Am J Ther*. 2017;24(5):e507–e516.

intervention with H_2-receptor antagonists, nonparticulate antacids, or proton pump inhibitors will reduce gastric volume, acidity, or both, thereby reducing the risk and severity of aspiration pneumonitis.

Preoperative Evaluation

A comprehensive preoperative evaluation of the obese surgical patient is critical to identify and address possible multisystem comorbidities, and to allow the development of an individualized perioperative care plan.[45–47] The presence of any of the following factors, (1) central obesity; (2) metabolic syndrome; and (3) peripheral oxygen saturation <95% breathing air, are important for risk prediction and can be assessed without recourse to complicated diagnostic testing.[48] Previous anesthetic experiences as detailed by the patient and previous anesthetic records are often useful sources of information.

Airway. Preoperative airway assessment is important in all patients but is especially so in those who are obese.[49] Both anatomic and physiologic changes contribute to difficult airway management in the obese. Anatomic changes associated with obesity that contribute to a potentially difficult airway include limitation of movement of the atlantoaxial joint and cervical spine by upper thoracic and low cervical fat pads; excessive tissue folds in the mouth and pharynx; short, thick neck; thick submental fat pad; suprasternal, presternal, and posterior cervical fat; and large breasts in females. Excess pharyngeal tissue deposited in the lateral pharyngeal walls may not be noticed during routine airway examination. The history obtained from the patient and examination of previous records may help predict airway difficulties.

Obesity is an accepted risk factor for difficult mask ventilation and airway management. With adequate positioning and airway resources available, most obese patients can be adequately and safely managed. However, the closed claims database revealed that obesity was a risk factor in 68% of claims associated with difficult endotracheal intubation in the United States.[50] Patients who are morbidly obese (i.e., BMI >40) are four times as likely to experi-
3 ence a complication related to airway management.[51] Although OSA contributes to difficult mask ventilation in the obese,[49] a neck circumference of ≥40 cm is the biggest predictor of difficult mask ventilation, difficult laryngoscopy, and difficult endotracheal intubation.[52]

Cardiopulmonary. Cardiopulmonary evaluation should focus on issues peculiar to the obese patient including evaluation for systemic hypertension, pulmonary hypertension, signs of right and/or left ventricular failure, and ischemic heart disease. Hypertension is common resulting from increased sympathetic activation and the proinflammatory state. 2017 Guidelines from the American Heart Association documented hypertension as a modifiable cardiovascular risk factor.[53] Recommendations include systolic blood pressure of <120 mmHg and diastolic pressures of <80 mmHg.[53] It may be difficult to detect signs of cardiac failure such as elevated jugular venous pressure, pathologic heart sounds, pulmonary crackles, hepatomegaly, and peripheral edema because of excess adiposity. Pulmonary hypertension is more common in this patient population because of chronic pulmonary impairment. The common symptoms of pulmonary hypertension are exertional dyspnea, fatigue, and syncope (which collectively reflect an inability to increase cardiac output during activity). Further cardiac testing may be individually required, based on these initial clinical findings.[54] Tricuspid regurgitation on echocardiography is the most useful confirmatory test of pulmonary hypertension but should be combined with clinical evaluation. An ECG may demonstrate signs of right ventricular hypertrophy such as tall precordial R waves, right axis deviation, and right ventricular strain. The sensitivity of the ECG increases as the pulmonary artery pressure increases. Chest radiographs may show evidence of underlying lung disease and prominent pulmonary arteries.

Evidence of OSA and OHS should be obtained preoperatively 4
because they are frequently associated with difficult airway management and increased perioperative pulmonary complications. A history of hypertension or a neck circumference >40 cm correlates with an increased probability of OSA. OSA is a legitimate reason to delay elective surgery for a proper evaluation.[23] OSA patients should generally be treated as inpatients; however, outpatient surgery can be considered under certain circumstances, including mild OSA, use of local or regional anesthesia with minimal sedation, availability of a 23-hour observation postanesthesia care unit, and when patients can resume oral medication at the time of discharge. OSA patients using a CPAP device at home should be instructed to bring it with them to the hospital and it may be needed postoperatively. The possibility of invasive monitoring, prolonged intubation, and postoperative mechanical ventilation should be discussed with obese patients. Arterial blood gas measurements help evaluate ventilation, as well as the need for perioperative oxygen administration and postoperative ventilation. Routine pulmonary function tests and liver function tests are not cost-effective in asymptomatic obese patients.

Metabolic. Metabolic and nutritional abnormalities are common in these patients. The high prevalence of insulin resistance and diabetes in obese patients justifies the need of considering glycemia checks preoperatively, and correcting abnormalities if present. Preoperative evaluation should include assessment of therapies for glycemia control, last time and dose of preoperative administration, and usual glucose values for a specific patient. Electrolytes should be checked before surgery, particularly in patients with poor compliance to medications or acutely ill patients. Other nutritional deficiencies include vitamin B12, iron, calcium, and folate. Vitamin and nutritional deficiencies can lead to a collective form of postoperative polyneuropathy, known as acute postgastric reduction surgery (APGARS) neuropathy, a polynutritional multisystem disorder characterized by protracted postoperative vomiting, hyporeflexia, and muscular weakness. Differential diagnoses of this disorder include thiamine deficiency (Wernicke encephalopathy, beriberi), vitamin B12 deficiency, and Guillain–Barré syndrome. Close attention to dosing and monitoring of neuromuscular blocking agents is recommended in cases of suspected or diagnosed APGARS neuropathy. Chronic vitamin K deficiency may lead to coagulation abnormalities, requiring administration of vitamin K analog or fresh-frozen plasma. Patients scheduled for repeat bariatric surgery should be screened preoperatively for long-term metabolic and nutritional abnormalities.

Hematology. Morbid obesity is a known risk factor for perioperative thromboembolic events, including sudden death from acute pulmonary embolism. Thromboprophylaxis guidelines exist, especially for patients undergoing bariatric surgery,[55] but preoperative evaluation should confirm these plans. Guidelines from the American Society of Chest Physicians recommend, in patients undergoing bariatric surgery, the combination of intermittent pneumatic compression devices with heparin (unfractionated or low molecular weight heparin), and warn that greater doses in obese patients may be needed than in nonobese ones.[56] Prolonged postoperative regimens (1 to 3 weeks) are being explored in bariatric patients.[57] Four important risk factors, namely venous stasis disease, BMI ≥60, central obesity, and OHS and/or OSA, are significant in the development of postoperative DVT, and if present, preoperative prophylactic placement of an inferior vena cava filter should be considered. A combination of short duration of surgery, lower extremity pneumatic compression, and routine early ambulation may preclude mandatory heparin anticoagulation, except in patients with a history of previous DVT, a known hypercoagulable state, or a significant family history of DVT.

Intraoperative Considerations

Equipment and Monitoring

Specially designed tables or two regularly sized operating room tables may be required for safe anesthesia and surgery in obese patients. Regular operating room tables have a maximum weight limit of approximately 200 kg, but operating room tables capable of holding up to 455 kg, with a greater width or side accessories to accommodate the extra girth, are available. Strapping obese patients to the operating room table in combination with a malleable beanbag helps keep them from falling off the operating room table.

Supine positioning causes ventilatory impairment and inferior vena cava and aortic compression in obese patients. FRC and oxygenation are decreased further with supine positioning. Head-down positioning, often required during bariatric procedures, further worsens FRC and should be avoided if possible. Simply changing the obese patient from a sitting to supine position can cause a significant increase in oxygen consumption and cardiac output. The head-up position provides the longest safe apnea period during induction of anesthesia.[48] by precluding hypoxemia if intubation is delayed. Both intraoperative positive end-expiratory pressure (PEEP) and the head-up position significantly decrease the alveolar–arterial oxygen tension difference and increase total respiratory compliance to a similar degree, but the head-up position results in lower airway pressures. However, both interventions decrease cardiac output significantly, partially counteracting the beneficial effects on oxygenation. Prone positioning, rarely required in the obese patient, should be correctly performed with freedom of abdominal movement to prevent detrimental effects on lung compliance, ventilation, and arterial oxygenation. Lateral decubitus positioning allows for better diaphragmatic excursion and should be favored over prone positioning whenever the surgical procedure permits. Particular care should be paid to protecting pressure areas because pressure sores, neural injuries, and rhabdomyolysis may occur. Brachial plexus and lower extremity nerve injuries are frequent. Carpal tunnel syndrome is the most common mononeuropathy after bariatric surgery. Other reported neurologic complications include encephalopathy (Wernicke), optic neuropathy, and myelopathy associated with vitamin B12 and copper deficiencies.[58]

Monitoring the surgical obese patient poses additional challenges. Careful selection of proper size of blood pressure cuff and location is important for accurate detection of irregularities
5 in blood pressure. Blood pressure measurements can be falsely elevated if a cuff is too small. Cuffs with bladders that encircle a minimum of 75% of the upper arm circumference or, preferably, the entire arm, should be used. In the supine position, forearm measurements with a standard cuff can be used when upper arm measurements are challenging.[59] Although invasive arterial pressure monitoring is not routine for all patients, it may be indicated for the super morbidly obese patient, not only for those patients with cardiopulmonary disease, but also for those patients in whom the noninvasive blood pressure cuff does not fit properly. Central venous catheterization, though not routinely needed, may be required for intravenous access in patients with inadequate peripheral access for perioperative fluid management. Central venous catheters, pulmonary artery catheters and/or transesophageal echocardiography can be used selectively in patients with significant cardiopulmonary disease or in patients undergoing extensive surgery.

Airway Management

Adequate preoxygenation is vital in obese patients because of rapid desaturation after loss of consciousness related to increased oxygen consumption and decreased FRC. Although 100% oxygen increases the formation of atelectasis, it extends the nonhypoxic apnea period after induction of anesthesia. Recent recommendations encourage the addition of a head-up position during preoxygenation for prolonging the nonhypoxic apneic period in the obese patient.[60] The extra time gained may help preclude hypoxemia if intubation is delayed. The head-up position can be achieved with reversed Trendelenburg or semisitting position,[60] and may also help to prevent aspiration and facilitate visualization during laryngoscopy. Preoperative use of noninvasive positive pressure ventilation (NIPPV), CPAP, or oxygen administration during induction will also delay peri-induction hypoxemia.[61] Passive apneic oxygenation adjuvant techniques have been proposed to delay apneic hypoxemia, via oxygen supplementation by nasal cannula, high-flow nasal cannula (HFNC), or laryngeal mask airway (LMA).[62]

Obese patients are more likely than nonobese patients to present with difficult mask ventilation and intubation, especially if they have a short, thick neck and OSA.[49,52] If mask ventilation is needed, exhaled tidal volumes of obese patients may be greater when the patient is in a 25-degree head-up position compared to supine.[63] Holding the mask with two hands in the V-E position (with the operator's thumbs along the sides of the mask and the first and second fingers behind the angle of the mandible to perform a jaw thrust) may be more effective than the C-E position (with the thumbs and first fingers on the mask and the fourth and fifth fingers on the patients' mandible).[64] If a difficult intubation is anticipated, a strategy should be developed depending upon the type of surgery, skills of the anesthesiologist, and patient level of cooperation and condition.[25] The strategy should include plans for (1) awake intubation; (2) the patient who can be adequately ventilated but is difficult to intubate; (3) the patient who cannot be ventilated or intubated; and (4) emergency invasive airway rescue.[25] During awake intubation, sedative–hypnotic medications should be reduced to a minimum. Sedation with dexmedetomidine during awake intubation provides adequate anxiolysis and analgesia without respiratory depression.[65] Hypoxia and aspiration of gastric contents should be prevented at all costs during endotracheal intubation. An experienced colleague who is present or immediately available during induction and airway management can be helpful with mask ventilation or attempts at intubation. A surgeon capable of accessing the airway surgically should be readily available. A "ramped" position that elevates the obese 6
patient's upper body improves laryngoscopic view compared with the standard supine "sniffing" position. Towels or folded blankets under the shoulders and head can compensate for the exaggerated flexed position caused by posterior cervical fat (Fig. 45-5). The objective of this maneuver, known as "stacking," is to position the patient so that the tip of the chin is at a higher level than the chest to facilitate laryngoscopy and intubation.

Although direct laryngoscopy is used successfully in many obese patients, assuming optimal positioning has been achieved, the immediate availability of other intubating tools is highly recommended. These include videolaryngoscopes, intubating stylettes (e.g., Eschmann stylet, tube exchanger), LMAs, and fiberoptic bronchoscopes. Videolaryngoscopes have proven to be

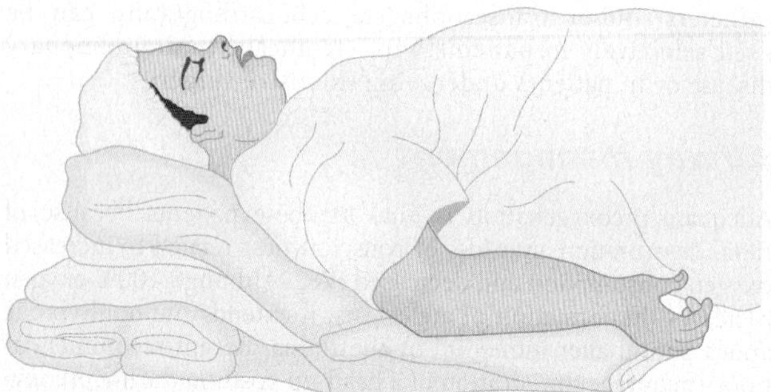

Figure 45-5 Ramped position with "stacking" of towels and blankets.

efficient tools for intubating obese patients, reducing the duration of intubation and the number of attempts, with a similar or better glottic view than standard direct laryngoscopy.[66] Multiple laryngoscopic attempts and repeated attempts at intubation are consistent with increased airway and hemodynamic complications. The closed claims data also support the recommendations to limit conventional intubation attempts to three before using other strategies.[50] LMAs can be useful for temporarily achieving airway patency in patients with difficult mask ventilation and intubation, or for placing a definitive endotracheal tube via an intubating LMA.[25]

Induction and Maintenance

Concerns of hypoxemia, gastric regurgitation, and aspiration during induction and intubation justify the common use of rapid sequence induction (RSI) strategies. Gastroesophageal reflux disease is relatively common in obese patients, and the incidence of regurgitation and severe pneumonitis in case of aspiration is increased in this population (as discussed earlier in physiology section). Findings suggest that unpremedicated, nondiabetic fasting obese surgical patients with no significant gastroesophageal pathology are unlikely to have high-volume, low-pH gastric contents after routine preoperative fasting and that routine preoperative fasting guidelines (6 hours for solids, 2 hours for clear liquids) may be safe in obese patients.[67] In any case, the use of an RSI versus standard induction should be routinely and carefully evaluated in obese patients and the final decision individualized based on the patient's risk of difficult mask ventilation, intubation, hypoxemia, and gastric aspiration during induction.

7 No systematic comparison of anesthetic agents or techniques is available in obese patients. Larger doses of induction agents may be required because blood volume, muscle mass, and cardiac output increase linearly with the degree of obesity. Any of the commonly available intravenous induction agents may be employed after taking into consideration problems peculiar to individual patients. An increased dose of succinylcholine is necessary because of an increase in activity of pseudocholinesterase. Myalgia is not frequently seen following succinylcholine in morbidly obese patients.[68] Succinylcholine is highly recommended for tracheal intubation, especially in obese patients in which airway management is considered challenging or with high risk of peri-induction hypoxemia or aspiration due to its rapid onset and limited duration of action. Rocuronium can also be considered for tracheal intubation. However, its duration of action is more prolonged than succinylcholine.

Continuous infusion of a short-acting intravenous agent, such as propofol, or any of the inhalation agents, or a combination, may be used to maintain anesthesia. Desflurane, sevoflurane, and isoflurane are minimally metabolized and are therefore useful agents in the obese patient, with desflurane possibly providing faster washout. The use of nitrous oxide (N_2O), despite its rapid elimination and analgesic properties, is limited by the high oxygen demand in this patient population. Short-acting opioids are preferred in obese patients to provide adequate analgesia but avoid postoperative respiratory depression. Remifentanil and fentanyl, carefully titrated to clinical effect, are the most common choices.[45] Dexmedetomidine, an α_2-agonist with sedative and analgesic properties, has no clinically significant adverse effects on respiration and is an attractive anesthetic adjunct in obese patients.[69] Furthermore, it reduces postoperative opioid analgesic requirements.[69]

Profound muscle relaxation is important during laparoscopic bariatric procedures to facilitate ventilation and to maintain an adequate working space for visualization and safe manipulation of laparoscopic instruments. It also facilitates extraction of excised tissues. Collapse of the pneumoperitoneum and tightening of the patient's musculature around port sites are early indications of inadequate muscle relaxation.[43] Vecuronium, rocuronium, and cisatracurium are useful nondepolarizing muscle-blocking agents for maintenance of muscle relaxation. Pneumoperitoneum should not be increased above 15 mmHg since intra-abdominal pressures of 20 mmHg or greater can cause caval compression and decrease cardiac output.[45] Cephalad displacement of the diaphragm and carina by the pneumoperitoneum during laparoscopy can cause a firmly secured endotracheal tube to displace into a main stem bronchus.

Anesthesia personnel may be asked to facilitate the proper placement of an intragastric balloon to help the surgeon size the gastric pouch, and also to facilitate performance of leak tests with saline or methylene blue through a nasogastric tube. Care should be taken to ensure a tight seal of the endotracheal tube cuff, otherwise, aspiration of saline or methylene blue can occur. All endogastric tubes should be completely removed (not just merely pulled back into the esophagus) before gastric division to avoid unplanned stapling and transection of these devices.

Fluid Management

Excess adipose tissue may mask peripheral perfusion, making fluid balance difficult to assess. Blood loss is usually greater in the obese than in the nonobese patient for the same type of surgery because technical difficulties in accessing the surgical site necessitate larger incisions and more extensive dissection. Because intravenous fluid requirements are generally greater than predicted, fluid management is particularly challenging in the obese patient. Normovolemia should be the goal, to avoid increased hemodynamic instability, postoperative nausea and vomiting, and acute tubular necrosis (ATN) from hypovolemia. ATN occurs in approximately 2% of patients undergoing bariatric surgery. Associated risk factors include BMI greater than 50 kg/m^2, prior history of renal disease, intraoperative hypotension, and prolonged surgical times.[70] Normovolemia also reduces the risk of hypervolemic complications such as decompensated congestive heart failure, peripheral tissue edema, and pulmonary complications. Rapid infusion of intravenous fluids should be avoided because pre-existing congestive cardiac failure is common in the obese patient. The use of IBW estimates and appropriate monitoring can help to avoid potential hyperhydration in morbidly obese patients. Preliminary findings demonstrate that during laparoscopic bariatric surgery, urine output does not correlate with the rate of intraoperative fluid administration,[71] and the total volume of fluids infused does not seem to affect the incidence of postoperative rhabdomyolysis.[72]

Mechanical Ventilation

Obesity makes titration of ventilatory settings challenging, since increasing weight does not imply a proportional growth of the lung. Obese patients are still likely to be exposed to high tidal volumes because of miscalculation of predicted or ideal body weight,[73,74] high airway pressures due to decreased respiratory system compliance, and low PEEP levels.[75] Although similar ventilatory parameters in nonobese patients can be used, it may be challenging to maintain plateau pressures 30 cmH_2O.[5] Greater inflation pressures may be tolerated in obese patients,[76] possibly because the pressure of extra adipose tissue on the chest wall acts against the inspiratory airway pressure, thus partially attenuating the lung overdistention that would otherwise occur. In any case, 6 to 8 mL/kg PBW tidal volumes are often recommended for obese patients.[77] Larger tidal volumes offer no added advantages during ventilation of anesthetized morbidly obese patients. Further increasing tidal volumes only increases the peak inspiratory airway pressure, end-expiratory (plateau) airway pressure, and lung compliance without significantly improving arterial oxygen tension.[78] No specific ventilatory mode (volume vs. pressure control ventilation [PCV]) has been found significantly better for oxygenation and CO_2 clearance in obese patients, although pressure modes have in some studies correlated with increased oxygenation.[79]

8 Positive PEEP is the only ventilatory parameter that has consistently been shown to improve respiratory function in obese subjects, although the ideal PEEP value is still unknown.Recruitment maneuvers in addition to the use of PEEP are the most effective ventilatory technique to prevent postoperative atelectasis in obese patients and are increasingly recommended.[77,80] These techniques for alveolar recruitment are clearly beneficial in obese patients, compared to nonobese ones.[79,81] Different methods for performing recruitment maneuvers exist. A simple one proposed by Pelosi et al. is a series of three short (6 seconds) inflations with PCV to administer a large tidal volume by reaching an inspiratory pressure of 40 to 55 cmH_2O.[82] Other recruitment techniques are summarized by Shah et al.[79] These higher-than-usual airway pressures may be needed to compensate for the decreased chest wall compliance and to achieve an adequate transpulmonary pressure. The combination of recruitment maneuvers and PEEP aims to open and maintain the patency of small airway units, therefore improving ventilation–perfusion matching and oxygenation. This practice in obese surgical patients leads to improved oxygenation and respiratory mechanics and reduced atelectasis,[83,84] although whether clinical outcomes overall are improved remains unresolved.[85] Recruitment maneuvers and PEEP can decrease venous return and cardiac output, although they are usually adequately tolerated in normovolemic morbidly obese patients.[78] Inspired oxygen fraction (FiO_2) should be titrated to the minimum levels that assure acceptable oxygenation levels while avoiding reabsorption atelectasis. Some experts recommend that the FiO_2 to be kept lower than 0.8 in obese patients.[82]

Emergence

9 Prompt but safe extubation reduces the likelihood that the morbidly obese patient will become ventilator dependent. This is especially important in patients with underlying cardiopulmonary disease. The patient should be preferably extubated in the semirecumbent position and recovered in the sitting position, which provide more favorable respiratory mechanics than the supine position.[82] Some institutions mandate the presence of two anesthesia providers for the emergence and extubation of morbidly obese patients. Supplemental oxygen should be administrated after extubation. An observation period of at least 5 minutes after extubation before transporting the patient away from the operating room is often recommended. The risk of hypoventilation in the immediate postoperative period, with the consequent hypercapnia with or without hypoxemia, is leading to the development of noninvasive monitoring techniques and the increasing use of CPAP.[23]

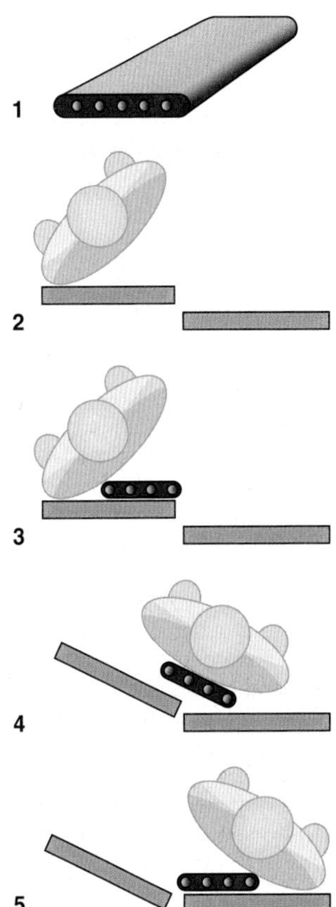

Figure 45-6 Illustration of the Walter Henderson maneuver. **1,** Patient transfer device (PTD; a.k.a. patient roller); **2,** patient tilted to slip roller underneath; **3,** roller slipped under patient; **4,** table tilted to roll patient "downhill" onto bed; **5,** patient rolled onto bed. (Reprinted with permission from Ogunnaike BO, Whitten CW. Bariatric surgery and the prevention of postoperative respiratory complications: In response. *Anesth Analg*. 2004;98(6):1810–1811.)

Lifting devices such as the HoverMatt (Patient Handling Technologies, Allentown, PA), the patient transfer device (PTD; Alimed, Dedham, MA), and gantry-style mechanical lifting devices that use slings are useful for transporting morbidly obese patients onto or off the operating room table. The PTD can be combined with the Walter Henderson maneuver (Fig. 45-6) to safely and gently transfer obese patients onto their postoperative beds.[86]

Monitored Anesthesia Care and Sedation

Monitoring of the adequacy of ventilation and oxygenation is extremely important in obese patients. Obese patients present a higher risk of sedation-induced respiratory depression, so careful titration of benzodiazepines, opioids, and propofol is mandatory to avoid hypercapnia and/or hypoxemia. Hypoxemia may require unplanned intubation, so a thorough airway examination and preparation for unintended airway management is critical even in MAC/sedation cases. The prevalence of closed claims related to adverse respiratory events during monitored anesthesia cases is increasing, compared to respiratory complications or airway management complications encountered during general anesthesia.[87] Obesity and suboptimal monitoring of pulse oximetry and/or end-tidal capnography are significant key factors in adverse events during MAC.

Regional Anesthesia and Analgesia

Neuraxial anesthetic techniques (spinal, epidural, combined spinal epidural [CSE]) or peripheral nerve blocks can be used alone or in combination with general anesthesia. Transversus abdominis plane (TAP) blocks or wound infusions are often effective for postoperative pain control.[88] With proper planning, these techniques may be used successfully and should be considered in the anesthetic plan for obese patients who are candidates for regional anesthesia. Regional techniques reduce opioid-related complications but there are other distinct advantages: (1) minimal or reduced manipulation of the airway; (2) administration of fewer medications with cardiopulmonary depression; (3) reduced risk of postoperative nausea and vomiting; (4) better postoperative pain control; and (5) improved postoperative outcomes. When epidural anesthesia is combined with general anesthesia, time to tracheal extubation may be reduced in patients receiving a combined technique compared to general anesthesia alone. However, there is an increased risk of block failure in obese patients compared to those of normal weight, and these patients also experience an increased risk of complications.[89] Intravenous access should always be secured prior to block placement in case of local anesthetic systemic toxicity or a high spinal.

Neuraxial Anesthesia

Physiologic changes associated with neuraxial anesthesia. Neuraxial anesthesia can produce serious cardiopulmonary compromise in obese patients undergoing surgery, necessitating careful monitoring. Because pulmonary mechanics, lung volumes, FRC, oxygenation, and ventilation are altered in these individuals, supine and Trendelenburg positioning during neuraxial anesthesia can lead to deterioration of lung volumes and further reductions in FRC. FRC may fall below closing capacity, promoting small airway collapse, atelectasis, ventilation–perfusion mismatch, and hypoxia, especially during supine and Trendelenburg positioning.[90] It is often helpful to measure the oxygen saturation in the sitting and supine positions to indicate the degree of pulmonary reserve prior to initiating neuraxial anesthesia. The excess weight of the abdominal wall can compress the vena cava, causing decreased cardiac preload, reflex tachycardia, and decreased cardiac output. Early observations suggest that spinal anesthesia in obese patients increases the risk for hypotension and cardiac arrest. During supine positioning, circulatory changes can contribute to these arrests.[91]

Despite these important considerations, use of neuraxial techniques can offer important advantages when compared to general anesthesia alone. Parenteral opioid administration can be hazardous in these patients because of increased sensitivity to opioids, risk of hypoxemia, a high incidence of sleep apnea, and increased incidence of adverse respiratory events following surgery. The American Society of Anesthesiologists has published guidelines for the care of patients with OSA and recommends that regional anesthetic techniques should be considered to reduce or eliminate the requirements for systemic opioids in patients with sleep apnea.[23]

Positioning and placement. Positioning is an important step in placement of a successful neuraxial anesthetic. Spinal or epidural placement in the sitting position will assist with identification of the midline. The patient's back should be parallel to the edge of the bed to prevent lateral needle deviation away from the midline. Lateral deviation of the midline will increase the depth to the epidural or spinal spaces and can result in block failure and an increased risk for intraoperative conversion to general anesthesia in less-than-ideal circumstances. Anatomic landmarks are often obscured in these patients. If spinal processes cannot be appreciated with deep palpation, a line can be drawn from the cervical vertebral spinal process to the uppermost portion of the gluteal cleft. This line approximates the midline of the patient over the vertebral column. Ultrasound imaging can also be helpful to identify spinal processes and has been shown to significantly reduce the number of needle passes and decrease the time for spinal block placement in morbidly obese patients undergoing orthopedic surgery.[92] Since the iliac crests may also be difficult to appreciate, the patient's skin folds can be used to aid in drawing a line perpendicular to the vertical line so that the intersection point can serve as a reasonable spinal or epidural needle insertion guide.

Neuraxial anesthetic placement can be particularly difficult, especially when bony landmarks are nonpalpable, there is limited back flexion, and there are false losses of resistance due to fat deposition. It is often difficult to predict the depth to the epidural space but there is a general correlation with BMI. Prepuncture ultrasonography may be useful to facilitate epidural placement in obese parturients to assist in predicting the depth to the epidural space.[93] However, ultrasound has limitations in this patient population. The image quality can be compromised due to fat overlying the epidural space and the distance to the epidural space may be inaccurate if the subcutaneous tissue is compressed. In some cases, a long 25-gauge needle can be used for infiltration of local anesthetic as well as to identify spinous processes. Questioning the patient is often helpful in determining whether needle placement is correctly midline or incorrectly lateral (e.g., "Does it feel like I'm in the middle of your back?"). A recent study demonstrated that obese women were less likely to identify the midline by pinprick compared to nonobese women. However, both groups of women were correct 99% of the time in identifying whether a stimulus (fingertip vs. pinprick) was to the right or left of the midline.[94] In most cases, standard neuraxial needles (9 to 10 cm) are usually of sufficient length if placement is midline. However, longer needles (16 cm) are sometimes needed in extremely obese parturients. These needles can cause serious injury by overpenetration, so they should only be used after careful assessment of the midline and once standard-length needles are determined to be inadequate.

Spinal anesthesia. Single-injection spinal anesthesia is a popular neuraxial anesthetic technique but there are concerns about technical difficulties, exaggerated spread of local anesthetic, hypotension, and an inability to prolong the block, especially in the obese patient. Spinal anesthesia is reasonable if the airway examination is normal, there is no cardiopulmonary disease, and the surgery is expected to be less than 90 minutes. It is often easier to insert the spinal needle when a large gauge stiff epidural needle is used as a guide for the smaller flexible spinal needle.

Decreased cerebral spinal fluid volumes have been confirmed in obese patients by magnetic resonance imaging,[95] suggesting that the effective dose of spinal local anesthetic is reduced in obese patients when they receive the same anesthetic as a nonobese patient. The decreased spinal fluid volume results from displacement of the cerebral spinal fluid by soft tissue movement into the intervertebral foramen caused by an increase in abdominal pressure. This results in a direct positive correlation between the height of the block and the degree of obesity when patients receive the same volume and dose of spinal bupivacaine in the sitting position. Higher levels of spinal anesthesia have been demonstrated in obese patients and smaller volumes of bupivacaine are needed in obese individuals to achieve similar sensory levels. When supine, the large buttocks of obese patients may elevate the caudal end of the vertebral column, effectively creating a Trendelenburg position and exaggerating the cephalad spread of spinal anesthesia. In order to avoid a high block when hyperbaric bupivacaine is used, a ramp can be placed under the patient's chest to elevate the cervical and thoracic spines to normalize this Trendelenburg effect. Although there are reports of no clinical differences in the height of sensory block after spinal anesthesia in obese compared to nonobese parturients, spinal anesthesia should be performed with caution because of the immediate consequences of extensive blockade and also the hazards of intraoperative induction of general anesthesia in the event of prolonged surgery.

Epidural anesthesia. Epidural anesthesia offers several advantages over single-injection spinal anesthesia including titratable dosing of local anesthetics, ability to prolong the block, decreased risk of excessive motor block, more controllable hemodynamic changes, and availability for postoperative analgesia. Incremental dosing of epidural-administered local anesthetics will reduce the risk of hypotension and high block. However, studies have demonstrated that epidural anesthesia fails more often than spinal or CSE techniques[96] in laboring patients, with increased maternal BMI contributing to the rate of failure of neuraxial techniques.

Catheter dislodgment is another potential problem in obese patients. Before securing the epidural catheter, a patient should move from an upright sitting position to a lateral position.[97] In this study by Hamilton et al., the changes in epidural catheter distance to skin with patient position modifications (sitting flexed to up, up to lateral, flexed to lateral) averaged a maximum of 0.67 to 1.04 cm (parturients with BMI <25 and >30, respectively). The changes in epidural catheter depth in this study were significantly increased with the BMI of patients, and the maximum observed changes in distance to skin were also significantly increased with the BMI (with >4-cm change in one obese patient).[97] Because the ligamentum flavum has a mild grip on the epidural catheter, repositioning allows the epidural catheter to be pulled into the subcutaneous fat, sometimes by several centimeters. After repositioning, the catheter is subsequently taped in place without adjusting the catheter. This maneuver is helpful in reducing the incidence of catheter dislodgement and block failure.

In cases of inadvertent dural puncture, a catheter may be threaded into the subarachnoid (intrathecal) space for continuous spinal analgesia, which offers benefits in reliability and density consistent with a single-injection spinal. Converting to a continuous spinal anesthetic does not appear to affect the subsequent rate of postdural puncture headache or the need for an epidural blood patch.[98] Each case must be handled individually. Intrathecal catheters must be carefully marked so that they are never mistaken for an epidural catheter. Accidental administration of an epidural dose of local anesthetic through a spinal catheter can produce the immediate and disastrous complications a high spinal such as respiratory compromise, loss of airway patency, and unconsciousness. Higher levels of spinal anesthesia may result from the reduced CSF volume in obese patients.[95]

CSE. CSE anesthesia is an alternative to either conventional spinal or epidural anesthesia alone. However, there is concern that CSE is technically more complicated and that the epidural catheter is "unproven" during the duration of spinal analgesia, creating the risk of a delayed conversion to general anesthesia if the epidural catheter is nonfunctional. However, a large retrospective study of 2,395 labor analgesia procedures revealed that the CSE technique did not delay recognition of epidural catheter failures.[99] Even if the patient does not receive a "spinal dose" during CSE placement, the return of CSF in the spinal needle is itself confirmation of correct midline needle placement. This additional information increases the likelihood that the epidural catheter placement will be satisfactory, producing a bilateral block, improved sacral spread, and onset of anesthesia/analgesia.

Peripheral Nerve Block

The use of peripheral nerve blocks with and without general anesthesia has been increasing for surgical procedures. Case reports have described the use of oblique subcostal TAP catheters as an alternative to epidural analgesia after upper abdominal surgery in obese patients.[100] The dosing of local anesthetics during regional anesthesia can be challenging in the obese. Too large of a dose may increase the risk of complications such as hypotension, systemic toxicity, or respiratory compromise related to diaphragmatic hemiparesis. However, if the dose is too small, there is a risk of block failure. The maximum safe dose of local anesthetic for a peripheral nerve block or local infiltration should be based on IBW rather than actual weight due to the risk of local anesthetic systemic toxicity.

Peripheral nerve blocks can be technically challenging in obese patients. Placement may be complicated by difficult positioning, obscure anatomic landmarks, and inadequate needle length. There may be an increased failure rate compared to techniques performed in patients of normal weight. Early studies determined that the risk of block failure increased with the patient's BMI, although it should be noted that these blocks were all performed using a nerve stimulator rather than with ultrasound guidance.[89] However, a later retrospective review of continuous peripheral nerve blocks performed with ultrasound guidance found no differences in catheter insertion time or success rates in patients with obesity compared with patients of normal weight.[101] Ultrasound guidance may be a helpful tool to increase block success as well as safety,[102] decrease procedure time,[103] and decrease the minimum effective dose of local anesthetic solutions.[104] A greater penetration depth of ultrasound is needed in the obese for visualization of the target nerve structures. Low-frequency transducers allow greater tissue penetration, but high-frequency transducers produce the best images.[105] Consequently, the quality of ultrasound images in the obese may be inferior to those obtained in nonobese patients. Successful use of ultrasound for peripheral nerve blocks requires training and experience. Several societies have recommended education and training guidelines for ultrasound-guided regional anesthesia.[106]

Postoperative Considerations

Ventilatory Evaluation and Management

There is an increased incidence of atelectasis in morbidly obese patients after general anesthesia, which persists into the postoperative period. Consequently, initiation of CPAP or bilevel positive airway pressure (BiPAP) has been advocated. The use of NIPPV does not seem to increase the incidence of major anastomotic leakage after gastric bypass surgery, despite a theoretical risk of gastric insufflation. Adequate analgesia, use of a properly fitted elastic binder for abdominal support, early ambulation, deep breathing exercises, and incentive spirometry are all useful adjuncts to avoid postoperative hypoventilation and atelectasis. Pulse oximetry and arterial blood gases should be monitored when they are indicated. Postoperative CPAP may improve oxygenation but does not facilitate CO_2 elimination.

Table 45-4 Summary of Practice Guidelines for the Perioperative Management of Patients with Obstructive Sleep Apnea: A Report by the American Society of Anesthesiologists Task Force on Perioperative Management of Patients with Obstructive Sleep Apnea[25]

- Regional anesthetic techniques should be considered to reduce or eliminate the requirements for systemic opioids in patients with OSA.
- If neuraxial anesthesia is planned, the benefits and risks of using an opioid or opioid-local anesthetic mixture as compared to local anesthetic alone must be considered.
- If patient-controlled systemic opioids are used, continuous background infusions should be avoided or used with extreme caution.
- Nonsteroidal anti-inflammatory agents and other modalities should be considered to reduce opioid requirements.
- Supplemental oxygen should be administered continuously to all patients who are at increased perioperative risk from OSA until they are able to maintain their baseline oxygen saturation while breathing room air.
- Hospitalized patients at increased risk of respiratory compromise from OSA should be monitored with continuous pulse oximetry after discharge from the recovery room.

OSA, obstructive sleep apnea.

Postoperative Analgesia

Pain management is an important part of the postoperative care plan of obese patients. The goal of pain management in these individuals is not only to provide adequate analgesia but also ensure early mobilization and adequate respiratory function. Mobilization in these individuals is often difficult but it is critically important for the prevention of complications. Pressure ulcerations, pulmonary emboli, deep venous thrombosis, and pneumonia are some of the common complications that can be prevented by early mobilization. Plans for pain management should include the following: (1) multimodal analgesics; (2) regional anesthesia/analgesia techniques; (3) early mobilization; (4) supplemental oxygen; and (5) elevation of the head of the bed. Besides delivery of a safe analgesic technique, adequate postoperative monitoring is required to ensure safety.

Obese patients with OSA have an increased likelihood of postoperative pulmonary complications.[20] All of these complications occur more commonly in patients with known OSA. Opioids are known to increase the risk of central apnea but patients with sleep
10 apnea are at particular risk for opioid-induced apnea.[23] Because of the risk of hypoventilation and hypoxemia in obese patients with and without sleep apnea, postoperative pain management should include opioid-sparing multimodal analgesic techniques to reduce the risk of respiratory depression. The American Society of Anesthesiologists practice guidelines encourages the use of regional analgesic techniques instead of systemic opioids in the postoperative pain management of patients with sleep apnea. Those guidelines are summarized in Table 45-4. Regional anesthetic techniques are known to reduce the risk of opioid-related complications.[107] However, these techniques will be contraindicated in some patients.

Monitoring

11 Obese patients who have received either neuraxial or parenteral opioids require careful postoperative monitoring. In most cases, routine admission to intensive care or high acuity care units is unnecessary since admission to these units has not been shown to reduce the risk of pulmonary complications or change perioperative outcome. Patients with a history of sleep apnea treated with noninvasive positive airway pressure should be encouraged to bring their own equipment to the hospital to reduce the risk of respiratory depression. All patients receiving neuraxial opioids should be monitored for adequacy of ventilation using common clinical signs such as respiratory rate, depth of respiration (assessed without disturbing a sleeping patient), oxygenation (e.g., pulse oximetry when appropriate), and level of consciousness.[108]

Ambulatory Anesthesia

Outpatient surgery can be considered under certain circumstances. Identifying obese patients who are suitable candidates for ambulatory surgery depends upon early identification of patient comorbidities, the invasiveness of the procedure, planned anesthetic technique (e.g., local or regional anesthesia with minimal sedation), postoperative pain management as well as the skill of the surgeon and anesthesiologist (Table 45-5).[48,109]

The American College of Surgeons National Surgical Quality Improvement Program (NSQIP) database identified risk factors for morbidity and mortality within 72 hours after ambulatory surgery.[110] Although the incidence of morbidity and mortality was only 0.1% in nearly 250,000 cases, independent risk factors for perioperative morbidity included high BMI, chronic obstructive pulmonary disease, hypertension, history of TIA/stroke, previous cardiac surgery, and longer surgical times. In the cohort, unplanned postoperative intubation, pneumonia, and wound disruption were the most commonly identified comorbidities. Others have determined that increased BMI, ASA ≥3, age >80 years, and length of surgery >1 hour, all increased the risk for unplanned hospital admission. Because increased BMI is a contributor for increased perioperative risk, exclusion criteria should be developed for patients undergoing ambulatory surgery. A systematic review determined that BMI alone did not increase the risk for perioperative complications or unexpected admission after ambulatory surgery, but the authors caution that most super-obese patients (i.e., BMI ≥50 kg/m^2) are not candidates for ambulatory surgery.[111]

Because many morbidly obese patients are diagnosed with sleep-disordered breathing, these patients may be considered for ambulatory procedures if their co-morbid conditions are optimized, and postoperative pain control is easily achieved with nonopioid techniques. The morbidly obese and those with OSA present unique and increasingly frequent challenges to ambulatory practices. The problem is further compounded in that many patients with OSA do not carry a formal diagnosis and many are obese. These patients are likely to cause major anesthetic problems throughout the perioperative period. Ambulatory surgical patients with propensity for OSA demonstrate an increased number of laryngoscopy attempts, difficult laryngoscopic grade views, and the use of fiber-optic intubation. These patients may also have respiratory insufficiency soon after extubation. Examination

Table 45-5 Factors to Consider When Scheduling Obese Patients for Ambulatory Surgery[48]

	Patient Factors	Anesthetic Factors	Surgical Factors
Appropriate for ambulatory surgery	• Usually BMI < 50 kg/m^2 • Good functional capacity • Comorbid conditions optimized (e.g., OSA treated with CPAP/NIV) • VTE prophylaxis	• Adequate preoperative preparation • Regional anesthesia? • Pain control is easily achieved with nonopioid techniques • Availability of a 23-h observation postanesthesia care unit • Experienced anesthesia team	• Noninvasive surgery • Adequate time scheduled for surgery and time for discharge • Adequate equipment
Inappropriate for ambulatory surgery	• Poor functional capacity • Metabolic syndrome • Inadequately treated HTN, cardiovascular disease • Symptomatic/untreated respiratory disease (untreated OSA, low O_2 saturation) • Previous VTE	High likelihood for admission due to inadequate pain control	Prolonged procedure

BMI, body mass index; CPAP, continuous positive airway pressure; OSA, obstructive sleep apnea; NIV, non-invasive ventilation; HTN, hypertension; VTE, venous thromboembolism.

Adapted from Wynn-Hebden A, Bouch DC. Anaesthesia for the obese patient. *BJA Educ*. 2020;20:388–395.

of large databases has demonstrated increased risk for emergency intubation, respiratory failure, mechanical ventilation, aspiration pneumonia, atrial fibrillation, and acute respiratory distress syndrome (ARDS).[112,113] These patients are more likely to suffer from respiratory arrest with preoperative sedation or postoperative analgesia because they are particularly sensitive to the respiratory depressant effects of even small dosages of sedatives or analgesics. Data suggest that patients who have a pre- or postoperative diagnosis of sleep apnea are twice as likely to have respiratory complications compared to controls. However, patients with a known preoperative diagnosis of OSA and established CPAP usage were less likely to experience cardiovascular complications compared with patients who were diagnosed postoperatively.[114] OSA patients who use a CPAP device at home should be instructed to bring it on the day of surgery as it may be needed in the immediate postoperative period, and should be used for several days afterward.[115] Some recommend that a postoperative observational unit with close monitoring of oxygen saturation or an intensive care unit setting should be used for monitoring OSA patients postoperatively.[116] The possibility of invasive monitoring, prolonged intubation, and postoperative mechanical ventilation should be discussed with obese patients.

Critical Care and Resuscitation

Caring for critically ill obese patients poses the same challenges as during surgery, in terms of equipment, monitoring, and multiple comorbidities.[76] In addition, the nutritional status of the critically ill obese patient is often paradoxical and difficult to address. Hyperglycemia from pre-existing diabetes or a stress-induced state is common and should be corrected because hyperglycemia is associated with a higher mortality rate. Obese patients are more likely to become ventilator dependent than nonobese patients. Although BMI has been associated with an increased risk of developing acute lung injury (ALI) and ARDS,[74,117] the effect on clinical outcomes is still being explored.[74] The relative contributions to the risk of obesity itself versus its commonly associated comorbidities (e.g., diabetes) are unclear. The search for the optimal ventilatory management in obese patients is increasingly using concepts of personalized respiratory system mechanics, esophageal manometry, or novel imaging techniques such as electrical impedance tomography (EIT).[118,119]

The possible need for cardiopulmonary resuscitation should be entertained when caring for the morbidly obese critically ill patient. There are both equipment and technical concerns. Chest compressions may not be effective and mechanical compression devices may be required. The maximum 400 J of energy on regular defibrillators is sufficient for morbidly obese patients because their chest wall is usually not much thicker, but the higher transthoracic impedance from the fat may require several attempts. Airway management by conventional means may be very difficult and direct visualization of anatomic landmarks can be extremely challenging should a "can't intubate, can't ventilate" situation occur and require emergency cricothyroidotomy. Tracheostomy, percutaneous cricothyrotomy, transtracheal jet ventilation, and retrograde wire intubation are time-consuming and technically difficult procedures in such emergency situations and should be reserved as final options and be performed by experienced practitioners.

Morbidity and Mortality

Pre-existing disease impacts the risk of perioperative adverse events, and patients with obesity and its associated comorbidities are at increased risk for morbidity and mortality postoperatively.[120] Because of the higher risk of postoperative complications than in nonobese patients, outpatient surgery in this population is controversial and should be individualized.[48]

The NSQIP database was queried from 2012 to 2016 to evaluate perioperative risk in obese patients undergoing nonbariatric surgery.[121] Over 1.3 million cases were analyzed to assess the impact of BMI on postoperative outcomes. The study reported an increasing risk of perioperative morbidity, infectious, and critical care complications with increasing BMI compared to normal BMI. Other common postoperative adverse events included respiratory complications (i.e., atelectasis, pneumonia), vascular complications (i.e., thrombophlebitis, deep venous thrombosis), and wound complications (i.e., infection, dehiscence).Obese patients present a higher risk of perioperative pulmonary complications including unplanned intubation or ventilation at >48 hours postoperatively,[121] especially if preoperative respiratory conditions (e.g., OSA) are present.[20,45] Sequential compression devices (SCDs), routine early ambulation, and careful perioperative anticoagulation decrease the risk of thromboembolism.[122] Some known contributing factors to the risk of infection are hyperglycemia or diabetes,[123] longer duration of surgical procedures,[123] hypoperfusion or low tissular oxygen tension,[124] and low tissular antibiotic concentration. Rhabdomyolysis is also more common in morbidly obese patients undergoing laparoscopic procedures when compared with the equivalent open approach, especially when the procedure is prolonged. An obese patient with previously diagnosed metabolic syndrome has a significantly greater risk of perioperative morbidity and mortality than an obese patient with no metabolic syndrome features.[125]

Finally, the NSQIP study reported relative odds of procedure-adjusted mortality of 2.31 and 2.63 in the super obesity (BMI 50.0 to 59.9 kg/m^2) and super–super obesity (BMI: ≥60.0 kg/m^2) groups, respectively.[121]

For further review and interactivities, please see the videos and narrative interactive clinical vignettes (NICVs) accessible in the complimentary eBook bundled with this text. Access instructions are located on the inside front cover.

REFERENCES

1. Obesity: preventing and managing the global epidemic. Report of a WHO consultation. *World Health Organ Tech Rep Ser*. 2000;894:i–xii, 1–253.
2. WHO. WHO Fact Sheet Obesity and Overweight. Accessed May 27, 2022. https://www.who.int/news-room/fact-sheets/detail/obesity-and-overweight
3. Hales CM, Carroll MD, Fryar CD, Ogden CL. Prevalence of obesity and severe obesity among adults: united states, 2017–2018. *NCHS Data Brief*. 2020;(360):1–8.
4. Ng M, Fleming T, Robinson M, et al. Global, regional, and national prevalence of overweight and obesity in children and adults during 1980–2013: a systematic analysis for the Global Burden of Disease Study 2013. *The Lancet*. 2014;384(9945):766–781. Doi:10.1016/s0140-6736(14)60460-8
5. Acute Respiratory Distress Syndrome Network; Brower RG, Matthay MA, Morris A, et al. Ventilation with lower tidal volumes as compared with traditional tidal volumes for acute lung injury and the acute respiratory distress syndrome. *N Engl J Med*. 2000;342(18):1301–8. doi: 10.1056/NEJM200005043421801.
6. Leykin Y, Miotto L, Pellis T. Pharmacokinetic considerations in the obese. *Best Pract Res Clin Anaesthesiol*. 2011;25(1):27–36.
7. Leitzmann MF, Moore SC, Koster A, et al. Waist circumference as compared with body-mass index in predicting mortality from specific causes. *PloS One*. 2011;6(4):e18582.
8. Lagerros YT, Rössner S. Obesity management: what brings success? *Therap Adv Gastroenterol*. 2013;6:77–88.
9. Hemmingsson E, Johansson K, Eriksson J, Sundström J, Neovius M, Marcus C. Weight loss and dropout during a commercial weight-loss program including a very-low-calorie diet, a low-calorie diet, or restricted normal food: observational cohort study. *Am J Clin Nutr*. 2012;96(5):953–961.
10. Apovian CM, Aronne LJ, Bessesen DH, et al; Endocrine Society. Pharmacological management of obesity: an Endocrine Society clinical practice guideline. *J Clin Endocrinol Metab*. 2015;100(2):342–362
11. Aronne LJ, Wadden TA, Peterson C, Winslow D, Odeh S, Gadde KM. Evaluation of phentermine and topiramate versus phentermine/topiramate extended-release in obese adults. *Obesity (Silver Spring)*. 2013;21(11):2163–2171.
12. Carroll FI, Blough BE, Mascarella SW, Navarro HA, Lukas RJ, Damaj MI. Bupropion and bupropion analogs as treatments for CNS disorders. *Adv Pharmacol*. 2014;69:177–216.
13. Wadden TA, Hollander P, Klein S, et al; NN8022-1923 Investigators. Weight maintenance and additional weight loss with liraglutide after low-calorie-diet-induced weight loss: the SCALE Maintenance randomized study. *Int J Obes (Lond)*. 2013;37(11):1443–1451.
14. Yun JW. Possible anti-obesity therapeutics from nature–a review. *Phytochemistry*. 2010;71(14–15):1625–1641.
15. Abe A, Kaye AD, Gritsenko K, Urman RD, Kaye AM. Perioperative analgesia and the effects of dietary supplements. *Best Pract Res Clin Anaesthesiol*. 2014;28(2):183–189.
16. Arterburn D, Powers JD, Toh S, et al. Comparative effectiveness of laparoscopic adjustable gastric banding vs laparoscopic gastric bypass. *JAMA Surg*. 2014;149(12):1279–1287.
17. Sinha AC, Singh PM, Bhat S. Are we operating too late? Mortality analysis and stochastic simulation of costs associated with bariatric surgery: reconsidering the BMI Threshold. *Obes Surg*. 2015.
18. Yao, G., Kang, L., Li, J. et al. Effective weight control via an implanted self-powered vagus nerve stimulation device. *Nat Commun*. 2018;9:5349. https://doi.org/10.1038/s41467-018-07764-z
19. Steier J, Lunt A, Hart N, Polkey MI, Moxham J. Observational study of the effect of obesity on lung volumes. *Thorax*. 2014;69(8):752–759.
20. Memtsoudis SG, Besculides MC, Mazumdar M. A rude awakening–the perioperative sleep apnea epidemic. *N Engl J Med*. 2013;368(25):2352–2353.
21. Abrishami A, Khajehdehi A, Chung F. A systematic review of screening questionnaires for obstructive sleep apnea. *Can J Anaesth*. 2010;57(5):423–438.
22. Yeh PS, Lee YC, Lee WJ, et al. Clinical predictors of obstructive sleep apnea in Asian bariatric patients. *Obes Surg*. 2010;20(1):30–35.
23. American Society of Anesthesiologists Task Force on Perioperative Management of patients with obstructive sleep apnea. Practice guidelines for the perioperative management of patients with obstructive sleep apnea: an updated report by the American Society of Anesthesiologists Task Force on Perioperative Management of patients with obstructive sleep apnea. *Anesthesiology*. 2014;120(2):268–286.
24. Chirinos JA, Gurubhagavatula I, Teff K, et al. CPAP, weight loss, or both for obstructive sleep apnea. *N Engl J Med*. 2014;370(24):2265–2275.
25. Apfelbaum JL, Hagberg CA, Connis RT, et al. 2022 American Society of Anesthesiologists Practice guidelines for management of the difficult airway. *Anesthesiology*. 2022;136(1):31–81.
26. Porhomayon J, Nader ND, Leissner KB, El-Solh AA. Respiratory perioperative management of patients with obstructive sleep apnea. *J Intensive Care Med*. 2014;29(3):145–153.
27. Marik PE, Desai H. Characteristics of patients with the "malignant obesity hypoventilation syndrome" admitted to an ICU. *J Intensive Care Med*. 2013;28(2):124–130.
28. Chau EH, Lam D, Wong J, Mokhlesi B, Chung F. Obesity hypoventilation syndrome: a review of epidemiology, pathophysiology, and perioperative considerations. Review. *Anesthesiology*. 2012;117(1):188–205.
29. Engeli S, Böhnke J, Gorzelniak K, et al. Weight loss and the renin-angiotensin-aldosterone system. *Hypertension*. 2005;45(3):356–362.
30. Finer N. Medical consequences of obesity. *Medicine*. 2011;39(1):18–23.
31. Birgel M, Gottschling-Zeller H, Röhrig K, Hauner H. Role of cytokines in the regulation of plasminogen activator inhibitor-1 expression and secretion in newly differentiated subcutaneous human adipocytes. *Arterioscler Thromb Vasc Biol*. 2000;20(6):1682–1687.
32. Nilsson M, Johnsen R, Ye W, Hveem K, Lagergren J. Obesity and estrogen as risk factors for gastroesophageal reflux symptoms. *JAMA*. 2003;290(1):66–72.
33. American Society of Anesthesiologists Committee. Practice guidelines for preoperative fasting and the use of pharmacologic agents to reduce the risk of pulmonary aspiration: application to healthy patients undergoing elective procedures: an updated report by the American Society of Anesthesiologists Committee on Standards and Practice Parameters. *Anesthesiology*. 2011;114(3):495–511.
34. Cheymol G. Effects of obesity on pharmacokinetics implications for drug therapy. *Clin Pharmacokinet*. 2000;39(3):215–231.
35. Suneja M, Kumar AB. Obesity and perioperative acute kidney injury: a focused review. *J Crit Care*. 2014;29(4):694.e1–696.e6.
36. Kastorini CM, Milionis HJ, Esposito K, Giugliano D, Goudevenos JA, Panagiotakos DB. The effect of Mediterranean diet on metabolic syndrome and its components: a meta-analysis of 50 studies and 534,906 individuals. *J Am Coll Cardiol*. 2011;57(11):1299–1313.
37. Tzimas P, Petrou A, Laou E, Milionis H, Mikhailidis DP, Papadopoulos G. Impact of metabolic syndrome in surgical patients: should we bother? *British journal of anaesthesia*. 2015;115(2):194–202.
38. Alberti KGMM, Eckel RH, Grundy SM, et al; International Diabetes Federation Task Force on Epidemiology and Prevention, National Heart, Lung, and Blood Institute, American Heart Association, World Heart Federation, International Atherosclerosis Society, International Association for the Study of Obesity. Harmonizing the metabolic syndrome: a joint interim statement of the International Diabetes Federation Task Force on Epidemiology and Prevention; National Heart, Lung, and Blood Institute; American Heart Association; World Heart Federation; International Atherosclerosis Society; and International Association for the Study of Obesity. *Circulation*. 2009;120(16):1640–1645.
39. Frezza EE, Wachtel M. Metabolic syndrome: a new multidisciplinary service line. *Obes Surg*. 2011;21(3):379–385.
40. Friesen JHP. Lean-scaled weight: a proposed weight scalar to calculate drug doses for obese patients. *Can J Anaesth*. 2013;60(2):214–215.
41. Hall JE. The kidney, hypertension, and obesity. *Hypertension*. 2003;41(3 Pt 2):625–633.
42. Monk TG, Rietbergen H, Woo T, Fennema H. Use of sugammadex in patients with obesity: a pooled analysis. *Am J Ther*. 2017; 24(5):e507–e516.
43. Ogunnaike BO, Jones SB, Jones DB, Provost D, Whitten CW. Anesthetic considerations for bariatric surgery. *Anesth Analg*. 2002;95(6):1793–1805.
44. Ferraz ÁAB, de Siqueira LT, Campos JM, de Araújo GC, Martins Filho ED, Ferraz EM. ANTIBIOTIC PROPHYLAXIS IN BARIATRIC SURGERY: a continuous infusion of cefazolin versus ampicillin/sulbactam and ertapenem. *Arq Gastroenterol*. 2015;52(2):83–87.

45. Schumann R. Anaesthesia for bariatric surgery. *Best Pract Res Clin Anaesthesiol*. 2011;25(1):83–93.
46. Bein B, Scholz J. Anaesthesia for adults undergoing non-bariatric surgery. *Best Pract Res Clin Anaesthesiol*. 2011;25(1):37–51.
47. Schug SA, Raymann A. Postoperative pain management of the obese patient. *Best Pract Res Clin Anaesthesiol*. 2011;25(1):73–81.
48. Wynn-Hebden A, Bouch DC. Anaesthesia for the obese patient. *BJA Educ*. 2020;20(11):388–395.
49. Heidegger T. Management of the difficult airway. *N Engl J Med*. 2021;384(19):1836–1847.
50. Joffe AM, Aziz MF, Posner KL, Duggan LV, Mincer SL, Domino KB. Management of difficult tracheal intubation: a closed claims analysis. *Anesthesiology*. 2019;131(4):818–829.
51. Cook TM, Woodall N, Frerk C; Fourth National Audit Project. Major complications of airway management in the UK: results of the Fourth National Audit Project of the Royal College of Anaesthetists and the Difficult Airway Society. Part 1: anaesthesia. *Br J Anaesth*. 2011;106(5):617–631.
52. Moon TS, Fox PE, Somasundaram A, et al. The influence of morbid obesity on difficult intubation and difficult mask ventilation. *J Anesth*. 2019;33(1):96–102.
53. Whelton PK, Carey RM, Aronow WS, et al. 2017 ACC/AHA/AAPA/ABC/ACPM/AGS/APhA/ASH/ASPC/NMA/PCNA guideline for the prevention, detection, evaluation, and management of high blood pressure in adults: a report of the American College of Cardiology/American Heart Association Task Force on Clinical Practice Guidelines. *Hypertension*. 2018;71(6):e13–e115.
54. Katkhouda N, Mason RJ, Wu B, Takla FS, Keenan RM, Zehetner J. Evaluation and treatment of patients with cardiac disease undergoing bariatric surgery. *Surg Obes Relat Dis*. 2012;8(5):634–640.
55. Stenberg E, Dos Reis Falcao LF, O'Kane M, et al. Correction to: guidelines for perioperative care in bariatric surgery: Enhanced Recovery After Surgery (ERAS) Society recommendations: a 2021 update. *World J Surg*. 2022;46(4):752.
56. Geerts WH, Bergqvist D, Pineo GF, et al. Prevention of venous thromboembolism: American College of Chest Physicians Evidence-Based Clinical Practice Guidelines (8th Edition). *Chest*. 2008;133(6 Suppl):381S–453S.
57. Magee CJ, Barry J, Javed S, Macadam R, Kerrigan D. Extended thromboprophylaxis reduces incidence of postoperative venous thromboembolism in laparoscopic bariatric surgery. *Surg Obes Relat Dis*. 2010;6(3):322–325.
58. Juhasz-Pocsine K, Rudnicki SA, Archer RL, Harik SI. Neurologic complications of gastric bypass surgery for morbid obesity. *Neurology*. 2007;68(21):1843–1850.
59. Leblanc ME, Auclair A, Leclerc J, et al. Blood pressure measurement in severely obese patients: validation of the forearm approach in different arm positions. *Am J Hypertens*. 2019;32(2):175–185.
60. Couture EJ, Provencher S, Somma J, Lellouche F, Marceau S, Bussières JS. Effect of position and positive pressure ventilation on functional residual capacity in morbidly obese patients: a randomized trial. *Can J Anaesth*. 2018;65(5):522–528.
61. Delay JM, Sebbane M, Jung B, et al. The effectiveness of noninvasive positive pressure ventilation to enhance preoxygenation in morbidly obese patients: a randomized controlled study. *Anesth Analg*. 2008;107(5):1707–1713.
62. Wong DT, Dallaire A, Singh KP, et al. High-flow nasal oxygen improves safe apnea time in morbidly obese patients undergoing general anesthesia: a randomized controlled trial. *Anesth Analg*. 2019;129(4):1130–1136.
63. Chang JE, Seol T, Hwang JY. Body position and the effectiveness of mask ventilation in anaesthetised paralysed obese patients: a randomised cross-over study. *Eur J Anaesthesiol*. 2021;38(8):825–830.
64. Fei M, Blair JL, Rice MJ, et al. Comparison of effectiveness of two commonly used two-handed mask ventilation techniques on unconscious apnoeic obese adults. *Br J Anaesth*. 2017;118(4):618–624.
65. Abdelmalak B, Makary L, Hoban J, Doyle DJ. Dexmedetomidine as sole sedative for awake intubation in management of the critical airway. *J Clin Anesth*. 2007;19(5):370–373.
66. Maassen R, Lee R, Hermans B, Marcus M, van Zundert A. A comparison of three videolaryngoscopes: the Macintosh laryngoscope blade reduces, but does not replace, routine stylet use for intubation in morbidly obese patients. *Anesth Analg*. 2009;109(5):1560–1565.
67. Maltby JR, Pytka S, Watson NC, Cowan RAM, Fick GH. Drinking 300 mL of clear fluid two hours before surgery has no effect on gastric fluid volume and pH in fasting and non-fasting obese patients. *Can J Anaesth*. 2004;51(2):111–115.
68. Lemmens HJM, Brodsky JB. The dose of succinylcholine in morbid obesity. *Anesth Analg*. 2006;102(2):438–442.
69. Feld JM, Hoffman WE, Stechert MM, Hoffman IW, Ananda RC. Fentanyl or dexmedetomidine combined with desflurane for bariatric surgery. *J Clin Anesth*. 2006;18(1):24–28.
70. Ricciardi R, Town RJ, Kellogg TA, Ikramuddin S, Baxter NN. Outcomes after open versus laparoscopic gastric bypass. *Surg Laparosc Endosc Percutan Tech*. 2006;16(5):317–320.
71. Matot I, Paskaleva R, Eid L, et al. Effect of the volume of fluids administered on intraoperative oliguria in laparoscopic bariatric surgery: a randomized controlled trial. *Arch Surg*. 2012;147(3):228-234.
72. Wool DB, Lemmens HJ, Brodsky JB, Solomon H, Chong KP, Morton JM. Intraoperative fluid replacement and postoperative creatine phosphokinase levels in laparoscopic bariatric patients. *Obes Surg*. 2010;20(6):698–701.
73. Bender SP, Paganelli WC, Gerety LP, et al. Intraoperative lung-protective ventilation trends and practice patterns: a report from the Multicenter Perioperative Outcomes Group. *Anesth Analg*. 2015;121(5):1231–1239.
74. Anzueto A, Frutos-Vivar F, Esteban A, et al; Ventila group. Influence of body mass index on outcome of the mechanically ventilated patients. *Thorax*. 2011;66(1):66–73.
75. Ball L, Hemmes SNT, Serpa Neto A, et al. Intraoperative ventilation settings and their associations with postoperative pulmonary complications in obese patients. *British journal of anaesthesia*. 2018;121(4):899–908.
76. Lewandowski K, Lewandowski M. Intensive care in the obese. *Best Pract Res Clin Anaesthesiol*. 2011;25(1):95–108.
77. Fernandez-Bustamante A, Hashimoto S, Serpa Neto A, Moine P, Vidal Melo MF, Repine JE. Perioperative lung protective ventilation in obese patients. *BMC Anesthesiol*. 2015;15:56.
78. Bohm SH, Thamm OC, von Sandersleben A, et al. Alveolar recruitment strategy and high positive end-expiratory pressure levels do not affect hemodynamics in morbidly obese intravascular volume-loaded patients. *Anesth Analg*. 2009;109(1):160–163.
79. Shah U, Wong J, Wong DT, Chung F. Preoxygenation and intraoperative ventilation strategies in obese patients: a comprehensive review. *Curr Opin Anaesthesiol*. 2015.
80. Aldenkortt M, Lysakowski C, Elia N, Brochard L, Tramèr MR. Ventilation strategies in obese patients undergoing surgery: a quantitative systematic review and meta-analysis. *Br J Anaesth*. 2012;109(4):493–502.
81. Prove Network Investigators for the Clinical Trial Network of the European Society of Anaesthesiology, Hemmes SN, Gama de Abreu M, Pelosi P, Schultz MJ. High versus low positive end-expiratory pressure during general anaesthesia for open abdominal surgery (PROVHILO trial): a multicentre randomised controlled trial. *Lancet*. 2014;384(9942):495–503.
82. Pelosi P, Gregoretti C. Perioperative management of obese patients. *Best Pract Res Clin Anaesthesiol*. 2010;24(2):211–225.
83. Costa Souza GM, Santos GM, Zimpel SA, Melnik T. Intraoperative ventilation strategies for obese patients undergoing bariatric surgery: systematic review and meta-analysis. *BMC Anesthesiol*. 2020;20(1):36.
84. Simon P, Girrbach F, Petroff D, et al; PROBESE Investigators of the Protective Ventilation Network and the Clinical Trial Network of the European Society of Anesthesiology. Individualized versus fixed positive end-expiratory pressure for intraoperative mechanical ventilation in obese patients: a secondary analysis. *Anesthesiology*. 2021;134(6):887–900.
85. Writing Committee for the PROBESE Collaborative Group of the PROtective VEntilation Network (PROVEnet) for the Clinical Trial Network of the European Society of Anaesthesiology; Bluth T, Serpa Neto A, Schultz MJ, et al. Effect of intraoperative high positive end-expiratory pressure (peep) with recruitment maneuvers vs low peep on postoperative pulmonary complications in obese patients: a randomized clinical trial. *JAMA*. 2019;321(23):2292–2305.
86. Rosenblatt MA, Reich DL, Roth R. Bariatric surgery and the prevention of postoperative respiratory complications. *Anesth Analg*. 2004;98(6):1810; author replies 1810–1811.
87. Metzner J, Posner KL, Lam MS, Domino KB. Closed claims' analysis. *Best Pract Res Clin Anaesthesiol*. 2011;25(2):263–276.
88. Budiansky AS, Margarson MP, Eipe N. Acute pain management in morbid obesity an evidence based clinical update. *Surg Obes Relat Dis*. 2017;13(3):523–532.
89. Nielsen KC, Guller U, Steele SM, Klein SM, Greengrass RA, Pietrobon R. Influence of obesity on surgical regional anesthesia in the ambulatory setting: an analysis of 9,038 blocks. *Anesthesiology*. 2005;102(1):181–187.
90. Damia G, Mascheroni D, Croci M, Tarenzi L. Perioperative changes in functional residual capacity in morbidly obese patients. *Br J Anaesth*. 1988;60(5):574–578.
91. Tsueda K, Debrand M, Zeok SS, Wright BD, Griffin WO. Obesity supine death syndrome: reports of two morbidly obese patients. *Anesth Analg*. 1979;58(4):345–347.
92. Chin KJ, Perlas A, Chan V, Brown-Shreves D, Koshkin A, Vaishnav V. Ultrasound imaging facilitates spinal anesthesia in adults with difficult surface anatomic landmarks. *Anesthesiology*. 2011;115(1):94–101.
93. Balki M, Lee Y, Halpern S, Carvalho JCA. Ultrasound imaging of the lumbar spine in the transverse plane: the correlation between estimated and actual depth to the epidural space in obese parturients. *Anesth Analg*. 2009;108(6):1876–1881.
94. Butcher M, George RT, Ip J, Campbell JP, Yentis SM. Identification of the midline by obese and non-obese women during late pregnancy. *Anaesthesia*. 2014;69(12):1351–1354.
95. Hogan QH, Prost R, Kulier A, Taylor ML, Liu S, Mark L. Magnetic resonance imaging of cerebrospinal fluid volume and the influence of body habitus and abdominal pressure. *Anesthesiology*. 1996;84(6):1341–1349.
96. Bloom SL, Spong CY, Weiner SJ, et al; National Institute of Child Health and Human Development Maternal-Fetal Medicine Units Network. Complications of anesthesia for cesarean delivery. *Obstet Gynecol*. 2005;106(2):281–287.
97. Hamilton CL, Riley ET, Cohen SE. Changes in the position of epidural catheters associated with patient movement. *Anesthesiology*. 1997;86(4):778–784; discussion 29A.
98. Russell IF. A prospective controlled study of continuous spinal analgesia versus repeat epidural analgesia after accidental dural puncture in labour. *Int J Obstet Anesth*. 2012;21(1):7–16.
99. Booth JM, Pan JC, Ross VH, Russell GB, Harris LC, Pan PH. Combined spinal epidural technique for labor analgesia does not delay recognition of epidural catheter failures: a single-center retrospective cohort survival analysis. *Anesthesiology*. 2016;125(3):516–524.

100. Niraj G, Kelkar A, Fox AJ. Oblique sub-costal transversus abdominis plane (TAP) catheters: an alternative to epidural analgesia after upper abdominal surgery. *Anaesthesia.* 2009;64(10):1137–1140.
101. Brodsky JB, Mariano ER. Regional anaesthesia in the obese patient: lost landmarks and evolving ultrasound guidance. *Best Pract Res Clin Anaesthesiol.* 2011;25(1):61–72.
102. Chantzi C, Saranteas T, Zogogiannis J, Alevizou N, Dimitriou V. Ultrasound examination of the sciatic nerve at the anterior thigh in obese patients. *Acta Anaesthesiol Scand.* 2007; 51(1):132.
103. Brull R, Lupu M, Perlas A, Chan VWs, McCartney CJL. Compared with dual nerve stimulation, ultrasound guidance shortens the time for infraclavicular block performance. *Can J Anaesth.* 2009;56(11):812–818.
104. Casati A, Baciarello M, Di Cianni S, et al. Effects of ultrasound guidance on the minimum effective anaesthetic volume required to block the femoral nerve. *Br J Anaesth.* 2007;98(6):823–827.
105. Sites BD, Brull R, Chan VW, et al. Artifacts and pitfall errors associated with ultrasound-guided regional anesthesia. Part II: a pictorial approach to understanding and avoidance. *Reg Anesth Pain Med.* 2007;32(5):419–433.
106. Narouze SN, Provenzano D, Peng P, et al; American Society of Regional Anesthesia and Pain Medicine, European Society of Regional Anaesthesia and Pain Therapy, Asian Australasian Federation of Pain Societies. The American Society of Regional Anesthesia and Pain Medicine, the European Society of Regional Anaesthesia and Pain Therapy, and the Asian Australasian Federation of Pain Societies Joint Committee recommendations for education and training in ultrasound-guided interventional pain procedures. *Reg Anesth Pain Med.* 2012;37(6):657–664.
107. von Ungern-Sternberg BS, Regli A, Reber A, Schneider MC. Effect of obesity and thoracic epidural analgesia on perioperative spirometry. *Br J Anaesth.* 2005;94(1):121–127.
108. American Society of Anesthesiologists Task Force on Neuraxial O; Horlocker TT, Burton AW, Connis RT, et al. Practice guidelines for the prevention, detection, and management of respiratory depression associated with neuraxial opioid administration. *Anesthesiology.* 2009;110(2):218–230.
109. Abdullah HR, Chung F. Perioperative management for the obese outpatient. *Current Opin Anaesthesiol.* 2014;27(6):576–582.
110. Mathis MR, Naughton NN, Shanks AM, et al. Patient selection for day case-eligible surgery: identifying those at high risk for major complications. Research Support, N.I.H., Extramural. *Anesthesiology.* 2013;119(6):1310–1321.
111. Joshi GP, Ahmad S, Riad W, Eckert S, Chung F. Selection of obese patients undergoing ambulatory surgery: a systematic review of the literature. *Anesth Analg.* 2013;117(5):1082–1091.
112. Memtsoudis S, Liu SS, Ma Y, et al. Perioperative pulmonary outcomes in patients with sleep apnea after noncardiac surgery. Comparative Study Research Support, N.I.H., Extramural Research Support, Non-U.S. Gov't Research Support, U.S. Gov't, P.H.S. *Anesth Analg.* 2011;112(1): 113–121.
113. Mokhlesi B, Hovda MD, Vekhter B, Arora VM, Chung F, Meltzer DO. Sleep-disordered breathing and postoperative outcomes after elective surgery: analysis of the nationwide inpatient sample. Comparative Study Research Support, N.I.H., Extramural Research Support, Non-U.S. Gov't. *Chest.* 2013;144(3):903–914.
114. Mutter TC, Chateau D, Moffatt M, Ramsey C, Roos LL, Kryger M. A matched cohort study of postoperative outcomes in obstructive sleep apnea: could preoperative diagnosis and treatment prevent complications? Research Support, N.I.H., Extramural Research Support, Non-U.S. Gov't. *Anesthesiology.* 2014;121(4):707–718.
115. Joshi GP, Ankichetty SP, Gan TJ, Chung F. Society for Ambulatory Anesthesia consensus statement on preoperative selection of adult patients with obstructive sleep apnea scheduled for ambulatory surgery. *Anesth Analg.* 2012;115(5):1060–1068.
116. Seet E, Chung F. Management of sleep apnea in adults – functional algorithms for the perioperative period: continuing professional development. *Can J Anaesth.* 2010;57(9):849–864.
117. Gong MN, Bajwa EK, Thompson BT, Christiani DC. Body mass index is associated with the development of acute respiratory distress syndrome. *Thorax.* 2010;65(1):44–50.
118. Kacmarek RM, Wanderley HV, Villar J, Berra L. Weaning patients with obesity from ventilatory support. *Curr Opin Crit Care.* 2021;27(3):311–319.
119. De Jong A, Wrigge H, Hedenstierna G, et al. How to ventilate obese patients in the ICU. *Intensive Care Med.* 2020;46(12):2423–2435. Doi:10.1007/s00134-020-06286-x
120. Bilimoria KY, Liu Y, Paruch JL, et al. Development and evaluation of the universal ACS NSQIP surgical risk calculator: a decision aid and informed consent tool for patients and surgeons. *J Am Coll Surg.* 2013;217(5):833 842 e1–e3.
121. Gupta M, Dugan A, Chacon E, et al. Detailed perioperative risk among patients with extreme obesity undergoing nonbariatric general surgery. *Surgery.* 2020;168(3):462–470.
122. Gonzalez QH, Tishler DS, Plata-Munoz JJ, et al. Incidence of clinically evident deep venous thrombosis after laparoscopic Roux-en-Y gastric bypass. *Surg Endosc.* 2004;18(7):1082–1084.
123. Cheadle WG. Risk factors for surgical site infection. *Surg Infect (Larchmt).* 2006;7(Suppl 1): S7–S11.
124. Kabon B, Rozum R, Marschalek C, et al. Supplemental postoperative oxygen and tissue oxygen tension in morbidly obese patients. *Obes Surg.* 2010;20(7):885–894.
125. Tung A. Anaesthetic considerations with the metabolic syndrome. *Br J Anaesth.* 2010; 105(Suppl 1):i24–i33.

46 The Liver: Surgery and Anesthesia

RANDOLPH H. STEADMAN • VICTOR W. XIA • MICHELLE Y. BRAUNFELD

KEY POINTS

1 The liver is the largest internal organ, accounting for 2% of the total body mass of adults. It receives 25% of the cardiac output via a dual afferent blood supply. The portal vein supplies 75% of the hepatic blood flow, the hepatic artery supplies the remaining 25%. Because of the higher oxygen content in the hepatic artery, each vessel provides roughly 50% of the hepatic oxygen supply.

2 The liver plays a preeminent role in the intermediary metabolism of nutrients (glucose, nitrogen, and lipids) and the detoxification of chemicals, including lipophilic medications. Liver dysfunction affects the metabolism of nutrients and xenobiotics, and negatively impacts nearly every other organ system.

3 Portal hypertension, the end result of hepatic injury and fibrotic changes, results in portosystemic shunts that bypass the liver's metabolic and detoxification capabilities. When nitrogenous waste and other substances normally cleared by the liver enter the central circulation, hepatic encephalopathy ensues.

4 Additional complications of portal hypertension include variceal hemorrhage, ascites, and hepatorenal syndrome. Cardiac sequelae include hyperdynamic circulation due to decreased systemic vascular resistance, which results in an increase in cardiac output.

5 Perioperative complications encountered by cirrhotic patients include liver failure, postoperative bleeding, infection, and renal failure. Patients with a model for end-stage liver disease (MELD) score of less than 11 have a low postoperative mortality and represent an acceptable surgical risk. End-stage liver disease patients with a risk of postoperative liver failure should have elective abdominal surgery at institutions with a liver transplant program. In patients with a MELD score of 20 or higher (or Child Class C), high mortality risk contraindicates elective procedures until after liver transplantation.

6 Medical management undertaken to optimize cirrhotic patients undergoing surgery should be directed toward treating active infection, minimizing vasoactive infusions, optimizing central blood volume and renal status, minimizing ascites, and improving encephalopathy and coagulopathy.

7 The perioperative risk of patients with end-stage liver disease depends more on the operative site and the degree of liver impairment than the anesthetic technique.

Hepatic Function in Health

The liver is the largest internal organ and is the body's metabolic headquarters. It weighs 1.5 kg or about 2% of the total body weight in an adult. The functional unit of the liver is the lobule, a structure roughly 1 mm × 2 mm that consists of plates of hepatocytes located in a radial distribution about a central vein. The afferent blood supply from the portal vein and hepatic arteriole enters at the periphery of the lobule. Bile, formed in the hepatocytes, flows into canaliculi located between the plates of hepatocytes and drains into bile ducts located at the periphery of the lobule next to portal venules and hepatic arterioles. The large pores in the endothelial lining, the sinusoids, allow plasma and its proteins to move readily into the tissue spaces surrounding hepatocytes, an area known as the spaces of Disse. This fluid drains into the lymphatic system. The liver generates about half of the body's lymph (Fig. 46-1).

The liver receives approximately 25% of the cardiac output via 1
a dual supply. The portal venules conduct blood from the portal vein, which drains the gastrointestinal tract. The portal vein supplies 75% of the liver inflow, or about 1 L/min. The hepatic arterioles supply the remaining 25% of the hepatic blood flow.

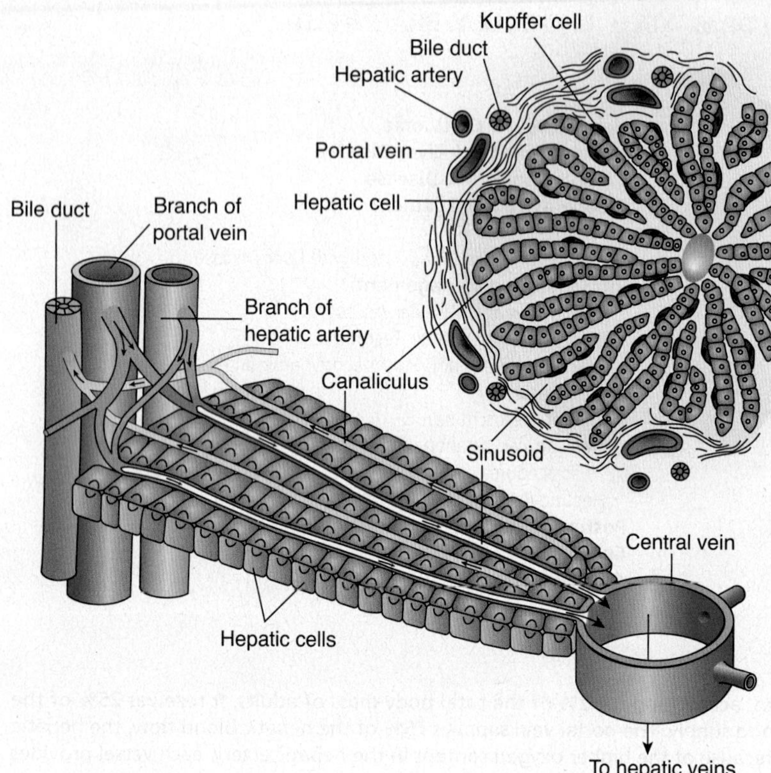

Figure 46-1 A magnified cross-section of a liver lobule **(right)** with its component cells and structures is juxtaposed to a 90-degree rotated view of a portion of this cross-section **(left)** showing the mixing of hepatic portal and arterial blood in the hepatic sinusoids. The sinusoids empty into the central vein, which sends blood to the hepatic vein and from there into the vena cava. (Adapted with permission from Porth CM. Disorders of hepatobiliary and exocrine pancreas function. *Essentials of Pathophysiology: Concepts of Altered Physical States*. 4th ed. Wolters Kluwer;2015:726.)

Due to the higher oxygen content of arterial blood, each vessel contributes about 50% of the hepatic oxygen supply.

The liver's high blood flow is due to low vascular resistance in the portal vein. The average portal vein pressure is 8 to 10 mmHg, which exceeds hepatic venous pressure by 4 to 5 mmHg. However, when injured hepatocytes are replaced by fibrous tissue, blood flow is impeded and portal venous pressure increases. A hepatic venous pressure gradient (HVPG) greater than 5 mmHg is abnormal and defines portal hypertension.[1] Sympathetic innervation from T3 to T11 controls resistance in the hepatic venules. Changes in compliance in the hepatic venous system contribute to the regulation of cardiac output and blood volume. In the presence of reduced portal venous flow, the hepatic artery can increase flow by as much as 100% to maintain hepatic oxygen delivery. The reciprocal relationship between flow in the two afferent vessels is termed the "hepatic arterial buffer response."[2]

The microcirculation of the liver lobule is divided into three zones that receive varying oxygen content.[3] Zone 1 receives oxygen-rich blood from the adjacent portal vein and hepatic artery. As blood moves through the sinusoid, it passes from the intermediate zone 2 into zone 3, which surrounds the central vein. Blood entering zone 3 is oxygen poor. Pericentral hepatocytes have a greater quantity of cytochrome P450 enzymes and are the site of anaerobic metabolism. Hypoxia and reactive metabolic intermediates from biotransformation affect zone 3 more prominently than other zones.

Due to its ability to distend, the liver is capable of storing up to 1 L of blood. The liver serves as a reservoir capable of accepting blood or releasing blood at times of low blood volume. The liver also stores vitamins, particularly vitamins B_{12} (1-year supply), D (3-month supply), and A (10-month supply). Excess body iron is transported via apoferritin to the liver for storage as ferritin, which is released when circulating iron levels are low. Thus, the liver apoferritin system serves as a blood iron buffer.

Reticuloendothelial cells called Kupffer cells line the venous sinusoids. These macrophages phagocytize bacteria that enter the sinusoids from the intestines. Less than 1% of bacteria that enter the liver pass through to the systemic circulation.

The liver is involved in energy production and storage of nutrients absorbed from the intestines. The liver aids in blood glucose regulation through its glucose buffer function. This is accomplished by storing glucose as glycogen, converting other carbohydrates (principally fructose and galactose) to glucose, and synthesizing glucose from amino acids and triglyceride (gluconeogenesis). In patients with altered liver function, blood glucose concentration can rise several fold higher than the postprandial levels found in patients with normal hepatic function. 2

The liver synthesizes fat, cholesterol, phospholipids, and lipoproteins. It also efficiently metabolizes fat, converting fatty acids to acetyl coenzyme A (CoA), an excellent source of energy, which can be diverted to the citric acid cycle to liberate energy for the liver. The liver generates more acetyl-CoA than it consumes. The excess is packaged as acetoacetic acid for use elsewhere in the body. The majority of cholesterol synthesized in the liver is converted to bile salts and secreted in the bile. The remainder is distributed to the rest of the body where it is used to form cellular membranes and other vital structures. Fat synthesis from protein and carbohydrates occurs almost exclusively in the liver, and the liver is responsible for most fat metabolism.

The liver also plays a key role in protein metabolism. The liver synthesizes all of the plasma proteins with the exception of γ-globulins, which are formed in plasma cells. The liver is capable of forming 15 to 50 g of protein per day, an amount sufficient to replace the body's entire supply of protein in several weeks. Albumin is the major protein synthesized by the liver and is the primary determinant of plasma oncotic pressure. The liver also synthesizes the nonessential amino acids from keto acids, which are also synthesized in the liver.

The liver is capable of deamination of amino acids, which is required for energy production or the conversion of amino acids to carbohydrates or fats. Deamination produces ammonia, which is toxic. Intestinal bacteria are an additional source of ammonia. The liver removes ammonia through the formation of urea.

All of the blood clotting factors, with the exception of factors III (tissue thromboplastin), IV (calcium), and VIII (von Willebrand factor), are synthesized in the liver. Vitamin K is required for the synthesis of prothrombin (factor II) and factors VII, IX, and X.

Hepatocytes produce roughly 500 mL of bile daily. Between meals, the high pressure in the sphincter of Oddi diverts bile to the gallbladder for storage. The gallbladder holds 35 to 50 mL of bile in concentrated form. The presence of fat in the duodenum causes release of the hormone cholecystokinin from duodenal mucosa, which reaches the gallbladder via circulation and stimulates gallbladder contraction. Bile contains bile salts, bilirubin, and cholesterol. Bile salts act as a detergent, solubilizing fat into micelles, which are absorbed. Bile salts return to the liver via the portal vein, completing the enterohepatic circulation. Bile salts are needed for fat absorption, and cholestasis can result in steatorrhea and vitamin K deficiency.

The liver has the unique ability to restore itself after injury or partial hepatectomy. As much as two-thirds of the liver can be removed with regeneration of the remaining liver in a matter of weeks.[4] Hepatocyte growth factor, produced by mesenchymal cells in the liver, and other growth factors, such as epidermal growth factor (EGF), cytokines, tumor necrosis factor (TNF), and interleukin-6, are involved in stimulating regeneration. Growth factor-β, a known inhibitor of hepatocyte proliferation, is involved in halting the regenerative process, which appears to be related to the ratio of liver-to-body weight.[5] Inflammation, such as with a viral infection of the liver, impairs regeneration.

Assessment of Hepatic Function

A number of laboratory tests are available to assess the liver. Collectively termed *liver function tests* (LFTs), many, including aspartate aminotransferase (AST) and alanine aminotransferase (ALT), do not evaluate function but rather are markers of cellular injury. Increased serum levels of these enzymes, AST (formerly serum glutamic oxaloacetic transaminase; SGOT) and ALT (formerly serum glutamic pyruvic transaminase; SGPT), occur in many types of hepatic disease. Because AST is also found in nonhepatic tissues (including the heart, skeletal muscle, kidney, and brain), elevations are not specific for hepatic disease. In contrast, ALT is primarily localized to the liver.

Fatty liver and chronic infections are associated with mild (several fold) elevations of AST and ALT. Acute hepatitis produces larger increases, but the highest concentrations, which can exceed 50 times normal, are seen with acute hepatic necrosis. Absolute levels of these enzymes are not always helpful, as declining values may indicate either recovery or a lack of surviving hepatocytes. The AST/ALT ratio may be helpful in differentiating alcoholic liver disease, in which the ratio is typically greater than 2, from viral hepatitis, which is associated with a ratio lower than 1.

Indices of bile flow obstruction include serum levels of alkaline phosphatase (AP), 5′-nucleotidase (5′-NT), γ-glutamyl transferase (GGT), and bilirubin. AP isoenzymes are found in multiple organs including the liver, bone, kidney, intestines, placenta, and leukocytes. Normally, most circulating AP originates from liver and bone. Hepatic AP is concentrated in the microvilli of bile canaliculi and the sinusoidal surface of hepatocytes. Elevations of serum AP disproportionate to changes in AST and ALT occur with obstructions to bile flow. However, AP elevations may originate from other tissues, including the placenta during pregnancy. Although 5′-NT is also found in many tissues, elevations are highly specific for hepatobiliary obstruction. Elevations of 5′-NT may reflect the detergent action of bile salts on plasma membranes, a requirement for its release. Because 5′-NT is specific for liver diseases, measurement of 5′-NT is useful to determine whether elevated AP is of hepatic origin. Serum GGT is the most sensitive laboratory indicator of biliary tract disease but it is less specific than 5′-NT and has largely been replaced by 5′-NT.

Bilirubin originates primarily from the breakdown of hemoglobin released from senescent red blood cells. Serum bilirubin levels are determined by the van den Bergh reaction, which separates bilirubin into two fractions: A lipid-soluble, indirect-reacting form (unconjugated bilirubin) and a water-soluble, direct-reacting form (conjugated bilirubin). Elevated levels of unconjugated bilirubin indicate an excess production of bilirubin (hemolysis) or a decrease in the uptake and conjugation of bilirubin by hepatocytes. Conjugated bilirubin is elevated by impaired intrahepatic excretion or extrahepatic obstruction. Even with complete biliary tract obstruction, the bilirubin rarely exceeds 35 mg/dL because of renal excretion of conjugated bilirubin.

Tests of hepatic synthetic function focus on the measurement of serum albumin and coagulation testing. Although the liver is the primary site of albumin synthesis, excessive protein losses (enteropathy, burns, nephrotic syndrome) can also result in low albumin levels. Because of its 3-week half-life, serum albumin is not a reliable indicator of acute liver disease. In contrast, the prothrombin time (PT) and international normalized ratio (INR) are sensitive indicators of hepatic disease because of the short half-life of factor VII. The PT depends upon sufficient intake of vitamin K, which in turn depends upon adequate biliary secretion of bile salts. In patients with biliary obstruction, the PT can be prolonged despite preserved hepatic function. Other conditions that can affect the PT in the absence of liver disease include congenital coagulation factor deficiencies, consumptive coagulopathies such as disseminated intravascular coagulation (DIC), and warfarin therapy. Factor Xa inhibitors, including rivaroxaban and apixaban, also prolong PT, but PT and INR are not reliable tests for monitoring these agents.[6]

A number of other tests exist to assess hepatic function, though their use in the United States is limited primarily to research applications. Indocyanine green (ICG) elimination estimates hepatic blood flow and hepatocellular function due to the high extraction ratio of ICG (>70%). The MEGX test measures the conversion of lidocaine to monoethylglycinexylidide (MEGX) via hepatic demethylation.

Ancillary tests to confirm specific diagnoses include serologic tests for the various hepatitis viruses, autoantibodies (for the diagnosis of primary biliary cirrhosis [PBC]), ceruloplasmin (Wilson disease), ferritin (hemochromatosis), α_1-antitrypsin (α_1-antitrypsin deficiency), and α-fetoprotein (hepatocellular carcinoma [HCC]). Serum ammonia is useful for following patients with hepatic encephalopathy (HE).

Hepatobiliary Imaging

Selection of the appropriate imaging technique depends on the differential diagnosis and whether a concurrent therapeutic intervention is planned. Plain radiography has a limited role in the evaluation of liver disease. Abdominal X-rays can be useful to detect calcified or gas-containing lesions. Examples include calcified gallstones, chronic calcific pancreatitis, gas-containing liver abscesses, portal venous gas, and emphysematous cholecystitis.

Ultrasonography is the primary screening test for hepatic parenchymal disease and extrahepatic biliary disease. It is the method of choice for detecting gallstones, the presence of ascites, and portal or hepatic vein thrombosis. Its major limitations are its dependence on the operator's skill and its inability to penetrate bone or air, including bowel gas.

Radioisotope scanning has largely been replaced by computed tomography (CT) scanning. However, it is still used in patients with suspected acute cholecystitis. Radioisotopes visualized in the gallbladder rule out obstruction of the cystic duct, whereas visualization of the biliary tree and common bile duct without the gallbladder indicates cystic duct obstruction and the presence of cholecystitis.

CT scanning supplements ultrasonography, providing information on the liver texture, gallbladder disease, bile duct dilatation, and mass lesions of the liver and pancreas. CT provides more resolution than ultrasonography and is less operator dependent. Lesions can be biopsied under CT guidance. The disadvantages of CT include radiation exposure and cost.

Magnetic resonance imaging (MRI) is increasingly being used for the evaluation of hepatobiliary disease. MRI is superior to CT for the assessment of malignant focal liver lesions and diffuse liver disease.[7] MRI is also useful for the evaluation of biliary disease. MRI offers the advantages of avoiding radiation exposure and the risk of contrast-induced nephropathy. The primary disadvantage is the need for breath-hold sequences, which can require sedation or anesthesia in young and/or uncooperative patients.

Percutaneous transhepatic cholangiography (THC) is the percutaneous injection of contrast into the bile ducts under fluoroscopic guidance. It can be used to determine the site and cause of biliary obstruction and to evaluate whether cholangiocarcinoma is surgically resectable. It can also be used for balloon dilatation of biliary strictures and/or placement of an internal stent or external drain. Endoscopic retrograde cholangiopancreatography (ERCP) uses endoscopy to visualize the ampulla of Vater and selectively inject contrast material into the pancreatic and common bile ducts. ERCP has the advantage over THC of not requiring a dilated biliary tree to achieve a high probability of success. ERCP permits sphincterotomy and stone extraction, biopsy, brushings, balloon dilatation, and stent insertion.

Liver Biopsy

Liver biopsy continues to have a role in the evaluation of patients with liver disease. It is the method of choice to determine whether liver damage is due to necrosis, inflammation, steatosis, or fibrosis. The presence of coagulopathy or thrombocytopenia may contraindicate percutaneous liver biopsy, although transjugular liver biopsy is often performed under these conditions.

Hepatic and Hepatobiliary Diseases

Liver disease may be the result of a variety of causes, which include developmental or genetic defects, metabolic abnormalities, autoimmune diseases, infectious diseases, neoplasm, alcohol, environmental toxins, and drug toxicity. A report from the National Vital Statistics System for the year 2017 lists liver disease as the 11th leading cause of death in the United States, responsible for almost 42,000 deaths in that year.[8] A recent publication exploring the epidemiology of chronic liver disease (CLD) suggests the prevalence of liver disease is almost 36%, and largely attributable to the ubiquity of nonalcoholic fatty liver disease (NAFLD).[9] The rise in prevalence of NAFLD has paralleled the increases in known risk factors for obesity and type 2 diabetes, suggesting that it will only continue to increase.

Liver disease can be divided into two main groups on the basis of the primary anatomy affected. Processes may be considered primarily hepatocellular (parenchymal) or biliary. Progressive biliary disease may eventually lead to fibrotic changes and cirrhosis, but it is characteristic of the biliary diseases that cholestasis precedes hepatocellular dysfunction. In hepatocellular diseases, evidence of cholestasis and synthetic dysfunction appear synchronously (Table 46-1). The fact that hepatocellular function is

Table 46-1 Blood Tests and the Differential Diagnosis of Hepatic Dysfunction

	Bilirubin Overload (Hemolysis)	Parenchymal Dysfunction	Cholestasis
Aminotransferases	Normal	Increased (may be normal or decreased in advanced stages)	Normal (may be increased in advanced stages)
Alkaline phosphatase	Normal	Normal	Increased
Bilirubin	Increased	Increased	Increased
	Unconjugated	Conjugated	Conjugated
Serum proteins	Normal	Decreased	Normal (may be decreased in advanced stages)
Prothrombin time	Normal	Decreased (may be normal in early stages)	Normal (may be prolonged in advanced stages)
Blood urea nitrogen	Normal	Normal (may be decreased in advanced stages)	Normal
Sulfobromophthalein/indocyanine green	Normal	Retention	Normal or retention

From Gelman S. Anesthesia and the liver. In: Barash P, Cullen B, Stoelting R, eds. *Clinical Anesthesia*. 3rd ed. Lippincott-Raven;1997:1011.

preserved until late in the course of cholestatic disease is a disadvantage for patients with cholestatic liver disease awaiting liver transplantation.

Liver disease may also be described as acute or chronic. The most common causes for acute liver disease are drug toxicity and infection. Acute illnesses may resolve spontaneously, segue into chronic disease, or result in acute liver failure (ALF). Although the primary cause of ALF in the United States was once infectious (presumed acute hepatitis A and B), drug toxicity—particularly acetaminophen toxicity—is currently the leading cause of this condition in the Western world. Other causes of acute liver dysfunction include infection, alcoholic hepatitis, nonacetaminophen drug toxicity, and pregnancy-related hepatic diseases. The most common causes for CLD are chronic viral hepatitis, alcoholic liver disease, and NAFLD. Although the prevalence rates of chronic viral hepatitis and alcoholic liver disease have been relatively stable or decreasing over the past 10 years, the prevalence of NAFLD has grown significantly and appears to be linked to the current epidemic of obesity and type 2 diabetes.[9] The most important consequences of CLD are portal hypertension, cirrhosis, and malignancy.

Acute Liver Failure

ALF (previously termed fulminant hepatic failure) is defined as the appearance of encephalopathy together with coagulopathy, usually an INR 1.5 or more, in a patient who has no previous history of liver disease and who has had an illness of shorter than 26 weeks' duration. Although further distinctions in duration of disease, such as hyperacute and subacute, were once used, they are no longer considered useful for prognosis and have been abandoned. ALF is a rare entity with an incidence of about 2,000 cases per year in the United States. Drug-related toxicity accounts for over half of the cases of ALF in the United States. Of these drug-related cases, over 80% are the result of acetaminophen ingestion. In descending order, the next most common causes are idiopathic, acute viral hepatitis, autoimmune, and ischemic.[10] The natural history of adult ALF in the United States is one of spontaneous recovery in approximately 45% of patients, liver transplantation in 25%, and death without transplantation in 30%.[10] Etiology has a significant bearing on outcome, with the more favorable prognosis for patients with acetaminophen overdose, ischemic injury, and hepatitis A and poorer prognosis for those with nonacetaminophen drug-induced liver injury (DILI), acute hepatitis B, Wilson disease, and autoimmune hepatitis.[11]

Patients with no previous history of liver disease who present with signs or symptoms and laboratory evidence of significant hepatitis should have an INR measured and undergo a careful mental status examination. An INR of 1.5 or more and any evidence of encephalopathy should lead to admission to the hospital for ALF. History should include questions about potential infectious or toxic exposures and a detailed review of recent medications or ingestions. Questions should include details about herbal and nutritional supplements because these have been associated with ALF as well. Except for the finding of encephalopathy, physical examination may be unrevealing. In particular, evidence of CLD should not be present, as the patient should not have had adequate time to develop the stigmata of portal hypertension and cirrhosis. Acute decompensation of CLD or "acute on chronic" liver disease is a separate condition with different etiologies, therapy, and prognostic indicators.

Standard initial laboratory tests are indicated in Table 46-2.[11] Further laboratory and investigative studies are directed by the history, for example, radiologic imaging or ultrasound for suspected hepatic vein thrombosis. Although etiologies of ALF are heterogeneous, there are manifestations that are common to all

Table 46-2 Initial Laboratory Analysis of Suspected Acute Liver Failure

Prothrombin time/INR
Chemistries
Sodium, potassium, chloride, bicarbonate, calcium, magnesium, phosphate glucose
AST, ALT, alkaline phosphatase, GGT, total bilirubin, albumin creatinine, blood urea nitrogen
Arterial blood gas
Arterial lactate
Complete blood count
Blood type and screen
Acetaminophen level
Toxicology screen
Viral hepatitis serologies
Anti-HAV IgM, HBSAg, anti-HBc IgM, anti-HEV,[a] anti-HCV[b]
Ceruloplasmin level[c]
Pregnancy test (females)
Ammonia (arterial if possible)
Autoimmune markers
ANA, ASMA, immunoglobulin levels
HIV status[d] Amylase and lipase

[a]If clinically indicated.
[b]Done to recognize potential underlying infection.
[c]Done only if Wilson disease is a consideration (e.g., in patients less than 40 y without another obvious explanation for acute liver failure); in this case uric acid level and bilirubin to alkaline phosphatase ratio may be helpful as well.
[d]Implications for potential liver transplantation.
INR, international normalized ratio; AST, aspartate aminotransferase; ALT, alanine aminotransferase; GGT, gamma-glutamyl transferase; HAV, hepatitis A virus; IgM, immunoglobulin M; HBSAg, hepatitis B surface antigen; HEV, hepatitis E virus; HCV, hepatitis C virus; ANA, antinuclear antibody; ASMA, antismooth muscle antibody.
Adapted with permission from Polson J, Lee WM. AASLD position paper: the management of acute liver failure. *Hepatology*. 2005;41:1179.

patients who have massive hepatic necrosis. The most serious, and often the proximate cause of death, is acute cerebral edema and intracranial hypertension. Effects on other organ systems include coagulopathy, circulatory dysfunction and hypotension, acute kidney injury, and metabolic derangements. Encephalopathy is a necessary finding to diagnose ALF. Encephalopathy is graded on a I to IV scale and is described in Table 46-3. The presence of cerebral edema is directly related to the depth of encephalopathy. The incidence of cerebral edema is almost negligible in stage I to stage II coma but increases to 25% to 35% with stage III and 75% with stage IV. As with the encephalopathy of cirrhosis, the underlying mechanism is not completely understood but hyperammonemia plays a significant role. Ammonia, which is toxic, is generally metabolized via the urea cycle in the liver. The brain has no cells capable of utilizing the urea cycle and thus must resort

Table 46-3 Grades of Encephalopathy

I. Changes in behavior with minimal change in level of consciousness
II. Gross disorientation, drowsiness, possibly asterixis, inappropriate behavior
III. Marked confusion, incoherent speech, sleeping most of the time but arousable to vocal stimuli
IV. Comatose, unresponsive to pain, decorticate, or decerebrate posturing

Note: Some patients will overlap grades; clinical judgment is required.
Adapted from Conn HO, Leevy CM, Vhlahcevic ZR, et al. Comparison of lactulose and neomycin in the treatment of chronic portal-systemic encephalopathy: a double blind controlled trial. *Gastroenterology*. 1977;72:573.

Table 46-4 ICP Management Protocol

Initiate in rapid stepwise fashion for ICP >20 mmHg for >5 min
Keep CPP >60 mmHg with norepinephrine or phenylephrine infusion
Mannitol 1 g/kg IV bolus, may repeat if serum osmolarity <320 mOsm/kg
Hyperventilation to target PCO_2 30–35 mmHg
Hypothermia using cooling blanket to core temperature of 33°–34°C
Initiate neuromuscular blockade if needed with cisatracurium 0.2 mg/kg IV bolus, 3 μg/kg/min infusion—adjust to 2/4 on train of four
Pentobarbital 5 mg/kg bolus, repeated 3–5 mg/kg boluses as necessary—titrate to ICP effect
3% saline: Calculate dose to achieve serum sodium in 145–155 mEq/L range

ICP, intracranial pressure; CPP, cerebral perfusion pressure; IV, intravenous.
Adapted with permission from Raschke RA, Curry SC, Rempe S, et al. Results of a protocol for the management of patients with fulminant liver failure. *Crit Care Med*. 2008;36:2244.

to detoxifying ammonia by synthesizing glutamine from ammonia and glutamate within astrocytes. Glutamine is osmotically active and results in osmotic astrocyte edema. Other contributors to the observed cerebral edema may include a systemic inflammatory response and the loss of cerebral autoregulation, which leads to cerebral hyperemia. Potential targets for therapy include osmotic and mechanical reduction of cerebral edema, elimination of ammonia, manipulation of cerebral blood flow and metabolism, and reduction of the inflammatory response.

General measures to reduce cerebral edema include maintaining the patient in a 30-degree head-up position and making sure the head is in neutral position so as not to impede venous return. Once a patient is intubated, muscle relaxants should be considered to minimize rises in intracranial pressure (ICP) from coughing, bucking, and shivering. Mannitol can be used to induce an osmotic diuresis but may have limited utility in the patient with compromised renal function. Another option may be hypertonic saline, ideally targeting a serum sodium of 145 to 155 mEq/L.[12]

Although hyperventilation may acutely reduce the cerebral hyperemia associated with ALF, the response is short lived. There is no evidence that chronic hyperventilation affords any decrease in episodes of intracranial hypertension or any survival benefit. Current recommendations are to maintain normocarbia and to reserve hyperventilation for response to acute rises in ICP. Barbiturates can be used to decrease cerebral metabolism; however, their use may be limited by hypotension.

Although there are no absolute associations between a specific ammonia level and the presence of cerebral edema, it has been observed that cerebral edema is uncommon when ammonia levels are <75 μM, but is likely at >200 μM.[11] Ammonia can be eliminated by the administration of lactulose or nonabsorbable antibiotics such as rifaximin or neomycin; however, there is no evidence to support their use in the setting of ALF. Furthermore, neomycin is specifically contraindicated because of the risk of nephrotoxicity. Renal replacement therapy has been successfully used to reduce ammonia levels and is associated with reduced mortality. For this reason, it is considered a therapeutic cornerstone in some institutions.[13]

Corticosteroids have not been shown to be effective in ALF, but there may be a place for prophylactic antibiotics to prevent sepsis and minimize the inflammatory mediator burden in specific clinical settings.

The optimal method by which to monitor the presence and progression of cerebral edema and intracranial hypertension is controversial. Serial head CTs are often obtained for patients who progress to stage III or stage IV coma, but they are not reliable for diagnosing or quantitating intracranial hypertension. CT can, however, provide information on structural abnormalities such as intracranial hemorrhage. Although many centers will place an ICP monitor to guide therapy in patients with stage III to stage IV coma, there are no randomized controlled studies to support this practice. Furthermore, placement of an ICP is not a benign procedure, frequently entailing aggressive correction of coagulopathy and multiple trips to the operating room. Nonetheless, many believe that ICP monitors are invaluable for guiding acute therapy and for helping to determine who may no longer be a viable candidate for transplantation. In addition to measuring ICP, these monitors allow calculation of cerebral perfusion pressure (CPP = MAP − ICP), which should be kept between 60 and 80 mmHg. An effective protocol for managing intracranial hypertension in patients with stage III or stage IV encephalopathy has been described (Table 46-4) and resulted in a 95% response to treatment of episodes of ICP greater than 20 mmHg. Furthermore, in this prospective series, ICP was monitored in all patients, and no patients died of isolated cerebral edema. The authors used a protocol that included activated recombinant factor VII (rFVIIa) to correct coagulopathy prior to ICP placement. Significant bleeding complications from ICP monitoring were not encountered.[14]

Predicting outcomes in patients with liver disease is difficult. The two most widely used prognostic models are the Clichy or Paul Brousse Hospital criteria and the King's College Hospital criteria. The Clichy criteria recommend transplantation for patients in stage III or stage IV coma on the basis of age and factor V levels. The transplantation threshold is 20% factor V activity for patients under 30 years or 30% factor V activity for patients above 30 years.[15] There is no distinction made for the etiology of ALF, which is felt to be a weakness of these criteria. The King's College Hospital (Table 46-5) criteria account for the improved spontaneous outcomes of patients who have ALF on the basis of acetaminophen toxicity.[16] Although the positive predictive value of the King's College Hospital criteria has been shown to be clinically acceptable in ALF patients, the negative predictive value drops below 50% in patients with nonacetaminophen-related ALF.[17] Thus, patients who fail to fulfill these criteria include a number of patients who will die without being properly considered for transplantation. Modifications to the King's College Hospital criteria to improve performance have been proposed, such as consideration of serum lactate levels.[13] Other potential scoring models include the MELD score, the Sequential Organ Failure Assessment

Table 46-5 King's College Selection Criteria for Liver Transplantation According to the Etiology of Acute Liver Failure

Etiology	Selection Criteria for Transplantation
Acetaminophen	Arterial pH <7.30 despite normal intravascular filling pressures (irrespective of grade of encephalopathy) OR Prothrombin time >100 s + serum creatinine >300 μmol/L in patients in grade III or IV encephalopathy
Nonacetaminophen	Prothrombin time >100 s (irrespective of grade of encephalopathy) OR Any three of the following (irrespective of grade of encephalopathy): Non-A, non-B hepatitis (cryptogenic), halothane hepatitis, or other drug toxicity Age <10 y or >40 y Jaundice to encephalopathy interval >7 d Prothrombin time >50 s Serum bilirubin >300 μmol/L

Adapted with permission from O'Grady JG, Alexander GJ, Hayllar KM, et al. Early indicators of prognosis in fulminant liver failure. *Gastroenterology.* 1989;97:439.

(SOFA), and the Acute Physiology and Chronic Health Evaluation II (APACHE II).[18,19]

An elevated INR is a necessary finding for the diagnosis of ALF; however, clinically significant spontaneous bleeding is uncommon. Traditional standard of care recommends correction of thrombocytopenia to 50,000/mm^3 or more and INR to 1.5 or less for the bleeding patient or the patient about to undergo an invasive procedure. However, it has become clear that conventional coagulation studies such as INR and platelet count are poor predictors of bleeding complications of invasive procedures in patients with ALF or CLD.[20] Small studies suggest that whole blood viscoelastic studies are more accurate predictors of bleeding in both high- and low-risk invasive procedures;[21] however, they have not yet been validated for this purpose. Specific treatment thresholds for the nonbleeding patient are difficult to define, but it is suggested that prophylactic therapy not be undertaken except in anticipation of an invasive procedure. One exception may be a platelet count of 10,000/mm^3 or less.[11] Occasionally, rFVIIa or prothrombin complex concentrate is used to correct a resistant INR abnormality or to avoid fluid overload. It should be kept in mind that these agents carry a thrombotic risk and are contraindicated when the etiology of ALF is associated with hypercoagulability, such as pregnancy or Budd–Chiari syndrome.

Hypotension in ALF may be the result of several days of gastrointestinal losses, poor intake, or myocardial dysfunction, but likely includes a component of decreased arterial tone as liver necrosis progresses. The hypotensive ALF patient should undergo volume status and cardiac function assessment prior to consideration of inotropes or vasopressors. Vasopressors may be used either to treat systemic hypotension or to maintain an adequate CPP. On the basis of recommendations for septic patients, either norepinephrine or dopamine may be used. Although the use of arginine vasopressin (AVP) and its analogues was once avoided because of fears of further increasing ICP, more recent evidence suggests that these drugs increase cerebral blood flow but not ICP and are therefore safe.[11]

Acute Hepatitis

The most common causes of acute viral hepatitis are, collectively, the five identified viral hepatitides: A (HAV), B (HBV), C (HCV), D (HDV or delta-virus), and E (HEV). HAV and HBV have been well characterized and vaccines have been developed to prevent their transmission. As a result of widespread vaccination, the incidence of new cases of HAV and HBV has decreased steadily worldwide. Unfortunately, the same cannot be said for HCV, for which there is no currently available vaccine. The number of reported new cases of HCV is decreasing but this is likely the result of better screening of transfused blood products and the adoption of universal precautions. HDV is a single-strand RNA genome that requires the helper function of HBV for virion assembly and so must occur either as a coinfection or as a superinfection with HBV. HEV is a small RNA virus that has been responsible for several epidemics of hepatitis, primarily in underdeveloped countries with poor sanitation.

The diagnosis of acute hepatitis is made on the basis of classic signs and symptoms, together with laboratory studies to assess liver damage and serologic assays. Symptoms can be nonspecific, such as fatigue, poor appetite, nausea, vomiting, and abdominal pain, and many infections are subclinical. Signs may include jaundice, or a serum-sickness–type presentation with fever, arthralgia or arthritis, and rash that results from circulating hepatitis antigen–antibody complexes. Incubation periods can be several weeks to even months, and patients may undergo surgery without awareness of illness. For this reason, viral hepatitis should be part of the differential diagnosis when there is any evidence of postoperative liver injury.

HAV is a picornavirus that is spread primarily by the fecal–oral route or via contaminated food or water. HAV has a wide range of manifestation from asymptomatic disease (particularly in children) to ALF. ALF is rare (<1%) and is more likely than other causes to result in spontaneous recovery (69%) in patients without underlying liver disease. There is no chronic disease state associated with HAV.

HBV is a DNA virus that is spread via parenteral, cutaneous, or mucosal exposure to infected blood or body fluids. HBV surface antigen (HBsAg) is the hallmark of active HBV infection and usually appears during the incubation period, 1 to 10 weeks after exposure. ALF caused by acute HBV infection occurs in less than 1% of cases but has only a 20% rate of spontaneous recovery. Maintenance of seropositivity for HBsAg for more than 6 months after recovery suggests chronic infection and occurs in 2% to 5% of infected adults.

HDV infection occurs in conjunction with HBV infection and is estimated to be present in 5% of patients with chronic HBV. Two types of HDV infection are described: coinfection with acute HBV and superinfection on top of chronic HBV. Both types cause severe illness and may cause ALF.

HCV, once referred to as non-A, non-B hepatitis until its identification in 1989, is transmitted primarily parenterally. Because of the identification of HCV, the ability to serologically screen blood products for its presence has all but eliminated it as a source of posttransfusion hepatitis. Causes of transmission are often not identifiable, but the most commonly known risk factor is parenteral drug use. HCV has a high rate of progression to chronic disease (50% to 85%) and a risk of developing cirrhosis ranging from 5% to 25% over 25 to 30 years.[22]

Alcoholic Hepatitis

Alcoholic hepatitis is the syndrome marked by the development of jaundice and liver dysfunction in the setting of heavy alcohol use. Encephalopathy may be present in severe alcoholic hepatitis and, if so, portends a poorer prognosis. Laboratory studies show moderate serum aminotransferase elevations (<300 IU/mL), with AST being elevated more than ALT. The AST:ALT ratio is more than 2 in about 70% of patients with alcoholic hepatitis. Elevations of serum creatinine are particularly ominous as they may indicate impeding hepatorenal syndrome (HRS).

A history of excessive alcohol use is supportive of the diagnosis of alcoholic hepatitis, but up to 20% of these patients may have a coexisting cause of liver disease. Although liver biopsy is not required to make the diagnosis of alcoholic hepatitis, it is important to investigate other potential causes of acute liver disease.

The key component of therapy for alcoholic hepatitis is abstinence. For those patients with severe alcoholic hepatitis, medical therapy should also be considered. This consists of nutritional therapy that takes into account not only protein–calorie nutrition but vitamin and mineral deficiencies as well.

Drug-Induced Liver Injury

Often considered as an afterthought when a patient presents with new abnormalities in liver-related laboratory studies, DILI is a significant cause of morbidity and mortality. Although the process of diagnosing DILI is not well defined and it is largely a diagnosis of exclusion, DILI should always be considered when formulating the differential diagnosis of patients presenting with liver abnormalities. Moreover, DILI is a serious problem for the pharmaceutical industry, as it is the most common reason for regulatory actions such as failure of approval, removal from market, or restrictions on indications for use. Nonacetaminophen drug-induced idiosyncratic liver injury accounts for 11% to 13% of cases of ALF and, with a 20% rate of survival with supportive care, has a poorer than average rate of spontaneous recovery.[10]

The liver is commonly involved in drug toxicity because of its central role in drug metabolism. Drugs may either be directly hepatotoxic or propagate toxic metabolites, most often as products of phase I drug metabolism and the cytochrome P450 enzyme.[23] Cell injury follows via cell stress, mitochondrial injury, or immune-mediated mechanisms. Cell stress may result from glutathione depletion or the binding of reactive metabolites to intracellular enzymes, proteins, or lipids. Mitochondrial injury may result from the uncoupling of mitochondrial respiration with the depletion of adenosine triphosphate (ATP) and accumulation of reactive oxygen species (ROS). Immune-mediated injury may result from the binding of reactive metabolites to cell structures, creating antigenic entities that can invoke the formation of antibodies against the cell structures themselves.

Perhaps the best known potentially hepatotoxic drug in anesthesia is halothane. Halothane was introduced to patient care in 1956 and was widely used because of its lack of flammability, potency, and patient tolerance. However, reports of postoperative liver injury began to appear shortly thereafter and, by 1963, over 300 cases of "halothane hepatitis" had been reported. The National Academy of Sciences produced a retrospective epidemiologic study on the use of halothane from these reports. The National Halothane Study reviewed cases of fatal hepatic necrosis from among 34 centers in the United States occurring within 6 weeks of the administration of a general anesthetic. Of the 856,000 anesthetics reviewed, about 255,000 involved halothane, and 82 cases of fatal hepatic necrosis were identified. Sixty-three of these cases could be ascribed to an identifiable clinical factor, leaving 19 with otherwise unexplained hepatic necrosis. Fourteen of the 19 had received a halothane anesthetic but did not have consistent histologic findings. Uncertainty over the direct association between halothane and the cases of fatal hepatic necrosis, together with the calculated incidence of 1 in 35,000 anesthetics even if such association did exist, led to the conclusion that halothane overall had a good safety record. The possible association with repeated exposure to halothane did not go unrecognized, and there was an editorial recommendation that halothane be avoided in patients with a history of unexplained fever and jaundice following a general anesthetic.

It is generally agreed that halothane hepatitis is composed of two different manifestations. A relatively mild, self-limited form is characterized by elevations in liver-related laboratory studies without evidence of liver failure. This may occur in up to 20% of patients after halothane exposure. A proposed mechanism for this hepatocellular damage is the combination of halothane degradation products and hypoxia caused by imbalance in the hepatic oxygen supply–demand relationship. There is strong evidence that the severe, fulminant form of halothane hepatitis is an immune-mediated process. The association with repeated halothane exposure and the appearance of rash and eosinophilia support this hypothesis. Furthermore, circulating IgG antibodies against liver proteins, modified by the reactive trifluoroacetyl (TFA) metabolite of halothane, have been identified in the sera of patients with clinical halothane hepatitis.[24] Although other halogenated inhalational anesthetics that produce TFA metabolites such as enflurane, isoflurane, and desflurane have been associated with acute hepatic failure, the occurrence of hepatitis attributed to these agents is very rare. Because halothane is by far the most extensively metabolized of these agents (20% halothane metabolized vs. 2% enflurane, 0.2% isoflurane, and 0.01% desflurane) the production of TFA metabolites would seem to correlate with the incidence of associated hepatitis. Indeed, an animal study examining the extent of hepatic tissue trifluoroacetylation after exposure to halogenated anesthetics showed that halothane produced significantly more tissue acylation than enflurane, isoflurane, or desflurane.[25]

Pregnancy-Related Liver Diseases

Abnormalities in liver studies occur in 3% to 5% of pregnancies. Although many causes reflect underlying hepatic or biliary disease, the most common causes are one of the five acute, pregnancy-related conditions: hyperemesis gravidarum; intrahepatic cholestasis of pregnancy; preeclampsia; preeclampsia complicated by hemolysis, low platelet count, and elevated liver enzymes (HELLP syndrome); and acute fatty liver of pregnancy (AFLP; Table 46-6). Hyperemesis gravidarum is a feature of the first trimester of pregnancy and is characterized by vomiting of sufficient severity to warrant intravenous (IV) hydration. Risk factors include hyperthyroidism, molar pregnancy, and multiple pregnancies.[26] Liver enzymes are increased in about 50% of patients (up to 20-fold elevation), but bilirubin is usually normal or minimally elevated.[27] It is important to distinguish hyperemesis from acute viral hepatitis or from drug toxicity. Therapy is primarily supportive and the condition usually resolves by the second trimester.

Intrahepatic cholestasis of pregnancy usually presents in the second to third trimester. The proposed etiology is interference with bile acid transport across the canalicular membrane, resulting in serum bile acid elevation and pruritus. In addition to modest increases in bilirubin (usually <5 mg/dL) aminotransferases may also be elevated up to 20-fold, and serum bile acids may be elevated up to 100-fold.[27] As with hyperemesis gravidarum, treatment is primarily supportive, aimed at relieving pruritus. Unlike

Table 46-6 Distinguishing Features of Intrahepatic Cholestasis of Pregnancy, HELLP Syndrome, and Acute Fatty Liver of Pregnancy (AFLP)

	Cholestasis of Pregnancy	HELLP	AFLP
Pregnancies	0.1% (United States)	0.2–0.6%	0.005–0.01%
Onset	25–32 wks	Third trimester or postpartum	Third trimester or postpartum
Family history	Often	No	Occasionally
Presence of preeclampsia	No	Yes	50%
Typical clinical features	Pruritus, mild jaundice, elevated bile acids, decreased vitamin K	Hemolysis, thrombocytopenia (<50,000 often)	Liver failure with coagulopathy, encephalopathy hypoglycemia, DIC
Aminotransferases	Mild to 10- to 20-fold elevation	Mild to 10- to 20-fold elevation	300–500 typical but variable elevation
Bilirubin	<5 mg/dL	<5 mg/dL unless massive necrosis	Often <5 mg/dL, higher if severe
Hepatic imaging	Normal	Hepatic infarcts, hematomas, rupture	Fatty infiltration
Histology	Normal–mild cholestasis, no necrosis	Patchy/extensive necrosis and hemorrhage	Microvesicular fat in zone 3
Maternal mortality	0%	1–25%	7–18%
Fetal/perinatal mortality	0.4–1.4%	11%	9–23%
Recurrence in subsequent pregnancies	45–70%	4–19%	α-Subunit, long-chain 3-hydroxyacyl-CoA dehydrogenase (LCHAD) defect—yes No fatty acid oxidation defect—rare

DIC, disseminated intravascular coagulation.
Adapted with permission from Hay JE. Liver disease in pregnancy. *Hepatology*. 2008;47:1067.

hyperemesis, intrahepatic cholestasis of pregnancy may be associated with chronic placental insufficiency, premature labor, and sudden fetal death. Therefore, pregnancies complicated by intrahepatic cholestasis of pregnancy are considered high risk.

The three remaining uniquely pregnancy-related conditions all present in the third trimester. Preeclampsia is diagnosed by the triad of hypertension, edema, and proteinuria. Elevation of aminotransferases is indicative of severe preeclampsia. The appearance of microangiopathic hemolytic anemia (MAHA), elevated liver enzymes, and low platelet count in the preeclamptic patient comprises the HELLP syndrome and occurs in 20% of severely preeclamptic patients. MAHA is the result of vascular endothelial injury with subsequent fibrin deposition and platelet consumption. This also leads to areas of hepatic infarction and subsequent hemorrhage, which may coalesce into large hematomas and lead to capsular rupture and intraperitoneal bleeding. Laboratory studies show elevated aminotransferases, up to 10- to 20-fold, and modest increases in bilirubin. A peripheral smear will show the characteristic schistocytes and burr cells of MAHA. Platelet count may be used to distinguish between mild, moderate, and severe HELLP, with platelet counts of 100,000 to 150,000/mm^3, 50,000 to 100,000/mm^3, and less than 50,000/mm^3, respectively.

Abdominal CT imaging is the preferred study to detect major hepatic complications of infarct, hematoma, or rupture. Contained hepatic hemorrhage can be managed conservatively with correction of volume deficit and coagulopathy. Capsular rupture or rapid extension of a hematoma is life-threatening and demands more aggressive treatment for control of bleeding, usually emergency laparotomy. Rarely, there may be an indication for transplantation for the patient in whom bleeding cannot be controlled. Delivery is definitive therapy for HELLP syndrome. Therapy remains the same regardless of timing of presentation, and most patients will quickly improve after delivery.

AFLP is the result of rapid microvesicular fatty infiltration of the liver resulting in acute portal hypertension and encephalopathy. Although the exact mechanism of AFLP is unknown, there is an association between it and abnormalities in the enzymes involved in β-oxidation of fatty acids. Symptoms are similar to severe preeclampsia and HELLP syndrome; however, the AFLP patient may additionally have laboratory and clinical findings more unique to liver failure, such as hypoglycemia, elevated ammonia, asterixis, and encephalopathy.

Arrangements for rapid delivery should follow diagnosis of AFLP, as recovery can only follow delivery. Recovery may be prolonged in patients who are severely ill upon presentation, and there is a role for transplantation in the patient who continues to progress to ALF after delivery.

Chronic Hepatocellular Disease

CLD is a major public health burden in the United States, with an increase in prevalence of 25% in the period from 1988 to 1994 to almost 36% in the period from 2013 to 2016.[9] From 2013 to 2016, the prevalences of the most common causes of CLD in the United States were hepatitis B 0.35%, hepatitis C 2.7%, alcoholic liver disease 1.0%, and NAFLD 32.0%.[9] Notably, the increase in CLD between 1988 and 2016 was almost entirely attributable to an increase in NAFLD.

Cirrhosis and Portal Hypertension

3 Cirrhosis is the end product of the long course of CLD, during which there have been either steady or recurrent episodes of parenchymal inflammation and necrosis with resultant disruption of normal hepatic architecture (NICV 46-1). Areas of fibrosis and regenerative nodules replace the normal arrangement of hepatic lobules. Blood flow through the liver is disrupted as well, with the formation of shunts between afferent (portal venous and hepatic arterial) and efferent (hepatic venous) vessels. Increased resistance to blood flow through the liver leads to portal hypertension. Severe portal hypertension is generally defined as a HVPG of >10 to 12 mmHg. At this point CLD becomes a systemic illness affecting other organ systems.[28]

Hemostasis

Hemostasis is a dynamic process that is the product of interaction between coagulation, platelets, and fibrinolysis, resulting in the formation and revision of clot. Liver disease affects all three of these components, both quantitatively and qualitatively.

The liver is the site of synthesis for all procoagulant and anticoagulant factors, with the exception of tissue thromboplastin (III), calcium (IV), and von Willebrand factor (VIII). It is also the site for clearance of activated factors.

Cirrhotic patients are customarily considered to have a bleeding diathesis on the basis of abnormalities in conventional tests of coagulation such as PT and partial thromboplastin time (PTT). However, such tests reflect the activity of only a portion of the procoagulant factors and do not consider the concomitant decrease in anticoagulant factors, which are not customarily measured. It is the balance of procoagulant and anticoagulant forces, not the isolated measurement of either portion of the coagulation system, that indicates the effective generation of thrombin.[29] Not surprisingly, PT and PTT abnormalities correlate poorly with bleeding complications following invasive procedures, such as liver biopsy.[30] In fact, there is evidence that, should one account for differences in the anticoagulant levels between normal and cirrhotic patients by adding thrombomodulin (an activator of the anticoagulant protein C) to the PT assay, normal and cirrhotic patients generate the same amounts of thrombin.[29,31] Thus, one may conclude that the decreased levels of protein C in cirrhotic patients balance the decreased levels of procoagulants, leaving thrombin generation in vivo unaltered.

Even more counterintuitive is the increasing evidence that cirrhotic patients not only have normal thrombin generation but may actually also have a procoagulant imbalance on the basis of reduced levels of the anticoagulants protein C and antithrombin III, together with an increase in FVIII and von Willebrand factor.[29,32] Clinically, this is supported by studies reporting not only the lack of protection of liver disease against the formation of venous thromboembolism (VTE)[33] but also an increased risk of VTE formation associated with the presence of cirrhotic and noncirrhotic liver disease.[34]

The cholestatic diseases (e.g., PBC, sclerosing cholangitis) may eventually progress to cirrhosis, but until that happens, the coagulopathy of these diseases has a different nature from that of hepatocellular dysfunction. The coagulopathy of biliary disease is characterized by functional deficiencies in the vitamin K–dependent procoagulants II, VII, IX, and X and anticoagulants protein C and protein S. Vitamin K is a fat-soluble cofactor necessary for the final step in the production of these factors, carboxylation of the precursor produced by the liver. Bile salts are necessary for absorption of vitamin K, and impaired bile secretion in cholestasis results in vitamin K deficiency. Parenteral vitamin K can correct this deficiency and return coagulation to normal as long as the liver is still capable of manufacturing adequate amounts of factor precursors. It cannot, however, correct the coagulopathy of hepatocellular dysfunction.

Dysfibrinogenemia has been described in acute, chronic, and neoplastic liver disease and is the most common qualitative defect of coagulation factors, occurring in 70% to 80% of cirrhotics. Its presence does not appear to be related to the severity of hepatic dysfunction, but instead to be associated with hepatic tissue regeneration. Excess sialic acid residues on the fibrinogen interfere with the enzymatic activity of thrombin and cause abnormal polymerization of fibrin monomers. Thus, although serum fibrinogen levels may be adequate, function is not accurately reflected.

Platelets provide primary hemostasis by interaction with the vessel wall at the site of injury and the formation of a physical plug. Thrombocytopenia is a well-known feature of cirrhosis. Estimates of incidence range from 30% to 64% in chronic cirrhotics, but platelet counts below 30,000/mm^3 are rare.[35] Because the liver is the primary site of thrombopoietin production, decreased levels of thrombopoietin contribute. Other factors include immunologic mechanisms, direct bone-marrow suppression, and consumptive processes such as DIC. However, the primary cause of thrombocytopenia is splenic sequestration in the setting of portal hypertension. Up to 90% of the platelet population may be sequestered in the spleen. Elevated levels of von Willebrand factor are felt to compensate for decreased platelet counts, augmenting the platelet–endothelial cell interaction on vessel walls.

A second function of platelets is to promote thrombin generation. Activated platelets provide negatively charged phospholipids on their surfaces, which act as receptors for the assembly of coagulation factors, thus promoting coagulation. A series of assays measuring thrombin generation concluded that platelet counts below a threshold of 100,000/mm^3 negatively correlated with thrombin production. It was further estimated that the minimum platelet count necessary to support near-normal thrombin generation was 56,000/mm^3.[31] This information provides further support to the use of platelet transfusion in the bleeding patient with platelet counts in and below that range. Platelet transfusions are not indicated in the absence of bleeding.

The fibrinolytic system limits and revises clot formation. The initial step is activation of plasmin from plasminogen by enzymes such as tissue plasminogen activator (tPA). Plasmin consumes fibrin, producing fibrin degradation products such as D-dimer. The fibrinolytic system in cirrhotic patients has many abnormalities which may account for accelerated fibrinolysis, which has a reported incidence of 30% to 46% in patients with end-stage liver disease.[36] The liver is the site of tPA clearance, and elevated tPA levels have been noted in patients with cirrhosis.[37] Furthermore, the liver is the site of synthesis for plasmin inhibitors, such as plasmin activator inhibitor-1 (PAI-1) and thrombin-activatable fibrinolysis inhibitor (TAFI). However, as with the process of coagulation, what matters is the balance of these factors that promote and inhibit fibrinolysis and where their net forces lie. Commonly used studies for assessing the presence and severity of accelerated fibrinolysis include the euglobulin clot lysis time (ECLT) and viscoelastic whole blood testing (VET). A clot lysis index in VET has been defined as the ratio of the clot amplitude at a defined period of time in the assay, to the clot maximum amplitude (MA). A ratio less than the assay's normal range indicates the presence of accelerated fibrinolysis and suggests the need for an antifibrinolytic agent such as epsilon aminocaproic acid or tranexamic acid in the presence of otherwise unexplained bleeding.

DIC is primarily a thrombotic diathesis, followed by widespread secondary fibrinolysis. As factors are consumed, DIC becomes a bleeding diathesis of factor and platelet deficiencies. Whether or not DIC is a feature of stable CLD is controversial. Because cirrhosis shares common laboratory abnormalities with DIC, standard laboratory values cannot distinguish between consumption and decreased synthesis and so have little utility. More recent approaches to answer this question have utilized assays for substances that would be expected to be elevated as the result of excessive thrombin production, the sine qua non of DIC. These include the cleaved by-products of coagulation factor activation such as prothrombin fragment F1 + 2, fibrinopeptide A, and thrombin–antithrombin (TAT) complexes. Elevation of these would suggest that low levels of procoagulation factors are the result of consumption rather than underproduction.

It is generally agreed on the basis of examination of these special assays that overt DIC is probably not a feature of stable CLD. However, an entity called "accelerated intravascular coagulation and fibrinolysis (AICF)" has been described. This may be considered a low-grade consumptive process that occurs in less than 30% of cirrhotics, primarily in those with severe, decompensated disease. Although it may not have immediate clinical consequence, patients who exhibit this phenomenon are considered at increased risk to progress to DIC in the presence of a known stimulus, such as sepsis or spontaneous bacterial peritonitis (SBP).

Cardiac Manifestations

4 The cirrhotic patient typically has a hyperdynamic circulation, characterized by a high cardiac output, low arterial blood pressure, and low systemic vascular resistance. On examination, the patient is warm and appears well-perfused despite systolic arterial pressures in the 80s and 90s. Although pulmonary arterial pressures may be mildly elevated, the pulmonary vascular resistance (PVR) is usually within the normal range. Consideration of the formula for calculating PVR (mean pulmonary artery pressure, mPAP, minus pulmonary capillary wedge divided by cardiac output) reveals the explanation: the cardiac output is elevated proportionally to the transpulmonary gradient (the numerator in the equation). Although these patients have an elevated intravascular volume, this is not usually reflected in an elevated wedge pressure. This is due to sequestration of this volume into the massively dilated and collateralized splanchnic vascular bed. Thus, the effective circulating volume is reduced, which has consequences on other organ systems as well.

At the heart of these circulatory changes is portal hypertension. Portal hypertension causes local production of vasodilators such as natriuretic peptides, vasoactive intestinal peptide, endotoxin, glucagon, and especially nitric oxide.[38] Elevated production of nitric oxide has been observed to precede the formation of the hyperdynamic circulation in cirrhosis, and inhibition of nitric oxide formation has been shown to increase arterial pressure in cirrhotic patients. Furthermore, there is reduced circulatory responsivity to sympathetic stimulation primarily due to overproduction of vasodilators.[39]

In addition to hyperdynamic circulation, the cirrhotic patient may have a combination of other cardiac functional abnormalities that are not immediately apparent in the baseline state. These abnormalities comprise four key components of a condition termed "cirrhotic cardiomyopathy." They include: (1) the aforementioned increase in cardiac output and decrease in peripheral vascular resistance; (2) systolic and diastolic dysfunction; (3) cardiac resistance to β-adrenergic stimulation; and (4) electrophysiologic abnormalities.

Historically, cirrhosis has not been associated with cardiomyopathy because the hyperdynamic circulation was presumed to reflect cardiac vigor and the few patients who had overt dilated cardiomyopathy were thought to be manifesting alcoholic cardiomyopathy. However, elevated cardiac output is only a consequence of the profound decrease in afterload resulting from the dilated peripheral circulation. Systolic incompetence is revealed by physiologic or pharmacologic stress and is manifested by an inability to increase cardiac output in response to exercise and an inability to increase ejection fraction despite an increase in end-diastolic volume. Furthermore, the severity of cardiac dysfunction seems to be directly correlated with the severity of liver disease.[40]

Diastolic dysfunction has been described in cirrhotic patients as well. Diastolic dysfunction renders cirrhotic patients very sensitive to changes in cardiac filling making them vulnerable to both heart failure and prerenal insufficiency.

Autonomic dysfunction is another characteristic of the altered cirrhotic cardiovascular system. Chronotropic and hemodynamic incompetence in response to various challenges such as sustained handgrip, ice water hand submersion, Valsalva maneuver, and tilt table testing has demonstrated autonomic neuropathy in 43% of cirrhotic patients. Although apparently unrelated to autonomic dysfunction, prolonged QTc interval is also observed in cirrhotic patients with an incidence ranging from 30% in Child's A to 60% in Child's C patients (see later).[41] This should be kept in mind when treating these patients with drugs known to prolong the QT interval.

Coronary artery disease (CAD) in cirrhotic patients has become an area of interest particularly as the application of liver transplantation has expanded to include older patients with comorbidities. Risk factors for CAD in cirrhotic patients are similar to those of other patient populations: hypertension, dyslipidemia, age, gender, and obesity. However, nonalcoholic steatohepatitis (NASH) has been recognized as an increasingly important cause for transplantation and carries with it both the cardiac disease risks of its attendant maladies, obesity and diabetes, and a chronic inflammatory state. The optimal test for identifying cirrhotic patients with significant CAD is unclear. Because many of these patients cannot exercise, pharmacologic stress testing is most commonly employed. Unfortunately, studies investigating the predictive value of noninvasive functional testing, particularly dobutamine stress echocardiography, have generally shown poor sensitivity and variable quality of negative predictive value (75% to 89%).[42] Thus, among liver transplantation candidates, consideration should be given to proceeding with coronary angiography if the patient is judged to have a high likelihood of CAD.[43] For less complex surgeries, however, this may not be warranted.

Renal Dysfunction

The hallmarks of renal dysfunction in cirrhosis are the seemingly inappropriate avid retention of sodium and free water, together with renal hypoperfusion and consequent decreased glomerular filtration. The extreme manifestation of this is the HRS, a prerenal functional abnormality that is the renal response to the circulatory abnormalities of advanced cirrhosis. Renal function is an important risk factor for mortality, a fact that is emphasized by its presence as one of only three variables used in calculating the MELD score, the primary predictor of 3-month mortality for patients on the liver transplantation waiting list.

Although the most dramatic and unique renal manifestation of CLD is the HRS, cirrhotic patients are also at high risk for more prosaic causes of renal dysfunction, such as parenchymal renal disease, sepsis, nephrotoxicity, and hypovolemia. It is important to remember that HRS is a diagnosis of exclusion and that other possible potentially treatable causes must be ruled out because therapies will differ.

Despite the fact that the cirrhotic patient's liver disease predominates, one should be mindful of any comorbidities that exist. Glomerulonephritis and diabetic nephropathy are not infrequent findings. NAFLD, the most common nonviral cause of adult CLD, is associated with type II diabetes. Immune complex nephropathies such as IgA nephropathy and membranous proliferative glomerulonephropathy are associated with chronic hepatitis C infection.[44] In addition, some underlying causes of liver failure are directly associated with renal dysfunction. These include such diseases as amyloidosis, systemic lupus erythematosus, autoimmune hepatitis, polycystic liver disease, and Alagille syndrome.

The cirrhotic circulatory system is characterized by marked sympathetic stimulation, and activation of the renin–angiotensin–aldosterone and vasopressin systems in response to the loss of effective circulating volume to the massively dilated splanchnic vasculature of portal hypertension. These systems combine to save salt and water and reduce renal perfusion. Elevated levels of renal prostaglandins help to maintain renal perfusion. Thus, cirrhotic patients are very sensitive to the prostaglandin inhibition of nonsteroidal anti-inflammatory medications. Aminoglycosides, angiotensin-converting enzyme inhibitors, and angiotensin receptor blockers are other drug groups associated with nephrotoxicity in cirrhotic patients. Despite the expectation that contrast administration would be nephrotoxic, there is no evidence to support that concern.[45]

Cirrhotic patients are at risk for hypovolemia from a number of causes, including gastrointestinal bleeding, diuretic use, and diarrhea resulting from lactulose or rifaximin administration. Unfortunately, it can be difficult to assess intravascular volume status in patients who are total–body volume overloaded, whose measured central filling pressures may reflect transmitted elevated intra-abdominal pressures because of ascites, and whose measured serum creatinine levels are poor estimates of GFR due to decreased muscle mass. Nonetheless, pursuit of a diagnosis by discontinuing diuretics and providing volume expansion with albumin can help differentiate hypovolemia from the other prerenal etiology of interest, HRS. Failure for creatinine to improve in response to such measures is strongly suggestive of HRS as the underlying cause.

HRS is the end-stage renal manifestation of the systemic circulatory derangement of cirrhosis. It is considered a functional derangement, primarily on the basis of successful transplantation of kidneys from HRS patients. Although it is often invoked in the differential diagnosis of acute renal dysfunction in cirrhotic patients, it accounts for only about 23% of the cases of acute kidney injury in hospitalized cirrhotic patients.[46] Nonetheless, in cirrhotic patients with ascites, the incidence of HRS is 18% at 1 year and 39% at 5 years.

The generally agreed-upon criteria for diagnosing HRS are those proposed by the International Ascites Club.[47] Two manifestations of HRS are recognized, and the terminology for them has recently changed as understanding of the disease processes has changed. Previously HRS was divided into Type I and Type II manifestations. Type I was characterized by rapid progression of renal failure and a high mortality rate but was potentially reversible with treatment. Type II followed a slow and inexorable progression that paralleled the worsening of the patient's underlying liver disease. What was once called Type 1 and Type 2 HRS are now called HRS-AKI (acute kidney injury) and HRS-CKD (chronic kidney disease).

HRS AKI is characterized by the fulfilment of standard AKI criteria (an absolute increase in serum Cr of at least 0.3 mg/dL within 48 h or 1.5 × baseline Cr level within the last 7 d) in a cirrhotic patient, in whom structural renal abnormalities have been excluded. Notably, this definition allows diagnosis (and thus therapy) to begin at an earlier juncture than that of Type I HRS, which required a serum creatinine of at least 2.5 mg/dL for diagnosis. Often a precipitating cause such as SBP, sepsis, gastrointestinal bleeding, or surgical stress can be identified and should be addressed as rapidly as possible. Nephrotoxic drugs should be discontinued and a trial of volume expansion considered.

HRS-CKD is defined as a reduction in estimated GFR <60 mL/1.73 m^2 per minute for at least 3 months. HRS-CKD is more indolent and may be considered the expected consequence of continuous and progressive activity of the circulatory homeostatic triad of the sympathetic, renin–angiotensin–aldosterone and vasopressin systems in an attempt to compensate for the progressive loss of effective circulating blood volume to the increasingly dilated splanchnic vasculature. The most compelling clinical problem in these patients is refractory ascites.

Although profound renal vasoconstriction is the proximate cause of HRS, therapy aimed at directly increasing renal perfusion by the use of prostaglandins, dopamine agonists, or endothelin antagonists has been unsuccessful. More effective has been therapy targeting the underlying pathology that leads to the renal vasoconstrictive response, that is, reduction of portal hypertension and/or splanchnic vasodilation.

Vasoconstrictors such as AVP or its analogues, somatostatin or its analogues, and α-agonists such as norepinephrine and midodrine, combined with volume expansion, have shown efficacy in reversing HRS-AKI (typically defined as a reduction in creatinine to 1.5 mg/dL). AVP and its analogues are particularly attractive, because they interact with V1 receptors, which mediate vasoconstriction and are particularly well represented in the splanchnic circulation. Choices among these therapies are to some extent dictated by drug availability because, for example, terlipressin is not available in the United States. Terlipressin is perhaps the most studied vasopressor for HRS and is effective in 40% to 60% of HRS-AKI patients.[48] If reversal of HRS-AKI is successful and therapy is withdrawn, recurrence is uncommon. Although response to vasopressor plus volume expansion has been observed in HRS-CKD, recurrence after withdrawal of therapy is the rule.

Placement of a transjugular intrahepatic portal shunt (TIPS) lowers portal pressures and would be expected to decompress the splanchnic circulation, returning volume directly to the central circulation. Although pilot studies have shown TIPS capable of reversing both types of HRS, it has limited application primarily because of the exclusionary criteria used in these studies; for example, Child–Pugh score above 12, active infection, and serum bilirubin above 5 mg/dL, as well as risk of de novo development or worsening of HE. Furthermore, even when initially successful, there is a high rate of shunt stenosis and migration.

Liver transplantation is the definitive therapy for HRS. For patients with HRS who are transplant candidates, renal replacement therapy is the typical bridge to transplantation. In countries where terlipressin is available, terlipressin plus albumin volume expansion is also a bridge option. There is some sense that, if allowed to continue, HRS that requires renal replacement therapy may not be reversible. In the First International Liver Transplantation Society Expert Panel Consensus on Renal Insufficiency in Liver Transplantation, it was recommended that patients who had received dialysis at least twice weekly for more than 6 weeks prior to transplantation be considered for combined liver–kidney transplantation.[49]

Pulmonary Complications

Pulmonary complications have long been associated with portal hypertension with or without intrinsic hepatic disease. Estimates of as high as 50% to 70% of patients with CLD complain of shortness of breath.[50] There are many commonplace mechanisms underlying pulmonary abnormalities observed in patients with liver disease. The differential diagnoses include ventilation–perfusion abnormalities associated with underlying obstructive airway disease, fluid retention, pleural effusion, and decreased lung capacities secondary to large volume ascites. α_1-Antitrypsin disease is a metabolic syndrome that has both lung and liver manifestations, similar to cystic fibrosis. In addition, there are two types of vascular abnormalities unique to the setting of portal hypertension that carry significant morbidity and mortality. These abnormalities have been termed hepatopulmonary syndrome (HPS) and portopulmonary hypertension (POPH). Their severity may even overshadow the underlying liver disease, so much so that their presence and severity influences candidacy for liver transplantation.

HPS consists of the triad of liver dysfunction, otherwise unexplained hypoxemia, and intrapulmonary vascular dilation (IPVD) that may be present in up to 20% of patients who present for liver transplantation. The diagnostic criteria for HPS are as follows[51]:

- Oxygenation defect: Partial pressure of oxygen below 80 mmHg or alveolar–arterial oxygen gradient of at least 15 mmHg while breathing ambient air
- Pulmonary vascular dilatation: Positive findings on contrast-enhanced echocardiography or abnormal uptake in the brain (>6%) with radioactive lung-perfusion scanning
- Liver disease: Portal hypertension (most common) with or without cirrhosis

IPVDs are of two types. Type I lesions are more common and are manifested as precapillary dilations at the alveolar level. Type II lesions are larger dilations that are more centrally located in the lungs and behave as anatomic shunts. Demonstration of IPVD may be made by agitated saline contrast-enhanced echocardiography or by technetium-labeled microaggregated albumin (TcMAA). In the absence of HPS, microbubbles and albumin microaggregates injected into the venous circulation are trapped by the pulmonary capillary bed. The delayed (>3 cardiac cycles) appearance of microbubbles in the left atrium or increased (>5%) extrapulmonary uptake of TcMAA suggest direct arteriovenous communication in the lungs and the presence of IPVDs. Type I IPVDs are functional rather than true anatomic shunts. IPVDs result in a massive increase in pulmonary capillary diameter, from 8 to 15 μm to 50 to 500 μm. This, together with the usually hyperdynamic circulation of the cirrhotic patient, allows insufficient time for oxygen diffusion through the entire stream of capillary blood. This results in a central stream of poorly oxygenated blood that is functionally shunted. This lesion is easily correctable with the administration of oxygen, because increased FiO_2 increases oxygen diffusion through the dilated capillary. In fact, failure of 100% oxygen to correct the PaO_2 to greater than 150 mmHg is suggestive of the presence of true anatomic or type II shunt.[52] Also of interest is the unique positional oxygenation change that occurs with this syndrome, called orthodeoxia. Because IPVDs predominate in the bases of the lungs, standing worsens hypoxemia and the supine position improves oxygenation as blood is redistributed from the bases to the apices.

The natural history of HPS is usually one of progressive hypoxemia. The pathogenesis of HPS is poorly understood, hampering the development of effective therapy. Suspected contributing factors include nitric oxide, splanchnic endotoxemia, decreased clearance of inflammatory mediators, and angiogenesis. Genetic factors are thought to contribute also. Postliver-transplantation correction of hypoxemia is almost universal, although it may take up to a year.[53]

Table 46-7 Criteria for Portopulmonary hypertension (POPH)

- Clinical evidence of portal hypertension with or without hepatic disease
- mPAP >20 mmHg at rest
- mPAOP < 15 mmHg
- PVR >240 dynes/sec/cm^5 or 3 Wood units

Adapted from Simonneau G, Montani D, Celermajer D, et al. Haemodynamic definitions and updated clinical classification of pulmonary hypertension. *Eur Respir J* 2019;53:1801913.

mPAP, mean pulmonary arterial pressure; PVR, pulmonary vascular resistance; mPAOP, mean pulmonary artery occlusion pressure

POPH is defined as pulmonary hypertension that exists in a patient who has portal hypertension with no other known cause. The specific diagnostic criteria are shown in Table 46-7.

Severity of POPH is graded by mPAP, with mild, moderate, and severe POPH defined as less than 35 mmHg, 35 to 50 mmHg, and more than 50 mmHg, respectively. Traditionally, pulmonary hypertension was defined as mPAP ≥25 mmHg. In the 6th World Symposium on Pulmonary Hypertension in 2018, the cut-off of mPAP was lowered to 20 mmHg. However, there is still some concern that this new definition includes otherwise healthy individuals in which current treatments may not be of benefit.[54]

The occurrence of POPH is 2% in a population of patients with known portal hypertension,[55] as compared to 0.13% in an unselected population.[56] Among liver transplant candidates, the prevalence is 4% to 6%.[57] The occurrence of POPH is unrelated to the severity of the underlying liver disease or portal hypertension, with one epidemiologic study documenting a distribution of 51% Child's A, 38% Child's B, and 11% Child's C patients among a population of patients sent to a referral center with the diagnosis of POPH.[58] Female patients as well as patients with underlying autoimmune hepatitis are at increased risk for POPH, and patients with chronic hepatitis C are at decreased risk.[57,58]

Similar to HPS patients, symptoms of POPH are nonspecific, commonly consisting of dyspnea, generalized weakness, and decreased exercise tolerance. Although HPS and POPH may coexist, such an occurrence is uncommon and POPH patients may have only a modest decrease in PaO_2 if at all. The single best screening study for POPH is the 2D transthoracic echocardiography (TTE). TTE allows estimation of right ventricular systolic pressure (RVSP) by the velocity of the tricuspid regurgitant jet. TTE screening has a sensitivity of 97% and a specificity of 77% in diagnosing moderate to severe POPH in patients undergoing pretransplantation workup.[59] However, right-sided cardiac catheterization is necessary, both to confirm elevated pressures and to measure PVR.

Therapy includes conventional measures such as diuresis, as well as some specific vasodilator therapy. Calcium channel blockers, often used in other patients with pulmonary hypertension, are contraindicated in this population because they promote mesenteric vasodilation and worsen portal hypertension. Other drugs used include prostanoids, phosphodiesterase inhibitors, and endothelin antagonists. Reported success with these modalities is on the basis of case reports or case series, and no one therapy has emerged as definitive. Nonetheless, one goal of therapy is to make the patient transplant eligible by reducing mPAP and PVR into an acceptable range.

Epoprostenol (PgI) has been shown to reduce pulmonary pressures in POPH and has been documented to have a survival benefit in pulmonary hypertension.[60] Epoprostenol also has an antiplatelet effect and promotes vascular remodeling. However, it must be administered as a continuous infusion via central access with little tolerance for interruption of the infusion. It has also been associated with splenomegaly and worsening thrombocytopenia, sufficient to limit its use. The phosphodiesterase inhibitor sildenafil has also shown ability to reduce pulmonary pressures at 3 months, but without a sustained response at 12 months.[61] Nonetheless, it may be useful in combination therapy or it may provide a window for transplantation. The endothelin antagonists bosentan and ambrisentan, have both been documented to decrease PVR and increase CO over a sustained period.[62]

The role of liver transplantation in the treatment of POPH is not well defined because outcomes of transplantation are not predictable. Some patients have resolution of POPH with transplant, some may have no or incomplete resolution and continue to require medical therapy, and some may experience worsening POPH. Nonetheless, it is an option for a select group of patients whose pulmonary hemodynamics and cardiac function suggest they will tolerate the procedure. Evaluation of the patient for potential transplantation must include a right heart catheterization to measure mPAP and calculate PVR. Patients with mPAP less than 35 mmHg can be expected to tolerate transplant and do well postoperatively. Those with mPAP 35 mmHg or more and elevated PVR may be considered if they respond to therapy sufficiently to reduce their mPAP below 35 mmHg and PVR below 240 dynes/sec/cm[5].[62]

Hepatic Encephalopathy

HE is a serious, albeit reversible, neuropsychiatric complication that is a feature of both CLD and acute liver disease. The manifestations range from subtle, subclinical abnormalities that can only be discerned by formal psychometric tests (minimal HE) to clearly evident neurologic and behavioral derangements that are easily diagnosed at the bedside (overt HE). Although HE can appear as the result of portal–systemic shunting without intrinsic liver disease, the onset of HE is generally associated with advanced hepatocellular disease. Moreover, even minimal HE can affect the patient's ability to maintain employment, drive a car, perform daily activities, and interact with family. The fact that HE is frequently reversible emphasizes the importance of identifying and treating this condition.

The diagnosis of overt HE encompasses two sets of criteria: neuropsychologic and neuromotor. Neuropsychologic assessment focuses on level of consciousness, attention and ability to follow commands, and effect. This is most often graded on a I to IV scale (Table 46-3). Physical examination may elicit asterixis or other evidence of hyperreflexiveness such as clonus or Babinski sign. Other focal findings can include nystagmus or decerebrate posturing. However, focal neurologic findings should prompt appropriate imaging to rule out structural neurologic lesions because these patients are at risk for intracranial bleeding and are not immune to other neurologic pathologies such as ischemic brain disease, abscess, and tumor.

It is generally agreed that HE is the result of the failure of the liver to adequately metabolize certain substances that when accumulated are neurotoxic, rather than failure to synthesize substances critical to normal neurotransmission. The proposed World Congress definitions support this by recognizing a type of HE that is associated with normal hepatocellular function but shunting of blood around the liver (type B). Historically, HE has been attributed to hyperammonemia resulting from inadequate hepatic metabolism of ammonia. Although ammonia continues to be considered an important contributor, severity of HE does not necessarily correlate with ammonia levels. This may be explained by recent investigations which have provided evidence for a multitude of other factors and mechanisms contributing to HE, including other gut-derived neurotoxins, γ-aminobutyric acid (GABA) and other endogenous GABA receptor agonists, oxidative stress, inflammatory mediators, hyponatremia, and abnormal serotonin and histamine neurotransmission.[63] Nonetheless, ammonia and its effect on astrocytes play a central role in the pathogenesis of HE. MRI studies of patients with CLD and HE demonstrate a low-grade cerebral edema. However, in contradistinction to the cerebral edema associated with ALF, intracranial hypertension is rare.[64]

The initial step in evaluating the patient with liver disease who presents with encephalopathy is to rule out causes other than HE. The differential diagnosis includes other metabolic encephalopathies such as uremia, sepsis, glucose and electrolyte abnormalities, and endocrinopathies. Sepsis is a well-known precipitating factor for HE via inflammatory mediators such as TNF-α, and cytokines IL-1 and IL-6. Structural and vascular CNS lesions or CNS infections should also be considered. Because cirrhotic patients are exquisitely sensitive to sedative medications and have impaired hepatic (and often renal) metabolism, careful search for possible drug-related encephalopathy should be undertaken. Once other potential causes have been eliminated, the next step should be a systematic search for an underlying cause or precipitating factor (Table 46-8). Once identified, treatment or elimination should commence as soon as possible and may be sufficient for clinical improvement.

If addressing the underlying cause does not produce improvement, the next step is to employ therapy designed to either reduce the production of or increase the excretion of ammonia. Historically, the nonabsorbable disaccharide lactulose has been the mainstay of therapy and remains the first-line drug for treating HE.[65] Although the basis for its benefit is unclear, there are two proposed mechanisms for its salutary effect. First, anaerobic bacteria in the colon ferment lactulose to produce weak acids and acidify the colon. This acid milieu converts ammonia into ammonium, which is poorly absorbed. Secondly, it is proposed that this acid milieu is also cathartic, and that catharsis augments reduced absorption.

Although simple reduction in protein intake seems an intuitive solution, in fact protein restriction may be harmful for

Table 46-8 Precipitating Factors in Hepatic Encephalopathy
Constipation
Dehydration
Gastrointestinal bleeding
Bowel obstruction or ileus
Infection—e.g. spontaneous bacterial peritonitis, sepsis
Excessive dietary protein
Hypokalemia
Hypoglycemia
Hypothyroidism
Hypoxia
Metabolic alkalosis
Anemia
Azotemia/uremia
Hepatic malignancy
Transjugular intrahepatic portal shunt, surgical shunt
Vascular occlusion

cirrhotic patients who tend to have little nutritional reserve due to poor intake and who have likely lost nutritional ground with every hospitalization. Practice guidelines for the treatment of HE patients recommend a normal protein intake (1 to 1.5 g/kg/d), preferably in the form of plant-based rather than animal protein because of its higher calorie to nitrogen ratio.[65]

Zinc is a cofactor in the urea cycle and may be a dietary deficiency in cirrhotic patients. Although it is unclear which patients might benefit, practice guidelines recommend consideration of chronic zinc supplementation for HE patients.

Ascites

Ascites is the most common complication of cirrhosis leading to hospitalization. The occurrence of ascites marks a threshold in the nature of the underlying liver disease and is associated with a 70% mortality rate within 5 years.[66] Thus, the current recommendation is that patients who present with ascites and who are potential candidates for liver transplantation should be referred for liver transplantation evaluation. Not all ascites is hepatic in nature; about 15% has a nonhepatic etiology. Nonhepatic causes include malignancy, cardiac failure, renal disease, pancreatitis, and tuberculosis. Perhaps the most expeditious study to define the nature of new-onset ascites is a paracentesis. In particular, the serum–ascites albumin gradient (SAAG) is extremely useful for delineating portal hypertensive ascites from other causes. It is calculated as the difference between simultaneously measured serum and ascites albumin levels. A SAAG 1.1 mg/dL or more indicates portal hypertension with 97% accuracy. Standard initial therapy for portal hypertensive ascites is salt restriction (2 g/d) and diuretics. Hyponatremia is common among cirrhotic patients with ascites and generally does not warrant fluid restriction unless the serum sodium level is below 120 to 125 mEq/L. Rapid correction of hyponatremia is undesirable because cirrhotic patients are particularly at risk for osmotic demyelination syndrome (ODS), a potentially devastating neurologic complication. Current recommendations allow an increase of 4 to 6 mEq/L per day, not to exceed 8 mEq/L in 24 hours for patients with advanced liver disease.[66] This requires careful choices of IV fluids and medication diluents, particularly if one must compensate for administration of blood products which carry a high obligate sodium load. Consideration may be given to using a prothrombin complex instead of FFP and 25% albumin instead of 5% albumin to reduce exogenous sodium administration.

Refractory ascites, defined as ascites that is immutable to sodium restriction, maximum doses of diuretics, and paracentesis, heralds another change in the nature of the underlying cirrhosis. It is the hallmark complication of type II HRS and indicates increased disease severity. Once patients become refractory to maximum standard medical therapy, the 6-month mortality is 21%.[67] Therapeutic options for patients are limited and include serial paracentesis, liver transplantation, TIPS placement, and peritoneovenous shunt. Although current practice is to replace albumin when ascitic fluid is drained, this practice is not well supported by randomized prospective trials. The reasons for using albumin replacement include preventing paracentesis-induced circulatory dysfunction, minimizing electrolyte disturbances, minimizing the nutritional impact of albumin loss, and preventing renal impairment. Current recommendations are that patients with drainage volumes less than 5 L do not need albumin replacement; for larger volume paracentesis, 6 to 8 g albumin/L replacement may be considered.[66] TIPS placement can generally be expected to improve quality of life by obviating the need for serial paracentesis, but this must be balanced against an increase in encephalopathy and the high incidence of shunt malfunction.[68]

Peritoneovenous shunting is an older intervention that has generally fallen into disuse because of associated complications and lack of survival benefit. However, for patients who cannot easily travel for serial paracentesis and who are not candidates for TIPS or transplantation, this may be the only option.

Infections of ascitic fluid are sufficiently common that the American Association for the Study of Liver Diseases recommends paracentesis for all hospitalized patients with ascites. SBP is diagnosed when the polymorphonuclear (PMN) leukocyte count in ascitic fluid is 250 cells/mm^3 or more in the absence of any other identifiable intra-abdominal source. Bacterial translocation from the bowel is the most common source of SBP, although nosocomial infection from bacteremia associated with invasive procedures occurs as well. Because cell counts are available more quickly than culture results, the decision to treat is made empirically on that basis. Patients should immediately be treated with a broad-spectrum antibiotic. Sepsis may develop rapidly in these patients and SBP is a recognized precipitating factor for type I HRS. Because of this, timely administration of antibiotics in this fragile population is so important that empiric antibiotics are warranted even for patients who do not meet the diagnostic ascitic fluid PMN cell count but who exhibit signs and symptoms suggesting infection such as fever, abdominal pain, evidence of worsening hepatic or renal function, and otherwise unexplained worsening encephalopathy.

Varices

Varices, particularly esophageal varices, are one of the end results of portal hypertension. In cirrhosis, increases in portal pressure result from distorted hepatic architecture left in the wake of inflammatory insults. Fibrosis and regenerative nodules cause impedance to splanchnic flow through the liver and lead to formation of portosystemic collaterals, particularly with the gastric and esophageal venous systems. Progression of portal hypertension leads to increased local production of nitric oxide and, eventually, massive splanchnic vasodilation. Thus, portal hypertension becomes a problem of not only impedance to flow but also a massive increase in flow to the liver. Rupture of the high-pressure collaterals that are formed is a highly lethal and feared complication of portal hypertension.

Portal hypertension is diagnosed by measurement of the wedged hepatic venous pressure (WHVP). Although this is not a direct measure of portal pressure, WHVP has been demonstrated to correlate well with it. WHVP is measured by advancing a catheter into a hepatic vein to wedge position. To correct for the contribution of increased intra-abdominal pressure from ascites, a free hepatic venous pressure or an inferior vena caval pressure should be subtracted from the measured WHVP to give the HVPG. A normal HVPG is 3 to 5 mmHg. Patients with esophageal varices can be expected to have HVPGs of at least 10 to 12 mmHg.

Esophagogastroduodenoscopy is the gold-standard procedure for diagnosing varices. Presence of varices correlates with the severity of the underlying liver disease, with incidence increasing from 40% in Child's A patients to 85% in Child's C patients.

Nonselective β-blockers reduce portal pressure by two mechanisms: a decrease in cardiac output (β_1) and splanchnic vasoconstriction (β_2). Acute variceal bleed should be managed with a combination of volume resuscitation, correction of severe coagulopathy, pharmacologic manipulation of portal pressure, and endoscopic variceal ligation. The temptation to vigorously volume resuscitate and completely correct all coagulation abnormalities should be resisted. Because bleeding is, to some extent, a pressure-related phenomenon, aggressive volume replacement may lead to resistant or recurrent bleeding. The goal instead should be adequate resuscitation to maintain a hemoglobin level of 8 mg/dL and consideration of blood product transfusion to improve significant abnormalities in platelet count and INR. Elective intubation for airway protection is often warranted in these patients. Medications to reduce portal pressure include vasopressin and its analogues and somatostatin and its analogues. Although β-blockers can reduce portal pressures, their effect on systemic pressures makes them undesirable in this setting. Early endoscopic variceal ligation in combination with pharmacotherapy is the preferred treatment for acute variceal bleed.

Hepatocellular Carcinoma

Worldwide, primary liver cancer is the second leading cause of cancer-related deaths.[69] Of the primary liver cancers, hepatocellular cancer (HCC) is the most common, accounting for 75% of the diagnoses. Risk factors include chronic viral hepatitis infection, hemochromatosis, and cirrhosis of any provenance. The prevalence of underlying cirrhosis in patients with HCC is 80% to 90%. Even if the HCC patient does not have cirrhosis, there is almost always an underlying chronic hepatitis/chronic necroinflammatory state that seems to be a key ingredient for HCC.

Surgical resection is the optimal treatment for HCC for those patients who have sufficient hepatic reserve. Unfortunately, many patients with HCC have cirrhosis and are unable to tolerate resection. In the United States, fewer than 5% of patients are candidates for resection. Liver transplantation can be an option for those patients who are not resection candidates but whose disease can be expected to have transplant outcomes similar to that of other indications for transplant. There are several established criteria to identify those patients, the earliest being the Milan criteria (one tumor no larger than 5 cm or 3 tumors, no larger than 3 cm each). Other established criteria have attempted to refine appropriate selection for liver transplantation by manipulating size, number, and associated tumor marker levels in their constructs.[70]

Patients who are neither surgical candidates nor transplant candidates may be managed by radiofrequency ablation or chemoembolization of their tumors. In addition, some centers use these therapies to maintain transplant eligibility for patients on the waiting list.

Nonalcoholic Fatty Liver Disease

NAFLD describes a range of conditions characterized by excessive fat deposition in the liver. NAFLD ranges in severity from simple fat deposition (steatosis) to fat deposition together with inflammation and hepatocellular necrosis (steatohepatitis or NASH). Primary NAFLD is associated with insulin resistance and its attendant manifestations, which are components of the metabolic syndrome: obesity, central adiposity, type II diabetes, arterial hypertension, and hypertriglyceridemia. In fact, it is often referred to as the hepatic manifestation of the metabolic syndrome. Unsurprisingly, NAFLD is the most common cause of elevated liver enzymes in adults.[71] NAFLD may coexist with other hepatic pathologies and exacerbates damage when it appears together with chronic hepatitis C, hemochromatosis, or alcoholic liver disease.[72] Within the disease spectrum of NAFLD, only NASH is associated with the serious consequences of HCC and cirrhosis. The gold standard for distinguishing NASH from other NAFLD is liver biopsy with the key features of macrovesicular steatosis, lobular inflammation, hepatocyte ballooning, and often perisinusoidal fibrosis. The prevalence of NASH in the United States is estimated to be 3% to 5%.[71]

Chronic Cholestatic Disease

Biliary obstruction increases pressures in the bile ducts, leading to reflux of bile into the liver sinusoids where it may also communicate with the vascular system. Serum levels of bilirubin, bile salts, and AP (which is synthesized by the biliary epithelium) rise. If bacteria are present in bile, the patient is at risk for infectious complications such as ascending cholangitis, hepatic abscess, and sepsis. Cholestasis and hyperbilirubinemia are associated with an increased incidence of acute kidney injury. This may be mediated by endotoxemia, as the result of both sepsis and loss of bile salts to the vascular space. Bile salts are normally secreted into the intestine where they prevent bacterial overgrowth and bind endotoxin, thereby preventing its absorption into the portal circulation. Loss of intestinal bile salts because of biliary obstruction may cause portal and systemic endotoxemia, leading to kidney injury. Kidney injury may additionally be exacerbated by the induced diuresis, as well as impairment of myocardial contractility, resulting from elevated serum levels of bile salts. It has also been noted that patients who come to transplant for the chronic cholestatic diseases, PBC and primary sclerosing cholangitis (PSC), have evidence of preserved or hypercoagulability on the basis of increased incidence of portal venous thrombosis, elevated levels of thrombin–antithrombin (TAT) complexes, and thromboelastographic indices consistent with hypercoagulability.

Chronic cholestatic disease in the adult population is primarily the result of immunologic mechanisms resulting in PBC or PSC. These diseases are frequently associated with other autoimmune pathology.

PBC is a disease characterized by the progressive destruction of small intrahepatic bile ducts, together with portal inflammation that eventually leads to cirrhosis. The laboratory hallmark of PBC is the antimitochondrial antibody, which is present in 95% of patients. Liver biopsy confirms diagnosis and allows histologic disease staging. The typical disease course is one of steady progressive loss of small bile ducts together with increasing fibrosis, leading to cirrhosis over the course of 10 to 20 years. Ursodeoxycholic acid, which may have immunomodulatory effects, is the only drug demonstrated to retard progression of the disease and offer survival benefit. Liver transplantation is the most definitive therapy, but is associated with a recurrence rate of 10% to 35%.[73]

PSC is a progressive inflammatory disease of the medium and large intra- and extrahepatic bile ducts. The diagnostic studies of choice are ERCP and magnetic resonance cholangiopancreatography (MRCP), which reveal the characteristic beaded pattern of the biliary tree caused by multiple stenotic lesions. PSC has an extremely high association with inflammatory bowel disease (IBD), primarily ulcerative colitis but occasionally Crohn disease. It is also associated with other autoimmune diseases, such as insulin-dependent diabetes and psoriasis. Other contributors to the morbidity of PSC are recurrent bacterial cholangitis, cholangiocarcinoma, and, particularly in those patients with coexisting IBD, colon carcinoma. Over the average 15-year disease course of PSC, 15% to 30% of patients are likely to develop cholangiocarcinoma, which carries a very poor prognosis and may cause ineligibility for transplant.[74] Liver transplantation is the most definitive therapy for PSC but is associated with disease recurrence.

Preoperative Management

Hepatic Evaluation

The evaluation of hepatic function begins with a thorough history, starting with an inquiry into risk factors and the presence of symptoms attributable to CLD. Prior episodes of jaundice, particularly in relationship to surgical procedures and anesthesia, should be investigated. Alcohol consumption, use of recreational or illicit drugs, medications (including herbal products), presence of tattoos, sexual promiscuity, consumption of raw seafood, and a history of travel to areas in which hepatitis is endemic should be sought. Symptoms of fatigue, anorexia, weight loss, nausea, vomiting, easy bruising, pruritus, dark-colored urine, biliary colic, abdominal distention, and gastrointestinal bleeding warrant further investigation for the presence of liver disease.

Physical examination findings suggestive of active liver disease include icterus, palmar erythema, spider angiomas, gynecomastia, hepatosplenomegaly, ascites, testicular atrophy, petechiae, ecchymoses, and asterixis.

In the absence of findings suggestive of liver disease, routine laboratory tests to assess hepatocellular integrity and hepatic synthetic function are not warranted. Routine laboratory testing may yield false-positive results, and true-positive results are infrequent in asymptomatic patients. In a study of over 7,600 surgical patients who underwent routine preoperative screening, liver-enzyme tests were abnormal in 11 asymptomatic patients, roughly 1 of 700 (0.1%). Of the patients with elevations, 3 (1 in 2,500 or 0.04%) developed jaundice.[75]

Because the normal range for laboratory tests is defined as the mean plus or minus two standard deviations, 5% of normal patients can be expected to fall outside the normal range, with 2.5% following above the upper limit of normal. As a result, minor elevations of liver enzymes—those less than three times the normal range—may be of no clinical importance.[76] The recommended approach is to avoid testing liver enzymes in asymptomatic patients. Nonetheless, in the presence of abnormal results (in an asymptomatic patient) the safest approach is to repeat testing; in the absence of elevations greater than three times the upper limits of normal, it is reasonable to proceed with surgery.

In patients with more substantial elevations of liver enzymes, causes include alcohol abuse, medications, chronic hepatitis B and C, NASH, autoimmune hepatitis, hemochromatosis, Wilson disease, and α_1-antitrypsin deficiency. Nonhepatic causes include celiac sprue and muscle diseases. Medications include selected antibiotics, antiepileptic drugs, lipid-lowering agents, nonsteroidal anti-inflammatory agents, and sulfonylureas. Herbal medications and drugs of abuse are also associated with liver enzyme abnormalities.

Perioperative Risk Associated with Liver Disease

In patients with known liver disease, the etiology of hepatic dysfunction should be determined. Based on retrospective, small case series from the 1960s and 1970s, acute hepatitis confers a prohibitive risk for elective surgery. In a series of 36 patients with undiagnosed hepatitis who underwent laparotomy (for suspected biliary obstruction or hepatic malignancy) nearly one-third died. All patients with acute hepatitis, due to either virus or alcohol, died. The majority of patients suffered complications that included bacterial peritonitis, wound dehiscence, and hepatic failure.[77]

With improved diagnostic testing, which includes serologic testing for hepatitis C, ultrasound testing for gallstones, and improved imaging techniques for hepatic cancer, it is far more likely today that accurate diagnoses can be made preoperatively. As a result, laparotomies are unlikely in patients with unsuspected hepatitis. In the absence of accumulating evidence, consensus opinion is that elective surgery should be postponed in patients with acute hepatitis.[78]

Table 46-9 Modified Child–Pugh Score

	Points[a]		
Presentation	1	2	3
Albumin (g/dL)	>3.5	2.8–3.5	<2.8
Prothrombin time			
Seconds prolonged	<4	4–6	>6
International normalized ratio	<1.7	1.7–2.3	>2.3
Bilirubin (mg/dL)[b]	<2	2–3	>3
Ascites	Absent	Slight–moderate	Tense
Encephalopathy	None	Grade I–II	Grade III–IV

[a]Class A = 5 to 6 points; B = 7 to 9 points; C = 10 to 15 points.
[b]Cholestatic diseases (e.g., primary biliary cirrhosis) produce bilirubin elevations that are disproportionate to the hepatic dysfunction. Thus, the following adjustments should be made: Assign 1 point for a bilirubin level of 4 mg/dL; 2 points for bilirubin concentrations between 4 and 10 mg/dL; and 3 points for bilirubin >10 mg/dL.

In patients with CLD, it is not feasible to postpone surgery until recovery. A number of studies have investigated the risk of surgery in patients with cirrhosis.[79] Early studies identified various components of the Child–Turcotte–Pugh score, as well as the composite score, as important prognostic factors for perioperative mortality.

Child and Turcotte first described their classification system in 1964. They identified five factors—albumin, bilirubin, ascites, encephalopathy, and nutritional status—as important prognostic factors for patients with cirrhosis. Each of the factors was categorized according to three levels of severity and combined to generate a composite score leading to an assignment of one of three classes of severity (class A, B, or C, with C representing the most severe hepatic dysfunction). In 1972, Pugh modified the score, replacing nutritional status with PT (Table 46-9). The score was originally designed for patients undergoing portosystemic shunt procedures but has subsequently been applied to patients with cirrhosis undergoing other surgeries. In studies conducted over multiple decades, the modified Child score performed similarly in predicting postoperative mortality: 10% in Child A, 17% to 30% in Child B, and 60% to 80% in Child C.[79] As a comparison, the 3-month mortality for hospitalized patients not undergoing surgery was 4% for Child A, 14% for Child B, and 51% for Child C.

The MELD (Model for End-Stage Liver Disease) score was originally designed to predict mortality for patients undergoing transjugular intrahepatic portocaval shunt (TIPS) procedures.[80] Subsequently, it was identified as an improvement over the Child score for the allocation of organs for liver transplant candidates due to its replacement of the subjective elements of the Child score (ascites, encephalopathy) with more objective ones, INR and creatinine. The MELD score is a useful predictor of 90-day wait list mortality in liver transplant candidates.[81] The MELD score weighs the continuous variables linearly or logarithmically instead of assigning arbitrary categories, as is the case with the Child score: MELD score = $9.57 \times \log_e$ (creatinine mg/dL) + $3.78 \times \log_e$ (bilirubin mg/dL) + $11.2 \times \log_e$ (INR) + 6.43.

The MELD score appears to predict perioperative mortality of 5
cirrhotic patients. In a single-center study of 140 surgical procedures, the *c*-statistic for the MELD score's ability to predict 30-day

mortality was 0.72. A *c*-statistic of 0.5 indicates predictive ability similar to chance (a 50:50 likelihood of predicting the outcome), whereas a *c*-statistic of 0.7 and higher is considered useful. In the cohort of patients undergoing abdominal surgery, the *c*-statistic improved to 0.80. In this study, a MELD score between 25 and 30 was associated with a 30-day mortality of 50% after abdominal surgery.[82] Each point in the MELD score up to a score of 20 equated to an additional 1% mortality; each MELD point over 20 equated to an additional 2% mortality. A larger study of 772 cirrhotics found similar results; a MELD score of 25 was associated with a 30-day mortality of 50%. Other than the MELD score, other important predictors of perioperative mortality in cirrhotics were age (age >70 equated to 3 MELD points) and coexisting disease (ASA physical status > IV equated to 5 MELD points).[83] The perioperative complications encountered by cirrhotic patients include liver failure, postoperative bleeding, infection, and renal failure. These authors concluded that patients with a MELD score of less than 11 have a low postoperative mortality and represent an acceptable surgical risk. However, based on the list of complications, the authors recommend that these patients should preferably have surgery at institutions with a liver transplant center. In patients with a MELD score of 20 or higher, the high mortality risk contraindicates elective procedures until after liver transplantation.[83]

In 2021, a collaborative between the Department of Veterans Affairs (Veterans Outcomes and Costs Associated with Liver Disease, VOCAL) and University of Pennsylvania derived the VOCAL-Penn score from over 4,700 surgeries in 3,700 patients. The score consisted of nine variables, using only bilirubin from the MELD score in addition to eight other variables, including surgery category.[84] The c-statistic for the VOCAL-Penn score, 0.86, surpassed previous scoring systems. The calculator is available online (www.vocalpennscore.com).

6 Medical management undertaken to optimize cirrhotic patients undergoing surgery should be directed toward treating active infection, optimizing central blood volume and renal status while minimizing ascites, and improving encephalopathy and coagulopathy. However, there is little evidence to support specific goal-directed targets for preoperative care. The perioperative risk depends more on the operative site (as evidenced by the VOCAL-Penn score) and the degree of liver impairment than the anesthetic technique. Upper abdominal surgery (cholecystectomy), when compared to hysterectomy, was associated with liver-enzyme abnormalities, whereas the anesthetic technique (halothane, enflurane, or fentanyl) was not. In a retrospective study of 733 cirrhotic patients mortality was associated with a number of factors in addition to the Child score: male gender, the presence of ascites, cryptogenic cirrhosis (vs. other etiologies), elevated creatinine, preoperative infection, higher ASA physical status, and surgery on the respiratory system.[85] The presence of each additional factor conferred additional risk. For instance, 1-year mortality in patients with six risk factors was over 80%, whereas mortality with two risk factors was approximately 30%.

In addition to optimizing medical management, efforts should be made to minimize surgical risk through the consideration of less invasive surgery. Gallstones are twice as common in cirrhotic patients as in patients without cirrhosis. Laparoscopic surgery appears safe in patients with Child–Pugh A and B cirrhosis. Uncontrolled retrospective studies have suggested a lower mortality and shorter hospital stay; however, Child's C patients may benefit from percutaneous drainage of the gallbladder rather than a laparoscopic approach.[86] In a series of over 4,200 laparoscopic cholecystectomies from Taiwan, the group with cirrhosis ($n = 226$) had a mortality of approximately 1:100, whereas mortality was 1:2,000 for those without cirrhosis.[87] Meta-analyses of randomized trials in cirrhotic patients showed the laparoscopic approach was associated with less blood loss, shorter operative time, and shorter hospitalization compared to an open approach.[88,89] Preoperative decompression of portal hypertension by TIPS may improve outcomes in patients with severe portal hypertension.[90] However, TIPS is associated with increases in pulmonary artery pressure and can worsen encephalopathy.

Intraoperative Management

Monitoring and Vascular Access

In addition to routine noninvasive monitors, the need for arterial pressure monitoring should be considered for patients with end-stage liver disease. The decision is based on the presence of preoperative systemic hypotension due to vasodilation, anticipated blood loss, the need for intraoperative laboratory studies, coexisting disease, and age. Arterial cannulation should be considered in patients undergoing liver resection. The usefulness of CVP monitoring to predict fluid responsiveness has been questioned.[91] Some experts have abandoned CVP monitoring in the setting of liver resection. In our practice we do not place a CVP catheter exclusively for monitoring. Pulmonary artery catheterization is used for patients with known or suspected pulmonary artery hypertension and for patients with a low cardiac ejection fraction. Transesophageal echocardiography (TEE) is a sensitive monitor for the assessment of preload, contractility, ejection fraction, regional wall motion abnormalities, and emboli. In a small series of patients with esophageal varices, TEE universally aided in diagnosis and was not associated with bleeding complications, although transgastric views were avoided to minimize esophageal manipulation.[92] Other authors have confirmed the safety of TEE in this population.[93] Viscoelastic coagulation testing using thromboelastography (TEG) or thromboelastometry, if available, may be a useful guide for coagulation management.[29] Viscoelastic tests reflect the overall effects of altered levels of endogenous pro- and anticoagulant factors, which may be in balance if both are reduced proportionally. Recently, the clinical significance of an abnormal PT as a predictor of bleeding risk has been questioned because this test reflects only procoagulant factor levels rather than the rebalanced hemostatic system, which may be capable of normal thrombin generation.

Selection of Anesthetic Technique

Neuraxial versus General Anesthesia

The effect of neuraxial anesthesia on hepatic blood flow appears related to alterations of systemic blood pressure. More recent studies support the conclusion that hepatic blood flow is reduced by epidural anesthesia and interestingly, further reduced by an infusion of norepinephrine.[94] However, other studies suggest that vasopressors (ephedrine and dopamine) restore hepatic blood flow. Despite this confusing picture, high (T-5) neuraxial blocks appear to reduce hepatic blood flow, and this effect may not be reversed when block-related hypotension is corrected with catecholamines. Thus, avoidance of high neuraxial block and hypotension seems prudent in patients with advanced liver disease.

Standard contraindications to neuraxial blockade should be considered and weighed against the procedure's benefits on a case-by-case basis. Many patients with advanced hepatic disease may not warrant consideration for neuraxial techniques due to coagulopathy and/or thrombocytopenia. Nerve blockade may be appropriate even when neuraxial blockade is contraindicated. The transversus abdominis plane (TAP) and quadratus lumborum

(QL) blocks have been used successfully for abdominal surgery, including hepatobiliary procedures.[95,96]

Volatile Anesthetics

Volatile anesthetics decrease hepatic blood flow, albeit to a variable degree.

Halothane, still in use in developing countries, is more likely than other inhaled anesthetics to cause cardiovascular depression and results in the greatest reduction of hepatic blood flow. At anesthetic concentrations of 1 MAC, isoflurane and sevoflurane produce very little reduction in hepatic blood flow. However, desflurane appears to more substantially decrease hepatic blood flow at 1 MAC, causing a 30% reduction at this anesthetic depth. Animal studies suggest desflurane preserves total hepatic blood flow. At higher anesthetic concentrations, isoflurane results in a dose-dependent reduction in hepatic blood flow beyond that seen at 1 MAC. This dose-dependent reduction in hepatic blood flow does not occur with sevoflurane. In animal studies, both sevoflurane and isoflurane maintain the hepatic arterial buffer response, which increases hepatic arterial blood flow in the presence of reductions of portal blood flow.

In addition to variable effects on hepatic blood flow, concern exists regarding the production of reactive intermediates during the metabolism of volatile anesthetics. Halothane hepatitis, described earlier in this chapter, is largely responsible for these concerns. However, there is little evidence to suggest that other volatile anesthetics are responsible for hepatic complications. With the exception of sevoflurane, volatile anesthetics undergo metabolism that yields reactive TFA intermediates. These bind to hepatic proteins and produce an immunologic reaction. However, the incidence of liver injury correlates with the extent to which inhaled anesthetics undergo oxidative metabolism. Although 20% of halothane and 2.5% of enflurane are metabolized to TFA intermediates, the corresponding percentages for isoflurane and desflurane are 0.2% and 0.02%, respectively.[25]

Although there is a lack of evidence supporting a role for current volatile anesthetics in causing hepatic injury, several reports describe instances when repeated exposure to halogenated anesthetics was associated with hepatic dysfunction. Because there is no pathognomonic liver pathology, the diagnosis is based on the exclusion of other causes and a history of recent exposure. The potential for toxic metabolites seems related to the degree of in vivo biotransformation of the various halogenated anesthetics. Nonetheless, desflurane, which undergoes the least biotransformation, has been implicated in a case of hepatotoxicity in a patient who may have been sensitized by previous halothane exposure.[97]

Sevoflurane undergoes more extensive metabolism than isoflurane or desflurane, rapidly producing detectable plasma concentrations of fluoride and hexafluoroisopropanol (HFIP), which are conjugated by the liver and excreted by the kidney. In distinction to the other agents, sevoflurane does not produce reactive TFA metabolites or fluoroacetylated liver proteins. This fact led to the suggestion that patients sensitized to other volatile anesthetics could be safely anesthetized with sevoflurane.[98] Indeed, despite the more extensive metabolism, there is no evidence that sevoflurane's metabolites, including compound A (produced in a reaction with carbon dioxide absorbents), produce hepatic injury.[99] However, there are sporadic reports of ALF occurring after sevoflurane exposure.[100,101] Although the cause in this case is not certain, this report suggests that patients who are sensitized to one volatile anesthetic (i.e., evidence of hepatic injury following prior exposure) should not subsequently receive any other fluorinated anesthetic.

Nitrous Oxide

Nitrous oxide administration has not been shown to cause hepatocellular injury in the absence of hepatic hypoxemia. In patients with mild alcoholic hepatitis, techniques that incorporated nitrous oxide were not associated with biochemical worsening. Due to sympathomimetic effects, nitrous oxide can lead to decreased hepatic blood flow, and inhibition of methionine synthase can occur after even brief exposures. However, the clinical significance of these effects is unclear, although prolonged or repeated exposure could induce a vitamin B_{12} deficiency.[102]

Intravenous Anesthetics

IV anesthetics such as propofol, etomidate, and midazolam, do not appear to alter hepatic function when given for a short duration during minor procedures. The effects of IV anesthetics after prolonged infusions and in patients with advanced liver disease are not well studied. A rare syndrome of lactic acidosis, lipemia, rhabdomyolysis, hyperkalemia, myocardial failure, and death, first reported in children in the 1990s, was described after lengthy infusions of propofol. Patients on prolonged (>48 h), high dose (>5 mg/kg/h) propofol infusions should be monitored for worsening lactic acidosis and escalating vasopressor requirements. In the event of such findings, propofol should be discontinued and continuous hemofiltration considered.[103]

There is no evidence that opioids have an effect on hepatic function that is independent of hepatic blood flow. All opioids increase sphincter of Oddi pressure. Some authors have suggested that morphine causes spasm in the sphincter of Oddi, but a review failed to show a differential effect, concluding that morphine may be preferred over meperidine for the treatment of patients with acute pancreatitis due to less risk of seizures.[104]

Pharmacokinetic and Pharmacodynamic Alterations

The decreased functional mass of hepatocytes and reduced hepatic blood flow due to portocaval shunts lead to reduced metabolism of drugs that rely on hepatic metabolism for clearance.

Factors that affect hepatic clearance include blood flow to the liver, the fraction of the drug unbound to plasma proteins, and intrinsic clearance. Drugs with a low extraction ratio (less than 0.3) have restrictive hepatic clearance. Clearance of drugs in this class is affected by protein binding, the induction or inhibition of hepatic enzymes, age, and hepatic pathology, but clearance is not significantly affected by hepatic blood flow. Drugs with a high extraction ratio (greater than 0.7) undergo extensive first-pass metabolism, which alters their bioavailability after oral administration. Regardless of the route of administration, drugs with high extraction ratios are significantly affected by alteration in hepatic blood flow, which can occur with hemodynamic changes or hepatic inflow clamping during liver resection. High extraction ratio drugs tend to have short elimination half-lives (e.g., propranolol $t_{1/2} = 3.9$ hours).

Benzodiazepines are an example of a class of drugs with a low extraction ratio. As is commonly the case for drugs with low extraction ratios, the elimination half-lives can be long (diazepam $t_{1/2} = 43$ hours). Studies have shown conflicting effects of cirrhosis on the metabolism of midazolam, possibly due to changes in protein binding. As hepatic protein synthesis declines with advancing liver disease, the drug fraction bound to protein decreases. Because only the unbound drug is available for metabolism by hepatic enzymes, the elimination may be unaffected despite a reduction in intrinsic hepatic clearance. Bilirubin and bile acids can increase the unbound drug fraction by displacing drugs from protein binding sites. An increase in the free fraction of a drug leads to enhanced effects. The volume of distribution can increase with an increase in the unbound drug. The complex interactions that affect pharmacokinetics in patients with end-stage liver disease can result in unpredictable effects. However, the altered pharmacodynamic effects that occur in patients with encephalopathy frequently lead to an increased sensitivity to sedatives and analgesics.

Opioid metabolism is reduced in patients with liver disease. Dosing intervals should be increased to avoid drug accumulation. Prolonged elimination is more prominent with morphine and meperidine than the shorter duration synthetic opioids, although contradictory data exist that suggest pharmacokinetics is not significantly altered by liver disease. The clearance of the meperidine metabolite normeperidine is reduced in liver disease, which can lead to neurotoxicity. The elimination of a single IV opioid bolus is less affected than that of a continuous infusion due to redistribution to storage sites. Remifentanil, rapidly hydrolyzed by blood and tissue esterases, is an exception among the opioids as its elimination is independent of both hepatic function and the duration of infusion. The pharmacodynamic effects of opioids are altered by liver disease, which argues for a dose reduction in patients with advanced disease because of the ability to precipitate or worsen encephalopathy.

Most induction agents, including ketamine, etomidate, propofol, and thiopental, are highly lipophilic and have high extraction ratios. Although elimination should be prolonged in the presence of liver disease, clearance in cirrhotics is similar to normal patients. However, the pharmacodynamic effects are more pronounced, and in some cases, as with dexmedetomidine and the benzodiazepines, the duration of action can be prolonged.

The intermediate duration neuromuscular blocking agents metabolized by the liver, vecuronium and rocuronium, exhibit a prolonged duration of action in patients with liver disease. Pancuronium's action is also prolonged. Despite this, a resistance to the initial dose of neuromuscular blocker typically occurs due to elevated γ-globulin concentrations and an increase in the volume of distribution (due to edema and/or ascites). Atracurium and cisatracurium undergo organ-independent elimination. Their durations of action are not affected by liver disease. However, their metabolite, laudanosine, is eliminated by the liver but neurotoxicity has not been reported.[105] In cirrhotic patients, succinylcholine metabolism is altered due to reduced plasma cholinesterase activity; however, the clinical impact is rarely significant.

Vasopressors

In contrast to the increased response to sedatives, patients with liver disease exhibit a reduced response to endogenous vasoconstrictors, including angiotensin II, AVP, and norepinephrine.[106]

Hyporesponsiveness to catecholamines may be modulated by the release of nitric oxide, prostacyclin, and other endothelial-derived factors in response to humoral and mechanical stimuli.[107]

Volume Resuscitation

The selection of fluid and blood products for volume resuscitation is, in general, similar in patients with and without liver disease. However, in end-stage liver disease, serum albumin function is quantitatively and qualitatively decreased.[108] Albumin has three major indications in the treatment of cirrhotic patients.[109] The first is after large volume (4 to 5 L) paracentesis, which is relevant for intra-abdominal surgery. The second is in the presence of SBP to prevent renal impairment, specifically in patients with bilirubin greater than 4 mg/dL or creatinine greater than 1 mg/dL. The third is the presence of HRS-AKI, where its use is beneficial in conjunction with splanchnic vasoconstrictors.

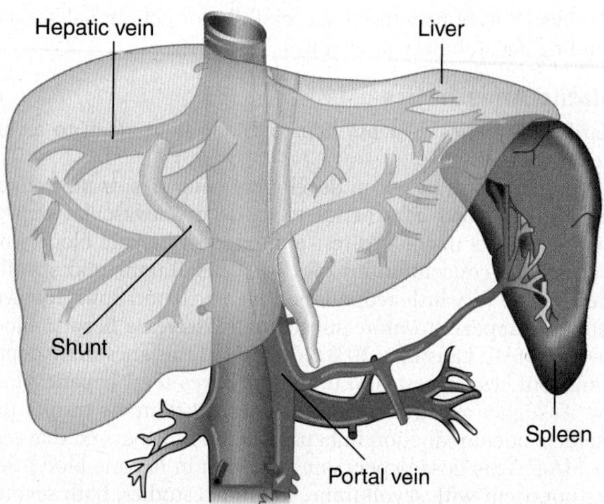

Figure 46-2 Transjugular intrahepatic portosystemic shunt procedure. A stent (or stents) is passed through the internal jugular vein over a wire into the hepatic vein. The wire and stent or stents are then advanced into the portal vein, after which blood can pass through the portal vein into the hepatic vein and bypass and decompress dilated esophageal veins.

Transjugular Intrahepatic Portosystemic Shunt Procedure

TIPS creates a connection between the portal and systemic circulations using a minimally invasive technique (Fig. 46-2). The indication is to decompress portal hypertension in the setting of esophageal varices and/or intractable ascites.

Sedation is commonly used to facilitate placement, though some proceduralists prefer general anesthesia, as it limits patient movement, controls diaphragmatic excursion, and reduces the risk of aspiration. In patients with recent variceal bleeding, volume resuscitation may be necessary. Due to coagulopathy, patients may require clotting factors and/or platelets before the procedure.[110,111] Complications include pneumothorax or vascular injury during access to the jugular vein. Dysrhythmias can occur during catheter insertion due to stimulation of the endocardium. Providers should be prepared for the possibility of hemorrhage, which can occur in the presence of extrahepatic artery or portal vein puncture. TIPS increases venous return, which can unmask undiagnosed cardiac dysfunction or pulmonary hypertension, two conditions with increased prevalence in patients with CLD.

Hepatic Resection

In the late 1800s, the first gastrectomies and cholecystectomies were performed in Europe, but surgery on the liver was regarded as dangerous, if not impossible. In 1908, Pringle described the technique of digital compression of the hepatic hilar vessels to control bleeding, which was a significant advance. Lortat-Jacob is credited with performing the first right hepatectomy in 1952. Another advance occurred in 1957 when segmental liver anatomy was described by Couinaud and others (Fig. 46-3).

Despite these advances, hepatic surgery was associated with operative mortality rates of 20% or more as recently as the 1980s (1 Video 46-1 and 2 Video 46-2). Hemorrhage was a significant cause of morbidity and mortality. Persistence, along with further advances in surgery, anesthesia, and intensive care led to

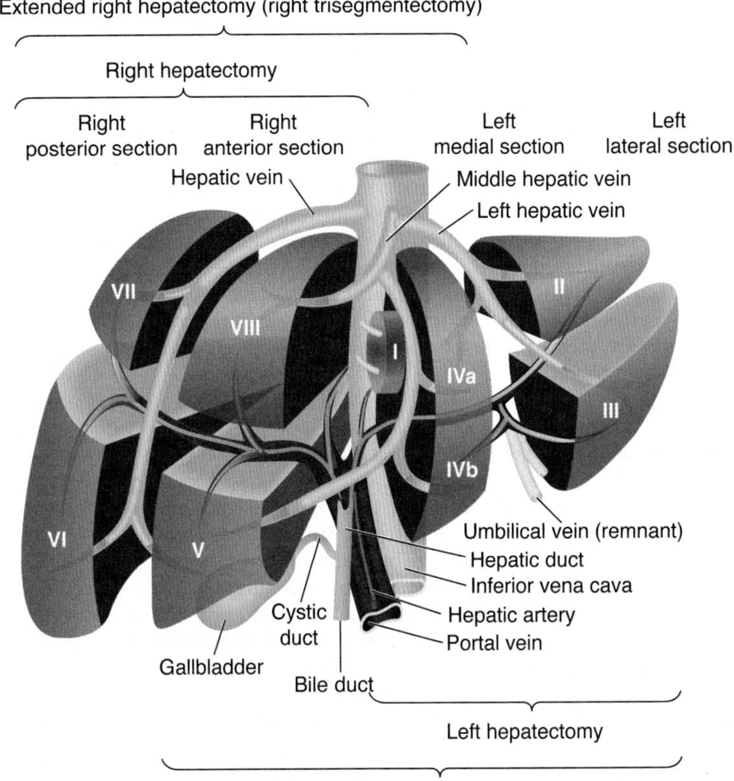

Figure 46-3 Schematic depiction of Couinaud segmental liver anatomy and the normal portal venous structures.

a reduction in mortality. Today, hepatic resections are performed with mortality rates of 5% or less. Partial hepatectomy in normal, noncirrhotic livers is associated with mortality rates of 1% to 2%. The percentage of patients requiring major hepatectomy (resection of three or more liver segments) for primary or secondary cancer appears to be decreasing; however, the perioperative mortality of major hepatectomy appears unchanged over time.[112] Further improvements in outcome are most likely to come from efforts to preserve parenchyma and prevent abdominal infection.

Improved surgical technique with avoidance of the thoracoabdominal approach (which was associated with high morbidity) contributes to improved outcomes. Smooth fracture of liver parenchyma accompanied by bipolar coagulation made parenchymal transection possible. New transection techniques using ultrasonic dissectors, high-pressure water jets, and/or harmonic scalpels may be helpful, but they have not been proven to be superior to conventional clamp crush techniques.[113] Preoperative imaging techniques delineate variations in portal, arterial, and bile duct anatomy.

Transfusion is necessary in less than 20% of patients. Yet, bleeding remains a major complication, and the hepatic veins are a significant source of blood loss. Maintaining CVP at a normal or even low (<5 cm H_2O) level has been suggested as a technique to limit blood loss.[114] However, some question the necessity of a low CVP technique given that blood loss is less significant in the current era. Whether a low CVP is deleterious to renal function is of uncertain clinical relevance.[115] Whether CVP is a reliable monitor of fluid responsiveness in liver surgery has also been questioned.[91] Two single-center series of living liver donors concluded that CVP is not a predictor of blood loss during hepatic resection.[116] A recent meta-analysis also concluded that optimal methods to lower CVP are uncertain and low CVP does not necessarily reduce morbidity.[114]

Vasopressors have a direct effect on splanchnic vessels, reducing splanchnic pressure and thereby decreasing blood loss.[117] Portal triad clamping (of the afferent vessels) and total vascular occlusion (of the afferent vessels plus the supra- and infrahepatic vena cava) are both effective in decreasing blood loss during hepatic resection. Portal triad clamping is better tolerated hemodynamically and has little effect on liver function if it is intermittent. Ischemic preconditioning (10-minute inflow occlusion, followed by a 10-minute reperfusion period) followed by continuous inflow clamping for up to 75 minutes was equally effective to intermittent inflow clamping (15-minute periods followed by 5-minute reperfusion) with regard to protection against postoperative liver injury in noncirrhotic patients undergoing hepatic resection. Ischemic preconditioning plus continuous clamping resulted in less blood loss than intermittent clamping.[118]

Air embolism, a known complication of hepatic resection, is more common when there is needed for a large hepatectomy (such as a right lobectomy), when the tumor is near the vena cava, or involves portal vessels. Low CVP may increase the risk of venous air embolism, though this has not been substantiated.

Even in patients with normal preoperative coagulation profiles, the INR and platelet count can be abnormal after liver resection. The severity of the derangement correlates with the extent of the resection, usually peaks on postoperative day 1 or 2 and takes 5 or more days to resolve. This has implications for choice of postoperative pain management technique, including the use of neuraxial analgesia. Some authors advise against preoperative epidural catheter placement, whereas others recommend correcting coagulation abnormalities prior to catheter removal.[119] Based on viscoelastic testing, a brief period of hypercoagulability may be present after liver resection despite a prolonged PT.[120] A large database review of >27,000 hepatopancreatobiliary surgeries showed no effect of epidural analgesia on mortality or morbidity, but a 0.5 day increase in length of stay.[121] Alternatives that avoid epidural catheter placement include intrathecal opioid combined with IV analgesics, and local anesthesia infusion systems.[122] Erector spinae plane blocks and posterior QL blocks appear equally effective in providing postoperative analgesia after laparoscopic liver resection.[123]

Surgical techniques for hepatic resection continue to evolve, though indications for newer procedures are not always clearly defined. Examples include minimally invasive liver surgery, thermal ablation of hepatic tumors, and portal vein embolization to induce hypertrophy of the remnant liver. Despite this, complications are common after hemihepatectomy (52% of 144 patients); these include pleural effusions, biliary leakage, wound dehiscence, ascites, and, intra-abdominal abscess.[124] In this series, a higher preoperative MELD score was associated with the development of complications.

Postoperative Liver Dysfunction

Postoperative liver dysfunction is characterized by the presence of asymptomatic elevation of hepatic transaminases, jaundice, and/or symptoms suggestive of liver failure, such as encephalopathy. Mild elevations of liver enzymes can occur after surgery, particularly upper abdominal procedures. Elevations that are less than several times the upper limit of normal are frequently transient and do not require rigorous investigation. More severe elevations suggest hepatocellular injury, which may have several etiologies, including hypoxemia, viral or bacterial insult, trauma, and chemical toxicity.

Asymptomatic, mild elevations of hepatic enzymes are common within hours after surgery, but they do not usually persist for more than 2 days. Such elevations were more common after halothane than enflurane administration (incidence of 50% vs. 20%, respectively); they are rare in patients without hepatic dysfunction and with the use of newer inhaled anesthetics.[125]

Persistent jaundice or more severe elevations of hepatic enzymes requires investigation. Hepatic hypoxemia can occur due to several mechanisms, including cardiopulmonary etiologies (pneumonia, atelectasis, heart failure), hypoperfusion (secondary to shock), anemia, or fever (Table 46-10). Surgery itself decreases hepatic blood flow. Reabsorption of surgical or traumatic hematomas and transfusion of red blood cells are major causes of postoperative jaundice. Ten percent of transfused red cells hemolyze within 24 hours of transfusion. The bilirubin load per unit transfused is 250 mg. The liver may take time to clear this significant bilirubin load.

Table 46-10 Causes of Postoperative Liver Dysfunction

Hepatocellular
Drugs
Anesthetics
Ischemia
Shock, hypotension, iatrogenic injury
Viral hepatitis
Cholestasis
Benign postoperative cholestasis
Sepsis
Bile duct injury
Drugs
Antibiotics, antiemetics
Choledocholithiasis or pancreatitis
Cholecystitis
Gilbert syndrome

Table 46-11 Causes of Hyperbilirubinemia

Unconjugated (Indirect)
Excessive bilirubin production (hemolysis)
Immaturity of enzyme systems
Physiologic jaundice of newborn
Jaundice of prematurity
Inherited defects
Gilbert syndrome
Crigler–Najjar syndrome
Drug effects
Conjugated (Direct)
Hepatocellular disease (hepatitis, cirrhosis, drugs)
Intrahepatic cholestasis (drugs, pregnancy)
Benign postoperative jaundice, sepsis
Congenital conjugated hyperbilirubinemia
Dubin–Johnson syndrome
Rotor syndrome
Obstructive jaundice
Extrahepatic (calculus, stricture, neoplasm)
Intrahepatic (sclerosing cholangitis, neoplasm, primary biliary cirrhosis)

Adapted from Friedman L, Martin P, Munoz S. Liver function tests and the objective evaluation of the patient with liver disease. In: Zakim D, Boyer T, eds. *Hepatology: A Textbook of Liver Disease*. 3rd ed. WB Saunders;1996:791.

Unconjugated hyperbilirubinemia suggests hemolysis, an inherited disorder such as Gilbert syndrome, or the less common Crigler–Najjar syndrome. In both syndromes, the absence or marked decrease of bilirubin glucuronyltransferase produces an unconjugated hyperbilirubinemia. Surgical and anesthetic problems are uncommon in patients with Gilbert and Crigler–Najjar syndromes. Hemoglobinopathies (e.g., sickle cell disease), erythrocyte metabolism defects (e.g., glucose-6-phosphate dehydrogenase deficiency), transfusion reactions, and prosthetic heart valves can also cause hemolysis.

If over 50% of bilirubin is conjugated, hepatocellular dysfunction is likely. Hypoxemia, toxic reactions, unsuspected preexisting liver disease, trauma, and congenital disorders should be considered (Table 46-11). Dubin–Johnson and Rotor syndromes are congenital disorders associated with a defect in bilirubin excretion, which causes a conjugated bilirubinemia. Surgery can worsen these syndromes.

The nature and site of the surgical procedure is an important risk factor for postoperative liver failure.[78] Abdominal surgery appears to reduce hepatic blood flow significantly. Abdominal traction can elevate prostaglandin levels, which may be a causal factor. Not surprisingly, hepatic resection is a risk factor for postoperative liver failure. The indication for resection in many patients is HCC, which is associated with chronic hepatitis or cirrhosis. The functional reserve of the remnant hepatic parenchyma is difficult to estimate in the cirrhotic liver. In a series of over 700 hepatic resections, patients with obstructive jaundice due to malignancy had a higher postoperative mortality (21%) than those with cirrhosis (8.7%), whereas patients with a normal liver had a postresection mortality of 1%.[126] When renal failure accompanies hyperbilirubinemia, the mortality exceeds 50%. Low intestinal levels of bile salts appear to promote the absorption of endotoxin from the gastrointestinal tract, whereas vasoconstrictive inflammatory mediators can precipitate renal hypoperfusion.

Cardiac surgery in patients with cirrhosis is not well tolerated. Cardiopulmonary bypass exacerbates preexisting hepatic disease by unknown mechanisms. The overall perioperative mortality in patients with cirrhosis was 31%; the mortality was 80% in patients with Child's B cirrhosis.[127] A systematic review of cardiac surgery in cirrhotic patients reported 1-year mortality of 27%, 66%, and 79% in Child's A, B, and C patients, respectively, results that are similar to those published a decade earlier.[128] For comparison, the mortality in patients without cirrhosis is approximately 2%.[129]

Conclusions

In patients with new-onset liver disease, elective surgery should be postponed until the course of the disease is known. In patients with preexisting liver disease, the severity of the disease should be characterized to assess risk. In patients with MELD scores of 20 or higher, or Child Class C, elective high-risk procedures (abdominal and cardiac surgery) should be deferred until after liver transplantation. Patients with MELD scores of less than 11 represent an acceptable risk. End-stage liver disease patients with a risk of postoperative liver failure should have elective abdominal surgery at institutions with a liver transplant program. Although no anesthetic technique is universally preferred, the presence of coagulopathy may contraindicate neuraxial regional techniques. The chosen technique should be designed to maintain splanchnic, hepatic, and renal perfusion. When surgery is unavoidable in patients with advanced liver disease, transfer to a liver transplant center should be considered in order to facilitate pretransplant evaluation and listing.

Acknowledgments

We gratefully acknowledge the contributions of previous edition authors, Brian S. Kaufman and J. David Roccaforte, as portions of their chapter have been retained in this revision.

For further review and interactivities, please see the videos and narrative interactive clinical vignettes (NICVs) accessible in the complimentary eBook bundled with this text. Access instructions are located on the inside front cover.

REFERENCES

1. Bochnakova T. Hepatic venous pressure gradient. *Clin Liver Dis (Hoboken)*. 2021;17(3):144–148. doi:10.1002/cld.1031
2. Eipel C, Abshagen K, Vollmar B. Regulation of hepatic blood flow: the hepatic arterial buffer response revisited. *World J Gastroenterol*. 2010;16(48):6046–6057. doi:10.3748/wjg.v16.i48.6046
3. Qin L, Crawford J. Anatomy and cellular functions of the liver. In: *Zakim and Boyer's Hepatology: A Textbook of Liver Disease*. 7th ed. Elsevier; 2018:2–19.
4. Olthoff KM. Hepatic regeneration in living donor liver transplantation. *Liver Transpl*. 2003;9(10 Suppl 2):S35–S41. doi:10.1053/jlts.2003.50229
5. Viebahn CS, Benseler V, Holz LE, et al. Invading macrophages play a major role in the liver progenitor cell response to chronic liver injury. *J Hepatol*. 2010;53(3):500–507. doi:10.1016/j.jhep.2010.04.010
6. Ofek F, Bar Chaim S, Kronenfeld N, Ziv-Baran T, Berkovitch M. International normalized ratio is significantly elevated with rivaroxaban and apixaban drug therapies: a retrospective study. *Clin Ther*. 2017;39(5):1003–1010. doi:10.1016/j.clinthera.2017.04.007
7. Balci NC, Befeler AS, Leiva P, Pilgram TK, Havlioglu N. Imaging of liver disease: comparison between quadruple-phase multidetector computed tomography and magnetic resonance imaging. *J Gastroenterol Hepatol*. 2008;23(10):1520–1527. doi:10.1111/j.1440-1746.2008.05434.x
8. Kochanek KD, Murphy SL, Xu JQ, Arias E. Deaths: Final data for 2017. National Vital Statistics Reports; vol 68 no 9. Hyattsville, MD: National Center for Health Statistics. 2019.
9. Younossi ZM, Stepanova M, Younossi Y, et al. Epidemiology of chronic liver diseases in the USA in the past three decades. Gut. 2020;69(3):564–568. doi: 10.1136/gutjnl-2019-318813.
10. Lee WM, Squires RH, Nyberg SL, Doo E, Hoofnagle JH. Acute liver failure: Summary of a workshop. *Hepatology*. 2008;47(4):1401–1415. doi:10.1002/hep.22177
11. Lee WM, Stravitz RT, Larson AM. Introduction to the revised American Association for the Study of Liver Diseases Position Paper on acute liver failure 2011. *Hepatology*. 2012;55(3):965–967. doi:10.1002/hep.25551
12. Murphy N, Auzinger G, Bernel W, Wendon J. The effect of hypertonic sodium chloride on intracranial pressure in patients with acute liver failure. *Hepatology*. 2004;39(2):464–470. doi:10.1002/hep.20056
13. Vasques F, Cavazza A, Bernal W. Acute liver failure. *Curr Opin Crit Care*. 2022;28(2):198–207. doi:10.1097/MCC.0000000000000923
14. Raschke RA, Curry SC, Rempe S, et al. Results of a protocol for the management of patients with fulminant liver failure. *Crit Care Med*. 2008;36(8):2244–2248. doi:10.1097/CCM.0b013e31818029a3
15. Bismuth H, Samuel D, Castaing D, et al. Orthotopic liver transplantation in fulminant and subfulminant hepatitis. The Paul Brousse experience. *Ann Surg*. 1995;222(2):109–119. doi:10.1097/00000658-199508000-00002
16. Cholongitas E, Theocharidou E, Vasianopoulou P, et al. Comparison of the sequential organ failure assessment score with the King's College Hospital criteria and the model for end-stage liver disease score for the prognosis of acetaminophen-induced acute liver failure. *Liver Transplant*. 2012;18(4):405–412. doi:10.1002/lt.23370
17. Riordan SM, Williams R. Mechanisms of hepatocyte injury, multiorgan failure, and prognostic criteria in acute liver failure. *Semin Liver Dis*. 2003;23(3):203–215. doi:10.1055/s-2003-42639
18. Flamm SL, Yang Y-X, Singh S, Falck-Ytter YT; AGA Institute Clinical Guidelines Committee. American Gastroenterological Association Institute Guidelines for the diagnosis and management of acute liver failure. *Gastroenterology*. 2017;152(3):644–647. doi:10.1053/j.gastro.2016.12.026
19. Rovegno M, Vera M, Ruiz A, Benítez C. Current concepts in acute liver failure. *Ann Hepatol*. 2019;18(4):543–552. doi:10.1016/j.aohep.2019.04.008
20. Lisman T, Bakhtiari K, Pereboom IT, Hendriks HG, Meijers JC, Porte RJ. Normal to increased thrombin generation in patients undergoing liver transplantation despite prolonged conventional coagulation tests. *J Hepatol*. 2010;52(3):355–361.
21. De Pietri L, Bianchini M, Montalti R, et al. Thrombelastography-guided blood product use before invasive procedures in cirrhosis with severe coagulopathy: a randomized, controlled trial. *Hepatology*. 2016;63(2):566–573. doi:10.1002/hep.28148
22. Ghany MG, Strader DB, Thomas DL, Seeff LB; American Association for the Study of Liver Diseases. Diagnosis, management, and treatment of hepatitis C: an update. *Hepatology*. 2009;49(4):1335–1374. doi:10.1002/hep.22759
23. Watkins PB, Seeff LB. Drug-induced liver injury: summary of a single topic clinical research conference. *Hepatology*. 2006;43(3):618–631. doi:10.1002/hep.21095
24. Kenna JG, Satoh H, Christ DD, Pohl LR. Metabolic basis for a drug hypersensitivity: antibodies in sera from patients with halothane hepatitis recognize liver neoantigens that contain the trifluoroacetyl group derived from halothane. *J Pharmacol Exp Ther*. 1988;245(3):1103–1109.
25. Njoku D, Laster MJ, Gong DH, Eger EI 2nd, Reed GF, Martin JL. Biotransformation of halothane, enflurane, isoflurane, and desflurane to trifluoroacetylated liver proteins: association between protein acylation and hepatic injury. *Anesth Analg*. 1997;84(1):173–178. doi:10.1097/00000539-199701000-00031
26. Fell DB, Dodds L, Joseph KS, Allen VM, Butler B. Risk factors for hyperemesis gravidarum requiring hospital admission during pregnancy. *Obstet Gynecol*. 2006;107(2 Pt 1):277–284. doi:10.1097/01.AOG.0000195059.82029.74
27. Bacq Y. Liver diseases unique to pregnancy: a 2010 update. *Clin Res Hepatol Gastroenterol*. 2011;35(3):182–193. doi:10.1016/j.clinre.2010.11.011
28. Ripoll C. Hepatic venous pressure gradient and outcomes in cirrhosis. *J Clin Gastroenterol*. 2007;41 Suppl 3:S330–S335. doi:10.1097/MCG.0b013e318150d0f4
29. Tripodi A. Tests of coagulation in liver disease. *Clin Liver Dis*. 2009;13(1):55–61. doi:10.1016/j.cld.2008.09.002
30. Segal JB, Dzik WH, Transfusion Medicine/Hemostasis Clinical Trials Network1. Paucity of studies to support that abnormal coagulation test results predict bleeding in the setting of invasive procedures: an evidence-based review. *Transfusion (Paris)*. 2005;45(9):1413–1425. doi:10.1111/j.1537-2995.2005.00546.x
31. Tripodi A, Primignani M, Chantarangkul V, et al. Thrombin generation in patients with cirrhosis: the role of platelets. *Hepatology*. 2006;44(2):440–445. doi:10.1002/hep.21266
32. Lisman T, Bongers TN, Adelmeijer J, et al. Elevated levels of von Willebrand Factor in cirrhosis support platelet adhesion despite reduced functional capacity. *Hepatology*. 2006;44(1):53–61. doi:10.1002/hep.21231
33. Northup PG, McMahon MM, Ruhl AP, et al. Coagulopathy does not fully protect hospitalized cirrhosis patients from peripheral venous thromboembolism.: CME. *Am J Gastroenterol*. 2006;101(7):1524–1528. doi:10.1111/j.1572-0241.2006.00588.x
34. Søgaard KK, Horváth-Puhó E, Grønbaek H, Jepsen P, Vilstrup H, Sørensen HT. Risk of venous thromboembolism in patients with liver disease: a nationwide population-based case-control study. *Am J Gastroenterol*. 2009;104(1):96–101. doi:10.1038/ajg.2008.34

35. Amitrano L, Guardascione MA, Brancaccio V, Balzano A. Coagulation disorders in liver disease. *Semin Liver Dis*. 2002;22:83–96.
36. Kujovich JL. Hemostatic defects in end stage liver disease. *Crit Care Clin*. 2005;21(3):563–587. doi:10.1016/j.ccc.2005.03.002
37. Puoti C, Bellis L, Guarisco R, et al. Quantitation of tissue polypeptide antigen (TPA) in hepatic and systemic circulation in patients with chronic liver diseases. *J Gastroenterol Hepatol*. 2009;24(12):1847–1851. doi:10.1111/j.1440-1746.2009.05916.x
38. Moller S, Henriksen JH. Cardiovascular complications of cirrhosis. *Gut*. 2008;57(2):268–278. doi:10.1136/gut.2006.112177
39. Schepke M, Heller J, Paschke S, et al. Contractile hyporesponsiveness of hepatic arteries in humans with cirrhosis: evidence for a receptor-specific mechanism. *Hepatology*. 2001;34(5):884–888. doi:10.1053/jhep.2001.28794
40. Wong F, Girgrah N, Graba J, Allidina Y, Liu P, Blendis L. The cardiac response to exercise in cirrhosis. *Gut*. 2001;49(2):268–275.
41. Puthumana L, Chaudhry V, Thuluvath PJ. Prolonged QTc interval and its relationship to autonomic cardiovascular reflexes in patients with cirrhosis. *J Hepatol*. 2001;35(6):733–738.
42. Raval Z, Harinstein ME, Skaro AI, et al. Cardiovascular risk assessment of the liver transplant candidate. *J Am Coll Cardiol*. 2011;58(3):223–231. doi:10.1016/j.jacc.2011.03.026
43. Wray CL. Liver transplantation in patients with cardiac disease. *Semin Cardiothorac Vasc Anesth*. 2018;22(2):111–121.
44. McGuire BM, Julian BA, Bynon JS, et al. Brief communication: glomerulonephritis in patients with hepatitis C cirrhosis undergoing liver transplantation. *Ann Intern Med*. 2006;144(10):735–741. doi:10.7326/0003-4819-144-10-200605160-00007
45. Guevara M, Fernández-Esparrach G, Alessandria C, et al. Effects of contrast media on renal function in patients with cirrhosis: a prospective study. *Hepatology*. 2004;40(3):646–651. doi:10.1002/hep.20373
46. Garcia-Tsao G, Parikh CR, Viola A. Acute kidney injury in cirrhosis. *Hepatology*. 2008;48(6):2064–2077. doi:10.1002/hep.22605
47. Salerno F, Guevara M, Bernardi M, et al. Refractory ascites: pathogenesis, definition and therapy of a severe complication in patients with cirrhosis. *Liver Int*. 2010;30(7):937–947. doi:10.1111/j.1478-3231.2010.02272.x
48. Solà E, Ginès P. Renal and circulatory dysfunction in cirrhosis: current management and future perspectives. *J Hepatol*. 2010;53(6):1135–1145. doi:10.1016/j.jhep.2010.08.001
49. Charlton MR, Wall WJ, Ojo AO, et al. Report of the first international liver transplantation society expert panel consensus conference on renal insufficiency in liver transplantation. *Liver Transpl*. 2009;15(11):S1–S34. doi:10.1002/lt.21877
50. Palma DT, Fallon MB. The hepatopulmonary syndrome. *J Hepatol*. 2006;45(4):617–625. doi:10.1016/j.jhep.2006.07.002
51. Rodríguez-Roisin R, Krowka MJ. Hepatopulmonary syndrome–a liver-induced lung vascular disorder. *N Engl J Med*. 2008;358(22):2378–2387. doi:10.1056/NEJMra0707185
52. Krowka MJ, Plevak DJ, Findlay JY, Rosen CB, Wiesner RH, Krom RA. Pulmonary hemodynamics and perioperative cardiopulmonary-related mortality in patients with portopulmonary hypertension undergoing liver transplantation. *Liver Transpl*. 2000;6:443–450.
53. Iyer VN, Swanson KL, Cartin-Ceba R, et al. Hepatopulmonary syndrome: favorable outcomes in the MELD exception era. *Hepatology*. 2013;57(6):2427–2435. doi:10.1002/hep.26070
54. Simonneau G, Montani D, Celermajer DS, et al. Haemodynamic definitions and updated clinical classification of pulmonary hypertension. *Eur Respir J*. 2019;53(1):1801913. doi:10.1183/13993003.01913-2018
55. Hadengue A, Benhayoun MK, Lebrec D, Benhamou JP. Pulmonary hypertension complicating portal hypertension: prevalence and relation to splanchnic hemodynamics. *Gastroenterology*. 1991;100(2):520–528.
56. McDonnell PJ, Toye PA, Hutchins GM. Primary pulmonary hypertension and cirrhosis: are they related? *Am Rev Respir Dis*. 1983;127(4):437–441. doi:10.1164/arrd.1983.127.4.437
57. Kawut SM, Krowka MJ, Trotter JF, et al. Clinical risk factors for portopulmonary hypertension. *Hepatology*. 2008;48(1):196–203. doi:10.1002/hep.22275
58. Le Pavec J, Souza R, Herve P, et al. Portopulmonary hypertension: survival and prognostic factors. *Am J Respir Crit Care Med*. 2008;178(6):637–643. doi:10.1164/rccm.200804-613OC
59. Kim W, Krowka MJ, Plevak DJ, et al. Accuracy of Doppler echocardiography in the assessment of pulmonary hypertension in liver transplant candidates. *Liver Transpl*. 2000;6(4):453–458. doi:10.1053/jlts.2000.7573
60. Soulaidopoulos S, Goulis I, Cholongitas E. Pulmonary manifestations of chronic liver disease: a comprehensive review. *Ann Gastroenterol*. 2020;33(3):237–249. doi:10.20524/aog.2020.0474
61. Reichenberger F, Voswinckel R, Steveling E, et al. Sildenafil treatment for portopulmonary hypertension. *Eur Respir J*. 2006;28(3):563–567. doi:10.1183/09031936.06.00030206
62. Krowka MJ, Fallon MB, Kawut SM, et al. International Liver Transplant Society Practice Guidelines: diagnosis and management of hepatopulmonary syndrome and portopulmonary hypertension. *Transplantation*. 2016;100(7):1440–1452. doi:10.1097/TP.0000000000001229
63. Bass NM, Mullen KD, Sanyal A, et al. Rifaximin treatment in hepatic encephalopathy. *N Engl J Med*. 2010;362(12):1071–1081.
64. Cudalbu C, Taylor-Robinson SD. Brain edema in chronic hepatic encephalopathy. *J Clin Exp Hepatol*. 2019;9(3):362–382. doi:10.1016/j.jceh.2019.02.003
65. Blei AT. Pathophysiology of brain edema in fulminant hepatic failure, revisited. *Metab Brain Dis*. 2001;16:85–94.
66. Biggins SW, Angeli P, Garcia-Tsao G, et al. Diagnosis, evaluation, and management of ascites, spontaneous bacterial peritonitis and hepatorenal syndrome: 2021 Practice Guidance by the American Association for the Study of Liver Diseases. *Hepatology*. 2021;74(2):1014–1048. doi:10.1002/hep.31884
67. Ginès P, Cárdenas A, Arroyo V, Rodés J. Management of cirrhosis and ascites. *N Engl J Med*. 2004;350(16):1646–1654. doi:10.1056/NEJMra035021
68. D'Amico G, Luca A, Morabito A, Miraglia R, D'Amico M. Uncovered transjugular intrahepatic portosystemic shunt for refractory ascites: a meta-analysis. *Gastroenterology*. 2005;129(4):1282–1293. doi:10.1053/j.gastro.2005.07.031
69. McGlynn KA, Petrick JL, El-Serag HB. Epidemiology of hepatocellular carcinoma. *Hepatology*. 2021;73 Suppl 1:4–13. doi:10.1002/hep.31288
70. Lozanovski VJ, Ramouz A, Aminizadeh E, et al. Prognostic role of selection criteria for liver transplantation in patients with hepatocellular carcinoma: a network meta-analysis. *BJS Open*. 2022;6(1):zrab130. doi: 10.1093/bjsopen/zrab130
71. Vernon G, Baranova A, Younossi ZM. Systematic review: the epidemiology and natural history of non-alcoholic fatty liver disease and non-alcoholic steatohepatitis in adults. *Aliment Pharmacol Ther*. 2011;34(3):274–285. doi:10.1111/j.1365-2036.2011.04724.x
72. Ratziu V, Bellentani S, Cortez-Pinto H, Day C, Marchesini G. A position statement on NAFLD/NASH based on the EASL 2009 special conference. *J Hepatol*. 2010;53(2):372–384. doi:10.1016/j.jhep.2010.04.008
73. El-Masry M, Puig CA, Saab S. Recurrence of non-viral liver disease after orthotopic liver transplantation. *Liver Int*. 2011;31(3):291–302. doi:10.1111/j.1478-3231.2010.02434.x
74. McGill JM, Kwiatkowski AP. Cholestatic liver diseases in adults. *Am J Gastroenterol*. 1998;93(5):684–691. doi:10.1111/j.1572-0241.1998.206_a.x
75. Schemel WH. Unexpected hepatic dysfunction found by multiple laboratory screening. *Anesth Analg*. 1976;55(6):810–812. doi:10.1213/00000539-197611000-00013
76. Kasarala G, Tillmann HL. Standard liver tests. *Clin Liver Dis (Hoboken)*. 2016;8(1):13–18. doi:10.1002/cld.562
77. Powell-Jackson P, Greenway B, Williams R. Adverse effects of exploratory laparotomy in patients with unsuspected liver disease. *Br J Surg*. 1982;69(8):449–451. doi:10.1002/bjs.1800690805
78. Friedman LS. Surgery in the patient with liver disease. *Trans Am Clin Climatol Assoc*. 2010;121:192–204; discussion 205.
79. Neeff H, Mariaskin D, Spangenberg H-C, Hopt UT, Makowiec F. Perioperative mortality after non-hepatic general surgery in patients with liver cirrhosis: an analysis of 138 operations in the 2000s using Child and MELD Scores. *J Gastrointest Surg*. 2011;15(1):1–11. doi:10.1007/s11605-010-1366-9
80. Malinchoc M, Kamath PS, Gordon FD, Peine CJ, Rank J, ter Borg PC. A model to predict poor survival in patients undergoing transjugular intrahepatic portosystemic shunts. *Hepatology*. 2000;31(4):864–871. doi:10.1053/he.2000.5852
81. Freeman RB Jr, Wiesner RH, Harper A, et al. The new liver allocation system: moving toward evidence-based transplantation policy. *Liver Transplant*. 2002;8(9):851–858. doi:10.1053/jlts.2002.35927
82. Northup PG, Wanamaker RC, Lee VD, Adams RB, Berg CL. Model for end-stage liver disease (MELD) predicts nontransplant surgical mortality in patients with cirrhosis. *Ann Surg*. 2005;242(2):244–251. doi:10.1097/01.sla.0000171327.29262.e0
83. Teh SH, Nagorney DM, Stevens SR, et al. Risk factors for mortality after surgery in patients with cirrhosis. *Gastroenterology*. 2007;132(4):1261–1269. doi:10.1053/j.gastro.2007.01.040
84. Mahmud N, Fricker Z, Hubbard RA, et al. Risk prediction models for post-operative mortality in patients with cirrhosis. *Hepatology*. 2021;73(1):204–218. doi:10.1002/hep.31558
85. Ziser A, Plevak DJ, Wiesner RH, Rakela J, Offord KP, Brown DL. Morbidity and mortality in cirrhotic patients undergoing anesthesia and surgery. *Anesthesiology*. 1999;90(1):42–53. doi:10.1097/00000542-199901000-00008
86. Currò G, Iapichino G, Melita G, Lorenzini C, Cucinotta E. Laparoscopic cholecystectomy in Child-Pugh class C cirrhotic patients. *JSLS*. 2005;9(3):311–315.
87. Yeh CN, Chen MF, Jan YY. Laparoscopic cholecystectomy in 226 cirrhotic patients. Experience of a single center in Taiwan. *Surg Endosc*. 2002;16(11):1583–1587. doi:10.1007/s00464-002-9026-0
88. Cheng Y, Xiong XZ, Wu S-J, Lin Y-X, Cheng N-S. Laparoscopic vs. open cholecystectomy for cirrhotic patients: a systematic review and meta-analysis. *Hepatogastroenterology*. 2012;59(118):1727–1734. doi:10.5754/hge11688
89. Wang SY, Yeh CN, Jan YY, Chen MF. Management of gallstones and acute cholecystitis in patients with liver cirrhosis: what should we consider when performing surgery? *Gut Liver*. 2021;15(4):517–527. doi:10.5009/gnl20052
90. Azoulay D, Buabse F, Damiano I, et al. Neoadjuvant transjugular intrahepatic portosystemic shunt: a solution for extrahepatic abdominal operation in cirrhotic patients with severe portal hypertension. *J Am Coll Surg*. 2001;193(1):46–51. doi:10.1016/s1072-7515(01)00911-5
91. Marik PE, Baram M, Vahid B. Does Central Venous Pressure Predict Fluid Responsiveness? A systematic review of the literature and the tale of seven mares. *Chest*. 2008;134(1):172–178. doi:10.1378/chest.07-2331

92. Spier BJ, Larue SJ, Teelin TC, et al. Review of complications in a series of patients with known gastro-esophageal varices undergoing transesophageal echocardiography. *J Am Soc Echocardiogr*. 2009;22(4):396–400. doi:10.1016/j.echo.2009.01.002
93. Myo Bui CC, Worapot A, Xia W, et al. Gastroesophageal and hemorrhagic complications associated with intraoperative transesophageal echocardiography in patients with model for end-stage liver disease score 25 or higher. *J Cardiothorac Vasc Anesth*. 2015;29(3):594–597. doi:10.1053/j.jvca.2014.10.030
94. Meierhenrich R, Wagner F, Schütz W, et al. The effects of thoracic epidural anesthesia on hepatic blood flow in patients under general anesthesia. *Anesth Analg*. 2009;108(4):1331–1337. doi:10.1213/ane.0b013e3181966e6f
95. Niraj G, Kelkar A, Jeyapalan I, et al. Comparison of analgesic efficacy of subcostal transversus abdominis plane blocks with epidural analgesia following upper abdominal surgery. *Anaesthesia*. 2011;66(6):465–471. doi:10.1111/j.1365-2044.2011.06700.x
96. Ökmen K, Metin Ökmen B, Sayan E. Ultrasound-guided lateral versus posterior Quadratus Lumborum Block for postoperative pain after laparoscopic cholecystectomy: a randomized controlled trial. *Turk J Surg*. 2019;35(1):23–29. doi:10.5578/turkjsurg.4161
97. Berghaus TM, Baron A, Geier A, Lamerz R, Paumgartner G. Hepatotoxicity following desflurane anesthesia. *Hepatology*. 1999;29(2):613–614. doi:10.1002/hep.510290211
98. Martin JL. [Volatile anesthetics and liver injury: a clinical update or what every anesthesiologist should know]. *Can J Anaesth*. 2005;52(2):125–129. doi:10.1007/BF03027715
99. Obata R, Bito H, Ohmura M, et al. The effects of prolonged low-flow sevoflurane anesthesia on renal and hepatic function. *Anesth Analg*. 2000;91(5):1262–1268. doi:10.1097/00000539-200011000-00039
100. Lehmann A, Neher M, Kiessling A-H, Isgro F, Koloska A, Boldt J. Case report: fatal hepatic failure after aortic valve replacement and sevoflurane exposure. *Can J Anaesth*. 2007;54(11): 917–921. doi:10.1007/BF03026797
101. Masin-Spasovska J, Dimitrovski K, Stavridis S, et al. Acute fulminant hepatatis in kidney transplant recipient after repeated sevoflurane anesthesia–a case report and literature review. *Curr Drug Saf*. 2013;8(2):141–144. doi:10.2174/15748863113089990026
102. Edigin E, Ajiboye O, Nathani A. Nitrous oxide-induced B12 deficiency presenting with myeloneuropathy. *Cureus*. 2019;11(8):e5331. doi:10.7759/cureus.5331
103. Hemphill S, McMenamin L, Bellamy MC, Hopkins PM. Propofol infusion syndrome: a structured literature review and analysis of published case reports. *Br J Anaesth*. 2019;122(4): 448–459. doi:10.1016/j.bja.2018.12.025
104. Thompson DR. Narcotic analgesic effects on the sphincter of Oddi: a review of the data and therapeutic implications in treating pancreatitis. *Am J Gastroenterol*. 2001;96(4):1266–1272. doi:10.1111/j.1572-0241.2001.03536.x
105. Szakmany T, Woodhouse T. Use of cisatracurium in critical care: a review of the literature. *Minerva Anestesiol*. 2015;81(4):450–460.
106. Wagener G, Kovalevskaya G, Minhaz M, Mattis F, Emond JC, Landry DW. Vasopressin deficiency and vasodilatory state in end-stage liver disease. *J Cardiothorac Vasc Anesth*. 2011;25(4):665–670. doi:10.1053/j.jvca.2010.09.018
107. Vanhoutte PM, Shimokawa H, Feletou M, Tang EHC. Endothelial dysfunction and vascular disease - a 30th anniversary update. *Acta Physiol (Oxf)*. 2017;219(1):22–96. doi:10.1111/apha.12646
108. Alves de Mattos A. Current indications for the use of albumin in the treatment of cirrhosis. *Ann Hepatol*. 2011;10 Suppl 1:S15–S20.
109. Bernardi M, Ricci CS, Zaccherini G. Role of human albumin in the management of complications of liver cirrhosis. *J Clin Exp Hepatol*. 2014;4(4):302–311. doi:10.1016/j.jceh.2014.08.007
110. Davidson JC, Rahim S, Hanks SE, et al. Society of Interventional Radiology Consensus Guidelines for the Periprocedural Management of Thrombotic and Bleeding Risk in Patients Undergoing Percutaneous Image-Guided Interventions-Part I: Review of Anticoagulation Agents and Clinical Considerations: Endorsed by the Canadian Association for Interventional Radiology and the Cardiovascular and Interventional Radiological Society of Europe. *J Vasc Interv Radiol JVIR*. 2019;30(8):1155–1167. doi:10.1016/j.jvir.2019.04.016
111. Patel IJ, Rahim S, Davidson JC, et al. Society of Interventional Radiology Consensus Guidelines for the Periprocedural Management of Thrombotic and Bleeding Risk in Patients Undergoing Percutaneous Image-Guided Interventions-Part II: Recommendations: Endorsed by the Canadian Association for Interventional Radiology and the Cardiovascular and Interventional Radiological Society of Europe. *J Vasc Interv Radiol*. 2019;30(8):1168–1184.e1. doi:10.1016/j.jvir.2019.04.017
112. Kingham TP, Correa-Gallego C, D'Angelica MI, et al. Hepatic parenchymal preservation surgery: decreasing morbidity and mortality rates in 4,152 resections for malignancy. *J Am Coll Surg*. 2015;220(4):471–479. doi:10.1016/j.jamcollsurg.2014.12.026
113. Clavien P-A, Petrowsky H, DeOliveira ML, Graf R. Strategies for safer liver surgery and partial liver transplantation. *N Engl J Med*. 2007;356(15):1545–1559. doi:10.1056/NEJMra065156
114. Hughes MJ, Ventham NT, Harrison EM, Wigmore SJ. Central venous pressure and liver resection: a systematic review and meta analysis. *HPB (Oxford)*. 2015;17(10):863–871. doi:10.1111/hpb.12462
115. Correa-Gallego C, Berman A, Denis SC, et al. Renal function after low central venous pressure-assisted liver resection: assessment of 2116 cases. *HPB (Oxford)*. 2015;17(3):258–264. doi:10.1111/hpb.12347
116. Kim YK, Chin JH, Kang SJ, et al. Association between central venous pressure and blood loss during hepatic resection in 984 living donors. *Acta Anaesthesiol Scand*. 2009;53(5):601–606. doi:10.1111/j.1399-6576.2009.01920.x
117. Massicotte L, Perrault MA, Denault AY, et al. Effects of phlebotomy and phenylephrine infusion on portal venous pressure and systemic hemodynamics during liver transplantation. *Transplantation*. 2010;89(8):920–927. doi:10.1097/TP.0b013e3181d7c40c
118. Petrowsky H, McCormack L, Trujillo M, Selzner M, Jochum W, Clavien PA. A prospective, randomized, controlled trial comparing intermittent portal triad clamping versus ischemic preconditioning with continuous clamping for major liver resection. *Ann Surg*. 2006;244(6):921–928; discussion 928–930. doi:10.1097/01.sla.0000246834.07130.5d
119. Elterman KG, Xiong Z. Coagulation profile changes and safety of epidural analgesia after hepatectomy: a retrospective study. *J Anesth*. 2015;29(3):367–372. doi:10.1007/s00540-014-1933-4
120. Barton JS, Riha GM, Differding JA, et al. Coagulopathy after a liver resection: is it over diagnosed and over treated? *HPB (Oxford)*. 2013;15(11):865–871. doi:10.1111/hpb.12051
121. Kone LB, Maker VK, Banulescu M, Maker AV. Epidural analgesia is associated with prolonged length of stay after open HPB surgery in over 27,000 patients. *J Gastrointest Surg*. 2021;25(7):1716–1726. doi:10.1007/s11605-020-04751-y
122. Lee SH, Gwak MS, Choi SJ, et al. Prospective, randomized study of ropivacaine wound infusion versus intrathecal morphine with intravenous fentanyl for analgesia in living donors for liver transplantation. *Liver Transplant*. 2013;19(9):1036–1045. doi:10.1002/lt.23691
123. Kang R, Lee S, Kim GS, et al. Comparison of analgesic efficacy of erector spinae plane block and posterior quadratus lumborum block in laparoscopic liver resection: a randomized controlled trial. *J Pain Res*. 2021;14:3791–3800. doi:10.2147/JPR.S343366
124. Alghamdi T, Abdel-Fattah M, Zautner A, Lorf T. Preoperative model for end-stage liver disease score as a predictor for posthemihepatectomy complications. *Eur J Gastroenterol Hepatol*. 2014;26(6):668–675. doi:10.1097/MEG.0000000000000035
125. Aronsohn A, Jensen D. Hepatobiliary manifestations of critically ill and postoperative patients. *Clin Liver Dis*. 2011;15(1):183–197. doi:10.1016/j.cld.2010.09.004
126. Belghiti J, Hiramatsu K, Benoist S, Massault P, Sauvanet A, Farges O. Seven hundred forty-seven hepatectomies in the 1990s: an update to evaluate the actual risk of liver resection. *J Am Coll Surg*. 2000;191(1):38–46. doi:10.1016/s1072-7515(00)00261-1
127. Morimoto N, Okada K, Okita Y. Results of cardiac surgery in advanced liver cirrhosis. *Gen Thorac Cardiovasc Surg*. 2013;61(2):79–83. doi:10.1007/s11748-012-0175-3
128. Jacob KA, Hjortnaes J, Kranenburg G, de Heer F, Kluin J. Mortality after cardiac surgery in patients with liver cirrhosis classified by the Child-Pugh score. *Interact Cardiovasc Thorac Surg*. 2015;20(4):520–530. doi:10.1093/icvts/ivu438
129. Abramov D, Tamariz MG, Fremes SE, et al. Trends in coronary artery bypass surgery results: a recent, 9-year study. *Ann Thorac Surg*. 2000;70(1):84–90. doi:10.1016/s0003-4975(00)01249-2

47 Endocrine Function

JEFFREY J. SCHWARTZ • SHAMSUDDIN AKHTAR

KEY POINTS

1. The major risk of anesthesia in the poorly controlled thyrotoxic patient is thyroid storm, which must be aggressively treated with β-blockers, iodide, and antithyroid drugs.
2. Asymptomatic or mild hypothyroidism does not appear to significantly increase anesthetic risk and is not a contraindication to surgery. Moderate to severe hypothyroidism should be corrected before surgery to prevent multisystem complications.
3. Patients who have received corticosteroids for more than 3 weeks in the past year may have adrenal suppression; supplemental steroids in the perioperative period should be considered.
4. Preoperative preparation of the pheochromocytoma patient with α-blockers decreases intraoperative hemodynamic instability.
5. Pheochromocytoma manipulation is associated with severe hypertension that should be treated aggressively with nitroprusside, phentolamine, or other rapidly acting vasodilators.
6. The major perioperative risks to the diabetic patient come from unrecognized or poorly managed coexisting diseases, especially coronary artery disease.
7. Very tight control of perioperative blood glucose levels appears to increase the risk of hypoglycemic complications without clearly reducing the risk of hyperglycemic complications.
8. Endotracheal intubation may be unpredictably difficult in patients with acromegaly.

Thyroid Gland

The thyroid gland secretes thyroid hormones, thyroxine (T_4) and 3,3′,5-triiodothyronine (T_3), which are the major regulators of cellular metabolic activity. Thyroid hormones exert a variety of actions by regulating the synthesis and activity of various proteins. They are necessary for proper cardiac, pulmonary, and neurologic function during both health and illness.

Thyroid Metabolism and Function

The production of thyroid hormone is initiated by the active uptake and concentration of iodide in the thyroid gland (Fig. 47-1). Dietary iodine is reduced to iodide in the gastrointestinal (GI) tract. Circulating iodide is taken up by the thyroid gland, where it is bound to tyrosine residues to form various iodotyrosines. After organification, monoiodotyrosine or diiodotyrosine is coupled enzymatically by thyroid peroxidase to form either T_3 or T_4. These hormones are attached to the thyroglobulin protein and stored as colloid in the gland. The release of T_3 and T_4 from the gland is accomplished through proteolysis from the thyroglobulin and diffusion into the circulation. Thyrotropin (thyroid-stimulating hormone [TSH]) is produced in the anterior pituitary gland, and its secretion is regulated by thyrotropin-releasing hormone produced in the hypothalamus. TSH is responsible for maintaining the uptake of iodide and proteolytic release of thyroid hormone. Excess iodide inhibits the synthesis and secretion of thyroid hormone. Circulating thyroid hormone inhibits thyrotropin-releasing hormone and TSH secretion in a classic negative-feedback loop. The thyroid gland is solely responsible for the daily secretion of T_4 (80 to 100 μg/d). The half-life of T_4 in the circulation is about 7 days.

Approximately 80% of T_3 is produced by the extrathyroidal deiodination of T_4 and 20% is produced by direct thyroid secretion. The half-life of T_3 is 24 to 30 hours. Most of the effects of thyroid hormones are mediated by the more potent and less protein-bound T_3. The degree to which these hormones are protein bound in the circulation is the major factor influencing their activity and degradation. T_4 is metabolized by monodeiodination to either T_3 or reverse T_3 (rT_3). T_3 is biologically active, whereas rT_3 is inactive. The major fraction of circulating hormone is bound to thyroxine-binding globulin (TBG), with a smaller fraction

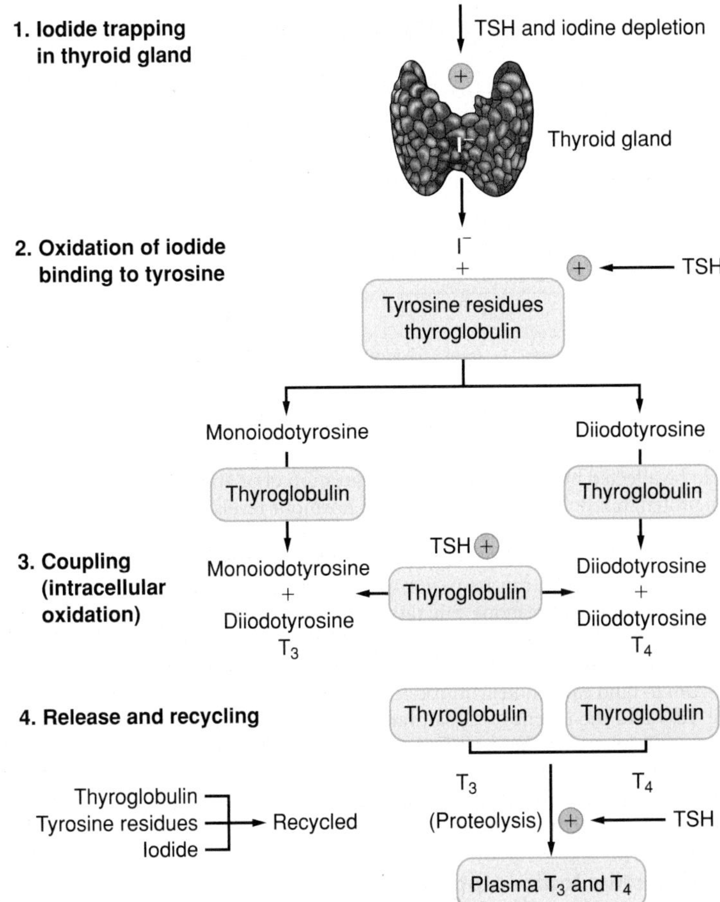

Figure 47-1 Thyroid hormone biosynthesis consists of four stages: (1) organification, (2) binding, (3) coupling, and (4) release. TSH, thyroid-stimulating hormone; T_3, triiodothyronine; T_4, thyroxine.

bound to albumin and transthyretin. Less than 0.1% is present as free, unbound hormone. Changes in serum-binding protein concentrations have a major effect on total T_3 and T_4 serum concentrations. The plasma normally contains 5 to 12 μg/dL of T_4 and 60 to 180 ng/dL of T_3. Many drugs can affect thyroid function, including amiodarone and dopamine.[1]

Although thyroid hormone is important to many aspects of growth and function, the anesthesiologist is most often concerned with the cardiovascular manifestations of thyroid disease.[2] Thyroid hormone affects tissue responses to sympathetic stimuli and increases the intrinsic contractile state of cardiac muscle. β-Adrenergic receptors are increased in number, and cardiac α-adrenergic receptors are decreased by thyroid hormone.[3]

Tests of Thyroid Function

Thyroid-Stimulating Hormone

The current immunochemiluminometric assays for TSH are sensitive and specific enough to be recommended as the first test in evaluating suspected thyroid dysfunction. TSH is often higher than 20 μIU/mL in primary hypothyroidism (normal 0.4 to 4.5 μIU/mL). Conversely, depressed TSH levels signal the presence of hyperthyroidism. Subclinical hypothyroidism is a condition characterized by elevated TSH and normal T_4 levels. A low TSH level in a clinically hypothyroid patient indicates disease at the pituitary or hypothalamic level. The goal of thyroid replacement therapy is to normalize TSH levels.[3] Starvation, fever, stress, corticosteroids, and T_3 or T_4, all can depress TSH levels.

Serum Thyroxine

The serum T_4 assay is a standard test for evaluation of thyroid gland function (Table 47-1). The total T_4 is elevated in approximately 90% of patients with hyperthyroidism, and it is low in 85% of those who are hypothyroid. The total concentration of T_4 is measured by an automated immunoassay. The serum T_4 concentration is influenced by thyroid hormone protein–binding capacity. An increase or decrease in TBG levels or in protein binding may therefore alter the total T_4 but not the concentration of free T_4. Because of the effect of TBG on circulating total T_4, T_4 levels should never be used alone to evaluate thyroid disease. Elevations in the TBG concentration are the most common cause of hyperthyroxinemia in euthyroid patients. Increases in TBG due to acute liver disease, pregnancy, or drugs (oral contraceptives, exogenous estrogens, clofibrate, opioids) may be the causative factor. Because total T_4 can be misleadingly high in euthyroidism or normal in hypothyroidism, some measure of free thyroid hormone activity (free T_4) should also be used.

Serum Triiodothyronine

Serum T_3 levels are not commonly measured but can be evaluated to detect disease in patients with clinical evidence of hyperthyroidism in the absence of elevated T_4. In these cases, T_3 may be the only thyroid hormone produced in excess. T_3 concentrations may be depressed by factors that impair the peripheral conversion of T_4 to T_3 (nonthyroidal illness, previously known as sick euthyroid syndrome). In 50% of hypothyroid patients, the serum T_3 concentration is low; in the remaining 50%, it is normal.

Table 47-1 Tests of Thyroid Gland Function

	T_4	T_3	THBR	TSH
Hyperthyroidism	Elevated	Elevated	Elevated	Normal or low
Primary hypothyroidism	Low	Low or normal	Low	Elevated
Secondary hypothyroidism	Low	Low	Low	Low
Nonthyroidal illness (decreased peripheral conversion of T_4 to T_3)	Normal	Low	Normal	Normal
Pregnancy	Elevated	Normal	Low	Normal

T_4, total serum thyroxine; T_3, serum triiodothyronine; THBR, thyroid hormone binding rate; TSH, thyroid-stimulating hormone.

Tests for Assessing Thyroid Hormone Binding

Because conventional assays measure total hormone levels, which can be affected by changes in the concentration of or abnormalities in protein binding without affecting free hormone levels, it is necessary to correct for thyroid-binding proteins to accurately interpret total thyroxine levels. Most commonly, a "direct" measurement of unbound T_3 and T_4 can be performed; in actuality, these tests do not measure free hormone but rather try to account for binding abnormalities. An older test calculates the free T_3 or T_4 index using the T_3 resin uptake test which measures the ability of the patient's serum to bind exogenously introduced T_3. This reflects the amount of TBG and the extent of T_3 saturation on TBG. The T_3 uptake is inversely related to the degree of unsaturated TBG. Indirect measurement of free hormone levels can be calculated by multiplying the total hormone level by the thyroid hormone binding ratio, which can be calculated from the T_3-resin uptake.

Radioactive Iodine Uptake

The thyroid gland has the ability to concentrate large amounts of inorganic iodide. The oral administration of radioactive iodine (^{131}I or ^{123}I) can be used to indicate thyroid gland activity. Thyroid uptake is elevated in hyperthyroidism unless the hyperthyroidism is caused by thyroiditis, in which case the uptake is low or absent. Because of overlap in values, it is difficult to distinguish patients who are euthyroid from those who are hypothyroid. Radioactive iodine uptake may be increased by a variety of factors, including dietary iodine deficiency, renal failure, and congestive heart failure. Because uptake is under TSH control, elevated, free T_4 levels and corticosteroids decrease radioactive iodide uptake. Functioning ("hot") thyroid tissue is rarely malignant. Nonfunctioning ("cold") tissue may be malignant or benign.

Hyperthyroidism

Hyperthyroidism results from the exposure of tissues to excessive amounts of thyroid hormone (Table 47-2). The most common cause is the multinodular diffuse goiter of Graves disease. This typically occurs between the ages of 20 and 40 years and occurs predominantly in women. Most patients with this condition demonstrate a syndrome characterized by diffuse glandular enlargement, ophthalmopathy, dermopathy, and clubbing of the fingers. A thyroid-stimulating autoantibody may be present. Thyroid adenoma is the second most common cause of hyperthyroidism. Another cause of increased thyroid hormone synthesis is thyroiditis. Subacute thyroiditis frequently follows a respiratory illness and is characterized by a firm, painful gland. This type of thyroiditis is frequently treated with anti-inflammatory agents. Rarely, subacute thyroiditis may occur in a patient with a normal-sized, painless gland. Hashimoto thyroiditis is a chronic autoimmune disease that usually produces hypothyroidism but may occasionally produce hyperthyroidism. Hyperthyroidism may also be associated with pregnancy, ^{131}I therapy, thyroid carcinoma, trophoblastic tumors, or TSH-secreting pituitary adenomas. Iatrogenic hyperthyroidism may follow thyroid hormone replacement or may occur after iodide exposure (angiographic contrast media) in patients with chronically low iodide intake (Jod–Basedow phenomenon). The antiarrhythmic agent amiodarone is iodine rich and is another cause of iodine-induced thyrotoxicosis.[4]

The manifestations of hyperthyroidism are weight loss, diarrhea, skeletal muscle weakness and stiffness, warm and moist skin, heat intolerance, and nervousness. Cardiovascular manifestations include increased left ventricular contractility and ejection fraction, tachycardia, elevated systolic blood pressure, decreased diastolic blood pressure, increased myocardial oxygen consumption, and decreased vascular resistance. Hypercalcemia, thrombocytopenia, and mild anemia may be present. Elderly patients may present with heart failure, atrial fibrillation, or other cardiac dysrhythmias. They may also present with apathetic hyperthyroidism characterized by depression and withdrawal, without the usual systemic signs or symptoms.

Treatment and Anesthetic Considerations

The most important goal in managing the hyperthyroid patient is to make the patient euthyroid before surgery, if possible. The

Table 47-2 Causes of Hyperthyroidism

Intrinsic thyroid disease
- Hyperfunctioning thyroid adenoma
- Toxic multinodular goiter

Abnormal TSH stimulator
- Graves disease
- Trophoblastic tumor

Disorders of hormone storage or release
- Thyroiditis

Excess production of thyroid-stimulating hormone
- Pituitary thyrotropin (rare)

Extrathyroidal source of hormone
- Struma ovarii
- Functioning follicular carcinoma

Exogenous thyroid
- Iatrogenic
- Iodine induced

TSH, thyroid-stimulating hormone.

drugs propylthiouracil and methimazole are thiourea derivatives that inhibit organification of iodide and the synthesis of thyroid hormone.[5] Propylthiouracil also decreases the peripheral conversion of T_4 to T_3. Normal thyroid glands usually contain a store of hormone that is large enough to maintain a euthyroid state for several months, even if synthesis is abolished. Therefore, hyperthyroid patients are unlikely to be regulated to a euthyroid state with antithyroid drugs alone in less than 6 to 8 weeks. Toxic reactions from these drugs are uncommon but include skin rash, nausea, fever, agranulocytosis, hepatitis, and arthralgias.

Inorganic iodide inhibits iodide organification and thyroid hormone release—the Wolff–Chaikoff effect. Iodide is also effective in reducing the size and vascularity of the hyperplastic gland and has a role in the preparation of the patient for emergency thyroid surgery. Antithyroid drugs should be started before iodide treatment because of the possibility of worsening the thyrotoxicosis.

β-Adrenergic antagonists are effective in attenuating the manifestations of excessive sympathetic activity and should be used in all hyperthyroid patients unless contraindicated. β-Adrenergic blockade alone does not inhibit hormone synthesis; however, propranolol does impair the peripheral conversion of T_4 to T_3 over 1 to 2 weeks. Propranolol given over 12 to 24 hours decreases tachycardia, heat intolerance, anxiety, and tremor. Any β-blocker may be used, and long-acting agents are more convenient. The combination of propranolol (in doses titrated to effect) plus potassium iodide (two to five drops every 8 hours) is frequently used before surgery to ameliorate cardiovascular symptoms and reduce circulating concentrations of T_4 and T_3. Preoperative preparation usually requires 7 to 14 days.

Heart failure secondary to poorly controlled paroxysmal atrial fibrillation may improve with slowing of the ventricular rate, but abnormalities of left ventricular function secondary to hyperthyroidism may not be corrected with the use of β-antagonists. If a hyperthyroid patient with clinically apparent disease requires emergency surgery, β-adrenergic blockade should be administered to achieve a heart rate below 90 beats per minute. β-Blockers do not prevent thyroid storm. Glucocorticoids such as dexamethasone (8 to 12 mg/d) are used in the management of severe thyrotoxicosis because they reduce thyroid hormone secretion and the peripheral conversion of T_4 to T_3.

Radioactive iodine therapy is an effective treatment for some patients with thyrotoxicosis.[6] However, it should not be administered to patients who are pregnant because it crosses the placenta and may destroy the fetal thyroid. A side effect of radioiodine therapy is hypothyroidism; 10% to 60% of cases occur in the first year of therapy and an additional 2% occur per year thereafter.

A variety of anesthetic techniques and drugs have been used for hyperthyroid patients undergoing surgery. All antithyroid medications are continued through the morning of surgery. The goal of intraoperative management is to achieve a depth of anesthesia that prevents an exaggerated sympathetic response to surgical stimulation while avoiding the administration of medication that stimulates the sympathetic nervous system. It is best to avoid using ketamine for induction, even when a patient is clinically euthyroid. Hypotension that occurs during surgery is best treated with direct-acting vasopressors rather than a medication that provokes the release of catecholamines. The incidence of myasthenia gravis is increased in hyperthyroid patients; thus, the initial dose of muscle relaxant should be reduced, and a twitch monitor should be used to titrate subsequent doses. Minimum alveolar concentration (MAC) requirement for anesthesia is not affected by hyperthyroidism. Regional anesthesia is an excellent alternative when appropriate; however, epinephrine-containing solutions should be avoided.

Table 47-3 Management of Thyroid Storm

IV fluids
Sodium iodide, 250 mg PO or IV q6h
Propylthiouracil, 200–400 mg PO or via NGT q6h
Hydrocortisone, 50–100 mg IV q6h
Propranolol, 10–40 mg PO q4–6h, or esmolol infusion to treat hyperadrenergic signs
Cooling blankets and acetaminophen and meperidine (25–50 mg) IV q4–6h may be used to prevent shivering
Bile acid sequestrants (e.g., cholestyramine 4 g PO q6h) may be used as adjunctive therapy

NGT, nasogastric tube.

Thyroid storm is a life-threatening exacerbation of hyperthy- 1
roidism that most commonly develops in the undiagnosed or untreated hyperthyroid patient because of the stress of surgery or nonthyroid illness.[7] Operating on an acutely hyperthyroid gland may provoke thyroid storm, although this is probably not due to mechanical release of hormone.[8] Its manifestations include hyperthermia, tachycardia, dysrhythmias, myocardial ischemia, congestive heart failure, agitation, and confusion. Thyroid storm must be distinguished from, or considered with, pheochromocytoma, malignant hyperthermia, and light anesthesia. Although free T_4 levels are often markedly elevated, no laboratory test is diagnostic. Treatment involves large doses of propylthiouracil and supportive measures to control fever and restore intravascular volume (Table 47-3). Invasive hemodynamic monitoring is especially useful in guiding the treatment of patients with significant left ventricular dysfunction (Table 47-3). Again, it is essential to remove or treat the precipitating event.

Anesthesia for Thyroid Surgery

Thyroidectomy as an alternative to prolonged medical therapy for hyperthyroidism is used less frequently now than in the past (1 Video 47-1). Indications include failed medical therapy, underlying cancer, and symptomatic goiter. It is usually performed under general endotracheal anesthesia, although the use of the laryngeal mask airway is increasing.[9] Use of a laryngeal mask airway allows real-time visualization of vocal cord function because the patient is allowed to breathe spontaneously. Limited thyroidectomy may also be performed under bilateral superficial cervical plexus block. The anesthesiologist must be prepared to manage an unexpected difficult intubation because the incidence of difficult intubation during goiter surgery is 5% to 8%.[10] Thyroid cancer increases the risk of difficult intubation, but the size of the goiter is not predictive. Large goiters, especially if associated with evidence of significant airway obstruction or tracheal deviation, may warrant securing the airway while the patient is awake. Large substernal goiters can behave as anterior mediastinal masses and cause intrathoracic airway obstruction after induction of general anesthesia. Computed tomography (CT) or magnetic resonance imaging (MRI) should be reviewed prior to surgery. Minimally invasive procedures such as robot-assisted transaxillary[11] and transoral thyroidectomies are being performed with increasing frequency. Nasal intubations are required for the transoral approach. Complications after thyroidectomy include recurrent laryngeal nerve (RLN) damage, tracheal compression secondary to hematoma or tracheomalacia, and hypoparathyroidism. Pneumothorax may occur during resection of substernal goiters. Hypoparathyroidism secondary to the inadvertent surgical removal of parathyroid glands is most frequently seen after total thyroidectomy. The symptoms of hypocalcemia develop within

24 to 96 hours after surgery.[12] Laryngeal stridor progressing to laryngospasm may be one of the first indications of hypocalcemic tetany. Intravenous (IV) administration of calcium chloride or calcium gluconate is warranted in this situation. Magnesium levels should also be monitored and corrected if low. Bilateral RLN injury is rare but necessitates immediate reintubation. Unilateral nerve injury is more common and is often transient.[13] Unilateral damage to the RLN is characterized by hoarseness and a paralyzed vocal cord, whereas bilateral injury causes stridor or aphonia (see Chapter 28). It is wise to evaluate vocal cord function before and after surgery by laryngoscopy or by asking the patient to phonate by saying the sound for "E." Some surgeons elect to monitor RLN function intraoperatively. A nerve stimulator may be used by the surgeon to stimulate suspicious structures and note contraction of the laryngeal muscles. Alternatively, the nerve integrity monitor (NIM; Medtronic Xomed) endotracheal tube can be used. This endotracheal tube has two pairs of electrodes embedded in the shaft just above the cuff. When properly positioned, the electrodes will be in contact with the vocal cords and an electromyographic signal can be monitored. Muscle relaxants and topical laryngeal anesthesia must be avoided to obtain accurate signals during surgery. Succinylcholine or a small dose of rocuronium can be used to facilitate intubation. Care must be taken that the NIM tube is still positioned properly after the head and neck have been manipulated for optimal surgical exposure.[14] Postoperative extubation of the trachea should be performed under optimal conditions. Intraoperative laryngeal nerve injury or collapse of the tracheal rings from previous weakening may mandate emergency reintubation.

Hypothyroidism

Hypothyroidism is a relatively common disease (0.3% to 5% of the adult population) that results from inadequate circulating levels of T_4, T_3, or both.[15] The development of hypothyroidism is often slow and progressive, making the clinical diagnosis difficult, especially in more subtle cases. Hypofunctioning of the thyroid gland has many causes (Table 47-4). Primary failure of the thyroid gland refers to decreased production of thyroid hormone, despite adequate TSH production, and accounts for 95% of all cases of thyroid dysfunction. The remainder of the cases are caused by either hypothalamic or pituitary disease (secondary hypothyroidism) and are associated with other pituitary deficiencies.

Table 47-4 Causes of Hypothyroidism

Primary hypothyroidism
• Autoimmune
• Irradiation to the neck
• Previous ^{131}I therapy
• Surgical removal
• Thyroiditis (Hashimoto disease)
• Severe iodine depletion
• Medications (iodines, propylthiouracil, methimazole)
• Hereditary defects in biosynthesis
• Congenital defects in gland development
• Infiltrative disorders (e.g., amyloidosis, sarcoidosis)
Secondary or tertiary hypothyroidism
• Hypopituitarism
• Hypothalamic disease

Adapted from Jameson J, Mandel SJ, Weetman AP. Hypothyroidism. In: Loscalzo J, Fauci A, Kasper D, et al. eds. *Harrison's Principles of Internal Medicine*. 21st ed. McGraw Hill; 2022. https://accessmedicine.mhmedical.com/content.aspx?bookid=3095§ionid=263546550

A lack of thyroid hormone produces a variety of signs and symptoms. Early findings are often nonspecific. A history of radioiodine therapy, external neck irradiation, or the presence of a goiter should increase suspicion. There is a generalized reduction in metabolic activity resulting in lethargy, slow mental functioning, cold intolerance, and slow movements. The cardiovascular manifestations of hypothyroidism reflect the importance of thyroid hormone for myocardial contractility and catecholamine function. Patients exhibit bradycardia, decreased cardiac output, and increased peripheral resistance.[16] The accumulation of a cholesterol-rich pericardial fluid produces low voltage on the electrocardiogram (ECG). Heart failure only rarely occurs in the absence of coexisting heart disease. Angina pectoris itself is unusual in hypothyroidism but can appear when thyroid hormone treatment is initiated. Ventilatory responsiveness to hypoxia and hypercapnia is depressed in hypothyroid patients. This depression is potentiated by sedatives, opioids, and general anesthesia. Postoperative ventilatory failure requiring prolonged ventilation is rarely seen in hypothyroid patients in the absence of coexisting lung disease, obesity, or myxedema coma. Other abnormalities found in hypothyroidism include anemia, coagulopathy, hypothermia, sleep apnea, and impaired renal free water clearance with hyponatremia. Decreased GI motility can contribute to postoperative ileus. In longstanding or severe disease, the stress response may be blunted and adrenal depression may occur.

Treatment and Anesthetic Considerations

Symptomatic hypothyroidism is treated with hormone replacement therapy.[17] Untreated hypothyroidism in pregnant patients is associated with an increased incidence of spontaneous abortion and mental and physical abnormalities in the offspring; therefore, treatment of hypothyroid women who are pregnant is also important. Controversy remains regarding the preoperative anesthetic management of the hypothyroid patient. Given the multisystem effects of thyroid hormone, it seems logical to recommend that all hypothyroid surgical candidates be restored to a euthyroid state before surgery. However, there is limited evidence to suggest that hypothyroid patients are unusually sensitive to anesthetic drugs, have prolonged recovery times, or have a higher incidence of perioperative cardiovascular instability or collapse.

No increase in serious complications in patients with mild or moderate hypothyroidism undergoing general anesthesia has been noted.[18] One study identified a higher incidence of intraoperative hypotension and postoperative GI and neuropsychiatric complications in mild and moderately hypothyroid patients undergoing noncardiac surgery, but still concluded there were no compelling clinical reasons to postpone surgery in these patients.[19] Surgery in severely hypothyroid patients should be postponed when possible until these patients are at least partially treated. 2

The management of hypothyroid patients with symptomatic coronary artery disease is somewhat controversial.[20] The need for thyroid hormone replacement therapy must be weighed against the risk of precipitating myocardial ischemia. Several studies and a literature review found no differences in the frequency of intraoperative or postoperative complications when mild or moderate hypothyroid patients underwent cardiac surgery. In symptomatic patients or unstable patients with cardiac ischemia, thyroid replacement should probably be delayed until after coronary revascularization.

Most anesthetic medications may be used without difficulty in hypothyroid patients. Ketamine has been proposed as the ideal induction agent because it stimulates the sympathetic nervous

Table 47-5 Management of Myxedema

Tracheal intubation and controlled ventilation as needed
Levothyroxine, 200–300 µg IV over 5–10 min initially, and 100 mcg IV q24h
Hydrocortisone, 100 mg IV, then 25 mg IV q6h
Fluid and electrolyte therapy as indicated by serum electrolyte levels
Cover to conserve body heat; no warming blankets

system. The maintenance of anesthesia may be safely achieved with either IV or inhaled anesthetics. There appears to be little, if any, decrease in the MAC for volatile agents. Regional anesthesia is a good choice in the hypothyroid patient, provided intravascular volume is well-maintained. Monitoring is directed toward the early recognition of hypotension, congestive heart failure, or hypothermia. Scrupulous attention should be paid to maintaining normal body temperature.

Myxedema coma represents a severe form of hypothyroidism characterized by stupor or coma, hypoventilation, hypothermia, hypotension, and hyponatremia. This is a medical emergency with a high mortality rate (25% to 50%) and, as such, requires aggressive therapy (Table 47-5). Only lifesaving surgery should proceed in the face of myxedema coma. IV thyroid replacement is initiated as soon as the clinical diagnosis is made. An IV loading dose of T_4 (sodium levothyroxine, 200 to 300 mcg) is given initially and followed by a maintenance dose of T_4, 50 to 200 mcg/d intravenously.[21] Alternatively, T_3 may be used because it has a more rapid onset. Improvements in heart rate, blood pressure, and body temperature may occur within 24 hours. However, replacement therapy with either form of thyroid hormone may precipitate myocardial ischemia. There is also an increased likelihood of acute primary adrenal insufficiency in these patients, and they should receive stress doses of hydrocortisone. Steroid replacement should continue until normal adrenal function can be confirmed.

Parathyroid Glands

Calcium Physiology

The normal adult body contains approximately 1 to 2 kg of calcium (Ca^{2+}), of which 99% is in the skeleton.[22] Plasma calcium is present in three forms: (1) a protein-bound fraction (50%); (2) an ionized fraction (45%); and (3) a diffusible but nonionized fraction (5%) that is complexed with phosphate, bicarbonate, and citrate. It is the ionized fraction that is physiologically active and homeostatically regulated. The normal total serum calcium concentration is 8.8 to 10.4 mg/dL. Albumin binds approximately 90% of the protein-bound fraction of calcium, and total serum Ca^{2+} consequently depends on albumin levels. In general, an increase or decrease in albumin of 1 g/dL is associated with a parallel change in total serum Ca^{2+} of 0.8 mg/dL. The serum-ionized Ca^{2+} concentration is affected by temperature and blood pH through alterations in Ca^{2+} binding to albumin. Acidosis decreases protein binding (increases ionized Ca^{2+}), and alkalosis increases protein binding (decreases ionized Ca^{2+}). The concentration of free Ca^{2+} ion is of critical importance in regulating skeletal and cardiac muscle contraction, coagulation, neurotransmitter release, endocrine secretion, and a variety of other cellular functions. Consequently, the maintenance of serum Ca^{2+} concentration is subject to tight hormonal control by parathyroid hormone (PTH) and vitamin D (Fig. 47-2).

PTH acts to maintain the extracellular fluid Ca^{2+} concentration through direct effects on bone resorption and renal Ca^{2+} resorption in the distal tubule and indirectly through its effects on the synthesis of 1,25-dihydroxyvitamin D. The renal effects of PTH include phosphaturia and bicarbonaturia, in addition to enhanced Ca^{2+} and magnesium resorption. Most evidence suggests that rapid changes in blood Ca^{2+} levels are primarily the result of hormonal effects on bone and, to a lesser extent, on renal Ca^{2+} clearance, whereas maintenance of overall Ca^{2+} balance depends more on the indirect effects of the hormone on intestinal calcium absorption.

PTH secretion is primarily regulated by the serum-ionized Ca^{2+} concentration. This negative-feedback mechanism is exquisitely sensitive at maintaining calcium levels in a normal range. Release of PTH is also influenced by phosphate, magnesium, and catecholamine levels. Acute hypomagnesemia directly stimulates PTH release, whereas chronic magnesium depletion appears to inhibit proper functioning of the parathyroid gland. The plasma phosphate concentration has an indirect influence on PTH secretion by causing reciprocal changes in the serum-ionized Ca^{2+} concentration.

Vitamin D is absorbed from the GI tract and can be produced enzymatically by ultraviolet irradiation of the skin. Vitamin D (cholecalciferol) is made from cholesterol metabolites and is inactive. Calciferol is hydroxylated in the liver to 25-hydroxycholecalciferol (25-OHD); in the kidney, it is further hydroxylated to 1,25-dihydroxycholecalciferol [1,25$(OH)_2$D] or 24,25-dihydroxycholecalciferol [24,25$(OH)_2$D]. 25-OHD is the major circulating form of vitamin D. The synthesis of this form is not regulated by a hormone or by Ca^{2+} or phosphate levels. 1,25$(OH)_2$D and 24,25$(OH)_2$D are the major active metabolites of vitamin D, and their production is reciprocally regulated at the kidney. Hypocalcemia and hypophosphatemia cause an increased production of 1,25$(OH)_2$D and a decreased production of 24,25$(OH)_2$D. 1,25$(OH)_2$D stimulates bone, kidney, and intestinal absorption of calcium and phosphate. Vitamin D deficiency can lead to decreased intestinal absorption of Ca^{2+} and secondary hyperparathyroidism.

Hyperparathyroidism

Primary hyperparathyroidism is due to a benign parathyroid adenoma (90% of cases) or hyperplasia (9%) and very rarely due to a parathyroid carcinoma.[23] Primary hyperparathyroidism may also exist as part of a multiple endocrine neoplastic (MEN) syndrome. Hyperplasia usually involves all four glands. Although most patients with primary hyperparathyroidism are hypercalcemic, most are asymptomatic at the time of diagnosis. When symptoms occur, they usually result from the hypercalcemia that accompanies the disease. Primary hyperparathyroidism occurring during pregnancy is associated with a high maternal and fetal morbidity rate (50%). The placenta allows the fetus to concentrate calcium, promoting fetal hypercalcemia and leading to hypoparathyroidism in the newborn. Pregnant women with primary hyperparathyroidism are usually treated with surgery.

Hypercalcemia is responsible for a broad spectrum of signs and symptoms. Nephrolithiasis is the most common manifestation, occurring in 60% to 70% of patients. Polyuria and polydipsia are also common complaints. An increase in bone turnover may lead to generalized demineralization and subperiosteal bone resorption; however, only a small group of patients (10% to 15%) have clinically significant bone disease. Patients may experience generalized skeletal muscle weakness and fatigability, epigastric discomfort, peptic ulceration, or constipation. Psychiatric manifestations include depression, memory loss, confusion, or psychosis. Between 20% and 50% of patients are

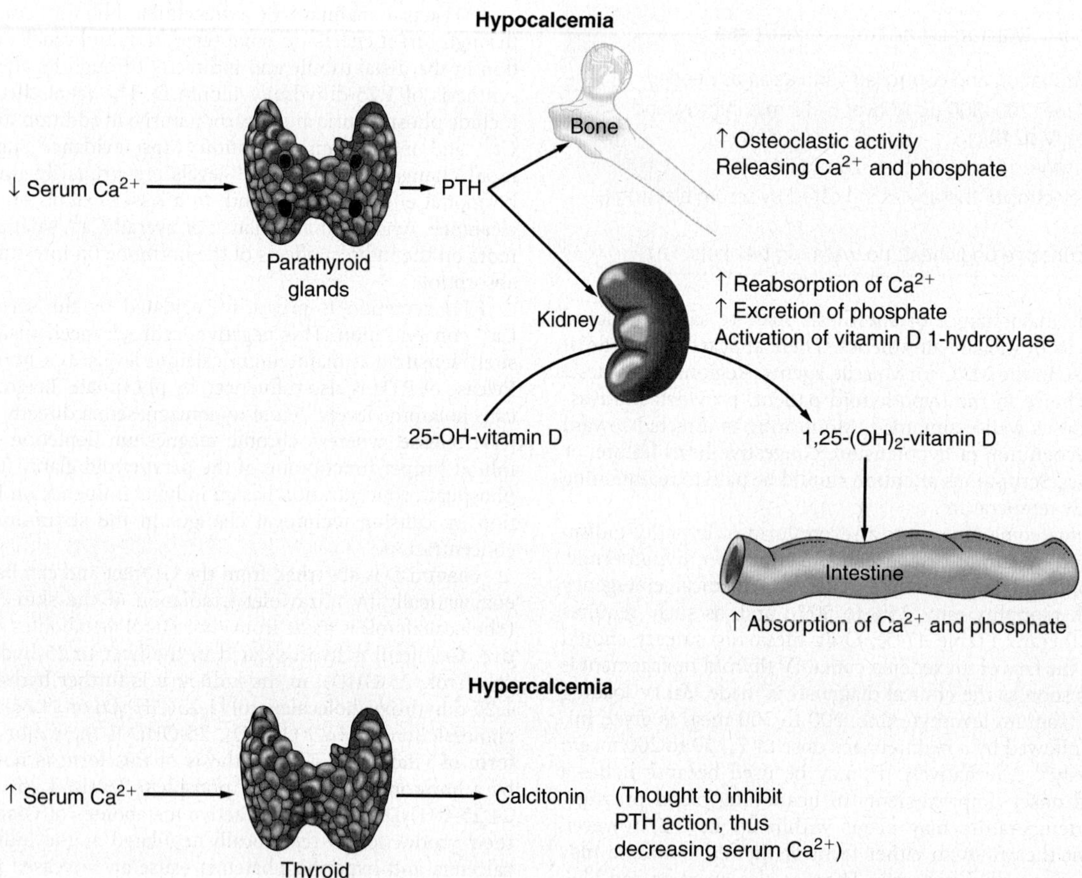

Figure 47-2 Parathyroid hormone (PTH) and vitamin D metabolism and action. 25-OH, 25-hydroxycholecalciferol; 1,25-$(OH)_2$, 1,25-dihydroxycholecalciferol. (Reprinted with permission from McClatchey KD. *Clinical Laboratory Medicine*. 2nd ed. Lippincott Williams & Wilkins; 2002.)

hypertensive at diagnosis, but this usually resolves with successful treatment of the disease. Cardiac function is enhanced in the early stages of hypercalcemia. Calcium flux into the cells is reflected in the plateau phase of the action potential (phase 2). As extracellular calcium increases, the inward flux is more rapid, and phase 2 is shortened (see Chapter 12). The corresponding ECG change is a shorter QT interval. Cardiac contractility may increase until a level between 15 and 20 mg/dL is reached. At this point, there is prolongation of the PR segment and QRS complex that can result in heart block or bundle branch block. Bradycardia also occurs.

An elevated serum Ca^{2+} concentration should warrant consideration of the diagnosis of primary hyperparathyroidism. The serum phosphate concentration is nonspecific, with many patients having normal or near-normal levels. The reported incidence of hyperchloremic acidosis varies widely in primary hyperparathyroidism, but most patients usually have a serum chloride concentration greater than 102 mEq/L. Rarely does a patient with hypercalcemia secondary to ectopic PTH production (malignancy) present with hyperchloremic acidosis. The definitive diagnosis of primary hyperparathyroidism is made by measuring elevated, or inappropriately normal, PTH levels in the presence of hypercalcemia. An elevated nephrogenous cyclic adenosine monophosphate is noted in over 90% of patients with primary hyperparathyroidism.

Hypercalcemia may also result from the ectopic production of PTH or PTH-like substances from lung, genitourinary, breast, GI, or lymphoproliferative malignancies. Tumors may also produce hypercalcemia through direct bone resorption or the production of osteoclast-activating factor. In the absence of a clinically obvious neoplasm, there may be difficulty in differentiating between PTH-producing malignancies and primary hyperparathyroidism. PTH fragments from malignant tissue differ from native PTH, so precise laboratory identification may aid in distinguishing between ectopic PTH production and primary hyperparathyroidism.

Secondary hyperparathyroidism represents an increase in parathyroid function due to conditions that produce hypocalcemia or hyperphosphatemia. Chronic renal disease is a common cause of hyperphosphatemia (due to decreased phosphate excretion) and decreased vitamin D metabolism. The hypocalcemia that results leads to an increased production of PTH. GI disorders accompanied by malabsorption may also lead to a secondary increase in parathyroid activity. Tertiary hyperparathyroidism refers to the development of hypercalcemia in a patient who has had prolonged secondary hyperparathyroidism that has caused adenomatous changes in the parathyroid gland and unregulated PTH production.

Treatment and Anesthetic Considerations

Surgery is the treatment of choice for the patient with symptomatic disease. However, there is controversy surrounding the choice of treatment in the asymptomatic patient. It is not clear whether untreated asymptomatic primary hyperparathyroidism that does not progress causes long-term complications. Nevertheless, surgery is often chosen over medical therapy because it offers definitive treatment and is generally safe.

Preoperative preparation focuses on the correction of intravascular volume and electrolyte irregularities. It is particularly important to evaluate the patient with chronic hypercalcemia for abnormalities of the renal, cardiac, or central nervous systems. Emergency treatment of hypercalcemia is undertaken before surgery when the serum Ca^{2+} concentration exceeds 15 mg/dL (7.5 mEq/L). Lowering of the serum Ca^{2+} concentration is initially accomplished by expanding the intravascular volume and establishing a sodium diuresis. This is achieved with the IV administration of normal saline and, if necessary, furosemide. Rehydration alone is capable of lowering the serum Ca^{2+} level by at least 2 mg/dL. Hydration dilutes the serum Ca^{2+}, and sodium diuresis promotes Ca^{2+} excretion through an inhibition of sodium and Ca^{2+} resorption in the proximal renal tubule. Hypokalemia and hypomagnesemia may result.

Another element in the treatment of hypercalcemia is the correction of hypophosphatemia. Hypophosphatemia increases GI absorption of Ca^{2+}, stimulates the breakdown of bone, and impairs the uptake of Ca^{2+} by bone. Low serum phosphate levels impair cardiac contractility and may contribute to congestive heart failure. Hypophosphatemia also causes skeletal muscle weakness, hemolysis, and platelet dysfunction.

Other medications that have a role in lowering the serum Ca^{2+} include bisphosphonates, mithramycin, calcitonin, and glucocorticoids. Bisphosphonates are pyrophosphate analogs that inhibit osteoclast action. They are the drugs of choice for severe hypercalcemia. Toxic effects include fever and hypophosphatemia. Calcitonin is useful in transiently lowering the serum Ca^{2+} level by 2 to 4 mg/dL through direct inhibition of osteoclastic bone resorption. The advantages of calcitonin are the mild side effects (urticaria, nausea) and the rapid onset of action. However, calcitonin resistance usually develops within 24 to 48 hours. Glucocorticoids are effective in lowering the serum Ca^{2+} concentration in several conditions (sarcoidosis, some malignancies, hyperthyroidism, vitamin D intoxication) through their actions on osteoclast bone resorption, GI absorption of calcium, and urinary calcium excretion. Glucocorticoids are usually of no benefit in the treatment of primary hypercalcemia. Finally, hemodialysis or peritoneal dialysis can be used to lower the serum Ca^{2+} level when alternative regimens are ineffective or contraindicated.

There is no evidence that a specific anesthetic drug or technique has advantages over another. A thorough knowledge of the clinical manifestations attributable to hypercalcemia is of the greatest value in choosing an anesthetic technique. Special monitoring is usually not required. There is an increased requirement for vecuronium, and probably all nondepolarizing muscle relaxants during onset of neuromuscular blockade.[24] However, because of the unpredictable response to neuromuscular blocking drugs, a conservative approach to muscle paralysis makes sense. Careful positioning of the osteopenic patient is necessary to avoid pathologic bone fractures.

Anesthesia for Parathyroid Surgery

General anesthesia is most commonly used for parathyroid surgery. An endotracheal tube is usually used to secure the airway, but supraglottic airways can be used successfully. Minimally invasive parathyroidectomy is superior to conventional bilateral cervical exploration in patients with sporadic primary hyperparathyroidism[25] and can be performed under monitored anesthesia care with bilateral cervical plexus block.[26] Some centers use an intraoperative rapid PTH assay to help determine when a hyperfunctioning gland has been removed. A freely back-flowing IV catheter is needed for frequent sampling. There is *in vitro*, but no clinical evidence that propofol interferes with the assay; however, some surgeons prefer that propofol not be used within 15 minutes of an assay.[27] Postoperative complications include RLN injury, bleeding, and transient or complete hypoparathyroidism. Unilateral RLN is characterized by hoarseness and usually requires no intervention. Bilateral RLN injury is a rare complication, producing aphonia and requiring immediate tracheal intubation.

After successful parathyroidectomy, a decrease in the serum Ca^{2+} level should be observed within 24 hours. Patients with significant preoperative bone disease may have hypocalcemia after removal of the PTH-secreting gland(s). This "hungry bone" syndrome is the result of rapid remineralization of bone. Thus, serum Ca^{2+}, magnesium, and phosphorus levels should be closely monitored until stable. The serum Ca^{2+} nadir usually occurs within 3 to 7 days.

Hypoparathyroidism

An underproduction of PTH or resistance of the end-organ tissues to PTH results in hypocalcemia (<8 mg/dL).[28] The normal physiologic response to hypocalcemia is an increase in PTH secretion and $1,25(OH)_2D$ synthesis, with an increase in Ca^{2+} mobilization from bone, GI absorption, and renal tubule reclamation. The most common cause of acquired PTH deficiency is unintentional removal of the parathyroid glands during thyroid or parathyroid surgery. Other causes of acquired hypoparathyroidism include ^{131}I therapy for thyroid disease, neck trauma, granulomatous disease, or an infiltrating process (malignancy or amyloidosis). Severe hypomagnesemia (<0.8 mEq/L) from any cause can produce hypocalcemia by suppressing PTH secretion and interfering with PTH action. Renal insufficiency leads to phosphorus retention and impaired $1,25(OH)_2D$ synthesis, which results in hypocalcemia. These patients are commonly treated with vitamin D, which increases intestinal calcium absorption and suppresses secondary increases in PTH secretion. Hypocalcemia due to pancreatitis and burns results from the suppression of PTH and from the sequestration of calcium.

Clinical Features and Treatment

The clinical features of hypoparathyroidism are a manifestation of hypocalcemia. Neuronal irritability and skeletal muscle spasms, tetany, or seizures reflect a reduced threshold of excitation. Latent tetany may be demonstrated by eliciting the Chvostek or Trousseau sign. A Chvostek sign is a contracture of the facial muscle produced by tapping the facial nerve as it passes through the parotid gland. A Trousseau sign is a contraction of the fingers and wrist after application of a blood pressure cuff inflated above the systolic blood pressure for approximately 3 minutes. Other common complaints of hypocalcemia include fatigue, depression, paresthesias, and skeletal muscle cramps. The acute onset of hypocalcemia after thyroid or parathyroid surgery may manifest as stridor and apnea. Cardiovascular manifestations of hypocalcemia include congestive heart failure, hypotension, and a relative insensitivity to the effects of β-adrenergic agonists (see Chapter 12). Delayed ventricular repolarization results in a prolonged QT interval on the ECG. Although prolongation of the QT interval may be a reliable sign of hypocalcemia in an individual patient, the ECG is relatively insensitive for the detection of hypocalcemia.

The treatment of hypoparathyroidism consists of electrolyte replacement. The objective is to have the patient's clinical symptoms under control before anesthesia and surgery. Hypocalcemia caused by magnesium depletion is treated by correcting the magnesium deficit. Serum phosphate excess is corrected by the removal of phosphate from the diet and the oral administration of phosphate-binding resins (aluminum hydroxide). The urinary excretion of phosphate can be increased with a saline volume infusion. Ca^{2+} deficiencies are corrected with Ca^{2+} supplements or vitamin D analogs. Patients with severe symptomatic hypocalcemia are treated with IV calcium gluconate (10 to 20 mL of 10% solution, diluted) given slowly over several minutes and followed by a continuous infusion (0.5 to 1.5 mg/kg/h) of elemental Ca^{2+}. The correction of serum Ca^{2+} levels should be monitored by measuring serum Ca^{2+} concentrations and following clinical symptoms. When oral or IV calcium is inadequate to maintain a normal serum-ionized calcium level, vitamin D is added to the regimen.

Adrenal Cortex

The adrenal cortex functions to synthesize and secrete three types of hormones. Endogenous and dietary cholesterol is used in the adrenal biosynthesis of glucocorticoids (cortisol), mineralocorticoids (aldosterone and 11-deoxycorticosterone), and androgens (dehydroepiandrosterone). Cortisol and aldosterone are the two essential hormones, whereas adrenal androgens are of relatively minor physiologic significance in adults. The major biologic effects of adrenal cortical hyperfunction or hypofunction occur due to cortisol or aldosterone excess or deficiency. Abnormal function of the adrenal cortex may render a patient unable to respond appropriately during a period of surgical stress or critical illness.

Glucocorticoid Physiology

Cortisol (hydrocortisone) is the most potent endogenous glucocorticoid and is produced by the inner portions of the adrenal cortex. Cortisol is produced under the control of adrenocorticotropic hormone (ACTH; corticotropin), a polypeptide synthesized and released by the anterior pituitary gland. Glucocorticoids exert their biologic effects by diffusing into the cytoplasm of target cells and combining with specific high-affinity receptor proteins.

The daily production of endogenous cortisol is approximately 10 mg. The maximal output is rarely more than 200 mg. Most of the circulating hormone is bound to the α-globulin cortisol-binding globulin. It is the relatively small amount of free hormone that exerts the biologic effects. Endogenous glucocorticoids are inactivated primarily by the liver and are excreted in the urine as 17-hydroxycorticosteroids. Cortisol is also filtered at the glomerulus and may be excreted unchanged in the urine. Although the rate of cortisol secretion is decreased by approximately 30% in the elderly patient, plasma cortisol levels remain in a normal range because of a corresponding decrease in hepatic and renal clearance.

Cortisol secretion is directly controlled by ACTH, which in turn is regulated by the corticotropin-releasing factor from the hypothalamus. ACTH is synthesized in the pituitary gland from a precursor molecule that also produces β-lipotropin and β-endorphin. The secretion of ACTH and corticotropin-releasing factor is governed chiefly by glucocorticoids, the sleep–wake cycle, and stress. Cortisol is the most potent regulator of ACTH secretion, acting by a negative-feedback mechanism to maintain cortisol levels in a physiologic range. ACTH release follows a diurnal pattern, with maximal activity occurring soon after awakening. This diurnal pattern of activity occurs in normal subjects and in those with adrenal insufficiency. Psychological or physical stress (trauma, surgery, intense exercise) also promotes ACTH release, regardless of the level of circulating cortisol or the time of day.

Cortisol has multiple effects on intermediate carbohydrate, protein, and fatty acid metabolism, as well as maintenance and regulation of immune and circulatory function. Glucocorticoids enhance gluconeogenesis, elevate blood glucose, and promote hepatic glycogen synthesis. The catabolic effect of glucocorticoids is partially blocked by insulin. The net effect on protein metabolism is enhanced degradation of muscle tissue and negative nitrogen balance. In supraphysiologic amounts, glucocorticoids suppress growth hormone secretion and impair somatic growth. The anti-inflammatory actions of cortisol relate to its effect in stabilizing lysosomes and promoting capillary integrity. Cortisol also antagonizes leukocyte migration inhibition factor, thus reducing white cell adherence to vascular endothelium and diminishing leukocyte response to local inflammation. Phagocytic activity does not decrease, although the killing potential of macrophages and monocytes is diminished. Other diverse actions include the facilitation of free water clearance, maintenance of blood pressure, a weak mineralocorticoid effect, promotion of appetite, stimulation of hematopoiesis, and induction of liver enzymes.

Mineralocorticoid Physiology

Aldosterone is the most potent mineralocorticoid produced by the adrenal gland. This hormone binds to receptors in sweat glands, the alimentary tract, and the distal convoluted tubule of the kidney. Aldosterone is a major regulator of extracellular volume and potassium homeostasis through the resorption of sodium and the secretion of potassium by these tissues. The major regulators of aldosterone release are the renin–angiotensin system and serum potassium levels (Fig. 47-3). The juxtaglomerular apparatus that

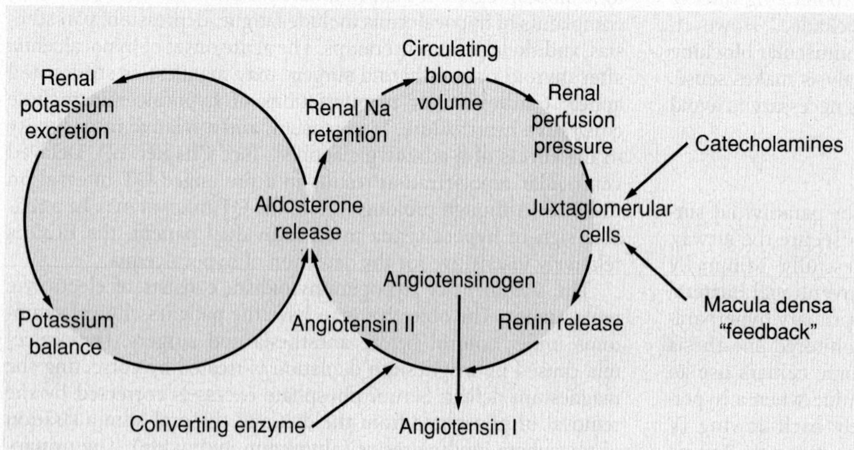

Figure 47-3 Interrelationship of the volume and potassium feedback loops on aldosterone secretion. (Adapted from Petersdorf RG. *Harrison's Principles of Internal Medicine.* 10th ed. McGraw-Hill; 1983.)

surrounds the renal afferent arterioles produces renin in response to decreased perfusion pressures and sympathetic stimulation. Renin splits the hepatic precursor angiotensinogen to form the decapeptide angiotensin I, which is then altered enzymatically by angiotensin-converting enzyme (primarily in the lung) to form the octapeptide angiotensin II. Angiotensin II is the most potent vasopressor produced in the body. It directly stimulates the adrenal cortex to produce aldosterone. The renin–angiotensin system is the body's most important regulator of volume status. Other stimuli that increase the production of aldosterone include hyperkalemia and, to a limited degree, hyponatremia, prostaglandin E, and ACTH.

Glucocorticoid Excess (Cushing Syndrome)

Cushing syndrome, caused by either overproduction of cortisol by the adrenal cortex or exogenous glucocorticoid therapy, is a syndrome characterized by truncal obesity, hypertension, hyperglycemia, increased intravascular fluid volume, hypokalemia, fatigability, abdominal striae, osteoporosis, and muscle weakness. Most endogenous cases of Cushing syndrome are due to bilateral adrenal hyperplasia secondary to ACTH produced by an anterior pituitary microadenoma or nonendocrine tumor (e.g., of the lung, kidney, or pancreas). In approximately 20% to 25% of patients, Cushing syndrome is caused by the primary overproduction of cortisol and other adrenal steroids by an adrenal neoplasm. These tumors are usually unilateral and approximately half are malignant. When Cushing syndrome occurs in patients older than 60 years of age, the most likely cause is an adrenal carcinoma or ectopic ACTH produced from a nonendocrine tumor. Overall, the most common cause of Cushing syndrome is the prolonged administration of exogenous glucocorticoids to treat a variety of illnesses.

The signs and symptoms of Cushing syndrome follow from the known actions of glucocorticoids. Truncal obesity and thin extremities reflect increased muscle wasting and a redistribution of fat in facial, cervical, and truncal areas. Impaired calcium absorption and a decrease in bone formation may result in osteopenia. Sixty percent of patients have hyperglycemia, but overt diabetes mellitus (DM) occurs in less than 20%. Hypertension and fluid retention are seen in most patients. Profound emotional changes, ranging from emotional lability to frank psychosis, may be present. An increased susceptibility to infection reflects the immunosuppressive effects of corticosteroids. Hypokalemic alkalosis without distinctive physical findings is common when adrenal hyperplasia is caused by ectopic ACTH production from a nonendocrine tumor.

The laboratory diagnosis of hyperadrenocorticism is based on a variable elevation in plasma and urinary cortisol levels, urinary 17-hydroxycorticosteroids, and plasma ACTH. Once the diagnosis is established, simultaneous measurement of plasma ACTH and cortisol levels can determine whether the Cushing syndrome is due to primary pituitary or adrenal disease.[29]

Alternatively, a dexamethasone suppression test can be used. Patients with pituitary adenomas frequently show depression in cortisol and 17-hydroxycorticosteroid levels when a high dose of dexamethasone is administered because the tumor retains some negative-feedback control. This response is not observed in patients with adrenal tumors.

Anesthetic Management

General considerations for the preoperative preparation of the patient include treating hypertension, diabetes, and normalizing intravascular fluid volume and electrolyte concentrations. Diuresis with the aldosterone antagonist spironolactone helps mobilize fluid and normalize potassium concentration. Careful positioning of the osteopenic patient is important to avoid fractures. Intraoperative monitoring requirements should be based on the patient's cardiac reserve and consideration of the site and extent of the proposed surgery. When either unilateral or bilateral adrenalectomy is planned, glucocorticoid replacement therapy is initiated at a dose equal to full replacement of adrenal output during periods of extreme stress (see Steroid Replacement during the Perioperative Period). The total dosage is reduced by approximately 50% per day until a daily maintenance dose is achieved (20 to 30 mg/d). Hydrocortisone given in doses of this magnitude exerts significant mineralocorticoid activity, and additional exogenous mineralocorticoid is usually not necessary during the perioperative period. After bilateral adrenalectomy, most patients require 0.05 to 0.1 mg/d of fludrocortisone (9-α-fluorohydrocortisone) starting around day 5 to provide mineralocorticoid activity. Slightly higher doses may be needed if prednisone is used for glucocorticoid maintenance because it has little intrinsic mineralocorticoid activity. The fludrocortisone dose is reduced if congestive heart failure, hypokalemia, or hypertension develops. For the patient with a solitary adrenal adenoma, unilateral adrenalectomy may be followed by normalization of function in the contralateral gland over time. Treatment plans should therefore be individualized. The production of glucocorticoids or ACTH by a neoplasm may not be eliminated if the tumor is unresectable. These patients often need continuous medical therapy with steroid inhibitors such as metyrapone to control their symptoms.

There are no specific recommendations regarding the use of a particular anesthetic technique or medication in patients with hyperadrenocorticism. When significant skeletal muscle weakness is present, a conservative approach to the use of muscle relaxants is warranted. Etomidate has been used for temporizing medical treatment of severe Cushing syndrome because of its inhibition of steroid synthesis.

Mineralocorticoid Excess

Hypersecretion of the major adrenal mineralocorticoid aldosterone increases the renal tubular exchange of sodium for potassium and hydrogen ions. This leads to hypertension, hypokalemic alkalosis, skeletal muscle weakness, and fatigue. Possibly as many as 1% of unselected hypertensive patients have primary hyperaldosteronism. The increase in renal sodium reabsorption and extracellular volume expansion is partly responsible for the high incidence of diastolic hypertension in these patients. Patients with primary hyperaldosteronism (Conn syndrome) characteristically do not have edema. Secondary aldosteronism results from an elevation in renin production. The diagnosis of primary or secondary hyperaldosteronism should be entertained in the nonedematous hypertensive patient with persistent hypokalemia who is not receiving potassium-wasting diuretics. Hyposecretion of renin that fails to increase appropriately during volume depletion or salt restriction is an important finding in primary aldosteronism. The measurement of plasma renin levels is useful in distinguishing primary from secondary hyperaldosteronism. It is of limited value in differentiating patients with primary aldosteronism from those with other causes of hypertension because renin activity is also suppressed in approximately 25% of patients with essential hypertension.

Anesthetic Considerations

Preoperative preparation for the patient with primary aldosteronism is directed toward restoring the intravascular volume and normalizing electrolyte concentrations. Hypertension and hypokalemia may be controlled by restricting sodium intake and administration of the aldosterone antagonist spironolactone. This diuretic works slowly to produce an increase in potassium levels, with dosages in the range of 25 to 100 mg every 8 hours. Total body potassium deficits are difficult to estimate and may be greater than 300 mEq. Whenever possible, potassium should be replaced slowly to allow equilibration between intracellular and extracellular potassium stores. The usual complications of chronic hypertension also need to be assessed and treated.

Adrenal Insufficiency (Addison Disease)

The undersecretion of adrenal steroid hormones may develop as the result of a primary inability of the adrenal gland to produce sufficient hormone quantities or due to a deficiency in the production of ACTH.

Clinically, primary adrenal insufficiency is usually not apparent until at least 90% of the adrenal cortex has been destroyed. Historically, the predominant cause of primary adrenal insufficiency was tuberculosis; today, the most frequent cause of Addison disease is idiopathic secondary to autoimmune destruction of the gland. Autoimmune destruction of the adrenal cortex causes both glucocorticoid and mineralocorticoid deficiencies. A variety of other conditions presumed to have an autoimmune pathogenesis may also occur concomitantly with idiopathic Addison disease. Hashimoto thyroiditis in association with autoimmune adrenal insufficiency is termed Schmidt syndrome. Other possible causes of adrenal gland destruction include certain bacterial, fungal, and advanced human immunodeficiency virus infections; metastatic cancer; sepsis; and hemorrhage. Secondary adrenal insufficiency occurs when the anterior pituitary fails to secrete a sufficient quantity of ACTH. Pituitary failure may result from tumor, infection, surgical ablation, or radiation therapy. Pituitary surgery may cause transient adrenal insufficiency requiring supplemental glucocorticoids.[30]

Patients receiving chronic corticosteroid therapy will not generally have frank adrenal insufficiency; however, they may have hypothalamic–pituitary–adrenal (HPA) suppression and develop acute adrenal insufficiency during the stress of the perioperative period. Relative adrenal insufficiency is a common finding in critically ill surgical patients with hypotension requiring vasopressors.[31] Therefore, a patient with signs of chronic glucocorticoid excess can have findings of acute adrenal insufficiency.

Clinical Presentation

The cardinal symptoms of idiopathic Addison disease include chronic fatigue, muscle weakness, anorexia, weight loss, nausea, vomiting, and diarrhea. Hypotension is almost always encountered in the disease process. Female patients may exhibit decreased axillary and pubic hair growth because of reduced adrenal androgen secretion. An acute crisis can present as abdominal pain, severe vomiting and diarrhea, hypotension, decreased consciousness, and shock. Diffuse hyperpigmentation occurs in most patients with primary adrenal insufficiency and is secondary to the compensatory increase in ACTH and β-lipotropin. These hormones stimulate an increase in melanocyte production. Mineralocorticoid deficiency is characteristically present in primary adrenal disease; as a result, there is a reduction in urine sodium conservation. Hyperkalemia may be a cause of life-threatening cardiac dysrhythmias. Adrenal insufficiency secondary to pituitary disease is not associated with cutaneous hyperpigmentation or mineralocorticoid deficiency. Salt and water balance is usually maintained unless severe fluid and electrolyte losses overwhelm the subnormal aldosterone secretory capacity. Organic lesions of pituitary origin require a diligent search for coexisting hormone deficiencies. The term "critical illness-related corticosteroid insufficiency" (CIRCI) has been used to describe relative or absolute adrenal insufficiency in critically ill patients.[32] Theses may not present with classic symptoms of adrenal insufficiency. The clinical picture may resemble that of sepsis without a source of infection. A high degree of suspicion should exist in any patient who has cardiovascular instability without a defined cause.[33,34]

Diagnosis

The patient's pituitary–adrenal responsiveness should be determined when the diagnosis of primary or secondary adrenal insufficiency is suspected. Biochemical evidence of impaired adrenal or pituitary secretory reserve unequivocally confirms the diagnosis. Patients who are clinically stable may undergo testing before treatment is initiated. Those believed to have acute adrenal insufficiency should receive immediate therapy.

Plasma cortisol levels are measured before and 30 and 60 minutes after the IV administration of 250 mcg of synthetic ACTH. There are multiple determinants of adequate adrenal reserve; usually, the plasma cortisol level rises to at least 18 mcg/dL 60 minutes after the injection of synthetic ACTH.[35] Patients with adrenal insufficiency usually demonstrate little or no adrenal response.

Treatment and Anesthetic Considerations

Normal adults secrete about 10 mg of cortisol and 0.1 mg of aldosterone per day. Glucocorticoid therapy is usually given twice daily in a dosage sufficient to meet physiologic requirements. A typical regimen in the unstressed patient may consist of prednisone 5 mg in the morning and 2.5 mg in the evening, or hydrocortisone 20 mg in the morning and 10 mg in the evening. The daily glucocorticoid dosage is typically 50% higher than basal adrenal output to cover the patient for mild stress. Replacement dosages are adjusted in response to the patient's clinical symptoms or the occurrence of intercurrent illnesses. Daily mineralocorticoid replacement is also administered; most patients require 0.05 to 0.1 mg/d of fludrocortisone. The mineralocorticoid dose may be reduced if severe hypokalemia, hypertension, or congestive heart failure develops, or the dose may be increased if postural hypotension is present.

Secondary adrenal insufficiency often occurs in the presence of multiple hormone deficiencies. A decrease in ACTH production results in decreased secretion of cortisol and adrenal androgens, but aldosterone control by more dominant mechanisms remains intact. A liberal salt diet is encouraged. Glucocorticoid substitution follows the same guidelines previously outlined for primary adrenal insufficiency.

Immediate therapy of acute adrenal insufficiency is mandatory, regardless of the etiology, and consists of electrolyte resuscitation and steroid replacement (Table 47-6). Initial therapy begins with the rapid IV administration of an isotonic crystalloid solution. A dose of 100 mg of hydrocortisone is administered as an IV bolus over several minutes. Steroid replacement is continued during the first 24 hours with 100 mg of IV hydrocortisone given every 8 hours or by continuous infusion. If the patient is stable, the

Table 47-6 Management of Acute Adrenal Insufficiency

Hydrocortisone, 100 mg IV bolus, followed by hydrocortisone, 100 mg q6h for 24 h
Fluid and electrolyte replacement as indicated by vital signs, serum electrolyte levels, and serum glucose

steroid dose is reduced starting on the second day. If the patient continues to be hemodynamically unstable after fluid resuscitation, inotropic support may be necessary. Invasive monitoring can be valuable as a guide to both diagnosis and therapy.

Steroid Replacement during the Perioperative Period

Perioperatively, patients with adrenal insufficiency and those with HPA suppression from chronic steroid use require additional corticosteroids to mimic the increased output of the normal adrenal gland during stress. The normal adrenal gland can secrete up to 100 mg/m^2 of cortisol per day or more during the perioperative period.[36] The pituitary–adrenal axis is usually considered to be intact if a plasma cortisol level higher than 19 mcg/dL is measured during acute stress, but there is no precise threshold. The degree of adrenal responsiveness has been correlated with the duration of surgery and the extent of surgical trauma. In previous research, the mean maximal plasma cortisol level during major surgery (colectomy, hip osteotomy) was 47 mcg/dL. Minor surgical procedures (herniorrhaphy) resulted in mean maximal plasma cortisol levels of 28 mcg/dL. Adrenal activity may also be affected by the choice of anesthetic technique. Regional anesthesia during surgery of the lower abdomen and extremities is effective in postponing the elevation in cortisol levels.[37] Deep general anesthesia may also suppress the elevation of stress hormones such as ACTH and cortisol during surgical procedures.

Although symptoms indicative of clinically significant adrenal insufficiency have been reported during the perioperative period, these clinical findings have rarely been documented in direct association with glucocorticoid deficiency.[38] There is evidence in adrenally suppressed primates that subphysiologic steroid replacement causes perioperative hemodynamic instability and increased mortality.

3 Identifying which patients require steroid supplementation can be difficult. Though recommended by some, provocative testing with ACTH stimulation is too costly to justify compared with the risk of brief steroid supplementation. HPA suppression can occur after five daily doses of prednisone of at least 20 mg but in general, doses of steroids given for less than 3 weeks are not associated with HPA suppression. Daily morning doses of prednisone less than 5 mg are also not associated with HPA suppression. Recovery of HPA function occurs gradually and can take up to 9 to 12 months. HPA suppression is uncommon but can occur with topical, regional, and inhaled steroids depending on dose. Alternate-day therapy decreases the risk of HPA suppression.

There is no proven optimal regimen for perioperative steroid replacement (Table 47-7).[39] For minor outpatient surgeries, patients should take their usual morning steroid dose and no supplementation is needed. For surgeries associated with moderate stress, such as joint replacement, a common regimen involves patients taking their usual morning steroid dose, then supplementing with hydrocortisone 50 mg IV at induction, followed by hydrocortisone 25 mg IV every 8 hours for six doses, along with resumption of usual home regimen on the second postoperative day. For major surgeries (e.g., coronary artery bypass graft), patients are instructed to take their usual morning steroid dose, then supplemented with hydrocortisone 100 mg IV at induction, followed by hydrocortisone 50 mg every 8 hours for at least six doses. This regimen is tapered over the second or third postoperative day until patients can resume their usual home steroid regimen. A low-dose cortisol replacement program using an IV infusion of 25 mg of cortisol before the induction of anesthesia, followed by a continuous infusion of cortisol (100 mg) in the next 24 hours, has also been advocated (Fig. 47-4). This low-dose cortisol replacement program was used in patients with proven adrenal insufficiency and resulted in plasma cortisol levels as high as those seen in healthy control subjects subjected to a comparable operative stress. One study with a limited number of patients found no problems with cardiovascular instability if patients received their usual dose of steroids.[40] An extensive review concluded that the best evidence was that patients should receive their usual daily dose but no supplementation.[41] No conclusive evidence supports an increased incidence of infection or

Table 47-7 Management Options for Steroid Replacement in the Perioperative Period Based on Degree of Surgical Stress
For minor surgeries, take usual morning steroid dose. No supplementation is needed
For moderate surgeries, take usual morning steroid dose. Administer 50 mg hydrocortisone IV prior to induction and 25 mg q8h for 24–36 h
For major surgeries, take usual morning steroid dose. Administer 100 mg IV hydrocortisone IV prior to induction and 50 mg IV q8h for 24–36 h

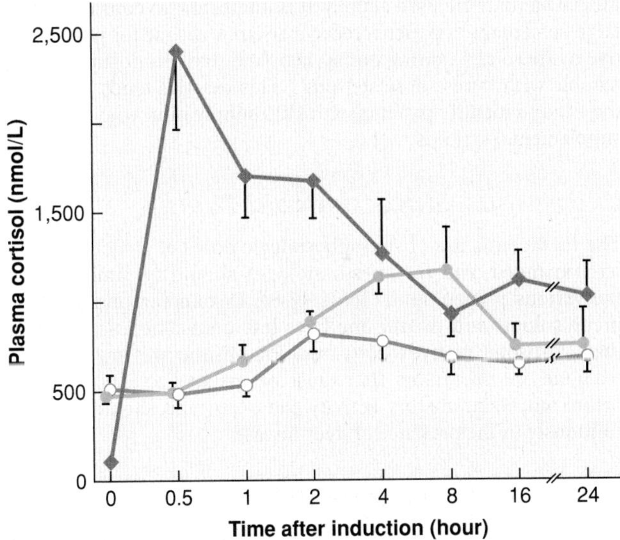

Figure 47-4 Plasma cortisol concentrations (mean ± SEM) were measured in three groups of patients undergoing elective surgery. Group I control patients, $n = 8$ (*closed circles*), had never received corticosteroids. Group II patients, $n = 8$ (*open circles*), received preoperative corticosteroids with a normal response to preoperative adrenocorticotropic hormone (ACTH; corticotropin) stimulation testing. These patients and control patients received no corticosteroid substitution during the perioperative period. Group III, $n = 6$ (*closed diamonds*), consisted of patients receiving long-term corticosteroid therapy with an abnormal response to ACTH stimulation testing during the perioperative period. These patients (group III) received intravenous (IV) cortisol, 25 mg, after the induction of anesthesia plus a continuous IV infusion of cortisol, 100 mg, during the next 24 hours. Plasma cortisol levels in group III were significantly lower than in the other two groups before the induction of anesthesia. After IV administration of cortisol to group III patients, plasma concentrations were significantly higher than in groups I and II for the next 2 hours ($p < 0.01$). Thereafter, the mean plasma concentrations were similar for all groups. There were no clinical signs of circulatory insufficiency in any group. (Reprinted from Symreng T, Karlberg BE, Kagedol B, et al. Physiological cortisol substitution of long-term steroid-treated patients undergoing major surgery. *Br J Anaesth*. 1981;53:949. Copyright © 1981 Elsevier. With permission.)

Table 47-8 Glucocorticoid Preparations

Generic Name	Anti-inflammatory	Mineralocorticoid	Approximate Equivalent Dose (mg)
Short-acting			
Hydrocortisone	1.0	1.0	20.0
Cortisone	0.8	0.8	25.0
Prednisone	4.0	0.25	5.0
Prednisolone	4.0	0.25	5.0
Methylprednisolone	5.0	—	4.0
Intermediate-acting			
Triamcinolone	5.0	—	4.0
Long-acting			
Dexamethasone	30.0	—	0.75

Relative milligram comparisons with cortisol. The glucocorticoid and mineralocorticoid properties of cortisol are set as 1.0.

abnormal wound healing when supraphysiologic doses of supplemental steroids are used acutely. It is interesting to consider that a large percentage of patients receive dexamethasone for postoperative nausea and vomiting prophylaxis and that this dosing is comparable with "stress dose steroids." This practice tends to negate the need to identify patients with HPA suppression who will need supplemental steroids.

Exogenous Glucocorticoid Therapy

The therapeutic use of supraphysiologic doses of glucocorticoids has expanded, and the anesthesiologist should be familiar with the various preparations (Table 47-8). Dexamethasone, methylprednisolone, and prednisone have less mineralocorticoid effect than cortisone or hydrocortisone. Prednisone and methylprednisolone are precursors that must be metabolized by the liver before anti-inflammatory activity can occur and should be used cautiously in the presence of liver disease.

Mineralocorticoid Insufficiency

Isolated mineralocorticoid insufficiency has been reported as a congenital biosynthetic defect, after unilateral adrenalectomy for removal of an aldosterone-secreting adenoma, during protracted heparin therapy, and in patients with a deficiency in renin production. This syndrome is commonly seen in patients with mild renal failure and longstanding DM. A feature common to all patients with hypoaldosteronism is a failure to increase aldosterone production in response to salt restriction or volume contraction.

Most patients present with hypotension, hyperkalemia that may be life-threatening, and a metabolic acidosis that is out of proportion to the degree of coexisting renal impairment. Patients with low renin secretion, hypoaldosteronism, and renal dysfunction respond to ACTH stimulation. Nonsteroidal anti-inflammatory drugs, which inhibit prostaglandin synthesis, may further inhibit renin release and exacerbate the condition. Patients with isolated hypoaldosteronism are given fludrocortisone orally in a dose of 0.05 to 0.1 mg/d. Patients with low renin secretion usually require higher doses to correct the electrolyte abnormalities. Caution should be observed in patients with hypertension or congestive heart failure. An alternative approach in these patients is the administration of furosemide alone or in combination with mineralocorticoid.

Adrenal Medulla

The adrenal medulla is derived embryologically from neuroectodermal cells. As a specialized part of the sympathetic nervous system, the adrenal medulla synthesizes and secretes the catecholamines epinephrine (80%) and norepinephrine (20%). Preganglionic fibers of the sympathetic nervous system bypass the paravertebral ganglia and pass directly from the spinal cord to the adrenal medulla. The adrenal medulla is analogous to a postganglionic neuron, although the catecholamines secreted by the medulla function as hormones, and not as neurotransmitters (see chapter 13, Video 13-1).

The synthesis of norepinephrine begins with hydroxylation of tyrosine to dopa (Fig. 47-5, 2 Video 47-2). This rate-limiting step in catecholamine biosynthesis is regulated such that synthesis is coupled to release. In the adrenal medulla and in those rare central neurons using epinephrine as a neurotransmitter, most of the norepinephrine is converted to epinephrine by the enzyme phenylethanolamine-*N*-methyltransferase. It is likely that the capacity of the adrenal medulla to synthesize epinephrine is influenced by the flow of glucocorticoid-rich blood from the adrenal cortex through the intra-adrenal portal system because a high concentration of glucocorticoid can induce the enzyme phenylethanolamine-*N*-methyltransferase.

In the adrenal medulla, catecholamines are stored in chromaffin granules complexed with adenosine triphosphate and Ca^{2+}. The normal adrenal releases epinephrine and norepinephrine by exocytosis in response to stimulation by preganglionic sympathetic neurons. The circulatory half-life (10 to 30 seconds) of these catechols is considerably longer than the brief receptor activity of norepinephrine released as a neurotransmitter from postganglionic sympathetic nerve endings. Biotransformation of circulating norepinephrine and epinephrine is accomplished chiefly by the enzyme catechol-*O*-methyltransferase, located in the liver and kidney. Monoamine oxidase is of less importance in the metabolism of circulating catechols. Metanephrine and vanillylmandelic acid are the major end products of catecholamine metabolism. These metabolites and a small amount of unchanged catecholamine (1%) appear in the urine.

The outflow of postganglionic sympathetic neurotransmitters and circulating catecholamine from the adrenal medulla is coordinated by higher cortical centers connected to the brainstem. The

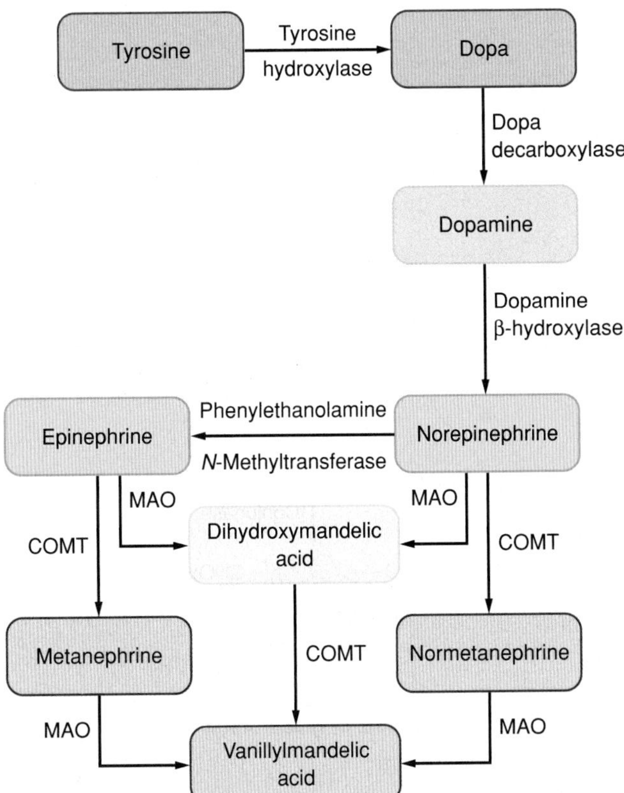

Figure 47-5 Synthesis and metabolism of endogenous catecholamines. COMT, catechol-*O*-methyltransferase; MAO, monoamine oxidase. (Adapted from Stoelting RK, Dierdorf SF, eds. Anesthesia and co-existing Disease. Churchill-Livingstone; 1983. Copyright © 1983 Elsevier. With permission.)

intrinsic activity of the brainstem sympathetic areas is modulated by higher cortical functions, emotional reactions (anger, fear), and various physiologic stimuli, including changes in the physical and chemical properties of the extracellular fluid (e.g., hypoglycemia, hypotension). The adrenal medulla and sympathetic nervous system are often stimulated together in a generalized fashion, although there are many physiologic conditions in which they act independently.

Pheochromocytoma

The only important endocrine disease process associated with the adrenal medulla is pheochromocytoma (NICV 47-2). These tumors produce, store, and secrete catecholamines. Paragangliomas are tumors that arise from autonomic ganglia and behave pathophysiologically like pheochromocytomas.[42] Most pheochromocytomas secrete both epinephrine and norepinephrine, with the fraction of secreted norepinephrine being greater than that secreted by the normal gland. Although pheochromocytomas occur in less than 0.2% of hypertensive patients, it is important to rule out this condition in patients with clinically suspect symptoms because surgical extirpation is curative in over 90% of patients and complications are often lethal in undiagnosed cases. Postmortem series have reported high perioperative mortality rates in undiagnosed patients undergoing relatively minor surgical procedures. Most deaths are from cardiovascular causes. Perioperative morbidity is related to tumor size and the degree of catecholamine secretion.[43]

Most (85% to 90%) pheochromocytomas are solitary tumors localized to a single adrenal gland, usually the right. Approximately 10% of adults and 25% of children have bilateral tumors. The tumor may also originate in extra-adrenal sites (10%), anywhere along the paravertebral sympathetic chain; however, 95% of tumors are in the abdomen, and a small percentage are in the thorax, urinary bladder, or neck. Malignant spread of these highly vascular tumors occurs in approximately 10% of cases.

In approximately 5% of cases, this tumor is inherited as a familial autosomal dominant trait. It may be part of the polyglandular syndrome referred to as MEN IIA or IIB. Type IIA includes medullary carcinoma of the thyroid, parathyroid hyperplasia, and pheochromocytoma; type IIB consists of medullary carcinoma of the thyroid, pheochromocytoma, and neuromas of the oral mucosa. Pheochromocytomas may also arise in association with von Recklinghausen neurofibromatosis or von Hippel–Lindau disease (retinal and cerebellar angiomatosis). The pheochromocytoma of the familial syndromes is rarely extra-adrenal or malignant. Bilateral tumors occur in approximately 75% of cases. When these patients present with a single adrenal pheochromocytoma, the chances of subsequent development of a second adrenal pheochromocytoma are sufficiently high that bilateral adrenalectomy should be considered. Every member of a MEN family should be considered at risk for pheochromocytoma.

Clinical Presentation

Pheochromocytoma may occur at any age, but it is most common in young to middle adult life. The clinical manifestations are mainly due to the pharmacologic effects of the catecholamines released from the tumor. These tumors are not innervated, and catecholamine release is independent of neurogenic control. Most patients have sustained hypertension, although occasionally it is paroxysmal.[44] When true paroxysms occur, the blood pressure may rise to alarmingly high levels, placing the patient at risk for cerebrovascular hemorrhage, heart failure, dysrhythmias, or myocardial infarction. Headache, palpitations, tremor, profuse sweating, and either pallor or flushing may accompany an attack. Pheochromocytoma can masquerade as malignant hyperthermia. Physical examination of the patient with pheochromocytoma may be unrevealing during the period between attacks, unless the patient presents with symptoms and signs of sequelae related to longstanding hypertension. A catecholamine-induced cardiomyopathy may be accompanied by heart failure and cardiac dysrhythmias. Paroxysms are often unprovoked but may be precipitated by displacement of the abdominal contents or, in the case of a tumor in the bladder, by micturition.

Diagnosis

Biochemical determination of free catecholamine and catecholamine metabolites in the urine is the most common screening test used to establish the diagnosis of pheochromocytoma.[45] Urinary normetanephrine and unconjugated norepinephrine and epinephrine levels are measured in a 24-hour urine collection and are expressed as a function of the creatinine clearance (Fig. 47-6). Excess production of catecholamines is diagnostic for pheochromocytoma. Free catecholamines represent less than 1% of the originally released hormone, and urinary levels are not always significantly elevated. Hence, differentiation from normal subjects may be difficult. A change in the ratio of unconjugated epinephrine to norepinephrine may be the only biochemical finding. Certain drugs interfere with urinary assays, and some patients with paroxysmal hypertension have normal values between attacks.

Although routine laboratory data are unlikely to provide specific diagnostic insight, ECG, chest radiograph, and complete

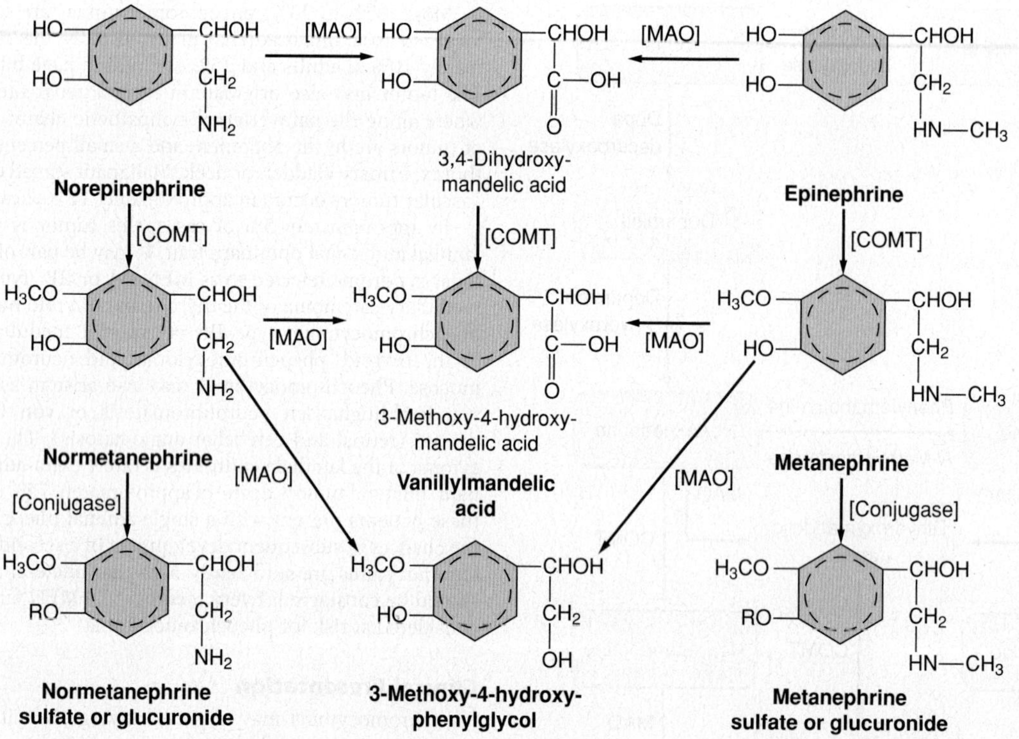

Norepinephrine → [MAO] → 3,4-Dihydroxy-mandelic acid ← [MAO] ← Epinephrine

[COMT] [COMT] [COMT]

Normetanephrine → [MAO] → 3-Methoxy-4-hydroxy-mandelic acid / Vanillylmandelic acid ← [MAO] ← Metanephrine

[Conjugase] [MAO] [MAO] [Conjugase]

Normetanephrine sulfate or glucuronide; 3-Methoxy-4-hydroxy-phenylglycol; Metanephrine sulfate or glucuronide

Figure 47-6 Catabolism of norepinephrine and epinephrine.

blood cell count can provide valuable information about end-organ damage to the clinician who entertains the diagnosis. Left ventricular hypertrophy and nonspecific T-wave changes are two of the more common ECG findings. Evidence of acute myocardial infarction or tachyarrhythmia has also been reported. The chest radiograph may reveal cardiomegaly, and the blood count often shows an elevated hematocrit consistent with a reduced intravascular volume and hemoconcentration. Standardized imaging methods such as CT and MRI are used in the noninvasive localization of these tumors.[46] Ultrasound and MRI are especially useful in pregnant patients. ^{123}I-labeled metaiodobenzylguanidine scintigraphy is also effective in localizing recurrent or extra-adrenal masses.

Anesthetic Considerations

Preoperative Preparation

4 Perioperative mortality rates have decreased from a high of 45% to between 0% and 3% for excision of pheochromocytoma following the introduction of α-antagonists for preoperative therapy. Perioperative blood pressure fluctuations, myocardial infarction, congestive heart failure, cardiac dysrhythmias, and cerebral hemorrhage, all appear to be reduced in frequency when the patient has been treated before surgery with α-blockers and the intravascular fluid compartment has been re-expanded.[47] Extended treatment with α-antagonists is also effective in treating the clinical manifestations of catecholamine myocarditis. However, α-blocker therapy has never been studied in a controlled way, and there are some groups that question its necessity due to the availability of potent titratable vasodilators for intraoperative use.[48] A list of drugs frequently used in the management of pheochromocytoma is given in Table 47-9.

α-Adrenergic blockade is initiated once the diagnosis of pheochromocytoma is established (see Chapter 13). Phenoxybenzamine, a long-acting (24 to 48 hours), noncompetitive presynaptic (α_2) and postsynaptic (α_1) blocker, has traditionally been used at doses of 10 mg every 8 hours. Increments are added until the blood pressure is controlled and paroxysms disappear. Most patients need between 80 and 200 mg/d. The absorption after oral administration is variable, and side effects are common. Certain cardiovascular reflexes such as the baroreceptor reflex are blunted, and postural hypotension may occur. Selective competitive α_1-blockers, such as doxazosin, terazosin, and prazosin, can also be used effectively with fewer side effects. Because postural hypotension can be pronounced with the commencement of therapy, the initial 1-mg dose is given at bedtime. Postural changes are also seen with maintenance therapy. A comparison of patients with pheochromocytoma receiving phenoxybenzamine or prazosin has shown both drugs to be equally effective in controlling blood pressure. Although the optimal period of preoperative treatment has not been established, most clinicians recommend beginning α-blockade therapy at least 10 to 14 days before the proposed surgery; however, periods as short as 3 to 5 days have been used.[49] During this time, the contracted intravascular volume and hematocrit return toward normal and the blood pressure is stabilized. Despite the possibility of hypotension after vascular isolation of the tumor, most clinicians continue α-blockers until the morning of surgery. Calcium channel blockers can also be used alone or in combination with α-blockers.

β-Adrenergic blockade is occasionally added after α-blockade has been established. This addition is considered in patients with persistent tachycardia or cardiac dysrhythmias that may be caused by nonselective α-blockade or epinephrine-secreting tumors. β-Blockers should not be given until adequate α-blockade is ensured to avoid the possibility of unopposed α-mediated vasoconstriction. There is no clear preoperative advantage of one β-antagonist over another, although the short half-life of esmolol may allow better control of heart rate and arrhythmias in the

Table 47-9 Drugs Used in the Management of Pheochromocytoma

Drug	Action	Preoperative Blood Pressure Control	Pressor Crisis	Comment
Phentolamine	Nonselective α-antagonist	—	1–5 mg IV; 0.5–1 mg/min IV	Short duration of action ~5 min
Phenoxybenzamine	Nonselective α-antagonist	20 mg/d PO up to 160 mg/d in divided doses	—	Long half-life; may accumulate
Doxazosin (terazosin dosing similar)	Selective α_1-antagonist	1 mg/d PO up to 8 mg/d PO	—	"First-dose phenomenon" may cause syncope
Propranolol	Nonselective β-antagonist	40 mg/d PO up to 480 mg/d in divided doses to control tachycardia	1–2 mg IV bolus	Should not be given prior to α-blockade
Atenolol	Selective β_1-antagonist	50–100 mg/d PO	—	Long-acting drug eliminated unchanged by kidney
Esmolol	Selective β_1-antagonist	—	250–500 µg/kg IV loading followed by maintenance infusion 25–250 µg/kg/min	Short-acting; elimination half-life ~9 min
Labetalol	α-antagonist and β-antagonist	200 mg/d PO in divided doses up to 800 mg/d	10 mg IV bolus	A much weaker α-blocker than β-blocker; may cause hypertensive response
Nitroprusside	Direct vasodilator	—	0.5–1.5 µg/kg/min initially, increased to maximum of 8 µg/kg/min; titrate to effect	Powerful vasodilator; short-acting
Magnesium sulfate	Direct vasodilator and membrane stabilizer	—	2–4 g IV bolus followed by 1–2 g/h and additional 1–2 g boluses as needed	May potentiate neuromuscular blockade
Nicardipine	Calcium channel antagonist	—	5 mg/h increased to max of 15 mg/h titrate to effect	Long elimination half-life
α-Methyltyrosine	Inhibitor of biosynthesis of catecholamine	1–4 g/d PO in divided doses	—	Suitable for patients who are not candidates for surgery; may be nephrotoxic

perioperative setting. Labetalol, a β-adrenergic antagonist with α-blocking activity, is effective as a second-line medication, but can increase blood pressure when used alone.

α-Methyltyrosine is an agent that inhibits the enzyme tyrosine hydroxylase, the rate-limiting step in catecholamine biosynthesis. This medication is generally reserved for patients with metastatic disease or for situations in which surgery is contraindicated and long-term medical therapy is required though some institutions are including it as part of preoperative preparation. When α-methyltyrosine is used in combination with α-adrenergic–blocking agents, there is a significant reduction in catecholamine biosynthesis.

Unrecognized pheochromocytoma during pregnancy may be life-threatening to the mother and fetus. Although the safety of adrenergic-blocking agents during pregnancy has not been established, these agents probably improve fetal survival in pregnant patients with pheochromocytoma. The trend is to perform surgery during the first trimester or at the time of cesarean delivery.[50] There is no reason to terminate an early pregnancy, but the patient should be aware of the risk of spontaneous abortion resulting from abdominal surgery to remove the tumor.

Perioperative Anesthetic Management

Symptomatic patients continue to receive medical therapy until tachycardia, cardiac dysrhythmias, and paroxysmal elevations in blood pressure are well controlled. If it is not possible to initiate α-blocking therapy before surgery or if the patient has received less than 48 hours of intensive treatment, it may be necessary to infuse nitroprusside during the induction of anesthesia. A low-dose infusion is often initiated in anticipation of the marked blood pressure elevations that can occur with laryngoscopy and surgical stimulation.

Most patients with solitary tumors without evidence of metastases or local invasion undergo a laparoscopic or robotic minimally invasive retroperitoneal approach. If the surgeon needs to assess for bilateral disease or the dissection is too difficult, then the procedure can be converted to an open one. During laparoscopic surgery, creation of pneumoperitoneum may cause release of catecholamines and large changes in hemodynamics; these changes can be controlled with a vasodilator.[51] Cortical-sparing adrenalectomies are becoming more common to preserve adrenal function.

Continuous intra-arterial blood pressure monitoring is required for managing the patient with pheochromocytoma. Central venous access can be useful in anticipation of the potential need to administer vasoactive medications. The need for more intensive monitoring is dictated by the presence of absence of coexisting cardiopulmonary disease.

5 Although there is no clear advantage to one anesthetic technique over another, drugs that are known to liberate histamine are avoided. Dopamine antagonists such as droperidol and metoclopramide can provoke catecholamine release and should not be used. A sedative–hypnotic, in combination with an opioid analgesic, is often selected for induction. It is extremely important to achieve an adequate depth of anesthesia before proceeding with laryngoscopy to minimize the sympathetic nervous system response to this maneuver. Maintenance is achieved with an opioid analgesic and a potent inhalation agent. Manipulation of the tumor may produce a marked elevation in blood pressure. Acute hypertensive crises are treated with IV infusions of nitroprusside or phentolamine or any vasodilator mentioned later. Phentolamine is a short-acting α-adrenergic antagonist that may be given as an IV bolus (2 to 5 mg) or by continuous infusion. Tachydysrhythmia is controlled with IV boluses of propranolol (1-mg increments) or by a continuous infusion of the ultrashort-acting selective β_1-adrenergic antagonist esmolol. The disadvantage of long-acting β-blockers may be persistence of bradycardia and hypotension after the tumor is removed. Even esmolol may be problematic because there are cases of cardiac arrest after clamping of the venous drainage in patients receiving large doses of esmolol. Almost every vasodilator has been tried and recommended as an adjuvant to control hypertension. Magnesium sulfate given as an infusion with intermittent boluses has been administered successfully.[52] Nicardipine, clevidipine,[53] nitroglycerin, diltiazem, fenoldopam, and prostaglandin E_1 have all been used anecdotally. The reduction in blood pressure that may occur after ligation of the tumor's venous supply can be dangerously abrupt and should be anticipated through close communication with the surgical team. Restitution of any intravascular fluid deficit is the initial therapy in this situation. After replenishment of the intravascular volume, if the patient remains hypotensive, phenylephrine is administered. Norepinephrine or vasopressin may also be needed.[53] After surgery, catecholamine levels return to normal over several days. Approximately 75% of patients become normotensive within 10 days. Hypoglycemia must be watched for as insulin levels rise from loss of catecholamine-induced β-cell suppression.

Diabetes Mellitus

A fasting glucose level below 100 mg/dL is considered normal. Individuals with documented fasting glucose levels above 126 mg/dL (HbA1c ≥6.5%) are considered diabetic, whereas those with levels between 100 and 125 mg/dL (HbA1c 5.7 to 6.4) are considered prediabetic.[54] Other definitions include glucose ≥200 mg/dL after 2 hours of glucose challenge during an oral glucose tolerance test (OGTT), or random glucose ≥200 mg/dL with presentation of hyperglycemia symptoms. An estimated 9.4% of the adult U.S. population have DM and about 40 million Americans have prediabetes.[55] DM is the most commonly occurring endocrine disease found in surgical patients, and 25% to 50% of diabetics will require surgery at some point in their lives. Although the most serious complications of DM are related to its character as a chronic disease, it can cause difficulties in the short-term management of acute illness. DM can remain clinically unapparent until exacerbated by the stress of trauma or surgery.[56] Some observational studies report that hyperglycemia is present in 32% to 38% of patients in community hospitals, 41% of critically ill patients with acute coronary syndromes, and 80% of patients after cardiac surgery.[57] In these reports, approximately one-third of nonintensive care unit (non-ICU) patients and approximately 80% of ICU patients had no history of diabetes before admission.[57]

Knowledge of the physiology of glucose metabolism and the stress response is important for understanding the principles of treatment of DM and the specific pathologic entities that comprise the clinical picture of DM.

Classification

DM primarily manifests as a disease of glucose metabolism; however, it significantly affects lipid and protein metabolism and has an impact on a wide range of endocrine functions. Despite a variety of etiologic factors, its hallmark is an absolute or relative insulin deficiency.

DM is classified into four broad types: type 1 diabetes, type 2 diabetes, gestational DM, and diabetes due to other causes.[54]

Type 1 DM is due to pancreatic β-cell destruction, usually leading to absolute insulin deficiency. It accounts for 5% to 10% of DM cases and is distinguished from type 2 DM, which accounts for the remaining 90% to 95% of DM cases. Most patients with type 1 DM experience the onset of disease early in life. Consequently, this form was also formerly referred to as juvenile-onset diabetes. However, type 1 DM and type 2 DM are heterogeneous diseases in which clinical presentation and disease progression may vary considerably. The traditional paradigms of type 2 DM presenting only in adults and type 1 DM only in children are no longer accurate, as both diseases occur in both cohorts.[58] Classification is important for determining therapy. Hyperglycemia in patients with type 1 DM cannot be controlled with diet or oral hypoglycemic agents; rather, it mandates treatment with insulin as there is an absolute deficiency of insulin. It is difficult to maintain an optimal glucose level in patients with type 1 DM. They are more likely to become ketotic and sustain progressive end-organ complications.[54]

Patients with type 2 DM, also formerly called adult-onset diabetes, typically experience a gradual onset of the disease later in life. It is due to a progressive loss of insulin secretion in the background of insulin resistance. However, the type 2 form can occur in young people, and conversely, many older adults can acquire a severe and brittle form of type 1 DM. Because of the obesity epidemic, many adolescents and teenagers are presenting more frequently with type 2 DM.[54] Patients with type 2 DM are often overweight and have resistance to the effects of insulin (commonly referred to as insulin resistance); hence, they may have normal or even elevated levels of insulin initially. In milder forms, type 2 DM can be treated with diet, lifestyle modifications, and oral hypoglycemic agents. Because these patients are relatively resistant to ketosis, their disease may not be clinically apparent until exacerbated by the stress of surgery or intercurrent illness.

Other types of DM can be a result of a disease that damages the pancreas and thus impairs insulin secretion. Pancreatic surgery, chronic pancreatitis, cystic fibrosis, and hemochromatosis can damage the pancreas and impair insulin secretion sufficiently to produce clinical DM. DM can also result from one of the endocrine diseases that produces a hormone that opposes the action of insulin. Hence, a patient with a glucagonoma, pheochromocytoma, or acromegaly may develop diabetes. An increased effect of glucocorticoids, from either Cushing disease or steroid or tacrolimus therapy (after organ transplantation), may also oppose the effect of insulin enough to elicit clinical diabetes and would certainly complicate the management of pre-existing diabetes. Thiazide diuretic and atypical antipsychotics (clozapine, olanzapine, risperidone, ziprasidone, quetiapine) increase the risk of diabetes.[59] Treatment of human immunodeficiency virus/acquired immunodeficiency syndrome, genetic defects in β-cell function, and genetic defects in insulin action can also induce diabetes (monogenic diabetes).[54]

Gestational diabetes is typically diagnosed in the second or third trimester of pregnancy and may presage future type 2 DM. Specific tests and diagnostic criteria are used to diagnose gestational diabetes; these include the glucose challenge test and the oral glucose challenge test.[54]

Physiology

Insulin has multiple and complex interactions with lipid, protein, and glucose metabolism. It also has many nonmetabolic functions.[60] For our purposes, it is easiest to regard the effects of insulin on glucose metabolism as primary and to view its effects on other metabolic functions only as they relate to glucose.

Insulin is a protein produced by the β cells of the islets of Langerhans in the pancreas. The basal rate of insulin secretion is about 1 unit/h, which can increase by 5- to 10-fold after ingestion of food. Normal production in the adult human is approximately 40 to 50 units/d. Insulin acts through its specific receptor on cells. The half-life of insulin in the circulation is 5 minutes. However, clinically, it appears to have a longer duration of action, due to delays in binding and release from the cellular receptors.[61] These facts lead us to the important principle that once a high level of insulin saturates all the binding sites, insulin will not have a more potent effect, just a more long-lasting effect.

Insulin is metabolized in the liver and kidneys. In patients with hepatic dysfunction, the loss of gluconeogenesis and a prolongation of insulin effect increase the risk of hypoglycemia. Similarly, in patients with renal disease, the action of insulin is prolonged. As such, they are more prone to hypoglycemia, and exogenous insulin should be administered judiciously.

Insulin release is related to a number of events. First, glucose and amino acids directly stimulate insulin release. The mechanism involves interaction with other hormones (glucagon, cortisol, etc.), and hormones from the GI tract that are released during enteral feeding (glucagon-like peptide-1 [GLP-1]) and glucose-dependent insulinotropic peptide (GIP). Through vagal stimulation, the autonomic nervous system also increases insulin release, as does β-adrenergic stimulation and α-adrenergic blockade. Nitric oxide stimulates insulin secretion, and potassium depletion decreases insulin secretion. Factors secreted by skeletal myocytes, adipocytes (e.g., leptin, resistin, adiponectin), and bone also influence glucose homeostasis.

The most fundamental action of insulin is to stimulate cellular uptake of glucose in skeletal muscle cells, adipose tissue, and cardiac cells. This is particularly important in skeletal muscle cells, where muscle activity also increases glucose uptake and is an important variable in the management of the physically active diabetic patient. The brain, liver, and immune cells are exceptions, where insulin does not affect glucose transport. Hence, the patient with diabetes has hyperglycemia because of inadequate cellular uptake of glucose in muscle and adipose tissue. Along with glucose, potassium enters the cells under the influence of insulin, so the diabetic patient is also likely to have an imbalance of potassium concentrations across cell membranes.

Other important metabolic functions of insulin include the stimulation of glycogen formation, as well as the suppression of gluconeogenesis and lipolysis. The patient with insulin deficiency has low glycogen stores and active gluconeogenesis. This implies that in the diabetic patient, because of an absence of glycogen, protein must be broken down to make glucose. Insulin also increases the uptake of amino acids into muscle cells. Hence, an insulin deficiency leads to catabolism and negative nitrogen balance.

Fat metabolism is also abnormal in the diabetic state, with acceleration of lipid catabolism and increased formation of ketones. A deficiency of insulin leads to increased fatty acid liberation from adipose tissue. These fatty acids have multiple metabolic effects, including interference with carbohydrate phosphorylation in muscle, which leads to further hyperglycemia. Low concentrations of insulin, which may be inadequate to prevent hyperglycemia, are often sufficient to block lipolysis. This effect explains the common clinical situation in which a patient is hyperglycemic without being ketotic.

Glucagon is a polypeptide released from the α cells of the pancreas and acts both to stimulate the release of insulin and to oppose some of its effects. It has both a direct and an indirect ability to increase circulating glucose levels. In some patients, after total pancreatic resection, glucose balance is not as poor as might be expected because of the concomitant absence of glucagon. Glucagon release is stimulated by hypoglycemia, epinephrine, and cortisol and is suppressed by glucose ingestion.

The metabolic effects of stress are intricately involved with the same pathways as those involved in DM. During stress, elevations in the circulating levels of cortisol, glucagon, catecholamines, and growth hormone act to stimulate gluconeogenesis and glycogenolysis and cause hyperglycemia. In addition, glucagon and adrenergic stimulation exert a suppressive effect on insulin release. Furthermore, inflammatory mediators released during stress enhance the release of counter-regulatory hormones and directly affect the intracellular signaling pathways of insulin, culminating in significant insulin resistance.[62,63] Hence, mild hyperglycemia may occur in the stressed patient who does not have DM. In a patient with minimal or subclinical DM before the stressful episode, stress-induced hyperglycemia may become difficult to manage and may require the use of insulin.

Diagnosis

For decades, the diagnosis of diabetes was based on plasma glucose criteria, either the fasting plasma glucose (FPG) or the 2-hour value in the 75-g OGTT. In 2009, the criteria to diagnose DM was amended and now includes hemoglobin A1c (HbA1c) above 6.5%.[54] The correlation of HbA1c percentages and average plasma glucose levels is presented in Figure 47-7. Other criteria for diagnosing DM are listed in Table 47-10. As with most diagnostic tests, a test result suggested that the presence of diabetes should be repeated to rule out laboratory error, unless the diagnosis is clear on clinical grounds.[54,64]

Treatment

Patients with type 1 DM require exogenous insulin to survive. Further, the risk of microvascular complications can be decreased if glycemic control is maintained near normal levels of blood glucose (HbA1c <7%).[54,65] Patients may be on a range of doses and regimens. These include multiple-component insulin regimens, multiple daily injections (MDIs), or continuous subcutaneous (SC) insulin infusion (CSII).[54] Intensive treatment of hyperglycemia in *newly* diagnosed patients may reduce long-term cardiovascular disease rates; however, intensive glycemic control

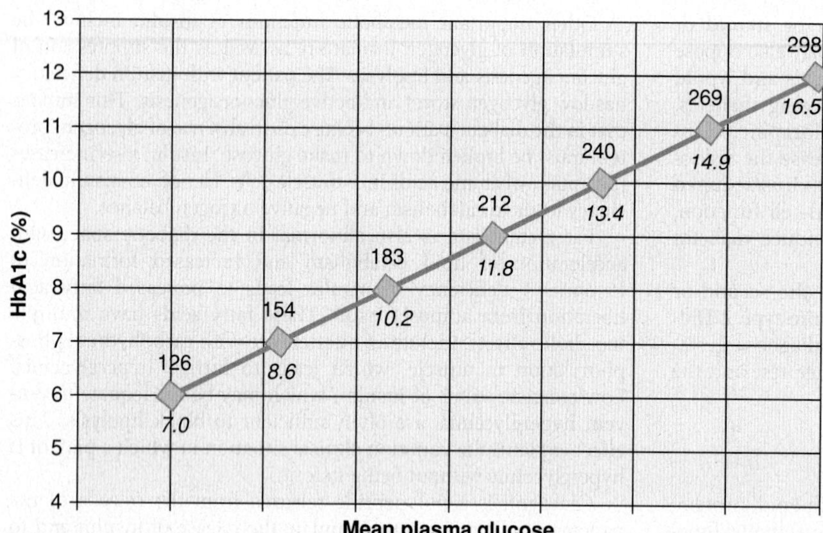

Figure 47-7 Correlation of hemoglobin A1c with average glucose. (Mean plasma glucose values above the line are in mg/dL and below the line and italic are in mmol/dL.) Estimates are based on 2,700 glucose measurements over 3 months per A1c measurement in 507 adults with type 1, type 2, and no diabetes. The correlation between A1c and average glucose was 0.92. (Data from Nathan DM, Kuenen J, Borg R, et al. Translating the A1C assay into estimated average glucose values. *Diabetes Care*. 2008; 31(8):1473–1478.)

(HbA1c <6.5% for 3.5 to 5.6 years) in patients with longstanding diabetes (8 to 11 years) has shown no reduction in cardiovascular outcomes.[66] Furthermore, intensive insulin therapy (IIT) prior to and during pregnancy reduces the risk of fetal malformations and morbidity.[54]

Patients with type 2 DM may initially be treated with diet/lifestyle modification, exercise, and metformin therapy.[67] Metformin is a biguanide that decreases hepatic glucose output and enhances the sensitivity of both hepatic and peripheral tissues to insulin.[68] If this fails to control glucose levels or the diabetes worsens, therapy with insulin and additional oral agents is indicated.[54] The goal is to decrease HbA1c levels below 7% safely, without causing hypoglycemia. Each new class of noninsulin agents added to initial therapy is expected to reduce HbA1c by 0.9% to 1.1%.[69] Selected properties of noninsulin glucose-lowering drugs are noted in Table 47-11. Sulfonylureas (glibornuride, gliclazide, glimepiride, glipizide, gliquidone, glyburide, glyclopyramide) and glinides (repaglinide, nateglinide, mitiglinide) enhance β-cell insulin secretion. Rosiglitazone (Avandia) and pioglitazone (Actos) are thiazolidinediones that increase insulin sensitivity. α-Glucosidase inhibitors (acarbose, miglitol, voglibose) decrease postprandial glucose absorption. Amylin analogs (pramlintide) suppress glucagon secretion and slow gastric emptying. Incretin mimetics (exenatide, semaglutide), as the name implies, emulate natural incretin hormones (GLP-1, glucose-dependent insulinotropic polypeptide [GIP]) and increase insulin production, inhibit glucagon secretion, and decrease glucose absorption. Dipeptidylpeptidase-4 inhibitors (alogliptin, linagliptin, saxagliptin, sitagliptin, vildagliptin) also slow degradation of incretin hormones, increase endogenous incretin hormone levels, and improve postprandial hyperglycemia. Sodium-glucose cotransporter 2 (SGLT2) inhibitors (canagliflozin, dapagliflozin, empagliflozin, ertugliflozin) provide insulin-dependent glucose lowering by blocking glucose reabsorption in the proximal renal tubule via SGLT2 inhibition. There is an increased risk of ketoacidosis in patients with type 1 and type 2 DM who are treated with SGLT2 inhibitors.[70] Bariatric surgery may be considered for adults with a body mass index higher than 35 kg/m^2 and type 2 diabetes, especially if the diabetes or associated comorbidities are difficult to control with lifestyle and pharmacologic therapy.[54] The American Diabetes Association (ADA) clinical guidelines state that metabolic surgery should be considered in individuals with type 2 DM and a body mass index >30 kg/m^2 if hyperglycemia is inadequately controlled despite optimal medical therapy.[71]

Table 47-10 Criteria for the Diagnosis of Diabetes

Criteria
A1c ≥6.5%. The test should be performed in a laboratory using a method that is certified and standardized.[a]
Fasting plasma glucose ≥126 mg/dL (7 mmol/L). Fasting is defined as no caloric intake for at least 8 h.[a]
2-h plasma glucose ≥200 mg/dL (11.1 mmol/L) during an oral glucose tolerance test. The test should be performed as described by the World Health Organization, using a glucose load containing the equivalent of 75 g anhydrous glucose dissolved in water.[a]
In a patient with classic symptoms of hyperglycemia or hyperglycemic crisis, a random plasma glucose ≥200 mg/dL (11.1 mmol/L).

[a]In the absence of unequivocal hyperglycemia, result should be confirmed by repeat testing.

Adapted from Surks MI, Sievert R. Drugs and thyroid function. *N Engl J Med*. 1995;333:1688–1694.

Anesthetic Management

Successful management of diabetic patients is as dependent on, or more dependent on, chronic complication management than acute hyperglycemia.

Preoperative

Preoperative evaluation and management has three important goals: One is determining end-organ complications of DM. This requires a thorough history and physical, a recent ECG, blood urea nitrogen, potassium, creatinine, glucose, and urinalysis. Second is determining the patient's glucose-lowering regimen. Preoperative counseling needs to be tailored to the patient's glucose-lowering regimen. The third goal is to determine the patient's current glycemic control and the need for preoperative intervention to control glucose levels.

End-Organ Complications of Diabetes

Atherosclerosis develops earlier and is more widespread in diabetic patients compared with nondiabetics. Manifestations include 6

Table 47-11 Properties of Selected Glucose-Lowering Drugs

Class	Compounds	Mechanism	Actions
Biguanides	Metformin	Activate AMP-kinase	Decrease hepatic glucose production Decrease intestinal glucose absorption Increase insulin action
Sulfonylureas (second generation)	Glibenclamide/glyburide Glipizide Gliclazide Glimepiride	Close KATP channels on β-cell plasma membranes	Increase insulin secretion
Meglitinides (glinides)	Repaglinide Nateglinide	Close KATP channels on β-cell plasma membranes	Increase insulin secretion
Thiazolidinediones (glitazones)	Pioglitazone Rosiglitazone	Activate the nuclear transcription factor PPAR-γ	Increase peripheral insulin sensitivity
α-Glucosidase inhibitors	Acarbose Miglitol	Inhibit intestinal α-glucosidase	Intestinal carbohydrate digestion (consequently, absorption is slowed)
GLP-1 receptor agonists (incretin mimetics)	Exenatide Semaglutide Liraglutide Albiglutide Dulaglutide	Activate GLP-1 receptors (β-cells/endocrine pancreas; brain/autonomous nervous system)	Increase insulin secretion (glucose dependent) Decrease glucagon secretion (glucose dependent) Slow gastric emptying Increase satiety
DPP-4 inhibitors (incretin enhancers)	Sitagliptin Vildagliptin Saxagliptin Linagliptin Alogliptin	Inhibit DPP-4 activity, increasing postprandial, endogenously released, active incretin hormone concentration	Increase active GLP-1 concentration Increase active GIP concentration Increase insulin secretion Decrease glucagon secretion
Bile acid sequestrants	Colesevelam	Bind bile acids in the intestinal tract, increasing bile acid production	Decrease hepatic glucose production Increase incretin levels
Dopamine-2 agonists	Bromocriptine	Activate dopaminergic receptors	Alter hypothalamic regulation of metabolism Increase insulin sensitivity
SGLT2 inhibitors	Canagliflozin Dapagliflozin Empagliflozin	Inhibits SGLT2 in the proximal nephron	Block glucose reabsorption by the kidney, increasing glucosuria
Amylin mimetics	Pramlintide	Activates amylin receptors in the pancreas	Decrease glucagon secretion Slow gastric emptying Increase satiety

AMP, adenosine monophosphate; DPP, dipeptidyl peptidase; GLP, glucagon-like peptide; KATP, adenosine triphosphate potassium; PPAR, peroxisome proliferator-activated receptor; SGLT, sodium-glucose transport protein.

Derived from American Diabetes Association. Standards of medical care in diabetes–2016. *Diabetes Care*. 2016;39(Suppl 1):S1–S119.

coronary artery disease, peripheral vascular disease, cerebrovascular disease, and renovascular disease. The incidence of postoperative myocardial infarction is increased in diabetic patients, and the perioperative complication rate is higher. Coronary artery disease can manifest at a young age or atypically in type 1 diabetics. Silent myocardial ischemia and infarction occur more commonly in diabetic patients, perhaps because of sensory neuropathy of the visceral afferents to the heart. DM may be associated with a cardiomyopathy in the face of angiographically normal coronary arteries, possibly with diffuse disease in arteries too small to be visualized. The American College of Cardiology/American Heart Association guidelines recognize DM as a risk factor when evaluating patients for noncardiac surgery.[72] Preoperative hyperglycemia, as documented by increased HbA1c, has consistently been associated with poor perioperative outcomes in a variety of clinical situations.[61,73]

Diabetic nephropathy occurs in 20% to 40% of patients with diabetes and is the leading cause of end-stage renal disease (ESRD). Albuminuria usually precedes a steady decline in renal function. Microalbuminuria (30 to 299 mg/24 h) has been shown to be the earliest stage of diabetic nephropathy in type 1 DM and a marker for development of nephropathy in type 2 DM.[52,74]

Patients with diabetes can develop heterogeneous neuropathies with diverse clinical manifestations. Most common among the neuropathies are chronic sensorimotor distal symmetric polyneuropathy and autonomic neuropathy.[75] Cardiovascular autonomic neuropathy is clinically the most important. It presents as resting tachycardia, exercise intolerance, and orthostatic hypotension. Autonomic function may be tested by measuring the beat-to-beat variation in heart rate during breathing, heart rate response to a Valsalva maneuver, and orthostatic changes in diastolic blood pressure and heart rate. Diabetic patients with autonomic neuropathy are at increased risk for intraoperative hypotension requiring vasopressor support, as well as perioperative cardiorespiratory arrest.[76–78] There may be an exaggerated pressor response to tracheal intubation.[79] Autonomic neuropathy also predisposes to intraoperative hypothermia.[80]

In addition, diabetic patients may have GI neuropathies (e.g., esophageal enteropathy, gastroparesis, constipation, diarrhea, fecal incontinence). They may have delayed gastric emptying and therefore they may be at increased risk of pulmonary aspiration of gastric contents. Autonomic function tests can predict the presence of solid food particles in gastric contents, but not increased gastric volume or acidity. Metoclopramide or erythromycin may be useful in emptying the stomach of solid food.[54]

In up to 40% of juvenile patients with DM presenting for renal transplantation, direct laryngoscopy can be difficult.[81] This may be due to diabetic stiff joint syndrome, a frequent complication of type 1 DM, leading to decreased mobility of the atlanto-occipital joint. The "prayer sign," an inability to approximate the palmar surfaces of the interphalangeal joints, is associated with stiff joint syndrome and may predict difficult laryngoscopy. Diabetic patients are at an increased risk of cognitive decline, dementia, fractures, cancer, obstructive sleep apnea, and hearing disorders.[54]

Determining Glucose-Lowering Regimen and Preoperative Counseling

Though specific protocols vary from institution to institution, a typical protocol recommended by ADA follows.[82] Patients who are on oral antihyperglycemic medications are advised to discontinue these medications the night before surgery. No oral hypoglycemic medications are administered or advised on the morning of surgery. Medications are reinstituted after the patient has resumed a normal diet. Patients who are on sulfonylureas are particularly at risk for developing hypoglycemia. Metformin should be withheld on the day of surgery. Though metformin has been associated with severe lactic acidosis during episodes of hypotension, poor perfusion, or hypoxia, similar perioperative outcomes have been reported in patients who have undergone surgery without discontinuing metformin.[83] SGLT2 inhibitors must be discontinued 3 to 4 days before surgery.

For patients who are taking short- or long-acting insulin preparations, adjustment of the insulin should take into account the timing of their insulin regimen (Table 47-12). Patients who take both evening and morning doses of insulin should take their usual dose of evening short-acting insulin but reduce their intermediate- or long-acting insulin dose by 20% the night before surgery. On the morning of surgery, they should omit their morning short-acting insulin and reduce the intermediate by 50%—or long-acting dose by 20% (and take this only if the fasting glucose is >120 mg/dL).[54] If patients are using a premixed insulin, they are instructed to reduce their evening dose by 20% and hold insulin completely on the morning of the procedure.[82] Patients with type 1 DM need some basal insulin at all times. An increasing number of patients with DM in the United States are receiving

Table 47-12 Properties of Common Insulin Preparations

Insulin/Insulin Analog Preparation	Onset	Peak	Duration
Lispro, aspart, glulisine (SC)	10–15 min	0.5-1.5 h	3–5 h
Regular (SC)	0.5–1 h	2–3 h	4–8 h
Regular (IV)	15 min	15–30 min	0.5–1 h
NPH (SC)	2–4 h	4–10 h	10–16 h
Glargine (SC)	2–4 h	none	20–24 h
Detemir (SC)	1–4 h	none	12–24 h
Degludec (SD)	1–9 h	none	42 h

IV, intravenous; SC, subcutaneous; SD, standard deviation.
Adapted from Powers AC, Fowler MJ, Rickels MR. Diabetes Mellitus: Management and Therapies. In: Loscalzo J, Fauci A, Kasper D, et al. eds. *Harrison's Principles of Internal Medicine*. 21st ed. McGraw Hill; 2022.

CSII therapy (also called insulin pump therapy) to achieve optimal glucose control. Insulin pumps have been safely utilized during surgery. It is recommended that pump basal insulin dose be reduced by 20% to 25%.[54] Blood glucose should be checked every hour if the pump is continued during surgery and at least every 2 to 4 hours while the patient is taking nothing by mouth.

Preoperative Glycemic Control

It is axiomatic that the patient should attain the best possible preoperative glucose control; however, no randomized controlled study has documented that achieving a certain glycemic range preoperatively for a certain period of time improves perioperative outcomes.[84] Despite the lack of high-quality evidence, an HbA1c level <8% is now being recommended for adult patients with diabetes undergoing elective surgical procedures.[85] Similarly, the European Society of Cardiology recommends that elective noncardiac surgery be postponed in patients with an HbA1c ≥8.5%, if it is "safe and practical."[86] Currently, no evidence-based guidelines exist regarding when to cancel a surgical procedure due to hyperglycemia. Providers need to weigh several issues when considering this question. First, the urgency of surgery should be considered. Second, the presence of an unstable metabolic state such as diabetic ketoacidosis (DKA) should be ruled out. Elective surgery in an unstable metabolic state is not recommended (see "Emergencies"). Another consideration is that the hyperglycemia may be caused by the illness for which the patient has presented for surgery (e.g., wound infection, intra-abdominal sepsis, osteomyelitis). Providers must therefore assess the patient for stability, the need for the procedure, the risks of the procedure, and the ability of the patient to achieve glucose control if the surgery is postponed. Some institutions have used a cutoff value of 300 mg/dL as a trigger in the preoperative area for evaluation for ketoacidosis. In other institutions, it is left to the discretion of the physician.[82] However, it is recommended to postpone nonurgent or elective surgery if there is an acute rise in glucose to above 400 mg/dL.[87]

Intraoperative

The details of the anesthetic plan depend intimately on the end-organ complications present. Invasive monitoring may be indicated for the patient with heart disease, awake intubation may be necessary if a difficult intubation is predicted, fluid management and drug choices may depend on renal function, and aspiration must be considered if there is gastroparesis.

Blood glucose levels should be measured before, during, and after surgery. Blood glucose should be monitored every 4 to 6 hours while the patient is *nil per os*.[54] The need for additional measurements is determined by the duration and magnitude of surgery, as well as the brittleness of the diabetes. Hourly measurements are reasonable in high-risk patients, especially those receiving continuous insulin through either an insulin pump or infusion.

The standard glucose dosage for an adult patient is 5 to 10 g/h (100 to 200 mL of 5% dextrose solution hourly). Intraoperative administration of glucose should be guided by the patient's glucose level. Routine administration of additional glucose-containing IV fluids is not recommended. It is best to separately record dextrose administration and fluids administered.

Monitoring of the patient who arrives in the operating room with a significant metabolic impairment such as DKA is similar to management in the medical ICU, and should include hourly determinations of blood glucose, arterial pH, electrolytes, and fluid balance. Frequent reassessments with medical consultation as necessary guide the use of fluids and electrolytes, especially potassium, insulin, phosphate, and glucose.

Another area of monitoring that is extremely important in the diabetic patient is positioning on the operating table. Injuries to the limbs or nerves are more likely in the patient who arrives in the operating room already compromised by diabetic peripheral vascular disease or neuropathy. The peripheral nerves may already be partly ischemic and therefore particularly vulnerable to pressure or stretch injuries.

Hyperglycemia and Perioperative Outcomes

Prior to 2001, little attention was paid to the control of hyperglycemia in the perioperative period or in the acute phase of critical illness managed in the ICU. Permissive or stress-induced hyperglycemia was generally accepted as the norm. Stress-induced hyperglycemia is defined as a transient response to the stress of an acute injury or illness.[57] Observational studies have reported a significant prevalence of hyperglycemia in hospitalized patients. Seventy percent of diabetic patients with acute coronary syndrome and 80% of cardiac surgery patients in the perioperative period may develop hyperglycemia.[67] Hyperglycemia in a hospital setting is defined as any blood glucose higher than 140 mg/dL.[85] Hyperglycemia significantly impairs chemotaxis, phagocytosis, generation of reactive oxygen species, and intracellular killing of bacteria.[88] Vascular reactivity is also decreased by hyperglycemia and is proposed to be related to decreased nitric oxide production. Acute hyperglycemia has also been shown to lead to poor outcomes in the setting of myocardial infarction and stroke.[88]

In surgical patients, *post*operative hyperglycemia is associated with an increased risk of infection, renal and pulmonary complications, and also mortality (Fig. 47-8).[61,89–93] Many studies have addressed the effects of hyperglycemia *peri*operatively and confirmed similar associations.[84,94–96] One study demonstrated that for every 20 mg/dL increase in the mean intraoperative glucose, the risk of an adverse outcome increased by more than 30%.[94]

Two other glycemic factors are also associated with poor perioperative outcomes. Hypoglycemia is a rare occurrence compared to hyperglycemia, but it is associated with increased mortality.[97,98] Finally, glucose variability (changes in the measured level of blood glucose) is an independent predictor of mortality.[99] This indicates that measures of glycemia, other than glucose concentration, may be important in the pathophysiology of hyperglycemia. Three different methods of expression of glucose variability are utilized: standard deviation (SD) of glucose, the mean amplitude of glycemic excursion (MAGE), and the glycemic lability index (GLI). MAGE is the mean of absolute values of any change in glucose (consecutive values) that are more than 1 SD of the entire set of glucose values. GLI is the squared difference between consecutive glucose measures per unit of actual time between those samples. Of these three methods, the GLI may be the best discriminator for mortality.[100]

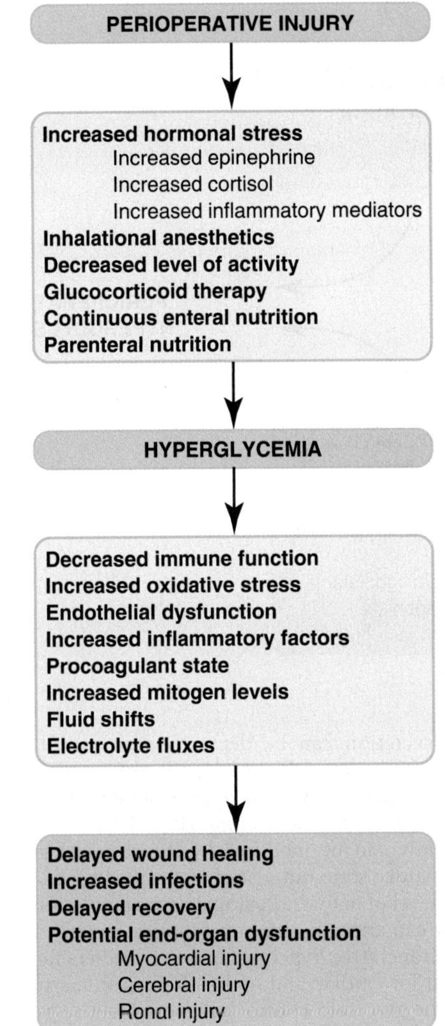

Figure 47-8 Relation among perioperative injury, hyperglycemia, and outcomes. (Reprinted with permission from Akhtar S, Barash PG, Inzucchi SE. Scientific principles and clinical implications of perioperative glucose regulation and control. *Anesth Analg*. 2010;110[2]:478–497.)

Perioperative Glycemic Control

Many factors influence glucose levels in the perioperative period (Fig. 47-9). Endogenous insulin secretions, exogenous insulin administration, insulin resistance, endogenous glucose production, exogenous glucose administration, and overall glucose consumption are some of the key factors that determine a patient's glucose levels.

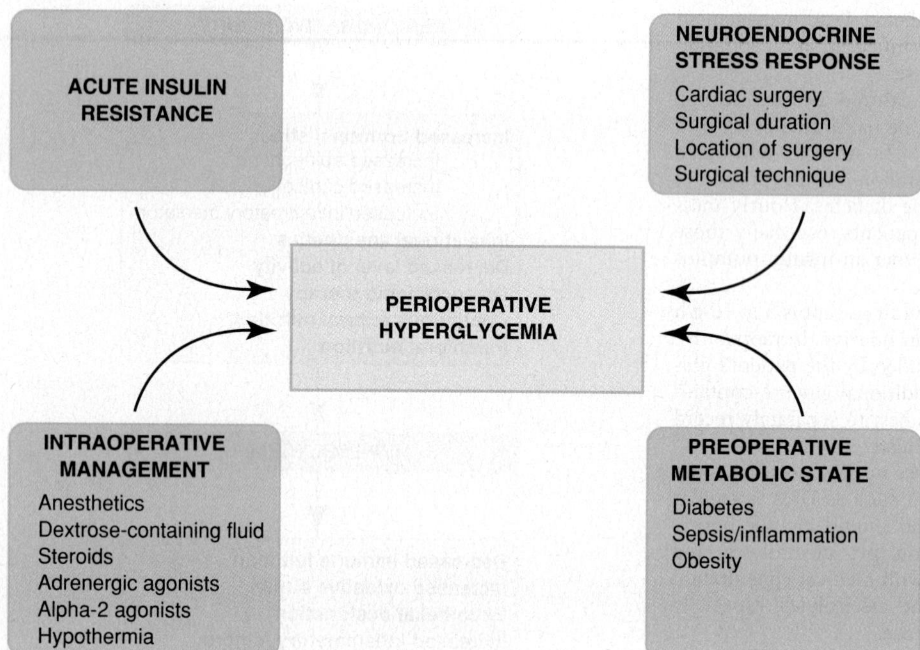

Figure 47-9 Modulators of perioperative hyperglycemia. (Reprinted with permission from Akhtar S, Barash PG, Inzucchi SE. Scientific principles and clinical implications of perioperative glucose regulation and control. *Anesth Analg*. 2010;110[2]:478–497.)

Insulin secretion can be decreased because of the direct effects of anesthetics, whereas significant insulin resistance develops postoperatively. The degree of insulin resistance is directly related to surgical trauma (Fig. 47-10). Insulin resistance not only can be modified by the stress of surgery and the inflammatory state but also may be affected by nutritional intake and level of activity. Postoperative ambulation and physical activity can alter glucose consumption acutely. Intraoperative and postoperative hyperglycemia are predictable in patients who present for cardiac and high-risk noncardiac surgery and/or have poor glycemic control preoperatively (e.g., diabetics, or patients who have an ongoing metabolic insult secondary to trauma or sepsis).[61]

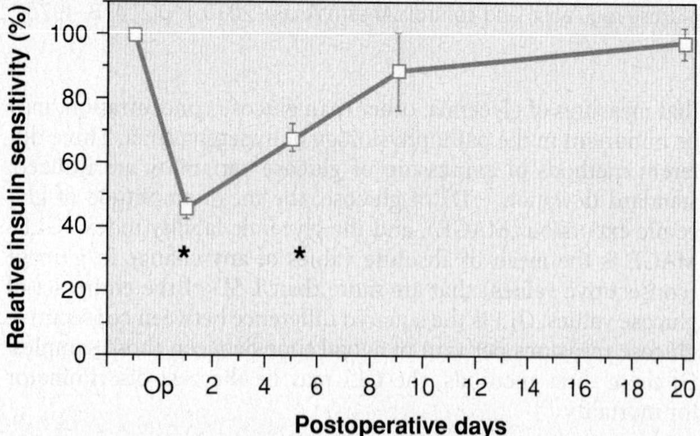

Figure 47-10 Time course for postoperative insulin resistance in patients undergoing open cholecystectomy. Relative insulin sensitivity represented as a percentage that is calculated as postoperative insulin sensitivity/perioperative insulin sensitivity × 100. Insulin sensitivity was determined within 5 days preoperatively and at days 1 ($n = 9$), 5, 9, and 20 ($n = 5$) postoperatively. *Statistically significant difference. Op, day of the operation. (Reprinted with permission from Thorell A, Efendic S, Gutnaik M, Häggmark T, Ljungqvist O. Insulin resistance after abdominal surgery. *Br J Surg*. 1994;81:59–63.)

Glycemic Goals

In 2001, van den Berghe et al.[101] published a landmark paper that demonstrated a mortality benefit of tight glucose control in critically ill patients in the surgical ICU. From this study originated the concept of IIT as a means of normalizing elevated glucose levels in critically ill patients. IIT was defined by a target glucose range of 80 to 110 mg/dL, and standard care implied a target glucose range of 180 to 200 mg/dL.[101] Although the study by van den Berghe et al. was a single-center, nonblinded trial, other retrospective studies also supported their findings and many centers adopted IIT protocols for management of hyperglycemia in the ICU. Furthermore, numerous studies documented clinical benefit of glycemic control in patients who underwent cardiac surgery.[61] However, most of the evidence was from prospective observational or retrospective studies. Over the course of the next few years, several studies comparing IIT to standard care failed to demonstrate a difference with respect to mortality. The IIT groups also demonstrated high incidences of hypoglycemia (8% to 28%), which was six times higher than the control group.[102–105]

The largest study to date, the NICE-SUGAR study, a multicenter, multinational randomized controlled trial, compared the effect of intensive glycemic control (target 81 to 108 mg/dL, mean blood glucose attained 115 mg/dL) to standard glycemic control (target 144 to 180 mg/dL, mean blood glucose attained 144 mg/dL) on outcomes among 6,104 critically ill participants, almost all of whom required mechanical ventilation.[106] Surprisingly, 90-day mortality was significantly higher in the intensive versus the conventional group in both surgical and medical patients, as was mortality from cardiovascular causes. Severe hypoglycemia was also more common in the intensively treated group (6.8% vs. 0.5%). The results of this study were in stark contrast to the van den Berghe et al. study, which reported a 42% relative reduction in ICU mortality in critically ill surgical patients treated to a target blood glucose of 80 to 110 mg/dL. 7

One situation where tight glucose control with insulin may be beneficial is in patients who are administered exogenous glucose via total parenteral nutrition.[107] This was the case in the van den

Table 47-13 Current Recommendations for Glycemic Control in Critically Ill Patients

Organization	Year	Patient Population	Treatment Threshold (mg/dL)	Target Glucose Level (mg/dL)
Society of Thoracic Surgeons	2009	Cardiac surgery in ICU	150	150–180
Institute for Healthcare Improvement	2009	ICU patients	180	<180
American College of Physicians	2011	ICU patients	180	140–180
Surviving Sepsis Campaign	2013	ICU patients	180	<180
European Society of Cardiology	2014	Patients after major noncardiac surgery	180	140–180
American Diabetes Association	2016	ICU patients	180	140–180

Berghe et al. study, where patients received significant exogenous glucose early in the ICU. Furthermore, the control group in the NICE-SUGAR trial had reasonably good blood glucose management and was maintained at a mean glucose of 144 mg/dL, only 29 mg/dL above the intensively managed patients. Accordingly, this study's findings do not negate the concept that glycemic control in the ICU is important. However, they do strongly suggest that it may not be necessary to target blood glucose values to a highly stringent target of less than 110 mg/dL, and it may be dangerous to control glucose too tightly.

Several studies published after the NICE-SUGAR trial underscored the findings of that investigation. Annane et al.[108] found no reduction in mortality and increased hypoglycemia in a randomized controlled trial of IIT with glucocorticoids in the treatment of septic shock. The control group was given standard insulin therapy plus glucocorticoids. Meta-analyses of randomized trials investigating IIT demonstrated no overall effect on mortality and increased hypoglycemia rates in the IIT groups compared with controls.[107,109–111] An observational cohort study published prior to the NICE-SUGAR trial compared outcomes before and after institution of an IIT policy. Hypoglycemia was increased and no survival benefit was noted with the institution of IIT.[112] ADA recommends a target range 80 to 180 mg/dL for blood glucose in the perioperative period; in general, tighter glycemic targets are not advised.[54]

In summary, association between perioperative hyperglycemia and poor outcomes is strong. Though hyperglycemia develops frequently in patients who undergo cardiac or high-risk noncardiac surgery, the value of controlling glucose levels tightly *intraoperatively* has not been proven. Poor glycemic control is probably a marker of significant metabolic perturbation, which is beyond the regulatory capacity of the body. Given that in the NICE-SUGAR trial the standard insulin therapy control group (140 to 180 mg/dL range) had similar outcomes (if not better) than the IIT group, the 140 to 180 mg/dL range is now generally accepted as the new goal. In 2009, the American Association of Clinical Endocrinologists (AACE) and the ADA released formal recommendations for the management of hyperglycemia in the ICU.[113] The recommended threshold to initiate an insulin infusion is no higher than 180 mg/dL. Once insulin therapy has been initiated, the 140 to 180 mg/dL goal range is targeted.

In addition to the AACE/ADA, various other professional organizations have published guidelines for the management of glucose levels in the ICU.[114] The Surviving Sepsis Campaign[115] recommends maintaining glucose levels below 180 mg/dL; the Institute for Healthcare Improvement target is less than 180 mg/dL; the 2014 European Society of Cardiology guidelines for perioperative cardiac management in noncardiac surgery patients do take into account the results of the NICE-SUGAR study and recommend maintaining glucose levels less than 180 mg/dL in postsurgery patients.[86] The Society of Thoracic Surgeons (for cardiac surgery) targets 150 to 180 mg/dL, whereas the guidelines from the American College of Physicians recommend keeping glucose below 180 mg/dL in critically ill patients (Table 47-13).[116]

Hyperglycemia in hospitalized patients has been defined as blood glucose above 140 mg/dL (7.8 mmol/L). In noncritically ill hospitalized patients, the goal is to keep the glucose level between 80 and 180 mg/dL.[54] This should ideally be achieved by basal plus bolus insulin dosing rather than sliding scale insulin. Practitioners should also keep in mind that target glucose levels for terminally ill, elderly, frail, and nursing home patients have not been established. There is consensus that in these populations, the risk of hypoglycemia outweighs the risk of hyperglycemia and less stringent targets may be more appropriate.[52,54,117]

Management of Perioperative Hyperglycemia

In view of the complex nature of glycemic control in the perioperative period, maintaining glucose levels within a specific range can be demanding. The narrower the desired glycemic range, the more resource intensive the protocol will be.

There are multiple insulin preparations with varying duration of actions that can be administered in many ways.[118] The simplest way is to administer short-acting insulin subcutaneously. Only a few studies have studied this route, and they have not been very successful in maintaining glucose in the desired range (40% to 60% of the time) and achieving it in a timely manner. In the perioperative setting, the state of peripheral perfusion is extremely variable, and vasoconstriction is very common, often secondary to hypovolemia or hypothermia. Hence, absorption of any drug administered subcutaneously can be erratic and unreliable. Similarly, sliding scale protocols have also been disappointing and are strongly discouraged in the management of hyperglycemia in hospitalized patients.[118] Most study protocols that have demonstrated desirable glycemic control in the acute care setting have used continuous IV insulin infusion combined with IV bolus injections. Targeted glucose levels are achieved successfully and promptly using these dynamic scale protocols combined with frequent blood glucose determinations. Once a certain requirement of insulin in a 24-hour period is known, the patient can be transitioned to basal–bolus insulin protocol. This requires giving a certain amount of long-acting insulin (which provides a fraction of basal insulin requirement), supplemented by three or four doses of short-acting insulin bolus based on blood glucose measurements.[57] A randomized controlled trial has shown that basal–bolus treatment improved glycemic control and reduced hospital complications compared with sliding scale insulin in general surgery patients with type 2 diabetes.[119]

Blood glucose can be determined by central laboratory, blood–gas analysis machines, or various point-of-care testing devices that use capillary blood (fingerstick). Point-of-care devices are most commonly used in many acute care areas for glucose monitoring and management. Practitioners should keep in mind that the accuracy of these handheld meters can vary by 20%.[120] Glucose meter analysis (arterial and capillary blood) may provide higher glucose values, whereas blood–gas meter analysis of arterial blood may yield lower glucose values compared with central laboratory values. The hemodynamic state of the patient may also affect the accuracy of the blood glucose measurement by the point-of-care devices. Furthermore, whole blood glucose values and plasma glucose values are different, and the same is true for arterial and venous blood. Therefore, a real possibility exists of overdosing or underdosing a patient with insulin. Hence, aberrant glucose values should be verified by central laboratory measurements, and practitioners should be aware of the performance of the point-of-care devices used in their institutions.[121] Because of the coronavirus disease 2019 pandemic, continuous glucose monitoring (CGM) devices have been approved for use in the hospital setting.[122] Studies are currently underway to assess the effectiveness of this approach, which may lead to the routine use of these devices in the inpatient setting.[123]

Type 1 Diabetes

Type 1 diabetics require exogenous insulin or they will rapidly develop ketoacidosis and its complications. This can be achieved by administering one-half to two-thirds of the patient's usual intermediate-acting insulin subcutaneously on the morning of surgery. In addition to this basal insulin, a regular insulin sliding scale (RISS) can be added and titrated to blood glucose measurement.[124] Alternatively, an insulin infusion of 0.5 to 2 units/h can meet basal metabolic needs and be adjusted to maintain blood glucose at the desired level.[118] With either method, a slow glucose infusion (5% dextrose in water at 75 to 125 mL/h) will prevent hypoglycemia while the patient is fasting.

Type 2 Diabetes

Patients who are on oral antihyperglycemic medications are advised to discontinue their medications the night (or sometimes a few days) before surgery. No oral hypoglycemic medications are administered on the morning of surgery. Patients on chronic insulin are treated based on their insulin regimen. Perioperative glucose control can be achieved by insulin infusion titrated to blood glucose or basal long-acting insulin supplemented by a RISS. The use of a RISS as the sole method of control is to be discouraged because it can predispose to wide fluctuations in glucose level.[57]

Postoperatively, as the patient resumes oral intake, therapy can be transitioned to the patient's chronic regimen. Patients with type 2 diabetes who have had a gastric bypass procedure may have rapid resolution of glucose intolerance and will often need their oral agents and insulin reduced or even discontinued in the postoperative period. This effect appears to be due to changes in the incretin hormones such as GIP and GLP-1 rather than weight loss itself.[125]

Emergencies

Hyperglycemic hyperosmolar state (HHS) and DKA represent two extremes in the spectrum of decompensated DM. DKA is more common than HHS and accounts for 1% of diabetes-related emergencies. The mortality rate for HHS (10% to 20%) is greater than the mortality from DKA (5%).[126] Patients may present with a diabetic emergency, or the condition may develop perioperatively because of stress, trauma, or infection.[127]

Hyperglycemic Hyperosmolar State

An occasional elderly patient with minimal or mild DM may present with remarkably high blood glucose levels (>600 mg/dL) and profound dehydration (9 to 12 L). It is often precipitated by concurrent illnesses such as MI, stroke, sepsis, pneumonia, and other serious infections. Patients with HHS usually have enough endogenous insulin activity to prevent lipolysis and ketosis; even with blood sugar concentrations of 1,000 mg/dL, they are not in ketoacidosis. It takes only *one-tenth* as much insulin to suppress lipolysis as it does to stimulate glucose utilization. Presumably, it is the combination of an impaired thirst response and decreased fluid intake in the presence of relative insulin deficiency that allows the hyperglycemia to develop. Hyperglycemia induces an osmotic diuresis that also contributes to intravascular volume depletion. Marked hyperosmolarity may lead to coma and seizures, and increased plasma viscosity predisposes patients to intravascular thrombosis. HHS responds quickly to rehydration and small doses of insulin. If there are no cardiovascular contraindications, 1 to 2 L (or 15 to 30 mL/kg) of normal saline should be infused over 1 hour. Insulin, by bolus or infusion, should be administered after initial volume has been administered.[128] Administering insulin before adequate fluid replacement can result in cardiovascular collapse. Insulin-mediated glucose uptake moves water out of the intravascular space and into cells, causing severe hypovolemia. With rapid correction of the hyperosmolarity, cerebral edema is a risk, and recovery of mental acuity may be delayed after the blood glucose level and circulating volume have been normalized.[129] HHS tends to have a substantially higher mortality than DKA, 15% versus 1% respectively, in some clinical series.

Diabetic Ketoacidosis

DKA is defined by the biochemical triad of ketonemia, hyperglycemia, and acidemia.[130] If the diabetic patient has insufficient insulin to block lipolysis and the metabolism of free fatty acids, the metabolic by-products acetoacetate and β-hydroxybutyrate accumulate. These ketone bodies are organic acids and cause a metabolic acidosis with an increased unmeasured anion gap.[131] Patients often present because of intercurrent illness, trauma, or the untoward cessation of insulin therapy. Although hyperglycemia is almost always present, the degree of hyperglycemia does not correlate with the severity of acidosis. Blood sugar levels are often in the 250- to 600-mg/dL range. Occasionally, the serum glucose is only minimally elevated (euglycemic DKA). This has been seen in patients treated with SGLT2 inhibitors The patient is chronically dehydrated because of the combination of the hyperglycemia-induced osmotic diuresis and the nausea and vomiting typical of this syndrome. Because leukocytosis, abdominal pain, GI ileus, and mildly elevated amylase levels are all common in ketoacidosis, an occasional patient is misdiagnosed as having an intra-abdominal surgical problem. Cerebral edema, an extremely serious complication of DKA, is seen most frequently in children.

Diagnostic criteria for DKA include ketonemia or significant ketonuria; blood glucose above 250 mg/dL or known DM; and anion-gap metabolic acidosis (serum bicarbonate below 18 mmol/L or arterial pH less than 7.3).[132] Treatment of DKA includes insulin administration and fluid and electrolyte replacement (Table 47-14). Route of administration of insulin is determined by the severity of DKA. Mild to moderate DKA can be treated with subcutaneously administered insulin analogs. However, severe DKA requires IV insulin administration. Typically, a

Table 47-14 Management of Diabetic Ketoacidosis

Regular insulin, 10-unit IV bolus, followed by an insulin infusion nominally at (blood glucose/150) units/h
Isotonic IV fluids as guided by vital signs and urine output; anticipate 4–10 L deficit
When urine output is more than 0.5 mL/kg/h, give potassium chloride, 10–40 mEq/h (with continuous electrocardiographic monitoring when the rate is >10 mEq/h)
When serum glucose is decreased to 250 mg/dL, add dextrose 5% at 100 mL/h
Consider sodium bicarbonate if pH <6.9

continuous infusion is started at 0.1 unit/kg/h as long as serum potassium is above 3.3 mEq/L. If the blood glucose does not fall by 10% in the first hour, a bolus of 0.1 unit/kg is administered. Another alternative is to administer 0.1 unit/kg as a bolus followed by an infusion at 0.1 unit/kg/h. When blood glucose levels decrease below 250 mg/dL, glucose should be added to the IV fluid while insulin therapy continues. Fluid requirements can be marked; 1 to 2 L of normal saline, or equivalent, should be given over 1 to 2 hours. After the first hour, they may need to be continued at 15 to 20 mL/kg/h. Further deficits can be replaced more gradually with Ringer's lactate or 0.45% normal saline. In euglycemic DKA associated with SGLT2 inhibitor use, the pharmacologic effect of these medications may persist for 10 to 14 days following discontinuation of therapy. Relapse of ketoacidosis is common if nutritional intake has not advanced during this time (e.g., in the postoperative setting). Potassium replacement is a key concern in patients with DKA. Because of the diuresis, the total body potassium stores are reduced (estimated deficit [3 to 5 mEq/kg]). However, acidosis by itself causes a shift of potassium ions out of cells. Thus, the serum potassium concentration may be normal or even slightly elevated while the patient is acidotic. As soon as the metabolic acidosis is corrected, the potassium ions shift back into the cells. Furthermore, insulin also shifts the potassium intracellularly. Consequently, the serum potassium concentration can decline acutely. Therefore, early and vigorous potassium replacement is required, with the exception of those patients with renal failure. Hypophosphatemia also occurs with the correction of the acidosis and, if severe, may cause impairment of ventilation, resulting from skeletal muscle weakness. Instead of DKA, the diabetic patient with a metabolic acidosis may have lactic acidosis, which results from poor tissue perfusion or sepsis. It is diagnosed by the presence of an increased serum lactate concentration without an elevated ketone concentration. Several studies have shown that the use of bicarbonate in patients with DKA made no difference in resolution of acidosis or time to discharge.[133] Its use is not generally indicated unless the patient is hemodynamically unstable with pH below 7.1 or has a pH below 6.9 even without hemodynamic instability. Venous thrombosis, upper GI bleeding, and acute respiratory distress syndrome occasionally complicate DKA.

DKA must also be distinguished from the syndrome of alcoholic ketoacidosis. This typically occurs in the poorly nourished alcoholic patient after acute intoxication. Except for the presence of chemical ketoacidosis, alcoholic ketoacidosis is not clinically related in any way to DM. The alcoholic patient may be hypoglycemic or mildly hyperglycemic. The predominant ketone in this syndrome is β-hydroxybutyrate, which tends to react less sensitively in the standard laboratory nitroprusside reaction measurement of ketones. Hence, the diagnosis may be obscured. Administration of dextrose and parenteral fluids is the specific treatment for alcoholic ketoacidosis; insulin is not indicated (except in the rare circumstance in which the patient also has clear-cut DM).

Hypoglycemia

Hypoglycemia is a major limiting factor in the glycemic management of diabetic patients. The precise level at which symptomatic hypoglycemia occurs is variable. The normal, fasted patient may have blood sugar levels no higher than 50 mg/dL without symptoms. However, the diabetic patient who has a chronically elevated blood sugar level may be symptomatic at levels significantly above this glucose concentration. Hypoglycemia is almost impossible to diagnose clinically in the unconscious patient.

Hypoglycemia is classified into three levels. Level 1 hypoglycemia is defined as a glucose concentration <70 mg/dL but greater than 54 mg/dL. Level 2 hypoglycemia is defined as a blood glucose concentration <54 mg/dL. It is the threshold at which neuroglycopenic symptoms begin to occur and requires immediate treatment. Level 3 hypoglycemia is defined as a severe event characterized by altered mental and/or physical functioning that requires assistance from another person for recovery.[134]

Hypoglycemia results in activation of the sympathetic nervous system and autonomic symptoms, including sweating, palpitations, tremor, and hunger. Neuroglycopenic symptoms include behavioral and cognitive impairment, drowsiness, speech difficulty, blurred vision, seizures, coma, and death. Many of the autonomic as well as the early neurologic symptoms are notably absent in the intubated, sedated, critically ill, or anesthetized patient. In the anesthetized patient, these signs of sympathetic hyperactivity can easily be misinterpreted as inadequate or "light" anesthesia. Furthermore, in patients being treated with β-adrenergic–blocking agents or in patients with advanced diabetic autonomic neuropathy, the sympathetic hyperactivity of hypoglycemia may be blunted. Thus, the clinical diagnosis of hypoglycemia in the surgical patient may be difficult to make, and only a high degree of suspicion and frequent blood glucose checks can prevent this complication. Treatment of hypoglycemia is with 25 g of IV dextrose (50 mL of dextrose 50% in water) or 1 mg of intramuscular glucagon if the patient is not alert, and 8 ounces of juice in the alert patient. The goal is to achieve a blood glucose level above 100 mg/dL.

Hypoglycemia is more likely to occur in the diabetic surgical patient if insulin or sulfonylureas are given without supplemental glucose. With renal insufficiency, the action of insulin and oral hypoglycemic agents is prolonged.

Pituitary Gland

The pituitary gland is located below the base of the brain in a bony structure called the sella turcica. The pituitary gland and the hypothalamus together form a central unit that regulates the release of various hormones. The pituitary gland is divided into two components. The *anterior pituitary* (adenohypophysis) secretes prolactin, growth hormone, gonadotropins (luteinizing hormone and follicle-stimulating hormone), TSH, and ACTH. The *posterior pituitary* (neurohypophysis) secretes the hormones vasopressin and oxytocin. Hormone release from the anterior and posterior pituitary is regulated by the hypothalamus. Regulatory peptides or preformed hormones from the hypothalamus are transported to the pituitary gland through vascular or tissue connections.

Anterior Pituitary

Hyposecretion of anterior pituitary hormones is usually due to compression of the gland by tumor. This may begin as an isolated deficiency, but it usually develops into multiglandular dysfunction. Male impotence or secondary amenorrhea in women is an early manifestation of panhypopituitarism. Panhypopituitarism after postpartum hemorrhagic shock (Sheehan syndrome) is due to necrosis of the anterior pituitary gland. Radiation therapy delivered to the sella turcica or nearby structures and surgical hypophysectomy is another cause of panhypopituitarism. Panhypopituitarism is treated with specific hormone replacement therapy, which should be continued in the perioperative period. Stress doses of corticosteroids are necessary for patients receiving steroid replacement because of inadequate ACTH.

The hypersecretion of various anterior pituitary hormones is usually caused by an adenoma. Excess prolactin secretion with galactorrhea is a common hormonal abnormality associated with pituitary adenoma. Cushing disease may occur secondary to excess ACTH production. Gigantism or acromegaly may occur due to excess growth hormone production in the child or adult, respectively.[135] Excessive secretion of TSH is rare.

Acromegaly in the adult patient may pose several problems for the anesthesiologist. Hypertrophy occurs in skeletal, connective, and soft tissues.[136] The tongue and epiglottis are enlarged, making the patient susceptible to upper airway obstruction. The incidence of difficult intubation is 20% to 30% and may be clinically unpredictable.[137] Hoarseness may reflect thickening of the vocal cords or paralysis of an RLN due to stretching. Dyspnea or stridor is associated with subglottic narrowing. Peripheral nerve or artery entrapment, hypertension, and DM are other common findings. The anesthetic management of these patients is complicated by distortion of the facial anatomy and upper airway. Induction of general anesthesia may put the patient at increased risk if mask fit is improper or vocal cord visualization is impaired. When the preoperative history suggests upper airway or vocal cord involvement, it is prudent to consider intubation of the trachea while the patient is awake.

Posterior Pituitary

The posterior pituitary, or neurohypophysis, is composed of terminal nerve endings that extend from the ventral hypothalamus. Vasopressin (antidiuretic hormone [ADH]) and oxytocin are the two principal hormones secreted by the posterior pituitary. Both hormones are synthesized in the supraoptic and paraventricular nuclei of the hypothalamus. They are bound to inactive carrier proteins, neurophysins, and transported by axons to membrane-bound storage vesicles located in the posterior pituitary. ADH is a nonapeptide that circulates as a free peptide after its release. The primary functions of ADH are maintenance of extracellular fluid volume and regulation of plasma osmolality. Oxytocin elicits contraction of the uterus and promotes milk secretion and ejection by the mammary glands.

Vasopressin (ADH)

ADH promotes resorption of solute-free water by increasing cell membrane permeability to water alone. The target sites for ADH are the collecting tubules of the kidneys. A decrease in free water clearance causes a decrease in serum osmolality and a corresponding increase in circulating blood volume. Under normal conditions, the primary stimulus for the release of ADH is an increase in serum osmolality.

Osmoreceptors located in the hypothalamus are sensitive to changes in the normal serum osmolality of as little as 1% (normal osmolality is approximately 285 mOsm/L). Stretch receptors in the left atrium and perhaps pulmonary veins, which are sensitive to moderate reductions in the blood volume, are also capable of stimulating ADH secretion. The need to restore plasma volume may at times override osmotic inhibition of ADH release. Various physiologic and pharmacologic stimuli also influence the secretion of ADH. Positive-pressure ventilation of the lungs, stress, anxiety, hyperthermia, β-adrenergic stimulation, and any histamine-releasing stimulus can promote the release of ADH.

ADH also has other actions. It can increase blood pressure by constricting vascular smooth muscle. This activity is most significant in the splanchnic, renal, and coronary vascular beds, and provides the rationale for administering exogenous vasopressin in the management of hemorrhage due to esophageal varices. Caution must be taken when this drug is used in patients with coronary artery disease. ADH (even in small doses) can precipitate myocardial ischemia through vasoconstriction of the coronary arteries. It is unclear whether selective arterial infusion is safer than systemic administration with respect to cardiac and vascular side effects. ADH is also often used in vasodilatory shock as an adjuvant to other pressor agents.

ADH also promotes hemostasis through an increase in the level of circulating von Willebrand factor and factor VIII. Desmopressin (DDAVP), an analog of ADH, is commonly used to treat some types of von Willebrand disease (see Chapter 17). DDAVP is also frequently used to reverse the coagulopathy of renal failure.

Diabetes Insipidus

Diabetes insipidus results from inadequate secretion of ADH or resistance on the part of the renal tubules to ADH (nephrogenic diabetes insipidus). Failure to secrete adequate amounts of ADH results in polydipsia, hypernatremia, and a high output of poorly concentrated urine. Hypovolemia and hypernatremia may become so severe as to be life-threatening. This disorder usually occurs after destruction of the pituitary gland by intracranial trauma, infiltrating lesions, or surgery, especially neurosurgery and in particular hypophysectomy (see Chapter 37).[138] It can appear intraoperatively or in the immediate postoperative period. Patients in whom diabetes insipidus develops secondary to severe head trauma or subarachnoid hemorrhage often have impending brain death or are presenting for organ retrieval. Treatment of diabetes insipidus depends on the extent of the hormonal deficiency. During surgery, the patient with complete diabetes insipidus can be treated with DDAVP or vasopressin infusion combined with administration of an isotonic crystalloid solution.[139] The serum sodium and plasma osmolality are measured on a regular basis and therapeutic changes are made accordingly. If diabetes insipidus occurs postoperatively, free access to water is often all that is needed. If persistent or severe, DDAVP administered intranasally has prolonged antidiuretic activity (12 to 24 hours). Nonhormonal agents that have antidiuretic effects include the oral hypoglycemic chlorpropamide, carbamazepine, clofibrate, and, paradoxically, thiazide diuretics though these are rarely used.

Inappropriate Secretion of Antidiuretic Hormone

Inappropriate and excessive secretion of ADH may occur in association with many diverse pathologic processes, including head injuries, intracranial tumors, pulmonary infections, small cell carcinoma of the lung, and hypothyroidism (see Chapter 37). Surgery and trauma can cause transiently elevated ADH levels. The clinical manifestations occur due to dilutional hyponatremia, decreased serum osmolality, and a reduced urine output with a high osmolality. Weight gain, skeletal muscle weakness, and mental confusion or convulsions are presenting symptoms. Peripheral edema and hypertension are rare because volume regulation via the renin–angiotensin system is intact. The diagnosis of the syndrome of inappropriate ADH secretion is one of exclusion; other causes of hyponatremia must be ruled out first. The prognosis is related to the underlying cause of the syndrome.

The treatment for patients with mild or moderate water intoxication is restriction of fluid intake to 800 mL/d. Patients with severe water intoxication associated with hyponatremia (sodium <120 mEq/L) and central nervous system symptoms may require more aggressive therapy, with the IV administration of a hypertonic saline solution. This may be administered in conjunction with furosemide. The use of isotonic and hypertonic saline can be very nuanced and may actually worsen hyponatremia depending on the urine osmolarity. Caution must be observed in patients with poor left ventricular function. Too-rapid correction of hyponatremia may induce osmotic demyelination and cause permanent brain damage. Serum sodium should not be raised by more than 8 mEq/L in 24 hours. Other drugs that may be used in the patient with the syndrome of inappropriate ADH are demeclocycline and lithium. Demeclocycline interferes with the ability of the renal tubules to concentrate urine. Lithium is usually not used because of the high incidence of toxicity. Vasopressin-2 receptor antagonists, such as tolvaptan, may be useful in specific situations.

Endocrine Response to Surgical Stress

Anesthesia, surgery, and trauma elicit a generalized endocrine metabolic response characterized by an increase in the plasma levels of cortisol, ADH, renin, catecholamines, and endorphins and by metabolic changes such as hyperglycemia and a negative nitrogen balance.[140,141] There is also an increase in inflammatory markers such as C-reactive protein which would not be generally considered part of an endocrine response. Various neural and humoral factors (e.g., pain, anxiety, acidosis, local tissue factors, hypoxia) play a role in activating this stress response. There is an acute response to critical illness that is characterized by normal pituitary function, but target organ insensitivity. During the chronic phase of critical illness, there is generalized endocrine hypofunction probably of a hypothalamic origin.

The induction of anesthesia increases the levels of circulating catecholamines and is a form of metabolic stress. Regional anesthesia can block part, but not all, of the metabolic stress response during surgery, probably by blockade of the neural communication from the surgical area.[142] It is theorized that the persistently high levels of circulating catecholamines in trauma and critical illness lead to stress hyperglycemia through a direct inhibition of insulin release. Bypass of the gut hormonal actions in patients receiving IV glucose feedings, especially if given in large amounts, contributes to the impairment of insulin release during illness and can create a particularly difficult management problem for diabetic patients.

Endorphins are a group of endogenous peptides with opioid activity that have been isolated from the central nervous system. It is well documented that β-endorphin is released from the anterior pituitary, where it is contained as part of β-lipoprotein, a 91-chain amino acid, which is a cleavage product of the precursor peptide for ACTH. Large increases in the central nervous system and plasma concentrations of endorphins in response to emotional or surgical stimuli suggest that these substances play a role in the body's response to stress. These substances modulate painful stimuli by binding to opiate receptors located throughout the brain and spinal cord.

Numerous experiments have focused on the stress response and its relation to the depth of anesthesia. Regional anesthesia and general anesthesia appear to blunt the release of various stress hormones during the period of surgical stimulation in a dose-dependent fashion. Historically, anesthesiologists have relied on the indirect measurement of hemodynamic variables such as blood pressure and heart rate to evaluate the level of autonomic activity in response to anesthesia and surgery. It is assumed that the physiologic manifestations of stress are potentially harmful, especially in patients with limited functional reserve. Aspects of the stress response may affect oncologic outcomes after cancer surgery. As such, anesthetic techniques and pain management strategies are designed to limit this neurohormonal response in the hope of providing the patient with the best prognosis. Further investigations are needed to assess the impact of these efforts on perioperative, and long-term morbidity and mortality.

For further review and interactivities, please see the videos and narrative interactive clinical vignettes (NICVs) accessible in the complimentary eBook bundled with this text. Access instructions are located on the inside front cover.

REFERENCES

1. Surks MI, Sievert R. Drugs and thyroid function. *N Engl J Med.* 1995;333:1688–1694.
2. Deegan RJ, Furman WR. Cardiovascular manifestations of endocrine dysfunction. *J Cardiothorac Vasc Anesth.* 2011;25:705–720.
3. Klein I, Danzi S. Thyroid disease and the heart. *Circulation.* 2007;116:1725–1735.
4. Danzi S, Klein I. Amiodarone-induced thyroid dysfunction. *J Intensive Care Med.* 2015:30; 179–185.
5. Cooper DS. Antithyroid drugs. *N Engl J Med.* 2005;352:905–917.
6. De Leo S, Lee SY, Braverman LE. Hyperthyroidism. *Lancet.* 2016;388:906–918.
7. Smallridge RC. Metabolic and anatomic thyroid emergencies: a review. *Crit Care Med.* 1992; 20:276–291.
8. Chiha M, Samarasinghe S, Kabaker AS. Thyroid storm: an updated review. *J Intensive Care Med.* 2015;30(3):131–140.
9. Chun BJ, Bae JS, Lee SH, Joo J, Kim ES, Sun DI. A prospective randomized controlled trial of the laryngeal mask airway versus the endotracheal intubation in the thyroid surgery: evaluation of postoperative voice, and laryngopharyngeal symptom. *World J Surg.* 2015;39:1713–1720.
10. Bouaggad A, Nejmi SE, Bouderka MA, Abbassi O. Prediction of difficult tracheal intubation in thyroid surgery. *Anesth Analg.* 2004;99:603–606.
11. Boccara G, Guenoun T, Aidan P. Anesthetic implications for robot-assisted transaxillary thyroid and parathyroid surgery: a report of twenty cases. *J Clin Anesth.* 2013;25:508–512.
12. Szubin L, Kacker A, Kakani R, Komisar A, Blaugrund S. The management of post-thyroidectomy hypocalcemia. *Ear Nose Throat J.* 1996;75:612–614, 616.
13. Wagner HE, Seiler C. Recurrent laryngeal nerve palsy after thyroid gland surgery. *Br J Surg.* 1994;81:226–228.
14. Dionigi G, Chiang FY, Dralle H, et al. Safety of neural monitoring in thyroid surgery. *Int J Surg.* 2013;11:S120–S126.
15. Lindsay RS, Toft AD. Hypothyroidism. *Lancet.* 1997;349:413–417.
16. Stathatos N, Wartofsky L. Perioperative management of patients with hypothyroidism. *Endocrinol Metab Clin North Am.* 2003;32:503–518.
17. Toft AD. Thyroxine therapy. *N Engl J Med.* 1994;331:174–180.
18. Bennett-Guerrero E, Kramer DC, Schwinn DA. Effect of chronic and acute thyroid hormone reduction on perioperative outcome. *Anesth Analg.* 1997;85:30–36.
19. Ladenson PW, Levin AA, Ridgway EC, Daniels GH. Complications of surgery in hypothyroid patients. *Am J Med.* 1984;77:261–266.
20. Whitten CW, Latson TW, Klein KW, Elmore J, Spencer R, Duggar P. Anesthetic management of a hypothyroid cardiac surgical patient. *J Cardiothorac Vasc Anesth.* 1991;5:156–159.
21. Weinberg AD, Ehrenwerth J. Anesthetic considerations and perioperative management of patients with hypothyroidism. *Adv Anesth.* 1987;4:185–212.
22. Mihai R, Farndon JR. Parathyroid disease and calcium metabolism. *Br J Anaesth.* 2000;85: 29–43.
23. Fraser WD. Hyperparathyroidism. *Lancet.* 2009;374:145–158.
24. Roland EJ, Wierda JM, Eurin BG, Roupie E. Pharmacodynamic behaviour of vecuronium in primary hyperparathyroidism. *Can J Anaesth.* 1994;41:694–698.
25. Udelsman R, Lin Z, Donovan P. The superiority of minimally invasive parathyroidectomy based on 1650 consecutive patients with primary hyperparathyroidism. *Ann Surg.* 2011;253: 585–591.

26. Shindo ML, Rosenthal JM, Lee T. Minimally invasive parathyroidectomy using local anesthesia with intravenous sedation and targeted approaches. *Otolaryngol Head Neck Surg.* 2008;138:381–387.
27. Kivela JE, Sprung J, Richards ML, et al. Effects of propofol on intraoperative parathyroid hormone monitoring in patients with primary hyperparathyroidism undergoing parathyroidectomy: a randomized control trial. *Can J Anaesth.* 2011;58:525–531.
28. Gafni RI, Collins MT. Hypoparathyroidism. *N Engl J Med.* 2019;380:1738–1747.
29. Vaughan ED Jr. Diseases of the adrenal gland. *Med Clin North Am.* 2004;88:443–466.
30. Inder WJ, Hunt PJ. Glucocorticoid replacement in pituitary surgery: guidelines for perioperative assessment and management. *J Clin Endocrinol Metab.* 2002;87:2745–2750.
31. Rivers EP, Gaspari M, Saad GA, et al. Adrenal insufficiency in high-risk surgical ICU patients. *Chest.* 2001;119:889–896.
32. Téblick A, Gunst J, Van den Berghe G. Critical illness-induced corticosteroid insufficiency: what it is not and what it could be. *J Clinical Endocrinol Metab.* 2022;107:2057–2064
33. Axelrod L. Perioperative management of patients treated with glucocorticoids. *Endocrinol Metab Clin North Am.* 2003;32:367–383.
34. Annane D, Pastores SM, Rochwerg B, et al. Guidelines for the diagnosis and management of critical illness-related corticosteroid insufficiency (CIRCI) in critically ill patients (part I): Society of Critical Care Medicine (SCCM) and European Society of Intensive Care Medicine (ESICM) 2017. *Crit Care Med.* 2017;45(12):2078–2088.
35. Charmandari E, Nicolaides NC, Chrousos GP. Adrenal insufficiency. *Lancet.* 2014;383;2152–2167.
36. Coursin DB, Wood KE. Corticosteroid supplementation for adrenal insufficiency. *JAMA.* 2002;287:236–240.
37. Engquist A, Brandt MR, Fernandes A, Kehlet H. The blocking effect of epidural analgesia on the adrenocortical and hyperglycemic responses to surgery. *Acta Anaesthesiol Scand.* 1977;21:330–335.
38. Salem M, Tainsh RE Jr, Bromberg J, Loriaux DL, Chernow B. Perioperative glucocorticoid coverage: a reassessment 42 years after emergence of a problem. *Ann Surg.* 1994;219:416–425.
39. Liu MM, Reidy AB, Saatee S, Collard CD. Perioperative steroid management: approaches based on current evidence. *Anesthesiology.* 2017;127:166–172
40. Glowniak JV, Loriaux DL. A double-blind study of perioperative steroid requirements in secondary adrenal insufficiency. *Surgery.* 1997;121:123–129.
41. Marik PE, Varon J. Requirement of perioperative stress doses of corticosteroids: a systematic review of the literature. *Arch Surg.* 2008;143(12):1222–1226.
42. Berends AMA, Kerstens MN, Lenders JWM, Timmers HJLM. Approach to the patient: perioperative management of the patient with pheochromocytoma or sympathetic paraganglioma. *J Clin Endocrinol Metab.* 2020;105(9):dgaa441.
43. Kinney MAO, Warner ME, van Heerden JA, et al. Perianesthetic risks and outcomes of pheochromocytoma and paraganglioma resection. *Anesth Analg.* 2000;91:1118–1123.
44. Kinney MAO, Narr BJ, Warner MA. Perioperative management of pheochromocytoma. *J Cardiothorac Vasc Anesth.* 2002;16:359–369.
45. Chen H, Sippel RS, O'Dorisio MS, Vinik AI, Lloyd RV, Pacak K; North American Neuroendocrine Tumor Society (NANETS). The North American Neuroendocrine Tumor Society consensus guideline for the diagnosis and management of neuroendocrine tumors: pheochromocytoma, paraganglioma, and medullary thyroid cancer. *Pancreas.* 2010;39:775–783.
46. Neumann HPH, Young WF Jr, Eng C. Pheochromocytoma and paraganglioma. *N Engl J Med.* 2019;381:552–565.
47. Lenders JWM, Duh QY, Eisenhofer G, et al. Pheochromocytoma and paraganglioma: an Endocrine Society clinical practice guideline. *J Clin Endocrinol Metab.* 2014;99:1915–1942.
48. Schimmack S, Kaiser J, Probst P, Kalkum E, Diener MK, Strobel O. Meta-analysis of α-blockade versus no blockade before adrenalectomy for phaeochromocytoma. *Br J Surg.* 2020;107(2):e102–e108.
49. Pacak K. Preoperative management of the pheochromocytoma patient. *J Clin Endocrinol Metab.* 2007;92:4069–4079.
50. Patel D, Phay JE, Yen TWF, et al. Update on pheochromocytoma and paraganglioma from the SSO Endocrine and Head and Neck Disease Site Working Group, part 2 of 2: perioperative management and outcomes of pheochromocytoma and paraganglioma. *Ann Surg Oncol.* 2020;27(5):1338–1347.
51. Joris JL, Hamoir EE, Hartstein GM, et al. Hemodynamic changes and catecholamine release during laparoscopic adrenalectomy for pheochromocytoma. *Anesth Analg.* 1999;88:16–21.
52. James MF, Cronjé L. Pheochromocytoma crisis: the use of magnesium sulfate. *Anesth Analg.* 2004;99:680–686.
53. Lord MS, Augoustides JGT. Perioperative management of pheochromocytoma: focus on magnesium, clevidipine, and vasopressin. *J Cardiothorac Vasc Anesth.* 2012;26:526–531.
54. American Diabetes Association Professional Practice Committee. 2. Classification and diagnosis of diabetes: Standards of Medical Care in Diabetes-2022. *Diabetes Care.* 2022;45(Suppl 1): S17–S38.
55. Tsao CW, Aday AW, Almarzooq ZI, et al. Heart disease and stroke statistics—2022 update: a report from the American Heart Association. *Circulation.* 2022;145:e153–e639.
56. Corathers SD, Falciglia M. The role of hyperglycemia in acute illness: supporting evidence and its limitations. *Nutrition.* 2011;27(3):276–281.
57. Smiley D, Umpierrez GE. Management of hyperglycemia in hospitalized patients. *Ann N Y Acad Sci.* 2010;1212:1–11.
58. Dabelea D, Rewers A, Stafford JM, et al; SEARCH for Diabetes in Youth Study Group. Trends in the prevalence of ketoacidosis at diabetes diagnosis: the SEARCH for diabetes in youth study. *Pediatrics.* 2014:133;e938–e945.
59. Erickson SC, Le L, Zakharyan A, et al. New-onset treatment-dependent diabetes mellitus and hyperlipidemia associated with atypical antipsychotic use in older adults without schizophrenia or bipolar disorder. *J Am Geriatr Soc.* 2012;60:474–479.
60. Kim JA, Montagnani M, Koh KK, Quon MJ. Reciprocal relationships between insulin resistance and endothelial dysfunction: molecular and pathophysiological mechanisms. *Circulation.* 2006;113(15):1888–1904.
61. Akhtar S, Barash PG, Inzucchi SE. Scientific principles and clinical implications of perioperative glucose regulation and control. *Anesth Analg.* 2010;110(2):478–497.
62. Bagry HS, Raghavendran S, Carli F. Metabolic syndrome and insulin resistance: perioperative considerations. *Anesthesiology.* 2008;108(3):506–523.
63. Biddinger SB, Kahn CR. From mice to men: insights into the insulin resistance syndromes. *Annu Rev Physiol.* 2006;68:123–158.
64. Sacks DB, Arnold M, Bakris GL, et al. Guidelines and recommendations for laboratory analysis in the diagnosis and management of diabetes mellitus. *Clin Chem.* 2011;57(6):e1–e47.
65. Nathan DM. Diabetes: advances in diagnosis and treatment. *JAMA.* 2015:314;1052–1062.
66. Skyler JS, Bergenstal R, Bonow RO, et al; American Diabetes Association, American College of Cardiology Foundation, American Heart Association. Intensive glycemic control and the prevention of cardiovascular events: implications of the ACCORD, ADVANCE, and VA diabetes trials: a position statement of the American Diabetes Association and a scientific statement of the American College of Cardiology Foundation and the American Heart Association. *Diabetes Care.* 2009:32;187–192.
67. Qaseem A, Humphrey LL, Sweet DE, Starkey M, Shekelle P; Clinical Guidelines Committee of the American College of Physicians. Oral pharmacologic treatment of type 2 diabetes mellitus: a clinical practice guideline from the American College of Physicians. *Ann Intern Med.* 2012;156(3):218–231.
68. Bailey CJ, Turner RC. Metformin. *N Engl J Med.* 1996;334(9):574–579.
69. Bennett WL, Maruthur NM, Singh S, et al. Comparative effectiveness and safety of medications for type 2 diabetes: an update including new drugs and 2-drug combinations. *Ann Intern Med.* 2011;154(9):602–613.
70. FDA Drug Safety Communication. FDA revises labels of SGLT2 inhibitors for diabetes to include warnings about too much acid and serious urinary tract infections. *FDA website.* Accessed March 4, 2016. www.fda.gov/Drugs/DrugSafety/ucm475463.htm
71. American Diabetes Association Professional Practice Committee. 8. Obesity management for the treatment of type 2 diabetes: Standards of Medical Care in Diabetes-2022. *Diabetes Care.* 2022;45(Suppl 1):S113–S124.
72. Fleisher LA, Fleischmann KA, Auerbach AD, et al; American College of Cardiology, American Heart Association. 2014 ACC/AHA guideline on perioperative cardiovascular evaluation and management of patients undergoing noncardiac surgery: a report of the American College of Cardiology Foundation/American Heart Association Task Force on practice guidelines. *J Am Coll Cardiol.* 2014;64:e77–e137.
73. Pichardo-Lowden A, Gabbay RA. Management of hyperglycemia during the perioperative period. *Curr Diab Rep.* 2012;12(1):108–118.
74. Garg JP, Bakris GL. Microalbuminuria: marker of vascular dysfunction, risk factor for cardiovascular disease. *Vasc Med.* 2002;7(1):35–43.
75. Freeman R. Not all neuropathy in diabetes is of diabetic etiology: differential diagnosis of diabetic neuropathy. *Curr Diab Rep.* 2009;9(6):423–431.
76. Charlson ME, MacKenzie CR, Gold JP. Preoperative autonomic function abnormalities in patients with diabetes mellitus and patients with hypertension. *J Am Coll Surg.* 1994;179(1): 1–10.
77. Latson TW, Ashmore TH, Reinhart DJ, Klein KW, Giesecke AH. Autonomic reflex dysfunction in patients presenting for elective surgery is associated with hypotension after anesthesia induction. *Anesthesiology.* 1994;80(2):326–337.
78. Page MM, Watkins PJ. Cardiorespiratory arrest and diabetic autonomic neuropathy. *Lancet.* 1978;1(8054):14–16.
79. Vohra A, Kumar S, Charlton AJ, Olukoga AO, Boulton AJ, McLeod D. Effect of diabetes mellitus on the cardiovascular responses to induction of anaesthesia and tracheal intubation. *Br J Anaesth.* 1993;71(2):258–261.
80. Kitamura A, Hoshino T, Kon T, Ogawa R. Patients with diabetic neuropathy are at risk of a greater intraoperative reduction in core temperature. *Anesthesiology.* 2000;92(5):1311–1318.
81. Hogan K, Rusy D, Springman SR. Difficult laryngoscopy and diabetes mellitus. *Anesth Analg.* 1988;67(12):1162–1165.
82. American Diabetes Association Professional Practice Committee. 16. Diabetes care in the hospital: Standards of Medical Care in Diabetes—2022. *Diabetes Care.* 2022;45(Suppl 1): S244–S253.
83. Duncan AI, Koch CG, Xu M, et al. Recent metformin ingestion does not increase in-hospital morbidity or mortality after cardiac surgery. *Anesth Analg.* 2007;104(1):42–50.
84. King JT Jr, Goulet JL, Perkal MF, Rosenthal RA. Glycemic control and infections in patients with diabetes undergoing noncardiac surgery. *Ann Surg.* 2011;253(1):158–165.

85. Korytkowski MT, Muniyappa R, Antinori-Lent K,et al. Management of hyperglycemia in hospitalized patients in non-critical care setting: an Endocrine Society clinical practice guideline. *J Clin Endocrinol Metab*. 2022;107:2101–2128.
86. Halvorsen S, Mehilli J, Cassese S, et al. 2022 ESC Guidelines on cardiovascular assessment and management of patients undergoing non-cardiac surgery: Developed by the task force for cardiovascular assessment and management of patients undergoing non-cardiac surgery of the European Society of Cardiology (ESC) Endorsed by the European Society of Anaesthesiology and Intensive Care (ESAIC). *Eur Heart J*. 2022;43(39):3826–3924. doi: 10.1093/eurheartj/ehac270.
87. Alexanian SM, McDonnell ME, Akhtar S. Creating a perioperative glycemic control program. *Anesthesiol Res Pract*. 2011;2011:465974.
88. Inzucchi SE. Clinical practice: management of hyperglycemia in the hospital setting. *N Engl J Med*. 2006;355(18):1903–1911.
89. Vriesendorp TM, Morélis QJ, Devries JH, Legemate DA, Hoekstra JB. Early post-operative glucose levels are an independent risk factor for infection after peripheral vascular surgery: a retrospective study. *Eur J Vasc Endovasc Surg*. 2004;28(5):520–525.
90. Pomposelli JJ, Baxter JK 3rd, Babineau TJ, et al. Early postoperative glucose control predicts nosocomial infection rate in diabetic patients. *JPEN J Parenter Enteral Nutr*. 1998;22(2):77–81.
91. Swenne CL, Lindholm C, Borowiec J, Schnell AE, Carlsson M. Peri-operative glucose control and development of surgical wound infections in patients undergoing coronary artery bypass graft. *J Hosp Infect*. 2005;61(3):201–212.
92. Noordzij PG, Boersma E, Schreiner F, et al. Increased preoperative glucose levels are associated with perioperative mortality in patients undergoing noncardiac, nonvascular surgery. *Eur J Endocrinol*. 2007;156(1):137–142.
93. Schmeltz LR, DeSantis AJ, Thiyagarajan V, et al. Reduction of surgical mortality and morbidity in diabetic patients undergoing cardiac surgery with a combined intravenous and subcutaneous insulin glucose management strategy. *Diabetes Care*. 2007;30(4):823–828.
94. Gandhi GY, Nuttall GA, Abel MD, et al. Intraoperative hyperglycemia and perioperative outcomes in cardiac surgery patients. *Mayo Clin Proc*. 2005;80(7):862–866.
95. Frisch A, Chandra P, Smiley D, et al. Prevalence and clinical outcome of hyperglycemia in the perioperative period in noncardiac surgery. *Diabetes Care*. 2010;33(8):1783–1788.
96. Polito A, Thiagarajan RR, Laussen PC, et al. Association between intraoperative and early postoperative glucose levels and adverse outcomes after complex congenital heart surgery. *Circulation*. 2008;118(22):2235–2242.
97. Krinsley J, Preiser JC. Intensive insulin therapy to control hyperglycemia in the critically ill: a look back at the evidence shapes the challenges ahead. *Crit Care*. 2010;14(6):330.
98. Zoungas S, Patel A, Chalmers J, et al; ADVANCE Collaborative Group. Severe hypoglycemia and risks of vascular events and death. *N Engl J Med*. 2010;363(15):1410–1418.
99. Krinsley JS. Glycemic variability: a strong independent predictor of mortality in critically ill patients. *Crit Care Med*. 2008;36(11):3008–3013.
100. Mackenzie IMJ, Whitehouse T, Nightingale PG. The metrics of glycaemic control in critical care. *Intensive Care Med*. 2011;37(3):435–443.
101. van den Berghe G, Wouters P, Weekers F, et al. Intensive insulin therapy in critically ill patients. *N Engl J Med*. 2001;345(19):1359–1367.
102. van den Berghe G, Wilmer A, Hermans G, et al. Intensive insulin therapy in the medical ICU. *N Engl J Med*. 2006;354(5):449–461.
103. Arabi YM, Dabbagh OC, Tamim HM, et al. Intensive versus conventional insulin therapy: a randomized controlled trial in medical and surgical critically ill patients. *Crit Care Med*. 2008;36(12):3190–3197.
104. Brunkhorst FM, Engel C, Bloos F, et al; German Competence Network Sepsis (SepNet). Intensive insulin therapy and pentastarch resuscitation in severe sepsis. *N Engl J Med*. 2008; 358(2):125–139.
105. Preiser JC, Devos P, Ruiz-Santana S, et al. A prospective randomised multi-centre controlled trial on tight glucose control by intensive insulin therapy in adult intensive care units: the Glucontrol study. *Intensive Care Med*. 2009;35(10):1738–1748.
106. NICE-SUGAR Study Investigators; Finfer S, Chittock DR, Su SYS, et al. Intensive versus conventional glucose control in critically ill patients. *N Engl J Med*. 2009;360(13):1283–1297.
107. Marik PE, Preiser JC. Toward understanding tight glycemic control in the ICU: a systematic review and metaanalysis. *Chest*. 2010;137(3):544–551.
108. Annane D, Cariou A, Maxime V, et al. Corticosteroid treatment and intensive insulin therapy for septic shock in adults: a randomized controlled trial. *JAMA*. 2010;303(4):341–348.
109. COIITSS Study Investigators; Griesdale DE, de Souza RJ, van Dam RM, et al. Intensive insulin therapy and mortality among critically ill patients: a meta-analysis including NICE-SUGAR study data. *CMAJ*. 2009;180(8):821–827.
110. Kansagara D, Fu R, Freeman M, Wolf F, Helfand M. Intensive insulin therapy in hospitalized patients: a systematic review. *Ann Intern Med*. 2011;154(4):268–282.
111. Buckleitner AM, Martínez-Alonso M, Hernández M, Solà I, Mauricio D. Perioperative glycaemic control for diabetic patients undergoing surgery (review). *Cochrane Database Syst Rev*. 2012;9:CD007315.
112. Treggiari MM, Karir V, Yanez ND, Weiss NS, Daniel S, Deem SA. Intensive insulin therapy and mortality in critically ill patients. *Crit Care*. 2008;12(1):R29.
113. Moghissi ES, Korytkowski MT, DiNardo M, et al; American Association of Clinical Endocrinologists, American Diabetes Association. American Association of Clinical Endocrinologists and American Diabetes Association consensus statement on inpatient glycemic control. *Endocr Pract*. 2009;15(4):353–369.
114. Schricker T, Lattermann R. Perioperative catabolism. *Can J Anesth*. 2015;62:182–193.
115. Evans L, Rhodes A, Alhazzani W, et al. Surviving sepsis campaign: international guidelines for management of sepsis and septic shock 2021. *Intensive Care Med*. 2021;47(11): 1181–1247.
116. Qaseem A, Humphrey LL, Chou R, Snow V, Shekelle P, Clinical Guidelines Committee of the American College of Physicians. Use of intensive insulin therapy for the management of glycemic control in hospitalized patients: a clinical practice guideline from the American College of Physicians. *Ann Intern Med*. 2011;154(4):260–267.
117. Sinclair AJ, Paolisso G, Castro M, Bourdel-Marchasson I, Gadsby R, Mañas LR; European Diabetes Working Party for Older People. European Diabetes Working Party for Older People 2011 clinical guidelines for type 2 diabetes mellitus: executive summary. *Diabetes Metab*. 2011;37(Suppl 3):S27–S38.
118. Moghissi E, Inzucchi S. The evolution of glycemic control in the hospital setting. In: Draznin B, ed. *Managing Diabetes and Hyperglycemia in the Hospital Setting*. American Diabetes Association; 2016:1–10.
119. Umpierrez GE, Smiley D, Jacobs S, et al. Randomized study of basal-bolus insulin therapy in the inpatient management of patients with type 2 diabetes undergoing general surgery (RABBIT 2 surgery). *Diabetes Care*. 2011;334:256–261.
120. Rice MJ, Pitkin AD, Coursin DB. Review article: glucose measurement in the operating room: more complicated than it seems. *Anesth Analg*. 2010;110(4):1056–1065.
121. Maerz LL, Akhtar S. Perioperative glycemic management in 2011: paradigm shifts. *Curr Opin Crit Care*. 2011;17(4):370–375.
122. U.S. Food and Drug Administration. Enforcement Policy for Non-Invasive Remote Monitoring Devices Used to Support Patient Monitoring During the Coronavirus Disease 2019 (COVID-19) Public Health Emergency (Revised). 2020. https://www.fda.gov/media/136290/download
123. American Diabetes Association Professional Practice Committee. 7. Diabetes technology: Standards of Medical Care in Diabetes–2022. *Diabetes Care*. 2022;45(Suppl1):S97–S112.
124. Coursin DB, Connery LE, Ketzler JT. Perioperative diabetic and hyperglycemic management issues. *Crit Care Med*. 2004;32(4 Suppl):S116–S125.
125. Cummings DE, Overduin J, Foster-Schubert KE. Gastric bypass for obesity: mechanisms of weight loss and diabetes resolution. *J Clin Endocrinol Metab*. 2004;89(6):2608–2615.
126. Gosmanov AR, Gosmanova EO, Kitabchi AE. Hyperglycemic crises: diabetic ketoacidosis (DKA) and hyperglycemic hyperosmolar state (HHS). In: DeGroot LJ, Beck-Peccoz P, Chrousos G, et al., eds. *Endotext*. MDText.com; 2015.
127. Nyenwe EA, Kitabchi AE. Evidence-based management of hyperglycemic emergencies in diabetes mellitus. *Diabetes Res Clin Pract*. 2011;94(3):340–351.
128. Scott AR; Joint British Diabetes Societies (JBDS) for Inpatient Care, JBDS hyperosmolar hyperglycaemic guidelines group. Management of hyperosmolar hyperglycaemic state in adults with diabetes. *Diabet Med*. 2015;32:714–724.
129. Pasquel FJ, Umpierrez GE. Hyperosmolar hyperglycemic state: a historic review of the clinical presentation, diagnosis, and treatment. *Diabetes Care*. 2014;37:3124–3131.
130. Savage MW, Dhatariya KK, Kilvert A, et al; Joint British Diabetes Societies. Joint British Diabetes Societies guideline for the management of diabetic ketoacidosis. *Diabet Med*. 2011; 28(5):508–515.
131. Kamel KS, Halperin ML. Acid-base problems in diabetic ketoacidosis. *N Engl J Med*. 2015;372: 546–554.
132. Peterson C, Fox JA, Devallis P, Rizzo R, Mizuguchi KA. Starvation in the midst of cardiopulmonary bypass: diabetic ketoacidosis during cardiac surgery. *J Cardiothorac Vasc Anesth*. 2012;26:910–916.
133. Duhon B, Attridge RL, Franco-Martinez AC, Maxwell PR, Hughes DW. Intravenous sodium bicarbonate therapy in severely acidotic diabetic ketoacidosis. *Ann Pharmacother*. 2013;47:970–975.
134. American Diabetes Association Professional Practice Committee. 6. Glycemic targets: Standards of Medical Care in Diabetes–2022. *Diabetes Care*. 2022;45(Suppl1):S83–S96.
135. Colao A, Grasso LFS, Giustina A. et al. Acromegaly. *Nat Rev Dis Primers*. 2019;5:20.
136. Appleby I, John R, Hirsch N. Pituitary disease and anaesthesia. *Anaesth Intensive Care Med*. 2020;21:312–316.
137. Kapoor I, Mahajan C, Prabhakar H. Assessment of airway in patients with acromegaly undergoing surgery: predicting successful tracheal intubation. *J Neuroanaesthesiol Crit Care*. 2021;8:40–44.
138. Nemergut EC, Dumont AS, Barry UT, Laws ER. Perioperative management of patients undergoing transsphenoidal pituitary surgery. *Anesth Analg*. 2005;101:1170–1181.
139. Devin JK. Hypopituitarism and central diabetes insipidus perioperative diagnosis and management. *Neurosurg Clin North Am*. 2013;23:679–689.
140. Burton D, Nicholson G, Hall G. Endocrine and metabolic response to surgery. *Continuing Ed Anaesthesia Crit Care Pain*. 2004:4;144–147.
141. Langouche L, van den Berghe G. The dynamic neuroendocrine response to critical illness. *Endocrinol Metab Clin North Am*. 2006;35:777–791.
142. Fant F, Tina E, Sandblom D, et al. Thoracic epidural analgesia inhibits the neuro-hormonal but not the acute inflammatory stress response after radical retropubic prostatectomy. *Br J Anaesth*. 2013;110:747–757.

48 Anesthesia for Otolaryngologic Surgery

RAYMOND S. PARK • JAMES M. PEYTON

KEY POINTS

1. The restricted spaces in the airway require an understanding and cooperative relationship between surgeon and anesthesiologist and the use of specially adapted equipment suitable to these cramped areas.
2. Despite only mild-to-moderate tonsillar enlargement on physical examination, children with obstructive sleep apnea have upper airway obstruction while awake and apnea during sleep. The clinician should not underestimate the severity of the problem based on tonsillar size alone.
3. Patients with Obstructive Sleep Apnea have increased sensitivity to opioids, and consequently, the dose administered should be reduced by as much as 50%.
4. Post-tonsillectomy hemorrhage may result in unappreciated large volumes of swallowed blood originating from the tonsillar fossa. These patients must be considered to have a full stomach, and anesthetic precautions addressing this situation must be taken.
5. The middle ear and sinuses are air-filled, nondistensible cavities. During procedures in which the eardrum is replaced, or perforation is patched, nitrous oxide should be discontinued or, if this is not possible, limited to a maximum of 50% during the application of the tympanic membrane graft to avoid pressure-related displacement.
6. During functional endoscopic sinus surgical procedures, systemic absorption of vasoconstrictive agents may cause hypertension, bradycardia, tachycardia, and arrhythmias. Preoperative evaluation should include a thorough investigation of the patient's cardiovascular status. Rapid response by the anesthesiologist to these effects is necessary for preventing complications.
7. Patients with a history of head and neck cancer may have undergone prior chemotherapy that can impact specific organ systems or radiation, leading to fibrosis and ankylosis of the temporomandibular joint, rendering direct laryngoscopy difficult.
8. Facial trauma is commonly associated with other injuries such as cervical spine and head injuries that can affect patient care beyond airway management.

Evaluating the Airway

Air flows through the upper respiratory passages, into the trachea, bronchi, bronchioles, and alveoli in the healthy human. Airflow occurs seemingly without either thought or effort, and the actual work of respiration in the unobstructed airway is minimal. However, airway obstruction due to malformation, tumor, infection, or trauma may significantly alter the clinical presentation and make gas exchange laborious and energy-consuming. The increased work of breathing can leave the patient exhausted, incapable of maintaining adequate gas exchange, and finally succumbing to ventilatory failure. Significant obstruction and anatomic distortion may be present in a patient with minimal evidence of disease because clinically evident upper airway obstruction is a late sign. It is a most distressing experience for the anesthesiologist to discover an obstructed upper airway during anesthetic induction unexpectedly or attempted tracheal intubation.

In the presence of tumor, other mass lesions, or infection in the airway, it may be helpful to obtain a radiologic evaluation of the airway with plain films of the tracheal and laryngeal air columns, computed tomography (CT), or magnetic resonance imaging (MRI) studies of the airway. Significant anatomic distortion may be appreciated and help the anesthesiologist determine the most appropriate technique for securing the airway.

Anesthesia for Pediatric Ear, Nose, and Throat Surgery

The safe management of the pediatric patient undergoing surgery on the ear, nose, and throat is particularly challenging for the anesthesiologist. The restricted spaces in the child's airway require a considerate and cooperative relationship between surgeon and 1 anesthesiologist and the use of specially adapted equipment suitable to these cramped areas.

Tonsillectomy and Adenoidectomy

Untreated adenoidal hyperplasia may lead to nasopharyngeal obstruction, causing failure to thrive, speech disorders, obligate mouth breathing, sleep disturbances, orofacial abnormalities with an upper airway narrowing, and dental abnormalities. Surgical removal of the adenoids is usually accompanied by tonsillectomy; however, purulent adenoiditis, despite adequate medical therapy, and recurrent otitis media with effusion secondary to adenoidal hyperplasia are improved with adenoidectomy alone.

Tonsillectomy is one of the more commonly performed pediatric surgical procedures.[1] The major indications for surgery are chronic or recurrent acute tonsillitis, peritonsillar abscess, tonsillar hyperplasia, and obstructive sleep apnea syndrome. In addition, patients with cardiac valvular disease are at risk for endocarditis from recurrent streptococcal bacteremia secondary to infected tonsils. Tonsillar hyperplasia may lead to chronic airway obstruction resulting in sleep apnea, carbon dioxide (CO_2) retention, cor pulmonale, failure to thrive, swallowing disorders, and speech abnormalities. These risks are eliminated with the removal of the tonsils.

Obstruction of the oropharyngeal airway by hypertrophied tonsils leading to apnea during sleep is an important clinical entity referred to as *obstructive sleep apnea syndrome (OSAS)*. Despite only mild-to-moderate tonsillar enlargement on physical examination, these patients have upper airway obstruction while awake and apnea during sleep. The treatment goals are to relieve the airway obstruction and increase the cross-sectional area of the pharynx.[2] Some patients require continuous nasal positive airway pressure during sleep, whereas others may require a tracheostomy to bypass the chronic upper airway obstruction that is present. The two most frequent levels of obstruction during sleep are at the soft palate and the base of the tongue.[3,4] Most children have tremendous improvement in their symptoms after tonsillectomy.

In children with long standing hypoxemia and hypercarbia, increased airway resistance can lead to cor pulmonale (Fig. 48-1). Patients may have electrocardiographic evidence of right ventricular hypertrophy and radiographic evidence consistent with cardiomegaly. Each apneic episode causes increased pulmonary artery pressure with significant systemic and pulmonary artery hypertension, leading to ventricular dysfunction and cardiac dysrhythmias.[5] These patients often have dysfunction in the medulla or hypothalamic areas of the central nervous system, causing persistently elevated CO_2, despite relief of airway obstruction as well as a hyperreactive pulmonary vascular bed. The increased pulmonary vascular resistance and myocardial depression in response to hypoxia, hypercarbia, and acidosis are far greater than expected for that degree of physiologic alteration in the normal population. Cardiac enlargement is frequently reversible with surgical removal of the tonsils and adenoids.

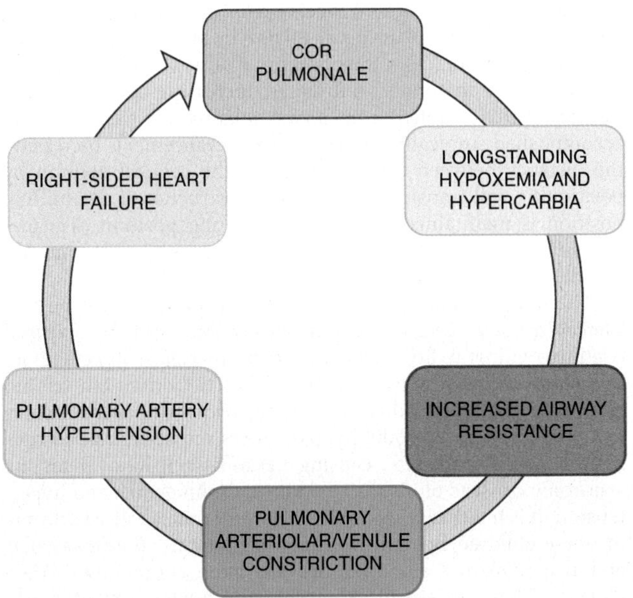

Figure 48-1 Events leading to cor pulmonale.

Preoperative Evaluation

A thorough history is the basis for the preoperative evaluation. Seek a history of sleep-disordered breathing (SDB). Begin the physical examination with observation of the patient. Note the presence of audible respirations, mouth breathing, nasal quality of the speech, and chest retractions. Mouth breathing may be the result of chronic nasopharyngeal obstruction. An elongated face, retrognathic mandible, and a high-arched palate may be present. Inspect the oropharynx to evaluate tonsillar size to determine the ease of mask ventilation and tracheal intubation (Fig. 48-2). The presence of wheezing or rales on auscultation of the chest may be a lower respiratory component of upper airway infection. Inspiratory stridor or prolonged expiration may indicate partial airway obstruction from hypertrophied tonsils or adenoids.

Consider measuring of hematocrit and coagulation parameters. Because patients requiring tonsillectomy and adenoidectomy have frequent infections, the parent should be questioned about the current use of antibiotics, antihistamines, or other medicines. Many nonprescription cold medications and antihistamines contain aspirin, which may affect platelet function, and this potential anticoagulation should be considered. Chest radiographs and electrocardiograms (ECGs) are not required unless specific abnormalities are elicited during the history, such as recent pneumonia, bronchitis, upper respiratory infection (URI), or history consistent with cor pulmonale, which is seen in children with OSAS. An echocardiogram may be indicated in those children with a history of cardiac abnormalities.

Sleep-Disordered Breathing and Obstructive Sleep Apnea

SDB is a spectrum of disorders ranging from primary snoring to OSAS. SDB affects 10% of the population, but only 1% to 4% will progress to OSAS. OSAS is characterized by periodic, partial, or complete obstruction of the upper airway during sleep.[6–9] Proper screening and diagnosis of obstructive sleep apnea before surgery for both children and adults is essential in reducing the associated risks. Several methods for assessing OSAS exist and can be broadly characterized as polysomnography (PSG), which refers to formal sleep studies based in a hospital or at home, nocturnal oximetry, and clinical questionnaires.[10] The STOP-BANG questionnaire has been developed to screen adult patients for obstructive sleep apnea. It includes information on Snoring, daytime somnolence and Tiredness, Observation of apnea during sleep, and elevations in Blood pressure. Predicting risk in children, however, is far more complicated.[11,12] The STBUR questionnaire has been proposed as an alternative for pediatric patients. It evaluates Snoring, Trouble Breathing, and Un-Refreshed after sleep and has the potential to be a reliable predictor of children at risk for perioperative respiratory events.[13]

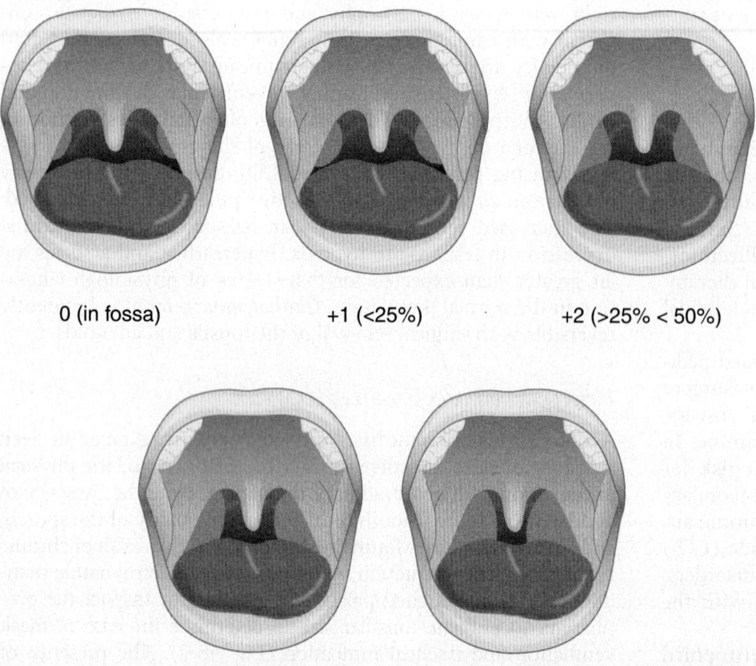

Figure 48-2 Classification of tonsil size, including the percentage of oropharyngeal area occupied by hypertrophied tonsils.

The role of polysomnography for most children is controversial. The decision to order a polysomnography is influenced by test availability, patient medical history, patient age, clinician practice patterns, and caregiver preference. In an American Academy of Pediatrics (AAP) statement on diagnosis and management of OSAS, the authors conclude that while few of the screening techniques for OSAS have sufficient sensitivity and specificity to reliably provide a clinical diagnosis, there is inadequate infrastructure to provide PSG for all patients with suspected OSAS. Therefore, PSG is recommended in situations where alternative screening and testing methods are inconclusive. Alternatively, the American Academy of Otolaryngology-Head and Neck Surgery (AAO-HNS) only recommends PSG in cases where there is a discordance between tonsillar size and reported OSAS symptoms. A 2017 survey showed that only 3.5% of pediatric otolaryngologists referred greater than 90% of children with OSAS for polysomnography before adenotonsillectomy.[14]

Repetitive arousal from sleep to restore airway patency is a common feature, as are episodic sleep-associated oxygen desaturation, hypercarbia, and cardiac dysfunction resulting from airway obstruction. Individuals who experience obstruction during sleep may have snoring loud enough to be heard through closed doors or observed pauses in breathing during sleep. They may awaken from sleep with a choking sensation. Parents report restless sleep in affected children and frequent somnolence or fatigue while awake despite adequate sleep hours. These children fall asleep easily in nonstimulating environments and are difficult to arouse at the usual awakening time. Type 1 OSAS is characterized by lymphoid hyperplasia without obesity, whereas type 2 OSAS patients are obese with minimal lymphoid hyperplasia. Approximately 10% of OSAS is present in preschool and school-aged children and is thought to decline after 9 years of age.

Obesity changes craniofacial anthropometric characteris-
2 tics. Therefore, a body mass index of 95% for age or greater is a predisposing physical characteristic that increases the risk of developing OSAS.[15,16] Children with craniofacial abnormalities, including a small maxilla and mandible, a large tongue for a given mandibular size, and a thick neck have a similar increased risk. Many of these children have syndromes that are associated with additional comorbidities. Anatomic nasal obstruction and Class 4 touching tonsils reduce the oropharyngeal cross-sectional area, which constitutes an additional risk. Pharyngeal size is determined by the soft-tissue volume inside the bony enclosure of the mandible; an anatomic imbalance between the upper airway soft-tissue volume and craniofacial size will result in obstruction. Neural mechanisms control the magnitude of pharyngeal muscle contraction, and the interaction between the anatomical balance and neural mechanisms determines pharyngeal airway size. Increased neural mechanisms can compensate for the anatomic imbalance in obstructive sleep apnea patients during wakefulness. When these neural mechanisms are suppressed during sleep or anesthesia, pharyngeal dilator muscles do not contract maximally, and therefore the pharyngeal airway severely narrows because of the anatomical imbalance. Increasing bony enclosure size will provide relief from airway obstruction. This is only accomplished surgically by mandibular advancement. Increasing the distance between the mentum and the cervical column by positioning will transiently relieve the obstruction if the sniffing position is maintained. Similarly, the sitting position displaces excessive soft tissue outside the bony enclosure through the submandibular space.

The long-term effects of OSAS are not limited to the airway. Increased body mass index and obesity may lead to increased cognitive vulnerability, as illustrated by increased hyperactivity frequency and C-reactive protein levels. OSAS duration has no relation to the reversibility of neurobehavioral impairment since many believe that episodic hypoxia alters the prefrontal cortex's neurochemical substrate, causing neuronal cell loss. Metabolic syndrome consists of insulin resistance, dyslipidemia, and hypertension. It is felt that OSAS is a risk factor for metabolic syndrome in obese children but not in nonobese patients. Cardiovascular and hemodynamic comorbidities are more common in OSAS patients. These consist of altered blood pressure regulation and alterations in sympathetic activity and reactivity. Also present are endothelial dysfunction and initiation and propagation of inflammatory response facilitated by increases in C-reactive protein levels. Systemic inflammation using interleukins as a marker is a component of OSAS in both obese and nonobese children and is reversed after tonsillectomy. Systemic hypertension, changes in left ventricular geometry, and intermittent hypoxia leading to pulmonary artery hypertension are well-described comorbidities present in patients with OSAS.

The mainstay of the management is the surgical removal of tonsils and adenoids, which carries a near 80% success rate in resolving OSAS.[17] Additional options include expansion pharyngoplasty, supraglottoplasty, mandibular distraction osteogenesis (MDO), and uvulopharyngopalatoplasty. MDO addresses OSAS in patients with craniofacial abnormalities such as Treacher Collins syndrome and Pierre Robin Sequence. MDO has been shown to significantly improve or completely resolve OSAS in this patient population in 92% of patients.[18] In addition, MDO has been associated with improved modified Cormack and Lehane view on direct laryngoscopy in patients with Pierre Robin Sequence.[19] Recurrence may occur in children with craniofacial abnormalities and others. If the surgical intervention does not resolve the problem, nocturnal continuous positive airways pressure (CPAP) is the next treatment modality.

Tonsillotomy, or partial tonsillectomy, is being increasingly utilized as an alternative therapy in patients with OSAS due to evidence suggesting lower rates of postsurgical hemorrhage and decreased pain compared with tonsillectomy.[20,21] However, with tonsillotomy, there remains concern for tonsillar regrowth necessitating additional surgeries and inferior treatment of OSAS due to subtotal removal of tonsillar tissue.[20] A recent Cochrane review looking at tonsillotomy versus tonsillectomy in children concluded that tonsillotomy probably results in a faster return to normal activity and a slight reduction in postoperative complications requiring medical intervention in the first week after surgery. There were insufficient data to determine the long-term effects on symptoms or recurrence of OSAS, reoperation rates, and quality of life.[22] For patients with severe or refractory OSAS where corrective surgery is being considered or patients with persistent OSAS after surgery, drug-induced sleep endoscopy (DISE) can be performed to characterize the anatomic basis of obstruction (see Chapter 23, NICV 23-1). One study found that compared with clinical examination alone, information from DISE resulted in a change in surgical plan in 78% of cases.[23]

During DISE, patients are sedated to reproduce obstructive symptoms that occur during sleep. The objectives of sedation include maintenance of spontaneous respiration, and as these patients are at high risk of obstruction, timely emergence is important for safe recovery and discharge. Coincident with these goals, agents with a rapid offset such as propofol and dexmedetomidine infusion are typically used with or without ketamine bolus.[24] By nature, these patients are at increased risk of obstruction with sedation. The anesthesiologist should have equipment immediately available such as oral and nasal airways and supraglottic airway (SGA) such as a laryngeal mask airway (LMA), to bypass and relieve the obstruction. Once the patient is sedated, nasal endoscopic evaluation is performed to evaluate the upper airway for specific areas of obstruction that would be potentially corrected by surgical intervention. Currently, there are no data demonstrating that the choice of anesthetic agents used during DISE changes the results of the procedure, and hence surgical decision making and the eventual outcome of the corrective surgery. Surgeons remain concerned that certain drugs (volatile agents and propofol) may cause too much airway collapse, while ketamine may cause an increase in muscle tone. Dexmedetomidine has been touted as an ideal agent for these procedures, but this alters sleep architecture by decreasing the proportion of rapid eye movement (REM) to non–rapid eye movement (NREM) sleep, and OSAS predominantly occurs during REM sleep. There is no ideal drug combination that reproduces natural sleep conditions. Clear communication between the surgical and anesthesia teams regarding desired anesthetic depth is more important than the medications used.

Anesthetic Management

The goals of the anesthetic management for tonsillectomy and adenoidectomy are to render the child unconscious, to provide the surgeon with optimal operating conditions, to establish intravenous access to provide a route for volume expansion and medications when necessary, and to provide rapid emergence so that the patient is awake and able to protect the recently instrumented airway. Premedication may be used sparingly as sedative premedication should be avoided in children with obstructive sleep apnea, intermittent obstruction, or very large tonsils. The use of an antisialagogue may minimize secretions in the operative field.

Anesthesia is commonly induced with a volatile anesthetic agent, oxygen, and nitrous oxide (N_2O) by mask. Parental presence in the operating room (OR) during mask induction may be helpful in the anxious unpremedicated child. Tracheal intubation is best accomplished under deep inhalation anesthesia or aided by a short-acting nondepolarizing muscle relaxant. Many clinicians may choose to eliminate the neuromuscular-blocking agent in favor of enhancing the depth of anesthesia with the use of propofol. Acetaminophen can be used as part of a multimodal pain regimen to reduce opioid consumption, particularly for patients having surgery to treat OSAS. One study demonstrated that patients undergoing adenotonsillectomy who received fentanyl 1 to 2 mcg/kg and either acetaminophen 15 mg/kg intravenously or 40 mg/kg rectally had a median time to postoperative rescue analgesia of 7 and 10 hours, respectively.[25] The addition of 0.5 to 1 mcg/kg of dexmedetomidine infused during the procedure may help to attenuate emergence delirium in toddlers after the anesthetic.[26] Although intraoperative nonsteroidal anti-inflammatory drugs should be avoided intraoperatively to decrease the risk of postoperative hemorrhage; these agents are safe and effective in the postacute recovery period. They are recommended as part of the standard analgesic regimen by the American Academy of Otolaryngology–Head and Neck Surgery (AAO-HNS)[27,28] and the recent Prospect guidelines on pain relief following adenotonsillectomy.[29] Due to the increased opioid sensitivity of patients with OSAS, the standard dose of opioids should be reduced by 50%.[30] Codeine should be avoided due to the possibility of rapid metabolism and conversion and, due to these concerns, carries a black box warning from the FDA for use in pediatric patients undergoing tonsillectomy.[30–32] Use of codeine in this patient population is also strictly contraindicated in the AAO-HNS guidelines for pediatric tonsillectomy.[27] Blood in the pharynx may enter the trachea during the surgical procedure.

For this reason, the supraglottic area may be packed with petroleum gauze, or a cuffed endotracheal tube may be used. If a cuffed endotracheal tube is selected, careful attention to the inflation pressure of the cuff is essential if postextubation croup is to be avoided. Monitoring consists of a precordial stethoscope, ECG, automated blood pressure, pulse oximetry, and end-tidal capnography.

Emergence from anesthesia should be rapid, and the child should be alert before transfer to the recovery area. The child should be awake and able to clear blood or secretions from the oropharynx as efficiently as possible before removing the endotracheal tube. Maintenance of airway and pharyngeal reflexes are essential in preventing aspiration, laryngospasm, and airway obstruction. There is no difference in the incidence of airway complications on emergence between patients who are extubated awake or deeply anesthetized.[33]

The use of the LMA for adenotonsillectomy was described in 1990; however, it was not until the widespread availability of a streamlined, flexible model that it was routinely used for this purpose.[34,35] There is an emerging trend to use the flexible LMA for tonsillectomy, which protects the vocal cords from blood or secretions that may be present in the oropharynx.[36] The wide, rigid tube of the standard LMA model does not fit under the mouth gag and is easily compressed or dislodged during full mouth opening. The flexible model has a soft, reinforced shaft that easily fits under the mouth gag without becoming dislodged or compressed. Adequate surgical access can be achieved, and the lower airway is protected from exposure to blood during the procedure.[37,38] Since the cuff is larger and occupies a more significant percentage of the posterior hypopharynx; there is a greater risk of airway fire if the electrocautery touches the LMA. Insertion is possible after the intravenous administration of propofol or when sufficient depth of anesthesia is achieved using a volatile agent administered by a face mask. The same depth of anesthesia should be obtained during insertion of the LMA as would be required for performing laryngoscopy and endotracheal intubation. Assisted ventilation is safe and effective if care is taken to avoid excessive peak inspiratory pressure that may also lead to gastric insufflation.

Tonsillar enlargement can make LMA insertion difficult therefore care in placement is essential. Maneuvers to overcome this include increased head extension, lateral insertion of the mask, anterior displacement of the tongue, pressure on the tip of the LMA using the index finger as it negotiates the pharyngeal curve, or use of the laryngoscope if all else fails. Dislodgment of the device does not occur during extreme head extension, assuming good position and ventilation were obtained before changes in head position.[39]

Advantages of the LMA over traditional endotracheal intubation are a decrease in postoperative stridor and laryngospasm and an increase in immediate postoperative oxygen saturation. If the child is breathing spontaneously at a regular rate and depth, the LMA may be removed before emergence from anesthesia. The oropharynx should be gently suctioned with a soft, flexible catheter, the LMA removed, an oral airway inserted if necessary, and the respirations assisted with 100% oxygen delivered by a face mask. If the practitioner wants to remove the LMA when the child has emerged from anesthesia, it should be removed as soon as possible after the return to consciousness. In addition, it may be appropriate to pass a nasogastric tube through the suction port of a second-generation LMA, or an LMA without a gastric port, beyond the cuff to empty the stomach after surgery.

Complications

Post-tonsillectomy mortality within the first 48 hours in both children and adults has been reported to be increased in patients who are obese, have a neurologic impairment, or cardiopulmonary compromise.[40] The incidence of emesis after tonsillectomy ranges from 30% to 65%.[41] Whether emesis is due to irritant blood in the stomach or stimulation of the gag reflex by inflammation and edema at the surgical site remains unclear. Central nervous system stimulation from the gastrointestinal tract, as may be seen with gastric distention from the introduction of swallowed or insufflated air, may trigger the emetic center of the brain. Decompressing the stomach with an orogastric tube may help prevent this response. Treatment with ondansetron 0.10 to 0.15 mg/kg, either with or without dexamethasone, 0.5 mg/kg, is very effective in reducing post-tonsillectomy nausea and vomiting, pain, and time to oral intake.[42] There is concern that dexamethasone is associated with an increased risk of postoperative bleeding; however, this has not been consistently observed. Therefore, the AAO-HNSF currently recommends administering a single dose of intraoperative dexamethasone during tonsillectomy surgery in children. Dehydration secondary to poor oral intake because of nausea, vomiting, or pain can occur after tonsillectomy in 1% of cases. Vigorous intravenous hydration during surgery can offset the physiologic effects of lower postoperative fluid intake.

The most severe complication of tonsillectomy is postoperative hemorrhage, which occurs at a frequency of 0.1% to 8.1%. The recent increased popularity of coblation tonsillectomy may result in an incidence of post-tonsillectomy hemorrhage up to 11.1%.[43,44] Approximately 75% of postoperative tonsillar hemorrhage occurs within 6 hours of surgery. Most of the remaining 25% occurs within the first 24 hours of surgery, although bleeding may be noted until the sixth postoperative day, thus the "six hours or six days" guideline. Sixty-seven percent of postoperative bleeding originates from the tonsillar fossa, 26% in the nasopharynx, and 7% in both.[40] Initial attempts to control bleeding may be made using pharyngeal packs and cautery. If this fails, patients must return to the OR for exploration and surgical hemostasis. 4

Unappreciated large volumes of blood originating from the tonsillar bed may be swallowed. Patients must be considered to have a full stomach, and anesthetic precautions addressing this situation must be taken. A rapid-sequence induction accompanied by cricoid pressure and a styletted endotracheal tube is controversial but may be of benefit in some circumstances. Because the amount of blood swallowed can be considerable, blood pressure must be checked in erect and supine positions to exclude orthostatic changes resulting from decreases in vascular volume. Intravenous access and hydration must be established before the induction of anesthesia. A variety of laryngoscope blades, endotracheal tubes, and functioning suction apparatus should be prepared in duplicate because blood in the airway may impair visualization of the vocal cords and cause plugging of the endotracheal tube. In situations where ongoing bleeding has complicated endotracheal intubation, the use of SGA has been described as a rescue technique to provide oxygenation and ventilation.[45,46]

Pain after adenoidectomy is usually minimal, but pain after a tonsillectomy may be severe. This contributes to poor fluid intake and the overall discomfort of patients. An increase in postoperative pain medication requirements has been noted in patients having laser or electrocautery as part of the operative tonsillectomy compared with those who have had sharp surgical dissection and ligation of blood vessels to achieve hemostasis. Intraoperative administration of corticosteroids may decrease edema formation and subsequent patient discomfort. Although infiltration of the peritonsillar space with local anesthetic and epinephrine effectively reduces intraoperative blood loss, it does not significantly decrease postoperative pain.[47]

Peritonsillar abscess, or quinsy tonsil, is a condition that may require immediate surgical intervention to relieve potential or existing airway obstruction. An acutely infected tonsil may undergo abscess formation, producing a large mass in the lateral pharynx that can interfere with swallowing and breathing (Figs. 48-3 through 48-5). Fever, pain, and trismus are frequent symptoms. Treatment consists of surgical drainage of the abscess, either with or without tonsillectomy, and intravenous antibiotic therapy. Although the airway seems compromised, the peritonsillar abscess is usually fixed in the lateral pharynx. It does not usually interfere with the patient's ventilation by face mask after induction of general anesthesia. Visualization of the vocal cords should not be impaired because the pathologic process is

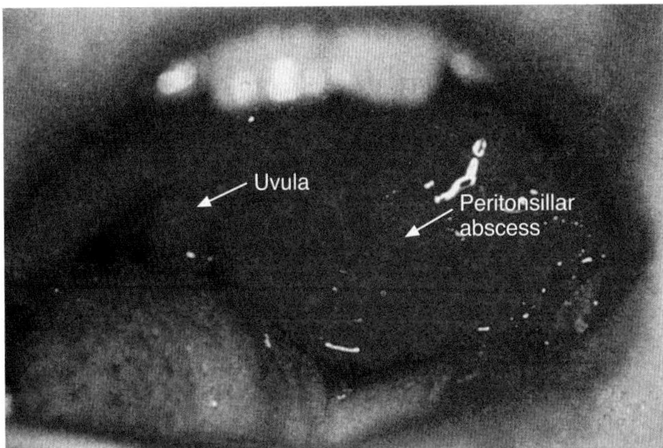

Figure 48-3 Patient with a peritonsillar abscess on the left side. Note the displacement of the uvula. (Courtesy of Michael Cunningham, MD, Boston, MA.)

supraglottic and well above the laryngeal inlet. Laryngoscopy must be carefully performed, avoiding manipulation of the larynx and surrounding structures. Intubation should be gentle because the tonsillar area is tense and friable, and inadvertent rupture of the abscess can occur, leading to spillage of purulent material into the trachea. A head-down position may be helpful during laryngoscopy to decrease the risk of purulent aspiration in the event of abscess rupture.

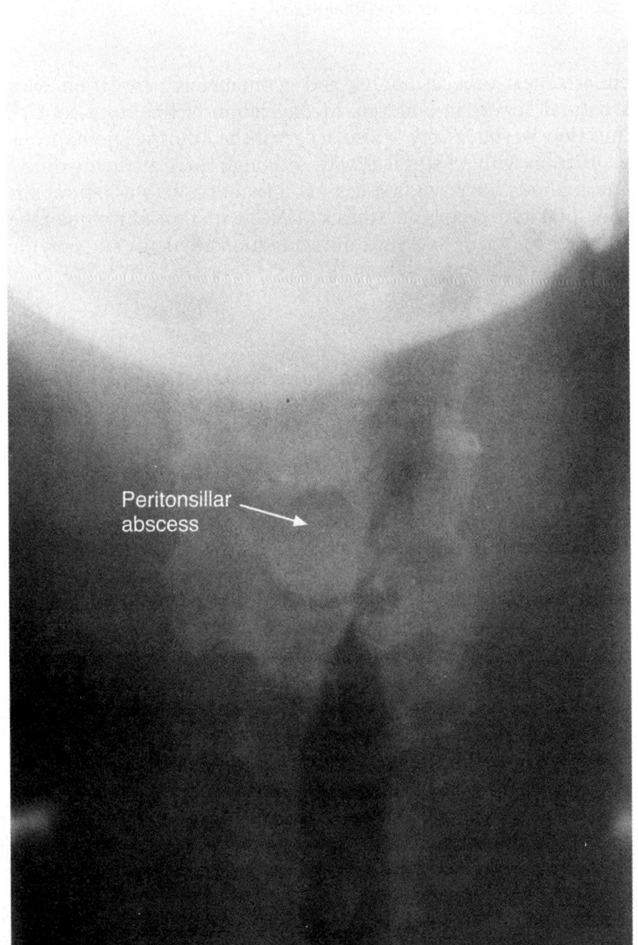

Figure 48-4 Neck radiograph of a patient with a peritonsillar abscess (*arrow*).

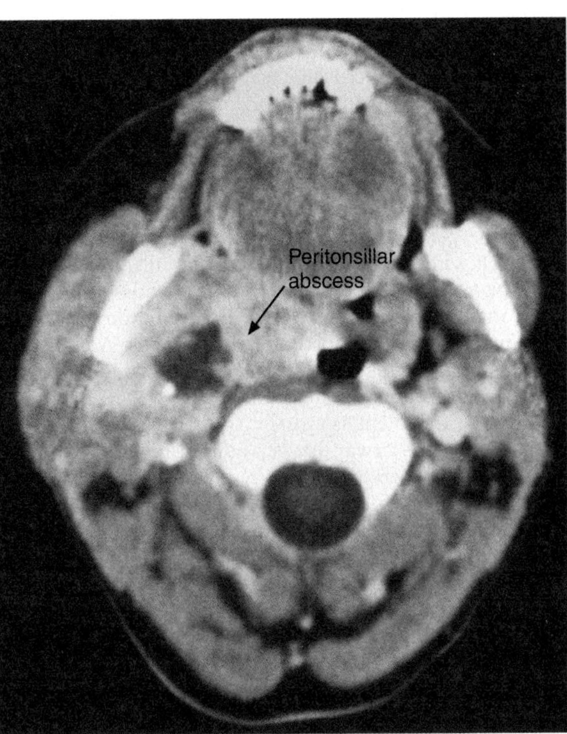

Figure 48-5 Computed tomography scan of a patient with a peritonsillar abscess (*arrow*).

Acute postoperative pulmonary edema is an infrequent but potentially life-threatening complication encountered when airway obstruction is suddenly relieved. One proposed mechanism is that during inspiration before adenotonsillectomy, the generated negative intrapleural pressure causes an increase in venous return, enhancing pulmonary blood volume. In a healthy child without airway obstruction, pleural pressure ranges from −2.5 cm to −10 cm H_2O during inspiration. Intrapleural pressure generated in a child with airway obstruction can be as much as −30 cm H_2O, which disrupts the capillary walls of the pulmonary microvasculature when transmitted to the interstitial peribronchial and perivascular spaces. Concurrent with a negative transpulmonary gradient is an increase in venous return to the right side of the heart, thus increasing preload, which in the setting of "leaky capillaries" facilitates transudation of fluid into the alveolar space. To counterbalance this negative gradient, positive intrapleural and alveolar pressures are generated during exhalation, decreasing pulmonary venous return and blood volume. This phenomenon is similar to an expiratory "grunt" mechanism in which the trans pleural pressures generated are identical to those present during a Valsalva maneuver.

The rapid relief of airway obstruction results in decreased airway pressure, an increase in venous return, pulmonary hydrostatic pressure, hyperemia, and finally, pulmonary edema. The all-important counterbalance of the expiratory grunt in limiting pulmonary venous return is lost when the obstruction is relieved. Contributing factors are the increased volume load on both ventricles and the inability of the pulmonary lymphatic system to remove acutely large amounts of fluid. The anesthesiologist may attempt to prevent this situation during induction of anesthesia by applying moderate amounts of continuous positive pressure to the airway, thus allowing time for circulatory adaptation to occur. This physiologic sequence is like that in patients with severe acute airway obstruction secondary to epiglottitis or laryngospasm.

Negative-pressure pulmonary edema is signaled by the appearance of frothy pink fluid in the endotracheal tube of an intubated patient or the presence of a decreased oxygen saturation, wheezing, dyspnea, and increased respiratory rate in the immediate postoperative period in a previously extubated patient. Mild cases may present with minimal symptoms. The differential diagnosis of negative-pressure pulmonary edema includes aspiration of gastric contents, adult respiratory distress syndrome, congestive heart failure, volume overload, and anaphylaxis. A chest radiograph illustrating diffuse, usually bilateral interstitial pulmonary infiltrates and an appropriate clinical history will confirm the diagnosis.[48,49] Treatment is usually supportive, with the maintenance of a patent airway, oxygen administration, and diuretic therapy in cases where patients may have concurrent hypervolemia. In severe cases, endotracheal intubation and mechanical ventilation with positive end-expiratory pressure may be necessary. Resolution is usually rapid and may occur within hours of inception. Most cases resolve within 24 hours without treatment. There is no reliable method for predicting which children will experience this clinical syndrome after their airway obstruction has been resolved.

Adenoidectomy patients may be safely discharged on the same day after recovering from anesthesia. Although most tonsillectomy patients previously required postoperative admission to the hospital for observation, administration of analgesics, and hydration, many centers are discharging tonsillectomy patients on the day of surgery without adverse outcomes, and this trend will likely continue.[49] Patients should be observed for early hemorrhage for 4 to 6 hours and be free from significant nausea, vomiting, and pain before discharge. The ability to take fluid by mouth is not a requirement for discharge home. However, intravenous hydration must be adequate to prevent dehydration. Excessive somnolence and severe vomiting are indications for hospital admission.

There are patients for whom early discharge is not advised, and those patients should be admitted to the hospital after a tonsillectomy. The characteristics of such patients are listed in Table 48-1. A recent recommendation by the AAP recommends that children who exhibit oxygen saturation <80% in the post-tonsillectomy recovery period be admitted to an inpatient unit and monitored for respiratory depression.[50] Despite the removal of hypertrophied lymphoid tissue in the hypopharynx, some children remain at risk for postoperative obstruction, particularly in the subgroup of patients with severe OSAS.[51,52] Admission to an intensive care unit (ICU) is controversial and reserved for those children with very severe OSAS, comorbidities that cannot be managed on the floor, and children who have demonstrated significant airway obstruction and desaturation in the initial postoperative period that required intervention beyond repositioning and oxygen supplementation.[53]

Table 48-1 Tonsillectomy and Adenoidectomy Inpatient Guidelines: Recommendation of the American Academy of Otolaryngology—Head and Neck Surgery

Admit patients to the hospital after adenotonsillectomy if they meet any of the following criteria:

- Age ≤3 yrs
- Severe OSAS with an apnea–hypopnea index of 10 or more obstructive events/hour, oxygen saturation nadir <80% or both
- Abnormal coagulation values with or without an identified bleeding disorder in the patient or family
- Systemic disorders that put the patient at increased preoperative cardiopulmonary, metabolic, or general medical risk
- Child with craniofacial or other airway abnormalities including, but not limited to, syndromic disorders such as Treacher Collins syndrome, Crouzon syndrome, Goldenhar syndrome, Pierre Robin anomalad, CHARGE syndrome, achondroplasia, and, most prominently, Down syndrome, as well as isolated airway abnormalities such as choanal atresia and laryngotracheal stenosis
- When extended travel time, weather conditions, and home social conditions are not consistent with close observation, cooperation, and ability to return to the hospital quickly at the discretion of the attending physician

CHARGE, coloboma of the eye, *h*eart defects, *a*tresia of the choanae, *r*etardation of growth and/or development, *g*enital and/or urinary abnormalities, and *e*ar abnormalities.

Laryngology

There have been significant advances in knowledge regarding voice disorders and strategies for managing them. This developed in adult practice, and the subspeciality of phoniatrics emerged. This expertise is now prevalent in surgeons for pediatric and adult patient populations. The most common disorder is vocal nodules resulting from laryngeal hyperfunction producing hoarseness. Papillomatosis of the vocal cords is another cause of voice disorder and vocal fold paralysis.[54] Treatment of papillomatosis includes laser ablation, easily performed with a laser reflective endotracheal tube in adults, and spontaneous ventilation with a natural airway in children. Medialization of the vocal cord or injection laryngoplasty is also accomplished during spontaneous ventilation with a natural airway. Although there are many different methods for providing general anesthesia with a natural airway, total intravenous anesthesia (TIVA) with topicalization of the vocal cords during spontaneous ventilation offers the surgeon the best view of the surgical field.[55]

Ear Surgery

The ear and its associated structures are target organs for many pathologic conditions. General anesthesia for ear surgery has its own set of unique considerations that must be addressed.

Myringotomy and Tube Insertion

Chronic serous otitis in children can lead to hearing loss. Drainage of accumulated fluid in the middle ear is an effective treatment for this condition. Myringotomy, which creates an opening in the tympanic membrane for fluid drainage, may be performed alone. During healing, the drainage path may become occluded; therefore, ventilation tube placement is usually included. The insertion of a small plastic tube in the tympanic membrane serves as a vent for the ostium. It allows for continued drainage of the middle ear until the tubes are naturally extruded in 6 months to 1 year or surgically removed at an appropriate time.

Myringotomy and tube insertion are relatively short, and anesthesia may be effectively accomplished with a potent inhalation agent, oxygen, and nitrous oxide (N_2O) administered by a face mask. Premedication is not recommended because most sedative drugs used for premedication will far outlast the duration of the surgical procedure. Patients with chronic otitis frequently have accompanying recurrent upper respiratory tract infections (URIs). Because tracheal intubation is not required for routine patients, the criteria for cancellation of surgery and anesthesia may differ for this procedure. Insertion of myringotomy tubes may be undertaken in most children with a concomitant URI, provided that this can be completed with facemask anesthesia and endotracheal intubation is avoided. There is no significant difference in perioperative morbidity between asymptomatic patients and those fulfilling URI criteria.[56,57] It is recommended that patients with URI symptoms receive supplemental postoperative oxygen. Analgesic options for myringotomy tubes include intranasal or intramuscular medications, though the use of dual therapy with fentanyl and ketorolac compared with single-agent administration was associated with superior analgesia without clinically significant increases in the post anesthesia care unit PACU time or postoperative nausea and vomiting (PONV).[58]

Middle Ear and Mastoid

Tympanoplasty and mastoidectomy are two of the most common procedures performed on the middle ear and accessory structures (NICV 48-1). To gain access to the surgical site, the head is positioned on a headrest lower than the operative table, and extreme degrees of lateral rotation may be required. Excessive tension on the heads of the sternocleidomastoid muscles must be avoided. The laxity of the cervical spine ligaments and the immaturity of the odontoid process in children make them especially prone to C1 to C2 subluxation.

Ear surgery often involves surgical identification and preservation of the facial nerve, which requires isolation of the nerve by the surgeon and verification of its function using electrical stimulation (Fig. 48-6, 1 Video 48-1). This is accomplished by brainstem auditory-evoked potential and electrocochleogram monitoring, which requires that complete muscle relaxation be avoided.[59] If an opioid-relaxant technique is chosen, however, at least 30% of the muscle response should be preserved as determined by a twitch monitor. This fact suggests that it is not mandatory to avoid skeletal muscle relaxants in the anesthetic management of patients undergoing surgical procedures when monitoring facial nerve function is necessary.

Bleeding must be kept to a minimum during surgery of the small structures of the middle ear. Prevention of excessive increases in blood pressure and normotension can help improve the surgical field. Relative hypotension can also be effective, though careful consideration should be given to the risks of lowered blood pressure against the potential benefit of reduced surgical bleeding, as even short periods of intraoperative hypotension have been associated with perioperative morbidity, including acute kidney injury, myocardial infarction, stroke, and postoperative delirium.[60–63] Additional contraindications to this technique include patients with intracranial hypertension, hypovolemia, or a history of vascular, cerebrovascular, or another end-organ disease.[64] Concentrated epinephrine solution, often 1:1,000, can be injected into the area of the tympanic vessels to produce vasoconstriction. However, concentrations as low as 1:400,000 may give equivalent reductions in local blood flow with less potential for adverse effects from the inadvertent intravascular injection.[65,66] Close attention should be paid to the volume of injected epinephrine to avoid dysrhythmias and wide swings in blood pressure.

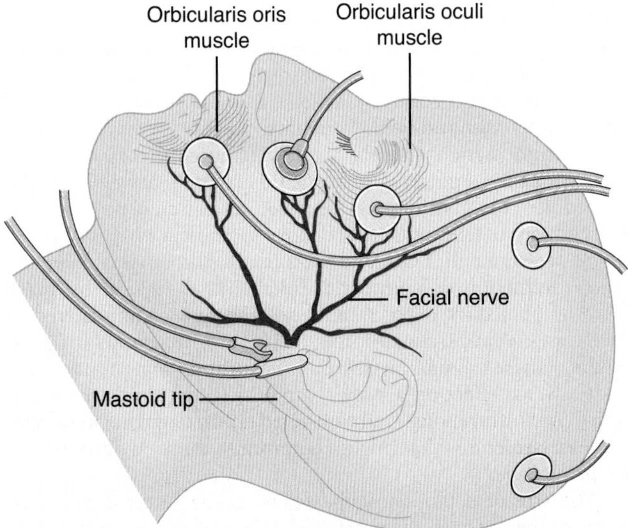

Figure 48-6 Illustration of the facial nerve and monitoring electrodes. (Courtesy of Steve Ronner, Ph.D., Boston, MA.)

The middle ear and sinuses are air-filled, nondistensible cavities. 5 An increase in the volume of gas in these structures increases pressure. N_2O diffuses along a concentration gradient into the air-filled middle ear spaces more rapidly than nitrogen moves out. Passive venting occurs at 20 to 30 cm H_2O pressure. The use of N_2O results in pressures exceeding the eustachian tube's ability to vent the middle ear within 5 minutes, leading to pressure buildup.[67] During procedures in which the eardrum is replaced or perforation is patched, N_2O should be discontinued or, if this is not possible, limited to a maximum of 50% during the application of the tympanic membrane graft to avoid pressure-related displacement.

N_2O is quickly reabsorbed after it is discontinued, creating a void in the middle ear with resulting negative pressure. This negative pressure may result in serous otitis, disarticulation of the ossicles in the middle ear (especially the stapes), and hearing impairment, which may last up to 6 weeks after surgery. The use of N_2O is related to a high incidence of PONV, which is a direct result of negative middle ear pressure during recovery. The vestibular system is stimulated by traction placed on the round window by the negative pressure created. Although all patients have the potential for nausea and vomiting after surgery, children younger than 3 years seem to be most affected. If N_2O cannot be avoided, vigorous use of antiemetics is warranted.

Airway Surgery

Airway surgery is a potentially high-risk surgical intervention that requires the surgical and anesthesia teams to work seamlessly together. For anesthesiologists to manage children requiring airway surgery, they need to understand the pathology and the surgical approach to determine the anesthetic requirements. Clear communication and trust between providers are vital components of sharing the airway, and the requirements of the surgical technique may dictate several aspects of the anesthetic.

The methods used to manage the airway and allow oxygenation during shared airway surgery are[68]:

1. Spontaneous breathing.
2. Positive pressure ventilation via an endotracheal tube (often a small microlaryngsocopy tube) inserted in the proximal trachea.
3. Jet ventilation—may be supraglottic or subglottic/transtracheal.
4. Apneic oxygenation using humidified, high-flow nasal oxygen delivery systems or intermittent ventilation.
5. Cross-field ventilation with an endotracheal or endobronchial tube within the distal airway.
6. Extracorporeal membrane oxygenation (ECMO)/cardiopulmonary bypass (CPB).

Table 48-2 Causes of Stridor

Supraglottic Airway	Larynx	Subglottic Airway
Laryngomalacia	Laryngocele	Tracheomalacia
Vocal cord paralysis	Infection (tonsillitis, peritonsillar abscess)	Vascular ring
Subglottic stenosis	Foreign body	Foreign body
Hemangiomas	Choanal atresia	Infection (croup, epiglottitis)
Cysts	Cyst Mass Large tonsils Large adenoids Craniofacial abnormalities	

Some operations can be performed using direct laryngoscopic exposure of the airway alone. Other cases may require laryngeal suspension to enable full surgical access to the airway.

Stridor

Noisy breathing due to obstructed airflow is known as *stridor.* Inspiratory stridor results from upper airway obstruction; expiratory stridor results from lower airway obstruction; biphasic stridor is present with midtracheal lesions. The evaluation of a patient with stridor begins with a thorough history. The age of onset suggests a cause: Laryngotracheomalacia is usually present at or shortly after birth, whereas cysts or mass lesions develop later in life (Table 48-2). Vocal cord paralysis may be congenital or acquired. Acquired vocal cord paralysis may be due to iatrogenic injury sustained during surgery, neurologic abnormalities such as Arnold–Chiari malformation, local invasion by tumors, and specific chemotherapy regimens. Information indicating positions that make the stridor better or worse should be obtained, and placing a patient in a position that allows gravity to aid in reducing obstruction can be of benefit during anesthetic induction.

Physical examination reveals the general condition of a patient and the degree of airway compromise. Laboratory examination may include an assessment of hemoglobin, a chest radiograph, and barium swallow, which can aid in identifying lesions that may be compressing the trachea. Other radiologic examinations such as MRI and CT scans may be indicated in isolated instances but are not routinely ordered. Specific notes of the signs and symptoms listed in Table 48-3 should be made.

Laryngomalacia is the most common cause of stridor in infants. It is most often due to a long epiglottis that prolapses

Table 48-3 Clinical Component of the Evaluation of Patients with Stridor

Respiratory rate	Chest retractions
Heart rate	Nasal flaring
Wheezing	Level of consciousness
Cyanosis	

posteriorly and prominent arytenoid cartilages with redundant aryepiglottic folds obstructing the glottis during inspiration.[69] Many times, laryngomalacia will improve as patients grow older, though patients with severe obstructive symptoms may need surgical intervention.

Though most patients with unilateral vocal cord paralysis (UVCP) are stridulous, they rarely have signs of overt airway obstruction, as would be the case with bilateral cord paralysis. Younger children with UVCP may have a weak cry and frequent aspirations from a lack of ability to oppose their vocal cords and protect their airway fully. In contrast, older patients may only have hoarseness symptoms and poor vocal projection.

The definitive diagnosis for both laryngomalacia and UVCP is obtained by direct laryngoscopy and rigid or flexible bronchoscopy. The preliminary examination is usually carried out in the surgeon's office. A small, flexible fiberoptic bronchoscope is inserted through the nares into the oropharynx, and the movement of the vocal cords is observed. Alternatively, it may be accomplished in the OR before anesthetic induction in an awake patient or a lightly anesthetized patient during spontaneous respiration. Patients must be breathing spontaneously so that the vocal cords can move freely. After deepening anesthesia and topicalization of the vocal cords is performed using 1% to 2% lidocaine, a rigid bronchoscope is inserted through the vocal cords, and the subglottic area is inspected; the lower trachea and bronchi are evaluated with a rigid or flexible fiberoptic bronchoscope. Treatment for laryngomalacia and UVCP can be performed with direct laryngoscopy and bronchoscopy. During supraglottoplasty, redundant tissue is removed in a targeted manner to improve airflow mechanics. Interventional therapy for UVCP aims to medialize the paralyzed cord so that it can make contact with the contralateral functioning vocal cord and allow for airway protection. This can be accomplished with periodic injection laryngoplasty or more permanent interventions such as medicalization thyroplasty and reinnervation procedures. Reinnervation procedures do not return vocal cord mobility but restore tone such that the vocal cord assumes a more medial position.[70]

Bronchoscopy

Small infants may be brought into the OR unpremedicated. Older children and adults may experience respiratory depression and worsening airway obstruction if heavy premedication is administered, so only light sedation is suggested. The airway must be protected from aspiration of gastric contents during prolonged airway manipulation; therefore, premedication with the full regimen of acid aspiration prophylaxis may be indicated.

The anesthetic goals are analgesia, an unconscious patient, and a "quiet" surgical field. Coughing, bucking, or straining during instrumentation with the rigid bronchoscope may cause difficulty for the surgeon and damage the patient's airway. After the procedure, patients should be returned to consciousness quickly, with airway reflexes intact. For most patients, a pulse oximeter, blood pressure cuff, ECG, and precordial stethoscope are applied before induction of anesthesia. Inhalation induction by mask is accompanied by oxygen and a volatile agent administered in increasing concentrations in children and intravenous drugs in adults. Patients should be placed in the position that produces the least adverse effect on airway symptoms (often the sitting position). An intravenously administered antisialagogue may help decrease secretions that might compromise the view through the bronchoscope.

The size of a bronchoscope refers to the internal diameter. Because the external diameter may be significantly greater than in an endotracheal tube of similar size (Table 48-4), care must be taken to select a bronchoscope of proper outer diameter to avoid

Table 48-4 Comparison of External Diameter of Standard Endotracheal Tubes Versus Rigid Bronchoscope

Endotracheal Tube	Rigid Bronchoscope	
Internal Diameter (mm)	*Internal Diameter (mm)*	*External Diameter (mm)*
2.5	3.5	4.2
3	4.3	5
3.5	4.9	5.7
4	5.5	6.7
5	6.8	7.8
6	8.2	8.2

damage to the laryngeal structures. A rigid bronchoscope can be used for ventilation of the lungs during the airway examination. It is inserted through the vocal cords, and ventilation is accomplished through a side port, which can be attached to the anesthesia circuit. During ventilation with the viewing telescope in place, high resistance may be encountered due to partial occlusion of the lumen. High fresh gas flow rates, large tidal volumes, and high inspired volatile anesthetic concentrations are often necessary to compensate for leaks around the ventilating bronchoscope and the increased resistance encountered when the viewing telescope is in place. Manual ventilation at higher-than-normal rates is most effective in achieving adequate ventilation. Adequate time for exhalation must be provided for passive recoil of the chest.[71]

An alternative ventilation method is jet ventilation, which involves intermittent bursts of oxygen delivered under pressure (see Chapter 28, Video 28-4).[72,73] Intermittent flow is accomplished using a programmed jet ventilator but can alternatively be accomplished with manual controls. Jet ventilation techniques are associated with the additional risks of pneumothorax or pneumomediastinum due to rupture of alveolar blebs or a bronchus.[74] Because ventilation may be intermittent and suboptimal; oxygen should be used as the carrier gas during the bronchoscopic examination. Intravenous drugs that cause excessive respiratory depression should be avoided. It is wise to ask the surgeon if the movement of the vocal cords will be required after the procedure or if tracheal or bronchial dynamics will be evaluated during the procedure so that the anesthetic may be planned accordingly (i.e., spontaneous respirations preserved during light levels of anesthesia vs. no respiratory efforts and the use of short-acting muscle relaxants).

Maintenance of anesthesia can be accomplished with a volatile anesthetic augmented by propofol infusion (100 to 300 mcg/kg/min) or during open airway surgery where controlled administration of volatile anesthetic agents is not possible, with TIVA. Techniques using propofol infusions supplemented by ketamine, dexmedetomidine, and opiates (particularly remifentanil) have been described.[68,75] After rigid bronchoscopy, a tracheal tube can be placed in the trachea to control the airway during anesthesia recovery, or the anesthesia team can manage the airway without a tracheal tube if they feel one is not needed. An additional advantage of placing an endotracheal tube is that if the surgeon should want to examine the distal airways, a small, flexible fiberoptic bronchoscope can be passed through the endotracheal tube, but this is also possible via other airway adjuncts such as a supraglottic airway device.

Pediatric Airway Emergencies

Upper airway emergencies may be life-threatening and demand immediate treatment. Rapid respiratory failure can occur in patients with croup, epiglottitis, or foreign-body aspiration, and few clinical situations are more challenging to the anesthesiologist.

Epiglottitis

Acute epiglottitis is one of the most feared infectious diseases in children and adults and results from *Haemophilus influenzae* type B (2 Video 48-2, NICV 48-2). A conservative estimate of the incidence of epiglottitis is 10 to 40 cases per million people in the United States. Since 1985, with the widespread vaccination against *H. influenzae* type B (Hib), the most common organism related to epiglottitis, the overall incidence of the disease among children has dropped dramatically. It can progress with extreme rapidity from sore throat to airway obstruction to respiratory failure and ultimately to death if proper diagnosis and intervention are not rapidly implemented. Patients are usually between 2 and 7 years of age, although epiglottitis has been reported in younger children and adults. Epiglottitis in the very young (younger than 1 year) is unusual and occurs in only about 4% of cases, and in adults, it peaks between ages 20 and 40 years. Vaccination against *H. influenzae* type B polysaccharide is now recommended before 2 years of age to provide immunity before pediatric patients' most significant period of vulnerability.

Characteristic signs and symptoms of acute epiglottitis include sudden onset of fever, dysphagia, drooling, thick, muffled voice, and preference for the sitting position with the head extended and leaning forward. Retractions, labored breathing, and cyanosis may be observed in cases in which respiratory obstruction is present. However, the patient may be pale and toxic in the early stages without respiratory distress. *Supraglottitis* may be a more appropriate designation because it is the tissues of the supraglottic structures—from the vallecula to the arytenoids—involved in the infectious process. At no time, especially in the emergency department or radiography suite, should direct visualization of the epiglottis be attempted in the unanesthetized patient due to the risk of laryngospam. The differential results from negative pressure inside and the atmospheric pressure outside the extrathoracic airway, resulting in slight narrowing during everyday inspiration. The pressure differential on inspiration is exaggerated in the patient with airway obstruction. This dynamic collapse of the airway may become life-threatening in the struggling, agitated patient, and every attempt should be made to keep the patient calm. Blood draws, intravenous catheter insertion, excessive manipulation of the patient, and sedation should be avoided before securing the airway to avoid the possibility of total obstruction.

If the clinical situation allows, oxygen should be administered by mask, and lateral radiographs of the soft tissues in the neck may be obtained. Thickening of the aryepiglottic folds and swelling of the epiglottis may be noted (the "thumbprint" sign). The radiologic examination should be carried out only if skilled personnel and adequate equipment accompany the patient. The patient with severe airway compromise should proceed from the emergency department directly to the operating suite, accompanied by the anesthesiologist and surgeon. Parental presence in this situation may calm an anxious and frightened child.

In all cases of epiglottitis, an artificial airway is established using tracheal intubation. In some centers in which personnel experienced in the management of the compromised airway are not available, tracheostomy is a less-favored alternative. The child is kept in the sitting position in the OR while monitors are placed. A pulse oximeter and the availability of capnography are essential;

a precordial stethoscope may be helpful. If it is believed to be helpful, one parent may accompany the child and remain in the OR during the induction of general anesthesia. The OR must be prepared with equipment and personnel for laryngoscopy, rigid bronchoscopy, and tracheostomy. Standard blade video laryngoscopy should be considered to optimize first attempt success and allow for a common shared airway view with other anesthesia and surgical providers to identify the airway due to potentially distorted anatomy secondary to inflammation. Anesthetic induction is accomplished by inhalation of oxygen and increasing concentrations of sevoflurane. After loss of consciousness occurs, intravenous access should be secured, and the child lowered into the supine position. Laryngoscopy followed by oral tracheal intubation is then accomplished usually without muscle relaxants. The endotracheal tube should be at least one size (0.5 mm) smaller than would typically be chosen, and a stylet is often helpful. Once the surgeon has examined the larynx, noting the appearance of the epiglottis, aryepiglottic folds, and surrounding tissues, tissue and blood cultures are taken, and antibiotic therapy is initiated. The child is then transferred to the ICU for continued observation. Sedation is appropriate at this time. Tracheal extubation is usually attempted 48 to 72 hours later in the OR when a significant leak around the tracheal tube is present and visual inspection of the larynx by flexible fiberoptic bronchoscopy confirms reduction in swelling of the epiglottis and surrounding tissues.

Laryngotracheobronchitis

Laryngotracheobronchitis (LTB), or croup, occurs in children from 6 months to 6 years of age but is primarily seen in children younger than 3 years. It is usually viral in etiology, and its onset is more insidious than epiglottitis. The child presents with low-grade fever, inspiratory stridor, and a "barking" cough. Radiologic examination confirms the diagnosis, and subglottic narrowing of the airway column secondary to circumferential soft-tissue edema produces the "steeple" sign characteristic of LTB. Approximately 6% of patients with LTB require admission to the hospital. Treatment includes cool, humidified mist and oxygen therapy, usually administered in a tent for mild-to-moderate cases. More severe cases of LTB are accompanied by tachypnea, tachycardia, and cyanosis. Racemic epinephrine administered by a nebulizer is beneficial. A great deal of controversy has surrounded the use of steroids, but the current opinion is that a short course of steroids may be helpful. In rare circumstances, thick secretions are present in the airway, and the child requires intubation to allow pulmonary toilet and suctioning to be performed. Management in the ICU and extubation are carried out in the same fashion as epiglottitis.

Foreign-Body Aspiration

A significant cause of morbidity and mortality in children and adults is the aspiration of a foreign body. Any history of coughing, choking, or cyanosis while eating should suggest the possibility of foreign-body aspiration. Peanuts, popcorn, jelly beans, and hot dogs are some of the ingested items most commonly associated with pulmonary aspiration. Any patient who presents to the emergency department with refractory wheezing should be suspected of this diagnosis. Physical findings include decreased breath sounds, tachypnea, stridor, wheezing, and fever. These signs indicate an obstructive process with inflammation present in the airway. Some foreign bodies are identifiable on radiologic examination; however, 90% are radiolucent, and air trapping, infiltrate, and atelectasis are noted.

The most common site of foreign-body aspiration is the main stem bronchus, the right being more frequent than the left (Fig. 48-7). Food particles comprise the majority of aspirated items; however, beads, pins, and small toys are not unusual. Each type of aspirated item has potential complications associated with it. Vegetable items expand with moisture encountered in the respiratory tract. They can fragment into multiple pieces, thus creating a situation in which the original foreign body is in one bronchus and, with coughing, a fragment is dislodged and transported to the other bronchus. Oil-containing objects, such as peanuts, cause a chemical inflammation, and sharp objects cause bleeding in addition to the obstruction.

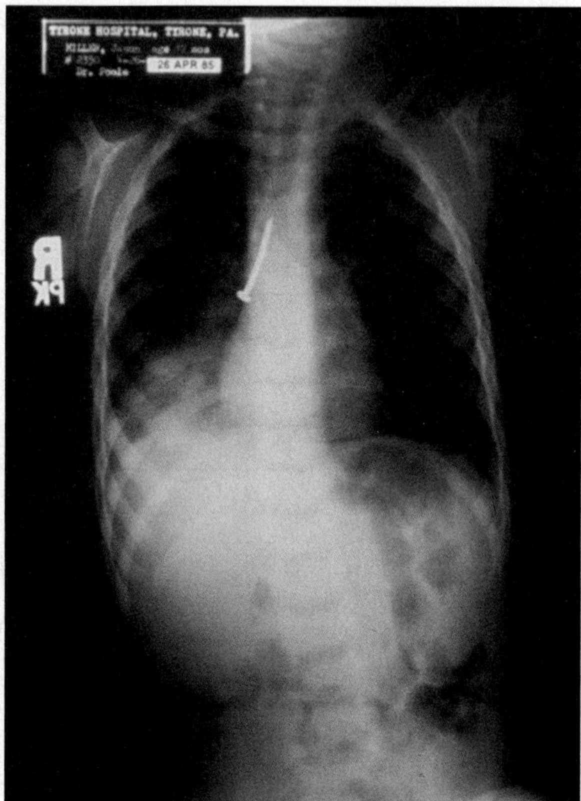

Figure 48-7 Aspirated foreign body in the right mainstem bronchus.

All aspirated foreign bodies in the airway should be removed in the OR and considered emergencies. No sedation should be administered to patients before removal of the foreign body. If the patient has recently eaten, full-stomach precautions must be taken, and anesthesia should be induced intravenously (topical anesthetic cream may be applied to the skin before intravenous catheter insertion in small children) by rapid sequence and gentle cricoid pressure maintained during intubation of the trachea. If the child has not eaten recently, anesthesia may be induced by inhalation of sevoflurane in oxygen by mask. Inhalation induction can be prolonged secondary to airway obstruction, and N_2O should be avoided to prevent air trapping distal to the obstruction. After the evacuation of the stomach by an orogastric tube, the airway may be given over to the surgeon, who introduces a rigid bronchoscope and removes the aspirated object.

Spontaneous ventilation may potentially minimize the risk of distal translocation of the foreign body and pressure accumulation due to a ball/valve effect. The risk of this complication should be balanced against the potential for complications that a controlled ventilation technique may avoid with muscle relaxation, including laryngospasm, patient movement, and coughing/vomiting. In addition, the anesthetic depth required to maintain spontaneous ventilation while avoiding patient movement may predispose the patient to hypotension. A study that retrospectively analyzed complications for rigid bronchoscopy cases for foreign-body removal comparing spontaneous with controlled ventilation did not find a more significant association with a complication with either technique.[76] Ventilation via the bronchoscope requires careful attention. Hypoxia and hypercarbia may occur because of inadequate ventilation caused by a massive leak around the bronchoscope or, more commonly, the inability to provide adequate gas exchange through a narrow-lumen bronchoscope fitted with an internal telescope. These conditions are remedied by frequent removal of the telescope and withdrawal of the bronchoscope to the mid trachea, allowing adequate ventilation. Bronchospasm may occur during the respiratory tract examination and should be treated with increasing depths of anesthesia, nebulized albuterol, or intravenous bronchodilators. Although rare, pneumothorax should be suspected if acute deterioration occurs during the procedure.

Once the foreign body has been removed, the entire tracheobronchial tree is examined to detect additional objects or fragments. Often, vigorous irrigation and suctioning distal to the obstruction are required to remove secretions and prevent the possibility of postobstructive pneumonia. Steroids are administered if the inflammation of the airway mucosa is observed. Close postoperative observation of the patient is required so that early intervention may be instituted in the event of respiratory compromise secondary to airway edema or infection.

Pediatric and Adult Surgery

Specific surgical procedures are commonly performed in adults and children, including nasal surgery and laser airway surgery.

Laser Surgery of the Airway

One of the most significant advances in airway surgery has been the use of the laser (*l*ight *a*mplification by *s*timulated *e*mission of *r*adiation) (3 Video 48-3). For use in the airway, the laser provides precision in targeting lesions, minimal bleeding and edema, preservation of surrounding structures, and rapid healing. The laser consists of a tube with reflective mirrors at either end and an amplifying medium to generate electron activity, resulting in light production (NICV 48-3).[77] The CO_2 laser is the most widely used in medical practice, having particular application in the treatment of laryngeal or vocal cord papillomas, laryngeal webs, resection of redundant subglottic tissue, and coagulation of hemangiomas. The laser is beneficial for the surgeon because the invisible beam of light affords an unobstructed view of the lesion during resection. The energy emitted by a CO_2 laser is absorbed by water contained in blood and tissues. Human tissue is approximately 80% water, and laser energy absorbed by tissue water rapidly increases the temperature, denaturing protein and vaporizing the target tissue. The thermal energy of the laser beam cauterizes capillaries as it vaporizes tissues; thus, bleeding and postoperative edema are minimized.

The properties that give the laser a high degree of specificity also supply the route by which a misdirected laser beam may cause injury to a patient or unprotected OR personnel. The eyes are especially vulnerable, and all OR personnel should wear laser-specific eye goggles with side protectors to prevent injury. Because of the limited penetration (0.01 mm) of the CO_2 laser may cause damage only to the cornea. Other lasers, such as the neodymium–yttrium-aluminum-garnet (Nd: YAG), have deeper penetration and may cause retinal injury and scarring. The eyes of a patient undergoing laser treatment must be protected by taping them shut, followed by applying wet gauze pads and a metal shield. Any stray laser beam is absorbed by the damp gauze, preventing the penetration of the eyes. Laser radiation increases the temperature of the absorbent material, and flammable objects such as surgical drapes must be kept away from the path of the laser beam. To avoid cutaneous burns from deflected beams, wet towels should be applied to the exposed skin of the face and neck when the laser is being used in the airway. Laser smoke plumes may cause damage to the lungs; interstitial pneumonia has been reported with long-term exposure. In addition, it has been postulated that cancer cells and virus particles, including human immunodeficiency virus, are vaporized during laser application, and the resultant smoke plume, if inhaled, may be a vehicle for spread. The use of specially designed surgical masks for filtering laser smoke is recommended.

Most anesthetic techniques are suitable for laser surgery, provided that patients are immobile and the laser beam can be directed at a target that is entirely still and in full view (NICV 48-4). Both N_2O and oxygen support combustion; therefore, the primary gas for anesthetic maintenance should consist of blended air and oxygen or helium and oxygen. A pulse oximeter should ensure adequate oxygenation at the lowest possible inspired oxygen concentration. Anesthesia during laser surgery may be administered with or without an endotracheal tube. The choice of endotracheal tube used during laser surgery can affect the technique's safety. All standard polyvinyl chloride (PVC) endotracheal tubes are flammable and can ignite and vaporize, producing hydrochloric acid when in contact with the laser beam. Cuffed endotracheal tubes should be inflated with sterile saline. Methylene blue has been added so that a cuff rupture from a misdirected laser spark is readily detected by the blue dye and extinguished by the saline.[78] Endotracheal tubes have been manufactured specifically for use during laser surgery. Some have a double cuff to protect the airway in the event of a cuff rupture, and some have a unique matte finish that effectively prevents reflected laser beam scattering; some have both. Nonreflective flexible metal endotracheal tubes are also specifically manufactured for use during laser surgery. The outer diameter of each size of metal laser tube is considerably greater than the PVC counterpart, especially in the small sizes used for pediatric anesthesia (Table 48-5).

An apneic technique is preferred by some surgeons, especially when working on the airway of small infants and children. The advantage of this technique is an open surgical field to the absence of an endotracheal tube, which may obscure the surgical field. In this circumstance, a child is anesthetized and rendered immobile using a muscle relaxant or deep inhalation of a volatile anesthetic.

Table 48-5 Comparison of Standard Plastic Versus Metal Endotracheal Tubes

	External Diameter (mm)	
Internal Diameter (mm)	***Plastic***	***Metal***
3 (uncuffed)	4.3	5.2
3.5 (uncuffed)	4.9	5.7
4 (uncuffed)	5.5	6.1
4.5 (cuffed)	6.2	7
5 (cuffed)	6.8	7.5
5.5 (cuffed)	7.5	7.9
6 (cuffed)	8.2	8.5

The patient's trachea is not intubated, and the airway is given over to the surgeon, who uses the laser for brief periods. Between laser applications, the patient's lungs are ventilated by a mask. Because apnea is a component of this technique, it is prudent to ventilate the lungs with oxygen. Although this technique has been widely used with safety, there is a greater potential for debris and resected material to enter the trachea and the potential for airway trauma due to repeated endotracheal intubation.

A jet ventilator is a modification of the apneic technique that does not require tracheal intubation but does provide for oxygenation; ventilation during laser surgery uses a jet ventilator. The operating laryngoscope is fitted with a catheter that delivers oxygen through a variable pressure reducing valve. Additional room air is entrained, and the patient's lungs are ventilated with this combination of gases. This technique produces a quiet surgical field because large chest excursions of the diaphragm are eliminated, and ventilation is uninterrupted. In morbidly obese patients and those with severe small airway disease, adequate ventilation is difficult to impossible, and an alternative method should be used. Apneic oxygenation using a high-flow humidified oxygen source has also been described in adults and children. This has been able to maintain oxygenation for significant periods without the need to interrupt surgery to maintain oxygen saturation.[79–81]

The final technique that may be used is spontaneous ventilation without an endotracheal tube (Fig. 48-8). A surgical laryngoscope fitted with an oxygen insufflation port is inserted into the larynx. Anesthesia may be induced with a volatile agent by mask but is maintained with total intravenous agents without muscle relaxant in the spontaneously breathing patient. Propofol may be infused with or without short-acting narcotic, other adjuncts such as dexmedetomidine or ketamine, and the vocal cords may be sprayed with 4% lidocaine to decrease reactivity. This technique is advantageous because more extended periods of uninterrupted laser application may be provided. Disadvantages include the absence of complete airway control, limited protection from laryngospasm, limited protection from debris entering the airway, vocal cords' motion, and difficult scavenging.

Nasal Surgery

During nasal surgery, close communication between the anesthesiologist and the otorhinolaryngologist is essential for a successful outcome and avoiding major complications. Functional endoscopic sinus surgery (FESS) is the most common procedure performed in the nasal area. Historically, nasal procedures were completed under topical or local anesthesia with sedation so that the patient could signal the surgeon if problems arose.[82] As endoscopic nasal surgery grew more extensive in scope and duration, general anesthesia became preferred, and local anesthesia with sedation was reserved for the more straightforward cases.

To achieve optimal surgical field visualization, bleeding must be kept to a minimum. Current anesthetic practice includes vasoconstrictors, the elevation of the head, and avoiding excessive increases in blood pressure. Preoperative evaluation of the patient

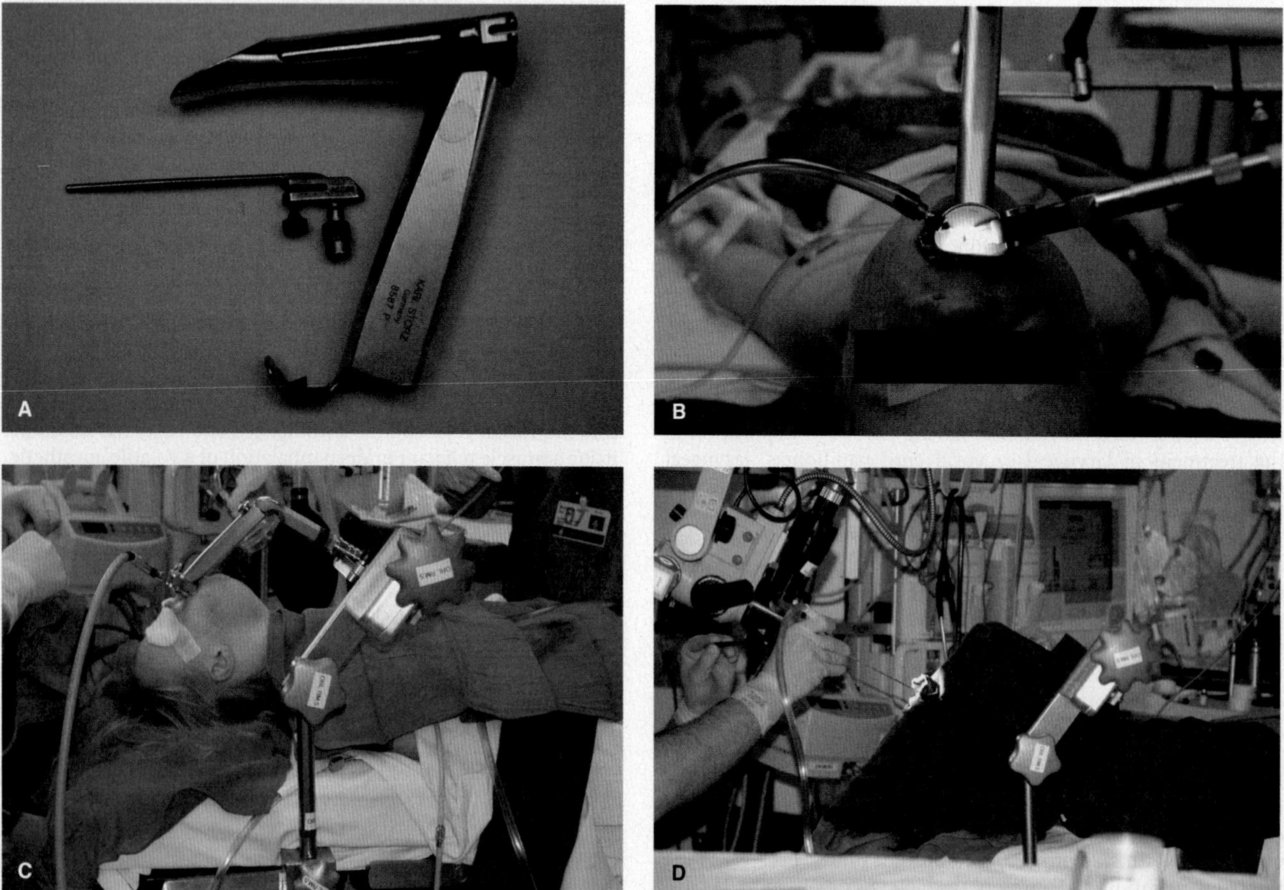

Figure 48-8 **A:** The surgical laryngoscope and the jet ventilator needle. **B:** The surgical view of the laryngoscope positioned in the patient's pharynx and connected to a continuous flow of oxygen through the jet ventilator needle. **C:** View of the anesthetized, spontaneously breathing patient. **D:** Laser-aided resection of vocal cord lesion.

includes a focused cardiovascular history to document coronary artery disease, peripheral artery disease, and cardiac arrhythmias, which might be exacerbated by using sympathomimetic agents used for local vasoconstriction. Positive findings may alter the degree of head elevation, use of topical constrictors, the anesthetic technique, and the lower limit of blood pressure that can be safely tolerated.

6 Intranasal vasoconstriction has been accomplished using local anesthetics combined with cocaine, epinephrine, and phenylephrine. Systemic absorption of these agents can cause hypotension, hypertension, bradycardia, tachycardia, and arrhythmias.[83,84] For patients on beta-blocker or calcium channel–blocker therapy, alpha-agonist–induced hypertension may lead to pulmonary edema and cardiac failure. Prompt treatment is needed to prevent serious complications.

The patient is positioned with the head elevated 15 degrees to facilitate venous drainage. This position may give some modest hypotension; however, there is the potential for venous pooling in the lower extremities. General anesthesia is maintained with inhalation-based or TIVA. TIVA may also have the added benefit of reducing both coughing on emergence and PONV.

Skull Base Surgery

Skull base surgery may be considered the logical extension of nasal surgery involving the practice of otorhinolaryngology, neurosurgery, and anesthesiology. Most adult patients undergoing skull base surgery have malignant tumors, with a smaller group of patients having benign tumors, congenital malformations, or other abnormalities. These patients often require radiologic procedures to determine the location and extent of the lesion before surgery. Noninvasive tests include CT and MRI scans to ascertain the extent of bony and soft-tissue abnormalities. In contrast, more invasive angiography may be needed to determine tumor location and blood supply. These studies may then be used to program intraoperative localizing systems to help guide the surgical dissection.[85] Finally, embolization of lesions may be performed a day or 2 before surgery to shrink the lesion and decrease blood loss during the operative procedure.[86]

7 Special attention during the preoperative assessment should be given to prior surgical procedures, which may affect the airway, chemotherapy, and radiation treatment.[87] Previous surgical procedures may alter a previously accessible airway, requiring advanced airway management techniques to intubate the trachea. Prior chemotherapy can have anesthetic implications depending on the agents used. Patients who have received cardiotoxic agents whose effects are dose-dependent may require a cardiac evaluation, including an echocardiogram. Decreased cardiac function may impact the type of anesthetic agents used and require invasive blood pressure monitoring with an arterial catheter. Prior treatment with neurotoxic agents may reduce the dose of muscle relaxants or cause their duration of action to be prolonged, requiring neuromuscular monitoring. Prior radiation therapy usually does not cause systemic problems unless the pituitary gland is damaged, which can give rise to the issues of panhypopituitarism leading to hypothyroidism, hypoadrenocorticism, and diabetes insipidus. Prior radiation therapy may lead to fibrosis and ankylosis of the temporomandibular joint, rendering direct laryngoscopy difficult. Previous radiation to the operative site may also increase blood loss and poor wound healing. Secondary radiation fibrosis may also make surgical dissection more difficult and time-consuming. It may also necessitate the use of free or vascularized grafts to close the surgical site. The location of the donor site and potential anastomotic sites must also be considered when positioning the patient.

Close attention must be paid to evaluating the head and neck during the physical examination. Usually, these patients do not have a difficult airway or require special techniques for intubation. Oral intubation is the preferred route for lesions requiring a midline surgical approach. If the lesion does not cross the midline, an oral or nasal approach may be used. Nasal endotracheal tubes may be secured using a heavy suture through the nasal septum and around the tube. Oral endotracheal tubes may be secured by either wiring the endotracheal tube to the teeth, suturing it to the gingival periosteum, or using a circummandibular wire.

There are two noteworthy points for anesthetic consideration: The use of muscle relaxation and blood conservation strategies. Like other procedures in which the facial nerve is at risk for injury or transection during dissection, it is necessary to avoid paralysis to periodically stimulate the facial nerve to verify its integrity. Muscle relaxants may be given if nerve stimulation is no longer required. Minimizing blood loss and a plan for replacement with blood products must be considered. If there is anticipation for large-volume blood loss, various approaches can be utilized to potentially reduce the need for transfusion. Anemia identified preoperatively can be treated with iron and erythropoietin. Acute normovolemic hemodilution can be used to minimize blood loss during the procedure. Recently, antithrombolytic therapy has been used successfully in craniofacial procedures and may be of benefit in these cases.[88,89] Directed donor or autologous blood donation have been used to minimize or decrease the exposure to allogenic blood products. Blood salvage techniques, such as cell saver, are usually not appropriate. Most surgical sites are not reached through sterile approaches and would also be relatively contraindicated in surgeries involving resection of tumors.

Upper Airway Infections

Infectious processes of the upper airway can occur in the adult and present the same problems of airway compression, distortion, and compromise. Inflammation of the upper airway caused mainly by gram-negative bacteria may present the same symptoms as epiglottitis in the pediatric age group. While these patients present with fever, chills, drooling, and difficulty speaking and swallowing, they do not usually appear with critical airways from swelling. These same symptoms may occur with Ludwig's angina and generalized cellulitis of the submandibular region.[90] The infection is often the result of dental abscesses and extends into the submandibular, submental, and sublingual areas. Involvement of the sublingual spaces pushes the tongue upward and backward and can lead to asphyxiation due to airway obstruction. Should this occur, emergent surgical interventions may be required to drain the abscess and relieve the airway obstruction.

Airway management can be very difficult in these cases.[91] Awake tracheostomy with local anesthesia has been considered the safest for these patients (see Chapter 28, Video 28-19). If an awake tracheostomy is performed, positive-pressure ventilation should be avoided until proper tracheal tube placement is confirmed, as insufflation into a false or blind passage can lead to significant patient morbidity. Alternative intubation techniques include fiberoptic nasal intubation and direct laryngoscopy after inhalational anesthesia. These patients require care in an ICU, whether they have a tracheotomy or an endotracheal tube once the abscess has been drained, as increased swelling may develop. The trachea should not be extubated until there is some resolution of the swelling.

Maxillofacial Trauma

Traumatic disruption of the bony, cartilaginous, and soft-tissue components of the face and upper airway challenges the anesthesiologist to recognize the nature and extent of the injury and consequent anatomic alteration, create a plan for securing the airway safely, implement the plan without doing further damage, maintain the airway during the administration of an anesthetic, and determine when and how to extubate the patient's trachea. Also necessary is creating a comfortable environment for both surgeon and anesthesiologist in a limited workspace.

It is conventional to divide the facial skeleton into thirds. The lower third consists of the mandible, subdivisions of midline symphysis, body, angle, ramus, condyle, and coronoid process. The mandible has a unique horseshoe shape that causes forces to gather at its points of vulnerability, often distant from the point of impact. As a result, fractures of the mandible typically occur posteriorly where the cortex is also thinner, at the angle of the mandible, the ramus, and the condyle.[92,93] With a condylar fracture, there is potential for TMJ involvement and resulting limitations in jaw mobility. Another common point of fracture is in the body of the mandible at the level of the first or second molar. Clinical experience indicates that this distribution occurs after high-velocity, high-impact trauma, such as an automobile accident. After trauma inflicted by a fist, a blunt weapon, or a fall, there is a greater tendency to fracture the symphysis, parasymphysis, and body.[94] Fractures of the mandible typically do not extend into the skull base. The middle third contains the zygomatic arch of the temporal bone, blending into the zygomaticomaxillary complex, the maxillae, nasal bones, and orbits. The force from a blow to the midface, especially from in front and above, does not follow a normal vector of force dispersion and redistribution. Instead, it creates an abnormal shearing force, which may tear the facial skeleton from the cranial skeleton and extend the fracture into the skull base. Therefore, in any patient with severe midfacial trauma, a fracture of the bottom of the skull must be considered. The superior third consists of the frontal bone.

In 1901, Rene LeFort of Lille, France, determined the common lines of midface fracture, which are thus eponymous and called LeFort I, LeFort II, and LeFort III fractures.

The LeFort I fracture is a horizontal fracture of the maxilla, passing above the floor of the nose but involving the lower third of the septum, mobilizing the palate, maxillary alveolar process, and the lower third of the pterygoid plates and parts of the palatine bones. The fractured segment may be displaced posteriorly or laterally or rotated about a vertical axis. The LeFort II fracture is pyramidal, beginning at the junction of the thick upper part of the nasal bone. The thinner portion forms the upper margin of the anterior nasal aperture. The fracture crosses the medial wall of the orbit, including the lacrimal bone beneath the zygomaticomaxillary suture, crosses the lateral wall of the antrum, and passes posteriorly through the pterygoid plates. The fractured segment may be displaced posteriorly or rotated about an axis. In a LeFort III fracture, the fracture line parallels the base of the skull, separating the midfacial skeleton from the cranium base. The fracture line passes through the base of the nose, ethmoid bone, and the orbital plates. The cribriform plate of the ethmoid may or may not be fractured.

The fracture line crosses the lesser wing of the sphenoid, then down to the pterygomaxillary fissure and sphenopalatine fossa. From the inferior orbital fissure base, the fracture extends laterally and upward to the frontozygomatic suture and downward and backward to the root of the pterygoid plates. A LeFort III fracture results from massive force applied to the midface. The zygomata are displaced, using rotational force to the zygomatic arches. The arches are usually fractured as a result.

In a patient with a LeFort III fracture, the midface is mobilized and often distracted posteriorly. The normal convexity of the face becomes concave, giving rise to the characteristic "dish face deformity" of a LeFort III fracture. Even if this facial concavity is not clinically evident, a LeFort III fracture should be suspected if the incisive edges of the maxillary and mandibular teeth are opposed instead of the normal position in which the maxillary incisors shingle over the mandibular incisors. This apposition serves as a subtle clue to minimal posterior displacement of the midface.

Nasotracheal intubation is contraindicated in LeFort II or III fractures where the cribriform plate of the ethmoid bone may be involved. Foreign material from the nasopharynx may result in causing meningitis or, even more devastating, the endotracheal tube can enter the cranial cavity. Even positive-pressure bag and mask ventilation can force foreign material or air into the skull.[95] Radiographic studies should be done before nasotracheal intubation whenever trauma to the skull base is suspected.

In the patient with facial trauma, concomitant injuries may not be apparent. One study revealed that in patients with maxillofacial injury due to low-velocity, low-impact blows, 4% had additional major life-threatening injuries, and 10% had other minor injuries. With high-velocity, high-impact accidents, 32% had major additional injuries, and 31% had additional minor injuries.[96] Of great importance, cervical spine fractures occurred in 1.2% of high-velocity injuries. Multiple studies have reported cervical spine and significant head injury in patients with facial skeletal trauma, with an incidence as high as 10.8% and 88.7%, respectively.[97,98] The area of cervical injury is frequently related to the site of maxillofacial trauma. Upper face injuries are associated with mid-to-lower cervical spine injuries, while unilateral mandibular injuries involve the upper cervical spine.[97]

To the extent that the patient's clinical situation allows, the degree of facial trauma and concomitant injuries should be assessed. This information should be incorporated into any plan for airway management. Patients with known or suspected cervical spine injuries should have appropriate protective precautions during airway management. Intubating patients with facial trauma can be challenging due to distorted or even disrupted anatomy that can also be obscured by blood, emesis, and displaced teeth.[99] For cases in which there is a concern for difficult intubation, traditional direct laryngoscopy should not be chosen as the primary airway management technique due to its low success rate.[100,101] Advanced airway techniques, such as video laryngoscopy or intubation with a flexible fiberoptic bronchoscope, should be considered.[102,103] This can be done as an awake or minimally sedated technique in cooperative patients, but uncooperative patients may need to be sedated or anesthetized before intubation. Surgical airway placement may be required for patients with extensive airway injury that does not permit intubation or for conditions such as laryngotracheal disruption that can be worsened with conventional intubation techniques such as direct laryngoscopy.[104]

If a patient cannot open their mouth during the preoperative evaluation, one must ascertain if the restriction to mouth opening results from pain, trismus, mechanical problem, or some combination of the three. Simple fractures of the mandible can be very painful; however, once the patient is anesthetized, the mouth can be opened, and tracheal intubation can proceed without difficulty. There may be mechanical interference with opening from injury to the temporomandibular area either directly or indirectly. Direct trauma to the mandibular condyle or zygomatic arch may cause fractures that interfere with the normal function of the TM joint. Indirect trauma is caused by transmittal of force up the body and ramus to the condyles. Compression fractures of condyles in the glenoid fossa and greenstick fractures may impede opening.

Trismus, a spasm of the muscles of mastication, can result from trauma or infection and interfere with mouth opening. It, too, is usually overcome by general anesthesia and muscle relaxation.

The caveat here is that some degree of joint immobility will occur should the trismus be long-standing. If a facial infection causes the trismus, the affected muscles may become edematous and swell, causing a mechanical interference with opening.

Acknowledgments

We gratefully acknowledge the contributions of previous edition authors, Alexander Gotta, Charles Nargozian, and Lynne R Ferrari, as portions of their chapter have been retained in this revision.

For further review and interactivities, please see the videos and narrative interactive clinical vignettes (NICVs) accessible in the complimentary eBook bundled with this text. Access instructions are located on the inside front cover.

REFERENCES

1. Cullen, KA, Hall MJ, Golosinskiy A. Ambulatory surgery in the United States, 2006. *Natl Health Stat Report*. 2009;(11):1–25.
2. Section on Pediatric Pulmonology, S.o.O.S.A.S.A.A.o.P. Clinical practice guideline: diagnosis and management of childhood obstructive sleep apnea syndrome. *Pediatrics*. 2002; 109(4):704–712.
3. Myatt, HM, Beckenham EJ. The use of diagnostic sleep nasendoscopy in the management of children with complex upper airway obstruction. *Clin Otolaryngol Allied Sci*. 2000; 25(3):200–208.
4. Chaban, R, Cole P, Hoffstein V. Site of upper airway obstruction in patients with idiopathic obstructive sleep apnea. *Laryngoscope*. 1988;98(6 Pt 1):641–647.
5. Blum, RH, McGowan FX. Chronic upper airway obstruction and cardiac dysfunction: anatomy, pathophysiology and anesthetic implications. *Pediatric Anesthesia*. 2004;14(1):75–83.
6. Lerman, J. Unraveling the mysteries of sleep-disordered breathing in children. *Anesthesiology*. 2006;105(4):645–647.
7. Gross, JB, Bachenberg KL, Benumof JL, et al. Practice guidelines for the perioperative management of patients with obstructive sleep apnea: a report by the American Society of Anesthesiologists Task Force on Perioperative Management of patients with obstructive sleep apnea. *Anesthesiology*. 2006;104(5):1081–1093; quiz 1117–1118.
8. Brown, KA. Outcome, risk, and error and the child with obstructive sleep apnea. In: *Pediatric Anesthesia*. Blackwell Publishing Ltd.; 2011:771–780.
9. Patino, M, Sadhasivam S, Mahmoud M. Obstructive sleep apnoea in children: perioperative considerations. *Br J Anaesth*. 2013;111 Suppl 1:i83–i95.
10. Ohn, M, Eastwood P, von Ungern-Sternberg BS. Preoperative identification of children at high risk of obstructive sleep apnea. *Paediatr Anaesth*. 2019.
11. Chung, F, Yegneswaran B, Liao P, et al. STOP Questionnaire. *Anesthesiology*. 2008;108(5): 812–821.
12. Chung, SA, Yuan H, Chung F. A systemic review of obstructive sleep apnea and its implications for anesthesiologists. *Anesth Analg*. 2008;107(5):1543–1563.
13. Tait, AR, Voepel-Lewis T, Christensen R, O'Brien LM. The STBUR questionnaire for predicting perioperative respiratory adverse events in children at risk for sleep-disordered breathing. *Paediatr Anaesth*. 2013;23(6):510–516.
14. Friedman, NR, Ruiz AG, Gao D, Jensen A, Mitchell RB. Pediatric obstructive sleep-disordered breathing: updated polysomnography practice patterns. *Otolaryngol Head Neck Surg*. 2019; 161(3):529–535.
15. Tsuiki, S, Isono S, Ishikawa T, Yamashiro Y, Tatsumi K, Nishino T. Anatomical balance of the upper airway and obstructive sleep apnea. *Anesthesiology*. 2008;108(6):1009–1015.
16. Coté, CJ, Posner KL, Domino KB. Death or neurologic injury after tonsillectomy in children with a focus on obstructive sleep apnea: houston, we have a problem!. *Anesth Analg*. 2014: 1276–1283.
17. Marcus, CL, Moore RH, Rosen CL, et al. A randomized trial of adenotonsillectomy for childhood sleep apnea. *N Engl J Med*. 2013;368(25):2366–2376.
18. Resnick, CM, Calabrese CE, Sahdev R, Padwa BL. Is tongue-lip adhesion or mandibular distraction more effective in relieving obstructive apnea in infants with robin sequence? *J Oral Maxillofac Surg*. 2019;77(3):591–600.
19. Heffernan, CB, Calabrese CE, Resnick CM. Does mandibular distraction change the laryngoscopy grade in infants with Robin sequence? *J Oral Maxillofac Surg*. 2019;77(2):371–379.
20. Acevedo, JL, Shah RK, Brietzke SE. Systematic review of complications of tonsillotomy versus tonsillectomy. In: *Otolaryngology—Head and Neck Surgery*. SAGE Publications; 2012: 871–879.
21. Windfuhr, JP, Savva K, Dahm JD, Werner JA. Tonsillotomy: facts and fiction. *Eur Arch Otorhinolaryngol*. 2015;272(4):949–969.
22. Blackshaw, H, Springford LR, Zhang LY, Wang B, Venekamp RP, Schilder AG. Tonsillectomy versus tonsillotomy for obstructive sleep-disordered breathing in children. *Cochrane Database Syst Rev*. 2020;4:CD011365.
23. Eichler, C, Sommer JU, Stuck BA, Hörmann K, Maurer JT. Does drug-induced sleep endoscopy change the treatment concept of patients with snoring and obstructive sleep apnea? In: *Sleep Breath*. Springer-Verlag; 2013:63–68.
24. Truong, MT, Woo VG, Koltai PJ. Sleep endoscopy as a diagnostic tool in pediatric obstructive sleep apnea. *Int J Pediatr Otorhinolaryngol*. 2012;76(5):722–727.
25. Capici, F, Ingelmo PM, Davidson A, et al. Randomized controlled trial of duration of analgesia following intravenous or rectal acetaminophen after adenotonsillectomy in children. In: *British Journal of Anaesthesia*. Oxford University Press; 2008:251–255.
26. Pestieau, SR, Quezado ZM, Johnson YJ, et al. High-dose dexmedetomidine increases the opioid-free interval and decreases opioid requirement after tonsillectomy in children. *Can J Anesth/J Can Anesth*. 2011;58(6):540–550.
27. Mitchell, RB, Archer SM, Ishman SL, et al. Clinical practice guideline: tonsillectomy in children (update). *Otolaryngol Head Neck Surg*. 2019;160(1_suppl):S1–S42.
28. Losorelli SD, Scheffler P, Qian ZJ, Lin HC, Truong MT. Post-tonsillectomy ibuprofen: Is there a dose-dependent bleeding risk? *Laryngoscope*. 2021.
29. Aldamluji, N, Burgess A, Pogatzki-Zahn E, Raeder J, Beloeil H, PROSPECT Working Group collaborators. PROSPECT guideline for tonsillectomy: systematic review and procedure-specific postoperative pain management recommendations. *Anaesthesia*. 2021;76(7): 947–961.
30. Brown, KA, Laferriere A, Lakheeram I. Recurrent hypoxemia in children is associated with increased analgesic sensitivity to opiates, in *Anesthesiology*. 2006;105(4):665–669.
31. Kuehn, BM. FDA: no codeine after tonsillectomy for children. *JAMA*. 2013;309(11):1100.
32. Voronov, P, Przybylo HJ, Jagannathan N. Apnea in a child after oral codeine: a genetic variant - an ultra-rapid metabolizer. *Paediatr Anaesth*. 2007;17(7):684–687.
33. Patel, RI, Hannallah RS, Norden J, Casey WF, Verghese ST. Emergence airway complications in children: a comparison of tracheal extubation in awake and deeply anesthetized patients. *Anesth Analg*. 1991;73(3):266–270.
34. Alexander, CA. A modified Intavent laryngeal mask for ENT and dental anaesthesia. *Anaesthesia*. 1990;45(10):892–893.
35. Haynes, SR, Morton NS. The laryngeal mask airway: a review of its use in paediatric anaesthesia. *Pediatric Anesthesia*. 1993;3(2):65–73.
36. Johr, M. Anaesthesia for tonsillectomy. *Curr Opin Anaesthesiol*. 2006;19(3):260–261.
37. Williams, PJ, Bailey PM. Comparison of the reinforced laryngeal mask airway and tracheal intubation for adenotonsillectomy. *Br J Anaesth*. 1993;70(1):30–33.
38. Nair, I, Bailey PM. Review of uses of the laryngeal mask in ENT anaesthesia. *Anaesthesia*. 1995;50(10):898–900.
39. Goudsouzian, NG, Cleveland R. Stability of the laryngeal mask airway during marked extension of the head. *Pediatric Anesthesia*. 1993;3(2):117–119.
40. Goldman, JL, Baugh RF, Davies L, et al. Mortality and major morbidity after tonsillectomy: etiologic factors and strategies for prevention. *Laryngoscope*. 2013;123(10):2344–2353.
41. Gunter, JB, McAuliffe JJ, Beckman EC, Wittkugel EP, Spaeth JP, Varughese AM. A factorial study of ondansetron, metoclopramide, and dexamethasone for emesis prophylaxis after adenotonsillectomy in children. *Pediatric Anesthesia*. 2006;16(11):1153–1165.
42. Czarnetzki, C. Dexamethasone and risk of nausea and vomiting and postoperative bleeding after tonsillectomy in children. *JAMA*. 2008;300(22):2621.
43. Windfuhr, J, Chen Y, Remmert S. Hemorrhage following tonsillectomy and adenoidectomy in 15,218 patients. *Otolaryngol Head Neck Surg*. 2005;132(2):281–286.
44. Windfuhr, JP, Deck JC, Remmert S. Hemorrhage following coblation tonsillectomy. *Ann Otol Rhinol Laryngol*. 2005;114(10):749–756.
45. Jagannathan, N, Wong DT. Successful tracheal intubation through an intubating laryngeal airway in pediatric patients with airway hemorrhage. *J Emerg Med*. 2011;41(4):369–373.
46. Go, WH, Kim KT, Kim JY, Choe WJ, Kim JW. The use of laryngeal mask airway in pediatric patient with massive post-tonsillectomy hemorrhage. *Korean J Anesthesiol*. 2012;63(2): 177–178.
47. Broadman, LM, Patel RI, Feldman BA, Sellman GL, Milmoe G, Camilon F. The effects of peritonsillar infiltration on the reduction of intraoperative blood loss and post-tonsillectomy pain in children. *Laryngoscope*. 1989;99(6):578–581.
48. Mehta, VM, Har-El G, Goldstein NA. Postobstructive pulmonary edema after laryngospasm in the otolaryngology patient. *Laryngoscope*. 2006;116(9):1693–1696.
49. Brigger, M, Brietzke S. Outpatient tonsillectomy in children: a systematic review. *Otolaryngol Head Neck Surg*. 2006;135(1):1–7.
50. Marcus, CL, Brooks LJ, Draper KA, et al. Diagnosis and management of childhood obstructive sleep apnea syndrome. *Pediatrics*. 2012;130(3):576–584.
51. Nixon, GM, Kermack AS, McGregor CD, et al. Sleep and breathing on the first night after adenotonsillectomy for obstructive sleep apnea. *Pediatr Pulmonol*. 2005;39(4):332–338.
52. Brown, KA, Brouillette RT. The elephant in the room: lethal apnea at home after adenotonsillectomy. In *Anesth Analg*. 2014;1157–1159.
53. Statham, MM, Elluru RG, Buncher R, Kalra M. Adenotonsillectomy for obstructive sleep apnea syndrome in young children. *Arch Otolaryngol Head Neck Surg*. 2006;132(5):476.

54. Possamai, V, Hartley B. Voice disorders in children. *Pediatr Clin North Am*. 2013;60(4):879–892.
55. Malherbe, S, Whyte S, Singh P, Amari F, King A, Ansermino JM. Total intravenous anesthesia and spontaneous respiration for airway endoscopy in children–a prospective evaluation. *Paediatr Anaesth*. 2010;20(5):434–438.
56. Tait, AR, Malviya S. Anesthesia for the child with an upper respiratory tract infection: still a dilemma? *Anesth Analg*. 2005;100(1):59–65.
57. Tait, AR, Malviya S, Voepel-Lewis T, Munro HM, Seiwert M, Pandit UA. Risk factors for perioperative adverse respiratory events in children with upper respiratory tract infections. *Anesthesiology*. 2001;95(2):299–306.
58. Stricker, PA, Muhly WT, Jantzen EC, et al. Intramuscular fentanyl and ketorolac associated with superior pain control after pediatric bilateral myringotomy and tube placement surgery: a retrospective cohort study. *Anesth Analg*. 2017;124(1):245–253.
59. Levine, RA. Monitoring auditory evoked potentials during cerebellopontine angle tumor surgery: relative value of electrocochleography, brainstem auditory evoked potentials, and cerebellopontine angle recordings. In: *Intraoperative Neurophysiologic Monitoring in Neurosurgery*. Springer Science + Business Media; 1991:193–204.
60. Sun, LY, Wijeysundera DN, Tait GA, Beattie WS. Association of intraoperative hypotension with acute kidney injury after elective noncardiac surgery. *Anesthesiology*. 2015;515–523.
61. Bijker, JB, Persoon S, Peelen LM, et al. Intraoperative hypotension and perioperative ischemic stroke after general surgery: a nested case-control study. *Anesthesiology*. 2012;116(3): 658–664.
62. van Waes, JA, van Klei WA, Wijeysundera DN, van Wolfswinkel L, Lindsay TF, Beattie WS. Association between intraoperative hypotension and myocardial injury after vascular surgery. *Anesthesiology*. 2016;124(1):35–44.
63. Wachtendorf, LJ, Azimaraghi O, Santer P, et al. Association between intraoperative arterial hypotension and postoperative delirium after noncardiac surgery: a retrospective multicenter cohort study. *Anesth Analg*. 2022;134(4):822–833.
64. Lavoie, J. Blood transfusion risks and alternative strategies in pediatric patients. In: *Pediatric Anesthesia*. Blackwell Publishing Ltd.; 2011:14–24.
65. Gessler, EM, Hart AK, Dunlevy TM, Greinwald JH Jr. Optimal concentration of epinephrine for vasoconstriction in ear surgery. In: *The Laryngoscope*. John Wiley & Sons, Inc; 2001: 1687–1690.
66. Dunlevy, TM, O'Malley TP, Postma GN. Optimal concentration of epinephrine for vasoconstriction in neck surgery. In: *The Laryngoscope*. John Wiley & Sons, Inc.; 1996:1412–1414.
67. Casey, WF, Drake-Lee AB. Nitrous oxide and middle ear pressure. *Anaesthesia*. 1982;37(9): 896–900.
68. Bradley, J, Lee GS, Peyton J. Anesthesia for shared airway surgery in children. *Paediatr Anaesth*. 2020.
69. Zalzal, GH. Stridor and airway compromise. *Pediatr Clin North Am*. 1989;36(6):1389–1402.
70. Butskiy, O, Mistry B, Chadha NK. Surgical interventions for pediatric unilateral vocal cord paralysis: a systematic review. *JAMA Otolaryngol Head Neck Surg*. 2015;141(7):654–660.
71. Soriano, SG, Kim C, Jones DT. Surgical airway, rigid bronchoscopy, and transtracheal jet ventilation in the pediatric patient. *Anesthesiol Clin North America*. 1998;16(4):827–838.
72. Cook, TM, Alexander R. Major complications during anaesthesia for elective laryngeal surgery in the UK: a national survey of the use of high-pressure source ventilation. *Br J Anaesth*. 2008;101(2):266–272.
73. Mausser, G, Friedrich G, Schwarz G. Airway management and anesthesia in neonates, infants and children during endolaryngotracheal surgery. *Paediatr Anaesth*. 2007;17(10):942–947.
74. Jaquet, Y, Monnier P, Van Melle G, Ravussin P, Spahn DR, Chollet-Rivier M. Complications of different ventilation strategies in endoscopic laryngeal surgery: a 10-year review. *Anesthesiology*. 2006;104(1):52–59.
75. Wang, JT, Peyton J, Hernandez MR. Anesthesia for pediatric rigid bronchoscopy and related airway surgery: tips and tricks. *Paediatr Anaesth*. 2022;32(2):302–311.
76. Litman, RS, Ponnuri J, Trogan I. Anesthesia for tracheal or bronchial foreign body removal in children: an analysis of ninety-four cases. *Anesth Analg*. 2000;91(6):1389–1391.
77. Hermens, JM, Bennett MJ, Hirshman CA. Anesthesia for laser surgery. *Anesth Analg*. 1983;62(2):218–229.
78. Apfelbaum, JL, Caplan RA, Barker SJ, et al. Practice advisory for the prevention and management of operating room fires: an updated report by the American Society of Anesthesiologists Task Force on Operating Room Fires. *Anesthesiology*. 2013;118(2):271–290.
79. Humphreys, S, Lee-Archer P, Reyne G, Long D, Williams T, Schibler A. Transnasal humidified rapid-insufflation ventilatory exchange (THRIVE) in children: a randomized controlled trial. *Br J Anaesth*. 2017;118(2):232–238.
80. Nekhendzy, V, Saxena A, Mittal B, et al. The safety and efficacy of transnasal humidified rapid-insufflation ventilatory exchange for laryngologic surgery. *Laryngoscope*. 2020;130(12): E874–E881.
81. Patel, A, Nouraei SA. Transnasal Humidified Rapid-Insufflation Ventilatory Exchange (THRIVE): a physiological method of increasing apnoea time in patients with difficult airways. *Anaesthesia*. 2015;70(3):323–329.
82. Lee, WC, Kapur TR, Ramsden WN. Local and regional anesthesia for functional endoscopic sinus surgery. *Annal Otol Rhinol Laryngol*. 1997;106(9):767–769.
83. Groudine, SB, Hollinger I, Jones J, DeBouno BA. New York State Guidelines on the topical use of phenylephrine in the operating room. *Anesthesiology*. 2000;92(3):859–864.
84. John, G, Low JM, Tan PE, van Hasselt CA. Plasma catecholamine levels during functional endoscopic sinus surgery. *Clin Otolaryngol*. 1995;20(3):213–215.
85. Cartellieri, M, Vorbeck F, Kremser J. Comparison of six three-dimensional navigation systems during sinus surgery. *Acta Otolaryngol*. 2001;121(4):500–504.
86. Gruber, A, Bavinzski G, Killer M, Richling B. Preoperative embolization of hypervascular skull base tumors. *Minim Invasive Neurosurg*. 2000. 43(2):62–71.
87. Rees, CA, Wu X, Eisen EA, Pastel DA, Halter RJ, Paydarfar JA. Radiation exposure alters airway deformability and bony structure displacement during laryngoscopy. *Laryngoscope Investig Otolaryngol*. 2019;4(6):609–616.
88. Goobie, SM, Meier PM, Pereira LM, et al. Efficacy of tranexamic acid in pediatric craniosynostosis surgery. *Anesthesiology*. 2011;114(4):862–871.
89. Henry, DA, Carless PA, Moxey AJ, et al. Anti-fibrinolytic use for minimising perioperative allogeneic blood transfusion. *Cochrane Database Syst Rev*. 2011;(3):CD001886.
90. Greenberg, SL, Huang J, Chang RS, Ananda SN. Surgical management of Ludwig's angina. *ANZ J Surg*. 2007;77(7):540–543.
91. Kulkarni, AH, Pai SD, Bhattarai B, Rao ST, Ambareesha M. Ludwig's angina and airway considerations: a case report. *Cases J*. 2008;1(1):19.
92. Huelke, DF, Patrick LM. Mechanics in the production of mandibular fractures: strain-gauge measurements of impacts to the chin. *J Dent Res*. 1964;43(3):437–446.
93. Nahum, AM. The biomechanics of facial bone fracture. *Laryngoscope*. 1975;85(1):140–156.
94. Olson, RA, Fonseca RJ, Zeitler DL, Osbon DB. Fractures of the mandible: a review of 580 cases. *J Oral Maxillofac Surg*. 1982;40(1):23–28.
95. Dacosta, A, Billard JL, Gery P, Vermesch R, Bertrand M, Bertrand JC. Posttraumatic intracerebral pneumatocele after ventilation with a mask: case report. *J Trauma*. 1994;36(2): 255–257.
96. Luce, EA, Tubb TD, Moore AM. Review of 1,000 major facial fractures and associated injuries. *Plast Reconstr Surg*. 1979;63(1):26–30.
97. Mithani, SK, St-Hilaire H, Brooke BS, Smith IM, Bluebond-Langner R, Rodriguez ED. Predictable patterns of intracranial and cervical spine injury in craniomaxillofacial trauma: analysis of 4786 patients. *Plast Reconstr Surg*. 2009;1293–1301.
98. Mulligan, RP, Mahabir RC. The prevalence of cervical spine injury, head injury, or both with isolated and multiple craniomaxillofacial fractures. *Plast Reconstr Surg*. 2010;1647–1651.
99. Stephens, CT, Kahntroff S, Dutton RP. The success of emergency endotracheal intubation in trauma patients: a 10-year experience at a major adult trauma referral center. *Anesth Analg*. 2009;866–872.
100. Fiadjoe, JE, Nishisaki A, Jagannathan N, et al. Airway management complications in children with difficult tracheal intubation from the Pediatric Difficult Intubation (PeDI) registry: a prospective cohort analysis. *Lancet Respir Med*. 2016;4(1):37–48.
101. Heidegger, T. Management of the difficult airway. *N Engl J Med*. 2021;384(19):1836–1847.
102. Park, R, Peyton JM, Fiadjoe JE, et al. The efficacy of GlideScope(R) videolaryngoscopy compared with direct laryngoscopy in children who are difficult to intubate: an analysis from the paediatric difficult intubation registry. *Br J Anaesth*. 2017;119(5):984–992.
103. Peyton, J, Park R, Staffa SJ, et al. A comparison of videolaryngoscopy using standard blades or non-standard blades in children in the Paediatric Difficult Intubation Registry. *Br J Anaesth*. 2021;126(1):331–339.
104. Jain, U, McCunn M, Smith CE, Pittet JF. Management of the traumatized airway. *Anesthesiology*. 2015.

49 Anesthesia for Ophthalmologic Surgery

STEVEN GAYER • ALECIA L. S. STEIN

KEY POINTS

1 Cataract surgery is one of the most frequently performed surgical procedures worldwide but represents just one aspect of the various ophthalmic subspecialties, which include cornea, retina, glaucoma, uveitis, strabismus, oculoplastic, and oncology surgeries.

2 Eye surgery patients are often at the extremes of age, ranging from premature babies with retinopathy of prematurity to nonagenarians with multiple coexisting diseases in which age-related anesthetic considerations are key.

3 With intraocular procedures, globe akinesia, patient movement, and control of intraocular pressure (IOP) are important variables; however, with extraocular surgery, the significance of IOP fades and elicitation of the oculocardiac reflex becomes a concern.

4 Inhalation anesthetics cause dose-related reductions in IOP. The exact mechanisms are unknown, but postulated causes include depression of a control center in the diencephalon, reduction of aqueous humor production, enhancement of aqueous outflow, and/or relaxation of the extraocular muscles.

5 The oculocardiac reflex is triggered by pressure on the globe and by traction on the extraocular muscles as well as on the conjunctiva or on the orbital structures. This reflex, whose afferent limb is trigeminal and efferent limb is vagal, may also be elicited by performing a regional eye block, by ocular trauma, and by direct pressure on tissue remaining in the orbital apex after enucleation.

6 Ophthalmic drugs may significantly alter the patient's reaction to anesthesia. Similarly, anesthetic drugs and maneuvers may dramatically influence intraocular dynamics.

7 Several anesthetic options are available for the many types of ocular procedures, including general anesthesia, retrobulbar (intraconal) block, peribulbar (extraconal) anesthesia, sub-Tenon block, topical analgesia, and intracameral injection.

8 The complications of ophthalmic anesthesia can be both vision- and life-threatening.

1 Cataract surgery is one of the most frequently performed surgical procedures, with more than 3 million performed annually in the United States and over 20 million conducted worldwide.[1] Nonetheless, cataract surgery is just one aspect of the various ophthalmic surgical subspecialties, which include cornea, retina, glaucoma, uveitis, strabismus, oculoplastic, and oncologic surgeries. As the population expands and ages, these case volumes will surely continue to increase.[1–3]

Caring for patients undergoing ophthalmic surgery presents many unique challenges for the anesthesiologist (Table 49-1). In addition to possessing technical expertise, the anesthesiologist must have detailed knowledge of ocular anatomy, physiology, and pharmacology. It is essential to appreciate that ophthalmic drugs may significantly alter the reaction to anesthesia and that concomitantly anesthetic drugs and maneuvers may dramatically influence intraocular dynamics. Patients undergoing ophthalmic surgery may represent extremes of age. They may have coexisting diseases (e.g., diabetes mellitus, coronary artery disease, essential hypertension, chronic lung disease, renal insufficiency/failure), and they are likely to be elderly. Indeed, the elderly constitute the most rapidly growing subset of the U.S. population, with the census projecting that by 2030, one in five Americans will be age 65 or older. Furthermore, "the elderly" is a uniquely vulnerable group with reduced functional reserve and a myriad of age-related diseases. 2

Table 49-1 Requirements of Ophthalmic Surgery

Requirements of Ophthalmic Surgery
Safety
Akinesia
Analgesia
Minimal bleeding
Avoidance or obtundation of oculocardiac reflex
Control of intraocular pressure
Awareness of drug interactions
Smooth emergence

3 One must be knowledgeable about the numerous surgical procedures that are unique to ophthalmology. Although the list of ocular surgical interventions is lengthy, these procedures may, in general, be classified as *extraocular* or *intraocular.* This distinction is important because anesthetic considerations are different for these two major surgical categories. For example, with intraocular procedures, globe akinesia, patient movement, and control of intraocular pressure (IOP) are important variables; however, with extraocular surgery, the significance of IOP fades and elicitation of the oculocardiac reflex becomes a concern.

Anatomy of the Eye

The anesthesiologist should be knowledgeable about ocular anatomy as a basis for learning ophthalmic regional anesthesia and to enhance one's understanding of the range of ophthalmic procedures (Fig. 49-1). Pertinent components of ocular anatomy include the bony orbit, the eye itself, extraocular muscles, innervation, vasculature, the eyelids, and the lacrimal system.

The orbit is a bony pyramidal cavity housing the globe and its associated structures in the skull. The walls of the orbit are composed of the following bones: frontal, zygomatic, greater wing of the sphenoid, maxilla, palatine, lacrimal, and ethmoid. A familiarity with the surface relationships of the orbital rim aids performance of regional blocks.

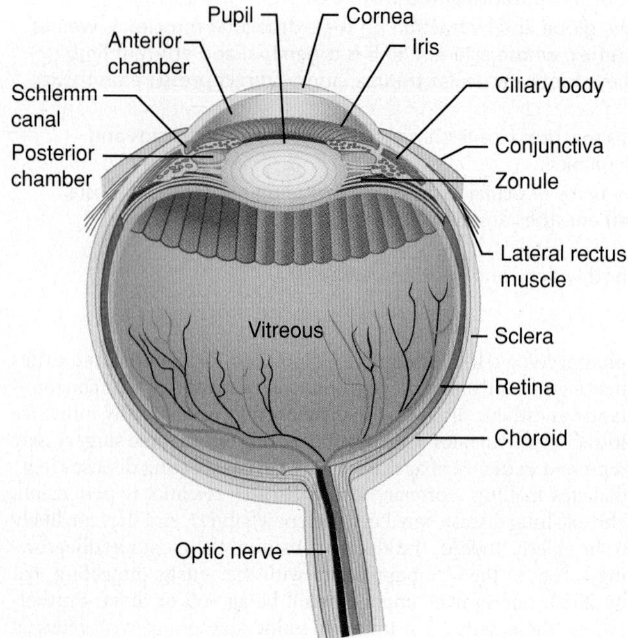

Figure 49-1 Diagram of ocular anatomy.

The optic foramen, located at the orbital apex, transmits the optic nerve and the ophthalmic artery as well as the sympathetic nerves from the carotid plexus. The superior orbital fissure transmits the superior and inferior branches of the oculomotor nerve; the lacrimal, frontal, and nasociliary branches of the trigeminal nerve; the trochlear and abducens nerves; and the superior and inferior ophthalmic veins. The inferior orbital or sphenomaxillary fissure contains the infraorbital and zygomatic nerves and communication between the inferior ophthalmic vein and the pterygoid plexus. The infraorbital foramen, located about 4 mm below the orbital rim in the maxilla, transmits the infraorbital nerve, artery, and vein. The lacrimal fossa contains the lacrimal gland in the superior temporal orbit. The supraorbital notch, located at the junction of the medial one-third and temporal two-thirds of the superior orbital rim, transmits the supraorbital nerve, artery, and vein. The supraorbital notch, the infraorbital foramen, and the lacrimal fossa are all clinically palpable.

The globe is a large sphere with part of a smaller sphere incorporated in the anterior surface, constituting a structure with two different radii of curvature. Structurally, the eye is composed of three layers: sclera, uveal tract, and retina. The fibrous outer layer, or *sclera,* is protective, providing rigidity to maintain eye shape. Anteriorly, the cornea, is highly avascular and transparent, permitting light to pass into the internal ocular structures. The double-spherical shape of the eye exists because the corneal arc of curvature is steeper than the scleral arc of curvature such that the focusing of rays of light to form a retinal image commences at the cornea.

The *uveal tract,* or middle layer of the globe, is vascular and in direct apposition to the sclera. It is composed of the iris, ciliary body, and choroid. The iris includes the pupil, which controls the amount of light entering the eye by contractions of three sets of muscles. The iris dilator is sympathetically innervated; the iris sphincter and the ciliary muscle have parasympathetic innervation. Posterior to the iris lays the ciliary body, which produces aqueous humor (see Formation and Drainage of Aqueous Humor, later). The ciliary muscles, situated in the ciliary body, adjust the shape of the lens to accommodate focusing at various distances. Large vessels and a network of small vessels and capillaries known as the *choriocapillaris* constitute the choroid, which supplies nutrition to the outer part of the retina.

The *retina* is a neurosensory membrane composed of 10 layers that convert light impulses into neural impulses. These neural impulses are then carried through the optic nerve to the brain. A potential space, known as the *suprachoroidal space,* separates the sclera from the uveal tract. This potential space, however, may become blood-filled during an expulsive or suprachoroidal hemorrhage. The vitreous cavity fills the globe centrally. It is filled with a gelatinous substance known as *vitreous humor.* This material is adherent to the most anterior 3 mm of the retina as well as to large blood vessels and the optic nerve. The vitreous humor may pull on the retina, causing retinal tears and retinal detachment.

The crystalline lens, located posterior to the pupil, refracts rays of light passing through the cornea and pupil to focus images on the retina. The ciliary muscle, whose contractile state causes tautness or relaxation of the lens zonules, regulates the thickness of the lens.

In addition, six extraocular muscles move the eye within the orbit. The bilobed lacrimal gland provides most of the tear film, which serves to maintain a moist anterior surface on the globe. The lacrimal drainage system—composed of the puncta, canaliculi, lacrimal sac, and lacrimal duct—drains into the nose below the inferior turbinate. Blockage of this system occurs frequently, necessitating procedures ranging from lacrimal duct probing to dacryocystorhinostomy, which involves anastomosis of the lacrimal sac to the nasal mucosa.

Covering the surface of the globe and lining the eyelids is a mucous membrane called the *conjunctiva*. Because drugs are absorbed across the membrane, it is a popular site for administration of ophthalmic drugs.

The eyelids consist of four layers: the conjunctiva, the cartilaginous tarsal plate, a muscle layer composed mainly of the orbicularis and the levator palpebrae, and the skin. The eyelids protect the eye from foreign objects; through blinking, the tear film produced by the lacrimal gland is spread across the surface of the eye, keeping the cornea moist.

Blood supply to the eye and orbit is by means of branches of both the internal and external carotid arteries. Venous drainage of the orbit is accomplished through the multiple anastomoses of the superior and inferior ophthalmic veins. Venous drainage of the eye is achieved mainly through the central retinal vein. All these veins empty directly into the cavernous sinus.

The sensory and motor innervations of the eye and its adnexa are very complex, with multiple cranial nerves supplying branches to various ocular structures. A branch of the oculomotor nerve supplies a motor root to the ciliary ganglion, which in turn supplies the sphincter of the pupil and the ciliary muscle. The trochlear nerve supplies the superior oblique muscle. The abducens nerve supplies the lateral rectus muscle. The trigeminal nerve constitutes the most complex ocular and adnexal innervation. In addition, the zygomatic branch of the facial nerve eventually divides into an upper branch, supplying the frontalis and the upper lid orbicularis, whereas the lower branch supplies the orbicularis of the lower lid.

Physiology of Intraocular Pressure

The eye is a complex organ which functions through a series of intricate physiologic processes. While comprehensive discussion of the entire physiologic makeup of the eye is not the focus of this text, the formation and drainage of aqueous humor and the resulting influence on IOP is among the most essential components of ocular physiology to the anesthesiologist. Understanding this fundamental aspect of ocular physiology is necessary to appreciate how various anesthetic agents and manipulations impact IOP.

Formation and Drainage of Aqueous Humor

Two-thirds of the aqueous humor is formed in the posterior chamber by the ciliary body in an active secretory process involving both carbonic anhydrase and cytochrome oxidase systems (Fig. 49-2). The remaining third is formed by passive filtration of aqueous humor from the vessels on the anterior surface of the iris.

At the ciliary epithelium, sodium is actively transported into the aqueous humor in the posterior chamber. Bicarbonate and chloride ions passively follow the sodium ions. This active mechanism results in the osmotic pressure of the aqueous humor being many times greater than that of plasma. It is this disparity in osmotic pressure that leads to an average rate of aqueous humor production of 2 μL/min.

Aqueous humor flows from the posterior chamber through the pupillary aperture and into the anterior chamber, where it mixes with the aqueous formed by the iris. During its journey into the anterior chamber, the aqueous humor bathes the avascular lens and, once in the anterior chamber, it also bathes the corneal endothelium. The aqueous humor then flows to the peripheral anterior chamber and exits the eye through the cobweblike trabecular meshwork, Schlemm canal, and episcleral venous system. A network of connecting venous channels eventually leads to the superior vena cava and the right atrium. Thus, obstruction of venous return at any point from the eye to the right side of the heart impedes aqueous drainage, elevating IOP accordingly.

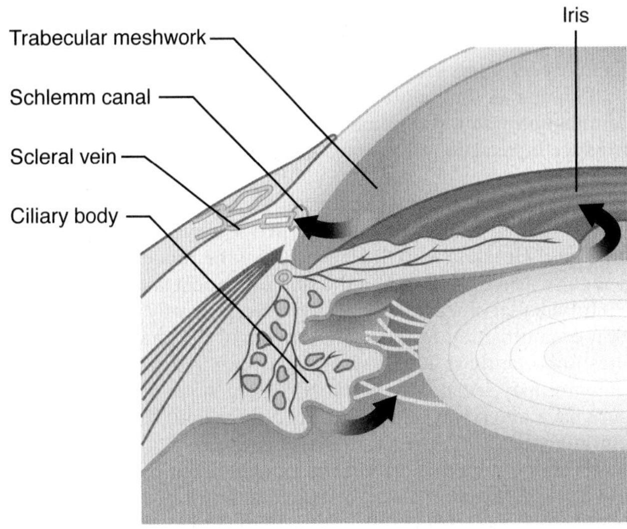

Figure 49-2 Ocular anatomy concerned with control of intraocular pressure.

Intraocular Pressure Regulation

IOP normally varies between 10 and 21.7 mmHg and is considered abnormal above 22 mmHg. This level varies from 1 to 2 mmHg with each cardiac contraction. Also, a diurnal variation of 2 to 5 mmHg is observed, with a higher value noted on awakening. This higher awakening pressure has been ascribed to vascular congestion, pressure on the globe from closed lids, and mydriasis—all of which occur during sleep.

During anesthesia, a rise in IOP can produce permanent visual loss. If the IOP is already elevated, a further increase can trigger acute glaucoma. If penetration of the globe occurs when the IOP is excessively high, rupture of a blood vessel with subsequent hemorrhage may transpire. IOP becomes atmospheric once the eye cavity has been entered, and any sudden rise in pressure may lead to prolapse of the iris and lens, and loss of vitreous. Thus, proper control of IOP is critical.

Three main factors influence IOP: (1) external pressure on the eye. This occurs with contraction of the orbicularis oculi muscle and the tone of the extraocular muscles, venous congestion of orbital veins (as may occur with vomiting and coughing), and conditions such as orbital tumor; (2) scleral rigidity; and (3) changes in intraocular contents that are semisolid (lens, vitreous, or intraocular tumor) or fluid (blood and aqueous humor). Although these factors affect IOP, the major control of intraocular tension is exerted by the fluid content, especially the aqueous humor.

Sclerosis of the sclera, not uncommonly seen in the elderly, may be associated with decreased scleral compliance and increased IOP. Other degenerative changes of the eye linked with aging can also influence IOP, the most significant being a hardening and enlargement of the crystalline lens. When these degenerative changes occur, they may lead to anterior displacement of the lens–iris diaphragm. A resultant shallowness of the anterior chamber angle may then occur, reducing access to the trabecular meshwork by the aqueous. This process is usually gradual, but if rapid lens engorgement occurs, angle-closure glaucoma may transpire abruptly.

Changes in the nature of the vitreous that affect the amount of unbound water also influence IOP. Myopia, trauma, and aging produce liquefaction of vitreous gel and a subsequent increase in unbound water, which may lower IOP by facilitating fluid removal. However, under different circumstances, the opposite may occur; that is, the hydration of more normal vitreous may be associated with elevation of IOP. Hence, it may be prudent to produce a slightly dehydrated state in the surgical patient with glaucoma.

Intraocular blood volume, determined primarily by vessel dilation or contraction in the spongy layers of the choroid, contributes importantly to IOP. Although changes in arterial or venous pressure may secondarily affect IOP, excursions in arterial pressure have much less importance than do venous fluctuations. In chronic arterial hypertension, ocular pressure returns to normal levels after a period of adaptation brought about by compression of vessels in the choroid as a result of increased IOP. Thus, a feedback mechanism reduces the total volume of blood, keeping IOP relatively constant in patients with systemic hypertension.

However, if venous return from the eye is disturbed at any point from the Canal of Schlemm to the right atrium, IOP increases substantially. Trendelenburg position, a cervical collar, and even a tight necktie can produce increased intraocular blood volume and distention of orbital vessels as well as attenuated aqueous drainage.[4] Straining, vomiting, or coughing greatly increases venous pressure and raises IOP as much as 40 mmHg or more. Laryngoscopy and tracheal intubation may also elevate IOP, even without any visible reaction to intubation, especially if the patient coughs. Topical anesthesia of the larynx may attenuate the systemic hypertensive response to laryngoscopy but does not reliably prevent associated increases in IOP.[5] Ordinarily, the pressure elevation from such increases in blood volume or venous pressure dissipates rapidly. However, if the coughing or straining occurs during ocular surgery when the eye is open, as in penetrating keratoplasty (corneal transplant), the result may be a disastrous expulsive hemorrhage, at worst, or a disconcerting loss of vitreous, at best.

Despite the notable role of venous pressure, scleral rigidity, and vitreous composition, maintenance of IOP is determined primarily by the rate of aqueous formation and the rate of aqueous humor outflow. The most important influence on formation of aqueous humor is the difference in osmotic pressure between aqueous humor and plasma. This fact is illustrated by the equation:

$$\text{IOP} = K[(\text{OPaq} - \text{OPpl}) + \text{CP}] \quad (49\text{-}1)$$

where K is the coefficient of outflow, OPaq is the osmotic pressure of aqueous humor, OPpl is the osmotic pressure of plasma, and CP is the capillary pressure. Hypertonic solutions such as mannitol are used to lower IOP because a small change in the solute concentration of plasma can markedly influence the formation of aqueous humor and hence IOP.

Fluctuations in aqueous humor outflow may also produce a dramatic alteration in IOP. The most significant factor controlling aqueous humor outflow is the diameter of Fontana space within the trabecular meshwork, as illustrated by the equation:

$$A = \frac{r^2(\text{Piop} - \text{Pv})}{8\eta L} \quad (49\text{-}2)$$

where A is the volume of aqueous outflow per unit of time, r is the radius of Fontana spaces, Piop is the IOP, Pv is the venous pressure, η is the viscosity, and L is the length of Fontana spaces. When the pupil dilates, the volume within the trabecular meshwork (Fontana space) narrows, resistance to outflow increases, and IOP rises. Because mydriasis is undesirable in both closed-angle glaucoma and open-angle glaucoma, miotics are applied conjunctivally in patients with glaucoma.

Intraocular Pressure Dysregulation: Glaucoma

Dysregulation of aqueous humor homeostasis is a serious state that if left untreated can progress to optic nerve dysfunction and loss of vision—the disease state termed glaucoma. Glaucoma classification is varied and complex—including acquired versus congenital, high-IOP versus normal pressure, acute versus chronic, and open-angle versus closed-angle. Angle-closure glaucoma may be either acute or chronic; notably, acute angle-closure glaucoma is an urgent condition requiring rapid intervention and presents with a tense painful eye, whereas chronic angle-closure disease is far more common and often asymptomatic.

With open-angle glaucoma, the elevated IOP exists within an anatomically open anterior chamber angle. It is believed that sclerosis of trabecular tissue results in impaired aqueous humor filtration and drainage. Treatment strategies seek to decrease aqueous production, increase trabecular meshwork outflow, and/or decrease episcleral venous pressure (see section on anesthetic implications of ophthalmic medications). Closed-angle glaucoma is characterized by the peripheral iris moving into direct contact with the posterior corneal surface, mechanically obstructing aqueous humor outflow. People who have a narrow angle between the iris and the posterior cornea are predisposed to this condition. In these patients, mydriasis can produce such increased thickening of the peripheral iris that corneal touching occurs, closing the angle. Another mechanism producing acute closed-angle glaucoma is swelling of the crystalline lens. In this case, pupillary block occurs, with the edematous lens blocking the flow of aqueous humor from the posterior to the anterior chamber. This situation can also develop if the lens is traumatically dislocated anteriorly, physically blocking the anterior chamber.

The systemic use of anticholinergics in usual doses is safe for glaucomatous eyes. Atropine in the clinical dose range has no effect on IOP in either open-angle or closed-angle glaucoma. When 0.4 mg of atropine is given parenterally to a 70-kg person, approximately 0.0001 mg is absorbed by the eye.[6] Garde et al.[7] reported, however, that scopolamine has a greater mydriatic effect than atropine and recommended not using scopolamine in patients with known or suspected closed-angle glaucoma.

Equation 49-2, describing the volume of aqueous outflow per unit of time, clearly demonstrates that outflow is exquisitely sensitive to fluctuations in venous pressure. Because a rise in venous pressure produces an increased volume of ocular blood and decreased aqueous outflow, it is obvious that considerable elevation of IOP occurs with any maneuver that increases venous pressure. Hence, in addition to preoperative instillation of miotics, consider avoiding IOP-elevating maneuvers such as overhydration, constriction around the patient's neck, prolonged Trendelenburg or prone position, and hypercapnia, which may induce choroidal vascular congestion.

Substantive increases in IOP are encountered during robotic-assisted laparoscopic procedures such as prostatectomy or hysterectomy. However, Awad et al. found no difference between IOP at induction versus 45 minutes to 1 hour after emergence from anesthesia. Three months following surgery, they noted no significant difference in ocular parameters (visual acuity, retinal nerve fiber thickness, ganglion cell complex girth) in patients without preexisting ophthalmic disease.[8] The optic nerve may, however, be at risk in some advanced glaucoma patients kept in prolonged steep Trendelenburg position coupled with abdominal CO_2 insufflation.

In these situations, one may contemplate preoperative ophthalmology consultation and intraoperative prophylactic administration of acetazolamide and/or mannitol.[9]

A small percentage of glaucoma patients experience a marked decrement in vision following surgery, termed visual field "wipe out." Although no distinct etiology is known, several surgical, anesthetic, and postoperative reasons have been postulated. Proposed, but not validated, anesthesia mechanisms include pressure on the optic nerve or its circulation by local anesthetic, blood, or a compression device; direct optic nerve injury by a needle; and hypoperfusion of the optic nerve due to hypotension during general anesthesia or vasoconstrictors admixed with local anesthetic.

Primary congenital glaucoma is classified according to age of onset, with the infantile type presenting any time after birth until 3 years of age. The juvenile type presents between the ages of 37 months and 30 years. Moreover, childhood glaucoma may also occur in conjunction with various eye diseases or developmental anomalies such as aniridia, mesodermal dysgenesis syndrome, and retinopathy of prematurity.

Successful management of infantile glaucoma depends critically on early diagnosis. Presenting symptoms include photophobia, blepharospasm, excessive tearing, and irritability. Ocular enlargement, termed *buphthalmos*, or "ox eye," and corneal haziness secondary to edema are common. If glaucoma develops after 3 years of age buphthalmos is rare because the eye is much less elastic by then.

As infantile glaucoma is frequently associated with obstructed aqueous humor outflow, management often requires surgical creation, by goniotomy or trabeculotomy, of a route for aqueous humor to flow into the canal of Schlemm. However, advanced disease may be unresponsive to even multiple goniotomies, and the more radical trabeculectomy or some other variety of filtering procedure may be necessary.

The juvenile form of glaucoma, in which the cornea and eye size are normal, is commonly associated with a family history of open-angle glaucoma and is treated similarly to primary open-angle glaucoma.

In cases of pediatric secondary glaucoma, goniotomy and filtering may be unsuccessful, whereas cyclocryotherapy may affect a reduction in IOP, pain, and corneal edema. Here, the ciliary body is destroyed with a cryoprobe cooled to −70 °C, thus dramatically decreasing aqueous formation.

It is essential to appreciate that the high IOP frequently encountered in infantile glaucoma can be significantly reduced when a surgical plane of general anesthesia is achieved. Some clinicians maintain that ketamine is a useful drug to use for examination under anesthesia when infantile glaucoma is part of the differential diagnosis because ketamine does not appear to spuriously lower IOP measurement, moreover, even normal infants sporadically have pressures in the mid-20s. Hence, diagnosis is not based exclusively on the numerical pressure recorded under anesthesia. Other factors such as corneal edema and increased corneal diameter, tears in Descemet membrane, and cupping of the optic nerve are considered in making the diagnosis. If these aberrations are noted, surgical intervention may be mandatory, even in the setting of a reputedly normal IOP.

Factors Influencing Intraocular Pressure

Ventilation and Temperature

Hyperventilation decreases IOP, whereas asphyxia, administration of carbon dioxide, and hypoventilation have been shown to elevate IOP. Hypothermia lowers IOP. On initial consideration, hypothermia might be expected to raise IOP because of the associated increase in viscosity of aqueous humor. However, hypothermia is linked with decreased formation of aqueous humor and with vasoconstriction; hence, the net result is a reduction in IOP.

Airway Management

Airway management may impact IOP significantly. Direct Laryngoscopy and intubation can raise IOP severalfold as can an eventful extubation. This is of particular concern for traumatic eye injuries and glaucoma patients. Sufficient depth of anesthesia upon airway insertion should be assured. A "smooth" emergence without bucking is requisite. Video laryngoscopy may raise IOP to a lesser extent than the traditional direct instrumentation approach.[10] Inserting a supraglottic airway may be associated with minimal effect on IOP, depending on the depth of anesthesia when the device is inserted. For this reason, the supraglottic airway is often preferred for ophthalmic surgery. For some, however, an endotracheal tube provides greater reassurance when the anesthesiologist has less access to the patient's head.

Anesthetic Agents

Inhalation anesthetics cause dose-related decreases in IOP. 4
Nitrous oxide, when combined with sevoflurane and remifentanil had no independent effect.[11] Sevoflurane and propofol decrease IOP equally during nonophthalmic surgery.[12] Moreover, virtually all CNS depressants, including propofol and etomidate, dexmedetomidine, barbiturates, neuroleptics, opioids, and hypnotics, lower IOP at dose ranges for sedation and general anesthesia in both normal and glaucomatous eyes.[13] The exact mechanisms are unknown, but postulated causes include depression of a central nervous system (CNS) control center in the diencephalon, reduction of aqueous humor production, enhancement of aqueous humor outflow, or relaxation of the extraocular muscles.[6]

Controversy surrounds the issue of ketamine's effect on IOP. Administered intravenously or intramuscularly, ketamine initially was believed to increase IOP significantly, as measured by indentation tonometry.[14] Corssen and Hoy[15] reported a slight but statistically significant increase in IOP that appeared unrelated to changes in blood pressure or depth of anesthesia. However, nystagmus made proper positioning of the tonometer difficult and may have resulted in less-than-accurate measurements. Conflicting results arose from a study in which 2 mg/kg of ketamine given intravenously to adults failed to have a significant effect on IOP.[16] Furthermore, several pediatric studies reported no increase in IOP with ketamine.[17,18]

Some of the confusion may arise from differences in premedication practices and from the use of different instruments to measure IOP. More recent studies have used applanation tonometry rather than indentation tonometry. There is insufficient convincing evidence to support the notion that ketamine precipitates significant increase in IOP. Notably, though, ketamine's proclivity to cause nystagmus and blepharospasm makes it a less-than-optimal agent for many types of ophthalmic surgery.

Other Medications

Hypertonic Solutions

Intravenous (IV) administration of hypertonic solutions such as dextran, urea, mannitol, and sorbitol elevates plasma osmotic pressure, thereby decreasing aqueous humor formation and reducing IOP. Mannitol's onset, peak (30 to 45 minutes), and duration of action (5 to 6 hours) are similar to those of urea. However,

IV mannitol has fewer side effects than urea. Moreover, both drugs may produce acute intravascular volume overload. Sudden expansion of plasma volume secondary to efflux of intracellular water into the vascular compartment places a heavy workload on the kidneys and heart, and can cause dilution of plasma sodium, hypertension, and congestive heart failure. Furthermore, subsequent mannitol-associated diuresis with volume depletion may trigger hypotension.

Acetazolamide

IV administration of acetazolamide inactivates carbonic anhydrase and interferes with the sodium pump. The resultant decrease in aqueous humor formation lowers IOP. However, the action of acetazolamide is not limited to the eye, and systemic effects include loss of sodium, potassium, and water secondary to the drug's renal tubular effects. Such electrolyte imbalances may then be linked to cardiac dysrhythmias during general anesthesia.

An advantage of acetazolamide is its relative ease of administration. Whereas large volumes of hypertonic solutions must be infused to reduce IOP, acetazolamide is easily dispensed from a single small vial. Acetazolamide may also be given orally, and topical carbonic anhydrase inhibitors are commercially available.

Neuromuscular Blocking Drugs

Both nondepolarizing and depolarizing neuromuscular blocking agents impact IOC through direct and indirect mechanisms. All nondepolarizing neuromuscular agents given in equipotent ED95 doses directly lower IOP by relaxing the extraocular muscles (Fig. 49-3).[19] However, it is important to note that if paralysis of the respiratory muscles is accompanied by inadequate ventilation, the associated elevation in arterial CO_2 may supervene to increase IOP.

In contrast, depolarizing agents such as succinylcholine lead to an increase in IOP. This phenomenon may be clinically relevant in situations where the external structure of the globe is compromised, such as in trauma of the eye or following recent corneal transplantation, and in the surgically open eye. Lincoff et al.[20] first reported extrusion of vitreous after succinylcholine administration to a patient with a surgically open eye. An average peak IOP increase of about 9 mmHg is produced within 1 to 4 minutes of an intubating dose of succinylcholine which returns to baseline typically within 7 minutes.[21] The ocular hypertensive effect of succinylcholine has been attributed to several mechanisms, including the tonic contraction of extraocular muscle fasciculation,[6] choroidal vascular dilation, and relaxation of orbital smooth muscle. One study speculates that the primary mechanism of the IOP increase is the result of a cycloplegic action which produces a deepening of the anterior chamber and increased outflow resistance.[22] The investigators proposed that

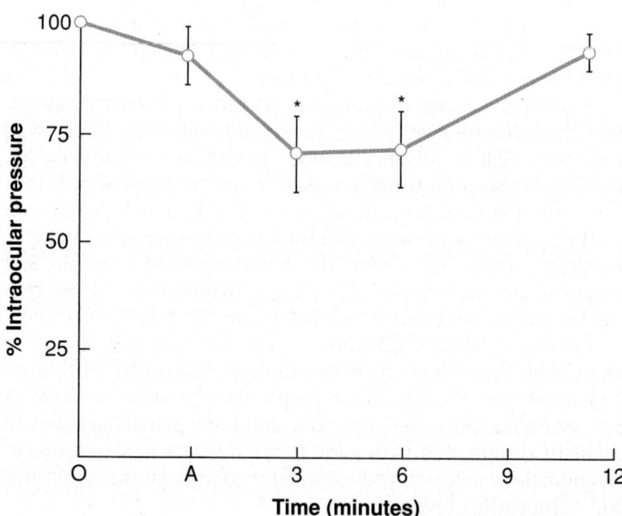

Figure 49-3 Mean intraocular pressure after administration of thiopental, 3 to 4 mg/kg, and pancuronium, 0.08 mg/kg at 0. *A*, loss of lid reflex; * = $P < .05$. (Adapted with permission from Litwiller RW, DiFazio CA, Rushia EF. Pancuronium and intraocular pressure. *Anesthesiology*. 1975;42:750–752.)

changes in extraocular muscle tone alone do not contribute substantially to the ocular pressure surge because the phenomenon was still present in an experimental setup with the extraocular muscles detached.

A variety of methods have been advocated to prevent succinylcholine-induced elevations in IOP. However, although some attenuation of the increase results, none of these techniques consistently and completely block the ocular hypertensive response. Prior administration of such drugs as acetazolamide, narcotics, β-blockers, and nondepolarizing neuromuscular blocking drugs have been suggested. Pretreatment with a small defasciculating dose of nondepolarizing drug may be effective.

In 1968, using indentation tonometry, Miller et al.[23] reported that pretreatment with small amounts of gallamine or *d*-tubocurarine prevented succinylcholine-associated increases in IOP. However, in 1978, using the more sensitive applanation tonometer, Meyers et al.[24] were unable to consistently circumvent the ocular hypertensive response after similar pretreatment therapy (Table 49-2). In addition, Verma[25] claimed that a "self-taming" technique in which a small dose of succinylcholine is administered prior to induction was protective, but in a controlled study using applanation tonometry, Meyers et al.[26] challenged this claim. Although IV pretreatment with lidocaine, 1 to 2 mg/kg, may blunt the hemodynamic response to laryngoscopy,[5,27]

Table 49-2 Effects of Succinylcholine on Intraocular Pressure: Double-Blind *d*-Tubocurarine or Gallamine Pretreatment

		Intraocular Pressure (mmHg, MEAN ± SE)		
Pretreatment[a]	**Mean Age (y)**	***Baseline***	***3 min after Pretreatment***	***1 min after Succinylcholine***[b]
d-Tubocurarine	13.4	13 ± 1	12.3 ± 1.2	24 ± 1.3
Gallamine	8.7	10.9 ± 1.1	10.6 ± 1	23.4 ± 2.3

[a]*d*-Tubocurarine, 0.09 mg/kg, or gallamine, 0.3 mg/kg.
[b]1 to 1.5 mg/kg intravenously.
Reprinted with permission from Meyers EF, Krupin T, Johnson M, et al. Failure of nondepolarizing neuromuscular blockers to inhibit succinylcholine-induced increased intraocular pressure: a controlled study. *Anesthesiology*. 1978;48:149–151.

such a therapy does not reliably prevent the ocular hypertensive response associated with succinylcholine and intubation.[28] However, Grover et al.[29] claimed that pretreatment with lidocaine, 1.5 mg/kg intravenously, 1 minute before induction with thiopental and succinylcholine offered protection from IOP increases because of succinylcholine and may therefore be of value in rapid-sequence induction for open eye injuries (NICV 49-1 and Video 49-1).

See further discussion in the later section, "Open-Eye, Full-Stomach" Encounters as to why it may no longer be valid to recommend that succinylcholine be used with reluctance in ocular surgery.

Oculocardiac Reflex

5 Bernard Aschner and Giuseppe Dagnini first described the oculocardiac reflex in 1908 (NICV 49-2). This reflex bradycardia is triggered by pressure on the globe and by traction on the extraocular muscles as well as on the conjunctiva or the orbital structures. Moreover, the reflex may also be elicited by performance of an eye block, by ocular trauma, and by direct pressure on tissue remaining in the orbital apex after enucleation.[30] The afferent limb is trigeminal and the efferent limb is vagal. Although the most common manifestation of the oculocardiac reflex is sinus bradycardia, a wide spectrum of cardiac dysrhythmias may occur, including junctional rhythm, ectopic atrial rhythm, atrioventricular blockade, ventricular bigeminy, multifocal premature ventricular contractions, wandering pacemaker, idioventricular rhythm, asystole, and ventricular tachycardia.[31] This reflex may appear during either local or general anesthesia; however, hypercarbia and hypoxemia are believed to augment the incidence and severity of the problem, as may shallow anesthetic depth.

Reports on the incidence of the oculocardiac reflex are remarkable in their striking variability. Berler[32] reported an incidence of 50%, but other sources quote rates ranging from 16% to 82%. Commonly, those articles disclosing a higher incidence included study population children, who tend to have more vagal tone.

A variety of maneuvers to abolish or obtund the oculocardiac reflex have been promulgated. None of these methods have been consistently effective, safe, and reliable. Regional anesthesia can block the afferent limb of the reflex but is not without other potential complications. Inclusion of intramuscular anticholinergic drugs such as atropine or glycopyrrolate in the usual premedication regimen for oculocardiac reflex prophylaxis is ineffective.[33] Atropine given intravenously within 30 minutes of surgery may reduce the incidence of the reflex. For pediatric strabismus surgery, however, some anesthesiologists administer IV atropine, 0.02 mg/kg, just before commencing surgery.[34] Alternatively, glycopyrrolate, 0.01 mg/kg administered intravenously, may be associated with less tachycardia than atropine in this setting. Moreover, some anesthesiologists claim that prior IV administration of atropine may yield more serious and refractory cardiac dysrhythmias than the reflex itself. Clearly, atropine may be considered a potential myocardial irritant. A variety of cardiac dysrhythmias[35] and several conduction abnormalities,[36] including ventricular fibrillation, ventricular tachycardia, and left bundle branch block, have been attributed to IV atropine.

It is generally believed that the prophylactic measures, fraught with inherent hazards, are usually not indicated in adults. If a cardiac dysrhythmia appears, the surgeon should be asked to immediately cease operative manipulation. Next, the patient's anesthetic depth and ventilatory status are evaluated. Commonly, heart rate and rhythm return to baseline within 20 seconds after institution of these measures. Moreover, Moonie et al.[37] noted that the reflex is attenuated with repeated manipulation. Bradycardia is less likely to recur, probably secondary to fatigue of the reflex arc at the level of the cardioinhibitory center (tachyphylaxis). However, if the initial cardiac dysrhythmia is especially serious or if the reflex tenaciously recurs, atropine should be administered intravenously.

Direct intra-arterial chemotherapy may be indicated for infants and children with retinoblastoma. This so-called superselective ophthalmic artery chemotherapy is conducted under general anesthesia in a dedicated interventional radiology suite. The procedure involves insertion of a microcatheter into the ophthalmic artery with subsequent infusion of high-concentration chemotherapeutic agent, typically melphalan, directly to the retina and choroid via the ciliary and central retinal artery branches. Serious adverse cardiopulmonary responses to cannulation of the ophthalmic artery or injection of the agent have been described.[38] These responses are characterized by abrupt drop in end-tidal CO_2 with concomitant chest wall rigidity noted as markedly reduced lung compliance akin to acute bronchospasm, profound hypoxia, systemic hypotension, and bradycardia. Harris reported an approximate 40% overall incidence,[39] whereas Phillips et al.,[38] who did not encounter the reaction during initial treatment, noted a 39% occurrence during the second or subsequent catheterization. Yamane et al.[40] confronted bradycardia with such frequency that they considered it to be an indicator of successful ophthalmic artery cannulation. Preoperative IV atropine did not alter the incidence or severity of the reaction. It is postulated that superselective ophthalmic artery chemotherapy may trigger a trigeminal-afferent autonomic reflex response akin to the oculocardiac reflex. The phenomenon has been referred to as a trigeminocardiac reflex (TCR) because the stimulus is decidedly posterior to the globe. Harris proposes that "trigeminal afferents, particularly in these young patients, act as exquisitely sensitive baroreceptors to the increased pressure during microcatheter insertion and infusion."[39] Analogous to the oculocardiac reflex, the TCR is often self-limited and is suppressed by removal of the stimulus, in this case, withdrawal of the catheter from the ophthalmic artery. Profound or refractory TCR is treated by ceasing catheter advancement, 100% oxygen, employing higher airway pressures, and administration of IV boluses of 0.5 to 1.0 mcg/kg epinephrine.[41]

Anesthetic Implications of Ophthalmologic Medications

There is considerable potential for drug interactions during 6
administration of anesthesia for ocular surgery. Topical ophthalmic drugs may produce undesirable systemic effects or may have deleterious anesthetic implications. Systemic absorption of topical ophthalmic drugs may occur from either the conjunctiva or the nasal mucosa after drainage through the nasolacrimal duct. In addition, from spillover, some percutaneous absorption through the immature epidermis of the premature infant may transpire. Occluding the nasolacrimal duct by pressing on the inner canthus of the eye after each drop instillation greatly decreases systemic absorption. Some of the potentially concerning topical ocular drugs include anticholinesterases, cocaine, cyclopentolate, epinephrine, phenylephrine, and timolol. In addition, intraocular sulfur hexafluoride and other intraocular gases have important anesthetic ramifications. Furthermore, certain ophthalmic drugs given systemically may produce untoward sequelae germane to anesthetic management. Drugs in this category include glycerol, mannitol, and acetazolamide.

Parasympathomimetic Agents

Echothiophate, also known as *phospholine iodide,* is a long-acting anticholinesterase miotic that lowers IOP by decreasing resistance to the outflow of aqueous humor. It has been used to treat glaucoma refractory to other therapies and for children with accommodative esotropia. It may prolong the action of succinylcholine by reducing plasma pseudocholinesterase activity by 95% following absorbtion into the systemic circulation after conjunctival instillation. Moreover, normal enzyme activity does not return until 4 to 6 weeks after discontinuation of the drug.[42] Hence, the anesthesiologist may anticipate prolonged apnea after a dose of succinylcholine. In addition, a delay in metabolism of ester local anesthetics may be expected.

Pilocarpine is a cholinergic agonist that increases trabecular outflow. It can precipitate bronchospasm, hypertension, and tachydysrhythmias. A lower-concentration version, available for treatment of mild presbyopia, may decrease vision, cause headache, and increase risk of retinal detachment.

Cocaine

Cocaine, introduced to ophthalmology in 1884 by Koller, has limited topical ocular use because it can cause corneal pitting and erosion. However, as the only local anesthetic that inherently produces vasoconstriction and shrinkage of mucous membranes, cocaine has been used in nasal packs for dacryocystorhinostomy. The drug is so well absorbed from mucosal surfaces that achieved plasma concentrations are comparable to direct IV injection. Because cocaine interferes with catecholamine uptake, it has a sympathetic nervous system potentiating effect.

The usual maximal dose of cocaine used in clinical practice is 200 mg for a 70-kg adult, or 3 mg/kg. Although 1 g is considered to be the usual lethal dose for an adult, considerable variation occurs. Furthermore, systemic reactions may appear with as little as 20 mg. Meyers[43] described two cases of cocaine toxicity during dacryocystorhinostomy, underscoring that cocaine is contraindicated in hypertensive patients or in patients receiving drugs such as tricyclic antidepressants or monoamine oxidase inhibitors. In addition, sympathomimetics, such as epinephrine or phenylephrine, should not be given with cocaine. The use of cocaine has largely been abandoned owing to its toxicity profile and potential for drug abuse. So-called pseudococaine solutions consisting of lidocaine 4%, oxymetazoline 0.05%, and peppermint oil are nearly as effective.

Obviously, before administering cocaine or another potent vasoconstrictor for dacryocystorhinostomy, doses of dilute solutions should be meticulously calculated and carefully administered. If serious cardiovascular effects occur, labetalol should be used to counteract them[44] β-Blocking agents should not be administered in this situation owing to the potential to exacerbate hypertension as a result of unopposed α-adrenergic stimulation. Labetalol offers the advantages of combined α-blockade and β-blockade. In addition, labetalol is preferable to esmolol because of its longer duration of action. It is important to appreciate, however, that labetalol has not been shown to reverse coronary artery vasoconstriction in humans. In the setting of cocaine-associated chest pain and/or myocardial infarction, β-blockers should not be administered acutely, rather, nitroglycerin should be given.

Cyclopentolate

Cyclopentolate is a mydriatic agent that may cause cycloplegia and CNS toxicity, including dysarthria, disorientation, and frank psychotic reactions. Purportedly, CNS dysfunction is more likely to follow use of the 2% solution as opposed to the 1% solution. Cases of convulsions in children after ocular instillation of cyclopentolate have been reported. PACU staff must be alerted that it can lead to drowsiness in order to reduce the potential for incorrect differential diagnosis following eye surgery.[45] Hence, for pediatric use, 0.5% to 1% solutions are recommended.

Phenylephrine

Pupillary dilation and capillary decongestion are reliably produced by topical phenylephrine. Although systemic effects secondary to topical application of prudent concentration/doses are rare,[46] hypertension, headache, tachycardia, and tremulousness have been reported. Cardiac dysrhythmias, severe myocardial ischemia, and even myocardial infarction may develop after topical 10% eye drops in patients with coronary artery disease. Those with cerebral aneurysms may be susceptible to cerebral hemorrhage after phenylephrine in this concentration. In general, a safe systemic level follows absorption from either the conjunctiva or the nasal mucosa after drainage by the tear ducts. However, phenylephrine should not be given in the eye after surgery has begun and venous channels are patent.

Children are especially vulnerable to overdose and may respond in a dramatic and adverse fashion to phenylephrine drops. Hence, the use of only 2.5%, rather than 10%, phenylephrine is recommended in infants and the elderly, and the frequency of application should be strictly limited in these patient populations.

Beta-adrenergic Antagonists

Timolol, a nonselective β-adrenergic blocking drug, historically has been a popular antiglaucoma drug. Carteolol, levobunolol, and metipranolol are more recent medications in this class. Because significant conjunctival absorption may occur, nonselective β-adrenergic antagonists should be administered with caution to patients with known obstructive airway disease, congestive heart failure, or greater than first-degree heart block. Life-threatening asthmatic crises have been reported after the administration of timolol drops to some patients with chronic, stable asthma.[47] The development of severe sinus bradycardia, sick sinus syndrome, and cardiac arrest has been reported after timolol.[48] Moreover, timolol has been implicated in the exacerbation of myasthenia gravis[49] and in the production of postoperative apnea in neonates and young infants.[50]

In contrast to nonselective β-adrenergic blocking drugs, betaxolol, a β_1-blocker, is said to be more oculospecific and have minimal systemic effects.[51] However, patients receiving an oral β-blocker and betaxolol should be observed for potential additive effect on known systemic effects of β-blockade. Caution should be exercised in patients receiving catecholamine-depleting drugs. Although betaxolol has produced only minimal effects in patients with obstructive airway disease, caution should be exercised in the treatment of patients with excessive restriction of pulmonary function. Moreover, betaxolol is contraindicated in patients with sinus bradycardia, congestive heart failure, greater than first-degree heart block, cardiogenic shock, and overt myocardial failure.

Alpha-adrenergic Agonists

Apraclonidine and brimonidine effect IOP by decreasing aqueous production or increasing uveoscleral outflow. Side effects include hypotension, headache, and somnolence.

Table 49-3 Differential Solubilities of Gases

Gas	Blood–Gas Partition Coefficients
Perfluoropropane	0.001
Sulfur hexafluoride	0.004
Nitrogen	0.015
Nitrous oxide	0.468

Intraocular Perfluorocarbons

For retinal detachment, a relatively insoluble expandable gas may be injected into the vitreous to mechanically tamponade reattachment. By varying the concentration, volume, and type of gas used, bubbles can be produced that last from 5 to 70 days before being completely absorbed. Nitrous oxide is manyfold more diffusible than perfluorocarbons, can readily expand the size of a gas bubble, and so should be discontinued 15 minutes prior to injection of a gas bubble.

Should the patient need another operation of any sort, it must be remembered that perfluorocarbons may linger in the eye for a protracted period.[52] If nitrous oxide is administered during this interval, the bubble can rapidly expand, risking retinal and optic nerve ischemia secondary to central retinal artery occlusion (CRAO). Nitrous oxide should be avoided for 5 days after air injection, for 10 days after sulfur hexafluoride injection, and for 70 days following perfluoropropane (Table 49-3).[53] A MedicAlert bracelet is placed on the patient to warn against administration of nitrous oxide during the window of vulnerability (see section on Retinal Detachment Surgery).

Systemic Ophthalmic Drugs

In addition to topical and intraocular therapies, various ophthalmic drugs given systemically may result in complications of concern to the anesthesiologist. These systemic drugs include glycerol, mannitol, and acetazolamide. The first two decrease IOP by dehydrating the vitreous, the latter decreases aqueous production. Oral glycerol may be associated with nausea/vomiting and risk of aspiration, hyperglycemia, mental confusion, and seizure activity.

The recommended IV dose of mannitol for eye surgery is up to 1 g/kg, however, at Bascom Palmer Eye Institute, a more typical total dose is 12.5 g given slowly. Serious systemic problems may result from rapid infusion of large doses of mannitol. These complications include renal failure, congestive heart failure, pulmonary congestion, electrolyte imbalance (particularly glucose), hypotension or hypertension, myocardial ischemia, and, rarely, allergic reactions. Clearly, the patient's renal and cardiovascular status must be assessed before mannitol therapy.

Acetazolamide, a carbonic anhydrase inhibitor decreases aqueous production. Due to its renal tubular effects, it should be considered contraindicated in patients with marked hepatic or renal dysfunction or in those with low sodium levels or abnormal potassium values. Electrolyte imbalances can trigger serious cardiac dysrhythmias. Furthermore, people with chronic lung disease may be vulnerable to the development of severe acidosis with long-term acetazolamide therapy. Topical carbonic anhydrase inhibitors appear to be relatively free of clinically important systemic effects.

Anesthesia Management

Preoperative Evaluation

Patients undergoing ophthalmic surgery may represent extremes of age. They may have coexisting diseases (e.g., diabetes mellitus, coronary artery disease, essential hypertension, chronic lung disease, renal insufficiency/failure), and they are likely to be elderly. Indeed, the elderly constitute the most rapidly growing subset of the U.S. population, with the census projecting that by 2030, one in five Americans will be age 65 or older. Furthermore, the elderly are a uniquely vulnerable group with reduced functional reserve and a potential myriad of age-related diseases.

Preoperative preparation and evaluation begins with the establishment of rapport and communication among the anesthesiologist, the surgeon, and the patient. Most patients realize that surgery and anesthesia entail inherent risks, and they appreciate a candid explanation of potential complications, balanced with information concerning probability or frequency of adverse sequelae. Such an approach also fulfills the medicolegal responsibilities of the physician to obtain informed consent.

The preoperative evaluation also provides a forum for the anesthesiologist to set patient expectations for the intraoperative experience. Many American patients anticipate being unconscious and insensate during eye surgery. These patients should be informed that the nature of the procedure dictates field avoidance, the surgeon at the patient's head and airway, the anesthesiologist at the patient's side; obliging preservation of a patent, functional airway and sufficient mental capacity to remain relatively still. Intraoperative awareness is expected. Postoperative recall of surgery may or may not be suppressed by the amnestic effects of agents administered during the procedure.

A history and physical examination are the foundation of safe patient care. Questionnaires in lieu of medical evaluation lack sensitivity to detect pertinent medical issues.[54] A complete list of medications, both systemic and topical, must be obtained so potential drug interactions can be anticipated and essential medication administered. A history of any allergies to medicines, foods, or tape should be documented. Knowledge of any personal or family history of adverse reactions to anesthesia is mandatory. For eye surgery, requisite laboratory data is typically not required. Indeed, the American Society of Anesthesiologists (ASA) task force on preoperative evaluation concluded that routine preoperative tests are commonly not useful in assessing and managing patients' perioperative experience. Schein et al.,[55] for example, demonstrated that "routine" testing does not improve cataract patient safety or outcome. Some physicians and laypersons misinterpreted the results and conclusions of this investigation, believing that patients having cataract surgery need no preoperative evaluation. It is crucial to note that all patients in this trial received regular medical care and were evaluated by a physician preoperatively. Patients whose medical status indicated a need for preoperative laboratory tests were excluded from the study. Clearly, testing should be based on the results of the history and physical examination. The favorable economic impact of a "targeted" approach is obvious, because "routine" testing for annual U.S. cataract operations neither decreases adverse events nor improves outcomes but is estimated to cost $150 million.[56] The Society for Ambulatory Anesthesia recommends no preoperative testing prior to cataract surgery unless there is an indication independent of the procedure.[57]

The dilemma whether to continue or suspend antithrombotic therapy prior to surgery is not unique to the ophthalmic patient population. Many elderly eye surgery patients are on antiplatelet or anticoagulant therapy because of a history of coronary or vascular pathology. These individuals are at higher risk for perioperative hemorrhagic events, including retrobulbar hemorrhage, circumorbital hematoma, intravitreous bleeding, and hyphema. Although prior discontinuation of antithrombotic agents may diminish the potential for perioperative ocular bleeding, such strategy may increase the risk of adverse events like myocardial ischemia, infarction, cerebrovascular accident, and deep venous thrombosis.

The consensus of studies exploring this controversial issue suggest that cataract and other ophthalmic procedures can be safely performed under regional anesthesia without discontinuing antithrombotic agents.[58–61] A multicenter study of almost 20,000 elderly cataract patients attempted to establish the risks and benefits of continuing aspirin or warfarin therapy.[60] Despite the large population studied, the rate of complications was so low that absolute differences in risk were minimal. Patients who continued therapy did not have more ocular hemorrhage; those who discontinued treatment did not have a greater incidence of medical events. A meta-analysis of 11 studies revealed that continuing warfarin therapy for cataract patients was associated with an increased risk of bleeding, but almost all instances were self-limiting and not clinically relevant. No patient had bleeding-related compromise of visual acuity.[62,63]

Articles in the *Annals of Surgery*[64] and the *New England Journal of Medicine*[65] categorized retina surgery as being distinctly apart from other ophthalmic procedures owing to the high risk for intraoperative hemorrhage. However, contemporary ophthalmic literature suggests otherwise.[66,67] Retrospective studies of hemorrhagic complications in patients undergoing retina surgery taking antithrombotics demonstrate equivalent or higher rates of bleeding compared to controls. Nonetheless, in nearly all of these studies bleeding did not cause long-term visual sequelae; most were self-limited vitreous hemorrhages that rarely required returning to the operating room. Evolving surgical techniques including smaller gauge vitrectomy may further decrease the risk of perioperative hemorrhage.

Regional anesthesia for eye surgery also presents another bleeding risk. Traditionally, some physicians held that patients taking antithrombotic medications should not receive a regional eye block owing to increased hemorrhagic risk. Others express preference for sub-Tenon's over extraconal block. Significantly, there are no data that conclusively substantiate a contradiction to conduction anesthesia. In most papers, risks have been shown to be comparable regardless of antithrombotic continuation or interruption.[62,68] A recent review of the literature confirms the absence of sight-threatening complications associated with regional anesthesia blocks in patients on single antiplatelet agents or anticoagulants.[69]

The direct antithrombotic agents such as the anticoagulants dabigatran, rivaroxaban, and apixaban, as well as the antiplatelet medications prasugrel and ticagrelor, add further complication because their efficacy cannot be monitored with conventional clotting assays.

The continuing evolution of this debate emphasizes the need to evaluate the systemic risk of stopping antithrombotic agents against the consequences associated with potential surgical/anesthetic hemorrhage. Most studies are of a retrospective nature and have varying degrees of scientific rigor. Sight-threatening bleeding is sufficiently rare that it would require an enormous sample size in order to render adequate statistical power. Most patients should continue their antithrombotic medication regimens prior to ophthalmic surgery.[57]

Another area of potential concern involves coronary artery disease patients with bare-metal or drug-eluting stents. Although bare-metal stents are susceptible to in-stent restenosis, drug-eluting stents are more vulnerable to stent thrombosis, a complication with a high mortality rate. Thus, patients with drug-eluting stents are typically on dual antiplatelet therapy for extended periods of time. The emerging consensus is that the risk of thrombotic complications in patients with drug-eluting stents appears to outweigh the risk of bleeding complications. Therefore, given current information, a convincing case can be made for continuing dual antiplatelet therapy in the perioperative period and for delaying elective surgery for 30 days after bare-metal stent insertion and for 6 months following drug-eluting stent placement.[63,70,71] Recognizing that the stress response to cataract surgery is more muted and the systemic inflammatory response is minimal, the Society for Ambulatory Anesthesia recommends that patients with coronary stents can have cataract surgery 30 days after stent placement, provided that antiplatelet therapy has been uninterrupted.[57]

Eye surgery patients are often at the extremes of age, ranging from premature babies with retinopathy of prematurity to nonagenarians. Hence, special age-related considerations such as altered pharmacokinetics and pharmacodynamics apply. In addition, elderly patients frequently have multiple comorbidities, including thyroid dysfunction, cardiopulmonary, and renal diseases. Hypertension is encountered in most geriatric patients. Those with poorly controlled blood pressure should not receive dilating eye drops, such as phenylephrine, without consulting an anesthesiologist. Systemic absorption of high concentrations (e.g., 10% phenylephrine) or improperly instilled mydriatics can precipitate a hypertensive crisis with potentially devastating consequences.

As our society becomes increasingly geriatric, the number of ophthalmic surgery patients presenting with cardiac implantable electronic devices (CIEDs) grows. The type of CIED, indication for implantation, and residual battery life should be ascertained prior to surgery.[72] The potential responses to a magnet, number of pacing or tachydysrrhythmic events, or shocks delivered may also be determined. There is debate as to suitability of patients with certain CIEDs in free-standing ambulatory surgical facilities.[73] Novel and evolving devices are increasingly complex and may require real-time access to a cardiac device team.[74]

The theoretical possibility of eye injury from patient movement in the event of implantable cardioverter defibrillator (ICD) discharge during surgery exists. Although there is a broad spectrum of ophthalmic surgical procedures, the majority of cases do not employ electrocautery or use minimal bipolar cautery. For some, such as small-incision extracapsular clear-corneal cataract surgery, no cautery is used. Thus, there is low risk of electromagnetic interference precipitating device discharge. Despite millions of procedures performed each year, there have not been any case reports of ICD activation during ophthalmic surgery and none of the device manufacturers have documented such an incident.[75,76] A retrospective survey of ophthalmic anesthesia providers found that over 80% did not use a magnet to reprogram or inactivate an ICD before surgery.[75]

Perioperative movement is a possible cause of patient eye injury and potential anesthesiologist liability. An analysis of ophthalmic monitored anesthesia care (MAC) closed claims cases that resulted in blindness or poor visual outcome found that more than 80% were associated with inadequate anesthesia and/or patient movement either during the block or intraoperatively.[77] Cough, orthopnea, and restlessness are the most common precipitators of excessive motion. Propofol sedation for eye block is associated with sneezing. Midazolam, fentanyl, and alfentanil given prior to propofol abate the sneeze reflex.[78] Intraoperative movement during general anesthesia may also induce dire visual consequences. Because most ophthalmic surgical procedures are elective, should an enhanced risk of perioperative movement be noted during the preoperative assessment, the prudent course may be to postpone surgery until the patient is in optimal condition to remain relatively still[79] or to perform the procedure under general anesthesia. Deliberate patient selection is requisite in order to prescribe the optimal anesthesia care plan.

The anesthesiologist must be aware of the anesthetic implications of congenital and metabolic diseases with ocular manifestations. Diabetic patients often present with ocular complications, and the anesthesiologist must be knowledgeable about the systemic disturbances of physiology that affect these patients. Indeed, the list of congenital and metabolic diseases associated with ocular pathologic effects that have important anesthetic implications is lengthy. A partial summary includes syndromes such as Crouzon, Apert, Goldenhar (oculoauriculovertebral dysplasia), Sturge–Weber, Marfan, Lowe (oculocerebrorenal syndrome), Down (trisomy 21), Wagner–Stickler, and Riley–Day (familial dysautonomia). Other diseases in this category are homocystinuria, myotonia dystrophica, and sickle cell disease.[80]

Anesthesia Options

The requirements of ophthalmic surgery include safety, akinesia, analgesia, minimal bleeding, avoidance or obtundation of the oculocardiac reflex, prevention of intraocular hypertension, awareness of drug interactions, and suppression of vomiting, coughing, or retching (Table 49-1). Moreover, the exigencies of ophthalmic anesthesia mandate that the anesthesiologist be positioned remote from the patient's airway, sometimes creating logistic problems.

7 A number of anesthetic options exist, including general anesthesia, retrobulbar (intraconal) block, peribulbar (extraconal) anesthesia, sub-Tenon block, topical anesthesia, and intracameral injection. General anesthesia is typically administered for infants and children. Some adolescent and most adult patients can be cared for with regional or topical anesthesia and MAC, with or without sedation. The choice of anesthesia technique should be individualized on the basis of the patient's needs and preferences, the nature and duration of the procedure, the resources and capabilities of the facility, and the preferences and skills of the anesthesiologist and the surgeon. Broader factors that influence anesthesia choice include cultural expectations, traditional institutional practices, cost, availability of personnel and facilities, and the specifics of the health care delivery system.[81]

The retrobulbar block has traditionally been the most popular regional anesthetic technique for eye surgery. Since the mid-1990s, owing to a presumed superior safety profile, peribulbar injection is preferred in the United States, whereas the sub-Tenon block is favored in the United Kingdom and New Zealand[82] Topical analgesia has prevailed for cataract surgery.[83] Although cataract surgery embodies the majority of eye procedures, there are a variety of other subspecialty operations, including corneal transplant and procedures for glaucoma, strabismus, and tumor, as well as oculoplastic, orbital, vitreoretinal, and eye trauma procedures. Most of these continue to be accomplished primarily with a regional eye block and sedation,[84] albeit some warrant general anesthesia.

From the late 19th century, when Koller demonstrated the effectiveness of cocaine to abate the pain associated with eye surgery, conduction anesthesia had been the purview of eye surgeons. Lundy introduced orthopedic regional anesthesia techniques at Mayo Clinic in 1924, however, they did not become established as an integral part of routine anesthesia practice until the 1970s. In a 1994 survey of anesthesiology and ophthalmology programs, no formal training or education in ophthalmic regional anesthesia techniques was provided to anesthesia residents in most academic programs.[85] This survey concluded that anesthesiologists who perform ophthalmic blocks should have knowledge of orbital anatomy and ocular risk factors.

Anesthesiologists have had increasing interest in administering ocular anesthesia. Many ophthalmologists and administrators encourage anesthesiologists to administer the blocks to facilitate operating room efficiency. In reply to a recent survey, nearly 75% of Massachusetts ophthalmologists who use eye blocks indicated that they rely on anesthesiologists to perform them.[86] A recent national survey of retinal subspecialists revealed that anesthesiologists administer the regional anesthetic in a substantial portion of vitreoretinal surgery cases.[87]

Yet, to date, anesthesiology residents receive minimal or no ophthalmic anesthesia training, and must rely on postgraduate education such as workshops conducted at major regional and national meetings.[88] Anesthesiologists who perform eye blocks should have didactic and hands-on training, including identification of higher-risk eyes and management of complications.[86]

When a regional anesthetic of the orbit is administered, by either the anesthesiologist or the ophthalmologist, sedation may be administered before performance of the block and/or initiation of surgery. It is the responsibility of the anesthesia service or its delegates to monitor the patient's vital signs and be vigilant for the oculocardiac reflex, signs of brainstem anesthesia or intravascular injection of local anesthetics, and the need for airway support or other interventions.

Side of Anesthesia and Surgery

In an attempt to ensure proper patient, side, site, and procedure selection, The Joint Commission held a "Wrong Site Summit" in 2003 in which they developed the initial universal protocol for preventing wrong site, wrong procedure, wrong person surgery (NICV 49-3). The policy is tripartite, involving preoperative verification, marking of the intended site, and a "time-out" immediately before the start of a procedure.[89] Patient involvement and effective communication are key components.

Ophthalmologic surgery and regional anesthesia confer greater risk than many other surgical procedures owing to the potential for laterality errors. Patients (and medical staff) may be confused as to the side, site, or actual procedure. Sedatives or anesthetic agents may enhance the likelihood of error. Some patients, such as children and infants, may lack the competence to intervene. Similarity of names can be conducive to mistakes. Procedural factors may be contributory; a wrong side may be draped or prepared, a patient's cap may obscure a clearly marked surgical site. Human factors play a key role in the problem. Failure to cross-check consent forms, patient charts, and patients occasionally still occurs. Our distraction-rich environment, coupled with dysfunctional oral/written communication and lack of proper adherence to safety protocols, also plays a role.

Anesthesia Techniques

In the past, ophthalmic procedures commonly involved large ocular incisions. General endotracheal anesthesia, with deep and sustained neuromuscular paralysis and placement of sandbags to surround the patient's head, were typical strategies to ensure perioperative immobility. Currently, general anesthesia typically is reserved for children and adults who are unable to communicate, cooperate, or remain suitably stationary. Supraglottic airways (SGAs) have been increasingly accepted as a means to secure the airway in patients with minimal risk for aspiration who are having eye surgery with general anesthesia.[90] The SGA is not only safe and effective in this setting but also offers the advantage of less increase in IOP on insertion and removal than is encountered

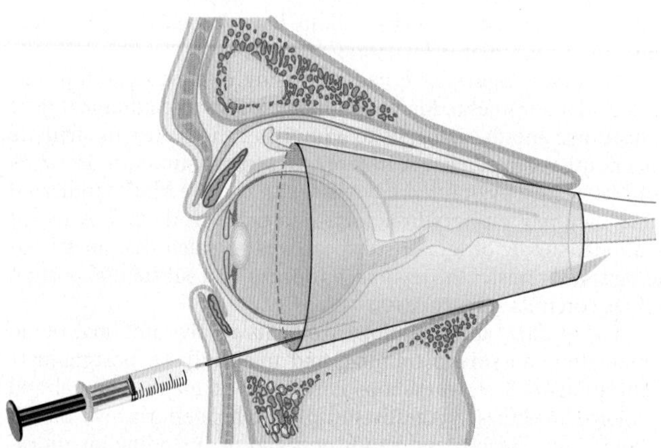

Figure 49-4 Intraconal (retrobulbar) block and schematic representation of the intraorbital muscle cone.

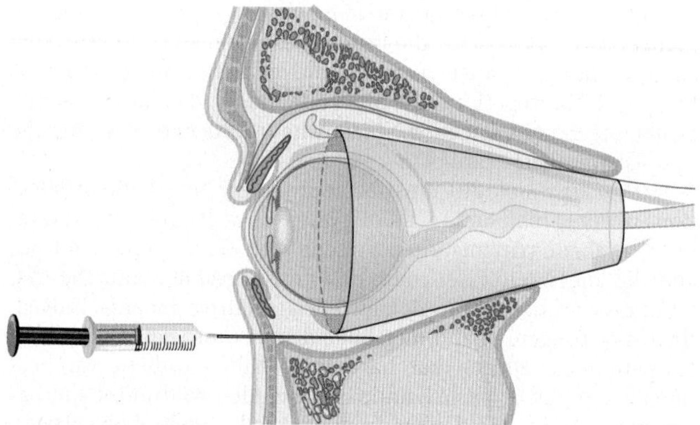

Figure 49-6 Extraconal (peribulbar) block and schematic representation of the intraorbital muscle cone.

with an endotracheal tube.[91] Similarly, less bucking and coughing on emergence and during the recovery phase have been noted.[92] Vigilance must be maintained to detect intraoperative displacement of the SGA. In addition, intraoperative laryngospasm in infants and neonates may occur with an SGA.

Maneuvers to suppress the surge in IOP from straining and coughing upon emergence from general endotracheal anesthesia should be considered. These include deep extubation, and/or administration of lidocaine, narcotics, or dexmedetomidine. A 0.25 to 1.0 mcg/kg dose of dexmedetomidine administered 15 minutes prior to emergence from general anesthesia decreases coughing and agitation in a dose-dependent fashion.[93]

Retrobulbar (Intraconal) and Peribulbar (Extraconal) Blocks

In 1844, Knapp described one of the first techniques for ophthalmic regional anesthesia.[94] In the early 20th century, Atkinson[95] introduced the retrobulbar block, a practical needle-based means to achieve analgesia and profound akinesia of the globe. For a retrobulbar block, the needle tip is situated behind (retro) the globe (bulbar). The peribulbar block, a more recently introduced needle-based technique, varies from the retrobulbar block in terms of the depth and angulation of needle placement within the orbit. Here, the needle tip is placed around (peri) the globe (bulbar). The terminology is inadequate because "retro" and "peri" only vaguely describe the difference between the two techniques. The four rectus muscles, along with connective tissue septae, create a defined compartment known as the *orbital cone*, which extends from the rectus muscle origins around the optic foramen at the apex of the orbit to the attachment of the muscles onto the globe anteriorly. Retrobulbar blocks are accomplished by directing a needle through the eyelid or via the conjunctiva toward the orbital apex with sufficient depth and angulation such that the needle passes through the muscle cone (Figs. 49-4 and 49-5).[96] Local anesthetic is then instilled. The term intraconal injection is therefore a better, more descriptive name for the procedure than the older, retrobulbar block.[97] Intra- and extraconal needle-based blocks are useful as main anesthetic technique in adults or for an opioid-reducing multimodal adjunct to postoperative analgesia in children, where they may be safely performed following induction of general anesthesia.[98]

Cadaveric dissections have shown that there is no complete intermuscular septum encircling the rectus muscles, linking them together to form an impermeable conal compartment behind the globe.[99] Ripart et al.[100] clearly demonstrated that extraconal injections of dye into cadaveric specimens diffused into the intraconal space, and solutions placed within the cone distributed to the extraconal space. Thus, the peribulbar or, more properly termed, extraconal block is executed by directing a needle through the eyelid or via the conjunctiva to less depth and with minimal angulation, parallel to the globe, toward the greater wing of the sphenoid bone (Figs. 49-6 and 49-7). Local anesthetic instilled in this extraconal space will eventually penetrate toward the optic nerve and other structures, establishing conduction anesthesia. The extraconal

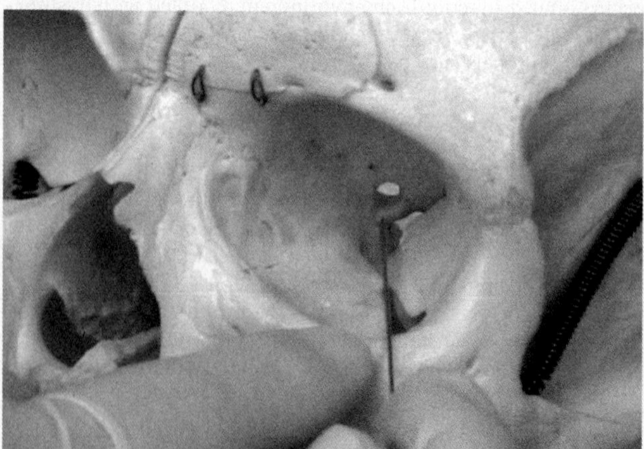

Figure 49-5 Needle placement for intraconal (retrobulbar) block.

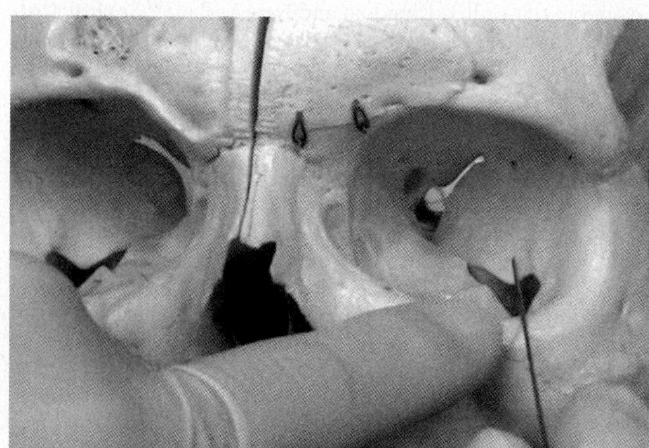

Figure 49-7 Needle placement for extraconal (peribulbar) block.

block may be theoretically safer because the needle tip is kept at a greater distance from vital intraorbital structures and brain.

The didactic classification of block nomenclature based on the relationship of the needle and the muscle cone is a useful means to conceptualize the differences between two types of needle-based eye blocks. It is important to emphasize, though, that needle path cannot always be predicted by clinical evaluation alone. Radiologic studies have shown that some percentage of intraconal blocks administered by experienced physicians are, in fact, extraconal, and vice versa.[101]

Again, a retrobulbar block is more precisely described as an intraconal injection. It positions local anesthetics deep within the orbit proximate to the nerves and muscle origins. Thus, it requires low volume, has rapid onset, and yields intense depth of anesthesia. The peribulbar or, more accurately labeled, extraconal block is placed further from the optic and other orbital nerves, requires larger volumes of local anesthetic, and has longer latency of onset. The needle entry point for both blocks is at the same inferotemporal location. The junction of the lateral third and medial two-thirds of the inferior orbital rim in line with the lateral limbal margin has been the conventional access point. However, locating the needle entry point more laterally may serve to decrease the likelihood of injecting local anesthetics into the delicate inferior rectus or inferior oblique muscles. This is important because intramuscular injection of anesthetics has been postulated as a potential cause of postoperative strabismus.[102] Medial approaches at the caruncle have also been popularized.[103] Supplementation of anesthesia with an injection above the globe may not be prudent because the preponderance of vessels lie in the superior orbit. In addition, the belly of the superior oblique muscle and the trochlear muscle can be encountered superonasally.

Katsev et al.[104] demonstrated that the tips of commonly used 1.5-in (38-mm) needles can reach critical structures in the densely packed apex of the orbit in almost 20% of classic retrobulbar blocks. Consequently, needles 1.25 in (31-mm) or shorter are appropriate. Controversy exists over the advantages of sharp versus dull needles. Dull needles may require more force to penetrate the globe. However, sharp needles are less painful to insert and may cause less damage in the face of inadvertent globe puncture.[105] In the past, patients were asked to gaze superonasally while a block was conducted. Unsold et al.[106] found that this maneuver caused the optic nerve to stretch directly in the path of the incoming needle during intraconal injection, exposing it to risk of needle trauma. Patients should be instructed to maintain gaze in the neutral position, leaving the optic nerve lax within the orbit in the course of needle insertion.[107] Elevations in IOP after an eye block can be minimized by application of gentle noncontinuous digital pressure or use of an ocular decompression device.[108]

Akinesia of the eyelids is obtained by blocking the branches of the facial nerve supplying the orbicularis muscle. Lid akinesia is often a direct consequence of the larger volume of local anesthetic used for extraconal blocks. Intraconal blocks, in contrast, often leave the orbicularis oculi fully functional. Thus, a facial nerve block is performed in conjunction with retrobulbar block to prevent squeezing of the eyelid, which could result in extrusion of intraocular contents during corneal transplantation, for example. Since facial nerve block was first used for ophthalmic surgery by Van Lint in 1914, numerous methods of facial nerve blockade have been described. These techniques block the facial nerve after its exit point from the skull in the stylomastoid foramen. Moving distally to proximally to the foramen, the techniques include the Van Lint, Atkinson, O'Brien, and Nadbath–Rehman methods. Although each has advantages and disadvantages, the Nadbath–Rehman approach can potentially produce the most serious systemic consequences. With this approach, a 27-gauge, 12-mm needle is inserted between the mastoid process and the posterior border of the mandibular ramus. Because of the proximity of the jugular foramen (10 mm medial to the stylomastoid foramen) to the injection site, ipsilateral paralysis of cranial nerves IX, X, and XI can occur, producing hoarseness, dysphagia, pooling of secretions, agitation, respiratory distress, or laryngospasm. Moreover, because the Nadbath–Rehman block produces complete hemifacial akinesia, which interferes with oral intake, this approach is not recommended for outpatients.

Table 49-4 Complications of Needle-based Ophthalmic Anesthesia

Stimulation of oculocardiac reflex arc
Superficial hemorrhage → circumorbital hematoma
Retrobulbar hemorrhage ± retinal perfusion compromise → loss of vision
Globe penetration ± intraocular injection → retinal detachment, loss of vision
Trauma to optic nerve or orbital cranial nerves → loss of vision
Optic nerve sheath injection → orbital epidural anesthesia
Extraocular muscle injury, leading to postoperative strabismus, diplopia
Intra-arterial injection, producing immediate convulsions
Central retinal artery occlusion
Inadvertent brainstem anesthesia → contralateral amaurosis, mydriasis, muscle paresis
Neurocardiopulmonary compromise

Complications associated with needle-based ophthalmic anesthetics may be local or systemic and may result in blindness or even death (Table 49-4). Bleeding may be superficial or deep, arterial or venous. Superficial hemorrhage may produce an unsightly circumorbital hematoma. Retrobulbar hemorrhage, when arterially based, may produce precipitous bleeding and a palpable, dramatic increase in IOP, as well as globe proptosis and entrapment of the upper lid. With the globe's vascular supply in jeopardy, the patient's long-term ultimate visual acuity may be quickly compromised. Consultation with an ophthalmologist should be immediately sought, and fundoscopic examination, tonometric measurement of IOP, ultrasound to assess presence/location of blood, and even a lateral canthotomy may be warranted. Continuous ECG monitoring is indicated because the oculocardiac reflex may occur as blood extravasates from the muscle cone. The decision to proceed with surgery in the presence of a mild or moderate hemorrhage depends on numerous factors, including the degree of bleeding, the nature of the planned ophthalmologic surgery, and the patient's condition.

Penetration of the sclera is a distinct, although rare, possibility with needle-based anesthesia techniques. Mechanical trauma, with potential retinal detachment, and local anesthetic–induced chemical injury to delicate retina tissue can occur. Blindness or very poor vision may be the result. Globe puncture is defined as a single entry into the eye, whereas perforation is caused by two full-thickness wounds—an entry and a subsequent exit. The globe's posterior pole is the most commonly penetrated area. Risk factors for posterior pole needle injury include presence of an elongated globe, recessed orb, and/or atypical-shaped eye. The anteroposterior distance of an eye may be long because of myopia or presence of globe-enveloping intraorbital hardware such as a scleral buckle. Some patients have an abnormal outpouching of the eye, termed *staphyloma.* Most staphylomata are located at the posterior of the globe, surrounding the juncture of the eye with the optic nerve.[109]

By definition, an intraconal (retrobulbar) anesthetic is administered by purposefully angling the needle steeply and deeply within the orbit behind the globe. If the globe is longer than one assumes, it is at greater risk of penetration or puncture by the needle. In one study, ultrasound detection determined that the tip of the needle, placed in classic retrobulbar fashion, can be much closer to the posterior pole of the globe than presupposed by physicians.[110] Extraconal (peribulbar) anesthesia entails shallower placement of the needle without directing the needle inward toward the orbital apex; thus, it is associated with a lower incidence of globe needle injury. Be aware, however, that it is still possible to engage the needle with sclera laterally. The risk of penetrating the sclera with a needle is also inversely proportional to the anesthesiologist's education and experience. This notion is affirmed by several reports of globe injuries rendered by inadequately educated or trained personnel in the early 1990s.[111]

Appropriate preanesthesia evaluation includes direct interrogation concerning myopia or previous scleral buckle surgery, because both imply increased globe length. Bayes et al.[112] showed that a history of correction for myopia as a child or young adult was both highly sensitive and highly specific for having an elongated axial length. Physical examination of surface anatomy should note the position of the globe within the orbit and whether enophthalmos is present. A recessed eye is at greater risk of needle-tip misadventure. The most important laboratory examination is the preoperative ultrasound. For patients undergoing cataract surgery, an ultrasound is *always* performed to calculate the appropriate intraocular lens to insert intraoperatively. In addition, it reveals the length and shape of the eye. An axial length greater than 26 mm confers greater risk of penetration or perforation. In the event that the ultrasound report is not found in the patient's chart, the anesthesiologist should inquire about the results before embarking on a needle-based block.

In the future, portable real-time ultrasonography may have a role in reducing the risk of penetrating injury (Fig. 49-8).[113] Needle-based eye blocks are "blind" techniques primarily dependent on surface anatomy landmarks to position the needle correctly. Ultrasound-guided direct visualization of the needle, the orbital anatomy, and the spread of local anesthetic may improve the quality and safety of these blocks.[114]

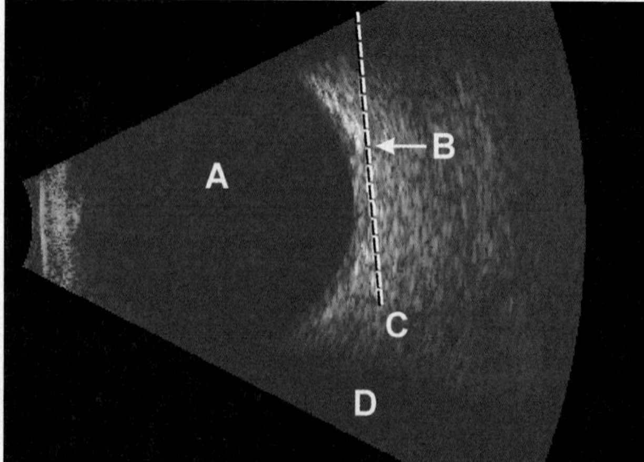

Figure 49-8 Ultrasound-guided block with overlay. **A:** Globe. **B:** Needleshaft. **C:** Needle tip. **D:** Optic nerve.

The eye is easily accessible, and its geometry and surrounding elements are relatively straightforward. Additionally, the tissue contents of the orbit lack gas-filled or osseous structures, making this a suitable area for ultrasonic imaging. Sonography of the eye, however, is not without risk. Owing to potential thermal and mechanical bioeffects, the U.S. Food and Drug Administration has imposed stricter physical parameters for ophthalmic ultrasound. In particular, limits on mechanical index and thermal index have been reduced to 0.23 and less than 1, respectively. Commercial ultrasound transducers marketed to anesthesiologists may not comply with these recommendations. A rabbit model study comparing thermal and mechanical changes induced by exposure to ophthalmic- and nonophthalmic-rated transducers showed significant changes in intraorbital temperature after moderate exposure to a nonophthalmic-rated device, emphasizing the need to ensure that proper eye-appropriate ultrasound equipment is employed for these blocks.[115]

Brainstem anesthesia and inadvertent intravascular injection of local anesthetics are two additional potentially devastating consequences of needle-based ocular anesthesia. In the course of accidental intravascular arterial injection, local anesthetics flow from the needle via a branch of the ophthalmic artery in retrograde fashion to the internal carotid artery and then to the circle of Willis. Rapid redistribution of local anesthetic to the brain results in immediate onset of convulsions. Cardiopulmonary instability may also occur.

Although the incidence of brainstem anesthesia is rare, it is even less common with extraconal versus intraconal blocks. Brainstem anesthesia is a consequence of the direct spread of local anesthetic agents to the brain along the meningeal sheath surrounding the optic nerve. In contradistinction to intra-arterial injection, symptoms are typically not immediate. There is a continuum of sequelae dependent on the concentration and volume of drug that gains access centrally, as well as the specific areas into which the anesthetic spreads (Fig. 49-9).[116] Nicoll et al.[117]

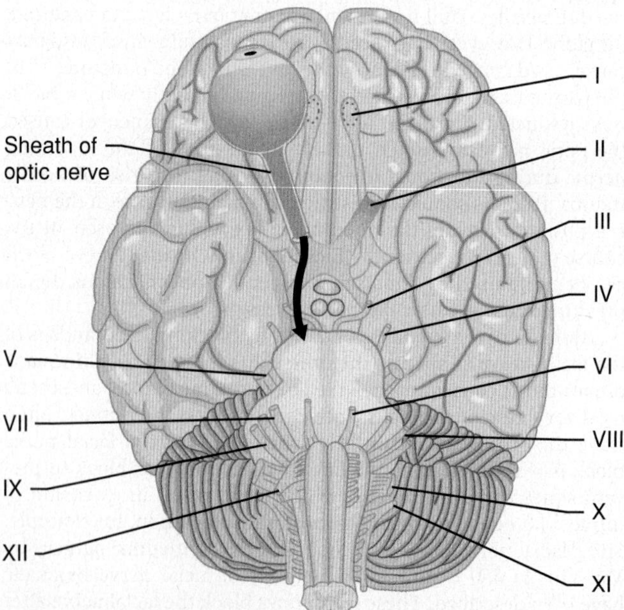

Figure 49-9 Base of the brain and the path that local anesthetic agents might follow if inadvertently injected into the subarachnoid space. This route includes the cranial nerves, pons, and midbrain. (Adapted from Javitt JC, Addiego R, Friedberg HL, et al. Brain stem anesthesia after retrobulbar block. *Ophthalmology.* 1987;94:718. Copyright © 1987 Elsevier. With permission.)

reported 16 cases of apparently central spread of anesthetics in a series of 6,000 intraconal blocks. Eight patients developed respiratory arrest. Examination of the conscious patient's contralateral, nonblocked eye for amaurosis, mydriasis, and extraocular muscle paresis may confirm the diagnosis of brainstem anesthesia. The abducens and oculomotor nerves are more commonly affected than the superior oblique muscle's trochlear nerve. Other protean CNS signs may include violent shivering, eventual loss of consciousness, apnea, and hemiplegia, paraplegia, quadriplegia, or hyperreflexia. Blockade of cranial nerves VIII to XII results in deafness, vertigo, vagolysis, dysphagia, aphasia, and loss of neck muscle power. It is axiomatic that personnel skilled in airway maintenance and ventilatory and circulatory support should be immediately available whenever ophthalmic anesthetic blocks are administered.

Cannula-based Techniques

Turnbull performed the first sub-Tenon block in 1884 by incising conjunctiva, opening Tenon capsule and instilling cocaine drops. Cannula-based ophthalmic regional anesthesia was formally described bySwan[118] in 1956 and then rediscovered and popularized in the 1990s as another practical means to achieve analgesia and akinesia of the globe, while offering potential advantages in certain circumstances over needle-based blocks.[119] Imaging studies have shown that local anesthetics instilled beneath Tenon capsule spread into the posterior orbit.[120] The block is accomplished by inserting a blunt cannula through a small incision in the conjunctiva and Tenon capsule, with subsequent infusion of local anesthetics (Fig. 49-10). Onset of analgesia is rapid. The ultimate extent of globe akinesia is proportional to the volume of local anesthetic injected. One large prospective study by Guise[121] of 6,000 such blocks found this technique to be highly effective. Advantages, particularly for very myopic patients who have elongated axial lengths, include decreased risk of posterior pole penetration or perforation because needles are not placed into the posterior orbit.

After application of topical anesthetic, the episcleral space can be accessed from all quadrants by forceps and blunt-tipped scissors; however, the incision is most commonly made in the inferonasal quadrant. The cannula is guided through the opening with the aid of a toothless forceps. It is common for some portion of the local anesthetic to sublux out of the incision site. Conjunctival bleeding, chemosis, and ballooning of the conjunctiva are also common. Fortunately, these are cosmetic issues that rarely affect outcome. Guise[121] estimated the incidence of minor hemorrhage to be below 10% and had to abandon only one case because of a large subconjunctival hemorrhage that was not sight-threatening. Thus, the sub-Tenon block may be a prudent ocular anesthesia technique for the anticoagulated patient at risk for retrobulbar hemorrhage.

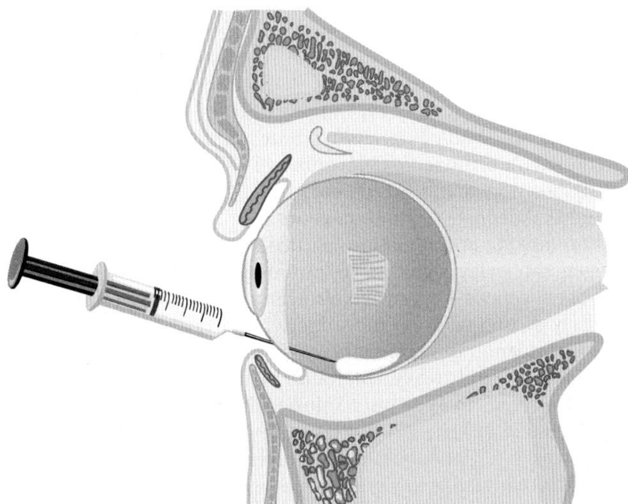

Figure 49-10 Sub-Tenon (episcleral) block with blunt cannula.

Sub-Tenon blocks are employed less frequently in North America than in Europe, perhaps in part due to anesthesiologists' reticence to use scissors to cut through conjunctiva and Tenon capsule. Variations of sub-Tenon blocks include use of ultrashort cannulae (6 mm) and needle-based episcleral block techniques.[122] An incisionless sub-Tenon block, using a triport cannula without scissors has been pioneered by Allman et al.[123] A recent modification to the technique, also omitting the scissors, employs a reusable metal or disposable plastic conjunctival probe to create a small tunnel into the sub-Tenon space.[124] This simplifies the block technique, creates a more consistent form-fitting aperture into the tunnel and diminishes the time required to perform the procedure. Use of a metallic lacrimal dilator in lieu of scissors for incisionless sub-Tenon block is associated with less local anesthetic chemosis and postoperative subconjunctival hemorrhage.[125]

Major complications of sub-Tenon anesthesia include globe perforation,[126] hemorrhage, rectus muscle trauma, postoperative strabismus, orbital cellulitis, optic nerve neuritis, and brainstem anesthesia.[127] More complications are reported with longer (18- to 25-mm) rigid metallic cannulae. Shorter (12 mm), more flexible plastic cannulae may be preferable; however, they are associated with a higher incidence of conjunctival hemorrhage and chemosis. There has been a report of a death associated with a sub-Tenon block, potentially secondary to central spread of local anesthetic.[128] However, the definitive pathogenesis remains an enigma.[129]

Topical Analgesia

Ophthalmologists have also been returning to a technique that was popularized during the late 1800s and early 1900s—the use of topical anesthetic agents, particularly when the surgical incision is made through clear cornea. Indeed, surface analgesia was the technique of choice for cataract surgery until the evolution of effective needle-based methods of regional anesthesia and improved safety of general anesthesia in the 1930s. Multiple advances in cataract surgery that have enabled faster operations with greater control and less trauma have allowed ophthalmologists to re-examine the use of topical anesthesia for this procedure.

Fully anticoagulated patients may be excellent candidates for topical analgesia, as are monocular patients who are spared the trauma of prolonged local anesthetic–induced postoperative amaurosis. Potential disadvantages of topical anesthesia include eye movement during surgery, patient anxiety or discomfort, and, rarely, allergic reactions. Patient selection is critical and should be restricted to individuals who are alert and able to follow instructions, and who can refrain from eye movement and lid squeezing. Patients who are demented or photophobic, or who cannot communicate, may be inappropriate candidates, as are those with active infection. Similarly, regional anesthesia may be more suitable for patients with dense cataracts or small pupils who may require significant iris manipulation or those for whom large scleral incisions are anticipated.

Topical analgesia can be achieved with local anesthetic drops or gels. Anesthetic gels produce greater levels of drug in the anterior chamber than equal doses of drops and may afford superior surface analgesia.[130] Concerns about increased potential for postoperative endophthalmitis with gel-based topical analgesia exist because gels might theoretically form a barrier to bactericidal agents. Therefore, if administered, gels should be applied after antiseptic solutions, taking care to apply anesthetic drops before the use of caustic bactericidal preps.

Analgesia can be supplemented with intracameral injection of 0.1 to 0.2 mL of 1% preservative-free lidocaine into the anterior chamber. So-called shugarcaine, an intracameral admixture of preservative-free lidocaine and bisulfite-free epinephrine in salt solution, provides analgesia, dilates the pupil, and stabilizes the iris.[131] It is often employed for cataract surgery patients with benign prostatic hyperplasia who typically exhibit symptoms of floppy iris intraoperatively. This syndrome has strong association with oral α_1-selective adrenergic antagonists, particularly the α_{1a} class that includes tamsulosin and silodosin. It manifests as a triad of poor pupillary dilation, floppy iris tissue, and a tendency for the iris to prolapse during surgery, resulting in a higher rate of cataract surgical complications.[132] Of note, symptoms can persist for over a year after discontinuation of α_1 antagonists.

Choice of Local Anesthetics, Block Adjuvants, and Adjuncts

Anesthetics for ocular surgery are selected on the basis of onset and duration needed. Fast-onset, brief-duration local anesthetics are optimal for procedures such as cataract surgery or pterygium excision. Longer-acting agents are indicated for lengthier operations such as vitreoretinal surgery. Ophthalmic anesthesia has a tradition of mixing different local anesthetics to produce a block with shorter latency of onset yet longer duration of effect, although clinically there may not be true advantage to combining agents.[133,134] The concentration of each of the combined local anesthetics becomes diluted, affording less individual drug permeation into the nerve. Additionally, depending on the pH and pKa of the local anesthetics, admixing drugs may lower one agent's pH, decreasing the unionized portion of anesthetic available to penetrate the nerve.[134] Bupivacaine 0.75% concentration has been shown to have potential to cause extraocular muscle toxicity. Lower concentrations do not have such a propensity.[135] Ropivacaine 0.75% or 1%, either alone or admixed with lidocaine, is an effective agent for eye block that has less cardiotoxic effects than 0.75% bupivacaine.[136,137]

Sodium bicarbonate, morphine, clonidine, midazolam, and even vecuronium have been used as local anesthetic adjuvants in ophthalmic surgery. Epinephrine, the most common vasoconstrictor additive, may prolong the block by delaying washout of drug from the orbit. There is concern, however, that epinephrine may compromise retinal perfusion[138]; it is best avoided in patients with glaucomatous optic nerve damage.

Without question, however, hyaluronidase has been the most popular ancillary agent used to modify ocular local anesthetic actions since it was introduced by Atkinson in 1949. It acts by hydrolyzing hyaluronic acid, a natural substance that binds cells together, keeping them cohesive. Thus, hyaluronidase, in doses of 0.75 to 300 International Units per milliliter increases tissue permeability, serves to promote dispersion of local anesthetics through tissues within the orbit, reduces the increase in orbital pressure associated with the volume of injected anesthetics, and enhances the quality of orbital blockade.[139] Furthermore, hyaluronidase may reduce the risk of local anesthetic–induced extraocular muscle injury because clustered increases of postoperative diplopia were reported after national shortages of the drug in 1998 and 2000.[140] Studies since that time have supported these findings.[141] However, it is possible that technique was altered in response to the absence of hyaluronidase by placing needles deeper, using more injections, or depositing larger volumes of local anesthetics. Perhaps as a consequence of past national shortages, many facilities choose to obtain hyaluronidase from local compounding labs. In recent years, tainted medications from compounding facilities have led to multiple deaths due to fungal meningitis in chronic pain patients and permanent blindness in macular degeneration patients. Hyaluronidase is currently widely available in a human recombinant formulation, obviating the need for compounded formulations.

Digital pressure and mechanical devices have been used to soften the globe prior to surgery. Essentially, they are all variations on a ball, balloon, or bag theme. The Super Pinky ball and the Honan Intraocular Pressure Reducer (The Lebanon Corporation, Lebanon, Indiana) are examples 106. Immediately after administration of regional orbital anesthesia, the compression device may be positioned on the eye for 5 to 20 minutes. Reduction of IOP to below baseline levels is not uncommon. However, excessive pressure on the globe by these devices may impede blood flow, causing ischemic optic neuropathy (ION) or CRAO, possibly leading to blindness.[142] The Honan device addresses this potentially catastrophic complication with a pneumatic bellows that maintains even compression of the globe coupled to a manometric gauge that indicates a numeric value of applied pressure. A safety valve limits the amount of inflation of the bellows. With the increasing popularity of smaller incisions, lower-profile prosthetic lenses, and topical analgesia for cataract surgery, there is less need for IOP-reducing devices.

General Principles of Monitored Anesthesia Care

Many advocate the IV administration of an appropriate agent immediately prior to ocular regional anesthesia to provide comfort and amnesia. Polypharmacy and deep sedation in the form of high doses of opioids, benzodiazepines, and hypnotics may be unwise because of the pharmacologic vagaries in the geriatric population and the attendant risks of respiratory depression, airway obstruction, hypotension, CNS aberrations, and prolonged recovery time. This undesirable technique has all the disadvantages of a general anesthetic in the absence of an endotracheal tube or SGA without the advantage of controllability that general anesthesia offers. After the block has been performed, the patient should be relaxed but sufficiently responsive to avoid head movement associated with snoring or sudden abrupt movement on awakening. Perioperative patient movement is a leading cause of patient eye injury and anesthesiologist liability.[77] Clearly, patients under monitored sedation must be capable of remaining relatively still, responding rationally to commands, and maintaining airway patency. Undersedation should likewise be avoided because tachycardia and hypertension may have deleterious effects, especially in patients with coronary artery disease. Curiously, a significant fraction of patients who have had cataract extraction on both eyes perceive the second eye surgery as being longer in duration, more painful, and/or generally more unpleasant.[143] Moreover, patients with orthopedic deformities or arthritis must be meticulously positioned and given comfortable padding on the operating table. Adequate ventilation about the face is essential to avoid carbon dioxide accumulation, particularly because supplemental oxygen can delay signs of desaturation and hypoventilation.[144] Use of exogenous oxygen can also contribute to surgical fire, particularly during oculoplastic surgery performed with electrocautery. Consider air or mixed air/oxygen instead of oxygen for these procedures. Tightly occluded drapes may also promote accumulation of oxygen. In fact, burn injuries during facial surgery with supplemental oxygen account for nearly one-third of MAC closed claims cases.[145] Patients must be comfortably warm because the hazards of shivering in patients having delicate eye surgery are well known. Further, shivering causes a risk for patients with coronary artery disease. Continuous ECG monitoring is vital, lest performance of the ophthalmic regional block, pressure on the orbit, or tugging on the extraocular muscles stimulates the oculocardiac reflex arc and produces dangerous cardiac dysrhythmias. Likewise, pulse oximetry is essential. The adequacy of the sedated patient's ventilation should be assessed by clinical signs as well as exhaled carbon dioxide. Unequivocally, MAC should reflect "maximum anesthesia caution, not minimal anesthesiology care."[146]

Studies have confirmed that most cataract operations performed in the United States are conducted with the patient under some form of local anesthesia (either retrobulbar, peribulbar, sub-Tenon, intracameral, or topical analgesia), with monitoring equipment used in 97% of cases and an anesthesiologist present in 78% of cases.[147] An international survey of ophthalmologists reported routine use of anesthesia-trained personnel in 96% and 97% of cases in the United States and Australia, respectively.[148] On the other side of the spectrum, ophthalmologists from Malaysia and Thailand had anesthesia monitoring 31% and 18% of the time, respectively.

An important study by Rosenfeld et al.[149] assessed the need for MAC in cataract surgery. These investigators prospectively studied the incidence and nature of interventions required by anesthesia personnel in 1,006 consecutive cataract operations (both phacoemulsification and extracapsular techniques were included) performed under peribulbar block. They also analyzed germane information, including patient demographic data, medical history, and preoperative laboratory tests, for ability to predict those patients at greatest risk for intervention. They found that 37% of patients required some type of intervention and that in general the majority of those interventions could not have been predicted before surgery. Patients younger than 60 years required intervention in over 60% of cases. The interventions ranged from minor forms, such as verbal reassurance and hand holding, to administering such IV medications as supplemental sedation or antihypertensive, pressor, or antiarrhythmic agents, or to providing respiratory assistance. Although hypertension, lung disease, renal disease, and a diagnosis of cancer were related to interventions, these four conditions combined accounted for only a small portion of the needed interventions. Moreover, although many of the interventions were relatively minor, several were more serious, and 30% were considered (by the involved anesthesia personnel) to be critical to the success of the operation. The investigators concluded that MAC by qualified anesthesia personnel is reasonable and justified and contributes to the quality of patient care when cataract surgery is performed with local anesthesia. Fung et al.[150] examined satisfaction scores for community-based cataract surgery via topical anesthesia and discovered that patients' value and regard for the anesthesiologist's role actually increased from the preoperative to the postoperative interview. In view of the fact that topical anesthesia produces analgesia that is less profound and provides operating conditions that are less ideal than regional or general anesthesia, it seems likely that anesthesia care is equally appropriate to provide comfort, support, and indicated drugs for these patients as well. For both ethical and surgical reasons, the ophthalmologist's attention must not be distracted from the microsurgical field.

Anesthetic Management in Specific Situations

"Open-Eye, Full-Stomach" Encounters

The anesthesiologist involved in caring for a patient with a penetrating eye injury and a full stomach confronts special challenges. The risk of aspiration and choice of airway must be weighed against the risk of blindness in the injured eye that could result from elevated IOP and extrusion of ocular content resulting from use of certain medications or coughing or bucking on induction. In cases of polytrauma, attention should be given to note presence of other injuries.

Although regional anesthesia is often a valuable alternative for the management of nonfasted trauma patients, this option had traditionally been considered contraindicated with penetrating eye injuries because of the potential to extrude intraocular contents via pressure generated by injection of local anesthetics. Needle instrumentation of the orbit, squeezing of the eyelids, and pressure due to bleeding are additional reasons that regional anesthesia was typically avoided in open-globe scenarios. Nonetheless, case reports of successful use of ophthalmic blocks in this setting have been published.[151] Recognizing that there are several distinct permutations of eye injuries, Scott et al.[152] developed techniques to safely block patients with *select* open-globe injuries. In a 4-year period, 220 disrupted eyes were repaired via regional anesthesia. A significant number of injuries were caused by intraocular foreign bodies and dehiscence of cataract or corneal transplant incisions. Blocked eyes tended to have more anterior, smaller wounds than those repaired via general anesthesia. There was no outcome difference—that is, change of visual acuity from initial evaluation until final examination—between the eyes repaired via regional versus general anesthesia. Moreover, combined topical anesthesia and sedation for *selected* patients with open-globe injuries has also been reported.[153] Ophthalmologists' shift from the hospital operating room suite to ambulatory surgery facilities and specialty eye-care surgery centers has unbound their ties to hospitals. Many no longer maintain hospital privileges, creating impetus to operate on eye injury patients on an ambulatory surgical basis in their own facilities. For some patients, general anesthesia in an ambulatory center may confer an unacceptable level of systemic risk. In those scenarios, selection of regional or topical anesthesia for repair of traumatic eye injuries may be a prudent alternative.

Nonetheless, general anesthesia remains the more commonly accepted modality for many traumatic eye injury patients. A recent survey of retina subspecialists indicated that general anesthesia was used in 90% of corneal ruptured globe cases, 94% of scleral ruptured globe procedures and 62% of surgery for intraocular foreign body.[87] Since all but a small subset of these emergent open-globe injuries will undergo general anesthesia, avoiding significant fluctuation of IOP in combination with choice of the safest induction technique that addresses any aspiration risk in the unfasted patient is paramount. Depending on the severity of globe compromise, most cases are urgent but may proceed once appropriate fasting times have passed. In those cases, smooth IV induction without paralysis and insertion of a supraglottic airway is a safe way to proceed. In those cases which cannot wait, a standard IV induction with a neuromuscular blocking agent to facilitate tracheal intubation is the choice approach in those with existing venous access. Confirmation of appropriate depth of anesthesia and the onset of neuromuscular blockade with quantitative neuromuscular monitoring will ensure a controlled induction without coughing or straining and the associated extreme IOP elevation. Additionally, utilizing a rapid sequence induction technique and performance of the Sellick maneuver may afford some protection from aspiration of gastric contents.

Succinylcholine offers the distinct advantages of swift onset, maximal intubating conditions, and brief duration of action, but its associated IOP elevation confers a theoretical risk of vitreal expulsion when the globe integrity is compromised. Although the advisability of this technique has been debated,[154] the few reports attributing such occurrences to succinylcholine have many confounders which make true causation difficult.[155] The 1957 watershed article of Lincoff et al.[20] states: "Various communications have been received from ophthalmologists who have used succinylcholine in surgery. This includes several reports of cases in which succinylcholine was given to forestall impending vitreous prolapse only to have a prompt expulsion of vitreous occur." Under such desperate circumstances, it is extremely difficult to attribute the expulsion of vitreous directly to succinylcholine.[154]

Rocuronium, with its rapid onset, is a useful drug in these circumstances, provided a "rapid onset" dose (1.2 mg/kg intravenously) is administered. Its prolonged duration of action, especially when administered at the higher dosage, is a feature that had been considered disadvantageous as compared with succinylcholine. With sugammadex reversal recovery of over 90% train-of-four responses may be accomplished in less than 120 seconds.[156] Thus, a new paradigm for the "open-globe, full-stomach" scenario may entail rapid-sequence induction with high-dose rocuronium to achieve swift onset of intubating conditions, followed by quick termination of neuromuscular blocking effect by sugammadex if one cannot intubate or cannot ventilate.[157]

When confronted with a patient whose airway anatomy or anesthetic history suggests potential difficulties, the anesthesiologist should consult with the ophthalmologist concerning the probability of saving the injured eye. In selected instances, general anesthesia may be avoided by using topical or regional anesthesia. If this approach is not feasible, awake fiberoptic laryngoscopy and intubation may be the safest option, realizing that substantial increases in IOP may occur if the patient gags or coughs. These risks, which can be minimized by thorough topical anesthesia of the airway, assume relative unimportance when balanced against the risk of being unable to ventilate and oxygenate the patient.

Intraocular Surgery

Advances in both anesthesia and in technology permit a level of controlled intraocular manipulation that was previously not possible (Table 49-5).

Table 49-5 Concerns with Various Ocular Procedures

Procedure	Concerns
Strabismus repair	Oculocardiac reflex Oculogastric reflex Forced duction testing Malignant hyperthermia
Intraocular surgery	Proper control of IOP Akinesia Drug interactions Associated systemic disease
Retinal detachment surgery	Nitrous oxide interaction with air, sulfur hexafluoride, or perfluorocarbon gas bubble Venous air embolism Oculocardiac reflex Proper control of IOP

IOP, intraocular pressure.

Proper control of IOP is crucial for intraocular procedures such as glaucoma drainage surgery, open-sky vitrectomy, penetrating keratoplasty (corneal transplantation), and traditional intracapsular cataract extraction. Before scleral incision (when IOP becomes equal to atmospheric pressure), a low-normal IOP is essential because abrupt decompression of a hypertensive eye could result in iris or lens prolapse, vitreous loss, or expulsive choroidal hemorrhage. Available data have not demonstrated a major difference in the rate of complications such as vitreous loss and iris prolapse between local anesthesia and general anesthesia.

Maximal pupillary dilation is important for many types of intraocular surgery and can be induced by continuous infusion of epinephrine 1:200,000 in a balanced salt solution, delivered through a small-gauge needle placed in the anterior chamber. Almost simultaneous with its administration, the drug is removed by aspiration from the chamber. The iris usually dilates immediately on contact with the epinephrine infusion, and drug uptake is presumably limited by the associated intense vasoconstriction of the iris and ciliary body. However, epinephrine may also be potentially absorbed by drainage through the canal of Schlemm into the venous system or by spillover of the infusion into the conjunctival vessels or drainage to the nasal mucosa.

Retinal Detachment Surgery

Surgery to repair retinal detachments may involve various procedures. Externally, a synthetic silicone band may be implanted around the globe in order to produce localized or encircling scleral force to approximate and reattach the retina (Table 49-5). During globe manipulation, rotation of the globe with traction on the extraocular muscles may elicit the oculocardiac reflex. The anesthesiologist must be vigilant about potential cardiac dysrhythmias. IV acetazolamide or mannitol to lower IOP may be requested to soften the globe during buckling.

Furthermore, internal tamponade of a retinal break may be accomplished by vitrectomy with fluid/air exchange, the surgical removal of vitreous humor with subsequent replacement by air plus an expandable gas such as sulfur hexafluoride into the globe's posterior segment. Because of blood gas partition coefficient differences, the administration of nitrous oxide may enhance the internal tamponade effect of the perfluorocarbon intraoperatively, only to be followed by a dramatic drop in IOP and volume on discontinuation of nitrous oxide. The injected bubble, in the presence of concomitant administration of nitrous oxide, can cause a rapid and dramatic rise in IOP, reaching a peak within 20 minutes[157,158] (see earlier section on Intraocular Perfluorocarbons). Because the resultant rise in IOP may compromise retinal circulation, Stinson and Donlon[158] recommended cessation of nitrous oxide administration 15 minutes before gas injection to prevent significant changes in the volume of the intravitreous gas bubble. Furthermore, Wolf et al.[53] stated that if a patient requires anesthesia after intravitreous gas injection, nitrous oxide should be omitted for 5 days after an air injection and for 10 days after sulfur hexafluoride injection. In cases in which perfluoropropane has been injected, the nitrous oxide proscription should be in effect for longer than 70 days. Alternatively, silicone oil, a vitreous substitute, may be injected to achieve internal tamponade of a retinal break. Moreover, it should be pointed out that cervicofacial subcutaneous emphysema and pneumomediastinum have been reported after the injection of pressurized gas during retinal detachment surgery.[159] Although the precise mechanism of injury remains speculative, it was hypothesized that the pressure indicator for the perfluorocarbon gas injection may have malfunctioned.

It should be emphasized that resorption time is not always uniform or predictable. For example, a diabetic 19-year-old woman was injected with sulfur hexafluoride 25 days before subsequent surgery and a diabetic 37-year-old man was injected with perfluoropropane gas 41 days before subsequent surgery. Both were given intraoperative nitrous oxide and developed CRAO and permanent blindness in the affected eye.[160] Because the pressure in the retinal arterial vessels is lower in patients with diabetes, the elderly, and those with atherosclerosis, these patients are likely at higher risk for this devastating complication.[161,162] The international distributors of medical-grade gases, in cooperation with American distributors and the FDA, provide warning bracelets for patients who receive intraocular gas injection to alert health professionals to the presence of the bubble and the need to avoid nitrous oxide administration.

Vitrectomy with fluid/air exchange is generally considered to be a low-risk procedure with negligible mortality; however, beginning in 2005, the anesthesiology and ophthalmology literature have reported multiple cases of sudden death during retina surgery.[163,164] For 30 years, procedural access into the vitreous cavity was achieved by incision through the pars plana portion of the sclera with subsequent direct suturing of the infusion line into the scleral wall. Plain sclerotomy was supplanted by cannulated sclerotomy beginning in 2002, 3 years prior to the first reported case of venous air embolism during retina surgery. This latter technique involves introduction of an unsutured cannula via an insertion trocar, a significant time-saving maneuver that also allows for sutureless wound closure at the conclusion of surgery. Morris et al. theorized that accidental creation of a choroidal detachment combined with displacement or slippage of the unsecured cannula into the suprachoroidal space may lead to entry of air under continuous pressure during fluid/air exchange through a torn vortex vein with subsequent transmission to the systemic venous circulation.[163] They note that an infusion pressure of 40 mmHg into a 25-gauge line can produce air flow (against atmospheric) of 350 cc/min through a globe whose total volume is approximately 5 to 6 cc! A lethal air embolism can occur with as little as 200 to 300 cc. In vitro and in vivo studies have confirmed venous air embolism from air introduced into the choroid blood flow or vortex draining veins via a malpositioned infusion cannula as the likely mechanism.[163,165] Fatal air embolism has also been reported during endoresection of choroidal melanoma and in repair of traumatic globe injuries.[166]

Most retina surgery now occurs in ambulatory facilities that are not typically capable of effective resuscitation from profound venous air embolism. It is important for anesthesiologists to confirm that vitreoretinal surgeons are aware of this rare phenomenon. A team approach formal timeout with verbal confirmation of proper infusion cannula position prior to and during air infusion throughout fluid/air exchange vitrectomy is prudent and potentially lifesaving.[167] Anesthesiologists may note the infusion cannula position and the surgeon's requested air infusion pressure settings during surgery. Although nasal cannula end-tidal CO_2 measurements are qualitative, a precipitous decline, accompanied by hypotension or dysrhythmia may indicate need for immediate intervention with cardiopulmonary support and prompt transfer to a higher-acuity hospital-intensive care setting capable of extracorporeal membrane oxygenation.

Anesthesiologists are sometimes faced with the unpopular duty of triaging the order of unscheduled cases. Clearly salvage of life takes priority over salvage of limb, but where do nonelective eye operations fit in? A rhegmatogenous retinal detachment is the most common posterior segment emergency. It occurs when a break or tear in the retina allows vitreous fluid to dissect underneath the retina. There are two types: fovea-sparing and fovea-involving. For the former, the macula remains attached, preserving central vision and retaining high likelihood of ultimately achieving excellent visual acuity following surgery. In fovea-involving detachments, the macula is separated, so the prognosis for ultimate visual acuity of 20/40 or better is much lower. Although it seems logical that the sooner the retina is reattached, the better the prognosis, clinical evidence suggests that duration of macular detachment has little to no effect on visual outcome so long as the repair is accomplished within about 1 week. It is generally considered safe to delay surgery to the next available elective surgical slot.[168] Fovea-sparing detachments, however, are more urgent, though still not emergent, and can likely be deferred for 1 to 3 days following the detachment without affecting ultimate visual acuity.[169]

There is debate regarding the urgency of removal of an intraocular foreign body. Studies have suggested that surgery within 72 hours reduces the incidence of vision-threatening endophthalmitis. Recent literature challenges this guiding principle, because not a single case of endophthalmitis or other deleterious side effects arose during Operation Iraqi Freedom and Operation Enduring Freedom despite a 21-day median time to foreign body removal.[170]

Strabismus Surgery

Approximately 3% of the population has strabismus, or misalignment of the visual axes, resulting in diplopia, amblyopia, or loss of stereopsis (Table 49-5). Indeed, strabismus corrective surgery is the most common pediatric ocular operation performed in the United States, entailing a variety of techniques to weaken an extraocular muscle by moving its insertion on the globe (recession) or to strengthen it by eliminating a short strip of the tendon or muscle (resection).

Infantile strabismus occurs within the first 6 months of life and is often observed in the neonatal period. Although most patients with strabismus are healthy, normal children, the incidence of strabismus is increased in those with CNS dysfunction such as cerebral palsy and meningomyelocele with hydrocephalus. Moreover, strabismus may be acquired secondary to oculomotor nerve trauma or sensory abnormalities such as cataracts or refractive aberrations.

In addition to the well-known propensity of strabismus surgery to trigger the oculocardiac reflex (previously discussed), strabismus or ptosis patients are thought to have an increased incidence of malignant hyperthermia.[171] This observation is consistent with the impression that people susceptible to malignant hyperthermia often have localized areas of skeletal muscle weakness or other musculoskeletal abnormalities. Although recent studies have challenged this belief, anesthesiologists providing care for eye muscle surgery patients must be cognizant of the theoretically enhanced risk. Other aspects of strabismus surgery of interest to anesthesiologists include succinylcholine-induced interference with the forced duction test (FDT) and an increased incidence of postoperative nausea and vomiting.

Ophthalmologists occasionally use an intraoperative maneuver, FDT, to inform their surgical treatment plan by delineating whether the malalignment is due to muscle paresis or a restrictive force. To perform the FDT, the surgeon grasps the sclera of the anesthetized eye with forceps near the corneal limbus and moves the eye into each field of gaze, concomitantly assessing the tissue and its elastic properties.

In strabismus surgery where the ophthalmologist intends to utilize the FDT, there is research to suggest that use of succinylcholine alters the FDT response, prolonging its return to baseline by approximately 20 to 30 minutes. France et al.[172] quantitated the magnitude and duration of change of the FDT after succinylcholine administration. They demonstrated that quantification of the force necessary to rotate the globe remained notably increased over control for 15 minutes, even though the rise in IOP and the skeletal muscle paralysis lasted less than 5 minutes. Whenever possible, succinylcholine should be avoided in patients undergoing repeat strabismus surgery[173] or in the event of succinylcholine use, the FDT should wait until at least 20 minutes after such administration.[174] In reality, current anesthetic management of strabismus surgery in children really does not require use of any paralytic and succinylcholine use in children is not routine and typically reserved for emergency situations such as breaking laryngospasm.

The SGA has gained significant popularity for strabismus surgery in the United States, provided the patient is at minimal risk for aspiration. The laryngeal mask airway can be inserted without the use of muscle relaxants, causes less hemodynamic perturbation, and is associated with less straining and coughing on removal. Alternatively, in adult strabismus patients, the surgery can be accomplished in most patients with monocular disease with an eye block and sedation. Both techniques, regional plus sedation and SGA airway use without paralysis in the cases where general anesthesia is warranted make the interaction between succinylcholine and the FDT less of a concern in current clinical practice.

Vomiting after eye muscle surgery is common, giving credibility to the existence of the oculogastric reflex. Eberhart et al.'s four-point scale for risk of postoperative vomiting in pediatric patients includes surgery longer than 30 minutes, age over 3, history of postoperative emesis, and *strabismus surgery*.[175] The administration of droperidol, 0.075 mg/kg at induction of anesthesia before manipulation of the eye, has been shown to reduce the incidence of vomiting after strabismus surgery to a clinically acceptable level of approximately 10% without prolonging recovery time.[176] Moreover, a lower dose of droperidol, 0.02 mg/kg intravenously, administered immediately after anesthetic induction in patients with strabismus may decrease both the incidence and severity of nausea and vomiting.[177] Many physicians stopped using droperidol owing to the FDA's "black box" warning about QT-interval prolongation. However, the droperidol doses used for postoperative nausea and vomiting are extremely low and unlikely to be associated with notable cardiovascular events. Indeed, considerable concern has been expressed about the quality and quantity of evidence and the validity of the FDA conclusion.[178]

Prophylactic IV administration of a serotonin receptor antagonist such as ondansetron, dolasetron, granisetron, or palonosetron is also efficacious. Newer classes of antiemetics are now available. The NK1 receptor antagonist, aprepitant, has a 40-hour half-life and may be administered in oral form preoperatively or parenterally upon induction of anesthesia. Amisulpride, an antipsychotic at high doses, is a nonsedating dopamine receptor antagonist not associated with QTc prolongation or extrapyramidal side effects. It is currently approved for adult patients. Combination therapy consisting of one or two antiemetics, each with a different mechanism of action, plus a glucocorticoid such as dexamethasone has been shown to be efficacious and safe in patients at high risk for postoperative nausea and vomiting.[178] The lower incidence of emesis after strabismus surgery associated with a total IV technique with propofol must be balanced against the higher incidence of oculocardiac reflex and bradycardia.[178,179] In addition, avoiding narcotics may be helpful, although a recent paper found no difference in postoperative nausea or vomiting in children who received a remifentanil–sevoflurane mixture versus sevoflurane without the narcotic.[180] One study demonstrates that the nonopioid analgesic ketorolac, in a dose of 0.75 mg/kg intravenously, provides analgesia comparable with that of morphine in pediatric patients with strabismus, but with a much lower incidence of nausea and vomiting in the first 24 hours.[181] The intraoperative administration of an eye block during pediatric vitreoretinal surgery has been shown to eliminate the need for opioids perioperatively.[182]

Principles of Laser Therapy

In 1957, in a laboratory at Columbia University, the first design for the laser was born. The invention has revolutionized industry, refined scientific measurements, provided therapy for countless medical and surgical conditions, and inspired 13 Nobel Prizes. The principle is based on the consequences of a photon meeting an electron in an excited state. Sometimes the collision produces a second photon that has the same color and direction as the original. When repeated on a large scale, this process creates an orderly beam of light. The term *laser* was coined to describe this photon-cloning effect, and the acronym signifies light amplified by stimulated emission of radiation.

Laser radiation has many notable properties. Because it is monochromatic, all the photons have the same wavelength, energy, and frequency. It is coherent, with all the photons in phase. Moreover, laser radiation is collimated, so its beam is nondivergent. These properties allow the precision that is associated with laser surgery. The amount of radiant energy (joules) absorbed by tissues is the product of power (watts) multiplied by duration (seconds). Surgical lasers typically are used in either a continuous or a pulsed mode.

The effect that a particular laser beam exerts on tissue depends predominantly on its wavelength and power density. A specific laser's wavelength depends on its lasing medium, which also gives the laser its name. In general, the longer the wavelength, the more strongly absorbed the light. The converse is true; the shorter the wavelength, the more scattered the light. The power of the laser beam is converted to heat at a shallow depth. Coherent light of high-power density excels in cutting or vaporizing tissue. Lower-power densities are used to photocoagulate tissue and promote hemostasis. Of course, another variable that can be manipulated to produce a given effect is the duration of contact between laser beam and tissue. Additional uses of lasers of low-power density include the photoactivation of systemically administered dyes to precisely treat localized disease sites, such as with age-related macular degeneration.

Lasers are used to treat a wide spectrum of eye conditions, including three of the most common causes of visual loss in the United States: diabetic retinopathy, glaucoma, and age-related macular degeneration. The use of lasers expanded to include the rapidly growing field of refractive surgery. Argon, krypton, diode, dye-tuned, neodymium: yttrium-aluminum-garnet (Nd:YAG), and excimer lasers are among those commonly used for ophthalmic surgery. Owing to concerns that indirect exposure to laser energy could cause ocular damage to operating room personnel, staff working with or near the laser wear protective goggles designed to block the particular wavelength of light emitted by the laser in use.

The argon laser emits blue-green light with a wavelength of approximately 488 to 515 nm (approximately 0.5 μm). This laser has low maximum power and is easily transmitted by fiberoptic bundles. Light from the argon laser is strongly absorbed by hemoglobin, melanin, and other pigments, rendering it useful in retinal detachment surgery to photocoagulate or cauterize pigment epithelium and the adjacent neurosensory retina, thus creating an adhesion between the retina and the "wall of the eye" to keep the retina attached. This photocoagulative property of the argon and similar lasers achieves its therapeutic effect in the treatment of diabetic retinopathy by focal and controlled necrosis of a limited amount of ischemic retina. The argon laser is also used with some efficacy to treat the late complications that can develop in the natural history of retinal vein occlusion. Because emissions of the argon laser can penetrate the cornea and lens, causing severe retinal damage, personnel in the vicinity of the argon laser should wear orange protective goggles.

The Nd:YAG, commonly called the *YAG laser*, emits light in the infrared range (wavelength 1,064 nm [1.06 μm]) and is useful in posterior lens capsule surgery. The Nd:YAG laser has high-power density and is efficacious in creating an opening in opacified posterior capsule membranes that develop in approximately one-third of cases after phacoemulsification or other extracapsular cataract surgery. Personnel working in the vicinity of this laser should wear green goggles and realize that their ability to detect cyanosis will be impaired.

An excimer laser (sometimes, and more correctly, called an *exciplex laser*) is a form of high-power, ultraviolet chemical laser frequently used in the delicate refractive surgery commonly referred to as *laser corrective surgery* or *LASIK*. The term *excimer* is short for "excited dimer," and *exciplex* is short for "excited complex." An excimer laser generally uses a combination of inert gas (argon, krypton, or xenon) and a reactive gas (fluorine or chlorine). Under appropriate conditions of electrical stimulation, a pseudomolecule called a *dimer* is generated, which can exist only in an energized state and gives rise to laser light in the ultraviolet range, typically with wavelengths of 125 to 200 nm. The ultraviolet light from an excimer laser is well absorbed by biologic matter and organic compounds. Instead of burning or cutting material, the excimer laser supplies enough energy to disrupt the molecular bonds of surface tissue through ablation. This property allows removal of exceptionally fine layers of surface material with almost no heating or change to neighboring tissue. These lasers are usually operated with a pulse rate of around 100 Hz and a pulse duration of 10 ns, although some may operate as high as 8 kHz and 30 ns.

Age-related macular degeneration is the most common cause of blindness in the elderly and has become alarmingly prevalent. The treatment of the generally more severe wet form of age-related macular degeneration has interestingly progressed over the years from the initial photocoagulation of the neovascular membrane that develops in the central retina or macula. Cauterization obliterates this membrane but can also damage the adjacent healthy macular tissue. The next modality used to treat age-related macular degeneration was the cold laser to photoactivate an intravenously injected drug, verteporfin, which chemically changed on light exposure of 693 nm in the presence of oxygen. By precisely applying the cold laser light to the area of the neovascular membrane, the photoactivated verteporfin produced highly reactive oxygen radicals and "selectively" necrosed the diseased tissue. Because of ill effects on nearby healthy tissue, this approach has been superseded by a more effective, nonlaser treatment with intravitreous injection of monoclonal antibody drugs such as ranibizumab (FDA-approved) or bevacizumab (off-label).

Postoperative Ocular Complications

Postoperative eye complications in nonocular surgery range from corneal abrasion with minor visual disturbances to serious visual disturbances including total vision loss from insults occurring at various points of the visual pathway. An analysis of 60,965 patients undergoing nonocular surgery from 1988 to 1992, the incidence of eye injury was 0.056% (34 patients).[183] A more recent analysis[184] of 75,120 patients found an incidence of 0.023%. In both studies, corneal abrasion was by far the primary complication noted (21 out 34 and 17 of 23, respectively). Other reported injuries included conjunctivitis, blurry vision, red eye, chemical injury, direct ocular trauma, and blindness. Independent risk factors for greater relative risk of ocular injury were protracted surgical procedures, lateral intraoperative positioning, head or neck surgery, general anesthesia. A specific mechanism of injury could be identified in only 21% of cases.

Analysis of the Anesthesia Closed Claims Project database over the last several decades show that the most recent representation of claims related to all eye injuries (from ocular and nonocular surgeries) are 4% to 5% of all surgical anesthesia-based claims and yet have resulted in some of the largest financial recompense.[185] Eye-related injury claims peaked in the 1970–80s at 5% to 6% of claims and have been trending downward to 4% since the 1990s and 2000s. Further analysis demonstrates that the proportion of claims related to eye surgery that are related to needle-based ophthalmic blocks and patient movement make up the majority of events (29% and 13%, respectively) increasing from 2% in the 1980s to 7% in the 1990s but have decreased in the past decade.[186] The reported injuries were typically permanent with more than half of the claims resulted in vision loss. As sub-Tenon and topical anesthesia for cataract removal became more common, there has been a commiserate decrease in claims from needle trauma related to eye blocks.[186] Of note, since the 1990s only 3% of eye surgery claims were for wrong eye procedures and none have been reported to the closed claims database since 2002.[187] When claims related to needle-based ophthalmic blocks are excluded, injuries to the visual pathway comprise 4% of all closed claims.

Common postoperative complications after nonocular surgery include corneal abrasions and minor vision disturbances from various surface irritants (*see below*) and are typically transient. Permanent postoperative vision loss (POVL) is a far more rare but devastating complication that has been associated with certain types of surgery, including complex spinal surgery in the prone position, operations involving extracorporeal circulation, and head and neck surgery and is discussed in a later subsection (see Postoperative Vision Loss).[188]

Surface Injuries

Corneal Abrasion

Although the most common ocular complication of general anesthesia is corneal abrasion,[189] the incidence varies widely, depending on the perioperative circumstances (NICV 49-4). In a prospective study, Cucchiara and Black[190] found a 0.17% incidence of corneal abrasion in 4,652 neurosurgical patients whose eyes were protected, whereas Batra and Bali[189] a decade earlier reported a 44% incidence of corneal abrasion when eyes were left unprotected and partly open. A more recent study of over 100,000 nonophthalmologic procedures found an incidence of 0.15%, which decreased to 0.079% following a teaching initiative.[191] Deljou et al. reported significant increased risk with longer duration of general anesthesia and with nonsupine surgical positioning.[192]

A variety of mechanisms can result in corneal abrasion, including damage from the face mask, surgical drapes, or spilled solutions. During tracheal intubation, watch bands or hospital identification badges on lanyards or clipped to the laryngoscopist's scrub pocket can traumatize the cornea. Ocular injury may also occur from loss of pain sensation, obtundation of protective corneal reflexes, and decreased tear production during anesthesia. Therefore, it may be prudent to tape the eyelids closed immediately after induction and during mask ventilation and laryngoscopy. In addition to taping the eyelids, applying protective goggles and instilling petroleum-based ointments into the conjunctival sac may provide protection. Disadvantages of ointments include occasional allergic reactions; flammability, which may make their use undesirable during surgery around the face and contraindicated during laser surgery; and blurred vision in the early postoperative period. The blurring and foreign body sensation associated with ophthalmic ointments may increase the incidence of postoperative corneal abrasions if they trigger excessive rubbing of the eyes while the patient is still emerging from anesthesia. Even water-based (methylcellulose) ointments may be irritating and cause scleral erythema. Accordingly, it is standard of care to secure the eyelids closed with tape during general anesthesia. For procedures above the clavicle, ocular occluders or hard eye goggles may be indicated. Special attention should also be devoted to frequent checking of the eyes during procedures on a prone patient to ensure that they are free from pressure.

The typical presentation of corneal abrasion is unilateral eye pain with tearing or photophobia and the sensation of a foreign body. Pain is typically exacerbated by blinking and ocular movement. Diagnosis may be confirmed by inspection of the eye for a foreign body such as an eyelash and/or pain relief upon instilling a single eyedrop of short-acting local anesthetic, typically proparacaine. Consider ophthalmologic consultation if pain is not relieved, symptoms are bilateral, or pupillary reflexes are abnormal (see postsurgical acute glaucoma section below). Traditional treatment included patching the injured eye, however, this may delay wound healing. Local anesthetics may also delay wound healing and can cause keratitis so are not indicated. Instead, limited duration topical NSAIDs may be used for pain management. Routine topical antibiotics are controversial. Although permanent sequelae are possible, healing usually occurs within 72 hours.

Chemical Injury

Spillage of solutions during skin preparation may result in chemical damage to the eye. The FDA has reported serious corneal damage from eye contact with Hibiclens, a 4% chlorhexidine gluconate solution formulated with a detergent. Again, with meticulous attention to detail, this misadventure is preventable. Treatment consists of liberal bathing of the eye with balanced salt solution to remove the offending agent. After surgery, it may be desirable to have an ophthalmologist examine the eye to document any residual injury or lack thereof.

Photic Injury

Direct or reflected light beams may permanently damage the eye. For patients undergoing nonocular laser surgery, the potential for serious injury to the cornea or retina from certain laser beams requires that the patient's eyes be protected with moist gauze pads and metal shields and that operating room personnel wear protective glasses. These goggles must be appropriately tinted for the specific wavelength they are intended to block. Clear goggles may be worn when working with the carbon dioxide laser, whereas for work with the argon, Nd:YAG, or Nd:YAG-KTP (potassium titanyl phosphate) laser, the goggles must be tinted orange, green, or orange-red, respectively.

Postoperative Vision Loss

Vision loss in the perioperative period can range from mild and transient to permanent complete blindness. Mild visual disturbances such as photophobia or diplopia are common and typically transient in nature. Blurred vision in the early postoperative period may also reflect the residual effects of petroleum-based ophthalmic ointments or ocular effects of anticholinergic drugs administered (see subsection *Corneal Abrasion*). Unfortunately, not all postoperative visual disturbances self-resolve and rarely, patients awake with deficits of visual field and even complete blindness—a devastating patient outcome.

POVL can result from injury occurring at any point along the visual pathway—from the cornea to the visual cortex of the occipital lobe. Historically, the occurrence of POVL was not widely appreciated and such cases were typically attributed to infarcts impacting the visual cortex or from globe compression and resulting in cortical blindness or CRAO, respectively. Only until an uptick in reports reporting complication of POVL from spine surgery in the prone position leading to injury of the optic nerve, or ION, did general awareness begin to increase. These increasing cases of major vision loss were being noted at a time when such spinal fusion procedure cases were rapidly surging and had more than doubled than those of the decade prior.[193] The first national data set at this time put the incidence of postoperative vision loss after spine surgery in the prone position at 0.017%.[194] As a result, the American Society of Anesthesiology (ASA) Committee on Professional Liability and the ASA Closed Claim Project to establish the POVL Registry to identify risk factors of POVL.[188] Analysis of the first 93 cases revealed significant information about the etiology and risk factors that led to much advancement in the awareness and reduction of POVL, specifically ION, following major spine surgery[195] The various causes of POVL are discussed in further detail below.

Postsurgical Acute Glaucoma

Acute angle-closure glaucoma provokes an abrupt increase in IOP, manifesting as a painful eye with potential for permanent compromise of vision. It typically occurs spontaneously but has been reported, albeit rarely, after spinal and general anesthesia. Acute angle-closure glaucoma caused by pupillary block is a serious, multifactorial disease. Risk factors include genetic predisposition, shallow anterior chamber depth, increased lens thickness, small corneal diameter, female gender, and advanced age. Those patients considered at risk should undergo a preoperative ophthalmic evaluation and perioperative miotic therapy. After surgery, these patients should be scrupulously watched for red eye or a fixed dilated pupil, as well as for complaints of pain and blurred vision. One study[196] explored possible precipitating events in at-risk patients and found no evidence that the type of anesthetic agent, the duration of surgery, the volume of parenteral fluids, or the intraoperative blood pressure were related to the development of acute angle-closure glaucoma.

Despite its seriousness, acute angle-closure glaucoma may be difficult to recognize.[197] Physicians should be knowledgeable about this potential complication because diagnostic delay may detrimentally affect visual outcome and cause permanent optic nerve damage. The clinician's challenge is discerning whether a painful eye is due to a corneal abrasion or acute angle-closure glaucoma. The former typically is not vision-threatening, while the latter is truly emergent, requiring timely ophthalmologic consultation to confirm the diagnosis and acutely decrease IOP with systemic and topical therapy.

Hemorrhagic Retinopathy

Valsalva retinopathy is a retinal hemorrhage associated with forceful exhalation against a closed airway, as in turbulent emergence or with protracted vomiting. It has been reported with intraoperative Valsalva maneuvers, bucking on the endotracheal tube, coughing, and sneezing.[198] Fortunately, these venous hemorrhages are usually self-limiting and resolve completely in days to a few months. Because no visual changes occur unless the macula is involved, most cases are asymptomatic. However, if bleeding into the optic nerve occurs, resulting in optic atrophy, or if the hemorrhage is massive, permanent visual impairment may ensue. In some instances of massive hemorrhage, vitrectomy may be beneficial.

Retinal venous hemorrhage has also been described after injections of local anesthetics, steroids, or saline into the lumbar epidural space.[199] The patients all received large injections (≥40 mL) into the epidural space prior to developing blurry vision or headaches. On funduscopic examination, retinal hemorrhage was consistently observed. Eight of the nine patients described had complete recovery. It is believed that the hemorrhage is produced by rapid epidural injection, which causes a sudden increase in intracranial pressure. It is possible that obesity, hypertension, coagulopathies, pre-existing elevated cerebrospinal fluid pressure (as seen in pseudotumor cerebri), and such retinal vascular diseases as diabetic retinopathy may be risk factors. Caution is recommended when injecting drugs or fluid into the epidural space; a slow injection rate and using the minimal volume necessary to accomplish the desired objective are recommended. Of note, cases of valsalva retinopathy have occurred with sneezing, screaming, weightlifting, inflating balloons, sexual intercourse, and more.[200]

Retinal bleeding may also originate from the arterial circulation, often associated with extraocular trauma. Funduscopic examination reveals cotton–wool exudates, a condition known as *Purtscher retinopathy* which should be ruled out when a trauma patient complains of postanesthetic visual loss. It is associated with a poor prognosis, and most patients sustain permanent visual impairment.

Retinal Ischemia

Retinal ischemia or infarction may also result from direct ocular trauma secondary to external pressure exerted by an ill-fitting anesthetic mask, especially in a hypotensive setting, from embolism during cardiac surgery, or from the intraocular injection of a large volume of sulfur hexafluoride or other gases in the presence of high concentrations of nitrous oxide. It may also result from increased ocular venous pressure associated with impaired venous drainage or elevated IOP.

The importance of carefully positioning patients and scrupulously monitoring external pressure on the eye cannot be overemphasized, especially when the patient is in the prone or jackknife position. When the head is dependently positioned, venous pressure may be elevated. If external pressure is applied to the globe from improper head support, perfusion pressure to the eye is likely to be reduced. An episode of systemic hypotension in this setting could further decrease perfusion pressure and thereby decrease intraocular blood flow, resulting in possible retinal ischemia.

It is imperative that a padded or foam headrest be used for procedures done with patients in the prone position. The patient's eyes must be in the opening of this headrest, and they should be checked at frequent intervals for pressure. Alternatively, Mayfield tongs can be used. During some spine procedures, a steep head-down position may be employed to decrease surgical venous bleeding and enhance procedural exposure. This position, in combination with deliberate hypotension and infusion of large quantities of crystalloid, may increase the risk of compromising the ocular circulation. It seems prudent to avoid combining these three risk factors to any significant degree.

Occlusion of the central retinal artery (CRAO) or of its branches is an important, and frequently preventable, causes of postoperative visual loss. CRAO is most commonly reported following spinal, nasal, sinus, or neck surgery, as well as coronary artery bypass graft (CABG) surgery, but most cases of POVL following spine surgery are due to ION rather than CRAO.[188] In addition to external pressure on the eye, causes can include emboli from carotid plaques or other sources as well as vasospasm or thrombosis after radical neck surgery complicated by hemorrhage and hypotension and after intranasal injection of α-adrenergic agonists. Several cases have followed intra-arterial injections of corticosteroids or local anesthetics in branches of the external carotid artery, with possible retrograde embolization to the ocular blood supply.[201] Mabry[202] suggested that the mechanism of injury involves positioning the needle intra-arterially to produce retrograde flow into the branches of the ophthalmic artery, as well as the perfusion pressure that must be overcome during the injection. Therefore, when injecting in the nasal and sinus areas, topical vasoconstrictors should be applied to decrease the size of the vascular bed, and a small (25-gauge) needle on a low-volume syringe should be used to minimize injection pressure. Moreover, because some cases have followed injections of corticosteroids combined with other drugs, it is believed that this practice may predispose to formation of drug crystals and therefore should be discouraged.

Signs of central retinal arterial occlusion including proptosis, chemosis, hyphema, corneal abrasion, and lid bruising are apparent. Pathognomonic findings on funduscopic examination reveal a pale, edematous retina and a cherry-red spot. Platelet-fibrin, cholesterol, calcific, or crystalloid emboli may be found in narrowed retinal arterioles. Embolic or arteritic causes may be discovered via echocardiogram, carotid ultrasound, and temporal artery biopsy. Computed tomography (CT) and magnetic resonance imaging (MRI) studies are usually negative.

Prevention is much more successful than treatment. It may be possible to apply ocular massage (contraindicated if glaucoma is a possibility) to dislodge an embolus to more peripheral sites, and IV acetazolamide and 5% carbon dioxide inhalation have been used to increase retinal blood flow. The prognosis, however, typically is poor, and approximately 50% of patients with central retinal arterial occlusion eventually have optic atrophy.

Postoperative Ischemic Optic Neuropathy

ION in the nonsurgical setting is the most common cause of sudden-onset visual loss in patients older than 50 years of age. ION can be classified as arteritic or nonarteritic and the vascular insult can occur at the anterior or posterior segment of the optic nerve: anterior and posterior ION, respectively.[203] ION, both anterior and posterior, is the most common cause of POVL and those undergoing CABG and long-prone spinal-fusion surgeries are at greater risk than other types of surgery.[204] Risk factors for ION after spine prone surgery include male gender, obesity, use of Wilson surgical frame, longer duration of anesthesia, elevated levels of blood loss and lower proportion of colloid to crystalloid fluid administration.[203]

Anterior Ischemic Optic Neuropathy

The pathophysiology of anterior ION is likely multifactorial but has not been completely established. The primary mechanism is likely to involve temporary states of low blood flow through the vessels supplying the anterior portion of the optic nerve, although intra-axonal edema and disturbed autoregulation to the optic nerve head may also play a role.[204] Coexisting systemic disease, especially involving the cardiovascular system and (to a lesser extent) the endocrine system, is common in patients in whom anterior ION develops. Male gender also strongly predominates. Other risk factors for postoperative anterior ION include CABG and other thoracovascular operations, as well as spinal surgery. Although massive bleeding, anemia, and hypotension are commonly described intraoperative risk factors, a retrospective survey of surgeons who perform spinal fusion surgery disclosed that hypotension and anemia were equally prevalent in patients in whom ION developed and in those in whom it did note.[204]

Other risk factors are increased IOP or orbital venous pressure. Although emboli may also play a role, anterior ION is not usually caused by emboli because emboli preferentially lodge in the central retinal artery rather than in the short posterior ciliary arteries that supply the anterior optic nerve.

Increased IOP caused by extrinsic compression of the eye decreases retinal blood flow, which can produce both retinal and optic nerve injuries.

Moreover, increased IOP can result from large infusions of crystalloid when the head is steeply dependent, as during many spinal operations.[205] Increased orbital venous pressure results in a decreased perfusion pressure gradient to the optic nerve head. Interestingly, one patient who had ION despite perioperative normotension had marked facial edema after surgery of protracted duration.[205] Similarly, a study in cardiac surgery patients revealed that increases in IOP correlated with the degree of hemodilution and the use of crystalloid priming solution.[206] Patients with anterior ION were more likely to have significant weight gain within 24 hours of open-heart surgery, again suggesting the role of elevated ocular venous pressure in impeding blood flow to the optic nerve.[206]

According to Roth and Gillesberg,[201] a complex interaction of factors such as ocular venous pressure, hemodilution, hypotension, release of endogenous vasoconstrictors, and individual risk factors such as atherosclerosis and aberrant optic nerve circulation may be implicated in the development of anterior ION. Therefore, specific recommendations for preventative strategies are elusive. However, external pressure on the eyes must be meticulously avoided. It also seems prudent to minimize time in the prone position when the head is notably dependent. In patients with pre-existing cardiovascular disease, significant hypertension, or glaucoma, it seems advisable to maintain systemic blood pressure as close to baseline as possible.[201]

Patients with anterior ION typically have painless visual loss that may not be noted until the first postoperative day (or possibly later), an afferent pupillary defect, altitudinal field defects, and optic disc edema or pallor. MRI or CT initially shows enlargement of the optic nerve. However, optic atrophy is detected by MRI later.

The prognosis for anterior ION varies but is often grim. Although there is no recognized treatment for anterior ION, Williams et al.[207] reviewed the various therapies that may be instituted. These include IV acetazolamide, furosemide, mannitol, and steroids. Maintaining the head-up position could be helpful if increased ocular venous pressure is operative. Surgical optic nerve sheath fenestration or decompression is not only ineffective but may actually be harmful.[208]

Posterior Ischemic Optic Neuropathy

The posterior optic nerve has a less luxuriant blood supply than the anterior optic nerve. Most perioperative ION cases associated with spine surgery occur in the posterior optic nerve where there is poor collateral flow, rendering the nerve vulnerable to prolonged pathophysiologic changes in blood flow. In contrast to anterior ION, relatively few cases have been reported after CABG, and posterior ION appears to be less related to coexisting cardiovascular disease. Approximately 11% of cases were associated with cardiopulmonary bypass procedures. As with anterior ION, male patients outnumber female patients substantially. Many cases have been associated with surgery involving the neck, nose, sinuses, or spine. In approximately one-third of cases reported, facial edema has been noted.[201]

Posterior ION is produced by reduced oxygen delivery to the retrolaminar part of the optic nerve. Compression of the pial vessels (supplied by small collaterals from the ophthalmic artery) or embolic phenomena have been postulated to produce ischemia.[201]

A hypoxic insult in this region results in a slower development of ischemic damage, so a symptom-free period often precedes the loss of vision. In some patients, the onset of symptoms may be delayed several days. Typical findings include an afferent pupillary defect or nonreactive pupil. Disc edema is not a feature of posterior ION because of its retro-orbital position. CT scan in the early postoperative period may reveal enlargement of the intraorbital portion of the optic nerve. Bilateral blindness is more common with posterior ION than with anterior ION, indicating involvement of the optic chiasm. Concomitant disease of the eye or ocular blood supply may be related to posterior ION.[201] Some cases may show partial improvement spontaneously, but often no improvement is noted. Steroids may be considered for treatment. Preventive strategies are as outlined for anterior ION.

A review of the first 6 years of cases submitted to the ASA Postoperative Visual Loss Registry found that spinal surgery patients at greatest risk for ION and visual compromise include those with predisposing patient-specific factors, surgery exceeding 6 hours' duration, and blood loss of more than a liter.[186] In the 83 reported cases, there was no causative evidence of traumatic eye injury from edema or direct pressure on the globe. Mean blood pressure and hematocrit varied widely among those who developed postoperative blindness. However, 34% of cases had the lowest mean arterial blood pressure or systolic blood pressure at least 40% below baseline, and in only 6% of cases were the mean arterial or systolic pressures less than 20% below baseline. The ASA practice advisory for perioperative visual loss associated with spine surgery concludes that there is no established "transfusion threshold" and that deliberate intraoperative hypotension during surgery has not been proven as contributory to postoperative loss of vision.[209] The consultants and specialty society members, however, expressed concern about the use of deliberate hypotension in high-risk patients and recommended that the use of this technique be determined on a case-by-case basis. Further, they recommended that high-risk patients should be positioned so that their heads are level with or higher than the heart, if possible. Patients' heads should be maintained in a neutral forward position, avoiding neck flexion, extension, lateral flexion, or rotation, if possible. Finally, consideration should be given to using *staged* spine procedures to avoid excessively protracted periods in the prone position for high-risk patients.[210]

In 2012, the first multicenter study to identify risk factors for ION patients compared with patients without ION after prone spinal fusion surgery using detailed perioperative data was published.[211] Cases with anterior and posterior ION were combined. After multivariate analysis, risk factors for ION after spinal fusion surgery included male sex, obesity, Wilson frame use, prolonged anesthesia duration, greater estimated blood loss, and lower-percent colloid administration. No statistically significant independent effect on ION of older age, hypertension, atherosclerosis, smoking, or diabetes was identified. These findings suggest that the etiology of ION may be more heavily influenced by intraoperative factors than by any known pre-existing comorbidities or vasculopathy. Fully half of the risk factors strongly support the speculation that acute venous congestion of the optic canal is a potential contributor to ION in this setting.[212] Perhaps over time, investigators will be able to determine what role, if any, an inflammatory response, either locally or systemically, plays in the genesis of ION.[212]

Cortical Blindness

Brain injury rostral to the optic nerve may cause cortical blindness. The impairment is produced by damage to the visual path beyond the lateral geniculate nucleus or the visual cortex in the occipital lobe. Similar to anterior ION, cortical blindness is a significant concern in patients undergoing CABG, and systemic disease is often present. Emboli and sustained profound hypotension are common causes. Other events implicated in the pathophysiology include cardiac arrest, hypoxemia, intracranial hypertension, exsanguinating hemorrhage, vascular occlusion, thrombosis, and vasospasm.

Differential diagnostic features include a normal optic disc on fundoscopy and normal pupillary responses. There is, however, loss of optokinetic nystagmus with normal eye motility. CT and MRI are helpful in delineating the extent of brain infarction associated with cortical blindness. Occipital lesions are frequently bilateral, and CT findings typically indicate posterior cerebral artery thrombosis, basilar artery occlusion, posterior cerebral artery branch occlusion, or watershed infarction. Lesions after CABG often include the parieto-occipital area.

Whereas most cases of ION do not improve significantly or completely, visual recovery from cortical blindness in previously healthy patients may be considerable but prolonged. Preventive strategies include maintenance of adequate systemic perfusion pressure and, in cardiac surgery, minimizing manipulation of the aorta, meticulous removal of air and particulate matter during valvular procedures, and use of an arterial line filter in selected patients during bypass.

Other Complications

Postcataract Ptosis

Ptosis after cataract surgery is not uncommon, and multiple factors have been implicated in its etiology.[213,214] These include the presence of a pre-existing ptosis, injection of anesthetic solution into the upper lid when performing facial nerve block, injection of local anesthesia through the upper eyelid at the 12 o'clock position, ocular compression or massage, use of the eyelid speculum, placement of a superior rectus bridle suture with traction on the superior rectus–levator complex, creation of a large conjunctival flap, prolonged or tight patching in the postoperative period, and postoperative eyelid edema. Feibel et al.[175] believed that the development of postcataract ptosis is multifactorial and that no single aspect of cataract surgery is the sole contributor. Taylor et al.[214] used MRI immediately after diagnosis of diplopia in four patients who received extraconal block. They found peribulbar edema consistent with direct local anesthetic–induced myotoxicity after presumed inadvertent intramuscular injection. Although local anesthetics are clearly myotoxic, the local anesthetic injection cannot be isolated as the primary factor because postsurgical ptosis is also seen in patients undergoing surgery with general anesthesia.

Acknowledgments

We gratefully acknowledge the contributions of previous edition author, Kathryn E. McGoldrick, as portions of their chapter have been retained in this revision.

For further review and interactivities, please see the videos and narrative interactive clinical vignettes (NICVs) accessible in the complimentary eBook bundled with this text. Access instructions are located on the inside front cover.

REFERENCES

1. National Eye Institute. Statistics and data. Accessed June 16, 2022 https://www.nei.nih.gov/eyedata.
2. Eye Health Statistics, American Academy of Ophthalmology. Accessed February 14th, 2023. https://www.aao.org/newsroom/eye-health-statistics
3. Varma R, Vajaranant TS, Burkemper B, et al. Visual impairment and blindness in adults in the United States: Demographic and Geographic Variations from 2015 to 2050. *JAMA Ophthalmol.* 2016;134(7):802–809.
4. Teng C, Gurses-Ozden R, Liebmann JM, Tello C, Ritch R. Effect of a tight necktie on intraocular pressure. *Br J Ophthalmol.* 2003;87:946–948.
5. Stoelting RK. Circulatory changes during direct laryngoscopy and tracheal intubation: influence of duration of laryngoscopy with or without prior lidocaine. *Anesthesiology.* 1977;47:381–384.
6. Duncalf D, Foldes FF. Effect of anesthetic drugs and muscle relaxants on intraocular pressure. In: Smith RB, ed. *Anesthesia in Ophthalmology.* Little Brown; 1973:21.
7. Garde JF, Aston R, Endler GC, et al. Racial mydriatic response to belladonna preparations. *Anesth Analg.* 1978;57:572–576.
8. Awad H, Bai M, Ramadan ME, et al. The effect of increased intraocular pressure during steep Trendelenburg positioning in robotic prostatectomy and hysterectomy on structural and functional ocular parameters. *Anesth Analg.* 2020;130(4):975–982.
9. Gayer S, Gedde SJ. Intra-operative management of increased intraocular pressure in a patient with glaucoma undergoing robotic prostatectomy in Trendelenburg position. *A A Case Rep.* 2016;6:17–18.
10. Ozkan AS, Akbas S. Comparison of the effects of the McGrath MAC, C-MAC, and Macintosh laryngoscopes on the intraocular pressures of non-ophthalmic patients: a prospective, randomized, clinical trial. *Anaesth Crit Care Pain Med.* 2021;40(6):100974.
11. Goyagi T, Sato T, Horiguchi T, Nishikawa T. The effect of nitrous oxide on the intraocular pressure in patients undergoing abdominal surgery under sevoflurane and remifentanil anesthesia. *Open J Anesthesiol.* 2016;6:85.
12. Sator-Katzenschlager S, Deusch E, Dolezal S, et al. Sevoflurane and propofol decrease intraocular pressure equally during nonophthalmic surgery and recovery. *Br J Anaesth.* 2002; 89:764–766.
13. Kelly DJ, Farrell SM. Physiology and role of intraocular pressure in contemporary anesthesia. *Anes Analg.* 2018;126(5):1551–1562.
14. Yoshikawa K, Murai Y. Effect of ketamine on intraocular pressure in children. *Anesth Analg.* 1971;50:199–202.
15. Corssen G, Hoy JE. A new parenteral anesthetic—CI581: its effect on intraocular pressure. *J Pediatr Ophthalmol.* 1967;4:20.
16. Peuler M, Glass DD, Arens JF. Ketamine and intraocular pressure. *Anesthesiology.* 1975;43: 575–578.
17. Ausinsch B, Rayburn RL, Munson ES, Levy NS. Ketamine and intraocular pressure in children. *Anesth Analg.* 1976;55:773–775.
18. Drayna PC, Estrada C, Wang W, et al. Ketamine is not associated with elevation of intraocular pressure during procedural sedation. *Am J Emerg Med.* 2012;30:1215–1218.
19. Litwiller RW, Difazio CA, Rushia EL. Pancuronium and intraocular pressure. *Anesthesiology.* 1975;42:750–752.
20. Lincoff HA, Breinin GM, DeVoe AG. Effect of succinylcholine on the extraocular muscles. *Am J Ophthalmol.* 1957;44:440–444.
21. Pandey K, Badolas RP, Kumar S. Time course of intraocular hypertension produced by suxamethonium. *Br J Anaesth.* 1972;44:191–196.
22. Kelly RE, Dinner M, Turner LS, Haik B, Abramson DH, Daines P. Succinylcholine increases intraocular pressure in the human eye with the extraocular muscles detached. *Anesthesiology.* 1993;79:948–952.
23. Miller RD, Way WL, Hickey RF. Inhibition of succinylcholine-induced increased intraocular pressure by nondepolarizing muscle relaxants. *Anesthesiology.* 1968;29:123.
24. Meyers EF, Krupin T, Johnson M, Zink H. Failure of nondepolarizing neuromuscular blockers to inhibit succinylcholine-induced increased intraocular pressure: a controlled study. *Anesthesiology.* 1978;48:149–151.
25. Verma RS. "Self-taming" of succinylcholine-induced fasciculations and intraocular pressure. *Anesthesiology.* 1979;50:245–247.
26. Meyers EF, Singer P, Otto A. A controlled study of the effect of succinylcholine self-taming on IOP. *Anesthesiology.* 1980;53:72–74.
27. Stoelting RK. Blood pressure and heart rate changes during short duration laryngoscopy for tracheal intubation: influences of viscous or intravenous lidocaine. *Anesth Analg.* 1978;57:197–199.
28. Smith RB, Babinski M, Leano N. Effect of lidocaine on succinylcholine-induced rise in IOP. *Can Anaesth Soc J.* 1979;26:482–483.
29. Grover VK, Lata K, Sharma S, Kaushik S, Gupta A. Efficacy of lignocaine in the suppression of the intraocular pressure response to suxamethonium and tracheal intubation. *Anaesthesia.* 1989;44:22–25.
30. Nicholson D, Kossler A, Topping K, Stary CM. Exaggerated oculocardiac reflex elicited by local anesthetic injection of an empty orbit: a case report. *A A Case Rep.* 2017;9(12):337–338.
31. Alexander JP. Reflex disturbances of cardiac rhythm during ophthalmic surgery. *Br J Ophthalmol.* 1975;59:518–524.
32. Berler DK. Oculocardiac reflex. *Am J Ophthalmol.* 1963;12(56):954–959.
33. Mirakur RK, Clarke RS, Dundee JW, McDonald JR. Anticholinergic drugs in anaesthesia: a survey of their present position. *Anaesthesia.* 1978;33:133–138.
34. Steward DJ. Anticholinergic premedication for infants and children. *Can Anaesth Soc J.* 1983; 30:325–328.

35. Massumi RA, Mason DT, Amsterdam EA, et al. Ventricular fibrillation and tachycardia after intravenous atropine for treatment of bradycardias. *N Engl J Med*. 1972;287:336–338.
36. McGoldrick KE. Transient left bundle branch block during local anesthesia. *Anesthesiol Rev*. 1981;8(6):36.
37. Moonie GT, Rees DI, Elton D. Oculocardiac reflex during strabismus surgery. *Can Anaesth Soc J*. 1964;11:621–632.
38. Phillips TJ, McGuirk SP, Chahat HK, et al. Autonomic cardio-respiratory reflex reactions and super selective ophthalmic arterial chemotherapy for retinoblastoma. *Pediatric Anesth*. 2013; 23:940–945.
39. Harris EA. Autonomic cardio-respiratory reflex reactions and super selective ophthalmic arterial chemotherapy for retinoblastoma (letter). *Pediatric Anesth*. 2014;24:230–231.
40. Yamane T, Kaneko A, Mohri M. The technique of ophthalmic arterial infusion therapy for patients with intraocular retinoblastoma. *Int J Clin Oncol*. 2004;9:69–73.
41. Scharoun JH, Han JH, Gobin P. Anesthesia for ophthalmic artery chemosurgery. *Anesthesiology*. 2017;126;165–172.
42. Ellis EP, Esterdahl M. Echothiophate iodide therapy in children: effect upon blood cholinesterase levels. *Arch Ophthalmol*. 1967;77:598–601.
43. Meyers EF. Cocaine toxicity during dacryocystorhinostomy. *Arch Ophthalmol*. 1980;98: 842–843.
44. Gay GR, Loper KA. Control of cocaine-induced hypertension with labetalol (letter). *Anesth Analg*. 1988;67:92.
45. Wakayama A, Nishina S, Miki A, et al. Incidence of side effects of topical atropine and cyclopentolate hydrochloride for cycloplegia in Japanese children: a multicenter study. *Jpn J Ophthalmol*. 2018;62:531–536.
46. Brown MM, Brown GC, Spaeth GL. Lack of side effects from topically administered 10% phenylephrine eye drops: a controlled study. *Arch Ophthalmol*. 1980;98:487–489.
47. Jones FL, Eckberg NL. Exacerbation of asthma by timolol. *N Engl J Med*. 1979;301:170.
48. Maenpaa J, Pelkonen O. Cardiac safety of ophthalmic timolol. *Expert Opin Drug Saf*. 2016;15: 1549–1561.
49. Shavitz SA. Timolol and myasthenia gravis. *JAMA*. 1979;242:1611–1612.
50. Bailey PL. Timolol and postoperative apnea in neonates and young infants. *Anesthesiology*. 1984;61:622.
51. Vinker S, Kaiserman I, Waitman DA, Blackman S, Kitai E. Prescription of ocular beta-blockers in patients with obstructive pulmonary disease: does a central electronic medical record make a difference? *Clin Drug Investig*. 2006;26:495–500.
52. Lee EJK. Use of nitrous oxide causing severe visual loss 37 days after retinal surgery. *Br J Anaesth*. 2004;93:464–464.
53. Wolf GL, Capriano C, Hartung J. Effects of nitrous oxide on gas bubble volume in the anterior chamber. *Arch Ophthalmol*. 1985;103:418–419.
54. Marcus EN, Gayer S, Anderson DR. Medical evaluation of patients before ocular surgery (editorial). *Am J Ophthalmol*. 2003;136:338–339.
55. Schein OD, Katz J, Bass EB, et al. The value of routine preoperative medical testing before cataract surgery. *N Engl J Med*. 2000;342:168–175.
56. Chen CL, Lin GA, Bardash NT, et al. Preoperative medical testing in Medicare patients undergoing cataract surgery. *N Engl J Med*. 2015;372(16):1530–1538.
57. Sweitzer B, Rajan N, Schell D, Gayer S, Eckert S, Joshi GP. Preoperative care for cataract surgery: The Society for Ambulatory Anesthesia (SAMBA) position statement. *Anesth Analg*. 2021:133(6):1431–1436.
58. Charles S, Rosenfeld PJ, Gayer S. Medical consequences of stopping anticoagulants prior to intraocular surgery or intravitreal injections. *Retina*. 2007;27(7):813–815.
59. Feitl ME, Krupin T. Retrobulbar anesthesia. *Ophthalmol Clin North Am*. 1990;3:83.
60. Katz J, Feldman MA, Bass EB, et al. Risks and benefits of anticoagulant and antiplatelet medication use before cataract surgery. *Ophthalmology*. 2003;110:1784–1788.
61. Kumar CM, Seet E. Stopping antithrombotics during regional anesthesia and eye surgery: crying wolf? *Br J Anaesth*. 2017;118:154–158.
62. Jamula E, Anderson J, Douketis JD. Safety of continuing warfarin therapy during cataract surgery: a systematic review and meta-analysis. *Thomb Res*. 2009;124:292–299.
63. Douketis JD, Berger PB, Dunn AS, et al. The perioperative management of antithrombotic therapy: American College of Chest Physicians Evidence-Based Clinical Practice Guidelines (8th ed). *Chest*. 2008;133(6 suppl):299S–339S.
64. Gertein NS, Schulman WH, Petersen TR, et al. Should more patients continue aspirin therapy perioperatively? Clinical impact on aspirin withdrawal syndrome. *Ann Surg*. 2012;255: 811–819.
65. Baron TH, Kamath PS, McBane RD. Management of antithrombotic therapy in patients undergoing invasive procedures. *N Engl J Med*. 2013;368:2113–2124.
66. McClellan AJ, Flynn HW, Smiddy WE, Gayer SI. The use of perioperative antithrombotic agents in posterior segment ocular surgery. *Am J Ophthalmol*. 2014;158:858–859.
67. McClellan AJ, Flynn HW, Gayer S. A novel issue for vitreoretinal surgeons. *Retina*. 2016;36: 245–246.
68. Kallio H, Paloheimo M, Maunuksela E. Haemorrhage and risk factors associated with retrobulbar/peribulbar block: a prospective study in 1383 patients. *Br J Anaesth*. 2000; 85(5): 708–711.
69. Makuloluwa AK, Tiew S, Briggs M. Peri-operative management of ophthalmic patients on anti-thrombotic agents: a literature review. *Eye*. 2019;33:1044–1059.
70. American Society of Anesthesiologists Committee on Standards and Practice Parameters. Practice alert for the perioperative management of patients with coronary artery stents: a report by the American Society of Anesthesiologists Committee on Standards and Practice Parameters. *Anesthesiology*. 2009;110:22–23.
71. Hawn MT, Graham LA, Richman JS, Itani KM, Henderson WG, Maddox TM. Risk of major adverse cardiac events following noncardiac surgery in patients with coronary stents. *JAMA*. 2013;310(14):1462–1472.
72. Practice advisory for the perioperative management of patients with cardiac implantable electronic devices: pacemakers and implantable cardioverter defibrillators 2020. An updated report by the American Society of Anesthesiologists taskforce on perioperative management of patients with cardiac implantable electronic devices. *Anesthesiology*. 2020;132;225–252.
73. Rosero EB, Rajan N, Joshi GP. Pro-con debate: are patients with a cardiovascular implantable electronic device suitable to receive care in a free-standing ambulatory surgery center? *Anesth Analg*. 2022;134(5):919–992.
74. Coursin DB, Scuderi PE. The 6Ps: prior planning prevents problems and poor performance. *Anesth Analg*. 2022;134(5):916–991.
75. Bayes J. A survey of ophthalmic anesthetists on managing pacemakers and implanted cardiac defibrillators. *Anesth Analg*. 2006;103:1615–1616.
76. Stoller GL. Ophthalmic surgery and the implantable cardioverter defibrillator. *Arch Ophthalmol*. 2006;124:123–125.
77. Bhananker SM, Posner KL, Cheney FW, Caplan RA, Lee LA, Domino KB. Injury and liability associated with monitored anesthesia care: a closed claims analysis. *Anesthesiology*. 2006;104:228–234.
78. Tao JP. Sneezing reflex associated with intravenous sedation and periocular anesthetic injection. *Am J Ophthalmol*. 2009;147(1):183–184.
79. Gayer S. Key components of risk associated with ophthalmic anesthesia. *Anesthesiology*. 2006;105:859.
80. McGoldrick KE. Ocular pathology and systemic diseases. In: McGoldrick KE, ed. *Anesthetic Implications: Anesthesia for Ophthalmic and Otolaryngologic Surgery*. WB Saunders; 1992:210.
81. Kumar CM, Seet E, Eke T, Irwin MG, Joshi GP. Peri-operative considerations for sedation-analgesia during cataract surgery: a narrative review. *Anaesthesia*. 2019;74:1601–1610.
82. NICE. National Institute for Health and Care Excellence. Cataracts in adults: management. NICE Guideline [NG77]. Published October 26, 2017.
83. Leaming DV. Practice styles and preferences of ASCRS members: 2002 survey. *J Cataract Refract Surg*. 2003;29:1412–1420.
84. Gayer S, Flynn HW Jr. Sub-Tenon's injection for local anesthesia in posterior segment surgery (discussion). *Ophthalmology*. 2000;107:41–46.
85. Miller-Meeks MJ, Bergstrom T, Karp KO. Prevalent attitudes regarding residency training in ocular anesthesia. *Ophthalmology*. 1994;101:1353–1356.
86. Nanji KC, Roberto SA, Morley MG, Bayes J. Preventing adverse events in cataract surgery: recommendations from a Massachusetts expert panel. *Anesth Analg*. 2018;126:1537–1547.
87. Yannuzzi NA, Sridhar J, Flynn HW, et al. *Ophthalmology Retina*. 2019;3(9):804–805.
88. Smith MP, Sprung J, Zura A, et al. A survey of exposure to regional anesthesia techniques in American anesthesia residency training programs. *Reg Anesth Pain Med*. 1999;24(1):11–16.
89. Universal protocol for preventing wrong site, wrong procedure, wrong person surgery. *Joint Commission on Accreditation of Healthcare Organizations website*. Accessed December 16, 2015. http://www.jointcommission.org/standards_information/up.aspx
90. Wainwright AC. Positive pressure ventilation and the laryngeal mask airway in ophthalmic anaesthesia. *Br J Anaesth*. 1995;75:249–250.
91. Lamb K, James MF, Janicki PK. The laryngeal mask airway for intraocular surgery: effects on intraocular pressure and stress responses. *Br J Anaesth*. 1992;69:143–147.
92. Thomson KD. The effect of the laryngeal mask airway on coughing after eye surgery under general anesthesia. *Ophthalmic Surg*. 1992;23:630–631.
93. Aouad MT, Zeeni C, Al Nawwar RA, et al. Dexmedetomidine for improved quality of emergence from general anesthesia: a dose finding study. *Anesth Analg*. 2019;129(6):1504–1511.
94. Knapp H. On cocaine and its use in ophthalmic and general surgery. *Arch Ophthalmol*. 1884; 13:402.
95. Atkinson WS. Retrobulbar injection of anesthetic within the muscular cone. *Arch Ophthalmol*. 1936;16:494.
96. Gayer S. Ophthalmic anesthesia: more than meets the eye. In: Schwartz AJ, ed. *American Society of Anesthesiologists Refresher Courses in Anesthesiology*. Lippincott Williams & Wilkins; 2006:55.
97. Gayer S, Kumar CM. Ophthalmic regional anesthesia techniques. *Minerva Anestesiol*. 2008; 74:23–33.
98. Jean YK, Kam D, Gayer S, Palte HD, Stein ALS. Regional anesthesia for pediatric ophthalmic surgery: a review of the literature. *Anesth Analg*. 2020;130(5):1351–1363.
99. Korneef L. The architecture of the musculofibrous apparatus in the human orbit. *Acta Morphol Neerl Scand*. 1977;15:35–64.
100. Ripart J, Lefrant JY, de la Coussaye JE, Prat-Pradal D, Vivien B, Eledjam JJ. Peribulbar versus retrobulbar anesthesia for ophthalmic surgery. *Anesthesiology*. 2001;94:56–62.

101. Carneiro HM, Tiexeira KI, de Avila MP, Limongi RM, Magacho L. Comparison of needle path, anesthetic dispersion, and quality of anesthesia in retrobulbar and peribulbar blocks. *Reg Anesth Pain Med*. 2016;41(1):37–42.
102. Capó H, Roth E, Johnson T, Muñoz M, Siatkowski RM. Vertical strabismus after cataract surgery. *Ophthalmology*. 1996;103:918–921.
103. Ripart J, Lefrant J, Lalourcey L, et al. Medial canthus (caruncle) single injection periocular anesthesia. *Anesth Analg*. 1996;83:1234–1238.
104. Katsev DA, Drews RC, Rose BT. An anatomic study of retrobulbar needle path length. *Ophthalmology*. 1989;96:1221–1224.
105. Waller SG, Taboada J, O'Connor P. Retrobulbar anesthesia risk: do sharp needles really perforate the eye more easily than blunt needles? *Ophthalmology*. 1993;100:506–510.
106. Unsold R, Stanley JA, DeGroot J. The CT topography of retrobulbar anesthesia. *Graefes Arch Clin Exp Ophthalmol*. 1981;217:125–136.
107. Vohra SB. A review of the directions of gaze during intraocular anesthetic blocks. *Ophthal Surg Lasers Imag*. 2012;43:162–168.
108. Gayer S, Denham D, Alarakhia K, et al. Ocular decompression devices: liquid mercury balloon versus the tungsten powder balloon. *Am J Ophthalmol*. 2006;142:500–501.
109. Ohno-Matsui K. Proposed classification of posterior staphylomas based on analysis of eye shape by three-dimensional magnetic resonance imaging and wide field fundus imaging. *Ophthalmology*. 2014;121:1798–1809.
110. Birch A, Evans M, Redembo E. The ultrasonic localization of retrobulbar needles during retrobulbar block. *Ophthalmology*. 1995;102:824–826.
111. Grizzard WS, Kirk NM, Pavan PR, Antworth MV, Hammer ME, Roseman RL. Perforating ocular injuries caused by anesthesia personnel. *Ophthalmology*. 1991;98:1011–1016.
112. Bayes J, Zheng H, Rosow CE. Early use of eyeglasses for myopia predicts long axial length of the eye. *Anesth Analg*. 2010;110:119–121.
113. Gayer S. Ocular ultrasound guided anesthesia. In: Singh AD, Hayden BC, eds. *Ophthalmic Ultrasonography*. Elsevier; 2012:195–200.
114. Sadler A, McLeod G, McHardy PG, Wilkinson T. Ultrasound detection of iatrogenic injury during peribulbar eye block: a cadaveric study. *Reg Anesth Pain Med*. 2020;45:740–743.
115. Palte HD, Gayer S, Arrieta E, et al. Are ultrasound-guided ophthalmic blocks injurious to the eye? A comparative rabbit model study of two ultrasound devices evaluating intraorbital thermal and structural changes. *Anesth Analg*. 2012;115(1):194–201.
116. Chin YC, Kumar CM. Brainstem anesthesia revisited: mechanism, presentation and management. *Trends Anesth Crit Care*. 2013;3:252–256.
117. Nicoll JM, Acharya PA, Ahlen K, Baguneid S, Edge KR. Central nervous system complications after 6000 retrobulbar blocks. *Anesth Analg*. 1987;66:1298–1302.
118. Swan KC. New drugs and techniques for ocular anesthesia. *Trans Am Acad Ophthalmol Otolaryngol*. 1956;60:368–375.
119. Gayer S, Cass GD. Sub-Tenon techniques should be one option among many. *Anesthesiology*. 2004;100:196.
120. Niemi-Murola L, Krootila K, Kivisaari R, Kangasmäki A, Kivisaari L, Maunuksela EL. Localization of local anesthetic solution by magnetic resonance imaging. *Ophthalmology*. 2004;111:342–347.
121. Guise PA. Sub-Tenon anesthesia: a prospective study of 6000 blocks. *Anesthesiology*. 2003;98:964–968.
122. Ripart J, Metge L, Prat-Pradal D, Lopez FM, Eledjam JJ. Medial canthus single-injection episcleral (sub-Tenon) anesthesia: computed tomography imaging. *Anesth Analg*. 1998;87:42.
123. Allman KG, Theron AD, Byles DB. A new technique of incisionless, minimally invasive sub-Tenon's anaesthesia. *Anaesthesia*. 2008;63(7):782–783.
124. Palte HD, Gayer S. A novel technique for minimally invasive sub-Tenon's anesthesia. *Reg Anesth Pain Med*. 2019;44(1):131–132.
125. Coban-Karatas M, Yalcin-Cok O, Kumar CM. Lacrimal dilator-facilitated incisionless versus standard sub-Tenon's block: a randomized, prospective and non inferiority comparative study. *Eye*. 2020;35:1961–1966.
126. Frieman BJ, Friedberg MA. Globe perforation associated with sub-Tenon's anesthesia. *J Ophthalmol*. 2001;131:520–521.
127. Ruschen H, Bremner FD, Carr C. Complications after sub-Tenon's eye block. *Anesth Analg*. 2003;96:273–277.
128. Quantock C, Goswami T. Death potentially secondary to sub-Tenon's block. *Anaesthesia*. 2007;62:175–177.
129. Palte HD, Gayer S. Death after a sub-Tenon's block. *Anaesthesia*. 2007;62:531.
130. Bardocci A, Lofoco G, Perdicaro S, Ciucci F, Manna L. Lidocaine 2% gel versus lidocaine 4% unpreserved drops for topical anesthesia in cataract surgery: a randomized controlled trial. *Ophthalmology*. 2003;110:144.
131. Shugar JK. Use of epinephrine for IFIS prophylaxis. *J Cataract Refract Surg*. 2006;32:1074–1075.
132. Bell CM, Hatch WV, Fischer HD, et al. Association between tamsulosin and serious ophthalmic adverse events in older man following cataract surgery. *JAMA*. 2009;301(19):1991–1996.
133. Jaichandran VV, Raman R, Gella L, Sharma T. Local anesthetic agents for vitreoretinal surgery. No advantage to mixing solutions. *Ophthalmology*. 2015;122:1030–1033.
134. Nestor CC, Ng C, Sepulveda P, Irwin MG. Pharmacological and clinical implications of local anaesthetic mixtures: a narrative review. *Anaesthesia*. 2020;77:339–350.
135. Zhang C, Phamonvaechavan R, Rajan A, Poon DY, Topcu-Yilmaz P, Guyton DL. Concentration-dependent bupivacaine myotoxicity in rabbit extraocular muscle. *J AAPOS*. 2010;14:323–327.
136. Borazan M, Karalezli A, Oto S, Algan C, Aydin Akova Y. Comparison of bupivacaine 0.5% and lidocaine 2% mixture with levobupivacaine 0.75% and ropivacaine 1% in peribulbar anaesthesia for cataract surgery with phacoemulsification. *Acta Ophthal Scand*. 2007;85:844–847.
137. Uy H, de Jesus AA, Paray AA, Flores JD, Felizar LB. Ropivacaine-lidocaine versus bupivacaine-lidocaine for retrobulbar anesthesia in cataract surgery. *J Cataract Refract Surg*. 2002;28:1023–1026.
138. Netland PA, Harris A. Color Doppler ultrasound measurements after topical and retrobulbar epinephrine in primate eyes. *Invest Ophthalmol Vis Sci*. 1997;38:2655–2661.
139. Adams L. Adjuvants to local anaesthesia in ophthalmic surgery. *Br J Ophthalmol*. 2011;95(10):1345–1349.
140. Brown SM, Coats DK, Collins ML, Underdahl JP. Second cluster of strabismus cases after periocular anesthesia without hyaluronidase. *J Cataract Refract Surg*. 2001;27:1872–1875.
141. Hamada S, Devys JM, Xuan TH, et al. Role of hyaluronidase in diplopia after peribulbar anesthesia for cataract surgery. *Ophthalmology*. 2005;112(5):879–882.
142. Jay WM, Aziz MZ, Green K. Effect of intraocular pressure reducer on ocular and optic nerve blood flow in phakic rabbit eyes. *Acta Ophthalmol*. 1986; 64:52–57.
143. Adatia FA, Munro M, Jivraj I, Ajani A, Braga-Mele R. Documenting the subjective patient experience of first versus second cataract surgery. *J Cataract Refract Surg*. 2015; 41:116–121.
144. Downs JB. Has oxygen administration delayed appropriate respiratory care? Fallacies regarding oxygen therapy. *Respir Care*. 2003;48:611.
145. Mehta SP, Bhananker SM, Posner KL, Domino KB. Operating room fires: a closed claims analysis. *Anesthesiology*. 2013;118:1133–1139.
146. Hug CC. MAC should stand for maximum anesthesia caution, not minimal anesthesiology care (editorial). *Anesthesiology*. 2006;104:221–223.
147. Norregaard JC, Schein OD, Bellan L, et al. International variation in anesthesia care during cataract surgery: results from the International Cataract Surgery Outcomes Study. *Arch Ophthalmol*. 1997;115:1304–1308.
148. Eichel R, Goldberg I. Anaesthesia techniques for cataract surgery: a survey of delegates to the Congress of the International Council of Ophthalmology, 2002. *Clin Experiment Ophthalmol*. 2005;33:469–472.
149. Rosenfeld SI, Litinsky SM, Snyder DA, Plosker H, Astrove AW, Schiffman J. Effectiveness of monitored anesthesia care in cataract surgery. *Ophthalmology*. 1999;106:1256–1260.
150. Fung D, Cohen MM, Stewart S, Davies A. What determines patient satisfaction with cataract care under topical local anesthesia and monitored sedation in a community hospital setting? *Anesth Analg*. 2005;100:1644–1650.
151. Gayer S. Rethinking anesthesia strategies for patients with traumatic eye injuries: alternatives to general anesthesia. *Curr Anesth Crit Care*. 2006;17:191.
152. Scott IU, McCabe CM, Flynn HW Jr, et al. Local anesthesia with intravenous sedation for surgical repair of selected open globe injuries. *Am J Ophthalmol*. 2002;134:707–711.
153. Boscia F, La Tegola MG, Columbo G, Alessio G, Sborgia C. Combined topical anesthesia and sedation for open-globe injuries in selected patients. *Ophthalmology*. 2003;110:1555–1559.
154. McGoldrick KE. The open globe: Is an alternative to succinylcholine necessary? (editorial). *J Clin Anesth*. 1993;5:1–4.
155. Amadasun FE, Isesele TO. Vitreous humour extrusion after suxamethonium induction of anaesthesia in a polytraumatized patient: a case report. *Case Rep Med*. 2010;2010:913763.
156. de Boer H, Driessen JJ, Marcus MA, Kerkkamp H, Heeringa M, Klimek M. Reversal of rocuronium-induced (1.2 mg/kg) neuromuscular block by sugammadex: a multicenter dose-finding and safety study. *Anesthesiology*. 2007;107:239–244.
157. Kopman AF. Sugammadex: a revolutionary approach to neuromuscular antagonism (editorial). *Anesthesiology*. 2006;104:631–633.
158. Stinson TW, Donlon JV. Interaction of SF6 and air with nitrous oxide. *Anesthesiology*. 1979;51:S16.
159. Colson JD. Cervicofacial subcutaneous emphysema and pneumomediastinum after retinal detachment surgery: just another monitored anesthesia eye case. *J Clin Anesth*. 2011;23:410.
160. Seaberg RR, Freeman WR, Goldbaum MH, Manecke GR Jr. Permanent postoperative vision loss associated with expansion of intraocular gas in the presence of a nitrous oxide-containing anesthetic. *Anesthesiology*. 2002;97:1309–1310.
161. Dallinger S, Findl O, Strenn K, Eichler HG, Wolzt M, Schmetterer L. Age dependence of choroidal blood flow. *J Am Geriatr Soc*. 1998;46:484–487.
162. Recchia FM, Brown GC. Systemic disorders associated with retinal vascular occlusion. *Curr Opin Ophthalmol*. 2000;11:462–467.
163. Ledowski T, Kiese F, Jeglin S, Scholz J. Possible air embolism during eye surgery. *Anesth Analg*. 2005;100(6):1651–1652.
164. Morris RE, Boyd GL, Sapp MR, et al. Ocular venous air embolism (OVAE): a review. *J Vitreoretin Dis*. 2019;3(2):99–106.
165. Gayer S, Palte HD, Albini T, et al. In vivo porcine model of venous air embolism during pars plana vitrectomy. *Am J Ophth*. 2016;171:139–144.
166. Rojanaporn D, Tipsuriyaporn B, Chulalaksiriboon P, Virankabutra T, Morakul S, Damato B. Fatal air embolism after choroidal melanoma endoresection without air infusion: a case report. *Ocul Oncol Pathol*. 2021;7:321–325.

167. Iyer PG, Gayer S, Albini TA, Flynn HW. Venous air embolism: a rare but serious complication of fluid-gas exchange during pars plana vitrectomy. *Am J Ophthalmol.* 2021:227;A3–A4.
168. Wykoff CC, Flynn HW, Scott IU. What is the optimal timing for rhegmatogenous retinal detachment repair? *JAMA Ophthalmol.* 2013;131(11):1399–1400.
169. Wykoff CC, Smiddy WE, Mathen T, Schwartz SG, Flynn HW Jr, Shi W. Fovea-sparing retinal detachments: time to surgery and visual outcomes. *Am J Ophthalmol.* 2010;150:205–210.
170. Colyer MH, Weber ED, Weichel ED, et al. Delayed intraocular foreign body removal without endophthalmitis during Operations Iraqi Freedom and Enduring Freedom. *Ophthalmology.* 2007;114(8):1439–1447.
171. Li G, Brady JE, Rosenberg H, Sun LS. Excess comorbidities associated with malignant hyperthermia diagnosis in pediatric hospital discharge records. *Pediatr Anesth.* 2011;21:958–963.
172. France NK, France TD, Wordburn JD Jr, Burbank DP. Succinylcholine alteration of the forced duction test. *Ophthalmology.* 1980;87:1282–1287.
173. Jampolsky A. Strabismus: surgical overcorrections. *Highlights Ophthalmol.* 1965;8:78.
174. Dell R, Williams B. Anaesthesia for strabismus surgery: a regional survey. *Br J Anaesth.* 1999; 82:761–763.
175. Eberhart LH, Geldner G, Kranke P, et al. The development and validation of a risk score to predict the probability of postoperative vomiting in pediatric patients. *Anesth Analg.* 2004;99: 1630–1637.
176. Lerman MD, Eustis S, Smith DR. Effect of droperidol pretreatment on postanesthetic vomiting in children undergoing strabismus surgery. *Anesthesiology.* 1986;65:322–325.
177. Brown RE, James DG, Weaver RG, Wilhoit RD, Bauman LA. Low-dose droperidol versus standard-dose droperidol for prevention of postoperative vomiting after pediatric strabismus surgery. *J Clin Anesth.* 1991;3:306–309.
178. Gan TJ, Belani KG, Bergese S, et al. Fourth Consensus Guidelines for the management of postoperative nausea and vomiting. *Anesth Analg.* 2020;131:411–448.
179. Watcha MF, Simeon RM, White PF, Stevens JL. Effect of propofol on the incidence of postoperative vomiting after strabismus surgery in pediatric outpatients. *Anesthesiology.* 1991;75:204–209.
180. Oh AY, Kim JH, Hwang JW, Do SH, Jeon YT. Incidence of postoperative nausea and vomiting after pediatric strabismus surgery with sevoflurane or remifentanil–sevoflurane. *Br J Anaesth.* 2010;104:756–760.
181. Munro HM, Riegger LQ, Reynolds PI, Wilton NC, Lewis IH. Comparison of the analgesic and emetic properties of ketorolac and morphine for paediatric outpatient strabismus surgery. *Br J Anaesth.* 1994;72:624–628.
182. Yao L, Zhao H, Jiang B, Feng Y. Retrobulbar block in pediatric vitreoretinal surgery eliminates the need for intraoperative fentanyl and postoperative analgesia: a randomized controlled study. *Reg Anesth Pain Med.* 2017;42(4):521–526.
183. Roth S, Thisted RA, Erickson JP, et al. Eye injuries after nonocular surgery: a study of 60,965 anesthetics from 1988–1992. *Anesthesiology.* 1996;85:1020–1027.
184. Yu HD, Chou AH, Yang MW, Chang CJ. An analysis of perioperative eye injuries after nonocular surgery. *Acta Anaesthesiologica Taiwanica.* 2010;48(3):122–129.
185. Gild WA, Posner KL, Caplan RA, et al. Eye injuries associated with anesthesia. *Anesthesiology.* 1992;76:204–208.
186. Lee LA, Posner KL, Domino KB, Caplan RA, Cheney FW. Injuries associated with regional anesthesia in the 1980s and 1990s: a closed claims analysis. *Anesthesiology.* 2004;101:143–152.
187. Lee L, Posner KL, Domino KB. Trends in injuries to the visual pathways and medicolegal payments from the Closed Claims Project Database. Presented at: Anesthesiology 2013 Annual Meeting; October 12–16, 2013; San Francisco, CA. Abstract A2058.
188. Lee LA, Roth S, Posner KL, et al. The American Society of Anesthesiologists Postoperative Visual Loss Registry: analysis of 93 spine surgery cases with postoperative visual loss. *Anesthesiology.* 2006;105:652–659.
189. Batra YK, Bali M. Corneal abrasions during general anesthesia. *Anesth Analg.* 1977;56:363–365.
190. Cucchiara R, Black S. Corneal abrasion during anesthesia and surgery. *Anesthesiology.* 1988; 69:978–979.
191. Martin DP, Weingarten TN, Gunn PW, et al. Performance improvement system and perioperative corneal injuries. *Anesthesiology.* 2009;111:320–326.
192. Deljou A, Weingarten TN, Mahr MA, Sprung J, Martin DP. Postoperative corneal injuries: incidence and risk factors. *Anesthesia and analgesia.* 2018;129(3):737–742.
193. Deyo RA, Nachemson A, Mirza SK. Spinal-fusion surgery—the case for restraint. *N Engl J Med.* 2004;350(7):722–726.
194. Shen Y, Drum M, Roth S. The prevalence of perioperative visual loss in the United States: a 10-year study from 1996 to 2005 of spinal, orthopedic, cardiac, and general surgery. *Anesth Analg* 2009;109:1534–1545.
195. Rubin DS, Parakati I, Lee LA, Moss HE, Joslin CE, Roth S. Perioperative visual loss in spine fusion surgery: ischemic optic neuropathy in the United States from 1998 to 2012 in the Nationwide Inpatient Sample. *Anesthesiology.* 2016;125(3):457–464.
196. Drance SM. Angle-closure glaucoma among Canadian Eskimos. *Can J Ophthalmol.* 1973;8: 252–254.
197. Gayer S. Prone to blindness: answers to postoperative visual loss. *Anesth Analg.* 2010;112: 11–12.
198. Pollack AL, McDonald HR, Ai E, et al. Massive suprachoroidal hemorrhage during pars plana vitrectomy associated with valsalva maneuver. *American Journal ophthalmology.* 2001;132: 383–387.
199. Purdy EP, Ajimal GS. Vision loss after lumbar epidural steroid injection. *Anesth Analg.* 1988; 86:119–122.
200. Honemann C, Brandt L. Valsalva retinopathy: a rare complication following general anesthesia. *A A Case Rep.* 2015;5(12):231–233.
201. Roth S, Gillesberg I. Injuries to the visual system and other sense organs. In: Benumof JL, Saidman LJ, eds. *Anesthesia and Perioperative Complications.* 2nd ed. Mosby; 1999:377.
202. Mabry RL. Visual loss after intranasal corticosteroid injection. *Arch Otolaryngol.* 1981;107: 484–486.
203. Biousse V, Newman NJ. Ischemic optic neuropathies. *N Engl J Med.* 2015;372:2428–2436.
204. Myers MA, Hamilton SR, Bogosian AJ, et al. Visual loss as a complication of spinal surgery. *Spine.* 1997;22:1325–1329.
205. Dilger JA, Tetzlaff JE, Bell GR, Kosmorsky GS, Agnor RC, O'Hara JF Jr. Ischemic optic neuropathy after spinal fusion. *Can J Anaesth.* 1998;45:63–66.
206. Shapira OM, Kimmel WA, Lindsey PS, Shahian DM. Anterior ischemic optic neuropathy after open heart operations. *Ann Thorac Surg.* 1996;61:660–666.
207. Williams EL, Hart WM, Tempelhoff R. Postoperative ischemic optic neuropathy. *Anesth Analg.* 1995;80:1018–1029.
208. The Ischemic Optic Neuropathy Decompression Trial Research Group. Optic nerve decompression surgery is not effective and may be harmful. *JAMA.* 1995;273:625.
209. American Society of Anesthesiologists Task Force on Perioperative Visual Loss. Practice advisory for perioperative visual loss associated with spine surgery: an updated report by the American Society of Anesthesiologists Task Force on Perioperative Visual Loss. *Anesthesiology.* 2012;116:274–285.
210. American Society of Anesthesiologists Task Force on Perioperative Visual Loss. Practice advisory for perioperative visual loss associated with spine surgery 2019: an updated report by the American Society of Anesthesiologists Task Force on Perioperative Visual Loss, the North American Neuro-Ophthalmology Society, and the Society for Neuroscience in Anesthesiology and Critical Care. *Anesthesiology.* 2019;130:12–30.
211. The Postoperative Visual Loss Study Group. Risk factors associated with ischemic optic neuropathy after spinal fusion surgery. *Anesthesiology.* 2012;116:15–24.
212. Warner M. Cracking open the door on perioperative visual loss (editorial). *Anesthesiology.* 2012;116:1–2.
213. Feibel RM, Custer PL, Gordon MO. Postcataract ptosis: a randomized, double-masked comparison of peribulbar and retrobulbar anesthesia. *Ophthalmology.* 1993;100:660–665.
214. Taylor G, Devys JM, Heran F, Plaud B. Early exploration of diplopia with magnetic resonance imaging after peribulbar anaesthesia. *Br J Anaesth.* 2004;92:899–901.

50 The Renal System and Anesthesia for Urologic Surgery

MARK STAFFORD-SMITH • ANGELA L. POLLAK • CATHERINE M. KUHN • JAMIE R. PRIVRATSKY

KEY POINTS

1. Kidney filtration and reabsorption are susceptible to alterations by surgical illness and anesthesia. Autoregulation of renal blood flow (RBF) is effective over a wide range of mean arterial pressures (50 to 150 mmHg). Autoregulation of urine flow does not occur, but a linear relationship between mean arterial pressure above 50 mmHg and urine output is observed.
2. Kidney medullary blood flow is low (2% of total RBF) but central to the kidneys' ability to concentrate urine. During periods of reduced kidney perfusion, the metabolically active medullary thick ascending limb may be especially vulnerable to ischemic injury.
3. The physiologic response to surgical stress invokes intrinsic mechanisms for sodium and water conservation. Kidney cortical vasoconstriction causes a shift in perfusion toward juxtamedullary nephrons, a decrease in glomerular filtration rate, and retention of salt and water result.
4. The stress response may induce a decrease in RBF and glomerular filtration rate, causing afferent arteriolar vasoconstriction. If this situation is not reversed, ischemic damage to the kidney may result in acute renal failure (ARF).
5. Anesthetic-induced reductions in RBF have been described for many agents but are usually clinically insignificant and reversible. Likewise, anesthetic agents have not been shown to interfere with the kidney response to physiologic stress.
6. Isolated ARF carries a mortality of up to 60% in surgical patients, with acute tubular necrosis being the cause of ARF in most of these patients.
7. Surgical patients with nondialysis-dependent chronic kidney disease are at higher risk of developing end-stage renal disease. The single most reliable predictor of new postoperative need for dialysis is preoperative kidney insufficiency.
8. Overall, there are no conclusive comparative studies demonstrating superior kidney protection or improved kidney outcome with general versus regional anesthesia.
9. Maintaining adequate intravascular volume and hemodynamic stability with aggressive management of kidney hypoperfusion is a basic principle of anesthetic care to prevent acute kidney injury.
10. Urologic patients are often elderly, have numerous comorbidities, and require critical evaluation prior to any urologic procedure.
11. Combining epidural with general anesthetic techniques for some major urologic surgeries may offer advantages for accelerated recovery, improved analgesia, and even better outcomes, but these techniques must be conducted with respect for other perioperative issues, including thromboprophylaxis for prevention of deep venous thrombosis.

12 Watchful waiting, minimally invasive principles, and technologic innovation (e.g., laparoscopy, robotics) have changed the favored approach to many kidney, bladder, and prostate disorders, in some cases reducing the number of high-risk surgeries, in others creating other safer less morbid alternate treatments.

13 Absorption of irrigating solution related most often to transurethral prostate or bladder tumor resections can cause "TUR syndrome," a condition that, while becoming less common, has the potential to be serious and even life threatening during the several hours following surgery. Knowledge of specific concerns relevant to the different irrigating solutions, and vigilance of the anesthesiologist to factors that minimize absorption, recognition of signs and symptoms, and appropriate treatment are key to favorable outcomes with this condition.

The kidney plays a central role in implementing and controlling a variety of homeostatic functions; these include tight control of extracellular fluid volume and composition, and efficient excretion of uremic toxins in the urine. Acute kidney injury (AKI) disturbs such functions, and can occur because of systemic inflammation, nephrotoxin exposure, or as the consequence of prolonged reduction in kidney oxygen delivery due to surgical or medical disease; practically speaking several factors are often identified. The first part of this chapter reviews kidney physiology and pathophysiologic states as they relate to anesthetic practice, and then addresses strategies to recognize and manage patients at risk for AKI and renal failure. The second part describes current urologic procedures and their attendant anesthetic management issues.

Kidney Anatomy and Physiology

Gross Anatomy

The two normal *kidneys* are reddish-brown organs and are ovoid in outline, but the medial margin is deeply indented and concave at its middle where a wide, vertical cleft (the hilus) transmits structures entering and leaving the kidney (Fig. 50-1). The *hilus* lies at approximately the level of the first lumbar vertebra. The kidneys lie in the paravertebral gutters, behind the peritoneum, with the right kidney resting slightly lower than the left one due to the presence of the liver. At its upper end, the ureter has dilated to give rise to the *renal pelvis*, which passes through the hilus into the kidney proper. There it is continuous with several short funnel-like tubes (calyces) that unite it with the kidney parenchyma. The renal blood vessels lie anterior to the pelvis of the kidney, but some branches may pass posteriorly. Kidney pain sensation is conveyed back to spinal cord segments T10 through L1 by sympathetic fibers. Sympathetic innervation is supplied by preganglionic fibers from T8 to L1. The vagus nerve provides parasympathetic innervation to the kidney, and the S2 to S4 spinal segments supply the ureters.

Each kidney is enclosed in a thick, fibrous capsule, itself surrounded by a fatty capsule that fills the space inside a loosely applied renal (Gerota) fascia. The developing kidney is first formed in the pelvis and then ascends to its final position on the posterior abdominal wall. During its ascent, the kidney receives blood supply from several successive sources, such that an accessory renal artery from the aorta may be found entering the lower pole of the kidney. When first formed, the rudimentary kidneys are close together and may fuse to give rise to a horseshoe kidney. This organ is unable to ascend, "held in place" by the inferior mesenteric artery, and thus when present it remains forever a pelvic organ.

The *bladder* is located in the retropubic space and receives its innervation from sympathetic nerves originating from T11 to L2, which conduct pain, touch, and temperature sensations, whereas bladder stretch sensation is transmitted via parasympathetic fibers from segments S2 to S4. Parasympathetics also provide the bladder with most of its motor innervation.

The *prostate, penile urethra*, and *penis* also receive sympathetic and parasympathetic fibers from the T11 to L2 and S2 to S4 segments, respectively. The pudendal nerve provides pain sensation to the penis via the dorsal nerve of the penis. Sensory innervation of the *scrotum* is via cutaneous nerves, which project to lumbosacral segments, whereas testicular sensation is conducted to lower thoracic and upper lumbar segments. While the *female urethra* is much shorter than the male urethra (4 vs. 20 cm), sources of autonomic innervation are the same.

Ultrastructure

Inspection of the cut surface of the kidney reveals the paler *cortex*, adjacent to the capsule, and the darker, conical pyramids of the kidney *medulla* (Fig. 50-1). The pyramids are radially striated and are covered with cortex, extending into the kidney as the renal columns. *Collecting tubules* from each lobe of the kidney (pyramid and its covering of cortex) discharge urine into the calyceal system via renal papillae at the entrance of each pyramid into the calyx proper. These collecting tubules originate deep within the radial striations (medullary rays) of the kidney and convey urine formed in the structural units of the kidneys, the *nephrons*. The parenchyma of each kidney contains approximately 1×10^6 tightly packed nephrons, each one consisting of a tuft of capillaries (the *glomerulus*) invaginated into the blind, expanded end (glomerular corpuscle) of a long tubule that leaves the renal corpuscle to form the proximal convoluted tubule in the cortex. This leads into the straight tubule, which loops down into the medullary pyramid (*loop of Henle*) and hence back to the cortex to become continuous with the distal convoluted tubule. This then opens into a collecting duct that is common to a number of nephrons and passes through the pyramid to enter the lesser calyx at the papilla. It is in these parts of the nephron (proximal tubule, loop of Henle, distal tubule, and collecting duct) that urine is formed, concentrated, and conveyed to the ureters. The distal convoluted tubule comes into very close contact with the afferent glomerular arteriole, and the modified cells of each form the *juxtaglomerular apparatus*, a complex physiologic feedback control mechanism contributing in part to the precise control of intra- and extrarenal hemodynamics that is a hallmark feature of the normally functioning kidney.

As is the case for the kidney tubules, the vasculature of the kidney is highly organized. The renal artery enters the kidney at the hilum and then divides many times before producing the arcuate arteries that run along the boundary between cortex and outer medulla. Interlobular arteries branch from arcuate arteries toward the outer kidney surface, giving rise as they pass through the cortex to numerous afferent arterioles, each leading to a single glomerular capillary tuft. The barrier where filtration from the vascular to tubular space within the glomerulus occurs is highly specialized and includes fenestrated negatively charged capillary endothelial cells and tubular epithelial cells (podocytes) separated by a basement membrane. Normally, selective permeability permits approximately 25% of the plasma elements to pass into the Bowman capsule; only cells and proteins >60 to 70 kDa cannot cross. However, abnormalities of this barrier can occur with

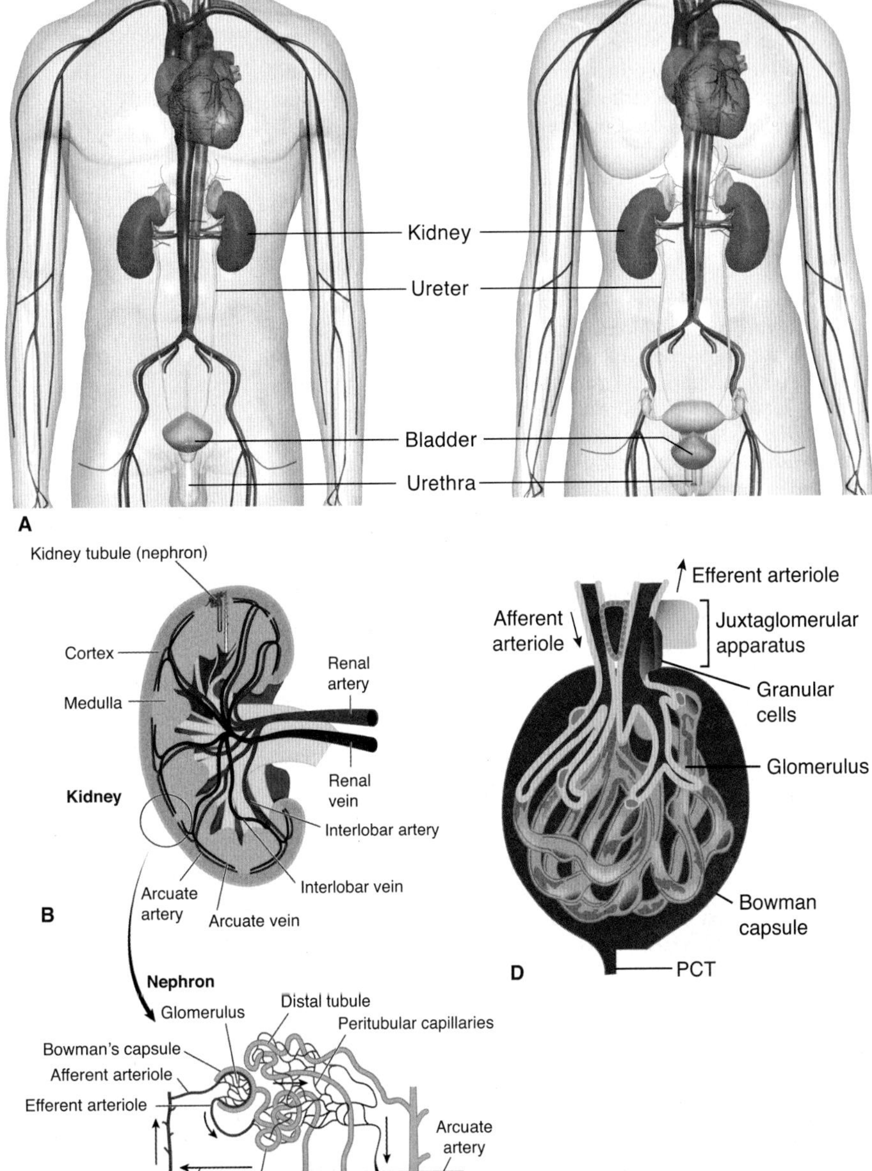

Figure 50-1 The gross anatomy (**A**) and internal structure of the genitourinary system and kidney. Internal organization of the kidney includes cortex and medulla regions and the vasculature. Renal vascularity and unique supply of the glomerulus and nephron. There are two distinct capillary networks in series that determine renal perfusion and glomerularfiltration. The blood supply to the renal parenchyma is supplied by branches that arise distal to theglomerulus (**B, C**). (**D**); 20% of plasma that enters the glomerulus passes through the specialized capillary wall into the Bowman capsule and enters the tubule to be processed and generate urine. PCT, proximal convoluted tubule, DCT, distal convoluted tubule. (A: LifeART image copyright © 2023. Lippincott Williams & Wilkins. All rights reserved; B,C: From Jones RA, Vasanawala S, Grattan-Smith D. Perfusion and Dynamic Contrast-Enhanced Imaging to Study Renal Function. In: Bammer R, ed. *MR and CT Perfusion and Pharmacokinetic Imaging: Clinical Applications and Theoretical Principles*. Wolters Kluwer; 2017:1123–1135. Figure 75.1.)

disease that may permit filtration of much larger proteins and even red blood cells; these changes manifest as the *nephrotic syndrome* (proteinuria >3.5 g/24 hr) or *glomerulonephritis* (hematuria and proteinuria). The glomerular capillaries exit Bowman capsule and merge to form the efferent arteriole and peritubular capillaries that nourish the tubules. The kidney vasculature is unusual in having this arrangement of two capillary beds joined in series by arterioles. Blood supply to the entire tubular system comes from the glomerular efferent arteriole, which branches into an extensive capillary network. Some of these peritubular capillaries, the *vasa recta*, descend deep into the medulla to parallel the loops of Henle. The vasa recta then return in a cortical direction with the loops, join other peritubular capillaries, and empty into the cortical veins.

Correlation of Structure and Function

Because kidney tissue makes up only 0.4% of body weight but receives 25% of cardiac output, the kidneys are by far the most highly perfused major organs in the body, and this facilitates plasma filtration at rates as high as 125 to 140 mL/min in young adults. As highlighted the functions of the kidney are many and varied, including waste filtration, endocrine and exocrine activities, immune and metabolic functions, and maintenance of physiologic homeostasis. As well as tight regulation of extracellular solutes such as sodium, potassium, hydrogen, bicarbonate, and glucose, the kidney also generates ammonia and glucose and eliminates nitrogenous and other metabolic wastes including urea, creatinine, bilirubin, and other uremic toxins (i.e., substances that have toxic effects when they accumulate due to kidney impairment). Finally, circulating hormones secreted by the kidney influences red blood cell generation, calcium homeostasis, and systemic blood pressure.

The kidney fulfills its dual roles of toxin excretion and body fluid management by filtering large amounts of fluid and solutes from the blood and secreting waste products into the tubular fluid. Effects on the normal filtration and reabsorption processes of comorbid disease, surgery, and anesthesia are the focus of the next section.

Glomerular Filtration

Production of urine begins with water and solute filtration from plasma flowing into the glomerulus via the afferent arteriole. The *glomerular filtration rate* (GFR) is a measure of glomerular function expressed as milliliters of plasma filtered per minute. The *ultrafiltration constant* (Kf) is directly related to glomerular capillary permeability and glomerular surface area. The two major determinants of filtration pressure are glomerular capillary pressure (P_{GC}) and glomerular oncotic pressure (p_{GC}). P_{GC} is directly related to renal artery pressure and is heavily influenced by arteriolar tone at points upstream (afferent) and downstream (efferent) from the glomerulus. An increase in afferent arteriolar tone, as occurs with intense sympathetic or angiotensin II stimulation, causes filtration pressure and GFR to fall. Milder degrees of sympathetic or angiotensin activity cause a selective increase in efferent arteriolar tone, which tends to increase filtration pressure and GFR. The p_{GC} is directly dependent on plasma oncotic pressure. Afferent arteriolar dilatation enhances GFR by increasing glomerular flow, which in turn elevates glomerular capillary pressure. Recent general revisions of Starling's original formula to incorporate the newly appreciated importance of the endothelial glycocalyx layer also appear to be relevant to glomerular filtration, particularly for pathologic states that involve proteinuria (e.g., diabetic nephropathy).[1–3]

Autoregulation of Kidney Blood Flow and Glomerular Filtration Rate

Renal blood flow (RBF) *autoregulation* maintains relatively constant rates of RBF and glomerular filtration over a wide range of arterial blood pressure. Kidney autoregulation of blood flow and filtration is accomplished primarily by local feedback signals that
1 modulate glomerular arteriolar tone to protect the glomeruli from excessive perfusion pressure (Fig. 50-2).

In health, autoregulation of RBF is effective over a wide range of systemic arterial pressures. Several mechanisms for regulating blood flow to the glomerulus have been described, and all involve modulation of afferent glomerular arteriolar tone. The *myogenic reflex theory* holds that an increase in arterial pressure causes the afferent arteriolar wall to stretch and then constrict (by reflex); likewise, a decrease in arterial pressure causes reflex afferent arteriolar dilatation. The other proposed mechanism of RBF autoregulation is a phenomenon called *tubuloglomerular feedback*, which is also responsible for autoregulation of GFR.

Tubuloglomerular feedback allows the composition of distal tubular fluid to influence glomerular function through actions involving the juxtaglomerular apparatus. When RBF falls, the related decrease in GFR causes less chloride delivery to the juxtaglomerular apparatus, which in turn induces afferent arteriole dilation. As a result, glomerular flow and pressure then increase, and GFR returns to previous levels. Chloride also acts as the feedback signal for control of efferent arteriolar tone. When GFR falls, declining chloride delivery to the juxtaglomerular apparatus triggers release of *renin*, which ultimately causes the formation of *angiotensin II*. In response to angiotensin, efferent arteriolar constriction increases glomerular pressure, which increases glomerular filtration. It is important to realize that autoregulation of urine flow does not occur, and that above a mean arterial pressure of 50 mmHg there is a linear relationship between mean arterial pressure and urine output.

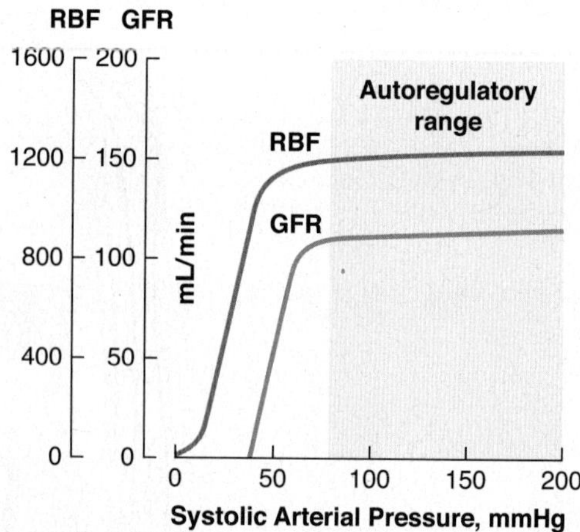

Figure 50-2 Renal blood flow (RBF) autoregulation maintains RBF and glomerular filtration rate (GFR) relatively constant with changes in systolic blood pressure from about 80 to 200 mmHg.

Tubular Reabsorption of Sodium and Water

Active, energy-dependent reabsorption of sodium begins almost immediately as the glomerular filtrate enters the proximal tubule. Here, an adenosine triphosphatase pump drives the sodium into tubular cells while chloride ions passively follow. Glucose, amino acid, and other organic compound reabsorption are strongly coupled to sodium in the proximal tubule. Normally, the proximal tubule reabsorbs two-thirds of the filtered sodium. Notably, no active sodium transport occurs in the loop of Henle until the medullary thick ascending limb is reached. Cells of the medullary thick 2
ascending limb are metabolically active in their role of reabsorbing sodium and chloride and have a high oxygen consumption compared with the thin portions of the descending and ascending limbs.

Reabsorption of water is a passive, osmotically driven process tied to the reabsorption of sodium and other solutes. Water reabsorption also depends on peritubular capillary pressure; high capillary pressure opposes water reabsorption and tends to increase urine output. The proximal tubule reabsorbs approximately 65% of filtered water in an isosmotic fashion with sodium and chloride. The descending limb of the loop of Henle allows water to follow osmotic gradients into the kidney interstitium. However, the thin ascending limb and medullary thick ascending limb are relatively impermeable to water and play a key role in the production of concentrated urine. Only 15% of filtered water is reabsorbed by the loop of Henle; the remaining filtrate volume flows into the distal tubule. There, and in the collecting duct, water reabsorption is controlled entirely by *antidiuretic hormone* (ADH) secreted by the pituitary gland. Conservation of water and excretion of excess solute by the kidneys would be impossible without the ability to produce concentrated urine. This is accomplished by establishing a hyperosmotic medullary interstitium and regulation of water permeability of the distal tubule and collecting duct via the action of ADH.

ADH increases the water permeability of the collecting ducts and allows for passive diffusion of water (under considerable osmotic pressure) back into the circulation. The posterior pituitary gland releases ADH in response to an increase in either extracellular sodium concentration or extracellular osmolality. In addition, ADH release can be triggered by an absolute or relative reduction in intravascular fluid volume. The arterial baroreceptors 3 are activated when hypovolemia leads to a decrease in blood pressure, whereas atrial receptors are stimulated by a decline in atrial filling pressure. Both circulatory reflex systems stimulate release of ADH from the pituitary and cause retention of water by the kidney in an effort to return the intravascular volume toward normal. ADH also causes kidney cortical vasoconstriction when it is released in large amounts, such as during the physiologic stress response to trauma, surgery, or other critical illness. This induces a shift of RBF to the hypoxia-prone kidney medulla.

The Renin–Angiotensin–Aldosterone System

Renin release by the afferent arteriole may be triggered by hypotension, decreased tubular chloride concentration, or by sympathetic stimulation. Renin enhances *angiotensin II* production, which in turn induces renal efferent arteriolar vasoconstriction. Angiotensin II also promotes ADH release from the posterior pituitary, sodium reabsorption by the proximal tubule, and aldosterone release by the adrenal medulla. *Aldosterone* stimulates the distal tubule and collecting duct to reabsorb sodium (and water), resulting in intravascular volume expansion. Sympathetic nervous system stimulation may also directly cause release of aldosterone. This leads to kidney cortical vasoconstriction, a decrease in GFR, and salt and water retention.

Kidney Vasodilator Mechanisms

Opposing the saline retention and vasoconstriction observed in stress states are the actions of *atrial natriuretic peptide* (ANP), *nitric oxide*, and the kidney *prostaglandin* system. ANP is released by the cardiac atria in response to increased stretch under conditions of volume expansion. Both natriuresis and aquaresis increase as ANP blocks reabsorption of sodium in the distal tubule and collecting duct. ANP also increases GFR, causes systemic vasodilatation, inhibits the release of renin, opposes production and action of angiotensin II, and decreases aldosterone secretion.[4,5] Likewise, nitric oxide produced in the kidney opposes the kidney vasoconstrictor effects of angiotensin II and the adrenergic nervous system, promotes sodium and water excretion, and participates in tubuloglomerular feedback.[6]

Prostaglandins are produced by the kidney as part of a complex system that modulates RBF and opposes the actions of ADH and the renin–angiotensin–aldosterone system.[7] Stress states, kidney ischemia, and hypotension stimulate the production of kidney prostaglandins through the enzymes phospholipase A_2 and cyclooxygenase. Prostaglandins produced by cyclooxygenase activity cause dilatation of renal arterioles (antiangiotensin II), whereas their distal tubular effects result in an increase in sodium and water excretion (anti-ADH and aldosterone). The kidney prostaglandin system is important in maintaining RBF and sodium and water excretion during times of high physiologic stress and poor kidney perfusion.[7]

Clinical Assessment of the Kidney

Most agree that immediate perioperative measures such as urine output correlate poorly with perioperative kidney function[8]; however, much about the kidneys can be learned from knowing how effectively they clear circulating substances and inspection of the urine (i.e., urinalysis).

Kidney Function Tests

Filtration is a useful method to clinically assess kidney function. As a key indicator of disease, knowledge of limited filtration capacity is important to guide drug dosing for agents cleared by the kidneys and helps with preoperative risk stratification. Also, acute declines in filtration capacity indicate kidney injury and predict a more complicated clinical course.[5] *GFR*, as previously mentioned, refers to the plasma volume filtered per unit time by the kidneys, and normal values range from 90 to 140 mL/min. Normal GFRs relate to the patient age, size, and sex. In general, GFR declines 10% per decade after age 30 and is approximately 10 mL/min higher in men than women. A GFR below 60 mL/min meets criteria for chronic kidney disease (CKD) and is considered impaired, while values lower than 15 mL/min are often associated with uremic symptoms and may require dialysis.

An "ideal" substance to assess GFR through its clearance from the circulation must have specific properties, including a steady supply, free filtration, and no tubular reabsorption or excretion; ideally, it is also cheap and easy to measure. Unfortunately, the perfect ideal substance is yet to be identified. The "gold standard" GFR tools involve expensive and cumbersome measurements (e.g., inulin, ^{51}Cr-EDTA or ^{99}Tc-DTPA clearance), while the most practical and inexpensive test involves an imperfect "ideal" substance, *creatinine*. However, despite creatinine's limitations, its relatively steady supply from muscle metabolism, modest tubular secretion, and proven usefulness in numerous clinical settings make it the most used kidney filtration marker currently available. Although more ideal substances and other "early biomarkers" of AKI are being evaluated as clinical tools, current candidates (e.g., cystatin C) have yet to replace creatinine. The reader is referred to recent reviews on this subject.[9,10]

Estimates of GFR (eGFR) can be made by determining *creatinine clearance* (CrCl) from urine and blood creatinine tests. In stable, critically ill patients, 2-hour urine collections are sufficient to calculate CrCl,[11] using the following formula:

$$\text{CrCl (mL/min)} = (U_{cr}\ \text{(mg/dL)} \times V\ \text{(mL)}) \,/\, (P_{cr}\ \text{(mg/dL)} \times \text{time (min)})$$

where U_{Cr} = urine creatinine, V = total volume of urine collected, P_{Cr} = plasma creatinine, time = collection time.

However, if patient characteristics are known, GFR can also be estimated from a single steady-state serum creatinine value. Notably, predictive formulas are developed using data from stable (nonsurgical) populations, and factors such as fluid shifts, hemodilution, and hemorrhage add an "unsteadiness" to perioperative estimates of GFR using serum creatinine.

Nonetheless, serum creatinine remains, so far, an unsurpassed perioperative tool, particularly to reflect *trends* of change in kidney filtration and to predict outcome, even during the perioperative period.[12–14] The most commonly used models for estimating kidney function are the Cockroft–Gault, Modification of Diet in Renal Disease (MDRD), and Chronic Kidney Disease Epidemiology Collaboration (CKD-EPI) equations. Of the predictive formulas, the Cockroft–Gault equation is one of the oldest and estimates clearance of creatinine.[15] The Cockroft–Gault equation uses patient sex, age (years), weight (kg), and serum creatinine (mg/dL):

$$\text{Cockroft–Gault eGFR (mL/min)} = (140 - \text{age}) \times \text{weight (kg)} / (\text{Cr} \times 72)(\times 0.85 \text{ for female patients})$$

The Modification of Diet in Renal Disease (MDRD) equation is most applicable for estimating GFR in stable CKD.[16] The MDRD method tends to significantly underestimate measured GFR, particularly in healthy patients with GFR >60 mL/min/m^2. An abbreviated MDRD formula is available that can estimate GFR measured in milliliters per minute per 1.73 m^2:

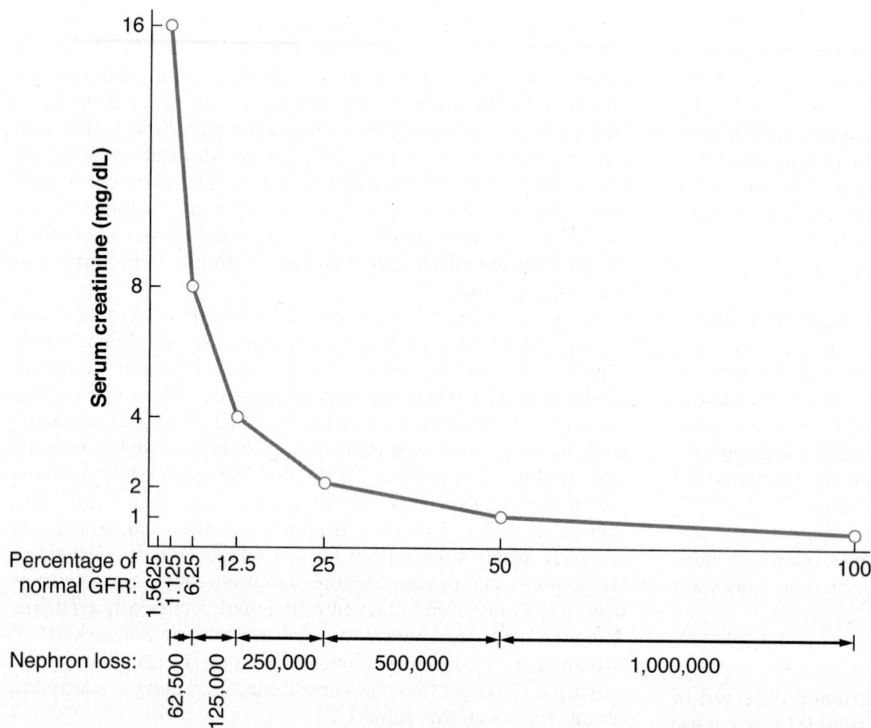

Figure 50-3 The nonlinear relationship between changes in kidney filtration and serum creatinine level means that a large reduction (e.g., 75%, 120 to 30 mL/min) in glomerular filtration rate (GFR) may be associated with a modest rise in serum creatinine. Proportional reductions in GFR and (approximate) nephron loss (x-axis) have an inverse logarithmic relationship with serum creatinine concentration (y-axis). (Modified from Faber MD, Kupin WL, Krishna G, et al. In: Lazarus JM, Brenner BM, eds. *Acute Renal Failure: The Differential Diagnosis of ARF*. 3rd ed. Churchill Livingstone, 1993:133)

$$\text{GFR} = 186 \times (\text{serum creatinine} - \text{mg/dL})^{-1.154} \times (\text{age})^{-0.203}$$
$$(\times\, 0.742 \text{ for female patients})$$
$$(\times\, 1.210 \text{ for black patients})$$

The National Kidney Foundation (NKF) and the American Society of Nephrology (ASN) task force now recommend the use of the 2021 CKD-EPI creatinine equation for estimation of GFR.[17] This version of the equation no longer includes race as a variable to recognize diversity within communities of color and potential consequences of clinical decision making that disproportionately affects one racial group. The 2021 CKD-EPI creatinine formula was found to be the most accurate estimation of GFR when compared to the gold standard.[18] The NKF-ASN task force also recommends the increased use of serum cystatin C, another filtration marker, in conjunction with creatinine to improve accuracy of GFR estimation particularly in patients with extremes of body habitus and thus serum creatinine values. However, serum cystatin C is not a test readily available in all laboratories.

Some consensus definitions for significant perioperative kidney dysfunction exist. The Society of Thoracic Surgeons defines postoperative AKI as either a new requirement for dialysis or a rise in serum creatinine to >2 mg/dL involving at least a 50% increase in serum creatinine above baseline.[19] Another definition requires a creatinine rise of >25% or 0.5 mg/dL (44 mmol/L) within 48 hours.[20] Two previous AKI definitions included the Acute Dialysis Quality Initiative (ADQI) and the Acute Kidney Injury Network (AKIN) definition. The ADQI Group definition for critically ill patients grades AKI by an acute creatinine rise of 50% as risk, 100% as injury, or 200% as *f*ailure (the RIFLE criteria).[21] The AKIN definition, a 1.5-fold or 0.3 mg/dL (≥26.4 mmol/L) creatinine rise within a 48-hour period or more than 6 hours of oliguria (>0.5 mL/kg/hr), is a modification of its RIFLE predecessor.[21,22] The most current consensus definition for AKI comes from Kidney Disease Improving Global Outcomes (KDIGO): an increase in serum creatinine by ≥0.3 mg/dL (≥26.5 μmol/L) within 48 hours; or increase in serum creatinine to ≥1.5 times baseline, which is known or presumed to have occurred within the prior 7 days; or urine volume <0.5 mL/kg/hr for 6 hours.[23] Notably, serum creatinine does not usually rise significantly until GFR rates fall below 50 mL/min, so preoperative serum creatinine levels may fall within the normal range in patients even with some degree of existing kidney dysfunction (Fig. 50-3).

Blood urea nitrogen (BUN) is sometimes used to assess kidney function but possesses few of the characteristics of an ideal substance for such a task. Tubular urea transport changes with some conditions (e.g., dehydration), and urea generation can be highly variable, particularly during the postoperative period (i.e., catabolic state). In addition, hemodilution (e.g., cardiopulmonary bypass [CPB]) may affect circulating BUN levels.

Urinalysis and Urine Characteristics

Urine inspection can reveal abnormal cloudiness, color, and unexpected odors. Detailed descriptions of urine examination are available[24]; therefore, only a summary is provided here. Cloudy urine is due to suspended elements such as white or red blood cells and/or crystals. Lightly centrifuged urine sediment will normally contain 80 ± 20 mg of protein per day and up to two red blood cells per high-power field (400×); higher levels of red blood cells or protein reflect abnormal kidney function. Urine protein electrophoresis can differentiate proteinuria from a glomerular (filtering), tubular (reuptake), overflow (supply that saturates the reuptake system), or tissue (e.g., kidney inflammation) abnormality.[25] Notably, intraoperative use of lysine analog antifibrinolytic agents causes a temporary reversible tubular proteinuria. In contrast, color changes reflect dissolved substances; this occurs most commonly with dehydration, but other causes include food colorings, drugs, and liver disease (e.g., bilirubin). Unusual odors are less common but can also be diagnostic (e.g., maple syrup urine disease). Chromogenic "dipstick" chemical tests can determine urine pH and provide a semiquantitative analysis of protein, blood, nitrites, leukocyte esterase, glucose, ketones, urobilinogen, and bilirubin. In addition, microscopy can identify crystals, cells, tubular casts, and bacteria.

Urine *specific gravity* (the weight of urine relative to distilled water) normally ranges between 1.001 and 1.035, and can be used as a surrogate for osmolarity (normal 50 to 1,000 mOsm/kg), with 1.010 reflecting a specific gravity similar to that of plasma. High specific gravity (>1.018) implies preserved kidney concentrating ability, unless high levels of glucose, protein, or contrast dye injection have raised specific gravity without significantly changing osmolarity.

Although poor urine output (e.g., <400 mL urine/24 hr) may reflect hypovolemia or impending *prerenal* renal failure, a majority of perioperative AKI episodes develop in the absence of oliguria.[4] The normal response to hypovolemia is kidney solute retention; fluid and electrolyte retention produces a concentrated urine with a low sodium content (<20 mEq/L). In contrast, impaired concentrating ability due to AKI causes urine to approach plasma osmolarity (isosthenuria) with a higher sodium content (>40 mEq/L). The kidneys' ability to retain electrolytes is also reflected in the *fractional excretion of sodium* (FE_{Na}), a test that uses a spot sample of urine and blood to compare sodium and creatinine excretion; this test can be useful to distinguish hypovolemia and kidney injury:

$$FE_{Na} = U_{Na}/P_{Na} \times P_{Cr}/U_{Cr} \times 100$$

where U_{Na} = urine sodium, P_{Na} = plasma sodium, U_{Cr} = urine creatinine, and P_{Cr} = plasma creatinine.

FE_{Na} <1% implies that sodium is being normally conserved while values above 1% are consistent with acute tubular necrosis (ATN).

Perioperative Nephrology

Pathophysiology

Altered kidney function can be thought of as a clinical continuum ranging from the normal compensatory changes seen during stress to frank renal failure. Clinically, there is considerable overlap between compensated and decompensated kidney dysfunctional states. The kidney under stress reacts in a predictable manner to help restore intravascular volume and maintain blood pressure. The sympathetic nervous system reacts to trauma, shock, or pain by releasing norepinephrine, which acts much like angiotensin II on the renal arterioles. Norepinephrine also activates the renin–
5 angiotensin–aldosterone system and causes ADH release. The net result of modest activity of the stress response system is a shift of blood flow from the kidney cortex to the medulla, avid sodium and water reabsorption, and decreased urine output (i.e., acute kidney "success"). A more intense stress response may induce a decrease in RBF and GFR by causing afferent arteriolar constriction. If this extreme situation is not reversed, ischemic damage to the kidney may result, and AKI and failure may become clinically manifest.

Electrolyte Disorders

Disorders of Sodium Balance

Hyponatremia is the most commonly occurring electrolyte disorder[26,27] (see also Chapter 14). Symptoms rarely occur unless sodium values are <125 mmol/L, and these include a spectrum ranging from anorexia, nausea, and lethargy to convulsions, dysrhythmias, coma, and even death due to osmotic brain swelling.[28–30] Hyponatremia may occur in the setting of an expanded (e.g., transurethral resection [TUR] syndrome), normal, or contracted extracellular fluid volume, and both volume status and urinary sodium concentration are key markers in differentiating the large number of potential causes of hyponatremia. If water excess is a reason for hyponatremia, a dilute urine with a sodium concentration >20 mmol/L is expected. Conversely, avid kidney sodium retention (urine sodium <20 mmol/L) suggests sodium loss as a cause. If hyponatremia is acute, the risk of neurologic complications is higher, and cautious treatment is indicated to prevent cerebral edema and seizures. This should be accomplished with intravenous hypertonic saline and furosemide to enhance water excretion and prevent sodium overload (see transurethral resection syndrome section).

Hypernatremia (serum sodium >145 mmol/L) is generally the result of sodium gain or water loss, most commonly the latter. Dehydration of brain tissue can cause symptoms ranging from confusion to convulsions and coma. In cases of hypernatremia, laboratory studies often show evidence of hemoconcentration (increased hematocrit and serum protein concentrations). In addition, urine output is usually low (<500 mL/day) and hyperosmolar (>1,000 mOsm), with very low urinary sodium concentration and evidence of prerenal failure (elevations of BUN and serum creatinine). Occasionally, the urine is not maximally concentrated, suggesting an osmotic diuresis or an intrinsic kidney disorder such as diabetes insipidus. The primary goal of treatment is restoration of serum tonicity, which can be achieved with isotonic or hypotonic parenteral fluids and/or diuretics unless irreversible kidney injury is present, in which situation dialysis may be necessary.

Disorders of Potassium Balance

Even minor variations in serum potassium concentration can lead to symptoms such as skeletal muscle weakness, gastrointestinal ileus, myocardial depression, malignant ventricular dysrhythmias, and asystole. Nearly 98% of total body potassium is intracellular. Circulating potassium levels are tightly controlled via kidney and gastrointestinal excretion and reabsorption, but potassium also moves between the intra- and extracellular compartments under the influence of insulin and β_2-adrenoceptors. In the kidney, 70% of potassium reabsorption occurs in the proximal tubule and another 15% to 20% in the loop of Henle. The collecting duct is responsible for potassium excretion under the influence of aldosterone.

Hypokalemia may be due to a net potassium deficiency or transfer of extracellular potassium to the intracellular space. Notably, total body depletion may exist even with normal extracellular potassium levels (e.g., diabetic ketoacidosis). Causes of hypokalemia include extrarenal loss (e.g., vomiting, diarrhea), kidney loss (impaired processing due to drugs, hormones, or inherited kidney abnormalities), potassium shifts between the extra- and intracellular spaces (e.g., insulin therapy), and, occasionally, inadequate intake. Clinical manifestations of hypokalemia include ECG changes (flattened T waves—"no pot, no T," U waves, prodysrhythmic state) and skeletal muscle weakness. Hypokalemia treatment involves supplementation by either intravenous or oral route; however, extreme caution should be used with intravenous potassium administration since overly rapid delivery can cause hyperkalemic cardiac arrest.

If a patient has *hyperkalemia* (elevated serum potassium level >5.5 mEq/L), it is important to consider the duration of the condition since chronic hyperkalemia is far better tolerated than an acute rise. Other than laboratory artifacts (e.g., hemolyzed sample), causes of hyperkalemia include abnormal kidney excretion, abnormal cellular potassium release, or abnormal distribution between the intracellular and the extracellular space. Clinical manifestations of acute hyperkalemia include a range of ECG changes that can be clearly observed with the infusion of high potassium cardioplegia immediately following aortic cross clamp application during cardiac surgery. Peaked T waves, ST-segment depression, and shortened QT interval are soon followed by manifestations of severe hyperkalemia including QRS complex widening, prolonged PR interval, disappearance of the P wave, sine wave QRS, ventricular fibrillation, and asystole.

Disorders of Calcium, Magnesium, and Phosphorus

Most of a grown adult's 1 to 2 kg of calcium is in bone (98%), with the remaining 2% in one of the three forms: Ionized, chelated, or protein-bound. Normal serum calcium values range between 8.5 and 10.2 mg/dL, but only the ionized fraction (50%) is biologically active and precisely regulated. Ionized extracellular calcium concentration (iCa^{++}) is controlled by the combined actions of parathyroid hormone (PTH), calcitonin, and vitamin D and further modulated by dietary and environmental factors. The clinical manifestations of *hypocalcemia* include cramping, digital numbness, laryngospasm, carpopedal spasm, bronchospasm, seizures, and respiratory arrest. A positive Chvostek sign (facial muscle twitching in response to tapping the facial nerve) or Trousseau sign (carpal spasm induced by brachial artery occlusion) are the classic hallmarks of hypocalcemia but in practice are often absent. Mental status changes, including irritability, depression, and impaired cognition, may also occur. Cardiac manifestations include QT interval prolongation and dysrhythmias. Hypocalcemia may be due to several mechanisms, including a decrease in PTH secretion or action, reduced vitamin D synthesis or action, resistance of bone to PTH or vitamin D effects, or calcium sequestration. Acute hypocalcemia due to citrate toxicity can develop from rapid infusion of citrate-stored packed red blood cells, particularly with citrate accumulation during the anhepatic phase of liver transplant procedures. Parathyroidectomy, either selectively or as a complication of thyroidectomy during neck surgery, can acutely reduce PTH levels and precipitate hypocalcemia. Citrate used for regional anticoagulation with chronic dialysis can also cause hypocalcemia and may also lead to hypomagnesemia from decreased PTH secretion. Hypocalcemia due to reduced serum protein levels is physiologically unimportant. Clinical symptoms of *hypercalcemia* correlate with its acuity and include constipation, nausea and vomiting, drowsiness, lethargy, weakness, stupor, and coma. Cardiovascular manifestations may include hypertension, shortened QT interval, heart block, and other dysrhythmias. The most frequent causes of hypercalcemia are primary hyperparathyroidism and malignancy. Other causes include thiazide (increased kidney calcium reabsorption) or lithium (inhibits PTH release) therapy and rarer medical conditions including granulomatous disease, thyrotoxicosis, and multiple endocrine neoplasia (MEN) types I and II.

Magnesium is a multifunctional cation that is found primarily in the intracellular space. As extracellular magnesium represents only 0.3% of total (mainly intracellular) stores, normal serum levels (1.6 to 2.2 mg/dL) are a poor reflection of total body magnesium. *Hypomagnesemia* (<1.6 mg/dL) may sometimes be asymptomatic, but clinically important problems can and do manifest, including neuromuscular, cardiac, neurologic, and related electrolytic (hypokalemia and hypocalcemia) abnormalities. Causes of hypomagnesemia can be divided in four broad categories: Decreased intake, gastrointestinal loss, kidney loss, and redistribution. Nutritional hypomagnesemia can result from malabsorption syndromes in patients receiving parenteral nutrition, and it is also present in 25% of alcoholics. Redistribution occurs with acute pancreatitis, administration of catecholamines, and in "hungry bone syndrome" after parathyroidectomy.[31] Magnesium can be supplemented orally or via the parenteral route. Clinical manifestations of *hypermagnesemia* (>4 to 6 mg/dL) are serious and potentially fatal. Minor symptoms include hypotension, nausea, vomiting, facial flushing, urinary retention, and ileus. In more extreme cases, flaccid skeletal muscular paralysis, hyporeflexia, bradycardia, bradydysrhythmias, respiratory depression, coma, and cardiac arrest may occur. Hypermagnesemia generally occurs in two clinical settings: compromised kidney function (GFR <20 mL/min) and excessive magnesium intake (e.g., excessive intravenous therapy in preeclampsia). Although mild hypermagnesemia in the setting of normal kidney function can be treated with supportive care and withdrawal of the cause, in some cases dialysis is necessary.

Phosphorus is a major intracellular anion that plays a role in regulation of glycolysis, ammoniagenesis, and calcium homeostasis and is an essential component of adenosine triphosphate and red blood cell 2,3-diphosphoglyceric acid synthesis. *Hypophosphatemia* is clinically more important than hyperphosphatemia and can result in symptoms including muscle weakness, respiratory failure, and difficulty in weaning critically ill patients from mechanical ventilation when serum levels are <0.32 mmol/L. In addition, low phosphate levels may diminish oxygen delivery to tissues and rarely cause hemolysis. Hypophosphatemia can result from intracellular redistribution (from catecholamine therapy), from inadequate intake or absorption secondary to alcoholism or malnutrition, or from increased kidney or gastrointestinal losses.[32] Intravenous and oral supplementation can be used to treat hypophosphatemia. *Hyperphosphatemia* (>5 mg/dL) is generally related to accompanying hypocalcemia although increased phosphate levels may also lead to calcium precipitation and decreased intestinal calcium absorption. Significantly elevated serum phosphate levels are most commonly due to reduced excretion from kidney insufficiency but can also result from excess intake or redistribution of intracellular phosphorus. Treatment of chronic hyperphosphatemia includes dietary phosphate restriction and oral phosphate binders.

Acid–Base Disorders

The primary determinant of serum pH is the balance between plasma bicarbonate (HCO_3^-) concentration and the PCO_2 in the extracellular space. Acid–base homeostasis involves tight regulation of HCO_3^- and $PaCO_2$. Primary extracellular pH derangements due to abnormal bicarbonate reabsorption and proton (H^+) elimination by the kidney lead to metabolic acidosis or alkalosis, while factors that abnormally affect respiratory drive influence $PaCO_2$, leading to respiratory acidosis or alkalosis. Because combined problems are often seen in perioperative critically ill patients, an approach to both "pure" and "mixed" acid–base disorders is presented here.

Metabolic Acidosis

The *anion gap* (AG) represents the total serum concentration of unmeasured anions and can be calculated as $AG = (Na^+ + K^+) - (HCO_3^- + Cl^-)$. It allows differentiation of the causes of metabolic acidosis into normal AG (12 ± 4) and increased AG (>16 mmol/L) varieties. Conditions that cause an increase in negatively charged ions other than bicarbonate and chloride (e.g., lactate, salicylate) increase the AG. In contrast, non-AG metabolic acidosis results from kidney or gastrointestinal HCO_3^- loss and is associated with high chloride levels (hyperchloremic metabolic acidosis). The usual compensatory response to all types of metabolic acidoses is hyperventilation, which leads to a partial pH correction toward normal. Winter formula predicts expected $PaCO_2$ for a metabolic acidosis as follows: $PaCO_2 = (1.5 \times HCO_3^-) + 8$.

Metabolic Alkalosis

Metabolic alkalosis is a common primary acid–base disturbance associated with increased plasma HCO_3^-. Increased extracellular HCO_3^- is due to a net loss of H^+ and/or addition of HCO_3^-. The most common cause of metabolic alkalosis is gastrointestinal acid loss due to vomiting or nasogastric suctioning; the resulting hypovolemia leads to secretion of renin and aldosterone and enhanced absorption of HCO_3^-. Thiazides and loop diuretics both induce a net loss of chloride and free water and can cause a volume "contraction" alkalosis.

Respiratory Acidosis

If the lungs fail to eliminate CO_2, hypercapnia and respiratory acidosis result, characterized by increased $PaCO_2$ and decreased blood pH. Acute and chronic causes can be differentiated by examining arterial pH, $PaCO_2$, and HCO_3^- values. In the early phase of respiratory acidosis, increased $PaCO_2$ stimulates kidney generation and secretion of H^+. The kidneys continue to adapt to the increased pH through greater titratable acid excretion (e.g., ammonium) and HCO_3^- generation. Therefore, acute respiratory acidosis is characterized by an elevated $PaCO_2$, acidemia, and a relatively normal HCO_3^-. In contrast, chronic respiratory acidosis is associated with an elevated HCO_3^- (often accompanied by a relatively normal pH) due to kidney compensation.

Respiratory Alkalosis

Increased minute ventilation is the primary cause of respiratory alkalosis, characterized by decreased $PaCO_2$ and increased pH. Patients with acute, uncompensated respiratory alkalosis have normal plasma HCO_3^-. In chronic respiratory alkalosis, kidney compensation leads to decreased plasma HCO_3^-. The causes of respiratory alkalosis relate to abnormal respiratory drive from stimulants or toxins (e.g., salicylate, caffeine, nicotine, progesterone), central nervous system abnormalities (e.g., anxiety, stroke, increased intracranial pressure), pulmonary abnormalities (e.g., pulmonary embolism, pneumonia), mechanical hyperventilation, or systemic conditions such as liver failure and sepsis.

Mixed Acid–Base Disorders

It is not uncommon for a metabolic derangement to coexist with a respiratory derangement, particularly in intensive care patients. A general approach to the diagnosis of mixed acid–base disorders requires a step-wise approach that begins with a focused history and physical examination. An arterial blood gas and a concurrent serum chemistry panel (including Na^+, K^+, Cl^-, and total CO_2 concentrations) should also be obtained, and the use of an acid–base map may help differentiate simple from mixed disorders (Fig. 50-4).

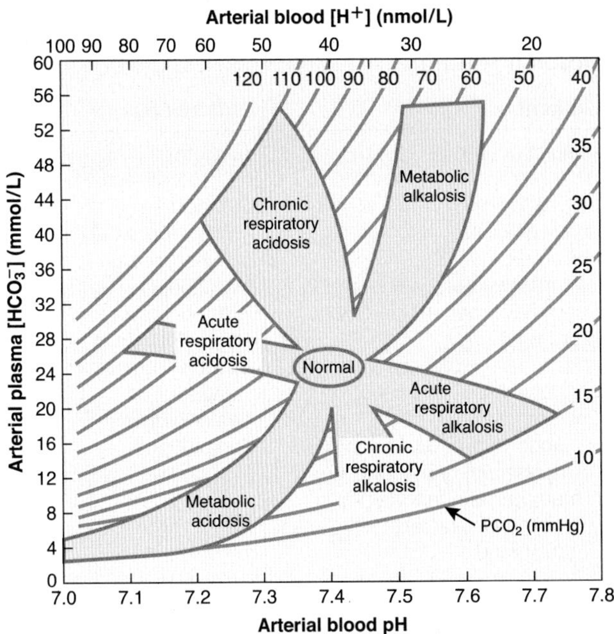

Figure 50-4 Acid–base map. Plotting the PCO_2 and H^+ (from the arterial blood gas) against plasma HCO_3^- (from the serum chemistry panel) for a patient can identify simple acid–base disorders. When mixed disorders exist, values may fall outside the shaded areas. (Reprinted with permission from DuBose TD Jr. Acid-base disorders. In: Brenner BM, ed., *Brenner & Rector's The Kidney*. 7th ed. Philadelphia, PA: WB Saunders; 2004:938.)

Acute Kidney Conditions

Acute Kidney Injury

Acute kidney injury (AKI) is now the preferred term for an acute deterioration in kidney function. It is associated with a decline in glomerular filtration and results in inability of the kidneys to excrete nitrogenous and other wastes. This manifests as an accumulation of creatinine and urea in the blood (uremia) and is often accompanied by reduced urine production, although nonoliguric forms of postoperative AKI are common.[33] In surgical patients, ATN is the most common cause of AKI. AKI frequently occurs in the setting of critical illness with multiple organ failure when the
6 mortality is alarmingly high (up to 80%).[34] Notably, extracorporeal kidney support appears to have little impact in altering the generally poor outcome associated with AKI in critically ill surgical patients.[34] Even studies that advocate the use of extracorporeal technology report mortality of between 50% and 70%.[29,30,35–37]

AKI can be caused by *prerenal* factors causing kidney hypoperfusion, *intrinsic* kidney causes, or *postrenal* causes (obstructive uropathy). There are many pathophysiologic similarities between the various causes of kidney injury.

Prerenal Azotemia

Prerenal azotemia is the increase in BUN associated with kidney hypoperfusion or ischemia that has not yet caused kidney parenchymal damage. The metabolically active cells of the medullary thick ascending limb of the loop of Henle are especially vulnerable to hypoxic damage because of their relatively high oxygen consumption.[38] AKI ensues when necrosis of tubular cells releases debris into the tubules, causing flow obstruction, increased tubular back pressure, and leak of tubular fluid. Often, prerenal AKI is precipitated in patients with pre-existing kidney vasoconstriction (e.g., volume depletion, heart failure, or sepsis) by nephrotoxin exposure or further reductions in cardiac output.

Intrinsic Acute Kidney Injury

The term *intrinsic* not only implies a primary kidney cause of AKI but also includes AKI due to ischemia, nephrotoxins, and kidney parenchymal diseases. ATN remains the most common ischemic lesion and represents an extension of prerenal azotemia, whereas cortical necrosis may follow a massive renovascular insult such as prolonged suprarenal aortic clamping or renal artery embolism. Nephrotoxins often act in concert with hypoperfusion or underlying kidney vasoconstrictive states to damage kidney tubules or the microvasculature. Several common nephrotoxins, some of which are difficult to avoid in a hospitalized patient population, are listed in Table 50-1.

Postrenal Acute Kidney Injury (Obstructive Uropathy)

Downstream obstruction of the urinary collecting system is the least common pathway to established AKI, accounting for <10% of cases.[39] Because it can generally be corrected, it is extremely important to exclude with a kidney ultrasound examination as a source of AKI. The obstructing lesion may occur at any level of the collecting system, from the kidney pelvis to the distal urethra. Intraluminal

Table 50-1 Nephrotoxins Commonly Found in the Hospital Setting

Exogenous	Endogenous
Antibiotics (aminoglycosides, cephalosporins, amphotericin B, sulfonamide, tetracyclines, vancomycin) Anesthetic agents (methoxyflurane, enflurane) Nonsteroidal anti-inflammatory drugs (aspirin, ibuprofen, naproxen, indomethacin, ketorolac) Chemotherapeutic–immunosuppressive agents (cisplatinum, cyclosporin A, methotrexate, mitomycin, nitrosoureas, tacrolimus) Contrast media	Calcium (hypercalcemia) Uric acid (hyperuricemia and hyperuricosuria) Myoglobin (rhabdomyolysis) Hemoglobin (hemolysis) Bilirubin (obstructive jaundice) Oxalate crystals Paraproteins

pressure rises and is eventually transmitted back to the glomerulus, thereby reducing glomerular filtration pressure and rate.

Nephrotoxins and Perioperative Acute Kidney Injury

Nephrotoxin exposure is a common occurrence in hospitalized patients and frequently plays a role in the cause of AKI in this population. Nephrotoxins may take the form of drugs, nontherapeutic chemicals, heavy metals, poisons, and endogenous compounds (Table 50-1). The nephrotoxins most likely to contribute to kidney dysfunction/failure in the perioperative period are certain antimicrobial and chemotherapeutic–immunosuppressive agents, radiocontrast media, nonsteroidal anti-inflammatory drugs (NSAIDs), and the endogenous heme pigments myoglobin and hemoglobin. These diverse groups of kidney toxins share a common pathophysiologic characteristic: they disturb either kidney oxygen delivery or oxygen utilization and thereby promote kidney ischemia.

Antimicrobial and chemotherapeutic–immunosuppressive agents are effective because they are cellular toxins. When these drugs are filtered, reabsorbed, secreted, and eventually excreted by the kidney, toxic concentrations in kidney cells can be reached. The aminoglycoside antibiotics and amphotericin B are particularly difficult to avoid because they are effective antimicrobials, with few available alternatives. Their effect can be additive with other nephrotoxic factors causing impairment of kidney function. Hypovolemia, fever, kidney vasoconstriction, and concomitant therapy with other nephrotoxic agents should be avoided wherever possible. Electrolyte disorders such as hypercalcemia, hypomagnesemia, hypokalemia, and metabolic acidosis can further enhance nephrotoxic damage to the kidney.

Cyclosporin A and tacrolimus are indispensable components of many immunosuppressive drug regimens, but in combination with other nephrotoxins and clinical factors, they can cause acute and exacerbate chronic kidney injuries in transplant recipients.[36]

Yacoub and colleagues suggest that angiotensin-converting enzyme (ACE) inhibitors and angiotensin receptor blockers (ARBs) should not be given for 48 hours prior to routine cardiac surgery. In their meta-analysis of 29 retrospective studies (>50,000 procedures) these authors linked chronic ACE inhibitor or ARB use until the day of surgery with higher mortality risk (20%; $P = .005$) and AKI rates (17%; $P = .04$).[40] ACE inhibitors and ARBs are also associated with increased AKI risk in patients receiving diuretic therapy; those with volume depletion, CHF, or diabetes; and in the elderly.[41,42] Finally, while ACE inhibitors and ARBs are sometimes prescribed to slow the progression of CKD, their use with NSAIDs and other nephrotoxic agents such as cyclosporine, tacrolimus, and aprotinin are also associated with increased perioperative AKI risk.[41,43,44]

Discontinuing loop diuretic therapy on the day prior to surgery should also receive careful consideration. Two studies have linked chronic diuretic therapy with postoperative AKI,[45,46] with one differentiating loop (not thiazide) diuretics as having higher AKI and mortality risk.[46] Other retrospective studies report high furosemide dose as a risk factor for AKI following contrast exposure during coronary angiography and then subsequent off-pump cardiac surgery.[47] Short-term furosemide also worsened AKI in one randomized cardiac surgery trial and a retrospective study of noncardiac surgery patients.[48,49]

In contradistinction, patients taking statins prior to their CABG (but not isolated valve) surgery had lower dialysis and mortality rates in a meta-analysis of 17 studies (>47,000 patients) addressing this issue.[50]

Radiocontrast media might pose a threat to kidney function of patients with diabetic nephropathy, pre-existing kidney vasoconstriction (heart failure, hypovolemia), or kidney insufficiency.[51] Radiocontrast dye has effects on kidney function that develop 24 to 48 hours after exposure and peak at 3 to 5 days. Measures that may prevent AKI or lessen the severity of kidney damage include prehydration, smaller contrast doses, and judicious withholding of other nephrotoxins, such as NSAIDs. Hu and colleagues concluded that nonemergent cardiac procedures should be delayed for 24 hours after contrast administration to reduce the incidence of postoperative AKI in their meta-analysis of eight retrospective studies (>11,000 patients receiving dye within three days preoperatively).[52] However, it should be noted that a meta-analysis and a large retrospective propensity-matched cohort analysis of emergency room patients found no association with contrast administration and AKI incidence for patients undergoing diagnostic computed tomography (CT) scans.[53,54] Thus, administration of limited doses of newer contrast agents for diagnostic CT scans appears to be relatively AKI risk-free; although caution should still be exercised in patients receiving large contrast loads during angiography—ideally such exposures should be separated from surgery by at least 24 hours.

NSAIDs produce reversible inhibition of prostaglandin synthesis and are well-known nephrotoxins.[55] Except in cases of massive overdose, NSAIDs produce kidney dysfunction only in patients with coexisting kidney hypoperfusion or vasoconstriction. Advanced age, hypovolemia, end-stage hepatic disease, heart failure, sepsis, chronic renal insufficiency, and major surgery are risk factors for development of NSAID-induced AKI.[56]

Myoglobin and hemoglobin are both capable of causing AKI in critically ill surgical patients. Myoglobin seems to be a more potent nephrotoxin than hemoglobin because it is more readily filtered at the glomerulus and can be reabsorbed by the kidney tubules, where it chelates nitric oxide and thus induces medullary vasoconstriction and ischemia.[57] Hypovolemia and acidemia potentiate the toxicity of both pigments. Reduced intravascular volume causes a decrease in RBF and GFR, which results in a smaller volume of tubular fluid with a relatively higher concentration of pigment. There is also evidence suggesting that pigment precipitation inside the tubular lumen is enhanced under acidotic conditions and that tubular obstruction plays a role in the pathogenesis of AKI.[57,58]

Preventive treatment of pigment-induced AKI is directed at increasing RBF and tubular (urine) flow while correcting any existing acidosis. These goals may be accomplished by expanding the intravascular fluid volume with crystalloid infusion, stimulating an osmotic diuresis with mannitol, and increasing the urine pH with intravenous bicarbonate therapy.[59] Adequate systemic resuscitation from shock is a prerequisite if AKI is to be avoided, especially in massive crush injuries and electrical burns. Though high-quality evidence for its efficacy is lacking, forced mannitol-alkali diuresis is recommended as the second step in the preventive treatment of myoglobinuria, with urine flow rates of up to 300 mL/hr and a urine pH of >6.5 advocated for patients with massive crush injuries.[59]

The nephrotoxicity of volatile agents remains controversial. Inhalation anesthetics such as enflurane, isoflurane, and sevoflurane can generate free fluoride ions during their metabolism, which (when levels are >50 mM/L) may cause polyuric AKI by interfering with tubular concentrating ability. However, peak fluoride levels during administration of these agents seldom reach toxic levels, and there are few reports describing volatile agent–induced nephrotoxicity.[60] The potential of sevoflurane-induced nephrotoxicity has been related to the production of compound A during prolonged, low fresh gas flow, sevoflurane anesthesia.[61] Although there are insufficient data to conclude that sevoflurane-induced kidney injury occurs in the human population, even during low gas flow anesthesia, it is probably prudent to maintain a fresh gas flow of at least 2 L/min formation during sevoflurane anesthesia.[62]

Fluid selection for resuscitation has also been associated with nephrotoxicity. Evidence of increased rates of renal replacement therapy in critically ill and septic patients receiving hydroxyethyl starches resulted in the elimination of these fluids from routine clinical practice.[63,64] Crystalloid selection, between balanced solutions (such as lactated Ringer solution and Plasma-Lyte A) versus 0.9% "normal" saline also impacts kidney associated adverse events. In noncritically ill patients, balanced crystalloids were associated with lower incidences of major adverse kidney events within 30 days than normal saline.[65] In critically ill adults, use of balanced crystalloids also resulted in lower rates of new renal replacement therapy or persistent kidney dysfunction, when compared with normal saline.[66] In addition, excessive use of normal saline (termed "chloride-liberal" strategy) was attributed with higher risks of AKI and renal replacement therapy compared to a chloride-restrictive strategy in a prospective study of 1,543 critically ill patients.[67]

Not only the fluid type, but also the amount can influence the development of AKI. It is well known that kidney hypoperfusion can lead to AKI, however, fluid overload can also worsen kidney injury through intra-abdominal hypertension and venous and interstitial congestion within the kidney.[68] In addition, a meta-analysis examining kidney function in randomized controlled perioperative goal-directed therapy (GDT) studies revealed a very modest role for fluid management in effective GDT protocols, with the most effective reduction in AKI rates coming from significant inotropic intervention and less fluid resuscitation.[69] Thus, optimal fluid management in the perioperative period, both in the type and amount of fluid, has significant effects on kidney function.

Chronic Kidney Disease

Patients with nondialysis-dependent CKD are at increased risk of developing *end-stage renal disease* (ESRD). ESRD is the term used to describe a clinical syndrome characterized by kidney dysfunction that would prove fatal without renal replacement therapy. These patients have GFR values <25% of normal. Less impaired kidney function may be categorized as chronic renal insufficiency (25% to 40% of normal GFR) or decreased kidney reserve (60% to 75% of normal GFR). Patients with decreased kidney reserve are sometimes asymptomatic and frequently do not have elevated blood levels of creatinine or urea. However, established kidney insufficiency often results in patently abnormal serum creatinine and BUN values, but nocturia (due to reduced concentrating ability) may be the only symptom.

Table 50-2 Factors Contributing to Hyperkalemia in Chronic Renal Failure

Potassium Intake
Increased dietary intake
Exogenous IV supplementation
Potassium salts of drugs
Sodium substitutes
Blood transfusion
Gastrointestinal hemorrhage
Potassium Release from Intracellular Stores
Increased catabolism, sepsis
Metabolic acidosis
β-Adrenergic blocking agents
Digitalis intoxication (Na–K-ATPase inhibition)
Insulin deficiency
Succinylcholine
Potassium Excretion
Acute decrease in GFR
Constipation
Potassium-sparing diuretics
Angiotensin-converting enzyme inhibitors (decreased aldosterone secretion)
Heparin (decreased aldosterone effect)

IV, intravenous; Na–K-ATPase, Na–K-adenosine triphosphatase; GFR, glomerular filtration rate.

The *uremic syndrome* represents an extreme form of chronic renal failure, which occurs as the surviving nephron population and GFR decreases below 10% of normal. It results in inability of the kidney to perform its two major functions: Regulation of the volume and composition of the extracellular fluid and excretion of waste products. Water balance in ESRD becomes difficult to manage because the number of functioning nephrons is too small either to concentrate or to fully dilute the urine. This results in failure both to conserve water and to excrete excess water. Patients with uremic syndrome often require frequent or continuous dialysis.

Life-threatening hyperkalemia may occur in CKD because of slower-than-normal potassium clearance. Situations predisposing patients with kidney failure to hyperkalemia are presented in Table 50-2. Derangements in calcium, magnesium, and phosphorus metabolism are also commonly seen in CKD (Table 50-3).

Metabolic acidosis occurs in two forms in ESRD: A hyperchloremic, normal AG acidosis and a high AG acidosis from inability to excrete titratable acids. Both render patients susceptible to an endogenous acid load such as may occur in shock states, hypovolemia, or with an increase in catabolism.

Cardiovascular complications of the uremic syndrome are primarily due to volume overload, high renin–angiotensin activity, autonomic nervous system hyperactivity, acidosis, and electrolyte disturbances. Hypertension due to extracellular fluid volume expansion, autonomic factors, and hyperreninemia is an almost universal finding in ESRD. Together with volume overload, acidemia, anemia, and possibly the presence of high-flow arteriovenous fistulae created for dialysis access, hypertension may contribute to the development of myocardial dysfunction and

Table 50-3 The Uremic Syndrome

Water Homeostasis
Extracellular fluid expansion
Electrolyte and Acid–base
Hyponatremia
Hyperkalemia
Hypercalcemia or hypocalcemia
Hyperphosphatemia
Hypermagnesemia
Metabolic acidosis
Cardiovascular
Heart failure
Hypertension
Pericarditis
Myocardial dysfunction
Dysrhythmias
Respiratory
Pulmonary edema
Central hyperventilation
Hematologic
Anemia
Platelet hemostatic defect
Immunologic
Cell-mediated and humoral immunity defects
Gastrointestinal
Delayed gastric emptying, anorexia, nausea, vomiting, hiccups, upper gastrointestinal tract inflammation/hemorrhage
Neuromuscular
Encephalopathy, seizures, tremors, myoclonus
Sensory and motor polyneuropathy
Autonomic dysfunction, decreased baroreceptor responsiveness, dialysis-associated hypotension
Endocrine Metabolism
Renal osteodystrophy
↓ Glucose intolerance
Hypertriglyceridemia, ↑ atherosclerosis

heart failure. Pericarditis may occur secondary to uremia or dialysis, with pericardial tamponade developing in 20% of the latter group.[70] Pulmonary problems associated with CKD are limited to changes in lung water and control of ventilation. Pulmonary edema and restrictive pulmonary dysfunction are commonly seen in patients with kidney failure and are usually responsive to dialysis. Hypervolemia, heart failure, reduced serum oncotic pressure, and increased pulmonary capillary permeability are relevant factors in the development of pulmonary edema. Chronic metabolic acidosis may also be responsible for the hyperventilation seen in patients with ESRD, but increased lung water and poor pulmonary compliance can also stimulate hyperventilation.

The anemia of CKD occurs as a result of reduced levels of erythropoietin, red cell damage, ongoing gastrointestinal blood loss, and iron or vitamin deficiencies. Platelet dysfunction may aggravate blood loss, but it is responsive to dialysis, cryoprecipitate administration, and desmopressin acetate (or 1-deamino-8-D-arginine vasopressin [DDAVP]). Acquired defects in both cellular and humoral immunity probably account for the high prevalence of serious infections (60%) and high mortality from sepsis in CKD (30%).

Drug Prescribing in Renal Failure

If a drug depends solely on the kidney for clearance, then a simple approach to prescribing might involve a calculated percentage reduction in drug dosage that matches the reduction in GFR. Although GFR can be accurately measured, an estimated clearance derived from serum creatinine is usually adequate for these purposes. Unfortunately, clearance of most medications involves a more complex combination of both hepatic and kidney functions, and drug level measurement or algorithms for specific drugs are often recommended.

AKI may affect absorption of a drug. For example, a reduced first-pass effect through the gastrointestinal tract and liver is associated with increased serum levels of oral β-blockers and opioids in patients with AKI. Also, an increase in the volume of distribution is seen in most patients with CKD due to increased plasma volume and decreased plasma protein binding. However, plasma protein binding is highly variable, with acidic drugs having reduced binding and basic agents (e.g., amide local anesthetics) having increased binding. Importantly, for drugs with less binding, "normal" drug levels may reflect dangerously high active (unbound) drug levels. For example, therapeutic phenytoin levels are typically reported as being in the range of 10 to 20 mg/mL normally but 4 to 10 mg/mL in cases of renal failure. Finally, hepatic metabolism of drugs is difficult to predict in the setting of renal failure because some hepatic enzymes are inhibited whereas others are induced, and accompanying liver disorders may alter the relationship of drug clearance with GFR.

Anesthetic Agents in Renal Failure

Halogenated volatile anesthetics, with the historically important exceptions of methoxyflurane and possibly enflurane, do not directly cause kidney dysfunction or interfere with the normal compensatory mechanisms activated by the stress response. Though now rarely used except as an inhaled analgesic in some countries, nephrotoxicity of methoxyflurane appears to be due to its metabolism, which results in release of the fluoride ions believed responsible for the kidney injury.[71] It has been suggested that kidney, not hepatic, metabolism of methoxyflurane may be responsible for generating fluoride ions locally that contribute to nephrotoxicity.[72] Enflurane nephrotoxicity may also occur[73] but is of minor clinical importance, even in patients with pre-existing kidney dysfunction. Although direct anesthetic effects on the kidney are usually not harmful, indirect effects may combine with hypovolemia, shock, nephrotoxin exposure, or other kidney vasoconstrictive states to produce kidney dysfunction. If the chosen anesthetic technique causes a protracted reduction in cardiac output or sustained hypotension that coincides with a period of intense kidney vasoconstriction, kidney dysfunction or failure could result. This is true for either general or regional anesthesia. There are no comparative studies demonstrating superior kidney protection or improved kidney outcome with general versus regional anesthesia.

Significant kidney impairment may affect the disposition, metabolism, and excretion of the commonly used anesthetic agents. Inhalation anesthetics are, of course, an exception to the rule that drugs with central nervous system activity (which generally are lipid soluble) must be converted to more hydrophilic compounds by the liver before being excreted by the kidney. The water-soluble metabolites of agents that are not inhaled may accumulate in renal failure and display prolonged pharmacodynamic effects if they possess even a small percentage of the pharmacologic activity of the parent drug. Drugs that are eliminated unchanged by the kidneys (e.g., certain nondepolarizing muscle relaxants, the cholinesterase inhibitors, many antibiotics, digoxin) have a prolonged elimination half-life when given to patients with kidney failure. Many drugs used in anesthesia are highly protein-bound and may demonstrate exaggerated clinical effects when protein binding is reduced by uremia.

Induction Agents and Sedatives

Although now rarely used, sodium thiopental serves as a good illustrative example of how reduced protein binding in CKD may affect the clinical use of an anesthetic agent. Burch and Stanski[74] showed that the free fraction of an induction dose of thiopental is almost doubled in patients with renal failure. This accounts for the exaggerated clinical effects seen with thiopental in CKD patients and the substantial reduction in the necessary induction dose of this agent in uremic patients when compared with patients with normal kidney function.

Ketamine is less extensively protein-bound than thiopental, and renal failure appears to have less influence on its free fraction. Redistribution and hepatic metabolism are largely responsible for termination of the anesthetic effects, with <3% of the drug excreted unchanged in the urine. Norketamine, the major metabolite, has one-third the pharmacologic activity of the parent drug and is further metabolized before it is excreted by the kidney.[75]

Etomidate, although only 75% protein-bound in normal patients, has a larger free fraction in patients with ESRD.[76] The decrease in protein binding does not seem to alter the clinical effects of an etomidate anesthetic induction in patients with renal failure.

Propofol undergoes extensive, rapid hepatic biotransformation to inactive metabolites that are renally excreted. Its pharmacokinetics appear to be unchanged in patients with renal failure,[77] and there are no reports of prolongation of its effects in ESRD.

The benzodiazepines, as a group, are extensively protein-bound. CKD increases the free fraction of benzodiazepines in the plasma, and this potentiates their clinical effect. Certain benzodiazepine metabolites are pharmacologically active and have the potential to accumulate with repeated administration of the parent drug to anephric patients. For example, 60% to 80% of midazolam is excreted as its (active) α-hydroxy metabolite,[78] which accumulates during long-term infusions in patients with renal failure.[78] AKI appears to slow the plasma clearance of midazolam, whereas repeated diazepam or lorazepam administration in CKD may carry a risk of active metabolite-induced sedation. Alprazolam is one of the few drugs related to anesthesia practice that has undergone pharmacodynamic studies in patients with CKD. Schmith et al.[79] found that when decreased protein binding and increased free fraction of alprazolam are taken into account, patients with CKD are actually more sensitive to its sedative effects than healthy persons.

Dexmedetomidine is primarily metabolized in the liver. Volunteers with kidney impairment receiving dexmedetomidine experienced a longer-lasting sedative effect than subjects with normal kidney function. The most likely explanation is that less protein binding of dexmedetomidine occurs in subjects with kidney dysfunction.[80]

Opioids

Single-dose studies of the pharmacokinetics of morphine in renal failure demonstrate no alteration in its disposition. However, chronic administration results in accumulation of its 6-glucuronide metabolite, which has potent analgesic and sedative effects.[81] There is also a decrease in protein binding of morphine in ESRD, which mandates a reduction in its initial dose. Meperidine is remarkable for its neurotoxic, renally excreted metabolite (normeperidine) and is not recommended for use in patients with poor kidney function. Hydromorphone is metabolized to hydromorphone-3-glucuronide, which is excreted by the kidneys. This active metabolite accumulates in patients with renal failure and may cause cognitive dysfunction and myoclonus.[82] Codeine also has the potential for causing prolonged narcosis in patients with renal failure and cannot be recommended for long-term use.[81]

Fentanyl appears to be a better choice of opioid for use in ESRD because of its lack of active metabolites, unchanged free fraction, and short redistribution phase.[83] Small-to-moderate doses, titrated to effect, are well tolerated by uremic patients.

Alfentanil has been shown to have reduced protein binding but no change in its elimination half-life or clearance in ESRD and is extensively metabolized to inactive compounds.[84] Therefore, caution should be exercised in administering a loading dose, but the total dose and infusion dose should be similar to those for patients with normal kidney function. The free fraction of sufentanil is unchanged in ESRD; however, its pharmacokinetics are variable, and it has been reported to cause prolonged narcosis.[85]

Remifentanil is rapidly metabolized by blood and tissue esterases to a weakly active (about 4,600 times less potent) *m*-opioid agonist and renally excreted metabolite, remifentanil acid. Renal failure has no effect on the clearance of remifentanil, but elimination of the principal metabolite, remifentanil acid, is markedly reduced. However, the clinical implications of this metabolite are likely limited.[86]

Muscle Relaxants

Muscle relaxants are the most likely group of drugs used in anesthetic practice to produce prolonged effects in ESRD because of their dependence on kidney excretion (Table 50-4). Only succinylcholine, atracurium, *cis*-atracurium, and mivacurium appear to have minimal kidney excretion of the unchanged parent compound. Most nondepolarizing muscle relaxants must be either hepatically excreted or metabolized to inactive forms in order to terminate their activity. Some muscle relaxants have renally excreted, active metabolites that may contribute to their prolonged duration of action in patients with ESRD. Although the following discussion focuses on the pharmacology of individual muscle relaxants, coexisting acidosis and electrolyte disturbances, as well as drug therapy (e.g., aminoglycosides, diuretics, immunosuppressants, magnesium-containing antacids), may alter the pharmacodynamics of muscle relaxants in patients with renal failure.[87]

Succinylcholine has a long history of use in CKD that has been somewhat confused by conflicting reports of plasma cholinesterase activity in renal failure.[88,89] Provided the serum potassium concentration is not dangerously elevated, its use can be justified as part of a rapid-sequence anesthesia induction technique because its duration of action in ESRD is not significantly prolonged. However, use of a continuous succinylcholine infusion often raises concerns since the major metabolite, succinylmonocholine, is weakly active and excreted by the kidney. The rise in serum potassium following succinylcholine administration (0.5 mEq/L in normal subjects) implies that levels of this electrolyte should be normalized to the best extent possible in patients with renal failure, but clinical suggests that the potassium rise following succinylcholine administration of is usually well tolerated in patients with *chronically* elevated serum potassium levels. Use of the long-acting muscle relaxants doxacurium, pancuronium, and pipecuronium might also be questioned in patients with known kidney insufficiency. In a single-dose study of doxacurium, Cook et al.[90] demonstrated an increased elimination half-life, reduced plasma clearance, and prolonged duration of effect in patients with renal failure. Similar findings have been reported for the pharmacokinetics of pipecuronium. Intermediate-acting muscle relaxants (atracurium, *cis*-atracurium, vecuronium, and rocuronium) have a distinct advantage in ESRD because of their shorter duration. The risk of a clinically significant, prolonged block is much reduced. Atracurium and its derivative, *cis*-atracurium, undergo

Table 50-4 Nondepolarizing Muscle Relaxants in Renal Failure

Drug	% Renal Excretion	Half-life (hr) Normal/ ESRD	Renally Excreted Active Metabolite	Use in ESRD
d-Tubocurarine	60	1.4–2.2	–	Avoid
Metocurine	45–60	6/11.4	–	Avoid
Pancuronium	30	2.3/4–8	+	Avoid
Gallamine	>85	2.5/6–20	–	Avoid
Pipecuronium	37	1.8–2.3/4.4	+	Avoid
Doxacurium	30	1.7/3.7	–	Avoid
Vecuronium	30	0.9/1.4	+	Avoid infusion
Rocuronium	30	1.2–1.6/1.6–1.7	–	Variable duration
Atracurium/*cis*-atracurium	<5	0.3/0.4	–	Normal
Mivacurium	<7	2 min/2 min	–	Duration 1.5 × normal
Rapacuronium	<12	0.5/0.5	++	Normal single dose

ESRD, end-stage renal disease.

enzymatic ester hydrolysis and spontaneous nonenzymatic (Hoffman) degradation with minimal kidney excretion of the parent compound. Their elimination half-life, clearance, and duration of action are not affected by renal failure,[91] nor have they been reported to cause prolonged clinical effects in ESRD. These characteristics strongly support their use in patients with kidney disease. One potential concern is that an atracurium metabolite, laudanosine, may cause seizures in experimental animals and may accumulate with repeated dosing or continuous infusion.[92] However, this has not been realized in intensive care patients with renal failure receiving prolonged infusions of atracurium. Consistent with its greater potency and lower dosing requirements, *cis*-atracurium metabolism results in lower laudanosine blood levels than does atracurium in ESRD patients.

Initial reports suggested that the pharmacokinetics of vecuronium are unchanged in renal failure, but it has subsequently emerged that its duration of action is prolonged as a result of reduced plasma clearance and increased elimination half-life.[91] An intubating dose lasts approximately 50% longer in patients with ESRD.[93] In addition, the active metabolite, 3-desmethylvecuronium accumulates in anephric patients receiving a continuous vecuronium infusion, producing a prolonged neuromuscular blockade.

Rocuronium has a pharmacokinetic profile in normal subjects similar to that of vecuronium.[94] Single-dose pharmacokinetic studies in patients with renal failure have reported conflicting results. Szenohradszky et al.[95] reported that renal failure increased the volume of distribution and elimination half-life of rocuronium but had no effect on its clearance. Cooper et al.[96] found that its clearance was reduced, and the duration of block was widely variable in patients with renal failure, although the mean duration of relaxation and spontaneous recovery was not statistically different from that in control subjects.

The short-acting muscle relaxant mivacurium is enzymatically eliminated by plasma pseudocholinesterase at a somewhat slower rate than succinylcholine. Low pseudocholinesterase activity correlates with slower recovery from a bolus dose of mivacurium in anephric patients.[89] The maintenance infusion dose has been reported to be both lower[97] and similar[98] to that in normal control subjects.

The pharmacokinetics of the clinically available anticholinesterases are affected by renal failure.[99] They have a prolonged duration of action in ESRD because of their heavy reliance on renal excretion. The anticholinergic agents atropine and glycopyrrolate, used in conjunction with the anticholinesterases, are similarly excreted by the kidney. Therefore, no dosage alteration of the anticholinesterases is required when antagonizing neuromuscular blockade in patients with reduced kidney function.

Sugammadex provides a novel approach to the reversal of muscle relaxants. This agent is a modified γ-cyclodextrin that encapsulates aminosteroidal neuromuscular blocking agents (e.g., rocuronium, vecuronium, pancuronium), which leads to a swift decline of free muscle relaxant in the plasma and rapid reversal.[100] Several studies have revealed that sugammadex-rocuronium complexes are cleared more slowly in patients with ESRD and recovery to a train-of-four ratio of 0.9 is prolonged. Despite this altered pharmacokinetic profile of sugammedex, the reversal of neuromuscular blockade by sugammadex was found to still be effective and safe in patients with ESRD as compared with patients with normal kidney function.[101,102]

Diuretic Drugs: Effects and Mechanisms

When salt or water intake exceeds renal and extrarenal losses fluid overload results, leading to excess total body water and usually sodium. Fluid overload may be evenly distributed among the body compartments (e.g., congestive heart failure), or the interstitial space may be increased (i.e., edema) while the circulating blood volume may be normal or even decreased (e.g., posttraumatic or postoperative). Edema results when Starling forces favor passage of fluid into the interstitial space. Fluid overload due to a variety of chronic conditions (congestive heart failure, renal failure, or hepatic cirrhosis) may be first recognized during preoperative assessment and may require that elective surgery be delayed for treatment to reduce operative risk. The first line of therapy for fluid overload that includes all body compartments involves restriction of salt and water ingestion; however, diuretic therapy is often indicated.

The Physiologic Basis of Diuretic Action

Diuretics are typically grouped according to their site and mechanism of action (Fig. 50-5). Under normal conditions, kidney function assures that <1% of the filtered Na^+ load enters the urine

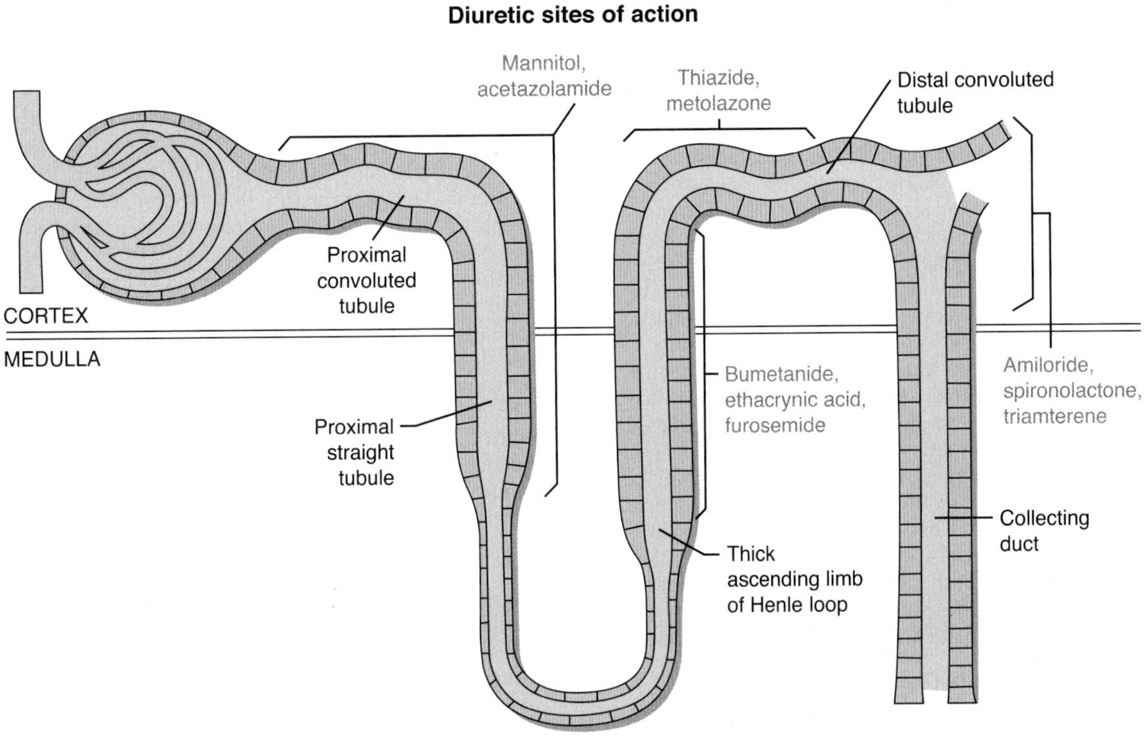

Diuretic sites of action

Figure 50-5 Site of action of commonly available diuretics. (From Mende CW. *Current issues in diuretic therapy*. Hosp Pract. 1990;25(suppl 1):15, reprinted by permission of the Taylor & Francis Ltd, http://www.tandfonline.com.)

(i.e., the FE_{Na} is <1%). The Na^+/K^+-ATPase pump on the basolateral surface (blood side) of kidney tubular cells is primarily responsible for active pumping of Na^+ out of cells into blood in exchange for K^+. This pump causes a net movement of positive charge out of the cell (2 K^+ in, for every 3 Na^+ out) creating an electrochemical gradient that also causes Na^+ to enter the luminal (urine) side of the cell. Kidney tubular cells in different portions of the nephron have different luminal "systems" to allow this Na^+ influx. These systems are the sites of action where the different diuretics work.

Proximal Tubule Diuretics

In the proximal tubule, a specialized luminal transporter exchanges protons (H^+) for sodium ions; the result is sodium reabsorption and acidification of the urine. The excreted H^+ combines with bicarbonate (HCO_3^-) in the tubule to form carbonic acid: $H^+ + HCO_3^- \rightarrow H_2CO_3$. Carbonic acid converts to water (H_2O) and carbon dioxide (CO_2) in a reaction catalyzed by carbonic anhydrase: $H_2CO_3 \rightarrow H_2O + CO_2$. The same enzyme, carbonic anhydrase, allows this reaction to occur in reverse within tubular cells, converting H_2CO_3 to HCO_3^- and H^+, generating more H^+ for countertransport with Na^+, and releasing bicarbonate that passes into the circulation. Carbonic anhydrase inhibitors are drugs that inhibit this enzyme; the net effect of these agents is that sodium and bicarbonate, that would otherwise have been reabsorbed, remain in the urine and result in an alkaline diuresis.

Although patients may develop a metabolic acidosis when taking these agents, compensatory processes in the tubules accommodate the effects of carbonic anhydrase inhibitors so that their long-term use rarely causes this problem. However, these agents can be useful, for example, with contraction alkalosis from aggressive diuresis with loop diuretics (see later discussion); administration of these drugs can reduce $PaCO_2$ and improve PaO_2 for patients with little accompanying change in blood pH. Specific uses for carbonic anhydrase inhibitors include the treatment of mountain sickness, open-angle glaucoma, and to increase respiratory drive in patients with central sleep apnea.[103,104]

Osmotic Diuretics

Substances such as mannitol that are freely filtered at the glomerulus but poorly reabsorbed by the kidney tubule will cause an osmotic diuresis. In the water-permeable segments of the proximal tubule and loop of Henle, fluid reabsorption occurs, and filtered mannitol is concentrated. Eventually oncotic pressure in the tubular fluid resists further fluid reabsorption. Mannitol also draws water from cells into the plasma and effectively increases RBF.

Mannitol has been widely used for the treatment of increased intracranial pressure but also as a strategy to prevent AKI (see Chapter 36). Although animal studies warranted hope, apart from AKI prophylaxis in kidney transplantation, there is no evidence to suggest mannitol is effective either for the prevention or treatment of AKI.[105–107] Even in cadaveric kidney transplant recipients, the data are modest to support a beneficial effect.[108] In a controlled trial of mannitol prophylaxis in patients with mild chronic renal failure, it was less effective than hydration alone for prevention of contrast-associated nephropathy.[106] Mannitol therapy is not without complications. As mannitol shifts water between fluid compartments, there can be effects on plasma and intracellular electrolyte concentrations, including hyponatremia and hypochloremia and intracellular increases in K^+ and H^+. Patients with normal kidney function quickly correct these changes, but patients with kidney impairment may develop significant circulatory overload with hemodilution and pulmonary edema, hyperkalemic metabolic acidosis, central nervous system depression, and even severe hyponatremia requiring urgent hemodialysis.[109]

Loop Diuretics

The electrochemical gradient established by the Na^+/K^+-ATPase in the loop of Henle drives the transport of one Na^+, one K^+, and two Cl^- ions into the tubule cells from the tubular fluid. Because the thick ascending limb segment of the loop of Henle is water-impermeable, reabsorption of solute concentrates the interstitium and dilutes the tubular fluid. Loop diuretics, such as furosemide, bumetanide, and torsemide, directly inhibit the electroneutral transporter, preventing salt reabsorption from occurring. Because 25% of filtered NaCl is normally reabsorbed in the loop of Henle, loop diuretics cause a large salt load to pass to the distal convoluted tubule that is beyond the extra reserve of this tubular segment to reabsorb; consequently, large volumes of dilute urine ensue.

Loop diuretics are a first-line therapeutic modality for treatment of acute decompensated congestive heart failure. Although loop diuretics have no proven mortality benefit, they reduce left ventricular filling pressures and very effectively relieve the symptoms of congestion, pulmonary edema, extremity swelling, and hepatic congestion. Adverse effects of loop diuretics include hypokalemia, hyponatremia, and also AKI. Heart failure patients with atrial fibrillation may also be prescribed digitalis, which in combination with furosemide, can lead to hypokalemia-induced dysrhythmias. Loop diuretics, especially furosemide, may cause ototoxicity particularly in patients with kidney insufficiency.[110]

Distal Convoluted Tubule Diuretics

Distal convoluted tubule diuretics, such as thiazides (e.g., hydrochlorothiazide) and metolazone, act in the early part of this segment to block the NaCl cotransport mechanism across apical plasma membranes. Because the distal tubule is relatively water-impermeable, net NaCl absorption causes urinary dilution. Clinically, distal convoluted tubule diuretics are used for the treatment of hypertension (often as sole therapy), volume overload disorders, and to relieve the symptoms of edema in pregnancy.

Adverse reactions associated with distal tubule diuretics include electrolyte disturbances and volume depletion. Hydrochlorothiazide specifically has been associated with a number of other side effects including pancreatitis, jaundice, diarrhea, and aplastic anemia.

Distal (Collecting Duct) Acting Diuretics

Unlike in the more proximal nephron segments, NaCl absorption in the collecting duct cells is not electroneutral. That is, a net electrical gradient is maintained both by the Na^+/K^+-ATPase Na^+ ion channels and in the luminal membranes. As a result, the tubule lumen is negatively charged with respect to the blood. This normally causes K^+ secretion into the tubular lumen through K^+-specific ion channels. Distal K^+-sparing diuretics (e.g., amiloride and triamterene) directly inhibit luminal Na^+ entry, blocking this mechanism, and resulting in a K^+-"sparing" effect. In addition, H^+ secretion is inhibited.

A second class of distal-acting, potassium-sparing diuretics is the competitive aldosterone antagonists (e.g., spironolactone and eplerenone). Ordinarily, the mineralocorticoid hormone aldosterone is released by the body in response to angiotensin II or hyperkalemia. Aldosterone normally stimulates Na^+ reabsorption and K^+ excretion by the collecting duct. Inhibition of the aldosterone effect by these drugs causes a mild natriuresis and K^+ retention. Distal K^+-sparing agents are used primarily for K^+-sparing diuresis (e.g., in patients with volume overload receiving digitalis or with hypokalemic alkalosis). In addition, these drugs are especially useful in treating disorders involving secondary hyperaldosteronism, such as cirrhosis with ascites. Spironolactone treatment has been shown to improve survival with volume overload and left ventricular dysfunction or heart failure.[111] Hyperkalemia and hyperkalemic, hyperchloremic metabolic acidoses are significant complications of the injudicious use of spironolactone, triamterene, or amiloride.

Dopaminergic Agonists

Intravenous infusion of low-dose dopamine (1 to 3 mg/kg/min) is natriuretic owing primarily to a modest increase in the GFR and reduction in proximal Na^+ reabsorption mediated by dopamine type 1 (DA_1) receptors.[112] Fenoldopam is a selective DA_1 receptor agonist with little cardiac stimulation. At higher doses, the pressor response to dopamine is beneficial in patients with hypotension, but it has little or no kidney effect in critically ill or septic patients.[112,113] The so-called "renal-dose" dopamine for the treatment of AKI, although widely used, has not been demonstrated to have significant renoprotective properties in numerous studies[114–116] and can cause worsened splanchnic oxygenation, impaired gastrointestinal function, impaired endocrine and immunologic system function, blunting of ventilatory drive, and increased risk of postcardiac surgery atrial fibrillation.[117–119]

SGLT2 Inhibitors

Sodium-glucose co-transporter 2 inhibitors (SGLT2 inhibitors) were developed for the treatment of hyperglycemia in type 2 diabetes mellitus but have been found to have additional benefits such as weight loss, reducing cardiovascular events, as well as protective kidney effects.[120] SGLT2 inhibitors work at the level of the proximal tubule to prevent the reabsorption of approximately 90% of filtered glucose. In addition to promoting kidney excretion of glucose, SGLT2 inhibitors lower glomerular capillary hypertension and hyperfiltration leading to improved cortical oxygenation and less tubular glucotoxicity and it is by this mechanism that SGLT2 inhibitors are thought to be kidney protective and preserve glomerular filtration rate. Recent studies have demonstrated that some SGLT2 inhibitors are effective at slowing the progression of kidney disease and lowering the risk of kidney failure and death in people with CKD, regardless of the presence or absence of type 2 diabetes.[121] Of consideration, AKI is an adverse event that can occur with initiation of SGLT inhibitor therapy, but is reversible with discontinuation. Perioperatively, current FDA recommendation is to discontinue taking SLGT2 inhibitors 3 to 4 days prior to elective surgery to prevent the serious euglycemic ketoacidosis.[122] More studies are necessary to fully elucidate the patient populations that would benefit from these agents as well as better understand their role, and when to discontinue these medications perioperatively.

High Renal-Risk Surgical Procedures

Cardiac Surgery

Cardiac operations requiring CPB can be expected to result in AKI or renal failure in up to 7% of patients.[123,124] There are numerous risk factors associated with the development of postoperative AKI in this population (Fig. 50-6).[125] Interestingly, patients with preoperative CKD appear to tolerate surgery and CPB remarkably well.[126] Kidney ischemia-reperfusion, inflammatory mediators, and toxin exposure are considered to be primary pathologic mechanisms involved in AKI. Kidney risk factors contributing to each of these mechanisms include preoperative left ventricular dysfunction, duration of CPB, pulse pressure hypertension,[127] and aprotinin therapy.[128]

Although some retrospective studies suggest "beating heart" off pump coronary artery bypass grafting lowers kidney risk compared with the traditional CPB techniques,[129] randomized studies have been inconclusive. However, despite the fact that pulsatile

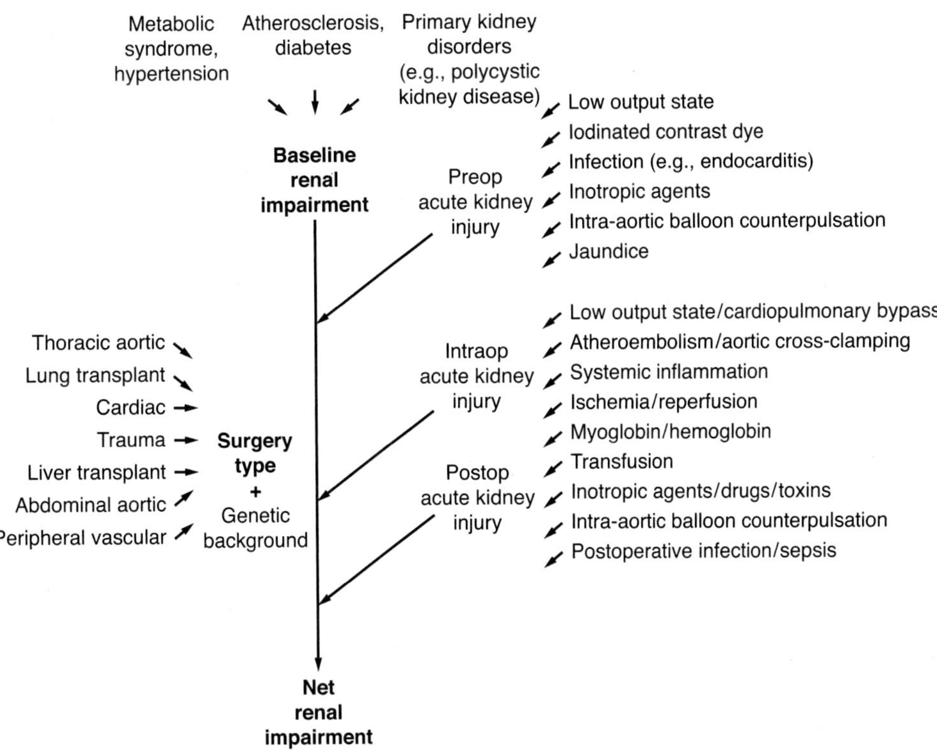

Figure 50-6 Clinical risk factors that predict perioperative acute kidney injury and kidney dysfunction. Preop, preoperative; Intraop, intraoperative; postop, postoperative. (Reprinted with permission from Stafford-Smith M, Patel UD, Phillips-Bute BG, et al. Acute kidney injury and chronic kidney disease after cardiac surgery. *Adv Chronic Kidney Dis.* 2008;15:257–277.)

CPB suppresses plasma renin activity, postoperative kidney function in patients with normal kidneys undergoing pulsatile or nonpulsatile CPB is equivalent.

Numerous agents have been used intraoperatively without success in attempts to protect the kidney during cardiac surgery. Mannitol use during CPB is partly aimed at avoiding hemoglobin-induced AKI, by promoting urine flow and reducing kidney cell swelling. Dopamine is infused at low doses (<5 mg/kg/min) as a kidney vasodilator without benefit. Costa et al.[130] administered low-dose dopamine during CPB to patients with preoperative kidney dysfunction and were able to induce a saluresis without affecting GFR or protecting the kidney from ischemic injury. Dopexamine improved CrCl and systemic oxygen delivery in one cardiac surgery study,[131] but a systemic review of 21 randomized, controlled trials failed to confirm benefit.[132] Other studies examining the kidney protective effects of fenoldopam, ANP, and insulin-like growth factor-1 in this population have not shown a consistently protective effect.

Noncardiac Surgery

Several common noncardiac surgical procedures can compromise previously normal kidney function. Emergency surgery has been reported as a risk factor for AKI, with trauma surgery figuring as a prominent subgroup of emergency procedures.[133] ATN is the typical kidney lesion associated with trauma, and it may be produced by a number of ischemic mechanisms. Most often, hypovolemic shock, pigmenturia, multiple organ failure, or exogenous nephrotoxins are responsible for sequential or simultaneous insults to the kidney. AKI that develops in the trauma patient may be characterized by an early oliguric picture related to inadequate volume resuscitation, or by a later, sometimes nonoliguric syndrome associated with multiple organ failure, nephrotoxin exposure, or sepsis. The outcomes of these two posttraumatic AKI scenarios are dramatically different. The early form is associated with high mortality rates, whereas only 20% to 30% of patients will die in the case of nonoliguric AKI.[134] Not surprisingly, trauma victims with pre-existing kidney insufficiency experience much higher mortality than previously healthy patients.[135]

9

Preventing AKI in patients presenting for emergency surgery begins with proper management of intravascular volume depletion and shock. Restoring euvolemia while maintaining cardiac output and systemic oxygen delivery is an important goal. Urine flow, once established, is maintained at ≥0.5 mL/kg/hr. Invasive hemodynamic monitoring may be required to manage intraoperative cardiovascular instability due to surgical manipulation, blood loss, fluid shifts, and anesthetic effects, although noninvasive measures of volume status are often sufficient to monitor more straightforward fluid resuscitation. Nephrotoxin exposure should be kept to a minimum in the unstable trauma victim. Radiocontrast media, NSAIDs, and myoglobin pose the greatest threat in this patient group. There is no place for either furosemide or mannitol therapy in the early, resuscitative phase of trauma management, except in the case of head injury with elevated intracranial pressure or when massive rhabdomyolysis is suspected.

Vascular surgery requiring aortic clamping has deleterious effects on kidney function regardless of the level of clamp placement. Suprarenal clamping results in an attenuated ATN-like lesion.[136] Infrarenal clamping causes a smaller, short-lived reduction in GFR and is associated with a lower risk of AKI, whereas surgery involving the thoracic aorta has a 25% incidence of AKI.[137] Two major predictors of AKI following aortic surgery are pre-existing kidney dysfunction and perioperative hemodynamic instability.[138] Olsen et al.[139] reported in a large series of patients undergoing abdominal aortic aneurysm repair that the overall incidence of AKI was 12%. Patients who had emergency surgery for ruptured aneurysm had a very high incidence of hemodynamic instability, and AKI developed in 26%; in contrast, elective aortic surgery was associated with good hemodynamic control and a 4% incidence of renal failure. Atheromatous renal artery emboli and prolonged aortic clamp time may contribute to ischemic kidney injury in these patients.

The endovascular approach (endostent) has mostly replaced conventional intra-abdominal surgery in many centers. The etiology of AKI after endovascular and open repair of aortic aneurysm is multifactorial (kidney ischemia, atheroembolism, hemodynamic instability). Although hemodynamic changes during endovascular procedures on the aorta may be less dramatic than those accompanying open repair, endovascular-treated patients may be exposed to substantial amounts of radiocontrast dye, which can exacerbate postoperative kidney dysfunction, especially in those with pre-existing kidney insufficiency. Nonetheless, comparisons of surgical and femoral transcatheter procedures, such as for abdominal aortic aneurysm repair indicate considerably lower rates of postoperative AKI and dialysis.[140]

Most historical efforts to preserve perioperative kidney function have centered on diuretic and kidney vasodilator therapies, although a large body of evidence no longer supports the use of either intravenous mannitol or dopamine to prevent AKI in this setting. More recently, some advocate for the general adoption of a collective of perioperative kidney best practices, termed the "KDIGO bundle." Although such an intervention has received little critical appraisal to date, following cardiac surgery, a single center trial showed benefit while a multicenter randomized feasibility trial did not identify reduced AKI rates in 278 patients.[141] These results suggest further adequately powered, multi-center randomized studies are needed to draw firm conclusions. The hope is that earlier AKI recognition, through a future generation of "early biomarker" tests may facilitate prompt recognition of AKI risk or diagnosis, much earlier than serum creatinine allows, to improve the effectiveness of current interventions.

As previously discussed, patients with hepatic failure or cholestatic jaundice are particularly susceptible to AKI. When the serum conjugated bilirubin exceeds 8 mg/dL, endotoxins from the gastrointestinal tract are absorbed into the portal circulation, causing intense kidney vasoconstriction. Intravenous mannitol and/or oral administration of bile salts in the preoperative period may limit kidney dysfunction in patients with cholestatic jaundice. This phenomenon may contribute to the high incidence of AKI after liver transplantation and biliary surgery. AKI occurs in up to two-thirds of liver transplant recipients.[142] Many liver transplant candidates have overt hepatorenal syndrome, kidney dysfunction, and presumably underlying kidney vasoconstriction. When such patients are exposed to intraoperative hemodynamic instability, massive transfusion, and nephrotoxins, AKI frequently follows.[143]

Anesthetic Considerations for Urologic Procedures

A review of urologic surgical procedures is outlined below, including sections on nephrectomy, cystectomy, prostatectomy, TUR procedures, and therapies for urolithiasis. For each section, general disease principles and treatment rationales are briefly discussed, perioperative management and potential complications reviewed, and then important aspects related to specific procedures within
10 the section highlighted (e.g., simple vs. radical nephrectomy). Selected additional topics are outlined at the end of the section. Notably, a deliberate approach has been taken to minimize repetition by referring the reader to other chapter sections whenever appropriate.

Nephrectomy

Nephrectomy procedures involve partial, radical, or simple resection of the kidney. Each year in the United States, there are approximately 46,000 nephrectomies for benign or malignant disease, and an additional 6,000 donor surgeries for renal transplant. While radical nephrectomy is the standard for resectable kidney cancer, simple nephrectomy is typical for benign disease. Some kidney tumors invade the renal vein extending as far as the inferior vena cava or right atrium; these tumors require additional procedures to safely retrieve their intravascular component. Kidney transplant donor nephrectomy involves simple nephrectomy with measures to avoid organ trauma and optimize graft function. The so-called "nephron sparing" or partial nephrectomy is indicated for limited benign disease but increasingly is being considered for wider indications including selected cancerous lesions.

The approach and incision for nephrectomy are based on surgical priorities and surgeon preference. Retroperitoneal approaches require a flank incision and lateral decubitus positioning with flank extension (Fig. 50-7), allowing access to the kidney without breaching the peritoneal cavity. This approach has obvious advantages in reducing infection risk but also simplifies procedures involving prior abdominal surgery or obesity. Challenges related to the retroperitoneal approach include access to the vena cava, risk of unintentional pneumothorax, and the adverse effects of lateral decubitus position and flank extension on respiratory vital capacity, which can be reduced up to 20% (see Chapter 28).

Anterior approaches to nephrectomy involve supine positioning and breach of the peritoneal cavity through midline, subcostal, or thoracoabdominal incisions that provide direct access to both the kidney and major vascular structures. Although transperitoneal approaches add the risk of visceral injury and peritonitis, they improve access to the kidney pedicle (e.g., trauma, hemorrhage) with best access to both kidneys being through midline incisions (e.g., bilateral nephrectomy for end-stage polycystic kidney disease). The thoracoabdominal approach enters both the peritoneal and pleural spaces and rarely may require single-lung ventilation.

In recent years, *laparoscopic* retro- and transperitoneal approaches to nephrectomy have surpassed their open equivalents in popularity, particularly for simple and donor procedures, but these techniques are even being used for "nephron-sparing" partial nephrectomy. Other recent innovations include robotic-assisted, single port laparoscopic, and even transvaginal minimally invasive nephrectomies.

Preoperative Considerations

Recruits for donor nephrectomy surgery are typically healthy individuals; however, perioperative risk for other nephrectomy procedures often relates to the indication for surgery. Although smoking and obesity are the most important risk factors for kidney cancer, many other cardiovascular risk factors are also strongly associated with kidney cancer risk including advanced age, male sex, chronic or ESRD, and hypertension. Hence, protocols for assessment and management of perioperative cardiac risk are particularly relevant to nephrectomy surgery.[144]

Simple nephrectomy for infectious indications is uncommon but most often involves diabetic patients and can be grouped into two categories. Elective procedures involve irreversible kidney damage due to chronic pyelonephritis (e.g., xanthogranulomatous).[145] In contrast, emergent procedures are associated with very high mortality rates (up to 43%) and generally involve critically ill patients with acute emphysematous pyelonephritis unresponsive to antibiotics.

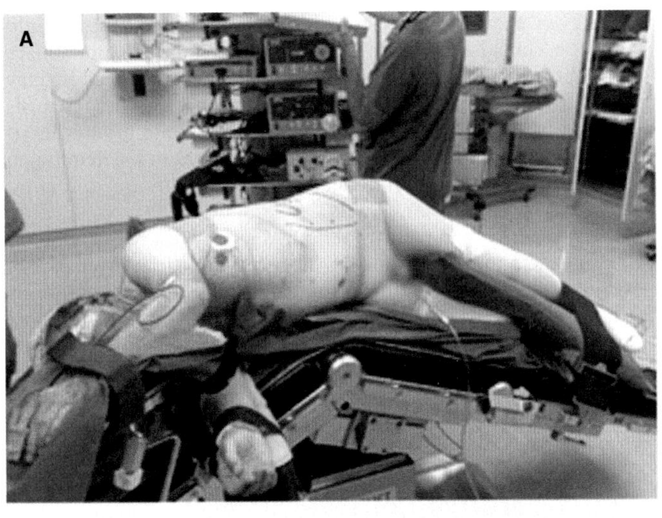

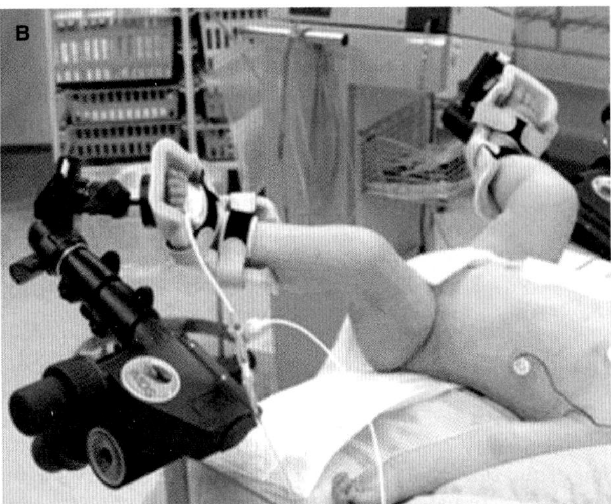

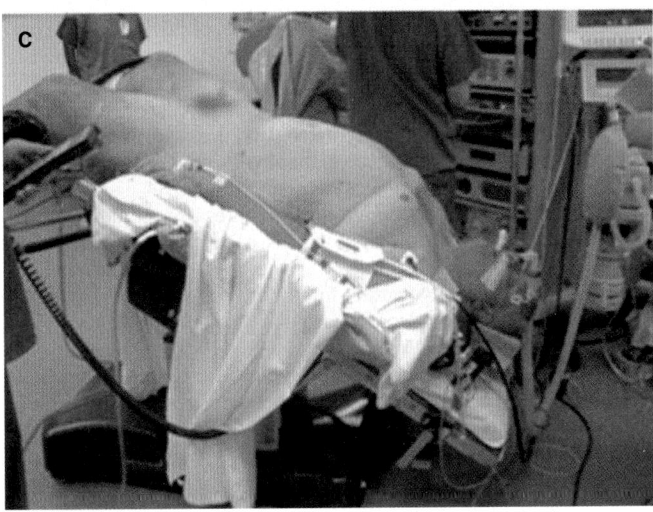

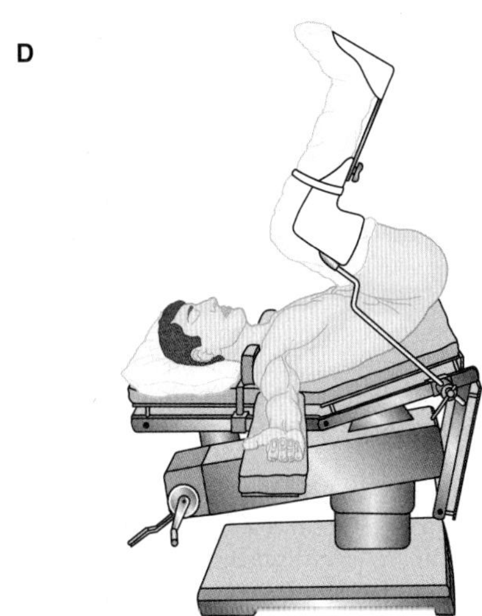

Figure 50-7 Common positioning options for urologic surgery include right lateral decubitus with waist extension (**A**), lithotomy (**B**), supine with steep (30 to 45 degrees) Trendelenburg (**C**), and exaggerated lithotomy (**D**).

Several hereditary conditions that are associated with kidney cancer also have attributes that must be considered in anesthetic planning[146]; for example, individuals with Birt–Hogg–Dubé syndrome have pulmonary cysts that increase the risk of intraoperative spontaneous pneumothorax, while patients with von Hippel–Lindau syndrome, the commonest of these disorders, have high rates of pheochromocytoma and neuroendocrine tumors.

Ten to 40% of patients presenting with kidney cancer have associated paraneoplastic syndromes.[147] Beyond fever, cachexia, and weight loss, these subdivide into endocrine and nonendocrine categories. Tumor-related endocrine effects include hypercalcemia (PTH-like effects), hypertension (renin), anemia/polycythemia (erythropoietin), nonmetastatic hepatic dysfunction (Stauffer syndrome), galactorrhea, Cushing syndrome, and ectopic insulin and glucagon production, while nonendocrine effects include amyloidosis, neuromyopathies, vasculopathy, nephropathy, coagulopathy, and elevated prostaglandin levels. Of kidney cancers presenting with hypercalcemia, 50% are paraneoplastic in origin. Kidney tumors may also be associated with a hypercoagulable state; sudden intraoperative clot formation has been reported.[148]

As with most major urologic surgeries, other investigations for nephrectomy surgery include routine ECG, chest x-ray, complete blood cell count, electrolyte profile with serum BUN and creatinine, liver function tests, serum calcium assessment, bleeding profile, and urine analysis. Although normal serum creatinine level and evidence of contralateral function by intravenous pyelogram are sometimes considered sufficient assessment to predict adequate postoperative kidney function, a noninvasive differential kidney scan (iodine-131 or technetium-99m computerized isotope renograph) is often performed for more precise prediction of postoperative GFR.

Urologic surgery patients often present with additional disease workup that can provide a wealth of information beyond routine studies and assessment of their urinary tract. Abdominal CT scans detail tumor size, location, and invasion of the kidney collecting system or perirenal fat, while MRI is most valuable to assess for vena caval and/or cardiac chamber involvement.

Standard recommended preoperative management of chronic drug therapies is all that is necessary for most nephrectomy procedures, although dose adjustment may be considered if significant changes in kidney function are anticipated.

Intraoperative Considerations

Preparation for even the most "straightforward" nephrectomy surgery demands sufficient monitoring and vascular access to respond to complications, most notably significant hemorrhage, an uncommon but ever-present risk in such procedures. Beyond standard monitoring and two large bore peripheral intravenous catheters, requirements for intravascular access and additional monitoring are dictated by patient condition and complexity of the procedure and may include a peripheral intra-arterial catheter for continuous blood pressure recording and repeated blood gas assessment and sometimes central venous access.

While central venous line placement is not essential for most nephrectomy surgeries, patient and procedural factors such as comorbidities (e.g., cardiac history) and bleeding risk (e.g., tumor extension into venous structures) may warrant such access. If placement of a central venous catheter is deemed necessary, selection of the side *ipsilateral* to the nephrectomy surgery for subclavian or internal jugular central venous puncture should be considered to minimize the risk of bilateral pneumothorax.

Assessment of infection, bony metastases, and bleeding risk may influence the decision to include neuraxial procedures in the anesthesia plan. Sometimes spinal imaging from CT and MRI scans can provide added detail useful when contemplating epidural catheter placement. If a lumbar or thoracic epidural catheter is placed, this is usually done prior to anesthesia induction to allow for a meaningful test dose sequence and to facilitate pre-incision administration of epidural opiates. Varied opinions regarding intraoperative local anesthetic dosing of the epidural catheter involve concerns over hemodynamic stability and the likelihood of significant blood loss during the procedure.

Neuraxial injection or catheter placement prior to anesthesia induction (e.g., epidural catheter insertion) can be followed by placement of intra-arterial and central venous access after anes-
11 thesia induction in most cases. Bladder catheter placement is essential for all nephrectomy procedures; urinary output monitoring provides information on intravascular volume status in the absence of central venous pressure monitoring, avoids the possibility of urinary retention, and also provides valuable information postoperatively regarding kidney function, bleeding sources, and the possibility of clot-related urinary tract obstruction. Noninvasive cardiac output monitoring (e.g., esophageal Doppler, stroke volume variation, pulse pressure variation) techniques may be useful in selected patients.

Anesthesia induction agent selection to achieve hypnosis, paralysis, and blunting of the hemodynamic intubation response should be matched to any use of regional anesthesia, the anticipated duration of the procedure, and the patient's kidney function. Intraoperative and postoperative pain management can be accomplished by intravenous or other opioid therapies such as patient-controlled analgesia, neuraxial analgesia or truncal blocks.[149,150] Strategic use of analgesic strategies (e.g., multimodal analgesia, truncal blocks, continuous epidural analgesia), may attenuate postoperative neuroendocrine responses, resolve ileus sooner and improve postoperative ventilatory mechanics, potentially improving survival following major urologic surgery.[151]

Potential intraoperative complications include injury to major blood vessels (e.g., inferior vena cava, aorta), gastrointestinal organs (e.g., spleen, liver, pancreas), and unrecognized entry into the pleural space with resultant pneumothorax. Complications associated with hemorrhage during nephrectomy are uncommon but mandate preparatory steps beyond monitoring and generous intravenous access. Confirmation that blood products are present or readily available should occur immediately prior to surgery. Routine fluid and patient warming technology and even a rapid transfusion device for selected cases should also be considered. Since unexplained changes in pulmonary mechanics or hypotension during a nephrectomy procedure may reflect diaphragmatic injury and pneumothorax, such changes should be discussed with the surgeon to facilitate prompt intervention. This may require direct repair of a rent in the diaphragm as well as needle decompression of a pneumothorax and chest tube insertion.

Particularly in the setting of limited kidney reserve, in addition to consideration of transfusion "triggers" and strict avoidance of unjustifiable blood product administration, a note of caution is warranted regarding the potential for resuscitation "overshoot" in response to acute hemorrhage. Strict attention to appropriate monitors during fluid resuscitation and appropriate use of arterial blood gas assessment, assisted by good communication with the surgeon, will help avoid the risk of pulmonary edema from fluid overload.

Postoperative Considerations

Nephrectomy is associated with high rates of postoperative complications, particularly following radical nephrectomy. Added to standard concerns, such as hemorrhage and unrecognized visceral injury, are atelectasis, ileus, superficial and deep wound infections, temporary or permanent renal failure, and incisional hernia. The most common radical nephrectomy complications are adjacent organ (bowel, spleen, liver, diaphragm, or pancreas) and vascular injury. Overall complication rates are similar whether an open or laparoscopic approach is used.[152–154] Bleeding commonly requires transfusion.[155–157] Other less common major complications include myocardial infarction, congestive heart failure, pulmonary embolism, cerebrovascular accident, pneumonia, and thrombophlebitis.

Given the loss of kidney tissue, a logical extension of nephrectomy would be the need to adjust postoperative dosing of drug therapies to accommodate the anticipated decrease in GFR associated with an approximate 50% reduction in functioning nephrons. While a drop in GFR can be anticipated, notably adaptation of the remaining kidney usually results in a postnephrectomy modest 25% decline.

The pain of nephrectomy, laparoscopic or open, is significant. Analgesia can be achieved with epidural or spinal analgesia strategies, systemic opioids, and nonopioid adjuncts. Recent findings of improved recovery using epidural analgesia for major abdominal surgeries[158] have not been assessed specifically for nephrectomy surgery.

Specific Procedures

Simple and Donor Nephrectomies

Simple nephrectomy is sufficient intervention for irreversible nonmalignant disease such as untreatable infection, unsalvageable kidney trauma, or a nonfunctioning kidney due to calculi or hypertensive disease. Up to 86% of patients with hypertension that is presumed to be renovascular in origin with noncorrectable unilateral renal artery disease have improved hypertension control after simple nephrectomy.

During donor procedures, several steps are added to simple nephrectomy, including administration of drugs intravenously just prior to explant to achieve low-level anticoagulation (e.g., 3,000 USP heparin units) and forced diuresis (e.g., mannitol 12.5 g, furosemide 40 mg), extension of (laparoscopic) incisions to assure atraumatic organ extraction, and postharvest protamine administration. Procured organs are infused with cold preservative (e.g., University of Wisconsin or histidine–tryptophan–ketoglutarate solutions) and stored on ice and/or cold machine perfused. Just over one-third of kidney transplants in the United States are from living donors and, compared to cadavers, living kidney donation is associated with improved short- and long-term outcomes (i.e., recipient and graft survival).

Radical Nephrectomy

Renal cell carcinoma is the main indication for radical nephrectomy and accounts for 90% to 95% of kidney neoplasms and 3% of all malignancies in adults. With the exception of hereditary syndromes with high tumor rates (see above), a positive family history incurs a two- to threefold increased risk of kidney cancer, but such individuals constitute only 2% of radical nephrectomies. Hematuria, a palpable mass and flank pain, is the classic triad at presentation, but nowadays kidney tumors are more often (approximately 72%) diagnosed incidentally during workup for other nonurologic problems. Occasionally, tumors declare due to signs or symptoms of vena caval involvement such as dilated abdominal veins (left) varicocele, lower extremity edema, or pulmonary embolism. Symptomatic tumors usually reflect more advanced disease and are more often associated with metastasis and a poor prognosis. Transitional cell cancers of the upper urothelial tract (ureters, renal pelvis) are also treated by radical nephrectomy with resection of the associated ureter including a cuff of bladder tissue. Up to one-third of kidney cancer patients have metastases at diagnosis, but many are still candidates for surgery.

Radical nephrectomy involves renal artery and vein ligation with subsequent removal *en bloc* of the kidney, perinephric fat, Gerota fascia, proximal ureter, and often the adjacent adrenal gland. Lymph node dissection is then performed from the diaphragm to the aortic bifurcation. Most kidney cancers stay within Gerota fascia and can be completely removed, but a disappointing 20% to 30% of patients with successful surgery still have their disease return. Although radical nephrectomy is standard for central and large tumors, the value of nephron-sparing partial nephrectomy for early-stage and small renal cell cancers is being evaluated. While nonsurgical therapies are available, renal cell cancers are resistant to radiation and chemotherapy. Blood loss during radical nephrectomy is highly dependent on the location and extent of the tumor. Laparoscopic innovations have reduced bleeding for all types of nephrectomy surgeries.

Radical Nephrectomy with Inferior Vena Cava Tumor Thrombus

Between 4% and 10% of patients with renal cell carcinoma have the so-called "tumor thrombus" extension beyond the kidney either limited to the renal vein or extending into the inferior vena cava. Although often restricted to the vessel lumen, the thrombus may become adherent to the vessel wall,[159] and right atrial involvement is present in 1% of cases. Radical nephrectomy procedures involving resection of tumor thrombus are particularly challenging due to their risk of sudden major bleeding and potential for acute hemodynamic instability (e.g., inferior vena cava clamping or tumor pulmonary embolism).

Kidney tumors with IVC thrombus are classified by the extent of tumor thrombus within the IVC and right atrium (levels I to IV; Fig. 50-8) and require different procedures in addition to radical nephrectomy.[160] In general, thrombus extraction can occur with simple proximal and distal caval control alone for tumors that go no further than the infrahepatic IVC. As thrombus extends into the intrahepatic IVC or higher, isolating the vessel to extract the thrombus becomes more challenging and ultimately can only be achieved safely using CPB with or without aortic crossclamping and cardiac arrest. In addition to sternotomy incision, such procedures require standard heparin anticoagulation and employ an added circuit venous line filter to trap tumor fragments (Fig. 50-8). Other interventions used at some institutions in the treatment of kidney tumor caval thrombus include venovenous bypass, inferior vena cava filter insertion, and even deep hypothermic circulatory arrest.

Appropriate considerations when monitoring these complex procedures include radial arterial catheterization, central venous and rarely pulmonary artery catheter placement, and intraoperative transesophageal echocardiography (Fig. 50-8). In cases where supradiaphragmatic tumor thrombus is present, placement of a pulmonary artery catheter prior to thrombus resection is contraindicated due to risk of embolization of tumor fragments. If the thrombus extends into the suprahepatic IVC, hepatic mobilization with Pringle maneuver (clamping of the hepatoduodenal ligament to interrupt blood flow through the hepatic artery and portal vein) may be required, generally for less than 30 minutes.[161] Additional preparation includes all steps standard for procedures involving CPB (see Chapter 38), including large bore peripheral intravenous access, vasoactive infusions, fluid, and blood products. Preoperative therapeutic embolization of the tumor is sometimes also used in cases of arterial thrombus, extensive parasitic vessel formation, or with anticipated difficulty in isolating the renal artery. Despite the potential for significant blood loss, cell saver technology use is discouraged due to the potential for returning tumor cells to the circulation.

"Nephron-Sparing" Partial Nephrectomy

Minimizing unnecessary loss of healthy tissue is a logical part of surgical planning for any kidney resection. Partial nephrectomy is often sufficient for benign tumors, but this procedure is also becoming an alternate to radical nephrectomy for some cancerous renal cell tumors, particularly when kidney parenchyma must be preserved; examples include bilateral tumors, CKD, tumors in a single remaining kidney, or where the contralateral kidney is at risk for future disease or tumor. Even when the contralateral kidney is normal, studies are now demonstrating comparable long-term results with nephron-sparing partial nephrectomy procedures as with radical nephrectomy for patients with a single, localized small tumor (<4 cm) and even medium-sized (<7 cm) peripherally located tumors. Limitations of partial nephrectomy include a higher perioperative risk of bleeding and urine leak, and a local tumor recurrence rate of 1% to 6%.

Laparoscopic and Robotic Nephrectomies

Laparoscopic and robotic techniques can be applied to retroperitoneal and transperitoneal approaches and all types of nephrectomies (i.e., radical, simple, or partial). Compared to open approaches, these minimally invasive strategies employ access through small airtight ports. Insufflation of carbon dioxide into the peritoneal cavity or retroperitoneal space is used to separate structures and enhance visibility. In recent years, laparoscopic techniques have surpassed open nephrectomies in popularity, particularly for simple and radical procedures. Laparoscopic approaches to radical nephrectomy are even being successfully employed in the treatment of locally invasive kidney cancer. Laparoscopic partial nephrectomy is technically more demanding than its open counterpart and currently involves temporary clamping of the kidney hilum to optimize visibility during excision and minimize blood loss. The warm ischemic time related to clamping can cause AKI, particularly if the duration exceeds 30 minutes.[162,163]

Some studies have reported comparisons of equivalent open and laparoscopic procedures. Laparoscopic radical nephrectomy

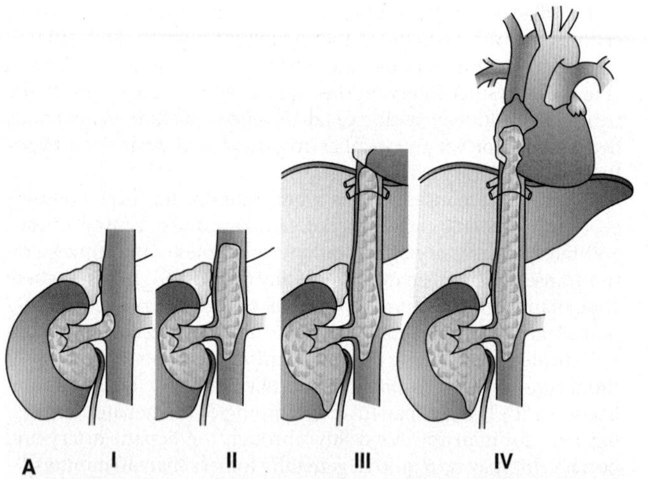

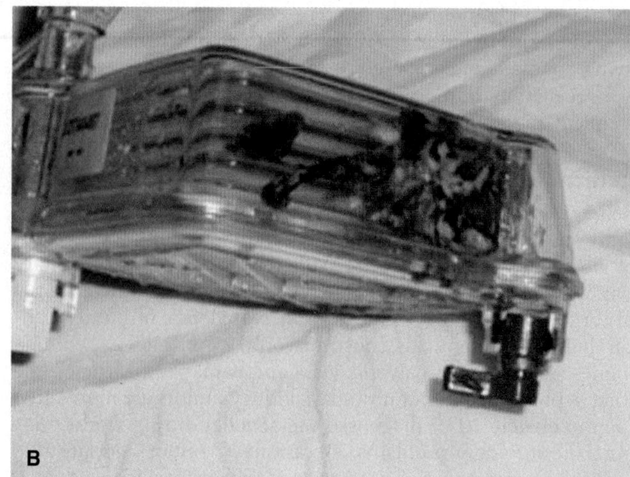

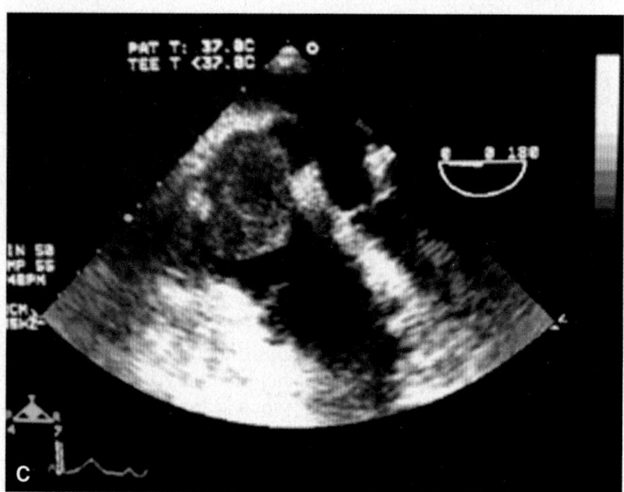

Figure 50-8 Radical nephrectomy with inferior vena cava thrombus removal for renal cell carcinoma is a major operative procedure. Surgical complexity is predicted by the extent of intravascular tumor thrombus, as classified by the most proximal level of tumor extension (levels I to IV; **A**). Evidence of thrombus emboli in the venous filter following cardiopulmonary bypass (**B**) highlights the friability of intravascular renal cell carcinoma thrombus. Intraoperative transesophageal echocardiography demonstrates right atrial extension of a renal cell tumor (**C**). (A: reprinted with permission from Nesbitt JC, Soltero ER, Dinney CP, et al. Surgical management of renal cell carcinoma with inferior vena cava tumor thrombus. *Ann Thorac Surg*. 1997;63:1592–1600.)

for cancer involves smaller incisions, less blood loss, decreased postoperative analgesic requirement, shorter hospital stay and convalescent period, and similar long-term outcomes when compared with open radical nephrectomy.[164,165] Likewise, laparoscopic "nephron-sparing" partial nephrectomy results in less bleeding and a shorter hospital stay, and for selected tumors has 5- and 10-year outcomes similar to those of open partial nephrectomy.[166,167] Laparoscopic donor nephrectomy has no adverse effects on the success of kidney transplant but is associated with less pain and analgesic requirement, faster hospital discharge, and better quality of life compared with open donor nephrectomy.[168] Institutional experience with laparoscopic and robotic assistance with nephrectomy procedures may influence anesthetic planning and the perceived need for invasive procedures (e.g., central venous cannulation).

Traditional open nephrectomy is associated with a significant incidence of chronic pain ranging from 5% to 26%.[169,170] The hope is that laparoscopic approaches will reduce the incidence of chronic pain syndromes. The perceived differences between laparoscopic and open nephrectomy procedures have influenced clinical practice including anesthesia planning for postoperative pain management. Compared to open nephrectomy, the reduced pain and shorter recovery times have meant that epidural anesthesia is less likely to be selected for laparoscopic approaches, with postoperative pain control for these procedures provided by a multimodal strategy involving opiates and appropriate nonopioid adjuncts. NSAIDs are rarely used to avoid their potential nephrotoxic effects. Recent small studies have reported good success with continuous local anesthetic infusions via catheters placed in the rectus and retroperitoneal sheaths intraoperatively (across the intercostal, ilioinguinal, and ileohypogastric nerves). Benefits include reduced pain levels, opioid requirements, nausea, time to recovery and discharge, and cost.[171,172]

Robotic approaches to nephrectomy surgery are widely used in some countries, but have very similar considerations to laparoscopic nephrectomy in terms of issues such as pneumoperitoneum. Notably, robotic nephrectomy has specific positioning requirements due to the robotic equipment, and care must be taken to assure that the robotic arms do not cause pressure injury to the patient. Depending on the experience of the surgical team, robotic procedures may also take more time. Notably, the role of robot assistance is also being similarly explored and developed for several other major urologic surgeries (e.g., partial nephrectomy, radical cystectomy, pyeloplasty, and radical cystectomy).[173]

Physiology of Pneumoperitoneum

Despite potential surgical advantages of laparoscopic surgery, the consequences of pneumoperitoneum, most notably systemic CO_2 absorption and obstruction of venous return from the lower body, are important particularly for patients with cardiopulmonary disease (Table 50-5)[174] (see Chapter 33). These include an average 30% decrease in cardiac output with the institution of

Table 50-5 Physiology of CO_2 Pneumoperitoneum in the Trendelenburg Position

Organ System	Effect
Cardiovascular	↑ Systemic vascular resistance ↑ Mean arterial pressure ↑ Myocardial oxygen consumption ↓ Renal, portal, and sphlanchnic flow
Respiratory	↑ Ventilation–perfusion mismatch ↓ Functional residual capacity ↓ Vital capacity ↓ Compliance ↑ Peak airway pressure Pulmonary congestion and edema Hypercarbia, respiratory acidosis
Central nervous system	↑ Intracranial pressure ↑ Cerebral blood flow ↑ Intraocular pressure Catecholamine release
Endocrine	Activation of renin–angiotensin system
Others	Gastroesophageal regurgitation Venous air embolism Neuropraxia, especially brachial Tracheal tube displacement Facial and airway edema

Reprinted with permission from Irvine M, Patil V. Anaesthesia for robot-assisted laparoscopic surgery. *Continuing Education in Anaesthesia, Critical Care & Pain*. 2009;9:125–129.

pneumoperitoneum which, due to an associated increase in systemic vascular resistance (afterload), is often accompanied by little change or even an increase (up to 16%) in mean arterial blood pressure. Systemic vascular resistance and cardiac output usually return to near-normal values over the 10 minutes following institution of pneumoperitoneum. Preoperative fluid loading, with additional preinduction colloid boluses before institution of pneumoperitoneum, result in higher stroke volume and urine output compared to standard intraoperative fluid regimens, but studies are lacking regarding any evidence of improved outcome using this strategy.[175]

A strategy involving hydration and limiting insufflation pressures to below 12 mmHg is advocated. Presumably related to derangements of kidney perfusion, pneumoperitoneum insufflation pressures of >15 mmHg have been associated with postoperative AKI. Following laparoscopic donor nephrectomy, some donors develop oliguria despite hemodynamic stability and liberal fluid management strategies. The etiology of this is unclear, but it is usually self-limited. Urine output of >2 mL/kg/hr is reassuring, although there is no clear evidence that the diuretic effects of furosemide, mannitol, "renal dose" dopamine, fenoldopam, or ANP analogs are of any value in protecting the kidney.[176]

Other effects of pneumoperitoneum include restricted diaphragmatic excursion, acid–base abnormalities due to systemic absorption of CO_2, neurohumoral responses, and the potential for venous gas embolism. Reductions in pulmonary compliance and functional residual capacity, combined with CO_2 absorption, often cause respiratory acidosis. Cephalad displacement of the abdominal contents, particularly in obese patients, can also add atelectasis and ventilation–perfusion mismatch. Cardiac valvular dysfunction has been reported during laparoscopic nephrectomy,[177] and cardiac ischemia can develop in "at-risk" patients with coronary artery disease. There is also an immediate increase in intracranial pressure with the institution of the pneumoperitoneum.

Hemodynamic instability or hypoxia that occurs with CO_2 insufflation due to the above-mentioned perturbations must be addressed, and a small number of patients will require conversion to an open surgical approach. However, despite the numerous disturbances, a majority of patients can be safely managed through episodes of pneumoperitoneum with appropriate circulatory support, thoughtful ventilator management, and good communication between surgeon and anesthesiologist that includes a willingness to adjust CO_2 insufflation pressures. Notably, adequate neuromuscular blockade plays a role in keeping insufflation pressures at the lowest level required to achieve optimal surgical exposure.

Offsetting advantages of laparoscopic approaches are risks also seen in settings other than nephrectomy including trauma during trocar placement (approx. 0.5%) and increased rates of postoperative deep venous thrombosis.

Cystectomy and Other Major Bladder Surgeries

Cystectomy surgery involves removal of all or part of the urinary bladder. While radical cystectomy is standard for most muscle-invasive malignant disease, simple cystectomy is primarily for benign bladder disease. Of the 69,250 cases of bladder cancer expected in 2011 in the United States, approximately 90% will undergo a surgical procedure for their disease. Radical cystectomy combines bladder removal with resection of other pelvic organs and lymph nodes. Partial or simple cystectomy and transurethral resection of bladder tumor (TURBT) (see transurethral resection procedures section) are other procedures used in the treatment of benign and malignant bladder diseases.

In removing the entire bladder, simple and radical cystectomy procedures oblige a companion surgery to allow for future urine collection. The so-called "diversion procedures" involve redirecting the ureters, most commonly to a pouch fashioned from ileum (ileal conduit), that passively drains urine into a bag through a stoma on the patient's abdominal wall. Alternate options include the so-called "continent" diversion reconstructive procedures which are becoming more popular. Since diversion surgeries can make future diagnosis of appendicitis difficult, some surgeons routinely also perform an appendectomy as part of urinary diversion procedures.

Supine or modified lithotomy positioning (Fig. 50-7) and midline incision with avoidance of the umbilicus are standard for open cystectomy surgery; however, a transverse abdominal incision is occasionally used. Much like nephrectomy surgery, both retroperitoneal and transperitoneal approaches are feasible for cystectomy, and laparoscopic and robotic-assisted techniques are becoming popular both for cystectomy and diversion procedures.

Preoperative Considerations

The most common patients presenting for cystectomy are those with bladder cancer. Approximately 90% have transitional cell tumors, and approximately 90% of these have already invaded muscle at diagnosis. Bladder tumors occasionally present with urinary retention but are generally diagnosed by hematuria (microscopic or macroscopic) with or without voiding symptoms such as urgency, frequency, and dysuria. Prior to cystectomy, patients have usually undergone one or several cystoscopies for tumor biopsy or resection, and many have already received radiation and chemotherapy.

Risk factors for bladder cancer and atherosclerosis overlap, and perioperative protocols for cardiac risk assessment and management are relevant to cystectomy surgery.[144] Smoking history is most important, doubling the risk of bladder cancer, while occupational exposures in the leather, dye, and rubber industry and drinking water with high arsenic levels also contribute. Men are about four times more likely than women to be diagnosed with bladder cancer with white men twice as likely as African American men. The average patient presenting with bladder cancer is 65 years old. Paraneoplastic syndromes similar to those seen with kidney cancer have been reported with bladder cancer but are relatively rare.

Intraoperative Considerations

Anesthetic management for cystectomy is similar to that for nephrectomy surgery (see above), including preparation for the potential for major bleeding. Although patients strictly could undergo cystectomy surgery with epidural anesthesia alone, this is rarely chosen due to the extended duration of surgery. Particular attention should be paid to the approach to assessment of intravascular volume during cystectomy surgery given the considerable potential for bleeding and hypovolemia and the absence of meaningful urine output data. Combining intraoperative epidural analgesia with a general anesthetic for cystectomy may reduce bleeding and improve postoperative analgesia without otherwise affecting complication rates.[178]

A trend in radical cystectomy has been toward the use of fast-track protocols (e.g., Enhanced Recovery After Surgery [ERAS]). Made popular by their use in colorectal surgeries, such protocols include a variety of evidence-based preoperative, intraoperative, and postoperative management strategies aimed at achieving early return of gastrointestinal function and good pain control, and by thus minimizing the surgical stress response and reducing end-organ dysfunction, improving overall recovery following major surgery. The use of such pathways is most recognized to significantly reduce time to discharge and incidence of postoperative complications following colorectal surgery. Although recent studies caution that colorectal ERAS protocols may be associated with significant increased risk of developing postoperative AKI, it remains unclear if this is associated with increased long-term morbidity and mortality.[179] Nonetheless, cumulative evidence of improved outcomes with implementation of ERAS protocols for cystectomy generally supports the use of this approach, and do not seem to add risk of AKI.[180,181]

For radical cystectomy, for example ERAS Society recommendations start with preoperative counseling, education, and optimization. Avoidance of oral mechanical bowel preparation is recommended. Rather than prolonged fasting prior to surgery, the patient can consume a light meal 6 hours prior to surgery, water up until 2 hours before surgery, and a carbohydrate drink for preoperative hydration and glucose and insulin optimization. After arrival in the preoperative area, a multimodal analgesic regimen (often involving truncal blocks or thoracic epidural catheter insertion for regional analgesia, and a minimal approach to systemic opioid administration) is started, along with venous thromboembolism prophylaxis using subcutaneous heparin injection. Intraoperatively, a minimally invasive surgical approach is employed whenever possible. End-organ function is optimized through a goal-directed fluid management strategy involving noninvasive cardiac output monitoring.[182] Postoperatively, return of gastrointestinal function is encouraged through early mobilization and oral diet, and avoidance of nasogastric intubation.[183]

Postoperative Considerations

Simple cystectomy with diversion procedure involves a more limited dissection of pelvic structures relative to radical cystectomy and is generally associated with considerably less blood loss and lower complication rates.[184] Following radical cystectomy with diversion, some patients will require admission to an intensive care unit. Average blood loss ranges between 560 and 3,000 mL, and transfusion is common. Hospital lengths of stay can be long but vary considerably among centers. The mortality rate for radical cystectomy with diversion procedure is approximately 1%, and perioperative complications are common (27.3%).[185] Early problems include acute pyelonephritis following ureteral catheter removal, ileus, injury to local structures such as the obturator nerve (adductor palsy and gait disturbance), and impaired lymph drainage (lymphocele, leg edema).

Specific Procedures

Partial Cystectomy

Nonmalignant indications for partial bladder resection include bladder endometriosis and benign tumors (e.g., lymphangioma). Wherever partial cystectomy will suffice, the effects of added surgery and poorer quality of life associated with a urinary diversion procedure can be eliminated. Hence, the current interest in methods to identify bladder cancer patients for whom partial cystectomy with pelvic lymph node dissection may be as good a treatment as radical cystectomy. Selective "bladder-sparing" protocols that use responsiveness of a tumor to chemotherapy and radiation therapy as a guide to surgical decision making appear to successfully identify about one-third of the patients whose long-term outcome with partial cystectomy are equivalent to radical cystectomy, without the need for a diversion procedure.[173]

Simple and Radical Cystectomy

Simple cystectomy is indicated for benign disease such as neurogenic bladder, refractory bladder pain syndrome (interstitial cystitis), bladder damage from radiation, and refractory incontinence.

Radical cystectomy involves resection of the bladder and related pelvic structures including pelvic lymphadenectomy of obturator and iliac nodes. In the male, the bladder en bloc is removed with pelvic peritoneum, prostate and seminal vesicles, ureteric remnants, and a small piece of membranous urethra, and in the female, the uterus, ovaries, fallopian tubes, vaginal vault, and urethra. Alternate terminology to radical cystectomy for these major procedures includes the following: In the male, "radical cystoprostatectomy" and, in the female, "radical cystectomy with pelvic exenteration."

Ileal Conduit and Other Diversion Procedures

The concept of ileal conduit surgery is relatively straightforward, involving creation of an ileal pouch that is attached to both ureters and the abdominal wall as a stoma. In contrast, continent diversion procedures are numerous and diverse in their approaches to urine collection and drainage. Continent urinary diversions can be categorized into (1) ureterosigmoidostomy, (2) continent cutaneous diversions, and (3) "neobladder" diversions to the native urethra.[186] Ureterosigmoidostomy is only occasionally used and involves tunneling the ureters to the sigmoid colon, with urine storage and elimination being through the rectum. Continent cutaneous reservoirs resemble ileal conduit surgery, but the stomal attachment to the abdominal wall is modified to produce a valve mechanism, with urine drainage achieved by intermittent catheter drainage. Many continent cutaneous variants exist that involve the use of different bowel segments as the source for the reservoir (e.g., ileum, ileocecum, ascending colon, sigmoid colon, or transverse colon). Finally, continent orthotopic diversions involve "neobladder" construction from terminal ileum, cecum, or sigmoid colon, which is attached to

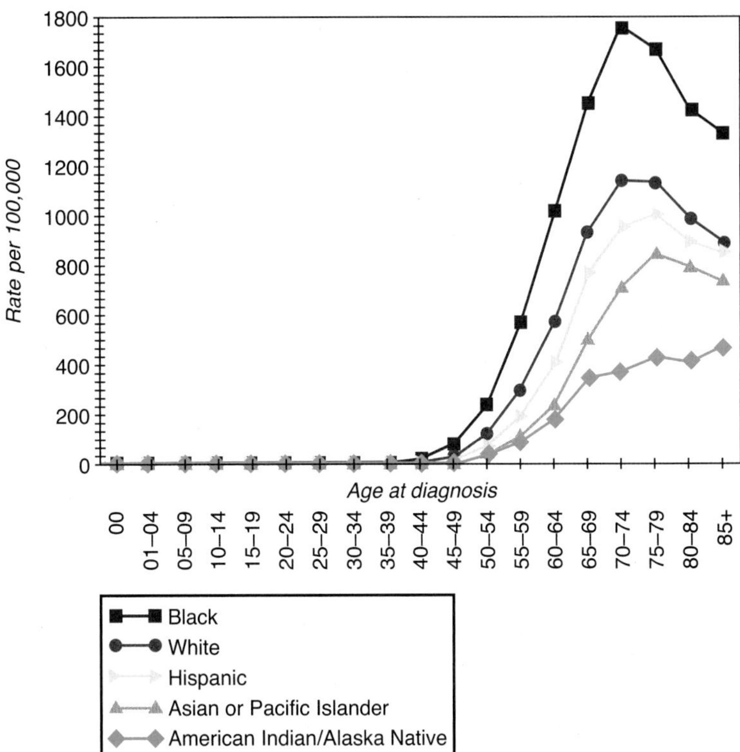

Figure 50-9 Crude incidence rates for prostate cancer, by race/ethnicity. (From www.seer.cancer.gov, accessed March 2012.)

proximal urethra and its intact rhabdosphincter mechanism. Notably, all urinary diversion procedures involve extensive dissection and are considerably more challenging if the patient has received preoperative radiation therapy. Complications of urinary diversion surgery include bowel obstruction, urinary tract infection, deep venous thrombosis and pulmonary embolism, pneumonia, upper urinary tract damage, and skin breakdown around the stoma.

After recovery, patients with urinary diversions are vulnerable to conditions that require subsequent surgeries; these include problems at the stoma site (e.g., stricture, hernia, prolapse, retraction 5% to 10%), fistulae between urinary tract and bowel (3%), bowel obstruction, reservoir or other genitourinary stone diseases (5%), impotence, primary tumor recurrence, and even bowel cancer in the bladder pouch. In addition, postradical cystectomy bladder cancer victims are subjected to frequent surveillance procedures due to their high risk for future upper urinary tract urothelial malignancies (3%) and may require radical nephroureterectomy.

Anesthetic considerations for patients who present with existing diversion procedures include metabolic and electrolyte abnormalities such as hyperchloremic metabolic acidosis (common), hypokalemia, hypocalcemia and hypomagnesemia, and high rates of urinary tract infection and pyelonephritis. In addition, these individuals frequently suffer from chronic diarrhea and may have problems related to malabsorption (e.g., vitamin B_{12} deficiency).

Prostatectomy

Almost all procedures involving complete resection of the prostate (i.e., prostatectomy) are for adenocarcinoma of the prostate, since nonmalignant surgical disease of the prostate is typically so amenable to TUR (see the next section). Despite prostate cancer being a disease limited to men, it is the second most common cancer in most countries with an incidence that increases significantly with age and is approximately 50% more common in African American men than in Caucasian men (Fig. 50-9).[187]

Current evidence-based opinion on the optimal management of prostate cancer is rapidly evolving, including the relative value of intervention (i.e., hormonal, cryo-, chemo-, internal and external radiation therapy, highly focused ultrasound ablation, and surgery) compared to an expanded role for "watchful waiting" in low-risk groups, as identified by measures such as tumor aggressiveness (e.g., Gleason score) and biomarkers (e.g., prostate-specific antigen levels). A second related concept is also emerging—that prostate cancer may exist in clinically significant (approximately 15%) and "insignificant" forms.[188] In general, surgical approaches are likely in younger men, while elderly patients who may die from disorders other than their prostate cancer are being more frequently advised to pursue nonsurgical therapy.

Prostatectomy can be performed using retropubic or perineal approaches and is amenable to endoscopic techniques with or without robotic assistance. The retropubic approach requires the patient to be supine with the bed extended and in Trendelenburg position (Fig. 50-7) and allows access to the prostate gland and related lymph nodes from behind the pubic symphysis (and the best chance of sparing the neurovascular bundle), using either a vertical midline or Pfannenstiel (horizontal low suprapubic) incision. In contrast, the perineal approach requires the patient be in exaggerated lithotomy and steep Trendelenburg position (Fig. 50-7), with an incision between the scrotum and the anal sphincter that provides adequate access to the prostate (but not lymph nodes).

Preoperative Considerations

Beyond advanced age, relatively few factors predict likelihood of contracting prostate cancer. Family history more than doubles the chances of the disease, while African American descent increases the risk by approximately 50% (Fig. 50-9). Otherwise, factors such as smoking, obesity, diet, history of vasectomy, prostatitis, or sexually transmitted diseases have little or no effect on prostate cancer risk. Due to the advanced age of the population presenting for prostatectomy, an emphasis on comorbid disease in preoperative evaluation is particularly relevant. Paraneoplastic syndromes similar to those seen with kidney cancer are occasionally evident in prostate cancer patients.

Intraoperative Considerations

Anesthetic management for open prostatectomy is similar to that for cystectomy surgery (see above), including attentiveness to the potential for major bleeding. Epidural catheter placement is usually in the low thoracic spinal region, guided in part by the chosen option for anesthesia, including spinal/epidural alone, general alone, or combined spinal/epidural and general anesthesia. A surgical block to at least the T10 level is required for procedures performed using neuraxial block alone. In one study, patients experienced 33% less pain when preemptive epidural dosing occurred prior to incision.[189] Radical prostatectomy may take longer than the duration of a single-dose spinal anesthetic, so epidural or combined spinal–epidural is recommended. Notably, a neuraxial alone strategy for perineal prostatectomy is likely to be poorly tolerated due to the uncomfortable exaggerated lithotomy and head-down positioning requirements. Exaggerated lithotomy position for prostatectomy has also been associated in some studies with higher rates of neurologic injury (21% with transient sensory or motor deficit); patients appearing to be at greater risk when surgery lasts longer than 180 minutes.[190,191] In addition, even with general anesthesia, some patients tolerate the exaggerated lithotomy–head-down position for perineal prostatectomy poorly due to elevated ventilation pressures and impaired oxygenation.

As with cystectomy surgery, the approach to intravascular volume assessment during prostatectomy must consider the potential for bleeding and hypovolemia and limited meaningful urine output data; the need for arterial and/or pressure central venous monitoring should be guided by patient comorbidities. Neuraxial anesthesia for prostatectomy has been associated with decreased blood loss in some studies.[192] However, any blood-sparing benefits of neuraxial anesthesia appear to be lost when it is combined with mechanical ventilation (and general anesthesia), possibly due to the effect of increased intrathoracic pressure on prostatic venous pressures.[193] Notably, breaching of the rich prostatic venous plexuses also creates the potential for acute hemodynamic instability from major venous air embolism, which has been reported during both retropubic and perineal prostatectomy approaches; suspicion of this complication warrants immediate steps to flood the surgical field and alter patient positioning to raise venous pressures above atmospheric, in addition to other standard resuscitation measures.[194]

Postoperative Considerations

Simple prostatectomy requires a limited dissection relative to radical prostatectomy and is generally associated with less blood loss and lower complication rates. Nonetheless, most radical prostatectomy patients are not admitted to an intensive care unit. Average blood loss for radical prostatectomy surgery is between 500 and 1,500 mL,[195] and approximately 10% of patients will require a perioperative blood transfusion.[196] In addition to vascular injury, other common serious intraoperative complications include bowel or ureteral injury. The mortality rate for radical prostatectomy is less than 1%. Impaired lymph drainage (lymphocele, leg edema) is associated in some studies with increased rates of postoperative deep venous thrombosis and pulmonary embolism.[196]

Transversus abdominis plane local anesthetic blocks are used at some institutions for pain management to facilitate retropubic prostatectomy fast tracking recovery protocols[197]; ultrasound guidance for these procedures can minimize procedure-related risk of adjacent structure injury (e.g., bowel).

Specific Procedures

Simple Prostatectomy

Simple open prostatectomy is occasionally required for resection of very large prostate glands affected by benign prostatic hypertrophy (BPH),[198] but, in the era of medical therapies such as α-1 selective adrenergic receptor blockers and 5-α reductase inhibitors, this is an infrequent procedure. Currently, retropubic prostatectomy is the most common approach in the United States.

Radical Prostatectomy

Radical prostatectomy involves removal of the entire prostate gland, seminal vesicles, and generally the surrounding nerves and veins. The part of the urethra within the prostate gland's transition zone is also removed. Preservation of one or both cavernous nerves (part of the neurovascular bundle on each side of the prostate) can improve post surgery quality of life (i.e., reduced urinary incontinence and erectile dysfunction) but limits the extent of possible resection. Notably, the incidence of positive margins with tumor resection during radical prostatectomy is significant (~30%). The value of more aggressive resection with sural nerve grafting to address erectile dysfunction remains unclear.[199] Controversial early data on the association of epidural anesthesia and analgesia with lower rates of cancer recurrence[200] have not been substantiated in more recent reports.

Laparoscopic and Robotic Prostatectomy

Minimally invasive laparoscopic and robotic-assisted approaches to prostatectomy are gaining popularity and most urologic procedures can now be performed using a minimally invasive robotic approach (see Chapter 43) (1 Video 50-1).[201] Robot-assisted laparoscopic radical prostatectomy is the most performed robotic surgery and this approach comprises over 80% of prostatectomies performed in the United States.[202] Robotic prostatectomy is performed in the steep Trendelenburg position with CO_2 pneumoperitonium. While these techniques are characterized by less pain, shorter hospital stays, faster recovery, and improved patient satisfaction,[203] they also present added challenge for the anesthesiologist, including prolonged procedure duration, the risk of hypothermia, occult blood loss, and the physiologic stresses of pneumoperitoneum and exaggerated Trendelenburg with or without lithotomy positioning.

Laparoscopic and robotic prostatectomy procedures require general anesthesia with endotracheal intubation. Standard monitoring and adequate intravenous access must be established prior to patient positioning since access after positioning is very difficult (Fig. 50-10). Pulse oximeter probe placement should avoid the ear lobe to anticipate the potential for inaccurate readings in this location, presumably related to the venous engorgement with head-down positioning and pneumoperitoneum.[204] Intra-arterial and central venous monitoring are not routine but may be indicated based on patient comorbidities. As with all robotic surgeries, due to the fixed position of the robot arms, movements such as coughing can cause injury internally or at port sites, so care must be taken to maintain adequate depth of anesthesia and neuromuscular blockade. Exaggerated Trendelenburg positioning is required for the procedure, and some practitioners deliberately refrain from dosing epidural catheters to avoid cephalad spread of epidural drugs during the procedure.

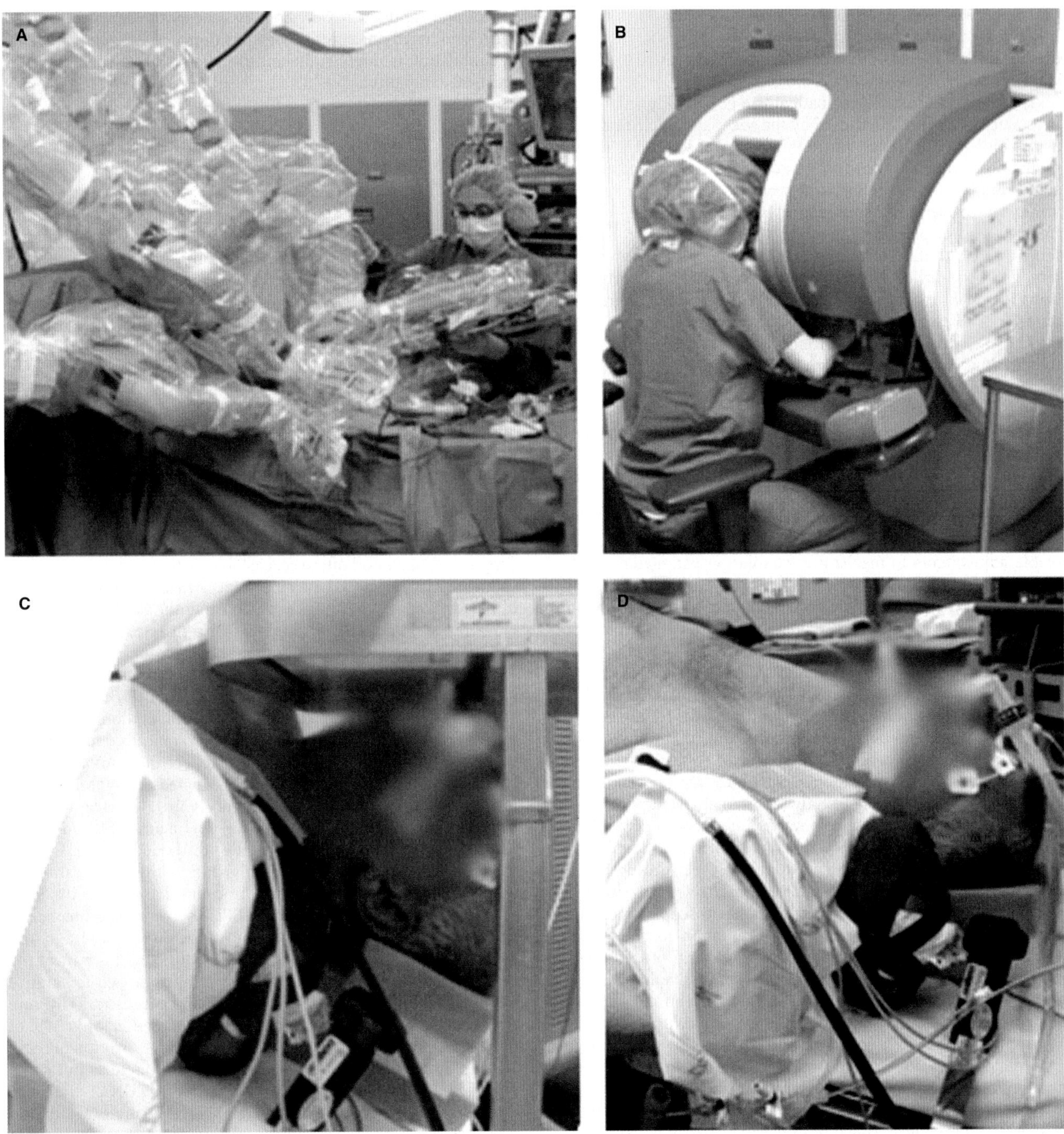

Figure 50-10 Images from a robotic radical prostatectomy procedure highlights the significant difficulty in accessing patients after the robot is docked (**A**), the remote location of the surgeon (**B**), the utility of a carefully placed Mayo stand to protect the patient's face and endotracheal tube (**C**), and the value of shoulder support padding to avoid pressure injuries (**D**).

Steep Trendelenburg (30 to 45 degrees head-down) to facilitate pelvic access during laparoscopic and robotic prostatectomy procedures increases the risk of several important complications (Fig. 50-7). To prevent sliding, patients must be well situated on the operating table (e.g., within a vacuum bean bag) then firmly secured (e.g., tape, safety belt). Arms should be placed on angled armboards *prior* to lowering the end table section during lithotomy positioning to minimize the risk of pinched or crushed fingers. The patient's arms are generally tucked at the side, and pressure points carefully padded. Additional padding should distribute localized pressure from shoulder braces, which sometimes support a significant fraction of the patient's body weight (Fig. 50-10). Beyond brachial plexus protection with shoulder padding, attention should be paid to radial (at the humerus), ulnar (at the elbow), and lateral femoral cutaneous (by the lithotomy leg holders) nerves to minimize axonal injuries. Finally, since oral ulceration and even conjunctival burns have been attributed to lithotomy-related reflux of gastric contents, steps such as preoperative antacid therapy, stomach drainage by orogastric tube, and waterproof eye taping should all be considered.[205]

Lack of easy access to the patient is a concern during robotic prostatectomy, primarily caused by the sheer size of current robot arms (Fig. 50-10). Hence, positioning preparation must be thorough and completed prior to robot docking. A Mayo instrument stand directly above the patient's head can help prevent robotic arms from causing pressure-related facial injuries and/or endotracheal tube displacement (Fig. 50-10).[206] Operating room staff must also be trained for robot emergencies, particularly timely removal of the device. Notably, while cardioversion and defibrillation are possible with the robot docked, cardiopulmonary resuscitation with chest compressions is nearly impossible.

The physiology of steep Trendelenburg positioning is well tolerated by healthy patients (NICV 50-1),[207] but this cannot be assumed for those with serious comorbidities. Adding to the stresses of head-down positioning during laparoscopic prostatectomy are the effects of CO_2 pneumoperitoneum (see nephrectomy section; Table 50-5). Although no formal guidelines exist, additional monitoring for patients with cardiac disease (e.g., compensated congestive heart failure) may be justified to assess responses to position-related intravascular volume shifts. Respiratory effects of robotic prostatectomy are numerous and often require considerable adjustments to mechanical ventilation parameters. Endotracheal tube cuff location should be just beyond the vocal cords, to minimize the potential for developing a mainstem intubation with the cephalad shift of the diaphragm and mediastinum from the combination of head-down and pneumoperitoneum.[204] The related encroachment of abdominal contents on the diaphragm also has significant effects on pulmonary function, particularly in obese patients, including reductions in functional residual capacity, vital capacity, and overall lung compliance that translate into the need for higher peak airway pressures for equivalent tidal volumes. In addition, obese patients experience greater ventilation; perfusion mismatching. One study reported an average 8% lower tidal volumes, 22% higher respiratory rates, and a 38% higher peak inspiratory pressures to maintain similar end-tidal carbon dioxide levels but lower oxygen saturation levels, during robotic compared to open retropubic radical prostatectomy.[208] Interestingly, CO_2 insufflation for retroperitoneal laparoscopic procedures requires greater increases in minute ventilation to compensate for absorbed CO_2 than equivalent transperitoneal procedures.[205] Tolerance of mildly elevated CO_2 levels (permissive hypercarbia) during some phases of the surgery may be a good strategy in some patients but is potentially ill-advised for patients with CKD where even mild respiratory acidosis can be associated with significant hyperkalemia.[209] Transcranial Doppler[210] and cerebral oximetry[207] to monitor intracranial perfusion have been suggested for patients with cerebrovascular disease. Potential adverse effects on intraocular pressure of head-down positioning in at-risk patients (e.g., poorly controlled glaucoma) have not been rigorously studied. Despite all these physiologic perturbations, the need to convert from laparoscopic/robotic assisted to open techniques for major urologic procedures is remarkably infrequent.[205]

During robotic prostatectomy, one of the major surgical steps involves reanastomosis of the severed urethral ends after prostate gland resection, this is often made more complicated by urine from the bladder neck spilling directly into the operative field, obscuring the surgeon's view and impeding progress. Anticipation of this problem by the anesthesiologist can assist the surgeon through cautious fluid restriction, particularly prior to urethral anastomosis. A generally restrictive approach to fluid administration may also attenuate the development of mild facial, periorbital, and even occasionally laryngeal edema associated with prolonged steep lithotomy position.[204,205] However, edema accumulation is rarely sufficient to threaten airway patency after tracheal extubation.

Transurethral Surveillance and Resection Procedures

Transurethral endoscopy is a commonly used, relatively noninvasive surgical tool in the armamentarium of the urologist, that can play an important role in the management and treatment of urothelial cancers (e.g., cystoscopy/ureteroscopy surveillance, TURBT), urolithiasis (e.g., ureteroscopic stent placement, basket stone retrieval), and BPH (e.g., transurethral resection of the prostate [TURP]). Despite the benign and noninvasive appearance of transurethral tissue resection surgeries (TURBT, TURP), these procedures are occasionally associated with significant morbidity and even mortality.

Cystoscopy and TURBT procedures are used in the surveillance, staging, and management of transitional cell bladder cancers (see cystectomy section). For patients with superficial cancers that do not invade the bladder muscle, bladder biopsy and subsequent TURBT may be curative, but such patients require ongoing cystoscopy surveillance and often receive biologic therapies (e.g., Bacillus Calmette–Guerin [BCG] vaccine) that reduce the recurrence rate of bladder cancer, presumably by boosting the immune response. Nonetheless, about 50% of patients with a resected bladder cancer will develop another bladder or ureteral cancer in the future.

TURP is a mainstay, and even "gold standard" therapy to alleviate urine obstructive symptoms related to BPH. BPH describes 12
the smooth muscle and epithelial cell proliferation within the transition zone of the prostate that histologically characterizes this disorder. The symptoms of BPH reflect the combination of bladder outlet obstruction (static) and increased smooth muscle tone (dynamic). While TURP surgery with electrocautery has been for many decades central to the treatment of BPH, a proliferation of other options explains the steady decrease in the use of TURP for BPH treatment, partly due to the significant side effects that can occur with this procedure (e.g., incontinence, impotence). Medical therapy for BPH is common, directed at both static and dynamic components of the disease (α-1 adrenergic antagonists and α-1A reductase inhibitors), and is part of the current more conservative watchful waiting approach to surgical treatment of BPH. Numerous alternate procedures to TURP are now being used for BPH; in 2005, TURP represented only 39% of BPH procedures compared to 81% in 1999.[211] Description of these alternate procedures is beyond the scope of this text, but some of these include transurethral needle ablation (TUNA), transurethral microwave thermal therapy (TUMT), transurethral ablation prostatectomy (TURAPY), holmium laser ablation of the prostate (HoLAP), interstitial laser coagulation (ILC), ultrasound/high intensity focused ultrasound (HIFU), and water intensity hyperthermia (WIT).

Positioning concerns for cystoscopy, TURBT, and TURP are the same as for other procedures in lithotomy position (Fig. 50-10) and in particular relate to adequate padding of pressure points and avoidance of peroneal nerve compression.

Preoperative Considerations

Patients presenting for TURP are likely to be elderly and may have other serious comorbidities. Cardiovascular and pulmonary status should be carefully assessed to evaluate the patient's ability to tolerate the intravascular volume changes associated with the procedure. Patients on anticoagulant therapy may not be candidates for spinal anesthesia, depending on the indication for anticoagulation. The risk of stopping the anticoagulant perioperatively may or may not be worth the advantages of spinal anesthesia for a particular patient. Decisions about this should be made in conjunction with the surgeon, as the risk of postoperative bleeding following TURP will likely dictate an interval of normal coagulation or bridging treatment with short-acting anticoagulants such as heparin.

Intraoperative Considerations

Choice of anesthetic technique for cystoscopy, TURBT, and TURP procedures should be tailored to the individual and can be performed safely with either general or regional anesthesia.[212] Neuraxial block allows the patient to remain awake and may hasten the diagnosis of bladder or prostatic capsule perforation and the TUR syndrome and may also decrease blood loss compared with general anesthesia.[213,214] For ambulatory surgery patients, care must be taken in the selection of spinal anesthetic medications so as to avoid prolonged anesthetic duration and delayed discharge from the facility. Combined spinal–epidural techniques or general anesthesia may have advantages if the length of surgery is unpredictable. Notably, the lower central venous pressure associated with regional anesthesia may actually increase the likelihood of significant irrigation fluid absorption.[215]

Hypothermia can complicate TURP procedures: Body temperature decreases approximately 1° C/hr of surgery, and shivering occurs in 16% of patients who receive room-temperature irrigation fluids. Hypothermia does not develop if irrigation solutions are warmed to body temperature.[216]

Approximately 2.5% of patients require transfusion during TURP surgery. Average blood loss is 2 to 4 mL/min,[217] but individual bleeding rates can be difficult to assess due to mixing with irrigating fluid. The patient's vital signs may be useful to guide transfusion,[218] but, with prolonged resections, serial assessments of hemoglobin level are advisable.

Surgical perforation of the prostatic capsule occurs in 2% of TURP procedures, usually resulting in extraperitoneal fluid extravasation. Awake patients with a neuraxial anesthetic may complain during surgery of new-onset pain localized to the lower abdomen and back.[218,219] Bladder perforation during TURBT more commonly results in extravasation of fluid intraperitoneally and may produce abdominal distension and complaints of abdominal and shoulder pain in awake patients.[220] Notably, evidence of perforation often only becomes clear postoperatively.

Postoperative Considerations

Although abnormal bleeding after TURP occurs in fewer than 1% of resections,[217] 2% to 3% of patients will require transfusion perioperatively.[221,222] Blood loss following TURBT is usually less than 100 mL, although postoperative hemorrhage can rarely occur. Thromboplastin, a thrombogenic stimulant found in high concentrations in prostate cancer cells, can rarely trigger disseminated intravascular coagulation.[218] Another cause of post-TURP bleeding is release of prostatic tissue plasminogen activators. These factors convert plasminogen to plasmin, causing fibrinolysis. Treatment of these conditions is supportive and may include transfusion of coagulation factors and platelets.[223] Prophylactic administration of antifibrinolytics (e.g., tranexamic acid) demonstrated some success, but has not gained widespread acceptance as standard practice.[224] Nevertheless, it may be considered in cases of refractory bleeding.

As outlined above, bladder, prostatic capsule, or urethral perforation are uncommon but serious complications that may manifest postoperatively with or without symptoms of TUR syndrome (see later). Fever related to TURP procedures may indicate bacteremia secondary to spread of bacteria through open prostatic venous sinuses, particularly with a history of infectious prostatitis.

The most common complications following TURP surgery are the need for urinary recatheterization (4%), prostatic capsule perforation (2%), and postoperative hemorrhage requiring transfusion (1%).[225] The 30-day mortality following TURP is 0.2%[219,226–229] and most commonly relates to serious cardiac and respiratory complications.[230]

Specific Procedures

Cystoscopy and Ureteroscopy

While surveillance cystoscopy is often performed under local anesthesia outside the operating room with minimal monitoring or sedation and without the involvement of anesthesia personnel, some cystoscopy and most ureteroscopy procedures, particularly for those patients with comorbidities, occur in the operating room setting. Cystoscopy and ureteroscopy are rarely associated with significant complications, and perioperative considerations should generally parallel those for the disease being screened for or managed (see related sections).

Transurethral Bladder Tumor Resection

During any simple cystoscopy or ureteroscopy procedure, abnormal tissue may require one or more planned or unanticipated diagnostic biopsies or biopsy/resections. As outlined above (see cystectomy section), risk factors for bladder cancer and atherosclerosis overlap and cardiac risk assessment is relevant to TURBT surgery.[231] A serious intraoperative complication of TURBT is bladder perforation by the rigid cystoscope during tissue resection, which occasionally occurs due to unexpected patient movement. For this reason, muscle relaxation is preferred during general anesthesia, particularly in lateral wall resections where the obturator nerve may be stimulated by electrocautery, producing a violent contraction of the ipsilateral thigh muscles. Neuraxial anesthesia to the T9 to T10 dermatomal level also provides adequate anesthesia for the procedure and prevents the obturator reflex. Regional anesthesia may also facilitate detection of bladder perforation. Postoperative pain is usually minimal and responds well to nonopiate and opiate medications.

Transurethral Prostate Resection (TURP)

Standard procedure during TURP surgery involves inserting a "resectoscope," a specialized endoscopy instrument with an electrode capable of both coagulating and cutting tissue, into the urethra then bladder, and the tissue protruding into the prostatic urethra is then resected.[232] There has been much recent interest in the use of lasers rather than electrocautery to resect excess prostate tissue. A variety of different lasers have been utilized. Laser techniques have advantages over traditional electrocautery approaches particularly related to traditional irrigation fluid restrictions: Laser resection has no requirement for a nonconductive fluid, so 0.9% saline may be used, avoiding complications of absorption related to hypo-osmolarity and solute toxicity (see TUR syndrome below). Furthermore, the potential for systemic absorption may be reduced due to the lower irrigation infusion rates and pressures necessary for laser procedures.[233,234] Lasers also have coagulative properties, resulting in less blood loss and lower rates of transfusion.

Table 50-6 Properties of Commonly used Irrigating Solutions for Transurethral Resection Procedures

Solution	Osmolality (mOsm/L)	Advantages	Disadvantages
Distilled water	0	Improved visibility	Hemolysis Hemoglobinemia Hemoglobinuria Hyponatremia
Glycine (1.5%)	200	Less likelihood of TUR syndrome	Transient postoperative visual syndrome Hyperammonemia Hyperoxaluria
Sorbitol (3.3%)	165	Same as glycine	Hyperglycemia, possible lactic acidosis Osmotic diuresis
Mannitol (5%)	275	Isosmolar solution Not metabolized	Osmotic diuresis Possibility of acute intravascular volume expansion

TURP, transurethral resection of the prostate.
Adapted from Krongrad A, Droller MJ. Complications of transurethral resection of the prostate. In: Marshall FF, ed. *Urologic Complications: Medical and Surgical, Adult and Pediatric*. 2nd ed. St. Louis: Mosby-Year Book; 1990:5. Copyright © 1990 Elsevier. With permission.

Irrigating Solutions and Transurethral Resection Syndrome

Key to a surgeon's endoscopic view during transurethral procedures is a visually clear irrigating solution, infused with a pump or via gravity (and drained away) to flush out blood and resected tissue and keep space between structures. Safety characteristics of the irrigating solution are important since, with tissue resection or urinary tract injury, significant amounts of the fluid may inadvertently enter the circulation; for example, during TURP through openings in the venous plexus or retroperitoneal rents in the prostatic capsule or consequent to perforation of the urinary bladder into the peritoneal space during TURBT. Other procedures where inadvertent perforation can cause the TUR syndrome include cystoscopy, ureteroscopy (URS), percutaneous nephrolithotomy (PNL), and laser vaporization of the prostate.

13 The spectrum of morbidities associated with irrigating solution absorption are termed the TUR syndrome. A variety of nonconductive *nonelectrolytic* solutions are in common use. The crystalloids have current-dispersing properties due to their ionic characteristics that make them unsuitable for use with unipolar electrocautery. When absorbed in significant amounts, nonelectrolytic irrigation solutions combine electrolyte disturbances with hypervolemia. Notably, newer transurethral *bipolar* electrocautery and laser techniques now allow irrigation with isotonic crystalloid solutions (e.g., 0.9% saline), but until these technologies totally replace unipolar electrocautery, nonconducting osmotically active irrigating solutions will continue to be used, each variant having its own concerns (Table 50-6).[211]

It is, therefore, important that the anesthesiologist be aware of solutions used for transurethral procedures at their own institution, since TUR syndrome for each irrigating solution has its own profile (Table 50-6). Nonetheless, *TUR syndrome* historically describes a common cluster of symptoms related to hypervolemic water intoxication; the principal components are (a) excessive volume expansion (respiratory distress, congestive heart failure, pulmonary edema, hypertension, bradycardia, hypotension, etc.), (b) hyponatremia (mental confusion, nausea, etc.; Table 50-7), and (c) other problems specific to each of the irrigating solutions.[235–237] Notably, any future trend toward limiting irrigation to physiologic solutions (e.g., 0.9% saline), should eliminate all but the hypervolemic component of the TUR syndrome.

Of available irrigating solutions, distilled water is rarely utilized due to its hypotonicity. Water intoxication with distilled water rapidly causes severe hyponatremia, leading to hemolysis, hemoglobinemia, and renal failure. Sorbitol and glucose solutions cause hyperglycemia when they are absorbed. Glycine, an amino acid normally metabolized to ammonia, may cause a depressed mental status and even coma (due to hyperammonemia) that can last 24 to 48 hours postoperatively.[238,239] Also reported with glycine are blurred vision, minimally or nonreactive pupils, and transient blindness.[240,241] Since glycine has structural similarities to aminobutyric acid, these visual disturbances are thought to reflect neurotransmitter-mediated brainstem or cranial nerve inhibition rather than cerebral edema.[241]

Absorption of very large amounts of irrigant (>2 L) is usually required to manifest the TUR syndrome (NICV 50-2). The incidence of symptomatic TUR syndrome is highest during TURP procedures where it may be as high as 1.4%.[221] Typically, intraoperative irrigation infusion rates of 300 mL/min are used during TURP procedures for optimal surgical visualization.[230] Some intravascular absorption is to be expected; rates of 20 mL/min are typical, but these can reach as high as 200 mL/min.[242] Factors that predict increased irrigation fluid absorption during a TURP procedure include the number and size of open venous sinuses (i.e., greater blood loss implies greater potential for irrigation

Table 50-7 Signs and Symptoms of Acute Hyponatremia

Serum Na^+ (mEq/L)	CNS Changes	ECG Changes
120	Confusion Restlessness	Possible widening of QRS complex
115	Somnolence Nausea	Widened QRS complex Elevated ST segment
110	Seizures Coma	Ventricular tachycardia or fibrillation

CNS, central nervous system; ECG, electrocardiogram.
Adapted with permission from Springer: Jensen V. The TURP syndrome. *Can J Anaesth*. 1991;38:90.

absorption), surgical disruption of the prostatic capsule, longer duration of resection, higher hydrostatic pressure of the irrigating fluid, and lower venous pressure at the irrigant–blood interface.[217]

To minimize fluid absorption, procedural guidelines include limiting resection time to <1 hour and suspending the irrigating fluid bag no more than 30 cm above the operating table at the beginning and 15 cm in the final stages of resection.[217,243] In addition, avoidance of hypotonic intravenous fluids and treatment of regional anesthesia-induced hypotension with judicious use of intravenous vasopressor agents rather than intravenous fluids should be considered.

Symptomatic TUR syndrome is much less common following TURBT (and usually related to symptoms of bladder perforation), but it is important to be aware of the possibility of its occurrence since it may present somewhat differently due to the slower rate of fluid absorption.[220] Most notably, the time course of symptoms following bladder perforation during TURBT reflects the slower absorption from the abdominal cavity, compared to direct prostatic venous plexus entry with TURP. For example, nadir serum sodium values are generally reached between 1 and 6 hours following TURP, whereas TUR syndrome following TURBT occurs between 2 and 9 hours postoperatively.[220]

Clinical manifestations of the TUR syndrome range from mild (restlessness, nausea, shortness of breath, dizziness) to severe (seizures, coma, hypertension, bradycardia, cardiovascular collapse). In the awake patient with a regional block, a classic triad of symptoms has been described that consists of an increase in both systolic and diastolic pressures associated with an increase in pulse pressure, bradycardia, and mental status changes.[218,235]

Early symptoms associated with TUR syndrome are mostly related to acute intravascular volume expansion, independent of changes in serum osmolality and sodium.[237] Initial hypertension and bradycardia from acute volume overload may evolve into left heart failure, pulmonary edema, and even cardiovascular collapse.[244] With the continued absorption of hypotonic irrigation fluid, cerebral edema as a consequence of dilutional hyponatremia may develop. Rapid change, as opposed to a specific low threshold serum sodium concentration, is responsible for most of the signs and symptoms of TUR syndrome (Table 50-7).[235]

When neurologic or cardiovascular complications of TURP procedures are recognized intraoperatively, prompt intervention is necessary (Table 50-8). First, the surgeon should be informed of the patient's status change so that the procedure can be completed or terminated as quickly as possible. The hallmark of patient treatment is to restore extracellular tonicity. Although the traditional recommended rate of serum sodium correction is 0.5 mEq/L/hr, this is for chronic hyponatremia, and no established rate for correction of acute hyponatremia exists. Symptomatic patients with serum sodium concentrations <120 mEq/L should have their extracellular tonicity corrected with hypertonic saline. Sodium chloride in a 3% solution should be infused at a rate no greater than 100 mL/hr. Serum electrolytes should be followed closely, and the hypertonic saline discontinued when the patient is asymptomatic or serum sodium concentration exceeds 120 mEq/L. Treatment with hypertonic saline has been associated with development of demyelinating central nervous system lesions (central pontine myelinolysis) due to rapid increases in plasma osmolality, and this approach should be reserved for patients with severe, life-threatening symptoms.[245] The demyelination is the result of excessive shrinkage of brain cells after rapid hydration with hyperosmolar solution as the brain cells have extruded important osmoles to compensate for the chronic hypotonicity. Notably, reports of demyelination after correction of acute symptomatic hyponatremia are rare, and there are no reports of demyelination after treatment of acute TUR syndrome.[237]

Table 50-8 Treatment of the Transurethral Resection Syndrome

Ensure oxygenation and circulatory support
Notify surgeon and terminate procedure as soon as possible
Consider insertion of invasive monitors if cardiovascular instability occurs
Send blood to laboratory for evaluation of electrolytes, creatinine, glucose, and arterial blood gases
Obtain 12-lead electrocardiogram
Treat mild symptoms (with serum Na^+ concentration >120 mEq/L) with fluid restriction and loop diuretic (furosemide)
Treat severe symptoms (if serum Na^+ <120 mEq/L) with 3% sodium chloride IV at a rate <100 mL/hr
Discontinue 3% sodium chloride when serum Na^+ >120 mEq/L

Therapies for Urolithiasis

Stone disease of the urinary tract, urolithiasis, can be subdivided on the basis of the location of the stone into nephrolithiasis (kidney), ureterolithiasis (ureter), or cystolithiasis (bladder). Nephrolithiasis is a common clinical problem, with an increasing incidence. The lifetime prevalence of nephrolithiasis is 10% in men and 5% in women. Up to 50% of patients with an initial stone episode will have a recurrence within 5 years.[246]

The composition of kidney stones varies (Table 50-9). The most common type of stones contain calcium and are radio-opaque. Stones form when the concentration of stone-forming salts in the urine is elevated (e.g., oxalate) or when the level of stone inhibitors in the urine is low (e.g., citrate). This results in supersaturation of the urine with salts, allowing crystals to form and grow, particularly in situations where urine volume is low. This pathophysiology explains the principles of the medical management of kidney stones: Increasing urine volume and maneuvers to restore urinary salt balance, through dietary and medical treatment.[247,248]

The preferred diagnostic modality for urolithiasis is helical noncontrast CT scan which can identify radio-opaque and radiolucent stones in the entire urinary system and determine whether hydronephrosis is present. Ultrasound imaging is also informative for stones in the kidney and proximal ureter but cannot image the distal ureter and may miss smaller stones. Compared to helical CT and ultrasonography, plain radiographs (Kidney–Ureter–Bladder, KUB) provide no additional information about obstruction or hydronephrosis and can miss stones in the kidney or ureter. Intravenous pyelography is rarely used since it offers no added information compared to other diagnostic modalities and exposes the patient to radiation and contrast-related kidney injury.[248]

Patients with kidney stones typically present with intermittent or continuous moderate to severe colicky pain in the ipsilateral flank and upper abdomen. Testicular or labial pain is more typical with distal ureteric stones. Occasionally, patients present with painless urinary infection or hematuria. Conservative nonsurgical therapy for smaller stones consists of analgesics (e.g., NSAIDs and/or opiates) and aggressive fluid administration to promote

Table 50-9 Spectrum of Kidney Stones Types: Composition, Frequency, and Causes

Stone Composition	Frequency	Mechanism
Calcium oxalate or Calcium phosphate	70–80%	Hypercalciuria • High sodium and protein diet • Hypercalcemia, e.g., hyperparathyroidism • Chronic metabolic acidosis Low urine output • Chronic dehydration Hyperuricosuria • High purine, high protein intake • Gout Hyperoxaluria • Low dietary calcium • High oxalate diet • Genetic Low urine citrate • Chronic metabolic acidosis • Renal tubular acidosis • Inflammatory bowel disease
Uric Acid	10–15%	Low urine pH Chronic metabolic acidosis Hyperuricosuria Obesity Lesch–Nyhan syndrome
Magnesium ammonium phosphate (struvite)	10–15%	Urinary infections (urea-splitting bacteria), e.g., Proteus, Klebsiella, Staphylococcus, Pseudomonas, Providentia, and *Corynebacterium urealyticum*
Cystine	<1%	Cystinuria—autosomal recessive
Others: Indinavir Triamterene Xanthine	<1%	Antiretroviral drug for HIV Potassium-sparing diuretic Xanthine oxidase inhibitor therapy, e.g., allopurinol

Modified from Hall PM. Nephrolithiasis: Treatment, causes, and prevention. *Cleve Clin J Med*. 2009;76:583–591; Brown P. Management of urinary tract infections associated with nephrolithiasis. *Curr Infect Dis Rep*. 2010;12:450–454.

urine flow and passage of the stone. The so-called "medical expulsive therapy" (MET) to promote ureter relaxation and the spontaneous passage of small ureteral stones involves treatment with calcium-channel blockers (e.g., nifedipine), α-blockers (e.g., tamsulosin), and sometimes, corticosteroids.[248,249] The likelihood of stone passage without surgery relates to the size of the stone, its location, and the presence or absence of urinary system anatomic abnormalities such as strictures. If stones do not pass spontaneously or respond to MET, various surgical options can be considered, as discussed above (Fig. 50-11).

Preoperative Considerations

Anesthetic planning for urolithiasis surgery should include standard considerations (NICV 50-3). Typical calcium salt stone disease presents in the third to fifth decades of life[248] and is commonly associated with comorbidities such as obesity, hypertension, and hyperparathyroidism. Patients with renal failure or CKD should be assessed for the sequelae of these conditions, including platelet dysfunction, anemia, and electrolyte abnormalities. Bladder stones are often diagnosed in patients with poor voiding capacity, for example, paraplegic patients, and the associated perioperative concerns for these patients should be addressed. Although paraplegic patients with sensory deficits below T6 lack pain perception for cystoscopy procedures, they are at risk for *autonomic hyperreflexia* and require anesthesia to block the afferent stimulation that can provoke this reaction (e.g., bladder distension). This can be achieved with deeper levels of general anesthesia or regional anesthesia.[250] Patients with idiopathic hypercalciuria are often treated with thiazide diuretics, and serum potassium should be assessed preoperatively.[248]

Perioperative opioid analgesic dosing for urolithiasis procedures can be challenging. Patients with recurrent nephrolithiasis may be receiving chronic opioid therapy and demonstrate tolerance intra- and postoperatively. In contrast, when severe colic is alleviated by surgery for an opioid naive patient already treated with opiates, postoperative somnolence is quite common. Renal colic is often associated with nausea and vomiting, and preoperative aspiration prophylaxis should be considered.

Unless open surgery is planned, there is rarely a need for blood transfusion for stone surgery. Selection of appropriate monitors should be dictated by patient comorbidities, as significant blood loss or fluid shifts are unusual with these procedures. However, if difficulty achieving vascular access during a procedure is anticipated (e.g., percutaneous nephrolithotripsy), there should be a low threshold for establishing central access prior to the procedure. Antibiotic prophylaxis is important, particularly with infected stones or pyelonephritis. When lasers are required, appropriate eye protection should be provided for the perioperative team and patient.

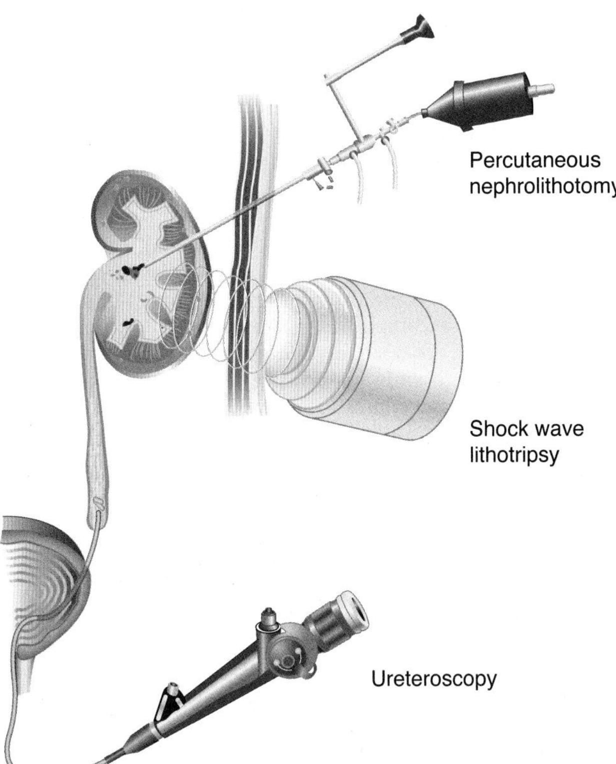

Figure 50-11 Urinary tract stones: Intervention choices. (Reprinted with permission from: Samplaski M, Irwin B, Desai M. Less-invasive ways to remove stones from thekidneys and ureters. *Cleve Clin J Med* 2009; 76(10) 592-598. Copyright © 2023 Cleveland Clinic Foundation. All rights reserved.)

Intraoperative Considerations

Compared with other more invasive urologic procedures, stone surgeries generally do not involve large amounts of blood loss or fluid shifts, with the possible exception of percutaneous nephrolithotripsy (see later). Information about anesthetic choice and potential intraoperative issues is discussed in the individual sections below and in the sections on nephrectomy and transurethral surgery elsewhere in this chapter. Monitoring decisions and anesthetic choices should be made on the basis of patient comorbidity, and intraoperative care should focus on those as well.

Postoperative Considerations

Postoperative concerns for urolithiasis procedures are generally minor. Interestingly, patients with severe renal colic prior to less-invasive surgeries (e.g., URS) may have less or no pain postoperatively with relief of their urinary obstruction and stone retrieval. However, immediately following urinary tract instrumentation, many patients experience rather uncomfortable bladder and ureteral spasms. These spasms are typically more responsive to NSAIDs, oxybutynin, and belladonna and opium suppositories than to parenteral opioids.

Occasionally, open surgery is required for upper urinary tract stone removal, with postoperative concerns comparable to nephrectomy patients having similar incisions; these include pain, which may be sufficient to require epidural analgesia, and monitoring requirements to ensure that adequate resuscitation related to any blood loss has occurred.

Monitoring the adequacy of urine output and maintaining any urinary irrigation or drainage system (e.g., stents, three-way Foley catheters) to promote clearance of blood in the urinary system is important, as clots or stone fragments can cause acute urinary obstruction.

After extraction or lithotripsy of stones, particularly struvite stones or in the setting of pyelonephritis, patients may develop a pattern of rigors, hypotension, and fever, which can lead to shock. Urine culture results can be misleading in predicting which patients will develop sepsis since urine below the level of a stone may be clean, yet urine upstream of the stony obstruction may be infected. A sepsis picture can be noted during the procedure but is more likely to occur postoperatively. Indications of intravascular bacterial seeding from infected urine needs prompt attention with blood cultures, fluids and resuscitation, and institution of appropriate antibiotic therapy to prevent more serious sequelae of a sepsis syndrome. The potential acuity of this situation should not be underestimated, as even healthy ASA 1 to 2 patients can develop systemic inflammatory response syndrome (SIRS) and require aggressive resuscitation and intensive care.[251]

Specific Procedures

Shock Wave Lithotripsy

Shock wave lithotripsy (SWL) is best suited for intranephric stones that are small to moderate in size but can be used for proximal ureteral stones as well (NICV 50-4). The principle of SWL is to use focused sound waves to break the stone into pieces small enough to pass through the ureters, bladder, and urethra during normal urination. This requires transmission of the sound wave beam via an interface with the patient's body. Early SWL was conducted via immersion in a water bath, which created this interface. In addition to the significant positioning maneuvers associated with this procedure, patients are prone to hypothermia during the procedure. Dysrhythmias can be a special problem as the transmission of the ultrasonic pulse is timed and triggered by the ECG. Significant respiratory and hemodynamic changes are associated with immersion and emergence from the water bath, which can be problematic particularly for patients with cardiopulmonary disease.[252] Modern "dry" SWL uses a smaller water-filled coupling device to provide an interface with the patient, which simplifies the procedure considerably. Newer SWL machines also have a more tightly focused sound beam and can deliver the required energy at pressures in each acoustic pulse that are less painful for the patient. These advances allow most procedures to be conducted in an outpatient setting, with topical local anesthesia and analgesia/sedation provided with combinations of nonsteroidal anti-inflammatory medications and opiates. General anesthesia and/or deep sedation are rarely required.

Several factors affect the likelihood of success of SWL. Since increased distance from beam to stone reduces the effectiveness of SWL, this procedure is less successful in obese patients.

Extremely hard stones (such as cysteine and calcium oxalate) are more resistant to lithotripsy and may best be addressed with other treatment modalities.[253] Patients may require more than one treatment for complete stone comminution. As pulse counts increase, so does the risk of kidney injury and even subcapsular hematoma.[247] SWL is the least-invasive and most commonly performed procedure for the management of stone disease, however, even for this approach several relative and absolute contraindications exist (Table 50-10).

Percutaneous Nephrolithotomy

PNL is useful for the management of larger intranephric stones, especially those resistant to SWL, staghorn calculi, and some proximal ureteral stones. PNL requires initial placement of a ureteral

Table 50-10 Contraindications to Shock Wave Lithotripsy

Absolute contraindications	Bleeding disorder or anticoagulation Pregnancy
Relative contraindications	Large calcified aortic or renal artery aneurysms Untreated urinary tract infection Obstruction distal to the renal calculi Pacemaker, ICD, or neurostimulation implant Morbid obesity

ICD, implantable cardioverter-defibrillator.

stent via cystoureteroscopy performed in the lithotomy position. This stent will prevent ureteral obstruction as fragments of stone pass through the ureter following PNL. Following stent placement, the patient is repositioned to an oblique prone position for percutaneous puncture of the kidney pelvis under fluoroscopic guidance, which is followed by placement of a nephrostomy tube to facilitate placement of a nephroscope for stone extraction with forceps or other instruments. Large stones may require use of an ultrasound or laser probe, also placed via the nephrostomy, to fragment them to facilitate removal. The combination of fluoroscopy and direct vision of the kidney pelvis and ureters with nephro- and ureteroscopy is used to ensure that complete removal of the stone(s) has been achieved. Large volumes of irrigation are used to cool the ultrasound probe and wash away the debris, making TUR syndrome an occasional complication of PNL. Because of the large irrigant volume, blood loss can be underappreciated, and unexplained hemodynamic instability during these procedures is often a manifestation of blood loss. Published rates of transfusion during or after PNL range from 5% to 14%.[254] Pneumothorax, though rare, is a possible complication of the procedure depending on the approach used for insertion of the nephroscope.

General anesthesia with endotracheal intubation allows for a secure airway for positioning into the prone position and is most commonly used in many centers; however, spinal anesthesia can also be used.[255] For certain patients, local infiltration with sedation may even suffice.[256]

Ureteroscopy for Removal of Stones

Ureteroscopy for removal of stones (URS) is the procedure of choice for midureteral and distal ureteral stones that have failed conservative management. It is also indicated for treatment of bilateral ureteral stones and can be considered in patients for whom cessation of anticoagulation is not advisable. Morbidly obese patients for whom SWL is not advised are also candidates for this procedure.[247] Although more invasive than SWL, URS generally achieves a higher stone-free rate and can be used to remove stones in all portions of the ureter. Newer technology has allowed smaller, more flexible ureteroscopes, and lasers are now incorporated to facilitate stone disintegration. Various "basket" and other retrieval devices can be inserted through the ureteroscope. The postoperative complications from ureterosopic stone retrieval include perforation of the ureter (5%) and stricture formation (<2%) and rarely TUR syndrome.[257] The procedure can be performed using urethral local anesthesia with intravenous sedation and monitored anesthesia care, spinal, or general anesthesia.

The previous section addresses anesthetic concerns related to cystoscopy and ureteroscopy.

Open and Laparoscopic Pyelolithotomy or Nephrectomy

With the advent of the previously discussed modalities for the treatment of urolithiasis, the use of laparoscopic or open surgery for removal of stones has declined considerably, and they should not be considered first-line treatment for stone disease. Patients who have failed SWL or PNL or who require open surgery for other indications are candidates for open treatment of stone disease. This can be accomplished laparoscopically (retroperitoneal or transperitoneal) or open, depending on the capabilities of the surgeon. Compared with less-invasive approaches, both laparoscopic and open procedures result in more postoperative pain, longer hospital stays and recovery and are associated with higher complication rates.

Urogynecology, Pregnancy-Related and other Miscellaneous Urologic Procedures

A variety of urogynecologic procedures that treat pelvic floor prolapse are directed at symptomatic improvement of stress incontinence. These procedures are relatively noninvasive, often accomplished using a transvaginal approach with the patient in the lithotomy position, and frequently performed as outpatient procedures with same-day discharge home. Anesthesia can be accomplished with local infiltration accompanied by heavy sedation and monitored anesthetic care, neuraxial anesthesia using spinal or combined spinal/epidural local anesthetic injection, or general anesthesia. Local preferences may dictate anesthetic choice, as suggested by reports from some centers regarding the selection of spinal anesthesia that describe on the one hand improved patient and surgeon satisfaction,[258] and on the other a four-fold higher urinary retention rate[259] and 1 hour longer post-anesthesia care unit stay.

Renal colic is the most common nonobstetric cause of abdominal pain requiring hospitalization in pregnant women.[247] Medical management of these patients must consider the fetal gestational age regarding decisions about appropriate analgesics (e.g., NSAIDs in the third trimester may cause premature closure of the fetal ductus arteriosus and adverse kidney effects). Diagnostic tests preferably avoid ionizing radiation and favor the use of ultrasound whenever possible. Interventions in pregnant patients with symptomatic nephrolithiasis have traditionally been limited to ureteral stents to relieve pain and prevent obstruction, with definitive therapy delayed postpartum; however, the need for repeated stent exchanges is common. More recent data support the safety and efficacy of URS for stone removal during pregnancy. SWL is contraindicated in pregnancy.[260,261]

Surgical urologic issues related to the obstetrical patient are uncommon, with the exception of inadvertent injury to the ureter or bladder during cesarean section which, if recognized, should be repaired intraoperatively.[262] Ureteral stenting is also occasionally required to enable ureter identification during a cesarean/hysterectomy procedure for placenta accreta or percreta.[263]

Impotence Surgery and Medication

The impotence drugs sildenafil (Viagra), tadalafil (Cialis), and vardenafil (Levitra) all inhibit cyclic GMP (cGMP)-specific phosphodiesterase type 5 (PDE 5) in vascular smooth muscle

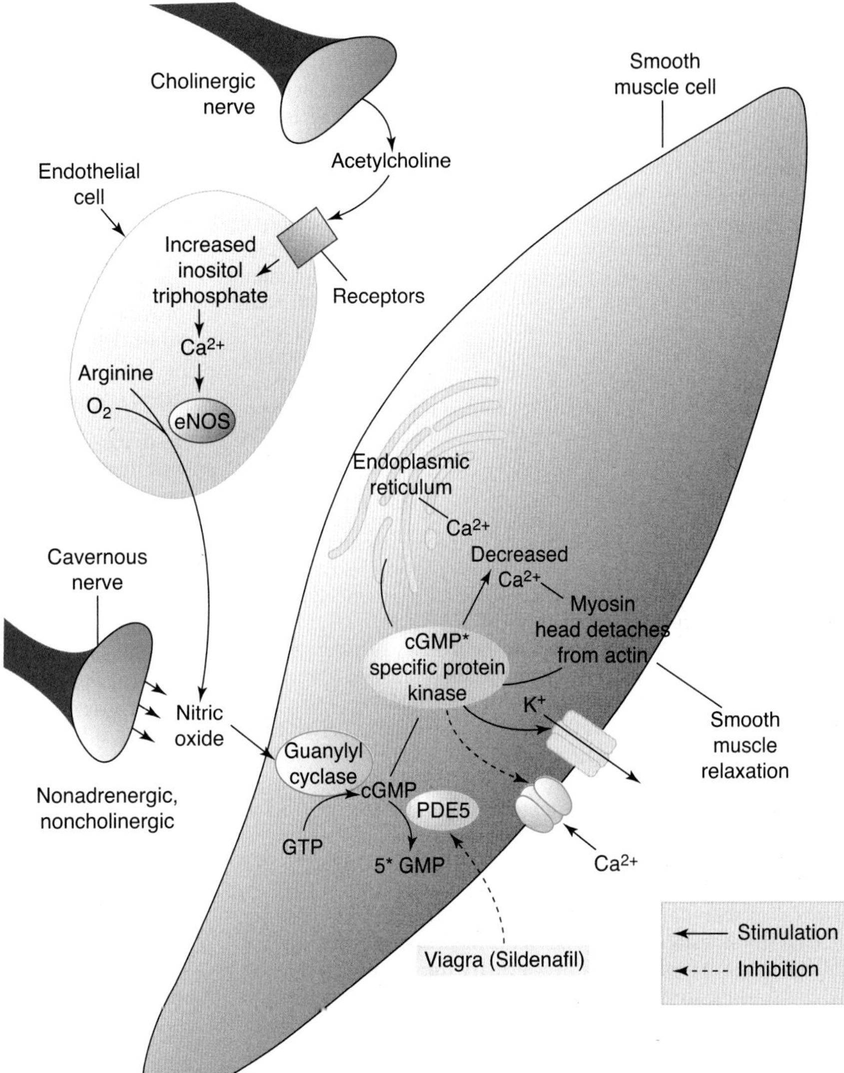

Figure 50-12 Nitric oxide–mediated vascular smooth muscle relaxation, including the inhibiting effects of sildenafil on cyclic GMP-specific phosphodiesterase type 5 (PDE 5). (From Metabolism of Amino Acids and Other Nitrogenous Compounds : Nitric Oxide and Viagra Cutting Edge Article. In: Boyer RF. Concepts in Biochemistry. 2nd ed. *John Wiley & Sons Publishers*, Inc; 2003. Figure 2.)

(Fig. 50-12). Blocking PDE 5 impairs cGMP breakdown, the mediator of nitric oxide effects that produce erectile responses to sexual stimulation through penile arterial vasodilation and corpus cavernosum smooth muscle relaxation. These agents have effects on other vessels and can be a useful treatment for pulmonary artery hypertension (trade names; sildenafil—Revatio, tadalfil—Adcirca).

Rational perioperative management of PDE 5 inhibitor agents is important. Notably, while impotence therapies should be discontinued before surgery to minimize the risk of hypotension, pulmonary hypertension therapies must continue throughout the perioperative period. Although inhaled nitric oxide therapy can safely be used with PDE 5 inhibitors since its effects are limited to the pulmonary vasculature, whenever these agents are combined with systemic nitric oxide donors such as nitroglycerin or sodium nitroprusside, exaggerated hypotensive responses are likely due to their dramatic potentiation of the peripheral vasodilator effects of nitric oxide.

Erectile dysfunction refractory to medical therapies can be treated by penile prosthesis implantation. Most prostheses are inflatable, with a secondary fluid reservoir and/or pump either behind the abdominal wall or inside the scrotum. Semirigid prostheses that do not involve pumps or reservoirs are also available, but these are less commonly used. Although penile implant procedures are relatively noninvasive, many recipients are elderly with multiple comorbidities, including vascular disease and diabetes. Traditionally, implantation has been performed under general or neuraxial anesthesia, but regional block (combined proximal dorsal nerve block and crural block) with sedation and monitored anesthesia care is also suitable if an abdominal incision is not required.[264]

Pediatric Surgical Urologic Disorders

The anesthesiologist caring for a pediatric patient undergoing a urologic procedure must first and foremost have a strong grasp of concepts of pediatric anesthesiology. General anesthesia is typical for these procedures, although a caudal block may provide good postoperative pain control (see Chapter 42).

Nephrectomy and Adrenalectomy

Many adult urologic procedures are also performed in children, although frequently for different indications. Nephrectomy, for example, is used to treat Wilms tumor and nonfunctioning kidney due to obstructive uropathy, stone disease, vesicoureteral reflux, or multicystic dysplastic kidney. Pediatric nephrectomy is amenable to open or laparoscopic approaches with general anesthesia.[265]

Adrenalectomy for neuroblastoma (28%), pheochromocytoma (21%), or adenoma (14%) can most often be achieved laparoscopically, although conversion to an open procedure, most often necessary due to tumor adherence to surrounding organs, is more common than in adults (10%).[266]

As for adults, the preoperative workup and preparation of patients with pheochromocytoma should be thorough. Since inherited syndromes such as neurofibromatosis, von Hippel–Lindau disease, tuberous sclerosis, Sturge–Weber syndrome, and MEN are commonly associated with pediatric pheochromocytoma, other related characteristics of these conditions should also be considered in preoperative preparation.[267] As for adult pheochromocytoma, preoperative therapy with α-1 adrenergic blocking agents (e.g., phenoxybenzamine) is recommended (see Chapter 46).[268]

Reconstructive Urologic Procedures

A number of urologic procedures related to congenital urologic deformities are performed almost exclusively on children. Many of these procedures are reconstructive in nature, intended to functionally repair a defect present at birth.

Bladder exstrophy, where part of the urinary bladder remains outside the body through a defect in the abdominal wall, occurs in 1 per 10,000 to 50,000 live births with a 2:1 male:female ratio.[269] Associated abnormalities are frequently present in the pelvic bones and external genitalia. Repair requires one or more of the following three procedures in a staged fashion, with primary closure of the abdominal wall and osteotomy usually occurring before 4 months of age, epispadias repair between 8 and 24 months of age, and bladder neck reconstruction at 40 to 60 months.[270]

Repair of ureteropelvic junction obstruction (UPJO) and ureterovesical reimplantation to treat vesicoureteral reflux requires general anesthesia and may be performed open or laparoscopically. Reconstruction of the lower urinary tract is more frequently achieved using an open approach, although laparoscopy is beginning to gain favor.

Posterior urethral valves (PUVs) are persistent embryonic membranes that cause bladder outlet obstruction and can lead to incomplete emptying, bladder hypertrophy, and even kidney insufficiency or failure. PUVs occur exclusively in males, with an incidence of 1 to 2 per 10,000 male births and may be diagnosed before or after birth by ultrasound. While temporary treatment involves catheterization and antibiotics to prevent infection, definitive surgical repair is required, usually in the early postnatal period. Nonetheless, approximately one-third of the patients with PUV develop end-stage renal disease and require dialysis and/or kidney transplantation.[271]

Undescended testis (cryptorchidism) affects 2% to 4% of male newborns. Cryptorchidism that persists at 1 year of age (1%) requires surgical repair (orchiopexy) normally as an outpatient procedure under general anesthesia.[272]

Hypospadius, an abnormal location of the urethral meatus on the ventral aspect of the penis resulting from incomplete embryologic development, occurs in 0.3% to 0.8% of male infants. Surgical repair is most commonly performed around 6 months of age as an outpatient procedure under general anesthesia, often supplemented with caudal analgesia. More complex repairs may require a second staged procedure around 12 months.

Circumcision of newborns is usually accomplished under ring block or local anesthetic infiltration without the presence of an anesthesiologist, although in older children general anesthesia with or without neuraxial anesthesia may be more appropriate.

Urologic Surgical Emergencies

Urologic emergencies are relatively rare, but three urologic emergency surgeries are worthy of mention. *Testicular torsion* requires emergency attention due to the high risk, if otherwise untreated, for infarction or gangrene which would require orchiectomy. In contrast, patients with *Fournier Gangrene* and *sepsis* associated with nephrolithiasis are noteworthy since emergent definitive surgical therapy is the most effective way to reverse their infectious process and improve their prognosis. These latter patients are generally very seriously ill, and often the anesthesiologist provides ongoing resuscitation and applies critical care principles while delivering anesthetic care.

Testicular Torsion

Testicular torsion has a bimodal incidence, in the neonatal period and during early pubertal to teenage years (NICV 50-5). Testicular torsion affects approximately 1 in 4,000 young men, and 65% of cases occur in teenagers. When the spermatic cord twists, venous outflow from a testicle is obstructed, and eventually this compromises arterial flow, leading to ischemia and infarction.[273] Patients with testicular torsion present with acute scrotal pain and tenderness, most cases not involving a history of trauma. A predisposing anatomic "bell-clapper deformity," which allows the testes to rotate freely in the tunica vaginalis, is the most common cause of this problem. Other risk factors include testicular tumors, a history of cryptorchidism, and an increase in testicular volume (e.g., puberty). Common misdiagnoses include epididymitis/orchitis, incarcerated hernia, and varicocele.[273] Absence of the cremasteric reflex is usually present on physical examination, and Doppler ultrasonography demonstrates decreased or absent blood flow. Equivocal physical examination findings dictate surgical exploration.

Apart from the considerable pain that torsion causes, the most important priority is the viability of the testicle. Testicular torsion requires immediate intervention, as viability decreases significantly with the duration of testicular ischemia. Success in saving the testicle relates to the timing from symptom onset to de-torsion, with success rates of 90%, 50%, and 10% with delays of 6, 12, and greater than 24 hours, respectively.[274]

Anesthesia for testicular torsion surgery must respect its emergent nature, including the likelihood that the patient has not fasted. Regional or general anesthesia is appropriate, but spinal anesthesia is relatively contraindicated due to the high risk of postdural puncture headache in the young population where the problem is most often manifested.

Fournier Gangrene

Fournier gangrene is a form of necrotizing fasciitis affecting the genitalia. It presents most commonly in older men, and frequently associated comorbidities include diabetes mellitus, morbid obesity, and immune suppression.[275] Minor genital trauma is often the inciting event, but rapid widespread inflammation, infection, and ultimately polymicrobial sepsis characterize the condition. Fournier gangrene patients often present with already established septic shock warranting the emergent status for surgery, but fluid resuscitation and institution of broad-spectrum antibiotic therapy (commonly staphylococci, streptococci, enterobacteriaceae, and anaerobes) are also priorities.[276] Surgical management consists of incision, drainage, and debridement of affected tissue. Hyperbaric oxygen therapy is also employed at some centers[277,278] but does not replace emergent surgical debridement. Morbidity and mortality are significant, with advanced age and presence of septic shock at presentation portending the highest risk.[279]

Anesthetic planning must incorporate assessment of the degree of sepsis and hemodynamic status of the patient. General anesthesia with endotracheal intubation and positive pressure ventilation is standard. Intra-arterial and central venous access are often indicated to facilitate resuscitation of the patient. Transfusion may be necessary since the extensive tissue resection can involve significant blood loss. Patients often require postoperative intensive care admission to manage the sequelae of sepsis and often undergo repeated procedures for additional debridement, wound care, and eventually wound closure.[276]

Emergency Treatment of Nephrolithiasis

Most patients who require surgical or interventional treatment of nephrolithiasis can be managed electively, but patients with infection associated with urinary tract obstruction, AKI, bilateral obstructing stones, intractable pain or vomiting, or obstruction in a solitary (native or transplanted) kidney should be managed urgently to avoid sepsis and preserve kidney function.[253] Procedures indicated for these conditions to alleviate obstruction include cystoscopy with stent insertion, percutaneous nephrostomy, and very rarely, open pyelolithotomy or nephrectomy for definitive treatment related to stones unsuccessfully treated by less-invasive interventions. Identification of patients who have infected urine and obstruction is important as they are at high risk of developing sepsis, which can manifest preoperatively, intraoperatively, or postoperatively. As with any infection, the principles of drainage and institution of appropriate antibiotic therapy are paramount, and in the presence of complete urinary obstruction, antibiotic therapy alone is insufficient treatment. If the urinary tract can be decompressed with a stent or nephrostomy, definitive management can be postponed until the patient has responded to antibiotic therapy.[247] Patients with nephrolithiasis complicated by urinary tract infection are at higher risk for infection with antibiotic-resistant pathogens, which requires targeted antibiotic therapy.[280]

Another category of patients requiring urgent surgery are patients with declining kidney function in the setting of urinary obstruction (e.g., ureteral obstruction from renal papillary necrosis, blood clots, or urethral obstruction due to blood clots or stricture).[246] Other situations (e.g., obstructed solitary or transplanted kidney, hemorrhage, and blood clots) may dictate urgent, rather than elective, surgery to relieve the urinary obstruction and preserve kidney function, though in the absence of infection this group of patients may not be as acutely ill.

Anesthetic considerations for emergent nephrolithiasis surgery are similar to those for equivalent elective procedures (see above). Additional considerations include the potential need for more invasive monitoring, for example, direct arterial blood pressure monitoring in the setting of sepsis. Similarly, hemodynamically unstable septic patients often have ongoing needs for fluid resuscitation, pharmacologic support of the circulation, and in the setting of deteriorating kidney function may require alterations from standard anesthetic agent selections. Since evidence of sepsis may not manifest until the postoperative period, raised awareness for such concerns should continue through into the postanesthetic recovery period.

For further review and interactivities, please see the videos and narrative interactive clinical vignettes (NICVs) accessible in the complimentary eBook bundled with this text. Access instructions are located on the inside front cover.

REFERENCES

1. Woodcock TE, Woodcock TM. Revised starling equation and the glycocalyx model of transvascular fluid exchange: an improved paradigm for prescribing intravenous fluid therapy. *Br J Anaesth.* 2012;108(3):384–394.
2. Singh A, Satchell SC, Neal CR, McKenzie EA, Tooke JE, Mathieson PW. Glomerular endothelial glycocalyx constitutes a barrier to protein permeability. *J Am Soc Nephrol.* 2007;18(11):2885–2893.
3. Garsen M, Rops AL, Rabelink TJ, Berden JH, van der Vlag J. The role of heparanase and the endothelial glycocalyx in the development of proteinuria. *Nephrol Dial Transplant.* 2014;29(1):49–55.
4. Alpert RA, Roizen MF, Hamilton WK, et al. Intraoperative urinary output does not predict postoperative renal function in patients undergoing abdominal aortic revascularization. *Surgery.* 1984;95(6):707–711.
5. Conlon PJ, Stafford-Smith M, White WD, et al. Acute renal failure following cardiac surgery. *Nephrol Dial Transplant.* 1999;14(5):1158–1162.
6. Levin A. Cystatin C, serum creatinine, and estimates of kidney function: searching for better measures of kidney function and cardiovascular risk. *Ann Intern Med.* 2005;142(7):586–588.
7. Grubb A, Bjork J, Lindstrom V, Sterner G, Bondesson P, Nyman U. A cystatin C-based formula without anthropometric variables estimates glomerular filtration rate better than creatinine clearance using the Cockcroft-Gault formula. *Scand J Clin Lab Invest.* 2005;65(2):153–162.
8. Alpert MA, Govindarajan G, Del Rosario ML, Reisin E. The role of the renin-angiotensin system in the pathophysiology, prevention, and treatment of renal impairment in patients with the cardiometabolic syndrome or its components. *J Cardiometab Syndr.* 2009;4(1):57–62.
9. Srisawat N, Murugan R, Kellum JA. Repair or progression after AKI: a role for biomarkers? *Nephron Clin Pract.* 2014;127(1-4):185–189.
10. Wasung ME, Chawla LS, Madero M. Biomarkers of renal function, which and when? *Clin Chim Acta.* 2015;438:350–357.
11. Sladen RN, Endo E, Harrison T. Two-hour versus 22-hour creatinine clearance in critically ill patients. *Anesthesiology.* 1987;67(6):1013–1016.
12. Bloor GK, Welsh KR, Goodall S, Shah MV. Comparison of predicted with measured creatinine clearance in cardiac surgical patients. *J Cardiothorac Vasc Anesth.* 1996;10(7):899–902.
13. Gowans EM, Fraser CG. Biological variation of serum and urine creatinine and creatinine clearance: ramifications for interpretation of results and patient care. *Ann Clin Biochem.* 1988;25(Pt 3):259–263.
14. Morgan DB, Dillon S, Payne RB. The assessment of glomerular function: creatinine clearance or plasma creatinine? *Postgrad Med J.* 1978;54(631):302–310.
15. Cockcroft DW, Gault MH. Prediction of creatinine clearance from serum creatinine. *Nephron.* 1976;16(1):31–41.
16. Levey AS, Bosch JP, Lewis JB, Greene T, Rogers N, Roth D. A more accurate method to estimate glomerular filtration rate from serum creatinine: a new prediction equation. Modification of Diet in Renal Disease Study Group. *Ann Intern Med.* 1999;130(6):461–470.
17. Delgado C, Baweja M, Crews DC, et al. A unifying approach for GFR estimation: Recommendations of the NKF-ASN Task Force on reassessing the inclusion of race in diagnosing kidney disease. *Am J Kidney Dis.* 2022;79(2):268–288.e1.
18. Michels WM, Grootendorst DC, Verduijn M, Elliott EG, Dekker FW, Krediet RT. Performance of the Cockcroft-Gault, MDRD, and new CKD-EPI formulas in relation to GFR, age, and body size. *Clin J Am Soc Nephrol.* 2010;5(6):1003–1009.
19. Ferguson TB Jr, Dziuban SW Jr, Edwards FH, et al. The STS National Database: current changes and challenges for the new millennium. Committee to Establish a National Database in Cardiothoracic Surgery, The Society of Thoracic Surgeons. *Ann Thorac Surg.* 2000;69(3):680–691.
20. Barrett BJ, Parfrey PS. Prevention of nephrotoxicity induced by radiocontrast agents. *N Engl J Med.* 1994;331(21):1449–1450.
21. Bellomo R, Ronco C, Kellum JA, Mehta RL, Palevsky P. Acute renal failure – definition, outcome measures, animal models, fluid therapy and information technology needs: the Second International Consensus Conference of the Acute Dialysis Quality Initiative (ADQI) Group. *Crit Care.* 2004;8(4):R204–R212.
22. Mehta RL, Kellum JA, Shah SV, et al.; Acute Kidney Injury Network. Acute kidney injury network: report of an initiative to improve outcomes in acute kidney injury. *Crit Care.* 2007;11(2):R31.
23. Kidney Disease: Improving Global Outcomes (KDIGO) Acute Kidney Injury Work Group. KDIGO clinical practice guideline for acute kidney injury. *Kidney inter.* 2012;2(Suppl 1):1–138.
24. Greenberg A, ed. *Primer on Kidney Diseases.* 4th ed. Elsevier Saunders; 2005.
25. Stafford-Smith M. Antifibrinolytic agents make alpha1- and beta2-microglobulinuria poor markers of post cardiac surgery renal dysfunction. *Anesthesiology.* 1999;90:928–929.
26. Anderson RJ, Chung HM, Kluge R, Schrier RW. Hyponatremia: a prospective analysis of its epidemiology and the pathogenetic role of vasopressin. *Ann Intern Med.* 1985;102(2):164–168.
27. Verbalis JG. Hyponatremia: epidemiology, pathophysiology, and therapy. *Curr Opin Nephrol Hypertens.* 1993;2(4):636–652.

28. Arieff AI. Hyponatremia, convulsions, respiratory arrest, and permanent brain damage after elective surgery in healthy women. *N Engl J Med*. 1986;314(24):1529–1535.
29. Arieff AI, Ayus JC, Fraser CL. Hyponatraemia and death or permanent brain damage in healthy children. *BMJ*. 1992;304(6836):1218–1222.
30. Ayus JC, Wheeler JM, Arieff AI. Postoperative hyponatremic encephalopathy in menstruant women. *Ann Intern Med*. 1992;117(11):891–897.
31. Witteveen JE, van Thiel S, Romijn JA, Hamdy NA. Hungry bone syndrome: still a challenge in the post-operative management of primary hyperparathyroidism: a systematic review of the literature. *Eur J Endocrinol*. 2013;168(3):R45–R53.
32. Amanzadeh J, Reilly RF Jr. Hypophosphatemia: an evidence-based approach to its clinical consequences and management. *Nat Clin Pract Nephrol*. 2006;2(3):136–148.
33. Anderson RJ, Linas SL, Berns AS, et al. Nonoliguric acute renal failure. *N Engl J Med*. 1977;296(20):1134–1138.
34. Doi K, Rabb H. Impact of acute kidney injury on distant organ function: recent findings and potential therapeutic targets. *Kidney Int*. 2016;89(3):555–564.
35. Bagshaw SM, Laupland KB, Doig CJ, et al. Prognosis for long-term survival and renal recovery in critically ill patients with severe acute renal failure: a population-based study. *Crit Care*. 2005;9(6):R700–R709.
36. Wilkinson A, Cohen D. Renal failure in the recipients of nonrenal solid organ transplants. *J Am Soc Nephrol*. 1999;10(5):1136–1144.
37. Uchino S, Kellum JA, Bellomo R, et al. Acute renal failure in critically ill patients: a multinational, multicenter study. *JAMA*. 2005;294(7):813–818.
38. Alonso A, Lau J, Jaber B, Weintraub A, Sarnak M. Prevention of radiocontrast nephropathy with N-acetylcysteine in patients with chronic kidney disease: a meta-analysis of randomized, controlled trials. *Am J Kidney Dis*. 2004;43(1):1–9.
39. Liano F, Pascual J. Epidemiology of acute renal failure: a prospective, multicenter, community-based study. Madrid Acute Renal Failure Study Group. *Kidney Int*. 1996;50(3):811–818.
40. Yacoub R, Patel N, Lohr JW, Rajagopalan S, Nader N, Arora P. Acute kidney injury and death associated with renin angiotensin system blockade in cardiothoracic surgery: a meta-analysis of observational studies. *Am J Kidney Dis*. 2013;62(6):1077–1086.
41. Knight EL, Glynn RJ, McIntyre KM, Mogun H, Avorn J. Predictors of decreased renal function in patients with heart failure during angiotensin-converting enzyme inhibitor therapy: results from the studies of left ventricular dysfunction (SOLVD). *Am Heart J*. 1999;138(5 Pt 1): 849–855.
42. Schoolwerth AC, Sica DA, Ballermann BJ, Wilcox CS; Council on the Kidney in Cardiovascular D, the Council for High Blood Pressure Research of the American Heart Association. Renal considerations in angiotensin converting enzyme inhibitor therapy: a statement for healthcare professionals from the Council on the Kidney in Cardiovascular Disease and the Council for High Blood Pressure Research of the American Heart Association. *Circulation*. 2001;104(16):1985–1991.
43. Adhiyaman V, Asghar M, Oke A, White AD, Shah IU. Nephrotoxicity in the elderly due to co-prescription of angiotensin converting enzyme inhibitors and nonsteroidal anti-inflammatory drugs. *J R Soc Med*. 2001;94(10):512–514.
44. Kincaid EH, Ashburn DA, Hoyle JR, Reichert MG, Hammon JW, Kon ND. Does the combination of aprotinin and angiotensin-converting enzyme inhibitor cause renal failure after cardiac surgery? *Ann Thorac Surg*. 2005;80(4):1388–1393; discussion 93.
45. Metz LI, LeBeau ME, Zlabek JA, Mathiason MA. Acute renal failure in patients undergoing cardiothoracic surgery in a community hospital. *WMJ*. 2009;108(2):109–114.
46. Reynolds A, White W, Stafford-Smith M, et al. The relationship of loop diuretics with acute kidney injury and mortality after cardiac surgery. *Anesth Analg*. 2013;116(suppl):SCA3.
47. Zhang Y, Ye N, Chen YP, Cheng H. Relation between the interval from coronary angiography to selective off-pump coronary artery bypass grafting and postoperative acute kidney injury. *Am J Cardiol*. 2013;112(10):1571–1575.
48. Lassnigg A, Donner E, Grubhofer G, Presterl E, Druml W, Hiesmayr M. Lack of renoprotective effects of dopamine and furosemide during cardiac surgery. *J Am Soc Nephrol*. 2000;11(1): 97–104.
49. Kheterpal S, Tremper KK, Englesbe MJ, et al. Predictors of postoperative acute renal failure after noncardiac surgery in patients with previously normal renal function. *Anesthesiology*. 2007;107(6):892–902.
50. Singh I, Rajagopalan S, Srinivasan A, et al. Preoperative statin therapy is associated with lower requirement of renal replacement therapy in patients undergoing cardiac surgery: a meta-analysis of observational studies. *Interact Cardiovasc Thorac Surg*. 2013;17(2):345–352.
51. Rudnick M, Feldman H. Contrast-induced nephropathy: what are the true clinical consequences? *Clin J Am Soc Nephrol*. 2008;3(1):263–272.
52. Hu Y, Zhong Q. Contrast-induced nephropathy may constitute a marker of underlying limited renal reserve for cardiac surgical procedures? *Ann Thorac Surg*. 2013;95(5):1841.
53. Aycock RD, Westafer LM, Boxen JL, Majlesi N, Schoenfeld EM, Bannuru RR. Acute kidney injury after computed tomography: a meta-analysis. *Ann Emerg Med*. 2018;71(1):44–53.e4.
54. Hinson JS, Ehmann MR, Fine DM, et al. Risk of acute kidney injury after intravenous contrast media administration. *Ann Emerg Med*. 2017;69(5):577–586.e4.
55. Taber SS, Mueller BA. Drug-associated renal dysfunction. *Crit Care Clin*. 2006;22(2):357–374, viii.
56. Huerta C, Castellsague J, Varas-Lorenzo C, Garcia Rodriguez L. Nonsteroidal anti-inflammatory drugs and risk of ARF in the general population. *Am J Kidney Dis*. 2005;45(3):531–539.
57. Oh KJ, Lee HH, Lee JS, et al. Reversible renal vasoconstriction in a patient with acute renal failure after exercise. *Clin Nephrol*. 2006;66(4):297–301.
58. Melli G, Chaudhry V, Cornblath DR. Rhabdomyolysis: an evaluation of 475 hospitalized patients. *Medicine (Baltimore)*. 2005;84(6):377–385.
59. Singh D, Chander V, Chopra K. Rhabdomyolysis. *Methods Find Exp Clin Pharmacol*. 2005;27(1):39–48.
60. Eichhorn JH, Hedley-Whyte J, Steinman TI, Kaufmann JM, Laasbert LH. Renal failure following enflurane anesthesia. *Anesthesiology*. 1976;45(5):557–560.
61. Eger EI, Gong D, Koblin DD, et al. Dose-related biochemical markers of renal injury after sevoflurane versus desflurane anesthesia in volunteers. *Anesth Analg*. 1997;85(5):1154–1163.
62. Conzen PF, Kharasch ED, Czerner SF, et al. Low-flow sevoflurane compared with low-flow isoflurane anesthesia in patients with stable renal insufficiency. *Anesthesiology*. 2002;97(3):578–584.
63. Myburgh JA, Finfer S, Bellomo R, et al. Hydroxyethyl starch or saline for fluid resuscitation in intensive care. *N Engl J Med*. 2012;367(20):1901–1911.
64. Perner A, Haase N, Guttormsen AB, et al. Hydroxyethyl starch 130/0.42 versus Ringer's acetate in severe sepsis. *N Engl J Med*. 2012;367(2):124–134.
65. Self WH, Semler MW, Wanderer JP, et al.; SALT-ED Investigators. Balanced crystalloids versus saline in noncritically ill adults. *N Engl J Med*. 2018;378(9):819–828.
66. Semler MW, Self WH, Wanderer JP, et al.; SMART Investigators and the Pragmatic Critical Care Research Group. Balanced crystalloids versus saline in critically ill adults. *N Engl J Med*. 2018;378(9):829–839.
67. Yunos NM, Bellomo R, Hegarty C, Story D, Ho L, Bailey M. Association between a chloride-liberal vs chloride-restrictive intravenous fluid administration strategy and kidney injury in critically ill adults. *JAMA*. 2012;308(15):1566–1572.
68. Prowle JR, Kirwan CJ, Bellomo R. Fluid management for the prevention and attenuation of acute kidney injury. *Nat Rev Nephrol*. 2014;10(1):37–47.
69. Prowle JR, Chua HR, Bagshaw SM, Bellomo R. Clinical review: volume of fluid resuscitation and the incidence of acute kidney injury – a systematic review. *Crit Care*. 2012;16(4):230.
70. Gunukula SR, Spodick DH. Pericardial disease in renal patients. *Semin Nephrol*. 2001;21(1):52–56.
71. Crandell WB, Pappas SG, Macdonald A. Nephrotoxicity associated with methoxyflurane anesthesia. *Anesthesiology*. 1966;27(5):591–607.
72. Kharasch ED, Hankins DC, Thummel KE. Human kidney methoxyflurane and sevoflurane metabolism. Intrarenal fluoride production as a possible mechanism of methoxyflurane nephrotoxicity. *Anesthesiology*. 1995;82(3):689–699.
73. Mazze RI, Calverley RK, Smith NT. Inorganic fluoride nephrotoxicity: prolonged enflurane and halothane anesthesia in volunteers. *Anesthesiology*. 1977;46(4):265–271.
74. Burch PG, Stanski DR. Decreased protein binding and thiopental kinetics. *Clin Pharmacol Ther*. 1982;32(2):212–217.
75. Gan TJ. Pharmacokinetic and pharmacodynamic characteristics of medications used for moderate sedation. *Clin Pharmacokinet*. 2006;45(9):855–869.
76. Carlos R, Calvo R, Erill S. Plasma protein binding of etomidate in patients with renal failure or hepatic cirrhosis. *Clin Pharmacokinet*. 1979;4(2):144–148.
77. Kirvela M, Olkkola KT, Rosenberg PH, Yli-Hankala A, Salmela K, Lindgren L. Pharmacokinetics of propofol and haemodynamic changes during induction of anaesthesia in uraemic patients. *Br J Anaesth*. 1992;68(2):178–182.
78. Vinik HR, Reves JG, Greenblatt DJ, Abernethy DR, Smith LR. The pharmacokinetics of midazolam in chronic renal failure patients. *Anesthesiology*. 1983;59(5):390–394.
79. Schmith VD, Piraino B, Smith RB, Kroboth PD. Alprazolam in end-stage renal disease. II. Pharmacodynamics. *Clin Pharmacol Ther*. 1992;51(5):533–540.
80. De Wolf AM, Fragen RJ, Avram MJ, Fitzgerald PC, Rahimi-Danesh F. The pharmacokinetics of dexmedetomidine in volunteers with severe renal impairment. *Anesth Analg*. 2001;93(5): 1205–1209.
81. Chan GL, Matzke GR. Effects of renal insufficiency on the pharmacokinetics and pharmacodynamics of opioid analgesics. *Drug Intell Clin Pharm*. 1987;21(10):773–783.
82. Babul N, Darke AC, Hagen N. Hydromorphone metabolite accumulation in renal failure. *J Pain Symptom Manage*. 1995;10(3):184–186.
83. Murphy EJ. Acute pain management pharmacology for the patient with concurrent renal or hepatic disease. *Anaesth Intensive Care*. 2005;33(3):311–322.
84. Davis PJ, Stiller RL, Cook DR, Brandom BW, Davis JE, Scierka AM. Effects of cholestatic hepatic disease and chronic renal failure on alfentanil pharmacokinetics in children. *Anesth Analg*. 1989;68(5):579–583.
85. Wiggum DC, Cork RC, Weldon ST, Gandolfi AJ, Perry DS. Postoperative respiratory depression and elevated sufentanil levels in a patient with chronic renal failure. *Anesthesiology*. 1985;63(6):708–710.
86. Pitsiu M, Wilmer A, Bodenham A, et al. Pharmacokinetics of remifentanil and its major metabolite, remifentanil acid, in ICU patients with renal impairment. *Br J Anaesth*. 2004;92(4):493–503.
87. Szenohradszky J, Caldwell JE, Wright PM, et al. Influence of renal failure on the pharmacokinetics and neuromuscular effects of a single dose of rapacuronium bromide. *Anesthesiology*. 1999;90(1):24–35.
88. Ryan DW. Preoperative serum cholinesterase concentration in chronic renal failure. Clinical experience of suxamethonium in 81 patients undergoing renal transplant. *Br J Anaesth*. 1977;49(9):945–949.

89. Cook DR, Freeman JA, Lai AA, et al. Pharmacokinetics of mivacurium in normal patients and in those with hepatic or renal failure. *Br J Anaesth*. 1992;69(6):580–585.
90. Cook DR, Freeman JA, Lai AA, et al. Pharmacokinetics and pharmacodynamics of doxacurium in normal patients and in those with hepatic or renal failure. *Anesth Analg*. 1991;72(2):145–150.
91. Della Rocca G, Pompei L, Coccia C, et al. Atracurium, cisatracurium, vecuronium and rocuronium in patients with renal failure. *Minerva Anestesiol*. 2003;69(7-8):605–611, 12, 5.
92. Fahey MR, Rupp SM, Canfell C, et al. Effect of renal failure on laudanosine excretion in man. *Br J Anaesth*. 1985;57(11):1049–1051.
93. Lynam DP, Cronnelly R, Castagnoli KP, et al. The pharmacodynamics and pharmacokinetics of vecuronium in patients anesthetized with isoflurane with normal renal function or with renal failure. *Anesthesiology*. 1988;69(2):227–231.
94. Robertson EN, Driessen JJ, Booij LH. Pharmacokinetics and pharmacodynamics of rocuronium in patients with and without renal failure. *Eur J Anaesthesiol*. 2005;22(1):4–10.
95. Szenohradszky J, Fisher DM, Segredo V, et al. Pharmacokinetics of rocuronium bromide (ORG 9426) in patients with normal renal function or patients undergoing cadaver renal transplantation. *Anesthesiology*. 1992;77(5):899–904.
96. Cooper RA, Maddineni VR, Mirakhur RK, Wierda JM, Brady M, Fitzpatrick KT. Time course of neuromuscular effects and pharmacokinetics of rocuronium bromide (Org 9426) during isoflurane anaesthesia in patients with and without renal failure. *Br J Anaesth*. 1993;71(2):222–226.
97. Phillips BJ, Hunter JM. Use of mivacurium chloride by constant infusion in the anephric patient. *Br J Anaesth*. 1992;68(5):492–498.
98. Blobner M, Jelen-Esselborn S, Schneider G, et al. Effect of renal function on neuromuscular block induced by continuous infusion of mivacurium. *Br J Anaesth*. 1995;74(4):452–454.
99. Morris RB, Cronnelly R, Miller RD, Stanski DR, Fahey MR. Pharmacokinetics of edrophonium in anephric and renal transplant patients. *Br J Anaesth*. 1981;53(12):1311–1314.
100. Epemolu O, Bom A, Hope F, Mason R. Reversal of neuromuscular blockade and simultaneous increase in plasma rocuronium concentration after the intravenous infusion of the novel reversal agent Org 25969. *Anesthesiology*. 2003;99(3):632–637; discussion 6A.
101. Staals LM, Snoeck MM, Driessen JJ, et al. Reduced clearance of rocuronium and sugammadex in patients with severe to end-stage renal failure: a pharmacokinetic study. *Br J Anaesth*. 2010;104(1):31–39.
102. Kim YS, Lim BG, Won YJ, Oh SK, Oh JS, Cho SA. Efficacy and safety of sugammadex for the reversal of rocuronium-induced neuromuscular blockade in patients with end-stage renal disease: a systematic review and meta-analysis. *Medicina (Kaunas)*. 2021;57(11):1259.
103. Larson EB, Roach RC, Schoene RB, Hornbein TF. Acute mountain sickness and acetazolamide. Clinical efficacy and effect on ventilation. *JAMA*. 1982;248(3):328–332.
104. White DP, Zwillich CW, Pickett CK, Douglas NJ, Findley LJ, Weil JV. Central sleep apnea. Improvement with acetazolamide therapy. *Arch Intern Med*. 1982;142(10):1816–1819.
105. Conger JD. Interventions in clinical acute renal failure: what are the data? *Am J Kidney Dis*. 1995;26(4):565–576.
106. Solomon R, Werner C, Mann D, D'Elia J, Silva P. Effects of saline, mannitol, and furosemide to prevent acute decreases in renal function induced by radiocontrast agents. *N Engl J Med*. 1994;331(21):1416–1420.
107. *National Kidney Foundation's Primer on Kidney Diseases*. 6th ed. Elsevier Saunders; 2014.
108. Better OS, Rubinstein I, Winaver JM, Knochel JP. Mannitol therapy revisited (1940-1997). *Kidney Int*. 1997;52(4):886–894.
109. Borges HF, Hocks J, Kjellstrand CM. Mannitol intoxication in patients with renal failure. *Arch Intern Med*. 1982;142(1):63–66.
110. Gallagher KL, Jones JK. Furosemide-induced ototoxicity. *Ann Intern Med*. 1979;91(5):744–745.
111. Pitt B, Zannad F, Remme WJ, et al. The effect of spironolactone on morbidity and mortality in patients with severe heart failure. Randomized Aldactone Evaluation Study Investigators. *N Engl J Med*. 1999;341(10):709–717.
112. Jose PA, Felder RA. What we can learn from the selective manipulation of dopaminergic receptors about the pathogenesis and treatment of hypertension? *Curr Opin Nephrol Hypertens*. 1996;5(5):447–451.
113. Bellomo R, Cole L, Ronco C. Hemodynamic support and the role of dopamine. *Kidney Int Suppl*. 1998;66:S71–S74.
114. Marik PE. Low-dose dopamine: a systematic review. *Intensive Care Med*. 2002;28(7):877–883.
115. Kellum JA, Decker JM. Use of dopamine in acute renal failure: a meta-analysis. *Crit Care Med*. 2001;29(8):1526–1531.
116. Prins I, Plotz FB, Uiterwaal CS, van Vught HJ. Low-dose dopamine in neonatal and pediatric intensive care: a systematic review. *Intensive Care Med*. 2001;27(1):206–210.
117. Holmes CL, Walley KR. Bad medicine: low-dose dopamine in the ICU. *Chest*. 2003;123(4):1266–1275.
118. Argalious M, Motta P, Khandwala F, et al. "Renal dose" dopamine is associated with the risk of new-onset atrial fibrillation after cardiac surgery. *Crit Care Med*. 2005;33(6):1327–1332.
119. Denton MD, Chertow GM, Brady HR. "Renal-dose" dopamine for the treatment of acute renal failure: scientific rationale, experimental studies and clinical trials. *Kidney Int*. 1996;50(1):4–14.
120. Vallon V, Verma S. Effects of SGLT2 inhibitors on kidney and cardiovascular function. *Annu Rev Physiol*. 2021;83:503–528.
121. Heerspink HJL, Stefánsson BV, Correa-Rotter R, et al.; DAPA-CKD Trial Committees and Investigators. Dapagliflozin in patients with chronic kidney disease. *N Engl J Med*. 2020;383(15):1436–1446.
122. Thiruvenkatarajan V, Meyer EJ, Nanjappa N, Van Wijk RM, Jesudason D. Perioperative diabetic ketoacidosis associated with sodium-glucose co-transporter-2 inhibitors: a systematic review. *Br J Anaesth*. 2019;123(1):27–36.
123. Abel RM, Buckley MJ, Austen WG, Barnett GO, Beck CH Jr, Fischer JE. Etiology, incidence, and prognosis of renal failure following cardiac operations. Results of a prospective analysis of 500 consecutive patients. *J Thorac Cardiovasc Surg*. 1976;71(3):323–333.
124. Swaminathan M, Shaw A, Phillips-Bute B, et al. Trends in acute renal failure associated with coronary artery bypass graft surgery in the United States. *Crit Care Med*. 2007;35(10):2286–2291.
125. Filsoufi F, Rahmanian PB, Castillo JG, Chikwe J, Carpentier A, Adams DH. Early and late outcomes of cardiac surgery in patients with moderate to severe preoperative renal dysfunction without dialysis. *Interact Cardiovasc Thorac Surg*. 2008;7(1):90–95.
126. Bechtel JF, Detter C, Fischlein T, et al. Cardiac surgery in patients on dialysis: decreased 30-day mortality, unchanged overall survival. *Ann Thorac Surg*. 2008;85(1):147–153.
127. Aronson S, Fontes ML, Miao Y, Mangano DT. Risk index for perioperative renal dysfunction/failure: critical dependence on pulse pressure hypertension. *Circulation*. 2007;115(6):733–742.
128. Mangano DT, Tudor IC, Dietzel C. The risk associated with aprotinin in cardiac surgery. *N Engl J Med*. 2006;354(4):353–365.
129. Hix JK, Thakar CV, Katz EM, Yared JP, Sabik J, Paganini EP. Effect of off-pump coronary artery bypass graft surgery on postoperative acute kidney injury and mortality. *Crit Care Med*. 2006;34(12):2979–2983.
130. Costa P, Ottino GM, Matani A, et al. Low-dose dopamine during cardiopulmonary bypass in patients with renal dysfunction. *J Cardiothorac Anesth*. 1990;4(4):469–473.
131. Berendes E, Mollhoff T, Van Aken H, et al. Effects of dopexamine on creatinine clearance, systemic inflammation, and splanchnic oxygenation in patients undergoing coronary artery bypass grafting. *Anesth Analg*. 1997;84(5):950–957.
132. Renton MC, Snowden CP. Dopexamine and its role in the protection of hepatosplanchnic and renal perfusion in high-risk surgical and critically ill patients. *Br J Anaesth*. 2005;94(4):459–467.
133. Novis BK, Roizen MF, Aronson S, Thisted RA. Association of preoperative risk factors with postoperative acute renal failure. *Anesth Analg*. 1994;78(1):143–149.
134. Stene JK. Renal failure in the trauma patient. *Crit Care Clin*. 1990;6(1):111–119.
135. Cachecho R, Millham FH, Wedel SK. Management of the trauma patient with pre-existing renal disease. *Crit Care Clin*. 1994;10(3):523–536.
136. Myers BD, Miller DC, Mehigan JT, et al. Nature of the renal injury following total renal ischemia in man. *J Clin Invest*. 1984;73(2):329–341.
137. Godet G, Fleron MH, Vicaut E, et al. Risk factors for acute postoperative renal failure in thoracic or thoracoabdominal aortic surgery: a prospective study. *Anesth Analg*. 1997;85(6):1227–1232.
138. Svensson LG, Coselli JS, Safi HJ, Hess KR, Crawford ES. Appraisal of adjuncts to prevent acute renal failure after surgery on the thoracic or thoracoabdominal aorta. *J Vasc Surg*. 1989;10(3):230–239.
139. Olsen PS, Schroeder T, Perko M, et al. Renal failure after operation for abdominal aortic aneurysm. *Ann Vasc Surg*. 1990;4(6):580–583.
140. Schermerhorn ML, O'Malley AJ, Jhaveri A, Cotterill P, Pomposelli F, Landon BE. Endovascular vs. open repair of abdominal aortic aneurysms in the Medicare population. *N Engl J Med*. 2008;358(5):464–474.
141. Zarbock A, Küllmar M, Ostermann M, et al. Prevention of cardiac surgery-associated acute kidney injury by implementing the KDIGO guidelines in high-risk patients identified by biomarkers: The PrevAKI-Multicenter Randomized Controlled Trial. *Anesth Analg*. 2021;133(2):292–302.
142. Yalavarthy R, Edelstein CL, Teitelbaum I. Acute renal failure and chronic kidney disease following liver transplantation. *Hemodial Int*. 2007;11(Suppl 3):S7–S12.
143. Lopez Lago AM, Fernandez Villanueva J, Garcia Acuna JM, Paz ES, Vizoso EF, Perez EV. Evolution of hepatorenal syndrome after orthotopic liver transplantation: comparative analysis with patients who developed acute renal failure in the early postoperative period of liver transplantation. *Transplant Proc*. 2007;39(7):2318–2319.
144. Fleisher LA, Beckman JA, Brown KA, et al. ACC/AHA 2007 Guidelines on Perioperative Cardiovascular Evaluation and Care for Noncardiac Surgery: Executive Summary: A Report of the American College of Cardiology/American Heart Association Task Force on Practice Guidelines (Writing Committee to Revise the 2002 Guidelines on Perioperative Cardiovascular Evaluation for Noncardiac Surgery): Developed in Collaboration With the American Society of Echocardiography, American Society of Nuclear Cardiology, Heart Rhythm Society, Society of Cardiovascular Anesthesiologists, Society for Cardiovascular Angiography and Interventions, Society for Vascular Medicine and Biology, and Society for Vascular Surgery. *Circulation*. 2007;116(17):1971–1996.
145. Khaira HS, Shah RB, Wolf JS Jr. Laparoscopic and open surgical nephrectomy for xanthogranulomatous pyelonephritis. *J Endourol*. 2005;19(7):813–817.
146. Richard S, Lidereau R, Giraud S. The growing family of hereditary renal cell carcinoma. *Nephrol Dial Transplant*. 2004;19(12):2954–2958.
147. Palapattu GS, Kristo B, Rajfer J. Paraneoplastic syndromes in urologic malignancy: the many faces of renal cell carcinoma. *Rev Urol*. 2002;4(4):163–170.
148. Galvez JA, Clebone A, Garwood S, Popescu WM. Fatal intraoperative cardiac thrombosis in a patient with renal cell carcinoma. *Anesthesiology*. 2011;114(5):1212.

149. Zayed M, Allers K, Hoffmann F, Bantel C. Transversus abdominis plane block in urological procedures: A systematic review and meta-analysis. *Eur J Anaesthesiol*. 2021;38(7):758–767.
150. Koo CH, Ryu JH. Anesthetic considerations for urologic surgeries. *Korean J Anesthesiol*. 2020;73(2):92–102.
151. Wijeysundera DN, Beattie WS, Austin PC, Hux JE, Laupacis A. Epidural anaesthesia and survival after intermediate-to-high risk non-cardiac surgery: a population-based cohort study. *Lancet*. 2008;372(9638):562–569.
152. Dunn MD, Portis AJ, Shalhav AL, et al. Laparoscopic versus open radical nephrectomy: a 9-year experience. *J Urol*. 2000;164(4):1153–1159.
153. Permpongkosol S, Link RE, Su LM, et al. Complications of 2,775 urological laparoscopic procedures: 1993 to 2005. *J Urol*. 2007;177(2):580–585.
154. Pareek G, Hedican SP, Gee JR, Bruskewitz RC, Nakada SY. Meta-analysis of the complications of laparoscopic renal surgery: comparison of procedures and techniques. *J Urol*. 2006;175(4): 1208–1213.
155. Gill IS, Matin SF, Desai MM, et al. Comparative analysis of laparoscopic versus open partial nephrectomy for renal tumors in 200 patients. *J Urol*. 2003;170(1):64–68.
156. Simmons MN, Gill IS. Decreased complications of contemporary laparoscopic partial nephrectomy: use of a standardized reporting system. *J Urol*. 2007;177(6):2067–2073; discussion 73.
157. Turna B, Frota R, Kamoi K, et al. Risk factor analysis of postoperative complications in laparoscopic partial nephrectomy. *J Urol*. 2008;179(4):1289–1294; discussion 94–95.
158. Lassen K, Soop M, Nygren J, et al. Consensus review of optimal perioperative care in colorectal surgery: Enhanced Recovery After Surgery (ERAS) Group recommendations. *Arch Surg*. 2009;144(10):961–969.
159. Schefft P, Novick AC, Straffon RA, Stewart BH. Surgery for renal cell carcinoma extending into the inferior vena cava. *J Urol*. 1978;120(1):28–31.
160. Neves RJ, Zincke H. Surgical treatment of renal cancer with vena cava extension. *Br J Urol*. 1987;59(5):390–395.
161. Nesbitt JC, Soltero ER, Dinney CP, et al. Surgical management of renal cell carcinoma with inferior vena cava tumor thrombus. *Ann Thorac Surg*. 1997;63(6):1592–600.
162. Porpiglia F, Renard J, Billia M, et al. Is renal warm ischemia over 30 minutes during laparoscopic partial nephrectomy possible? One-year results of a prospective study. *Eur Urol*. 2007;52(4):1170–1178.
163. Desai MM, Gill IS, Ramani AP, Spaliviero M, Rybicki L, Kaouk JH. The impact of warm ischaemia on renal function after laparoscopic partial nephrectomy. *BJU Int*. 2005;95(3):377–383.
164. Eskicorapci SY, Teber D, Schulze M, Ates M, Stock C, Rassweiler JJ. Laparoscopic radical nephrectomy: the new gold standard surgical treatment for localized renal cell carcinoma. *ScientificWorldJournal*. 2007;7:825–836.
165. Permpongkosol S, Chan DY, Link RE, et al. Long-term survival analysis after laparoscopic radical nephrectomy. *J Urol*. 2005;174(4 Pt 1):1222–1225.
166. Russo P. Is laparoscopic partial nephrectomy as effective as open partial nephrectomy in patients with renal cell carcinoma? *Nat Clin Pract Urol*. 2008;5(1):12–13.
167. Gill IS, Kavoussi LR, Lane BR, et al. Comparison of 1,800 laparoscopic and open partial nephrectomies for single renal tumors. *J Urol*. 2007;178(1):41–46.
168. Nicholson ML, Elwell R, Kaushik M, Bagul A, Hosgood SA. Health-related quality of life after living donor nephrectomy: a randomized controlled trial of laparoscopic versus open nephrectomy. *Transplantation*. 2011;91(4):457–461.
169. Waller JR, Hiley AL, Mullin EJ, Veitch PS, Nicholson ML. Living kidney donation: a comparison of laparoscopic and conventional open operations. *Postgrad Med J*. 2002;78(917): 153–157.
170. Owen M, Lorgelly P, Serpell M. Chronic pain following donor nephrectomy–a study of the incidence, nature and impact of chronic post-nephrectomy pain. *Eur J Pain*. 2010;14(7):732–734.
171. Biglarnia AR, Tufveson G, Lorant T, Lennmyr F, Wadstrom J. Efficacy and safety of continuous local infusion of ropivacaine after retroperitoneoscopic live donor nephrectomy. *Am J Transplant*. 2011;11(1):93–100.
172. Panaro F, Gheza F, Piardi T, et al. Continuous infusion of local anesthesia after living donor nephrectomy: a comparative analysis. *Transplant Proc*. 2011;43(4):985–987.
173. Yates DR, Vaessen C, Roupret M. From Leonardo to da Vinci: the history of robot-assisted surgery in urology. *BJU Int*. 2011;108(11):1708–1713; discussion 14.
174. Branche PE, Duperret SL, Sagnard PE, Boulez JL, Petit PL, Viale JP. Left ventricular loading modifications induced by pneumoperitoneum: a time course echocardiographic study. *Anesth Analg*. 1998;86(3):482–487.
175. Mertens zur Borg IR, Di Biase M, Verbrugge S, Ijzermans JN, Gommers D. Comparison of three perioperative fluid regimes for laparoscopic donor nephrectomy: A prospective randomized dose-finding study. *Surg Endosc*. 2008;22(1):146–150.
176. Feltracco P, Ori C. Anesthetic management of living transplantation. *Minerva Anestesiol*. 2010;76(7):525–533.
177. Fahy BG, Barnas GM, Nagle SE, Flowers JL, Njoku MJ, Agarwal M. Changes in lung and chest wall properties with abdominal insufflation of carbon dioxide are immediately reversible. *Anesth Analg*. 1996;82(3):501–505.
178. Ozyuvaci E, Altan A, Karadeniz T, Topsakal M, Besisik A, Yucel M. General anesthesia versus epidural and general anesthesia in radical cystectomy. *Urol Int*. 2005;74(1):62–67.
179. Koerner CP, Lopez-Aguiar AG, Zaidi M, et al. Caution: increased acute kidney injury in Enhanced Recovery after Surgery (ERAS) protocols. *Am Surg*. 2019;85(2):156–161.
180. Lee G, Patel HV, Srivastava A, Ghodoussipour S. Updates on enhanced recovery after surgery for radical cystectomy. *Ther Adv Urol*. 2022;14:17562872221109022.
181. Lone Z, Zhang A, Benidir T, et al. The role of enhanced recovery after surgery protocols in the development of acute kidney injury following radical cystectomy. *Urol Oncol*. 2022;40(10): 453.e1–453.e7.
182. Gan TJ, Soppitt A, Maroof M, et al. Goal-directed intraoperative fluid administration reduces length of hospital stay after major surgery. *Anesthesiology*. 2002;97(4):820–826.
183. Cerantola Y, Valerio M, Persson B, et al. Guidelines for perioperative care after radical cystectomy for bladder cancer: Enhanced Recovery After Surgery (ERAS((R))) society recommendations. *Clin Nutr*. 2013;32(6):879–887.
184. Rowley MW, Clemens JQ, Latini JM, Cameron AP. Simple cystectomy: outcomes of a new operative technique. *Urology*. 2011;78(4):942–945.
185. Novotny V, Hakenberg OW, Wiessner D, et al. Perioperative complications of radical cystectomy in a contemporary series. *Eur Urol*. 2007;51(2):397–401; discussion 401–402.
186. Mullen R, Scollay JM, Hecht G, McPhillips G, Thompson AM. Death within 48 h–adverse events after general surgical procedures. *Surg*. 2012;10(1):1–5.
187. www.seer.cancer.gov.
188. Ploussard G, Epstein JI, Montironi R, et al. The contemporary concept of significant versus insignificant prostate cancer. *Eur Urol*. 2011;60(2):291–303.
189. Gottschalk A, Smith DS, Jobes DR, et al. Preemptive epidural analgesia and recovery from radical prostatectomy: a randomized controlled trial. *JAMA*. 1998;279(14):1076–1082.
190. Price DT, Vieweg J, Roland F, et al. Transient lower extremity neurapraxia associated with radical perineal prostatectomy: a complication of the exaggerated lithotomy position. *J Urol*. 1998;160(4):1376–1378.
191. Keller H. Re: Transient lower extremity neurapraxia associated with radical perineal prostatectomy: a complication of the exaggerated lithotomy position. *J Urol*. 1999;162(1):171.
192. Salonia A, Crescenti A, Suardi N, et al. General versus spinal anesthesia in patients undergoing radical retropubic prostatectomy: results of a prospective, randomized study. *Urology*. 2004;64(1):95–100.
193. Malhotra V. Anesthesia considerations radical prostatectomy. *Rev Mex de Anestesiol*. 2006;29(S1):89–92.
194. Memtsoudis SG, Malhotra V. Catastrophic venous air embolus during prostatectomy in the Trendelenburg position. *Can J Anaesth*. 2003;50(10):1084–1085.
195. Whalley DG, Berrigan MJ. Anesthesia for radical prostatectomy, cystectomy, nephrectomy, pheochromocytoma, and laparoscopic procedures. *Anesthesiol Clin North Am*. 2000;18(4): 899–917, x.
196. Klevecka V, Burmester L, Musch M, Roggenbuck U, Kroepfl D. Intraoperative and early postoperative complications of radical retropubic prostatectomy. *Urol Int*. 2007;79(3):217–225.
197. Dudderidge T, Doyle P, Mayer E, et al. Evolution of care pathway for laparoscopic radical prostatectomy. *J Endourol*. 2012;26(6):660–665.
198. Sutherland DE, Perez DS, Weeks DC. Robot-assisted simple prostatectomy for severe benign prostatic hyperplasia. *J Endourol*. 2011;25(4):641–644.
199. White WM, Kim ED. Interposition nerve grafting during radical prostatectomy: cumulative review and critical appraisal of literature. *Urology*. 2009;74(2):245–250.
200. Biki B, Mascha E, Moriarty DC, Fitzpatrick JM, Sessler DI, Buggy DJ. Anesthetic technique for radical prostatectomy surgery affects cancer recurrence: a retrospective analysis. *Anesthesiology*. 2008;109(2):180–187.
201. Mikhail D, Sarcona J, Mekhail M, Richstone L. Urologic robotic surgery. *Surg Clin North Am*. 2020;100(2):361–378.
202. Giri S, Sarkar DK. Current status of robotic surgery. *Indian J Surg*. 2012;74(3):242–247.
203. Fuchs KH. Minimally invasive surgery. *Endoscopy*. 2002;34(2):154–159.
204. Irvine M, Patil V. Anaesthesia for robot-assisted laparoscopic surgery. Continuing Education in Anaesthesia, *Crit Care Pain*. 2009;9(4):125–129.
205. Conacher ID, Soomro NA, Rix D. Anaesthesia for laparoscopic urological surgery. *Br J Anaesth*. 2004;93(6):859–864.
206. Pathan H, Gulati S. A case of airway occlusion in robotic surgery. *J Robotic Surg*. 2007;1:169–170.
207. Kalmar AF, Foubert L, Hendrickx JF, et al. Influence of steep Trendelenburg position and CO(2) pneumoperitoneum on cardiovascular, cerebrovascular, and respiratory homeostasis during robotic prostatectomy. *Br J Anaesth*. 2010;104(4):433–439.
208. Gainsburg DM, Wax D, Reich DL, Carlucci JR, Samadi DB. Intraoperative management of robotic-assisted versus open radical prostatectomy. *JSLS*. 2010;14(1):1–5.
209. Sladen RN. Anesthetic considerations for the patient with renal failure. *Anesthesiol Clin North Am*. 2000;18(4):863–882, x.
210. Colomina MJ, Godet C, Pellise F, Bago J, Villanueva C. Transcranial Doppler monitoring during laparoscopic anterior lumbar interbody fusion. *Anesth Analg*. 2003;97(6):1675–1679.
211. Rocco B, Albo G, Ferreira RC, et al. Recent advances in the surgical treatment of benign prostatic hyperplasia. *Ther Adv Urol*. 2011;3(6):263–272.
212. Reeves MD, Myles PS. Does anaesthetic technique affect the outcome after transurethral resection of the prostate? *BJU Int*. 1999;84(9):982–986.
213. Mackenzie AR. Influence of anaesthesia on blood loss in transurethral prostatectomy. *Scott Med J*. 1990;35(1):14–16.
214. McGowan SW, Smith GF. Anaesthesia for transurethral prostatectomy. A comparison of spinal intradural analgesia with two methods of general anaesthesia. *Anaesthesia*. 1980;35(9):847–853.

215. Gehring H, Nahm W, Baerwald J, et al. Irrigation fluid absorption during transurethral resection of the prostate: spinal vs. general anaesthesia. *Acta Anaesthesiol Scand*. 1999;43(4):458–463.
216. Allen TD. Body temperature changes during prostatic resection as related to the temperature of the irrigating solution. *J Urol*. 1973;110(4):433–435.
217. Hatch PD. Surgical and anaesthetic considerations in transurethral resection of the prostate. *Anaesth Intensive Care*. 1987;15(2):203–211.
218. Krongrad A, Droller M. Complications of transurethral resection of the prostate. In: Marshall F, eds. *Urologic Complications: Medical and Surgical, Adult and Pediatric*. 2nd ed. Mosby-Year Book; 1990:305.
219. Mebust WK, Holtgrewe HL, Cockett AT, Peters PC. Transurethral prostatectomy: immediate and postoperative complications. A cooperative study of 13 participating institutions evaluating 3,885 patients. *J Urol*. 1989;141(2):243–247.
220. Dorotta I, Basali A, Ritchey M, O'Hara JF Jr, Sprung J. Transurethral resection syndrome after bladder perforation. *Anesth Analg*. 2003;97(5):1536–1538.
221. Reich O, Gratzke C, Bachmann A, et al. Morbidity, mortality and early outcome of transurethral resection of the prostate: a prospective multicenter evaluation of 10,654 patients. *J Urol*. 2008;180(1):246–249.
222. Ahyai SA, Gilling P, Kaplan SA, et al. Meta-analysis of functional outcomes and complications following transurethral procedures for lower urinary tract symptoms resulting from benign prostatic enlargement. *Eur Urol*. 2010;58(3):384–397.
223. Ansell J. Acquired bleeding disorders. In: Rippe J, Irwin R, Alpert J, Dalen J, eds. *Intensive Care Medicine*. 2nd ed. Little, Brown; 1991:1013.
224. Rannikko A, Petas A, Taari K. Tranexamic acid in control of primary hemorrhage during transurethral prostatectomy. *Urology*. 2004;64(5):955–958.
225. Wasson JH, Reda DJ, Bruskewitz RC, Elinson J, Keller AM, Henderson WG. A comparison of transurethral surgery with watchful waiting for moderate symptoms of benign prostatic hyperplasia. The Veterans Affairs Cooperative Study Group on Transurethral Resection of the Prostate. *N Engl J Med*. 1995;332(2):75–79.
226. Melchior J, Valk WL, Foret JD, Mebust WK. Transurethral prostatectomy: computerized analysis of 2,223 consecutive cases. *J Urol*. 1974;112(5):634–642.
227. Perrin P, Barnes R, Hadley H, Bergman RT. Forty years of transurethral prostatic resections. *J Urol*. 1976;116(6):757–758.
228. Fuglsig S, Aagaard J, Jonler M, Olesen S, Norgaard JP. Survival after transurethral resection of the prostate: a 10-year followup. *J Urol*. 1994;151(3):637–639.
229. Matani Y, Mottrie AM, Stockle M, Voges GE, Fichtner J, Hohenfellner R. Transurethral prostatectomy: a long-term follow-up study of 166 patients over 80 years of age. *Eur Urol*. 1996;30(4):414–417.
230. Fitzpatrick JM. Minimally invasive and endoscopic management of benign prostatic hyperplasia. In: Wein A, Kavoussi L, Novick A, Partin A, Peters C, eds. *Campbell-Walsh Urology*. 9th ed. Saunders Elsevier; 2007:2803.
231. Gettman M, Segura J. Indications and outcomes of ureteroscopy for urinary stones. Stoller M, Meng M, eds. Humana Press; 2004.
232. Freiha F, Deem S, Pearl RG. Urology: transurethral resection of the protate (TURP). In: Jaffe RA, Samuels SI, eds. *Anesthesiologist's Manual of Surgical Procedures*. Raven Press; 1994:553.
233. Shah HN, Kausik V, Hegde S, Shah JN, Bansal MB. Evaluation of fluid absorption during holmium laser enucleation of prostate by breath ethanol technique. *J Urol*. 2006;175(2):537–540.
234. Akata T, Yoshimura H, Matsumae Y, et al. Changes in serum Na+ and blood hemoglobin levels during three types of transurethral procedures for the treatment of benign prostatic hypertrophy. *Masui*. 2004;53(6):638–644.
235. Jensen V. The TURP syndrome. *Can J Anaesth*. 1991;38(1):90–96.
236. Agin C. Anesthesia for transurethral prostate surgery. In: Lebowitz P, eds. *Anesthesia for Urologic Surgery*. Brown; 1993:25.
237. Gravenstein D. Transurethral resection of the prostate (TURP) syndrome: a review of the pathophysiology and management. *Anesth Analg*. 1997;84(2):438–446.
238. Roesch RP, Stoelting RK, Lingeman JE, Kahnoski RJ, Backes DJ, Gephardt SA. Ammonia toxicity resulting from glycine absorption during a transurethral resection of the prostate. *Anesthesiology*. 1983;58(6):577–579.
239. Hoekstra PT, Kahnoski R, McCamish MA, Bergen W, Heetderks DR. Transurethral prostatic resection syndrome–a new perspective: encephalopathy with associated hyperammonemia. *J Urol*. 1983;130(4):704–707.
240. Ovassapian A, Joshi CW, Brunner EA. Visual disturbances: an unusual symptom of transurethral prostatic resection reaction. *Anesthesiology*. 1982;57(4):332–334.
241. Barletta JP, Fanous MM, Hamed LM. Temporary blindness in the TUR syndrome. *J Neuroophthalmol*. 1994;14(1):6–8.
242. Hahn RG, Ekengren JC. Patterns of irrigating fluid absorption during transurethral resection of the prostate as indicated by ethanol. *J Urol*. 1993;149(3):502–506.
243. Rippa A. Transurethral resection of the prostate: aids and accessories. In: Smith A, eds. *Smith's Textbook of Endourology*. Quality Medical; 1996:1190.
244. Hahn RG, Stalberg HP, Ekengren J, Rundgren M. Effects of 1.5% glycine solution with and without 1% ethanol on the fluid balance in elderly men. *Acta Anaesthesiol Scand*. 1991;35(8):725–730.
245. Black R. Disorders of plasma sodium and plasma potassium. In: Rippe J, Irwin R, Alpert J, Dalen J, eds. *Intensive Care Medicine*. 2nd ed. Little, Brown; 1991:794.
246. Hall PM. Nephrolithiasis: treatment, causes, and prevention. *Cleve Clin J Med*. 2009;76(10): 583–591.
247. Preminger GM, Tiselius HG, Assimos DG, et al. 2007 Guideline for the management of ureteral calculi. *Eur Urol*. 2007;52(6):1610–1631.
248. Hollingsworth JM, Rogers MA, Kaufman SR, et al. Medical therapy to facilitate urinary stone passage: a meta-analysis. *Lancet*. 2006;368(9542):1171–1179.
249. Auge BK, Preminger GM. Update on shock wave lithotripsy technology. *Curr Opin Urol*. 2002;12(4):287–290.
250. Lambert DH, Deane RS, Mazuzan JE Jr. Anesthesia and the control of blood pressure in patients with spinal cord injury. *Anesth Analg*. 1982;61(4):344–348.
251. Mariappan P, Tolley DA. Endoscopic stone surgery: minimizing the risk of post-operative sepsis. *Curr Opin Urol*. 2005;15(2):101–105.
252. Abbott MA, Samuel JR, Webb DR. Anaesthesia for extracorporeal shock wave lithotripsy. *Anaesthesia*. 1985;40(11):1065–1072.
253. Samplaski MK, Irwin BH, Desai M. Less-invasive ways to remove stones from the kidneys and ureters. *Cleve Clin J Med*. 2009;76(10):592–598.
254. Stoller ML, Lee KL, Schwartz BF, Viele MK. Autologous blood use in percutaneous nephrolithotomy. *Urology*. 1999;54(3):444–449.
255. Mehrabi S, Karimzadeh Shirazi K. Results and complications of spinal anesthesia in percutaneous nephrolithotomy. *Urol J*. 2010;7(1):22–25.
256. Aravantinos E, Karatzas A, Gravas S, Tzortzis V, Melekos M. Feasibility of percutaneous nephrolithotomy under assisted local anaesthesia: a prospective study on selected patients with upper urinary tract obstruction. *Eur Urol*. 2007;51(1):224–227; discussion 8.
257. Johnson DB, Pearle MS. Complications of ureteroscopy. *Urol Clin North Am*. 2004;31(1): 157–171.
258. Foon R, Toozs-Hobson P, Cooper G. Anaesthesia for incontinence surgery: spinal anaesthesia or sedation? *J Obstet Gynaecol*. 2010;30(6):605–608.
259. Wohlrab KJ, Erekson EA, Korbly NB, Drimbarean CD, Rardin CR, Sung VW. The association between regional anesthesia and acute postoperative urinary retention in women undergoing outpatient midurethral sling procdures. *Am J Obstet Gynecol*. 2009:571.e1–e5.
260. Lifshitz DA, Lingeman JE. Ureteroscopy as a first-line intervention for ureteral calculi in pregnancy. *J Endourol*. 2002;16(1):19–22.
261. Ulvik NM, Bakke A, Hoisaeter PA. Ureteroscopy in pregnancy. *J Urol*. 1995;154(5):1660–1663.
262. Yossepowitch O, Baniel J, Livne PM. Urological injuries during cesarean section: intraoperative diagnosis and management. *J Urol*. 2004;172(1):196–199.
263. Belfort MA. Placenta accreta. *Am J Obstet Gynecol*. 2010;203(5):430–439.
264. Hsu GL, Hsieh CH, Chen HS, et al. The advancement of pure local anesthesia for penile surgeries: can an outpatient basis be sustainable? *J Androl*. 2007;28(1):200–205.
265. Casale P, Kojima Y. Robotic-assisted laparoscopic surgery in pediatric urology: an update. *Scand J Surg*. 2009;98(2):110–119.
266. St Peter SD, Valusek PA, Hill S, et al. Laparoscopic adrenalectomy in children: a multicenter experience. *J Laparoendosc Adv Surg Tech A*. 2011;21(7):647–649.
267. Waguespack SG, Rich T, Grubbs E, et al. A current review of the etiology, diagnosis, and treatment of pediatric pheochromocytoma and paraganglioma. *J Clin Endocrinol Metab*. 2010;95(5):2023–2037.
268. Ein SH, Pullerits J, Creighton R, Balfe JW. Pediatric pheochromocytoma. A 36-year review. *Pediatr Surg Int*. 1997;12(8):595–598.
269. Meinhardt H. Computational modelling of epithelial patterning. *Curr Opin Genet Dev*. 2007;17(4):272–280.
270. Baird AD, Nelson CP, Gearhart JP. Modern staged repair of bladder exstrophy: a contemporary series. *J Pediatr Urol*. 2007;3(4):311–315.
271. Nasir AA, Ameh EA, Abdur-Rahman LO, Adeniran JO, Abraham MK. Posterior urethral valve. *World J Pediatr*. 2011;7(3):205–216.
272. Barthold JS, Gonzalez R. The epidemiology of congenital cryptorchidism, testicular ascent and orchiopexy. *J Urol*. 2003;170(6 Pt 1):2396–2401.
273. Ringdahl E, Teague L. Testicular torsion. *Am Fam Physician*. 2006;74(10):1739–1743.
274. Davenport M. ABC of general surgery in children. Acute problems of the scrotum. *BMJ*. 1996;312(7028):435–437.
275. Paty R, Smith AD. Gangrene and Fournier's gangrene. *Urol Clin North Am*. 1992;19(1):149–162.
276. Norton KS, Johnson LW, Perry T, Perry KH, Sehon JK, Zibari GB. Management of Fournier's gangrene: an eleven year retrospective analysis of early recognition, diagnosis, and treatment. *Am Surg*. 2002;68(8):709–713.
277. Korhonen K, Hirn M, Niinikoski J. Hyperbaric oxygen in the treatment of Fournier's gangrene. *Eur J Surg*. 1998;164(4):251–255.
278. Mindrup SR, Kealey GP, Fallon B. Hyperbaric oxygen for the treatment of fournier's gangrene. *J Urol*. 2005;173(6):1975–1977.
279. Corcoran AT, Smaldone MC, Gibbons EP, Walsh TJ, Davies BJ. Validation of the Fournier's gangrene severity index in a large contemporary series. *J Urol*. 2008;180(3):944–948.
280. Brown P. Management of urinary tract infections associated with nephrolithiasis. *Curr Infect Dis Rep*. 2010;12(6):450–454.

51 Anesthesia for Orthopedic Surgery

SARAH S. JOO • ELLEN M. SOFFIN • STEPHEN C. HASKINS • MEGHAN A. KIRKSEY

KEY POINTS

1 Optimal anesthetic management for orthopedic surgery requires expertise in regional anesthesia and analgesia techniques.
2 Regional anesthesia can provide physiologic benefits and facilitate recovery compared to general anesthesia.
3 General anesthesia is appropriate for surgeries not amenable to and/or patients with contraindications to regional techniques.
4 Orthopedic surgery patients may have limited mobility and may require special attention to avoid positioning-related injury.
5 Patients presenting for spine surgery should be evaluated carefully for potential airway challenges and/or impaired respiratory function.
6 Major spine surgery frequently involves significant bleeding, and a blood conservation strategy should be considered as part of the anesthetic plan.
7 Intraoperative monitoring of spinal cord function should be used for surgeries where the cord is at risk of injury.
8 Catastrophic venous air embolism during spine surgery may present as unexplained hypotension with high end-tidal nitrogen and low end-tidal carbon dioxide.
9 Nerve injury may result from surgical trauma and/or nerve blockade in the setting of pre-existing neurologic deficits.
10 In the sitting position, for every 20 cm of difference in height of the head from the heart, there is a 15-mmHg difference in mean arterial pressure.
11 Ephedrine, atropine, and glycopyrrolate should be available for management of hypotensive bradycardic events occurring during surgery in the beach chair position.
12 Interscalene blocks cause hemidiaphragmatic paresis and can cause respiratory compromise in patients with reduced pulmonary function.
13 Venous thromboembolism is a common complication of lower extremity orthopedic surgery performed with inadequate thromboprophylaxis.
14 The American Society of Regional Anesthesia has released guidelines for safe use of regional anesthesia in the setting of antithrombotic or thrombolytic therapy.

Introduction

1 Perioperative management of the patient undergoing orthopedic surgery involves knowledge of orthopedic surgical techniques and associated complications, including nerve injury. Expertise in regional anesthetic techniques for both surgical anesthesia and postoperative analgesia is of paramount importance. Appropriate patient positioning produces optimal surgical conditions while avoiding complications related to stretch, pressure, and hemodynamic changes. Orthopedic procedures can be associated with large-volume blood loss; therefore, one must be familiar with tourniquet use, controlled intraoperative hypotension, blood salvage techniques, use of antifibrinolytics, fluid resuscitation (see Chapter 16), transfusions, and related complications (see Chapter 17).

Orthopedic surgical patients benefit greatly from early mobilization and rehabilitation, both of which can be expedited by specific anesthetic techniques and proactive postoperative analgesia. A multimodal approach, often utilizing neuraxial and/or peripheral nerve blocks, can enhance recovery and improve functional outcomes. Patients undergoing major orthopedic surgery are at high risk for venous thromboembolism (VTE). Knowledge of current pharmacologic and mechanical methods of thromboprophylaxis is required, and regional techniques must be optimized to minimize associated bleeding risk.

Preoperative Assessment

All patients should undergo medical and laboratory testing appropriate to their medical history and planned procedure (see Chapter 23). Preoperative assessment of the orthopedic patient must include special attention to potential airway difficulties, considerations relating to mobility and intraoperative positioning, and medication history related to opioid dependence and anticoagulation status. Cardiopulmonary symptoms and exercise tolerance may be difficult to assess in this population because of limitations in mobility. As a result, pharmacologic functional cardiovascular testing and formal pulmonary function testing may be warranted in patients with concerning risk factors. Overall, patients undergoing orthopedic procedures are considered at intermediate risk for perioperative cardiac complications.

Patients with rheumatoid arthritis often require orthopedic surgery and merit special attention. Rheumatoid arthritis can affect the pulmonary, cardiac, and musculoskeletal systems. Airway management can be challenging in these patients. Involvement of the cervical spine and temporomandibular joints results in limited neck range of motion and mouth opening. Atlantoaxial instability, with subluxation of the odontoid process, can lead to spinal cord injury during neck extension. Patients on chronic steroid therapy may require perioperative steroid replacement.

All medications should be reviewed during a preoperative visit with detailed instructions as to which medications to hold and which to continue until surgery. Patients taking opioids may have developed tolerance and opioid-induced hyperalgesia. Although abrupt cessation of opioids is not advised, weaning of chronic opioids under the direction of a pain management specialist prior to elective surgery may be beneficial. Antihypertensives without a significant rebound effect may be held on the day of surgery if there is concern for excessive intraoperative hypotension or renal injury related to angiotensin-converting enzyme inhibitors or angiotensin receptor blockers. A plan for management of anticoagulants must be agreed upon by the medical and surgical teams and communicated clearly to the patient. Anesthetic techniques must take into account the specifics of each patient's anticoagulation status and plan.

Preoperative evaluation should include a standard focused physical examination (see Chapter 23). Orthopedic patients may have coexisting disease or trauma requiring special attention to distorted airway anatomy or limited neck mobility. Proposed sites of needle placement for regional anesthesia and line placement should be assessed for evidence of infection and anatomic abnormalities. A brief neurologic examination with documentation of pre-existing deficits is crucial. Potential positioning difficulties related to body habitus, joint pain or instability, fractures, and/or fusions should be considered. Preoperative education regarding the surgical procedure, anesthetic/analgesic options, and postoperative rehabilitation plan should be provided.

Selection of Anesthetic Technique

2 Many orthopedic surgical procedures, because of their localized peripheral sites, lend themselves to regional anesthesia (RA) techniques. Neural structures may be blocked at the peripheral nerve, plexus, or neuraxial level (see Chapters 35 and 36). RA offers several advantages over general anesthesia including enhanced rehabilitation, accelerated hospital discharge, improved analgesia, decreased nausea and vomiting, less respiratory and cardiac depression, improved perfusion, reduced blood loss, and decreased risk of infection and thromboembolism. It is important to communicate potential benefits and encourage RA when appropriate.

The optimal regional technique and local anesthetic depend 3
on factors including surgery duration, indication for postoperative sympathectomy, and desired degree and duration of postoperative sensory/motor block to allow for active or passive physical therapy. General anesthesia is appropriate for orthopedic surgery at sites not amenable to regional and in patients with contraindications to regional techniques owing to factors such as anticoagulation status, infection at the needle insertion site, pre-existing nerve injury or disease, and patient refusal. Of note, a contraindication to one regional technique may not preclude the use of another. For example, coagulopathy may prevent the use of neuraxial or deep plexus blocks, but a superficial peripheral nerve block may be appropriate. In contrast, a neuraxial block may be safer in a patient with pre-existing peripheral neuropathy.

Anesthesia for Spine Surgery

Preoperative Assessment

Preoperative evaluation for spine surgery should assess involve- 4
ment of the respiratory, cardiovascular, and neurologic systems. Difficult airways are common in patients presenting for surgery involving the upper thoracic or cervical spine; therefore, airway evaluation should focus on restricted neck movement, cervical spine stability, and exacerbation of symptoms with movement or position. Both clinical and radiographic assessment of cervical spine stability should be discussed with the surgeon prior to neck manipulation. The decision to secure the airway awake, asleep, or with advanced airway devices should be made prior to surgery and the patient counseled accordingly. Awake tracheal intubation is preferred when assessing for neurologic function prior to use of a traction device.

Patients presenting for spine surgery often have impaired 5
respiratory function (1 Video 51-1). Scoliosis can cause restrictive lung disease, neuromuscular diseases can be associated with recurrent chest infections, and patients with spinal cord injury may already be ventilator dependent. Physical examination and history should focus on functional impairment. Chest radiograph, arterial blood gas, and pulmonary function tests may be indicated in patients with restrictive pulmonary disease. A preoperative vital capacity less than 30% to 35% of predicted is associated with prolonged postoperative ventilation after scoliosis surgery.[1] Optimization of pulmonary function targets treatment of reversible causes with the use of preoperative physical therapy, antibiotics, and bronchodilators as indicated.

Cardiac dysfunction is often associated with spine pathology and may be a primary manifestation of the disease as seen in muscular dystrophies. Rarely, scoliosis can cause cor pulmonale secondary to chronic hypoxemia and pulmonary hypertension. An electrocardiogram (ECG) and echocardiogram should be obtained to assess left ventricular function and pulmonary arterial pressures. Dobutamine stress echocardiography may be necessary to assess cardiac function in patients with limited exercise tolerance or mobility.

Neurologic deficits of spine patients generally relate to the underlying disease and should be discussed in detail with the patient and surgeon and documented. With cervical spine surgery, extra care must be taken to avoid injury during tracheal intubation and positioning. Neuromuscular diseases increase risk of aspiration during airway manipulation. In patients with spinal cord injury, spinal shock and autonomic dysreflexia are of particular concern.

Positioning for Spine Surgery

Positioning for spine surgery depends on the level and approach of the procedure. Patients may be transitioned between supine, lateral, and prone positions intraoperatively. Overall goals of positioning are to (1) pad as needed to protect peripheral nerves, bony prominences, and the eyes, (2) avoid displacement of unstable fractures during surgery, and (3) ensure low venous pressures and thereby minimize blood loss at the surgical site. Low venous pressures can be facilitated by maintaining a free abdomen and reverse Trendelenburg position.

The posterior approach to spine surgery requires prone positioning (Fig. 51-1, see Chapter 29, Videos 29-1 and 29-5). Pressure on the abdomen causes inferior vena cava compression, increasing bleeding from valveless epidural veins, reducing cardiac output, and increasing the risk of lower limb thrombosis.[2] Therefore, adequate foam padding should be placed under the chest (below the axillae) and the anterior superior iliac spines. The arms should not be abducted to more than 90 degrees and should be positioned with slight internal rotation to reduce the risk of brachial plexus stretching. With the elbow flexed in the prone position, the ulnar nerve is at particular risk of pressure-related injury and should be protected. The eyes should be taped closed; appropriate positioning with a ProneView (Mizuho OSI, Union City, CA) or Mayfield fixator will avoid pressure on the eyes/orbits while maintaining a neutral neck position.

The anterior approach to the thoracolumbar spine can be achieved in the supine or lateral position. For scoliosis surgery, the convexity of the curve is usually uppermost, and removal of one or more ribs may be necessary for surgical exposure. Placement of a double-lumen endotracheal tube to collapse the lung on the operative side may be required for surgery above T8 in the lateral position.

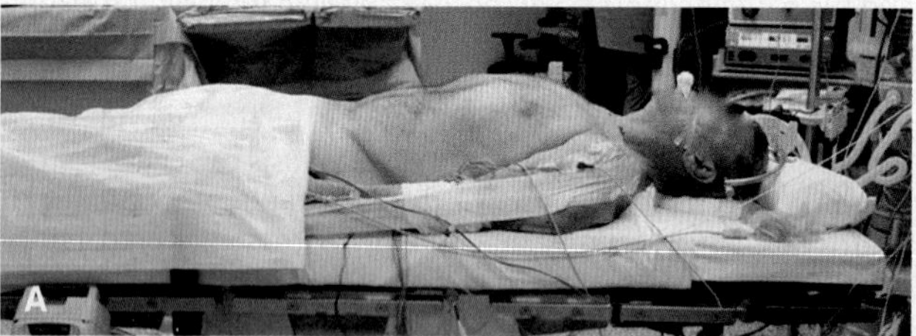

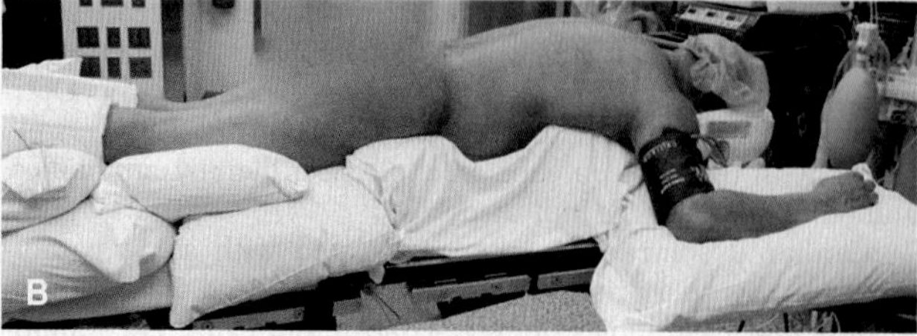

Figure 51-1 Positioning for spine surgery. **A:** Supine positioning for anterior approach. The neck is maintained in a neutral-flexed position and the head is supported with a round foam pillow or other supportive devices. The shoulders are taped in caudal traction to aid exposure. In-line traction is applied via Gardner-Wells tongs. **B:** Prone positioning for posterior approach. The head and neck are neutral with the face supported on a head frame (ProneView) to avoid any direct pressure to the eyes. The shoulders are abducted to less than 90 degrees. The forearms are placed on padded supports at the level of the mattress to minimize direct pressure on the ulnar nerve at the elbow. The pelvis and chest are supported to minimize intra-abdominal pressure.

For cervical spine surgery, anterior approaches require the supine position and posterior approaches require prone positioning (Fig. 51-1). The patient may be positioned with the head 180 degrees away from the anesthetic machine to allow surgical access. Therefore, extensions may be needed for breathing circuits and intravascular lines, and it may be necessary to place venous access in the patient's foot. Endotracheal tubes must be carefully secured without disruption of the surgical field. The head may be supported on a padded head ring or the "horseshoe" of a Mayfield attachment. If neck traction is required, it is generally achieved by placing pins and weights onto the outer skull. Reverse Trendelenburg minimizes venous bleeding and provides countertraction. Venous pooling in the lower limbs and carotid artery retraction can cause swift and significant hemodynamic changes; therefore, an arterial line is advisable. Because the arms will typically be tucked at the sides, the arterial line should be placed prior to positioning.

Blood Conservation

The frequency of transfusion in adult spine surgery ranges from 6
50% to 81%.[3] Most of the blood loss during spinal instrumentation and fusion occurs with decortication and is proportional to the number of vertebral levels involved.

Patients may become coagulopathic perioperatively, owing to fibrinolysis or dilution of coagulation factors and/or platelets. The detailed mechanisms of coagulopathy and the role of factor testing during spine surgery are poorly defined. However, it appears that a significant deviation from baseline of either the prothrombin time or activated partial thromboplastin time is predictive of bleeding and may be used to guide transfusion therapy.[4] A rare cause of bleeding during spine surgery is trauma to the aorta, vena cava, or iliac vessels. Unexplained rapidly evolving hypotension with signs of hypovolemia should alert the anesthesiologist to this possibility, and close communication with the surgical team is vital.

Measures to decrease blood loss and transfusion requirements during major spine surgery include preoperative autologous donation, proper positioning, the use of intraoperative blood salvage, and the administration of antifibrinolytics such as tranexamic acid (TXA) (see Chapter 17). Recent data indicate that TXA not only reduces surgical bleeding and transfusion requirements but also does so without increased incidence of pulmonary embolism (PE), deep venous thrombosis (DVT), or myocardial infarction.[5,6]

Spinal Cord Monitoring

Intraoperative monitoring (IOM) of spinal cord function is now 7
considered mandatory for all surgeries in which the cord is at risk of injury. Risk is incurred when corrective forces are applied to the spine, osteotomies are made, or the spinal canal is surgically invaded. Data suggest that IOM may substantially reduce the incidence of motor deficits or paraplegia after cervical surgery and scoliosis surgery.[7–9] There are three main methods of IOM: the wake-up test, somatosensory evoked potential (SSEP) monitoring, and motor evoked potential (MEP) recording.

The wake-up test involves intraoperative awakening of the patient after completion of spinal instrumentation to assess motor function of upper and lower extremities. If there is satisfactory movement of the hands but not the feet, then distraction on the rod is released one notch and the wake-up test repeated. Surgical anesthesia can be achieved with a volatile anesthetic, nitrous oxide, and opioids, with or without propofol. Opioids are important for analgesia and tolerance of the endotracheal tube while the patient is awake. Although recall of the event occurs in only 0% to 20% of patients and is rarely viewed as unpleasant,[10] it is important to describe the wake-up test prior to surgery to minimize anxiety should the patient have recall.

The wake-up test has a number of disadvantages, including the risk that an uncooperative patient could move, dislodge the endotracheal tube, or even fall from the table. In addition, the wake-up test assesses function only at the time it is performed and has the potential to provide false reassurance after instrumentation but prior to an unexpected neurologic injury. Thus, the wake-up test is most suitable if other monitoring techniques are not available or equivocal or if they fail.

SSEPs assess the dorsal column pathways of proprioception and vibration that are supplied by the posterior spinal artery. SSEPs are altered by neural injury, volatile anesthetics, hypercarbia, hypoxia, hypotension, and hypothermia.[11] Motor pathways are supplied by the anterior spinal artery and are monitored by MEPs. MEPs are considered technically more difficult to use, in part because they are impeded by use of muscle relaxants. If both SSEP and MEP are to be monitored during spine surgery, a suitable anesthetic regimen would include an ultrashort-acting opioid infusion with a low-dose inhaled anesthetic or total intravenous anesthesia with monitoring of the electroencephalogram or bispectral index to minimize the potential for intraoperative awareness (see Chapter 37).

Postoperative paraplegia has occurred despite preservation of intraoperative SSEPs; however, MEPs in combination with SSEPs may increase the early detection of spinal cord ischemia.[12] Acute alterations in signal amplitude or latency can signify spinal cord compromise and may be the result of direct trauma, ischemia, compression, or hematoma. If changes occur, it is recommended that surgery be discontinued, blood pressure returned to normal or 20% above normal, and volatile agents decreased or discontinued. Arterial blood gases can help rule out a metabolic derangement. If the signal does not return to normal, the surgeon should release distraction on the cord. A wake-up test can be performed at this time to definitively exclude neurologic deficits.

Spinal Cord Injury

Patients presenting with a traumatic spinal cord injury should be examined immediately to assess for signs of respiratory insufficiency, airway obstruction, rib fractures, and chest wall or facial trauma. Spinal cord function above the level of the injury should be determined. If the muscles controlled by the C5 nerve roots (deltoid, biceps, brachialis, and brachioradialis) are flaccid, partial diaphragmatic paralysis should also be expected.

Patients requiring spine stabilization surgery may present with spinal shock, which occurs immediately after the injury and lasts up to 3 weeks. Injuries at or above T5 are associated with hypotension due to a physiologic sympathectomy and loss of tone from the splanchnic vascular beds. Lesions above the cardiac accelerator fibers (T1 to T4) cause bradycardia. Hypotension due to spinal injury is poorly responsive to intravenous fluids and vasopressors, and excessive fluid administration may contribute to the development of pulmonary edema.

With complete cord transection above T5, following recovery from spinal shock, 85% of patients go on to exhibit autonomic hyperreflexia. The syndrome can also occur with injuries at lower levels and is characterized by severe paroxysmal hypertension with bradycardia from the baroreceptor reflex, dysrhythmias, and cutaneous vasoconstriction below and vasodilation above the level of the injury. Episodes are typically precipitated by distention of the bladder or rectum but can be induced by any noxious stimulus including surgery. Treatment involves removal of the stimulus, deepening of anesthesia, and administration of direct-acting vasodilators. Untreated, the hypertensive crisis may progress to seizures, intracranial hemorrhage, or myocardial infarction.

Ventilatory impairment increases with higher levels of spinal injury. A high cervical lesion that includes the diaphragmatic segments (C3 to C5) results in respiratory failure and death without mechanical ventilation. Lesions between C5 and T7 cause significant alterations in respiratory function due to loss of abdominal and intercostal support. Flaccid thoracic muscles can lead to paradoxic respirations and a vital capacity reduction of 60%. Inability to cough and effectively clear secretions causes atelectasis and increased risk of infection.

Succinylcholine can be administered safely for the first 48 hours after spinal cord injury. After that time, a proliferation of acetylcholine receptors in the muscle can cause hypersensitivity to depolarizing muscle relaxants leading to marked hyperkalemia.[13] Maximal hyperkalemia risk from succinylcholine occurs between 4 weeks and 5 months after spinal injury. Serum potassium levels may rise as high as 14 mEq/L, causing ventricular fibrillation and cardiac arrest. Although succinylcholine should be avoided in all patients with spinal cord injury after 48 hours, nondepolarizing paralytic agents can be used.

Patients with spinal cord injury are poikilothermic, owing to disruption of sympathetic pathways carrying temperature sensation and subsequent loss of vasoconstriction below the level of injury. Normothermia can be achieved by applying exogenous heat to the skin, increasing ambient air temperature, warming intravenous fluids, and humidifying gases.

Scoliosis

Scoliosis involves a lateral and rotational deformity of the spine and occurs in up to 4% of the population. Most cases are idiopathic (70%), with a male-to-female ratio of 1:4. Surgery is considered when the Cobb angle, a measure of curvature, exceeds 50 degrees in the thoracic or 40 degrees in the lumbar spine. The goal of surgery is to halt progression of the condition and partially correct the deformity, preventing further respiratory and cardiovascular deterioration.

Scoliosis can cause chronic hypoxia, hypercapnia, and pulmonary vascular constriction resulting in irreversible pulmonary vascular changes, pulmonary hypertension, and, eventually, right ventricular hypertrophy and cor pulmonale. Thus, untreated idiopathic scoliosis can progress rapidly and is often fatal by the fourth or fifth decade of life. Scoliosis is also often associated with congenital heart conditions, including mitral valve prolapse, coarctation of the aorta, and cyanotic heart disease, suggesting a common embryonic insult or collagen defect.

Although the long-term effect of scoliosis repair is to halt the decline in respiratory function, pulmonary function acutely deteriorates for 7 to 10 days after surgery. Preoperative vital capacity is a reliable prognostic indicator of respiratory reserve, and postoperative ventilator support is likely to be required for patients with a vital capacity less than 40% of predicted.

Anesthetic considerations for surgical correction of scoliosis by spinal fusion and instrumentation include management in the prone position, hypothermia during long procedures with extensive exposure, and replacement of blood and fluid losses (see Chapter 29, Video 29-4). Adequate hemodynamic monitoring and venous access are essential. An arterial line allows for close hemodynamic monitoring and assessment of blood gases, whereas a central venous catheter may be helpful in evaluating blood and fluid management and can be used to aspirate air in the case of venous air embolism. Patients with evidence of pulmonary hypertension or severe coexistent cardiovascular or pulmonary disease may require a pulmonary artery catheter.

Muscular Disorders

Muscular dystrophy and cerebral palsy are important causes of scoliosis. Duchenne muscular dystrophy (DMD) has an incidence of 1:3,300 male births and is inherited as a sex-linked recessive condition affecting skeletal, cardiac, and smooth muscle. Patients with DMD lack a membrane cytoskeletal protein, dystrophin, and typically present between the ages of 2 and 6 years, with progressive weakness of proximal muscle groups. Up to one-third have intellectual impairment. DMD patients have a high incidence of cardiac abnormalities (50% to 70%). In the later stages of the disease, dilated cardiomyopathy may occur in association with mitral valve incompetence. Up to 50% of patients have cardiac conduction defects predisposing to dysrhythmias that can, in some cases, lead to cardiac arrest during spine surgery. Patients with DMD are sensitive to nondepolarizing neuromuscular blocking agents, and hyperkalemia may occur with use of succinylcholine. In general, the prognosis of scoliosis associated with neuromuscular disease is worse than that of idiopathic scoliosis, and these patients frequently require postoperative ventilatory support.

Degenerative Vertebral Column Disease

Spinal stenosis, spondylosis, and spondylolisthesis are all forms of degenerative vertebral column disease, causing pain and/or progressive neurologic symptoms requiring surgical intervention.

Patients presenting with degenerative conditions affecting the cervical spine should undergo preoperative assessment of symptoms, and a comprehensive airway examination should be performed as described earlier. Intraoperatively, procedures performed by the anterior approach rely on a surgical incision at the border of the sternocleidomastoid muscle, near critical anatomic structures. Lateral retraction of the carotid artery may endanger cerebral perfusion, particularly in the elderly patient. Retraction of the esophagus and trachea medially may cause pharyngeal laceration, laryngeal edema, and recurrent laryngeal nerve paralysis. Cerebrospinal fluid leaks and trauma to the vertebral artery have also been reported.

General anesthesia is preferred for nearly all degenerative thoracic and cervical procedures because of the high spinal level that would be required with a regional technique. General anesthesia ensures airway control, is associated with greater patient acceptance, and can be used for prolonged operations. For lower thoracic and lumbar spine surgery, either general anesthesia or neuraxial anesthesia (NA) may be safely administered. A recent meta-analysis of randomized trials comparing general to spinal anesthesia concluded that spinal anesthesia was associated with lower blood loss and lower early pain scores and shorter length of hospital stay, whereas general anesthesia was associated with higher surgeon satisfaction.[14]

Postoperative Care of the Spine Patient

Most patients can be extubated immediately after spine surgery if the procedure was uncomplicated and preoperative vital capacity values were acceptable. Postoperative ventilation may be required in patients with neuromuscular disorders, severe restrictive pulmonary dysfunction with a preoperative vital capacity of less than 35% of predicted, right ventricular failure, obesity, or sleep apnea. Patients with prolonged procedures, thoracic cavity invasion, or blood loss greater than 30 mL/kg^{-1} may require postoperative ventilation.[15] In the event of significant blood loss requiring aggressive resuscitation, particularly in the prone position, facial and laryngeal edema may compromise an uncontrolled airway and extubation is not advisable. Residual opioid or muscle relaxant may lead to hypoventilation or apnea, especially in patients with neuromuscular disease. Neurologic status must also be monitored closely to determine appropriateness for extubation.

Postoperative mechanical ventilation may be maintained for a few hours, with the head of the bed elevated when possible, until hypothermia and metabolic derangements have been corrected and facial and airway edema have improved. Aggressive postoperative pulmonary therapy, including incentive spirometry, is necessary to avoid postextubation atelectasis and pneumonia. Careful monitoring of systemic pressures, urine output, and wound drainage is essential to ensure adequate resuscitation and absence of significant postoperative hemorrhage.

After spine surgery, analgesia traditionally includes systemic opioids. Adequate and safe opioid administration can often be accomplished using patient-controlled analgesia devices with or without background infusions. Side effects of opioids can include respiratory depression, sedation, and gastrointestinal ileus. These concerns are amplified after major spine surgery when respiratory status may be compromised. Neurologic status must be followed closely and bowel dysmotility is common.

Multimodal analgesia within "enhanced recovery after surgery" pathways is increasingly being used for postoperative pain management after spine surgery and can be effective for reducing pain scores, opioid consumption, opioid-related side effects, and length of hospital stay.[16] Historically, options for regional analgesia for spine surgery patients were limited to local anesthetic wound infiltration or intrathecal morphine.[17] More recently, field and fascial plane blocks are being applied to spine surgery care, including transversus abdominis plane block,[18,19] erector spinae plane block,[20,21] and thoracolumbar interfascial plane block.[22] The addition of nonopioid analgesics to analgesic regimens, including nonsteroidal anti-inflammatories, corticosteroids, and acetaminophen can also reduce opioid use, improve analgesia, and decrease opioid-related side effects (Table 51-1). Anticonvulsant medications should be considered on a case-by-case basis, given recent evidence related to risk of harm without evidence of clear analgesic benefit in anticonvulsant-naive patients.[23] Historically, nonsteroidal anti-inflammatory drugs were avoided after complex spine surgery because of effects on bone remodeling and solid fusion. More recent data suggest that a short course of low-dose nonselective nonsteroidal anti-inflammatory is reasonable.[24] However, the surgical team should be consulted prior to initiating therapy.

Complications of Spine Surgery

Venous air embolus (VAE) is a catastrophic event that is a particular risk during laminectomy because of the large amount of exposed bone and location of the surgical site above the level of the heart. VAE presents as unexplained hypotension with an increase in the end-tidal nitrogen concentration or a precipitous fall in the end-tidal carbon dioxide concentration. Prompt diagnosis and treatment increase patient survival with VAE. Prevention and management measures include intravascular volume expansion, careful positioning, positive end-expiratory pressure, and jugular venous compression. Treatment includes flooding the surgical site with saline, controlling sites of air entry, repositioning the patient with the surgical site below the right atrium, aspiration of air from a multiorifice central venous catheter, cessation of inhaled nitrous oxide, and resuscitation with oxygen, intravenous fluids, and inotropic agents. Massive embolism may necessitate supine repositioning and cardiopulmonary resuscitation.

Table 51-1 Multimodal Analgesia for Orthopedic Surgery

Drug Name	Mechanism of Action	Common Side Effects	Additional Considerations
Paracetamol/Acetaminophen			
Acetaminophen	COX inhibition (predominantly COX-2)	Hepatoxicity	Avoid in liver disease and alcoholism
NSAIDs			
Ketorolac, meloxicam, ibuprofen	COX-1/2 inhibition	Nephrotoxicity Gastritis May impair bone healing	Avoid in renal impairment and/or inflammatory bowel disease
Celecoxib	Selective COX-2 inhibition	Nephrotoxicity Gastritis	Avoid in renal impairment and coronary artery disease Avoid in patients with sulfa allergy
Nontraditional Opioids			
Methadone	Opioid agonist, NMDA receptor antagonist, inhibits reuptake of NE	Drowsiness, sedation, constipation, dizziness, nausea/vomiting	Promotility bowel regimen required
Tramadol, tapentadol	Weak μ-opioid agonist, inhibits reuptake of NE		Tramadol also blocks reuptake of 5-HT; opioid receptor binding affinity is 6000 times less than morphine
Miscellaneous			
Ketamine	NMDA receptor antagonist	Tachycardia, dysphoria	Avoid with increased ICP, asthma; Transdermal patch or infusion
Lidocaine	Blocks Na^+-gated channels, thereby blocking nerve conduction	Hepatic dysfunction	Transdermal patch or infusion
Dexmedetomidine	α-2 adenoreceptor agonist	Bradycardia Hypotension	Infusion only

COX, cyclooxygenase; ICP, intracranial pressure; NE, norepinephrine; NMDA, *N*-methyl-D-aspartate; NSAIDs, nonsteroidal anti-inflammatory drugs.

Vision loss is a rare, nonfatal yet catastrophic complication associated with spine surgery. The etiology of vision loss can be optic neuropathy, retinal artery occlusion, or cerebral ischemia. Most cases are associated with complex instrumented fusions,[25] significant sustained intraoperative hypotension, anemia, large intraoperative blood loss, and prolonged surgery.[26]

The American Society of Anesthesiologists (ASA) Postoperative Visual Loss Registry reported on 93 cases of visual loss after spine surgery submitted anonymously to the ASA Closed Claims Study. Ischemic optic neuropathy was the most common cause of visual loss and accounted for 83 of 93 cases.[25] Risk factors for ischemic optic neuropathy after spinal surgery include male sex, obesity, Wilson frame use, long anesthetic duration, large blood loss, and use of noncolloid fluids.[27]

Upper Extremity Surgery

Orthopedic surgical procedures to the upper extremity are well suited for regional anesthetic techniques. Peripheral nerve block adjuvants that prolong nerve block duration can provide significant postoperative analgesia.[28] Continuous catheter techniques can also provide sustained analgesia and facilitate early mobilization.

9 The benefits of regional anesthesia for upper extremity surgery are well established. However, many orthopedic patients may have concurrent central or peripheral neuropathy and upper extremity surgical procedures may involve peripheral nerves with these pre-existing deficits. Physicians must be cognizant of the increased risk of nerve injury resulting from "double-crush syndrome" in the setting of surgical trauma and nerve blockade. The decision to perform regional anesthesia in a patient with pre-existing neurologic deficits or who is at risk for perioperative neurapraxia should be made on an individual basis after discussion with the patient and surgeon. Meticulous regional anesthetic technique with ultrasound guidance, appropriate use of local anesthetic solutions, careful patient positioning, and serial postoperative neurologic examinations may reduce the incidence of postoperative neurologic dysfunction.

Local anesthetic selection is based on the duration and degree of sensory or motor block required. The patient should be informed of the anticipated block duration prior to surgery and instructed to protect the extremity until block resolution. If there is a possibility of block resolution overnight, it is not unreasonable to recommend that the patient commence oral pain medication at bedtime, even while numb, to minimize the risk of sudden and severe pain overnight. It should also be noted that rarely supraclavicular, superior trunk, and infraclavicular blocks are complicated by pneumothorax that may not manifest until 6 to 12 hours after surgery. Although these blocks are routinely performed safely for inpatient and ambulatory surgeries, each patient should be told to contact their surgeon immediately if any respiratory difficulties develop postoperatively.

Surgery to the Shoulder and Upper Arm

Reconstructive shoulder surgeries, including open shoulder surgery and shoulder arthroscopies, present unique management and positioning considerations to the anesthesiologist (see Chapter 55, Video 55-5). For arthroscopies, nerve injury can occur from stretching due to traction and direct trauma from portal placement, with reported rates of injury ranging from less than 0.1% to 10%.[29] For total shoulder replacements, the incidence of neurologic complications is reported to be between 0.8% to 4.3%.[29] An institutional review of 1,569 patients who underwent total shoulder arthroplasty (TSA) between 1993 and 2007 revealed a 2.2% rate of perioperative nerve injury.[30] It is notable that although a significant percentage of TSA-associated nerve injuries occur at the level of the brachial plexus, this study found a lower rate of perioperative nerve injury in patients who received interscalene blocks (ISBs).[30] It is important to communicate both the risk of nerve injury after major shoulder surgery and the lack of evidence that brachial plexus nerve blocks contribute significantly to this risk.

Nerve injury can also be associated with trauma. Axillary nerve and brachial plexus injuries are most often associated with proximal humerus fractures, and radial nerve palsy can be associated with humeral shaft fractures. This highlights the need for careful examination and documentation of deficits prior to use of a regional anesthetic and clear communication with patients regarding current evidence about associated risks and benefits.

Surgical Approach and Positioning

Surgical procedures to the upper arm and shoulder are typically performed with the patient sitting in the "beach chair" or, less commonly, lying in the lateral decubitus position (see Chapter 29). In either position, the patient's head, neck, and hips must be secured to prevent lateral movement during surgical manipulation, with frequent reassessment throughout the case. Excessive rotation or flexion of the head away from the operative side results in stretch injury to the brachial plexus. Care must be taken to avoid pressure on the eyes and ears. Access to the patient's face and airway is often limited, so any airway devices and connections must be carefully secured. In spontaneously breathing patients with unsecured airways, good airflow must be maintained to minimize carbon dioxide rebreathing and pockets of oxygen that present a fire safety risk.

10 Positioning generally depends on the specifics of the surgery and surgeon preference. The lateral position has been associated with increased rates of neurapraxia from stretch injuries and is a challenging position from which to convert from an arthroscopic to an open procedure should this become necessary.[31] The beach chair position allows for easy conversion to open procedures, improved intra-articular visualization and orientation, and decreased brachial plexus traction injury. However, there is a risk for lateral femoral cutaneous nerve injury, with higher risk in patients with higher body mass index.[32]

The beach chair position also presents several hemodynamic challenges for the anesthesiologist. Venous pooling in the legs can cause hypotension and decreased cardiac output. Blood pressure at the head will be lower than at the arm or leg, with every 20 cm of height difference equating to an approximately 15-mmHg difference in mean arterial pressure (Fig. 51-2). Association between hypotension and cerebral desaturation has been reported, and there have been case reports of catastrophic neurologic injuries (e.g., cerebral and spinal cord ischemia, vision loss) in the sitting position. Studies suggest an imbalance in supply and demand of cerebral oxygenation in the beach chair position, but an association between these variables of cerebral oxygenation and adverse outcomes has not been clearly shown.[33] Further research is needed to define the incidence of adverse neurologic outcomes and optimal monitoring and prevention strategies.

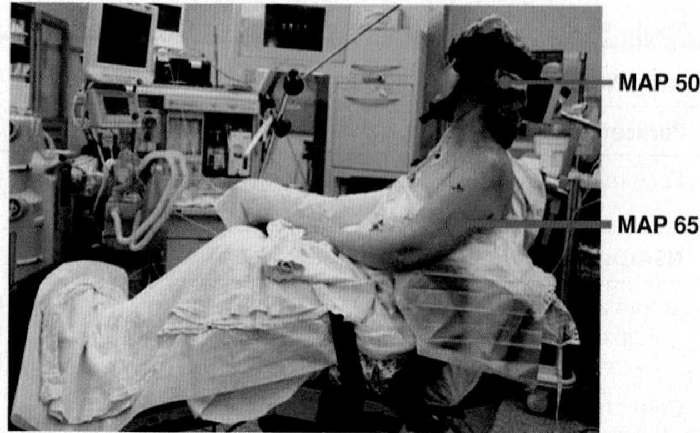

Figure 51-2 Positioning for upper extremity surgery: beach chair position. The patient is placed semi-recumbent with the head, neck, and torso supported in neutral position by a head harness and padding. Hips are flexed to 45 to 60 degrees and the knees to 30 degrees resting on a knee pillow. The chair is in 10 to 15 degrees of Trendelenburg. Pressure points are padded and the eyes are protected. The nonoperative arm is placed on an arm support. The major risk during surgery in the beach chair position is hypotension; for every 1-cm rise above the heart, there is a 0.75-mmHg drop in mean arterial pressure (MAP). Thus, a 20-cm rise in the head causes a 15-mmHg fall in cerebral MAP.

Up to 24% of patients undergoing surgery in the beach chair 11
position under general or regional anesthesia can experience hemodynamically significant hypotensive bradycardic events (HBEs).[34] Although usually brief and resolving spontaneously, these episodes can lead to severe asystolic cardiac events if prompt treatment is not initiated. The exact etiology of HBE is unknown; however, it is hypothesized that ventricular underfilling induces the Bezold–Jarisch reflex. Studies have found that intraoperative use of epinephrine, fentanyl, hydralazine, propofol, and dexmedetomidine is associated with increased risk of HBE.[35–37] In contrast, preincision administration of ondansetron or metoprolol may significantly decrease this risk.[38,39] Ephedrine, atropine, and glycopyrrolate have been used successfully to manage such events and should be immediately available when patients are undergoing surgery in the beach chair position.

A tourniquet cannot be used during proximal upper extremity procedures, and significant blood loss may occur. Moreover, patients are at risk of sudden hemodynamic instability from embolic syndromes caused by fat, air, and/or cement. Arterial cannulation for continuous direct blood pressure measurement and monitoring of hemoglobin concentration should be considered, particularly during TSA and humeral fracture reduction/fixation.

Anesthetic Management

Surgery to the shoulder and humerus may be performed under regional anesthesia, general anesthesia, or a combined approach. With careful positioning and appropriate sedation, interscalene, superior trunk, or supraclavicular blockade alone can provide excellent surgical anesthesia (Table 51-2). General anesthesia without a nerve block should be considered in patients with a preexisting brachial plexopathy or significant cervical spine disease because of the risk of perioperative exacerbation of neurologic deficits. With general anesthesia, the airway can be secured with either a supraglottic airway or an endotracheal tube. A supraglottic

Table 51-2 Regional Techniques for Upper Extremity Surgery

Block	Nerves Blocked	Applications	Comments
Interscalene	Brachial plexus: C5, C6, C7	Shoulder Humerus Partial coverage of lateral clavicle	May not cover inferior trunk/ulnar nerve (may not be adequate for hand–forearm surgery)
Superior Trunk	Brachial plexus: C5, C6	Shoulder Humerus Elbow	High rate of ipsilateral phrenic nerveparalysis Common Horner syndrome and recurrent laryngeal nerve palsy
Suprascapular	Brachial plexus: C5, C6	Shoulder Humerus	Less potential risk of ipsilateral phrenic nerve paralysis Analgesia noninferior to ISB for shoulder surgery Risk of pneumothorax
Supraclavicular	Brachial plexus: C5, C6, C7	Shoulder Humerus Elbow Forearm Wrist Hand	Less potential risk of ipsilateral phrenic nerve paralysis Anterior approach analgesia noninferior to ISB for shoulder surgery Posterior approach combined with axillary nerve block inferior to ISB for shoulder surgery Risk of pneumothorax Analgesia inferior to ISB for shoulder surgery Highest risk of pneumothorax
Infraclavicular	Radial, ulnar, median, and axillary nerves	Distal humerus Elbow Forearm Wrist Hand	Musculocutaneous nerve may be spared Intercostobrachial nerve not blocked; separate block may be required for surgery Risk of pneumothorax
Axillary	Radial, ulnar, median	Elbow Forearm Wrist Hand	Musculocutaneous nerve can be blocked separately and reliably at this level with ultrasound guidance

airway can be adequate for the beach chair position—it has the advantage of spontaneous respirations that decrease the reduction of venous return and hypotension that could be seen with positive pressure ventilation. A major disadvantage of supraglottic airway use or deep sedation with nasal cannula is the difficulty in accessing the airway during the case in the event of device dislodgement or respiratory insufficiency.

12 Utilization of regional techniques for analgesia after shoulder surgeries has gradually increased over the past decade. Regional anesthesia has been shown to reduce opioid use and opioid-related side effects, improve postoperative pain control, facilitate time to discharge, reduce complications and readmission rates, and improve patient satisfaction.[40–42] A combination of regional and general anesthesia may be chosen to attain optimal analgesia while concurrently securing a patient's airway, providing neuromuscular relaxation (i.e., glenoid exposure, shoulder stabilization procedures), or providing anesthesia for a surgical field extending outside of the block dermatomes.

The ISB is the most used peripheral nerve block for shoulder surgery. Historically, it was noted that ISB caused ipsilateral diaphragmatic paresis in 100% of patients.[43] With a functioning contralateral diaphragm, this leads to a 25% loss of pulmonary function. However, if the contralateral diaphragm is significantly impaired, complete respiratory failure will occur, and, therefore, bilateral ISB blocks should be avoided. Low-volume ISBs in combination with general anesthesia for elective shoulder surgery not only provide good analgesic efficacy, but also rarely result in unilateral phrenic nerve palsy that is clinically significant in healthy patients because ventilation is supported by accessory and intercostal muscles. However, ISB should be used with caution in patients with severe pulmonary disease, as the loss of diaphragmatic function may cause such patients to need supplemental oxygen or ventilation support postoperatively. Care should also be taken when considering ISB in patients with decreased functional reserve capacity, such as those with obesity or sleep apnea, because they are also at increased risk of clinically significant reductions in pulmonary function. Diaphragmatic paresis, when it occurs, is present for the duration of the block, so extra caution should be used when considering administration of adjuvants that will prolong these blocks. ISB can also cause transient Horner syndrome (ipsilateral ptosis, miosis, anhidrosis, and enopthalmos) and recurrent laryngeal nerve blockade (hoarseness). These side effects can be concerning for patients and should be part of the preoperative consent.

While the ISB continues to be the gold standard for many anesthesiologists, concerns about its effect on respiratory function and its safety profile[44] have led to the exploration of other peripheral nerve blocks for the shoulder performed more distally along the brachial plexus.

The supraclavicular block (SCB) is an alternative to the ISB that has fewer side effects. However, compared to the ISB, the SCB may require larger volumes of local anesthetic to achieve adequate analgesia, as there is a concern that the SCB may not cover the more proximal suprascapular nerve with smaller volumes. Moreover, the incidence of phrenic nerve palsy after SCB remains clinically significant, though less common than with ISB.[45,46] One recently developed alternative to the ISB or SCB is the superior trunk block, which is composed of the C5 and C6 nerve roots that track distally to form the superior trunk and then branch into the major nerves that innervate the shoulder. As a low-volume block slightly distal to the level of the ISB, this technique provides effective analgesia and preserves hemidiaphragmatic function.

The suprascapular nerve provides a portion of sensory innervation to the shoulder. In a large multicenter, double-blind study of 136 patients, a selective subomohyoid anterior suprascapular nerve block was shown to provide noninferior analgesia to the ISB in patients undergoing ambulatory arthroscopic surgery.[47] The posterior suprascapular nerve block combined with the axillary nerve block, on the other hand, is inferior to ISB for analgesia for major shoulder surgeries, as it does not provide adequate coverage of the lateral pectoral, subscapular, and musculocutaneous nerves.

Surgery to the Elbow, Wrist, and Hand

In patients without contraindications, surgery in the areas of the distal humerus, elbow, forearm, wrist, and hand can be performed with supraclavicular, infraclavicular, or axillary nerve blocks (Table 51-2). Infraclavicular and supraclavicular approaches to the brachial plexus are the most reliable and provide consistent anesthesia to the four major peripheral nerves of the brachial plexus. The medial aspect of the upper arm, supplied by the intercostobrachial nerve, is generally spared by infraclavicular and axillary blocks and may be blocked by a subcutaneous injection of local anesthetic immediately distal to the axilla for the prevention of tourniquet pain.

Minor hand procedures such as carpal tunnel release, reduction of phalanx fractures, and superficial wound debridements without a tourniquet may require only local infiltration or peripheral blockade at the midhumeral, elbow, or wrist level. Intravenous regional anesthesia (Bier block) using a double tourniquet is an alternative technique for short surgeries in the hand and forearm, but does not provide postoperative analgesia.

Postoperative Regional Analgesia

Peripheral nerve blocks are associated with earlier discharge and decreased risk of hospital admission following rotator cuff repair.[41] For TSA, peripheral nerve blocks improve pain management with no increase in complications or resource usage.[48] Brachial plexus catheters may be inserted using interscalene, infraclavicular, and axillary approaches, and are typically left in place for 2 to 3 days without adverse effects. Indwelling perineural catheters may decrease both opioid requirements and opioid-related side effects, and also improve rehabilitation.

Lower Extremity Surgery

Orthopedic surgeries involving the lower extremity are among the most commonly performed operations in the United States. Demand for total joint arthroplasty of the hip and knee is rising due to increased life expectancy and emphasis on improving quality of life. General anesthesia or regional anesthesia can be utilized for surgery on the lower extremities. The mortality and morbidity benefits of a neuraxial technique are somewhat controversial; however, with an increasing trend toward ambulatory total joint replacement, there is evidence that regional anesthesia improves readiness for discharge, improves same-day discharge, and can reduce readmissions.[49,50]

When compared to general anesthesia, a large database study revealed that neuraxial techniques for total hip arthroplasty (THA) and total knee arthroplasty (TKA) are associated with lower 30-day mortality, decreased incidence of thromboembolic events, less blood loss, and lower transfusion requirements, along with decreases in length of stay (LOS), cost, and in-hospital complications (NICV 51-1).[51] However, both a systemic review of THA and TKA patients and a randomized controlled trial in hip fracture patients revealed no significant difference in morbidity and mortality between the general anesthesia and NA.[52,53] Peripheral nerve block anesthesia and analgesia are associated with improved outcomes after TKA and THA.[54]

A significant complication of orthopedic lower extremity surgery is perioperative DVT formation and VTE. Knowledge of anticoagulant dose and timing is essential to prevent the rare yet devastating complication of an epidural hematoma as a result of neuraxial technique (Table 51-3) (see Venous Thromboembolism and Thromboprophylaxis).[55]

Surgery to the Hip and Pelvis

Primary partial hip arthroplasties or THAs are frequently performed, with almost 600,000 operations each year in the United States alone.[56] The majority of hip fracture and arthroplasty patients are in the geriatric population and present with multiple comorbidities; therefore, optimal perioperative conditions are essential for these patients.

Surgical Approach and Positioning

The anterior surgical approach for hip arthroplasty is gaining favor because it is tissue sparing, allowing for a smaller incision and the potential for less pain, faster recovery, and improved mobility (Fig. 51-3). However, most surgery to the hip and femur is performed using a posterior approach. The patient is placed in the lateral decubitus position with the arms neutral and abducted/flexed less than 90 degrees for this approach. An axillary roll is placed to prevent compression of the brachial plexus and axillary artery (Fig. 51-3). The airway should be accessed with the patient supine before surgical positioning when performing general anesthesia. A neuraxial anesthetic can be performed with the patient sitting or in the lateral position. The cervical spine and head must be kept neutral during positioning. Mild airway obstruction often improves in the lateral decubitus position; however, the airway should be secured prior to lateral positioning if there are any significant concerns.

Anesthesia Technique

While general anesthesia is still commonly performed, evidence supports the use of NA for hip or femur surgery given the potential for improved morbidity and readiness for discharge.[49–51,53] NA, when performed properly and with adherence to anticoagulation guidelines, is low risk; however, exact complication estimates are elusive given extensive variability in practice contexts and patient populations. Patients with coagulation abnormalities, spinal stenosis, and older age are at higher risk of adverse outcomes after NA, and hematomas are less likely to occur with subarachnoid techniques compared to epidurals.[57]

For hip fracture surgery, neuraxial techniques may decrease hospital LOS, but their overall mortality benefit is controversial.[58] Hip fracture patients tend to be frail, often presenting with comorbidities that are difficult to optimize; however, surgery performed within 48 hours of admission will decrease inpatient mortality and the development of pressure sores. Therefore, surgery should be performed as soon as is safely possible.

Extra care should be taken when considering the impact of NA-associated sympathectomy and hypotension in patients with significant comorbidities, particularly severe aortic stenosis. Prior to epidural or spinal anesthesia, a fluid bolus will help avoid a precipitous drop in blood pressure. Slow and controlled dosing through an epidural catheter can also prevent rapid hypotension.

Table 51-3 Summary of ASRA Practice Advisory Guidelines for Neuraxial Anesthesia and Antithrombotics

Agent	American Society of Regional Anesthesia Guidelines for Neuraxial Anesthesia
Warfarin	Stop at least 5 d prior to neuraxial block, confirm normalization of INR prior to needle insertion. Recommend against the concurrent use of medications that affect other components of the clotting mechanism (e.g., ASA, NSAIDs, thienopyridines, UFH, LMWH). Catheters should be removed with INR <1.5. Removal with INR between 1.5 and 3.0 merits caution. Warfarin dose should be held or reduced for INR >3.0. Continue neurologic assessment at least 24 h after catheter removal.
Antiplatelets	
ASA	No contraindications
Cangrelor	Stop for a minimum of 3 h. Wait 8 h after neuraxial block or catheter removal before administration of drug.
Cilostazol	Stop for a minimum of 48 h. Wait 6 h after neuraxial block or catheter removal before administration of drug.
Clopidogrel	Stop for 5–7 d prior to neuraxial block. If neuraxial considered between 5 and 7 d, restoration of platelet function should be confirmed.
Dipyridamole	Stop for a minimum of 24 h. Wait 6 h after neuraxial block or catheter removal before administration of drug.
Prasugrel	Stop for 7–10 d prior to neuraxial block. If loading dose administered, wait 6 h after neuraxial block or catheter removal before administration of drug.
Ticagrelor	Stop for 5–7 d prior to neuraxial block. If loading dose administered, wait 6 h after neuraxial block or catheter removal before administration of drug.
Ticlopidine	Stop for 10 d prior to neuraxial block. If loading dose administered, wait 6 h after neuraxial block or catheter removal before administration of drug.
Platelet Glycoprotein IIb/IIIa Receptor Antagonists	
Abciximab	Avoid until normal platelet function has recovered. Time to normal platelet aggregation is 24–48 h.
Eptifibatide	Avoid until normal platelet function has recovered. Time to normal platelet aggregation is 4–8 h.
Tirofiban	Avoid until normal platelet function has recovered. Time to normal platelet aggregation is 4–8 h.
Heparins	
LMWH	Preoperatively: Wait 12 h after prophylactic dose, 24 h after treatment dose. Postoperatively: Catheters should be removed at least 4 h prior to initiation of twice-daily dosing regimens. For single daily dosing of LMWH, catheters can be maintained but should only be removed 12 h after last dose.
Subcutaneous UFH	5,000 units twice or three times daily: 4–6 h or assessment of coagulation status. 7,500–10,000 units twice daily: 12 h and assessment of coagulation status. Therapeutic dose: 24 h and assessment of coagulation status. Therapeutic dose not recommended with use of an indwelling catheter. Restart immediately after catheter removal. Check platelet count if >4 d on heparin.
Intravenous UFH	Discontinue 4–6 h and check normal coagulation status. Restart 1 h after neuraxial block or catheter removal. Check platelet count if >4 d on heparin.
Thrombin and Xa Inhibitors	
Fondaparinux	No recommendation on timing prior to neuraxial block. Recommend neuraxial blocks occur under conditions used in clinical trials (single needle pass, atraumatic needle placement, avoidance of indwelling catheters). Wait 6 h after catheter removal before restarting drug.
Dabigatran	Stop for 120 h (5 d) prior to neuraxial block. However, depending on renal function, the medication can be safely held for 72–120 h. See guidelines for details.[55] Wait 6 h after neuraxial block or catheter removal before administration of drug.
Apixaban	Stop for 72 h prior to neuraxial block. Wait at least 6 h after neuraxial block or catheter removal before administration of drug.
Betrixaban	Stop for 72 h prior to neuraxial block. Wait at least 5 h after neuraxial block or catheter removal before administration of drug
Edoxaban	Stop for 72 h prior to neuraxial block. Wait 6 h after neuraxial block or catheter removal before administration of drug.
Rivaroxaban	Stop for 72 h prior to neuraxial block. Wait 6 h after neuraxial block or catheter removal before administration of drug.
Thrombolytics/fibrinolytics/ direct thrombin inhibitors	Neuraxial techniques contraindicated except in unusual circumstances.

ASA, aspirin; INR, international normalized ratio; LMWH, low–molecular-weight heparin; NSAIDs, nonsteroidal anti-inflammatory drugs; UFH, unfractionated heparin.

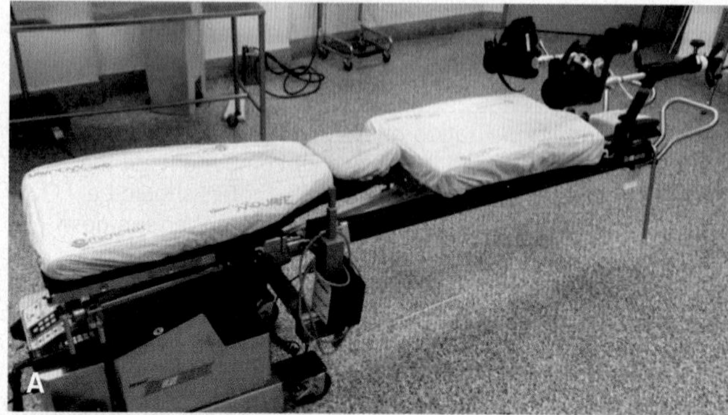
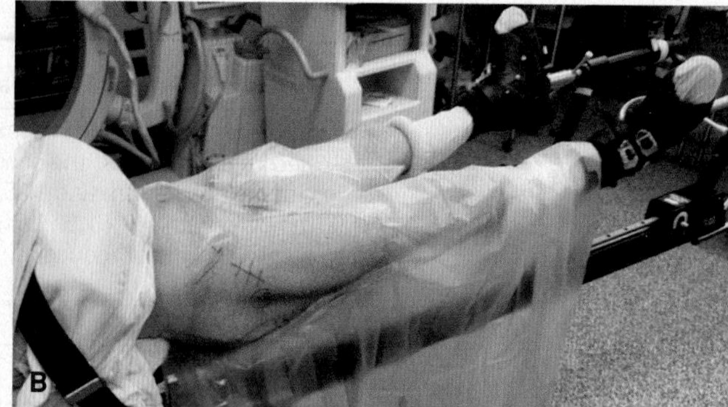
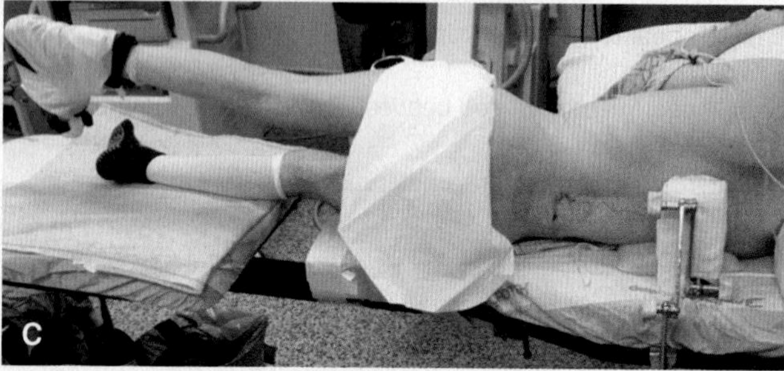
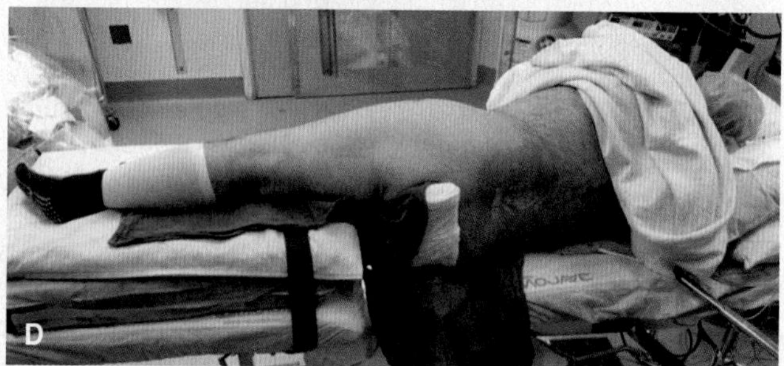

Figure 51-3 Positioning for hip surgery. **A:** The Mizuho OSI Hana trauma table utilized for anterior total hip arthroplasty. **B:** Patient positioned for anterior total hip arthroplasty on Mizuho OSI Hana trauma table. A padded post is placed between the legs to allow for traction, dislocation, and rotation of the femoral head. **C:** Lateral positioning for hip arthroscopy. The surgical leg is placed in a boot for traction, dislocation, and rotation of the femoral head from the acetabulum. **D:** Lateral positioning for total hip arthroplasty. An inflatable axillary roll prevents pressure on the axillary artery and brachial plexus.

A lumbar plexus block (LPB) or psoas compartment block is an anatomically deep block that provides a potent analgesic for hip surgery. The needle depth increases the risk of unintentional vascular puncture; therefore, the LPB is avoided in anticoagulated patients. It should also be noted that performing an LPB can rarely result in unintentional intrathecal or intravascular injection. Femoral nerve block (FNB) is a useful alternative; however, quadriceps weakness may increase postoperative fall risk during rehabilitation.[59] Use of LPB or FNB nerve catheters may decrease postoperative opioid requirements and opioid-related side effects.

Fascial plane blocks present additional analgesic options for hip surgery.[60] The quadratus lumborum block (QLB), pericapsular nerve group (PENG) block, and suprainguinal fascia iliaca blocks, all offer the benefit of being fully or partially motor sparing in comparison to traditional LPB and FNBs. However, the relative novelty of the blocks, along with contradictory evidence regarding the analgesic benefits, make it unclear if the fascial plane blocks will ultimately replace the more traditional "gold standard" peripheral nerve blocks.

As THA surgical technique has evolved to include smaller implants, smaller incisions, and less cementing, recovery has become faster and less painful. As a result, some surgeons perform injections of a "cocktail" that may contain a local anesthetic, epinephrine, a nonsteroidal anti-inflammatory, a corticosteroid, or an antibiotic into the periarticular space. While such infiltration techniques perform better than placebo, it does not appear that they outperform peripheral nerve blocks.[61]

Blood Loss and Transfusion

Deliberate hypotension using NA during hip surgery decreases blood loss and intraoperative transfusion needs compared to general anesthesia[62,63]; however, its practice is controversial.[64–66] The wide use of the antifibrinolytic agent TXA, both intravenously or topically in the perioperative setting, has been demonstrated to be safe and to decrease blood loss and transfusion requirements in joint arthroplasty, even in high-risk patients.[67] Maintaining normothermia improves intraoperative coagulation.

Ambulatory Hip Surgery

Hip arthroscopy is a common procedure to repair labral tears and treat hip dysplasia and femoroacetabular impingement. Patients are placed in either the supine or lateral position (Fig. 51-3). Maximal relaxation is necessary while the leg is placed in traction to facilitate dislocation of the femoral head from the acetabulum to access the hip joint. Relaxation can be achieved by spinal, epidural, or general anesthesia.

A potentially life-threatening complication of hip arthroscopy is the extravasation of the arthroscopy fluid from the hip joint into the peritoneal cavity. In extreme cases, intra-abdominal fluid extravasation (IAFE) can cause abdominal compartment syndrome resulting in hemodynamic instability, cardiovascular collapse, and, in tragic circumstances, death. Iliopsoas tenotomy with concomitant high pump pressures is a risk factor for IAFE. Treatment ranges from clinical observation to diuresis and, in severe cases, abdominal laparotomy. IAFE should be considered in a hemodynamically unstable patient experiencing severe abdominal or pelvic pain postoperatively. Point-of-care ultrasound (POCUS) can diagnose IAFE using the focused assessment with sonography in trauma (FAST) examination.[68] Hip arthroscopy is a painful procedure, and an LPB can improve postoperative analgesia but may prolong recovery.[69] Fascial plane blocks such as the QLB and PENG have demonstrated mixed analgesic efficacy in hip arthroscopy.

Surgery to the Knee

Total Knee Arthroplasty

Over 700,000 TKAs are performed each year in the United States.[56] Because TKA involves the cutting and cementing of two long bones, the femur, and tibia, these procedures have a painful recovery with a high incidence of chronic pain following both primary and revision procedures. It is important to create an appropriate postoperative analgesia plan to ensure mobility and facilitate range-of-motion therapy.

Positioning and Blood Loss

Knee arthroplasties and arthroscopies are performed supine to allow easy access to and evaluation of the knee joint in extension and flexion. A thigh tourniquet will minimize bleeding and improve surgical visualization; however, the tourniquet may not optimally compress the arteries in patients with severe atherosclerosis. Tourniquets should be used with caution in patients with active infections or thromboses in the lower extremity as exsanguination may cause systemic spread. The antifibrinolytic TXA can be safely utilized to decrease blood loss and blood transfusion.[70] As described earlier for hip surgery, controlled hypotension is a controversial option if a tourniquet cannot be applied.

Analgesia for Total Knee Arthroplasty

The optimal analgesia for TKA is a complex and evolving topic (Table 51-4). Regional anesthesia improves patient pain outcomes compared to traditional opioid regimens. Epidural catheters with a continuous infusion of dilute local anesthetic and low-dose opioids can provide excellent pain control, particularly when paired with patient-controlled epidural analgesia. Management of an epidural catheter for postoperative analgesia must account for pharmacologic venous thromboprophylaxis. Ultrasound-guided regional anesthesia has led to a significant increase in the use of peripheral nerve blocks and catheters as components of postoperative analgesic regimens. Intrathecal morphine can be utilized in addition to peripheral nerve blocks for postoperative analgesia; however, prolonged postoperative monitoring is required due to the risk of delayed respiratory depression. A balanced multimodal analgesic regimen can include pharmacologic treatment with anti-inflammatories, acetaminophen, opioids, and medications that manage neuropathic components of pain, such as pregabalin. Such a multimodal approach can maximize analgesic efficacy while minimizing side effects.

The femoral, sciatic, and obturator nerves provide sensation to the knee joint. The most commonly utilized peripheral nerve blocks are the LPB, fascia iliaca (3-in-1 block), FNB, and adductor canal (or saphenous) nerve blocks (see Chapter 36). These blocks can be combined with a sciatic nerve block, an obturator nerve block, or an infiltration between the popliteal artery and the capsule of the posterior knee (IPACK) block. Literature and clinical practice continue to evolve regarding which blocks or combination of blocks best facilitate rehabilitation and postoperative mobilization, thereby reducing time to hospital discharge, enhancing cost-effectiveness, and reducing the risk for complications such as ambulation-related falls.

Historically, FNB was currently considered the peripheral nerve block of choice for TKA analgesia because it has a low complication profile and is easy to perform with nerve stimulation or ultrasound guidance. However, although its correlation is disputed, one drawback to FNB is quadriceps weakness (up to 80%) and associated fall risk.

Recently, motor-sparing blocks such as the adductor canal block (ACB) have demonstrated a similar analgesic profile to FNB, but with the added benefit of increased mobility by sparing quadriceps strength. Performing the block requires ultrasound guidance and the use of a low local anesthetic volume within the adductor canal can minimize motor blockade of the vastus medialis.

Table 51-4 Anesthetic Techniques and Nerve Blocks for Lower Extremity Surgery

Procedure	Anesthetic (*Optimal Anesthetic)	Nerve Block Options (*Preferred Blocks)
• Partial or total hip arthroplasty • Hip fracture surgery • Hip arthroscopy	• ***Neuraxial** • General anesthesia	• Lumbar plexus (psoas compartment) block • Femoral nerve block • Fascia iliaca block • Supra inguinal fascia iliaca block • Fascial plane locks (Quadratus Lumborum Block and Pericapsular Nerve Group Block)
• Partial or total knee arthroplasty	• ***Neuraxial** • General anesthesia	• Femoral nerve block (FNB) • ***Adductor canal block (ACB) or saphenous nerve block** • Lumbar plexus (psoas compartment) block • Sciatic nerve block (in combination with ACB) • Selective tibial nerve block (in combination with ACB) • Obturator nerve block (in combination with ACB) • Interspace between the popliteal artery and posterior capsule of the knee (IPACK) block (in combination with ACB)
• Anterior cruciate ligament reconstruction	• Neuraxial • General anesthesia	• ***Adductor canal block (ACB) or saphenous nerve block** • Interspace between the popliteal artery and posterior capsule of the knee (IPACK) block (in combination with ACB) • Femoral nerve block
• Bunionectomy • Hammer toe correction • Midfoot fusion • Ankle fracture • Achilles tendon repair	• Neuraxial • General anesthesia • Ankle block (surgery involving toes)	• ***Popliteal fossa sciatic nerve block** • Ankle block • ***Adductor canal block (ACB) or saphenous nerve block** (in combination with popliteal fossa sciatic nerve block)

The sciatic nerve provides sensation to the posterior compartment of the knee and, in combination with an FNB, can reduce opioid consumption after TKA.[71] Sciatic nerve blockade causes a "foot drop" that can increase postoperative fall risk and delay diagnosis of common peroneal nerve palsy, a complication seen with large valgus corrections of the knee. A selective tibial nerve block is an alternative that provides similar analgesia without the corresponding foot drop.[72]

As noted above, the IPACK block is a motor-sparing alternative to the sciatic nerve block for posterior knee pain[73,74] that targets the 12 articular branches of both the anterior and posterior knee capsule. These blocks have demonstrated analgesic efficacy when performed in addition to ACB or periarticular injections. Transient foot drops are rare but can occur if local anesthesia is deposited near the sciatic nerve.

Periarticular injections (local infiltration technique) with cocktails of medications (see Surgery to the Hip and Pelvis, Anesthesia Technique) performed by the surgeon can reduce LOS and improve resting pain scores compared to placebo; however, they do not seem to provide greater benefit than regional anesthesia techniques. Liposomal bupivacaine can be added to periarticular injections to prolong the effect of the local anesthetic, although the benefit of liposomal bupivacaine over standard local anesthetics is not conclusive and both the safety profile and cost should be considered.

Ambulatory Knee Surgery

Ambulatory knee surgery has increased because health care costs have encouraged outpatient management of less complex cases. An optimal anesthetic in this setting has a rapid onset and fast offset with minimal side effects to prevent prolonged postanesthesia care unit stays or unexpected overnight admissions. NA results in a lower rate of nausea and vomiting than general anesthesia and can improve readiness to discharge. However, in a practice with rapid turnover time or limited postanesthesia care unit capacity, the need to wait for block resolution may not be practical. In such settings, general anesthesia with multimodal antinausea prophylaxis may be appropriate.

In performing a spinal anesthetic in an ambulatory setting, a short-to-intermediate–acting local anesthetic should be utilized. Intrathecal lidocaine causes a high rate of transient neurologic symptoms (TNS) and is rarely used. Historically, the reported incidence of TNS with 1.5% mepivacaine was also significant; however, with the ubiquitous use of anti-inflammatories such as ketorolac and dexamethasone for antiemetic prophylaxis, the incidence is quite low.[75] TNS is rare with 2% chloroprocaine and 0.5% bupivacaine, although bupivacaine may not be appropriate for ambulatory cases owing to its longer duration. Short-acting narcotics (e.g., fentanyl) can be added to spinal blocks to increase anesthetic potency, but the resulting pruritus may not be tolerated. In a large multicenter retrospective study of ambulatory TKA, there was no difference in complications associated with anesthetic type, however, NA was associated with higher same-day discharge, lower pain, lower opioid use, and a lower incidence of postoperative nausea and vomiting.[50]

Anterior cruciate ligament (ACL) reconstruction is a common ambulatory procedure performed with a cadaveric allograft or an autograft from the patellar tendon or hamstring. The autograft is preferred in younger and more active patients, but the patellar tendon and hamstring grafts cause significant postoperative pain. An epidural or spinal block can provide intraoperative anesthesia in combination with an FNB, ACB, or catheters for analgesia. However, FNB is not superior to multimodal analgesia and may prolong discharge. In addition, quadriceps weakness can be a complication of ACL reconstructions owing to muscle atrophy and activation failure, and FNB may cloud the clinical picture. An ACB can provide similar analgesia to an FNB after ACL surgery without causing quadriceps weakness.[76] The IPACK block may provide analgesic benefit for ACL surgery as well, although more randomized controlled trials are needed to determine the utility.

Surgery to the Foot and Ankle

Innervation of the foot and ankle is provided by the femoral nerve (via the saphenous nerve) and the sciatic nerve (via the posterior tibial, sural, and deep and superficial peroneal nerves) (see Chapter 22, Video 22.2). Anesthesia for foot surgery can be performed with an ankle block or a sciatic nerve block in the popliteal fossa with a saphenous nerve block as needed for coverage of the medial foot and ankle (see Chapter 36). Some surgeons prefer ankle blocks to avoid the foot drop caused by a sciatic nerve block. A neuraxial or general anesthetic may be required to minimize patient movement and facilitate use of a thigh tourniquet.

Surgery to the foot and ankle can cause severe pain, and regional anesthesia provides optimal postoperative analgesia, particularly in outpatient settings. Long-acting local anesthetics such as bupivacaine and ropivacaine can provide up to 24 hours of analgesia. The addition of adjuvants like preservative-free dexamethasone can consistently extend analgesia beyond 24 hours.[28] Local anesthetic infusion through an indwelling catheter can also prolong analgesia with minimal opioid-related side effects, including in the outpatient setting.[77] Peripheral nerve catheters may be challenging for noncompliant patients or those with limited access to follow-up care. In the outpatient setting, care must be taken to prevent accidental trauma to an anesthetized extremity, and patients should be instructed on how to best protect the limb upon discharge.

Pediatric Orthopedic Anesthesia

Pediatric patients present with a variety of orthopedic conditions, including congenital deformities, trauma, infections, and malignancies (see Chapter 43). Orthopedic procedures may be performed under regional, general, or a combination of anesthetic techniques depending on patient age, operative site, positioning, and surgical duration.

The Pediatric Regional Anesthesia Network database has established the safety of regional anesthetic blocks and catheters in children despite wide variability in local anesthetic doses.[78–80] Upper and lower extremity blocks may be performed with similar safety profiles in children who are awake as in those who are receiving sedation or general anesthesia. The anatomic differences between the pediatric and adult spine and spinal cord must be appreciated, and caudal blocks should be considered for lower extremity surgery in very young children (see Chapter 35).

Special Considerations in Orthopedics

Amputation

Following amputation, many patients experience phantom limb pain, phantom limb sensations, and/or stump pain that can be chronic, debilitating, and difficult to manage. Adequate analgesia administered for at least 2 to 3 days preoperatively and continued postoperatively with either intravenous patient-controlled analgesia or epidural may reduce incidence of phantom limb pain.[81,82]

Microvascular Surgery

Microvascular surgery is often required for restoration of blood flow following orthopedic trauma. Microvascular surgery can take many hours to perform, often requiring general anesthesia to maintain patient comfort and prevent movement. Mechanical ventilation can help avoid vasoconstriction caused by hyperoxia and hypocarbia as well as by hypercarbia-induced catecholamine release. Moreover, optimal anesthetic management for microvascular surgery utilizes regional techniques that provide sympathectomy (maximizing vasodilation) and diminish the stress response (minimizing vasospasm and thrombotic risk).[83] Maintenance of normothermia is essential to minimize vasoconstriction, and volume replacement is recommended at a rate of 3.5 to 6 mL/kg per hour.[84] Permissive hemodilution to a hematocrit of 30% can be considered for optimization of blood viscosity, and oxygen-carrying capacity. Vasopressors may be beneficial for maintenance of flap flow; however, their use must be discussed with the surgical team prior to initiation due to concerns for potential flap ischemia. Postoperative local anesthetic neuraxial and/or perineural infusions are recommended to help maintain adequate perfusion postoperatively.[85,86] Antithrombotics, including unfractionated and low–molecular-weight heparins, are often used to prevent graft thrombosis and must be taken into consideration when managing catheter insertion and removal postoperatively.

Acute Compartment Syndrome

Acute compartment syndrome (ACS) occurs when soft tissue pressures in a closed extremity compartment exceed capillary perfusion pressure, resulting in ischemic tissue damage. ACS is often first heralded by symptoms of pain out of proportion to injury; therefore, the excellent analgesic benefits of RA techniques must be weighed against the potential risk of delayed diagnosis of compartment syndrome. While the severity of ACS-related pain can often "break through" the analgesic effects of low-dose neuraxial or perineural local anesthetic infusions, there are several cases in which nerve blocks were reported to have masked episodes of ACS. Use of RA should be discussed with the surgical team and patient when ACS is a potential concern, and minimum effective doses/concentrations of local anesthetics should be used when performing RA in this setting.[87] Recent guidelines suggest that particular vigilance should be maintained for the following surgeries: tibial shaft fractures, high tibial and low femoral osteotomies, high-energy tibial plateau fractures, dual midshaft forearm fractures, and high-energy single-bone forearm fractures.[88]

Tourniquets

Tourniquets are often used to minimize blood loss and provide a bloodless operating field for extremity orthopedic surgery. The cuff should be large enough to comfortably encircle the limb, and the width should be more than half the limb diameter. Damage to underlying vessels, nerves, and muscles can be caused by excessively high tourniquet pressures and/or prolonged inflation times. In general, a cuff pressure 100 mmHg above a patient's measured systolic pressure is adequate for the thigh and 50 mmHg above systolic pressure is adequate for the arm. The duration of safe tourniquet inflation is generally considered to be 2 hours; however, a perfusion break followed by repeat exsanguination may be considered if longer total tourniquet times are required. Breakthrough bleeding during tourniquet inflation is often due to intramedullary blood flow in long bones or small arterial vessels between the two bones of a distal extremity and cannot be resolved by tourniquet overinflation.

Tourniquet pain can become significant over time and can be mitigated with opioids and/or hypnotics or definitively managed by tourniquet deflation. Transient systemic metabolic acidosis, increased arterial carbon dioxide levels, and a drop in systemic blood pressure can be expected with tourniquet deflation and are generally well tolerated in healthy patients. Special care should be taken at the time of tourniquet deflation in patients with significant comorbidities who may be susceptible to such changes.

Fat Embolus Syndrome/Bone Cement Implantation Syndrome

Fat embolism syndrome (FES) is a constellation of symptoms commonly including hypoxemia, petechial rash, and cognitive changes that is associated with significant fat embolism from traumatic injuries, surgery involving long-bone fractures, and bilateral arthroplasty (NICV 51-2). The symptoms of FES are thought to result from microvascular occlusion as well as the inflammatory response to trauma and embolized fat.[89] The incidence of FES in isolated long-bone fractures is 0.5% to 0.9%, with symptoms ranging from mild dyspnea to frank coma that typically occur 24 to 48 hours after the injury; however, fulminant episodes can occur within hours of traumatic injury.[89] Major and minor clinical and laboratory criteria for FES diagnosis are listed in Table 51-5, as classified by Gurd and Schonfeld.[90,91] Early fixation and corticosteroid use in long-bone fracture patients may be beneficial in preventing the syndrome.[92] Management of FES is largely supportive and may require early mechanical ventilation and the associated mortality rate is high, with estimates ranging from 10% to 20%.

Bone cement implantation syndrome (BCIS) is a poorly defined syndrome of hypoxemia, hypotension, and/or altered mental status observed in patients undergoing fracture repair or arthroplasty with cementation (NICV 51-3). The syndrome is defined as occurrence of these events in temporal proximity to cementation, prosthesis insertion, joint reduction, or tourniquet deflation, with its severity defined by degree of hypoxemia and hypotension.[93] Although BCIS has historically been attributed to circulation of methyl methacrylate cement monomers, it has since been shown that monomer levels are too low to account for the severity of observed signs and symptoms. It is likely that the syndrome overlaps extensively with FES and results from embolization of fat and other debris that is exacerbated by high-pressure intramedullary expansion of cement. Such embolization can trigger a cascade of endothelial damage, histamine release, and complement activation that contributes to the severity of FES and BCIS.[93] Invasive monitoring with an arterial line can improve rapid detection of clinically significant hemodynamic changes when cemented implants are being placed. Central venous pressure and pulmonary artery catheter placement may be considered in medically fragile patients in whom cementation cannot be avoided.

Venous Thromboembolism and Thromboprophylaxis

Without chemical prophylaxis, DVT develops in 40% to 80% of orthopedic patients.[94] Between 1% and 10% of patients show clinical evidence of PE, and fatal PE occurs in 0.2% to 5% of patients.[94] Over the last few decades, the incidence of DVT and PE has decreased dramatically with appropriate mechanical and/or pharmacologic thromboprophylaxis, advances in anesthetic and surgical techniques, and early mobilization.[95] Recently, rates of DVT and PE for hip and knee arthroplasty have been reported to be less than 1%.[96]

Table 51-5 Criteria for Fat Embolism Syndrome[90,91]

Gurd's Criteria	Major	Minor	Laboratory
Requires 1 major and 4 minor/laboratory signs	Petechiae (axillary/subconjunctival)	Tachycardia	Microglobulinemia (required for diagnosis)
	Hypoxemia	Fever	Thrombocytopenia
	Depressed consciousness	Retina: fat emboli	Anemia
	Pulmonary edema	Sputum: fat globules	Elevated erythrocyte sedimentation rate
		Urine: fat globules	
Schonfeld Fat Embolism Index	**Criteria**	**Points**	
Requires 5 or more points	Petechial rash	5	
	Diffuse alveolar infiltrates	4	
	Hypoxemia	3	
	Confusion	1	
	Fever	1	
	Tachycardia	1	
	Tachypnea	1	

Given the significant risk of thromboembolism following orthopedic surgery (NICV 51-4), many medical societies have issued guidelines for VTE prophylaxis following orthopedic surgery, including the American Academy of Orthopedic Surgeons,[97] American College of Chest Physicians,[98] and the American Society of Hematology.[99] All of these guidelines recommend a form of VTE prophylaxis, but there is no agreement on the type or duration.[100] All recommend more potent prophylaxis in patients with risk factors for VTE, especially if there is a prior history of VTE. All suggest the use of mechanical prophylaxis with intermittent pneumatic compression unless contraindicated. Recently, the International Consensus Meeting convened an international group of experts from various specialties including anesthesiology, cardiology, hematology, internal medicine, and orthopedics to generate VTE guidelines for orthopedic surgery.[101]

14 Caution must be taken when considering use of RA in patients who are receiving preoperative anticoagulation, as well as those who will require postoperative anticoagulation for DVT prophylaxis. The American Society of Regional Anesthesia updated its practice advisory in 2018 for the use of regional anesthesia in the setting of antithrombotic or thrombolytic therapy for minimizing the risk of clinically significant hematomas in at-risk patients.[55] A summary of recommendations in its fourth edition for neuraxial blockade in the setting of anticoagulants is presented in Table 51-3. It is generally recommended that the same guidelines be followed when deep plexus blocks are performed or peripheral nerve blocks are being placed near poorly compressible vessels.

For further review and interactivities, please see the videos and narrative interactive clinical vignettes (NICVs) accessible in the complimentary eBook bundled with this text. Access instructions are located on the inside front cover.

REFERENCES

1. Jenkins JG, Bohn D, Edmonds JF, Levison H, Barker GA. Evaluation of pulmonary function in muscular dystrophy patients requiring spinal surgery. *Crit Care Med.* 1982;10(10):645–649.
2. Edgcombe H, Carter K, Yarrow S. Anaesthesia in the prone position. *Br J Anaesth.* 2008;100(2):165–183.
3. Elgafy H, Bransford RJ, McGuire RA, Dettori JR, Fischer D. Blood loss in major spine surgery: are there effective measures to decrease massive hemorrhage in major spine fusion surgery? *Spine (Phila Pa 1976).* 2010;35(9 Suppl):S47–S56.
4. Tse EY, Cheung WY, Ng KFJ, Luk KDK. Reducing perioperative blood loss and allogeneic blood transfusion in patients undergoing major spine surgery. *J Bone Joint Surg Am.* 2011;93(13):1268–1277.
5. Zhao Y, Xi C, Xu W, Yan J. Role of tranexamic acid in blood loss control and blood transfusion management of patients undergoing multilevel spine surgery: A meta-analysis. *Medicine (Baltimore).* 2021;100(7):e24678.
6. Lu VM, Ho YT, Nambiar M, Mobbs RJ, Phan K. The perioperative efficacy and safety of antifibrinolytics in adult spinal fusion surgery: a systematic review and meta-analysis. *Spine (Phila Pa 1976).* 2018;43(16):E949–E958.
7. Epstein NE, Danto J, Nardi D. Evaluation of intraoperative somatosensory-evoked potential monitoring during 100 cervical operations. *Spine (Phila Pa 1976).* 1993;18(6):737–747.
8. Nuwer MR, Dawson EG, Carlson LG, Kanim LE, Sherman JE. Somatosensory evoked potential spinal cord monitoring reduces neurologic deficits after scoliosis surgery: results of a large multicenter survey. *Electroencephalogr Clin Neurophysiol.* 1995;96(1):6–11.
9. Fehlings MG, Brodke DS, Norvell DC, Dettori JR. The evidence for intraoperative neurophysiological monitoring in spine surgery: does it make a difference? *Spine (Phila Pa 1976).* 2010;35(9 Suppl):S37–S46.
10. Pathak KS, Brown RH, Nash CL Jr, Cascorbi HF. Continuous opioid infusion for scoliosis fusion surgery. *Anesth Analg.* 1983;62(9):841–845.
11. Pathak KS, Ammadio M, Kalamchi A, Scoles PV, Shaffer JW, Mackay W. Effects of halothane, enflurane, and isoflurane on somatosensory evoked potentials during nitrous oxide anesthesia. *Anesthesiology.* 1987;66(6):753–757.
12. Schwartz DM, Auerbach JD, Dormans JP, et al. Neurophysiological detection of impending spinal cord injury during scoliosis surgery. *J Bone Joint Surg Am.* 2007;89(11):2440–2449.
13. Martyn JA, White DA, Gronert GA, Jaffe RS, Ward JM. Up-and-down regulation of skeletal muscle acetylcholine receptors. Effects on neuromuscular blockers. *Anesthesiology.* 1992;76(5):822–843.
14. De Cassai A, Geraldini F, Boscolo A, et al. General anesthesia compared to spinal anesthesia for patients undergoing lumbar vertebral surgery: a meta-analysis of randomized controlled trials. *J Clin Med.* 2020;10(1):102.
15. Vedantam R, Lenke LG, Bridwell KH, Haas J, Linville DA. A prospective evaluation of pulmonary function in patients with adolescent idiopathic scoliosis relative to the surgical approach used for spinal arthrodesis. *Spine (Phila Pa 1976).* 2000;25(1):82–90.
16. Soffin EM, Beckman JD, Tseng A, et al. Enhanced recovery after lumbar spine fusion: a randomized controlled trial to assess the quality of patient recovery. *Anesthesiology.* 2020;133(2):350–363.
17. Steel T, Jones R, Crossman J, Sheehy J, Bentivoglio P, Pell M. Intraoperative wound infiltration with bupivacaine in patients undergoing lumbar spine surgery. *J Clin Neurosci.* 1998;5(3):298–303.

18. Soffin EM, Freeman C, Hughes AP, et al. Effects of a multimodal analgesic pathway with transversus abdominis plane block for lumbar spine fusion: a prospective feasibility trial. *Eur Spine J*. 2019;28(9):2077–2086.
19. Reisener MJ, Hughes AP, Okano I, et al. The association of transversus abdominis plane block with length of stay, pain and opioid consumption after anterior or lateral lumbar fusion: a retrospective study. *Eur Spine J*. 2021;30(12):3738–3745.
20. Asar S, Sarı S, Altinpulluk EY, Turgut M. Efficacy of erector spinae plane block on postoperative pain in patients undergoing lumbar spine surgery. *Eur Spine J*. 2022;31(1):197–204.
21. Soffin EM, Okano I, Oezel L, et al. Impact of ultrasound-guided erector spinae plane block on outcomes after lumbar spinal fusion: a retrospective propensity score matched study of 242 patients. *Reg Anesth Pain Med*. 2022;47(2):79–86.
22. Ahiskalioglu A, Yayik AM, Doymus O, et al. Efficacy of ultrasound-guided modified thoracolumbar interfascial plane block for postoperative analgesia after spinal surgery: a randomized-controlled trial. *Can J Anaesth*. 2018;65(5):603–604.
23. Verret M, Lauzier F, Zarychanski R, et al; Canadian Perioperative Anesthesia Clinical Trials (PACT) Group. Perioperative use of gabapentinoids for the management of postoperative acute pain: a systematic review and meta-analysis. *Anesthesiology*. 2020;133(2):265–279.
24. Sivaganesan A, Chotai S, White-Dzuro G, McGirt MJ, Devin CJ. The effect of NSAIDs on spinal fusion: a cross-disciplinary review of biochemical, animal, and human studies. *Eur Spine J*. 2017;26(11):2719–2728.
25. Lee LA, Roth S, Posner KL, et al. The American Society of Anesthesiologists Postoperative Visual Loss Registry: analysis of 93 spine surgery cases with postoperative visual loss. *Anesthesiology*. 2006;105(4):652–659; quiz 867–868.
26. Warner ME, Warner MA, Garrity JA, MacKenzie RA, Warner DO. The frequency of perioperative vision loss. *Anesth Analg*. 2001;93(6):1417–1421, table of contents.
27. Postoperative Visual Loss Study Group. Risk factors associated with ischemic optic neuropathy after spinal fusion surgery. *Anesthesiology*. 2012;116(1):15–24.
28. Kirksey MA, Haskins SC, Cheng J, Liu SS. Local anesthetic peripheral nerve block adjuvants for prolongation of analgesia: a systematic qualitative review. *PLoS One*. 2015;10(9):e0137312.
29. Dwyer T, Henry PDG, Cholvisudhi P, Chan VWS, Theodoropoulos JS, Brull R. Neurological complications related to elective orthopedic surgery: part 1: common shoulder and elbow procedures. *Reg Anesth Pain Med*. 2015;40(5):431–442.
30. Sviggum HP, Jacob AK, Mantilla CB, Schroeder DR, Sperling JW, Hebl JR. Perioperative nerve injury after total shoulder arthroplasty: assessment of risk after regional anesthesia. *Reg Anesth Pain Med*. 2012;37(5):490–494.
31. Li X, Eichinger JK, Hartshorn T, Zhou H, Matzkin EG, Warner JP. A comparison of the lateral decubitus and beach-chair positions for shoulder surgery: advantages and complications. *J Am Acad Orthop Surg*. 2015;23(1):18–28.
32. Holtzman AJ, Glezos CD, Feit EJ, Gruson KI. Prevalence and risk factors for lateral femoral cutaneous nerve palsy in the beach chair position. *Arthroscopy*. 2017;33(11):1958–1962.
33. Murphy GS, Greenberg SB, Szokol JW. Safety of beach chair position shoulder surgery: a review of the current literature. *Anesth Analg*. 2019;129(1):101–118.
34. Neal JM, Gerancher JC, Hebl JR, et al. Upper extremity regional anesthesia: essentials of our current understanding, 2008. *Reg Anesth Pain Med*. 2009;34(2):134–170.
35. Sia S, Sarro F, Lepri A, Bartoli M. The effect of exogenous epinephrine on the incidence of hypotensive/bradycardic events during shoulder surgery in the sitting position during interscalene block. *Anesth Analg*. 2003;97(2):583–588.
36. Song SY, Son SH, Kim SO, Roh WS. Intravenous fentanyl during shoulder arthroscopic surgery in the sitting position after interscalene block increases the incidence of episodes of bradycardia hypotension. *Korean J Anesthesiol*. 2011;60(5):344–350.
37. Ryu T, Kim BJ, Woo SJ, et al. Retrospective analysis of risk factors of hypotensive bradycardic events during shoulder arthroscopic surgery under interscalene blockade in the sitting position. *Korean J Anesthesiol*. 2020;73(6):542–549.
38. Nallam SR, Dara S. Effect of intravenous ondansetron on reducing the incidence of hypotension and bradycardia events during shoulder arthroscopy in sitting position under interscalene brachial plexus block: a prospective randomized trial. *Indian J Anaesth*. 2015;59(6):353–358.
39. Liguori GA, Kahn RL, Gordon J, Gordon MA, Urban MK. The use of metoprolol and glycopyrrolate to prevent hypotensive/bradycardic events during shoulder arthroscopy in the sitting position under interscalene block. *Anesth Analg*. 1998;87(6):1320–1325.
40. Chan JJ, Cirino CM, Vargas L, et al. Peripheral nerve block use in inpatient and outpatient shoulder arthroplasty: a population-based study evaluating utilization and outcomes. *Reg Anesth Pain Med*. 2020;45(10):818–825.
41. Danninger T, Stundner O, Rasul R, et al. Factors associated with hospital admission after rotator cuff repair: the role of peripheral nerve blockade. *J Clin Anesth*. 2015;27(7):566–573.
42. Warrender WJ, Syed UAM, Hammoud S, et al. Pain management after outpatient shoulder arthroscopy: a systematic review of randomized controlled trials. *Am J Sports Med*. 2017;45(7):1676–1686.
43. Urmey WF, Talts KH, Sharrock NE. One hundred percent incidence of hemidiaphragmatic paresis associated with interscalene brachial plexus anesthesia as diagnosed by ultrasonography. *Anesth Analg*. 1991;72(4):498–503.
44. Lee LA, Posner KL, Kent CD, Domino KB. Complications associated with peripheral nerve blocks: lessons from the ASA Closed Claims Project. *Int Anesthesiol Clin*. 2011;49(3):56–67.
45. Guo CW, Ma JX, Ma XL, et al. Supraclavicular block versus interscalene brachial plexus block for shoulder surgery: a meta-analysis of clinical control trials. *Int J Surg*. 2017;45:85–91.
46. Tedore TR, Lin HX, Pryor KO, et al. Dose-response relationship between local anesthetic volume and hemidiaphragmatic paresis following ultrasound-guided supraclavicular brachial plexus blockade. *Reg Anesth Pain Med*. 2020;45(12):979–984.
47. Abdallah FW, Wijeysundera DN, Laupacis A, et al. Subomohyoid anterior suprascapular block versus interscalene block for arthroscopic shoulder surgery: a multicenter randomized trial. *Anesthesiology*. 2020;132(4):839–853.
48. Stundner O, Rasul R, Chiu YL, et al. Peripheral nerve blocks in shoulder arthroplasty: how do they influence complications and length of stay? *Clin Orthop Relat Res*. 2014;472(5):1482–1488.
49. Duque M, Schnetz MP, Yates AJ Jr, et al. Impact of neuraxial versus general anesthesia on discharge destination in patients undergoing primary total hip and total knee replacement. *Anesth Analg*. 2021;133(6):1379–1386.
50. Yap E, Wei J, Webb C, Ng K, Behrends M. Neuraxial and general anesthesia for outpatient total joint arthroplasty result in similarly low rates of major perioperative complications: a multicentered cohort study. *Reg Anesth Pain Med*. 2022;47(5):294–300.
51. Memtsoudis SG, Sun X, Chiu YL, et al. Perioperative comparative effectiveness of anesthetic technique in orthopedic patients. *Anesthesiology*. 2013;118(5):1046–1058. Erratum in: *Anesthesiology*. 2016 Sep;125(3):610.
52. Johnson RL, Kopp SL, Burkle CM, et al. Neuraxial vs general anaesthesia for total hip and total knee arthroplasty: a systematic review of comparative-effectiveness research. *Br J Anaesth*. 2016;116(2):163–176.
53. Neuman MD, Feng R, Carson JL, et al; REGAIN Investigators. Spinal anesthesia or general anesthesia for hip surgery in older adults. *N Engl J Med*. 2021;385(22):2025–2035.
54. Memtsoudis SG, Cozowicz C, Bekeris J, et al. Anaesthetic care of patients undergoing primary hip and knee arthroplasty: consensus recommendations from the International Consensus on Anaesthesia-Related Outcomes after Surgery group (ICAROS) based on a systematic review and meta-analysis. *Br J Anaesth*. 2019;123(3):269–287.
55. Horlocker TT, Vandermeuelen E, Kopp SL, Gogarten W, Leffert LR, Benzon HT. Regional anesthesia in the patient receiving antithrombotic or thrombolytic therapy: American Society of Regional Anesthesia and Pain Medicine Evidence-Based Guidelines (Fourth Edition). *Reg Anesth Pain Med*. 2018;43(3):263–309.
56. Most Common Operations in Hospital Inpatient Stays – HCUP Fast Stats. Accessed June 5, 2022. https://www.hcup-us.ahrq.gov/faststats/NationalProceduresServlet
57. Neal JM, Barrington MJ, Brull R, et al. The second ASRA practice advisory on neurologic complications associated with regional anesthesia and pain medicine: executive summary 2015. *Reg Anesth Pain Med*. 2015;40(5):401–430.
58. Neuman MD, Rosenbaum PR, Ludwig JM, Zubizarreta JR, Silber JH. Anesthesia technique, mortality, and length of stay after hip fracture surgery. *JAMA*. 2014;311(24):2508–2517.
59. Johnson RL, Kopp SL, Hebl JR, Erwin PJ, Mantilla CB. Falls and major orthopaedic surgery with peripheral nerve blockade: a systematic review and meta-analysis. *Br J Anaesth*. 2013; 110(4):518–528.
60. Kim DH, Kim SJ, Liu J, Beathe J, Memtsoudis SG. Fascial plane blocks: a narrative review of the literature. *Reg Anesth Pain Med*. 2021;46(7):600–617.
61. Jiménez-Almonte JH, Wyles CC, Wyles SP, et al. Is Local Infiltration Analgesia Superior to Peripheral Nerve Blockade for Pain Management After THA: A Network Meta-analysis. *Clin Orthop Relat Res*. 2016;474(2):495–516.
62. Guay J. The effect of neuraxial blocks on surgical blood loss and blood transfusion requirements: a meta-analysis. *J Clin Anesth*. 2006;18(2):124–128.
63. Sharrock NE, Bading B, Mineo R, Blumenfeld JD. Deliberate hypotensive epidural anesthesia for patients with normal and low cardiac output. *Anesth Analg*. 1994;79(5):899–904.
64. Jiang J, Zhou R, Li B, Xue F. Is deliberate hypotension a safe technique for orthopedic surgery?: a systematic review and meta-analysis of parallel randomized controlled trials. *J Orthop Surg Res*. 2019;14(1):409.
65. Sessler DI, Bloomstone JA, Aronson S, et al; Physiology group, Preoperative blood pressure group, Intraoperative blood pressure group, Postoperative blood pressure group. Perioperative Quality Initiative consensus statement on intraoperative blood pressure, risk and outcomes for elective surgery. *Br J Anaesth*. 2019;122(5):563–574.
66. Liu J, Zhong H, DeMeo D, et al. Controlled hypotension during neuraxial anesthesia is not associated with increased odds of in-hospital common severe medical complications in patients undergoing elective primary total hip arthroplasty – a retrospective case control study. *PLoS One*. 2021;16(4):e0248419.
67. Poeran J, Chan JJ, Zubizarreta N, Mazumdar M, Galatz LM, Moucha CS. Safety of tranexamic acid in hip and knee arthroplasty in high-risk patients. *Anesthesiology*. 2021;135(1):57–68.
68. Haskins SC, Desai NA, Fields KG, et al. Diagnosis of intraabdominal fluid extravasation after hip arthroscopy with point-of-care ultrasonography can identify patients at an increased risk for postoperative pain. *Anesth Analg*. 2017;124(3):791–799.
69. Schroeder KM, Donnelly MJ, Anderson BM, Ford MP, Keene JS. The analgesic impact of preoperative lumbar plexus blocks for hip arthroscopy. A retrospective review. *Hip Int*. 2013; 23(1):93–98.
70. Fillingham YA, Ramkumar DB, Jevsevar DS, et al. Tranexamic acid in total joint arthroplasty: the endorsed clinical practice guides of the American Association of Hip and Knee Surgeons,

American Society of Regional Anesthesia and Pain Medicine, American Academy of Orthopaedic Surgeons, Hip Society, and Knee Society. *Reg Anesth Pain Med.* 2019;44(1):7–11.

71. Abdallah FW, Brull R. Is sciatic nerve block advantageous when combined with femoral nerve block for postoperative analgesia following total knee arthroplasty? A systematic review. *Reg Anesth Pain Med.* 2011;36(5):493–498.
72. Sinha SK, Abrams JH, Arumugam S, et al. Femoral nerve block with selective tibial nerve block provides effective analgesia without foot drop after total knee arthroplasty: a prospective, randomized, observer-blinded study. *Anesth Analg.* 2012;115(1):202–206.
73. Kandarian B, Indelli PF, Sinha S, et al. Implementation of the IPACK (Infiltration between the Popliteal Artery and Capsule of the Knee) block into a multimodal analgesic pathway for total knee replacement. *Korean J Anesthesiol.* 2019;72(3):238–244.
74. Kim DH, Beathe JC, Lin Y, et al. Addition of infiltration between the popliteal artery and the capsule of the posterior knee and adductor canal block to periarticular injection enhances postoperative pain control in total knee arthroplasty: a randomized controlled trial. *Anesth Analg.* 2019;129(2):526–535.
75. Wyles CC, Pagnano MW, Trousdale RT, et al. More Predictable Return of Motor Function with Mepivacaine Versus Bupivacaine Spinal Anesthetic in Total Hip and Total Knee Arthroplasty: A Double-Blinded, Randomized Clinical Trial. *J Bone Joint Surg Am.* 2020;102(18):1609–1615.
76. Chisholm MF, Bang H, Maalouf DB, et al. Postoperative analgesia with saphenous block appears equivalent to femoral nerve block in ACL reconstruction. *HSS J.* 2014;10(3):245–251.
77. Ilfeld BM, Morey TE, Wang RD, Enneking FK. Continuous popliteal sciatic nerve block for postoperative pain control at home: a randomized, double-blinded, placebo-controlled study. *Anesthesiology.* 2002;97(4):959–965.
78. Polaner DM, Taenzer AH, Walker BJ, et al. Pediatric Regional Anesthesia Network (PRAN): a multi-institutional study of the use and incidence of complications of pediatric regional anesthesia. *Anesth Analg.* 2012;115(6):1353–1364.
79. Walker BJ, Long JB, De Oliveira GS, et al. Peripheral nerve catheters in children: an analysis of safety and practice patterns from the pediatric regional anesthesia network (PRAN). *Br J Anaesth.* 2015;115(3):457–462.
80. Suresh S, De Oliveira GS Jr. Local anaesthetic dosage of peripheral nerve blocks in children: analysis of 40 121 blocks from the Pediatric Regional Anesthesia Network database. *Br J Anaesth.* 2018;120(2):317–322.
81. Katsuly-Liapis I, Georgakis P, Tierry C. Preemptive extradural analgesia reduces the incidence of phantom pain in lower limb amputees. *British Journal of Anaesthesia.* 1996;76 Suppl 2:125: A410.
82. Karanikolas M, Aretha D, Tsolakis I, et al. Optimized perioperative analgesia reduces chronic phantom limb pain intensity, prevalence, and frequency: a prospective, randomized, clinical trial. *Anesthesiology.* 2011;114(5):1144–1154.
83. Hagau N, Longrois D. Anesthesia for free vascularized tissue transfer. *Microsurgery.* 2009; 29(2):161–167.
84. Motakef S, Mountziaris PM, Ismail IK, Agag RL, Patel A. Emerging paradigms in perioperative management for microsurgical free tissue transfer: review of the literature and evidence-based guidelines. *Plast Reconstr Surg.* 2015;135(1):290–299.
85. Kurt E, Ozturk S, Isik S, Zor F. Continuous brachial plexus blockade for digital replantations and toe-to-hand transfers. *Ann Plast Surg.* 2005;54(1):24–27.
86. Taras JS, Behrman MJ. Continuous peripheral nerve block in replantation and revascularization. *J Reconstr Microsurg.* 1998;14(1):17–21.
87. Marhofer P, Halm J, Feigl GC, Schepers T, Hollmann MW. Regional anesthesia and compartment syndrome. *Anesth Analg.* 2021;133(5):1348–1352.
88. Dwyer T, Burns D, Nauth A, Kawam K, Brull R. Regional anesthesia and acute compartment syndrome: principles for practice. *Reg Anesth Pain Med.* 2021;46(12):1091–1099.
89. Rothberg DL, Makarewich CA. Fat embolism and fat embolism syndrome. *J Am Acad Orthop Surg.* 2019;27(8):e346–e355.
90. Gurd AR. Fat embolism: an aid to diagnosis. *J Bone Joint Surg Br.* 1970;52(4):732–737.
91. Schonfeld SA, Ploysongsang Y, DiLisio R, et al. Fat embolism prophylaxis with corticosteroids. A prospective study in high-risk patients. *Ann Intern Med.* 1983;99(4):438–443.
92. Bederman SS, Bhandari M, McKee MD, Schemitsch EH. Do corticosteroids reduce the risk of fat embolism syndrome in patients with long-bone fractures? A meta-analysis. *Can J Surg.* 2009; 52(5):386–393.
93. Donaldson AJ, Thomson HE, Harper NJ, Kenny NW. Bone cement implantation syndrome. *Br J Anaesth.* 2009;102(1):12–22.
94. Geerts WH, Pineo GF, Heit JA, et al. Prevention of venous thromboembolism: the Seventh ACCP Conference on Antithrombotic and Thrombolytic Therapy. *Chest.* 2004;126(3 Suppl): 338S–400S.
95. Lu N, Salvati EA. Multimodal prophylaxis for venous thromboembolic disease after total hip and knee arthroplasty: current perspectives. *Chin J Traumatol.* 2010;13(6):362–369.
96. Warren JA, Sundaram K, Anis HK, Kamath AF, Higuera CA, Piuzzi NS. Have venous thromboembolism rates decreased in total hip and knee arthroplasty? *J Arthroplasty.* 2020; 35(1):259–264.
97. Mont MA, Jacobs JJ. AAOS clinical practice guideline: preventing venous thromboembolic disease in patients undergoing elective hip and knee arthroplasty. *J Am Acad Orthop Surg.* 2011;19(12):777–778.
98. Falck-Ytter Y, Francis CW, Johanson NA, et al. Prevention of VTE in orthopedic surgery patients: Antithrombotic Therapy and Prevention of Thrombosis, 9th ed: American College of Chest Physicians Evidence-Based Clinical Practice Guidelines. *Chest.* 2012;141(2 Suppl): e278S–e325S.
99. Anderson DR, Morgano GP, Bennett C, et al. American Society of Hematology 2019 guidelines for management of venous thromboembolism: prevention of venous thromboembolism in surgical hospitalized patients. *Blood Adv.* 2019;3(23):3898–3944.
100. Muscatelli SR, Charters MA, Hallstrom BR. Time for an update? A look at current guidelines for venous thromboembolism prophylaxis after hip and knee arthroplasty and hip fracture. *Arthroplast Today.* 2021;10:105–107.
101. ICM-VTE General Delegates. Recommendations from the ICM-VTE: general. *J Bone Joint Surg Am.* 2022;104(Suppl 1):4–162.

52 Transplant Anesthesia

CHRISTINE CHOI • GERARD R. MANECKE • SCOTT LINDBERG • RANDOLPH H. STEADMAN

KEY POINTS

1. Brain death is declared when the clinical picture is consistent with irreversible cessation of all brain functions.
2. Anesthesiologists have a significant role to play in organ procurement and should consult with local organ procurement personnel for protocols to optimize healthy graft retrieval.
3. Extended criteria organs, including donation after cardiac death (DCD), are used because of ongoing organ shortage; cold ischemia times should be minimized for extended criteria donor organs.
4. Living kidney and liver donors must be healthy and without significant cardiopulmonary, neurologic, or psychiatric disease, diabetes, obesity, or hypertension.
5. Renal transplant recipients are often anemic, with hyperdynamic cardiac indices.
6. For renal transplantation, the major anesthetic consideration is maintenance of renal blood flow, typically achieved with volume expansion using balanced salt solutions rather than vasopressors.
7. Patients with end-stage liver disease have multiorgan dysfunction with secondary cardiac, pulmonary, renal, and neurologic complications.
8. Liver transplantation is traditionally described in three phases: dissection, anhepatic phase, and neohepatic phase, with graft reperfusion marking the start of the neohepatic phase.
9. Intraoperative management of lung transplant patients should focus on fluid and ventilatory strategies designed to minimize acute lung injury and primary graft dysfunction.
10. Mechanical circulatory support devices are increasingly common in patients presenting for heart transplantation.
11. Nonischemic cardiomyopathy has replaced ischemic cardiomyopathy as the most common indication for heart transplantation.
12. For all transplant recipients, antibiotic, antiviral, antifungal, immunosuppressive, and disease-specific drug regimens should be disrupted minimally in the perioperative period.

Transplantation begins with the donor, and an anesthesiologist's exquisite attention to the details of organ donor management affects the life of multiple organ recipients. Most anesthesiologists will have little experience managing donors, and high-quality literature in this area is lacking, so experienced personnel from local organ procurement organizations (OPOs) should be consulted. The United Network of Organ Sharing (UNOS; www.unos.org) was created by the 1984 National Organ Transplant Act to manage the Organ Procurement and Transplant Network (OPTN) for efficient and equitable distribution of donated organs. The system for organ placement received a technology upgrade in 2006 with the launch of DonorNet, an electronic resource for matching and distribution of organs around the United States. Speed of placement is important because brain-dead donors are unstable, and it is particularly important to transplant extended criteria donor (ECD) grafts with minimal cold ischemia times. In general, maximum cold ischemia times are ideally less than 6 hours for heart or lung grafts, 12 hours for livers, and up to 36 hours for kidneys. The UNOS website data contain center- and region-specific transplant databases, regularly updated. The Scientific Registry of Transplant Recipients (www.ustransplant.org) is also a source of transplant data for clinicians, patients, and researchers.

About 180,000 patients were on solid-organ transplant waiting lists in the United States in 2020. Of this number on the waiting list, 78% were awaiting kidneys, 14% livers, 5% hearts,

Table 52-1 Transplant Activity by Organ (2020)

Organ	# Waitlist Candidates	# Transplants Performed
Kidney	141,341	23,642 total 78% deceased donor 22% living donor
Liver	25,200	8,906 total 94% deceased donor 6% living donor
Pancreas	999	87
Pancreas-kidney	3,054	827
Small bowel	371	91
Heart	8,473	3,715
Lung	4,208	2,597

Data from Israni AK. OPTN/SRTR 2020 annual data report: Introduction. *Am J Transplant*. 2022;22 Suppl 2:11–20.

2% lungs, 0.5% pancreas, and 0.2% intestines.[1] Donation has not kept pace with demand. A total of over 40,000 transplants were reported in the United States in 2020 (Table 52-1). The waitlist additions for organs declined in 2020, likely due to the COVID-19 pandemic. Despite this, waitlist additions exceeded the number of transplants performed for all organs. The kidney waitlist is six times greater than the number of kidney transplants performed, the liver list is three times greater than the number of liver transplants performed, and the heart and lung waitlists are each double the number of transplants performed.[1] The ongoing gap between need for and availability of donor organs continues to push practice changes to increase the donor pool and more equitably distribute organs, including use of grafts from "donation after cardiac death" (DCD) donors as well as paired kidney donations (kidney swaps), and new modifications to the Model for End-Stage Liver Disease (MELD) scoring. Patient survival varies by organ (Table 52-2).

Table 52-2 Patient Survival (%) by Organ and Years Post Transplant (For Transplants Performed between 2008 and 2015)

Organ	1 y (%)	3 y (%)	5 y (%)
Kidney	97.1	93.0	86.5
Liver	91.8	83.8	76.2
Pancreas	91.0	87.5	79.8
Pancreas–kidney	97.5	94,8	88.9
Small bowel	82.8	68.9	58.9
Heart	90.9	85.6	78.6
Lung	87.9	70.5	56.1
Heart/lung	80.9	58.3	50.2

Data from https://optn.transplant.hrsa.gov/data/view-data-reports/national-data/

Anesthetic Management of Organ Donors

Brain-Dead Donors (Donation after Neurologic Determination of Death)

Brain-dead, heart-beating donors (DBD donors) deserve expert intensive care unit (ICU) and anesthetic management because they contribute life to many transplant recipients.[2] Particular attention should be paid to communication because anesthesiologists may be interacting with unfamiliar personnel from OPOs and surgical procurement teams.

Brain death is declared when the clinical picture is consistent 1
with irreversible cessation of all brain functions (NICV 52-1).[3] Legal and medical brain death criteria differ from state to state, but all require permanent absence of both cerebral and brainstem functions. Potential reversible causes of coma such as hypothermia, hypotension, hypoglycemia, drug or toxin intoxications, and acid–base or electrolyte imbalances must be corrected prior to declaration of brain death. Clinical or neurologic imaging evidence consistent with irreversible brain damage must be present. Brain-dead donors are unresponsive to sensory stimuli and have no brainstem reflexes, including ventilatory drive with apnea testing, but may have complex motor activity originating from the spinal cord or peripheral nerves. If the clinical criteria are incomplete, then ancillary testing such as cerebral angiography, transcranial doppler, and/or electroencephalography can be obtained to confirm the clinical examination. Physicians involved in the transplant recipient process should not be involved in the declaration of brain death of a donor. Hospitals should incorporate the most recent recommendations of the Quality Standards Subcommittee of the American Academy of Neurology for brain death assessment.[4]

Brain death is associated with two distinct hemodynamic stages with wide swings in hormone levels, systemic inflammation, and oxidant stress, all of which negatively impact donor organ function. The initial autonomic storm caused by catecholamine surge leads to tachycardia, hypertension, and acute myocardial dysfunction. It is associated with ischemia and ischemic-reperfusion injury. The second stage of brainstem death is characterized by profound hypotension and relative hypovolemia due to subsequent pituitary failure, deactivation of the sympathetic nervous system, and brain herniation.[2] Cardiac output (CO) and intravascular volume should be optimized to ensure adequate end-organ perfusion during this state of hypovolemic shock, and the use of invasive hemodynamic monitoring tools is recommended. Recommended fluid resuscitation goals include a mean arterial pressure above 60 mmHg, minimum urine output of 1 mL/kg/h, maintenance of left ventricular (LV) ejection fraction of 45%, and only low doses of vasopressors. Dopamine has been traditionally recommended as first-line vasopressor of choice. Vasopressin is a common alternative as it reduces pressor requirement, protects lung function, and increases the rate of successful organ procurement.[5,6] Norepinephrine or phenylephrine are reserved for severe circulatory shock as high-dose catecholamines can be detrimental to organ procurement. Fluid resuscitation goals must be individualized on a case-by-case basis as aggressive fluid resuscitation is favored for kidney preservation while conservative fluid resuscitation is favored for lung preservation.[2] Once pituitary failure ensues, hormone therapy may help stabilize donors hemodynamically and thereby extend the donor pool,[7] but there is little deep research on hormone replacement therapy and clinical practice varies widely. Central diabetes insipidus is common due to compression of the pituitary from brainstem herniation. Vasopressin has been shown to improve organ procurement rate and is now recommended in donors with hypotension despite adequate intravascular volume resuscitation.[5] Desmopressin can be used in those donors with less hemodynamic instability. Thyroid hormone replacement seems to improve heart transplant outcomes and is recommended for cardiac donors with LV ejection fraction less than 45%.[7,8] Hormone therapy regimens include triiodothyronine (4 μg IV bolus then 3 μg/h infusion, though its use is not well supported by meta-analyses) and desmopressin (1 unit IV bolus then 0.5 to 4 units/h infusion) to maintain systemic vascular resistance (SVR) at 800 to 1,200 dyne-sec/cm^5.[9,10] Corticosteroid replacement with methylprednisolone is often used to reduce the inflammatory response, and the use of high-dose corticosteroid has been reported to improve lung procurement rates with less vasopressor requirement.[11,12] Insulin infusion to maintain blood glucose at 120 to 180 mg/dL is also recommended, and recent studies support glucose control for maintaining donor kidney graft quality.[13] Thromboprophylaxis is important because of the high incidence of deep vein thrombosis and pulmonary emboli in critically ill patients.

Other medications that should be available for the donor operation are broad-spectrum antibiotics, mannitol and loop diuretics, and heparin. A lung-protective ventilatory strategy is important in lung donors, with tidal volumes of 6 to 8 mL/kg and positive end-expiratory pressure (PEEP) adjusted to minimize the required fraction of inspired oxygen (FiO_2).[14]

Anesthetic management during organ procurement has similar goals as management of the donor in the ICU. UNOS has created a resource for managing organ donors in an effort to improve donor care and, therefore, the function of donated organs.[2] The procurement teams, who may come from several centers, may have discrepant requests depending on the organs to be procured. The transport of ventilated donors to the operating room (OR) often requires PEEP support. If more complex ventilator settings are used in the ICU, they should be continued during transport and in the OR.

2 The mainstay of donor management is the maintenance of euvolemia and perfusion; therefore, central venous pressure (CVP) monitoring is commonplace. CVP is maintained at 6 to 12 mmHg, and when pulmonary artery (PA) catheters are used to assess cardiac function, pulmonary capillary wedge pressure is maintained at lower than 12 mmHg. Surgeons procuring the lungs will want to keep the CVP low, and diuretics may be requested just prior to collection of the lungs. Conversely, surgeons procuring kidneys usually want high filling pressures. Efforts should be made to maintain serum sodium levels below 155 mmol/L as higher levels are associated with poor liver graft function.[15] Donor oxygenation, perfusion, and normothermia are all important anesthetic goals, and the precise end points of therapy require coordination and communication with the various surgical teams. In general, arterial PCO_2 is maintained at 30 to 35 mmHg. Brain-dead patients may have intact spinal reflexes, so they may require neuromuscular blockade during organ procurement.

Donor lungs are more susceptible to injury in brain-dead patients before procurement than other organs, likely from contusion, aspiration, or edema with fluid resuscitation. Consequently, many multiorgan donors do not meet the idealized strict criteria for lung donation. Extended criteria are used for donor lungs because of ongoing shortages.[16,17] For example, a review of UNOS data showed that lung donors less than 64 years old show no major differences from those less than 55 years old.[18] Acceptance of some lungs from donors with a smoking history is another example of working outside the strict criteria. Sputum Gram stains and cultures are routinely obtained on all lung donors and antibiotics for a donor with a positive Gram stain can lower the risk of posttransplant infection. Prior to lung removal, surgeons will perform bronchoscopy. Glucocorticoids may be requested, and prostaglandin E_1 may be requested to improve circulation of the lung preservation solution. Evidence of aspiration seen on bronchoscopy, bilateral pulmonary infiltrates, or persistent purulent secretions are criteria for donor exclusion.[19] Ischemic times should still be less than 6.5 hours.[20] In addition to the usual immunologic criteria, donor–recipient compatibility is based on height and/or total lung capacity. DCD donors are still useful for lung transplantation, and ex vivo lung perfusion is emerging as a way to extend the lung donor pool.

Donor heart history is very important in identifying heart donors, and electrocardiography and echocardiography are mandatory. The ideal heart donor is less than 50 years old and hemodynamically stable. Presence of major chest trauma, cardiac disease, active infection, prolonged cardiac arrest, malignancy, human immunodeficiency virus (HIV) or hepatitis, or intracardiac injections moves the donor from ideal to marginal status. The overall health status of the donor prior to determination of brain death can facilitate a directed laboratory evaluation, which may include cardiac catheterization. Younger donors, short ischemic time, low donor inotrope requirement, and oversized organs are preferred for recipients with pulmonary hypertension. Human leukocyte antigen (HLA) typing and ABO blood group compatibility are determined. The donor heart size should be within 20% to 30% of the recipient's heart size.

For heart retrieval, the surgeons perform a pericardiotomy, and the aortic root is cannulated for infusion of cardioplegia solutions. Following ligation of the great veins, the heart is compressed and exsanguinated, cardioplegia is given to induce cardiac arrest, and the aorta is cross clamped. After cardiectomy, the donor heart is preserved in cold ice slush. For donors who provide both lungs and the heart to a single recipient, a combined cardiopulmonary surgical extraction is performed. Surgical techniques have been developed to allow three recipients from one thoracic donor: two single-lung transplants and a heart transplant. The heart is removed first, leaving a small cuff of left atrium attached to the lungs. The harvesting team will ask for systemic heparinization just prior to exsanguination and excision. Cardioplegia is administered, the heart stops ejecting, and the heart is removed. The trachea is transected and the lungs are removed *en bloc* for later separation.

A shortage of available donors has led to increased use of marginal (extended criteria) donors and separate alternate transplant lists of recipients who consent to accept ECDs. An increased risk of primary graft dysfunction (PGD) is the main reason to avoid marginal donors. Marginal donors are typically used for patients who do not meet the standard recipient criteria, with advanced age a common reason for alternative listing. Common donor factors that lead to marginal status are abnormal hepatitis screening tests, LV dysfunction or coronary artery disease, advanced age, and DCD.

Donation after Cardiac Death (Donation after Circulatory Determination of Death)

In 2007, U.S. hospitals were mandated by The Joint Commission, 3
in collaboration with OPOs, to develop DCD policies and protocols in response to organ donor shortages. The OPTN policies provide general guidelines and minimum requirements for DCD. UNOS also provides an excellent quick general reference on DCD available at https://www.unos.org/wp-content/uploads/unos/Critical_Pathway_DCD_Donor.pdf. However, individualized DCD protocols are developed in collaboration with the transplant

and donor hospitals, and the local OPO. Therefore, DCD protocols are not uniform throughout the United States. DCD donors accounted for 30.2% of donors in the United States in 2021,[21] highlighting the need to optimize DCD protocols further. Pediatric DCD donors also provide quality organs for transplantation, and the American Academy of Pediatrics has endorsed their use.[22]

DCD donors typically have severe brain damage considered not recoverable but may have brain electrical activity. The decision to withdraw life-sustaining treatment must be made by the patient's surrogate independently and prior to the OPO initiating discussion of potential organ donation. The OPO is responsible for obtaining informed consent for the organ donation and for facilitating any preorgan recovery procedures, such as drug administration or vascular cannulation. The withdrawal of life support is timed to maximize the function of organs from these donors. Typically, end-of-life care is provided by the same medical team responsible for the care of the donor in the ICU. The organ recovery team is prohibited from being present for the withdrawal of life-sustaining treatment, may not guide the palliative process, and is prohibited from declaring the death of the donor. Death is defined by the cessation of respiration and circulation (i.e., arterial monitoring showing no pulse pressure, or Doppler monitoring showing no flow) after withdrawal of futile treatment measures. An authorized member from the donor hospital team declares death.

Suitable DCD donors are those in whom death is anticipated within 1 to 2 hours of withdrawal of life support. A plan for the donor's care should be in place if the patient does not die within the anticipated time frame, and ideally, care should be transferred back to the team that knows the patient and family. Predicting death within an hour of withdrawal of support is not an exact science, so evaluation tools to help predict which patients will die within this time frame are useful (Table 52-3).[23] For death to be declared, circulation and respiration must be absent for a minimum of 2 minutes before the start of organ recovery. A scoring system for predicting the death of pediatric DCD donors has also been developed and validated.[24]

Organ recovery started more than 5 minutes after respiratory and circulatory arrest may compromise donor organ quality, but this limit has been extended with reasonable transplant outcomes. The major goal of surgical management during procurement is to limit warm ischemia time through rapid cooling techniques and minimal in situ dissection.

Table 52-3 UNOS Consensus Committee Criteria for Prediction of DCD Death within 60 Minutes of Withdrawal of Life-Sustaining Treatment

- Apnea
- Respiratory rate <8 or >30 breaths/min
- Dopamine ≥15 μg/kg/min
- Left or right ventricular assist device
- Venoarterial or venovenous extracorporeal membrane oxygenation
- Positive end-expiratory pressure ≥10 and SaO_2 ≤92%
- FiO_2 ≥0.5 and SaO_2 ≤92%
- Norepinephrine or phenylephrine ≥0.2 μg/kg/min
- Pacemaker-unassisted heart rate <30
- IABP 1:1 or dobutamine or dopamine ≥10 μg/kg/min and CI ≤2.2 L/min/m²
- IABP 1:1 and CI ≤1.5 L/min/m²

CI, cardiac index; DCD, donation after cardiac death; IABP, intra-aortic balloon pump; SaO_2, arterial oxygen saturation; UNOS, United Network of Organ Sharing.

No major differences in intraoperative events during the transplant procedure between DCD and DBD kidney grafts have been reported. DCD kidneys have an increased risk of delayed graft function, increasing costs, but long-term function is not reduced; DCD livers generally have worse survival than DBD livers.[2] DCD hearts have been gaining popularity in the United States and preliminary data show promising results.

Living Kidney Donors

Safety and comfort are the primary considerations in the care of living donors. Living donors must be healthy and without significant cardiopulmonary, neurologic, or psychiatric disease; diabetes; obesity; or hypertension. Renal function must be normal, with no history of renal stones or proteinuria. The vast majority of living kidney grafts are retrieved laparoscopically with only a small number of these robotically assisted. As many as 21% of donors experience perioperative complications, with about 3% classified as severe.[25] Enhanced recovery protocols and diligent anesthetic practice are effective to reduce complications and improve quality of recovery.[26] Renal blood flow is decreased by both anesthesia and laparoscopic insufflation of the peritoneum, so a variety of fluid regimens have been suggested to blunt prerenal damage to the kidneys. Fluid loading overnight before surgery (vs. fluid administration starting with surgery) is associated with better creatinine clearance acutely during the procedure, and some suggest a colloid bolus just before pneumoperitoneum. Central venous access is rarely warranted in donor nephrectomy. CVP does not accurately reflect volume status with the patient in lateral decubitus position and with pneumoperitoneum. Nitrous oxide is contraindicated for laparoscopic donor nephrectomy because distended bowel can crowd the surgical field. 4

For open nephrectomy, the patient is positioned in the lateral decubitus position with the bed flexed to expose and arch the flank. Donors are almost always managed with general anesthesia. Donor nephrectomy should be an uncomplicated procedure, and most donors are extubated in the OR at the end of the case. Epidural and combined epidural–spinal techniques (supplemented with intravenous propofol) as well as general–epidural combined techniques were common in the past but have mainly been replaced by fascial plane blocks. Postoperative pain following donor nephrectomy can be severe, and patient-controlled analgesia is often used. The pain can still be severe enough to limit respiratory effort and mobilization of the patient. A survey of 333 donors found that nearly 25% reported pain more than a year after donation, and 17% reported a functional limitation.[27] Early complications include pulmonary conditions (atelectasis, pneumothorax, pneumonia), urinary tract infections, and wound problems. Long-term complications include reduced renal function, hypertension, albuminuria, and psychiatric issues (anxiety, depression). Some centers admit donors to a step-down or medical ICU for a day after surgery, but the total hospital stay is usually only 2 to 4 days. Bladder catheters are removed on postoperative day 1. Patients should be advised that full recovery (i.e., feeling normal) takes 4 to 6 weeks, especially after an open procedure. Fortunately, perioperative mortality is rare but cannot be denied as a possible outcome during preoperative patient discussions.

Living Liver Donors

Living liver donors have traditionally been employed in patients who are unlikely to receive MELD score prioritization, but increasingly living donors are being used for recipients with acute liver failure (ALF) (see Chapter 46, Video 46-1).[28] Left lobe

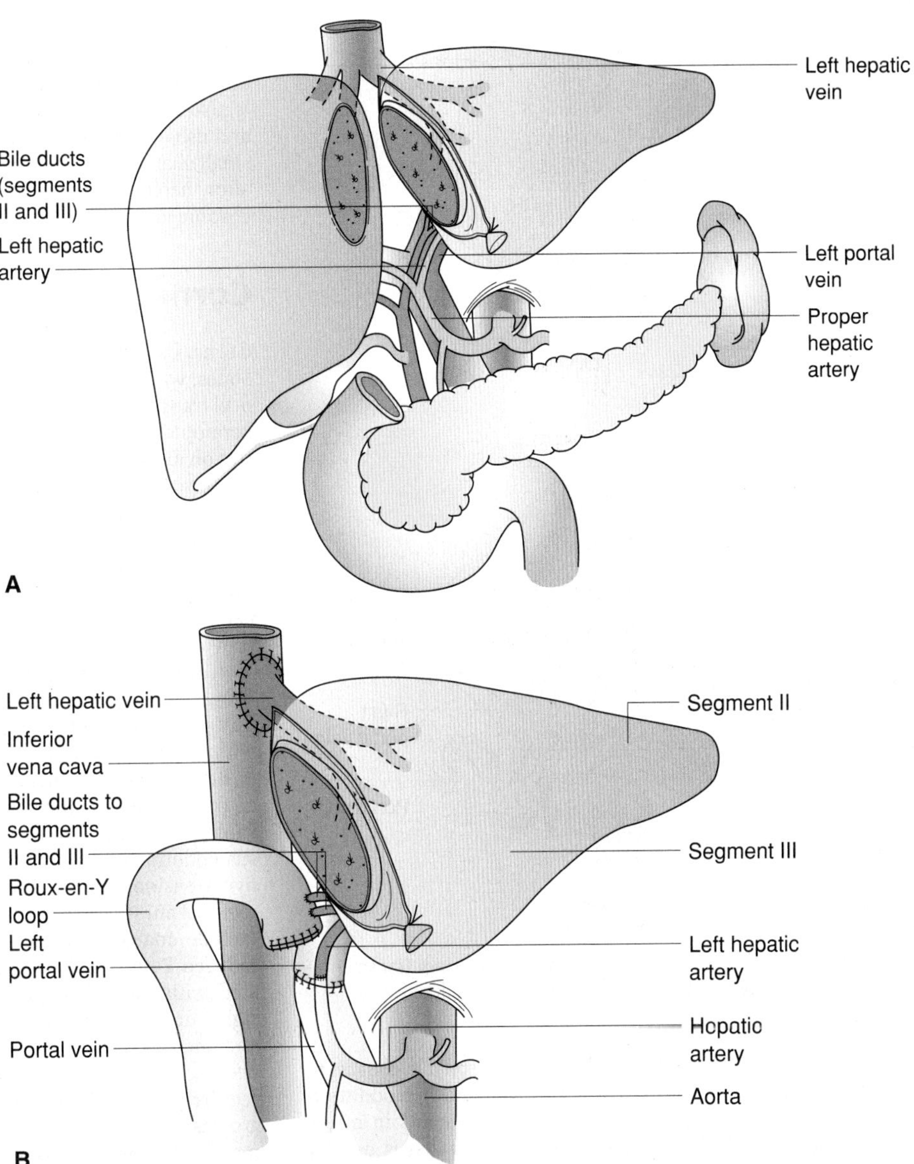

Figure 52-1 Left lateral segment (segments II and III) living donor transplantation. **A:** Donor operation. **B:** Recipient operation complete.

liver donation (segments II and III) is usually done in the context of adult-to-pediatric donation with recipients smaller than 15 kg. Left lateral segmentectomy is generally well tolerated (Fig. 52-1). Nonetheless, living left lobe donors must be healthy and without a history of or risk for thromboembolic disease. By comparison, donor right hepatectomy needed for adult-to-adult liver transplantation is a major procedure (Fig. 52-2) and carries significant risk. The residual liver volume of the donor must be greater than 35% of original volume to prevent "small for size" syndrome in the donor. Because the risk for this syndrome is increased in older donors or in patients with cholestatic or hepatocellular disease, adult-to-adult living donors should have no liver disease. Mortality after liver donation in the United States has been estimated to be as high as 1.7%. The Korean experience with more than 10,000 donations found 53 mortalities after donation with a median follow-up of nearly 6 years. The most common cause of death was suicide, accounting for 35% of mortality, followed by cancer and traffic accident.[29] Donors have no benefit from surgery, so any risk is significant and efforts to improve safety and support for donors should be continued. Serious complication rates are high for right liver donors (up to a third of donors depending on the center), including air embolism, atelectasis, pneumonia, respiratory depression, and biliary tract damage. Enhanced recovery protocols have demonstrated improvements in complication rates and overall quality of recovery, but many controversies remain.[30]

Large liver resections may require virtually complete hepatic vascular occlusion (cross-clamping of the hepatic pedicle usually without cava clamping). Not unexpectedly, venous return falls significantly. Without the collaterals developed by patients with chronic liver disease, normal donors may experience significant hypotension when the hepatic pedicle is cross clamped. Blood pressure is maintained largely through reflex increases in endogenous vasopressin and norepinephrine levels. For these reasons, volume loading is reasonable prior to clamping, but institutional practices vary widely. Some centers try to reduce blood loss by maintaining low CVP, whereas CVP monitoring is not routine in other centers. Sufficiently powered studies to prove that the benefits of low CVP (reduced transfusion requirements) outweigh the risks (renal compromise, air embolism) are unlikely to be performed, and institutional practices vary widely. If vasopressors are

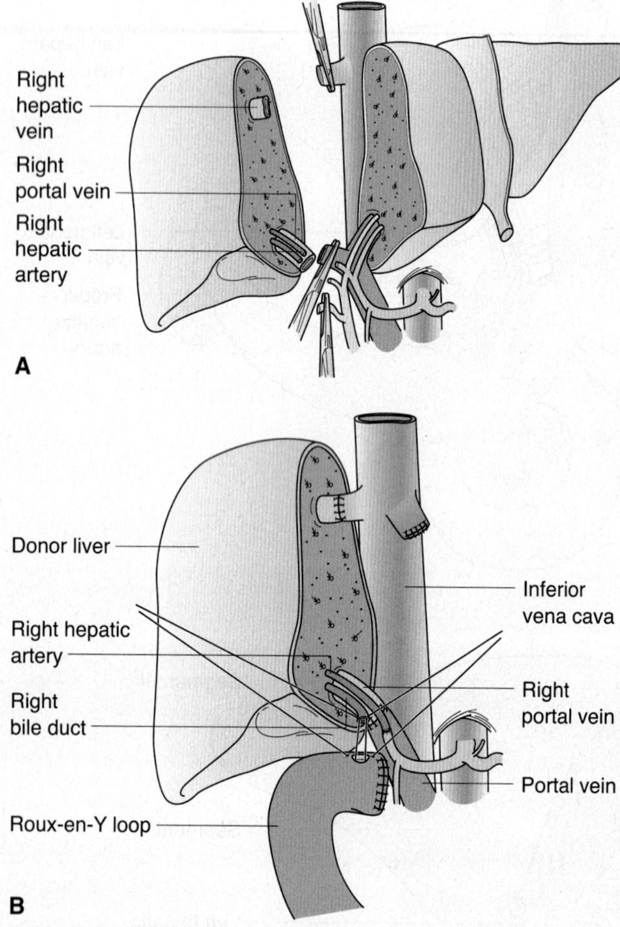

Figure 52-2 Right lobe (segments V to VIII) living donor transplantation. **A:** Donor operation. **B:** Recipient operation completed.

needed, vasopressin and norepinephrine are reasonable choices to enhance normal endogenous reflexes. Isovolemic hemodilution has been reported to reduce transfusion requirements in major hepatic resections. At experienced centers, blood loss is usually less than 1 L, and transfusion is rare. Blood salvage is useful and some centers offer autologous donation programs for donors, which can reduce the need for allogeneic blood transfusions. Availability of transesophageal echocardiography (TEE) to guide volume management in challenging cases may obviate the need for central venous access for monitoring. Many centers routinely avoid central lines if adequate peripheral access can be obtained. Most donors can be extubated safely in the OR at the end of the case. Hypothermia is a preventable reason for not extubating in the OR. An important aspect of enhanced recovery protocols is regional analgesia and narcotic avoidance. Many techniques have been used in living donor resections, such as epidurals, intrathecal narcotics, subcostal transversus abdominis plane (TAP) blocks, and erector spinae plane blocks. No quality studies exist comparing techniques. While epidural analgesia has demonstrated superior pain control, concerns for postoperative coagulopathy and epidural hematoma risk have limited its adoption. Laparoscopic and robot-assisted techniques are becoming more common, but issues such as prolonged warm ischemia time remain a barrier to widespread adoption of these techniques.[31]

Hypophosphatemia (with excessive loss of phosphate in the urine) is common after hepatectomy and should be treated with sodium phosphate infusions to maintain phosphate levels of 3.5 to 5.4 mg/dL, unless patients have significant renal compromise (creatinine clearance <50 mL/h). International normalized ratio (INR) is also abnormal in the postoperative period after liver resection and usually returns to baseline levels within 5 to 7 days, although small changes in liver function tests can persist for up to 3 months after hepatectomy. Some living liver donors can experience chronic low platelet counts after hepatectomy.

Corneal Transplantation

Corneas are the most common tissue transplanted in the United States, with around 49,000 transplants performed in 2021.[32] Corneal transplant, or keratoplasty, may be full thickness (penetrating keratoplasty, involving all five corneal layers), or partial thickness (involving the anterior or deep layers). Anesthetic goals include analgesia and akinesia, avoidance of increased intraocular pressure, the oculocardiac reflex, and postoperative nausea and vomiting (PONV).[33] Cornea graft recipients are often elderly, but routine preoperative testing does not decrease adverse events or improve outcomes.[34] Perioperative discontinuation of anticoagulants should be undertaken in consultation with the prescribing provider.

Corneal surgery can be performed under topical anesthesia (often with IV sedation), regional anesthesia, or general anesthesia (see Chapter 49). General anesthesia is preferred for patients with cognitive dysfunction, tremor, claustrophobia, or inability to lie flat, and for longer surgeries involving complex pathology of the anterior chamber. An increased risk of PONV is a disadvantage of general anesthesia. The use of laryngeal masks versus endotracheal intubation may reduce the potential for ocular hypertension from postoperative coughing. The advantages of regional anesthesia (retrobulbar, peribulbar, or sub-Tenon blocks) include analgesia, akinesia, ablation of the oculocardiac reflex, reduced PONV, and quicker recovery. Disadvantages are associated with the risk of local anesthetic injection, which include sight-threatening hemorrhage, infection, total spinal anesthesia, and increased intraocular pressure due to the volume of local anesthetic. Avoidance of elevations in intraocular pressure may require head-up positioning. In less invasive partial thickness keratoplasty, Trendelenburg position may rarely be requested. The major intraoperative complications of corneal transplantation are extrusion of ocular content and expulsive choroidal hemorrhage. Rejection of corneal allografts is the most common cause of graft loss in the first year after transplantation.

Renal Transplantation

Preoperative Considerations

The allocation of deceased donor (DD) kidneys in the United States changed in 2014 with the implementation of the Kidney Donor Profile Index (KDPI), a percentile score from 0% to 100% intended to provide the best grafts to patients with the longest predicted posttransplant survival. Lower scores are associated with longer estimated graft function. The KDPI is based upon the Kidney Donor Risk Index (KDRI), in which lower KDRI scores are associated with longer estimated graft function. The KDRI combines 10 donor factors in a single number that estimates the likelihood of graft failure after DD kidney transplant. The 10 donor factors (age, height, weight, ethnicity, history of hypertension, history of diabetes, cause of death, creatinine, hepatitis C status, and DCD status) included in the KDRI provide more granularity

Table 52-4 Diagnoses of Kidney Transplant Recipients (2018)

Diagnosis	Patients on List (%)
Diabetes	25.6
Hypertension	22.9
Glomerulonephritis	21.6
Other or unknown	29.9

Data from adr.usrds.org (accessed April 2022)

in evaluating donor grafts than prior systems. This system was intended to provide shorter wait times for higher-risk candidates who are willing to accept grafts with shorter estimated half-lives. A Living Kidney Donor Profile Index (LKDPI), proposed in 2016, compares the quality of live donor kidneys to each other and to DD kidneys.[35]

Postimplementation evaluation of the new kidney allocation system has shown that a higher percentage of kidney offers were transplanted (fewer grafts were declined) and the median KDRI of those grafts was higher compared to historical controls.[36] The new allocation system appears to be achieving its goal of improving longevity matching and broadening access for previously disadvantaged populations, including highly sensitized patients and those with an extended time on dialysis.[37] The cost of improved equity is an increase in cold ischemia times as kidneys are shipped over longer distances. Despite this, there is a lower risk of graft loss (HR = 0.90).[38] Kidney allocation is much more complicated than liver allocation; updated rules for kidney allocation can be found at optn.transplant.hrsa.gov.

Chronic kidney disease (CKD), a low estimated glomerular filtration rate (eGFR) or proteinuria, affects more than one in seven U.S. adults, or about 15% of the population.[39] End-stage renal disease (ESRD), requiring long-term dialysis or kidney transplantation, affects over 750,000 in the United States. Approximately 70% of this number are on dialysis and 30% have received transplants. In 2021, a total of over 24,000 kidney transplants were performed in the United States. Of these, 76% came from DDs and 24% came from living donors.[21] The most common recipient age group was 50 to 64 years. The proportion of candidates receiving transplants within 5 years ranged from 17% to 54% by state.[40] In 2020, 138,800 individuals were waiting for a kidney transplant; over 4,800 patients died while waiting for a kidney transplant, and another 3,800 became too sick to undergo transplantation.[40]

Diseases treated with renal transplants are shown in Table 52-4. Many of these underlying diagnoses are also risk factors for coronary artery disease, so preoperative evaluation is focused on cardiovascular function, but a comprehensive medical workup is essential.

5 About half the mortality of patients on dialysis is due to heart failure. Cardiovascular disease is the leading cause of death (and therefore graft loss) after renal transplantation.[41] Therefore, cardiovascular risk factor modification is imperative before and after transplantation, including management of hypertension and hyperlipidemia. Renal transplant recipients are often anemic, with hyperdynamic cardiac indices. Patients older than 50 years (with or without risk factors for coronary disease) are generally screened with dobutamine stress tests or myocardial scintigraphy. The interval at which these studies are repeated in patients listed for transplantation varies between centers. Peripheral vascular disease should also be assessed. Hypercoagulable states are common in patients with renal disease and deserve detailed evaluation so that they can be managed perioperatively.[42] Graft thrombosis is the main cause of graft failure in the first year.

All solid-organ transplant candidates are screened for tumors (mammography, Papanicolaou test, colonoscopy, prostate-specific antigen) and infection (dental evaluation, viral serologies). Patients should have good control of their diabetes before transplantation and have an evaluation for psychiatric stability and social support. Severe heart, lung, or liver disease; active malignancy; active or untreatable infections; active drug use; and uncontrolled psychiatric disease are exclusion criteria for renal transplantation.

Dialysis-dependent patients should be dialyzed before surgery to avoid intraoperative hyperkalemia, fluid overload, and acidosis. Cadaveric grafts can be safely transplanted after 24 hours of cold ischemia time, and potentially after 36 hours, allowing scheduling of preoperative dialysis. Delayed graft function is associated with longer cold ischemia times, particularly in high KDRI grafts.[43] Delayed graft function increases length of stay and hospital costs; however, DCD and DBD donor kidney transplants are associated with similar graft survival.[44]

Intraoperative Procedures

Most renal transplantation is done under general anesthesia, although the use of epidural or spinal anesthesia is technically possible. The entire surgery should take less than 3 hours.

While patients with epidurals reportedly have better postoperative pain relief, concerns over uremic platelet dysfunction and residual heparin from preoperative dialysis have limited the use of regional anesthesia for kidney transplantation.[45] The patient's preoperative medication lists should be reviewed; antihypertensives are common in this population. Although recommendations vary and renal transplant patients have not been well studied, consideration should be given to maintaining β-blockers and withholding angiotensin II receptor blockers before transplantation.[46]

Rapid-sequence induction (preceded by oral sodium bicitrate) is indicated in diabetic patients with gastroparesis. Rocuronium is useful for patients in whom rapid-sequence induction is indicated, but the duration of block may be prolonged in patients with ESRD. In general, the long-acting nondepolarizing muscle relaxants are avoided and shorter-acting agents such as cisatracurium (cleared by Hoffman elimination) are used. A bladder catheter is placed. Before incision, antibiotics are given. A central venous catheter may be placed to facilitate administration of immunosuppressant drugs and CVP monitoring, but this practice varies by institutional protocol and good peripheral access alone may be sufficient.

Incision is usually in the lower right abdomen to facilitate placement of the graft in the iliac fossa. The recipient iliac artery and vein are used for graft vascularization, followed by connection of the ureter to the recipient bladder. If the kidney is too large for the iliac fossa, it can be positioned in the retroperitoneal space. Iliac vessels may be used for anastomoses, or the aorta and inferior vena cava may be required.

The major anesthetic consideration is maintenance of renal 6
blood flow. No data are available to determine whether inhaled versus balanced intravenous techniques are better at preserving graft perfusion. Similarly, the choice of inhaled gas has not been shown to significantly affect posttransplant renal function. Isoflurane, sevoflurane, and desflurane are all used to manage renal transplant patients. Morphine effect is prolonged in the setting of ESRD, and high doses of meperidine can cause accumulation of its toxic metabolite, normeperidine, in these patients. Fentanyl, alfentanil, and sufentanil pharmacokinetics are clinically normal, though heterogeneity in pharmacokinetics in this population

warrants increased vigilance for postoperative respiratory depression. Remifentanil metabolite accumulation may occur in ESRD; however, remifentanil metabolites have very low opioid activity and infusions of up to 12 hours are unlikely to produce prolonged opioid effects.

Hypertensive renal transplant patients often require antihypertensive drugs perioperatively. Calcium channel blockers have been best studied for renal protection of cyclosporine-treated hypertensive transplant patients. After surgery, angiotensin-converting enzyme inhibitors are increasingly used, and α-blockers may be as effective as calcium channel blockers.[47] Typical hemodynamic goals during transplant are systolic pressure greater than 90 mmHg, mean systemic pressure greater than 60 mmHg, and often CVP greater than 10 mmHg despite the fact that CVP is not a reliable marker of fluid status.[48] More reliable indicators of hypovolemia are variations in systolic blood pressure and pulse pressure on the arterial line waveform during mechanical ventilation. Hypotension associated with pulse pressure variation greater than 13% is likely to respond to fluid.[49] These goals are usually achievable without vasopressors, using isotonic fluids and adjustment of anesthetic doses. Hemodynamic management varies widely among centers, so close communication between surgeon and anesthesiologist is imperative. Balanced salt solutions (Ringer's lactate, Plasma Lyte) are the crystalloid of choice for kidney transplantation as they are associated with less acidosis and hyperkalemia when compared with normal saline. Starch solutions should be avoided as they increase the risk of renal injury. Evidence is lacking to support the routine use of albumin during kidney transplantation.[48] Dopamine does not reliably improve renal function in this setting. The selective dopamine-1 receptor agonist fenoldopam is used in some centers to improve renal blood flow during kidney transplantation although evidence supporting improved outcomes is lacking.

Once the vascular anastomoses are started (typically the renal vein followed by the renal artery), diuresis is initiated (both mannitol and furosemide are often given). Heparin and verapamil should also be available in the OR. In some centers, anesthesiologists are asked to administer the first doses of immunosuppression. Usually, a glucocorticoid is administered as a bolus before reperfusion. In addition, antilymphocyte preparations are typically administered shortly before or after reperfusion, via slow infusion to avoid hypotension. The most commonly used induction agents for kidney transplantation are either T-cell depleting or interleukin (IL)-2 receptor-blocking antibodies combined with lower doses of standard immunosuppressive therapy (compared to high-dose standard immunosuppressives alone). For patients at high risk of rejection, rabbit antithymocyte globulin (rATG, a T-cell antibody) is often selected for induction. For patients who cannot tolerate rATG due to hypotension, leukopenia, or thrombocytopenia, or who are at lower risk of rejection, the IL-2 antibody basiliximab is often selected. Patients at high risk of rejection include those with a mismatch of one or more HLAs, panel reactive antibody greater than 20%, donor-specific antibody, blood group incompatibility, delayed graft function, and/or longer cold ischemia times (>24 hours). Younger recipients and older donors are also at increased risk of rejection. Conventional immunosuppression typically includes calcineurin inhibitors (cyclosporine or tacrolimus) and glucocorticoids. A kidney graft is defective in concentrating urine and reabsorbing sodium, so attention to electrolytes is important.

Glucose control is also important for patients undergoing transplantation. Aside from avoidance of hypoglycemia and hyperglycemia, evidence for precise perioperative targets has not been established.[50] Nonetheless, blood glucose values between 100 to 180 mg/dL are reasonable during renal transplantation.

Although renal transplant patients are often anemic coming to surgery, transfusion is rarely required in the OR. Many patients may be receiving erythropoietin preoperatively. Because of immunosuppression, if cytomegalovirus (CMV)-negative patients receiving a CMV-negative organ are transfused, CMV-negative blood is preferred. Leukocyte filters are also effective in preventing CMV transmission but are probably inferior to CMV-negative blood.[51]

Most surgical complications of renal transplantation are not recognized in the OR. The common postoperative complications are ureteral obstruction and fistulae, vascular thromboses, lymphoceles, wound complications, and bleeding. Vascular complications can lead to early graft loss.

Patient-controlled analgesia is a good choice for postoperative pain management, and despite prolonged action, morphine can be used safely if patients are well monitored. Nonsteroidal anti-inflammatory agents and cyclooxygenase-2 inhibitors are contraindicated. Pain can be severe, prompting some centers to explore combination blocks (ilioinguinal–iliohypogastric and intercostal nerve blocks)[52] or TAP blocks[53] for posttransplant pain control. Chronic pain after kidney transplantation is common,[54] suggesting that more attention should be given to early postoperative pain management.

In children, the most common causes of ESRD requiring transplantation are congenital (largely anatomic developmental) anomalies. Kidney size mismatch can complicate the surgery in small children. Adult donor kidneys may have to be placed in the retroperitoneum of small children. Although chronic peritoneal dialysis may help expand the abdominal volume, attention to peak inspiratory pressures at closure is important, and increased airway pressures should be reported to the surgical team. Pediatric renal transplantation is associated with somewhat lower rates of success than adult transplantation, with vascular thromboses of the grafts more common in younger children as well as problems with adherence to immunosuppressive regimens.

Liver Transplantation

Preoperative Considerations

In June of 2013, Share 35 was initiated for liver transplantation to allocate donor livers to higher acuity patients (with MELD scores >35), resulting in sicker patients presenting for transplant (NICV 52-2). The program mandated extended regional sharing of livers and intestines to liver–intestine candidates. Though overall mortality after liver transplantation did not change with Share 35, some regions experienced poorer outcomes. Hyponatremia in liver transplant recipients is associated with increased mortality on the waiting list, especially in less sick patients. For this reason, the MELD score was modified in January 2016 to include sodium, the first score change since its implementation in 2002.[101] 7

MELD is calculated as follows:

$$10 \times [(0.957 \times \ln(\text{serum creatinine})] + [(0.378 \times \ln(\text{serum bilirubin})] + [1.12 \times \ln(\text{INR})] + 6.43$$

MELD-Na is MELD − Na − [0.025 × MELD × (140 − Na)] + 140. Sodium (Na) values for this formula are capped at lower and upper limits of 125 and 140 mmol/L, respectively.

Mathematical modeling suggests that this change will save about 60 lives per year. In keeping with federal legislation and the final rule, UNOS continues to refine the allocation of donor organs, with the goals of improving access to life-saving transplants and maximizing the utility of a limited organ supply. The

Table 52-5 Multisystem Complications of End-Stage Liver Disease

System	Consequence
Central Nervous System	
Encephalopathy (confusion to coma)	Fatigue Blood–brain barrier disruption and intracranial hypertension (acute liver failure)
Pulmonary	
Respiratory alkalosis Reduced diffusing capacity	Hypoxemia/hepatopulmonary syndrome
Pulmonary hypertension	Reduced right heart function
Cardiovascular	
Reduced systemic vascular resistance Diastolic dysfunction Prolonged QT interval Blunted responses to inotropes Blunted responses to vasopressors Diabetes	Hyperdynamic circulation
Gastrointestinal	
Gastrointestinal bleeding from varices Ascites Delayed gastric emptying	
Hematologic	
Decreased synthesis of clotting factors Hypersplenism (pancytopenia) Impaired fibrinolytic mechanisms	Risk of massive surgical bleeding
Renal	
Hepatorenal syndrome	Impaired renal excretion of drugs
Hyponatremia	
Endocrine	
Glucose intolerance	
Osteoporosis	Fracture susceptibility
Nutritional/metabolic	Muscle wasting and weakness
Other	
Poor skin integrity; pruritus Increased volume of distribution for drugs	
Decreased citrate metabolism	Calcium requirement with rapid fresh frozen plasma infusion

latest revision occurred in 2022 with the implementation of geographic acuity circles, which removed donor service area and regions from allocation.

Liver transplant programs vary considerably in the number of transplants performed. The number of transplants performed in a given center is only a percentage of patients evaluated for liver transplantation. The anesthesiologist's input into the workup of liver transplant candidates is essential for decisions regarding listing and optimal preparation of patients for transplantation. Patients with ESLD have multiorgan dysfunction with cardiac, pulmonary, and renal compromise because of their liver disease (Table 52-5). Furthermore, many liver transplant recipients are more than 60 years old. Common diagnoses leading to liver transplantation are shown in Table 52-6. With the availability of pharmacologic cures for hepatitis C, the number of these patients requiring transplantation has been steadily declining since 2012. In addition, the high efficacy of these drugs has been increasingly used to expand the donor pool, as hepatitis C donors may now be used in hepatitis C–negative recipients, with treatment of the viral infection initiated immediately after transplantation.

Table 52-6 Diagnoses Leading to Liver Transplantation in Adults

Hepatocellular Disease
Hepatitis C
Laennec cirrhosis (alcoholic)
Combined hepatitis C virus/Laennec cirrhosis
Autoimmune hepatitis
Cryptogenic (idiopathic) cirrhosis
Hepatitis B
Small hepatocellular carcinoma (usually with other hepatocellular diseases)
Nonalcoholic steatohepatitis

Cholestatic Disease
Primary biliary cirrhosis
Primary sclerosing cholangitis

Acute Liver Failure
Viral (unknown)
Acute hepatitis viruses (A, B, C)
Drug-induced liver failure
Wilson disease

Pediatric patients are prioritized for transplant using pediatric end-stage liver disease (PELD) score, calculated as follows:

$$10 \times [(0.48 \times \ln(\text{serum bilirubin})) + 1.857 \times \ln(\text{INR})] - [0.687 \times \ln(\text{serum albumin})] + 0.436 \text{ (if} <12 \text{ months)} + 0.667 \text{ (if history of growth failure)}$$

For pediatric patients, PELD point exception requests are frequently made where the disease severity is not represented by the PELD score. These exceptions increase the chance of organ allocation in patients with diagnoses such as urea cycle disorders, organic acidemia, and hepatoblastoma.

Patients with ALF are given priority for donor livers, followed by patients with the highest MELD/PELD score and compatible blood group. All liver transplant patients are screened for infectious diseases including HIV, CMV, and Epstein–Barr virus. As for other solid-organ transplants, major infection and malignancy may exclude patients from consideration for transplantation. Several centers have had good experience transplanting HIV-positive patients (kidney or liver), though these patients have somewhat increased mortality compared to HIV-negative controls. Nonetheless, in HIV-positive patients with high MELD, transplantation confers a survival benefit.[55]

Renal dysfunction is common in patients undergoing liver transplantation. Even a small increase in serum creatinine in these patients suggests significant renal dysfunction; hence, creatinine is emphasized in MELD scoring.

Difficult decisions about patient candidacy are common in evaluating liver transplant candidates. Several are discussed here to highlight the need for regular involvement of a transplant anesthesiologist in the candidacy evaluation process. Patients with ESLD generally have very low SVR, high cardiac index, and increased mixed venous oxygen saturation. Liver disease is not protective against coronary artery disease. Because cardiovascular disease is the most common cause of 30-day mortality following liver transplantation, a rigorous cardiac workup is warranted. Cardiac evaluation protocols vary among centers due to varying expertise and capabilities. Transplant programs should work with anesthesiology and cardiology groups to establish an evaluation protocol that stratifies and mitigates cardiac risk.[56] Many programs use dobutamine stress echocardiography or myocardial stress scintigraphy, although the effectiveness of diagnosing coronary artery disease in these patients is not well established.[57] Patients with evidence of significant coronary lesions usually require cardiac catheterization to identify stenoses amenable to angioplasty preoperatively. These studies can be done safely even in patients with significant renal dysfunction. Patients with severe coronary artery disease that is unamenable to revascularization are generally not candidates for liver transplantation. Functional assessment of patients in addition to laboratory and imaging studies is important, and one study found that achieving a distance of less than 250 meters on a 6-minute walk test is an independent predictor of death on the transplant waiting list.[58]

Every effort should be made to maximize therapy for coronary artery disease and other heart diseases before transplantation. Patients with hypertrophic obstructive cardiomyopathy (HOCM) and LV outflow tract obstruction can be treated with alcohol ablation of the septum before surgery to improve cardiac function during transplantation. HOCM patients can benefit particularly from TEE monitoring because PA capillary wedge pressure does not accurately reflect LV volume in this population. Patients with a patent foramen ovale may be at risk for intraoperative stroke, and some centers work with cardiologists to close larger shunts noninvasively before surgery. Nonalcoholic steatohepatitis is increasingly an indication for liver transplantation and may be associated with increased major postoperative cardiac events.[59]

Patients presenting with portopulmonary hypertension (POPH) are particularly challenging to manage during transplantation. The diagnosis of POPH is made by a mean pulmonary artery pressure (mPAP) of 25 mmHg or higher, mean pulmonary capillary wedge pressure less than 15 mmHg, and pulmonary vascular resistance (PVR) greater than 240 dyne-sec/cm^5 (3 Wood units) in the setting of liver disease. In the sixth World Symposium on Pulmonary Hypertension in 2018, the cut-off of mPAP has been lowered to 20 mmHg for diagnosis of pulmonary hypertension.[60] Echocardiography is also used to screen patients for POPH and intracardiac shunts. Systolic PA pressure estimates are made by capturing the maximum velocity of regurgitant flow across the tricuspid valve. If moderate-to-severe pulmonary hypertension (estimated systolic PA pressure >50 mmHg) is suggested, right heart catheterization is needed for direct pressure measurements. Multiple case reports and small retrospective reviews demonstrate that patients with POPH are at substantial risk of perioperative death. There is general agreement that a mean PA pressure greater than 50 mmHg is an absolute contraindication to liver transplantation. Patients with PA pressures between 35 and 50 mmHg and PVR greater than 250 dyne-sec/cm^5 are also likely at increased risk. Efforts to lower PA pressure before transplantation pay off and considerably reduce the risk of transplantation.[61] Epoprostenol is the usual first-line therapy for POPH and is effective in lowering PA pressures significantly in many patients, but it requires home IV delivery. Intraoperative use of epoprostenol is complicated by its platelet inhibitory effects. Inhaled iloprost has been used in Europe for POPH patients with good results. Sildenafil is also useful for treatment of POPH and can be given via nasogastric tube during surgery. Controlling PA pressures is critical in patients with the most severe POPH, and patients have been successfully managed with the mixed endothelin antagonist bosentan or the selective endothelin-A receptor antagonist ambrisentan or imatinib. Right heart dysfunction that does not reverse after treatment of primary pulmonary hypertension is considered a contraindication to liver transplantation. Inhaled nitric oxide (iNO) can be useful for managing PA pressures during liver transplantation.

PFTs are often abnormal in ESLD, with most patients showing reduced diffusion capacity for carbon monoxide. Hepatopulmonary syndrome (HPS, a widened alveolar–arterial gradient in room air owing to liver disease) can lead to severe hypoxemia. Contrast echocardiography is used to diagnose intrapulmonary vasodilation using agitated saline. The microbubbles act as a contrast. If intracardiac shunts are present, bubbles promptly appear in the LV. The delayed appearance of bubbles (> three heartbeats after injection) suggests intrapulmonary shunting consistent with HPS. Once a contraindication to transplantation, HPS is now an indication for transplantation because it is the only therapy that can reverse the underlying physiology. If HPS is severe and unresponsive to oxygen, transplantation is risky because the immediate perioperative period may be complicated by frank graft hypoxia and failure. Fortunately, most patients with HPS have some element of physiologic ventilation–perfusion mismatch, are oxygen responsive, and can be safely transplanted.

Some patients with refractory ascites and normal renal function can have relief from ascites with terlipressin treatment. The U.S. Food and Drug Administration (FDA) approved terlipressin in 2013 (orphan status) for treatment of ascites. Terlipressin is used in many countries outside of the United States for treatment of hepatorenal syndrome (HRS). The CONFIRM trial showed an improved recovery of renal function with terlipressin and albumin.[62] In 2020, the FDA declined to approve terlipressin for the treatment of HRS due primarily to the failure to demonstrate a survival benefit.

Recently, a large number of new drugs for the treatment of hepatitis C have entered the market,[63] including protease inhibitors, viral polymerase inhibitors, viral replication complex inhibitors, new interferon formulations, and new ribavirin formulations. Drug–drug interactions with the new anti–hepatitis C virus drugs are just being reported. Telaprevir inhibits CYP3A and induces a significant reduction in oral clearance of midazolam (and limits its oxidation) in liver microsomes. Protease inhibitors used to treat HIV can interact with midazolam to cause prolonged sedation. Even in the absence of these drug–drug interactions, metabolism of benzodiazepines may be compromised in patients with ESLD; even typical doses may precipitate hepatic encephalopathy and are best avoided.

Intraoperative Procedures

The duration of liver transplant surgery varies considerably depending on the complexity of the case. On average, liver transplants take 6 or more hours. In some situations, patients can be extubated at the end of the case but predicting easy versus difficult cases is not an exact science. Consequently, intensive preparation for surgery is important. Rapid-sequence induction of general anesthesia is indicated because patients with ESLD often have gastroparesis in addition to increased intra-abdominal pressure from ascites. For anticipated difficult cases, many centers place two arterial catheters; one in the radial artery and the other one in the femoral artery (left femoral if a kidney transplant is planned). PA catheters are still used in many centers to follow PVR, and TEE is increasingly used for monitoring volume status, particularly for patients with cardiac disease undergoing transplantation (see Chapter 27). Major hemorrhagic complications in patients with esophageal varices are rare, but fear of these complications has limited TEE use in some centers. For difficult cases, adequate access for rapid intravenous infusions should be obtained prior to skin incision. Before surgical incision, blood product availability must be confirmed. A rapid infusion system with the ability to deliver at least 500 mL/min of warmed blood should be primed and in the room. Normothermia, essential for optimal hemostasis, should be maintained with fluid warmers and convective air blankets over the legs and upper body. Bladder catheters and nasogastric tubes are placed in all patients.

8 Liver transplantation is traditionally described in three phases: dissection phase, anhepatic phase, and neohepatic phase, with reperfusion of the graft marking the start of the neohepatic phase. The major issues during the first phase of transplantation are hemostatic management, metabolic optimization, and renal protection. The major anesthetic goals of this phase are treatment of bleeding, management of potassium levels, and maintenance of CO and intravascular volume for renal protection. Some centers advocate low CVP management of liver transplant patients to reduce blood loss,[64] but this technique may not be tolerated by patients with higher MELD scores and marginal renal function. An abdominal incision in patients with massive ascites causes a rapid paracentesis, and albumin infusion is warranted to prevent postparacentesis circulatory dysfunction. Cirrhotics often have very low albumin levels as well as poorly functioning albumin.

Coagulation

Although standard laboratory coagulation studies have not been shown to predict bleeding, they are still valuable for coagulation management. The use of viscoelastic testing has become widespread. Though many transplants can be done with minimal transfusions, predicting bleeding is difficult, and anesthesiologists should be prepared for massive transfusion. Fresh frozen plasma (FFP) is used to maintain an INR of <2.0 in patients with anticipated or ongoing bleeding. Rapid infusion of FFP can quickly lead to ionized hypocalcemia because of the citrate load that is not metabolized by a diseased liver. Infusion of calcium chloride ($CaCl_2$), adjusted to ionized Ca^{2+} levels, is better at maintaining constant calcium (Ca^{2+}) levels than are intermittent boluses. Use of calcium boluses will cause wide calcium swings and overuse of calcium. At this time, there is not sufficient U.S. experience with prothrombin complex concentrates[65] in liver transplant recipients to know the place for these products, though their use has become common in Europe. Platelet transfusion has traditionally been used to maintain platelet counts above 50,000/mm^3; however, platelet transfusion has been associated with worse graft and patient survival.[66] Importantly, we find that maintaining fibrinogen above 150 mg/dL with cryoprecipitate is critical for hemostasis and obviates the need for platelet transfusions in most patients. Cell-saver blood may also be used to limit allogeneic transfusions, although it is generally not used in patients with hepatocellular carcinoma.

Many other factors contribute to poor hemostasis in liver transplant patients besides poor clotting factor synthesis, including renal failure, infection, endothelial dysfunction, and high portal pressures.[67] This complexity in the etiology of underlying bleeding problems is likely a factor in our inability to predict bleeding during liver transplantation.

In addition to complex coagulopathies of ESLD, many patients with liver disease have a superimposed hypercoagulable state (see Chapter 17). For example, patients with autoimmune liver diseases may have antiphospholipid antibodies. Many authors have suggested that the coagulation status of cirrhotics is "balanced" when reduced levels of procoagulant factors are offset by reduced levels of endogenous anticoagulant factors such as ADAMTS-13, antithrombin, protein C, and plasminogen. This rebalancing is tenuous as further reductions in procoagulants or anticoagulants can tip the balance in the direction of bleeding or thrombosis. In addition, elevated von Willebrand factor and factor VIII can contribute to prohemostatic changes in patients with liver disease.[67] Experienced transplant anesthesiologists recognize that both coagulopathy and hypercoagulability can cause simultaneous and serious problems—two diseases rather than a balanced system, and hemorrhage can coexist with simultaneous thrombosis. In addition to monitoring discrete parts of the coagulation profile to guide transfusion therapies, it is important to look at a measure of whole-blood clotting to assess thrombotic potential. Most centers use viscoelastic tests, thromboelastography (TEG), or thromboelastometry (ROTEM) to help sort out complex coagulation disturbances and their evolution during liver transplantation, to help with interpretation of standard laboratory tests of coagulation, and to get a picture of overall clotting and fibrinolysis status. If viscoelastic testing indicates normal or hypernormal whole-blood clotting in the presence of high INR and low fibrinogen and platelets (and usually elevated D-dimers), this pattern is a caution that the patient may have a clinically significant hypercoagulable state. In patients with a history of thrombotic events, a formal hypercoagulability workup should be done as part of liver transplant evaluation. Under these circumstances, the authors' approach is to avoid pharmacologic procoagulant or antifibrinolytic drugs. For the majority of patients with coagulopathy dominated by synthetic dysfunction, thrombocytopenia, and hypofibrinogenemia, whole-blood clotting is delayed. If these patients have insufficient hemostasis, many centers supplement transfusion therapy with antifibrinolytic agents. Considerable center-dependent variation in the use and dosing of antifibrinolytics makes generalizations difficult. Both lysine analog plasmin inhibitors (epsilon-aminocaproic acid and tranexamic acid) have been documented to be safe[68] in most coagulopathic patients during liver transplantation, provided there is no evidence or history of hypercoagulability. There is some evidence that they may reduce transfusion. Fibrinolysis acutely worsens immediately after reperfusion to varying degrees, depending largely on the amount of tissue plasminogen activator released from the graft. A (re)bolus of an antifibrinolytic may be helpful to maintain hemostasis once this postreperfusion exacerbation of fibrinolysis is documented.

Activated factor VII can be used during liver transplantation but is usually reserved for rescue of refractory critical bleeding unresponsive to more standard management because of its expense and the risk of thrombosis. When this drug is given, INR rapidly normalizes, although the amount of circulating clotting factors does not change, complicating interpretation of laboratory coagulation studies. Recombinant factor VII administration is also useful for surgical hemostasis for placement of intracranial pressure (ICP) monitors in patients with ALF and for selected patients undergoing liver transplantation with difficult red cell crossmatches or in patients who refuse transfusion on religious grounds.

Pulmonary embolism is an unusual complication of liver transplantation, reflecting the complex coagulation imbalance of ESLD and liver transplantation. If diagnosed promptly, low-dose tissue

Table 52-7 Diagnostic Criteria for Hepatorenal Syndrome versus Other Etiology of Renal Dysfunction

Presence of ascites
No improvement following discontinuation of diuretics
No improvement after 48 h of albumin supplementation (1 g/kg/d)
No signs of shock
No recent nephrotoxic medications
No signs of kidney disease (proteinuria, microhematuria, normal renal ultrasound)

From Gupta K, Bhurwal A, Law C, et al. Acute kidney injury and hepatorenal syndrome in cirrhosis. *World J Gastroenterol.* 2021;27(26):3984–4003.

plasminogen activator (0.5 to 4 mg) delivered into the CVP port of a pulmonary artery catheter (PAC) can lyse the clot quickly.

Perioperative renal dysfunction is a major challenge in liver transplantation and can be exacerbated by hypovolemia and anesthetic-induced impairment of renal blood flow. Post–liver transplant renal dysfunction is associated with the baseline level of preoperative renal dysfunction and liver disease, as well as intraoperative hemodynamic instability and graft quality.[69] Creatinine levels can significantly underestimate the degree of renal dysfunction, especially in ESLD patients with significant muscle wasting.[70] HRS is defined as renal dysfunction due to chronic liver disease or ALF. It is considered a diagnosis of exclusion with specific criteria (Table 52-7). HRS classification was updated in 2015 by the International Club of Ascites: HRS type 1 and HRS type 2 were renamed HRS-AKI (acute kidney injury) and HRS-CKD (chronic kidney disease). HRS-AKI is defined as conditions meeting the six criteria for HRS and an increase in serum Cr of 0.3 mg/dL from baseline in 48 hours, or 1.5 times baseline Cr within 7 days. This departs from diagnostic criteria for HRS type 1 by removing the requirement for an absolute value of Cr greater than 2.5 mg/dL.[71] Acute kidney injury prevention best practices include spontaneous bacterial peritonitis (SBP) prophylaxis, intravenous albumin administration if SBP is present, and antibiotic prophylaxis for gastrointestinal bleeding.[72] In addition, a large-volume (>5 L) drainage of ascites with incision should be accompanied by albumin therapy to prevent renal decompensation, with recommended albumin doses of 6 to 8 g/L of ascites drained. Importantly, higher doses of albumin are associated with better survival in type 1 HRS. Norepinephrine may be useful for HRS because of relief of splanchnic vasodilatation, though the data are sparse. The α_1-agonist midodrine in combination with octreotide is useful for improving renal function in some patients. No prospective trials have been done to support the use of one vasopressor over another during transplantation, and intraoperative pharmacologic renal support is largely guided by the hepatology literature. Dopamine is not useful for preserving renal function during liver transplantation. The most important consideration for patients with HRS is to ensure adequate volume replacement before instituting diuresis in the OR.

The *anhepatic phase* begins when the liver is functionally excluded from the circulation. Historically, the vena cava is clamped above (suprahepatic) and below (infrahepatic) the liver, and the portal vein and hepatic artery are clamped. With complete caval cross-clamping, venous return falls by 50% to 60%, often resulting in hypotension. Venovenous bypass (VVB) may be used to increase venous return and therefore CO, to increase renal and gut perfusion, and to decompress portal pressures for a better surgical field. VVB is rarely used in centers where surgeons use cava-sparing techniques, and hemodynamics during the anhepatic period can be managed with volume loading and vasopressors as needed. VVB carries potential complications, including arm lymphedema, air embolism, and vascular injury, and its benefit is limited when anhepatic times are short. Surgical techniques that preserve caval flow (e.g., piggyback technique) are standard in most U.S. centers and make intraoperative management significantly easier, but anesthesiologists should be familiar with managing both surgical situations.

Reperfusion of the graft is the most dynamic, eventful time of the liver transplant. Communication between the surgical and anesthesia teams is essential in precise preparation for reperfusion. Caval clamps are removed first, and the integrity of the caval anastomoses is ensured. Caval reperfusion is usually hemodynamically well tolerated. However, portal vein reperfusion often results in hemodynamic instability. The original descriptions of reperfusion syndrome emphasized (often severe) hypotension and bradycardia with portal reperfusion.[73] Now, with flushing techniques that precede reperfusion and changes in preservation solution, bradycardia is less common. Typically, reperfusion is associated with hypotension (further drop of already low SVR), which may or may not require treatment. The authors' preparation for reperfusion is to hyperventilate to induce a respiratory alkalemia that will offset the acid load from the graft and to administer 1,000 mg of $CaCl_2$ *precisely at the time of portal reperfusion* to counteract the effects of high potassium concentration on the heart. If, despite these preparations, T waves on electrocardiogram (ECG) become elevated, $CaCl_2$ is repeated. Some anesthesiologists prefer to treat ECG changes only after they are diagnosed, but because the acid load and potassium of reperfusion can be anticipated, the authors' practice is to counteract these prophylactically. Lidocaine, atropine, norepinephrine, and epinephrine are available at the time of reperfusion in case of ventricular dysrhythmias, bradyarrhythmias, or severe hypotension. Hepatic artery unclamping is usually hemodynamically uncomplicated. Advancement in the storage of organs continues to mitigate the sequalae of reperfusion. In 2021, the FDA approved two machine perfusion devices for the preservation of livers for transplantation. Early experience with these devices has demonstrated improved postreperfusion hemodynamics.[74]

Microemboli and right ventricular (RV) dysfunction are common at reperfusion, and intracardiac thromboemboli are not rare.[75] Intracardiac emboli and biventricular dysfunction are associated with adverse postoperative cardiac events.[75] Methylene blue is used by some to counteract the vasoplegic state of reperfusion, but its effects on outcome are unknown.[76] On the other hand, a study in which iNO was given during the entire transplant suggested significant acute benefits (decreased hepatocyte apoptosis) and earlier graft recovery, including faster coagulation factor synthesis. Attempts to precondition the reperfused graft were analyzed in a well-designed trial, which showed no difference with propofol versus sevoflurane preconditioning.[77]

In the *neohepatic phase*, calcium is not required after the acute effects of reperfusion wane; lack of an ongoing calcium requirement, even when FFP is infused rapidly, is early indication of graft metabolic function. During the neohepatic phase, the base deficit improves with graft metabolism of citrate and lactate. Within the first hour after reperfusion, the CO decreases as SVR increases to prereperfusion levels as the graft metabolizes the vasoactive substances that were unleashed at reperfusion. In addition, the graft appearance should be noted. It should have a smooth edge and no evidence of engorgement. Bile is made in the first half-hour after reperfusion in a well-functioning graft. Renal function can improve after reperfusion, probably because of graft metabolism of renal vasoconstrictors. ECD grafts are often slow to function metabolically in the OR. (For these and other classes of ECD livers, cold ischemia times should be limited, which can significantly affect the OR schedule.) Fibrinolysis after reperfusion may require antifibrinolytic agents. ROTEM may be more sensitive than TEG in detecting fibrinolysis,[78] but the decision to add or increase antifibrinolytics after reperfusion should be made by assessing surgical hemostasis as well as point-of-care tests.

During the neohepatic period, biliary anastomoses are completed and sources of surgical bleeding are corrected. Drains are placed and the abdomen is closed. Fast-tracking protocols for liver transplant patients are common in experienced centers.

Pediatric Liver Transplantation

Indications for pediatric liver transplantation differ considerably from those of adults, with biliary atresia (44%) and inborn errors of metabolism (34%) being the most common indications.[79] POPH is rare in children, but biliary atresia is associated with cardiac defects and situs inversus. Children younger than 1 year of age with inherited liver disease are often very small for their age. In small children, a radial artery catheter and at least one large (18-g) peripheral intravenous line are placed after induction of anesthesia. Surgeons may place tunneled central lines before incision, which are useful for intraoperative transfusions, postoperative administration of drugs, and CVP monitoring. Children with previous Kasai operations for biliary atresia may have massive bleeding during dissection because of adhesions. Small children receiving large grafts may have respiratory compromise with abdominal closure. Because hepatic artery thrombosis (HAT) is a more common complication in children than adults, some centers choose to have the INR at the end of surgery in the 1.8 to 2 range; postoperative aspirin and alprostadil are often used to prevent HAT. If flow is inadequate (by poor Doppler signals) in the artery after anastomosis, intraoperative reanastomosis or a new anastomosis may be required acutely. Aortic cross-clamping may be necessary for these anastomoses. Biliary complications are also common in pediatric transplant recipients, especially those receiving adult left lateral segment grafts, with HAT a significant contributor to biliary complications. Use of split livers (one liver for two patients) puts a strain on transplant teams but is important for extending the donor pool.[80]

Acute Liver Failure

Anesthetic considerations for adults and children with ALF are focused on protection of the brain (see Chapter 37) so in many ways, management is opposite that of chronic liver failure, in which the kidneys are the most fragile organ requiring protection during liver transplantation. Patients with a diagnosis of ALF should be managed in the ICU, because they can have a rapidly progressive course of elevated ICP, leading to herniation and death. It is important to develop a detailed multidisciplinary protocol for managing these patients. ALF is much less common than chronic liver disease and so a single center may have little experience with managing this presentation. ICP monitoring in patients with ALF is contentious. While some centers consider it useful in managing these patients, it has not been demonstrated to improve outcomes, and placement risks intracranial bleeding. Some centers have gained expertise in transcranial Doppler monitoring in place of invasive ICP monitoring[81] thereby avoiding the risk of ICP monitoring in coagulopathic patients.

Anesthetic management of these patients starts in the ICU, with intubation as needed for airway protection in the setting of encephalopathy or for initiation of therapeutic hypothermia. Mild hypothermia (core temperature 34 °C to 35 °C) is used in some centers for ALF, though recent retrospective analysis suggests no benefit.[82] The head is positioned midline and the head of the bed raised. Mild hyperventilation is also commonly used to manage ICP but is best used as a rescue therapy. Mannitol is used for osmotherapy to an end point of 310 to 315 mOsm/L for serum osmolality. Hypertonic saline is also useful for lowering ICP in some patients, with a target serum Na of 145 to 155 mEq/L.[83] Liver-assist devices used to bridge patients with ALF to transplantation have not generally shown benefit.

It is important to avoid all cerebral vasodilating anesthetics, including all inhaled agents. With decreased availability of barbiturates, propofol is commonly used. Patients may come to the OR on *N*-acetylcysteine, a glutathione donor. When antihypertensive therapy is required, labetalol does not cause significant cerebral vasodilation in these patients. Acute cerebral vasodilatation often occurs with reperfusion. The management of intracranial hypertension and cerebral edema is based on very small studies of patients with ALF and on adaptations of studies directed at the control of intracranial hypertension in other settings (see Chapter 37).

Pancreas and Islet Transplantation

The majority of pancreas transplants (about 85%) are done as simultaneous pancreas and kidney transplants from a single DD. Pancreata grafted in these procedures have historically had better long-term survival than grafts done after kidney transplantation or as independent pancreas grafts. Independent pancreas grafts are usually performed for patients with type 1 diabetes, who have frequent metabolic complications (hypoglycemia) but preserved renal function. With proper donor selection and aggressive attention to targeted antibiotic coverage, better graft survival rates after isolated pancreas transplant have been reported. Nonetheless, pancreas transplantation is becoming less frequent and islet transplantation has increased, likely because pancreas transplants are associated with higher rates of surgical and postoperative complications. Optimal immunosuppression for islet transplantation, to ward off both allo- and autoimmunity, remains a significant problem. Encapsulation of islets to create a barrier to immune cells has also been a surprisingly hard problem.[84]

The preoperative assessment of pancreas/islet transplant recipients focuses on the end-organ complications of type 1 diabetes (see Chapter 47). Monitoring will depend on cardiac status, but generally, patients do not require PA catheters and have been evaluated for cardiac disease as part of the transplant workup. Nonetheless, cardiovascular disease is present in many patients undergoing pancreas transplantation, although they tend to be younger than liver transplant recipients.

The major difference between pancreas transplantation and other procedures is that strict attention to control of blood glucose is indicated to protect newly transplanted β cells from hyperglycemic damage. No formula for controlling blood glucose has emerged as a standard of intraoperative management. In general, if adult patients arrive with glucose above 250 mg/dL, 10 units of insulin can be given intravenously, followed by an infusion of insulin. The infusion starting rate varies, depending on the initial blood glucose level. Once blood glucose levels are controlled (<140 mg/dL), intravenous 5% dextrose (about 100 mL/h) should also be infused as the insulin infusion is continued to prevent hypoglycemia. The most important issue is to check the response to insulin frequently and adjust infusions as necessary. Little literature exists for a patient with an implanted insulin pump, though more than 400,000 have been implanted in the United

States.[85] Protocols for patients undergoing surgery with insulin pumps emphasize preadmission contact with an endocrinologist and documentation of pump status from preoperative to postoperative settings. A reasonable recommendation is to continue to use the pump at basal rates in these patients as long as its operation is reviewed and blood glucose levels are monitored regularly during surgery.

Islet transplants were revived by the Edmonton protocol, published in 2000.[86] The major changes introduced included a glucocorticoid-free immunosuppression regimen and immediate transplantation of islets after isolation. Since that time, islets have been cultured after isolation in many centers, which makes surgical scheduling easier. Islets are generally infused into the portal circulation; acute portal hypertension may result from the infusion. This surgery should not be complicated by significant blood loss.

Small Bowel and Multivisceral Transplantation

Indications for intestinal transplantation include impending liver failure in patients with intestinal failure (or short-gut syndromes requiring total parenteral nutrition [TPN]), frequent severe dehydration in patients with intestinal failure, and severe complications of central lines for TPN (sepsis, thrombosis of central veins). Patients who develop liver failure from TPN for intestinal failure are candidates for combined liver–intestine transplantation, and the presence of a liver in the graft may have a protective effect on the bowel graft.[87] In these cases, liver failure should be irreversible, and biopsy findings are often required to corroborate this conclusion in patients without overt ESLD. In general, intestinal transplantation is usually performed only in patients with life-threatening complications of intestinal failure, mostly in children, but increasingly in adult recipients.

A major hurdle for these transplants is line placement adequate for transfusion of blood products and fluids, often needed during these long cases. Anesthesiologists should review angiographic studies to determine venous patency before attempting central line placement. Ultrasound devices are helpful in identifying the known patent vessels for cannulation, but surgical cutdowns or interventional radiologic techniques for venous access may be necessary, including transhepatic or intraoperative renal vein catheterization. Superior vena cava or inferior vena cava obstruction may require preoperative intervention (surgical and/or lytic) for adequate vascular access for surgery.[88] Antibiotic regimens should be continued during the surgery. Nitrous oxide, as in liver transplantation, should be avoided.

Common complications of intestinal failure include dehydration and electrolyte abnormalities, gastric acid hypersecretion, pancreatic insufficiency, bone disease, and TPN-induced liver failure.[89] Because electrolyte abnormalities are common, they should be monitored continuously during surgery and appropriate replacement instituted. Because enteral feeding will not be possible until weeks after surgery, TPN should be continued in the perioperative period.

Like reperfusion of liver grafts, intestinal graft reperfusion is associated with an acute release of acid and potassium from the graft and a postreperfusion syndrome. Anticipatory bicarbonate and $CaCl_2$ administration are useful to counteract the effects of acid and potassium on the heart. After reperfusion, coagulopathy may worsen and is usually managed by reassessment of INR, fibrinogen, and platelet counts, and correction with blood products. Epidural anesthesia may be useful for pain management.[90]

Composite Tissue Allografts

Upper extremity and face transplants are extremely complex procedures performed only in a few centers. More than 130 patients have received hand or arm transplants, with the longest survivor 11 years posttransplant. Since 2021, more than 45 patients have received full or partial face transplants (hopkinsmedicine.org). For face donors, surgeons prefer to procure the face first, before other organs are procured. The graft recovery is complex, with isolation of motor and sensory nerves as well as venous and arterial vessels. Multiple surgeons are involved in both graft recovery and implantation. Recipient nose and mouth deformities will certainly require individualized airway care. Protocols for these patients are just being developed, but the choice of anesthetic and fluid management is directed at preventing microvasculature constriction and postoperative edema.

Anesthesiologists should be involved in perioperative protocol development for these new procedures from the initial planning stages of a program. Well-planned regional nerve blocks can be very useful for upper extremity transplants and other anesthesia-specific concerns can be addressed in advance.[91] Limb transplant recipients may be heparinized. Bilateral limb allografts expose the recipient to two reperfusion events. The common feature of these grafts is that they contain multiple organs (blood vessels, nerves, muscle, skin). Multiple anastomoses imply a very long surgical procedure. Composite tissue recipients require intense immunosuppression, in part because the skin is highly antigenic, and some immunosuppressants that are unfamiliar to anesthesiologists may be administered intraoperatively. In addition to complex triple-drug immunosuppression, donor marrow infusions may be used in an effort to induce tolerance to the allograft. Preparation for massive blood loss in these cases is essential.

Face grafting also may require massive transfusion, and blood loss may be difficult to quantify because of bleeding into the drapes. The surgery can be very prolonged. Common complications include postoperative renal dysfunction, acute respiratory distress syndrome, and jugular vein thrombosis. These cases are immunologically extremely complex.[92]

Lung Transplantation

Lung transplantation is accepted therapy for end-stage pulmonary and pulmonary vascular disease to improve longevity and quality of life. The Department of Health and Human Services OPTN reports more than 46,000 lung transplant procedures in the United States since 1988, and the 2020 Registry of the International Society for Heart and Lung Transplantation (ISHLT) reports 69,200 lung transplants performed worldwide since 1988.[93] The median waiting time has improved recently with OPTN data from 2011 to 2014 showing a range between 100 and 400 days. However, many patients die awaiting transplant because of the shortage of suitable organs. Over the past 20 years, there has been a slow but steady improvement in overall outcome in lung transplantation. Data compiled by OPTN from 2008 to 2015 reveal median 1-year survival rate of 87.7%, 3-year survival of 71.8%, and 5-year survival of 58.6% for double-lung transplant recipients. The media survival is 6.2 years with better long-term survival for bilateral lung transplants than single-lung transplantation (median 7.1 vs. 4.5 years).[93,94] In the past, the most common indication for lung transplantation was chronic obstructive pulmonary disease. However, since 2007, interstitial lung disease (ILD) including idiopathic interstitial pneumonia (IIP) and non-IIP ILD has become the leading indication with that number increasing every year

(32.4% and 8.1%, respectively) worldwide.[93,95] This trend is even more noticeable in North America where ILD now accounts for 47% of lung transplants compared to 38% just over a decade ago.[95] COPD (30.1%), cystic fibrosis (CF) (15.2%), and α-1-antitrypsin deficiency (4.7%) are the other indications for lung transplants.[95]

The surgical options for lung transplantation are single-lung transplant, *en bloc* double, sequential double, cadaveric or living donor lobar transplantation, and combined heart–lung transplantation. The ISHLT registry for 2019 indicates a continued increase in double-lung transplants over the past two decades, with a relatively stable number of single-lung transplants, a trend likely related to reports of improved outcome after double-lung transplantation.[95] Double-lung transplantation is most commonly used in patients with pulmonary vascular disease and CF, although its use is increasing in chronic obstructive pulmonary disease and interstitial lung disease. Single-lung transplantation is favored for those with emphysema because of good short-term outcomes, with the added advantage of leaving a donor lung for another recipient. Lung transplant centers vary in applying single- or double-lung transplant and the procedure indications are still debated. Double-lung transplantation, however, is indicated if a single-lung transplantation would allow a continuing pathologic process to jeopardize either the native or transplanted lung. For example, the presence of pulmonary infection, as in CF, in the native lung would likely spread to the transplanted lung. In pulmonary hypertension, the remaining pulmonary vascular disease in the native lung would result in progressive pulmonary hypertension and thus hypertensive vasculopathy in a transplanted lung. Finally, a severely emphysematous lung, with its high compliance, would be at risk for air trapping and barotrauma when coexisting with a transplanted lung with normal compliance.

While the use of cardiopulmonary bypass (CPB) and extracorporeal membrane oxygenation (ECMO) has been avoided in the past, there has recently been a growing trend of use of CPB and in particular ECMO. Perioperative complications and immediate postoperative mortality tend to be higher in those patients who received ECMO.[96,97] However, there seems to be no difference in overall primary graft function, and mid- and long-term outcomes.[96,97] Some studies have even shown superior survival rate at 1, 3, and 5 years, and advocate for routine prophylactic use of ECMO.[98] CPB should be always available for lung transplants no matter the indication. The use of Ex-Vivo lung perfusion machine is on the rise with the potential to expand the donor pool.[99]

Recipient Selection

International Guidelines for the Selection of Lung Transplant Candidates were updated in 2021 by consensus agreement of several thoracic societies (summarized in Table 52-8). In general, patients should be considered for lung transplantation if they meet the following criteria; clinically and physiologically advance lung disease for which medical therapy is insufficient, patients are at high risk (>50%) of death from lung disease without transplantation, high likelihood (>80%) of surviving at least 5 years post transplantation given adequate graft function.[100] Ideally, referral for lung transplant should begin prior to the urgent need of transplantation to give sufficient time for patients to undergo adequate pretransplant evaluations and address modifiable risk factors. Underlying disease will also influence the timing of referral. Contraindications to lung transplantation are based on risk factors for poor posttransplant outcomes (Table 52-9). Patients with severe cardiac disease can be considered for combined heart–lung transplantation but are not candidates for isolated lung transplant. A Lung Allocation System, developed by the United Network for Organ Sharing, is used, with candidates given a lung allocation score to determine their waitlist status. This system weighs the net benefit of transplant and clinical urgency, with higher scores indicating greater potential benefit and higher urgency.[101]

Patient evaluation requires a multidisciplinary approach. Patients are screened for malignancy, prior and/or current

Table 52-8 Lung Recipient Selection Guidelines

General Indications
Chronic, end-stage lung disease
High risk of death (>50%) from lung disease within 2 y
High chance of 5-y survival (>80%) from general medical perspective assuming normal graft function
Disease-specific Indications
Chronic Obstructive Pulmonary Disease
BODE index score of 5–6 with increased mortality risk factors
FEV_1 <20–25% of predicted value
Pulmonary artery to aorta diameter >1 on CT scan
Clinical deterioration despite maximal medical therapy
Poor quality of life
Interstitial Lung Disease
Any form of pulmonary fibrosis with FVC <80% predicted or DLCO <40% predicted
Chronic O_2 requirement at rest or exertion
Rapid disease progression despite medical therapy
Cystic Fibrosis
FEV_1 <40% with limited 6 min walk distance, hypoxemia/hypercapnia, pulmonary hypertension, massive hemoptysis, etc.
FEV_1 <25% predicted
Rapid decline in lung function or acute worsening of symptoms
Chronic respiratory failure with hypoxemia and hypercapnia, hemoptysis, mechanical ventilation
Pulmonary hypertension
Worsening nutritional status, weight loss BMI <18 kg/m^2
Frequent exacerbations or hospitalizations
Pulmonary Hypertension
ESC/ERS intermediate or high risk, REVEAL risk score >8 despite appropriate medical therapy
Severe RV dysfunction despite medical therapy
IV or SC prostacyclin therapy
Worsening disease despite maximal medical therapy
Secondary liver of kidney dysfunction due to PAH
Pediatric
NYHA class III or IV
Rapid decline in FEV_1 for those with CF
IV or SC prostacyclin therapy for those with PAH
Disease unresponsive to maximal medical therapy
Diminished growth

FEV_1, forced expiratory volume in 1 second; NYHA, New York Heart Association; PAH, pulmonary arterial hypertension; SC, subcutaneous; IV, intravenous; ESC/ERS, European Society of Cardiology/European Respiratory Society; RV, right ventricle; BMI, body mass index; FVC, forced vital capacity; DLCO, diffusing capacity for carbon monoxide; BODE index, BMI, airflow limitation (forced expiratory volume in one second), dyspnea and 6-min walk distance.

From Leard LE, Holm AM, Valapour M, et al. Consensus document for the selection of lung transplant candidates: An update from the International Society for Heart and Lung Transplantation. *J Heart Lung Transplant*. 2021;40(11):1349–1379.

Table 52-9 Risk Factors for Poor Lung Transplant Outcomes

Absolute contraindication	Lack of patient willingness or acceptance of transplant Malignancy with high risk of recurrence of death GFR <40 mL/min/1.73 m^2 ACS or MI within 30 d Stroke within 30 d Liver cirrhosis Acute liver failure Acute renal failure Septic shock Active extrapulmonary or disseminated infection Active TB infection Active HIV infection with detectable viral load Limited functional status Progressive cognitive impairment Habit of nonadherence Active substance abuse or dependence
Risk factors for high or substantially increased risk of poor outcome	Age >70 y Cardiac comorbidity (CAD, LVEF <40%, severe CVA) Severe esophageal dysmotility Hematologic disorders difficult to treat BMI >35 kg/m^2 or <16 kg/m^2 Limited functional status Psychosocial limitations Infection with specific species (*Burkholderia cenocepacia, Myocobacterium abscessus*, etc.) Hepatitis B or C with detectable viral load ECMO Retransplant
General risk factors	Age 65–70 y old GFR 40–60 mL/min/1.73 m^2 History of CAD or LVEF 40–50% Peripheral vascular disease Connective tissue disease Severe GERD or esophageal dysmotility Pancytopenia Osteoporosis BMI 30–35 or 16–17 Frailty, poor nutritional status Poorly controlled diabetes Substance use (marijuana, vaping) Previous thoracic surgery HIV with nondetectable viral load

From Leard LE, Holm AM, Valapour M, et al. Consensus document for the selection of lung transplant candidates: An update from the International Society for Heart and Lung Transplantation. *J Heart Lung Transplant*. 2021;40(11):1349–1379.

infections, and vaccination status. Gastric esophageal reflux and gastric emptying are assessed through esophagogastroduodenoscopy and swallow studies as aspiration can be detrimental for new graft function. Pulmonary function testing, lung volume plethysmograph, arterial blood gas, and 6-minute walk tests are performed to evaluate patient's pulmonary status. Cardiac evaluation includes left and right heart catheterization and transthoracic echocardiography (TTE). Lung transplantation is not advocated for acute disease processes, such as acute respiratory distress syndrome. However, there are a limited but growing number of case reports for lung transplants being performed for those patients with the novel SARS-CoV-2 virus. Specific age limits were recommended in the past; however, current guidelines list age more than 65 years as a risk factor only. CF is associated with complex chronic pulmonary infections and colonization with microbial flora that can negatively affect transplant outcomes. However, even colonization with *Burkholderia cenocepacia or gladioli* is now considered to be only a relative contraindication and most CF patients can be successfully transplanted despite chronic bacterial infections.[100]

It is not uncommon for candidates to be on the waitlist for an extended period of time. Therefore, it is essential to review recent laboratory and functional data as disease progression may have resulted in change in status since the original workup. Lung transplant candidates have poor pulmonary status and are frequently receiving multiple therapies including oxygen, inhaled bronchodilators, steroids, and pulmonary vasodilators. It is critical to confirm the ABO compatibility of the donor and recipient prior to surgery.

Intraoperative Management

Lung transplant patients are understandably anxious. However, they have minimal pulmonary reserve, and sedation must be given carefully under monitored conditions. After determining oxygen saturation, slow incremental dosing of a short-acting benzodiazepine (0.25 to 2.0 mg of midazolam) may be used for anxiolysis. Premedication with narcotics such as fentanyl must be administered with extreme caution, if at all, because of their ventilatory depressant effect. Because these procedures are done on an urgent or emergent basis, the patient often presents with a full stomach. Use of metoclopramide, histamine-2 antagonists, and a nonparticulate antacid are usually warranted.

Lung transplant recipients are often chronically intravascularly volume depleted, and chronic pulmonary hypertension is common. These factors predispose the patients to hypotension and decreased CO upon anesthetic induction. Having a preinduction arterial line for invasive blood pressure monitoring is crucial. Many patients are unable to rest in a supine or in Trendelenburg position during the preinduction phase. Placement of a single large-bore peripheral intravenous catheter is usually adequate for initiation of the anesthetic, with central venous access achieved after induction. Induction of anesthesia with a pharmacologic agent that will ensure hemodynamic stability such as etomidate is advised. Rapid sequence induction is often performed to reduce aspiration risk. A single-lumen tube is adequate for an *en bloc*, double-lung transplant using CPB, but lung isolation is necessary for other surgical approaches. Lung isolation can be achieved with a double-lumen tube or a single-lumen tube with a bronchial blocker, depending on the type of lung transplant. The double-lumen tube, compared to bronchial blockade techniques, is less prone to dislodgement, improves deflation of the operative lung during dissection, allows better suctioning of secretions, and permits the application of continuous positive airway pressure to the operative lung if indicated. A bronchial blocker is more easily dislodged with surgical manipulation and requires repositioning midsurgery in the case of a bilateral sequential procedure. A left-sided double-lumen tube is preferred because a right-sided tube may be difficult to position relative to the right upper lobe bronchus. Once the patient is intubated, a TEE probe is typically inserted to monitor the patient's cardiac status throughout the surgical duration. Central venous access is achieved. Placement of a PAC is often warranted for monitoring CO and PVR, with a catheter capable of continuous CO and mixed venous oxygenation saturation (MVO_2) preferred.

Maintenance of anesthesia is achieved using a balanced anesthetic technique of volatile anesthetics, neuromuscular blockers, opioids, and other adjuvant analgesic medications. Concerns about hemodynamic instability in this patient population may restrict the anesthetic doses that can be administered, and this may increase the risk of awareness. Monitoring with processed electroencephalography may thus be useful; anesthetic management guided by bispectral index monitoring has been associated with a reduction of the incidence of intraoperative awareness. Muscle relaxation can be maintained with nondepolarizing neuromuscular blocking agents such as rocuronium or vecuronium that are associated with minimal hemodynamic side effects. Nitrous oxide is rarely used because it may exacerbate bullous emphysematous disease, pulmonary hypertension, or intraoperative hypoxemia. Broad-spectrum antibiotics are initiated prior to surgical incision given the high infection risk. Induction of an immunosuppressive regimen can be started intraoperatively or postoperatively. Monoclonal antibodies (basiliximab) and polyclonal agents (antilymphocyte, antithymocyte globulin) are the two main immunosuppressant agents used.

During the early phases of surgical exposure, normocarbia is maintained on two-lung ventilation with a lung-protective tidal volume ventilation strategy of 6 to 8 mL/kg of ideal body weight. Patients are typically maintained on 100% FiO_2 in anticipation of one-lung ventilation to follow. During one-lung ventilation, a decrease in tidal volume to 4 to 5 mL/kg of ideal body weight is recommended with peak airway pressures not to exceed 30 cmH_2O. FiO_2 may be titrated to maintain oxygen saturation above 88%. However, hypoxia is common during this period and any weaning from 100% FiO_2 may be unattainable. Strategies to improve oxygenation and ventilation are discussed in detail in Chapter 38: these include the application of PEEP to the dependent lung and CPAP to the nondependent lung. The I:E ratio may be adjusted. Modern anesthesia machines can be adjusted to pressure-controlled ventilation or other advanced ventilatory modes. PA clamping of the nonventilated lung can be performed by the surgeon in refractory hypoxia. CPB or venovenous (VV)/venoarterial (VA) ECMO is indicated during lung transplantation if adequate oxygenation cannot be maintained despite ventilatory and pharmacologic maneuvers and PA clamping. Other indications for CPB include inability to provide adequate ventilation, or RV failure.

Hemodynamic instability is not uncommon during the surgical procedure, especially during PA clamping, partial left atrium clamping for pulmonary vein cuff anastomosis, and reperfusion. Hypotension can be treated with direct α-agonist agents such as norepinephrine or phenylephrine. Vasopressin is a good choice as it does not increase PVR. Lung transplant recipients often have reduced RV function due to underlying pulmonary hypertension. Inotropic agents such as epinephrine, dobutamine, and milrinone can be used if RV dysfunction is noted. iNO or epoprostenol may also be used if RV dysfunction is suspected from a rise in PA pressure. Mechanical circulatory support (MCS) systems should always be available in case hemodynamic stability becomes difficult to achieve with pharmacologic agents alone. Due to the risk of pulmonary edema and PGD, a conservative fluid resuscitation strategy is recommended. Colloid administration is preferred over crystalloid for volume resuscitation, with careful attention paid to the total amount of fluids being administered. The transfusion of blood products, especially in large volumes, is generally avoided due to a high risk of subsequent PGD. Vasoactive drugs should be used to maintain hemodynamics, and fluids should be administered as intermittent boluses while keeping CVP less than 7 cmH_2O. CO monitoring using PAC, or minimally invasive techniques such as esophageal Doppler or pulse contour analysis, is useful for guiding fluid administration while assuring adequate CO. Lung recipients are susceptible to pulmonary hypertension and RV dysfunction or failure during single-lung ventilation. Optimizing oxygenation and ventilation does not always improve RV function, and vasodilator and/or inotropic support may be required. iNO is an option for improving respiratory and right heart function.

While the use of specific mechanical circulatory devices is largely institutionally dependent, the mechanical circulatory devices that can be employed during lung transplants include VV ECMO, VA ECMO, and CPB. In patients with normal cardiac function and limited hemodynamic instability but refractory hypoxemia, VV ECMO may suffice. VA ECMO or full CPB may be necessary in those with limited cardiac reserve, severe hemodynamic instability, and refractory hypoxemia. ECMO has the advantage of needing less anticoagulation. There is also growing data to suggest that VA ECMO is noninferior to CPB with lower rates of PGD, bleeding complications, need for dialysis, and a shorter intubation period and overall hospital stay.[102–104]

After pneumonectomy, the surgeon will size the donor vascular tissue to the recipient vessels and sequentially anastomose the atrial/pulmonary vein patch, bronchus, and PA. The donor lung is kept cold with ice in the surgical field until reperfusion. Once the donor lungs are transplanted and vascular anastomosis completed, reinflation of the lungs ensues with several recruitment breaths followed by the reinitiation of lung protective ventilation with low tidal volumes. The surgical anastomotic site is checked with a bronchoscope, often by the anesthesiologist. Methylprednisolone is administered prior to reperfusion of the graft. TEE is useful to assess pulmonary venous drainage and PA blood flow patterns and velocities in the transplanted lung. Systemic hypotension can occur during reperfusion but it is usually not as significant as is seen with liver graft reperfusion. Along with *ex vivo* perfusion, Perfadex, a low–molecular-weight dextran solution, improves early graft function and is used widely for preservation during procurement. There can nonetheless be reperfusion injury to the lung presenting as pulmonary edema. PEEP and lung protective strategies are particularly useful in this scenario. Particular attention should be paid to eliminating excessive peak airway pressures and PEEP to avoid disruption of the surgical anastomoses. High FiO_2 has been associated with PGD. The FiO_2 is quickly weaned down (typically to about 40% to 50% FiO_2) and titrated to maintain SpO_2 above 92%. Once surgical closure is completed, unless there is a contraindication, the double-lumen tube is exchanged for a single-lumen tube (preferably larger than 8.0 mm in internal diameter) to promote ease of management in the ICU. The large diameter facilitates postoperative bronchopulmonary toilet and diagnostic bronchoscopy, as needed. Significant oropharyngeal edema, high PEEP requirement, or a need for differential lung ventilation justifies leaving the double-lumen tube in place postoperatively to allow improvement in clinical status prior to endotracheal tube exchange. In the absence of contraindications, consideration of early extubation should be discussed with the surgeon so narcotic use can be minimized and multimodal analgesia can be used.

Lung-transplant recipients recover in the ICU postprocedure. They are typically extubated within 24 hours of surgery, provided their clinical condition is stable. Postoperative pain control can be challenging. Thoracic epidural catheters are placed preoperatively at some centers, especially in patients who are believed unlikely to require CPB with its associated anticoagulation. Another option is to place the epidural in the early postoperative period, after coagulopathies are corrected. The epidural can be placed using light sedation during weaning from mechanical ventilation, allowing better neurologic monitoring and pain control prior to tracheal extubation. Other options for postoperative pain relief include postoperative paravertebral blocks, and intercostal nerve blocks performed intraoperatively. Multimodal analgesic techniques, including patient-controlled analgesia, dexmedetomidine infusion, intravenous acetaminophen, and nonsteroidal anti-inflammatory agents, are now standard components of enhanced recovery after surgery programs.[105]

Single-Lung Transplantation

9 Single-lung transplantation accounts for about 15% to 20% of all lung transplants. Single-lung transplantation can be performed via anterior or posterior lateral thoracotomy, or midline sternotomy. A lateral thoracotomy approach is often preferred due to better exposure of the hilum of the lung. Prior to ligation of the PA and vein, the PA may be temporarily clamped to assess the rise in PA pressure. If the PA pressure rise is excessive and RV dysfunction is noted, then MCS with either CPB or ECMO will be needed. If this is the case, the patient must be positioned to allow rapid access to either the aorta and right atrium or the femoral artery and vein. This can be accomplished via either anterior thoracotomy with partial sternotomy or lateral thoracotomy with decreased angulation of the hips to allow access to the femoral vessels. Determination of the operative side is based on preoperative ventilation–perfusion studies and prior thoracic surgeries. The lung with poorer function is typically the one replaced.

Double-Lung Transplantation

Bilateral double lung transplant accounts for about 80% of adult lung transplants and 97% of pediatric lung transplants.[106,107] Bilateral lung transplant is typically performed in the supine position, using a transverse thoracosternotomy ("clamshell" incision) approach. The arms can be suspended on a padded bar above the patient or tucked at the sides. If the arms are suspended, care must be taken to avoid stretching the brachial plexi. These cases can also be performed via midline sternotomy or bilateral anterior thoracotomy. *En bloc* double-lung transplantation requires CPB, and a single-lumen endotracheal tube is sufficient. Bilateral sequential transplantation requires lung isolation, preferably via a double-lumen endotracheal tube. Bilateral sequential transplantation is now the preferred procedure because a tracheal anastomosis is unnecessary and there is less surgical bleeding. Most centers electively institute ECMO or CPB for this procedure if preoperative pulmonary hypertension is present, and urgent ECMO or CPB if difficulties in oxygenation, ventilation, or RV dysfunction develop. Typically, the more severely diseased lung is transplanted first. If the disease is homogenous, the right lung is often transplanted first. Serial implantation implies a longer ischemic time for the second lung, but this has not been shown to adversely affect outcome. Once the first allograft is in, one-lung ventilation and perfusion can be resumed in the allograft while the contralateral side is transplanted. Once the contralateral side transplant is complete, chest tubes can be placed. MCS, if used, will be weaned off. Chest closure will ensue. At the conclusion of the case, the double-lumen tube should be exchanged for a single-lumen tube, provided it is safe to do so. Tube exchange over an airway exchange catheter is recommended as airway swelling during the surgical case can lead to difficult intubating conditions. The clamshell incision is extensive and can cause significant postoperative pain. A thoracic epidural may be very useful for managing postoperative pain.

Pediatric Lung Transplantation

The Registry of the ISHLT pediatric report indicates 2,323 lung transplants were performed between 1992 and 2018.[107] Pediatric lung transplantation has increased over the past 15 years, with adolescents undergoing the majority of the procedures. The most common diagnoses are CF (although the number of CF recipients has declined in Europe and elsewhere between 2010 and 2018), congenital heart disease, COPD, and idiopathic pulmonary fibrosis/hypertension. Overall survival is similar for pediatric and adult populations. There appeared to be age-related survival differences, with infants doing better than adolescents in the past. However, survival in adolescents (age 11 to 17 years) has improved drastically compared to previous decades.[107,108] Overall, survival rates are about 85% at 1 year and about 70% at 5 years. Regardless of mortality outcome, quality of life still appears to be improved by lung transplantation in many patients. The role of lung transplantation in the treatment of CF deserves further study to determine firm indications and the optimal age and pretransplant diagnosis and status. Most pediatric patients receive double-lung transplantation with CPB via a clamshell incision, with a single-lumen endotracheal tube. Central and arterial access is necessary for perioperative monitoring.

Primary Graft Dysfunction

Lung transplant complications include PGD, acute and chronic graft rejection, airway and vascular anastomotic site complications, pleural complications, and infections. The most common causes of acute transplanted lung failure are acute graft rejection, inadequate pulmonary venous drainage, and PGD. The etiology of PGD, a major cause of posttransplant morbidity and mortality, is multifactorial and complex. PGD, defined as allograft dysfunction within 72 hours of transplantation, is graded on a scale of 0 to 3.[109] Grade 3 is defined as Pao_2/Fio_2 less than 200 with radiographic infiltrates consistent with pulmonary edema. Grade 3 PGD is associated with significantly high 30-day mortality.[110] Grades 1 and 2 are also associated with infiltrates, but are less severe, with Pao_2/Fio_2 ratios greater than 300 and between 200 and 300, respectively. Grade 0 is essentially a normal lung, in which the Pao_2/Fio_2 ratio is greater than 300 and there are no pulmonary infiltrates. Recipient risk factors for PGD include female sex, African American race, obesity, idiopathic pulmonary fibrosis, sarcoidosis, and idiopathic pulmonary arterial hypertension. Donor risk factors include history of smoking, heavy alcohol use, lung contusions, or aspiration along with older age. Surgical risk factors include long ischemic time and massive transfusion. The role of CPB as a contributing factor to PGD is unclear, with conflicting results. The transplant literature does not show a correlation between fluid management in the OR and outcome, although management of pulmonary transplant patients as if they have acute lung injury with a protective strategy as described earlier is recommended. Severe, life-threatening PGD has been successfully managed with ECMO.[111]

Inhaled Nitric Oxide

iNO therapy may be used to decrease PVR and improve oxygenation (see Chapter 38). iNO has an extremely short duration of action in vivo, rapidly inactivated by reacting with heme, resulting in methemoglobin. Because iNO is preferentially delivered to ventilated areas, vascular relaxation in these areas leads to improved blood flow and hence improvements in ventilation–perfusion matching and oxygenation. Rapid inactivation of iNO in the pulmonary vasculature prevents its systemic distribution and avoids systemic vasodilatation and hypotension.

The relative merits of routine intraoperative use of iNO versus restricted use of iNO remain subject to debate. iNO can decrease PVR, improve oxygenation, decrease inflammatory response to surgery or trauma, impede microbial growth, and its hemodynamic effect is limited only to the pulmonary system. Proponents argue that the use of iNO in the recipient, and possibly even the donor, takes advantage of the immunomodulatory and antimicrobial activities of NO to reduce recipient lung injury.[112] Opponents argue that iNO use should be limited as data seem to show no benefit to iNO in preventing reperfusion injury or PGD.[113,114] NO may mediate other clinically beneficial effects through activation of guanylate cyclase in platelets to attenuate platelet aggregation and adhesion.[115] Early initiation of iNO post lung transplant in recipients with pulmonary hypertension has shown efficacy in preventing acute graft rejection.[116] The authors recommend that the use of iNO should be based on specific clinical circumstances.

Heart–Lung Transplant (Adult and Pediatric)

The first successful combined heart—lung transplantation was performed in 1981. Heart–lung transplantation is the least common intrathoracic transplant procedure with the ISHLT reporting a total of 1,532 adult heart—lung transplants performed between January 1992 to December 2018.[117] ISHLT reports 733 pediatric heart—lung transplantation performed during the same time frame.[118] Bilateral sequential lung transplant has largely replaced heart–lung transplantation, and improved pharmacologic management of pulmonary hypertension and RV failure obviates the need for the heart–lung procedure. Because indications for lung transplantation have evolved to replace heart–lung transplant for diagnoses such as primary pulmonary hypertension and CF, congenital heart disease and idiopathic pulmonary hypertension are now the most common indications for heart–lung transplantation.[117]

Anesthetic management of heart–lung transplant patients is similar to that of isolated heart or lung transplant patients. Because a tracheal anastomosis is performed, a single-lumen endotracheal tube is sufficient. The endotracheal tube is either removed or withdrawn above the suture line during CPB to facilitate the tracheal anastomosis. Inotropes may be needed for RV dysfunction immediately after bypass. Pulmonary reperfusion injury can also occur, requiring management of acute lung injury as described for lung transplantation.

Heart Transplantation

Since Christian Barnard performed the first successful heart transplant in South Africa in 1967, the procedure has become accepted practice for treatment of heart failure recalcitrant to medical therapy. In this section, anesthetic considerations for patients undergoing heart transplantation, as well as a brief overview of mechanical circulatory devices for heart failure are discussed. Over 84,297 individuals have received heart transplants in the United States since 1988 (data provided by OPTN). The median wait time for status 1A patients is 87 days while wait times for status 1B and 2 patients range from 250 to 726 days. Currently, more than 3,400 patients await heart transplants. Overall 1-year survival has improved from 74% in the early 1980s to 90% currently. The 5-year survival for primary transplantation is currently 79%. Nonischemic cardiomyopathy is the leading cause of heart transplants, followed closely by ischemic cardiomyopathy from coronary artery disease. The number of patients with congenital heart disease, hypertrophic cardiomyopathy, and restrictive cardiomyopathy from amyloidosis presenting for cardiac transplantation has steadily increased over the years. As the population ages and the use of cardiac transplantation and mechanical assist devices expands, increasing numbers of patients will present for transplantation, management of previous transplantation, or for mechanical assist devices.

Short-, Intermediate-, and Long-Term Mechanical Circulatory Support Systems

Survival rates for patients with congestive heart failure (CHF) have improved over the years with advancement in medical therapy. However, the 1-year mortality rate remains at 21% for men and 17% for women, and 5-year mortality remains at 50% for men and 46% for women.[119] The general management of heart failure centers around the modification of causes and associated comorbidities through pharmacologic therapy and lifestyle changes. However, those patients who are refractory to medical treatment may be offered cardiac implantable electronic devices (CIEDs) and MCS devices. Patients with end-stage heart failure who have mechanical cardiac support experience better survival and quality of life than those receiving medical management alone.[120] MCS devices may be offered to the patient as a bridge-to-recovery, bridge-to-transplantation, or destination therapy. MCS can be categorized into short-term versus intermediate- to long-term devices. Short-term MCS include the intra-aortic balloon pump (IABP), percutaneous MCS (such as Impella or Tandem Heart), and ECMO. Intermediate- to long-term devices include ventricular assist devices (VADs). The purpose of these devices is to provide hemodynamic support by augmenting the work of the native LV and RV.

IABPs are placed into the descending thoracic aorta and serve to augment coronary perfusion pressure during diastole through inflation of the balloon pump. During systole, the IABP provides afterload reduction by a vacuum effect created by the rapidly deflating balloon. If further LV systolic function augmentation is needed, then a percutaneous MCS such as the Impella can be placed. The Impella (Abiomed, Danvers, MA) is a catheter-based co-axial pump device that is inserted across the aortic valve. It pumps blood from the LV to the aorta and helps decompress the failing LV. The TandemHeart (Cardiac Assist Inc., Pittsburgh, PA) is a percutaneous VAD placed for short-term hemodynamic circulatory support (Fig. 52-3). The left-sided cannula is advanced from the femoral vein into the left atrium by puncturing the interatrial septum. It provides left atrial to iliac artery bypass and is powered by a centrifugal pump located externally. If additional mechanical support is needed, then an ECMO device can be instituted. ECMO can be initiated through percutaneous cannulation in the femoral vein/artery or internal jugular vein, or through central cannulation via median sternotomy. ECMO has the advantage of being able to provide oxygenation and ventilation through a membrane oxygenator in addition to the ventricular support provided by an IABP or Impella.

LVADs vary in significant ways, and it is important to understand the specifics of the LVAD being used. Variations include flow pattern (pulsatile or nonpulsatile), requirement for anticoagulation (none, aspirin, warfarin), filling pattern, power source (battery or alternating current), potential for electromagnetic interference, and impact of dysrhythmias and defibrillation on the device. Acetone-containing products and Betadine should be avoided near these devices because they can damage the cannula or drive lines. There are currently three generations of LVADs that are commercially available. First-generation LVADs are pulsatile positive displacement pumps that provided excellent

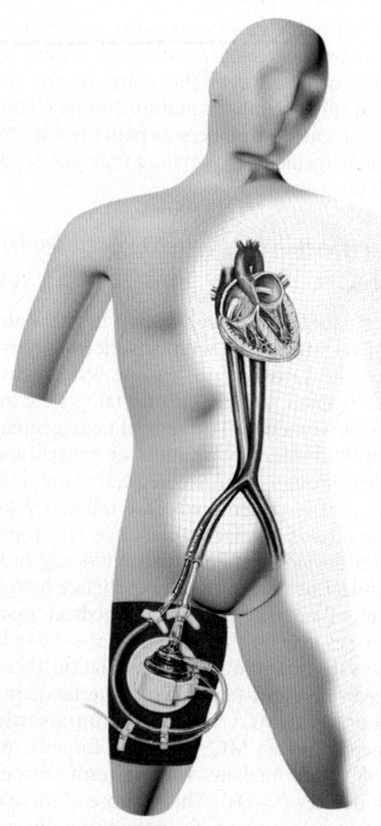

Figure 52-3 TandemHeart percutaneous ventricular assist device. Cannulas are placed percutaneously into the femoral vein and femoral artery, and the drive mechanism and power supply are external. The femoral venous line is placed across the atrial septum so as to drain the left atrium. Minimally invasive placement is a significant advantage of this system. (Courtesy TandemLife, Inc.)

hemodynamic support and improved mortality. Examples of first-generation devices include HeartMate I, Thoratec (Abbott Laboratories, Pleasanton, CA), paracorporeal ventricular assist device (PVAD), and Novacor (Baxter Healthcare Corporation, Berkeley, CA). However, due to limited durability and complication rates, these are now rarely used. Second- and third-generation devices are continuous-flow devices with a smaller size and a single moving part. These are silent, have increased durability, and are easier to implant. Second-generation devices use continuous axial flow and include Heartmate II (Abbott Laboratories, Pleasanton, CA) and the Jarvik 2000 (Jarvik Heart Inc., New York, NY). With Heartmate II (Fig. 52-4), the flow pump sits outside the LV in between the inflow and outflow cannula. It can generate up to 10 L/min of flow. The Jarvik 2000 flow pump sits at the LV apex and can generate up to 7 L/min of flow. Third-generation LVADs (Fig. 52-4) use continuous centrifugal flow and include Heartmate 3 (Abbott Laboratories, Pleasanton, CA) and HeartWare (Medtronic, Dublin, Ireland). They are generally known for their long durability (5 to 10 years), low thromboembolic risks, and even more compact size compared to second-generation devices. The HeartWare has a single moving impeller that is hydrodynamically suspended in the housing chamber which is attached at the LV apex. The impeller can spin up to a rate of 4,000 rpm and generate up to 10 L/min of flow. The Heartmate 3 uses a magnetically levitating centrifugal rotor which is directly implanted into the LV apex. The centrifugal pump can spin at rate of 3,000 to 9,000 rpm and generate up to 10 L/min of flow. The relative benefits of these devices are mixed. When comparing HeartWare to HeartMate II, HeartWare seemed to have a higher rate of complication including strokes and RV failure, while patients receiving the HeartMate II had higher rates of device failure and malfunction.[121] Both devices showed similar improvement in functional status and survival. The MOMENTUM 3 trial found higher survival, free of disabling strokes, and lower reoperation rates or replacement of device due to device malfunction for HeartMate 3 compared to HeartMate II.[122,123] The SynCardia total artificial heart (SynCardia Systems, Tucson, AZ) is the only singular device that is currently used for implantation worldwide for biventricular support. However, the Thoratec PVAD can be implanted into both the right and left ventricle (BiVAD) to support biventricular function.

As VADs become more common, it is crucial for anesthesiologists to be familiar with the anesthetic management of patients with VADs undergoing cardiac and noncardiac surgery. Patients presenting for initial device placement are in various stages of decompensated heart failure and require advanced monitoring, often with an arterial line and either PA or central venous catheter. Careful titration of inotropic agents and vasopressors may be necessary during the procedure. TEE is vital for VAD placement to confirm the correct positioning of guide wires, and is also indicated to evaluate for valve pathologies and intracardiac shunts that may complicate LVAD placement and to guide intraoperative management of volume status and vasoactive medications. A repeated TEE examination is performed after device placement to confirm proper cannula placement and flow.

For patients with LVADs presenting for noncardiac surgery, a preoperative evaluation of the LVAD parameters, anticoagulation status, and comorbidities will be important. The make and model of the device, implantation date, pump speed, flow, and power along with pulsatility index (PI) should be noted prior to the operation. Once in the OR, the LVAD should be switched from battery power to a wall electrical power outlet through the power base unit. The power base unit displays the parameters of the LVAD. Over time, many patients gain some degree of arterial pulsatility such that a noninvasive blood pressure cuff may be used. If a blood pressure measurement is not obtainable through noninvasive means, then placement of an arterial line is necessary. Ultrasound guidance will generally be necessary for line placement as pulses may not be palpable. The focus of intraoperative hemodynamic management is to maintain preload and afterload for proper functioning of the LVAD. Pump speed is the only adjustable variable on the LVAD and is described in revolutions per minute (RPM). Pump flow is measured in L/min and is calculated based on the pump speed and the pressure gradient across the LVAD pump. Pump power is measured in watts (W) and is dependent upon pump flow. An increase in pump flow generally correlates to an increase in power. A sudden decrease in power can indicate a pump malfunction, mechanical disruption, or thrombosis within the pump system. PI is used to describe the contribution of the native LV to the overall CO. High PI indicates a degree of LV contribution to CO whereas low PI indicates minimal native LV contractility or low intravascular volume. To maintain hemodynamic stability in patients with an LVAD, maintenance of adequate preload and afterload along with adjustment of pump speed is necessary, and avoidance of arrhythmias is crucial. Without adequate preload, the LV walls may be sucked down ("suction event") into the inflow cannula, potentially leading to deadly arrhythmias. Without sufficient afterload, end-organ perfusion may be compromised. However, with too much afterload, LVAD pump flow may decrease leading to stasis of blood in the LV. A rule of thumb is to maintain the patient's MAP within 10% of baseline or at least above 70 mmHg.

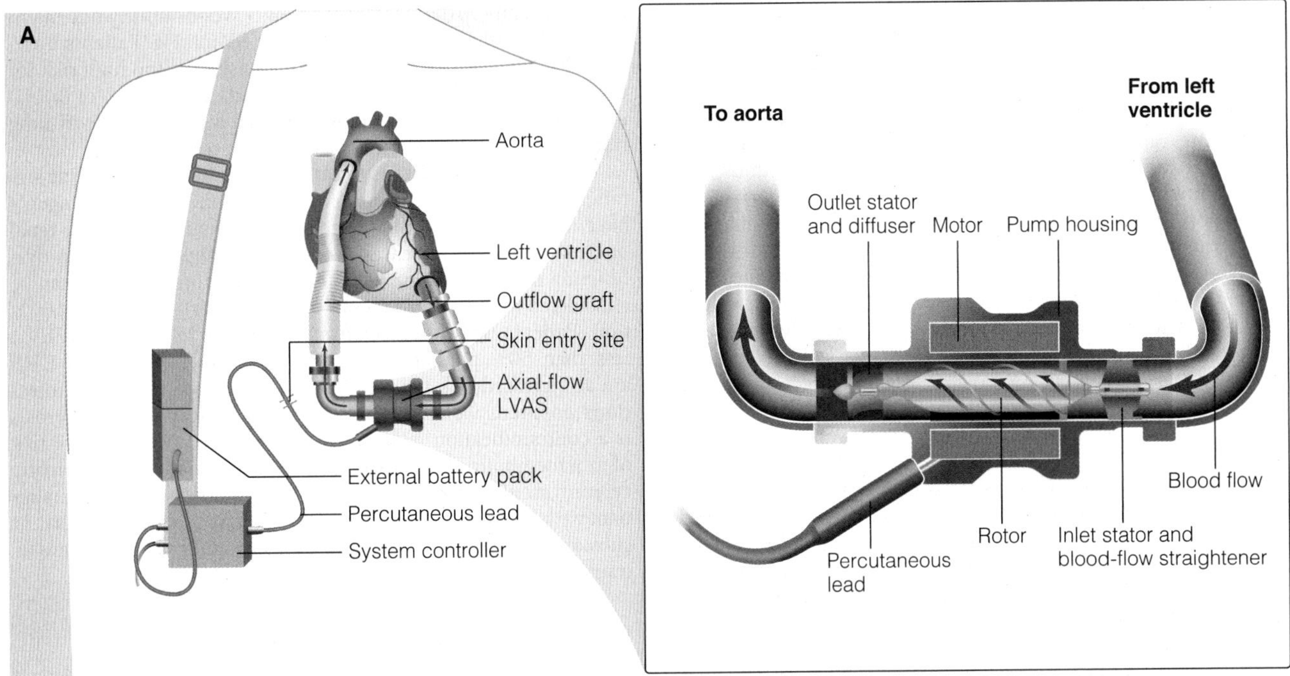

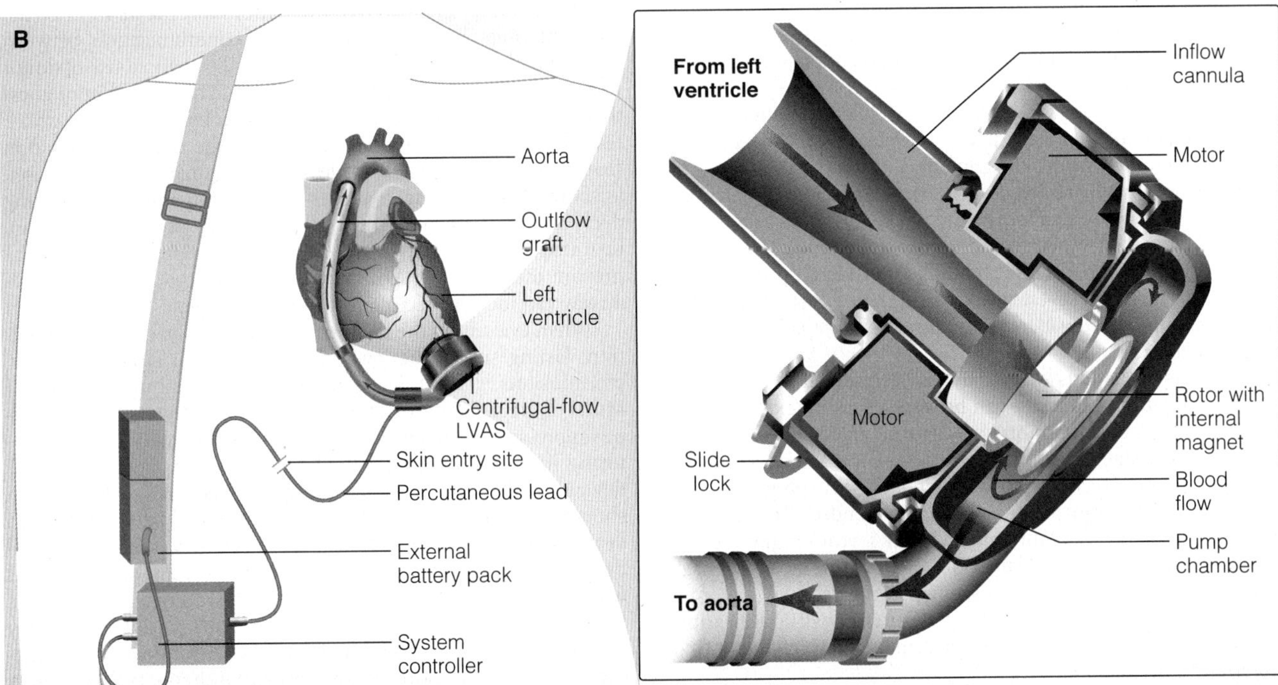

Figure 52-4 **A:** Axial flow pump VAD (HeartMate II). The axial flow pump sits outside the heart. **B**: Centrifugal flow pump VAD (HeartMate 3 and HeartWare). The centrifugal pump is attached to the apex of the left ventricle. (Reprinted by permission from Lee MSL, Altman NL, Branch-Elliman W. Expanding use of new technology creates new challenges in preventing and managing infections: a review of diagnostic and management considerations for infections among patients with long-term invasive devices for advanced heart failure. *Curr Infect Dis Rep*. 2020;22(16). Figure 1.)

An individual familiar with the device should be present to assist with management and troubleshooting if the clinician does not have sufficient experience.

11 Besides MCS systems, many medical interventions exist to extend the life of patients awaiting donors. Pharmacologic options for management of CHF include angiotensin-converting enzyme inhibitors, β-blockers, diuretics, and digoxin. Intravenous inotropic support is common although its use has gone down with the rise in the use of MCS. For transplants performed in 2010 to 2018, 35.7% of recipients were receiving intravenous inotropic

support compared to 43.4% (January 2001 to December 2009) and 46.7% (January 1992 to December 2000) during the previous decades.[124] The use of MCS has increased during the same time period; VAD use has increased from 18.9% (January 2001 to December 2009) to 40.4% (January 2010 to December 2018).[124] In addition, cardiac resynchronization therapy (CRT) has been shown to reduce morbidity and mortality in patients with LV systolic dysfunction, prolonged QRS duration, and New York Heart Association Class III or IV heart failure despite optimal pharmacologic therapy.[125] Many patients presenting for heart transplantation have had a CRT device placed as part of their management, frequently with implantable cardioverter–defibrillator capability as well. CRT can improve symptoms, exercise tolerance, and quality of life in properly selected patients as well as improve survival.[126]

Recipient Selection

More than 5 million Americans have CHF, with the incidence increasing with age. Of these, only about 3,000 per year are listed for heart transplantation. The ISHLT consensus guidelines for the selection of patients for heart transplantation were published in 2006 and updated in 2016.[127,128] In general, patients are referred for transplant evaluation if they have one of the following conditions: New York Heart Association (NYHA) Class IV heart failure despite optimal medical therapy, cardiogenic shock on maximal pharmacologic and MCS, restrictive or hypertrophic cardiomyopathy, intractable life-threatening arrhythmias, or severe ischemic heart disease not amenable to surgical or percutaneous interventions.[128] Those patients with congenital heart disease that is not amenable to palliative surgery or other interventions may also be referred for transplantation.[128] The age limit for transplant referral has remained at 70 although carefully selected patients over 70 years of age may be considered. The maximum BMI allowed has been increased from 30 kg/m^2 to 35 kg/m^2. Assessment of frailty has been newly added as a criterion for recipient selection. The ISHLT also advocates for the use of MCS systems as a bridge to transplant candidacy. Surgical correction of coronary artery disease or valvular heart disease should be considered prior to listing, and patients with severe mitral regurgitation and low ejection fraction should be considered for mitral valve repair instead of transplantation.

Prognosis in patients with CHF has been linked to functional capacity. Functional capacity can be assessed using exercise testing, and oxygen consumption (VO_2) during maximal exercise.[129] In patients on a stable medical regimen, maximal VO_2 less than 10 to 12 mL/kg/min is associated with a poor 1-year prognosis and referral for cardiac transplantation is recommended. Patients with VO_2 more than 14 mL/kg/min have a better 1-year prognosis with medical therapy than transplantation. Heart failure survival prognosis score (HFSS) may also be used to prognosticate HF patients. There is evidence that the HFSS may be better in risk stratification and prognostication, especially in those patients receiving device therapy.[130]

There are several contraindications to cardiac transplantation. Severe, irreversible pulmonary hypertension is a relative contraindication to transplant because of subsequent RV failure in the newly transplanted heart. Right heart catheterization is performed to determine the transpulmonary gradient (the difference between mean PA pressure and pulmonary capillary wedge pressure) and PVR. A transpulmonary gradient above 16 mmHg or PVR (the ratio of transpulmonary gradient to CO) greater than 5 Woods units is considered relative contraindication for cardiac transplant. To optimize patient condition while awaiting transplant referral, pulmonary vasodilators, inotropic agents, and diuretics may be used to attempt to decrease PVR below 3 Woods units while maintaining a systolic blood pressure above 85 mmHg. Patients unresponsive to these therapies are often considered too high risk for cardiac transplantation and may be candidates for LVAD or BiVAD insertion as destination therapy, although a combined heart-lung transplant may be an alternative treatment option.

Other contraindications to cardiac transplantation include significant noncardiac disease. Because immunosuppressive agents have renal and hepatic side effects, the presence of intrinsic renal or hepatic disease increases the risk of perioperative organ dysfunction or failure. Some patients with multiorgan disease can be considered for combined heart–kidney or heart–liver transplantation. Patients with forced expiratory volume in 1 second (FEV_1) less than 50% predicted despite optimal management of CHF are at increased risk for ventilatory failure and respiratory infections posttransplant. The presence of significant atherosclerosis is a contraindication because of the increased perioperative risk of atheroembolic complications. Severe debilitating symptomatic cerebrovascular disease, severe systemic illness such as malignancy with limited life expectancy, inadequate social support, or substance abuse issues may also be contraindications for cardiac transplantation.

Preanesthetic Considerations

Donor heart function worsens with donor cold ischemia times above 6 hours. For this reason, the timing of transplantation depends on when the donor surgery can be done, frequently during night hours. Preoperative evaluation and preparation of the recipient must be expeditious. Close communication between the donor and recipient teams facilitates the optimal use of donor organs while minimizing ischemia times. The induction of anesthesia and surgical incision of the recipient begin when the donor team has evaluated the donor and made the final determination that the organ is acceptable. Ideally, the recipient heart is excised as soon as the donor heart arrives at the recipient hospital. Timing decisions are based on travel distance and the time necessary to transport the donor organ, as well as the time it will take to prepare the recipient. A history of prior sternotomy or difficult airway can increase recipient preparation time.

When evaluating the recipient, a few issues need special attention: fasting status, the level of cardiovascular support (inotropic infusions, chronic medications for heart failure, presence of MCS), anticoagulation status, antibiotic prophylaxis and immunosuppressive regimen, and presence of hemodynamic monitoring lines or antiarrhythmic devices, such as pacemaker, CRT device, or defibrillator. Cardiac transplants tend to happen on short notice so patients often will not have had adequate time to fast. Rapid sequence induction will be necessary if the patient's nil per os (NPO) status is inadequate. It is not uncommon for patients waiting for cardiac transplantation to be receiving intravenous inotropic support with dobutamine or milrinone. Patients may also be on chronic inhaled or intravenous pulmonary vasodilators to lower PVR. Inotropic support and pulmonary vasodilators should be continued into the OR as abrupt cessation may have hemodynamic consequences. If the patient is receiving hemodynamic support through an MCS, extra care should be taken while transporting the patient to the OR and an expert familiar with the management of the particular MCS should accompany the patient to the OR. Transplant recipients are often anticoagulated with a vitamin K antagonist or direct-acting oral anticoagulant (DOAC). Anticoagulation status should be assessed with laboratory values such as prothrombin time and INR, and reversal of anticoagulation with intravenous vitamin K, prothrombin complex concentrate, or other DOAC-specific agents should be anticipated.

Obtaining a baseline coagulation test with TEG or ROTEM is useful when managing coagulation status. An adequate supply of blood products should be verified. Antibiotic prophylaxis should be confirmed with the surgical team. Typically, a broad-spectrum antibiotic such as vancomycin and a cephalosporin will be administered prior to surgical incision. The immunosuppressive regimen is individualized and institution dependent. The need for preoperative immunosuppression with corticosteroids or other agents should be confirmed with the surgical team prior to surgical incision. Antiarrhythmic devices must be interrogated and reprogrammed to a mode that will not be affected by electrocautery interference. If the patient has had multiple previous central lines, then ultrasound evaluation of the central vessels may be helpful to determine vessel patency. Recent chest radiographs and laboratory studies must be reviewed to assess pulmonary, hepatic, and renal compromise associated with CHF.

Many anesthetic management issues related to the care of the heart transplant patient are similar to those for open-heart surgeries (see Chapter 39), but notable differences are the strictest attention to sterility and immunosuppression, poorer hemodynamic status of transplant candidates, and issues related to early donor heart function and denervation.

Invasive arterial pressure monitoring should be obtained prior to induction and defibrillator pads should be placed. Large-bore intravenous access, whether central or peripheral, is necessary for administration of resuscitation medications and volume during induction. Inotropes should be readily available prior to induction. Dobutamine, epinephrine, milrinone, norepinephrine, dopamine, vasopressin, and phenylephrine have all been used effectively in the perioperative management of heart transplant patients. If the patient has been on chronic intravenous inotropic therapy, this should be continued during induction. A balanced induction technique with an emphasis on hemodynamic stability should be used. Placement of a PAC is favored by many centers and can be typically placed postinduction along with central venous access. Appropriate antibiotics and immunosuppressive therapy are given prior to surgical incision.

Presence of an LVAD or prior sternotomy increases the length of the procedure and its associated risks. Where possible, old medical records should be reviewed to determine if the patient has had prior aprotinin exposure. Epsilon-aminocaproic acid (EACA) or tranexamic acid can be used as an antifibrinolytic agent to decrease perioperative bleeding. Packed red blood cells should be immediately available prior to incision, particularly in repeat sternotomy. The CMV status of the donor and recipient is needed to determine whether CMV-negative packed red blood cells should be ordered. Availability of plasma, platelets, and cryoprecipitate should be confirmed at the start of the procedure. The surgical team may elect to place arterial and venous access sheaths in the femoral artery and vein prior to surgical incision in case CPB needs to be emergently initiated.

Intraoperative Management

The choice of anesthetic technique should be focused on minimizing cardiovascular instability and complications. High-dose narcotic techniques can be safely used for induction. Balanced anesthetic maintenance techniques with benzodiazepines, lower doses of narcotics, intravenous anesthetic agents, and inhalation anesthetics can be used,[131] and early extubation using ultra fast-track protocols has been successful.[132] Cerebral oximetry and processed EEG monitoring are useful to assess global perfusion and depth of anesthesia. Neuromuscular blockade with a nondepolarizing agent is recommended. Hypotension may not respond to ephedrine or phenylephrine, and other inotropes and vasopressors such as epinephrine, norepinephrine, and vasopressin should be instituted rapidly in such cases.

A comprehensive TEE examination should be performed after induction of anesthesia and after weaning from CPB once the new donor heart has been transplanted. Early diagnosis of hemodynamic deterioration can facilitate rapid therapy and hemodynamic stability. The native heart can be monitored prior to CPB for changes in ventricular function or an increase in valvular regurgitation. If the recipient has a MCS device, then the placement of the device and integrity of the surrounding structures should be noted. There is an increased risk of intracardiac thrombus in the native recipient heart, so the left atrium and ventricle should be thoroughly examined and surgical manipulation of the heart should be minimized prior to aortic cross-clamping if thrombus is noted.

Median sternotomy is performed for orthotopic heart transplantation. In the classic biatrial approach, the atria are transected at the grooves, and the right and left atria are anastomosed individually along with pulmonary and aortic vascular anastomoses. However, the bicaval approach (Fig. 52-5), in which anastomoses are created in the superior and inferior vena cava rather than the right atrium, preserves tricuspid valve function and normal conduction in the right atrium. A meta-analysis revealed favorable early and late outcomes using the bicaval technique, so this technique is now performed frequently and is becoming the standard approach.[133]

Heparin dosing is similar to that for other CPB procedures. Cannulation of the aorta is performed high along the ascending aorta, near the aortic arch. The superior and inferior venae cava are cannulated individually. By encircling the cava with tourniquets, all blood flow is directed through the cannula into the bypass circuit, and the surgical field is bloodless. After initiation of CPB, the recipient heart is dissected and excised, except for the left atrial tissue "cuff" encompassing the pulmonary veins. Prior to resection of the native heart, the PAC should be withdrawn from the surgical field. The catheter can be readvanced after removal of the superior cava cannula. Maintenance of CPB and weaning from CPB are associated with the same issues as for other cardiac surgical procedures. Air should be evacuated prior to weaning from CPB. The ischemic time for the donor heart starts with aortic cross-clamping during the harvest and ends with removal of the cross-clamp from the recipient aorta.

Prior to weaning from CPB, the heart is reevaluated with TEE, with attention to ventricular and valvular function. Intracardiac shunts should be ruled out. Anastomotic sites should be evaluated and pleural effusions should be noted. Because the donor heart is denervated, normal physiologic feedback controlling inotropy and chronotropy is lost. A direct-acting cardiac β-receptor agonist such as isoproterenol or epinephrine is used frequently to increase graft heart rate. Use of temporary epicardial pacing is sometimes needed until the β-receptor agonist has had adequate time to reach maximal effect. Severe vasoplegia may be present and multiple vasopressor agents may be necessary to maintain hemodynamic stability. Residual atrial tissue, in the case of biatrial technique, may continue to have electrical activity, and can lead to two P waves noted on ECG (one from native atrial tissue, one from donor). The native P wave has no physiologic effect on the donor heart.

Inotrope selection for weaning from CPB is similar to other cardiac surgical procedures (see Chapter 39). Special consideration should be given to recipients with preoperative pulmonary hypertension, donor hearts with long ischemic times, or donor hearts that are deemed marginal. The risk of donor right heart failure is increased in these cases. The donor right heart is not accustomed to high pulmonary resistance and may fail acutely. Therapy

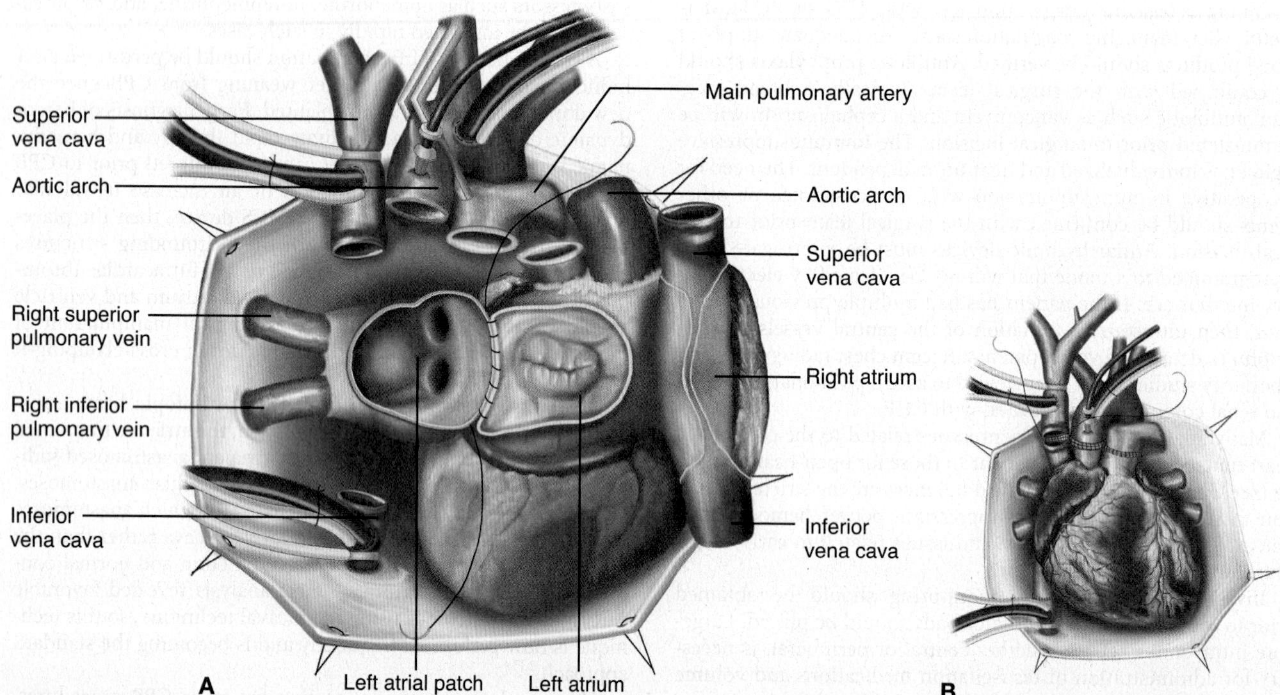

Figure 52-5 Anatomy of bicaval orthotopic heart transplant. **A:** A recipient left atrial patch including the four pulmonary veins remains in the recipient. Anastomoses are performed at the superior and inferior vena cava, aorta, pulmonary artery, and left atrium. **B:** The completed transplantation. (Modified with permission from Lima B, Gonzalez-Stawinski GV. Heart transplants: bicaval versus biatrial techniques. In: Grover FL, Mack MJ, eds. *Master Techniques in Surgery: Cardiac Surgery*. Wolters Kluwer; 2016:409–418.)

for graft right heart failure is similar to therapy for right heart failure in other cardiac cases. The goal is to improve contractility and decrease PVR. If intravenous agents do not facilitate weaning from CPB, iNO and inhaled prostacyclin (iloprost) have been shown to be beneficial in this population.[134] Primary (no identifiable cause) or secondary (identifiable cause such as hyperacute graft rejection or surgical complication) graft dysfunction may be noted while trying to wean from CPB. MCS systems such as ECMO or IABP may be used if weaning from CPB fails after multiple attempts and despite maximal pharmacologic intervention.

Once the patient is weaned from CPB, hemostasis of the surgical field is achieved, chest tubes are placed, and the sternotomy is closed. Patients will remain intubated and sedated at the conclusion of the surgical procedure and will be recovered in the ICU posttransplant. Patients are typically extubated within 24 hours if no immediate perioperative complications such as hemodynamic instability, bleeding, or respiratory issues are present.

Pediatric Heart Transplantation

The International Thoracic Organ Transplant Registry reports over 15,726 pediatric heart transplants performed worldwide since 1992[135] and UNOS reports over 11,200 pediatric heart transplants performed since 1988;[21] about 60% are performed in children less than 1 year or over 11 years old. Congenital heart disease or idiopathic/viral cardiomyopathy are the two leading causes of pediatric heart transplantation, making up about 75% of these patients, with retransplantation due to graft failure an increasing indication. The median age of the recipient has gone up from 6 to 7 years of age over the past decade. Pediatric patients receiving cardiac transplant now present with higher rates of prior cardiac surgery and increased use of intravenous inotropic agents and MCS systems (including ECMO and VADs).[135] One-year survival has risen from 87% during 2000 to 2005 to 92% during 2012 to 2017.[135]

Preoperative evaluation focuses on cardiopulmonary status and the particulars of the cardiac physiology in congenital heart disease patients (see Chapter 39). Palliative procedures may have been performed prior to transplant, and reoperation increases surgical risk. Central venous catheters and intra-arterial catheters are placed routinely, usually after induction. After an inhalation induction, anesthetic management frequently involves high-dose narcotics and intermittent benzodiazepines.

Marginal donors are, not surprisingly, also being used for pediatric heart grafts, including size mismatches, high donor inotrope requirement, prolonged ischemic time, and ABO mismatch.[136] Although ABO-incompatible transplantation is contraindicated in the adult population, it is more successful in infant recipients.[137,138] Hyperacute rejection does not occur because of the immaturity of the immune system and the absence of antibodies to various antigens, including blood group antigens. For ABO mismatched grafts, recipient isohemagglutinin titers are obtained pretransplantation and plasma exchange is performed during CPB. Four-year follow-up data show similar morbidity and mortality compared with ABO-compatible recipients, and waiting list survival is improved because of expansion of the donor pool.

Cardiac Transplantation from Donation after Circulatory Determination of Death

Despite advancements in medical management of heart failure and MCS systems, there remains a global shortage of organs for transplantation and many patients die while awaiting organ availability. The concept of organ transplantation from donation after circulatory determination of death (DCDD or DCD) donors is not new, and DCD liver, kidney, and pancreas transplants are not uncommon in the United States. However, there were only 12 DCD cardiac transplants in the United States between 2010 to 2019, with most DCD heart transplants performed in European countries. Recently, there has been a steady increase in cardiac transplants from DCD donors in the United States with 349 DCD cardiac transplants performed in 2020 and 2021. While logistical and ethical/legal concerns exist, multiple professional societies including UNOS, ISHLT, and SCCM have published statements in support of DCD heart transplants.[139]

There are two main mechanisms by which the DCD heart can be procured: direct procurement and perfusion (DPP) and normothermic regional perfusion (NRP). DPP involves removal of the heart after declaration of death and evaluation of the organ *ex situ* in an organ perfusion machine such as the TransMedics Organ Care System (TransMedics, Andover, MA). NRP involves ligation of the aortic arch vessels to achieve cessation of blood flow to the brain after declaration of circulatory death, followed by reestablishment of circulatory flow through CPB or ECMO, and evaluation of the organ function *in situ* in the organ donor. Both methods have been used successfully with promising results in different countries and institutions.[140,141] The method used for organ recovery is dependent upon institutional preference and local regulations. Management of the donor is under the responsibility of the ICU team. Once the donor is declared dead by the ICU team, then the procurement team is allowed to prepare the donor's body for procurement. Management of the recipient is as mentioned in the previous section.

Management of the Transplant Patient for Nontransplant Surgery

As the population of transplant recipients has increased, the incidence of elective or emergent nontransplant surgery in these patients has grown. These patients cannot always return to the transplant center for surgery, so anesthesiologists outside transplant centers often encounter these patients. For solid-organ recipients, evaluation of patients is centered on the function of the grafted organ. In renal and liver transplant patients, the level of renal dysfunction will often determine the choice of drugs such as antibiotics and neuromuscular blockers, and dose modification or avoidance of drugs undergoing renal excretion may be necessary. A major consideration for renal transplant recipients is maintenance of renal perfusion with adequate systemic arterial pressure and volume replacement. Thus, a low threshold should be used in employing advanced monitoring such as intra-arterial pressure and minimally invasive CO with stroke volume variation. In major surgeries with large fluid shifts, or situations in which major organ function is tenuous, CVP monitoring should be considered. Likewise, TEE may be very useful to monitor cardiac function and intravenous volume status. The use of PA pressure monitoring is generally reserved for patients in whom pulmonary hypertension is a significant clinical problem that must be managed with medications such as iNO or a prostaglandin. Signs of infection may be masked in transplant patients by immunosuppression, so any signs of sepsis or systemic inflammatory response should be addressed and managed aggressively. Failing, rejected, or reinfected liver grafts are often accompanied by deterioration of renal function. In these cases, preserving renal function can be challenging, and every effort should be made to do so, as discussed above.

For all transplant recipients, antibiotic, antiviral, antifungal, and immune suppression regimens should be disrupted as little as possible in the perioperative period. The types of infection to which transplant recipients are susceptible change over time, with donor-derived and hospital-acquired infections predominating in the first posttransplant month. Infections acquired by transplant patients in months 2 to 6 versus later after transplantation are also distinct, and these patterns should guide antibiotic prophylaxis and perioperative diagnostic procedures. Infectious disease specialists are important consultants for perioperative transplant patients.

Commonly used immunosuppressive agents and the perioperative considerations they present are listed in Table 52-10. Immunosuppressive agents are given in three phases: induction (at the time of transplant), maintenance (ongoing, indefinite), and for signs of transplant rejection (usually a high "pulse" dose of immunosuppression). When recipients present for nontransplant surgery, they will most often be in the maintenance phase, although surgeries during the induction or rejection phases may present as well. Immunosuppressive medications increase the risk of perioperative infection not only of the surgical wound, but of intravascular catheters, urinary catheters, and the bronchopulmonary system. Strict aseptic technique should be used in the placement of all vascular catheters, especially those placed centrally. The immunosuppressive regimen should be clearly determined, as should the perioperative implications of these medications, as medication levels may need to be monitored perioperatively. Significant intraoperative fluid shifts can cause an acute decrease in cyclosporine or tacrolimus blood levels. Because these medications have narrow therapeutic windows, consideration should be given to repeat testing of drug levels on the day of surgery. Consultation with the primary transplant team is advised. Virtually all liver diseases can recur in grafted livers, including autoimmune diseases, fatty liver, and hepatitis C. The degree of liver dysfunction from recurrent disease should be evaluated by hepatologists and by using standard laboratory tests.

Most anesthetic and antinociceptive medications can safely be provided to transplant recipients, although nonsteroidal anti-inflammatory medications (NSAIDs), such as ketorolac, should be avoided as many transplant recipients have underlying renal dysfunction related to immunosuppressive agents that could be exacerbated by NSAIDs. NSAIDs also increase the risk of gastrointestinal hemorrhage in patients already at risk for this complication from chronic steroid use. Particular attention to hepatic and renal function should be used when administering muscle relaxants. Benzylisoquinoline muscle relaxants, such as cisatracurium, that do not rely on renal or hepatic elimination may be advisable in patients with impaired hepatic or renal function.

Regional and general anesthetic techniques have both been used successfully in posttransplant patients, and the choice of anesthetic technique should be guided by the usual factors governing that decision. The advantages of regional anesthetic techniques in lung transplant patients include minimization of airway manipulation and decreased infection risk. Nasal intubation should be avoided because of the potential risk for infection presented by nasal flora. In addition to standard monitors, invasive monitors should be used if warranted based on the surgical procedure and the general health status of the patient.

Most lung transplants are now achieved with bronchial instead of tracheal anastomoses, the risk of tracheal suture line stenosis or disruption with manipulation is markedly diminished. Lung transplant recipients with a tracheal anastomosis have a diminished or absent cough reflex because the transplant is denervated below the level of the suture line. These patients are at increased risk of retained secretions and pneumonia, and

Table 52-10 Common Immunosuppressive Agents Administered to Transplant Recipients

General Class	Mechanism	Example Medication	Common Side Effects, Perioperative Considerations
Corticosteroids	Immune suppression by sequestration of CD4 T cells in reticuloendothelial system and inhibiting transcription of cytokines	Prednisone	Electrolyte abnormalities, impaired tissue integrity, impaired wound healing, gastrointestinal bleeding, hyperglycemia
Antimetabolites	Cell cycle arrest	Azathioprine Cyclophosphamide	Azathioprine: hepatic dysfunction, pancreatitis, renal dysfunction, glucose intolerance, enhanced neuromuscular blockade
Calcineurin inhibitors	↓ IL-2 production by activated T cells	Tacrolimus Cyclosporine	Cyclosporine: hypertension, renal dysfunction, enhanced neuromuscular blockade. Tacrolimus: hypertension, renal dysfunction. Both metabolized by cytochrome P-450 system (CYP3A4-may affect metabolism of intravenous agents such as benzodiazepines, fentanyl, and propofol)
Polyclonal antibodies	↓ T-cell activity	Rabbit antithymocyte globulin (thymoglobulin)	Anemia, myelosuppression, thrombocytopenia
Anti-CD3 monoclonal antibodies	↓ T-cell activity	Muromonab-CD3	Leukopenia, bronchospasm, pulmonary edema, fever chills. Less commonly used now in favor of Thymoglobulin, which has fewer side effects
Anti-CD52 monoclonal antibodies	↓ T-cell activity	Alemtuzumab	Fever, chills (usually during first few weeks of treatment)
Anti-IL-2 receptor monoclonal antibodies	↓ IL-2 activity	Daclizumab	Upper respiratory infection
Target of rapamycin (TOR) inhibitors	Cell cycle arrest	Sirolimus	Impaired wound healing, myelosuppression, capillary leak syndromes

have increased airway hyperreactivity and bronchospasm. Comparison of preoperative pulmonary function testing, arterial blood gas, and chest x-ray results with prior studies can help diagnose acute infection or rejection, and provide information about overall lung function in patients who have received single-lung transplants. Significant decreases in FEV_1, vital capacity, and total lung capacity and an obstructive pattern may indicate acute rejection, or other pulmonary problems such as chronic obstructive pulmonary disease or pneumonia. Arterial blood gas in the presence of rejection will show an increased alveolar–arterial oxygen gradient compared to stable baseline gases, along with perihilar infiltration on chest x-ray. However, rejection and infection can be difficult to distinguish clinically. If the patient is suspected of having an active pulmonary process, consultation with a pulmonologist for a possible diagnostic bronchoscopy should be considered prior to surgery. Patients who present for surgery with signs of acute rejection or infection may benefit from delay of surgery to optimize their status. Both rejection and infection in the face of surgery are associated with increased risk of morbidity and mortality.

Transplanted hearts are denervated, which affects perioperative management significantly. The transplanted heart cannot respond to indirect-acting agents and so medications with combined indirect and direct effects, such as dopamine and ephedrine, will have reduced efficacy. Clinical maneuvers that depend upon the ordinary innervation of the heart, such as carotid massage and Valsalva maneuver, will have no immediate hemodynamic effect. The β-receptor effects of epinephrine and norepinephrine are exaggerated in heart transplant recipients versus their α effects. Isoproterenol, being a direct β_1 agonist, may be particularly useful in managing bradydysrhythmias and depressed myocardial function in cardiac transplant recipients. Dobutamine and dopamine may also be useful, with epinephrine and norepinephrine usually reserved for cases of cardiogenic shock. ECG analysis and monitoring may show two P waves, one from a residual cuff of native right atrial tissue and one from the right atrium of the transplanted heart. The native P wave will not conduct to the implanted heart, and these nonconducted P waves should not be confused with complete heart block. Because the denervated heart does not reflexively compensate for the hemodynamic changes induced by regional anesthetics and general anesthesia, direct-acting sympathomimetics are the most effective means of treating hemodynamic depression from anesthetics in cardiac transplant recipients.

Preoperative evaluation of heart transplant recipients should focus on cardiac functional status. Significant rejection will present with symptoms of heart failure. All heart transplant patients should be evaluated with ECG and TTE prior to surgery. New findings should be discussed with the cardiology consultant to determine the need for stress testing or myocardial biopsy. Invasive monitors should be placed only when warranted by the clinical status and surgical procedure. Use of TEE, CVP, or minimally invasive CO monitoring such as esophageal Doppler or arterial pulse wave CO can be helpful in managing fluids, vasopressors, and inotropic support.

For additional information please see NICV 52-3 in the eBook bundled with this text.

Acknowledgment

Marie Csete, M.D., Ph.D., and Dalia Banks, M.D. for their contributions to the previous edition of this chapter.

For further review and interactivities, please see the videos and narrative interactive clinical vignettes (NICVs) accessible in the complimentary eBook bundled with this text. Access instructions are located on the inside front cover.

REFERENCES

1. Israni AK. OPTN/SRTR 2020 annual data report: introduction. *Am J Transplant*. 2022;22 Suppl 2:11–20.
2. Kotloff RM, Blosser S, Fulda GJ, et al; Society of Critical Care Medicine/American College of Chest Physicians/Association of Organ Procurement Organizations Donor Management Task Force. Management of the potential organ donor in the ICU: Society of Critical Care Medicine/American College of Chest Physicians/Association of Organ Procurement Organizations Consensus Statement. *Crit Care Med*. 2015;43:1291–1325.
3. A definition of irreversible coma. Report of the Ad Hoc Committee of the Harvard Medical School to Examine the Definition of Brain Death. *JAMA*. 1968;205:337–340.
4. Wijdicks EFM, Varelas PN, Gronseth GS, Greer DM; American Academy of Neurology. Evidence-based guideline update: determining brain death in adults: report of the Quality Standards Subcommittee of the American Academy of Neurology. *Neurology*. 2010;74:1911–1918.
5. Plurad DS, Bricker S, Neville A, Bongard F, Putnam B. Arginine vasopressin significantly increases the rate of successful organ procurement in potential donors. *Am J Surg*. 2012;204:856–860;discussion 860–861.
6. Callahan DS, Neville A, Bricker S, et al. The effect of arginine vasopressin on organ donor procurement and lung function. *J Surg Res*. 2014;186:452–457.
7. Rosendale JD, Kauffman HM, McBride MA, et al. Aggressive pharmacologic donor management results in more transplanted organs. *Transplantation*. 2003;75:482–487.
8. Venkateswaran RV, Steeds RP, Quinn DW, et al. The haemodynamic effects of adjunctive hormone therapy in potential heart donors: a prospective randomized double-blind factorially designed controlled trial. *Eur Heart J*. 2009;30:1771–1780.
9. Novitzky D, Cooper DK, Rosendale JD, Kauffman HM. Hormonal therapy of the brain-dead organ donor: experimental and clinical studies. *Transplantation*. 2006;82:1396–1401.
10. Zaroff JG, Rosengard BR, Armstrong WF, et al. Consensus conference report: maximizing use of organs recovered from the cadaver donor: cardiac recommendations, March 28–29, 2001, Crystal City, Va. *Circulation*. 2002;106:836–841.
11. Pinsard M, Ragot S, Mertes PM, et al. Interest of low-dose hydrocortisone therapy during brain-dead organ donor resuscitation: the CORTICOME study. *Crit Care*. 2014;18:R158.
12. McElhinney DB, Khan JH, Babcock WD, Hall TS. Thoracic organ donor characteristics associated with successful lung procurement. *Clin Transplant*. 2001;15:68–71.
13. Olmos A, Feiner J, Hirose R, et al. Impact of a quality improvement project on deceased organ donor management. *Prog Transplant*. 2015;25:351–360.
14. Mascia L, Pasero D, Slutsky AS, et al. Effect of a lung protective strategy for organ donors on eligibility and availability of lungs for transplantation: a randomized controlled trial. *JAMA*. 2010;304:2620–2627.
15. Schnuelle P, Gottmann U, Hoeger S, et al. Effects of donor pretreatment with dopamine on graft function after kidney transplantation: a randomized controlled trial. *JAMA*. 2009; 302:1067–1075.
16. Orens JB, Boehler A, de Perrot M, et al; Pulmonary Council, International Society for Heart and Lung Transplantation. A review of lung transplant donor acceptability criteria. *J Heart Lung Transplant*. 2003;22:1183–1200.
17. Chaney J, Suzuki Y, Cantu E 3rd, van Berkel V. Lung donor selection criteria. *J Thorac Dis*. 2014;6:1032–1038.
18. Baldwin MR, Peterson ER, Easthausen I, et al. Donor age and early graft failure after lung transplantation: a cohort study. *Am J Transplant*. 2013;13:2685–2695.
19. Klein AS, Messersmith EE, Ratner LE, Kochik R, Baliga PK, Ojo AO. Organ donation and utilization in the United States, 1999–2008. *Am J Transplant*. 2010;10:973–986.
20. Thabut G, Mal H, Cerrina J, et al. Graft ischemic time and outcome of lung transplantation: a multicenter analysis. *Am J Respir Crit Care Med*. 2005;171:786–791.
21. Available at: https://optn.transplant.hrsa.gov/data/view-data-reports/national-data/#
22. Committee on Hospital Care, Section on Surgery, and Section on Critical Care. Policy statement–pediatric organ donation and transplantation. *Pediatrics*. 2010;125:822–828.
23. DeVita MA, Brooks MM, Zawistowski C, Rudich S, Daly B, Chaitin E. Donors after cardiac death: validation of identification criteria (DVIC) study for predictors of rapid death. *Am J Transplant*. 2008;8:432–441.
24. Das A, Anderson IM, Speicher DG, Speicher RH, Shein SL, Rotta AT. Validation of a pediatric bedside tool to predict time to death after withdrawal of life support. *World J Clin Pediatr*. 2016;5: 89–94.
25. Sterkenburg A, Kulu Y, Mieth M, et al. Long-term surgical outcome and risk factors in living kidney donors. *Transplant Proc*. 2020;52:722–730.
26. Byrne MHV, Mehmood A, Summers DM, Hosgood SA, Nicholson ML. A systematic review of living kidney donor enhanced recovery after surgery. *Clin Transplant*. 2021;35(7):e14384.
27. Zorgdrager M, van Londen M, Westenberg LB, et al. Chronic pain after hand-assisted laparoscopic donor nephrectomy. *Br J Surg*. 2019;106:711–719.
28. Goldaracena N, Spetzler VN, Marquez M, et al. Live donor liver transplantation: a valid alternative for critically ill patients suffering from acute liver failure. *Am J Transplant*. 2015; 15:1591–1597.
29. Hong SK, Choe S, Yi N-J, et al. Long-term survival of 10,116 Korean live liver donors. *Ann Surg*. 2021;274:375–382.
30. Agarwal V, Divatia JV. Enhanced recovery after surgery in liver resection: current concepts and controversies. *Korean J Anesthesiol*. 2019;72:119–129.
31. Marubashi S, Nagano H. Laparoscopic living-donor hepatectomy: review of its current status. *Ann Gastroenterol Surg*. 2021;5:484–493.
32. The 2021 Eye Bank Association of America Statistical Report, available at https://restoresight.org/statistical-report/ (accessed Apr 2022).
33. Chua AWY, Chua MJ, Kam PCA. Recent advances and anaesthetic considerations in corneal transplantation. *Anaesth Intensive Care*. 2018;46:162–170.
34. Chen CL, Lin GA, Bardach NS, et al. preoperative medical testing in Medicare patients undergoing cataract surgery. *N Engl J Med*. 2015;372:1530–1538.
35. Massie AB, Leanza J, Fahmy LM, et al. A risk index for living donor kidney transplantation. *Am J Transplant*. 2016;16:2077–2084.
36. Philipse E, Lee APK, Bracke B, et al. Does Kidney Donor Risk Index implementation lead to the transplantation of more and higher-quality donor kidneys? *Nephrol Dial Transplant*. 2017; 32:1934–1938.
37. Stewart DE, Kucheryavaya AY, Klassen DK, Turgeon NA, Formica RN, Aeder MI. Changes in deceased donor kidney transplantation one year after KAS implementation. *Am J Transplant*. 2016;16:1834–1847.
38. Samoylova ML, Shaw BI, Irish W, et al. Decreased graft loss following implementation of the kidney allocation score (KAS). *Am J Surg*. 2020;220:1278–1283.
39. CDC report on chronic kidney disease in the United States, 2021, available at: https://www.cdc.gov/kidneydisease/publications-resources/CKD-national-facts.html (accessed Apr 2022).
40. Lentine KL, Smith JM, Hart A, et al. OPTN/SRTR 2020 annual data report: kidney. *Am J Transplant*. 2022;22:21–136.
41. Aziz F, Jorgenson M, Garg N, et al. New approaches to cardiovascular disease and its management in kidney transplant recipients. *Transplantation*. 2022;106(6):1143–1158.
42. Parajuli S, Lockridge JB, Langewisch ED, Norman DJ, Kujovich JL. Hypercoagulability in kidney transplant recipients. *Transplantation*. 2016;100:719–726.
43. Helanterä I, Ibrahim HN, Lempinen M, Finne P. Donor age, cold ischemia time, and delayed graft function. *Clin J Am Soc Nephrol*. 2020;15:813–821.
44. Müller AK, Breuer E, Hübel K, et al. Long-term outcomes of transplant kidneys donated after circulatory death. *Nephrol Dial Transplant*. 2022;37(6):1181–1187.
45. Ricaurte L, Vargas J, Lozano E, Díaz L; Organ Transplant Group. Anesthesia and kidney transplantation. *Transplant Proc*. 2013;45:1386–1391.
46. Spiro MD, Eilers H. Intraoperative care of the transplant patient. *Anesthesiol Clin*. 2013;31: 705–721.
47. Weir MR, Burgess ED, Cooper JE, et al. Assessment and management of hypertension in transplant patients. *J Am Soc Nephrol*. 2015;26:1248–1260.
48. Wagener G, Bezinover D, Wang C, et al. Fluid management during kidney transplantation: a consensus statement of the Committee on Transplant Anesthesia of the American Society of Anesthesiologists. *Transplantation*. 2021;105:1677–1684.
49. Teboul J-L, Monnet X, Chemla D, Michard F. Arterial pulse pressure variation with mechanical ventilation. *Am J Respir Crit Care Med*. 2019;199:22–31.
50. Lo C, Toyama T, Oshima M, et al. Glucose-lowering agents for treating pre-existing and new-onset diabetes in kidney transplant recipients. *Cochrane Database Syst Rev*. 2020;8(8): CD009966.

51. Mabilangan C, Burton C, Nahirniak S, O'Brien S, Preiksaitis J. Transfusion-transmitted and community-acquired cytomegalovirus infection in seronegative solid organ transplant recipients receiving seronegative donor organs. *Am J Transplant.* 2020;20:3509–3519.
52. Shoeibi G, Babakhani B, Mohammadi SS. The efficacy of ilioinguinal-iliohypogastric and intercostal nerve co-blockade for postoperative pain relief in kidney recipients. *Anesth Analg.* 2009;108:330–333.
53. Singh PM, Borle A, Makkar JK, Trisha A, Sinha A. Evaluation of transversus abdominis plane block for renal transplant recipients–a meta-analysis and trial sequential analysis of published studies. *Saudi J Anaesth.* 2018;12:261.
54. Davison SN, Rathwell S, Ghosh S, George C, Pfister T, Dennett L. The prevalence and severity of chronic pain in patients with chronic kidney disease: a systematic review and meta-analysis. *Can J Kidney Health Dis.* 2021;8:205435812199399.
55. Zarinsefat A, Gulati A, Shui A, et al. Long-term outcomes following kidney and liver transplant in recipients with HIV. *JAMA Surg.* 2022;157:240.
56. Barman PM, VanWagner LB. Cardiac risk assessment in liver transplant candidates: current controversies and future directions. *Hepatology.* 2021;73:2564–2576.
57. Robertson M, Chung W, Liu D, et al. Cardiac risk stratification in liver transplantation: results of a tiered assessment protocol based on traditional cardiovascular risk factors. *Liver Transpl.* 2021;27:1007–1018.
58. Carey EJ, Steidley DE, Aqel BA, et al. Six-minute walk distance predicts mortality in liver transplant candidates. *Liver Transpl.* 2010;16:1373–1378.
59. VanWagner LB, Serper M, Kang R, et al. Factors associated with major adverse cardiovascular events after liver transplantation among a national sample. *Am J Transplant.* 2016;16: 2684–2694.
60. Simonneau G, Montani D, Celermajer DS, et al. Haemodynamic definitions and updated clinical classification of pulmonary hypertension. *Eur Respir J.* 2019;53:1801913.
61. Jose A, Shah SA, Anwar N, Jones CR, Sherman KE, Elwing JM. Pulmonary vascular resistance predicts mortality and graft failure in transplantation patients with portopulmonary hypertension. *Liver Transpl.* 2021;27:1811–1823.
62. Wong F, Pappas SC, Curry MP, et al; CONFIRM Study Investigators. Terlipressin plus albumin for the treatment of type 1 hepatorenal syndrome. *N Engl J Med.* 2021;384:818–828.
63. Wang LS, D'Souza LS, Jacobson IM. Hepatitis C-a clinical review. *J Med Virol.* 2016;88: 1844–1855.
64. Carrier FM, Ferreira Guerra S, Coulombe J, et al. Intraoperative phlebotomies and bleeding in liver transplantation: a historical cohort study and causal analysis. *Can J Anaesth.* 2022;69: 438–447.
65. Ghadimi K, Levy JH, Welsby IJ. Prothrombin complex concentrates for bleeding in the perioperative setting. *Anesth Analg.* 2016;122:1287–1300.
66. Chin JL, Hisamuddin SH, O'Sullivan A, Chan G, McCormick PA. Thrombocytopenia, platelet transfusion, and outcome following liver transplantation. *Clin Appl Thromb Hemost.* 2016; 22:351–360.
67. Tripodi A, Mannucci PM. The coagulopathy of chronic liver disease. *N Engl J Med.* 2011;365: 147–156.
68. Nicolau-Raducu R, Ku TC, Ganier DR, et al. Epsilon-aminocaproic acid has no association with thromboembolic complications, renal failure, or mortality after liver transplantation. *J Cardiothorac Vasc Anesth.* 2016;30:917–923.
69. Caragata R, Wyssusek KH, Kruger P. Acute kidney injury following liver transplantation: a systematic review of published predictive models. *Anaesth Intensive Care.* 2016;44:251–261.
70. Francoz C, Glotz D, Moreau R, Durand F. The evaluation of renal function and disease in patients with cirrhosis. *J Hepatol.* 2010;52:605–613.
71. Gupta K, Bhurwal A, Law C, et al. Acute kidney injury and hepatorenal syndrome in cirrhosis. *World J Gastroenterol.* 2021;27:3984–4003.
72. Pena Polanco NA, Martin P, Carrion AF. Advances in the management of renal dysfunction in patients with cirrhosis. *Gastroenterol Hepatol (N Y).* 2021;17:211–220.
73. Aggarwal S, Kang Y, Freeman JA, Fortunato FL Jr, Pinsky MR. Postreperfusion syndrome: hypotension after reperfusion of the transplanted liver. *J Crit Care.* 1993;8:154–160.
74. Angelico R, Perera MTPR, Ravikumar R, et al. Normothermic machine perfusion of deceased donor liver grafts is associated with improved postreperfusion hemodynamics. *Transplant Direct.* 2016;2:e97.
75. Shillcutt SK, Ringenberg KJ, Chacon MM, et al. Liver transplantation: intraoperative transesophageal echocardiography findings and relationship to major postoperative adverse cardiac events. *J Cardiothorac Vasc Anesth.* 2016;30:107–114.
76. Hosseinian L, Weiner M, Levin MA, Fischer GW. Methylene blue: magic bullet for vasoplegia? *Anesth Analg.* 2016;122:194–201.
77. Beck-Schimmer B, Bonvini JM, Schadde E, et al. Conditioning with sevoflurane in liver transplantation: results of a multicenter randomized controlled trial. *Transplantation.* 2015;99:1606–1612.
78. Abuelkasem E, Lu S, Tanaka K, Planinsic R, Sakai T. Comparison between thrombelastography and thromboelastometry in hyperfibrinolysis detection during adult liver transplantation. *Br J Anaesth.* 2016;116:507–512.
79. Wagenaar AE, Tashiro J, Sola JE, Ekwenna O, Tekin A, Perez EA. Pediatric liver transplantation: predictors of survival and resource utilization. *Pediatr Surg Int.* 2016;32:439–449.
80. Nemes B, Gámán G, Polak WG, et al. Extended-criteria donors in liver transplantation Part II: reviewing the impact of extended-criteria donors on the complications and outcomes of liver transplantation. *Expert Rev Gastroenterol Hepatol.* 2016;10:841–859.
81. Rajajee V, Williamson CA, Fontana RJ, Courey AJ, Patil PG. Noninvasive intracranial pressure assessment in acute liver failure. *Neurocrit Care.* 2018;29:280–290.
82. Karvellas CJ, Todd Stravitz R, Battenhouse H, Lee WM, Schilsky ML, US Acute Liver Failure Study Group. Therapeutic hypothermia in acute liver failure: a multicenter retrospective cohort analysis. *Liver Transpl.* 2015;21:4–12.
83. Kandiah PA, Olson JC, Subramanian RM. Emerging strategies for the treatment of patients with acute hepatic failure. *Curr Opin Crit Care.* 2016;22:142–151.
84. Farney AC, Sutherland DER, Opara EC. Evolution of islet transplantation for the last 30 years. *Pancreas.* 2016;45:8–20.
85. Mackey PA, Thompson BM, Boyle ME, et al. Update on a quality initiative to standardize perioperative care for continuous subcutaneous insulin infusion therapy. *J Diabetes Sci Technol.* 2015;9:1299–1306.
86. Shapiro AM, Lakey JR, Ryan EA, et al. Islet transplantation in seven patients with type 1 diabetes mellitus using a glucocorticoid-free immunosuppressive regimen. *N Engl J Med.* 2000; 343:230–238.
87. Loo L, Vrakas G, Reddy S, Allan P. Intestinal transplantation: a review. *Curr Opin Gastroenterol.* 2017;33:203–211.
88. Kapur S, Paik E, Rezaei A, Vu DN. Where there is blood, there is a way: unusual collateral vessels in superior and inferior vena cava obstruction. *Radiographics.* 2010;30:67–78.
89. Rege A, Sudan D. Intestinal transplantation. *Best Pract Res Clin Gastroenterol.* 2016;30: 319–335.
90. Dalal A. Intestinal transplantation: the anesthesia perspective. *Transplant Rev (Orlando).* 2016;30:100–108.
91. Lang RS, Gorantla VS, Esper S, et al. Anesthetic management in upper extremity transplantation: the Pittsburgh experience. *Anesth Analg.* 2012;115:678–688.
92. Shokri T, Saadi R, Wang W, Reddy L, Ducic Y. Facial transplantation: complications, outcomes, and long-term management strategies. *Semin Plast Surg.* 2020;34:245–253.
93. Chambers DC, Zuckermann A, Cherikh WS, et al; International Society for Heart and Lung Transplantation. The International Thoracic Organ Transplant Registry of the International Society for Heart and Lung Transplantation: 37th adult lung transplantation report—2020; focus on deceased donor characteristics. *J Heart Lung Transplant.* 2020;39: 1016–1027.
94. Chambers DC, Cherikh WS, Goldfarb SB, et al; International Society for Heart and Lung Transplantation. The International Thoracic Organ Transplant Registry of the International Society for Heart and Lung Transplantation: thirty-fifth adult lung and heart-lung transplant report—2018; focus theme: multiorgan Transplantation. *J Heart Lung Transplant.* 2018;37: 1169–1183.
95. Chambers DC, Cherikh WS, Harhay MO, et al; International Society for Heart and Lung Transplantation. The International Thoracic Organ Transplant Registry of the International Society for Heart and Lung Transplantation: Thirty-sixth adult lung and heart–lung transplantation report—2019; focus theme: donor and recipient size match. *J Heart Lung Transplant.* 2019;38:1042–1055.
96. Ius F, Sommer W, Tudorache I, et al. Five-year experience with intraoperative extracorporeal membrane oxygenation in lung transplantation: Indications and midterm results. *J Heart Lung Transplant.* 2016;35:49–58.
97. Ius F, Aburahma K, Boethig D, et al. Long-term outcomes after intraoperative extracorporeal membrane oxygenation during lung transplantation. *J Heart Lung Transplant.* 2020; 39:915–925.
98. Hoetzenecker K, Schwarz S, Muckenhuber M, et al. Intraoperative extracorporeal membrane oxygenation and the possibility of postoperative prolongation improve survival in bilateral lung transplantation. *J Thorac Cardiovasc Surg.* 2018;155:2193–2206.e3.
99. Cypel M, Yeung JC, Liu M, et al. Normothermic ex vivo lung perfusion in clinical lung transplantation. *N Engl J Med.* 2011;364:1431–1440.
100. Leard LE, Holm AM, Valapour M, et al. Consensus document for the selection of lung transplant candidates: an update from the International Society for Heart and Lung Transplantation. *J Heart Lung Transplant.* 2021;40:1349–1379.
101. Davis SQ, Garrity ER Jr. Organ allocation in lung transplant. *Chest.* 2007;132:1646–1651.
102. Bermudez CA, Shiose A, Esper SA, et al. Outcomes of intraoperative venoarterial extracorporeal membrane oxygenation versus cardiopulmonary bypass during lung transplantation. *Ann Thorac Surg.* 2014;98:1936–1942; discussion 1942–1933.
103. Machuca TN, Collaud S, Mercier O, et al. Outcomes of intraoperative extracorporeal membrane oxygenation versus cardiopulmonary bypass for lung transplantation. *J Thorac Cardiovasc Surg.* 2015;149:1152–1157.
104. Martin AK, Jayaraman AL, Nabzdyk CG, et al. Extracorporeal membrane oxygenation in lung transplantation: analysis of techniques and outcomes. *J Cardiothorac Vasc Anesth.* 2021; 35:644–661.
105. Wick EC, Grant MC, Wu CL. Postoperative multimodal analgesia pain management with nonopioid analgesics and techniques: a review. *JAMA Surg.* 2017;152:691–697.

106. Chambers DC, Perch M, Zuckermann A, et al; International Society for Heart and Lung Transplantation. The International Thoracic Organ Transplant Registry of the International Society for Heart and Lung Transplantation: thirty-eighth adult lung transplantation report-2021; focus on recipient characteristics. *J Heart Lung Transplant*. 2021;40:1060–1072.
107. Hayes D Jr, Harhay MO, Cherikh WS, et al; International Society for Heart and Lung Transplantation. The International Thoracic Organ Transplant Registry of the International Society for Heart and Lung Transplantation: twenty-fourth pediatric lung transplantation report-2021; focus on recipient characteristics. *J Heart Lung Transplant*. 2021;40:1023–1034.
108. Paraskeva MA, Edwards LB, Levvey B, et al. Outcomes of adolescent recipients after lung transplantation: an analysis of the International Society for Heart and Lung Transplantation Registry. *J Heart Lung Transplant*. 2018;37:323–331.
109. Snell GI, Yusen RD, Weill D, et al. Report of the ISHLT Working Group on Primary Lung Graft Dysfunction, part I: definition and grading-a 2016 Consensus Group statement of the International Society for Heart and Lung Transplantation. *J Heart Lung Transplant*. 2017;36:1097–1103.
110. Diamond JM, Arcasoy S, Kennedy CC, et al. Report of the International Society for Heart and Lung Transplantation Working Group on Primary Lung Graft Dysfunction, part II: epidemiology, risk factors, and outcomes-a 2016 Consensus Group statement of the International Society for Heart and Lung Transplantation. *J Heart Lung Transplant*. 2017;36:1104–1113.
111. Van Raemdonck D, Hartwig MG, Hertz MI, et al. Report of the ISHLT Working Group on primary lung graft dysfunction Part IV: prevention and treatment: a 2016 Consensus Group statement of the International Society for Heart and Lung Transplantation. *J Heart Lung Transplant*. 2017;36:1121–1136.
112. Meyer KC, Love RB, Zimmerman JJ: The therapeutic potential of nitric oxide in lung transplantation. *Chest*. 1998;113:1360–1371.
113. Botha P, Jeyakanthan M, Rao JN, et al. Inhaled nitric oxide for modulation of ischemia-reperfusion injury in lung transplantation. *J Heart Lung Transplant*. 2007;26:1199–1205.
114. Ardehali A, Laks H, Levine M, et al. A prospective trial of inhaled nitric oxide in clinical lung transplantation. *Transplantation*. 2001;72:112–115.
115. Beghetti M, Sparling C, Cox PN, Stephens D, Adatia I. Inhaled NO inhibits platelet aggregation and elevates plasma but not intraplatelet cGMP in healthy human volunteers. *Am J Physiol Heart Circ Physiol*. 2003;285:H637–H642.
116. Cornfield DN, Milla CE, Haddad IY, Barbato JE, Park SJ. Safety of inhaled nitric oxide after lung transplantation. *J Heart Lung Transplant*. 2003;22:903–907.
117. Chambers DC, Cherikh WS, Harhay MO, et al; International Society for Heart and Lung Transplantation. The International Thoracic Organ Transplant Registry of the International Society for Heart and Lung Transplantation: thirty-sixth adult lung and heart-lung transplantation report-2019; focus theme: donor and recipient size match. *J Heart Lung Transplant*. 2019; 38:1042–1055.
118. Hayes D Jr, Cherikh WS, Chambers DC, et al; International Society for Heart and Lung Transplantation. The International Thoracic Organ Transplant Registry of the International Society for Heart and Lung Transplantation: twenty-second pediatric lung and heart-lung transplantation report-2019; focus theme: donor and recipient size match. *J Heart Lung Transplant*. 2019: 38:1015–1027.
119. Roger VL, Weston SA, Redfield MM, et al. Trends in heart failure incidence and survival in a community-based population. *JAMA*. 2004;292:344–350.
120. Rose EA, Gelijns AC, Moskowitz AJ, et al; Randomized Evaluation of Mechanical Assistance for the Treatment of Congestive Heart Failure (REMATCH) Study Group. Long-term use of a left ventricular assist device for end-stage heart failure. *N Engl J Med*. 2001;345: 1435–1443.
121. Rogers JG, Pagani FD, Tatooles AJ, et al. Intrapericardial left ventricular assist device for advanced heart failure. *N Engl J Med*. 2017;376:451–460.
122. Mehra MR, Naka Y, Uriel N, et al; MOMENTUM 3 Investigators. A fully magnetically levitated circulatory pump for advanced heart failure. *N Engl J Med*. 2017;376:440–450.
123. Mehra MR, Uriel N, Naka Y, et al; MOMENTUM 3 Investigators. A fully magnetically levitated left ventricular assist device - final report. *N Engl J Med*. 2019;380:1618–1627.
124. Khush KK, Hsich E, Potena L, et al; International Society for Heart and Lung Transplantation. The International Thoracic Organ Transplant Registry of the International Society for Heart and Lung Transplantation: thirty-eighth adult heart transplantation report - 2021; focus on recipient characteristics. *J Heart Lung Transplant*. 2021;40:1035–1049.
125. McAlister FA, Ezekowitz J, Hooton N, et al. Cardiac resynchronization therapy for patients with left ventricular systolic dysfunction: a systematic review. *JAMA*. 2007;297:2502–2514.
126. Goldenberg I, Kutyifa V, Klein HU, et al. Survival with cardiac-resynchronization therapy in mild heart failure. *N Engl J Med*. 2014;370:1694–1701.
127. Mehra MR, Kobashigawa J, Starling R, et al. Listing criteria for heart transplantation: International Society for Heart and Lung Transplantation guidelines for the care of cardiac transplant candidates–2006. *J Heart Lung Transplant*. 2006;25:1024–1042.
128. Mehra MR, Canter CE, Hannan MM, et al; International Society for Heart Lung Transplantation (ISHLT) Infectious Diseases, Pediatric and Heart Failure and Transplantation Councils. The 2016 International Society for Heart Lung Transplantation listing criteria for heart transplantation: a 10-year update. *J Heart Lung Transplant*. 2016;35:1–23.
129. Fleg JL, Piña IL, Balady GJ, et al. Assessment of functional capacity in clinical and research applications: an advisory from the Committee on Exercise, Rehabilitation, and Prevention, Council on Clinical Cardiology, American Heart Association. *Circulation*. 2000;102: 1591–1597.
130. Goda A, Lund LH, Mancini D: The Heart Failure Survival Score outperforms the peak oxygen consumption for heart transplantation selection in the era of device therapy. *J Heart Lung Transplant*. 2011;30:315–325.
131. Demas K, Wyner J, Mihm FG, Samuels S. Anaesthesia for heart transplantation. A retrospective study and review. *Br J Anaesth*. 1986;58:1357–1364.
132. Kianfar AA, Ahmadi ZH, Mirhossein SM, et al. Ultra fast-track extubation in heart transplant surgery patients. *Int J Crit Illn Inj Sci*. 2015;5:89–92.
133. Zijderhand CF, Veen KM, Caliskan K, et al. Biatrial versus bicaval orthotopic heart transplantation: a systematic review and meta-analysis. *Ann Thorac Surg*. 2020;110:684–691.
134. Kieler-Jensen N, Lundin S, Ricksten SE. Vasodilator therapy after heart transplantation: effects of inhaled nitric oxide and intravenous prostacyclin, prostaglandin E1, and sodium nitroprusside. *J Heart Lung Transplant*. 1995;14:436–443.
135. Singh TP, Cherikh WS, Hsich E, et al; International Society for Heart and Lung Transplantation. The International Thoracic Organ Transplant Registry of the International Society for Heart and Lung Transplantation: Twenty-fourth pediatric heart transplantation report — 2021; focus on recipient characteristics. *J Heart Lung Transplant*. 2021;40:1050–1059.
136. Singh TP, Hsich E, Cherikh WS, et al; International Society for Heart and Lung Transplantation. The International Thoracic Organ Transplant Registry of the International Society for Heart and Lung Transplantation: 23rd pediatric heart transplantation report-2020; focus on deceased donor characteristics. *J Heart Lung Transplant*. 2020;39:1028–1037.
137. Kohler S, Engmann R, Birnbaum J, et al. ABO-compatible retransplantation after ABO-incompatible infant heart transplantation: absence of donor specific isohemagglutinins. *Am J Transplant*. 2014;14:2903–2905.
138. Irving CA, Gennery AR, Carter V, et al. ABO-incompatible cardiac transplantation in pediatric patients with high isohemagglutinin titers. *J Heart Lung Transplant*. 2015;34: 1095–1102.
139. Gries CJ, White DB, Truog RD, et al; American Thoracic Society Health Policy Committee. An official American Thoracic Society/International Society for Heart and Lung Transplantation/ Society of Critical Care Medicine/Association of Organ and Procurement Organizations/ United Network of Organ Sharing Statement: ethical and policy considerations in organ donation after circulatory determination of death. *Am J Respir Crit Care Med*. 2013;188: 103–109.
140. Messer S, Page A, Axell R, et al. Outcome after heart transplantation from donation after circulatory-determined death donors. *J Heart Lung Transplant*. 2017;36:1311–1318.
141. Chew HC, Iyer A, Connellan M, et al. Outcomes of donation after circulatory death heart transplantation in Australia. *J Am Coll Cardiol*. 2019;73:1447–1459.

53 Anesthesia for Trauma and Burns

PUDKRONG K. AICHOLZ • JOSHUA M. TOBIN

KEY POINTS

1 Perioperative care of acutely injured, hemorrhaging patients requires both timely operative control and well-balanced resuscitation based on understanding the mechanism of each injury, pathophysiology of trauma, and trauma-induced coagulopathy.

2 Airway management in traumatized patients is generally achieved by rapid sequence induction with manual in-line stabilization to minimize movement of cervical spine, in conjunction with either direct or video laryngoscopy.

3 In "cannot intubate, cannot ventilate" situations, invasive airway access by cricothyroidotomy should be promptly undertaken.

4 Vasopressor use during early trauma resuscitation for correction of blood pressure has not been shown to improve outcomes and is associated with high mortality risk.

5 Neurologic injury is a leading cause of death in trauma. Prevention of secondary injury caused by hypotension and hypoxemia is important for improvement of long-term outcome following traumatic brain injury.

6 The cornerstone of trauma resuscitation is "hemostatic" blood products administration with emphasis on plasma:erythrocyte (RBC) ratios, as well as platelet:RBC ratios greater than 1:2, preferably closer to 1:1.

7 Group O whole blood with low hemagglutinin (anti-A and anti-B) titer offers logistical advantages over blood component therapy and has been increasingly used during initial trauma resuscitation. Early data showed similar survival benefits and safety profile of this to component therapy.

8 Viscoelastic hemostatic assays (VHA) are increasingly utilized for trauma resuscitation. However, VHA-guided resuscitation has not shown survival benefit over traditional coagulation tests.

9 Compared to adults, perioperative considerations in pediatric trauma include a predominance of blunt and traumatic brain injury; airway anatomical differences; and varying respiratory, cardiovascular and hematologic physiology.

10 Major burns can cause systemic pathophysiologic effects correlating to severity of burn injury, manifesting in two temporal phases: (1) burn shock phase (24 to 48 hours after injury) characterized by intravascular volume loss resulting in reduced circulatory volume and possible organ hypoperfusion, and (2) hypermetabolic phase (48 to 72 hours after injury) characterized by hyperdynamic circulation, increased body temperature, oxygen consumption and drug metabolism.

11 Inhalational injury increases mortality of burn-injured patients. It can occur as thermal and chemical injury to the upper airway, noxious chemical injury to the lower airway (tracheobronchial-alveolar), and systemic toxicity from toxic gases. A high index of suspicion and repeated monitoring is crucial, as patients can require early tracheal intubation to prevent airway obstruction.

What Is Trauma Anesthesia?

1 Trauma is the leading cause of death in young Americans and the leading cause of years-of-life lost. Surgical correction of hemorrhage is of no utility in a poorly resuscitated patient, and an elegant resuscitation in a patient in whom bleeding is not controlled is equally useless. The role of the anesthesiologist in trauma is to guide the resuscitation of the trauma patient in the operating room (and increasingly in the interventional radiology suite). Effective resuscitation prepares the patient for the next step on the continuum of care, often in the intensive care unit (ICU). The trauma anesthesiologist is as a resuscitation consultant[1]; equal parts teammate, clinical pharmacologist, applied physiologist, procedural expert, and respectful skeptic.

Defining the training and quantifying the clinical benefit of trauma anesthesia, however, can be challenging. When trauma resuscitation practices were compared between critical care trained anesthesiologists, and noncritical care anesthesiologists, critical care trained anesthesiologists administered more crystalloid, less albumin, fewer vasopressors, and more fresh frozen plasma (FFP).[2] Mortality, however, was no different between the two groups.

Standardization of care can offer some benefit and checklists can contribute to that standardization. Checklists decrease inpatient complications and death.[3] Checklists are especially useful in an emergency, but they require leadership to implement.[4,5] Checklists offer the opportunity to "plug holes" in resuscitation with a methodical approach to a series of step-wise processes. Failure can be conceptualized as a "Swiss cheese" model in which several smaller errors must align, similar to slices of Swiss cheese, to enable a serious error. The trajectory for failure is mathematically described as a Bethe Lattice [$N_k = z(z - 1)^{k-1}$ for $k > 0$].[6]

Stanford University developed an emergency manual of cognitive aids for use during crisis resource management in anesthesiology and it is available at http://emergencymanual.stanford.edu. Specific checklists for trauma anesthesia have been developed. Tobin et al. developed a template for care in critically injured patients[7] that places impactful stages of resuscitation in a logical order throughout the continuum of care from induction, thorough anesthetic management to ICU transition. A cognitive aid adapted the Tobin checklist into a visually appealing multicolored format.[8]

This chapter will describe trauma anesthesia fundamentals, including airway management, transfusion, and resuscitation practices. A systematic approach to trauma anesthesia will consider pulmonary, cardiovascular, and neurologic topics. Monitoring of resuscitation, as well as evaluation of the trauma patient overall will be discussed. Special populations will be described including pediatric and burn patients.

Airway

Medications useful during an emergency anesthetic resuscitation are described in Table 53-1. Rapid sequence induction (RSI) and direct laryngoscopy are safe in trauma. In an analysis of 6,088 patients over 10 years at a level I trauma center; 98.6% were successfully intubated via the orotracheal route, while only 0.3% required a surgical airway.[9] Similarly, in a Norwegian system of prehospital critical care, prehospital anesthesiologists successfully intubated 99.2% of patients.[10]

A gum elastic bougie can be inserted into the glottic opening during laryngoscopy and followed with a "tube over stylet" technique to properly place an endotracheal tube in challenging airways. This approach has been adopted for use in emergent or challenging airways. A randomized control trial evaluated 1,102 patients intubated with a bougie or with a stylet.[11] The investigators found no difference between the two approaches regarding successful first-attempt intubation, severe hypoxemia, esophageal intubation, pneumothorax or injury to oropharyngeal structures. Nevertheless, the bougie approach has been adopted by some prehospital and emergency services with reported anecdotal success. Manual in-line stabilization (MILS) is frequently undertaken during emergency airway management in trauma to stabilize the cervical spine during intubation. Interestingly, cervical spine injury during intubation is not common. Of 81 patients with vertebral body fractures, 26 required airway management and 22 were intubated via the orotracheal route (the remaining 4 were intubated via the nasotracheal route).[12] There was no subsequent neurologic

Table 53-1 Common Anesthetic Medications Used during Resuscitation

Medication	Dose	Mechanism of Action	Comments
Sedative/Hypnotics			
Propofol	1–3 mg/kg	GABA-A agonist	Can drop SVR
Ketamine	1–2 mq/kq	NMDA antagonist	Maintains airway reflexes and SVR
Etomidate	0.6 mg/kg	GABA-A agonist	Single doses for induction can suppress hypothalamic–pituitary–adrenal axis
Neuromuscular Blocking Agents			
Succinylcholine	1–2 mg/kg	Depolarizing neuromuscular relaxant	Can cause life-threatening hyperkalemia in burns and spinal cord injury
Rocuronium	0.6–1.2 mg/kg	Nondepolarizing muscle relaxant	Can be effectively used as NMB in rapid sequence induction
Cis-Atracurium	0.1–0.2 mg/kg	Nondepolarizing muscle relaxant	Eliminated by Hofmann degradation. Useful in renal insufficiency/failure
Vecuronium	0.1 mg/kg	Nondepolarizing muscle relaxant	Longer duration NMB
Adjuncts			
Tranexamic acid	1 g over 10 minutes, then 1 g over 8 hrs	Synthetic lysine derivative/ antifibrinolytic	Improvement in mortality when given within 3 hrs of injury
Vasopressin	5–20 IU	Potent vasoconstrictor	Shunts blood to cerebral, cardiac, and pulmonary vascular beds
Calcium Chloride	1 g	Facilitates smooth muscle contraction	Used to restore low calcium levels during massive transfusion
Hydrocortisone	100 mg	Potent mineralocorticoid	Treats adrenal suppression seen in critical illness

GABA-A, gamma-aminobutyric acid-A; SVR, systemic vascular resistance; NMB, neuromuscular blockade.

deficit in any of these patients. Of 69 patients with documented high spinal cord injury, 29 required tracheal intubation, of which 26 were intubated orotracheally (3 were intubated via the nasotracheal route). There was no worsening of neurologic deficit in any of these patients, again demonstrating that orotracheal intubation, even in cases of documented cervical spine or cord pathology, is safe.

MILS is used to minimize movement of the cervical spine, regardless of documented injury. One investigation of subluxation, angulation, and distraction in a cadaveric model found that MILS did not have a significant impact on maximal motion using either direct laryngoscopy (DL) or the Bullard laryngoscope (a precursor to video laryngoscopy [VL]).[13] Alternatively, other work shows a seeming contradiction. A cadaver model was used to measure angular rotation, axial distraction, and anterior–posterior displacement at the C5–6 disk space.[14] MILS produced significantly less movement than a cervical spine collar. When used as part of a culture of good communication within the intubating team, MILS is an easy, low-cost technique that can be used to remind the laryngoscopist to manipulate the cervical spine as little as possible.

Ruling out cervical spine injury as soon as clinically feasible is important in early management of the trauma airway. Patients who remain in cervical collar immobilization for 48 hours can show signs of ligamentous edema on MRI scan, even without initial spine injury. Leaving a trauma patient in a cervical collar that is unnecessary for several days may condemn them to 6 weeks or longer of unneeded cervical immobilization. Cervical spine evaluation can be undertaken promptly with a series of questions assessing: (1) if there are any high-risk factors necessitating radiography (i.e., age over 65 years, dangerous mechanism, paresthesias)?; (2) are there any low-risk factors that allow safe assessment of range-of-motion (i.e., simple rear-end motor vehicle accident, sitting in the emergency department, ambulation since the accident, delayed onset of neck pain, absence of mid-line tenderness)?; and (3) can the patient actively rotate the head 45 degrees to the left and right?[15] This "Canadian C-Spine Rule" is 100% sensitive and 45% specific in identifying cervical spine injuries.

The National Emergency X-ray Radiography Utilization Study (NEXUS) Group also investigated the use of simple, noninvasive assessment criteria to rule out cervical spine injury in 34,069 patients who suffered blunt trauma and underwent radiography of the cervical spine.[16] Five criteria—(1) no midline tenderness, (2) no focal neurologic deficit, (3) normal alertness, (4) no intoxication, (5) no distracting injury—were 99% sensitive in detecting cervical spine injury, with a negative predictive value of 99.8%.

Video Laryngoscopy

VL affords an improved view of the vocal cords. It is less clear, however, if VL offers an advantage over DL during tracheal intubation. A meta-analysis of 17 trials comprising 2,000 patients showed no difference in successful first attempts at intubation or time to intubation.[17] Non-experts (e.g., medical students, paramedic students, nurses) intubated 200 patients following familiarization training on manikins.[18] The use of VL did have greater overall success and faster time to intubation; however, there was no difference in these metrics by the time the fifth patient was intubated. In trauma, VL did not improve mortality when compared to DL.[19] A total of 623 patients were randomized to DL or VL. Not only was there no difference in mortality, but there was higher median intubation duration in the VL group. Subgroup analysis found higher mortality in patients suffering from traumatic brain injury (TBI). This may have been related to more frequent occurrences of oxygen saturation less than 80% in patients with TBI. VL was compared to DL in an intensive care setting. First-attempt success was no different between 186 patients randomized to the VL arm and 185 patients randomized to the DL arm (67.7% vs. 70.3%, $P = .6$).[20] The median time to successful tracheal intubation was 3 minutes in both groups. Severe life-threatening complications were higher in the VL group (9.5% vs. 2.8%, $P = .01$).

Trimmel et al. compared 326 tracheal intubations by prehospital physicians with either VL or DL. First-attempt success was higher with DL (96.2% vs. 61.9%, $P < .001$).[21] A second-attempt crossover methodology was also used (i.e., failure with VL was followed by attempt with DL) and demonstrated 95.3% second-attempt success with DL compared to 66.7% second-attempt success with VL. Failure to advance the endotracheal tube into the trachea and impaired visualization due to blood were cited as factors contributing to VL failure.

A Cochrane report on VL versus DL evaluating 64 studies concluded that there was no difference in first-attempt success, reduction in hypoxia or mortality.[22] Overall, there was no evidence that VL "reduces the number of intubation attempts or the incidence of hypoxia or respiratory complications...[or] affects time required for intubation."

Supraglottic Airways

Supraglottic airways (SGAs) are sometimes used in trauma. Laryngeal mask airways were used in 15 trauma patients that were entrapped and unable to be intubated.[23] A supraglottic device was used successfully in 57 trauma patients either as a rescue device or as a primary device for less experienced providers.[24] There are substantial limitations to the use of SGAs in trauma, however. The SGA does not definitively secure the airway, offers limited protection against the risk of aspiration, and provides challenges to positive pressure ventilation in noncompliant lungs. In one case report of ventilation following drowning, peak pressure adequate for ventilation was unable to be generated, resulting in air insufflation into the stomach.[25]

The intubating SGA airway offers an alternative airway technique in trauma and has been used with success in a morbidly obese patient with chest trauma.[26]

Cricothyroidotomy

In the event of a can't intubate, can't ventilate situation, cricothyroidotomy may be the option remaining to secure the airway. While cricothyroidotomy can be a relatively straight-forward, albeit emergency procedure, it is associated with significant complication rates. In a prospective observational study of 282 trauma patients requiring airway management in a combat setting, 17 patients required cricothyroidotomy.[27] Four of those 17 cricothyroidotomies failed (failure rate of 23.5%). Compared to medics, physicians intubated the majority of these patients requiring prehospital airway management, had the highest rates of success, and the lowest rates of complications. Similar work by another group found that prehospital cricothyroidotomy failed to cannulate the trachea in 26% of cases.[28] Notably, 66% of patients undergoing percutaneous cricothyroidotomy died. The majority of patients (82%) requiring cricothyroidotomy had gunshot wounds to the face, neck, or head. As noted previously, more highly trained providers (e.g., physicians, physician assistants) had lower failure rates than medics (15% vs. 33%). When indicated, cricothyroidotomy should be committed to and promptly undertaken. The "scalpel-finger-tube" approach has been described.[29] The use of a bougie rather than a finger may further aid the swift and efficient passage of an endotracheal tube and is recommended by the Difficult Airway Society.

Pulmonary

Ventilatory strategies can be broadly categorized as decelerating flow patterns (i.e., pressure control) and constant flow patterns (i.e., volume target/volume control). Given the challenges in accurately measuring dynamic ventilator volumes in the clinical setting, the mathematical integral of flow is typically used to calculate volumes. Low lung volume ventilation is a widely acknowledged strategy to limit lung injury in critically ill patients. The well-known Adult Respiratory Distress Syndrome (ARDS) Net trial demonstrated a mortality benefit (31% vs. 39%, $P = .007$) in patients ventilated with lower tidal volumes of 6 mL/kg, as well as more ventilator free days in the same group (12 days vs. 10 days, $P = .007$).[30] Lower tidal volume ventilation was used as part of an approach allowing permissive hypercarbia and both a ladder of escalating fraction of inspired oxygen (F_IO_2) and positive end-expiratory pressure (PEEP).

Guldner et al. authored an excellent review of intraoperative ventilator management[31] that focused on lung-protective strategies including recruitment maneuvers, as well as a proposed protocol for lung protection in the operating room. Historically, alveolar recruitment was obtained via a sustained Valsalva maneuver, typically holding PEEP at a ~30 cm H_2O for approximately 30 seconds. This tends to divert gas to healthy compliant tissue and does not recruit atelectatic lung tissue. As described in the Guldner review, a more effective strategy cycles increasing levels of PEEP over tidal volume ventilation in a step wise pattern (i.e., PEEP changes of 10-15-20-15-10 over 3 tidal volume breaths each). This proposed lung-protective ventilatory strategy essentially applies low lung volume ventilation to healthy lungs in the operating room, where the objective is to avoid lung injury and/or alveolar recruitment before it occurs.

Low tidal volume ventilation initiated in the operating room before lung injury was evaluated in 20 reports including over 2,800 patients.[32] Low lung volume ventilation was associated with decreased lung injury development (RR 0.33, CI 0.23–0.47) and decreased mortality (RR 0.64, CI 0.46–0.89). Lower tidal volumes were also associated with a lower incidence of pulmonary infection and lower mean hospital length of stay (LOS). In other work, Serpa Neto et al. compared protective ventilatory strategies to conventional ventilation strategies.[33] Postoperative pulmonary complications (e.g., postoperative lung injury, pulmonary infection, barotrauma) were evaluated in a review of 15 randomized controlled trials. Lung-protective ventilation with lower tidal volumes was associated with fewer postoperative pulmonary complications compared to conventional ventilation strategies (adjusted RR 0.64, CI 0.46–0.88, $P < .01$); however, the same benefit was not observed when comparing a low tidal volume + low PEEP strategy to a low tidal volume + high PEEP strategy (adjusted RR 0.93, CI 0.64–1.37, $P = .72$). While postoperative pulmonary complications and tidal volume were related in this study, complications and PEEP were not.

Transfusion-associated circulatory overload (TACO) can occur following massive transfusion and presents challenges to ventilatory management in trauma patients. Transudative flow of fluid to the interstitium contributes to decreased lung compliance. TACO is characterized by respiratory distress and hydrostatic pulmonary edema within 6 hours of blood transfusion.[34] Patients may present with volume overload, lung crackles, and generalized sequelae of positive fluid balance. Risk factors include history of hemorrhagic shock, chronic renal failure, heart failure, and positive fluid balance per hour. TACO may respond to diuresis; however, any diuretic therapy in hemorrhagic shock must be carefully evaluated in the context of volume loss from bleeding.

TACO and transfusion-related acute lung injury (TRALI) can present with similar clinical pictures of respiratory embarrassment following blood transfusion. TACO generally presents with hydrostatic pulmonary edema, whereas TRALI presents more commonly as pulmonary permeability edema related to an inflammatory-immune response.[35] Brain natriuretic peptide and leukocyte antibody testing may offer a technique to distinguish TACO and TRALI; however, more work is needed to elucidate the pathogenesis of these two entities.[36]

Cardiovascular

It is appealing in many clinical settings to correct low blood pressure resulting from blood loss with vasopressor support. Unfortunately, this has not been shown to improve outcome in trauma patients. One investigation evaluated 1,349 trauma patients, 351 of whom received vasopressor support from either, dopamine, epinephrine, phenylephrine, norepinephrine, or vasopressin.[37] Mortality was significantly worse in those patients who received vasopressors (43.6% vs. 4.2%, $P < .01$).

Other work looked at mortality in 921 severely injured blunt trauma patients who survived 48 hours and were treated with norepinephrine, vasopressin, dopamine, or phenylephrine.[38] Early vasopressor use was associated with an 80% higher risk of mortality (hazard ratio 1.81, CI 1.1–2.9, $P = .013$). It is notable that the 95% confidence interval for the hazard ratio crossed unity in the vasopressin group. While this does not imply that vasopressin improved mortality, it was not statistically significantly associated with worsened mortality.

Vasopressin is a potent vasoconstrictor that acts on most of the vascular distribution, with the notable exception of cerebral, pulmonary, and cardiac vascular beds. It amplifies the neuroendocrine response, and is more potent than norepinephrine or angiotensin II, while maintaining efficacy in hypoxia and severe acidosis. Animal models of vasopressin use in hemorrhagic shock have shown impressive results. In a porcine model of liver injury, animals were resuscitated with either vasopressin, placebo or crystalloid resuscitation.[39] Mean arterial pressure (MAP) was higher in the vasopressin group (58 mmHg vs. 32 mmHg, $P < .05$), vasopressin improved abdominal blood flow but did not cause further blood loss, and all vasopressin animals survived until bleeding was controlled plus an additional 60 minutes. All animals in the other treatment arms died. Another porcine model of liver injury compared vasopressin, epinephrine, and placebo.[40] MAP was higher in the vasopressin group compared to the epinephrine and placebo groups at 2.5 minutes (82 mmHg vs. 23 mmHg vs. 11 mmHg, $P < .001$) as well as at 10 minutes (42 mmHg vs. 10 mmHg vs. 6 mmHg, $P < .001$). Hepatic and renal artery blood flow was higher in the vasopressin group, and all (7/7) animals in the vasopressin group survived to bleeding control plus an additional 60 minutes, compared to none (0/14) of the animals in the other groups.

Vasopressin use in humans with traumatic hemorrhagic shock has also been encouraging. In one case report a 41-year-old woman suffered a fall from a height of 15 m, sustaining multiple blunt trauma injuries and hemorrhagic shock.[41] She was transfused with packed red blood cells (PRBCs) and fresh frozen plasma (FFP) during transfer to a trauma center. Intravenous fluids and norepinephrine were initiated at arrival, but she remained hemodynamically unstable. A vasopressin infusion, together with emergency interventional radiology coiling of bleeding pelvic vasculature, stabilized the patient. Despite orthopedic, liver, and traumatic brain injuries, the patient was discharged from the ICU after 39 days with no neurologic deficit. The Arginine Vasopressin during the Early Resuscitation of Traumatic Shock (AVERT) trial randomized trauma patients with hemorrhagic who had received 6 units of PRBCs to receive a vasopressin bolus of 4 units followed by assignment to either a vasopressin infusion or placebo.[42] The vasopressin group required fewer blood products (1.4 L vs. 2.9 L, $P = .01$), however, without a difference in crystalloid or vasopressor use. Both groups had similar mortality and complications, although the vasopressin group experienced fewer DVTs (5/44 vs. 16/47, $P = .02$). Thus, recent evidence to support vasopressin treatment of traumatic hemorrhagic shock is encouraging.

Methylene blue has been used to restore blood pressure in vasoplegic patients (e.g., cardiopulmonary bypass, burns), although supporting evidence is unclear.[43] Methylene blue inhibits guanylyl cyclase, interrupts cGMP pathways and antagonizes the vasodilatory effect of nitric oxide (NO) on the endothelium. In a retrospective study of 226 vasoplegic patients following cardiopulmonary bypass,[44] those who received methylene blue had worse mortality, renal failure, and hyperbilirubinemia. While methylene blue may be useful as a rescue therapy, its use as a first-choice agent is not currently supported by a wide body of literature.

Vasopressor use must be interpreted in the context of the underlying pathophysiology of hemorrhagic shock. While increasing the blood pressure in a hypotensive patient is appealing, the approach underestimates the role that tissue perfusion plays in hemorrhagic shock. Tissue perfusion is likely more closely linked to blood flow than to blood pressure. Recent work has attempted to describe the circulatory system in terms of an electrical circuit to better model behavior of the complex interactions between tissues beds.[45] One challenge of such a model is matching the pulsatile arterial system (similar to an alternating current circuit) to the more dampened, high-capacitance venous system (similar to a direct current circuit). Current computer modeling tools may offer an approach to describe such phenomenon mathematically and may suggest new therapies for hemorrhagic shock.

Hypotensive Resuscitation

During hypotensive resuscitation of trauma patients, low blood pressure is tolerated until surgical control of bleeding is undertaken. Cowell described this approach over one hundred years ago,[46] based on the concept that higher, or even normal, blood pressure will exacerbate blood loss in patients in whom bleeding has not been controlled (i.e., "pop the clot"). It has been difficult, however, to demonstrate a clear benefit of hypotensive resuscitation. A prospective investigation of 110 trauma patients randomized to a target resuscitation systolic blood pressure of either 100 mmHg or 70 mmHg reported identical mortality in each group (4/55).[47] A larger, multicenter study compared outcomes 1,216 patients with an injury severity score (ISS) greater than 15 who received at least 500 mL of prehospital crystalloid to those receiving less than 500 mL.[48] In normotensive patients, the larger crystalloid infusion increased the risk of mortality (HR 2.5, CI 1.3–4.9, $P < .01$) and worsened coagulopathy (OR 2.2, CI 1.01–4.9, $P = .04$). However, in patients who were hypotensive, the larger crystalloid infusion raised the emergency department systolic blood pressure. Furthermore for each 1 mmHg increase in systolic blood pressure, survival increased by 2% (OR 1.02, CI 1.01–1.03, $P < .01$).

The definition of hypotension can be challenging to quantify. Walsh et al. evaluated 33,330 noncardiac surgery patients to develop an empirical definition of hypotension.[49] They found that the risk of acute kidney injury (defined as an elevation of creatinine to 1.5 times the baseline) and myocardial injury (defined as elevations in troponin or CK-MB isoenzymes) increased with a MAP less than 55 mmHg. Longer durations of lower blood pressure increased the risk for end-organ dysfunction.

Neurologic

Neurologic injury is a leading cause of death in trauma. Hypoten- 5
sion and hypoxemia have detrimental effects following TBI. In an analysis of 717 patients with a Glasgow Coma Scale (GCS) less than 8; a systolic blood pressure less than 90 mmHg or a partial pressure of oxygen (PaO_2) less than 60 mmHg increased mortality by 150%,[50] ascribed largely to hypotension. In TBI patients it is important to maintain sufficient cerebral-perfusion pressure (CPP) to support metabolic energetics—a potentially challenging goal in patients with associated injuries. For example, the abdominal trauma surgeon may request a lower MAP, while the neurotrauma surgeon may request a higher MAP. In these cases, the trauma anesthesiologist serves as a focal point for the discussion of cooperative management of complex multitrauma patients.

Decompressive craniectomy can be used to lower intracranial pressure (ICP) in patients with severe TBI unresponsive to standard ICP therapies (see Chapter 37). However, in one decompressive craniectomy was associated with similar rates of death at 6 months (19% vs. 18%)[51] despite resulting in fewer interventions for elevated ICP, shorter ICU LOS, and less time with an elevated ICP. The decompressive craniectomy group also had worse scores on the Glasgow Outcome Scale score (OR 1.84, CI 1.05–3.24, $P = .03$) and higher odds of having an unfavorable outcome (OR 2.21, 95% CI 1.14–4.26, $P = .02$). Placement of a ventriculostomy catheter has been suggested to help with such TBI decision-making; however, when compared to imaging with computed tomography (CT)[52] no differences in functional outcomes were reported.

Steroids are another therapeutic option for TBI. In an investigation of over 10,000 patients with TBI and Glasgow Coma Scale (GCS) score less than 14 within 8 hours of injury,[53] patients who received 48 hours of either methylprednisolone (compared to placebo) had a higher relative risk of both death within 2 weeks and death/disability at 6 months (RR 1.18, CI 1.09–1.27, $P = .001$). A Cochrane review of steroid treatment in TBI evaluating 20 trials with over 12,000 patients found significant heterogeneity, making the authors unable to calculate a pooled result estimate of the risk of death.[54] The authors noted that the largest trial (accounting for 80% of all randomized patients in the review) did find an increased risk of death with steroid use (RR 1.15, CI 1.07–1.24). The review showed no significant increased risk of infection or gastrointestinal bleeding.

Hyperosmolar therapy with either mannitol or hypertonic saline can be used as an osmotic diuretic to decrease ICP following TBI. By facilitating its osmotic shift from brain tissue into the vasculature, fluid is then eliminated via the urine. Animal studies have found that 10% sodium chloride lowered ICP and increased CPP compared to 20% mannitol.[55] A systemic review reported that both treatments facilitate diuresis.[56] Upadhyay et al. evaluated 200 pediatric ICU patients with raised ICP who were treated with mannitol or 3% saline.[57] Using MAP as a surrogate for ICP they found that 3% saline lowered MAP and decreased coma hours compared to mannitol. The use of hypertonic saline further avoided the risk of renal failure sometimes seen with the use of mannitol. A review of hyperosmolar therapy for raised ICP noted the risk of renal failure with the use of mannitol, possibly related to hypovolemia, while also noting that 3% saline should be administered via central venous access.[58] The review references the Brain Trauma Foundation recommendation for mannitol.

Prevention of secondary brain injury by maintaining cerebral perfusion and oxygenation is critically important in improving long-term outcome following TBI. Post-traumatic seizure prophylaxis in the first 7 days following injury is advocated by the Brain Trauma Foundation.[59,60] Phenytoin, a sodium channel blocker, has been investigated thoroughly over the past several decades for prevention of post-traumatic seizures. Levetiracetam binds to the synaptic vesicle protein SV2A and offers comparable efficacy but does not require frequent checking of medication levels.[61]

Resuscitation

Transfusion

6 The cornerstone of trauma resuscitation is blood product administration. Massive transfusion is defined as transfusion of more than 10 units of whole blood in 24 hours, an estimated blood loss of greater than 150 mL/hr, or the transfusion of greater than 5 units of whole blood in 3 hours.[62] In the military conflicts of the first two decades of the 21st century, empiric administration of FFP was employed in trauma resuscitation, often in a ratio of 1 unit PRBC to 1 unit of FFP. A retrospective review of the military experience evaluated 246 patients at a Combat Support Hospital.[63] Mortality was improved in patients with ratios closer to unity (1:8 = 65% mortality, 1:2.5 = 34%, 1:1.4 = 19%, $P < .001$). Subsequent civilian trauma reports showed similarly improved survival with transfusion ratios for both FFP:PRBC and platelet:PRBC that approached unity.[64] Ratios closer to 1:1 were associated with decreased truncal hemorrhage and increased 6-hour, 24-hour, and 30-day survival, as well as increased ICU-free days, ventilator-free days, and hospital-free days.

However, improvement in survival with ratios closer to 1:1 was potentially confounded by survivor bias. Patients who received FFP had lived long enough to receive the thawed blood product (potentially as long as 45 minutes).[65] In observational studies, early deaths may have be disproportionately over-represented by the low FFP:PRBC ratio cohort, with early survivors surviving long enough to receive more FFP.

In an attempt to define the optimal transfusion ratio, Davenport et al. reported the maximal hemostatic effect to be at FFP:PRBC ratios of 1:2–3:4.[66] FFP:PRBC transfusion ratios >1:1 conferred no benefit, while any hemostatic effect of balanced FFP to PRBC ratios seemed to be limited to coagulopathic patients. The Pragmatic Randomized Optimum Platelet and Plasma Ratio study (PROPPR) was designed to better define the benefit of 1:1 transfusion ratios.[67] Plasma-to-platelet-to-PRBC ratios of 1:1:1 and 1:1:2 were prospectively compared in patients who received more than 10 units of PRBC in the first 24 hours after injury. There was no difference in 24-hour or 30-day mortality; however, in the 1:1:1 group (i.e., more plasma) exsanguination was significantly decreased and more patients achieved hemostasis. More liberal use of FFP raised the potential issue of volume overload or coagulation hyper-responsiveness; however, there was no difference between the groups in ARDS, multiorgan failure, thromboembolic events, or sepsis.

The safety and efficacy of plasma use in the prehospital trauma setting was investigated in the PAMPer study.[68] A total of 501 patients were randomized to either plasma or standard care groups. The plasma group experienced lower mortality (23.2% vs. 33%, CI −18.6 to −1, $P = .03$), suggesting benefit to early administration of blood products. As in the PROPPR study there was no difference in a variety of complications, including multiorgan failure, acute lung injury, ARDS, infection, allergic reaction, or transfusion related reaction. Interestingly, some European militaries have long used dried plasma preparations. The French have used a pH-buffered, freeze-dried plasma product pooled from 8 to 10 donors with a 2-year shelf-life and have encountered no adverse events. Similarly, the German military has used "LyoPlas," a single donor product with a shelf life of 18 months. This is a type-specific product and must be reconstituted with a buffering solution.

Whole Blood Resuscitation

Whole blood (WB) resuscitation was historically used in military and combat trauma settings, mainly as "fresh" WB collected from a "walking blood bank."[69] WB resuscitation has recently gained more application in the civilian setting. Many level-1 trauma cen- 7
ters across the United States are incorporating low-titer group O whole blood (LTOWB) for initial trauma resuscitation.[70,71] Despite some military experiences suggesting a survival benefit of fresh WB compared to separate component therapy, fresh WB carries a risk of infectious disease transmission and is not FDA-approved.[72,73] LTOWB has low hemagglutinin (anti-A and anti-B) titers and has emerged as a more practical solution, with cold storage increasing shelf-life to 21 to 35 days.[69]

Since group O red blood cells are compatible with all blood types, major acute hemolytic transfusion reactions (i.e., major mismatch) are eliminated for LTOWB. Concerns remain for minor hemolytic transfusion reactions between donor's anti-A and anti-B hemagglutinin and recipient's red cells, requiring use of only donors with low titer (usually defined as less than 200 to 256 dilution).[74,75] Some institutions set a predefined maximum transfusion units of WB.[71]

Numerous studies both in military and civilian settings have reported no evidence of increased hemolytic reactions for WB recipients[76] when compared to either component therapy or LTOWB,[74,77] or between group O and non–group O recipients of LTOWB.[78,79] This has led many authors to conclude that WB has a similar safety profile to component therapy.[69,75,80]

Whole blood provides a potential practical advantage over component therapy by utilizing a single larger bag that delivers a more concentrated and balanced hemostatic product that requires less time to prepare. Whole blood therapy, however, has not shown a significant difference in survival compared to individual components, with systematic reviews noting large heterogeneity in methodology of studies and stressing the need for a large randomized controlled trial on the topic.[76,80,81]

Several cautions are important when considering LTOWB resuscitation. LTOWB use in females, especially those younger than 50 years old, requires selecting only Rh-negative WB to avoid the risk of Rh alloimmunization (anti-D conversion) in Rh-negative recipients and subsequent potential hemolytic disease in future newborns. In addition, the total volumes of WB are usually larger than that of PRBCs (approximately 500 vs. 250 to 350 mL).[74] To mitigate the risk of TACO, clinicians should frequently reassess resuscitation status to avoid volume overload. Also, leukoreduction might be applied to WB in an effort to decrease platelet concentration and aggregation.[82–84] Lastly, WB older than 2 weeks may have reduced and variable hemostatic function, necessitating additional component therapy.[69]

Adjuncts

Tranexamic acid is a synthetic antifibrinolytic that inhibits lysine binding sites on plasminogen. The resultant decrease in plasmin limits degradation of fibrin clot. It has been used for many years in obstetric and orthopedic practice, and found recent increased use in trauma care. In the CRASH-2 trial (a multicenter, prospective, randomized trial that included over 20,000 patients),[85] administration of tranexamic acid decreased all-cause mortality and death due to bleeding, with no increase in vascular occlusive events. The benefit of tranexamic acid use was seen when administered within 3 hours of injury. Interestingly, there was no difference in blood transfusions, and one criticism of the study has been that a relatively modest number of patients received blood products. The MATTERs study looked at 896 consecutive trauma admissions, of whom 293 received tranexamic acid.[86] Although patients who received tranexamic acid were more severely injured, they experienced lower mortality. Those patients who received more than 10 units of PRBCs in a 24-hour period benefited the most from antifibrinolysis.

The use of tranexamic acid for all trauma patients has been called into question, however, as impaired fibrinolysis can potentially worsen mortality.[87] In a study of 180 trauma patients, fibrinolytic shutdown was identified in 64% of patients (mortality 17%), physiologic fibrinolysis was seen in 18% of patients (mortality 3%), and hyperfibrinolysis was seen in 18% of patients (mortality 44%). The authors caution against use of tranexamic acid in all patients and suggest careful selection of patients who may benefit. CRASH-3 evaluated the potential risk of antifibrinolytics in over 12,000 TBI patients[88] without major extracranial bleeding. In patients with mild-to-moderate TBI, tranexamic acid lowered the risk of TBI-related death (RR 0.78, CI 0.64–0.95). More specifically, patients with reactive pupils had a decreased risk of TBI-related death (RR 0.87, CI 0.77–0.98). Beneficial effect was not apparent in patients with severe TBI. The risk of vascular occlusive events and seizures was no different between groups.

Calcium is a divalent cation required as a cofactor in multiple bioenergetic pathways. The citrate preservative in blood products can chelate calcium, lowering its concentration and contributing to hypotension.[89] The impact of hypocalcemia in trauma patients is unclear. Hypocalcemia increased mortality in 352 trauma patients who experienced critical bleeding and required massive transfusion. Trauma patients are also frequently hypocalcemic on admission (i.e., before transfusion). In one study, nearly 75% of 212 severely injured trauma patients (mean ISS = 34) were hypocalcemic (ionized calcium < 1.15 mmol/L) or severely hypocalcemic (ionized calcium < 0.9 mmol/L) prior to transfusion[90]; however, survival was not significantly different from similarly injured trauma patients who were normocalcemic. In other work, mortality was worse in 591 trauma patients admitted to a level I trauma center who presented with low calcium (15.5%) compared to high calcium (8.7%).[91] Multiple transfusions and massive transfusion were also elevated in the low calcium group. Multivariable logistic regression analysis showed that an ionized calcium concentration less than 1 mmol/L was independently predictive of the need for massive transfusion (OR 2.2, CI 1.05–5).

Prothrombin Complex Concentrate (PCC) offers a hemostatic effect with a lower volume than FFP. PCC is targeted to factors II, IX, and X (3 factor PCC [3-PCC]), or factors II, VII, IX, and X (4 factor PCC [4-PCC]). Either formulation can decrease administered volume, decrease the risk of TACO, and limit the risk of hydrostatic pulmonary edema. PCC also contains variable amounts of protein C, protein S, and heparin. Lyophilized PCC allows reconstitution rather than thawing, and provides 25 times the concentration of clotting factors.[92] Doses of 25 units/kg are targeted to reverse coagulopathy. Fibrinogen is available in FFP, cryoprecipitate, and fibrinogen concentrate, and can decrease blood product use.[93] Fibrinogen can correct hypofibrinogenemia due to dilutional coagulopathy, disseminated intravascular coagulation (DIC), and liver failure.[94] In a prospective study of 63 patients, fibrinogen reduced PRBC and FFP use in bleeding patients; however, three venous and one arterial nonfatal thrombotic events were noted.

Estrogen can help to correct uremic platelet dysfunction and gastrointestinal bleeding. Although its mechanism of action is uncertain, it appears to act by decreasing production of L-arginine, resulting in decreases in NO, guanylyl cyclase, and cGMP. This affect may lead to increase in thromboxane A2 and ADP, leading to formation of a platelet plug. Estrogen may also decrease antithrombin III (ATIII) and protein S, as well as increase factor VII. Desmopressin has been used to treat uremic platelet dysfunction by releasing factor VII from storage sites, thereby minimizing the effects of dysfunctional von Willebrand Factor (vWF).

Steroids

Adrenal insufficiency in critical illness is well described, thus hydrocortisone and its attendant intense mineralocorticoid activity can be used to improve sensitivity to catecholamines, decrease inflammatory markers, and decrease vasopressor requirements. The CORTICUS trial evaluated 251 sepsis patients in a randomized controlled trial receiving hydrocortisone at a dose of 50 mg,[95] finding no mortality benefit. Adrenal insufficiency has also been described in trauma, although treatment effects are unclear.[96] In one study of 34 trauma patients receiving cosyntropin immediately following injury, 47% were nonresponders (defined as an increase in cortisol of <9 mcg/dL) and 24% remained as nonresponders after 1 week. Mortality was similar in both groups; however nonresponders had a longer duration of norepinephrine infusion. In another study, stepwise dosing of phenylephrine was evaluated before and after administration of 50 mg of hydrocortisone. Hydrocortisone was found to decrease the ED50 by 37% and increased sensitivity to phenylephrine in trauma patients at the end of the resuscitation period (i.e., hours after the trauma).[97] A randomized controlled trial in 150 trauma patients[98] treated with hydrocortisone (200 mg × 5 days, 100 mg × 1 day, 50 mg × 1 day) reported no difference in mortality (absolute difference 3%, 95% CI –5 to 11, $P = .44$). However, the hospital-acquired pneumonia was less frequent (HR 0.51, 95% CI 0.3–0.83, $P = .007$) and ventilator-free days increased by 4 days in the hydrocortisone group (95% CI 2–7, $P = .001$).

Crystalloid Therapy

Blood is the ideal fluid with which to resuscitate a trauma patient in hemorrhagic shock. There may be instances, however, in which crystalloid may be used in small quantities. It is important to understand the effect of these fluids in the context of ongoing metabolic derangements. Chloride-rich solutions can contribute to hyperchloremic metabolic acidosis and worsen acid–base status in trauma patients. In a prospective, open-label study, critically ill patients received either chloride-rich solutions (e.g., 0.9% saline, 4% succinylated gelatin solution, 4% albumin) or chloride-poor solutions (e.g., lactated solution, Plasma-Lyte, chloride-poor 20% albumin).[99] Those receiving lower chloride content solutions experienced a higher rate of renal injury, as well as higher use of renal replacement therapy (RRT). There was no difference between in hospital mortality, ICU or hospital LOS, or the need for RRT following discharge.

Conversely, a meta-analysis evaluating the use of low chloride content solutions in critically ill patients found no statistically significant difference in mortality or the use of RRT.[100] in a randomized controlled trial comparing Plasma-Lyte to 0.9% sodium chloride as resuscitative fluids in the first 24 hours following trauma,[101] Plasma-Lyte was associated with improved base excess, improved pH, and lower serum chloride, but without a significant difference in mortality, resource utilization, or urine output. Another randomized controlled trial compared balanced multielectrolyte solution to 0.9% saline in critically ill patients and found no difference in mortality, new need for RRT, or serum creatinine.[102] There was also no difference in adverse events between the study groups.

Together these data suggest that there is either no difference in outcome among critically ill patients resuscitated with chloride-rich solutions (e.g., 0.9% saline) versus balanced salt solutions (e.g., Plasma-Lyte), or that there may be a benefit to balanced salt solutions. Either way, there is no physiologic advantage to chloride-rich solutions. It remains important to emphasize that the ideal resuscitative fluid in hemorrhagic shock is blood.

Bicarbonate

Lactic acidosis is a common feature of hemorrhagic shock. Treatment of lactic acidosis with sodium bicarbonate may actually worsen intracellular acidosis, however, despite improving serum pH.[103] No controlled studies have shown an improvement in hemodynamics attributable to sodium bicarbonate. The use of bicarbonate in resuscitation is dependent upon adequate renal function, as bicarbonate helps primarily in the elimination of hydrogen ion (and potassium) via the urine. Ultimately, there is no convincing evidence to support the use of bicarbonate in trauma patients with lactic acidosis.

Renal

Urine output is one of the most sensitive, though nonspecific measures of resuscitation in the operating room. A urine output of 0.5 to 1 mL/kg/hr is thought to suggest adequate renal perfusion. In trauma, hypovolemia can lead to a prerenal syndrome due to hypoperfusion and acute tubular necrosis, resulting in decreased urine output. Tubular obstruction by necrotic cells at the pars recta can occur at the nephron's proximal tubule and Loop of Henle, while intratubular casts can precipitate when myoglobin reacts with Tamm-Horsfall tubular protein.[104] Rhabdomyolysis following trauma can also contribute to acute kidney injury (AKI); however. serum myoglobin alone is not an indication forRRT. Acute tubular necrosis is best treated with prompt fluid administration decrease the incidence of post-traumatic AKI.[105]

Low-dose dopamine can increase renal and mesenteric blood flow in some experimental models. The use of such renal dose dopamine to treat renal failure, however, has not been correlated with improvement in a number of markers for renal function.[106] Furthermore, low-dose dopamine can worsen splanchnic oxygenation, as well as impair gastrointestinal function, endocrine function, and immunologic function. A meta-analysis found that low-dose dopamine did not prevent mortality onset of acute renal failure or the need for RRT.[107]

Diuretic therapy may mask ongoing AKI in trauma patients by facilitating urine output at the expense of renal cellular dysfunction.[108] AKI determines the response to furosemide, rather than furosemide defining the degree of AKI. Furosemide also can result in alkalosis, as well as contribute to hypovolemia and hypokalemia, which can lead to dysrhythmias such as atrial fibrillation. The combination of bicarbonate and mannitol (BIC/MAN) has been used historically to treat renal failure and was evaluated in a review of 2,083 trauma patients.[109] There was no difference in RRT or mortality in patients with a creatine kinase greater than 5,000 U/L who had received BIC/MAN therapy. Thus, the best approach to treat low urine output in the context of hemorrhagic shock is with fluid resuscitation and RRT, as indicated by RIFLE criteria.[110]

Measures of Resuscitation

Evaluation of the adequacy of resuscitation during ongoing hemorrhagic shock presents challenges. Sudden drops in end-tidal carbon dioxide ($ETCO_2$) suggest an increase in dead-space ventilation. In hemorrhagic shock, precipitous drops in $ETCO_2$ represent a substantial perfusion deficit and are an early indicator of impending cardiovascular collapse. Mathematical modeling of data from patients who suffered cardiac arrest evaluated $ETCO_2$ in the context of a return of spontaneous circulation (ROSC).[111] A higher peak $ETCO_2$, larger area under the $ETCO_2$ curve and rising $ETCO_2$ slope all correlated positively with ROSC. A cumulative maximum $ETCO_2$ of greater than 20 mmHg between 5 and 10 minutes postintubation predicted ROSC with a sensitivity of 0.88 and specificity of 0.77 ($P < 0.001$). The utility of $ETCO_2$ in trauma care was examined in 106 trauma patients. Arterial blood gas samples were collected in the operating room during surgery.[112] An $ETCO_2$ of 27 mmHg or greater was associated with 5% mortality, whereas an $ETCO_2$ less than 24 mmHg was associated with 68% mortality.

The base deficit attempts to isolate the metabolic contribution to acid–base status, and is the amount of base required to bring 1 L of whole blood at 37°C and a partial pressure of CO_2 of 40 mmHg to a pH of 7.4. It serves as a rapidly obtainable and dynamic measure of resuscitation that accurately reflects the state of resuscitation in trauma patients, and is superior to pH at assessing the effectiveness of resuscitation.[113] As with any variable measured during a dynamic process, a single value is less important than its trend.

In 1,191 trauma patients, base deficit was associated with need for blood transfusion (OR 0.8, $P < .001$).[114] Worsening base deficit was associated with lower blood pressure, higher ISS, and increased transfusion requirements. In addition, severely deranged base deficit (<–10 mmHg) was associated with significantly worse mortality than normal (2 to –2), mild (–3 to –5), or moderate (–6 to –9) base deficit derangement. A base deficit classification system has been proposed which defines Class I shock as base deficit <2, Class II as base deficit 2–6, Class III as base deficit 6 to 10, and Class IV as base deficit >10.[115] This system was more predicative than traditional Advanced Trauma Life Support (ATLS) classification systems at predicting the need for blood transfusion and mortality.

Stroke volume variability (SVV) evaluates the difference in maximum/minimum stroke volumes divided by the mean stroke volume calculated from a floating average over 30 seconds ($SVV = [SV_{max} - SV_{min}]/SV_{mean}$). The stroke volume is calculated from the area under the function defined by the arterial line waveform.[116] When evaluated as a measure of the adequacy of resuscitation, SVV > 9.5% predicted a 5% increase in stroke volume with administration of a 100 mL bolus of fluid.[117] Fluid responders correlated with SVV, but not with heart rate or central venous pressure (CVP). The area under the receiver operator characteristic (ROC) was 0.87 for SVV, 0.59 for heart rate, and 0.49 for CVP. An area under the ROC of 0.5 suggests no correlation between measured metrics.

The use of CVP to guide fluid therapy has been called into question. Marik et al. investigated CVP as a metric to guide fluid therapy in a meta-analysis.[118] They found that the area under the ROC for correlation "between the CVP and change in cardiac performance following an intervention that altered cardiac preload" was 0.56 for all studies reviewed, 0.56 for ICU-only studies reviewed, and 0.56 for studies reviewed from the operating room. There is little evidence to support the use of CVP as a metric for fluid responsiveness and/or resuscitation.

Table 53-2 Assessment of Blood Consumption

Penetrating Mechanism?	yes/no
Systolic Blood Pressure <90 mmHg?	yes/no
Heart Rate >120 beats per minute?	yes/no
Positive FAST Exam?	yes/no
If 2 or more YES answers, then activate Massive Transfusion Protocol	

The assessment of blood consumption (ABC) score can be used to predict the need for massive transfusion.[119] Four variables are assessed quickly, noninvasively, and without laboratory support; penetrating mechanism of injury, positive FAST (abdominal ultrasound) examination, systolic blood pressure <90 mmHg, heart rate >120 beats per minute (Table 53-2). A positive response to two or more variables is 75% sensitive and 86% specific for predicting the need for massive transfusion.

Viscoelastic Testing

The complex pathophysiology and temporal dynamics of trauma-induced coagulopathy (TIC) call for tests that yield timely and specific results that can be used to diagnose, monitor, and guide therapy. The objective is to achieve adequate blood coagulation and reduce hemorrhagic mortality, while minimizing unnecessary risk and costs of blood product transfusion.[120]

Traditionally, conventional coagulation tests (CCTs) including prothrombin time (PT), international normalized ratio (INR), activated partial thromboplastin time (aPTT), Clauss fibrinogen level, and platelet counts have been the standard tests for TIC.[121] Although there is no standard definition,[122] studies most commonly define TIC as INR of >1.2 (or PT > 18 seconds)[123] and are associated with worsened hemorrhage and mortality.[124–126] More recent studies, however, have shown that INR or PT may be prolonged in samples with adequate coagulation factor activity levels. Thus, INR is increasingly recognized more as a biomarker for injury severity rather than for dysfunctional hemostasis.

Point-of-care (POC) coagulation tests are increasingly utilized for trauma resuscitation due in part to their rapid turn-around time (Fig. 53-1). Viscoelastic hemostatic assays (VHA) are widely used and studied. VHA devices are available from many manufacturers using different reagents, test mechanics, and results parameters (see Chapter 17). They share the commonalities of being POC and of quantifying the increasing viscosity of whole blood as the blood clot forms.[127] VHA tracings typically represent four phases of clot kinetics: initiation, propagation, clot strength, and fibrinolysis.[128] Figure 53-2 depicts schematic tracings and parameters of the two most commonly use VHA devices—thromboelastography (TEG) and rotational thromboelastometry (ROTEM). The corresponding hemostatic component of choice for resuscitation during each phase of coagulation is displayed.

Theoretically VHA addresses many limitations of CCT. Results of VHA are prompt. Although VHA devices require 15 to 45 minutes to complete the test, actionable results can be obtained as early as 5 minutes. Several groups have shown strong correlation between early clot amplitudes and both maximum clot firmness as well as massive transfusion.[129–131] Some institutions utilize a rapid emergency hemorrhage panel as an alternative to POC testing. Careful attention to logistical issues (e.g., immediate movement of the sample to the testing area, limiting checks for hemolysis and rapid centrifugation) can reduce turn-around-times of CCT to those comparable to VHA.[132]

CCT cannot reliably identify hyperfibrinolysis, whereas VHA can identify both hyperfibrinolysis (associated with early TIC) and fibrinolytic shutdown (mostly occurring hours later).[133] Studies have shown increased mortality and more complications with both hyperfibrinolysis and fibrinolytic shutdown identified on VHA. This is typically from hemorrhage in hyperfibrinolysis and thrombosis in fibrinolytic shutdown.[134–138]

While conventional platelet counting only measures the quantity of platelets, the phase of clot strength in VHA reflects both the quantity and function of platelet and fibrinogen, with platelets accounting for 70% to 80% of the peak resistance curve[133,139] (Fig. 53-2, MA or MCF). However, differentiating preinjury and postinjury platelet dysfunction requires additional assays with different reagents (e.g., ROTEM/TEG platelet mapping). Other POC devices that can determine platelet function and detect different inhibitors include Multiplate (Roche Diagnostics International Ltd.) and Verifynow (Accumetrics, CA).[120]

To distinguish the hemostatic effects of fibrinogen from that of platelets, both VHA devices have assays containing different platelet inhibitors—functional fibrinogen TEG and FIBTEM. A strong correlation between both tests and the gold-standard laboratory-based Clauss method have been confirmed both in trauma and nontrauma population.[140–142] While pathophysiologic rationale supports using POC VHA in trauma patients, survival benefit of VHA is still questionable. Two earlier systematic reviews limited to trauma patients found little to no evidence of to support an association between VHA and survival.[143,144] Interestingly, recent Cochrane and Eastern Association for the Surgery of Trauma (EAST) reviews recommended VHA for the potential benefits of reduced blood product transfusions and mortality.[145,146] However, studies included for these reviews had low level of evidence and populations were not limited to trauma. The most recent multicenter trial comparing VHA-guided versus CCT-guided resuscitation (ITACTIC study)[147] reported no difference in clinical outcomes, including the rate of massive transfusion or mortality. However, TIC was less prevalent in the study (25%) and overall massive transfusion rate was low (27%). This raises the concern that the population studied may not have been coagulopathic enough to identify the benefit of VHA (Table 53-3).

Table 53-3 Comparison of Conventional Coagulation Test and Viscoelastic Hemostatic Assays

	Conventional Coagulation Test	Viscoelastic Test
Turnaround time	15–60 min[a]	20–40 min[b]
Costs	Less	More
Perform on	Citrated plasma	Whole blood
Detect hyperfibrinolysis	No	Yes
Detect hypercoagulation	No	Yes
Detect Warfarin	Yes	Unreliable
Detect DOAC	No	Nonspecific
Detect primary hemostasis abnormality	No	No

[a]With emergency hemorrhage panel.
[b]Actionable results within 5–10 min.

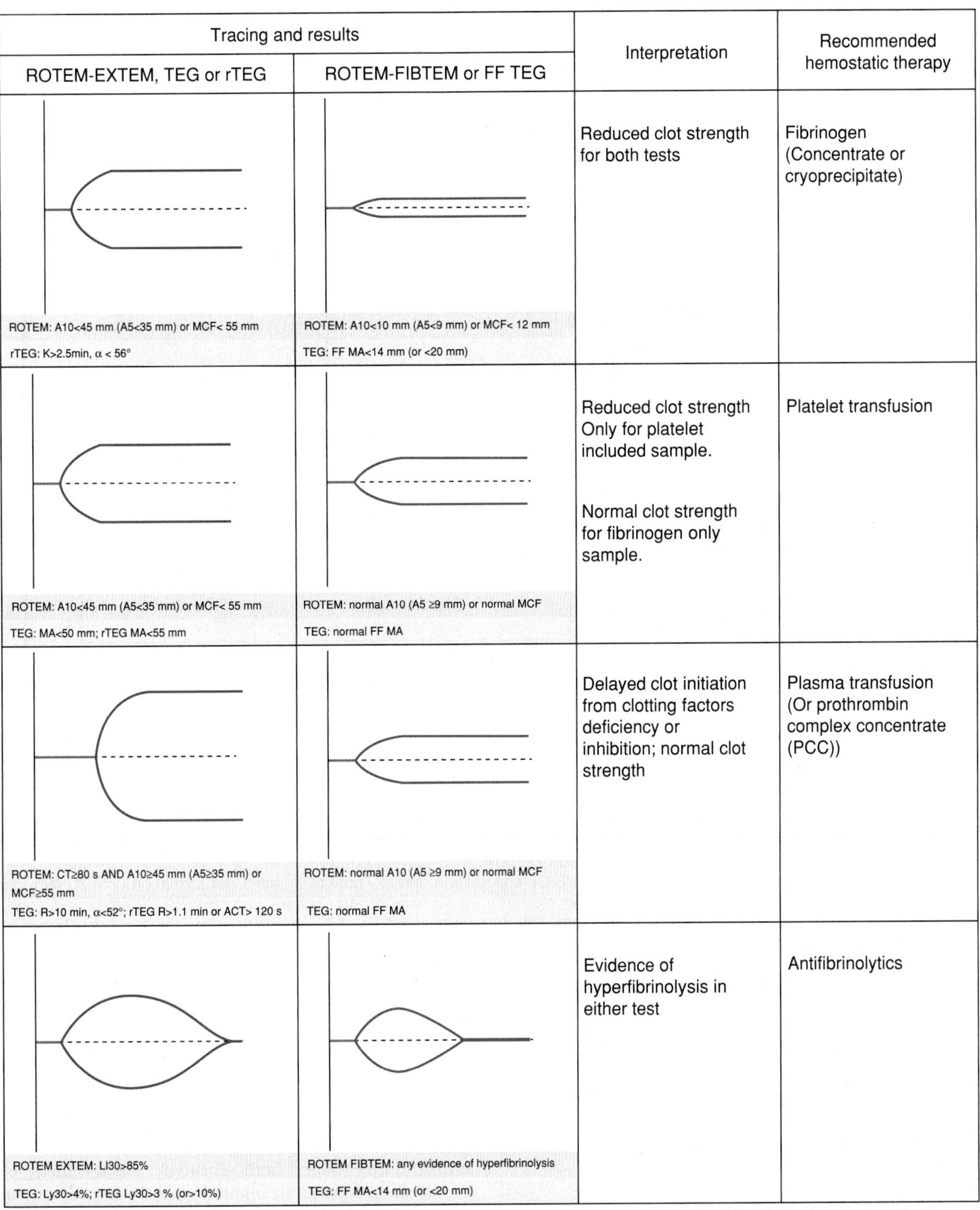

Tracing and results		Interpretation	Recommended hemostatic therapy
ROTEM-EXTEM, TEG or rTEG	ROTEM-FIBTEM or FF TEG		
ROTEM: A10<45 mm (A5<35 mm) or MCF< 55 mm rTEG: K>2.5min, α < 56°	ROTEM: A10<10 mm (A5<9 mm) or MCF< 12 mm TEG: FF MA<14 mm (or <20 mm)	Reduced clot strength for both tests	Fibrinogen (Concentrate or cryoprecipitate)
ROTEM: A10<45 mm (A5<35 mm) or MCF< 55 mm TEG: MA<50 mm; rTEG MA<55 mm	ROTEM: normal A10 (A5 ≥9 mm) or normal MCF TEG: normal FF MA	Reduced clot strength Only for platelet included sample. Normal clot strength for fibrinogen only sample.	Platelet transfusion
ROTEM: CT≥80 s AND A10≥45 mm (A5≥35 mm) or MCF≥55 mm TEG: R>10 min, α<52°; rTEG R>1.1 min or ACT> 120 s	ROTEM: normal A10 (A5 ≥9 mm) or normal MCF TEG: normal FF MA	Delayed clot initiation from clotting factors deficiency or inhibition; normal clot strength	Plasma transfusion (Or prothrombin complex concentrate (PCC))
ROTEM EXTEM: LI30>85% TEG: Ly30>4%; rTEG Ly30>3 % (or>10%)	ROTEM FIBTEM: any evidence of hyperfibrinolysis TEG: FF MA<14 mm (or <20 mm)	Evidence of hyperfibrinolysis in either test	Antifibrinolytics

Figure 53-1 POC coagulation testing. Schematic examples of viscoelastic tracings and recommended treatment strategies. ACT, activated clotting time; A5, amplitude at 5 minutes after coagulation start; A10, amplitude at 10 minutes after coagulation start; CT, coagulation time; K, time from initial clot formation until 20 mm amplitude; Li30, Lysis index percent reduction in amplitude from maximum clot firmness 30 minutes after coagulation time; LY30, percent reduction of area under the curve at 30 minutes compared to maximum amplitude; MA, maximum amplitude; MCF, maximum clot firmness; R, reaction time.

Several limitations exist for VHA, including cost effectiveness. A retrospective study showed that while costing less than one-tenth of viscoelastic tests, POC INR testing correlated well with both the TEG values and blood product transfusion.[148] Most physicians are also less familiar with VHA and there is a steep learning curve in both performing and interpreting VHA tests. Older VHA devices also have high intra- and interoperator variability.[143,149] However, newer devices are cartridge-based and automated, thus associated with lower variability.[150] Importantly, these in vitro tests measure only secondary hemostasis. Thus,

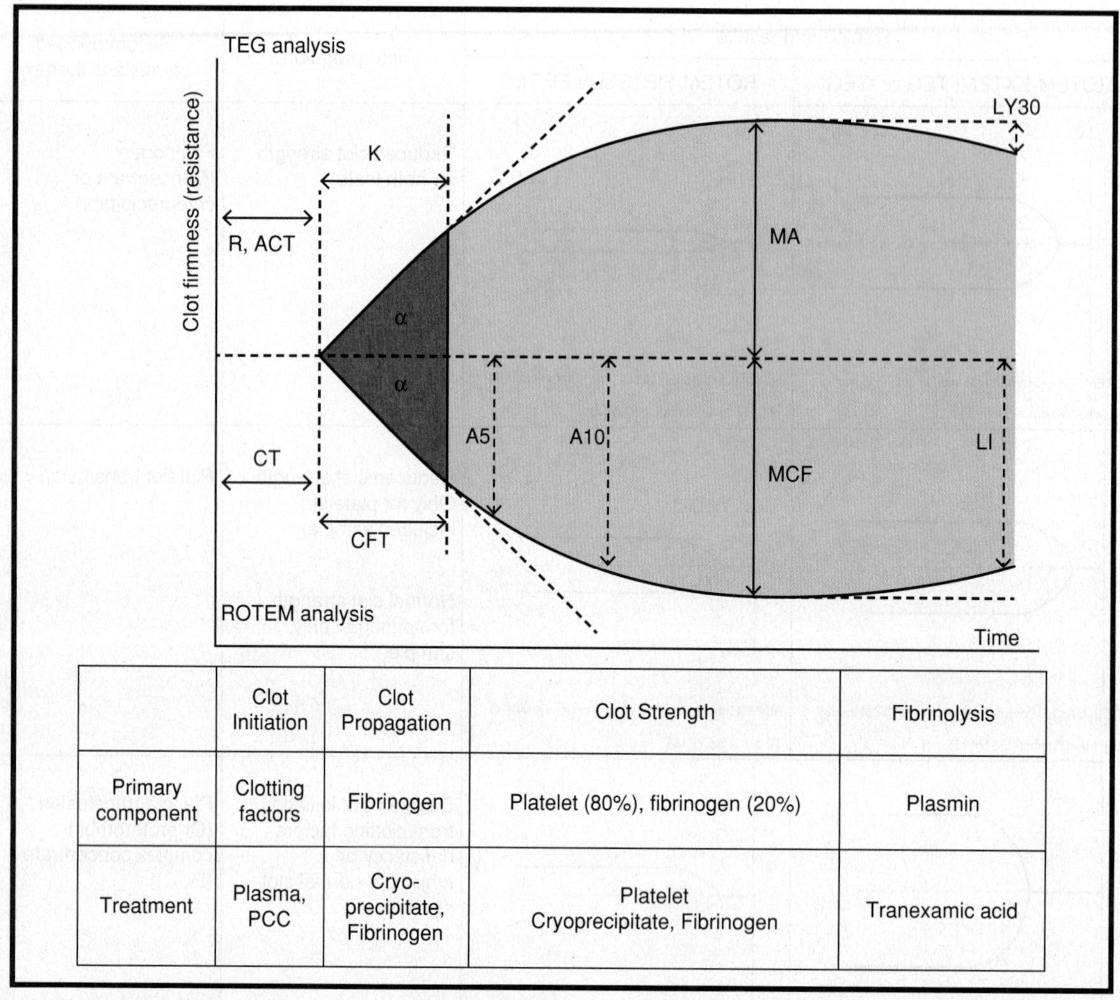

	Clot Initiation	Clot Propagation	Clot Strength	Fibrinolysis
Primary component	Clotting factors	Fibrinogen	Platelet (80%), fibrinogen (20%)	Plasmin
Treatment	Plasma, PCC	Cryo-precipitate, Fibrinogen	Platelet Cryoprecipitate, Fibrinogen	Tranexamic acid

Figure 53-2 Schematic tracing and parameters of TEG and ROTEM. ACT, activated clotting time; A5, amplitude at 5 minutes after coagulation start; A10, amplitude at 10 minutes after coagulation start; CT, coagulation time; K, time from initial clot formation until 20 mm amplitude; Li30, Lysis index percent reduction in amplitude from maximum clot firmness 30 minutes after coagulation time; LY30, percent reduction of area under the curve at 30 minutes compared to maximum amplitude; MA, maximum amplitude; MCF, maximum clot firmness; R, reaction time.

they cannot detect pathology with primary hemostasis, such as von Willebrand disease, nor depict the function of vascular endothelium on in vivo hemostasis. Samples are also heated to body temperature and recalcified, masking the effect of hypothermia and hypocalcemia on hemostasis. In addition, while VHA may be useful for detection of coagulation abnormality found with direct oral anticoagulants (DOACs), these assays cannot differentiate the effects of DOACs from TIC.[151,152]

Point-of-Care Ultrasound

Point-of-Care ultrasound (PoCUS) is commonly defined as the use of ultrasonography at the bedside to guide a procedure or to rapidly answer specific goal-oriented diagnostic clinical questions.[153] Diagnostic use of the US is a key competency in the practice of trauma anesthesia. This is reflected in the recent American Board of Anesthesiology (ABA) content guidelines and the American Society of Anesthesiologists educational programs.[154,155]

Focused Assessment with Sonography for Trauma (FAST) has long been a part of ATLS adjuncts to the primary trauma survey[156] (Fig. 53-3). The primary goal is to evaluate the presence of pathologic free fluid (anechoic) in the pericardial, peritoneal and pleural cavities; thus the standard FAST examination includes four views[157]: subxiphoid (pericardial), right flank (hepato-renal), left flank (perisplenic), suprapubic (pelvic).[158] Extended FAST (E-FAST) also evaluates the anterior thoracic view to assist with identifying pneumothoraces (see below).[159]

A large randomized study demonstrated that FAST reduced the time to surgery, CT imaging use, and hospital stay.[160] Systematic reviews found both sensitivity and specificity of FAST for detecting injuries in blunt thoracoabdominal trauma to be relatively high (74% to 82% and 96% to 99%, respectively).[161,162] While specificity remained high (94% to 100%) in blunt trauma, FAST was found less sensitive (as low as 28%) for penetrating trauma.[163] Limitations of FAST include poor detection of bowel, retroperitoneal, diaphragmatic, and pancreatic injuries. These factors highlight the importance of further investigation, typically using CT scan to rule out specific injuries when FAST is negative and index of suspicion is high.

Ultrasound has been increasingly studied and used to assist with airway management (Fig. 53-4). Ultrasound can be used in trauma care to predict difficult airways, to identify the cricothyroid membrane, to facilitate rapid front-of-neck access in expected

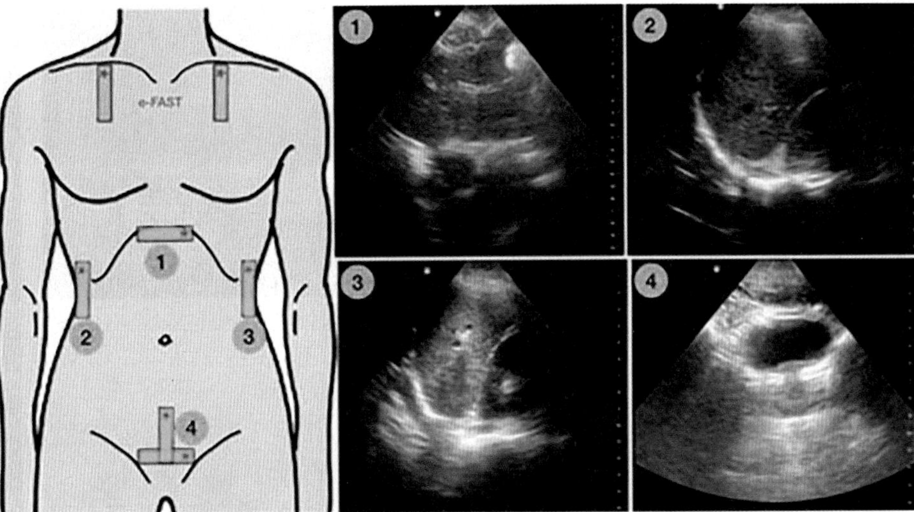

Figure 53-3 FAST exam. Probe placements and images obtained through each window of Focal Assessment with Sonography in Trauma (FAST) examination. The drawing on the left shows locations and orientation of ultrasound probes. Ultrasonographic images on the right show normal structures and views (negative study) corresponding to each window; subxiphoid cardiac view (1), right upper quadrant (RUQ, Morrison's pouch, 2), left upper quadrant (LUQ, 3), suprapubic (4). E-FAST adds on anterior thoracic views on both sides to detect pneumothorax. (Right ultrasonographic figures courtesy of Kamonwon Lenghong, MD, FTCEP.)

difficult airways, and to confirm endotracheal (vs. esophageal) tube position, especially in low cardiac output state where capnography can be less reliable.[164–168]

PoCUS for detection of pneumothorax (PTX) has been extensively applied in different clinical scenarios. A recent meta-analysis found superior sensitivity and specificity of thoracic PoCUS (91% and 99%, respectively) for detection of pneumothorax in trauma patients compared to chest x-ray (47% and 100%).[169] A high-frequency linear probe is used in the parasagittal orientation to visualize the least dependent portion of the lungs (the anterior chest wall in supine patients). The resulting image usually shows ribs shadows and bright hyperechoic line of the pleura between and underneath the ribs (Fig. 53-5). Lung movements from breathing typically show as "lung sliding sign," a dynamic "shimmering" horizontal movement along the visceral and parietal pleural surface. Findings suggestive of PTX include absence of lung sliding, or the "barcode sign" (examined in M-mode ultrasound), as well as a lung transition point between presence and absence of lung sliding.[170,171]

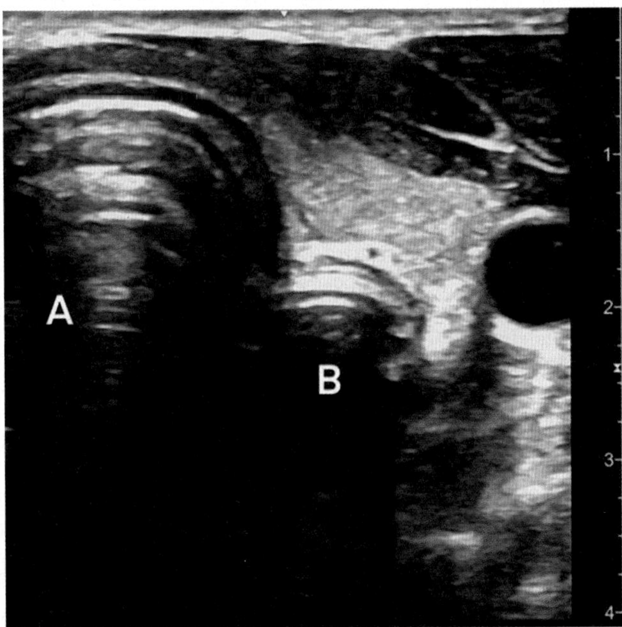

Figure 53-4 Esophageal intubation. Ultrasound finding of esophageal intubation. (*A*) The trachea is seen as a hypoechoic acoustic shadow below the hyperechoic horseshoe-shaped tracheal cartilage (tissue–air interface). Lateral to the trachea, the esophagus (*B*) (normally donut shaped with thick wall) is seen as a dilated structure with hyperechoic curved line surrounded by a thin muscular layer and distal hypoechoic shadow; characteristic of "double trachea sign." (Courtesy of Rajen Nathwani MD, University of Washington, Seattle WA.)

Conversely, the detection of a pleural effusion, often associated with hemothorax in trauma patients, is evaluated at the most dependent portion of the thorax (mid-to-posterior axillary line in supine patients). Effusions are seen as an anechoic collection between visceral and parietal pleura or diaphragm.[172] The most specific sign is the "extension of the thoracic spine" sign, where the spine can be visualized above the diaphragm.[173] One meta-analysis reported acceptable sensitivity and specificity (67% and 99%) of US for detecting hemothorax.

In addition to evaluation of pericardial fluid examined under subxiphoid view of e-FAST, ultrasound can be applied to evaluate other cardiovascular physiology and pathology. Focused Cardiac Ultrasound (FOCUS) is a time-sensitive, concise echocardiographic examination done in conjunction with other hemodynamic parameters.[174] It has emerged as the "21st century stethoscope" increasingly utilized in various critical conditions including trauma care.[175,176] Using either transthoracic echocardiography (TTE) or transesophageal echocardiography (TEE), FOCUS primarily assesses for pericardial effusion, intravascular status, ventricular size, and function (see Appendix 7).

Intraoperatively, TEE is more useful than TTE due to less interference over the surgical field and better image quality.[177] In addition to the above assessments, TEE can also be used to assess blunt traumatic aortic injury with high sensitivity and specificity.[178] One case series describing rescue TEE use in unstable trauma patients found that TEE findings changed management in 49% of the patients, with fluid challenge and initiation of inotropic supports being most common.[179] TEE is absolutely contraindicated in patients with esophageal injury, and should be performed with extreme caution in patients with severe coagulopathy and cervical spine pathology.[180]

Future

Many emergency medical service (EMS) systems in Europe and Australasia deploy anesthesiology or emergency medicine

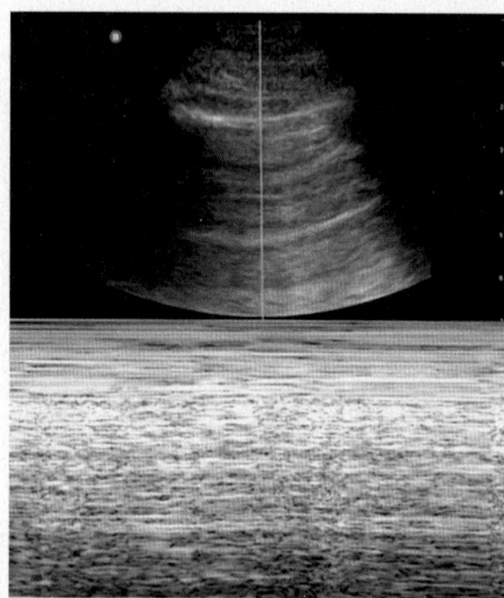

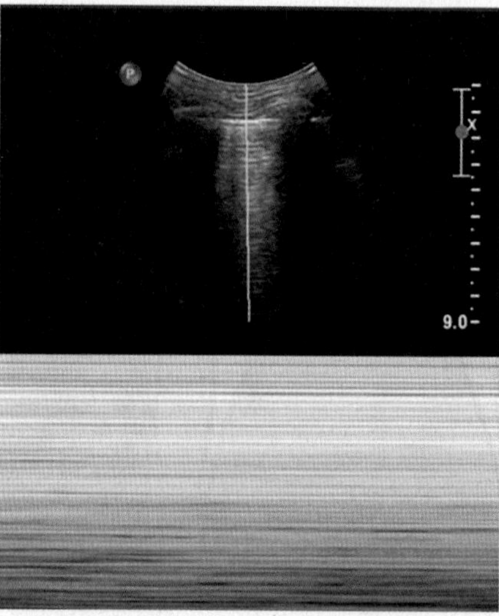

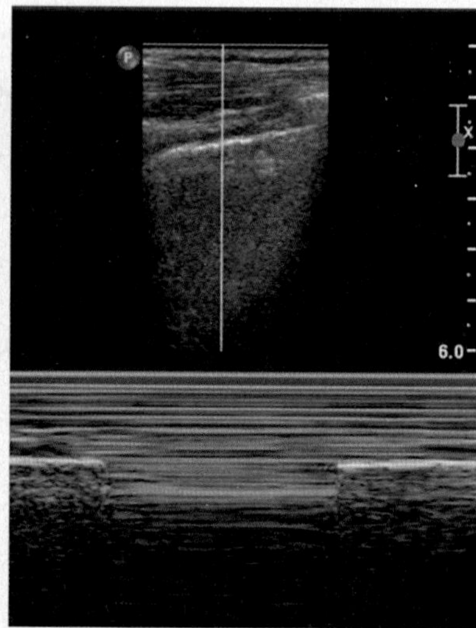

Figure 53-5 Lung ultrasound. Anterior chest wall ultrasound in B (**top**) and M (**bottom**) modes. **Left:** normal lung sliding with seashore sign. **Middle:** loss of lung sliding with barcode or stratosphere sign. **Right:** lung point sign. (Courtesy of Rathachai Kaewlai, MD and Kamonwon Lenghong, MD, FTCEP.)

physicians, partnered with advanced practice paramedics, to the prehospital scenes of seriously injured patients and on critical care transportation missions.[1] A growing body of literature demonstrates the advantage "bringing the trauma bay to the injured."[181–183] Future trauma system design must consider the advantage of advanced prehospital trauma care.

The perimorbid presentation of severely injured patients presents challenges to resuscitation and trauma surgery. A combined effort of prehospital care, damage control surgery, targeted resuscitation, interventional radiology, and critical care management offers the best chance for success. In some centers extracorporeal membrane oxygenation (ECMO) is used to manage cardiopulmonary collapse.[184] Heparin-bonded ECMO circuits (which can decrease the need for systemic anticoagulation), the increasing familiarity of ICU staff with the management of ECMO, and the ability to "buy time" in the dying process all offer potential for the more common use of ECMO in severe trauma.

Immunotherapy

As the role of inflammation in trauma becomes more clearly defined, the trauma anesthesiologist must understand the immune implications of severe injury and an understanding of potential therapeutic options. The inflammatory-immune response to the stress of trauma may offer an opportunity to influence the development and progression of end organ injury.[185] For example, immunomodulating diets may decrease infection, anti-high mobility group box 1 antibody therapy may play a role in acute lung injury during hemorrhage, and a refined understanding of role of FFP in protecting the endothelium from inflammation are all potential future therapies.

Further therapies to attenuate the inflammatory response and potentially improve outcome in hemorrhagic shock include Adenosine, Lidocaine, Magnesium (ALM) therapy. Adenosine is an endogenous nucleoside important in the supply/demand relationship of bioenergetics, lidocaine is a class IB antiarrhythmic, and magnesium is involved in ionic regulation as well as cellular bioenergetics.[186] Together ALM produces a polarizing cardioplegia (–80 mV) that does not arrest the heart, in distinction to the potassium-rich depolarizing cardioplegia (–50 mV) often used in cardiac surgery. It has been hypothesized that this creates "natural hibernators" by decreasing action potential duration through opening of potassium channels with adenosine, inhibiting sodium fast channels in phase 0 with lidocaine, and protecting from ischemia reperfusion and postoperative arrhythmia with magnesium. ALM corrects hyperfibrinolysis in rats, acting at the endothelial thrombomodulin-thrombin complex. There is a shift in thrombin substrate from a Protein C pathway toward the Thrombin Activatable Fibrinolysis Inhibitor (TAFI) pathway.

ALM was compared to saline, sham or no treatment in a rat model of TBI.[187] The ALM subjects all survived and showed improved cardiac function and cerebral blood flow, as well as a decrease in proinflammatory cytokines (IL1b, TNF alpha). There was also an increase in anti-inflammatory cytokines in the brain (IL10, IL4) and a decrease in brain injury markers (neuron-specific enolase, HMGB1). Another rat model of liver injury was used to approximate noncompressible hemorrhage.[188] ALM subjects had undetectable levels of IL1 alpha, and below baseline levels of IL1 beta, IL2, IL6, TNF alpha during the bolus phase of the protocol. During the infusion phase of the protocol, the ALM subjects had levels of biomarkers similar to the sham group. ADP-platelet aggregation and collagen platelet aggregation were improved with ALM. In comparison, non-ALM subjects were unable to aggregate platelets, had decreased fibrinogen levels, and were hypocoagulable. ALM may act to create a "permissive environment" for healing without overexpression of the inflammatory response by releasing IL1 leading to induction and amplification of inflammation for healing. Overexpression can result in excessive inflammation and potential multiorgan failure, whereas the opposite may offer therapeutic benefit. While ALM appears encouraging in hemorrhagic shock, it has not been demonstrated in any human trials to improve outcome.

Special Populations

Pediatrics

Injury is the leading cause of death among children and adolescents in the United States,[189] accounting for years of potential life loss that surpass other major diseases. While the basic tenets of trauma assessment and resuscitation share similarities

in children and adults, there are some unique considerations in
9 pediatrics. Approximately 90% of all pediatric trauma are blunt injuries, most commonly as a result of motor vehicle crashes and falls.[190,191] Nearly 75% of pediatric trauma patients are associated with TBI, which in turn accounts for 70% of mortality.[192] Obtundation caused by TBI and other physiologic abnormalities can lead to airway obstruction and respiratory compromise that can lead to secondary injury to the traumatized brain, as well as to cardiac arrest. This stresses the significance and priority of airway and ventilation management in this population.

Pediatric anatomical features include a smaller oral cavity, relatively large tongue and soft tissue, and more anterior larynx, all of which can make airway management challenging (see Chapter 43).[193] Larger head-to-body ratios and a prominent occiput typically cause neck flexion in supine position, potentiating airway obstruction. Children also have reduced respiratory reserve due to increased oxygen consumption and reduced functional residual capacity (FRC), making them prone to hypoxia. A full stomach should be assumed in all pediatric trauma patients regardless of reported fasting time.[194,195] Similar to adult trauma, the preferred method of airway management is RSI with restriction of cervical motion.[156] Up to 35% of spinal cord injury in children can present as spinal cord injury without radiographic abnormality (SCIWORA).[196]

A child's weight and age not only guide airway equipment sizes and drug doses, but also with calculating fluid and blood volumes. A length-based resuscitation tape (i.e., Broselow tape) can be used to determine a pediatric patient's weight appropriate medication doses and equipment sizes.

In "cannot intubate, cannot ventilate" (CICV) situations when ventilation with a SGA has also failed, emergency invasive pathway should be considered. In children younger than 10 to 12 years, due to smaller size of the airway and proximity to the vocal cords, needle cricothyroidotomy is preferable over surgical cricothyroidotomy due to less potential damage to the surrounding structures.[197]

Differences in cardiovascular physiology also play a role in pediatric trauma resuscitation. A child's physiologic reserve can help maintain normal blood pressures even with a drop of up to 30% to 40% of circulatory volume. Tachycardia, capillary refill and level of consciousness are therefore more sensitive indicators of early hypovolemic shock. The knowledge of age-specific normal physiologic ranges is crucial. Importantly, mean systolic blood pressure (SBP) in children is approximately 90 mmHg plus 2-times age in years, while the lower limit (5th percentile) of SBP is approximately 70 mmHg plus 2-times age in years.[198] Total blood volume differs across age groups, ranging from 90 mL/kg for a full-term neonate, 85 mL/kg for 1 to 6 months old, 75 mL/kg for children 6 months to 5 years, and 70 mL/kg for 5 years and older.[199]

Venous access can be challenging in traumatized children. If unsuccessful after two attempts of percutaneous peripheral venous catheter insertion, intraosseous needle placement should be considered. Preferred sites in pediatrics include anteromedial tibia and distal femur.[200] With low body mass-to-body surface area ratios, children can develop hypothermia precipitously. Prevention of hypothermia and the associated coagulation abnormality is crucial in this population.

Many trauma resuscitation strategies used in adults are still under debate for pediatric populations. For example, extrapolation of adult evidence like damage control resuscitation with 1:1:1 ratio has not shown benefit in children.[201,202] while tranexamic acid has only shown survival benefit in children suffering injury in a combat setting.[203] This leaves a question of applicability among the majority of blunt pediatric trauma patients. Limited evidence of viscoelastic tests in injured children also has not shown survival benefit.[204,205] Lastly, evidence suggests that hypotensive resuscitation might be harmful in children due to the small gap between their baseline BP and cerebral autoregulatory limit.[206,207]

Burns

Burns are a significant public health problem, with 11 million people suffering new burns each year globally[208] and an estimated 180,000 deaths.[209] Trauma anesthesia often involves many facets of care for these patients including airway and pain management, resuscitation, and intraoperative management.

Major burns result in multiorgan systemic pathophysiologic 10
effects that can occur from the onset of injuries to long after healing of wounds. These effects, typically correlated in severity with area of burn injury, occur in two temporal phases. Burn shock (ebb phase) is the early phase that typically persists for 24 to 48 hours after injury and is characterized by intravascular (plasma) volume loss into both injured and noninjured tissue,[210] resulting in reduced circulatory volume and hemoconcentration. Cardiac output can fall up to 60% from baseline.[211] Coupled with increased systemic vascular resistance, this can lead to impaired tissue and organ perfusion.[212] The hypermetabolic state (flow phase) follows, typically starting 48 to 72 hours after injury. Inflammatory cytokines and other damage-associated molecular patterns (DAMPs) propel this phase, resulting in systemic vasodilation,[213] hyperdynamic circulation, increased basal body temperature, oxygen consumption, and muscle protein catabolism. These effects can last up to years after burn injury,[214] highlighting the essence of nutritional support in burn care including intensive care and perioperative periods.

Burns can be classified in various approaches. Burn depth, according to skin destruction, is categorized as superficial burns (epidermis), partial-thickness burns (part of dermis) and full-thickness burns (entire dermis).[215] Partial-thickness burns are subclassified into superficial and deep partial thickness. The former requires less time to heal and usually without scarring or functional impairment, and the latter requires surgical debridement and grafting.[216]

Present in 2% to 14% of admitted burn patients, inhalation 11
injury significantly increases mortality above that predicted by extent of skin burn.[215,217,218] Distinct types of inhalation injury, can occur concurrently, including thermal and chemical injury to the upper airway (supraglottic), noxious chemical injury to the lower airway (tracheobronchial-alveolar), and systemic toxicity from toxic gasses.

Due to efficient heat exchange and protective reflexes of the respiratory tract, true thermal injuries are usually limited to the upper airway.[219] This can lead to mucosal edema and swelling of the structures, and ultimately to upper airway obstruction. Similar to fluid leak during the ebb phase, mucosal edema can progress over the early hours of active fluid resuscitation, stressing the value of high index of suspicion, repeated clinical observation and monitoring for diagnosis and management of this condition, particularly related to airway patency.

Conversely, the lower respiratory tract and lung parenchyma are vulnerable to respiratory irritants from chemical byproducts of combustion. The assault can cause loss of surfactant, airway ciliary dysfunction, sloughing of mucosal epithelium, release of inflammatory mediators which in turn cause bronchoconstriction, increased exudative loss into interstitium and cast formation.[219,220] Overall, these factors potentiate loss of hypoxic pulmonary vasoconstriction[221] and increase risks of bronchospasm, lower airway obstruction, atelectasis, and pneumonia.[212]

While there is no standard for diagnosis and grading of inhalational injury, a combination of traditional clinical findings including history and physical examination with additional testing are most commonly used. Likelihood of inhalation injury rises when burns occur in an enclosed space, when the patient was unconscious at the scene and with larger cutaneous burns. Pertinent physical examination findings include deep facial burns, soot on and swelling of the oro/nasopharynx, carbonaceous sputum, hoarse voice and inability to swallow. Flexible bronchoscopy (FB) is one of the most common modalities used to aid in diagnosis and severity stratification and was found to have high accuracy.[222] One study also found FB diagnosis of inhalation injury useful for predicting mortality and ICU LOS.[223] Other additional diagnostic tests include chest CT,[224] virtual bronchoscopy,[225] xenon ventilation-perfusion scan,[222] and pulmonary function tests.[226] Of note, patients with inhalation injury can present fully conscious with a patent airway, and initial chest x-ray lacks reliability to detect this condition.[227]

For additional information please see NICVs 53-1–53-3 and Videos 53-1–53-3 in the eBook bundled with this text.

For further review and interactivities, please see the videos and narrative interactive clinical vignettes (NICVs) accessible in the complimentary eBook bundled with this text. Access instructions are located on the inside front cover.

REFERENCES

1. Tobin JM. Anesthesiologist as resuscitation consultant. *Int Anesthesiol Clin.* 2017;55:1–3.
2. Bardes JM, Biswas S, Strumwasser AM, et al. Comparison of trauma resuscitation practices by critical care anesthesiologists and non-critical care anesthesiologists. *J Clin Anesth.* 2020;65:109890.
3. Haynes AB, Weiser TG, Berry WR, et al. A surgical safety checklist to reduce morbidity and mortality in a global population. *N Engl J Med.* 2009;360:491–499.
4. Walker IA, Reshamwalla S, Wilson IH. Surgical safety checklists: do they improve outcomes? *Br J Anaesth.* 2012;109:47–54.
5. Hunter DN, Finney SJ. Follow surgical checklists and take time out, especially in a crisis. *BMJ.* 2011;343:d8194.
6. Reason J. The contribution of latent human failures to the breakdown of complex systems. *Philos Trans R Soc Lond B Biol Sci.* 1990;327:475–484.
7. Tobin JM, Grabinsky A, McCunn M, et al. A checklist for trauma and emergency anesthesia. *Anesth Analg.* 2013;117:1178–1184.
8. Behrens V, Dudaryk R, Nedeff N, Tobin JM, Varon AJ. The ryder cognitive aid checklist for trauma anesthesia. *Anesth Analg.* 2016;122:1484–1487.
9. Stephens CT, Kahntroff S, Dutton RP. The success of emergency endotracheal intubation in trauma patients: a 10-year experience at a major adult trauma referral center. *Anesth Analg.* 2009;109:866–872.
10. Sollid SJ, Lossius HM, Soreide E. Pre-hospital intubation by anaesthesiologists in patients with severe trauma: an audit of a Norwegian helicopter emergency medical service. *Scand J Trauma Resusc Emerg Med.* 2010;18:30.
11. Driver BE, Semler MW, Self WH, et al. Effect of use of a bougie vs endotracheal tube with stylet on successful intubation on the first attempt among critically ill patients undergoing tracheal intubation: a randomized clinical trial. *JAMA.* 2021;326:2488–2497.
12. Shatney CH, Brunner RD, Nguyen TQ. The safety of orotracheal intubation in patients with unstable cervical spine fracture or high spinal cord injury. *Am J Surg.* 1995;170:676–679; discussion 9–80.
13. Turner CR, Block J, Shanks A, Morris M, Lodhia KR, Gujar SK. Motion of a cadaver model of cervical injury during endotracheal intubation with a Bullard laryngoscope or a Macintosh blade with and without in-line stabilization. *J Trauma.* 2009;67:61–66.
14. Gerling MC, Davis DP, Hamilton RS, et al. Effects of cervical spine immobilization technique and laryngoscope blade selection on an unstable cervical spine in a cadaver model of intubation. *Ann Emerg Med.* 2000;36:293–300.
15. Stiell IG, Wells GA, Vandemheen KL, et al. The Canadian C-spine rule for radiography in alert and stable trauma patients. *JAMA.* 2001;286:1841–1848.
16. Hoffman JR, Mower WR, Wolfson AB, Todd KH, Zucker MI. Validity of a set of clinical criteria to rule out injury to the cervical spine in patients with blunt trauma. National Emergency X-Radiography Utilization Study Group. *N Engl J Med.* 2000;343:94–99.
17. Griesdale DE, Liu D, McKinney J, Choi PT. Glidescope((R)) video-laryngoscopy versus direct laryngoscopy for endotracheal intubation: a systematic review and meta-analysis. *Can J Anaesth.* 2012;59(1):41–52.
18. Nouruzi-Sedeh P, Schumann M, Groeben H. Laryngoscopy via Macintosh blade versus GlideScope: success rate and time for endotracheal intubation in untrained medical personnel. *Anesthesiology.* 2009;110:32–37.
19. Yeatts DJ, Dutton RP, Hu PF, et al. Effect of video laryngoscopy on trauma patient survival: a randomized controlled trial. *J Trauma Acute Care Surg.* 2013;75:212–219.
20. Lascarrou JB, Boisrame-Helms J, Bailly A, et al. Video laryngoscopy vs direct laryngoscopy on successful first-pass orotracheal intubation among ICU patients: a randomized clinical trial. *JAMA.* 2017;317:483–493.
21. Trimmel H, Kreutziger J, Fitzka R, et al. Use of the glidescope ranger video laryngoscope for emergency intubation in the prehospital setting: a randomized control trial. *Crit Care Med.* 2016;44:e470–e476.
22. Lewis SR, Butler AR, Parker J, Cook TM, Schofield-Robinson OJ, Smith AF. Videolaryngoscopy versus direct laryngoscopy for adult patients requiring tracheal intubation: a Cochrane Systematic Review. *Br J Anaesth.* 2017;119:369–383.
23. Hulme J, Perkins GD. Critically injured patients, inaccessible airways, and laryngeal mask airways. *EMJ.* 2005;22:742–744.
24. Schalk R, Meininger D, Ruesseler M, et al. Emergency airway management in trauma patients using laryngeal tube suction. *Prehosp Emerg Care.* 2011;15:347–350.
25. Baker PA, Webber JB. Failure to ventilate with supraglottic airways after drowning. *Anaesth Intensive Care.* 2011;39:675–677.
26. Bindra T, Nihalani SK, Bhadoria P, Wadhawan S. Use of intubating laryngeal mask airway in a morbidly obese patient with chest trauma in an emergency setting. *J Anaesthesiol Clin Pharmacol.* 2011;27:544–546.
27. Adams BD, Cuniowski PA, Muck A, De Lorenzo RA. Registry of emergency airways arriving at combat hospitals. *J Trauma.* 2008;64:1548–1554.
28. Mabry RL. An analysis of battlefield cricothyrotomy in Iraq and Afghanistan. *J Spec Oper Med.* 2012;12:17–23.
29. Paix BR, Griggs WM. Emergency surgical cricothyroidotomy: 24 successful cases leading to a simple 'scalpel-finger-tube' method. *Emerg Med Australas.* 2012;24:23–30.
30. Acute Respiratory Distress Syndrome Network; Brower RG, Matthay MA, Morris A, Schoenfeld D, Thompson BT, Wheeler A. Ventilation with lower tidal volumes as compared with traditional tidal volumes for acute lung injury and the acute respiratory distress syndrome. *N Engl J Med.* 2000;342:1301–1308.
31. Guldner A, Kiss T, Serpa Neto A, et al. Intraoperative protective mechanical ventilation for prevention of postoperative pulmonary complications: a comprehensive review of the role of tidal volume, positive end-expiratory pressure, and lung recruitment maneuvers. *Anesthesiology.* 2015;123:692–713.
32. Serpa Neto A, Cardoso SO, Manetta JA, et al. Association between use of lung-protective ventilation with lower tidal volumes and clinical outcomes among patients without acute respiratory distress syndrome: a meta-analysis. *JAMA.* 2012;308:1651–1659.
33. Serpa Neto A, Hemmes SN, Barbas CS, et al. Protective versus conventional ventilation for surgery: a systematic review and individual patient data meta-analysis. *Anesthesiology.* 2015;123:66–78.
34. Murphy EL, Kwaan N, Looney MR, et al. Risk factors and outcomes in transfusion-associated circulatory overload. *Am J Med.* 2013;126:357e29–38.
35. Semple JW, Rebetz J, Kapur R. Transfusion-associated circulatory overload and transfusion-related acute lung injury. *Blood.* 2019;133:1840–1853.
36. Skeate RC, Eastlund T. Distinguishing between transfusion related acute lung injury and transfusion associated circulatory overload. *Curr Opin Hematol.* 2007;14:682–687.
37. Plurad DS, Talving P, Lam L, Inaba K, Green D, Demetriades D. Early vasopressor use in critical injury is associated with mortality independent from volume status. *J Trauma.* 2011;71:565–670; discussion 70–72.
38. Sperry JL, Minei JP, Frankel HL, et al. Early use of vasopressors after injury: caution before constriction. *J Trauma.* 2008;64:9–14.
39. Raedler C, Voelckel WG, Wenzel V, et al. Treatment of uncontrolled hemorrhagic shock after liver trauma: fatal effects of fluid resuscitation versus improved outcome after vasopressin. *Anesth Analg.* 2004;98:1759–1766.
40. Voelckel WG, Raedler C, Wenzel V, et al. Arginine vasopressin, but not epinephrine, improves survival in uncontrolled hemorrhagic shock after liver trauma in pigs. *Crit Care Med.* 2003;31:1160–1165.
41. Krismer AC, Wenzel V, Voelckel WG, et al. Employing vasopressin as an adjunct vasopressor in uncontrolled traumatic hemorrhagic shock. Three cases and a brief analysis of the literature. *Anaesthesist.* 2005;54:220–224.
42. Sims CA, Holena D, Kim P, et al. Effect of low-dose supplementation of arginine vasopressin on need for blood product transfusions in patients with trauma and hemorrhagic shock: a randomized clinical trial. *JAMA Surg.* 2019;154:994–1003.
43. Farina Junior JA, Celotto AC, da Silva MF, Evora PR. Guanylate cyclase inhibition by methylene blue as an option in the treatment of vasoplegia after a severe burn. A medical hypothesis. *Med Sci Monit.* 2012;18:HY13-7.
44. Weiner MM, Lin HM, Danforth D, Rao S, Hosseinian L, Fischer GW. Methylene blue is associated with poor outcomes in vasoplegic shock. *J Cardiothorac Vasc Anesth.* 2013;27:1233–1238.

45. Tobin JM. Toward an electrical analog of the cardiovascular system in hemorrhage. *Cardiovasc Eng Technol*. 2021;12:526–529.
46. Cowell EM. Nature and treatment of wound shock and allies conditions. *JAMA*. 1918;70:607–621.
47. Dutton RP, Mackenzie CF, Scalea TM. Hypotensive resuscitation during active hemorrhage: impact on in-hospital mortality. *J Trauma*. 2002;52:1141–1146.
48. Brown JB, Cohen MJ, Minei JP, et al. Goal-directed resuscitation in the prehospital setting: a propensity-adjusted analysis. *J Trauma Acute Care Surg*. 2013;74:1207–1212; discussion 12–14.
49. Walsh M, Devereaux PJ, Garg AX, et al. Relationship between intraoperative mean arterial pressure and clinical outcomes after noncardiac surgery: toward an empirical definition of hypotension. *Anesthesiology*. 2013;119:507–515.
50. Chesnut RM, Marshall LF, Klauber MR, et al. The role of secondary brain injury in determining outcome from severe head injury. *J Trauma*. 1993;34:216–222.
51. Cooper DJ, Rosenfeld JV, Murray L, et al. Decompressive craniectomy in diffuse traumatic brain injury. *N Engl J Med*. 2011;364:1493–1502.
52. Chesnut RM, Temkin N, Carney N, et al. A trial of intracranial-pressure monitoring in traumatic brain injury. *N Engl J Med*. 2012;367:2471–2481.
53. Roberts I, Yates D, Sandercock P, et al. Effect of intravenous corticosteroids on death within 14 days in 10008 adults with clinically significant head injury (MRC CRASH trial): randomised placebo-controlled trial. *Lancet*. 2004;364:1321–1328.
54. Alderson P, Roberts I. Corticosteroids for acute traumatic brain injury. *Cochrane Database Syst Rev*. 2005;2005(1):CD000196.
55. da Silva JC, de Lima Fde M, Valenca MM, de Azevedo Filho HR. Hypertonic saline more efficacious than mannitol in lethal intracranial hypertension model. *Neurol Res*. 2010;32:139–143.
56. Boone MD, Oren-Grinberg A, Robinson TM, Chen CC, Kasper EM. Mannitol or hypertonic saline in the setting of traumatic brain injury: what have we learned? *Surg Neurol Int*. 2015;6:177.
57. Upadhyay P, Tripathi VN, Singh RP, Sachan D. Role of hypertonic saline and mannitol in the management of raised intracranial pressure in children: a randomized comparative study. *J Pediatr Neurosci*. 2010;5:18–21.
58. Ropper AH. Hyperosmolar therapy for raised intracranial pressure. *N Engl J Med*. 2012;367:746–752.
59. Brain Trauma Foundation; American Association of Neurological Surgeons; Congress of Neurological Surgeons; Joint Section on Neurotrauma and Critical Care, AANS/CNS; Bratton SL, Chestnut RM, Ghajar J, et al. Guidelines for the management of severe traumatic brain injury. XIII. Antiseizure prophylaxis. *J Neurotrauma*. 2007;24(Suppl 1):S83–S86.
60. Torbic H, Forni AA, Anger KE, Degrado JR, Greenwood BC. Use of antiepileptics for seizure prophylaxis after traumatic brain injury. *Am J Health Syst Pharm*. 2013;70:759–766.
61. Abou-Khalil B. Levetiracetam in the treatment of epilepsy. *Neuropsychiatr Dis Treat*. 2008;4:507–523.
62. Malone DL, Hess JR, Fingerhut A. Massive transfusion practices around the globe and a suggestion for a common massive transfusion protocol. *J Trauma*. 2006;60:S91–S96.
63. Borgman MA, Spinella PC, Perkins JG, et al. The ratio of blood products transfused affects mortality in patients receiving massive transfusions at a combat support hospital. *J Trauma*. 2007;63:805–813.
64. Holcomb JB, Wade CE, Michalek JE, et al. Increased plasma and platelet to red blood cell ratios improves outcome in 466 massively transfused civilian trauma patients. *Ann Surg*. 2008;248:447–458.
65. Ho AM, Dion PW, Yeung JH, et al. Prevalence of survivor bias in observational studies on fresh frozen plasma:erythrocyte ratios in trauma requiring massive transfusion. *Anesthesiology*. 2012;116:716–728.
66. Davenport R, Curry N, Manson J, et al. Hemostatic effects of fresh frozen plasma may be maximal at red cell ratios of 1:2. *J Trauma*. 2011;70:90–95; discussion 5–6.
67. Holcomb JB, Tilley BC, Baraniuk S, et al. Transfusion of plasma, platelets, and red blood cells in a 1:1:1 vs a 1:1:2 ratio and mortality in patients with severe trauma: the PROPPR randomized clinical trial. *JAMA*. 2015;313:471–482.
68. Sperry JL, Guyette FX, Adams PW. Prehospital plasma during air medical transport in trauma patients. *N Engl J Med*. 2018;379:1783.
69. Cap AP, Beckett A, Benov A, et al. Whole blood transfusion. *Mil Med*. 2018;183:44–51.
70. Muldowney M, Aichholz P, Nathwani R, Stansbury LG, Hess JR, Vavilala MS. Advances in hemorrhage control resuscitation. *Curr Opin Anaesthesiol*. 2022;35:176–181.
71. Yazer MH, Spinella PC, Anto V, Dunbar NM. Survey of group A plasma and low-titer group O whole blood use in trauma resuscitation at adult civilian level 1 trauma centers in the US. *Transfusion*. 2021;61:1757–1763.
72. Spinella PC, Perkins JG, Grathwohl KW, Beekley AC, Holcomb JB. Warm fresh whole blood is independently associated with improved survival for patients with combat-related traumatic injuries. *J Trauma*. 2009;66:S69–S76.
73. Nessen SC, Eastridge BJ, Cronk D, et al. Fresh whole blood use by forward surgical teams in Afghanistan is associated with improved survival compared to component therapy without platelets. *Transfusion*. 2013;53(Suppl 1):107S–113S.
74. Hazelton JP, Cannon JW, Zatorski C, et al. Cold-stored whole blood: a better method of trauma resuscitation? *J Trauma Acute Care Surg*. 2019;87:1035–1041.
75. Black JA, Pierce VS, Kerby JD, Holcomb JB. The Evolution of blood transfusion in the trauma patient: whole blood has come full circle. *Semin Thromb Hemost*. 2020;46:215–220.
76. Jackson B, Murphy C, Fontaine MJ. Current state of whole blood transfusion for civilian trauma resuscitation. *Transfusion*. 2020;60(Suppl 3):S45–S52.
77. Seheult JN, Anto V, Alarcon LH, Sperry JL, Triulzi DJ, Yazer MH. Clinical outcomes among low-titer group O whole blood recipients compared to recipients of conventional components in civilian trauma resuscitation. *Transfusion*. 2018;58:1838–1845.
78. Seheult JN, Triulzi DJ, Alarcon LH, Sperry JL, Murdock A, Yazer MH. Measurement of haemolysis markers following transfusion of uncrossmatched, low-titre, group O+ whole blood in civilian trauma patients: initial experience at a level 1 trauma centre. *Transfus Med*. 2017;27:30–35.
79. Leeper CM, Yazer MH, Cladis FP, Saladino R, Triulzi DJ, Gaines BA. Use of uncrossmatched cold-stored whole blood in injured children with hemorrhagic shock. *JAMA Pediatr*. 2018;172:491–492.
80. Malkin M, Nevo A, Brundage SI, Schreiber M. Effectiveness and safety of whole blood compared to balanced blood components in resuscitation of hemorrhaging trauma patients – A systematic review. *Injury*. 2021;52:182–188.
81. Crowe E, DeSantis SM, Bonnette A, et al. Whole blood transfusion versus component therapy in trauma resuscitation: a systematic review and meta-analysis. *J Am Coll Emerg Physicians Open*. 2020;1:633–641.
82. Remy KE, Yazer MH, Saini A, et al. Effects of platelet-sparing leukocyte reduction and agitation methods on in vitro measures of hemostatic function in cold-stored whole blood. *J Trauma Acute Care Surg*. 2018;84:S104–S114.
83. Thomas KA, Shea SM, Yazer MH, Spinella PC. Effect of leukoreduction and pathogen reduction on the hemostatic function of whole blood. *Transfusion*. 2019;59:1539–1548.
84. Morris MC, Veile R, Friend LA, et al. Effects of whole blood leukoreduction on platelet function and hemostatic parameters. *Transfus Med*. 2019;29:351–357.
85. Shakur H, Roberts I, Bautista R, et al. Effects of tranexamic acid on death, vascular occlusive events, and blood transfusion in trauma patients with significant haemorrhage (CRASH-2): a randomised, placebo-controlled trial. *Lancet*. 2010;376:23–32.
86. Morrison JJ, Dubose JJ, Rasmussen TE, Midwinter MJ. Military Application of Tranexamic Acid in Trauma Emergency Resuscitation (MATTERs) Study. *Arch Surg*. 2012;147:113–119.
87. Moore HB, Moore EE, Gonzalez E, et al. Hyperfibrinolysis, physiologic fibrinolysis, and fibrinolysis shutdown: the spectrum of postinjury fibrinolysis and relevance to antifibrinolytic therapy. *J Trauma Acute Care Surg*. 2014;77:811–817; discussion 7.
88. CRASH-3 trial collaborators. Effects of tranexamic acid on death, disability, vascular occlusive events and other morbidities in patients with acute traumatic brain injury (CRASH-3): a randomised, placebo-controlled trial. *Lancet*. 2019;394:1713–1723.
89. Ho KM, Leonard AD. Concentration-dependent effect of hypocalcaemia on mortality of patients with critical bleeding requiring massive transfusion: a cohort study. *Anaesth Intensive Care*. 2011;39:46–54.
90. Vivien B, Langeron O, Morell E, et al. Early hypocalcemia in severe trauma. *Crit Care Med*. 2005;33:1946–1952.
91. Magnotti LJ, Bradburn EH, Webb DL, et al. Admission ionized calcium levels predict the need for multiple transfusions: a prospective study of 591 critically ill trauma patients. *J Trauma*. 2011;70:391–395; discussion 5–7.
92. Tanaka KA, Esper S, Bolliger D. Perioperative factor concentrate therapy. *Br J Anaesth*. 2013;111(Suppl 1):i35–i49.
93. Levy JH, Szlam F, Tanaka KA, Sniecienski RM. Fibrinogen and hemostasis: a primary hemostatic target for the management of acquired bleeding. *Anesth Analg*. 2012;114:261–274.
94. Gollop ND, Chilcott J, Benton A, Rayment R, Jones J, Collins PW. National audit of the use of fibrinogen concentrate to correct hypofibrinogenaemia. *Transfus Med*. 2012;22:350–355.
95. Sprung CL, Annane D, Keh D, et al. Hydrocortisone therapy for patients with septic shock. *N Engl J Med*. 2008;358:111–124.
96. Hoen S, Asehnoune K, Brailly-Tabard S, et al. Cortisol response to corticotropin stimulation in trauma patients: influence of hemorrhagic shock. *Anesthesiology*. 2002;97:807–813.
97. Hoen S, Mazoit JX, Asehnoune K, et al. Hydrocortisone increases the sensitivity to alpha1-adrenoceptor stimulation in humans following hemorrhagic shock. *Crit Care Med*. 2005;33:2737–2743.
98. Roquilly A, Mahe PJ, Seguin P, et al. Hydrocortisone therapy for patients with multiple trauma: the randomized controlled HYPOLYTE study. *JAMA*. 2011;305:1201–1209.
99. Yunos NM, Bellomo R, Hegarty C, Story D, Ho L, Bailey M. Association between a chloride-liberal vs chloride-restrictive intravenous fluid administration strategy and kidney injury in critically ill adults. *JAMA*. 2012;308:1566–1572.
100. Kawano-Dourado L, Zampieri FG, Azevedo LCP, et al. Low-versus high-chloride content intravenous solutions for critically ill and perioperative adult patients: a systematic review and meta-analysis. *Anesth Analg*. 2018;126:513–521.
101. Young JB, Utter GH, Schermer CR, et al. Saline versus Plasma-Lyte A in initial resuscitation of trauma patients: a randomized trial. *Ann Surg*. 2014;259:255–262.
102. Finfer S, Micallef S, Hammond N, et al. Balanced multielectrolyte solution versus saline in critically ill adults. *N Engl J Med*. 2022;386:815–826.

103. Forsythe SM, Schmidt GA. Sodium bicarbonate for the treatment of lactic acidosis. *Chest.* 2000;117:260–267.
104. Petejova N, Martinek A. Acute kidney injury due to rhabdomyolysis and renal replacement therapy: a critical review. *Crit Care.* 2014;18:224.
105. Butkus DE. Post-traumatic acute renal failure in combat casualties: a historical review. *Mil Med.* 1984;149:117–124.
106. Holmes CL, Walley KR. Bad medicine: low-dose dopamine in the ICU. *Chest.* 2003;123: 1266–1275.
107. Kellum JA, M Decker J. Use of dopamine in acute renal failure: a meta-analysis. *Crit Care Med.* 2001;29:1526–1531.
108. Ho KM, Power BM. Benefits and risks of furosemide in acute kidney injury. *Anaesthesia.* 2010;65:283–293.
109. Brown CV, Rhee P, Chan L, Evans K, Demetriades D, Velmahos GC. Preventing renal failure in patients with rhabdomyolysis: do bicarbonate and mannitol make a difference? *J Trauma.* 2004;56:1191–1196.
110. Bellomo R, Ronco C, Kellum JA, Mehta RL, Palevsky P, Acute Dialysis Quality Initiative w. Acute renal failure – definition, outcome measures, animal models, fluid therapy and information technology needs: the Second International Consensus Conference of the Acute Dialysis Quality Initiative (ADQI) Group. *Crit Care.* 2004;8:R204–R212.
111. Einav S, Bromiker R, Weiniger CF, Matot I. Mathematical modeling for prediction of survival from resuscitation based on computerized continuous capnography: proof of concept. *Acad Emerg Med.* 2011;18:468–475.
112. Tyburski JG, Collinge JD, Wilson RF, Carlin AM, Albaran RG, Steffes CP. End-tidal CO2-derived values during emergency trauma surgery correlated with outcome: a prospective study. *J Trauma.* 2002;53:738–743.
113. Connelly CR, Schreiber MA. Endpoints in resuscitation. *Curr Opin Crit Care.* 2015;21: 512–519.
114. Davis JW, Dirks RC, Kaups KL, Tran P. Base deficit is superior to lactate in trauma. *Am J Surg.* 2018;215:682–685.
115. Mutschler M, Nienaber U, Brockamp T, et al. Renaissance of base deficit for the initial assessment of trauma patients: a base deficit-based classification for hypovolemic shock developed on data from 16,305 patients derived from the TraumaRegister DGU(R). *Crit Care.* 2013;17:R42.
116. Vakily A, Parsaei H, Movahhedi MM, Sahmeddini MA. A system for continuous estimating and monitoring cardiac output via arterial waveform analysis. *J Biomed Phys Eng.* 2017;7: 181–190.
117. Berkenstadt H, Margalit N, Hadani M, et al. Stroke volume variation as a predictor of fluid responsiveness in patients undergoing brain surgery. *Anesth Analg.* 2001;92:984–989.
118. Marik PE, Cavallazzi R. Does the central venous pressure predict fluid responsiveness? An updated meta-analysis and a plea for some common sense*. *Crit Care Med.* 2013;41: 1774–1781.
119. Nunez TC, Voskresensky IV, Dossett LA, Shinall R, Dutton WD, Cotton BA. Early prediction of massive transfusion in trauma: simple as ABC (assessment of blood consumption)? *J Trauma.* 2009;66:346–352.
120. Francis RCE, Theurl I, Maegele M, Graw JA. Point-of-Care diagnostics of coagulation in the management of bleeding and transfusion in trauma patients. *Curr Opin Anaesthesiol.* 2020;33:246–252.
121. Tantry US, Hartmann J, Neal MD, et al. The role of viscoelastic testing in assessing peri-interventional platelet function and coagulation. *Platelets.* 2022;33:520–530.
122. Moore EE, Moore HB, Kornblith LZ, et al. Trauma-induced coagulopathy. *Nat Rev Dis Primers.* 2021;7:30.
123. Wirtz MR, Baumann HM, Klinkspoor JH, Goslings JC, Juffermans NP. Viscoelastic testing in trauma. *Semin Thromb Hemost.* 2017;43:375–385.
124. Frith D, Goslings JC, Gaarder C, et al. Definition and drivers of acute traumatic coagulopathy: clinical and experimental investigations. *J Thromb Haemost.* 2010;8:1919–1925.
125. Maegele M, Lefering R, Yucel N, et al. Early coagulopathy in multiple injury: an analysis from the German Trauma Registry on 8724 patients. *Injury.* 2007;38:298–304.
126. Peltan ID, Vande Vusse LK, Maier RV, Watkins TR. An International normalized ratio-based definition of acute traumatic coagulopathy is associated with mortality, venous thromboembolism, and multiple organ failure after injury. *Crit Care Med.* 2015;43:1429–1438.
127. Johannsen S, Brohi K, Johansson PI, et al. Getting hit by the bus around the world – a global perspective on goal directed treatment of massive hemorrhage in trauma. *Curr Opin Anaesthesiol.* 2021;34:537–543.
128. Sayce AC, Neal MD, Leeper CM. Viscoelastic monitoring in trauma resuscitation. *Transfusion.* 2020;60(Suppl 6):S33–S51.
129. Kelly JM, Rizoli S, Veigas P, Hollands S, Min A. Using rotational thromboelastometry clot firmness at 5 minutes (ROTEM((R)) EXTEM A5) to predict massive transfusion and in-hospital mortality in trauma: a retrospective analysis of 1146 patients. *Anaesthesia.* 2018;73: 1103–1109.
130. Laursen TH, Meyer MAS, Meyer ASP, et al. Thrombelastography early amplitudes in bleeding and coagulopathic trauma patients: Results from a multicenter study. *J Trauma Acute Care Surg.* 2018;84:334–341.
131. Scala E, Coutaz C, Gomez F, Alberio L, Marcucci C. Comparison of ROTEM sigma to standard laboratory tests and development of an algorithm for the management of coagulopathic bleeding in a tertiary center. *J Cardiothorac Vasc Anesth.* 2020;34:640–649.
132. Chandler WL, Ferrell C, Trimble S, Moody S. Development of a rapid emergency hemorrhage panel. *Transfusion.* 2010;50:2547–2552.
133. Brill JB, Brenner M, Duchesne J, et al. The role of TEG and ROTEM in damage control resuscitation. *Shock.* 2021;56:52–61.
134. Kim JS, Wang IJ, Yeom SR, et al. Usefulness of rotational thromboelastometry as a mortality predictor of hyperfibrinolysis in patients with severe trauma. *Acute Crit Care.* 2018;33: 162–169.
135. Veigas PV, Callum J, Rizoli S, Nascimento B, da Luz LT. A systematic review on the rotational thrombelastometry (ROTEM(R)) values for the diagnosis of coagulopathy, prediction and guidance of blood transfusion and prediction of mortality in trauma patients. *Scand J Trauma Resusc Emerg Med.* 2016;24:114.
136. Barrett CD, Moore HB, Vigneshwar N, et al. Plasmin thrombelastography rapidly identifies trauma patients at risk for massive transfusion, mortality, and hyperfibrinolysis: A diagnostic tool to resolve an international debate on tranexamic acid? *J Trauma Acute Care Surg.* 2020;89:991–998.
137. Moore HB, Moore EE, Huebner BR, et al. Fibrinolysis shutdown is associated with a fivefold increase in mortality in trauma patients lacking hypersensitivity to tissue plasminogen activator. *J Trauma Acute Care Surg.* 2017;83:1014–1022.
138. Stettler GR, Moore EE, Moore HB, et al. Redefining postinjury fibrinolysis phenotypes using two viscoelastic assays. *J Trauma Acute Care Surg.* 2019;86:679–685.
139. Moore HB, Moore EE, Chapman MP, et al. Viscoelastic measurements of platelet function, not fibrinogen function, predicts sensitivity to tissue-type plasminogen activator in trauma patients. *J Thromb Haemost.* 2015;13:1878–1887.
140. Baksaas-Aasen K, Van Dieren S, Balvers K, et al. Data-driven development of ROTEM and TEG Algorithms for the management of trauma hemorrhage: a prospective observational multicenter study. *Ann Surg.* 2019;270:1178–1185.
141. Khunakanan S, Akaraborworn O, Sangthong B, Thongkhao K. Correlation between maximum clot firmness in FIBTEM and fibrinogen level in critical trauma patients. *Crit Care Res Pract.* 2019;2019:2756461.
142. de Vries JJ, Veen CSB, Snoek CJM, Kruip M, de Maat MPM. FIBTEM clot firmness parameters correlate well with the fibrinogen concentration measured by the Clauss assay in patients and healthy subjects. *Scand J Clin Lab Invest.* 2020;80:600–605.
143. Hunt H, Stanworth S, Curry N, et al. Thromboelastography (TEG) and rotational thromboelastometry (ROTEM) for trauma induced coagulopathy in adult trauma patients with bleeding. *Cochrane Database Syst Rev.* 2015;2015(2):CD010438.
144. Da Luz LT, Nascimento B, Shankarakutty AK, Rizoli S, Adhikari NK. Effect of thromboelastography (TEG(R)) and rotational thromboelastometry (ROTEM(R)) on diagnosis of coagulopathy, transfusion guidance and mortality in trauma: descriptive systematic review. *Crit Care.* 2014;18:518.
145. Wikkelso A, Wetterslev J, Moller AM, Afshari A. Thromboelastography (TEG) or thromboelastometry (ROTEM) to monitor haemostatic treatment versus usual care in adults or children with bleeding. *Cochrane Database Syst Rev.* 2016;2016(8):CD007871.
146. Bugaev N, Como JJ, Golani G, et al. Thromboelastography and rotational thromboelastometry in bleeding patients with coagulopathy: Practice management guideline from the Eastern Association for the Surgery of Trauma. *J Trauma Acute Care Surg.* 2020;89:999–1017.
147. Baksaas-Aasen K, Gall LS, Stensballe J, et al. Viscoelastic haemostatic assay augmented protocols for major trauma haemorrhage (ITACTIC): a randomized, controlled trial. *Intensive Care Med.* 2021;47:49–59.
148. Goodman MD, Makley AT, Hanseman DJ, Pritts TA, Robinson BR. All the bang without the bucks: defining essential point-of-care testing for traumatic coagulopathy. *J Trauma Acute Care Surg.* 2015;79:117–124; discussion 24.
149. Anderson L, Quasim I, Steven M, et al. Interoperator and intraoperator variability of whole blood coagulation assays: a comparison of thromboelastography and rotational thromboelastometry. *J Cardiothorac Vasc Anesth.* 2014;28:1550–1557.
150. Gurbel PA, Bliden KP, Tantry US, et al. First report of the point-of-care TEG: A technical validation study of the TEG-6S system. *Platelets.* 2016;27:642–649.
151. Korpallova B, Samos M, Bolek T, et al. ROTEM Testing for Direct Oral Anticoagulants. *Semin Thromb Hemost.* 2021;47:815–823.
152. Spahn DR, Bouillon B, Cerny V, et al. The European guideline on management of major bleeding and coagulopathy following trauma: fifth edition. *Crit Care.* 2019;23:98.
153. Zimmerman J. Overview of perioperative uses of ultrasound. *UpToDate*; 2021.
154. OSCE Content Outline. https://www.theaba.org/pdfs/OSCE_Content_Outline.pdf.
155. Diagnostic POCUS Certificate Program. https://www.asahq.org/education-and-career/educational-and-cme-offerings/pocus; Accessed March 26, 2022.
156. ATLS Subcommittee; American College of Surgeons' Committee on Trauma; International ATLS working group. Advanced trauma life support (ATLS(R)): the ninth edition. *J Trauma Acute Care Surg.* 2013;74:1363–1366.
157. Pariyadath M. Emergency ultrasound in adults with abdominal and thoracic trauma. *UpToDate*; 2021.

158. Bahner D, Blaivas M, Cohen HL, et al. AIUM practice guideline for the performance of the focused assessment with sonography for trauma (FAST) examination. *J Ultrasound Med.* 2008;27:313–318.
159. American Institute of Ultrasound in Medicine; American College of Emergency Physicians. AIUM practice guideline for the performance of the focused assessment with sonography for trauma (FAST) examination. *J Ultrasound Med.* 2014;33:2047–2056.
160. Melniker LA, Leibner E, McKenney MG, Lopez P, Briggs WM, Mancuso CA. Randomized controlled clinical trial of point-of-care, limited ultrasonography for trauma in the emergency department: the first sonography outcomes assessment program trial. *Ann Emerg Med.* 2006;48:227–235.
161. Nishijima DK, Simel DL, Wisner DH, Holmes JF. Does this adult patient have a blunt intra-abdominal injury? *JAMA.* 2012;307:1517–1527.
162. Stengel D, Leisterer J, Ferrada P, Ekkernkamp A, Mutze S, Hoenning A. Point-of-care ultrasonography for diagnosing thoracoabdominal injuries in patients with blunt trauma. *Cochrane Database Syst Rev.* 2018;12:CD012669.
163. Quinn AC, Sinert R. What is the utility of the Focused Assessment with Sonography in Trauma (FAST) exam in penetrating torso trauma? *Injury.* 2011;42:482–487.
164. Kristensen MS, Teoh WH, Graumann O, Laursen CB. Ultrasonography for clinical decision-making and intervention in airway management: from the mouth to the lungs and pleurae. *Insights Imaging.* 2014;5:253–279.
165. Ezri T, Gewurtz G, Sessler DI, et al. Prediction of difficult laryngoscopy in obese patients by ultrasound quantification of anterior neck soft tissue. *Anaesthesia.* 2003;58:1111–1114.
166. Srinivasarangan M, Akkamahadevi P, Balkal VC, Javali RH. Diagnostic accuracy of ultrasound measurements of anterior neck soft tissue in determining a difficult airway. *J Emerg Trauma Shock.* 2021;14:33–37.
167. You-Ten KE, Desai D, Postonogova T, Siddiqui N. Accuracy of conventional digital palpation and ultrasound of the cricothyroid membrane in obese women in labour. *Anaesthesia.* 2015;70:1230–1234.
168. Gottlieb M, Holladay D, Peksa GD. Ultrasonography for the confirmation of endotracheal tube intubation: a systematic review and meta-analysis. *Ann Emerg Med.* 2018;72:627–636.
169. Chan KK, Joo DA, McRae AD, et al. Chest ultrasonography versus supine chest radiography for diagnosis of pneumothorax in trauma patients in the emergency department. *Cochrane Database Syst Rev.* 2020;7:CD013031.
170. Kuo F BH, Deng Y. Role of point-of-care ultrasound in the early stages of trauma care. *Curr Anesthesiol Rep.* 2020;10:69–79.
171. Heinz ER VA. Point-of-care ultrasound for the trauma anesthesiologist. *Curr Anesthesiol Rep.* 2022:1–9.
172. Kruisselbrink R, Chan V, Cibinel GA, Abrahamson S, Goffi A. I-AIM (Indication, acquisition, interpretation, medical decision-making) framework for point of care lung ultrasound. *Anesthesiology.* 2017;127:568–682.
173. Vargas CA, Quintero J, Figueroa R, Castro A, Watts FA. Extension of the thoracic spine sign as a diagnostic marker for thoracic trauma. *Eur J Trauma Emerg Surg.* 2021;47:749–755.
174. Haskins SC, Tanaka CY, Boublik J, Wu CL, Sloth E. Focused cardiac ultrasound for the regional anesthesiologist and pain specialist. *Reg Anesth Pain Med.* 2017;42:632–644.
175. Gillman LM, Kirkpatrick AW. Portable bedside ultrasound: the visual stethoscope of the 21st century. *Scand J Trauma Resusc Emerg Med.* 2012;20:18.
176. Labovitz AJ, Noble VE, Bierig M, et al. Focused cardiac ultrasound in the emergent setting: a consensus statement of the American Society of Echocardiography and American College of Emergency Physicians. *J Am Soc Echocardiogr.* 2010;23:1225–1230.
177. Leichtle SW, Singleton A, Singh M, Griffee MJ, Tobin JM. Transesophageal echocardiography in the evaluation of the trauma patient: a trauma resuscitation transesophageal echocardiography exam. *J Crit Care.* 2017;40:202–206.
178. Shiga T, Wajima Z, Apfel CC, Inoue T, Ohe Y. Diagnostic accuracy of transesophageal echocardiography, helical computed tomography, and magnetic resonance imaging for suspected thoracic aortic dissection: systematic review and meta-analysis. *Arch Intern Med.* 2006;166:1350–1356.
179. Griffee MJ, Singleton A, Zimmerman JM, Morgan DE, Nirula R. The effect of perioperative rescue transesophageal echocardiography on the management of trauma patients. *A A Case Rep.* 2016;6:387–390.
180. Giron-Arango L, D'Empaire PP. Is there a role for transesophageal echocardiography in the perioperative trauma patient? *Curr Anesthesiol Rep.* 12(2):210–216.
181. Carroll SL, Dye DW, Smedley WA, et al. Early and prehospital trauma deaths: who might benefit from advanced resuscitative care? *J Trauma Acute Care Surg.* 2020;88:776–782.
182. Apodaca A, Olson CM Jr, Bailey J, Butler F, Eastridge BJ, Kuncir E. Performance improvement evaluation of forward aeromedical evacuation platforms in Operation Enduring Freedom. *J Trauma Acute Care Surg.* 2013;75:S157–S163.
183. Tobin JM, Reid C, Burns BJ. Multidisciplinary prehospital critical care. *J Trauma Acute Care Surg.* 2020;89:e188–e189.
184. Strumwasser A, Tobin JM, Henry R, et al. Extracorporeal membrane oxygenation in trauma: a single institution experience and review of the literature. *Int J Artif Organs.* 2018;41:845–853.
185. Tobin JM, Gavitt BJ, Nomellini V, Dobson GP, Letson HL, Shackelford SA. Immunotherapeutic options for inflammation in trauma. *J Trauma Acute Care Surg.* 2020;89:S77–S82.
186. Dobson GP, Letson HL. Adenosine, lidocaine, and $Mg2^+$ (ALM): from cardiac surgery to combat casualty care–teaching old drugs new tricks. *J Trauma Acute Care Surg.* 2016;80:135–145.
187. Letson HL, Dobson GP. Adenosine, lidocaine, and $Mg2^+$ (ALM) resuscitation fluid protects against experimental traumatic brain injury. *J Trauma Acute Care Surg.* 2018;84:908–916.
188. Letson H, Dobson G. Adenosine, lidocaine and $Mg2^+$ (ALM) fluid therapy attenuates systemic inflammation, platelet dysfunction and coagulopathy after non-compressible truncal hemorrhage. *PLoS One.* 2017;12:e0188144.
189. Cunningham RM, Walton MA, Carter PM. The major causes of death in children and adolescents in the United States. *N Engl J Med.* 2018;379:2468–2475.
190. Tracy ET, Englum BR, Barbas AS, Foley C, Rice HE, Shapiro ML. Pediatric injury patterns by year of age. *J Pediatr Surg.* 2013;48:1384–1388.
191. Bradshaw CJ, Bandi AS, Muktar Z, et al. International study of the epidemiology of paediatric trauma: PAPSA research study. *World J Surg.* 2018;42:1885–1894.
192. Lam WH, MacKersie A. Paediatric head injury: incidence, aetiology and management. *Paediatr Anaesth.* 1999;9:377–385.
193. Adewale L. Anatomy and assessment of the pediatric airway. *Paediatr Anaesth.* 2009;19 (Suppl 1):1–8.
194. Ivashkov Y, Bhananker SM. Perioperative management of pediatric trauma patients. *Int J Crit Illn Inj Sci.* 2012;2:143–148.
195. Schmitz B, Albrecht S. Pediatric trauma anesthesia. *Curr Opin Anaesthesiol.* 2002;15:187–191.
196. Leonard J. Spinal cord injury without radiographic abnormality (SCIWORA) in children. In: Bachur RG, Wiley JF, eds. *UpToDate;* 2020.
197. Okada Y, Ishii W, Sato N, Kotani H, Iiduka R. Management of pediatric 'cannot intubate, cannot oxygenate'. *Acute Med Surg.* 2017;4:462–466.
198. Lee L. Trauma management: unique pediatric considerations. *UpToDate;* 2021.
199. Riley AA, Arakawa Y, Worley S, Duncan BW, Fukamachi K. Circulating blood volumes: a review of measurement techniques and a meta-analysis in children. *ASAIO J.* 2010;56:260–264.
200. Fiser DH. Intraosseous infusion. *N Engl J Med.* 1990;322:1579–1581.
201. Cannon JW, Johnson MA, Caskey RC, Borgman MA, Neff LP. High ratio plasma resuscitation does not improve survival in pediatric trauma patients. *J Trauma Acute Care Surg.* 2017;83:211–217.
202. Nosanov L, Inaba K, Okoye O, et al. The impact of blood product ratios in massively transfused pediatric trauma patients. *Am J Surg.* 2013;206:655–660.
203. Eckert MJ, Wertin TM, Tyner SD, Nelson DW, Izenberg S, Martin MJ. Tranexamic acid administration to pediatric trauma patients in a combat setting: the pediatric trauma and tranexamic acid study (PED-TRAX). *J Trauma Acute Care Surg.* 2014;77:852–858; discussion 8.
204. Vogel AM, Radwan ZA, Cox CS Jr, Cotton BA. Admission rapid thrombelastography delivers real-time "actionable" data in pediatric trauma. *J Pediatr Surg.* 2013;48:1371–1376.
205. Deng Q, Hao F, Wang Y, Guo C. Rotation thromboelastometry (ROTEM) enables improved outcomes in the pediatric trauma population. *J Int Med Res.* 2018;46:5195–5204.
206. Clebone A. Pediatric trauma transfusion and cognitive aids. *Curr Opin Anaesthesiol.* 2018;31:201–206.
207. Michelet D, Arslan O, Hilly J, et al. Intraoperative changes in blood pressure associated with cerebral desaturation in infants. *Paediatr Anaesth.* 2015;25:681–688.
208. Stokes MAR, Johnson WD. Burns in the Third World: an unmet need. *Ann Burns Fire Disasters.* 2017;30:243–246.
209. Burns. https://www.who.int/news-room/fact-sheets/detail/burns; ccessed March 31, 2022.
210. Guilabert P, Usua G, Martin N, Abarca L, Barret JP, Colomina MJ. Fluid resuscitation management in patients with burns: update. *Br J Anaesth.* 2016;117:284–296.
211. Sharar S. Anesthesia for patients with burn injuries. *UpToDate;* 2021.
212. Bittner EA, Shank E, Woodson L, Martyn JA. Acute and perioperative care of the burn-injured patient. *Anesthesiology.* 2015;122:448–464.
213. Crum RL, Dominic W, Hansbrough JF, Shackford SR, Brown MR. Cardiovascular and neurohumoral responses following burn injury. *Arch Surg.* 1990;125:1065–1069.
214. Jeschke MG, Gauglitz GG, Kulp GA, et al. Long-term persistance of the pathophysiologic response to severe burn injury. *PLoS One.* 2011;6:e21245.
215. Advanced burn life support course. 2018. http://ameriburn.org/wp-content/uploads/2019/08/2018-abls-providermanual.pdf
216. Rice P. Assessment and classification of burn injury. *UpToDate;* 2021.
217. Klein MB, Goverman J, Hayden DL, et al. Benchmarking outcomes in the critically injured burn patient. *Ann Surg.* 2014;259:833–841.
218. Lionelli GT, Pickus EJ, Beckum OK, Decoursey RL, Korentager RA. A three decade analysis of factors affecting burn mortality in the elderly. *Burns.* 2005;31:958–963.
219. Holley AD, Reade MC, Lipman J, Cohen J. There is no fire without smoke! Pathophysiology and treatment of inhalational injury in burns: a narrative review. *Anaesth Intensive Care.* 2020;48:114–122.
220. Enkhbaatar P, Pruitt BA Jr, Suman O, et al. Pathophysiology, research challenges, and clinical management of smoke inhalation injury. *Lancet.* 2016;388:1437–1446.

221. Walker PF, Buehner MF, Wood LA, et al. Diagnosis and management of inhalation injury: an updated review. *Crit Care.* 2015;19:351.
222. Hunt JL, Agee RN, Pruitt BA Jr. Fiberoptic bronchoscopy in acute inhalation injury. *J Trauma.* 1975;15:641–649.
223. Ching JA, Ching YH, Shivers SC, Karlnoski RA, Payne WG, Smith DJ Jr. An analysis of inhalation injury diagnostic methods and patient outcomes. *J Burn Care Res.* 2016;37:e27–e32.
224. Yamamura H, Kaga S, Kaneda K, Mizobata Y. Chest computed tomography performed on admission helps predict the severity of smoke-inhalation injury. *Crit Care.* 2013;17:R95.
225. Gore MA, Joshi AR, Nagarajan G, Iyer SP, Kulkarni T, Khandelwal A. Virtual bronchoscopy for diagnosis of inhalation injury in burnt patients. *Burns.* 2004;30:165–168.
226. Cao L, Zhang XG, Wang JG, et al. Pulmonary function test findings in patients with acute inhalation injury caused by smoke bombs. *J Thorac Dis.* 2016;8:3160–3167.
227. El-Helbawy RH, Ghareeb FM. Inhalation injury as a prognostic factor for mortality in burn patients. *Ann Burns Fire Disasters.* 2011;24:82–88.

Section 9

POSTANESTHETIC MANAGEMENT, CRITICAL CARE, AND PAIN MANAGEMENT

54 Postanesthesia Recovery

MICHAEL A. FOWLER • KEITH A. HOWELL

KEY POINTS

1. Postoperative planning begins when a patient is scheduled for surgery. With emerging protocols for Enhanced Recovery After Surgery (ERAS), specific evidence-based and best practice structure for patient care has the goal of providing care that is coordinated with the surgical team to provide the best outcomes and reduce unnecessary use of resources.
2. The level of PACU care depends on the type/approach of surgery, type of anesthetic, intraoperative course of events, as well as patient pre-existing and evolving comorbidities. Typical recovery settings include inpatient recovery, ambulatory recovery (phase I for more intensive needs and phase II for less intensive needs), short stay (23-hour admit), and recovery from specific procedures (e.g., computed tomography, magnetic resonance imaging, invasive radiology, cardiac, pediatric, and radiation procedures).
3. The transfer of care to a PACU nurse includes assuring that the patient has had appropriate monitoring applied, admission vital signs taken, a direct and thorough report received that allows for rapid evaluation should complications arise, as well as a nurse capable of handling the acuity of the patient's medical/surgical problems.
4. Relative hypovolemia should be evaluated and managed in PACU based on the patient's comorbidities, preoperative status (i.e., bowel preparation, postdialysis), type and duration of surgery, blood loss, and urine output.
5. Postoperative analgesia should be individualized to requirements and expectations. A multimodal approach includes the appropriate use of nonsteroidal anti-inflammatory drugs, narcotics, adjuncts, regional and local anesthetics, as well as anxiety relief and appropriate emotional support.
6. Discharge criteria should be tailored to the individual patient's underlying disease, recovery course, and postdischarge level of care.
7. The cardiac risks during the postoperative stay include myocardial ischemia, which may be minimized with continued use of beta-blockers, analgesia, nitrates, supplemental oxygen, adequate circulating volume, oxygen-carrying capacity, heart rate control, and an understanding of hypercoagulable states.

8 The respiratory risks of a patient must take into account the preoperative respiratory disease status. Residual anesthetics, residual muscle relaxants, opioids, and sedatives all impair responsiveness to increasing CO_2 and decreasing O_2 levels. Pain itself can decrease respiration and minute ventilation, leading to CO_2 retention and hypoxemia. Supplemental O_2 application alone does not guarantee hypoxemia will not occur.

9 The evaluation of a patient's ability to void may be affected by type of surgery (i.e., genitourinary surgery, hernia repairs) or type of anesthetic (i.e., regional, neuraxial, or opioids).

10 Glycemic monitoring and control should persist as a continuum from intraoperative management. Good glycemic control may help with fighting infection, improve wound healing, which can result in better surgical outcomes. Hypoglycemia occurs because of preoperative fasting, intraoperative administration of insulin, as well as the patient using programmable insulin pumps.

11 Hypothermia can lead to an increased length of stay in PACU, lethargy, decreased minute ventilation, decreased strength, and increased cardiac demand. It is important to assure that the patient is dry and insulated. The use of air warming blankets, warming mats, and intravenous fluid warmers all minimize hypothermia.

12 Many elderly patients experience a varied degree of postoperative confusion, delirium, or cognitive dysfunction in the PACU. Many pediatric patients also experience postemergence delirium leading to increased length of stay in the PACU.

13 Postoperative nausea and vomiting is a major cause of patient discomfort and dissatisfaction, as well as an aspiration risk and causes prolonged PACU stay.

Postanesthesia Recovery

Each patient recovering from an anesthetic has circumstances that require an individualized problem-oriented approach. Postanesthesia recovery must continue to adapt to meet the needs of the changing perioperative landscape, advances in technology, changing surgical techniques; and to respond to improved evidence-based research. Dissemination of anesthesia services beyond the perisurgical arena brought changes and greater demands on recovery units.

Standards for Postanesthesia Care

Standards for Postanesthesia Care were first approved by the ASA House of Delegates originating from the Standards and Practice Parameters Committee for Postanesthesia Care on October 12, 1988. The five standards of postoperative care were last amended on October 23, 2019. These standards are used to determine who needs managed recovery, the types and levels of recovery, who is responsible for patient care and how the patient should be monitored prior to discharge from the postanesthesia care unit (PACU).[1]

Value and Economics of Postanesthesia Care Unit

The quality of postanesthesia care is composed of many variables such as tracking of complications, time per patient spent in recovery, overall clinical outcomes, and patient satisfaction. The value of postanesthesia care is a measure of the quality of care provided compared with the amount of resources spent per patient outcome. The PACU helps to use resources efficiently by having trained staff who routinely care for postsurgical patients, thereby recognizing/preventing complications, and by having physicians instituting appropriate and timely therapies.

The actual cost of PACU care incorporates costs of staffing, space, disposables, and hardware (resource utilization). Triage and discharge policies affect both how many admissions occur and what resources each admission consumes. Nurse staffing continues to be the largest direct cost in the PACU. The mix of nursing staff, experience of nurses, staffing ratios, and the complexity and duration of PACU stay affect the overall personnel cost per admission. The level of monitoring provided affects the capital expenditure for equipment, and disposable items account for operating expenditures. The patient acuity mix also determines needs for staffing and equipment such as ventilators, additional monitors, intravenous pumps, patient warming devices and patient-controlled analgesia pumps. The type of physician coverage—such as dedicated coverage versus on-demand coverage—can affect response time, efficiency of care, costs, and patient outcomes. The use of routine postoperative diagnostic testing and therapies without evidence-based need can lead to unnecessary treatments, increasing cost per patient and possible worse patients' outcomes.

Cost comparisons between institutions are difficult because charges and cost factors vary widely across institutions, in different regions of the United States, and between countries. They constantly change over time. Regulatory requirements, standards of care, medical-legal climates, and institutional requirements vary greatly between regions and even between facilities in the same locale. It is difficult to establish cost-effectiveness goals of a single PACU because of the differing requirements of individual patients having the same procedures. This difference can be the result of levels of patient comorbidities, level of procedure complexity, surgeon, type of anesthetic, as well as patient perception and expectations. These are just some of the factors that can determine the type of care needed postoperatively. Continued pressures from many fronts to contain costs and maximize cost-effectiveness force each surgical facility to continually evaluate the value of its PACU care to each individual patient.

PACU medical directors are challenged to optimize clinical results while minimizing expenditures. Innovative PACU practices should guarantee safe care, minimize cost, and fulfill regulatory and institutional requirements. Medical professionals (physicians, nursing, and support staff) must work in concert to identify practices that are wasteful versus those that have proven yield/benefit. The impact of many PACU-proposed interventions on clinical outcomes is not easily substantiated by controlled scientific analysis. Useless or routine testing, unjustifiable therapy, and inappropriate PACU admissions should be eliminated. However, using a more expensive therapy may generate real savings by decreasing additional therapies, testing, admissions, or length of stay. Another important element essential for patient safety and efficiency in the PACU is communication with the intraoperative anesthesiology service. Communication is perhaps the least expensive tool in medicine and the one most universally proven to be involved in human error events. Utilization of PACU resources is directly related to anesthetic duration and technique. In one study, 22.1% of 37,000 patients had a minor anesthesia-related event or complication that prolonged PACU stays and consumed PACU resources.[2] Another study showed how postoperative adverse events increase the amount of nursing resources needed in the PACU.[3] Close coordination between the PACU and the anesthesiology service should reduce the frequency and impact of such events.

1 Continued collaboration with surgical teams and developing Enhanced Recovery After Anesthesia (ERAS) protocols might create an opportunity to shorten the length of stay in the PACU. Providers in the recovery unit must be aware of these protocols and manage patients accordingly. Observed change is frequently seen by reducing transportation delays, persistence of pain or nausea, waiting for space, or surgeon discharge delays.[4] Cost-saving measures in other areas may also increase the cost of PACU care; for example, fast-tracking to discharge to home rather than to a hospital bed. The cost savings of not occupying a hospital bed is offset by an increase in PACU stay and therefore greater consumption of PACU resources.[5] The savings may be a cost savings for the patient and beneficial for the facility as a whole but at a greater expense to the PACU. True savings are only realized when operational changes yield a decrease in expenditures for staff, supplies, or equipment. For example, patients who can bypass the PACU create a savings opportunity only if paid nursing hours are reduced or if more surgical cases are covered with the same hours. With the use of less invasive surgical techniques combined with innovative anesthetic techniques, such as regional anesthetics, shorter PACU stays can result in real savings opportunities. However, the areas of scheduling, clerical, or maintenance tasks must not consume excess staffing hours without savings realized. Finally, trimming costs could entail an increase in unwanted risk to patients. Standardized or consistent handoffs between anesthesia providers and PACU staff can maximize best patient care while minimizing costs. Differentiating between cost-effective postanesthesia care and unsafe practice remains a matter of constant professional judgment and debate daily in most PACUs.

Levels of Postoperative/Postanesthesia Care

With continued demand to increase overall health care efficiency, caution must be taken to provide the most appropriate care for each patient. As anesthesia services expand to cover a variety of patient types in ever-increasing areas outside the operating room,
2 selecting the correct type of recovery is essential. For the many differing anesthesia areas ranging from inpatient surgery, ambulatory surgery, to off-site procedures, the level of postoperative care that a patient requires is determined by the degree of underlying illness, comorbidities, and the duration as well as the type of anesthesia and surgery. These factors are used to assess the risk of postoperative complications. Less invasive surgeries or procedures combined with shorter-duration anesthetic regimens facilitate high levels of arousal and minimal cardiovascular and respiratory depression at the end of surgery.

Using a less intensive postanesthesia setting for selected patients can reduce costs for a surgical procedure and allow the facility to divert scarce PACU resources to patients with greater needs. Alert patients are more satisfied when spared the unnecessary assessments in interventions of PACU care. Amenities such as recliners, reading material, television, music, and food improve perceptions (emotional satisfaction) without affecting quality or safety. Earlier reunion with family or visitors in the low-intensity setting is desirable assuming that postoperative care is safe and appropriate. This aspect is especially important in the pediatric population.

Creation of separate PACUs for inpatients, ambulatory, or non-operating room anesthesia (NORA) patients is one possible way to streamline PACU care for appropriately triaged patients. Phase I recovery would be reserved for more intense recovery and would require more one-on-one care for staff. Phase II recovery should be less intensive and is appropriate for patients after less invasive procedures requiring less attention from nursing while recovering. If separation of different phases of care is not possible, then providing the appropriate level of monitoring and coverage to the degree of postoperative impairment achieves similar results in a single PACU area. However, care equal to a full-intensity PACU must always be available, given the incidence of complications after anesthesia and surgery.[6] As the aging population generates an increase in the complexity of surgical care in the face of tighter control of resources, maintaining appropriate PACU capacity and safety by observing applicable PACU guidelines and standards will be increasingly important.[7,8] Major complications occur in 3% to 17% of inpatient surgery procedures and require treatment after admission to the PACU. Most patients spend 1 hour or less in the PACU. Staff for typical patient type following surgery remain prepared with continued education and simulations to ensure unit training and up to date patient care.[9]

Postanesthetic Triage

Patients must be carefully evaluated to determine which level of care is appropriate. Triage should be based on clinical condition, length/type of procedure and anesthetic, and the potential for complications that require intervention. Alternatives to PACU care must be used in a nondiscriminatory fashion. Arbitrary criteria based on age, American Society of Anesthesiologists (ASA) classification, ambulatory versus inpatient versus off-site procedure status, or type of insurance should not be used for determining the level of recovery care. An individual patient undergoing a specific procedure or anesthetic should receive the same appropriate level of postoperative care whether the procedure is performed in a hospital operating room, an ambulatory surgical center, an endoscopy room, an invasive radiology suite, or an outpatient office. In accordance with the ASA Standards of Post Anesthesia Care, Standard I, an anesthesiologist familiar with the patient can determine which level of care is required or if time in a recovery area is needed. If doubt exists about a patient's safety in a lower intensity setting, the patient should be admitted to a higher level of care for recovery. Patient safety should always be favored over concerns of cost.

After superficial procedures using local infiltration, minor blocks, or sedation, patients can almost always recover with less intensive monitoring and coverage. Healthy patients undergoing more extensive procedures (e.g., hernia repairs, arthroscopic procedures, minor orthopedic procedures) under local, plexus, or peripheral nerve blockade might also bypass phase I recovery and go directly to phase II. The increasing use of continuous peripheral nerve catheters for surgery has shortened PACU time and can eliminate many hospital admissions.[10] Innovative anesthetic techniques, advanced surgical techniques, and use of bispectral index monitoring help facilitate fast-track postoperative care.[11]

For more intensive procedures and patients with greater acuity, bypassing the PACU and direct admission to intensive care units (ICUs) can reduce demands on the PACU as well as decreasing the number of hand offs, thereby reducing risk for errors. Direct ICU admission still requires proper postoperative reporting to the accepting unit including how to communicate with the surgical service and anesthesiologist. These ICUs must be trained and prepared to receive immediate postoperative patients as well as meet the standards of the PACU.

Safety in the Postanesthesia Care Unit

Every PACU should have medical oversight in the form of a Medical Director. The PACU Medical Director must ensure the PACU environment is as safe as possible for both patients and staff. Beyond usual safety policies, maintain staffing and training to ensure appropriate coverage and skill mix are available to deal with unforeseen crises. Incidence of adverse events in the PACU correlates with nursing workload and staff availability.[3] Ideally, all staff should have PACU certification, and staffing ratios should never fall below acceptable standards.[8] Less skilled or training staff must be appropriately supervised, and a sufficient number of certified personnel must always be available to handle worst-case scenarios.

The PACU staff protects patients who are temporarily incompetent and preserves patients' rights to observance of advanced directives and to informed consent for additional procedures. The staff is obligated to optimize each patient's privacy, dignity, and to minimize the psychological impact of unpleasant or frightening events. Observance of procedures for handwashing, sterility, and infection control should be strictly enforced.[12] Medical Directors must safeguard against potential for personal assault of patients during recovery such as unwarranted restraints and procedures without consent. Access to the PACU should be strictly controlled. With increasing acceptance of reuniting patients with family or others, safety and privacy issues must be continually addressed.

The PACU environment must also be safe for professionals. Air handling should guarantee that personnel are not exposed to unacceptable levels of trace anesthetic gases, although trace gas monitoring is not necessary. Ensure that staff members receive appropriate vaccinations, including those for hepatitis B, influenza, and others required by their institution. Practitioners must adhere to policies for radiation safety, infection control, disposal of sharps, universal precautions for blood-borne diseases, and safeguarding against exposure to pathogens such as methicillin-resistant *Staphylococcus*, vancomycin-resistant *Enterococcus*, *Clostridium difficile*, or tuberculosis. Personal protective equipment (PPE) such as gloves and eye protection must be worn to protect both the patient and provider. Having masks, gowns, and appropriate particulate respiratory equipment easily accessible is needed for particular cases. Following current infection control policies and guidelines are essential for patient and staff safety. Ensure that sufficient help is available to avoid injury while lifting and positioning patients or while dealing with emergency situations. Precise documentation and clear delineation of responsibility is essential for proper care of patients and can protect staff against unnecessary medicolegal exposure.

Admission to the Postanesthesia Care Unit

Every patient admitted to a PACU should have vital signs, airway patency, peripheral oxygen saturation, ventilatory rate/character, and level of pain recorded and periodically monitored.[7] Assessment with periodic recording every 5 minutes for the first 15 minutes and every 15 minutes thereafter is a minimum. Document temperature, level of consciousness, mental status, neuromuscular function, hydration status, degree of nausea on admission/discharge, and more frequently if appropriate, are also minimum standards of care. Every patient should be continuously monitored with a pulse oximeter and at least a single-lead electrocardiogram (ECG). Extra leads, particularly precordial V3–6, are appropriate if left ventricular ischemia is likely. Capnography is necessary for patients receiving mechanical ventilation or those at risk for compromised ventilatory function. Transduction and recorded output from invasive monitors such as arterial, central venous or pulmonary arterial catheters must be accomplished. Diagnostic (laboratory) testing should be ordered only for specific indications or part of a designed recovery protocol.

Anesthesiology providers should manage the patient in the 3
PACU until a PACU nurse secures admission vital signs, attaches appropriate monitors, and care is transferred with a complete report to the nursing staff. A succinct but thorough report that includes sufficient information to allow rapid evaluation and intervention for postoperative complications must be legibly recorded using a standardized format printed on the PACU record (Table 54-1). This report should be similar to the OR timeout. Providing patient identification, procedure performed, anesthetic type, and continuing therapies. Documentation of the time and amount of all neuromuscular relaxants, respiratory depressant medications, and reversal agents should be included. Outlined orders, specific therapeutic end points, and, most importantly, how to contact the responsible anesthesiologist all must be transmitted. The anesthesiologist should never transfer responsibility to PACU personnel until the patient's airway status, ventilation, and hemodynamics are appropriate for the caregivers to whom they entrust the patient's care. Leaving a patient in the hands of someone unfamiliar or incapable of adequately handling the acuity of the medical situation in a rush to perform "the next case" may constitute abandonment of care. Check the function of indwelling cannulae, intravenous catheters, monitors and verify medication type and rates of any intravenous infusions before completing transfer of care.

Postoperative Pain Management

Relief of surgical pain with minimal side effects is a major goal during PACU care and a top priority for patients.[7,13–15] Periodically assess and document level of pain throughout recovery. The Joint Commission for Accreditation of Health Organizations mandated that a numerical pain scale or visual scale be used with periodic recording and an acceptable score for discharge. Inadequate postoperative analgesia is a major source of preoperative fear and ultimate dissatisfaction for surgical patients. In addition to improving comfort, analgesia reduces sympathetic nervous system response, thereby avoiding hypertension, tachycardia, and dysrhythmias.
In hypovolemic patients the sympathetic nervous system activity 4
may well mask relative hypovolemia. Administration of analgesics can precipitate hypotension in an apparently stable patient, especially if direct or histamine-induced vasodilation occurs. It is important to assess a tachycardic patient with low or normal blood pressure who complains of pain carefully before giving analgesics that might precipitate or accentuate hypotension.

The actual degree of postoperative pain can be difficult to establish. Severity of pain varies among surgical procedures and anesthetic techniques. Staff members may be relatively ineffective at quantifying level of discomfort. Patients are often able to communicate despite having received sedative hypnotic drugs. Furthermore, patients may be impaired in their communication abilities coming into the hospital or may be affected by the entire medical experience, and thereby may be afraid to express

Table 54-1 Components of a Postanesthesia Care Unit Admission Report

Preoperative History/Procedures
- Medication allergies or reactions
- Pertinent earlier surgical procedures
- Underlying medical illness
- Chronic medications
- Acute problems (e.g., ischemia, acid–base status, dehydration)
- Premedications (e.g., antibiotics and time given, β-adrenergic blockers, antiemetics)
- Preoperative pain control (e.g., nerve blocks, adjunct medications, narcotics)
- Preoperative pain assessment (chronic and acute pain scores)
- NPO status

Intraoperative Factors
- Surgical procedure
- Type of anesthetic
- Type and difficulty of airway management
- Relaxant/reversal status
- Time and amount of opioids administered
- Type and amount of intravenous fluids administered
- Estimated blood loss
- Urine output
- Unexpected surgical or anesthetic events
- Intraoperative vital sign ranges
- Intraoperative laboratory findings
- Drugs given (e.g., steroids, diuretics, antibiotics, vasoactive medications, antiemetics)

Assessment and Report of Current Status
- Airway patency
- Ventilatory adequacy
- Level of consciousness
- Level of pain
- Heart rate and heart rhythm
- Endotracheal tube position
- Systemic pressure
- Intravascular volume status
- Function of invasive monitors
- Size and location of intravenous catheters
- Anesthetic equipment (e.g., epidural catheters, peripheral nerve catheters)
- Overall impression

Postoperative Instructions
- Expected airway and ventilatory status
- Acceptable vital sign ranges
- Acceptable urine output and blood loss
- Surgical instructions (e.g., positioning, wound care)
- Anticipated cardiovascular problems
- Orders for therapeutic interventions
- Diagnostic tests to be secured
- Therapeutic goals and end points before discharge
- Location of responsible physician

NPO, nothing by mouth.

their needs. Inexperienced nurses overestimate a patient's pain, whereas more experienced nurses tend to underestimate the pain.[16] Either error can lead to inappropriate treatment. Use of a numeric pain scale yields more reliable results but requires that a patient be willing to communicate. A wide divergence can exist between a patient's cognitive perception of pain and sympathetic nervous system response, related to psychological, cultural, and cardiovascular differences among individuals. Some patients perceive severe pain with minimal sympathetic nervous system activity, whereas others exhibit hypertension and tachycardia with minimal complaint of discomfort. The best measure of analgesia is the patient's perception. Heart rate, respiratory rate and depth, sweating, nausea, and vomiting all may be signs of pain but their absence or presence is not in itself reliable as a measure of the presence of pain.

Careful identification of patient subgroups, assessment of individual analgesic requirements, and implementation of a planned, multimodal approach will provide seamless pain control through and beyond the PACU interval.[17] In a study of postoperative pain in 10,008 ambulatory patients, only 5.3% related severe pain in the PACU and 1.7% in the discharge area (Fig. 54-1). However,

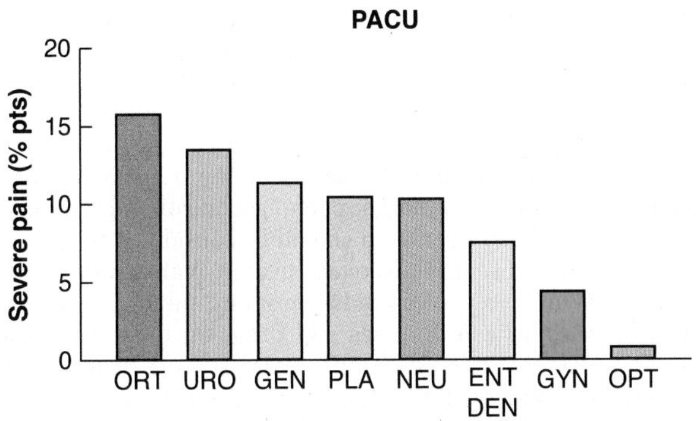

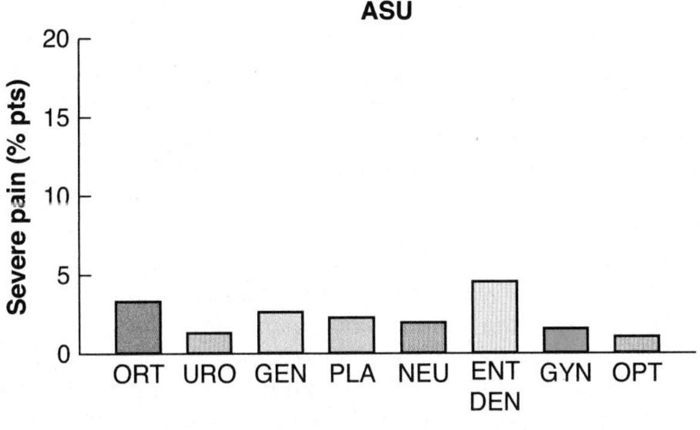

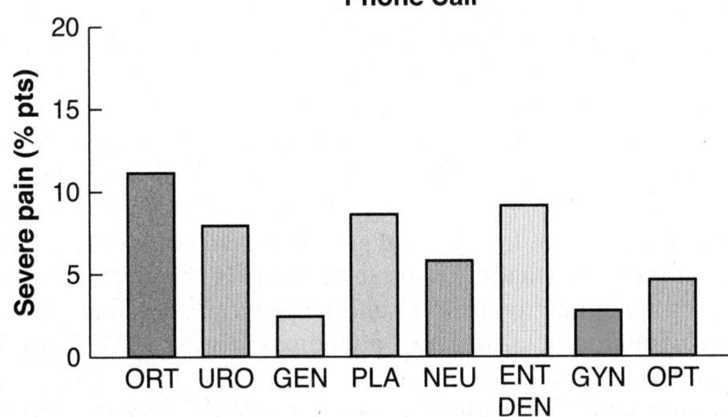

Figure 54-1 Percentage of patients experiencing severe pain in the postanesthesia care unit (PACU), the ambulatory surgery unit (ASU), and during phone call follow-up at 24 hours. ORT, orthopedics; URO, urology; GEN, general; PLA, plastics; NEU, neurology; ENT, ear, nose, throat; DEN, dental; GYN, gynecology; OPT, ophthalmology. (Reprinted with permission from Chung F, Ritchie E, Su J. Postoperative pain in ambulatory surgery. *Anesth Analg*. 1997;85:808.)

a much higher percentage of patients relate that moderate-to-severe pain recurs after discharge.[18,19] To avoid masking signs of an unrelated condition or a surgical complication, ascertain that the nature and intensity of pain are appropriate for the surgical procedure. The central nervous system (CNS) signs of hypoxemia, acidemia, or cerebral hypoperfusion often mimic those of pain, especially during emergence. Administration of parenteral analgesics or sedatives can acutely worsen hypoventilation, airway obstruction, or hypotension, causing sudden deterioration. Evaluating orientation, the level of arousal, and cardiovascular or pulmonary status usually identifies such patients. With the continued opioid crisis, opioid use disorder (OUD) patients on maintenance plans of methadone or opioid agonist/antagonist (buprenorphine/naloxone) can present with pain control challenges. Knowing if patients have received their daily treatment doses helps aid in managing post procedure acute pain. It is recommended to continue the preoperative dose of the patient's maintenance plan. Even patients who have continued with their daily maintenance treatment, a higher dose of opioids may be expected. To adequately control pain, opioids should be continuous or scheduled rather than on a needed basis. Undertreatment of pain predisposes these patients to decreased responsiveness to opioid therapy. An aggressive plan including nonsteroidal anti-inflammatory drugs, acetaminophen, gabapentinoids, alpha 2 agonist, and regional anesthesia should be considered.[20]

5 Surgical pain can be effectively treated with a multimodal approach. While usage of opioids continues, the use of regional and local anesthetic techniques and drugs such as acetaminophen, NSAIDs, neuroleptics, alpha agonists have proven to be effective in reducing pain. Sufficient analgesia is the end point, even if large doses of opioids are necessary in tolerant patients. Short-acting opioids are useful to expedite discharge and minimize nausea in ambulatory settings,[21] although duration of analgesia can be a problem. During intravenous titration of opioids, assess for incremental respiratory or cardiovascular depression. Oral and transdermal analgesics have a limited role in the PACU but are helpful for ambulatory patients transitioning to PACU discharge. Rectal analgesics are sometimes useful in small children. Interventions such as repositioning, reassurance, or extubation also help minimize discomfort.

Other analgesic modalities provide pain relief in and beyond the PACU.[22] Titration if intravenous opioids in the PACU is important for smooth transition to intravenous patient-controlled analgesia. Injection of opioids into the epidural or subarachnoid space during anesthesia or in the PACU yields prolonged postoperative analgesia in selected patients.[23,24] Nausea and pruritus are troubling side effects, and immediate or delayed ventilatory depression can occur related to vascular uptake and cephalad spread in cerebrospinal fluid. Nausea should resolve with antiemetics, whereas pruritus and ventilatory depression often respond to naloxone infusion. Addition of local anesthetic or clonidine enhances analgesia and decreases the risk of side effects from epidural opioids, although local anesthetics add risk of hypotension or motor blockade. Epidural analgesia is effective after thoracic or abdominal procedures and helps wean obese patients or those with chronic obstructive pulmonary disease (COPD) from mechanical ventilation.

Continuous flow catheters with pressure delivery systems of local anesthetics have been used intrawound to reduce pain and opioid requirements, increase patient satisfaction, and reduce length of hospital stay.[25] These same delivery systems have been safely used with continuous peripheral nerve catheters for in hospital as well as outpatient use.[26,27] With the use of ultrasound-guided techniques for catheter placement, appropriately selected outpatients can safely receive the pain control benefits of regional anesthesia.[10] However, extensive written and oral postoperative instructions must be provided, with systems in place for 24-hour access by patients for catheter-related complications.

Placement of long-acting regional analgesic blocks reduces pain, controls sympathetic nervous system activity, and often improves ventilation.[22] After shoulder procedures, interscalene block yields almost complete pain relief with only moderate inconvenience from motor impairment. Paralysis of the ipsilateral diaphragm can impair postoperative ventilation in patients with marginal reserve, although the impact is small in most patients.[28] Suprascapular nerve block might be an alternative to avoid this potentially serious side effect. The continued evolving regional anesthesia techniques and types of nerve blocks can be useful in the postoperative setting for either supplementing inadequate previous coverage or regional anesthesia not part of original anesthetic plan. Caudal analgesia or paravertebral blocks can also be effective in children after inguinal or genital procedures, whereas infiltration of local anesthetic into joints, soft tissues, or incisions decreases the intensity of pain. Other modalities, such as guided imagery, hypnosis, transcutaneous nerve stimulation, music, massage, or acupuncture, have limited utility for surgical pain but may provide a positive patient experience.

Use of patient-controlled analgesia, spinal opioids, or neural blockade mandates anticipation of risk beyond the PACU. The plan for extended postoperative analgesia should be prepared before induction of surgical anesthesia, and then orient the anesthetic and PACU care toward that plan. These plans should be in agreement with the patient, surgeon, and anesthesiologist. If one analgesic modality proves inadequate, take particular care when implementing a second technique.

Fear, anxiety, and confusion often accentuate postoperative pain during recovery, especially after general anesthesia. Titration of an intravenous sedative such as midazolam may attenuate this psychogenic component. It is important to distinguish between requirements for analgesia and for anxiolysis. Opioids are poor sedatives and anxiolytics, whereas benzodiazepines are poor analgesics. However, when pain control modalities appear larger than what might be anticipated, one should consider the possibility that anxiety is playing a large role in the dysphoric event in the PACU.

Discharge Criteria 6

Before discharge from the postoperative unit to a lower level of care, each patient should be sufficiently oriented to assess their physical condition and be able to summon assistance. Airway reflexes and motor function must be adequate to maintain patency and prevent aspiration. One should ensure that ventilation and oxygenation are acceptable, with sufficient reserve to cover minor deterioration in unmonitored settings. Blood pressure, heart rate, and indices of peripheral perfusion should be relatively constant for at least 15 minutes and appropriately near baseline. Achieving normal body temperature is not an absolute requirement, but there should be resolution of shivering. Acceptable analgesia must be achieved and nausea/vomiting appropriately controlled. Patients should be observed for at least 15 minutes after the last intravenous opioid or sedative is administered to assess peak effects and side effects. If regional anesthetics have been administered, longer observation could be appropriate to assess effectiveness and rule out local toxicity. One should monitor oxygen saturation for 15 minutes after discontinuation of supplemental oxygen to detect hypoxemia and rule out likely complications of surgery (e.g., bleeding, vascular compromise, pneumothorax) or of underlying conditions (e.g., hypertension, myocardial ischemia,

Table 54-2 Two Most Commonly Used Postanesthesia Care Unit Discharge Criteria Systems

Modified Aldrete Scoring System	Postanesthetic Discharge Scoring System
Respiration 2 = Able to take deep breath and cough 1 = Dyspnea/shallow breathing 0 = Apnea	**Vital signs** 2 = BP + pulse within 20% preop baseline 1 = BP + pulse within 20–40% preop baseline 0 = BP + pulse >40% preop baseline
O_2 saturation 2 = Maintains SpO_2 >92% on room air 1 = Needs O_2 inhalation to maintain O_2 saturation >90% 0 = O_2 saturation <90% even with supplemental oxygen	**Activity** 2 = Steady gait, no dizziness or meets preop level 1 = Requires assistance 0 = Unable to ambulate
Consciousness 2 = Fully awake 1 = Arousable on calling 0 = Not responding	**Nausea and vomiting** 2 = Minimal/treated with PO medication 1 = Moderate/treated with parenteral medication 0 = Severe/continues despite treatment
Circulation 2 = BP ± 20 mmHg preop 1 = BP ± 20–50 mmHg preop 0 = BP ± 50 mmHg preop	**Pain** Controlled with oral analgesics and acceptable to patient: 2 = Yes 1 = No
Activity 2 = Able to move four extremities voluntary or on command 1 = Able to move two extremities 0 = Unable to move extremities Score ≥9 for discharge	**Surgical bleeding** 2 = Minimal/no dressing changes 1 = Moderate/up to two dressing changes required 0 = Severe/more than three dressing changes required Score ≥9 for discharge

BP, blood pressure; PO, oral.

hyperglycemia, bronchospasm). One should also document a brief neurologic assessment to assure that the patient is at their baseline and review results of diagnostic tests. If these generic criteria cannot be met, postponement of discharge or transfer to a specialized unit is advisable. There is no demonstrable benefit from a mandatory minimum duration of PACU care.

Scoring systems such as the Modified Aldrete Score or Postanesthesia Discharge Scoring System (Table 54-2) are two commonly used systems for patient assessment and attempt to simplify and standardize patient discharge criteria. Fixed PACU discharge criteria must be used with caution because variability among patients is tremendous. Scoring systems that quantify physical status or establish thresholds for vital signs are useful for assessment but cannot replace individual evaluation.[29,30] Ideally, each patient should be evaluated for discharge by an anesthesiologist using a consistent set of criteria, considering the severity of underlying disease, the anesthetic and recovery course, and the level of care at the destination (Table 54-2). A plan for the continued management of likely postdischarge symptoms such as pain, nausea, headache, dizziness, drowsiness, and fatigue must be made prior to discharge.[19] The use of postanesthesia discharge criteria reduces discharge delays for inpatients versus a traditional method of physician examination only with no observable difference in safety.[31]

Postoperative Evaluation

The Centers for Medicare and Medicaid Services (CMS) have instituted compliance policies for those entities that participate in the Medicare and Medicaid programs. The policy for postanesthesia follow-up requires a written follow-up that is performed by an individual that is qualified to administer anesthesia no later than 48 hours post procedure. The timeframe starts as soon as the patient arrives in the recovery area or ICU. The evaluation should be performed only after the patient has sufficiently recovered from anesthesia and is able to participate and answer questions or perform simple tasks. The postanesthesia evaluation must contain the following elements:

- Respiratory function, including respiratory rate, airway patency, and oxygen saturation
- Cardiovascular function, including pulse rate and blood pressure
- Mental status
- Temperature
- Pain
- Nausea and vomiting
- Postoperative hydration

Cardiovascular Complications

The purpose of this section is to focus on events unique to recovering patients rather than review all possible cardiovascular events one might encounter in the PACU. In the PACU, some reflexes previously blunted by general anesthetics, sedatives, and opioids return toward baseline, revealing an unexpected cardiovascular compromise. Perhaps the two most common types of patients to encounter troubles will be the patient with coronary artery disease and the patient with congestive heart failure. Patients in the PACU may not complain of angina due to residual anesthetics and pain medications. The first sign of myocardial ischemia may well be hypotension, and the use of sedation techniques that cause hypotension, for example using drugs like dexmedetomidine, may cloud the picture of a patient's cardiac disease.

The most common sign of myocardial ischemia is tachycardia. Tachycardia is very often a reaction to, not the cause of, myocardial ischemia. Not all tachycardia heralds myocardial ischemia, however, in a patient who seems at risk for coronary artery disease, new-onset tachycardia that is not caused by pain should be taken seriously. The ECG may show classic ST-T wave elevation or depression depending on lead placement and area of ischemia. But the lack of ST-T wave elevation does not rule out coronary artery disease. Transmural myocardial infarctions outside the PACU show no ECG diagnostic changes 10% to 30% of the time. So, the clinician must be especially suspicious of a series of hemodynamic changes in a person at risk for coronary 7 artery disease. Early intervention with nitrates, opioids, beta-blockers, and even anticoagulants may save a life. Cardiology should be involved to gain immediate and timely access to the cardiac catheterization laboratory or for angiolytic drug therapy. With increasing use of bare metal and drug eluding stents (DES), recognition that patients who have stopped antiplatelet therapy and are in postoperative hypercoagulable states can quickly occlude these stents. Proactive intervention requires quick recognition and response. Involvement and communication with the surgical service must be immediate and decisions especially as to anticoagulation and lytic therapy should be made among several services in consultation.

Congestive heart failure is epidemic in our ever-aging population. The outpatient cardiology services have an expanding armamentarium of new inotropic/vasodilator therapy, devices, and interventions that allow patients to compensate for their congestive heart failure. It is helpful to know not only the ejection fraction but also the activities of daily living, exercise tolerance, and other risk indices. The ejection fraction is only an estimate of the fractional shortening of the myocardial actin and myosin fibrils. Although it is a useful estimate of severity of impairment, one is struck by how stable some patients may be with a large, dilated heart contracting at a 15% ejection fraction. They are compensated but have little reserve. The potential problems of bleeding, volume shifts, and respiratory compromise in the PACU could quickly cause decompensation. There are also no absolute numbers with regard to fluid restriction but precaution should be taken when giving fluid challenges. The use of transesophageal echocardiography and transthoracic echo, may be of great use in the PACU. Within a very few minutes, a puzzling hypotensive situation might be explained by an echocardiogram. The echocardiogram allows rapid viewing of myocardial contractility, regional wall motion, volume status, and valvular dysfunction.

With evolving cardiac treatments and less invasive techniques, specialized PACU care can be as safe and more cost effective than ICU admission. The natural extension is to establish some highly specialized PACUs that function as step-down or short-term ICUs. In a study of 85 prospective patients[32] undergoing "off-pump" coronary artery bypass graft procedures, the patients were extubated in 12 ± 2 minutes after the chest was closed. They were then taken to a special part of the PACU where they were monitored for a number of hours (up to 480 minutes in some situations). Patients were then either discharged to the cardiac floors or sent to an ICU. Of the 85 patients in this study, only 4 failed the PACU stay and had to be admitted to an ICU. Bradycardia was the cause for failure in three cases and there was one case of myocardial infarction. Two patients later returned to the ICU from the cardiac ward; one patient had atrial fibrillation and another case of myocardial infarction. During the same time 304 patients who were not undergoing off-pump coronary artery bypass graft surgery were admitted to the cardiac ICU. The cost for PACU stay was $5,140.00 less than for an ICU-admitted patient. Although this study seems quite favorable, the two groups of patients were not comparable.

High-risk vascular and thoracic surgery patients have shown that they could each be adequately cared for in an adequately staffed and prepared PACU.[33] Hospitals can improve its patient throughput by putting more resources into expanded PACU care and less into ICU services. Nursing reviews are available to give input as to how to structure such new units.[34,35]

Anesthesiology services are in increased demand throughout most hospitals. The PACU will likely need to prepare to care for those patients. Some facilities may elect to have separate recovery facilities and staff different from the traditional operating room PACU. Invasive cardiology suites provide ablation techniques for dysrhythmias, automated implantable defibrillators are placed in hybrid suites, operating rooms, or catheterization laboratories and the possibility of percutaneous valve replacements as well as some hybrid and percutaneous coronary revascularization procedures. If these patients require deep sedation or general anesthesia, the patient will also require PACU care.

Cardiac implantable electrical devices such as cardiac pacemakers and cardioverter-defibrillators are commonplace in many postanesthetic patients. Knowledge of the device type and how it was managed during anesthetics is important for safe post procedure care. Continuous monitoring of cardiac rate and rhythm consistent with ASA standard monitors should be performed throughout the immediate post procedure period. Cardiac implantable devices that were reprogrammed should be restored to preoperative ambulatory settings before the patient is discharged from a monitored setting. Backup pacing and cardioversion/defibrillation equipment should be immediately available. Interrogation of devices should be performed if emergency surgery was performed without appropriate device interrogation prior to the operation, if there was significant electromagnetic interference close proximity to the device, suspicion that antitachycardia therapy might have been disabled rather than suspended, or if antitachycardia therapy was observed or if concern of electronic device malfunction is suspected. For cardiac devices not interrogated during the immediate postoperative period, they should be interrogated within 30 days after the procedure.[36]

The cardiac patient is common today. New procedures and pressure to ever streamline operating room care is pressuring the PACU to become more and more a cardiac mini-ICU. The smart PACU medical director and hospital administrator will see that with targeted resources, patients may well be safely cared for in a more cost-effective manner with quicker throughput by using a PACU approach.

Postoperative Pulmonary Dysfunction

Mechanical, hemodynamic, and pharmacologic factors related to surgery and anesthesia impair ventilation, oxygenation, and airway maintenance.[37] Heavy smoking, obesity, sleep apnea, severe asthma, and COPD increase the risk of postoperative ventilatory events.[38] Preoperative pulmonary function testing has limited predictive value for postoperative complications,[39] perhaps with the exception of postoperative bronchospasm in smokers.[40]

Inadequate Postoperative Ventilation

In PACU patients, mild respiratory acidemia due to decreased minute ventilation is expected; thus elevated $PaCO_2$ does not necessarily indicate inadequate postoperative ventilation. Inadequate ventilation should be suspected when (1) respiratory acidemia occurs coincident with tachypnea, anxiety, dyspnea, labored ventilation, or increased sympathetic nervous system activity;

(2) hypercarbia reduces the arterial pH below 7.30; or (3) $PaCO_2$ progressively increases with a progressive decrease in arterial pH.

Inadequate Respiratory Drive

8 During early recovery from anesthesia, residual effects of intravenous and inhalation anesthetics blunt the ventilatory responses to both hypercarbia and hypoxemia. Sedatives augment depression from opioids or anesthetics.

Hypoventilation and hypercarbia can evolve insidiously during transfer and admission to the PACU. Although effects of intraoperative medications are usually waning, the peak depressant effect of an intravenous opioid given just before transfer occurs in the PACU. Coincident depression of medullary centers that regulate the sympathetic nervous system can blunt signs of acidemia or hypoxemia such as hypertension, tachycardia, and agitation, concealing hypoventilation. Patients might communicate lucidly and even complain of pain while experiencing significant opioid-induced hypoventilation. One must decide between an acceptable level of postoperative ventilatory depression and a tolerable level of pain or agitation. Patients with abnormal CO_2/pH responses from morbid obesity, chronic airway obstruction, or sleep apnea are more sensitive to respiratory depressants.[41] Children with active or recent upper respiratory infection are more prone to breath-holding, severe cough, and arterial desaturations below 90% during recovery, especially if they have a history of reactive airway disease, secondhand smoke exposure, or have undergone intubation and/or airway surgery.[42] If hypoventilation from opioids is excessive, forced arousal and careful titration (20 to 40 μg at a time) of intravenous naloxone reverses respiratory depression without affecting analgesia. Flumazenil (0.1 mg titrated to effect up to 1.5 mg) directly reverses depressant effects of benzodiazepines on ventilatory drive but is usually not needed.

The abrupt diminution of a noxious stimulus (e.g., tracheal extubation, placement of a postoperative block) may promote hypoventilation or airway obstruction by altering the balance between arousal from discomfort and depression from medication. Intracranial hemorrhage or edema sometimes presents with hypoventilation, especially after posterior fossa craniotomy. Bilateral carotid body injury after endarterectomy can ablate peripheral hypoxic drive. Chronic respiratory acidemia from COPD alters CNS sensitivity to pH and makes hypoxic drive dominant, but hypoventilation from supplemental oxygen rarely occurs.

Increased Airway Resistance

High resistance to gas flow through airways increases work of breathing and CO_2 production. If inspiratory muscles cannot generate sufficient pressure gradients to overcome resistance, alveolar ventilation fails to match CO_2 production and progressive respiratory acidemia occurs.

In postoperative patients, increased upper airway resistance is caused by obstruction in the pharynx (posterior tongue displacement, change in anteroposterior and lateral dimensions from soft tissue collapse), in the larynx (laryngospasm, laryngeal edema), or in the large airways (extrinsic compression from hematoma, tumor, or tracheal stenosis). Weakness from residual neuromuscular relaxation,[43] myasthenia gravis or myasthenic syndromes can contribute, but it is seldom the primary cause of airway compromise. If the airway is clear of vomitus or foreign bodies, simple maneuvers such as improving the level of consciousness, lateral positioning, chin lift, mandible elevation, or placement of an oropharyngeal or nasopharyngeal airway usually relieve obstruction. A nasopharyngeal airway may be better tolerated when the patient

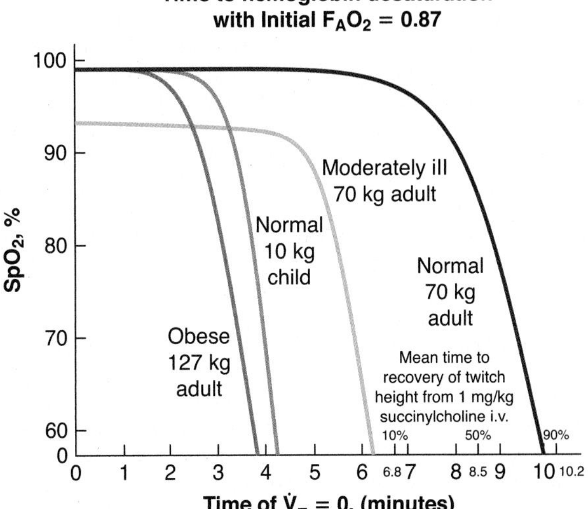

Figure 54-2 Rate of SpO_2 decline after onset of apnea. (Reprinted with permission from Benumof JL, Dagg R, Benumof R. Critical hemoglobin desaturation will occur before return to an unparalyzed state following 1 mg/kg intravenous succinylcholine. *Anesthesiology*. 1997; 87:979.)

has functional gag reflexes. Acute extrinsic upper airway compression (e.g., an expanding neck hematoma) must be relieved.

During emergence, stimulation of the pharynx or vocal cords by secretions, blood, foreign matter, or extubation can generate laryngospasm.[44] Laryngeal constrictor muscles occlude the tracheal inlet and reduce gas flow. Patients who smoke or are chronically exposed to smoke have irritable airway conditions, have copious secretions, or have undergone upper airway surgery are at higher risk.[37,42] Laryngospasm can usually be overcome by providing gentle positive pressure (10 to 20 mmHg continuous) in the oropharynx by mask with 100% O_2. Prolonged laryngospasm is relieved with a small dose of succinylcholine (e.g., 0.1 mg/kg) or deepening sedation with propofol. In most situations, an intubating dosage of succinylcholine should not be used to break postoperative laryngospasm. As little as 5 to 10 mg of succinylcholine can break the laryngospasm. Unless assisted ventilation is provided, declining PAO_2 causes serious hypoxemia before spontaneous ventilation resumes (Fig. 54-2).[45] If the functional residual capacity (FRC) is abnormally reduced, the decreased volume of O_2 available in the lungs accelerates the development of hypoxemia. Severe laryngeal obstruction can occur secondarily because of acute hypocalcemia after parathyroid excision.

Soft-tissue edema worsens airway obstruction, especially in children and adults recovering from procedures on the neck. Nebulized vasoconstrictors like epinephrine help somewhat, but steroids have little effect acutely. Patients with C1 esterase inhibitor deficiency can develop severe angioneurotic edema after even slight trauma to the airway. Pathologic airway obstruction (e.g., severe edema, epiglottitis, retropharyngeal abscess, encroaching tumors) might require emergency tracheal intubation, but airway manipulation is dangerous because minor trauma from intubation attempts can convert a marginal airway into a total obstruction. Judgment by the individual anesthesiologist regarding timing, patient status, available equipment along with airway management skills all play a part of the decision as to where when and how to intubate. Sedatives or muscle relaxants used to facilitate intubation can worsen obstruction by compromising the patient's volitional efforts to maintain the airway and by eliminating spontaneous ventilation (1 Video 54-1). Equipment and personnel necessary for emergency cricothyroidotomy or tracheostomy should be available. Needle cricothyroidotomy using a 14-gauge intravenous catheter or a commercially available kit permits oxygenation and marginal ventilation until the airway is secured, especially if jet ventilation with 100% oxygen is used.

Reduction of cross-sectional area in small airways increases overall airway resistance because resistance varies inversely with the fourth power of radius during turbulent flow. Pharyngeal or tracheal stimulation from secretions, suctioning, aspiration, or a tracheal tube can trigger a reflex constriction of bronchial smooth muscle in emerging patients with reactive airways. Histamine release precipitated by medication or allergic reactions also increases airway smooth muscle tone. Decreased radial traction on small airways reduces cross-sectional area in patients with COPD or with decreased lung volume secondary to obesity, surgical manipulation, excessive lung water, or splinting. Preoperative spirometric evidence of increased airway resistance predicts an increased risk of postoperative bronchospasm.[40] Smokers and patients with bronchospastic conditions are at highest risk.[46] If ventilatory requirements are increased by warming, hyperthermia, or work of breathing, high flow rates convert laminar flow to higher-resistance turbulent flow. Prolonged expiratory time or audible turbulent air flow (wheezing) during forced vital capacity expiration often unmasks subclinical airway resistance. Resistance is higher during expiration because intermediate-diameter airways are compressed by positive intrathoracic pressure. High airway resistance does not always cause wheezing because flow might be so impeded that no sound is produced. Signs of increased resistance mimic those of decreased pulmonary compliance. Spontaneously breathing patients exhibit accessory muscle recruitment, labored ventilation, and increased work of breathing with either condition, except that patients with decreased lung compliance tend to be tachypneic whereas those with increased airway resistance tend to have more normal respiratory rates.

The treatment of small airway resistance is directed at an underlying etiology. One must eliminate laryngeal or airway stimulation. Patients often respond to their pre-existing regimen of their inhalers. Levalbuterol or metaproterenol nebulized in oxygen resolves postoperative bronchospasm with minimal tachycardia. Nebulized racemic epinephrine effectively relaxes smooth muscle, but side effects of tachycardia and flushing can be seen. Isoproterenol has also been nebulized with good results. Intramuscular or sublingual terbutaline can be added. Administration of steroid therapy offers little acute improvement, but may prevent later recurrence. Bronchospasm that is resistant to β_2-sympathomimetic medication may improve with an anticholinergic medication such as atropine or ipratropium. If bronchospasm is life-threatening, an intravenous epinephrine infusion yields profound bronchodilation. Increased small airway resistance caused by mechanical factors (e.g., loss of lung volume, retained secretions, pulmonary edema) usually does not resolve with bronchodilators. Restoration of lung volume with incentive spirometry or deep tidal ventilation increases radial traction on small airways. Reducing left ventricular filling pressures might relieve airway resistance caused by increased lung water, although interstitial fluid accumulation can persist. Also, extended contraction of airway smooth muscle obstructs venous and lymphatic flow, leading to airway wall edema that resolves slowly.

Decreased Compliance

Reduced pulmonary compliance increases the elastic work of breathing. In the extreme, low compliance causes progressive respiratory muscle fatigue, hypoventilation, and respiratory acidemia. Parenchymal changes also affect compliance. Reduction of FRC leads to small airway closure and distal lung collapse, requiring greater energy expenditure to re-expand the lung. Pulmonary edema increases the lung's weight and inertia and elevates surface tension by interfering with surfactant activity, making expansion more difficult. Pulmonary contusion or hemorrhage interferes with lung expansion, as do restrictive lung diseases, skeletal abnormalities, intrathoracic lesions, hemothorax, pneumothorax, or cardiomegaly. Obesity affects pulmonary compliance, especially when adipose tissue compresses the thoracic cage or increases intra-abdominal pressure in supine or lateral positions. Extrathoracic factors such as tight muscles of the chest or abdominal dressings and gas in the stomach or bowel reduce chest wall compliance. Most notably after intra-abdominal laparoscopic procedures, retained CO_2 may impair diaphragm movement. The CO_2 has the capability to dissecting into the thorax creating either a pneumothorax or pneumomediastinum, which is usually a self-limited event as the CO_2 is relatively rapidly absorbed. There is usually no need for chest tube intervention. An intra-abdominal tumor, hemorrhage, ascites, bowel obstruction, or pregnancy impairs diaphragmatic excursion and reduces compliance.

Work of breathing is improved by resolving problems that reduce compliance. Allowing patients to recover in a semi-sitting (semi-Fowler) position reduces work of breathing. Incentive spirometry and chest physiotherapy help restore lung volume, as does positive end-expiratory pressure (PEEP) or continuous positive airway pressure (CPAP). In patients with COPD and highly compliant lungs, positive airway pressure might force the rib cage and diaphragms toward their excursion limits, accentuating inspiratory muscular effort.

Neuromuscular and Skeletal Problems

Postoperative airway obstruction and hypoventilation are accentuated by incomplete reversal of neuromuscular relaxation. Residual paralysis compromises airway patency, ability to overcome airway resistance, airway protection, and ability to clear secretions.[47] Intraoperative use of shorter-acting relaxants might decrease the incidence of residual paralysis but does not eliminate the problem. Marginal reversal can be more dangerous than near-total paralysis because a weak, agitated patient exhibiting uncoordinated movements and airway obstruction is more easily identified. A somnolent patient exhibiting mild stridor and shallow ventilation from marginal neuromuscular function might be overlooked, allowing insidious hypoventilation and respiratory acidemia or regurgitation with aspiration to occur. PACU staff should be aware of patients who have received nondepolarizing muscle relaxants but no reversal agents because they often exhibit low levels of residual paralysis.[48] Safety of techniques designed to avoid reversal of short- and intermediate-duration relaxants has not been substantiated, and reversal of nondepolarizing relaxants is recommended.[7] The selective relaxant binding agent, γ-cyclodextrins (i.e., sugammadex), is a reversal drug that can avoid the side effects of other anticholinesterases and anticholinergics.[49] Patients with neuromuscular abnormalities such as myasthenia gravis, Eaton–Lambert syndrome, periodic paralysis, or muscular dystrophies exhibit exaggerated or prolonged responses to muscle relaxants. Even without relaxant administration, these patients can exhibit postoperative ventilatory insufficiency. Medications potentiate neuromuscular relaxation (e.g., antibiotics, furosemide, propranolol, phenytoin), as does hypocalcemia or hypermagnesemia.

Diaphragmatic contraction is compromised in some postoperative patients, forcing more reliance on intercostal muscles, and reducing the ability to overcome decreased compliance or increased ventilatory demands. Impairment of phrenic nerve function from interscalene block, trauma, or thoracic and neck operations can "paralyze" one or rarely both diaphragms.[28] Adequate ventilation will normally be maintained with only one diaphragm, and marginal ventilation by external intercostal muscles alone. However, with high work of breathing, muscle weakness, or increased ventilatory demands, a nonfunctional diaphragm impairs minute ventilation. Thoracic spinal or epidural blockade interferes with intercostal muscle function and reduces ventilatory reserve, especially in patients with COPD. Abnormal motor neuron function (e.g., Guillain–Barré syndrome, cervical spinal cord trauma), flail chest, or severe kyphosis or scoliosis can cause postoperative ventilatory insufficiency.

Simple tests help assess mechanical ability to ventilate. The ability to sustain head elevation in a supine position, a forced vital capacity of 10 to 12 mL/kg, an inspiratory pressure more negative than –25 cm H_2O, and train-of-four assessment imply that strength of ventilatory muscles is adequate to sustain ventilation and to take a large enough breath to cough. However, none of these clinical end points reliably predicts recovery of airway protective reflexes,[48] and failure on these tests does not necessarily indicate the need for assisted ventilation.

The use of noninvasive mechanical ventilation techniques such as CPAP or bilevel positive airway pressure (BiPAP) may help prevent intubation or reintubation. By using these noninvasive airway techniques, patients can often overcome some of the above discussed issues interfering with normal respiration. Units other than ICUs are able to manage these patients therefore offloading the burden of the ICU.

Occasionally, a clinical picture suggests ventilatory insufficiency when ventilation is adequate. Voluntary limitation of chest expansion to avoid pain (splinting) causes labored, rapid, shallow breathing characteristic of inadequate ventilation. Splinting seldom causes actual hypoventilation and usually improves with analgesia and repositioning. Ventilation with small tidal volumes due to thoracic restriction or reduced compliance seems to generate afferent input from pulmonary stretch receptors, leading to dyspnea, labored breathing, and accessory muscle recruitment despite appropriate minute ventilation. Occasional large, "satisfying" lung expansions often relieve these symptoms. Finally, spontaneous hyperventilation to compensate for a metabolic acidemia might generate tachypnea or labored breathing, which can be mistaken for ventilatory insufficiency.

Increased Dead Space

Ventilation of unperfused dead space or of poorly perfused alveoli with high ventilation/perfusion $\dot{V}/\dot{Q}$ ratios is less effective in removing CO_2. Expansion of dead space volume or reduction of tidal volume increases the fraction of each breath wasted in dead space ($\dot{V}_D/\dot{V}_T$) and the amount of CO_2 from the previous exhalation that is rebreathed. A proportionally larger increase in total minute ventilation is required to meet any increase in CO_2 production. Patients with high $\dot{V}_D/\dot{V}_T$ are at greater risk for postoperative ventilatory failure.

Occasionally, an acute increase in dead space contributes to respiratory acidemia in postoperative patients. Although upper airway dead space is reduced after tracheal intubation and tracheostomy, excessive tubing volume or valve reversal in breathing circuits promotes rebreathing of CO_2. PEEP or CPAP elevates physiologic dead space, especially in patients with high pulmonary compliance. Pulmonary embolization of air, thrombus, or cellular debris increases physiologic dead space, although impact on CO_2 excretion is often compensated by accelerated minute ventilation from hypercarbic and hypoxic drives or reflex responses. Decreased cardiac output can increase $\dot{V}_D/\dot{V}_T$ by decreasing perfusion to well-ventilated, nondependent lung. Irreversible increases in dead space occur if adult respiratory distress syndrome (ARDS) destroys pulmonary microvasculature.

Increased Carbon Dioxide Production

Carbon dioxide production varies directly with metabolic rate, body temperature, and substrate availability. During anesthesia, CO_2 production falls to approximately 60% of the normal 2 to 3 mL/kg/min as hypothermia lowers metabolic activity and neuromuscular relaxation reduces tonic muscle contraction. Therefore, during recovery, metabolic rate and CO_2 production can increase by 40%. Shivering, high work of breathing, infection, sympathetic nervous system activity, or rapid carbohydrate metabolism during intravenous hyperalimentation accelerates CO_2 production. Malignant hyperthermia generates CO_2 production many times greater than normal, which rapidly exceeds ventilatory reserve and causes severe respiratory and metabolic acidemia. Even mild increases of CO_2 production can precipitate respiratory acidemia if low compliance, airway resistance, or neuromuscular paralysis interfere with ventilation. With the exception of adjusting hyperalimentation, improving work of breathing, reducing shivering, or treating hyperthermia, there is little yield from addressing CO_2 production in PACU patients.

Inadequate Postoperative Oxygenation

Systemic arterial partial pressure of oxygen (PaO_2) is the best indicator of pulmonary oxygen transfer from alveolar gas to pulmonary capillary blood. Arterial hemoglobin saturation monitored by pulse oximetry yields less information on alveolar-arterial gradients and is not helpful in assessing impact of hemoglobin dissociation curve shifts or carboxyhemoglobin.[50] Evaluation of metabolic acidemia or mixed-venous oxygen content yields insight into peripheral oxygen delivery and utilization. Adequate arterial oxygenation does not mean that cardiac output, arterial perfusion pressure, or distribution of blood flow will maintain tissue oxygenation. Sepsis, hypotension, anemia, or hemoglobin dissociation abnormalities can generate tissue ischemia despite adequate oxygenation.

In postoperative patients, the acceptable lower limit for PaO_2 varies with individual patient characteristics. A PaO_2 below 65 to 70 mmHg causes significant hemoglobin desaturation, although tissue oxygen delivery might be maintained at lower levels. Maintaining PaO_2 between 80 and 100 mmHg (saturation 93% to 97%) ensures adequate oxygen availability. Little benefit is derived from elevating PaO_2 above 110 mmHg because hemoglobin is fully saturated, and the amount of additional oxygen dissolved in plasma is negligible. During mechanical ventilation, a spontaneous breathing trial or PaO_2 above 80 mmHg with 0.4 FIO_2 and 5 cm H_2O CPAP[50] usually predicts sustained adequate oxygenation after tracheal extubation.

Distribution of Ventilation

Loss of dependent lung volume commonly causes $\dot{V}/\dot{Q}$ mismatching (shunt effect) and hypoxemia. A reduction in FRC decreases radial traction on small airways, leading to collapse and distal atelectasis that can worsen for 36 hours after surgery.[51] Reduced ventilation in dependent lung is particularly damaging because gravity directs pulmonary blood flow to dependent areas. Obese patients sustain large decreases in FRC during surgery. Older patients normally exhibit some airway closure at end expiration, and those with COPD have more severe closure that is exacerbated by small reductions in FRC. Retraction, packing, manipulation, or peritoneal insufflation during upper abdominal surgery reduces FRC, as does compression from leaning surgical assistants.[52] Prone, lithotomy, or Trendelenburg positions are also create atelectasis, especially in obese patients. Right upper lobe collapse secondary to partial right main stem intubation is a frequently overlooked cause of hypoxemia. During one-lung anesthesia, the weight of unsupported mediastinal contents, pressure from abdominal contents on the dependent diaphragm, and lung compression all reduce dependent lung volume. Gravity and lymphatic obstruction promote interstitial fluid accumulation and further $\dot{V}/\dot{Q}$ mismatching. This "down lung syndrome" may appear as unilateral pulmonary edema on the chest film.

Postoperatively, acute pulmonary edema from hydrodynamic forces (overhydration, ventricular dysfunction, airway obstruction), or increased capillary permeability (ARDS, transfusion-related acute lung injury, drug reactions) leads to hypoxemia by interfering with both $\dot{V}/\dot{Q}$ matching and diffusion of oxygen. Strong inspiratory efforts against an obstructed airway decrease FRC and promote negative pressure pulmonary edema. Small airway occlusion from compression, retained secretions, or aspiration leads to distal hypoventilation and hypoxemia, as does main stem intubation. Pneumothorax or hemothorax also reduce lung volume.

Conservative measures that restore lung volume often improve oxygenation. If possible, patients should recover in a semi-sitting or reverse Trendelenburg position to reduce abdominal pressure on the diaphragms. Pain with ventilation encourages shallow breathing, so analgesia helps maintain FRC, especially with upper abdominal or chest wall incisions. Deep ventilation, cough, chest physiotherapy, and incentive spirometry may help expand FRC, mobilize secretions, and accustom a patient to incisional discomfort, but actual efficacy is debated.[53,54] For serious postoperative reduction of FRC, positive pressure is effective. CPAP (5 to 7 cm H_2O) or bilevel CPAP can be delivered by face mask for several hours until factors promoting loss of lung volume resolve. If hypoxemia is severe or patient finds the CPAP or bilevel mask intolerable, tracheal intubation is usually required. Intubation for delivery of CPAP or bilevel ventilation does not mandate positive pressure ventilation. Ventilatory requirements should be assessed independently, considering $PaCO_2$, arterial pH, and work of breathing. Usually, 5 to 10 cm H_2O of CPAP or PEEP improves PaO_2 without risking hypotension, increased intracranial pressure, or barotrauma. If PaO_2 does not improve, one must re-evaluate the etiology. An occasional patient with ARDS or pulmonary contusion might require expiratory pressures in excess of 10 cm H_2O for improved oxygenation.

Tracheal intubation eliminates normal expiratory resistance and the "physiologic PEEP" (2 to 5 cm H_2O) that helps maintain lung volume during spontaneous ventilation. Exposing an intubated trachea to ambient pressure may cause a gradual reduction in FRC. Healthy, slender patients will often tolerate short periods of intubation without positive pressure, but generally it is prudent to use 5 cm H_2O CPAP for intubated postoperative patients.

Distribution of Perfusion

Poor distribution of pulmonary blood flow also interferes with $\dot{V}/\dot{Q}$ matching and oxygenation. Flow distribution is primarily determined by hydrodynamic factors (PA and venous pressures, vascular resistance), which are affected by gravity, airway pressure, lung volume, and cardiac dynamics. Flow distribution is modulated by hypoxic pulmonary vasoconstriction (HPV), which diverts flow from air spaces that exhibit low PaO_2. In postoperative patients, position affects oxygenation if gravity forces blood flow to areas with reduced ventilation. For example, placing a poorly ventilated lung in a dependent position can reduce PaO_2. Postoperative changes in PA pressure, airway pressure, and lung volume also have complex effects on blood flow distribution that can adversely affect $\dot{V}/\dot{Q}$ matching. Residual inhalation anesthetics, vasodilators, and sympathomimetics directly affect vascular tone and HPV, partially explaining larger alveolar–arterial oxygen gradients after general anesthesia. Patients with liver cirrhosis exhibit poor $\dot{V}/\dot{Q}$ matching caused by small arteriovenous shunts that form throughout their lungs. Circulating endotoxin impairs HPV, contributing to hypoxemia in septic patients.

In the PACU, few interventions are useful to improve $\dot{V}/\dot{Q}$ matching by changing the distributions pulmonary blood flow. However, avoiding placing an atelectatic or diseased lung in a dependent position can be helpful. Placing poorly ventilated parenchyma in a nondependent position could improve $\dot{V}/\dot{Q}$ matching, but positioning a diseased lung in an "up" position may promote drainage of purulent material into the unaffected lung. Avoiding vasodilatory medications may improve PaO_2 but benefits from these medications usually outweigh drawbacks from impaired HPV.

Inadequate Alveolar P_AO_2

Postoperative hypoxemia is occasionally caused by a global reduction of P_AO_2, usually from inadequate ventilation, and marked increase in P_ACO_2 (see the alveolar gas equation in Chapter 15 Respiratory Function in Anesthesia). Hypoventilation must be severe to cause hypoxemia based on the alveolar gas equation. Apnea, airway obstruction, soft-tissue edema, or laryngospasm as well as very high small airway resistance all lead to rapid depletion of alveolar oxygen, and preclude effective ventilation. If cessation of ventilation does occur, the rate of P_AO_2 decline varies with age, body habitus, degree of underlying illness, and initial P_AO_2[45] (Fig. 54-3). Hypoxemia might also occur if opioids or residual anesthetic levels severely depress ventilatory drive. Partial airway obstruction does not usually reduce P_AO_2, especially when patients are receiving supplemental oxygen. Increasing the oxygen content of the FRC with supplemental oxygen safeguards against hypoxemia from hypoventilation or airway obstruction, and eliminates the use of the pulse oximeter as a monitor of hypoventilation. Rarely, excessive concentrations of eliminated gases reduce P_AO_2. After general anesthesia, rapid outpouring of nitrous oxide displaces alveolar gas and can lower P_AO_2 if a patient is hypoventilating or breathing ambient air, but this "diffusion hypoxia" usually occurs before PACU admission. Volume displacement of oxygen could also occur during severe hypercarbia in a patient breathing ambient air, although acidemia is often a greater problem.

Reduced Mixed Venous PO_2

Mixed-venous partial pressure of oxygen ($P\bar{v}O_2$) is affected by arterial oxygen content, cardiac output, distribution of peripheral blood flow, and tissue oxygen extraction. If arterial oxygen content decreases or tissue extraction increases, $P\bar{v}O_2$ falls. The lower the $P\bar{v}O_2$ in blood that is shunted or flows through low $\dot{V}/\dot{Q}$ units, the greater the reduction of PaO_2. Blood with a low $P\bar{v}O_2$ also extracts larger volumes of oxygen from alveolar gas, amplifying the effect of hypoventilation or airway obstruction on P_AO_2. Very low $P\bar{v}O_2$ increases the risk of resorption atelectasis in poorly ventilated alveoli. In postoperative patients, shivering, infection, and hypermetabolism lower $P\bar{v}O_2$ by increasing peripheral oxygen extraction. Low cardiac output and hypotension also lower $P\bar{v}O_2$ by decreasing tissue oxygen delivery. Supplemental oxygen reduces the impact of low $P\bar{v}O_2$ on alveolar oxygen extraction and on arterial oxygenation.

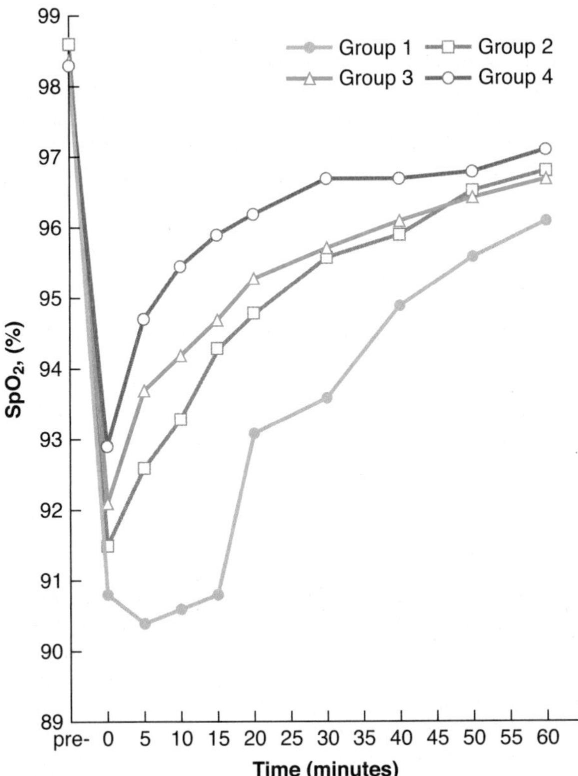

Figure 54-3 SpO_2 versus postanesthesia care unit time in patients spontaneously ventilating in room air after general anesthesia (Group 1, 0 to 1 year of age; group 2, 1 to 3 years; group 3, 3 to 14 years; group 4, 14 to 58 years). (Reprinted with permission from Xue FS, Huang YG, Tong SY, et al. A comparative study of early postoperative hypoxemia in infants, children, and adults undergoing elective plastic surgery. *Anesth Analg* 1996;83:709.)

Obstructive Sleep Apnea

Obstructive sleep apnea (OSA) is a syndrome in which patients exhibit a period of partial or complete obstruction of the upper airway (see Chapter 23, NICV 23-7). This obstruction in turn interrupts sleep patterns, resulting in daytime hypersomnolence, decreased ability to concentrate, increased irritability, as well as aggressive and distractible behavior in children. The airway obstruction may cause episodic oxygen desaturation, hypercarbia, and possibly lead to cardiac dysfunction. It is estimated that 9% of women and 24% of men in the United States show disordered breathing while asleep, and 2% of women and 4% of men show overt symptoms of OSA.[55] A more recent study of urban patients showed a 5-year incidence of about 7.5% of moderate-to-severe sleep disordered breathing (SDB) and approximately 16% for mild-to-moderate SDB. Incidence was influenced by age, sex, BMI, waist hip ratio, and serum cholesterol concentration. Predominance in men diminishes with increased age and by 50 years of age, incidence between men and women are similar.[56] In February 2014, the ASA Task Force on Perioperative Management of Patients with Obstructive Sleep Apnea issued guidelines based on the ASA scoring system for OSA and classifying patients as having mild, moderate, or severe OSA based on the apnea-hypopnea index (AHI) the number of apnea and hypopnea events per hour of sleep.[57]

Mild OSA	AHI	5–14 events/hr
Moderate OSA	AHI	15–29 events/hr
Severe OSA	AHI	>30 events/hr

The perioperative management of the OSA patient must start preoperatively with a well-planned anesthetic taking into account the type, location, and recovery of surgery. Postoperative management concerns include analgesia, oxygenation, patient positioning, and monitoring. Regional anesthesia with minimal sedation is best for recovery versus increased use of opioids. Supplemental oxygen should be used immediately postoperatively. Patients who use CPAP or noninvasive positive pressure ventilation should use these therapies in the PACU. The use of high-flow nasal cannula oxygenation (HFNCO) is widely used in the ICU setting and may be beneficial to the OSA patient when other modalities are not readily available. HFNCO delivers flows of up to 60 L/min to improve respiratory distress and reduce the need for intubation by more comfortably providing a higher FIO_2, adjusting FIO_2, and heated/humidified air.[58] Positioning should be used to minimize the patients' ability to obstruct the airway, which can be limited based on the type of surgery. Adult OSA patients show improvement in AHI scores while in lateral, prone, and sitting positions compared with supine. With regard to monitoring, there is agreement among the consultants on the ASA Task Force that pulse oximetry should be used until the patients' oxygen saturation remains above 90% on room air while sleeping. The use of telemetry for monitoring pulse oximetry, ECG, or ventilation can be beneficial in reducing adverse postoperative events and should be used on a patient need basis. With increasing studies of OSA, the increased standardization of information regarding this patient population will lead to greater evidence-based treatment and supported clinical care.

Anemia

Preoperative hematocrit and intraoperative hemorrhage determine a patient's red cell mass and oxygen-carrying capacity after surgery. Reduction of hematocrit caused by dilution has less impact. The hematocrit at which oxygen delivery becomes insufficient to match tissue needs varies with cardiac reserve, oxygen consumption, hemoglobin dissociation, PaO_2, and blood flow distribution. The actual level at which shock, lack of tissue oxygen delivery, occurs is known as the *critical* DO_2 level. For animals and humans who have normal myocardial function and are euvolemic, critical DO_2 requires at least 3 to 3.5 g/dL hemoglobin concentration. Of course, hemoglobin this low is not an appropriate transfusion trigger. However, it does illustrate the large excess of hemoglobin available to meet metabolic O_2 demands. Each patient has a minimum hematocrit below which tissues use inefficient anaerobic metabolism, generating a lactic acidemia. Patients with vascular disease are at increased risk of vital organ ischemia as hematocrit falls. Work from the ASA and the cardiac anesthesia/surgery societies (Society of Thoracic surgeons and Society of Cardiovascular Anesthesiologists) have published guidelines for transfusion and blood product management. It is well accepted now that patients who are stable, not bleeding, and euvolemic may tolerate a hemoglobin of 6.0 g/dL. Transfusion may be of some benefit between 6 and 8 g/dL and it is rarely of use above 10 g/dL.

Supplemental Oxygen

The incidence of hypoxemia in postoperative patients is high. In PACU patients placed on room air, 30% of patients younger than 1 year of age, 20% aged 1 to 3 years, 14% aged 3 to 14 years, and 7.8% of adults had hemoglobin saturations fall below 90%, with many falling below 85%[59] (Fig. 54-3). Clinical observation and assessment of cognitive function do not accurately screen for hypoxemia, so monitoring with pulse oximetry is essential throughout PACU admission.[60] One cannot predict which patients

Table 54-3 Common Oxygen Delivery Systems with Correlating O_2 Flow Rates to Delivered FiO_2 Ranges

System	O_2 Flow Rate (L/min)	FiO_2
Nasal cannula	1	0.21–0.24
	2	0.23–0.28
	3	0.27–0.32
	4	0.31–0.36
	5	0.35–0.40
	6	0.39–0.44
Simple mask	5	0.30–0.40
	8	0.40–0.60
Partial rebreathing mask	10	0.50–0.65
Nonrebreathing mask	10–15	0.60–near 1.00

will become hypoxemic or when hypoxemia will occur. Patients with lung disease or obesity, those recovering from thoracic or upper abdominal procedures, and those with preoperative hypoxemia are at increased risk.[61] Postoperative hypoxemia occurs in children, especially those with respiratory infections or chronic adenotonsillar hypertrophy. Hypoxemia occurs frequently after regional anesthesia.[24]

Supplemental oxygen should be administered only to patients at high risk of hypoxemia or with low SpO_2 readings (Table 54-3). However, some recommend supplemental oxygen be administered in the PACU during initial recovery and perhaps during transport to the PACU.[7] Supplemental oxygen does not address underlying causes of hypoxemia in postoperative patients, its use does not guarantee that hypoxemia will not occur, and it is likely to mask hypoventilation.[62] Although oxygen might cause minor mucosal drying, routine humidification is of little benefit unless intubation bypasses natural humidification. Oxygen apparatus can increase the risk of corneal abrasion during emergence.

Perioperative Aspiration

During anesthesia, depression of airway reflexes places patients at risk for intraoperative or postoperative pulmonary aspiration that may manifest in the PACU. Pulmonary morbidity from perioperative aspiration varies with the type and volume of the aspirate. Although aspiration of gastric contents is most widely feared, surgical patients also experience other aspiration syndromes.

Aspiration of clear oral secretions during induction, face mask ventilation, or emergence is common and usually insignificant. Cough, mild tracheal irritation, or transient laryngospasm are immediate sequelae, although large-volume aspiration predisposes to infection, small airway obstruction, or pulmonary edema. Aspiration of blood secondary to trauma, epistaxis, or airway surgery generates marked changes on the chest radiograph that are out of proportion with clinical signs. Aspirated "sterile" blood causes minor airway obstruction but is rapidly cleared by mucociliary transport, resorption, and phagocytosis. Massive blood aspiration or aspiration of clots obstructs airways, interferes with oxygenation, and leads to fibrinous changes in air spaces and to pulmonary hemochromatosis from iron accumulation in phagocytic cells. Secondary infection is a threat, especially if tissue or purulent matter is also aspirated.

Aspiration of food, small objects, pieces of teeth, or dental appliances causes persistent cough, diffuse reflex bronchospasm, airway obstruction with distal atelectasis, or pneumonia. Complications are often localized and treated with antibiotics and supportive care once the foreign matter is expelled or removed. Secondary thermal, chemical, or traumatic airway injury from aspirated objects can occur. Of course, complete upper airway or tracheal obstruction by an aspirated object is a life-threatening emergency.

Aspiration of acidic gastric contents during vomiting or regurgitation causes chemical pneumonitis characterized initially by diffuse bronchospasm, hypoxemia, and atelectasis.[63] The morbidity increases directly with volume and inversely with the pH of the acidic aspirate. Aspiration of partially digested food worsens and prolongs pneumonitis, especially if vegetable matter is present. Food particles mechanically obstruct airways and are a nidus for secondary bacterial infection. In serious cases, epithelial degeneration, interstitial and alveolar edema, and hemorrhage into air spaces rapidly progresses to ARDS with high-permeability pulmonary edema. Destruction of pneumocytes, decreased surfactant activity, hyaline membrane formation, and emphysematous changes can follow, leading to $\dot{V}/\dot{Q}$ mismatching and reduced compliance. Destruction of microvasculature increases pulmonary vascular resistance and dead space ventilation.

The incidence of serious aspiration is relatively low in PACU patients, but the risk is still significant. Frequency of postoperative vomiting remains high, especially if gas has accumulated in the stomach. Protective airway reflexes such as cough, swallowing, and laryngospasm are suppressed by depressant medications such as inhalation anesthetics, sedatives, and opiates, so observe carefully patients with decreased levels of consciousness. Persisting effects of laryngeal nerve blocks or topical local anesthetics used to reduce airway irritability decrease postoperative airway protection, as does residual sedation. Reflexes are also impaired by residual neuromuscular paralysis.[48,64] Patients can sustain airway patency and spontaneous ventilation, pass a head lift test, have a tactile train-of-four T4/T1 ratio >0.7, and still have impaired airway reflexes from residual paralysis. The T4/T1 ratio should exceed 0.9 before reflexes are completely competent.[64] Risk of aspiration also increases if reversal is omitted. Hypotension, hypoxemia, or acidemia cause both emesis and obtundation, increasing aspiration risk.

In the PACU, vigilance against aspiration is important. Trendelenburg position might promote regurgitation but aids in airway clearance if regurgitation or vomiting occurs. Head elevation in unconscious patients should be avoided because it creates a gravitational gradient from pharynx to lung. High-risk patients should not have the trachea extubated until airway reflexes are restored. Even though a patient is awake and able to follow commands they may well still have depressed gag reflex for some considerable number of hours after surgery/anesthesia. The introduction of opioids and other sedatives may turn a situation of relatively good airway protection into one of potential aspiration. Aspiration of acidic fluid can still occur around an inflated tracheal tube cuff, so one should frequently monitor the upper airway for secretions or vomitus. One should avoid cuff deflation until extubation because the rigid tube impairs laryngospasm, swallowing, and other protective reflexes. The pharynx should be suctioned and the trachea extubated at end inspiration with positive airway pressure to promote expulsion of material trapped below the cords but above the inflated cuff. Observation is essential after extubation because airway reflexes might be temporarily impaired. Anatomic distortion in the airway from soft-tissue trauma or surgical intervention interferes with airway protection. Mandibular fixation makes expulsion of vomitus, blood, or secretions difficult, so equipment for release of mandibular fixation available should be available.

Discovery of gastric secretions in the pharynx mandates immediate lateral head positioning (assuming cervical spine integrity) and suction of the airway. If airway reflexes are compromised, tracheal intubation is often appropriate. After intubation, the trachea is suctioned through the tracheal tube before positive pressure ventilation; this avoids widely disseminating aspirated material into distal airways. Instillation of saline or alkalotic solutions is not recommended. Assessing the pH of tracheal aspirate is useless because buffering is immediate. Checking pharyngeal aspirate pH is more accurate but of little practical value. Suspicion that aspiration has occurred mandates 24 to 48 hours of monitoring for development of aspiration pneumonitis. If the likelihood of aspiration is small in an ambulatory patient, outpatient follow-up can be done, assuming hypoxemia, cough, wheezing, or radiographic abnormalities do not appear within 4 to 6 hours. The patient should receive explicit instructions to contact a medical facility at the first appearance of malaise, fever, cough, chest pain, or other symptoms of pneumonitis. If the likelihood of aspiration is high, the patient should be admitted to the hospital. Fluffy infiltrates may appear on the chest radiograph any time within 24 hours. Hypoxemia might develop quickly or evolve insidiously as injury progresses, so frequent pulse oximetry monitoring is important.

If hypoxemia, increased airway resistance, consolidation, or pulmonary edema evolves, the patient should be supported with supplemental oxygen and CPAP. Mechanical ventilation may be necessary. Steroids yield no improvement and may increase the risk of bacterial super infection. Bacterial infection does not always follow aspiration, so prophylactic antibiotics merely promote colonization by resistant organisms. If bacterial infection is apparent, antibiotic therapy should be instituted based on culture results. If cultures are equivocal, use of broad-spectrum antibiotics with coverage for gram-negative rods and anaerobes, including *Bacteroides fragilis,* is recommended. Overall therapy is similar to that for ARDS. Pulmonary edema from increased capillary permeability should not be treated with diuretics unless high filling pressures or hypervolemia exist.

Postoperative Renal Complications

9 Ability to Void

The ability to void should be assessed because opioids and autonomic side effects of regional anesthesia interfere with sphincter relaxation and promote urine retention. Urinary retention is common after urologic, inguinal, and genital surgery, and retention frequently delays discharge.[4] Observation after these surgeries is needed to determine if inability to urinate is a possible surgical complication. Neither the patient nor staff can accurately estimate bladder volume through sensation or palpation. An ultrasonic bladder scan helps assess bladder volume before discharge and avoid the archaic practice of routine "straight catheterization." It is reasonable to discharge select ambulatory patients from the facility and inpatients to a floor before they void.[7,65,66] When inpatients are transferred prior to voiding, urination should be monitored to avoid complications from urinary retention. If urinary retention persists beyond a prescribed interval (10 to 12 hours after discharge), the patient should be instructed to contact a health care facility. High return rates after urologic procedures are related to urinary retention.[67]

Renal Tubular Function

Analysis of urine yields information about postoperative renal tubular function. Urine color is not useful for assessing concentrating ability, but it does assist recognition of hematuria, hemoglobinuria, or pyuria. Urine osmolarity (reflecting the number of particles in solution) is a more reliable index of tubular function than specific gravity, which is affected by molecular weight of solutes. An osmolarity >450 mOsm/L indicates intact tubular concentrating ability. A urine sodium concentration far below or a potassium concentration above serum concentrations also indicates tubular viability, as does acidification or alkalinization of urine. Osmolarity, electrolyte, and pH values close to those in serum may indicate poor tubular function or acute tubular necrosis.

Inorganic fluoride released during metabolism of certain inhalation anesthetics can cause a transient reduction of tubular concentrating ability after long anesthetics. Higher fluoride levels cause renal tubular necrosis. Interaction of sevoflurane with dry carbon dioxide absorbents (often found in first cases or peripheral locations) generates compound A, a vinyl ether that degrades to release inorganic fluoride. Although transient impairment of protein retention and concentrating ability may occur, use of sevoflurane does not seriously affect renal function.

Oliguria

Oliguria (≤0.5 mL/kg/hr) occurs frequently during recovery and usually reflects an appropriate renal response to hypovolemia. The stress response of surgery also increases antidiuretic hormone (ADH), which can lead to decreased urine output. However, decreased urine output might indicate abnormal renal function. The acceptable degree and duration of oliguria vary with baseline renal status, the surgical procedure, and the anticipated postoperative course. In patients without catheters, one should assess interval since last voiding, and bladder volume to help differentiate oliguria from inability to void. One should check indwelling urinary catheters for kinking, for obstruction by blood clots or debris, and for the catheter tip being positioned above the urinary level in the bladder, and aggressively evaluate oliguria if intraoperative events could jeopardize renal function (e.g., aortic cross-clamping, severe hypotension, possible ureteral ligature, massive transfusion). Systemic blood pressure must be adequate for renal perfusion, based on preoperative pressures. Administration of desmopressin for hematologic purposes seldom affects postoperative urinary output. After urine is sent for electrolyte and osmolarity determinations, a 300 to 500 mL intravenous crystalloid bolus helps assess whether oliguria represents a renal response to hypovolemia, provided no diuretics were administered intraoperatively. If urine output does not improve, consider a larger bolus or a diagnostic trial of furosemide, 5 mg intravenously. Furosemide increases urine output if oliguria reflects tubular resorption of fluid. Patients receiving chronic diuretic therapy might require a diuretic to maintain postoperative urine output.

Persistence of oliguria despite hydration, adequate perfusion pressure, and a furosemide challenge increases the likelihood of acute tubular necrosis, ureteral obstruction, renal artery or vein occlusion, or inappropriate ADH secretion. Cystoscopy, intravenous pyelography, angiography, or radionuclide scanning may help clarify renal status. Osmotic or loop diuretics may be useful to attenuate renal damage. The use of low-dose dopamine or dobutamine has not proven to improve renal function. Fenoldopam used perioperatively has shown to reduce the risk of acute kidney injury for select high-risk cardiac surgical patients.[68] Consultation with a nephrologist is prudent.

Polyuria

Relying on high postoperative urinary output to gauge intravascular volume status or renal viability can be misleading. Profuse urine output often reflects generous intraoperative fluid administration, but osmotic diuresis caused by hyperglycemia and glycosuria is another common cause, particularly if glucose-containing crystalloid solutions are infusing. Polyuria might also reflect intraoperative diuretic administration. However, sustained polyuria (4 to 5 mL/kg/hr) can indicate abnormal regulation of water clearance or high-output renal failure, especially if urinary losses compromise intravascular volume and systemic blood pressure. Diabetes insipidus occurs secondary to intracranial surgery, pituitary ablation, head trauma, or increased intracranial pressure. A urine specific gravity of ≤1.005 and a urine osmolality <200 mOsm/kg are the hallmark of diabetes insipidus. See Chapter 37 Anesthesia for Neurosurgery for discussion of diabetes insipidus.

Metabolic Complications

Postoperative Acid–Base Disorders

Categorization of postoperative acid–base abnormalities into primary and compensatory disorders is difficult because rapidly changing pathophysiology can often generate multiple primary disorders.

Respiratory Acidemia

Respiratory acidemia is frequently encountered in PACU patients because anesthetics, opioids, and sedatives promote hypoventilation by depressing CNS sensitivity to pH and $PaCO_2$. In awake, spontaneously breathing patients with adequate analgesia, hypercarbia, and acidemia are usually mild ($PaCO_2$ 45 to 50 mmHg, pH 7.36 to 7.32). Deeply sedated patients exhibit more profound acidemia. Patients with residual neuromuscular paralysis, increased airway resistance, or decreased pulmonary compliance might not sustain adequate ventilation despite an intact CNS drive, especially if CO_2 production is elevated by fever, shivering, or hyperalimentation. The kidneys require hours to generate a compensatory metabolic alkalosis, so compensation for acute postoperative respiratory acidemia is limited.

Symptoms of respiratory acidemia include agitation, confusion, and tachypnea. Sympathetic nervous system response to low pH causes hypertension, tachycardia, and dysrhythmias. Respiratory acidemia caused by CNS depression often produces less intense signs of sympathetic nervous system activity. In patients with head injury, intracranial tumors, or cerebral edema, respiratory acidemia increases cerebral blood flow and intracranial pressure. At very low pH, catecholamines cannot interact with adrenergic receptors, so heart rate and blood pressure decrease precipitously. Treatment consists of correcting the imbalance between CO_2 production and alveolar ventilation. Raising the level of consciousness by the judicious reversal of opioids or benzodiazepines improves ventilatory drive. It is important to ensure that the patient does not have increased airway resistance or residual neuromuscular blockade. If spontaneous ventilation cannot maintain CO_2 excretion, tracheal intubation and mechanical ventilation are necessary. Reducing CO_2 production by controlling fever or shivering may be helpful.

Metabolic Acidemia

Evaluation of acute postoperative metabolic acidemia is relatively straightforward (Table 54-4). Occasionally, ketoacidosis occurs in diabetic patients. During ketoacidosis, serum glucose levels are elevated and ketones are detectable in blood or urine. Patients with renal failure or renal tubular acidosis usually exhibit a preoperative metabolic acidemia. Large volumes of saline infusions during surgery can generate a mild hyperchloremic, metabolic acidemia, but use of lactated Ringer solution avoids this problem.[69] Rarely, a patient manifests acidemia from toxic ingestion of aspirin or methanol. Once these unusual causes are excluded, postoperative metabolic acidemia almost always represents lactic acidemia secondary to insufficient delivery or utilization of oxygen in peripheral tissues. Peripheral hypoperfusion is often caused by low cardiac output (hypovolemia, cardiac failure, dysrhythmia) or peripheral vasodilation (sepsis, catecholamine depletion, sympathectomy). Arteriolar constriction from hypothermia or pressor administration reduces tissue perfusion and induces abnormal blood flow distribution. Hypoxemia, severe anemia, impaired hemoglobin dissociation, CO poisoning, and inability to use oxygen in the mitochondria (cyanide or arsenic poisoning) also generate lactic acidemia.

Table 54-4 Causes of Acidemia

Causes
Normal anion gap acidosis
GI loss of bicarbonate
Diarrhea
Urinary diversion
GI fistulas or drains
Renal loss of bicarbonate
Renal tubular acidosis
Renal insufficiency
Recovery phase of ketoacidosis
Increased anion gap acidosis
Ketoacidosis (diabetic, alcoholic, severe cachexia)
Lactic acidosis (seizures, neuroleptic malignant syndrome, MH, severe asthma, pheochromocytoma, cardiogenic shock, hypovolemia, severe anemia, regional ischemia, sepsis, hypoglycemia)
Respiratory acidosis

GI, gastrointestinal; MH, malignant hyperthermia.

A spontaneously breathing patient will increase minute ventilation in response to metabolic acidemia and quickly generate a respiratory alkalosis to compensate for metabolic acidemia. However, general anesthetics and analgesics suppress this ventilatory response. The sympathetic response to acute postoperative metabolic acidemia is often milder than the response to respiratory acidemia because hydrogen and bicarbonate ions cross the blood–brain barrier with more difficulty than CO_2. Treatment consists of resolving the condition causing accumulation of metabolic acid. For example, ketoacidosis is treated with intravenous potassium, insulin, and glucose. Improving cardiac output or systemic blood pressure will reduce lactic acid production, as will rewarming. If conditions causing lactate accumulation are improved and acidemia is mild, renal excretion of hydrogen ions will restore normal pH. For severe or progressive acidemia, intravenous bicarbonate or calcium gluconate helps restore pH.

Respiratory Alkalemia

Pain or anxiety during emergence causes hyperventilation and acute respiratory alkalemia. Excessive mechanical ventilation also generates respiratory alkalemia, especially if hypothermia or paralysis has decreased CO_2 production. Pathologic causes of "central" hyperventilation include sepsis, cerebrovascular accident, or paradoxic CNS acidosis (an imbalance of bicarbonate concentration across the blood–brain barrier caused by prolonged hyperventilation). Acute respiratory alkalemia can generate confusion, dizziness, atrial dysrhythmias, and abnormal cardiac conduction. Alkalemia decreases cerebral blood flow, causing hypoperfusion and even stroke in patients with cerebrovascular disease. If the alkalemia is severe, reduced serum ionized calcium concentration precipitates muscle fasciculation or hypocalcemic tetany. Very high pH depresses cardiovascular, CNS, and catecholamine receptor functions. Metabolic compensation for acute respiratory alkalemia is limited because time constants for bicarbonate excretion are large. Treatment necessitates reducing alveolar ventilation, usually by administering analgesics and sedatives for pain and anxiety. Rebreathing of CO_2 has little application in the PACU.

Metabolic Alkalemia

Metabolic alkalemia is rare in PACU patients unless vomiting, gastric suctioning, dehydration, alkaline ingestion, or potassium-wasting diuretics caused an alkalemia that existed before surgery. Excessive intraoperative bicarbonate administration causes postoperative metabolic alkalemia, but alkalemia from metabolism of lactate or citrate usually does not appear within the first 24 hours. Respiratory compensation through retention of CO_2 is rapid but limited because hypoventilation eventually causes hypoxemia. Hydration and correction of hypochloremia and hypokalemia allow the kidney to excrete excess bicarbonate.

Glucose Disorders and Control

10 Adequate glucose control has been recommended to reduce morbidity in a variety of postsurgical patients. The control of glucose in diabetic and nondiabetic patients has shown to reduce complications and hospital length of stay and improve patient outcomes. However, the potential for hypoglycemia and coma should not be discounted. Insulin therapy should be based on serum glucose levels and requires careful and timely monitoring of blood glucose levels to avoid hypoglycemia, including clear and concise hand off of information when patients care is transferred. Urine glucose measurements should be reserved to assess osmotic diuresis and estimate renal transport thresholds by comparison with serum levels. Many diabetic patients present with insulin pumps. It is important to know if these devices were continued through the perioperative period or when to appropriately reinstitute therapy in the PACU.

Hyperglycemia

Glucose infusions and stress responses commonly elevate serum glucose levels after surgery. For most patients during anesthesia, glucose should not be included in maintenance intravenous solutions. Moderate postoperative hyperglycemia (150 to 250 mg/dL) resolves spontaneously and has little adverse effect in the nondiabetic patient. Higher glucose levels cause glycosuria with osmotic diuresis and interfere with serum electrolyte determinations. Severe hyperglycemia increases serum osmolality to a point that cerebral disequilibrium and hyperosmolar coma occur. Type I diabetic patients are at risk for ketoacidosis. Potassium replacement and serial blood glucose determinations are essential.

Hypoglycemia

Hypoglycemia in the PACU can be caused by endogenous insulin secretion or by excessive or inadvertent insulin administration. Serious postoperative hypoglycemia is rare and easily treated with intravenous 50% dextrose followed by glucose infusion. Either sedation or excessive sympathetic nervous system activity masks signs and symptoms of hypoglycemia after anesthesia. Diabetic patients and especially patients who have received insulin therapy intraoperatively must have serum glucose levels measured to avoid the serious problems related to hypoglycemia. Extreme care with documenting and reporting the use of insulin is paramount to provide safe and appropriate care.

Electrolyte Disorders

Hyponatremia

Postoperative hyponatremia occurs if free water is infused during surgery or if sodium-free irrigating solution is absorbed during transurethral prostatic resection or hysteroscopy. Accumulation of serum glycine or its metabolite, ammonia, might exacerbate symptoms. Free water retention is also caused by inappropriate ADH secretion, prolonged labor induction with oxytocin, or respiratory uptake of nebulized droplets. Theoretically, excessive infusion of isotonic saline leads to excretion of hypertonic urine, desalination, and iatrogenic hyponatremia. Symptoms of moderate hyponatremia include agitation, disorientation, visual disturbances, and nausea, whereas severe hyponatremia causes unconsciousness, impaired airway reflexes, and CNS irritability that progress to grand mal seizures. Therapy includes intravenous normal saline and intravenous furosemide to promote free water excretion. Infusion of hypertonic saline may be useful for severe hyponatremia, but with diligence not to increase serum sodium by 0.5 mEq/hr to avoid CNS lesions or pulmonary edema. Serum sodium concentration and osmolarity should be measured every 2 to 4 hours during hypertonic saline therapy.

Hypokalemia

Postoperative hypokalemia is often inconsequential but might generate serious dysrhythmias, especially in patients taking digoxin. A potassium deficit caused by chronic diuretic therapy, nasogastric suctioning, or vomiting often underlies hypokalemia. Urinary and hemorrhagic losses, dilution, and insulin therapy generate acute hypokalemia that worsens during respiratory alkalemia. Excess sympathetic nervous system activity, infusion of calcium, or β-mimetic medications exacerbates effects of hypokalemia. Adding potassium to peripheral intravenous fluids often restores serum concentration, but concentrated solutions infused through a central catheter may be necessary. It is deceiving to think that 10 to 30 mEq of potassium will correct low potassium levels. Potassium is an intracellular ion and a plasma potassium deficit is indicative of a far greater intracellular deficit. It is the intracellular-to-extracellular ratio that may well be important, and rapid changes can contribute to as dysrhythmias as can mild hypokalemia alone.

Hyperkalemia

A high serum potassium level raises the suspicion of spurious hyperkalemia from a hemolyzed specimen or from sampling near an intravenous catheter containing potassium or banked blood. Postoperative hyperkalemia occurs after excessive potassium infusion or in patients with renal failure or malignant hyperthermia. Acute acidemia exacerbates hyperkalemia. Treatment with intravenous insulin and glucose acutely lowers potassium, whereas intravenous calcium counters myocardial effects. Hemodialysis may be necessary for high potassium levels or symptomatic patients.

Calcium and Magnesium

Although underlying parathyroid disease or massive fluid replacement reduces total body and ionized calcium, symptomatic hypocalcemia seldom occurs in the PACU. A rare patient might exhibit upper airway obstruction from hypocalcemia after parathyroid excision. Reduction of the ionized fraction by acute alkalemia may cause myocardial conduction and contractility abnormalities, decreased vascular tone, or tetany. Transfusion of blood containing chelating agents (e.g., citrate) rarely causes symptomatic hypocalcemia. Administration of calcium chloride or calcium gluconate to hypocalcemic patients improves cardiovascular dynamics.

Magnesium plays a key role in restoration of neuromuscular function after surgery and in maintenance of cardiac rhythm and conduction. Hypermagnesemia is rare because the kidneys effectively excrete excessive magnesium. Obstetric patients who have been receiving magnesium for tocolysis or control of severe pregnancy-induced hypertension can present with postoperative hyporeflexia, and at higher serum levels will show prolonged atrioventricular conduction or complete heart block. Treatment entails intravenous calcium and diuretics.

Miscellaneous Complications

Incidental Trauma

Each patient admitted to the PACU should be carefully evaluated for traumatic complications. Discovery of a complication necessitates careful documentation, notification of physicians responsible for extended care, consultation with specialists, and follow-up.

Ocular Injuries and Visual Changes

Corneal abrasion caused by drying or inadvertent eye contact is a common intraoperative eye injury (see Chapter 49, NICV 49-4). The incidence of this type of injury in a nonophthalmic patient is estimated to be between 0.034% and 0.17%, with the higher incidence related to prone or lateral positioning.[70] Corneal injury can occur during emergence in the PACU from patients rubbing their eyes, if a rigid oxygen face mask rides up on the eye, if the eye is rubbed with a pulse oximeter probe, or from eye make-up being rubbed in the eyes. Abrasions cause tearing, decreased visual acuity, pain, and photophobia. Fluorescein staining aids diagnosis. Abrasions usually heal spontaneously within 72 hours without scarring, but severe injury can cause cataract formation and impair vision. There is no standard treatment for corneal abrasions, but symptomatic treatment includes artificial tears, topical antibiotics, topical analgesics, and eye closure. Daily follow-up with patients with corneal abrasions should be done to verify healing and rule out other causes of eye pain. If the patient is not improved in 48 hours, the patient should be referred to an ophthalmologist.

Visual acuity is often impaired after anesthesia. Autonomic side effects of medications impair accommodation, and residual ocular lubricants cloud vision. Impairment of retinal perfusion by ocular compression generates postoperative visual disturbances ranging from loss of acuity to permanent blindness.[71,72] Ischemic optic atrophy can also occur in the absence of external compression.[73] Risk of blindness is higher after long procedures in the prone position, as well as in patients with vascular disease, pre-existing hypertension, diabetes, and sickle cell anemia. A significant percentage of postoperative patients suffer deficits in acuity unrelated to ocular trauma, some of whom require permanent refractive adjustment.[74] Anesthesiologists should be alert for visual impairment and check acuity when assessing patients at higher risk for ischemic optic atrophy.

Hearing Impairment

Hearing impairment after anesthesia and surgery is relatively common.[75] Although impairment is often subclinical, patients sometimes experience decreased auditory acuity, tinnitus, or roaring. The incidence of detectable hearing impairment is particularly high after dural puncture for spinal anesthesia (8% to 16%), and varies with needle size, needle type, and patient age. Impairment can be unilateral or bilateral and usually resolves spontaneously. Hearing loss also occurs after general anesthesia for both noncardiac and cardiac surgery, and is often related to disruption of the round window or tympanic membrane rupture. Eustachian tube inflammation and otitis secondary to endotracheal intubation can also impact hearing.

Oral, Pharyngeal, and Laryngeal Injuries

Laryngoscope blades, surgical instruments, rigid oral airways, and dentition can all cause trauma of oral soft tissues. Lip, tongue, or gum abrasions are treated with an ice pack and analgesia. Penetrating injuries caused by tissue entrapment between teeth and rigid devices may require topical antibiotics. After a traumatic tracheal intubation, hematoma or edema might cause partial upper airway obstruction. Nebulized racemic epinephrine often improves stridor more quickly than steroids. Dental damage can occur during airway manipulations or during emergence if a patient bites on a rigid oral airway or forcefully clenches their teeth. It is important to document tooth or dental appliance damage, obtain a dental consultation, and observe for signs of foreign body aspiration.[76]

Sore throat and/or hoarseness after tracheal intubation occur in 20% to 50% of patients, depending on the degree of trauma during laryngoscopy and oropharyngeal suctioning, the duration of intubation, and the type of endotracheal tube. Mucosal irritation also presents as an unquenchable dryness in mouth and throat. The use of local anesthetic ointments to lubricate endotracheal tubes may cause additional mucosal irritation. Topical viscous lidocaine attenuates irritation from nasogastric tubes but may increase risk of aspiration during recovery. In children, the severity of postextubation laryngeal edema or tracheitis varies with age, intubation duration, and degree of trauma or tube movement. Most recover with cool mist therapy, but nebulized racemic epinephrine and dexamethasone may be needed in more severe cases. Laryngoscopy and intubation can also cause hypoglossal, lingual, or recurrent laryngeal nerve damage, vocal cord evulsion, desquamation of laryngeal or tracheal mucosa, edema or ulceration, and tracheal perforation. Postoperative sore throat and dysphagia also occurs without intubation, related to use of laryngeal mask airways,[77] oral airways, trauma from suctioning, or drying from nonhumidified gases. Neck and jaw soreness is commonly seen after face mask anesthetics.

Nerve Injuries

Nerve injuries caused by improper positioning during anesthesia generate serious long-term complications.[78] Spinal cord injury can be caused by positioning for intubation or by hematoma accumulation after placement of neuraxial anesthetics. Peripheral nerve compression during general or regional anesthesia sometimes causes permanent sensory and motor deficits, as do stretch injuries from hyperextension of an extremity.[79] Any bruising or skin breakdown noted postoperatively should prompt evaluation for underlying nerve damage. Many postoperative neuropathies have no identifiable cause. This is particularly true for ulnar neuropathy, which may be related to subtle positioning problems, pre-existing impairment, or sensitivity of the nerve to ischemia.[80]

Every complaint of nonsurgical pain, numbness, or weakness from a postoperative patient should be carefully evaluated. In the event of neuropathic weakness, electromyographic studies may determine the location of the lesion and possible reversibility of the nerve deficit. Sensory neuropathies rarely last longer than 5 days and should be referred to a neurologist if the deficit exceeds this time or if it progresses.[81]

Postdural puncture headache may first occur in the PACU, although most appear within 24 to 48 hours. Headache is more frequent after difficult subarachnoid anesthetics with multiple attempts and after inadvertent dural puncture during attempted epidural placement. Subarachnoid air bubbles from loss-of-resistance testing may contribute. In the PACU, treatment is supportive with hydration, analgesics, and positioning. In severe cases, early intervention with the definitive treatment of epidural blood patch might be considered. Nerve injury secondary to needle contact or intraneuronal injection during placement of regional anesthesia is rare but does occur.[79,82] In one study, 6.3% of 4,767 patients experienced paresthesia during placement of spinal anesthesia, but only 0.126% had persisting symptoms.[83] In the PACU, patients often complain of pain, focal numbness, residual paresthesia, or dysesthesia. Symptoms are usually transient. One should administer analgesia, reassure the patient, document findings, and follow for the possibility of an evolving neurologic deficit.

During recovery from spinal anesthesia, some patients exhibit lower extremity discomfort, buttock pain, and other signs of sacral or lumbar neurologic irritation. This problem is more common in obese patients, after procedures in lithotomy position, and after spinal anesthesia with 5% lidocaine.[82] Symptoms are transient and treated supportively. Rarely, a patient exhibits headache and meningeal signs caused by chemical meningitis after injection of a spinal drug that is contaminated or outside the acceptable pH range.

Soft-Tissue and Joint Injuries

If pressure points are improperly padded, soft-tissue ischemia and necrosis can occur, especially with lateral or prone positioning. Prolonged scalp pressure causes localized alopecia, whereas entrapment of ears, breasts, genitalia, or skin folds causes inflammation or necrosis. Regional ischemia from major arterial compression is rare. Thermal, electrical, or chemical burns from cautery equipment, preparatory solutions, or adhesives also occur. Extravasation of intravenous medications or fluids can cause sloughing, localized chemical neuropathy, or compartment syndromes. Excessive joint or muscle extension leads to postoperative backache, joint pain, stiffness, and even joint instability. After regional anesthesia, extremities must be properly secured and padded to prevent nerve injury.

Skeletal Muscle Pain

Postoperative muscle pain can be caused by many intraoperative factors. Prolonged lack of motion or unusual muscle stretch during positioning often contributes to muscle stiffness and aching. Postoperative myalgia has been reported to range between 5% and 83% of patients after the use of succinylcholine,[84] while the pathogenesis of this myalgia remains unclear.[82,85] Acute myalgia also occurs after administration of other muscle relaxants and in patients receiving no relaxant. Delayed-onset muscle fatigue can appear days after surgery and resolves spontaneously.

Hypothermia and Shivering

Although intraoperative temperature maintenance is a goal, patients still exhibit postoperative hypothermia (NICV 54-1). Rate of heat loss is similar during general or regional anesthesia, but rewarming is slower after regional anesthesia because residual vasodilation and paralysis impede heat generation and retention. Cachectic, traumatized, or burned patients experience greater temperature reduction, as do infants because of a low ratio of body mass-to-surface area.

Hypothermia complicates and prolongs care in the PACU.[86] 11 Average PACU stay is increased by 40 to 90 minutes for hypothermic patients.[87] Postoperative hypothermia increases sympathetic nervous system activity with increased epinephrine and norepinephrine levels,[88] elevates peripheral vascular resistance, and decreases venous capacitance. Risk of myocardial ischemia[89] and dysrhythmia from mechanical myocardial stimulation is increased. Vasoconstriction interferes with the reliability of pulse oximetry and intra-arterial pressure monitoring. Hypoperfusion jeopardizes marginal tissue grafts and promotes tissue hypoxia and metabolic acidemia. The higher affinity of hemoglobin compromises oxygen unloading to hypothermic tissues. Platelet sequestration, decreased platelet function, and reduced clotting factor function contribute to coagulopathy. Moderate hyperglycemia occurs, cellular immune responses are compromised, and postoperative infection rates increase.[90] A decrease in the minimal alveolar concentration of inhalation anesthetics (5% to 7% per 1°C cooling) accentuates residual sedation. Low perfusion and impaired biotransformation might increase the duration of neuromuscular relaxants and sedatives. Moderate hypothermia (28° to 32°C) is associated with cardiac dysrhythmias. Severe hypothermia (≤28°C) interferes with cardiac rhythm generation and impulse conduction. On ECG, the PR, QRS, or QT intervals lengthen, and J waves appear. Spontaneous ventricular fibrillation occurs at temperatures <28°C.

During emergence, hypothalamic regulation generates shivering to increase endogenous heat production.[91] Shivering increases the risk of incidental trauma, disrupts medical devices, and interferes with ECG and pulse oximetry monitoring. Oxygen consumption and CO_2 production can increase 200%. Associated increases in minute ventilation and cardiac output might precipitate ventilatory failure in patients with limited reserve or myocardial ischemia in those with coronary artery disease.[89] Shivering is accentuated by tremors related to emergence from inhalation anesthesia. Tremors exhibit clonic and tonic components, and likely reflect decreased cortical influence on spinal cord reflexes.

Restoration of normothermia is an important goal during recovery. Supplemental oxygen should be instituted and forced-air warming devices are most useful for treating hypothermia. Intravenous fluids and blood should be warmed. For most patients, shivering from mild-to-moderate hypothermia is uncomfortable but self-limited, and needs no treatment other than rewarming and reassurance. Many medications have been recommended to suppress shivering, but meperidine is most efficacious in conjunction with rewarming.[7] Fentanyl has also been used with patients in whom meperidine is contraindicated. Withholding reversal of relaxants in ventilated, sedated patients attenuates shivering but increases rewarming time. If temperature is near normal (>96°F) and shivering is resolved, transfer from PACU to an inpatient floor or a discharge area is acceptable.

The Surgical Care Improvement Project, sponsored by CMS, The Joint Commission (TJC), and other national partners, is a program that uses several quality measures to help improve the safety and outcomes of surgical patients. One of those measures important to anesthesiologists is maintaining patients' temperatures above 36°C. While this measure really begins with care in the operating room, the PACU has a 15-minute period from admission to have a measured patient temperature of at least 36°C. Maintaining normothermia has been shown to reduce wound infections in surgical patients, producing better outcomes and reducing length of stay.

Hyperthermia

Hyperthermia is relatively uncommon in the PACU. Occasionally, a patient exhibits short-lived hyperthermia from close draping or aggressive intraoperative heat preservation. Postoperative fever sometimes reflects a pre-existing infection (e.g., sinusitis, upper respiratory or urinary tract infection) or an infection exacerbated by the surgical procedure (e.g., resection of infected tonsils or appendix, abscess drainage, urinary tract manipulation). Elevated temperature might indicate a drug or transfusion reaction. Muscarinic blocking agents such as atropine interfere with cooling and might contribute to fever, but they are seldom the cause in adults. Other hypermetabolic states such as thyroid storm must be considered. High fever occurs with malignant hyperthermia, but signs such as metabolic acidemia, tachycardia, muscle rigidity, dysrhythmia, and tachypnea usually establish the diagnosis first.

Ambient cooling, chest physiotherapy, incentive spirometry, and antipyretics are usually sufficient to treat postoperative fever. One should withhold offending medications or blood products if a drug or transfusion reaction is suspected and notify the physician responsible for extended care to ensure postdischarge evaluation. For therapies for thyroid storm, see Chapter 47 Endocrine Function, and for malignant hyperthermia see Chapter 24 Rare Coexisting Diseases.

Persistent Sedation

Approximately 90% of patients regain consciousness within 15 minutes of admission to the PACU; unconsciousness persisting for a greater period is considered prolonged (NICV 54-2).[92] Even a highly susceptible patient should respond to a stimulus within 30 to 45 minutes after a reasonably conducted anesthetic. In a patient with prolonged sedation, one should research the level of preoperative responsiveness to uncover intoxication with drugs and alcohol or pre-existing mental dysfunction. One should note the time and amount of preoperative and intraoperative sedative medications, and review any unusual intraoperative events. The rate and character of spontaneous ventilation helps judge residual opioid effect, bradypnea being pathognomonic for opioid effect. Physical assessment should include a tactile stimulus such as a light skin pinch, which elicits greater arousal than verbal stimulation, perhaps because sensory input is amplified through the reticular activating system. Diagnostic value of pupillary response is low.

Residual sedation from inhalation anesthetics might cause prolonged unconsciousness, especially after long procedures, in obese patients, or when high concentrations are continued through the end of surgery. Prolonged sedation is less likely after anesthesia with low solubility agents such as sevoflurane or desflurane. Premedications that have sedative effects (e.g., diphenhydramine, hydroxyzine, promethazine, droperidol, lorazepam, midazolam, meclizine, and scopolamine) contribute to postoperative somnolence. Sedation from intraoperative opioid or sedative administration is dose-related. Opioids are the only drugs that cause bradypnea; thus, regardless of what other drug effects, if the respiratory rate is <14 to 16, then opioids are clearly affecting the patient's level of consciousness. To assess sedation from opioids, one can administer low-dose intravenous naloxone (0.04-mg increments every 2 minutes, up to 0.2 mg). With careful titration, respiratory depression and sedation can be reversed without dangerous reversal of analgesia. If unconsciousness is related to residual opioid effect, ventilatory rate and arousal will increase with ≤0.2 mg of intravenous naloxone, unless a patient has received a massive opioid overdose.

Flumazenil (0.2 mg intravenously per minute to a total of 1.0 mg), a competitive benzodiazepine antagonist, differentiates sedation from midazolam and diazepam, although duration of action is short. Risk of inducing seizures must be considered in reversing chronic benzodiazepine users. Neither naloxone nor flumazenil should be used as a routine element of postoperative care.[7] Pharmacologic reversal should be reserved for specific indications in individual patients. Administration of intravenous physostigmine (0.5 to 1 mg) counteracts but does not reverse sedation caused by inhalation anesthetics, other sedatives, and anticholinergics. If administration of naloxone, flumazenil, or physostigmine does not improve the level of consciousness, unconsciousness is most likely not related to reversible residual anesthetic medications. However, it is still possible that an unrecognized, preoperative overdose with depressant oral drugs (i.e., anticholinergic and antihistamines) is responsible.

The increasing use of dexmedetomidine for sedation cases, can lead to persistent sedation in the PACU. These patients are usually easy to arouse and follow commands readily. They tend to have less respiratory depression unless other respiratory depressant medications have also been given. The minimal effect on respiratory drive by dexmedetomidine allows safe discharge from the PACU as long as the destination of the patient is sufficient to care for the level of sedation.

Profound residual neuromuscular paralysis could mimic unconsciousness by precluding any motor response to stimuli. This phenomenon could occur after gross overdosage, if reversal agents are omitted, in patients with unrecognized neuromuscular disease, with phase II blockade from succinylcholine, or its use in a patient with pseudocholinesterase deficiency. Observation of purposeful motion, spontaneous ventilation, or reflex muscular movement eliminates residual paralysis as an explanation; low-energy peripheral nerve stimulation will help with the diagnosis of residual muscle relaxation. CNS depression secondary to intravenous local anesthetic toxicity or inadvertent subarachnoid injection can mimic postoperative coma. Children who were exhausted before surgery are often difficult to arouse after anesthesia, especially if sleep patterns are disrupted by emergency surgery at night. Hypothermia below 33°C impairs consciousness and increases the depressant effect of medications. Core temperatures below 30°C can cause fixed pupillary dilation, areflexia, and coma. A serum glucose level will eliminate severe hypoglycemia or hyperglycemic hyperosmolar coma as causes. Suspicion that unresponsiveness is caused by hypoglycemia indicates an immediate empiric trial of intravenous 50% dextrose. Hyposmolar states (<260 mOsm/L) such as acute hyponatremia (Na <125 mEq/L) are ruled out by checking serum electrolyte and osmolarity. Arterial blood gas analysis reveals CO_2 narcosis ($PaCO_2$ >80 to 100 mmHg) as well as carboxyhemoglobin levels for carbon monoxide poisoning. A patient may also be feigning unresponsiveness or having a hysterical reaction that presents as unconsciousness is a diagnosis of exclusion.

If a diagnosis remains elusive, consult a neurologist for a thorough neurologic evaluation. Occasionally, unresponsiveness reflects subclinical grand mal seizures secondary to delirium tremens or an underlying seizure disorder. Cerebral anoxia from hypoperfusion or prolonged profound hypoxemia must be considered. In injured patients or those recovering from intracranial surgery, evaluate for unrecognized head trauma, intracerebral hemorrhage, or increased intracranial pressure. Patients sometimes awaken very slowly after long intracranial procedures.[93] Cerebral thromboembolism is another possibility in patients who have undergone internal jugular or subclavian cannulation.

Patients with atrial fibrillation, carotid bruits, or hypercoagulable states are also at increased risk of thromboembolism. Paradoxic air or fat embolism through a right-to-left intracardiac shunt should be considered. After cardiac, proximal major vascular, or invasive neck surgery, risk of postoperative stroke ranges from 2.2% to 5.2%.[94] Postoperative cerebrovascular accidents in other patients are rare, showing a 0.03% to 0.08% incidence in the fourth decade but increasing to 3% to 4% by the eighth decade, and usually become evident after the PACU interval.[95]

Altered Mental Status

Recovering patients sometimes exhibit inappropriate mental reactions, ranging from lethargy and confusion to physical combativeness and extreme disorientation (NICV 54-3).

Emergence Reactions

Aside from the disturbance to staff and other patients, a stormy emergence reaction has significant medical consequences. The risk of incidental trauma increases, including contusion or fracture, corneal abrasion, and sprains from struggling. Thrashing jeopardizes suture lines, orthopedic fixations, vascular grafts, drains, tracheal tubes, and vascular catheters. Agitated patients manifest high levels of sympathetic nervous system tone, tachycardia, and hypertension. Less appreciated is the risk of injury to staff struggling to protect a combative patient.

For a short period after regaining consciousness, some patients appear unable to appropriately process sensory input. Most exhibit somnolence, slight disorientation, and sluggish mental reactions that rapidly clear. Others experience wide emotional swings such as weeping or escalating resistance to positioning and restraint. Predicting which patients will have adverse psychological reactions is difficult. Emergence delirium, which is prevalent in children and young adults, is difficult to predict preoperatively and does not appear to be related to specific types of anesthesia.[96] In young children, anxiety is heightened by parental separation. Heightened anxiety seems to be the one consistent factor in predicting emergence delirium.[97] Many therapies have been tried to prevent or stop emergence delirium in pediatric patients without much success; however, the use of dexmedetomidine has shown promise in reducing this phenomenon without increasing time to extubate or time to discharge.[98] Ketamine and propofol have also been used with some success.[99] Very young children may react inappropriately to sound when hearing acutely improves after myringotomies. Patients with reduced mental capacity, psychiatric disorders, organic brain dysfunction, or hostile preoperative interactions manifest those problems after surgery. Inability to speak secondary to oral fixation or tracheal intubation generates frustration or fear that exaggerates emergence reactions. Ethnic, cultural, and psychological characteristics play some role. A language barrier or a new postoperative hearing impairment accentuates an emergence reaction because input from PACU staff might not be understood. The incidence of stormy emergence is probably higher after procedures with high emotional significance. Recall of intraoperative events can generate severe panic and anxiety during emergence.[100] In patients who abuse alcohol, opioids, cocaine, or other illicit drugs, intoxication or withdrawal can elicit bizarre emergence behavior. Disorientation, paranoia, and combativeness occur after use of scopolamine as a premedication or antiemetic, which can be treated with intravenous physostigmine. Ketamine can cause dysphoria and hallucination, although acute reactions are rare. Etomidate can be a cause of restlessness.

Pain amplifies agitation, confusion, and aggressive behavior during emergence[101]; therefore, it is helpful to ensure adequate postoperative analgesia early in the PACU course. Urinary urgency or gastric distention from trapped gas generates discomfort and agitation, as do tight dressings, painful phlebotomy, and poor positioning. Endotracheal or nasogastric tubes and urinary catheters are also uncomfortable. Check for unusual pain sources such as corneal abrasion, entrapment of body parts, infiltrated vascular catheters, or small devices left beneath a patient. Nausea, dizziness, and pruritus are distressing during emergence. Some patients struggle to move from a supine into a more comfortable semi-sitting or lateral position, especially those with gastroesophageal reflux, pulmonary congestion, or obesity. Emerging patients often resist physical restraint. Residual paralysis elicits agitation or uncoordinated motions that make a patient appear disoriented and combative. Observation of weakness or a peculiar flopping nature of voluntary motion helps in the diagnosis. However, patients can appear fully recovered by head lift and train-of-four monitoring but still perceive impaired swallowing, visual acuity, and sense of strength.[102]

Combativeness, confusion, or disorientation might reflect respiratory dysfunction. Moderate hypoxemia often presents with clouded mentation, disorientation, and agitation resembling that caused by pain. Respiratory acidemia elicits profound agitation, although acidemia caused by ventilatory center depression generates less agitation because higher CNS functions are also depressed. Hypercarbia is more likely to cause lethargy or somnolence. Limitation of inspiratory volume by chest dressings, gastric distention, or splinting causes a vague dissatisfaction with lung inflation similar to air hunger. This sensation also occurs during mechanical ventilation with low delivered volumes and is probably mediated by stretch receptors in the lung. Inability to generate a forceful cough or clear secretions causes distress, as well as high work of breathing. Interstitial pulmonary edema elicits symptoms of air hunger before airway flooding occurs. Agitation can be profound, even with adequate ventilation and oxygenation.

Metabolic abnormalities interfere with lucidity. Lactic acidemia causes anxiety and mild disorientation; acute hyponatremia clouds the sensorium; and hypoglycemia causes first agitation and then diminished responsiveness. Seizure activity might mimic agitation and combativeness. Seizures should be higher in the differential diagnosis in patients with epilepsy, head trauma, and chronic alcohol or cocaine abuse. Cerebral hypoperfusion can produce disorientation, agitation, and combativeness, which can be seen after head trauma or space-occupying lesions. Action such as increasing the mean arterial pressure might be required to assure cerebral perfusion pressure.

There are few interventions that prevent combative emergence reactions.[97] Altered mental status is treated supportively because most emergence reactions often disappear within 10 to 15 minutes. Verbal reassurances that surgery is completed and that the patient is doing well are invaluable. One should use the patient's name frequently with reassurance of well-being, and stress the time and location. When practical, one should allow patients to choose their own position and provide adequate analgesia. In selected cases, parenteral sedation relieves fear or anxiety and smoothes emergence. Identifying whether a patient is reacting to pain or to anxiety is important. Benzodiazepines and barbiturates are ineffective analgesics, whereas opioids are poor sedatives. One should not administer sedative or analgesic medications if altered mental status might reflect a physiologic abnormality such as hypoxemia, hypoglycemia, hypotension, or acidemia, and use restraints only if a patient's or staff's safety is jeopardized.

Delirium and Cognitive Decline

A high percentage of elderly patients (5% to 50%) experience some degree of postoperative confusion, delirium, or cognitive 12 decline.[103,104] Patients exhibit fluctuations in level of consciousness and orientation, or deterioration of memory, mental functions, and acquisition of new information. Delirium may be exhibited by two subtypes, hypoactive predominates while a smaller percentage is hyperactive. The problem may be related to exacerbation of central cholinergic insufficiency by narcotics, sedatives, or anticholinergics. However, stress of surgery, fever, pain, emesis, sleep deprivation, and loss of routine undoubtedly contribute. Presence of pre-existing dementia, cognitive abnormalities, organic brain syndrome, or hearing and visual impairment predicts postoperative delirium, as does evidence of physical infirmity such as high ASA physical status or lack of stress response to surgery. Cognitive dysfunction also occurs at lower incidence (15% greater than control) in younger patients, more frequently resolves within 3 months, and may be related to inactivity during recuperation.[105] Although signs often appear on the first to third postoperative day, onset is often evident in the PACU.

Overall, recovery of cognitive function is slower in the elderly.[106] Because older patients are often skilled at concealing declining capabilities, careful assessment of preoperative capabilities helps identify deficits that affect postoperative status. Postoperative lethargy, clouded sensorium, or delirium sometimes reflects an acute physiologic change. Hyperosmolarity from hyperglycemia or hypernatremia as well as hyponatremia can alter consciousness. Cerebral fluid shifts with decreased mentation occur in patients on dialysis and after rapid correction of severe dehydration. Patients receiving atropine premedication or chronic meperidine therapy might exhibit anticholinergic-induced delirium. Disorientation or clouded sensorium can reflect chronic use of psychogenic drugs, premedication with long-acting sedatives, or unrecognized intoxication. Life-threatening conditions such as seizures, hypoxemia, hypoglycemia, hypotension, acidemia, or cerebrovascular accident sometimes present with confusion, disorientation, inability to vocalize, or reduced level of consciousness, especially if earlier signs and symptoms are misinterpreted.

While there is no anesthetic technique known to be better at avoiding postoperative delirium, there are things to avoid that might reduce the incidence.[107] Avoiding known factors such as benzodiazepines, anticholinergics and meperidine will reduce a patient's risk.[108] Setting protocols to enhance a safe and efficient recovery begins with the initial planning of surgery. Recovery in the PACU should be aware of and implement these protocols to remain consistent with the continuum of care. Pain management is a major factor for reducing the incidence of delirium. Patients should be properly hydrated, remove catheters that are no longer needed, restore cognitive stimulation with returning eye glasses and hearing aids, reorientation and frequent human interaction may aid in limiting or reducing delirium.

13 Postoperative Nausea and Vomiting

Postoperative nausea and vomiting (PONV) and postoperative discharge nausea and vomiting (PDNV) continue to be a significant challenge to be avoided after many types of anesthetics (NICV 54-4). Not only is PONV considered by many patients the most unpleasant aspect following an anesthetic, many describe this as their greatest fear of subsequent anesthetics.[109] Patients are often more concerned about PONV than pain or other risks associated with anesthesia and surgery. In addition to patients' dissatisfaction with nausea and vomiting, there exist medical risks (increased abdominal pressure, increased central venous pressure, aspiration of gastric contents, sympathetic nervous system response with increasing blood pressure and heart rate as well as parasympathetic responses producing bradycardia and hypotension). PONV represents a significant burden to be avoided due to patient satisfaction and safety as well as the economic impact of prolonged PACU stays and unanticipated admissions.

The incidence of PONV varies with many potential causes. Patients often experience nausea and emesis after discharge from the PACU which may coincide with increased oral intake or waning effect of antiemetics. Surgeries associated with a higher risk of PONV are eye procedures, peritoneal or intestinal irritation, ear-nose-throat procedures especially with middle ear manipulation, dental and cosmetic procedures. Patient groups at increased are those with a previous history of PONV or motion sickness, menstruating females, children over the age of two, obesity, and nonsmokers.[110] Perioperative factors that may increase the incidence include no PO intake (starvation, dehydration), autonomic imbalance, pain, and the effects of anesthetics on the chemotactic center.

Incidence of PONV is lower following regional rather than general anesthesia especially with a decreased use of opioids.[111] The use of nonopioid analgesics may reduce the frequency of emesis while providing adequate pain control. Induction agents such as propofol and barbiturates are associated with reduced incidence compared to etomidate and ketamine. A total intravenous anesthetic (TIVA) technique with propofol greatly reduces PONV incidence compared to a pure inhalation anesthetic. There is little significant difference among inhalation agents, although sevoflurane and desflurane might generate slightly higher rates of nausea. The choice of anticholinergic reversal agents may be a contributing factor but remains unclear to what degree.

Several interventions have been evaluated and can be implemented to reduce the incidence of PONV. The use of meclizine 25 mg preoperatively for patients predisposed to motion sickness is effective. Prophylaxis with 5-HT3 receptor antagonists (i.e., ondansetron) prior to emergence significantly reduces incidence and is cost effective. Dexamethasone also has antiemetic effects and can be used effectively with other prophylactic agents. Hydration is effective, easy, and cost effective. The use of droperidol prophylaxis decreased due to a 2001 FDA black box warning with prolonged QT on ECG as well as manufacturing challenges beginning in 2013. The FDA letter regarding the use of droperidol did not address the usual prophylaxis dose of 0.625 mg, but recommended ECG monitoring for 2 to 3 hours after administration. Clarification on the use of droperidol came in 2008 stating that the black box warning only pertained to those doses approved by the FDA as indicated on the product label which is for 2.5 mg or greater.[112] In September of 2011, the FDA came out with a similar safety announcement regarding prolonged QT with the use of ondansetron, which appeared in the literature in 2005. There were no recommendations regarding routine ECG monitoring with the use of ondansetron but caution and monitoring should be used with those patients with known prolonged QT syndromes.[113] The need for rescue therapy in the PACU should use a different class of drug than that used prophylactically. Use of 5-HT3 antagonists is useful only after 6 hours of initial dose. Promethazine, dimenhydrinate, droperidol, metoclopramide, and intramuscular ephedrine have been useful for rescue therapy as well as isopropyl alcohol swab aromatherapy.[114] Rescue with nonselective antihistamines (i.e., promethazine) is effective but caution is advised in patients where increased sedation can be problematic such as children and patients with OSA. Acupuncture, acupressure, and TENS therapy can provide relief; but, due to provider proficiency, patient acceptance and proven efficacy compared to antiemetic medications, these methods are less frequently used.[115] More serious causes of nausea and vomiting such as hypotension, hypoxia, hypoglycemia, increased intracranial pressure, or gastric bleeding should be considered in appropriate patients.

For further review and interactivities, please see the videos and narrative interactive clinical vignettes (NICVs) accessible in the complimentary eBook bundled with this text. Access instructions are located on the inside front cover.

REFERENCES

1. Standards for Postanesthesia Care (Approved by House of Delegates on October 12, 1988 and last amended on October 23, 2019). https://www.asahq.org/standards-and-guidelines/standards-for-postanesthesia-care
2. Bothner U, Georgieff M, Schwilk B. The impact of minor perioperative anesthesia-related incidents, events, and complications on postanesthesia care unit utilization. *Anesth Analg*. 1999;89:506.
3. Cohen MM, O'Brien-Pallas LL, Copplestone C, Wall R, Porter J, Rose DK. Nursing workload associated with adverse events in the postanesthesia care unit. *Anesthesiology*. 1999;91:1882.
4. Pavlin DJ, Rapp SE, Polissar NL, Malmgren JA, Koerschgen M, Keyes H. Factors affecting discharge time in adult outpatients. *Anesth Analg*. 1998;87:816.
5. Song D, Chung F, Ronayne M, Ward B, Yogendran S, Sibbick C. Fast-tracking (bypassing the PACU) does not reduce nursing workload after ambulatory surgery. *Br J Anaesth*. 2004;93:768.
6. Hines R, Barash PG, Watrous G, O'Connor T. Complications occurring in the postanesthesia care unit: A survey. *Anesth Analg*. 1992;74:503.
7. American Society of Anesthesiologists Task Force on Postanesthetic Care. Practice guidelines for postanesthetic care: A report by the American Society of Anesthesiologists Task Force on Postanesthetic Care. *Anesthesiology*. 2002;96:742.
8. Sullivan EE. Standards of perianesthesia nursing practice 2002. *J Perianesth Nurs*. 2002;17:275.
9. Preston N, Gregory M. Patient recovery and the post anaesthesia care unit. *Anaesth Intensive Care Med*. 2015;16(9):443–445.
10. Swenson JD, Bay N, Loose E, et al. Outpatient management of continuous peripheral nerve catheters placed using ultrasound guidance: An experience in 620 patients. *Anesth Analg*. 2006;103:1436.
11. Apfelbaum JL, Walawander CA, Grasela TH, et al. Eliminating intensive postoperative care in same-day surgery patients using short-acting anesthetics. *Anesthesiology*. 2002;97:66K.
12. Pittet D, Stephan F, Hugonnet S, Akakpo C, Souweine B, Clergue F. Hand-cleansing during postanesthesia care. *Anesthesiology*. 2003;99:530.
13. Macario A, Weinger M, Carney S, Kim A. Which clinical anesthesia outcomes are important to avoid the perspective of patients. *Anesth Analg*. 1999;89:652.
14. Strassels SA, Chen C, Carr DB. Postoperative analgesia: Economics, resource use, and patient satisfaction in an urban teaching hospital. *Anesth Analg*. 2002;94:130.
15. Apfelbaum JL, Chen C, Mehta SS, Gan TJ. Postoperative pain experience: Results from a national survey suggest postoperative pain continues to be undermanaged. *Anesth Analg* 2003;97:534.
16. Rundshagen I, Schnabel K, Standl T, Schulte am Esch J. Patients' vs nurses' assessments of postoperative pain and anxiety during patient- or nurse-controlled analgesia. *Br J Anaesth*. 1999;82:374.
17. American Society of Anesthesiologists Task Force on Acute Pain Management. Practice guidelines for acute pain management in the perioperative setting: An updated report by the American Society of Anesthesiologists Task Force on Acute Pain Management. *Anesthesiology*. 2004;100:1573.
18. Chung F, Ritchie E, Su J. Postoperative pain in ambulatory surgery. *Anesth Analg*. 1997;85:808.
19. Wu CL, Berenholtz SM, Pronovost PJ, Fleisher LA. Systematic review and analysis of postdischarge symptoms after outpatient surgery. *Anesthesiology*. 2002;96:994.
20. Sritapan Y, Clifford S, Bautista A. Perioperative Management of Patients on Buprenorphine and Methadone: A Narrative Review. *Balkan Med J*. 2020;37(5):247–252.
21. Peng PW, Sandler AN. A review of the use of fentanyl analgesia in the management of acute pain in adults. *Anesthesiology*. 1999;90:576.
22. White PF. The role of non-opioid analgesic techniques in the management of pain after ambulatory surgery. *Anesth Analg*. 2002;94:577.
23. Gwirtz KH, Young JV, Byers RS, et al. The safety and efficacy of intrathecal opioid analgesia for acute postoperative pain: Seven years' experience with 5,969 surgical patients at Indiana University Hospital. *Anesth Analg*. 1999;88:599.
24. de Leon-Casasola OA, Lema MJ. Postoperative epidural opioid analgesia: What are the choices? *Anesth Analg*. 1996;83:867.
25. Baig MK, Zmora O, Derdemezi J, Weiss EG, Nogueras JJ, Wexner SD. Use of the ON-Q pain management system is associated with decreased postoperative analgesic requirement: Double blind randomized placebo pilot study. *J Am Coll Surg*. 2006;202:297.
26. Capdevila X, Pirat P, Bringuier S, et al. Continuous peripheral nerve blocks in hospital wards after orthopedic surgery: A multicenter prospective analysis of the quality of postoperative analgesia and complications in 1,416 patients. *Anesthesiology*. 2005;103:1035.
27. Ilfeld BM, Enneking FK. Continuous peripheral nerve blocks at home: A review. *Anesth Analg*. 2005;100:1822.
28. Casati A, Fanelli G, Cedrati V, Berti M, Aldegheri G, Torri G. Pulmonary function changes after interscalene brachial plexus anesthesia with 0.5% and 0.75% ropivacaine: A double-blinded comparison with 2% mepivacaine. *Anesth Analg*. 1999;88:587.
29. Aldrete JA. The post-anesthesia recovery score revisited. *J Clin Anesth*. 1995;7:89.
30. White PF, Song D. New criteria for fast-tracking after outpatient anesthesia: A comparison with the modified Aldrete's scoring system. *Anesth Analg*. 1999;88:1069.
31. Brown I, Jellish WS, Kleinman B, et al. Use of postanesthesia discharge criteria to reduce discharge delays for inpatients in the postanesthesia care unit. *J Clin Anesth*. 2008;20(3):175–179.
32. Noiseux N, Bracco D, Prieto I, Hemmerling TM. Do patients after off-pump coronary artery bypass grafting need the intensive care unit? A prospective audit of 85 patients. *Interact Cardiovasc Thorac Surg*. 2008;7:32.
33. Schweizer A, Khatchatourian G, Hohn L, Spiliopoulos A, Romand J, Licker M. Opening of a new postanesthesia care unit: Impact on critical care utilization and complications following major vascular and thoracic surgery. *J Clin Anesth*. 2002;14:486.
34. Heland M, Retsas A. Establishing a cardiac surgery recovery unit within the post anaesthesia care unit. *Collegian*. 1999;6:10.
35. Baltimore JJ. Perianesthesia care of cardiac surgery patients: A CPAN review. *J Perianesth Nurs*. 2001;16:246.
36. Practice Advisory for the Perioperative Management of Patients with Cardiac Implantable Electronic Devices: Pacemakers and Implantable Cardioverter–Defibrillators 2020: An Updated Report by the American Society of Anesthesiologists Task Force on Perioperative Management of Patients with Cardiac Implantable Electronic Devices. *Anesthesiology*. 2020;132:225–252.
37. Rose DK, Cohen MM, Wigglesworth DF, DeBoer DP. Critical respiratory events in the postanesthesia care unit, patient, surgical, and anesthetic factors. *Anesthesiology*. 1994;81:410.
38. Schwilk B, Bothner U, Schraag S, Georgieff M. Perioperative respiratory events in smokers and nonsmokers undergoing general anaesthesia. *Acta Anaesthesiol Scand*. 1997;41:348.
39. Ballantyne JC, Carr DB, deFerranti S, et al. The comparative effects of postoperative analgesic therapies on pulmonary outcome: Cumulative meta-analyses of randomized, controlled trials. *Anesth Analg*. 1998;86:598.
40. Warner DO, Warner MA, Offord KP, Schroeder DR, Maxson P, Scanlon PD. Airway obstruction and perioperative complications in smokers undergoing abdominal surgery. *Anesthesiology*. 1999;90:372.
41. Strauss SG, Lynn AM, Bratton SL, Nespeca MK. Ventilatory response to CO_2 in children with obstructive sleep apnea from adenotonsillar hypertrophy. *Anesth Analg*. 1999;89:328.
42. Tait AR, Malviya S, Voepel-Lewis T, Munro HM, Seiwert M, Pandit UA. Risk factors for perioperative adverse respiratory events in children with upper respiratory tract infections. *Anesthesiology*. 2001;95:299.
43. D'Honneur G, Lofaso F, Drummond GB, et al. Susceptibility to upper airway obstruction during partial neuromuscular block. *Anesthesiology*. 1998;88:371.
44. Asai T, Koga K, Vaughan RS. Respiratory complications associated with tracheal intubation and extubation. *Br J Anaesth*. 1998;80:767.
45. Benumof JL, Dagg R, Benumof R. Critical hemoglobin desaturation will occur before return to an unparalyzed state following 1 mg/kg intravenous succinylcholine. *Anesthesiology*. 1997; 87:979.
46. Warner DO, Warner MA, Barnes RD, et al. Perioperative respiratory complications in patients with asthma. *Anesthesiology*. 1996;85:460.
47. Berg H, Roed J, Viby-Mogensen J, et al. Residual neuromuscular block is a risk factor for postoperative pulmonary complications. A prospective, randomised, and blinded study of postoperative pulmonary complications after atracurium, vecuronium and pancuronium. *Acta Anaesthesiol Scand*. 1997;41:1095.
48. Debaene B, Plaud B, Dilly MP, Donati F. Residual paralysis in the PACU after a single intubating dose of nondepolarizing muscle relaxant with an intermediate duration of action. *Anesthesiology*. 2003;98:1042.
49. de Boer HD, Driessen JJ, Marcus MA, Kerkkamp H, Heeringa M, Klimek M. Reversal of rocuronium-induced (1.2 mg/kg) profound neuromuscular block by sugammadex: A multicenter, dose-finding and safety study. *Anesthesiology*. 2007;107:239.
50. Stoller JK, Kester L. Respiratory care protocols in postanesthesia care. *J Perianesth Nurs*. 1998;13:349.
51. Rothen HU, Sporre B, Engberg G, Wegenius G, Hedenstierna G. Airway closure, atelectasis and gas exchange during general anaesthesia. *Br J Anaesth*. 1998;81:681.
52. Karayiannakis AJ, Makri GG, Mantzioka A, Karousos D, Karatzas G. Postoperative pulmonary function after laparoscopic and open cholecystectomy. *Br J Anaesth*. 1996;77:448.
53. Thomas JA, McIntosh JM. Are incentive spirometry, intermittent positive pressure breathing, and deep breathing exercises effective in the prevention of postoperative pulmonary complications after upper abdominal surgery? A systematic overview and meta-analysis. *Phys Ther*. 1994;74:3.
54. Overend TJ, Anderson CM, Lucy SD, Bhatia C, Jonsson BI, Timmermans C. The effect of incentive spirometry on postoperative pulmonary complications: A systematic review. *Chest*. 2001;120:971.
55. Young T, Palta M, Dempsey J, Skatrud J, Weber S, Badr S. The occurrence of sleep-disordered breathing among middle-aged adults. *N Engl J Med*. 1993;328:1230.

56. Tishler PV, Larkin EK, Schluchter MD, Redline S. Incidence of sleep-disordered breathing in an urban adult population: the relative importance of risk factors in the development of sleep-disordered breathing. *JAMA*. 2003;289(17):2230–2237.
57. American Society of Anesthesiologists Task force on Perioperative Management of Patients with Obstructive sleep apnea. Practice guidelines for the perioperative management of patients with obstructive sleep apnea: an updated report by the American Society of Anesthesiologists Task Force on Perioperative Management of patients with obstructive sleep apnea. *Anesthesiology*. 2014;120:268–286.
58. Carullo PC, Phillips DP, Abuelkasem E, Hilmi IA. The perioperative application of high flow nasal cannula: a single center experience. *J Anesth Crit Care Open Acess*. 2020;12(1):1–5.
59. Xue FS, Huang YG, Tong SY, et al. A comparative study of early postoperative hypoxemia in infants, children and adults undergoing elective plastic surgery. *Anesth Analg*. 1996;83:709.
60. Moller JT, Johannessen NW, Espersen K, et al. Randomized evaluation of pulse oximetry in 20,802 patients: II. perioperative events and postoperative complications. *Anesthesiology*. 1993;78:445.
61. Xue FS, Li BW, Zhang GS, et al. The influence of surgical sites on early postoperative hypoxemia in adults undergoing elective surgery. *Anesth Analg*. 1999;88:213.
62. Moller JT, Wittrup M, Johansen SH. Hypoxemia in the postanesthesia care unit: An observer study. *Anesthesiology*. 1990;73:890.
63. Ng A, Smith G. Gastroesophageal reflux and aspiration of gastric contents in anesthetic practice. *Anesth Analg*. 2001;93:494.
64. Eriksson LI, Sundman E, Olsson R, et al. Functional assessment of the pharynx at rest and during swallowing in partially paralyzed humans: Simultaneous videomanometry and mechanomyography of awake human volunteers. *Anesthesiology*. 1997;87:1035.
65. Mulroy MF, Salinas FV, Larkin KL, Polissar NL. Ambulatory surgery patients may be discharged before voiding after short-acting spinal and epidural anesthesia. *Anesthesiology*. 2002;97:315.
66. Marshall SI, Chung F. Discharge criteria and complications after ambulatory surgery. *Anesth Analg*. 1999;88:508.
67. Twersky R, Fishman D, Homel P. What happens after discharge? Return hospital visits after ambulatory surgery. *Anesth Analg*. 1997;84:319.
68. Cogliati AA, Vellutini R, Nardini A, et al. Fenoldopam infusion for renal protection in high-risk cardiac surgery patients: A randomized clinical study. *J Cardiothorac Vasc Anesth*. 2007;21:847.
69. Waters JH, Gottlieb A, Schoenwald P, Popovich MJ, Sprung J, Nelson DR. Normal saline versus lactated Ringer's solution for intraoperative fluid management in patients undergoing abdominal aortic aneurysm repair: An outcome study. *Anesth Analg*. 2001;93:817.
70. Moos DD, Lind DM. Detection and treatment of perioperative corneal abrasions. *J Perianesth Nurs*. 2006;21:332.
71. Myers MA, Hamilton SR, Bogosian AJ, Smith CH, Wagner TA. Visual loss as a complication of spine surgery. A review of 37 cases. *Spine*. 1997;22:1325.
72. Warner ME, Warner MA, Garrity JA, MacKenzie RA, Warner DO. The frequency of perioperative vision loss. *Anesth Analg*. 2001;93:1417.
73. Williams EL, Hart WM Jr, Tempelhoff R. Postoperative ischemic optic neuropathy. *Anesth Analg*. 1995;80:1018.
74. Warner ME, Fronapfel PJ, Hebl JR, et al. Perioperative visual changes. *Anesthesiology*. 2002; 96:855.
75. Sprung J, Bourke DL, Contreras MG, Warner ME, Findlay J. Perioperative hearing impairment. *Anesthesiology*. 2003;98:241.
76. Warner ME, Benenfeld SM, Warner MA, Schroeder DR, Maxson PM. Perianesthetic dental injuries: Frequency, outcomes, and risk factors. *Anesthesiology*. 1999;90:1302.
77. Brimacombe J, Holyoake L, Keller C, et al. Pharyngolaryngeal, neck, and jaw discomfort after anesthesia with the face mask and laryngeal mask airway at high and low cuff volumes in males and females. *Anesthesiology*. 2000;93:26.
78. Practice advisory for the prevention of perioperative peripheral neuropathies: A report by the American Society of Anesthesiologists Task Force on Prevention of Perioperative Peripheral Neuropathies. *Anesthesiology*. 2000;92:1168.
79. Cheney FW, Domino KB, Caplan RA, Posner KL. Nerve injury associated with anesthesia: A closed claims analysis. *Anesthesiology*. 1999;90:1062.
80. Warner MA, Warner DO, Matsumoto JY, Harper CM, Schroeder DR, Maxson PM. Ulnar neuropathy in surgical patients. *Anesthesiology*. 1999;90:54.
81. Warner MA. Perioperative neuropathies. *Mayo Clin Proc*. 1998;73:567.
82. Auroy Y, Benhamou D, Bargues L, et al. Major complications of regional anesthesia in France: The SOS regional anesthesia hotline service. *Anesthesiology*. 2002;97:1274.
83. Horlocker TT, McGregor DG, Matsushige DK, Schroeder DR, Besse JA. A retrospective review of 4,767 consecutive spinal anesthetics: Central nervous system complications. Perioperative outcomes group. *Anesth Analg*. 1997;84:578.
84. Schreiber JU, Mencke T, Biedler A, et al. Postoperative myalgia after succinylcholine: No evidence for an inflammatory origin. *Anesth Analg*. 2003;96:1640.
85. Bettelli G. Which muscle relaxants should be used in day surgery and when. *Curr Opin Anaesthesiol*. 2006;19:600.
86. Sessler DI. Complications and treatment of mild hypothermia. *Anesthesiology*. 2001;95:531.
87. Lenhardt R, Marker E, Goll V, et al. Mild intraoperative hypothermia prolongs postanesthetic recovery. *Anesthesiology*. 1997;87:1318.
88. Sun LS, Adams DC, Delphin E, et al. Sympathetic response during cardiopulmonary bypass: Mild versus moderate hypothermia. *Crit Care Med*. 1997;25:1990.
89. Frank SM, Fleisher LA, Breslow MJ, et al. Perioperative maintenance of normothermia reduces the incidence of morbid cardiac events. A randomized clinical trial. *JAMA*. 1997;277:1127.
90. Ammori JB, Sigakis M, Englesbe MJ, O'Reilly M, Pelletier SJ. Effect of intraoperative hyperglycemia during liver transplantation. *J Surg Res*. 2007;140:227.
91. De Witte J, Sessler DI. Perioperative shivering: Physiology and pharmacology. *Anesthesiology*. 2002;96:467.
92. Zelcer J, Wells DG. Anaesthetic-related recovery room complications. *Anaesth Intensive Care*. 1987;15:168.
93. Schubert A, Mascha EJ, Bloomfield EL, DeBoer GE, Gupta MK, Ebrahim ZY. Effect of cranial surgery and brain tumor size on emergence from anesthesia. *Anesthesiology*. 1996;85:513.
94. Wong GY, Warner DO, Schroeder DR, et al. Risk of surgery and anesthesia for ischemic stroke. *Anesthesiology*. 2000;92:425.
95. Kim J, Gelb AW. Predicting perioperative stroke. *J Neurosurg Anesthesiol*. 1995;7:211.
96. Vlajkovic GP, Sindjelic RP. Emergence delirium in children: Many questions, few answers. *Anesth Analg*. 2007;104:84.
97. Voepel-Lewis T, Malviya S, Tait AR. A prospective cohort study of emergence agitation in the pediatric postanesthesia care unit. *Anesth Analg*. 2003;96:1625.
98. Isik B, Arslan M, Tunga AD, Kurtipek O. Dexmedetomidine decreases emergence agitation in pediatric patients after sevoflurane anesthesia without surgery. *Paediatr Anaesth*. 2006;16:748.
99. Abu-Shahwan I, Chowdary K. Ketamine is effective in decreasing the incidence of emergence agitation in children undergoing dental repair under sevoflurane general anesthesia. *Paediatr Anaesth*. 2007;17:846.
100. Schwender D, Kunze-Kronawitter H, Dietrich P, Klasing S, Forst H, Madler C. Conscious awareness during general anaesthesia: Patients' perceptions, emotions, cognition and reactions. *Br J Anaesth*. 1998;80:133.
101. Lynch EP, Lazor MA, Gellis JE, Orav J, Goldman L, Marcantonio ER. The impact of postoperative pain on the development of postoperative delirium. *Anesth Analg*. 1998;86:781.
102. Kopman AF, Yee PS, Neuman GG. Relationship of the train-of-four fade ratio to clinical signs and symptoms of residual paralysis in awake volunteers. *Anesthesiology*. 1997;86:765.
103. Cook DJ, Rooke GA. Priorities in perioperative geriatrics. *Anesth Analg*. 2003;96:1823.
104. Zakriya KJ, Christmas C, Wenz JFS, Franckowiak S, Anderson R, Sieber FE. Preoperative factors associated with postoperative change in confusion assessment method score in hip fracture patients. *Anesth Analg*. 2002;94:1628.
105. Johnson T, Monk T, Rasmussen LS, et al. Postoperative cognitive dysfunction in middle-aged patients. *Anesthesiology*. 2002;96:1351.
106. Dodds C, Allison J. Postoperative cognitive deficit in the elderly surgical patient. *Br J Anaesth*. 1998;81:449.
107. Card E, Pandharipande P, Tomes C, et al. Emergence from general anaesthesia and evolution of delirium signs in the post-anaesthesia car unit. *Br J Anaesth*. 2015;115:411–417.
108. Neufeld KJ, Leotsakos JM, Sieber FE, et al. Outcomes of early delirium diagnosis after general anesthesia in the elderly. *Anesth Analg*. 2013;117:471–478.
109. Kerger H, Turan A, Kredel M, et al. Patients' willingness to pay for anti-emetic treatment. *Acta Anaesthesiol Scand*. 2007;51:38.
110. Sinclair DR, Chung F, Mezei G. Can postoperative nausea and vomiting be predicted? *Anesthesiology*. 1999;91:109.
111. Williams BA, Kentor ML, Vogt MT, et al. Economics of nerve block pain management after anterior cruciate ligament reconstruction: Potential hospital cost savings via associated postanesthesia care unit bypass and same-day discharge. *Anesthesiology*. 2004;100:697.
112. Rappaport BA. FDA response to droperidol black box warning editorials. *Anesth Analg*. 2008;106(5):1585.
113. Charbit B, Albaladejo P, Funck-Brentano C, Legrand M, Samain E, Marty J. Prolongation of QTc interval after postoperative nausea and vomiting treatment by droperidol or ondansetron. *Anesthesiology*. 2005;102(6):1094–1100.
114. Gan TJ, Belani KG, Bergese S, et al. Fourth Consensus Guidelines for the Management of Postoperative Nausea and Vomiting [published correction appears in Anesth Analg. 2020 Nov;131(5):e241]. *Anesth Analg*. 2020;131(2):411–448.
115. Lee A, Done ML. The use of nonpharmacologic techniques to prevent postoperative nausea and vomiting: A meta-analysis. *Anesth Analg*. 1999;88:1362.

55 Acute Pain Management

STEPHEN M. MACRES • USHA SALDANHA • JON Y. ZHOU • ROBERT BISHOP • AMY CHEN

KEY POINTS

1 Inadequate relief of postoperative pain has adverse physiologic effects that can contribute to significant morbidity and mortality, resulting in the delay of patient recovery and return to daily activities.

2 The pain pathway is not "hard wired" and nociceptive input is not passively transmitted from the periphery to the brain. Tissue injury tends to fuel neuroplastic changes within the nervous system, which results in both peripheral and central sensitization.

3 In order for preventive analgesia to be successful, three critical principles must be adhered to: (1) The depth of analgesia must be adequate to block all nociceptive input during surgery, (2) the analgesic technique must be extensive enough to include the entire surgical field, and (3) the duration of analgesia must include both the surgical and postsurgical periods.

4 The various opioid analgesics available today have distinct pharmacologic differences that we can credit to their intricate interaction with the classical three main opioid receptors mu, delta, and kappa (μ, δ, and κ). The opioid receptors are members of a G protein–coupled (guanosine triphosphate regulatory proteins) receptor family, which signals via a second messenger such as cyclic adenosine monophosphate or an ion channel.

5 Opioid-sparing multimodal pharmacotherapy, regional anesthesia techniques, and the continuous monitoring of patient ventilation with pulse oximetry and capnography can decrease the risk of opioid-related respiratory depression, particularly in high-risk individuals.

6 The therapeutic benefit of nonsteroidal anti-inflammatory drugs is believed to be mediated through the inhibition of cyclooxygenase enzymes, types 1 and 2, which convert arachidonic acid to prostaglandins.

7 Short-term use of parecoxib and valdecoxib in patients following coronary artery bypass surgery is associated with an increased risk of thromboembolic events. The authors, therefore, do not recommend prescribing a cyclooxygenase-2 inhibitor for patients with a known history of coronary artery disease or cerebrovascular disease.

8 The five variables associated with all modes of patient-controlled analgesia include (1) bolus dose, (2) incremental (demand) dose, (3) lockout interval, (4) background infusion rate, and (5) 1- and 4-hour limits. A typical patient-controlled analgesia regimen in an otherwise healthy adult would be an incremental dose of 1 to 2 mg of morphine with an 8- to 10-minute lockout. The authors do not recommend a background infusion of opioid in the opioid-naive patient.

9 Epidural analgesia is a critical component of multimodal perioperative pain management and improved patient outcome. Meta-analyses investigating the efficacy of epidural analgesia found epidural analgesia to be superior to systemically administered opioids.

10 The opioid-dependent patient is often identified just moments prior to surgery and the anesthesia team needs to be innovative. The anesthesiologist needs to be flexible enough to tailor an individual anesthetic that incorporates a multimodal approach, combining regional anesthesia with general anesthesia and nonopioid coanalgesics with opioid analgesics. Opioids remain the mainstay of perioperative pain management, and an adequate dose of opioid needs to be maintained to avoid precipitating withdrawal symptoms.

11 Perioperative management of the opioid-tolerant patient requires prudent use of both opioid and nonopioid analgesics as well as the application of site-specific regional anesthesia/analgesia.

12 Establishing a successful perioperative pain management service begins with an institutional commitment to support the service. The team must be built around a physician leader with training and experience in pain medicine. There must be other anesthesiologists available to support the service.

Globally, over 300 million surgical procedures are performed each year, and many are performed in the inpatient setting.[1] Appropriate management of acute perioperative pain using multimodal opioid-sparing analgesia is therefore crucial. In 2012, the American Society of Anesthesiologists developed treatment guidelines for acute postoperative pain, which was updated and amended in a document promulgated by the American society of Pain Medicine, the American Society of Regional Anesthesia (ASRA), and the American Society of Anesthesiologists in 2016.[2] Soon thereafter, the U.S. Health and Human Services (HHS) Pain Management Best Practices Inter-Agency Task Force published acute pain guidelines that emphasized the importance of opioid-sparing multimodal management of acute perioperative pain.[3] Despite significant advances in our knowledge and treatment of acute pain and dissemination of these guidelines, significant deficits continue to persist, and the management of acute postoperative pain is still less than optimal.

Inadequate relief of postoperative pain has adverse physiologic effects that can contribute to significant morbidity and mortality, resulting in the delay of patient recovery and return to daily activities.[4] In addition, poor postoperative pain control contributes to patient dissatisfaction with the surgical experience and may have adverse psychological consequences.[5] Poorly managed postoperative pain can also increase the incidence of persistent postoperative pain conditions. Because aggressive management of acute postoperative pain is so beneficial, guidelines continue to be updated and we are fortunate that a multisociety collaborative effort was undertaken in 2021, which developed seven guiding principles for the management of acute perioperative pain (Table 55-1).[6]

1 The inadequate relief of postoperative pain has adverse physiologic effects that can contribute to significant morbidity and mortality, resulting in the delay of patient recovery and return to daily activities.[4] In addition, poor postoperative pain control contributes to patient dissatisfaction with the surgical experience and may have adverse psychological consequences.[5] Poorly managed postoperative pain can also increase the incidence of persistent postoperative pain conditions.

Table 55-1 Guiding Principles for Acute Perioperative Pain Management

1. Conduct a preoperative evaluation including assessment of medical and psychologic conditions, concomitant medications, history of chronic pain, substance abuse disorder, and previous postoperative treatment regimens and responses, to guide the perioperative pain management plan.
2. Use a validated pain assessment tool to track responses to postoperative pain treatments and adjust treatment plans accordingly.
3. Offer multimodal analgesia, or the use of a variety of analgesic medications and techniques combined with nonpharmacologic interventions, for the treatment.
4. Provide patient- and family-centered individually tailored education to the patient (and/or responsible caregiver), including information on treatment options for managing postoperative.
5. Provide education to all patients (adult) and primary caregivers on the pain treatment plan, including proper storage and disposal of opioids and tapering.
6. Adjust the pain management plan based on adequacy of pain relief and presence of adverse events.
7. Have access to consultation with a pain specialist for patients who have inadequately controlled postoperative pain or are at high risk of inadequately controlled postoperative.

Reproduced with Mariano ER, Dickerson DM, Szokol JW, et al. A multisociety organizational consensus process to define guiding principles for acute perioperative pain management. *Reg Anesth Pain Med.* 2022;47:118–127, with permission from BMJ Publishing Group Ltd.

Acute Pain Defined

Acute pain is defined as "an unpleasant sensory and emotional experience associated with, or resembling that associated with, actual or potential tissue damage."[7] In general, acute pain resolves within 1 month. However, poorly managed acute pain that might occur following surgery can produce pathophysiologic processes in both the peripheral and central nervous systems that have the potential to produce chronicity.[5] Acute pain–induced change in the central nervous system is known as *neuronal plasticity*. This can cause sensitization of the nervous system, resulting in allodynia and hyperalgesia. Surgical procedures that can be associated with chronic painful conditions include amputation of a limb, lateral thoracotomy, inguinal herniorrhaphy, abdominal hysterectomy, saphenous vein stripping, open cholecystectomy, nephrectomy, and mastectomy.[5]

Anatomy of Acute Pain

The nociceptive pathway is an afferent (Fig. 55-1, 1 Video 55-1) three-neuron, dual-ascending (i.e., anterolateral and dorsal column medial lemniscal pathways) system, with descending modulation

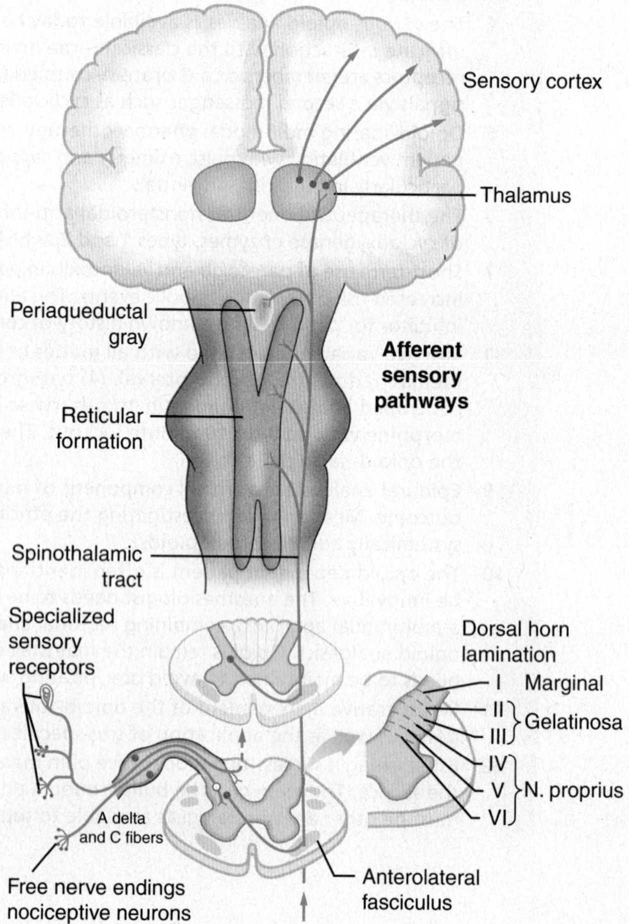

Figure 55-1 Afferent nociceptive pathway.

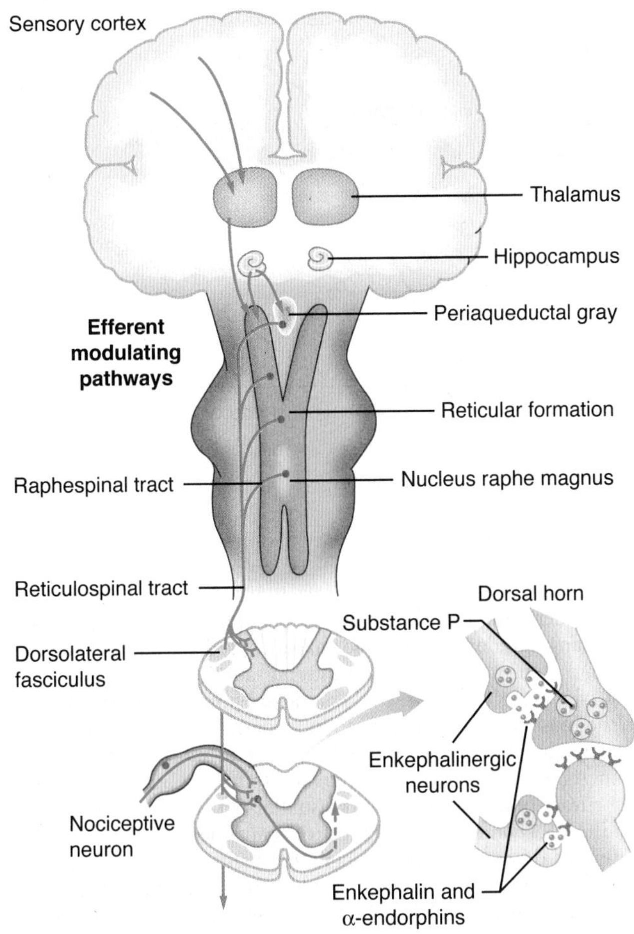

Figure 55-2 Efferent pathways involved in nociceptive regulation.

Table 55-2 Primary Afferent Nerves

Fiber Class[a]	Velocity	Effective Stimuli
Aβ (myelinated) (12–20 μ dia)	Group II (>40–50 m/s)	Low-threshold mechanoreceptors Specialized nerve endings (Pacinian corpuscles)
Aδ (myelinated) (1–4 μ dia)	Group III (10 < x < 40 m/s)	Low-threshold mechanical or thermal High-threshold mechanical or thermal Specialized nerve endings
C (unmyelinated) (0.5–1.5 μ dia)	Group IV (<2 m/s)	High-threshold thermal, mechanical, and chemical Free nerve endings

[a]Aβ/Aδ/C is the Erlanger–Gasser classification and refers to axon size; II/III/IV is the Lloyd–Hunt classification and is defined on conduction velocity in muscle afferents. Because of the relationship between size and state of myelination with conduction velocity, these designations are often used interchangeably.

Reprinted with permission from Warfield CA, Bajwa ZH, eds. *Principles and Practice of Pain Medicine*. 2nd ed. McGraw-Hill; 2004:14. Table 1.1.

(Fig. 55-2) from the cortex, thalamus, and brainstem.[8] Nociceptors are free nerve endings located in skin, muscle, bone, and connective tissue with cell bodies located in the dorsal root ganglia. The first-order neurons that make up the dual ascending system have their origins in the periphery as A delta (Aδ) and polymodal C fibers (Table 55-2). Aδ fibers transmit "first pain," which is described as sharp or stinging in nature and is well localized. Polymodal C fibers transmit "second pain," which is more diffuse in nature and is associated with the affective and motivational aspects of pain. First-order neurons synapse on second-order neurons in the dorsal horn primarily within laminas I, II, and V, where they release excitatory amino acids and neuropeptides (Figs. 55-3 and 55-4). Some fibers can ascend or descend in the Lissauer tract prior to terminating on neurons that project to higher centers. Second-order neurons consist of nociceptive-specific and wide dynamic-range (WDR) neurons. Nociceptive-specific neurons are located primarily in lamina I, respond only to noxious stimuli, and are thought to be involved in the sensory-discriminative aspects of pain. WDR neurons are predominately located in laminae IV, V, and VI, respond to both nonnoxious and noxious input, and are involved with the affective–motivational component of pain. Axons of both nociceptive-specific and WDR neurons ascend the spinal cord via the dorsal column–medial lemniscus and the anterior lateral spinothalamic tract to synapse on third-order neurons in the contralateral thalamus, which then project to the somatosensory cortex, where nociceptive input is perceived as pain (Fig. 55-1).

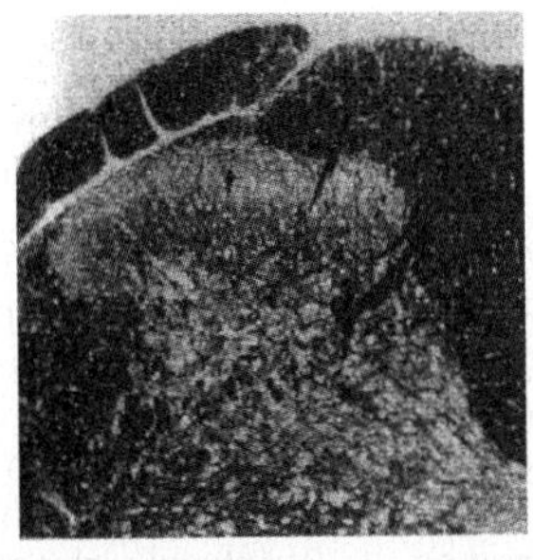

Figure 55-3 Schematic on the right showing the Rexed lamination and the approximate organization of the approach of the afferent to the spinal cord as they enter at the dorsal root entry zone and then penetrate into the dorsal horn to terminate in laminae I and II (A/C) or penetrate more deeply to loop upward to terminate as high as the dorsum of lamina III (Aβ). Inset on the left shows the histologic appearance of the left dorsal quadrant, and large, myelinated axons. (Reprinted with permission from Warfield CA, Bajwa ZH, eds. *Principles and Practice of Pain Medicine*. 2nd ed. McGraw-Hill; 2004:17. Figure 1.5.)

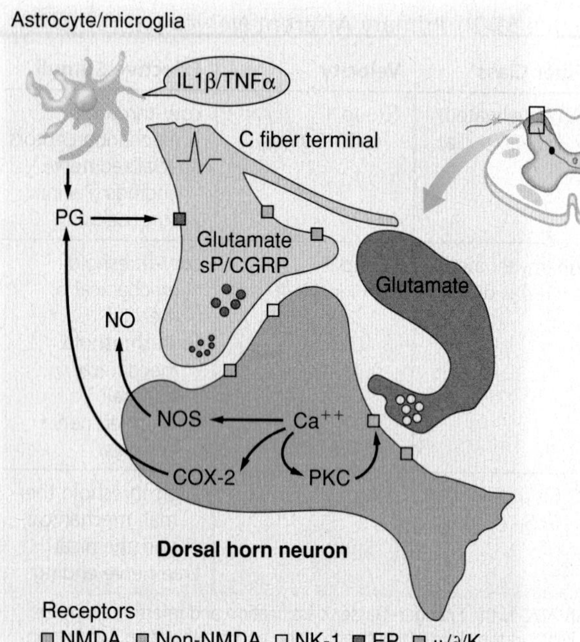

Figure 55-4 Schematic summarizing the organization of dorsal horn systems that contribute to the processing of nociceptive information. (1) Primary afferent C fibers release peptide (e.g., substance P [sP], calcitonin gene–related peptide [CGRP], and so on) and excitatory amino acid (glutamate) products. Small dorsal root ganglion (DRG) cells, as well as some postsynaptic elements, contain nitric oxide synthase (NOS) and are able, upon depolarization, to release NO (nitric oxide). (2) Peptides and excitatory amino acids evoke excitation in second-order neurons. For glutamate, direct monosynaptic excitation is mediated by non–*N*-methyl-D-aspartate (NMDA) receptors (i.e., acute primary afferent excitation of WDR neurons is not mediated by the NMDA or neurokinin 1 [NK-1] receptor). (3) Interneurons excited by afferent barrage induce excitation in second-order neurons via an NMDA receptor. This leads to a marked increase in intracellular Ca^2+ and the activation of kinases and phosphorylating enzymes. Prostaglandins (PGs) generated by cyclooxygenase-2 (COX-2) and NO by NOS are formed and released. These agents diffuse extracellularly and facilitate transmitter release (retrograde transmission) from primary and nonprimary afferent terminals, either by a direct cellular action (e.g., NO) or by an interaction with a specific class of receptors (e.g., EP receptors for prostanoids). (4) Non-neuronal sources of prostaglandins may include activated astrocytes and microglia that are stimulated by circulating cytokines, which are released secondary to peripheral nerve injury and inflammation. Terminal excitability can be altered by activation of a variety of receptors located on the sensory terminal, including those for, μ-, δ-, and κ-opioids. (Reprinted with permission from Warfield CA, Bajwa ZH, eds. *Principles and Practice of Pain Medicine*. 2nd ed. McGraw-Hill; 2004:17. Figure 1.6.)

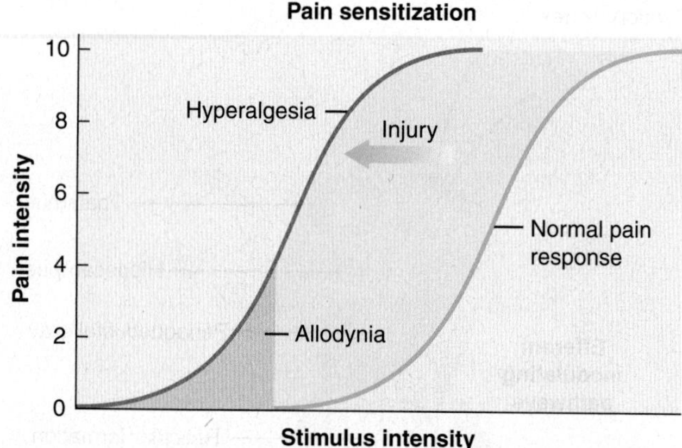

Figure 55-5 Pain sensitization. (Courtesy of Dave Klemm.)

Pain Processing

2 A key development in our understanding of pain processing is that the pain pathway is not "hard wired" and nociceptive input is not passively transmitted from the periphery to the brain (2 Video 55-2).[9] Tissue injury tends to fuel neuroplastic changes within the nervous system, which results in both peripheral and central sensitization. Clinically, this can manifest as *hyperalgesia,* which is defined as an exaggerated pain response to a normally painful stimulus, and *allodynia,* which is defined as a painful response to a typically nonpainful stimulus (Fig. 55-5).[9]

The four elements of pain processing include (1) transduction, (2) transmission, (3) modulation, and (4) perception (Fig. 55-6, 3 Video 55-3). *Transduction* is the event whereby noxious thermal, chemical, or mechanical stimuli are converted into an action potential. *Transmission* occurs when the action potential is conducted through the nervous system via the first-, second-, and third-order neurons, which have cell bodies located in the dorsal root ganglion, dorsal horn, and thalamus, respectively. *Modulation* of pain transmission involves altering afferent neural transmission along the pain pathway. The dorsal horn of the spinal cord is the most common site for modulation of the pain pathway, and modulation can involve either *inhibition* or *augmentation* of the pain signals.[8] Examples of *inhibitory* spinal modulation include (1) release of inhibitory neurotransmitters such as γ-amino butyric acid (GABA) and glycine by intrinsic spinal neurons, and (2) activation of descending efferent neuronal pathways from the motor cortex, hypothalamus, periaqueductal gray matter, and the nucleus raphe magnus, which results in the release of norepinephrine, serotonin, and endorphins in the dorsal horn. Spinal modulation, which results in *augmentation* of pain pathways, is manifested as central sensitization, which is a consequence of neuronal plasticity. The phenomenon of "wind-up" is a specific example of central plasticity that results from repetitive C-fiber stimulation of WDR neurons in the dorsal horn. *Perception* of pain is the final common pathway, which results from the integration of painful input into the somatosensory and limbic cortices. In general, traditional analgesic therapies have only targeted pain *perception.* A *multimodal approach* to pain therapy should target all four elements of the pain-processing pathway.

Chemical Mediators of Transduction and Transmission

Tissue damage following surgical procedures leads to the activation of small nociceptive nerve endings and local inflammatory cells (e.g., macrophages, mast cells, lymphocytes, and platelets) in the periphery. Antidromic release of substance P and glutamate from small nociceptive afferents results in vasodilation, extravasation of plasma proteins, and stimulation of inflammatory cells to release numerous algogenic substances (Table 55-3 and Fig. 55-7). This chemical milieu will both directly produce pain transduction via nociceptor stimulation as well as facilitate pain transduction by increasing the excitability of nociceptors. *Peripheral sensitization* of polymodal C fibers and high-threshold mechanoreceptors by these chemicals leads to *primary hyperalgesia,* which is an exaggerated response to pain at the site of injury.

As is the case in the periphery, the dorsal horn of the spinal cord contains numerous transmitters and receptors involved in

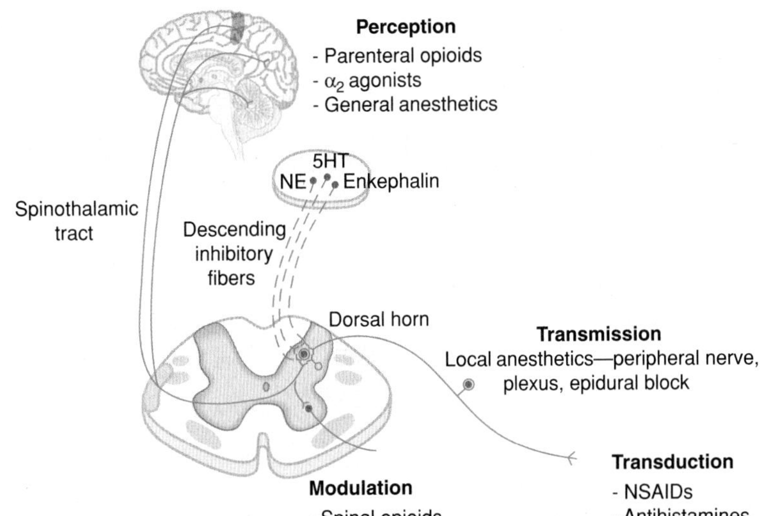

Figure 55-6 The four elements of pain processing: transduction, transmission, modulation, and perception. 5HT, serotonin; NE, norepinephrine; NMDA, *N*-methyl-D-aspartate; NSAIDs, nonsteroidal anti-inflammatory drugs; CCK, cholecystokinin; NO, nitric oxide.

pain processing. Three classes of transmitter compounds integral to pain transmission include (1) the excitatory amino acids glutamate and aspartate, (2) the excitatory neuropeptides substance P and neurokinin A, and (3) the inhibitory amino acids glycine and GABA. The various pain receptors include (1) the *N*-methyl-D-aspartate (NMDA), (2) the α-amino-3-hydroxy-5-methylisoxazole-4-propionic acid (AMPA), (3) the kainate receptor, and (4) the metabotropic receptor (Fig. 55-8).

The AMPA and kainate receptors, which are sodium channel dependent, are essential for fast synaptic afferent input. On the other hand, the NMDA receptor, which is calcium channel dependent is only activated following prolonged depolarization of the cell membrane. Release of substance P into the spinal cord will remove the magnesium block on the channel of the NMDA receptor, giving glutamate free access to the NMDA receptor. Repetitive C-fiber stimulation of WDR neurons in the dorsal horn at intervals of 0.5 to 1 Hz can precipitate the occurrence of windup and *central sensitization* (Fig. 55-9). This leads to *secondary hyperalgesia*, which, by definition, is an increased pain response evoked by stimuli outside the area of injury.

Table 55-3 Algogenic Substances

Substance	Source	Effect
Bradykinin	Macrophages and plasma kininogen	Activates nociceptors
Serotonin	Platelets	Activates nociceptors
Histamine	Platelets and mast cells	Produces vasodilation, edema, and pruritus Potentiates the response of nociceptors to bradykinin
Prostaglandin	Tissue injury and cyclooxygenase pathway	Sensitizes nociceptors
Leukotriene	Tissue injury and lipooxygenase pathway	Sensitizes nociceptors
Excess H+ ions	Tissue injury and ischemia	Increases pain and hyperalgesia associated with inflammation
Cytokines (e.g., interleukins and tissue necrosis factor)	Macrophages	Excites and sensitizes nociceptors
Adenosine	Tissue injury	Pain and hyperalgesia
Neurotransmitters (e.g., glutamate and substance P)	Antidromic release by peripheral nerve terminals following tissue injury	Substance P activates macrophages and mast cells Glutamate activates nociceptors
Nerve growth factor	Macrophages	Stimulates mast cells to release histamine and serotonin Induces heat hyperalgesia Sensitizes nociceptors

Adapted from Dougherty PM, Raja SN. Neurochemistry of Somatosensory and Pain Processing. In: Benzon HT, Raja SN, Molloy RE, et al., eds. *Essentials of Pain Medicine and Regional Anesthesia*. 2nd ed. Philadelphia, PA: Elsevier; 2005:7. Copyright © 2005 Elsevier. With permission.

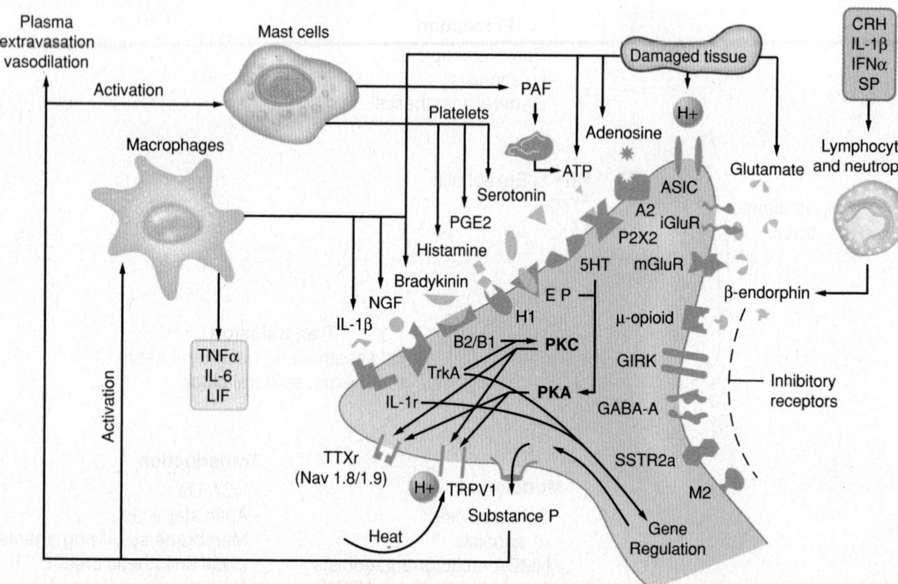

Figure 55-7 Schematic of the neurochemistry of somatosensory processing at peripheral sensory nerve endings. (Adapted from Dougherty PM, Raja SN. Neurochemistry of Somatosensory and Pain Processing. In: Benzon HT, Raja SN, Molloy RE, et al., eds. *Essentials of Pain Medicine and Regional Anesthesia*. 2nd ed. Philadelphia, PA: Elsevier; 2005:8. Copyright © 2005 Elsevier. With permission.)

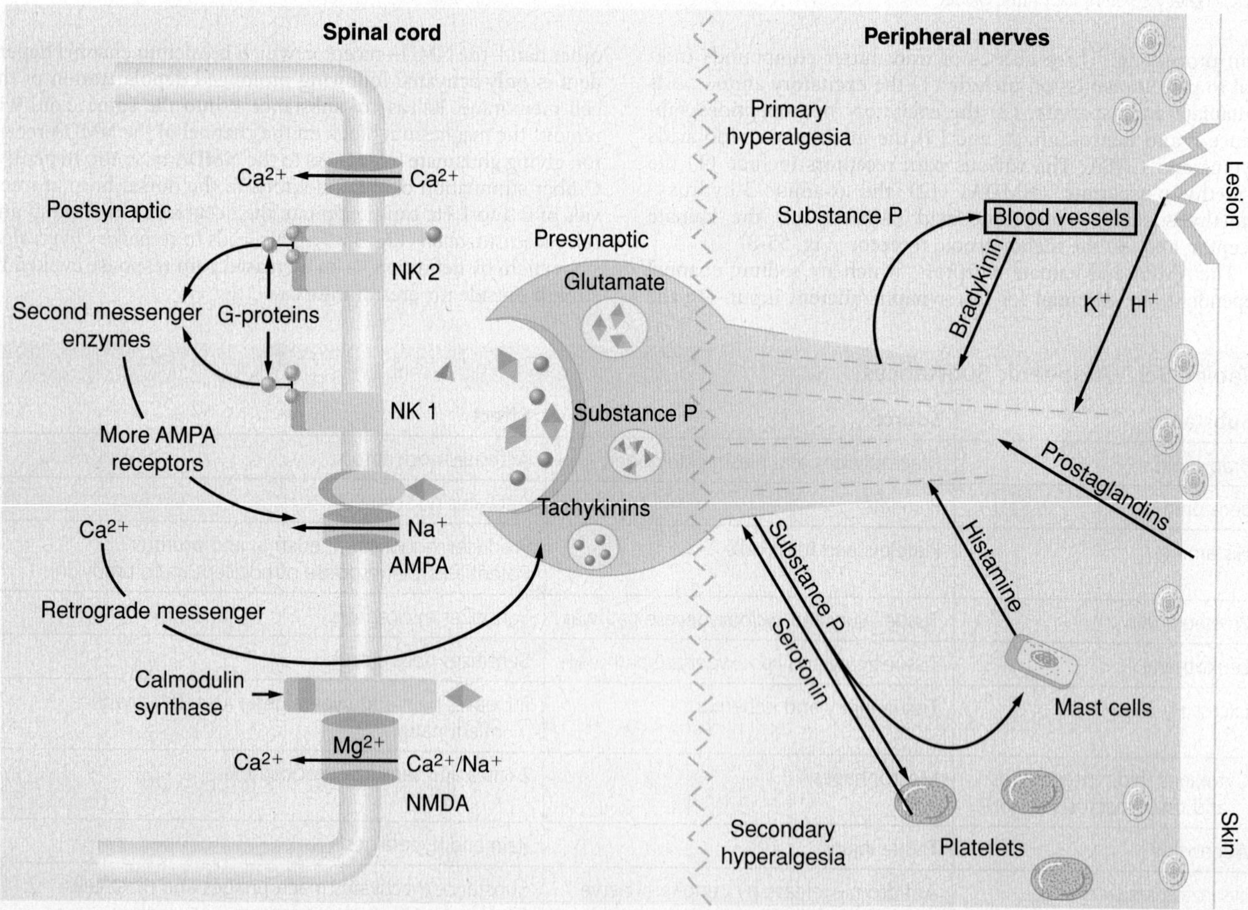

Figure 55-8 Schematic representation of peripheral and spinal mechanism involved in neuroplasticity. Primary hyperalgesia results from tissue release of toxic substances. These toxic substances spread to adjacent tissues, prolonging the hyperalgesic state (secondary hyperalgesia). As C fiber terminals increase in frequency of release of neurotransmitters, such as glutamate, substance P, tachykinins, brain-derived neurotrophic factor, and calcitonin gene–related peptide, the effects of these neurotransmitters are summated, resulting in prolonged depolarizations of second-order neurons (wind-up). Function changes at the second-order neuron occur as a result of neurotransmitter binding to postsynaptic receptors, which results in activity-dependent plasticity of the spinal cord. AMPA, α-amino-3-hydroxy-5-methyl-4-isoxazole propionic acid; NK, neurokinin; NMDA, *N*-methyl-D-aspartate.

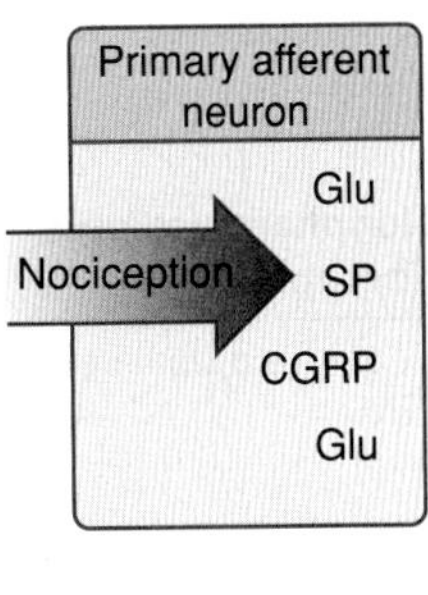

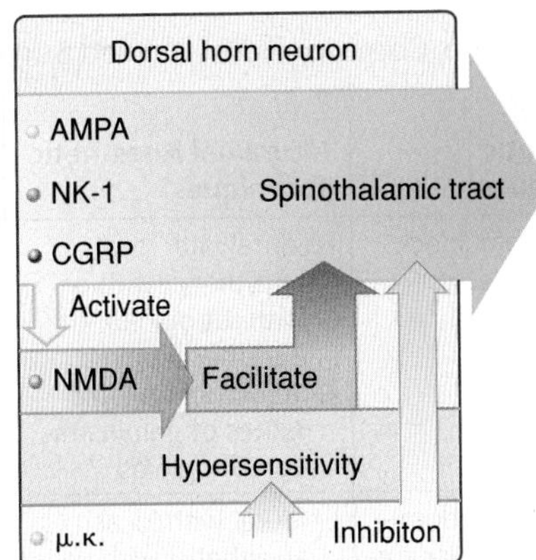

Figure 55-9 Primary nociceptive transmission in the spinal cord. Primary afferent nociceptive input is transmitted via α-amino-3-hydroxy-5-methyl-4-isoxazole propionic acid (AMPA), neurokinin-1 (NK1), and calcitonin gene–related peptide (CGRP) synapses, whose signals work their way to the thalamus. Glutaminergic (*N*-methyl-D-aspartate [NMDA]) synapses do not participate significantly in primary nociceptive transmission, but instead play a crucial role in spinal sensitization. Accordingly, even after complete NMDA blockade in the spinal cord, primary afferent nociceptive information is transmitted to the thalamus. NMDA antagonists thus have an antihyperalgesic rather than an analgesic effect in the spinal cord. Glu, glutamate; SP, substance P. (Adapted with permission from the International Association for the Study of Pain. Pain control updates. *IASP Newletter*. 2005;13[2]:3.)

The Surgical Stress Response

Although similar, postoperative pain and the surgical stress response are not the same. Surgical stress causes release of cytokines (e.g., interleukin-1, interleukin-6, and tumor necrosis factor-α) and precipitates adverse neuroendocrine and sympathoadrenal responses, resulting in detrimental physiologic responses, particularly in high-risk patient.[5]

The increased secretion of catabolic hormones such as cortisol, glucagon, growth hormone, and catecholamines and the decreased secretion of anabolic hormones such as insulin and testosterone characterize the neuroendocrine response. This results in hyperglycemia and a negative nitrogen balance, the consequences of which include poor wound healing, muscle wasting, fatigue, and impaired immunocompetency. The sympathoadrenal response has detrimental effects on numerous organ systems[10]; these are listed in Table 55-4.

Preventive Analgesia

3 Preventive analgesia includes any antinociceptive regimen delivered at any time during the perioperative period that will attenuate pain-induced sensitization. The term "preventive analgesia" replaces the older terminology "preemptive analgesia," which is defined as an analgesic regimen that is administered prior to surgical incision and is more effective at pain relief than the same regimen administered after surgery. Although use of the term preemptive analgesia has been popular in the past, evidence of its clinical benefit in humans has been mixed and the term should be considered obsolete.[11] The goal of preventive analgesia is to block the development of sustained pain. Theoretically, this occurs by preventing NMDA receptor activation in the dorsal horn that is associated with wind-up, facilitation, central sensitization expansion of receptive fields, and long-term potentiation, all of which can lead to a chronic pain state.[9] In order for preventive analgesia to be successful, three critical principles must be adhered to: (1) the depth of analgesia must be adequate enough to block all nociceptive input during surgery, (2) the analgesic technique must be extensive enough to include the entire surgical field and (3) the duration of analgesia must include both the surgical and postsurgical periods. Patients with pre-existing chronic pain may not respond as well to these techniques because of pre-existing sensitization of the nervous system.[11]

Table 55-4 Consequences of Poorly Managed Acute Pain[5,10]

Cardiovascular	Tachycardia, hypertension, and increase in cardiac workload
Pulmonary	Respiratory muscle spasm (splinting), decrease in vital capacity, atelectasis, hypoxia, and increased risk of pulmonary infection
Gastrointestinal	Postoperative ileus
Renal	Increased risk of oliguria and urinary retention
Coagulation	Increased risk of thromboemboli
Immunologic	Impaired immune function
Muscular	Muscle weakness and fatigue. Limited mobility can increase the risk of thromboembolism
Psychological	Anxiety, fear, and frustration results in poor patient satisfaction

Strategies for Acute Pain Management

Most postoperative pain is nociceptive in character, but there are a small percentage of patients who can experience neuropathic pain postoperatively. It is critical to recognize this fact because patients with neuropathic pain are at increased risk of progressing to a chronic pain state. Neuropathic pain is a result of accidental nerve injury secondary to cutting, traction, compression, or entrapment.[5] Clinical features may include continuous burning, paroxysmal shooting, or electric pain with associated allodynia, hyperalgesia, and dysesthesias. There can be a delay in the onset of the pain, and it can follow a nondermatomal distribution. Surgical procedures that are a relatively high risk for neuropathic pain include limb amputations, breast surgery, gallbladder surgery, thoracic surgery, and inguinal hernia repair.[5] Nociceptive pain responds best to opioids, nonsteroidal anti-inflammatory drugs (NSAIDs), para-aminophenol agents, and regional anesthesia techniques.[12] Neuropathic pain, on the other hand, may benefit from the addition of the nonopioid analgesic adjuvants such as the NMDA receptor antagonists, α_2-agonists, and the α_2–δ subunit calcium channel ligands, which will be discussed in detail. The recommended components for multimodal perioperative pain management of routinely performed surgical procedures are listed in Table 55-5.[2] The reader is also referred to an excellent and timely review of fascial plane chest wall blocks for coronary artery bypass surgery by Kelava M and colleagues.[13] For specific dosing recommendations of both opioids and nonopioid analgesics during preoperative, intraoperative, and postoperative phases of care, refer to Tables 55-6 to 55.8.[14]

Table 55-5 Options for Components of Multimodal Therapy for Commonly Performed Surgeries

Type of Surgery	Systemic Pharmacologic Therapy	Local, Intra-articular, or Topical Techniques[a]	Regional Anesthetic Techniques[a]	Neuraxial Anesthetic Techniques[a]	Nonpharmacologic Therapies
Thoracotomy	Opioids[b] NSAIDs[c] and/or acetaminophen Gabapentin or pregabalin[c] IV ketamine[d]		Paravertebral block Consider erector spinae block	Epidural with local anesthetic (with or without opioid), or intrathecal opioid Note: Avoid multiple routes of adminstration of opioids	Cognitive modalities TENS
Open laparotomy	Opioids[b] NSAIDs[c] and/or acetaminophen Gabapentin or pregabalin[c] IV ketamine IV lidocaine infusion	Local anesthetic at incision	Transversus abdominis plane block for incision below the umbilicus. Rectus sheath block for midline incision	Epidural with local anesthetic (with or without opioid), or intrathecal opioid Note: Avoid multiple routes of adminstration of opioids	Cognitive modalities TENS
Total hip replacement	Opioids[b] NSAIDs[c] and/or acetaminophen Gabapentin or pregabalin[c] IV ketamine[d]	Intra-articular local anesthetic and/or opioid	Site-specific regional anesthetic technique with local anesthetic (e.g., fascia iliaca block or PENG block)	Epidural with local anesthetic (with or without opioid), or intrathecal opioid Note: Avoid multiple routes of adminstration of opioids	Cognitive modalities TENS
Total knee replacement	Opioids[b] NSAIDs[c] and/or acetaminophen Gabapentin or pregabalin[c] IV ketamine[d]	Intra-articular local anesthetic and/or opioid	Site-specific regional anesthetic technique with local anesthetic (Adductor canal block, local infiltration, and iPACK block)	Epidural with local anesthetic (with or without opioid), or intrathecal opioid Note: Avoid multiple routes of administration of opioids	Cognitive modalities TENS
Spinal fusion	Opioids[b] Acetaminophen[e] Gabapentin or pregabalin[c] IV ketamine[d]	Local anesthetic at incision	Erector spinae plane block for lumbar spine surgery	Epidural with local anesthetic (with or without opioid), or intrathecal opioid Note: Avoid multiple routes of administration of opioids	Cognitive modalities TENS
Cesarean section	Opioids[b] NSAIDs[c] and/or acetaminophen	Local anesthetic at incision	Transversus abdominal plane block	Epidural with local anesthetic (with or without opioid), or intrathecal opioid Note: Avoid multiple routes of administration of opioids	Cognitive modalities TENS
Coronary artery bypass grafting	Opioids[b] Acetaminophen Gabapentin or pregabalin[c] IV ketamine[d]		Fascial plane chest wall blocks[13]	Note: Avoid multiple routes of administration of opioids	Cognitive modalities TENS

Blank cells indicate techniques generally not used for the procedure in question.
[a]Intra-articular, peripheral regional, and neuraxial techniques typically not used together.
[b]Use IV PCA when parenteral route needed for more than a few hours and patients have adequate cognitive function to understand the device and safety limitations.
[c]May be administered preoperatively.
[d]On the basis of panel consensus, primarily consider for use in opioid-tolerant or otherwise complex patients.
[e]Use as adjunctive treatments.
NSAIDs, nonsteroidal anti-inflammatory drugs; TENS, transcutaneous electrical nerve stimulation.
Reprinted from Chou R, Gordon DB, de Leon-Casasola OA, et al. Management of postoperative pain: a clinical practice guideline from the American Pain Society, the American Society of Regional Anesthesia and Pain Medicine, and the American Society of Anesthesiologists' Committee on Regional Anesthesia, Executive Committee, and Administrative Council. *J Pain*. 2016;17(2):131–157. Copyright © 2016 Elsevier. With permission.

Table 55-6 Guidelines for Preoperative Analgesia

Drug	Dosing Guidelines	Comments
Acetaminophen	975 mg IV adult dose	Avoid in patients with acute decompensated liver failure.
Celecoxib	400 mg po for age <65 y 200 mg po for age >65 y	Avoid in patients with pre-existing renal failure.
Gabapentin	300 mg po for age <65 y 100–300 mg po for age >65 y	Adjust dose in patients with renal failure since the drug is 100% cleared by the kidneys.

Adapted from Hyland SJ, Brockhaus KK, Vincent WR, et al. Perioperative pain management and opioid stewardship: a practical guide. *Healthcare*. 2021; 9(3):333.

Table 55-7 Guidelines for Intraoperative Multimodal Analgesia

Drug	Dosing (Intravenous)	Benefits	Comments
Lidocaine	Dosing is based on ideal body weight. Bolus: 0.5–1.5 mg/kg Infusion: 1–1.5 mg/kg/h The infusion may be continued postoperatively on a monitored floor per institution protocol.	Opioid sparing and hastens bowel recovery.	Avoid in patients with cardiac abnormalities, seizure disorder, electrolyte imbalance, and pregnancy. Do not combine with local anesthetic based regional anesthesia or topical lidocaine patches.
Ketamine	Bolus: 0.1–0.35 mg/kg Infusion: 0.1–1 mg/kg/h May consider postoperative infusion in a monitored setting per institution protocol.	Opioid sparing. Useful in the opioid-tolerant patient.	Avoid in patients with psychiatric disturbance, cardiovascular or hepatic disease and in pregnancy.
Magnesium	Bolus: 1–3 g Infusion: 0.5–1 g	Opioid sparing	Avoid in: Renal insufficiency, neuromuscular disorders, electrolyte imbalance, bradyarrhythmias, hypotension, and hemodynamic compromise.
Dexmedetomidine	Bolus: 0.5–0.6 mcg/kg Infusion: 0.3–1 mcg/kg/h	Opioid sparing Useful perineural adjunct for nerve block.	Monitor carefully. Hypotension and bradycardia are common side effects
Esmolol	Bolus: 500 mcg/kg Infusion: 5–50 mcg/kg/min	Maybe opioid sparing but evidence is limited.	Avoid in patients who are receiving concomitant β-blocking or AV nodal blocking therapies.
Dexamethasone	1–10 mg (usual dosing range is 0.1–0.2 mg/kg) once at the beginning of the case.	Opioid sparing Anti-emetic Anti-inflammatory Useful perineural adjunct for nerve block.	Systemic administration can cause hyperglycemia and demargination of white cells.
Methadone	0.1–0.3 mg/kg (do not exceed 30 mg) once at the beginning of the case	Methadone has NMDA receptor antagonist effects and may be helpful with neuropathic pain much like ketamine.	Causes QTc prolongation. Plasma half-life is long so you must monitor for respiratory depression.

NOTE: mg, milligram; mcg, microgram.
Adapted from Hyland SJ, Brockhaus KK, Vincent WR, et al. Perioperative pain management and opioid stewardship: a practical guide. *Healthcare*. 2021; 9(3):333.

Table 55-8 Guidelines for Postoperative Inpatient Analgesia

Drug	Dosing Guidelines	Comments
Acetaminophen (APAP)	650 mg po q4h while awake or, 975 mg po q6h.	Consider intravenous dosing in the patient who is npo.
Anti-inflammatory		
Celecoxib	100–200 mg po q12–24h	COX-II inhibitors may be preferred over ibuprofen
Meloxicam		No current recommendations
Ibuprofen	400 mg po TID or q6h with meals	
Ketorolac	15 mg IV q 6 h × 24 h	Not recommended for more than 5 d. Adjust dose in renal failure.
Gabapentinoid		
Gabapentin	100 mg po TID or 100 mg po at breakfast and lunch then 300 mg po at qhs.	May be dosed just at bedtime particularly if the drug causes too much sedation during the day.
Pregabalin	25–50 mg po BID	Although gabapentinoids are opioid sparing, they can cause excessive sedation and respiratory depression when combined with opioids. Be judicious when combining the two drugs.
Oxycodone	Opioid-naivepatient: 5-mg po q4h prn moderate to severe pain.	Opioid-tolerant patient: initial dosing should take into account the patients daily oral morphine equivalent.
Hydrocodone	Same dosing as with oxycodone	In the United States, this product is combined with acetaminophen. Avoid concurrent dosing with po or IV acetaminophen.
NMDA Receptor Antagonist		
Ketamine	Bolus dose: 0.1–0.35 mg/kg or 5–10 mg IVP once or q2h PRN for refractory pain. Consult acute pain service for specific guidelines.	Continuous infusion: 0.05—0.35 mg/kg/h (0.83—5.83 mcg/kg/min) May be administered postoperatively on a monitored floor per institution protocol.

Adapted from Hyland SJ, Brockhaus KK, Vincent WR, et al. Perioperative pain management and opioid stewardship: a practical guide. *Healthcare*. 2021; 9(3):333.

Assessment of Acute Pain

The need for assessment of the patient in pain is illustrated by the postoperative patient who is said to be relatively pain free, but who, on inspection, is lying almost completely still in bed (4 Video 55-4). Too often, such a patient has had a recent cursory evaluation that included the traditional verbal analog score (VAS) 0 to 10 scale ("on a scale of 0 to 10, with 0 being no pain and 10 being the worst pain you can imagine, how much pain are you in" from which the patient reported a low VAS score of 1/10) (Fig. 55-10). The treating team took that to be reassuring information and moved along. No one asked the patient about pain with movement, breathing, moving bowels, and so forth, all potentially important functional goals for the postoperative course that may be undermined by untreated pain.

A variety of well-studied pain measurement scales exist that can be helpful yet are not definitive. Unidimensional instruments such as the familiar numerical pain scale already mentioned, the visual analog scale, and the "faces" (Fig. 55-10) pain-rating scale can provide some degree of guidance about a patient's experience of pain, but all of these are completely subjective and are open to wide variation between subjects and within subjects at different times.

Multidimensional instruments, such as the Mcgill Pain Questionnaire or the Brief Pain Inventory, provide a broader picture of a patient's experience, but are usually more cumbersome to administer and, in the end, suffer the same limitations as all other attempts to measure pain. A number of tools to assess cancer-related and noncancer chronic pain have been advanced and validated.[15] Most of these focus on persistent background pain and do not help identify intermittent or breakthrough pain. Several assessment scales specifically address breakthrough or episodic pain. The Breakthrough Pain Questionnaire was introduced by Portenoy and Hagen to assess breakthrough pain in cancer patients and has also been studied in patients with acute noncancer pain, for which it can offer a picture of both breakthrough and background pain states.[16]

Ultimately, we are left with a maxim first attributed to Dr John Bonica, the father of pain medicine: "Pain is what a patient says it is." The best way to begin assessing a patient's pain is to *ask* about it and *listen* to the answers. Attempts to reduce the experience to finite details may lead to failure to ask the right questions, distance us from our patients, focus us away from the whole person, and, potentially, miss golden diagnostic clues that could lead to effective interventions.

Effective treatment of acute pain requires assessment as well as vigilant reassessment to determine if the primary goals are met, adversity has occurred, or changes are necessary.

Acute pain may be viewed as breakthrough, intermittent, or background in nature (Table 55-9). The assessment process for

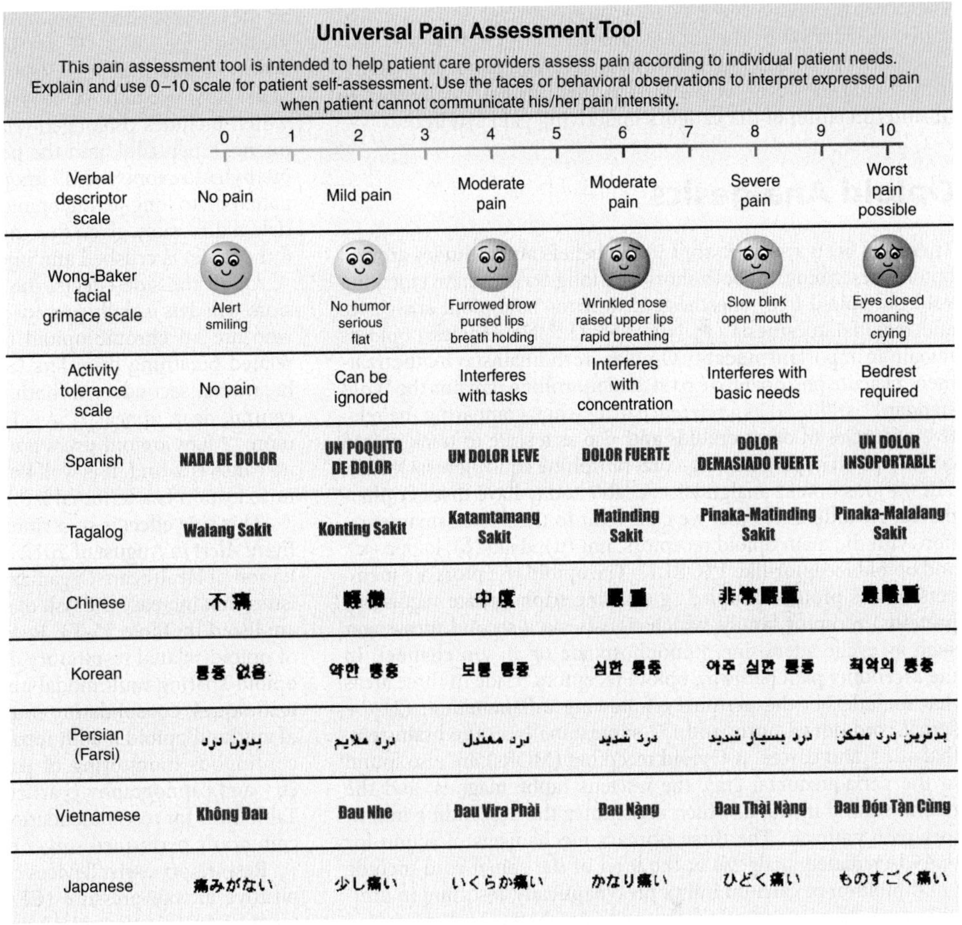

Universal Pain Assessment Tool

This pain assessment tool is intended to help patient care providers assess pain according to individual patient needs. Explain and use 0–10 scale for patient self-assessment. Use the faces or behavioral observations to interpret expressed pain when patient cannot communicate his/her pain intensity.

	0	2	4	6	8	10
Verbal descriptor scale	No pain	Mild pain	Moderate pain	Moderate pain	Severe pain	Worst pain possible
Wong-Baker facial grimace scale	Alert smiling	No humor serious flat	Furrowed brow pursed lips breath holding	Wrinkled nose raised upper lips rapid breathing	Slow blink open mouth	Eyes closed moaning crying
Activity tolerance scale	No pain	Can be ignored	Interferes with tasks	Interferes with concentration	Interferes with basic needs	Bedrest required
Spanish	NADA DE DOLOR	UN POQUITO DE DOLOR	UN DOLOR LEVE	DOLOR FUERTE	DOLOR DEMASIADO FUERTE	UN DOLOR INSOPORTABLE
Tagalog	Walang Sakit	Konting Sakit	Katamtamang Sakit	Matinding Sakit	Pinaka-Matinding Sakit	Pinaka-Malalang Sakit
Chinese	不痛	輕微	中度	嚴重	非常嚴重	最嚴重
Korean	통증 없음	약한 통증	보통 통증	심한 통증	아주 심한 통증	최악의 통증
Persian (Farsi)	بدون درد	درد ملایم	درد معتدل	درد شدید	درد بسیار شدید	بدترین درد ممکن
Vietnamese	Không Đau	Đau Nhe	Đau Vira Phài	Đau Nặng	Đau Thậi Nặng	Đau Độu Tận Cùng
Japanese	痛みがない	少し痛い	いくらか痛い	かなり痛い	ひどく痛い	ものすごく痛い

Figure 55-10 Linear verbal analog score and "faces" pain assessment tool.

each of these is relatively similar and will help to resolve the related condition into broad pathophysiologic groups such as cancer versus noncancer, and nociceptive versus neuropathic, or mixed pain states. Such an approach supports a rational process for developing a useful differential diagnosis and approach. Table 55-10 lists the common features of pain that are usually reviewed during the assessment for acute pain. A thorough physical examination must also be performed with particular attention to the neurologic examination, which may offer clues to aberrant neural processing. Such neurologic findings may indicate nerve injury, alerting the astute clinician to a neuropathic rather than a nociceptive pain state that requires a different analgesic approach.[17] A provocative physical examination may include examination of the affected areas with maneuvers that may provoke pain such as range of motion testing, walking, and coughing.

Table 55-9 Three Classes of Acute Pain

Class	Description
Breakthrough	Pain that escalates above a persistent background pain
Transitory and intermittent	Pain that is episodic in the absence of background pain
Background	Pain that is persistent but may vary over time

Table 55-10 Features of Pain Commonly Addressed During Assessment

Onset of pain
Temporal pattern of pain
Site of pain
Radiation of pain
Quality (character) of pain
Intensity (severity) of pain
Exacerbating factors (what makes the pain start or get worse?)
Relieving factors (what prevents the pain or makes it better?)
Response to analgesics (including attitudes and concerns about opioids)
Response to other interventions
Associated physical symptoms
Associated psychological symptoms
Interference with activities of daily living
Oral morphine equivalent (OME)

The benefits of provocative testing must outweigh the associated suffering incurred by the patient. Medical imaging is also a common part of the acute pain workup. Overemphasis on imaging data should, however, be avoided as this can potentially lead to misinterpretation of the patient's underlying pain syndrome.

Opioid Analgesics

4 There has been a seismic shift in the beliefs and attitudes around opioid prescribing, for both short- and long-term use. An emerging field of "opioid-free" anesthesia prioritizes nonopioid analgesics and regional anesthesia (NICV 55-1).[18] Nonetheless, opioids remain an important modality. Opioids are the mainstay for the treatment of acute postoperative pain, and morphine remains the "gold standard": still used as a reference drug when comparing the relative potencies of other opioids and also as a scale to track opioid consumption in patients (e.g., oral morphine equivalents: OMEs). The various opioid analgesics available today have distinct pharmacologic differences that we can credit to their intricate interaction with the main opioid receptors: mu (μ), delta (δ), kappa (κ), and opioid receptor-like 1 (ORL1). The opioid receptors are members of a G protein–coupled (guanosine triphosphate regulatory proteins) receptor family, which signals via a second messenger such as cyclic adenosine monophosphate or an ion channel. In the ascending pain pathway, opioid receptors reside in three areas that include (1) the periphery, following inflammation; (2) the spinal cord dorsal horn; and (3) supraspinally in the brainstem, thalamus, and cortex. μ-Opioid receptors (MORs) are also found in the periaqueductal gray, the nucleus raphe magnus, and the rostral ventral medulla, which constitutes the descending inhibitory pain pathway. The three primary mechanisms of action for opioid-mediated analgesia at the level of the spinal cord include (1) inhibition of calcium influx presynaptically, resulting in inhibition of depolarization of the cell membrane and decreased release of neurotransmitters and neuropeptides into the synaptic cleft, (2) enhanced potassium efflux from the cell postsynaptically, resulting in hyperpolarization of the cell and a decrease in signal transmission, and (3) activation of a descending inhibitory pain circuit via inhibition of GABAergic transmission in the brainstem. Peripheral opioid receptors, which mediate analgesia, are located on primary afferent neurons. Activation of these receptors inhibits the release of pronociceptive and proinflammatory substances like substance P, which accounts for the analgesic and anti-inflammatory effects. The "broad-spectrum" opioid, methadone, also has NMDA receptor antagonist properties and inhibits the reuptake of serotonin and norepinephrine, which may make it useful in the treatment of neuropathic pain.

There is great diversity in the available routes of administration of opioid analgesics. Table 55-11 is a list of relevant pharmacokinetic data. Table 55-12 offers equianalgesic dosing guidelines for the various opioids. The reader is referred to the section, in this chapter, on Perioperative Pain Management of the Opioid Dependent Patient for a detailed discussion of incomplete cross-tolerance between the different opioids and dosing considerations.

Common adverse side effects associated with opioid therapy include nausea, vomiting, constipation, urinary retention, delirium, hallucinations, myoclonus, falls, hypotension, aspiration pneumonia, dizziness, sedation, and respiratory depression. Opioid-related adverse effects have the potential to increase the utilization of health care resources, which can have far-reaching consequences. In a recent retrospective review of 402 patients undergoing orthopedic surgery, the authors concluded that constipation, emesis, and confusion were associated with significant increase in postoperative hospital length of stay (p-LOS) and, of all the adverse effects, opioid-induced constipation (OIC) had the greatest effect on p-LOS.[19] Unfortunately, tolerance rarely develops to the constipating effects of the opioids. Numerous different pharmacologic approaches have been developed to combat OIC, which includes prolonged-release formulations that contain naloxone, tapentadol, and the peripherally acting MOR antagonists methylnaltrexone and alvimopan.[20] The benefit of the addition of naloxone to long-acting opioids such as oxycodone is the reduced risk of diversion, given that the opioid is immediately antagonized if the tablet is crushed and injected or snorted.

Of all the side effects, the most serious is respiratory depression, which is usually preceded by sedation. During sleep, patients who are on chronic opioid therapy develop a variety of sleep-related breathing disorders (SRBDs) which manifest as irregular breathing, secondary to both obstructive sleep apnea (OSA) and central sleep apnea (CSA). Hypoxia and hypercapnia are common. "Many opioid users are found dead in bed and at autopsy, no cause is found. It is well known that the sine qua non of opioid intoxication is a terminal lethal apnea."[21]

This side effect is so serious, in fact, that it generated a *Sentinel* 5
Event Alert in August of 2012 by the Joint Commission on Accreditation of Healthcare Organizations (JCAHO).[22] Patient characteristics that increase the risk of sedation and respiratory depression are listed in Table 55-13. Recommendations to decrease the risk of opioid-related respiratory depression include the liberal use of opioid-sparing multimodal pharmacotherapy, regional anesthesia techniques, consolidating routes of administration (e.g., removal of epidural opioid if additional IV opioids are prescribed) and the continuous monitoring of patient ventilation with pulse oximetry and capnography (particularly in high-risk individuals). See Table 55-5 for recommendations for multimodal therapy for some commonly performed surgeries.

Respiratory assist devices can also be very helpful. Continuous positive airway pressure (CPAP) is recommended for the treatment of OSA in the opioid-dependent patient. However, patients can fail CPAP and CSA can emerge. These patients may be better candidates for either a bilevel device with backup rate or an adaptive servoventilation (ASV) device. A more comprehensive discussion of this topic is beyond the scope of this chapter and the reader is referred to the excellent review by Javaheri and Randerath.[21]

Other disconcerting side effects associated with the chronic use of opioids include opioid-induced hyperalgesia (OIH) and immune modulation. OIH is a relatively rare phenomenon whereby patients who are receiving opioids suddenly and paradoxically become more sensitive to pain despite continued treatment with opioids. Evidence suggests that OIH is more likely to develop following high doses of phenanthrene opioids such as morphine.[23] Changing the opioid to a phenyl piperidine derivative such as fentanyl may thwart OIH. There is also evidence that coadministration of an NMDA receptor antagonist can abolish opioid-induced tolerance and OIH.[23] Finally, opioid analgesics have profound immunomodulatory effects, which include inhibition of cellular and humoral immune functions, depressed natural killer cell activity, promotion of angiogenesis, and inhibition of apoptosis. Such effects can be beneficial or deleterious depending upon the clinical situation.[24,25]

Morphine is the prototype opioid and is the reference drug to which all other analgesics are compared in terms of potency. Although the plasma half-life of the drug is approximately 2 hours, its analgesic duration of action is closer to 4 to 5 hours. Morphine undergoes hepatic glucuronidation to morphine-6-glucuronide and morphine-3-glucuronide, both of which are cleared by the kidney. Morphine-6-glucuronide is an active metabolite of morphine and is thought to be responsible for most of the analgesia associated with chronic dosing of the drug. Morphine-3-glucuronide, on

Table 55-11 Opioid Analgesic Pharmacokinetics[34]

Drug	Onset of Effect	Peak Effect	Duration of Effect	Elimination t½	VD (L/kg)	Protein Binding (%)	Metabolism Pathway	Active Metabolites	Major Excretion Pathway
Alfentanil	Immediate	1.5–2 min	<10 min	1.5–1.85 h	0.4–1	92%	Liver	—	Urine
Buprenorphine multiple formulations available: (IV, IM, sublingual, buccal, implantable, subcutaneous, transdermal)	Intramuscular 15 min Intravenous (IV) is faster	1 h IV is sooner	6 h (IM)	1.2–7.2 h (mean 2.2 h) following IV administration of 0.3 mg		96%	Liver (CYP3A4) N-dealkylation to norbuprenorphine		Feces and urine
Codeine	Oral: 10–30 min, IV: 15 min	0.5–1 h	Oral: 4–6 h, IV: 5 h	2.5–3 h	—	—	Liver	Morphine	Urine
Fentanyl injection	IV: immediate, IM: 7–8 min	—	IV: 0.5–1 h, IM: 1–2 h	3.65 h	4	Alters with increasing ionization	Liver	—	Urine
Fentanyl transdermal	—	24–72 h	72 h	≈17 h	6	Decreases with increasing ionization	Liver: CYP3A4	—	Urine
Fentanyl transmucosal	—	—	—	7 h	4	80–85%	Liver: CYP3A4	—	Urine
Hydromorphone	IM/SC: 15 min	0.5–1 h	IR: 4–5 h, ER: 24 h, IM/	IR: 2.3 h, ER: 18.6 h	≈4	8–20%	Liver: glucuronidation	—	Urine
	Oral: 30 min	Subcutaneous: 4–5 h	IM/subcutaneous: 2 6 h						
Levorphanol	IM: 15–30 min	Oral: 1 h	—	IV: 11–16 h	IV: 10–13	40%	—	—	—
Meperidine	—	—	2–4 h	3–6 (parent), <20 h (normeperidine)	60–80%	Liver	Normeperidine	—	
Methadone	Parenteral: 10–20 min	—	4 h	8–59 h	2–6	85–90%	Liver primarily CYP3A4 and to lesser extent CYP2D6	—	Urine and fecal
	Oral: 30–60 min								
Morphine sulfate	IM/SC: 10–30 min	Epidural: 10–15 min, Oral: 1 h	Subcutaneous/ IM: 4–5 h	1.5–2 h	1–6	20–35%	Liver: glucuronidation	Morphine-6-glucuronide	Urine
Oxycodone	Within 60 min	—	IR: 3–4 h CR: 12 h	IR: 3.2 h, CR: 4.5 h	2.6	45%	Liver: Somewhat involves CYP2D6	Noroxycodone and oxymorphone	Urine
Oxymorphone	Parenteral: 5–10 min	—	Parenteral: 3–6 h	1.3 h	≈3	—	Liver	—	Urine
Propoxyphene* (due to cardiotoxic effects, the drug has been withdrawn from the U.S. market)	—	2–2.5 h	—	6–12 h (parent), 30–36 h (norpropoxyphene)	—	80%	Liver	Norpropoxyphene	Urine
Remifentanil	Rapid	—	—	10–20 min	0.35	70%	Hydrolysis by esterases	—	Urine
Sufentanil	IV: immediate, Epidural: 10 min	—	Epidural: 1.7 h	2.7 h	—	91–93%, 79% in neonates	Liver and small intestine	—	—
Tramadol	—	—	2 h (tramadol), 3 h (M1, active metabolite)	6.3 h (tramadol), 7.4 h (M1, active metabolite)	2.6–2.9	20%	Liver: CYP2D6 and CYP3A4	O-desmethyl-tramadol (M1) via CYP2D6	Urine

CR, controlled release; CT, cytochrome; ER, extended release; IM, intramuscular; IR, mmediate release; IV, intravenous; SC, subcutaneous.

Table 55-12 Opioid Equianalgesic Dosing[115–117]

Drug	Dosage	
	IV/IM/SQ	Oral (mg)
Morphine	10 mg (IV)	30
Buprenorphine	0.3 mg (IV)	NA
Hydromorphone (Dilaudid)	1.5–2 mg	6–8
Hydrocodone (Vicodin)	NA	30–45
Oxymorphone (Opana IR and ER)	1 mg	10
Oxycodone (Percocet, Oxycontin)	10–15 mg	20
Levorphanol (Levo-Dromoran)	2 mg	4
Fentanyl	100 μg	NA
Meperidine (Demerol)	100 mg	300
Codeine	100 mg	200
Methadone	The conversion ratio for methadone is variable.	

ER, extended release; IM, intramuscular; IR, immediate release; IV, intravenous; SQ, subcutaneous.

This table should serve as a general guideline when dosing opioid analgesics. Numerous resources are available in the literature and online. Always consult an acute pain specialist if you have questions about managing an opioid-dependent patient.

the other hand, is considered to be devoid of analgesic activity. With chronic dosing, these metabolites can accumulate and can be particularly problematic in patients with renal failure. Dosing adjustment is therefore necessary, and monitoring of side effects is important. Morphine-6-glucuronide contributes to side effects such as drowsiness, nausea and vomiting, coma, and respiratory depression. Morphine-3-glucuronide, on the other hand, is thought to cause agitation, myoclonus, delirium, and hyperalgesia.

Hydromorphone is a semisynthetic opioid that has four to six times the potency of morphine. It is available for oral, rectal, parenteral, and neuraxial administration. *Hydrocodone* is the most widely prescribed opioid analgesic in the United States. It has weak affinity for the μ-receptor; however, demethylation by the CYP2D6 enzyme converts hydrocodone into hydromorphone, which has stronger μ-receptor binding. Patients with the extensive metabolizer (EM) phenotype report better opioid effects and fewer adverse opioid effects than the patients with the poor metabolizer (PM) phenotype. Point-of-care, phenotype-based dosing strategies would preclude prescribing hydrocodone to patients with the PM phenotype. Whereas the oral bioavailability of the drug is reported to be 20% to 50%, its bioavailability via the subcutaneous route is 78%, making it the ideal drug for long-term subcutaneous administration in the opioid-tolerant patient. Like morphine, hydromorphone is biotransformed in the liver. The active metabolites are dihydromorphine and dihydroisomorphine and the inactive metabolite is hydromorphone-3-glucuronide. Although hydromorphone has traditionally been the preferred opioid for patients with acute pain and impaired kidney function, evidence suggests that hydromorphone-3-glucuronide can accumulate in those with renal failure and may contribute to side effects such as neuroexcitation and cognitive impairment. Opioid-related side effects such as nausea, vomiting, sedation, cognitive impairment, and pruritus are reported to be less intense with hydromorphone than morphine. In fact, the incidence of pruritus following neuraxial administration of hydromorphone is reported to be approximately 5% versus the 11% to 77% range reported for neuraxial morphine.[26]

Codeine is an opioid agonist that has both analgesic and antitussive properties. In the United States, codeine is available for oral, subcutaneous, and intramuscular administration. As previously

Table 55-13 Risk Factors for Opioid-Induced Respiratory Depression

Surgical and Patient Risk Factors	Comorbidities as Risk Factors	Perioperative Risk Factors
First 24 h after surgery	Diagnosed OSA Suspected OSA	Concomitant use of sedatives
Orthopedic general and transplant surgery	Renal disease	PCA
Elderly >60 y	Pulmonary disease (including COPD)	Excessive dose of opioids
Females	Cardiac disease (including CAD, CHF, arrhythmias)	Multiple route of administration
ASA 3 and 4	Diabetes mellitus	Multiple prescribes
Opioid dependent	Obesity	Two or more opioids
Genetic polymorphism	Hypertension Neurologic disease (stroke, dementia) Liver disease PACU respiratory events Hypoventilation Apnea Desaturation Sedation/analgesia mismatch	Excessive sedation Inadequate monitoring Hyperoxemia Patient on O_2 during respiratory depression

ASA, American Society of Anesthesiologists; CAD, coronary artery disease, CHF, congestive heart failure; COPD, chronic obstructive pulmonary disease; OSA, obstructive sleep apnea; PACU, postanesthesia care unit; PCA, patient-controlled analgesia.

Reprinted with permission from Gupta K, Prasad A, Nagappa M, et al. Risk factors for opioid-induced respiratory depression and failure to rescue. *Current Opinion in Anesthesiology*. 2018;31(1):110–119.

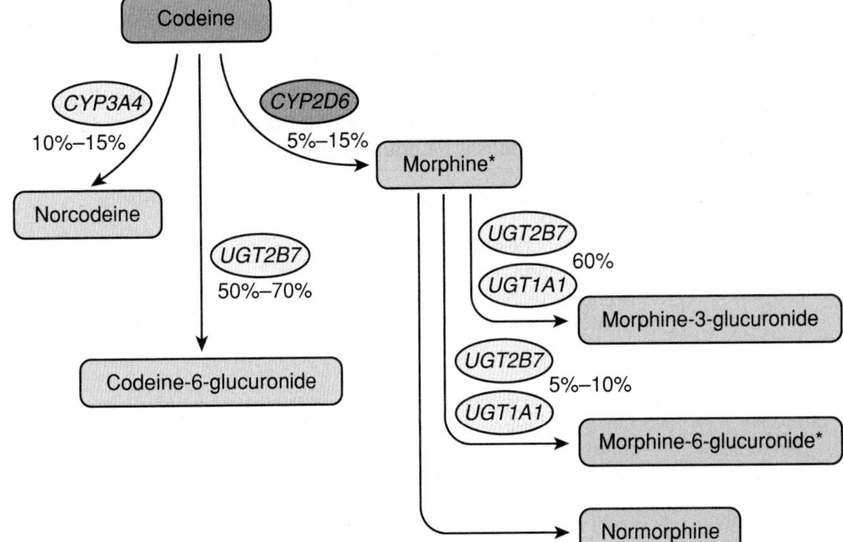

Figure 55-11 Codeine metabolism pathway in an individual with cytochrome P450 2D6 (CYP2D6) extensive metabolism. *Asterisks* denote active metabolites. (Adapted with permission from Crews KR, Gaedigk A, Dunnenberger HM, et al. Clinical Pharmacogenetics Implementation Consortium guidelines for cytochrome P450 2D6 genotype and codeine therapy: 2014 update. *Clin Pharmacol Ther*. 2014;95(4):376–382. Copyright © 2014 American Society for Clinical Pharmacology and Therapeutics.)

mentioned, codeine is a prodrug that is devoid of analgesic activity and requires metabolic conversion by the CYP2D6 enzyme into morphine, which has a 200-fold greater affinity for the MOR than the parent drug codeine. In *EMs*, O-demethylation of the drug by the CYP2D6 enzyme accounts for only 5% to 10% clearance of codeine; however, this conversion to morphine is critical for opioid activity (Fig. 55-11). In *PMs* and *ultrarapid* metabolizers, codeine is contraindicated because of lack of efficacy in the former and the potential for toxicity in the latter (Table 55-14).[27] Whereas slow metabolizers of codeine display poor analgesia from the drug, rapid metabolizers can experience toxicity from the active metabolite, morphine (Fig. 55-11).

Oxycodone (Oxycontin, Percocet) is used for the treatment of both acute and chronic pain and in the United States, the drug is only available for oral administration. Oxycodone is predominantly metabolized by CYP3A4 to inactive metabolites; however, approximately 11% of an oxycodone dose is cleared by CYP2D6 to produce the minor metabolite oxymorphone, which is reported to be eight times as potent as the parent drug.[27] It is theoretically possible that toxicity or overdose could occur in CYP2D6 ultrarapid metabolizers or in patients who are concomitantly taking a CYP3A4 inhibitor (e.g., diltiazem, verapamil) (Fig. 55-12).

Fentanyl, a synthetic opioid chemically related to the phenylpiperidines, is a relatively selective μ-receptor agonist, which is considered to have 80 times the potency of morphine following intravenous (IV) administration. It is extensively metabolized in the liver to norfentanyl and other inactive metabolites, which are excreted in the urine and bile. Fentanyl is therefore suitable for patients in renal failure. The drug is available for IV, subcutaneous, transdermal, transmucosal, and neuraxial administration.

Sufentanil, alfentanil, and *remifentanil* are analogs of fentanyl that have analgesic effects like those of morphine and the other μ-receptor agonists. *Sufentanil* has approximately 1,000 times the potency of morphine and is primarily used in the operating room either intravenously or neuraxially.[28] Like fentanyl, sufentanil is very lipophilic and, although their pharmacokinetic and pharmacodynamic profiles are similar, sufentanil has a smaller volume of distribution and shorter elimination half-life.[28] The high intrinsic potency of sufentanil makes it an excellent choice for epidural analgesia in the opioid-dependent patient.[29] *Alfentanil* has approximately 10 times the potency of morphine and, like sufentanil, is used primarily in the operating room. *Remifentanil* is an ultra–short-acting synthetic opioid. The potency of the drug is approximately equal to that of fentanyl. Remifentanil is rapidly degraded by tissue and plasma esterases, which accounts for its incredibly short terminal elimination half-life of 10 to 20 minutes.[28] Rapid clearance and lack of accumulation make this a very desirable opioid in the operative setting, particularly during neurosurgery when remifentanil is combined with propofol as part of a total intravenous anesthetic (TIVA). Remifentanil in a patient-controlled analgesia (PCA) modality has been used successfully in laboring women. It can be considered as a "second-line" analgesic option if neuraxial analgesia is contraindicated or unsuccessful.[30] A disadvantage of remifentanil is that discontinuation of an infusion results in rapid loss of analgesia. For surgical cases that have been maintained on remifentanil and have a reasonable expectation of postoperative pain, a bridging dose of a longer-acting opioid may be required. There is also evidence to suggest that remifentanil infusions may be associated with the development of OIH. Further studies are clearly needed to better define this phenomenon.

Meperidine, a phenylpiperidine, is a synthetic MOR agonist with a short half-life. The drug is recommended for the short-term management of acute pain only and has no role in the management of chronic pain. The drug is biotransformed by the liver to normeperidine, a potentially neurotoxic metabolite, which has a 12- to 16-hour half-life. Repetitive dosing of meperidine can cause accumulation of normeperidine, which may precipitate tremulousness, myoclonus, and seizures. It is therefore recommended that the total daily IV dose in an otherwise healthy adult without renal or central nervous system disease should not exceed 600 mg/d and should not be administered for longer than 48 hours.[31] We do not recommend the use of meperidine for IV PCA. The drug is contraindicated in patients receiving monoamine oxidase inhibitors (MOAs), as this may precipitate a syndrome characterized by muscle rigidity, hyperpyrexia, and seizures. Meperidine has some local anesthetic activity and has been used in neuraxial anesthesia for cesarean section in patients with true amide allergy, although the evidence is largely limited to case reports.[32]

Methadone is a relatively inexpensive synthetic opioid considered to be a broad-spectrum opioid because it is a (1) μ-receptor agonist, (2) NMDA antagonist, and (3) inhibitor of monoamine transmitter reuptake, making it potentially useful for the treatment of neuropathic pain. The drug is well absorbed from the gastrointestinal tract with a reported bioavailability approximating 80%.

Table 55-14 Assignment of Likely Codeine Metabolism Phenotypes Based on Cytochrome P450 2D6 (*CYP2D6*) Diplotypes

Phenotype	Implications for Codeine Metabolism	Recommendations for Codeine Therapy	Classification of Recommendation for Codeine Therapy[a]	Considerations for Alternative Opioids
Ultrarapid metabolizer	Increased formation of morphine following codeine administration, leading to higher risk of toxicity	Avoid codeine use due to potential for toxicity.	Strong	Alternatives that are not affected by this CYP2D6 phenotype include morphine and nonopioid analgesics. Tramadol and, to a lesser extent, hydrocodone and oxycodone are not good alternatives because their metabolism is affected by CYP2D6 activity.[b,c]
Extensive metabolizer	Normal morphine formation	Use label-recommended age- or weight-specific dosing.	Strong	—
Intermediate metabolizer	Reduced morphine formation	Use label-recommended age- or weight-specific dosing. If no response, consider alternative analgesics such as morphine or a nonopioid.	Moderate	Monitor tramadol use for response.
Poor metabolizer	Greatly reduced morphine formation following codeine administration, leading to insufficient pain relief	Avoid codeine use due to lack of efficacy.	Strong	Alternatives that are not affected by this CYP2D6 phenotype include morphine and nonopioid analgesics. Tramadol and, to a lesser extent, hydrocodone and oxycodone are not good alternatives because their metabolism is affected by CYP2D6 activity; these agents should be avoided.[b,c]

[a]Rating scheme is described in Supplementary Data online.
[b,c]There is substantial evidence for decreased efficacy of tramadol in poor metabolizers and a single case report of toxicity in an ultrarapid metabolizer with renal impairment following tramadol use postsurgery. Use of other analgesics in CYP2D6 poor and ultrarapid metabolizers may therefore be preferable. Some other opioid analgesics, such as hydrocodone and oxycodone, are metabolized by CYP2D6. To avoid treatment complications, opioids that are not metabolized by CYP2D6 including morphine, oxymorphone, buprenorphine, fentanyl, methadone, and hydromorphone, along with nonopioid analgesics, may be considered as alternatives for use in CYP2D6 poor and ultrarapid metabolizers.
Reprinted with permission from Crews KR, Gaedigk A, Dunnenberger HM, et al. Clinical Pharmacogenetics Implementation Consortium guidelines for cytochrome P450 2D6 genotype and codeine therapy: 2014 update. *Clin Pharmacol Ther*. 2014;95(4):376–382. Copyright © 2014 American Society for Clinical Pharmacology and Therapeutics.

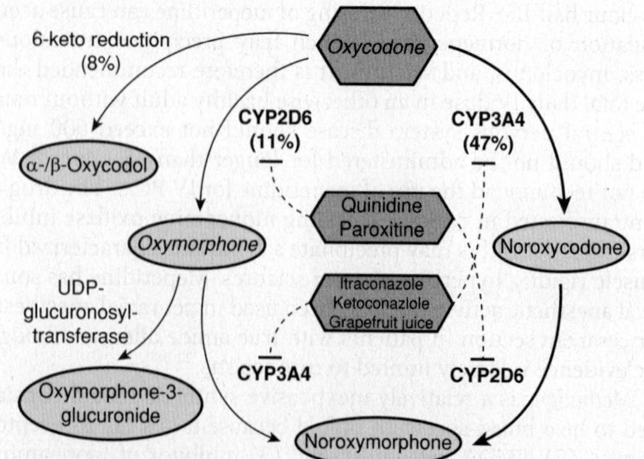

Figure 55-12 Oxycodone metabolism. (Adapted with permission from Landau R, Bollag LA, Kraft JC. Pharmacogenetics and anaesthesia: the value of genetic profiling. *Anaesthesia*. 2012;67(2):165–179. Copyright © 2011 The Association of Anaesthetists of Great Britain and Ireland.)

The drug is extensively metabolized in the liver by the cytochrome P450 (CYP450) system to inactive metabolites, which are cleared in the bile and urine; unlike morphine, it is generally not necessary to adjust the dosage of methadone in patients with renal insufficiency. Methadone has an elimination half-life of 22 hours and, following a single dose, the duration of analgesia is approximately 3 to 6 hours. With repetitive dosing, however, methadone can accumulate. Slow tissue release into the blood stream can result in a long elimination half-life of up to 128 hours and duration of analgesia of 8 to 12 hours. This long half-life explains the potential risk for cumulative toxicity and therefore the importance of monitoring for side effects such as excessive sedation and confusion following the initiation of an around-the-clock dosing regimen. *Methadone* is subject to genetic polymorphism secondary to modifications by genetic variations in CYP2D6, the opioid receptor mu-1 (OPRM1), and the ABCB1 drug transport protein. Methadone fatalities are associated with the slow metabolizer phenotype.

Buprenorphine is a highly lipophilic partial MOR agonist, κ-receptor (KOR) antagonist, and ORL1 agonist (NICV 55-2). It is a lipophilic opioid with moderate intrinsic activity and a high affinity for the MOR. The elimination half-life of the drug following IV administration is 1.2 to 7.2 hours (mean 2.2 hours). The terminal half-life of the drug following sublingual administration, however, is considerably longer secondary to sequestration of the drug in the oral mucosa and buccal fat. The drug is metabolized in the liver by the CYP3A4 enzyme to norbuprenorphine, a weak μ-agonist responsible for respiratory depression. Buprenorphine and norbuprenorphine are rapidly conjugated via phase II reaction to buprenorphine-3-glucuronide and norbuprenorphine-3-glucuronide and neither metabolite decreases respiratory rate. In humans, buprenorphine is reported to have a ceiling effect for respiratory depression but not for analgesia. Buprenorphine is reported to be effective in a broader variety of pain phenotypes than fentanyl. In animal models, it has proven to be efficacious in the treatment of neuropathic pain and in a human pain model, it can block secondary hyperalgesia and central sensitization. Buprenorphine also produces less constipation and less cognitive dysfunction than other MOR agonists and does not prolong the QTc interval like methadone.[33]

Buprenorphine is an excellent alternative for the treatment of acute pain in the patient who cannot tolerate morphine secondary to allergy or other sensitivity. In the adult patient, the parenteral dose of buprenorphine is 300 micrograms (mcg), which is equivalent to 10 mg of morphine.[34] The recommended dosing interval is every 6 hours. Additional routes of administration include intramuscular, neuraxial, subcutaneous, sublingual, buccal, and transdermal.

A novel (off-label) route of administration of buprenorphine is the perineural application of the drug with local anesthetic. To prolong the duration of a single injection peripheral nerve block at the brachial and lumbar plexuses, buprenorphine may be combined with a long-acting local anesthetic (bupivacaine or ropivacaine) with clonidine and dexamethasone and is referred to as *multimodal perineural analgesia*. This multimodal four-drug combination is reported to provide upward of 40 hours of analgesia, which is vastly superior to less than 12 to 16 hours with a single long-acting local anesthetic. This single injection technique can be useful in austere environments or in situations which preclude placement of a continuous perineural catheter. The block can be performed quickly and offers an inexpensive alternative to a continuous perineural catheter.[35]

Tramadol (Ultram) and *Tapentadol (Nucynta)* are orally active, centrally acting synthetic analgesics possessing a novel mechanism of action which combines μ-receptor agonist activity with monoamine reuptake inhibition. Whereas tramadol inhibits reuptake of both norepinephrine and serotonin, tapentadol only inhibits the reuptake of norepinephrine. Tramadol is a prodrug which is metabolized in the liver by the CYP450 CYP2D6 system to the active metabolite O-desmethyltramadol (M1), which has 200 times greater μ-receptor affinity, greater potency, and longer half-life than the parent drug. This can be significant because there can be an attenuated analgesic effect in the 5% to 15% of the population that has decreased CYP2D6 activity, as is the case with codeine. PMs display incomplete analgesia. The frequency of PMs varies by ethnicity and is reported to be 8% in Whites, 2% to 7% in African Americans, and 0% to 0.5% in Asian populations. Tapentadol, on the other hand, is metabolized in the liver to an inactive metabolite via phase II glucuronidation and the drug does not require enzymatic conversion to an active drug. As such, tapentadol offers a distinct advantage over tramadol in terms of reduced variability in analgesia secondary to genetic polymorphism. Tapentadol metabolism will also not be subject to drug/drug interactions at the level of the CYP2D6 enzyme.[27,36]

Tramadol is indicated for mild to moderately severe acute pain. The drug is available as 50-mg tablets. The recommended adult dose is 50–100 mg orally, q 4–6 h, not to exceed 400 mg in 24 hours. The drug is also available in extended-release formulations and a combination product with acetaminophen. Tapentadol is indicated for moderate to severe acute pain. It is available as 50-mg, 75-mg, and 100-mg tablets, which can be dosed every 4 to 6 hours, not to exceed 700 mg on the first day of dosing and 600 mg every day thereafter. Tapentadol IR 50 and 75 mg provides postoperative analgesia like oxycodone IR 10 mg and with fewer gastrointestinal side effects. Advantages of tapentadol over tramadol include (1) lack of CYP450 drug interactions, (2) lower risk of seizures and serotonin syndrome, (3) superior analgesia, (4) fewer GI side effects and (5) less variation in individual drug response secondary to genetic polymorphism.[37]

Both drugs should be administered with caution in patients at risk for respiratory depression. In addition, both drugs have the potential to produce serotonin syndrome (mental status changes, autonomic instability, and neuromuscular aberrations), particularly if administered with serotonergic drugs (selective serotonin reuptake inhibitors [SSRIs], selective norepinephrine uptake inhibitors, tricyclic antidepressants [TCAs], MAOs inhibitors, and triptans). Caution is advised when dosing these drugs in patients with a seizure disorder.

Finally, opioid rotation is a very useful technique to restore analgesic sensitivity in the highly tolerant patient, and methadone is a common choice for opioid rotation. Because cross-tolerance is incomplete, the calculated equianalgesic dose of any new opioid is always lower than expected. One must be particularly cautious, however, when converting from morphine to methadone as the morphine/methadone equianalgesic ratio appears to be curvilinear; whereas the oral morphine-to-methadone conversion ratio is 3:1 at morphine doses of less than 100 mg/d, the ratio is 20:1 at morphine doses of more than 1,000 mg/d.[38] (Table 55-15). Always

Table 55-15 Conversion Ratios from Morphine to Methadone

Daily Chronic Oral Morphine Dose		Conversion Ratio (Oral Morphine: Oral Methadone)	
<100 mg	(e.g., 90 mg PO morphine)	3:1	(e.g., 30 mg PO methadone)
100–300 mg	(e.g., 300 mg PO morphine)	5:1	(e.g., 60 mg PO methadone)
300–600 mg	(e.g., 600 mg PO morphine)	10:1	(e.g., 60 mg PO methadone)
600–800 mg	(e.g., 720 mg PO morphine)	12:1	(e.g., 60 mg PO methadone)
800–1,000 mg	(e.g., 900 mg PO morphine)	15:1	(e.g., 60 mg PO methadone)
>1,000 mg	(e.g., 1,200 mg PO morphine)	20:1	(e.g., 60 mg PO methadone)

PO, by mouth. Always consult an acute pain expert when dosing methadone or converting from one opioid analgesic to another.
From Hawley P, Chow L, Fyles G, et al. Clinical Outcomes of Start-Low, Go-Slow Methadone Initiation for Cancer-Related Pain: What's the Hurry? *J Palliat Med* 2017;20:1244-51.

Table 55-16 Methadone Drug Interactions

Clinical Significance	Increase Methadone Concentration/Effects	Decrease Methadone Concentration/Effects
Documented clinical effects	Ciprofloxacin (Cipro), diazepam (Valium), ethanol (acute use), fluconazole (Diflucan), urinary alkalinizers	Amprenavir (Agenerase), efavirenz (Sustiva), nelfinavir (Viracept), nevirapine (Viramune), phenobarbital, phenytoin (Dilantin), rifampin (Rifadin), ritonavir (Norvir), urinary acidifiers
Documented enzyme effects	Cimetidine (Tagamet), fluoxetine (Prozac)	Carbamazepine (Tegretol)
Clinical effects uncertain	Omeprazole (Prilosec), quinidine, paroxetine (Paxil)	
Predicted interaction	Delavirdine (Rescriptor), grapefruit juice, or fruit	Ethanol (chronic use)
No current clinical evidence	Ketoconazole (Nizoral), macrolide antibiotics (erythromycin, clarithromycin [Biaxin], troleandomycin [TAO]), tricyclic antidepressants, verapamil (Calan)	

seek expert advice when dosing methadone. There are numerous drug interactions with methadone, as shown in Table 55-16. Whereas inhibition of methadone metabolism will theoretically provoke toxicity, induction of methadone metabolism could potentially precipitate inadequate analgesia or even withdrawal symptoms. Frequent adjustments of the methadone dosage may therefore be required if medications are added to or eliminated from a patient's drug regimen. A rare side effect associated with methadone is a pause-dependent dysrhythmia associated with bradycardia, QT prolongation, and Torsades de pointe.

Biased Opioid Ligands

The "opioid crisis" has accelerated the search for a therapeutic alternative capable of providing analgesia while devoid of the adverse side effects associated with contemporary opioids such as constipation, pruritus, respiratory depression, physical dependence, tolerance, and euphoria. In an effort to develop a safer opioid analgesic with fewer adverse side effects, research has focused on the development of biased agonists at the opioid receptor. Activation of the opioid receptor results in G-protein activation, which results in inhibition of cAMP production, activation of G-protein coupled inwardly rectifying potassium channels (GIRK) and inhibition of calcium channels, and β-arrestin-2 recruitment. Evidence suggests that G-protein activation mediates the analgesic effects of opioids, whereas β-arrestin-2 mediates the adverse effects of opioids (Fig. 55-13). A biased agonist would therefore preferentially activate the G-protein rather than the β-arrestin pathway. This hypothesis, however, has been challenged and some studies have suggested that the perceived bias may be due to the agonist's low intrinsic activity or unique pharmacokinetic profile. Notwithstanding the controversy over mechanism of action, the putative G-protein biased compound TRV-130 (oliceridine) was recently approved by the Food and Drug Administration (FDA) in August of 2020 for the treatment of moderate to severe acute pain. An IV dose of 1 mg of oliceridine is reported to be equianalgesic to 5 mg of IV morphine. Recommended adult-dosing guidelines are 1 to 2 mg IV every 1 to 3 hours as needed, not to exceed 27 mg in any 24-hour period of time. The drug is extensively metabolized by the liver via the CYP450 system, primarily CYP3A4 and CYP2D6, to inactive metabolites. No dosage adjustment is necessary in patients with mild to moderate hepatic dysfunction or end-stage renal disease, though careful dosing should be undertaken in the patient with severe hepatic disease. When compared to morphine, oliceridine may have a lower risk of gastrointestinal and respiratory complications, although a dose-dependent increase in respiratory depression has been reported. Prudence, therefore, dictates close monitoring of the patient in the same fashion as with traditional opioids. Unfortunately, oliceridine displays reward-enhancing effects similar to both morphine and oxycodone and therefore can be subject to abuse.[39] The "holy grail" for analgesia will be to create pure G-protein biased compounds that are antinociceptive with significantly reduced side effects, and predictable half-lives, that are available in various routes for administration. Biased opioid ligands are a step in the right direction, but further research is warranted before we can fully embrace them as the analgesic panacea.

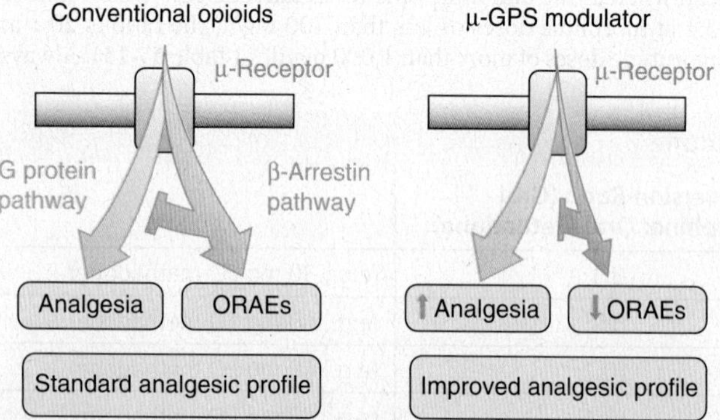

Figure 55-13 Biased Opioid Ligand. Mechanism of action: conventional opioids versus μ-GPS modulators. ORAEs, opioid-related adverse events. (Reprinted with Viscusi ER. Improving the therapeutic window of conventional opioids: novel differential signaling modulators. *Reg Anesth Pain Med.* 2019;44:32–37, with permission from BMJ Publishing Group Ltd.)

Nonopioid Analgesic Adjuncts

6

The *NSAIDs* are among the most commonly used drugs in the world because of their anti-inflammatory, analgesic, and antipyretic effects (Table 55-17). The therapeutic benefit of NSAIDs is believed to be mediated through the inhibition of cyclooxygenase (COX) enzymes (prostaglandin H_2 [PGH_2] synthetases), types 1 and 2, which convert arachidonic acid to PGH_2. The COX enzyme consists of two active sites: (1) the COX site and (2) the

Table 55-17 Nonopioid Analgesics (Adult Dosing Guidelines)[31,34]

Drug	Route	Half-life (h)	Dose (mg)	Comments
Para-aminophenols				
Acetaminophen	PO and IV	2	500–1,000 mg q4–6h Maximum daily dose (MDD) in the healthy adult is 4,000 mg. Intravenous dosing guidelines: Adult >50 kg: 1 g q4–6h not to exceed 4 g/d Adult <50 kg: 15 mg/kg q4–6h not to exceed 3 g/d. Pedi >33 kg: 15 mg/kg q4–6h not to exceed 3 g/d. Pedi 10–33 kg: 15 mg/kg q4–6h not to exceed 2 g/d	Hepatotoxicity can occur in chronic alcoholics receiving therapeutic doses Administer intravenous formulation over 15 min
Salicylates				
Acetylsalicylic acid	PO	0.25	500–1,000 mg q4–6h MDD is 4,000 mg in the healthy adult	Salicylic acid has a $T_{1/2}$ 2–3 h at low doses and >20 h at higher doses. Because of the risk of Reyes syndrome avoid the use of aspirin in children <12 y old
Diflunisal	PO	8–12	500 mg q8–12h	Decrease the dose in the elderly to 500–1,000 mg/d
Choline magnesium trisalicylate	PO	9–17	Loading dose (LD) = 1,000 mg 1,000–1,500 mg q12h	Unlike aspirin does not increase bleeding time; MDD = 2,000–3,000 mg
NSAIDs Propionic Acids				
Ibuprofen Intravenous formulation (Caldolor) available in the United States in 2009.	PO and IV	2	400 mg q4–6h	Intravenous ibuprofen: Infuse over 30 minutes to avoid phlebitis Limit adult dose to 3,200 mg/day
Naproxen	PO	12–15	250 mg q6–8h	LD = 500 mg; MDD = 1,500 mg
Ketoprofen	PO	2.1	25–50 mg q6–8h	MDD = 300 mg
Oxaprozin	PO	42–50	600 mg q12–24h	MDD = 1,200 mg
Indolacetic Acids				
Indomethacin	PO	2	25 mg q8–12h	MDD = 200 mg
Sulindac	PO	7.8	150 mg q12h	MDD = 400 mg Active metabolite has a half-life of 16 h
Etodolac	PO	7.3	300–400 mg q8–12h	MDD = 1,000 mg
Pyrrolacetic Acids				
Ketorolac	IV	6	30 mg initially followed by 15–30 mg q6–8h not to exceed 5 d	MDD = 120 mg; hypovolemia should be corrected prior to administration Decrease the dose in the elderly (>65 y of age) and in renal failure
Phenylacetic Acids				
Diclofenac potassium	PO	2	50 mg q8h	MDD = 150 mg
Enolic Acids (Oxicams)				
Meloxicam	PO IV	15–20	7.5–15 mg q24h 30 mg once per day	COX-2 selectivity similar to celecoxib
Piroxicam	PO	50	20–40 mg q24h	
Naphthylalkanone				
Nabumetone	PO	22.5	500–750 mg q8–12h	LD = 1,000 mg MDD = 2,000 mg Active metabolite has half-life = 22.5 h
COX-2 Inhibitor				
Celecoxib	PO	11	100–200 mg q12h	LD = 400 mg; MDD = 400 mg Avoid this drug in patients with coronary heart disease, cerebrovascular disease, or in patients allergic to sulfonamides

PO, by mouth; IV, intravenously; COX-2, cyclooxygenase; LD, loading dose; MDD, maximum daily dose.

peroxidase site. NSAIDs mediate their effects by binding to the COX site.

COX-1 is the constitutive enzyme that produces prostaglandins, which are important for general "house-keeping" functions such as gastric protection and hemostasis. COX-2, on the other hand, is the inducible form of the enzyme that produces prostaglandins that mediate pain, inflammation, fever, and carcinogenesis. Prostaglandin E_2 is the key mediator of both peripheral and central pain sensitization. Peripherally, prostaglandins do not directly mediate pain; rather, they contribute to hyperalgesia by sensitizing nociceptors to other mediators of pain sensation such as histamine and bradykinin.[40] Centrally, prostaglandins enhance pain transmission at the level of the dorsal horn by (1) increasing the release of substance P and glutamate from first-order pain neurons, (2) increasing the sensitivity of second-order pain neurons, and by inhibiting the release of neurotransmitters from the descending pain-modulating pathways.

NSAIDs have proved effective in the treatment of postoperative pain. In addition, they are opioid-sparing and can significantly decrease the incidence of opioid-related side effects such as postoperative nausea and vomiting and sedation.[41] Unlike the opioids, NSAIDs exhibit a "ceiling effect" with respect to maximum analgesic effects. Parenteral NSAIDs such as ketorolac are commonly employed as part of a multimodal approach for acute perioperative pain management. The optimal dose of ketorolac for postoperative pain control is 15 to 30 mg intravenously every 6 to 8 hours, not to exceed 5 days. The dose should be decreased in patients with renal failure. Recently, in 2020, the FDA approved a COX-2 preferential NSAID, IV meloxicam, that is administered as a once-a-day dosing regimen (30 to 60 mg IV) for perioperative pain.[42]

Despite the benefits of NSAIDs in the perioperative period, they are not without some significant side effects. Platelet dysfunction, gastrointestinal ulceration, and an increased risk of nephrotoxicity are several reasons why the nonselective NSAIDs may be avoided in the perioperative period. The risk of nephrotoxicity is increased in patients with hypovolemia, congestive heart failure, and chronic renal insufficiency.[40] The COX-2–selective inhibitors were developed to minimize these side effects. The COX-2–specific inhibitor celecoxib (Celebrex) is available in the United States. Rofecoxib (Vioxx) and valdecoxib (Bextra), also released in the same period, were recalled by the manufacturers because of concerns about adverse cardiovascular risks. Celecoxib is the only COX-2–specific inhibitor currently available in the United States for acute postoperative pain. The recommended oral loading dose is 400 mg followed by 200 mg orally every 12 hours for several days.

Because prostaglandins play a crucial role in renal function through their effect on blood flow, natriuresis, and glomerular filtration, both traditional NSAIDs and COX-2 inhibitors can cause fluid retention and hypertension.

7 The authors do not recommend prescribing a COX-2 inhibitor for patients with a known history of coronary artery disease or cerebrovascular disease. Both COX-1 and COX-2 play significant roles in bone fusion following fracture and the use of traditional NSAIDs has been found to inhibit the healing process, particularly following lumbar spinal fusion surgery. The effect of COX-2 inhibitors on bone fusion following orthopedic procedures continues to be controversial, and no recommendations can be made at this time.

The *para-aminophenol* derivative acetaminophen (paracetamol) has both analgesic and antipyretic properties, like aspirin, but it is devoid of any anti-inflammatory effects. The drug is primarily a centrally acting inhibitor of the COX enzyme with minimal peripheral effects. Acetaminophen neither enters the active site of the COX enzyme nor binds to the COX site. Instead, it prevents COX activation by reducing heme at the peroxidase site of the enzyme. In addition, there may be modulation of descending inhibitory serotoninergic pathways and the drug may act on the opioid, cannabinoid, transient receptor potential of vanilloid type 1 ($TRPV_1$), and NMDA receptors.[43] Acetaminophen is devoid of many of the side effects generally associated with the NSAIDs, such as gastrointestinal ulceration, impaired platelet function, adverse cardiorenal effects, and impairment of bone fusion following orthopedic procedures. Acetaminophen is opioid sparing and can be used in conjunction with an NSAID as part of a multimodal analgesic program. The combination of acetaminophen with an NSAID is thought to provide analgesia that is superior to using either drug alone.[44] In adults, 2 g of oral acetaminophen is equivalent to 200 mg of celecoxib.

IV acetaminophen (Ofirmev) was released in the United States in November of 2010. The drug is available as a 1 g (1,000 mg/100 mL) infusion that does not require reconstitution and can be infused through a peripheral IV line over 15 minutes. However, in patients that can tolerate oral intake, oral dosing may be more cost-effective without any decrease in analgesic effect. IV dosing is most effective in patients that are not able to tolerate oral intake or who have had recent abdominal surgery with expected delay in gastric absorption.[45] See Table 55-17 for dosing guidelines.

NMDA receptor antagonists, such as ketamine and dextromethorphan, may be useful analgesic adjuncts. Excitatory neurotransmitter stimulation of the NMDA receptor is believed to be involved in the development and maintenance of several adverse phenomena including (1) persistent postoperative pain, (2) hypersensitivity, windup, and allodynia, (3) opioid-induced tolerance, and (4) OIH. *Low-dose IV ketamine* has proven to be very effective in the management of perioperative pain. Numerous meta-analyses have described the opioid-sparing effect of the drug, and although the magnitude of the effect varies from one study to the next, it appears that the use of perioperative IV ketamine, for up to 48 hours postoperatively, can reduce opioid consumption by upward of 40%.[46] IV ketamine also reduces pain scores and no major complications have been reported following 48 hours of continuous infusion. Low-dose IV ketamine is defined by the recent ASRA consensus guidelines as a bolus dose of ketamine that is 0.35 mg/kg or less or an infusion that is 1.0 mg/kg/h or less.[47] The primary mechanism of action of ketamine is NMDA receptor blockade, but additionally, the drug interacts with opioidergic, cholinergic, and monoaminergic receptors and blocks sodium channels.[48] In 2018, the ASRA released expert consensus guidelines supporting the use of subanesthetic IV ketamine for patients undergoing painful surgery, for opioid-tolerant patients undergoing any surgery, for patients with opioid tolerance with sickle cell crisis, and for patients with OSA. Contraindications for using subanesthetic ketamine include poorly controlled cardiovascular disease, pregnancy, active psychosis, and severe liver disease.[47]

NMDA receptor antagonists may act synergistically when combined with an opioid. However, the combination of ketamine (1 mg/mL) with morphine (1 mg/mL) administered as an IV PCA to patients following major abdominal surgery does not significantly improve pain relief.[49] In patients with morphine-resistant pain, however, the combination of 250 μg/kg of ketamine plus 15 μg/kg of morphine, as a bolus dose, has been reported to provide significant analgesia.[48] The ideal IV PCA morphine–ketamine combination ratio is 1:1 with an 8-minute lockout.[50] Ketamine is not recommended as the sole IV agent in a PCA for routine use.

Dextromethorphan, the d-isomer of the codeine analog levorphanol, is a noncompetitive NMDA receptor antagonist that has been used for many years as an antitussive. Dextromethorphan does not have a direct analgesic effect; rather, analgesia is likely mediated by its NMDA receptor antagonism. The drug can be administered orally, intravenously, and intramuscularly. A sustained-release suspension is available that contains dextromethorphan (30 mg/5 mL), which is marketed as Delsym. Following oral administration, dextromethorphan is metabolized to dextrorphan. This metabolite accounts for most of the side effects, the most common of which are nausea and vomiting. Dextromethorphan has been shown to both inhibit secondary hyperalgesia following peripheral burn injury and causes a reduction in the temporal summation of pain. The preoperative administration of 150 mg of oral dextromethorphan can reduce the PCA morphine requirements of patients undergoing abdominal hysterectomy and the preincisional administration of 120 mg of intramuscular dextromethorphan provides analgesia in patients undergoing elective upper abdominal surgery. Finally, a randomized double-blind, placebo-controlled study has demonstrated that dextromethorphan dosed 200 mg orally every 8 hours (e.g., 2 hours prior to surgery, then 8 hours and 16 hours thereafter) can provide a modest reduction in morphine consumption following knee surgery.[51] Because dextromethorphan can trigger histamine release and is generally only available in oral liquid form, the use of it as an adjunct to treat moderate to severe perioperative pain is not as common compared to IV ketamine.[52]

The α_2-*adrenergic agonists* clonidine (half-life 9 to 12 hours) and dexmedetomidine (half-life 2 hours) may be administered perioperatively to provide analgesia, sedation, and anxiolysis. The presynaptic activation of α_2-receptors results in decreased release of norepinephrine that is believed to mediate analgesia. Whereas clonidine is a selective partial agonist for the α_2-adrenoreceptor, dexmedetomidine is superselective for this receptor. Their respective α_2/α_1 binding ratios are 220:1 for clonidine versus 1,620:1 for dexmedetomidine. Analgesia is mediated supraspinally (locus coeruleus), spinally (substantia gelatinosa), and peripherally. Dexmedetomidine is reported to have greater affinity for the 2A subtype of the receptor, which may account for the drug's superior analgesic properties compared to clonidine. Clonidine can be administered orally, transdermally, intravenously, perineurally, and neuraxially for perioperative pain management. Premedication with 5 μg/kg of oral clonidine in patients undergoing knee surgery can decrease the use of PCA morphine and decrease the incidence of postoperative nausea and vomiting. In addition, the combination of oral clonidine, 3 to 5 μg/kg with 0.2 mg/24 hours of transdermal clonidine can decrease postoperative PCA morphine requirement by 50% following prostatectomy surgery. In a double-blind, placebo-controlled study involving total knee arthroplasty (TKA), investigators demonstrated that the addition of 25 μg of intrathecal clonidine to a bupivacaine (15 mg) and morphine (250 μg) spinal anesthetic cocktail could reduce postoperative morphine use and improve VAS pain scores at 24 hours.[53] In combination with a local anesthetic, clonidine in doses of 0.5 to 1.0 μg/kg may enhance the efficacy and increase the duration of perineural blocks. A four-drug combination including bupivacaine (2.5 mg/mL), clonidine (3 μg/mL), buprenorphine (18 μg/mL), and dexamethasone (66 μg/mL) has been reported to provide greater than 24 hours of postoperative analgesia.[35] Side effects from clonidine include sedation, hypotension, and bradycardia if the dose exceeds 150 μg.

Dexmedetomidine is a potent and highly selective α_2-adrenoreceptor agonist which demonstrates cardioprotective, neuroprotective, and renoprotective effects against hypoxic/ischemic injury.[54] Dexmedetomidine is a useful and safe adjunct in numerous clinical situations, such as (1) premedication prior to intubation and extubation, (2) procedural sedation, (3) awake intubation, (4) awake craniotomies, (5) an adjuvant to regional anesthesia, and (6) as part of a multimodal protocol for intraoperative and postoperative analgesia. See Table 55-18 for dosing guidelines. Dexmedetomidine does not decrease gut motility and prevents postoperative nausea and vomiting and shivering. In the intensive care unit (ICU), dexmedetomidine has proven to be a very useful drug that decreases central nervous system sympathetic outflow in a dose-dependent manner. It provides adequate sedation without significant respiratory depression and analgesia that is opioid sparing. Unlike propofol and midazolam, dexmedetomidine is not a GABAergic drug, has no anticholinergic effects and promotes more physiologic sleep pattern attributes, which attenuates neurocognitive impairment (delirium and agitation) and promotes early extubation and shorter length of stay (LOS) in the ICU.[55] The most frequently observed adverse effects associated with the use of dexmedetomidine are bradycardia and hypotension, which can be adequately treated with atropine, glycopyrrolate, and ephedrine.

Table 55-18 Dexmedetomidine Dosing Guidelines

Route	Dose
Intravenous	Loading dose: 1 μg/kg over 10–20 min
Maintenance dose: 0.2–0.7 μg/kg/h	
Intramuscular	2.5 μg/kg as premedication
Spinal	0.1–0.2 μg/kg
Epidural	1–2 μg/kg
Peripheral nerve block	1 μg/kg
Buccal	1–2 μg/kg
Intranasal	1–2 μg/kg

Reprinted with permission from Naaz S, Ozair E. Dexmedetomidine in current anaesthesia practice: a review. *J Clin Diagn Res.* 2014;8(10):GE01–GE04.

The *gabapentinoids* (α_2–δ subunit calcium channel ligands) *gabapentin* (Neurontin) and *pregabalin* (Lyrica) are indicated for the treatment of partial-onset seizures, neuropathic pain (e.g., postherpetic neuralgia), and other chronic pain states such as fibromyalgia. A growing body of evidence supports the use of these drugs during the perioperative period to decrease postoperative pain and opioid use. There is a decreased incidence of postoperative delirium, vomiting, pruritus, and urinary retention associated with the perioperative use of these drugs, probably secondary to their opioid-sparing effects. Furthermore, because the gabapentinoids can prevent the establishment of surgery-induced central sensitization, these drugs may play a role in preventing the transition from acute pain to chronic pain. Common side effects associated with these drugs include sedation, headache, dizziness, and visual disturbances.[56,57]

Compared to traditional analgesics, which decrease afferent input from the site of tissue injury, the gabapentinoids decrease the hyperexcitability of dorsal horn neurons caused by tissue damage.[58] Although structurally similar to GABA, these drugs are not GABAergic and do not bind $GABA_A$, $GABA_B$, or $GABA_C$ radioligand sites or allosteric GABA receptor sites. The gabapentinoids have two antinociceptive mechanisms of action: modulation of the calcium-induced release of glutamate centrally in the dorsal horn and activation of descending noradrenergic pathways in the spinal cord and brain (Fig. 55-14).[57]

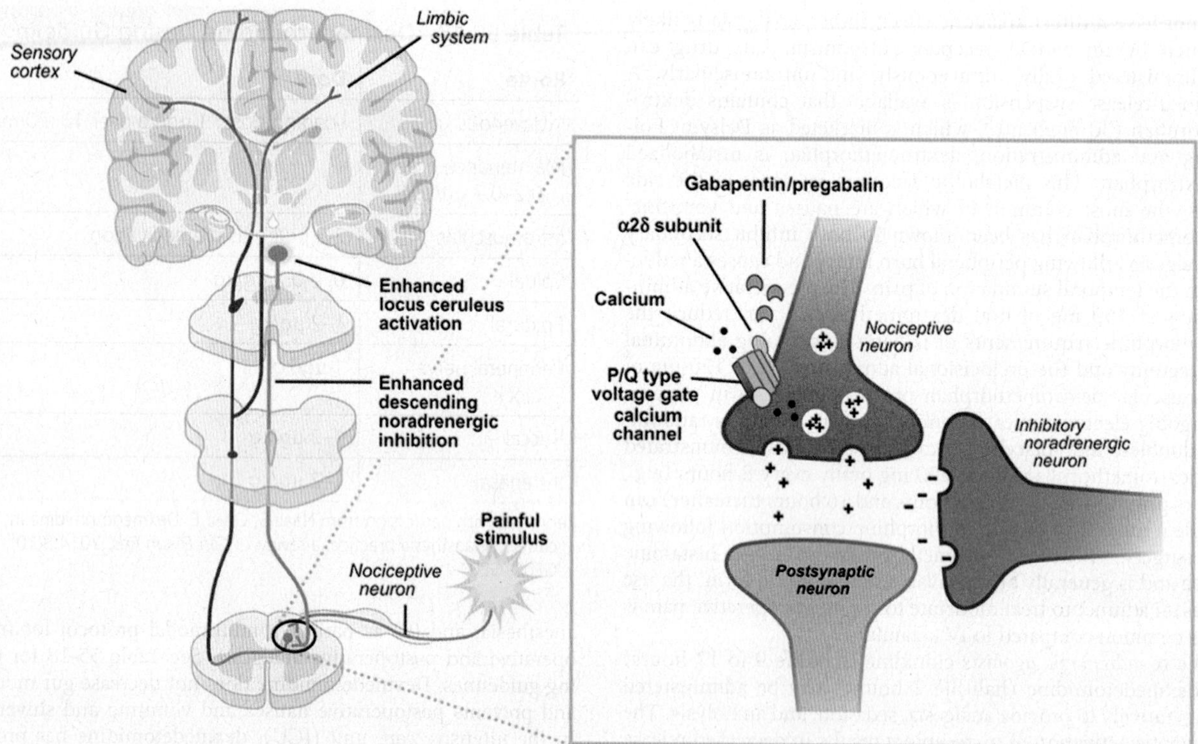

Figure 55-14 Hypothesized mechanisms of action of gabapentin. Gabapentin binds to the α-2δ subunit of voltage-gated P/Q type calcium channels. This binding appears to modulate the function and traffic of these channels, which appear on the synaptic bulb of presynaptic neurons. Calcium influx through these channels after a pain-evoked action potential is believed to trigger the fusion of synaptic vesicles with the neuronal membrane and consequent release of neurotransmitters in the dorsal horn of the spinal cord. Gabapentin may exert its analgesic effect by inhibiting or modulating this process. In addition, gabapentin may exert an analgesic effect by activating descending inhibitory noradrenergic pathways that regulate neurotransmission of pain signals in the dorsal horn of the spinal cord. (Reprinted with permission from Schmidt PC, Ruchelli G, Mackey SC. Perioperative gabapentinoids: choice of agent, dose, timing, and effects on chronic postsurgical pain. *Anesthesiology*. 2013;119(5):1215–1221.)

When administered orally, both gabapentin and pregabalin are absorbed by amino acid carrier systems in the small intestine. The gastrointestinal absorption of gabapentin occurs only in the duodenum through a saturable transport system, such that increasing dose results in decreasing bioavailability. Consequently, increased doses of gabapentin result in incrementally smaller increases in plasma drug concentration (e.g., nonlinear pharmacokinetics).[59] Pregabalin, on the other hand, is absorbed throughout the small intestines through a nonsaturable transport system and has a linear pharmacokinetic profile (dose-independent absorption) and is more potent than gabapentin. Gabapentin oral absorption is significantly impaired by antacids, including Bicitra. Both drugs are renally excreted and undergo insignificant liver metabolism.

Gabapentinoids can increase the risk of postoperative sedation and may, in combination with opioid analgesics, place the patient at an increased risk for postoperative respiratory depression. The optimal perioperative dosing regimen and treatment duration remain unclear. In a retrospective study[60] of patients undergoing total hip and knee arthroplasty, premedication of patients with greater than 300 mg of gabapentin, as part of a multimodal analgesic regimen that included a preoperative dose of sustained release oxycodone, was associated with an increased risk of postoperative respiratory depression. In another placebo-controlled crossover study, the combination of pregabalin and remifentanil produced additive analgesia but potentiated respiratory depression and produced greater cognitive side effects.[61] Thus, in the opioid-naive patient, the preoperative dose of gabapentin should rarely exceed 300 mg orally and gabapentinoids should not be combined with a preoperative dose of sustained release opioid. Only in rare circumstances, such as in the opioid-dependent patient or in the patient at increased risk for chronic postsurgical pain (e.g., thoracotomy), should higher doses of gabapentinoids be contemplated.[57] See Tables 55-6 and 55-8 for dosing guidelines.

Gabapentin has been included in many enhanced recovery after surgery (ERAS) protocols as either a one-time dose or several doses perioperatively. However, a meta-analysis of 281 trials with 24,682 patients demonstrated that gabapentin was associated with lower pain scores at 6 hours postoperatively, but that the difference was not clinically significant. Thus, while it is the consensus that gabapentinoids are opioid sparing and effective in attenuating pain, the role of gabapentin as a regular adjunct for optimizing perioperative pain control is inconclusive.[62]

Following IV administration, the local anesthetic lidocaine has been shown to be analgesic, antihyperalgesic, and anti-inflammatory.[63,64] In vitro studies indicate that the beneficial effects of IV lidocaine are mediated by inhibitory actions on voltage-gated sodium channels, voltage-gated calcium channels, potassium channels, G protein–coupled receptors (GPCRs), NMDA receptors, and the glycinergic system.[65] The perioperative infusion of lidocaine has been shown to not only improve postoperative analgesia in patients recovering from laparoscopic colectomy but to also decrease postoperative opioid requirements, attenuate postoperative ileus, and accelerate time to discharge from the hospital.[63,65,66] The ideal perioperative dosing of systemic lidocaine has yet to be clearly defined, although a bolus dose of 1.5 to 2.0 mg/kg followed by an infusion of 1.5 to 2 mg/kg/h has been recommended for the treatment of pain.[65] An initial bolus dose is recommended to shorten the time needed to achieve a plasma steady state within a goal serum concentration therapeutic range of 1 to 5 mcg/mL. Serum concentrations greater than 5 mcg/mL are associated with cardiovascular and central nervous system toxicity. In contrast, the time at which the infusion is stopped does not appear to be of great importance. Stopping lidocaine infusions earlier than 60 minutes before skin closure versus letting the infusion run for more than 60 minutes after skin closure produced no statistical differences in pain scores, LOS, time to bowel movement, or nausea and vomiting.[67] Lidocaine infusion is contraindicated in any patient with arrhythmia, heart failure, coronary artery disease, Stokes–Adams disease (cardiovascular syncope), or heart block. IV lidocaine should also not be infused concurrently with any other local anesthetics including peripheral nerve blocks or topical lidocaine patches due to the additive effect of local anesthetics and the increased risk of local anesthetic systemic toxicity (LAST).[68] If a peripheral nerve block is warranted, it should be performed at least 6 hours (i.e., 4 half-lives) after the lidocaine infusion is stopped.

Recent meta-analyses indicate that the perioperative administration of IV *magnesium* may also be an effective adjunct in the treatment of perioperative pain.[69,70] IV magnesium infusion decreases pain scores, is opioid sparing in the first 24 hours following surgery and is devoid of any serious adverse effects. In a trial of 50 patients undergoing scoliosis surgery, the combination of intraoperative IV magnesium (bolus dose: 50 mg/kg over 30 minutes, maintenance dose: 8 mg/kg/h) with low-dose ketamine (bolus dose: 0.2 mg/kg, maintenance dose: 0.15 mg/kg/h) versus low-dose ketamine alone decreased postoperative morphine consumption and improved sleep and patient satisfaction scores.[71] The mechanism of analgesia is thought to be mediated by NMDA receptor antagonism as well as regulation of calcium influx into the cell, resulting in suppression of neuropathic pain and inhibition of central sensitization, potentially making this drug useful in the opioid-tolerant patient.

The *glucocorticoids* are well known for their analgesic, anti-inflammatory, and antiemetic effects. Inhibition of cytosolic phospholipase A_2 upstream from the lipoxygenase and COX enzymes in the prostaglandin cascade most certainly accounts for both their anti-inflammatory and analgesic effects by inhibiting leukotriene and prostaglandin production. The mechanism of the antiemetic effect of the corticosteroids is less clearly understood but appears to be centrally mediated.[72] In combination with a gabapentinoid, acetaminophen, and an NSAID, dexamethasone is considered a useful component of a multimodal drug strategy to effectively attenuate postsurgical pain. The recommended preoperative IV dose is 0.11 to 0.2 mg/kg. Dexamethasone causes perineal irritation in 50% to 70% of individuals following rapid administration, and so dilution in 50 mL of normal saline and administration over 10 minutes prior to surgery is preferred.[73] Acute perioperative pain management can be challenging in the opioid-tolerant patient; high-dose IV dexamethasone, combined with a proton pump inhibitor, has been recommended as a useful therapeutic option.[74] Dexamethasone has also been administered via the perineural route as part of a four-drug cocktail. It is the opinion of the authors that the perineural dose of dexamethasone should not exceed 1 to 2 mg per nerve plexus.[75]

Methods of Analgesia

Patient-Controlled Analgesia

PCA is any technique of pain management that allows the patients to administer their own analgesia on demand. We will highlight some important aspects of PCA as a complete review of PCA is beyond the scope of this chapter; we refer the reader to excellent reviews on this topic.[76,77] In the United States, the most common drugs administered via PCA are morphine, hydromorphone, and fentanyl. Hydromorphone is recommended as an alternative in renal failure; however, fentanyl might be a better choice as it has no active metabolites. Meperidine is not recommended for use in an IV PCA secondary to accumulation of its potentially toxic metabolite normeperidine. 8

The five variables associated with all modes of PCA include (1) bolus dose, (2) incremental (demand) dose, (3) lockout interval, (4) background infusion rate, and (5) 1- and 4-hour limits. A typical PCA regimen in an otherwise healthy adult would be an incremental dose of 1 to 2 mg of morphine with an 8- to 10-minute lockout (Table 55-19). The authors do not recommend a background infusion of opioid in the opioid-naive patient. Background

Table 55-19 Patient-Controlled Analgesia (PCA) Regimens for Opioid-Naive Adult Patients: Commonly-Prescribed Dose Ranges

Drug	Concentration	Demand (PCA) Dose Range	Lockout Interval	Maximum in 4 h
Morphine	1 mg/mL	0.5–2 mg	5–10 minutes	30 mg
Hydromorphone	0.2 mg/mL	0.1–0.4 mg	10 min	6 mg
Fentanyl	10 mcg/mL	5–20 mcg	4–10 min	300 mcg

- This PCA regimen should be used after achieving adequate pain control in the acute postoperative period. Initial postoperative pain control should be performed in a monitored setting such as the PACU or ICU. IV opioids may be used for initial pain control if titrated carefully to analgesic effect while monitoring respiration and oxygenation. For example, hydromorphone may be administered by a PACU nurse from 0.1 to 0.4 mg IV bolus every 5 to 10 minutes until adequate analgesia before initiating PCA.
- Dosing should be individualized according to patient-specific factors, clinical situation, comorbidities, and concurrent medications. Lower doses and continuous pulse oximetry and end-tidal carbon dioxide monitoring are recommended during the early postoperative period, in older adults, and in patients with increased risk for respiratory depression, hypoxia, and/or opioid accumulation (eg, due to obstructive airway disease, sleep apnea, obesity, low body weight, frailty, renal and/or hepatic impairment, or use with other medications with sedating and/or respiratory depressant properties).
- The use of a continuous infusion (basal opioid infusion) is not recommended in patients who are not mechanically-ventilated.
- PCA dose ranges and other details shown in the table are suggestions only; protocols will vary by institution. For additional detail, refer to the individual Lexicomp drug information monographs included with UpToDate.

PACU: Postanesthesia care unit; ICU: Intensive care unit; IV: intravenous.

Adapted from Mariano E. Management of acute perioperative pain in adults. In: Fishman S, ed. *UpToDate*. Waltham, MA. (Accessed on September 3, 2022)August 30, 2022. https://www.uptodate.com/contents/management-of-acute-perioperative-pain-in-adults#H2.

Table 55-20 Relative Risk Factors Associated with the Use of Patient-Controlled Analgesia

Pulmonary disease
Obstructive sleep apnea
Renal or hepatic dysfunction
Congestive heart failure
Closed head injury
Altered mental status
Lactating mothers

infusions should be reserved for patients with chronic malignant or nonmalignant pain who are opioid tolerant, or patients with persistent pain who have failed a trial of incremental PCA dosing. Prudence dictates consultation with an expert in the management of the opioid-tolerant patient. In the elderly, the dose of the PCA should be decreased. The relative risk factors for use of an opioid PCA are listed in Table 55-20. If more than two risk factors exist, it may be appropriate to avoid using a PCA in the standard dosing regimen and administer opioids only as needed.

Opioid-related side effects include nausea and vomiting, pruritus, sedation, respiratory depression, and confusion. Consensus guidelines for the treatment of nausea and vomiting include prescribing various combinations of dopamine antagonists, serotonin antagonists, neurokinin 1 (NK1) receptor antagonists, glucocorticoids, anticholinergics, and antihistamines as well as nonpharmacologic prophylaxis.[78] In addition, the perioperative systemic administration of an α_2-agonist (e.g., dexmedetomidine), which is both analgesic and opioid sparing, has been shown to reduce the incidence of postoperative nausea and vomiting.[79] Pruritus can be ameliorated with the use of diphenhydramine, hydroxyzine, or a low dose of an opioid antagonist (e.g., naloxone) or mixed agonist–antagonist (e.g., nalbuphine). Excessive sedation and the risk of respiratory depression may respond to a change in the opioid. The use of a multimodal analgesic technique, for example, incorporating the use of a regional anesthetic (e.g., epidural or peripheral nerve blockade), an NSAID, acetaminophen, or other nonopioid analgesics such as an NMDA receptor antagonist or an α_2–δ subunit calcium channel ligand, will have an opioid-sparing effect which will reduce the risk of these adverse side effects.

Neuraxial Analgesia

Although opioid analgesics have been prescribed to patients for many centuries, the exact mechanism of action was not completely understood until 1971, when the opioid receptor was discovered. Within 5 years' time, Yaksh[80] reported that morphine could produce spinally mediated analgesia in a rat model. Soon thereafter, in 1979 and 1981, respectively, Wang[81] and then Onofrio[82] reported significant pain relief following the neuraxial administration of morphine in patients with severe cancer-related pain. The intrathecal administration of opioids, or the epidural administration of opioids plus a local anesthetic, can achieve significant pain relief for patients.

9 *Epidural analgesia* is a critical component of multimodal perioperative pain management and improved patient outcomes. Meta-analysis investigating the efficacy of epidural analgesia found epidural analgesia to be superior to systemically administered opioids.[83] The efficacy of an epidural technique is determined by factors that include (1) appropriate catheter placement relative to the level of the incision site (i.e., *congruency*), (2) choice of analgesic drugs, (3) rates of infusion, (4) duration of epidural analgesia, and (5) type of pain assessment (rest versus dynamic). Ideally, the epidural catheter is positioned *congruent* with the surgical incision (Fig. 55-15). Thoracic epidural catheter placement is recommended for both thoracic and upper abdominal surgical procedures because of the observed improvement in coronary artery blood flow, and the reduction in pulmonary complications and the duration of postoperative ileus. The optimal duration of epidural analgesia has not been determined, but recommendations are that the infusion be continued for at least 2 to 4 days. Epidural infusions lasting less than 24 hours do not appear to offer any clear cardiovascular advantages.

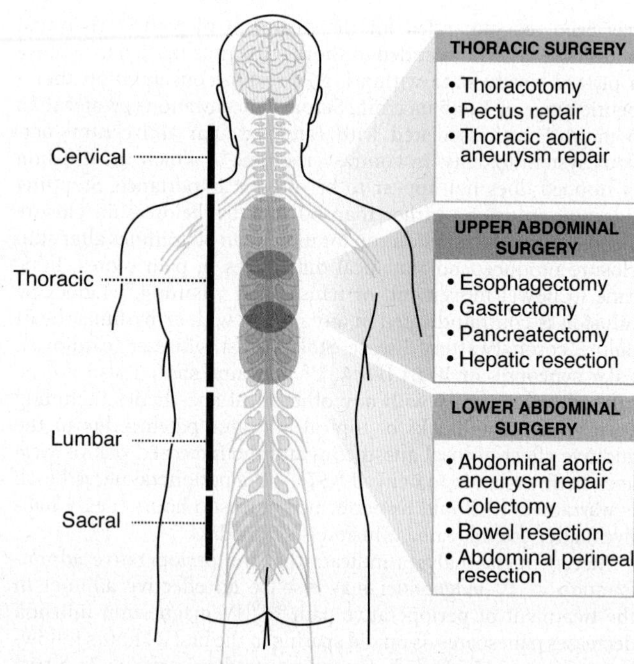

Figure 55-15 Schematic of the adult spine. Regions of the spine that can be used to insert thoracic epidural catheters in a variety of surgeries are shown. The *green shaded oval* in the thoracic spine represents the region for insertion for patients undergoing thoracic surgical procedures. The *blue shaded oval* depicts the area of insertion for patients undergoing upper abdominal surgery. The *pink shaded oval* represents the area of insertion for patients undergoing lower abdominal surgery. (Reprinted with permission from Manion SC, Brennan TJ, Riou B, et al. Thoracic Epidural Analgesia and Acute Pain Management. *Anesthesiology*. 2011;115:181–188.)

Epidurally administered opioids have the distinct advantage of producing analgesia without causing significant sympatholytic effect or motor blockade. Analgesia occurs by way of a *spinal mechanism* and then through a *supraspinal mechanism* following systemic adsorption. The spinal mechanism occurs following diffusion of the drug into the spinal fluid and is determined by meningeal permeability. Opioids with intermediate lipophilicity (e.g., hydromorphone, alfentanil, and meperidine) can easily move between the aqueous and lipid regions of the arachnoid membrane and therefore have high meningeal permeability. However, morphine has greater bioavailability in the spinal cord than alfentanil, fentanyl, and sufentanil.[84] Sufentanil may be considered the epidural opioid of choice in the opioid-tolerant patient taking more than 250 mg/d of oral morphine because of its high intrinsic activity.

In general, the epidural administration of hydrophilic opioids tends to have a slow onset, long duration, and a mechanism of action that is primarily spinal in nature whereas the epidural administration of lipophilic opioids has a quick onset, short duration, and a mechanism of action that is primarily supraspinal secondary to rapid systemic uptake. However, the data are controversial and the primary site of action of lipophilic opioids such as fentanyl may be determined by the mode of administration. Bolus administration of fentanyl appears to have a segmental analgesic effect whereas epidural infusion of fentanyl appears to have a nonsegmental (systemic) effect. There are some data, however, that suggest that there can be significant spinal mechanisms of action of the lipophilic opioids, particularly with the thoracic epidural infusion of fentanyl.

The combination of a local anesthetic and an opioid in the epidural space is believed to have a synergistic effect.[83] Local anesthetics have the unique ability to block the stress response by blocking afferent input to the spinal cord. Although bupivacaine plus fentanyl may be the most common combination, bupivacaine plus morphine is a reasonable option. Hydromorphone plus bupivacaine also makes very good sense as this combination has all the advantages of a hydrophilic opioid with excellent meningeal permeability. Although epidural infusions may consist of just a hydrophilic opioid, this is not a common practice at our institution. We place the epidural *congruent* with the surgical incision and, as a rule, the infusion consists simply of local anesthetic. This is particularly beneficial for the patient who may not tolerate opioid-related side effects such as pruritus. Table 55-21 contains epidural dosing guidelines. It is not recommended to administer opioids by multiple simultaneous routes because of the potential for additive respiratory depressant effects. A systemic opioid (e.g., PCA) should not be used in combination with a neuraxial opioid (e.g., epidural morphine).

Clonidine is another adjuvant medication that is reported to enhance analgesia. Clonidine (2 μg/mL) can be combined with an opioid and a local anesthetic and is usually infused at a rate of 5 to 20 μg/h. Side effects that limit its clinical usefulness, however, include hypotension, bradycardia, and sedation. An epidural infusion consisting of ropivacaine 0.2%, fentanyl 5 μg/mL, and clonidine 2 μg/mL infused at a rate of 3 to 7 mL/h following a TKA has been reported to cause no significant sedation in this dosage range.[85]

Intrathecal analgesia with a variety of drugs is a widely accepted practice for the treatment of both acute and chronic pain. Opioid

Table 55-21 Guidelines for Adult Epidural Catheter Dosing Regimen[a,b]

Catheter Placement	Surgical Dermatome		
	Lumbar (e.g., total knee arthroplasty or lower extremity bypass surgery)	Low thoracic (e.g., exploratory laparotomy, xiphopubic incision)	Mid-to-high thoracic (e.g., thoracotomy, sternotomy)
Lumbar T_{12}–caudal	Catheter congruent with incision! Bupivacaine 0.05–0.1% or ropivacaine 0.1–0.2% with or without opioid: Fentanyl 2–5 μg/mL or morphine 0.1 mg/mL or hydromorphone 0.02 mg/mL	Catheter/incision incongruency! [c]May consider bupivacaine or ropivacaine with a hydrophilic opioid. *This is not ideal!* [d]Hydrophilic opioids are required! Morphine 0.1 mg/mL or hydromorphone 0.02 mg/mL	Not applicable
Low thoracic T_8 to T_{12}	Not applicable	Catheter congruent with incision! Bupivacaine 0.05–0.1% or ropivacaine 0.1–0.2% with or without opioid: Fentanyl 2–5 μg/mL or morphine 0.1 mg/mL or hydromorphone 0.02 mg/mL	Catheter/incision incongruency! May consider bupivacaine or ropivacaine with an opioid but *this is not ideal!* Lipophilic Fentanyl 2–5 μg/mL. *This is not the ideal opioid!* [d]Hydrophilic opioids are a better choice! 1. Morphine 0.1 mg/mL or 2. hydromorphone 0.02 mg/mL
Mid-to-high thoracic T_4 to T_8	Not applicable	Not applicable	Catheter Congruent with surgical incision! Bupivacaine 0.05–0.1% or ropivacaine 0.1–0.2% with or without opioid: fentanyl 2–5 μg/mL or morphine 0.1 mg/mL or hydromorphone 0.02 mg/mL

Use caution: Multiple *routes of administration of opioids (e.g., PCA plus epidural) is not recommended! The risk of respiratory depression is increased*

[a]Rate of infusion, 2–10 mL/h. Recommended adult dose for epidural bupivacaine. Do not exceed 400 mg/24 h!

[b]May consider Clonidine 1–2 μg/mL in the epidural. Remember hypotension, bradycardia, and sedation are common at doses greater than 14 μg/h.

[c]Local anesthetic efficacy is diminished if the catheter placement is not congruent with the surgical incision!

[d]Hydrophilic opioids provide a broad band of analgesia! Morphine is the gold standard. Epidural hydromorphone may cause less pruritus. The authors prefer to place epidurals that are congruent with the surgical incision and administer local anesthetic without additional opioid.

Table 55-22 Intrathecal Analgesia Dosing Guidelines[31,86,118,a]

Surgical Procedure	Intrathecal Drug Dose
Labor analgesia	Sufentanil 2.5–5 µg
Cesarean section (C-section)	Morphine 100 µg. The addition of clonidine 60 µg is synergistic and can increase the duration of spinal analgesia after C-section but also increases intraoperative sedation and hypotension.
Outpatient knee arthroscopy	Fentanyl 10–25 µg will improve intraoperative analgesia without prolonging postoperative motor blockade. The authors do not, however, recommend the use of intrathecal opioids for outpatient surgery. We prefer motor-sparing nerve blocks for postoperative pain control (e.g., anterior cruciate ligament [ACL] repair). Patients are discharged home with an elastomeric pump that contains a local anesthetic, which can supply 48–72 h of postoperative analgesia.
Total knee arthroplasty (TKA)	Morphine 100 µg has been recommended for inpatients. The authors avoid the use of intrathecal morphine and prefer to provide opioid-sparing analgesia with the application of targeted motor-sparing peripheral nerve blockade. Patients are discharged home with an elastomeric pump that contains a local anesthetic, which can supply 48–72 h of postoperative analgesia.
Total hip arthroplasty (THA)	Morphine 100 µg has been recommended, however, the authors currently avoid the use of intrathecal opioids and provide opioid free postoperative analgesia by placing a fascia iliaca block, a pericapsular nerve group block (PENG), or a quadratus lumborum block.
Thoracotomy and major abdominal surgery	Although doses of morphine as high as 500 µg have been recommended in the past, the authors advise against its use since the incidence of side effects such as nausea and vomiting, urinary retention, pruritus, and **respiratory depression** increase significantly with doses >300 µg. We suggest the use of alternative techniques for acute pain management such as placement of a thoracic epidural, paravertebral block, or erector spinae plane block.

[a]50–100 µg of intrathecal hydromorphone approximates 100–200 µg of intrathecal morphine.[118]

analgesics, including morphine, hydromorphone, meperidine, methadone, fentanyl, and sufentanil, are commonly administered for this purpose.[86] Their distribution within the intrathecal space following administration is complex. Hydrophilic opioids (e.g., morphine) penetrate the spinal cord and bind to specific pre- and postsynaptic receptors within the dorsal horn. They traverse the dura slowly, bind to epidural fat poorly, and slowly enter the plasma. They tend to have a slow onset of action, long duration, and provide a broad band of analgesia. Delayed respiratory depression is more common with hydrophilic opioids secondary to rostral spread.[86] Lipophilic opioids (e.g., fentanyl), on the other hand, tend to bind to nonspecific receptors in the white matter.

Table 55-23 Intrathecal Analgesia: Other Dosing Guidelines[86,119]

Intrathecal Drug	Dosing	Comments
Clonidine	15–45 µg improves the quality of spinal blockade in outpatient surgery	Side effects increase significantly at intrathecal doses >150 µg
Epinephrine	0.1–0.6 mg	Not recommended for outpatient surgery
	Dose-related increase time for: 1. Return of motor function 2. Return of micturition	

They rapidly cross the dura and are quickly sequestered into epidural fat and swiftly enter the systemic circulation. In general, lipophilic opioids tend to have a rapid onset of action, short duration, and a narrow band of analgesia. Delayed respiratory depression is less of a problem with the lipophilic opioids. Other side effects associated with intrathecal opioids include nausea and vomiting, urinary retention, and pruritus (refer to Table 55-22 for dosing guidelines).

Other useful analgesic additives include the α_2-agonists, NSAIDs, NMDA receptor antagonists, acetylcholinesterase inhibitors, adenosine, epinephrine, and benzodiazepines. The α_2-agonists alter pain transmission by binding to pre- and postsynaptic receptors within the dorsal horn of the spinal cord. Evidence suggests that intrathecal clonidine is synergistic with spinal local anesthetics, prolongs sensory and motor blockades, and causes less urinary retention than intrathecal morphine.[86] Intrathecal clonidine does not cause respiratory depression or pruritus. Intrathecal doses of 150 mcg, however, are reported to increase the incidence of hypotension, bradycardia, and nausea (refer to Table 55-23 for additional dosing recommendations).[86] Anecdotal reports suggest that the neuraxial administration of an NSAID, either accidentally or intentionally, is both safe and effective. Further investigation for the treatment of postoperative pain is required to define the role of intrathecal NSAIDs as well as the acetylcholinesterase inhibitors, NMDA receptor antagonists, adenosine, and benzodiazepines. No recommendations can be made at this time.

The Opioid-Dependent Patient

Although this discussion focuses on the patient with chronic pain syndromes, these strategies for perioperative pain management are easily adaptable to other opioid-dependent populations. Formerly, chronic pain had been defined as "pain without apparent biologic value that has persisted beyond the normal tissue healing time usually taken to be three months" (International Association for the Study of Pain) and "pain of a duration or intensity that adversely affects the function or well-being of the patient" (American Society of Anesthesiologists). Recently, however, the definition has been further subdivided into *chronic primary pain* and *chronic secondary pain syndromes*. "Chronic primary pain is defined as pain in one or more anatomical regions that persists or recurs for longer than 3 months and is associated with significant emotional distress or functional disability (interference with activities of daily life and participation in social roles) and that cannot be better accounted for by another chronic pain condition." On the other hand, "chronic secondary pain syndromes are linked to other diseases as the underlying cause, for which pain may initially be regarded as a symptom." These can include chronic cancer-related pain, chronic postsurgical or post traumatic pain, chronic neuropathic pain, chronic headache and orofacial pain, chronic visceral pain, and chronic musculoskeletal pain.[87] Chronic pain is often associated with anxiety and depression, which may require treatment with various anxiolytics, antidepressants, anticonvulsants, antiarrhythmics, and skeletal muscle relaxants in addition to opioids. Symptoms unique to chronic pain include tight musculature, limited range of motion, lack of energy, sleep disturbance, irritability, and social withdrawal. Associated psychiatric diagnoses may include hypochondriasis and psychosis.

Since the late 1990s, the percentage of patients with chronic pain for whom chronic opioids have been prescribed has increased dramatically and the United States has led the way. The reason for this is considered to be twofold: (1) more aggressive and compassionate treatment of chronic pain of malignant origin in cancer patients who are surviving longer and (2) to a much larger extent, the willingness of the medical community to treat pain of nonmalignant origin, such as osteoarthritis, with opioids.[88] The goal of opioid therapy for chronic pain was to improve pain, function, and quality of life. Unfortunately, evidence suggests that despite the increased use of opioids for chronic nonmalignant pain, there has been no corresponding reductions in the rates of disability or improvements in health status.[89] Unacceptable opioid side effects and concerns about adverse hormonal effects and immune modulation from long-term exposure caused some patients to abandon therapy. The long-term adverse consequences of chronic opioid use included physical dependence, the potential for withdrawal symptoms upon abrupt discontinuation of the opioid and the development of OIH and tolerance.

Tragically, during this same period, the liberal use of opioids for the treatment of both acute and chronic pain has resulted in an opioid crisis of unprecedented proportions. Since 1999, more than 600,000 individuals in the United States and Canada have died from an opioid overdose and the most recent data from the Centers for Disease Control and Prevention (cdc.gov/nchs) estimates that "overdose deaths from opioids increased to 75,673 in the 12-month period ending in April 2021, up from 56,064 the year before."

The opioid crisis has occurred in three waves. The first wave, which began in the 1990s, is attributed to the excessive prescribing of the drug Oxycontin™ in the mistaken belief, secondary to deceptive marketing practices, that it was somehow less addictive than other opioids. The second wave occurred in 2010 when drug traffickers started to market their product (e.g., heroin) to individuals addicted to prescription opioids. Finally, the third wave began in 2014, when illicit drug manufacturers contaminated counterfeit pharmaceutical pills with fentanyl. The COVID-19 pandemic has only served to exacerbate the problem.[90]

The U.S. FDA defines opioid tolerance as the use of the oral morphine equivalent of greater than or equal to 60 mg a day for 7 days or longer.[91] Recent evidence suggests that the opioid-tolerant patient can potentially have a complicated hospital course resulting in an increased hospital LOS and a high readmission rate.[91] A multimodal approach to acute pain management is highly recommended for the opioid-tolerant patient.

Definitions

Physical dependence is a "physiologic state of adaptation to a specific psychoactive substance characterized by the emergence of a *withdrawal syndrome* during abstinence, which may be relieved in total or in part by re-administration of the substance." Opioid *withdrawal* is characterized by an increased sympathetic and parasympathetic response that results in hypertension, tachycardia, diaphoresis, abdominal cramping, and diarrhea. *Tolerance* is a rightward shift of the dose–response curve and is "a state in which an increased dosage of a psychoactive substance is needed to produce a desired effect." Escalating doses of opioid may also be explained by an underlying progression of the disease state or by the development of OIH. Tolerance can be innate or acquired. Innate tolerance is a genetically predetermined sensitivity to a drug, whereas acquired tolerance can have a pharmacokinetic, learned, or pharmacodynamic basis. Pharmacokinetic tolerance involves a diminution in the effects of a drug because of changes in distribution and metabolism usually secondary to enzyme induction of the CYP450 system, which results in accelerated metabolism. Learned tolerance refers to compensatory behavior that masks intoxication. Pharmacodynamic tolerance refers to neuroadaptive changes that occur following chronic exposure to opioids, which may involve receptor desensitization secondary to receptor downregulation, internalization, and uncoupling of opioid receptors from G proteins. Opioids exhibit *cross-tolerance* to each other, but the degree of cross-tolerance varies widely and is often incomplete.[92] Clinicians use incomplete cross-tolerance to their advantage to restore analgesic sensitivity in highly tolerant patients through opioid rotation.[92] Because cross-tolerance is incomplete, analgesia is restored with the new opioid at more than 50% below the predicted equianalgesic dose.[92]

Differential tolerance commonly occurs in patients who are receiving chronic opioids, and this puts them at an increased risk for adverse consequences, particularly respiratory depression. "The concept of differential tolerance development means that different targets of opioid drugs do not develop tolerance at the same speed and to the same degree."[93] Whereas tolerance develops fastest to the analgesic effects of opioids, tolerance for the respiratory depressant effects and gastrointestinal effects can be significantly delayed. This can therefore place the opioid-tolerant patient at significant risk for respiratory depression during the postoperative period when their pain is appropriately treated with opioids.[93] It must be stressed that the development of tolerance or physical dependence in no way implies that the patient is addicted to an opioid. The American Society of Addiction Medicine defines ***addiction*** as "a treatable, chronic medical disease involving complex interactions among brain circuits, genetics, the environment, and an individual's life experiences. People with addiction use substances or engage in behaviors that become compulsive and often continue despite harmful consequences." (Available online: https://www.asam.org/quality-care/definition-of-addiction. Accessed February 13, 2022.)

The Transitional Pain Service

Since the quality of acute perioperative pain management in opioid-dependent patients can be unpredictable and frequently disjointed, the development of a transitional pain service (TPS) has been recommended. The TPS is a multidisciplinary group that uses a multimodal approach to pain management to "bridge the gap between acute and chronic pain" in complex surgical patients such as those with chronic pain (e.g., sickle cell disease), chronic opioid use (e.g., failed back syndrome), and opioid use disorder (OUD). A variety of therapeutic interventions can be provided throughout the surgical continuum by a TPS which will benefit the patient (Table 55-24). Various staffing models have been described in the literature[94]: the "high-intensity" model used at the Toronto General Hospital employs five anesthesiologists and various support staff for a total of 16 FTEs, and the "low-intensity" model practiced at the Veterans Administration Medical Center (VAMC) in Salt Lake City employs one acute pain–trained anesthesiologist with several support staff for a total of 5 full-time equivalent (FTEs). The VAMC group recently published a retrospective cohort study comparing patients receiving primary or revision orthopedic surgery prior to instituting a TPS and after instituting a TPS,[95] revealing that implementation of a TPS can significantly reduce the overall use of opioids following orthopedic surgery. An economic analysis of the ratio of savings to cost utilizing this "low-intensity" approach has been shown to have a positive economic impact (Fig. 55-16).[94] A TPS does not have to be a separate entity *per se* and can certainly be located within a pre-existing perioperative surgical home customized to the institution where resources can be shared to reduce expenses.

Table 55-24 A List of Potential Pharmacologic, Procedural, and Nonpharmacologic Interventions that May be Provided by a Transitional Pain Service

Potential Interventions	Description
Pharmacologic	Opioid-weaning assistance before and/or after surgery and perioperative multimodal opioid-sparing analgesia
Procedural	
Neuromodulation	Peripheral nerve neuromodulation, transcutaneous electrical nerve stimulation
Peripheral nerve blockade/ cryoneurolysis	Ambulatory continuous perineural nerve blocks, peripheral nerve cryoneurolysis
Acupuncture	Therapeutic technique developed within traditional Chinese medicine using small-diameter needle stimulation
Nonpharmacologic	
Pain-coping skills applications	Electronic health applications
Sensory therapy	Music, visual, distraction, and relaxation techniques
Psychological interventions	Cognitive–behavioral therapy, biofeedback, counseling

Adapted from Sun EC, Mariano ER, Narouze S, et al. Making a business plan for starting a transitional pain service within the US healthcare system. *Reg Anesth Pain Med.* 2021;46(8):727–731.

Management of the Opioid-Dependent Patient

Patients who are receiving opioids preoperatively are at an increased risk during the perioperative period for adverse outcomes. Prudence, therefore, dictates that the clinicians caring for the patient query their state's prescription drug monitoring program (PDMP). In California, this is referred to as the Controlled Substance Utilization Review and Evaluation System (CURES). Physicians can easily run a Patient Activity Report (PAR) to confirm the drug prescribed, the dose, and dispensing date as well as the name of the patient, the prescribing physician, and the pharmacy. Since the risk is dose dependent, it is useful to categorize preoperative opioid use into three groups (O-NET): *opioid naive, opioid exposed, and opioid tolerant* (Fig. 55-17). The opioid-naive patient is defined as having received no opioids in the previous 90 days. The opioid-exposed patient has a history of <60 mg/d oral morphine equivalent in the previous 90 days. The opioid-tolerant patient is defined as having received >60 mg/d

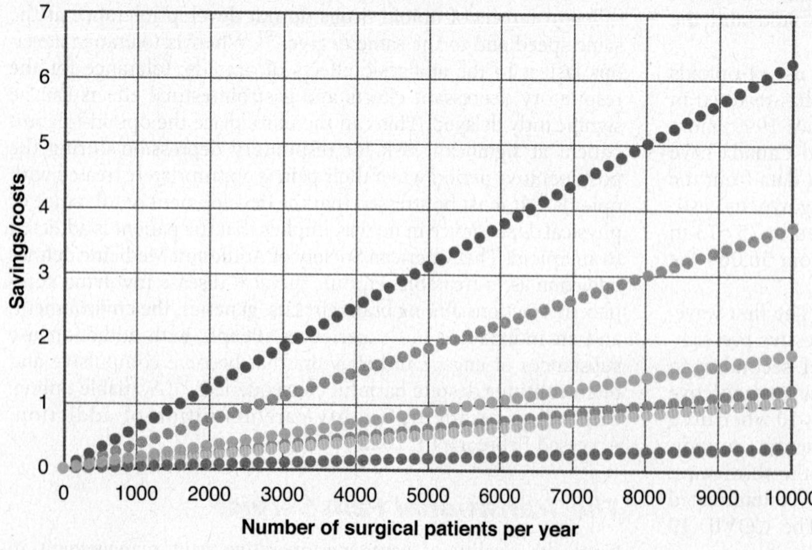

Figure 55-16 Opioid-naive, opioid-exposed, and opioid-tolerant patients. (Reprinted with Sun EC, Mariano ER, Narouze S, et al. Making a business plan for starting a transitional pain service within the US healthcare system. *Reg Anesth Pain Med.* 2021;46(8):727–731, with permission from BMJ Publishing Group Ltd.)

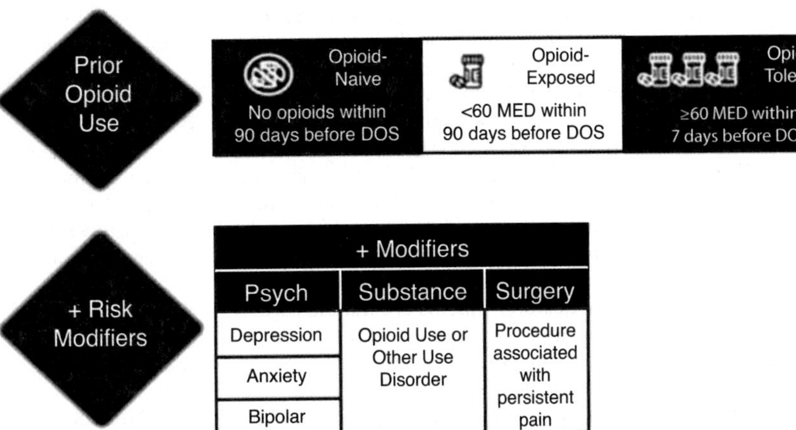

Figure 55-17 Low-risk, moderate-risk, and high-risk categories based on comorbidities and type of surgery. (Derived from Edwards DA, Hedrick TL, Jayaram J, et al. American Society for Enhanced Recovery and Perioperative Quality Initiative Joint Consensus Statement on Perioperative Management of Patients on Preoperative Opioid Therapy. *Anesth Analg*. 2019;129:553–566. In: Hyland SJ, Wetshtein AM, Grable SJ, Jackson MP. Acute Pain Management Pearls: A Focused Review for the Hospital Clinician. Healthcare (Basel). 2022 Dec 22;11(1):34. Figure 3. Copyright © 2022 by the authors. https://creativecommons.org/licenses/by/4.0/)

oral morphine equivalent in the 7 days prior to surgery. Opioid-tolerant patients have a greater likelihood of a complicated hospital course, which may manifest through delayed wound healing, increased surgical reintervention, prolonged hospital stays, higher readmission rates, greater health care costs, and increased mortality. Patients can be further stratified into low-, moderate- and high-risk categories based on comorbidities and type of surgery (Fig. 55-17). Identifying and managing modifiable risks factors prior to surgery has the potential to improve surgical outcome as well as improve the surgical experience for the patient.[96] See Table 55-25.

10 The onus for the identification of the opioid-dependent patient rests with the patient's surgical team, preoperative evaluation staff, and the anesthesia team.[97] Ideally, the patient and the health care teams will formulate a perioperative pain management plan prior to surgery, and, depending upon availability, the patient can be seen and evaluated by the institution's TPS where appropriate procedural interventions can be recommended (Table 55-24). Often, however, the opioid-dependent patient is identified just moments prior to surgery and the anesthesia team needs to be innovative.[29] The ideal perioperative pain management strategy in the opioid-dependent patient will involve a multimodal approach that employs regional analgesia techniques (neuraxial or peripheral nerve blockade), when appropriate, in conjunction with systemic nonopioid medications. Opioids, however, remain the mainstay of perioperative pain management and an adequate dose of opioid needs to be maintained to avoid precipitating withdrawal symptoms.

Table 55-25 Perioperative Management of the Patient Taking Preoperative Opioids

1. **Categorize and define preoperative opioid use:**
   - Define the patient as opioid *naive, exposed, or tolerant*.
2. **Risk stratification of the patient:**
   - Use O-NET classification system (see figure) to risk stratify the patient.
3. **Optimize patient management according to the O-NET criteria:**
   - Consult perioperative pain specialist prior to surgery in high-risk patients.
   - Consider a preoperative opioid taper to the lowest effective dose.
   - Optimize psychosocial comorbidities.
   - Do not discontinue buprenorphine or methadone if the patient is receiving these medications for medication treatment of opioid use disorder (MOUD).
4. **Strategies for perioperative pain management of the moderate- to high-risk patient:**
   - Use multimodal analgesia pain management strategies that include the use of regional anesthesia techniques when applicable.
5. **Is opioid free management possible?**
   - This may be possible. Opioid-free management is a shared decision between the patient and the perioperative physician that can be tailored to the type of surgery and specific regional anesthetic technique.
6. **Strategy for managing postoperative pain:**
   - Optimize nonopioid analgesics.
   - Use the lowest effective opioid dose.
   - Avoid escalation of the opioid dose.
   - Use regional anesthesia that is procedure specific and opioid sparing. Use a continuous nerve block technique when indicated.
7. **Strategy for managing postoperative opioids at the time of discharge:**
   - Limit the amount of the discharge opioid prescription to an amount that is appropriate for the expected pain.
   - If the patient has been managed in the hospital with a continuous nerve block technique, consider continuing the infusion as an outpatient.

Reprinted with permission from Edwards DA, Hedrick TL, Jayaram J, et al. American Society for Enhanced Recovery and Perioperative Quality Initiative Joint Consensus Statement on Perioperative Management of Patients on Preoperative Opioid Therapy. *Anesthesia & Analgesia*. 2019;129(2):553–566.

11 *Preoperative management* of the patient involves determining the patient's "baseline" opioid requirement. On the day of surgery, the patient should be instructed to take their normal opioid dose. If for some reason, the patient neglects to take the opioid on the day of surgery, the anesthesiologist can administer an equivalent dose preoperatively. The opioid-dependent patient has increased opioid requirements, which are reported to be 30% to 100% greater than an opioid-naive patient[88] and perioperative dosages may have to be carefully increased. However, chronic use of opioids also produces *differential opioid tolerance* which can potentially place the opioid-tolerant patient at an increased risk for respiratory depression when larger doses of opioids are administered. We suggest that the patient's baseline opioid regimen be continued during their hospital admission and that acute perioperative pain be managed with nonpharmacological approaches such as the application of heat, cold, or splinting, as indicated, in addition to prescribing nonopioid analgesics and regional anesthesia (e.g., neuraxial and peripheral nerve blockade) when appropriate. Short-acting opioids may be prescribed for breakthrough pain that fails to respond to the above interventions.

Patients prescribed transdermal fentanyl patches are usually instructed to maintain their fentanyl patch into the operating room and this can serve as their baseline opioid requirement. In the case of major surgery, or when the risk of major blood loss or sepsis is significant, patients may be instructed to discontinue their transdermal patch and an IV fentanyl infusion can be initiated instead to maintain adequate plasma concentrations. Patients maintained on methadone should continue their baseline dose throughout the perioperative period. In the United States, methadone is available for both oral and IV administration. Patients receiving more than 200 mg of methadone per day can develop a prolonged QT interval, which places them at risk for Torsades de Pointes. It is therefore recommended that a baseline ECG be obtained for comparison. Patients who are maintained on the partial opioid agonist buprenorphine may continue to receive the drug for postoperative pain control; morphine, hydromorphone, or fentanyl may be administered to supplement analgesia as required.[98] Full antagonists (e.g., naloxone and naltrexone) and the partial agonists–antagonists (e.g., nalbuphine, pentazocine, and butorphanol) should be avoided because they will precipitate withdrawal symptoms in opioid-dependent patients.

Because it is well documented that the use of systemic nonopioid analgesics is opioid sparing in the opioid-naive patient, it is reasonable to apply this experience to the opioid-tolerant patient. Any multimodal protocol for the perioperative care of the opioid-tolerant patient should include some combination of gabapentin or pregabalin, an NSAID or selective cyclooxygenase (COX-2) inhibitor, acetaminophen, dexamethasone, an NMDA receptor antagonist, α_2-receptor agonists, lidocaine, and magnesium.[99]

Both *gabapentin* and *pregabalin* bind to the α-2δ subunit of voltage-gated P/Q-type calcium channels in the dorsal horn of the spinal cord and, by modulating the release of excitatory neurotransmitters from activated nociceptors, these drugs are believed to inhibit pain transmission and central sensitization.[57] They are both recommended for the treatment of perioperative pain in the opioid-tolerant patient.[74] Although gabapentin and pregabalin have similar mechanisms of action, pregabalin may be the preferred drug because of superior bioavailability and better diffusion into the central nervous system.[74]

The *NSAIDs* (e.g., ibuprofen and naproxen) have displayed proven efficacy for the treatment of postoperative pain and their opioid-sparing effect accounts for a significant reduction in opioid-related side effects, especially postoperative nausea, and vomiting. Likewise, the analgesic effects of the *selective COX-2 inhibitors* are analogous to the NSAIDs. The recommended dose of celecoxib that reduces both postoperative pain and decreases opioid requirement is 400 mg orally 2 hours prior to surgery.[74,100]

Acetaminophen is an effective adjuvant in the treatment of postoperative pain. It has an opioid-sparing effect, and can potentially decrease the incidence of postoperative nausea and vomiting. The mechanism of action of the drug is elusive but is thought to involve inhibition of the COX enzyme via interaction at the peroxidase site, modulation of the descending inhibitory serotoninergic pathways, and opioid agonist effects. There is also some evidence that acetaminophen interacts with the endocannabinoid system, $TRPV_1$, and NMDA receptors,[101] which may make this drug particularly efficacious in the opioid-tolerant patient. Acetaminophen may be administered orally or intravenously. The IV route offers the advantage of earlier and higher peak plasma levels compared to oral acetaminophen, resulting in superior cerebrospinal fluid levels. The recommended adult dose in patients above 50 kg is 1,000 mg intravenously every 6 hours. The first dose may be administered just prior to surgery and continued postoperatively for as long as the patient is unable to tolerate oral intake. A single systematic qualitative review of 21 trials demonstrated that the combination of an NSAID with acetaminophen produces analgesia that is superior to either drug alone.[44] Finally, dexamethasone may be beneficial in the opioid-dependent patient, secondary to decreased neurotransmitter release and decreased production of the NMDA receptor antagonist kynurenic acid.[74] The recommended preoperative IV dose is 0.11 to 0.2 mg/kg.[73] Doses as high as 0.2 mg/kg have been administered as part of a multimodal analgesic strategy.[74]

Intraoperative management of the opioid-dependent patient requires the prudent use of fentanyl, morphine, or hydromorphone to provide effective intraoperative anesthesia, postoperative analgesia and to prevent opioid withdrawal. This requires the administration of the patients' baseline opioid requirement plus their intraoperative requirements secondary to surgical stimulation. Exact opioid dosing guidelines do not exist, but because of receptor downregulation, secondary to chronic opioid administration, intraoperative opioid doses may need to be increased 30–50% compared to the opioid naive patient. Opioid rotation takes advantage of the fact that a new opioid will bind a different opioid receptor subtype and be metabolized differently, and thus a new opioid may be useful in the surgical setting. Following the cancer pain model, the dose of the new opioid should be less than 50% of the calculated equianalgesic dose because of incomplete cross-tolerance.[92] Although this new opioid may be administered for several days postoperatively, prudence dictates that a physician or pharmacist well versed in pain management should convert the patient to an appropriate oral opioid regimen for discharge from the hospital.

The optimal intraoperative dose of opioid varies considerably from patient to patient. Monitoring intraoperative vital signs such as heart rate, pupil size, and respiratory rate can be useful and allows the clinician to avoid the negative consequences of opioid overdosing or underdosing. It can be clinically informative to reverse neuromuscular blockade toward the end of a general anesthetic and allow the patient to breathe spontaneously while still anesthetized. Patients with a respiratory rate greater than 20 breaths per minute and significantly dilated pupils require additional opioid. Titrating fentanyl, morphine, or hydromorphone to a respiratory rate of 12 to 14 breaths per minute and a moderately miotic pupil is recommended prior to emergence.

Activation of the NMDA receptor by the second messenger protein kinase C (PKC) is reported to play a critical role in the development of opioid tolerance.[74] Inhibition of the NMDA receptor with the NMDA receptor antagonist ketamine can be a useful strategy in this patient population because it is reported to be effective at reversing morphine tolerance and restoring its effectiveness as an analgesic.[88] The recommended intraoperative dose of ketamine for the opioid-tolerant patient is 0.5 mg/kg as a bolus dose at the beginning of the case, followed by 10 mcg/kg/min as an infusion for the duration of the case.[102] Low-dose ketamine may be continued into the postoperative period for up to 48 hours without any serious complications.

The α_2-adrenoreceptor agonists (e.g., dexmedetomidine and clonidine) have moderate analgesic effects and opioid-sparing effects in the opioid-naive patient. In the perioperative setting, they are sedating and anxiolytic and can decrease the stress response to surgery and mitigate postoperative shivering, nausea, vomiting, and agitation. The α_2-adrenoreceptor agonists may be particularly valuable in the treatment of the opioid-tolerant patient because they attenuate opioid withdrawal symptoms and can reduce postoperative opioid requirements and pain.[97,103]

IV lidocaine has been gaining acceptance as part of a multimodal approach to perioperative pain management, particularly in the patient receiving abdominal surgery or in the patient in whom regional anesthesia is contraindicated. Systemic lidocaine displays analgesic, anti-inflammatory, and anti-hyperalgesic properties, which are mediated by inhibition of voltage-dependent sodium channels, NMDA receptors, and GPCRs. Indirect blockade of the NMDA receptor through inhibition of PKC potentially makes this a useful drug in the opioid-tolerant patient.[104]

Like ketamine, IV magnesium is an NMDA receptor antagonist that can suppress neuropathic pain, potentiate morphine analgesia, attenuate morphine tolerance,[69] and abolish the development of hyperalgesia and central sensitization.[71] Because magnesium and ketamine bind to different sites on the NMDA receptor, it has been posited that the combination of the two drugs may enhance analgesia through a "superadditive effect."[105] Future studies should focus on an ideal dosing regimen to maximize analgesia while decreasing drug-related side effects in the treatment of acute perioperative pain in the opioid-tolerant patient.[106]

Postoperative management of the opioid-dependent patient can be very challenging. Ideally, the optimal amount of opioid has been administered to the patient during the intraoperative period, allowing them to emerge from anesthesia comfortably sedated and pain free. On arrival to the recovery room, IV opioids may be administered on an "as-needed" basis; however, initiation of an IV PCA opioid with both a basal and an incremental (bolus) dose will minimize the risk of breakthrough pain. The recommended basal infusion should equate to the patient's hourly preoperative oral opioid dose requirement as this will avoid precipitating withdrawal symptoms. A reasonable initial value for the bolus dose is an amount equal to that administered during 1 hour of the background infusion. For example, a patient taking 90 mg of oral morphine per day (e.g., 30 mg orally every 8 hours) equates to 30 mg of IV morphine per day, which can be administered as a basal morphine infusion of 1.25 mg/h. The recommended bolus dose (i.e., the demand dose) should be one-half of the patient's hourly dose: approximately 0.6 mg in this example. A lockout interval of 10 minutes is a reasonable starting point. Prudence dictates that the patient be constantly monitored for oversedation and respiratory depression. The PCA can be programmed with hourly or 4-hour dose limits to increase safety. Consultation with an expert in acute perioperative pain management, however, is strongly advised when managing these patients. Basal infusions are not required for patients who are maintained on their transdermal fentanyl patches as these provide adequate basal analgesia. Therefore, a fentanyl PCA with a bolus dose and an appropriate lockout interval may be all that is required. Patients recovering from same-day surgery will be initially treated with IV doses of opioids in the recovery room. They can be quickly transitioned to an oral regimen consisting of their baseline opioid requirement plus an appropriate amount of short-acting opioid for breakthrough pain consistent with the invasiveness of the surgery.[99]

Nonopioid analgesics should be part of any multimodal perioperative pain management strategy in the opioid-dependent patient. Low-dose IV ketamine may be continued into the postoperative period, although specific dosing recommendations are not available at this time. In a single case report involving an opioid-dependent trauma patient, ketamine was administered postoperatively at a starting dose of 10 μg/kg/min and then gradually tapered to 2.5 μg/kg/min over 45 minutes. This regimen provided significant pain control and was opioid sparing. The ketamine infusion was continued for 7 days without any adverse sequelae.[107]

Regional anesthesia is highly recommended in the opioid-dependent patient. Peripheral nerve blockade (either single injection or continuous catheter) or epidural analgesia can be very useful as part of a multimodal pain regimen. However, we do not recommend administering neuraxial opioids in this patient population: the patient's baseline opioid dose as well as the opioid for breakthrough pain should be delivered systemically. Because of the risk of respiratory depression, we do not recommend administering opioids by multiple routes simultaneously. A physician well versed in acute and chronic pain management who is comfortable with the equianalgesic dosing of opioids should, ideally, be involved in the care of the patient. Careful monitoring of these patients for excessive sedation or respiratory depression is mandatory, and staff in the recovery room and on the postsurgical units should be alerted to the potential risk for respiratory depression.

Special Populations

Patients with OUD who are receiving medication treatment of opioid use disorder (MOUD) are a unique population of patients who merit special consideration in the management of perioperative pain. Medications that are approved by the FDA for the treatment of OUD include *methadone, buprenorphine, and naltrexone*. Discontinuation of methadone or buprenorphine, prior to surgery, is not recommended. Patients receiving maintenance methadone preoperatively should continue that dose during the perioperative period. It may be dosed once daily or divided into three doses given at 8-hour intervals for better analgesia. Serious side effects associated with methadone include QT interval prolongation, cardiac arrhythmias (e.g., torsades de pointes), and respiratory depression secondary to its long half-life.

In the United States, buprenorphine has received FDA approval for the management of acute pain, OUD, and chronic pain. Buprenorphine is a partial mu receptor agonist, kappa receptor antagonist, and nociceptin opioid receptor (ORL-1) agonist. Buprenorphine is a very effective analgesic with a ceiling effect on respiratory depression, which makes it a potentially safer alternative to methadone for the management of OUD. Buprenorphine is available in routes of administration that include parenteral, transdermal, sublingual, buccal films, subcutaneous, and subdermal implants. Expert opinion recommends that buprenorphine should not be routinely discontinued prior to surgery. Consultation with an expert in acute pain management of the opioid-tolerant patient is highly recommended.

Naltrexone is a semisynthetic opioid antagonist that is derived from oxymorphone via substitution of the n-methyl with a methylcyclopropyl group. Naltrexone is used in both alcohol- and opioid-dependent patients who are highly motivated to remain abstinent. The drug is available as a once-daily 50-mg oral dose or a once-monthly 380-mg depot injection of naltrexone embedded within a biodegradable biosphere matrix (Vivitrol™). Perioperative management of these patients requires holding the oral formulation for 3 days prior to surgery and, ideally, scheduling surgery for at least 4 weeks after the last dose of depot naltrexone. These patients can experience opioid receptor upregulation due to chronic opioid antagonism with naltrexone, which places them at increased risk for opioid-related side effects such as respiratory depression. A full discussion of this topic is beyond the scope of this chapter and the reader is referred to some excellent reviews on the subject.[14,108]

Organization of Perioperative Pain Management Services

Despite the availability of effective analgesics and nonpharmacologic techniques, acute postoperative pain continues to be an unresolved worldwide problem.[109,110] The effective management of acute perioperative pain is a crucial component of good perioperative care and recovery from surgery. Poorly managed postoperative pain is associated with poor outcomes including increased hospital LOS, poor sleep, increased time to first ambulation, increased opioid use, delirium in the elderly, cardiopulmonary and thromboembolic complications, and potentially increasing costs to the health care system. The inadequate management of acute postoperative pain increases the risk of progression to chronic postoperative surgical pain (CPSP) following certain surgical procedures (Table 55-26).

There is good evidence that the overall incidence of moderate-to-severe pain in surgical patients is about 25% to 40% despite the availability of pain treatment.[111] There are considerable barriers that challenge the establishment and/or effectiveness of acute pain teams in managing patients across the continuum of care. A major obstacle to the establishment of postoperative pain services is its cost in a privatized health system, wherein limited reimbursement for postoperative care discourages the establishment of a service. The value of an acute perioperative pain service (APPS), apart from its benefit for patient care, comes from the added value of reducing hospital costs by improving surgical outcome and by facilitating patient recovery and early discharge.[112] Depending on the reimbursement model, this added value could make an APPS a persuasive investment despite the upfront expenditures required to provide the service. The APPS provides direct patient care such as the management of continuous epidural and regional catheter infusions and other modalities and can play a leading role in patient education and the education of other physicians, nurses, and caregivers to ensure their competence in effectively assessing, managing, and meeting a patient's needs. A proactive APPS would ideally provide the surgical patient with a continuum of care that spans the pre- to postoperative phases of treatment. The primary goal is to reduce the variability of acute pain management by using "protocol-based systems that optimizes resource utilization while improving patient care."[113] Although it is convenient to regard postoperative pain primarily as acute pain caused by tissue injury associated with surgery, this may exclude other important factors that contribute to a patient's suffering following surgery. Acute postsurgical pain can also be caused by prolonged patient positioning or pressure effects from prolonged immobility. Many patients presenting for elective surgery may also suffer chronic pain from underlying illness or injury (e.g., degenerative diseases or malignancy) which may contribute significantly to the intensity of the postoperative pain experienced by the patient. Postoperative pain remains a substantial problem that is often masked by a patient's acceptance of pain as a natural consequence of surgery. Other common patient barriers include cultural and language barriers, personal experience or the experiences of friends and relatives, stoicism, and/or opiophobia. For these reasons, postoperative pain management begins preoperatively with patient education to alleviate the attendant anxiety, apprehension, and fear of surgery, to understand the patient's fears and concerns, and to come to an agreement with the patient that pain control is an expected goal of care. Education is also the key to changing the attitudes of other caregivers to effectively treat their patient's pain. In developing a perioperative pain service, it is important to bear in mind that the importance of effective perioperative pain management extends well beyond the mere establishment of

Table 55-26 Prevalence of Chronic Postsurgical Pain in Common Surgeries in the United States[11,22–24]

	Any Intensity (%)	Moderate–severe Intensity (%)	Prevalence (%); Prevalence if Restricted to a Severe Pain Rating	Number of Operations in U.S. Nonfederal Community Hospitals[a] in 2014[7]
Amputation of limb	3–85%	5–10%	Up to 85%[8]	Not available
Arthroplasty, knee	13–44%	15%	44% (15%)[9]	723,086
Caesarean section	6–55%	5–10%	Up to 12%[10]	1,142,680
Cholecystectomy	3–50%[11]	Not reported	Not reported	300,245
Craniotomy	0–65%[12]	25%	12–16%[13]	Not available
Hip replacement	27%	6%	27% (15%)[9]	487,625
Inguinal hernia repair	5–63%	2–4%	6–29%[14]	Not available
Laminectomy and spinal fusion	10–40%	4–6[15]	5–36%[16,17]	564,911
Mastectomy	11–57%	5–10%	22%[18]	Not available
Coronary artery bypass graft	30–50%	5–10%	28% (4%)[19]	160,240
Thoracotomy	5–65%	10%	48%[20,21]	Not available

[a]Nonfederal community hospitals account for 786 874 (87%) of 902 202 hospital beds in the United States.

Reprinted from Glare P, Aubrey KR, Myles PS. Transition from acute to chronic pain after surgery. *Lancet*. 2019;393(10180):1537–1546. Table 1.

dedicated personnel. It must also encompass a leadership role in transforming the institutional culture to elevate the relief of pain and suffering to its place as a primary goal of patient care.[114]

12 The key component to establishing a successful perioperative pain management service is an institutional commitment to support the service. The team must be built around a physician leader with training and experience in pain medicine. This leader is responsible for the development and implementation of clinical pathways and protocols that enhance recovery following surgery. These protocols must include pain assessment tools that are suitable for use across the continuum of care. The ideal structure of the APPS may consist of midlevel providers (registered nurses and nurse practitioners), who can follow these protocolized pain management pathways, with an anesthesiologist as the physician leader in a supervisory role. Depending on the needs of the institution, other members of the team may include acute pain fellows, residents, interns, and medical students as well as a pharmacist and an anesthesia technician. Other anesthesiologists must be available to participate in the supervisory role to ensure continuity of service.

Conclusion

Standardized acute perioperative pain management strategies that optimize patient care through the judicious use of opioids and procedure-specific techniques should be incorporated into all enhanced recovery protocols.[6] Perioperative acute pain management must incorporate evidence-based and opioid stewardship strategies that emphasize the judicious use of opioids and procedure-specific regional anesthesia techniques that can mitigate the risk of opioid-related adverse drug events. Communication, cooperation, and collaboration among health care providers is paramount if we are to achieve the goal of optimal patient care. Accomplishing this requires integration of information and systems from disparate disciplines within medicine. It challenges physicians to acquire a patient-focused perspective that provides the patient with a pleasant perioperative experience and enhanced recovery following surgery. In doing so, clinicians will be challenged to construct systems within hospitals, such as a transitional pain service and addiction specialist consultation, to support positive outcome benefits to patients. The cost of ignoring pain and suffering has been widely cited to be in the billions of dollars each, but the cost in suffering is immeasurable.

For additional information please see Chapter 36, Videos 36.1, 36.4, 36-6, 36.8-36.10 and 5 Video 55-5 in the eBook bundled with this text.

For further review and interactivities, please see the videos and narrative interactive clinical vignettes (NICVs) accessible in the complimentary eBook bundled with this text. Access instructions are located on the inside front cover.

REFERENCES

1. Meara JG, Leather AJ, Hagander L, et al. Global Surgery 2030: evidence and solutions for achieving health, welfare, and economic development. *Lancet*. 2015;386:569–624.
2. Chou R, Gordon DB, de Leon-Casasola OA, et al. Management of postoperative pain: a clinical practice guideline from the American Pain Society, the American Society of Regional Anesthesia and Pain Medicine, and the American Society of Anesthesiologists' Committee on Regional Anesthesia, Executive Committee, and Administrative Council. *J Pain*. 2016;17:131–157.
3. U.S. Department of Health and Human Services (2019, May). *Pain Management Best Practices Inter-Agency Task Force Report*: Updates, Gaps, Inconsistencies, and Recommendations. Retrieved from U.S. Department of Health and Human Services website: https://www.hhs.gov/ash/advisory-committees/pain/reports/index.html.
4. Wu CL, Naqibuddin M, Rowlingson AJ, Lietman SA, Jermyn RM, Fleisher LA. The effect of pain on health-related quality of life in the immediate postoperative period. *Anesth Analg*. 2003;97:1078–1085.
5. Joshi GP, Ogunnaike BO. Consequences of inadequate postoperative pain relief and chronic persistent postoperative pain. *Anesthesiol Clin North Am*. 2005;23:21–36.
6. Mariano ER, Dickerson DM, Szokol JW, et al. A multisociety organizational consensus process to define guiding principles for acute perioperative pain management. *Reg Anesth Pain Med*. 2022;47:118–127.
7. Raja SN, Carr DB, Cohen M, et al. The revised International Association for the Study of Pain definition of pain: concepts, challenges, and compromises. *Pain*. 2020;161:1976–1982.
8. Raja SN, Dougherty PM. Anatomy and physiology of somatosensory and pain processing. In *SPEC—Essentials of Pain Medicine and Regional Anesthesia (Reprint)*. Elsevier Inc.; 2005:1–6. https://doi.org/10.1016/B978-0-443-06651-1.50005-8.
9. Wilder-Smith OHG, Arendt-Nielsen L. Postoperative hyperalgesia: its clinical importance and relevance. *Anesthesiology*. 2006;104:601–607.
10. Rowlingson J. Update on acute pain management. *Anesth Analg*. 2006.
11. Lavand'homme P. From preemptive to preventive analgesia: time to reconsider the role of perioperative peripheral nerve blocks? *Reg Anesth Pain Med*. 2011;36:4–6.
12. Taylor D. Improving outcomes in acute pain management: optimizing patient selection. *MedScape Neurology*. 2004.
13. Kelava M, Alfirevic A, Bustamante S, Hargrave J, Marciniak D. Regional anesthesia in cardiac surgery: an overview of fascial plane chest wall blocks. *Anesth Analg*. 2020;131:127–135.
14. Hyland SJ, Brockhaus KK, Vincent WR, et al. Perioperative pain management and opioid stewardship: a practical guide. *Healthcare (Basel)*. 2021;9:333.
15. Caraceni A, Cherny N, Fainsinger R, et al. Pain measurement tools and methods in clinical research in palliative care: recommendations of an Expert Working Group of the European Association of Palliative Care. *J Pain Symptom Manage*. 2002;23:239–255.
16. Portenoy RK, Bennett DS, Rauck R, et al. Prevalence and characteristics of breakthrough pain in opioid-treated patients with chronic noncancer pain. *J Pain*. 2006;7:583–591.
17. Bennett M. The LANSS Pain Scale: the Leeds assessment of neuropathic symptoms and signs. *Pain*. 2001;92:147–157.
18. Lavand'homme P, Estebe JP. Opioid-free anesthesia: a different regard to anesthesia practice. *Curr Opin Anaesthesiol*. 2018;31:556–561.
19. Pizzi LT, Toner R, Foley K, et al. Relationship between potential opioid-related adverse effects and hospital length of stay in patients receiving opioids after orthopedic surgery. *Pharmacotherapy*. 2012;32:502–514.
20. Camilleri M. Opioid-induced constipation: challenges and therapeutic opportunities. *Am J Gastroenterol*. 2011;106:835–842.
21. Javaheri S, Randerath W. Opioid-induced central sleep apnea: mechanisms and therapies. *Sleep Medicine Clinics*. 2014;9:49–56.
22. Safe use of opioids in hospitals. *Sentinel Event Alert*. 2012;8:1–5.
23. Angst MS, Clark JD. Opioid-induced hyperalgesia: a qualitative systematic review. *Anesthesiology*. 2006;104:570–587.
24. Budd K. Pain management: is opioid immunosuppression a clinical problem? *Biomed Pharmacother*. 2006;60:310–317.
25. Gupta K, Kshirsagar S, Chang L, et al. Morphine Stimulates Angiogenesis by Activating Proangiogenic and Survival-promoting Signaling and Promotes Breast Tumor Growthl. *Cancer Res*. 2002;62:4491–4498.
26. Sarhill N, Walsh D, Nelson K. Hydromorphone: Pharmacology and clinical applications in cancer patients. *Support Care Cancer*. 2001;9:84–96.
27. Crews KR, Gaedigk A, Dunnenberger HM, et al; Clinical Pharmacogenetics Implementation Consortium. Clinical Pharmacogenetics Implementation Consortium guidelines for cytochrome P450 2D6 genotype and codeine therapy: 2014 update. *Clin Pharmacol Ther*. 2014;95:376–382.
28. Mahajan G, Fishman SM. Chapter 11 - major opioids in pain management. In: Benzon HT, Raja SN, Molloy RE, Liu SS, Fishman SM, eds. *Essentials of Pain Medicine and Regional Anesthesia*. 2nd ed. Churchill Livingstone; 2005:94–105.
29. Mitra S, Sinatra RS. Perioperative management of acute pain in the opioid-dependent patient. *Anesthesiology*. 2004;101:212–227.
30. Ronel I, Weiniger CF. Non-regional analgesia for labour: remifentanil in obstetrics. *BJA Educ*. 2019;19:357–361.
31. American Pain Society. *Principles of Analgesic Use in the Treatment of Acute Pain and Cancer Pain*. American Pain Society; 2003.
32. Nguyen Thi TV, Orliaguet G, Ngû TH, Bonnet F. Spinal anesthesia with meperidine as the sole agent for cesarean delivery. *Reg Anesth*. 1994;19:386–389.
33. Davis MP. Twelve reasons for considering buprenorphine as a frontline analgesic in the management of pain. *J Support Oncol*. 2012;10:209–219.
34. *Drug Facts and Comparisons*. Wolters Kluwer Health; 2011.
35. Williams BA, Butt MT, Zeller JR, Coffee S, Pippi MA. Multimodal perineural analgesia with combined bupivacaine-clonidine-buprenorphine-dexamethasone: safe in vivo and chemically compatible in solution. *Pain Med*. 2015;16:186–198.

36. Frampton JE. Tapentadol immediate release: a review of its use in the treatment of moderate to severe acute pain. *Drugs*. 2010;70:1719–1743.
37. eMedExpert. Difference between Tramadol and Tapentadol. 2015.
38. Hawley P, Chow L, Fyles G, Shokoohi A, O'Leary MJ, Mittelstadt M. Clinical Outcomes of Start-Low, Go-Slow Methadone Initiation for Cancer-Related Pain: What's the Hurry? *J Palliat Med*. 2017;20:1244–1251.
39. Tan HS, Habib AS. Oliceridine: a novel drug for the management of moderate to severe acute pain - a review of current evidence. *J Pain Res*. 2021;14:969–979.
40. Katz JA. Chapter 16—NSAIDs and COX-2-selective inhibitors. In: Benzon HT, Raja SN, Molloy RE, Liu SS, Fishman SM, eds. *Essentials of Pain Medicine and Regional Anesthesia*. 2nd ed. Churchill Livingstone; 2005:141–158.
41. Marret E, Kurdi O, Zufferey P, Bonnet F. Effects of nonsteroidal antiinflammatory drugs on patient-controlled analgesia morphine side effects: meta-analysis of randomized controlled trials. *Anesthesiology*. 2005;102:1249–1260.
42. Viscusi ER, Gan TJ, Bergese S, et al. Intravenous meloxicam for the treatment of moderate to severe acute pain: a pooled analysis of safety and opioid-reducing effects. *Reg Anesth Pain Med*. 2019;44:360.
43. Smith HS. Perioperative intravenous acetaminophen and NSAIDs. *Pain Med*. 2011;12:961–981.
44. Ong CK, Seymour RA, Lirk P, Merry AF. Combining paracetamol (acetaminophen) with nonsteroidal antiinflammatory drugs: a qualitative systematic review of analgesic efficacy for acute postoperative pain. *Anesth Analg*. 2010;110:1170–1179.
45. Jibril F, Sharaby S, Mohamed A, Wilby KJ. Intravenous versus oral acetaminophen for pain: systematic review of current evidence to support clinical decision-making. *Can J Hosp Pharm*. 2015;68:238–247.
46. Jouguelet-Lacoste J, La Colla L, Schilling D, Chelly JE. The use of intravenous infusion or single dose of low-dose ketamine for postoperative analgesia: a review of the current literature. *Pain Med*. 2015;16:383–403.
47. Schwenk ES, Viscusi ER, Buvanendran A, et al. Consensus guidelines on the use of intravenous ketamine infusions for acute pain management from the American Society of Regional Anesthesia and Pain Medicine, the American Academy of Pain Medicine, and the American Society of Anesthesiologists. *Reg Anesth Pain Med*. 2018;43:456–466.
48. Weinbroum AA. A single small dose of postoperative ketamine provides rapid and sustained improvement in morphine analgesia in the presence of morphine-resistant pain. *Anesth Analg*. 2003;96:789–795.
49. Reeves M, Lindholm DE, Myles PS, Fletcher H, Hunt JO. Adding ketamine to morphine for patient-controlled analgesia after major abdominal surgery: a double-blinded, randomized controlled trial. *Anesth Analg*. 2001;93:116–120.
50. Sveticic G, Gentilini A, Eichenberger U, Luginbühl M, Curatolo M. Combinations of morphine with ketamine for patient-controlled analgesia: a new optimization method. *Anesthesiology*. 2003;98:1195–1205.
51. Wadhwa A, Clarke D, Goodchild CS, Young D. Large-dose oral dextromethorphan as an adjunct to patient-controlled analgesia with morphine after knee surgery. *Anesth Analg*. 2001; 92:448–454.
52. Weinbroum AA, Rudick V, Paret G, Ben-Abraham R. The role of dextromethorphan in pain control. *Can J Anaesth*. 2000;47:585–596.
53. Sites BD, Beach M, Biggs R, et al. Intrathecal clonidine added to a bupivacaine-morphine spinal anesthetic improves postoperative analgesia for total knee arthroplasty. *Anesth Analg*. 2003;96:1083–1088.
54. Afonso J, Reis F. Dexmedetomidine: current role in anesthesia and intensive care. *Rev Bras Anestesiol*. 2012;62:118–133.
55. Pasin L, Landoni G, Nardelli P, et al. Dexmedetomidine reduces the risk of delirium, agitation and confusion in critically Ill patients: a meta-analysis of randomized controlled trials. *J Cardiothorac Vasc Anesth*. 2014;28:1459–1466.
56. Clarke H, Bonin RP, Orser BA, Englesakis M, Wijeysundera DN, Katz J. The prevention of chronic postsurgical pain using gabapentin and pregabalin: a combined systematic review and meta-analysis. *Anesth Analg*. 2012;115:428–442.
57. Schmidt PC, Ruchelli G, Mackey SC, Carroll IR. Perioperative gabapentinoids: choice of agent, dose, timing, and effects on chronic postsurgical pain. *Anesthesiology*. 2013;119:1215–1221.
58. Zhang J, Ho KY, Wang Y. Efficacy of pregabalin in acute postoperative pain: a meta-analysis. *Br J Anaesth*. 2011;106:454–462.
59. Gilron I. Gabapentin and pregabalin for chronic neuropathic and early postsurgical pain: current evidence and future directions. *Curr Opin Anaesthesiol*. 2007;20:456–472.
60. Weingarten TN, Jacob AK, Njathi CW, Wilson GA, Sprung J. Multimodal analgesic protocol and postanesthesia respiratory depression during phase I recovery after total joint arthroplasty. *Reg Anesth Pain Med*. 2015;40:330–336.
61. Myhre M, Diep LM, Stubhaug A. Pregabalin has analgesic, ventilatory, and cognitive effects in combination with remifentanil. *Anesthesiology*. 2016;124:141–149.
62. Verret M, Lauzier F, Zarychanski R, et al; Canadian Perioperative Anesthesia Clinical Trials (PACT) Group. Perioperative use of gabapentinoids for the management of postoperative acute pain: a systematic review and meta-analysis. *Anesthesiology*. 2020;133:265–279.
63. Kaba A, Laurent SR, Detroz BJ, et al. Intravenous lidocaine infusion facilitates acute rehabilitation after laparoscopic colectomy. *Anesthesiology*. 2007;106:11–18.
64. Ventham NT, Kennedy ED, Brady RR, et al. Efficacy of intravenous lidocaine for postoperative analgesia following laparoscopic surgery: a meta-analysis. *World J Surg*. 2015;39: 2220–2234.
65. van der Wal SE, van den Heuvel SA, Radema SA, et al. The in vitro mechanisms and in vivo efficacy of intravenous lidocaine on the neuroinflammatory response in acute and chronic pain. *Eur J Pain*. 2016;20:655–674.
66. Herroeder S, Pecher S, Schönherr ME, et al. Systemic lidocaine shortens length of hospital stay after colorectal surgery: a double-blinded, randomized, placebo-controlled trial. *Ann Surg*. 2007;246:192–200.
67. Khan JS, Yousuf M, Victor JC, Sharma A, Siddiqui N. An estimation for an appropriate end time for an intraoperative intravenous lidocaine infusion in bowel surgery: a comparative meta-analysis. *J Clin Anesth*. 2016;28:95–104.
68. Foo I, Macfarlane AJR, Srivastava D, et al. The use of intravenous lidocaine for postoperative pain and recovery: international consensus statement on efficacy and safety. *Anaesthesia*. 2021;76:238–250.
69. Albrecht E, Kirkham KR, Liu SS, Brull R. Peri-operative intravenous administration of magnesium sulphate and postoperative pain: a meta-analysis. *Anaesthesia*. 2013;68:79–90.
70. De Oliveira GS, Jr., Castro-Alves LJ, Khan JH, McCarthy RJ. Perioperative systemic magnesium to minimize postoperative pain: a meta-analysis of randomized controlled trials. *Anesthesiology*. 2013;119:178–190.
71. Jabbour HJ, Naccache NM, Jawish RJ, et al. Ketamine and magnesium association reduces morphine consumption after scoliosis surgery: prospective randomised double-blind study. *Acta Anaesthesiol Scand*. 2014;58:572–579.
72. Koç S, Memis D, Sut N. The preoperative use of gabapentin, dexamethasone, and their combination in varicocele surgery: a randomized controlled trial. *Anesth Analg*. 2007;105: 1137–1142.
73. De Oliveira GS, Jr., Almeida MD, Benzon HT, McCarthy RJ. Perioperative single dose systemic dexamethasone for postoperative pain: a meta-analysis of randomized controlled trials. *Anesthesiology*. 2011;115:575–588.
74. Mahathanaruk M, Hitt J, de LeonCasasola OA. Perioperative management of the opioid tolerant patient for orthopedic surgery. *Anesthesiol Clin*. 2014;32:923–932.
75. Williams BA, Ibinson JW, Mangione MP, et al. Research priorities regarding multimodal peripheral nerve blocks for postoperative analgesia and anesthesia based on hospital quality data extracted from over 1,300 cases (2011–2014). *Pain*. 2014;16:7–12.
76. Macintyre PE. Safety and efficacy of patient-controlled analgesia. *Br J Anaesth*. 2001;87:36–46.
77. Mariano E. Management of acute perioperative pain in adults. In: Fishman S, ed. *UpToDate*. UpToDate. Accessed on September 3, 2022.
78. Gan TJ, Belani KG, Bergese S, et al. Fourth consensus guidelines for the management of postoperative nausea and vomiting. *Anesth Analg*. 2020;131:411–48.
79. Blaudszun G, Lysakowski C, Elia N, Tramèr MR. Effect of perioperative systemic α2 agonists on postoperative morphine consumption and pain intensity: systematic review and meta-analysis of randomized controlled trials. *Anesthesiology*. 2012;116:1312–1322.
80. Yaksh TL, Rudy TA. Analgesia mediated by a direct spinal action of narcotics. *Science*. 1976; 192:1357–1358.
81. Wang JK, Nauss LA, Thomas JE. Pain relief by intrathecally applied morphine in man. *Anesthesiology*. 1979;50:149–151.
82. Onofrio BM, Yaksh TL, Arnold PG. Continuous low-dose intrathecal morphine administration in the treatment of chronic pain of malignant origin. *Mayo Clin Proc*. 1981;56:516–520.
83. Block BM, Liu SS, Rowlingson AJ, Cowan AR, Cowan JA, Jr., Wu CL. Efficacy of postoperative epidural analgesia: a meta-analysis. *JAMA*. 2003;290:2455–2463.
84. Bernards CM, Shen DD, Sterling ES, et al. Epidural, cerebrospinal fluid, and plasma pharmacokinetics of epidural opioids (part 1): differences among opioids. *Anesthesiology*. 2003;99: 455–465.
85. Förster GJ, Rosenberg PH. Small dose of clonidine mixed with low-dose ropivacaine and fentanyl for epidural analgesia after total knee arthroplasty. *Br J Anaesth*. 2004;2004:670–677.
86. Rathmell JP, Lair TR, Nauman B. The role of intrathecal drugs in the treatment of acute pain. *Anesth Analg*. 2005;101:S30–S43.
87. Treede RD, Rief W, Barke A, et al. Chronic pain as a symptom or a disease: the IASP Classification of Chronic Pain for the International Classification of Diseases (ICD-11). *Pain*. 2019; 160:19–27.
88. Schug SA. Acute pain management in the opioid-tolerant patient. *Pain Manag*. 2012;2: 581–591.
89. Sites BD, Beach ML, Davis MA. Increases in the use of prescription opioid analgesics and the lack of improvement in disability metrics among users. *Reg Anesth Pain Med*. 2014;39: 6–12.
90. Humphreys K, Shover CL, Andrews CM, et al. Responding to the opioid crisis in North America and beyond: recommendations of the Stanford-Lancet Commission. *Lancet*. 2022; 399:555–604.
91. Gulur P, Williams L, Chaudhary S, Koury K, Jaff M. Opioid tolerance–a predictor of increased length of stay and higher readmission rates. *Pain Physician*. 2014;17:E503–E507.
92. Pasternak GW. Incomplete cross tolerance and multiple mu opioid peptide receptors. *Trends Pharmacol Sci*. 2001;22:576–591.

93. Hayhurst CJ, Durieux ME. Differential opioid tolerance and opioid-induced hyperalgesia: a clinical reality. *Anesthesiology*. 2016;124:483–488.
94. Sun EC, Mariano ER, Narouze S, et al. Making a business plan for starting a transitional pain service within the US healthcare system. *Reg Anesth Pain Med*. 2021;46:727–731.
95. Buys MJ, Bayless K, Romesser J, et al. Opioid use among veterans undergoing major joint surgery managed by a multidisciplinary transitional pain service. *Reg Anesth Pain Med*. 2020;45:847–852.
96. Edwards DA, Hedrick TL, Jayaram J, et al; POQI-4 Working Group. American Society for Enhanced Recovery and Perioperative Quality Initiative joint consensus statement on perioperative management of patients on preoperative opioid therapy. *Anesth Analg*. 2019; 129:553–566.
97. Carroll IR, Angst MS, Clark JD. Management of perioperative pain in patients chronically consuming opioids. *Reg Anesth Pain Med*. 2004;29:576–591.
98. Khanna IK, Pillarisetti S. Buprenorphine - an attractive opioid with underutilized potential in treatment of chronic pain. *J Pain Res*. 2015;8:859–870.
99. Carr DaC D. Management of acute pain in the patient chronically using opioids for non-cancer pain. In: Fishman S, Abrahm, Janet, ed. *UpToDate*. UpToDate. Accessed September 3, 2022.
100. Derry S, Moore RA. Single dose oral celecoxib for acute postoperative pain in adults. *Cochrane Database Syst Rev*. 2013;10:CD004233.
101. Smith HS. Potential analgesic mechanisms of acetaminophen. *Pain Physician*. 2009;12:269–280.
102. Loftus RW, Yeager MP, Clark JA, et al. Intraoperative ketamine reduces perioperative opiate consumption in opiate-dependent patients with chronic back pain undergoing back surgery. *Anesthesiology*. 2010;113:639–646.
103. Ramaswamy S, Wilson JA, Colvin L. Non-opioid-based adjuvant analgesia in perioperative care. *Contin Educ Anaesth Crit Care Pain*. 2013;13:152–157.
104. Couceiro M, Lima L, Couceiro L, Valença M. Intravenous lidocaine to treat postoperative pain. *Revista Dor*. 2014;15.
105. Liu HT, Hollmann MW, Liu WH, Hoenemann CW, Durieux ME. Modulation of NMDA receptor function by ketamine and magnesium: Part I. *Anesth Analg*. 2001;92:1173–1181.
106. Naidu R, Flood P. Magnesium: is there a signal in the noise? *Anesthesiology*. 2013;119:13–15.
107. Haller G, Waeber JL, Infante NK, Clergue F. Ketamine combined with morphine for the management of pain in an opioid addict. *Anesthesiology*. 2002;96:1265–1266.
108. Kohan L, Potru S, Barreveld AM, et al. Buprenorphine management in the perioperative period: educational review and recommendations from a multisociety expert panel. *Reg Anesth Pain Med*. 2021;46:840–859.
109. Buvanendran A, Fiala J, Patel KA, Golden AD, Moric M, Kroin JS. The incidence and severity of postoperative pain following inpatient surgery. *Pain Med*. 2015;16:2277–2283.
110. Gan TJ, Habib AS, Miller TE, White W, Apfelbaum JL. Incidence, patient satisfaction, and perceptions of post-surgical pain: results from a US national survey. *Curr Med Res Opin*. 2014;30:149–160.
111. Dolin SJ, Cashman JN, Bland JM. Effectiveness of acute postoperative pain management: I. Evidence from published data. *Br J Anaesth*. 2002;89:409–423.
112. Stadler M, Schlander M, Braeckman M, Nguyen T, Boogaerts JG. A cost-utility and cost-effectiveness analysis of an acute pain service. *J Clin Anesth*. 2004;16:159–167.
113. Zaccagnino MP, Bader AM, Sang CN, Correll DJ. The perioperative surgical home: a new role for the acute pain service. *Anesth Analg*. 2017;125:1394–1402.
114. Berry PH, Dahl JL. The new JCAHO pain standards: implications for pain management nurses. *Pain Manag Nurs*. 2000;1:3–12.
115. Portenoy RK, Mehta Z, Ahmed E. Cancer pain managemet with opioids: optmizing analgesia. In: Abrahm J, ed. *UpToDate*. UpToDate. Accessed September 4, 2022).
116. Kishner S, Schraga ED. Opioid equivalents and conversions. *Medscape*; 2022. https://emedicine.medscape.com/article/2138678-overview?
117. Calculating total daily dose of opioids for safer dosage. Published March 14, 2016. Accessed September 4, 2022. https://www.cdc.gov/drugoverdose/pdf/calculating_total_daily_dose-a.pdf
118. Sharpe EE, Molitor RJ, Arendt KW, et al. Intrathecal morphine versus intrathecal hydromorphone for analgesia after cesarean delivery: a randomized clinical trial. *Anesthesiology*. 2020;132:1382–1391.
119. Liu SS, McDonald SB. Current issues in spinal anesthesia. *Anesthesiology*. 2001;94:888–906.

56 Chronic Pain Management

ROBERT W. HURLEY • ARIANA M. NELSON • HONORIO T. BENZON • STEVEN P. COHEN

KEY POINTS

1. Under normal conditions, A delta and C fibers transmit nociceptive information (pain) to the spinal cord from free nerve endings in the periphery. In chronic pain conditions, the A beta fibers, which normally transmit non-noxious information, also participate in nociceptive transmission.
2. Radicular symptoms of pain, paresthesia, and numbness in a dermatomal distribution in the presence of objective signs of weakness, diminished reflexes, and positive straight-leg raise are secondary to pathology or dysfunction of the spinal nerve roots.
3. Most randomized controlled studies evaluating efficacy of epidural steroid injections confirm temporary relief of radicular pain. Studies on thermal rhizotomy of the medial branch nerves for relief of facet syndrome show benefit of 3- to 12-month duration. These therapies mitigate use of opioids.
4. Postherpetic neuralgia is typically managed pharmacologically, although interventional techniques may be used in refractory cases.
5. Antidepressants and antiepileptics are effective for treatment of neuropathic pain syndromes. Antiepileptics are first-line treatment due to a more favorable side-effect profile and speed of therapeutic effect, but efficacy is improved when combined with an antidepressant.
6. Complex regional pain syndrome that does not respond to nerve blocks, physical therapy, and/or pharmacologic management may respond to spinal cord stimulation.
7. Pain secondary to cancer is generally managed most effectively with a combination of antiepileptic, antidepressant, and opioid pharmacologic agents in addition to interventional procedures.
8. Neurolysis of the visceral sympathetic system for pain secondary to abdominal or pelvic cancer relieves pain, decreases opioid consumption, and improves patient quality of life.
9. Vertebroplasty and kyphoplasty are indicated for vertebral compression fractures, although some studies question their efficacy.
10. Spinal cord stimulation is effective in patients with failed back syndrome and complex regional pain syndrome and is likely effective in treatment of angina and critical limb ischemia.
11. Intrathecal drug delivery systems are valuable options in cancer pain patients in whom opioids are ineffective at high doses or cause intolerable side effects. Chronic noncancer pain patients have improved outcomes if using no or minimal opioids prior to initiation of intrathecal therapy.

Anatomy, Physiology, and Neurochemistry of Somatosensory Pain Processing

Primary Afferents and Peripheral Stimulation

A variety of mechanical, thermal, electrical, or chemical stimuli can result in the sensation and perception of pain (see Chapter 55, Video 55-2). Information about these painful or noxious stimuli is transmitted to higher brain centers by receptors and neurons that are often distinct from those that carry innocuous somatic sensory information. The mammalian somatosensory system is subserved by four groups of afferent fibers differentiated by their anatomy, rate of transmission, and sensory modality transduced (Table 56-1).

The heavily myelinated large-diameter A beta (Aβ) fibers have specialized encapsulated nerve endings, which transduce innocuous or low-threshold mechanical stimulation. The activation of Aβ fibers may contribute to the mechanism of pain relief achieved with transcutaneous electrical nerve stimulators (TENS). Aβ fibers may also participate in pain signaling by adopting a "phenotype" similar to that of a C fiber (*vide infra*).[1]

1 The next groups of fibers represent the specialized sensory neurons that respond to actual or potential tissue damage, the *nociceptors*. The lightly myelinated medium-diameter A delta (Aδ) fibers and the unmyelinated small-diameter C fibers have free nerve endings that transduce noxious or high-threshold thermal, mechanical, and chemical stimulation. Patients with a mutation of the tyrosine kinase protein A, which is a component of the nerve growth factor receptor, fail to develop Aβ, Aδ, or C fibers and have no ability to sense pain. Unlike receptors in the Aβ fibers, the Aδ and C fibers respond to stimulation of their receptive fields in a characteristic manner with slow adaptation and residual firing following the withdrawal of the stimulus. Although these two fiber groups respond similarly to stimulation, they mediate different aspects of pain sensation. The rapidly conducting Aδ fibers mediate the "first" pain or *epicritic pain*, which is well localized and is characterized as sharp or prickling. The slowly conducting C fibers mediate the "second" pain or *protopathic pain*, which temporally follows the epicritic pain and is poorly localized or diffuse and is characterized as burning or dull.

The majority of Aδ and C nociceptors are polymodal and therefore are responsible for the transduction of noxious stimuli of different modalities. Nociceptive nerve endings are also located in muscle, the fascia, and adventitia of blood vessels, the knee joint, the dura, and the viscera. The primary afferent peripheral (distal) terminals express a variety of specific transducer channels that are sensitive over a range of stimulus intensities. When they are activated by the appropriate stimulus (thermal, chemical, or mechanical) these channels activate voltage-sensitive cation channels (e.g., sodium [Nav] and calcium [Cav]) and initiate an action potential. The sodium channel is of special interest following the discovery of its involvement in patients who are insensitive to pain. An epidemiologic study identified three Pakistani families with congenital insensitivity to pain. All were found to possess nonsense mutations of the *SCN9A* gene, resulting in truncation of the Nav1.7 isoform of the sodium channel.[2] Other mutations of this gene result in the impaired inactivation of this channel, which causes paroxysmal hyperexcitability resulting in erythromelalgia, a rare and extremely painful condition affecting the extremities.

The understanding of the molecular underpinning of the sensory processing of pain has primarily come from studying the transient receptor potential (TRP) channels. The cloning and characterization of the "capsaicin" receptor of the TRP family of nonselective cation channels expanded the field immensely.[3] Members of this molecular family transduce thermal, mechanical, and chemical information in the periphery. The capsaicin receptor named *TRP vanilloid 1* (TRPV1), which responds to capsaicin and other vanilloid compounds and is also activated by acid and heat, is localized to nociceptors and provides an excellent example of the integration of multiple sensory modalities within a single neuron.[3] Mice lacking the TRPV1 receptor are deficient in their response to thermal but not mechanical or other noxious stimuli. These data suggest that this member of the family of TRP channels may play a role in the integration of noxious chemical and thermal stimuli while having relatively less to do with mechanical transduction. Despite this clear involvement of the TRP channel family in the sensory process of nociception, drug development targeting these channels has not resulted in any successful analgesic therapies.[4]

Table 56-1 Primary Afferent Fibers and Their Function

Modality	Receptor	Fiber Type	Conduction Velocity and Diameter	Rate of Adaptation	Function
Proprioceptive	Golgi and Ruffini endings, muscle spindle afferents	Aα	70–120 m/s 15–20 μm	Slow and rapid	Muscle tension, length, and velocity
Mechanosensitive	Meissner, Ruffini, Pacinian corpuscles, and Merkel disc	Aβ	40–70 m/s 5–15 μm	Rapid (slow—Merkel)	Touch, flutter, motion, pressure, vibration
Thermoreceptive	Free nerve endings	Aδ	10–35 m/s 1–5 μm	Slow	Innocuous cold
	Free nerve endings	C	0.5–1 m/s <1 μm	Slow	Innocuous warmth
Nociceptive	Free nerve endings	Aδ	10–35 m/s 1–5 μm	Slow	Sharp pain
	Free nerve endings	C	0.5–1 m/s <1 μm	Slow	Burning pain

Neurochemistry of Peripheral Nerve and the Dorsal Root Ganglion

The nociceptive primary afferents, the Aδ and C fibers, represent the principal target of pharmacologic manipulation to treat pain. Glutamate receptors, as well as opioid, substance P, somatostatin, and vanilloid receptors, have been identified on the peripheral endings of these nerve fibers. Although the transmission of acute nociceptive information is primarily by the Aδ and C fibers, a subset of the Aδ and C fibers are *thermoreceptors* that transduce innocuous cold and warm information, respectively. The cell bodies of primary afferents, regardless of the structure they innervate, make up the *dorsal root ganglia* (DRG) located just outside the spinal cord within the bony foramen.

Primary afferent activation results in a postsynaptic excitatory event in the spinal cord. Glutamate is the primary neurotransmitter serving this function. Acute activation events are mediated by the α-amino-3-hydroxy-5-methyl-4-isoxazole propionic acid (AMPA)-type glutamate receptor present on the dorsal horn neurons. This receptor produces a robust but brief depolarization of the postsynaptic membrane by increasing sodium conductance and augmenting the activation of the *N*-methyl-D-aspartate (NMDA)-type glutamate receptor. In addition to glutamate, populations of primary afferents contain and release a variety of neuropeptides, including substance P, calcitonin gene–related peptide, adenosine triphosphate, adenosine, galanin, and somatostatin and growth factors, including brain-derived nerve growth factor.

Neurobiology of the Spinal Cord and Spinal Trigeminal Nucleus

Primary afferent fibers enter the gray matter of the spinal cord through the *dorsal root entry zone* and innervate the spinal cord. Most heavily myelinated primary afferent fibers (Aα, Aβ) carrying sensory information, including tactile, pressure, and vibratory sense, enter in dorsal roots, traverse across the top of the dorsal horn of the spinal cord (Lissauer tract), and ascend ipsilaterally within the dorsal column and provide collateral branches into the gray matter of the dorsal horn. The small-diameter, lightly myelinated and unmyelinated fibers transmitting temperature and nociceptive information enter Lissauer tract and innervate the gray matter of the spinal cord. Unlike the heavily myelinated fibers, these fibers may also ascend rostrally or descend caudally through Lissauer tract before they innervate adjacent spinal levels.

The gray matter of the spinal cord is made up of synaptic terminations of primary afferents and the second-order neurons that form the first stage of processing and integration of sensory information. The gray matter of the spinal cord is divided into 10 laminae based on histologic appearance. The dorsal horn includes laminae I to VI and represents the primary sensory complement of the spinal cord (Fig. 56-1). The ventral horn, including laminae VII to IX and lamina X, is involved in somatic motor and autonomic functions, respectively. *Somatic* C fiber nociceptive afferent endings primarily terminate in the laminae I and II of the same and/or one to two adjacent spinal segments from which they entered from the periphery, whereas *visceral* C fiber nociceptive afferents can terminate in the dorsal horn more than five segments rostrally or caudally. They terminate in the ipsilateral laminae I, II, V, X, and in contralateral laminae V and X. Therefore, visceral afferents have a wider branching pattern and the nociceptive information they transmit is less localizable to a particular area of the body.

In addition to the primary afferent endings, neurons of the descending pathways and local interneurons also innervate the superficial dorsal horn (laminae I and II). The outer marginal layer or lamina I contains interneurons and cells that send axonal projections to the brainstem and midbrain structures. The substantia gelatinosa, or lamina II, also contains excitatory and inhibitory interneurons but fewer projection neurons. Laminae III and IV contain interneurons and the second-order neurons that make up the dorsal column pathways relaying non-nociceptive sensory and proprioceptive information. Laminae IV to VI contain interneurons and a modest portion of nociceptive projection neurons that distribute input to the brainstem and thalamus.

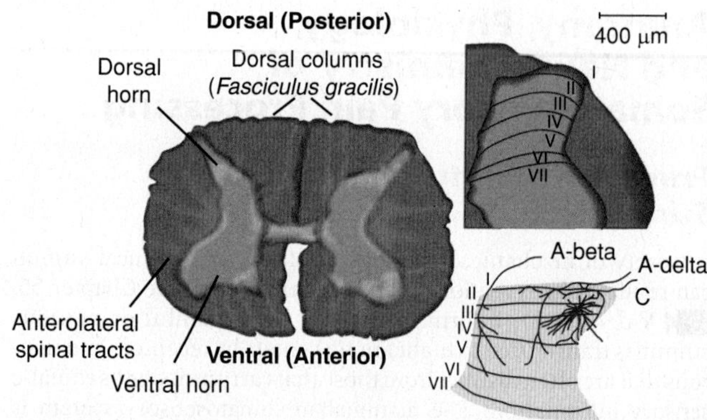

Figure 56-1 Histologic sections and schematic diagrams of the spinal dorsal horn. The histologic section at left is from the lumbar segment of the spinal cord. It is labeled to show the relationship between the major spinal somatosensory structures. The histologic section at right is from the rat lumbar spinal cord. The *outer heavy lines* show the boundary of the spinal gray matter and the *inner heavy lines* show the boundaries of Rexed laminae. These boundaries are established by the histologic characteristics of each zone, and the layers are identified by the Roman numerals. The drawing at the bottom illustrates the pattern of primary afferent innervation to the nonhuman primate spinal dorsal horn. The large myelinated (A-beta) fibers segregate to the dorsal aspect of an entering root and then track medially in the dorsal horn and terminate in layers III to V. The small myelinated (A-delta) fibers and C fibers that carry nociceptive information segregate ventrally in the entering roots, course laterally in the dorsal horn, and then largely terminate in the superficial layers (I and II) of the dorsal horn. (Adapted from Raja SN, Dougherty PM. Anatomy and physiology of somatosensory and pain processing. In: Benzon HT, Raja SN, Molloy RE, et al., eds. *Essentials of Pain Medicine and Regional Anesthesia*. 2nd ed. Elsevier-Churchill Livingstone; 2005:3. Copyright © 2005 Elsevier. With permission.)

Nociceptive somatic input is primarily transmitted by second-order lamina I, IV, and V projection neurons as the contralateral spinothalamic tract (STT) pathway, which travels to numerous brainstem regions and the thalamus. There is a nociceptive visceral processing area in laminae III, IV, V, VII, and X. The visceral nociceptive input is relayed by second-order neurons whose axons travel within the dorsal column. Like the fibers transmitting non-noxious sensory information, these fibers remain uncrossed until relayed with the crossed medial lemniscal fibers to the thalamus. The visceral pain information transmitted by the ventral STT is likely originating from cells also receiving somatic nociceptive input. Nociceptive and non-nociceptive sensory information from the head, neck, and dura transmitted via the trigeminal nerve innervates the dorsal horn of the spinal trigeminal nucleus in the caudal medulla. The organization and neurotransmitter complement of the spinal trigeminal nucleus is like that of the spinal dorsal horn.

Neurobiology of Ascending Pathways

Dorsal Column Tracts

The dorsal column contains the axons of second-order spinal cord projection neurons in addition to the ascending axons of primary afferent neurons relaying touch, pressure, and vibratory sensation. Second-order dorsal column cells in the central visceral processing region of the spinal cord around lamina X also respond to noxious visceral stimulation and converge on some of the thalamic cells receiving nociceptive information from the skin and other somatic structures.

Spinothalamic Tract

STT neurons are the primary relay cells providing nociceptive input from the spinal cord to supraspinal levels. The axons of STT cells cross the midline of the spinal cord through the anterior white commissure and ascend primarily in the contralateral and anterolateral tracts. The axons of STT cells terminate primarily in the posterior complex of the thalamus, including the ventral posterior lateral and ventral posterior medial nuclei. Non-noxious sensory input from the same body region converges on the same target thalamic neurons providing somatotopic encoding for localization of the input onto the cortical representation of the specific body region, permitting localization of the source of nociceptive input. The STT cells receiving noxious somatic input are predominantly situated in lamina I and the lateral aspect of the dorsal horn in laminae IV to V. However, other STT neurons are scattered throughout the deep dorsal horn, intermediate region, including lamina X, and even in lamina VII of the ventral horn. These STT cells receive both somatic and visceral nociceptive information.

Spinohypothalamic, Limbic, and Cortical Connections

Pain is a sensory experience but also possesses an affective component to the perception of noxious stimuli. Pain can variably provoke fear, anxiety, and depression, resulting in autonomic responses, including increased heart rate and blood pressure as well as the endocrine stress response. These responses to noxious stimuli are mediated by the spinohypothalamic and spinoamygdalar pathways. In addition to their affective function, these regions are also thought to be involved in antinociception. Ascending axonal projections of these pathways arise predominantly from the spinal cord laminae I and X.

Neurobiology of Descending Pathways

The primary components of this descending pain inhibition system, but certainly not all-inclusive, is the "triad" of the periaqueductal gray (PAG), the rostral ventral medulla (RVM), and the dorsolateral pontine tegmentum (DLPT).[5] The PAG is an important site for the production of antinociception following electrical or chemical activation, or the injection of opioid receptor agonists. The endogenous opioid enkephalin is present within this nucleus, and opioid receptors of each subtype are present in this region. The PAG provides dense projections to the RVM, the locus coeruleus, and A7 nuclei. Although the RVM can function as a relay nucleus in the production of antinociception by more cephalad midbrain structures, including the PAG, it also has a primary role in the suppression of nociceptive transmission at the level of the spinal cord. The suppression of nociceptive reflex behavior is mediated by the axons of RVM neurons that descend within the dorsolateral funiculus and terminate bilaterally in laminae I, II, V, VI, and VII of the spinal cord. Anatomic studies have shown that these axons terminate coincident with interneurons of the dorsal horn that are related to nociceptive transmission.[6] Consistent with the anatomic terminations of the RVM axons, physiologic studies have shown that stimulation of the RVM results in the inhibition of a population of nociceptive-specific neurons within the dorsal horn as well as selective inhibition of the nociceptive responses of wide-dynamic range neurons. The DLPT is also an important component of spinal cord nociceptive modulation. It contains all of the noradrenergic neurons that project to the RVM and the spinal cord, and electrical stimulation of the DLPT sites produces spinal cord α_2-adrenergic receptor–mediated analgesia.[7]

Neurobiology of Supraspinal Structures Involved in Higher Cortical Processing

Higher cortical centers play a role in the perception of painful stimuli as well as the integration of the sensory-discriminative and affective components of the noxious stimulation. The localization of the neural structures involved in this perception and integration is still in its adolescence. The development of positron emission tomography (PET) and functional magnetic resonance imaging (fMRI) technologies has moved this research forward. These imaging technologies produce indirect evidence of neural activity related to pain stimulation including the primary and secondary somatosensory cortexes, the anterior cingulate gyrus, the insula, and the prefrontal cortex. As the primary and secondary cortexes are known to be somatosensory processing regions, the imaging studies are consistent with a sensory-discriminative role of these structures. The insula and frontal cortex may contribute to memory and learning of events related to painful stimuli. The anterior cingulate cortex is thought to be involved in the analysis of the emotional significance of the painful input.

Transition from Acute to Persistent or Chronic Nociception

Pain sensation is unique among the somatosensory modalities in that it does not rapidly adapt to prolonged stimulation as do the other sensory modalities, such as fine touch (see Chapter 55, Video 55-1). In fact, continued stimulation may produce greater noxious sensation or reduce the stimulus threshold or intensity that is necessary for the appreciation of the sensation as noxious. For instance, previously innocuous thermal or mechanical stimulation (e.g., warm water of a shower or the light touch of a towel) may be perceived as painful following a prior noxious stimulus (e.g., sunburn). This is termed *allodynia.* Another example of an altered pain state that may follow an acute injury is that of *hyperalgesia,* in which a previously noxious stimulus is perceived as more painful (Table 56-2). The sensation of increased intensity of noxious stimulation at the site of the injury is the result of the sensitization of the peripheral nociceptors.

Persistent C fiber, but not Aβ fiber, stimulation as can occur with tissue injury and inflammation, has been shown to enhance the response to subsequent stimulation and augment the size of the receptive field of the respective dorsal horn neuron. Therefore, afferent input from adjacent dermatomal areas now produces neuronal excitation. Furthermore, non-noxious stimulation becomes increasingly able to activate these neurons. This general phenomenon has come to be termed *wind-up* or *central sensitization.*[8] This activation is thought to explain the allodynia and hyperalgesia observed surrounding the site of injury in the acute, subacute phases and be contributory to these phenomena in the chronic phase of pain.

In addition to the alteration of the chemical milieu surrounding the primary afferent distal terminal that results from injury or persistent high-intensity stimulation, axonal sprouting and the formation of a neuroma may occur. The neuroma may have an altered complement of ion channels, including an upregulation of sodium channels or a downregulation of potassium channels, which has the net result of increasing neuronal excitability and

Table 56-2 Definitions

Paresthesia	Abnormal sensation due to neural insult, severe symptoms may be termed dysesthesia
Hyperalgesia	Higher severity of pain than anticipated due to noxious stimulus
Allodynia	Pain due to non-noxious stimulus
Radicular pain	Pain in distribution of a dermatome
Radiculitis	Inflammation of the nerve root; symptoms vary but are in dermatomal distribution
Radiculopathy	Sensory or motor deficit in the distribution of a dermatome
Spondylosis	Degenerative change in the spine
Spondylolysis	Fracture in the osseous bridge between adjacent spine segments due to trauma or degeneration
Spondylolisthesis	Shift of a vertebral body out of alignment with adjacent spinal segments. Can only occur in presence of spondylolysis.

increasing nociceptive transmission. It has been shown that, following nerve damage, an increase in the expression of sodium channels occurs in the neuroma and the DRG. Numerous sodium channels exist on primary afferents; Nav1.8 and 1.9 subtypes are primarily found on C fiber DRG cells. Genetic "knock-down" or removal of the Nav1.8 channel had no effect on baseline pain thresholds; however, it reversed nerve injury–evoked nociception.[9] Also following nerve damage, potassium currents have been shown to be reduced, suggesting a reduction in these channels contributing to spontaneous nociceptive activity. Consistent with this notion, it has been observed that potassium channel antagonists increase and potassium channel agonists decrease ectopic firing after peripheral nerve injury.[10]

Neuromas of injured primary afferents have altered sensitivity to several humoral factors, including cytokines, prostaglandins, and catecholamines. These factors are released from a variety of cell types, including inflammatory cells and neuronal support cells. Cytokines directly activate the nerve and neuroma through receptors that become expressed in the membrane after the nerve injury. A molecule that has been shown to have a prominent role following nerve damage is tumor necrosis factor subunit *alpha* (TNF-α). Shortly after injury, TNF-α decreases potassium conductance, increasing neuronal excitability, whereas the long-term changes may be produced through the activation of second messenger systems, resulting in altered protein production. Application of TNF-α to the peripheral nerve results in hyperalgesia and systemic delivery of antibodies to TNF-α or TNF-α–binding protein reduces neuropathic pain. Prostaglandins are also released from inflammatory cells following nerve and tissue damage. They can enhance the opening of Nav1.8 channels by acting though receptors on the afferent terminal.

Although acute noxious stimuli are transmitted to the spinal cord via Aδ and C fibers, the presence of allodynia is thought to be mediated by the activation of large-diameter Aβ fibers through what has been termed a *phenotypic* switch.[1] Prior to peripheral injury, the Aβ fibers, unlike the C fibers, do not express substance P. However, following injury these fibers can express this neuropeptide, which implicates Aβ fibers in the transmission of noxious peripheral stimulation. This provides further support for the involvement of somatic Aβ fibers in at least some form of the allodynic pain states. Furthermore, the blockade of Aβ fibers results in a reduction in light-touch–evoked allodynia. This phenotypic switch of Aβ fibers may represent another avenue for therapeutic intervention; however, the remaining barrier is differentiating between Aβ fibers involved in noxious versus non-noxious sensory information.

The transition from acute or subacute to chronic pain likely involves an interaction between central mechanisms and peripheral mechanisms. Central mechanisms include changes of the supraspinal structures and descending inhibitory pathways.[11] Peripheral mechanisms include altered activity of receptors and primary afferents described above. This interaction is demonstrated in studies in which chronic neuropathic pain is briefly extinguished by peripheral nerve blocks[12] and post-stroke neuropathic pain is reduced when the peripheral nerves serving the pain location were anesthetized.[13] These changes are due to multiple influences including ongoing peripheral input resulting in phenotypic changes from gene transcription and expression in the DRG, as well as responses to injury from non-neuronal cells including immune cells, glial cells, keratinocytes, cancer cells, and stem cells resulting in a chronic neuroinflammation.[14] These factors provide additional targets for future therapies to reduce the acute to chronic pain transition.

Management of Common Pain Syndromes

Spine Pain: Radicular Pain Syndromes

Spine pain is most common in the low back and can be due to radicular pain/radiculopathy from a herniated disc or spinal/foraminal stenosis, spondylosis, internal disc disruption, or myofascial pain syndrome. Sacroiliac joint (SIJ) syndrome and piriformis syndrome ordinarily cause buttock pain but can present as lower back pain or mimic radicular pain. Other sources of spine pain include metastases and vertebral body fractures.[15]

Spine and radicular pain secondary to a herniated disc is due 2
to nerve root irritation and subsequent inflammatory processes but the presence of a herniated disc does not automatically result in pain. Up to 36% of the general population and up to 53% of pregnant women may experience an asymptomatic herniated disc. If symptomatic, the patient usually presents with spine pain and radicular symptoms in the distribution of the involved nerve root. Paresthesia, loss of sensation, reduced muscle strength, and diminished reflexes may also be evident in the affected dermatomal distribution. Follow-up studies of patients with a herniated disc often show spontaneous regression, absence of symptoms in the presence of additional abnormalities, and partial or complete resolution without surgical treatment.[16]

Herniated nucleus pulposus results in local release of cytokines and other inflammatory mediators that cause a chemical radiculitis. Disc cells express TNF-α, which, when applied to spinal nerve roots, can cause changes like those observed after application of disc material. Although selective inhibition of TNF-α may reduce the intraneural edema, a randomized controlled trial demonstrated that injection of a TNF-α inhibitor in a pain-generating disc did not reduce pain or disability scores of patients.[17] Similarly, studies evaluating use of disease-modifying antirheumatic drugs for spine and radicular pain are low quality or demonstrate either inconclusive or short-term benefits.[18]

Physical therapy, NSAIDs, acetaminophen, and short courses of muscle relaxants are effective first-line agents in treating spine pain. Antiepileptics are not effective in treating low back pain or lumbosacral radicular pain.[19] Duloxetine was noted to be superior to placebo in treating the neuropathic component of chronic low back pain.[20]

3 Epidural steroid injections (ESIs) may be considered for patients with spine pain that do not respond to noninterventional management. Steroids have antinociceptive and anti-inflammatory effects related to phospholipase A_2 inhibition. The local application of methylprednisolone blocks transmission of C fibers but not Aβ fibers. Most controlled studies have demonstrated moderate-term efficacy of ESIs for treatment of radicular pain[21,22] and a decreased need for operative intervention.[23,24] The relief provided by ESIs can minimize the need for opioids and NSAIDs and their related side effects, but should only be offered when consideration is given for the natural history of spine pain, which typically improves over time. ESIs should be a component, but not the sole modality, of nonsurgical management of spine pain.

Fluoroscopy should be used to guide ESI to assure insertion of the needle at the affected vertebral level and document appropriate flow of the injectate. Reassessment should be carried out 2 to 3 weeks after the initial injection. The rote practice of multiple ESIs in a patient, with a short interval between injections, is not advised. If there is no response to an initial injection, it can be repeated once because some patients require a second injection for therapeutic response. If there is partial response, up to three injections may be performed.

Epidural placement via an interlaminar (IL) approach deposits steroid into the posterior epidural space whereas the transforaminal (TF) approach traverses the intervertebral foramina to access the anterolateral epidural space, which deposits steroid closer to the nerve root (Fig. 56-2). Controlled studies that compare the two approaches show similar moderate-duration efficacy, especially if the IL approach is paramedian, which deposits steroid in the lateral posterior epidural space, closer to the anterolateral site of nerve insult than the midline approach.

Complications of ESIs related to the technique include needle trauma, vasospasm, and infection and are relatively more common with cervical/thoracic than lumbar/sacral injections. Other complications of ESI may be due to the injected agent, vehicle, or additives. Glucocorticoids reduce the hypoglycemic effect of insulin and interfere with blood glucose control in patients with diabetes mellitus. ESIs also cause dose-related suppression of the hypothalamic pituitary adrenal axis that resolves in most cases within 1 to 2 weeks but can persist for greater than 3 weeks.[25,26] In patients over 40 years of age, repeatedly injected steroids may reduce bone density due to cumulative effects on bone metabolism, which can increase the risk of vertebral fractures.[27] A significant decrease in bone mineral density in postmenopausal women may be associated with a cumulative methylprednisolone dose of greater than 200 mg over a 1-year period or greater than 400 mg over 3 years.[28]

Studies show that the lowest effective dose for lumbar IL ESI is 40 mg of methylprednisolone, for TF ESI is 10 mg of triamcinolone acetate, and for TF ESI is 4 mg of dexamethasone phosphate.[29,30] These lowest effective steroid doses, or their pharmacologic equivalent, should be employed for ESIs to reduce adverse effects. Appropriate clinical assessment, documentation of benefits, and an adequate interval should be observed before ESI is repeated.

Injury to the CNS can occur with ESIs because needle injection targets are near vertebral and radicular arteries, which are then vulnerable to trauma or unintentional injection of the steroid resulting in occlusion or vasospasm of the vessels. Methylprednisolone acetate theoretically carries the highest risk as it has the largest particles, while triamcinolone has marginally smaller particles and betamethasone the smallest (Fig. 56-3). However, a 2021 report showed the same incidence of adverse events for particulate and nonparticulate steroids, although the study included patients who had non-TF injections.[31] These adverse events have also been described after injection of local anesthetic or dye, without steroid.[32]

Dexamethasone has no identifiable particles and therefore appears ideal for TF ESIs. However, it is easily washed out from the epidural space hence its use in IL injection can be questioned. The efficacy of nonparticulate dexamethasone is similar to the particulate steroids although it may require more injections.[33]

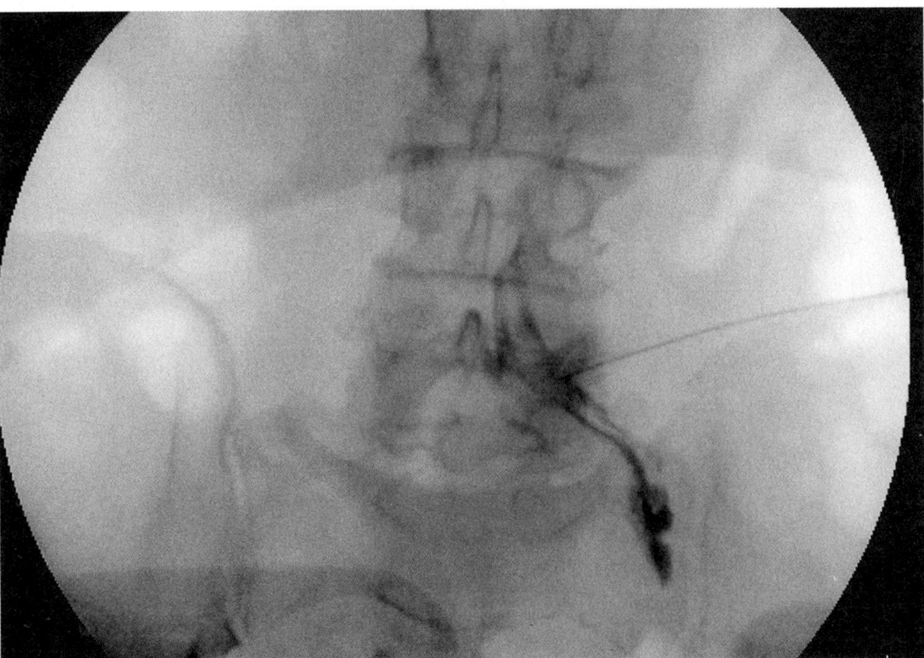

Figure 56-2 Right L5 transforaminal epidural injection. Note the spread of the contrast medium proximally into the lateral epidural space and distally along the nerve root.

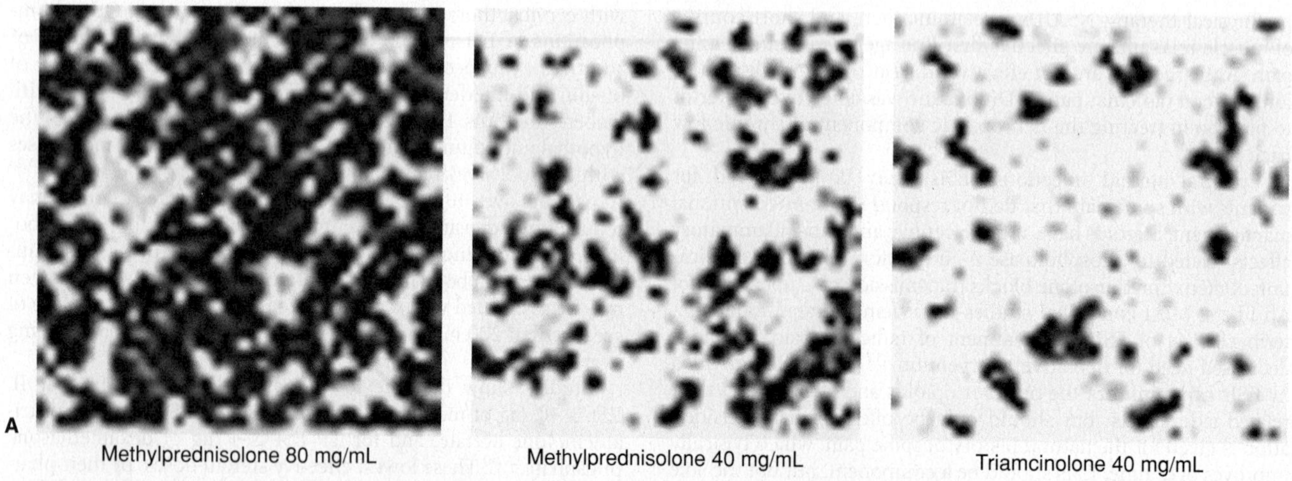

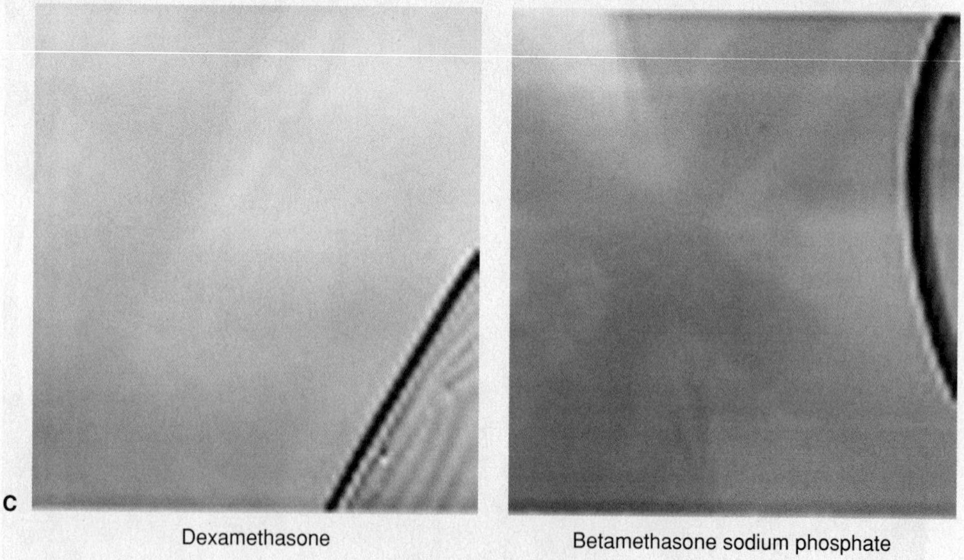

A

Methylprednisolone 80 mg/mL

Methylprednisolone 40 mg/mL

Triamcinolone 40 mg/mL

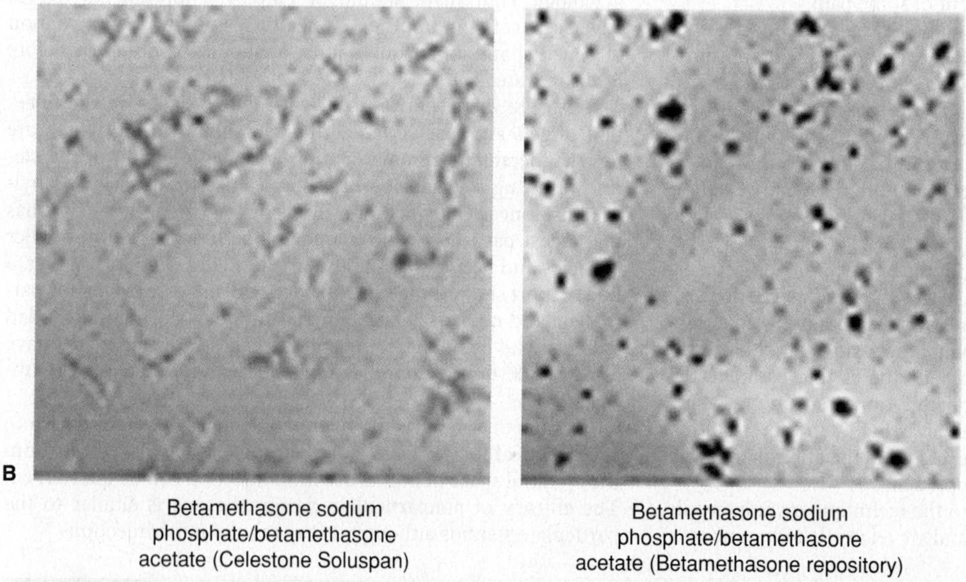

B

Betamethasone sodium phosphate/betamethasone acetate (Celestone Soluspan)

Betamethasone sodium phosphate/betamethasone acetate (Betamethasone repository)

C

Dexamethasone

Betamethasone sodium phosphate

Figure 56-3 **A:** Typical microscopic appearances of methylprednisolone, 80 mg/mL and 40 mg/mL, and triamcinolone 40 mg/mL. The particles are amorphous in appearance. **B:** The particles of commercial betamethasone (Celestone Soluspan) are rod-like and lucent, whereas those of the compounded betamethasone (betamethasone repository) are amorphous. **C:** Note that dexamethasone is pure liquid. (Adapted with permission from Benzon HT, Chew TL, McCarthy R, et al. Comparison of the particle sizes of the different steroids and the effect of dilution: a review of the relative neurotoxicities of the steroids. *Anesthesiology*. 2007; 106:331–338.)

In a 2015 report, a multispecialty working group, together with several national organizations, made recommendations to improve the safety of ESIs.[34] These include the following:

1. IL ESIs should be performed using image guidance with appropriate anteroposterior, lateral, or contralateral oblique views, and contrast media.
2. Cervical IL ESI should be performed at C6–C7 or C7–T1 but not at more superior levels.
3. TF ESIs should be performed by injecting contrast medium under real-time fluoroscopy and/or digital subtraction imaging, using an anteroposterior view, before injection.
4. Particulate steroids should not be used in cervical TF ESIs.
5. There are situations in which a particulate steroid may be used in lumbar TF ESIs.

ESIs are more effective in patients with acute radicular symptoms; they are not effective in patients with chronic lumbar radiculopathy. The efficacy of ESIs in spinal stenosis, when combined with local anesthetic, may last up to 3 months.[35] The evidence for epidural local anesthetic alone in spinal stenosis, without steroid, is low but may be entertained in view of the side effects of steroids.[36]

Low Back Pain: Facet Syndrome

Patients with low back pain secondary to facet pathology exhibit pain in the low back that radiates to the ipsilateral posterior thigh and usually terminates at the knee. On physical examination, there may be paraspinal tenderness and reproduction of pain with extension–rotation maneuvers of the back. The diagnosis of facet syndrome is achieved by a combination of the patient's history, physical examination findings, and a positive response to prognostic medial branch blocks (MBBs) (Fig. 56-4) or facet joint injections (Fig. 56-5). For MBBs, some investigators recommend the use of local anesthetics with different durations of effect (e.g., lidocaine and bupivacaine) and to correlate the duration of relief with the known duration of effect of the drug. This reduces false-positive prognostic outcome of MBBs and permits more judicious patient selection for progression to radiofrequency ablation (RFA), however does increase the false-negative rate.

There are no published steroid dose–response studies in facet intra-articular injection, but existing literature suggests the minimum effective dose per joint to be 10- to 20-mg methylprednisolone or triamcinolone, 3-mg betamethasone, or 2-mg dexamethasone. Patients may have a response to facet joint injections for up to 6 months,[37] a response that is more likely in patients with acute facet joint inflammation (e.g., positive findings on SPECT imaging).[38] It is therefore advisable to wait for diminution of pain relief (to less than 50%), after facet joint injection, before performing medial branch RFA after the local anesthetic injection procedures.

Guidelines recommend MBBs rather than intra-articular facet injections as the predictive tool before lumbar or cervical RFA based on better face validity, high failure rate for intra-articular injections, and studies demonstrating better outcomes when MBBs are used to identify candidates for RFA.[39,40] Controlled studies have shown improvements after RFA of the lumbar medial branches that lasted 3 to 12 months.[41,42] For cervical facet syndrome, a 2016 systematic review showed that a majority of the patients were pain free at 6 months and over one-third were pain-free at 1 year.[43] A Cochrane review of 12 studies noted moderate evidence supporting facet joint RFA compared to placebo over the short-term and low-quality evidence supporting the efficacy of RFA over steroid injections.[44]

Buttock Pain: Sacroiliac Joint Syndrome and Piriformis Syndrome

The pain of SIJ syndrome is in the region of the affected SIJ and the medial buttock. The pain may radiate to the groin, posterior thigh, and occasionally below the knee. Physical examination usually reveals tenderness over the sacroiliac sulcus, reduction in joint mobility, and reproduction of the pain when the affected SIJ is stressed. There are multiple tests for SIJ dysfunction which include the FABER (flexion, abduction, and external rotation) or

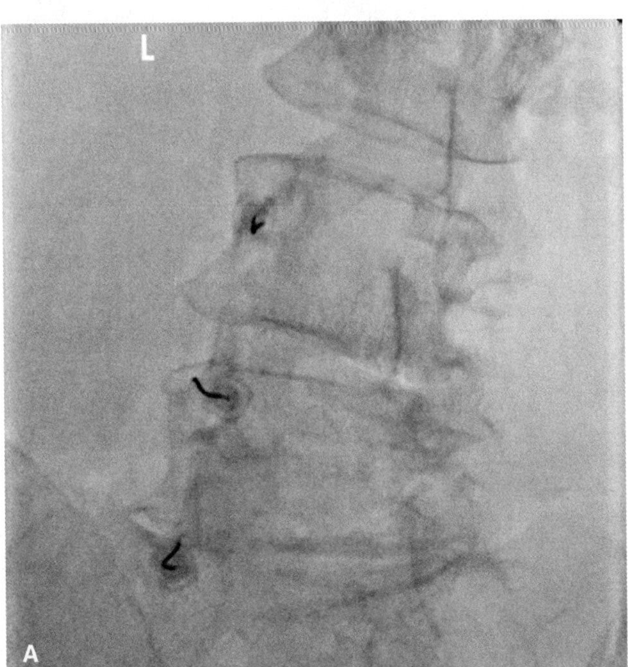

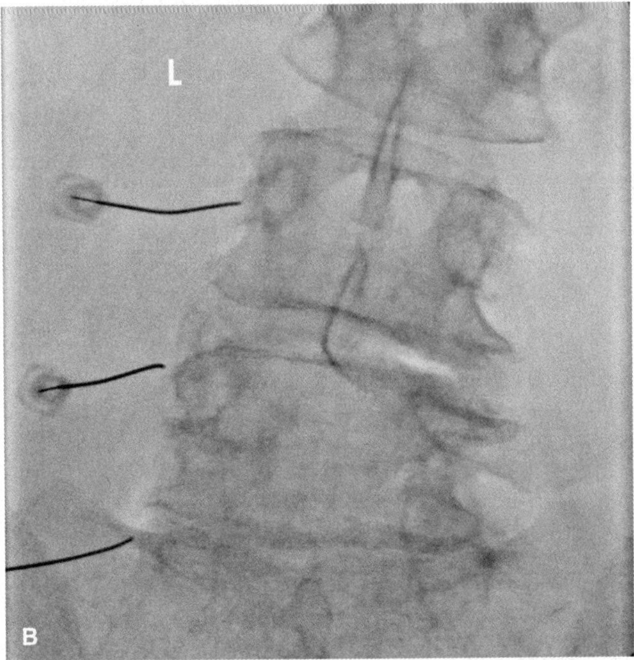

Figure 56-4 Medial branch block of L4/5 and L5/S1 facet joints with 22-gauge 3.5-in needle. **A:** Placement at the location of the MB nerve of L3, L4, and the L5 primary dorsal ramus (top to bottom, respectively) in the 25-degree oblique view. **B:** Anterior–posterior view of the needle placement.

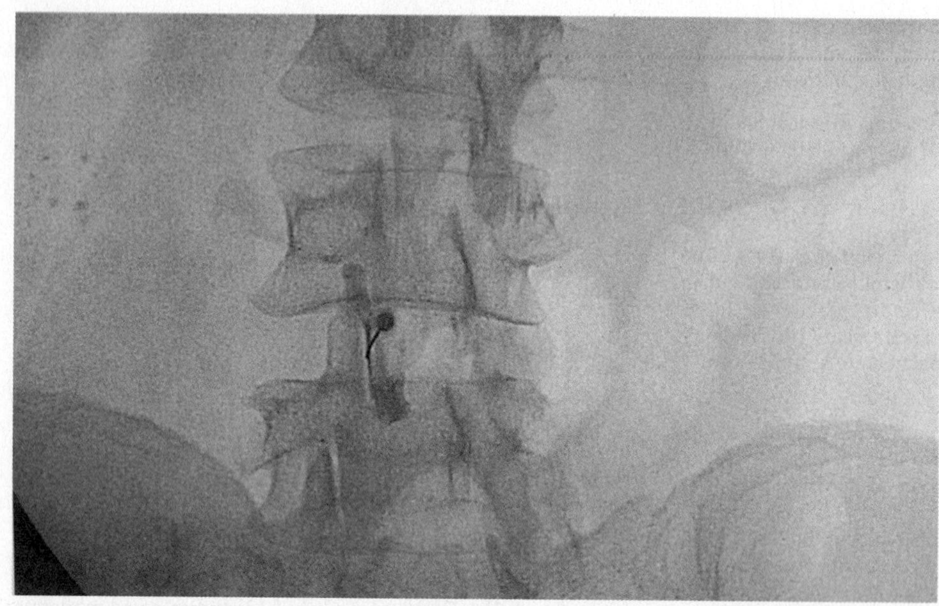

Figure 56-5 Left L4 to L5 facet joint injection. The injection of 5 mL of contrast medium demonstrates the extent of the joint capsule.

Patrick's, Gaenslen's, Yeoman's, iliac (gapping) distraction, iliac compression, thigh thrust (posterior SIJ shear), sacral thrust, and Gillet (stork) tests. The presence of symptoms and physical examination findings suggestive of SIJ syndrome, pain on three of the provocative tests, and a positive response to SIJ injection are adequate to make the diagnosis of SIJ dysfunction.

The treatments for SIJ dysfunction include physical therapy, manipulation, intra-articular steroid injections (Fig. 56-6), RFA, and surgical fusion of the joint. Physical therapy and chiropractic manipulations are used extensively; however, there is no large outcome study validating their use. Intra-articular injections of steroid (40 to 60 mg of methylprednisolone or other depot steroid) and local anesthetic into the SIJ may result in up to 2 to 3 months of relief. Fluoroscopy guidance is more accurate than landmark-based techniques and better than ultrasound, especially in obese patients. Combined intra- and extra-articular injections appear to be more effective,[45] which may be due to the extra-articular location of some nociceptors.[46] There are no dose–response studies but 40 mg appears to be the lowest effective intra-articular dose. Cranial spread observed with a dye study (Fig. 56-7) improves

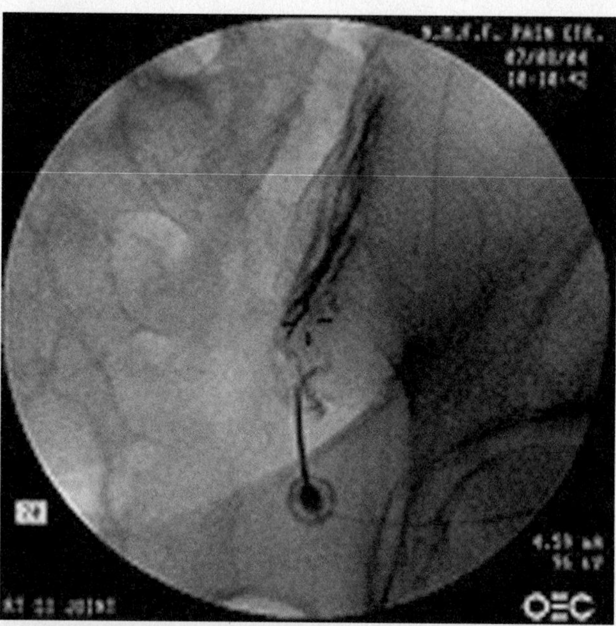

Figure 56-6 Sacroiliac joint injection. Note the spread of the contrast medium along the joint. (Adapted from Benzon HT, Nader A. Hip, sacroiliac joint, and piriformis injections. In: Benzon HT, Rathmell J, Wu C, et al., eds. *Raj's Practical Management of Pain*. 4th ed. Mosby Elsevier; 2008:1070. Copyright © 2008 Elsevier. With permission.)

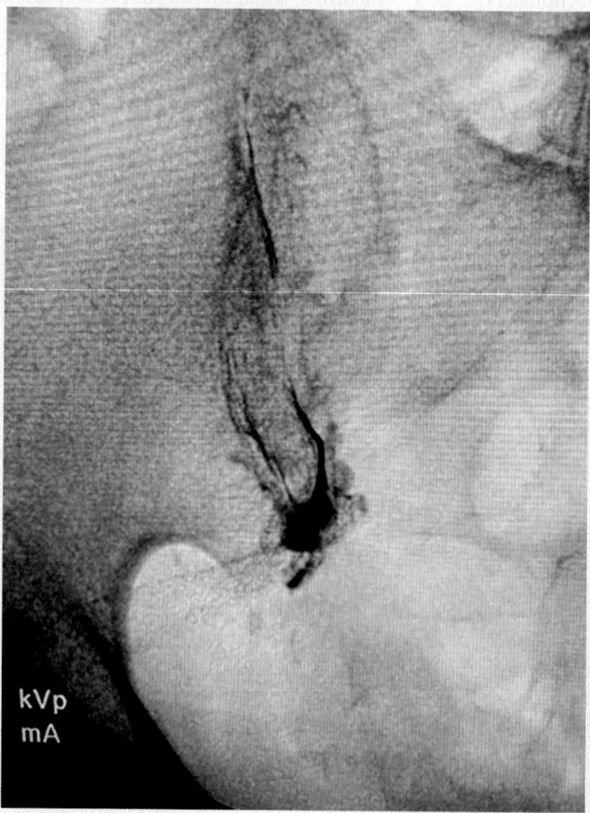

Figure 56-7 Sacroiliac joint injection with needle entry at inferior margin of the joint and cranial spread of contrast dye.

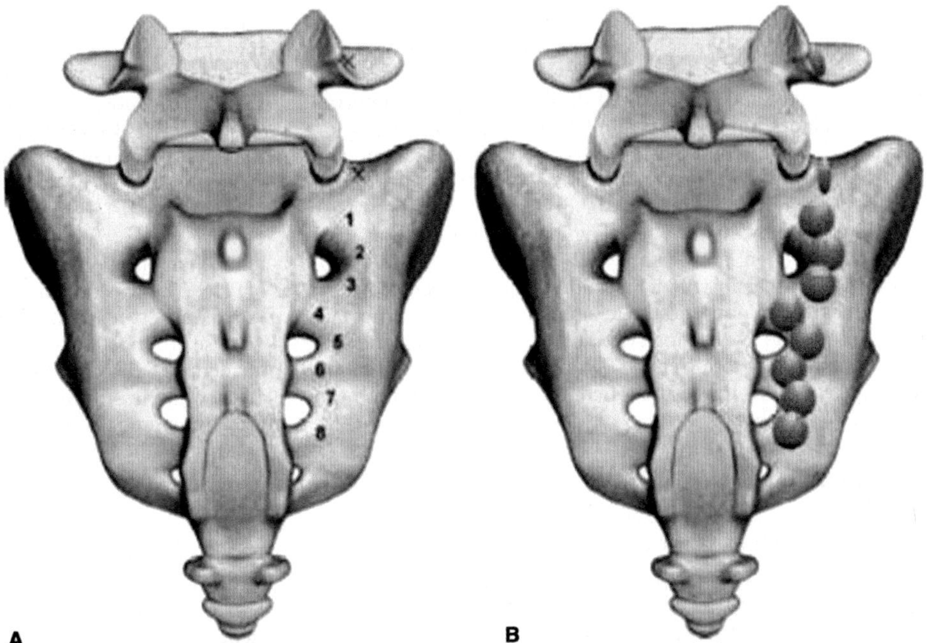

Figure 56-8 Target points (**A**) and expected lesions (**B**) from water-cooled radiofrequency denervation at the right L5 medial branch and the S1, S2, and S3 lateral branches. (Adapted with permission from Cohen SP, Hurley RW, Buckenmaier CC 3rd, et al. Randomized placebo-controlled study evaluating lateral branch radiofrequency denervation for sacroiliac joint pain. *Anesthesiology*. 2008;109:279–288.)

short-term efficacy and relief that may last 9 months when two to three intra-articular injections are given in 1 year.

Local anesthetic blockade of the sensory innervation of the dorsal portion of the SIJ, the primary dorsal ramus of L5 and the lateral branches of the dorsal rami of S1 to S3, can be performed when the relief from the SIJ injection is temporary. Relief from the local anesthetic block may last weeks to months when combined with physical therapy. Thermal radiofrequency (RF) lesioning of the lateral branches is performed for a more lasting relief. Denervation of the lower portion of the SI joint may be achieved by the creation of bipolar RF strip lesions along the dorsal border of the SI joint in a "leapfrog" manner. The use of a multi-lesion probe (Simplicity II, NeuroTherm) along the posterior sacral plate lateral to the foramina can be effective for at least 6 months in approximately 50% of patients.[47] A water-cooled RF technique (Fig. 56-8) is also effective because it produces larger lesions capable of capturing the variable innervation along the lateral border of the sacral foramina.[48]

Piriformis Syndrome

Piriformis syndrome, another pain syndrome that originates in the buttocks, comprises 5% of patients referred for the treatment of back and leg pain. It occurs after trauma, surgery, and infection, or from compression of one of the components of the sciatic nerve as it runs between two divisions of the piriformis muscle.[49] Patients with piriformis syndrome complain of buttock pain with or without radiation to the ipsilateral leg. The buttock pain usually extends from the sacrum to the greater trochanter of the femur, whereas irritation of the sciatic nerve results in buttock pain that radiates to the ipsilateral leg. Prolonged sitting, as in driving or biking, or rising from a sitting position aggravates the pain. The pain is aggravated by hip flexion, adduction, and internal rotation. Neurologic examination is typically negative. There may be leg numbness when the sciatic nerve is irritated; the straight-leg test may be normal or limited. Three signs confirm the presence of piriformis syndrome:[49] (1) The *Pace sign*, wherein there is pain and weakness on resisted abduction of the hip in a patient who is seated with the hip flexed; (2) the *Lasègue sign*, wherein there is pain on flexion, adduction, and internal rotation of the hip in a patient who is supine (note that some clinicians also classify pain on straight-leg raise the Lasègue sign); and (3) the *Freiberg sign*, wherein there is pain on forced internal rotation of the extended thigh. Note that the piriformis is an internal rotator of the flexed hip and an external rotator of the extended hip. The diagnosis of piriformis syndrome is made on clinical grounds. Electromyography may detect myopathic and neuropathic changes, including a delay in the H-reflex, with the affected leg in a flexed, adducted, and internally rotated (FADIR) position as compared with the same H-reflex in the normal anatomic position.

The treatment of piriformis syndrome includes physical therapy combined with medications such as muscle relaxants, anti-inflammatory drugs, and analgesics to reduce the spasm, inflammation, and pain. Local anesthetic and steroid injections into the piriformis muscle may break the pain/muscle spasm cycle. Techniques involving identification of the piriformis muscle include the use of CT guidance, use of a nerve stimulator, or combined fluoroscopy–nerve stimulator guidance. Similar efficacy of fluoroscopy and ultrasound-guided piriformis injections has been reported.[50] There appears to be no difference between lidocaine and lidocaine with betamethasone. If relief from the local anesthetic is transient, then the piriformis muscle may be injected with 100 units of botulinum toxin A in 2 to 3 mL of local anesthetic. Perisciatic injection of steroid, in addition to injection into the piriformis muscle may be performed when there is pain along the sciatic nerve.

Myofascial Pain Syndrome and Fibromyalgia

Myofascial pain syndrome is a painful regional syndrome characterized by the presence of active trigger point(s) in skeletal muscle (NICV 56-1). The trigger point can be observed as a palpable taut band and manipulation of the trigger point, by digital pressure or by penetration with a needle, may induce a twitch response. There is point tenderness in the taut band; pressure on the tender nodule induces pain that the patient recognizes as an experienced pain pattern, and there may be limitation to full passive range of motion of the affected muscle.

The management of myofascial pain syndrome includes repeated application of a cold spray over the trigger point in line with the involved muscle fibers, followed by gentle massage of the trigger point and stretching of the affected muscle. Physical therapy includes improving posture, body mechanics, relaxation techniques, trigger point massage, post-isometric relaxation, and reciprocal inhibition. A component of a multimodal treatment plan is local anesthetic injection or dry needling of the trigger point. Studies show that dry needling may be as effective as local anesthetic injection; however, the local anesthetic decreases procedural pain. Local anesthetic injection alone has been shown to be as effective as local anesthetic and steroid injection. Several injections at 2- to 3-week intervals, followed by physical therapy, may result in a long-term benefit. Botulinum toxin injections have been suggested but the results of clinical studies have not been uniform.

Fibromyalgia

The most recent[51] American College of Rheumatology criteria for classification of fibromyalgia, requires:

1. Generalized pain, defined as pain in at least 4 of 5 regions, is present.
2. Symptoms have been present at a similar level for at least 3 months.
3. Widespread pain index (WPI) ≥7 and symptom severity scale (SSS) score ≥5 OR WPI of 4–6 and SSS score ≥9.
4. Fibromyalgia is a valid diagnosis irrespective of other diagnoses. A diagnosis of fibromyalgia does not exclude the presence of other clinically important illnesses.

There is a strong genetic and familial component to the development of fibromyalgia. Family members of fibromyalgia patients are more likely to have irritable bowel syndrome, temporomandibular disorders, headaches, and a host of other regional pain syndromes.

Opioidergic activity is normal or increased in fibromyalgia, and levels of cerebrospinal fluid enkephalins are roughly twice as high in these patients compared to healthy controls. The increased activity of endogenous opioidergic systems explains clinicians' observations that opioids are ineffective in this syndrome. On the other hand, the principal metabolite of norepinephrine, 3-methoxy-4-hydroxyphenethylene glycol, is lower in the CSF of patients with fibromyalgia. This may explain the efficacy of drugs that raise levels of both serotonin and norepinephrine (tricyclic antidepressants [TCAs], duloxetine, milnacipran, tramadol).

The optimal treatment of fibromyalgia is a multifaceted program comprised of pharmacologic and nonpharmacologic therapy. Efficacious medications include serotonin and norepinephrine receptor inhibitors (SNRIs), duloxetine and milnacipran,[52] pregabalin, amitriptyline, gabapentin, and gamma-hydroxybutyrate (sodium oxybate). Effective nondrug treatment includes patient education, supportive therapy, exercise programs (specifically low-intensity low-impact programs), and cognitive-behavioral and operant-behavioral therapy.

Neuropathic Pain Syndromes

Herpes Zoster and Postherpetic Neuralgia

Some patients with acute herpes zoster have a prodrome of dermatomal pain before the skin eruptions (NICV 56-2). The pain of acute herpes zoster is usually moderate in severity and can be managed with analgesics, and the pain usually subsides with healing of the rash. About 10% to 15% of patients develop postherpetic neuralgia (PHN), commonly referred to as *shingles*, or pain that persists more than 3 months after resolution of the rash; the incidence rises from 30% to 50% in the elderly. The risk factors for the development of PHN include increased pain during the acute stage, greater severity of the skin lesion, older age, and the presence of a prodrome. The use of antiviral drugs (acyclovir, famciclovir, or valacyclovir) has been shown to hasten the healing of the rash, reduce the duration of viral shedding, and decrease the incidence of PHN. The selection of the antiviral medication is often driven by the frequency of administration and the cost, rather than efficacy. The use of varicella vaccine has become popular as it decreases the incidence of PHN,[53] a recent recombinant vaccine has increased efficacy and less decline over time compared with the previously used live attenuated virus vaccine.

Most of the studies on the efficacy of neuraxial and peripheral nerve blocks performed during the acute stage of herpes zoster have been either retrospective or case series. Prospective controlled studies have yielded conflicting results, although to be effective in preventing PHN, the blocks are preferably performed within 2 weeks of rash onset.

The mainstay of treatment for PHN is pharmacologic manage- 4
ment that includes antiepileptics, opioids, and antidepressants. 5
Although antidepressants are effective, their use is precluded by the frequent occurrence of side effects which include anticholinergic symptoms such as tachycardia, dry mouth, constipation, and prostatism in elderly males. Nortriptyline is preferred over amitriptyline because it is equally effective and better tolerated. Opioids and tramadol can be effective but can cause tolerance, dependence, and other issues. The antiepileptics gabapentin and pregabalin are usually effective in the management of PHN. Their side effects include somnolence, dizziness, and peripheral edema. Studies show that the combination of gabapentin with controlled-release morphine, and gabapentin with nortriptyline, were more effective and required lower daily dosages than with monotherapy of either drug.[54] Venlafaxine is an SNRI antidepressant that has fewer side effects but is less effective than TCAs. Based on efficacy, antidepressants are the first choice for neuropathic pain syndromes, followed by opioids, tramadol, and gabapentin/pregabalin. When quality of life, side effects, prevention of substance use disorder (SUD), and regulatory issues are considered in addition to pain relief, then gabapentin/pregabalin may be the preferred first-line agents. Topical medications including lidocaine patch or high-concentration capsaicin may be helpful for allodynia and localized pain.

The role of sympathetic blocks in reducing the pain of acute zoster and in preventing PHN has not been established. Intrathecal methylprednisolone with lidocaine, given once a week for four administrations, appears to be more effective in relieving PHN compared with intrathecal lidocaine or no treatment. However, a study that tried to confirm the efficacy of intrathecal steroid was suspended because of lack of efficacy.[55] Given conflicting efficacy studies and risks of the procedure, the use of intrathecal steroid as treatment for PHN is not conclusively recommended.[56] Studies on spinal cord stimulation (SCS) showed some benefit but were retrospective and did not use a control group.[57,58]

Diabetic Painful Neuropathy

Peripheral neuropathy may be present in approximately 65% of patients with insulin-dependent diabetes, most commonly distal symmetric polyneuropathy. The incidence of diabetic neuropathy increases with duration of diabetes, age, and degree of hyperglycemia; neuropathies generally develop after persistence of hyperglycemia for several years. The pathophysiology of diabetic neuropathy includes the polyol pathway, microvascular, and glycosylation end-product theories. All pathways result in chronic ischemia of the nerve.

The management of diabetic painful neuropathy (DPN) includes tight control of the patient's blood glucose, lifestyle modification, control of dyslipidemia (it may be associated with development of DPN) and pharmacologic therapy. The antiepileptics gabapentin and pregabalin appear to be effective in the management of DPN, with the efficacy of gabapentin enhanced by the addition of controlled-release morphine or nortriptyline.[54] The TCAs are more effective than SNRIs but given their more favorable side-effect profile, duloxetine is the most widely prescribed agent for DPN. The European Federation of Neurological Sciences Task Force and the International Association for the Study of Pain (IASP) Neuropathic Pain Special Interest group (NeuPSIG) recommend the SNRIs (duloxetine, milnacipran) as the first-choice drugs for the treatment of DPN.[59,60] The efficacy of tramadol and the opioids morphine and hydromorphone has not been established and the role of SCS requires further study.[61]

Human Immunodeficiency Virus Neuropathy

Symptomatic neuropathy occurs in 10% to 35% of patients who are seropositive for human immunodeficiency virus (HIV), and pathologic abnormalities exist in almost all patients with acquired immunodeficiency syndrome (AIDS). The sensory neuropathies associated with HIV include distal sensory polyneuropathy, the more common neuropathy related to viral infection, and antiretroviral toxic neuropathy (ATN) secondary to the treatment. The clinical features of HIV sensory neuropathy typically include painful allodynia and hyperalgesia. The onset is gradual and most commonly involves the lower extremities. The neuropathy and dysesthesia progress from the distal to the more proximal structures. There is minimal subjective or objective motor involvement, and this is generally limited to the intrinsic muscles of the foot.

There is no FDA-approved medication for HIV-related sensory neuropathy, instead the treatment is symptomatic and includes optimization of the patient's metabolic and nutritional status. The antiepileptics, particularly lamotrigine (300 mg/day), can be effective therapy for HIV sensory neuropathy as well as ATN. Gabapentin is also effective at doses of 1,200 to 3,600 mg/day. Topical lidocaine and high-dose capsaicin cream are also effective. Studies on the use of cannabis showed some efficacy but it was oflimited duration (5 days).[62,63]

Phantom Pain

Nearly all patients with amputated extremities experience nonpainful phantom sensations in the absent limb. The onset of phantom pain may be immediate but commonly occurs within the first few days following amputation. Approximately 50% of patients with pain experience a decrease in pain over time, whereas the other 50% report no change or an increase in pain over time. Phantom pain is caused by both peripheral and central factors. Peripheral mechanisms include neuromas, an increase in C fiber activity, and sodium channel activation. Central mechanisms include abnormal firing of spinal internuncial neurons and supraspinal involvement secondary to the development of new synaptic connections in the cerebral cortex.

Numerous prophylactic measures have, with variable success, been undertaken to reduce the incidence of phantom limb pain. These include perioperative epidural infusions of opioids and local anesthetics or clonidine, and continuous brachial plexus blockade with memantine. Treatment of phantom limb pain includes pharmacologic and nonpharmacologic measures and there is evidence for effective use of gabapentin, morphine, tramadol, intramuscular botulinum toxin, and epidural ketamine.[64] Nonpharmacologic measures include TENS, spinal cord stimulators, and biofeedback. A combination of pharmacologic treatment with physical, psychological, or behavioral intervention is the most effective approach. Percutaneous placement of a peripheral nerve stimulation (PNS) implant for 60 days has been shown to provide relief of lower extremity phantom limb pain for up to 12 months.[65]

Complex Regional Pain Syndrome

Complex regional pain syndrome (CRPS) is now considered nociplastic in nature, caused by ongoing inflammation and damage of tissues, in contrast to neuropathic pain, which is due to nerve damage (NICV 56-3). *CRPS type I* was originally termed *reflex sympathetic dystrophy*, whereas *CRPS type II* represents *causalgia*. The clinical features of CRPS type II are the same as in CRPS type I except there is a preceding nerve injury in CRPS II. The risk factors for the development of CRPS include previous trauma, nerve injury (for causalgia), previous surgery, work-related injuries, and female sex. The signs and symptoms of CRPS include spontaneous pain, hyperalgesia, allodynia, plus trophic, sudomotor, vasomotor abnormalities, and, finally, active and passive movement disorders. CRPS is a clinical diagnosis, and if made in accordance with the specific (Budapest) criteria, has very high sensitivity and specificity.[66]

6 Treatments for CRPS include sympathetic nerve blocks, physical therapy, and medications. Oral therapy includes gabapentin, memantine (an NMDA blocker), and alendronate. Intravenous infusions include ketamine and bisphosphonates[67] and intramuscular or subcutaneous calcitonin can also be used.[68] Ketamine can be given either as a 4- to 5-day infusion at 1 to 7 μg/kg/min or for 4 hours daily for 10 days at an infusion rate of 0.35 mg/kg/hr, although in either case liver enzymes should be serially monitored. Sympathetic blocks provide short-term relief, facilitating physical therapy, and can be performed in a series if there is over 50% relief from the first block.[69] Phenol neurolysis of the lumbar paravertebral sympathetic ganglia appears to be as effective as thermal RF. Injection of botulinum toxin A (76 IU) into the L2 and L3 sympathetic ganglia results in a greater increase in limb temperature and reduction in pain compared to levobupivacaine.[70] Note that the degree of temperature increase does not correlate with the amount of pain relief but with the magnitude of sympathetic block. SCS should be considered if the patient does not respond to other treatments.[71]

Cancer Pain

Cancer pain may be somatic, visceral, or neuropathic in origin (NICV 56-4). Somatic pain tends to be responsive to opioids, NSAIDs and neural blockade, visceral pain responds to sympathetic nerve blocks, and neuropathic pain is responsive to antiepileptics, TCAs, and SNRIs.

7 Management of cancer pain should be multifaceted and may include one or more of the following: (1) tumor-specific antineoplastic therapy, (2) multiple classes of pharmacologic analgesics, (3) interventional procedures, (4) behavioral and psychological interventions, and (5) palliative care. Opioids are the mainstay of treatment for cancer pain as most patients have a positive response when appropriate guidelines are followed. Advanced interventional treatments include neurolytic procedures targeting sympathetic ganglia and intrathecal opioids.

Neurolytic Blocks for Visceral Pain from Cancer

Celiac Plexus Block

The celiac plexus is a collection of ganglia that innervates all abdominal viscera except for the left side of the colon and the pelvis. It is anterior to the crura of the diaphragm and surrounds the abdominal aorta and the celiac and superior mesenteric arteries. The celiac plexus receives sympathetic fibers from the greater, lesser, and least splanchnic nerves, which are located retroperitoneally at the level of the T12 and L1 vertebrae and receives parasympathetic fibers from the vagus nerve.

Blockade of the celiac plexus can be achieved by antecrural and retrocrural injections (Fig. 56-9). Several percutaneous approaches have been described, including the posterior peri-aortic approach, the posterior transaortic approach, the transdiscal approach, and the anterior peri-aortic approach.[72] Fluoroscopy (Fig. 56-10), computed tomography (Fig. 56-11), and ultrasound guidance may assist the interventionalist in performing the blockade. In the fluoroscopy-guided procedure, the tip of the needle is directed toward the body of the L1 vertebrae. A diagnostic injection with local anesthetic may be used prior to neurolysis to predict efficacy. The use of local anesthetic provides superior results when combined with phenol for neurolysis. In general, 50% to 100% alcohol or 3% to 12% phenol is employed for the neurolytic block. The dosages of the neurolytic agents are 30 to 50 mL for the antecrural space, 15 to 30 mL for the retrocrural space, and 10 to 15 mL on each side for splanchnic nerve blockade.[72]

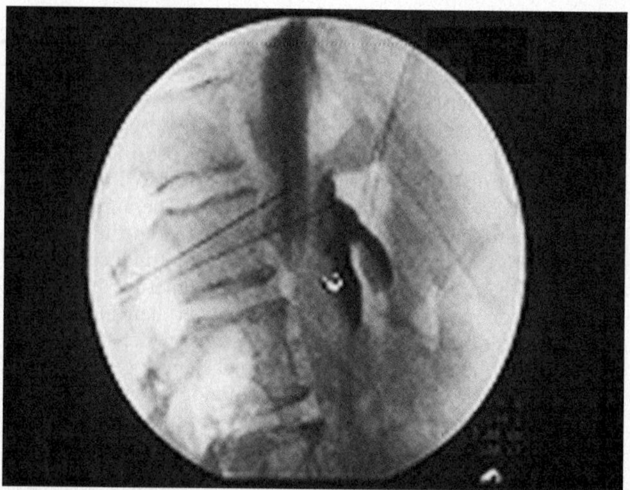

Figure 56-9 Retrocrural versus anterocrural approaches to neurolysis of the celiac plexus. Note that the tip of the needle is in the upper third of L1 and about 1 cm beyond the border of the vertebral body for the retrocrural technique; the spread of the contrast medium is cephalad. In contrast, the tip of the needle is the lower third of L1 and about 3 cm beyond the border of the vertebral body for the anterocrural technique; the spread of the contrast medium is caudad and in front of the aorta. (Adapted from de Leon-Casasola OA. Neurolysis of the sympathetic axis for cancer pain management. In: Benzon HT, Rathmell J, Wu C, et al., eds. *Raj's Practical Management of Pain*. 4th ed. Mosby Elsevier;2008;918. Copyright © 2008 Elsevier. With permission.)

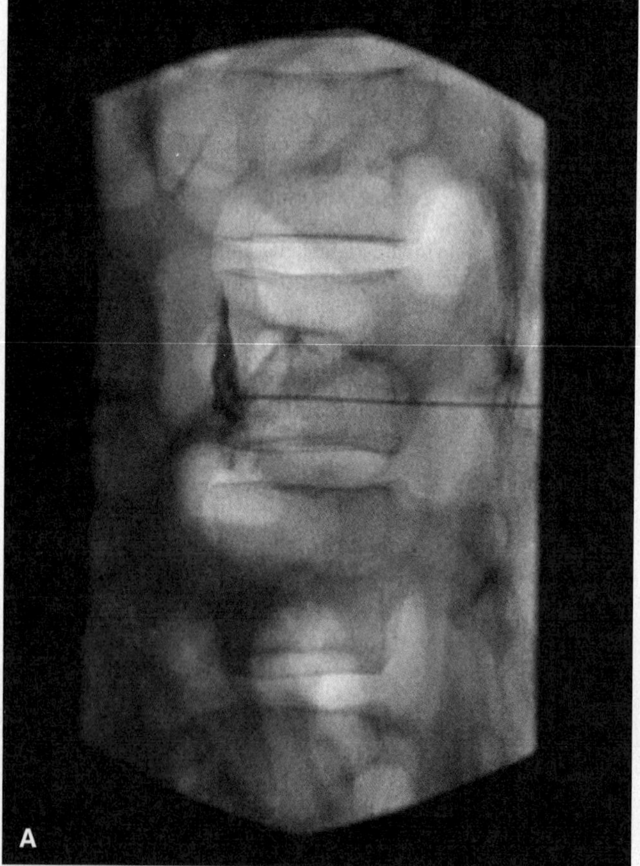

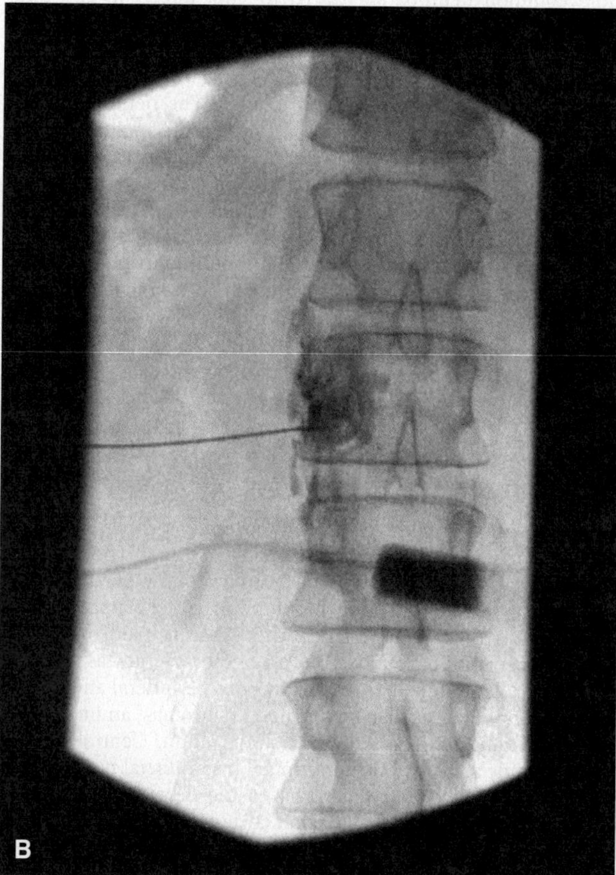

FIGURE 56-10 A, B: Splanchnic nerve block performed with fluoroscopic guidance. The greater, lesser and least splanchnic nerves form the celiac plexus.

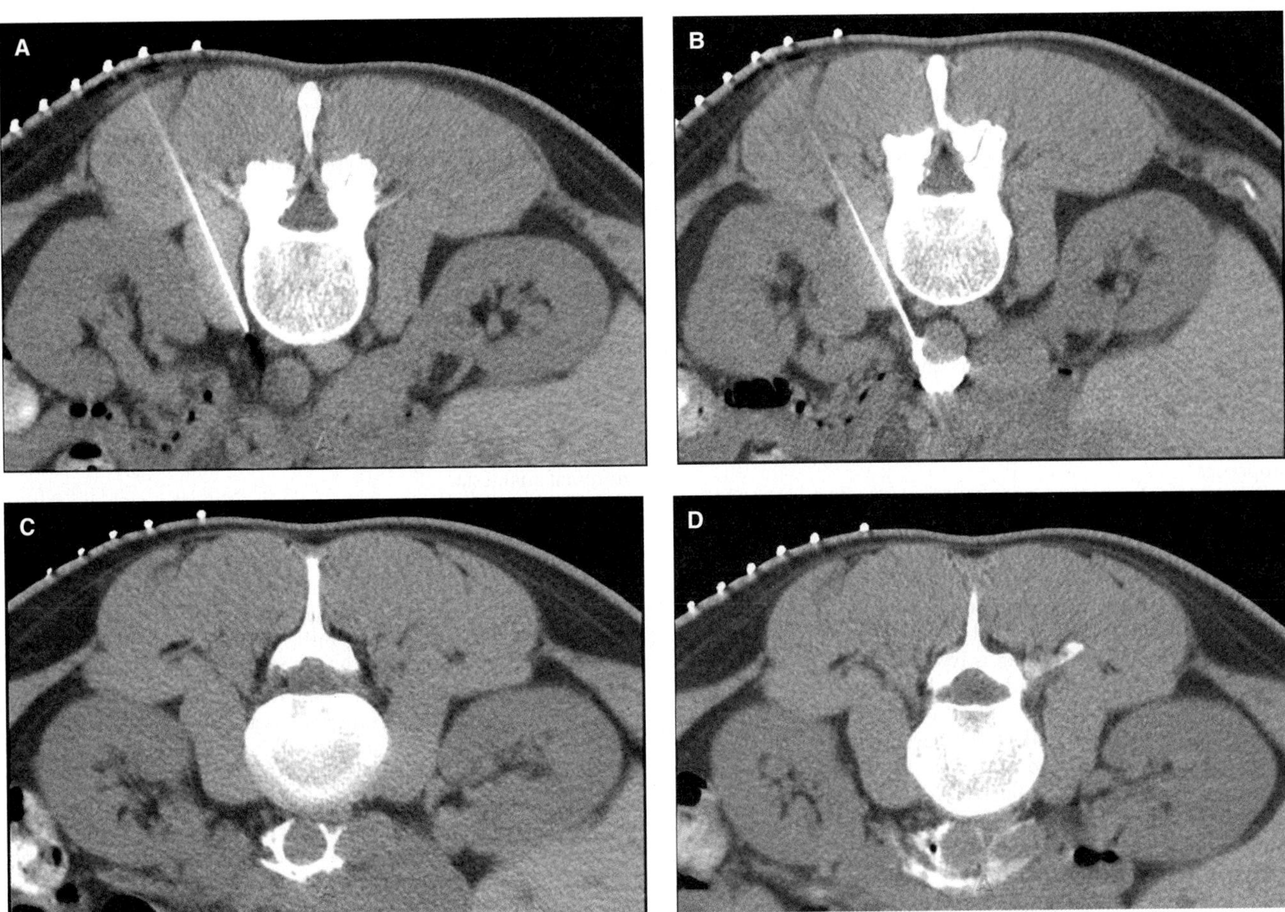

Figure 56-11 Celiac plexus block performed with CT guidance demonstrating peri-aortic spread of injectate.

There appears to be no difference in efficacy between approaches to celiac plexus blockade.[73] However, splanchnic neurolysis has been reported to have superior results compared to celiac plexus neurolysis for cancer of the pancreatic body and tail.[74] Complications from celiac plexus block include retroperitoneal hematoma, reactive pleurisy, hiccups, hematuria, abdominal aortic dissection, transient motor paralysis, and paraplegia. Paraplegia and transient motor paralysis may be due to spasm of the lumbar segmental arteries that perfuse the spinal cord, direct vascular or neurologic injury, or retrograde spread to the nerve roots or spinal cord. The most common side effects include back pain, diarrhea, and orthostatic hypotension.

8 The efficacy of celiac plexus neurolysis in improving quality of life and relieving pain from cancer of the upper abdomen has been substantiated in controlled studies. The European Association for Palliative Care (EAPC)[75] and the American Society of Pain and Neuroscience (ASPN)[76] both strongly endorse the use of celiac plexus block for treatment of pancreatic cancer pain.

Superior Hypogastric Plexus Block

Superior hypogastric plexus block is indicated for pelvic pain secondary to cancer and chronic nonmalignant conditions. The plexus is in the retroperitoneum, bilaterally extending from the lower third of the L5 vertebra to the upper third of the S1 vertebra. Fluoroscopy is used to guide two 7-cm needles in medial and caudal directions until the tips lie anterior to the L5 to S1 intervertebral disc space. Alternatively, a single needle can be used via the transdiscal approach. After injection of contrast medium, 6 to 8 mL of local anesthetic is administered for a diagnostic block while phenol or alcohol is employed for neurolysis. Anterior ultrasound-guided superior hypogastric plexus block is also effective in reducing pain and opioid requirement in pelvic pain especially in elderly patients and in the presence of bladder cancer.[77] Although large prospective controlled studies are lacking, the EAPC[75] and ASPN[76] endorse consideration of superior hypogastric plexus block for patients with intractable cancer-related pelvic pain.

Ganglion Impar Block

Pain in the perineal area associated with malignancies can be treated with neurolysis of the ganglion impar (Walther ganglion), a solitary retroperitoneal structure located anterior to the sacrococcygeal junction. Visceral afferents innervating the perineum, distal rectum, anus, distal urethra, vulva, and distal third of vagina converge at the ganglion. The trans-sacrococcygeal approach involves traversing the sacrococcygeal ligament until the tip of the needle is just anterior to the anterior portion of the sacrum. Local anesthetic (4 to 8 mL) is used for diagnostic block and 6% to 10% phenol or 50% alcohol is used for neurolysis. Despite a lack of controlled studies, ganglion impar blocks are considered effective and safe in relieving perineal pain secondary to cancer[78] and are recommended by ASPN.[76]

Pharmacologic Management of Pain

Opioids

Morphine is the standard for opioid therapy for cancer pain (see Chapter 20, Opioids). It has a variable oral bioavailability between 10% and 45%. The metabolites of morphine include morphine-6-glucuronide, which provides additional analgesia, and morphine-3-glucuronide, which contributes to adverse effects like hyperalgesia and tolerance. The *number needed to treat* (NNT) for 10 mg of morphine for postoperative pain is 2.9 and its *number needed to harm* (NNH) is 9.1. Hydromorphone, a μ-receptor agonist, is three to five times more potent than morphine when given orally and five to seven times more potent when given parenterally. Its 3- to 4-hour duration of analgesic effect is like that of morphine, but patients often prefer it for reasons that are not well characterized. Its metabolite, hydromorphone-3-glucoronide, is analogous to morphine-3-glucuronide in its absence of analgesic properties.

Methadone has a 35% to 100% bioavailability, high potency, and a long duration of action. Its other advantages include lack of an active metabolite, low cost, delayed withdrawal symptoms and salutary effects such as NMDA receptor antagonism and serotonin reuptake inhibition. Its potency compared with morphine ranges from 1:1 to 1:2 with acute dosing but can be 1:4 with chronic dosing. Although analgesic dosing is typically every 8 hours, methadone has a long and unpredictable half-life ranging from 5 to 130 hours that makes it difficult to achieve steady-state plasma concentrations, increasing the risk of accumulation. Due to this, accidental drug overdose deaths have historically been a concern with methadone use[79] but the safety margin has improved markedly due to adoption of slow uptitration strategies. There is even some evidence to support the safety of relaxing in-person restriction for provision of methadone to patients with SUD.[80] In addition to respiratory depression, methadone can cause cardiac side effects in the form of rhythm abnormalities, including QT prolongation and *torsades de pointes*. Most reports occurred in the setting of high-dose maintenance therapy (>120 mg daily) for the treatment of SUD; however, these complications have also been reported with lower doses. Experts recommend disclosure of the dysrythmogenic property of the drug, a screening ECG before initiation of therapy, follow-up ECGs in patients who are taking over 100 mg daily, and risk stratification. The risk should be discussed when the QTc interval is 450 to 500 msec and the methadone dose reduced or discontinued when the interval is greater than 500 msec.[81]

Many strong opioids are available in controlled-release (long-acting) and immediate-release (short-acting) formulations. Oxycodone is a prodrug and is converted by the enzyme cytochrome P450 2D6 to the biologically active oxymorphone (a μ-opioid agonist) and the inactive noroxycodone. It has high bioavailability (60%) and the controlled-release preparation of oxycodone has been implicated in high rates of SUD prior to its reformulation to include abuse-deterrent technologies. Fentanyl is a highly potent opioid that causes rapid development of tolerance. Oral controlled-release formulations do not exist, but it is available as a topical patch that is rotated every 72 hours and typically only prescribed for cancer pain and patients unable to use the gastrointestinal route of opioid administration. Fentanyl does not cause histamine release. Oxymorphone has greater affinity for the μ-receptor than morphine and little or no affinity to the κ-opioid receptor. When administered intravenously, it is 10 times more potent than morphine and has lower histamine release. Due to extensive first-pass hepatic metabolism, the bioavailability of oxymorphone is only 10% but high lipid solubility is responsible for rapid onset of analgesia. Concomitant use with alcohol is dangerous as this increases its plasma concentration by as much as 300%. Buprenorphine is a partial agonist at the μ-receptor, a κ-antagonist, and a weak δ-agonist. It has a rapid onset (30 minutes) when given orally and a long duration of action of 6 to 9 hours. Buprenorphine antagonizes full opioid agonists due to its high receptor binding affinity. Hydrocodone reaches peak serum concentrations within 1 to 2 hours and has a half-life of 2.5 to 4 hours.

The weak opioids include codeine, tramadol, and tapentadol. Codeine is transformed to morphine via the enzyme cytochrome P450 2D6 and has an NNT of 16.7. Genetic factors can alter the effect of these drugs. Approximately 9% of Caucasians do not have the enzyme to metabolize and experience analgesia from codeine. Asians have a lower rate of codeine O-demethylation, resulting in less morphine formation. Children under 12 years of age lack maturity of the enzyme and cannot convert the drug to morphine, and therefore experience the drug's side effects with minimal analgesia.

Tramadol is a weak opioid agonist and a monoaminergic drug with serotonin and norepinephrine reuptake inhibition activity. It has bioavailability of 80% to 90%, low abuse potential, low incidence of constipation, and minimal risk of respiratory depression, which is possibly limited to patients with severe renal failure. It has a dose-dependent efficacy, with NNTs of 8.5 for 50 mg, 5.3 for 75 mg, 4.8 for 100 mg, and 2.9 for 150 mg. The maximum dose of tramadol is 400 to 500 mg/day. Tapentadol is a more potent opioid agonist than tramadol and functions as a norepinephrine reuptake inhibitor but lacks serotonin activity. Tapentadol has side effects and adverse reactions that are like those of tramadol but has a higher risk of substance abuse and respiratory depression due to its increased opioid agonism. The oral equianalgesic doses of morphine 10 mg intravenously or 30 mg orally are (1) 200 mg of codeine, (2) 30 mg of hydrocodone, (3) 20 mg of oxycodone, (4) 150 mg of tramadol, and (5) 75 mg of tapentadol.

Opioids likely impair driving ability at any dose as even individuals receiving stable low daily doses of 20 mg of morphine or equivalent are at increased risk for motor vehicle collisions.[82] Increasing opioid dose by greater than 30% over a period of 2 days worsens cognitive performance, and stable daily doses higher than 120 mg increase motor vehicle accident risk markedly. Patients who recently initiated opioids, take moderate-to-high doses or recently increased their dose should be counseled as to the hazards of driving.

Opioids are commonly used for cancer pain, with long-acting opioids serving as the mainstay while being supplemented by short-acting formulations for breakthrough pain. Opioid monotherapy in cancer pain is rarely successful and adjuvants and procedural interventions are usually added for increased efficacy. The use of opioids for acute or short-term pain (<3 months) following surgery or traumatic injuries is well accepted and supported by the literature. The use of opioids for treatment of chronic (>3 months) of noncancer pain is controversial. To date, no controlled studies have established the efficacy of chronic opioid therapy for greater than 3 months[83] but it is likely to be effective for long-term analgesia in a small subset of patients. Due to the undesirable issues associated with the use of opioids, such as SUD, aberrant behaviors, and regulatory issues, opioids are a third-line drug for neuropathic pain. It should be noted that although individual studies show efficacy of opioids in low back pain in the short term, a meta-analysis did not show reduced pain when compared with a placebo or a nonopioid control group.[84] Opioids, in addition to NSAIDs and muscle relaxants, may be efficacious for the short-term relief of acute low back pain, but the long-term efficacy of opioids (≥16 weeks) is unclear and cannot be recommended.[83] When treating fibromyalgia, tramadol, tapentadol, or a tramadol/acetaminophen combination is the only opioids that have been shown to be more effective than placebo. Other opioids, including pure opioid agonists, should not be used in the treatment of fibromyalgia and chronic widespread pain. In general, prior to initiation of opioid therapy, the risks and benefits should be carefully assessed, goals established, and dosing re-addressed at regular intervals.[85]

Opioids have significant risks including tolerance, physical dependence, SUD, and opioid misuse. A body of evidence suggests that among chronic pain patients receiving opioid therapy, 6% to 37% will exhibit aberrant drug-related behaviors, 8% to 16% will abuse opioids, and 2% to 14% will develop SUD.[83] Factors predictive of increased risk for misuse include personal or family history of SUD, history of sexual abuse, younger age, major depression, and use of psychotropic medications. A subset of patients self-medicate with opioids to inappropriately manage depression independent of pain.[86]

Pharmacologic Treatment of Neuropathic Pain

First-line medication recommendations for neuropathic pain include antiepileptics, SNRIs, and TCAs. Second-line recommendations included capsaicin 8% patches, topical lidocaine, and tramadol. Botulinum toxin A and opioids are third-line medications, but strong opioids have been linked to worsened outcomes.[87]

Antiepileptics

Neuropathic pain is associated with functional changes in sodium and calcium channel subunit expression. In chronic nerve injury, redistribution, and alteration of subunit composition of sodium and calcium channels results in spontaneous firing at ectopic sites along the sensory pathway. Most antiepileptics are sodium channel blockers, inhibiting spontaneous activities at neuromas, DRG, and at the dorsal horn of the spinal cord, which explains their efficacy in neuropathic pain syndromes. Some antiepileptics also act on ion channel systems, including $GABA_A$ receptor agonists (topiramate and felbamate), $GABA_A$ transaminase blockers (vigabatrin), $GABA_A$ transport blockers (tiagabine), and glutamate receptor antagonists (felbamate and topiramate). The other types directly block calcium channels (lamotrigine), T-type calcium channels (topiramate and zonisamide) and α_2-delta subunits (gabapentin and pregabalin). Controlled studies have demonstrated the efficacy of the antiepileptics in several neuropathic pain syndromes including trigeminal neuralgia, PHN, DPN, HIV polyneuropathy, phantom limb pain, spinal cord injury (SCI) pain, and central poststroke pain.

Gabapentin is an effective drug in neuropathic pain (PHN, DPN, and SCI), multiple sclerosis pain, neuropathic cancer pain, and fibromyalgia. Gabapentin has a wide therapeutic range but considerable bioavailability variation among individuals and up to 50% of patients will experience adverse effects without any benefit.[88] Compared to gabapentin, pregabalin has a more linear pharmacokinetic profile and thus more consistent therapeutic dose range. Given their identical pharmacodynamics, pregabalin and gabapentin have similar indications and their most common side effect is drowsiness, which can be mitigated by slow uptitration. The popularity of gabapentin and pregabalin can be traced to their perceived low morbidity but they can increase risk of overdose if prescribed concomitantly with an opioid.[89]

Lamotrigine is effective in treatment of HIV polyneuropathy, pain from SCI, trigeminal neuralgia, and central poststroke pain. The most common side effect is rash, and use of lamotrigine is limited by the risk of Stevens–Johnson syndrome. Topiramate is

Table 56-3 Dosages (mg/day) of the Commonly Used Antidepressants and Anticonvulsants[a]

Antidepressants	Anticonvulsants
Amitriptyline: 10–300	Gabapentin: 900–3,600, tid
Doxepin: 30–300	Lamotrigine: 50–150
Nortriptyline: 50–150	Mexiletine: 300–1,350, tid
Desipramine: 25–300	Oxcarbazepine: 300–900, bid
Fluoxetine: 5–40	Pregabalin: 150–600, bid
Paroxetine: 20–40	Topiramate: 50–200, bid
Venlaflaxine: 37.5–300	
Duloxetine: 60–120, od or bid	
Milnacipran: 100–200 mg, 50–100 mg bid	

tid, three times a day; bid, twice a day; od, once daily.
[a]Unless indicated, dosing is once a day. Start with smallest possible dose and titrate to efficacy or side effects.

effective in migraine prophylaxis, similar to divalproex. Oxcarbazepine is similar in chemical structure to carbamazepine with fewer side effects and noted to be effective in trigeminal neuralgia; with rapid pain relief that may be noted within 24 to 48 hours. The recommended doses of the commonly used antiepileptics are in Table 56-3.

The side effects of antiepileptics include dizziness, fatigue, somnolence, weight gain due to peripheral edema (gabapentin and pregabalin); rash (lamotrigine); paresthesia, cognitive effects, weight loss (topiramate); hyponatremia; and low thyroid concentrations (oxcarbazepine).

Antidepressants

TCAs have a serotonergic effect (interference with serotonin reuptake and alteration of serotonin binding to receptors in neural tissue), a noradrenergic effect (interaction with α-receptors), an opioidergic effect, blockade of the NMDA receptor complex, inhibition of the uptake of adenosine, blockade of sodium and calcium channels and may have an anti-inflammatory effect. The NNTs of antidepressants are comparable to those of opioids and antiepileptics. Antidepressants also inhibit the histaminic, cholinergic, muscarinic, and nicotinic receptors, resulting in sedation, dry mouth, and urinary retention. TCAs, specifically amitriptyline and nortriptyline, have long been used to treat neuropathic pain but evidence to support this is minimal.[87]

In addition to their antidepressant action, SNRIs have an antinociceptive effect with duloxetine having increased selectivity for serotonin. Venlafaxine has increased serotonergic effects at lower doses but with greater noradrenergic activity above 215 mg/day. Duloxetine and milnacipran have preferential noradrenergic effect, longer half-lives (12 and 8 hours, respectively) and have no active metabolites. Duloxetine is effective in DPN and fibromyalgia and milnacipran provides moderate pain relief to patients with fibromyalgia. However, the most effective treatment of fibromyalgia is achieved with concomitant use of pregabalin and duloxetine.[90] The efficacy of the SNRIs in DPN and fibromyalgia, coupled with the improved side-effect profile (free of cholinergic, histaminic, and α-adrenergic receptor effects, and less potential for drug interactions) compared to TCAs is the basis for their more common prescription.

Table 56-4 Recommended Drugs for Chronic Pain Syndromes

Postherpetic Neuralgia	Diabetic Painful Neuropathy	Spinal Cord Injury	Fibromyalgia	Human Immunodeficiency Virus (HIV)
Pregabalin	Duloxetine	Pregabalin	Duloxetine	Lamotrigine
Gabapentin	Pregabalin	Gabapentin	Pregabalin	Gabapentin
Opioid	Gabapentin	Lamotrigine	Milnacipran	
Antidepressants	Antidepressants	IV lidocaine	Tramadol	
Tramadol	Mexilitine (±)			
Lidoderm patch (allodynia)				

TCAs have an NNT of 2.1 to 2.8 for treatment of PHN, 1.3 to 3.4 for DPN, and 1.7 for central pain. The side effects of antidepressants include cholinergic effects such as dry mouth, sedation, and urinary retention. Venlafaxine may cause hypertension and mania and may exacerbate seizures. When weaning off the medication, a gradual decrease is recommended for duloxetine to prevent agitation, anxiety, confusion, and hypomania. TCAs are more likely to cause weight gain compared with SNRIs. TCAs impair driving ability during the first week of treatment or during dose escalation, but in patients with long-term (>3 years) use of TCAs, driving abilities are not impaired.[91] The serotonin specific reuptake inhibitors (SSRIs) (citalopram, paroxetine) have minimal benefit in neuropathic pain. The recommended doses for the commonly used antidepressants are summarized in Table 56-3.

Lidocaine Patch, Capsaicin Patch, Mexiletine, and Cannabinoids

The 5% lidocaine patch delivers lidocaine locally at the site of neuropathic pain generation, limiting its systemic effects and reducing its interactions with other concomitantly administered medications; analgesia is by local sodium channel blockade and not by its systemic effects. The patch contains 700 mg of lidocaine in an adhesive vehicle. It is recommended that no more than three patches be applied concomitantly for a maximum of 12 hr/day. Pain relief typically occurs within a few days, but a minority of patients will experience delayed onset of analgesia; therefore a 2-week trial period is prudent. Some patients continue to experience relief between patch applications, but in patients with pain upon patch removal, duration of application should be extended to 16 to 18 hours. Only 3% of the total dose applied is absorbed systemically and the maximum plasma lidocaine concentration is usually achieved on the second day of use, with significantly lower concentrations than the cardiotoxic threshold.

Capsaicin has been shown to defunctionalize TRPV1 nerve endings and reduce epidermal nerve fiber density and is an effective treatment for the pain of PHN, DPN, and HIV neuropathy.[92] A higher-concentration capsaicin 8% patch is superior to both placebo and low-concentration (0.04%) capsaicin. Its NNT is 12 for 30% relief and analgesia may persist up to 12 weeks after one application. Due to burning sensation during initial placement, local anesthetic cream should be applied to the treatment area one hour prior to patch application. A 60-minute application of capsaicin is better tolerated and is similar in efficacy to 90-minute application. There is an increase in pain 20 to 30 minutes after application, which resolves 2 to 3 hours after removal of the patch. A maximum of four doses can be administered at intervals of 12 weeks.[93]

Mexiletine is an oral analog of lidocaine and can treat the pain of diabetic neuropathy, thalamic stroke, spasticity, and myotonia with modest efficacy however it is not well tolerated by most patients. A favorable response to intravenous lidocaine does not necessarily predict a similar response to mexiletine. The median recommended dose of mexiletine is 600 mg/per day.

Cannabinoids

Cannabinoids may be effective in neuropathic pain, but the lack of strong efficacy evidence in combination with the potential for misuse and mental health risks necessitates judicious patient selection.[94] A 2017 systematic review and meta-analysis of multiple studies revealed limited evidence for cannabis-based medication on pain reduction for chronic pain.[95] As of May 2022, the prescription and consumption of medical cannabis was legal in 37 states, four territories, and the District of Columbia, although federally illegal (Schedule I), which limits ability of investigators to study the benefits of cannabis. Dronabinol and nabilone, synthetic cannabinoids approved for nausea treatment, have shown no benefit in acute postsurgical pain in clinical trials. Dronabinol did reduce pain intensity in chronic pain patients who were opioid tolerant,[96] but had similar psychoactive effects to inhaled cannabis.[97]

Based on original studies, review articles, and meta-analysis publications, the recommended drugs for several different chronic pain syndromes are listed in Table 56-4.

Buprenorphine–Naloxone Therapy

Buprenorphine, an opioid partial agonist, is often combined with naloxone as an abuse deterrent formulation that may be offered as sublingual tablets, sublingual films, or buccal films. It has been noted to be effective in outpatient SUD treatment and offers several advantages over methadone maintenance programs. As opioids are associated with adverse physiologic and social consequences, buprenorphine /naloxone has been prescribed as an alternative therapy, even in patients without risk factors for SUD. Although it may provide inferior analgesia to other opioids,[98] in patients with opioid dependence or SUD, studies showed the drug to have some efficacy in treating chronic pain.[99]

Interventional Techniques

Use of Contrast for Interventional Pain Procedures

When performing interventional procedures, an iodimnated contrast medium is usually injected before the pain-relieving medication to assure correct needle placement and exclude off-target delivery. If there is a history of a previous hypersensitivity reaction to the contrast medium an alternative contrast agent may be indicated, such as a gadolinium-based contrast agent (GBCA). Several adverse events have been associated with the use of GBCAs, including nephrogenic systemic fibrosis, gadolinium brain deposition/retention, and encephalopathy/death from unintentional intrathecal injection. These events are associated with the gadolinium ion, a toxic lanthanide element. Linear GBCAs are less stable and release the gadolinium easier than the macrocyclic agents. GBCAs, especially linear agents, should be used with caution in patients with renal insufficiency. Gadolinium brain deposition can occur after two intravenous MRIs so the interventional pain physician should be aware, and document, previous diagnostic tests where contrast was used. Clinical sequelae from gadolinium brain retention have not been established. A multisociety practice advisory published in 2021 recommended against the use of a GBCA in IL and TF epidural injections.[100] Regarding hypersensitivity reactions, the unintentional use of the same ICM in patients who had an index reaction does not usually result in a repeat reaction. This is probably related to the extravascular injection of small volumes and the concomitant injection of steroid.

Thermal Annular Procedures

Intradiscal electrothermal therapy (IDET) is a procedure wherein a thermal resistance catheter is placed percutaneously in the posterolateral portion of the disc. Heat causes the collagen of the annulus fibrosis to contract. Two randomized sham-controlled studies examined IDET in discogenic pain patients, with one study showing significant improvements in pain scores and Oswestry Disability Index[101] and the other study finding no significant differences in pain or functional outcome between the IDET-treated and sham control groups.[102] The procedure was not approved by the U.S. Centers for Medicare and Medicaid Services, leading to a dramatic reduction in clinical use and research. Given the difficulty of navigating the IDET catheter in degenerated discs, a bilateral cooled RF approach—biacuplasty—was developed. A prospective study showed efficacy of biacuplasty compared to a sham control at 6 and 12 months[103] and an open-label trial showed it to be superior to conventional medical management.[104] Similar to other thermal annular procedures, third-party insurance coverage remains extremely limited.

Recent evidence suggests the vertebral bodies, in particular the endplates, may be a source of axial LBP. Endplates may fracture, thereby increasing communication with the relatively avascular disc, and there is upregulation of cyclooxygenase, calcitonin gene–related peptide (CGRP) and various prostaglandins in degenerated discs. This has led to efforts targeting the basivertebral nerve, which innervates trabecular bone of vertebral bodies. Several industry-sponsored randomized trials have demonstrated greater than 1-year pain reduction and functional improvement compared to standard of care and sham neurotomy after basivertebral nerve RFA,[105] but generalizing these findings to real-world populations, and identifying appropriate candidates remain as clinical challenges.

Minimally Invasive Lumbar Decompression Procedure

Spinal stenosis is narrowing of the spinal canal with compression of the nerve roots as demonstrated with an MRI or CT scan. Spinal canal narrowing can occur centrally, in the lateral recesses, or in the intervertebral foramina, and be secondary to hypertrophy or buckling of the ligamentum flavum, disc protrusions or spondylolisthesis, or hypertrophy of the facet joints. Pain from lumbosacral stenosis is typically located in the low back area, buttocks, thighs, and/or legs in combination with neurogenic claudication, especially with erect posture (due to smaller spinal canal diameter in this position) or ambulation. In a 3-year follow-up of nonsurgically treated patients published in 2022 it showed that one-third had improvement, 50% showed no change while 10% to 20% had worsening of symptoms.[35] The minimally invasive lumbar decompression (MILD) procedure is a minimally invasive method of spinal decompression. It is indicated in patients with low back pain and neurogenic claudication associated with MRI or CT evidence of central canal stenosis secondary to ligamentum flavum hypertrophy in the lumbar segments. The procedure involves a small percutaneous laminotomy and thinning of the ligamentum flavum to increase the critical diameter of the stenosed spinal canal. A one- or, more commonly, two-level decompression is performed. In contrast to surgical decompression with fusion wherein there is complete resection of the ligamentum flavum and bony posterior elements compressing the thecal sac and exiting nerve roots, the MILD procedure only partially debulks the ligamentum flavum. Although randomized studies have demonstrated superiority of MILD to ESIs[106] and as add-on therapy to conventional medical management[107] in central lumbar stenosis, utilization has been limited at the time this chapter was authored due to restrictions on payment by insurers.

Vertebroplasty and Kyphoplasty

Vertebroplasty and kyphoplasty are percutaneous interventional modalities used to treat vertebral compression fractures (VCFs), a condition usually secondary to osteoporosis in elderly patients and associated with significant morbidity and mortality. Most healed VCFs are asymptomatic; pain may be experienced in acute or subacute VCF with bending, lifting, prolonged sitting or standing, or when the patient attempts to stand from a seated position. The pain is usually a deep back pain and may occasionally be accompanied by radiculitis and/or paravertebral muscle spasm. Radiography shows osteopenia or decreased bone mass; MRI is the imaging modality of choice as it can detect bony edema associated with an acute fracture, which is the primary indication for vertebral augmentation.

Vertebroplasty involves the injection of polymethylmethacrylate (PMMA) into the affected vertebral body; *kyphoplasty* involves the insertion of a balloon prior to the injection of the cement. These procedures can lead to restoration of some of the decreased vertebral height in some patients, and improved strength of the vertebral body. Both procedures are performed under fluoroscopic guidance. Vertebral body access is obtained through a uni- or bipedicular approach. The entire vertebral body does not have to be filled with cement to achieve pain relief, with one study finding no association with the volume of injected cement and clinical outcomes.[108] Kyphoplasty involves the percutaneous introduction of a balloon into the vertebral body, inflation of the balloon (Fig. 56-12), then filling of the potential space created by the balloon with PMMA. The creation of potential space by the balloon allows the use of a more viscous PMMA than that used for vertebroplasty.

The complications of percutaneous vertebral augmentation include leakage of the PMMA, an increased risk of adjacent segment fractures, and complications related to the procedure. The factors that contribute to PMMA leakage include the level of injection, severity of fracture, and the amount of cement injected. Neurologic complications include radiculopathy, spinal claudication, and paraplegia. Kyphoplasty may be associated with a

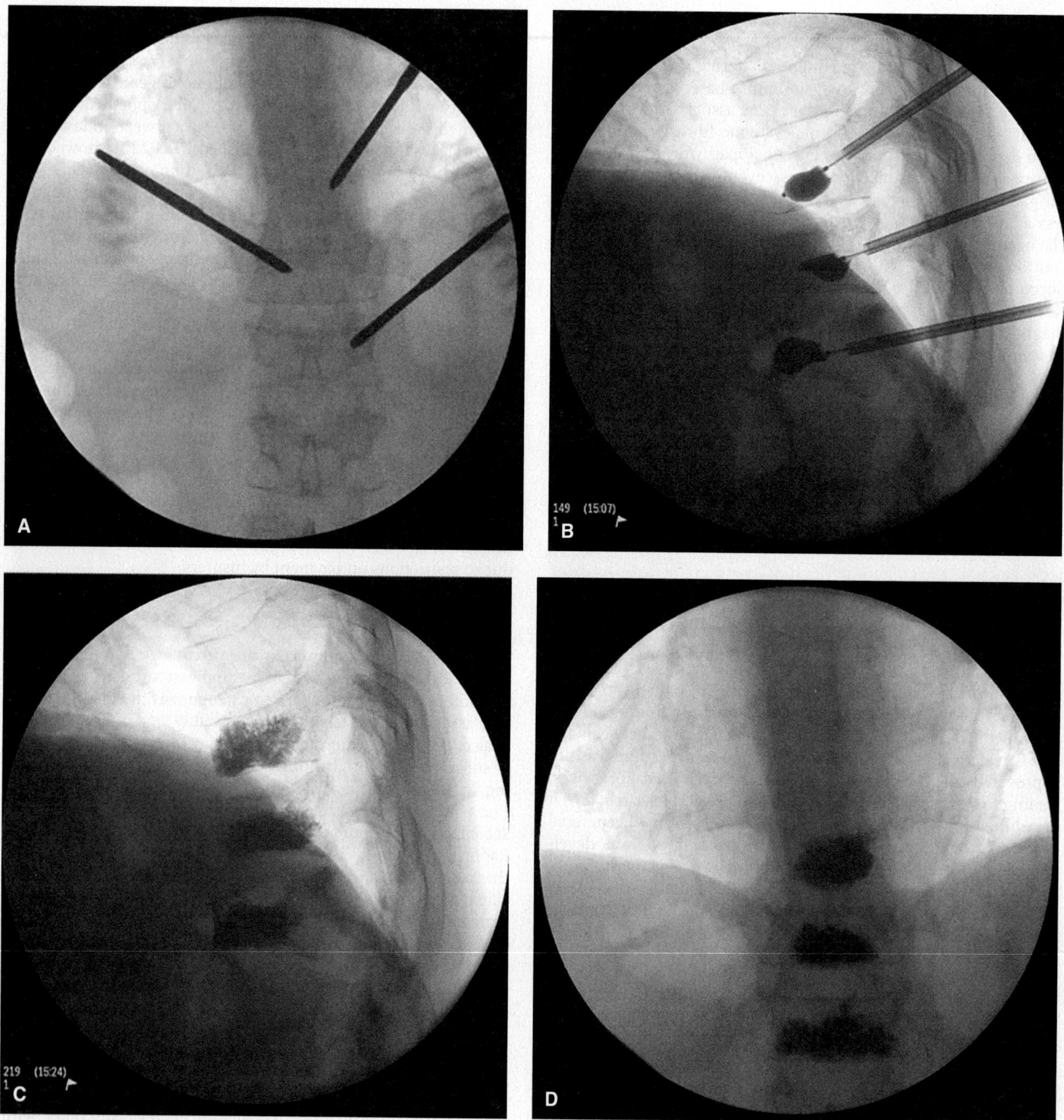

Figure 56-12 Kyphoplasty performed on T10, T11, and T12 spinal levels. **A:** Unipedicular approach at alternating levels. **B:** Balloon deployment in lateral view, **C:** PMMA deposition in lateral view, **D:** PMMA deposition in anterior/posterior view.

lower rate of cement extravasation because of the higher viscosity of the PMMA that is used, lower injection pressure employed, and the inflatable bone trap that seals pathways for cement leakage, though some have argued that this may limit the spread of cement to affected areas. Complications related to the procedure include infection, bleeding, and allergic reactions.

9 Although there have been reported benefits from vertebroplasty, controlled studies have found either no significant differences between vertebroplasty and sham procedures, or only small clinically questionable benefit.[109] Although the conduct of the studies was criticized, questions about the mechanisms and the effectiveness of this procedure remain unanswered. Two reports showed the superiority of balloon kyphoplasty for VCFs in patients with osteoporosis or cancer when compared with a control nonsurgical care group.[110,111] These two randomized studies were partly criticized, in that funding for the study came from the maker of the device, and one of the authors was affiliated with the company. A more recent (2018) systematic review comparing vertebroplasty and kyphoplasty found no significant differences in pain scores or function, though the latter was associated with increased vertebral

body height, decreased kyphotic wedge angle, and less cement leakage.[112]

Spinal Cord Stimulation

The analgesic effect of SCS may involve the *gate control theory*, neurotransmitter modulation in the spinal cord affecting pain pathways and suppression of sympathetic activity, with antidromic activity and supraspinal mechanisms also playing roles. It is hypothesized that SCS increases the input of large nerve fibers, thus closing the "gate" at the substantia gelatinosa of the dorsal horn of the spinal cord. SCS may alter the local neurochemistry of the dorsal horn, with decreased hyperexcitability of wide dynamic range neurons. SCS is associated with increased levels of the inhibitory neurotransmitter GABA and a decrease of the excitatory neurotransmitters glutamate and aspartate. In ischemic pain, the analgesia may be secondary to alteration of the sympathetic tone, leading to a more favorable oxygen supply-and-demand balance.

In the United States, SCS is approved as an aid in the management of failed back surgery syndrome, intractable low back and leg pain, complex regional pain syndrome and diabetic neuropathy, while in Europe it is also approved for refractory angina and limb ischemia. However, there are many clinical indications that are considered off-label, including placement of all cervical spine stimulators. Patients who failed conservative therapy and experience temporary pain relief from a stimulation trial that ranges from 5 days to 4 weeks, with no psychological contraindications, generally proceed to permanent implantation; conversion rates typically range from 50% to over 85%. Contraindications include systemic or local site of infection and abnormal coagulopathy. Complications include nerve and SCI, infection, hematoma, and lead breakage or migration.

10 Evidence generally supports the efficacy of SCS for treatment of persistent back and leg pain, though studies have yielded a wide range of outcomes, with those sponsored by industry demonstrating superior results.[113] In one systematic review evaluating SCS for neuropathic pain, the authors found conflicting evidence for efficacy against placebo, but low-to-moderate evidence for effectiveness against conventional medical management.[114] For diabetic neuropathy, a systematic review that contained two randomized trials found superiority for SCS compared to medical management.[115] In one large database review involving over 550,000 patients who received SCS for failed back surgery syndrome, the most common indication, the authors found either no or only small, clinically questionable reductions in chronic opioid therapy.[116] In general, SCS are more favorable for peripheral neuropathic pain than for nociceptive, central, or mixed pain conditions.

Modifications to SCS parameters, in particular frequency rate and pattern, have shown signs of improved effectiveness. High-frequency SCS at 10 kHz has shown superior pain relief in back and leg pain compared to conventional SCS (at low frequency 40 to 130 Hz) in long-term follow-up. Unlike conventional stimulation, SCS at 10 kHz is paresthesia free, which should theoretically lend itself to placebo-controlled trials. Burst SCS, which applies pulse trains of five consecutive waves of higher-frequency stimulation at 500 Hz, has been shown to result in improved back and leg pain control compared to tonic stimulation, in a mostly paresthesia-free fashion.[117] More recently, closed-loop SCS, which adjusts stimulation intensity to minimise the difference between the measured and target-evoked compound action potentials, has also been shown to be superior to conventional stimulation for back and leg pain.[118]

Studies examining the efficacy of SCS in CRPS have consisted of retrospective case series, prospective clinical studies, and two random controlled trials. One demonstrated superiority at 2 years for pain but not function compared to conventional medical management, but no significant benefit afterward,[71] while the other found short-term superiority of SCS compared to placebo, but no differences between various types and frequencies.[119] Criticisms of randomized trials that compare SCS to medical management include the robust placebo effect for invasive procedures and that most patients who receive SCS already failed medical management. For pain from peripheral ischemia and angina, there is some evidence in the form of randomized trials for modest effects on pain relief, relief of angina, and limb salvage.[120,121]

SCS electrodes are placed via a Touhy needle as shown in Figure 56-13.

Peripheral Nerve Stimulation

Electrical stimulation of a peripheral nerve can be used to treat neuropathic pain, ideally arising from a single nerve. When considering PNS it is important to distinguish between open and percutaneous PNS approaches. In open PNS, nerve stimulation is made feasible with a circumferential (cuff) electrode that requires surgical exposure of the target nerve. Application of high-frequency (10-kHz) alternating current using a cuff electrode around a peripheral nerve has been shown to result in reversible complete neuronal conduction block. In contrast, PNS involves the use of cylindrical percutaneous lead placed near the target nerve or in the subcutaneous area supplied by the target nerve. The former percutaneous approach requires target specificity and may be subject to lead migration and unwanted motor stimulation in mixed nerves. The latter approach is referred to as *peripheral nerve field stimulation* and is less target specific but also less technically challenging. Trials for PNS have consisted of electrical stimulation, local anesthetic nerve block, and pulsed RF. Of note, the use of temporary devices has been shown to provide sustained relief in some patients, presumably by reversing peripheral and central sensitization. Small industry-sponsored placebo-controlled trials and comparative-effectiveness studies have shown effectiveness in post-stroke shoulder pain, postamputation pain, low back pain, and post-traumatic neuropathy.[113] For the most common indication, the prevention of migraine headache by occipital nerve stimulation, the authors of a systematic review found a large effect size but substantial heterogeneity based on three sham-controlled trials, with the highest-quality study being negative for the primary outcome.[122]

Dorsal Root Ganglion Stimulation

A hybrid between SCS and PNS involves DRG stimulation. In DRG stimulation, special percutaneous leads are introduced, initially in the IL epidural space, and directed toward the adjacent target DRG. Advantages of this technique involve targeting unique dermatomes and difficult-to-target areas such as the foot, along with minimal-to-no positional changes in paresthesia intensity compared to conventional SCS. A recent comparative-effectiveness study involving 152 CRPS patients randomized to DRG stimulation or paresthesia-based SCS showed a significantly greater proportion of patients achieving 50% or more pain relief with DRG stimulation at a 12-month follow-up.[123]

Intrathecal Drug Delivery

Intrathecal drug delivery (IDD) enables opioids and other anal- 11
gesics to be directly deposited near the spinal cord receptors, resulting in analgesia at lower doses (Figs. 56-14 and 56-15). An additional mechanism for spinal opioids is the release of adenosine

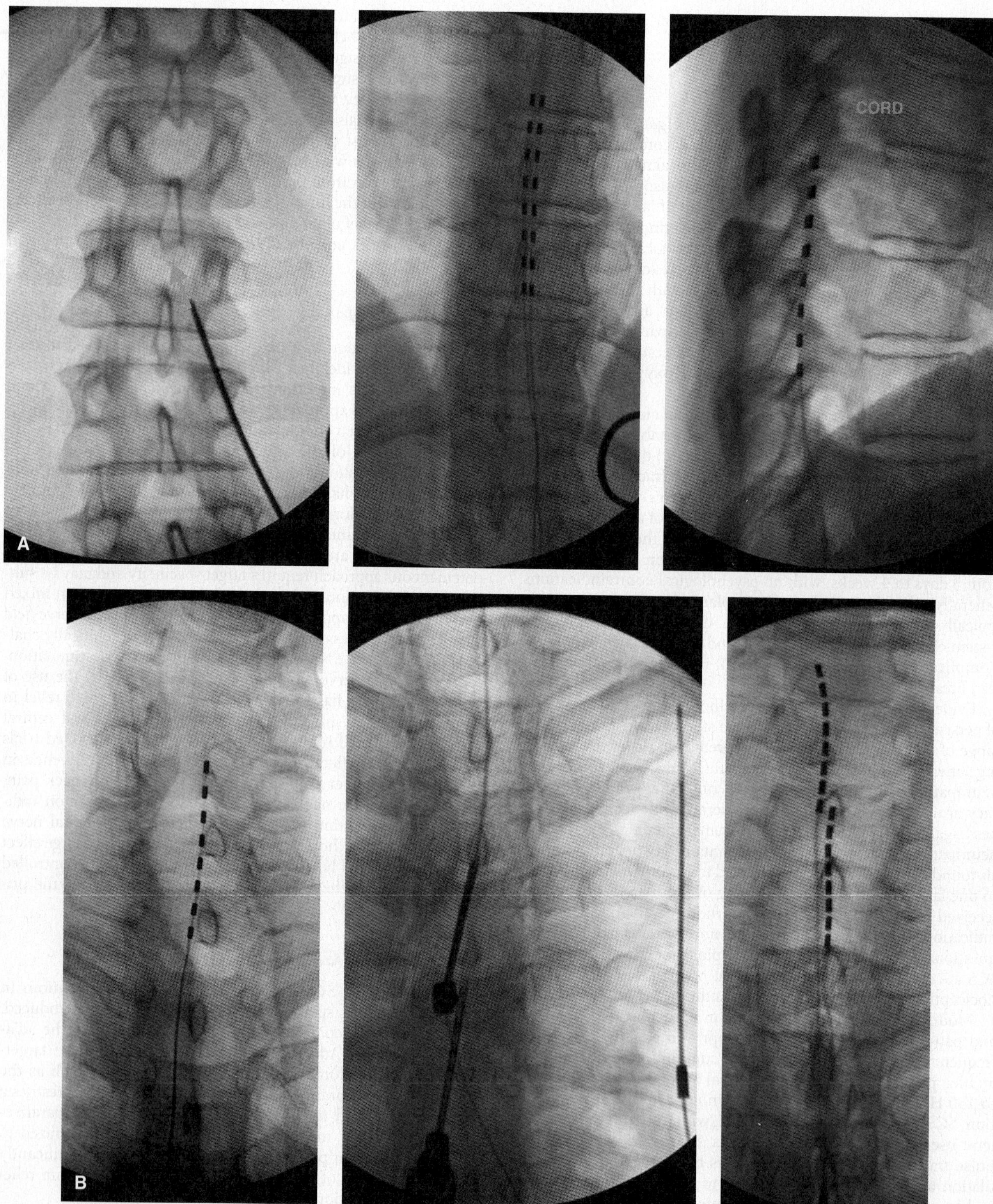

Figure 56-13 Placement of the epidural needle and the spinal cord electrodes at the thoracic (**A**) and cervical (**B**) levels.

into cerebrospinal fluid. IDD systems are valuable options in chronic pain patients who have not responded to other modalities and in whom oral or transdermal medications/opioids are ineffective at reasonable doses or cause certain unacceptable side effects such as gastrointestinal dysfunction for opioids, and sedation for opioids and baclofen. The top indication for IDD has historically been spinal pain, though recent guidelines recommending lower doses of opioids have translated to decreased utilization in chronic

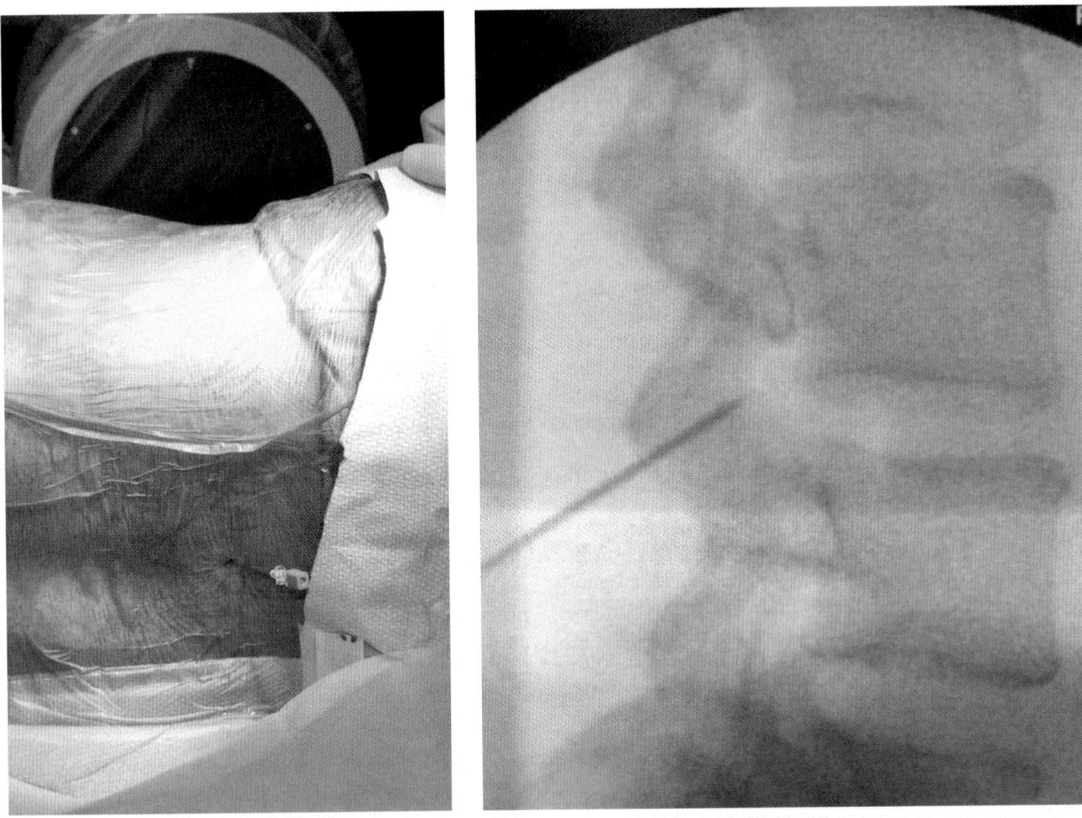

Figure 56-14 Placement of the intrathecal needle under fluoroscopy.

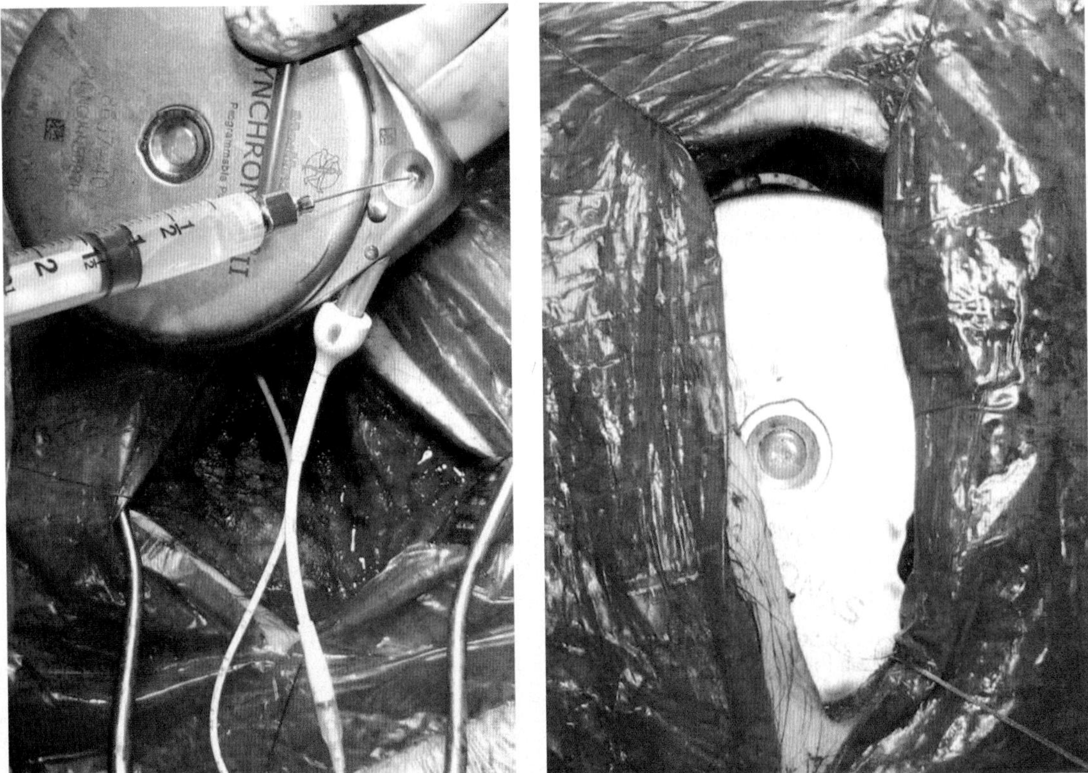

Figure 56-15 Connection of the intrathecal catheter to the programmable pump and confirmation of cerebrospinal fluid prior to placement in the pocket.

noncancer pain. IDD allows the drug to be directly deposited near the spinal cord receptors, bypassing the blood–brain barrier and the first-pass effect encountered by systemic medications. Hence, medications that have limited blood–brain barrier permeability and medications whose target receptors are in the spinal canal can be delivered more efficiently and at significantly lower doses. For morphine and baclofen, the oral:intrathecal equianalgesic doses are 300:1 and 100:1, respectively.

There are only two medications approved by the FDA for IDD for pain indications: preservative-free morphine and the synthetic peptide ziconotide, which is not available in any other formulation. According to recent polyanalgesic consensus guidelines, first-line medications for the treatment of chronic pain are ziconotide and morphine. Fentanyl, with or without bupivacaine, is considered less desirable.[124] Hydromorphone, with or without bupivacaine, is considered second line, with sufentanil, clonidine, baclofen and other adjuvants considered third-line or later therapy. Although baclofen is FDA-approved for the management of spasticity, it has a limited role in pain applications.

Patients receiving intrathecal opioids develop tolerance not unlike what is observed with systemic opioids. Side effects such as pruritus, urinary retention, myoclonus, and peripheral edema are more likely to occur with intrathecal than systemic administration of opioids. In addition, an 8% risk of developing an intrathecal catheter tip granuloma is unique to intrathecal opioid infusion. These are typically sterile inflammatory masses consisting of fibroblasts, macrophages, neutrophils, and monocytes. The incidence of granuloma formation is increased with higher doses and concentrations of morphine and hydromorphone, but not fentanyl. The development of granulomas is not mediated through opioid receptors and experiments suggest that granuloma formation may be related to dural mast cell degranulation occurring in response to morphine and hydromorphone but not fentanyl. Signs of granuloma formation include loss of analgesia, increased pain, loss of sensation, and other neurologic symptoms in the dermatome of the intrathecal catheter tip, and in later stages, paraplegia and loss of bowel and bladder function.

Considering the often-chronic nature of non-cancer pain and the longer duration of expected therapy compared to cancer pain, the risk of tolerance, hyperalgesia, and granuloma formation may be elevated in this population; hence, the placement of an intrathecal pump for non-cancer pain should be made only after a careful risk:benefit analysis. Although a small, randomized, controlled, double-blind trial performed in 15 people receiving intrathecal morphine for noncancer pain found higher pain scores and a higher dropout rate in patients allocated to a 20% weekly dose reduction over 10 weeks compared to those whose dose was maintained, the rapid tapering and short-term follow-up limit generalizability.[125]

Factors that should be considered before instituting IDD systems for noncancer pain include a patient's age (younger people are at higher risk of tolerance and hyperalgesia), comorbidities, pain location, pain type and frequency, baseline opioid consumption, and the response to a drug trial. Intrathecal trials may either be single-shot or involve longer time periods of epidural or intrathecal drug administration. Whereas several day intrathecal drug trials have higher face validity, consensus guidelines are neutral regarding preference.[124] Patients with well-localized pain may be better candidates for IDD given the limited spread of intrathecal medications past the catheter tip, and in individuals with lower body pain, bupivacaine may added as an adjuvant.

Complications of IDD systems can be divided into those related to the procedure/device and those related to the medications infused. Procedure/device-related complications include wound dehiscence, skin erosion over the device, infection, bleeding, CSF leak, seroma or hygroma collection, pump malfunction, catheter kinks or shearing, and overdose from "pocket" fills. Opioid-related complications include androgen deficiency, decreased testosterone levels and hypogonadism with increased risk of bone mineral deficiency, peripheral edema with morphine and hydromorphone, pruritus, urinary retention, and formation of an intrathecal granuloma. Bupivacaine may cause sensorimotor deficits and urinary retention and clonidine may cause hypotension. Withdrawal from failure to refill the pump on time may occur with opioids, clonidine, and baclofen, with fatal outcomes reported from baclofen withdrawal.

Summary

Chronic pain is the leading reason people seek medical care, with untreated pain associated with higher rates of psychosocial dysfunction, poverty, substance abuse, and even lower life expectancy. The proper treatment of pain is a unique field of medicine that is considered by some to be an independent specialty of medicine. The practice of chronic pain medicine requires comprehensive knowledge of basic science, pharmacology, and psychology; the ability to interpret imaging and other diagnostic tests; and psychomotor skill to accurately and safely perform interventional procedures. Chronic pain medicine is interdisciplinary in nature, and the physician's primary training in anesthesiology, physical medicine and rehabilitation, neurology, or psychiatry is enhanced by further fellowship training in pain medicine.

For further review and interactivities, please see the videos and narrative interactive clinical vignettes (NICVs) accessible in the complimentary eBook bundled with this text. Access instructions are located on the inside front cover.

REFERENCES

1. Neumann S, Doubell TP, Leslie T, Woolf CJ. Inflammatory pain hypersensitivity mediated by phenotypic switch in myelinated primary sensory neurons. *Nature*. 1996;384(6607):360–364.
2. Cox JJ, Reimann F, Nicholas AK, et al. An SCN9A channelopathy causes congenital inability to experience pain. *Nature*. 2006;444(7121):894–898.
3. Caterina MJ, Schumacher MA, Tominaga M, Rosen TA, Levine JD, Julius D. The capsaicin receptor: a heat-activated ion channel in the pain pathway. *Nature*. 1997;389(6653):816–824.
4. Koivisto AP, Belvisi MG, Gaudet R, Szallasi A. Advances in TRP channel drug discovery: from target validation to clinical studies. *Nat Rev Drug Discov*. 2022;21(1):41–59.
5. Basbaum AI, Fields HL. The origin of descending pathways in the dorsolateral funiculus of the spinal cord of the cat and rat: further studies on the anatomy of pain modulation. *J Comp Neurol*. 1979;187(3):513–531.
6. Basbaum AI, Clanton CH, Fields HL. Three bulbospinal pathways from the rostral medulla of the cat: an autoradiographic study of pain modulating systems. *J Comp Neurol*. 1978;178(2):209–224.
7. Clark FM, Proudfit HK. The projection of noradrenergic neurons in the A7 catecholamine cell group to the spinal cord in the rat demonstrated by anterograde tracing combined with immunocytochemistry. *Brain Res*. 1991;547(2):279–288.
8. Woolf CJ. Evidence for a central component of post-injury pain hypersensitivity. *Nature*. 1983;306(5944):686–688.
9. Lai J, Gold MS, Kim C-S, et al. Inhibition of neuropathic pain by decreased expression of the tetrodotoxin-resistant sodium channel, NaV1.8. *Pain*. 2002;95(1):143–152.
10. Munro G, Dalby-Brown W. Kv7 (KCNQ) channel modulators and neuropathic pain. *J Med Chem*. 2007;50(11):2576–2582.
11. Denk F, McMahon SB, Tracey I. Pain vulnerability: a neurobiological perspective. *Nat Neurosci*. 2014;17(2):192–200.
12. Vaso A, Adahan HM, Gjika A, et al. Peripheral nervous system origin of phantom limb pain. *Pain*. 2014;155(7):1384–1391.
13. Haroutounian S, Ford AL, Frey K, et al. How central is central poststroke pain? The role of afferent input in poststroke neuropathic pain: a prospective, open-label pilot study. *Pain*. 2018;159(7):1317–1324.
14. Ji RR, Chamessian A, Zhang YQ. Pain regulation by non-neuronal cells and inflammation. *Science*. 2016;354(6312):572–577.
15. Knezevic NN, Candido KD, Vlaeyen JWS, Van Zundert J, Cohen SP. Low back pain. *Lancet*. 2021;398(10294):78–92.

16. Borenstein DG, O'Mara JW Jr, Boden SD, et al. The value of magnetic resonance imaging of the lumbar spine to predict low-back pain in asymptomatic subjects: a seven-year follow-up study. *J Bone Joint Surg Am*. 2001;83(9):1306–1311.
17. Cohen SP, Wenzell D, Hurley RW, et al. A double-blind, placebo-controlled, dose-response pilot study evaluating intradiscal etanercept in patients with chronic discogenic low back pain or lumbosacral radiculopathy. *Anesthesiology*. 2007;107(1):99–105.
18. Malik KM, Nelson A, Benzon H. Disease-modifying antirheumatic drugs for the treatment of low back pain: a systematic review of the literature. *Pain Pract*. 2016;16(5):629–641.
19. Shanthanna H, Gilron I, Rajarathinam M, et al. Benefits and safety of gabapentinoids in chronic low back pain: a systematic review and meta-analysis of randomized controlled trials. *PLoS Med*. 2017;14(8):e1002369.
20. Schukro RP, Oehmke MJ, Geroldinger A, Heinze G, Kress HG, Pramhas S. Efficacy of duloxetine in chronic low back pain with a neuropathic component: a randomized, double-blind, placebo-controlled crossover trial. *Anesthesiology*. 2016;124(1):150–158.
21. Manchikanti L, Knezevic E, Knezevic NN, et al. Epidural injections for lumbar radiculopathy or sciatica: a comparative systematic review and meta-analysis of Cochrane review. *Pain Physician*. 2021;24(5):E539–e554.
22. Benzon HT, Huntoon MA, Rathmell JP. Improving the safety of epidural steroid injections. *JAMA*. 2015;313(17):1713–1714.
23. Riew KD, Yin Y, Gilula L, et al. The effect of nerve-root injections on the need for operative treatment of lumbar radicular pain. A prospective, randomized, controlled, double-blind study. *J Bone Joint Surg Am*. 2000;82(11):1589–1593.
24. Kleimeyer JP, Koltsov JCB, Smuck MW, Wood KB, Cheng I, Hu SS. Cervical epidural steroid injections: incidence and determinants of subsequent surgery. *Spine J*. 2020;20(11):1729–1736.
25. Abdul AJ, Ghai B, Bansal D, Sachdeva N, Bhansali A, Dhatt SS. Hypothalamic pituitary adrenocortical axis suppression following a single epidural injection of methylprednisolone acetate. *Pain Physician*. 2017;20(7):E991–e1001.
26. Habib G, Jabbour A, Salman J, Hakim G, Haddad H. The effect of epidural methylprednisolone acetate injection on the hypothalamic-pituitary-adrenal axis. *J Clin Anesth*. 2013;25(8):629–633.
27. Stout A, Friedly J, Standaert CJ. Systemic absorption and side effects of locally injected glucocorticoids. *Pm r*. 2019;11(4):409–419.
28. Kerezoudis P, Rinaldo L, Alvi MA, et al. The effect of epidural steroid injections on bone mineral density and vertebral fracture risk: a systematic review and critical appraisal of current literature. *Pain Med*. 2018;19(3):569–579.
29. Ahadian FM, McGreevy K, Schulteis G. Lumbar transforaminal epidural dexamethasone: a prospective, randomized, double-blind, dose-response trial. *Reg Anesth Pain Med*. 2011;36(6):572–578.
30. Van Boxem K, Rijsdijk M, Hans G, et al. Safe use of epidural corticosteroid injections: recommendations of the WIP Benelux Work Group. *Pain Pract*. 2019;19(1):61–92.
31. Eworuke E, Crisafi L, Liao J, et al. Risk of serious spinal adverse events associated with epidural corticosteroid injections in the Medicare population. *Reg Anesth Pain Med*. 2021;46(3):203–209.
32. Benzon HT, Chew TL, McCarthy RJ, Benzon HA, Walega DR. Comparison of the particle sizes of different steroids and the effect of dilution: a review of the relative neurotoxicities of the steroids. *Anesthesiology*. 2007;106(2):331–338.
33. Kennedy DJ, Plastaras C, Casey E, et al. Comparative effectiveness of lumbar transforaminal epidural steroid injections with particulate versus nonparticulate corticosteroids for lumbar radicular pain due to intervertebral disc herniation: a prospective, randomized, double-blind trial. *Pain Med*. 2014;15(4):548–555.
34. Rathmell JP, Benzon HT, Dreyfuss P, et al. Safeguards to prevent neurologic complications after epidural steroid injections: consensus opinions from a multidisciplinary working group and national organizations. *Anesthesiology*. 2015;122(5):974–984.
35. Katz JN, Zimmerman ZE, Mass H, Makhni MC. Diagnosis and management of lumbar spinal stenosis: a review. *JAMA*. 2022;327(17):1688–1699.
36. Jensen RK, Harhangi BS, Huygen F, Koes B. Lumbar spinal stenosis. *BMJ*. 2021;373:n1581.
37. Campos WK, Linhares MN, Sarda J, et al. Predictors of pain recurrence after lumbar facet joint injections. *Front Neurosci*. 2019;13:958.
38. Ackerman WE, 3rd, Ahmad M. Pain relief with intraarticular or medial branch nerve blocks in patients with positive lumbar facet joint SPECT imaging: a 12-week outcome study. *South Med J*. 2008;101(9):931–934.
39. Cohen SP, Bhaskar A, Bhatia A, et al. Consensus practice guidelines on interventions for lumbar facet joint pain from a multispecialty, international working group. *Reg Anesth Pain Med*. 2020;45(6):424–467.
40. Hurley RW, Adams MCB, Barad M, et al. Consensus practice guidelines on interventions for cervical spine (facet) joint pain from a multispecialty international working group. *Reg Anesth Pain Med*. 2022;47(1):3–59.
41. van Wijk RM, Geurts JW, Wynne HJ, et al. Radiofrequency denervation of lumbar facet joints in the treatment of chronic low back pain: a randomized, double-blind, sham lesion-controlled trial. *Clin J Pain*. 2005;21(4):335–344.
42. Nath S, Nath CA, Pettersson K. Percutaneous lumbar zygapophysial (Facet) joint neurotomy using radiofrequency current, in the management of chronic low back pain: a randomized double-blind trial. *Spine (Phila Pa 1976)*. 2008;33(12):1291–1297; discussion 1298.
43. Engel A, Rappard G, King W, Kennedy DJ. The effectiveness and risks of fluoroscopically-guided cervical medial branch thermal radiofrequency neurotomy: a systematic review with comprehensive analysis of the published data. *Pain Med*. 2016;17(4):658–669.
44. Maas ET, Ostelo RW, Niemisto L, et al. Radiofrequency denervation for chronic low back pain. *Cochrane Database Syst Rev*. 2015;2015(10):Cd008572.
45. Cohen SP, Bicket MC, Kurihara C, et al. Fluoroscopically guided vs landmark-guided sacroiliac joint injections: a randomized controlled study. *Mayo Clin Proc*. 2019;94(4):628–642.
46. Luukkainen RK, Wennerstrand PV, Kautiainen HH, Sanila MT, Asikainen EL. Efficacy of periarticular corticosteroid treatment of the sacroiliac joint in non-spondylarthropathic patients with chronic low back pain in the region of the sacroiliac joint. *Clin Exp Rheumatol*. 2002;20(1):52–54.
47. Schmidt PC, Pino CA, Vorenkamp KE. Sacroiliac joint radiofrequency ablation with a multilesion probe: a case series of 60 patients. *Anesth Analg*. 2014;119(2):460–462.
48. Cohen SP, Hurley RW, Buckenmaier CC 3rd, Kurihara C, Morlando B, Dragovich A. Randomized placebo-controlled study evaluating lateral branch radiofrequency denervation for sacroiliac joint pain. *Anesthesiology*. 2008;109(2):279–288.
49. Benzon HT, Katz JA, Benzon HA, Iqbal MS. Piriformis syndrome: anatomic considerations, a new injection technique, and a review of the literature. *Anesthesiology*. 2003;98(6):1442–1448.
50. Fowler IM, Tucker AA, Weimerskirch BP, Moran TJ, Mendez RJ. A randomized comparison of the efficacy of 2 techniques for piriformis muscle injection: ultrasound-guided versus nerve stimulator with fluoroscopic guidance. *Reg Anesth Pain Med*. 2014;39(2):126–132.
51. Wolfe F, Clauw DJ, Fitzcharles MA, et al. 2016 Revisions to the 2010/2011 fibromyalgia diagnostic criteria. *Semin Arthritis Rheum*. 2016;46(3):319–329.
52. Arnold LM, Lu Y, Crofford LJ, et al. A double-blind, multicenter trial comparing duloxetine with placebo in the treatment of fibromyalgia patients with or without major depressive disorder. *Arthritis Rheum*. 2004;50(9):2974–2984.
53. McGirr A, Widenmaier R, Curran D, et al. The comparative efficacy and safety of herpes zoster vaccines: a network meta-analysis. *Vaccine*. 2019;37(22):2896–2909.
54. Gilron I, Bailey JM, Tu D, Holden RR, Jackson AC, Houlden RL. Nortriptyline and gabapentin, alone and in combination for neuropathic pain: a double-blind, randomised controlled crossover trial. *Lancet*. 2009;374(9697):1252–1261.
55. Rijsdijk M, van Wijck AJ, Meulenhoff PC, Kavelaars A, van der Tweel I, Kalkman CJ. No beneficial effect of intrathecal methylprednisolone acetate in postherpetic neuralgia patients. *Eur J Pain*. 2013;17(5):714–723.
56. Dworkin RH, O'Connor AB, Kent J, et al. Interventional management of neuropathic pain: NeuPSIG recommendations. *Pain*. 2013;154(11):2249–2261.
57. Dong DS, Yu X, Wan CF, et al. Efficacy of short-term spinal cord stimulation in acute/subacute zoster-related pain: a retrospective study. *Pain Physician*. 2017;20(5):E633–E645.
58. Huang J, Yang S, Yang J, et al. Early treatment with temporary spinal cord stimulation effectively prevents development of postherpetic neuralgia. *Pain Physician*. 2020;23(2):E219–E230.
59. Attal N, Cruccu G, Baron R, et al. EFNS guidelines on the pharmacological treatment of neuropathic pain: 2010 revision. *Eur J Neurol*. 2010;17(9):1113–e1188.
60. Dworkin RH, O'Connor AB, Audette J, et al. Recommendations for the pharmacological management of neuropathic pain: an overview and literature update. *Mayo Clin Proc*. 2010;85(3 Suppl):S3–14.
61. Sills S. Treatment of painful polyneuropathies of diabetic and other origins with 10 kHz SCS: a case series. *Postgrad Med*. 2020;132(4):352–357.
62. Abrams DI, Jay CA, Shade SB, et al. Cannabis in painful HIV-associated sensory neuropathy: a randomized placebo-controlled trial. *Neurology*. 2007;68(7):515–521.
63. Ellis RJ, Toperoff W, Vaida F, et al. Smoked medicinal cannabis for neuropathic pain in HIV: a randomized, crossover clinical trial. *Neuropsychopharmacology*. 2009;34(3):672–680.
64. McCormick Z, Chang-Chien G, Marshall B, Huang M, Harden RN. Phantom limb pain: a systematic neuroanatomical-based review of pharmacologic treatment. *Pain Med*. 2014;15(2):292–305.
65. Gilmore CA, Ilfeld BM, Rosenow JM, et al. Percutaneous 60-day peripheral nerve stimulation implant provides sustained relief of chronic pain following amputation: 12-month follow-up of a randomized, double-blind, placebo-controlled trial. *Reg Anesth Pain Med*. 2019;44:637–645
66. Harden NR, Bruehl S, Perez R, et al. Validation of proposed diagnostic criteria (the "Budapest Criteria") for complex regional pain syndrome. *Pain*. 2010;150(2):268–274.
67. Nicol AL, Hurley RW, Benzon HT. Alternatives to opioids in the pharmacologic management of chronic pain syndromes: a narrative review of randomized, controlled, and blinded clinical trials. *Anesth Analg*. 2017;125(5):1682–1703.
68. Benzon HT, Liu SS, Buvanendran A. Evolving definitions and pharmacologic management of complex regional pain syndrome. *Anesth Analg*. 2016;122(3):601–604.
69. Zhu X, Kohan LR, Morris JD, Hamill-Ruth RJ. Sympathetic blocks for complex regional pain syndrome: a survey of pain physicians. *Reg Anesth Pain Med*. 2019. rapm-2019-100418. Online ahead of print.
70. Yoo Y, Lee CS, Kim J, Jo D, Moon JY. Botulinum toxin type A for lumbar sympathetic ganglion block in complex regional pain syndrome: a randomized trial. *Anesthesiology*. 2022;136(2):314–325.
71. Kemler MA, de Vet HC, Barendse GA, van den Wildenberg FA, van Kleef M. Spinal cord stimulation for chronic reflex sympathetic dystrophy–five-year follow-up. *N Engl J Med*. 2006;354(22):2394–2396.

72. Urits I, Jones MR, Orhurhu V, et al. A comprehensive review of the celiac plexus block for the management of chronic abdominal pain. *Curr Pain Headache Rep.* 2020;24(8):42.
73. Kwon HJ, Jang K, Leem JG, Shin JW, Kim DH, Choi SS. Factors associated with successful response to neurolytic celiac plexus block in patients with upper abdominal cancer-related pain: a retrospective study. *Korean J Pain.* 2021;34(4):479–486.
74. Süleyman Ozyalçin N, Talu GK, Camlica H, Erdine S. Efficacy of coeliac plexus and splanchnic nerve blockades in body and tail located pancreatic cancer pain. *Eur J Pain.* 2004;8(6):539–545.
75. Mercadante S, Klepstad P, Kurita GP, Sjøgren P, Giarratano A. Sympathetic blocks for visceral cancer pain management: a systematic review and EAPC recommendations. *Crit Rev Oncol Hematol.* 2015;96(3):577–583.
76. Aman MM, Mahmoud A, Deer T, et al. The American Society of Pain and Neuroscience (ASPN) Best Practices and Guidelines for the interventional management of cancer-associated pain. *J Pain Res.* 2021;14:2139–2164.
77. Kroll CE, Schartz B, Gonzalez-Fernandez M, et al. Factors associated with outcome after superior hypogastric plexus neurolysis in cancer patients. *Clin J Pain.* 2014;30(1):55–62.
78. Le Clerc QC, Riant T, Levesque A, et al. Repeated ganglion Impar Block in a cohort of 83 patients with chronic pelvic and perineal pain. *Pain Physician.* 2017;20(6):E823–E828.
79. Okie S. A flood of opioids, a rising tide of deaths. *N Engl J Med.* 2010;363(21):1981–1985.
80. Brothers S, Viera A, Heimer R. Changes in methadone program practices and fatal methadone overdose rates in Connecticut during COVID-19. *J Subst Abuse Treat.* 2021;131:108449.
81. Rajan J, Scott-Warren J. The clinical use of methadone in cancer and chronic pain medicine. *BJA Education.* 2015;16(3):102–106.
82. Gomes T, Redelmeier DA, Juurlink DN, Dhalla IA, Camacho X, Mamdani MM. Opioid dose and risk of road trauma in Canada. *JAMA Intern. Med.* 2013;173(3):196.
83. Chou R, Turner JA, Devine EB, et al. The effectiveness and risks of long-term opioid therapy for chronic pain: a systematic review for a National Institutes of Health Pathways to Prevention Workshop. *Ann Intern Med.* 2015;162(4):276–286.
84. Abdel Shaheed C, Maher CG, Williams KA, Day R, McLachlan AJ. Efficacy, tolerability, and dose-dependent effects of opioid analgesics for low back pain: a systematic review and meta-analysis. *JAMA Intern Med.* 2016;176(7):958–968.
85. Dowell D, Haegerich TM, Chou R. CDC Guideline for prescribing opioids for chronic pain–United States, 2016. *JAMA.* 2016;315(15):1624–1645.
86. Goesling J, Henry MJ, Moser SE, et al. Symptoms of depression are associated with opioid use regardless of pain severity and physical functioning among treatment-seeking patients with chronic pain. *J Pain.* 2015;16(9):844–851.
87. Falk J, Thomas B, Kirkwood J, et al. PEER systematic review of randomized controlled trials: management of chronic neuropathic pain in primary care. *Can Fam Physician.* 2021;67(5): e130–e140.
88. Wiffen PJ, Derry S, Bell RF, et al. Gabapentin for chronic neuropathic pain in adults. *Cochrane Database Syst Rev.* 2017;6(6):Cd007938.
89. Gomes T, Juurlink DN, Antoniou T, Mamdani MM, Paterson JM, van den Brink W. Gabapentin, opioids, and the risk of opioid-related death: a population-based nested case-control study. *PLoS Med.* 2017;14(10):e1002396.
90. Migliorini F, Maffulli N, Eschweiler J, Knobe M, Tingart M, Colarossi G. Pharmacological management of fibromyalgia: a Bayesian network meta-analysis. *Expert Rev Clin Pharmacol.* 2022;15(2):205–214.
91. van der Sluiszen N, Vermeeren A, van Dijken JH, et al. Driving performance and neurocognitive skills of long-term users of sedating antidepressants. *Hum Psychopharmacol.* 2021;36(1):1–12.
92. Kennedy WR, Vanhove GF, Lu S-p, et al. A randomized, controlled, open-label study of the long-term effects of NGX-4010, a high-concentration capsaicin patch, on epidermal nerve fiber density and sensory function in healthy volunteers. *J Pain.* 2010;11(6):579–587.
93. Simpson DM, Gazda S, Brown S, et al. Long-term safety of NGX-4010, a high-concentration capsaicin patch, in patients with peripheral neuropathic pain. *J Pain Symptom Manage.* 2010;39(6):1053–1064.
94. Waldfogel JM, Nesbit SA, Dy SM, et al. Pharmacotherapy for diabetic peripheral neuropathy pain and quality of life: a systematic review. *Neurology.* 2017;88(20):1958–1967.
95. Aviram J, Samuelly G. Systematic review efficacy of cannabis-based medicines for pain management: a systematic review and meta-analysis of randomized controlled trials. *Pain physician.* 2017;20:E755–E796.
96. Narang S, Gibson D, Wasan AD, et al. Efficacy of dronabinol as an adjuvant treatment for chronic pain patients on opioid therapy. *J Pain.* 2008;9(3):254–264.
97. Issa MA, Narang S, Jamison RN, et al. The subjective psychoactive effects of oral dronabinol studied in a randomized, controlled crossover clinical trial for pain. *Clin J Pain.* 2014; 30(6):472–478.
98. Chen KY, Chen L, Mao J. Buprenorphine–naloxone therapy in pain management. *Anesthesiology.* 2014;120(5):1262–1274.
99. Veldman S, van Beek M, van Rijswijk S, et al. Effects of opioid rotation to buprenorphine/naloxone on pain, pain thresholds, pain tolerance, and quality of life in patients with chronic pain and opioid use disorder. *Pain.* 2022;163(5):955–963.
100. Benzon HT, Maus TP, Kang HR, et al. The use of contrast agents in interventional pain procedures: a multispecialty and multisociety practice advisory on nephrogenic systemic fibrosis, gadolinium deposition in the brain, encephalopathy after unintentional intrathecal gadolinium injection, and hypersensitivity reactions. *Anesth Analg.* 2021;133(2):535–552.
101. Pauza KJ, Howell S, Dreyfuss P, Peloza JH, Dawson K, Bogduk N. A randomized, placebo-controlled trial of intradiscal electrothermal therapy for the treatment of discogenic low back pain. *Spine J.* 2004;4(1):27–35.
102. Freeman BJC, Fraser RD, Cain CMJ, Hall DJ, Chapple DCL. A randomized, double-blind, controlled trial: intradiscal electrothermal therapy versus placebo for the treatment of chronic discogenic low back pain. *Spine.* 2005;30(21):2369–2377.
103. Kapural L, Vrooman B, Sarwar S, et al. A randomized, placebo-controlled trial of transdiscal radiofrequency, biacuplasty for treatment of discogenic lower back pain. *Pain Med.* 2013;14(3): 362–373.
104. Desai MJ, Kapural L, Petersohn JD, et al. A prospective, randomized, multicenter, open-label clinical trial comparing intradiscal biacuplasty to conventional medical management for discogenic lumbar back pain. *Spine.* 2016;41(13):1065–1074.
105. Fischgrund JS, Rhyne A, Franke J, et al. Intraosseous basivertebral nerve ablation for the treatment of chronic low back pain: 2-year results from a prospective randomized double-blind sham-controlled multicenter study. *Int J Spine Surg.* 2019;13(2):110–119.
106. Staats PS, Chafin TB, Golovac S, et al. Long-term safety and efficacy of minimally invasive lumbar decompression procedure for the treatment of lumbar spinal stenosis with neurogenic claudication: 2-year results of MiDAS ENCORE. *Reg Anesth Pain Med.* 2018;43(7): 789–794.
107. Deer TR, Costandi SJ, Washabaugh E, et al. The MOTION study: a randomized controlled trial with objective real-world outcomes for lumbar spinal stenosis patients treated with the mild® procedure: one-year results. *Pain Med.* 2022;23(4):625–634.
108. Kaufmann TJ, Trout AT, Kallmes DF. The effects of cement volume on clinical outcomes of percutaneous vertebroplasty. *AJNR Am J Neuroradiol.* 2006;27(9):1933–1937.
109. Buchbinder R, Osborne RH, Ebeling PR, et al. A Randomized trial of vertebroplasty for painful osteoporotic vertebral fractures. *N Engl J Med.* 2009;361(6):557–568.
110. Wardlaw D, Cummings SR, Van Meirhaeghe J, et al. Efficacy and safety of balloon kyphoplasty compared with non-surgical care for vertebral compression fracture (FREE): a randomised controlled trial. *Lancet North Am Ed.* 2009;373(9668):1016–1024.
111. Berenson J, Pflugmacher R, Jarzem P, et al. Balloon kyphoplasty versus non-surgical fracture management for treatment of painful vertebral body compression fractures in patients with cancer: a multicentre, randomised controlled trial. *Lancet Oncol.* 2011;12(3):225–235.
112. Wang B, Zhao CP, Song LX, Zhu L. Balloon kyphoplasty versus percutaneous vertebroplasty for osteoporotic vertebral compression fracture: a meta-analysis and systematic review. *J Orthop Surg Res.* 2018;13(1):264.
113. Knotkova H, Hamani C, Sivanesan E, et al. Neuromodulation for chronic pain. *Lancet.* 2021; 397(10289):2111–2124.
114. Duarte RV, Nevitt S, McNicol E, et al. Systematic review and meta-analysis of placebo/sham controlled randomised trials of spinal cord stimulation for neuropathic pain. *Pain.* 2020; 161(1):24–35.
115. Duarte RV, Nevitt S, Maden M, et al. Spinal cord stimulation for the management of painful diabetic neuropathy: a systematic review and meta-analysis of individual patient and aggregate data. *Pain.* 2021;162(11):2635–2643.
116. Vu TN, Khunsriraksakul C, Vorobeychik Y, et al. Association of spinal cord stimulator implantation with persistent opioid use in patients with postlaminectomy syndrome. *JAMA Netw Open.* 2022;5(1):e2145876.
117. Kirketeig T, Schultheis C, Zuidema X, Hunter CW, Deer T. Burst spinal cord stimulation: a clinical review. *Pain Med.* 2019;20(Suppl 1):S31–S40.
118. Mekhail N, Levy RM, Deer TR, et al. Long-term safety and efficacy of closed-loop spinal cord stimulation to treat chronic back and leg pain (Evoke): a double-blind, randomised, controlled trial. *Lancet Neurol.* 2020;19(2):123–134.
119. Kriek N, Groeneweg JG, Stronks DL, de Ridder D, Huygen FJ. Preferred frequencies and waveforms for spinal cord stimulation in patients with complex regional pain syndrome: a multicentre, double-blind, randomized and placebo-controlled crossover trial. *Eur J Pain.* 2017; 21(3):507–519.
120. Ubbink DT, Vermeulen H, Spincemaille GH, Gersbach PA, Berg P, Amann W. Systematic review and meta-analysis of controlled trials assessing spinal cord stimulation for inoperable critical leg ischaemia. *Br J Surg.* 2004;91(8):948–955.
121. Tsigaridas N, Naka K, Tsapogas P, Pelechas E, Damigos D. Spinal cord stimulation in refractory angina. A systematic review of randomized controlled trials. *Acta Cardiol.* 2015;70(2): 233–243.
122. Moisset X, Pereira B, Ciampi de Andrade D, Fontaine D, Lantéri-Minet M, Mawet J. Neuromodulation techniques for acute and preventive migraine treatment: a systematic review and meta-analysis of randomized controlled trials. *J Headache Pain.* 2020;21(1):142.
123. Deer TR, Levy RM, Kramer J, et al. Dorsal root ganglion stimulation yielded higher treatment success rate for complex regional pain syndrome and causalgia at 3 and 12 months: a randomized comparative trial. *Pain* 2017;158:669–681.
124. Deer TR, Pope JE, Hayek SM, et al. The Polyanalgesic Consensus Conference (PACC): recommendations on intrathecal drug infusion systems best practices and guidelines. *Neuromodulation.* 2017;20(2):96–132.
125. Raphael JH, Duarte RV, Southall JL, Nightingale P, Kitas GD. Randomised, double-blind controlled trial by dose reduction of implanted intrathecal morphine delivery in chronic non-cancer pain. *BMJ Open.* 2013;3(7).

57 Critical Care Medicine

MATTHEW R. HALLMAN

KEY POINTS

1 Simple and inexpensive interventions in the intensive care unit (ICU), such as the utilization of checklists, protocols, and care bundles can result in substantial improvements in patient outcomes.

2 The goal of resuscitation in brain injury is to prevent continuing cerebral insult after a primary injury has already occurred. This is accomplished by restoring cerebral blood flow, maintaining adequate cerebral perfusion pressure, reducing intracranial pressure, evacuating space occupying lesions, and avoiding fever, hyperglycemia, and hypoxia.

3 "Triple-H" therapy consisting of hypertension, hypervolemia, and hemodilution is no longer recommended for the treatment of cerebral vasospasm in subarachnoid hemorrhage. Instead, maintenance of euvolemia and a controlled stepwise trial of blood pressure augmentation in patients with suspected vasospasm are recommended.

4 Administration of thrombolytic therapy (rtPA) to patients presenting within 4.5 hours of onset of acute ischemic stroke results in improved neurologic outcome.

5 There are four general types of shock: hypovolemic, cardiogenic, distributive, and obstructive. The 28-day mortality for septic and cardiogenic shock, two of the most common types encountered in the ICU, are 20% to 40% and 70% to 80%, respectively.

6 In patients with septic shock, early and aggressive use of fluid resuscitation, appropriate antibiotics, infectious source control, and vasopressors/inotropes as needed improves survival.

7 Despite strong regional, local, and individual biases, there is little evidence to suggest that the mode of mechanical ventilation contributes significantly to any major outcome measure, and the choice of mode is largely one of clinician preference.

8 Separation from mechanical ventilation in patients who are recovering from respiratory failure is accelerated by respiratory therapy–driven protocols and daily trials of spontaneous breathing.

9 Ventilation with low tidal volume (6 mL/kg) in patients with acute lung injury and acute respiratory distress syndrome reduces mortality, compared to traditional tidal volumes (12 mL/kg).

10 Red blood cell transfusion in the ICU should be restricted (transfusion threshold hemoglobin <7 g/dL) with the possible exception of patients with active bleeding, early septic shock, acute myocardial infarction, unstable angina, or primary neurologic or neurosurgical problems.

11 Available evidence suggests that practices favoring light sedation, bolus administration versus continuous infusion of sedatives, and daily trials of awakening in ICU patients result in a variety of benefits, including a shortened duration of mechanical ventilation, decreased time in the ICU, and reduced mortality.

12 Delay in treatment of nosocomial infections is associated with increased mortality. Treatment should not be delayed pending diagnostic evaluation; rather treatment should be started after culture specimens are sent, and antibiotics then "de-escalated" after 48 to 72 hours to ensure adequate initial antibiotic treatment, but avoid long-term overuse of antibiotics.

13 End-of-life care is an important aspect of ICU care, and good communication between medical teams, patients, and their family members is required to ensure that delivered care is consistent with patient values and preferences. Patients at high risk of death or severely impaired functional recovery should be offered care focused on comfort and not just curative treatment. Palliative care can also be offered in conjunction with curative care.

Introduction

Anesthesiologists and Critical Care Medicine

Historically, Critical Care Medicine (CCM) evolved as a specialty nearly simultaneously in Europe and North America but has followed different models in regard to the involvement of anesthesiologists. The first intensive care unit (ICU) in Europe may have been located in Denmark in the 1950s, and concurrently the first critical care physician, or "intensivist," may well have been an anesthesiologist.[1] Anesthesiologists continued to play a defining role in the development of CCM in most of Europe, Australia, New Zealand, Japan, and elsewhere, and comprise the majority of intensivists in many countries around the world today. In North America, anesthesiologists were also integral to the development of CCM as a specialty. However, in contrast to other countries, in the United States anesthesiologists have played a smaller role in the specialty, and today comprise a minority of the intensivist workforce.[2]

Although it has been suggested that the first ICU in North America was established at Johns Hopkins in 1923 to care for postoperative neurosurgical patients, it was not until the late 1950s and early 1960s that true multidisciplinary ICUs began to appear. Anesthesiologists played a natural role in the evolution of ICUs, given their familiarity with surgical resuscitation and mechanical ventilation. Early on, however, the concept of "intensivists" did not exist, and patients were often managed by their primary physician (be it a surgeon or internist) and nurses, with formal or informal consultation given by specialists, including anesthesiologists.

In the early 1960s, the first CCM training program was established at the University of Pittsburgh under the direction of an anesthesiologist, Peter Safar, and the concept of "intensivist" was born. As defined by Dr. Safar, the qualities and qualifications of such an individual should include inquisitiveness, thoughtfulness, and a high level of motivation, action orientation, diplomacy, and scientific training. In the late 1960s, a group including Dr. Safar and another anesthesiologist, Ake Grenvik, were instrumental in inaugurating the Society of Critical Care Medicine (SCCM). Anesthesiologists working through SCCM were instrumental in developing the board certification process for CCM, and in 1986 the first CCM Certification examination was administered by the American Board of Anesthesiology.[3]

Anesthesiology and Critical Care Medicine: The Future

A significant shortage of intensivists exists currently and is projected to continue.[2,4] This is driven by substantial evidence that intensivists increase the quality of ICU care and improve patient outcomes, while at the same time the aging population is increasing. Anesthesiology as a specialty is ideally suited to help alleviate this shortage. Anesthesiologists are hospital-based, have sound fundamental training in physiology, pharmacology, invasive procedures, and monitoring, and have excellent historical and contemporary role models for the anesthesiologist as intensivist. While it seems certain that anesthesiologists will continue to play an important role in CCM worldwide, the current conditions in the United States are ideally suited for anesthesiologists wishing to pursue careers in CCM.

Critical Care Medicine: A Systems and Processes Approach

Critical care encompasses all disciplines of medicine. It is clearly beyond the scope of a single chapter to provide detailed coverage of all aspects of critical illness, including physiology, pathophysiology, and management of disease. In addition, many critical care issues are commonly encountered by anesthesiologists who practice solely in the operating room and are covered in detail elsewhere in this text. Thus, this chapter will focus on topics that are relatively unique to the ICU, but are widely applicable to the care of critically ill or injured patients. The entire chapter focuses on evidence-based practices that may improve both patient outcomes and healthcare system performance in the perioperative setting.

Grading of levels of evidence and practice guidelines in an effort to improve clinical care has become standard practice. Several different grading systems exist, with no clear evidence that one is superior to another. Furthermore, given uncertainty about the methodology of grading systems and their effects on patient outcomes,[5] we have chosen not to include "grades" or levels of evidence in this chapter.

Processes of Care in the ICU

There is increasing pressure in medicine to deliver high-quality care. With the passage of the Affordable Care Act (ACA) in 2010, the U.S. federal government provided a definition of high-quality care and sought, among other things, to link quality care and reimbursement.[6] The six components of quality care according to the ACA are timely, effective, efficient, patient centered, equitable, and safe care. This legislation is rapidly changing many aspects of healthcare delivery in the United States, and the ICU is no exception.[7]

A primary way to improve quality across a system is to reduce variability within the system. Processes of care are evidence-based organizational and individual practices and structures that seek to improve the quality of care delivered by standardizing some aspects of healthcare delivery. Although the number of potential process targets is nearly limitless, there are only a few that are widely agreed to improve the quality of care.

Staffing

As advances in medical and surgical therapeutics have increased the complexity of care for an aging and increasingly ill population of patients, it has become increasingly clear that the involvement of intensivists in the management of the critically ill patient is desirable.[8] While numerous studies have suggested that mortality and other intermediate end-points such as ICU length of stay, duration of mechanical ventilation, and cost can be reduced when "high-intensity" physician staffing models that mandate management or comanagement by intensivists are used, the level of involvement is less clear. For example, the benefit of in-house nighttime attending physician intensivist staffing compared to daytime only in-house attending physician staffing may be dependent on other factors, but a consistent benefit has not been found.[9,10] The best staffing model for a given ICU likely depends on many factors that are not yet fully understood.

Patient outcomes appear to be further improved by the addition of multidisciplinary providers to intensivist-led teams. Examples include pharmacist participation in daily rounds, as well as the inclusion of nurses, dieticians, and respiratory therapists. These practices significantly reduce costs and medication-related adverse events, and are also associated with decreased patient mortality.[11]

Checklists

1 Despite the improvement in communication and information transfer that occurs with multidisciplinary teams, the high stress

Table 57-1 Suggested Daily Intensive Care Unit Checklist

- Adequate sedation and analgesia
- Spontaneous awakening trial
- Spontaneous breathing trial
- Mobility goal
- Nutrition/diet ordered
- Deep-venous thrombosis prophylaxis initiated
- Glucose control adequate
- Unnecessary labs and imaging discontinued
- Antibiotics discontinued
- Foley catheter removed
- Central venous catheter and arterial line removed
- Patient and family update, goals of care reviewed
- Plan of the day reviewed

and massive volume of information in the ICU environment can lead to errors. Checklists have been widely implemented on ICU rounds as cognitive aides that serve as daily reminders to evaluate a limited number of interventions, preventative measures, bundles, and processes of care that can improve outcomes. Their implementation is associated with a decrease in mortality and ICU length of stay, and they cost virtually nothing.[12] It has been suggested that a checklist prompting consideration of potential interventions is more important than the specific interventions or protocols that are subsequently enacted, especially in ICUs with high-intensity staffing models.[13] Considering these potential benefits and the minimal economic investment required for checklist implementation, their use is strongly recommended. In fact, many of the care processes in this chapter commonly appear on checklists and should be considered with every patient, every day. Suggested content for consideration and inclusion in a daily ICU checklist is listed in Table 57-1. Content might be added or removed based on local ICU considerations.

Protocols and Care Bundles

The use of standardized protocols and care bundles has targeted improved timeliness and appropriateness of treatment for a variety of common ICU diagnoses, as well as prevention of common complications. For example, implementing a standardized order set for patients with septic shock may lower 28-day mortality.[14] Similarly, implementing a simple ventilator care bundle may reduce the incidence of ventilator-associated pneumonia (VAP) and antibiotic utilization.[15] Other studies have shown reduced rates of central line–associated bloodstream infections (CLABSIs) by implementing protocols and bundles.[16] An important additional benefit of utilizing standardized care processes is an improved ability to track outcomes and engage in quality assurance (QA) and quality improvement (QI) programs.

Resource Management

In 2014 the Critical Care Societies Collaborative (CCSC) released a list of "Five Things Physicians and Patients Should Question" in critical care as part of the Choosing Wisely initiative to reduce unnecessary interventions that lack cost-effectiveness. At the top of the CCM list is a recommendation to not order diagnostic studies (chest x-rays, blood gases, blood chemistries, cell counts, and electrocardiograms) at regular intervals (e.g., daily) without clear clinical indications. Compared with a practice of ordering tests only to answer clinical questions, or when doing so will affect management, the routine ordering of tests increases costs, does not benefit patients and may in fact harm them.[17] Additional recommendations including restrictive transfusion thresholds, avoiding oversedation and parenteral nutrition (PN) unless clearly indicated, and discussing end-of-life issues are addressed in other sections of this chapter. This type of effort to minimize unnecessary interventions recognizes both the financial impact such practice decisions have on individual patients and the healthcare system overall, as well as the physician's role in providing not just effective, but efficient care.

Neurologic and Neurosurgical Critical Care

Neuromonitoring

There are many neuromonitoring techniques with both intraoperative and ICU applicability. Electroencephalogram (EEG), evoked potential monitors, near-infrared spectroscopy (NIRS), brain tissue oxygenation ($PbrO_2$), cerebral microdialysis, intracranial pressure (ICP) monitoring, transcranial Doppler (TCD) ultrasonography, and jugular venous saturation (SjO_2) monitoring may all help in assessing pathophysiologic processes and adjusting therapy. These techniques are discussed in Chapters 26, 37, and 53, and will not be discussed in detail here.

Diagnosis and Clinical Management of the Most Common Types of Neurologic Failure

Traumatic Brain Injury

Traumatic brain injury (TBI) results in nearly 2.5 million emergency department visits annually in the United States, and TBI is a diagnosis in over 30% of traumatic injury-related deaths.[18] Prognosis following TBI remains challenging. The most powerful predictors of poor outcome include age >45 years, poor pupillary reactivity, low postresuscitation Glasgow Coma Scale (GCS) with the motor component being most predictive, and unfavorable intracranial diagnosis as established by radiologic features on computed tomography (CT). Additional factors including hypotension (systolic blood pressures [SBP] <90 mmHg), hypoxia, anemia (hemoglobin <11 g/dL), and hyperglycemia (blood glucose >1,800 mg/dL) are also associated with poor outcomes, but to a lesser extent.[19]

The GCS (see Chapter 53) is the most widely used clinical measure of injury severity in patients with TBI. The advantages of this scale are that it provides an objective method of measuring consciousness, it has high intra- and inter-rater reliability across observers with a wide variety of experience, and it has an excellent correlation with outcome.[20] However, the GCS is not measurable in patients who are sedated or neuromuscularly blocked at admission, and is less accurate when only the partial score is used. TBI qualifies as severe when the GCS is 8 or less.

Pupillary dilatation and light reactivity are also useful predictors of neurologic outcome after TBI. When both pupils are dilated and unreactive the odds ratio of poor neurologic outcome or death is three to five times greater than when both pupils are reactive.[19]

Hypotension is also a strong predictor of poor outcome in TBI. The 4th edition of the Brain Trauma Foundation's Guidelines for the Management of Traumatic Brain Injury recommends SBP be maintained above 100 mmHg for patients ages 50 to 69, and above 110 mmHg for those ages 15 to 49 and above age 70 years.[21] The recommendation is not based on high-quality evidence, but is a change from prior recommendations to keep the SBP above 90 mmHg and reflects a growing recognition that delayed cerebral ischemia (DCI) is one of the most important contributors to poor outcome.

Radiologic imaging is important in the diagnosis and prognosis of patients with TBI. A number of CT-based scoring systems have been developed and correlated with outcome, but the amount of midline shift, presence of subarachnoid blood, compression of the third ventricle basal cistern and diffuse axonal injury patterns portend worse outcomes, while epidural hematomas generally have better outcomes.[19] In addition, it should be noted that about one-third to one-half of TBI patients present with no imaging lesion at admission, but develop delayed lesions, which are associated with substantially worse neurologic outcome.

The goal of resuscitation in traumatic and other types of brain injury is to prevent continuing cerebral insult after a primary injury has already occurred. The extent of the primary cerebral injury is usually determined by the mechanism of the trauma and duration of cerebral ischemia. A primary insult is often associated with intracranial hypertension and systemic hypotension which lead to decreased cerebral perfusion and brain ischemia. Concomitant hypoxemia aggravates brain hypoxia—especially in the presence of hyperthermia and seizures—which increases brain metabolic demand. The combined effect of these factors lead to secondary brain injury characterized by excitotoxicity, oxidative stress, and inflammation. The resulting cerebral ischemia may be the single most important secondary event to affect outcome following a cerebral insult. Prevention of secondary injury is the main goal of resuscitative efforts.

2 Traumatized areas of the brain manifest impaired autoregulation and disruption of the blood–brain barrier (1 Video 57-1). If space-occupying lesions or edema are present, these will contribute to reduced brain compliance, leading to increased ICP and consequent reduction in cerebral blood flow (CBF). The rationale for attempting to optimize cerebral perfusion pressure (CPP) arises from the assumption that cerebral regions surrounding the primary lesion may be close to the ischemic threshold. Therefore, the goals of neuroresuscitation are to restore CBF by maintenance of adequate CPP, reduction of ICP, evacuation of space-occupying lesions, initiation of therapies for cerebral protection, and avoidance of hypoxia.

Unfortunately, the ICU treatment of TBI is hindered by a lack of rigorous, randomized, controlled trials to prove benefit for many of the management strategies utilized today. The Brain Trauma Foundation Guidelines for the Management of Severe Traumatic Brain Injury represent the most comprehensive set of recommendations, but it should be noted that these guidelines are continually evolving as new evidence becomes available.[22] General guidelines for management of patients with severe TBI appears in Table 57-2. Basic principles of acute anesthetic management in TBI, including osmotherapy, are discussed further in Chapter 53; sedation, hyperventilation, hypothermia, corticosteroids, antiseizure prophylaxis, and the role of decompressive surgical intervention are discussed in further detail here.

Sedation of neurologically impaired patients is typically achieved with short-acting sedatives to allow for frequent assessment by neurologic examination.[23] Although no studies have investigated the effect of sedation on outcome in such patients, a common practice is to provide sedation with propofol, benzodiazepines, or dexmedetomidine in patients following TBI. These agents have favorable effects on cerebral oxygen balance, although propofol is more potent in this regard. Undesirable effects of sedatives can lead to a reduction in CPP due to hemodynamic depression, or to an increase in CBF and a simultaneous increase in ICP.

Table 57-2 ICU Management of Patients with Severe Traumatic Brain Injury

Basic principles applied to all patients, assuming initial surgical management	• Head elevation 30–45 degrees[a] • CPP 60–70 Torr ▪ Euvolemia, vasopressors as needed ▪ ICP <20 Torr ▪ Mannitol, hypertonic saline ▪ CSF drainage • SaO_2 ≥95%; $PaCO_2$ 35–40 Torr • Temperature ≤37°C • Glucose ▪ <180 mg/dL • Sedation and analgesia • Early enteral nutrition • Seizure, stress ulcer, and DVT prophylaxis
Refractory intracranial hypertension	• Optimized hyperventilation with SjO_2 and/or $PbrO_2$ monitoring
Consider one or all of these interventions, depending on individual circumstances	• Barbiturate coma • Mild therapeutic hypothermia (33°–35°C) • Decompressive craniectomy

[a]Unless contraindicated by spine injury, hemodynamic instability, or otherwise.
ICU, intensive care unit; CPP, cerebral perfusion pressure; ICP, intracranial pressure; CSF, cerebrospinal fluid; SaO_2, arterial oxygen saturation; $PaCO_2$, arterial carbon dioxide tension; DVT, deep venous thrombosis; SjO_2, jugular venous oxygen saturation; $PbrO_2$, brain tissue oxygen tension.

Propofol rapidly penetrates the central nervous system and has rapid elimination kinetics. Despite the induction of systemic hypotension, propofol decreases cerebral metabolism resulting in a coupled decline in CBF, with a consequent decrease in ICP. Propofol's favorable pharmacologic and neurophysiologic profile has led to its widespread use in neurointensive care, and high-dose propofol has been advocated as a substitute for barbiturate therapy in patients with refractory intracranial hypertension. However, prolonged (>24 hours), high-dose (>80 μg/kg/min) propofol administration has been associated with lactic acidosis, cardiac failure, and death (propofol infusion syndrome) in children and adults with TBI.[24] Thus, the use of high-dose propofol to control refractory intracranial hypertension is not recommended, and barbiturates should be considered if ICP is not controlled by moderate doses of propofol.

The mechanisms by which barbiturates exert their cerebral protective effect appear to be mediated by a reduction in ICP via alteration in vascular tone, reduction of cerebral metabolic rate, and inhibition of free radical peroxidation. Although barbiturates are effective at reducing ICP, their routine use in TBI does not appear beneficial, and may in fact result in excess mortality in patients with diffuse brain injury.[25,26] This effect may in part relate to the profound cardiovascular depressant effects of barbiturates. However, high-dose barbiturate therapy may be considered in hemodynamically stable, severe TBI patients with intracranial hypertension refractory to maximal medical and surgical ICP-lowering therapy.[21,27] In some patients, pentobarbital may induce cerebral hypoxia by reducing CBF in excess of metabolism, and therefore SjO_2 monitoring may be considered during barbiturate therapy.

The centrally acting α_2-agonist dexmedetomidine has both sedative and analgesic effects. Its most desirable property is that it can allow for a more interactive and awake patient than other sedatives. (See section on Sedation, later.) Although it has not been studied specifically in brain-injured patients, it has been shown that CBF–cerebral metabolic rate of oxygen ($CMRO_2$) coupling remains intact in healthy volunteers during dexmedetomidine infusion.[28]

Hyperventilation effectively reduces ICP by reducing CBF, but the role hyperventilation should play in routine management of TBI is not clear. There are concerns that hyperventilation may lead to critically low CBF and worsen cerebral ischemia.[29] Based on the available evidence, prolonged or prophylactic hyperventilation should be avoided after severe TBI, especially in the first 24 hours after the injury. Hyperventilation may be necessary for brief periods to reduce intracranial hypertension refractory to sedation, osmotic therapy, and cerebrospinal fluid (CSF) drainage, and should be guided by SjO_2 and/or $PbrO_2$.[21] A marked fall in either of these values suggests a harmful effect of hyperventilation, and that it should be reduced or discontinued.

Experimentally, hypothermia causes a reduction in cerebral metabolism by decreasing all cell functions related to neuronal electric activity and those responsible for cellular integrity. In addition, mild hypothermia has been shown to decrease the release of substrates associated with tissue injury such as glutamate and aspartate. However, numerous randomized trials of therapeutic mild hypothermia (33° to 35°C) in patients with TBI published over two decades and enrolling more than 1,000 total patients have failed to demonstrate a mortality benefit or improvement in neurologic outcome with hypothermia. In addition, a recent randomized, controlled trial of induced mild hypothermia for the treatment of refractory high ICP found worse outcomes at 6 months in the group treated with hypothermia.[30] Thus, induction of mild hypothermia in patients with TBI, either prophylactically or to treat high ICP, cannot be recommended.[21] Corticosteroids to reduce posttraumatic inflammatory injury in TBI were advocated for 30 years or more, but without convincing evidence of benefit. The Corticosteroid Randomization after Significant Head Injury (CRASH) study, published in 2004, prospectively randomized over 10,000 patients presenting with acute TBI to receive high-dose methylprednisolone or placebo for 48 hours after hospital admission.[31] Methylprednisolone administration was associated with an approximately 20% increase in the relative risk of death at 2 weeks in the entire cohort, and this detriment was evident across subgroups divided by severity and type of injury. Thus, high-dose corticosteroids should not be administered as therapy for acute TBI. Likewise, intravenous magnesium administration did not improve outcomes in patients with TBI, and might even have a negative effect in the treatment of significant brain injury.[32]

Anticonvulsants are effective at preventing early posttraumatic seizures within 7 days following TBI. However, the evidence does not indicate that prevention of early seizures improves outcome following TBI.[33] Seizures should therefore be treated on an as-needed basis, and prophylactic use of antiepileptic medications is typically not continued for more than 7 days.

Finally, it should be noted that use of albumin as fluid replacement therapy in patients with TBI has been associated with increased mortality in a subgroup analysis of a randomized controlled trial comparing saline and albumin.[34] Albumin appears to increase cerebral edema, possibly due to the hypoosmolar constitution of the specific albumin product used in this study, and the high oncotic pressure of albumin leaking from damaged blood vessels into surrounding parenchyma.

An additional third-tier therapy to control refractory elevated ICP is decompressive craniectomy (DC). While one large randomized trial of decompressive craniotomy for refractory high ICP in TBI showed worse outcomes in the craniectomy group, another large randomized trial of the same intervention with inclusion criteria that included a more sustained ICP elevation showed a survival benefit with craniectomy.[35,36] Current guidelines suggest that DC is a reasonable intervention in appropriately selected patients, but the benefit can be difficult to predict.

Subarachnoid Hemorrhage

The incidence of subarachnoid hemorrhage (SAH) in the United States varies from 7.5 to 12.1 cases per 100,000 of population. The rupture of an intracranial aneurysm most commonly causes SAH. Other causes of SAH include trauma, vertebral and carotid artery dissection, dural and spinal arteriovenous malformations, mycotic aneurysms, sickle cell disease, cocaine abuse, coagulation disorders, and pituitary apoplexy. Aneurysmal SAH is associated with considerable morbidity and mortality, with one-third of SAH patients dead before receiving medical attention, and only one-third of patients being functional survivors.[37] The leading causes of death and disability are the direct effect of the initial bleed, cerebral vasospasm with resulting stroke, and rebleeding. Although the number of early deaths may not have changed substantially, the overall case fatality rate of aneurysmal SAH has fallen over time, and is reported in the 40% to 50% range in most studies.[38,39] Approximately 40% to 50% of survivors have good neurologic outcome after SAH, as measured by the modified Rankin scale.[38] Severity of the initial bleed is the most important determinant of SAH outcome.

At the time of aneurysm rupture, a large hemorrhage results in a critical reduction in CBF due to an increase in ICP toward arterial diastolic values. The persistence of a no-flow pattern is associated with acute vasospasm and swelling of perivascular astrocytes, neuronal cells, and capillary endothelia. After SAH, injury to the posterior hypothalamus may stimulate release of norepinephrine from the adrenal medulla and sympathetic cardiac efferent nerves. The release of norepinephrine has been associated with ischemic changes in the subendocardium (neurogenic stunned myocardium or stress cardiomyopathy), cardiac dysrhythmias, and pulmonary edema.[40]

In survivors of the initial bleed, management emphasizes the prevention of DCI and early aneurysm control with either surgery or interventional neuroradiology (coiling). Approximately 10% to 23% of unsecured aneurysms will rebleed in the first 2 weeks, with approximately 6% occurring within the first 24 hours after the initial hemorrhage. Rebleeding is associated with a mortality rate of over 50%.[41] Early aneurysm occlusion substantially reduces the risk of this complication, and it is recommended that aneurysms be secured as early as possible and within 24 hours of rupture.[37]

With the improvement of the operative management, delayed neurologic deterioration due to cerebral vasospasm and DCI, cerebral edema, hydrocephalus, and the effects of fever and electrolyte abnormalities—has become an increasingly important cause of death and disability. In addition, patients can develop a number of medical problems related to either the SAH or associated critical illness.

Cerebral vasospasm after SAH is identified by angiography in up to 60% of patients, and is correlated with the amount and location of subarachnoid blood. A subsequent reduction in CBF is ultimately responsible for the appearance of DCI, which occurs in approximately one-third of patients suffering from SAH. DCI typically presents as altered consciousness and/or transient focal neurologic deficits beyond the first 3 days after aneurysm rupture, typically peaks in 7 to 10 days, and resolves over 10 to 14 days. If severe, vasospasm can result in cerebral infarction and persistent neurologic deficits, which contribute to considerable long-term morbidity.

TCD has been used to identify and quantify cerebral vasospasm on the basis that blood flow velocity increases as the diameter of the vessel decreases. Changes in measured velocities over time may be more reliable than absolute values in predicting symptomatic vasospasm, but there is poor correlation between TCD velocities and angiographic findings, especially for the posterior circulation.

Oral nimodipine (60 mg every 4 hours for 21 days) is recognized as an effective treatment to improve neurologic outcome (reduction of cerebral infarction and poor functional outcome) and mortality in SAH patients with vasospasm.[42,43] Because angiographic studies do not demonstrate a difference in the frequency of vasospasm compared with a placebo-treated group, the benefits of nimodipine have been attributed to a cytoprotective effect related to the reduced availability of intracellular calcium and improved microvascular collateral flow. Cilostazol, a phosphodiesterase inhibitor with vasodilatory and antiplatelet effects, is the only other pharmacologic therapy to have demonstrated improvements in long-term disability, but its use is currently not included in SAH guidelines. Other pharmacologic therapies to prevent or treat cerebral vasospasm including magnesium, nicardipine, fasudil (a rho kinase inhibitor and vasodilator) and clazosentan (a selective endothelin A receptor blocker) have shown the ability to reduce vasospasm and DCI, but have not been shown to improve disability or mortality. Although earlier studies suggested that statins may have a protective effect in preventing cerebral vasospasm and DCI, subsequent randomized trials have not substantiated this finding.

3 Hypervolemia, hypertension, and hemodilution (triple-H) therapy is historically one of the mainstays of prevention and treatment of cerebral ischemia associated with SAH-induced vasospasm, despite the lack of strong evidence for its effectiveness, especially for prophylactic use.[44] Triple-H therapy evolved from the observed association of hypovolemia with poor outcomes after SAH, CBF dysregulation, and the beneficial rheologic effects of anemia on CBF. However, current consensus guidelines recommend modification of this strategy to include maintenance of euvolemia, avoidance of intentional hemodilution, and a controlled trial of stepwise blood pressure augmentation in patients with suspected DCI.[37] In addition, discontinuation of nimodipine is recommended if its administration results in hypotension. Careful monitoring for cardiopulmonary complications of hemodynamic therapy is recommended.

Interventional neuroradiology with the use of balloon angioplasty can reverse or improve vasospasm-induced neurologic deficits if initiated early after the development of ischemic symptoms. Although observational data suggest a beneficial effect of angioplasty on long-term outcomes, these findings have not been confirmed in randomized, controlled trials, and the risks of angioplasty include intimal dissection, vessel rupture, ischemia, and infarction. Current guidelines recommend consideration of angioplasty in patients with symptomatic vasospasm who have failed medical management.

Hydrocephalus is another cause of neurologic dysfunction after SAH, occurring in 25% of patients surviving the hemorrhage. The presence of blood in the ventricular system obstructs ventricular drainage and CSF absorption sites (subarachnoid villi). Ventricular drainage is usually successful in improving neurologic symptoms due to hydrocephalus. A minority of patients will require a permanent ventriculoperitoneal shunt. Seizures also occur in 13% of patients with SAH, and are more common in patients with a neurologic deficit; thus, prophylactic anticonvulsant therapy may be considered in the immediate posthemorrhage period, but long-term use is not supported.[37]

Hyponatremia occurs in 10% to 34% of patients after SAH. Hyponatremia usually develops several days after the hemorrhage and is attributed to two main causes: (1) a syndrome of inappropriate antidiuretic hormone (SIADH), which is associated with euvolemia or mild hypervolemia and an excess of free water, or (2) cerebral "salt wasting" with depletion of sodium and water. The differentiation of these two entities is difficult but important, because SIADH is treated by free-water restriction, whereas cerebral salt wasting is treated with volume repletion and sodium administration. Thus, assessment of intravascular volume status is a key component when deciding on the treatment regimen for hyponatremia associated with SAH. Urine electrolyte analysis is not discriminative, as urine sodium is high in both disorders, particularly in association with intravenous saline administration.

Other medical complications are relatively common after SAH and include pneumonia, neurogenic pulmonary edema and acute lung injury (ALI), stress (Takotsubo) cardiomyopathy, sepsis, and venous thromboembolism (VTE). Fever is highly prevalent after SAH and is associated with poor outcomes. Although fever is often due to noninfectious causes after SAH, a rigorous search for infection is necessary. Fever control is recommended during the risk period for DCI, particularly in high-risk patients.

Acute Ischemic Stroke

Although the incidence of stroke has declined over the past few decades, stroke affects nearly 800,000 people annually, and was the fifth leading cause of death in the United States as of 2013.[49] Nearly 90% of strokes can be attributed to an ischemic mechanism such as atherosclerosis, thrombosis, cardioembolism, or hypotension. Other major causes of stroke are intracerebral and subarachnoid hemorrhage. Unusual causes of stroke such as carotid artery dissection, hypercoagulation syndromes, or infective endocarditis should be considered in younger patients without traditional risk factors for stroke. Transient ischemic attacks may precede stroke and should be considered as a warning sign. The prognosis after stroke varies depending on the size and location of the lesion. In patients with acute ischemic stroke, the duration of coma appears to be the most important predictor of outcome and successful therapy.

Rapid clot lysis and restoration of circulation via systemic 4 thrombolysis limit the extent of brain injury and improve outcome after thrombotic stroke. American Heart Association/American Stroke Association (AHA/ASA) guidelines recommend systemic thrombolysis using intravenous alteplase or tenecteplase to patients presenting with acute ischemic stroke within 3 hours of symptom onset (barring contraindications), and up to 4.5 hours after symptom onset in select individuals.[45,46]

Accumulating evidence suggests that mechanical thrombectomy as an adjunct to systemic thrombolysis offers additional outcome benefits to select patients with ischemic stroke. Thus, the AHA/ASA guidelines recommend stent retrieval of clot in patients who have received intravenous fibrinolytics within 4.5 hours of symptom onset if they have evidence of internal carotid or proximal middle cerebral artery (MCA) occlusion, and treatment can be initiated within 6 hours of symptom onset.[47] In addition, mechanical thrombectomy may be considered up to 24 hours from symptom onset in selected patients with a poor examination and imaging showing an anterior circulation stroke with a small ischemic core but large penumbra.[48,49]

Neither unfractionated nor low–molecular-weight heparin has been shown to prevent progression or reduce the rate of stroke recurrence when administered within 48 hours of the acute event, and therefore are not recommended. In general, heparin is only recommended for early secondary prophylaxis in patients with suspected cardiac embolism. Aspirin 325 mg has been shown to reduce the risk of early recurrent ischemic stroke. It is recommended within 24 to 48 hours of stroke onset in most patients, but it does increase the risk of hemorrhagic stroke. The frequency of deep venous thrombosis (DVT) in acute stroke is reduced by anticoagulants (e.g., low–molecular-weight heparin), but not by antiplatelet agents. However, it is unclear if the frequency of pulmonary embolism is also reduced.

The majority of patients with acute ischemic stroke present with severe arterial hypertension. In theory, permissive hypertension should be allowed after stroke because reduction of the CPP could compromise the viable brain surrounding the ischemic region (ischemic penumbra), although high-level evidence to support this recommendation is lacking. However, severe hypertension (blood pressure >220/120 mmHg) should be controlled because of increased risk of hemorrhagic transformation; a lower threshold is indicated after alteplase administration (blood pressure <185/110). If the stroke is accompanied by raised ICP due to cerebral edema, the principles of treatment of raised ICP discussed earlier for TBI similarly apply. Cytotoxic brain edema usually occurs 24 to 96 hours after acute ischemic stroke, and osmotherapy constitutes the basis of ICP reduction with possible hemicraniectomy in select patients (see later). Steroids are of no value in the treatment of ischemic stroke, and although some have advocated therapeutic hypothermia, there is insufficient evidence to recommend this approach in stroke outside of research settings. As with SAH, fever is associated with poor outcome after ischemic stroke, and close temperature monitoring and management are recommended. Hyperglycemia is also associated with poor outcome in ischemic stroke, and it is recommended to monitor and maintain blood glucose within the range of 140 to 180 mg/dL.[45]

Hemispheric MCA infarction with subsequent cerebral edema, increased ICP, and herniation (malignant MCA syndrome) is often fatal. Randomized trials demonstrated that hemicraniectomy improves survival in this setting.[50] However, this benefit may come at the expense of increased and often severe disability in survivors. This seems particularly true for patients greater than 60 years of age. Cerebellar infarction can likewise result in fatal brainstem compression due to local edema. Case series suggest that suboccipital craniectomy can be life-saving in this situation, and that patients can recover with acceptable functional outcomes.[51]

Anoxic Brain Injury

Anoxic brain injury most commonly occurs as a result of cardiac arrest, either in- or out-of-hospital. Of patients who survive their initial cardiac arrest, in-hospital mortality ranges from approximately 50% to 90%, and a high percentage of survivors suffer brain injury with significant long-term disability. The pathophysiology of anoxic brain injury is multifactorial, and includes excitatory neurotransmitter release, accumulation of intracellular calcium, and oxygen free radical generation. Unfortunately, pharmacologic therapies aimed at several of these pathways, including barbiturates, benzodiazepines, corticosteroids, calcium channel antagonists, and free radical scavengers have failed to improve the outcome of anoxic brain injury.

Mild therapeutic hypothermia (target temperature 33°C) has been widely applied to unconscious patients who survive initial resuscitation from cardiac arrest due to the belief it is neuroprotective. However, recent, well-conducted studies and meta-analyses have failed to show consistent benefit to this practice.[52] Instead, current guidelines suggest strict fever control with a target temperature of <37.5°C. For patients who are mildly hypothermic without intervention in the post-arrest period, they should not be actively rewarmed. This approach appears to result in similar neurologic outcomes and may reduce infectious and bleeding complications.[53]

Cardiovascular and Hemodynamic Aspects of Critical Care

Types of Shock

One of the most common and urgent requirements for critical care is the presence of shock. Shock is a state characterized by tissue oxygen delivery that is inadequate to meet demand. Often this is associated with circulatory instability and severe systemic hypotension. Shock states are commonly classified according to the primary cause of circulatory failure. Distributive (sometimes called vasodilatory) shock results from a reduction in systemic vascular resistance (SVR), often associated with an increased cardiac output (CO) as may happen in sepsis, anaphylaxis, or spinal cord injury. Cardiogenic shock results from left or right (or both) heart failure and is characterized by low CO and increased SVR. Hypovolemic shock is also associated with low CO and increased peripheral resistance, most commonly due to hemorrhage. Obstructive shock is characterized by an obstruction to forward flow such as may happen with a tension pneumothorax, pericardial tamponade, or pulmonary embolism. The most common form of shock encountered in the ICU depends on the type of ICU, but septic, cardiogenic, and hypovolemic shock are all common. Shock of all kinds is highly morbid and despite extensive research and aggressive management, the mortality from shock remains staggeringly high. Approximately 35% to 40% of patients die within 28 days of the onset of septic shock, and the mortality rate is 70% to 80% for patients with cardiogenic shock. The mortality from hypovolemic shock is highly variable and depends upon the etiology and the rapidity of recognition and treatment. Mortality from septic shock may be improving, as evidenced by the fact that control-group mortality in sepsis trials has decreased from 46% to approximately 20% between 2001[54] and 2014,[55–57] although this may reflect broader screening and inclusion of less sick patients than in past trials. Cardiogenic and septic shock are discussed in more detail in the following section, whereas the causes and treatment of hypovolemic and obstructive shock are discussed in Chapters 39 and 53. 5

Cardiogenic Shock

The hallmark of cardiogenic shock is primary pump failure, which itself may be caused by extensive myocardial infarction (MI), nonischemic cardiomyopathy, dysrhythmia, or mechanical complication (e.g., mitral regurgitation, ventricular septal defect). The pathophysiologic characteristics include a reduction in contractility, usually accompanied by dilatation of cardiac cavities and venous congestion. Determining the etiology of cardiogenic shock is of utmost importance because the treatment varies considerably based on the underlying mechanism. For example, the role of β-blockers in the management of nonischemic decompensated heart failure has evolved to be of increasing importance[58] and diuresis is frequently indicated, whereas in acute ischemic ST elevation MI (STEMI) β-blockers are critical and there is little role for acute diuresis. In addition to a thorough history and detailed physical exam, a chest radiograph (CXR), basic metabolic profile, complete blood count, 12-lead electrocardiogram (ECG), serum troponin measurements, B-type natriuretic peptide levels, and echocardiography should be obtained in all patients presenting with heart failure and are helpful in differentiating between the various etiologies.[59]

The onset of pump failure is associated with two compensatory mechanisms: a reflex vasoconstriction in systemic vessels causing an increase in left ventricle (LV) workload and myocardial oxygen demand, and a redistribution of blood volume toward the heart and the lungs.

Several studies have demonstrated that the incidence and severity of LV failure complicating acute MI are directly related to the extent of ventricular muscle necrosis. Consequently, therapy should minimize myocardial oxygen demand and raise oxygen delivery to the ischemic area. This goal is complicated by the fact that many resuscitative approaches to correct hypotension increase myocardial oxygen consumption (e.g., preload augmentation, inotropes, and vasopressors, as discussed later). In patients without hypotension, pharmacologic vasodilatation using nitroglycerin or sodium nitroprusside may reduce myocardial oxygen consumption and improve ventricular ejection by reducing LV afterload, and may also produce a shift of blood from the lungs to the periphery by reducing venous tone. Synthetic B-type natriuretic peptide (nesiritide) and dopamine agonists such as fenoldopam have similar effects, but have shown inconsistent benefit in large, randomized trials and are not recommended for routine management.[60,61] When pharmacologic interventions are not sufficient to restore hemodynamic stability, the use of mechanical support with the insertion of intra-aortic balloon pump counterpulsation and ventricular assist devices can help unload the ventricles (see Chapter 39).

In patients with MI, coronary reperfusion can be achieved with systemic thrombolysis or, preferably, primary percutaneous coronary intervention (PCI). The AHA/American College of Cardiology guidelines recommend treatment of STEMI by PCI within 90 minutes of presentation to PCI-capable centers, by thrombolytic therapy within 30 minutes of presentation to non–PCI-capable centers, or by rapid transfer under certain conditions of favorable timing.[62] Guidelines clearly favor PCI over fibrinolysis when both are feasible within the appropriate time frame. For patients with ischemia and cardiogenic shock, the addition of temporary mechanical support including intra-aortic balloon counterpulsation, intravascular microaxial LV assist devices, or venoarterial extra corporeal membrane oxygenation (VA-ECMO) may provide some benefit, but data on the use of LV assist devices (LVADs) in the setting of acute ischemic cardiogenic shock are limited.[63,64] These may be effective devices to bridge patients in shock until recovery or transplant.[65]

Management of cardiac failure related to specific valvular abnormalities is discussed in Chapter 39.

Septic Shock

Septic shock is a form of distributive shock associated with infection and the activation of the systemic inflammatory response (NICV 57-1). It is usually characterized by a high CO, low SVR, hypotension, and regional blood flow redistribution that result in tissue hypoperfusion. Other noninfectious causes of distributive shock include acute spinal cord injury, pancreatitis, burns, fulminant hepatic failure, multiple traumatic injuries, toxic shock syndrome, anaphylactic and anaphylactoid reactions, and drug or toxin reactions, including insect bites, transfusion reactions, and heavy metal poisoning. Septic shock is the most common shock syndrome, accounting for roughly two-thirds of shock patients in broad critical care populations.[66] Severe sepsis and septic shock account for at least 10% of ICU admissions, and septic shock is more common in the very young and very old, in men than in women, and in black patients than in white patients.

The definitions of sepsis and septic shock have evolved over time, but remain predicated on an underlying infectious cause of physiologic dysregulation (Table 57-3).

The initiating event in septic shock appears to be the interaction between organism-specific ligands on pathogens and ligand-specific receptors (e.g., toll-like receptors, nucleotide-binding oligomerization domain–like receptors, and others) on cells of the innate immune system. The resulting release of immune mediators sets in motion a complex series of events that results in altered gene expression, T-cell differentiation, complement activation, elaboration of procoagulant processes, and the production and release of other immunomodulatory cytokines. Together, these events produce the septic phenotype (e.g., microthrombi, endothelial dysfunction, capillary leak, vasodilatation, effective hypovolemia, hypoperfusion, and organ failure).[66]

Table 57-3 Definitions of Sepsis and Septic Shock

Sepsis: Life-threatening organ dysfunction caused by a dysregulated host-response to infection
An acute increase in the Sequential Organ Failure Assessment (SOFA) score ≥ 2 points as a result of infection
The full SOFA score includes assessment of PaO_2:FiO_2, bilirubin, urine output or serum creatine, hypotension, platelet count, and Glascow Coma Score[214]
A baseline SOFA of zero can be assumed in patients without known pre-existing organ dysfunction
Septic Shock: Persistent requirement for vasopressors to maintain MAP > 65 mmHg and serum lactate >2 mmol/L despite adequate intravascular volume resuscitation
Additional findings suggestive of possible infection:
Core temperature <36°C or >38°C
Tachycardia >90 beats/min
Tachypnea >22 breaths/min while breathing spontaneously
Hypotension: Systolic Blood Pressure <100 mmHg
Altered mental status
Hyperglycemia: serum glucose >140 mg/dL in the absence of diabetes
Plasma C reactive protein > two standard deviations above normal
Coagulopathy: International Normalized Ratio >1.5
Multiple Organ Dysfunction Syndrome: Presence of several altered organ functions in an acutely ill patient such that homeostasis cannot be maintained without intervention

Although the calculated CO often increases, and echocardiography often shows hyperdynamic LV function in early sepsis, this may be secondary to the decrease in SVR that is a hallmark of septic shock. LV contractility itself is depressed in many patients. A global decrease in cardiac contractility, combined with relative hypovolemia, may reduce oxygen delivery to tissues. Even in the case of normal or seemingly adequate CO and oxygen delivery, metabolic needs are increased during sepsis, and the ability of the tissues to extract and utilize oxygen may be impaired. Thus, a metabolic acidosis may be present despite normal levels of oxygen transport. A decrease in cellular oxygen extraction capacity may result from factors other than hypoperfusion, such as direct cellular damage by toxins and/or mediators or maldistribution of blood flow. The impact of impaired perfusion on organ function depends on individual susceptibility to hypoxia. Though hypoperfusion is the suspected cause of lactic acidosis in sepsis, various degrees of intermediary metabolic alterations may contribute to the increased lactate production independent of perfusion, or when tissue oxygen tension is normal.

The hallmark of treatment of septic shock includes early antimicrobial therapy and source control, restoration of organ perfusion by augmenting circulating volume, stroke volume, and/or oxygen carrying capacity, and the management of the expected consequences of sepsis, organ failure, and critical care (e.g., infections, acute kidney injury [AKI], and VTE) (NICV 57-2). These have been thoroughly investigated and discussed in the Surviving Sepsis Campaign Guidelines (summarized in Table 57-4), which provide an excellent review of the evidence for various components of therapy.[67]

Table 57-4 Management of Sepsis and Septic Shock

- Initiation of early goal–directed resuscitation should begin as soon as sepsis is suspected
- Obtain cultures to identify causative organisms before starting antibiotic therapy, and obtain imaging studies promptly to identify potential sources of infection
- Administer empiric broad-spectrum antibiotics within 1 hr of sepsis diagnosis, and reassess appropriateness of antimicrobial therapy upon availability of microbiology results
- Avoid using procalcitonin levels to decide when to start antimicrobial therapy, but procalcitonin levels may help in deciding when to stop antimicrobial therapy
- Search for and control infection sources promptly
- Use balanced crystalloids as initial fluid resuscitation with consideration given to adding albumin when large volumes of crystalloid are required
- Do not use hetastarch formulations
- Use an initial fluid resuscitation volume of at least 30 mL/kg in the first 3 hours with additional fluid challenges continuing as long as there is hemodynamic improvement as assessed by either static or dynamic assessment methods
- Serum lactate levels should be followed serially to aid in assessing the adequacy of resuscitation
- Norepinephrine is the preferred first-line vasopressor for a target MAP ≥ 65 mmHg
- Vasopressin may be added at a fixed rate as an adjunct to norepinephrine, but should not be used alone. The addition of vasopressin is recommended instead of further norepinephrine dose escalation when the norepinephrine dose reaches 0.25–0.5 μg/kg/min
- Epinephrine may be added when hypotension persists despite norepinephrine and vasopressin therapy
- Use of dopamine is recommended only in highly selected circumstances and should generally be avoided
- Consider adding dobutamine to norepinephrine or using epinephrine alone in low cardiac output states that persist despite adequate fluid resuscitation
- Levosimendan and terlipressin are not recommended
- Targeting supranormal values of oxygen delivery is not recommended
- Intravenous corticosteroids are recommended if shock persists despite adequate volume resuscitation and vasopressor therapy
- Target a hemoglobin of 7–9 g/dL in the absence of tissue hypoperfusion, coronary artery disease, or acute hemorrhage
- For mechanically ventilated patients with ARDS, use low tidal volume (6 cc/kg) ventilation, limit inspiratory plateau pressure to ≤30 cmH_2O, and apply positive end-expiratory pressure
- For patients with moderate-to-severe sepsis-induced ARDS, prone positioning for at least 12 hrs per day is recommended
- Neuromuscular blockade should be used to facilitate prone positioning in patients with moderate-to-severe ARDS, and a strategy of intermittent bolus dosing is preferred to continuous infusion
- For patients with severe sepsis-induced ARDS who fail mechanical ventilation, veno-venous ECMO is suggested if the treating team has the experience and resources
- Elevate of the head of the bed to a semirecumbent position unless contraindicated
- Avoid routine use of pulmonary artery catheters in patients with acute lung injury
- Use protocols for ventilation weaning and sedation/analgesia, with daily sedation interruption if using continuous infusion sedation
- Intensive Care Unit admission within 6 hours of diagnosis
- Use bicarbonate to correct arterial pH <7.2 in the setting of acute kidney injury
- Discuss goals of care and prognosis with patients and their families, and integrate the principles of palliative care to address patient and family suffering when appropriate

ARDS, acute respiratory distress syndrome; ECMO, extra corporeal membrane oxygenation.
Adapted from Singer M, Deutschman CS, Seymour CW, et al. The Third International Consensus Definitions for Sepsis and Septic Shock (Sepsis-3). *JAMA*. 2016;315(8):801–810.

Active screening protocols and resuscitation algorithms have enjoyed immense popularity and have been adopted widely, despite the lack of consistent benefit in organized trials[54–56,68] and poor adherence in evaluations of the implementation of care bundles.[69–71] Nevertheless, the practice of systematic, early, and aggressive attention, treatment, and monitoring has such tremendous face validity that these strategies are likely to remain the standard of care for some time.

Monitoring and Resuscitation in Shock States

The primary goal of monitoring patients in or at risk for shock is to identify and measure the presence of hemodynamic instability and inadequate tissue oxygen delivery, so that interventions can be undertaken to improve these perturbations. Invasive monitors used in shock states can be separated into those that assess hemodynamics and CO, and those that assess the degree to which the metabolic needs of the patient are being met.

Hemodynamic Monitoring

Adequate circulating volume is a necessary condition of adequate stroke volume and oxygen delivery, although assessing this volume is difficult (Chapter 26, Video 26-6). Intravascular pressure assessments such as the mean arterial pressure (MAP) and central venous pressure (CVP) have tremendous face validity, a historical track record, and are easy to measure and understand. However, these measures have their faults. Clinicians adhere poorly to MAP goals[72] and high-quality data linking active MAP management to improved outcomes remain elusive.[73] Moreover, given the typically poor correlation between various MAP measurement modalities,[74] its use as a proxy for hemodynamic information is suspect.[75] Similarly, the CVP is a poor predictor of whether a patient's stroke volume will respond to fluid.[76] Like monitoring CVP and MAP, the pulmonary artery catheter (PAC) has theoretical utility and is discussed at length in Chapter 26. However, despite the theoretical benefits, there are few data to support a positive effect of PAC utilization on mortality or other substantive outcome variables. Patient populations, including those with acute respiratory distress syndrome (ARDS), congestive heart failure, septic shock, and high-risk surgical patients, have all been the subject of investigations targeting the effect of PAC use on outcome.[77,78] These trials have all failed to show benefit, and PAC use has greatly waned.

Echocardiography

Both transthoracic echocardiography (TTE), and transesophageal echocardiography (TEE) provide accurate diagnostic information about dynamic ventricular function, valvular anatomy, pericardial anatomy, and intracardiac pressures. Although TEE has long been used in the operating room and is discussed in detail in Chapter 27, TTE use is becoming more widespread in the ICU as the size and cost of the equipment are decreasing. The major limitation of focused cardiac ultrasound is that it does not provide continuous monitoring. However, ultrasound training and equipment have become increasingly ubiquitous in a variety of specialties and subspecialties including anesthesiology and critical care medicine, making the availability of appropriately skilled providers more common. Both TTE and TEE applications are discussed in more detail in Appendix 6.

Dynamic Respiratory Indices

Positive pressure ventilation (PPV) has predictable effects on stroke volume in both normal subjects and critically ill patients, because it reduces venous return and increases right ventricular afterload. During PPV there is an inspiratory reduction in right ventricular stroke volume due to decreased venous return and a subsequent reduction in LV end-diastolic volume appearing during the expiratory phase of the respiratory cycle. Therefore, the LV stroke volume varies cyclically with ventilation and is paralleled by a similar variation in systolic blood pressure and pulse pressure. These effects are more pronounced in patients on the steeper part of the Frank–Starling curve where, by definition, patients will enjoy a larger increase in stroke volume for a given increase in LV end-diastolic volume (i.e., a fluid bolus).

The relationship between these respirophasic changes in stroke volume and position on the Frank–Starling curve can be exploited to make inferences about a patient's likely response to fluid administration. Several metrics to approximate these changes in stroke volume variation have been identified. These include systolic pressure variation (SPV) and pulse pressure variation, both of which utilize analysis of arterial waveforms. Thresholds indicating abnormal variation vary by device, but are generally in the range of 10% to 15%. The higher the degree of variation, the more stroke volume is changing with respiration, and, ultimately, the more likely the patient is to experience an increase in stroke volume with fluid administration. Compared to static measures such as CVP, systolic and pulse pressure variations are superior predictors of fluid responsiveness in patients with a variety of critical illnesses, including septic shock, ARDS and following cardiac surgery.[76,79]

It should be noted that the use of these metrics has only been validated in patients who are tracheally intubated and receiving PPV. Spontaneous or noninvasive ventilation is associated with a different set of hemodynamic effects, and their relationship to volume responsiveness is less clear. Furthermore, the majority of data were collected in patients receiving tidal volumes of at least 8 mL/kg, and patients need to be in a sinus rhythm; atrial fibrillation, and frequent ectopy will alter the variation in arterial waveform amplitude independent of respirophasic changes, thereby exaggerating variation. Finally, because such analysis requires patients be synchronous with mechanical ventilation, study patients were generally deeply sedated, if not paralyzed. These pitfalls may limit generalizability of findings to patients in current ICUs, where a more restrictive approach to sedation and tidal volumes is frequently employed. Finally, while dynamic respirophasic indices remain accurate in patients with open abdomens, they do not predict fluid responsiveness in patients with an open chest.[80,81]

Less-Invasive Cardiac Output Monitors

A host of less-invasive (relative to PAC) CO monitors have become commercially available in the past two decades. They all generally work by exploiting underlying physical properties and physiologic relationships that are sensitive to changes in blood volume and blood flow. In most cases, complex mathematical corrections are applied to adjust for various sources of error including a variety of anthropometric indices. These techniques include the analysis of systemic arterial pulse contours,[82] various dilutional techniques (similar to PAC thermodilution),[83] arterial Doppler-based techniques,[84] bioreactance-based techniques[85] and others. While detailed discussion of all such techniques and devices is beyond the scope of this chapter, it's important to note that all of these techniques suffer from two common limitations. First, their use is not associated with improvement in outcomes generally recognized as meaningful in the critically ill population. This may be at least partially attributable to the fact that the performance of all these devices tends to worsen in settings of actively changing hemodynamic conditions such as during active volume resuscitation and titration of vasopressors. Second, their output tends to lack agreement with "gold-standard" assessments of CO. For this reason, their regular use is not recommended, although they may have application in specific situations.

Metabolic Monitoring

Although an adequate circulation is necessary for resuscitation, occult hypoperfusion is possible in the setting of seemingly adequate hemodynamic conditions.[86] Once goals for an adequate circulation are met, metabolic goals can be addressed to detect and treat such cellular hypoperfusion, using lactate clearance and venous oximetry.

As the product of anaerobic metabolism, lactate is an indicator of insufficient oxygen delivery to cells. As elevated lactate levels decrease, improved perfusion is assumed, and organ function should improve. Clearance of lactate as a goal of resuscitation has been studied in patients with septic[87] and undifferentiated shock,[88] and current sepsis treatment guidelines recommend it be followed as a marker of improving tissue hypoperfusion.[67] There are also important limitations to using lactate levels as a marker of tissue hypoperfusion, especially in shock states. Lactate levels reflect both the production and elimination of lactate, and while it is assumed that decreasing lactate levels may indicate improved tissue perfusion, the failure of levels to fall does not necessarily indicate increased production. The liver and kidneys account for the majority of lactate elimination, and shock-induced dysfunction of either organ can greatly impede lactate clearance, even after production has returned to normal levels. In addition, catecholamines—particularly epinephrine—can increase hepatic glucose metabolism and can lead to increased lactate production (depending on the hepatic bioenergetic state) despite the lack of tissue hypoperfusion.[89]

Venous oximetry, or assessment of mixed venous oxygen saturation (SvO_2), aims to measure post-organ bed oxygenation as a way to infer the oxygen extraction ratio and make further inference about adequacy of oxygen delivery. Measurement requires a PAC, which requires technical skill and carries risk of complications. A somewhat less invasive and less costly alternative to placing a PAC for the measurement of SvO_2 is to measure $ScvO_2$ via a central venous catheter (CVC). $ScvO_2$ is approximately 5 mmHg higher than SvO_2 in critically ill patients, but correlates well with SvO_2 during changes in hemodynamic status.[90] Because $ScvO_2$ approximates true SvO_2, trends in $ScvO_2$ closely mimic trends in SvO_2.

The level of $ScvO_2$ has been associated with mortality in sepsis. Supranormal levels, whether present at the outset of treatment or after treatment, may be a marker of altered oxygen utilization and are associated with a high mortality.[91] The impact of venous oximetry on outcome, however, is mixed. Achieving $ScvO_2$ more than 70% was independently associated with improved mortality in a retrospective analysis of sepsis care bundles (the only care factor positively associated with mortality),[69] although a much larger and similar analysis did not find the same favorable association between $ScvO_2$ and mortality.[70] Moreover, three subsequent well-conducted attempts to replicate Rivers' initial trial failed to show benefit with the assessment of $ScvO_2$.[55–57]

An important observation about monitoring technology must be recognized. Any individual technique is vulnerable to bias, contraindications, and error. Given the high stakes and complexity of hemodynamic and metabolic assessment, the wisest approach is to understand the strengths and weaknesses of many possible strategies, apply the techniques most appropriate to a given patient with an eye toward possible bias, and interpret the information generated within the broader context of the patient's history, examination, and ever-changing clinical status.

Acute Respiratory Failure

Acute respiratory failure is characterized by a derangement in pulmonary gas exchange or an imbalance between the work of breathing and respiratory muscle capacity. It is usually accompanied by hypoxemia and/or hypercapnia. Indeed, in some cases respiratory failure may be caused by "nonrespiratory" issues (e.g., coma that results in the inability to protect the airway). Acute respiratory failure is a common phenomenon. Depending on the type of ICU, the majority of patients may be mechanically ventilated at any given time, and many critically ill patients are mechanically ventilated for some portion of their ICU stay. The treatment of acute respiratory failure is primarily supportive, typically necessitates supplemental oxygen, and often requires mechanical ventilation with or without tracheal intubation. Acute respiratory failure typically resolves when the initiating condition is adequately treated. The following subsections will discuss basic principles of mechanical ventilation, some of the more challenging types of respiratory failure, and potential therapeutic approaches to respiratory failure.

Principles of Mechanical Ventilation

While the first mechanical ventilators were negative pressure machines termed "iron lungs," contemporary mechanical ventilation in the ICU is PPV that includes both invasive positive pressure ventilation (IPPV, delivered to an intubated patient through an endotracheal or tracheostomy tube) and noninvasive positive pressure ventilation (NPPV, i.e., delivered to an nonintubated patient through a tight fitting mask) (2 Video 57-2). The simplest form of PPV provides a preset tidal volume (volume control) or inspiratory pressure (pressure control) and respiratory rate. Any breathing that the patient does above this preset minimum respiratory rate is either supported (assist-control [AC]) or not (intermittent mandatory ventilation [IMV]). However, ICU ventilators /have become increasingly powerful and complex, capable of delivering high inspiratory flows, and utilizing microprocessors that simultaneously monitor and respond to multiple characteristics of the respiratory circuit. Thus, ventilatory modes used today include pressure support ventilation, pressure control ventilation, volume control ventilation, pressure-regulated volume control ventilation, high-frequency ventilation, proportional assist ventilation, airway pressure release ventilation, synchronous IMV, and
7 others. Despite strong regional, local, and individual biases, there is little evidence to suggest that the mode of mechanical ventilation contributes significantly to any major outcome measure, and the choice of mode is largely one of clinician preference.

Mechanical PPV has been traditionally considered supportive therapy that is applied until the initiating cause of respiratory failure improves sufficiently for the patient to breathe without assistance. However, mechanical ventilation itself may also be injurious in certain settings. Traditionally, tidal volumes of 10 to 15 mL/kg were routinely used to ventilate patients in the ICU. The use of such "supraphysiologic" tidal volumes (normal resting tidal volumes are 5 to 7 mL/kg) evolved from the observation that the use of smaller-sized volumes was associated with the development of atelectasis and hypoxemia in anesthetized patients in the operating room. However, large tidal volumes can result in cardiovascular compromise, barotrauma, ventilator-induced or ventilator-associated lung injury (VILI or VALI), and excess mortality.

PPV results in increased intrathoracic pressure, reduces venous return, and results in reduced CO and blood pressure. In addition, PPV can result in alveolar overdistention and rupture which manifests as pneumothorax, pneumomediastinum, and subcutaneous emphysema (barotrauma). Both of these effects are amplified in patients with obstructive lung disease (asthma and chronic obstructive lung disease [COPD]) whose intrinsic limitations to expiratory flow lead to air trapping and the development of intrinsic positive end-expiratory pressure, or "auto-PEEP." Air trapping results in alveolar overdistention, increases the risk of barotrauma, and can contribute substantially to increased intrathoracic pressure and cardiovascular depression. Detection and quantification of auto-PEEP is requires actively holding exhalation for a prolonged interval (expiratory pause) with both inspiratory and expiratory ventilator valves closed. Auto-PEEP can also also be detected by observing a failure of expiratory flow to return to zero prior to initiation of the next breath.

The ventilatory strategy in these patients typically focuses on maximizing available expiratory time by limiting tidal volume and respiratory rate. Reducing inspiratory time further increases the proportion of each respiratory cycle available for expiration. This strategy is often associated with hypercapnia and respiratory acidosis, but does not appear to be harmful. The benefits of reduced air trapping and auto-PEEP outweigh this potential detriment. To decrease inspiratory time, the inspiratory flow rate must increase which results in increased peak airway pressure. However, most of the pressure is dissipated in the endotracheal tube and large airways and does not necessarily increase static (i.e., plateau) pressure. Importantly, mean airway pressures will fall with increased expiratory time. In order to accomplish these goals, deep sedation is often required, and rarely neuromuscular blockade must be used. The adoption of this type of ventilatory strategy in the 1980s and 1990s was associated with a dramatic reduction in mortality due to acute, severe asthma and respiratory failure, from as high as 23% to less than 5%.[92]

In contrast to barotrauma, VILI and VALI refer to microscopic injury to the lung due to overdistention (sometimes called volutrauma) and cyclic closing and reopening of alveoli (sometimes called atelectotrauma). VILI has been well demonstrated in numerous experimental models, is histologically similar to the features seen in lung injury of other causes, and is characterized by diffuse alveolar damage and increased microvascular permeability. In addition, VILI is associated with the systemic release of inflammatory mediators that may contribute to multiple organ failure. Clinically, patients felt to be at risk for VILI are those with abnormally low recruitable lung volumes, in particular those with ARDS. Thus, a "lung-protective" ventilatory strategy utilizing low tidal volume ventilation has been shown to reduce mortality when applied to patients with ARDS (see later). In addition, accumulating evidence suggests that the use of low tidal volume ventilation may reduce the risk of developing ARDS in critically ill patients.[93] Although tidal volumes of 10 to 12 mL/kg may still be indicated for some patients, in most cases an initial tidal volume of 8 mL/kg is appropriate, and volumes as low as 4 mL/kg may be appropriate in some cases. In addition, because lung volumes correlate with height rather than weight, tidal volume selection should be based on predicted or ideal body weight, rather than actual weight to avoid lung overdistention. Predicted body weight (PBW) can be calculated from the formula: PBW = 50 + 2.3 (height [inches] − 60) (males), or 45.5 + 2.3 (height [inches] − 60) (females).

Although mechanical ventilation generally implies PPV, NPPV, or continuous positive airway pressure (CPAP) can be delivered via a tight-sealing nasal or full-face mask. NPPV is applied using either standard ICU ventilators (typically set to pressure support or pressure control modes, with or without PEEP) or specially designed ventilators that deliver CPAP or bi-level positive airway pressure (Bi-PAP). These dedicated noninvasive ventilators generate high gas flow, can cycle between a high inspiratory pressure and a lower expiratory pressure, and can sense and respond to patient inspiratory effort. Originally developed for home ventilation in patients with obstructive sleep apnea and chronic respiratory failure, newer models are targeted for use in the ICU and incorporate monitoring packages that allow assessment of delivered tidal volumes and respiratory patterns. However, there is no evidence that the type of ventilator used for NPPV affects patient outcome, and the choice of equipment is typically based on availability and familiarity.

Compared to IPPV delivered through an endotracheal tube, NPPV has been associated with improved outcomes in a variety of settings including cardiogenic pulmonary edema, COPD exacerbation, respiratory failure in immunosuppressed patients, post-extubation respiratory failure in surgical patients, and as a supportive measure following extubation in patients with high-risk factors for failing extubation.[94] Improved outcomes are likely are attributable to avoidance of complications associated with tracheal intubation including a reduction in VAP and avoidance of sedating medications typically provided with IPV. However, NPPV is not without risk, and has been associated with increased complications, including a higher rate of myocardial infarction in patients with severe, worsening, or established respiratory failure. Therefore, NPPV is best and most safely utilized when patient characteristics are ideal, including an awake, cooperative patient (with the exception of rapidly reversible obtundation due to hypercarbia), a low risk for regurgitation and aspiration of gastric contents, and a high likelihood that the process resulting in respiratory failure is rapidly reversible.

Another alternative to tracheal intubation and mechanical ventilation for patients with acute hypoxemic respiratory failure is the provision of oxygen through high flow nasal cannulae (HFNC), wherein a high concentration of heated and humidified oxygen is delivered at flow rates from 40 to 60 L/min. This technique not only delivers high inspired oxygen fraction (FIO_2) but also generates low levels of PEEP and may reduce the work of breathing. Outcome benefits including decreased ICU utilization and improved mortality have been described for patients who receive a trial of HFNC before being intubated for acute hypoxemic respiratory failure due to a variety of causes including sepsis and SARS-CoV2 infection.[95]

8 "Weaning" from mechanical ventilation is better termed "liberation" or "separation" from ventilation, because weaning implies that ventilation must be gradually withdrawn (NICV 57-3). However, separation from mechanical ventilation is more a function of the resolution of the cause of respiratory failure than the technique used to withdraw ventilatory support.[96] The process of separation from mechanical ventilation is expedited when respiratory therapy–driven protocols are used that focus on daily assessment of the ability to breathe without assistance.[97] In addition to a reassuring performance on a spontaneous breathing trial, additional, generally accepted parameters indicating a readiness for extubation include improvement of the inciting process, adequate oxygenation, the ability to maintain a patent airway and manage secretions, and hemodynamic stability.

Acute Respiratory Distress Syndrome

ARDS is a syndrome of acute, hypoxemic respiratory failure marked pathologically by diffuse alveolar damage, with resulting increased lung permeability and diffuse alveolar edema.[98] ARDS can occur as a result of direct injury to the lung (e.g., aspiration or pneumonia), or in association with extrapulmonary infection (sepsis) or injury (e.g., multiple trauma). ARDS and diffuse alveolar damage are associated with an inflammatory cell infiltration of the lung, increased systemic markers of inflammation, and progression through exudative, fibroproliferative, and fibrotic phases of injury over days to weeks.

Table 57-5 Acute Respiratory Distress Syndrome

Timing	Acute, onset within 7 days of precipitating illness, injury or onset of respiratory symptoms
Imaging	Bilateral opacities on chest radiograph not fully explained by a focal process. On computed tomography bilateral and diffuse ground glass opacities with a heterogeneous distribution of consolidation (typically in dependent areas) and normal or hyperinflated parenchyma (typically in nondependent areas)
Etiology of radiographic opacities	Cannot be fully attributable to pulmonary edema from cardiac failure or volume overload, masses, atelectasis, or pleural effusions
Oxygenation	Mild: 200 mmHg $< PaO_2{:}FIO_2 \leq 300$ mmHg with PEEP or CPAP ≥ 5 cm H_2O Moderate: 100 mmHg $< PaO_2{:}FIO_2 \leq 200$ mmHg with PEEP ≥ 5 cm H_2O Severe: $PaO_2{:}FIO_2 \leq 100$ mmHg with PEEP ≥ 5 cm H_2O

$PaO_2{:}FIO_2$, ratio of partial pressure of oxygen on arterial blood gas to fraction of inspired oxygen; PEEP, positive end-expiratory pressure; CPAP, continuous positive airway pressure (can be delivered by noninvasive mode).
Adapted from The ARDS Definition Task Force. Acute respiratory distress syndrome: The Berlin definition. *JAMA*. 2012;307(23):2526–2533.

In order to better standardize the definition of ARDS for epidemiologic and research purposes, in 1994 a joint American-European Consensus Conference (AECC) proposed criteria for characterizing ARDS according to the severity of gas exchange abnormality, and distinguished ALI as a less severe version of ARDS, at least in terms of gas exchange. Another multinational consensus conference convened in 2011 to refine the definition of ARDS; the resulting "Berlin Definition" eliminated the "ALI" term, added more explicit criteria for the timing and presentation of the syndrome, and stratified ARDS into three grades of severity according to gas exchange criteria[99] (Table 57-5).

ARDS is highly prevalent in the ICU population and accounts for 10% to 15% of all ICU admissions.[100] Of predisposing factors, sepsis carries the highest risk (approximately 30%) and is the most common cause of ARDS. Mortality associated with ARDS is difficult to discern because of the widespread presence of comorbidities and concomitant acute illness and injury. Most patients who die with an ARDS diagnosis do so because of an underlying problem such as traumatic injury or sepsis. Far fewer patients die due to hypoxemia. Not surprisingly, ARDS mortality varies greatly with the population of patients studied; for example, ARDS mortality in trauma patients is 10% to 15%, whereas mortality in medical ICU patients is as high as 60%.

Clinically, ARDS is characterized by reduced static thoracic (lung and chest wall) compliance and severe impairment of gas exchange, including high intrapulmonary shunt and dead-space fraction. These mechanics and gas exchange abnormalities create a challenge in terms of optimizing mechanical ventilation, because maintenance of adequate oxygenation and carbon dioxide elimination are both problematic. In addition, although the ratio of PaO_2 to FIO_2 (P/F ratio) does not appear to predict mortality, high dead-space fraction does, and may reflect the extent of pulmonary vascular injury.[101] Pulmonary hypertension often develops as the syndrome progresses, and can complicate hemodynamic management.

Although ARDS appears to be a diffuse process by CXR, lung opacification is surprisingly heterogeneous when the lung is imaged by computed tomography. Areas of dense opacification are frequently confined to the posterior, dependent portion of the lung, leaving a small, relatively normal, recruitable volume available for ventilation. This low recruitable lung volume has been termed the "baby lung," and has important implications for ventilatory management in ARDS.

9 The treatment of ARDS is largely supportive, including aggressive treatment of inciting events, avoiding complications, and providing mechanical ventilatory support. Because mechanical ventilation can itself be injurious, a strategy of lung protective ventilation (LPV) should be utilized. This strategy includes utilizing lower tidal volumes (≤6 mL/kg of ideal body weight) to minimize overdistention of healthy alveoli, higher levels of PEEP in order to avoid end-expiratory alveolar collapse and reopening, limiting plateau pressure (30 cm H_2O or less) to avoid barotrauma, permissively allowing for mild-to-moderate hypercapnea (and associated respiratory acidosis), and minimizing FiO_2 with a target PaO_2 >55 mmHg and/or SpO_2 >88%. This strategy was shown to result in a relative mortality reduction of 22% when compared to a control group ventilated with tidal volumes of 12 mL/kg, and remains one of the only interventions that has been unequivocally proven to reduce mortality in patients with ARDS.[102]

Because ARDS is marked by high intrapulmonary shunt, hypoxemia is relatively unresponsive to oxygen therapy. Thus, strategies to recruit collapsed lung are necessary. This is most commonly achieved by using PEEP. The optimal balance between PEEP and FiO_2 has been long debated, but at this point there is no strong evidence to favor either a "high PEEP, low FiO_2" or a "minimal PEEP, high FiO_2" strategy.[103] Other maneuvers to promote recruitment of lung include the use of esophageal manometry to titrate PEEP and tidal volume, recruitment maneuvers or sigh breaths, pressure controlled ventilation, airway pressure release ventilation, inverse ratio ventilation (prolonged inspiratory time), prone positioning, and high-frequency ventilation. Of these techniques, prone positioning alone is associated with improved survival. A meta-analysis of seven randomized, controlled trials of patients with ARDS and ALI and a subsequent multicenter, randomized, controlled trial found a mortality benefit to prone positioning in patients with severe ARDS.[104,105] While prone positioning carries some risks associated with inadvertent dislodgment of vascular access, unintended extubation and pressure injury, it is recommended in patients with ARDS and a P/F ratio of ≤150.

Additional therapies that may have benefit for some patients include neuromuscular blockade and extracorporeal membrane oxygenation (ECMO). Although the use of neuromuscular blockade to facilitate mechanical ventilation of patients with ARDS has generally been on the decline due to fears of increased risk of critical illness myopathy, a French multicenter trial that randomized patients with severe ARDS (P/F ratio <150) to early treatment with cisatracurium versus placebo suggested a mortality benefit.[106] While a subsequent study failed to find a similar benefit, the low incidence of critical illness myopathy in both studies, along with the utility of neuromuscular blockade to facilitate mechanical ventilation in a subset of difficult to ventilate patients suggest there is still a role for these drugs.[107] Additional experimental data suggest that the benefits of neuromuscular blockade in ARDS may be due to anti-inflammatory effects of nicotinic receptor inhibition.[108]

The use of ECMO to support patients with severe ARDS has historically been controversial but experienced a resurgence in interest during the influenza pandemic of 2009, with some observational data suggesting a survival benefit to ECMO.[109] In addition, a UK-based multicenter trial published in 2009 randomized patients with severe ARDS to consideration for ECMO at a specialized referral center versus conventional treatment at their originating hospital. Patients randomized to ECMO consideration had an increased likelihood of disability-free survival at 6 months, although there were a number of concerns with the trial structure and results that limited widespread adoption of ECMO in ARDS.[110] A subsequent randomized clinical trial published in 2018 was stopped early for futility, but the 11% absolute reduction in 60-day mortality in the ECMO intervention group prompted widespread reconsideration of the utility of ECMO in severe, refractory ARDS at centers with adequate experience and resources to implement it.[111] While skepticism remains regarding the widespread use of ECMO for routine management of severe ARDS given the invasive nature of this approach, cost considerations, and need for transfer to specialized centers, some guidelines now suggest it be considered.[67] The primary risks of ECMO relate to bleeding, coagulation disorders, limb ischemia, vascular injuries related to cannulation, and infection.

A number of additional "rescue" therapies have been trialed for cases of severe ARDS that are refractory to established management techniques. While some of these therapies improve physiologic parameters, none have shown a survival benefit. One such therapy is high-frequency oscillatory ventilation, which has been compared to conventional ventilation for treatment of ARDS in a variety of studies including several multicenter, randomized controlled trials which failed to show improved outcomes.[112]

Inhaled vasodilators such as nitric oxide (iNO) and prostaglandins also variably and transiently improve oxygenation in ARDS by improving blood flow to ventilated alveoli. However, several randomized, prospective trials have failed to show any relevant long-term outcome benefits associated with iNO administration to patients with ARDS, and there is suggestion of an increased risk of renal injury.[113,114] Similarly prostaglandins have not shown significant outcome benefits and may be associated with systemic hypotension.[115]

Given that ARDS is marked by high permeability pulmonary edema, it is intuitive that administration of excessive fluids be avoided. Results from a randomized, controlled trial found that a conservative fluid management strategy that emphasized diuresis resulted in improved oxygenation, more ventilator-free days, and more days not in the ICU, but no significant difference in mortality compared to liberal fluid management.[116] Another intervention to facilitate reduction of lung water in ARDS is coadministration of albumin with diuretics.[117] Similar improvements in fluid balance and oxygenation were again demonstrated, but this study was underpowered to detect a more meaningful mortality difference. Although a small study suggested that administration of inhaled β-agonists might also enhance lung water clearance in patients with ARDS, a subsequent large randomized, controlled trial failed to show benefit to this therapy.[118]

An additional area of controversy in the management of patients with ARDS is the use of corticosteroids to halt the inflammatory and proliferative phases of injury. While some trials have suggested a mortality benefit, the generalizability of the results has been questioned for various reason including the homogeneity of ARDS etiology in the trial subjects.[119,120] This is important because patients with bacterial pneumonia or septic shock–associated ARDS have underlying processes that may independently benefit from steroids, whereas those with viral pneumonia or trauma-induced ARDS may not.[121] In contrast to patients with ARDS caused by seasonal influenza and H1N1 influenza that do not appear to benefit from steroids, patients with SARS-CoV2-associated ARDS have modestly lower mortality when treated with steroids.[122]

Table 57-6 Kidney Disease: Improving Global Outcomes (KDIGO) Classification of Acute Kidney Injury

Stage	Serum Creatinine	Urine Output	In-hospital Mortality Odds Ratio
1	↑ Serum Cr ≥1.5× baseline within 7 days OR ↑ Serum Cr ≥0.3 mg/dL within 48 h	<0.5 mL/kg/h for 6–12 hrs	2.5
2	↑ Serum Cr ≥2× baseline	<0.5 mL/kg/h for >12 hrs	5.4
3	↑ Serum Cr ≥3× baseline OR ↑ Serum Cr ≥4 mg/dL OR renal replacement therapy	<0.3 mL/kg/h for 24 hrs OR anuria × 12 hrs	10.1

OR, odds ratio.
Adapted from Kellum JA, Lameire N, Group KAGW. Diagnosis, evaluation, and management of acute kidney injury: a KDIGO summary (Part 1). *Crit Care.* 2013;17:204 and Mehta RL, Kellum JA, Shah SV, et al. Acute Kidney Injury Network: report of an initiative to improve outcomes in acute kidney injury. *Crit Care.* 2007;11(2):R31.

Taken together, these results suggest that some patients with ARDS may benefit from corticosteroid treatment; however, in order to maximize benefit and avoid harm, treatment decisions should be individualized and take into account ARDS etiology, timing and patient specific factors.

Acute Kidney Injury

AKI is reported to occur in up to 66% of critically ill patients.[123] In 2004, a consensus group proposed standard criteria for classifying the severity of renal injury and the associated outcomes.[124] The criteria, known as the RIFLE (risk of renal dysfunction, injury to the kidney, failure or loss of kidney function, and end-stage kidney disease) criteria, have been subsequently modified by the Acute Kidney Injury Network (AKIN) group, and most recently by the Kidney Disease: Improving Global Outcomes (KDIGO) group (Table 57-6).[125,126]

Despite the evolving definition of AKI, its incidence appears to be fairly stable over the past 20 years.[123] Moreover, the hospital mortality associated with AKI requiring dialysis has remained approximately 60% for nearly five decades.[127] This is discouraging when one considers reductions in mortality in association with other organ failures over the same time interval. The reasons for the lack of improvement in outcome are unclear, but likely include insensitive means for identifying patients with incipient renal failure and lack of effective preventive and therapeutic measures.

In the ICU, AKI occurs due to prerenal causes and tubular injury (acute tubular necrosis) in the vast majority of cases.[127] Other potential causes of AKI in the ICU include glomerulonephritis, vasculitis, interstitial nephritis, macro- and microvascular diseases (e.g., thrombotic thrombocytopenic purpura), toxins (nonsteroidal anti-inflammatory drugs, cisplatin, aminoglycosides, radiologic contrast, myoglobin, and hemoglobin), and urinary tract obstruction. The initial evaluation of AKI should focus on identifying easily correctable causes; thus, assessment of volume status utilizing functional hemodynamic monitoring, identification of nephrotoxic agents through careful history taking and medication review, urinalysis to identify possible glomerulonephritis or interstitial nephritis, and ultrasonography to rule out postrenal or obstructive sources of AKI are all important.

In incipient and established AKI, supportive care is the rule, with the focus on maintenance of euvolemia, avoidance of renal toxins, adjustment of medication doses, and monitoring of electrolytes and acid–base status. Pharmacologic approaches to the prevention and treatment of AKI have been uniformly disappointing. Current guidelines recommend against the use of low-dose dopamine, recombinant atrial natriuretic peptide, fenoldopam, colloid solutions, and diuretics for the prevention and treatment of AKI.[123] In the specific setting of contrast-induced nephropathy, the first intervention is avoidance of contrast exposure whenever possible. If contrast must be used, low- or iso-osmolar contrast agents, and pre- and postcontrast exposure intravascular volume expansion with crystalloid are recommended. Sodium bicarbonate solutions and *N*-acetyl cysteine are ineffective.[128]

Although hemodialysis (i.e., renal replacement therapy [RRT]) is typically considered a supportive measure in AKI, interest has focused on the potential for RRT to improve renal recovery and reduce mortality. Research on RRT in the ICU has focused on the type, intensity, and dose of dialysis, as well as the timing of initiation of RRT.

The intensity of RRT is determined by both the frequency of treatment and the degree of solute clearance per unit of time. Increased intensity of RRT has failed to improve outcomes in critically ill patients with AKI in two large, randomized clinical trials.[129,130] However, it should be noted that the prescribed intensity of RRT is seldom delivered in clinical practice owing to therapy interruptions for procedures or when filters require replacement. As such, efforts to ensure maximal delivery of the prescribed RRT dose are important. Early initiation of RRT has similarly failed to demonstrate a mortality benefit, and may in fact lead to more complications.[131]

Continuous renal replacement therapy (CRRT) (including continuous venovenous hemofiltration and hemodialysis) has long been known as a useful technique when hemodynamic instability is present. In contrast to intermittent hemodialysis, effective solute removal is possible with CRRT in the presence of arterial hypotension. Despite this theoretical advantage to CRRT, several studies, including a relatively large, multicenter randomized controlled trial, found no survival benefit to CRRT compared to intermittent hemodialysis.[132] The two techniques are considered equivalent.

Endocrine Aspects of Critical Care Medicine

Glucose Management in Critical Illness

Hyperglycemia is commonly encountered in critically ill patients and occurs in both diabetics and nondiabetics. Hyperglycemia results primarily because of increased glucose production and insulin resistance caused by inflammatory and hormonal mediators that are released in response to injury. Hyperglycemia may also be aggravated by various therapeutic and supportive interventions, including the use of corticosteroids and total PN. Although the risks of hyperglycemia for patients with diabetes who are ketosis-prone have long been appreciated, hyperglycemia is also detrimental to critically ill patients in a broader sense. Hyperglycemia is associated with increased risk of postoperative infection (wound and otherwise) and poor outcome in patients with stroke, acute MI, TBI, and AKI.[133]

Given these considerations, strict glycemic control in critically ill patients has been advocated as leading to multiple outcome benefits. A single randomized controlled trial of surgical patients published in 2001 found that intensive insulin therapy (goal glucose <110 mg/dL) reduced ICU mortality by approximately 50% compared to more conventional therapy (goal glucose <215 mg/dL).[134] Based largely on the results of this one trial there was widespread adoption of protocols to target blood glucose between 80 and 110 mg/dL. Unfortunately, the benefits of the initial trial were not reproduced in multiple subsequent trials, and in fact an increased risk of hypoglycemia and associated harm have been observed.[135] After an additional large, multicenter, multinational randomized controlled trial of intensive insulin therapy showed increased mortality in the tight glucose control group, the practice of maintaining blood glucose between 80 and 110 mg/dL was widely abandoned.[136] Current serum glucose targets are somewhat variable, but most agree that 140 to 180 mg/dL is an acceptable goal in most patients.

Adrenal Function in Critical Illness

The stress response to injury includes an increase in serum cortisol levels in most critically ill patients. However, adrenal insufficiency may also occur in critically ill patients for several reasons, including inhibition of adrenal stimulation or corticosteroid synthesis by drugs or cytokines and direct injury to or infection of the pituitary or adrenal glands.[137] Thus, adrenal insufficiency has been reported to occur with increased frequency in critically ill patients with trauma, burns, sepsis, and other conditions in comparison with the general population.

The diagnosis of adrenal insufficiency in critical illness is complicated by limitations of commonly used tests of adrenal function. Cortisol is highly protein bound, and serum proteins, including albumin, are commonly depressed in critically ill patients. Although total serum cortisol levels are low in critically ill patients with hypoproteinemia, free cortisol levels are elevated.[138] This suggests that older reports utilizing total serum cortisol levels in critically ill patients may overestimate the incidence of adrenal insufficiency. However, until free cortisol assays are more widely available, the diagnosis of adrenal insufficiency in critical illness must be based on clinical suspicion and total cortisol levels.

In addition to absolute adrenal insufficiency (low baseline cortisol and poor response to adrenocorticotropic hormone [ACTH] administration/stimulation), a condition of relative adrenal insufficiency (defined as an increase in serum cortisol of ≤9 μg/dL in response to ACTH administration, independent of the baseline cortisol level) has been described in patients in septic shock and with other illnesses. Low-normal baseline cortisol levels, high baseline cortisol levels, and a poor response to ACTH are all predictors of increased mortality in critical illness.[139]

Although high-dose corticosteroids for the treatment of septic shock are of no benefit, evidence suggests that lower doses (hydrocortisone 200 to 300 mg/day) can reduce dependency on vasopressors and shorten the duration of shock. Evidence for a mortality benefit is unclear, with some trials showing improved mortality and others showing lack of efficacy.[140–143] A 2019 meta-analysis suggests that there is evidence supporting a small 28-day (but not 90-day) mortality benefit with the use of low-dose hydrocortisone (200 to 300 mg/day or equivalent) in sepsis, but that the incidence of metabolic derangements is also increased.[144] Current guidelines suggest a trial of low-dose hydrocortisone only in patients with vasopressor-dependent septic shock.[67] There does not appear to be an increased risk of gastric ulceration, superinfection, or neuromuscular weakness according to this analysis, but hypernatremia and hyperglycemia are more common in patients receiving steroids.

Thyroid Function in Critical Illness

Measures of thyroid function, including levels of thyrotropin (TSH), T_3, and T_4, are deranged in the majority of critically ill patients. Depression of T_3 occurs within hours of injury or illness and can persist for weeks. TSH levels may be normal initially, but fall to inappropriately low levels as illness progresses. T_4 levels are also often low, but can be normal or high. Low hormone levels may occur for a variety of reasons, including altered binding and metabolism early in the course of illness, and depressed neuroendocrine function with more prolonged illness. In addition, certain drugs (e.g., dopamine) can depress thyroid function through central mechanisms.[145] Low thyroid hormone levels, particularly T_3, correlate with the severity of illness and are associated with an increased risk of death.[146]

It is controversial whether the observed abnormalities in thyroid hormones represent an appropriate response to illness or true hypothyroidism; thus, the terms "euthyroid sick syndrome" and "nonthyroidal illness" have been coined to describe thyroid function abnormalities in critical illness. Furthermore, it is not clear whether replacement of thyroid hormones is indicated or beneficial in critical illness. T_3 administration to brain-dead organ donors appears to improve hemodynamic stability, although randomized trials have found minimal or no benefit to T_3 or T_4 administration in patients undergoing cardiopulmonary bypass and cardiac surgery.[147] In addition, several small studies have found no benefit to T_3 or T_4 administration to patients with a variety of critical illnesses. Larger, randomized prospective trials are necessary to define the role of routine thyroid hormone supplementation in nonthyroidal illness.

Importantly, true hypothyroidism may be present in the critically ill, particularly in the geriatric population and should be considered in the face of refractory shock, adrenal insufficiency, unexplained coma, and prolonged, unexplained respiratory failure. True hypothyroidism is marked by an elevation of TSH (usually >25 mU/L) in the face of a low T_4 level.

Somatotropic Function in Critical Illness

Growth hormone (GH) levels are low in prolonged critical illness, and it has been conjectured that deficiencies of GH and insulin-like growth factor-1 (IGF-1) contribute to the muscle wasting seen in acute illness.[146] However, although small trials have found that GH administration can attenuate muscle catabolism in critical illness, a large, randomized trial found that administration of high-dose GH to critically ill patients resulted in increased mortality.[148] Thus, GH administration during critical illness cannot be advocated at this time, although further exploration of the benefits of smaller doses of GH may be warranted.

Anemia and Transfusion Therapy in Critical Illness

Anemia is a frequent if not obligate accompaniment of critical illness. The vast majority of patients admitted to the ICU are anemic at some point in their hospital stay, and approximately 40% to 50% of them will receive transfused blood.[149] Importantly, both anemia and the amount of transfused blood are independently associated with mortality.[150,151] However, this association does not denote cause and effect, particularly for anemia, which may just be a marker of the severity of illness.

The cause of anemia in critical illness is multifactorial and related to blood loss from the primary injury or illness, iatrogenic blood loss due to daily blood sampling, nutritional deficiencies, and marrow suppression.[152] Given that approximately 13% of ICU patients may have iron, folate or vitamin B_{12} deficiencies, these parameters should be checked when consideration is given to blood transfusion.

10 Treatment of anemia in critical illness is the source of considerable debate. In unstressed subjects, severe anemia (Hb of 5 g/dL or less) is amazingly well tolerated due to physiologic compensations that maintain oxygen delivery and extraction. However, it has long been assumed that critically ill patients have less efficient compensatory mechanisms and reduced physiologic reserve, and thereby require a higher Hb concentration than unstressed individuals. Historically, this has translated to a red blood cell (RBC) transfusion threshold at an Hb concentration of approximately 10 g/dL.

11 Transfusion of RBCs is not without risks including infection, transfusion-related acute lung injury (TRALI), transfusion-associated circulatory overload (TACO), transfusion-related immunomodulation (TRIM), microchimerism, and more (see Chapter 17 for a more complete discussion of transfusion risks). These negative effects of transfusion may help explain why the landmark TRICC (transfusion requirements in critical care) study found that 30-day mortality was not affected when a restrictive transfusion threshold (Hb <7 g/dL) was used, compared to a more conventional threshold of less than 10 g/dL.[153] Furthermore, a trend in mortality reduction favored the restrictive group, and various subgroups of patients (less than 55 years of age and less severely ill by APACHE [acute physiology and chronic health evaluation] scoring) had a significantly lower mortality when they were transfused using the restrictive strategy. A similar trial in pediatric patients found no mortality difference between restrictive and liberal transfusion strategies, suggesting that a restrictive strategy is safe in critically ill children.[154] Studies in patients with TBI and acute upper gastrointestinal (GI) hemorrhage confirm that restricting RBC transfusion to an Hb concentration of less than 7 g/dL reduces exposure to blood products, reduces complications, and in the case of upper GI hemorrhage improves survival.[155,156] Likewise, liberal RBC transfusion as part of goal-directed therapy that has been incorporated into the protocol for septic shock did not favorably affect outcomes.[57] These studies support clinical practice guidelines that recommend a restrictive transfusion practice in the ICU, with the possible exception of patients with active myocardial or cerebral ischemia.[149]

Alternatives to the transfusion of RBCs for treatment of anemia are not currently available for widespread use. Several hemoglobin-based oxygen carriers (HBOCs) have been studied in clinical trials involving trauma and surgery, but results have been mixed, and none are currently FDA approved for use. Compassionate use of HBOCs in patients who have refused blood transfusion for religious reasons has been reported.

Prevention of anemia in critical illness is an appealing alternative to transfusion. One simple and potentially cost-saving approach is to reduce the volume and frequency of blood draws in the ICU. As noted earlier, iatrogenic blood loss is a major factor in the development of anemia of critical illness. Another potential approach is the administration of recombinant erythropoietin and iron, but trials supporting their routine use have shown inconsistent results and they are not currently recommended.

Nutrition in the Critically Ill Patient

Critical illness can lead to hypermetabolic states, and if nutritional support is inadequate or delayed, patients are at immediate risk of malnutrition. Poor nutritional status is associated with increased mortality and morbidity among critically ill patients. Therefore, appropriate nutrition is an important aspect of critical care and adequate nutritional support should be considered a standard of care. What constitutes *adequate* nutritional support, however, remains less clear. Although prior guidelines recommended 80% to 100% of predicted caloric needs, research suggests no harm to intentional underfeeding (providing 20% to 50% of predicted caloric needs.[157] Current guidelines recommend providing between 12 and 25 kcal/kg as soon as possible during an ICU admission.[158] Although over 200 formulas have been promoted for predicting daily calorie requirements of the critically ill patient, the American Society for Parenteral and Enteral Nutrition (ASPEN) and SCCM guidelines do not specify any specific formula. It is acceptable to use a simple formula based on the patient's ideal body weight to calculate predicted caloric needs, of which 15% to 20% should be represented by proteins (1.2 to 2 g/kg/day).

Feeding intolerance due to high gastric residual volume can be improved by the administration of gastric prokinetic agents and positioning an enteric tube postpyloric. However, when compared to gastric feeding, postpyloric feeding does not result in a clinically significant reduction of pneumonia, ICU length of stay, or mortality.[159] In some patients, intermittent enteral feeding, as opposed to a continuous feeding regimen, may allow earlier attainment of the enteral calorie goal.[160]

Another way to reach calorie goals in patients with significant GI tract dysfunction is the use of PN. While there has been ongoing debate for decades regarding the timing of PN initiation, delayed initiation (days 7 to 10) has been associated with a decrease in infections, shorter duration of mechanical ventilation, less need for RRT, and cost savings.[161] Strategies to optimize delivery of Enteral Nutrition (EN) include starting at the target rate, use of feeding protocols with higher thresholds for gastric residuals volumes, use of motility agents, and small bowel feeding—and should be employed in patients without an absolute contraindication to EN prior to initiating PN. Additional strategies to minimize the risks of EN including head of the bed elevation should also be considered.

Among special enteral formulations, immunonutrition has been hypothesized to influence infectious morbidity and mortality in critically ill patients via a beneficial effect on GI immunologic function. This effect appears more likely in surgical patients, such as those with burns and those who are in trauma. Specific enteral formulations, particularly those with high concentrations of glutamine, have the strongest data to support their use[162] The use of various fatty acids is not supported by current guidelines.[158] Many disease states result in micronutrient deficiencies, and the administration of supplemental micronutrients (e.g., selenium, zinc, and vitamins A, C, and E) are generally considered safe. However, evidence supporting their use is of overall low quality and high risk of bias, and therefore should be interpreted with caution.[163]

A potential severe complication of resuming caloric intake through either EN or PN in malnourished patients is the development of refeeding syndrome. This is characterized by large and rapid intracellular shifting of phosphorous, potassium, magnesium, and thiamine. The resultant acute drop in serum electrolyte levels and can result in fatal cardiac dysrhythmias if not promptly recognized and treated. Nutrition should be initiated with caution and close monitoring in any malnourished patients.[164]

Sedation and Analgesia for the Critically Ill Patient

Goals and Assessment

Most patients in the ICU will experience some form of pain, agitation, or anxiety during their admission, and the indications for sedation and analgesia in the ICU are many. Although individual medications frequently provide multiple pharmacodynamic effects, including sedation, analgesia, and anxiolysis, it is helpful to think about these effects separately when selecting medications for an individual patient. For instance, painful procedures such as the insertion of indwelling catheters, endotracheal tubes, and thoracostomy tubes require analgesia, but often do not require anxiolysis or sedation. Conversely, agitated delirium or acute alcohol withdrawal do not require analgesia and are more appropriately treated with sedatives.

The goal of any sedation and analgesia strategy in the ICU is to provide enough medication to effectively treat patient symptoms, but to avoid adverse effects such as delirium, long-term cognitive deficits, and respiratory depression that are associated with overtreatment. The patient with an ideal level of sedation and analgesia is at reduced risk for dislodging catheters, removing monitoring devices, or falling out of bed. They are more likely to be synchronous with the mechanical ventilator, which improves oxygenation and reduces the risk of lung injury. They are also better able to participate with care, early mobilization, and physical and occupational therapy.

Assessing the adequacy of attempts to achieve these goals can be difficult. Several factors such as interindividual variability, evolving severity of disease and organ dysfunction, variably intense pain stimuli and multiple drug interactions influence the analgesic and sedative needs of ICU patients. Therefore, it is important to titrate medications according to established therapeutic goals and re-evaluate sedation requirements frequently. Several validated scales are available to assess sedation levels over time. The most commonly used are the Ramsay sedation scale, the Riker sedation–agitation scale (SAS), and the Richmond agitation–sedation scale (RASS). Features common to these scales are the ability to grade sedation over different depths and allow for indicators of agitation. There is no evidence that one scale is superior to another at this time, although the RASS has been more rigorously assessed for reliability and validity.[165] Similarly, there are a variety of validated pain scales. These scales are discussed in Chapter 55. The important point regarding assessment scales for pain, sedation, and delirium is that an assessment utilizing a validated scoring system should be made before and after every intervention to assess progress in achieving treatment goals.

Pharmacologic Management

Virtually any hypnotic-anxiolytic or opioid used in the operating room can be used in the ICU to provide sedation and analgesia, respectively. However, propofol, midazolam, and dexmedetomidine are the most used hypnotic-anxiolytics. Each of these drugs has advantages and disadvantages, and detailed discussions of their properties can be found in Chapters 19 and 20. Some important considerations of their use in the ICU environment are discussed here.

Dexmedetomidine is unique in that its mechanism of action is profoundly different from that of propofol and benzodiazepines. It provides sedation without inducing unresponsiveness or coma, may have some analgesic effects, and has little affect on respiratory drive. However, dexmedetomidine does not reliably provide deep sedation and does not reliably produce amnesia, making it inappropriate as a solo hypnotic-anxiolytic in patients requiring paralysis. In addition, it can produce significant bradycardia and hypotension which may limit its use in hemodynamically compromised patients.[166] Compared to propofol and midazolam, dexmedetomine does not shorten duration of mechanical ventilation or provide any mortality benefits.[167–169]

Propofol has become the most common sedative agent for mechanically ventilated ICU patients. It is equally efficacious but less expensive than dexmedetomidine, and is more effective in reliably inducing deep sedation. When compared to benzodiazapines, it is associated with a shorter duration of mechanical ventilation and less delirium.[170] However, it can cause myocardial depression and worsen hypotension. Because the current commercially available formulation is constituted in a lipid emulsion, it can also cause hypertriglyceridemia and a significant caloric load that should be accounted for when determining nutritional support levels. Propofol can also lead to the potentially lethal "propofol infusion syndrome," especially when used at high doses for long periods of time.

Benzodiazepines also produce deep sedation and amnesia, and have reduced potential to cause hemodynamic instability. In addition, they are also an inexpensive and effective treatment for alcohol withdrawal, which is a common coexisting diagnosis in critically ill patients.,

Opiates are a very common component of many ICU analgesia and sedation regimens, and can be used as single agents in certain types of patients (e.g., patients with acute postoperative pain, with uncomplicated respiratory failure requiring modest degrees of mechanical ventilation, or who require sedation but do not tolerate hypnotic-anxiolytic drugs).[171] Like dexmedetomidine, opiates do not reliably produce amnesia, and are not appropriate as single agents in patients who require paralysis. Morphine, hydromorphone and fentanyl are the most commonly used opioids to provide analgesia in the ICU. Morphine should be avoided in patients with renal failure due to active metabolites that accumulate in the presence of impaired renal function.

Additional adjunctive medications for treating pain in critically ill patients include acetaminophen, low-dose ketamine infusion (1 to 2 μg/kg/hr), non-steroidal anti-inflammatories (NSAIDs), gabapentin, pregabalin, and carbamazepine. All of these medications may have opioidsparing effects and should be considered in selected patients.[171]

Delirium and Neurocognitive Complications

Neurocognitive complications including delirium and prolonged cognitive dysfunction are associated with a number of sedative medications. They may be more common in patients treated with deeper levels of sedation. The distinguishing characteristics of delirium include an acute onset and fluctuating course, inattention, disorganized thinking, and altered level of consciousness. Structured screening instruments such as the Confusion

Assessment Method for the ICU (CAM-ICU) are available, and their use in concert with proactive screening regimens are recommended for the diagnosis of delirium in the ICU.[172]

Critically ill patients are often deeply sedated, in part due to concerns for patient comfort, but also because of potential benefits afforded by a reduction in the sympathoadrenal response to injury. However, available evidence from observational and randomized trials suggests that practices favoring light sedation, bolus administration versus continuous infusion of sedatives, and promoting daily trials of awakening in ICU patients result in a variety of benefits, including a shortened duration of mechanical ventilation, decreased time in the ICU, and reduced mortality.[173–176]

Nonpharmacologic techniques including the use of both verbal and written communication, frequent reorientation, maintenance of a day–night cycle and noise reduction strategies can be used to promote sleep, improve comfort and safety and to reduce delirium and confusion. Antipsychotic medications like haloperidol and quetiapine are used commonly to both treat or prevent delirium or agitation, and to promote sleep or treat insomnia. Guidelines specifically cite the lack of evidence for the use of quetiapine, haloperidol, and atypical antipsychotics for the prevention of delirium, and their routine use is not recommended.[171]

Depth of sedation may also play a role in long-term outcomes after discharge from the ICU and hospital. Increasing evidence suggests that patients admitted to the ICU are at risk of developing symptoms of posttraumatic stress disorder, delusional memories, and longer-term cognitive dysfunction.[177,178] Approximately one-third will have signs and symptoms of cognitive dysfunction persisting 12 months after discharge, but the association with sedative use is less certain.[179]

Complications in the ICU: Detection, Prevention, and Therapy

Nosocomial Infections

Nosocomial infections are a major source of morbidity and mortality in the critically ill (see Chapter 26, Video 26-9). At some level, nosocomial infections are unavoidable and occur because of the nature of intensive care—patients are critically ill with altered host defenses, they require invasive devices (endotracheal tubes, intravascular catheters, etc.) that provide portals of entry for infectious organisms, and they receive therapies that increase the risk of infection (e.g., glucocorticoids, PN). On the other hand, many nosocomial infections are preventable with relatively simple interventions.[180] This became more financially relevant in the United States in 2008, when the Center for Medicare and Medicaid Services (CMS) ceased reimbursing hospitals for treatment of preventable complications such as catheter-associated urinary tract infection (CAUTI) and catheter-related bloodstream infection (CRBSI).

Several types and sources of infections are relatively unique to ICU care and should be included in the differential diagnosis when signs suggestive of infection arise. These infections include sinusitis, VAP, CRBSI (also referred to as central line-associated bloodstream infection [CLABSI]), CAUTI, and invasive fungal infection.

Sinusitis

Radiographic sinusitis is common in critically ill patients with indwelling oral and nasal tubes. Nasotracheal intubation confers a greater risk than does orotracheal intubation of radiographic sinusitis, occurring in approximately 95% and 25% of patients with nasal and oral tubes after 1 week of intubation, respectively.[181] Several reports suggest that approximately 10% of radiographically diagnosed sinusitis is infected as determined by quantitative cultures, although the incidence may be higher. One study reported that bacterial sinusitis was responsible for 16% of fevers of unknown origin in a surgical ICU.[182] The organisms cultured from sinuses represent those that are responsible for other nosocomial infections, particularly VAP (staphylococcal species, enteric gram-negative bacteria, and nonlactose-fermenting gram-negative rods such as *Pseudomonas* and *Acinetobacter*). Bacterial sinusitis may predispose to the development of VAP, possibly because of microaspiration of infected secretions.

Prevention of sinusitis should focus on efforts to improve sinus drainage, including semirecumbent positioning and avoidance of nasal tubes. Bacterial sinusitis should be considered in patients with unexplained fever and leukocytosis in the ICU. If radiographic sinusitis is documented, any nasal tubes should be removed, and nasal irrigation and short-term administration of nasal decongestants should be considered. If the patient is severely ill, broad-spectrum antibiotic coverage should be considered. If these maneuvers do not result in resolution of signs and symptoms of sinusitis in 2 to 3 days, otolaryngologic consultation and consideration of sinus drainage procedures may be undertaken.

Ventilator-Associated Pneumonia

Tracheal intubation and mechanical ventilation increase the risk of nosocomial pneumonia, thus the term VAP. The likelihood of developing VAP increases with the duration of mechanical ventilation, but the precise incidence is difficult to define due to substantial variability in how VAP is defined. Because VAP is widely associated with increased morbidity, it is an obvious target for QI interventions. In an effort to facilitate the study of such interventions the Centers for Disease Control and Prevention (CDC) implemented a standardized ventilator-associated event (VAE) surveillance program through the National Healthcare Safety Network (NHSN) in 2013.[183] Possible and probable VAP are specifically defined within the larger category of VAE. Importantly, in an effort to remove the subjective variability inherent to interpretation of radiographic studies, this definition of VAP does not make use of radiologic data, nor was it intended to be a clinical definition. Recent studies show inconsistent overlap in VAP detection when the NHSN and traditional definitions are simultaneously applied to the same population, with more cases of VAP detected using lower respiratory tract culture-based clinical criteria (that typically include a radiographic component) than with the NHSN criteria.[184] Given this caveat, recent studies utilizing the NHSN definition put the incidence at less than 4% per mechanical ventilation episode.[185] This contrasts with an incidence greater than 15% at 1 week of ICU and greater than 20% at 2 weeks described in older studies, and likely reflects increasing adherence to best practices for VAP prevention as well as changing definitions.

Although the mortality in patients with VAP ranges between 30% and 70%, the attributable mortality (the number of patients who die because of VAP rather than with VAP) is more difficult to assess. This may be due to differences in the type of ICU, patient factors, diagnostic techniques across studies, or differences in the virulence of the causative pathogens. Although earlier work suggested an attributable mortality to VAP greater than 40%, more recent and rigorously conducted work suggests that the effect of VAP on mortality is minimal.[186]

VAP can be categorized as "early-onset," occurring within the first 48 to 72 hours of intubation/ventilation, or "late-onset," occurring thereafter (note that 4 days of mechanical ventilation is required in order for it to qualify as a VAE per the NHSN definition). Early-onset VAP is generally caused by organisms such as *Haemophilus influenzae, Streptococcus pneumoniae,* methicillin-sensitive *Staphylococcus aureus,* and other relatively antibiotic-sensitive oral flora that enter the trachea around the time of intubation. Late-onset VAP is associated with more virulent organisms such as methicillin-resistant *S. aureus, Pseudomonas aeruginosa,* and *Acinetobacter.* In general, early-onset organisms are associated with zero or low attributable mortality, whereas late-onset organisms, particularly *Pseudomonas* and *Acinetobacter* species, are associated with higher mortality.

There are a number of interventions that can reduce the incidence of VAP, some of which are relatively simple and inexpensive, and others that are costlier and/or associated with some risk. The simplest and least expensive interventions are strict handwashing between patients, and semirecumbent positioning of the patient (head-of-bed angle at 30 degrees or greater from horizontal). Considering their negligible risks, these practices should be rigorously applied in all ICUs.

The use of acid suppression therapy to prevent GI bleeding is more controversial. Acid-suppression therapies have been associated with increased VAP risk because they allow bacterial overgrowth in the stomach. Further, the risk of significant GI bleeding is very low in the ICU, even in high-risk patients (those with coagulopathy or on mechanical ventilation). Thus, GI acid suppression therapy may be reserved for high-risk patients, and sucralfate may be considered as an alternative agent to acid-suppressive regimens despite its potentially reduced effectiveness.

Somewhat more expensive interventions to reduce VAP that may be useful include specialized endotracheal tubes with subglottic suctioning ports and silver coatings. Although a meta-analysis supports the use of endotracheal tubes with subglottic suctioning ports to reduce the incidence of VAP and shorten both hospital and ICU length of stay, silver-coated tubes have not been proven beneficial in this regard.[187,188]

Given that aspiration of gastric and oropharyngeal organisms appears to be a mechanism for the development of VAP, intervening to "decontaminate" these sites may have benefits. Selective digestive decontamination (SDD) with nonabsorbable antimicrobial agents has been controversial for many years, but growing evidence supports the practice.[189] Limited oral decontamination with chlorhexidine is more commonplace and also likely reduces VAP incidence.[190]

An additional and important approach to reduce the overall mortality of VAP involves refinement of the diagnostic process and limitation of antibiotic therapy to avoid the development and proliferation of antibiotic resistant organisms. An invasive diagnostic strategy is likely more accurate than traditional clinical criteria to diagnose VAP. Invasive strategies typically involve collection of either tracheal aspirate specimens or bronchial–alveolar specimens using lavage or protected brushes, and then quantitating bacterial growth in the laboratory. Thus, VAP is diagnosed only when bacteria are seen within bronchoalveolar cells microscopically or when bacterial growth exceeds specific thresholds ($\geq 10^4$ colony-forming units/mL for bronchoalveolar lavage and $\geq 10^3$ colony-forming units/mL for protected brush specimens). Current Infectious Disease Society of America guidelines specify that tracheal aspirate specimens are preferred over bronchial–alveolar specimens for VAP diagnosis, although the data supporting this recommendation are conflicting and it is a "weak" recommendation.[191] It therefore seems appropriate to favor collection of tracheal aspirate specimens, but to recognize that bronchial-alveolar specimens may be appropriate for some patients.

12 It is clear that delay in treatment of nosocomial infections (including VAP) is associated with increased mortality. Treatment should not be delayed pending diagnostic evaluation; rather, treatment should be started after culture specimens are sent, if the clinical suspicion of VAP is high. Antibiotics can then be narrowed in spectrum or discontinued altogether depending on the results from quantitative cultures after 48 to 72 hours (Table 57-7). This approach is known as "de-escalating therapy" and is designed to ensure adequate initial antibiotic treatment, yet avoid overuse of antibiotics in the long term. Antibiotic selection should be predicated on hospital bacterial growth and resistance patterns. In general, for patients with early-onset VAP, antibiotics can be relatively narrow in spectrum and limited to a single agent. For late-onset VAP, broader spectrum antibiotics should be initiated and include

Table 57-7 Suggested Empiric Antibiotic Regimens for Common Intensive Care Unit Infections

Infection	Regimen
Ventilator-Associated Pneumonia	
• Early (<72 hrs of intubation and hospital admission)	Ceftriaxone PLUS azithromycin; consider adding vancomycin or linezolid if known history of MRSA
• Late (>72 hours of intubation or hospital admission)	Vancomycin OR linezolid AND cefepime; consider adding ciprofloxacin if high incidence of MDR GNRs
Bloodstream infections	Vancomycin OR linezolid AND cefepime
Urinary Tract Infections	
• Noncatheter-associated	Ceftriaxone
• Catheter-associated	Ceftazidime ADD vancomycin if GPCs on gram stain; CONSIDER meropenem instead of ceftazidime if concerned for MDR GNRs or ESBLs
C. difficile diarrhea	Vancomycin (oral dosing); IF shock, megacolon or ileus, then ADD IV metronidazole
Meningitis	
• Nonsurgical	Dexamethasone AND ceftriaxone AND vancomycin AND ampicillin AND acyclovir
• Postsurgical	Cefepime AND metronidazole AND vancomycin
Intra-abdominal Infections	
• Community-acquired	Ceftriaxone AND metronidazole
• Hospital-acquired	Vancomycin AND either piperacillin-tazobactam OR meropenem
Sepsis, site unknown	Vancomycin AND meropenem Consider adding ciprofloxacin if concern for MDR GNRs or ESBLs

MDR, multi-drug resistant; MRSA, methicillin-resistant *Staphylococcus aureus;* GNR, gram-negative rods; GPC, gram-positive cocci; ESBL, extended spectrum β-lactamase. Initial antibiotic regimen should take into account local antibiograms. Antibiotic regimens should be narrowed once culture results are available.

agents from two different classes—resistant gram-negative organisms and methicillin-resistant *S. aureus*.

The optimal duration of antibiotic therapy for VAP is not well defined, but 8 days of antibiotic therapy appears effective and results in more antibiotic-free days.[192] However, VAP caused by nonlactose–fermenting gram-negative rods (including *Pseudomonas*) have a higher infection recurrence rate with an initial 8-day course of therapy, thus longer courses can be considered.

Catheter-Related Bloodstream Infections

As strictly defined by the CDC, CRBSI includes the following criteria: (1) clinical suspicion of catheter-related infection (including low likelihood of infection elsewhere), plus (2) positive culture of blood drawn from the catheter or a segment of catheter, plus (3) matching positive blood culture drawn from another site, preferably by direct venotomy or arterial puncture. Given this strict definition, the incidence of CRBSI is less than 5% in most studies. However, the incidence of bacteremia is affected by several factors, including the conditions and technique of insertion, type and location of catheter, and the duration of catheterization, and can vary widely from study to study. The attributable mortality of CRBSI is approximately 11%, which is much lower than that for primary bacteremia or bacteremia associated with another site of infection.[193]

CRBSI is more likely when placement occurs under emergency conditions, and is reduced by the use of strict aseptic technique with full barrier precautions. This includes preinsertion handwashing, full gown and gloves, and the use of a large barrier drape.[16] In addition, skin cleansing with chlorhexidine is more effective than other agents at reducing catheter-related infection. Attention to these practices can dramatically reduce catheter-related infection. These simple interventions should be considered as standards of care.

CRBSI and bacteremia increase with the duration of catheterization, particularly for durations of greater than 2 days. However, routine catheter replacement at 3 or 7 days does not reduce the incidence of infection, and results in increased mechanical complications. Thus, routine guidewire exchange of catheters is not recommended.

Catheters coated with either antiseptics (chlorhexidine and silver sulfadiazine) or antibiotics (rifampin and minocycline) reduce bacterial colonization of catheters as well as bacteremia. This effect becomes manifest only after days 5 to 6 of the catheter being in place; thus, the CDC recommends the use of antimicrobial-coated catheters in patients with an expected duration of catheterization of greater than 5 days, particularly if the local rate of CRBSI is high.[194] However, more recent data suggest that although coated catheters reduced the incidence of colonization and CRBSI, they may not reduce the incidence of clinically diagnosed sepsis or mortality.[195] Ultimately, key of strategies to reduce CRBSI are to limit the duration of insertion, and the need for continued central venous catheterization should be reviewed daily. CRBSI may be insertion site-dependent, but adoption of these practices seem to be lessening the role that infectious concerns play when choosing a catheter insertion site.[196]

Catheter-related venous thrombosis occurs commonly and is associated with an increased risk of infection. Routine flushing of catheter ports with heparin reduces both the incidence of thrombosis and infection. However, heparin solutions contain antimicrobial preservatives and it is unclear if the heparin or the preservative is responsible for the beneficial effect. In addition, heparin may induce thrombocytopenia. Therefore, the CDC does not recommend the routine use of heparin flushing.[194]

Organisms commonly responsible for catheter-related bacteremia include *S. epidermidis* and *S. aureus*, enteric gram-negative bacteria, *P. aeruginosa* and *Acinetobacter*, and occasionally *Enterococcal* species. Although coagulase-negative staphylococci are commonly isolated from blood cultures in the ICU, they are rarely responsible for true infection. When catheter-related bacteremia is confirmed, the offending catheter should be removed and appropriate antibiotics continued for a minimum of 7 days. Longer courses should be considered for *S. aureus* bacteremia, given its predilection to cause endocarditis. Suspected CRBSI can be addressed by sending screening cultures drawn through the catheter and from a peripheral site. Guidewire exchange of the catheter with culture of the intracutaneous segment and tip can also be considered in this situation, but should a CRBSI be confirmed, the catheter should be removed, not exchanged. Depending on the patient's severity of illness, a strong suspicion of catheter-related bacteremia should trigger the institution of broad-spectrum antibiotic coverage, including coverage for methicillin-resistant staphylococcal species and nonlactose–fermenting gram-negative rods, until culture results return, with subsequent de-escalation of therapy. Similar to VAP, early appropriate antibiotic coverage of catheter-related bacteremia will likely reduce mortality, although this has not been systematically studied.

Urinary Tract Infection

The urinary tract is the second most common source of infection in the ICU, with infections occurring in up to one-third of patients. The incidence of CAUTI increases with the duration of bladder catheterization.[180] The responsible organisms are similar to those causing other nosocomial infections and include staphylococcal species, *Enterococcus*, enteric gram-negative bacteria, and nonlactose–fermenting gram-negative bacteria such as *Pseudomonas*. Bacteriuria is associated with bacteremia about 5% of the time. Similar to other ICU-acquired infections, CAUTIs are associated with increased mortality, although the attributable mortality is not clear.

Prevention of ICU-acquired CAUTI includes using careful handwashing and aseptic technique during catheter insertion and minimization of catheterization duration. The use of antimicrobial catheter coatings may also reduce the incidence of CAUTI, although the evidence is insufficient at this point to recommend general use of coated catheters.[197]

Invasive Fungal Infections

Invasive fungal infections in nonneutropenic patients are caused by *Candida* species in the vast majority of cases. Risk factors for *Candida* infection include the presence of CVCs, recent abdominal surgery, anastomotic leakage and GI perforation, dialysis-dependent renal failure, administration of PN, multiple broad-spectrum antibiotics, and steroids.[198] In addition to these factors, invasive *Aspergillus* and *Mucormycosis* are more typically associated with profound immunosuppression and diabetes, respectively.[199]

A significant clinical dilemma involves accurate and timely identification of invasive fungal infections. Positive cultures from sterile fluid remain the gold standard, but may take 72 to 96 hours to turn positive and may be positive in only 50% of autopsy-confirmed infections. To improve accuracy and timeliness of the diagnosis, a number of molecular and serologic techniques have been developed. β-D–glucan is present in the cell wall of *Candida* and *Aspergillus* species, as well as *Pneumocystis jiroveci*, and an assay detecting its presence is approximately 80% sensitive and specific. A number of promising whole blood-based polymerase chain reaction (PCR) tests have also recently become available, with sensitivities above 90% in published trials and results available within hours of sample collection. However, they are expensive and have not yet been proven in clinical practice. For diagnosis of *Aspergillus* and *Mucormycosis*, imaging with CT and magnetic resonance is invaluable, as biopsy and surgical debridement play an important role in management.[199]

Candida albicans is responsible for approximately 50% of invasive *Candida* infections in critically ill patients. *C. tropicalis, C. paraisopolis, C. glabrata,* and *C. krusei* account for the remainder.[198] In addition to simple bloodstream infection, *Candida* species are associated with CAUTI, postoperative peritonitis, and disseminated blood-borne infection. *Candida* is frequently cultured from the urine and sputum, but treatment is usually not necessary, as *Candida* pneumonia is unlikely and candiduria often clears without treatment, mostly with discontinuation of the bladder catheter. In addition, candiduria often recurs after initially successful antifungal therapy. True *Candida* peritonitis is also difficult to separate from contamination of culture specimens, but given that the mortality associated with *Candida* peritonitis is approximately 50%, treatment is warranted if clinical signs suggest infection. Similarly, candiduria and *Candida* in sputum cultures may be treated if there are systemic signs of infection, as colonization is a risk factor for invasive infection.

Disseminated blood-borne *Candida* infection can result in endophthalmitis, endocarditis, and hepatic and pulmonary abscesses. It is likely to occur when initial treatment of candidemia is delayed and is associated with a high mortality. Prevention of invasive *Candida* infection involves avoidance of risk factors, including limitation of intravascular catheterization, PN, and antibiotic administration. Prophylactic therapy with fluconazole may be effective at reducing the risk of invasive *Candida* infection in high-risk patients, but this strategy has not been associated with improved mortality in the nonneutropenic population, and may increase the incidence of invasive infection with more resistant species, such as *C. glabrata* and *C. krusei.* Prophylactic therapy should be reserved for only the high-risk patient. Empiric therapy should be considered in patients with a high likelihood of invasive *Candida* infection while awaiting culture results, as delay in treatment is associated with increased mortality. However, care should be taken to de-escalate therapy after several days in the absence of positive cultures or clinical response.

Documented *Candida* bloodstream infection should be treated aggressively, with therapy started promptly and continued for at least 2 weeks after the last positive blood culture. An ophthalmologic examination is warranted in patients with documented or suspected bloodstream infection, as patients with endophthalmitis may require longer courses of therapy. Intravascular catheters that are potential sources of bloodstream infection should be removed. Treatment of *Candida* infections has evolved over time, and current guidelines now recommend echinocandins such as caspofungin, micafungin, and anidulifungin as the first-line treatment in most settings. Liposomal amphotericin B is generally reserved for refractory, life-threatening infections such as fungal endocarditis, invasive *Aspergillosis* and *Mucormycosis.* In addition, surgical debridement plays a key role in management of *Mucormycosis.* Suggested empiric treatment of common ICU infections is outlined in Table 57-7.

Stress Ulceration and Gastrointestinal Hemorrhage

Gastric mucosal breakdown with resulting gastritis and ulceration (stress ulceration) can lead to GI bleeding in the ICU. Clinically significant GI bleeding results in hemodynamic instability and/or a sudden fall in hematocrit that results in blood transfusion. The incidence of clinically significant stress-related GI bleeding is relatively low—less than 5% in high-risk patients and less than 1% for low-risk patients.[200] The major risk factors for stress-related GI bleeding are mechanical ventilation and coagulopathy. Secondary risk factors among mechanically ventilated patients include renal failure, thermal injury, and possibly head injury, although the latter two factors have not been recently evaluated. Conversely, EN may protect against significant GI bleeding.

Stress ulcer prophylaxis (SUP) strategies include acid suppression agents such as histamine type 2 receptor antagonists, proton pump inhibitors, and cytoprotective agents such as sucralfate. However, the agent of choice and related benefits are controversial due to methodologic flaws in study designs, significant publication bias, and concerns about the potential for these medications to cause harm.[201,202] The potential for harm may be related to acid suppression favoring gastric colonizing bacterial overgrowth that may increase the risk of nosocomial pneumonia and *C. difficile* colitis. Because of the lack of clear benefit, potential for harm, and low rate of gastric bleeding in patients receiving EN, current evidence supports restricting their use to high-risk patients who are without EN for greater than 48 hours.

Venous Thromboembolism

VTE encompasses both DVT and pulmonary emoblism (PE), and occurs frequently in critically ill patients, with incidences of DVT of 10% to 30% and PE of 1.5% to 5%.[203] However, the reported incidence varies widely depending on the study design, DVT detection method, and patient population studied. Virtually all critically ill patients have one or more risk factors for VTE. Determination of VTE risk is important in that it will help in choosing prophylactic therapy and in determining the level of suspicion for VTE in individual patients (Table 57-8).

In addition to classic lower extremity DVT, upper extremity DVT occurs with increased frequency in the ICU population.[204] This is directly associated with the use of CVCs in the subclavian and internal jugular sites. Upper extremity DVT can result in PE in up to one-third of cases, with occasional fatalities. Catheter-related thrombosis is also associated with increased risk of CRBSI and bacteremia. Finally, upper extremity DVT is associated with considerable long-term morbidity, particularly related to post-thrombotic syndrome.

The literature supporting prophylactic measures to prevent VTE in the ICU population is relatively poor and generally shows differences only in intermediate end points (e.g., asymptomatic DVT), with no differences in the incidence of PE or death. In general, the risks of VTE prophylaxis, including heparin-induced thrombocytopenia and bleeding, must be weighed against the risk of VTE. It is generally agreed that high-risk patients without contraindications should receive pharmacologic prophylaxis, and low-risk patients with contraindications should receive mechanical prophylaxis with intermittent pneumatic compression devices. There are an ever-expanding number of medications that may be used for VTE chemoprophylaxis, but unfractionated heparin and low–molecular-weight heparin remain the most commonly used and most studied, with guidelines from professional societies updated regularly.[205] A number of validated scoring systems have been developed for both surgical and medical populations to assess VTE risk. In patients at high risk for DVT with contraindications to anticoagulation, the preventative placement of a vena cava filter may be considered, although there are few data to support this practice. To reduce CVC–associated thrombosis and infection, catheter tips should be positioned in the superior vena. Heparin bonding of catheters may also reduce local thrombosis. Importantly, it should be recognized that the incidence of VTE in patients receiving pharmacologic prophylaxis remains substantial, ranging between 5% and 30% depending on the therapy and population studied.

Table 57-8 Caprini Venous Thromboembolism Risk Assessment Model

1 Point	2 Points	3 Points	5 Points
Age 41–60 years	Age 61–74 yrs	Age >75 yrs	Stroke <1 mo
Minor surgery	Arthroscopic surgery	Personal history of VTE	Elective lower extremity arthroplasty
Body mass index >25 kg/m^2	Major open surgery >45 min	Family history of VTE	Hip, pelvis, or leg fracture
Swollen legs	Laparoscopic surgery >45 min	Any thrombophilia	Acute spinal cord injury <1 month
Varicose veins	Bed rest >72 h	Elevated serum homocysteine	Multiple trauma <1 month
Pregnant or postpartum <1 month	Immobilizing plaster cast	Heparin-induced thrombocytopenia	
History of miscarriage	Central venous access		
Oral contraceptives or hormone replacement therapy			
Sepsis <1 mo			
Serious lung disease <1 mo			
Abnormal pulmonary function			
Acute myocardial infarction			
Congestive heart failure <1 month			
History of inflammatory bowel disease			
Medical patient on bed rest			

High risk: ≥5 points
Intermediate risk: 3–4 points
Low risk: 1–2 points
Very low risk: 0 points

VTE, venous thromboembolism.
Adapted from Pollak AW, McBane RD 2nd. Succinct review of the new VTE prevention and management guidelines. *Mayo Clin Proc.* 2014;89:394–408. Copyright © 2014 Elsevier. With permission.

Given the high incidence of asymptomatic DVT in critically ill patients, a high index of suspicion for VTE must be maintained. However, despite the high incidence of DVT, routine screening studies for DVT do not appear to improve clinical outcomes in the ICU. Thus, VTE should be considered in critically ill patients in the face of relatively nonspecific findings, such as unexplained tachycardia, tachypnea, fever, asymmetric extremity edema, and gas exchange abnormalities, including high dead-space ventilation. Compression Doppler ultrasonography is the most commonly utilized test for diagnosis of DVT and has good positive and negative predictive value compared to contrast venography.[206] Helical chest CT has supplanted radionuclide ventilation–perfusion scanning as the primary test for the diagnosis of PE.[207] CT scanning can also be extended to include the extremities to diagnose DVT. However, ventilation–perfusion scanning and/or pulmonary angiography may have utility in specific circumstances, including in the presence of renal insufficiency (concerns about contrast-induced nephrotoxicity) or equivocal results on CT scan. In addition, pulmonary angiography may be the test of choice when the likelihood of PE is high and anticoagulation is contraindicated, necessitating immediate placement of a vena cava filter. D-Dimer levels are not useful in the ICU population because they are frequently elevated and nonspecific in critically ill patients.

The mainstay of treatment for VTE is either unfractioned or low–molecular-weight heparin, which should be started prior to confirmatory studies if clinical suspicion is high. In situations of hemodynamic compromise, the use of systemic thrombolytic therapy may be life-saving. However, if bleeding risk is elevated, catheter-directed thrombolysis and clot evacuation techniques, or open surgical thrombectomy, can be considered. Venoarterial ECMO may also provide support in cases of massive PE. The specific interventions are largely dependent on institutional capabilities and clinical circumstances.

For patients who have contraindications to anticoagulation or who have recurrent PE despite anticoagulation, vena cava filters can be placed in the superior or inferior vena cava, depending on DVT location. Ultimately, given the long-term thrombotic complications associated with these devices, patients with vena cava filters should be anticoagulated when no longer contraindicated, and the devices should be removed when they are no longer required.

ICU-Acquired Weakness

The term ICU-acquired weakness (ICUAW) encompasses a wide variety of neuromuscular abnormalities developing as a consequence of critical illness. ICUAW is characterized by weakness that is symmetrical and bilateral, occurs during an ICU stay, and is not attributable to another specific etiology. The spectrum of illness ranges from subjective muscle fatigue to flaccid quadriplegia. Although various studies have attempted to distinguish neuropathic from myopathic syndromes, resulting in a bewildering list of associated acronyms, it is likely that there is considerable overlap between the two in terms of risk factors, presentation, and prognosis.[208]

ICUAW is associated with prolonged duration of mechanical ventilation, ICU stay, hospital stay, and mortality. Prospective studies have shown that up to 11% of mechanically ventilated patients exhibit evidence of weakness at 24 hours. By 7 days the incidence may increase to 60%, and among those with ARDS and sepsis the number may be even higher. In addition to sepsis, factors strongly associated with the development of ICUAW include duration of illness and hyperglycemia. Although corticosteroid and neuromuscular blocking drug administration have classically been associated with ICUAW, more recent evidence suggests that their use in modern ICUs is not associated with ICUAW. This is likely due to contemporary practice of using shorter-acting agents in lower doses and for much shorter courses than was historically the case. Less specific contributors to the development of ICUAW include a catabolic nutritional state, systemic proinflammatory state, and generalized muscle unloading.

Prevention of ICUAW centers on avoidance or minimization of contributory risk factors, including long courses of high-dose steroids, prolonged neuromuscular blockade, and hyperglycemia. High-quality evidence in support of specific interventions to prevent ICUAW exists only for avoidance of hyperglycemia. There is moderate-quality evidence that early mobilization and physical therapy may be beneficial.[209–211]

The diagnosis of ICUAW should be entertained in all critically ill patients with unexplained weakness. Electrodiagnostic studies can help confirm the diagnosis and rule out other, potentially treatable causes of weakness such as Guillain–Barré syndrome. Muscle biopsy is confirmatory in cases of myopathy, but given its invasive nature, biopsy is not warranted outside of research settings.

End-of-Life Care in the ICU

13 Nearly 20% of patients in the United States die during a hospitalization with an ICU stay.[212] Consequently, the ICU is an important setting for delivering high-quality end-of-life care. Shared decision making and patient- and family-centered care require good communication between medical teams, patients, and their family members to ensure that delivered care is consistent with patient values and preferences. The Institute of Medicine Committee on Approaching Death released its report *Dying in America: Improving Quality and Honoring Individual Preferences Near the End of Life* in 2014. The report emphasizes the need for improved communication about end-of-life preferences between clinicians and patients in order to avoid unwanted treatment.[213] It is becoming more widely recognized that palliative care is one way to achieve this goal. Its implementation is associated with a higher quality of life, so much so that the CCSC Choosing Wisely campaign for critical care has recommended that patients at high risk of death or severely impaired functional recovery be offered care focused primarily on comfort, as an alternative to care focused primarily on a cure.[23] It is important to recognize that palliative care can also be offered in conjunction with curative care, and that intensivists play an important role in delivering palliative care in the ICU, in collaboration with palliative care specialists.

For further review and interactivities, please see the videos and narrative interactive clinical vignettes (NICVs) accessible in the complimentary eBook bundled with this text. Access instructions are located on the inside front cover.

REFERENCES

1. Berthelsen PG, Cronqvist M. The first intensive care unit in the world: Copenhagen 1953. *Acta Anaesthesiol Scand.* 2003;47(10):1190–1195.
2. Angus DC, Kelley MA, Schmitz RJ, White A, Popovich J, Jr. Caring for the critically ill patient. Current and projected workforce requirements for care of the critically ill and patients with pulmonary disease: can we meet the requirements of an aging population? *JAMA* .2000;284(21):2762–2770.
3. Spielman FJ. Critical care medicine: anesthesiology steps forward. *Bull Anesth Hist.* 2003;21(1):12–13.
4. Halpern NA, Pastores SM, Oropello JM, Kvetan V. Critical care medicine in the United States: addressing the intensivist shortage and image of the specialty. *Crit Care Med.* 2013;41(12):2754–2761.
5. Kavanagh BP. The GRADE system for rating clinical guidelines. *PLoS Med.* 2009;6(9):e1000094. (In eng).
6. Senate and House of Representatives of the United Statestat. Patient Protection and Affordable Care Act. 2010.
7. Dogra AP, Dorman T. Critical Care Implications of the Affordable Care Act. *Crit Care Med.* 2015;44(3):e168–173.
8. Weled BJ, Adzhigirey LA, Hodgman TM, et al. Critical Care Delivery: The Importance of Process of Care and ICU Structure to Improved Outcomes: An Update From the American College of Critical Care Medicine Task Force on Models of Critical Care. *Crit Care Med.* 2015;43(7):1520–1525.
9. Wallace DJ, Angus DC, Barnato AE, Kramer AA, Kahn JM. Nighttime intensivist staffing and mortality among critically ill patients. *N Engl J Med.* 2012;366(22):2093–2101.
10. Kerlin MP, Adhikari NK, Rose L, et al. An Official American Thoracic Society Systematic Review: The effect of nighttime intensivist staffing on mortality and length of stay among intensive care unit patients. *Am J Respir Crit Care Med.* 2017;195(3):383–393.
11. Stollings JL, Devlin JW, Lin JC, et al. Best Practices for Conducting Interprofessional Team Rounds to Facilitate Performance of the ICU Liberation (ABCDEF) Bundle. *Crit Care Med.* 2020;48(4):562–570.
12. Hales BM, Pronovost PJ. The checklist–a tool for error management and performance improvement. *J Crit Care.* 2006;21(3):231–235.
13. Vincent JL, Creteur J. Paradigm shifts in critical care medicine: the progress we have made. *Crit Care.* 2015;19(Suppl 3):S10.
14. Micek ST, Roubinian N, Heuring T, et al. Before-after study of a standardized hospital order set for the management of septic shock. *Crit Care Med.* 2006;34(11):2707–2713.
15. Morris AC, Hay AW, Swann DG, et al. Reducing ventilator-associated pneumonia in intensive care: impact of implementing a care bundle. *Crit Care Med.* 2011;39(10):2218–2224.
16. Pronovost P, Needham D, Berenholtz S, et al. An intervention to decrease catheter-related bloodstream infections in the ICU. *N Engl J Med.* 2006;355(26):2725–2732.
17. Collaborative CCS. Choosing wisely: five things physicians and patients should question. *American Board of Internal Medicine Foundation.* http://www.choosingwisely.org/clinician-lists#keyword=critical_care.
18. Centers for Disease Control and Prevention. CDC grand rounds: reducing severe traumatic brain injury in the United States. *MMWR Morb Mortal Wkly Rep.* 2013;62(27):549–552.
19. Collaborators MCT, Perel P, Arango M, et al. Predicting outcome after traumatic brain injury: practical prognostic models based on large cohort of international patients. *BMJ.* 2008;336(7641):425–429.
20. Teasdale G, Jennett B. Assessment of coma and impaired consciousness. A practical scale. *Lancet.* 1974;2(7872):81–84.
21. Carney N, Totten AM, O'Reilly C, et al. Guidelines for the Management of Severe Traumatic Brain Injury, Fourth Edition. *Neurosurgery.* 2017;80(1):6–15.
22. Guidelines for the management of severe traumatic brain injury. *J Neurotrauma.* 2007;24(Suppl 1):S1–106.
23. Mirski MA, Muffelman B, Ulatowski JA, Hanley DF. Sedation for the critically ill neurologic patient. *Crit Care Med.* 1995;23(12):2038–2053.
24. Cremer OL, Moons KG, Bouman EA, et al. Long-term propofol infusion and cardiac failure in adult head-injured patients. *Lancet.* 2001;357(9250):117–118.
25. Schwartz ML, Tator CH, Rowed DW, et al. The University of Toronto head injury treatment study: a prospective, randomized comparison of pentobarbital and mannitol. *Can J Neurol Sci.* 1984;11(4):434–440.
26. Ward JD, Becker DP, Miller JD, et al. Failure of prophylactic barbiturate coma in the treatment of severe head injury. *J Neurosurg.* 1985;62(3):383–388.
27. Eisenberg HM, Frankowski RF, Contant CF, Marshall LF, Walker MD High-dose barbiturate control of elevated intracranial pressure in patients with severe head injury. *J Neurosurg.* 1988;69(1):15–23.
28. Drummond JC, Dao AV, Roth DM, et al. Effect of dexmedetomidine on cerebral blood flow velocity, cerebral metabolic rate, and carbon dioxide response in normal humans. *Anesthesiology.* 2008;108(2):225–232.
29. Robertson CS, Valadka AB, Hannay HJ, et al. Prevention of secondary ischemic insults after severe head injury. *Crit Care Med.* 1999;27(10):2086–2095.

30. Andrews PJ, Sinclair HL, Rodriguez A, et al. Hypothermia for intracranial hypertension after traumatic brain injury. *N Engl J Med.* 2015;373(25):2403–2412.
31. Roberts I, Yates D, Sandercock P, et al. Effect of intravenous corticosteroids on death within 14 days in 10008 adults with clinically significant head injury (MRC CRASH trial): randomised placebo-controlled trial. *Lancet.* 2004;364(9442):1321–1328.
32. Temkin NR, Anderson GD, Winn HR, et al. Magnesium sulfate for neuroprotection after traumatic brain injury: a randomised controlled trial. *Lancet Neurol.* 2007;6(1):29–38.
33. Temkin NR, Dikmen SS, Wilensky AJ, et al. A randomized, double-blind study of phenytoin for the prevention of post-traumatic seizures. *N Engl J Med.* 1990;323(8):497–502.
34. Myburgh J, Cooper J, Finfer S, et al. Saline or albumin for fluid resuscitation in patients with traumatic brain injury. *N Engl J Med.* 2007;357(9):874–884.
35. Cooper DJ, Rosenfeld JV, Murray L, et al. Decompressive craniectomy in diffuse traumatic brain injury. *N Engl J Med.* 2011;364(16):1493–1502.
36. Hutchinson PJ, Kolias AG, Timofeev IS, et al. Trial of decompressive craniectomy for traumatic intracranial hypertension. *N Engl J Med.* 2016;375(12):1119–1130.
37. Connolly ES, Jr., Rabinstein AA, Carhuapoma JR, et al. Guidelines for the management of aneurysmal subarachnoid hemorrhage: a guideline for healthcare professionals from the American Heart Association/American Stroke Association. *Stroke.* 2012;43(6):1711–37.
38. Nieuwkamp DJ, Setz LE, Algra A, et al. Changes in case fatality of aneurysmal subarachnoid haemorrhage over time, according to age, sex, and region: a meta-analysis. *Lancet Neurol.* 2009; 8(7):635–642.
39. Etminan N, Chang HS, Hackenberg K, et al. Worldwide incidence of aneurysmal subarachnoid hemorrhage according to region, time period, blood pressure, and smoking prevalence in the population: a systematic review and meta-analysis. *JAMA Neurol.* 2019;76(5):588–597.
40. Kerro A, Woods T, Chang JJ. Neurogenic stunned myocardium in subarachnoid hemorrhage. *J Crit Care.* 2017;38:27–34.
41. van Donkelaar CE, Bakker NA, Veeger NJ, et al. Predictive factors for rebleeding after aneurysmal subarachnoid hemorrhage: rebleeding aneurysmal subarachnoid hemorrhage study. *Stroke.* 2015;46(8):2100–106.
42. Barker FG, 2nd, Ogilvy CS Efficacy of prophylactic nimodipine for delayed ischemic deficit after subarachnoid hemorrhage: a metaanalysis. *J Neurosurg.* 1996;84(3):405–414.
43. Dayyani M, Sadeghirad B, Grotta JC, et al. Prophylactic therapies for morbidity and mortality after aneurysmal subarachnoid hemorrhage: a systematic review and network meta-analysis of randomized trials. *Stroke.* 2022;53(6):1993–2005.
44. Treggiari MM, Walder B, Suter PM, Romand JA. Systematic review of the prevention of delayed ischemic neurological deficits with hypertension, hypervolemia, and hemodilution therapy following subarachnoid hemorrhage. *J Neurosurg.* 2003;98(5):978–984.
45. Powers WJ, Rabinstein AA, Ackerson T, et al. Guidelines for the Early Management of Patients With Acute Ischemic Stroke: 2019 Update to the 2018 Guidelines for the Early Management of Acute Ischemic Stroke: A Guideline for Healthcare Professionals From the American Heart Association/American Stroke Association. *Stroke.* 2019;50(12): e344–e418.
46. Powers WJ, Rabinstein AA, Ackerson T, et al. 2018 Guidelines for the Early Management of Patients With Acute Ischemic Stroke: A Guideline for Healthcare Professionals From the American Heart Association/American Stroke Association. *Stroke.* 2018;49(3):e46–e110.
47. Powers WJ, Derdeyn CP, Biller J, et al. 2015 American Heart Association/American Stroke Association Focused Update of the 2013 Guidelines for the Early Management of Patients With Acute Ischemic Stroke Regarding Endovascular Treatment: A Guideline for Healthcare Professionals From the American Heart Association/American Stroke Association. *Stroke.* 2015; 46(10):3020–3035.
48. Nogueira RG, Jadhav AP, Haussen DC, et al. Thrombectomy 6 to 24 hours after stroke with a mismatch between deficit and infarct. *N Engl J Med.* 2018;378(1):11–21.
49. Albers GW, Marks MP, Lansberg MG. Thrombectomy for stroke with selection by perfusion imaging. *N Engl J Med.* 2018;378(19):1849–1850.
50. Back L, Nagaraja V, Kapur A, Eslick GD. Role of decompressive hemicraniectomy in extensive middle cerebral artery strokes: a meta-analysis of randomised trials. *Intern Med J.* 2015;45(7):711–717.
51. Chen HJ, Lee TC, Wei CP. Treatment of cerebellar infarction by decompressive suboccipital craniectomy. *Stroke.* 1992;23(7):957–961.
52. Dankiewicz J, Cronberg T, Lilja G, et al. Hypothermia versus normothermia after out-of-hospital cardiac arrest. *N Engl J Med.* 2021;384(24):2283–2294.
53. Wyckoff MH, Greif R, Morley PT, et al. 2022 International Consensus on Cardiopulmonary Resuscitation and Emergency Cardiovascular Care Science With Treatment Recommendations: Summary From the Basic Life Support; Advanced Life Support; Pediatric Life Support; Neonatal Life Support; Education, Implementation, and Teams; and First Aid Task Forces. *Circulation.* 2022;146(25):e483–e557.
54. Rivers E, Nguyen B, Havstad S, et al. Early goal-directed therapy in the treatment of severe sepsis and septic shock. *N Engl J Med.* 2001;345:1368–1377.
55. Peake SL, Delaney A, Bailey M, et al. Goal-directed resuscitation for patients with early septic shock. *N Engl J Med.* 2014;371(16):1496–1506.
56. Mouncey P, Osborn TM, Power GS, et al. Trial of early, goal-directed resuscitation for septic shock. *N Engl J Med.* 2015;372:1301–1311.
57. Yealy DM, Kellum JA, Huang DT, et al. A randomized trial of protocol-based care for early septic shock. *N Engl J Med.* 2014;370(18):1683–1693.
58. Prins K, Neill, JM, Tyler, JO, et al. Effects of beta-blockade withdrawal in acute decompensated heart failure. *JACC: Heart Failure.* 2015;3:647–653.
59. Heidenreich PA, Bozkurt B, Aguilar D, et al. 2022 AHA/ACC/HFSA Guideline for the Management of Heart Failure: A Report of the American College of Cardiology/American Heart Association Joint Committee on Clinical Practice Guidelines. *J Am Coll Cardiol.* 2022;79(17): e263–e421.
60. O'Connor CM, Starling RC, Hernandez AF, et al. Effect of nesiritide in patients with acute decompensated heart failure. *N Engl J Med.* 2011;365(1):32–43.
61. Kelly J, Mentz RJ, Hasselbad V. Worsening heart failure during hospitalization for acute heart failure: insights from the Acute Study of Clinical Effectiveness of Nesiritide in Decompensated Heart Failure (ASCEND-HF). *Am Heart J.* 2015;170:298–305.
62. Writing Committee M, Lawton JS, Tamis-Holland JE, et al. 2021 ACC/AHA/SCAI Guideline for Coronary Artery Revascularization: A Report of the American College of Cardiology/American Heart Association Joint Committee on Clinical Practice Guidelines. *J Am Coll Cardiol.* 2022;79(2):e21–e129.
63. Dhruva SS, Ross JS, Mortazavi BJ, et al. Association of use of an intravascular microaxial left ventricular assist device vs intra-aortic balloon pump with in-hospital mortality and major bleeding among patients with acute myocardial infarction complicated by cardiogenic shock. *JAMA.* 2020;323(8):734–745.
64. Thiele H, Ohman EM, de Waha-Thiele S, Zeymer U, Desch S. Management of cardiogenic shock complicating myocardial infarction: an update 2019. *Eur Heart J.* 2019;40(32): 2671–2683.
65. Geller BJ, Sinha SS, Kapur NK, et al. Escalating and De-escalating Temporary Mechanical Circulatory Support in Cardiogenic Shock: A Scientific Statement From the American Heart Association. *Circulation.* 2022;146(6):e50–e68.
66. Angus D, van der Poll T. Severe sepsis and septic shock. *N Engl J Med.* 2013;369:840–851.
67. Evans L, Rhodes A, Alhazzani W, et al. Surviving Sepsis Campaign: International Guidelines for Management of Sepsis and Septic Shock 2021. *Crit Care Med.* 2021;49(11):e1063–e1143.
68. Investigators TP A randomized trial of protocol-based care for early septic shock. *N Engl J Med.* 2014;370:1683–1693.
69. Castellanos-Ortega A, Suberviola B, Garcia-Astudillo, LA, et al. Impact of the Surviving Sepsis Campaign protocols on hospital length of stay and mortality in septic shock patients: Results of a three-year follow-up quasi-experimental study. *Crit Care Med.* 2010;38: 1036–1043.
70. Levy M, Dellinger RP, Townsend SR, et al. The Surviving Sepsis Campaign: Results of an international guideline- based performance improvement program targeting severe sepsis. *Crit Care Med.* 2010;38:367–374.
71. Rhodes A, Phillips G, Beale R, et al. The Surviving Sepsis Campaign bundles and outcome: results from the International Multicentre Prevalence Study on Sepsis (the IMPreSS study). *Intensive Care Med.* 2015;41:1620–1628.
72. Takala J. Should we target blood pressure in sepsis? *Crit Care Med.* 2010;38(10):50–59.
73. Asfar P, Meziani F, Hamel JF, et al. High versus low blood-pressure target in patients with septic shock. *N Engl J Med.* 2014;370:1583–1593.
74. Wax D, Lin HM, Leibowitz AB. Invasive and concomitant noninvasive intraoperative blood pressure monitoring: observed differences in measurements and associated therapeutic interventions. *Anesthesiology.* 2011;115:973–978.
75. Magder S. The highs and lows of blood pressure: toward meaningful clinical targets in patients with shock. *Crit Care Med.* 2014;42:1241–1251.
76. Marik P, Cavallazzi R. Does the central venous pressure predict fluid responsiveness? An updated meta-analysis and a plea for some common sense. *Crit Care Med.* 2013;41:1774–1781.
77. Richard C, Warszawski J, Anguel N, et al. Early use of the pulmonary artery catheter and outcomes in patients with shock and acute respiratory distress syndrome: a randomized controlled trial. *JAMA.* 2003;290(20):2713–2720.
78. Sandham JD, Hull RD, Brant RF, et al. A randomized, controlled trial of the use of pulmonary-artery catheters in high-risk surgical patients. *N Engl J Med.* 2003;348(1):5–14.
79. Yang X, Du B. Does pulse pressure variation predict fluid responsiveness in critically ill patients? A systematic review and meta-analysis. *Crit Care.* 2014;18:650–657.
80. De Wall E, Rex S, Kruitwagen CL, Kalkman CJ, Buhre WF. Dynamic preload indicator fail to predict fluid responsiveness in open chest conditions. *Crit Care Med.* 2009;37:510–515.
81. Renner J, Gruenewald M, Hill M, et al. Non-invasive assessment of fluid responsiveness using CNAP technology is interchangeable with invasive arterial measurements during major open abdominal surgery. *Br J Anaesth.* 2017;118(1):58–67.
82. Monnet X, Anguel N, Naudin B, et al. Arterial pressure-based cardiac output in septic patients: different accuracy of pulse contour and uncalibrated pressure waveform devices. *Crit Care.* 2010;14:109.
83. Button D, Weibel L, Reuthebuch, O, et al. Clinical evaluation of the FloTrac/Vigileo system and two established continuous cardiac output monitoring devices in patients undergoing cardiac surgery. *Br J Anaesth.* 2007;99:329–339.
84. Scheeren TWL, Ramsay MAE. New developments in hemodynamic monitoring. *J Cardiothorac Vasc Anesth.* 2019;33(Suppl 1):S67–S72.

85. Kupersztych-Hagege E, Teboul JL, Artigas A, et al. Bioreactance is not reliable for estimating cardiac output and the effects of passive leg raising in critically ill patients. *Br J Anaesth*. 2013;111:961–966.
86. Abuleo G. Normotensive ischemic acute renal failure. *N Engl J Med*. 2007;357:797–805.
87. Jones A, Shapiro NI, Trzeciak S, et al. Lactate clearance vs central venous oxygen saturation as goals of early sepsis therapy: a randomized clinical trial. *JAMA*. 2010;303:739–746.
88. Jansen T, van Bommel J, Schoonderbeek FJ, et al. Early lactate-guided therapy in intensive care unit patients: a multicenter, open-label randomized controlled trial. *Am J Respir Crit Care Med*. 2010;182:752–761.
89. Hernandez G, Bellomo R, Bakker J. The ten pitfalls of lactate clearance in sepsis. *Intensive Care Med*. 2019;45(1):82–85.
90. Reinhart K, Kuhn HJ, Hartog C, Bredle DL. Continuous central venous and pulmonary artery oxygen saturation monitoring in the critically ill. *Intensive Care Med*. 2004;30(8):1572–1578.
91. Pope J, Jones AE, Gaieski DF. Multicenter study of central venous oxygen saturation (ScvO2) as a predictor of mortality in patients with sepsis. *Ann Emerg Med*. 2010;55:40–46.
92. Feihl F, Perret C. Permissive hypercapnia. How permissive should we be? *Am J Respir Crit Care Med*. 1994;150(6 Pt 1):1722–1737.
93. Determann RM, Royakkers A, Wolthuis EK, et al. Ventilation with lower tidal volumes as compared with conventional tidal volumes for patients without acute lung injury: a preventive randomized controlled trial. *Crit Care*. 2010;14(1):R1.
94. Rochwerg B, Brochard L, Elliott MW, et al. Official ERS/ATS clinical practice guidelines: noninvasive ventilation for acute respiratory failure. *Eur Respir J*. 2017;50(2).
95. Frat JP, Thille AW, Mercat A, et al. High-flow oxygen through nasal cannula in acute hypoxemic respiratory failure. *N Engl J Med*. 2015;372(23):2185–2196.
96. Esteban A, Frutos F, Tobin MJ, et al. A comparison of four methods of weaning patients from mechanical ventilation. Spanish Lung Failure Collaborative Group. *N Engl J Med*. 1995;332(6):345–350.
97. Girard TD, Alhazzani W, Kress JP, et al. An Official American Thoracic Society/American College of Chest Physicians Clinical Practice Guideline: Liberation from Mechanical Ventilation in Critically Ill Adults. Rehabilitation Protocols, Ventilator Liberation Protocols, and Cuff Leak Tests. *Am J Respir Crit Care Med*. 2017;195(1):120–133.
98. Schuster DP. What is acute lung injury? What is ARDS? *Chest*. 1995;107(6):1721–1726.
99. Force ADT, Ranieri VM, Rubenfeld GD, et al. Acute respiratory distress syndrome: the Berlin Definition. *JAMA*. 2012;307(23):2526–2533.
100. Meyer NJ, Gattinoni L, Calfee CS. Acute respiratory distress syndrome. *Lancet*. 2021;398(10300):622–637.
101. Nuckton TJ, Alonso JA, Kallet RH, et al. Pulmonary dead-space fraction as a risk factor for death in the acute respiratory distress syndrome. *N Engl J Med*. 2002;346(17):1281–1286.
102. Brower RG, Matthay MA, Morris A, et al. Ventilation with lower tidal volumes as compared with traditional tidal volumes for acute lung injury and the acute respiratory distress syndrome. The Acute Respiratory Distress Syndrome Network. *N Engl J Med*. 2000;342(18):1301–1308.
103. Santa Cruz R, Rojas JI, Nervi R, Heredia R, Ciapponi A. High versus low positive end-expiratory pressure (PEEP) levels for mechanically ventilated adult patients with acute lung injury and acute respiratory distress syndrome. *Cochrane Database Syst Rev*. 2013;6:CD009098.
104. Sud S, Friedrich JO, Taccone P, et al. Prone ventilation reduces mortality in patients with acute respiratory failure and severe hypoxemia: systematic review and meta-analysis. *Intensive Care Med*. 2010;36(4):585–599.
105. Guerin C, Reignier J, Richard JC, et al. Prone positioning in severe acute respiratory distress syndrome. *N Engl J Med*. 2013;368(23):2159–2168.
106. Papazian L, Forel JM, Gacouin A, et al. Neuromuscular blockers in early acute respiratory distress syndrome. *N Engl J Med*. 2010;363:1107–1116.
107. National Heart L, Blood Institute P, Moss M, et al. Early neuromuscular blockade in the acute respiratory distress syndrome. *N Engl J Med*. 2019;380(21):1997–2008.
108. Fanelli V, Morita Y, Cappello P, et al. Neuromuscular blocking agent cisatracurium attenuates lung injury by inhibition of nicotinic acetylcholine receptor-alpha1. *Anesthesiology*. 2016;124(1):132–140.
109. Noah MA, Peek GJ, Finney SJ, et al. Referral to an extracorporeal membrane oxygenation center and mortality among patients with severe 2009 influenza A(H1N1). *JAMA*. 2011;306(15):1659–1668.
110. Peek GJ, Mugford M, Tiruvoipati R, et al. Efficacy and economic assessment of conventional ventilatory support versus extracorporeal membrane oxygenation for severe adult respiratory failure (CESAR): a multicentre randomised controlled trial. *Lancet*. 2009;374(9698):1351–1363.
111. Combes A, Hajage D, Capellier G, et al. Extracorporeal membrane oxygenation for severe acute respiratory distress syndrome. *N Engl J Med*. 2018;378(21):1965–1975.
112. Maitra S, Bhattacharjee S, Khanna P, Baidya DK. High-frequency ventilation does not provide mortality benefit in comparison with conventional lung-protective ventilation in acute respiratory distress syndrome: a meta-analysis of the randomized controlled trials. *Anesthesiology*. 2015;122(4):841–851.
113. Taylor RW, Zimmerman JL, Dellinger RP, et al. Low-dose inhaled nitric oxide in patients with acute lung injury: a randomized controlled trial. *JAMA*. 2004;291(13):1603–1609.
114. Gebistorf F, Karam O, Wetterslev J, Afshari A. Inhaled nitric oxide for acute respiratory distress syndrome (ARDS) in children and adults. *Cochrane Database Syst Rev*. 2016;2016(6):CD002787.
115. Fuller BM, Mohr NM, Skrupky L, et al. The use of inhaled prostaglandins in patients with ARDS: a systematic review and meta-analysis. *Chest*. 2015;147(6):1510–1522.
116. Wiedemann HP, Wheeler AP, Bernard GR, et al. Comparison of two fluid-management strategies in acute lung injury. *N Engl J Med*. 2006;354(24):2564–2575. (In eng).
117. Martin GS, Moss M, Wheeler AP, et al. A randomized, controlled trial of furosemide with or without albumin in hypoproteinemic patients with acute lung injury. *Crit Care Med*. 2005;33(8):1681–1687. (In eng).
118. Matthay MA, Brower RG, Carson S, et al. Randomized, placebo-controlled clinical trial of an aerosolized beta-agonist for treatment of acute lung injury. *Am J Respir Crit Care Med*. 2011;184(5):561–568.
119. Steinberg KP, Hudson LD, Goodman RB, et al. Efficacy and safety of corticosteroids for persistent acute respiratory distress syndrome. *N Engl J Med*. 2006;354(16):1671–1684.
120. Meduri GU, Golden E, Freire AX, et al. Methylprednisolone infusion in early severe ARDS: results of a randomized controlled trial. *Chest*. 2007;131(4):954–963.
121. Lansbury LE, Rodrigo C, Leonardi-Bee J, Nguyen-Van-Tam J, Shen Lim W. Corticosteroids as adjunctive therapy in the treatment of influenza: an updated cochrane systematic review and meta-analysis. *Crit Care Med*. 2020;48(2):e98–e106.
122. Group RC, Horby P, Lim WS, et al. Dexamethasone in hospitalized patients with Covid-19. *N Engl J Med*. 2021;384(8):693–704.
123. Bellomo R, Kellum JA, Ronco C. Acute kidney injury. *Lancet*. 2012;380(9843):756–766.
124. Bellomo R, Ronco C, Kellum JA, Mehta RL, Palevsky P. Acute Dialysis Quality Initiative w. Acute renal failure - definition, outcome measures, animal models, fluid therapy and information technology needs: the Second International Consensus Conference of the Acute Dialysis Quality Initiative (ADQI) Group. *Crit Care*. 2004;8(4):R204–12.
125. Mehta RL, Kellum JA, Shah SV, et al. Acute Kidney Injury Network: report of an initiative to improve outcomes in acute kidney injury. *Crit Care*. 2007;11(2):R31.
126. Kellum JA, Lameire N, Group K. Diagnosis, evaluation, and management of acute kidney injury: a KDIGO summary (Part 1). *Crit Care*. 2013;17(1):204.
127. Singri N, Ahya SN, Levin ML. Acute renal failure. *JAMA*. 2003;289(6):747–751.
128. Weisbord SD, Gallagher M, Jneid H, et al. Outcomes after angiography with sodium bicarbonate and acetylcysteine. *N Engl J Med*. 2018;378(7):603–614.
129. Palevsky PM, Zhang JH, O'Connor TZ, et al. Intensity of renal support in critically ill patients with acute kidney injury. *N Engl J Med*. 2008;359(1):7–20.
130. Bellomo R, Cass A, Cole L, et al. Intensity of continuous renal-replacement therapy in critically ill patients. *N Engl J Med*. 2009;361(17):1627–1638.
131. STARRT-AKI Investigators, Canadian Critical Care Trials Group, Australian and New Zealand Intensive Care Society Clinical Trials Group, et al. Timing of Initiation of Renal-Replacement Therapy in Acute Kidney Injury. *N Engl J Med*. 2020;383(3):240–251.
132. Vinsonneau C, Camus C, Combes A, et al. Continuous venovenous haemodiafiltration versus intermittent haemodialysis for acute renal failure in patients with multiple-organ dysfunction syndrome: a multicentre randomised trial. *Lancet*. 2006;368(9533):379–385.
133. Dungan KM, Braithwaite SS, Preiser JC. Stress hyperglycaemia. *Lancet*. 2009;373(9677):1798–1807.
134. van den Berghe G, Wouters P, Weekers F, et al. Intensive insulin therapy in critically ill patients. *N Engl J Med*. 2001;345(19):1359–1367.
135. Wiener RS, Wiener DC, Larson RJ. Benefits and risks of tight glucose control in critically ill adults: a meta-analysis. *JAMA*. 2008;300(8):933–944.
136. Finfer S, Chittock DR, Su SY, et al. Intensive versus conventional glucose control in critically ill patients. *N Engl J Med*. 2009;360(13):1283–1297.
137. Cooper MS, Stewart PM. Corticosteroid insufficiency in acutely ill patients. *N Engl J Med*. 2003;348(8):727–734.
138. Hamrahian AH, Oseni TS, Arafah BM Measurements of serum free cortisol in critically ill patients. *N Engl J Med*. 2004;350(16):1629–1638.
139. Lipiner-Friedman D, Sprung CL, Laterre PF, et al. Adrenal function in sepsis: the retrospective Corticus cohort study. *Crit Care Med*. 2007;35(4):1012–1018.
140. Venkatesh B, Finfer S, Cohen J, et al. Adjunctive glucocorticoid therapy in patients with septic shock. *N Engl J Med*. 2018;378(9):797–808.
141. Annane D, Renault A, Brun-Buisson C, et al. Hydrocortisone plus fludrocortisone for adults with septic shock. *N Engl J Med*. 2018;378(9):809–818.
142. Sprung CL, Annane D, Didier K, et al. Hydrocortisone therapy for patients with septic shock. *N Engl J Med*. 2008;358(2):111–124.
143. Annane D, Sebille V, Charpentier C, et al. Effect of treatment with low doses of hydrocortisone and fludrocortisone on mortality in patients with septic shock. *JAMA*. 2002;288(7):862–871.
144. Fang F, Zhang Y, Tang J, et al. Association of Corticosteroid Treatment With Outcomes in adult patients with sepsis: a systematic review and meta-analysis. *JAMA Intern Med*. 2019;179(2):213–223.
145. Van den Berghe G, de Zegher F, Lauwers P. Dopamine and the sick euthyroid syndrome in critical illness. *Clin Endocrinol (Oxf)*. 1994;41(6):731–737.
146. Van den Berghe G, de Zegher F, Bouillon R. Clinical review 95: Acute and prolonged critical illness as different neuroendocrine paradigms. *J Clin Endocrinol Metab*. 1998;83(6):1827–1834.

147. Bennett-Guerrero E, Jimenez JL, White WD, et al. Cardiovascular effects of intravenous triiodothyronine in patients undergoing coronary artery bypass graft surgery. A randomized, double-blind, placebo- controlled trial. Duke T3 study group. *JAMA.* 1996;275(9):687–692.
148. Takala J, Ruokonen E, Webster NR, et al. Increased mortality associated with growth hormone treatment in critically ill adults. *N Engl J Med.* 1999;341(11):785–792.
149. Cable CA, Razavi SA, Roback JD, Murphy DJ. RBC transfusion strategies in the ICU: a concise review. *Crit Care Med.* 2019;47(11):1637–1644.
150. Vincent JL, Baron JF, Reinhart K, et al. Anemia and blood transfusion in critically ill patients. *JAMA.* 2002;288(12):1499–507.
151. Corwin HL, Gettinger A, Pearl RG, et al. The CRIT Study: Anemia and blood transfusion in the critically ill–current clinical practice in the United States. *Crit Care Med.* 2004;32(1):39–52.
152. Rodriguez RM, Corwin HL, Gettinger A, et al. Nutritional deficiencies and blunted erythropoietin response as causes of the anemia of critical illness. *J Crit Care.* 2001;16(1):36–41.
153. Hebert PC, Wells G, Blajchman MA, et al. A multicenter, randomized, controlled clinical trial of transfusion requirements in critical care. Transfusion Requirements in Critical Care Investigators, Canadian Critical Care Trials Group. *N Engl J Med.* 1999;340(6):409–417.
154. Lacroix J, Hebert PC, Hutchison JS, et al. Transfusion strategies for patients in pediatric intensive care units. *N Engl J Med.* 2007;356(16):1609–1619.
155. Robertson CS, Hannay HJ, Yamal JM, et al. Effect of erythropoietin and transfusion threshold on neurological recovery after traumatic brain injury: a randomized clinical trial. *JAMA.* 2014;312(1):36–47.
156. Villanueva C, Colomo A, Bosch A, et al. Transfusion strategies for acute upper gastrointestinal bleeding. *N Engl J Med.* 2013;368(1):11–21.
157. Arabi YM, Aldawood AS, Haddad SH, et al. Permissive underfeeding or standard enteral feeding in critically ill adults. *N Engl J Med.* 2015;372(25):2398–2408.
158. Compher C, Bingham AL, McCall M, et al. Guidelines for the provision of nutrition support therapy in the adult critically ill patient: The American Society for Parenteral and Enteral Nutrition. *JPEN J Parenter Enteral Nutr.* 2022;46(1):12–41.
159. Marik PE, Zaloga GP. Gastric versus post-pyloric feeding: a systematic review. *Crit Care.* 2003;7(3):R46–51.
160. MacLeod JB, Lefton J, Houghton D, et al. Prospective randomized control trial of intermittent versus continuous gastric feeds for critically ill trauma patients. *J Trauma.* 2007;63(1):57–61. (In eng).
161. Casaer MP, Mesotten D, Hermans G, et al. Early versus late parenteral nutrition in critically ill adults. *N Engl J Med.* 2011;365(6):506–517.
162. Chen QH, Yang Y, He HL, et al. The effect of glutamine therapy on outcomes in critically ill patients: a meta-analysis of randomized controlled trials. *Crit Care.* 2014;18(1):R8.
163. Berger MM, Shenkin A, Schweinlin A, et al. ESPEN micronutrient guideline. *Clin Nutr.* 2022;41(6):1357–1424.
164. da Silva JSV, Seres DS, Sabino K, et al. ASPEN Consensus Recommendations for Refeeding Syndrome. *Nutr Clin Pract.* 2020;35(2):178–195.
165. Ely EW, Truman B, Shintani A, et al. Monitoring sedation status over time in ICU patients: reliability and validity of the Richmond Agitation-Sedation Scale (RASS). *JAMA.* 2003;289(22):2983–2991.
166. Shehabi Y, Howe BD, Bellomo R, et al. Early sedation with dexmedetomidine in critically ill patients. *N Engl J Med.* 2019;380(26):2506–2517.
167. Riker RR, Shehabi Y, Bokesch PM, et al. Dexmedetomidine vs midazolam for sedation of critically ill patients: a randomized trial. *JAMA.* 2009;301(5):489–499.
168. Hughes CG, Mailloux PT, Devlin JW, et al. Dexmedetomidine or propofol for sedation in mechanically ventilated adults with sepsis. *N Engl J Med.* 2021;384(15):1424–1436.
169. Jakob S, Ruokonen, E, Grounds, RM, et al. Dexmedetomidine vs midazolam or propofol for sedation during prolonged mechanical ventilation: two randomized controlled trials. *JAMA.* 2012;307:1151–1160.
170. Garcia R, Salluh JIF, Andrade TR, et al. A systematic review and meta-analysis of propofol versus midazolam sedation in adult intensive care (ICU) patients. *J Crit Care.* 2021;64:91–99.
171. Devlin JW, Skrobik Y, Gelinas C, et al. Clinical Practice Guidelines for the Prevention and Management of Pain, Agitation/Sedation, Delirium, Immobility, and Sleep Disruption in Adult Patients in the ICU. *Crit Care Med.* 2018;46(9):e825–e873.
172. Ely EW, Inouye SK, Bernard GR, et al. Delirium in mechanically ventilated patients: validity and reliability of the confusion assessment method for the intensive care unit (CAM-ICU). *JAMA.* 2001;286(21):2703–2710.
173. Brook AD, Ahrens TS, Schaiff R, et al. Effect of a nursing-implemented sedation protocol on the duration of mechanical ventilation. *Crit Care Med.* 1999;27(12):2609–2615.
174. Kollef M, Levy NT, Ahrens TS, et al. The use of continuous i.v. sedation is associated with prolongation of mechanical ventilation. *Chest.* 1998;114:541–548.
175. Girard TD, Kress JP, Fuchs BD, et al. Efficacy and safety of a paired sedation and ventilator weaning protocol for mechanically ventilated patients in intensive care (Awakening and Breathing Controlled trial): a randomised controlled trial. *Lancet.* 2008;371(9607):126–134.
176. Kress J, Pohlman, AS, O'Connor, MF, Hall JB. Daily interruption of sedative infusions in critically ill patients undergoing mechanical ventilation. *N Engl J Med.* 2000;342:1471–1477.
177. Samuelson K, Lundberg D, Fridlund B. Memory in relation to depth of sedation in adult mechanically ventilated intensive care patients. *Intensive Care Med.* 2006;32(5):660–667.
178. Girard TD, Shintani AK, Jackson JC, et al. Risk factors for post traumatic stress disorder symptoms following critical illness requiring mechanical ventilation: a prospective cohort study. *Crit Care.* 2007;11(1):R28. (Research Support, N.I.H., Extramural).
179. Pandharipande P, Girard, TD, Jackson, JC, et al. Long-term cognitive impairment after critical illness. *N Engl J Med.* 2013;369:1306–1316.
180. Vincent JL. Nosocomial infections in adult intensive-care units. *Lancet.* 2003;361(9374): 2068–2077.
181. Rouby JJ, Laurent P, Gosnach M, et al. Risk factors and clinical relevance of nosocomial maxillary sinusitis in the critically ill. *Am J Respir Crit Care Med.* 1994;150(3):776–783.
182. van Zanten AR, Dixon JM, Nipshagen MD, et al. Hospital-acquired sinusitis is a common cause of fever of unknown origin in orotracheally intubated critically ill patients. *Crit Care.* 2005;9(5):R583–590. (In eng).
183. Magill SS, Klompas M, Balk R, et al. Developing a new, national approach to surveillance for ventilator-associated events: executive summary. *Chest.* 2013;144(5):1448–1452.
184. Klein Klouwenberg PM, van Mourik MS, Ong DS, et al. Electronic implementation of a novel surveillance paradigm for ventilator-associated events. Feasibility and validation. *Am J Respir Crit Care Med.* 2014;189(8):947–955.
185. Klompas M, Anderson D, Trick W, et al. The preventability of ventilator-associated events. The CDC Prevention Epicenters Wake Up and Breathe Collaborative. *Am J Respir Crit Care Med.* 2015;191(3):292–301.
186. Bekaert M, Timsit JF, Vansteelandt S, et al. Attributable mortality of ventilator-associated pneumonia: a reappraisal using causal analysis. *Am J Respir Crit Care Med.* 2011;184(10):1133–1139. (Research Support, Non-U.S. Gov't) (In eng).
187. Muscedere J, Rewa O, McKechnie K, et al. Subglottic secretion drainage for the prevention of ventilator-associated pneumonia: a systematic review and meta-analysis. *Crit Care Med.* 2011;39(8):1985–1991.
188. Tokmaji G, Vermeulen H, Muller MC, et al. Silver-coated endotracheal tubes for prevention of ventilator-associated pneumonia in critically ill patients. *Cochrane Database Syst Rev.* 2015;8:CD009201.
189. Hammond NE, Myburgh J, Seppelt I, et al. Association Between Selective Decontamination of the Digestive Tract and In-Hospital Mortality in Intensive Care Unit Patients Receiving Mechanical Ventilation: A Systematic Review and Meta-analysis. *JAMA.* 2022;328(19):1922–1934.
190. Zhao T, Wu X, Zhang Q, et al. Oral hygiene care for critically ill patients to prevent ventilator-associated pneumonia. *Cochrane Database Syst Rev.* 2020;12(12):CD008367.
191. Kalil AC, Metersky ML, Klompas M, et al. Management of Adults With Hospital-acquired and Ventilator-associated Pneumonia: 2016 Clinical Practice Guidelines by the Infectious Diseases Society of America and the American Thoracic Society. *Clin Infect Dis.* 2016;63(5):e61–e111.
192. Pugh R, Grant C, Cooke RP, Dempsey G. Short-course versus prolonged-course antibiotic therapy for hospital-acquired pneumonia in critically ill adults. *Cochrane Database Syst Rev.* 2015;8:CD007577.
193. Renaud B, Brun-Buisson C. Outcomes of primary and catheter-related bacteremia. A cohort and case-control study in critically ill patients. *Am J Respir Crit Care Med.* 2001;163(7): 1584–1590.
194. O'Grady NP, Alexander M, Burns LA, et al. Guidelines for the prevention of intravascular catheter-related infections. *Clin Infect Dis.* 2011;52(9):e162–193.
195. Chong HY, Lai NM, Apisarnthanarak A, Chaiyakunapruk N. Comparative Efficacy of Antimicrobial Central Venous Catheters in Reducing Catheter-Related Bloodstream Infections in Adults: Abridged Cochrane Systematic Review and Network Meta-Analysis. *Clin Infect Dis.* 2017;64(suppl_2):S131–S140.
196. Marik PE, Flemmer M, Harrison W. The risk of catheter-related bloodstream infection with femoral venous catheters as compared to subclavian and internal jugular venous catheters: a systematic review of the literature and meta-analysis. *Crit Care Med.* 2012;40(8):2479–2485.
197. Chenoweth CE. Urinary tract infections: 2021 update. *Infect Dis Clin North Am.* 2021;35(4): 857–870.
198. McCarty TP, White CM, Pappas PG. Candidemia and invasive candidiasis. *Infect Dis Clin North Am.* 2021;35(2):389–413.
199. Suleyman G, Alangaden GJ. Nosocomial fungal infections: epidemiology, infection control, and prevention. *Infect Dis Clin North Am.* 2021;35(4):1027–1053.
200. Cook DJ, Fuller HD, Guyatt GH, et al. Risk factors for gastrointestinal bleeding in critically ill patients. Canadian Critical Care Trials Group. *N Engl J Med.* 1994;330(6):377–381.
201. Australian PIft, New Zealand Intensive Care Society Clinical Trials Group AHSCCSCN, the Irish Critical Care Trials G, et al. Effect of Stress Ulcer Prophylaxis With Proton Pump Inhibitors vs Histamine-2 Receptor Blockers on In-Hospital Mortality Among ICU Patients Receiving Invasive Mechanical Ventilation: The PEPTIC Randomized Clinical Trial. *JAMA.* 2020;323(7):616–626.
202. Krag M, Perner A, Wetterslev J, et al. Stress ulcer prophylaxis versus placebo or no prophylaxis in critically ill patients. A systematic review of randomised clinical trials with meta-analysis and trial sequential analysis. *Intensive Care Med.* 2014;40(1):11–22.
203. Geerts W, Selby R. Prevention of venous thromboembolism in the ICU. *Chest.* 2003;124(6 Suppl):357S–363S.
204. Joffe HV, Goldhaber SZ. Upper-extremity deep vein thrombosis. *Circulation.* 2002;106(14): 1874–1880.

205. Holbrook A, Schulman S, Witt DM, et al. Evidence-based management of anticoagulant therapy: Antithrombotic Therapy and Prevention of Thrombosis, 9th ed: American College of Chest Physicians Evidence-Based Clinical Practice Guidelines. *Chest*. 2012;141(2 Suppl): e152S–84S.
206. Kearon C, Ginsberg JS, Hirsh J. The role of venous ultrasonography in the diagnosis of suspected deep venous thrombosis and pulmonary embolism. *Ann Intern Med*. 1998;129(12): 1044–1049.
207. Anderson DR, Kahn SR, Rodger MA, et al. Computed tomographic pulmonary angiography vs ventilation-perfusion lung scanning in patients with suspected pulmonary embolism: a randomized controlled trial. *JAMA*. 2007;298(23):2743–2753.
208. Hermans G, Van den Berghe G. Clinical review: intensive care unit acquired weakness. *Crit Care*. 2015;19:274.
209. Farhan H, Moreno-Duarte I, Latronico N, Zafonte R, Eikermann M. Acquired muscle weakness in the surgical intensive care unit: nosology, epidemiology, diagnosis, and prevention. *Anesthesiology*. 2016;124(1):207–234.
210. Hermans G, De Jonghe B, Bruyninckx F, Van den Berghe G. Interventions for preventing critical illness polyneuropathy and critical illness myopathy. *Cochrane Database Syst Rev*. 2014;1:CD006832.
211. Alhazzani W, Alenezi F, Jaeschke RZ, Moayyedi P, Cook DJ. Proton pump inhibitors versus histamine 2 receptor antagonists for stress ulcer prophylaxis in critically ill patients: a systematic review and meta-analysis. *Crit Care Med*. 2013;41(3):693–705.
212. Angus DC, Barnato AE, Linde-Zwirble WT, et al. Use of intensive care at the end of life in the United States: an epidemiologic study. *Crit Care Med*. 2004;32(3):638–643.
213. Committee on Approaching Death: Addressing Key End of Life Issues; Institute of Medicine. Dying in America: Improving Quality and Honoring Individual Preferences Near the End of Life. *Institute of Medicine*. http://www.nap.edu/read/18748/chapter/1.
214. Vincent JL, Moreno R, Takala J, et al. The SOFA (Sepsis-related Organ Failure Assessment) score to describe organ dysfunction/failure. On behalf of the Working Group on Sepsis-Related Problems of the European Society of Intensive Care Medicine. *Intensive Care Med*. 1996;22(7): 707–710.

58 Cardiopulmonary Resuscitation

ELIZABETH H. SINZ • CHARLES W. OTTO

KEY POINTS

1 Brain adenosine triphosphate is depleted after 4 to 6 minutes of no blood flow. It returns to nearly normal within 6 minutes of starting effective cardiopulmonary resuscitation (CPR).

2 The major components of resuscitation from cardiac arrest are airway, breathing, circulation, drugs, and electrical therapy (ABCDE).

3 Currently the two dominant theories for the mechanism of blood flow during closed-chest compressions are: cardiac pump and thoracic pump.

4 During CPR, myocardial perfusion is 20% to 50% of normal, whereas cerebral perfusion is maintained at 50% to 90% of normal.

5 Approximately 1.2% of adults admitted to U.S. hospitals suffer in-hospital cardiac arrest (IHCA). Outcomes from IHCA continue to improve with a current survival rate of 25%—significantly better than the outcomes from out-of-hospital cardiac arrest (OHCA), which carries a survival rate of 10%. The rate of survival after perioperative cardiac arrest is much higher—about 40%.

6 End-tidal carbon dioxide is an excellent noninvasive and readily available monitor of the effectiveness of closed-chest compressions.

7 Effective uninterrupted chest compressions and defibrillation should take precedence over medications when cardiac arrest is due to ventricular fibrillation or ventricular tachycardia. Effective chest compressions and epinephrine are the primary treatment for cardiac arrest with a nonshockable rhythm. The underlying cause of cardiac arrest should be identified concurrently and immediately reversed if possible.

8 Although there is limited evidence that vasopressors result in better early restoration of spontaneous circulation, there is no strong evidence that they improve long-term survival in cardiac arrest.

9 After vasopressors, the drugs most likely to be of benefit during CPR are those that help suppress ectopic ventricular rhythms.

10 Ventricular fibrillation is the most common electrocardiogram pattern found during witnessed sudden cardiac arrest in adults.

11 Untreated ventricular fibrillation is a time-sensitive model with three phases: electrical, circulatory, and metabolic.

12 In the pediatric age group, cardiac arrest is more likely related to progressive deterioration of respiratory and circulatory function and less likely to be a sudden event.

13 For optimal outcome, successful restoration of spontaneous circulation must be followed by correction of reversible causes of arrest, including immediate coronary reperfusion and aggressive supportive care.

14 Excellent teamwork and communication are key for leveraging procedural skills, resuscitation expertise, and diagnostic acumen during and after a cardiac arrest.

15 Patients have the right to place limitations on medical treatment, including establishing do-not-resuscitate orders, even while undergoing surgical procedures, particularly palliative procedures. Anesthesiologists must be prepared to provide informed consent that includes matching the patient's goals of care with requested limitations on resuscitative interventions.

Treatment of cardiac and respiratory arrest is an integral part of anesthesia practice. The American Board of Anesthesiology states in its *Policy Booklet for 2022* that the "clinical management and teaching of cardiac, pulmonary, and neurologic resuscitation" are among the activities that define the specialty of anesthesiology.[1] The cardiopulmonary physiology and pharmacology that form the basis of anesthesia practice are applicable to treating the victim of cardiac arrest. However, there is specialized knowledge relating to blood flow, ventilation, and pharmacology under the conditions of cardiac arrest that must be understood. In addition, it is important for anesthesiologists to differentiate the general term "resuscitation" as it applies to usual practice versus the specific use of this term in the context of cardiac arrest. This chapter concentrates on those aspects of cardiopulmonary resuscitation (CPR) that are different from the more common circumstances requiring cardiovascular support (e.g., shock, dysrhythmias).

History

Anesthesiologists have contributed many of the elements of modern CPR and continue to be active investigators and teachers in the field. Discoveries leading to current CPR practice have a long history recorded in many famous works.[2,3] The earliest reference may be the Bible story of Elisha breathing life back into the son of a Shunammite woman (2 Kings 4:34). In 1543, Andreas Vesalius[4] described tracheotomy and artificial ventilation. William Harvey's manual manipulation of the heart is well known. Early teaching of resuscitation was organized by the Society for the Recovery of Persons Apparently Drowned, founded in London in 1774.

Modern CPR developed primarily from the fortuitous assemblage of innovative clinicians and researchers in Baltimore in the 1950s and early 1960s. Building on the long history of contributions from around the world, these investigators laid the framework for current CPR practice. In the late 1950s, mouth-to-mouth ventilation was established as an effective means of artificial ventilation.[5–9] The internal defibrillator was developed in 1933,[10] but it was not applied successfully until 1947.[11] It was another decade before general use was made possible by the development of external cross-chest defibrillation.[12,13] Despite these advances, widespread resuscitation from cardiac arrest was not possible until Kouwenhoven et al.[14] described success with closed-chest cardiac massage in a series of patients. The final major component of modern CPR was added in 1963, when Redding and Pearson[15] described improved success of obtaining return of spontaneous circulation (ROSC) with administration of vasopressor drugs.

Scope of the Problem

Cardiovascular disease remains the most common cause of death in the industrialized world. Although cardiovascular mortality has been declining in the United States since the mid-1960s,[16,17] there are over 350,000 out-of-hospital cardiac arrests and over 290,000 in-hospital cardiac arrests (IHCAs) per year in the United States with survival rates of 10% and 25%, respectively. In 2019, there were 550,000 deaths due to ischemic heart disease.[18] Thus, CPR teaching and research tend to focus on myocardial ischemia as the primary cause of cardiac arrest. However, anesthesiologists are more likely than other practitioners to deal with cardiac arrest from causes other than myocardial infarction.[19,20] CPR is symptomatic therapy, aimed at sustaining vital organ function until natural cardiac function is restored. The details of effective resuscitation technique are critical to sustain the patient while searching for a remediable cause of the arrest, as this is essential for postresuscitation survival.

Brain adenosine triphosphate (ATP) is depleted after 4 to 1
6 minutes of no blood flow. It returns to nearly normal within 6 minutes of starting effective CPR. Studies in animals suggest that good neurologic outcome may be possible after 10- to 15-minute periods of normothermic cardiac arrest if good circulation is promptly restored.[21,22] In clinical practice, the severity of the underlying cardiac disease is the major determining factor in the success or failure of resuscitation attempts. Of those factors potentially under control of the rescuers, poor outcomes are associated with long arrest times before CPR is begun, prolonged ventricular fibrillation (VF) without definitive therapy, and inadequate coronary and cerebral perfusion during cardiac massage. In emergency medical services-treated out-of-hospital treated cardiac arrests (OHCA), CPR begun by bystanders can more than double survival.[23,24] Although efforts to provide layperson training, dispatch-assisted CPR, and other measures have had a positive impact,[25] bystanders provide CPR only about 40% of the time in sudden cardiac arrest. Optimal outcome from VF is obtained if basic life support (BLS) is begun within 4 minutes of arrest and defibrillation applied within 8 minutes.[26] The importance of early defibrillation has been known for decades and is emphasized in CPR training.[27,28] What is increasingly recognized is the tendency to interrupt chest compressions frequently during a resuscitation attempt and the severe detrimental effects of this practice. Studies of emergency medical systems (EMS) in the mid-2000s suggested that chest compressions were performed less than half of the time during a typical out-of-hospital resuscitation, being interrupted for pulse checks, intubations, starting intravenous catheters, defibrillation attempts, and moving the victim.[29,30] Because blood flow falls rapidly with cessation of compressions and resumes slowly with reinstitution of compressions, these interruptions are a major contributor to poor survival rates.

In a study in casinos, where arrests are typically "witnessed" on security cameras, victims that received the first defibrillation shock with an AED within 3 minutes of collapse, followed by an effective rapid-response EMS, had a resuscitation rate of 74%,[29] although the median reported survival to discharge with any first recorded rhythm is often much worse.[23] With an estimated 292,000 adult IHCAs and 15,200 pediatric in-hospital arrests each year in the United States,[31] rates for survival to discharge are about 25% in adults[32] and 40% in children,[33] although there is wide variability.[16,18,34,35] Within the hospital, the operating room (OR) is the location where CPR has the highest rate of success. In previous research, cardiac arrest has been reported to occur approximately seven times for every 10,000 anesthetics.[36] When cardiac arrest is anesthesia-related, resuscitation was successful approximately 90% of the time. However, data from the American College of Surgery National Surgical Quality improvement Program database includes a narrower subset of anesthetics with a wider variety of causes. This data reports a much higher incidence of perioperative cardiac arrest, with one event for every 203 surgical patients and over 70% of these patients dying within a month.[37]

Components of Resuscitation

The major components of resuscitation from cardiac arrest are air- 2
way, breathing, circulation, drugs, and electrical therapy (ABCDE). Traditionally, these have been divided into two categories: BLS and advanced cardiac life support (ACLS). BLS entails elements that can be performed without additional equipment—basic airway management, rescue breathing, and manual chest compressions. BLS has evolved with the increasing availability of public-access

automatic external defibrillators (AEDs) and the recognition that careful attention to uninterrupted, effective chest compressions improves outcome more than any advanced therapy. In fact, the foundation of proficient ACLS is immediate and exquisite BLS. In the following sections, each of the components involved in resuscitation will be reviewed separately, followed by a discussion of combining the elements to achieve the best outcome.

Airway Management

The problem of airway obstruction caused by the tongue in the unconscious patient is familiar to the anesthesiologist. The techniques used for airway maintenance during anesthesia are applicable to the cardiac arrest victim. The primary method recommended to the public is the same head tilt–chin lift method commonly employed in the OR.[38] The head is extended by pressure applied to the brow while the mandible is pulled forward by pressure on the front of the jaw, lifting the tongue away from the posterior pharynx. The jaw thrust maneuver (applying pressure behind the rami of the mandible) is an effective alternative. Properly inserted oropharyngeal or nasopharyngeal airways can be useful, recognizing the danger of inducing vomiting or laryngospasm in the semiconscious victim. Supraglottic airways (e.g., laryngeal mask airway, laryngeal tube, King airway, etc.; see Chapter 28) have approximately equal outcomes compared to tracheal intubation based on a review of multiple studies.[39] Tracheal intubation provides the best airway control, preventing aspiration, and allowing the most effective ventilation. However, it should not interfere with chest compressions unless absolutely necessary. In some patients, mask ventilation or a supraglottic airway may provide the best emergency management. When other methods of establishing an airway are unsuccessful, emergency front of neck access (eFONA, e.g., tracheotomy or cricothyroidotomy) may be necessary.[40] As airway experts, anesthesiologists should have a fundamental understanding of surgical airway management and basic skills to obtain emergency FONA if required.

Foreign-Body Airway Obstruction

In 2020, unintentional choking or suffocation accounted for 5,000 deaths in the United States, with the majority of deaths in the elderly, but also a significant number in young children.[41] Airway occlusion by a foreign object must be considered in any victim who suddenly stops breathing and becomes cyanotic and unconscious. It occurs most commonly during eating and is usually due to food—especially meat—impacting the laryngeal inlet at the epiglottis or in the vallecula. Poorly chewed pieces of food, poor dentition or dentures, and elevated blood alcohol levels are the most common factors contributing to choking. The signs of total airway obstruction are the lack of air movement despite respiratory efforts and the inability of the victim to speak or cough. Partial airway obstruction will result in rasping or wheezing respirations accompanied by coughing. If the victim has good air movement and can cough forcefully, no intervention is indicated. However, if the cough weakens or cyanosis develops, the patient must be treated as if complete obstruction is present.

Parents and friends have been pounding on the backs of choking victims for centuries. In 1974, Heimlich[42] proposed abdominal thrusts as a better method of relieving airway obstruction and, in 1976, Guildner et al.[38] reported that sternal thrusts were just as effective. Subsequently, there were multiple studies of these maneuvers. In clinical practice, Redding[43] observed that no maneuver was always successful and that each occasionally was successful when another had failed. Back blows are applied directly over the thoracic spine between the scapulae. They must be delivered with force. Placing the victim in a head-down position (e.g., leaning over a chair) may help move the obstruction into the pharynx. If the first attempt is unsuccessful, repeated attempts should be made because hypoxia-related muscular relaxation may eventually allow success.

For the awake victim, abdominal thrusts are applied in the erect position (sitting or standing). The rescuer reaches around the victim from behind, placing the fist of one hand in the epigastrium between the xiphoid and umbilicus. The fist is grasped with the other hand and pressed into the epigastrium with a quick upward thrust. In the unconscious, thrusts are applied by kneeling astride the victim, placing the heel of one hand in the epigastrium and the other on top of the first hand. Care must be taken to ensure the xiphoid is not pushed into the abdominal contents and that the thrust is in the midline.

Sternal thrusts are valuable in victims who are massively obese or have an advanced pregnancy. In the erect victim, the chest is encircled from behind, as in the abdominal maneuver, but the fist is placed in the midsternum. For the unconscious, thrusts are applied from the side of the supine victim with a hand position the same as for external cardiac compression.

Complications of thrust maneuvers include laceration of the liver and spleen, gastric rupture, fractured ribs, and regurgitation. Emergency FONA may be indicated, and prehospital providers are commonly trained to perform this procedure in a timely manner.[44] EMS should be summoned concurrently with dislodgement attempts.

Ventilation

The standard approach to the unresponsive victim is to follow opening of the airway with ventilation. When ventilation is provided in the nonclinical setting, mouth-to-mouth or mouth-to-nose ventilation is the most expeditious and effective method immediately available. Although inspired gas with this method will contain approximately 4% carbon dioxide and 17% oxygen (composition of exhaled air), it is sufficient to maintain viability. In the clinical setting, positive-pressure rescue breaths are provided using a bag-mask apparatus. Some clinicians carry a face mask for out-of-hospital mouth-to-mask use in an emergency.

Physiology of Ventilation during Cardiopulmonary Resuscitation

In the absence of an endotracheal tube, the distribution of gas between the lungs and stomach during positive-pressure ventilation will be determined by the relative impedance to flow into each (i.e., the opening pressure of the esophagus and the lung–thorax compliance). It is likely that esophageal opening pressure during cardiac arrest is no more than that found in anesthetized individuals (approximately 20 cm H_2O), and lung–thorax compliance is likely reduced. To avoid gastric insufflation, inspiratory airway pressures must be kept low.

Insufflation of air into the stomach during CPR leads to gastric distention, impeding ventilation and increasing the risk of regurgitation and gastric rupture. Avoiding gastric insufflation requires that peak inspiratory airway pressures stay below esophageal opening pressure. Partial airway obstruction by the tongue and pharyngeal tissues is a major cause of increased airway pressure contributing to gastric insufflation during CPR. Meticulous attention to airway management is necessary during rescue breathing. A tidal volume of 0.5 to 0.6 L will cause a noticeable rise in the chest wall in most adults. Each rescue breath should be given over 1 second during a pause in chest compressions.

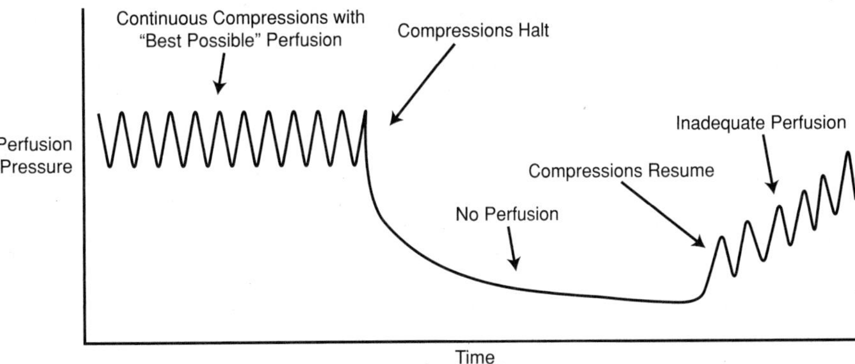

Figure 58-1 Perfusion abruptly decreases with cessation of chest compressions and returns gradually with resumption of compressions. (Reprinted from Cunningham LM, Mattu A, O'Connor RE, et al. Cardiopulmonary resuscitation for cardiac arrest: the importance of uninterrupted chest compressions in cardiac arrest resuscitation. *Am J Emerg Med.* 2012;30(8):1630–1638. Copyright © 2012 Elsevier. With permission. (Figure 2))

Techniques of Rescue Breathing

While maintaining an open airway with the head tilt–jaw lift technique, the hand on the forehead pinches the nose, the rescuer takes a normal breath, seals the victim's mouth with the lips, and exhales, watching for the chest to rise, indicating effective ventilation. For exhalation, the rescuer's mouth is removed from the victim, and the rescuer listens for escaping air while taking a breath. When both hands are being used in the jaw thrust maneuver of opening the airway, the cheek is used to seal the nose. For mouth-to-nose ventilation, the rescuer's lips surround the nose and the victim's lips are held closed. In some patients, the mouth must be allowed to open for exhalation with this technique. Give one breath over 1 second, take a normal breath, and give a second breath over 1 second. During CPR in adults and one-rescuer CPR in children, a pause for two breaths should be made after each 30 chest compressions. When there are two rescuers with a child victim, a pause for two breaths should be made after each 15 compressions.[45]

Several adjuncts to ventilation are available. Perhaps the most useful adjunct is a common mask, such as that used for anesthesia. The mask can be applied to the face and held in place with the thumbs and index fingers while the other fingers are used to apply jaw thrust. Breathing into the connector port of the mask provides ventilation. Masks are also available with one-way valves that direct the victim's exhaled gas away from the rescuer.

The self-inflating resuscitation bag and mask are the most common adjuncts used in rescue vehicles and hospitals. Although these devices have the advantages of noncontact and ability to use supplemental oxygen, they have been shown to be difficult for a single rescuer to apply properly to prevent substantial gas leak while maintaining a patent airway.[46] Tidal volumes with mouth-to-mouth and mouth-to-mask ventilation are often greater than those with the resuscitation bag. It is now recommended that if this device is used, two individuals manage the airway: one to hold the mask and maintain head position and one to squeeze the bag.[47] The self-inflating resuscitation bag can also be used with supraglottic airways and endotracheal tubes.

Tracheal intubation provides the best control of ventilation without concern for gastric distention. With a supraglottic airway or an endotracheal tube in place, breathing can proceed without synchronizing ventilation with chest compressions. Blood flow during CPR slows rapidly when chest compressions are stopped and recovers slowly when they are resumed (Fig. 58-1).[48–50] Consequently, advanced airway placement should be accomplished without stopping chest compressions if possible, and a supraglottic airway may be the best method to achieve this goal. Following placement, no pause in chest compressions should be made for ventilation, and one ventilation should be delivered no more than every 6 seconds. Positive-pressure ventilation increases intrathoracic pressure, reducing venous return and preload and worsening cardiac output during chest compressions.[51] Studies have not clearly demonstrated that any type of advanced airway management during resuscitation improves outcome over the self-inflating resuscitation bag and mask.[52]

Circulation

Physiology of Circulation during Closed-Chest Compression

The mechanism of blood flow during chest compressions is not fully elucidated. Two theories of the mechanism of blood flow during closed-chest compression have been dominant: the cardiac pump mechanism and the thoracic pump mechanism.[53,54] Additional theories have been proposed, including the lung pump theory, the left atrial pump theory, and the respiratory pump theory.[55] These mechanisms are not mutually exclusive, and which mechanism predominates in humans continues to be debated. 3

Cardiac Pump Mechanism

The cardiac pump mechanism was originally proposed by Kouwenhoven et al.[54] and Jude et al.[56] According to this theory, pressure on the chest compresses the heart between the sternum and the spine. Compression raises the pressure in the ventricular chambers, closing the atrioventricular valves and ejecting blood into the lungs and aorta. During the relaxation phase of closed-chest compression, expansion of the thoracic cage causes a subatmospheric intrathoracic pressure, facilitating blood return to the heart. The mitral and tricuspid valves open, allowing blood to fill the ventricles. Pressure in the aorta causes aortic valve closure and coronary artery perfusion. Chest compressions essentially replace the natural "squeeze" of heart muscle but the heart still functions as the pump.

The clinical implication of this mechanism is that it is critical to achieve an adequate compression depth to optimize the amount of blood ejected from the heart and equally important for full release after each compression to allow the heart to fill with blood.

Thoracic Pump Mechanism

In 1976, Criley et al.[57] reported a patient undergoing cardiac catheterization who simultaneously developed VF and an episode of cough-hiccups. With every cough-hiccup, a significant arterial pressure was noted. This led to the theory of a thoracic pump mechanism for blood flow during closed-chest compressions.[53] According to this theory, blood flows into the thorax during the relaxation phase of chest compressions in the same manner as that described for the cardiac pump mechanism. During the compression phase, all intrathoracic structures are compressed equally by the rise in intrathoracic pressure caused by sternal depression, forcing blood out of the chest. Backward flow through the venous system is prevented by valves in the subclavian and internal jugular veins and by dynamic compression of the veins at the thoracic outlet due to the increased intrathoracic pressure. Thicker, less compressible vessel walls prevent collapse on the arterial side, although arterial collapse will occur if intrathoracic pressure is raised enough.[58] The heart is a passive conduit with the atrioventricular valves remaining open during chest compressions. Because there is a significant pressure difference between the carotid artery and jugular vein, blood flow to the head is favored. The lack of valves in the inferior vena cava results in less resistance to backward flow, and pressures in the arteries and veins below the diaphragm are nearly equal. This is consistent with the fact that there is little blood flow to organs below the diaphragm.[59,60] One clinical correlate of this theory is that positive-pressure ventilation can adversely affect cardiac output, consistent with studies demonstrating increased mortality with excessive ventilations.

It seems clear that fluctuations in intrathoracic pressure play a significant role in blood flow during CPR. It is also likely that compression of the heart occurs under some circumstances. Factors that influence the mechanism probably include the compliance and configuration of the chest wall, size of the heart, force of the sternal compressions, duration of cardiac arrest, and other undiscovered factors. Recent investigations have demonstrated that younger patients are more often affected by cardiac pump issues while older patients are more affected by thoracic pump issues.[61]

Several other theories of blood flow mechanisms during CPR have been proposed, focusing on cardiopulmonary anatomy, pump action of the left atrium, and the vacuum effect created by the thorax. Variables such as time to initiate resuscitation, compression force and rate, body habitus, airway pressure, and presenting electrocardiogram also play a role. It is likely that the predominant mechanism of blood flow varies from victim to victim, perhaps with the predominant mechanisms changing during the resuscitation effort.[55]

Distribution of Blood Flow during Cardiopulmonary Resuscitation

4 Whatever the predominant mechanism, total body blood flow (cardiac output) is reduced from 10% to 33% of normal during experimental closed-chest cardiac massage. Similar severe reductions in flow are likely during clinical CPR in humans. Nearly all the blood flow is directed to organs above the diaphragm.[59,60] Myocardial perfusion is 20% to 50% of normal, whereas cerebral perfusion is maintained at 50% to 90% of normal. Abdominal visceral and lower extremity flow is reduced to 5% of normal. Total flow tends to decrease with time during CPR, but the relative distribution is not altered. Changes in CPR technique and the use of epinephrine may help sustain cardiac output over time.[60] Epinephrine improves blood flow to the brain and heart, whereas flow to organs below the diaphragm is unchanged or further reduced.

Gas Transport during Cardiopulmonary Resuscitation

During the low flow state of CPR, excretion of carbon dioxide (CO_2) (milliliters of CO_2 per minute in exhaled gas) is decreased from pre-arrest levels by approximately the same extent that cardiac output is reduced. This reduced CO_2 excretion is due primarily to shunting of blood flow away from the lower half of the body. The exhaled CO_2 reflects only the metabolism of the part of the body that is being perfused. In the nonperfused areas, CO_2 accumulates during CPR. When normal circulation is restored, the accumulated CO_2 is washed out, and a temporary increase in CO_2 excretion is observed.

Although CO_2 excretion is reduced during CPR, measurement of blood gases reveals an arterial respiratory alkalosis and a venous respiratory acidosis with a markedly elevated arteriovenous CO_2 difference.[62] The primary cause of these changes is the severely reduced cardiac output. Two factors account for the elevation of the venous partial pressure of CO_2 ($PvCO_2$). Buffering acid causes a reduction in serum bicarbonate, so the same blood CO_2 content results in a higher $PvCO_2$. In addition, the mixed venous CO_2 content is elevated. When flow to a tissue is reduced, all the CO_2 produced fails to be removed and CO_2 accumulates, raising the tissue partial pressure of CO_2. This allows more CO_2 to be carried in each aliquot of blood, and mixed venous CO_2 content increases. If flow remains constant, a new equilibrium is established in which all CO_2 produced in the tissue is removed but at a higher venous CO_2 content and partial pressure. In contrast to the venous blood, arterial CO_2 content and partial pressure ($PaCO_2$) are usually reduced during CPR. Although venous blood may have an increased CO_2, the marked reduction in cardiac output with maintained ventilation results in efficient CO_2 removal.

Decreased pulmonary blood flow during CPR causes a lack of perfusion to many nondependent alveoli. The alveolar gas of these lung units has no CO_2. Consequently, mixed alveolar CO_2 (i.e., end-tidal carbon dioxide [$ETCO_2$]) will be low and correlate poorly with arterial CO_2. However, $ETCO_2$ does correlate well with cardiac output during CPR.[63] As flow increases, more alveoli become perfused, there is less alveolar dead space, and $ETCO_2$ measurements rise.

Technique of Closed-Chest Compression

Cardiac arrest should be assumed in an unresponsive individual with abnormal or absent breathing. The community or institution emergency response system should immediately be activated and chest compressions begun. In emergency circumstances, it is difficult to detect a pulse, even in a major artery (carotid, femoral, axillary). No more than 10 seconds should be taken to check for a pulse and, if a pulse is not definitely felt, chest compressions should be started. Witnessed collapse with unresponsiveness in an adult in the absence of seizure activity is nearly always dysrhythmic cardiac arrest, and chest compressions should be started immediately.

Important considerations in performing closed-chest compressions are the position of the rescuer relative to the victim, the position of the rescuer's hands, and the rate and force of compression. The victim must be supine on a firm surface and the head level with the heart for adequate brain perfusion. The rescuer should stand or kneel next to the victim's side. Compressions are performed most effectively if the rescuer's hips are on the same level, or slightly above the level of the victim's chest.

Standard technique consists of the rhythmic application of pressure over the lower half of the sternum. The heel of one hand is placed on the lower sternum, and the other hand is placed on top of the first one. Great care must be taken to avoid pressing the xiphoid into the abdomen, which can lacerate the liver. Even with properly performed CPR, costochondral separation and rib fractures are common. Applying pressure on the ribs by improper hand placement increases these complications and risks puncturing the lung. Pressure on the sternum should be applied through the heel of the hand only, keeping the fingers free of the chest wall. The direction of force must be straight down on the sternum, with the arms straight and the elbows locked so the entire weight of the upper body is used to apply force. Inadequate chest recoil due to leaning on the chest during the relaxation phase has been demonstrated to be both common and deleterious to effective chest compressions. During relaxation, care must be taken to remove all pressure from the chest wall, but the hands should not lose contact with the chest wall.

The sternum must be depressed 5 to 6 cm (2 to 2½ in) in adults and teens. The duration of compression should be equal to that of relaxation, and the compression rate should be 100 to 120 times per minute. Push hard and push fast, minimizing interruptions in chest compressions. It is common practice to allow a brief pause for two 1-second breaths after every 30 compressions. However alternative approaches are in place, particularly in prehospital settings where the most common situation is an acute cardiac event and continuous chest compressions are performed until additional assistance is available. With an advanced airway in place, ventilations at a rate of 1 breath every 6 seconds should be interposed between compressions without a pause. It is important to avoid excessive ventilation in the patient with an advanced airway in place.

Alternative Methods of Circulatory Support

5 As currently practiced, CPR has limited success, with only approximately 40% of victims being admitted to the hospital and 10% surviving to discharge. Despite the occasional success of prolonged resuscitation, standard CPR will sustain most patients for only 15 to 30 minutes. If return of spontaneous circulation has not been achieved in that time, the outcome is dismal. Recognition of these limits and improved understanding of circulatory physiology during CPR have led to several proposals for alternatives to the standard techniques of closed-chest compression. The goals of the new methods are to provide better hemodynamics during CPR and thus improve survival and/or to extend the duration for which CPR can successfully support viability. Unfortunately, none of the alternatives has proved reliably superior to the standard technique.

Mechanical Chest Compression Devices

Following the description of "cough CPR" and the development of the thoracic pump theory, a pneumatic vest device was developed that would simulate the events of vigorous coughing.[64] The most common modification is the *load-distributing band (LDB)* device, which uses a pneumatically or electronically actuated circumferential constricting band and backboard.[65] A high-quality multicenter randomized controlled trial of the LDB versus manual CPR demonstrated equal survival to hospital discharge.[66] Case series also have used a number of piston-type devices to provide chest compressions with variable outcomes. The most commonly used is the *Lund University Cardiac Arrest System (LUCAS)* which is a gas (oxygen or air) or electric-powered piston that produces a consistent chest compression rate of 100/min and a compression depth of 5 cm and which incorporates a suction cup attached to the sternum to return the sternum to the starting position.[67] These devices can be useful in circumstances where manual compressions are difficult or dangerous to perform (e.g., in a moving ambulance, in the angiography suite, or during prolonged resuscitation attempts). However, it can take considerable time to deploy and remove the device, prolonging the time chest compressions are not being performed and worsening outcome. Their use requires a well-trained team that can minimize hands-off time while applying and removing the device.

Impedance Threshold Device

The impedance threshold device (ITD) is a valve that impedes air entry into the lungs during chest recoil of the relaxation phase of chest compressions, thus reducing intrathoracic pressure and increasing venous return to the thorax. Originally designed to be used with a cuffed endotracheal tube and active compression-decompression (ACD) CPR with a mechanical chest compression device (during which it would act to further increase the venous return of active decompression),[68] it can also be used with conventional CPR and a tight-fitting face mask or supraglottic airway.[69] Two randomized trials of OHCA comparing conventional CPR and the ITD with ACD CPR have shown improvement in short-term resuscitation.[68,70] One randomized trial of 8,718 OHCA victims undergoing standard CPR with an active versus sham ITD found no difference in short-term or long-term outcomes.[71] Although improved long-term survival has not been demonstrated, the ITD may be a useful adjunct for professionals trained in its use.

Invasive Techniques

In contrast to the closed-chest techniques, two invasive methods have been able to maintain cardiac and cerebral viability during long periods of cardiac arrest. In animal models, open-chest cardiac massage and extracorporeal CPR (ECPR) (cardiopulmonary bypass through the femoral artery and vein using a membrane oxygenator) can provide better hemodynamics, as well as better myocardial and cerebral perfusion, than closed-chest techniques.[72]

While open cardiac massage is primarily useful in situations where there are already personnel engaged with the skill set to perform this procedure, the increasing availability of emergency venoarterial extracorporeal membrane oxygenation (ECMO) has made extracorporeal cardiopulmonary resuscitation (ECPR) possible in many locations. ECPR provides perfusion and gas exchange while reversible causes of cardiac arrest are treated.[73] Predicting which patients will benefit from ECPR remains challenging, however younger patients with potentially reversible reasons for cardiac arrest and a short interval between arrest and initiation of CPR are most likely to benefit. Reversible causes can include acute coronary artery occlusion, pulmonary embolism, refractory VF, profound hypothermia, cardiac injury, cardiomyopathy, or drug intoxication. ECPR can also be a bridge to left ventricular assist device implantation or cardiac transplantation. Assessment for possible ECPR should be considered early and a request for assessment made after about 10 minutes of unsuccessful resuscitation[74] since observational studies[73] suggest that shorter time to ECPR initiation correlates with improved survival.[75] Excellent noninvasive CPR must be continued while ECPR is initiated.

Assessing the Adequacy of Circulation during Cardiopulmonary Resuscitation

The adequacy of closed-chest compression is frequently judged by palpation of a pulse in the carotid or femoral vessel. The palpable pulse primarily reflects systolic pressure and relates best to brain

Adult Cardiac Arrest Circular Algorithm

Start CPR
- Give oxygen
- Attach monitor/defibrillator

2 minutes

Return of Spontaneous Circulation (ROSC)

Check Rhythm

Post-Cardiac Arrest Care

If VF/pVT ***Shock***

Drug Therapy
IV/IO access
Epinephrine every 3-5 minutes
Amiodarone or lidocaine for refractory VF/pVT

Consider Advanced Airway
Quantitative waveform capnography

Treat Reversible Causes

Continuous CPR

Continuous CPR

Monitor CPR Quality

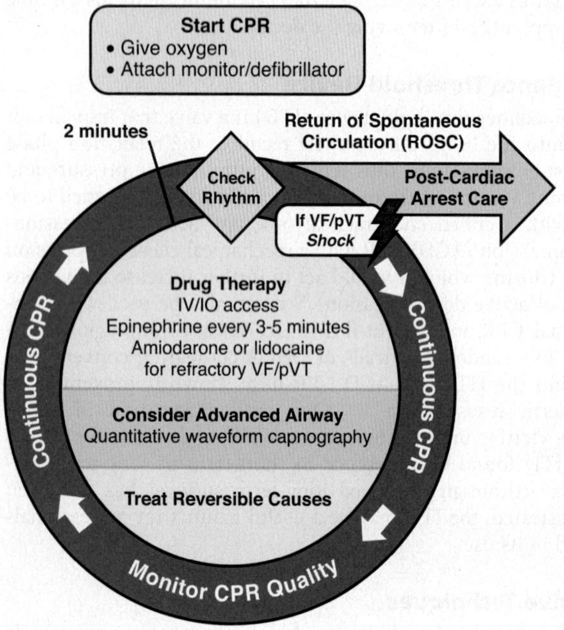

CPR Quality

- Push hard (at least 2 inches [5 cm]) and fast (100-120/min) and allow complete chest recoil.
- Minimize interruptions in compressions.
- Avoid excessive ventilation.
- Change compressor every 2 minutes, or sooner if fatigued.
- If no advanced airway, 30:2 compression-ventilation ratio.
- Quantitative waveform capnography
  – If $PETCO_2$ is low or decreasing, reassess CPR quality.

Shock Energy for Defibrillation

- **Biphasic:** Manufacturer recommendation (eg. initial dose of 120-200 J); if unknown, use maximum available. Second and subsequent doses should be equivalent, and higher doses may be considered.
- **Monophasic:** 360 J

Drug Therapy

- **Epinephrine IV/IO dose:** 1mg every 3-5 minutes
- **Amiodarone IV/IO dose:** First dose: 300 mg bolus. Second dose: 150 mg.
  or
- **Lidocaine IV/IO dose:** First dose: 1-1.5 mg/kg. Second dose: 0.5-0.75 mg/kg.

Advanced Airway

- Endotracheal intubation or supraglottic advanced airway
- Waveform capnography or capnometry to confirm and monitor ET tube placement
- Once advanced airway in place, give 1 breath every 6 seconds (10 breaths/min) with continuous chest compressions

Return of Spontaneous Circulation (ROSC)

- Pulse and blood pressure
- Abrupt sustained increase in $PETCO_2$ (typically ≥40 mm Hg)
- Spontaneous arterial pressure waves with intra-arterial monitoring

Reversible Causes

- Hypovolemia
- Hypoxia
- Hydrogen ion (acidosis)
- Hypo-/hyperkalemia
- Hypothermia
- Tension pneumothorax
- Tamponade, cardiac
- Toxins
- Thrombosis, pulmonary
- Thrombosis, coronary

Figure 58-2 Adult cardiac arrest circular algorithm. CPR, cardiopulmonary resuscitation; VF, ventricular fibrillation; VT, ventricular tachycardia; pVT, polymorphic ventricular tachycardia; IV, intravenous(ly); IO, intraosseous(ly); ET, endotracheal; $PETCO_2$, partial pressure of end tidal carbon dioxide; J, joules. (Reprinted with permission from 2020 American Heart Association Guidelines for CPR & ECC—Part 3: Adult Basic and Advanced Life Support. *Circulation*. 2020;142:S366–S468. © 2020 American Heart Association, Inc.)

perfusion. Cardiac output correlates better with mean pressure and coronary perfusion with diastolic pressure. In the femoral area, the palpable pulse is as likely to be venous as arterial. Whenever possible, more accurate means of monitoring the efficacy of chest compressions should be used such as $ETCO_2$ or arterial catheter if available. The importance of monitoring CPR quality is stressed in the AHA ACLS circular algorithm (Fig. 58-2).

Return of spontaneous circulation with an arrested heart greatly depends on restoring oxygenated blood flow to the myocardium. In experimental models, a minimum blood flow of 15 to 20 mL/min/100 g of myocardium has been shown to be necessary for successful resuscitation.[76] Obtaining such flow depends on closed-chest compressions developing adequate cardiac output and coronary perfusion pressure. Analogous to the beating heart, coronary perfusion during CPR occurs primarily in the relaxation phase (diastole) of chest compressions. In 1906, Crile and Dolley[77] suggested that a critical coronary perfusion pressure was necessary for successful resuscitation. This concept has been confirmed in numerous other reports.[60,76–86] During standard CPR, critical myocardial blood flow is associated with aortic diastolic pressure exceeding 40 mmHg. Because right atrial pressure can be elevated with some techniques, the aortic diastolic pressure minus the right atrial diastolic pressure is a more accurate reflection of coronary perfusion pressure. The critical coronary perfusion pressure is 15 to 25 mmHg. When invasive monitoring is available during CPR, adjustments in chest compression technique and epinephrine can ensure critical perfusion pressures are exceeded. Damage to the myocardium from underlying disease may preclude survival no matter how effective the CPR efforts. However, vascular pressures below critical levels are associated with poor results even in patients who may be salvageable (Table 58-1).

Although invasive pressure monitoring may be ideal, it is rarely available during CPR. $ETCO_2$ is readily available and is also an excellent noninvasive guide to the adequacy of closed-chest compressions.[87] CO_2 excretion during CPR with an endotracheal tube in place is flow-dependent rather than ventilation-dependent.

Table 58-1 Critical Variables Associated with Successful Resuscitation

Variable	Amount
Myocardial blood flow (mL/min/100 g)	>15–20
Aortic diastolic pressure (mmHg)	>40
Coronary perfusion pressure (mmHg)	>15–25
End-tidal carbon dioxide (mmHg)	>10

Because alveolar dead space is large in low-flow states, $ETCO_2$ is very low (frequently <10 mmHg). If blood flow improves with better CPR technique, more alveoli are perfused and $ETCO_2$ rises (usually to >20 mmHg with successful CPR). Often, the earliest sign of return of spontaneous circulation is a sudden increase in $ETCO_2$ to over 40 mmHg. Within a wide range of cardiac outputs during CPR, $ETCO_2$ correlates well with cardiac output,[88] coronary perfusion pressure,[89] and initial resuscitation.[90] $ETCO_2$ correlates with survival in human CPR and low $ETCO_2$ can predict a poor outcome.[91,92] Patients with $ETCO_2$ below 10 mmHg will not be resuscitated successfully. In the absence of invasive monitoring, whenever possible, $ETCO_2$ using continuous waveform capnography should be used to judge the effectiveness of chest compressions.[93] Attempts should be made to maximize the measured $ETCO_2$ by alterations in technique or drug therapy. It should be remembered that sodium bicarbonate administration liberates CO_2 into the blood and causes a temporary increase in $ETCO_2$. The elevation returns to baseline within 3 to 5 minutes of drug administration; for this period of time, $ETCO_2$ monitoring is not an accurate reflection of effectiveness of closed-chest compressions.

Pharmacologic Therapy

This discussion of drug therapy is confined to the use of drugs 7
during CPR attempts to restore spontaneous circulation. The 8
use of drugs to support the circulation when mechanical cardiac function is intact is discussed elsewhere (see Chapters 13 and 14). During cardiac arrest, drug therapy is secondary to other interventions. Effective uninterrupted chest compressions and defibrillation, if appropriate, should take precedence over medications. Establishing intravenous access and pharmacologic therapy should come as soon as possible but after these critical interventions are established. Although vasopressors are firmly established as improving survival in animal models, there is no strong evidence that they improve long-term survival in human cardiac arrest.[94,95] The most common drugs and the appropriate adult doses are shown in Table 58-2. In addition, pharmacologic and other therapeutic approaches for the treatment of bradycardia and tachycardia are shown in Figures 58-3 and 58-4. (See also 1 Video 58-1 and 2 Video 58-2.)

Routes of Administration

The preferred route of administration of drugs during CPR is intravenous. The most rapid and highest drug levels occur with administration into a central vein. However, peripheral intravenous administration is effective, and the antecubital and external jugular veins are preferred sites for starting an infusion during resuscitation because inserting a central catheter usually necessitates stopping CPR. Because of poor blood flow below the diaphragm during CPR, the distribution of intravenous drugs administered in the lower extremity may be extremely delayed. Even in the upper extremity, drugs may require 1 to 2 minutes to reach the central circulation. Onset of action may be accelerated if

Table 58-2 Adult Advanced Cardiac Life Support Drugs and Doses

Drug	Dose	Interval	Comment
Epinephrine	1 mg	Every 3–5 min or every other 2-min cycle of chest compressions	Target diastolic BP > 40 mmHg
Amiodarone	300 mg	May administer second dose of 150 mg after 5 minutes	
Lidocaine	1–1.15 mg/kg	Additional doses 0.5–0.75 mg/kg every 5 minutes	Maximum dose 3.0 mg/kg
Non-Routine Drugs	**Dose**	**Indications**	
Vasopressin	40 u	Known/suspected acidemia, prolonged resuscitation, or suspected pulmonary hypertension	Longer half-life than epinephrine
Sodium bicarbonate	1 mEq/kg	Acidemia, hyperkalemia, or overdose with tricyclic antidepressants or phenobarbital	Administration based on arterial pH of hyperkalemia
Calcium chloride	0.5–1.0 grams	Hypocalcemia (especially during large volume blood transfusion): hyperkalemia or hypermagnesemia; calcium channel blocker overdose	Repeat dosing based on ionized calcium levels or improved dynamics
Magnesium sulfate	1–2 grams	Torsades de pointes or known hypomagnesemia	
Lipid emulsion	1.5 ml/kg of 20% solution	Lipophilic drug toxicity such as local anesthetics (e.g. bupivacaine, tetracaine), beta-blockers (e.g. metoprolol, propranolol, pindolol), calcium-channel blockers (e.g. verapamil, diltiazem, nifedipine), or other lipophilic drugs (e.g. quetiapine, fluoxetine, lamotrigine, amitriptyline, bupropion, olanzapine)	Infuse 0.25 ml/kg min following bolus until toxin is cleared

Adult Bradycardia Algorithm

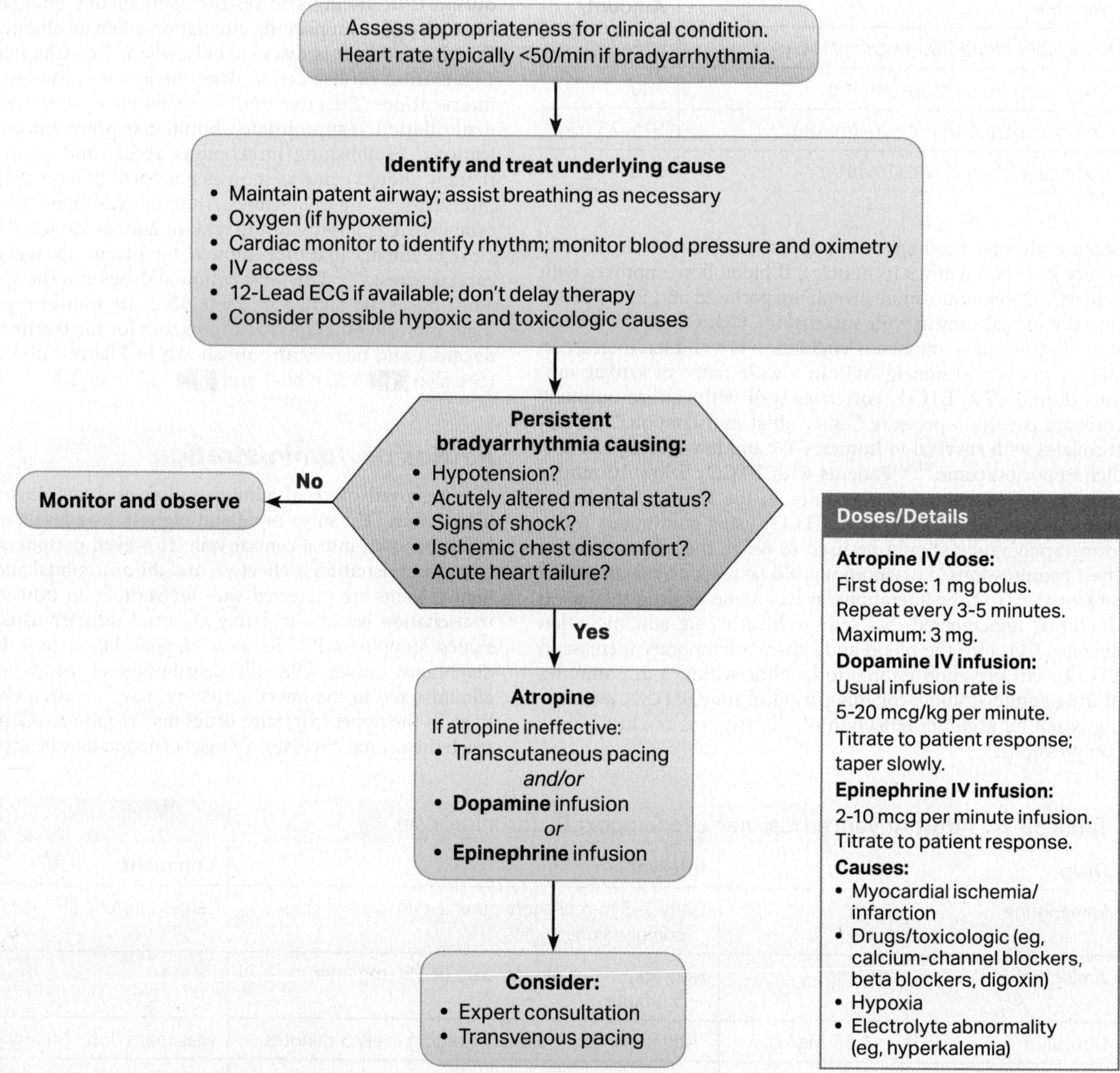

Figure 58-3 Adult bradycardia algorithm. ECG, electrocardiogram; IV, intravenous(ly). (Reprinted with permission, ACLS Advanced Cardiovascular Life Support Provider Manual. © 2020 American Heart Association, Inc.)

the drug bolus is followed by a 20- to 30-mL bolus of intravenous fluid.

Intraosseous (IO) administration of fluids and medications, especially into the proximal humerus, is a good alternative to intravenous cannulation, allowing drug delivery similar to that of intravenous administration.[96] IO access in the humerous may be rapidly obtained without stopping chest compressions, and administration at this site results in rapid transit to the central circulation. Flow rate via humeral IO access is about 100 cc/min under pressure, about six times the rate of tibial IO flow.[97] Care must be taken to avoid inadvertent dislodgement if the arm is repositioned or extended. Commercial kits are available to facilitate IO placement. Anesthesiologists should be familiar with IO access as a rapid alternative to venous access in an emergency and for a variety of other vascular access challenges.[98]

If IV or IO access cannot be established, the endotracheal tube is an alternative route for administration of epinephrine, vasopressin, lidocaine, and atropine. Sodium bicarbonate should not be given endotracheally. There are no data on endotracheal (ET) administration of amiodarone. The time to effect and drug levels achieved are inconsistent with endotracheal drug administration during CPR, so the optimal dose of drug is unknown using this route. In general, doses 2 to 2.5 times higher than the intravenous dose are recommended when this route is used. Better results may be obtained by flushing drug doses with 5 to 10 mL of normal saline. It is unclear whether intramuscular injection is better than simple instillation into the endotracheal tube.

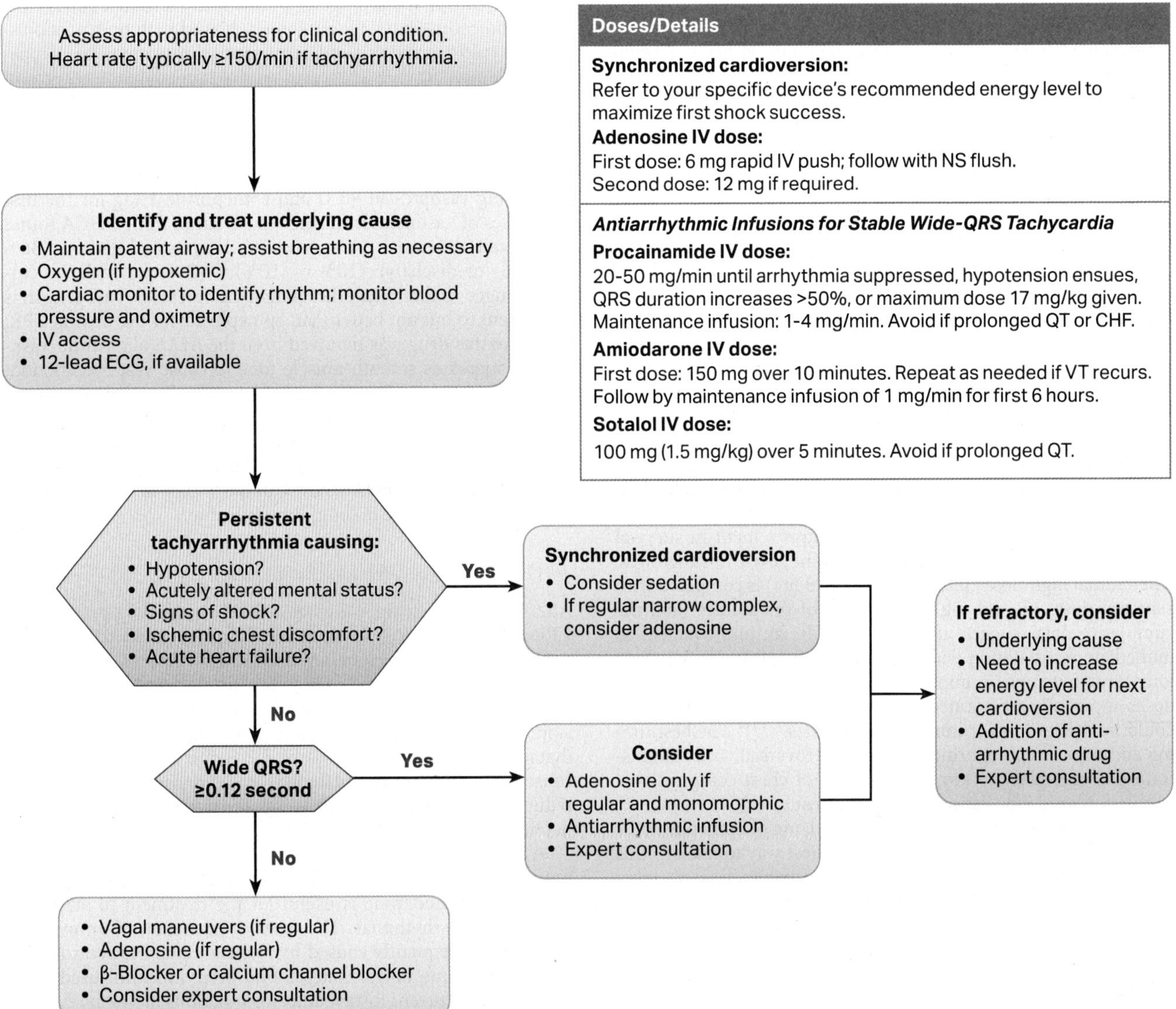

Figure 58-4 Adult tachycardia with a pulse algorithm. ECG, electrocardiogram; IV, intravenous(ly); CHF, congestive heart failure; J, joules; VT, ventricular tachycardia. (Reprinted with permission, ACLS Advanced Cardiovascular Life Support Provider Manual. © 2020 American Heart Association, Inc.)

Catecholamines and Vasopressors

Mechanism of Action

Epinephrine has been used in resuscitation since the 1890s and has been the vasopressor of choice in modern CPR since the studies of Redding and Pearson[15,99] in the 1960s. The efficacy of epinephrine lies entirely in its α-adrenergic properties[83] (see Chapter 13). Peripheral vasoconstriction leads to an increase in aortic diastolic pressure, causing an increase in coronary perfusion pressure and myocardial blood flow.[60,100,101] All strong α-adrenergic drugs (epinephrine, phenylephrine, methoxamine, dopamine, norepinephrine), regardless of β-adrenergic potency, are equally successful in aiding resuscitation, as are strong nonadrenergic vasopressors (vasopressin).[15,102–104] β-Adrenergic agonists without α activity (isoproterenol, dobutamine) are no better than placebo. α-Adrenergic blockade precludes resuscitation, whereas β-adrenergic blockade has no effect on the ability to restore spontaneous circulation.[80,81]

The β-adrenergic effects of epinephrine are potentially deleterious during cardiac arrest. In the fibrillating heart, epinephrine increases oxygen consumption and decreases the endocardial-to-epicardial blood flow ratio. Myocardial lactate production in the fibrillating heart is unchanged after epinephrine administration during CPR, suggesting that the increased coronary blood flow does not improve the oxygen supply-to-demand ratio. Large doses of epinephrine increase deaths in swine early after resuscitation because of tachyarrhythmias and hypertension, an effect partially offset by metoprolol administration. Despite these theoretical considerations, survival and neurologic outcome studies have shown no difference when epinephrine is used compared with a pure α-agonist (methoxamine or phenylephrine) during CPR in animals[99,105] or humans.[95,106]

Epinephrine

When added to chest compressions, epinephrine helps develop the critical coronary perfusion pressure necessary to provide enough myocardial blood flow for restoration of spontaneous circulation. With invasive monitoring present during CPR, an arterial diastolic pressure of 40 mmHg or coronary perfusion pressure of 20 mmHg must be obtained with good chest-compression technique and/or epinephrine therapy (Table 58-1). In the absence of such monitoring, the dose of epinephrine must be chosen empirically. Since the studies of Redding and Pearson[15,99] in the 1960s, the standard intravenous epinephrine dose used has been 0.5 to 1.0 mg. In the 1980s, animal studies suggested that higher doses of epinephrine might improve myocardial and cerebral perfusion and improve resuscitation success. Case reports and a series of children with historic controls were published, describing return of spontaneous circulation when large doses (0.1 to 0.2 mg/kg) of epinephrine were given to patients who had failed resuscitation with standard doses.

Subsequent outcome studies did not demonstrate conclusively that higher doses of epinephrine improve survival. Eight adult prospective randomized clinical trials involving more than 9,000 cardiac arrest patients found no improvement in survival to hospital discharge or neurologic outcome, even in subgroups, when initial high-dose epinephrine (5 to 18 mg) is compared with standard doses (1 to 2 mg).[106–113] Some of the studies (and the cumulative data) suggest that there may be an improvement in immediate resuscitation with high-dose epinephrine,[114] however long-term outcome is minimally improved at best.[115–118] High doses apparently are not needed early in most cardiac arrests and could be deleterious for long-term outcomes.[115,118] The best timing and dose of epinephrine remains controversial, and administration is secondary to key interventions of chest compressions, ventilation, or defibrillation in cardiac arrest.

Current recommendations are to give 1 mg of epinephrine IV every 3 to 5 minutes in the adult. The easiest way to manage this is to administer 1 mg of epinephrine approximately *every other* 2-minute cycle of CPR (i.e., about every 4 minutes). If this dose seems ineffective or in the setting of β-blocker or calcium channel blocker overdose, higher doses (3 to 7 mg) may be considered.

Vasopressin

Arginine vasopressin (antidiuretic hormone) has been used as an alternative to epinephrine in a dose of 40 U administered IV or IO (see Chapter 13). Vasopressin is a naturally occurring hormone that, when administered in high doses, is a potent nonadrenergic vasoconstrictor, acting by stimulation of smooth muscle V_1 receptors. The half-life in the intact circulation is 10 to 20 minutes and much longer than epinephrine during CPR. Animal studies have demonstrated that vasopressin is as effective as or more effective than epinephrine in maintaining vital organ blood flow during CPR. Repeated doses during prolonged CPR in swine were associated with significantly improved rates of neurologically intact survival compared with epinephrine and placebo. Postresuscitation myocardial depression and splanchnic blood flow reduction are more marked with vasopressin than epinephrine, but they are transient and can be treated with low doses of dopamine.[119] Clinical studies indicate that vasopressin is as effective as but not superior to epinephrine. A small randomized, blinded study comparing vasopressin and standard-dose epinephrine in 40 patients with out-of-hospital VF found improved 24-hour survival with vasopressin but no difference in return of spontaneous circulation or survival to hospital discharge.[120] A larger, clinical trial of 200 inpatients found no difference between the drugs in survival for 1 hour or to hospital discharge.[121] In this study, response times were short, indicating that CPR outcome achieved with both vasopressin and epinephrine in short-term cardiac arrest may be comparable. Compared with epinephrine, the hemodynamic effects of vasopressin are especially impressive during long cardiac arrests. Thus, vasopressin may find most use in prolonged resuscitation events, possibly due to its continued effectiveness in the setting of acidemia.[122,123] A multicenter, randomized study of 1,186 patients comparing vasopressin 40 U and epinephrine 1 mg for the first two doses of vasopressor during resuscitation from OHCA found no overall difference in survival to hospital admission (36% vs. 31%) or discharge (10% vs. 10%).[124] Overall, evidence currently suggests that, like other potent vasopressors, vasopressin is equivalent to but not better than epinephrine for use during CPR; therefore this drug was removed from the ACLS algorithm. Vasopressin increases smooth muscle tone to cause vasoconstriction, maintaining its potency despite acidosis and hypoxemia, in contrast to adrenergic pressors.[123] There may be a rationale for its use in cardiac arrest patients who are known to be acidemic pre-arrest or during prolonged cardiac arrest. The abysmal rate of recovery for this group of patients makes it unlikely that studies will reveal a statistical difference in long-term outcome.

Amiodarone and Lidocaine

After vasopressors, the drugs most likely to be of benefit during CPR are those that help suppress ectopic ventricular rhythms. Amiodarone and lidocaine are used during cardiac arrest to aid defibrillation when VF is refractory to electrical countershock therapy or when fibrillation recurs following successful conversion. Lidocaine, primarily an antiectopic agent with few hemodynamic effects, tends to reverse the reduction in VF threshold caused by ischemia or infarction. It depresses automaticity by reducing the slope of phase 4 depolarization and reducing the heterogeneity of ventricular refractoriness. 9

Amiodarone is a pharmacologically complex drug with sodium, potassium, calcium, and α-adrenergic and β-adrenergic blocking properties. Amiodarone is useful for the treatment of atrial and ventricular dysrhythmias. The initial formulation of intravenous amiodarone frequently caused hypotension and bradycardia due to the cosolvents polysorbate-80 and benzyl alcohol used in its preparation. Current intravenous formulations are hemodynamically and electrophysiologically inert and well tolerated.[125] There are three randomized, blinded, placebo-controlled clinical trials in shock-resistant cardiac arrest victims demonstrating improved survival to hospital with amiodarone treatment, although there was no difference in survival to discharge.[126–128] Although weak, this is more evidence of efficacy than exists for lidocaine.

When VF or pulseless ventricular tachycardia is recognized, defibrillation should be attempted (see Fig. 58-2). No antiarrhythmic agent has been shown to be superior to electrical defibrillation or more effective than placebo in the treatment of VF. Consequently, defibrillation should not be withheld or delayed to establish intravenous access or to administer drugs. When ventricular tachycardia or VF has not responded to or recurred following BLS, epinephrine, and defibrillation, amiodarone should be administered. In cardiac arrest, amiodarone is initially administered as a 300-mg rapid infusion. Supplemental infusions of 150 mg can be repeated as necessary for recurrent or resistant dysrhythmias to a maximum total daily dose of 2 g. (For dysrhythmias with an intact circulation, amiodarone is usually administered as 150 mg intravenously over 10 minutes, followed by a 1 mg/min infusion for

6 hours and 0.5 mg/min thereafter.) Lidocaine is no more effective than amiodarone in cardiac arrest but has few side effects. It is an alternative therapy in refractory fibrillation if amiodarone is not available. An initial bolus of 1 to 1.5 mg/kg should be given, and additional boluses of 0.5 to 0.75 mg/kg can be given every 5 to 10 minutes during CPR up to a total dose of 3 mg/kg.

Drugs Not Routinely Given during CPR

Atropine

Atropine sulfate enhances sinus node automaticity and atrioventricular conduction by its vagolytic effects. Although atropine has been given frequently during cardiac arrest associated with an electrocardiogram (ECG) pattern of asystole or slow pulseless electrical activity (PEA), neither animal nor human studies provide evidence that it actually improves outcome from asystolic or bradysystolic arrest.[129,130] The predominant cause of asystole and PEA is severe myocardial ischemia, and in particular situations (such as drowning and in the OR), this ischemia is typically due to profound hypoxia. Excessive parasympathetic tone probably contributes little to these rhythms during cardiac arrest in adults. Even in children, it is doubtful that parasympathetic tone plays a significant role during most arrests. Therefore, the most important treatment for asystole and PEA is effective chest compressions, ventilation, and epinephrine to improve coronary perfusion and myocardial oxygenation. There is no evidence that atropine is detrimental during cardiac arrest. However, routine use of atropine during cardiac arrest with these rhythms is unlikely to have benefit and is not recommended.

Sodium Bicarbonate

Although sodium bicarbonate was used commonly during CPR in the past, little evidence supports its efficacy. Use of sodium bicarbonate during resuscitation has been based on the theoretical considerations that acidosis lowers fibrillation threshold and impairs the physiologic response to catecholamines. But most studies have failed to demonstrate improved success of defibrillation or resuscitation with the use of bicarbonate.[131–136] The lack of effect of buffer therapy may be partially explained by the slow onset of metabolic acidosis during cardiac arrest. As measured by blood lactate or base deficit, acidosis does not become severe until 15 or 20 minutes of cardiac arrest.[62,137]

In contrast to the lack of evidence that buffer therapy during CPR improves survival, the adverse effects of excessive sodium bicarbonate administration are well documented. In the past, metabolic alkalosis, hypernatremia, and hyperosmolarity were common after administration of bicarbonate during resuscitation attempts.[137,138] These abnormalities are associated with low resuscitation rates and poor outcomes.

Intravenous sodium bicarbonate combines with a hydrogen ion to produce carbonic acid that dissociates into CO_2 and water. The partial pressure of CO_2 in blood is temporarily elevated until the excess CO_2 is eliminated through the lungs. Tissue acidosis during CPR is caused primarily by the low blood flow and accumulation of CO_2 in the tissues.[62] Therefore, concern has been expressed that the liberation of CO_2 by bicarbonate administration would only worsen the existing problem. This is of particular concern within myocardial cells and the brain. CO_2 readily diffuses across cell membranes and the blood–brain barrier, whereas bicarbonate diffuses much more slowly. Thus, it is possible that sodium bicarbonate administration could result in a paradoxical worsening of intracellular and cerebral acidosis by further raising intracellular and cerebral CO_2 without a balancing increase in bicarbonate. Direct evidence for this effect has not been found. Use of clinically relevant doses causes no change in spinal fluid acid–base status or myocardial intracellular pH during bicarbonate administration.[139,140] Therefore, paradoxical acidosis from sodium bicarbonate therapy remains a concern primarily on theoretical grounds.

Routine use of sodium bicarbonate is not recommended for patients in cardiac arrest. Current practice restricts its use to arrests associated with hyperkalemia, severe pre-existing metabolic acidosis, and tricyclic antidepressant or phenobarbital overdose. It may be considered for use in protracted resuscitation attempts after other modalities have been instituted and failed. When bicarbonate is used in these circumstances, the usual dose is 1 mEq/kg. However, dosing of sodium bicarbonate should be guided by blood–gas determination of acid–base status, whenever possible.

Calcium

With normal cardiovascular physiology, calcium increases myocardial contractility and enhances ventricular automaticity (see Chapter 12). Consequently, it has been advocated as a treatment for asystole and PEA. Early animal studies showed moderate success with calcium chloride in asphyxial arrest, although vasopressors were better.[15] In 1981, Dembo[141] reported dangerously high serum calcium levels (up to 18.2 mg/dL) during CPR and questioned the efficacy of calcium in cardiac arrest. Subsequently, several retrospective studies and prospective clinical trials during OHCA showed that calcium was no better than placebo in promoting resuscitation and survival from asystole or PEA.[142–146] Consequently, because of potentially deleterious effects, routine use of calcium is not recommended during CPR unless specific indications exist such as hyperkalemia, hypocalcemia, or calcium channel blocker toxicity. When calcium is administered, the chloride salt is recommended because it produces higher and more consistent levels of ionized calcium than other salts. The usual dose is 2 to 4 mg/kg of the 10% solution administered slowly intravenously. Calcium gluconate contains one-third as much molecular calcium as does calcium chloride and requires metabolism of gluconate in the liver.

Electrical Therapy

Electrical Pattern and Duration of Ventricular Fibrillation

VF is the most common ECG pattern found during witnessed sudden cardiac arrest in adults. The only consistently effective treatment is electrical defibrillation. The most important controllable determinant of failure to resuscitate a patient with VF is the duration of fibrillation.[147,148] Other important factors, such as underlying disease and metabolic status, are largely beyond the control of rescuers. Anesthesiologists are aware even from their initial training in cardiac anesthesia that the fibrillating heart has high oxygen consumption. In the setting of cardiac arrest, prolonged fibrillation worsens myocardial ischemia and decreases the time to irreversible cell damage, so the longer VF continues, the more difficult it is to defibrillate and the less likely is successful resuscitation.[80,149] If defibrillation occurs within 1 minute of fibrillation, CPR is unnecessary for resuscitation. Initial resuscitation success following out-of-hospital fibrillation and survival to hospital discharge are improved the earlier defibrillation is accomplished.[27,150] 10

The coarseness of the fibrillatory waves on the ECG may reflect the severity and duration of the myocardial insult and thus have prognostic significance.[151] However, the fibrillation amplitude seen on any one ECG lead varies with the orientation of that lead to the vector of the fibrillatory wave.[152] If the lead is oriented at right angles to the fibrillatory wave, a flat line can be seen. For this reason, the trace from a second lead should always be inspected before a decision is made not to defibrillate. Low-*amplitude* fibrillatory waveforms are less likely to be associated with successful resuscitation and more likely to convert to asystole following defibrillation.[151] Similarly, low-*frequency* fibrillatory waveforms are associated with poor outcomes; the median frequency of the waveform correlates with myocardial perfusion during CPR and with success of defibrillation.[153,154] Multiple studies in animals and humans have shown that analysis of the VF waveform can predict, with varying reliability, the success of defibrillation attempts.[148,151,154–158] It is not yet clear whether such waveform analysis can predict success of resuscitation or direct modification of therapy prospectively. Catecholamines with β-adrenergic activity increase the vigor of fibrillation and the amplitude of the electrical activity, leading to the practice of administering epinephrine to make it "easier" to defibrillate. However, experimental work has shown that manipulation of the electrical pattern with epinephrine does not influence the success of defibrillation or reduce the energy needed for defibrillation.[148,158] Consequently, defibrillation should not be delayed for drug administration.

Defibrillators: Energy, Current, and Voltage

Defibrillators derive power from a line source of alternating current or an integral battery. The typical defibrillator consists of a variable transformer that stores direct current in a capacitor, a switch to charge the capacitor, and discharge switches to complete the circuit from capacitor to electrodes. Defibrillators are classified by the current waveform delivered: monophasic (current flows in one direction between electrodes) or biphasic (current reverses direction between electrodes during the shock). Older defibrillators used a monophasic damped half-sinusoid or a monophasic truncated exponential waveform. However, all defibrillators currently on the market, including AEDs, deliver current in a truncated exponential (BTE), rectilinear (RLB), or pulsed biphasic waveform.

The AED is a device that monitors the ECG, recognizes VF, charges automatically, and gives a defibrillatory shock.[159] It has allowed the introduction of defibrillation into first-responder EMS networks and public-access defibrillation because minimally trained individuals can incorporate defibrillation into BLS skills, improving survival in out-of-hospital arrest by reducing time to delivery of the first shock.[26–28,160–162] The algorithms these devices use to detect VF are accurate with nearly perfect specificity. They will not defibrillate a nonfibrillatory rhythm. Sensitivity rates are somewhat lower. They sometimes have trouble recognizing low-amplitude VF and can misinterpret pacemaker spikes as QRS complexes. Unfortunately, rhythm analysis can require up to 90 seconds, during which chest compressions are not being given. This may adversely influence the outcome in some circumstances.

Some defibrillators measure transthoracic impedance prior to the shock by passing a low-voltage current through the chest during the charge cycle.[161,162] This technology allows current-based defibrillation by adjusting the delivered energy for the measured resistance, permitting the use of low-energy shocks in appropriate patients and identification of victims needing higher energy.[163] Several clinical studies have demonstrated no significant difference in outcome based on transthoracic impedance with impedance-compensating defibrillators.[164,165]

Defibrillation is accomplished by current passing through a critical mass of myocardium, causing simultaneous depolarization of the myofibrils. However, the output of defibrillators is indicated in energy units (joules or watt-seconds), not current (amperes). The relationships among energy, current, and impedance (resistance) are given by the following equations (standard units are indicated):

$$\text{Energy (joules)} = \text{Power (watts)} \times \text{Duration (seconds)} \quad (58\text{-}1)$$

$$\text{Power (watts)} = \text{Potential (volts)} \times \text{Current (amperes)} \quad (58\text{-}2)$$

$$\text{Current (amperes)} = \text{Potential (volts)}/\text{Resistance (ohms)} \quad (58\text{-}3)$$

$$\text{Current (amperes)} = \{\text{Energy (joules)}/[\text{Resistance (ohms)} \times \text{Duration (seconds)}]\}^{1/2} \quad (58\text{-}4)$$

From these equations, it can be determined that as the impedance between the paddle electrodes increases, the delivered energy is reduced. Because internal resistance is low, the primary determinant of delivered energy will be transthoracic impedance. When transthoracic impedance is high, actual delivered energy will be lower. Even at a constant delivered energy, the last equation above indicates that the delivered current (the critical determinant of defibrillation) will be reduced as impedance increases. At high impedance and relatively low-energy levels, current could be too low for defibrillation. Optimal results are obtained by keeping impedance as low as possible.

Transthoracic Impedance

Transthoracic impedance has been measured between 15 and 143 ohms in human defibrillation.[166] The average transthoracic impedance in human defibrillation is 70 to 80 ohms. Many of the important factors in minimizing transthoracic impedance are under the control of the rescuers. Resistance decreases with increasing electrode size; studies suggest that optimal paddle size may be 13 cm in diameter.[167,168] For adults, self-adhesive pad electrodes are most commonly 8 to 12 cm in diameter and work well in practice. Transthoracic impedance is slightly, but significantly, higher during inspiration than during exhalation,[169] since air is a poor electrical conductor. Resistance is probably of little clinical significance when reasonably proper technique and high-energy shocks are used.

Adverse Effects and Energy Requirements

Repeated defibrillation with high energy in animals can be associated with dysrhythmias, ECG changes suggesting myocardial damage, and morphologic evidence of myocardial necrosis.[170,171] Whether similar injuries occur in humans is less certain. Slight elevations in creatine kinase–MB fractions have been measured in patients following cardioversion with high energies.[172] A higher incidence of atrioventricular block has been observed in patients receiving high-energy shocks than in patients receiving low-energy shocks.[173] It seems likely that high-energy shocks, especially if repeated at close intervals, may result in myocardial damage. However, if energy is too low, the delivered current may be insufficient for defibrillation, especially when transthoracic impedance is high. There appears to be little risk of significant myocardial injury with currently recommended energy levels.

Older studies using monophasic waveform defibrillators found a general relationship between body size and energy requirements for defibrillation. Geddes et al.[174] observed that the current that is necessary for defibrillation in animals increased with increasing body mass. Children need less energy than adults, perhaps as low as 0.5 J/kg,[175] although the recommended dose is 2.0 to 4.0 J/kg, similar to that for adults.[45] Over the size range of adults, weight variability is not clinically significant and other factors are more important.[147]

Prior to 2005, the AHA recommendation for defibrillation with monophasic waveform devices was to use a stacked shock approach with an initial shock of 200 J followed immediately by a second shock at 200 to 300 J if the first was unsuccessful, followed by a third shock at 300 to 360 J if necessary.[176] However, the second and third shocks added limited incremental benefit and caused significant interruptions in chest compressions with reduced survival. Biphasic shocks terminate VF at lower energies than any of the monophasic waveforms[177] and have an 85% to 98% first-shock success.[178] Selected energies from 150 to 200 J are generally effective with biphasic truncated exponential waveforms, and a selected energy of 120 J is effective with a rectilinear biphasic waveform. AEDs have the energy dose preselected. Most manual biphasic devices display the effective dose range, and the user should select that dose. If the effective dose for a manual biphasic device is unknown, a dose of 200 J may be selected. This dose may not be optimal but falls within the effective dose range of nearly all biphasic devices. A single shock should be delivered with immediate resumption of chest compressions. If additional shocks are necessary, they may be given at the same or higher dose.

Putting It All Together

Since the mid-1970s, CPR has become widely practiced, facilitated by the efforts of the AHA, the International Red Cross, the European Resuscitation Council, and many other organizations around the world. The International Liaison Committee on Resuscitation, in conjunction with the AHA, periodically conducts an international review of the published science regarding CPR and emergency cardiac care. The resulting Consensus on Science and Treatment Recommendations[179] comprises the most complete evidence-based compilation of scientific data related to CPR practice. Individual organizations, including the AHA, use these data to develop guidelines for CPR practice. However, no common infrastructure exists that allows adoption of true international guidelines for CPR.

Following each consensus conference, the AHA refines and publishes specific guidelines for the teaching and practice of CPR in the United States.[45,180] These guidelines are developed because numerous individuals with varying levels of expertise (laypersons, emergency personnel, nurses, and physicians) need to be trained in a standardized approach if CPR is to be effective in saving lives. The AHA and other organizations also develop and sponsor courses at different levels of complexity for teaching CPR. The two levels of CPR care are referred to as *BLS* for ventilation and chest compressions with or without an AED, and *ACLS* for using all modalities available for resuscitation. Medical personnel must be well versed in both levels of care. BLS is also appropriate for laypersons. For IHCA, ACLS training of responders is associated with better outcomes, including significantly improved 1-year survival.[181]

The AHA guidelines and algorithms are carefully researched using the best evidence and experts available. For many years, survival rates were dismal and remained stagnant for decades in spite of multiple updates to guidelines for CPR practice and many courses for lay public and healthcare providers.[182] What has become clear is that improvements in the standard clinical process of CPR may be more important to increase survival than any new intervention.[183] Standardized quality control of CPR practice is mandatory during any clinical trial if meaningful results are to be achieved. A continuous quality improvement model may be more relevant to improved outcomes than the randomized control trial. More recent data show both overall improvement in outcomes and continued wide variability in patient outcome by location.[184,185]

In addition, there is increasing awareness that the single approach currently used for two pathophysiologically distinct entities (respiratory arrest and cardiac arrest) may not be optimal care for either. In the former, arrest occurs because of hypoxemia, and reoxygenating the blood by effective ventilation is mandatory for successful resuscitation. In the latter, arrest occurs because of cardiac dysrhythmia, usually with normal oxygenation, and attempts at ventilation during resuscitation, may in fact be harmful. Recognizing these issues, the AHA guidelines have been refined to emphasize the importance of assessing the quality of CPR efforts and stress the necessity of minimal interruptions in chest compressions throughout the resuscitation effort (see Fig. 58-2).

Time-Sensitive Model of Ventricular Fibrillation

Weisfeldt and Becker[186] have described untreated VF as a time- 11
sensitive model with three phases: electrical, circulatory, and metabolic. The *electrical phase* occurs during the first 4 to 5 minutes of the arrest, and early defibrillation is critical for success during this time. The *hemodynamic phase* follows for the next 10 to 15 minutes, when perfusing the myocardium and brain with oxygenated blood is critical. This is followed by what has been called the *metabolic phase*, when the ischemic injury to the heart is so great that it is not clear what interventions will be successful.

Prompt defibrillation during the electrical phase is when CPR has had the most dramatic effect and why public-access AEDs have proven beneficial. The longer VF continues, the more difficult it is to defibrillate and the less likely is successful resuscitation. AEDs have been employed successfully in many settings, including airplanes, airports, casinos, and in the community. The success of public-access defibrillation was dramatically demonstrated by the results of installing AEDs in Chicago airports where, over the first 2 years, there was a 55% 1-year neurologically intact survival rate.[187] Similarly, when AEDs were installed in Las Vegas casinos and security personnel were instructed in their use, there was a 53% survival to discharge (74% in patients who received the shock within 3 minutes of collapse).[29] If an arrest is witnessed and a defibrillator or AED is immediately available, then defibrillation should be the first priority in resuscitation. However, in the usual out-of-hospital rescue with emergency medical technicians or paramedics doing the defibrillation, a rapid response is to apply the first shock in 6 to 7 minutes, and the time to first shock frequently is more than 10 minutes. Similar delays occur during IHCAs, so many defibrillators now include an AED mode of operation to allow even nonclinical staff to defibrillate if necessary.

With the onset of VF and cessation of coronary perfusion, the high oxygen consumption of the fibrillating heart causes the rapid depletion of myocardial high-energy phosphates, reducing the time to irreversible cell damage. Myocardial ATP levels during VF correlate with the success of defibrillation and post-defibrillation contractile function.[188] By about 4 minutes, the ATP levels in the heart have fallen to levels that make restoration of normal contractile function problematic. Effective chest compressions help replete or delay reductions in ATP by generating an adequate coronary perfusion pressure to restore myocardial blood flow. Therefore, the most important intervention during the hemodynamic phase of cardiac arrest is producing coronary perfusion with chest compressions before any attempt to defibrillate. In the absence of prompt defibrillation, the most important intervention for neurologically normal survival from cardiac arrest is restoration and maintenance of cerebral and myocardial blood flow. Because perfusion pressures generated by chest compressions are quite low compared with the intact circulation, any interruption of chest compressions markedly reduces the chances for neurologically normal survival. Therefore, any intervention that interrupts chest compressions is strongly discouraged.

Bystander CPR and Basic Life Support

Restoration of cerebral and myocardial blood flow must begin at the scene of the cardiac arrest. There are many studies documenting improved survival if bystanders provide CPR to the victim while awaiting arrival of EMS. Unfortunately, the incidence of bystander CPR has been falling for three decades. The reasons for a bystander's reluctance to intervene are multiple but seem to be primarily lack of training, the complexity of the task, and fear of harm. Many of these concerns focus on the mouth-to-mouth ventilation part of the CPR intervention.[189–191] One survey indicated that only 15% of laypersons would perform CPR with mouth-to-mouth ventilation on a stranger. When given the option of doing chest compressions only, 68% indicated they would perform CPR on a stranger.[191]

If the airway remains patent during CPR, chest compressions cause substantial air exchange. Early studies in anesthetized, paralyzed humans suggested that the airway would not remain open in the unconscious,[5,9] leading to the teaching that airway control and artificial ventilation must accompany chest compressions. However, there are considerable data to suggest that eliminating mouth-to-mouth ventilation early in the resuscitation of witnessed fibrillatory cardiac arrest is not detrimental to outcome and may improve survival. Data from the Belgian Cardiopulmonary Resuscitation Registry (CPCR) have demonstrated that 14-day survival and neurologic outcome are the same if bystanders initiate full BLS or perform chest compressions only. Both are significantly better than if the bystanders only do mouth-to-mouth ventilation or attempt no CPR.[192,193] A Japanese study found better survival in victims who received bystander chest compression–only CPR than in those who received both chest compressions and mouth-to-mouth ventilation from bystanders.[194]

The necessity for ventilation during BLS has been studied in animal models. Since 1993, there have been six studies containing data from 169 swine demonstrating that in prolonged fibrillatory cardiac arrest, neurologically intact survival is the same with chest compression–only resuscitation as with idealized standard CPR (as recommended by the 2000 AHA guidelines[176]), with a 15:2 compression-to-ventilation ratio when compressions are interrupted for only 4 seconds to provide ventilation.[192,193,195–198] However, it has been demonstrated that a single lay rescuer interrupts chest compressions for an average of 16 seconds to deliver the two recommended mouth-to-mouth ventilations.[199] When the 15:2 compression-to-ventilation ratio with 16-second pauses for ventilation was tested in the swine model of prolonged fibrillatory arrest, standard CPR resulted in just 13% 24-hour survival compared with 73% in animals receiving chest compressions only.[200]

Recognizing the deleterious effects of prolonged pauses in chest compressions for ventilation, the 2005 AHA guidelines changed the compression-to-ventilation ratio from 15:2 to 30:2, recommending that ventilation be done in 2 to 4 seconds. When the 30:2 ratio with a more realistic 16-second pause for ventilations is compared with continuous chest compressions without ventilation in the animal model, the 24-hour neurologically normal survival is only 42% in the 30:2 group compared with 70% in the continuous compressions group.[201]

Based on these studies, the Save Hearts in Arizona Registry and Education (SHARE) program began a public education program stressing immediate call to 911 and continuous chest compressions without ventilation in the case of witnessed unexpected sudden collapse in adults. The major advantage of this program is that lay individuals can be taught chest compression-only CPR in a very short period with excellent retention. In Arizona between 2005 and 2009, the rate of bystander CPR increased from 28% to 40%, the rate of chest compression-only CPR among bystanders increased from 20% to 76%, and rate of survival to hospital discharge during those years was 7.8% for those receiving standard CPR and 13.3% for those receiving chest compression–only CPR.[202] The importance of minimizing interruptions in chest compressions was emphasized in a science advisory by the AHA recommending "hands-only CPR" for the lay public.[203] For well-trained healthcare providers operating within an organized EMS system, a randomized controlled trial of continuous chest compressions at 100/min with asynchronous ventilations at 10/min versus 30 compressions followed by a 5-second pause for two ventilations found no difference in survival or favorable neurologic function between the groups.[204]

Advanced Life Support

Recognizing that dysrhythmic arrest is most common in adults and the importance of establishing blood flow, AHA guidelines recommend that, CPR be initiated with chest compressions in the unresponsive individual before any attempt at ventilation when a single rescuer is present.[45] The principle of not interrupting chest compressions in order to maintain cerebral and myocardial perfusion applies to resuscitation attempts by healthcare providers as well as lay bystanders. The adverse hemodynamic consequences of interrupting chest compressions are well documented.[50,200] Blood flow stops almost immediately with cessation of chest compressions and returns slowly when they are resumed (Fig. 58-1). Several compressions are necessary before perfusion pressures return to the levels obtained before compressions were stopped.[49] This is particularly true for prolonged, repeated pauses for ventilation. But it is also relevant for the many other interruptions that occur during resuscitation: pulse checks, rhythm analysis, charging the defibrillator, stacked shocks, intubation, patient assessment, and intravenous line placement. Some reports have documented that paramedics spend only about half the time during a resuscitation doing chest compressions, mostly because they are following the standard guidelines.[30,205,206]

Chest compressions should be paused only when absolutely necessary and then for the shortest time possible. Intravenous line placement should not require cessation of chest compressions. Pulse checks occur only during pauses for rhythm analysis. Initial airway management may consist of insertion of an oropharyngeal airway and providing oxygen by mask with rescue breaths; assisted ventilation or intubation should be delayed until return of spontaneous circulation or until at least three cycles of compressions–rhythm analysis–shock are completed. A second rescuer's priorities should be obtaining intravenous access, delivering drugs, and relieving the individual giving chest compressions. If there are time and resources for airway management, ventilation and intubation are encouraged to take place while chest compressions continue.

Once ventilation begins, rescuers must be aware of the potentially deleterious effects of positive-pressure ventilation.[207,208] Positive-pressure ventilation increases intrathoracic pressure, reducing venous return, cardiac output, and coronary perfusion pressure and adversely affecting survival. These effects are amplified by the fact that physicians and paramedics often ventilate at rates that are many times the recommended 10 breaths per minute, even after extensive retraining.[205,207–209]

Rhythm Analysis and Defibrillation

As mentioned previously, after 4 to 5 minutes of VF, the myocardium is so depleted of high-energy phosphates that development of a normal contractile state is difficult, if not impossible. Therefore, chest compressions should begin immediately, ideally while an AED or defibrillator is being obtained. Compressions should continue until the defibrillator is in place and ready to analyze and shock the victim if indicated.[210,211] Pulse checks are done during the period of rhythm analysis occurring only after 2 minutes of high-quality CPR.

The interruption caused by stacked defibrillatory shocks was discussed previously. When combined with time for rhythm analysis and postshock pulse checks, this interruption may be unacceptably long or even fatal when an AED is in use instead of an experienced clinician interpreting the rhythm with a manual defibrillator.[212,213] The success rate of a single shock is more than 90% with the newer biphasic waveform units. Despite this success, the postshock pulse check detects a pulse in only 2.5% of the victims. Recognizing these concerns, the current AHA guidelines recommend a single shock with immediate resumption of chest compressions before the next pulse/rhythm check.

In prolonged VF arrest, successful defibrillation almost always results in asystole or PEA, as indicated by the extremely small number of victims with a pulse following shocks. In fact, the standard laboratory model for PEA is prolonged VF followed by defibrillation, all without chest compressions. Immediately restarting chest compressions after defibrillation to provide coronary perfusion nearly always results in reversion to a perfusing rhythm. The best chance for restoration of spontaneous circulation following defibrillation will be by immediately resuming chest compressions without waiting to check a pulse or reanalyze the ECG rhythm.

Attention to the quality of CPR and minimizing interruptions in chest compressions has led to significant improvements in survival from cardiac arrest over the past decade. In rural Rock and Walworth counties in Wisconsin, in the 3 years preceding a change, there were 92 witnessed out-of-hospital adult cardiac arrests with an initially shockable rhythm; 18 of these victims survived and 14 (15%) were neurologically intact. In the first 3 years of applying a minimal-interruption approach in these counties, there were 89 witnessed OHCAs; 42 (47%) of these patients survived and 35 (39%) were neurologically intact.[214] In two large metropolitan Arizona cities after institution of minimally interrupted cardiac resuscitation by the EMS, the rate of survival nearly tripled.[182,215] Among the 886 patients, survival to hospital discharge increased from 1.8% to 5.4%, and in the subgroup of 174 patients with witnessed cardiac arrest with VF, survival increased from 4.7% to 17.6%. These statistically significant results are encouraging in that they indicate a significant improvement in outcome from sudden cardiac death is possible with improved early resuscitative techniques.

Pediatric Cardiopulmonary Resuscitation

12 The principles of CPR discussed previously also apply to the child[15] in cardiac arrest. Arrest is less likely to be a sudden event and more likely related to progressive deterioration of respiratory and circulatory function in the pediatric age group. Airway and ventilation problems lead to asystole and PEA as the most common presenting rhythms. However, the consequences of myocardial and cerebral ischemia are the same as for the adult, and the basic approach to the unresponsive victim is similar. Although the higher incidence of respiratory arrest has led to emphasis on providing rescue breathing in children, the delay in providing ventilation is minimal when starting CPR with chest compressions, and this approach is recommended in an unresponsive pulseless child. The specific anatomic and physiologic considerations necessary for the child will be familiar to anesthesiologists. The special circumstance of neonatal resuscitation is discussed in Chapters 41 and 42.

The problem of airway management in the infant is well known to the anesthesiologist. Effective ventilation is especially critical because respiratory problems are frequently the cause for arrest. Mouth-to-mouth or mouth-to-nose and mouth (for infants) can be used as well as bag-valve-mask devices until intubation is possible. Cardiac compression in the infant is provided with two fingers on the midsternum or by encircling the chest with the hands and using the thumbs to provide compression. For the small child, compression can be provided with one hand on the midsternum. For both infants and children, compressions should be at least one-third the depth of the chest at a rate of 100 to 120/min. For a single rescuer, a 30:2 compression-to-ventilation ratio should be used and with two or more rescuers a 15:2 ratio is recommended.

The algorithm for pulseless arrest in the child is shown in Figure 58-5. Although defibrillation is less frequently necessary in children, the same principles apply as in the adult. However, the recommended starting energy is 2 J/kg, which is doubled if defibrillation is unsuccessful. Considerations for drug administration are the same as for the adult, except that the interosseous route in the anterior tibia is a particularly attractive option in small children. Drug therapy is similar to that of the adult but plays a larger role because electrical therapy is less often needed (Table 58-3). The pediatric algorithms for bradycardia and tachycardia are shown in Figures 58-6 and 58-7.

Postresuscitation Care

The major factors contributing to mortality following successful 13
resuscitation are progression of the primary disease and cerebral damage suffered as a result of the arrest. There is growing awareness that many potentially useful interventions during active CPR may not result in improved survival because of the lack of uniform supportive postresuscitation care, allowing progression to multisystem organ dysfunction and death. For optimal outcome, successful restoration of spontaneous circulation must be followed by correction of reversible causes of arrest, including immediate coronary reperfusion and aggressive supportive care (Fig. 58-8). Patients with successful restoration of spontaneous circulation should be transported to a facility with the capability of aggressive postarrest care, including percutaneous coronary intervention, targeted temperature management (TTM), and neurologic critical care. Order sets or checklists are commonly utilized to assist in the care of patients admitted to the intensive care unit for postresuscitation care.

Any cardiac arrest, even of brief duration, causes a generalized decrease in myocardial function similar to the regional hypokinesis seen following periods of regional ischemia. This is usually referred to as *global myocardial stunning* and can be mitigated with inotropic agents, if necessary. Active management following

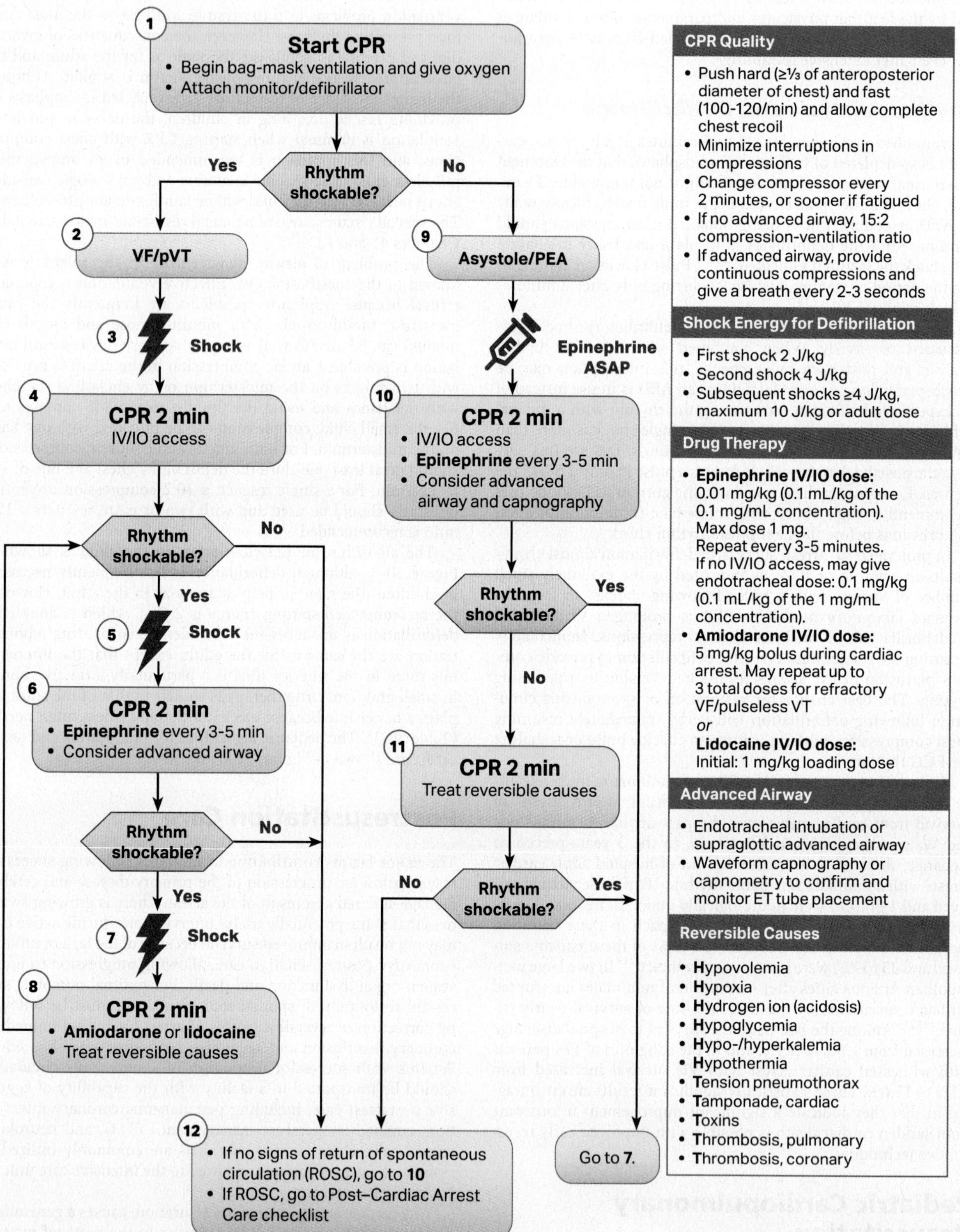

Figure 58-5 Pediatric cardiac arrest algorithm. CPR, cardiopulmonary resuscitation; VF, ventricular fibrillation; VT, ventricular tachycardia; PEA, pulseless electrical activity; IV, intravenous(ly); IO, intraosseous(ly); J, joules. (Reprinted with permission from 2020 American Heart Association Guidelines for CPR & ECC—Part 3: Adult Basic and Advanced Life Support. *Circulation*. 2020;142:S366–S468. © 2020 American Heart Association, Inc.)

Table 58-3 Medications for Pediatric Resuscitation

Drug	Dose	Remarks
Adenosine	0.1 mg/kg Repeat dose: 0.2 mg/kg (maximum 12 mg)	Monitor ECG during dosing Rapid IV/IO bolus with flush
Amiodarone	5 mg/kg IV/IO Maximum 15 mg/kg per day	Monitor ECG and blood pressure; adjust administration rate to urgency (IV push during cardiac arrest, more slowly over 20–60 min with perfusing rhythm). Expert consultation strongly recommended prior to use when patient has a perfusing rhythm. Use caution when administering with other drugs that prolong QT (obtain expert consultation). Hypotension is the most common side effect.
Atropine	0.02 mg/kg IV/IO/ ET[a] May repeat once Maximum single dose 0.5 mg in child	Higher doses may be given in the setting of organophosphate poisoning
Calcium chloride (10%)	20 mg/kg IV/IO (0.2 mL/kg)	Administer slowly
Calcium gluconate (10%)	60–100 mg/kg (0.6–1.0 mL/kg) IV/IO	Administer slowly
Epinephrine for bradycardia	IV/IO: 0.01 mg/kg (1:10,000, 0.1 mL/kg) ET: 0.1 mg/kg (1:1,000, 0.1 mL/kg)	
Epinephrine for pulseless arrest	IV/IO: 0.01 mg/kg (1:10,000, 0.1 mL/kg) ET: 0.1 mg/kg (1:1,000, 0.1 mL/kg) Subsequent doses: Repeat initial dose or may increase up to 10 times (0.1 mg/kg, 1:1,000, 0.1 mL/kg) Administer epinephrine every 3–5 min. IV/IO/ET doses as high as 0.2 mg/kg of 1:1,000 may be effective	
Glucose	0.5–1.0 g/kg IV/IO	Newborn: 5–10 mL/kg $D_{10}W$ Children: 2–4 mL/kg $D_{25}W$ Adolescents: 1–2 mL/kg $D_{50}W$
Lidocaine	Bolus: 1 mg/kg IV/IO	
	Infusion: 20–50 µg/kg/min	—
Magnesium sulfate	25–50 mg/kg IV/IO maximum dose 2 g	Over 10–20 min; faster in torsades de pointes
Naloxone	Full reversal: ≤5 yr or ≤20 kg: 0.1 mg/kg IV/IO/ET[a] ≥5 yr or >20 kg: 2 mg IV/IO/ET[a]	Use lower doses to reverse respiratory depression associated with therapeutic opioid use (1–5 mcg/kg titrate to effect)
Procainamide	15 mg/kg IV/IO over 30–60 min Adult dose: 20 mg/min IV infusion up to total maximum dose of 17 mg/kg	Monitor ECG and blood pressure Give slowly over 30–60 min Use caution when administering with other drugs that prolong QT
Sodium bicarbonate	1 mEq/kg IV/IO	Infuse slowly and ensure adequate ventilation

ECG, electrocardiogram; IV, intravenous; IO, intraosseous; ET, endotracheal.
[a]For endotracheal administration use higher doses (2 to 10 times the IV dose); dilute medication with normal saline to a volume of 3 to 5 mL and follow with several positive-pressure ventilations.
Reprinted with permission from Part 10: Pediatric Advanced Life Support. *Circulation*. 2000;102:I-291–I-342.

resuscitation appears to mitigate postischemic brain damage and improve neurologic outcomes. Although a significant number of patients have severe neurologic deficits following resuscitation, aggressive brain-oriented support does not seem to increase the proportion surviving in vegetative states.[216] A retrospective cohort study of postreturn of spontaneous circular (ROSC) patients at one center compared reasons for death for IHCA versus OHCA patients. IHCA patients were more likely to die due to comorbid withdrawal of life support (36% vs. 4%), refractory hemodynamic shock (25% vs. 17%) and sudden cardiac death (11% vs. 4%). OHCA patients were more likely to die due to neurologic withdrawal of support (73% vs. 27%) or respiratory failure (3% vs. 1%).[217]

When flow is restored following a period of global brain ischemia, in the ensuing 12 hours, three stages of cerebral reperfusion are seen. Immediately after resuscitation, there are multifocal

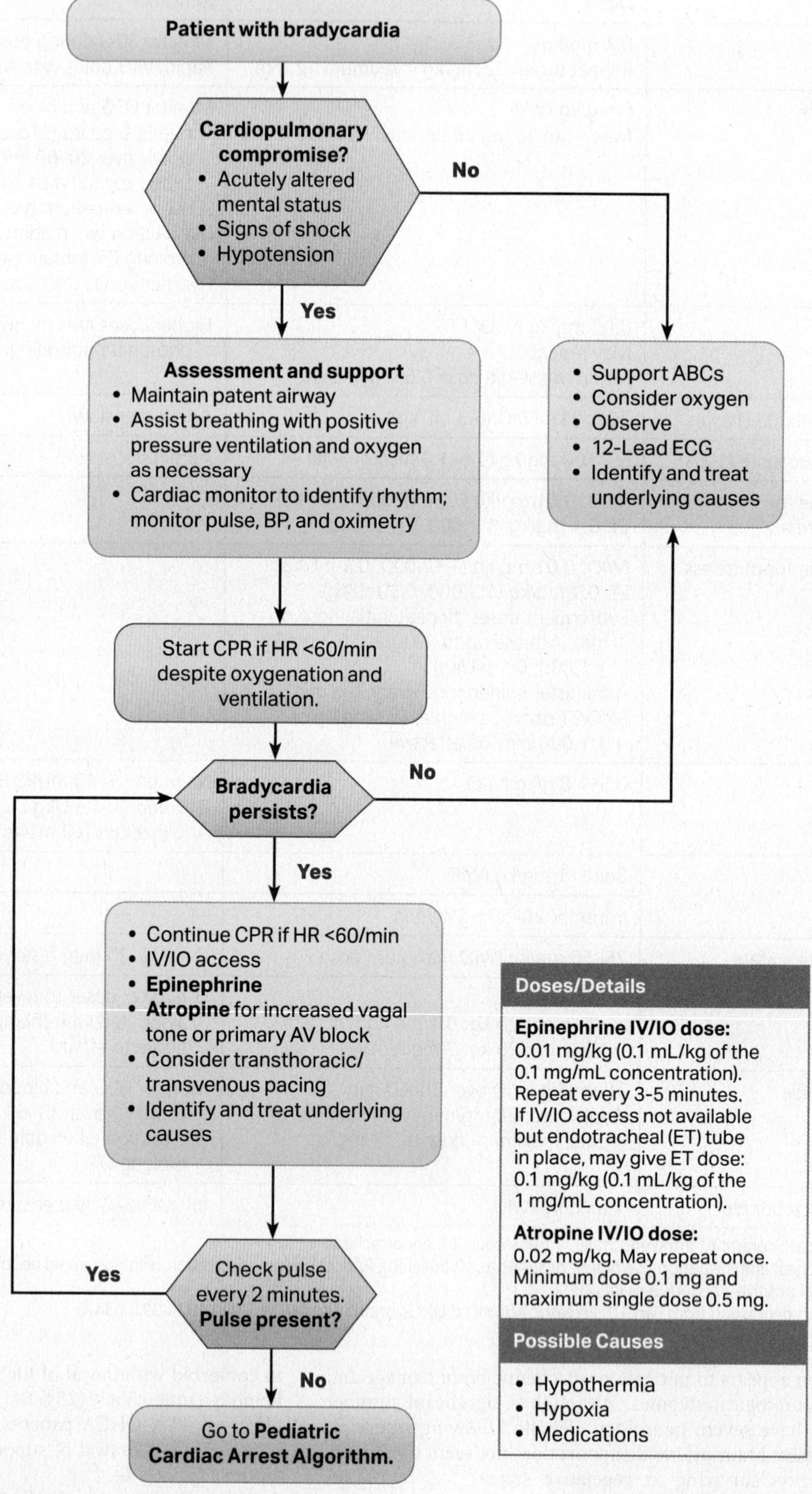

Figure 58-6 Pediatric bradycardia with a pulse algorithm. ABCs, airway, breathing, and circulation; ECG, electrocardiogram; CPR, cardiopulmonary resuscitation; HR, heart rate; IV, intravenous(ly); IO, intraosseous(ly); AV, atrioventricular. (Reprinted with permission from 2020 American Heart Association Guidelines for CPR & ECC—Part 4: Pediatric Basic and Advanced Life Support. *Circulation*. 2020;142:S469–S523. © 2020 American Heart Association, Inc.)

Pediatric Tachycardia With a Pulse Algorithm

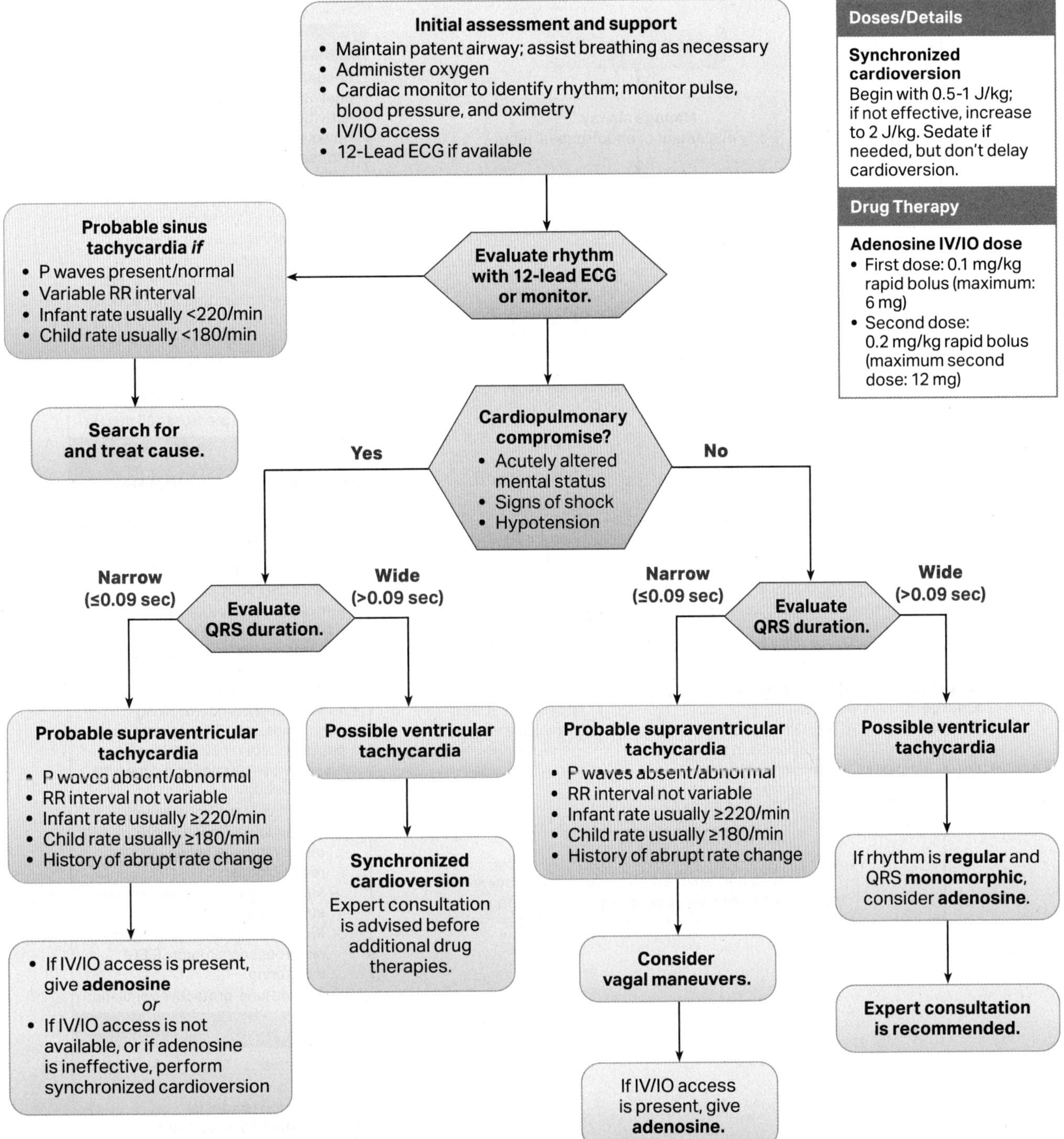

Figure 58-7 Pediatric tachycardia with a pulse algorithm. ECG, electrocardiogram; HR, heart rate; IV, intravenous(ly); IO, intraosseous(ly); J, joules. (Reprinted with permission from 2020 American Heart Association Guidelines for CPR & ECC—Part 4: Pediatric Basic and Advanced Life Support. *Circulation*.2020;142:S469–S523. © 2020 American Heart Association, Inc.)

areas of the brain with no reflow. Within 1 hour, there is global hyperemia followed quickly by prolonged global hypoperfusion. Elevation of intracranial pressure is unusual following resuscitation from cardiac arrest. However, severe ischemic injury can lead to cerebral edema and increased intracranial pressure in the ensuing days. Nonconvulsive seizures are common postresuscitation with or without therapeutic hypothermia.[218] Continuous or frequent electroencephalography (EEG) for diagnosis of seizure should be performed on comatose patients and treatment instituted if indicated.

ACLS Healthcare Provider Post–Cardiac Arrest Care Algorithm

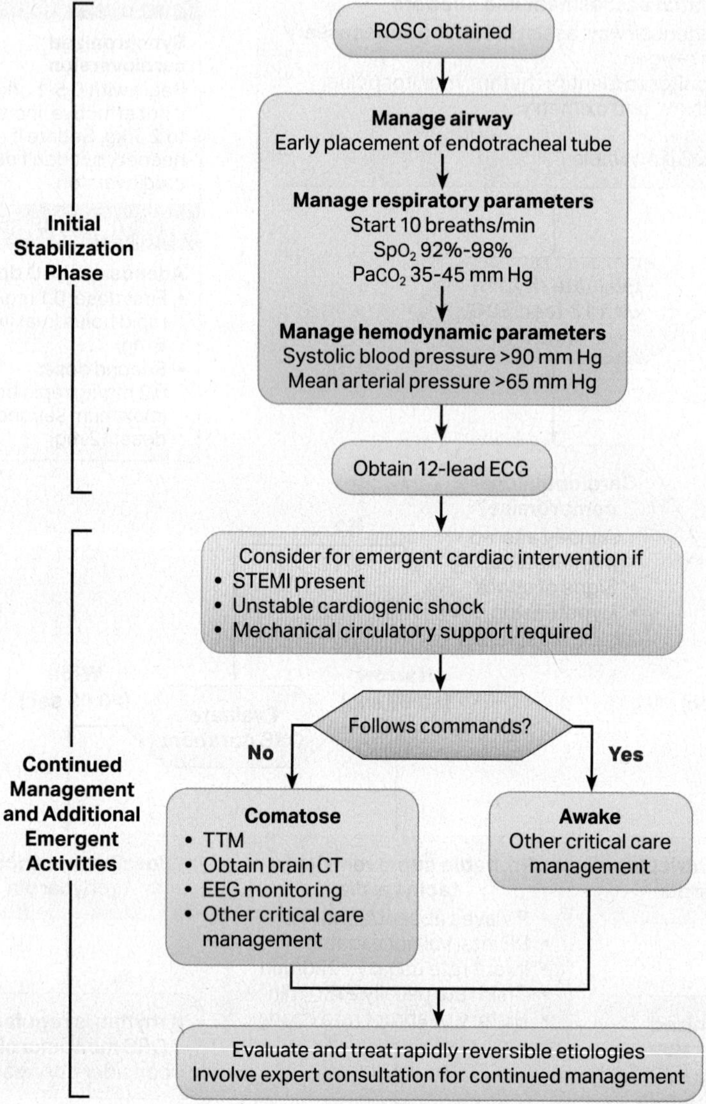

Initial Stabilization Phase

Resuscitation is ongoing during the post-ROSC phase, and many of these activities can occur concurrently. However, if prioritization is necessary, follow these steps:

- Airway management: Waveform capnography or capnometry to confirm and monitor endotracheal tube placement
- Manage respiratory parameters: Titrate FIO_2 for SpO_2 92%-98%; start at 10 breaths/min; titrate to $PaCO_2$ of 35-45 mm Hg
- Manage hemodynamic parameters: Administer crystalloid and/or vasopressor or inotrope for goal systolic blood pressure >90 mm Hg or mean arterial pressure >65 mm Hg

Continued Management and Additional Emergent Activities

These evaluations should be done concurrently so that decisions on targeted temperature management (TTM) receive high priority as cardiac interventions.

- Emergent cardiac intervention: Early evaluation of 12-lead electrocardiogram (ECG); consider hemodynamics for decision on cardiac intervention
- TTM: If patient is not following commands, start TTM as soon as possible; begin at 32-36°C for 24 hours by using a cooling device with feedback loop
- Other critical care management
  - Continuously monitor core temperature (esophageal, rectal, bladder)
  - Maintain normoxia, normocapnia, euglycemia
  - Provide continuous or intermittent electroencephalogram (EEG) monitoring
  - Provide lung-protective ventilation

H's and T's

Hypovolemia
Hypoxia
Hydrogen ion (acidosis)
Hypokalemia/**h**yperkalemia
Hypothermia
Tension pneumothorax
Tamponade, cardiac
Toxins
Thrombosis, pulmonary
Thrombosis, coronary

Figure 58-8 Adult post-cardiac arrest algorithm. SBP, systolic blood pressure; ECG, electrocardiogram; STEMI, ST elevation myocardial infarction; AMI, acute myocardial infarction; $PaCO_2$, arterial partial pressure of end-tidal carbon dioxide; FIO_2, fraction of inspired oxygen; SpO_2, oxygen saturation by pulse oximetry; IV, intravenous(ly); IO, intraosseous(ly). (Reprinted with permission from 2020 American Heart Association Guidelines for CPR & ECC—Part 3: Adult Basic and Advanced Life Support. *Circulation*. 2020;142:S366–S468. © 2020 American Heart Association, Inc.)

Postresuscitation support is focused on providing stable oxygenation and hemodynamics to minimize any further cerebral insult and to allow the patient time to recover from this massive physiologic insult. There is increasing recognition that following CPR, the comatose patient should be fully supported for at least 48 hours before neuroprognostication, and some studies support delaying for 72 hours postarrest.[219] Mechanical ventilation should be adjusted to ensure adequate oxygenation and ventilation without hyperventilation. Restlessness, coughing, or seizure activity should be aggressively treated. Control of shivering may require neuromuscular blockers. Oxygen free radicals are a major cause of reperfusion injury and postresuscitation hyperoxia may contribute to poor neurologic outcome.[220–222] Following return of spontaneous circulation, inspired oxygen should be titrated to maintain oxygen saturation by pulse oximetry between 94% and 99% as soon as possible. Hypocapnia ($PaCO_2$ <30 mmHg) should be avoided. Because cerebral autoregulation of blood flow is severely attenuated after cardiac arrest, both prolonged hypertension and hypotension are associated with worsened outcomes. Therefore, mean arterial pressure should be maintained at 90 to 110 mmHg. Hyperglycemia during cerebral ischemia is known to result in increased neurologic damage, but since glucose is the primary source of energy for brain metabolism, hypoglycemia must also be avoided. Although it is unknown if high serum glucose in the postresuscitation period influences outcome, it seems prudent to maintain glucose in the 120 to 180 mg/dL range. Specific pharmacologic therapy directed at brain preservation has not been shown to have further benefit. Although some animal trials of barbiturates have been promising, a large multicenter trial of thiopental found no improvement in neurologic status when this drug was given following cardiac arrest.[216] Calcium channel blockers have been shown to be equally unhelpful in human studies.[223]

In contrast to pharmacologic therapy, three more recent studies have demonstrated improved neurologic outcome with targeted temperature management (TTM), where a temperature between 32° and 36°C is maintained for 12 to 24 hours in cardiac arrest survivors who remain comatose after admission to the hospital.[221–226] The earlier trials used hypothermia and studied only patients whose initial rhythm was VF. These are the first studies to document improved neurologic outcome with a specific postarrest intervention, although it is still unclear exactly how TTM improves outcome. The International Liaison Committee on Resuscitation now recommends TTM for unconscious adult patients with return of spontaneous circulation after cardiac arrest at a constant temperature between 32° and 36°C for at least 24 hours.[227] For patients that suffer cardiac arrest in the OR, optimal management is not as clear. A multicenter retrospective study of intra-operative cardiac arrest patients showed no difference in 1-year favorable neurologic outcome among patients treated with TTM post-ROSC compared to those who did not; however, TTM was associated with a significantly higher rate of infection in this population.[228]

Prognosis

For the comatose survivor of CPR, the question of ultimate prognosis is important. Predicting poor neurologic outcome (death or vegetative state) is difficult. It is generally agreed that poor outcome should not be predicted any earlier than 48 hours after ROSC in patients not undergoing hypothermia and that time should be extended for those receiving hypothermia.[229] At this time point, most comatose patients with a poor outcome have either no response or only extensor posturing to painful stimuli. But the false-positive rate (a good outcome when a poor outcome is predicted) for this sign is high. So, decisions should not be made on this basis alone. Confirmatory signs that have nearly a 0% false-positive rate are the absence of a pupillary light reflex at 72 hours and absence of the N20 wave on somatosensory evoked potentials at 24 to 72 hours. Less reliable confirmatory signs include unreactive burst suppression or status epilepticus on electroencephalogram, status myoclonus (lasting >30 minutes) during first 72 hours after ROSC, diffuse anoxic injury on computed tomography or magnetic resonance imaging of the brain, and markedly and persistently elevated neuron-specific endolase.[230]

Resuscitation in the Operating Room

Unique Features and Special Circumstances

Cardiac arrest in the OR is often quite distinct from cardiac arrest in other settings. The patient is monitored, the arrest is witnessed, the cause is often known—sometimes even anticipated—and an entire resuscitative team is already present. Although the basic pathophysiology of cardiac arrest is the same, the interventions and order of interventions can often be tailored based on the most likely causes instead of simply following the standard algorithm. This is why cardiac arrest in the OR has a higher success rate compared to IHCA or OHCA generally.[231] Due to the increased incidence and need for specific treatment, there are some key events that anesthesiologists should be familiar with and ready to treat.[19,20] Being unprepared for uncommon events in the OR could be seen as a "Failure to Rescue," an important quality metric. This is "failure or delay in recognizing and responding to a hospitalized patient experiencing complications from a disease process or medical intervention."[231]

Arguably the most obvious causes for cardiac arrest in the OR are hypoxic or hemorrhagic arrest, and anesthesiologists have worked diligently to develop strategies and tools to deal with each. The AHA guidelines are designed to improve the chances of survival in the "unknown" patient who experiences cardiac arrest unexpectedly. The logic of these algorithms rests on what is the most likely cause of sudden death outside of the hospital and the efficacy of the available interventions for achieving ROSC and a good long-term outcome. Most adults in the United States with sudden OHCA are suffering from VF; the primary treatment is chest compressions and defibrillation. The most common type of cardiac arrest in the OR is PEA, which is notoriously more challenging and less treatable.

While anesthesiologists must be facile with the AHA guidelines, the guidelines alone are not adequate for successful resuscitation in an OR cardiac arrest. Cardiac arrest in the OR is not always sudden. Noticing and acting on early signs of deterioration are key for both the surgeon and anesthesiologist. For PEA arrest, the primary treatment is epinephrine and reversal/management of the underlying cause. This can be challenging when initial indicators of anaphylaxis, malignant hyperthermia, hyperkalemia, or hypocalcemia are difficult to discern in the anesthetized patient. Management of OR emergencies requires clear communication and a shared mental model,[232] especially for diagnoses of hemorrhagic shock, tension pneumothorax, cardiac tamponade, or cardiogenic shock from ischemia that require specific surgical and anesthetic interventions. Some diagnoses such as pulmonary embolism can be quite difficult to prove in the operative setting. Transesophageal echocardiogram can be quite useful in determining the underlying cause of unexpected or unresponsive hypotension but takes time and requires specially trained personnel.

Local anesthetic toxicity (LAST) is another potential cause of cardiac arrest in the OR. It can be due to a "high-spinal" from accidental overdose of local anesthetic into the cerebrospinal fluid via a spinal needle or misplaced catheter. LAST may also be related to high vascular concentration due to inadvertent intravascular injection during or after placement of a block. Because timely, targeted treatment is most efficacious, anesthesiologists must have a high index of suspicion and readiness to intervene when necessary.

Crisis Resource Management, Teamwork, and Communication

14 Anesthesiology was one of the first specialties to apply crisis resource management strategies from the airline industry to medical settings.[233] Although preparing for unexpected and rare events and managing crises is a key part of our role, unexpected cardiac arrest in the OR remains challenging as this requires the entire operative team to quickly redirect their focus to the priority of saving the patient's life. Precious time can be lost as the operative team overcomes its immediate surprise and disbelief to function as a code team. Planning, team leadership, and communication are crucial factors for optimal team performance.[234]

BLS skills are essential and must be initiated immediately. This can be challenging due to patient positioning, open surgical wounds, and unclear or unfamiliar roles. In order to provide optimal CPR in the OR, individuals and teams should regularly practice basic skills including chest compressions, defibrillation, and clear communication.[34,235] Guidelines and protocols should be created and tested to enhance the team's ability to get extra assistance, equipment, and medications. Teams can practice together to improve their readiness to respond and individuals can maintain their skills using simulators or simulated cases.

Ethical Issues: Do-Not-Resuscitate Orders in the Operating Room

15 Not long after the practice of CPR became widely accepted, healthcare professionals began to recognize that it was not always appropriate. The ethical principal of beneficence, or doing good for the patient, underlies all medical interventions. In many cases, CPR reverses sudden death and allows a person to recover, but for some people, CPR merely prolongs death or returns a person to an already miserable existence. This violates the ethical principal of nonmalfeasance and the longstanding fundamental admonition, *Primum non nocere* or "do no harm."

Because the outcome of CPR is not known until after it has been applied, CPR is standard medical care when an individual is unexpectedly found pulseless, making CPR the only medical intervention that requires an order not to receive it.[236,237] Patients, especially those who are elderly, have chronic disease, or have a terminal diagnosis are particularly concerned about inappropriate interventions, including CPR, that may only prolong rather than enhance their life. The patient's right to limit medical treatment is firmly established in modern medical practice based on the ethical principle of respect for patient autonomy. People have the right to place limitations on medical treatment even while undergoing other therapies, including surgical procedures. Such requests are generally accepted, even welcomed, by healthcare workers. However, the OR is one area of the hospital where Do Not Resuscitate (DNR) orders may cause conflict between medical personnel and patients.[238–240]

Since the early 1990s, the American Society of Anesthesiologists,[241] the American College of Surgeons,[242] and the Association of Operating Room Nurses[243] have had guidelines for patients coming to the OR with a DNR order in place.[244] The recommended approach is termed "reconsideration" of the DNR order. This is because the situation and expected outcome after a code in the OR is usually better compared to a code elsewhere.[36] Despite this guidance by all three of the major professional organizations related to perioperative care, and longstanding general agreement by ethicists on this issue, it is still widely assumed that pre-existing DNR orders are *automatically* rescinded in the OR setting. Although anesthesiologists may be uncomfortable talking to patients about resuscitation in the perioperative setting, it is neither ethical nor legal to automatically rescind a patient's DNR order simply because they are coming to the OR.

There are good reasons why a patient, even with a terminal diagnosis, would reject heroic measures such as resuscitation and still choose palliative therapy. If a surgical intervention will ameliorate symptoms or improve quality of life, there is no reason to withhold this treatment. Operative intervention may increase the risk of cardiac arrest, but that is certainly not a common or expected event.

At times, clinicians in the OR may perceive that their actions precipitated the cardiac event, therefore making them feel responsible for the patient's death and obligated to attempt to resuscitate the patient. The ethical principle that guides this situation is called the principle of double effect. This applies when the intention or goal of the procedure or anesthetic is to help the patient, but the anesthetic or procedure leads to death as an unintended result. It is the same ethical principal that allows the use of high doses of narcotics for palliative care of pain. Since every patient and situation is different, the best approach is a discussion with the patient or their representative about their goals of care.[245] The physician should exercise judgment to make the best recommendations that are in alignment with the patient's goals.

The term "resuscitation" can be confusing, since many routine interventions for patients under anesthesia could be considered resuscitative. Therefore, the specific interventions included in a DNR status must be clarified with specific allowance made for methods necessary to perform anesthesia and surgery. Many interventions commonly used in the OR (positive-pressure ventilation, vasopressors, antidysrhythmics, blood products) may be considered forms of resuscitation in other situations. The typical DNR order only affects what is to happen once the patient's heart stops. For example, mask ventilation would be permissible if needed temporarily, even for a patient with a DNI (do not intubate) order. Other measures short of chest compressions or defibrillation may still be permissible with a general DNR order and should be provided if the interventions are in alignment with meeting the patient's overall goals of care.

Despite these strong arguments for honoring a DNR request for an anesthetized patient, many OR personnel are uncomfortable managing a patient with a DNR order. Institutionally, these ethical conflicts should be addressed by adoption of clear policies.[246,247] Table 58-4 includes sample language that could be included in an institutional policy on DNR orders in the perioperative period.

It is reassuring to remember that limitations of care conversations are not needed for the vast majority of patients needing anesthetic care. Only patients who already have a DNR order or that request a DNR order just before surgery will require this discussion, which should be part of the consent for the procedure and the anesthetic. For the individual patient, conflicts can be resolved by communication among the patient, family, and other clinical caregivers. If there are limitations of interventions, these should be documented in the chart, both as a note with a description of the patient's goals of care and as an appropriate order. If an existing DNR order will be suspended, the duration of the suspension should be defined in the note and the order should be

Table 58-4 Sample Language for Management of a DNR Policy in the Perioperative Period

- When a patient with "Limited Support" or "Comfort Care" level of support orders will undergo a procedure in the operating room or elsewhere requiring anesthesiology services, their advance directive should be reviewed with the patient or, if the patient lacks decision-making capacity, the patient's health care agent/power of attorney, health care representative or legal guardian, and discussed with the surgeon, anesthesiologist, or other physician responsible for the patient's care.
- If there are modifications to the prior level of support designation, these changes should be entered in the patient's electronic medical record and communicated to the care team prior to the procedure.
- Orders for limited support are not automatically rescinded when a patient undergoes a procedure in the operating room.

changed in the chart so there is no confusion, especially in the postoperative period.

A full discussion of this topic may be found in "Ethical Guidelines for the Anesthesia Care of Patients with Do-Not-Resuscitate Orders or Other Directives that Limit Treatment" by the American Society of Anesthesiologists (ASA), which is available on the ASA website (www.asahq.org).

For further review and interactivities, please see the videos and narrative interactive clinical vignettes (NICVs) accessible in the complimentary eBook bundled with this text. Access instructions are located on the inside front cover.

REFERENCES

1. American Board of Anesthesiology. Policy Book. 2022. Available at https://www.theaba.org/wp-content/uploads/pdfs/Policy_Book.pdf. Accessed August 17, 2022.
2. *Resuscitation. An Historical Perspective.* A Catalogue of an Exhibit at The Annual American Society of Anesthesiologists in San Francisco, October 11-13, 1976. Available at https://www.woodlibrarymuseum.org/wp-content/uploads/rare-books/S_AHFO.pdf. Accessed February 19, 2023.
3. Brooks D. *Resuscitation: Care of the Critically Ill.* 2nd ed. Edward Arnold; 1986.
4. Vesalius A. De humani corporis fabrica libri septem. *Basileae: Ex Officina I. Oporini.* 1543;659 (i.e. 663).
5. Safar P, Escarraga LA, Elam JO. A comparison of the mouth-to-mouth and mouth-to-airway methods of artificial respiration with the chest-pressure arm-lift methods. *N Engl J Med.* 1958; 258(14):671–677.
6. Elam JO, Clements JA, Brown ES, Elton NW. Artificial respiration for the nerve gas casualty. *U S Armed Forces Med J.* 1956;7(6):797–810.
7. Gordon AS, Frye CW, Gittelson L, Sadove MS, Beattie EJ Jr. Mouth-to-mouth versus manual artificial respiration for children and adults. *J Am Med Assoc.* 1958;167(3):320–328.
8. Elam JO, Brown ES, Elder JD Jr. Artificial respiration by mouth-to-mask method; a study of the respiratory gas exchange of paralyzed patients ventilated by operator's expired air. *N Engl J Med.* 1954;250(18):749–754.
9. Safar P. Failure of manual artificial respiration. *Fed Proc.* 1958;17(1):139–139.
10. Hooker DR, Kouwenhoven WB, Langworthy OR. The effect of alternating electrical currents on the heart. *Am J Physiol.* 1933;103(2):444–454.
11. Beck CS, Pritchard WH, Feil HS. Ventricular fibrillation of long duration abolished by electric shock. *J Am Med Assoc.* 1947;135(15):985.
12. Zoll PM, Linenthal AJ, Gibson W, Paul MH, Norman LR. Termination of ventricular fibrillation in man by externally applied electric countershock. *N Engl J Med.* 1956;254(16): 727–732.
13. Kouwenhoven WB, Milnor WR, Knickerbocker GG, Chesnut WR Closed chest defibrillation of the heart. *Surgery.* 1957;42(3):550–561.
14. Kouwenhoven WB. Closed-chest cardiac massage. *JAMA.* 1960;174(17):2160–2160.
15. Redding JS, Pearson JW. Evaluation of drugs for cardiac resuscitation. *Anesthesiology.* 1963; 24:203–207.
16. Virani SS, Alonso A, Benjamin EJ, et al. Heart disease and stroke statistics-2020 update: A report from the American Heart Association. *Circulation.* 2020;141(9):e139–e596.
17. Rosamond W, Flegal K, Furie K, et al. Heart disease and stroke statistics—2008 update—A report from the American Heart Association Statistics Committee and Stroke Statistics Subcommittee. *Circulation.* 2008;117(4):E25–E146.
18. Tsao CW, Aday AW, Almarzooq ZI, et al. Heart Disease and Stroke Statistics-2022 Update: A Report From the American Heart Association. *Circulation.* 2022;145(8):e153–e639.
19. Moitra VK, Einav S, Thies KC, et al. Cardiac arrest in the operating room: resuscitation and management for the anesthesiologist: Part 1. *Anesth Analg.* 2018;126(3):876–888.
20. McEvoy MD, Thies KC, Einav S, et al. Cardiac arrest in the operating room: Part 2-special situations in the perioperative period. *Anesth Analg.* 2018;126(3):889–903.
21. Angelos M, Safar P, Reich H, A comparison of cardiopulmonary-resuscitation with cardiopulmonary bypass after prolonged cardiac-arrest in dogs - reperfusion pressures and neurologic recovery. *Resuscitation.* 1991;21(2–3):121–135.
22. Kern KB, Sanders AB, Janas W, et al. Limitations of open-chest cardiac massage after prolonged, untreated cardiac-arrest in dogs. *Ann Emerg Med.* 1991;20(7):761–767.
23. Chan PS, McNally B, Tang F, Kellermann A, CARES Surveillance Group. Recent trends in survival from out-of-hospital cardiac arrest in the United States. *Circulation.* 2014;130(21): 1876–1882.
24. Girotra S, van Diepen S, Nallamothu BK, et al. Regional Variation in out-of-hospital cardiac arrest survival in the United States. *Circulation.* 2016;133(22):2159–2168.
25. Blewer AL, Ho AFW, Shahidah N, et al. Impact of bystander-focused public health interventions on cardiopulmonary resuscitation and survival: a cohort study. *Lancet Public Health.* 2020; 5(8):e428–e436.
26. Weaver WD, Cobb LA, Hallstrom AP, Fahrenbruch C, Copass MK, Ray R. Factors influencing survival after out-of-hospital cardiac-arrest. *J Am Coll Cardiol.* 1986;7(4):752–757.
27. Eisenberg MS, Copass MK, Hallstrom AP, et al. Treatment of out-of-hospital cardiac arrests with rapid defibrillation by emergency medical technicians. *N Engl J Med.* 1980;302(25): 1379–1383.
28. Weaver WD, Hill D, Fahrenbruch CE, et al. Use of the automatic external defibrillator in the management of out-of-hospital cardiac-arrest. *N Engl J Med.* 1988;319(11):661–666.
29. Valenzuela TD, Roe DJ, Nichol G, Clark LL, Spaite DW, Hardman RG. Outcomes of rapid defibrillation by security officers after cardiac arrest in casinos. *N Engl J Med.* 2000;343(17): 1206–1209.
30. Valenzuela TD, Kern KB, Clark LL, et al. Interruptions of chest compressions during emergency medical systems resuscitation. *Circulation.* 2005;112(17):U1189–U1189.
31. Holmberg MJ, Ross CE, Fitzmaurice GM, et al. Annual incidence of adult and pediatric in-hospital cardiac arrest in the United States. *Circ Cardiovasc Qual Outcomes.* 2019;12(7): e005580.
32. Chan PS, Spertus JA, Kennedy K, Nallamothu BK, Starks MA, Girotra S. In-hospital cardiac arrest survival in the United States during and after the initial novel coronavirus disease 2019 pandemic surge. *Circ Cardiovasc Qual Outcomes.* 2022;15(2):e008420.
33. Holmberg MJ, Wiberg S, Ross CE, et al. Trends in survival after pediatric in-hospital cardiac arrest in the United States. *Circulation.* 2019;140(17):1398–1408.
34. Nallamothu BK, Guetterman TC, Harrod M, et al. How do resuscitation teams at top-performing hospitals for in-hospital cardiac arrest succeed? A qualitative study. *Circulation.* 2018;138(2):154–163.
35. Nadkarni VM, Larkin GL, Peberdy MA, et al. First documented rhythm and clinical outcome from in-hospital cardiac arrest among children and adults. *JAMA.* 2006;295(1):50–57.
36. Olsson GL, Hallen B. Cardiac-arrest during anesthesia - a computer-aided study in 250–543 anesthetics. *Acta Anaesthesiol Scand.* 1988;32(8):653–664.
37. Kazaure HS, Roman SA, Rosenthal RA, Sosa JA. Cardiac arrest among surgical patients: an analysis of incidence, patient characteristics, and outcomes in ACS-NSQIP. *JAMA Surg.* 2013; 148(1):14–21.
38. Guildner C. Manual techniques for opening an airway—critical-review. *Med Instrum.* 1980; 14(1):55–55.
39. Panchal AR, Berg KM, Hirsch KG, et al. 2019 American Heart Association focused update on advanced cardiovascular life support: Use of advanced airways, vasopressors, and extracorporeal cardiopulmonary resuscitation during cardiac arrest: An update to the American Heart Association guidelines for cardiopulmonary resuscitation and emergency cardiovascular care. *Circulation.* 2019;140(24):e881–e894.
40. Price TM, McCoy EP. Emergency front of neck access in airway management. *Bja Educ.* 2019;19(8):246–253.
41. Deaths in the home and community by age group and cause. National Safety Council Injury Facts 2020. https://injuryfacts.nsc.org/home-and-community/home-and-community-overview/deaths-in-the-home-and-community-by-age-group-and-cause/.
42. Heimlich HJ. Pop Goes Cafe Coronary. *Emerg Med.* 1974;6(6):154–155.
43. Redding JS. Choking controversy - Critique of evidence on the Heimlich maneuver. *Crit Care Med.* 1979;7(10):475–479.
44. Reardon RF, Robinson AE, Kornas R, et al. Prehospital surgical airway management: An NAEMSP position statement and resource document. *Prehosp Emerg Care.* 2022;26: 96–101.

45. Panchal AR, Bartos JA, Cabañas JG, et al. 2020 American Heart Association guidelines for cardiopulmonary resuscitation and emergency cardiovascular care. *Circulation*. 2020;142(16).
46. Harrison RR, Maull KI, Keenan RL, Boyan CP. Mouth-to-mask ventilation—a superior method of rescue breathing. *Ann Emerg Med*. 1982;11(2):74–76.
47. Jesudian MCS, Harrison RR, Keenan RL, Maull KI. Bag-valve-mask ventilation—2 rescuers are better than one - preliminary-report. *Crit Care Med*. 1985;13(2):122–123.
48. Berg RA, Sanders AB, Kern KB, et al. Adverse hemodynamic effects of interrupting chest compressions for rescue breathing during cardiopulmonary resuscitation for ventricular fibrillation cardiac arrest. *Circulation*. 2001;104(20):2465–2470.
49. Cunningham LM, Mattu A, O'Connor RE, Brady WJ. Cardiopulmonary resuscitation for cardiac arrest: the importance of uninterrupted chest compressions in cardiac arrest resuscitation. *Am J Emerg Med*. 2012;30(8):1630–1638.
50. Berg RA, Sanders AB, Kern KB, et al. Adverse hemodynamic effects of interrupting chest compressions for rescue breathing during cardiopulmonary resuscitation for ventricular fibrillation cardiac arrest. *Circulation*. 2001;104(20):2465–70.
51. Corp A, Thomas C, Adlam M. The cardiovascular effects of positive pressure ventilation. *BJA Educ*. 2021;21(6):202–209.
52. Callaway CW, Soar J, Aibiki M, et al. Part 4: Advanced life support 2015 international consensus on cardiopulmonary resuscitation and emergency cardiovascular care science with treatment recommendations. *Circulation*. 2015;132(16):S84–S145.
53. Babbs CF. New versus old theories of blood-flow during Cpr. *Crit Care Med*. 1980;8(3):191–195.
54. Kouwenhoven WB, Jude JR, Knickerbocker GG. Closed-Chest Cardiac Massage. *JAMA*. 1960;173(10):1064–1067.
55. Cipani S, Bartolozzi C, Ballo P, Sarti A. Blood flow maintenance by cardiac massage during cardiopulmonary resuscitation: Classical theories, newer hypotheses, and clinical utility of mechanical devices. *J Intensive Care Soc*. 2019;20(1):2–10.
56. Jude JR, Kouwenhoven WB, Knickerbocker GG. Cardiac arrest. Report of application of external cardiac massage on 118 patients. *JAMA*. 1961;178:1063–1070.
57. Criley JM, Blaufuss AH, Kissel GL. Cough-induced cardiac compression - self-administered form of cardiopulmonary resuscitation. *JAMA*. 1976;236(11):1246–1250.
58. Rudikoff MT, Maughan WL, Effron M, Freund P, Weisfeldt ML. Mechanisms of blood-flow during cardiopulmonary resuscitation. *Circulation*. 1980;61(2):345–352.
59. Holmes HR, Babbs CF, Voorhees WD, Tacker WA Jr, de Garavilla B. Influence of adrenergic-drugs upon vital organ perfusion during CPR. *Crit Care Med*. 1980;8(3):137–140.
60. Michael JR, Guerci AD, Koehler RC, et al. Mechanisms by which epinephrine augments cerebral and myocardial perfusion during cardiopulmonary resuscitation in dogs. *Circulation*. 1984;69(4):822–835.
61. Ewy GA. The mechanism of blood flow during chest compressions for cardiac arrest is probably influenced by the patient's chest configuration. *Acute Med Surg*. 2018;5(3):236–240.
62. Weil MH, Rackow EC, Trevino R, Grundler W, Falk JL, Griffel MI. Difference in acid-base state between venous and arterial blood during cardiopulmonary-resuscitation. *N Engl J Med*. 1986;315(3):153–156.
63. Sandroni C, De Santis P, D'Arrigo S. Capnography during cardiac arrest. *Resuscitation*. 2018;132:73–77.
64. Niemann JT, Rosborough JP, Niskanen RA, Criley JM. Circulatory support during cardiac-arrest using a pneumatic vest and abdominal binder with simultaneous high-pressure airway inflation. *Ann Emerg Med*. 1984;13(9):767–770.
65. Timerman S, Cardoso LF, Ramires JA, Halperin H. Improved hemodynamic performance with a novel chest compression device during treatment of in-hospital cardiac arrest. *Resuscitation*. 2004;61(3):273–280.
66. Wik L, Olsen JA, Persse D, et al. Manual vs. integrated automatic load-distributing band CPR with equal survival after out of hospital cardiac arrest. The randomized CIRC trial. *Resuscitation*. 2014;85(6):741–748.
67. Steen S, Liao Q, Pierre L, Paskevicius A, Sjöberg T. Evaluation of LUCAS, a new device for automatic mechanical compression and active decompression resuscitation. *Resuscitation*. 2002;55(3):285–299.
68. Plaisance P, Lurie KG, Payen D. Inspiratory impedance during active compression-decompression cardiopulmonary resuscitation—A randomized evaluation in patients in cardiac arrest. *Circulation*. 2000;101(9):989–994.
69. Aufderheide TP, Pirrallo RG, Provo TA, Lurie KG. Clinical evaluation of an inspiratory impedance threshold device during standard cardiopulmonary resuscitation in patients with out-of-hospital cardiac arrest. *Crit Care Med*. 2005;33(4):734–740.
70. Plaisance P, Lurie KG, Vicaut E, et al. Evaluation of an impedance threshold device in patients receiving active compression-decompression cardiopulmonary resuscitation for out of hospital cardiac arrest. *Resuscitation*. 2004;61(3):265–271.
71. Aufderheide TP, Nichol G, Rea TD, et al. A trial of an impedance threshold device in out-of-hospital cardiac arrest. *N Engl J Med*. 2011;365(9):798–806.
72. Debehnke DJ, Angelos MG, Leasure JE. Comparison of standard external Cpr, open-chest Cpr, and cardiopulmonary bypass in a canine myocardial infarct model. *Ann Emerg Med*. 1991;20(7):754–760.
73. Kim SJ, Kim HJ, Lee HY, Ahn HS, Lee SW. Comparing extracorporeal cardiopulmonary resuscitation with conventional cardiopulmonary resuscitation: A meta-analysis. *Resuscitation*. 2016;103:106–116.
74. Richardson ASC, Tonna JE, Nanjayya V, et al. Extracorporeal cardiopulmonary resuscitation in adults. Interim guideline consensus statement from the extracorporeal life support organization. *ASAIO J*. 2021;67(3):221–228.
75. Debaty G, Babaz V, Durand M, et al. Prognostic factors for extracorporeal cardiopulmonary resuscitation recipients following out-of-hospital refractory cardiac arrest. A systematic review and meta-analysis. *Resuscitation*. 2017;112:1–10.
76. Ralston SH, Voorhees WD, Babbs CF. Intrapulmonary epinephrine during prolonged cardiopulmonary resuscitation—Improved regional blood-flow and resuscitation in dogs. *Ann Emerg Med*. 1984;13(2):79–86.
77. Crile G, Dolley DH. An experimental research into the resuscitation of dogs killed by anesthetics and asphyxia. *J Exp Med*. 1906;8(6):713–725.
78. Redding JS. Abdominal compression in cardiopulmonary resuscitation. *Anesth Analg*. 1971;50(4):668–675.
79. Pearson JW, Redding JS. Influence of peripheral vascular tone on cardiac resuscitation. *Anesthesia Analgesia*. 1965;44(6):746–752.
80. Yakaitis RW, Otto CW, Blitt CD. Relative importance of alpha and beta adrenergic receptors during resuscitation. *Crit Care Med*. 1979;7(7):293–296.
81. Otto CW, Yakaitis RW, Blitt CD. Mechanism of action of epinephrine in resuscitation from asphyxial arrest. *Crit Care Med*. 1981;9(5):364–365.
82. Ditchey RV, Winkler JV, Rhodes CA. Relative lack of coronary blood flow during closed-chest resuscitation in dogs. *Circulation*. 1982;66(2):297–302.
83. Otto CW, Yakaitis RW. The role of epinephrine in CPR: a reappraisal. *Ann Emerg Med*. 1984;13(9 Pt 2):840–843.
84. Sanders AB, Ewy GA, Taft TV. Prognostic and therapeutic importance of the aortic diastolic pressure in resuscitation from cardiac-arrest. *Crit Care Med*. 1984;12(10):871–873.
85. Niemann JT, Criley JM, Rosborough JP, Niskanen RA, Alferness C. Predictive indexes of successful cardiac resuscitation after prolonged arrest and experimental cardiopulmonary resuscitation. *Ann Emerg Med*. 1985;14(6):521–528.
86. Paradis NA, Martin GB, Rivers EP, et al. Coronary perfusion-pressure and the return of spontaneous circulation in human cardiopulmonary resuscitation. *JAMA*. 1990;263(8):1106–1113.
87. Kalenda Z. Capnogram as a guide to the efficacy of cardiac massage. *Resuscitation*. 1978;6(4):259–263.
88. Weil MH, Bisera J, Trevino RP, Rackow EC. Cardiac-output and end-tidal carbon-dioxide. *Crit Care Med*. 1985;13(11):907–909.
89. Sanders AB, Atlas M, Ewy GA, Kern KB, Bragg S. Expired P-Co2 as an index of coronary perfusion-pressure. *Am J Emerg Med*. 1985;3(2):147–149.
90. Sanders AB, Ewy GA, Bragg S, Atlas M, Kern KB. Expired Pco2 as a prognostic indicator of successful resuscitation from cardiac-arrest. *Ann Emerg Med*. 1985;14(10):948–952.
91. Sanders AB, Kern KB, Otto CW, Milander MM, Ewy GA. End-tidal carbon dioxide monitoring during cardiopulmonary resuscitation. A prognostic indicator for survival. *JAMA*. 1989;262(10):1347–1351.
92. Levine RL, Wayne MA, Miller CC. End-tidal carbon dioxide and outcome of out-of-hospital cardiac arrest. *N Engl J Med*. 1997;337(5):301–306.
93. Kern KB, Sanders AB, Raife J, Milander MM, Otto CW, Ewy GA. A study of chest compression rates during cardiopulmonary resuscitation in humans. The importance of rate-directed chest compressions. *Arch Intern Med*. 1992;152(1):145–149.
94. Otto CW. Cardiovascular pharmacology. II: The use of catecholamines, pressor agents, digitalis, and corticosteroids in CPR and emergency cardiac care. *Circulation*. 1986;74(6 Pt 2):IV80–IV85.
95. Larabee TM, Liu KY, Campbell JA, Little CM. Vasopressors in cardiac arrest: a systematic review. *Resuscitation*. 2012;83(8):932–939.
96. Anson JA. Vascular access in resuscitation: is there a role for the intraosseous route? *Anesthesiology*. 2014;120(4):1015–1031.
97. Puga T, Montez D. Philbeck T, Davlantes C. Adequacy of intraosseous vascular access insertion sites for high-volume fluid infusion. *Crit Care Med*. 2016;44(12):143.
98. Anson JA, Sinz EH, Swick JT. The versatility of intraosseous vascular access in perioperative medicine: a case series. *J Clin Anesth*. 2015;27(1):63–67.
99. Redding JS, Pearson JW. Resuscitation from ventricular fibrillation. Drug therapy. *JAMA*. 1968;203(4):255–260.
100. Schleien CL, Dean JM, Koehler RC, et al. Effect of epinephrine on cerebral and myocardial perfusion in an infant animal preparation of cardiopulmonary resuscitation. *Circulation*. 1986;73(4):809–817.
101. Schleien CL, Koehler RC, Gervais H, et al. Organ blood flow and somatosensory-evoked potentials during and after cardiopulmonary resuscitation with epinephrine or phenylephrine. *Circulation*. 1989;79(6):1332–1342.
102. Redding JS, Pearson JW, Resuscitation from ventricular fibrillation - drug therapy. *JAMA*. 1968;203(4):255-&.
103. Otto CW, Yakaitis RW, Redding JS, Blitt CD. Comparison of dopamine, dobutamine, and epinephrine in Cpr. *Crit Care Med*. 1981;9(9):640–643.

104. Lindner KH, Prengel AW, Pfenninger EG, et al. Vasopressin improves vital organ blood flow during closed-chest cardiopulmonary resuscitation in pigs. *Circulation.* 1995;91(1):215–221.
105. Brillman J, Sanders A, Otto CW, Fahmy H, Bragg S, Ewy GA. Comparison of epinephrine and phenylephrine for resuscitation and neurologic outcome of cardiac arrest in dogs. *Ann Emerg Med.* 1987;16(1):11–17.
106. Lindner KH, Ahnefeld FW, Prengel AW. Comparison of standard and high-dose adrenaline in the resuscitation of asystole and electromechanical dissociation. *Acta Anaesthesiol Scand.* 1991;35(3):253–256.
107. Stiell IG, Hebert PC, Weitzman BN, et al. High-dose epinephrine in adult cardiac-arrest. *N Engl J Med.* 1992;327(15):1045–1050.
108. Brown CG, Martin DR, Pepe PE, et al. A comparison of standard-dose and high-dose epinephrine in cardiac-arrest outside the hospital. *N Engl J Med.* 1992;327(15):1051–1055.
109. Callaham M, Madsen CD, Barton CW, Saunders CE, Pointer J. A randomized clinical-trial of high-dose epinephrine and norepinephrine vs standard-dose epinephrine in prehospital cardiac-arrest. *JAMA.* 1992;268(19):2667–2672.
110. Choux C, Gueugniaud PY, Barbieux A, et al. Standard doses versus repeated high-doses of epinephrine in cardiac-arrest outside the hospital. *Resuscitation.* 1995;29(1):3–9.
111. Gueugniaud PY, Mols P, Goldstein P, et al. A comparison of repeated high doses and repeated standard doses of epinephrine for cardiac arrest outside the hospital. *N Engl J Med.* 1998; 339(22):1595–1601.
112. Lipman J, Wilson W, Kobilski S, et al. High-dose adrenaline in adult in-hospital asystolic cardiopulmonary-resuscitation - a double-blind randomized trial. *Anaesth Intensive Care.* 1993; 21(2):192–196.
113. Sherman BW, Munger MA, Foulke GE, Rutherford WF, Panacek EA. High-dose versus standard-dose epinephrine treatment of cardiac arrest after failure of standard therapy. *Pharmacotherapy.* 1997;17(2):242–247.
114. Jacobs IG, Finn JC, Jelinek GA, Oxer HF, Thompson PL. Effect of adrenaline on survival in out-of-hospital cardiac arrest: A randomised double-blind placebo-controlled trial. *Resuscitation.* 2011;82(9):1138–1143.
115. Perkins GD, Ji C, Achana F, et al. Adrenaline to improve survival in out-of-hospital cardiac arrest: the PARAMEDIC2 RCT. *Health Technol Assess.* 2021;25(25):1–166.
116. Lundin A, Rylander C, Karlsson T, Herlitz J, Lundgren P. Adrenaline, ROSC and survival in patients resuscitated from in-hospital cardiac arrest. *Resuscitation.* 2019;140:64–71.
117. Warren SA, Huszti E, Bradley SM, et al. Adrenaline (epinephrine) dosing period and survival after in-hospital cardiac arrest: a retrospective review of prospectively collected data. *Resuscitation.* 2014;85(3):350–358.
118. Sigal AP, Sandel KM, Buckler DG, Wasser T, Abella BS. Impact of adrenaline dose and timing on out-of-hospital cardiac arrest survival and neurological outcomes. *Resuscitation.* 2019;139: 182–188.
119. Prengel AW, Lindner KH, Keller A, Lurie KG. Cardiovascular function during the postresuscitation phase after cardiac arrest in pigs: A comparison of epinephrine versus vasopressin. *Crit Care Med.* 1996;24(12):2014–2019.
120. Lindner KH, Dirks B, Strohmenger HU, Prengel AW, Lindner IM, Lurie KG. Randomised comparison of epinephrine and vasopressin in patients with out-of-hospital ventricular fibrillation. *Lancet.* 1997;349(9051):535–537.
121. Stiell IG, Hébert PC, Wells GA, et al. Vasopressin versus epinephrine for inhospital cardiac arrest: a randomised controlled trial. *Lancet.* 2001;358(9276):105–109.
122. Landry DW, Oliver JA. The ATP-sensitive K+ channel mediates hypotension in endotoxemia and hypoxic lactic acidosis in dog. *J Clin Invest.* 1992;89(6):2071–2074.
123. Levy B, Fritz C, Tahon E, Jacquot A, Auchet T, Kimmoun A. Vasoplegia treatments: the past, the present, and the future. *Crit Care.* 2018;22(1):52.
124. Wenzel V, Krismer AC, Arntz HR, et al. A comparison of vasopressin and epinephrine for out-of-hospital cardiopulmonary resuscitation. *N Engl J Med.* 2004;350(2):105–113.
125. Van Herendael H, Dorian P. Amiodarone for the treatment and prevention of ventricular fibrillation and ventricular tachycardia. *Vasc Health Risk Manag.* 2010;6:465–472.
126. Kudenchuk PJ, Cobb LA, Copass MK, et al. Amiodarone for resuscitation after out-of-hospital cardiac arrest due to ventricular fibrillation. *N Engl J Med.* 1999;341(12):871–878.
127. Dorian P, Cass D, Schwartz B, Cooper R, Gelaznikas R, Barr A. Amiodarone as compared with lidocaine for shock-resistant ventricular fibrillation. *N Engl J Med.* 2002;346(12):884–890.
128. Kudenchuk PJ, Brown SP, Daya M, et al. Amiodarone, lidocaine, or placebo in out-of-hospital cardiac arrest. *N Engl J Med.* 2016;374(18):1711–1722.
129. Stueven HA, Tonsfeldt DJ, Thompson BM, Whitcomb J, Kastenson E, Aprahamian C. Atropine in asystole - human studies. *Ann Emerg Med.* 1984;13(9):815–817.
130. Coon GA, Clinton JE, Ruiz E. Use of atropine for brady-asystolic prehospital cardiac-arrest. *Ann Emerg Med.* 1981;10(9):462–467.
131. Guerci AD, Chandra N, Johnson E, et al. Failure of sodium-bicarbonate to improve resuscitation from ventricular-fibrillation in dogs. *Circulation.* 1986;74(6):75–79.
132. Federiuk CS, Sanders AB, Kern KB, Nelson J, Ewy GA. The effect of bicarbonate on resuscitation from cardiac-arrest. *Ann Emerg Med.* 1991;20(11):1173–1177.
133. Chang CY, Wu PH, Hsiao CT, Chang CP, Chen YC, Wu KH. Sodium bicarbonate administration during in-hospital pediatric cardiac arrest: A systematic review and meta-analysis. *Resuscitation.* 2021;162:188–197.
134. Touron M, Javaudin F, Lebastard Q, et al. Effect of sodium bicarbonate on functional outcome in patients with out-of-hospital cardiac arrest: a post-hoc analysis of a French and North-American dataset. *Eur J Emerg Med.* 2022;29(3):210–220.
135. Wang CH, Wu CY, Wu MC, et al. A retrospective study on the therapeutic effects of sodium bicarbonate for adult in-hospital cardiac arrest. *Sci Rep.* 2021;11(1):12380.
136. Wu KH, Chang CY, Chen YC, Chang CP, Hsiao CT, Weng HH. Effectiveness of sodium bicarbonate administration on mortality in cardiac arrest patients: A systematic review and meta-analysis. *J Emerg Med.* 2020;59(6):856–864.
137. Bishop RL, Weisfeldt ML, Sodium-bicarbonate Administration during cardiac-arrest—reply. *JAMA.* 1976;236(6):563–563.
138. Mattar JA, Weil MH, Shubin H, Stein L. Cardiac-arrest in critically III .2. hyperosmolal states following cardiac-arrest. *Am J Med.* 1974;56(2):162–168.
139. Sanders AB, Otto CW, Kern KB, Rogers JN, Perrault P, Ewy GA. Acid-base-balance in a canine model of cardiac-arrest. *Ann Emerg Med.* 1988;17(7):667–671.
140. Kette F, Weil MH, von Planta M, Gazmuri RJ, Rackow EC. Buffer agents do not reverse intramyocardial acidosis during cardiac resuscitation. *Circulation.* 1990;81(5):1660–1666.
141. Dembo DH. Calcium in advanced life support. *Crit Care Med.* 1981;9(5):358–359.
142. Harrison EE, Amey BD. The use of calcium in cardiac resuscitation. *Am J Emerg Med.* 1983; 1(3):267–273.
143. Stueven H, Thompson BM, Aprahamian C, Darin JC. Use of calcium in prehospital cardiac arrest. *Ann Emerg Med.* 1983;12(3):136–139.
144. Stueven HA, Thompson BM, Aprahamian C, Tonsfeldt DJ. Calcium chloride: reassessment of use in asystole. *Ann Emerg Med.* 1984;13(9 Pt 2):820–822.
145. Stueven HA, Thompson B, Aprahamian C, Tonsfeldt DJ, Kastenson EH. Lack of effectiveness of calcium-chloride in refractory asystole. *Ann Emerg Med.* 1985;14(7):630–632.
146. Vallentin MF, Granfeldt A, Meilandt C, et al. Effect of calcium vs. placebo on long-term outcomes in patients with out-of-hospital cardiac arrest. *Resuscitation.* 2022;179:21–24.
147. Kerber RE, Sarnat W. Factors influencing the success of ventricular defibrillation in man. *Circulation.* 1979;60(2):226–230.
148. Yakaitis RW, Ewy GA, Otto CW, Taren DL, Moon TE. Influence of time and therapy on ventricular defibrillation in dogs. *Crit Care Med.* 1980;8(3):157–163.
149. Sanders AB, Kern KB, Atlas M, Bragg S, Ewy GA. Importance of the duration of inadequate coronary perfusion-pressure on resuscitation from cardiac-arrest. *J Am Coll Cardiol.* 1985;6(1):113–118.
150. Weaver WD, Copass MK, Bufi D, Ray R, Hallstrom AP, Cobb LA. Improved neurologic recovery and survival after early defibrillation. *Circulation.* 1984;69(5):943–948.
151. Weaver WD, Cobb LA, Dennis D, Ray R, Hallstrom AP, Copass MK. Amplitude of ventricular fibrillation waveform and outcome after cardiac arrest. *Ann Intern Med.* 1985;102(1):53–55.
152. Ewy GA, Dahl CF, Zimmerman M, Otto C. Ventricular fibrillation masquerading as ventricular standstill. *Crit Care Med.* 1981;9(5):392.
153. Stewart AJ, Allen JD, Adgey AA. Frequency analysis of ventricular fibrillation and resuscitation success. *Q J Med.* 1992;85(306):761–769.
154. Brown CG, Griffith RF, Van Ligten P, et al. Median frequency–a new parameter for predicting defibrillation success rate. *Ann Emerg Med.* 1991;20(7):787–789.
155. Strohmenger HU, Lindner KH, Brown CG. Analysis of the ventricular fibrillation ECG signal amplitude and frequency parameters as predictors of countershock success in humans. *Chest.* 1997;111(3):584–589.
156. Povoas HP, Weil MH, Tang W, Bisera J, Klouche K, Barbatsis A. Predicting the success of defibrillation by electrocardiographic analysis. *Resuscitation.* 2002;53(1):77–82.
157. Strohmenger HU, Eftestol T, Sunde K, et al. The predictive value of ventricular fibrillation electrocardiogram signal frequency and amplitude variables in patients with out-of-hospital cardiac arrest. *Anesth Analg.* 2001;93(6):1428–1433.
158. Otto CW, Yakaitis RW, Ewy GA. Effect of epinephrine on defibrillation in ischemic ventricular fibrillation. *Am J Emerg Med.* 1985;3(4):285–291.
159. Cummins RO, Eisenberg M, Bergner L, Murray JA. Sensitivity, accuracy, and safety of an automatic external defibrillator—report of a field-evaluation. *Lancet.* 1984;2(8398): 318–320.
160. Cummins RO, Eisenberg MS, Litwin PE, Graves JR, Hearne TR, Hallstrom AP. Automatic external defibrillators used by emergency medical technicians—a controlled clinical-trial. *JAMA.* 1987;257(12):1605–1610.
161. Kerber RE, Kouba C, Martins J, et al. Advance prediction of trans-thoracic impedance in human defibrillation and cardioversion—importance of impedance in determining the success of low-energy shocks. *Circulation.* 1984;70(2):303–308.
162. Kerber RE, McPherson D, Charbonnier F, Kieso R, Hite P. Automated impedance-based energy adjustment for defibrillation—experimental studies. *Circulation.* 1985;71(1): 136–140.
163. Lerman BB, Dimarco JP, Haines DE. Current-based versus energy-based ventricular defibrillation—a prospective-study. *J Am Coll Cardiol.* 1988;12(5):1259–1264.
164. White RD, Blackwell TH, Russell JK, Snyder DE, Jorgenson DB. Transthoracic impedance does not affect defibrillation, resuscitation or survival in patients with out-of-hospital cardiac arrest treated with a non-escalating biphasic waveform defibrillator. *Resuscitation.* 2005; 64(1):63–69.

165. Chen B, Yin C, Ristagno G, et al. Retrospective evaluation of current-based impedance compensation defibrillation in out-of-hospital cardiac arrest. *Resuscitation*. 2013;84(5):580–585.
166. Kerber RE, Grayzel J, Hoyt R, Marcus M, Kennedy J. Trans-thoracic resistance in human defibrillation - influence of body-weight, chest size, serial shocks, paddle size and paddle contact pressure. *Circulation*. 1981;63(3):676–682.
167. Connell PN, Ewy GA, Dahl CF, Ewy MD. Transthoracic impedance to defibrillator discharge. Effect of electrode size and electrode-chest wall interface. *J Electrocardiol*. 1973;6(4):313–M.
168. Ewy GA, Taren D. Comparison of paddle electrode pastes used for defibrillation. *Heart Lung*. 1977;6(5):847–850.
169. Ewy GA, Hellman DA, McClung S, Taren D. Influence of ventilation phase on transthoracic impedance and defibrillation effectiveness. *Crit Care Med*. 1980;8(3):164–166.
170. Dahl CF, Ewy GA, Warner ED, Thomas ED. Myocardial necrosis from direct current countershock. Effect of paddle electrode size and time interval between discharges. *Circulation*. 1974;50(5):956–961.
171. Warner ED, Dahl C, Ewy GA. Myocardial injury from transthoracic defibrillator countershock. *Arch Pathol*. 1975;99(1):55–59.
172. Ehsani A, Ewy GA, Sobel BE. Effects of electrical countershock on serum creatine phosphokinase (CPK) isoenzyme activity. *Am J Cardiol*. 1976;37(1):12–18.
173. Weaver WD, Cobb LA, Copass MK, Hallstrom AP. Ventricular defibrillation – a comparative trial using 175-J and 320-J shocks. *N Engl J Med*. 1982;307(18):1101–1106.
174. Geddes LA, Tacker WA, Rosborough JP, Moore AG, Cabler PS. Electrical dose for ventricular defibrillation of large and small animals using precordial electrodes. *J Clin Invest*. 1974;53(1):310–319.
175. Gutgesell HP, Tacker WA, Geddes LA, Davis S, Lie JT, McNamara DG. Energy dose for ventricular defibrillation of children. *Pediatrics*. 1976;58(6):898–901.
176. Guidelines 2000 for Cardiopulmonary Resuscitation and Emergency Cardiovascular Care. Part 2: ethical aspects of CPR and ECC. *Circulation*. 2000;102(8 Suppl):I12–I21.
177. Bardy GH, Marchlinski FE, Sharma AD, et al. Multicenter comparison of truncated biphasic shocks and standard damped sine wave monophasic shocks fortransthoracic ventricular defibrillation. Transthoracic Investigators. *Circulation*. 1996;94(10):2507–2514.
178. Morrison LJ, Henry RM, Ku V, Nolan JP, Morley P, Deakin CD. Single-shock defibrillation success in adult cardiac arrest: a systematic review. *Resuscitation*. 2013;84(11):1480–1486.
179. Soar J, Maconochie I, Wyckoff MH, et al. 2019 International consensus on cardiopulmonary resuscitation and emergency cardiovascular care science with treatment recommendations: Summary from the basic life support; advanced life support; Pediatric life support; neonatal life support; education, implementation, and teams; and first aid task forces. *Circulation*. 2019;140(24):e826–e880.
180. Atkins DL, Sasson C, Hsu A, et al. 2022 Interim guidance to health care providers for basic and advanced cardiac life support in adults, children, and neonates with suspected or confirmed COVID-19: From the emergency cardiovascular care committee and get with the guidelines-resuscitation adult and pediatric task forces of the American Heart association in collaboration With the American Academy of Pediatrics, American Association for respiratory care, the society of critical care anesthesiologists, and American Society of anesthesiologists. *Circ Cardiovasc Qual Outcomes*. 2022;15(4):302–317.
181. Moretti MA, Cesar LA, Nusbacher A, Kern KB, Timerman S, Ramires JA. Advanced cardiac life support training improves long-term survival from in-hospital cardiac arrest. *Resuscitation*. 2007;72(3):458–465.
182. Rea TD, Eisenberg MS, Becker LJ, Murray JA, Hearne T. Temporal trends in sudden cardiac arrest: a 25-year emergency medical services perspective. *Circulation*. 2003;107(22):2780–2785.
183. Sanders AB., Cardiac arrest and the limitations of clinical trials. *N Engl J Med*. 2011;365(9):850–851.
184. Garcia RA, Girotra S, Jones PG, et al. Variation in out-of-hospital cardiac arrest survival across emergency medical service agencies. *Circ Cardiovasc Qual Outcomes*. 2022;15(6):e008755.
185. Rasmussen TP, Riley DJ, Sarazin MV, Chan PS, Girotra S. Variation across hospitals in in-hospital cardiac arrest incidence among Medicare beneficiaries. *JAMA Netw Open*. 2022;5(2):e2148485.
186. Weisfeldt ML., A three phase temporal model for cardiopulmonary resuscitation following cardiac arrest. *Trans Am Clin Climatol Assoc*. 2004;115:115–122; discussion 122.
187. Caffrey SL, Willoughby PJ, Pepe PE, Becker LB. Public use of automated external defibrillators. *N Engl J Med*. 2002;347(16):1242–1247.
188. Kern KB, Garewal HS, Sanders AB, et al. Depletion of myocardial adenosine triphosphate during prolonged untreated ventricular fibrillation: effect on defibrillation success. *Resuscitation*. 1990;20(3):221–229.
189. Ornato JP, Hallagan LF, McMahan SB, Peeples EH, Rostafinski AG. Attitudes of BCLS instructors about mouth-to-mouth resuscitation during the AIDS epidemic. *Ann Emerg Med*. 1990;19(2):151–156.
190. Brenner BE, Kauffman J. Reluctance of internists and medical nurses to perform mouth-to-mouth resuscitation. *Arch Intern Med*. 1993;153(15):1763–1769.
191. Locke CJ, Berg RA, Sanders AB, et al. Bystander cardiopulmonary resuscitation. Concerns about mouth-to-mouth contact. *Arch Intern Med*. 1995;155(9):938–943.
192. Bossaert L, Van Hoeyweghen R. Bystander cardiopulmonary resuscitation (CPR) in out-of-hospital cardiac arrest. The Cerebral Resuscitation Study Group. *Resuscitation*. 1989;17 Suppl:S55–S69; discussion S199–S206.
193. Van Hoeyweghen RJ, Bossaert LL, Mullie A, et al. Quality and efficiency of bystander CPR. Belgian Cerebral Resuscitation Study Group. *Resuscitation*. 1993;26(1):47–52.
194. group S-Ks. Cardiopulmonary resuscitation by bystanders with chest compression only (SOS-KANTO): an observational study. *Lancet*. 2007;369(9565):920–926.
195. Berg RA, Kern KB, Sanders AB, Otto CW, Hilwig RW, Ewy GA. Bystander cardiopulmonary resuscitation. Is ventilation necessary? *Circulation*. 1993;88(4 Pt 1):1907–1915.
196. Berg RA, Wilcoxson D, Hilwig RW, et al. The need for ventilatory support during bystander CPR. *Ann Emerg Med*. 1995;26(3):342–350.
197. Berg RA, Kern KB, Hilwig RW, et al. Assisted ventilation does not improve outcome in a porcine model of single-rescuer bystander cardiopulmonary resuscitation. *Circulation*. 1997;95(6):1635–1641.
198. Berg RA, Kern KB, Hilwig RW, Ewy GA. Assisted ventilation during 'bystander' CPR in a swine acute myocardial infarction model does not improve outcome. *Circulation*. 1997;96(12):4364–4371.
199. Assar D, Chamberlain D, Colquhoun M, et al. Randomised controlled trials of staged teaching for basic life support. 1. Skill acquisition at bronze stage. *Resuscitation*. 2000;45(1):7–15.
200. Kern KB, Hilwig RW, Berg RA, Sanders AB, Ewy GA. Importance of continuous chest compressions during cardiopulmonary resuscitation: improved outcome during a simulated single lay-rescuer scenario. *Circulation*. 2002;105(5):645–649.
201. Ewy GA, Zuercher M, Hilwig RW, et al. Improved neurological outcome with continuous chest compressions compared with 30:2 compressions-to-ventilations cardiopulmonary resuscitation in a realistic swine model of out-of-hospital cardiac arrest. *Circulation*. 2007;116(22):2525–2530.
202. Bobrow BJ, Spaite DW, Berg RA, et al. Chest compression-only CPR by lay rescuers and survival from out-of-hospital cardiac arrest. *JAMA*. 2010;304(13):1447–1454.
203. Sayre MR, Berg RA, Cave DM, et al. Hands-only (compression-only) cardiopulmonary resuscitation: a call to action for bystander response to adults who experience out-of-hospital sudden cardiac arrest: a science advisory for the public from the American Heart Association Emergency Cardiovascular Care Committee. *Circulation*. 2008;117(16):2162–2167.
204. Nichol G, Leroux B, Wang H, et al. Trial of continuous or interrupted chest compressions during CPR. *N Engl J Med*. 2015;373(23):2203–2214.
205. Wik L, Kramer-Johansen J, Myklebust H, et al. Quality of cardiopulmonary resuscitation during out-of-hospital cardiac arrest. *JAMA*. 2005;293(3):299–304.
206. Schmicker RH, Nichol G, Kudenchuk P, et al. CPR compression strategy 30:2 is difficult to adhere to, but has better survival than continuous chest compressions when done correctly. *Resuscitation*. 2021;165:31–37.
207. Aufderheide TP, Sigurdsson G, Pirrallo RG, et al. Hyperventilation-induced hypotension during cardiopulmonary resuscitation. *Circulation*. 2004;109(16):1960–1965.
208. Aufderheide TP, Lurie KG. Death by hyperventilation: a common and life-threatening problem during cardiopulmonary resuscitation. *Crit Care Med*. 2004;32(9 Suppl):S345–S351.
209. Milander MM, Hiscok PS, Sanders AB, Kern KB, Berg RA, Ewy GA. Chest compression and ventilation rates during cardiopulmonary resuscitation: the effects of audible tone guidance. *Acad Emerg Med*. 1995;2(8):708–713.
210. Cobb LA, Fahrenbruch CE, Walsh TR, et al. Influence of cardiopulmonary resuscitation prior to defibrillation in patients with out-of-hospital ventricular fibrillation. *JAMA*. 1999;281(13):1182–1188.
211. Wik L, Hansen TB, Fylling F, et al. Delaying defibrillation to give basic cardiopulmonary resuscitation to patients with out-of-hospital ventricular fibrillation: a randomized trial. *JAMA*. 2003;289(11):1389–1395.
212. Berg RA, Hilwig RW, Kern KB, Sanders AB, Xavier LC, Ewy GA. Automated external defibrillation versus manual defibrillation for prolonged ventricular fibrillation: lethal delays of chest compressions before and after countershocks. *Ann Emerg Med*. 2003;42(4):458–467.
213. Rea TD, Shah S, Kudenchuk PJ, Copass MK, Cobb LA. Automated external defibrillators: to what extent does the algorithm delay CPR? *Ann Emerg Med*. 2005;46(2):132–141.
214. Ewy GA, Kellum MJ, Bobrow BJ. Cardiocerebral resuscitation. Improving cardiac arrest survival with a new technique. *JEMS*. 2009;34(7):58–60, 63–65, 67; quiz 69.
215. Bobrow BJ, Clark LL, Ewy GA, et al. Minimally interrupted cardiac resuscitation by emergency medical services for out-of-hospital cardiac arrest. *JAMA*. 2008;299(10):1158–1165.
216. Brain Resuscitation Clinical Trial I Study Group. Randomized clinical-study of thiopental (Th) loading after cardiac-arrest. *Crit Care Med*. 1981;9(3):248–248.
217. Witten L, Gardner R, Holmberg MJ, et al. Reasons for death in patients successfully resuscitated from out-of-hospital and in-hospital cardiac arrest. *Resuscitation*. 2019;136:93–99.
218. Rittenberger JC, Popescu A, Brenner RP, Guyette FX, Callaway CW. Frequency and timing of nonconvulsive status epilepticus in comatose post-cardiac arrest subjects treated with hypothermia. *Neurocrit Care*. 2012;16(1):114–122.
219. Elmer J, Coppler PJ, Jones BL, Nagin DS, Callaway CW; University of Pittsburgh Post-Cardiac Arrest Service. Bayesian outcome prediction after resuscitation from cardiac arrest. *Neurology*. 2022;99(11):e1113–e1121.

220. Liu Y, Rosenthal RE, Haywood Y, Miljkovic-Lolic M, Vanderhoek JY, Fiskum G. Normoxic ventilation after cardiac arrest reduces oxidation of brain lipids and improves neurological outcome. *Stroke*. 1998;29(8):1679–1686.
221. Zwemer CF, Whitesall SE, D'Alecy LG. Cardiopulmonary-cerebral resuscitation with 100% oxygen exacerbates neurological dysfunction following nine minutes of normothermic cardiac arrest in dogs. *Resuscitation*. 1994;27(2):159–170.
222. Lipinski CA, Hicks SD, Callaway CW. Normoxic ventilation during resuscitation and outcome from asphyxial cardiac arrest in rats. *Resuscitation*. 1999;42(3):221–229.
223. A randomized clinical trial of calcium entry blocker administration to comatose survivors of cardiac arrest. Design, methods, and patient characteristics. The Brain Resuscitation Clinical Trial II Study Group. *Control Clin Trials*. 1991;12(4):525–545.
224. Hypothermia After Cardiac Arrest Study Group. Mild therapeutic hypothermia to improve the neurologic outcome after cardiac arrest. *N Engl J Med*. 2002;346(22):1756–1756.
225. Bernard SA, Gray TW, Buist MD, et al. Treatment of comatose survivors of out-of-hospital cardiac arrest with induced hypothermia. *N Engl J Med*. 2002;346(8):557–563.
226. Nielsen N, Wetterslev J, Cronberg T, et al. Targeted temperature management at 33°C versus 36°C after cardiac arrest. *N Engl J Med*. 2013;369(23):2197–2206.
227. Donnino MW, Andersen LW, Berg KM, et al. Temperature management after cardiac arrest an advisory statement by the advanced life support task force of the International Liaison Committee on Resuscitation and the American Heart Association Emergency Cardiovascular Care Committee and the Council on Cardiopulmonary, Critical Care, Perioperative and Resuscitation. *Circulation*. 2015;132(25):2448–2456.
228. Constant AL, Mongardon N, Morelot Q, et al. Targeted temperature management after intraoperative cardiac arrest: a multicenter retrospective study. *Intensive Care Med*. 2017;43(4):485–495.
229. Booth CM, Boone RH, Tomlinson G, Detsky AS. Is this patient dead, vegetative, or severely neurologically impaired? Assessing outcome for comatose survivors of cardiac arrest. *JAMA*. 2004; 291(7):870–879.
230. Callaway CW, Donnino MW, Fink EL, et al. Part 8: Post-Cardiac Arrest Care: 2015 American Heart Association Guidelines Update for Cardiopulmonary Resuscitation and Emergency Cardiovascular Care. *Circulation*. 2015;132(18 Suppl 2):S465–S482.
231. Hall KK, Shoemaker-Hunt S, Hoffman L, et al. In: *Making Healthcare Safer III: A Critical Analysis of Existing and Emerging Patient Safety Practices*. Agency for Healthcare Research and Quality (US); 2020.
232. Burian BK, Dismukes RK. Why we fail to rescue during critical events. *Anesthesiol Clin*. 2020;38(4):727–743.
233. Burden AR. High-fidelity simulation education and crisis resource management. *Anesthesiology clinics*. 2020;38(4):745–759.
234. Castelao EF, Russo SG, Riethmüller M, Boos M. Effects of team coordination during cardiopulmonary resuscitation: A systematic review of the literature. *J Crit Care*. 2013;28(4): 504–521.
235. Lemke DS, Young AL, Won SK, et al. Rapid-cycle deliberate practice improves time to defibrillation and reduces workload: A randomized controlled trial of simulation-based education. *AEM Educ Train*. 2021;5(4):e10702.
236. Bishop JP, Brothers KB, Perry JE, Ahmad A. Reviving the conversation around CPR/DNR. *Am J Bioeth*. 2010;10(1):61–67.
237. Van Norman G. Do not resuscitate during anesthesia and urgent procedures. *Ethics in Medicine*. 2022. https://depts.washington.edu/bhdept/ethics-medicine/bioethics-topics/detail/62.
238. Cohen CB, Cohen PJ. Do-not-resuscitate orders in the operating-room. *N Engl J Med*. 1991;325(26):1879–1882.
239. Walker RM. Dnr in the or - resuscitation as an operative risk. *JAMA*. 1991;266(17):2407–2412.
240. Waisel DB, Simon R, Truog RD, Baboolal H, Raemer DB. Anesthesiologist management of perioperative do-not-resuscitate orders: a simulation-based experiment. *Simul Healthc*. 2009;4(2):70–76.
241. American Society of Anesthesiologists. Committee on Ethics. Ethical Guidelines for the care of patient with do-not-resuscitate orders or other directives that limit treatment. 2018. Available at https://www.asahq.org/standards-and-guidelines/statement-on-ethical-guidelines-for-the-anesthesia-care-of-patients-with-do-not-resuscitate-orders. Accessed June 21, 2023.
242. Surgeons ACo. Statement on advance directives by paitnets: "Do Not Resuscitate" in the operating room. *Bull Am Coll Surg*. 2014;42–43.
243. Association of Operating Room Nurses. AORN position statement on perioperative care of patients with do-not-resuscitate or allow-natural-death orders. 2014. Available at https://aorn.org/docs/default-source/guidelines-resources/position-statements/patient-care/posstat-dnr-w-0620.pdf?sfvrsn=b4a9796d_1#:~:text=AORN%20Position%20Statement%20on%20Perioperative%20Care%20of%20Patients,of%20patients%20undergoing%20surgery%20or%20other%20invasive%20procedures1-5%3B. Accessed February 19, 2023.
244. Truog RD, Waisel DB, Burns JP, DNR in the OR: a goal-directed approach. *Anesthesiology*. 1999;90(1):289–295.
245. Truog RD, Waisel DB, Do-not-resuscitate orders: from the ward to the operating room; from procedures to goals. *Int Anesthesiol Clin*. 2001;39(3):53–65.
246. Margolis JO, McGrath BJ, Kussin PS, Schwinn DA. Do not resuscitate (Dnr) orders during surgery - ethical foundations for institutional policies in the United-States. *Anesth Analg*. 1995;80(4):806–809.
247. Waisel DB, Burns JP, Johnson JA, Hardart GE, Truog RD. Guidelines for perioperative do-not-resuscitate policies. *J Clin Anesth*. 2002;14(6):467–473.

59 Disaster Preparedness

JOSEPH H. MCISAAC III • CARIN A. HAGBERG • MICHAEL J. MURRAY

KEY POINTS

1. There are certain principles that are common to all disaster events, independent of their etiology. As a group, anesthesiologists are well prepared to assist their communities in planning for and in caring for patients who sustain injury or harm from such events.
2. Often overlooked during emergency preparedness and disaster management training is the development of a family plan and a personal preparedness plan. The former is important whether one lives alone; has a pet, family, or friends living with them, or has legal responsibility for a loved one (elderly parents, disabled person). A plan should be in place that provides care for and information to loved ones.
3. Anesthesiologists' basic understanding of physiology and pharmacology, airway skills, fluid resuscitation expertise, ability to manage ventilators, and provide anesthesia both in and out of the operating rooms, is invaluable.
4. If assigned to triage patients, the anesthesiologist will be expected to classify patients into four groups: Those requiring immediate care, delayed care, minimal care (first aid), and expectant (no care).
5. If a patient presents with life-threatening injury, the patient is treated first and decontaminated afterward; otherwise, all other patients are decontaminated in the triage area before they are evaluated and treated.
6. During a disaster, the anesthesiologist in charge of the schedule for the day should become the operating room medical director, co-locate with the operating room nurse in charge, and determine the status of ongoing cases. Surgeons in the midst of a procedure should be contacted and urged to finish as soon as possible. Elective cases should be postponed or cancelled.
7. In many disasters, infrastructure degradation plays a large part in reducing surgical capabilities at a time when demand is increased. Surgeons and anesthesiologists must consider what types of procedures can safely be undertaken and must prioritize care based on urgency and practicality.
8. There are three categories of biologic weapons. Category A are those weapons that are highly contagious, are associated with a high mortality rate, and have all the characteristics of a relatively ideal weapon of mass destruction.
9. The principle of disaster management following the release of ionizing radiation always involves containment (avoidance of bringing patients with material emitting ionizing radiation to the hospital). Therefore, as part of the containment process, to the extent possible, patients should be decontaminated at the site. Removal of clothing is critically important. β and γ rays and neutrons will no longer be present unless there is still material emitting this radiation on a person's clothing. Rather than guess whether radiation is still present it is best to disrobe patients and wash them with warm soapy water.
10. Orally administered potassium iodide can attenuate most radiation-induced thyroid effects, but must be given as quickly as possible because after 24 hours, there is little protective effect.
11. Because of the possibility of blast, thermal, and crush injuries that may occur along with radiation injury, the care of the injured may require the care of patients who have multiple combined injuries.
12. Patients who have sustained traumatic injury from an improvised explosive device but do not have third-degree burns should receive minimal amounts of intravenous crystalloid and should undergo "damage control resuscitation/surgery" as soon as possible.
13. Infrastructure degradation worsens the consequences of mass casualty events. Preparing to deliver care under austere circumstances, developing creative responses, and practicing (conducting simulations) regularly will mitigate the effects of a disaster and increase resilience for individuals, teams, and institutions.

Introduction

Hurricanes, the Boston Marathon bombing, the Asiana plane crash, the pandemics caused by COVID-19, and Ebola and Zika viruses are all events that entered our national consciousness, connoting vivid images of unfortunate circumstances. Although we cannot control, or even predict, the source of the next major disaster in the United States, it is far more likely to be Mother Nature and not an international terrorist who will be the force behind the destruction, but the latter scenario cannot be ignored. We can, however, control our preparedness and, therefore, our response to situations that result in mass casualties. As anesthesiologists, we have a responsibility not only to know our institution's disaster plan and our role therein but also to prepare our family members and ourselves so that we do not become unintended victims of the next disaster, which in turn would result in our unavailability to provide care during a disaster and in our becoming an additional burden to the healthcare system.

The World Association for Disaster and Emergency Medicine (WADEM) provides a useful diagram for defining disaster nomenclature (Fig. 59-1).[1] A *multiple casualty incident* (≤10 casualties arriving at a hospital simultaneously) typically refers to a situation that creates havoc within the hospital, but in these situations the hospital usually has the resources to manage the number of casualties arriving at its emergency department (ED). A *mass casualty event* (usually >10 casualties arriving at the ED) is one that has the potential to

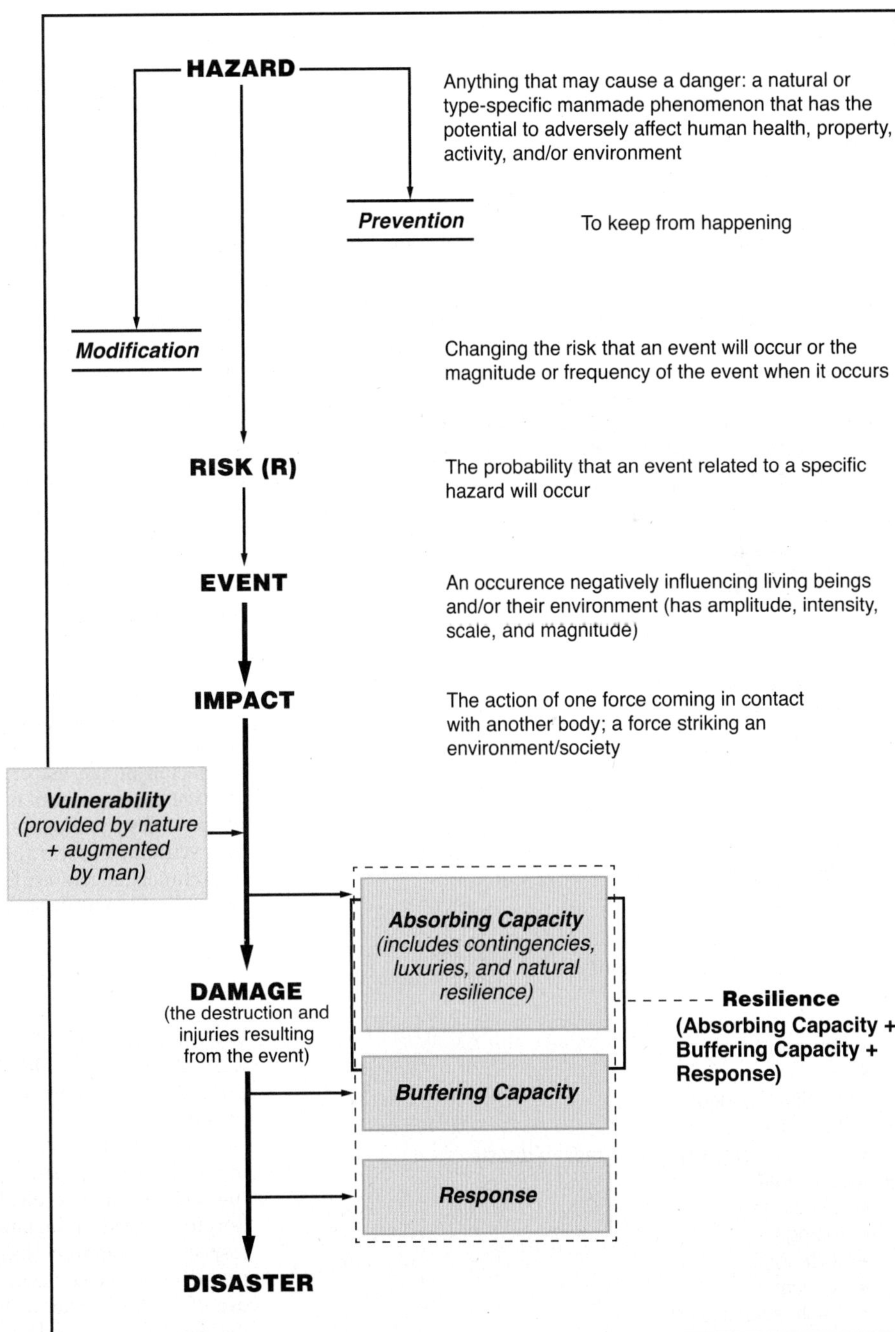

Figure 59-1 Diagrammatic descriptions of definitions. (Adapted with permission from Cambridge University Press, from Task Force on Quality Control of Disaster Management, World Association for Disaster and Emergency Medicine, Nordic Society for Disaster Medicine. Health disaster management: guidelines for evaluation and research in the Utstein style. Volume I. Conceptual framework of disasters. *Prehosp Disaster Med*. 2003;17 Suppl 3:1–177. World Association for Disaster and Emergency Medicine website. https://wadem.org/wp-content/uploads/2016/03/intro.pdf.)

overwhelm a hospital's ability to respond effectively. Certainly, the size of the hospital has bearing on how one defines a given situation, as larger hospitals have more resources to manage a larger number of casualties without being overwhelmed. Nonetheless, environmental factors also play a role in how effectively a hospital can respond to a situation. For example, a hospital's physical structure may be so damaged by an earthquake or a tornado that it is rendered inoperable, making it unsafe to provide care to its current patients, much less any new patients. As another example, flooding may result in the facility losing its external and emergency back-up electrical power supply—making it, for all practical purposes, inoperable.

Mass-casualty incidents and events may result from any number of disasters, most commonly from naturally occurring events, but they may also result from human activity, both intentional and unintentional. The Joint Commission (TJC) lists the most likely disasters for which a hospital should be prepared:

- Air disaster
- Violence/security/active shooter
- Hurricane
- Tornado
- Water crisis
- Winter storm

Shootings and chemical, biologic, radiologic, nuclear, and explosive (CBRNE) attacks comprise the most likely intentional events, whereas industrial accidents, vehicle collisions, collapse of stadiums or other public structures, and fires make up the most commonly encountered unintentional events (Table 59-1).

Table 59-1 Types of Disasters According to the Joint Commission on Accreditation of Healthcare Organizations

Natural
- **Meteorologic**
  - Hurricanes
  - Tornadoes
  - Floods
  - Mudslides
  - Extreme heat or cold
  - Forest fires
- **Geologic**
  - Earthquakes
  - Tsunamis
  - Volcanic eruptions
  - Lahars
- **Biologic**
  - Bacterial
  - Viral

Resulting from Human Activity
- **Unintentional**
  - Airplane/train/bus crash
  - Boat sinking
  - Fire
  - Nuclear accident
  - Industrial accident
  - Building collapses/sports stadium disaster
- **Intentional**
  - Chemical
  - Biologic
  - Radiologic
  - Nuclear
  - (High-yield) explosive

The first step in any disaster response plan is to mitigate or reduce risk. The 2015 Sendai Framework lays out a path for international collaboration on disaster risk reduction.[2] The United States is also cognizant of the benefits to its foreign policy by assisting in humanitarian missions. The U.S. Agency for International Development (USAID) spends a significant portion of its budget each year to provide humanitarian assistance in the wake of natural disasters such as floods, volcanic eruptions, and earthquakes. Of significance is that it spends just as much to mitigate the effects of future catastrophes.

The American Society of Anesthesiologists (ASA) recognized the importance of emergency preparedness and in the past decade established a Committee on Trauma and Emergency Preparedness (COTEP) and a Committee on Global Humanitarian Outreach (CGHO). The ASA has an extensive online set of resources to aid its members in emergency preparedness and disaster management.[3] As a member-driven organization, the ASA's development of these resources, for the most part, stems from members' requests to provide assistance during disasters (e.g., the 9–11 terrorist attack, numerous hurricanes and tornados, the 2010 Haitian earthquake, the Fukushima disaster, and the 2015 Nepal earthquake). ASA members who have been involved in relief efforts, including former or current military members and international members who have experienced terrorism on a more frequent basis, created a cacophony of voices calling for more education and training on how to prepare for a disaster and how to manage the victims of such disasters. Most residency program directors and anesthesiology residents would agree that although anesthesiologists are well prepared to manage individual patients, they lack the knowledge and education to manage the numbers of patients that might arise from a mass casualty event. There are entire books devoted to the topic and governments created large bureaucracies to address such events. This single book chapter does not provide adequate knowledge to cope with all contingencies.

However, there are certain principles that are common to all 1
such events, independent of their etiology, and as anesthesiologists we are well prepared to assist our communities in planning for and in caring for patients affected by a disaster. We must expend the energy to be better educated, as the initial response to any disaster always occurs at the local level; therefore, as anesthesiologists we must be prepared to provide assistance during such emergencies. Other physicians, hospital administrators, and nongovernment organizations (NGOs) all place anesthesia providers at the top of the list of healthcare workers who are needed to manage the sequelae of natural disasters and mass casualty events. In fact, anesthesiologists are in such demand that the NGO Doctors Without Borders (*Medecins san Frontieres*) waives its policy that clinicians commit for 9- to 18-month assignments; there is an option for anesthesia providers of 1- to 3-month assignments.[4]

Anesthesiologists have the requisite skills to assist in many types of disasters. We might be asked to provide anesthesia for an amputation to facilitate extrication from rubble, to start an intravenous (IV) infusion in someone debilitated by diarrhea or Ebola virus disease (EVD), or to provide ventilatory support to a COVID-19 patient. Although the clinical situations are not customary, these are services we provide on a daily basis to individual patients.

However, disasters and mass casualty events are not something in which we participate regularly; thus, education and training for these situations is critically important, beginning with preparation to respond to the most likely disasters that may occur in our respective geographic location. Even though natural and industrial disasters have occurred for millennia, the recent increasing use of CBRNE weapons by terrorists and in warfare emphasizes the need for increased preparedness.

However, time and time again history demonstrates that enthusiasm for education is high after an event and then tapers off; maintaining that enthusiasm is difficult and therefore most, if not all, healthcare facilities are not prepared to deal with mass casualty incidents, much less a mass casualty event, the exception being those facilities staffed by physicians with prior military training.[4–7] The majority of physicians most likely have not received adequate education to provide appropriate patient care in such situations. Rössler et al.[8] demonstrated that 24% of anesthesiologists who were deployed during humanitarian crises did not feel sufficiently prepared. Especially important for anesthesiologists who were deployed was the knowledge to repair and maintain anesthesia equipment, to perform peripheral nerve blocks using anatomic landmark techniques, to perform triage of mass casualties, and to treat patients with coexisting tropical disease.

In dealing with acts of terrorism, geography is not helpful in anticipating what might occur, but that is not to say that one cannot anticipate what to expect. One can learn from experience; terrorists have been successful, in their minds' eyes, with improvised explosive devices (IEDs), and even in those situations in which IEDs were not used, terrorists have chosen to use certain weapons of mass destruction (WMDs) more often than others. For example, a nerve agent, such as sarin, is most likely to be chosen as a chemical agent. Similarly, among biologic agents, anthrax, which was used in 2001, or smallpox would be the most likely choice because of the high lethality and infectivity associated with those two agents.[9,10] Twice in the past 20 years "dirty" bombs have either been planned or planted (and fortunately not used), so such devices would be the most likely source of radiation used by terrorists. However, to underscore what was stated here based on past experience, a natural or industrial event is more likely than a terrorist event.

One must also be cognizant that although they might never plan to participate in a humanitarian mission overseas and therefore thinks that there is no need to train to work in an austere environment, the environment may become very austere depending on the circumstances of the disaster in which one finds oneself. Any time a situation arises in which medical capability is significantly below standards to which we are accustomed in the United States, the anesthesiologist is practicing in an austere environment. This austerity might occur in a:

- Mass casualty event in which the number of cases overwhelms capacity
- Natural disaster in which the hospital is damaged or loses electricity or water
- Disaster (natural/industrial/terrorist) in which care is provided on site

As described above, graduates of anesthesiology training programs in North America have the potential to cope well in such situations, provided that they understand the basic requisites of disaster management, the focus of this chapter.

Preparation

Family Plan

2 To manage the numbers of casualties that would be expected during a mass casualty, one must be prepared.[11,12] Often overlooked during emergency preparedness and disaster management training is the development of a family plan and a personal preparedness plan. A family plan is important whether one lives alone; has a pet, family, or friends living with them; or has legal responsibility for a loved one (elderly parents, disabled person). There are a number of websites that guide one through the creation of such a plan (Appendix A).[3] During hurricane Katrina, about 35% of policemen and firemen did not show up for work, which should not be surprising.[13] These individuals may have had to evacuate a parent in an assisted living facility or children in a day care center. Just as the military requires service members to have a family care plan (a Last Will and Testament as well!), as critically important healthcare providers, we should also have family care plans. However, if you know that you will be unavailable during a disaster, then you have a responsibility to inform your employer or group of your personal situation. All family plans should include periodic family drills and updates. Plans might include situations such as what to do if there is a fire, what to do if parents do not make it home, the location of second copies of all-important documents, where to meet if the house or neighborhood is destroyed or not accessible. Many assume that they will be able to communicate with loved ones during a disaster but often cell phone towers are damaged or so many people are trying to use the system that the network is overwhelmed. Plan in advance so that you are prepared for these contingencies.

Just as service members have a duffel bag or sea bag packed with toiletries, bedding, change of clothes, money, flashlights, and battery-operated radio, those with such important roles as ours ideally should have a packed "bag" as well. In a hurricane, earthquake, flood, tornado, or huge solar flare, loss of electric power is very likely. ATMs, gas pumps, toll booths, and so on do not function without electricity—hence the need for some cash, flashlights, a battery-operated/wind-up radio (to stay abreast of the news)—and a vehicle that has a fuel tank that is not empty!

Government Plan

In September 2011, the U.S. Department of Homeland Security published its first edition of a 111-page document, the National Preparedness Goal.[14] Table 59-2 lists the multiple issues for which the Federal Emergency Management Agency (FEMA) must prepare, and with which agencies it must coordinate: the U.S. Departments of Justice, of Health and Human Services, of Agriculture, of Commerce, and of Defense. Of note is that within the "Response" section of the document, medical response is one of eleven types of responses for which the government has planned—a response which is under the auspices of the Department of Health and Human Services (DHHS). DHHS created and maintains a National Disaster Medical System (NDMS). Unfortunately, the system has not been adequately established and maintained. As highlighted by the U.S. response to the earthquake in Haiti in 2010, the DHHS maintained only three International Medical Surgical Response Teams (IMSuRT), teams that were established with the idea that they would provide care to U.S. citizens injured in areas of conflict. Unfortunately, only one was funded and equipped; and, prior to the earthquake in Haiti, it had been activated and used only once—namely, for the earthquake that occurred in 2003 in Bam, Iran. The IMSuRT has since morphed into a single, large unit called the Trauma and Critical Care Team (TCCT), distributed throughout the United States. Other teams that DHHS maintains in its NDMS are:

- Disaster Medical Assistance Team (DMAT) is a team that can rapidly mobilize a staff of physicians, nurses, and other support personnel and set up emergency facilities and pharmaceutical dispensaries geographically as close as possible to a disaster. The teams are self-sustaining for at least 72 hours before they require outside logistics. Just as the reserve military forces do, a DMAT is supposed to train one weekend per month. Not many surgeons and anesthesiologists have joined a DMAT, as the team does not have the capacity to perform surgical procedures!

Table 59-2 Issues for Which FEMA Must Prepare and Agencies with Which It Must Coordinate

Prevention	Protection	Mitigation	Response	Recovery
Forensics and attribution	Access control and identity verification	Community resilience	Critical transportation	Economic recovery
Intelligence and information sharing	Cybersecurity	Long-term vulnerability reduction	Environmental response/ health and safety	Health and social services
Interdiction and disruption	Intelligence and information sharing	Risk and disaster resilience assessment	Fatality management services	Housing
Screening, search, and detection	Interdiction and disruption Physical protective measures Risk management for protection programs and activities Screening, search, and detection Supply chain integrity and security	Threats and hazard identification	Infrastructure systems Mass care services Mass search and rescue operations On-scene security and protection Operational communications Public and private services and resources Public health and medical services Situational assessment	Infrastructure systems Natural and cultural resources

- Disaster Mortuary Team (DMORT), as the name implies, is a team that manages large numbers of dead bodies following a mass casualty event and that has the capacity to conduct forensic examinations.
- National Veterinary Response Team (NVRT) is a team established to provide veterinary services, as well as zoonotic disease surveillance.
- TCCT is a pool of specialists who would be activated during a crisis, whether domestic or international, and would have sufficient logistic support to ensure that the team could deploy to either a fixed facility or a field site. Once activated, TCCT members would be federal employees during their deployments for a minimum of 2 weeks and would be protected by workers' compensation laws, the federal tort claims act, and the Uniformed Services Employment and Reemployment Rights Act (USERRA). DHHS knows that many anesthesia providers do not have time for monthly drills or frequent call ups that the DMATs have. Although TCCT members would be encouraged to train with DMATs, participation in a TCCT requires far less of an investment in time. However, if activated, members of the teams would be expected to deploy or risk being dropped from the team and program.

Healthcare Agency Plans

In recent years, the United States has endured several notable events: the anthrax attacks of 2000 and 2001, the destruction of the World Trade Center Towers on September 11, 2001, the SARS epidemic of 2004, the 2020-present COVID-19 pandemic and the continued devastation caused by nature (hurricanes, earthquakes, tornadoes, floods, and fires) and terrorists. Subsequently, TJC, the Centers for Medicare and Medicaid Services (CMS), and the American Hospital Association (AHA) have more closely monitored and evaluated hospitals' and communities' emergency preparedness. In 2003, TJC published "Health Care at the Crossroads: Strategies for Creating and Maintaining Community-Wide Emergency Preparedness Systems."[15] The white paper has not been updated, but emergency preparedness is one of the standards TJC uses to accredit hospitals. Since 2003, TJC has hosted annual conferences and disseminates information to healthcare systems to help them be better prepared. One of TJC's most recent publications, "Requirements for Emergency Management Oversight," attempts to provide a clear description of leadership-level oversight of emergency management in general and critical access hospitals.[16] To ensure that Medicare and Medicaid patients receive appropriate care during a disaster, the CMS published a checklist that is meant to serve as a guide for healthcare facilities to prepare for and to plan for disasters and emergencies.[17]

Despite the best efforts of law enforcement, fire and rescue teams, and emergency medical agencies, hospitals will continue to play a vital role in helping communities respond to catastrophic events, whether natural, unintentional, or terrorist-initiated. TJC was proactive in recognizing that, "It is no longer sufficient to develop disaster plans and dust them off if a threat appears imminent. Rather a system of preparedness across communities must be in place every day."[15] Such a system is one that is best prepared to handle a surge in casualties or degradation of a facility's ability to handle any new patients following a disaster. The TJC acknowledged this need, despite decreasing healthcare resources, for what it describes as "surge capacity" within healthcare systems to handle potentially hundreds, if not thousands or more, of patients who might be victims of catastrophic events. By planning and drilling, the TJC hopes to reduce the appeal to terrorists of using WMD as an effective means of terrorism, and to help communities better respond to natural disasters. The white paper TJC published focused on three major areas:

- Enlisting the community to develop the local response.
- Focusing on the key aspects of the system that prepare the community to mobilize to care for patients, protect its staff, and serve the public.
- Establishing the accountabilities, oversight, leadership, and sustainment of a community-preparedness system.[15]

Although the guidelines are not mandatory or required by law, all hospitals aspire to have TJC accreditation and from that perspective, the white paper was important in that hospitals do have biannual drills of their emergency preparedness and disaster management plans, sometimes coordinating with local law enforcement agencies and health departments and emergency medical response teams, to create as realistic scenarios as possible. Unfortunately, the participation of anesthesiology departments in these drills is often minimal. Drills are usually held on weekdays during working hours, times during which it is often difficult to spare anesthesia providers. Because anesthesiology departments are fully staffed and completely operational during those hours, hospital administrators certify that they can handle the number of casualties coming through their ED. Unfortunately, the drills are not very realistic—for financial reasons, surgical procedures are never delayed or canceled, and the system is never tested at night or on weekends. At night, when there are minimal telecommunications personnel in place, how would a hospital mobilize its staff? Many have telephone "trees," but again, because they are not tested, many anesthesia providers have long since misplaced their contact information. Even if tested, how operational would the plan be during a major disaster when communication systems are overwhelmed? Short text messaging would be the best manner for departments to alert personnel to the disaster.

Other advantages to having anesthesiology departments participate in drills would be the establishment of trust with liaisons in the emergency response community and with local law enforcement agencies. How much better the outcome would have been if that had been the case in Moscow during the 2002 Nord-Ost siege when the Spetsnaz forces most likely used carfentanil against Chechen rebels without informing emergency response or hospital personnel, resulting in 170 deaths.[18]

Impediments to the establishment of effective response plans are not only financial but also based on a lack of awareness of what occurs during a disaster. As Israelis know from their years of dealing with suicide bombers, and as the Japanese found out during the release of sarin by an Aum Shinrikyo terrorist group in the Tokyo subway system in 1996, victims do NOT go to level I trauma centers, nor do they wait to be transported by emergency medical teams—they fan out in all directions to whatever healthcare facility they can find, and they do so on foot, by private vehicles, or by whatever means available.[19]

St. Luke's Hospital in Tokyo found itself inundated with close to 900 patients within 90 minutes after the subway sarin attacks. The ED lobby entrance (almost the entire first floor of the hospital) was crammed with patients, none of whom had been decontaminated. The ensuing chaos was difficult to manage and delayed treatment for those who needed it most. The affected patients required treatment best understood by anesthesiologists who use cholinesterase inhibitors daily and best administered by IV lines inserted by these same providers.

Depending on available staff, including how many of the providers will actually respond to a mass casualty event or disaster, there may be insufficient personnel available to cover all rooms in the facility's operating suites. In addition, other areas of the hospital will continue to require coverage, such as the obstetric ward, intensive care, radiology, and endoscopy suites for both disaster-related care and other emergencies. Creative staffing at higher ratios of coverage may be required to manage patient surges.

Other places anesthesia providers can assist in delivery of healthcare during a disaster include:

- Triage outside the hospital (who better to manage the pain or labored respiration of the expectant patient?)
- Decontamination (who better to evaluate for the presence of anticholinesterase [nerve] agents or cyanide toxicity?)
- Vascular access or airway management (made more difficult if wearing a hazard material, or HAZMAT, suit and even more difficult if one has never worn such a suit)
- Ventilator management in the intensive care unit (ICU) or in overflow areas of the hospital such as the postanesthesia care unit (PACU) of patients with respiratory failure caused by a nerve agent or biologic agent

Role of Anesthesiologist in Managing Mass Casualties

It is difficult to anticipate every situation in which anesthesiologists could be requested to assist in managing mass casualty situations. For example, on October 26, 2002, terrorists held 750 hostages at the Nord-Ost Theater in Moscow. Many believe that the authorities instilled nebulized or volatile carfentanil into the air ducts of the opera house, thereby immobilizing the terrorists. Unfortunately, because of the incapacitating effect of the carfentanil, the hostages became victims too. Patients were transported from the theater to hospitals without any treatment prior to arrival. Ideally, anesthesiologists or other healthcare providers with an opioid antagonist such as naloxone should have been readily available and present at the site to manage both casualties. Unfortunately, this was not the case.

Anesthesiologists' basic understanding of physiology and 3
pharmacology, airway skills, fluid resuscitation expertise, and ability to manage ventilators and provide anesthesia, both in and out of the operating rooms, is invaluable. In these mass casualty situations, many patients suffer burns, fractures, lacerations, soft tissue trauma, and amputations that will require triage, stabilization in the emergency room or in another facility near the emergency room, and possibly more definitive treatment in the operating room or in the ICU.

During a mass casualty event, an anesthesiologist may well be requested to provide anesthetic services in an area other than the operating room or ICU. They will not know where they will be working until they report to the hospital and the command and control center has developed a plan to manage the event.[20] The site of the command and control center is pre-established and outlined in the hospital's emergency preparedness plan, but typically it is within the hospital's ED or in close proximity. Other entrances to the hospital are typically closed during a mass casualty event for the purposes of maintaining control of the numbers of patients that might present and to allow for decontamination of patients, if necessary, avoiding exposure of hospital personnel to contagious agents or transferrable substances, such as nerve agents. The lack of such control and decontamination of the Tokyo subway sarin attack victims in 1995 resulted in a number of healthcare workers becoming ill by absorbing sarin from patients who had not been properly decontaminated.[19] Not only were they unable to work but they also became patients themselves, increasing the number of casualties requiring care and consuming resources.

Triage

If assigned to triage patients, the anesthesiologist will be expected 4
to classify patients into four groups—those requiring immediate care, delayed care, minimal care (first aid only), and expectant (no care, or comfort care only). The latter group includes those expected not to survive, or, because of the number of patients arriving, those for whom there are not adequate personnel or resources to adequately resuscitate without jeopardizing the lives of other patients who would not receive the care they require and for whom the prognosis is more favorable (Fig. 59-2). Experience has taught that initially triage officers are conservative; they try to save as many patients as possible, but over days, if not hours, they gain experience and become better at identifying patients for

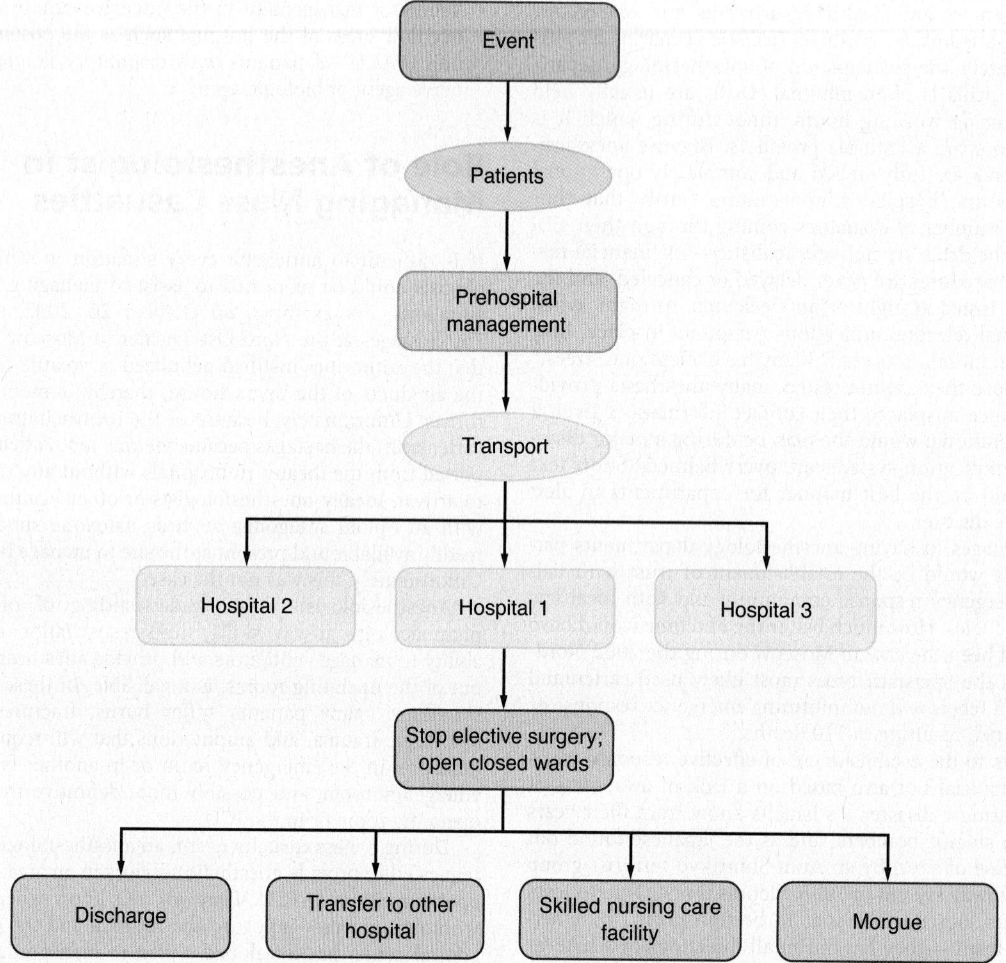

Figure 59-2 Surge capacity: How hospitals can deal with increased number of patients arriving at their emergency departments following a mass casualty event.

whom resources exist to improve outcome. In the future, technology may play a role,[21] but at present hospitals must rely on physicians' experience and, again, because of their knowledge of the hospitals resources in both the operating room (OR) and the ICU, they may well be the ideal triage officer. They will have to assess and decide if patients fall into one of the four groups. "Expectant" patients are usually transported to an area separate from the ED, where they receive comfort care. Such a site must be situated so that newly arriving patients are not exposed to the sight of dying patients. Anesthesiologists may well be assigned to provide such care because of expertise in managing airways, in establishing IV access for the administration of medications, and our familiarity with the available anxiolytic and analgesic medications. Some patients who may have been injured or affected during a disaster but who do not appear to require immediate treatment may require delayed care. Depending on the type exposure, some CBRNE casualties may require delayed therapy:

- Chemical (nerve) agents: If only headache, meiosis, rhinorrhea, and lacrimation after exposure, patients can be decontaminated (see later) and dismissed. Patients with dyspnea, bronchospasm, or arrhythmias will require treatment with atropine.
- Biologic agents: Fever, rash, dyspnea, cough. Antibiotics, antitoxins, antiviral agents, and supportive care.
- Radiation/nuclear: Nausea within 6 hours of exposure; because of the prevalence for those with this symptom, check leukocyte count, dismiss, and have the patient return in 48 hours for repeat check—if no change in count, no therapy is indicated. There are several new therapies in development for mitigation of the effects of radiation exposure.
- Explosive: If tympanic membranes are intact and SpO_2 is within normal limits, other injuries are unlikely.

Decontamination

In most situations, those with proper training decontaminate people in contact with chemical agents or radioactive materials—the decontamination is normally performed first and then patients are evaluated and triaged. The principle is to limit the exposure of the patient to the agent and prevent contamination of caregivers. Off-gassing of some chemical agents can be problematic, especially with large numbers of exposed patients awaiting decontamination. Consideration should be given to providing lightweight "escape hoods" (available from multiple vendors) to reduce respiratory exposure before decontamination can be performed. The decontamination process is usually fairly straightforward; clothes are removed and individuals are washed with copious amounts of water (the contaminated water and apparel can present quite a logistical challenge!); if individuals have been exposed to a chemical warfare agent, a dilute solution of sodium hypochlorite 0.5% (household bleach) can be used to hydrolyze the substance.

5 However, if a patient presents with life-threatening injury, the patient is treated first and decontaminated afterward. Patients with severe chemical agent poisoning may present with acute respiratory failure requiring emergency tracheal intubation. In this scenario, an anesthesiologist would be assigned to the decontamination station. For obvious reasons, the intubation would have to be performed with the anesthesiologist wearing a HAZMAT or a biohazard suit with multiple-layered gloves and a chemical protective mask. The suits are not insulated or cooled and if the decontamination is performed outside the hospital, the extremes of temperature can significantly hinder performance, as does the decreased manual dexterity, because of the gloves and the impairment in vision from the face hoods. Ideally, individuals with prior training would manage the airway intubation, but depending on circumstances, that may not happen. As many have learned from past experience, it is best to anticipate the unexpected, and to be flexible if the maximum numbers of patients are to be saved. Preparation of equipment and drugs before the arrival of contaminated patients decreases the difficulties with manual dexterity that are encountered while wearing the multiple-layered or rubber gloves. Consider securing the airway with a laryngeal mask airway, when indicated, rather than with a tracheal tube. Intraosseous cannulas are often easier to insert than IV cannulas when wearing HAZMAT personal protective equipment (PPE).

Emergency Department

Another place where an anesthesiologist might be assigned is the ED. While some level I trauma centers have an anesthesia team assigned to support the ED, many do not. Depending on the types of casualties, but especially for casualties from a violent explosion, anesthesiologists might be assigned to manage the airway and secure central venous access. Anesthesiologists should position themselves at the head of the bed and assume responsibility for the airway and venous access. For the former, it would be ideal to have two or three assistants (one providing in-line C-spine stabilization, another individual applying cricoid pressure, and a third individual administering medication). Sometimes it is necessary to remind ED physicians and trauma surgeons that "A" (airway) and "B" (breathing) come before "C" (circulation); certainly, the primary and secondary surveys can be conducted during this critical time point but ventilation and oxygenation must be assured. Often, all three can be conducted simultaneously.

In industrial accidents and fires, appropriate management of the airway has been critical. Patients with large-area burns will require IV access for provision of intravascular volume resuscitation. Depending on the event (burn vs. crush injury—protocols for fluid resuscitation vary), in patients with extensive soft tissue and skeletal muscle damage, alkalization of the urine (to prevent crystallization of myoglobin in the renal tubules) with volume resuscitation and diuresis may be organ and lifesaving.

Operating Room Management

6 COTEP developed and published a checklist to assist the anesthesiologist in charge of the operative suite in prioritizing tasks for the management of a mass casualty event (Table 59-3).[3] The first task is to open the facility's operating manual (Environment of Care Manual in TDJ parlance) to the appropriate annex for the disaster, which hopefully will be hospital specific. Next, the disaster call-in tree is activated. Experience has shown that a branching tree of phone numbers is far better than a linear list. The anesthesiologist in charge should become the operating room medical director, co-locate with the operating room nurse in charge, and determine the status of on-going cases. Surgeons in the midst

Table 59-3 Operating Room Procedures for Mass Casualty: Management Step by Step

Objective: To be able to manage the flow of patient care in operating rooms (ORs) during a mass casualty situation.

Steps: Indicate date and time for each item.

- Refer to facility's operations manual.
  Open up appropriate annex.
- Activate call-in tree.
  Assign an individual to activate. Use clerical personnel or automatic paging system, if available.
- Assess status of operating rooms.
  Determine staffing of ORs 0–2, 2–12, and 12–24 hours. Hold elective cases.
- Alert current ORs.
  Finish current surgical procedures as soon as possible and prepare to receive trauma.
- Assign staff.
  Set up for trauma/emergency cases.
- Anesthesia coordinator should become OR medical director.
  Work with OR nursing manager to facilitate communication and coordination of staff and facilities.
- Report OR status to hospital command center (HCC).
  Enter telephone, email address of HCC.
- Ensure adequate supplies.
  Coordinate with anesthesia techs/supply personnel to ensure adequate supplies of fluids, medications, disposables, etc.
- Contact the postanesthesia care unit.
  Accelerate transfer of patients to floors/ICUs in preparation for high volume of cases.
- Anesthesiologist should act as liaison in emergency department (ED).
  Send an experienced practitioner to the ED to act as a liaison (your eyes and ears) and keep communications open to anesthesia coordinator.
- Consider assembly of stat teams.
  Combination of anesthesia, surgical, nursing, respiratory personnel to triage, as needed.
- Hazardous material/weapons of mass destruction event.
  Review special personal protective procedures, such as decontamination and isolation techniques. Consider if part of the OR hallways should be considered "hot" or should have ventilation altered. Good resources include Chemical Hazards Emergency Medical Management and Radiation Emergency Medical Management websites.
- Coordinate with blood bank.
  Verify blood availability.
- Coordinate with other patient care areas.
  Intensive care units, obstetrics, pediatrics, etc. to ensure continuity of care for new and existing patients.

ICU, intensive care unit.
Developed by the Committee on Trauma and Emergency Preparedness.

of procedures should be contacted and urged to finish as soon as possible. Elective cases should be postponed or cancelled. A list of available rooms and staff should be rapidly assembled and transmitted to the hospital emergency operations center (HEOC). Determine realistic staffing for the next 0 to 2, 2 to 12, and 12 to 24 hours. Free staff should be directed to set up open rooms to receive trauma patients. Support staff can be directed to resupply (oversupply) locations in anticipation of heavy use. Coordination with the PACU, blood bank, and ICUs will improve patient movement and space availability. It is advisable to send a senior anesthesiologist, especially one with critical care experience, to the ED to act as a liaison between the ED and the OR. This physician should have their own dedicated communications link with the operating rooms to transmit timely intelligence on the nature and number of surgical cases anticipated. The liaison can also act as an advisor to the ED. Some larger institutions can consider sending teams to the ED to help with triage and initial management of casualties. If HAZMATS are involved, consideration should be given to appropriate secondary decontamination, isolation techniques, PPE, and antidotes needed.

7 In many types of disasters, infrastructure degradation plays a large part in reducing surgical capabilities at a time when demand is increased. Surgeons and anesthesiologists must consider what types of procedures can safely be undertaken and must prioritize care based on urgency and practicality. Closed reduction of fractures or external fixation may be the most suitable options, other than amputation, for the orthopedic surgeon. General surgeons may lose the ability to do robotic or laparoscopic intra-abdominal surgery, and many intrathoracic and intracranial procedures will be impractical. Wong et al.[22] showed that burn dressing changes and extensive wound debridements were the most frequent planned surgical procedures after acute trauma. Although early in a mass casualty event, elective procedures are cancelled or delayed, there will be a backlog of patients requiring surgery. Falls, burns, motor vehicle accidents, and childbirth will continue to occur, possibly with increased frequency, depending on the disaster. As the community's infrastructure degrades over time, hygiene and sanitation becomes a problem. Increased respiratory infections, gastrointestinal (GI) disease, and wound infections are likely to increase. Loss of electrical power, which can result in loss of heating, air conditioning, and water may make it difficult to maintain normal operative and postoperative conditions. Patients may present dehydrated and some authors suggest liberalization of fasting guidelines to reduce intraoperative fluid needs and improve postoperative wound healing.[23]

Chemical

Nerve Agents

Prior to the last century, it was unthinkable that rogue states or terrorists would use chemical agents. During the First World War, more than one million soldiers and civilians were exposed to chemical gas injuries, with over 100,000 of them dying. In 1935, Italy invaded Abyssinia (Ethiopia) and during that invasion, sprayed mustard gas from aircrafts. When Japan invaded China in 1937, mustard, phosgene, and hydrogen cyanide were used. In that same year, German chemical laboratories produced the first nerve agent, tabun. During 1963 to 1967, Egypt used phosgene and mustard agents in support of South Yemen during the civil war in that country. When Iraq attacked Iran in the 1980s, mustard and nerve agents were used. In all these examples, chemical agents were used by the military during armed conflict. The governments mentioned have all signed the Chemical Weapons Convention. January 2012 marked the end of an era as, in compliance with the Chemical Weapons Convention ratified by the Senate in 1997, the U.S. Army Chemical Materials Agency completed destruction of 27,000 tons of chemical weapons that it had manufactured and stored over the years.[24]

However, as one era ended another one had already begun. In 1994 and 1995, the use of the nerve agent sarin by the Japanese cult Aum Shinrikyo was a major turning point, because it was the first time that a terrorist group had used a nerve agent in a terrorist attack. More than 5,000 persons were evaluated at hospitals, approximately 1,000 of whom had been exposed to the nerve agent, and 18 died. Both sides in the ongoing Syrian Civil War that started in 2013 have used chemical agents, including chlorine, mustard agent, and sarin. The nerve agents are so named because of their mechanism of action. The G series agents (GA, GB, GD, GF) were developed but never used by Germany during 1930s. They are considered nonpersistent, lasting in the environment a few minutes to a few days. Both the Novichok and the V series agents (VE, VG, VM, VR, and VX) were manufactured by the USSR in 1980s. They persist in the environment and are 10 times more toxic that the G agents. VX is the only one ever fielded by the United States. Both types of agents have been used in assassinations in recent years.

Similar to organophosphate insecticides and to the anticholinesterase (AChE) drugs that anesthesiologists use daily, nerve agents inhibit AChE. This inhibition results in excessive amounts of acetylcholine (the reason why a cholinergic agent such as atropine or glycopyrrolate is administered anytime we inject an AChE, such as neostigmine) at preganglionic muscarinic and postganglionic muscarinic and nicotinic receptors, leading to copious secretions, meiosis, arrhythmias, bronchospasm, tonic muscle contractions, respiratory paralysis, seizures, and death. A cholinergic agent and competitive muscarinic blocker (i.e., atropine or glycopyrrolate) is administered to attenuate and block the muscarinic side effects of the agents.

When anticipating a nerve agent attack, U.S. military personnel pretreat themselves with low-dose pyridostigmine and don PPE; the latter prevents the agent from contacting and wetting skin from which it is readily absorbed, and low-dose pyridostigmine binds to AChE, preventing any nerve agent that is absorbed from binding to the enzyme. Pyridostigmine is a reversible drug that will be metabolized over time, whereas the nerve agents bind to AChE irreversibly.

U.S. military personnel carry syringes of atropine and of pralidoxime chloride (2-PAM-CL), an oxime that reactivates AChE by removing the nerve agent from its binding site on the enzyme. (Some NATO countries use other oximes.) Spontaneous reactivation of enzyme complex is variable, which partly accounts for differences in acute toxicity between the nerve agents. 2-PAM-CL is administered to reactivate the dialkylphosphonyl AChE enzyme more quickly.[25] The most optimistic estimates are that after exposure 30 minutes will elapse before casualties are transported to EDs, the diagnosis of nerve agent attack is made, and the oxime can be administered. Thirty minutes is optimistic, given that there have been deaths at chemical weapons manufacturing facilities within 2 minutes of accidental exposure. Toxicity of the nerve agents is not just related to which agent, but also to the dose of agent to which one is exposed, and the duration of exposure. However, if numbers of casualties arrive at a triage site outside a hospital ED, the sooner one administers an oxime, such as 2-PAM-CL, obidoxime, or HI-6, the better. Most of the nerve agents can be reversed with the exception of soman. With soman, aging of AChE occurs so fast that an oxime will have no effect, thus the need for pyridostigmine pretreatment. Even though aging occurs more slowly and reactivation occurs relatively rapidly in the case of nerve agents other than soman, early oxime administration is still clinically important in patients poisoned with these agents. Experimental studies on the treatment of nerve agent poisoning have to be interpreted with caution. Some studies have used prophylactic protocols, whereas the drugs concerned (atropine, oxime) would be given only to a civilian population after exposure. The experimental use of pyridostigmine before nerve agent exposure, although rational, is not of relevance in the civilian context. With the possible exception of the treatment of cyclosarin (GF) and soman poisoning, a review of available experimental evidence suggests that there are no clinically important differences between the different oximes in the treatment of nerve agent poisoning, if studies employing pretreatment with pyridostigmine are excluded.[25]

Limited experience (and lack of open literature) with novichok intoxication indicates that only prolonged treatment with antimuscarinics and supportive ventilation are useful therapies.

Diagnosis

Patients exposed to a nerve agent, either ingested, inhaled, or via the transdermal route, present with evidence of muscarinic site stimulation: airway, pupillary, and GI tract constriction; bradycardia; and activation of the glands within the eyes, nose, mouth, and sweat glands manifested by intense lacrimation, rhinorrhea, salivation, and sweating. The degree of exposure correlates with the amount of secretions produced. Nicotinic stimulation at preganglionic sites leads to tachycardia and hypertension, and at the nicotinic acetylcholine receptor on the neuromuscular junction, fasciculation, twitching, fatigue, and flaccid paralysis. The excessive parasympathetic activity leads to meiosis and loss of accommodation so that patients complain of blurred vision. Within the respiratory system, the increased parasympathetic activity leads to bronchorrhea and bronchoconstriction, which together with the respiratory muscle fatigue initially manifests as coughing, wheezing, and shortness of breath. The agent on the skin will produce localized sweating and fasciculation obvious to the naked eye. Within the cardiovascular system, activity within the muscarinic system leads to bradycardia, but depending on the degree of nicotinic activity in the preganglionic nodes, a patient's heart rate may be low, normal, or high. Within the GI tract, the increased parasympathetic activity leads to nausea, vomiting, diarrhea, and incontinence. This overall unopposed parasympathetic activity leads to a pneumonic of "DUMBBELS" (*d*iarrhea, *u*rination, *m*yosis, *b*ronchorrhea and *b*ronchoconstriction, *e*mesis, *l*acrimation, and *s*alivation).

Treatment

The toxicity of the nerve agents depends on the compound delivered, the dose that is delivered (LC), and the time (t) that an individual is exposed to that dose. For example, a patient exposed to 10 mg/m^3 of an agent for 10 minutes would have an LCt of 100 mg/min/m^3. The same could be achieved by being exposed to a concentration of 100 mg/m^3 for only 1 minute. The treatment for nerve agent poisoning is one with which every anesthesiologist is familiar. Atropine is a competitive muscarinic blocker. Pralidoxime chloride is the better long-term treatment as it reactivates AChE by removing the organophosphate compound. Atropine is administered at a dose of 2 to 6 mg or more and repeated every 5 to 10 minutes until secretions begin to decrease (i.e., until the patient is no longer salivating) and ventilation is improved. In severe casualties, 15 to 20 mg would not be unusual, and some casualties have required gram amounts of atropine. The U.S. military travels with automatic injectors containing 2 mg of atropine and 600 mg of 2-PAM-CL.

Depending on the extent of exposure, treatment differs. For minimal exposure, often seen with brief exposure to nerve agent vapor, patients may complain of headache and tightness in the chest and manifest myosis, rhinorrhea, and salivation. Individuals must be removed from further exposure, clothing removed, topical atropine applied to the eye if pain is significant, and wet decontamination must be performed if there was any liquid exposure. With moderate exposure, the same signs are present, but the patient demonstrates more severe rhinorrhea, complains of dyspnea, and on examination, there is evidence of bronchospasm and muscle fasciculation. Patients with moderate (and severe) poisoning require treatment with atropine and 2-PAM-CL intramuscularly. Casualties again must have their clothing removed and if they were exposed to liquid nerve agent, they need to go through a wet decontamination process. With severe exposure, the same symptoms as mentioned above are present, but now the patient manifests severe respiratory compromise, flaccid paralysis, incontinence, arrhythmias, and convulsions. After decontamination the patient will require repetitive doses of IV atropine, along with intramuscular 2-PAM-CL, IV benzodiazepines to treat the seizures (caused by the muscarinic effects of the nerve agents within the central nervous system [CNS][26]), and intubation and mechanical ventilation, depending on the degree of respiratory compromise.

With nerve agent casualties, decontamination is critical. It needs to be done as quickly as possible, first by leaving the area of exposure. As commented at the beginning of this chapter, healthcare and emergency workers in Japan became victims themselves by standing unprotected in the subway cars in which there was sarin.[19] Patients are decontaminated by removing their clothing and washing with copious amounts of water and 0.5% hypochlorite (dilute household bleach). The bleach is not as critical as washing with copious amounts of water. Depending on the number of casualties, EDs may coordinate with the fire department. For example, they might arrange fire trucks side-by-side with a "chamber" established between the two trucks in which individuals can disrobe and be sprayed with water as they walk through the chamber. From there, depending upon the severity of the symptoms, they would receive atropine, 2-PAM-CL, and further treatment.

Pulmonary Agents

The so-called pulmonary agents are, by nature, gases at room temperature, and almost any gas could be considered a pulmonary agent if released in sufficient quantity in a closed environment to displace oxygen, thereby causing exposed subjects to die by asphyxiation. Chlorine and phosgene are considered the classic pulmonary agents and the two most likely to be used by terrorists. If quantities are released that are sufficient to displace oxygen, then death results from asphyxia. In addition, these two gases are extremely toxic to the lungs; individuals who survive the acute exposure if they have inhaled even small amounts often develop acute lung injury or acute respiratory distress syndrome (ARDS). However, the treatment is no different from what a critical care anesthesiologist would provide in managing a patient with Silo Filler's Disease or Farmer's Lung, which develops after exposure to nitrogen dioxide when a farm worker opens or enters a silo that has inadequate ventilation. The treatment of the resulting noncardiogenic pulmonary edema from NO_2 or the pulmonary agents is supportive: mechanical ventilation using small tidal volumes (6 to 8 mL/kg), peak airway pressures (<30 cm H_2O), positive end expiratory pressure, and inspired oxygen concentrations of 50% to 60% or less.

Blood Agents

The third and final class of chemical toxins includes the blood agents—hydrogen cyanide and cyanogen chloride. Because of the instability of the latter, hydrogen cyanide is more likely to be used by terrorists in a closed environment as an aerosol. Again, anesthesiologists are familiar with this class of substances because of our clinical use of sodium nitroprusside as an intravascular vasodilator, which has cyanide as a metabolite. Cyanide inhibits cellular respiration by interrupting the oxidative electron transfer process in mitochondria. The treatment for cyanide toxicity is similar to what anesthesiologists would do for a patient who had an accidental overdose of sodium nitroprusside: IV thiosulfate and supportive care, including tracheal intubation, ventilation with 100% oxygen, and inotropes and vasopressors to stabilize the cardiovascular system.

Biologic

History

This section includes a discussion that considers the naturally occurring infectious agents, as well as those agents most likely to be used by terrorists. Many of the latter caused plagues in the past or were used as weapons. Infectious organisms have been used as biologic weapons since the dawn of history. Ghengis Khan is reported to have used cats infected with fleas bearing the plague to destroy towns in his conquest of Asia. In the 1770s, British forces distributed blankets that harbored smallpox virus to American Indians, killing more than 50% of the infected tribes. In World War II, Unit 731, a Japanese military unit, is reported to have dropped plague-infected fleas over populated areas of China, causing outbreaks of plague and killing several hundred thousand people.[27]

8 The ideal biologic weapon is one that has the greatest potential for adverse public health consequences, generating mass casualties, and with potential for easy large-scale dissemination that could cause mass hysteria and civil disruption. Such a weapon should be relatively easy to produce, inexpensive, highly infectious, and contagious, resulting in widespread morbidity and mortality. To be effective, there should be little or no natural immunity, which is currently the case with diseases such as smallpox, for which we no longer routinely vaccinate individuals, except in the military and in high-risk public health areas. There are three categories of biologic weapons (Table 59-4). Category A includes weapons that are highly contagious, that are associated with a high mortality rate, and that have all the characteristics of a relatively ideal weapon of mass destruction.

Table 59-4 Biologic Agents Used for Warfare

Category A: Highly contagious and fit all the characteristics of a relatively ideal biologic agent
Bacillus anthracis (anthrax)
Variola major (smallpox)
Yersinia pestis (plague)
Clostridium botulinum (botulism)
Francisella tularensis (tularemia)
Viral hemorrhagic fever (Ebola, Lassa, Marburg, Argentine)
Category B: Relatively easy to disseminate but have low mortality rates
Coxiella burnetii (Q fever)
Vibrio cholerae (cholera)
Burkholderia mallei (glanders)
Enteric pathogens (*E. coli* 0157:H7, *Salmonella, Shigella*)
Cholera, cryptosporidium
Various encephalitic viruses
Various biologic toxins
Category C: Emerging pathogens that might be engineered for biologic warfare
Various equine encephalitic viruses

Smallpox

The last case of naturally occurring smallpox in the world was reported in 1977 in Somalia.[28] In 1978, two laboratory workers were infected with the disease in the United Kingdom.[28] In 1980, the World Health Organization (WHO) announced that the world was free of this scourge. Terrorists might consider using smallpox as a weapon because an increasing number of people no longer carry immunity. Routine vaccination for smallpox is no longer performed, except in the military and for some public healthcare workers considered at high risk of contracting the disease (individuals whom the government would rely on to staff vaccination stations if there were a breakout).[28] Forty to eighty percent of patients exposed to the smallpox virus will become infected with the disease. Smallpox is highly infective, requiring only 10 to 100 organisms to infect an individual. The mortality rate is approximately 30% in unvaccinated patients and as high as 50% if smallpox occurs in communities that have no native immunity against smallpox. The protective effect of the smallpox vaccine decreases with time, but even at 20 years, the vaccine would provide some protection.

When an unvaccinated person is initially infected, they develop a prodrome of malaise, headache, and backache, with the onset of fever to as high as 40°C. The fever decreases over the next 3 or 4 days, at which time a rash develops. This progression is in contradistinction to chickenpox, in which the rash develops at the same time as the fever. Unlike chickenpox, smallpox has a predilection for the distal extremities and face, though no part of the body is spared. Also, all lesions in a patient with smallpox are at the same stage, whereas with chickenpox, lesions are at multiple different stages: papules, vesicles, pustules, and scabs. Most cases of smallpox are transmitted through aerosolized droplets that are inhaled, but clothes and blankets that have come in contact with pustules, until the scab falls off, are infectious; the organism can be transmitted in these linens.

Smallpox has probably been present in humans since 10,000 BC. It is transmitted human to human, and if used as a bioterrorism agent, would likely be dispersed by aerosols in the environment with the hope that multiple humans would be infected and would transmit the virus to other humans. There is evidence that the former Soviet Union developed transgenic smallpox viruses that are very infectious and for which the U.S. vaccine may not be completely protective. The time of onset after exposure to such a virus might be very short. Currently there are only two WHO-approved depositories of smallpox, at the Centers for Disease Control and Prevention (CDC) in Atlanta, Georgia, and at the Institute of Virus Preparations in Russia. With the collapse of the Soviet Union, there was a concern that some stores of smallpox made it into rogue countries that may have developed their own biologic weapons.

A look at how the WHO eradicated smallpox might be helpful in understanding how the United States has prepared to respond to smallpox as a biologic weapon. In the 18th century, 400,000 Europeans/year were dying from smallpox. Though only 1% of patients who survive smallpox become blind, it accounted for one-third of all cases of blindness in Europe. The WHO eradicated smallpox by identifying patients with smallpox and placing them in strict quarantine. Such patients are readily identified because of the presence of smallpox lesions on the face. Patients were quarantined and all their contacts were vaccinated, because there was a 3- to 7-day window with the naturally occurring virus before the patient developed symptoms and signs of smallpox.[29]

Vaccination against smallpox is controversial. The vaccine is made from a live vaccinia virus developed in calf lymph, but is not an attenuated smallpox virus itself. Smallpox is a member of the Orthodox genus of the poxviridae family of double-stranded deoxyribonucleic acid (DNA) viruses that also contain cowpox, monkey pox, and vaccinia. In the event of a documented case of smallpox, the CDC plans to quarantine the patient and immediate patient contacts within a certain geographic area would be vaccinated. There are stockpiles of vaccines placed strategically throughout the United States just for such an event. A bifurcated needle is dipped into the reconstituted vaccine and then 10 to 15 points of entry are made into the dermis of the upper deltoid. Because of the side effects of smallpox vaccinations, people with immunologic disorders, eczema (active or with a history of severe eczema), and pregnant or nursing women should not receive the vaccine. The CDC monitors for adverse side effects of vaccination; most are not serious, such as fever, rash, and malaise, although two cases of cardiomyopathy have been reported.[30] There is no plan to vaccinate the entire U.S. population following an isolated case.

Many obstacles have been overcome to develop second- and third-generation smallpox vaccines. Before 2001, the vaccine that was used, Dryvax (similar to what Jenner used in the 18th century), contained live attenuated virus and was the reason that immunocompromised individuals developed adverse events when vaccinated. From 2001 to the present, Acambis Modified Vaccinia Ankara (ACAM) has been used to vaccinate against smallpox. Dryvax and ACAM are fairly similar, though the latter may be a little safer to use than Dryvax, but not so much safer than when immunocompromised individuals are offered the vaccine. To avoid the dangers of a live vaccine, an inactive vaccine (modified vaccinia Ankara [MVA; Imvamune]) was developed[31]; the United States has a contract to purchase 20 million doses. The available evidence is that even immunocompromised individuals, such as those with HIV infection, might tolerate immunization. The CDC and the states' departments of health will implement their quarantine and vaccination plans should an index case or cluster cases occur.

Anthrax

Bacillus anthracis (anthrax) was probably used as a biologic weapon in the Middle Ages, when troops laying siege to a town would catapult infected animal carcasses over the ramparts into the inhabited areas. For reasons discussed later, this method was not a particularly effective method of infecting the native population. During the 20th century, several countries, including the United States, Great Britain, Russia, and Iraq, studied ways to "weaponize" anthrax. Normally, if anthrax spores are inhaled, they clump in the nasal pharynx. To be weaponized, *B. anthracis* must be finely ground so that it readily aerosolizes and can get to and deposit in the terminal bronchioles and alveoli.[32] Inhalation anthrax, which was relatively uncommon in the past, has an 80% fatality rate. One of the letters that was mailed in the anthrax attacks of 2001 contained 2 g of weapons-grade anthrax. With a median lethal dose (LD_{50}) of 1,000 spores, under optimal conditions, this was enough material to infect 50 million individuals. In a terrorist attack, for maximum effect, anthrax could be aerosolized and sprayed from airplanes or delivered through a dispersion device mounted on top of a missile. The attacks on North America in 2001 and the accidental release of spores at a biologic facility in the city of Sverdlovsk in the former Soviet Union in 1979 are illustrative of the potential of anthrax as a weapon. In the United States, 5 of 11 cases resulted in death (45% mortality rate); in the former Soviet Union, 66 of 77 died (86% mortality rate).[33] The Aum Shinrikyo also released anthrax spores in Tokyo in 1993. Fortunately, they used a nonpathogenic strain of anthrax and so there were no casualties.[32] As demonstrated in 2001 in the United States, terrorists are sophisticated enough that they might be successful in obtaining and releasing weapons-grade anthrax. Such attacks, even if detected early,[34] would create mass hysteria and greatly affect the entire country and world.[35]

Anthrax is a gram-positive, spore-forming bacillus that is transmitted to humans from contaminated animals, their byproducts, or carcasses. Spores may persist in soil for years. The disease is all but gone from North America, but is still prevalent in many developing countries, and herbivores, especially cattle, usually die within 24 to 48 hours of contracting the disease. The carcass has such a large number of organisms, that humans, who are relatively resistant to infection, can be exposed and contract the disease.[36]

There are three primary types of anthrax infection: Cutaneous, inhalation, and GI. Ninety-five percent of cases are cutaneous. From a public health perspective, inhalation anthrax is most concerning, as it usually affects 2,000 to 20,000 people worldwide per annum. People can be exposed through contact with animals in an agricultural or industrial setting (i.e., a rendering plant or tanning facility, or, as mentioned previously, in the production of biologic weapons).[37]

Anthrax has additional appeal to bioterrorists because inhalation anthrax is difficult to detect. It manifests as an influenza-like disease with fever, myalgias, malaise, and a nonproductive cough with or without chest pain.[38] After a few days, the patient appears to get better, but then a couple of days later the patient becomes much more ill with dyspnea, cyanosis, hemoptysis, stridor, and chest pain. The most notable finding on physical examination and laboratory testing is a widened mediastinum. Usually when a patient develops profound dyspnea, death ensues within 1 to 2 days. In the past, penicillin G was the treatment of choice, but since weaponized anthrax has been engineered to be resistant to penicillin G, ciprofloxacin or doxycycline is more commonly used. In the outbreaks in Florida, Washington DC, and New Jersey, contacts of infected patients or people exposed to the spores were treated with ciprofloxacin or doxycycline. A more recent study concluded that this drug regimen is the best strategy for managing a small-scale attack, as occurred in 2001.[39]

Plague

The oldest cases of *Yersinia pestis* (bubonic plague) were documented in China in the third century. *Y. pestis* has been thought to be the etiologic agent in multiple epidemics and three pandemics, the first of which was during the Roman emperor Justinian's reign; the second pandemic was during the 14th century—the Black Death—and killed one-third of the population of Europe; and the last was at the end of the 19th century and killed millions in China and India.[40] The first documented use of plague as a biologic weapon was in 1346 when the Tartars in their siege of the fortress at Kaffa catapulted infected corpses into the city.[27] Plague was used by Unit 731 to infect large areas of China, and as many as 200,000 Chinese may have died. More recently, the United States and Russia have studied *Y. pestis* as a bioagent, examining ways to aerosolize and ways to distribute the bacillus. Surprisingly, the organism is only viable for approximately 60 minutes after being distributed; if dispersed by an airplane, its viability would limit its infectivity for only 10 km from the dispersion site.

Y. pestis is a nonmotile, gram-positive bacillus. Rodents and fleas are its natural hosts, and they re-infect each other by fleas biting infected rodents. Soil can be contaminated and therefore rodents can acquire the disease simply by digging in an infected area. Humans are an accidental host and they usually acquire the disease from a fleabite, though rarely there can be direct inoculation of infected material into a person. Direct person-to-person transmission occurs with pneumonic plague.

There are two types of plague: bubonic and pneumonic. With bubonic plague, after a fleabite, there is a 2- to 6-day incubation period, at which time there is the sudden onset of fever, chills, weakness, and headache. Intense painful swelling occurs in the lymph nodes, usually in the groin, axilla, or neck. These swellings or buboes are typically oval in nature, 1 to 10 cm in diameter, and extremely tender. Up to 25% of patients will have pustules, papules, or skin lesions near these buboes. Without treatment, patients become septic, develop septic shock with cyanosis and gangrene in peripheral tissues, leading to the "black death" descriptor that was used during the pandemics in Europe. As mentioned, material from these buboes is infective only if inoculated into human tissue. However, patients who have bubonic plague can seed their lungs, in which case they develop pneumonic plague. During coughing, they aerosolize *Y. pestis,* which is highly contagious. Mortality for either form of the disease is above 50%. Diagnosis is made with a Gram stain or culture of organisms from blood, sputum, or buboes. The treatment of choice is streptomycin, but chloramphenicol and tetracycline are acceptable alternatives. Patients with pneumonic plague should be managed as one would manage a patient with drug resistance to tuberculosis, because the respiratory secretions are highly infectious. There is currently no vaccine against *Y. pestis.*

Tularemia

Francisella tularensis (tularemia) has some similarities to anthrax and plague, but is not nearly as dangerous. It was studied as a biologic weapon in the 20th century because it is highly infectious, requiring an inoculum of perhaps as small as only 10 organisms.[41] During World War II, tularemia developed in soldiers along the German-Russian front and was thought secondary to the use of *F. tularensis* as a biologic weapon. The fact that both armies were infected underscores one of the dangers of using infectious agents as biologic weapons. Often these are dispersed with aerosols, and despite the best predictions of air currents, they are notoriously unpredictable; with the shifting air currents, one's own troops could become infected. Unit 731 of the Japanese army also studied the use of *F. tularensis* as a biologic weapon, and the United States and Russia were known to have grown large quantities of *F. tularensis.*

F. tularensis is a gram-negative, pleomorphic rod. There are several animal hosts, with the cotton-tailed rabbit being one of the most susceptible. Normally, humans acquire *tularensis* through direct contact of an infected animal or from the bite of an infected tick or deerfly.[41] Occasionally, the ingestion of infected food or inhalation of a small amount of aerosol will initiate the disease. There are two strains of *F. tularensis,* Jellison A and B, with the B strain being relatively innocuous; in North America the A strain is quite virulent. Normally, a patient will develop a cutaneous ulcer at the site of entry after contact with an animal. As few as 10 or 50 organisms can invade the body through either hair follicles or mini abrasions. The incubation period is 2 to 6 days, at which time there is swelling and ulceration at the site of entry. As the swelling continues, the skin eventually breaks, creating an ulcer, which develops a necrotic base that becomes black as it scars. It is likely that *F. tularensis* would be delivered as an aerosol from an airplane, in which case, following inhalation, there is a 3- to 5-day incubation period, and then the onset of disease is marked with fever, pharyngitis, bronchitis, pneumonia, pleuritis, and hilar lymphadenopathy. Mortality rate for pneumonic tularemia is 5% to 15%.

The treatment of choice for tularemia is streptomycin, though gentamicin, tetracycline, and chloramphenicol have been used. There is concern that the former Soviet Union, perhaps the United States, and perhaps terrorists have engineered *F. tularensis* to be resistant to a number of agents. Prophylaxis with streptomycin, ciprofloxacin, or doxycycline has been recommended in the past for individuals exposed to the organism. There was a vaccine comprised of an attenuated whole organism strain, but it is no longer available.

Botulism

The first known work with *Clostridium botulinum* (botulism) as a biologic weapon was in World War II. Both the Germans and Japanese military and scientific communities experimented with *C. botulinum.* Unit 731 fed pure cultures of *C. botulinum* to Chinese captives with devastating effects. Both the United States and former Soviet Union are known to have produced large quantities of *C. botulinum* toxin, as have Iraq, Iran, Syria, and North Korea. In fact, after the first Gulf War, Iraq admitted to having over 19,000 L of concentrated botulism toxin, of which almost half was loaded on military weapons.[42] Nineteen thousand liters of botulinum toxin is enough to kill the world's population three times over! More recently, Aum Shinrikyo, the cult in Japan, dispersed aerosols of botulinum toxin on three different occasions in Japan. Fortunately, their dispersal methods were associated with multiple problems and no one was injured. Of concern is that a terrorist organization working with a rogue state could acquire and use botulinum as a bioterrorist weapon.

Botulism manifests as neuroparalysis caused by the toxin from *C. botulinum.* Unlike all the other biologic weapons mentioned previously, it is not caused by a live organism and, therefore, is not contagious. The organism from which botulinum toxin is derived is a gram-positive spore, which is an obligatory anaerobe, widely distributed in soil and in marine and agricultural products. Humans ingest *C. botulinum* without apparent effects until the organism begins to release toxins, of which there are several. Toxins are distributed from the GI tract, or from the lungs if inhaled, in the bloodstream to cholinergic nerve endings, where they block the release of acetylcholine at muscarinic and nicotinic receptors by inhibiting the intracellular fusion of the vesicles containing acetylcholine to nerve terminal membrane for release into the synaptic cleft. This mechanism is the exact opposite of the chemical nerve agents such as sarin, which result in an increase in the amount of acetylcholine at the cholinergic receptors, but the end result is the same. Patients develop a progressive weakness and a flaccid paralysis that begins in the extremities and progress until the respiratory muscles cease to contract. Of note, *C. botulinum* toxin is the most potent poison known to humans; the LD_{100} dose is only 1 pg.[43]

Shortly after ingestion or inhalation of the toxin, the incubation period is between 2 hours and 8 days, but most commonly between 12 and 36 hours.[44] As muscles become weak, patients develop diplopia, dysphonia, dysarthria, dysphagia, and eventually dyspnea and finally paralysis. Along with the effects noted within the skeletal muscle system caused by the lack of acetylcholine at the nicotinic receptor, muscarinic blockade results in decreased salivation, ileus, and urinary retention, again the opposite of what is seen with nerve agent poisoning.

Toxins can be removed through gastric lavage, use of cathartics, and with enemas. The treatment of patients includes the use of a trivalent antitoxin. Patients with profound respiratory embarrassment should have their airways protected and mechanical ventilation initiated. Without the use of antitoxin, it takes the patient 2 to 8 weeks to recover. The mortality rate is quoted as 5% to 10%.

Hemorrhagic Fevers

There are a number of viral hemorrhagic fevers that are listed as category A agents, including the arena viruses (Lassa fever and others), bunya viruses (hanta), flaviviruses (Dengue), and filoviruses (Ebola and Marburg). There are at least 18 viruses that cause human hemorrhagic fevers, which form a special group of viruses characterized by viral replication in lymphoid cells, after which patients develop fever and myalgia with an incubation of anywhere from 2 to 18 days, depending on the agent itself and the amount that is inhaled or inoculated across the dermis. They encompass syndromes that vary from febrile hemorrhagic fever with edema to septic shock, which rapidly leads to death. Both the United States and the former Soviet Union have experimented and have weaponized several of these viruses. Studies in nonhuman primates suggest that the agents are highly infectious, requiring only a few virions to produce illness.[44] The Aum Shinrikyo cult in Japan went to Africa in the 1990s to try to obtain an Ebola virus, which they planned to weaponize but fortunately, they were unsuccessful. There is no known incident where these agents have been used as a biologic weapon, but the natural outbreak of EVD during 2014–2015 spurred considerable investment in research and development into diagnostic tests and treatment with antivirals of the filoviruses (Ebola viruses and Marburg viruses).[45]

The viruses are single-stranded, ribonucleic acid (RNA) viruses that have a rodent or insect reservoir (bats are the natural reservoirs of Ebola virus)[46] and are communicated to humans by inhalation of an aerosol, through contact with an infected animal, or the bite of an infected insect. Humans are not a reservoir for the virus (NICV 59-1). The hemorrhagic fevers are contagious, and significant person-to-person transmission has occurred. The incubation period is within several days of contact or inhalation of the agent, at which time patients present with fever, myalgia, and evidence of a capillary leak (systemic leak or pulmonary edema), thrombocytopenia, and disseminated intravascular coagulation (DIC). The fatality rate, depending on the specific virus used, is anywhere from 2% to 60%. However, in the 2014–2015 EVD pandemic, as of March 3, 2016, the CDC and WHO reported that there had been 15,250 confirmed cases and that there were 11,316 deaths, for a fatality rate of about 75%.[47] There are no specific antiviral therapies for this class of viruses. Ribavirin, interferon-α, and hyperimmune globulin are often administered, with ribavirin being more protective against some of the viruses than others, but unfortunately one does not initially know what the etiologic agent is when the patient first presents.

Administration of convalescent serum and ZMapp (Mapp Biopharmaceutical, San Diego, CA, USA), a mixture of monoclonal antibodies, has been shown to be effective if treatment is begun early enough. In 2019, the U.S. Food and Drug Administration approved an Ebola vaccine, rVSV-ZEBOV, called Ervebo, for use in high-risk individuals.[48] Two antivirals have also been approved, a triple mixture of monoclonal antibodies atoltivimab, maftivimab, and odesivimab-ebgn and a single agent Ansuvimab-zykl.[49] The 2014–2015 outbreak demonstrated that Ebola presents a significant risk to healthcare workers, especially during the late stages of the disease. High-level PPE is required to be worn by healthcare workers whenever aerosols are generated, such as during suctioning, intubation, and bronchoscopy. Even flushing a toilet to dispose of bodily secretions has been shown to aerosolize viral particles. PPE is donned under observation prior to entering a patient's negative pressure isolation room. Proper doffing after patient contact is equally critical to avoid infection. The ASA website has an extensive protocol along with videos.[50] PPE can take as long as 30 minutes to put on and remove. Emergency intubation thus becomes impractical. All airway management should therefore be anticipatory. Elective surgery should be avoided. Every effort should be made to perform emergency procedures in the patient's isolation room. Equipment can be brought to the bedside and left afterward. If it is necessary to transport patients, staff must wear appropriate PPE and the patient, ideally, should be transported in an isopod. Intraoperative procedures should be established and practiced to avoid staff exposure.

Dengue fever, Chikungunya, and Zika virus disease have become increasingly prevalent across the tropics and subtropics. Dengue, Chikungunya, and Zika are viruses transmitted through *Aedes aegypti* and *Aedes albopictus* mosquitoes. In 2016, there was an outbreak of Zika in the Americas. Most infected patients were asymptomatic or had minor disease consisting of fever and rash. However, Zika virus infection has been associated with an increased incidence of microcephaly in babies born to infected mothers and an increase in Guillain–Barré disease. All three diseases can be transmitted through blood contamination and Zika virus has also been transmitted sexually. Current guidance suggests higher levels of PPE when participating in aerosol-generating procedures. Pregnant caregivers should consider higher levels of protection due to the apparent increased risk to the fetus from Zika infection.[51] At present, there is no vaccine for Zika virus infection and care of infected patients is supportive.

The Corona Virus Disease 2019 (COVID-19) pandemic of 2020–2022 is still ongoing at this writing. Whether it is naturally occurring or leaked from a lab is controversial, but it has to date killed close to 1 million people with more than 81 million cases confirmed in the United States alone. It has also drastically altered the world economy and disrupted supply chains.[52] Several vaccines have been produced and fielded, drastically reducing mortality of this rapidly mutating virus.[53] Remdesivir has also been approved as an antiviral agent with several other agents in development. COVID-19 has highlighted the need to stockpile PPE at local and regional levels, as well as the need to have the ability for rapid local manufacturing of medical supplies and devices. It has also highlighted the politicization of information, muddying the public health message, resulting in increased morbidity and mortality. COVID-19 highlighted the expertise of anesthesiologists who responded admirably to the surge of critically ill patients that overwhelmed hospital systems during the early waves of the pandemic.

Radiation—Nuclear

The greatest likelihood for dealing with patients who are exposed to ionizing radiation would come from a nuclear power plant or reactor accident, then from a terrorist action, and lastly from a detonation of a nuclear bomb. With respect to nuclear power plants, the U.S. Nuclear Regulatory Commission has not found that people living adjacent to the plants have increased rates of cancer; however, the commission continues to study the issue.[54] Unfortunately, that was not the case when there was release of radioactive material as has occurred in the past at Chernobyl, and most recently at the Fukushima Daiichi nuclear power plant in Japan following the earthquake and tsunami on March 11, 2011. It is claimed that the meltdown that occurred in Japan released only 10% as much radiation as occurred at Chernobyl.[55] In contrast, the cancer increase in the areas surrounding Fukushima was too low to detect.[56]

On April 26, 1986, workers at the Chernobyl nuclear power plant did not recognize or respond to evidence that one of the reactors was malfunctioning, with loss of cooling capacity and an explosion of the nuclear reactor.[57] Two workers died as a direct effect of the explosion, while those who remained in shielded areas survived unless they went to fight the fire, in which case they eventually died of radiation injury. Short-term γ and β emissions from the explosion and subsequent γ and β radiation from the reactor core debris killed many more, with long-term health effects to the entire community. Because of a lack of protective clothing and respirators, the radioactive material that exploded into the atmosphere rained down for several days, affecting many more workers and thousands of civilians. Primary sources of radiation were iodine-131, strontium-90, and cesium-137. During the subsequent 24 hours, 140,000 people were evacuated and potassium iodide tablets were distributed to as many people in the area as possible. Two hundred and thirty patients were subsequently hospitalized, with many patients succumbing to infections because of bone marrow suppression, and in those patients in whom bone marrow transplantation was attempted, 17 of 19 died because of associated radiation burns. All told, radiation burns caused 21 deaths. Oropharyngeal burns occurred in 28 patients. Over the next several years, the average radiation exposure around Chernobyl was four times normal due to residual ground contamination. Almost two decades later, the effects of Chernobyl continue to be felt in the immediate vicinity and in the area down-wind from the reactor site.[57] Ironically, a large number of Russian soldiers camped in the contaminated "Red Forest" near Chernobyl in 2022, during the Russian invasion of Ukraine. There are reports of large numbers of acute radiation cases that may have resulted in an unknown number of deaths.[58] The experience from Chernobyl reveals the kind of injuries that anesthesiologists can anticipate from nuclear accidents, including radiation burns, bone marrow suppression, the destruction of the lining of the GI tract, GI bleeding with translocation of bacteria, infection, sepsis, septic shock, and death. As evidenced by the experiences in Chernobyl, potassium iodide is indicated to protect the thyroid gland from taking up iodine-131, and other drugs are being considered, such as 5-androstenediol.

There have been other situations from which we can learn during which people have been exposed to ionizing radiation. On March 28, 1979, at the Three Mile Island nuclear power plant, the number 2 nuclear reactor overheated, and because the pressure relief valve failed to close, radioactive coolant was released into the containment facility.[59] As is often the case, there were numerous communication missteps, which resulted in the release of inconsistent information, generating genuine fear among individuals living nearby the nuclear power plant. There were no biologic effects of the event, but severe psychological sequelae did result.

On September 13, 1987, in Goiania, Brazil, a lead canister containing between 1,400 and 1,600 curies of cesium-137 contaminated 250 people; four of them died, and many others had short- and long-term health sequelae.[60] Mitigation efforts required the removal of 6,000 tons of clothing, furniture, dirt, trees, and other materials. The cesium had been left in a building in a lead canister when it was abandoned by its occupants; the canister was taken, opened by looters, and children played with the material.

Potential Sources of Ionizing Radiation Exposure

We are exposed to radiation on an annual basis from cosmic radiation, radon, medical devices, and in multiple stores and factories. In essence, half of our exposure comes from natural sources, with most of the remaining exposure originating from medical imaging and devices.[54] A chest radiograph leads to 5 to 10 millirem (mrem) of exposure, whereas a computed tomographic scan can result in 5,000 mrem of exposure.

Obviously, the greatest concern is the exposure to ionizing radiation that is unintentional—as occurred at the Chernobyl nuclear power plants. Intentional exposure threats are the result of military conflict or terrorism. With respect to the former, the two situations in which this occurred were in Hiroshima and Nagasaki in 1945. In Hiroshima, the bomb ("Little Boy") was only a 12.5-kiloton bomb, which killed an estimated 66,000 people and injured 69,000 more. The bomb that fell at Nagasaki ("Fat Boy") was a 22-kiloton plutonium implosion bomb, which killed between 39,000 and 74,000 people, with 75,000 people sustaining severe injuries. We learned from that experience that the majority of casualties are from the initial blast, fire, and the collapse of buildings. Radiation exposure subsequently killed many more. With any nuclear explosion, many individuals will be injured or die from the primary effect of the blast. Patients could have burn, crush, or radiation injury, or any combination thereof.

More recently, we have come to recognize that exposure to ionizing radiation may be as a result of terrorism. The most likely event will be the use of a dispersion device such as a conventional weapon or bomb surrounded with radionuclides such as cesium or strontium. In fact, in 1987, Iraq tested a 1-ton "dirty" bomb, and in 1996, Islamic terrorists in Chechnya placed a bomb packed with cesium-137 in a Moscow park that did not explode. While a radiation dispersion device remains the most likely event, terrorists could also target a nuclear power plant using a commercial jet, munitions, or internal sabotage.

Although a blast, crush, or thermal injury is readily apparent, the effects of ionizing radiation are usually not apparent. Anesthesiologists should be familiar with types of ionizing radiation, which include α particles, β particles, γ rays, x-rays, and neutrons. One also needs to understand how radiation is measured (Table 59-5). There are several methods, which take into account not only the decay rate of a radioactive isotope (becquerel [Bq] or a curie [Ci]) but also the dose absorbed, usually quantified as the amount absorbed by any type of tissue or material. The radiation-absorbed dose (rad or Gray [Gy]) is the international system of units (SI) method for denoting the amount of energy deposited in joules per kilogram. One Gy equals 100 rad. A sievert is the SI unit for measurement of *human* exposure to radiation in joules per kilogram, with 1 Sv = 100 rem (roentgen equivalent for man).

In a nuclear accident or catastrophe, patients could have several types of radiation exposure. They may receive external radiation from an x-ray–emitting device or from γ rays or β particles, they may be contaminated with debris emitting ionized radiation, or they might inhale gaseous radioactive material.[61] Some of this material can become incorporated into tissue as radioactive iodine isotopes would. In order to protect individuals, the distance from the source or explosion is important, as are the amount of shielding, the time one is exposed, and the amount of radioactive material to which one is exposed. Human tissue will block α particles (though if inhaled, α particles can penetrate up to 50 μm into the pulmonary epithelium material, leading to the development of lung cancer), but will not stop β particles or γ rays. Aluminum shields stop β particles, but γ rays can penetrate even concrete walls and lead is required to shield for both γ and x-rays.

The most likely injury from ionizing radiation is to those tissues that have the greatest turnover rate, that is, the sensitivity of tissues to radiation (from greatest to least) is for lymphoid, GI, reproductive, dermal, bone marrow, and nervous system tissue. In reality, the response of lymphoid and bone marrow to ionizing radiation cause the greatest problems. The thrombocytopenia, granulocytopenia, and the GI injury produce bleeding and bacterial translocation across the GI epithelium, the net result of which is sepsis and bleeding—the hallmarks of acute radiation syndrome, which lead to death.

Because ionizing radiation is invisible, affected individuals may appear normal. Patients who present with nausea, vomiting, diarrhea, and fever are likely to have severe acute radiation syndrome. Hypotension, erythema, and CNS dysfunction will manifest later.

Table 59-5 Radiation Exposure Terms

Term	Definition	Equivalence
Becquerel (Bq)	SI unit for measurement of radioactivity, defined as decay events per second 1 Bq = 1 disintegration per second	
Curie (Ci)	Traditional measure of radioactivity, as measured by radioactivity decay	1 Ci = 0.7×10^{10} disintegrations per second
Radiation-absorbed dose (rad)	Dose deposited by any type of radiation, in any type of tissue or material	1 rad = 0.01 Gy
Gray (Gy)	SI unit for the energy deposited by any type of radiation, in joules per kilogram	1 Gy = 100 rad
Roentgen equivalent man (rem)	Unit of human exposure to radiation	1 rem = 0.01 Sv
Sievert (Sv)	SI unit for measurement of human exposure to radiation, in joules per kilogram	1 Sv = 100 rem

SI, International System of units.

"Short-term" effects such as these, however, may not appear until days to weeks after the exposure, depending on the amount of exposure (as little as 0.75 to 1 Gy), whereas hematopoietic syndrome (severe lymphoid and bone marrow suppression) results from exposure to 3 to 6 Gy and may lead to death within 8 to 50 days. Long-term effects include thyroid cancer and psychological injury, as has been documented many times in the past.

Management

9 Should a radiation disaster occur, it would be followed by a huge coordinated local, state, and federal response, which at the federal level would include the U.S. Department of Homeland Security, the Department of Energy, the Department of Justice, FEMA, the Environmental Protection Agency, and the Nuclear Regulatory Commission. Of most importance, depending on the type of catastrophe, would be the immediate evacuation of the area. If evacuation, is impossible, a safe place should be sought within the home or building. The principles of disaster management always involve containment (avoid bringing patients with material emitting ionizing radiation to the hospital). Therefore, as part of the containment process, to the extent possible, patients should be decontaminated at the site. Removal of clothing is critically important. β and γ rays and neutrons will no longer be present on the patient unless there is still material emitting this radiation on a person's clothing. Rather than guess whether radiation is still present, it is best to disrobe patients. In previous mass casualty situations, maintenance of casualties' privacy has been a concern, but not one with an easy solution. Afterward, patients' skin should be washed with warm soapy water. Depending on the number of casualties, decontamination areas may have to be set up outside of hospitals, especially because individuals will arrive by private vehicles or on foot. Take care to isolate patients' personal belongings, giving the same consideration to biologic fluids—including saliva, blood, urine, and stool (all of which may be contaminated with radioisotopes and may therefore require special precautions when being handled)—as for clothing.

10 Potassium iodide can attenuate most of the radiation-induced thyroid effects, but must be given as quickly as possible because there is little protective effect if it is given more than 24 hours after exposure. Treatment is largely supportive, as these patients will develop acute radiation syndrome manifested by bleeding and sepsis. Treatment guidelines for management of postirradiation sepsis have been developed and advocated by the military.[62] The use of granulocyte colony–stimulating factor may be of benefit. Other treatments would include oral and GI decontamination using nasopharyngeal lavage, oral lavage and brushing, early stomach lavage, or administration of emetic and osmotic laxatives. Blocking agents include potassium iodide and strontium lactate. Mobilizing agents include ammonium chloride, calcium gluconate, and diuretics, which may enhance renal excretion. Chelation therapy that has been recommended includes calcium diethylenetriamine pentaacetic acid (DTPA) as an initial dose and then zinc-DTPA.[63] Granulocyte macrophage colony–stimulating factor and thrombopoietin or interleukin-11, though postulated, have not been proven to be of benefit. For individuals with a contaminated GI tract, selective decontamination may be helpful, though this again has not been demonstrated to be of benefit in this situation.[64]

Unfortunately, because of the possibility of blast, thermal, 11
and crush injuries, along with the radiation injury, the care of the injured may require the care of patients who have multiple combined injuries. The initial response should be as per the advanced trauma life support (ATLS) guidelines, which include an assessment of the airway, breathing, and circulation, and extent of trauma and then decontamination of the patient, after which the patient is stabilized and further evaluated. Wounds must be considered contaminated. "Dirty wounds" should not be closed but cleaned and debrided, excised, and observed. Unfortunately, in this situation, there is also the possibility that there may be the combined effects of a radiation-releasing event and the use of either chemical or biologic agents.[64] Because of the variety of types of terrorism, some of it reportedly government sponsored, communities and the U.S. government have had to plan for the detonation of a nuclear device on U.S. soil.[65,66]

Explosives

Management of traumatic injury is covered in Chapter 53, but a chapter on disaster management would not be complete without mentioning the use of explosive devices by terrorists. As the media reports daily, particularly in Afghanistan, the use of IEDs is the terrorist's favorite weapon. Patients have burns, fractures, lacerations, multiple shrapnel injuries, soft tissue trauma, and traumatic amputations. As the weapons have become more sophisticated and powerful, the extent of injuries has increased significantly. In 2012, U.S. military personnel experienced more multiple-than single-traumatic extremity amputations.[67]

12 Patients with any evidence of burns to the face or airway will require appropriate airway management. Patients should be intubated, awake if possible, because a significant number of these patients will have mild-to-moderate glottic edema at the time of intubation. Those patients with burns must be managed aggressively with respect to fluid resuscitation. With isolated total body surface injury, fluid resuscitation is aggressive. With polytrauma and no third-degree burns, "damage control resuscitation/surgery" is the norm.[68] The patient's body temperature is maintained and surgery is performed as soon as possible to stop the bleeding, thereby decreasing the need for blood products and the chances of developing a dilutional coagulopathy. Patients who do develop a coagulopathy appear to benefit from a ratio of packed red blood cells to fresh-frozen plasma to platelets of 1:1:1.[69,70] One study has demonstrated that tranexamic acid decreases the need for additional blood products. In patients with crush injury and markedly elevated creatine phosphokinase, alkalinization of the urine-forced diuresis may attenuate renal failure from myoglobinuria.

Leadership

Anesthesiologists are naturally placed to assume positions of leadership, but leadership is something that must be learned and developed through one's career. There are many resources available, from books to read, online videos, and courses of all lengths. The American Society of Anesthesiologists sponsors a Leadership Academy[71] offering online education complete with CME credits. The American Association for Physician Leaders sponsors a longer course resulting in the Certified Physician Executive designation.[72] There are also certificate programs from leading business schools as well as the Master of Business Administration (MBA) and Master of Healthcare Administration (MHA) degrees.

One particularly useful skill is the ability to communicate well during a crisis. According to the CDC, these principles are:

1. Be first. The first source of communication often becomes the source against which all others are measured.
2. Be right. Accuracy is critical to credibility.
3. Be credible. Honesty is fundamental to maintaining trust.
4. Express empathy. Emotion cannot be countered with facts. People must first know that their leaders care.
5. Promote action. Giving people something specific to do restores a sense of control over out-of-control circumstances.
6. Show respect. Lack of respect for a public in crisis undermines trust.[73]

Conclusion

Although it is unlikely that an anesthesiologist will be at the initial site of a natural or intentional disaster, it could happen. Most likely, anesthesiologists will become involved if the hospital at which they work provides care for a number of these patients. Anesthesiologists could find themselves involved in triage, in the ED, OR, or ICU.[74] As suggested for several of these situations, airway management and ventilator management may be critical, as would the establishment of intravascular access and volume resuscitation.

Obviously, it is critical to have a high index of suspicion if you are managing the index case, or two or more patients, with presenting signs and symptoms that are suggestive of the use of a biologic weapon. The individual who is the point of contact for the index case should notify the hospital infectious disease specialist and the local and state health departments. Factors that might indicate the intentional release of a biologic agent would include unusual temporal or geographic clustering of cases, an uncommon age distribution, or a significant number of cases (more than one) of acute flaccid paralysis that might suggest use of botulinum toxin.

If called to the hospital to be involved in managing such a catastrophe, the anesthesiologist must review basic decontamination and isolation techniques and, as mentioned previously, must follow those guidelines scrupulously. It is clear that anesthesiologists have the requisite training and experience to be of vital importance in managing such casualties. However, based on their training, they may not be emotionally prepared to manage these patients. They must remember that unlike their normal practice, they may have to triage patients, accept the fact that the standard of care may be different, and focus their efforts on interventions that will carry the greatest benefit for the greatest number of casualties.

This process begins when the anesthesiologist gets the call 13
at home or in the hospital regarding an impending mass casualty event. They must first report to the command and control center and, though most likely they may work in the operating room, they could also be used in the triage area in the ED or in the ICU. Of utmost importance is familiarity with the hospital's disaster plan. One must also develop one's own family care plan in anticipation of absence from the home for extended periods of time. Ensuring one's own safety through the appropriate use of protective devices to serve as barriers against radiologic, biologic, and chemical weapons is also of vital importance. Infrastructure degradation worsens the consequences of mass casualty events. Preparing to deliver care under austere circumstances, developing creative responses, and practicing (simulations) regularly will mitigate the effects of a disaster and increase resilience for individuals, teams, and institutions.

Appendix A. Disaster Preparedness Planning Guide for Families (from FEMA)

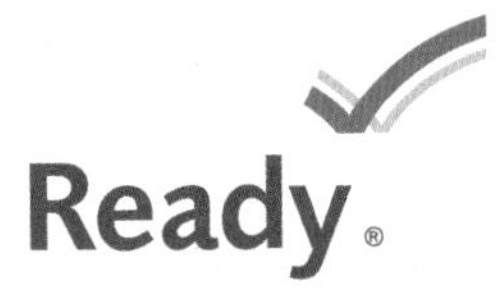

Family Emergency Plan

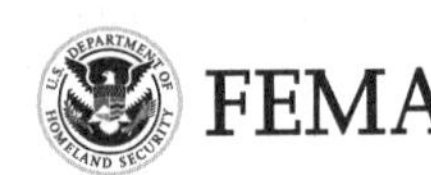

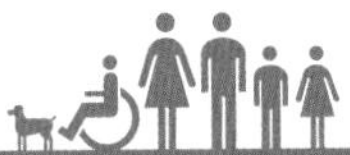

Make sure your family has a plan in case of an emergency. Before an emergency happens, sit down together and decide how you will get in contact with each other, where you will go, and what you will do in an emergency. Keep a copy of this plan in your emergency supply kit or another safe place where you can access it in the event of a disaster.

Out-of-Town Contact Name: ______ Telephone Number: ______

Email: ______

Neighborhood Meeting Place: ______ Telephone Number: ______

Regional Meeting Place: ______ Telephone Number: ______

Evacuation Location: ______ Telephone Number: ______

Fill out the following information for each family member and keep it up to date.

Name: ______ Social Security Number: ______
Date of Birth: ______ Important Medical Information: ______

Name: ______ Social Security Number: ______
Date of Birth: ______ Important Medical Information: ______

Name: ______ Social Security Number: ______
Date of Birth: ______ Important Medical Information: ______

Name: ______ Social Security Number: ______
Date of Birth: ______ Important Medical Information: ______

Name: ______ Social Security Number: ______
Date of Birth: ______ Important Medical Information: ______

Name: ______ Social Security Number: ______
Date of Birth: ______ Important Medical Information: ______

Write down where your family spends the most time: work, school, and other places you frequent. Schools, daycare providers, workplaces, and apartment buildings should all have site-specific emergency plans that you and your family need to know about.

Work Location One
Address: ______
Phone Number: ______
Evacuation Location: ______

Work Location Two
Address: ______
Phone Number: ______
Evacuation Location: ______

Work Location Three
Address: ______
Phone Number: ______
Evacuation Location: ______

Other places you frequent
Address: ______
Phone Number: ______
Evacuation Location: ______

School Location One
Address: ______
Phone Number: ______
Evacuation Location: ______

School Location Two
Address: ______
Phone Number: ______
Evacuation Location: ______

School Location Three
Address: ______
Phone Number: ______
Evacuation Location: ______

Other place you frequent
Address: ______
Phone Number: ______
Evacuation Location: ______

Important Information	Name	Telephone Number	Policy Number
Doctor(s):			
Other:			
Pharmacist:			
Medical Insurance:			
Homeowner's/Rental Insurance:			
Veterinarian/Kennel (for pets):			

Dial 911 for Emergencies

For further review and interactivities, please see the videos and narrative interactive clinical vignettes (NICVs) accessible in the complimentary eBook bundled with this text. Access instructions are located on the inside front cover.

REFERENCES

1. World Association for Disaster and Emergency Management (WADEM), Health Disaster Management. Guidelines for evaluation and research. http://wadem.org/guidelines.html. Published 2003. Accessed April 11, 2016.
2. United Nations. Sendai framework for disaster risk reduction 2015–2030. http://www.preventionweb.net/files/43291_sendaiframeworkfordrren.pdf. Published 2015. Accessed August 15, 2016.
3. American Society of Anesthesiologists (ASA), Committee on Trauma and Emergency Preparedness (COTEP). https://www.asahq.org/resources/resources-from-asa-committees/committee-on-trauma-and-emergency-preparedness. Published 2015. Accessed April 11, 2016.
4. Doctors Without Borders/Médecins Sans Frontières (MSF). Who we need. Doctors Without borders website. http://www.doctorswithoutborders.org/work-us/work-field/who-we-need/anesthesiologists-nurse-anesthetists. Published 2013. Accessed April 11, 2016.
5. Dara SI, Ashton RW, Farmer JC. Engendering enthusiasm for sustainable disaster critical care response: why this is of consequence to critical care professionals? *Crit Care.* 2005;9(2):125–127.
6. Gomez D, Haas B, Ahmed N, Tien H, Nathens A. Disaster preparedness of Canadian trauma centres: the perspective of medical directors of trauma. *Can J Surg.* 2011;54(1):9–16.
7. Ciraulo DL, Frykberg ER, Feliciano DV, et al. A survey assessment of the level of preparedness for domestic terrorism and mass casualty incidents among eastern association for the surgery of trauma members. *J Trauma.* 2004;56(5):1033–1039.
8. Rössler B, Marhofer P, Hüpfl M, Peterhans B, Schebesta K. Preparedness of anesthesiologists working in humanitarian disasters. *Disaster Med Public Health Prep.* 2013;7(4):408–412.
9. Moore ZS, Seward JF, Lane JM. Smallpox. *Lancet.* 2006;367(9508):425–435.
10. Tepper M, Whitehead J. Clinical predictors of bioterrorism-related inhalational anthrax. *Lancet.* 2005;365(9455):214.
11. Lynch DK. Plan ahead. *Anesth Analg.* 2010;110(3):653–654.
12. Merchant RM, Leigh JE, Lurie N. Health care volunteers and disaster response—first, be prepared. *N Engl J Med.* 2010;362(10):872–873.
13. Masterson L, Steffen C, Brin M, Kordick MF, Christos S. Willingness to respond: Of emergency department personnel and their predicted participation in mass casualty terrorist events. *J Emerg Med.* 2009;36(1):43–49.
14. US Department of Homeland Security (USDHS), Federal Emergency Management Agency (FEMA). National preparedness goal. http://www.fema.gov. Accessed April 11, 2016.
15. The Joint Commission on Accreditation of Healthcare Organizations (TJC). Health care at the crossroads: strategies for creating and sustaining community-wide emergency preparedness systems. http://www.jointcommission.org/assets/1/18/health_care_at_the_crossroads.pdf. Published 2003. Accessed April 11, 2016.
16. Joint Commission on Accreditation of Healthcare Organizations (TJC). Emergency management oversight requirements. http://www.jointcommission.org/assets/1/18/JCP0713_Emergency_Mgmt_Oversight.pdf. Published 2013. Accessed March 21, 2016.
17. US Department of Health and Human Services (DHHS). Emergency preparedness checklist. http//cms.gov/medicare/provider-enrollment-and certification/surveycertemergprep/downloads/sandc_epchecklist_provider.pdf. Published 2013. Accessed April 11, 2016.
18. Enserink M, Stone R. Questions swirl over knockout gas used in hostage crisis. *Science.* 2002;298:1150–1151.
19. Okumura T, Takasu N, Ishimatsu S, et al. Report on 640 victims of the Tokyo subway sarin attack. *Ann Emerg Med.* 1996;28(2):129–135.
20. Zane RD, Prestipino AL. Implementing the hospital emergency incident command system: an integrated delivery system's experience. *Prehosp Disaster Med.* 2004;19(4):311–317.
21. Goransson Nyberg A, Stricklin D, Sellstrom A. Mass casualties and healthcare following the release of toxic chemicals or radioactive material: contribution of modern biotechnology. *Int J Environ Res Public Health.* 2011;8(12):4521–4549.
22. Wong EG, Dominguez L, Trelles M, et al. Operative trauma in low-resource settings: the experience of Médecins Sans Frontières in environments of conflict, post conflict, and disaster. *Surgery.* 2015;157(5):850–856.
23. Jawa RS, Zakrison TL, Richards AT, Young DH, Heir JS. Facilitating safer surgery and anesthesia in a disaster zone. *Am J Surg.* 2012;204(3):406–409.
24. Chemical, Biological, Radiological and Nuclear Defense Information Analysis Center (CBRNIAC). U.S. Army Chemical Materials agency creates a safer tomorrow. *CBRNIAC Newsletter.* 2012;13(2):4–7.
25. Kassa J, Karasova JZ, Musilek K, Kuca K, Jung AY. A comparison of the neuroprotective efficacy of newly developed oximes (K117, K127) and currently available oxime (obidoxime) in tabun-poisoned rats. *Toxicol Mech Methods.* 2009;19(3):232–238.
26. Aroniadou-Anderjaska V, Figueiredo TH, Apland JP, Qashu F, Braga MF. Primary brain targets of nerve agents: the role of the amygdala in comparison to the hippocampus. *Neurotoxicology.* 2009;30(5):772–776.
27. Beeching NJ, Dance DA, Miller AR, Spencer RC. Biological warfare and bioterrorism. *BMJ.* 2002;324(7333):336–339.
28. Breman JG, Henderson DA. Diagnosis and management of smallpox. *N Engl J Med.* 2002;346(17):1300–1308.
29. Choo CW. The World Health Organization smallpox eradication programme. http://choo.fis.utoronto.ca/fis/courses/lis2102/KO.WHO.case.html. Published 2012. Accessed April 11, 2016.
30. Centers for Disease Control and Prevention (CDC). Smallpox vaccine adverse events among civilians—United States, March 4–10, 2003. *JAMA.* 2003;289(15):1921–1922.
31. Frey SE, Newman FK, Kennedy JS, et al. Clinical and immunologic responses to multiple doses of IMVAMUNE (modified vaccinia Ankara) followed by Dryvax challenge. *Vaccine.* 2007;25(51):8562–8573.
32. Inglesby TV, Henderson DA, Bartlett JG, et al. Anthrax as a biological weapon: medical and public health management. Working Group on Civilian Biodefense. *JAMA.* 1999;281(18):1735–1745.
33. Kalamas AG. Anthrax. *Anesthesiol Clin North Am.* 2004;22(3):533–540.
34. Janse I, Hamidjaja RA, Bok JM, van Rotterdam BJ. Reliable detection of *Bacillus anthracis*, *Francisella tularensis* and *Yersinia pestis* by using multiplex qPCR including internal controls for nucleic acid extraction and amplification. *BMC Microbiol.* 2010;10:314.
35. Martin G. Anthrax: lessons learned from the U.S. Capitol experience. *Mil Med.* 2003;168(9): 9–14.
36. Swartz MN. Recognition and management of anthrax: an update. *N Engl J Med.* 2001;345(22):1621–1626.
37. Dixon TC, Meselson M, Guillemin J, Hanna PC. Anthrax. *N Engl J Med.* 1999;341(11):815–826.
38. Shafazand S, Doyle R, Ruoss S, Weinacker A, Raffin TA. Inhalational anthrax: epidemiology, diagnosis, and management. *Chest.* 1999;116(5):1369–1376.
39. Schmitt B, Dobrez D, Parada JP, et al. Responding to a small-scale bioterrorist anthrax attack: cost-effectiveness analysis comparing pre-attack vaccination with postattack antibiotic treatment and vaccination. *Arch Intern Med.* 2007;167(7):655–662.
40. Prentice MB, Rahalison L. Plague. *Lancet.* 2007;369(9568):1196–1207.
41. Zietz BP, Dunkelberg H. The history of the plague and the research on the causative agent Yersinia pestis. *Int J Hyg Environ Health.* 2004;207(2):165–178.
42. Josko D. Botulin toxin: a weapon in terrorism. *Clin Lab Sci.* 2004;17(1):30–34.
43. Franz DR, Jahrling PB, McClain DJ, et al. Clinical recognition and management of patients exposed to biological warfare agents. *Clin Lab Med.* 2001;21(3):435–473.
44. Bhalla DK, Warheit DB. Biological agents with potential for misuse: a historical perspective and defensive measures. *Toxicol Appl Pharmacol.* 2004;199(1):71–84.
45. Kuhn JH, Dodd LE, Wahl-Jensen V, Radoshitzky SR, Bavari S, Jahrling PB. Evaluation of perceived threat differences posed by filovirus variants. *Biosecur Bioterror.* 2011;9(4):361–371.
46. Murray MJ. Ebola virus disease: a review of its past and present. *Anesth Analg.* 2015:121:798–809.
47. Centers for Disease Control and Prevention (CDC). 2014 Ebola outbreak in West Africa. http://www.cdc.gov/vhf/ebola/outbreaks/2014-west-africa/index.html. Published 2014. Accessed April 11, 2016.
48. Prevention and Vaccine | Ebola (Ebola Virus Disease). CDC. www.cdc.gov accessed 3-28-23.
49. Treatment | Ebola (Ebola Virus Disease). CDC. www.cdc.gov accessed 3-28-23.
50. American Society of Anesthesiologists (ASA), Committee on Trauma and Emergency Preparedness (COTEP). Ebola information. https://www.asahq.org/resources/clinical-information/ebola-information#4. Published 2016. Accessed April 11, 2016.
51. Centers for Disease Control and Prevention (CDC). Zika virus. http://www.cdc.gov/zika/index.html. Published 2016. Accessed March 4, 2016.
52. CDC COVID Data Tracker: Home. www.cdc.gov accessed 3-28-23.
53. Stay Up to Date with Your COVID-19 Vaccines. CDC. www.cdc.gov accessed 3-28-23.
54. US Nuclear Regulatory Commission, Office of Public Affairs. Fact sheet on biological effects of radiation. http://www.nrc.gov/Published. 2011. Accessed April 10, 2016.
55. Masamichi CN, Haruyasu N, Hiroaki T, et al. Preliminary estimation of release amounts of 131I and 137Cs accidentally discharged from the Fukushima Daiichi nuclear power plant into the atmosphere. *J Nucl Sci Tech.* 2011;(7):1129–1134.
56. Yamashita S, Suzuki S. Risk of thyroid cancer after the Fukushima nuclear power plant accident. *Respir Investig.* 2013;51(3): 128–133.
57. Shibata Y, Yamashita S, Masyakin VB, Panasyuk GD, Nagataki S. 15 years after Chernobyl: new evidence of thyroid cancer. *Lancet.* 2001;358(9297):1965–1966.
58. Image shows Russian troops camped in radioactive area during Chernobyl assault: NPR; Russian Troops Suffer 'Acute Radiation Sickness' After Digging Chernobyl Trenches (thedailybeast.com)
59. Collins DL. Human responses to the threat of or exposure to ionizing radiation at Three Mile Island, Pennsylvania, and Goiania, Brazil. *Mil Med.* 2002;167(2):137–138.
60. Collins DL, de Carvalho AB. Chronic stress from the Goiania 137Cs radiation accident. *Behav Med.* 1993;18(4):149–157.
61. Ibrahim SA, Simon SL, Bouville A, Melo D, Beck HL. Alimentary tract absorption (f1 values) for radionuclides in local and regional fallout from nuclear tests. *Health Phys.* 2010;99(2):233–251.

62. Brook I, Elliott TB, Ledney GD, Knudson GB. Management of postirradiation sepsis. *Mil Med.* 2002;167(2):105–106.
63. Knudson GB, Elliott TB, Brook I, et al. Nuclear, biological, and chemical combined injuries and countermeasures on the battlefield. *Mil Med.* 2002;167(2):95–97.
64. Shi C, Lu S. Radiation injuries. *Int J Low Extrem Wounds.* 2011;10(3):120–121.
65. Sternberg S. Experts plan for how to deal with nuclear terror strike. http://www.usatoday.com/news/nation/2011-03-15-nukemed14_ST_N.htm. Published March 15, 2011. Accessed April 10, 2016.
66. National Security Staff Interagency Policy Coordination, Subcommittee for Preparedness and Response to Radiological and Nuclear Threats. *Planning Guidance for Response to a Nuclear Detonation.* 2nd ed. US Environmental Protection Agency; 2010.
67. Zoroya G. IEDs contribute to increase in multiple amputations. http://www.usatoday.com/news/military/story/2012-06-04/IEDamputations-military-Afghanistan/55385376/1. Published June 4, 2012. Accessed. April 4, 2016.
68. Holcomb JB, Jenkins D, Rhee P, et al. Damage control resuscitation: directly addressing the early coagulopathy of trauma. *J Trauma.* 2007;62(2):307–310.
69. CRASH-2 Collaborators, Roberts I, Shakur H, Afolabi A, et al. The importance of early treatment with transexamic acid in bleeding trauma patients: an exploratory analysis of the CRASH-2 randomised controlled trial. *Lancet.* 2011;377(9771):1101.e1–1101.e2.
70. Borgman MA, Spinella PC, Perkins JG, et al. The ratio of blood products transfused affects mortality in patients receiving massive transfusions at a combat support hospital. *J Trauma.* 2007;63(4):805–813.
71. Leadership Academy | American Society of Anesthesiologists (asahq.org)
72. Earn Your Certified Physician Executive (CPE) | AAPL (physicianleaders.org)
73. 6 Principles of Crisis Communications From CDC (Plus Resource Materials) (prnewsonline.com) I don't have permission yet for the above quote.
74. Baker DJ. Management of casualties from terrorist chemical and biological attack: a key role for the anaesthetist. *Br J Anaesth.* 2002;89(2):211–214.

Section 10

APPENDICES

1. Formulas
2. Atlas of Electrocardiography
3. Pacemaker and Implantable Cardiac Defibrillator Protocols
4. American Society of Anesthesiologists Standards, Guidelines, and Statements
5. The American Society of Anesthesiologists Difficult Airway Algorithms
6. Herbal Medications
7. Atlas of Ultrasound and Echocardiography (eBook only)

APPENDIX 1
Formulas

Hemodynamic Formulas

Hemodynamic Variables: Calculations and Normal Values

Variable	*Calculation*	*Normal Values*
Cardiac index (CI)	CO/BSA	2.5–4.0 L/min/m^2
Stroke volume (SV)	CO × 1,000/HR	60–90 mL/beat
Stroke index (SI)	SV/BSA	40–60 mL/beat/m^2
Mean arterial pressure (MAP)	Diastolic pressure + ⅓ pulse pressure	80–120 mmHg
Systemic vascular resistance (SVR)	$\frac{MAP - \overline{CVP}}{CO} \times 79.9$	1,200–1,500 dyne-cm-sec^{-5}
Pulmonary vascular resistance (PVR)	$\frac{\overline{PAP} - \overline{PCWP}}{CO} \times 79.9$	100–300 dyne-cm-sec^{-5}
Right ventricular stroke work index (RVSWI)	$0.0136\ (\overline{PAP} - \overline{CVP}) \times SI$	5–9 g-m/beat/m^2
Left ventricular stroke work index (LVSWI)	$0.0136\ (MAP - \overline{PCWP}) \times SI$	45–60 g-m/beat/m^2

HR, heart rate; $\overline{CVP}$, mean central venous pressure; $\overline{PAP}$, mean pulmonary artery pressure; BSA, body surface area; CO, cardiac output; $\overline{PCWP}$, mean pulmonary capillary wedge pressure; MAP, mean arterial blood pressure.

Respiratory Formulas

	Normal Values (70 kg)
Alveolar oxygen tension $PAO_2 = (P_b - 47)\ FIO_2 - PACO_2$	110 mmHg ($FIO_2 = 0.21$)
Alveolar–arterial oxygen gradient $AaO_2 = PAO_2 - PaO_2$	<10 mmHg ($FIO_2 = 0.21$)
Arterial-to-alveolar oxygen ratio, a/A ratio	>0.75
Arterial oxygen content $CaO_2 = (SaO_2)\ (Hb \times 1.34) + PaO_2\ (0.0031)$	21 mL/100 mL
Mixed venous oxygen content $C\dot{V}O_2 = (S\dot{V}O_2)\ (Hb \times 1.34) + P\overline{V}O_2\ (0.0031)$	15 mL/100 mL
Arterial-venous oxygen content difference $aVO_2 = CaO_2 - C\overline{V}O_2$	4–6 mL/100 mL
Intrapulmonary shunt $\dot{Q}s/\dot{Q}t = (CCO_2 - CaO_2) / (CCO_2 - C\dot{V}O_2)$ $CCO_2 = (Hb \times 1.34) + (PAO_2 \times 0.0031)$	<5%
Physiologic dead space $\dot{V}d/\dot{V}t = (PaCO_2 - PECO_2) / PaCO_2$	0.33
Oxygen consumption $\dot{V}O_2 = CO\ (CaO_2 - C\dot{V}O_2)$	240 mL/min
Oxygen transport $O_2T = CO\ (CaO_2)$	1,000 mL/min

CaO_2, arterial oxygen content; $C\dot{V}O_2$, mixed venous oxygen content; CCO_2, pulmonary capillary oxygen content; CO, cardiac output; FIO_2, fraction inspired oxygen; O_2T, oxygen transport; P_B, barometric pressure; $\dot{Q}s/\dot{Q}t$, intrapulmonary shunt; $PACO_2$, alveolar carbon dioxide tension; $PaCO_2$, arterial carbon dioxide tension; PAO_2, alveolar oxygen tension; PaO_2, arterial oxygen tension; $PECO_2$, expired carbon dioxide tension; Vd, dead-space gas volume; $\dot{V}t$, tidal volume; $\dot{V}O_2$, oxygen consumption.

Lung Volumes and Capacities

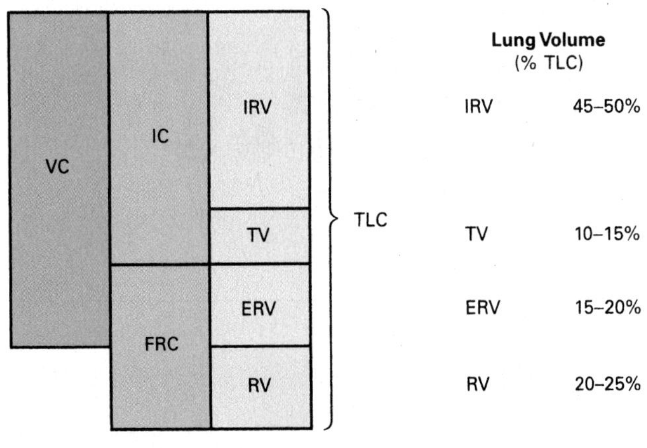

		Normal Values (70 kg)
Vital capacity	VC	4,800 mL
Inspiratory capacity	IC	3,800 mL
Functional residual capacity	FRC	2,400 mL
Inspiratory reserve volume	IRV	3,500 mL
Tidal volume	TV	1,500 mL
Expiratory reserve volume	ERV	1,200 mL
Residual volume	RV	1,200 mL
Total lung capacity	TLC	6,000 mL

APPENDIX 2
Atlas of Electrocardiography

GINA CLEOPATRA BADESCU

Lead Placement

	Electrode	
	Positive	***Negative***
Bipolar Leads		
I	LA	RA
II	LL	RA
III	LL	LA
Augmented Unipolar		
aVR	RA	LA, LL
aVL	LA	RA, LL
aVF	LL	RA, LA
Precordial		
V_1	4 ICS-RSB	
V_2	4 ICS-LSB	
V_3	Midway between V_2 and V_4	
V_4	5 ICS-MCL	
V_5	5 ICS-AAL	
V_6	5 ICS-MAL	

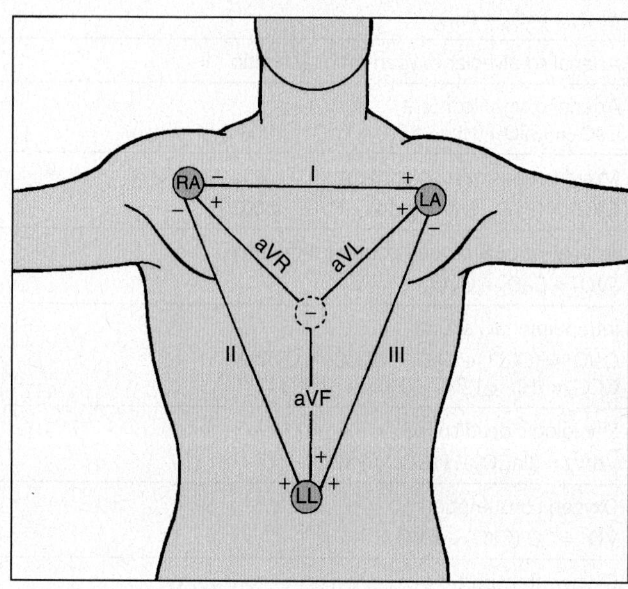

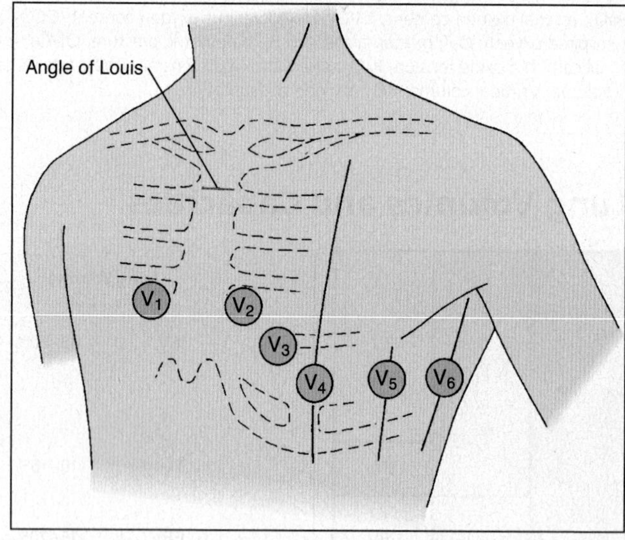

Abbrev.	Meaning
LA	Left arm
RA	Right arm
LL	Left leg
ICS	Intercostal space
RSB	Right sternal border
LSB	Left sternal border
MCL	Midclavicular line
AAL	Anterior axillary line
MAL	Midaxillary line

Sections and images of this appendix were developed, in part, for both Barash PG, Cullen BF, Cahalan MK, et al., eds. *Clinical Anesthesia*. 8th ed. Wolters Kluwer Health; 2016 and Kaplan JA, Reich DL, Savino JS, eds. *Kaplan's Cardiac Anesthesia: The Echo Era*. Elsevier; 2011, with permission of the editors and publishers.

The Normal Electrocardiogram—Cardiac Cycle

The normal electrocardiogram is composed of waves (P, QRS, T, and U) and intervals (PR, QRS, ST, and QT).

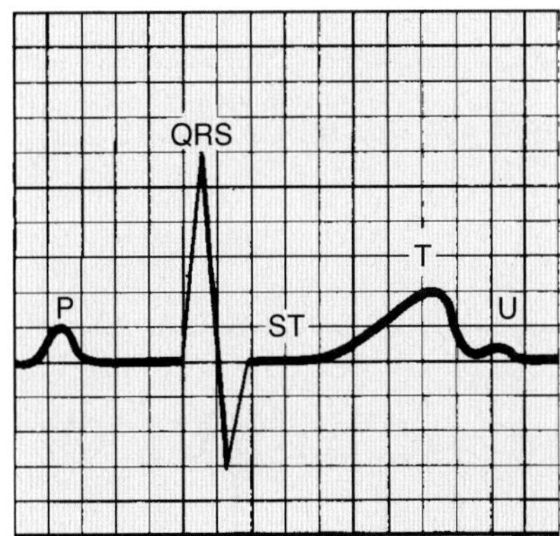

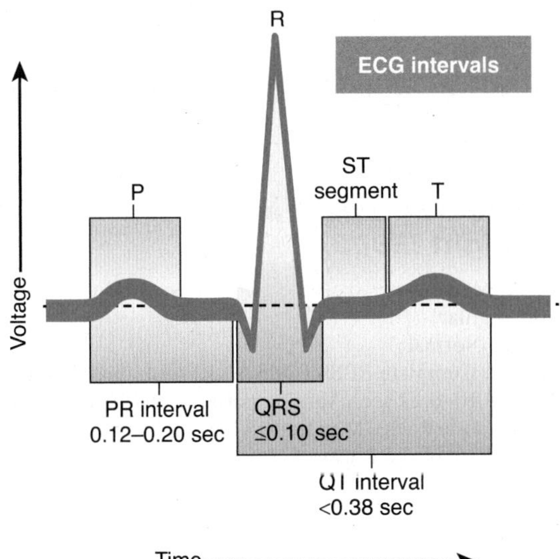

Video 1 Atrial Fibrillation

Rate: Variable (~150–200 beats/min)
Rhythm: Irregular
PR interval: No P wave; PR interval not discernible
QT interval: QRS normal

Note: Must be differentiated from atrial flutter: (1) absence of flutter waves and presence of fibrillatory line; (2) flutter usually associated with higher ventricular rates (>150 beats/min). Loss of atrial contraction reduces cardiac output (10%–20%). Mural atrial thrombi may develop. Considered controlled if ventricular rate is <100 beats/min.

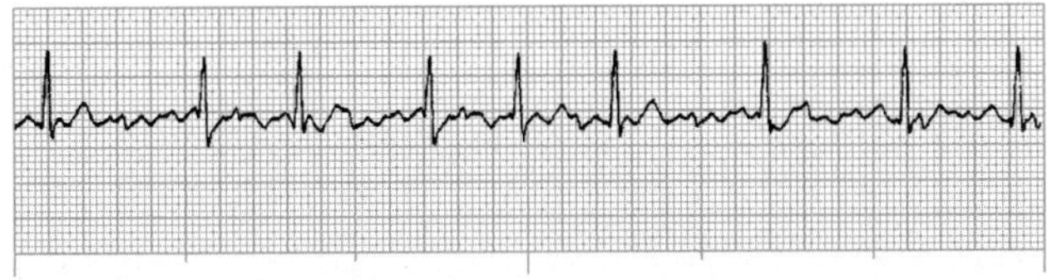

Video 2 Atrial Flutter

Rate: Rapid, atrial usually regular (250–350 beats/min); ventricular usually regular (<100 beats/min)
Rhythm: Atrial and ventricular regular
PR interval: Flutter (F) waves are saw-toothed. PR interval cannot be measured.
QT interval: QRS usually normal; ST segment and T waves are not identifiable.

Note: Vagal maneuvers will slow ventricular response, simplifying recognition of the F waves.

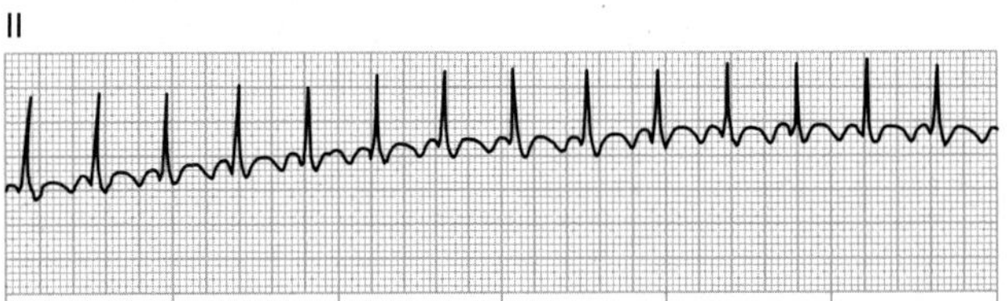

Video 3 Atrioventricular Block (First-Degree)

Rate: 60–100 beats/min
Rhythm: Regular
PR interval: Prolonged (>0.20 sec) and constant
QT interval: Normal

Note: Usually clinically insignificant; may be early harbinger of drug toxicity.

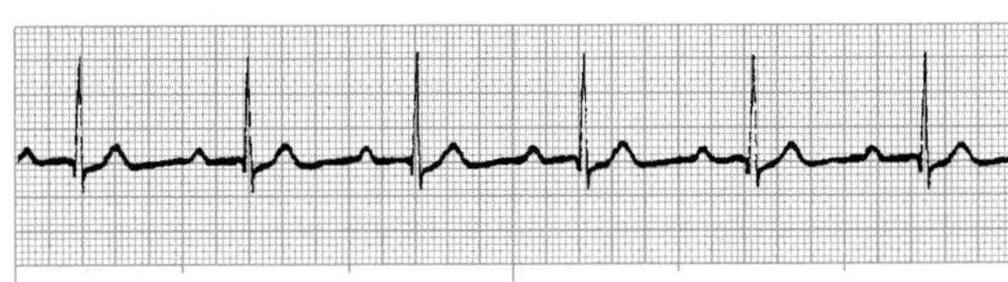

Video 4 Atrioventricular Block (Second-Degree), Mobitz Type I/ Wenckebach Block

Rate: 60–100 beats/min
Rhythm: Atrial regular; ventricular irregular
PR interval: P wave normal; PR interval progressively lengthens with each cycle until QRS complex is dropped (dropped beat). PR interval following dropped beat is shorter than normal.
QT interval: QRS complex normal but dropped periodically.

Note: Commonly seen in trained athletes and with drug toxicity.

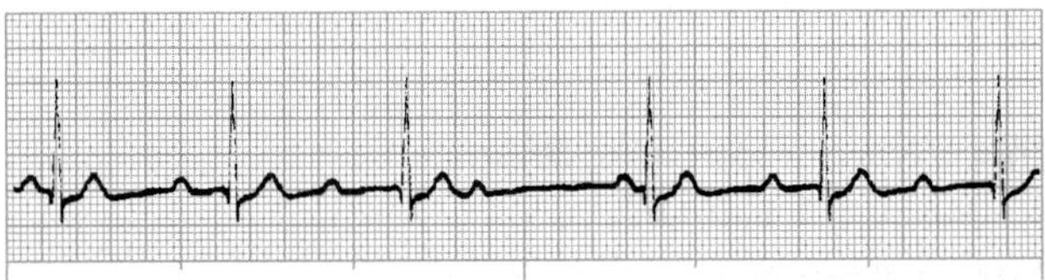

5 Video 5 Atrioventricular Block (Second-Degree), Mobitz Type II

Rate: <100 beats/min
Rhythm: Atrial regular; ventricular regular or irregular
PR interval: P waves normal, but some are not followed by QRS complex.
QT interval: Normal but may have widened QRS complex if block is at level of bundle branch. ST segment and T wave may be abnormal, depending on location of block.

Note: In contrast to Mobitz type I block, the PR and RR intervals are constant and the dropped QRS occurs without warning. The wider the QRS complex (block lower in the conduction system), the greater the amount of myocardial damage.

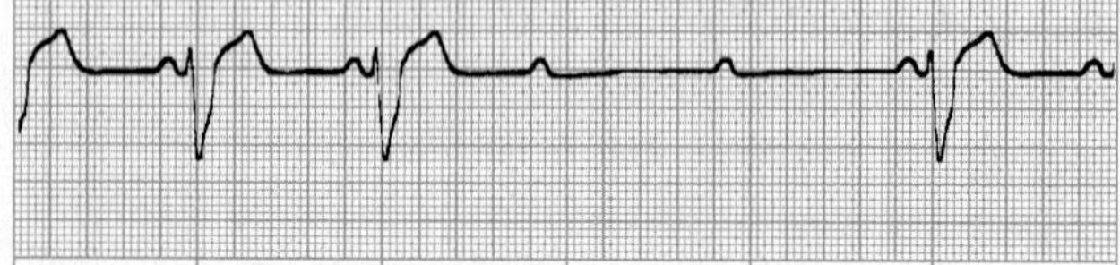

6 Video 6 Atrioventricular Block (Third-Degree), Complete Heart Block

Rate: <45 beats/min
Rhythm: Atrial regular; ventricular regular; no relationship between P wave and QRS complex.
PR interval: Variable because atria and ventricles beat independently.
QT interval: QRS morphology variable, depending on the origin of the ventricular beat in the intrinsic pacemaker system (atrioventricular junctional vs. ventricular pacemaker). ST segment and T wave normal.

Note: AV block represents complete failure of conduction from atria to ventricles (no P wave is conducted to the ventricle). The atrial rate is faster than ventricular rate. P waves have no relationship to QRS complexes (e.g., they are electrically disconnected). In contrast, with AV dissociation, the P wave is conducted through the AV node and the atrial and ventricular rate are similar. Immediate treatment with atropine or isoproterenol is required if cardiac output is reduced. Consideration should be given to insertion of a pacemaker. Seen as a complication of mitral valve replacement.

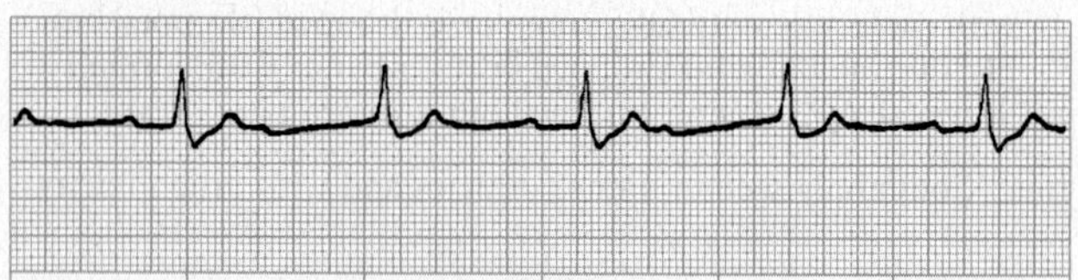

7 Video 7 Bundle Branch Block–Left (LBBB)

Rate: <100 beats/min
Rhythm: Regular
PR interval: Normal
QT interval: Complete LBBB (QRS >0.12 sec); incomplete LBBB (QRS = 0.10–0.12 sec); lead V_1 negative RS complex; I, aVL, V_6 wide R wave without Q or S component. ST segment and T-wave direction opposite direction of the R wave.

Note: LBBB does not occur in healthy patients and usually indicates serious heart disease with a poor prognosis. In patients with LBBB, insertion of a pulmonary artery catheter may lead to complete heart block.

Left Bundle Branch Block

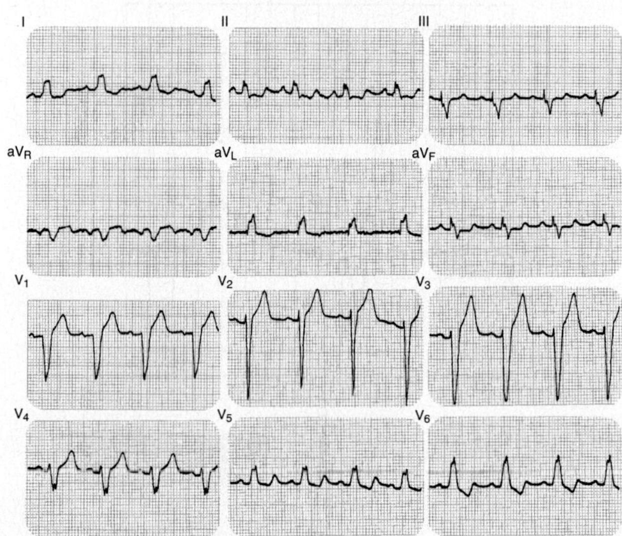

8 Video 8 Bundle Branch Block–Right (RBBB)

Rate: <100 beats/min
Rhythm: Regular
PR interval: Normal
QT interval: Complete RBBB (QRS >0.12 sec); incomplete RBBB (QRS = 0.10–0.12 sec). Varying patterns of QRS complex; rSR (V_1); RS, wide R with M pattern. ST segment and T wave opposite direction of the R wave.

Note: In the presence of RBBB, Q waves may be seen with a myocardial infarction.

Right Bundle Branch Block

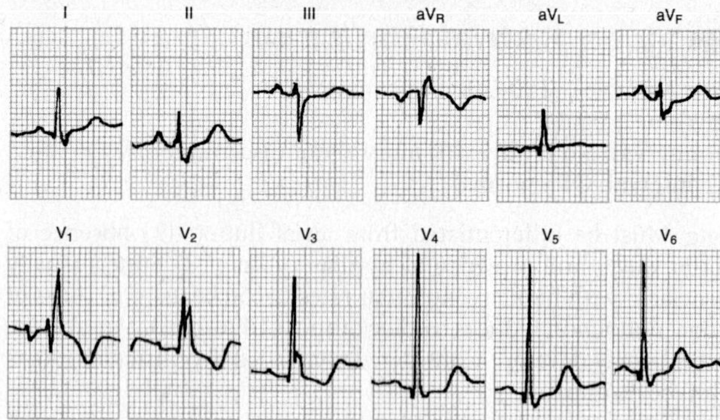

Coronary Artery Disease

9 *Video 9 Transmural Myocardial Infarction (TMI)*

Q waves seen on ECG, useful in confirming diagnosis, are associated with poorer prognosis and more significant hemodynamic impairment. Arrhythmias frequently complicate course. Small Q waves may be normal variant. For myocardial infarction (MI), Q waves >0.04 sec or depth exceeds one-third of R wave. For inferior wall MI, differentiate from RVH by axis deviation.

Myocardial Infarction

Anatomic Site	Leads	ECG Changes	Coronary Artery
Inferior	II, III, AVF	Q, ↑ ST, ↑ T	Right

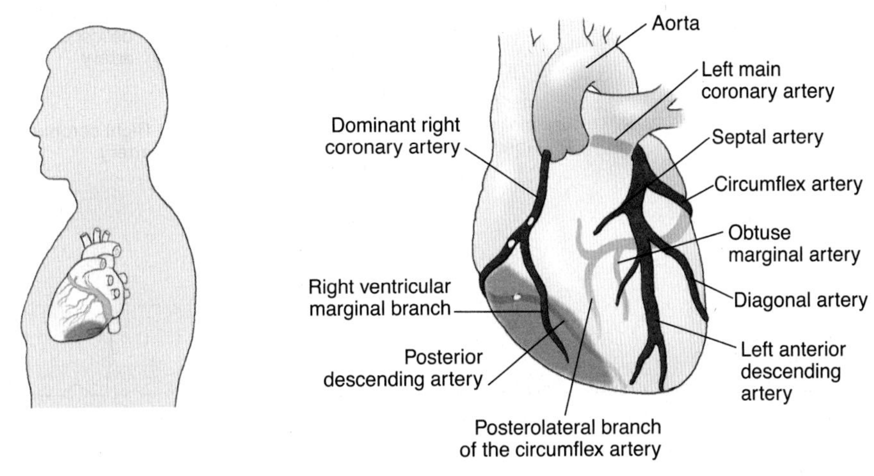

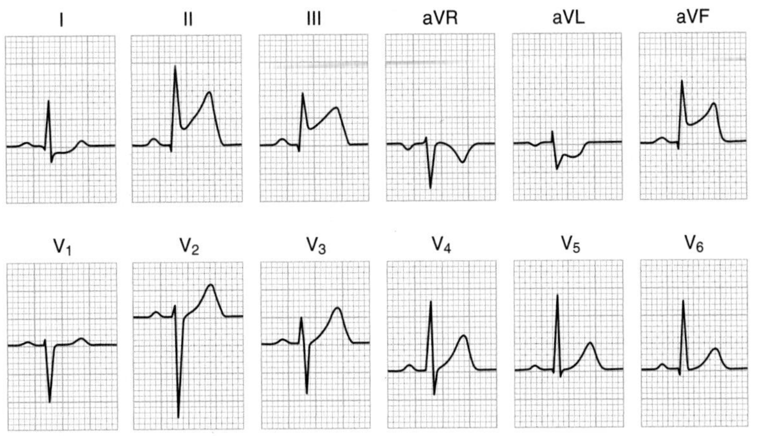

Myocardial Infarction			
Anatomic Site	**Leads**	**ECG Changes**	**Coronary Artery**
Posterior	V_1–V_2	↑ R, ↓ ST, ↓ T	Posterior descending

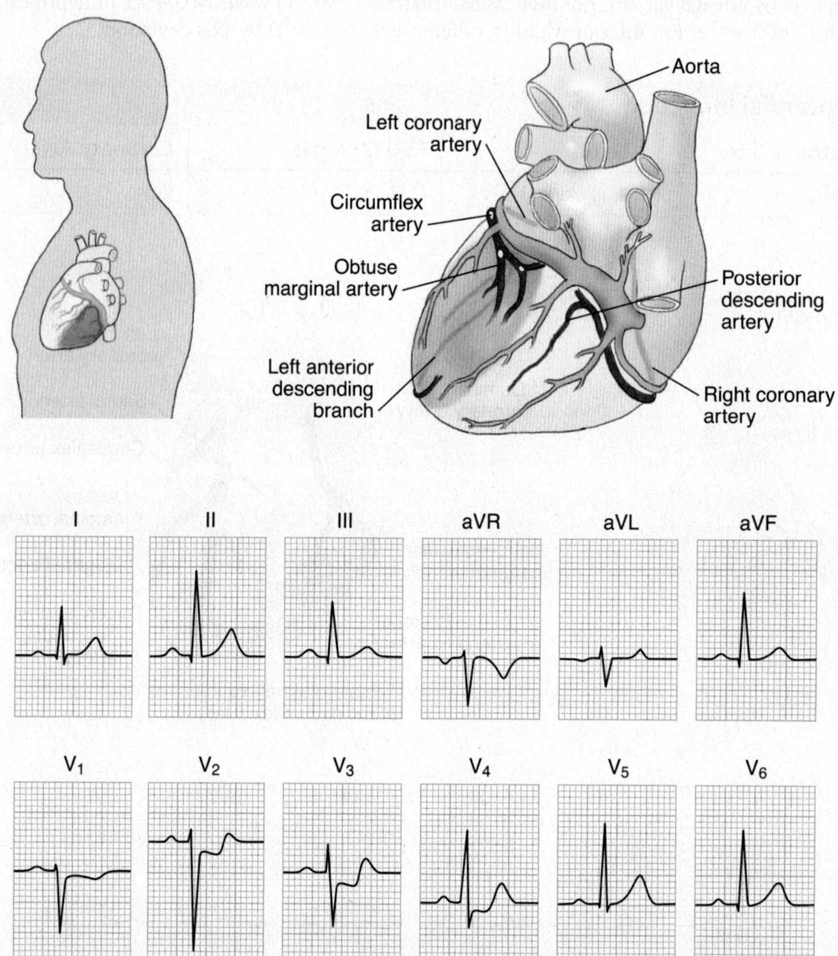

Myocardial Infarction			
Anatomic Site	**Leads**	**ECG Changes**	**Coronary Artery**
Lateral	I, aVL, V_5–V_6	Q, ↑ ST, ↑ T	Left circumflex

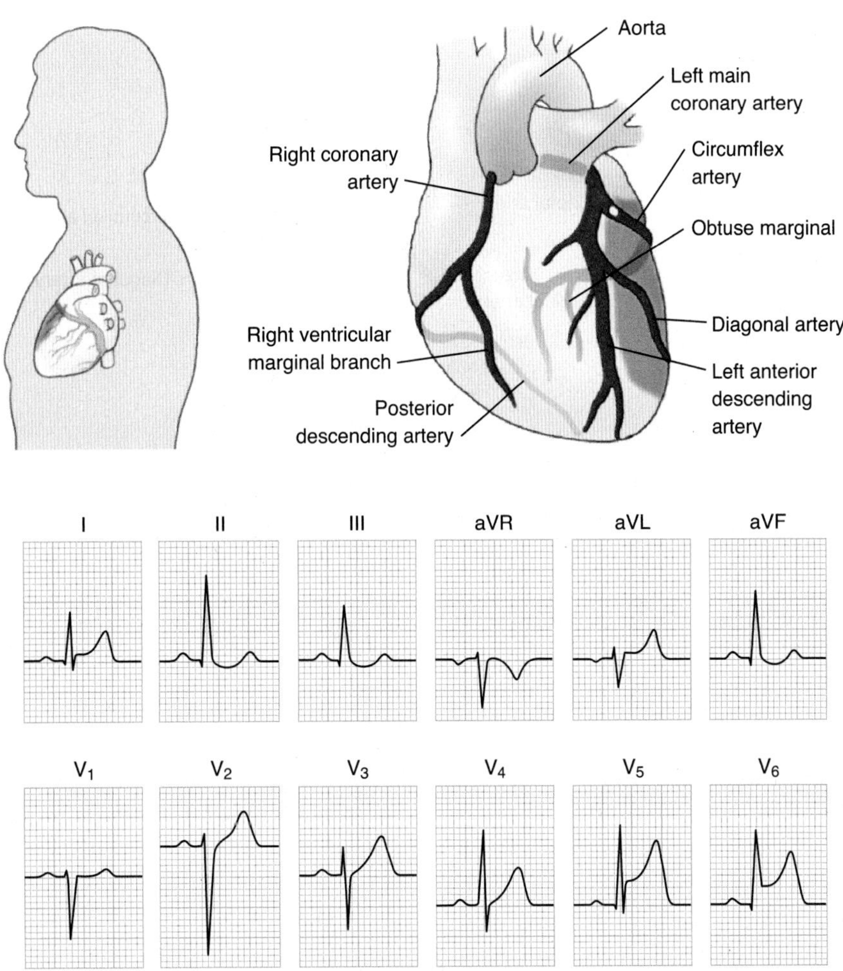

Myocardial Infarction			
Anatomic Site	**Leads**	**ECG Changes**	**Coronary Artery**
Anterior	I, aVL, V_1–V_4	Q, ↑ ST, ↑ T	Left anterior descending

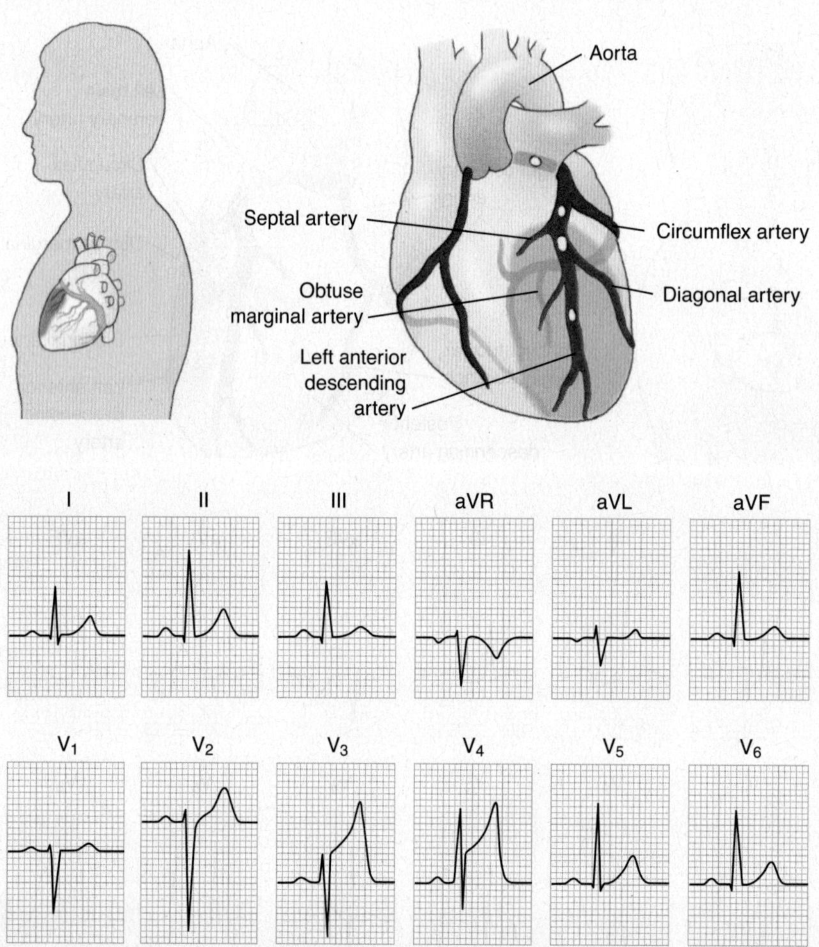

Myocardial Infarction			
Anatomic Site	**Leads**	**ECG Changes**	**Coronary Artery**
Anteroseptal	V_1–V_4	Q, ↑ ST, ↑ T	Left anterior descending

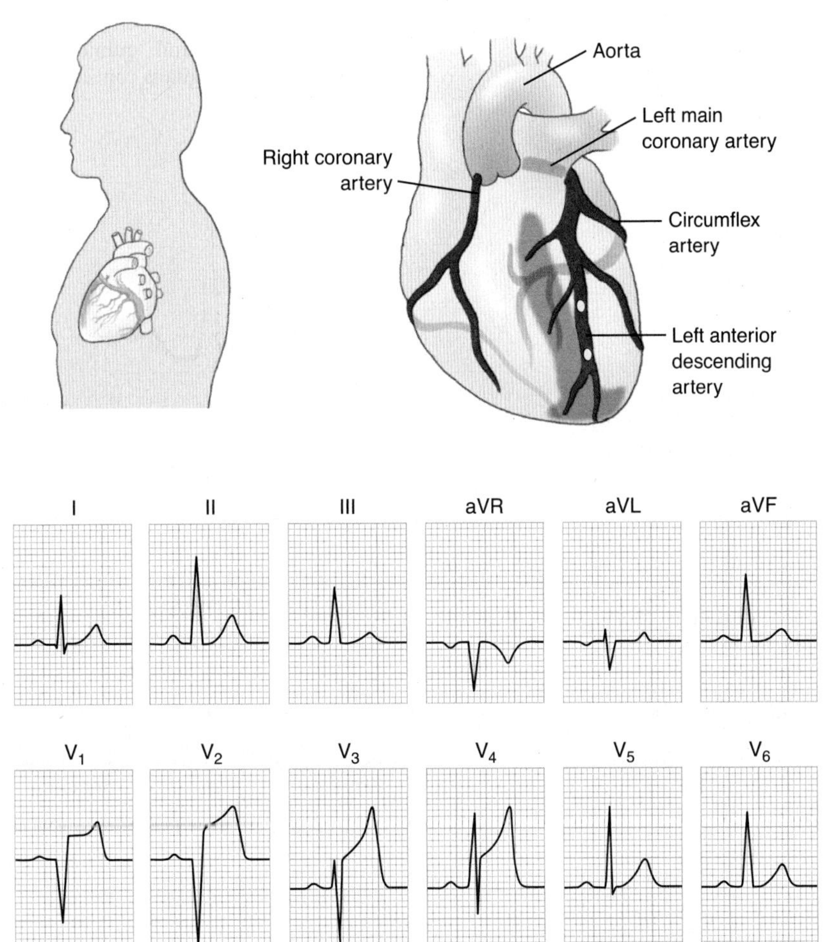

Video 10 Subendocardial Myocardial Infarction (SEMI)

Persistent ST-segment depression and/or T-wave inversion in the absence of Q wave. Usually requires additional laboratory data (e.g., isoenzymes) to confirm diagnosis. Anatomic site of coronary lesion is similar to that of TMI electrocardiographically.

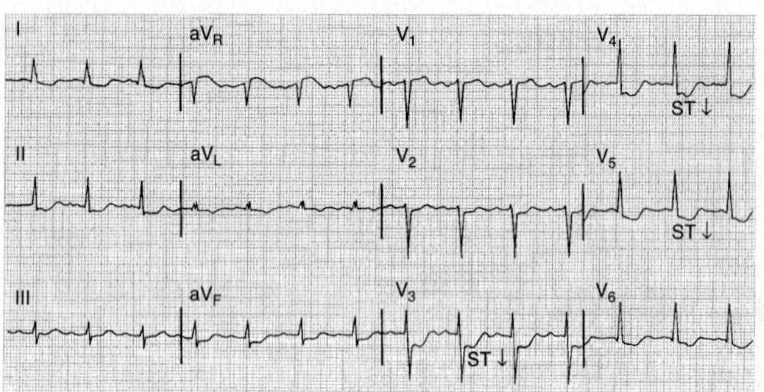

Video 11 Myocardial Ischemia

Rate: Variable

Video 12 **Rhythm:** Usually regular but may show atrial and/or ventricular arrhythmias.

PR interval: Normal

QT interval: ST segment depressed; J-point depression; T-wave inversion; conduction disturbances. (A) TP and PR intervals are baseline for ST-segment deviation. (B) ST-segment elevation. (C) ST-segment depression.

Note: Intraoperative ischemia usually is seen in the presence of "normal" vital signs (e.g., ±20% of preinduction values).

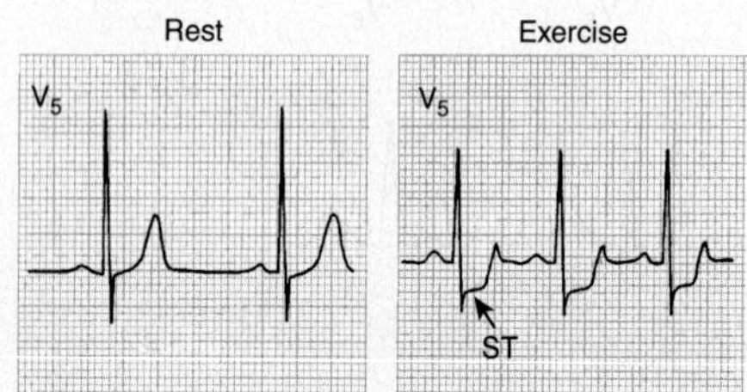

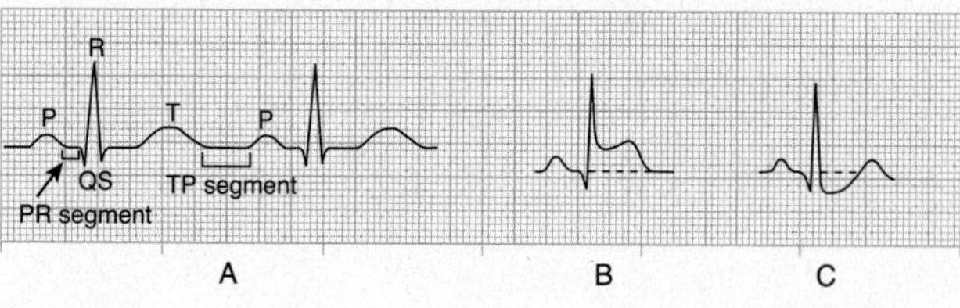

Video 13 Digitalis Effect

Rate: <100 beats/min

Rhythm: Regular

PR interval: Normal or prolonged

QT interval: ST-segment sloping ("digitalis effect")

Note: Digitalis toxicity can be the cause of many common arrhythmias (e.g., premature ventricular contractions, second-degree heart block). Verapamil, quinidine, and amiodarone cause an increase in serum digitalis concentration.

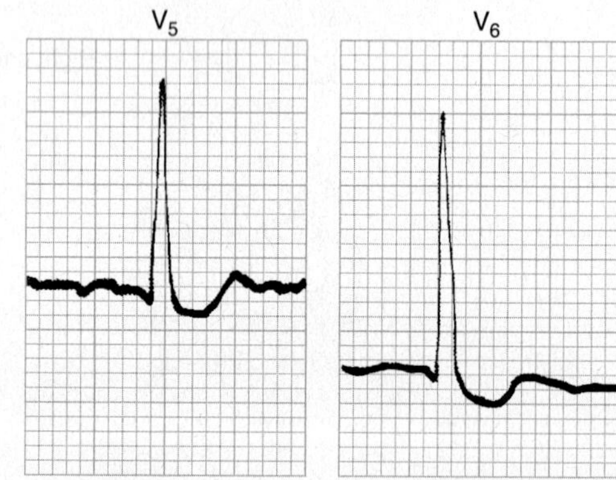

Electrolyte Disturbances

	↓ Ca^{2+}	↑ Ca^{2+}	↓ K^+	↑ K^+
Rate	<100 beats/min	<100 beats/min	<100 beats/min	<100 beats/min
Rhythm	Regular	Regular	Regular	Regular
PR interval	Normal	Normal/increased	Normal	Normal
QT interval	Increased	Decreased	Normal	Increased
Other			T wave flat U wave	T wave peaked

Note: ECG changes usually do not correlate with serum calcium. Hypocalcemia rarely causes arrhythmias in the absence of hypokalemia. In contrast, abnormalities in serum potassium concentration can be diagnosed by ECG. Similarly, in the clinical range, magnesium concentrations are rarely associated with unique ECG patterns. The presence of a U wave (>1.5 mm in height) can also be seen in left main coronary artery disease, with certain medications and long QT syndrome.

Calcium

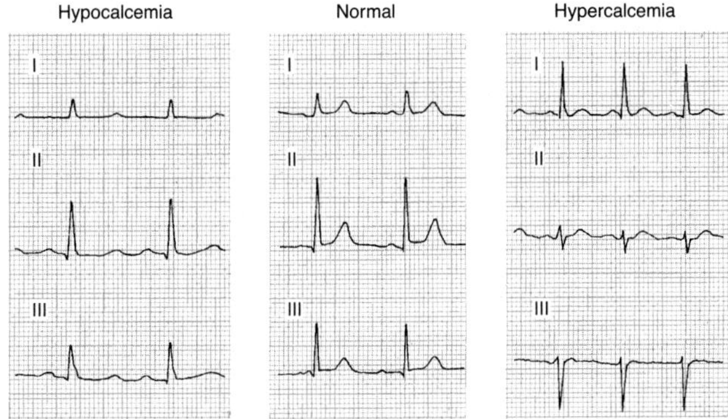

Video 14 Potassium

Hypokalemia (K^+ = 1.9 mEq/L)

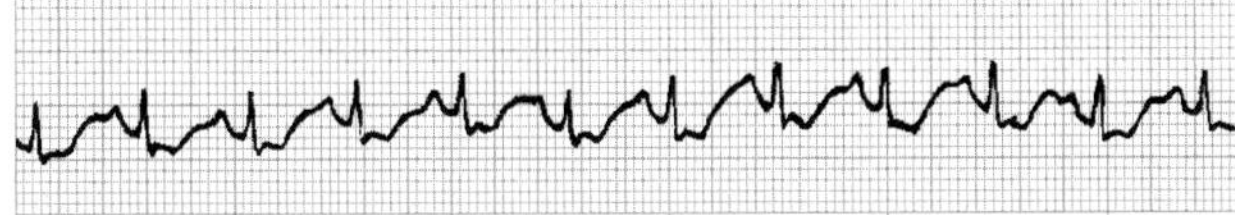

Hyperkalemia (K^+ = 7.9 mEq/L)

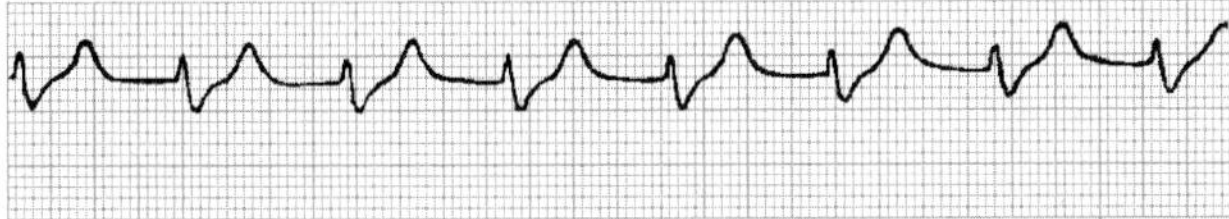

Hypothermia

Rate: <60 beats/min
Rhythm: Sinus
PR interval: Prolonged
QT interval: Prolonged

Note: Seen at temperatures below 33°C with ST-segment elevation (× point or Osborn wave). Tremor due to shivering or Parkinson disease may interfere with ECG interpretation and may be confused with atrial flutter. May represent normal variant of early ventricular repolarization. (*Arrow* indicates J point or Osborn waves.)

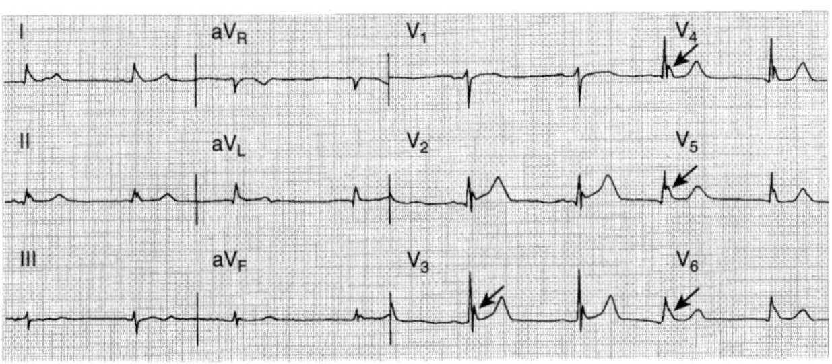

Multifocal Atrial Tachycardia

Rate: 100–200 beats/min
Rhythm: Irregular
PR interval: Consecutive P waves are of varying shape.
QT interval: Normal

Note: Seen in patients with severe lung disease. Vagal maneuvers have no effect. At heart rates <100 beats/min, it may appear as wandering atrial pacemaker. May be mistaken for atrial fibrillation. Treatment is of the causative disease process.

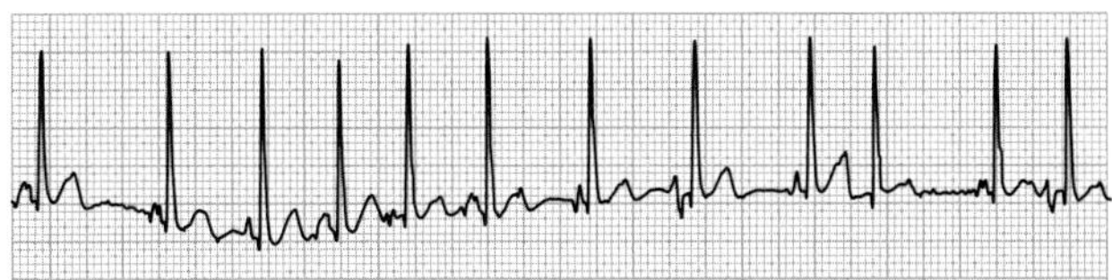

Video 15 Paroxysmal Atrial Tachycardia (PAT)

Rate: 150–250 beats/min
Rhythm: Regular
PR interval: Difficult to distinguish because of tachycardia obscuring P wave. P wave may precede, be included in, or follow QRS complex.
QT interval: Normal, but ST segment and T wave may be difficult to distinguish.

Note: Therapy depends on the degree of hemodynamic compromise. Carotid sinus massage, or other vagal maneuvers, may terminate rhythm or decrease heart rate. In contrast to management of PAT in awake patients, synchronized cardioversion, rather than pharmacologic treatment, is preferred in hemodynamically unstable anesthetized patients.

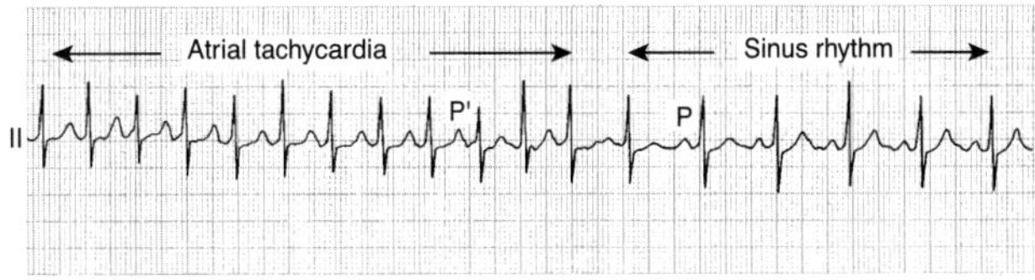

Video 16 Pericarditis

Rate: Variable
Rhythm: Variable
PR interval: Normal
QT interval: Diffuse ST and T-wave changes with no Q wave and seen in more leads than a myocardial infarction.

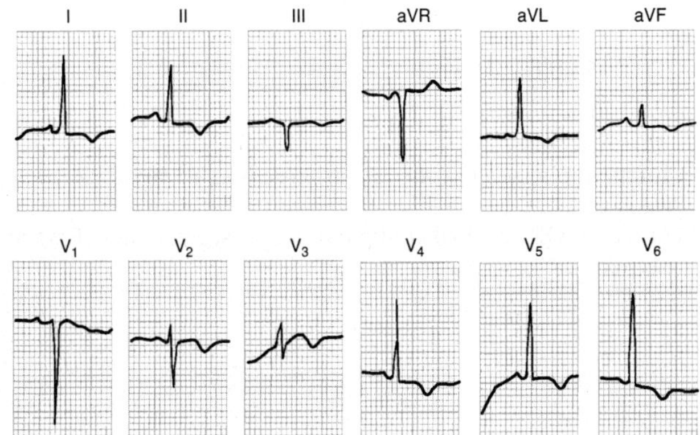

Pericardial Tamponade

Rate: Variable
Rhythm: Variable
PR interval: Low-voltage P wave
QT interval: Seen as electrical alternans with low-voltage complexes and varying amplitude of P, QRS, and T waves with each heart beat.

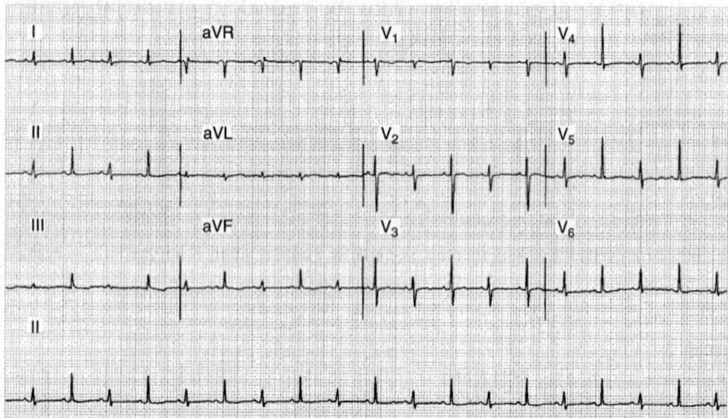

Pneumothorax

Rate: Variable
Rhythm: Variable
PR interval: Normal
QT interval: Normal

Note: Common ECG abnormalities include right-axis deviation, decreased QRS amplitude, and inverted T waves V_1–V_6. Differentiate from pulmonary embolus. May present as electrical alternans; thus, pericardial effusion should be ruled out.

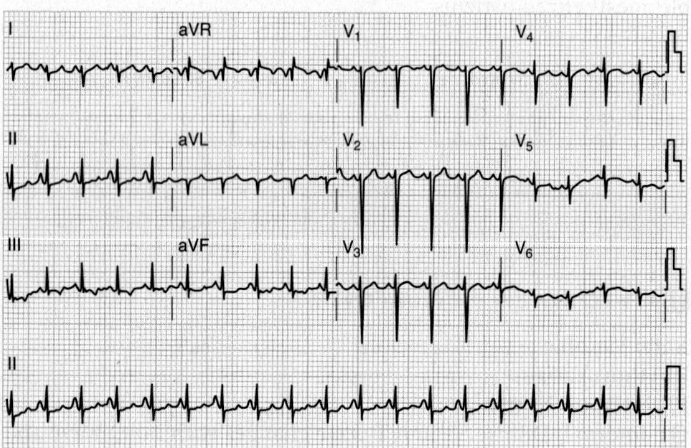

17 Video 17 Premature Atrial Contraction (PAC)

Rate: <100 beats/min
Rhythm: Irregular
PR interval: P waves may be lost in preceding T waves. PR interval is variable.
QT interval: QRS normal configuration; ST segment and T wave normal.

Note: Nonconducted PAC appearance similar to that of sinus arrest; T waves with PAC may be distorted by inclusion of P wave in the T wave.

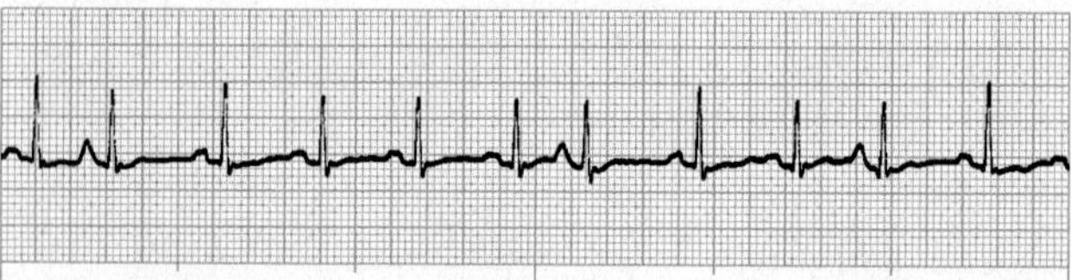

18 Video 18 Premature Ventricular Contraction (PVC)

19 Video 19 **Rate:** Usually <100 beats/min
Rhythm: Irregular
20 Video 20 **PR interval:** P wave and PR interval absent; retrograde conduction of P wave can be seen.
21 Video 21 22 Video 22 **QT interval:** Wide QRS (>0.12 sec); ST segment cannot be evaluated (e.g., ischemia); T wave opposite direction of QRS with compensatory pause. Fourth and eighth beats are PVCs.

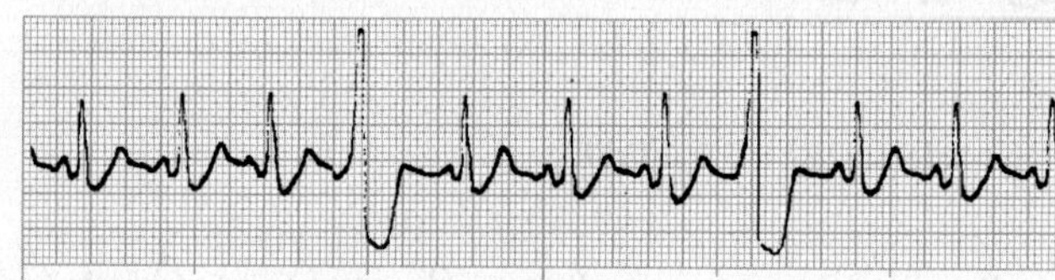

Pulmonary Embolus

Rate: >100 beats/min
Rhythm: Sinus
PR interval: P-pulmonale waveform
QT interval: Q waves in leads III and aVF

Note: Classic ECG signs S1Q3T3 with T-wave inversion also seen in V_1–V_4 and RV strain (ST depression V_1–V_4). May present with atrial fibrillation or flutter.

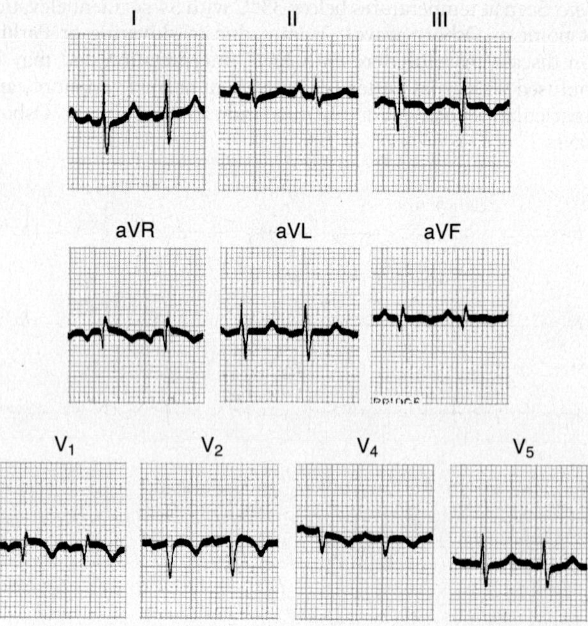

23 Video 23 Sinus Bradycardia

24 Video 24 **Rate:** <60 beats/min
Rhythm: Sinus
25 Video 25 **PR interval:** Normal
QT interval: Normal

Note: Seen in trained athletes as normal variant.

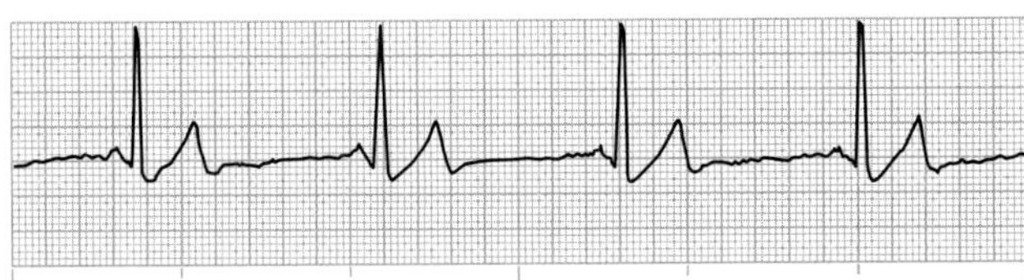

26 Video 26 Sinus Arrhythmia

Rate: 60–100 beats/min
Rhythm: Sinus
PR interval: Normal
QT interval: R-R interval variable

Note: Heart rate increases with inhalation and decreases with exhalation + 10%–20% (respiratory). Nonrespiratory sinus arrhythmia seen in elderly with heart disease. Also seen with increased intracranial pressure.

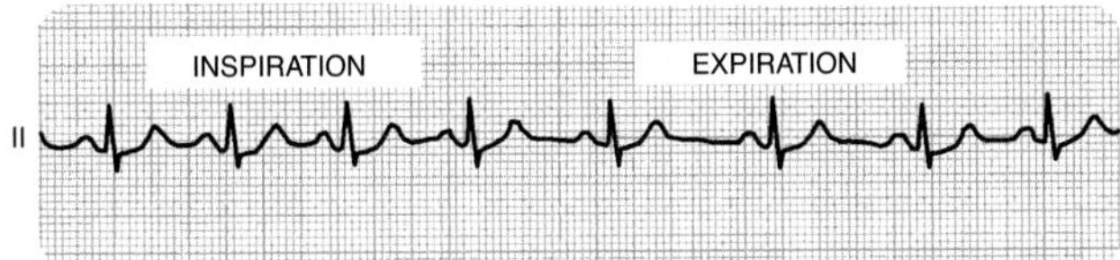

Sinus Arrest

Rate: <60 beats/min
Rhythm: Varies
PR interval: Variable
QT interval: Variable

Note: Rhythm depends on the cardiac pacemaker firing in the absence of sinoatrial stimulus (atrial pacemaker 60–75 beats/min; junctional 40–60 beats/min; ventricular 30–45 beats/min). Junctional rhythm most common. Occasional P waves may be seen (retrograde P wave).

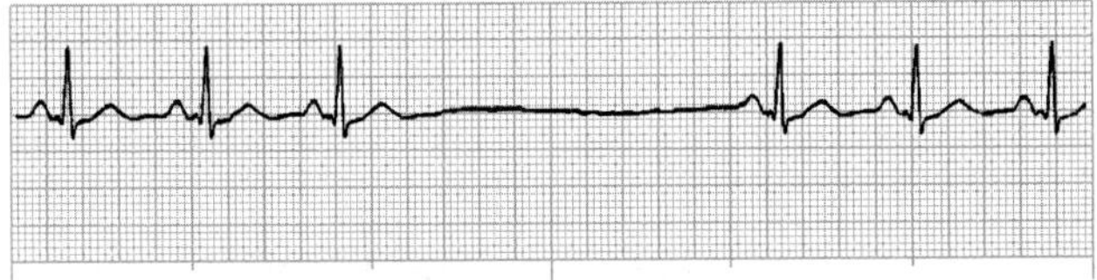

27 Video 27 Sinus Tachycardia

Rate: 100–160 beats/min
Rhythm: Regular
PR interval: Normal; P wave may be difficult to see.
QT interval: Normal

Note: Should be differentiated from paroxysmal atrial tachycardia (PAT). With PAT, carotid massage terminates arrhythmia. Sinus tachycardia may respond to vagal maneuvers but reappears as soon as vagal stimulus is removed.

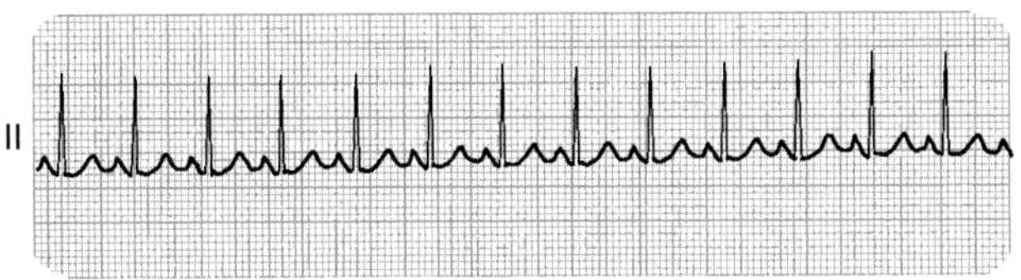

Subarachnoid Hemorrhage

Rate: <60 beats/min
Rhythm: Sinus
PR interval: Normal
QT interval: T-wave inversion is deep and wide. Prominent U waves are seen. Sinus arrhythmias are observed. Q waves may be seen and may mimic acute coronary syndrome.

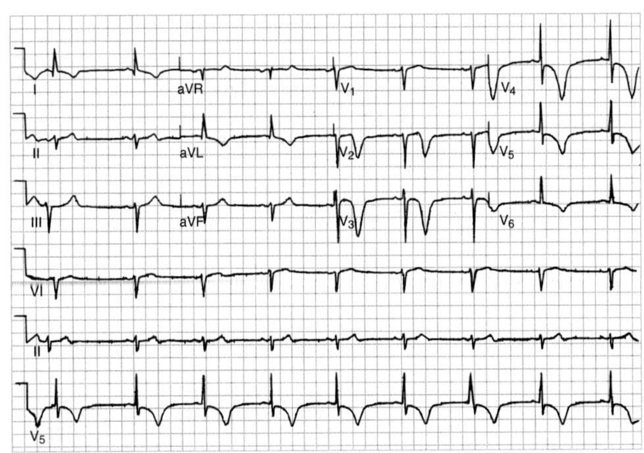

28 Video 28 Torsades de Pointes

Rate: 150–250 beats/min
Rhythm: No atrial component seen; ventricular rhythm regular or irregular.
PR interval: P wave buried in QRS complex.
QT interval: QRS complexes usually wide and with phasic variation twisting around a central axis (a few complexes point upward, then a few point downward). ST segments and T waves difficult to discern.

Note: Type of ventricular tachycardia associated with prolonged QT interval. Seen with electrolyte disturbances (e.g., hypokalemia, hypocalcemia, and hypomagnesemia) and bradycardia. Administering standard antiarrhythmics (lidocaine, procainamide, etc.) may worsen torsades de pointes. Prevention includes treatment of the electrolyte disturbance. Treatment includes shortening of the QT interval, pharmacologically or by pacing; unstable polymorphic VT is treated with immediate defibrillation.

Torsades de Pointes: Sustained

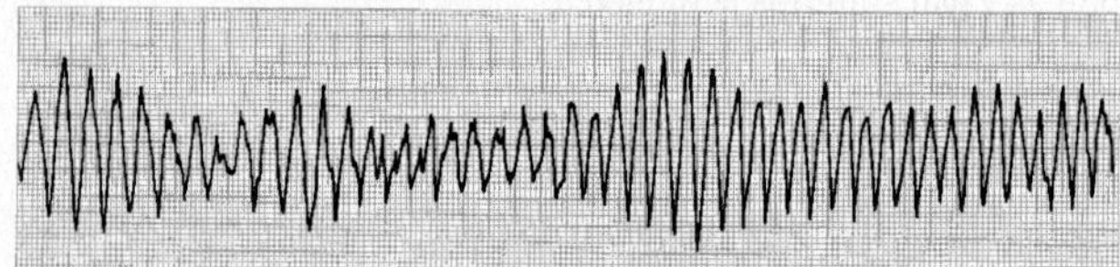

29 Video 29 Ventricular Fibrillation

Rate: Absent
Rhythm: None
PR interval: Absent
QT interval: Absent

Note: "Pseudoventricular fibrillation" may be the result of a monitor malfunction (e.g., ECG lead disconnect). Always check for carotid pulse before instituting therapy.

Coarse Ventricular Fibrillation

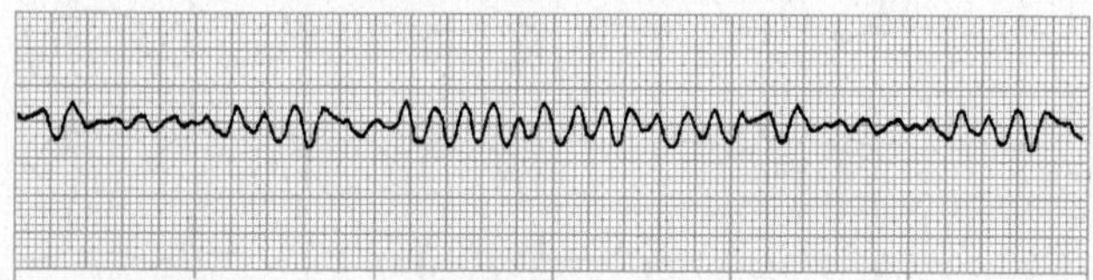

Fine Ventricular Fibrillation

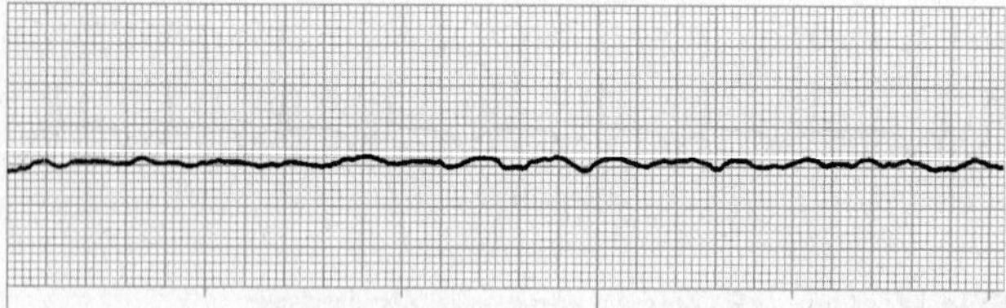

30 Video 30 Ventricular Tachycardia

Rate: 100–250 beats/min
Rhythm: No atrial component seen; ventricular rhythm irregular or regular.
PR interval: Absent; retrograde P wave may be seen in QRS complex.
QT interval: Wide, bizarre QRS complex. ST segment and T wave difficult to determine.

Note: In the presence of hemodynamic compromise, VT with a pulse is treated with immediate synchronized cardioversion, whereas VT without a pulse is treated with immediate defibrillation. If the patient is stable, with short bursts of ventricular tachycardia, pharmacologic management is preferred. Should be differentiated from supraventricular tachycardia with aberrancy (SVT-A). Compensatory pause and atrioventricular dissociation suggest a PVC. P waves and SR' (V_1) and slowing to vagal stimulus also suggest SVT-A.

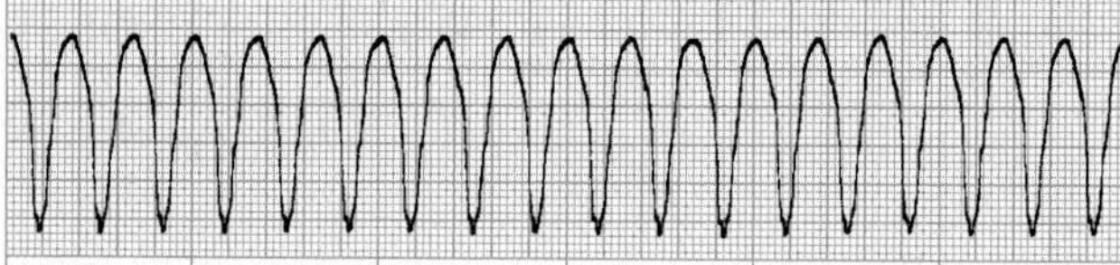

31 Video 31 Wolff–Parkinson–White Syndrome (WPW)

Rate: <100 beats/min
Rhythm: Regular
PR interval: P wave normal; PR interval short (<0.12 sec)
QT interval: Duration (>0.10 sec) with slurred QRS complex (delta wave). Type A has delta wave, RBBB, with upright QRS complex V_1. Type B has delta wave and downward QRS-V_1. ST segment and T wave usually normal.

Note: Digoxin should be avoided in the presence of WPW because it increases conduction through the accessory bypass tract (bundle of Kent) and decreases AV node conduction; consequently, ventricular fibrillation can occur.

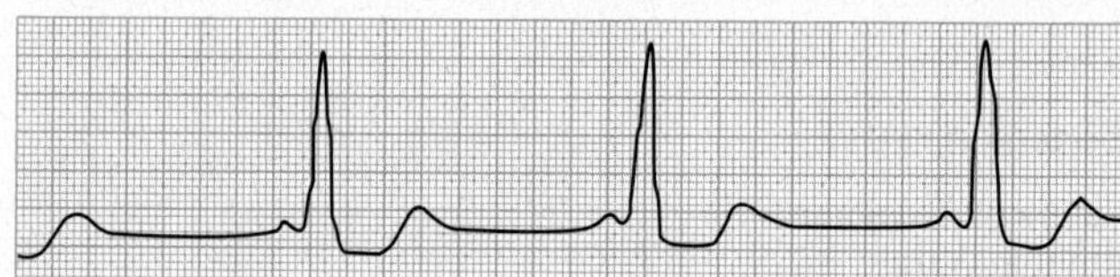

32 Video 32 Atrial Pacing

Pacemaker Tracings

Atrial pacing as demonstrated in this figure is used when the atrial impulse can proceed through the AV node. Examples are sinus bradycardia and junctional rhythms associated with clinically significant decreases in blood pressure. (*Arrows* are pacemaker spikes.)

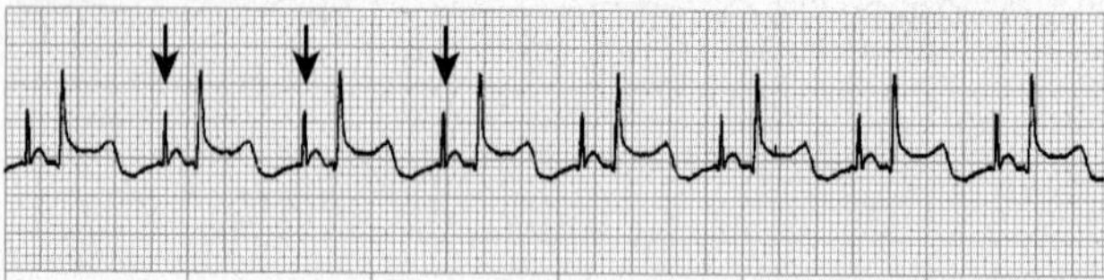

33 *Video 33 Ventricular Pacing*

In this tracing, ventricular pacing is evident by absence of atrial wave (P wave) and pacemaker spike preceding QRS complex. Ventricular pacing is employed in the presence of bradycardia secondary to AV block or atrial fibrillation. (*Arrows* are pacemaker spikes.)

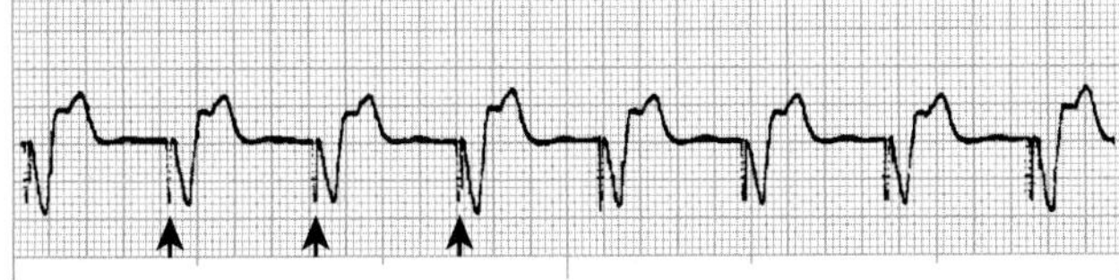

34 *Video 34 DDD Pacing*

DDD pacing, one of the most commonly used pacing modes, paces and senses both the right atrium and right ventricle (A-V sequential pacing). Each atrial and the right ventricular complex are preceded by a pacemaker spike.

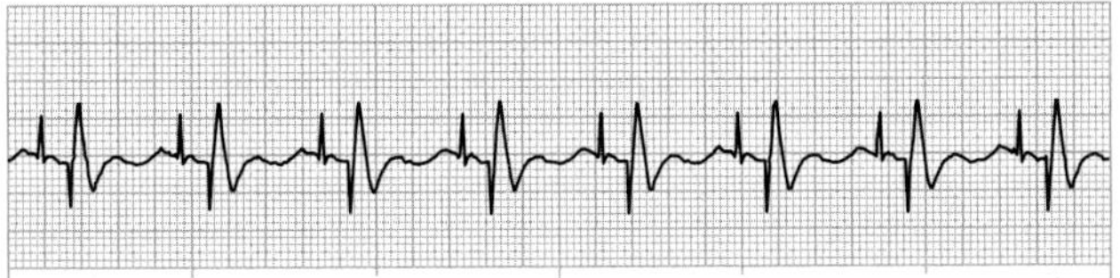

Acknowledgments

We gratefully acknowledge the contributions of previous edition authors, Benjamin M. Sherman, James R. Zaidan, and Paul G. Barash, as portions of their appendix have been retained in this revision.

Illustrations in this appendix are reprinted from Aehlert B. *ECGs Made Easy*. 4th ed. Mosby/Elsevier; 2011; Goldberger AL. *Clinical Electrocardiography: A Simplified Approach*. 7th ed. Mosby/Elsevier; 2006; Groh WJ, Zipes DP. Neurological disorders and cardiovascular disease. In: Bonow RO, Mann DL, Zipes DP, et al, eds. *Braunwald's Heart Disease: A Textbook of Cardiovascular Medicine*. 9th ed. Saunders/Elsevier; 2012; Huszar RJ. *Basic Dysrhythmias: Interpretation and Management*. 2nd ed. Mosby Lifeline; 1994; and Soltani P, Malozzi CM, Saleh BA, et al. Electrocardiogram manifestation of spontaneous pneumothorax. *Am J Emerg Med* 2009;27:750.e1–e5.

APPENDIX 3
Pacemaker and Implantable Cardiac Defibrillator Protocols

GINA CLEOPATRA BADESCU

Pacemakers

Pacemakers are devices that deliver electrical energy and control the patient's cardiac conduction system when necessary (Table A3-2).

Indications for Permanent Pacemaker Implantation

1. Sinus node dysfunction[1]
   - Patients with documented symptomatic bradycardia or chronotropic incompetence
   - Patients with bradycardia induced by essential medical regimen
   - Patients with syncopal episodes and induced sinus bradycardia or pauses on electrophysiologic studies
   - Patients with symptoms and heart rate less than 40 bpm
2. Atrioventricular node dysfunction
   - Third-degree or high-grade second-degree atrioventricular block (AVB) with symptomatic bradycardia or ventricular arrhythmias
   - Third-degree AVB or high-grade second-degree AVB with medication-induced bradycardia
   - Asymptomatic third-degree AVB with documented asystole longer than 3 seconds or longer than 5 seconds if atrial fibrillation is present
   - Third-degree AVB s/p AV node ablation, or postoperative third-degree AVB that is not expected to recover

Table A3-1 Abbreviation Table

Abbrev	Meaning	Abbrev	Meaning
3D	three dimensional	ICD	implantable cardiac defibrillators
ASA	American Society of Anesthesiologists	ILR	implantable loop recorder
ATP	antitachycardia pacing	LV	left ventricle
AV	atrioventricular	LVOT	left ventricular outflow tract
AVB	atrioventricular block	MRI	magnetic resonance imaging
BPEG	British Pacing and Electrophysiology Group	NASPE	North American Society of Pacing and Electrophysiology
bpm	beats per minute	NBG	N (NASPE), B (BPEG), G (GENERIC)
CAD	coronary artery disease	PG	pulse generator
CIED	cardiac implantable electronic devices	PP	external cardioversion-defibrillation pads or paddles
CPB	cardiopulmonary bypass	RA	right atrium
CRP	current return pad	R&R	rate and rhythm
CRT-D	cardiac resynchronization therapy–defibrillation	RF	radio frequency
CT	cautery tool	RT	radiation therapy
DCM	dilated cardiomyopathy	RV	right ventricle
ECG	electrocardiogram	SCD	sudden cardiac death
ECT	electroconvulsive therapy	SND	sinus node dysfunction
EF	ejection fraction	STEMI	ST-segment elevation myocardial infarction
EMI	electromagnetic interference	TUNA	transurethral needle ablation
HCM	hypertrophic cardiomyopathy	TURP	transurethral resection of prostate
HR	heart rate	VT	ventricular tachycardia
HRS	Heart Rhythm Society	VF	ventricular fibrillation
HV	HV interval		

Table A3-2 Generic Pacemaker Code: NASPE/BPEG Revised (2002)

Position I, Pacing Chamber(s)	Position II, Sensing Chamber(s)	Position III, Response(s) to Sensing	Position IV, Programmability	Position V, Multisite Pacing
O = none	O = none	O = none	O = none	O = none
A = atrium	A = atrium	I = inhibited	R = rate modulation	A = atrium
V = ventricle	V = ventricle	T = triggered		V = ventricle
D = dual (A + V)	D = dual (A + V)	D = dual (T + I)		D = dual (A + V)

NBG: N refers to North American Society of Pacing and Electrophysiology (NASPE), now called the Heart Rhythm Society (HRS); B refers to British Pacing and Electrophysiology Group (BPEG); and G refers to generic.

Reproduced with permission from Practice advisory for perioperative management of patients with cardiac rhythm management devices: pacemakers and implantable cardioverter-defibrillators. A report by the American Society of Anesthesiologists Task Force on Perioperative Management of Patients with Cardiac Rhythm Management Devices. *Anesthesiology*. 2011;114:247–261.

- Neuromuscular disorders with third-degree AVB: Erb dystrophy, Kearns–Sayre syndrome, myotonic muscular dystrophy
- Second-degree AVB with symptomatic bradycardia, or exercise-induced AVB

3. Bifascicular block and:
   - Type II second- or third-degree AVB
   - Alternating bundle branch block
   - Syncope
4. Second- or third-degree AVB after an ST elevation myocardial infarction (STEMI)
5. Hypersensitive carotid sinus syndrome and neurocardiogenic syncope
6. Cardiac transplantation patients who develop persistent inappropriate bradycardia
7. Other conditions:
   - Neuromuscular disease
   - Cardiac sarcoidosis with development of AVB
   - Central obstructive sleep apnea
8. Prevention and termination of certain arrhythmias (e.g., supraventricular tachycardia)
9. Hemodynamic indications:
   - Cardiac resynchronization therapy (CRT) in patients with ejection fraction (EF) below 35% and QRS greater than 120 msec
   - Hypertrophic cardiomyopathy and sinus node dysfunction (SND) or AV node dysfunction
10. Congenital heart diseases

Implantable Cardiac Defibrillators

Implantable cardiac defibrillators (ICDs) are rhythm management devices, which consist of a generator and a lead system.1 One lead is usually placed in the right atrium and the second lead in the right ventricular apex (Table A3-3). A specific type of ICD is the biventricular pacemaker, used for CRT. This device will have a third lead placed in the coronary sinus to pace the left ventricular (LV) lateral wall in synchrony with the right ventricle (RV), in the patient with EF below 35% and a QRS duration longer than 120 msec.[2]

Indications for ICD Implantation

1. Secondary prevention of sudden cardiac death (SCD) patients with a previous ventricular tachycardia/fibrillation (VT/VF) cardiac arrest
   - Patients with coronary artery disease (CAD) who survived one cardiac arrest (if >48 hours after an acute MI)
   - Patients with nonischemic dilated cardiomyopathy and
   - Hypertrophic cardiomyopathy
   - Arrhythmogenic right ventricular (RV) dysplasia
   - Genetic proarrhythmic syndromes with one prior episode of VT/VF; include long and short QT syndrome, Brugada syndrome, catecholaminergic polymorphic VT, idiopathic VF
   - Syncope with inducible sustained VT: when the arrhythmia is assumed to be the reason the syncope

Table A3-3 Generic Defibrillator Code (NBG): NASPE/BPEG

Position I, Shock Chamber(s)	Position II, Antitachycardia Pacing Chamber(s)	Position III, Tachycardia Detection	Position IV,[a] Antibradycardia Pacing Chamber(s)
O = none	O = none	E = electrogram	O = none
A = atrium	A = atrium	H = hemodynamic	A = atrium
V = ventricle	V = ventricle		V = ventricle
D = dual (A + V)	D = dual (A + V)		D = dual (A + V)

[a]For robust identification, position IV is expanded into its complete NBG code. For example, a biventricular pacing defibrillator with ventricular shock and antitachycardia pacing functionality would be identified as VVE-DDDRV, assuming that the pacing section was programmed DDDRV. Currently, no hemodynamic sensors have been approved for tachycardia detection (position III).

Reproduced with permission from Practice advisory for perioperative management of patients with cardiac rhythm management devices: pacemakers and implantable cardioverter-defibrillators. A report by the American Society of Anesthesiologists Task Force on Perioperative Management of Patients with Cardiac Rhythm Management Devices. *Anesthesiology*. 2011;114:247–261.

2. Primary prevention of SCD
   - Includes all the subgroups from the secondary prevention that are considered high risk but did not yet have an episode of VT/VF.

Potential Intraoperative Problems with CIEDs

Electromagnetic interference (EMI) with the device is more likely when electrocautery is used above the umbilicus in a patient with a CIED implanted in subclavicular region. For generators placed elsewhere (e.g., abdominal site), expert opinion also points to the 15-cm rule, which is a distance of 15 cm around the generator or cardiac leads with the highest risk of interference.[3]

EMI leads to:

1. Inhibition of pacemaker by EMI
2. Inappropriate delivery of antitachycardia therapy by ICD
3. Changes in lead parameters:
   - Atrial mode switching
   - Inappropriate ventricular sensing
   - Electrical reset
   - Increase in ventricular thresholds
4. "Runaway" pacemaker[4]
5. Pacemaker failure after direct contact with electrocautery and cardioversion
6. Conversion from VOO (Table A3-2) back to backup mode (reprogramming)
7. Transient of permanent loss of capture
8. Dislodgement of leads during atrial fibrillation ablation procedures[5]
9. Rate adaptive pacing (interaction of minute ventilation sensor with ECG/plethysmography)
10. Oversensing and inhibition with use of lithotripsy
11. Noise reversal mode
12. Myocardial burns
13. Radiofrequency ablation and therapeutic radiation are associated with a high risk of interference similar to EMI, due to long exposure to current. Grant et al. reported in a recent study that the most notable risk factor for malfunction of CIED in patients undergoing radiation therapy was neutron producing radiotherapy (RT). The incident CIED dose up to 5.4 Gy did not correlate with CIED malfunction, leading to the conclusion that it is possible that surgical relocation of the CIED may be minimized if nonneutron-producing RT is to be delivered.[6]
14. Scanning wand. A case report recently published by Plakke et al. documented a case of asystole induced by interference of the scanning wand with the temporary pacemaker with epicardial pacing wires placed routinely at separation from cardiopulmonary bypass.[7] Publication of this case report gave rise to a controversy, the manufacturer stating the scanning wand was used off-label, without properly following the instruction manual and placing most of the blame for the incident on the anesthesiologist.[8] This resulted in the provider's response of how responsibility is assigned with the use of this device.[9] This clearly begs the more important question of how do we get the healthcare providers appropriately educated on use of such devices.

General Principles of Perioperative Management of Patients with CIEDs

- The perioperative management of the patient with a CIED is via an individualized recommendation, made by the CIED team (electrophysiologist, cardiologist), in collaboration with members of the surgical/anesthesia team (perioperative team).[3] The recommendations should not be made by the industry representative without supervision by a physician who is qualified to manage these devices.
- The perioperative team should provide information to the CIED team regarding the upcoming procedure (Table A3-4).
- The CIED team should, in turn, provide information about the device and a recommendation for perioperative management of the device (Table A3-5).
- The patient with a pacemaker should have had an interrogation of the device in the 12 months prior to the surgical procedure, whereas the patient with an ICD should have had the device interrogated within 6 months prior to the scheduled procedure.
- The inactivation of the ICD or programming of a pacemaker to asynchronous mode is recommended when EMI is likely to occur.
- In patients in whom the ICD antiarrhythmia detection is turned off, the external defibrillator, with the pads positioned on the patient, is immediately available and ready to deliver therapy.
- In cases in which EMI is likely, the function of the CIED can be altered either by ferrous magnet or by reprogramming. See below for magnet response for ICD.
- Magnet response: Placing a magnet over a pacemaker generator will turn the pacemaker to asynchronous mode in most models.

Table A3-4 Essential Elements of the Information Given to the CIED Physician

- Type of procedure
- Anatomic location of surgical procedure
- Patient position during the procedure
- Will monopolar electrosurgery be used? (If so, anatomic location of EMI delivery.)
- Will other sources of EMI likely be present?
- Will cardioversion or defibrillation be used?
- Surgical venue (operating room, procedure suite, etc.)
- Anticipated postprocedural arrangements (anticipated discharge to home <23 hours, inpatient admission to critical care bed, telemetry bed)
- Unusual circumstances: Cardiothoracic or chest wall surgical procedure that could impair/damage or encroach upon the CIED leads, anticipated large blood loss, operation in close proximity to CIED

Reprinted with permission from Crossley GH, Poole JE, Rozner MA, et al. The Heart Rhythm Society (HRS)/American Society of Anesthesiologists (ASA) Expert Consensus Statement on the perioperative management of patients with implantable defibrillators, pacemakers and arrhythmia monitors: facilities and patient management this document was developed as a joint project with the American Society of Anesthesiologists (ASA), and in collaboration with the American Heart Association (AHA), and the Society of Thoracic Surgeons (STS). *Heart Rhythm*. 2011;8:1114–1154.

Table A3-5 Essential Elements of the Preoperative CIED Evaluation to Be Provided to the Operative Team

- Date of last device interrogation
- Type of device: Pacemaker ICD, CRT-D, CRT-P, ILR, implantable hemodynamic monitor
- Manufacturer and model
- Indication for device
  - Pacemaker: Sick sinus syndrome, AV block, syncope
  - ICD: Primary or secondary prevention
  - Cardiac resynchronization therapy
- Battery longevity documented as >3 months
- Are any of the leads <3 months old?
- Programming
  - Pacing mode and programmed lower rate
  - ICD therapy
    - Lowest heart rate for shock delivery
    - Lowest heart rate for ATP delivery
  - Rate-responsive sensor type, if programmed on
- Is the patient pacemaker dependent, and what is the underlying rhythm and heart rate if it can be determined?
- What is the response of this device to magnet placement
  - Magnet pacing rate for a pacemaker
  - Pacing amplitude response to magnet function
  - Will ICD detections resume automatically with removal of the magnet? Does this device allow for magnet application function to be disabled? If so, document programming of patient's device for this feature.
- Any alert status on CIED generator or lead
- Last pacing threshold: Document adequate safety margin with the date of that threshold

Reprinted with permission from Crossley GH, Poole JE, Rozner MA, et al. The Heart Rhythm Society (HRS)/American Society of Anesthesiologists (ASA) Expert Consensus Statement on the perioperative management of patients with implantable defibrillators, pacemakers and arrhythmia monitors: facilities and patient management this document was developed as a joint project with the American Society of Anesthesiologists (ASA), and in collaboration with the American Heart Association (AHA), and the Society of Thoracic Surgeons (STS). *Heart Rhythm*. 2011;8:1114–1154.

Placing a magnet over an ICD will suspend the arrhythmia detection. It will *not* switch the pacemaker function to asynchronous mode; therefore, in patients who are pacemaker dependent, the team must be aware of the risk of inhibition of the pacemaker by the EMI. If EMI is likely to occur, the recommendation is to reprogram the CIED prior to the case, by turning the arrhythmia detection function to off and program the pacemaker to asynchronous mode. Because a minority of models do not respond to magnet application in the fashion described above, it is always recommended to contact the manufacturer and confirm the response to magnet for the specific model one is dealing with.

- Complications related to application of magnet are rare. However, recent publication of a case report of three patients with intraoperative complications related to inadequate preoperative evaluation of the CIED and knowledge about response to magnet application underline the importance of following the ASA and HRS guidelines and gain knowledge about these issues preoperatively, as the complications are most of the time acute and severe.[10]

Risk Mitigation Strategies

- Use bipolar cautery where possible.[3]
- Use short bursts of monopolar cautery, 5 seconds or less.
- Place the return current pad in such a way to avoid crossing the generator.
- Have rescue equipment, including external pacemaker/defibrillator, immediately available for all patients with CIED.
- Activating the electrocautery in the area of the generator, even if the active electrode is not touching the patient, will cause interference.

Anesthesia Device Services

In the last few years, perioperative management of rhythm devices has become a more active focus of the Surgery and Anesthesia Departments in different institutions across the country. This is due to the increasing number of patients that present for surgery with one of these devices in place, posing real scheduling and management challenges, with the most concerning issue being scheduling delay. The Anesthesiology Department at the University of Washington evaluated management of CIED in the perioperative period by an Anesthesia Device Service (ADS) versus the Electrophysiology/Cardiology Service (EPCS) over a period of 4 years (2009–2013).[11]

The ADS was developed with help and training from the EPCS and managed 548 patients during this time, with no major complications or safety concerns and at the end of the 4 years obtained a slight reduction in the scheduling delays. Most errors made by the ADS were with restoration of the demand features postoperatively in the patients where the asynchronous mode was used during surgery, whereas the EPCS failed mostly at following the recommendations of the perioperative management of CIEDs by the HRS, published in 2011.[12]

The creation of such a service is a serious undertaking, necessitating training of anesthesiologists and a very close collaboration between the Anesthesiology and Cardiology Departments. However, it is conceivable that in the future this type of service will become an integral part of the perioperative surgical home, particularly in high-volume centers where the scheduling delays have a serious impact.

Table A3-6 and Figure A3-1 are examples of approaches to perioperative management of patients with CIEDs.[13]

Table A3-6 Example of a Stepwise Approach to the Perioperative Management of the Patient with a CIED

Perioperative Period	Patient/CIED Condition	Intervention
Preoperative evaluation	Patient has CIED Determine CIED type (PM, ICD, CRT)	Focused history Focused physical examination Manufacturer's CIED identification card Chest x-ray (no data available) Supplemental resources[a]
	Determine if patient is CIED-dependent for pacing function	Verbal history Bradyarrhythmia symptoms Atrioventricular node ablation No spontaneous ventricular activity[b]
	Determine CIED function	Comprehensive CIED evaluation[c] Determine if pacing pulses are present and create paced beats
Preoperative preparation	EMI unlikely during procedure EMI likely; CIED is PM	If EMI is unlikely, then special precautions are not needed Reprogram to asynchronous mode when indicated Suspend rate adaptive functions[d]
	EMI likely; CIED is ICD EMI likely; all CIED	Suspend antitachyarrhythmia functions. If patient is dependent on pacing function, then alter pacing function as above
	Intraoperative physiologic changes likely (e.g., bradycardia, ischemia)	Use bipolar cautery; ultrasonic scalpel Temporary pacing and cardioversion-defibrillation available Plan for possible adverse CIED–patient interaction
Intraoperative management	Monitoring	Electrocardiographic monitoring per ASA standard Peripheral pulse monitoring
	Electrocautery interference	CT/CRP no current through PG/leads Avoid proximity of CT to PG/leads Short bursts at lowest possible energy Use bipolar cautery; ultrasonic scalpel
	RF catheter ablation	Avoid contact of RF catheter with PG/leads RF current path far away from PG/leads Discuss these concerns with operator
	Lithotripsy	Do not focus lithotripsy beam near PG R-wave triggers lithotripsy? Disable atrial pacing
	MRI	Generally contraindicated If required, consult ordering physician, cardiologist, radiologist, and manufacturer
	Radiation therapy	PG/leads must be outside of RT field Possible surgical relocation of PG Verify PG function during/after RT course
	ECT	Consult with ordering physician, patient's cardiologist, a CIED service, or CIED manufacturer
Emergency defibrillation-cardioversion	ICD: magnet-disabled	Terminate all EMI sources Remove magnet to re-enable therapies Observe for appropriate therapies
	ICD: programming disabled	Programming to re-enable therapies or proceed directly with external cardioversion/defibrillation
	ICD: either of above	Minimize current flow through PG/leads PP as far as possible from PG PP perpendicular to major axis PG/leads To extent possible, PP in anterior-posterior location
	Regardless of CIED type	Use clinically appropriate cardioversion/defibrillation energy
Postoperative management	Immediate postoperative period Postoperative interrogation and restoration of CIED function	Monitor cardiac R&R continuously Back-up pacing and cardioversion/defibrillation capability Interrogation to assess function Settings appropriate?[e] Is CIED an ICD?[f] Use cardiology/PM-ICD service if needed

[a]Manufacturer's databases, pacemaker clinic records, cardiology consultation.
[b]With cardiac rhythm management device (CRMD) programmed VVI at lowest programmable rate.
[c]Ideally, CIED function assessed by interrogation, with function altered by reprogramming if required.
[d]Most times this will be necessary; when in doubt, assume so.
[e]If necessary, reprogram appropriate setting.
[f]Restore all antitachycardia therapies.

Reprinted with permission from Practice advisory for perioperative management of patients with cardiac rhythm management devices: pacemakers and implantable cardioverter-defibrillators. A report by the American Society of Anesthesiologists Task Force on Perioperative Management of Patients with Cardiac Rhythm Management Devices. *Anesthesiology*. 2011;114:247–261.

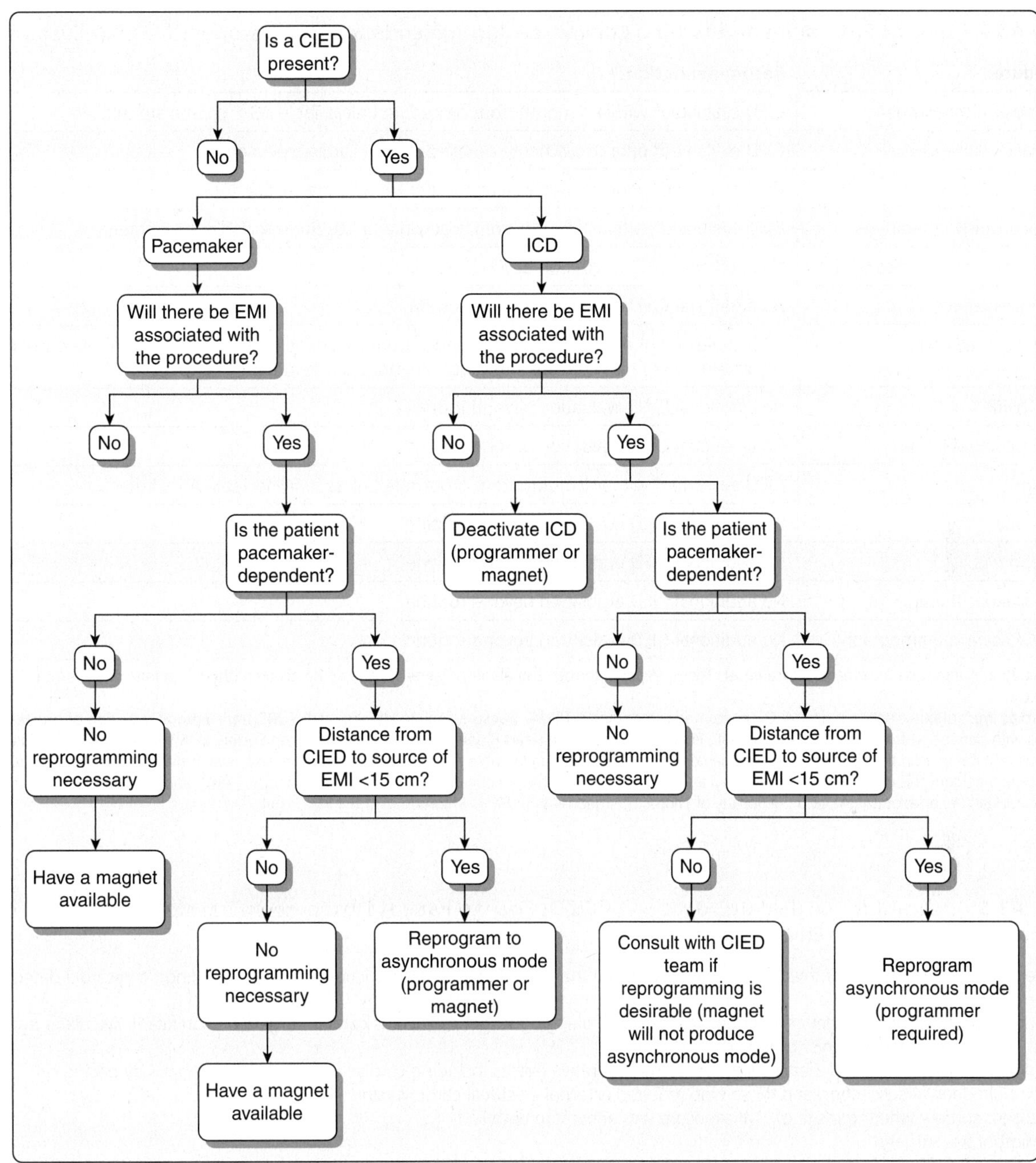

Figure A3-1 Example of an algorithm for perioperative management of patients with CIEDs. (Reprinted from Stone ME, Salter B, Fischer A. Perioperative management of patients with cardiac implantable electronic devices. *Br J Anaesth*. 2011;107(Suppl 1):i16–i26. Copyright © 2011 Elsevier. With permission.)

Recommendations for Postoperative Follow-Up of Patients with CIEDs (Tables A3-7 to A3-9)

Optimization of Pacing after Cardiopulmonary Bypass

Separation from CPB is usually associated with a conduction abnormality, from first-degree AV block, sinus bradycardia, to third-degree AV block, or interventricular delays.[14]

1. **Lead placement:** Right atrial (RA) lead: place at the cephalic atrial wall, between the atrial appendages. Right ventricular lead: place at the level of the right ventricle outflow tract (RVOT). For the patient with obstructive cardiomyopathy, the RV lead is better placed in the RV apex, for less dynamic obstruction of the LVOT. Biventricular pacing is initiated for patients with intraventricular conduction lesions and dyssynchrony of contraction. Place the LV lead at the basal posterolateral wall, and hook the two ventricular leads through a Y piece to the ventricular output of the temporary pacemaker box.
2. **Rate:** Program to obtain the best improvement in cardiac output and improvement in mixed venous saturation and arterial blood pressure.

Table A3-7 Specific Procedures and Writing Committee Recommendations on Postoperative CIED Evaluation

Procedure	Recommendation
Monopolar electrosurgery	CIED evaluated[a] within 1 month from procedure unless Table A3-8 criteria are fulfilled
External cardioversion	CIED evaluated[a] prior to discharge or transfer from cardiac telemetry
Radiofrequency ablation	CIED evaluated[a] prior to discharge or transfer from cardiac telemetry
Electroconvulsive therapy	CIED evaluated[a] within 1 month from procedure unless fulfilling Table A3-8 criteria
Nerve conduction studies (ENG)	No additional CIED evaluation beyond routine
Ocular procedures	No additional CIED evaluation beyond routine
Therapeutic radiation	CIED evaluated prior to discharge or transfer from cardiac telemetry; remote monitoring optimal; some instances may indicate interrogation after each treatment (see text)
TUNA/TURP	No additional CIED evaluation beyond routine
Hysteroscopic ablation	No additional CIED evaluation beyond routine
Lithotripsy	CIED evaluated[a] within 1 month from procedure unless fulfilling Table A3-8 criteria
Endoscopy	No additional CIED evaluation beyond routine
Iontophoresis	No additional CIED evaluation beyond routine
Photodynamic therapy	No additional CIED evaluation beyond routine
X-ray/CT scans/mammography	No additional CIED evaluation beyond routine

[a]This evaluation is intended to reveal electrical reset. Therefore, an interrogation alone is needed. This can be accomplished in person or by remote telemetry.

CIED, cardiac implantable electronic device; CT, computed tomography; TUNA, transurethral needle ablation; TURP, transurethral resection of prostate.

Reprinted with permission from Crossley GH, Poole JE, Rozner MA, et al. The Heart Rhythm Society (HRS)/American Society of Anesthesiologists (ASA) Expert Consensus Statement on the perioperative management of patients with implantable defibrillators, pacemakers and arrhythmia monitors: facilities and patient management this document was developed as a joint project with the American Society of Anesthesiologists (ASA), and in collaboration with the American Heart Association (AHA), and the Society of Thoracic Surgeons (STS). *Heart Rhythm*. 2011;8:1114–1154.

Table A3-8 Indications for the Interrogation of CIEDs Prior to Patient Discharge or Transfer from a Cardiac Telemetry Environment

- Patients with CIEDs reprogrammed prior to the procedure that left the device nonfunctional such as disabling tachycardia detection in an ICD.
- Patients with CIEDs who underwent hemodynamically challenging surgeries such as cardiac surgery or significant vascular surgery (e.g., abdominal aortic aneurysmal repair).[a]
- Patients with CIEDs who experienced significant intraoperative events including cardiac arrest requiring temporary pacing or cardiopulmonary resuscitation and those who required external electrical cardioversion.
- Emergent surgery where the site of EMI exposure was above the umbilicus
- Cardiothoracic surgery
- Patients with CIEDs who underwent certain types of procedures (Table A3-7) that emit EMI with a greater probability of affecting device function.
- Patients with CIEDs who have logistical limitations that would prevent reliable device evaluation within 1 month from their procedure

[a]The general purpose of this interrogation is to assure that reset did not occur. In these cases, a full evaluation including threshold evaluations is suggested.

CIED, cardiac implantable electrical device; EMI, electromagnetic interference; ICD, implantable cardiac defibrillator.

Reprinted with permission from Crossley GH, Poole JE, Rozner MA, et al. The Heart Rhythm Society (HRS)/American Society of Anesthesiologists (ASA) Expert Consensus Statement on the perioperative management of patients with implantable defibrillators, pacemakers and arrhythmia monitors: facilities and patient management this document was developed as a joint project with the American Society of Anesthesiologists (ASA), and in collaboration with the American Heart Association (AHA), and the Society of Thoracic Surgeons (STS). *Heart Rhythm*. 2011;8:1114–1154.

Table A3-9 Treatment of Pacemaker Failure

Rate	Possible Response
Adequate to maintain blood pressure	1. Oxygen, airway control 2. Place magnet over pacemaker 3. Atropine if sinus bradycardia
Severe bradycardia and hypotension	1. Oxygen, airway control 2. Place magnet over pacemaker 3. Other types of pacing if magnet does not activate the pacemaker (transcutaneous, esophageal, or transvenous) 4. Atropine if sinus bradycardia 5. Isoproterenol to increase ventricular rate
No escape rhythm	1. Cardiopulmonary resuscitation 2. Place magnet over pacemaker 3. Other types of pacing if magnet does not activate the pacemaker (transcutaneous, esophageal, or transvenous) 4. Isoproterenol to increase ventricular rate

Reprinted from Zaidan JR, Youngberg JA, Lake CL, et al., eds., *Cardiac, Vascular and Thoracic Anesthesia*. Churchill Livingstone; 2000.

3. **AV delay:** In patients with LV dysfunction, we can maximize the contribution of the atria to the preload. Use pulse wave Doppler through the mitral valve inflow, and modify the AV delay to obtain a clear E and A waveforms, and to ensure that the A wave finishes before the onset of the QRS; the closure of the mitral valve should happen at the end of the A wave, but before any diastolic mitral regurgitation.
4. **Pacing mode:** Three modes are explained here. In the patient with normal AV conduction, AAI mode allows for increase in HR and a physiologic depolarization of the ventricles. If inhibition by electrocautery is a concern, use asynchronous pacing in AOO mode (Table A3-2). For the patient with AV conduction delay, DOO or DDI should be used. DDI mode also avoids tracking of rapid atrial rates in case of post bypass atrial fibrillation.
5. **Biventricular pacing**[14,15] in patients with EF below 35% and QRS longer than 120 msec acute biventricular pacing improves torsion and mechanics of contraction, particularly in patients with mitral regurgitation due to papillary muscle dyssynchrony. Speckle-tracking, 3D echocardiography, M-mode definition of septal to wall motion delay, color Doppler tissue imaging, and analysis of segmental velocity are used to characterize ventricular dyssynchrony. Currently, available temporary pacemakers only allow biventricular pacing through a Y connection of the two ventricular epicardial wires to the ventricular output of the box. Acute CRT leads to an increase in myocardial performance with a slight decrease in myocardial oxygen consumption.

Acknowledgment

We gratefully acknowledge the contributions of previous edition authors, Benjamin M. Sherman, James R. Zaidan, and Paul G. Barash, as portions of their appendix have been retained in this revision.

REFERENCES

1. Stone KR, McPherson CA. Assessment and management of patients with pacemakers and implantable cardioverter defibrillators. *Crit Care Med.* 2004;32:S155–S165.
2. Epstein AE, Dimarco JP, Ellenbogen KA, et al. ACC/AHA/HRS 2008 guidelines for device-based therapy of cardiac rhythm abnormalities: executive summary. *Heart Rhythm.* 2008;5:934–955.
3. Crossley GH, Poole JE, Rozner MA, et al. The Heart Rhythm Society (HRS)/American Society of Anesthesiologists (ASA) Expert Consensus Statement on the perioperative management of patients with implantable defibrillators, pacemakers and arrhythmia monitors: facilities and patient management this document was developed as a joint project with the American Society of Anesthesiologists (ASA), and in collaboration with the American Heart Association (AHA), and the Society of Thoracic Surgeons (STS). *Heart Rhythm.* 2011;8:1114–1154.
4. Heller LI. Surgical electrocautery and the runaway pacemaker syndrome. *Pacing Clin Electrophysiol.* 1990;13:1084–1085.
5. Lakkireddy D, Patel D, Ryschon K, et al. Safety and efficacy of radiofrequency energy catheter ablation of atrial fibrillation in patients with pacemakers and implantable cardiac defibrillators. *Heart Rhythm.* 2005;2:1309–1316.
6. Grant JD, Jensen GL, Tang C, et al. Radiotherapy-induced malfunction in contemporary cardiovascular implantable electronic devices: clinical incidence and predictors. *JAMA Oncol.* 2015;1:624–632.
7. Plakke MJ, Maisonave Y, Daley SM, et al. Radiofrequency scanning for retained surgical items can cause electromagnetic interference and pacing inhibition if an asynchronous pacing mode is not applied. *A A Case Rep.* 2016;6:143–145.
8. Kane T. Editorial comment: manufacturer's response. *A A Case Rep.* 2016;6:142.
9. Rozner MA, Schultheis L, Schulman PM. The unstated Murphy's Law of the operating room: if something goes wrong, blame anesthesia. *A A Case Rep.* 2016;6:139–141.
10. Schulman PM, Rozner MA. Case report: use caution when applying magnets to pacemakers or defibrillators for surgery. *Anesth Analg.* 2013;117:422–427.
11. Rooke GA, Lombaard SA, Van Norman GA, et al. Initial experience of an anesthesiology-based service for perioperative management of pacemakers and implantable cardioverter defibrillators. *Anesthesiology.* 2015;123:1024–1032.
12. Rozner MA, Schulman PM. Creating an anesthesiologist-run pacemaker and defibrillator service: closing the perioperative care gap for these patients. *Anesthesiology.* 2015;123:990–992.
13. Stone ME, Salter A, Fischer G. Perioperative management of patients with cardiac implantable electronic devices. *Br J Anaesth.* 2011:107(Suppl 1):i16–i26.
14. Chua J, Schwarzenberger JA, Mahajan A. Optimization of pacing after cardiopulmonary bypass. *J Cardiothorac Vasc Anest.* 2012;26:291–301.
15. Wang DY, Richmond ME, Quinn TA, et al. Optimized temporary biventricular pacing acutely improves intraoperative cardiac output after weaning from cardiopulmonary bypass: a substudy of a randomized clinical trial. *J Thorac Cardiovasc Surg.* 2011;141:1002–1008.

APPENDIX 4
American Society of Anesthesiologists Standards, Guidelines, and Statements

Standards for Basic Anesthetic Monitoring
Developed By: Committee on Standards and Practice Parameters (CSPP)
Standard I
Standard II

Continuum of Depth of Sedation: Definition of General Anesthesia and Levels of Sedation/Analgesia
Committee of Origin: Quality Management and Departmental Administration

Basic Standards for Preanesthesia Care
Developed By: Committee on Standards and Practice Parameters (CSPP)

Standards for Postanesthesia Care
Developed By: Committee on Standards and Practice Parameters
Standard I
Standard II
Standard III
Standard IV
Standard V

Practice Advisory for the Prevention and Management of Operating Room Fires
APSF Fire Safety Algorithm[1]
Position on Monitored Anesthesia Care
Committee of Origin: Economics

Distinguishing Monitored Anesthesia Care (MAC) from Moderate Sedation/Analgesia (Conscious Sedation)
Committee of Origin: Economics

Ethical Guidelines for the Anesthesia Care of Patients with Do-Not- Resuscitate Orders or Other Directives that Limit Treatment
Committee of Origin: Ethics

Practice Guidelines for Preoperative Fasting and Use of Pharmacologic Agents to Reduce Risk of Pulmonary Aspiration: Application to Healthy Patients Undergoing Elective Procedures
Committee of Origin: Ethics

Standards for Basic Anesthetic Monitoring

Developed By: Committee on Standards and Practice Parameters (CSPP)

Last Affirmed: December 13, 2020 (last amended October 20, 2010) (original approval: October 21, 1986)

[1]This is not an ASA document but is included because of its relevance to fire safety (APSF Newsletter 2012;26:43, www.apsf.org).

These standards apply to all anesthesia care although, in emergency circumstances, appropriate life support measures take precedence. These standards may be exceeded at any time based on the judgment of the responsible anesthesiologist. They are intended to encourage quality patient care, but observing them cannot guarantee any specific patient outcome. They are subject to revision from time to time, as warranted by the evolution of technology and practice. They apply to all general anesthetics, regional anesthetics, and monitored anesthesia care. This set of standards addresses only the issue of basic anesthetic monitoring, which is one component of anesthesia care. In certain rare or unusual circumstances, (1) some of these methods of monitoring may be clinically impractical, and (2) appropriate use of the described monitoring methods may fail to detect untoward clinical developments. Brief interruptions of continual[2] monitoring may be unavoidable. These standards are not intended for application to the care of the obstetrical patient in labor or in the conduct of pain management.

Standard I

Qualified anesthesia personnel shall be present in the room throughout the conduct of all general anesthetics, regional anesthetics, and monitored anesthesia care.

Objective

Because of the rapid changes in patient status during anesthesia, qualified anesthesia personnel shall be continuously present to monitor the patient and provide anesthesia care. In the event there is a direct known hazard, for example, radiation, to the anesthesia personnel which might require intermittent remote observation of the patient, some provision for monitoring the patient must be made. In the event that an emergency requires the temporary absence of the person primarily responsible for the anesthetic, the best judgment of the anesthesiologist will be exercised in comparing the emergency with the anesthetized patient's condition and in the selection of the person left responsible for the anesthetic during the temporary absence.

Standard II

During all anesthetics, the patient's oxygenation, ventilation, circulation, and temperature shall be continually evaluated.

Oxygenation

Objective

To ensure adequate oxygen concentration in the inspired gas and the blood during all anesthetics.

[2]Note that "continual" is defined as "repeated regularly and frequently in steady rapid succession," whereas "continuous" means "prolonged without any interruption at any time."

Methods

1. Inspired gas: During every administration of general anesthesia using an anesthesia machine, the concentration of oxygen in the patient breathing system shall be measured by an oxygen analyzer with a low oxygen concentration limit alarm in use.[3]
2. Blood oxygenation: During all anesthetics, a quantitative method of assessing oxygenation such as pulse oximetry shall be employed.[4]
3. When the pulse oximeter is utilized, the variable pitch pulse tone and the low threshold alarm shall be audible to the anesthesiologist or the anesthesia care team personnel.[5] Adequate illumination and exposure of the patient are necessary to assess color.[6]

Ventilation

Objective

To ensure adequate ventilation of the patient during all anesthetics.

Methods

1. Every patient receiving general anesthesia shall have the adequacy of ventilation continually evaluated. Qualitative clinical signs such as chest excursion, observation of the reservoir breathing bag, and auscultation of breath sounds are useful. Continual monitoring for the presence of expired carbon dioxide shall be performed unless invalidated by the nature of the patient, procedure, or equipment. Quantitative monitoring of the volume of expired gas is strongly encouraged.[7]
2. When an endotracheal tube or laryngeal mask is inserted, its correct positioning must be verified by clinical assessment and by identification of carbon dioxide in the expired gas. Continual end-tidal carbon dioxide analysis, in use from the time of endotracheal tube/laryngeal mask placement, until extubation/removal or initiating transfer to a postoperative care location, shall be performed using a quantitative method such as capnography, capnometry, or mass spectroscopy.[8] When capnography or capnometry is utilized, the end-tidal CO_2 alarm shall be audible to the anesthesiologist or the anesthesia care team personnel.[9]
3. When ventilation is controlled by a mechanical ventilator, there shall be in continuous use a device that is capable of detecting disconnection of components of the breathing system. The device must give an audible signal when its alarm threshold is exceeded.
4. During regional anesthesia (with no sedation) or local anesthesia (with no sedation), the adequacy of ventilation shall be evaluated by continual observation of qualitative clinical signs. During moderate or deep sedation, the adequacy of ventilation shall be evaluated by continual observation of qualitative clinical signs and monitoring for the presence of exhaled carbon dioxide unless precluded or invalidated by the nature of the patient, procedure, or equipment.

Circulation

Objective

To ensure the adequacy of the patient's circulatory function during all anesthetics.

Methods

1. Every patient receiving anesthesia shall have the electrocardiogram continuously displayed from the beginning of anesthesia until preparing to leave the anesthetizing location.[10]
2. Every patient receiving anesthesia shall have arterial blood pressure and heart rate determined and evaluated at least every 5 minutes.[11]
3. Every patient receiving general anesthesia shall have, in addition to the above, circulatory function continually evaluated by at least one of the following: palpation of a pulse, auscultation of heart sounds, monitoring of a tracing of intra- arterial pressure, ultrasound peripheral pulse monitoring, or pulse plethysmography or oximetry.

Body Temperature

Objective

To aid in the maintenance of appropriate body temperature during all anesthetics.

Methods

Every patient receiving anesthesia shall have temperature monitored when clinically significant changes in body temperature are intended, anticipated, or suspected.

[3]Under extenuating circumstances, the responsible anesthesiologist may waive the requirements marked with a dagger (†); it is recommended that when this is done, it should be so stated (including the reasons) in a note in the patient's medical record.
[4]Under extenuating circumstances, the responsible anesthesiologist may waive the requirements marked with an dagger (†); it is recommended that when this is done, it should be so stated (including the reasons) in a note in the patient's medical record.
[5]Under extenuating circumstances, the responsible anesthesiologist may waive the requirements marked with a dagger (†); it is recommended that when this is done, it should be so stated (including the reasons) in a note in the patient's medical record.
[6]Under extenuating circumstances, the responsible anesthesiologist may waive the requirements marked with a dagger (†); it is recommended that when this is done, it should be so stated (including the reasons) in a note in the patient's medical record.
[7]Under extenuating circumstances, the responsible anesthesiologist may waive the requirements marked with a dagger (†); it is recommended that when this is done, it should be so stated (including the reasons) in a note in the patient's medical record.
[8]Under extenuating circumstances, the responsible anesthesiologist may waive the requirements marked with a dagger (†); it is recommended that when this is done, it should be so stated (including the reasons) in a note in the patient's medical record.
[9]Under extenuating circumstances, the responsible anesthesiologist may waive the requirements marked with a dagger (†); it is recommended that when this is done, it should be so stated (including the reasons) in a note in the patient's medical record.
[10]Under extenuating circumstances, the responsible anesthesiologist may waive the requirements marked with a dagger (†); it is recommended that when this is done, it should be so stated (including the reasons) in a note in the patient's medical record.
[11]Under extenuating circumstances, the responsible anesthesiologist may waive the requirements marked with a dagger (†); it is recommended that when this is done, it should be so stated (including the reasons) in a note in the patient's medical record.

Continuum of Depth of Sedation: Definition of General Anesthesia and Levels of Sedation/Analgesia[12]

Committee of Origin: Quality Management and Departmental Administration

(Approved by the ASA House of Delegates on October 13, 1999, and last amended on October 15, 2014)

	Minimal Sedation (Anxiolysis)	Moderate Sedation/ Analgesia (Conscious Sedation)	Deep Sedation/Analgesia	General Anesthesia
Responsiveness	Normal response to verbal stimulation	Purposeful[a] response to verbal or tactile stimulation	Purposeful[a] response following repeated or painful stimulation	Unarousable even with painful stimulus
Airway	Unaffected	No intervention required	Intervention may be required	Intervention often required
Spontaneous Ventilation	Unaffected	Adequate	May be inadequate	Frequently inadequate
Cardiovascular Function	Unaffected	Usually maintained	Usually maintained	May be impaired

[a]Reflex withdrawal from a painful stimulus is NOT considered a purposeful response.

Minimal Sedation (Anxiolysis) is a drug-induced state during which patients respond normally to verbal commands. Although cognitive function and physical coordination may be impaired, airway reflexes and ventilatory and cardiovascular functions are unaffected.

Moderate Sedation/Analgesia (Conscious Sedation) is a drug-induced depression of consciousness during which patients respond purposefully[13] to verbal commands, either alone or accompanied by light tactile stimulation. No interventions are required to maintain a patent airway, and spontaneous ventilation is adequate. Cardiovascular function is usually maintained.

Deep Sedation/Analgesia is a drug-induced depression of consciousness during which patients cannot be easily aroused but respond purposefully[14] following repeated or painful stimulation. The ability to independently maintain ventilatory function may be impaired. Patients may require assistance in maintaining a patent airway, and spontaneous ventilation may be inadequate. Cardiovascular function is usually maintained.

General Anesthesia is a drug-induced loss of consciousness during which patients are not arousable, even by painful stimulation. The ability to independently maintain ventilatory function is often impaired. Patients often require assistance in maintaining a patent airway, and positive pressure ventilation may be required because of depressed spontaneous ventilation or drug-induced depression of neuromuscular function. Cardiovascular function may be impaired.

Because sedation is a continuum, it is not always possible to predict how an individual patient will respond. Hence, practitioners intending to produce a given level of sedation should be able to rescue[15] patients whose level of sedation becomes deeper than initially intended. Individuals administering moderate sedation/analgesia (Conscious Sedation) should be able to rescue[16] patients who enter a state of deep sedation/analgesia, while those administering deep sedation/analgesia should be able to rescue[17] patients who enter a state of general anesthesia.

[12]Monitored Anesthesia Care (MAC) does not describe the continuum of depth of sedation rather it describes "a specific anesthesia service in which an anesthesiologist has been requested to participate in the care of a patient undergoing a diagnostic or therapeutic procedure."

[13]Reflex withdrawal from a painful stimulus is NOT considered a purposeful response.

[14]Reflex withdrawal from a painful stimulus is NOT considered a purposeful response.

[15]Rescue of a patient from a deeper level of sedation than intended is an intervention by a practitioner proficient in airway management and advanced life support. The qualified practitioner corrects adverse physiologic consequences of the deeper-than-intended level of sedation (such as hypoventilation, hypoxia, and hypotension) and returns the patient to the originally intended level of sedation. It is not appropriate to continue the procedure at an unintended level of sedation.

[16]Rescue of a patient from a deeper level of sedation than intended is an intervention by a practitioner proficient in airway management and advanced life support. The qualified practitioner corrects adverse physiologic consequences of the deeper-than-intended level of sedation (such as hypoventilation, hypoxia, and hypotension) and returns the patient to the originally intended level of sedation. It is not appropriate to continue the procedure at an unintended level of sedation.

[17]Rescue of a patient from a deeper level of sedation than intended is an intervention by a practitioner proficient in airway management and advanced life support. The qualified practitioner corrects adverse physiologic consequences of the deeper-than-intended level of sedation (such as hypoventilation, hypoxia, and hypotension) and returns the patient to the originally intended level of sedation. It is not appropriate to continue the procedure at an unintended level of sedation.

Basic Standards for Preanesthesia Care

Developed By: Committee on Standards and Practice Parameters (CSPP)

Last Affirmed: December 13, 2020 (original approval: October 14, 1987)

These standards apply to all patients who receive anesthesia care. Under exceptional circumstances, these standards may be modified. When this is the case, the circumstances shall be documented in the patient's record.

An anesthesiologist shall be responsible for determining the medical status of the patient and developing a plan of anesthesia care.

The anesthesiologist, before the delivery of anesthesia care, is responsible for the following:

1. Reviewing the available medical record.
2. Interviewing and performing a focused examination of the patient to:
   a. Discuss the medical history, including previous anesthetic experiences and medical therapy.
   b. Assess those aspects of the patient's physical condition that might affect decisions regarding perioperative risk and management.
3. Ordering and reviewing pertinent available tests and consultations as necessary for the delivery of anesthesia care.
4. Ordering appropriate preoperative medications.
5. Ensuring that consent has been obtained for the anesthesia care.
6. Documenting in the chart that the above has been performed.

Standards for Postanesthesia Care

Developed By: Committee on Standards and Practice Parameters

Last Amended: October 23, 2019 (original approval: October 27, 2004)

These standards apply to postanesthesia care in all locations. These standards may be exceeded based on the judgment of the responsible anesthesiologist. They are intended to encourage quality patient care but cannot guarantee any specific patient outcome. They are subject to revision from time to time as warranted by the evolution of technology and practice.

Standard I

All patients who have received general anesthesia, regional anesthesia, or monitored anesthesia care shall receive appropriate postanesthesia management.[18]

1. A postanesthesia care unit (PACU) or an area which provides equivalent postanesthesia care (e.g., a surgical intensive care unit) shall be available to receive patients after anesthesia care. All patients who receive anesthesia care shall be admitted to the PACU or its equivalent except by specific order of the anesthesiologist responsible for the patient's care.
2. The medical aspects of care in the PACU (or equivalent area) shall be governed by policies and procedures which have been reviewed and approved by the Department of Anesthesiology.
3. The design, equipment, and staffing of the PACU shall meet requirements of the facility's accrediting and licensing bodies.

Standard II

A patient transported to the PACU shall be accompanied by a member of the anesthesia care team who is knowledgeable about the patient's condition. The patient shall be continually evaluated and treated during transport with monitoring and support appropriate to the patient's condition.

Standard III

Upon arrival in the PACU, the patient shall be reevaluated and a verbal report provided to the responsible PACU nurse by the member of the anesthesia care team who accompanies the patient.

1. The patient's status on arrival in the PACU shall be documented.
2. Information concerning the preoperative condition and the surgical/anesthetic course shall be transmitted to the PACU nurse.
3. The member of the anesthesia care team shall remain in the PACU until the PACU nurse accepts responsibility for the nursing care of the patient.

Standard IV

The patient's condition shall be evaluated continually in the PACU.

1. The patient shall be observed and monitored by methods appropriate to the patient's medical condition. Particular attention should be given to monitoring oxygenation, ventilation, circulation, level of consciousness, and temperature. During recovery from all anesthetics, a quantitative method of assessing oxygenation such as pulse oximetry shall be employed in the initial phase of recovery.[19] This is not intended for application during the recovery of the obstetrical patient in whom regional anesthesia was used for labor and vaginal delivery.
2. An accurate written report of the PACU period shall be maintained. Use of an appropriate PACU-scoring system is encouraged for each patient on admission at appropriate intervals prior to discharge and at the time of discharge.
3. General medical supervision and coordination of patient care in the PACU should be the responsibility of an anesthesiologist.
4. There shall be a policy to assure the availability in the facility of a physician capable of managing complications and providing cardiopulmonary resuscitation for patients in the PACU.

[18]Refer to Perianesthesia Nursing Standards, Practice Recommendations and Interpretive Statements, published by ASPAN, for issues of nursing care.

[19]Under extenuating circumstances, the responsible anesthesiologist may waive the requirements marked with an asterisk (*); it is recommended that when this is done, it should be so stated (including the reasons) in a note in the patient's medical record.

Standard V

A physician is responsible for the discharge of the patient from the postanesthesia care unit.

1. When discharge criteria are used, they must be approved by the Department of Anesthesiology and the medical staff. They may vary depending upon whether the patient is discharged to a hospital room, to the intensive care unit, to a short-stay unit, or home.
2. In the absence of the physician responsible for the discharge, the PACU nurse shall determine that the patient meets the discharge criteria. The name of the physician accepting responsibility for discharge shall be noted on the record.

Practice Advisory for the Prevention and Management of Operating Room Fires (Fig. A4-1)

APSF Fire Safety Algorithm (Fig. A4-2)

Position on Monitored Anesthesia Care

Committee of Origin: Economics

(Approved by the House of Delegates on October 25, 2005, and last amended on October 17, 2018)

Monitored anesthesia care is a specific anesthesia service performed by a qualified anesthesia provider, for a diagnostic or therapeutic procedure. Indications for monitored anesthesia care include, but are not limited to, the nature of the procedure, the patient's clinical condition and/or the need for deeper levels of analgesia and sedation than can be provided by moderate sedation (including potential conversion to a general or regional anesthetic). Unlike monitored anesthesia care, moderate sedation is a proceduralist-directed service which does not include a qualified anesthesia provider's periprocedural assessment and has the inherent limitations that are policy directed for the non–anesthesia-qualified provider. Moderate sedation is a proceduralist-directed service that may be governed by separate institutional policies.

Monitored anesthesia care includes all aspects of anesthesia care—a preprocedure assessment and optimization, intraprocedure care and postprocedure management that is inherently provided by a qualified anesthesia provider as part of the bundled specific service. During monitored anesthesia care, the anesthesiologist provides or medically directs a number of specific services, including but not limited to:

- Preprocedural assessment and management of patient comorbidity and periprocedural risk
- Diagnosis and treatment of clinical problems that occur during the procedure
- Support of vital functions inclusive of hemodynamic stability, airway management and appropriate management of the procedure-induced pathologic changes as they affect the patient's coexisting morbidities
- Administration of sedatives, analgesics, hypnotics, anesthetic agents, or other medications as necessary for patient safety
- Psychological support and physical comfort
- Provision of other medical services as needed to complete the procedure safely

Monitored anesthesia care may include varying levels of sedation, awareness, analgesia, and anxiolysis as necessary. The qualified anesthesiologist provider of monitored anesthesia care must be prepared to convert to general anesthesia and respond to the pathophysiology (airway and hemodynamic changes) of procedure and position in the management in induction of general anesthesia when necessary. If the patient loses consciousness and the ability to respond purposefully, the anesthesia care is a general anesthetic, irrespective of whether airway instrumentation is required. Moderate Sedation/Analgesia on the other hand is a drug-induced depression of consciousness in which the patient responds purposefully to verbal commands, either alone or accompanied by light tactile stimulation. It is not anticipated that intervention will be required to maintain a patent airway and adequate spontaneous ventilation. Similarly, it is expected that cardiovascular function will be maintained without intervention.

Monitored anesthesia care is a physician service provided to an individual patient. Whereas "Moderate Sedation/Analgesia" is a service directed by the Proceduralist who is preoccupied in focusing on successfully completing the scheduled procedure. The Proceduralist may not be cognizant of ongoing pathophysiologic effects of sedatives given or procedure/position changes. Monitored anesthesia care should be subject to the same level of payment as general or regional anesthesia. Accordingly, the ASA Relative Value Guide provides for the use of proper base units, time and any appropriate modifier units as the basis for determining payment.

Distinguishing Monitored Anesthesia Care (MAC) from Moderate Sedation/Analgesia (Conscious Sedation)

Committee of Origin: Economics

(Approved by the ASA House of Delegates on October 27, 2004, last amended on October 21, 2009, and reaffirmed on October 17, 2018)

Moderate Sedation/Analgesia (Conscious Sedation; hereinafter known as Moderate Sedation) is a physician service recognized in the CPT procedural coding system. During Moderate Sedation, a physician supervises or personally administers sedative and/or analgesic medications that can allay patient anxiety and limit pain during a diagnostic or therapeutic procedure. During Moderate Sedation the responsible physician typically assumes the dual role of performing the procedure and supervising the sedation. Such drug-induced depression of a patient's level of consciousness to a "moderate" level of sedation, as defined in the Joint Commission (TJC) standards, is intended to facilitate the successful performance of the diagnostic or therapeutic procedure while providing patient comfort and cooperation. Physicians providing moderate sedation must be qualified to recognize "deep" sedation, manage its consequences and adjust the level of sedation to a "moderate" or lesser level. The continual appraisal of the effects of sedative or analgesic medications on the level of consciousness and on cardiac and respiratory function is an integral element of this service.

The American Society of Anesthesiologists has defined Monitored Anesthesia Care (see Position on Monitored Anesthesia Care, updated on October 17, 2018). This physician service can be distinguished from Moderate Sedation in several ways. An essential component of MAC is the periprocedural anesthesia assessment

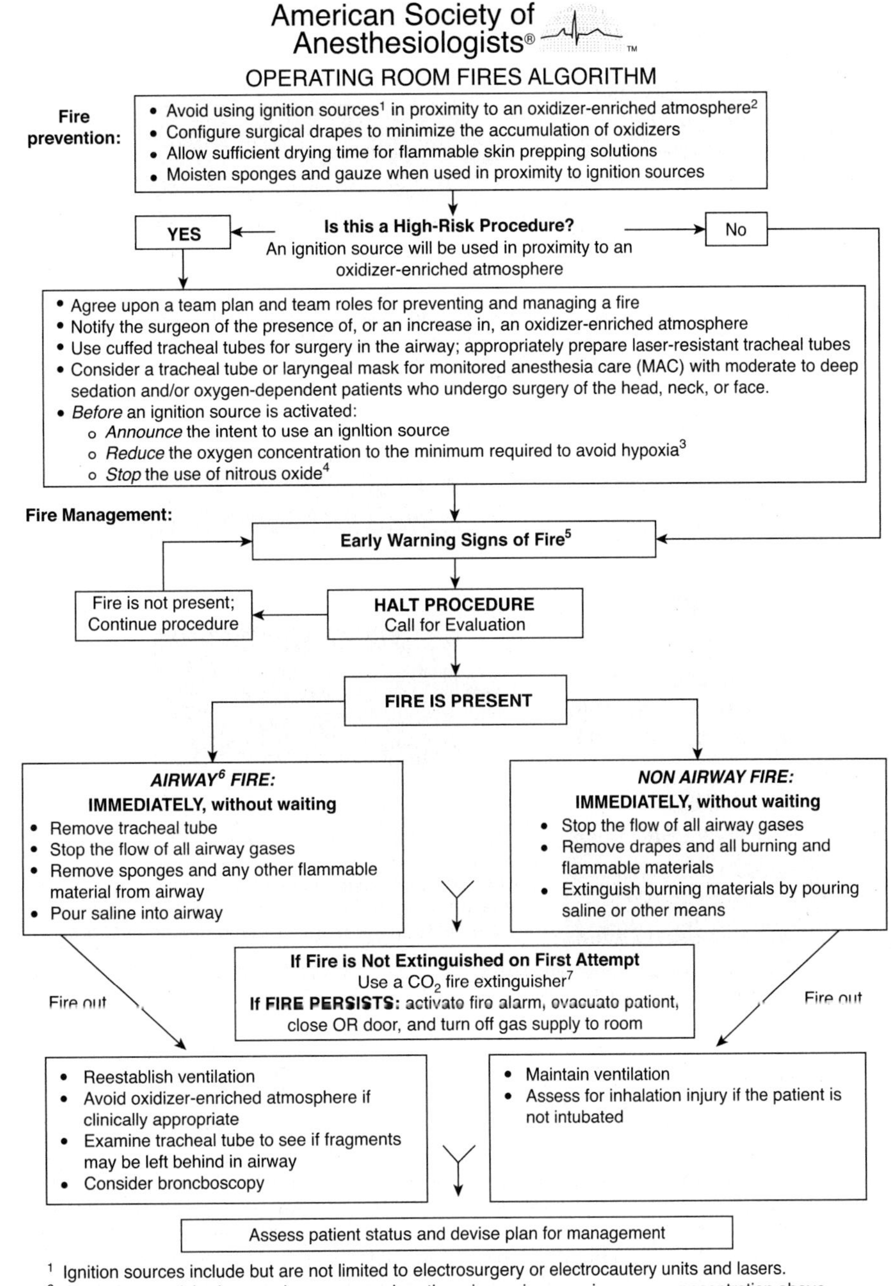

1 Ignition sources include but are not limited to electrosurgery or electrocautery units and lasers.
2 An oxidizer-enriched atmosphere occurs when there is any increase in oxygen concentration above room air level and/or the presence of any concentration of nitrous oxide.
3 After minimizing delivered oxygen, wait a period of time (e.g., 1-3 min) before using an ignition source. For oxygen-dependent patients, *reduce* supplemental oxygen delivery to the minimum required to avoid hypoxia. Monitor oxygenation with pulse oximetry, and if feasible, inspired, exhaled, and/or delivered oxygen concentration.
4 After stopping the delivery of nitrous oxide, wait a period of time (*e.g.*, 1-3 min) before using an ignition source.
5 Unexpected flash, flame, smoke or heat, unusual sounds (*e.g.*, a "pop," snap or "foomp") or odors, unexpected movement of drapes, discoloration of drapes or breathing circuit, unexpected patient movement or complaint.
6 In this algorithm, airway fire refers to a fire in the airway or breathing circuit.
7 A CO_2 fire extinguisher may be used on the patient if necessary.

Figure A4-1 Operating room fires algorithm. CO_2, carbon dioxide; OR, operating room. (Reprinted with permission from Caplan RA, Barker SJ, Connis RT, et al. Practice Advisory for the Prevention and Management of Operating Room Fires: An Updated Report by the American Society of Anesthesiologists Task Force on Operating Room Fires. *Anesthesiology*. 2013;118:271–290. https://doi.org/10.1097/ALN.0b013e31827773d2)

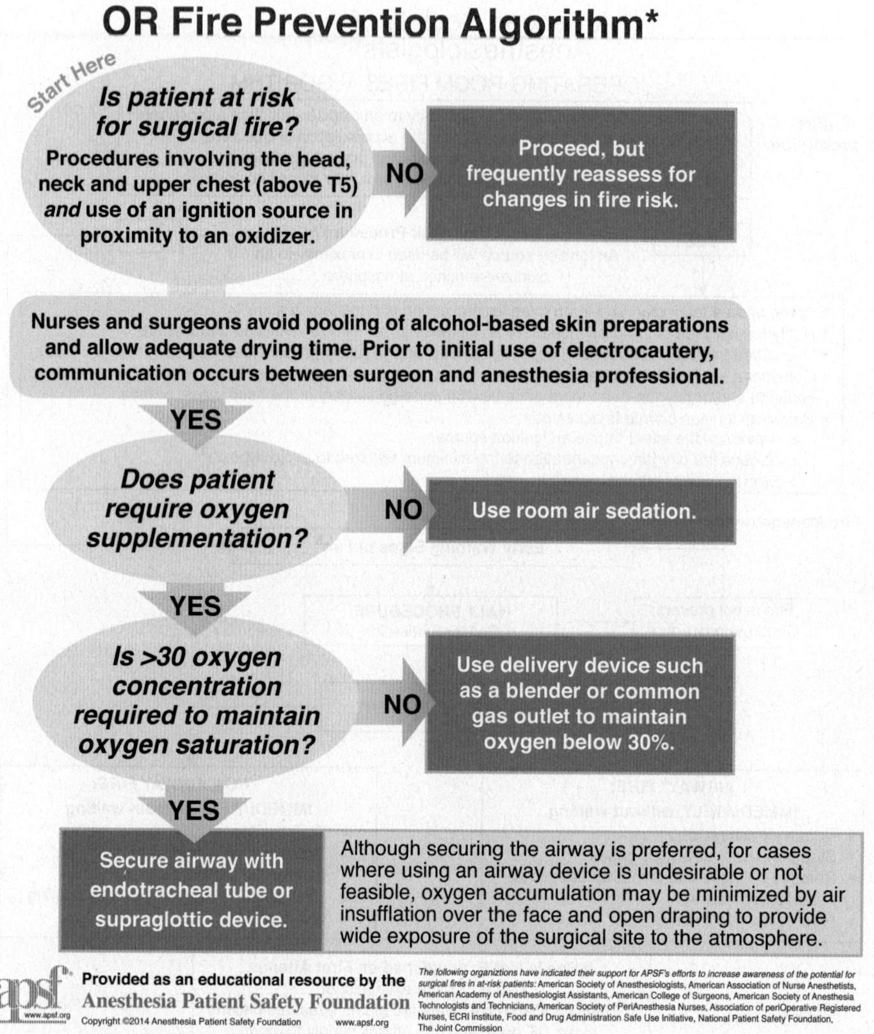

Figure A4-2 Fire Safety Algorithm. Note: This is not an ASA document but is included because of its relevance to fire safety. (Reprinted from Cowles C, Ehrenwerth J. Surgical Fire Prevention: A Review. Accessed June 9, 2021. https://www.apsf.org/article/surgical-fire-prevention-a-review/. Copyright © Anesthesia Patient Safety Foundation (APSF).)

and understanding of the patient's coexisting medical conditions and management of the patient's actual or anticipated physiologic derangements during a diagnostic or therapeutic procedure. While Monitored Anesthesia Care may include the administration of sedatives and/or analgesics often used for Moderate Sedation, the qualified anesthesia provider of MAC is focused exclusively and continuously on the patient for any attendant airway, hemodynamic and physiologic derangements. Further, the provider of MAC must be prepared and qualified to convert to general anesthesia. The proceduralist providing moderate sedation may have their attention diverted to their primary focus, the procedure. In addition, a provider's ability to intervene to rescue a patient's airway from any sedation-induced compromise is a prerequisite to the qualifications to provide Monitored Anesthesia Care. By contrast, Moderate Sedation is not expected to induce depths of sedation that would impair the patient's respiratory function or ability to maintain the integrity of their airway. These components of Monitored Anesthesia Care are unique aspects of an anesthesia service that are not part of Moderate Sedation.

The administration of sedatives, hypnotics, analgesics, as well as anesthetic drugs commonly used for the induction and maintenance of general anesthesia is often, but not always, a part of Monitored Anesthesia Care. In some patients who may require only minimal sedation, MAC is often indicated because even small doses of these medications could precipitate adverse physiologic responses that would necessitate acute clinical interventions and resuscitation. The attention of the proceduralist is focused on the completion of the procedure, not physiologic alterations. If a patient's condition and/or a procedural requirement is likely to require sedation to a "deep" level or even to a transient period of general anesthesia, only a practitioner privileged to provide anesthesia services should be allowed to manage the sedation. Due to the strong likelihood that "deep" sedation may, with or without intention, transition to general anesthesia, the skills of an anesthesia provider are necessary to manage the effects of general anesthesia on the patient as well as to return the patient quickly to a state of "deep" or lesser sedation.

Like all anesthesia services, Monitored Anesthesia Care includes an array of postprocedure responsibilities beyond the expectations of practitioners providing Moderate Sedation, including assuring a return to baseline consciousness, relief of pain, management of adverse physiologic responses or side effects from medications administered during the procedure, as well as the diagnosis and treatment of coexisting medical problems.

Monitored Anesthesia Care allows for the safe administration of a maximal depth of sedation in excess of that provided during Moderate Sedation. The ability to adjust the sedation level from full consciousness to general anesthesia during the course of a procedure provides maximal flexibility in matching sedation level to patient needs and procedural requirements. In situations where the procedure is more invasive or when the patient is especially fragile, optimizing sedation level is necessary to achieve ideal procedural conditions.

In summary, Monitored Anesthesia Care is a physician service that is clearly distinct from Moderate Sedation due to the expectations and qualifications of the provider who must be able to utilize all anesthesia resources to support life and to provide patient comfort and safety during a diagnostic or therapeutic procedure.

Ethical Guidelines for the Anesthesia Care of Patients with Do-Not-Resuscitate Orders or Other Directives that Limit Treatment

Committee of Origin: Ethics

(Approved by the ASA House of Delegates on October 17, 2001, and last amended on October 17, 2018)

These guidelines apply both to patients with decision-making capacity and also to patients without decision-making capacity who have previously expressed their preferences.

I. Given the diversity of published opinions and cultures within our society, an essential element of preoperative preparation and perioperative care for patients with do-not-resuscitate (DNR) orders or other directives that limit treatment is communication among involved parties. It is necessary to document relevant aspects of this communication.

II. Policies automatically suspending DNR orders or other directives that limit treatment prior to procedures involving anesthetic care may not sufficiently address a patient's rights to self- determination in a responsible and ethical manner. Such policies, if they exist, should be reviewed and revised, as necessary, to reflect the content of these guidelines.

III. The administration of anesthesia necessarily involves some practices and procedures that might be viewed as "resuscitation" in other settings. Prior to procedures requiring anesthetic care, any existing directives to limit the use of resuscitation procedures (i.e., do-not- resuscitate orders and/or advance directives) should, when possible, be reviewed with the patient or designated surrogate. As a result of this review, the status of these directives should be clarified or modified based on the preferences of the patient. One of the three following alternatives may provide for a satisfactory outcome in many cases.

A. Full Attempt at Resuscitation: The patient or designated surrogate may request the full suspension of existing directives during the anesthetic and immediate postoperative period, thereby consenting to the use of any resuscitation procedures that may be appropriate to treat clinical events that occur during this time.

B. Limited Attempt at Resuscitation Defined with Regard to Specific Procedures: The patient or designated surrogate may elect to continue to refuse certain specific resuscitation procedures (e.g., chest compressions, defibrillation, or tracheal intubation). The anesthesiologist should inform the patient or designated surrogate about which procedures are (1) essential to the success of the anesthesia and the proposed procedure, and (2) which procedures are not essential and may be refused.

C. Limited Attempt at Resuscitation Defined with Regard to the Patient's Goals and Values: The patient or designated surrogate may allow the anesthesiologist and surgical/procedural team to use clinical judgment in determining which resuscitation procedures are appropriate in the context of the situation and the patient's stated goals and values. For example, some patients may want full resuscitation procedures to be used to manage adverse clinical events that are believed to be quickly and easily reversible but to refrain from treatment for conditions that are likely to result in permanent sequelae, such as neurologic impairment or unwanted dependence upon life-sustaining technology.

IV. Any clarifications or modifications made to the patient's directive should be documented in the medical record. In cases where the patient or designated surrogate requests that the anesthesiologist use clinical judgment in determining which resuscitation procedures are appropriate, the anesthesiologist should document the discussion with particular attention to the stated goals and values of the patient.

V. Plans for postoperative/postprocedural care should indicate if or when the original, pre-existent directive to limit the use of resuscitation procedures will be reinstated. This occurs when the patient leaves the postanesthesia care unit or when the patient has recovered from the acute effects of anesthesia and surgery/procedure. Consideration should be given to whether continuing to provide the patient with a time-limited or event-limited postoperative/postprocedure trial of therapy would help the patient or surrogate better evaluate whether continued therapy would be consistent with the patient's goals.

VI. It is important to discuss and document whether there are to be any exceptions to the injunction(s) against intervention should there occur a specific recognized complication of the surgery/procedure or anesthesia.

VII. Concurrence on these issues by the primary physician (if not the surgeon/proceduralist of record), the surgeon/proceduralist, and the anesthesiologist is desirable. If possible, these physicians should meet together with the patient (or the patient's legal representative) when these issues are discussed. This duty of the patient's physicians is deemed to be of such importance that it should not be delegated. Other members of the healthcare team who are (or will be) directly involved with the patient's care during the planned procedure should, if feasible, be included in this process.

VIII. Should conflicts arise, the following resolution processes are recommended:

A. When an anesthesiologist finds the patient's or surgeon's/proceduralist's limitations of intervention decisions to be irreconcilable with one's own moral views, then the anesthesiologist should withdraw in a nonjudgmental fashion, providing an alternative for care in a timely fashion.

B. When an anesthesiologist finds the patient's or surgeon's/proceduralist's limitation of intervention decisions to be in conflict with generally accepted standards of care, ethical practice, or institutional policies, then the anesthesiologist should voice such concerns and present the situation to the appropriate institutional body.

C. If these alternatives are not feasible within the time frame necessary to prevent further morbidity or suffering, then in accordance with the American Medical Association's Principles of Medical Ethics, care should proceed with reasonable adherence to the patient's directives, being mindful of the patient's goals and values.

IX. A representative from the hospital's anesthesiology service should establish a liaison with surgical, procedural, and nursing services for presentation, discussion, and procedural application of these guidelines. Hospital staff should be made aware of the proceedings of these discussions and the motivations for them.

X. Modification of these guidelines may be appropriate when they conflict with local standards or policies and in those emergency situations involving patients lacking decision-making capacity whose intentions have not been previously expressed.

Practice Guidelines for Preoperative Fasting and Use of Pharmacologic Agents to Reduce Risk of Pulmonary Aspiration: Application to Healthy Patients Undergoing Elective Procedures

Committee of Origin: Ethics

(*Anesthesiology* March 2017, Vol. 126, 376–393)

A. Fasting Recommendations[a]	
Ingested Material	Minimum Fasting Period[c]
• Clear liquids[b]	2 h
• Breast milk	4 h
• Infant formula	6 h
• Nonhuman milk[d]	6 h
• Light meal[e]	6 h
• Fried foods, fatty foods, or meat	Additional fasting time (e.g., 8 or more hours) may be needed
B. Pharmacologic Recommendations	
Medication Type and Common Examples	Recommendation
Gastrointestinal stimulants:	
• Metoclopramide	May be used/no routine use
Gastric acid secretion blockers:	
• Climetidine	May be used/no routine use
• Famotidine	May be used/no routine use
• Ranitidine	May be used/no routine use
• Omeprazole	May be used/no routine use
• Lansoprazole	May be used/no routine use
Antacids:	
• Sodium citrate	May be used/no routine use
• Sodium bicarbonate	May be used/no routine use
• Magnesium trisilicate	May be used/no routine use
Antiemetics:	
• Ondansetron	May be used/no routine use
Anticholinergics:	
• Atropine	No use
• Scopolamine	No use
• Glycopyrrolate	No use
Combinations of the medications above:	No routine use

[a]These recommendations apply to healthy patients who are undergoing elective procedures. They are not intended for women in labor. Following the guidelines does not guarantee complete gastric emptying.
[b]The fasting periods noted above apply to all ages.
[c]Examples of clear liquids include water, fruit juices without pulp, carbonated beverages, clear tea, and black coffee.
[d]Since nonhuman milk is similar to solids in gastric emptying time, the amount ingested must be considered when determining an appropriate fasting period.
[e]A light meal typically consists of toast and clear liquids. Meals that include fried or fatty foods or meat may prolong gastric emptying time. Additional fasting time (e.g., 8 or more hours) may be needed in these cases. Both the amount and type of foods ingested must be considered when determining an appropriate fasting period.

APPENDIX 5
The American Society of Anesthesiologists Difficult Airway Algorithms

ASA Difficult Airway Algorithm: Adult Patients (Figure A5-1)

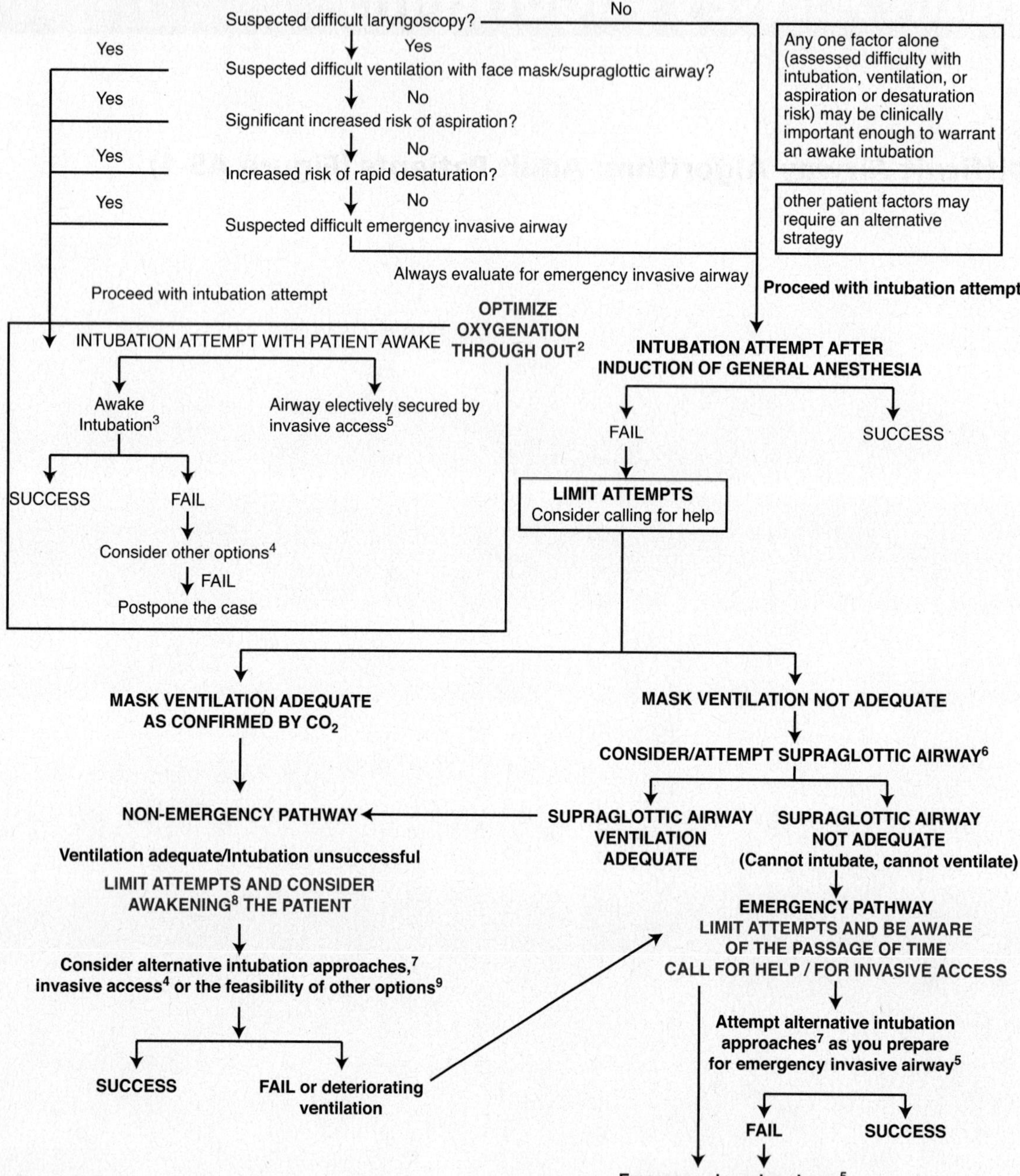

Figure A5-1 Difficult airway algorithm: Adult patients. [1]The airway manager's choice of airway strategy and techniques should be based on their previous experience; available resources, including equipment, availability, and competency of help; and the context in which airway management will occur. [2]Low- or high-flow nasal cannula, head elevated position throughout procedure. Noninvasive ventilation during preoxygenation. [3]Awake intubation techniques include flexible bronchoscope, videolaryngoscopy, direct laryngoscopy, combined techniques, and retrograde wire-aided intubation. [4]Other options include, but are not limited to, alternative awake technique, awake elective invasive airway, alternative anesthetic techniques, induction of anesthesia (if unstable or cannot be postponed) with preparations for emergency invasive airway, and postponing the case without attempting the above options. [5]Invasive airway techniques include surgical cricothyrotomy, needle cricothyrotomy with a pressure-regulated device, large-bore cannula cricothyrotomy, or surgical tracheostomy. Elective invasive airway techniques include the above and retrograde wire–guided intubation and percutaneous tracheostomy. Also consider rigid bronchoscopy and ECMO. [6]Consideration of size, design, positioning, and first versus second generation supraglottic airways may improve the ability to ventilate. [7]Alternative difficult intubation approaches include but are not limited to video-assisted laryngoscopy, alternative laryngoscope blades, combined techniques, intubating supraglottic airway (with or without flexible bronchoscopic guidance), flexible bronchoscopy, introducer, and lighted stylet or lightwand. Adjuncts that may be employed during intubation attempts include tracheal tube introducers, rigid stylets, intubating stylets, or tube changers and external laryngeal manipulation. [8]Includes postponing the case or postponing the intubation and returning with appropriate resources (e.g., personnel, equipment, patient preparation, awake intubation). [9]Other options include, but are not limited to, proceeding with procedure utilizing face mask or supraglottic airway ventilation. Pursuit of these options usually implies that ventilation will not be problematic. (Reprinted with permission from Apfelbaum JL, Hagberg CA, Connis RT, et al. 2022 American Society of Anesthesiologists Practice Guidelines for Management of the Difficult Airway. *Anesthesiology* 2022;136:31–81.)

ASA Difficult Airway Algorithm: Pediatric Patients (Figure A5-2)

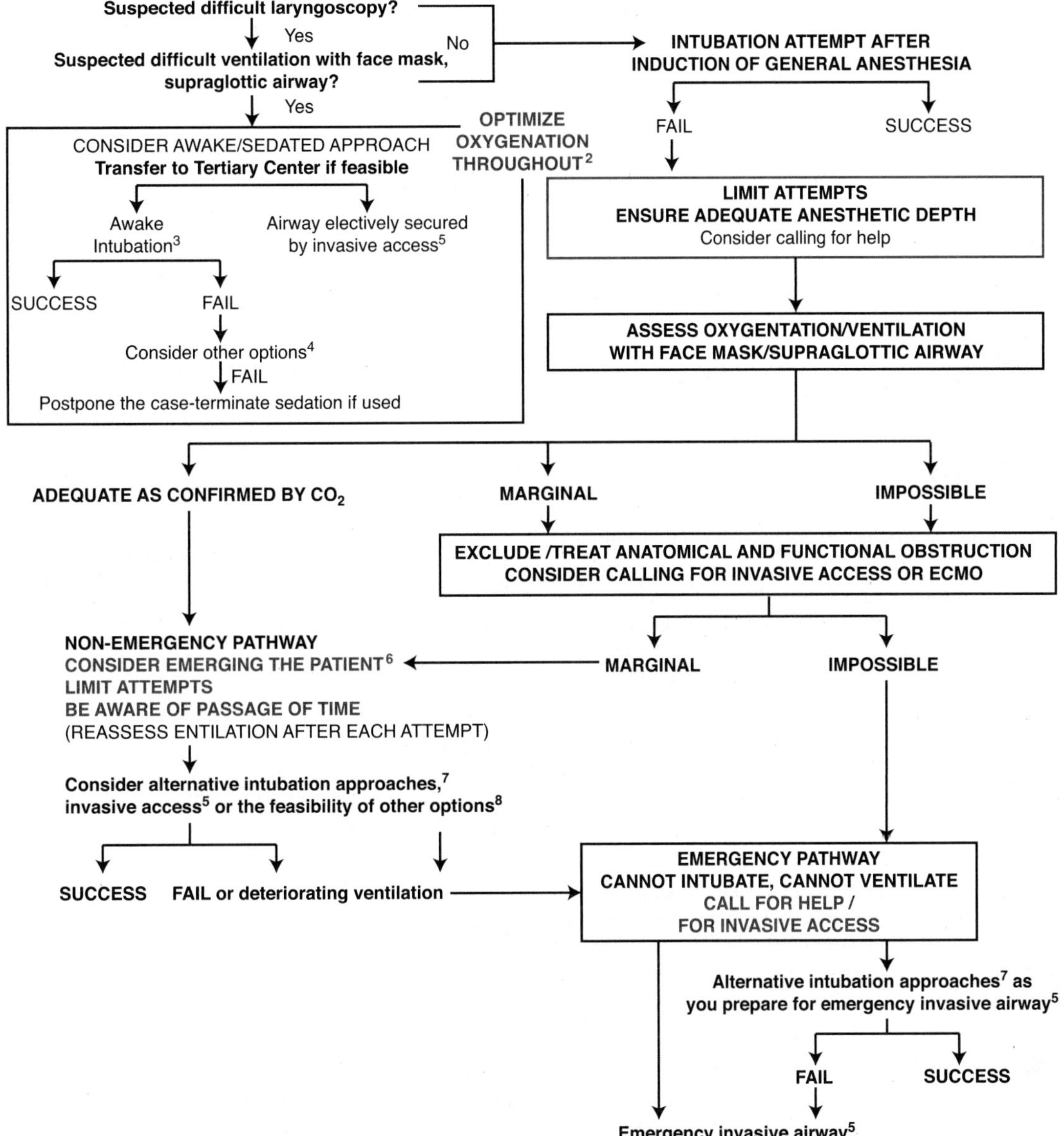

Figure A5-2 Difficult airway algorithm: Pediatric patients. [1]The airway manager's assessment and choice of techniques should be based on their previous experience; available resources, including equipment, availability, and competency of help; and the context in which airway management will occur. [2]Low- or high-flow nasal cannula, head elevated position throughout procedure. Noninvasive ventilation during preoxygenation. [3]Awake intubation techniques include flexible bronchoscope, videolaryngoscopy, direct laryngoscopy, combined techniques, and retrograde wire-aided intubation. [4]Other options include, but are not limited to, alternative awake technique, awake elective invasive airway, alternative anesthetic techniques, induction of anesthesia (if unstable or cannot be postponed) with preparations for emergency invasive airway, or postponing the case without attempting the above options. [5]Invasive airway techniques include surgical cricothyroidotomy, needle cricothyroidotomy if age-appropriate with a pressure-regulated device, large-bore cannula cricothyroidotomy, or surgical tracheostomy. Elective invasive airway techniques include the above and retrograde wire-guided intubation and percutaneous tracheostomy. Also consider rigid bronchoscopy and ECMO. [6]Includes postponing the case or postponing the intubation and returning with appropriate resources (e.g., personnel, equipment, patient preparation, awake intubation). [7]Alternative difficult intubation approaches include, but are not limited to, video-assisted laryngoscopy, alternative laryngoscope blades, combined techniques, intubating supraglottic airway (with or without flexible bronchoscopic guidance), flexible bronchoscopy, introducer, and lighted stylet. Adjuncts that may be employed during intubation attempts include tracheal tube introducers, rigid stylets, intubating stylets, or tube changers and external laryngeal manipulation. [8]Other options include, but are not limited to, proceeding with procedure utilizing face mask or supraglottic airway ventilation. Pursuit of these options usually implies that ventilation will not be problematic. Note: Developed in collaboration with the Society for Pediatric Anesthesia and the Pediatric Difficult Intubation Collaborative: John E. Fiadjoe, M.D., Thomas Engelhardt, M.D., Ph.D., F.R.C.A., Nicola Disma, M.D., Narasimhan Jagannathan, M.D., M.B.A., Britta S. von Ungern-Sternberg, M.D., Ph.D., D.E.A.A., F.A.N.Z.C.A., and Pete G. Kovatsis, M.D., F.A.A.P. (Reprinted with permission from Apfelbaum JL, Hagberg CA, Connis RT, et al. 2022 American Society of Anesthesiologists Practice Guidelines for Management of the Difficult Airway. *Anesthesiology* 2022;136:31–81.)

APPENDIX 6
Herbal Medications

STELLA HADDADIN

The authors and publisher have exerted every effort to ensure that the herbal medication selection in this appendix is in accord with current recommendations and practice at the time of publication.

Alfalfa

Uses: Diuretic, kidney, bladder and prostate conditions, hyperglycemia, asthma, arthritis, indigestion

Interaction/toxicity: Excessive use may interfere with anticoagulant therapy, potentiate drug-induced photosensitivity, and interfere with hormone therapy.

Angelica Root

Uses: Gastrointestinal spasm, loss of appetite, feeling of fullness, and flatulence

Interaction/toxicity: Can cause photodermatitis, claims to increase stomach acid, therefore interferes with antacids, sucralfate, H_2 antagonists, and proton pump inhibitors. Potentiates the effects and adverse effects of anticoagulants and antiplatelet drugs.

Anise

Uses: Dyspepsia and as a pediatric antiflatulent and expectorant

Interaction/toxicity: Excessive doses can prolong coagulation, increasing PT/INR because of coumarin contained in anise. An interaction exists with anticoagulant therapy, monoamine oxidase inhibitors (MAOIs), and hormone therapy. Catecholamine activity might increase blood pressure readings and increase heart rate.

Arnica Flower

Uses: Antiphlogistic, antiseptic, anti-inflammatory, analgesic

Interaction/toxicity: Potentiates anticoagulant and antiplatelet effect of drugs and possibly increases risk of bleeding.

Asafoetida

Uses: Chronic bronchitis, asthma, pertussis, hoarseness, hysteria, flatulent colic, chronic gastric, dyspepsia, irritable colon, and convulsions

Interaction/toxicity: Might increase the risk of bleeding, and excessive doses might interfere with blood pressure control. Can irritate GI tract and is contraindicated in patients with infectious or inflammatory GI conditions.

Bilberry

Uses: Peripheral vascular disease, diabetes, ophthalmologic diseases, peptic ulcer disease and scleroderma

Interaction/toxicity: Excessive use may interfere with coagulation and inhibit platelet aggregation; alters glucose regulation.

Bogbean

Uses: Rheumatism, loss of appetite, dyspepsia

Interaction/toxicity: Potentiates anticoagulant and antiplatelet drugs and possibly increases risk of bleeding.

Bromelain

Uses: Acute postoperative and posttraumatic conditions of swelling, especially of the nasal and paranasal sinuses, osteoarthritis

Interaction/toxicity: Potentiates anticoagulant and antiplatelet drugs and possibly increases risk of bleeding. Increases plasma and urine tetracycline level.

Cayenne

Uses: Muscle spasms, chronic pain

Interaction/toxicity: Overdose may cause hypothermia. May cause skin blisters.

Celery

Uses: Rheumatism, gout, hysteria, nervousness, weight loss as a result of malnutrition, loss of appetite, exhaustion, sedative, mild diuretic, urinary antiseptic, digestive aid, antiflatulent, blood purification

Interaction/toxicity: Potentiates anticoagulant and antiplatelet drugs and possibly increases risk of bleeding. There is an additive effect with drugs with sedative properties and may cause increase in phototoxic response to psoralen plus ultraviolet light A (PUVA) therapy because of its psoralen content.

Chamomile

Uses: Flatulence, nervous diarrhea, restlessness, insomnia, antispasmodic

Interaction/toxicity: Concomitant use with benzodiazepines might cause additive effects and side effects. Potentiates anticoagulant and antiplatelet drugs and possibly increases risk of bleeding. Is an inhibitor of the cytochrome P450 3A4 enzyme system.

Clove

Uses: Flatulence, nausea, and vomiting

Interaction/toxicity: Potentiates anticoagulant and antiplatelet drugs and possibly increases risk of bleeding.

Dandelion

Uses: Diuretic, GI disorders and anti-inflammatory effect

Interaction/toxicity: Excessive use may interfere with coagulation and inhibit platelet aggregation; alters glucose regulation. Do not use in the presence of biliary obstruction. Interactions with digoxin, lithium, insulin, oral hypoglycemics, cytochrome P450, ciprofloxacin, disulfram and metronidazole.

Danshen

Uses: Circulation problems, cardiovascular diseases, chronic hepatitis, abdominal masses, insomnia because of palpitations and tight chest, acne, psoriasis, eczema, aids in wound healing

Interaction/toxicity: Potentiates anticoagulant and antiplatelet drugs and possibly increases risk of bleeding. Increases the cardiovascular effects and side effects of digoxin.

Devil's Claw

Uses: Osteoarthritis, rheumatoid arthritis, gout, myalgia, fibrositis

Interaction/toxicity: Can affect heart rate, contractility of heart, and blood pressure. Might decrease blood glucose levels and have additive effects with medications used for diabetes. May cause an increase in gastric acid secretions.

Dong Quai

Uses: Gynecologic ailments, menopausal symptoms

Interaction/toxicity: Potentiates anticoagulant and antiplatelet drugs and possibly increases risk of bleeding.

Echinacea

Uses: Common colds, urinary tract infections

Interaction/toxicity: May cause hepatotoxicity especially with other concomitant hepatotoxins. Antagonizes steroids and immunosuppressants. May possess immunosuppressive activity after long-term use.

Ephedra

Uses: Diet aid, bacteriostatic, antitussive

Interaction/toxicity: May cause arrhythmias with inhalation anesthetics and cardiac glycosides. Life-threatening reaction with MAOIs. May cause depletion of catecholamines and lead to perioperative hemodynamic instability. Can cause death.

Fenugreek

Uses: Lower blood sugar in diabetics

Interaction/toxicity: Potentiates anticoagulant and antiplatelet drugs and possibly increases risk of bleeding. Inhibits corticosteroid drug activity, interferes with hormone therapy, can alter blood glucose control, and potentiate effect of MAOIs.

Feverfew

Uses: Migraine prophylaxis, antipyretic

Interaction/toxicity: Inhibit platelet activity. Potentiates anticoagulants. Abrupt withdrawal may cause rebound headaches. Uterine stimulant. Associated with serotonin syndrome.

Fish Oil

Uses: Cardiovascular disease, colon cancer, psychiatric disorders, diabetes, inflammatory disease, inflammatory bowel diseases, premenstrual syndrome and scleroderma

Interaction/toxicity: Excessive use may interfere with coagulation and inhibit platelet aggregation; alters glucose regulation; potentiates antihypertensive drugs.

Flaxseed Oil

Uses: Cardiovascular disease, colon cancer, psychiatric disorders, diabetes, inflammatory disease, inflammatory bowel diseases, breast cancer, and depression

Interaction/toxicity: Excessive use may interfere with coagulation and inhibit platelet aggregation; alters glucose regulation.

Garlic (Pertains to Supplement Product)

Uses: Lower lipids, antihypertensive, antiplatelet, antioxidant, antithrombolytic

Interaction/toxicity: Potentiates anticoagulants, especially in the presence of drugs that inhibit platelet function. Potentiates vasodilator drugs and antihypertensives. May decrease blood glucose levels as a result of increased serum insulin levels.

Ginger (Pertains to Supplement Product)

Uses: Antinauseant, antispasmodic

Interaction/toxicity: Inhibits thromboxane synthetase. Potentiates anticoagulants. May alter effects of calcium channel blockers.

Ginkgo

Uses: Circulatory stimulant, inhibit platelets

Interaction/toxicity: Potentiates anticoagulants, especially in the presence of aspirin, NSAIDs, heparin, and warfarin.

Ginseng

Uses: Antioxidant

Interaction/toxicity: Antagonize anticoagulants. Avoid use of sympathetic stimulants, which may result in tachycardia or hypertension. Possesses hypoglycemic effects. Potentiates digoxin and MAOIs.

Goldenseal

Uses: Diuretic, anti-inflammatory, hemostatic

Interaction/toxicity: May worsen edema and hypertension. Oxytocic possesses activity.

Grape Seed

Uses: Anti-oxidant, cardiovascular disorders, peripheral circulatory disorders, multiple sclerosis, Parkinson disease

Interaction/toxicity: Excessive use may interfere with coagulation and inhibit platelet aggregation; may inhibit xanthine oxidase.

Green Tea

Uses: Improves cognitive performance, lowers cholesterol and triglycerides, aids in the prevention of breast, bladder, esophageal, and pancreatic cancers. Decreased risk of Parkinson disease, gingivitis, obesity

Interaction/toxicity: Concomitant use might inhibit effect of adenosine and antagonize effect of warfarin. Because of the caffeine content, there is an increase in cardiac inotropic effects of beta-adrenergic agonist drugs, an increase in the effects and toxicity of clozapine, and an increased risk of agitation, tremors, and insomnia in combination with ephedrine. It might precipitate hypertensive crisis with MAOIs as well. Might reduce sedative effects of benzodiazepines.

Horse Chestnut

Uses: Scleroderma, peripheral vascular disorders, varicose veins and relieving pain, tiredness, tension, swelling in legs, itching, and edema

Interaction/toxicity: Excessive use may interfere with coagulation and inhibit platelet aggregation; phosphodiesterase inhibitor and alters glucose regulation. Potentiates anticoagulant and antiplatelet drugs and possibly increases risk of bleeding, hypoglycemic effects, might interfere with binding of protein binding drugs.

Kava-Kava

Uses: Anxiolytic, analgesic

Interaction/toxicity: Potentiates barbiturates, opioids, and benzodiazepines.

Licorice

Uses: Heal gastric and duodenal ulcers

Interaction/toxicity: May cause hypertension, hypokalemia, and edema.

Lovage Root

Uses: Used for inflammation of the lower urinary tract and prevention of kidney gravel; in "irrigation therapy," it is used as a mild diuretic

Interaction/toxicity: Might increase sodium retention and interfere with diuretic therapy.

Meadowsweet

Uses: Supportive therapy for colds

Interaction/toxicity: Can potentiate narcotic effects. Contains a salicylate constituent.

Onions

Uses: Loss of appetite, preventing atherosclerosis, dyspepsia, fever, colds, cough, tendency toward infection, and inflammation of the mouth and pharynx

Interaction/toxicity: May enhance antidiabetic drug effects and alter blood sugar control. Might enhance antiplatelet drug activity and increase bleeding risk.

Papain

Uses: Inflammation and swelling in patient with pharyngitis

Interaction/toxicity: Concomitant use with anticoagulant and antiplatelet drugs may increase risk of bleeding.

Parsley

Uses: Breath freshener, urinary tract infections, and kidney or bladder stones

Interaction/toxicity: Might interfere with oral anticoagulant therapy because of the vitamin K contained in parsley. May interfere with diuretic therapy by enhancing sodium retention. Might potentiate MAOI drug therapy.

Passion Flower

Uses: Generalized anxiety disorder

Interaction/toxicity: Concomitant use with barbiturates can increase drug-induced sleep time; can potentiate the effects of sedatives and tranquilizers, including sedative effects of antihistamines.

Quassia

Uses: Anorexia, indigestion, fever, mouthwash, as an anthelmintic for thread worms, nematodes, and ascaris

Interaction/toxicity: Stimulates gastric acid and might oppose effect of antacids and H_2 antagonists. Excessive doses might have additive effects with anticoagulant therapy with Coumadin. Concomitant use of potassium-depleting diuretics or stimulant laxative abuse might increase risk of cardiac glycoside toxicity as a result of potassium loss.

Red Clover

Uses: Hot flashes

Interaction/toxicity: Can increase the anticoagulant effects and bleeding risk because of its Coumarin content. May interfere with hormone replacement therapy or oral contraceptives, and may interfere with tamoxifen because of its potential estrogenic effects. Can inhibit cytochrome P450 (cyp450) 3A4.

Saw Palmetto

Uses: Benign prostatic hypertrophy, antiandrogenic

Interaction/toxicity: Potentiates birth control pills and estrogens. May cause hypertension.

St. John's Wort

Uses: Depression, anxiety

Interaction/toxicity: Possible interaction/toxicity with MAOIs and meperidine. May prolong anesthetic effects. Potentiates digoxin. May decrease effects of warfarin, steroids, and possibly benzodiazepines and calcium channel blockers.

Sweet Clover

Uses: Chronic venous insufficiency, including leg pain and heaviness, night-time leg cramps, itching and swelling, for supportive treatment of thrombophlebitis, lymphatic congestion, postthrombotic syndromes, and hemorrhoids

Interaction/toxicity: Use with hepatotoxic drugs might increase risk of hepatotoxicity. Concomitant use with anticoagulant and antiplatelet drugs may increase risk of bleeding.

Turmeric

Uses: Dyspepsia, jaundice, hepatitis, flatulence, abdominal bloating

Interaction/toxicity: Concomitant use with anticoagulant and antiplatelet drugs may increase risk of bleeding.

Valerian

Uses: Sedative, anxiolytic

Interaction/toxicity: Potentiates barbiturates and anesthetics. May blunt symptoms of benzodiazepine withdrawal.

Vitamin E

Uses: Vitamin E deficiency, heart disease

Interaction/toxicity: Concomitant use with anticoagulant and antiplatelet drugs may increase risk of bleeding. Might prevent tolerance to nitrates.

Willow Bark

Uses: Lower back pain, fever, rheumatic ailments, headache

Interaction/toxicity: Enough salicylate is present in willow bark to cause drug interactions common to salicylates or aspirin. Can impair effectiveness of beta-adrenergic blockers, probenecid, and sulfinpyrazone. Can increase effects, side effects, or toxicity of alcohol, anticoagulants, carbonic anhydrase inhibitors, heparin, methotrexate, NSAIDs, sulfonylureas, and valproic acid.

Index

Note: Page number followed by f or t indicates figure or table respectively.

C

E

F

J

K

O

T

W

X

Y

Z